DRUG INFORMATION HANDBOOK

A Clinically Relevant Resource for All Healthcare Professionals

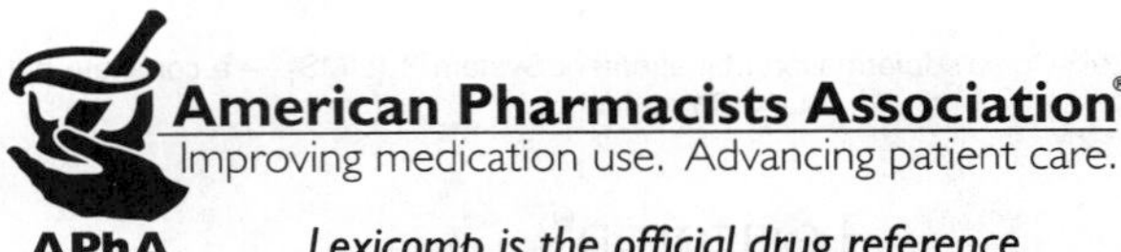

Lexicomp is the official drug reference for the American Pharmacists Association

23rd Edition

Lexicomp®

NOTICE

This data is intended to serve the user as a handy reference and not as a complete drug information resource. It does not include information on every therapeutic agent available. The publication covers over 1500 commonly used drugs and is specifically designed to present important aspects of drug data in a more concise format than is typically found in medical literature or product material supplied by manufacturers.

The nature of drug information is that it is constantly evolving because of ongoing research and clinical experience and is often subject to interpretation. While great care has been taken to ensure the accuracy of the information and recommendations presented, the reader is advised that the authors, editors, reviewers, contributors, and publishers cannot be responsible for the continued currency of the information or for any errors, omissions, or the application of this information, or for any consequences arising therefrom. Therefore, the author(s) and/or the publisher shall have no liability to any person or entity with regard to claims, loss, or damage caused, or alleged to be caused, directly or indirectly, by the use of information contained herein. Because of the dynamic nature of drug information, readers are advised that decisions regarding drug therapy must be based on the independent judgment of the clinician, changing information about a drug (eg, as reflected in the literature and manufacturer's most current product information), and changing medical practices. Therefore, this data is designed to be used in conjunction with other necessary information and is not designed to be solely relied upon by any user. The user of this data hereby and forever releases the authors and publishers of this data from any and all liability of any kind that might arise out of the use of this data. The editors are not responsible for any inaccuracy of quotation or for any false or misleading implication that may arise due to the text or formulas as used or due to the quotation of revisions no longer official.

Certain of the authors, editors, and contributors have written this book in their private capacities. No official support or endorsement by any federal or state agency or pharmaceutical company is intended or inferred.

The publishers have made every effort to trace any third party copyright holders, if any, for borrowed material. If they have inadvertently overlooked any, they will be pleased to make the necessary arrangements at the first opportunity.

If you have any suggestions or questions regarding any information presented in this data, please contact our drug information pharmacists at (330) 650-6506. Book revisions are available at our website at http://www.lexi.com/home/revisions/.

This manual was produced using Lexi-Comp's Information Management System™ (LIMS) — a complete publishing service of Lexi-Comp Inc.

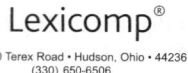

1100 Terex Road • Hudson, Ohio • 44236
(330) 650-6506

ISBN 978-1-59195-330-2 (North American Edition)

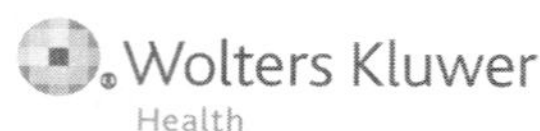

TABLE OF CONTENTS

DRUG INFORMATION HANDBOOK EDITORIAL ADVISORY PANEL

EDITORIAL ADVISORY PANEL

Tracy Hagemann, PharmD
Associate Professor
College of Pharmacy
The University of Oklahoma

JoEllen L. Hanigosky, PharmD
Clinical Coordinator
Department of Hematology/Oncology/Bone Marrow Transplant
Children's Hospital of Akron

Martin D. Higbee, PharmD
Associate Professor
Department of Pharmacy Practice and Science
The University of Arizona

Jane Hurlburt Hodding, PharmD
Executive Director, Inpatient Pharmacy Services and Clinical Nutrition Services
Long Beach Memorial Medical Center and Miller Children's Hospital

Mark T. Holdsworth, PharmD, BCOP
Associate Professor of Pharmacy & Pediatrics and *Pharmacy Practice Area Head*
College of Pharmacy
The University of New Mexico

Edward Horn, PharmD, BCPS
Clinical Specialist, Transplant Surgery
Allegheny General Hospital

Collin A. Hovinga, PharmD
Director of Research and *Associate Professor*
Dell Children's Medical Center
UT Austin School of Pharmacy

Darrell T. Hulisz, PharmD
Associate Professor
Department of Family Medicine
Case Western Reserve University

Douglas L. Jennings, PharmD, BCPS
Clinical Pharmacy Specialist, Cardiovascular Surgery
Jackson Memorial Hospital

Michael A. Kahn, DDS
Professor and Chairman
Department of Oral and Maxillofacial Pathology
Tufts University School of Dental Medicine

Jeannette Kaiser, MT, MBA
Medical Technologist
Akron General Medical Center

Julie J. Kelsey, PharmD
Clinical Specialist
Women's Health and Family Medicine
Department of Pharmacy Services
University of Virginia Health System

Patrick J. Kiel, PharmD, BCPS, BCOP
Clinical Pharmacy Specialist
Hematology and Stem Cell Transplant
Indiana University Simon Cancer Center

Polly E. Kintzel, PharmD, BCPS, BCOP
Clinical Pharmacy Specialist-Oncology
Spectrum Health

Michael Klepser, PharmD, FCCP
Professor of Pharmacy
Department of Pharmacy Practice
Ferris State University

Daren Knoell, PharmD
Associate Professor of Pharmacy Practice and Internal Medicine
Davis Heart and Lung Research Institute
The Ohio State University

David Knoppert, MScPhm, FCCP, MSc, FCSHP
Clinical Leader - Paediatrics
Pharmacy Services
London Health Sciences Centre
Children's Health Research Institute

Sandra Knowles, RPh, BScPhm
Drug Policy Research Specialist
Li Ka Shing Institute
St. Michael's Hospital

Jill M. Kolesar, PharmD, FCCP, BCPS
Associate Professor
School of Pharmacy
University of Wisconsin Paul P. Carbone Comprehensive Cancer Center

Susannah E. Koontz, PharmD, BCOP
Principal and Consultant
Pediatric Hematology/Oncology and Stem Cell Transplantation/Cellular Therapy
Koontz Oncology Consulting, LLC

Donna M. Kraus, PharmD, FAPhA, FPPAG, FCCP
Associate Professor of Pharmacy Practice and *Pediatric Clinical Pharmacist*
Departments of Pharmacy Practice and Pediatrics
University of Illinois

Daniel L. Krinsky, RPh, MS
Manager, MTM Services
Giant Eagle Pharmacy
Assistant Professor
Department of Pharmacy Practice
Northeast Ohio Medical University (NEOMED)

Tim T.Y. Lau, PharmD, ACPR, FCSHP
Pharmacotherapeutic Specialist in Infectious Diseases
Pharmaceutical Sciences
Vancouver General Hospital

Mandy C. Leonard, PharmD, BCPS
Assistant Professor
Cleveland Clinic Lerner College of Medicine of Case Western University
Assistant Director, Drug Information Services
The Cleveland Clinic Foundation

Jonathan Leung, PharmD, BCPS, BCPP
Neuropsychiatric Clinical Pharmacist
Mayo Clinic

John J. Lewin III, PharmD, BCPS
Clinical Specialist, Neurosciences Critical Care
The Johns Hopkins Hospital

Jeffrey D. Lewis, PharmD, MACM
Associate Dean and Associate Professor of Pharmacy Practice
Cedarville University School of Pharmacy

John Lindsley, PharmD, BCPS
Cardiology Clinical Pharmacy Specialist
The Johns Hopkins Hospital

Nicholas A. Link, PharmD, BCOP
Clinical Specialist, Oncology
Hillcrest Hospital

Curtis M. Rimmermann, MD, MBA, FACC
Gus P. Karos Chair
Clinical Cardiovascular Medicine
The Cleveland Clinic Foundation

Renee Rivard, PharmD
Consultant, Independent Medical Writer
Wolters Kluwer Health

P. David Rogers, PharmD, PhD, FCCP
Director, Clinical and Translational Therapeutics
University of Tennessee College of Pharmacy

James L. Rutkowski, DMD, PhD
Editor-in-Chief
Journal of Oral Implantology

Amy Rybarczyk, PharmD, BCPS
Pharmacotherapy Specialist, Internal Medicine
Akron General Medical Center

Jennifer K. Sekeres, PharmD, BCPS
Infectious Diseases Clinical Specialist
The Cleveland Clinic Foundation

Todd P. Semla, MS, PharmD, BCPS, FCCP, AGSF
National PBM Clinical Program Manager – Mental Health & Geriatrics
Department of Veterans Affairs
Pharmacy Benefits Management Services
Associate Professor, Clinical
Department of Medicine,
Psychiatry and Behavioral Health
Feinberg School of Medicine
Northwestern University

Chasity M. Shelton, PharmD, BCPS, BCNSP
Assistant Professor of Clinical Pharmacy
Department of Clinical Pharmacy
Neonatal Clinical Pharmacy Specialist
University of Tennessee Health Science Center

Vanessa Sherwood, BSc
Drug Information Pharmacist
IWK Pharmacy, Operations and Support Services

Pamela J. Sims, PharmD, PhD
Professor
Department of Pharmaceutical, Social, and Administrative Sciences
McWhorter School of Pharmacy
Samford University

Grant Sklar, PharmD, BCPS
Assistant Professor, Department of Pharmacy
and *Principal Clinical Pharmacist, General Medicine*
National University Hospital of Singapore

Joseph Snoke, RPh, BCPS
Manager
Core Pharmacology Group
Wolters Kluwer Health

Patricia L. Spenard, PharmD
Clinical Editor
Wolters Kluwer Health

Joni Lombardi Stahura, BS, PharmD, RPh
Pharmacotherapy Specialist
Wolters Kluwer Health

Kim Stevens, RN
Home Care
Samaritan Regional Health System

Stephen Marc Stout, PharmD, MS, BCPS
Pharmacotherapy Specialist
Wolters Kluwer Health

Dan Streetman, PharmD, RPh
Pharmacotherapy Specialist
Wolters Kluwer Health

Darcie-Ann Streetman, PharmD, RPh
Pharmacotherapy Specialist
Wolters Kluwer Health

Carol K. Taketomo, PharmD
Director of Pharmacy and Nutrition Services
Children's Hospital Los Angeles

Mary Temple-Cooper, PharmD
Pediatric Clinical Research Specialist
Hillcrest Hospital

Kelan Thomas, PharmD, MS, BCPS, BCPP
Assistant Professor of Pharmacy Practice
Touro University California, College of Pharmacy
Clinical Pharmacist
St. Helena Hospital Center for Behavioral Health Office

Elizabeth A. Tomsik, PharmD, BCPS
Senior Director
Content
Wolters Kluwer Health

Dana Travis, RPh
Pharmacotherapy Specialist
Wolters Kluwer Health

Jennifer Trofe-Clark, PharmD
Clinical Transplant Pharmacist
Hospital of The University of Pennsylvania

John N. van den Anker, MD, PhD, FCP, FAAP
Vice Chair of Pediatrics for Experimental Therapeutics
and *Chief and Professor of Evan and Cindy Jones Pediatric Clinical Pharmacology*
Children's National Medical Center
Professor of Pediatrics, Pharmacology & Physiology
George Washington University
School of Medicine and Health Sciences

Heather L. VandenBussche, PharmD
Professor of Pharmacy, Pediatrics
Pharmacy Practice
Ferris State University College of Pharmacy

Amy Van Orman, PharmD, BCPS
Pharmacotherapy Specialist
Wolters Kluwer Health

Kristin Watson, PharmD, BCPS
Assistant Professor, Cardiology
and *Clinical Pharmacist, Cardiology Service*
Heart Failure Clinic
University of Maryland Medical Center

David M. Weinstein, PhD, RPh
Director
Metabolism, Interactions, and Genomics Group
Wolters Kluwer Health

Anne Marie Whelan, PharmD
Associate Professor
College of Pharmacy
Dalhouise University

Greg Wiggers, PharmD, PhD
Pharmacotherapy Specialist
Wolters Kluwer Health

DESCRIPTION OF SECTIONS AND FIELDS USED IN THIS HANDBOOK

The *Drug Information Handbook, 23rd Edition* is divided into four sections.

The first section is a compilation of introductory text pertinent to the use of this book.

The drug information section of the handbook, in which all drugs are listed alphabetically, details information pertinent to each drug. Extensive cross-referencing is provided by U.S. brand names, Canadian brand names, and index terms.

The third section is an invaluable appendix which offers a compilation of tables, guidelines, nomograms, algorithms, and conversion information which can be helpful when considering patient care.

The last section of this handbook contains a Pharmacologic Category Index which lists all drugs in this handbook in their unique pharmacologic class.

The **Alphabetical Listing of Drugs** is presented in a consistent format and provides the following fields of information:

Generic Name	U.S. adopted name
Pronunciation	Phonetic pronunciation guide
Brand Names: U.S.	Trade names (manufacturer-specific) found in the United States. The symbol [DSC] appears after trade names that have been recently discontinued.
Brand Names: Canada	Trade names found in Canada
Index Terms	Other names or accepted abbreviations of the generic drug. May also include common brand names no longer available; this field is used to create cross-references to monographs.
Pharmacologic Category	Unique systematic classification of medications
Additional Appendix Information	Cross-reference to other pertinent drug information found in the appendix section of this handbook
Use	Information pertaining to FDA- or Canadian-approved indications for the drug
Unlabeled Use	Information pertaining to non-FDA-approved indications of the drug
Pregnancy Risk Factor	Five categories established by the FDA to indicate the potential of a systemically absorbed drug for causing risk to fetus
Pregnancy Considerations	A summary of human and/or animal information pertinent to or associated with the use of the drug as it relates to clinical effects on the fetus, newborn, or pregnant women
Breast-Feeding Considerations	Information pertinent to or associated with the human use of the drug as it relates to clinical effects on the nursing infant or postpartum woman
Prescribing and Access Restrictions	Provides information on any special requirements regarding the prescribing, obtaining or dispensing of drugs, including access restrictions pertaining to drugs with REMS elements and those drugs with access restrictions that are not REMS-related
Medication Guide Available	Identifies drugs that have an FDA-approved Medication Guide
Contraindications	Information pertaining to inappropriate use of the drug as dictated by approved labeling
Warnings/Precautions	Precautionary considerations, hazardous conditions related to use of the drug, and disease states or patient populations in which the drug should be cautiously used. Boxed warnings, when present, are clearly identified and are adapted from the FDA-approved labeling. Consult the product labeling for the exact black box warning through the manufacturer's or the FDA website.
Adverse Reactions	Side effects are grouped by percentage of incidence (if known) and/or body system; in the interest of saving space, <1% effects are grouped only by percentage.
Drug Interactions	
Metabolism/Transport Effects	If a drug has demonstrated involvement with cytochrome P450 enzymes, or other metabolism or transport proteins, this field will identify the drug as an inhibitor, inducer, or substrate of the specific enzyme(s) (eg, CYP1A2 or UGT1A1). CYP450 isoenzymes are identified as substrates (minor or major), inhibitors (weak, moderate, or strong), and inducers (weak or strong).
Avoid Concomitant Use	Designates drug combinations which should not be used concomitantly, due to an unacceptable risk:benefit assessment. Frequently, the concurrent use of the agents is explicitly prohibited or contraindicated by the product labeling
Increased Effect/Toxicity	Drug combinations that result in a increased or toxic therapeutic effect between the drug listed in the monograph and other drugs or drug classes
Decreased Effect	Drug combinations that result in a decreased therapeutic effect between the drug listed in the monograph and other drugs or drug classes

Ethanol/Nutrition/Herb Interactions	Presents a description of the interaction between the drug listed in the monograph and ethanol, food, or herb/nutraceuticals
Preparation for Administration	Provides information regarding the preparation of drug products prior to administration, including dilution, reconstitution, etc.
Storage/Stability	Information regarding storage and stability of commercially available products and products that have been reconstituted, diluted or otherwise prepared. Provides the time and conditions for which a solution or mixture will maintain potency.
Mechanism of Action	How the drug works in the body to elicit a response
Pharmacodynamics/ Kinetics	The magnitude of a drug's effect depends on the drug concentration at the site of action. The pharmacodynamics are expressed in terms of onset of action and duration of action. Pharmacokinetics are expressed in terms of absorption, distribution, protein binding, metabolism, bioavailability, half-life, time to peak serum concentration, and elimination.
Dosage	The amount of the drug to be typically given or taken during therapy for children and adults; also includes any dosing adjustment/comments for renal impairment or hepatic impairment and other suggested dosing adjustments (eg, hematological toxicity). The following age group definitions are utilized to characterize age-related dosing unless otherwise specified in the monograph: Neonate (0-28 days of age), infant (>28 days to 1 year of age), children (1-12 years of age), and adolescent (13-18 years of age).
Dietary Considerations	Specific dietary modifications and/or restrictions (eg, information about sodium content)
Usual Infusion Concentrations	Information describing the usual concentrations of drugs for continuous infusion administration in the pediatric and adult populations as appropriate. Concentrations are derived from the literature, manufacturer recommendation, or organizational recommendations (eg, the Institute for Safe Medication Practices [ISMP]) and are universally established. Institution-specific standard concentrations may differ from those listed.
Administration	Information regarding the recommended final concentrations, rates of administration for parenteral drugs, or other guidelines or relevant information to properly administer medications
Monitoring Parameters	Laboratory tests and patient physical parameters that should be monitored for safety and efficacy of drug therapy
Reference Range	Therapeutic and toxic serum concentrations listed including peak and trough levels
Test Interactions	Listing of assay interferences when relevant; (B) = Blood; (S) = Serum; (U) = Urine
Additional Information	Information about sodium content and/or pertinent information about specific brands
Product Availability	Provides availability information on products that have been approved by the FDA, but not yet available for use. Estimates for when a product may be available are included, when this information is known. May also provide any unique or critical drug availability issues.
Dosage Forms Considerations	More specific Information regarding product concentrations, ingredients, package sizes, amount of doses per container, and other important details pertaining to various formulations of medications
Dosage Forms	Information with regard to form, strength, and availability of the drug in the United States. **Note:** Additional formulation information (eg, excipients, preservatives) is included when available. Please consult labeling for further information.
Dosage Forms: Canada	Information with regard to form, strength, and availability of products that are uniquely available in Canada but currently are not available in the United States
Controlled Substance	Contains controlled substance schedule information as assigned by the United States Drug Enforcement Administration (DEA) or Canadian Controlled Substance Act (CDSA). CDSA information is only provided for drugs available in Canada and not available in the U.S.
Extemporaneous Preparations	Directions for preparing liquid formulations from solid drug products. May include stability information and references.

PREGNANCY CATEGORIES

Pregnancy Categories (sometimes referred to as pregnancy risk factors) are a letter system currently required under the *Teratogenic Effects* subsection of the product labeling. The system was initiated in 1979. The categories are required to be part of the package insert for prescription drugs that are systemically absorbed.

The categories are defined as follows:

A — Adequate and well-controlled studies in pregnant women have not shown that the drug increases the risk of fetal abnormalities.

B — Animal reproduction studies show no evidence of impaired fertility or harm to the fetus; however, no adequate and well-controlled studies have been conducted in pregnant women.
or
Animal reproduction studies have shown adverse events; however, studies in pregnant women have not shown that the drug increases the risk of abnormalities.

C — Animal reproduction studies have shown an adverse effect on the fetus. There are no adequate and well-controlled studies in humans and the benefits from the use of the drug in pregnant women may be acceptable, despite its potential risks.
or
Animal reproduction studies have not been conducted.

D — Based on human data, the drug can cause fetal harm when administered to pregnant women, but the potential benefits from the use of the drug may be acceptable, despite its potential risks.

X — Studies in animals or humans have demonstrated fetal abnormalities (or there is positive evidence of fetal risk based on reports and/or marketing experience) and the risk of using the drug in pregnant women clearly outweighs any possible benefit (for example, safer drugs or other forms of therapy are available).

The categories do not take into consideration nonteratogenic effects (that information is currently presented separately). In 2008, the Food and Drug Administration (FDA) proposed new labeling requirements which would eliminate the use of the pregnancy category system and replace it with scientific data and other information specific to the use of the drug in pregnant women. These proposed changes were suggested because the current category system may be misleading. For instance, some practitioners may believe that risk increases from category A to B to C to D to X, which is not the intent. In addition, practitioners may not be aware that some medications are categorized based on animal data, while others are based on human data. When the new labeling requirements are approved, product labeling will contain pregnancy and lactation subsections, each describing a risk summary, clinical considerations, and section for specific data.

For full descriptions of the current and proposed labeling requirements, refer to the following websites:

Labeling Requirements for Prescription Drugs and/or Insulin (Code of Federal Regulations, Title 21, Volume 4, Revised April 1, 2010). http://www.accessdata.fda.gov/scripts/cdrh/cfdocs/cfCFR/CFRSearch.cfm?fr=201.57

Content and Format of Labeling for Human Prescription Drug and Biological Products; Requirements for Pregnancy and Lactation Labeling (Federal Register, May 29, 2008). https://www.federalregister.gov/articles/2008/05/29/E8-11806/content-and-format-of-labeling-for-human-prescription-drug-and-biological-products-requirements-for

PREVENTING PRESCRIBING ERRORS

Prescribing errors account for the majority of reported medication errors and have prompted healthcare professionals to focus on the development of steps to make the prescribing process safer. Prescription legibility has been attributed to a portion of these errors and legislation has been enacted in several states to address prescription legibility. However, eliminating handwritten prescriptions and ordering medications through the use of technology [eg, computerized prescriber order entry (CPOE)] has been the primary recommendation. Whether a prescription is electronic, typed, or hand-printed, additional safe practices should be considered for implementation to maximize the safety of the prescribing process. Listed below are suggestions for safer prescribing:

- Ensure correct patient by using at least 2 patient identifiers on the prescription (eg, full name, birth date, or address). Review prescription with the patient or patient's caregiver.
- If pediatric patient, document patient's birth date or age and most recent weight. If geriatric patient, document patient's birth date or age.
- Prevent drug name confusion: For more information, see http://www.ismp.org/tools/confuseddrugnames.pdf.
  - Use TALLman lettering (eg, buPROPion, busPIRone, predniSONE, prednisoLONE). For more information, see http://www.fda.gov/drugs/drugsafety/medicationerrors/default.htm.
  - Avoid abbreviated drug names (eg, MSO_4, $MgSO_4$, MS, HCT, 6MP, MTX), as they may be misinterpreted and cause error.
  - Avoid investigational names for drugs with FDA approval (eg, FK-506, CBDCA).
  - Avoid chemical names such as 6-mercaptopurine or 6-thioguanine, as sixfold overdoses have been given when these were not recognized as chemical names. The proper names of these drugs are mercaptopurine or thioguanine.
  - Use care when prescribing drugs that look or sound similar (eg, look- alike, sound-alike drugs). Common examples include: Celebrex vs Celexa, hydroxyzine vs hydralazine, Zyprexa® vs Zyrtec.
- Avoid dangerous, error-prone abbreviations (eg, regardless of letter-case: U, IU, QD, QOD, µg, cc, @). Do not use apothecary system or symbols. Additionally, text messaging abbreviations (eg, "2Day") should never be used.
  - For more information, see http://www.ismp.org/tools/errorproneabbreviations.pdf.
- Always use a leading zero for numbers less than 1 (0.5 mg is correct and .5 mg is **incorrect**) and never use a trailing zero for whole numbers (2 mg is correct and 2.0 mg is **incorrect**).
- Always use a space between a number and its units as it is easier to read. There should be no periods after the abbreviations mg or mL (10 mg is correct and 10mg is **incorrect**).
- For doses that are greater than 1,000 dosing units, use properly placed commas to prevent 10-fold errors (100,000 units is correct and 100000 units is **incorrect**).
- Do not prescribe drug dosage by the type of container in which the drug is available (eg, do not prescribe "1 amp", "2 vials", etc).
- Do not write vague or ambiguous orders which have the potential for misinterpretation by other healthcare providers. Examples of vague orders to avoid: "Resume pre-op medications," "give drug per protocol," or "continue home medications."
- Review each prescription with patient (or patient's caregiver) including the medication name, indication, and directions for use.
- Take extra precautions when prescribing *high alert drugs* (drugs that can cause significant patient harm when prescribed in error). Common examples of these drugs include: Anticoagulants, chemotherapy, insulins, opioids, and sedatives.
  - For more information, see http://www.ismp.org/tools/institutionalhighalert.asp or http://www.ismp.org/communityRx tools/ambulatoryhighalert.asp.

To Err Is Human: Building a Safer Health System, Kohn LT, Corrigan JM, Donaldson MS, eds. Washington, D.C.: National Academy Press. 2000.

A Complete Outpatient Prescription[1]

A complete outpatient prescription can prevent the prescriber, the pharmacist, and/or the patient from making a mistake and can eliminate the need for further clarification. The complete outpatient prescription should contain:

- Patient's full name
- Medication indication
- Allergies
- Prescriber name and telephone or pager number
- For pediatric patients: Their birth date or age and current weight
- For geriatric patients: Their birth date or age
- Drug name, dosage form and strength
- For pediatric patients: Intended daily weight-based dose so that calculations can be checked by the pharmacist (ie, mg/kg/day or units/kg/day)
- Number or amount to be dispensed
- Complete instructions for the patient or caregiver, including the purpose of the medication, directions for use (including dose), dosing frequency, route of administration, duration of therapy, and number of refills.
- Dose should be expressed in convenient units of measure.
- When there are recognized contraindications for a prescribed drug, the prescriber should indicate knowledge of this fact to the pharmacist (ie, when prescribing a potassium salt for a patient receiving an ACE inhibitor, the prescriber should write "K serum leveling being monitored").

Upon dispensing of the final product, the pharmacist should ensure that the patient or caregiver can effectively demonstrate the appropriate administration technique. An appropriate measuring device should be provided or recommended. Household teaspoons and tablespoons should not be used to measure liquid medications due to their variability and inaccuracies in measurement; oral medication syringes are recommended.

For additional information, see http://www.ismp.org/Newsletters/acutecare/articles/20020601.asp

[1]Levine SR, Cohen MR, Blanchard NR, et al. Guidelines for preventing medication errors in pediatrics. *J Pediatr Pharmacol Ther.* 2001;6:426-442.

FDA NAME DIFFERENTIATION PROJECT: THE USE OF TALL-MAN LETTERS

Confusion between similar drug names is an important cause of medication errors. For years, The Institute For Safe Medication Practices (ISMP), has urged generic manufacturers to use a combination of large and small letters as well as bolding (ie, chlorpro**MAZINE** and chlorpro**PAMIDE**) to help distinguish drugs with look-alike names, especially when they share similar strengths. Recently the FDA's Division of Generic Drugs began to issue recommendation letters to manufacturers suggesting this novel way to label their products to help reduce this drug name confusion. Although this project has had marginal success, the method has successfully eliminated problems with products such as diphenhydr**AMINE** and dimenhy**DRINATE**. Hospitals should also follow suit by making similar changes in their own labels, preprinted order forms, computer screens and printouts, and drug storage location labels.

Lexi-Comp, Inc. Medical Publishing will use "Tall-Man" letters for the drugs suggested by the FDA or recommended by ISMP.

The following is a list of generic and brand name product names and recommended revisions.

Drug Product	Recommended Revision
acetazolamide	aceta**ZOLAMIDE**
alprazolam	**ALPRAZ**olam
amiloride	a**MIL**oride
amlodipine	am**LODIP**ine
aripiprazole	**ARIP**iprazole
atomoxetine	ato**MOX**etine
atorvastatin	atorva**STAT**in
Avinza	**AVIN**za
azacitidine	aza**CITID**ine
azathioprine	aza**THIO**prine
bupropion	bu**PROP**ion
buspirone	bus**PIR**one
carbamazepine	car**BAM**azepine
carboplatin	**CARBO**platin
cefazolin	ce**FAZ**olin
cefotetan	cefo**TE**tan
cefoxitin	cef**OX**itin
ceftazidime	cef**TAZ**idime
ceftriaxone	cef**TRIAX**one
Celebrex	Cele**BREX**
Celexa	Cele**XA**
chlordiazepoxide	chlordiaze**POXIDE**
chlorpromazine	chlorpro**MAZINE**
chlorpropamide	chlorpro**PAMIDE**
cisplatin	**CIS**platin
clobazam	clo**BAZ**am
clomiphene	clomi**PHENE**
clomipramine	clomi**PRAMINE**
clonazepam	clonaze**PAM**
clonidine	clo**NID**ine
clozapine	clo**ZAP**ine
cycloserine	cyclo**SERINE**
cyclosporine	cyclo**SPORINE**
dactinomycin	**DACTIN**omycin
daptomycin	**DAPTO**mycin
daunorubicin	**DAUNO**rubicin
dimenhydrinate	dimenhy**DRINATE**
diphenhydramine	diphenhydr**AMINE**
dobutamine	**DOBUT**amine
docetaxel	**DOCE**taxel
dopamine	**DOP**amine
doxorubicin	**DOXO**rubicin
duloxetine	**DUL**oxetine

Drug Product	Recommended Revision
ephedrine	e**PHED**rine
epinephrine	**EPINEPH**rine
epirubicin	**EPI**rubicin
eribulin	eri**BUL**in
fentanyl	fenta**NYL**
flavoxate	flavox**ATE**
fluoxetine	**FLU**oxetine
fluphenazine	flu**PHENAZ**ine
fluvoxamine	fluvoxa**MINE**
glipizide	glipi**ZIDE**
glyburide	gly**BURIDE**
guaifenesin	guai**FEN**esin
guanfacine	guan**FACINE**
Humalog	Huma**LOG**
Humulin	Humu**LIN**
hydralazine	hydr**ALAZINE**
hydrocodone	**HYDRO**codone
hydromorphone	**HYDRO**morphone
hydroxyzine	hydr**OXY**zine
idarubicin	**IDA**rubicin
infliximab	in**FLIX**imab
Invanz	**INV**anz
isotretinoin	**ISO**tretinoin
Klonopin	Klono**PIN**
Lamictal	La**MIC**tal
Lamisil	Lam**ISIL**
lamivudine	lami**VUD**ine
lamotrigine	lamo**TRI**gine
levetiracetam	Lev**ETIRA**cetam
levocarnitine	lev**OCARN**itine
lorazepam	**LOR**azepam
medroxyprogesterone	medroxy**PROGESTER**one
metformin	met**FORMIN**
methylprednisolone	methyl**PREDNIS**olone
methyltestosterone	methyl**TESTOSTER**one
metronidazole	metro**NIDAZOLE**
mitomycin	mito**MY**cin
mitoxantrone	Mito**XAN**trone
Nexavar	Nex**AVAR**
Nexium	Nex**IUM**
nicardipine	ni**CAR**dipine
nifedipine	**NIFE**dipine
nimodipine	ni**MOD**ipine
Novolin	Novo**LIN**
Novolog	Novo**LOG**
olanzapine	**OLANZ**apine
oxcarbazepine	**OX**carbazepine
oxycodone	oxy**CODONE**
Oxycontin	Oxy**CONTIN**
paclitaxel	**PACL**itaxel
paroxetine	**PAR**oxetine
pazopanib	**PAZOP**anib
pemetrexed	**PEME**trexed
penicillamine	penicill**AMINE**
pentobarbital	**PENT**obarbital
phenobarbital	**PHEN**obarbital
ponatinib	**PONAT**inib

FDA NAME DIFFERENTIATION PROJECT: THE USE OF TALL-MAN LETTERS

Drug Product	Recommended Revision
pralatrexate	**PRALA**trexate
prednisolone	predniso**LONE**
prednisone	predni**SONE**
Prilosec	Pri**LOSEC**
Prozac	**PRO**zac
quetiapine	**QUE**tiapine
quinidine	qui**NID**ine
quinine	qui**NINE**
rabeprazole	**RABE**prazole
Risperdal	Risper**DAL**
risperidone	risperi**DONE**
rituximab	ri**TUX**imab
romidepsin	romi**DEP**sin
romiplostim	romi**PLOS**tim
ropinirole	r**OPINIR**ole
Sandimmune	sand**IMMUNE**
Sandostatin	Sando**STATIN**
Seroquel	**SERO**quel
Sinequan	**SINE**quan
sitagliptin	sita**GLIP**tin
Solu-Cortef	Solu-**CORTEF**
Solu-Medrol	Solu-**MEDROL**
sorafenib	**SORA**fenib
sufentanil	**SUF**entanil
sulfadiazine	sulf**ADIAZINE**
sulfasalazine	sulfa**SALA**zine
sumatriptan	**SUMA**triptan
sunitinib	**SUNI**tinib
Tegretol	**TEG**retol
tiagabine	tia**GAB**ine
tizanidine	ti**ZAN**idine
tolazamide	**TOLAZ**amide
tolbutamide	**TOLBUT**amide
tramadol	tra**MAD**ol
trazodone	tra**ZOD**one
Trental	**TREN**tal
valacyclovir	val**ACY**clovir
valganciclovir	val**GAN**ciclovir
vinblastine	vin**BLAS**tine
vincristine	vin**CRIS**tine
zolmitriptan	**ZOLM**itriptan
Zyprexa	Zy**PREXA**
Zyrtec	Zyr**TEC**

FDA and ISMP lists of look-alike drug names with recommended tall man letter. http://www.ismp.org/tools/tallmanletters.pdf. Accessed January 6, 2011.
Name differentiation project. http://www.fda.gov/Drugs/DrugSafety/MedicationErrors/ucm164587.htm. Accessed January 6, 2011.
U.S. Pharmacopeia. USP quality review: use caution – avoid confusion. March 2001, No. 76. http://www.usp.org

ALPHABETICAL LISTING OF DRUGS

- **A-25 [OTC]** *see* Vitamin A *on page 2201*
- **A-200® Lice Treatment Kit [OTC]** *see* Pyrethrins and Piperonyl Butoxide *on page 1752*
- **A-200® Maximum Strength [OTC]** *see* Pyrethrins and Piperonyl Butoxide *on page 1752*
- **A+D® Original [OTC]** *see* Vitamin A and Vitamin D (Topical) *on page 2202*
- **A+D Prevent [OTC]** *see* Vitamin A *on page 2201*
- **A771726** *see* Teriflunomide *on page 2021*

Abacavir (a BAK a veer)

Brand Names: U.S. Ziagen

Brand Names: Canada Ziagen®

Index Terms Abacavir Sulfate; ABC

Pharmacologic Category Antiretroviral, Reverse Transcriptase Inhibitor, Nucleoside (Anti-HIV)

Use Treatment of HIV infections in combination with other antiretroviral agents

Pregnancy Risk Factor C

Pregnancy Considerations Adverse events have been observed in some animal reproduction studies. Abacavir crosses the human placenta. No increased risk of overall birth defects has been observed following first trimester exposure according to data collected by the antiretroviral pregnancy registry. Cases of lactic acidosis/hepatic steatosis syndrome related to mitochondrial toxicity have been reported in pregnant women with prolonged use of nucleoside analogues. It is not known if pregnancy itself potentiates this known side effect; however, women may be at increased risk of lactic acidosis and liver damage. In addition, these adverse events are similar to other rare but life-threatening syndromes which occur during pregnancy (eg, HELLP syndrome). Hepatic enzymes and electrolytes should be monitored in women receiving nucleoside analogues and clinicians should watch for early signs of the syndrome. In addition, mitochondrial dysfunction may develop in infants following *in utero* exposure. The pharmacokinetics of abacavir are not significantly changed by pregnancy and dose adjustment is not needed for pregnant women. The DHHS Perinatal HIV Guidelines consider abacavir to be an alternative NRTI in dual nucleoside combination regimens.

Regardless of CD4 count or HIV RNA copy number, all HIV-infected pregnant women should receive a combination antepartum antiretroviral (ARV) drug regimen; this includes women who require therapy for their own health, as well as women who do not yet require therapy for their own health. ARV therapy should be started as soon as possible if required for the woman's health. Although earlier initiation may be more effective in reducing the perinatal transmission of HIV, also consider maternal conditions (eg, nausea and vomiting) and the potential risks of first trimester fetal exposure for specific agents. Plasma HIV RNA levels should be assessed at ~34-36 weeks gestation in order to help determine mode of delivery. If ARV therapy must be interrupted for <24 hours during the peripartum period, stop then restart all medications simultaneously in order to decrease the chance of developing resistance. Long-term follow-up is recommended for all infants exposed to ARV medications.

Healthcare providers are encouraged to enroll pregnant women exposed to antiretroviral medications in the Antiretroviral Pregnancy Registry (1-800-258-4263 or www.APRegistry.com). Healthcare providers caring for HIV-infected women and their infants may contact the National Perinatal HIV Hotline (888-448-8765) for clinical consultation (DHHS [perinatal], 2012).

Breast-Feeding Considerations Maternal or infant antiretroviral therapy does not completely eliminate the risk of postnatal HIV transmission. In addition, multiclass-resistant virus has been detected in breast-feeding infants despite maternal therapy. Therefore, in the United States, where formula is accessible, affordable, safe, and sustainable, and the risk of infant mortality due to diarrhea and respiratory infections is low, complete avoidance of breast-feeding by HIV-infected women is recommended to decrease potential transmission of HIV (DHHS [perinatal], 2012).

Medication Guide Available Yes

Contraindications Hypersensitivity to abacavir or any component of the formulation (do not rechallenge patients who have experienced hypersensitivity to abacavir regardless of *HLA-B*5701* status); moderate-to-severe hepatic impairment

Warnings/Precautions Abacavir should always be used as a component of a multidrug regimen. **[U.S. Boxed Warning]: Serious and sometimes fatal hypersensitivity reactions have occurred.** Patients testing positive for the presence of the *HLA-B*5701* allele are at an increased risk for hypersensitivity reactions. Screening for *HLA-B*5701* allele status is recommended prior to initiating therapy or reinitiating therapy in patients of unknown status, including patients who previously tolerated therapy. Therapy is **not** recommended in patients testing positive for the *HLA-B*5701* allele. An allergy to abacavir should be reported in the patient's medical record (DHHS, 2013a). Reactions usually occur within 9 days of starting abacavir; ~90% occur within 6 weeks. Patients exhibiting symptoms from two or more of the following: Fever, skin rash, constitutional symptoms (malaise, fatigue, aches), respiratory symptoms (eg, pharyngitis, dyspnea, cough), and GI symptoms (eg, abdominal pain, diarrhea, nausea, vomiting) should discontinue therapy immediately and call for medical attention. Abacavir should be permanently discontinued if hypersensitivity cannot be ruled out, even when other diagnoses are possible and regardless of *HLA-B*5701* status. Abacavir SHOULD NOT be restarted because more severe symptoms may occur within hours, including LIFE-THREATENING HYPOTENSION AND DEATH. Fatal hypersensitivity reactions have occurred following the reintroduction of abacavir in patients whose therapy was interrupted (ie, interruption in drug supply, temporary discontinuation while treating other conditions). In some cases, signs of hypersensitivity may have been previously present, but attributed to other medical conditions (eg, acute onset respiratory diseases, gastroenteritis, reactions to other medications). If abacavir is restarted following an interruption in therapy, evaluate the patient for previously unsuspected symptoms of hypersensitivity. A higher incidence of severe hypersensitivity reactions may be associated with a 600 mg once daily dosing regimen.

[U.S. Boxed Warning]: Lactic acidosis and severe hepatomegaly with steatosis (sometimes fatal) have occurred with antiretroviral nucleoside analogues. Female gender, prior liver disease, obesity, and prolonged treatment may increase the risk of hepatotoxicity. May be associated with fat redistribution. Immune reconstitution syndrome may develop, resulting in the occurrence of an inflammatory response to an indolent or residual opportunistic infection during initial HIV treatment or activation of autoimmune disorders (eg, Graves' disease, polymyositis, Guillain-Barré syndrome) later in therapy; further evaluation and treatment may be required.

Use has been associated with an increased risk of myocardial infarction (MI) in observational studies; however, based on a meta-analysis of 26 randomized trials, the FDA has concluded there is not an increased risk. Consider using with caution in patients with risks for coronary heart disease and minimizing modifiable risk factors (eg, hypertension, hyperlipidemia, diabetes mellitus, and smoking) prior to use. Products may contain propylene glycol. Safety and efficacy in children <3 months of age have not been established.

Adverse Reactions Hypersensitivity reactions (which may be fatal) occur in ~5% of patients. Symptoms may include anaphylaxis, fever, rash (including erythema multiforme), fatigue, diarrhea, abdominal pain; respiratory symptoms (eg, pharyngitis, dyspnea, cough, adult respiratory distress syndrome, or respiratory failure); headache, malaise, lethargy, myalgia, myolysis, arthralgia, edema, paresthesia, nausea and vomiting, mouth ulcerations, conjunctivitis, lymphadenopathy, hepatic failure, and renal failure.

Note: Rates of adverse reactions were defined during combination therapy with other antiretrovirals (lamivudine and efavirenz **or** lamivudine and zidovudine). Only reactions which occurred at a higher frequency in adults (except where noted) than in the comparator group are noted. Adverse reaction rates attributable to abacavir alone are not available.

>10%:
- Central nervous system: Headache (7% to 13%)
- Gastrointestinal: Nausea (7% to 19%, children 9%)

1% to 10%:
- Central nervous system: Depression (6%), fever/chills (6%, children 9%), anxiety (5%)
- Dermatologic: Rash (5% to 6%, children 7%)
- Endocrine & metabolic: Triglycerides increased (2% to 6%)
- Gastrointestinal: Diarrhea (7%), vomiting (children 9%), amylase increased (2%)
- Hematologic: Thrombocytopenia (1%)
- Hepatic: AST increased (6%)
- Neuromuscular & skeletal: Musculoskeletal pain (5% to 6%)
- Miscellaneous: Hypersensitivity reactions (2% to 9%; may include reactions to other components of antiretroviral regimen), infection (ENT 5%)

<1% (Limited to important or life-threatening): Erythema multiforme, fat redistribution, GGT increased, hepatic steatosis, hepatomegaly, hepatotoxicity, immune reconstitution syndrome, lactic acidosis, MI, pancreatitis, Stevens-Johnson syndrome, toxic epidermal necrolysis

Drug Interactions

Metabolism/Transport Effects None known.

Avoid Concomitant Use There are no known interactions where it is recommended to avoid concomitant use.

Increased Effect/Toxicity

The levels/effects of Abacavir may be increased by: Ganciclovir-Valganciclovir; Ribavirin

Decreased Effect

The levels/effects of Abacavir may be decreased by: Protease Inhibitors

Ethanol/Nutrition/Herb Interactions Ethanol: Ethanol may increase the risk of toxicity.

Storage/Stability Store oral solution and tablets at controlled room temperature of 20°C to 25°C (68°F to 77°F). Oral solution may be refrigerated; do not freeze.

Mechanism of Action Nucleoside reverse transcriptase inhibitor. Abacavir is a guanosine analogue which is phosphorylated to carbovir triphosphate which interferes with HIV viral RNA-dependent DNA polymerase resulting in inhibition of viral replication.

Pharmacodynamics/Kinetics

Absorption: Rapid and extensive absorption

Distribution: V_d: 0.86 L/kg

Protein binding: 50%

Metabolism: Hepatic via alcohol dehydrogenase and glucuronyl transferase to inactive carboxylate and glucuronide metabolites

Bioavailability: 83%

Half-life elimination: 1.5 hours

Time to peak: 0.7-1.7 hours

Excretion: Primarily urine (as metabolites, 1.2% as unchanged drug); feces (16% total dose)

Dosage Oral:

Infants and Children ≥3 months to <16 years: 8 mg/kg body weight twice daily (maximum: 300 mg twice daily) in combination with other antiretroviral agents. **Note:** May consider 16-20 mg/kg once daily dosing (maximum: 600 mg/day) in stable patients with undetectable viral load and stable CD4 count (DHHS [pediatric], 2011)

U.S. manufacturer labeling: Alternative dosing to be considered for pediatric patients ≥14 kg who are able to swallow tablets:
- 14-21 kg: 150 mg (1/2 tablet) twice daily
- >21 kg to <30 kg: 150 mg (1/2 tablet) in the morning and 300 mg (1 tablet) in the evening
- ≥30 kg: 300 mg (1 tablet) twice daily

Adolescents ≥16 years and Adults: 300 mg twice daily or 600 mg once daily in combination with other antiretroviral agents (DHHS, 2013a; DHHS [pediatric], 2011)

Canadian labeling:

Infants and Children ≥3 months to 12 years: 8 mg/kg body weight twice daily (maximum: 300 mg twice daily) in combination with other antiretroviral agents

Adolescents >12 years and Adults: 300 mg twice daily in combination with other antiretroviral agents

Dosage adjustment in renal impairment: Canadian labeling (not in U.S. labeling): Use in ESRD or use of 600 mg once daily dosing is not recommended.

Dosage adjustment in hepatic impairment:

Mild impairment (Child-Pugh class A): 200 mg twice daily (oral solution is recommended)

Moderate-to-severe impairment (Child-Pugh class B or C): Use is contraindicated (has not been studied).

Dietary Considerations May be taken with or without food.

Administration May be administered with or without food.

Monitoring Parameters CBC with differential, serum creatine kinase, CD4 count, HIV RNA plasma levels, serum transaminases, triglycerides, serum amylase; *HLA-B*5701* genotype status prior to initiation of therapy and prior to reinitiation of therapy in patients of unknown *HLA-B*5701* status; signs and symptoms of hypersensitivity, particularly in patients untested for the *HLA-B*5701* allele

Additional Information Use regimens of abacavir and nevirapine with caution; both agents cause hypersensitivity reactions early in therapy (DHHS, 2013).

Hypersensitivity testing (*HLA-B*5701*): Prevalence of hypersensitivity reactions has been estimated at 5% to 8% in Caucasians and 2% to 3% in African-Americans. Pretherapy identification of *HLA-B*5701*-positive patients, and subsequent avoidance of abacavir therapy in these patients has been shown to reduce the occurrence of abacavir-mediated hypersensitivity reactions. An allergy to abacavir should be reported in the patient's medical record (DHHS, 2013). A skin patch test is in development for clinical screening purposes; however, only PCR-mediated genotyping methods are currently in clinical practice use for documentation of this susceptibility marker.

Dosage Forms Excipient information presented when available (limited, particularly for generics); consult specific product labeling.

Solution, Oral:

Ziagen: 20 mg/mL (240 mL) [contains methylparaben, propylene glycol, propylparaben, saccharin sodium; strawberry-banana flavor]

Tablet, Oral:

Ziagen: 300 mg [scored]

Generic: 300 mg

Abacavir and Lamivudine

(a BAK a veer & la MI vyoo deen)

Brand Names: U.S. Epzicom®

Brand Names: Canada Kivexa™

Index Terms Abacavir Sulfate and Lamivudine; Lamivudine and Abacavir

Pharmacologic Category Antiretroviral, Reverse Transcriptase Inhibitor, Nucleoside (Anti-HIV)

Use Treatment of HIV infections in combination with other antiretroviral agents

Pregnancy Risk Factor C

Medication Guide Available Yes

Dosage Oral: Adults: HIV: One tablet (abacavir 600 mg and lamivudine 300 mg) once daily

Dosage adjustment in renal impairment: Cl_{cr} <50 mL/minute: Use not recommended

Dosage adjustment in hepatic impairment: Use contraindicated.

Additional Information Complete prescribing information should be consulted for additional detail.

Dosage Forms Excipient information presented when available (limited, particularly for generics); consult specific product labeling.

Tablet:

Epzicom®: Abacavir 600 mg and lamivudine 300 mg

Abacavir, Lamivudine, and Zidovudine

(a BAK a veer, la MI vyoo deen, & zye DOE vyoo deen)

Brand Names: U.S. Trizivir®

Brand Names: Canada Trizivir®

Index Terms 3TC, Abacavir, and Zidovudine; Azidothymidine, Abacavir, and Lamivudine; AZT, Abacavir, and Lamivudine; Compound S, Abacavir, and Lamivudine; Lamivudine, Abacavir, and Zidovudine; ZDV, Abacavir, and Lamivudine; Zidovudine, Abacavir, and Lamivudine

Pharmacologic Category Antiretroviral, Reverse Transcriptase Inhibitor, Nucleoside (Anti-HIV)

Use Treatment of HIV infection (either alone or in combination with other antiretroviral agents) in patients whose regimen would otherwise contain the components of Trizivir®

Pregnancy Risk Factor C

Medication Guide Available Yes

Dosage Oral:

U.S. labeling: Adolescents ≥40 kg and Adults: One tablet twice daily. **Note:** Not recommended for patients <40 kg.

Canadian labeling: Adults ≥50 kg: One tablet twice daily. **Note:** Not recommended for patients <50 kg.

Dosage adjustment in renal impairment: Because lamivudine and zidovudine require dosage adjustment in renal impairment, Trizivir® should not be used in patients with Cl_{cr} <50 mL/minute

Dosage adjustment in hepatic impairment: Use is contraindicated.

Additional Information Complete prescribing information should be consulted for additional detail.

Dosage Forms Excipient information presented when available (limited, particularly for generics); consult specific product labeling.

Tablet, oral:

Trizivir®: Abacavir sulfate 300 mg, lamivudine 150 mg, and zidovudine 300 mg

Generic: Abacavir sulfate 300 mg, lamivudine 150 mg, and zidovudine 300 mg

◆ **Abacavir Sulfate** *see* Abacavir *on page* 18

◆ **Abacavir Sulfate and Lamivudine** *see* Abacavir and Lamivudine *on page* 20

Abatacept (ab a TA sept)

Brand Names: U.S. Orencia

Brand Names: Canada Orencia

Index Terms BMS-188667; CTLA-4Ig

Pharmacologic Category Antirheumatic, Disease Modifying; Selective T-Cell Costimulation Blocker

Use

Treatment of moderately- to severely-active adult rheumatoid arthritis (RA); may be used as monotherapy or in combination with other DMARDs

Treatment of moderately- to severely-active juvenile idiopathic arthritis (JIA); may be used as monotherapy or in combination with methotrexate

Note: Abatacept should **not** be used in combination with anakinra or TNF-blocking agents

Pregnancy Risk Factor C

Pregnancy Considerations Teratogenic effects were not observed in animal studies. There are no adequate and well-controlled studies in pregnant women. Due to the potential risk for development of autoimmune disease in the fetus, use during pregnancy only if clearly needed. A pregnancy registry has been established to monitor outcomes of women exposed to abatacept during pregnancy (1-877-311-8972).

Breast-Feeding Considerations Due to the potential for adverse reactions and possible effects on the developing immune system, breast-feeding is not recommended.

Contraindications There are no contraindications listed within the manufacturer's U.S. labeling.

Canadian labeling: Hypersensitivity to abatacept or any component of the formulation; patients with, or at risk of sepsis syndrome (eg, immunocompromised, HIV positive)

Warnings/Precautions Serious and potentially fatal infections (including tuberculosis and sepsis) have been reported, particularly in patients receiving concomitant immunosuppressive therapy. RA patients receiving a concomitant TNF antagonist experienced an even higher rate of serious infection. Caution should be exercised when considering the use of abatacept in any patient with a history of recurrent infections, with conditions that predispose them to infections, or with chronic, latent, or localized infections. Patients who develop a new infection while undergoing treatment should be monitored closely. If a patient develops a serious infection, abatacept should be discontinued. Screen patients for latent tuberculosis infection prior to initiating abatacept; safety in tuberculosis-positive patients has not been established. Treat patients testing positive according to standard therapy prior to initiating abatacept. Adult patients receiving abatacept in combination with TNF-blocking agents had higher rates of infections (including serious infections) than patients on TNF-blocking agents alone. The manufacturer does not recommend concurrent use with anakinra or TNF-blocking agents. Monitor for signs and symptoms of infection when transitioning from TNF-blocking agents to abatacept. Due to the effect of T-cell inhibition on host defenses, abatacept may affect immune responses against infections and malignancies; impact on the development and course of malignancies is not fully defined.

Use caution with chronic obstructive pulmonary disease (COPD), higher incidences of adverse effects (COPD exacerbation, cough, rhonchi, dyspnea) have been observed; monitor closely. Rare cases of hypersensitivity, anaphylaxis, or anaphylactoid reactions have been reported with intravenous administration; may occur with first infusion. Some reactions (hypotension, urticaria, dyspnea) occurred within 24 hours of infusion. Discontinue treatment if anaphylaxis or other serious allergic reaction occurs; medications for the treatment of hypersensitivity reactions should be available for immediate use. Patients should be screened for viral hepatitis prior to use; antirheumatic therapy may cause reactivation of hepatitis B. Patients should be brought up to date with all immunizations before initiating therapy. Live vaccines should not be given concurrently or within 3 months of discontinuation of therapy; there is no data available concerning secondary transmission of live vaccines in patients receiving therapy. Powder for injection may contain maltose, which may result in falsely-elevated serum glucose readings on the day of infusion. Higher incidences of infection and malignancy were observed in the elderly; use with caution.

Adverse Reactions **Note:** Percentages not always reported; COPD patients experienced a higher frequency of COPD-related adverse reactions (COPD exacerbation, cough, dyspnea, pneumonia, rhonchi)

>10%:

- Central nervous system: Headache (≤18%)
- Gastrointestinal: Nausea
- Respiratory: Nasopharyngitis (12%), upper respiratory tract infection
- Miscellaneous: Infection (adults 54%; children 36%), antibody development (2% to 41%)

1% to 10%:

- Cardiovascular: Hypertension (7%)
- Central nervous system: Dizziness (9%)
- Dermatologic: Skin rash (4%)
- Gastrointestinal: Dyspepsia (6%), abdominal pain, diarrhea
- Genitourinary: Urinary tract infection (6%)
- Immunologic: Immunogenicity (1% to 2%)
- Infection: Herpes simplex infection, influenza
- Local: Injection site reaction (3%)
- Neuromuscular & skeletal: Back pain (7%), limb pain (3%)
- Respiratory: Cough (8%), bronchitis, pneumonia, rhinitis, sinusitis
- Miscellaneous: Infusion-related reaction (≤9%), fever

<1% (Limited to important or life-threatening): Acute lymphocytic leukemia, anaphylactoid reaction, anaphylaxis, cellulitis, diverticulitis, dyspnea, exacerbation of arthritis, exacerbation of chronic obstructive pulmonary disease, hypersensitivity, hypotension, joint wear, malignant neoplasm (including malignant melanoma, malignant neoplasm of the bile duct, malignant neoplasm of bladder, malignant neoplasm of breast, malignant neoplasm of cervix, malignant neoplasm of kidney, malignant neoplasm of prostate, malignant neoplasm of skin, malignant neoplasm of thyroid, myelodysplastic syndrome, and uterine neoplasm), malignant neoplasm of lung, ovarian cyst, pruritus, pyelonephritis, rhonchi, urticaria, varicella, vasculitis (including hypersensitivity angiitis [cutaneous vasculitis and leukocytoclastic vasculitis]), wheezing

Drug Interactions

Metabolism/Transport Effects None known.

Avoid Concomitant Use

Avoid concomitant use of Abatacept with any of the following: Anakinra; Anti-TNF Agents; BCG; Belimumab; Natalizumab; Pimecrolimus; RiTUXimab; Tacrolimus (Topical); Tocilizumab; Tofacitinib; Vaccines (Live)

Increased Effect/Toxicity

Abatacept may increase the levels/effects of: Belimumab; Leflunomide; Natalizumab; Tofacitinib; Vaccines (Live)

The levels/effects of Abatacept may be increased by: Anakinra; Anti-TNF Agents; Denosumab; Pimecrolimus; RiTUXimab; Roflumilast; Tacrolimus (Topical); Tocilizumab; Trastuzumab

Decreased Effect

Abatacept may decrease the levels/effects of: BCG; Coccidioidin Skin Test; Sipuleucel-T; Vaccines (Inactivated); Vaccines (Live)

The levels/effects of Abatacept may be decreased by: Echinacea

Ethanol/Nutrition/Herb Interactions Herb/Nutraceutical: Avoid echinacea (has immunostimulant properties; consider therapy modifications).

Preparation for Administration Reconstitute each vial with 10 mL SWFI using the provided silicone-free disposable syringe (discard solutions accidentally reconstituted with siliconized syringe as they may develop translucent particles). Inject SWFI down the side of the vial to avoid foaming. The reconstituted solution contains 25 mg/mL abatacept. Further dilute (using a silicone-free syringe) in 100 mL NS to a final concentration of ≤10 mg/mL. Prior to adding abatacept to the 100 mL bag, the manufacturer recommends withdrawing a volume of NS equal to the abatacept volume required, resulting in a final volume of 100 mL. Mix gently; do not shake.

Storage/Stability

Prefilled syringe: Store at 2°C to 8°C (36°F to 46°F); do not freeze. Protect from light.

Powder for injection: Prior to reconstitution, store at 2°C to 8°C (36°F to 46°F); do not freeze. Protect from light. After dilution, may be stored for up to 24 hours at room temperature or refrigerated at 2°C to 8°C (36°F to 46°F). Must be used within 24 hours of reconstitution.

Mechanism of Action Selective costimulation modulator; inhibits T-cell (T-lymphocyte) activation by binding to CD80 and CD86 on antigen presenting cells (APC), thus blocking the required CD28 interaction between APCs and T cells. Activated T lymphocytes are found in the synovium of rheumatoid arthritis patients.

Pharmacodynamics/Kinetics

Bioavailability: SubQ: 78.6% (relative to I.V. administration)

Distribution: V_{ss}: 0.02-0.13 L/kg

Half-life elimination: 8-25 days

Dosage

Children 6-17 years: JIA: I.V.:

- <75 kg: 10 mg/kg, repeat dose at 2 and 4 weeks after initial infusion, and every 4 weeks thereafter
- ≥75 kg: Refer to adult I.V. dosing; maximum dose: 1000 mg

Adults: RA:

I.V.: Dosing is according to body weight:

- <60 kg: 500 mg
- 60-100 kg: 750 mg
- >100 kg: 1000 mg

I.V. regimen: Following the initial I.V. infusion, repeat I.V. dose (using the same weight-based dosing) at 2 weeks and 4 weeks after the initial infusion, and every 4 weeks thereafter.

SubQ regimen: Following the initial I.V. infusion (using the weight-based dosing), administer 125 mg subcutaneously within 24 hours of the infusion, followed by 125 mg subcutaneously once weekly thereafter. **Note:** Patients unable to receive I.V. infusions may omit the initial I.V. loading dose and initiate once weekly SubQ therapy directly.

Transitioning from I.V. therapy to SubQ therapy: Administer the first SubQ dose instead of the next scheduled I.V. dose.

Elderly: Refer to adult dosing; due to potential for higher rates of infections and malignancies, use caution.

Dosage adjustment for toxicity: Discontinue in patients who develop a serious infection.

Dosage adjustment in renal impairment: No dosage adjustment provided in manufacturer's labeling (has not been studied).

Dosage adjustment in hepatic impairment: No dosage adjustment provided in manufacturer's labeling (has not been studied).

Administration

I.V.: Infuse over 30 minutes. Administer through a 0.2-1.2 micron low protein-binding filter

SubQ: Allow prefilled syringe to warm to room temperature (for 30-60 minutes) prior to administration. Inject into the front of the thigh (preferred), abdomen (except for 2-inch area around the navel), or the outer area of the upper arms (if administered by a caregiver). Rotate injection sites (≥1 inch apart); do not administer into tender, bruised, red, or hard skin.

Monitoring Parameters Signs and symptoms of infection, signs and symptoms of hypersensitivity reaction; hepatitis and TB screening prior to therapy initiation

Test Interactions Contains maltose; may result in falsely elevated blood glucose levels with dehydrogenase pyrroloquinolinequinone or glucose-dye-oxidoreductase testing methods on the day of infusion. Glucose monitoring methods which utilize glucose dehydrogenase nicotine adenine dinucleotide (GDH-NAD), glucose oxidase, or glucose hexokinase are recommended.

Dosage Forms Excipient information presented when available (limited, particularly for generics); consult specific product labeling.

Solution, Subcutaneous [preservative free]:
Orencia: 125 mg/mL (1 mL)

Solution Reconstituted, Intravenous [preservative free]:
Orencia: 250 mg (1 ea)

◆ **Abbott-43818** *see* Leuprolide *on page 1189*

◆ **ABC** *see* Abacavir *on page 18*

◆ **ABCD** *see* Amphotericin B Cholesteryl Sulfate Complex *on page 122*

Abciximab (ab SIK si mab)

Brand Names: U.S. ReoPro

Brand Names: Canada ReoPro®

Index Terms 7E3; C7E3

Pharmacologic Category Antiplatelet Agent, Glycoprotein IIb/IIIa Inhibitor

Use Prevention of cardiac ischemic complications in patients undergoing percutaneous coronary intervention (PCI); prevention of cardiac ischemic complications in patients with unstable angina (UA)/non-ST-elevation myocardial infarction (NSTEMI) unresponsive to conventional therapy when PCI is scheduled within 24 hours

Note: Intended for use with aspirin and heparin, at a minimum.

Unlabeled Use To support PCI during ST-elevation myocardial infarction (STEMI) (administered at the time of primary PCI)

Pregnancy Risk Factor C

Pregnancy Considerations Animal reproduction studies have not been conducted. *In vitro* studies have shown only small amounts of abciximab to cross the placenta. It is not known whether abciximab can cause fetal harm when administered to a pregnant woman or can affect reproduction capacity.

Breast-Feeding Considerations It is not known if abciximab is excreted in breast milk. The manufacturer recommends that caution be exercised when administering abciximab to nursing women.

Contraindications Hypersensitivity to abciximab, murine proteins, or any component of the formulation; active internal hemorrhage or recent (within 6 weeks) clinically-significant GI or GU bleeding; history of cerebrovascular accident within 2 years or with significant neurological deficit; clotting abnormalities or administration of oral anticoagulants within 7 days unless prothrombin time (PT) is ≤1.2 times control PT value; thrombocytopenia (<100,000 cells/μL); recent (within 6 weeks) major surgery or trauma; intracranial tumor, arteriovenous malformation, or aneurysm; severe uncontrolled hypertension; history of vasculitis; use of dextran before PTCA or intent to use dextran during PTCA; concomitant use of another parenteral GP IIb/IIIa inhibitor

Warnings/Precautions Administration of abciximab is associated with increased frequency of major bleeding complications, including retroperitoneal bleeding, pulmonary bleeding, spontaneous GI or GU bleeding, and bleeding at the arterial access. Risk may be increased with patients weighing <75 kg, elderly patients (>65 years of age), history of previous GI disease, and recent thrombolytic therapy. When attempting I.V. access, avoid noncompressible sites (eg, subclavian or jugular veins).

The risk of major bleeds may increase with concurrent use of thrombolytics. Anticoagulation, such as with heparin, may contribute to the risk of bleeding. In serious, uncontrolled bleeding, abciximab and heparin should be stopped. Increased risk of hemorrhage during or following angioplasty is associated with unsuccessful PTCA, PTCA procedure >70 minutes duration, or PTCA performed within 12 hours of symptom onset for acute myocardial infarction. Prior to pulling the sheath, heparin should be discontinued for 3-4 hours and ACT ≤175 seconds or aPTT ≤50 seconds. Use standard compression techniques after sheath removal. Watch the site closely afterwards for further bleeding.

Administration of abciximab may result in human antichimeric antibody formation that can cause hypersensitivity reactions (including anaphylaxis), thrombocytopenia, or diminished efficacy. Readministration of abciximab within 30 days or in patients with human antichimeric antibodies (HACA) increases the incidence and severity of thrombocytopenia.

Adverse Reactions As with all drugs which may affect hemostasis, bleeding is associated with abciximab. Hemorrhage may occur at virtually any site. Risk is dependent on multiple variables, including the concurrent use of multiple agents which alter hemostasis and patient susceptibility.

>10%:
Cardiovascular: Hypotension (14%), chest pain (11%)
Gastrointestinal: Nausea (14%)
Hematologic: Minor hemorrhage (4% to 17%), major hemorrhage (1% to 14%)
Neuromuscular & skeletal: Back pain (18%)

1% to 10%:
Cardiovascular: Bradycardia (5%), peripheral edema (2%)
Central nervous system: Headache (7%)
Gastrointestinal: Vomiting (7%), abdominal pain (3%)
Hematologic: Thrombocytopenia: <100,000 cells/mm^3 (3% to 6%); <50,000 cells/mm^3 (0.4% to 2%)
Local: Pain at injection site (4%)

<1% (Limited to important or life-threatening): Abnormality in thinking, allergic reaction (possible), anaphylaxis (possible), arteriovenous fistula, bronchospasm, bullous skin disease, cellulitis, cerebrovascular accident, coma,

complete atrioventricular block, confusion, diabetes mellitus, embolism, hyperkalemia, incomplete atrioventricular block, inflammation, intestinal obstruction, intracranial hemorrhage, myalgia, nodal arrhythmia, pleural effusion, pneumonia, prostatitis, pruritus, pulmonary embolism, urinary retention, ventricular tachycardia, xerostomia

Drug Interactions

Metabolism/Transport Effects None known.

Avoid Concomitant Use

Avoid concomitant use of Abciximab with any of the following: Belimumab; Dextran

Increased Effect/Toxicity

Abciximab may increase the levels/effects of: Agents with Antiplatelet Properties; Anticoagulants; Belimumab; Collagenase (Systemic); Dabigatran Etexilate; Ibritumomab; Monoclonal Antibodies; Rivaroxaban; Salicylates; Thrombolytic Agents; Tositumomab and Iodine I 131 Tositumomab

The levels/effects of Abciximab may be increased by: Dasatinib; Dextran; Glucosamine; Herbs (Anticoagulant/Antiplatelet Properties); Ibrutinib; Multivitamins/Fluoride (with ADE); Multivitamins/Minerals (with ADEK, Folate, Iron); Multivitamins/Minerals (with AE, No Iron); Nonsteroidal Anti-Inflammatory Agents; Omega-3 Fatty Acids; Pentosan Polysulfate Sodium; Pentoxifylline; Prostacyclin Analogues; Tipranavir; Vitamin E

Decreased Effect

The levels/effects of Abciximab may be decreased by: Nonsteroidal Anti-Inflammatory Agents

Preparation for Administration Bolus dose: Aseptically withdraw the necessary amount of abciximab for the bolus dose into a syringe using a 0.2 or 5 micron low protein-binding syringe filter (or equivalent); the bolus should be administered 10-60 minutes before the procedure.

Continuous infusion: Aseptically withdraw amount required of abciximab for the infusion through a 0.2 or 5 micron low protein-binding syringe filter into a syringe; inject this into 250 mL of NS or D_5W to make solution. If a syringe filter was not used when preparing the infusion, administer using an in-line 0.2 or 0.22 micron low protein-binding filter.

Note: A standard concentration of 7.2 mg in 250 mL of NS or D_5W may also be prepared for all patients and administered at the standard dose (0.125 mcg/kg/minute; maximum: 10 mcg/minute) with a variable rate in mL/hour. Infuse for 12-24 hours via pump after bolus dose; length of therapy dependent on indication. Some institutions use a standard concentration of 9 mg in 250 mL of D_5W or NS.

Storage/Stability Vials should be stored at 2°C to 8°C (36°F to 46°F). Do not freeze or shake. After admixture, the prepared solution is stable for 12 hours.

The following stability information has also been reported: May store intact vials at 24°C to 28°C (76°F to 82°F) for up to 8 days (data on file [Eli Lilly, 2011]). However, the manufacturer recommends storage under refrigeration. Room temperature stability information should only be utilized in situations where the drug has been inadvertently exposed to prolonged room temperature.

Mechanism of Action Fab antibody fragment of the chimeric human-murine monoclonal antibody 7E3; this agent binds to platelet IIb/IIIa receptors, resulting in steric hindrance, thus inhibiting platelet aggregation

Pharmacodynamics/Kinetics

Onset: Rapid; platelet aggregation reduced to <20% of baseline at 10 minutes

Duration: Up to 72 hours for restoration of normal hemostasis (Schror, 2003)

Distribution: V_d: 0.07 L/kg (Schror, 2003)

Protein binding: Mostly bound to GP IIb/IIIa receptors on platelet surface

Metabolism: Unbound abciximab metabolized via proteolytic cleavage (Schror, 2003)

Half-life elimination: Plasma: ~30 minutes; dissociation half-life from GP IIb/IIIa receptors: up to 4 hours (Schror, 2003). **Note:** 29% and 13% of abciximab estimated to remain on GP IIb/IIIa receptors at 8 and 15 days, respectively (Mascelli, 1998). Platelet function may remain abnormal for up to 7 days post infusion (Osende, 2001).

Time to peak: Platelet inhibition: ~30 minutes (Mascelli, 1998)

Dosage

Percutaneous coronary intervention (PCI): I.V.: 0.25 mg/kg bolus administered 10-60 minutes prior to start of PCI followed by an infusion of 0.125 mcg/kg/minute (maximum: 10 mcg/minute) for 12 hours

Unstable angina/non-ST-elevation MI (UA/NSTEMI) unresponsive to conventional medical therapy with planned PCI within 24 hours: I.V.: 0.25 mg/kg bolus followed by an 18- to 24-hour infusion of 10 mcg/minute, concluding 1 hour after PCI.

ST-elevation myocardial infarction (STEMI) undergoing primary percutaneous coronary intervention (PCI) (unlabeled use; Kushner, 2009): I.V.:

Loading dose: 0.25 mg/kg bolus administered at the time of PCI

Maintenance infusion: 0.125 mcg/kg/minute (maximum: 10 mcg/minute) continued for up to 12 hours

Dosage adjustment in renal impairment: No dosage adjustment provided in manufacturer's labeling.

Dosage adjustment in hepatic impairment: No dosage adjustment provided in manufacturer's labeling.

Usual Infusion Concentrations: Adult I.V. infusion: 7.2 mg in 250 mL (concentration: 28.8 **mcg**/mL) **or** 9 mg in 250 mL (concentration: 36 **mcg**/mL) of D_5W or NS

Administration Abciximab is intended for coadministration with aspirin postangioplasty and heparin infused and weight adjusted to maintain a therapeutic bleeding time (eg, ACT 300-500 seconds). Solution must be filtered prior to administration. Do not shake the vial.

Monitoring Parameters Prothrombin time, activated partial thromboplastin time (aPTT), hemoglobin, hematocrit, platelet count, fibrinogen, fibrin split products, transfusion requirements, signs of hypersensitivity reactions, guaiac stools, Hemastix® urine. Platelet count should be monitored at baseline, 2-4 hours following bolus infusion, and at 24 hours (or prior to discharge, if before 24 hours). To minimize risk of bleeding:

Abciximab initiated 18-24 hours prior to PCI: Maintain aPTT between 60-85 seconds during the heparin/abciximab infusion period

During PCI: Maintain ACT between 200-300 seconds

Following PCI (if anticoagulation is maintained): Maintain aPTT between 50-75 seconds

Sheath removal should not occur until aPTT is ≤50 seconds or ACT ≤175 seconds.

Maintain bleeding precautions, avoid unnecessary arterial and venous punctures, use saline or heparin lock for blood drawing, assess sheath insertion site and distal pulses of affected leg every 15 minutes for the first hour and then every 1 hour for the next 6 hours. Arterial access site care is important to prevent bleeding. Care should be taken when attempting vascular access that only the anterior wall of the femoral artery is punctured, avoiding a Seldinger (through and through) technique for obtaining sheath access. Femoral vein sheath placement should be avoided unless needed. While the vascular sheath is in place, patients should be maintained on complete bedrest with the head of the bed at a 30° angle and the affected limb restrained in a straight position.

Observe patient for mental status changes, hemorrhage; assess nose and mouth mucous membranes, puncture sites for oozing, ecchymosis, and hematoma formation; and examine urine, stool, and emesis for presence of occult or frank blood; gentle care should be provided when removing dressings.

Dosage Forms Excipient information presented when available (limited, particularly for generics); consult specific product labeling.

Solution, Intravenous:

ReoPro: 2 mg/mL (5 mL)

◆ **Abelcet** *see* Amphotericin B (Lipid Complex) *on page 126*

◆ **Abelcet® (Can)** *see* Amphotericin B (Lipid Complex) *on page 126*

◆ **Abenol (Can)** *see* Acetaminophen *on page 28*

◆ **ABI-007** *see* PACLitaxel (Protein Bound) *on page 1546*

◆ **Abilify** *see* ARIPiprazole *on page 163*

◆ **Abilify Discmelt** *see* ARIPiprazole *on page 163*

◆ **Abilify Maintena** *see* ARIPiprazole *on page 163*

◆ **Abiraterone** *see* Abiraterone Acetate *on page 24*

Abiraterone Acetate (a bir A ter one AS e tate)

Brand Names: U.S. Zytiga

Brand Names: Canada Zytiga

Index Terms Abiraterone; CB7630

Pharmacologic Category Antiandrogen; Antineoplastic Agent, Antiandrogen

Use Prostate cancer: Treatment of metastatic, castration-resistant prostate cancer (in combination with prednisone)

Pregnancy Risk Factor X

Pregnancy Considerations Adverse effects were observed in animal reproduction studies at doses resulting in less systemic exposure than in humans. Adverse effects were also observed in the reproductive system of animals during toxicology and pharmacology studies. Based on the mechanism of action, abiraterone may cause fetal harm or fetal loss if administered during pregnancy. Abiraterone is not indicated for use in women and is specifically contraindicated in women who are or may become pregnant. It is not known if abiraterone is excreted in semen, therefore, men should use a condom and another method of birth control during treatment and for 1 week following therapy if having intercourse with a woman of reproductive age. Women who are or may become pregnant should wear gloves if contact with tablets may occur.

Breast-Feeding Considerations Not indicated for use in women

Contraindications Women who are or may become pregnant

Canadian labeling: Additional contraindication (not in U.S. labeling): Hypersensitivity to abiraterone acetate or any component of the formulation or container

Warnings/Precautions Hazardous agent - use appropriate precautions for handling and disposal (meets NIOSH, 2012 criteria). Significant increases in liver enzymes have been reported (higher likelihood in patients with baseline elevations), generally occurring in the first 3 months of treatment. May require dosage reduction or discontinuation. ALT, AST, and bilirubin should be monitored prior to treatment, every 2 weeks for 3 months and monthly thereafter; patients with hepatic impairment, elevations in liver function tests, or experiencing hepatotoxicity require more frequent monitoring (see dosage adjustment for hepatic impairment in Dosage and Monitoring Parameters). Evaluate liver function promptly with signs or symptoms of hepatotoxicity. The safety of retreatment after significant elevations (ALT or AST >20 times the upper limit of normal [ULN] and/or total bilirubin >10 times ULN) has not been evaluated. Avoid use in patients with pre-existing severe hepatic impairment; dosage reduction is recommended in patients with baseline moderate impairment. Canadian labeling (not in U.S. labeling) also recommends avoiding use in patients with pre-existing moderate hepatic impairment.

Concurrent infection, stress, or interruption of daily corticosteroids is associated with reports of adrenocortical insufficiency. Monitor closely for signs and symptoms of adrenocorticoid insufficiency, which could be masked by adverse events associated with mineralocorticoid excess. Diagnostic testing for adrenal insufficiency may be clinically indicated. Increased corticosteroid doses may be required before, during, and after stress. May cause increased mineralocorticoid levels, which may result in hypertension, hypokalemia and fluid retention (including grades 3 and 4 events). Concomitant administration with corticosteroids reduces the incidence and severity of these adverse events. Due to potential for hypertension, hypokalemia, or fluid retention, use with caution in patients with cardiovascular disease (particularly heart failure, recent MI, or ventricular arrhythmia); patients with left ventricular ejection fraction (LVEF) <50% or NYHA class III or IV heart failure were excluded from clinical trials. Monitor at least monthly for hypertension, hypokalemia, and fluid retention.

Abiraterone must be administered on an empty stomach (administer at least 1 hour before and 2 hours after any food). Potentially significant drug-drug interactions may exist, requiring dose or frequency adjustment, additional monitoring, and/or selection of alternative therapy. Avoid use with concomitant strong CYP3A4 inducers (dose modification is necessary if concomitant use cannot be avoided). Avoid concurrent administration with CYP2D6 substrates with a narrow therapeutic index (eg, thioridazine); if concurrent administration cannot be avoided, consider a dose reduction of the CYP2D6 substrate.

Adverse Reactions Note: Adverse reactions reported for use in combination with prednisone.

>10%:

Cardiovascular: Edema (25% to 27%), hypertension (9% to 22%; grades 3/4: 1% to 4%)

Central nervous system: Fatigue (39%), insomnia (14%)

Dermatologic: Bruise (13%)

Endocrine & metabolic: Increased serum triglycerides (63%), hyperglycemia (57%), hypernatremia (33%), hypokalemia (17% to 28%; grades 3/4: 3% to 5%), hypophosphatemia (24%; grades 3/4: 7%), hot flash (19% to 22%)

Gastrointestinal: Constipation (23%), diarrhea (18% to 22%), dyspepsia (6% to 11%)

Genitourinary: Urinary tract infection (12%)

Hematologic: Lymphocytopenia (38%; grades 3/4: 9%)

Hepatic: Increased serum ALT (11% to 42%; grades 3/4: 1% to 6%), increased serum AST (31% to 37%; grades 3/4: 2% to 3%)

Neuromuscular & skeletal: Joint swelling (30%, including joint discomfort), myalgia (26%)

Respiratory: Cough (11% to 17%), upper respiratory infection (5% to 13%), dyspnea (12%), nasopharyngitis (11%)

1% to 10%:

Cardiovascular: Cardiac arrhythmia (7%), chest pain (4%, including chest discomfort), cardiac failure (2%)

Central nervous system: Falling (6%)

Dermatologic: Skin rash (8%)

Genitourinary: Hematuria (10%), groin pain (7%), polyuria (7%), nocturia (6%)

Hepatic: Increased serum bilirubin (7%; grades 3/4: <1%)

Miscellaneous: Fever (9%)
Neuromuscular & skeletal: Bone fracture (6%)
<1% (Limited to important or life-threatening): Adrenocortical insufficiency

Drug Interactions

Metabolism/Transport Effects Substrate of CYP3A4 (major); **Note:** Assignment of Major/Minor substrate status based on clinically relevant drug interaction potential; **Inhibits** CYP1A2 (weak), CYP2C19 (moderate), CYP2C8 (strong), CYP2C9 (moderate), CYP2D6 (moderate), CYP3A4 (moderate), P-glycoprotein

Avoid Concomitant Use

Avoid concomitant use of Abiraterone Acetate with any of the following: Bosutinib; CYP3A4 Inducers (Strong); Ibrutinib; Ivabradine; Lomitapide; PAZOPanib; Pimozide; Pomalidomide; Silodosin; Simeprevir; Thioridazine; Tolvaptan; Topotecan; Ulipristal; VinCRIStine (Liposomal)

Increased Effect/Toxicity

Abiraterone Acetate may increase the levels/effects of: Afatinib; ARIPiprazole; Avanafil; Bosentan; Bosutinib; Budesonide (Systemic, Oral Inhalation); Carvedilol; Citalopram; Colchicine; CYP1A2 Substrates; CYP2C19 Substrates; CYP2C8 Substrates; CYP2C9 Substrates; CYP2D6 Substrates; CYP3A4 Substrates; Dabigatran Etexilate; Dofetilide; Eplerenone; Everolimus; FentaNYL; Fesoterodine; Halofantrine; Ibrutinib; Imatinib; Ivabradine; Ivacaftor; Lomitapide; Lurasidone; Metoprolol; Nebivolol; OxyCODONE; PAZOPanib; P-glycoprotein/ABCB1 Substrates; Pimecrolimus; Pimozide; Pioglitazone; Pomalidomide; Propafenone; Prucalopride; Ranolazine; Rivaroxaban; Salmeterol; Saxagliptin; Silodosin; Simeprevir; Thioridazine; Tolvaptan; Topotecan; Treprostinil; Ulipristal; Vilazodone; VinCRIStine (Liposomal); Zuclopenthixol

The levels/effects of Abiraterone Acetate may be increased by: Propafenone

Decreased Effect

Abiraterone Acetate may decrease the levels/effects of: Clopidogrel; Codeine; Ifosfamide; Tamoxifen; TraMADol

The levels/effects of Abiraterone Acetate may be decreased by: Bosentan; CYP3A4 Inducers (Strong); Dabrafenib; Deferasirox; Herbs (CYP3A4 Inducers); Spironolactone; Tocilizumab

Ethanol/Nutrition/Herb Interactions Food: Taking with food will increase systemic exposure. Management: Do not administer with food. Must be taken on an empty stomach, at least 1 hour before and 2 hours after food.

Storage/Stability Store at 20°C to 25°C (68°F to 77°F); excursions are permitted between 15°C and 30°C (59°F and 86°F).

Mechanism of Action Selectively and irreversibly inhibits CYP17 (17 alpha-hydroxylase/C17,20-lyase), an enzyme required for androgen biosynthesis which is expressed in testicular, adrenal, and prostatic tumor tissues. Inhibits the formation of the testosterone precursors dehydroepiandrosterone (DHEA) and androstenedione.

Pharmacodynamics/Kinetics

Distribution: V_{dss}: 19,669 ± 13,358 L
Protein binding: >99%; to albumin and alpha$_1$-acid glycoprotein
Metabolism: Abiraterone acetate is hydrolyzed to the active metabolite abiraterone; further metabolized to inactive metabolites abiraterone sulphate and N-oxide abiraterone sulphate via CYP3A4 and SULT2A1
Bioavailability: Systemic exposure is increased by food
Half-life elimination: 14.4-16.5 hours (Acharya, 2012)
Time to peak: 2 hours (Acharya, 2012)
Excretion: Feces (~88%); urine (~5%)

Dosage Prostate cancer, metastatic, castration-resistant: Adults: Oral: 1000 mg once daily (in combination with prednisone)

Dosage adjustment for concomitant strong CYP3A4 inducers: Avoid concomitant strong CYP3A4 inducers; if a strong CYP3A4 inducer must be administered concurrently, increase the abiraterone frequency to twice daily (eg, from 1000 mg once daily to 1000 mg twice daily). Upon discontinuation of the strong CYP3A4 inducer, reduce abiraterone back to the prior dose and frequency.

Dosage adjustment in renal impairment: No dosage adjustment necessary.

Dosage adjustment in hepatic impairment:

Hepatic impairment ***prior to*** treatment initiation:
Mild (Child-Pugh class A): No dosage adjustment necessary.
Moderate (Child-Pugh class B):
U.S. labeling: 250 mg once daily. Permanently discontinue if ALT and/or AST >5 times the upper limit of normal (ULN) or total bilirubin >3 times ULN during treatment.
Canadian labeling: Use is not recommended.
Severe (Child-Pugh class C): Avoid use

Hepatotoxicity ***during*** treatment:
U.S. labeling:
ALT and/or AST >5 times ULN or total bilirubin >3 times ULN: Withhold treatment until liver function tests return to baseline or ALT and AST ≤2.5 times ULN and total bilirubin ≤1.5 times ULN, then reinitiate at 750 mg once daily.
Recurrent hepatotoxicity on 750 mg/day: Withhold treatment until liver function tests return to baseline or ALT and AST ≤2.5 times ULN and total bilirubin ≤1.5 times ULN, then reinitiate at 500 mg once daily.
Recurrent hepatotoxicity on 500 mg once daily: Discontinue treatment
Canadian labeling:
ALT or AST >5 times ULN or total bilirubin >3 times ULN:
Withhold treatment until liver function tests normalize, then (when hepatic function returns to baseline) reinitiate at 500 mg once daily
Recurrent hepatotoxicity on 500 mg once daily: Discontinue treatment
ALT >20 times ULN (any time during treatment): Discontinue permanently.

Dietary Considerations Must be taken on an empty stomach, at least 1 hour before and 2 hours after food.

Administration Administer orally on an empty stomach, at least 1 hour before and 2 hours after food. Swallow tablets whole with water. Do not crush or chew.

Hazardous agent; use appropriate precautions for handling and disposal (meets NIOSH, 2012 criteria). Women who are or may become pregnant should wear gloves if handling the tablets.

Monitoring Parameters ALT, AST, and bilirubin prior to treatment, every 2 weeks for 3 months and monthly thereafter; if baseline moderate hepatic impairment (Child-Pugh class B), monitor ALT, AST, and bilirubin prior to treatment, weekly for the first month, every 2 weeks for 2 months then monthly thereafter. If hepatotoxicity develops during treatment (and only after therapy is interrupted and liver function tests have returned to safe levels), monitor ALT, AST, and bilirubin every 2 weeks for 3 months and monthly thereafter. Monitoring of testosterone levels is not necessary.

Monitor for signs and symptoms of adrenocorticoid insufficiency; if clinically indicated, consider appropriate diagnostics to confirm adrenal insufficiency. Monitor monthly for hypertension, hypokalemia, and fluid retention.

Dosage Forms Excipient information presented when available (limited, particularly for generics); consult specific product labeling.
Tablet, Oral:
Zytiga: 250 mg

◆ **ABLC** *see* Amphotericin B (Lipid Complex) *on page 126*

AbobotulinumtoxinA
(aye bo BOT yoo lin num TOKS in aye)

Brand Names: U.S. Dysport; Dysport (Glabellar Lines)
Index Terms Botulinum Toxin Type A
Pharmacologic Category Neuromuscular Blocker Agent, Toxin
Use Treatment of cervical dystonia in both toxin-naive and previously treated patients; temporary improvement in the appearance of moderate-severe glabellar lines associated with procerus and corrugator muscle activity
Pregnancy Risk Factor C
Medication Guide Available Yes
Dosage
Adults:
Cervical dystonia: I.M.: Initial: 500 units divided among affected muscles in toxin-naïve or toxin-experienced patients. May re-treat at intervals of ≥12 weeks
Dosage adjustments: Adjust dosage in 250-unit increments; do not administer at intervals <12 weeks; dosage range used in studies: 250-1000 units
Glabellar lines: Adults <65 years: I.M.: Inject 10 units (0.05 mL or 0.08 mL) into each of 5 sites (2 injections in each corrugator muscle and 1 injection in the procerus muscle) for a total dose of 50 units; do not administer at intervals <3 months; efficacy has been demonstrated up to 4 repeated administrations
Elderly:
Cervical dystonia: Refer to adult dosing.
Glabellar lines: Not recommended in patients ≥65 years of age

Dosage adjustment in renal impairment: No adjustment necessary
Dosage adjustment in hepatic impairment: No adjustment necessary
Additional Information Complete prescribing information should be consulted for additional detail.
Dosage Forms Excipient information presented when available (limited, particularly for generics); consult specific product labeling.
Solution Reconstituted, Intramuscular:
Dysport: 300 units (1 ea); 500 units (1 ea) [contains milk protein]
Dysport (Glabellar Lines): 300 units (1 ea) [contains albumin human, milk protein]

◆ **Abraxane** *see* PACLitaxel (Protein Bound) *on page 1546*
◆ **Abraxane for Injectable Suspension (Can)** *see* PACLitaxel (Protein Bound) *on page 1546*
◆ **Abreva [OTC]** *see* Docosanol *on page 644*
◆ **Absorica** *see* ISOtretinoin *on page 1129*
◆ **Abstral** *see* FentaNYL *on page 842*
◆ **ABT-335** *see* Fenofibrate and Derivatives *on page 837*
◆ **ABthrax** *see* Raxibacumab *on page 1791*
◆ **ABX-EGF** *see* Panitumumab *on page 1561*
◆ **AC 2993** *see* Exenatide *on page 815*
◆ **ACAM2000®** *see* Smallpox Vaccine *on page 1909*

Acamprosate (a kam PROE sate)

Brand Names: U.S. Campral
Brand Names: Canada Campral®
Index Terms Acamprosate Calcium; Calcium Acetylhomotaurinate
Pharmacologic Category GABA Agonist/Glutamate Antagonist
Use Maintenance of alcohol abstinence
Pregnancy Risk Factor C
Dosage Oral: Adults: Alcohol abstinence: 666 mg 3 times/day (a lower dose may be effective in some patients). **Note:** Treatment should be initiated as soon as possible following the period of alcohol withdrawal, when the patient has achieved abstinence and should be maintained if patient relapses.

Dosage adjustment in renal impairment:
Cl_{cr} 30-50 mL/minute: 333 mg 3 times/day
Cl_{cr} <30 mL/minute: Contraindicated in severe renal impairment.
Dosage adjustment in hepatic impairment:
Mild-to-moderate impairment: No dosage adjustments are recommended
Severe impairment: There are no dosage adjustments provided in manufacturer's labeling.
Additional Information Complete prescribing information should be consulted for additional detail.
Dosage Forms Excipient information presented when available (limited, particularly for generics); consult specific product labeling.
Tablet Delayed Release, Oral, as calcium:
Campral: 333 mg
Generic: 333 mg

◆ **Acamprosate Calcium** *see* Acamprosate *on page 26*

Acarbose (AY car bose)

Brand Names: U.S. Precose
Brand Names: Canada Glucobay™
Pharmacologic Category Antidiabetic Agent, Alpha-Glucosidase Inhibitor
Use Adjunct to diet and exercise to lower blood glucose in patients with type 2 diabetes mellitus (noninsulin dependent, NIDDM)
Pregnancy Risk Factor B
Pregnancy Considerations Adverse events have not been reported in animal reproduction studies. Low amounts of acarbose are absorbed systemically which should limit fetal exposure. Limited information is available describing pregnancy outcomes following maternal use of acarbose.

For women with diabetes, maternal hyperglycemia can be associated with adverse effects in the fetus, neonate, and mother. To prevent adverse events, prior to conception and throughout pregnancy, the maternal Hb A_{1c} should be kept close to normal but without causing significant hypoglycemia. The use of most oral antihyperglycemic agents in pregnant women is not recommended for routine management of GDM or type 2 diabetes mellitus in pregnant women; insulin is the drug of choice for the control of diabetes mellitus during pregnancy (ACOG, 2005; ADA, 2013; Kitzmiller, 2008; Metzger, 2007).
Breast-Feeding Considerations It is not known if acarbose is found in breast milk; however, low amounts of acarbose are absorbed systemically in adults, which may limit the amount that could distribute into breast milk. Although breast-feeding is encouraged for all women, including those with diabetes, the safety of acarbose during breast-feeding has not yet been established (Metzger, 2007). Breast-feeding is not recommended by the manufacturer.
Contraindications Hypersensitivity to acarbose or any component of the formulation; patients with diabetic ketoacidosis or cirrhosis; patients with inflammatory bowel

disease, colonic ulceration, partial intestinal obstruction, or in patients predisposed to intestinal obstruction; patients who have chronic intestinal diseases associated with marked disorders of digestion or absorption, and in patients who have conditions that may deteriorate as a result of increased gas formation in the intestine

Warnings/Precautions Acarbose given in combination with a sulfonylurea or insulin will cause a further lowering of blood glucose and may increase the hypoglycemic potential of the sulfonylurea or insulin. Treatment-emergent elevations of serum transaminases (AST and/or ALT) occurred in up to 14% of acarbose-treated patients in long-term studies. These serum transaminase elevations appear to be dose related and were asymptomatic, reversible, more common in females, and, in general, were not associated with other evidence of liver dysfunction. Fulminant hepatitis has been reported rarely. It may be necessary to discontinue acarbose and administer insulin if the patient is exposed to stress (ie, fever, trauma, infection, surgery). Use not recommended in patients with significant impairment (S_{cr} >2 mg/dL); use with caution in other patients with renal impairment.

Adverse Reactions

>10%:

Gastrointestinal: Diarrhea (31%) and abdominal pain (19%) tend to return to pretreatment levels over time; frequency and intensity of flatulence (74%) tend to abate with time

Hepatic: Transaminases increased (≤4%)

Postmarketing and/or case reports: Edema, erythema, exanthema, hepatitis, ileus/subileus, jaundice, liver damage, pneumatosis cystoides intestinalis, rash, thrombocytopenia, urticaria

Drug Interactions

Metabolism/Transport Effects None known.

Avoid Concomitant Use There are no known interactions where it is recommended to avoid concomitant use.

Increased Effect/Toxicity

Acarbose may increase the levels/effects of: Hypoglycemic Agents

The levels/effects of Acarbose may be increased by: Herbs (Hypoglycemic Properties); MAO Inhibitors; Neomycin; Pegvisomant; Salicylates; Selective Serotonin Reuptake Inhibitors

Decreased Effect

Acarbose may decrease the levels/effects of: Digoxin

The levels/effects of Acarbose may be decreased by: Corticosteroids (Orally Inhaled); Corticosteroids (Systemic); Loop Diuretics; Luteinizing Hormone-Releasing Hormone Analogs; Somatropin; Thiazide Diuretics

Ethanol/Nutrition/Herb Interactions Ethanol: Limit ethanol.

Storage/Stability Store at <25°C (77°F). Protect from moisture.

Mechanism of Action Competitive inhibitor of pancreatic α-amylase and intestinal brush border α-glucosidases, resulting in delayed hydrolysis of ingested complex carbohydrates and disaccharides and absorption of glucose; dose-dependent reduction in postprandial serum insulin and glucose peaks; inhibits the metabolism of sucrose to glucose and fructose

Pharmacodynamics/Kinetics

Absorption: <2% as active drug; ~35% as metabolites

Metabolism: Exclusively via GI tract, principally by intestinal bacteria and digestive enzymes; 13 metabolites identified (major metabolites are sulfate, methyl, and glucuronide conjugates)

Bioavailability: Low systemic bioavailability of parent compound; acts locally in GI tract

Half-life elimination: ~2 hours

Time to peak: Active drug: ~1 hour

Excretion: Urine (~34% as inactive metabolites, <2% parent drug and active metabolite); feces (~51% as unabsorbed drug)

Dosage Oral:

Adults: Dosage must be individualized on the basis of effectiveness and tolerance while not exceeding the maximum recommended dose

Initial dose: 25 mg 3 times/day with the first bite of each main meal; to reduce GI effects, some patients may benefit from initiating at 25 mg once daily with gradual titration to 25 mg 3 times/day as tolerated

Maintenance dose: Should be adjusted at 4- to 8-week intervals based on 1-hour postprandial glucose levels and tolerance until maintenance dose is reached. Dosage may be increased from 25 mg 3 times/day to 50 mg 3 times/day. Some patients may benefit from increasing the dose to 100 mg 3 times/day.

Maintenance dose ranges: 50-100 mg 3 times/day.

Maximum dose:

≤60 kg: 50 mg 3 times/day

>60 kg: 100 mg 3 times/day

Patients receiving sulfonylureas or insulin: Acarbose given in combination with a sulfonylurea or insulin will cause a further lowering of blood glucose and may increase the hypoglycemic potential of the sulfonylurea or insulin. If hypoglycemia occurs, appropriate adjustments in the dosage of these agents should be made.

Dosing adjustment in renal impairment:

Cl_{cr} ≥25 mL/minute: No dosage adjustment necessary. Although acarbose is primarily excreted unchanged, the increased plasma levels in renal impairment are not expected to affect efficacy (clinical response is localized to the GI tract); however, the effects on adverse effects are unknown.

Cl_{cr} <25 mL/minute or S_{cr} >2 mg/dL: Use not recommended (not adequately studied).

Dosing adjustment in hepatic impairment: No dosage adjustment provided in manufacturer's labeling.

Dietary Considerations Take with food (first bite of meal).

Administration Should be administered with the first bite of each main meal.

Monitoring Parameters Postprandial glucose, glycosylated hemoglobin levels, serum transaminase levels should be checked every 3 months during the first year of treatment and periodically thereafter, renal function (serum creatinine); blood pressure

Reference Range Recommendations for glycemic control in nonpregnant adults with diabetes (ADA, 2013):

Hb A_{1c}: <7% (a more aggressive [<6.5%] or less aggressive [<8%] Hb A_{1c} goal may be targeted based on patient-specific characteristics)

Preprandial capillary plasma glucose: 70-130 mg/dL

Peak postprandial capillary blood glucose: <180 mg/dL

Dosage Forms Excipient information presented when available (limited, particularly for generics); consult specific product labeling.

Tablet, Oral:

Precose: 25 mg, 50 mg, 100 mg

Generic: 25 mg, 50 mg, 100 mg

◆ **A-Caro-25 [OTC]** *see* Beta-Carotene *on page* 246

◆ **Accel-Amlodipine (Can)** *see* AmLODIPine *on page* 109

◆ **Accel-Clarithromycin (Can)** *see* Clarithromycin *on page* 446

◆ **Accel-Pioglitazone (Can)** *see* Pioglitazone *on page* 1649

◆ **Accolate** *see* Zafirlukast *on page* 2219

◆ **Accolate® (Can)** *see* Zafirlukast *on page* 2219

◆ **AccuNeb** *see* Albuterol *on page* 61

◆ **Accupril** *see* Quinapril *on page* 1761

◆ **Accutane** *see* ISOtretinoin *on page* 1129

◆ **Accutane® (Can)** *see* ISOtretinoin *on page* 1129

◆ **ACE** *see* Captopril *on page* 333

Acebutolol (a se BYOO toe lole)

Brand Names: U.S. Sectral

Brand Names: Canada Apo-Acebutolol®; Ava-Acebutolol; Mylan-Acebutolol; Mylan-Acebutolol (Type S); Nu-Acebutolol; Rhotral; Sandoz-Acebutolol; Sectral®; Teva-Acebutolol

Index Terms Acebutolol Hydrochloride

Pharmacologic Category Antiarrhythmic Agent, Class II; Antihypertensive; Beta-Blocker With Intrinsic Sympathomimetic Activity

Additional Appendix Information

Beta-Blockers *on page* 2294

Use Treatment of hypertension; management of ventricular arrhythmias

Unlabeled Use Treatment of chronic stable angina (**Note:** Not recommended for patients with prior MI)

Pregnancy Risk Factor B

Dosage Oral:

Adults:

Ventricular arrhythmias: Initial: 400 mg/day in 2 divided doses; maintenance: 600-1200 mg/day in divided doses; maximum: 1200 mg/day

Hypertension: 400-800 mg/day (larger doses may be divided); maximum: 1200 mg/day; usual dose range (JNC 7): 200-800 mg/day in 2 divided doses

Chronic stable angina (unlabeled use): Usual dose: 400-1200 mg/day in 2 divided doses (Gibbons, 2003); low doses (ie, 400 mg/day) may also be given as once daily (Pina, 1988)

Elderly: Consider dose reduction due to age-related increase in bioavailability; do not exceed 800 mg/day. In the management of hypertension, consider lower initial dose (eg, 200-400 mg/day) and titrate to response (Aronow, 2011).

Dosing adjustment in renal impairment:

Cl_{cr} 25-49 mL/minute: Reduce dose by 50%.

Cl_{cr} <25 mL/minute: Reduce dose by 75%.

Dosing adjustment in hepatic impairment: There are no dosage adjustments provided in manufacturer's labeling; use with caution.

Additional Information Complete prescribing information should be consulted for additional detail.

Dosage Forms Excipient information presented when available (limited, particularly for generics); consult specific product labeling.

Capsule, Oral, as hydrochloride:

Sectral: 200 mg [contains brilliant blue fcf (fd&c blue #1), fd&c yellow #6 (sunset yellow)]

Sectral: 400 mg [contains brilliant blue fcf (fd&c blue #1), fd&c red #40, fd&c yellow #6 (sunset yellow)]

Generic: 200 mg, 400 mg

Dosage Forms: Canada Excipient information presented when available (limited, particularly for generics); consult specific product labeling.

Tablet, Oral, as hydrochloride:

Sectral: 100 mg, 200 mg, 400 mg

◆ **Acebutolol Hydrochloride** *see* Acebutolol *on page* 28

◆ **Aceon** *see* Perindopril Erbumine *on page* 1622

◆ **Acephen [OTC]** *see* Acetaminophen *on page* 28

◆ **Acerola C 500 [OTC]** *see* Ascorbic Acid *on page* 172

◆ **Acetadote** *see* Acetylcysteine *on page* 36

◆ **Aceta-Gesic®** *see* Acetaminophen and Diphenhydramine *on page* 32

Acetaminophen (a seet a MIN oh fen)

Brand Names: U.S. Acephen [OTC]; APAP 500 [OTC]; Aspirin Free Anacin Extra Strength [OTC]; Cetafen Extra [OTC]; Cetafen [OTC]; Excedrin Tension Headache [OTC]; Feverall [OTC]; Little Fevers [OTC]; Mapap Arthritis Pain [OTC]; Mapap Children's [OTC]; Mapap Extra Strength [OTC]; Mapap Infant's [OTC]; Mapap Junior Rapid Tabs [OTC]; Mapap [OTC]; Non-Aspirin Pain Reliever [OTC]; Nortemp Children's [OTC]; Ofirmev; Pain & Fever Children's [OTC]; Pain Eze [OTC]; Q-Pap Children's [OTC]; Q-Pap Extra Strength [OTC]; Q-Pap Infant's [OTC]; Q-Pap [OTC]; RapiMed Children's [OTC]; RapiMed Junior [OTC]; Silapap Children's [OTC]; Silapap Infant's [OTC]; Triaminic Children's Fever Reducer Pain Reliever [OTC]; Tylenol 8 Hour [OTC]; Tylenol Arthritis Pain Extended Relief [OTC]; Tylenol Children's Meltaways [OTC]; Tylenol Children's [OTC]; Tylenol Extra Strength [OTC]; Tylenol Infant's Concentrated [OTC] [DSC]; Tylenol Jr. Meltaways [OTC]; Tylenol [OTC]; Valorin Extra [OTC]; Valorin [OTC]

Brand Names: Canada Abenol; Apo-Acetaminophen; Atasol; Novo-Gesic; Pediatrix; Tempra; Tylenol

Index Terms APAP (abbreviation is not recommended); N-Acetyl-P-Aminophenol; Paracetamol

Pharmacologic Category Analgesic, Miscellaneous

Use Treatment of mild-to-moderate pain and fever (analgesic/antipyretic)

I.V.: Additional indication: Management of moderate-to-severe pain when combined with opioid analgesia

Pregnancy Risk Factor C (intravenous)

Pregnancy Considerations Animal reproduction studies have not been conducted with intravenous acetaminophen, therefore, acetaminophen I.V. is classified as pregnancy category C. Acetaminophen crosses the placenta and can be detected in cord blood, newborn serum, and urine immediately after delivery. An increased risk of teratogenic effects has not been observed following maternal use of acetaminophen during pregnancy. Prenatal constriction of the ductus arteriosus has been noted in case reports following maternal use during the third trimester. The use of acetaminophen in normal doses during pregnancy is not associated with an increased risk of miscarriage or still birth; however, an increase in fetal death or spontaneous abortion may be seen following maternal overdose if treatment is delayed. Frequent maternal use of acetaminophen during pregnancy may be associated with wheezing and asthma in early childhood. The absorption may be delayed and the bioavailability of acetaminophen may be decreased in some women during pregnancy due to delayed gastric emptying.

Breast-Feeding Considerations Low concentrations of acetaminophen are excreted into breast milk and can be detected in the urine of nursing infants. Adverse reactions have generally not been observed; however, a rash caused by acetaminophen exposure was reported in one breast-feeding infant.

Contraindications Hypersensitivity to acetaminophen or any component of the formulation; severe hepatic impairment or severe active liver disease (Ofirmev™)

Warnings/Precautions [U.S. Boxed Warning]: Acetaminophen injection formulation has been associated with acute liver failure, at times resulting in liver transplant and death. Take care to avoid dosing errors; ensure that the dose in mg is not confused with mL, dosing in patients <50 kg is based on body weight, infusion pumps are properly programmed, and total daily dose of acetaminophen from all sources does not exceed the maximum daily limits.

Limit acetaminophen dose from all sources (prescription, OTC, combination products) and all routes of administration (I.V., oral, rectal) to <4 g/day (adults). In addition, chronic daily dosing may result in liver damage in some patients; hepatotoxicity is usually associated with excessive acetaminophen intake (>4 g/day in adults). Use with caution in patients with alcoholic liver disease; consuming ≥3 alcoholic drinks/day may increase the risk of liver damage. Use caution in patients with hepatic impairment or active liver disease. Use of I.V. formulation is contraindicated in patients with severe hepatic impairment or severe active liver disease. Use caution in patients with known G6PD deficiency; rare reports of hemolysis have occurred. Use caution in patients with chronic malnutrition and hypovolemia (I.V. formulation). Use caution in patients with severe renal impairment; consider dosing adjustments. Hypersensitivity and anaphylactic reactions have been reported; discontinue immediately if symptoms of allergic or hypersensitivity reactions occur. Rarely, acetaminophen may cause serious and potentially fatal skin reactions such as acute generalized exanthematous pustulosis, Stevens-Johnson syndrome (SJS), and toxic epidermal necrolysis (TEN). Discontinue treatment if severe skin reactions develop.

OTC labeling: When used for self-medication, patients should be instructed to contact healthcare provider if used for fever lasting >3 days or for pain lasting >10 days in adults or >5 days in children. OTC labeling limits the maximum daily dose to ≤3250 mg (dosage form specific).

Adverse Reactions Oral, Rectal: Frequency not defined:

Dermatologic: Skin rash

Endocrine & metabolic: Decreased serum bicarbonate, decreased serum calcium, decreased serum sodium, hyperchloremia, hyperuricemia, increased serum glucose

Genitourinary: Nephrotoxicity (with chronic overdose)

Hematologic & oncologic: Anemia, leukopenia, neutropenia, pancytopenia

Hepatic: Increased serum alkaline phosphatase, increased serum bilirubin

Hypersensitivity: Hypersensitivity reaction (rare)

Renal: Hyperammonemia, renal disease (analgesic)

I.V.:

>10%: Gastrointestinal: Nausea (adults 34%; children ≥5%), vomiting (adults 15%; children ≥5%)

1% to 10%:

Cardiovascular: Hypertension, hypotension, peripheral edema, tachycardia

Central nervous system: Headache (adults 10%; children ≥1%), insomnia (adults 7%; children ≥1%), agitation (children ≥5%), anxiety, fatigue, trismus

Dermatologic: Pruritus (children ≥5%), skin rash

Endocrine & metabolic: Hypervolemia, hypoalbuminemia, hypokalemia, hypomagnesemia, hypophosphatemia

Gastrointestinal: Constipation (children ≥5%), abdominal pain, diarrhea

Genitourinary: Oliguria (children ≥1%)

Hematologic & oncologic: Anemia

Hepatic: Increased serum transaminases

Local: Infusion site reaction (pain)

Neuromuscular & skeletal: Limb pain, muscle spasm

Ophthalmic: Periorbital edema

Respiratory: Atelectasis (children ≥5%), abnormal breath sounds, dyspnea, hypoxia, pleural effusion, pulmonary edema, stridor, wheezing

All formulations: <1% (Limited to important or life-threatening): Anaphylaxis, hypersensitivity reaction

Drug Interactions

Metabolism/Transport Effects **Substrate** of CYP1A2 (minor), CYP2A6 (minor), CYP2C9 (minor), CYP2D6 (minor), CYP2E1 (minor), CYP3A4 (minor); **Note:** Assignment of Major/Minor substrate status based on clinically relevant drug interaction potential; **Inhibits** CYP3A4 (weak)

Avoid Concomitant Use

Avoid concomitant use of Acetaminophen with any of the following: Pimozide

Increased Effect/Toxicity

Acetaminophen may increase the levels/effects of: ARIPiprazole; Busulfan; Dasatinib; Dofetilide; Imatinib; Lomitapide; Mipomersen; Pimozide; Prilocaine; Sodium Nitrite; SORAfenib; Vitamin K Antagonists

The levels/effects of Acetaminophen may be increased by: Dasatinib; Isoniazid; Metyrapone; Nitric Oxide; Probenecid; SORAfenib

Decreased Effect

The levels/effects of Acetaminophen may be decreased by: Anticonvulsants (Hydantoin); Barbiturates; CarBAMazepine; Cholestyramine Resin; Peginterferon Alfa-2b

Ethanol/Nutrition/Herb Interactions

Ethanol: Excessive intake of ethanol may increase the risk of acetaminophen-induced hepatotoxicity. Avoid ethanol or limit to <3 drinks/day.

Food: Rate of absorption may be decreased when given with food.

Herb/Nutraceutical: St John's wort may decrease acetaminophen levels.

Preparation for Administration Injectable solution may be administered directly from the vial without further dilution.

Doses <1000 mg (<50 kg): Withdraw appropriate dose from vial and transfer to a separate sterile container (eg, glass bottle, plastic I.V. container, syringe) for administration. Small volume pediatric doses (up to 600 mg [60 mL]) may be placed in a syringe and infused over 15 minutes via syringe pump.

Doses of 1000 mg (≥50 kg): Insert vented I.V. set through vial stopper.

Storage/Stability

Injection: Store intact vials at 20°C to 25°C (68°F to 77°F); do not refrigerate or freeze. Use within 6 hours of opening vial or transferring to another container. Discard any unused portion; single use vials only.

Oral formulations: Store at controlled room temperature.

Suppositories: Store at <27°C (80°F); do not freeze.

Mechanism of Action Although not fully elucidated, believed to inhibit the synthesis of prostaglandins in the central nervous system and work peripherally to block pain impulse generation; produces antipyresis from inhibition of hypothalamic heat-regulating center

Pharmacodynamics/Kinetics

Onset of action:

Oral: <1 hour

I.V.: Analgesia: 5-10 minutes; Antipyretic: Within 30 minutes

Peak effect: I.V.: Analgesic: 1 hour

Duration:

I.V., Oral: Analgesia: 4-6 hours

I.V.: Antipyretic: ≥6 hours

Absorption: Primarily absorbed in small intestine (rate of absorption dependent upon gastric emptying); minimal absorption from stomach; varies by dosage form

Distribution: ~1 L/kg at therapeutic doses

Protein binding: 10% to 25% at therapeutic concentrations; 8% to 43% at toxic concentrations

Metabolism: At normal therapeutic dosages, primarily hepatic metabolism to sulfate and glucuronide conjugates, while a small amount is metabolized by CYP2E1 to a highly reactive intermediate, N-acetyl-p-benzoquinone imine (NAPQI), which is conjugated rapidly with glutathione and inactivated to nontoxic cysteine and mercapturic acid conjugates. At toxic doses (as little as 4 g daily) ▶

glutathione conjugation becomes insufficient to meet the metabolic demand causing an increase in NAPQI concentrations, which may cause hepatic cell necrosis. Oral administration is subject to first pass metabolism.

Half-life elimination: Prolonged following toxic doses

Neonates: 7 hours (range: 4-10 hours)

Infants: ~4 hours (range: 1-7 hours)

Children: 3 hours (range: 2-5 hours)

Adolescents: ~3 hours (range: 2-4 hours)

Adults: ~2 hours (range: 2-3 hours); may be slightly prolonged in severe renal insufficiency (Cl_{cr}<30 mL/minute): 2-5.3 hours

Time to peak, serum: Oral: Immediate release: 10-60 minutes (may be delayed in acute overdoses); I.V.: 15 minutes

Excretion: Urine (<5% unchanged; 60% to 80% as glucuronide metabolites; 20% to 30% as sulphate metabolites; ~8% cysteine and mercapturic acid metabolites)

Dosage Note: No dose adjustment required if converting between different acetaminophen formulations. Limit acetaminophen dose from all sources (prescription and OTC) to <4 g daily (adults).

Oral: Note: OTC dosing recommendations may vary by product and/or manufacturer.

Infants and Children <12 years: 10-15 mg/kg/dose every 4-6 hours as needed; do **not** exceed 5 doses (2.6 g) in 24 hours; alternatively, the following age-based doses may be used; see table.

Children ≥12 years, Adolescents, and Adults:

Regular release: 325-650 mg every 4-6 hours or 1000 mg 3-4 times daily (maximum: 4 g daily)

Extended release: 1300 mg every 8 hours (maximum: 3.9 g daily)

Acetaminophen Pediatric Dosing (Oral)[1]

Weight (kg)	Weight (lbs)	Age	Dosage (mg)
2.7-5.3	6-11	0-3 mo	40
5.4-8.1	12-17	4-11 mo	80
8.2-10.8	18-23	1-2 y	120
10.9-16.3	24-35	2-3 y	160
16.4-21.7	36-47	4-5 y	240
21.8-27.2	48-59	6-8 y	320
27.3-32.6	60-71	9-10 y	400
32.7-43.2	72-95	11 y	480

[1]Manufacturer's recommendations; use of weight to select dose is preferred; if weight is not available, then use age. Manufacturer's recommendations are based on weight in pounds (OTC labeling); weight in kg listed here is derived from pounds and rounded; kg weight listed also is adjusted to allow for continuous weight ranges in kg. OTC labeling instructs consumer to consult with physician for dosing instructions in children under 2 years of age.

Rectal:

Infants and Children <12 years: 10-20 mg/kg/dose every 4-6 hours as needed; do **not** exceed 5 doses (2.6 g) in 24 hours. **Note:** Although the perioperative use of high-dose rectal acetaminophen (eg, 25-45 mg/kg/dose) has been investigated in several studies, its routine use remains controversial; optimal doses and dosing frequency to ensure efficacy and safety have not yet been established (Buck, 2001).

Children ≥12 years, Adolescents, and Adults: 325-650 mg every 4-6 hours or 1000 mg 3-4 times daily (maximum: 4 g daily)

I.V.:

Children 2-12 years: 15 mg/kg every 6 hours **or** 12.5 mg/kg every 4 hours; maximum single dose: 15 mg/kg/dose (≤750 mg/dose); maximum daily dose: 75 mg/kg/day (≤3.75 g daily)

Adolescents and Adults:

<50 kg: 15 mg/kg every 6 hours or 12.5 mg/kg every 4 hours; maximum single dose: 15 mg/kg/dose (750 mg/dose); maximum daily dose: 75 mg/kg/day (≤3.75 g daily)

≥50 kg: 650 mg every 4 hours or 1000 mg every 6 hours; maximum single dose: 1000 mg/dose; maximum daily dose: 4 g daily

Dosing interval in renal impairment:

Oral (Aronoff, 2007):

Children:

Cl_{cr} <10 mL/minute: Administer every 8 hours

Intermittent hemodialysis or peritoneal dialysis: Administer every 8 hours

CRRT: No adjustments necessary

Adults:

Cl_{cr} 10-50 mL/minute: Administer every 6 hours

Cl_{cr} <10 mL/minute: Administer every 8 hours

Intermittent hemodialysis or peritoneal dialysis: No adjustment necessary

CRRT: Administer every 8 hours

I.V.: Cl_{cr} ≤30 mL/minute: Use with caution; consider decreasing daily dose and extending dosing interval

Dosing adjustment/comments in hepatic impairment:

Oral: Use with caution. Limited, low-dose therapy is usually well tolerated in hepatic disease/cirrhosis. However, cases of hepatotoxicity at daily acetaminophen dosages <4 g daily have been reported. Avoid chronic use in hepatic impairment.

I.V.:

Mild-to-moderate impairment: Use with caution in hepatic impairment or active liver disease; manufacturer's labeling suggests a reduced total daily dosage may be warranted, although no specific dosage adjustments are provided.

Severe impairment: Use is contraindicated.

Dietary Considerations Some products may contain phenylalanine and/or sodium.

Administration

Suspension, oral: Shake well before pouring a dose.

Injection: For I.V. infusion only. May administer undiluted over 15 minutes.

Monitoring Parameters Serum APAP levels: Where acute overdose suspected and with long-term use in patients with hepatic disease; relief of pain or fever

Test Interactions Acetaminophen may cause false-positive urinary 5-hydroxyindoleacetic acid.

Additional Information In 2011, McNeil Consumer Healthcare announced it had voluntarily reduced the maximum doses and increased the dosing interval on the labeling of some of their acetaminophen OTC products in an attempt to protect consumers from inadvertent overdoses. For example, the maximum dose of Extra Strength Tylenol® OTC was lowered from 4 g/day to 3 g/day and the maximum dose of Regular Strength Tylenol® OTC was lowered from 3900 mg/day to 3250 mg/day. In addition, the dosing interval for Extra Strength Tylenol® OTC was increased from every 4-6 hours to every 6 hours. Healthcare professionals may still prescribe or recommend the 4 g/day maximum to patients (but are advised to use their own discretion and clinical judgment).

Dosage Forms Excipient information presented when available (limited, particularly for generics); consult specific product labeling. [DSC] = Discontinued product

Caplet, oral: 500 mg
Cetafen® Extra: 500 mg
Mapap® Extra Strength: 500 mg
Mapap® Extra Strength: 500 mg [scored]
Pain Eze: 650 mg
Tylenol®: 325 mg
Tylenol® Extra Strength: 500 mg
Caplet, extended release, oral:
Mapap® Arthritis Pain: 650 mg
Tylenol® 8 Hour: 650 mg
Tylenol® Arthritis Pain Extended Relief: 650 mg
Capsule, oral:
Mapap® Extra Strength: 500 mg
Captab, oral: 500 mg
Elixir, oral:
Mapap® Children's: 160 mg/5 mL (118 mL, 480 mL) [ethanol free; contains benzoic acid, propylene glycol, sodium benzoate; cherry flavor]
Gelcap, oral: 500 mg
Mapap®: 500 mg
Gelcap, rapid release, oral: 500 mg
Tylenol® Extra Strength: 500 mg
Geltab, oral: 500 mg
Excedrin® Tension Headache: 500 mg [contains caffeine 65 mg/geltab]
Injection, solution [preservative free]:
Ofirmev™: 10 mg/mL (100 mL)
Liquid, oral: 160 mg/5 mL (120 mL, 473 mL); 500 mg/5 mL (240 mL)
APAP 500: 500 mg/5 mL (237 mL) [ethanol free, sugar free; cherry flavor]
Mapap® Extra Strength: 500 mg/5 mL (237 mL) [contains propylene glycol, sodium 9 mg/15 mL, sodium benzoate; cherry flavor]
Q-Pap Children's: 160 mg/5 mL (118 mL, 473 mL) [ethanol free; contains propylene glycol, sodium 2 mg/5 mL, sodium benzoate; cherry flavor]
Q-Pap Children's: 160 mg/5 mL (118 mL) [ethanol free; contains propylene glycol, sodium 2 mg/5 mL, sodium benzoate; grape flavor]
Silapap Children's: 160 mg/5 mL (118 mL, 237 mL, 473 mL) [ethanol free, sugar free; contains propylene glycol, sodium benzoate; cherry flavor]
Tylenol® Extra Strength: 500 mg/15 mL (240 mL) [ethanol free; contains propylene glycol, sodium benzoate; cherry flavor]
Solution, oral: 160 mg/5 mL (5 mL, 10 mL, 20 mL)
Pain & Fever Children's: 160 mg/5 mL (118 mL, 473 mL) [ethanol free, sugar free; contains propylene glycol, sodium 1 mg/5 mL, sodium benzoate; cherry flavor]
Solution, oral [drops]: 80 mg/0.8 mL (15 mL [DSC])
Little Fevers™: 80 mg/mL (30 mL) [dye free, ethanol free, gluten free; contains propylene glycol, sodium benzoate; berry flavor]
Q-Pap Infant's: 80 mg/0.8 mL (15 mL) [ethanol free; contains propylene glycol; fruit flavor]
Silapap Infant's: 80 mg/0.8 mL (15 mL, 30 mL) [ethanol free; contains propylene glycol, sodium benzoate; cherry flavor]
Suppository, rectal: 120 mg (12s); 325 mg (12s); 650 mg (12s)
Acephen™: 120 mg (12s, 50s, 100s); 325 mg (6s, 12s, 50s, 100s); 650 mg (12s, 50s, 100s)
Feverall®: 80 mg (6s, 50s); 120 mg (6s, 50s); 325 mg (6s, 50s); 650 mg (50s)
Suspension, oral: 160 mg/5 mL (5 mL, 10.15 mL, 20.3 mL)
Mapap® Children's: 160 mg/5 mL (118 mL) [ethanol free; contains propylene glycol, sodium benzoate; cherry flavor]
Mapap® Infant's: 160 mg/5 mL (59 mL) [dye free, ethanol free; contains propylene glycol, sodium benzoate; cherry flavor]
Nortemp Children's: 160 mg/5 mL (118 mL) [ethanol free; contains propylene glycol, sodium benzoate; cotton candy flavor]
Pain & Fever Children's: 160 mg/5 mL (60 mL) [ethanol free; contains propylene glycol, sodium benzoate; cherry flavor]
Q-Pap Children's: 160 mg/5 mL (118 mL) [ethanol free; contains sodium 2 mg/5 mL, sodium benzoate; bubblegum flavor]
Q-Pap Children's: 160 mg/5 mL (118 mL) [ethanol free; contains sodium 2 mg/5 mL, sodium benzoate; cherry flavor]
Q-Pap Children's: 160 mg/5 mL (118 mL) [ethanol free; contains sodium 2 mg/5 mL, sodium benzoate; grape flavor]
Tylenol® Children's: 160 mg/5 mL (120 mL) [dye free, ethanol free; contains propylene glycol, sodium benzoate; cherry flavor]
Tylenol® Children's: 160 mg/5 mL (120 mL) [ethanol free; contains propylene glycol, sodium 2 mg/5 mL, sodium benzoate; bubblegum flavor]
Tylenol® Children's: 160 mg/5 mL (60 mL, 120 mL) [ethanol free; contains propylene glycol, sodium 2 mg/5 mL, sodium benzoate; cherry flavor]
Tylenol® Children's: 160 mg/5 mL (120 mL) [ethanol free; contains propylene glycol, sodium 2 mg/5 mL, sodium benzoate; grape flavor]
Tylenol® Children's: 160 mg/5 mL (120 mL) [ethanol free; contains propylene glycol, sodium 2 mg/5 mL, sodium benzoate; strawberry flavor]
Suspension, oral [drops]:
Tylenol® Infant's Concentrated: 80 mg/0.8 mL (30 mL [DSC]) [dye free; contains propylene glycol; cherry flavor]
Tylenol® Infant's Concentrated: 80 mg/0.8 mL (15 mL [DSC], 30 mL [DSC]) [ethanol free; contains sodium benzoate; cherry flavor]
Tylenol® Infant's Concentrated: 80 mg/0.8 mL (15 mL [DSC], 30 mL [DSC]) [ethanol free; contains sodium benzoate; grape flavor]
Syrup, oral:
Triaminic™ Children's Fever Reducer Pain Reliever: 160 mg/5 mL (118 mL) [contains benzoic acid, sodium 6 mg/5 mL; bubblegum flavor]
Triaminic™ Children's Fever Reducer Pain Reliever: 160 mg/5 mL (118 mL) [contains sodium 5 mg/5 mL, sodium benzoate; grape flavor]
Tablet, oral: 325 mg, 500 mg
Aspirin Free Anacin® Extra Strength: 500 mg
Cetafen®: 325 mg
Mapap®: 325 mg
Non-Aspirin Pain Reliever: 325 mg
Q-Pap: 325 mg [scored]
Q-Pap Extra Strength: 500 mg [scored]
Tylenol®: 325 mg
Tylenol® Extra Strength: 500 mg
Valorin: 325 mg [sugar free]
Valorin Extra: 500 mg [sugar free]
Tablet, chewable, oral: 80 mg
Mapap® Children's: 80 mg [fruit flavor]
Tablet, orally disintegrating, oral: 80 mg, 160 mg
Mapap® Children's: 80 mg [bubblegum flavor]
Mapap® Children's: 80 mg [grape flavor]
Mapap® Junior Rapid Tabs: 160 mg [bubblegum flavor]
RapiMed® Children's: 80 mg [gluten free, sugar free; bubblegum flavor]
RapiMed® Children's: 80 mg [gluten free, sugar free; wild grape flavor]
RapiMed® Junior: 160 mg [gluten free, sugar free; bubblegum flavor]
RapiMed® Junior: 160 mg [gluten free, sugar free; wild grape flavor]

Tylenol® Children's Meltaways: 80 mg [scored; bubblegum flavor]
Tylenol® Children's Meltaways: 80 mg [scored; grape flavor]
Tylenol® Jr. Meltaways: 160 mg [bubblegum flavor]
Tylenol® Jr. Meltaways: 160 mg [grape flavor]

◆ **Acetaminophen and Butalbital** *see* Butalbital and Acetaminophen *on page 305*

◆ **Acetaminophen and Chlorpheniramine** *see* Chlorpheniramine and Acetaminophen *on page 412*

Acetaminophen and Codeine

(a seet a MIN oh fen & KOE deen)

Brand Names: U.S. Capital® and Codeine; Tylenol® with Codeine No. 3; Tylenol® with Codeine No. 4

Brand Names: Canada ratio-Emtec-30; ratio-Lenoltec; Triatec-30; Triatec-8; Triatec-8 Strong; Tylenol Elixir with Codeine; Tylenol No. 1; Tylenol No. 1 Forte; Tylenol No. 2 with Codeine; Tylenol No. 3 with Codeine; Tylenol No. 4 with Codeine

Index Terms Codeine and Acetaminophen; Emtec; Tylenol #2; Tylenol #3; Tylenol Codeine

Pharmacologic Category Analgesic Combination (Opioid)

Use Relief of mild-to-moderate pain

Pregnancy Risk Factor C

Dosage Doses should be adjusted according to severity of pain and response of the patient. Adult doses ≥60 mg codeine fail to give commensurate relief of pain but merely prolong analgesia and are associated with an appreciably increased incidence of side effects. Oral:

Children: Analgesic:
- Codeine: 0.5-1 mg codeine/kg/dose every 4-6 hours
- Acetaminophen: 10-15 mg/kg/dose every 4 hours up to a maximum of 2.6 g/24 hours for children <12 years; **alternatively, the following can be used:**
  - 3-6 years: 5 mL 3-4 times/day as needed of elixir
  - 7-12 years: 10 mL 3-4 times/day as needed of elixir
  - >12 years: 15 mL every 4 hours as needed of elixir

Adults:
- Antitussive: Based on codeine (15-30 mg/dose) every 4-6 hours (maximum: 360 mg/24 hours based on codeine component)
- Analgesic: Based on codeine (30-60 mg/dose) every 4-6 hours (maximum: 4000 mg/24 hours based on acetaminophen component)
  - 1-2 tablets every 4 hours to a maximum of 12 tablets/24 hours

Dosing adjustment in renal impairment: See individual agents.

Dosing adjustment in hepatic impairment: Use with caution. Limited, low-dose therapy is usually well tolerated in hepatic disease/cirrhosis; however, cases of hepatotoxicity at daily acetaminophen dosages <4 g/day have been reported. Avoid chronic use in hepatic impairment.

Additional Information Complete prescribing information should be consulted for additional detail.

Dosage Forms Excipient information presented when available (limited, particularly for generics); consult specific product labeling.

Solution, oral [C-V]: Acetaminophen 120 mg and codeine phosphate 12 mg per 5 mL (5 mL, 10 mL, 12.5 mL, 15 mL, 120 mL, 480 mL)

Suspension, oral [C-V]:
- Capital® and Codeine: Acetaminophen 120 mg and codeine phosphate 12 mg per 5 mL (480 mL) [alcohol free; contains propylene glycol, sodium benzoate; fruit punch flavor]

Tablet, oral [C-III]: Acetaminophen 300 mg and codeine phosphate 15 mg; acetaminophen 300 mg and codeine phosphate 30 mg; acetaminophen 300 mg and codeine phosphate 60 mg
- Tylenol® with Codeine No. 3: Acetaminophen 300 mg and codeine phosphate 30 mg [contains sodium metabisulfite]
- Tylenol® with Codeine No. 4: Acetaminophen 300 mg and codeine phosphate 60 mg [contains sodium metabisulfite]

Dosage Forms: Canada Excipient information presented when available (limited, particularly for generics); consult specific product labeling. **Note:** In countries outside of the U.S., some formulations of Tylenol® with Codeine include caffeine.

Caplet:
- ratio-Lenoltec No. 1, Tylenol No. 1: Acetaminophen 300 mg, codeine phosphate 8 mg, and caffeine 15 mg
- Tylenol No. 1 Forte: Acetaminophen 500 mg, codeine phosphate 8 mg, and caffeine 15 mg

Solution, oral:
- Tylenol Elixir with Codeine: Acetaminophen 160 mg and codeine phosphate 8 mg per 5 mL (500 mL) [contains alcohol 7%, sucrose 31%; cherry flavor]

Tablet:
- ratio-Emtec, Triatec-30: Acetaminophen 300 mg and codeine phosphate 30 mg
- ratio-Lenoltec No. 1: Acetaminophen 300 mg, codeine phosphate 8 mg, and caffeine 15 mg
- ratio-Lenoltec No. 2, Tylenol No. 2 with Codeine: Acetaminophen 300 mg, codeine phosphate 15 mg, and caffeine 15 mg
- ratio-Lenoltec No. 3, Tylenol No. 3 with Codeine: Acetaminophen 300 mg, codeine phosphate 30 mg, and caffeine 15 mg
- ratio-Lenoltec No. 4, Tylenol No. 4 with Codeine: Acetaminophen 300 mg and codeine phosphate 60 mg
- Triatec-8: Acetaminophen 325 mg, codeine phosphate 8 mg, and caffeine 30 mg
- Triatec-8 Strong: Acetaminophen 500 mg, codeine phosphate 8 mg, and caffeine 30 mg

Controlled Substance C-III; C-V

Acetaminophen and Diphenhydramine

(a seet a MIN oh fen & dye fen HYE dra meen)

Brand Names: U.S. Aceta-Gesic®; Excedrin PM® [OTC]; Goody's PM® [OTC]; Legatrin PM® [OTC]; Mapap PM [OTC]; Percogesic® Extra Strength [OTC]; TopCare® Pain Relief PM [OTC]; Tylenol® PM [OTC]; Tylenol® Severe Allergy [OTC]

Index Terms Diphenhydramine and Acetaminophen

Pharmacologic Category Analgesic, Miscellaneous

Use Aid in the relief of insomnia accompanied by minor pain

Dosage Oral: Adults: 50 mg of diphenhydramine HCl (76 mg diphenhydramine citrate) at bedtime or as directed by physician; do not exceed recommended dosage; not for use in children <12 years of age

Dosing adjustment in hepatic impairment: Use with caution. Limited, low-dose therapy is usually well tolerated in hepatic disease/cirrhosis; however, cases of hepatotoxicity at daily acetaminophen dosages <4 g/day have been reported. Avoid chronic use in hepatic impairment.

Additional Information Complete prescribing information should be consulted for additional detail.

Dosage Forms Excipient information presented when available (limited, particularly for generics); consult specific product labeling.

Caplet, oral:
- Excedrin PM®: Acetaminophen 500 mg and diphenhydramine citrate 38 mg

Legatrin PM®: Acetaminophen 500 mg and diphenhydramine hydrochloride 50 mg
Mapap PM: Acetaminophen 500 mg and diphenhydramine hydrochloride 25 mg
Percogesic® Extra Strength: Acetaminophen 500 mg and diphenhydramine hydrochloride 12.5 mg
TopCare® Pain Relief PM: Acetaminophen 500 mg and diphenhydramine citrate 25 mg
Tylenol® PM: Acetaminophen 500 mg and diphenhydramine hydrochloride 25 mg
Tylenol® Severe Allergy: Acetaminophen 500 mg and diphenhydramine hydrochloride 12.5 mg
Captab, oral: Acetaminophen 500 mg and diphenhydramine hydrochloride 25 mg
Gelcap, rapid release, oral:
Tylenol® PM: Acetaminophen 500 mg and diphenhydramine hydrochloride 25 mg
Geltab, oral: Acetaminophen 500 mg and diphenhydramine hydrochloride 25 mg
Excedrin® PM: Acetaminophen 500 mg and diphenhydramine citrate 38 mg
Tylenol® PM: Acetaminophen 500 mg and diphenhydramine hydrochloride 25 mg
Liquid, oral:
Tylenol® PM: Acetaminophen 500 mg and diphenhydramine hydrochloride 25 mg per 15 mL (240 mL) [contains sodium benzoate; vanilla flavor]
Powder for solution, oral:
Goody's PM®: Acetaminophen 500 mg and diphenhydramine citrate 38 mg [contains potassium 41.9 mg and sodium 3.15 mg per powder]
Tablet, oral: Acetaminophen 500 mg and diphenhydramine hydrochloride 25 mg
Aceta-Gesic®: Acetaminophen 325 mg and diphenhydramine hydrochloride 12.5 mg
Excedrin® PM: Acetaminophen 500 mg and diphenhydramine citrate 38 mg

◆ **Acetaminophen and Hydrocodone** *see* Hydrocodone and Acetaminophen *on page 1006*
◆ **Acetaminophen and Oxycodone** *see* Oxycodone and Acetaminophen *on page 1538*

Acetaminophen and Pseudoephedrine

(a seet a MIN oh fen & soo doe e FED rin)

Brand Names: U.S. Ornex® Maximum Strength [OTC]; Ornex® [OTC]
Brand Names: Canada Contac® Cold and Sore Throat, Non Drowsy, Extra Strength; Dristan® N.D.; Dristan® N.D., Extra Strength; Sinutab® Non Drowsy; Sudafed® Head Cold and Sinus Extra Strength; Tylenol® Decongestant; Tylenol® Sinus
Index Terms Pseudoephedrine and Acetaminophen; Pseudoephedrine Hydrochloride and Acetaminophen
Pharmacologic Category Alpha/Beta Agonist; Analgesic, Miscellaneous
Use Temporary relief of nasal congestion, and minor aches and pains associated with colds, flu, sinusitis, or allergies
Dosage Oral:
Children 6-11 years (Ornex®): One caplet every 4-6 hours as needed (maximum: 4 caplets/day)
Children ≥12 years and Adults (Ornex®, Ornex® Maximum Strength): Two caplets every 4-6 hours as needed (maximum: 8 caplets/day)

Dosing adjustment in hepatic impairment: Use with caution. Limited, low-dose therapy is usually well tolerated in hepatic disease/cirrhosis; however, cases of hepatotoxicity at daily acetaminophen dosages <4 g/day have been reported. Avoid chronic use in hepatic impairment.

Additional Information Complete prescribing information should be consulted for additional detail.
Dosage Forms Excipient information presented when available (limited, particularly for generics); consult specific product labeling.
Caplet:
Ornex®: Acetaminophen 325 mg and pseudoephedrine hydrochloride 30 mg
Ornex® Maximum Strength: Acetaminophen 500 mg and pseudoephedrine hydrochloride 30 mg

Acetaminophen and Tramadol

(a seet a MIN oh fen & TRA ma dole)

Brand Names: U.S. Ultracet®
Brand Names: Canada Apo-Tramadol/Acet®; CO Tramadol/Acet; JAMP-ACET-Tramadol; Mar-Tramadol/Acet; Pat-Tramadol/Acet; TEVA-Tramadol/Acetaminophen; Tramacet; Tramaphen-Odan
Index Terms Tramadol Hydrochloride and Acetaminophen
Pharmacologic Category Analgesic Combination (Opioid); Analgesic, Miscellaneous
Use Short-term (≤5 days) management of acute pain
Pregnancy Risk Factor C
Dosage Oral: Adults: Acute pain: Two tablets every 4-6 hours as needed for pain relief (maximum: 8 tablets/day); treatment should not exceed 5 days
Dosage adjustment in renal impairment: Cl_{cr} <30 mL/minute: Maximum of 2 tablets every 12 hours; treatment should not exceed 5 days
Dosage adjustment in hepatic impairment: Use is not recommended.
Additional Information Complete prescribing information should be consulted for additional detail.
Dosage Forms Excipient information presented when available (limited, particularly for generics); consult specific product labeling.
Tablet, oral: Acetaminophen 325 mg and tramadol hydrochloride 37.5 mg
Ultracet®: Acetaminophen 325 mg and tramadol hydrochloride 37.5 mg

Acetaminophen, Aspirin, and Caffeine

(a seet a MIN oh fen, AS pir in, & KAF een)

Brand Names: U.S. Anacin® Advanced Headache Formula [OTC]; Excedrin® Extra Strength [OTC]; Excedrin® Migraine [OTC]; Fem-Prin® [OTC]; Goody's® Extra Strength Headache Powder [OTC]; Goody's® Extra Strength Pain Relief [OTC]; Pain-Off [OTC]; Vanquish® Extra Strength Pain Reliever [OTC]
Index Terms Aspirin, Acetaminophen, and Caffeine; Aspirin, Caffeine and Acetaminophen; Caffeine, Acetaminophen, and Aspirin; Caffeine, Aspirin, and Acetaminophen
Pharmacologic Category Analgesic, Miscellaneous
Use Relief of mild-to-moderate pain; mild-to-moderate pain associated with migraine headache
Dosage Oral: Adults:
Analgesic:
Based on **acetaminophen** component:
Mild-to-moderate pain: 325-650 mg every 4-6 hours as needed; do **not** exceed 4 g/day
Mild-to-moderate pain associated with migraine headache: 500 mg/dose (in combination with 500 mg aspirin and 130 mg caffeine) every 6 hours while symptoms persist; do not use for longer than 48 hours
Based on **aspirin** component:
Mild-to-moderate pain: 325-650 mg every 4-6 hours as needed; do **not** exceed 4 g/day

Mild-to-moderate pain associated with migraine headache: 500 mg/dose (in combination with 500 mg acetaminophen and 130 mg caffeine) every 6 hours while symptoms persist; do not use for longer than 48 hours

Product labeling:

Excedrin® Extra Strength, Excedrin® Migraine: Children >12 years and Adults: 2 doses every 6 hours (maximum: 8 doses/24 hours)

Note: When used for migraine, do not use for longer than 48 hours

Goody's® Extra Strength Headache Powder: Children >12 years and Adults: 1 powder, placed on tongue or dissolved in water, every 4-6 hours (maximum: 4 powders/24 hours)

Goody's® Extra Strength Pain Relief Tablets: Children >12 years and Adults: 2 tablets every 4-6 hours (maximum: 8 tablets/24 hours)

Vanquish® Extra Strength Pain Reliever: Children >12 years and Adults: 2 tablets every 4 hours (maximum: 12 tablets/24 hours)

Dosing adjustment in hepatic impairment: Use with caution. Limited, low-dose therapy is usually well tolerated in hepatic disease/cirrhosis; however, cases of hepatotoxicity at daily acetaminophen dosages <4 g/day have been reported. Avoid chronic use in hepatic impairment.

Additional Information Complete prescribing information should be consulted for additional detail.

Dosage Forms Excipient information presented when available (limited, particularly for generics); consult specific product labeling.

Caplet:

Excedrin® Extra Strength, Excedrin® Migraine: Acetaminophen 250 mg, aspirin 250 mg, and caffeine 65 mg

Vanquish® Extra Strength Pain Reliever: Acetaminophen 194 mg, aspirin 227 mg, and caffeine 33 mg

Geltab (Excedrin® Extra Strength, Excedrin® Migraine): Acetaminophen 250 mg, aspirin 250 mg, and caffeine 65 mg

Powder (Goody's® Extra Strength Headache Powder): Acetaminophen 260 mg, aspirin 520 mg, and caffeine 32.5 mg [contains lactose]

Tablet:

Anacin® Advanced Headache Formula: Acetaminophen 250 mg, aspirin 250 mg, and caffeine 65 mg

Excedrin® Extra Strength, Excedrin® Migraine, Pain-Off: Acetaminophen 250 mg, aspirin 250 mg, and caffeine 65 mg

Fem-Prin®: Acetaminophen 194.4 mg, aspirin 226.8 mg, and caffeine 32.4 mg

Goody's® Extra Strength Pain Relief: Acetaminophen 130 mg, aspirin 260 mg, and caffeine 16.25 mg

◆ **Acetaminophen, Butalbital, and Caffeine** *see* Butalbital, Acetaminophen, and Caffeine *on page 305*

◆ **Acetasol® HC** *see* Acetic Acid, Propylene Glycol Diacetate, and Hydrocortisone *on page 35*

◆ **Acetazolam (Can)** *see* AcetaZOLAMIDE *on page 34*

AcetaZOLAMIDE (a set a ZOLE a mide)

Brand Names: U.S. Diamox Sequels

Brand Names: Canada Acetazolam; Diamox®

Pharmacologic Category Anticonvulsant, Miscellaneous; Carbonic Anhydrase Inhibitor; Diuretic, Carbonic Anhydrase Inhibitor; Ophthalmic Agent, Antiglaucoma

Use Treatment of glaucoma (chronic simple open-angle, secondary glaucoma, preoperatively in acute angle-closure); drug-induced edema or edema due to congestive heart failure (adjunctive therapy; I.V. and immediate release dosage forms); centrencephalic epilepsies (I.V. and immediate release dosage forms); prevention or amelioration of symptoms associated with acute mountain sickness (immediate and extended release dosage forms)

Unlabeled Use Metabolic alkalosis; respiratory stimulant in stable hypercapnic COPD

Pregnancy Risk Factor C

Dosage Note: I.M. administration is not recommended because of pain secondary to the alkaline pH

Children:

Altitude illness:

Prevention: Oral: 2.5 mg/kg/dose every 12 hours started either the day before (preferred) or on the day of ascent and may be discontinued after staying at the same elevation for 2-3 days or if descent initiated; maximum dose: 125 mg/dose (Luks, 2010). **Note:** The International Society for Mountain Medicine does not recommend prophylaxis in children except in the rare circumstance of unavoidable rapid ascent or in children with known previous susceptibility to acute mountain sickness (Pollard, 2001).

Treatment: Oral: 2.5 mg/kg/dose every 8-12 hours; maximum dose: 250 mg/dose. **Note:** With high altitude cerebral edema, dexamethasone is the primary treatment; however, acetazolamide may be used adjunctively with the same treatment dose (Luks, 2010; Pollard, 2001).

Epilepsy: Oral: 8-30 mg/kg/day in divided doses. A lower dosing range of 4-16 mg/kg/day in 1-4 divided doses has also been recommended; maximum dose: 30 mg/kg/day or 1 g/day (Oles, 1989; Reiss, 1996). **Note:** Minimal additional benefit with doses >16 mg/kg/day. **Extended release capsule is not recommended for treatment of epilepsy.**

Adults:

Altitude illness: Oral: Manufacturer's labeling: 500-1000 mg/day in divided doses every 8-12 hours (immediate release tablets) or divided every 12-24 hours (extended release capsules). These doses are associated with more frequent and/or increased side effects. Alternative dosing has been recommended:

Prevention: 125 mg twice daily; beginning either the day before (preferred) or on the day of ascent; may be discontinued after staying at the same elevation for 2-3 days or if descent initiated (Basnyat, 2006; Luks, 2010). **Note:** In situations of rapid ascent (such as rescue or military operations), 1000 mg/day is recommended by the manufacturer. The Wilderness Medical Society recommends consideration of using dexamethasone in addition to acetazolamide in these situations (Luks, 2010).

Treatment: 250 mg twice daily. **Note:** With high altitude cerebral edema, dexamethasone is the primary treatment; however, acetazolamide may be used adjunctively with the same treatment dose (Luks, 2010).

Edema: Oral, I.V.: 250-375 mg once daily

Epilepsy: Oral: 8-30 mg/kg/day in divided doses. A lower dosing range of 4-16 mg/kg/day in 1-4 divided doses has also been recommended; maximum dose: 30 mg/kg/day or 1 g/day (Oles, 1989; Reiss, 1996). **Note:** Minimal additional benefit with doses >16 mg/kg/day. **Extended release capsule is not recommended for treatment of epilepsy.**

Glaucoma:

Chronic simple (open-angle): Oral, I.V.: 250 mg 1-4 times/day or 500 mg extended release capsule twice daily

Secondary or acute (closed-angle): Oral, I.V.: Initial: 250-500 mg; maintenance: 125-250 mg every 4 hours (250 mg every 12 hours has been effective in short-term treatment of some patients)

Metabolic alkalosis (unlabeled use): I.V.: 500 mg as a single dose; reassess need based upon acid-base status (Marik, 1991; Mazur, 1999)

Respiratory stimulant in stable hypercapnic COPD (unlabeled use): Oral: 250 mg twice daily (Wagenaar, 2003)

Elderly: Oral: Initial doses should begin at the low end of the dosage range.

Dosage adjustment in renal impairment: Note: Use is contraindicated in marked renal impairment; creatinine clearance cutoff not specified in manufacturer's labeling.

Cl_{cr} 10-50 mL/minute: Administer every 12 hours

Cl_{cr} <10 mL/minute: Avoid use

Hemodialysis: Moderately dialyzable (20% to 50%)

Peritoneal dialysis: Supplemental dose is not necessary (Schwenk, 1994)

Dosage adjustment in hepatic impairment: Use contraindicated in patients with cirrhosis or marked liver disease or dysfunction.

Additional Information Complete prescribing information should be consulted for additional detail.

Dosage Forms Excipient information presented when available (limited, particularly for generics); consult specific product labeling.

Capsule Extended Release 12 Hour, Oral:

Diamox Sequels: 500 mg

Generic: 500 mg

Solution Reconstituted, Injection [preservative free]:

Generic: 500 mg (1 ea)

Tablet, Oral:

Generic: 125 mg, 250 mg

Acetic Acid (a SEE tik AS id)

Index Terms Ethanoic Acid

Pharmacologic Category Otic Agent, Anti-infective; Topical Skin Product

Use Irrigation of the bladder; periodic irrigation of indwelling catheters; treatment of superficial bacterial infections of the external auditory canal

Pregnancy Risk Factor C

Dosage

Irrigation: Adults: (**Note:** Dosage of an irrigating solution depends on the capacity or surface area of the structure being irrigated):

For continuous irrigation of the urinary bladder with 0.25% acetic acid irrigation, the rate of administration will approximate the rate of urine flow; usually 500-1500 mL/24 hours

For periodic irrigation of an indwelling urinary catheter to maintain patency, about 50 mL of 0.25% acetic acid irrigation is required

Otic:

Children ≥3 years: Otitis externa: Insert saturated wick; keep moist 24 hours; remove wick and instill 5 drops 3-4 times/day. **Note:** 3-4 drops may be sufficient in children due to the smaller capacity of the ear canal.

Adults: Otitis externa: Insert saturated wick; keep moist 24 hours; remove wick and instill 5 drops 3-4 times/day

Additional Information Complete prescribing information should be consulted for additional detail.

Dosage Forms Excipient information presented when available (limited, particularly for generics); consult specific product labeling.

Solution, Irrigation:

Generic: 0.25% (250 mL, 500 mL, 1000 mL)

Solution, Otic:

Generic: 2% (15 mL, 60 mL)

◆ **Acetic Acid, Hydrocortisone, and Propylene Glycol Diacetate** *see* Acetic Acid, Propylene Glycol Diacetate, and Hydrocortisone *on page* 35

Acetic Acid, Propylene Glycol Diacetate, and Hydrocortisone

(a SEE tik AS id, PRO pa leen GLY kole dye AS e tate, & hye droe KOR ti sone)

Brand Names: U.S. Acetasol® HC; VoSol® HC

Index Terms Acetic Acid, Hydrocortisone, and Propylene Glycol Diacetate; Hydrocortisone, Acetic Acid, and Propylene Glycol Diacetate; Propylene Glycol Diacetate, Acetic Acid, and Hydrocortisone

Pharmacologic Category Otic Agent, Anti-infective

Use Treatment of superficial infections of the external auditory canal caused by organisms susceptible to the action of the antimicrobial, complicated by swelling

Dosage Children ≥3 years and Adults: Otic: Instill 3-5 drops in ear(s) every 4-6 hours

Additional Information Complete prescribing information should be consulted for additional detail.

Dosage Forms Excipient information presented when available (limited, particularly for generics); consult specific product labeling.

Solution, otic [drops]: Acetic acid 2%, propylene glycol diacetate 3%, and hydrocortisone 1% (10 mL)

Acetasol® HC: Acetic acid 2%, propylene glycol diacetate 3%, and hydrocortisone 1% (10 mL) [contains benzethonium chloride]

VoSol® HC: Acetic acid 2%, propylene glycol diacetate 3%, and hydrocortisone 1% (10 mL) [contains benzethonium chloride]

◆ **Acetoxymethylprogesterone** *see* MedroxyPROGESTERone *on page* 1278

Acetylcholine (a se teel KOE leen)

Brand Names: U.S. Miochol-E

Brand Names: Canada Miochol®-E

Index Terms Acetylcholine Chloride

Pharmacologic Category Cholinergic Agonist; Ophthalmic Agent, Miotic

Use Produces complete miosis in cataract surgery, keratoplasty, iridectomy, and other anterior segment surgery where rapid miosis is required

Contraindications Hypersensitivity to acetylcholine chloride or any component of the formulation

Warnings/Precautions During cataract surgery, use only after lens is in place. Open under aseptic conditions only; do not gas sterilize. Systemic effects rarely occur but can cause problems for patients with acute cardiac failure, bronchial asthma, peptic ulcer, hyperthyroidism, GI spasm, urinary tract obstruction, and Parkinson's disease.

Adverse Reactions Frequency not defined.

Cardiovascular: Bradycardia, flushing, hypotension

Ocular: Clouding, corneal edema, decompensation

Respiratory: Dyspnea

Miscellaneous: Diaphoresis

Drug Interactions

Metabolism/Transport Effects None known.

Avoid Concomitant Use There are no known interactions where it is recommended to avoid concomitant use.

Increased Effect/Toxicity

The levels/effects of Acetylcholine may be increased by: Acetylcholinesterase Inhibitors; Beta-Blockers

Decreased Effect There are no known significant interactions involving a decrease in effect.

Preparation for Administration Reconstitute in an aseptic environment immediately before use.

Storage/Stability Store unopened vial at 4°C to 25°C (39°F to 77°F); prevent from freezing. Prepare solution immediately before use and discard unused portion. Acetylcholine solutions are unstable. Only use if solution is clear and colorless.

Mechanism of Action Causes contraction of the sphincter muscles of the iris, resulting in miosis and contraction of the ciliary muscle, leading to accommodation spasm

Pharmacodynamics/Kinetics

Onset of action: Rapid

Duration: ~6 hours

Dosage Adults: Intraocular: 0.5-2 mL of 1% injection (5-20 mg) instilled into anterior chamber before or after securing one or more sutures

Dosage adjustment in renal impairment: No dosage adjustment provided in manufacturer's labeling.

Dosage adjustment in hepatic impairment: No dosage adjustment provided in manufacturer's labeling.

Administration Ophthalmic: Open under aseptic conditions only. Attach filter before irrigating eye. Instill into anterior chamber before or after securing one or more sutures; instillation should be gentle and parallel to the iris face and tangential to the pupil border; in cataract surgery, acetylcholine should be used only after delivery of the lens.

Dosage Forms Excipient information presented when available (limited, particularly for generics); consult specific product labeling.

Solution Reconstituted, Intraocular, as chloride:

Miochol-E: 20 mg (1 ea) [contains mannitol]

◆ **Acetylcholine Chloride** *see* Acetylcholine *on page 35*

Acetylcysteine (a se teel SIS teen)

Brand Names: U.S. Acetadote

Brand Names: Canada Acetylcysteine Injection; Acetylcysteine Solution; Mucomyst®; Parvolex®

Index Terms *N* Acetylcysteine; *N*-Acetyl-L-cysteine; *N*-Acetylcysteine; Acetylcysteine Sodium; Mercapturic Acid; Mucomyst; NAC

Pharmacologic Category Antidote; Mucolytic Agent

Additional Appendix Information

Contrast Media Reactions, Premedication for Prophylaxis *on page 2373*

Use Antidote for acute acetaminophen poisoning; repeated supratherapeutic ingestion (RSTI) of acetaminophen; adjunctive mucolytic therapy in patients with abnormal or viscid mucous secretions in acute and chronic bronchopulmonary diseases; pulmonary complications of surgery and cystic fibrosis; diagnostic bronchial studies

Unlabeled Use Prevention of contrast-induced renal dysfunction (oral, I.V.); distal intestinal obstruction syndrome (DIOS, previously referred to as meconium ileus equivalent)

Pregnancy Risk Factor B

Pregnancy Considerations Adverse events were not observed in animal reproduction studies. Based on limited reports using acetylcysteine to treat acetaminophen poisoning in pregnant women, acetylcysteine has been shown to cross the placenta and may provide protective levels in the fetus.

Acetylcysteine may be used to treat acetaminophen overdose in during pregnancy (Wilkes, 2005). In general, medications used as antidotes should take into consideration the health and prognosis of the mother; antidotes should be administered to pregnant women if there is a clear indication for use and should not be withheld because of fears of teratogenicity (Bailey, 2003).

Breast-Feeding Considerations It is not known if acetylcysteine is excreted in breast milk. The manufacturer recommends that caution be exercised when administering acetylcysteine to nursing women. Based on its pharmacokinetics, the drug should be nearly completely cleared 30 hours after administration; therefore, nursing women may consider resuming nursing 30 hours after dosing is complete.

Contraindications Hypersensitivity to acetylcysteine or any component of the formulation

Warnings/Precautions

Inhalation: Since increased bronchial secretions may develop after inhalation, percussion, postural drainage, and suctioning should follow. If bronchospasm occurs, administer a bronchodilator; discontinue acetylcysteine if bronchospasm progresses.

Intravenous: Acute flushing and erythema have been reported; usually occurs within 30-60 minutes and may resolve spontaneously. Serious anaphylactoid reactions have also been reported and are more commonly associated with I.V. administration, but may also occur with oral administration (Mroz, 1997). When used for acetaminophen poisoning, the incidence is reduced when the initial loading dose is administered over 60 minutes. The acetylcysteine infusion may be interrupted until treatment of allergic symptoms is initiated; the infusion can then be carefully restarted. Treatment for anaphylactoid reactions should be immediately available. Use caution in patients with asthma or history of bronchospasm as these patients may be at increased risk. Conversely, patients with high acetaminophen levels (>150 mg/dL) may be at a reduced risk for anaphylactoid reactions (Pakravan, 2008; Sandilands, 2009; Waring, 2008).

Acute acetaminophen poisoning: Acetylcysteine is indicated in patients with a serum acetaminophen level that indicates they are at "possible" risk or greater for hepatotoxicity when plotted on the Rumack-Matthew nomogram. There are several situations where the nomogram is of limited use. Serum acetaminophen levels obtained <4 hours postingestion are not interpretable; patients presenting late may have undetectable serum concentrations, despite having received a toxic dose. The nomogram is less predictive of hepatic injury following an acute overdose with an extended release acetaminophen product. The nomogram also does not take into account patients who may be at higher risk of acetaminophen toxicity (eg, alcoholics, malnourished patients, concurrent use of CYP2E1 enzyme-inducing agents [eg, isoniazid]). Nevertheless, acetylcysteine should be administered to any patient with signs of hepatotoxicity, even if the serum acetaminophen level is low or undetectable. Patients who present >24 hours after an acute ingestion or patients who present following an acute ingestion at an unknown time may be candidates for acetylcysteine therapy; consultation with a poison control center or clinical toxicologist is highly recommended.

Repeated supratherapeutic ingestion (RSTI) of acetaminophen: The Rumack-Matthew nomogram is not designed to be used following RSTIs. In general, an accurate past medical history, including a comprehensive acetaminophen ingestion history, in conjunction with AST concentrations and serum acetaminophen levels, may give the clinician insight as to the patient's risk of acetaminophen toxicity. Some experts recommend that acetylcysteine be administered to any patient with "higher than expected" serum acetaminophen levels or serum acetaminophen level >10 mcg/mL, even in the absence of hepatic injury; others recommend treatment for patients with laboratory evidence and/or signs and symptoms of hepatotoxicity (Hendrickson, 2006; Jones, 2000). Consultation with a poison control center or a clinical toxicologist is highly recommended.

Adverse Reactions

Inhalation: Frequency not defined.

Central nervous system: Drowsiness, chills, fever

Gastrointestinal: Vomiting, nausea, stomatitis

Local: Irritation, stickiness on face following nebulization

Respiratory: Bronchospasm, rhinorrhea, hemoptysis
Miscellaneous: Acquired sensitization (rare), clamminess, unpleasant odor during administration

Intravenous:

>10%: Miscellaneous: Anaphylactoid reaction (8% to 18%; shorter infusion periods [eg, <60 minutes] associated with increased incidence)

1% to 10%:

Cardiovascular: Flushing (1% to 8%), tachycardia (1% to 4%), edema (1% to 2%)
Dermatologic: Urticaria (6% to 8%), rash (2% to 4%), pruritus (1% to 4%)
Gastrointestinal: Vomiting (2% to 10%), nausea (1% to 6%)
Respiratory: Pharyngitis (≤1%), rhinorrhea (≤1%), rhonchi (≤1%), throat tightness (≤1%)

<1% (Limited to important or life-threatening): Anaphylaxis, angioedema, bronchospasm, chest tightness, cough, dizziness, dyspnea, headache, hypotension, respiratory distress, stridor, wheezing

Oral (Bebarta, 2010; Mroz, 1997):

Cardiovascular: Hypotension, tachycardia
Dermatologic: Angioedema, pruritus, urticaria
Gastrointestinal: Nausea, vomiting
Respiratory: Bronchospasm

Drug Interactions

Metabolism/Transport Effects None known.

Avoid Concomitant Use There are no known interactions where it is recommended to avoid concomitant use.

Increased Effect/Toxicity There are no known significant interactions involving an increase in effect.

Decreased Effect There are no known significant interactions involving a decrease in effect.

Preparation for Administration

Oral: Treatment of acetaminophen poisoning: Dilute the 20% solution 1:3 with a cola, orange juice, or other soft drink to prepare a 5% solution. Use within 1 hour of preparation.

Solution for injection (Acetadote): Acetaminophen poisoning: I.V.:

Loading dose: Dilute 150 mg/kg in D_5W 200 mL.
Second dose: Dilute 50 mg/kg in D_5W 500 mL.
Third dose: Dilute 100 mg/kg in D_5W 1000 mL.

Note: To avoid fluid overload in patients <40 kg and those requiring fluid restriction, decrease volume of D_5W proportionally (see table in dosing section). Discard unused portion.

Solution for inhalation: The 20% solution may be diluted with sodium chloride or sterile water; the 10% solution may be used undiluted.

Intravenous administration of solution for inhalation (unlabeled route): Using D_5W, dilute acetylcysteine 20% oral solution to a 3% solution.

Storage/Stability

Solution for injection (Acetadote): Store unopened vials at room temperature, 20°C to 25°C (68°F to 77°F). Following reconstitution with D_5W, solution is stable for 24 hours at room temperature. A color change may occur in opened vials (light pink or purple) and does not affect the safety or efficacy.

Solution for inhalation: Store unopened vials at room temperature; once opened, store under refrigeration and use within 96 hours. A color change may occur in opened vials (light purple) and does not affect the safety or efficacy.

Mechanism of Action Exerts mucolytic action through its free sulfhydryl group which opens up the disulfide bonds in the mucoproteins thus lowering mucous viscosity.

In patients with acetaminophen toxicity, acetylcysteine acts as a hepatoprotective agent by restoring hepatic glutathione, serving as a glutathione substitute, and enhancing the nontoxic sulfate conjugation of acetaminophen.

The presumed mechanism in preventing contrast-induced nephropathy is its ability to scavenge oxygen-derived free radicals and improve endothelium-dependent vasodilation.

Pharmacodynamics/Kinetics

Onset of action: Inhalation: 5-10 minutes
Duration: Inhalation: >1 hour
Distribution: 0.47 L/kg
Protein binding: 83%
Half-life elimination:

Reduced acetylcysteine: 2 hours
Total acetylcysteine: Adults: 5.6 hours; Newborns: 11 hours

Time to peak, plasma: Oral: 1-2 hours
Excretion: Urine

Dosage

Acetaminophen poisoning: **Note:** Only the 72-hour oral and 21-hour I.V. regimens are FDA-approved. Ideally, in patients with an acute acetaminophen ingestion, treatment should begin within 8 hours of ingestion or as soon as possible after ingestion. In patients who present following RSTI and treatment is deemed appropriate, acetylcysteine should be initiated immediately. Regardless of the treatment regimen selected, serum acetaminophen levels, liver function, and clinical status should be evaluated during and prior to the end of the treatment regimen to determine if treatment discontinuation is appropriate. In patients who continue to experience symptoms of hepatotoxicity or elevated liver function tests at the conclusion of a 72-hour oral or 21-hour I.V. regimen, extending the treatment course may be appropriate; however, when and to which patients additional doses should be administered is unclear. Possible candidates for extended therapy include patients with a suspected massive overdose, concomitant ingestion of other substances, or patients with pre-existing liver disease. In patients with persistently elevated acetaminophen levels, persistently elevated liver function tests, or an elevated INR, additional acetylcysteine should be administered. Typically, an additional "third dose" or "third bag" (I.V.: 100 mg/kg [maximum: 10 g] infused over 16 hours) is administered; however, this dose may be inadequate in some patients (Rumack, 2012). Consultation with a poison control center or clinical toxicologist is highly recommended to determine optimal patient care.

Children and Adults:

Oral: **Note:** Consultation with a poison control center or clinical toxicologist is highly recommended when considering the discontinuation of oral acetylcysteine prior to the conclusion of a full 18-dose course of therapy.

72-hour regimen: Consists of 18 doses; total dose delivered: 1330 mg/kg

Loading dose: 140 mg/kg
Maintenance dose: 70 mg/kg every 4 hours; repeat dose if emesis occurs within 1 hour of administration

I.V. (Acetadote):

21-hour regimen: Consists of 3 doses; total dose delivered: 300 mg/kg

Loading dose: 150 mg/kg (maximum: 15 **g**) infused over 60 minutes
Second dose: 50 mg/kg (maximum: 5 **g**) infused over 4 hours
Third dose: 100 mg/kg (maximum: 10 **g**) infused over 16 hours

Note: The fluid volume should be reduced in patients weighing <40 kg according to the following table:

Acetadote Dosing / Fluid Volume Guidelines for Patients ≤40 kg

Body Weight (kg)	Loading Dose 150 mg/kg over 1 h		Second Dose 50 mg/kg over 4 h		Third Dose 100 mg/kg over 16 h	
	Acetadote (mL)	D_5W (mL)	Acetadote (mL)	D_5W (mL)	Acetadote (mL)	D_5W (mL)
40	30	100	10	250	20	500
30	22.5	100	7.5	250	15	500
21	15.75	100	5.25	250	10.5	500
20	15	60	5	140	10	280
15	11.25	45	3.75	105	7.5	210
10	7.5	30	2.5	70	5	140
5	3.75	15	1.25	35	2.5	70

Obesity: In patients who weigh >100 kg, the following dosing regimen is recommended: I.V. (Acetadote):
21-hour regimen: Consists of 3 doses; total dose delivered: 30 **g**
Loading dose: 15 **g** infused over 60 minutes
Second dose: 5 **g** infused over 4 hours
Third dose: 10 **g** infused over 16 hours

Adjuvant therapy in respiratory conditions: **Note:** Patients should receive an aerosolized bronchodilator 10-15 minutes prior to acetylcysteine.
Inhalation, nebulization (face mask, mouth piece, tracheostomy): Acetylcysteine 10% and 20% solution (dilute 20% solution with sodium chloride or sterile water for inhalation); 10% solution may be used undiluted
Infants: 1-2 mL of 20% solution or 2-4 mL of 10% solution until nebulized given 3-4 times/day
Children and Adults: 3-5 mL of 20% solution or 6-10 mL of 10% solution until nebulized given 3-4 times/day; dosing range: 1-10 mL of 20% solution or 2-20 mL of 10% solution every 2-6 hours
Inhalation, nebulization (tent, croupette): Children and Adults: Dose must be individualized; may require up to 300 mL solution/treatment
Direct instillation: Adults:
Into tracheostomy: 1-2 mL of 10% to 20% solution every 1-4 hours
Through percutaneous intratracheal catheter: 1-2 mL of 20% or 2-4 mL of 10% solution every 1-4 hours via syringe attached to catheter

Diagnostic bronchogram: Nebulization or intratracheal: Adults: 1-2 mL of 20% solution or 2-4 mL of 10% solution administered 2-3 times prior to procedure

Prevention of contrast-induced nephropathy (CIN) (unlabeled use): Adults: Oral: 600-1200 mg twice daily for 2 days (beginning the day before the procedure); may be given as powder in capsules (some centers use solution, diluted in cola beverage or juice). **Note:** No longer recommended for use prior to percutaneous coronary intervention; instead adequate hydration is preferred (Levine, 2011).

Dosage adjustment in renal impairment: Oral, I.V.: No dosage adjustment provided in manufacturer's labeling.
Dosage adjustment in hepatic impairment:
Oral: No dosage adjustment provided in manufacturer's labeling.
I.V.: No dosage adjustment required.

Administration
Inhalation: Acetylcysteine is incompatible with tetracyclines, erythromycin, amphotericin B, iodized oil, chymotrypsin, trypsin, and hydrogen peroxide. Administer separately. Intermittent aerosol treatments are commonly given when patient arises, before meals, and just before retiring at bedtime.
Oral: Treatment of acetaminophen poisoning, administer orally as a 5% solution. Use within 1 hour of preparation. The unpleasant odor (sulfur-like) becomes less noticeable as treatment progresses. If patient vomits within 1 hour of dose, readminister. (**Note:** It is helpful to put the acetylcysteine on ice, in a cup with a cover, and drink through a straw; alternatively, administer via an NG tube).
I.V. (Acetadote): Acetaminophen poisoning:
Loading dose: Administer over 60 minutes.
Second dose: Administer over 4 hours.
Third dose: Administer over 16 hours.
If the commercial I.V. form is unavailable, the solution for inhalation has been used; each dose should be infused through a 0.2 micron Millipore filter (in-line) over 60 minutes (Yip, 1998); intravenous administration of the solution for inhalation is not USP 797-compliant.
Note: Undiluted injection, solution (Acetadote) is hyperosmolar (2600 mOsmol/L); when the diluent volume is decreased for patients <40 kg or requiring fluid restriction, the osmolarity of the solution may remain higher than desirable for intravenous infusion. To ensure tolerance of the infusion, osmolarity should be adjusted to a physiologically safe level (eg, ≥150 mOsmol/L in children).
Acetadote concentration: 7 mg/mL
Osmolarity in D_5W: 343 mOsmol/L
Osmolarity in 1/2NS: 245 mOsmol/L
Osmolarity in SWFI: 91 mOsmol/L
Acetadote concentration: 24 mg/mL
Osmolarity in D_5W: 564 mOsmol/L
Osmolarity in 1/2NS: 466 mOsmol/L
Osmolarity in SWFI: 312 mOsmol/L

Monitoring Parameters Acetaminophen poisoning: Monitor patient for the development of anaphylaxis or anaphylactoid reactions; monitor serum acetaminophen levels, AST, ALT, bilirubin, PT, INR, serum creatinine, BUN, serum glucose, hemoglobin, hematocrit, and electrolytes. Assess patient for nausea, vomiting, and skin rash following oral administration. Reassess LFTs for possible hepatotoxicity every 4-6 hours. An early elevation in the INR may be related to acetylcysteine therapy (Schmidt, 2002).
Acute ingestion: Obtain the first acetaminophen level 4 hours postingestion (or as soon as possible thereafter); plot on the Rumack-Matthew nomogram. In patients who have ingested an extended release formulation of acetaminophen or have coingested an agent known to delay gastric emptying, obtain a repeat serum acetaminophen measurement 4-6 hours following the first measurement if the original level (taken at 4-8 hours postingestion) when plotted on the Rumack-Matthew nomogram indicated that treatment was not necessary.

Dosage Forms Excipient information presented when available (limited, particularly for generics); consult specific product labeling.
Injection, solution [preservative free]: 20% (30 mL)
Acetadote: 20% [200 mg/mL] (30 mL)
Solution, for inhalation/oral: 10% [100 mg/mL] (10 mL, 30 mL); 20% [200 mg/mL] (10 mL, 30 mL)
Solution, for inhalation/oral [preservative free]: 10% [100 mg/mL] (4 mL, 10 mL); 20% [200 mg/mL] (4 mL, 10 mL, 30 mL)

◆ **Acetylcysteine Injection (Can)** *see* Acetylcysteine *on page 36*

◆ **Acetylcysteine, Methylcobalamin, and Methylfolate** *see* Methylfolate, Methylcobalamin, and Acetylcysteine *on page 1335*

◆ **Acetylcysteine, Methylfolate, and Methylcobalamin** *see* Methylfolate, Methylcobalamin, and Acetylcysteine *on page 1335*

Acitretin (a si TRE tin)

Brand Names: U.S. Soriatane

Brand Names: Canada Soriatane®

Pharmacologic Category Retinoid-Like Compound

Use Treatment of severe psoriasis

Pregnancy Risk Factor X

Pregnancy Considerations [U.S. Boxed Warning]: Not for use by women who are pregnant or intend to become pregnant. Acitretin is teratogenic in humans. Severe birth defects have been reported when conception occurred during treatment or after therapy was complete. Patients should not get pregnant for at least 3 years after discontinuation. In addition, because ethanol forms a teratogenic metabolite and would increase the duration of teratogenic potential, ethanol should not be consumed during treatment or for 2 months after discontinuation. The Do Your P.A.R.T. (Pregnancy Prevention Actively Required During and After Treatment) program explains teratogenic risks and requirements expected of females of childbearing potential. Limited amounts of acitretin are found in seminal fluid; although it appears this poses little risk to a fetus, the actual risk of teratogenicity is not known. Any pregnancy which occurs during treatment, or within 3 years after treatment is discontinued, should be reported to the manufacturer at 1-888-784-3335 or to the FDA at 1-800-FDA-1088.

Breast-Feeding Considerations Acitretin should not be given prior to or during nursing due to the potential for adverse effects in the nursing infant.

Medication Guide Available Yes

Contraindications Hypersensitivity to acitretin, other retinoids, or any component of the formulation; patients who are pregnant or intend on becoming pregnant; severe hepatic or renal dysfunction; chronically-elevated blood lipid levels; concomitant use with methotrexate or tetracyclines

Acitretin is contraindicated in females of childbearing potential unless all of the following conditions apply.

1) Patient has severe psoriasis unresponsive to other therapy or if clinical condition contraindicates other treatments.
2) Patient must have two negative urine or serum pregnancy tests prior to therapy.
3) Patient must have pregnancy test repeated monthly during therapy. After discontinuation of therapy, a pregnancy test must be repeated every 3 months for at least 3 years.
4) Patient must commit to using two effective forms of birth control starting 1 month prior to acitretin treatment and for 3 years after discontinuation. Prescriber must counsel patient about contraception every month during therapy and every 3 months following discontinuation for at least 3 years.
5) Patient is reliable in understanding and carrying out instructions.
6) Patient has received, and acknowledged, understanding of a careful oral and printed explanation of the hazards of fetal exposure to acitretin and the risk of possible contraception failure. Patient must sign an agreement/informed consent document stating that she understands these risks and that she should not consume ethanol during therapy or for 2 months after discontinuation.

Warnings/Precautions Hazardous agent - use appropriate precautions for handling and disposal (NIOSH, 2012). **[U.S. Boxed Warning]: Not for use by women who want to become pregnant;** patient should not get pregnant for at least 3 years after discontinuation. The Do Your P.A.R.T. (Pregnancy Prevention Actively Required During and After Treatment) program explains teratogenic risks and requirements expected of females of childbearing potential to prevent pregnancies from occurring during use and 3 years following discontinuation; this should be used to educate patients and healthcare providers. **[U.S. Boxed Warning]: Female patients should abstain from ethanol or ethanol-containing products during therapy and for 2 months after discontinuation. [U.S. Boxed Warning]: All patients should be advised not to donate blood during therapy or for 3 years following completion of therapy. [U.S. Boxed Warning]: Changes in transaminases occur in up to 1/3 of patients.** Monitor for hepatotoxicity; discontinue if significant elevations of liver enzymes occur. Use with caution in patients at risk of hypertriglyceridemias. Lipid changes including, increased triglycerides, increased cholesterol, and decreased HDL are common (up to 66%). Pseudotumor cerebri has been reported (rarely); may occur with the use of tetracyclines and acitretin independently. Discontinue if visual changes occur. May cause adverse effects to the eyes and vision, including a decrease in night vision or decreased tolerance to contact lenses. Use caution when operating vehicles at night; discontinue if visual changes occur. Patients receiving long-term treatment should be periodically examined for bony abnormalities; risk vs benefit of therapy should be considered if abnormalities occur. Depression, including thoughts of self-harm have been reported; use with caution in patients with a history of mental illness. May be photosensitizing; minimize sun or other UV exposure to treated areas. The risk of burning is increased with phototherapy; decreased doses are required. Transient worsening of psoriasis may initially occur; patients should be advised that it may take 2-3 months to achieve the full benefits of treatment. Not indicated for the treatment of acne. **[U.S. Boxed Warning]: All patients must be provided with a medication guide each time acitretin is dispensed. Female patients must also sign an informed consent prior to therapy.** Safety and efficacy for pediatric patients have not been established; growth potential may be affected.

Adverse Reactions

>10%:

Central nervous system: Hyperesthesia (10% to 25%)

Dermatologic: Cheilitis (>75%), alopecia (50% to 75%), skin peeling (50% to 75%), dry skin (25% to 50%), nail disorder (25% to 50%), pruritus (25% to 50%), erythematous rash (10% to 25%), paronychia (10% to 25%), skin atrophy (10% to 25%), sticky skin (10% to 25%)

Endocrine & metabolic: Hypertriglyceridemia (50% to 75%), fasting blood sugar increased (25% to 50%), HDL decreased (25% to 50%), hypercholesterolemia (25% to 50%), fasting blood sugar decreased (10% to 25%), magnesium increased/decreased (10% to 25%), phosphorus increased (10% to 25%), potassium increased (10% to 25%), sodium increased (10% to 25%)

Gastrointestinal: Xerostomia (10% to 25%)

Hematologic: Reticulocytes increased (25% to 50%), haptoglobin increased (10% to 25%), hematocrit decreased (10% to 25%), hemoglobin decreased (10% to 25%), neutrophils increased (10% to 25%), WBC increased/decreased (10% to 25%)

Hepatic: Liver function tests increased (25% to 50%), alkaline phosphatase increased (10% to 25%), direct bilirubin increased (10% to 25%), GGTP increased (10% to 25%)

Neuromuscular & skeletal: CPK increased (25% to 50%), arthralgia (10% to 25%), paresthesia (10% to 25%), rigors (10% to 25%), spinal hyperostosis progression (10% to 25%)

Ocular: Xerophthalmia (10% to 25%)

Renal: WBC in urine (25% to 50%), acetonuria (10% to 25%), hematuria (10% to 25%), RBC in urine (10% to 25%), uric acid increased (10% to 25%)

Respiratory: Rhinitis (25% to 50%), epistaxis (10% to 25%)

1% to 10%:

Cardiovascular: Edema, flushing

Central nervous system: Depression, fatigue, headache, insomnia, pain, somnolence

Dermatologic: Bullous eruption, cold/clammy skin, dermatitis, fissures, hair texture change, psoriasiform rash, purpura, pyogenic granuloma, rash, seborrhea, skin odor, sunburn, ulcers

Endocrine & metabolic: Calcium increased or decreased, chloride increased or decreased, hot flashes, iron increased/decreased, phosphorus decreased, potassium decreased, sodium decreased

Gastrointestinal: Abdominal pain, anorexia, appetite increased, diarrhea, gingival bleeding, gingivitis, nausea, saliva increased, stomatitis, taste disturbance, thirst, tongue disorder, ulcerative stomatitis

Hematologic: Haptoglobin decreased, hematocrit increased, hemoglobin increased, neutrophils decreased, RBC increased/decreased, reticulocytes decreased

Hepatic: Total bilirubin increased

Neuromuscular & skeletal: Arthritis, arthrosis, back pain, Bell's palsy, hypertonia, myalgia, osteodynia, peripheral joint hyperostosis

Ocular: Blepharitis, blurred vision, cataract, conjunctivitis, corneal epithelial abnormality, diplopia, eye pain, eyebrow or eyelash loss, night blindness, photophobia

Otic: Earache, tinnitus

Renal: Albumin decreased/increased, BUN increased, creatinine increased, glycosuria, proteinuria

Respiratory: Sinusitis

Miscellaneous: Diaphoresis increased

<1% (Limited to important or life-threatening): Abnormal gait, acne, aggression, anal disorder, anxiety, bleeding time increased, bone disorder, breast pain, chalazion, chest pain, ceruminosis, cirrhosis, conjunctival hemorrhage, constipation, corneal lesions, corneal ulceration, cough, cyanosis, cyst, deafness, diplopia, dizziness, dyspepsia, dysphonia, dysuria, ectropion, eczema, esophagitis, ethanol intolerance, fever, flu-like syndrome, fungal infection, furunculosis, gastritis, gastroenteritis, glossitis, gum hyperplasia, hair discoloration, healing impaired, hemorrhage, hemorrhoids, hepatic dysfunction, hepatitis, herpes simplex, hyperkeratosis, hypertrichosis, hypoesthesia, intermittent claudication, itchy eyes, jaundice, lacrimation abnormal, laryngitis, leukorrhea, libido decreased, malaise, melena, MI, migraine, moniliasis, muscle weakness, myopathy with peripheral neuropathy, nail fragility, nervousness, neuritis, olecranon bursitis, otitis media, pancreatitis, papilledema, peripheral ischemia, pharyngitis, photosensitivity, pseudotumor cerebri, recurrent sties, scaling of skin, scleroderma, skin fragility or thinning, skin hypertrophy, skin nodule, spinal hyperostosis (new lesion), sputum increased, suicidal thoughts, taste loss, tendonitis, tenesmus, thromboembolism, tongue ulceration, urticaria, vaginitis, vulvovaginitis, wart, weight gain

Drug Interactions

Metabolism/Transport Effects None known.

Avoid Concomitant Use

Avoid concomitant use of Acitretin with any of the following: Alcohol (Ethyl); Methotrexate; Multivitamins/Fluoride (with ADE); Multivitamins/Minerals (with ADEK, Folate, Iron); Multivitamins/Minerals (with AE, No Iron); Tetracycline Derivatives; Vitamin A

Increased Effect/Toxicity

Acitretin may increase the levels/effects of: Methotrexate; Porfimer; Vitamin A

The levels/effects of Acitretin may be increased by: Alcohol (Ethyl); Multivitamins/Fluoride (with ADE); Multivitamins/Minerals (with ADEK, Folate, Iron); Multivitamins/Minerals (with AE, No Iron); Tetracycline Derivatives; Vitamin A

Decreased Effect

Acitretin may decrease the levels/effects of: Contraceptives (Estrogens); Contraceptives (Progestins)

Ethanol/Nutrition/Herb Interactions

Ethanol: Use leads to formation of etretinate, a teratogenic metabolite with a prolonged half-life. Management: Female patients must avoid ethanol or ethanol-containing products concomitantly or within 2 months after discontinuing acitretin.

Food: Absorption increased when administered with food. Management: Take with food; avoid ingestion of additional sources of vitamin A (in excess of RDA).

Storage/Stability Store between 15°C to 25°C (59°F to 77°F). Avoid high temperatures and humidity. Protect from light.

Mechanism of Action Binds to and activates all nuclear subtypes (alpha, beta, and gamma) of retinoid X receptors (RXR) and retinoic acid receptors (RAR) to inhibit the expression of the pro-inflammatory cytokines interleukin-6 (IL-6), migration inhibitory factor-related protein-8 (MRP-8), and interferon-gamma (markers of hyperproliferation and abnormal keratinocyte differentiation). Resulting actions are anti-inflammatory and antiproliferative, and keratinocyte differentiation is normalized in the epithelium.

Pharmacodynamics/Kinetics Etretinate has been detected in serum for up to 3 years following therapy, possibly due to storage in adipose tissue.

Onset of action: May take 2-3 months for full effect; improvement may be seen within 8 weeks.

Absorption: Oral: ~72% absorbed when given with food

Protein binding: >99% bound, primarily to albumin

Metabolism: Metabolized to *cis*-acitretin; both compounds are further metabolized. Concomitant ethanol use leads to the formation of etretinate (active).

Half-life elimination: Acitretin: 49 hours (range: 33-96); *cis*-acitretin: 63 hours (range: 28-157); etretinate: 120 days (range: up to 168 days)
Time to peak: 2-5 hours
Excretion: Feces (34% to 54%); urine (16% to 53%)

Dosage Oral: Adults: Individualization of dosage is required to achieve maximum therapeutic response while minimizing side effects

Initial therapy: Therapy should be initiated at 25-50 mg/day, given as a single dose with the main meal
Maintenance doses of 25-50 mg/day may be given after initial response to treatment; the maintenance dose should be based on clinical efficacy and tolerability
American Academy of Dermatology recommends: 10-50 mg/day as a single dose; doses ≤25 mg/day are used to decrease side effects (Menter, 2009)

Dosing adjustment in renal impairment: There are no dosage adjustments provided in manufacturer's labeling.
Hemodialysis: Not removed by hemodialysis

Dosing adjustment in hepatic impairment: There are no dosage adjustments provided in manufacturer's labeling.

Dietary Considerations Take with food. Avoid ingestion of additional sources of exogenous vitamin A (in excess of RDA); use of ethanol and ethanol-containing products is contraindicated.

Administration Administer with food, preferably with the main meal of the day.

Hazardous agent; use appropriate precautions for handling and disposal (NIOSH, 2012).

Monitoring Parameters Lipid profile (baseline and at 1- to 2-week intervals for 4-8 weeks); liver function tests (baseline, and at 1- to 2-week intervals until stable, then as clinically indicated); blood glucose in patients with diabetes; bone abnormalities (with long-term use); pregnancy tests (2 negative tests prior to therapy initiation, monthly during treatment, and every 3 months for ≥3 years after discontinuation of therapy)

The American Academy of Dermatology recommends: CBC and renal function tests (baseline and then every 12 weeks); liver function tests (every 2 weeks for the first 8 weeks, then every 6-12 weeks thereafter) (Menter, 2009)

Additional Information Female patients are required to use two forms of birth control, at least one of which is a primary form, unless they have undergone a hysterectomy or are postmenopausal. Both forms of birth control must be used simultaneously for at least 1 month prior to therapy and for at least 3 years after discontinuation. Primary forms of birth control include tubal ligation, partner's vasectomy, IUD, or hormonal birth control products. Microdosed progestin products, referred to as "mini-pills," have been shown to be less effective when used with acitretin, and are not recommended. Secondary forms of contraception include diaphragms, latex condoms and cervical caps, all if used with a spermicide.

Dosage Forms Excipient information presented when available (limited, particularly for generics); consult specific product labeling.
Capsule, Oral:
Soriatane: 10 mg, 17.5 mg, 25 mg [contains edetate calcium disodium]
Generic: 10 mg, 17.5 mg, 25 mg

◆ **Aclaro** *see* Hydroquinone *on page* 1017
◆ **Aclaro PD** *see* Hydroquinone *on page* 1017
◆ **Aclasta (Can)** *see* Zoledronic Acid *on page* 2235
◆ **Aclovate** *see* Alclometasone *on page* 63

Acrivastine and Pseudoephedrine

(AK ri vas teen & soo doe e FED rin)

Brand Names: U.S. Semprex®-D

Index Terms Pseudoephedrine Hydrochloride and Acrivastine

Pharmacologic Category Alkylamine Derivative; Alpha/Beta Agonist; Decongestant; Histamine H_1 Antagonist; Histamine H_1 Antagonist, Second Generation

Use Relief of symptoms associated with seasonal allergic rhinitis

Pregnancy Risk Factor B

Dosage Oral: Children ≥12 years and Adults: One capsule every 4-6 hours (maximum: 4 doses/24 hours); treatment for >14 days has not been evaluated

Dosing adjustment in renal impairment: Avoid use in patients with Cl_{cr} ≤48 mL/minute.

Dosing adjustment in hepatic impairment: There are no dosage adjustments recommended in manufacturer's labeling.

Additional Information Complete prescribing information should be consulted for additional detail.

Dosage Forms Excipient information presented when available (limited, particularly for generics); consult specific product labeling.
Capsule:
Semprex®-D: Acrivastine 8 mg and pseudoephedrine hydrochloride 60 mg

◆ **Act® [OTC]** *see* Fluoride *on page* 880
◆ **ACT-D** *see* DACTINomycin *on page* 531
◆ **Actemra** *see* Tocilizumab *on page* 2080
◆ **ActHIB®** *see* *Haemophilus* b Conjugate Vaccine *on page* 981
◆ **Acthrel** *see* Corticorelin *on page* 493
◆ **Acticin** *see* Permethrin *on page* 1624
◆ **Actidose-Aqua [OTC]** *see* Charcoal, Activated *on page* 401
◆ **Actidose/Sorbitol [OTC]** *see* Charcoal, Activated *on page* 401
◆ **Actifed® (Can)** *see* Triprolidine and Pseudoephedrine *on page* 2131
◆ **Actigall** *see* Ursodiol *on page* 2142
◆ **Actimmune** *see* Interferon Gamma-1b *on page* 1108
◆ **Actimmune® (Can)** *see* Interferon Gamma-1b *on page* 1108
◆ **Actinomycin** *see* DACTINomycin *on page* 531
◆ **Actinomycin D** *see* DACTINomycin *on page* 531
◆ **Actinomycin CI** *see* DACTINomycin *on page* 531
◆ **Actiq** *see* FentaNYL *on page* 842
◆ **Activase** *see* Alteplase *on page* 85
◆ **Activase rt-PA (Can)** *see* Alteplase *on page* 85
◆ **Activated Carbon** *see* Charcoal, Activated *on page* 401
◆ **Activated Charcoal** *see* Charcoal, Activated *on page* 401
◆ **Activated Ergosterol** *see* Ergocalciferol *on page* 733
◆ **Activated Factor XIII** *see* Factor XIII Concentrate (Human) *on page* 829
◆ **Activated PCC** *see* Anti-inhibitor Coagulant Complex (Human) *on page* 147
◆ **Activella** *see* Estradiol and Norethindrone *on page* 763
◆ **Act® Kids [OTC]** *see* Fluoride *on page* 880
◆ **Actonel** *see* Risedronate *on page* 1824
◆ **Actonel® (Can)** *see* Risedronate *on page* 1824
◆ **Actonel® DR (Can)** *see* Risedronate *on page* 1824

Acyclovir (Systemic) (ay SYE kloe veer)

Brand Names: U.S. Zovirax

Brand Names: Canada Apo-Acyclovir; Mylan-Acyclovir; Nu-Acyclovir; ratio-Acyclovir; Teva-Acyclovir; Zovirax

Index Terms Aciclovir; ACV; Acycloguanosine

Pharmacologic Category Antiviral Agent

Additional Appendix Information

Dosing Considerations for the Critically-Ill Patient With Morbid Obesity *on page 2379*

Use Treatment of genital herpes simplex virus (HSV) and HSV encephalitis

Unlabeled Use Prevention of HSV reactivation in HIV-positive patients; prevention of HSV reactivation in hematopoietic stem cell transplant (HSCT); prevention of HSV reactivation during periods of neutropenia in patients with cancer; prevention of varicella zoster virus (VZV) reactivation in allogenic HSCT; prevention of CMV reactivation in low-risk allogeneic HSCT; treatment of disseminated HSV or VZV in immunocompromised patients with cancer; empiric treatment of suspected encephalitis in immunocompromised patients with cancer; treatment of initial and prophylaxis of recurrent mucosal and cutaneous herpes simplex (HSV-1 and HSV-2) infections in immunocompromised patients

Pregnancy Risk Factor B

Pregnancy Considerations Teratogenic effects were not observed in animal reproduction studies. Acyclovir has been shown to cross the human placenta (Henderson, 1992). Results from a pregnancy registry, established in 1984 and closed in 1999, did not find an increase in the number of birth defects with exposure to acyclovir when compared to those expected in the general population. However, due to the small size of the registry and lack of long-term data, the manufacturer recommends using during pregnancy with caution and only when clearly needed. Acyclovir may be appropriate for the treatment of genital herpes in pregnant women (CDC, 2010).

Breast-Feeding Considerations Acyclovir is excreted in breast milk. The manufacturer recommends that caution be exercised when administering acyclovir to nursing women. Limited data suggest exposure to the nursing infant of ~0.3 mg/kg/day following oral administration of acyclovir to the mother. Nursing mothers with herpetic lesions near or on the breast should avoid breast-feeding (Gartner, 2005).

Contraindications Hypersensitivity to acyclovir, valacyclovir, or any component of the formulation

Warnings/Precautions Use with caution in immunocompromised patients; thrombocytopenic purpura/hemolytic uremic syndrome (TTP/HUS) has been reported. Use caution in the elderly, pre-existing renal disease (may require dosage modification), or in those receiving other nephrotoxic drugs. Renal failure (sometimes fatal) has been reported. Maintain adequate hydration during oral or intravenous therapy. Use I.V. preparation with caution in patients with underlying neurologic abnormalities, serious hepatic or electrolyte abnormalities, or substantial hypoxia.

Varicella-zoster: Treatment should begin within 24 hours of appearance of rash; oral route not recommended for routine use in otherwise healthy children with varicella, but may be effective in patients at increased risk of moderate-to-severe infection (>12 years of age, chronic cutaneous or pulmonary disorders, long-term salicylate therapy, corticosteroid therapy).

Adverse Reactions

Oral:

>10%: Central nervous system: Malaise (≤12%)

1% to 10%:

Central nervous system: Headache (≤2%)

Gastrointestinal: Nausea (2% to 5%), vomiting (≤3%), diarrhea (2% to 3%)

Parenteral:

1% to 10%:

Dermatologic: Hives (2%), itching (2%), rash (2%)

Gastrointestinal: Nausea/vomiting (7%)

Hepatic: Liver function tests increased (1% to 2%)

Local: Inflammation at injection site or phlebitis (9%)

Renal: BUN increased (5% to 10%), creatinine increased (5% to 10%), acute renal failure

All forms: <1% (Limited to important or life-threatening): Abdominal pain, aggression, agitation, anemia, anorexia, ataxia, coma, confusion, consciousness decreased, delirium, desquamation, disseminated intravascular coagulopathy (DIC), dizziness, dysarthria, encephalopathy, fatigue, fever, gastrointestinal distress, hallucinations, hematuria, hemolysis, hepatitis, hyperbilirubinemia, hypotension, insomnia, jaundice, leukocytoclastic vasculitis, leukocytosis, leukopenia, lymphadenopathy, mental depression, myalgia, neutrophilia, pain, psychosis, renal failure, renal pain, seizure, somnolence, sore throat, thrombocytopenia, thrombocytopenic purpura/hemolytic uremic syndrome (TTP/HUS), thrombocytosis, visual disturbances

Drug Interactions

Metabolism/Transport Effects None known.

Avoid Concomitant Use

Avoid concomitant use of Acyclovir (Systemic) with any of the following: Zoster Vaccine

Increased Effect/Toxicity

Acyclovir (Systemic) may increase the levels/effects of: Mycophenolate; Tenofovir; Zidovudine

The levels/effects of Acyclovir (Systemic) may be increased by: Mycophenolate

Decreased Effect

Acyclovir (Systemic) may decrease the levels/effects of: Zoster Vaccine

Ethanol/Nutrition/Herb Interactions Food: Does not affect absorption of oral acyclovir.

Preparation for Administration Powder for injection: Reconstitute acyclovir 500 mg powder with SWFI 10 mL; do not use bacteriostatic water containing benzyl alcohol or parabens. For intravenous infusion, dilute in D_5W, D_5NS, $D_5$1/4NS, $D_5$1/2NS, LR, or NS to a final concentration ≤7 mg/mL. Concentrations >10 mg/mL increase the risk of phlebitis.

Storage/Stability

Capsule, tablet: Store at controlled room temperature of 15°C to 25°C (59°F to 77°F); protect from moisture.

Injection: Store powder at controlled room temperature of 15°C to 25°C (59°F to 77°F). Reconstituted solutions remain stable for 12 hours at room temperature. Do not refrigerate reconstituted solutions or solutions diluted for infusion as they may precipitate. Once diluted for infusion, use within 24 hours.

Mechanism of Action Acyclovir is converted to acyclovir monophosphate by virus-specific thymidine kinase then further converted to acyclovir triphosphate by other cellular enzymes. Acyclovir triphosphate inhibits DNA synthesis and viral replication by competing with deoxyguanosine triphosphate for viral DNA polymerase and being incorporated into viral DNA.

Pharmacodynamics/Kinetics

Absorption: Oral: 15% to 30%

Distribution: V_d: 0.8 L/kg (63.6 L): Widely (eg, brain, kidney, lungs, liver, spleen, muscle, uterus, vagina, CSF)

Protein binding: 9% to 33%

Metabolism: Converted by viral enzymes to acyclovir monophosphate, and further converted to diphosphate then triphosphate (active form) by cellular enzymes

Bioavailability: Oral: 10% to 20% with normal renal function (bioavailability decreases with increased dose)

Half-life elimination: Terminal: Neonates: 4 hours; Children 1-12 years: 2-3 hours; Adults: 3 hours

Time to peak, serum: Oral: Within 1.5-2 hours

Excretion: Urine (62% to 90% as unchanged drug and metabolite)

Dosage

Genital herpes simplex virus (HSV) infection:

I.V.: Children ≥12 years and Adults (immunocompetent): Initial episode, severe: 5 mg/kg/dose every 8 hours for 5-7 days **or** 5-10 mg/kg/dose every 8 hours for 2-7 days, follow with oral therapy to complete at least 10 days of therapy (CDC, 2010)

Oral:

Children, immunocompetent:

Initial episode (unlabeled use): 40-80 mg/kg/day divided into 3-4 doses for 5-10 days (maximum: 1000 mg daily) (*Red Book*, 2012)

Chronic suppression (unlabeled use): Children ≥12 years: 800 mg daily in 2 divided doses for ≤12 continuous months (*Red Book*, 2012)

Children, immunocompromised (unlabeled use; CDC, 2009): Initial episode:

Children <45 kg: 60 mg/kg/day divided into 3 doses for 5-14 days (maximum: 1200 mg daily)

Adolescents: 400 mg twice daily for 5-14 days

Adults:

Initial episode: 200 mg 5 times daily while awake for 10 days **or** 400 mg 3 times daily for 7-10 days (CDC, 2010)

Recurrence: 200 mg 5 times daily while awake for 5 days (per manufacturer's labeling; begin at earliest signs of disease)

Alternatively, the following regimens are also recommended by the CDC: 400 mg 3 times daily for 5 days; 800 mg twice daily for 5 days; 800 mg 3 times daily for 2 days (CDC, 2010)

Chronic suppression: 400 mg twice daily or 200 mg 3-5 times daily, for up to 12 months followed by re-evaluation (per manufacturer's labeling)

Herpes zoster (shingles):

Oral: Adults (immunocompetent): 800 mg 5 times daily for 7-10 days

I.V.:

Children <12 years (immunocompromised): 20 mg/kg/dose every 8 hours for 7 days

Children ≥12 years and Adults (immunocompromised): 10 mg/kg/dose or 500 mg/m^2/dose every 8 hours for 7 days

HSV encephalitis: I.V.:

Children 3 months to 12 years: 20 mg/kg/dose every 8 hours for 10 days (per manufacturer's labeling); dosing for 14-21 days also reported

Children ≥12 years and Adults: 10 mg/kg/dose every 8 hours for 10 days (per manufacturer's labeling); 10-15 mg/kg/dose every 8 hours for 14-21 days also reported

Mucocutaneous HSV:

I.V.:

Children <12 years (immunocompromised): Treatment: 10 mg/kg/dose every 8 hours for 7 days

Children ≥12 years and Adults (immunocompromised): Treatment: 5-10 mg/kg/dose every 8 hours for 7 days (Leflore, 2000); dosing for up to 14 days also reported

Oral (unlabeled use): Adults (immunocompromised): 400 mg 5 times daily for 7 days (Leflore, 2000)

Neonatal HSV: I.V.: Infants: Birth to 3 months: 10 mg/kg/dose every 8 hours for 10 days (manufacturer's labeling); 20 mg/kg/dose every 8 hours for 14 (skin and mucous membrane disease) to 21 days (CNS disease) (CDC, 2010)

Orolabial HSV (unlabeled use): Oral:

Children 1-6 years (immunocompetent, gingivostomatitis): Treatment of primary infection: 15 mg/kg/dose (maximum: 200 mg per dose) 5 times daily for 7 days, initiated within 72 hours of symptom onset (Amir, 1997)

Adults (immunocompetent):

Treatment: 200-400 mg 5 times daily for 5 days (Cernik, 2008; Leflore, 2000; Spruance, 1990) for episodic/recurrent treatment; for initial treatment, limited data are available, 200 mg 5 times daily or 400 mg 3 times daily for 7-10 days has been recommended by some clinicians.

Chronic suppression: 400 mg 2 times daily (has been clinically evaluated for up to 1 year) (Cernik, 2008; Rooney, 1993)

Varicella-zoster (chickenpox): Begin treatment within the first 24 hours of rash onset:

Oral: **Note:** The CDC HIV guidelines recommended duration of therapy is 7-10 days or until no new lesions for 48 hours (for patients with mild varicella and no or moderate immune suppression).

Children ≥2 years and ≤40 kg (immunocompetent): 20 mg/kg/dose (maximum: 800 mg per dose) 4 times daily for 5 days

Children >40 kg and Adults (immunocompetent): 800 mg 4 times daily for 5 days

I.V.:

Manufacturer's labeling (immunocompromised):

Children <12 years: 20 mg/kg/dose every 8 hours for 7 days

Children ≥12 years and Adults: 10 mg/kg/dose every 8 hours for 7 days

CDC HIV guidelines (immunocompromised):

Children <1 year: 10 mg/kg/dose every 8 hours for 7-10 days or until no new lesions for 48 hours

Children ≥1 year: 10 mg/kg/dose or 500 mg/m^2/dose every 8 hours for 7-10 days or until no new lesions for 48 hours

Adolescents and Adults: 10-15 mg/kg/dose every 8 hours for 7-10 days

Varicella-zoster acute retinal necrosis infection in HIV-exposed/-positive (unlabeled use; CDC, 2009): I.V.: Infants and Children: 10-15 mg/kg/dose every 8 hours for 10-14 days, followed by valacyclovir for 4-6 weeks

Prevention of HSV reactivation in HIV-positive patient (unlabeled use): Oral:
Children: 20 mg/kg/dose twice daily (maximum: 400 mg per dose) (CDC, 2009)
Adults: 400-800 mg 2-3 times daily (CDC, 2010)

Prevention of HSV reactivation in HSCT (unlabeled use): *CDC recommendations:* **Note:** Start at the beginning of conditioning therapy and continue until engraftment or until mucositis resolves (~30 days)
Oral: Adults: 200 mg 3 times daily
I.V.:
Children: 250 mg/m^2/dose every 8 hours or 125 mg/m^2/dose every 6 hours
Adults: 250 mg/m^2/dose every 12 hours

Prevention of VZV reactivation in allogeneic HSCT (unlabeled use): *NCCN guidelines:* Oral: Adults: 800 mg twice daily

Prevention of CMV reactivation in low-risk allogeneic HSCT (unlabeled use): *NCCN guidelines:* **Note:** Requires close monitoring (due to weak activity); not for use in patients at high risk for CMV disease: Oral: Adults: 800 mg 4 times daily

Treatment of disseminated HSV or VZV or empiric treatment of suspected encephalitis in immunocompromised patients with cancer: (unlabeled use): *NCCN guidelines:* I.V.: Adults: 10-12 mg/kg/dose every 8 hours

Treatment of episodic HSV infection in HIV-positive patient (unlabeled use): Oral: Adults: 400 mg 3 times daily for 5-10 days (CDC, 2010)

Dosage adjustment in renal impairment:
Oral:
Cl_{cr} 10-25 mL/minute/1.73 m^2: Normal dosing regimen 800 mg 5 times daily: Administer 800 mg every 8 hours
Cl_{cr} <10 mL/minute/1.73 m^2:
Normal dosing regimen 200 mg 5 times daily or 400 mg every 12 hours: Administer 200 mg every 12 hours
Normal dosing regimen 800 mg 5 times daily: Administer 800 mg every 12 hours
I.V.:
Cl_{cr} 25-50 mL/minute/1.73 m^2: Administer recommended dose every 12 hours
Cl_{cr} 10-25 mL/minute/1.73 m^2: Administer recommended dose every 24 hours
Cl_{cr} <10 mL/minute/1.73 m^2: Administer 50% of recommended dose every 24 hours
Intermittent hemodialysis (IHD) (administer after hemodialysis on dialysis days): Dialyzable (60% reduction following a 6-hour session): I.V.: 2.5-5 mg/kg every 24 hours (Heintz, 2009). **Note:** Dosing dependent on the assumption of 3 times weekly, complete IHD sessions.
Peritoneal dialysis (PD): Administer 50% of normal dose once daily; no supplemental dose needed
Continuous renal replacement therapy (CRRT) (Heintz, 2009; Trotman, 2005): Drug clearance is highly dependent on the method of renal replacement, filter type, and flow rate. Appropriate dosing requires close monitoring of pharmacologic response, signs of adverse reactions due to drug accumulation, as well as drug concentrations in relation to target trough (if appropriate). The following are general recommendations only (based on dialysate flow/ultrafiltration rates of 1-2 L/hour and minimal residual renal function) and should not supersede clinical judgment:
CVVH: I.V.: 5-10 mg/kg every 24 hours
CVVHD/CVVHDF: I.V.: 5-10 mg/kg every 12-24 hours

Note: The higher end of dosage range (eg, 10 mg/kg every 12 hours for CVVHDF) is recommended for viral meningoencephalitis and varicella-zoster virus infections.

Dosage adjustment in hepatic impairment: Oral, I.V.: No dosage adjustment provided in manufacturer's labeling; use caution in patients with severe impairment.

Dosing in obesity: Obese patients should be dosed using ideal body weight

Dietary Considerations May be taken with or without food. Some products may contain sodium.

Administration
Oral: May be administered with or without food.
I.V.: Avoid rapid infusion; infuse over 1 hour to prevent renal damage; maintain adequate hydration of patient; check for phlebitis and rotate infusion sites. Avoid I.M. or SubQ administration.

Monitoring Parameters Urinalysis, BUN, serum creatinine, liver enzymes, CBC

Dosage Forms Excipient information presented when available (limited, particularly for generics); consult specific product labeling.
Capsule, Oral:
Zovirax: 200 mg
Generic: 200 mg
Solution, Intravenous, as sodium [strength expressed as base]:
Generic: 50 mg/mL (10 mL, 20 mL)
Solution Reconstituted, Intravenous, as sodium [strength expressed as base]:
Generic: 500 mg (1 ea); 1000 mg (1 ea)
Suspension, Oral:
Zovirax: 200 mg/5 mL (473 mL) [banana flavor]
Generic: 200 mg/5 mL (473 mL)
Tablet, Oral:
Zovirax: 400 mg, 800 mg
Generic: 400 mg, 800 mg

Acyclovir (Topical) (ay SYE kloe veer)

Brand Names: U.S. Zovirax
Brand Names: Canada Zovirax®
Index Terms Aciclovir; ACV; Acycloguanosine; Sitavig®
Pharmacologic Category Antiviral Agent, Topical
Use Treatment of herpes labialis (cold sores), mucocutaneous HSV in immunocompromised patients
Pregnancy Risk Factor B
Dosage Topical:
Genital HSV: Adults (immunocompromised): Ointment: Initial episode: 1/2" ribbon of ointment for a 4" square surface area every 3 hours (6 times/day) for 7 days
Herpes labialis (cold sores): Children ≥12 years and Adults: Cream: Apply 5 times/day for 4 days
Mucocutaneous HSV: Ointment: Adults (non-life-threatening, immunocompromised): 1/2" ribbon of ointment for a 4" square surface area every 3 hours (6 times/day) for 7 days

Additional Information Complete prescribing information should be consulted for additional detail.

Product Availability
Sitavig®: FDA approved April 2013; anticipated availability is currently unknown
Sitavig® buccal tablets are indicated for the treatment of recurrent herpes labialis (cold sores) in immunocompetent adults.

Dosage Forms Excipient information presented when available (limited, particularly for generics); consult specific product labeling.
Cream, External:
Zovirax: 5% (5 g) [contains cetostearyl alcohol, propylene glycol]

Ointment, External:
Zovirax: 5% (30 g)
Generic: 5% (5 g, 15 g, 30 g)

◆ **ACZ885** *see* Canakinumab *on page 326*
◆ **AD32** *see* Valrubicin *on page 2153*
◆ **Adacel®** *see* Diphtheria and Tetanus Toxoids, and Acellular Pertussis Vaccine *on page 630*
◆ **Adacel®-Polio (Can)** *see* Diphtheria and Tetanus Toxoids, Acellular Pertussis, and Poliovirus Vaccine *on page 629*
◆ **Adagen** *see* Pegademase Bovine *on page 1585*
◆ **Adagen® (Can)** *see* Pegademase Bovine *on page 1585*
◆ **Adalat® XL® (Can)** *see* NIFEdipine *on page 1455*
◆ **Adalat CC** *see* NIFEdipine *on page 1455*

Adalimumab (a da LIM yoo mab)

Brand Names: U.S. Humira; Humira Pen; Humira Pen-Crohns Starter; Humira Pen-Psoriasis Starter

Brand Names: Canada Humira

Index Terms Antitumor Necrosis Factor Alpha (Human); D2E7; Human Antitumor Necrosis Factor Alpha

Pharmacologic Category Antirheumatic, Disease Modifying; Gastrointestinal Agent, Miscellaneous; Monoclonal Antibody; Tumor Necrosis Factor (TNF) Blocking Agent

Use

Ankylosing spondylitis: Treatment of ankylosing spondylitis (may be used in combination with methotrexate or other nonbiologic disease-modifying antirheumatic drugs (DMARDS)

Crohn's disease: Treatment of active Crohn's disease (moderate-to-severe) in patients with inadequate response to conventional treatment, or patients who have lost response to or are intolerant of infliximab

Juvenile idiopathic arthritis: Treatment of active juvenile idiopathic arthritis (moderate-to-severe); may be used alone or in combination with methotrexate

Plaque psoriasis: Treatment of chronic plaque psoriasis (moderate-to-severe) when systemic therapy is required and other agents are less appropriate

Psoriatic arthritis: Treatment of active psoriatic arthritis; may be used alone or in combination with methotrexate or other DMARDs

Rheumatoid arthritis: Treatment of active rheumatoid arthritis (moderate-to-severe); may be used alone or in combination with methotrexate or other DMARDs

Ulcerative colitis: Treatment of active ulcerative colitis (moderate-to-severe) in patients unresponsive to immunosuppressants (Note: Efficacy in patients that are intolerant to or no longer responsive to other TNF blockers has not been established.)

Canadian labeling: Additional use (not in U.S. labeling): Crohn's disease, pediatric: Treatment of adolescents with active Crohn's disease (moderate-to-severe) who have had an inadequate response to conventional treatment and/or other TNF blockers

Pregnancy Risk Factor B

Pregnancy Considerations Adverse events were not observed in animal reproduction studies. Adalimumab crosses the placenta and can be detected in cord blood at birth at concentrations higher than those in the maternal serum. In one study of pregnant women with inflammatory bowel disease, adalimumab was found to be measurable in a newborn for up to 11 weeks following delivery. Maternal doses of adalimumab were 40 mg every other week (n=9) or 40 mg weekly (n=1) and the last dose was administered 0.14-8 weeks prior to delivery (median 5.5 weeks) (Mahadevan, 2013). If therapy for inflammatory bowel disease is needed during pregnancy, adalimumab should be discontinued before 30 weeks gestation in order to decrease exposure to the newborn. In addition, the administration of live vaccines should be postponed until anti-TNF concentrations in the infant are negative (Habal, 2012; Mahadeven, 2013; Zelinkova, 2013).

Women exposed to adalimumab during pregnancy for the treatment of an autoimmune disease (eg, inflammatory bowel disease) may contact the OTIS Autoimmune Diseases Study at 877-311-8972.

Breast-Feeding Considerations Low concentrations of adalimumab may be detected in breast milk but are unlikely to be absorbed by a nursing infant. The manufacturer recommends caution be used if administered to a nursing woman.

Medication Guide Available Yes

Contraindications There are no contraindications listed within the FDA-approved labeling.

Canadian labeling: Hypersensitivity to adalimumab or any component of the formulation; severe infection (eg, sepsis, tuberculosis, opportunistic infection); moderate-to-severe heart failure (NYHA class III/IV)

Warnings/Precautions [U.S. Boxed Warnings]: Patients should be evaluated for latent tuberculosis infection with a tuberculin skin test prior to therapy. Treatment of latent tuberculosis should be initiated before adalimumab is used. Tuberculosis (disseminated or extrapulmonary) has been reactivated while on adalimumab. Most cases have been reported within the first 8 months of treatment. **Patients with initial negative tuberculin skin tests should receive continued monitoring for tuberculosis throughout treatment; active tuberculosis has developed in this population during treatment.** Rare reactivation of hepatitis B virus (HBV) has occurred in chronic virus carriers; use with caution; evaluate prior to initiation and during treatment.

[U.S. Boxed Warning]: Patients receiving adalimumab are at increased risk for serious infections which may result in hospitalization and/or fatality; infections usually developed in patients receiving concomitant immunosuppressive agents (eg, methotrexate or corticosteroids) and may present as disseminated (rather than local) disease. Active tuberculosis (or reactivation of latent tuberculosis), invasive fungal (including aspergillosis, blastomycosis, candidiasis, coccidioidomycosis, histoplasmosis, and pneumocystosis) and bacterial, viral or other opportunistic infections (including legionellosis and listeriosis) have been reported in patients receiving TNF-blocking agents, including adalimumab. Monitor closely for signs/symptoms of infection. Discontinue for serious infection or sepsis. Consider risks versus benefits prior to use in patients with a history of chronic or recurrent infection. Consider empiric antifungal therapy in patients who are at risk for invasive fungal infection and develop severe systemic illness. Caution should be exercised when considering use in the elderly or in patients with conditions that predispose them to infections (eg, diabetes) or residence/travel from areas of endemic mycoses (blastomycosis, coccidioidomycosis, histoplasmosis), or with latent or localized infections. Do not initiate adalimumab therapy with clinically important active infection. Patients who develop a new infection while undergoing treatment should be monitored closely. There is limited experience with patients undergoing surgical procedures while on therapy; consider long half-life with planned procedures and monitor closely for infection.

[U.S. Boxed Warning]: Lymphoma and other malignancies (some fatal) have been reported in children and adolescent patients receiving TNF-blocking agents, including adalimumab. Half the cases are lymphomas (Hodgkin and non-Hodgkin) and the other cases are ▶

varied, but include malignancies not typically observed in this population. Most patients were receiving concomitant immunosuppressants. **[U.S. Boxed Warning]: Hepatosplenic T-cell lymphoma (HSTCL), a rare T-cell lymphoma, has also been reported primarily in patients with Crohn's disease or ulcerative colitis treated with adalimumab and who received concomitant azathioprine or mercaptopurine; reports occurred predominantly in adolescent and young adult males.** Rare cases of lymphoma have also been reported in association with adalimumab. A higher incidence of nonmelanoma skin cancers was noted in adalimumab treated patients, when compared to the control group. Impact on the development and course of malignancies is not fully defined. May exacerbate pre-existing or recent-onset central or peripheral nervous system demyelinating disorders. Consider discontinuing use in patients who develop peripheral or central nervous system demyelinating disorders during treatment.

May exacerbate pre-existing or recent-onset demyelinating CNS disorders. Worsening and new-onset heart failure (HF) has been reported; use caution in patients with decreased left ventricular function. Use caution in patients with HF (Canadian labeling contraindicates use in NYHA III/IV). Patients should be brought up to date with all immunizations before initiating therapy. No data are available concerning the effects of adalimumab on vaccination. Live vaccines should not be given concurrently. No data are available concerning secondary transmission of live vaccines in patients receiving adalimumab. Rare cases of pancytopenia (including aplastic anemia) have been reported with TNF-blocking agents; with significant hematologic abnormalities, consider discontinuing therapy. Positive antinuclear antibody titers have been detected in patients (with negative baselines) treated with adalimumab. Rare cases of autoimmune disorder, including lupus-like syndrome, have been reported; monitor and discontinue adalimumab if symptoms develop. May cause hypersensitivity reactions, including anaphylaxis; monitor. Infection and malignancy has been reported at a higher incidence in elderly patients compared to younger adults; use caution in elderly patients. Potentially significant drug-drug interactions may exist, requiring dose or frequency adjustment, additional monitoring, and/or selection of alternative therapy. The packaging (needle cover of prefilled syringe) may contain latex. Product may contain polysorbate 80. According to the Centers for Disease Control and Prevention (CDC), pen-shaped injection devices should never be used for more than one person (even when the needle is changed) because of the risk of infection. The injection device should be clearly labeled with individual patient information to ensure that the correct pen is used (CDC, 2012).

Adverse Reactions

>10%:

- Central nervous system: Headache (12%)
- Dermatologic: Skin rash (6% to 12%)
- Hematologic & oncologic: Positive ANA titer (12%)
- Immunologic: Antibody development (3% to 26%; significance unknown)
- Infection: Serious infection (adults 1.4-6.7 events/100 person years; children 2 events/100 person years [Burmester, 2012])
- Local: Injection site reaction (12% to 20%; includes erythema, itching, hemorrhage, pain, swelling)
- Neuromuscular & skeletal: Increased creatine phosphokinase (15%)
- Respiratory: Upper respiratory tract infection (17%), sinusitis (11%)

5% to 10%:

- Cardiovascular: Hypertension (5%)
- Endocrine & metabolic: Hyperlipidemia (7%), hypercholesterolemia (6%)
- Gastrointestinal: Nausea (9%), abdominal pain (7%)
- Genitourinary: Urinary tract infection (8%), hematuria (5%)
- Hepatic: Increased serum alkaline phosphatase (5%)
- Hypersensitivity: Hypersensitivity reaction (children 6%; adults 1%)
- Local: Injection site reaction (8%; other than erythema, itching, hemorrhage, pain, swelling)
- Neuromuscular & skeletal: Back pain (6%)
- Respiratory: Flu-like symptoms (7%)
- Miscellaneous: Accidental injury (10%)

1% to 5%:

- Cardiovascular: Atrial fibrillation, cardiac arrest, cardiac arrhythmia, cardiac failure, chest pain, coronary artery disease, deep vein thrombosis, hypertensive encephalopathy, myocardial infarction, palpitations, pericardial effusion, pericarditis, peripheral edema, subdural hematoma, syncope, tachycardia, vascular disease
- Central nervous system: Confusion, myasthenia, paresthesia
- Dermatologic: Alopecia, cellulitis, erysipelas
- Endocrine & metabolic: Dehydration, ketosis, menstrual disease, parathyroid disease
- Gastrointestinal: Cholecystitis, cholelithiasis, diverticulitis, esophagitis, gastroenteritis, gastrointestinal hemorrhage, vomiting
- Genitourinary: Cystitis, pelvic pain
- Hematologic & oncologic: Adenoma, agranulocytosis, carcinoma (including breast, gastrointestinal, skin, urogenital), granulocytopenia, leukopenia, malignant lymphoma, malignant melanoma, pancytopenia, paraproteinemia, polycythemia
- Hepatic: Hepatic necrosis
- Infection: Herpes zoster, sepsis
- Neuromuscular & skeletal: Arthralgia, arthritis, arthropathy, bone fracture, limb pain, multiple sclerosis, muscle cramps, myasthenia, osteonecrosis, septic arthritis, synovitis, systemic lupus erythematosus, tendon disease, tremor
- Ophthalmic: Cataract
- Renal: Nephrolithiasis, pyelonephritis
- Respiratory: Asthma, bronchospasm, dyspnea, pleural effusion, pneumonia, respiratory depression, tuberculosis (including reactivation of latent infection; disseminated, miliary, lymphatic, peritoneal, and pulmonary)
- Miscellaneous: Abnormal healing, fever, postoperative complication (infection)

<1% (Limited to important or life-threatening): Abscess (limb, perianal), anal fissure, anaphylactoid reaction, anaphylaxis, angioedema, aplastic anemia, appendicitis, bacterial infection, basal cell carcinoma, cerebrovascular accident, cervical dysplasia, circulatory shock, cytopenia, dermal ulcer, endometrial hyperplasia, erythema multiforme, fixed drug eruption, fulminant necrotizing fasciitis, fungal infection, Guillain-Barre syndrome, hepatic failure, hepatitis B (reactivation), herpes simplex infection, histoplasmosis, hypersensitivity angiitis, increased serum transaminases, interstitial pulmonary disease (eg, pulmonary fibrosis), intestinal obstruction, intestinal perforation, leukemia, liver metastases, lupus-like syndrome, lymphadenopathy, lymphocytosis, malignant neoplasm of ovary, meningitis (viral), Merkel cell carcinoma, mycobacterium avium complex, myositis (children and adolescents), neutropenia, optic neuritis, pancreatitis, pharyngitis (children and adolescents), protozoal infection, psoriasis (including new onset, palmoplantar, pustular, or exacerbation), pulmonary embolism, respiratory failure, sarcoidosis, septic shock, skin granuloma (annulare; children and adolescents), Stevens-Johnson syndrome,

streptococcal pharyngitis (children and adolescents), testicular neoplasm, thrombocytopenia, vasculitis (systemic), viral infection

Drug Interactions

Metabolism/Transport Effects None known.

Avoid Concomitant Use

Avoid concomitant use of Adalimumab with any of the following: Abatacept; Anakinra; BCG; Belimumab; Canakinumab; Certolizumab Pegol; InFLIXimab; Natalizumab; Pimecrolimus; Rilonacept; Tacrolimus (Topical); Tocilizumab; Tofacitinib; Vaccines (Live)

Increased Effect/Toxicity

Adalimumab may increase the levels/effects of: Abatacept; Anakinra; Belimumab; Canakinumab; Certolizumab Pegol; InFLIXimab; Leflunomide; Natalizumab; Rilonacept; Tofacitinib; Vaccines (Live)

The levels/effects of Adalimumab may be increased by: Abciximab; Denosumab; Pimecrolimus; Roflumilast; Tacrolimus (Topical); Tocilizumab; Trastuzumab

Decreased Effect

Adalimumab may decrease the levels/effects of: BCG; Coccidioidin Skin Test; CycloSPORINE (Systemic); Sipuleucel-T; Theophylline Derivatives; Vaccines (Inactivated); Vaccines (Live); Warfarin

The levels/effects of Adalimumab may be decreased by: Echinacea

Ethanol/Nutrition/Herb Interactions Herb/nutraceutical: Echinacea may decrease the therapeutic effects of adalimumab; avoid concurrent use.

Storage/Stability Store under refrigeration at 2°C to 8°C (36°F to 46°F); do not freeze. Protect from light.

Mechanism of Action Adalimumab is a recombinant monoclonal antibody that binds to human tumor necrosis factor alpha (TNF-alpha), thereby interfering with binding to TNFα receptor sites and subsequent cytokine-driven inflammatory processes. Elevated TNF levels in the synovial fluid are involved in the pathologic pain and joint destruction in immune-mediated arthritis. Adalimumab decreases signs and symptoms of psoriatic arthritis, rheumatoid arthritis, and ankylosing spondylitis. It inhibits progression of structural damage of rheumatoid and psoriatic arthritis. Reduces signs and symptoms and maintains clinical remission in Crohn's disease and ulcerative colitis; reduces epidermal thickness and inflammatory cell infiltration in plaque psoriasis.

Pharmacodynamics/Kinetics

Distribution: V_d: 4.7-6 L; Synovial fluid concentrations: 31% to 96% of serum

Bioavailability: Absolute: 64%

Half-life elimination: Terminal: ~2 weeks (range: 10-20 days)

Time to peak, serum: SubQ: 131 ± 56 hours

Excretion: Clearance increased in the presence of anti-adalimumab antibodies; decreased in patients ≥40 years of age

Dosage SubQ:

Children ≥4 years: Juvenile idiopathic arthritis (JIA):

U.S. labeling:

15 kg to <30 kg: 20 mg every other week

≥30 kg: 40 mg every other week

Canadian labeling: 24 mg/m² (maximum dose: 40 mg) every other week

Adolescents ≥13 years and ≥40 kg: Crohn's disease:

Canadian labeling:

Initial: 160 mg (given as 4 injections on day 1 **or** given as 2 injections daily over 2 consecutive days), then 80 mg 2 weeks later (day 15; given as 2 injections on the same day). **Note:** 40 mg per injection.

Maintenance: 20 mg every other week beginning week 4 (day 29); may consider increasing dose to 40 mg every other week for disease flare or inadequate response. Potential benefits of continued therapy should be reassessed if inadequate response at 12 weeks.

Adults:

Ankylosing spondylitis: 40 mg every other week

Crohn's disease:

Initial: 160 mg (given as 4 injections on day 1 **or** given as 2 injections daily over 2 consecutive days), then 80 mg 2 weeks later (day 15). **Note:** 40 mg per injection.

Maintenance: 40 mg every other week beginning day 29. **Note:** Some patients may require 40 mg every week as maintenance therapy (Lichtenstein, 2009).

Plaque psoriasis:

Initial: 80 mg as a single dose

Maintenance: 40 mg every other week beginning 1 week after initial dose

Psoriatic arthritis: 40 mg every other week

Rheumatoid arthritis: 40 mg every other week; patients not taking methotrexate may increase dose to 40 mg every week

Ulcerative colitis:

Initial: 160 mg (given as 4 injections on day 1 **or** given as 2 injections daily over 2 consecutive days), then 80 mg 2 weeks later (day 15). **Note:** 40 mg per injection.

Maintenance: 40 mg every other week beginning day 29. **Note:** Only continue maintenance dose in patients demonstrating clinical remission by 8 weeks (day 57) of therapy.

Dosage adjustment in renal impairment: No dosage adjustment provided in manufacturer's labeling (has not been studied).

Dosage adjustment in hepatic impairment: No dosage adjustment provided in manufacturer's labeling (has not been studied).

Administration For SubQ injection (into thigh or lower abdomen, avoiding areas within 2 inches of navel); rotate injection sites. Do not use if solution is discolored or contains particulate matter. Do not administer to skin which is red, tender, bruised, or hard. Needle cap of the prefilled syringe may contain latex. Prefilled pens and syringes are available for use by patients (self-administration); the vial is intended for institutional use only. Vials do not contain a preservative; discard unused portion.

Monitoring Parameters Monitor improvement of symptoms and physical function assessments. Latent TB screening prior to initiating and during therapy; signs/symptoms of infection (prior to, during, and following therapy); CBC with differential; signs/symptoms/worsening of heart failure; HBV screening prior to initiating (all patients), HBV carriers (during and for several months following therapy); signs and symptoms of hypersensitivity reaction; symptoms of lupus-like syndrome; signs/symptoms of malignancy (eg, splenomegaly, hepatomegaly, abdominal pain, persistent fever, night sweats, weight loss), including periodic skin examination.

Dosage Forms Excipient information presented when available (limited, particularly for generics); consult specific product labeling.

Kit, Subcutaneous [preservative free]:

Humira: 20 mg/0.4 mL, 40 mg/0.8 mL [contains polysorbate 80]

Humira Pen: 40 mg/0.8 mL [contains polysorbate 80]

Humira Pen-Crohns Starter: 40 mg/0.8 mL [contains polysorbate 80]

Humira Pen-Psoriasis Starter: 40 mg/0.8 mL [contains polysorbate 80]

Dosage Forms: Canada Also refer to Dosage Forms. Excipient information presented when available (limited, particularly for generics); consult specific product labeling.

Injection, solution [pediatric, preservative free]:

Humira®: 40 mg/0.8 mL (0.8 mL) [vial] [contains polysorbate 80]

◆ **Adamantanamine Hydrochloride** *see* Amantadine *on page 92*

Adapalene (a DAP a leen)

Brand Names: U.S. Differin

Brand Names: Canada Differin®; Differin® XP

Pharmacologic Category Acne Products; Topical Skin Product, Acne

Use Treatment of acne vulgaris

Pregnancy Risk Factor C

Dosage Topical: Children >12 years and Adults: Apply once daily at bedtime

Additional Information Complete prescribing information should be consulted for additional detail.

Dosage Forms Excipient information presented when available (limited, particularly for generics); consult specific product labeling.

Cream, External:

Differin: 0.1% (45 g)

Generic: 0.1% (45 g)

Gel, External:

Differin: 0.1% (45 g)

Differin: 0.3% (45 g) [contains edetate disodium, methylparaben, propylene glycol]

Generic: 0.1% (45 g)

Lotion, External:

Differin: 0.1% (59 mL) [contains methylparaben, propylene glycol, propylparaben]

Adapalene and Benzoyl Peroxide

(a DAP a leen & BEN zoe il peer OKS ide)

Brand Names: U.S. Epiduo®

Brand Names: Canada Tactuo™

Index Terms Benzoyl Peroxide and Adapalene

Pharmacologic Category Acne Products; Topical Skin Product; Topical Skin Product, Acne

Use Topical treatment of acne vulgaris

Pregnancy Risk Factor C

Dosage Topical: Children ≥9 years, Adolescents, and Adults: Apply once daily to affected areas after skin has been cleaned and dried

Additional Information Complete prescribing information should be consulted for additional detail.

Dosage Forms Excipient information presented when available (limited, particularly for generics); consult specific product labeling.

Gel, topical:

Epiduo®: Adapalene 0.1% and benzoyl peroxide 2.5% (45 g)

◆ **Adcetris** *see* Brentuximab Vedotin *on page 278*

◆ **Adcetris™ (Can)** *see* Brentuximab Vedotin *on page 278*

◆ **Adcirca** *see* Tadalafil *on page 1983*

◆ **ADD 234037** *see* Lacosamide *on page 1159*

◆ **Addaprin [OTC]** *see* Ibuprofen *on page 1032*

◆ **Adderall** *see* Dextroamphetamine and Amphetamine *on page 589*

◆ **Adderall XR** *see* Dextroamphetamine and Amphetamine *on page 589*

Adefovir (a DEF o veer)

Brand Names: U.S. Hepsera

Brand Names: Canada Hepsera™

Index Terms Adefovir Dipivoxil; Bis-POM PMEA

Pharmacologic Category Antiviral Agent

Use Treatment of chronic hepatitis B with evidence of active viral replication (based on persistent elevation of ALT/AST or histologic evidence), including patients with lamivudine-resistant hepatitis B

Pregnancy Risk Factor C

Pregnancy Considerations Adverse events were observed in some animal reproduction studies. Pregnant women exposed to adefovir should be registered with the pregnancy registry (800-258-4263).

Breast-Feeding Considerations It is not known if adefovir is excreted in breast milk. Due to the potential for serious adverse reactions in the nursing infant, a decision should be made whether to discontinue nursing or to discontinue the drug, taking into account the importance of treatment to the mother.

Contraindications Hypersensitivity to adefovir or any component of the formulation

Warnings/Precautions [U.S. Boxed Warning]: Use with caution in patients with renal dysfunction or in patients at risk of renal toxicity (including concurrent nephrotoxic agents or NSAIDs). Chronic administration may result in nephrotoxicity. Dosage adjustment is required in adult patients with renal dysfunction or in patients who develop renal dysfunction during therapy; no data available for use in children ≥12 years or adolescents with renal impairment. Not recommended as first line therapy of chronic HBV due to weak antiviral activity and high rate of resistance after first year. May be more appropriate as second-line agent in treatment-naïve patients. Combination therapy with lamivudine in nucleoside-naïve patients has not been shown to provide synergistic antiviral effects. In patients with lamivudine-resistant HBV, switching to adefovir monotherapy was associated with a higher risk of adefovir resistance compared to adding adefovir to lamivudine therapy (Lok, 2009).

Calculate creatinine clearance before initiation of therapy. Consider alternative therapy in patients who do not respond to adefovir monotherapy treatment. **[U.S. Boxed Warning]: May cause the development of HIV resistance in patients with unrecognized or untreated HIV infection.** Determine HIV status prior to initiating treatment with adefovir. **[U.S. Boxed Warning]: Fatal cases of lactic acidosis and severe hepatomegaly with steatosis have been reported with the use of nucleoside analogues alone or in combination with other antiretrovirals.** Female gender, obesity, and prolonged treatment may increase the risk of hepatotoxicity. Treatment should be discontinued in patients with lactic acidosis or signs/symptoms of hepatotoxicity (which may occur without marked transaminase elevations). **[U.S. Boxed Warning]: Acute exacerbations of hepatitis may occur (in up to 25% of patients) when antihepatitis therapy is discontinued.** Exacerbations typically occur within 12 weeks and may be self-limited or resolve upon resuming treatment; risk may be increased with advanced liver disease or cirrhosis. Monitor patients following discontinuation of therapy. Safety and efficacy in children <12 years of age have not been established. Do not use concurrently with tenofovir (Viread®) or any product containing tenofovir (eg, Truvada®, Atripla®, Complera®).

Adverse Reactions

>10%:

Central nervous system: Headache (24% to 25%)

Gastrointestinal: Abdominal pain (15%), diarrhea (up to 13%)

Hepatic: Hepatitis exacerbation (up to 25% within 12 weeks of adefovir discontinuation)
Neuromuscular & skeletal: Weakness (up to 25%)
Renal: Hematuria (grade ≥3: 11%)

1% to 10%:
Dermatologic: Rash, pruritus
Endocrine & metabolic: Hypophosphatemia (<2 mg/dL: 1% and 3% in pre-/post-liver transplant patients, respectively)
Gastrointestinal: Flatulence (up to 8%), dyspepsia (5% to 9%), nausea, vomiting
Neuromuscular & skeletal: Back pain (up to 10%)
Renal: Serum creatinine increased (≥0.5 mg/dL: 2% to 3% in compensated liver disease; incidence may be higher in patients with decompensated cirrhosis or in liver transplant recipients), renal failure

Note: In liver transplant patients with baseline renal dysfunction, frequency of increased serum creatinine has been observed to be as high as 32% to 51% at 48 and 96 weeks post-transplantation, respectively; considering the concomitant use of other potentially nephrotoxic medications, baseline renal insufficiency, and predisposing comorbidities, the role of adefovir in these changes could not be established.

Respiratory: Cough (6% to 8%), rhinitis (up to 5%)

Postmarketing and/or case reports: Fanconi syndrome, hepatitis, myopathy, nephrotoxicity, osteomalacia, pancreatitis, proximal renal tubulopathy

Drug Interactions

Metabolism/Transport Effects None known.

Avoid Concomitant Use

Avoid concomitant use of Adefovir with any of the following: Tenofovir

Increased Effect/Toxicity

Adefovir may increase the levels/effects of: Tenofovir

The levels/effects of Adefovir may be increased by: Ganciclovir-Valganciclovir; Ribavirin; Tenofovir

Decreased Effect

Adefovir may decrease the levels/effects of: Tenofovir

Ethanol/Nutrition/Herb Interactions

Ethanol: Should be avoided in hepatitis B infection due to potential hepatic toxicity.

Food: Does not have a significant effect on adefovir absorption.

Storage/Stability Store controlled room temperature of 25°C (77°F).

Mechanism of Action Acyclic nucleotide reverse transcriptase inhibitor (adenosine analog) which interferes with HBV viral RNA-dependent DNA polymerase resulting in inhibition of viral replication.

Pharmacodynamics/Kinetics

Distribution: 0.35-0.39 L/kg
Protein binding: ≤4%
Metabolism: Prodrug; rapidly converted to adefovir (active metabolite) in intestine
Bioavailability: 59%
Half-life elimination: 7.5 hours; prolonged in renal impairment
Time to peak: 1.75 hours
Excretion: Urine (45% as active metabolite within 24 hours)

Dosage Oral: Children ≥12 years and Adults: 10 mg once daily

Treatment duration (AASLD practice guidelines): Adults:
Hepatitis Be antigen (HBeAg) positive chronic hepatitis: Treat ≥1 year until HBeAg seroconversion and undetectable serum HBV DNA; continue therapy for ≥6 months after HBeAg seroconversion
HBeAg negative chronic hepatitis: Treat >1 year until hepatitis B surface antigen (HBsAg) clearance

Note: Patients not achieving a <2 log decrease in serum HBV DNA after at least 6 months of therapy should either receive additional treatment or be switched to an alternative therapy (Lok, 2009).

Dosage adjustment in renal impairment: Adult recommendations only (no dosage adjustment recommendations available for patients <18 years with renal impairment):
Cl_{cr} ≥50 mL/minute: No dosage adjustment necessary
Cl_{cr} 20-49 mL/minute: 10 mg every 48 hours
Cl_{cr} 10-19 mL/minute: 10 mg every 72 hours
Hemodialysis: 10 mg every 7 days (following dialysis)

Dosage adjustment in hepatic impairment: No adjustment required

Dietary Considerations May be taken without regard to food.

Administration May be administered without regard to food.

Monitoring Parameters HIV status (prior to initiation of therapy); serum creatinine (prior to initiation and during therapy; every 3 months in patients with medical conditions which predispose to renal insufficiency and in all patients treated for >1 year; more frequent monitoring required if pre-existing real insufficiency detected [Lok, 2009]); LFTs for several months following discontinuation of adefovir; HBV DNA (every 3-6 months during therapy); HBeAg and anti-HBe

Additional Information Adefovir dipivoxil is a prodrug, rapidly converted to the active component (adefovir). It was previously investigated as a treatment for HIV infections (at dosages substantially higher than the approved dose for hepatitis B). The NDA was withdrawn, and no further studies in the treatment of HIV are anticipated (per manufacturer).

Dosage Forms Excipient information presented when available (limited, particularly for generics); consult specific product labeling.

Tablet, Oral, as dipivoxil:
Hepsera: 10 mg
Generic: 10 mg

◆ **Adefovir Dipivoxil** *see* Adefovir *on page* 48
◆ **Adempas** *see* Riociguat *on page* 1822
◆ **Adenocard** *see* Adenosine *on page* 49
◆ **Adenoscan** *see* Adenosine *on page* 49

Adenosine (a DEN oh seen)

Brand Names: U.S. Adenocard; Adenoscan

Brand Names: Canada Adenocard; Adenosine Injection, USP; PMS-Adenosine

Index Terms 9-Beta-D-Ribofuranosyladenine

Pharmacologic Category Antiarrhythmic Agent, Miscellaneous; Diagnostic Agent

Additional Appendix Information

Adult ACLS Algorithms *on page* 2363
Dosing Considerations for the Critically-Ill Patient With Morbid Obesity *on page* 2379
Pediatric ALS (PALS) Algorithms *on page* 2359

Use

Adenocard: Treatment of paroxysmal supraventricular tachycardia (PSVT) including that associated with accessory bypass tracts (Wolff-Parkinson-White syndrome); when clinically advisable, appropriate vagal maneuvers should be attempted prior to adenosine administration; **not effective for conversion of atrial fibrillation, atrial flutter, or ventricular tachycardia**

Adenoscan: Pharmacologic stress agent used in myocardial perfusion thallium-201 scintigraphy

Unlabeled Use

ACLS/PALS Guidelines (2010): Stable, narrow-complex regular tachycardias; unstable narrow-complex regular tachycardias while preparations are made for synchronized direct-current cardioversion; stable regular monomorphic, wide-complex tachycardia as a therapeutic (if SVT) and diagnostic maneuver

Adenoscan: Acute vasodilator testing in pulmonary artery hypertension

Pregnancy Risk Factor C

Pregnancy Considerations Animal reproduction studies have not been conducted. Adenosine is an endogenous substance and adverse fetal effects would not be anticipated. Case reports of administration during pregnancy have indicated no adverse effects on fetus or newborn attributable to adenosine (Blomström-Lundqvist, 2003). ACLS guidelines suggest use is safe and effective in pregnancy (Neumar, 2010).

Breast-Feeding Considerations Adenosine is endogenous in breast milk (Sugawara, 1995).

Contraindications Hypersensitivity to adenosine or any component of the formulation; second- or third-degree AV block, sick sinus syndrome, or symptomatic bradycardia (except in patients with a functioning artificial pacemaker); use in patients with atrial fibrillation/flutter with underlying Wolff-Parkinson-White (WPW) syndrome (Fuster, 2006); asthma (ACLS, 2010)

In addition to the above, Adenoscan should be avoided in patients with known or suspected bronchoconstrictive or bronchospastic lung disease.

Warnings/Precautions ECG monitoring required during use. Equipment for resuscitation and trained personnel experienced in handling medical emergencies should always be immediately available. Adenosine decreases conduction through the AV node and may produce first-, second-, or third-degree heart block. Patients with preexisting S-A nodal dysfunction may experience prolonged sinus pauses after adenosine; use caution in patients with first-degree AV block or bundle branch block. Use is contraindicated in patients with high-grade AV block, sinus node dysfunction or symptomatic bradycardia (unless a functional artificial pacemaker is in place). Rare, prolonged episodes of asystole have been reported, with fatal outcomes in some cases. Use caution in patients receiving other drugs which slow AV node conduction (eg, digoxin, verapamil). Potentially significant interactions may exist, requiring dose or frequency adjustment, additional monitoring, and/or selection of alternative therapy.

There have been reports of atrial fibrillation/flutter after adenosine administration in patients with PSVT associated with accessory conduction pathways; has also been reported in patients with or without a history of atrial fibrillation undergoing myocardial perfusion imaging with adenosine infusion. Adenosine may also produce profound vasodilation with subsequent hypotension. When used as a bolus dose (PSVT), effects are generally self-limiting (due to the short half-life of adenosine). However, when used as a continuous infusion (pharmacologic stress testing), effects may be more pronounced and persistent, corresponding to continued exposure; discontinue infusion in patients who develop persistent or symptomatic hypotension. Adenosine infusions should be used with caution in patients with autonomic dysfunction, stenotic valvular heart disease, pericarditis, pleural effusion, carotid stenosis (with cerebrovascular insufficiency), or uncorrected hypovolemia. Use caution in elderly patients; may be at increased risk of hemodynamic effects, bradycardia, and/or AV block.

Avoid use in patients with bronchoconstriction or bronchospasm (eg, asthma); mild-to-moderate exacerbations have been reported following use in a limited number of patients with asthma. Per the ACLS guidelines, use considered contraindicated in patients with asthma. Use caution in patients with obstructive lung disease not associated with bronchoconstriction (eg, emphysema, bronchitis); respiratory compromise has occurred during use. Immediately discontinue therapy if severe respiratory difficulty is observed.

Adenocard: Transient AV block is expected. Administer as a rapid bolus, either directly into a vein or (if administered into an I.V. line), as close to the patient as possible (followed by saline flush). Dose reduction recommended when administered via central line (ACLS, 2010). When used in PSVT, at the time of conversion to normal sinus rhythm, a variety of new rhythms may appear on the ECG. Watch for proarrhythmic effects (eg, polymorphic ventricular tachycardia) during and shortly after administration/termination of arrhythmia. Benign transient occurrence of atrial and ventricular ectopy is common upon termination of arrhythmia. Adenosine does not convert atrial fibrillation/flutter to normal sinus rhythm; however, may be used diagnostically in these settings if the underlying rhythm is not apparent. Use in patients with atrial fibrillation/flutter with underlying WPW syndrome is considered to be contraindicated since ventricular fibrillation may result (Fuster, 2006). Use with extreme caution in heart transplant recipients; adenosine may cause prolonged asystole; reduction of initial adenosine dose is recommended (ACLS, 2010); considered by some to be contraindicated in this setting (Delacrétaz, 2006). Avoid use in irregular or polymorphic wide-complex tachycardias; may cause degeneration to ventricular fibrillation (ACLS, 2010). When used for PSVT, dosage reduction recommended when used with concomitant drugs which potentiate the effects of adenosine (carbamazepine, dipyridamole)

Adenoscan: Drugs which antagonize adenosine (theophylline [includes aminophylline], caffeine) should be withheld for five half-lives prior to adenosine use. Avoid dietary caffeine for at least 12 hours prior to pharmacologic stress testing (Henzlova, 2006). Withhold dipyridamole-containing medications for at least 24 hours prior to pharmacologic stress testing (Henzlova, 2006).

Cardiovascular events: Cardiac arrest (fatal and nonfatal), myocardial infarction (MI), and sustained ventricular tachycardia requiring resuscitation have occurred following Adenoscan use. Avoid use in patients with signs or symptoms of unstable angina, acute myocardial ischemia, or cardiovascular instability due to possible increased risk of significant cardiovascular consequences. Appropriate measures for resuscitation should be available during use. In addition, systolic and diastolic pressure increases have been observed with Adenoscan infusion. In most instances, blood pressure increases resolved spontaneously within several minutes; occasionally, hypertension lasted for several hours.

Pulmonary artery hypertension: Acute vasodilator testing (not an approved use): Use with extreme caution in patients with concomitant heart failure (LV systolic dysfunction with significantly elevated left heart filling pressures) or pulmonary veno-occlusive disease/pulmonary capillary hemangiomatosis; significant decompensation has occurred with other highly selective pulmonary vasodilators resulting in acute pulmonary edema.

Adverse Reactions Note: Frequency varies based on use; higher frequency of infusion-related effects, such as flushing and lightheadedness/dizziness, were reported with continuous infusion (Adenoscan®).

>10%:

Cardiovascular: Cardiac arrhythmia (transient and new arrhythmia after cardioversion; eg, atrial premature contractions, atrial fibrillation, premature ventricular contractions; 55%), chest pressure (and discomfort; 7% to 40%)

Central nervous system: Headache (2% to 18%), dizziness (2% to 12%)

Dermatologic: Facial flushing (18% to 44%)

Gastrointestinal: Gastrointestinal distress (13%)

Neuromuscular & skeletal: Neck discomfort (includes throat, jaw; <1% to 15%)

Respiratory: Dyspnea (12% to 28%)

1% to 10%:

Cardiovascular: Atrioventricular block (infusion 6%; third-degree <1%), depression of ST segment on electrocardiogram (3%), hypotension (<1% to 2%), chest pain, palpitations

Central nervous system: Nervousness (2%), numbness (≤2%), paresthesia (≤2%), apprehension

Dermatologic: Diaphoresis

Gastrointestinal: Nausea (3%)

Neuromuscular & skeletal: Upper extremity discomfort (≤4%)

Respiratory: Hyperventilation

<1% (Limited to important or life-threatening): Asystole (prolonged), atrial fibrillation, blurred vision, bradycardia, bronchospasm, burning sensation, increased intracranial pressure, injection site reaction, loss of consciousness, myocardial infarction, respiratory arrest, seizure, torsades de pointes, transient hypertension, ventricular fibrillation, ventricular tachycardia

Drug Interactions

Metabolism/Transport Effects None known.

Avoid Concomitant Use There are no known interactions where it is recommended to avoid concomitant use.

Increased Effect/Toxicity

The levels/effects of Adenosine may be increased by: CarBAMazepine; Digoxin; Dipyridamole; Nicotine

Decreased Effect

The levels/effects of Adenosine may be decreased by: Caffeine; Theophylline Derivatives

Ethanol/Nutrition/Herb Interactions Food: Adenosine's therapeutic effect may be decreased if used concurrently with caffeine. Management: Avoid food or drugs with caffeine for at least 12 hours prior to pharmacologic stress testing.

Storage/Stability Store at controlled room temperature of 15°C to 30°C (59°F to 86°F). Do **not** refrigerate; crystallization may occur (may dissolve by warming to room temperature).

Mechanism of Action

Antiarrhythmic actions: Slows conduction time through the AV node, interrupting the re-entry pathways through the AV node, restoring normal sinus rhythm

Myocardial perfusion scintigraphy: Adenosine also causes coronary vasodilation and increases blood flow in normal coronary arteries with little to no increase in stenotic coronary arteries; thallium-201 uptake into the stenotic coronary arteries will be less than that of normal coronary arteries revealing areas of insufficient blood flow.

Pharmacodynamics/Kinetics

Onset of action: Rapid

Duration: Very brief

Metabolism: Blood and tissue to inosine then to adenosine monophosphate (AMP) and hypoxanthine

Half-life elimination: <10 seconds

Dosage

Adenocard: **Rapid I.V. push (over 1-2 seconds) via peripheral line, followed by a normal saline flush:**

Infants and Children:

Paroxysmal supraventricular tachycardia: Manufacturer's recommendation: I.V.:

<50 kg: Initial: 0.05-0.1 mg/kg (maximum initial dose: 6 mg). If conversion of PSVT does not occur within 1-2 minutes, may increase dose by 0.05-0.1 mg/kg. May repeat until sinus rhythm is established or to a maximum single dose of 0.3 mg/kg or 12 mg. Follow each dose with normal saline flush.

≥50 kg: Refer to Adult dosing

Pediatric advanced life support (PALS, 2010): Treatment of SVT: I.V., I.O.: Initial: 0.1 mg/kg (maximum initial dose: 6 mg); if not effective within 1-2 minutes, administer 0.2 mg/kg (maximum single dose: 12 mg). Follow each dose with ≥5 mL normal saline flush.

Adults: Paroxysmal supraventricular tachycardia: I.V. (peripheral line; see **Note**): Initial: 6 mg; if not effective within 1-2 minutes, 12 mg may be given; may repeat 12 mg bolus if needed (maximum single dose: 12 mg). Follow each dose with 20 mL normal saline flush. **Note:** Initial dose of adenosine should be reduced to 3 mg if patient is currently receiving carbamazepine or dipyridamole, has a transplanted heart or if adenosine is administered via central line (ACLS, 2010).

Adenoscan:

Pharmacologic stress testing: Continuous I.V. infusion via peripheral line: 140 mcg/kg/minute for 6 minutes using syringe or volumetric infusion pump; total dose: 0.84 mg/kg. Thallium-201 is injected at midpoint (3 minutes) of infusion.

Acute vasodilator testing in pulmonary artery hypertension (unlabeled use): I.V.: Initial: 50 mcg/kg/minute increased by 50 mcg/kg/minute every 2 minutes to a maximum dose of 500 mcg/kg/minute (Schrader, 1992) **or** to a maximum dose of 250 mcg/kg/minute (McLaughlin, 2009); acutely assess vasodilator response

Dosage adjustment in renal impairment: No dosage adjustment provided in manufacturer's labeling. However, adenosine is not renally eliminated.

Dosage adjustment in hepatic impairment: No dosage adjustment provided in manufacturer's labeling. However, adenosine is not hepatically eliminated.

Dietary Considerations Avoid dietary caffeine for at least 12 hours prior to pharmacologic stress testing.

Administration

Adenocard: For rapid bolus I.V. use only; administer I.V. push over 1-2 seconds at a peripheral I.V. site as proximal as possible to trunk (not in lower arm, hand, lower leg, or foot); follow each bolus with a rapid normal saline flush (infants and children ≥5 mL; adults 20 mL). Use of 2 syringes (one with adenosine dose and the other with NS flush) connected to a T-connector or stopcock is recommended. If administered via **central line** in adults, reduce initial dose (ACLS, 2010).

Adenoscan: For I.V. infusion only via peripheral line

Monitoring Parameters ECG, heart rate, blood pressure; consult individual institutional policies and procedures

Dosage Forms Excipient information presented when available (limited, particularly for generics); consult specific product labeling.

Solution, Intravenous:

Adenocard: 6 mg/2 mL (2 mL); 12 mg/4 mL (4 mL)

Adenoscan: 3 mg/mL (20 mL, 30 mL)

Generic: 6 mg/2 mL (2 mL); 12 mg/4 mL (4 mL)

Solution, Intravenous [preservative free]:

Generic: 3 mg/mL (20 mL, 30 mL); 6 mg/2 mL (2 mL); 12 mg/4 mL (4 mL)

- ◆ Adenosine Injection, USP (Can) *see* Adenosine *on page 49*
- ◆ ADH *see* Vasopressin *on page 2172*
- ◆ Adipex-P *see* Phentermine *on page 1632*
- ◆ A&D Jr. [OTC] *see* Vitamin A and Vitamin D (Systemic) *on page 2202*
- ◆ ADL-2698 *see* Alvimopan *on page 91*

Ado-Trastuzumab Emtansine

(a do tras TU zoo mab em TAN seen)

Brand Names: U.S. Kadcyla

Index Terms T-DM1; Trastuzumab Emtansine; Trastuzumab-DM1; Trastuzumab-MCC-DM1

Pharmacologic Category Antineoplastic Agent, Anti-HER2; Antineoplastic Agent, Antimicrotubular; Antineoplastic Agent, Monoclonal Antibody

Use Treatment of HER2-positive, metastatic breast cancer in patients who previously received trastuzumab and a taxane, separately or in combination, and have either received prior therapy for metastatic disease or developed disease recurrence during or within 6 months of completing adjuvant therapy.

Pregnancy Risk Factor D

Pregnancy Considerations Animal reproduction studies have not been conducted. **[U.S. Boxed Warning]: Exposure to ado-trastuzumab emtansine may cause embryo-fetal death. Effective contraception must be used in women of reproductive potential.** Oligohydramnios, pulmonary hypoplasia, skeletal malformations and neonatal death were observed following trastuzumab exposure during pregnancy (trastuzumab is the antibody component of ado-trastuzumab emtansine). The DM1 component of the ado-trastuzumab emtansine formulation is toxic to rapidly dividing cells and is also expected to cause fetal harm. Pregnancy status should be verified prior to therapy. Effective contraception is recommended during therapy and for 6 months after treatment for women of childbearing potential.

If ado-trastuzumab emtansine exposure occurs during pregnancy, healthcare providers should report the exposure to the Genentech Adverse Event Line (888-835-2555). Women exposed to ado-trastuzumab emtansine during pregnancy are encouraged to enroll in MotHER Pregnancy Registry (1-800-690-6720).

Breast-Feeding Considerations It is not known if ado-trastuzumab emtansine is excreted into breast milk. Endogenous immunoglobulins are found in breast milk. Due to the potential for serious adverse reactions in the nursing infant, the decision to discontinue ado-trastuzumab emtansine or discontinue breast-feeding during treatment should take in account the benefits of treatment to the mother.

Contraindications There are no contraindications in the manufacturer's labeling.

Warnings/Precautions Hazardous agent - use appropriate precautions for handling and disposal (meets NIOSH, 2012 criteria).

[U.S. Boxed Warning]: May result in left ventricular ejection fraction (LVEF) reductions. Evaluate left ventricular function (in all patients) prior to and at least every 3 months during treatment; withhold for clinically significant left ventricular function decreases. Treatment interruption or dosage reductions are required inpatients who develop LVEF declines. Use has not been studied in patients with LVEF <50% at baseline, with symptomatic CHF, serious arrhythmia, or recent history (within 6 months) of MI or unstable angina.

[U.S. Boxed Warning]: Serious hepatotoxicity, including liver failure and death, has been reported. Monitor transaminases and bilirubin at baseline and prior to each dose. Increases (transaminases or total bilirubin) may require dose reductions or discontinuation. Hepatotoxicity is typically manifested by asymptomatic and transient increases in transaminases, although fatal cases of drug induced liver injury and hepatic encephalopathy have occurred; may be confounded by comorbidities or concomitant hepatotoxic medications. Use has not been studied in patients with baseline serum transaminases >2.5 times ULN or bilirubin >1.5 times ULN. Cases of nodular regenerative hyperplasia (NRH), a rare liver disorder characterized by widespread benign transformation of hepatic parenchyma into small regenerative nodules, have been observed (by biopsy). NRH may develop into noncirrhotic portal hypertension. Consider NRH in patients with clinical symptoms of portal hypertension without associated transaminase elevations or manifestations of cirrhosis. Permanently discontinue if histopathology confirms NRH.

[U.S. Boxed Warning]: Exposure to ado-trastuzumab emtansine may cause embryo-fetal death. Effective contraception must be used in women of reproductive potential. Pregnancy status should be verified prior to therapy; effective contraception is recommended during therapy and for 6 months after treatment for women of childbearing potential.

Infusion reactions (flushing, chills, fever, bronchospasm, dyspnea, wheezing, hypotension, and/or tachycardia) have been reported. After termination of infusion, these reactions generally resolved within several hours to a day. Medications for the treatment of reactions should be available for immediate use. Monitor closely for infusion reactions, especially during initial infusion. If reaction occurs, decrease infusion rate; for severe infusion reactions, interrupt infusion; permanently discontinue for life-threatening reactions. Serious allergic/anaphylactic reaction was observed (rare). Use is not recommended in patients who had trastuzumab permanently discontinued due to infusion reaction or hypersensitivity (has not been evaluated).

Thrombocytopenia may occur; the incidence of thrombocytopenia may be higher in patients of Asian ancestry; monitor platelet count at baseline and prior to each dose; may require treatment interruption or dose reduction. Monitor closely if at bleeding risk due to thrombocytopenia and/or concomitant anticoagulant use. Neutropenia and anemia have also occurred. Local reactions (erythema, irritation, pain, swelling, or tenderness) secondary to extravasation have been noted; these were generally mild and typically occurred within 24 hours of infusion; monitor infusion site during infusion for possible infiltration. Sensory peripheral neuropathy has been reported, usually grade 1; monitor for signs and symptoms of neuropathy; may require treatment interruption and/or dose reduction. Interstitial lung disease (ILD), including pneumonitis has been reported; some cases resulted in acute respiratory distress syndrome and/or fatalities; permanently discontinue with diagnosis of ILD or pneumonitis. Signs and symptoms of pneumonitis include dyspnea, cough, fatigue, and pulmonary infiltrates; may or may not occur in correlation with infusion reaction. Patients with dyspnea at rest (due to advance malignancy complications or comorbidity) may be at increased risk for pulmonary toxicity.

[U.S. Boxed Warning]: Ado-trastuzumab emtansine and conventional trastuzumab are NOT interchangeable. Verify product label prior to reconstitution and administration to prevent medication errors. Potentially significant drug-drug or drug-food interactions may exist, requiring dose or frequency adjustment, additional monitoring, and/or selection of alternative therapy. Establish HER2 overexpression or gene amplification status prior to treatment; has only been studied in patients with evidence of HER2 overexpression, either as 3+ IHC (Dako Herceptest™) or FISH amplification ratio ≥2 (Dako *HER2* FISH pharmDx™ test); there is only limited data on patients with breast cancer positive by FISH and 0 or 1+ by IHC.

Adverse Reactions

>10%:

Central nervous system: Fatigue (36%), headache (28%), fever (19%), insomnia (12%)

Dermatologic: Skin rash (12%)

Gastrointestinal: Nausea (40%), constipation (27%), diarrhea (24%), abdominal pain (19%), vomiting (19%), xerostomia (17%), stomatitis (14%)

Hematologic: Thrombocytopenia (31%; grades 3/4: 15%; Asians grades 3/4: 45%), anemia (14%; grades 3/4: 4%)

Hepatic: Increased serum aspartate aminotransferase (98%; grades 3/4: <8%), increased serum alanine aminotransferase (82%; grades 3/4: <6%), increased serum transaminases (29%), increased serum bilirubin (17%)

Neuromuscular & skeletal: Musculoskeletal pain (36%), peripheral neuropathy (21%; grades 3/4: 2%), arthralgia (19%), weakness (18%), myalgia (14%)

Respiratory: Epistaxis (23%), cough (18%), dyspnea (12%)

1% to 10%:

Cardiovascular: Peripheral edema (7%), hypertension (5%; grades 3/4: 1%), left ventricular systolic dysfunction (2%)

Central nervous system: Dizziness (10%), chills (8%)

Dermatologic: Pruritus (6%)

Endocrine & metabolic: Hypokalemia (10%; grades 3/4: 3%)

Gastrointestinal: Dyspepsia (9%), dysgeusia (8%)

Genitourinary: Urinary tract infection (9%)

Hematologic: Neutropenia (7%; grades 3/4: 2%)

Hepatic: Increased serum alkaline phosphatase (5%)

Local: Infusion related reaction (1%)

Ocular: Blurred vision (5%), conjunctivitis (4%), dry eye syndrome (4%), lacrimation (3%)

Respiratory: Pneumonitis (≤1%)

Miscellaneous: Antibody development (5%), hypersensitivity (2%)

<1% (Limited to important or life-threatening): Anaphylaxis, hepatic encephalopathy, hepatic nodular regenerative hyperplasia, hepatotoxicity, portal hypertension

Drug Interactions

Metabolism/Transport Effects **Substrate** of CYP3A4 (major); **Note:** Assignment of Major/Minor substrate status based on clinically relevant drug interaction potential

Avoid Concomitant Use

Avoid concomitant use of Ado-Trastuzumab Emtansine with any of the following: BCG; Belimumab; CloZAPine; CYP3A4 Inhibitors (Strong); Fusidic Acid (Systemic); Natalizumab; Pimecrolimus; Tacrolimus (Topical); Tofacitinib; Vaccines (Live)

Increased Effect/Toxicity

Ado-Trastuzumab Emtansine may increase the levels/effects of: Belimumab; CloZAPine; Leflunomide; Natalizumab; Tofacitinib; Vaccines (Live); Vitamin K Antagonists

The levels/effects of Ado-Trastuzumab Emtansine may be increased by: Abciximab; CYP3A4 Inhibitors (Moderate); CYP3A4 Inhibitors (Strong); Dasatinib; Denosumab; Fusidic Acid (Systemic); Ivacaftor; Luliconazole; Mifepristone; Pimecrolimus; Roflumilast; Simeprevir; Tacrolimus (Topical); Trastuzumab

Decreased Effect

Ado-Trastuzumab Emtansine may decrease the levels/effects of: BCG; Cardiac Glycosides; Coccidioidin Skin Test; Sipuleucel-T; Vaccines (Inactivated); Vaccines (Live); Vitamin K Antagonists

The levels/effects of Ado-Trastuzumab Emtansine may be decreased by: Echinacea

Preparation for Administration Hazardous agent; use appropriate precautions for handling and disposal (meets NIOSH, 2012 criteria). Check vial labels to assure appropriate product is being reconstituted (ado-trastuzumab emtansine and conventional trastuzumab are different products and are **NOT** interchangeable).

Slowly inject sterile water for injection into the vial (5 mL for 100 mg vial or 8 mL for 160 mg vial) to a reconstituted concentration of 20 mg/mL. Gently swirl vial until completely dissolved. Reconstituted solution will be clear or slightly opalescent (there should be no visible particles) and colorless to pale brown. Dilute for infusion by adding to 250 mL sodium chloride 0.9%; gently invert bag to mix (do not shake).

Storage/Stability Store intact vials refrigerated at 2°C to 8°C (36°F to 46°F). Do not freeze or shake intact vials, reconstituted solution, or solutions diluted for infusion. Reconstituted vials do not contain preservative and should be used immediately, although may be stored for up to 24 hours at 2°C to 8°C (36°F to 46°F). Solutions diluted for infusion should be used immediately, although may be stored at 2°C to 8°C (36°F to 46°F) for up to 24 hours prior to use. This storage time is additional to the time allowed for the reconstituted vials.

Mechanism of Action Ado-trastuzumab emtansine is a HER2-antibody drug conjugate which incorporates the HER2 targeted actions of trastuzumab with the microtubule inhibitor DM1 (a maytansine derivative). The conjugate, which is linked via a stable thioether linker, allows for selective delivery into HER2 overexpressing cells, resulting in cell cycle arrest and apoptosis.

Pharmacodynamics/Kinetics

Distribution: V_d: 3.13 L

Protein binding: DM1: 93%

Metabolism: DM1 undergoes hepatic metabolism via CYP3A4/5

Half-life elimination: ~4 days

Time to peak: Near the end of the infusion

Dosage

Note: Do not substitute ado-trastuzumab emtansine for or with conventional trastuzumab; products are different and are **NOT** interchangeable.

Breast cancer, metastatic, HER2+: Adults: I.V.: 3.6 mg/kg every 3 weeks until disease progression or unacceptable toxicity; Maximum dose: 3.6 mg/kg

Missed doses: If a planned dose is missed or delayed, administer as soon as possible (at the dose and rate most recently tolerated), do not wait until the next planned cycle. Then adjust schedule to maintain a 3-week interval between doses.

Dosage adjustment in renal impairment:

Cl_{cr} ≥30 mL/minute: No dosage adjustment necessary.

Cl_{cr} <30 mL/minute: No dosage adjustment provided in the manufacturer's labeling (has not been studied).

Dosage adjustment in hepatic impairment: No dosage adjustment provided in the manufacturer's labeling (has not been studied).

Dosage adjustment for toxicity: Note: After a dose reduction is implemented, do not re-escalate dose.

Infusion-related reaction: Slow infusion rate or interrupt infusion. Permanently discontinue if life-threatening infusion reactions occur.

Dose levels for dosage reductions and/or discontinuation:
Starting dose: 3.6 mg/kg
First dose reduction: Reduce dose to 3 mg/kg
Second dose reduction: Reduce dose to 2.4 mg/kg
Further reductions necessary: Discontinue treatment.

Hematologic toxicity:
Grade 3 thrombocytopenia (platelets 25,000/mm^3 to <50,000/mm^3): Withhold treatment until platelet count recovers to ≤ grade 1 (platelets ≥75,000/mm^3), then resume treatment at the same dose level.
Grade 4 thrombocytopenia (platelets <25,000/mm^3): Withhold treatment until platelet count recovers to ≤ grade 1 (platelets ≥75,000/mm^3), then resume treatment with one dose level reduction.

Cardiotoxicity:
LVEF >45%: Continue treatment.
LVEF 40% to ≤45% and decrease is <10% points from baseline: Continue treatment and repeat LVEF assessment within 3 weeks.
LVEF 40% to ≤45% and decrease is ≥10% points from baseline: Withhold treatment and repeat LVEF assessment within 3 weeks; if repeat LVEF has not recovered to within 10% points from baseline, discontinue treatment.
LVEF <40%: Withhold treatment and repeat LVEF assessment within 3 weeks; if repeat LVEF is confirmed <40%, discontinue treatment.
HF (symptomatic): Discontinue treatment.

Hepatotoxicity:
Grade 2 ALT, AST elevations (>2.5 to ≤5 times ULN): Continue at same dose level.
Grade 3 ALT, AST elevations (>5 to ≤20 times ULN): Withhold until ALT, AST recover to ≤ grade 2, then resume with one dose level reduction.
Grade 4 ALT, AST elevations (>20 times ULN): Permanently discontinue treatment.
Grade 2 hyperbilirubinemia (>1.5 to ≤3 times ULN): Withhold until bilirubin recovers to ≤ grade 1 (≤1.5 times ULN), then resume at the same dose level.
Grade 3 hyperbilirubinemia (>3 to ≤10 times ULN): Withhold until bilirubin recovers to ≤ grade 1, then resume with one dose level reduction.
Grade 4 hyperbilirubinemia (>10 times ULN): Permanently discontinue treatment.
Concomitant ALT, AST >3 times ULN and total bilirubin >2 times ULN: Permanently discontinue treatment.
Nodular regenerative hyperplasia: Permanently discontinue treatment.

Peripheral neuropathy, grade 3 or 4: Temporarily discontinue until resolves to ≤ grade 2.

Pulmonary toxicity: Interstitial lung disease or pneumonitis: Permanently discontinue.

Administration Check label to ensure appropriate product is being administered (ado-trastuzumab emtansine and conventional trastuzumab are different products and are **NOT** interchangeable).

Infuse over 90 minutes (first infusion) or over 30 minutes (subsequent infusions if prior infusions were well tolerated) through a 0.22 micron inline nonprotein adsorptive polyethersulfone filter. Do not administer I.V. push or bolus. Do not administer with other medications.

Closely monitor infusion site during administration. Monitor patient during infusion for signs of infusion-related reactions (eg, fever, chills); monitor for at least 90 minutes following initial infusion and (if tolerated) for at least 30 minutes following subsequent infusions.

Hazardous agent; use appropriate precautions for handling and disposal (meets NIOSH, 2012 criteria).

Monitoring Parameters Platelet count (at baseline and prior to each dose), transaminases and bilirubin (at baseline and prior to each dose); pregnancy status; HER2 expression status. Evaluate left ventricular function (prior to and at least every 3 months during treatment; for LVEF <40% or 40% to 45% with ≥10% absolute decrease below baseline value, reassess within 3 weeks). Monitor infusion site during infusion for possible infiltration; monitor for infusion reactions (during infusion and for 90 minutes after initial infusion and for 30 minutes after subsequent infusions); signs and symptoms of neuropathy; pulmonary toxicity

Dosage Forms Excipient information presented when available (limited, particularly for generics); consult specific product labeling.
Solution Reconstituted, Intravenous [preservative free]:
Kadcyla: 100 mg (1 ea); 160 mg (1 ea) [contains mouse protein (murine) (hamster)]

- ◆ **Adoxa** *see* Doxycycline *on page 668*
- ◆ **Adoxa Pak 1/100** *see* Doxycycline *on page 668*
- ◆ **Adoxa Pak 1/150** *see* Doxycycline *on page 668*
- ◆ **Adoxa Pak 2/100** *see* Doxycycline *on page 668*
- ◆ **Adrenaclick** *see* EPINEPHrine (Systemic, Oral Inhalation) *on page 714*
- ◆ **Adrenalin** *see* EPINEPHrine (Systemic, Oral Inhalation) *on page 714*
- ◆ **Adrenaline** *see* EPINEPHrine (Systemic, Oral Inhalation) *on page 714*
- ◆ **ADR (error-prone abbreviation)** *see* DOXOrubicin *on page 661*
- ◆ **Adria** *see* DOXOrubicin *on page 661*
- ◆ **Adriamycin** *see* DOXOrubicin *on page 661*
- ◆ **Adrucil** *see* Fluorouracil (Systemic) *on page 882*
- ◆ **Adsorbent Charcoal** *see* Charcoal, Activated *on page 401*
- ◆ **Advagraf (Can)** *see* Tacrolimus (Systemic) *on page 1976*
- ◆ **Advair® (Can)** *see* Fluticasone and Salmeterol *on page 897*
- ◆ **Advair Diskus®** *see* Fluticasone and Salmeterol *on page 897*
- ◆ **Advair® HFA** *see* Fluticasone and Salmeterol *on page 897*
- ◆ **Advate** *see* Antihemophilic Factor (Recombinant) *on page 144*
- ◆ **Advicor®** *see* Niacin and Lovastatin *on page 1450*
- ◆ **Advil [OTC]** *see* Ibuprofen *on page 1032*
- ◆ **Advil® (Can)** *see* Ibuprofen *on page 1032*
- ◆ **Advil® Children's (Can)** *see* Ibuprofen *on page 1032*
- ◆ **Advil® Cold & Sinus [OTC]** *see* Pseudoephedrine and Ibuprofen *on page 1748*
- ◆ **Advil® Cold & Sinus (Can)** *see* Pseudoephedrine and Ibuprofen *on page 1748*
- ◆ **Advil® Cold & Sinus Daytime (Can)** *see* Pseudoephedrine and Ibuprofen *on page 1748*
- ◆ **Advil Junior Strength [OTC]** *see* Ibuprofen *on page 1032*
- ◆ **Advil Migraine [OTC]** *see* Ibuprofen *on page 1032*
- ◆ **AEGR-733** *see* Lomitapide *on page 1232*
- ◆ **Aerius® (Can)** *see* Desloratadine *on page 575*
- ◆ **Aerius® Kids (Can)** *see* Desloratadine *on page 575*

Afatinib (a FA ti nib)

Brand Names: U.S. Gilotrif
Index Terms Afatinib Dimaleate; BIBW 2992

Pharmacologic Category Antineoplastic Agent, Tyrosine Kinase Inhibitor; Epidermal Growth Factor Receptor (EGFR) Inhibitor

Use Nonsmall cell lung cancer (NSCLC): First-line treatment of metastatic NSCLC in patients with known EGFR exon 19 deletions or exon 21 (L858R) substitution mutations as detected by an approved test; **Note:** First-line treatment in patients with metastatic NSCLC with EGFR mutations other than exon 19 deletion or exon 21 (L858R) substitution has not been evaluated.

Pregnancy Risk Factor D

Pregnancy Considerations Adverse events were observed in animal reproduction studies. Based on its mechanism of action, afatinib is expected to cause fetal harm if used during pregnancy. Women of reproductive potential should use highly-effective contraception during therapy and for at least 2 weeks after treatment has been discontinued.

Breast-Feeding Considerations It is not known if afatinib is excreted into breast milk. Due to the potential for serious adverse reactions in the nursing infant, the manufacturer recommends a decision be made whether to discontinue nursing or to discontinue the drug, taking into account the importance of treatment to the mother.

Contraindications There are no contraindications listed within the manufacturer's labeling.

Warnings/Precautions Hazardous agent – use appropriate precautions for handling and disposal (meets NIOSH, 2012 criteria). Cutaneous reactions (eg, acneiform rash, erythema, and rash) are common; grade 3 reactions (characterized by bullous, blistering, and exfoliating lesions) and palmar-plantar erythrodysesthesia syndrome were also seen in clinical trials. May require therapy interruption and dosage reduction; discontinue if life-threatening cutaneous lesions occur. In clinical trials, diarrhea and stomatitis frequently occurred in patients treated with afatinib; diarrhea was observed in the majority of patients and typically appeared within the first 6 weeks of therapy. Dehydration and renal impairment may occur as a consequence of diarrhea; monitor closely. Patients may require antidiarrheal therapy (eg, loperamide); initiate at the onset of diarrhea and continue until free of loose bowel movements for 12 hours. May necessitate therapy interruption and dosage reduction.

Keratitis was reported rarely in clinical trials; monitor for signs/symptoms of keratitis (eg, acute or worsening eye inflammation, blurred vision, eye pain, lacrimation, light sensitivity, red eye). Interrupt therapy in patients with suspected keratitis and consider discontinuation if diagnosis of ulcerative keratitis is confirmed (permanently discontinue for persistent ulcerative keratitis). Use with caution in patients with a history of keratitis, severe dry eye, ulcerative keratitis, or who wear contact lens (risk factor for keratitis and ulceration). Interstitial lung disease (ILD) or ILD-like reactions occurred in a small percentage of patients treated with afatinib (some fatal). ILD incidence appeared to be higher in Asian as compared to non-Asian patients. Monitor closely for signs/symptoms of ILD (eg, acute respiratory distress syndrome, allergic alveolitis, lung infiltration, pneumonitis). Interrupt therapy for suspected ILD; discontinue therapy with confirmed diagnosis.

Hepatic function test abnormalities (some fatal) were observed in clinical trials. Monitor liver function tests periodically; may require therapy interruption and dosage reduction. Discontinue if severe hepatic impairment occurs during therapy. Closely monitor patients with moderate-to-severe renal impairment, may require dosage adjustments if not tolerated. Potentially significant drug-drug interactions may exist, requiring dose or frequency adjustment, additional monitoring, and/or selection of alternative therapy.

Adverse Reactions

>10%:

- Dermatologic: Acneiform eruption (90%; grade 3: 16%), paronychia (58%; grade 3: 11%), xeroderma (31%), pruritus (21%), cheilitis (12%)
- Endocrine & metabolic: Weight loss (17%; grade 3: 1%), hypokalemia (11%; grades 3/4: 4%)
- Gastrointestinal: Diarrhea (96%; grade 3: 15%), stomatitis (71%; grade 3: 9%), decreased appetite (29%; grade 3: 4%)
- Genitourinary: Cystitis (13%; grade 3: 1%)
- Hepatic: Increased serum transaminases (8% to 11%; grade 3: 2%)
- Ophthalmic: Conjunctivitis (11%)
- Respiratory: Epistaxis (17%), rhinorrhea (11%)
- Miscellaneous: Fever (12%)

1% to 10%:

- Central nervous system: Fatigue (<2%)
- Dermatologic: Palmar-plantar erythrodysesthesia (7%)
- Gastrointestinal: Vomiting (<5%)
- Renal: Renal insufficiency (6%; grade 3: >1%)
- Respiratory: Pneumonitis (>1%; Asian descent: 2%)

<1% (Limited to important or life-threatening): Keratitis, pneumonia, sepsis

Drug Interactions

Metabolism/Transport Effects Substrate of BCRP, P-glycoprotein; **Inhibits** BCRP, P-glycoprotein

Avoid Concomitant Use There are no known interactions where it is recommended to avoid concomitant use.

Increased Effect/Toxicity

Afatinib may increase the levels/effects of: Porfimer; Vitamin K Antagonists

The levels/effects of Afatinib may be increased by: P-glycoprotein/ABCB1 Inhibitors

Decreased Effect

Afatinib may decrease the levels/effects of: Cardiac Glycosides; Vitamin K Antagonists

The levels/effects of Afatinib may be decreased by: P-glycoprotein/ABCB1 Inducers

Ethanol/Nutrition/Herb Interactions

Food: Administration with a high-fat meal decreases C_{max} by 50% and AUC by 39% as compared to the fasted state. Management: Take at least 1 hour before or 2 hours after a meal.

Storage/Stability Store at 25°C (77°F); excursions permitted to 15°C to 30°C (59°F to 86°). Dispense in original bottle; protect from high humidity and light.

Mechanism of Action Highly selective blocker of the ErbB family, including EGFR (ErbB1), HER2 (ErbB2), and HER4 (ErbB4); covalently and irreversibly binds to the intracellular tyrosine kinase domain, resulting in tumor growth inhibition and tumor regression

Pharmacodynamics/Kinetics

Absorption: Decreased with high-fat meals

Protein binding: ~95%

Metabolism: Covalently adducted to proteins and nucleophilic small molecules (minimal enzymatic metabolism) (Wind, 2013)

Bioavailability: Tablets: 92% (as compared to an oral solution)

Half-life elimination: 37 hours

Time to peak: 2-5 hours

Excretion: Feces (85%); urine (4%); primarily as unchanged drug

Dosage Nonsmall cell lung cancer (NSCLC), metastatic, with EGFR exon 19 deletions or exon 21 (L858R) substitution mutations: Adults: Oral: 40 mg once daily until disease progression or unacceptable toxicity

Missed doses: Do not take a missed dose within 12 hours of next dose

Dosage adjustment for concomitant therapy:

P-gp inhibitors: If concomitant therapy is not tolerated, reduce afatinib daily dose by 10 mg. Upon discontinuation of the P-gp inhibitor, resume previous dose as tolerated.

P-gp inducers: Increase afatinib daily dose by 10 mg if on chronic concomitant therapy with a P-gp inducer. Resume previous dose 2 to 3 days after discontinuation of P-gp inducer.

Dosage adjustment for toxicity: Note: Permanently discontinue for intolerability or severe reaction occurring at a dose of 20 mg daily

Cardiovascular: Permanently discontinue for symptomatic left ventricular dysfunction.

Dermatologic: Withhold therapy for prolonged (>7 days) or intolerable Grade 2 or higher cutaneous reactions. Upon improvement to baseline or ≤ Grade 1, resume therapy at 10 mg per day less than previous dose. Discontinue permanently for life-threatening bullous, blistering, or exfoliative skin lesions.

Gastrointestinal: Greater than or equal to Grade 2 diarrhea that persists for ≥2 consecutive days despite antidiarrheal therapy: Interrupt therapy until resolution to ≤ Grade 1, then resume at 10 mg per day less than previous dose.

Ocular: Interrupt therapy for suspected keratitis; consider discontinuation if diagnosis of ulcerative keratitis is confirmed. Permanently discontinue for persistent ulcerative keratitis.

Pulmonary: Interrupt therapy for suspected interstitial lung disease (ILD); permanently discontinue if diagnosis is confirmed.

Other toxicity: Withhold therapy for ≥ Grade 3 adverse reactions. Upon improvement to baseline or ≤ Grade 1, resume therapy at 10 mg per day less than previous dose.

Dosage adjustment for renal impairment:

Pre-existing mild impairment (Cl_{cr} ≥60 mL/minute): No dosage adjustment necessary.

Pre-existing moderate-to-severe impairment (Cl_{cr} <60 mL/minute): No dosage adjustment provided in manufacturer's labeling (has not been studied in patients with severe impairment [Cl_{cr} <30 mL/minute]); closely monitor and adjust dose if necessary.

Renal toxicity during treatment: If ≥ Grade 2 renal toxicity occurs, withhold therapy. Upon improvement to baseline or ≤ Grade 1, resume therapy at 10 mg per day less than previous dose.

Dosage adjustment for hepatic impairment:

Pre-existing mild-to-moderate impairment (Child Pugh class A or B): No dosage adjustment necessary.

Pre-existing severe impairment (Child Pugh class C): No dosage adjustment provided in manufacturer's labeling (has not been studied); closely monitor and adjust dose if necessary.

Hepatotoxicity during treatment: Withhold therapy for ≥ Grade 3 hepatic dysfunction. Upon improvement to baseline or ≤ Grade 1, resume therapy at 10 mg per day less than previous dose. Permanently discontinue for severe afatinib-induced hepatic impairment.

Dietary Considerations Take at least 1 hour before or 2 hours after a meal.

Administration Administer orally at least 1 hour before or 2 hours after a meal. Do not take a missed dose within 12 hours of the next dose. Hazardous agent; use appropriate precautions for handling and disposal (meets NIOSH, 2012 criteria).

Monitoring Parameters Liver and renal function (periodically); monitor for skin toxicity, diarrhea, signs/symptoms of dehydration; monitor for signs/symptoms of interstitial lung disease (eg, acute respiratory distress syndrome, allergic alveolitis, lung infiltration, pneumonitis) and keratitis (eg, acute or worsening eye inflammation, blurred vision, eye pain, lacrimation, light sensitivity, red eye).

Dosage Forms Excipient information presented when available (limited, particularly for generics); consult specific product labeling.

Tablet, Oral:

Gilotrif: 20 mg

Gilotrif: 30 mg, 40 mg [contains fd&c blue #2 (indigotine)]

◆ **Afatinib Dimaleate** *see* Afatinib *on page* 54

◆ **Afeditab CR** *see* NIFEdipine *on page* 1455

◆ **Afinitor** *see* Everolimus *on page* 807

◆ **Afinitor Disperz** *see* Everolimus *on page* 807

◆ **AFirm 1X [OTC]** *see* Vitamin A *on page* 2201

◆ **AFirm 2X [OTC]** *see* Vitamin A *on page* 2201

◆ **AFirm 3X [OTC]** *see* Vitamin A *on page* 2201

Aflibercept (Ophthalmic) (a FLIB er sept)

Brand Names: U.S. Eylea

Index Terms AVE 0005; AVE 005; AVE-0005; VEGF Trap; VEGF Trap-Eye

Pharmacologic Category Ophthalmic Agent; Vascular Endothelial Growth Factor (VEGF) Inhibitor

Use Treatment of neovascular (wet) age-related macular degeneration (AMD); treatment of macular edema following central retinal vein occlusion (CRVO)

Pregnancy Risk Factor C

Pregnancy Considerations Adverse events were observed in animal reproduction studies.

Breast-Feeding Considerations It is not known if aflibercept (ophthalmic) is excreted in breast milk. Breast-feeding is not recommended by the manufacturer.

Contraindications Hypersensitivity to aflibercept or any component of the formulation; current ocular or periocular infection; active intraocular inflammation

Warnings/Precautions Administer injection using proper aseptic technique. Hypersensitivity may present as severe intraocular inflammation; instruct patients to report intraocular inflammation that increases with severity; rare hypersensitivity reactions (including anaphylaxis) have been associated with another VEGF inhibitor, pegaptanib, occurring within several hours of use; monitor closely. Equipment and appropriate personnel should be available for monitoring and treatment of anaphylaxis. Intravitreal injections may be associated with endophthalmitis, retinal detachment, increased intraocular pressure, infections, or thromboembolic events (eg, nonfatal stroke/MI, vascular death); postprocedure monitoring for these adverse effects should be completed.

Adverse Reactions

>10%: Ocular: Conjunctival hemorrhage (12% to 25%), eye pain (9% to 13%)

1% to 10%:

Local: Injection site pain (3%), injection site hemorrhage (1%)

Ocular: Intraocular pressure increased (5% to 8%), cataract (7%), vitreous detachment (6%), vitreous floaters (5% to 6%), conjunctival hyperemia (4% to 5%), corneal erosion (4% to 5%), foreign body sensation (3%), lacrimation increased (3%), retinal pigment epithelium detachment (3%), blurred vision (1% to 2%), retinal pigment epithelium tear (2%), eyelid edema (1%), corneal edema (1%)

Miscellaneous: Aflibercept antibodies (1% to 3%)

<1% (Limited to important or life-threatening): Endophthalmitis, hypersensitivity, intraocular inflammation, retinal detachment, retinal tear, thromboembolic events, traumatic cataract

Drug Interactions

Metabolism/Transport Effects None known.

Avoid Concomitant Use There are no known interactions where it is recommended to avoid concomitant use.

Increased Effect/Toxicity There are no known significant interactions involving an increase in effect.

Decreased Effect There are no known significant interactions involving a decrease in effect.

Storage/Stability Store at 2°C to 8°C (36°F to 46°F); do not freeze. Store in original container prior to use; protect from light.

Mechanism of Action Aflibercept is a recombinant fusion protein that acts as a decoy receptor for vascular endothelial growth factor-A (VEGF-A) and placental growth factor (PlGF). Decoy receptor binding prevents VEGF-A and PlGF from binding and activating endothelial cell receptors, thereby suppressing neovascularization and slowing vision loss.

Pharmacodynamics/Kinetics

Absorption: Low levels are detected in the serum following intravitreal injection

Half-life elimination: Plasma: 5-6 days

Dosage Intravitreal: Adults:

Age-related macular degeneration (AMD): 2 mg (0.05 mL) every 4 weeks for 3 months, then every 8 weeks thereafter

Macular edema following central retinal vein occlusion (CRVO): 2 mg (0.05 mL) every 4 weeks

Dosage adjustment in renal impairment: No dosage adjustment necessary

Dosage adjustment in hepatic impairment: No dosage adjustment provided in manufacturer's labeling (has not been studied); however, no adjustment expected due to minimal systemic absorption

Administration For ophthalmic intravitreal injection only. Remove contents from vial using a 5 micron, 19-gauge 1 1/2 inch filter needle (supplied) attached to a 1 mL syringe (supplied). Discard filter needle and replace with a sterile 30 gauge 1/2 inch needle (supplied) for intravitreal injection procedure (do not use filter needle for intravitreal injection). Depress plunger to expel excess air and medication (plunger tip should align with the 0.05 mL marking on syringe). Adequate anesthesia and a topical broad-spectrum antimicrobial agent should be administered prior to the procedure.

Monitoring Parameters Intraocular pressure immediately following injection; signs of infection/inflammation (for first week following injection); retinal perfusion; endophthalmitis; visual acuity

Dosage Forms Excipient information presented when available (limited, particularly for generics); consult specific product labeling.

Solution, Intraocular [preservative free]:

Eylea: 2 mg/0.05 mL (0.05 mL) [contains mouse protein (murine) (hamster)]

◆ **Aflibercept I.V.** *see* Ziv-Aflibercept (Systemic) *on page 2233*

◆ **Afluria** *see* Influenza Virus Vaccine (Inactivated) *on page 1078*

◆ **Afluria Preservative Free** *see* Influenza Virus Vaccine (Inactivated) *on page 1078*

◆ **Afrin Saline Nasal Mist [OTC]** *see* Sodium Chloride *on page 1914*

◆ **AG-013736** *see* Axitinib *on page 204*

Agalsidase Beta (aye GAL si days BAY ta)

Brand Names: U.S. Fabrazyme

Brand Names: Canada Fabrazyme®

Index Terms Alpha-Galactosidase-A (Recombinant); r-h α-GAL

Pharmacologic Category Enzyme

Use Replacement therapy for Fabry disease

Pregnancy Risk Factor B

Dosage I.V.: Children ≥8 years and Adults: 1 mg/kg every 2 weeks

Dosage adjustment in toxicity: Patient with IgE antibodies to agalsidase beta (rechallenge): 0.5 mg/kg every 2 weeks at an initial maximum infusion rate of 0.01 mg/minute; may gradually escalate dose (to maximum of 1 mg/kg every 2 weeks) and/or infusion rate (doubling the infusion rate every 30 minutes to a maximum rate of 0.25 mg/minute) as tolerated.

Dosage adjustment in renal impairment: No dosage adjustment required.

Dosage adjustment in hepatic impairment: No dosage adjustment provided in manufacturer's labeling.

Additional Information Complete prescribing information should be consulted for additional detail.

Dosage Forms Excipient information presented when available (limited, particularly for generics); consult specific product labeling.

Solution Reconstituted, Intravenous:

Fabrazyme: 5 mg (1 ea); 35 mg (1 ea) [contains mouse protein (murine) (hamster)]

◆ **Aggrastat** *see* Tirofiban *on page 2072*

◆ **Aggrenox®** *see* Aspirin and Dipyridamole *on page 182*

◆ **AGN 1135** *see* Rasagiline *on page 1786*

◆ **$AgNO_3$** *see* Silver Nitrate *on page 1896*

◆ **Agriflu (Can)** *see* Influenza Virus Vaccine (Inactivated) *on page 1078*

◆ **Agrylin** *see* Anagrelide *on page 136*

◆ **AHF (Human)** *see* Antihemophilic Factor (Human) *on page 143*

◆ **AHF (Human)** *see* Antihemophilic Factor/von Willebrand Factor Complex (Human) *on page 146*

◆ **AHF (Recombinant)** *see* Antihemophilic Factor (Recombinant) *on page 144*

◆ **Ahi-Temozolomide Capsules (Can)** *see* Temozolomide *on page 2005*

◆ **A-hydroCort** *see* Hydrocortisone (Systemic) *on page 1008*

◆ **A-Hydrocort** *see* Hydrocortisone (Systemic) *on page 1008*

◆ **A-hydroCort** *see* Hydrocortisone (Topical) *on page 1011*

◆ **AICC** *see* Anti-inhibitor Coagulant Complex (Human) *on page 147*

◆ **AIDS222089** *see* Bedaquiline *on page 229*

◆ **Airomir™ (Can)** *see* Albuterol *on page 61*

◆ **AJ-Cisplatin (Can)** *see* CISplatin *on page 437*

◆ **AJ-PIP/TAZ (Can)** *see* Piperacillin and Tazobactam *on page 1653*

◆ **AK Cide Oph (Can)** *see* Sulfacetamide and Prednisolone *on page 1957*

◆ **AK-Fluor** *see* Fluorescein *on page 880*

◆ **Akne-Mycin** *see* Erythromycin (Topical) *on page 744*

◆ **AK Pentolate Oph Soln (Can)** *see* Cyclopentolate *on page 504*

◆ **AK-Poly-Bac™** *see* Bacitracin and Polymyxin B *on page 220*

◆ **AK Sulf Liq (Can)** *see* Sulfacetamide (Ophthalmic) *on page 1956*

◆ **ALA** *see* Aminolevulinic Acid *on page 100*

◆ **5-ALA** *see* Aminolevulinic Acid *on page 100*

◆ **Ala Cort** *see* Hydrocortisone (Topical) *on page 1011*

◆ **Alagesic LQ** *see* Butalbital, Acetaminophen, and Caffeine *on page 305*

◆ **Alamag [OTC]** *see* Aluminum Hydroxide and Magnesium Hydroxide *on page 90*

◆ **Alamag Plus [OTC]** *see* Aluminum Hydroxide, Magnesium Hydroxide, and Simethicone *on page 90*

◆ **Ala Scalp** *see* Hydrocortisone (Topical) *on page 1011*

◆ **Alavert [OTC]** *see* Loratadine *on page 1240*

◆ **Alavert™ Allergy and Sinus [OTC]** *see* Loratadine and Pseudoephedrine *on page 1242*

◆ **Alaway [OTC]** *see* Ketotifen (Ophthalmic) *on page 1156*

◆ **Alaway Childrens Allergy [OTC]** *see* Ketotifen (Ophthalmic) *on page 1156*

Albendazole (al BEN da zole)

Brand Names: U.S. Albenza

Pharmacologic Category Anthelmintic

Use Treatment of parenchymal neurocysticercosis caused by *Taenia solium* and cystic hydatid disease of the liver, lung, and peritoneum caused by *Echinococcus granulosus*

Unlabeled Use Albendazole has activity against *Ascaris lumbricoides* (roundworm); *Ancylostoma caninum*; *Ancylostoma duodenale* and *Necator americanus* (hookworms); cutaneous larva migrans; *Enterobius vermicularis* (pinworm); *Giardia duodenalis* (giardiasis); *Gnathostoma spinigerum*; *Gongylonema* sp; *Mansonella perstans* (filariasis); *Oesophagostomum bifurcum*; *Opisthorchis sinensis* (liver fluke); *Trichinella spiralis* (Trichinellosis); visceral larva migrans (toxocariasis); activity has also been shown against the liver fluke *Clonorchis sinensis*, *Giardia lamblia*, *Cysticercus cellulosae*, and *Echinococcus multilocularis*. Albendazole has also been used for the treatment of intestinal microsporidiosis (*Encephalitozoon intestinalis*), disseminated microsporidiosis (*E. hellem*, *E. cuniculi*, *E. intestinalis*, *Pleistophora* sp, *Trachipleistophora* sp, *Brachiola vesicularum*), and ocular microsporidiosis (*E. hellem*, *E. cuniculi*, *Vittaforma corneae*).

Pregnancy Risk Factor C

Pregnancy Considerations Adverse events were observed in animal reproduction studies. Albendazole should not be used during pregnancy, if at all possible. The manufacturer recommends a pregnancy test prior to therapy in women of reproductive potential. Women should be advised to avoid pregnancy for at least 1 month following therapy. Discontinue if pregnancy occurs during treatment.

Breast-Feeding Considerations Albendazole excretion into breast milk was studied following a single oral 400 mg dose in breast-feeding women 2 weeks to 6 months postpartum (n=33). Mean albendazole concentrations 6 hours after the dose were 63.7 ± 11.9 ng/mL (maternal serum) and 31.9 ± 9.2 ng/mL (milk). An active and inactive metabolite was also detected in breast milk (Abdel-tawab, 2009). The manufacturer recommends that caution be exercised when administering albendazole to nursing women.

Contraindications Hypersensitivity to albendazole, benzimidazoles, or any component of the formulation

Warnings/Precautions Reversible elevations in hepatic enzymes have been reported; patients with abnormal LFTs and hepatic echinococcosis are at an increased risk of hepatotoxicity. Discontinue therapy if LFT elevations are >2 times the upper limit of normal; may consider restarting treatment with frequent monitoring of LFTs when hepatic enzymes return to pretreatment values. Agranulocytosis, aplastic anemia, granulocytopenia, leukopenia, and pancytopenia have occurred leading to fatalities (rare); use with caution in patients with hepatic impairment (more susceptible to hematologic toxicity). Discontinue therapy in all patients who develop clinically significant decreases in blood cell counts.

Neurocysticercosis: Corticosteroids (eg, dexamethasone or prednisolone) should be administered before or upon initiation of albendazole therapy to minimize inflammatory reactions and prevent cerebral hypertension. Anticonvulsant therapy should be used concurrently during the first week of therapy to prevent seizures. These measures are important to minimize neurological symptoms which may result from uncovering of pre-existing neurocysticercosis when using albendazole to treat other conditions. If retinal lesions exist, weigh risk of further retinal damage due to albendazole-induced changes to the retinal lesion vs benefit of disease treatment.

Adverse Reactions

>10%:

Central nervous system: Headache (11% neurocysticercosis; 1% hydatid)

Hepatic: LFTs increased (16% hydatid; <1% neurocysticercosis)

1% to 10%:

Central nervous system: Intracranial pressure increased (≤2%), dizziness (≤1%), fever (≤1%), vertigo (≤1%), meningeal signs (1%)

Dermatologic: Alopecia (<1% to 2%)

Gastrointestinal: Abdominal pain (≤6%), nausea/vomiting (4% to 6%)

<1% (Limited to important or life-threatening symptoms): Acute liver failure, acute renal failure, aplastic anemia, agranulocytosis, erythema multiforme, granulocytopenia, hepatitis, hypersensitivity reaction, leukopenia, neutropenia, pancytopenia, rash, Stevens-Johnson syndrome, thrombocytopenia, urticaria

Drug Interactions

Metabolism/Transport Effects Substrate of CYP1A2 (minor), CYP3A4 (minor); **Note:** Assignment of Major/Minor substrate status based on clinically relevant drug interaction potential

Avoid Concomitant Use There are no known interactions where it is recommended to avoid concomitant use.

Increased Effect/Toxicity

The levels/effects of Albendazole may be increased by: Grapefruit Juice

Decreased Effect

The levels/effects of Albendazole may be decreased by: Aminoquinolines (Antimalarial)

Ethanol/Nutrition/Herb Interactions Food: Albendazole serum levels may be increased if taken with a fatty meal (increases the oral bioavailability by up to 5 times). Management: Should be administered with a high-fat meal (peanuts or ice cream).

Storage/Stability Store between 20°C and 25°C (68°F to 77°F)

Mechanism of Action Active metabolite, albendazole sulfoxide, causes selective degeneration of cytoplasmic microtubules in intestinal and tegmental cells of intestinal helminths and larvae; glycogen is depleted, glucose uptake and cholinesterase secretion are impaired, and desecratory substances accumulate intracellulary. ATP production decreases causing energy depletion, immobilization, and worm death.

Pharmacodynamics/Kinetics

Absorption: Poor; may increase up to 5 times when administered with a fatty meal

Distribution: Well inside hydatid cysts and CSF

Protein binding: 70%

Metabolism: Hepatic; extensive first-pass effect; pathways include rapid sulfoxidation to active metabolite (albendazole sulfoxide [major]), hydrolysis, and oxidation

Half-life elimination: 8-12 hours

Time to peak, serum: 2-5 hours

Excretion: Urine (<1% as active metabolite); feces

Dosage Oral:

Infants and Children: Microsporidiosis (other than *Enterocytozoon bienuesi* or *V. corneae*), disseminated or intestinal infection (HIV-positive, unlabeled use): 15 mg/kg/day (maximum: 800 mg/day) in 2 divided doses continued until immune reconstitution after HAART initiation (CDC, 2009)

Children:

Cysticercus cellulosae (unlabeled use): 15 mg/kg/day (maximum: 800 mg/day) in 2 divided doses for 8-30 days; may be repeated as necessary

Echinococcus granulosus (tapeworm) (unlabeled use): 15 mg/kg/day (maximum: 800 mg) divided twice daily for 1-6 months

Giardia duodenalis (giardiasis) (unlabeled use): 10 mg/kg/day for 5 days (Yereli, 2004)

Children and Adults:

Neurocysticercosis:

<60 kg: 15 mg/kg/day in 2 divided doses (maximum: 800 mg/day) for 8-30 days

≥60 kg: 800 mg/day in 2 divided doses for 8-30 days

Note: Give concurrent anticonvulsant and corticosteroid (eg, dexamethasone or prednisolone) therapy during first week.

Hydatid:

<60 kg: 15 mg/kg/day in 2 divided doses (maximum: 800 mg/day)

≥60 kg: 800 mg/day in 2 divided doses

Note: Administer dose for three 28-day cycles with a 14-day drug-free interval in between each cycle.

Ancylostoma caninum, *Ascaris lumbricoides* (roundworm), *Ancylostoma duodenale* (hookworm), and *Necator americanus* (hookworm) (unlabeled use): 400 mg as a single dose

Clonorchis sinensis (Chinese liver fluke) (unlabeled use): 10 mg/kg/day for 7 days

Cutaneous larva migrans (unlabeled use): 400 mg once daily for 3 days

Enterobius vermicularis (pinworm) (unlabeled use): 400 mg as a single dose; repeat in 2 weeks

Gnathostoma spinigerum (unlabeled use): 800 mg/day in 2 divided doses for 21 days

Gongylonemiasis (unlabeled use): 400 mg once daily for 3 days

Mansonella perstans (unlabeled use): 800 mg/day in 2 divided doses for 10 days

Oesophagostomum bifurcum (unlabeled use): 400 mg as a single dose (Ziem, 2004)

Trichinella spiralis (Trichinellosis) (unlabeled use): 800 mg/day in 2 divided doses for 8-14 days plus corticosteroids for severe symptoms

Visceral larva migrans (toxocariasis) (unlabeled use): 800 mg/day in 2 divided doses for 5 days

Adults:

Cysticercus cellulosae (unlabeled use): 800 mg/day in 2 divided doses for 8-30 days; may be repeated as necessary

Disseminated microsporidiosis (unlabeled use): 800 mg/day in 2 divided doses

Echinococcus granulosus (tapeworm) (unlabeled use): 800 mg/day in 2 divided doses for 1-6 months

Giardia duodenalis (giardiasis) (unlabeled use): 400 mg once daily for 5 days

Intestinal microsporidiosis (*E. intestinalis*) (unlabeled use): 800 mg/day in 2 divided doses for 21 days

Ocular microsporidiosis (unlabeled use): 800 mg/day in 2 divided doses, in combination with fumagillin

Dosage adjustment in renal impairment: No dosage adjustment provided in the manufacturer's labeling (has not been studied). However, the need for adjustment not likely since albendazole is primarily eliminated by hepatic metabolism.

Dosage adjustment in hepatic impairment: No dosage adjustment provided in manufacturer's labeling. However, patients with underlying liver disease may be more at risk for adverse effects.

Dietary Considerations Should be taken with a high-fat meal.

Administration Should be administered with a high-fat meal. Administer anticonvulsant and corticosteroid therapy during first week of neurocysticercosis therapy. If patients have difficulty swallowing, tablets may be crushed or chewed, then swallowed with a drink of water.

Monitoring Parameters Monitor fecal specimens for ova and parasites for 3 weeks after treatment; if positive, retreat; LFTs and CBC with differential at start of each 28-day cycle and every 2 weeks during therapy (more frequent monitoring for patients with liver disease); ophthalmic exam (patients with neurocysticercosis); pregnancy test

Dosage Forms Excipient information presented when available (limited, particularly for generics); consult specific product labeling.

Tablet, Oral:

Albenza: 200 mg [contains saccharin sodium]

◆ **Albenza** *see* Albendazole *on page 58*

◆ **Albuked 5** *see* Albumin *on page 59*

◆ **Albuked 25** *see* Albumin *on page 59*

Albumin (al BYOO min)

Brand Names: U.S. Albuked 25; Albuked 5; Albumin-ZLB; Albuminar-25; Albuminar-5; AlbuRx; Albutein; Buminate; Flexbumin; Human Albumin Grifols; Kedbumin; Plasbumin-25; Plasbumin-5

Brand Names: Canada Alburex® 25; Alburex® 5; Albutein 25%; Albutein 5%; Buminate-25%; Buminate-5%; Plasbumin®-25; Plasbumin®-5

Index Terms Albumin (Human); Normal Human Serum Albumin; Normal Serum Albumin (Human); Salt Poor Albumin; SPA

Pharmacologic Category Blood Product Derivative; Plasma Volume Expander, Colloid

Use Plasma volume expansion and maintenance of cardiac output in the treatment of certain types of shock or impending shock; may be useful for burn patients, ARDS, and cardiopulmonary bypass; other uses considered by some investigators (but not proven) are retroperitoneal surgery, peritonitis, and ascites; unless the condition responsible for hypoproteinemia can be corrected, albumin can provide only symptomatic relief or supportive treatment

Note: Nutritional supplementation is not an appropriate indication.

Unlabeled Use In patients with cirrhosis, administered with diuretics to help facilitate diuresis; large volume paracentesis; volume expansion in dehydrated, mildly hypotensive patients with cirrhosis; to prevent renal impairment and reduce mortality associated with spontaneous bacterial peritonitis (SBP) in patients with cirrhosis

Pregnancy Risk Factor C

Pregnancy Considerations Animal reproduction studies have not been conducted. Albumin is used for the treatment of ovarian hyperstimulation syndrome (ASRM, 2008). Use for other indications may be considered in pregnant women when contraindications to nonprotein colloids exist (Liumbruno, 2009).

Breast-Feeding Considerations Endogenous albumin is found in breast milk.

Contraindications Hypersensitivity to albumin or any component of the formulation; patients with severe anemia or cardiac failure

Warnings/Precautions Use with caution in patients with hepatic or renal failure because of added protein load; rapid infusion of albumin solutions may cause vascular overload. All patients should be observed for signs of hypervolemia such as pulmonary edema. Use with caution in those patients for whom sodium restriction is necessary. Avoid 25% concentration in preterm infants due to risk of intraventricular hemorrhage. Packaging may contain natural latex rubber.

Adverse Reactions Frequency not defined.

Cardiovascular: Congestive heart failure (precipitation), edema, hypertension, hypotension, tachycardia

Central nervous system: Chills, headache

Dermatologic: Pruritus, skin rash, urticaria

Endocrine & metabolic: Hypervolemia

Gastrointestinal: Nausea, vomiting

Hypersensitivity: Anaphylaxis

Respiratory: Bronchospasm, pulmonary edema

Miscellaneous: Fever

Drug Interactions

Metabolism/Transport Effects None known.

Avoid Concomitant Use There are no known interactions where it is recommended to avoid concomitant use.

Increased Effect/Toxicity There are no known significant interactions involving an increase in effect.

Decreased Effect There are no known significant interactions involving a decrease in effect.

Preparation for Administration If 5% human albumin is unavailable, it may be prepared by diluting 25% human albumin with 0.9% sodium chloride or 5% dextrose in water. Do not use sterile water to dilute albumin solutions, as this has been associated with hypotonic-associated hemolysis.

Storage/Stability Store at a temperature ≤30°C (86°F); do not freeze. Do not use solution if it is turbid or contains a deposit; use within 4 hours after opening vial; discard unused portion.

Mechanism of Action Provides increase in intravascular oncotic pressure and causes mobilization of fluids from interstitial into intravascular space

Dosage I.V.:

5% should be used in hypovolemic patients or intravascularly-depleted patients

25% should be used in patients in whom fluid and sodium intake must be minimized

Dose depends on condition of patient:

Children: Hypovolemia: 0.5-1 g/kg/dose (10-20 mL/kg/dose of albumin 5%); maximum dose: 6 g/kg/day

Adults: Usual dose: 25 g; initial dose may be repeated in 15-30 minutes if response is inadequate; no more than 250 g should be administered within 48 hours

Hypovolemia: 5% albumin: 0.5-1 g/kg/dose; repeat as needed. **Note:** May be considered after inadequate response to crystalloid therapy and when nonprotein colloids are contraindicated. The volume administered and the speed of infusion should be adapted to individual response.

Large-volume paracentesis (>5 L) (unlabeled use): 25% albumin: 5-8 g for every liter removed (Garcia-Compeán, 1993; Moore, 2003) **or** 50 g total for paracentesis >5 L (ATS, 2004). **Note:** Administer soon after the procedure to avoid postprocedural complications (eg, hypovolemia, hyponatremia, renal impairment) (Moore, 2003).

SBP in patients with cirrhosis (unlabeled use): 25% albumin: Initial: 1.5 g/kg, followed by 1 g/kg on day 3 (in conjunction with appropriate antimicrobial therapy) (ATS, 2004; Sort, 1999). **Note:** Clinical trial employed albumin 20%; however, the difference in concentration compared with 25% albumin is deemed to be clinically inconsequential.

Dosage adjustment in renal impairment: No dosage adjustment provided in manufacturer's labeling; use with caution.

Dosage adjustment in hepatic impairment: No dosage adjustment provided in manufacturer's labeling.

Dietary Considerations Some products may contain potassium and/or sodium.

Administration For I.V. administration only. Use within 4 hours after opening vial; discard unused portion. In emergencies, may administer as rapidly as necessary to improve clinical condition. After initial volume replacement:

5%: Do not exceed 2-4 mL/minute in patients with normal plasma volume; 5-10 mL/minute in patients with hypoproteinemia

25%: Do not exceed 1 mL/minute in patients with normal plasma volume; 2-3 mL/minute in patients with hypoproteinemia

Rapid infusion may cause vascular overload. Albumin 25% may be given undiluted or diluted in normal saline. May give in combination or through the same administration set as saline or carbohydrates. Do not use with ethanol or protein hydrolysates, precipitation may form.

Monitoring Parameters Blood pressure, pulmonary edema, hematocrit

Additional Information Albumin 5% and 25% solutions contain 130-160 mEq/L sodium and are considered isotonic with plasma. Dilution of albumin 25% solution with sterile water produces a hypotonic solution; administration of such can cause hemolysis and/or renal failure. An albumin 5% solution is osmotically equivalent to an equal volume of plasma, whereas a 25% solution is osmotically equivalent to 5 times its volume of plasma. Albumin solutions are heated to 60°C for 10 hours, decreasing any possible risk of viral hepatitis transmission. To date, there have been no reports of viral transmission using these products.

Dosage Forms Excipient information presented when available (limited, particularly for generics); consult specific product labeling.

Solution, Intravenous:

Albumin-ZLB: 5% (250 mL, 500 mL); 25% (50 mL, 100 mL)

Albuminar-5: 5% (250 mL, 500 mL)

Albuminar-25: 25% (50 mL, 100 mL)

AlbuRx: 5% (250 mL, 500 mL)

Albutein: 25% (50 mL, 100 mL)

Buminate: 5% (250 mL, 500 mL); 25% (20 mL)

Human Albumin Grifols: 25% (50 mL, 100 mL)

Plasbumin-5: 5% (50 mL, 250 mL)

Plasbumin-25: 25% (20 mL, 50 mL, 100 mL)

Generic: 5% (50 mL); 25% (50 mL, 100 mL)

Solution, Intravenous [preservative free]:

Albuked 5: 5% (250 mL)

Albuked 25: 25% (50 mL, 100 mL)

Albutein: 5% (250 mL, 500 mL); 25% (50 mL, 100 mL)

Flexbumin: 25% (50 mL, 100 mL)

Kedbumin: 25% (50 mL, 100 mL)

Plasbumin-5: 5% (50 mL, 250 mL)

Plasbumin-25: 25% (20 mL, 50 mL, 100 mL)

Generic: 5% (100 mL, 250 mL, 500 mL); 25% (50 mL, 100 mL)

◆ **Albuminar-5** *see* Albumin *on page 59*

◆ **Albuminar-25** *see* Albumin *on page 59*

◆ **Albumin-Bound Paclitaxel** *see* PACLitaxel (Protein Bound) *on page 1546*

◆ **Albumin (Human)** *see* Albumin *on page 59*

◆ **Albumin-Stabilized Nanoparticle Paclitaxel** *see* PACLitaxel (Protein Bound) *on page 1546*

◆ **Albumin-ZLB** *see* Albumin *on page 59*

◆ **Alburex® 5 (Can)** *see* Albumin *on page 59*

- ◆ **Alburex® 25 (Can)** *see* Albumin *on page* 59
- ◆ **AlbuRx** *see* Albumin *on page* 59
- ◆ **Albutein** *see* Albumin *on page* 59
- ◆ **Albutein 5% (Can)** *see* Albumin *on page* 59
- ◆ **Albutein 25% (Can)** *see* Albumin *on page* 59

Albuterol (al BYOO ter ole)

Brand Names: U.S. AccuNeb; ProAir HFA; Proventil HFA; Ventolin HFA; VoSpire ER

Brand Names: Canada Airomir™; Apo-Salvent®; Apo-Salvent® AEM; Apo-Salvent® CFC Free; Apo-Salvent® Sterules; Dom-Salbutamol; Mylan-Salbutamol Respirator Solution; Mylan-Salbutamol Sterinebs P.F.; Novo-Salbutamol HFA; Nu-Salbutamol; PHL-Salbutamol; PMS-Salbutamol; ratio-Ipra-Sal; ratio-Salbutamol; Sandoz-Salbutamol; Teva-Salbutamol; Teva-Salbutamol Sterinebs P.F.; Ventolin®; Ventolin® Diskus; Ventolin® HFA; Ventolin® I.V. Infusion; Ventolin® Nebules P.F.

Index Terms Albuterol Sulfate; Salbutamol; Salbutamol Sulphate

Pharmacologic Category $Beta_2$ Agonist

Use Treatment or prevention of bronchospasm in patients with reversible obstructive airway disease; prevention of exercise-induced bronchospasm

Pregnancy Risk Factor C

Pregnancy Considerations Adverse events were observed in some animal reproduction studies. Albuterol crosses the placenta (Boulton, 1997). Congenital anomalies (cleft palate, limb defects) have rarely been reported following maternal use during pregnancy. Multiple medications were used in most cases, no specific pattern of defects has been reported, and no relationship to albuterol has been established. The amount of albuterol available systemically following inhalation is significantly less in comparison to oral doses.

Uncontrolled asthma is associated with adverse events on pregnancy (increased risk of perinatal mortality, preeclampsia, preterm birth, low birth weight infants). Albuterol is the preferred short acting beta agonist when treatment for asthma is needed during pregnancy (NAEPP, 2005; NAEPP, 2007).

Albuterol may affect uterine contractility. Maternal pulmonary edema and other adverse events have been reported when albuterol was used for tocolysis. Albuterol is not approved for use as a tocolytic; use caution when needed to treat bronchospasm in pregnant women. Use of the injection (Canadian product; not available in the U.S.) is specifically contraindicated in women during the first or second trimester who may be at risk of threatened abortion.

Breast-Feeding Considerations It is not known if albuterol is excreted into breast milk. The amount of albuterol available systemically following inhalation is significantly less in comparison to oral doses. According to the manufacturer, the decision to continue or discontinue breast-feeding during therapy should take into account the risk of exposure to the infant and the benefits of treatment to the mother. The use of beta-2-receptor agonists are not considered a contraindication to breast feeding (NAEPP, 2005).

Contraindications Hypersensitivity to albuterol or any component of the formulation

Injection formulation (Canadian labeling; product not available in U.S.): Hypersensitivity to albuterol or any component of the formulation; tachyarrhythmias; risk of abortion during first or second trimester

Warnings/Precautions Optimize anti-inflammatory treatment before initiating maintenance treatment with albuterol. Do not use as a component of chronic therapy without an anti-inflammatory agent. Only the mildest forms of asthma (Step 1 and/or exercise-induced) would not require concurrent use based upon asthma guidelines. Patient must be instructed to seek medical attention in cases where acute symptoms are not relieved or a previous level of response is diminished. The need to increase frequency of use may indicate deterioration of asthma, and treatment must not be delayed.

Use caution in patients with cardiovascular disease (arrhythmia or hypertension or HF), convulsive disorders, diabetes, glaucoma, hyperthyroidism, or hypokalemia. Beta-agonists may cause elevation in blood pressure, heart rate, and result in CNS stimulation/excitation. $Beta_2$-agonists may increase risk of arrhythmia, increase serum glucose, or decrease serum potassium.

Immediate hypersensitivity reactions (urticaria, angioedema, rash, bronchospasm) have been reported. Do not exceed recommended dose; serious adverse events, including fatalities, have been associated with excessive use of inhaled sympathomimetics. Rarely, paradoxical bronchospasm may occur with use of inhaled bronchodilating agents; this should be distinguished from inadequate response. All patients should utilize a spacer device or valved holding chamber when using a metered-dose inhaler; in addition, face masks should be used in children <4 years of age.

Adverse Reactions Incidence of adverse effects is dependent upon age of patient, dose, and route of administration.

Cardiovascular: Angina pectoris, atrial fibrillation, cardiac arrhythmia, chest discomfort, chest pain, extrasystoles, flushing, hypertension, hypotension, palpitations, supraventricular tachycardia, tachycardia

Central nervous system: Central nervous system stimulation, dizziness, drowsiness, headache, insomnia, irritability, migraine, nervousness, nightmares, restlessness, seizure, vertigo

Dermatologic: Diaphoresis, skin rash, urticaria

Endocrine & metabolic: Hyperglycemia, hypokalemia, lactic acidosis

Gastrointestinal: Diarrhea, dysgeusia, dyspepsia, gastroenteritis, nausea, vomiting, xerostomia

Genitourinary: Difficulty in micturition

Hematologic & oncologic: Lymphadenopathy

Hypersensitivity: Anaphylaxis, angioedema, hypersensitivity reaction

Local: Pain at injection site

Neuromuscular & skeletal: Muscle cramps, musculoskeletal pain, tremor, weakness

Otic: Otitis media

Respiratory: Bronchospasm, cough, epistaxis, exacerbation of asthma, laryngitis, oropharyngeal edema, oropharyngeal irritation, pharyngitis, rhinitis, upper respiratory tract inflammation, viral upper respiratory tract infection

<1% (Limited to important or life-threatening): Glossitis, hoarseness, ischemic heart disease, metabolic acidosis, pulmonary edema, throat irritation, tongue ulcer

Drug Interactions

Metabolism/Transport Effects None known.

Avoid Concomitant Use

Avoid concomitant use of Albuterol with any of the following: Beta-Blockers (Nonselective); Iobenguane I 123

Increased Effect/Toxicity

Albuterol may increase the levels/effects of: Atosiban; Loop Diuretics; Sympathomimetics; Thiazide Diuretics

The levels/effects of Albuterol may be increased by: AtoMOXetine; Cannabinoids; MAO Inhibitors; Tricyclic Antidepressants

Decreased Effect

Albuterol may decrease the levels/effects of: Iobenguane I 123

The levels/effects of Albuterol may be decreased by: Beta-Blockers (Beta1 Selective); Beta-Blockers (Nonselective); Betahistine

Ethanol/Nutrition/Herb Interactions

Food: Avoid or limit caffeine (may cause CNS stimulation).

Herb/Nutraceutical: Avoid ephedra, yohimbe (may cause CNS stimulation). Avoid St John's wort (may decrease the levels/effects of albuterol).

Preparation for Administration Solution for nebulization: To prepare a 2.5 mg dose, dilute 0.5 mL of solution to a total of 3 mL with normal saline; also compatible with cromolyn or ipratropium nebulizer solutions.

Storage/Stability

HFA aerosols: Store at 15°C to 25°C (59°F to 77°F).

Ventolin® HFA: Discard when counter reads 000 or 12 months after removal from protective pouch, whichever comes first. Store with mouthpiece down.

Infusion solution (Canadian labeling; product not available in U.S.): Ventolin® I.V.: Store at 15°C to 30°C (59°F to 86°F). Protect from light. After dilution, discard unused portion after 24 hours.

Solution for nebulization (0.5%): Store at 2°C to 25°C (36°F to 77°F).

AccuNeb®: Store at 2°C to 25°C (36°F to 77°F). Do not use if solution changes color or becomes cloudy. Use within 1 week of opening foil pouch.

Syrup: Store at 20°C to 25°C (68°F to 77°F).

Tablet: Store at 20°C to 25°C (68°F to 77°F).

Tablet, extended release: Store at 20°C to 25°C (68°F to 77°F)

Mechanism of Action Relaxes bronchial smooth muscle by action on beta$_2$-receptors with little effect on heart rate

Pharmacodynamics/Kinetics

Onset of action: Peak effect:

Nebulization/oral inhalation: 0.5-2 hours

CFC-propelled albuterol: 10 minutes

Ventolin® HFA: 25 minutes

Oral: 2-3 hours

Duration: Nebulization/oral inhalation: 3-4 hours; Oral: 4-6 hours

Metabolism: Hepatic to an inactive sulfate

Half-life elimination: Inhalation: 3.8 hours; Oral: 3.7-5 hours

Excretion: Urine (30% as unchanged drug)

Dosage

Oral:

Children: Bronchospasm:

2-6 years: 0.1-0.2 mg/kg/dose 3 times/day; maximum dose not to exceed 12 mg/day (divided doses)

6-12 years: 2 mg/dose 3-4 times/day; maximum dose not to exceed 24 mg/day (divided doses)

Extended release: 4 mg every 12 hours; maximum dose not to exceed 24 mg/day (divided doses)

Children >12 years and Adults: Bronchospasm (treatment): 2-4 mg/dose 3-4 times/day; maximum dose not to exceed 32 mg/day (divided doses)

Extended release: 8 mg every 12 hours; maximum dose not to exceed 32 mg/day (divided doses). A 4 mg dose every 12 hours may be sufficient in some patients, such as adults of low body weight.

Elderly: Bronchospasm (treatment): 2 mg 3-4 times/day; maximum: 8 mg 4 times/day

Metered-dose inhaler (90 mcg/puff):

Children ≤4 years *(NIH Guidelines, 2007)*:

Quick relief: 2 puffs every 4-6 hours as needed

Exacerbation of asthma (acute, severe): 4-8 puffs every 20 minutes for 3 doses, then every 1-4 hours as needed

Exercise-induced bronchospasm (prevention): 1-2 puffs 5 minutes prior to exercise

Children 5-11 years *(NIH Guidelines, 2007)*:

Bronchospasm, quick relief: 2 puffs every 4-6 hours as needed

Exacerbation of asthma (acute, severe): 4-8 puffs every 20 minutes for 3 doses, then every 1-4 hours as needed

Exercise-induced bronchospasm (prevention): 2 puffs 5-30 minutes prior to exercise

Children ≥12 years and Adults:

Bronchospasm, quick relief *(NIH Guidelines, 2007)*: 2 puffs every 4-6 hours as needed

Exacerbation of asthma (acute, severe) *(NIH Guidelines, 2007)*: 4-8 puffs every 20 minutes for up to 4 hours, then every 1-4 hours as needed

Exercise-induced bronchospasm (prevention) *(NIH Guidelines, 2007)*: 2 puffs 5-30 minutes prior to exercise

Metered-dose inhaler (100 mcg/puff): Airomir™ (Canadian availability):

Children 6-11 years:

Bronchospasm:

Acute treatment: 1 puff; additional puffs may be necessary if inadequate relief however patients should be advised to promptly consult healthcare provider or seek medical attention if no relief from acute treatment

Maintenance: 1 puff; may increase to maximum of 1 puff 4 times daily

Exercise-induced bronchospasm (prevention): 1 puff 30 minutes prior to exercise

Children ≥12 years and Adults:

Bronchospasm:

Acute treatment: 1-2 puffs; additional puffs may be necessary if inadequate relief however patients should be advised to promptly consult healthcare provider or seek medical attention if no relief from acute treatment

Maintenance: 1-2 puffs 3-4 times daily (maximum: 8 puffs daily)

Exercise-induced bronchospasm (prevention): 2 puffs 30 minutes prior to exercise

Solution for nebulization:

Children 2-12 years (AccuNeb®): Bronchospasm: 0.63-1.25 mg 3-4 times daily as needed

Children ≤4 years *(NIH Guidelines, 2007)*:

Quick relief: 0.63-2.5 mg every 4-6 hours as needed

Exacerbation of asthma (acute, severe): 0.15 mg/kg (minimum: 2.5 mg) every 20 minutes for 3 doses, then 0.15-0.3 mg/kg (maximum: 10 mg) every 1-4 hours as needed **or** 0.5 mg/kg/hour by continuous nebulization

Children 5-11 years *(NIH Guidelines, 2007)*:

Quick relief: 1.25-5 mg every 4-8 hours as needed

Exacerbation of asthma (acute, severe): 0.15 mg/kg (minimum: 2.5 mg) every 20 minutes for 3 doses, then 0.15-0.3 mg/kg (maximum: 10 mg) every 1-4 hours as needed **or** 0.5 mg/kg/hour by continuous nebulization

Children ≥12 years and Adults:

Bronchospasm: 2.5 mg 3-4 times daily as needed

Quick relief *(NIH Guidelines, 2007)*: 1.25-5 mg every 4-8 hours as needed

Exacerbation of asthma (acute, severe) *(NIH Guidelines, 2007)*: 2.5-5 mg every 20 minutes for 3 doses then 2.5-10 mg every 1-4 hours as needed, **or** 10-15 mg/hour by continuous nebulization

I.V. continuous infusion: Adults (Canadian labeling; product not available in U.S.): Severe bronchospasm and status asthmaticus: Initial: 5 mcg/minute; may increase up to 10-20 mcg/minute at 15- to 30-minute intervals if needed

Dosage adjustment in renal impairment: Use with caution in patients with renal impairment. No dosage adjustment required (including patients on hemodialysis, peritoneal dialysis, or CRRT; Aronoff, 2007).

Dosage adjustment in hepatic impairment: No dosage adjustment provided in manufacturer's labeling.

Administration

Metered-dose inhaler: Shake well before use; prime prior to first use, and whenever inhaler has not been used for >2 weeks or when it has been dropped, by releasing 3-4 test sprays into the air (away from face). Airomir™ Canadian product labeling recommends releasing a minimum of 4 test sprays when priming. HFA inhalers should be cleaned with warm water at least once per week; allow to air dry completely prior to use. A spacer device or valved holding chamber is recommended for use with metered-dose inhalers.

Solution for nebulization: Concentrated solution should be diluted prior to use. Blow-by administration is not recommended, use a mask device if patient unable to hold mouthpiece in mouth for administration.

Infusion solution (Canadian labeling; product not available in U.S.): Do not inject undiluted. Reduce concentration by at least 50% before infusing. Administer as a continuous infusion via infusion pump.

Oral: Do not crush or chew extended release tablets.

Monitoring Parameters FEV_1, peak flow, and/or other pulmonary function tests; blood pressure, heart rate; CNS stimulation; serum glucose, serum potassium; asthma symptoms; arterial or capillary blood gases (if patients condition warrants)

Test Interactions Increased renin (S), increased aldosterone (S)

Additional Information The 2007 National Heart, Lung, and Blood Institute Guidelines for the Diagnosis and Management of Asthma do not recommend the use of oral systemic albuterol as a quick-relief medication and do not recommend regularly scheduled daily, chronic use of inhaled beta-agonists for long-term control of asthma.

Dosage Forms Considerations

ProAir HFA 8.5 g canisters and Proventil HFA 6.7 g canisters contain 200 inhalations.

Ventolin HFA 18 g canisters contain 200 inhalations and the 8 g canisters contain 60 inhalations.

Dosage Forms Excipient information presented when available (limited, particularly for generics); consult specific product labeling.

Aerosol Solution, Inhalation:
- ProAir HFA: 108 (90 Base) MCG/ACT (8.5 g)
- Proventil HFA: 108 (90 Base) MCG/ACT (6.7 g)
- Ventolin HFA: 108 (90 Base) MCG/ACT (8 g, 18 g)

Nebulization Solution, Inhalation:
- Generic: 0.63 mg/3 mL (3 mL); (2.5 MG/3ML) 0.083% (3 mL); (5 mg/mL) 0.5% (20 mL)

Nebulization Solution, Inhalation [preservative free]:
- AccuNeb: 0.63 mg/3 mL (3 mL); 1.25 mg/3 mL (3 mL)
- Generic: 0.63 mg/3 mL (3 mL); 1.25 mg/3 mL (3 mL); (2.5 MG/3ML) 0.083% (3 mL); (5 mg/mL) 0.5% (1 ea); 0.083% (3 mL)

Syrup, Oral:
- Generic: 2 mg/5 mL (473 mL)

Tablet, Oral:
- Generic: 2 mg, 4 mg

Tablet Extended Release 12 Hour, Oral:
- VoSpire ER: 4 mg [contains fd&c blue #1 aluminum lake, fd&c yellow #10 aluminum lake]
- VoSpire ER: 8 mg
- Generic: 4 mg, 8 mg

Dosage Forms: Canada Excipient information presented when available (limited, particularly for generics); consult specific product labeling.

Aerosol, for oral inhalation:
- Airomir™: 100 mcg/inhalation (3.7 g) [chlorofluorocarbon free; 100 metered actuations]
- Airomir™: 100 mcg/inhalation (6.7 g) [chlorofluorocarbon free; 200 metered actuations]

Injection, solution, as sulphate:
- Ventolin® I.V.: 1 mg/1mL (5 mL)

◆ **Albuterol and Ipratropium** *see* Ipratropium and Albuterol *on page 1113*

◆ **Albuterol Sulfate** *see* Albuterol *on page 61*

◆ **Alcaine** *see* Proparacaine *on page 1733*

◆ **Alcaine® (Can)** *see* Proparacaine *on page 1733*

◆ **Alcalak [OTC]** *see* Calcium Carbonate *on page 318*

Alclometasone (al kloe MET a sone)

Brand Names: U.S. Aclovate

Index Terms Alclometasone Dipropionate

Pharmacologic Category Corticosteroid, Topical

Additional Appendix Information

Topical Corticosteroids *on page 2299*

Use Treatment of inflammation of corticosteroid-responsive dermatosis (low to medium potency topical corticosteroid)

Pregnancy Risk Factor C

Dosage Note: Therapy should be discontinued when control is achieved; if no improvement is seen within 2 weeks, reassessment of diagnosis may be necessary.

Topical:
- Children ≥1 year: Apply thin film to affected area 2-3 times/day; do not use for >3 weeks
- Adults: Apply a thin film to the affected area 2-3 times/day

Additional Information Complete prescribing information should be consulted for additional detail.

Dosage Forms Excipient information presented when available (limited, particularly for generics); consult specific product labeling.

Cream, External, as dipropionate:
- Aclovate: 0.05% (15 g, 60 g) [contains cetearyl alcohol, propylene glycol]
- Generic: 0.05% (15 g, 45 g, 60 g)

Ointment, External, as dipropionate:
- Generic: 0.05% (15 g, 45 g, 60 g)

◆ **Alclometasone Dipropionate** *see* Alclometasone *on page 63*

◆ **Alcortin A** *see* Iodoquinol and Hydrocortisone *on page 1109*

◆ **Aldactone** *see* Spironolactone *on page 1946*

◆ **Aldara** *see* Imiquimod *on page 1057*

◆ **Aldara® (Can)** *see* Imiquimod *on page 1057*

Aldesleukin (al des LOO kin)

Brand Names: U.S. Proleukin

Brand Names: Canada Proleukin®

Index Terms IL-2; Interleukin 2; Interleukin-2; Lymphocyte Mitogenic Factor; Recombinant Human Interleukin-2; T-Cell Growth Factor; TCGF; Thymocyte Stimulating Factor

Pharmacologic Category Antineoplastic Agent, Miscellaneous; Biological Response Modulator

Use Treatment of metastatic renal cell cancer, metastatic melanoma

Unlabeled Use Treatment of acute myeloid leukemia (AML)

Pregnancy Risk Factor C

Pregnancy Considerations Maternal toxicity and embryocidal effects were noted in animal studies. There are no adequate and well-controlled studies in pregnant women; use during pregnancy only if benefits to the mother outweigh potential risk to the fetus. Contraception is recommended for fertile males or females using this medication.

Breast-Feeding Considerations Due to the potential for serious adverse reactions in the nursing infant, breast-feeding should be discontinued during treatment.

Contraindications Hypersensitivity to aldesleukin or any component of the formulation; patients with abnormal thallium stress or pulmonary function tests; patients who have had an organ allograft. **Retreatment is contraindicated** in patients who have experienced sustained ventricular tachycardia (≥5 beats), uncontrolled or unresponsive cardiac arrhythmias, chest pain with ECG changes consistent with angina or MI, cardiac tamponade, intubation >72 hours, renal failure requiring dialysis for >72 hours, coma or toxic psychosis lasting >48 hours, repetitive or refractory seizures, bowel ischemia/perforation, or GI bleeding requiring surgery.

Warnings/Precautions Hazardous agent; use appropriate precautions for handling and disposal (NIOSH, 2012).

[U.S. Boxed Warning]: High-dose aldesleukin therapy has been associated with capillary leak syndrome (CLS), characterized by vascular tone loss and extravasation of plasma proteins and fluid into extravascular space. CLS results in significant hypotension and reduced organ perfusion which may be severe and can result in death; CLS onset is immediately after treatment initiation. Cardiac arrhythmia, angina, MI, respiratory insufficiency (requiring intubation), gastrointestinal bleeding or infarction, renal insufficiency, edema and mental status changes are also associated with CLS. Monitor fluid status and organ perfusion status carefully; consider fluids and/or pressor agents to maintain organ perfusion. **[U.S. Boxed Warning]: Therapy should be restricted to patients with normal cardiac and pulmonary functions as defined by thallium stress and formal pulmonary function testing.** Extreme caution should be used in patients with a history of prior cardiac or pulmonary disease and in patients who are fluid-restricted or where edema may be poorly tolerated. Withhold treatment for signs of organ hypoperfusion, including altered mental status, reduced urine output, systolic BP <90 mm Hg or cardiac arrhythmia. Once blood pressure is normalized, may consider diuretics for excessive weight gain/edema. Recovery from CLS generally begins soon after treatment cessation. Perform a thorough clinical evaluation prior to treatment initiation; exclude patients with significant cardiac, pulmonary, renal, hepatic, or central nervous system impairment from treatment. Patients with a more favorable performance status prior to treatment initiation are more likely to respond to aldesleukin treatment, with a higher response rate and generally lower toxicity.

[U.S. Boxed Warning]: Should be administered under the supervision of an experienced cancer chemotherapy physician in a facility with cardiopulmonary or intensive specialists and intensive care facilities available. Adverse effects are frequent and sometimes fatal. May exacerbate pre-existing or initial presentation of autoimmune diseases and inflammatory disorders; exacerbation and/or new onset have been reported with aldesleukin and interferon alfa combination therapy. Patients should be evaluated and treated for CNS metastases and have a negative scan prior to treatment; new neurologic symptoms and lesions have been reported in patients without pre-existing evidence of CNS metastases (symptoms generally improve upon discontinuation, however, cases with permanent damage have been reported). Mental status changes (irritability, confusion, depression) can occur and may indicate bacteremia, sepsis, hypoperfusion, CNS malignancy, or CNS toxicity. May cause seizure; use with caution in patients with seizure disorder.

[U.S. Boxed Warning]: Impaired neutrophil function is associated with treatment; patients are at risk for disseminated infection (including sepsis and bacterial endocarditis), and central line-related gram-positive infections. Treat pre-existing bacterial infection appropriately prior to treatment initiation. Monitor for signs of infection or sepsis during treatment. Antibiotic prophylaxis which has been associated with a reduced incidence of staphylococcal infections in aldesleukin studies includes the use of oxacillin, nafcillin, ciprofloxacin, or vancomycin.

[U.S. Boxed Warning]: Withhold treatment for patients developing moderate-to-severe lethargy or somnolence; continued treatment may result in coma. Standard prophylactic supportive care during high-dose aldesleukin treatment includes acetaminophen to relieve constitutional symptoms and an H_2 antagonist to reduce the risk of GI ulceration and/or bleeding. May impair renal or hepatic function; patients must have a serum creatinine ≤1.5 mg/dL prior to treatment. Concomitant nephrotoxic or hepatotoxic agents may increase the risk of renal or hepatic toxicity. Enhancement of cellular immune function may increase the risk of allograft rejection in transplant patients. An acute array of symptoms resembling aldesleukin adverse reactions (fever, chills, nausea, rash, pruritus, diarrhea, hypotension, edema, and oliguria) were observed within 1-4 hours after iodinated contrast media administration, usually when given within 4 weeks after aldesleukin treatment, although has been reported several months after aldesleukin treatment. The incidence of dyspnea and severe urogenital toxicities is potentially increased in elderly patients.

Adverse Reactions

>10%:

Cardiovascular: Hypotension (71%; grade 4: 3%), peripheral edema (28%), tachycardia (23%), edema (15%), vasodilation (13%), supraventricular tachycardia (12%; grade 4: 1%), cardiovascular disorder (11%; includes blood pressure changes, HF and ECG changes)

Central nervous system: Chills (52%), confusion (34%; grade 4: 1%), fever (29%; grade 4: 1%), malaise (27%), somnolence (22%), anxiety (12%), pain (12%), dizziness (11%)

Dermatologic: Rash (42%), pruritus (24%), exfoliative dermatitis (18%)

Endocrine & metabolic: Acidosis (12%; grade 4: 1%), hypomagnesemia (12%), hypocalcemia (11%)

Gastrointestinal: Diarrhea (67%; grade 4: 2%), vomiting (19% to 50%; grade 4: 1%), nausea (19% to 35%), stomatitis (22%), anorexia (20%), weight gain (16%), abdominal pain (11%)

Hematologic: Thrombocytopenia (37%; grade 4: 1%), anemia (29%), leukopenia (16%)

Hepatic: Hyperbilirubinemia (40%; grade 4: 2%), AST increased (23%; grade 4: 1%)

Neuromuscular & skeletal: Weakness (23%)

Renal: Oliguria (63%; grade 4: 6%), creatinine increased (33%; grade 4: 1%)

Respiratory: Dyspnea (43%; grade 4: 1%), lung disorder (24%; includes pulmonary congestion, rales, and rhonchi), cough (11%), respiratory disorder (11%; includes acute respiratory distress syndrome, infiltrates and pulmonary changes)

Miscellaneous: Antibody formation (66% to 74%), infection (13%; grade 4: 1%)

1% to 10%:

Cardiovascular: Arrhythmia (10%), cardiac arrest (grade 4: 1%), MI (grade 4: 1%), ventricular tachycardia (grade 4: 1%)

Central nervous system: Coma (grade 4: 2%), stupor (grade 4: 1%), psychosis (grade 4: 1%)

Gastrointestinal: Abdomen enlarged (10%)
Hematologic: Coagulation disorder (grade 4: 1%; includes intravascular coagulopathy)
Hepatic: Alkaline phosphatase increased (10%)
Renal: Anuria (grade 4: 5%), acute renal failure (grade 4: 1%)
Respiratory: Rhinitis (10%), apnea (grade 4: 1%)
Miscellaneous: Sepsis (grade 4: 1%)

<1% (Limited to important or life-threatening): Allergic interstitial nephritis, anaphylaxis, angioedema, asthma, atrial arrhythmia, AV block, blindness (transient or permanent), bowel infarction/necrosis/perforation, bradycardia, bullous pemphigoid, capillary leak syndrome, cardiomyopathy, cellulitis, cerebral edema, cerebral lesions, cerebral vasculitis, cholecystitis, colitis, crescentic IgA glomerulonephritis, Crohn's disease exacerbation, delirium, depression (severe; leading to suicide), diabetes mellitus, duodenal ulcer, encephalopathy, endocarditis, extrapyramidal syndrome, hemorrhage (including cerebral, gastrointestinal, retroperitoneal, subarachnoid, subdural), hepatic failure, hepatitis, hepatosplenomegaly, hypertension, hyperuricemia, hypothermia, hyperthyroidism, inflammatory arthritis, injection site necrosis, insomnia, intestinal obstruction, intestinal perforation, leukocytosis, malignant hyperthermia, meningitis, myocardial ischemia, myocarditis, myopathy, myositis, neuralgia, neuritis, neuropathy, neutropenia, NPN increased, oculobulbar myasthenia gravis, optic neuritis, organ perfusion decreased, pancreatitis, pericardial effusion, pericarditis, peripheral gangrene, phlebitis, pneumonia, pneumothorax, pulmonary edema, pulmonary embolus, respiratory acidosis, respiratory arrest, respiratory failure, rhabdomyolysis, scleroderma, seizure, Stevens-Johnson syndrome, stroke, syncope, thrombosis, thyroiditis, tracheoesophageal fistula, transient ischemic attack, tubular necrosis, ventricular extrasystoles

Drug Interactions

Metabolism/Transport Effects None known.

Avoid Concomitant Use

Avoid concomitant use of Aldesleukin with any of the following: CloZAPine; Corticosteroids

Increased Effect/Toxicity

Aldesleukin may increase the levels/effects of: CloZAPine; Hypotensive Agents

The levels/effects of Aldesleukin may be increased by: Contrast Media (Non-ionic); Interferons (Alfa)

Decreased Effect

The levels/effects of Aldesleukin may be decreased by: Corticosteroids

Ethanol/Nutrition/Herb Interactions Ethanol: May increase CNS adverse effects.

Preparation for Administration Hazardous agent; use appropriate precautions for handling and disposal (NIOSH, 2012). Reconstitute vials with 1.2 mL SWFI (preservative free) to a concentration of 18 million units (1.1 mg)/1 mL (sterile water should be injected towards the side of the vial). Gently swirl; do not shake. Further dilute with 50 mL of D_5W. Smaller volumes of D_5W should be used for doses ≤1.5 mg; avoid concentrations <30 mcg/mL and >70 mcg/mL (an increased variability in drug delivery has been seen). Plastic (polyvinyl chloride) bags result in more consistent drug delivery and are recommended. Filtration may result in loss of bioactivity. Addition of 0.1% albumin has been used to increase stability and decrease the extent of sorption if low final concentrations cannot be avoided.

Storage/Stability Store intact vials under refrigeration at 2°C to 8°C (36°F to 46°F). Protect from light. Plastic (polyvinyl chloride) bags result in more consistent drug delivery and are recommended. According to the manufacturer, reconstituted vials and solutions diluted for infusion are stable for 48 hours at room temperature or refrigerated although refrigeration is preferred because they do not contain preservatives. Do not freeze. Solution diluted with D_5W to a concentration of 220 mcg/mL and repackaged into tuberculin syringes was reported to be stable for 14 days refrigerated.

Mechanism of Action Aldesleukin is a human recombinant interleukin-2 product which promotes proliferation, differentiation, and recruitment of T and B cells, natural killer (NK) cells, and thymocytes; causes cytolytic activity in a subset of lymphocytes and subsequent interactions between the immune system and malignant cells; can stimulate lymphokine-activated killer (LAK) cells and tumor-infiltrating lymphocytes (TIL) cells.

Pharmacodynamics/Kinetics

Distribution: V_d: 4-7 L; primarily in plasma and then in the lymphocytes
Metabolism: Renal (metabolized to amino acids)
Half-life elimination: I.V.: Initial: 6-13 minutes; Terminal: 80-120 minutes
Excretion: Urine (primarily as metabolites)

Dosage Consider premedication with an antipyretic to reduce fever, an H_2 antagonist for prophylaxis of gastrointestinal irritation/bleeding, antiemetics, and antidiarrheals; continue for 12 hours after the last aldesleukin dose. Antibiotic prophylaxis is recommended to reduce the incidence of infection.

Children: I.V.: AML (unlabeled use): 9 million units (9 x 10^6 units)/m^2/day continuous infusion over 24 hours daily for 4 days; repeat 4 days later with 1.6 million units (1.6 x 10^6 units)/m^2/day continuous infusion over 24 hours daily for 10 days (Lange, 2008)

Adults: I.V.:

Renal cell carcinoma: 600,000 units/kg every 8 hours for a maximum of 14 doses; repeat after 9 days for a total of 28 doses per course; retreat if tumor shrinkage observed (and if no contraindications) at least 7 weeks after hospital discharge date

or

Unlabeled dosing: 720,000 units/kg every 8 hours for up to 12 doses; repeat with a second cycle 10-15 days later (Klapper, 2008)

Melanoma:

Single-agent use: 600,000 units/kg every 8 hours for a maximum of 14 doses; repeat after 9 days for a total of 28 doses per course; retreat if tumor shrinkage observed (and if no contraindications) at least 7 weeks after hospital discharge date

or

Unlabeled dosing: 720,000 units/kg every 8 hours for 12-15 doses; repeat with a second cycle ~14 days after the first dose of the initial cycle (Smith, 2008)

Combination biochemotherapy (unlabeled use): 9 million units/m^2/day continuous infusion over 24 hours for 4 days every 3 weeks for up to 4 cycles (Atkins, 2008) **or** 9 million units/m^2/day continuous infusion over 24 hours days 5 to 8, 17 to 20, and 26 to 29 every 42 days for up to 5 cycles (Eton, 2002) **or** 9 million units/m^2/day continuous infusion over 24 hours for 4 days every 3 weeks for 6 cycles (Legha, 1998)

Dosage adjustment in renal impairment: No specific recommendations by manufacturer. Use with caution.

Dosage adjustment for toxicity: Withhold or interrupt a dose for toxicity; do not reduce the dose.

Cardiovascular toxicity:

Atrial fibrillation, supraventricular tachycardia, or bradycardia that is persistent, recurrent, or requires treatment: Withhold dose; may resume when asymptomatic with full recovery to normal sinus rhythm.

Systolic BP <90 mm Hg (with increasing pressor requirements): Withhold dose; may resume treatment when systolic BP ≥90 mm Hg and stable or pressor requirements improve.

Any ECG change consistent with MI, ischemia or myocarditis (with or without chest pain), or suspected cardiac ischemia: Withhold dose; may resume when asymptomatic, MI/myocarditis have been ruled out, suspicion of angina is low, or there is no evidence of ventricular hypokinesia.

CNS toxicity: Mental status change, including moderate confusion or agitation: Withhold dose; may resume when resolved completely.

Dermatologic toxicity: Bullous dermatitis or marked worsening of pre-existing skin condition: Withhold dose; may treat with antihistamines or topical products (do not use topical steroids); may resume with resolution of all signs of bullous dermatitis.

Gastrointestinal: Stool guaiac repeatedly >3-4+: Withhold dose; may resume with negative stool guaiac.

Hepatotoxicity: Signs of hepatic failure, encephalopathy, increasing ascites, liver pain, hypoglycemia: Withhold dose and discontinue treatment for balance of cycle; may initiate a new course if indicated only after at least 7 weeks past resolution of all signs of hepatic failure (including hospital discharge).

Infection: Sepsis syndrome, clinically unstable: Withhold dose; may resume when sepsis syndrome has resolved, patient is clinically stable, and infection is under treatment.

Renal toxicity:

Serum creatinine >4.5 mg/dL (or ≥4 mg/dL with severe volume overload, acidosis or hyperkalemia): Withhold dose; may resume when <4 mg/dL and fluid/electrolyte status is stable.

Persistent oliguria or urine output <10 mL/hour for 16-24 hours with rising serum creatinine: Withhold dose; may resume when urine output >10 mL/hour with serum creatinine decrease of >1.5 mg/dL or normalization.

Respiratory toxicity: Oxygen saturation <90%: Withhold dose; may resume when >90%.

Retreatment with aldesleukin is contraindicated with the following toxicities: Sustained ventricular tachycardia (≥5 beats), uncontrolled or unresponsive cardiac arrhythmias, chest pain with ECG changes consistent with angina or MI, cardiac tamponade, intubation >72 hours, renal failure requiring dialysis for >72 hours, coma or toxic psychosis lasting >48 hours, repetitive or refractory seizures, bowel ischemia/perforation, or GI bleeding requiring surgery

Administration Administer as I.V. infusion over 15 minutes (do not administer with an inline filter). Allow solution to reach room temperature prior to administration. Flush before and after with D_5W, particularly if maintenance I.V. line contains sodium chloride. May also be administered by SubQ injection (unlabeled route)

Hazardous agent; use appropriate precautions for handling and disposal (NIOSH, 2012).

Monitoring Parameters

Baseline and periodic: CBC with differential and platelets, blood chemistries including electrolytes, renal and hepatic function tests, and chest x-ray; pulmonary function tests and arterial blood gases (baseline), thallium stress test (prior to treatment)

Monitoring during therapy should include daily (hourly if hypotensive) vital signs (temperature, pulse, blood pressure, and respiration rate), weight and fluid intake and output; in a patient with a decreased blood pressure, especially systolic BP <90 mm Hg, cardiac monitoring for rhythm should be conducted. If an abnormal complex or rhythm is seen, an ECG should be performed; vital signs in these hypotension patients should be taken hourly and central venous pressure (CVP) checked; monitor for change in mental status, and for signs of infection.

Additional Information 18 x 10^6 units = 1.1 mg protein

Dosage Forms Excipient information presented when available (limited, particularly for generics); consult specific product labeling.

Solution Reconstituted, Intravenous [preservative free]:
Proleukin: 22,000,000 units (1 ea)

◆ Aldex® CT *see* Diphenhydramine and Phenylephrine *on page 625*

◆ Aldomet *see* Methyldopa *on page 1333*

◆ Aldroxicon I [OTC] *see* Aluminum Hydroxide, Magnesium Hydroxide, and Simethicone *on page 90*

◆ Aldroxicon II [OTC] *see* Aluminum Hydroxide, Magnesium Hydroxide, and Simethicone *on page 90*

◆ Aldurazyme *see* Laronidase *on page 1176*

◆ Aldurazyme® (Can) *see* Laronidase *on page 1176*

Alemtuzumab (ay lem TU zoo mab)

Brand Names: Canada MabCampath®

Index Terms Anti-CD52 Monoclonal Antibody; Campath-1H; Humanized IgG1 Anti-CD52 Monoclonal Antibody; Lemtrada; MoAb CD52; Monoclonal Antibody Campath-1H; Monoclonal Antibody CD52

Pharmacologic Category Antineoplastic Agent, Monoclonal Antibody; Monoclonal Antibody

Use Campath®: Treatment (as a single agent) of B-cell chronic lymphocytic leukemia (B-CLL)

Unlabeled Use Conditioning regimen in stem cell transplant; prophylaxis of graft-versus-host disease (GVHD); treatment of steroid-refractory GVHD; treatment of T-cell prolymphocytic leukemia; treatment of autoimmune hemolytic anemia (CLL-induced); immunosuppressant in solid organ transplant (induction and steroid-refractory rejection); treatment of relapsed-remitting multiple sclerosis

Pregnancy Risk Factor C

Pregnancy Considerations Human IgG is known to cross the placental barrier; therefore, alemtuzumab may also cross the barrier and cause fetal B- and T-lymphocyte depletion. Use during pregnancy only if the benefit to the mother outweighs the potential risk to the fetus. Effective contraception is recommended during and for at least 6 months after treatment for women of childbearing potential and men of reproductive potential.

Breast-Feeding Considerations Human IgG is excreted in breast milk; therefore, alemtuzumab may also be excreted in milk. Due to the potential for serious adverse reactions in the nursing infant, the decision to discontinue alemtuzumab or to discontinue breast-feeding should take into account the importance of treatment to the mother and the half-life of alemtuzumab.

Prescribing and Access Restrictions As of September 4, 2012, alemtuzumab (Campath®) is no longer commercially available in the United States (or Europe); a restricted distribution program will allow access (free of charge) for appropriate patients. Information on necessary documentation and requirements is available at Campath Distribution Program (1-877-422-6728) or Genzyme Medical Information (1-800-745-4447, option 2).

Contraindications There are no contraindications listed in the manufacturer's labeling

Warnings/Precautions [U.S. Boxed Warning]: Serious infections (bacterial, viral, fungal, and protozoan) have been reported. Administer prophylactic medications against PCP pneumonia and herpes viral infections during treatment and for at least 2 months following last dose or until $CD4^+$ counts are ≥200 cells/μL (whichever is later). Severe and prolonged lymphopenia may occur;

CD4+ counts usually return to ≥200 cells/µL within 2-6 months; however, CD4+ and CD8+ lymphocyte counts may not return to baseline levels for more than 1 year. Monitor for CMV infection (during and for at least 2 months after completion of therapy). Withhold treatment during serious infections; may be reinitiated upon resolution of infection. Monitor for CMV infection (during and for at least 2 months after completion of therapy); initiate appropriate antiviral treatment and withhold alemtuzumab for CMV infection or confirmed CMV viremia (withhold alemtuzumab during CMV antiviral treatment).

[U.S. Boxed Warning]: Serious and potentially fatal infusion-related reactions may occur; monitor for infusion reaction; withhold treatment for grade 3 or 4 infusion reactions. Gradual escalation to the recommended maintenance dose is required at initiation and with treatment interruptions (for ≥7 days) to minimize infusion-related reactions. Infusion reaction symptoms may include acute respiratory distress syndrome, anaphylactic shock, angioedema, bronchospasm, cardiac arrest, cardiac arrhythmias, chills, dyspnea, fever, hypotension, myocardial infarction, pulmonary infiltrates, rash, rigors, syncope, or urticaria. The incidence of infusion reaction is highest during the first week of treatment. Premedicate with acetaminophen and an oral antihistamine. Medications for the treatment of reactions should be available for immediate use. Use caution and carefully monitor blood pressure in patients with ischemic heart disease and patients on antihypertensive therapy. Reinitiate with gradual dose escalation if treatment is withheld ≥7 days.

[U.S. Boxed Warning]: Serious and fatal cytopenias (including pancytopenia, bone marrow hypoplasia, autoimmune hemolytic anemia, and autoimmune idiopathic thrombocytopenia) have occurred. Single doses >30 mg or cumulative weekly doses >90 mg are associated with an increased incidence of pancytopenia. Severe prolonged myelosuppression, hemolytic anemia, pure red cell aplasia, bone marrow aplasia, and bone marrow hypoplasia have also been reported with use at the normal dose for the treatment of B-CLL. Discontinue for serious hematologic or other serious toxicity (except lymphopenia) until the event resolves. Permanently discontinue if autoimmune anemia or autoimmune thrombocytopenia occurs. Patients receiving blood products should only receive irradiated blood products due to the potential for transfusion-associated GVHD during lymphopenia.

Immune thrombocytopenia (ITP) or idiopathic thrombocytopenic purpura has been reported in 6 patients receiving alemtuzumab for the treatment of relapsed-remitting multiple sclerosis (RMSS); some cases were severe, with 1 fatality (Cuker, 2011). The median time to onset was 24.5 months from initial alemtuzumab exposure and 10.5 months from the last dose. In 4 cases, ITP was treated with standard ITP management and responses were observed within 1 week. After the initial case was discovered, patients in the RMSS study were instructed to report abnormal bleeding, bruising or petechial rash and blood counts were monitored monthly.

Patients should not be immunized with live, viral vaccines during or recently after treatment. The ability to respond to any vaccine following therapy is unknown.

Adverse Reactions Adverse reactions reported with Campath®:

>10%:

- Cardiovascular: Hypotension (16%), hypertension (14%), dysrhythmia (14%)
- Central nervous system: Fever (69%), chills (53%), headache (14%), dysthesias, fatigue
- Dermatologic: Urticaria (16%), rash (13%)
- Gastrointestinal: Abdominal pain, anorexia, mucositis, nausea, vomiting
- Hematologic: Lymphopenia (grades 3/4: 97%), neutropenia (77%; grade 3/4: 42% to 64% [median onset: 31 days, median duration: 28-37 days]), anemia (76%; grade 3/4: 12% to 38% [median onset: 31 days, median duration 8 days]), thrombocytopenia (71%; grade 3/4: 13% to 52% [median onset: 9 days; median duration: 14-21 days])
- Local: Injection site reaction (SubQ administration: 90%)
- Neuromuscular & skeletal: Musculoskeletal pain
- Respiratory: Dyspnea (14%)
- Miscellaneous: Infection (50% to 74%; grades 3/4: 5% to 21%; includes bacterial, fungal, protozoan, viral), CMV viremia (55%), infusion reactions (grades 3/4: 10% to 35%), CMV infection (16%), sepsis (grades 3/4/5: 3% to 10%)

1% to 10%:

- Cardiovascular: Tachycardia (10%)
- Central nervous system: Insomnia (10%), anxiety (8%)
- Dermatologic: Erythema (4%)
- Gastrointestinal: Diarrhea (10%)
- Hematologic: Neutropenic fever (grades 3/4: 5% to 10%)
- Neuromuscular & skeletal: Tremor (3%)
- Respiratory: Bronchospasm

<1% (Limited to important or life-threatening): Acute respiratory distress syndrome, anaphylactoid shock, angioedema, aplastic anemia, arrhythmia, bleeding, bone marrow aplasia, bone marrow hypoplasia, bruising, cardiac arrest, cardiac insufficiency, cardiomyopathy, chronic inflammatory demyelinating polyradiculoneuropathy (CIDP), ejection fraction decreased, Epstein-Barr virus, Epstein-Barr virus-associated lymphoproliferative disorder, Goodpasture's syndrome, Graves' disease, Guillain-Barré syndrome, hemolytic anemia, HF, immune thrombocytopenia (ITP), MI, optic neuropathy, pallor, petechia, *Pneumocystis jirovecii* pneumonia (PCP), progressive multifocal leukoencephalopathy (PML), pulmonary infiltrates, pure red cell aplasia, purpura, respiratory arrest, serum sickness, syncope, transfusion-associated GVHD, tumor lysis syndrome, virus reactivation (latent), weakness

Drug Interactions

Metabolism/Transport Effects None known.

Avoid Concomitant Use

Avoid concomitant use of Alemtuzumab with any of the following: BCG; Belimumab; CloZAPine; Natalizumab; Pimecrolimus; Tacrolimus (Topical); Tofacitinib; Vaccines (Live)

Increased Effect/Toxicity

Alemtuzumab may increase the levels/effects of: Belimumab; CloZAPine; Leflunomide; Natalizumab; Tofacitinib; Vaccines (Live)

The levels/effects of Alemtuzumab may be increased by: Abciximab; Denosumab; Pimecrolimus; Roflumilast; Tacrolimus (Topical); Trastuzumab

Decreased Effect

Alemtuzumab may decrease the levels/effects of: BCG; Coccidioidin Skin Test; Sipuleucel-T; Vaccines (Inactivated); Vaccines (Live)

The levels/effects of Alemtuzumab may be decreased by: Echinacea

Ethanol/Nutrition/Herb Interactions Herb/Nutraceutical: Echinacea may diminish the therapeutic effect of alemtuzumab.

Preparation for Administration Campath®: Dilute for infusion in 100 mL NS or D_5W. Compatible in polyvinylchloride (PVC) bags. Gently invert the bag to mix the solution. Do not shake prior to use.

Storage/Stability Campath®: Prior to dilution, store intact (30 mg/1 mL) vials at 2°C to 8°C (36°F to 46°F); do not freeze (if accidentally frozen, thaw in refrigerator prior to administration). Do not shake; protect from light. Following dilution, store at room temperature or refrigerate; protect from light; use within 8 hours. Discard unused portion in the vial.

Mechanism of Action Binds to CD52, a nonmodulating antigen present on the surface of B and T lymphocytes, a majority of monocytes, macrophages, NK cells, and a subpopulation of granulocytes. After binding to $CD52^+$ cells, an antibody-dependent lysis of malignant cells occurs.

Pharmacodynamics/Kinetics

Distribution: V_d: I.V.: 0.18 L/kg (range: 0.1-0.4 L/kg)

Metabolism: Clearance decreases with repeated dosing (due to loss of CD52 receptors in periphery), resulting in a sevenfold increase in AUC after 12 weeks of therapy.

Half-life elimination: I.V.: 11 hours (following first 30 mg dose; range: 2-32 hours); 6 days (following the last 30 mg dose; range: 1-14 days)

Dosage Adults: **Note: Dose escalation is required;** usually accomplished in 3-7 days. Single doses >30 mg or cumulative doses >90 mg/week increase the incidence of pancytopenia. Pretreatment (with acetaminophen 500-1000 mg and diphenhydramine 50 mg) is recommended prior to the first dose, with dose escalations, and as clinically indicated; I.V. hydrocortisone may be used for severe infusion-related reactions. Reinitiate with gradual dose escalation if treatment is withheld ≥7 days.

Dose escalation: Initial: 3 mg daily beginning on day 1; if tolerated (infusion reaction ≤grade 2), increase to 10 mg daily; if tolerated (infusion reaction ≤grade 2), may increase to maintenance of 30 mg per dose 3 times weekly if required for maintenance dose.

B-cell chronic lymphocytic leukemia (B-CLL): I.V.: Gradually escalate to a maintenance of 30 mg per dose 3 times weekly on alternate days for a total duration of therapy of up to 12 weeks (Hillmen, 2007; Keating, 2002)

B-CLL (unlabeled route): SubQ: Initial: 3 mg on day 1; if tolerated 10 mg on day 3; if tolerated increase to 30 mg on day 5; maintenance: 30 mg per dose 3 times weekly for a maximum of 18 weeks (Lundin, 2002) **or** 3 mg on day 1; if tolerated 10 mg on day 2; if tolerated 30 mg on day 3, followed by 30 mg per dose 3 times weekly for 4-12 weeks (Stilgenbauer, 2009)

Autoimmune cytopenias, CLL-induced, refractory (unlabeled use): I.V., SubQ: Gradually escalate to a maintenance of 10-30 mg per dose 3 times weekly for 4-12 weeks (Karlsson, 2007; Osterborg, 2009)

Graft versus host disease (GVHD), acute, steroid refractory, treatment (unlabeled use): I.V.: 10 mg daily for 5 consecutive days, then 10 mg weekly on days 8, 15, and 22 if CR not achieved (Martinez, 2009) **or** 10 mg weekly until symptom resolution (Schnitzler, 2009)

Multiple sclerosis, relapsed-remitting (RRMS; unlabeled use): I.V.: 12 mg daily for 5 consecutive days, followed 12 months later by 12 mg daily for 3 consecutive days; may receive an additional 12 mg daily for 3 consecutive days 12 months later (CAMMS223, 2008; Coles, 2012)

Renal transplant, induction (unlabeled use): I.V.: 30 mg as a single dose at the time of transplant (Hanaway, 2011)

Stem cell transplant (allogeneic) conditioning regimen (unlabeled use): I.V.: 20 mg daily for 5 days (in combination with fludarabine and melphalan) beginning 8 days prior to transplant (Mead, 2010) **or** beginning 7 days prior to transplant (Van Besien, 2009)

T-cell prolymphocytic leukemia (T-PLL; unlabeled use): I.V.: Initial test dose 3 mg or 10 mg, followed by dose escalation to 30 mg per dose 3 times weekly as tolerated until maximum response (Dearden, 2001) **or** Initial dose: 3 mg day 1, if tolerated increase to 10 mg day 2, if tolerated increase to 30 mg on day 3 (days 1, 2, and 3 are consecutive days), followed by 30 mg per dose every Monday, Wednesday, Friday for a total of 4-12 weeks (Keating, 2002)

Dosage adjustment for nonhematologic toxicity:

Note: If treatment is withheld ≥7 days, reinitiate at 3 mg with re-escalation to 10 mg and then 30 mg.

Grade 3 or 4 infusion reaction: Withhold infusion

Serious infection or other serious adverse reaction: Withhold alemtuzumab until resolution

Autoimmune anemia or autoimmune thrombocytopenia: Discontinue alemtuzumab

Dosage adjustment for hematologic toxicity (severe neutropenia or thrombocytopenia, not autoimmune):

Note: If treatment is withheld ≥7 days, reinitiate at 3 mg with re-escalation to 10 mg and then 30 mg.

ANC <250/mm³ and/or platelet count ≤25,000/mm³:

First occurrence: Withhold treatment; resume at 30 mg per dose when ANC ≥500/mm³ and platelet count ≥50,000/mm³

Second occurrence: Withhold treatment; resume at 10 mg per dose when ANC ≥500/mm³ and platelet count ≥50,000/mm³

Third occurrence: Discontinue alemtuzumab.

Patients with a baseline ANC ≤250/mm³ and/or a baseline platelet count ≤25,000/mm³ at initiation of therapy: If ANC and/or platelet counts decrease to ≤50% of the baseline value:

First occurrence: Withhold treatment; resume at 30 mg per dose upon return to baseline values

Second occurrence: Withhold treatment; resume at 10 mg per dose upon return to baseline values

Third occurrence: Discontinue alemtuzumab.

Dosage adjustment in renal impairment: No dosage adjustment provided in the manufacturer's labeling (has not been studied).

Dosage adjustment in hepatic impairment: No dosage adjustment provided in the manufacturer's labeling (has not been studied).

Administration Administer by I.V. infusion over 2 hours. Premedicate with diphenhydramine 50 mg and acetaminophen 500-1000 mg 30 minutes before each infusion. Hydrocortisone (I.V.) has been effective in decreasing severe infusion-related events. Start anti-infective prophylaxis. Other drugs should not be added to or simultaneously infused through the same I.V. line. Do not give I.V. push or bolus. Compatible in polyvinylchloride (PVC) or polyethylene lined administration sets.

SubQ (unlabeled route): SubQ administration has been studied (Lundin, 2002; Stilgenbauer, 2009); an increased rate of injection site reactions has been observed, with only rare incidences of chills or infusion-like reactions typically observed with I.V. infusion. A longer dose escalation time (1-2 weeks) may be needed due to injection site reactions (Lundin, 2002). Premedicate with diphenhydramine 50 mg and acetaminophen 500-1000 mg 30 minutes before dose. The subQ route should **NOT** be used for the treatment of T-PLL (Deardon, 2011).

Monitoring Parameters Vital signs; carefully monitor BP especially in patients with ischemic heart disease or on antihypertensive medications; CBC with differential and platelets (weekly, more frequent if worsening); signs and symptoms of infection; CD4+ lymphocyte counts (after treatment until recovery); CMV antigen (routinely during and for 2 months after treatment). Monitor closely for infusion reactions (including hypotension, rigors, fever, shortness of breath, bronchospasm, chills, and/or rash); consider TSH at baseline and then every 2-3 months during alemtuzumab treatment (Hamnvik, 2011).

Test Interactions May interfere with diagnostic serum tests that utilize antibodies.

Alendronate (a LEN droe nate)

Brand Names: U.S. Binosto; Fosamax

Brand Names: Canada Alendronate-70; Alendronate-FC; Apo-Alendronate®; Auro-Alendronate; CO Alendronate; Dom-Alendronate; Fosamax®; JAMP-Alendronate; Mint-Alendronate; Mylan-Alendronate; PHL-Alendronate; PMS-Alendronate; PMS-Alendronate-FC; Q-Alendronate; Ran-Alendronate; ratio-Alendronate; Riva-Alendronate; Sandoz-Alendronate; Teva-Alendronate

Index Terms Alendronate Sodium; Alendronic Acid Monosodium Salt Trihydrate; MK-217

Pharmacologic Category Bisphosphonate Derivative

Use Treatment of osteoporosis in postmenopausal females (Fosamax®, Binosto®); prevention of osteoporosis in postmenopausal females (Fosamax®); treatment of osteoporosis in males (Fosamax®, Binosto®); treatment of Paget's disease of the bone in patients who are symptomatic, at risk for future complications, or with alkaline phosphatase ≥2 times the upper limit of normal (Fosamax®); treatment of glucocorticoid-induced osteoporosis in males and females with low bone mineral density who are receiving a daily dosage ≥7.5 mg of prednisone (or equivalent) (Fosamax®)

Pregnancy Risk Factor C

Pregnancy Considerations Adverse events were observed in animal reproduction studies. It is not known if bisphosphonates cross the placenta, but fetal exposure is expected (Djokanovic, 2008; Stathopoulos, 2011). Bisphosphonates are incorporated into the bone matrix and gradually released over time. The amount available in the systemic circulation varies by dose and duration of therapy. Theoretically, there may be a risk of fetal harm when pregnancy follows the completion of therapy; however, available data have not shown that exposure to bisphosphonates during pregnancy significantly increases the risk of adverse fetal events (Djokanovic, 2008; Levy, 2009; Stathopoulos, 2011). Until additional data is available, most sources recommend discontinuing bisphosphonate therapy in women of reproductive potential as early as possible prior to a planned pregnancy; use in premenopausal women should be reserved for special circumstances when rapid bone loss is occurring (Bhalla, 2010; Pereira, 2012; Stathopoulos, 2011). Because hypocalcemia has been described following *in utero* bisphosphonate exposure, exposed infants should be monitored for hypocalcemia after birth (Djokanovic, 2008; Stathopoulos, 2011).

Breast-Feeding Considerations It is not known if alendronate is excreted into breast milk. The manufacturer recommends that caution be exercised when administering alendronate to nursing women.

Medication Guide Available Yes

Contraindications Hypersensitivity to alendronate, other bisphosphonates, or any component of the formulation; hypocalcemia; abnormalities of the esophagus (eg, stricture, achalasia) which delay esophageal emptying; inability to stand or sit upright for at least 30 minutes; increased risk of aspiration (effervescent tablets; oral solution)

Warnings/Precautions Use caution in patients with renal impairment (not recommended for use in patients with Cl_{cr} <35 mL/minute); hypocalcemia must be corrected before therapy initiation; ensure adequate calcium and vitamin D intake. May cause irritation to upper gastrointestinal mucosa. Esophagitis, dysphagia, esophageal ulcers, esophageal erosions, and esophageal stricture (rare) have been reported; risk increases in patients unable to comply with dosing instructions. Use with caution in patients with dysphagia, esophageal disease, gastritis, duodenitis, or ulcers (may worsen underlying condition). Discontinue use if new or worsening symptoms develop.

Osteonecrosis of the jaw (ONJ) has been reported in patients receiving bisphosphonates. Risk factors include invasive dental procedures (eg, tooth extraction, dental implants, boney surgery); a diagnosis of cancer, with concomitant chemotherapy or corticosteroids; poor oral hygiene, ill-fitting dentures; and comorbid disorders (anemia, coagulopathy, infection, pre-existing dental disease); risk may increase with duration of bisphosphonate use. Most reported cases occurred after I.V. bisphosphonate therapy; however, cases have been reported following oral therapy. A dental exam and preventative dentistry should be performed prior to placing patients with risk factors on chronic bisphosphonate therapy. The manufacturer's labeling states that discontinuing bisphosphonates in patients requiring invasive dental procedures may reduce the risk of ONJ. However, other experts suggest that there is no evidence that discontinuing therapy reduces the risk of developing ONJ (Assael, 2009). The benefit/risk must be assessed by the treating physician and/or dentist/surgeon prior to any invasive dental procedure. Patients developing ONJ while on bisphosphonates should receive care by an oral surgeon.

Atypical femur fractures have been reported in patients receiving bisphosphonates for treatment/prevention of osteoporosis. The fractures include subtrochanteric femur (bone just below the hip joint) and diaphyseal femur (long segment of the thigh bone). Some patients experience prodromal pain weeks or months before the fracture occurs. It is unclear if bisphosphonate therapy is the cause for these fractures, although the majority of cases have been reported in patients taking bisphosphonates. Patients receiving long-term (>3-5 years) therapy may be at an increased risk. Discontinue bisphosphonate therapy in patients who develop a femoral shaft fracture.

Severe (and occasionally debilitating) bone, joint, and/or muscle pain have been reported during bisphosphonate treatment. The onset of pain ranged from a single day to several months. Consider discontinuing therapy in patients who experience severe symptoms; symptoms usually resolve upon discontinuation. Some patients experienced recurrence when rechallenged with same drug or another bisphosphonate; avoid use in patients with a history of these symptoms in association with bisphosphonate therapy. In the management of osteoporosis, re-evaluate the need for continued therapy periodically; the optimal duration of treatment has not yet been determined. Consider discontinuing after 3-5 years of use in patients at low-risk for fracture; following discontinuation, re-evaluate fracture risk periodically.

Potentially significant drug-drug interactions may exist, requiring dose or frequency adjustment, additional monitoring, and/or selection of alternative therapy. Consult drug interactions database for more detailed information. Each effervescent tablet contains 650 mg of sodium (NaCl 1650 mg); use with caution in patients following a sodium-restricted diet.

Adverse Reactions Note: Incidence of adverse effects (mostly GI) increases significantly in patients treated for Paget's disease at 40 mg/day.

>10%: Endocrine & metabolic: Hypocalcemia (18%; transient, mild)

1% to 10%:

Central nervous system: Headache (≤3%)

Endocrine & metabolic: Hypophosphatemia (10%; transient, mild)

Gastrointestinal: Abdominal pain (1% to 7%), acid regurgitation (1% to 4%), dyspepsia (1% to 4%), nausea (1% to 4%), flatulence (≤4%), diarrhea (1% to 3%), gastroesophageal reflux disease (1% to 3%), constipation (≤3%), esophageal ulcer (≤2%), abdominal distension (≤1%), gastritis (≤1%), vomiting (≤1%), dysphagia (≤1%), gastric ulcer (1%), melena (1%)

Neuromuscular & skeletal: Musculoskeletal pain (≤6%), muscle cramps (≤1%)

<1% (Limited to important or life-threatening): Alopecia, anastomotic ulcer, angioedema, atrial fibrillation, dizziness, duodenal ulcer, dysgeusia, episcleritis, erythema, femur fracture (including diaphyseal, low-energy femoral shaft, and subtrochanteric fractures), erosive esophagitis, esophageal perforation, esophageal spasm, esophageal ulcer, esophagitis, exacerbation of asthma, femur fracture (including diaphyseal, low-energy femoral shaft, and subtrochanteric fractures), fever, flu-like symptoms, hypersensitivity reaction, hypocalcemia (symptomatic), joint swelling, lymphocytopenia, malaise, malignant neoplasm of esophagus, myalgia, oropharyngeal ulcer; ostealgia, myalgia, or arthralgia (occasionally severe, considered incapacitating in rare cases); osteonecrosis (jaw), peripheral edema, pruritus, scleritis (rare), skin photosensitivity (rare), skin rash, Stevens-Johnson syndrome, toxic epidermal necrolysis, urticaria, uveitis (rare), vertigo, weakness

Drug Interactions

Metabolism/Transport Effects None known.

Avoid Concomitant Use There are no known interactions where it is recommended to avoid concomitant use.

Increased Effect/Toxicity

Alendronate may increase the levels/effects of: Deferasirox; Phosphate Supplements

The levels/effects of Alendronate may be increased by: Aminoglycosides; Aspirin; Nonsteroidal Anti-Inflammatory Agents; Systemic Angiogenesis Inhibitors

Decreased Effect

The levels/effects of Alendronate may be decreased by: Antacids; Calcium Salts; Iron Salts; Magnesium Salts; Multivitamins/Minerals (with ADEK, Folate, Iron); Multivitamins/Minerals (with AE, No Iron); Proton Pump Inhibitors; Sucroferric Oxyhydroxide

Ethanol/Nutrition/Herb Interactions

Ethanol: May increase risk of osteoporosis and gastric irritation. Management: Avoid ethanol.

Food: All food and beverages interfere with absorption. Coadministration with caffeine may reduce alendronate efficacy. Coadministration with dairy products may decrease alendronate absorption. Beverages (especially orange juice, coffee, and mineral water) and food may reduce the absorption of alendronate as much as 60%. Management: Alendronate must be taken first thing in the morning and ≥30 minutes before the first food, beverage (except plain water), or other medication of the day.

Preparation for Administration Tablet, effervescent (Binosto®): Dissolve effervescent tablet in 120 mL of room temperature plain water (not mineral water or flavored water); wait ≥5 minutes after effervescence stops, then stir for 10 seconds and administer.

Storage/Stability

Oral solution: Store at 25°C (77°F), excursions permitted to 15°C to 30°C (59°F to 86°F). Do not freeze.

Tablet (Fosamax®): Store at room temperature of 15°C to 30°C (59°F to 86°F). Keep in well-closed container.

Tablet, effervescent (Binosto®): Store at 20°C to 25°C (68°F to 77°F), excursions permitted to 15°C to 30°C (59°F to 86°F). Protect from moisture. Store in original blister package until use.

Mechanism of Action A bisphosphonate which inhibits bone resorption via actions on osteoclasts or on osteoclast precursors; decreases the rate of bone resorption, leading to an indirect increase in bone mineral density. In Paget's disease, characterized by disordered resorption and formation of bone, inhibition of resorption leads to an indirect decrease in bone formation; but the newly-formed bone has a more normal architecture.

Pharmacodynamics/Kinetics

Distribution: 28 L (exclusive of bone)

Protein binding: ~78%

Metabolism: None

Bioavailability: Fasting: 0.6%; reduced up to 60% with coffee or orange juice

Half-life elimination: Exceeds 10 years

Excretion: Urine; feces (as unabsorbed drug)

Dosage Note: Consider discontinuing after 3-5 years of use for osteoporosis in patients at low-risk for fracture. Patients should receive supplemental calcium and vitamin D if dietary intake is inadequate.

Osteoporosis in postmenopausal females: Adults: Oral:

Prophylaxis: 5 mg once daily **or** 35 mg once weekly

Treatment: 10 mg once daily **or** 70 mg once weekly

Osteoporosis in males: Adults: Oral: 10 mg once daily **or** 70 mg once weekly

Osteoporosis secondary to glucocorticoids in males and females: Adults: Oral: Treatment: 5 mg once daily; a dose of 10 mg once daily should be used in postmenopausal females who are not receiving estrogen.

Paget's disease of bone in males and females: Adults: Oral: 40 mg once daily for 6 months

Retreatment: Relapses during the 12 months following therapy occurred in 9% of patients who responded to treatment. Specific retreatment data are not available. Following a 6-month post-treatment evaluation period, retreatment with alendronate may be considered in patients who have relapsed based on increases in serum alkaline phosphatase, which should be measured periodically. Retreatment may also be considered in those who failed to normalize their serum alkaline phosphatase.

Missed doses (once weekly): If a once-weekly dose is missed, it should be given the next morning after remembered; may then return to the original once-weekly schedule (original scheduled day of the week), however, do not give 2 doses on the same day.

Elderly: Refer to adult dosing.

Dosage adjustment in renal impairment:

Cl_{cr} ≥35 mL/minute: No dosage adjustment necessary.

Cl_{cr} <35 mL/minute: Use not recommended.

Dosage adjustment in hepatic impairment: No dosage adjustment necessary.

Dietary Considerations Ensure adequate calcium and vitamin D intake; if dietary intake is inadequate, dietary supplementation is recommended. Women and men should consume:

Calcium: 1000 mg/day (men: 50-70 years) **or** 1200 mg/day (women ≥51 years and men ≥71 years) (IOM, 2011; NOF, 2013)

Vitamin D: 800-1000 IU/day (men and women ≥50 years) (NOF, 2013). Recommended Dietary Allowance (RDA): 600 IU/day (men and women ≤70 years) **or** 800 IU/day (men and women ≥71 years) (IOM, 2011).

Administration Administer first thing in the morning and ≥30 minutes before the first food, beverage (except plain water), or other medication(s) of the day. Do not take with mineral water or with other beverages. Patients should be instructed to stay upright (not to lie down) for at least 30 minutes **and** until after first food of the day (to reduce esophageal irritation).

Oral solution: Administer oral solution, followed with at least 2 oz of plain water.

Tablet (Fosamax®): Must be taken with 6-8 oz of plain water.

Tablet, effervescent (Binosto®): Dissolve one tablet in 4 oz of room temperature plain water only; once effervescence stops, wait ≥5 minutes and stir the solution for ~10 seconds and then drink.

Monitoring Parameters
Osteoporosis: Bone mineral density (BMD) should be re-evaluated every 2 years (or more frequently) after initiating therapy (NOF, 2013); in patients with combined alendronate and glucocorticoid treatment, BMD should be made at initiation and repeated after 6-12 months; annual measurements of height and weight, assessment of chronic back pain; serum calcium and 25(OH)D; may consider monitoring biochemical markers of bone turnover

Paget's disease: Alkaline phosphatase; pain; serum calcium and 25(OH)D

Reference Range
Calcium (total): Adults: 9.0-11.0 mg/dL (2.05-2.54 mmol/L), may slightly decrease with aging

Phosphorus: 2.5-4.5 mg/dL (0.81-1.45 mmol/L)

Vitamin D: There is no clear consensus on a reference range for total serum 25(OH)D concentrations or the validity of this level as it relates clinically to bone health. In addition, there is significant variability in the reporting of serum 25(OH)D levels as a result of different assay types in use; however, the following ranges have been suggested:

Adults (IOM, 2011): Sufficient levels in practically all persons: ≥20 ng/mL (50 nmol/L); concern for risk of toxicity: >50 ng/mL (125 nmol/L)

Osteoporosis patients (NOF, 2013): Recommended level to reach and maintain: ~30 ng/mL (75 nmol/L)

Test Interactions Bisphosphonates may interfere with diagnostic imaging agents such as technetium-99m-diphosphonate in bone scans.

Dosage Forms Excipient information presented when available (limited, particularly for generics); consult specific product labeling.

Solution, Oral:
Generic: 70 mg/75 mL (75 mL)

Tablet, Oral:
Fosamax: 70 mg
Generic: 5 mg, 10 mg, 35 mg, 40 mg, 70 mg

Tablet Effervescent, Oral:
Binosto: 70 mg

- **Alendronate-70 (Can)** *see* Alendronate *on page 69*

Alendronate and Cholecalciferol
(a LEN droe nate & kole e kal SI fer ole)

Brand Names: U.S. Fosamax Plus D®

Brand Names: Canada Fosavance

Index Terms Alendronate Sodium and Cholecalciferol; Cholecalciferol and Alendronate; Vitamin D_3 and Alendronate

Pharmacologic Category Bisphosphonate Derivative; Vitamin D Analog

Use Treatment of osteoporosis in postmenopausal females; increase bone mass in males with osteoporosis

Pregnancy Risk Factor C

Medication Guide Available Yes

Dosage Osteoporosis: Adults: Oral: One tablet (alendronate 70 mg/cholecalciferol 2800 units **or** alendronate 70 mg/cholecalciferol 5600 units) once weekly. Consider discontinuing after 3-5 years of use for osteoporosis in patients at low-risk for fracture. Supplemental calcium and vitamin D may be necessary if dietary intake is inadequate.

Missed doses: If a once-weekly dose is missed, it should be given the next morning after remembered; may then return to the original once-weekly schedule (original scheduled day of the week), however, do not give 2 doses on the same day.

Dosage adjustment in renal impairment:
Cl_{cr} ≥35 mL/minute: No dosage adjustment necessary.
Cl_{cr} <35 mL/minute: Use is not recommended.

Dosage adjustment in hepatic impairment: Alendronate: No dosage adjustment necessary. Cholecalciferol: May not be adequately absorbed in patients who have malabsorption due to inadequate bile production.

Additional Information Complete prescribing information should be consulted for additional detail.

Dosage Forms Excipient information presented when available (limited, particularly for generics); consult specific product labeling.

Tablet:
Fosamax Plus D® 70/2800: Alendronate 70 mg and cholecalciferol 2800 units
Fosamax Plus D® 70/5600: Alendronate 70 mg and cholecalciferol 5600 units

- **Alendronate-FC (Can)** *see* Alendronate *on page 69*
- **Alendronate Sodium** *see* Alendronate *on page 69*
- **Alendronate Sodium and Cholecalciferol** *see* Alendronate and Cholecalciferol *on page 71*
- **Alendronic Acid Monosodium Salt Trihydrate** *see* Alendronate *on page 69*
- **Aler-Dryl [OTC]** *see* DiphenhydrAMINE (Systemic) *on page 622*
- **Alertec® (Can)** *see* Modafinil *on page 1390*
- **Alesse (Can)** *see* Ethinyl Estradiol and Levonorgestrel *on page 787*
- **Aleve [OTC]** *see* Naproxen *on page 1425*
- **Alfenta** *see* Alfentanil *on page 71*
- **Alfenta® (Can)** *see* Alfentanil *on page 71*

Alfentanil (al FEN ta nil)

Brand Names: U.S. Alfenta

Brand Names: Canada Alfentanil Injection, USP; Alfenta®

Index Terms Alfentanil Hydrochloride

Pharmacologic Category Analgesic, Opioid; Anilidopiperidine Opioid

Use Analgesic adjunct for the induction and maintenance of general anesthesia; analgesic component for monitored anesthesia care (MAC)

Pregnancy Risk Factor C

Pregnancy Considerations Adverse events were observed in some animal reproduction studies. Alfentanil is known to cross the placenta, which may result in severe respiratory depression in the newborn (Mattingly, 2003). When used for pain relief during labor, opioids may temporarily affect the heart rate of the fetus (ACOG, 2002). Use during labor and delivery is not recommended by the manufacturer.

Breast-Feeding Considerations Alfentanil is excreted into breast milk. Significant concentrations were observed in breast milk following administration of alfentanil 60 mcg/kg to nine women who underwent postpartum tubal ligation; concentrations were undetectable after 28 hours. The manufacturer recommends that caution be used if administered to nursing women. Parenteral opioids used during labor have the potential to interfere with a newborn's natural reflex to nurse within the first few hours after birth. Nursing infants exposed to large doses of opioids should be monitored for apnea and sedation (Montgomery, 2012).

Contraindications Hypersensitivity to alfentanil hydrochloride, to opioids, or any component of the formulation; increased intracranial pressure, severe respiratory depression

Warnings/Precautions Use with caution in patients with drug dependence, head injury, morbid obesity, acute asthma and respiratory conditions; hypotension has occurred in neonates with respiratory distress syndrome; use caution when administering to patients with bradyarrhythmias; inject slowly over 3-5 minutes (rapid I.V. infusion may result in skeletal muscle and chest wall rigidity, impaired ventilation, or respiratory distress/arrest); use of a nondepolarizing skeletal muscle relaxant may be required. Alfentanil may produce more hypotension compared to fentanyl, therefore, administer slowly and ensure patient has adequate hydration. Shares the toxic potentials of opioid agonists, and precautions of opioid agonist therapy should be observed. Should be administered by trained individuals. Safety and efficacy have not been established in children <12 years old.

Adverse Reactions

>10%:

Cardiovascular: Bradycardia, peripheral vasodilation

Central nervous system: Drowsiness, sedation, intracranial pressure increased

Endocrine & metabolic: Antidiuretic hormone release

Gastrointestinal: Nausea, vomiting, constipation

Ocular: Miosis

1% to 10%:

Cardiovascular: Cardiac arrhythmia, orthostatic hypotension

Central nervous system: Confusion, CNS depression

Ocular: Blurred vision

<1% (Limited to important or life-threatening): Convulsions, mental depression, paradoxical CNS excitation or delirium, dizziness, dysesthesia, rash, urticaria, itching, biliary tract spasm, urinary tract spasm, respiratory depression, bronchospasm, laryngospasm, physical and psychological dependence with prolonged use; cold, clammy skin

Drug Interactions

Metabolism/Transport Effects Substrate of CYP3A4 (major); **Note:** Assignment of Major/Minor substrate status based on clinically relevant drug interaction potential

Avoid Concomitant Use

Avoid concomitant use of Alfentanil with any of the following: Azelastine (Nasal); Conivaptan; Crizotinib; Enzalutamide; Fusidic Acid (Systemic); MAO Inhibitors; Paraldehyde

Increased Effect/Toxicity

Alfentanil may increase the levels/effects of: Alcohol (Ethyl); Alvimopan; Azelastine (Nasal); Beta-Blockers; Calcium Channel Blockers (Nondihydropyridine); CNS Depressants; Desmopressin; Diuretics; Hydrocodone; MAO Inhibitors; Metyrosine; Mirtazapine; Paraldehyde; Pramipexole; Propofol; ROPINIRole; Rotigotine; Selective Serotonin Reuptake Inhibitors; Zolpidem

The levels/effects of Alfentanil may be increased by: Amphetamines; Anticholinergics; Antifungal Agents (Azole Derivatives, Systemic); Antipsychotic Agents (Phenothiazines); Brimonidine (Topical); Cannabinoids; Cimetidine; Conivaptan; Crizotinib; CYP3A4 Inhibitors (Moderate); CYP3A4 Inhibitors (Strong); Dasatinib; Diltiazem; Doxylamine; Droperidol; Fluconazole; Fusidic Acid (Systemic); HydrOXYzine; Ivacaftor; Luliconazole; Macrolide Antibiotics; Magnesium Sulfate; MAO Inhibitors; Mifepristone; Perampanel; Simeprevir; Sodium Oxybate; Succinylcholine; Tapentadol

Decreased Effect

Alfentanil may decrease the levels/effects of: Pegvisomant

The levels/effects of Alfentanil may be decreased by: Ammonium Chloride; Enzalutamide; Mixed Agonist / Antagonist Opioids; Rifamycin Derivatives

Storage/Stability Store unopened ampuls at 20°C to 25°C (68°F to 77°F). Protect from light. For infusion, dilute in D_5W, NS, LR, or D_5NS to a concentration of 25-80 mcg/mL.

Mechanism of Action Binds with stereospecific receptors at many sites within the CNS, increases pain threshold, alters pain perception, inhibits ascending pain pathways; is an ultra short-acting opioid

Pharmacodynamics/Kinetics

Onset of action: Rapid

Duration (dose dependent): 30-60 minutes

Distribution: V_d: Newborns, premature: 1 L/kg; Children: 0.163-0.48 L/kg; Adults: 0.46 L/kg

Half-life elimination: Newborns, premature: 5.33-8.75 hours; Children: 40-60 minutes; Adults: 83-97 minutes

Dosage Doses should be titrated to appropriate effects; wide range of doses is dependent upon desired degree of analgesia/anesthesia

Children <12 years: Dose not established

Adults: Dose should be based on ideal body weight as follows (see table):

Alfentanil

Indication	Approx Duration of Anesthesia (min)	Induction Period (Initial Dose) (mcg/kg)	Maintenance Period (Increments/ Infusion)	Total Dose (mcg/kg)	Effects
Incremental injection	≤30	8-20	3-5 mcg/kg or 0.5-1 mcg/kg/min	8-40	Spontaneously breathing or assisted ventilation when required.
	30-60	20-50	5-15 mcg/kg	Up to 75	Assisted or controlled ventilation required. Attenuation of response to laryngoscopy and intubation.
Continuous infusion	>45	50-75	0.5-3 mcg/kg/min; average infusion rate 1-1.5 mcg/kg/min	Dependent on duration of procedure	Assisted or controlled ventilation required. Some attenuation of response to intubation and incision, with intraoperative stability.
Anesthetic induction	>45	130-245	0.5-1.5 mcg/kg/min or general anesthetic	Dependent on duration of procedure	Assisted or controlled ventilation required. Administer slowly (over 3 minutes). Concentration of inhalation agents reduced by 30% to 50% for initial hour.

Dosage adjustment in renal impairment: No dosage adjustment provided in manufacturer's labeling; use with caution.

Dosage adjustment in hepatic impairment: No dosage adjustment provided in manufacturer's labeling; use with caution.

Usual Infusion Concentrations: Adult I.V. infusion: 10 mg in 250 mL (total volume) (concentration: 40 **mcg/**mL) of D_5W or NS

Administration Administer I.V. slowly over 3-5 minutes or by I.V. continuous infusion.

Monitoring Parameters Respiratory rate, blood pressure, heart rate

Reference Range 100-340 ng/mL (depending upon procedure)

Additional Information Alfentanil may produce more muscle rigidity compared to fentanyl; therefore, be sure to administer slowly.

Dosage Forms Excipient information presented when available (limited, particularly for generics); consult specific product labeling.

Injectable, Injection [preservative free]:

Alfenta: 500 mcg/mL (2 mL, 5 mL)

Generic: 500 mcg/mL (2 mL, 5 mL)

Controlled Substance C-II

◆ **Alfentanil Hydrochloride** *see* Alfentanil *on page 71*

◆ **Alfentanil Injection, USP (Can)** *see* Alfentanil *on page 71*

◆ **Alferon N** *see* Interferon Alfa-n3 *on page 1104*

◆ **Alferon® N (Can)** *see* Interferon Alfa-n3 *on page 1104*

Alfuzosin (al FYOO zoe sin)

Brand Names: U.S. Uroxatral

Brand Names: Canada Apo-Alfuzosin®; Sandoz-Alfuzosin; Teva-Alfuzosin PR; Xatral

Index Terms Alfuzosin Hydrochloride

Pharmacologic Category Alpha$_1$ Blocker

Use Treatment of the functional symptoms of benign prostatic hyperplasia (BPH)

Unlabeled Use Facilitation of expulsion of ureteral stones

Pregnancy Risk Factor B

Pregnancy Considerations Adverese effects were not observed in animal reproduction studies.

Contraindications Hypersensitivity to alfuzosin or any component of the formulation; moderate or severe hepatic insufficiency (Child-Pugh class B and C); concurrent use with potent CYP3A4 inhibitors (eg, itraconazole, ketoconazole, ritonavir) or other alpha$_1$-blocking agents

Warnings/Precautions Not intended for use as an antihypertensive drug. May cause significant orthostatic hypotension and syncope, especially with first dose; anticipate a similar effect if therapy is interrupted for a few days, if dosage is rapidly increased, or used with antihypertensives (particularly vasodilators), PDE-5 inhibitors, nitrates or other medications which may result in hypotension. Discontinue if symptoms of angina occur or worsen. Alfuzosin has been shown to prolong the QT interval alone (minimal) and with other drugs with comparable effects on the QT interval (additive); use with caution in patients with known QT prolongation (congenital or acquired). Patients should be cautioned about performing hazardous tasks when starting new therapy or adjusting dosage upward. Discontinue if symptoms of angina occur or worsen. Rule out prostatic carcinoma before beginning therapy. Use caution with severe renal or mild hepatic impairment; contraindicated in moderate-to-severe hepatic impairment. Intraoperative floppy iris syndrome has been observed in cataract surgery patients who were on or were previously treated with alpha$_1$-blockers. Causality has not been established and there appears to be no benefit in discontinuing alpha-blocker therapy prior to surgery. May cause priapism. Contraindicated in patients taking strong CYP3A4 inhibitors or other alpha$_1$-blockers.

Adverse Reactions

1% to 10%:

Central nervous system: Dizziness (6%), fatigue (3%), headache (3%), pain (1% to 2%)

Gastrointestinal: Abdominal pain (1% to 2%), constipation (1% to 2%), dyspepsia (1% to 2%), nausea (1% to 2%)

Genitourinary: Impotence (1% to 2%)

Respiratory: Upper respiratory tract infection (3%), bronchitis (1% to 2%), pharyngitis (1% to 2%), sinusitis (1% to 2%)

<1% (Limited to important or life-threatening): Angina pectoris (pre-existing CAD), angioedema, atrial fibrillation, chest pain, edema, hepatic injury (including cholestatic), hypotension, intraoperative floppy iris syndrome (with cataract surgery), orthostatic hypotension, priapism, pruritus, syncope, tachycardia, thrombocytopenia

Drug Interactions

Metabolism/Transport Effects Substrate of CYP3A4 (major); **Note:** Assignment of Major/Minor substrate status based on clinically relevant drug interaction potential

Avoid Concomitant Use

Avoid concomitant use of Alfuzosin with any of the following: Alpha1-Blockers; CYP3A4 Inhibitors (Strong); Fusidic Acid (Systemic); Highest Risk QTc-Prolonging Agents; Ivabradine; Mifepristone; Protease Inhibitors; Telaprevir

Increased Effect/Toxicity

Alfuzosin may increase the levels/effects of: Alpha1-Blockers; Antihypertensives; Calcium Channel Blockers; Highest Risk QTc-Prolonging Agents; Moderate Risk QTc-Prolonging Agents; Nitroglycerin

The levels/effects of Alfuzosin may be increased by: Beta-Blockers; CYP3A4 Inhibitors (Moderate); CYP3A4 Inhibitors (Strong); Dasatinib; Fusidic Acid (Systemic); Ivabradine; Ivacaftor; Luliconazole; MAO Inhibitors; Mifepristone; Phosphodiesterase 5 Inhibitors; Protease Inhibitors; QTc-Prolonging Agents (Indeterminate Risk and Risk Modifying); Simeprevir; Telaprevir

Decreased Effect

Alfuzosin may decrease the levels/effects of: Alpha-/Beta-Agonists; Alpha1-Agonists

The levels/effects of Alfuzosin may be decreased by: Bosentan; CYP3A4 Inducers (Strong); Dabrafenib; Deferasirox; Herbs (CYP3A4 Inducers); Mitotane; Tocilizumab

Ethanol/Nutrition/Herb Interactions

Food: Food increases the extent of absorption. Management: Administer immediately following a meal at the same time each day.

Herb/Nutraceutical: St John's wort may decrease alfuzosin levels. Management: Avoid St John's wort.

Storage/Stability Store at room temperature of 25°C (77°F); excursions permitted to 15°C to 30°C (59°F to 86°F). Protect from light and moisture.

Mechanism of Action An antagonist of alpha$_1$-adrenoreceptors in the lower urinary tract. Smooth muscle tone is mediated by the sympathetic nervous stimulation of alpha$_1$-adrenoreceptors, which are abundant in the prostate, prostatic capsule, prostatic urethra, and bladder neck. Blockade of these adrenoreceptors can cause smooth muscles in the bladder neck and prostate to relax, resulting in an improvement in urine flow rate and a reduction in BPH symptoms.

Pharmacodynamics/Kinetics

Absorption: Decreased 50% under fasting conditions

Distribution: V_d: 3.2 L/kg

Protein binding: 82% to 90%

Metabolism: Hepatic, primarily via CYP3A4; metabolism includes oxidation, O-demethylation, and N-dealkylation; forms metabolites (inactive)

Bioavailability: 49% following a meal

Half-life elimination: 10 hours

Time to peak, plasma: 8 hours following a meal

Excretion: Feces (69%); urine (24%; 11% as unchanged drug)

Dosage Oral: Adults:

Benign prostatic hyperplasia (BPH): 10 mg once daily

Ureteral stones, expulsion (unlabeled use): 10 mg once daily, discontinue after successful expulsion (average time to expulsion 1-2 weeks) (Agrawal, 2009; Ahmed, 2010; Gurbuz, 2011). **Note:** Patients with stones >10 mm were excluded from studies.

Dosage adjustment in renal impairment: Bioavailability and maximum serum concentrations are increased by ~50% with mild (Cl_{cr} 60-80 mL/minute), moderate (Cl_{cr} 30-59 mL/minute), or severe (Cl_{cr} <30 mL/minute) renal impairment.

Note: Safety data is limited in patients with severe renal impairment (Cl_{cr} <30 mL/minute). Use with caution.

Dosage adjustment in hepatic impairment:

Mild hepatic impairment: Use has not been studied; use caution

Moderate or severe hepatic impairment (Child-Pugh class B or C): Clearance is decreased 1/3 to 1/4 and serum concentration is increased three- to fourfold; use is contraindicated

Dietary Considerations Take immediately following a meal at the same time each day.

Administration Tablet should be swallowed whole; do not crush or chew. Administer once daily (immediately following a meal); should be taken at the same time each day.

Monitoring Parameters Urine flow, blood pressure, PSA

Dosage Forms Excipient information presented when available (limited, particularly for generics); consult specific product labeling.

Tablet Extended Release 24 Hour, Oral, as hydrochloride:
Uroxatral: 10 mg
Generic: 10 mg

◆ Alfuzosin Hydrochloride *see* Alfuzosin *on page 73*

◆ Alglucosidase *see* Alglucosidase Alfa *on page 74*

Alglucosidase Alfa (al gloo KOSE i dase AL fa)

Brand Names: U.S. Lumizyme; Myozyme

Brand Names: Canada Myozyme®

Index Terms Alglucosidase; GAA; rhGAA

Pharmacologic Category Enzyme

Use

Lumizyme®: Replacement therapy for late-onset (noninfantile) Pompe disease without evidence of cardiac hypertrophy in patients 8 years and older

Myozyme®: Replacement therapy for infantile-onset Pompe disease

Pregnancy Risk Factor B

Prescribing and Access Restrictions As a requirement of the REMS program, access to this medication is restricted. Lumizyme® is available only through Lumizyme® ACE (Alglucosidase Alfa Control and Education) program; only trained and certified prescribers and healthcare facilities enrolled in the program may prescribe, dispense, or administer Lumizyme®. Patients must be enrolled in and meet all the conditions of the program to receive therapy. For enrollment, call 1-800-745-4447.

Access to Myozyme® is restricted by the manufacturer, and allowed only to patients <8 years of age with infantile-onset or late-onset Pompe disease (who are restricted from access to Lumizyme®) or to patients of any age with a diagnosis of infantile-onset Pompe disease or evidence of cardiac hypertrophy. To obtain Myozyme®, call 1-800-745-4447; no formal distribution program is established, but availability is controlled by Genzyme.

Dosage I.V.: Replacement therapy for Pompe disease:

Infantile-onset (Myozyme®):

Children 1 month to 3.5 years (at first infusion): 20 mg/kg over ~4 hours every 2 weeks

Children >3.5 years and Adults (unlabeled use): 20 mg/kg over ~4 hours every 2 weeks

Noninfantile, late-onset (Lumizyme®):

Children <8 years: Not recommended

Children ≥8 years and Adults: 20 mg/kg over ~4 hours every 2 weeks

Dosage adjustment in renal impairment: No dosage adjustment provided in the manufacturer's labeling.

Dosage adjustment in hepatic impairment: No dosage adjustment provided in the manufacturer's labeling.

Additional Information Complete prescribing information should be consulted for additional detail.

Dosage Forms Excipient information presented when available (limited, particularly for generics); consult specific product labeling.

Solution Reconstituted, Intravenous [preservative free]:
Lumizyme: 50 mg (1 ea) [contains polysorbate 80]
Myozyme: 50 mg (1 ea)

◆ Alimta *see* PEMEtrexed *on page 1601*

◆ Alinia *see* Nitazoxanide *on page 1463*

Aliskiren (a lis KYE ren)

Brand Names: U.S. Tekturna

Brand Names: Canada Rasilez

Index Terms Aliskiren Hemifumarate; SPP100

Pharmacologic Category Renin Inhibitor

Additional Appendix Information

Angiotensin Agents *on page 2280*

Use Hypertension: Treatment of hypertension, alone or in combination with other antihypertensive agents

Pregnancy Risk Factor D

Pregnancy Considerations [U.S. Boxed Warning]: Drugs that act on the renin-angiotensin system can cause injury and death to the developing fetus. Discontinue as soon as possible once pregnancy is detected. The use of drugs which act on the renin-angiotensin system are associated with oligohydramnios. Oligohydramnios, due to decreased fetal renal function, may lead to fetal lung hypoplasia and skeletal malformations. Use is also associated with anuria, hypotension, renal failure, skull hypoplasia, and death in the fetus/neonate. The exposed fetus should be monitored for fetal growth, amniotic fluid volume, and organ formation. Infants exposed *in utero* should be monitored for hyperkalemia, hypotension, and oliguria.

Breast-Feeding Considerations It is not known if aliskiren is excreted in breast milk. Due to the potential for serious adverse reactions in the nursing infant, a decision should be made whether to discontinue nursing or to discontinue the drug, taking into account the importance of treatment to the mother.

Contraindications

U.S. labeling: Concomitant use with an ACE inhibitor or ARB in patients with diabetes mellitus

Canada labeling: Additional contraindications (not in U.S. labeling): Hypersensitivity to aliskiren or any component of the formulation; history of angioedema with aliskiren, ACE inhibitors, or ARBs; hereditary or idiopathic angioedema; concomitant use with ACE inhibitors or ARBs in patients with GFR <60 mL/minute/1.73 m^2

Warnings/Precautions [U.S. Boxed Warning]: Drugs that act on the renin-angiotensin system can cause injury and death to the developing fetus. Discontinue as soon as possible once pregnancy is detected. Hypersensitivity reactions, including anaphylaxis and angioedema have been reported; since the effect of aliskiren on bradykinin levels is unknown, the risk of kinin-mediated etiologies of angioedema occurring is also unknown. Use with caution in any patient with a history of angioedema (of any etiology) as angioedema, some cases necessitating hospitalization and intubation, has been observed (rarely) with aliskiren use. Discontinue immediately following the occurrence of anaphylaxis or angioedema; do not readminister. Prolonged frequent monitoring may be required especially if tongue, glottis, or larynx are involved as they are associated with airway obstruction. Patients with a history of airway surgery may have a higher risk of airway obstruction. Early, aggressive, and appropriate management is critical. Hyperkalemia may occur (rarely) during monotherapy; risk may increase in patients with predisposing factors (eg, renal dysfunction, diabetes mellitus or concomitant use with ACE inhibitors, potassium-sparing diuretics, potassium supplements, and/or potassium-containing salts). Symptomatic hypotension may occur (rarely) during the initiation of therapy, particularly in volume or salt-depleted patients or with concomitant use of other agents acting on the renin-angiotensin-aldosterone system. If hypotension does occur, this is not a contraindication for further use; once blood pressure has been stabilized, aliskiren usually can be continued without difficulty. Use with caution or avoid in patients with deteriorating renal function or low renal blood flow (eg, renal artery stenosis, severe heart failure); may increase risk of developing acute renal failure and hyperkalemia. Concomitant use with an ACE inhibitor or ARB may increase risk of developing acute renal failure and should be avoided in patient with GFR <60 mL/minute. Use (monotherapy or combined with ACE inhibitors or ARBs) in patients with type 2 diabetes mellitus has demonstrated an increased incidence of renal impairment, hypotension, and hyperkalemia; use is contraindicated in patients with diabetes mellitus who are taking an ACE inhibitor or ARB. Potentially significant drug-drug interactions may exist, requiring dose or frequency adjustment, additional monitoring, and/or selection of alternative therapy.

Adverse Reactions

1% to 10%:

- Dermatologic: Skin rash (1%)
- Endocrine & metabolic: Hyperkalemia (monotherapy ≤1%; may be increased with concurrent ACE inhibitor or ARB)
- Gastrointestinal: Diarrhea (2%)
- Neuromuscular & skeletal: Increased creatine kinase (>300 increase%: 1%)
- Renal: Increased blood urea nitrogen (≤7%), increased serum creatinine (≤7%)
- Respiratory: Cough (1%)

<1% (Limited to important or life-threatening): Anaphylaxis, angina, angioedema, gastroesophageal reflux disease, hepatic insufficiency, increased liver enzymes, increased uric acid, myositis, periorbital edema, rhabdomyolysis, seizure, severe hypotension, Stevens-Johnson syndrome, toxic epidermal necrolysis

Drug Interactions

Metabolism/Transport Effects Substrate of CYP3A4 (minor), P-glycoprotein; **Note:** Assignment of Major/Minor substrate status based on clinically relevant drug interaction potential

Avoid Concomitant Use

Avoid concomitant use of Aliskiren with any of the following: CycloSPORINE (Systemic); Itraconazole

Increased Effect/Toxicity

Aliskiren may increase the levels/effects of: ACE Inhibitors; Amifostine; Angiotensin II Receptor Blockers; Antihypertensives; Hypotensive Agents; Obinutuzumab; RiTUXimab

The levels/effects of Aliskiren may be increased by: Alfuzosin; AtorvaSTATin; Brimonidine (Topical); Canagliflozin; CycloSPORINE (Systemic); Diazoxide; Heparin; Heparin (Low Molecular Weight); Herbs (Hypotensive Properties); Itraconazole; Ketoconazole (Systemic); MAO Inhibitors; Nonsteroidal Anti-Inflammatory Agents; Pentoxifylline; P-glycoprotein/ABCB1 Inhibitors; Phosphodiesterase 5 Inhibitors; Prostacyclin Analogues; Verapamil

Decreased Effect

Aliskiren may decrease the levels/effects of: Furosemide

The levels/effects of Aliskiren may be decreased by: Grapefruit Juice; Herbs (Hypertensive Properties); Methylphenidate; Nonsteroidal Anti-Inflammatory Agents; P-glycoprotein/ABCB1 Inducers; Yohimbine

Ethanol/Nutrition/Herb Interactions

Food: High-fat meals decrease absorption. Grapefruit juice may decrease the serum concentration of aliskiren. Management: Administer at the same time each day; may take with or without a meal, but consistent administration with regards to meals is recommended. Avoid concomitant use of aliskiren and grapefruit juice.

Herb/Nutraceutical: Some herbal medications may worsen hypertension (eg, licorice); others may increase the antihypertensive effect of aliskiren (eg, shepherd's purse). Management: Avoid bayberry, blue cohosh, cayenne, ephedra, ginger, ginseng (American), kola, licorice, and yohimbe. Avoid black cohosh, California poppy, coleus, golden seal, hawthorn, mistletoe, periwinkle, quinine, and shepherd's purse.

Storage/Stability Store at 25°C (77°F); excursions permitted to 15°C to 30°C (59°F to 86°F). Protect from moisture.

Mechanism of Action Aliskiren is a direct renin inhibitor, resulting in blockade of the conversion of angiotensinogen to angiotensin I. Angiotensin I suppression decreases the formation of angiotensin II (Ang II), a potent blood pressure-elevating peptide (via direct vasoconstriction, aldosterone release, and sodium retention). Ang II also functions within the Renin-Angiotensin-Aldosterone System (RAAS) as a negative inhibitory feedback mediator within the renal parenchyma to suppress the further release of renin. Thus, reductions in Ang II levels suppress this feedback loop, leading to further increased plasma renin concentrations (PRC) and subsequent activity (PRA). This disinhibition effect can be potentially problematic for ACE inhibitor and ARB therapy, as increased PRA could partially overcome the pharmacologic inhibition of the RAAS. As aliskiren is a direct inhibitor of renin activity, blunting of PRA despite the increased PRC (from loss of the negative feedback) may be clinically advantageous. The effect of aliskiren on bradykinin levels is unknown.

Pharmacodynamics/Kinetics

Onset of action: Maximum antihypertensive effect: Within 2 weeks

Absorption: Poor; absorption decreased by high-fat meal. Aliskiren is a substrate of P-glycoprotein; concurrent use of P-glycoprotein inhibitors may increase absorption.

Metabolism: Extent of metabolism unknown; *in vitro* studies indicate metabolism via CYP3A4

Bioavailability: ~3%

Half-life elimination: ~24 hours (range: 16-32 hours)

Time to peak, plasma: 1-3 hours

Excretion: Urine (~25% of absorbed dose excreted unchanged in urine); feces (unchanged via biliary excretion)

Dosage Oral:

Adults: Initial: 150 mg once daily; may increase to 300 mg once daily (maximum: 300 mg daily). **Note:** Prior to initiation, correct hypovolemia and/or closely monitor volume status in patients on concurrent diuretics during treatment initiation.

Elderly: No initial dosage adjustment required

Dosage adjustment in renal impairment:

Cl_{cr} ≥30 mL/minute: Initial: No dosage adjustment necessary.

Cl_{cr} <30 mL/minute: Initial: No dosage adjustment may be necessary (Vaidyanathan, 2007); however, risk of hyperkalemia and progressive renal dysfunction may occur; use with caution.

ESRD (requiring hemodialysis): Initial: No dosage adjustment may be necessary (Khadzhynov, 2012); however, with chronic therapy, risk of hyperkalemia is increased; use with extreme caution. **Note:** Hemodialysis eliminates a minimal fraction; does not significantly alter overall aliskiren exposure.

Dosage adjustment in hepatic impairment: Mild-to-severe: Initial: No dosage adjustment necessary.

Dietary Considerations May be taken with or without food; however, a high-fat meal reduces absorption. Consistent administration with regards to meals is recommended.

Administration Administer at the same time daily; may take with or without a meal, but consistent administration with regards to meals is recommended.

Monitoring Parameters Blood pressure; serum potassium, BUN, serum creatinine

Dosage Forms Excipient information presented when available (limited, particularly for generics); consult specific product labeling.

Tablet, Oral:

Tekturna: 150 mg, 300 mg

Aliskiren, Amlodipine, and Hydrochlorothiazide

(a lis KYE ren, am LOE di peen, & hye droe klor oh THYE a zide)

Brand Names: U.S. Amturnide™

Index Terms Aliskiren, Hydrochlorothiazide, and Amlodipine; Amlodipine Besylate, Aliskiren Hemifumarate, and Hydrochlorothiazide; Amlodipine, Aliskiren, and Hydrochlorothiazide; Amlodipine, Hydrochlorothiazide, and Aliskiren; Hydrochlorothiazide, Aliskiren, and Amlodipine; Hydrochlorothiazide, Amlodipine, and Aliskiren

Pharmacologic Category Antianginal Agent; Antihypertensive; Calcium Channel Blocker; Calcium Channel Blocker, Dihydropyridine; Diuretic, Thiazide; Renin Inhibitor

Use Treatment of hypertension (not for initial therapy)

Pregnancy Risk Factor D

Dosage Note: Not for initial therapy. Dose is individualized; combination product may be substituted for individual components in patients currently maintained on all three agents separately, used to switch a patient on any dual combination of the components who is experiencing dose-limiting adverse reactions from an individual component (to a lower dose of that component), or used as add-on therapy in patients not adequately controlled with any two of the following: Aliskiren, dihydropyridine calcium channel blockers, and thiazide diuretics.

Oral: Hypertension: Add-on/switch therapy/replacement therapy:

Adults: Aliskiren 150-300 mg and amlodipine 5-10 mg and hydrochlorothiazide 12.5-25 mg once daily; dose may be titrated after 2 weeks of therapy. Maximum recommended daily dose: Aliskiren 300 mg; amlodipine 10 mg; hydrochlorothiazide 25 mg

Elderly: Use of lower initial doses should be considered (use of individual components may be necessary).

Dosage adjustment in renal impairment:

Cl_{cr} ≥30 mL/minute: Initial: No dosage adjustment necessary.

Cl_{cr} <30 mL/minute: Initial: No dosage adjustment may be necessary (Vaidyanathan, 2007 [aliskiren]); however, risk of hyperkalemia and progressive renal dysfunction may occur with aliskiren; use with caution; hydrochlorothiazide is usually ineffective when Cl_{cr} <30 mL/minute and is contraindicated in patients who are anuric.

ESRD (requiring hemodialysis): Initial: No dosage adjustment may be necessary (Khadzhynov, 2012 [aliskiren]); however, risk of hyperkalemia is increased with chronic aliskiren therapy; use with extreme caution; hydrochlorothiazide is usually ineffective when Cl_{cr} <30 mL/minute and is contraindicated in patients who are anuric.

Dosage adjustment in hepatic impairment: Mild-to-severe: Use with caution and titrate slowly; amlodipine elimination prolonged; lower initial dose should be considered (possibly requiring use of the individual agents).

Additional Information Complete prescribing information should be consulted for additional detail.

Dosage Forms Excipient information presented when available (limited, particularly for generics); consult specific product labeling.

Tablet, oral:

Amturnide: Aliskiren 150 mg, amlodipine 5 mg, and hydrochlorothiazide 12.5 mg

Amturnide: Aliskiren 300 mg, amlodipine 5 mg, and hydrochlorothiazide 12.5 mg

Amturnide: Aliskiren 300 mg, amlodipine 5 mg, and hydrochlorothiazide 25 mg

Amturnide: Aliskiren 300 mg, amlodipine 10 mg, and hydrochlorothiazide 12.5 mg

Amturnide: Aliskiren 300 mg, amlodipine 10 mg, and hydrochlorothiazide 25 mg

Aliskiren and Hydrochlorothiazide

(a lis KYE ren & hye droe klor oh THYE a zide)

Brand Names: U.S. Tekturna HCT

Brand Names: Canada Rasilez HCT®

Index Terms Aliskiren Hemifumarate and Hydrochlorothiazide; Hydrochlorothiazide and Aliskiren

Pharmacologic Category Antihypertensive; Diuretic, Thiazide; Renin Inhibitor

Use Treatment of hypertension, including use as initial therapy in patients likely to need multiple antihypertensives for adequate control

Pregnancy Risk Factor D

Dosage Oral: **Note:** Dosage must be individualized. Combination product may be used as initial therapy or substituted for individual components in patients currently maintained on both agents separately or in patients not adequately controlled with monotherapy (using one of the agents or an agent within same antihypertensive class).

Adults: Hypertension:

Initial therapy: Aliskiren 150 mg and hydrochlorothiazide 12.5 mg once daily, dose may be titrated at 2- to 4-week intervals; maximum recommended daily doses: Aliskiren 300 mg; hydrochlorothiazide 25 mg

Add-on therapy: Initiate by adding the lowest available dose of the alternative component (aliskiren 150 mg or hydrochlorothiazide 12.5 mg); titrate to effect; maximum recommended daily doses: Aliskiren 300 mg; hydrochlorothiazide 25 mg

Replacement therapy: Substitute for the individually titrated components

Note: Prior to initiation, correct hypovolemia and/or closely monitor volume status in patients on concurrent diuretics during treatment initiation.

Elderly: No initial dosage adjustment required

Dosage adjustment in renal impairment:

Cl_{cr} ≥30 mL/minute: Initial: No dosage adjustment necessary.

Cl_{cr} <30 mL/minute: Initial: No dosage adjustment may be necessary (Vaidyanathan, 2007 [aliskiren]); however, risk of hyperkalemia and progressive renal dysfunction may occur with aliskiren; use with caution; hydrochlorothiazide is usually ineffective when Cl_{cr} <30 mL/minute and is contraindicated in patients who are anuric.

ESRD (requiring hemodialysis): Initial: No dosage adjustment may be necessary (Khadzhynov, 2012 [aliskiren]); however, risk of hyperkalemia is increased with chronic aliskiren therapy; use with extreme caution; hydrochlorothiazide is usually ineffective when Cl_{cr} <30 mL/minute and is contraindicated in patients who are anuric.

Dosage adjustment in hepatic impairment: Mild-to-severe: No dosage adjustment necessary.

Additional Information Complete prescribing information should be consulted for additional detail.

Dosage Forms Excipient information presented when available (limited, particularly for generics); consult specific product labeling.

Tablet:

Tekturna HCT:

150/12.5: Aliskiren 150 mg and hydrochlorothiazide 12.5 mg

150/25: Aliskiren 150 mg and hydrochlorothiazide 25 mg

300/12.5: Aliskiren 300 mg and hydrochlorothiazide 12.5 mg

300/25: Aliskiren 300 mg and hydrochlorothiazide 25 mg

- **Aliskiren Hemifumarate** *see* Aliskiren *on page 74*
- **Aliskiren Hemifumarate and Hydrochlorothiazide** *see* Aliskiren and Hydrochlorothiazide *on page 76*
- **Aliskiren, Hydrochlorothiazide, and Amlodipine** *see* Aliskiren, Amlodipine, and Hydrochlorothiazide *on page 76*
- **Alkeran** *see* Melphalan *on page 1286*
- **Alkeran® (Can)** *see* Melphalan *on page 1286*
- **All Day Allergy [OTC]** *see* Cetirizine *on page 396*
- **All Day Allergy Childrens [OTC]** *see* Cetirizine *on page 396*
- **All Day Pain Relief [OTC]** *see* Naproxen *on page 1425*
- **All Day Relief [OTC]** *see* Naproxen *on page 1425*
- **Allegra® (Can)** *see* Fexofenadine *on page 856*
- **Allegra-D® (Can)** *see* Fexofenadine and Pseudoephedrine *on page 858*
- **Allegra-D® 12 Hour** *see* Fexofenadine and Pseudoephedrine *on page 858*
- **Allegra-D® 24 Hour** *see* Fexofenadine and Pseudoephedrine *on page 858*
- **Allegra Allergy [OTC]** *see* Fexofenadine *on page 856*
- **Allegra Allergy Childrens [OTC]** *see* Fexofenadine *on page 856*
- **Allerdryl® (Can)** *see* DiphenhydrAMINE (Systemic) *on page 622*
- **Allerest** *see* Chlorpheniramine and Pseudoephedrine *on page 412*
- **Allergy [OTC]** *see* Loratadine *on page 1240*
- **Allergy Relief [OTC]** *see* DiphenhydrAMINE (Systemic) *on page 622*
- **Allergy Relief [OTC]** *see* Loratadine *on page 1240*
- **Allergy Relief Childrens [OTC]** *see* DiphenhydrAMINE (Systemic) *on page 622*
- **Allergy Relief For Kids [OTC]** *see* Loratadine *on page 1240*
- **Allernix (Can)** *see* DiphenhydrAMINE (Systemic) *on page 622*
- **Aller-Relief [OTC] (Can)** *see* Cetirizine *on page 396*
- **Allfen CD** *see* Guaifenesin and Codeine *on page 976*
- **Allfen CDX** *see* Guaifenesin and Codeine *on page 976*
- **Alli [OTC]** *see* Orlistat *on page 1516*
- **Alloprin® (Can)** *see* Allopurinol *on page 77*

Allopurinol (al oh PURE i nole)

Brand Names: U.S. Aloprim; Zyloprim

Brand Names: Canada Alloprin®; Novo-Purol; Zyloprim®

Index Terms Allopurinol Sodium

Pharmacologic Category Antigout Agent; Xanthine Oxidase Inhibitor

Additional Appendix Information

Desensitization Protocols *on page 2325*

Use

Oral: Management of primary or secondary gout (acute attack, tophi, joint destruction, uric acid lithiasis, and/or nephropathy); management of hyperuricemia associated with cancer treatment for leukemia, lymphoma, or solid tumor malignancies; management of recurrent calcium oxalate calculi (with uric acid excretion >800 mg/day in men and >750 mg/day in women)

I.V.: Management of hyperuricemia associated with cancer treatment for leukemia, lymphoma, or solid tumor malignancies

Pregnancy Risk Factor C

Pregnancy Considerations Adverse events were observed in some animal reproduction studies. Allopurinol crosses the placenta (Torrance, 2009). An increased risk of adverse fetal events has not been observed (limited data) (Hoeltzenbein, 2013).

Breast-Feeding Considerations Allopurinol and its metabolite are excreted into breast milk; the metabolite was also detected in the serum of the nursing infant (Kamilli, 1993). The manufacturer recommends caution be used when administering allopurinol to nursing women.

Contraindications Hypersensitivity to allopurinol or any component of the formulation

Warnings/Precautions Do not use to treat asymptomatic hyperuricemia. Has been associated with a number of hypersensitivity reactions, including severe reactions (vasculitis and Stevens-Johnson syndrome); discontinue at first sign of rash. Reversible hepatotoxicity has been reported; use with caution in patients with pre-existing hepatic impairment. Bone marrow suppression has been reported; use caution with other drugs causing myelosuppression. Caution in renal impairment, dosage adjustments needed. Use with caution in patients taking diuretics concurrently. Risk of skin rash may be increased in patients receiving amoxicillin or ampicillin. The risk of hypersensitivity may be increased in patients receiving thiazides, and possibly ACE inhibitors. Use caution with mercaptopurine or azathioprine; dosage adjustment necessary. Full effect on serum uric acid levels in chronic gout may take several weeks to become evident; gradual titration is recommended.

Adverse Reactions

Most commonly reported:

Dermatologic: Skin rash

Endocrine & metabolic: Gout (acute)

Gastrointestinal: Diarrhea, nausea

Hepatic: Increased liver enzymes, increased serum alkaline phosphatase

<1% (Limited to important or life-threatening): Ageusia, agranulocytosis, alopecia, angioedema, aplastic anemia, cataract, cholestatic jaundice, ecchymoses, eczematoid dermatitis, eosinophilia, exfoliative dermatitis, hepatic necrosis, hepatitis, hepatomegaly, hyperbilirubinemia, hypersensitivity reaction, leukocytosis, leukopenia, lichen planus, macular retinitis, myopathy, necrotizing angiitis, nephritis, neuritis, neuropathy, onycholysis, pancreatitis, purpura, renal failure, skin granuloma (annulare), Stevens-Johnson syndrome, thrombocytopenia, toxic epidermal necrolysis, toxic pustuloderma, uremia, vasculitis, vesicobullous dermatitis

Drug Interactions

Metabolism/Transport Effects None known.

Avoid Concomitant Use

Avoid concomitant use of Allopurinol with any of the following: Didanosine; Pegloticase; Tegafur

Increased Effect/Toxicity

Allopurinol may increase the levels/effects of: Amoxicillin; Ampicillin; Anticonvulsants (Hydantoin); AzaTHIOprine; Bendamustine; CarBAMazepine; ChlorproPAMIDE; Cyclophosphamide; Didanosine; Mercaptopurine; Pegloticase; Theophylline Derivatives; Vitamin K Antagonists

The levels/effects of Allopurinol may be increased by: ACE Inhibitors; Loop Diuretics; Thiazide Diuretics

Decreased Effect

Allopurinol may decrease the levels/effects of: Tegafur

The levels/effects of Allopurinol may be decreased by: Antacids

Ethanol/Nutrition/Herb Interactions

Ethanol: May decrease effectiveness.

Iron supplements: Hepatic iron uptake may be increased.

Vitamin C: Large amounts of vitamin C may acidify urine and increase kidney stone formation.

Preparation for Administration Reconstitute powder for injection with SWFI. Further dilution with NS or D_5W (50-100 mL) to ≤6 mg/mL is recommended.

Storage/Stability

Powder for injection: Store at controlled room temperature of 20°C to 25°C (68°F to 77°F). Following preparation, intravenous solutions should be stored at 20°C to 25°C (68°F to 77°F). Do not refrigerate reconstituted and/or diluted product. Must be administered within 10 hours of solution preparation.

Tablet: Store at controlled room temperature of 20°C to 25°C (68°F to 77°F). Protect from moisture and light.

Mechanism of Action Allopurinol inhibits xanthine oxidase, the enzyme responsible for the conversion of hypoxanthine to xanthine to uric acid. Allopurinol is metabolized to oxypurinol which is also an inhibitor of xanthine oxidase; allopurinol acts on purine catabolism, reducing the production of uric acid without disrupting the biosynthesis of vital purines.

Pharmacodynamics/Kinetics

Onset of action: Peak effect: 1-2 weeks

Absorption: Oral: ~80%; Rectal: Poor and erratic

Distribution: V_d: ~1.6 L/kg; V_{ss}: 0.84-0.87 L/kg; enters breast milk

Protein binding: <1%

Metabolism: ~75% to active metabolites, chiefly oxypurinol

Bioavailability: 49% to 53%

Half-life elimination:

Normal renal function: Parent drug: 1-3 hours; Oxypurinol: 18-30 hours

End-stage renal disease: Prolonged

Time to peak, plasma: Oral: 30-120 minutes

Excretion: Urine (76% as oxypurinol, 12% as unchanged drug)

Allopurinol and oxypurinol are dialyzable

Dosage Oral: **Note:** Doses >300 mg should be given in divided doses.

Management of hyperuricemia associated with chemotherapy:

Manufacturer's labeling:

Children <6 years: 150 mg/day

Children 6-10 years: 300 mg/day

Children >10 years and Adults: 600-800 mg/day in 2-3 divided doses

Alternative recommendations (unlabeled dosing; intermediate-risk for tumor lysis syndrome): Children and Adults: Intermediate-risk for tumor lysis syndrome: 10 mg/kg/day (maximum dose/day: 800 mg) in 3 divided doses **or** 50-100 mg/m^2 every 8 hours (maximum dose: 300 mg/m^2/day), begin 1-2 days before initiation of induction chemotherapy; may continue for 3-7 days after chemotherapy (Coiffier, 2008)

Gout (chronic): Adults:

Manufacturer's labeling: Mild: 200-300 mg/day; Severe: 400-600 mg/day; to reduce the possibility of acute gouty attacks, initiate dose at 100 mg/day and increase weekly to recommended dosage, also consider using low-dose colchicine or an NSAID to reduce the risk of a gouty attack. Maximum daily dose: 800 mg/day.

Alternative recommendations (unlabeled dosing): Initial: 100 mg/day, increasing the dose gradually every 4 weeks, while monitoring plasma uric acid levels to achieve a goal of <6 mg/dL; dosages of 600 mg/day and rarely, 900 mg/day may be required (McGill, 2010) **or** Initial: 100 mg/day, increasing the dose by 100 mg/day at 2-4 weeks intervals as required to achieve desired uric acid level of ≤6 mg/dL (EULAR gout guidelines; Zhang, 2006).

Recurrent calcium oxalate stones: Adults: 200-300 mg/day in single or divided doses

I.V.:

Management of hyperuricemia associated with chemotherapy: Note: Intravenous daily dose can be given as a single infusion or in equally divided doses at 6-, 8-, or 12-hour intervals.

Manufacturer's labeling:

Children: Starting dose: 200 mg/m^2/day beginning 1-2 days before chemotherapy

Adults: 200-400 mg/m^2/day (maximum: 600 mg/day) beginning 1-2 days before chemotherapy

Alternative recommendations (unlabeled dosing; intermediate-risk for tumor lysis syndrome): Children and Adults: 200-400 mg/m^2/day (maximum dose/day: 600 mg) in 1-3 divided doses beginning 1-2 days before the start of induction chemotherapy; may continue for 3-7 days after chemotherapy (Coiffier, 2008)

Note: Adequate fluid intake is desirable. A fluid intake sufficient to yield a daily urinary output of at least 2 L in adults is desirable.

Dosing adjustment in renal impairment:

Manufacturer's labeling: Oral, I.V.: Lower doses are required in renal impairment due to potential for accumulation of allopurinol and metabolites.

Cl_{cr} 10-20 mL/minute: 200 mg/day

Cl_{cr} 3-10 mL/minute: ≤100 mg/day

Cl_{cr} <3 mL/minute: 100 mg/dose at extended intervals

Alternative recommendations (unlabeled dosing):

Management of hyperuricemia associated with chemotherapy: Dosage reduction of 50% is recommended in renal impairment (Coiffier, 2008)

Gout: Oral:

Initiate therapy with 50-100 mg daily, and gradually increase to a maintenance dose to achieve a serum uric acid level of ≤6 mg/dL (with close monitoring of serum uric acid levels and for hypersensitivity) (Dalbeth, 2007).

Hemodialysis: Initial: 100 mg alternate days given post-dialysis, increase cautiously to 300 mg based on response. If dialysis is on a daily basis, an additional 50% of the dose may be required postdialysis (Dalbeth, 2007)

Dietary Considerations Should take oral forms after meals with plenty of fluid. Fluid intake should be administered to yield neutral or slightly alkaline urine and an output of ~2 L (in adults).

Administration

Oral: Do not initiate or discontinue allopurinol during an acute gout attack. Should administer oral forms after meals with plenty of fluid.

I.V.: The rate of infusion depends on the volume of the infusion; infuse maximum single daily doses (600 mg/day) over ≥30 minutes. Whenever possible, therapy should be initiated at 24-48 hours before the start of chemotherapy known to cause tumor lysis (including adrenocorticosteroids). I.V. daily dose can be administered as a single infusion or in equally divided doses at 6-, 8-, or 12-hour interval.

Monitoring Parameters CBC, serum uric acid levels, I & O, hepatic and renal function, especially at start of therapy; signs and symptoms of hypersensitivity

Reference Range Uric acid, serum: An increase occurs during childhood

Adults:

Males: 3.4-7 mg/dL or slightly more

Females: 2.4-6 mg/dL or slightly more

Target: ≤6 mg/dL

Values >7 mg/dL are sometimes arbitrarily regarded as hyperuricemia, but there is no sharp line between normals on the one hand, and the serum uric acid of those with clinical gout. Normal ranges cannot be adjusted for purine ingestion, but high purine diet increases uric acid. Uric acid may be increased with body size, exercise, and stress.

Dosage Forms Excipient information presented when available (limited, particularly for generics); consult specific product labeling.

Solution Reconstituted, Intravenous, as sodium [preservative free]:

Aloprim: 500 mg (1 ea)

Generic: 500 mg (1 ea)

Tablet, Oral, as sodium:

Zyloprim: 100 mg, 300 mg [scored]

Generic: 100 mg, 300 mg

Extemporaneous Preparations A 20 mg/mL oral suspension may be made with tablets and either a 1:1 mixture of Ora-Sweet® and Ora-Plus® or a 1:1 mixture of Ora-Sweet® SF and Ora-Plus® or a 1:4 mixture of cherry syrup concentrate and simple syrup, NF. Crush eight 300 mg tablets in a mortar and reduce to a fine powder. Add small portions of chosen vehicle and mix to a uniform paste; mix while adding the vehicle in incremental proportions to **almost** 120 mL; transfer to a calibrated bottle, rinse mortar with vehicle, and add quantity of vehicle sufficient to make 120 mL. Label "shake well". Stable for 60 days refrigerated or at room temperature (Allen, 1996; Nahata, 2004).

Allen LV Jr and Erickson MA 3rd, "Stability of Acetazolamide, Allopurinol, Azathioprine, Clonazepam, and Flucytosine in Extemporaneously Compounded Oral Liquids," *Am J Health Syst Pharm*, 1996, 53(16):1944-9.

Nahata MC, Pai VB, and Hipple TF, *Pediatric Drug Formulations*, 5th ed, Cincinnati, OH: Harvey Whitney Books Co, 2004.

◆ **Allopurinol Sodium** *see* Allopurinol *on page 77*

◆ **All-*trans* Retinoic Acid** *see* Tretinoin (Systemic) *on page 2117*

◆ **All-*trans* Vitamin A Acid** *see* Tretinoin (Systemic) *on page 2117*

◆ **Almacone® [OTC]** *see* Aluminum Hydroxide, Magnesium Hydroxide, and Simethicone *on page 90*

◆ **Almacone® Double Strength [OTC]** *see* Aluminum Hydroxide, Magnesium Hydroxide, and Simethicone *on page 90*

Almotriptan (al moh TRIP tan)

Brand Names: U.S. Axert

Brand Names: Canada Axert; Mylan-Almotriptan; Sandoz-Almotriptan

Index Terms Almotriptan Malate

Pharmacologic Category Antimigraine Agent; Serotonin 5-$HT_{1B, 1D}$ Receptor Agonist

Additional Appendix Information

Antimigraine Drugs: 5-HT_1 Receptor Agonists *on page 2288*

Use Acute treatment of migraine with or without aura in adults (with a history of migraine) and adolescents (with a history of migraine lasting ≥4 hours when left untreated)

Pregnancy Risk Factor C

Pregnancy Considerations Adverse events were observed in animal reproduction studies. Information related to almotriptan use in pregnancy is limited (Källén, 2011; Nezvalová-Henriksen, 2010; Nezvalová-Henriksen, 2012). Until additional information is available, other agents are preferred for the initial treatment of migraine in pregnancy (Da Silva, 2012; MacGregor, 2012; Williams, 2012).

Breast-Feeding Considerations It is not known if almotriptan is excreted in breast milk. The manufacturer recommends that caution be exercised when administering almotriptan to nursing women.

Contraindications Hypersensitivity to almotriptan or any component of the formulation; hemiplegic or basilar migraine; known or suspected ischemic heart disease (eg, angina pectoris, MI, documented silent ischemia, coronary artery vasospasm, Prinzmetal's variant angina); cerebrovascular syndromes (eg, stroke, transient ischemic attacks); peripheral vascular disease (eg, ischemic bowel disease); uncontrolled hypertension; use within 24 hours of another 5-HT_1 agonist; use within 24 hours of ergotamine derivatives and/or ergotamine-containing medications (eg, dihydroergotamine, ergotamine)

Warnings/Precautions Almotriptan is only indicated for the treatment of acute migraine headache; not indicated for migraine prophylaxis, or the treatment of cluster headaches, hemiplegic migraine, or basilar migraine. If a patient does not respond to the first dose, the diagnosis of acute migraine should be reconsidered.

Almotriptan should not be given to patients with documented ischemic or vasospastic CAD. Patients with risk factors for CAD (eg, hypertension, hypercholesterolemia, smoker, obesity, diabetes, strong family history of CAD, menopause, male >40 years of age) should undergo adequate cardiac evaluation prior to administration; if the cardiac evaluation is "satisfactory," the first dose of almotriptan should be given in the healthcare provider's office (consider ECG monitoring). All patients should undergo periodic evaluation of cardiovascular status during treatment. Cardiac events (coronary artery vasospasm, transient ischemia, myocardial infarction, ventricular tachycardia/fibrillation, cardiac arrest, and death), cerebral/subarachnoid hemorrhage, stroke, peripheral vascular ischemia, and colonic ischemia have been reported with 5-HT_1 agonist administration. Patients who experience sensations of chest pain/pressure/tightness or symptoms suggestive of angina following dosing should be evaluated for coronary artery disease or Prinzmetal's angina before receiving additional doses; if dosing is resumed and similar symptoms recur, monitor with ECG. Significant elevation in blood pressure, including hypertensive crisis, has also been reported on rare occasions following 5-HT_1 agonist administration in patients with and without a history of hypertension.

Transient and permanent blindness and partial vision loss have been reported (rare) with 5-HT_1 agonist administration. Almotriptan contains a sulfonyl group which is structurally different from a sulfonamide. Cross-reactivity in patients with sulfonamide allergy has not been evaluated; however, the manufacturer recommends that caution be exercised in this patient population. Use with caution in liver or renal dysfunction. Symptoms of agitation, confusion, hallucinations, hyper-reflexia, myoclonus, shivering, and tachycardia (serotonin syndrome) may occur with concomitant proserotonergic drugs (ie, SSRIs/SNRIs or triptans) or agents which reduce almotriptan's metabolism. Concurrent use of serotonin precursors (eg, tryptophan) is not recommended. If concomitant administration with SSRIs is warranted, monitor closely, especially at initiation and with dose increases. Efficacy has not been demonstrated in improvement of migraine-associated symptoms (eg, phonophobia, nausea, photophobia) in patients aged 12-17 years (Linder, 2008).

Adverse Reactions

1% to 10%:

Central nervous system: Somnolence (≤5%), dizziness (≤4%), headache (≤2%)

Gastrointestinal: Nausea (1% to 3%), vomiting (≤2%), xerostomia (1%)

Neuromuscular & skeletal: Paresthesia (≤1%)

<1% (Limited to important or life-threatening): Anaphylactic shock, angina, angioedema, breast pain, colitis, coronary artery vasospasm, hemiplegia, hypertension, myocardial ischemia, MI, neuropathy, rash, seizure, syncope, tachycardia, ventricular fibrillation, ventricular tachycardia, vertigo

Drug Interactions

Metabolism/Transport Effects Substrate of CYP2D6 (minor), CYP3A4 (minor); **Note:** Assignment of Major/Minor substrate status based on clinically relevant drug interaction potential

Avoid Concomitant Use

Avoid concomitant use of Almotriptan with any of the following: Ergot Derivatives; MAO Inhibitors

Increased Effect/Toxicity

Almotriptan may increase the levels/effects of: Antipsychotics; Ergot Derivatives; Metoclopramide; Serotonin Modulators

The levels/effects of Almotriptan may be increased by: Antipsychotics; CYP3A4 Inhibitors (Strong); Ergot Derivatives; MAO Inhibitors

Decreased Effect

The levels/effects of Almotriptan may be decreased by: Peginterferon Alfa-2b

Storage/Stability Store at 25°C (77°F); excursions permitted to 15°C to 30°C (59°F to 86°F).

Mechanism of Action Selective agonist for serotonin (5-HT_{1B} and 5-HT_{1D} receptors) in cranial arteries; causes vasoconstriction and reduces sterile inflammation associated with antidromic neuronal transmission correlating with relief of migraine

Pharmacodynamics/Kinetics

Absorption: Well absorbed

Distribution: V_d: ~180-200 L

Protein binding: ~35%

Metabolism: Via MAO type A oxidative deamination (~27% of dose) and CYP3A4 and 2D6 (~12% of dose) to inactive metabolites

Bioavailability: ~70%

Half-life elimination: 3-4 hours

Time to peak, plasma: 1-3 hours

Excretion: Urine (~75%; ~40% of total dose as unchanged drug); feces (~13% of total dose as unchanged drug and metabolites)

Dosage Oral: Children ≥12 years and Adults: Migraine: Initial: 6.25-12.5 mg in a single dose; if the headache returns, repeat the dose after 2 hours (maximum daily dose: 25 mg)

Note: The safety of treating more than 4 migraines/month has not been established.

Dosage adjustment with concomitant use of an enzyme inhibitor:

Patients receiving a potent CYP3A4 inhibitor: Initial: 6.25 mg in a single dose; maximum daily dose: 12.5 mg

Patients with renal impairment and concomitant use of a potent CYP3A4 inhibitor: Avoid use

Patients with hepatic impairment and concomitant use of a potent CYP3A4 inhibitor: Avoid use

Dosage adjustment in renal impairment: Severe renal impairment (Cl_{cr} ≤30 mL/minute): Initial: 6.25 mg in a single dose; maximum daily dose: 12.5 mg

Dosage adjustment in hepatic impairment: Initial: 6.25 mg in a single dose; maximum daily dose: 12.5 mg

Dietary Considerations May be taken without regard to meals.

Administration Administer without regard to meals.

Dosage Forms Excipient information presented when available (limited, particularly for generics); consult specific product labeling.

Tablet, Oral, as maleate:

Axert: 6.25 mg

Axert: 12.5 mg [contains fd&c blue #2 (indigotine)]

◆ Almotriptan Malate *see* Almotriptan *on page* 79

◆ Alocril *see* Nedocromil *on page* 1433

◆ Alocril® (Can) *see* Nedocromil *on page* 1433

◆ Alodox Convenience *see* Doxycycline *on page* 668

◆ Aloe Vesta Antifungal [OTC] *see* Miconazole (Topical) *on page* 1358

◆ Alomide *see* Lodoxamide *on page* 1231

◆ Alomide® (Can) *see* Lodoxamide *on page* 1231

◆ Aloprim *see* Allopurinol *on page* 77

◆ Alora *see* Estradiol (Systemic) *on page* 754

◆ Aloxi *see* Palonosetron *on page* 1554

Alpha-Galactosidase (AL fa ga lak TOE si days)

Brand Names: U.S. beano® Meltaways [OTC]; beano® [OTC]

Index Terms *Aspergillus niger*

Pharmacologic Category Enzyme

Use Prevention of flatulence and bloating attributed to a variety of grains, cereals, nuts, and vegetables

Dosage Oral: Children ≥12 years and Adults: Adjust dose according to the number of problem foods per meal:

Tablet, chewable (beano®): Usual dose: 2-3 tablets/meal

Tablet, orally disintegrating (beano® Meltaways): One tablet per meal

Dosage adjustment in renal impairment: No dosage adjustment provided in the manufacturer's labeling.

Dosage adjustment in hepatic impairment: No dosage adjustment provided in the manufacturer's labeling.

Additional Information Complete prescribing information should be consulted for additional detail.

Dosage Forms Excipient information presented when available (limited, particularly for generics); consult specific product labeling.

Tablet, chewable, oral:

beano®: 150 Galactosidase units [scored]

Tablet, orally disintegrating, oral:

beano® Meltaways: 300 Galactosidase units [strawberry flavor]

◆ Alpha-Galactosidase-A (Recombinant) *see* Agalsidase Beta *on page* 57

◆ Alphagan® (Can) *see* Brimonidine (Ophthalmic) *on page* 280

◆ 1α-Hydroxyergocalciferol *see* Doxercalciferol *on page* 660

◆ Alphanate® *see* Antihemophilic Factor/von Willebrand Factor Complex (Human) *on page* 146

◆ AlphaNine SD *see* Factor IX (Human) *on page* 825

◆ Alphaquin HP *see* Hydroquinone *on page* 1017

◆ AlphaTrex *see* Betamethasone *on page* 247

◆ **Alph-E [OTC]** *see* Vitamin E *on page 2202*

◆ **Alph-E-Mixed [OTC]** *see* Vitamin E *on page 2202*

◆ **Alph-E-Mixed 1000 [OTC]** *see* Vitamin E *on page 2202*

ALPRAZolam (al PRAY zoe lam)

Brand Names: U.S. ALPRAZolam Intensol; ALPRAZolam XR; Niravam; Xanax; Xanax XR

Brand Names: Canada Apo-Alpraz®; Apo-Alpraz® TS; Mylan-Alprazolam; NTP-Alprazolam; Nu-Alpraz; Teva-Alprazolam; Xanax TS™; Xanax®

Pharmacologic Category Benzodiazepine

Additional Appendix Information

Beers Criteria – Potentially Inappropriate Medications for Geriatrics *on page 2368*

Benzodiazepine Comparison Table *on page 2292*

Use Treatment of anxiety disorder (GAD); short-term relief of symptoms of anxiety; panic disorder, with or without agoraphobia; anxiety associated with depression

Unlabeled Use Anxiety in children

Pregnancy Risk Factor D

Pregnancy Considerations Benzodiazepines have the potential to cause harm to the fetus. Alprazolam and its metabolites cross the human placenta. Teratogenic effects have been observed with some benzodiazepines; however, additional studies are needed. The incidence of premature birth and low birth weights may be increased following maternal use of benzodiazepines; hypoglycemia and respiratory problems in the neonate may occur following exposure late in pregnancy. Neonatal withdrawal symptoms may occur within days to weeks after birth and "floppy infant syndrome" (which also includes withdrawal symptoms) has been reported with some benzodiazepines (Bergman, 1992; Iqbal, 2002; Wikner, 2007).

Breast-Feeding Considerations Benzodiazepines are excreted into breast milk. In a study of eight postpartum women, peak concentrations of alprazolam were found in breast milk ~1 hour after the maternal dose and the half-life was ~14 hours. Samples were obtained over 36 hours following a single oral dose of alprazolam 0.5 mg. Metabolites were not detected in breast milk. In this study, the estimated exposure to the breast-feeding infant was ~3% of the weight-adjusted maternal dose (Oo, 1995). Drowsiness, lethargy, or weight loss in nursing infants have been observed in case reports following maternal use of some benzodiazepines (Iqbal, 2002). Breast-feeding is not recommended by the manufacturer.

Contraindications Hypersensitivity to alprazolam or any component of the formulation (cross-sensitivity with other benzodiazepines may exist); narrow-angle glaucoma; concurrent use with ketoconazole or itraconazole

Warnings/Precautions Rebound or withdrawal symptoms, including seizures, may occur following abrupt discontinuation or large decreases in dose (more common in patients receiving >4 mg/day or prolonged treatment); the risk of seizures appears to be greatest 24-72 hours following discontinuation of therapy. Breakthrough anxiety may occur at the end of dosing interval. Use with caution in patients receiving concurrent CYP3A4 inhibitors, moderate or strong CYP3A4 inducers, and major CYP3A4 substrates; consider alternative agents that avoid or lessen the potential for CYP-mediated interactions. Use with caution in renal impairment or predisposition to urate nephropathy; has weak uricosuric properties. In older adults, benzodiazepines increase the risk of impaired cognition, delirium, falls, fractures, and motor vehicle accidents. Due to increased sensitivity in this age group, avoid use for treatment of insomnia, agitation, or delirium (Beers Criteria). Use with caution in or debilitated patients, patients with hepatic disease (including alcoholics) or respiratory disease, or obese patients.

Causes CNS depression (dose related) which may impair physical and mental capabilities. Patients must be cautioned about performing tasks that require mental alertness (eg, operating machinery or driving). Effects with other sedative drugs or ethanol may be potentiated. Benzodiazepines have been associated with falls and traumatic injury and should be used with extreme caution in patients who are at risk of these events.

Use caution in patients with depression, particularly if suicidal risk may be present. Episodes of mania or hypomania have occurred in depressed patients treated with alprazolam. May cause physical or psychological dependence. Acute withdrawal may be precipitated in patients after administration of flumazenil.

Benzodiazepines have been associated with anterograde amnesia. Paradoxical reactions have been reported with benzodiazepines, particularly in adolescent/pediatric or psychiatric patients. Does not have analgesic, antidepressant, or antipsychotic properties.

Adverse Reactions

>10%:

Central nervous system: Ataxia, cognitive dysfunction, depression, dizziness, drowsiness, dysarthria, fatigue, irritability, memory impairment, sedation

Endocrine & metabolic: Decreased libido, weight gain, weight loss

Gastrointestinal: Change in appetite, constipation, xerostomia

Genitourinary: Difficulty in micturition

Respiratory: Nasal congestion

1% to 10%:

Cardiovascular: Chest pain, hypotension, palpitations, sinus tachycardia, syncope

Central nervous system: Abnormal dreams, agitation, akathisia, altered mental status, confusion, depersonalization, derealization, disinhibition, disorientation, disturbance in attention, dystonia, fear, hallucination, headache, hypersomnia, hypoesthesia, insomnia, lethargy, malaise, nervousness, nightmares, paresthesia, restlessness, seizure, talkativeness, vertigo

Dermatologic: Dermatitis, diaphoresis, skin rash

Endocrine & metabolic: Increased libido, menstrual disease

Gastrointestinal: Abdominal pain, anorexia, diarrhea, dyspepsia, nausea, sialorrhea, vomiting

Genitourinary: Dysmenorrhea, sexual disorder, urinary incontinence

Hepatic: Increased liver enzymes, increased serum bilirubin, jaundice

Neuromuscular & skeletal: Arthralgia, back pain, dyskinesia, muscle cramps, muscle twitching, myalgia, tremor, weakness

Ophthalmic: Blurred vision

Respiratory: Allergic rhinitis, dyspnea, hyperventilation, upper respiratory tract infection

<1% (Limited to important or life-threatening): Amnesia, angioedema, diplopia, falling, galactorrhea, gynecomastia, hepatic failure, hepatitis, homicidal ideation, hyperprolactinemia, hypomania, mania, peripheral edema, sleep apnea, Stevens-Johnson syndrome, suicidal ideation, tinnitus

Drug Interactions

Metabolism/Transport Effects Substrate of CYP3A4 (major); **Note:** Assignment of Major/Minor substrate status based on clinically relevant drug interaction potential

Avoid Concomitant Use

Avoid concomitant use of ALPRAZolam with any of the following: Azelastine (Nasal); Conivaptan; Fusidic Acid (Systemic); Indinavir; Itraconazole; Ketoconazole (Systemic); OLANZapine; Paraldehyde; Sodium Oxybate

Increased Effect/Toxicity

ALPRAZolam may increase the levels/effects of: Alcohol (Ethyl); Azelastine (Nasal); Buprenorphine; CloZAPine; CNS Depressants; Hydrocodone; Methotrimeprazine; Metyrosine; Mirtazapine; Paraldehyde; Pramipexole; ROPINIRole; Rotigotine; Selective Serotonin Reuptake Inhibitors; Sodium Oxybate; Zolpidem

The levels/effects of ALPRAZolam may be increased by: Antifungal Agents (Azole Derivatives, Systemic); Aprepitant; Boceprevir; Brimonidine (Topical); Calcium Channel Blockers (Nondihydropyridine); Cimetidine; Conivaptan; Contraceptives (Estrogens); Contraceptives (Progestins); CYP3A4 Inhibitors (Moderate); CYP3A4 Inhibitors (Strong); Dasatinib; Doxylamine; Droperidol; Fosaprepitant; Fusidic Acid (Systemic); Grapefruit Juice; HydrOXYzine; Indinavir; Isoniazid; Itraconazole; Ivacaftor; Ketoconazole (Systemic); Luliconazole; Macrolide Antibiotics; Magnesium Sulfate; Methotrimeprazine; Mifepristone; OLANZapine; Perampanel; Protease Inhibitors; Proton Pump Inhibitors; Selective Serotonin Reuptake Inhibitors; Simeprevir; Tapentadol; Telaprevir

Decreased Effect

The levels/effects of ALPRAZolam may be decreased by: Bosentan; CarBAMazepine; CYP3A4 Inducers (Strong); Dabrafenib; Deferasirox; Herbs (CYP3A4 Inducers); Mitotane; Rifamycin Derivatives; Theophylline Derivatives; Tocilizumab; Yohimbine

Ethanol/Nutrition/Herb Interactions

Cigarette: Smoking may decrease alprazolam concentrations up to 50%.

Ethanol: Ethanol may increase CNS depression. Management: Avoid ethanol.

Food: Alprazolam serum concentration is unlikely to be increased by grapefruit juice because of alprazolam's high oral bioavailability. The C_{max} of the extended release formulation is increased by 25% when a high-fat meal is given 2 hours before dosing. T_{max} is decreased 33% when food is given immediately prior to dose and increased by 33% when food is given ≥1 hour after dose.

Herb/Nutraceutical: St John's wort may decrease alprazolam levels. Valerian, kava kava, and gotu kola may increase CNS depression. Management: Avoid St John's wort. Avoid valerian, kava kava, and gotu kola.

Storage/Stability

Immediate release tablets: Store at 20°C to 25°C (68°F to 77°F).

Extended release tablets: Store at 25°C (77°F); excursions permitted to 15°C to 30°C (59°F to 86°F).

Orally-disintegrating tablet: Store at room temperature of 20°C to 25°C (68°F to 77°F). Protect from moisture. Seal bottle tightly and discard any cotton packaged inside bottle.

Mechanism of Action Binds to stereospecific benzodiazepine receptors on the postsynaptic GABA neuron at several sites within the central nervous system, including the limbic system, reticular formation. Enhancement of the inhibitory effect of GABA on neuronal excitability results by increased neuronal membrane permeability to chloride ions. This shift in chloride ions results in hyperpolarization (a less excitable state) and stabilization.

Pharmacodynamics/Kinetics

Onset of action: Immediate release and extended release formulations: 1 hour

Duration: Immediate release: 5.1 ± 1.7 hours; Extended release: 11.3 ± 4.2 hours

Absorption: Extended release: Slower relative to immediate release formulation resulting in a concentration that is maintained 5-11 hours after dosing

Distribution: V_d: 0.9-1.2 L/kg

Protein binding: 80%; primarily to albumin

Metabolism: Hepatic via CYP3A4; forms two active metabolites (4-hydroxyalprazolam and α-hydroxyalprazolam)

Bioavailability: 90%

Half-life elimination:

Adults: 11.2 hours (Immediate release range: 6.3-26.9 hours; Extended release range: 10.7-15.8 hours); Orally-disintegrating tablet range: 7.9-19.2 hours)

Elderly: 16.3 hours (range: 9-26.9 hours)

Alcoholic liver disease: 19.7 hours (range: 5.8-65.3 hours)

Obesity: 21.8 hours (range: 9.9-40.4 hours)

Race: Asians: Increased by ~25% (as compared to Caucasians)

Time to peak, serum:

Immediate release: 1-2 hours

Extended release: ~9 hours (Glue, 2006); decreased by 1 hour when administered at bedtime (as compared to morning administration); decreased by 33% when administered with a high-fat meal; increased by 33% when administered ≥1 hour after a high-fat meal

Orally-disintegrating tablet: 1.5-2 hours; occurs ~15 minutes earlier when administered with water; decreased by 2 hours when administered with a high-fat meal

Excretion: Urine (as unchanged drug and metabolites)

Dosage Oral: **Note:** Treatment >4 months should be re-evaluated to determine the patient's continued need for the drug

Children: Anxiety (unlabeled use): Immediate release: Initial: 0.005 mg/kg/dose or 0.125 mg/dose 3 times/day; increase in increments of 0.125-0.25 mg, up to a maximum of 0.02 mg/kg/dose or 0.06 mg/kg/day (range of doses reported in one study: 0.375-3 mg/day) (Pfefferbaum, 1987). See "Dose Reduction" comment below.

Adults:

Anxiety: Immediate release: Initial: 0.25-0.5 mg 3 times/day; titrate dose upward every 3-4 days; usual maximum: 4 mg/day. Patients requiring doses >4 mg/day should be increased cautiously. Periodic reassessment and consideration of dosage reduction is recommended.

Panic disorder:

Immediate release: Initial: 0.5 mg 3 times/day; dose may be increased every 3-4 days in increments ≤1 mg/day. Mean effective dosage: 5-6 mg/day; some patients may require much as 10 mg/day

Extended release: 0.5-1 mg once daily; may increase dose every 3-4 days in increments ≤1 mg/day (range: 3-6 mg/day)

Switching from immediate release to extended release: Patients may be switched to extended release tablets by taking the total daily dose of the immediate release tablets and giving it once daily using the extended release preparation.

Preoperative anxiety (unlabeled use): 0.5 mg 60-90 minutes before procedure (De Witte, 2002)

Dose reduction: Abrupt discontinuation should be avoided. Daily dose may be decreased by 0.5 mg every 3 days; however, some patients may require a slower reduction. If withdrawal symptoms occur, resume previous dose and discontinue on a less rapid schedule.

Elderly: **Note:** Elderly patients may be more sensitive to the effects of alprazolam including ataxia and oversedation. The elderly may also have impaired renal function leading to decreased clearance. Titrate gradually, if needed and tolerated.

Immediate release: Initial: 0.25 mg 2-3 times/day

Extended release: Initial: 0.5 mg once daily

Dosing adjustment in renal impairment: No dosage adjustment provided in manufacturer's labeling; however, use caution

Dosing adjustment in hepatic impairment: Advanced liver disease:

Immediate release: 0.25 mg 2-3 times/day; titrate gradually if needed and tolerated

Extended release: 0.5 mg once daily; titrate gradually if needed and tolerated

Dietary Considerations Extended release tablet should be taken once daily in the morning.

Administration

Immediate release preparations: Can be administered sublingually if oral administration is not possible; absorption and onset of effect are comparable to oral administration (Scavone,1987; Scavone, 1992)

Extended release tablet: Should be taken once daily in the morning; do not crush, break, or chew.

Orally-disintegrating tablets: Using dry hands, place tablet on top of tongue and allow to disintegrate. If using one-half of tablet, immediately discard remaining half (may not remain stable). Administration with water is not necessary.

Monitoring Parameters Respiratory and cardiovascular status

Additional Information Not intended for management of anxieties and minor distresses associated with everyday life. Treatment longer than 4 months should be re-evaluated to determine the patient's need for the drug. Patients who become physically dependent on alprazolam tend to have a difficult time discontinuing it; withdrawal symptoms may be severe. To minimize withdrawal symptoms, taper dosage slowly; do not discontinue abruptly. Abrupt discontinuation after sustained use (generally >10 days) may cause withdrawal symptoms.

Dosage Forms Excipient information presented when available (limited, particularly for generics); consult specific product labeling.

Concentrate, Oral:

ALPRAZolam Intensol: 1 mg/mL (30 mL) [unflavored flavor]

Tablet, Oral:

Xanax: 0.25 mg [scored]

Xanax: 0.5 mg [scored; contains fd&c yellow #6 (sunset yellow)]

Xanax: 1 mg [scored; contains fd&c blue #2 (indigotine)]

Xanax: 2 mg [scored]

Generic: 0.25 mg, 0.5 mg, 1 mg, 2 mg

Tablet Dispersible, Oral:

Niravam: 0.25 mg, 0.5 mg, 1 mg, 2 mg [scored; orange flavor]

Generic: 0.25 mg, 0.5 mg, 1 mg, 2 mg

Tablet Extended Release 24 Hour, Oral:

ALPRAZolam XR: 0.5 mg

ALPRAZolam XR: 1 mg [contains fd&c yellow #10 (quinoline yellow)]

ALPRAZolam XR: 2 mg [contains fd&c blue #2 (indigotine)]

ALPRAZolam XR: 3 mg [contains fd&c blue #2 (indigotine), fd&c yellow #10 (quinoline yellow)]

Xanax XR: 0.5 mg

Xanax XR: 1 mg [contains fd&c yellow #10 (quinoline yellow)]

Xanax XR: 2 mg [contains fd&c blue #2 (indigotine)]

Xanax XR: 3 mg [contains fd&c blue #2 (indigotine), fd&c yellow #10 (quinoline yellow)]

Generic: 0.5 mg, 1 mg, 2 mg, 3 mg

Controlled Substance C-IV

Extemporaneous Preparations Note: Commercial oral solution is available (Alprazolam Intensol™: 1 mg/mL [dye free, ethanol free, sugar free; contains propylene glycol])

A 1 mg/mL oral suspension may be made with tablets and one of three different vehicles (a 1:1 mixture of Ora-Sweet® and Ora-Plus®, a 1:1 mixture of Ora-Sweet® SF and Ora-Plus®, or a 1:4 mixture of cherry syrup with Simple Syrup, NF). Crush sixty 2 mg tablets in a mortar and reduce to a fine powder. Add 40 mL of vehicle and mix to a uniform paste; mix while adding the vehicle in incremental proportions to **almost** 120 mL; transfer to a calibrated bottle, rinse mortar with vehicle, and add a quantity of vehicle sufficient to make 120 mL. Label "shake well" and "refrigerate". Stable for 60 days.

Nahata MC, Pai VB, and Hipple TF, *Pediatric Drug Formulations*, 5th ed, Cincinnati, OH: Harvey Whitney Books Co, 2004.

◆ **ALPRAZolam Intensol** *see* ALPRAZolam *on page 81*

◆ **ALPRAZolam XR** *see* ALPRAZolam *on page 81*

Alprostadil (al PROS ta dill)

Brand Names: U.S. Caverject; Caverject Impulse; Edex; Muse; Prostin VR

Brand Names: Canada Alprostadil Injection USP; Caverject®; Muse® Pellet; Prostin® VR

Index Terms PGE_1; Prostaglandin E_1

Pharmacologic Category Prostaglandin; Vasodilator

Use

Prostin VR Pediatric®: Temporary maintenance of patency of ductus arteriosus in neonates with ductal-dependent congenital heart disease until surgery can be performed. These defects include cyanotic (eg, pulmonary atresia, pulmonary stenosis, tricuspid atresia, Fallot's tetralogy, transposition of the great vessels) and acyanotic (eg, interruption of aortic arch, coarctation of aorta, hypoplastic left ventricle) heart disease.

Caverject®: Treatment of erectile dysfunction of vasculogenic, psychogenic, or neurogenic etiology; adjunct in the diagnosis of erectile dysfunction

Edex®, Muse®: Treatment of erectile dysfunction of vasculogenic, psychogenic, or neurogenic etiology

Unlabeled Use Treatment of pulmonary hypertension in infants and children with congenital heart defects with left-to-right shunts

Pregnancy Risk Factor X/C (Muse®)

Pregnancy Considerations Adverse events were observed in animal reproduction studies. Alprostadil is not indicated for use in women. The manufacturer of Muse® recommends a condom barrier when being used during sexual intercourse with a pregnant women.

Breast-Feeding Considerations Alprostadil is not indicated for use in women.

Contraindications Hypersensitivity to alprostadil or any component of the formulation; hyaline membrane disease or persistent fetal circulation and when a dominant left-to-right shunt is present; respiratory distress syndrome; conditions predisposing patients to priapism (sickle cell anemia, multiple myeloma, leukemia); patients with anatomical deformation of the penis, penile implants; use in men for whom sexual activity is inadvisable or contraindicated; pregnancy

Warnings/Precautions Use cautiously in neonates with bleeding tendencies. **[U.S. Boxed Warning]: Apnea may occur in 10% to 12% of neonates with congenital heart defects, especially in those weighing <2 kg at birth.** Apnea usually appears during the first hour of drug infusion. When used for patency of ductus arteriosus infuse for the shortest time at the lowest dose consistent with good patient care. Use for >120 hours has been associated with antral hyperplasia and gastric outlet obstruction.

When used in erectile dysfunction, priapism may occur; treat proloonged priapism (erection persisting for >4 hours) immediately to avoid penile tissue damage and permanent loss of potency; discontinue therapy if signs of penile fibrosis develop (penile angulation, cavernosal fibrosis, or Peyronie's disease). When used in erectile dysfunction (Muse®), syncope occurring within 1 hour of administration has been reported. The potential for drug-drug interactions may occur when Muse® is prescribed concomitantly with antihypertensives.

Adverse Reactions

Intraurethral:

>10%: Genitourinary: Penile pain, urethral burning

2% to 10%:

Central nervous system: Headache, dizziness, pain

Genitourinary: Vaginal itching (female partner), testicular pain, urethral bleeding (minor)

<2% (Limited to important or life-threatening): Tachycardia, perineal pain, leg pain

Intracavernosal injection:

>10%: Genitourinary: Penile pain

1% to 10%:

Cardiovascular: Hypertension

Central nervous system: Headache, dizziness

Genitourinary: Prolonged erection (>4 hours, 4%), penile fibrosis, penis disorder, penile rash, penile edema

Local: Injection site hematoma and/or bruising

<1% (Limited to important or life-threatening): Balanitis, injection site hemorrhage, priapism (0.4%)

Intravenous:

>10%:

Cardiovascular: Flushing

Central nervous system: Fever

Respiratory: Apnea

1% to 10%:

Cardiovascular: Bradycardia, hyper-/hypotension, tachycardia, cardiac arrest, edema

Central nervous system: Seizure, headache, dizziness

Endocrine & metabolic: Hypokalemia

Gastrointestinal: Diarrhea

Hematologic: Disseminated intravascular coagulation

Neuromuscular & skeletal: Back pain

Respiratory: Upper respiratory infection, flu syndrome, sinusitis, nasal congestion, cough

Miscellaneous: Sepsis, localized pain in structures other than the injection site

<1% (Limited to important or life-threatening): Anemia, anuria, bleeding, bradypnea, bronchial wheezing, cerebral bleeding, CHF, gastric regurgitation, hematuria, hyperbilirubinemia, hyperemia, hyperextension of neck, hyperirritability, hyperkalemia, hypoglycemia, hypothermia, jitteriness, lethargy, peritonitis, second-degree heart block, shock, stiffness, supraventricular tachycardia, thrombocytopenia, ventricular fibrillation

Drug Interactions

Metabolism/Transport Effects None known.

Avoid Concomitant Use

Avoid concomitant use of Alprostadil with any of the following: Phosphodiesterase 5 Inhibitors

Increased Effect/Toxicity

The levels/effects of Alprostadil may be increased by: Phosphodiesterase 5 Inhibitors

Decreased Effect There are no known significant interactions involving a decrease in effect.

Ethanol/Nutrition/Herb Interactions Ethanol: Avoid concurrent use (vasodilating effect).

Preparation for Administration

Caverject® Impulse™: Provided as a dual-chamber syringe with diluent in one chamber. To mix, hold syringe with needle pointing upward and turn plunger clockwise; turn upside down several times to mix. Device can be set to deliver specified dose, each device can be set at various increments.

Caverject® powder: Use only the supplied diluent for reconstitution (ie, bacteriostatic/sterile water with benzyl alcohol 0.945%).

Edex®: Reconstitute with NS.

Storage/Stability

Caverject® Impulse™: Store at controlled room temperature of 15°C to 30°C (59°F to 86°F). Following reconstitution, use within 24 hours and discard any unused solution.

Caverject® powder: The 5 mcg, 10 mcg, and 20 mcg vials should be stored at or below 25°C (77°F); The 40 mcg vial should be stored at 2°C to 8°C until dispensed. After dispensing, stable for up to 3 months at or below 25°C. Following reconstitution, all strengths should be stored at or below 25°C (77°F); do not refrigerate or freeze; use within 24 hours.

Caverject® solution: Prior to dispensing, store frozen at -20°C to -10°C (-4°F to -14°F). Once dispensed, may be stored frozen for up to 3 months, or under refrigeration at 2°C to 8°C (36°F to 46°F) for up to 7 days. Do not refreeze. Once removed from foil wrap, solution may be allowed to warm to room temperature prior to use. If not used immediately, solution should be discarded. Shake well prior to use.

Edex®: Store at controlled room temperature of 15°C to 30°C (59°F to 86°F); following reconstitution, use immediately and discard any unused solution.

Muse®: Refrigerate at 2°C to 8°C (36°F to 46°F); may be stored at room temperature for up to 14 days

Prostin VR Pediatric®: Refrigerate at 2°C to 8°C (36°F to 46°F). The following stability information has also been reported: May be stored at 20°C for up to 34 days or 30°C for up to 26 days (Cohen, 2007). Prior to infusion, dilute with D_5W or NS; use within 24 hours.

Mechanism of Action Causes vasodilation by means of direct effect on vascular and ductus arteriosus smooth muscle; relaxes trabecular smooth muscle by dilation of cavernosal arteries when injected along the penile shaft, allowing blood flow to and entrapment in the lacunar spaces of the penis (ie, corporeal veno-occlusive mechanism)

Pharmacodynamics/Kinetics

Onset of action: Rapid

Duration: <1 hour

Distribution: Insignificant following penile injection

Protein binding, plasma: 81% to albumin

Metabolism: ~75% by oxidation in one pass via lungs

Half-life elimination: 5-10 minutes

Excretion: Urine (90% as metabolites) within 24 hours

Dosage

Patent ductus arteriosus (Prostin VR Pediatric®):

I.V. continuous infusion into a large vein, or alternatively through an umbilical artery catheter placed at the ductal opening: 0.05-0.1 mcg/kg/minute with therapeutic response, rate is reduced to lowest effective dosage; with unsatisfactory response, rate is increased gradually; maintenance: 0.01-0.4 mcg/kg/minute

PGE_1 is usually given at an infusion rate of 0.1 mcg/kg/minute, but it is often possible to reduce the dosage to $1/2$ or even $1/10$ without losing the therapeutic effect.

Therapeutic response is indicated by increased pH in those with acidosis or by an increase in oxygenation (PO_2) usually evident within 30 minutes

Erectile dysfunction:

Caverject®, Edex®: Intracavernous: Individualize dose by careful titration; doses >40 mcg (Edex®) or >60 mcg (Caverject®) are not recommended: Initial dose must be titrated in physician's office. Patient must stay in the physician's office until complete detumescence occurs; if there is no response, then the next higher dose may be given within 1 hour; if there is still no response, a 1-day interval before giving the next dose is recommended; increasing the dose or concentration in the treatment of impotence results in increasing pain and discomfort

Vasculogenic, psychogenic, or mixed etiology: Initiate dosage titration at 2.5 mcg, increasing by 2.5 mcg to a dose of 5 mcg and then in increments of 5-10 mcg depending on the erectile response until the dose produces an erection suitable for intercourse, not lasting >1 hour; if there is absolutely no response to initial 2.5 mcg dose, the second dose may be increased to 7.5 mcg, followed by increments of 5-10 mcg

Neurogenic etiology (eg, spinal cord injury): Initiate dosage titration at 1.25 mcg, increasing to a dose of 2.5 mcg and then 5 mcg; increase further in increments 5 mcg until the dose is reached that produces an erection suitable for intercourse, not lasting >1 hour

Maintenance: Once appropriate dose has been determined, patient may self-administer injections at a frequency of no more than 3 times/week with at least 24 hours between doses

Muse® Pellet: Intraurethral:

Initial: 125-250 mcg

Maintenance: Administer as needed to achieve an erection; duration of action is about 30-60 minutes; use only two systems per 24-hour period

Elderly: Elderly patients may have a greater frequency of renal dysfunction; lowest effective dose should be used. In clinical studies with Edex®, higher minimally effective doses and a higher rate of lack of effect were noted.

Dosage adjustment in renal impairment: No dosage adjustment provided in manufacturer's labeling.

Dosage adjustment in hepatic impairment: No dosage adjustment provided in manufacturer's labeling.

Usual Infusion Concentrations: Pediatric I.V. infusion: 10 mcg/mL **or** 20 mcg/mL

Administration

Patent ductus arteriosus (Prostin VR Pediatric®): I.V. continuous infusion into a large vein or alternatively through an umbilical artery catheter placed at the ductal opening; manufacturer recommended maximum concentration for I.V. infusion: 20 mcg/mL

Erectile dysfunction: Use a 1/2 inch, 27- to 30-gauge needle. Inject into the dorsolateral aspect of the proximal third of the penis, avoiding visible veins; alternate side of the penis for injections.

Monitoring Parameters Arterial pressure, respiratory rate, heart rate, temperature, degree of penile pain, length of erection, signs of infection

Dosage Forms Excipient information presented when available (limited, particularly for generics); consult specific product labeling.

Kit, Intracavernosal:

Caverject Impulse: 10 mcg [contains benzyl alcohol]

Caverject Impulse: 20 mcg

Edex: 10 mcg, 20 mcg, 40 mcg

Pellet, Urethral:

Muse: 125 mcg (1 ea, 6 ea); 250 mcg (1 ea, 6 ea); 500 mcg (1 ea, 6 ea); 1000 mcg (1 ea, 6 ea)

Solution, Injection:

Prostin VR: 500 mcg/mL (1 mL) [contains benzyl alcohol]

Generic: 500 mcg/mL (1 mL)

Solution Reconstituted, Intracavernosal:

Caverject: 20 mcg (1 ea)

Caverject: 20 mcg (1 ea); 40 mcg (1 ea) [contains benzyl alcohol]

◆ **Alprostadil Injection USP (Can)** *see* Alprostadil *on page 83*

◆ **Alrex** *see* Loteprednol *on page 1250*

◆ **Alrex® (Can)** *see* Loteprednol *on page 1250*

◆ **Alsuma** *see* SUMAtriptan *on page 1969*

◆ **Altabax** *see* Retapamulin *on page 1800*

◆ **Altacaine** *see* Tetracaine (Ophthalmic) *on page 2034*

◆ **Altace** *see* Ramipril *on page 1778*

◆ **Altachlore [OTC]** *see* Sodium Chloride *on page 1914*

◆ **Altamist Spray [OTC]** *see* Sodium Chloride *on page 1914*

◆ **Altarussin [OTC]** *see* GuaiFENesin *on page 974*

◆ **Altaryl [OTC]** *see* DiphenhydrAMINE (Systemic) *on page 622*

◆ **Altavera** *see* Ethinyl Estradiol and Levonorgestrel *on page 787*

Alteplase (AL te plase)

Brand Names: U.S. Activase; Cathflo Activase

Brand Names: Canada Activase rt-PA; Cathflo Activase

Index Terms Alteplase, Recombinant; Alteplase, Tissue Plasminogen Activator, Recombinant; tPA

Pharmacologic Category Thrombolytic Agent

Use Management of ST-elevation myocardial infarction (STEMI) for the lysis of thrombi in coronary arteries; management of acute ischemic stroke (AIS); management of acute pulmonary embolism (PE)

Recommended criteria for treatment:

STEMI (ACCF/AHA; O'Gara, 2013): Ischemic symptoms within 12 hours of treatment or evidence of ongoing ischemia 12-24 hours after symptom onset with a large area of myocardium at risk or hemodynamic instability.

STEMI ECG definition: New ST-segment elevation at the J point in at least 2 contiguous leads of ≥2 mm (0.2 mV) in men or ≥1.5 mm (0.15 mV) in women in leads V_2-V_3 and/or of ≥1 mm (0.1 mV) in other contiguous precordial leads or limb leads. New or presumably new left bundle branch block (LBBB) may interfere with ST-elevation analysis and should not be considered diagnostic in isolation.

At non-PCI-capable hospitals, the ACCF/AHA recommends thrombolytic therapy administration when the anticipated first medical contact (FMC)-to-device time at a PCI-capable hospital is >120 minutes due to unavoidable delays.

AIS: Onset of stroke symptoms within 3 hours of treatment

Acute pulmonary embolism: Age ≤75 years: Documented massive PE (defined as acute PE with sustained hypotension [SBP <90 mm Hg for ≤15 minutes or requiring inotropic support], persistent profound bradycardia [HR <40 bpm with signs or symptoms of shock], or pulselessness); alteplase may be considered for submassive PE with clinical evidence of adverse prognosis (eg, new hemodynamic instability, worsening respiratory insufficiency, severe RV dysfunction, or major myocardial necrosis) and low risk of bleeding complications. **Note:** Not recommended for patients with low-risk PE (eg, normotensive, no RV dysfunction, normal biomarkers) or submassive acute PE with minor RV dysfunction, minor myocardial necrosis, and no clinical worsening (Jaff, 2011).

Cathflo® Activase®: Restoration of central venous catheter function

Unlabeled Use Acute ischemic stroke presenting 3-4.5 hours after symptom onset; acute peripheral arterial occlusion; infected parapneumonic effusion (with [adult] or without [pediatric] dornase alfa); prosthetic valve thrombosis; intra-arterial administration for patients who have contraindications to I.V. use (**Note:** Intra-arterial administration requires patient to be at an experienced stroke center with rapid access to cerebral angiography and qualified interventionalists)

Pregnancy Risk Factor C

Pregnancy Considerations Adverse events were observed in animal reproduction studies. The risk of bleeding may be increased in pregnant women. Information related to alteplase use in pregnancy is limited (Leonhardt, 2006; Li, 2012) and most guidelines consider pregnancy to be a relative contraindication for its use (Jaff, 2011; Jauch, 2013; O'Gara, 2013). Alteplase should not be withheld from pregnant women in life-threatening situations but should be avoided when safer alternatives are available (Bates, 2012; Li, 2012; Leonhardt, 2006; Vanden Hoek, 2010).

Breast-Feeding Considerations It is not known if alteplase is excreted in breast milk. The manufacturer recommends that caution be exercised when administering alteplase to nursing women.

Contraindications Hypersensitivity to alteplase or any component of the formulation

Treatment of STEMI or PE: Active internal bleeding; history of CVA; ischemic stroke within 3 months except when within 4.5 hours (Jaff, 2011; O'Gara, 2013); recent intracranial or intraspinal surgery or trauma; intracranial neoplasm; prior intracranial hemorrhage (Jaff, 2011; O'Gara, 2013); arteriovenous malformation or aneurysm; active bleeding (excluding menses) (O'Gara, 2013); known bleeding diathesis; severe uncontrolled hypertension; suspected aortic dissection (Jaff, 2011; O'Gara, 2013); significant closed head or facial trauma (Jaff, 2011; O'Gara, 2013) within 3 months with radiographic evidence of bony fracture or brain injury (Jaff, 2011)

Treatment of acute ischemic stroke: Evidence/history of intracranial hemorrhage or suspicion of subarachnoid hemorrhage on pretreatment evaluation; recent intracranial or intraspinal surgery; stroke or serious head injury within 3 months; uncontrolled hypertension at time of treatment (eg, >185 mm Hg systolic or >110 mm Hg diastolic); seizure at the onset of stroke; active internal bleeding; intracranial neoplasm; arteriovenous malformation or aneurysm; multilobar cerebral infarction (hypodensity >1/3 cerebral hemisphere); known bleeding diathesis including but not limited to current use of oral anticoagulants with an INR >1.7 (or PT >15 seconds), current use of direct thrombin inhibitors or direct factor Xa inhibitors with elevated sensitive laboratory tests (eg, aPTT, INR, platelet count, and ECT, TT, or appropriate factor Xa activity assays) (See **"Note"**; Jauch, 2013), administration of heparin within 48 hours preceding the onset of stroke with an elevated aPTT at presentation, or platelet count <100,000/mm^3.

Note: The AHA/ASA guidelines do allow the use of direct thrombin inhibitors (eg, dabigatran) or direct factor Xa inhibitors (eg, rivaroxaban) when sensitive laboratory tests (eg, aPTT, INR, platelet count, ECT, TT, or appropriate direct factor Xa activity assays) are normal or the patient has not received a dose of these agents for >2 days (assuming normal renal function).

Additional exclusion criteria within clinical trials:

Presentation <3 hours after initial symptoms (NINDS, 1995): Time of symptom onset unknown, rapidly improving or minor symptoms, major surgery within 2 weeks, GI or urinary tract hemorrhage within 3 weeks, aggressive treatment required to lower blood pressure, glucose level <50 or >400 mg/dL, and arterial puncture at a noncompressible site or lumbar puncture within 1 week.

Presentation 3-4.5 hours after initial symptoms (ECASS-III; Hacke, 2008; Jauch, 2013): Age >80 years, time of symptom onset unknown, rapidly improving or minor symptoms, current use of oral anticoagulants regardless of INR, glucose level <50 or >400 mg/dL, aggressive intravenous treatment required to lower blood pressure, major surgery or severe trauma within 3 months, baseline National Institutes of Health Stroke Scale (NIHSS) score >25 [ie, severe stroke], and history of both stroke and diabetes.

Warnings/Precautions The total dose should not exceed 90 mg for acute ischemic stroke or 100 mg for acute myocardial infarction or pulmonary embolism. Doses ≥150 mg associated with significantly increased risk of intracranial hemorrhage compared to doses ≤100 mg. Concurrent heparin anticoagulation may contribute to bleeding. In the treatment of acute ischemic stroke, concurrent use of anticoagulants was not permitted during the initial 24 hours of the <3 hour window trial (NINDS, 1995). The AHA/ASA does not recommend initiation of anticoagulant therapy within 24 hours of treatment with alteplase (Jauch, 2013). Initiation of SubQ heparin (≤10,000 units) or equivalent doses of low molecular weight heparin for prevention of DVT during the first 24 hours of the 3-4.5 hour window trial was permitted and did not increase the incidence of intracerebral hemorrhage (Hacke, 2008). For acute PE, withhold heparin during the 2-hour infusion period. Monitor all potential bleeding sites. Intramuscular injections and nonessential handling of the patient should be avoided. Venipunctures should be performed carefully and only when necessary. If arterial puncture is necessary, use an upper extremity vessel that can be manually compressed. If serious bleeding occurs, the infusion of alteplase and heparin should be stopped. Avoid aspirin for 24 hours following administration of alteplase; administration within 24 hours increases the risk of hemorrhagic transformation.

For the following conditions, the risk of bleeding is higher with use of thrombolytics and should be weighed against the benefits of therapy: Recent major surgery (eg, CABG, obstetrical delivery, organ biopsy, pregnancy, previous puncture of noncompressible vessels), prolonged CPR with evidence of thoracic trauma, lumbar puncture within 1 week, cerebrovascular disease, recent gastrointestinal or genitourinary bleeding, recent trauma, hypertension (systolic BP >175 mm Hg and/or diastolic BP >110 mm Hg), high likelihood of left heart thrombus (eg, mitral stenosis with atrial fibrillation), acute pericarditis, subacute bacterial endocarditis, hemostatic defects including ones caused by severe renal or hepatic dysfunction, significant hepatic dysfunction, pregnancy, diabetic hemorrhagic retinopathy or other hemorrhagic ophthalmic conditions, septic thrombophlebitis or occluded AV cannula at seriously infected site, advanced age (eg, >75 years), any other condition in which bleeding constitutes a significant hazard or would be particularly difficult to manage because of location. When treating acute MI or pulmonary embolism, use with caution in patients receiving oral anticoagulants. In the treatment of acute ischemic stroke (AIS) within 3 hours of symptom onset, the current use of oral anticoagulants is a contraindication per the manufacturer. According to the AHA/ASA, the current use of oral anticoagulants producing an INR >1.7, direct thrombin inhibitors, or direct factor Xa inhibitors with elevated sensitive laboratory tests are contraindications. However, alteplase may be administered to patients with AIS having received direct thrombin inhibitors (eg, dabigatran) or direct factor Xa inhibitors (eg, rivaroxaban) when sensitive laboratory tests (eg, aPTT, INR, platelet count, ECT, TT, or appropriate direct factor Xa activity assays) are normal or the patient has not received a dose of these agents for >2 days (assuming normal renal function). When treating AIS 3-4.5 hours after symptom onset, the use of alteplase should be avoided with current use of any oral anticoagulant regardless of INR (Jauch, 2013). In the treatment of STEMI, adjunctive use of parenteral anticoagulants (eg, enoxaparin, heparin, or fondaparinux) is recommended to improve vessel patency and prevent reocclusion and may also contribute to bleeding; monitor for bleeding (ACCF/AHA; O'Gara, 2013).

Coronary thrombolysis may result in reperfusion arrhythmias. Patients who present **within 3 hours** of stroke symptom onset should be treated with alteplase unless contraindications exist. A longer time window (**3-4.5 hours** after symptom onset) has been shown to be safe and efficacious for select individuals (Hacke, 2008; Jauch, 2013). Treatment of patients with minor neurological deficit or with rapidly improving symptoms is not recommended. Follow standard management for STEMI while infusing alteplase.

Cathflo® Activase®: When used to restore catheter function, use Cathflo® cautiously in those patients with known or suspected catheter infections. Evaluate catheter for other causes of dysfunction before use. Avoid excessive pressure when instilling into catheter.

Adverse Reactions As with all drugs which may affect hemostasis, bleeding is the major adverse effect associated with alteplase. Hemorrhage may occur at virtually any site. Risk is dependent on multiple variables, including the dosage administered, concurrent use of multiple agents which alter hemostasis, and patient predisposition. Rapid lysis of coronary artery thrombi by thrombolytic agents may be associated with reperfusion-related atrial and/or ventricular arrhythmia. **Note:** Lowest rate of bleeding complications expected with dose used to restore catheter function.

1% to 10%:
- Cardiovascular: Hypotension
- Central nervous system: Fever
- Dermatologic: Bruising (1%)
- Gastrointestinal: GI hemorrhage (5%), nausea, vomiting
- Genitourinary: GU hemorrhage (4%)
- Hematologic: Bleeding (0.5% major, 7% minor: GUSTO trial)
- Local: Bleeding at catheter puncture site (15.3%, accelerated administration)

<1% (Limited to important or life-threatening): Angioedema (orolingual), intracranial hemorrhage (0.4% to 0.87% when adult dose is ≤100 mg), retroperitoneal hemorrhage, pericardial hemorrhage, gingival hemorrhage, epistaxis, allergic reaction (anaphylaxis, anaphylactoid reactions, laryngeal edema, rash, and urticaria [<0.02%])

Additional cardiovascular events associated **with use in STEMI:** AV block, cardiogenic shock, heart failure, cardiac arrest, recurrent ischemia/infarction, myocardial rupture, electromechanical dissociation, pericardial effusion, pericarditis, mitral regurgitation, cardiac tamponade, thromboembolism, pulmonary edema, asystole, ventricular tachycardia, bradycardia, ruptured intracranial AV malformation, seizure, hemorrhagic bursitis, cholesterol crystal embolization

Additional events associated **with use in pulmonary embolism:** Pulmonary re-embolization, pulmonary edema, pleural effusion, thromboembolism

Additional events associated **with use in stroke:** Cerebral edema, cerebral herniation, seizure, new ischemic stroke

Drug Interactions

Metabolism/Transport Effects None known.

Avoid Concomitant Use There are no known interactions where it is recommended to avoid concomitant use.

Increased Effect/Toxicity

Alteplase may increase the levels/effects of: Anticoagulants; Dabigatran Etexilate

The levels/effects of Alteplase may be increased by: Agents with Antiplatelet Properties; Herbs (Anticoagulant/Antiplatelet Properties); Nonsteroidal Anti-Inflammatory Agents; Salicylates

Decreased Effect

The levels/effects of Alteplase may be decreased by: Aprotinin; Nitroglycerin

Ethanol/Nutrition/Herb Interactions Herb/Nutraceutical: Avoid cat's claw, dong quai, evening primrose, feverfew, red clover, horse chestnut, garlic, green tea, ginseng, ginkgo (all have additional antiplatelet activity).

Preparation for Administration

Activase®:

50 mg vial: Use accompanying diluent; mix by gentle swirling or slow inversion; do not shake. Vacuum is present in 50 mg vial. Final concentration: 1 mg/mL.

100 mg vial: Use transfer set with accompanying diluent (100 mL vial of sterile water for injection). No vacuum is present in 100 mg vial. Final concentration: 1 mg/mL.

Activase®: ST-elevation MI: Accelerated infusion: Bolus dose may be prepared by one of three methods:
1) Removal of 15 mL reconstituted (1 mg/mL) solution from vial
2) Removal of 15 mL from a port on the infusion line after priming
3) Programming an infusion pump to deliver a 15 mL bolus at the initiation of infusion

Activase®: Acute ischemic stroke: Bolus dose (10% of total dose) may be prepared by one of three methods:
1) Removal of the appropriate volume from reconstituted solution (1 mg/mL)
2) Removal of the appropriate volume from a port on the infusion line after priming
3) Programming an infusion pump to deliver the appropriate volume at the initiation of infusion

Cathflo® Activase®: Add 2.2 mL SWFI to vial; do not shake. Final concentration: 1 mg/mL.

Storage/Stability

Activase®: The lyophilized product may be stored at room temperature (not to exceed 30°C/86°F), or under refrigeration. Once reconstituted, it should be used within 8 hours.

Cathflo® Activase®: Store lyophilized product under refrigeration. Once reconstituted, it should be used within 8 hours.

Mechanism of Action Initiates local fibrinolysis by binding to fibrin in a thrombus (clot) and converts entrapped plasminogen to plasmin

Pharmacodynamics/Kinetics

Duration: >50% present in plasma cleared ~5 minutes after infusion terminated, ~80% cleared within 10 minutes; fibrinolytic activity persists for up to 1 hour after infusion terminated (Semba, 2000)

Excretion: Clearance (in patients with acute MI receiving accelerated regimen): Rapidly from circulating plasma (572 ± 132 mL/minute) (Tanswell, 1992), primarily hepatic; >50% present in plasma is cleared within 5 minutes after the infusion is terminated, ~80% cleared within 10 minutes (Semba, 2000)

Dosage

I.V. (Activase®):

ST-elevation myocardial infarction (STEMI): **Note:** Manufacturer's labeling recommends 3-hour infusion regimen; however, accelerated regimen preferred by the ACCF/AHA (O'Gara, 2013).

Accelerated regimen (weight-based):

Patients >67 kg: Total dose: 100 mg over 1.5 hours; administered as a 15 mg I.V. bolus over 1-2 minutes followed by infusions of 50 mg over 30 minutes, then 35 mg over 1 hour. Maximum total dose: 100 mg

Patients ≤67 kg: Infuse 15 mg I.V. bolus over 1-2 minutes followed by infusions of 0.75 mg/kg (not to exceed 50 mg) over 30 minutes then 0.5 mg/kg (not to exceed 35 mg) over 1 hour. Maximum total dose: 100 mg

Note: Thrombolytic should be administered within 30 minutes of hospital arrival. Administer concurrent aspirin, clopidogrel, and anticoagulant therapy (ie, unfractionated heparin, enoxaparin, or fondaparinux) with alteplase (O'Gara, 2013).

Acute massive or submassive pulmonary embolism (PE): 100 mg over 2 hours; may be administered as a 10 mg bolus followed by 90 mg over 2 hours as was done in patients with submassive PE (Konstantinides, 2002). **Note:** Not recommended for submassive PE with minor RV dysfunction, minor myocardial necrosis, and no clinical worsening or low-risk PE (ie, normotensive, no RV dysfunction, normal biomarkers) (Jaff, 2011).

Acute ischemic stroke: Within 3 hours of the onset of symptom onset (labeled use) **or** within 3-4.5 hours of symptom onset (unlabeled use; Hacke, 2008; Jauch, 2013): **Note:** Perform noncontrast-enhanced CT or MRI prior to administration. Initiation of anticoagulants (eg, heparin) or antiplatelet agents (eg, aspirin) within 24 hours after starting alteplase is not recommended; however, initiation of aspirin within 24-48 hours after stroke onset is recommended (Jauch, 2013). Initiation of SubQ heparin (≤10,000 units) or equivalent doses of low molecular weight heparin for prevention of DVT during the first 24 hours of the 3-4.5 hour window trial did not increase incidence of intracerebral hemorrhage (Hacke, 2008).

Recommended total dose: 0.9 mg/kg (maximum total dose: 90 mg)

Patients ≤100 kg: Load with 0.09 mg/kg (10% of 0.9 mg/kg dose) as an I.V. bolus over 1 minute, followed by 0.81 mg/kg (90% of 0.9 mg/kg dose) as a continuous infusion over 60 minutes.

Patients >100 kg: Load with 9 mg (10% of 90 mg) as an I.V. bolus over 1 minute, followed by 81 mg (90% of 90 mg) as a continuous infusion over 60 minutes.

Prosthetic valve thrombosis, right-sided (any size thrombus) or left-sided (thrombus area <0.8 cm^2), or left-sided (thrombus area ≥0.8 cm^2) when contraindications to surgery exist (unlabeled use) (Alpert, 2003; Guyatt, 2012; Roudaut, 2003):

High-dose regimen: Load with 10 mg, followed by 90 mg over 90-180 minutes (without heparin during infusion)

Low-dose regimen (preferred for very small adults): Load with 20 mg, followed by 10 mg/hour for 3 hours (without heparin during infusion)

Note: After successful administration of alteplase, heparin infusion should be introduced until warfarin achieves therapeutic INR (aortic: 3.0-4.0; mitral: 3.5-4.5) (Bonow, 2008). The 2012 ACCP guidelines for antithrombotic therapy make no recommendation regarding INR range after prosthetic valve thrombosis.

Intracatheter: Central venous catheter clearance (Cathflo® Activase® 1 mg/mL):

Patients <30 kg: 110% of the internal lumen volume of the catheter, not to exceed 2 mg/2 mL; retain in catheter for 0.5-2 hours; may instill a second dose if catheter remains occluded

Patients ≥30 kg: 2 mg (2 mL); retain in catheter for 0.5-2 hours; may instill a second dose if catheter remains occluded

Intra-arterial: Acute peripheral arterial occlusion (unlabeled use):

Weight-based regimen: 0.001-0.02 mg/kg/hour (maximum dose: 2 mg/hour) (Semba, 2000)

or

Fixed-dose regimen: 0.12-2 mg/hour (Semba, 2000)

Note: The ACC/AHA guidelines state that thrombolysis is an effective and beneficial therapy for those with acute limb ischemia (Rutherford categories I and IIa) of <14 days duration (Hirsch, 2006). The optimal dosage and concentration has not been established; a number of intra-arterial delivery techniques are employed with continuous infusion being the most common (Ouriel, 2004). The Advisory Panel to the Society for Cardiovascular and Interventional Radiology on Thrombolytic Therapy recommends dosing of ≤2 mg/hour and concomitant administration of subtherapeutic heparin (aPTT 1.25-1.5 times baseline) (Semba, 2000). Duration of alteplase infusion dependent upon size and location of the thrombus; typically between 6-48 hours (Disini, 2008).

Intrapleural: Complicated parapneumonic effusion (unlabeled use):

Children >3 months: 4 mg in 40 mL NS, first dose at time of chest tube placement with 1 hour dwell time, repeat every 24 hours for 3 days (total of 3 doses) **or** 0.1 mg/kg (maximum: 3 mg) in 10-30 mL NS, first dose after pigtail catheter (chest tube) placement, 0.75-1 hour dwell time, repeat every 8 hours for 3 days (total of 9 doses) (IDSA/PIDS, 2011)

Adults: 10 mg in 30 mL NS administered twice daily with a 1 hour dwell time for a total of 3 days; each dose followed in >2 hours by intrapleural dornase alfa (Rahman, 2011). Some clinicians suggest consideration of fibrinolytic use when patients have failed at least 24 hours of chest tube drainage and are poor surgical candidates (Hamblin, 2010).

Dosage adjustment in renal impairment: No dosage adjustment provided in manufacturer's labeling.

Dosage adjustment in hepatic impairment: No dosage adjustment provided in manufacturer's labeling.

Usual Infusion Concentrations: Pediatric I.V. infusion: 0.5 mg/mL **or** 1 mg/mL

Usual Infusion Concentrations: Adult I.V. infusion: 1 mg/mL

Note: Concentrations for some indications (eg, peripheral arterial occlusion) may require further dilution (eg, 0.1-0.2 mg/mL [Chan, 2001; Semba, 2000]) and a usual concentration may not be established.

Administration

Activase®: ST-elevation MI or acute ischemic stroke: Administer bolus dose (prepared by one of three methods) over 1 minute followed by infusion.

Infusion: Remaining dose for STEMI, AIS, or total dose for acute pulmonary embolism may be administered as follows: Any quantity of drug not to be administered to the patient must be removed from vial(s) prior to administration of remaining dose.

50 mg vial: Either PVC bag or glass vial and infusion set

100 mg vial: Insert spike end of the infusion set through the same puncture site created by transfer device and infuse from vial

If further dilution is desired, may be diluted in equal volume of 0.9% sodium chloride or D_5W to yield a final concentration of 0.5 mg/mL.

Cathflo® Activase®: Intracatheter: Instill dose into occluded catheter. Do not force solution into catheter. After a 30-minute dwell time, assess catheter function by attempting to aspirate blood. If catheter is functional, aspirate 4-5 mL of blood in patients ≥10 kg or 3 mL in patients <10 kg to remove Cathflo® Activase® and residual clots. Gently irrigate the catheter with NS. If catheter remains nonfunctional, let Cathflo® Activase® dwell for another 90 minutes (total dwell time: 120 minutes) and reassess function. If catheter function is not restored, a second dose may be instilled.

Parapneumonic effusion (unlabeled use): Intrapleural: Instill dose into chest tube and clamp drain. Although the optimum dwell time has not been determined, clinical trials more often have used either a 45 minute (Hawkins, 2004) or 1 hour (Rahman, 2011; St. Peter, 2009) dwell time; after dwell period, release clamp and connect chest tube to continuous suction.

Monitoring Parameters
Acute ischemic stroke (AIS): Baseline: Neurologic examination, head CT (without contrast), blood pressure, CBC, aPTT, PT/INR, glucose. During and after initiation: In addition to monitoring for bleeding complications, the 2013 AHA/ASA guidelines for the early management of AIS recommends the following:
Perform neurological assessments every 15 minutes during infusion and every 30 minutes thereafter for the next 6 hours, then hourly until 24 hours after treatment.
If severe headache, acute hypertension, nausea, or vomiting occurs, discontinue the infusion and obtain emergency CT scan.
Measure BP every 15 minutes for the first 2 hours of initiation then every 30 minutes for the next 6 hours, then hourly until 24 hours after initiation of alteplase. Increase frequency if a systolic BP is ≥180 mm Hg or if a diastolic BP is ≥105 mm Hg; administer antihypertensive medications to maintain BP at or below these levels.
Obtain a follow-up CT scan at 24 hours before starting anticoagulants or antiplatelet agents.
Central venous catheter clearance: Assess catheter function by attempting to aspirate blood.
ST-elevation MI: Baseline: Blood pressure, serum cardiac biomarkers, CBC, PT/INR, aPTT. During and after initiation: Assess for evidence of cardiac reperfusion through resolution of chest pain, resolution of baseline ECG changes, preserved left ventricular function, cardiac enzyme washout phenomenon, and/or the appearance of reperfusion arrhythmias; assess for bleeding potential through clinical evidence of GI bleeding, hematuria, gingival bleeding, fibrinogen levels, fibrinogen degradation products, PT and aPTT.

Reference Range Not routinely measured; literature supports therapeutic levels of 0.52-1.8 mcg/mL
Fibrinogen: 200-400 mg/dL
Activated partial thromboplastin time (aPTT): 22.5-38.7 seconds
Prothrombin time (PT): 10.9-12.2 seconds

Test Interactions Altered results of coagulation and fibrinolytic activity tests

Dosage Forms Excipient information presented when available (limited, particularly for generics); consult specific product labeling.
Solution Reconstituted, Injection:
Cathflo Activase: 2 mg (1 ea)
Solution Reconstituted, Intravenous:
Activase: 50 mg (1 ea); 100 mg (1 ea)

◆ **Alteplase, Recombinant** *see* Alteplase *on page 85*
◆ **Alteplase, Tissue Plasminogen Activator, Recombinant** *see* Alteplase *on page 85*
◆ **Alti-Doxazosin (Can)** *see* Doxazosin *on page 656*
◆ **Alti-Flurbiprofen (Can)** *see* Flurbiprofen (Systemic) *on page 892*
◆ **Alti-Ipratropium (Can)** *see* Ipratropium (Nasal) *on page 1112*
◆ **Alti-MPA (Can)** *see* MedroxyPROGESTERone *on page 1278*
◆ **Altoprev** *see* Lovastatin *on page 1250*

Aluminum Hydroxide
(a LOO mi num hye DROKS ide)

Brand Names: U.S. DermaMed [OTC]
Brand Names: Canada Amphojel®; Basaljel®
Pharmacologic Category Antacid; Antidote; Protectant, Topical
Use Treatment of hyperacidity; hyperphosphatemia; temporary protection of minor cuts, scrapes, and burns

Dosage
Oral:
Hyperphosphatemia:
Children: 50-150 mg/kg/24 hours in divided doses every 4-6 hours, titrate dosage to maintain serum phosphorus within normal range
Adults: Initial: 300-600 mg 3 times/day with meals
Antacid: Adults: 600-1200 mg between meals and at bedtime
Topical: Apply to affected area as needed; reapply at least every 12 hours
Dosage adjustment in renal impairment: Aluminum may accumulate in renal impairment.

Additional Information Complete prescribing information should be consulted for additional detail.

Dosage Forms Excipient information presented when available (limited, particularly for generics); consult specific product labeling.
Ointment, External:
DermaMed: (113 g)
Suspension, Oral:
Generic: 320 mg/5 mL (473 mL)

Aluminum Hydroxide and Magnesium Carbonate
(a LOO mi num hye DROKS ide & mag NEE zhum KAR bun nate)

Brand Names: U.S. Acid Gone Extra Strength [OTC]; Acid Gone [OTC]; Gaviscon® Extra Strength [OTC]; Gaviscon® Liquid [OTC]
Index Terms Magnesium Carbonate and Aluminum Hydroxide
Pharmacologic Category Antacid
Use Temporary relief of symptoms associated with gastric acidity
Dosage Oral: Adults:
Liquid:
Gaviscon® Regular Strength: 15-30 mL 4 times/day after meals and at bedtime
Gaviscon® Extra Strength: 15-30 mL 4 times/day after meals
Tablet (Gaviscon® Extra Strength): Chew 2-4 tablets 4 times/day
Dosage adjustment in renal impairment: Aluminum and/or magnesium may accumulate in renal impairment.

Additional Information Complete prescribing information should be consulted for additional detail.

Dosage Forms Excipient information presented when available (limited, particularly for generics); consult specific product labeling.
Liquid:
Acid Gone: Aluminum hydroxide 31.7 mg and magnesium carbonate 119.3 mg per 5 mL (360 mL)
Gaviscon®: Aluminum hydroxide 31.7 mg and magnesium carbonate 119.3 mg per 5 mL (355 mL) [contains sodium 0.57 mEq/5 mL and benzyl alcohol; cool mint flavor]
Gaviscon® Extra Strength: Aluminum hydroxide 84.6 mg and magnesium carbonate 79.1 mg per 5 mL (355 mL) [contains sodium 0.9 mEq/5 mL and benzyl alcohol; cool mint flavor]
Tablet, chewable:
Acid Gone Extra Strength: Aluminum hydroxide 160 mg and magnesium carbonate 105 mg
Gaviscon® Extra Strength: Aluminum hydroxide 160 mg and magnesium carbonate 105 mg [contains sodium 19 mg/tablet (1.3 mEq/tablet); cherry and original flavors]

Aluminum Hydroxide and Magnesium Hydroxide

(a LOO mi num hye DROKS ide & mag NEE zhum hye DROK side)

Brand Names: U.S. Alamag [OTC]; Mag-Al Ultimate [OTC]; Mag-Al [OTC]

Brand Names: Canada Diovol®; Diovol® Ex; Gelusil® Extra Strength; Mylanta™

Index Terms Magnesium Hydroxide and Aluminum Hydroxide

Pharmacologic Category Antacid

Use Antacid for symptoms related to hyperacidity associated with heartburn, hiatal hernia, upset stomach, peptic ulcer, peptic esophagitis, or gastritis

Dosage Oral: Children ≥12 years and Adults: OTC labeling:

Liquid (aluminum hydroxide 200 mg and magnesium hydroxide 200 mg per 5 mL): 10-20 mL 4 times/day (maximum: 80 mL/day)

Suspension (aluminum hydroxide 500 mg and magnesium hydroxide 500 mg per 5 mL): 10-20 mL 4 times/day, between meals and at bedtime (maximum: 45 mL/day)

Tablet (aluminum hydroxide 300 mg and magnesium hydroxide 150 mg): 1-2 tablets after meals or at bedtime, or as needed (maximum: 16 tablets/day)

Dosage adjustment in renal impairment: Aluminum and/or magnesium may accumulate in severe renal impairment.

Additional Information Complete prescribing information should be consulted for additional detail.

Dosage Forms Excipient information presented when available (limited, particularly for generics); consult specific product labeling. [DSC] = Discontinued product

Liquid, oral:

Mag-Al: Aluminum hydroxide 200 mg and magnesium hydroxide 200 mg per 5 mL (30 mL) [dye free, ethanol free, sugar free; contains propylene glycol, sodium 4 mg/5 mL; peppermint flavor]

Suspension, oral:

Mag-Al Ultimate: Aluminum hydroxide 500 mg and magnesium hydroxide 500 mg per 5 mL (20 mL) [contains propylene glycol, sodium 4 mg/5 mL; peppermint flavor]

Tablet, chewable:

Alamag: Aluminum hydroxide 300 mg and magnesium hydroxide 150 mg [contains phenylalanine 2.63 mg; wild cherry flavor]

Aluminum Hydroxide and Magnesium Trisilicate

(a LOO mi num hye DROKS ide & mag NEE zhum trye SIL i kate)

Brand Names: U.S. Gaviscon® Tablet [OTC]

Index Terms Magnesium Trisilicate and Aluminum Hydroxide

Pharmacologic Category Antacid

Use Temporary relief of hyperacidity

Dosage Oral: Adults: Chew 2-4 tablets 4 times/day or as directed by healthcare provider

Dosage adjustment in renal impairment: Aluminum and/or magnesium may accumulate in renal impairment.

Additional Information Complete prescribing information should be consulted for additional detail.

Dosage Forms Excipient information presented when available (limited, particularly for generics); consult specific product labeling. [DSC] = Discontinued product

Tablet, chewable: Aluminum hydroxide 80 mg and magnesium trisilicate 20 mg

Gaviscon®: Aluminum hydroxide 80 mg and magnesium trisilicate 20 mg [contains sodium 0.8 mEq/tablet; butterscotch flavor]

Aluminum Hydroxide, Magnesium Hydroxide, and Simethicone

(a LOO mi num hye DROKS ide, mag NEE zhum hye DROKS ide, & sye METH i kone)

Brand Names: U.S. Alamag Plus [OTC]; Aldroxicon I [OTC]; Aldroxicon II [OTC]; Almacone® Double Strength [OTC]; Almacone® [OTC]; Gelusil® [OTC]; Geri-Mox [OTC]; Maalox® Advanced Maximum Strength [OTC]; Maalox® Advanced Regular Strength [OTC]; Mi-Acid Maximum Strength [OTC] [DSC]; Mi-Acid [OTC]; Mintox Plus [OTC]; Mylanta® Classic Maximum Strength Liquid [OTC]; Mylanta® Classic Regular Strength Liquid [OTC]; Rulox [OTC]

Brand Names: Canada Diovol Plus®; Gelusil®; Mylanta® Double Strength; Mylanta® Extra Strength; Mylanta® Regular Strength

Index Terms Magnesium Hydroxide, Aluminum Hydroxide, and Simethicone; Simethicone, Aluminum Hydroxide, and Magnesium Hydroxide

Pharmacologic Category Antacid; Antiflatulent

Use Temporary relief of hyperacidity associated with gas; may also be used for indications associated with other antacids

Dosage Oral: Adults: 10-20 mL or 2-4 tablets 4-6 times/day between meals and at bedtime; may be used every hour for severe symptoms

Dosage adjustment in renal impairment: Aluminum and/or magnesium may accumulate in renal impairment.

Additional Information Complete prescribing information should be consulted for additional detail.

Dosage Forms Excipient information presented when available (limited, particularly for generics); consult specific product labeling. [DSC] = Discontinued product

Liquid, oral: Aluminum hydroxide 200 mg, magnesium hydroxide 200 mg, and simethicone 20 mg per 5 mL (360 mL); aluminum hydroxide 400 mg, magnesium hydroxide 400 mg, and simethicone 40 mg per 5 mL (360 mL)

Aldroxicon I: Aluminum hydroxide 200 mg, magnesium hydroxide 200 mg, and simethicone 20 mg per 5 mL (30 mL)

Aldroxicon II: Aluminum hydroxide 400 mg, magnesium hydroxide 400 mg, and simethicone 40 mg per 5 mL (30 mL)

Almacone®: Aluminum hydroxide 200 mg, magnesium hydroxide 200 mg, and simethicone 20 mg per 5 mL (355 mL) [contains benzyl alcohol, ethanol <0.5%, magnesium 83 mg/5 mL]

Almacone® Double Strength: Aluminum hydroxide 400 mg, magnesium hydroxide 400 mg, and simethicone 40 mg per 5 mL (360 mL)

Maalox® Advanced Maximum Strength: Aluminum hydroxide 400 mg, magnesium hydroxide 400 mg, and simethicone 40 mg per 5 mL (355 mL, 769 mL) [contains magnesium 167 mg/5 mL; cherry flavor]

Maalox® Advanced Maximum Strength: Aluminum hydroxide 400 mg, magnesium hydroxide 400 mg, and simethicone 40 mg per 5 mL (355 mL, 769 mL) [contains magnesium 167 mg/5 mL; lemon flavor]

Maalox® Advanced Maximum Strength: Aluminum hydroxide 400 mg, magnesium hydroxide 400 mg, and simethicone 40 mg per 5 mL (355 mL) [contains magnesium 167 mg/5 mL; mint flavor]

Maalox® Advanced Maximum Strength: Aluminum hydroxide 400 mg, magnesium hydroxide 400 mg, and simethicone 40 mg per 5 mL (355 mL) [contains magnesium 167 mg/5 mL; vanilla crème flavor]

Maalox® Advanced Regular Strength: Aluminum hydroxide 200 mg, magnesium hydroxide 200 mg, and simethicone 20 mg per 5 mL (360 mL, 780 mL) [contains magnesium 75 mg/5 mL, potassium 5 mg/5 mL, propylene glycol; mint flavor]

Mi-Acid: Aluminum hydroxide 200 mg, magnesium hydroxide 200 mg, and simethicone 20 mg per 5 mL (360 mL)

Mi-Acid Maximum Strength: Aluminum hydroxide 400 mg, magnesium hydroxide 400 mg, and simethicone 40 mg per 5 mL (360 mL)

Mylanta® Classic Maximum Strength: Aluminum hydroxide 400 mg, magnesium hydroxide 400 mg, and simethicone 40 mg per 5 mL (360 mL, 720 mL) [original, cherry, orange creme, and mint flavors]

Mylanta® Classic Regular Strength: Aluminum hydroxide 200 mg, magnesium hydroxide 200 mg, and simethicone 20 mg per 5 mL (360 mL) [original and mint flavors]

Suspension, oral: Aluminum hydroxide 225 mg, magnesium hydroxide 200 mg, and simethicone 25 mg per 5 mL (360 mL)

Geri-Mox: Aluminum hydroxide 200 mg, magnesium hydroxide 200 mg, and simethicone 25 mg per 5 mL (355 mL) [contains benzyl alcohol, magnesium 85 mg/5 mL; mint flavor]

Rulox: Aluminum hydroxide 200 mg, magnesium hydroxide 200 mg, and simethicone 25 mg per 5 mL (355 mL) [contains magnesium 85 mg/5 mL; mint flavor]

Tablet, chewable: Aluminum hydroxide 200 mg, magnesium hydroxide 200 mg, and simethicone 25 mg

Alamag Plus: Aluminum hydroxide 200 mg, magnesium hydroxide 200 mg, and simethicone 25 mg [contains magnesium 83 mg/tablet, phenylalanine 2.6 mg/tablet; cherry flavor]

Almacone®: Aluminum hydroxide 200 mg, magnesium hydroxide 200 mg, and simethicone 20 mg [dye free; contains magnesium 82 mg/tablet; peppermint flavor]

Gelusil®: Aluminum hydroxide 200 mg, magnesium hydroxide 200 mg, and simethicone 25 mg [peppermint flavor]

Mintox Plus: Aluminum hydroxide 200 mg, magnesium hydroxide 200 mg, and simethicone 25 mg [lemon crème flavor]

◆ **Aluminum Sucrose Sulfate, Basic** *see* Sucralfate *on page 1955*

Aluminum Sulfate and Calcium Acetate

(a LOO mi num SUL fate & KAL see um AS e tate)

Brand Names: U.S. Domeboro® [OTC]; Gordon Boro-Packs [OTC]; Pedi-Boro® [OTC]

Index Terms Calcium Acetate and Aluminum Sulfate

Pharmacologic Category Topical Skin Product

Use Astringent wet dressing for relief of inflammatory conditions of the skin; reduce weeping that may occur in dermatitis

Dosage Topical: Soak affected area in the solution 2-4 times/day for 15-30 minutes or apply wet dressing soaked in the solution for more extended periods; rewet dressing with solution 2-4 times/day every 15-30 minutes

Additional Information Complete prescribing information should be consulted for additional detail.

Dosage Forms Excipient information presented when available (limited, particularly for generics); consult specific product labeling.

Powder, for solution, topical: Aluminum sulfate 1191 mg and calcium acetate 839 mg per packet (12s)

Domeboro®: Aluminum sulfate tetradecahydrate 1347 mg and calcium acetate monohydrate 952 mg per packet (12s, 100s)

Gordon Boro-Packs: Aluminum sulfate 49% and calcium acetate 51% per packet (100s)

Pedi-Boro®: Aluminum sulfate tetradecahydrate 1191 mg and calcium acetate monohydrate 839 mg per packet (12s, 100s)

◆ **Alupent** *see* Metaproterenol *on page 1309*

◆ **Aluvea** *see* Urea *on page 2140*

◆ **Alvesco** *see* Ciclesonide (Systemic) *on page 421*

◆ **Alvesco® (Can)** *see* Ciclesonide (Systemic) *on page 421*

Alvimopan

(al VI moe pan)

Brand Names: U.S. Entereg

Index Terms ADL-2698; LY246736

Pharmacologic Category Gastrointestinal Agent, Miscellaneous; Opioid Antagonist, Peripherally-Acting

Use Postoperative ileus: To accelerate the time to upper and lower GI recovery following surgeries including partial bowel resection with primary anastomosis

Pregnancy Risk Factor B

Pregnancy Considerations Adverse events have not been observed in animal reproduction studies.

Breast-Feeding Considerations It is not known if alvimopan is excreted in breast milk. The manufacturer recommends that caution be exercised when administering alvimopan to nursing women.

Prescribing and Access Restrictions As a requirement of the REMS program, access to this medication is restricted. Only hospitals enrolled in the ENTEREG Access Support and Education (E.A.S.E.™) Program may administer this medication. Hospital staff must be educated on the need to limit to short-term (no more than 15 doses) and inpatient use. Hospitals may contact the E.A.S.E.™ program at 1-877-282-4786.

Contraindications Patients who have taken therapeutic doses of opioids for more than 7 consecutive days immediately prior to alvimopan

Warnings/Precautions [U.S. Boxed Warning]: For short-term (≤15 doses) hospital use only. Only hospitals that have registered through the ENTEREG Access Support and Education (E.A.S.E.™) Program and met all requirements may use. It will not be dispensed to patients who have been discharged from the hospital. Use not recommended in patients with complete bowel obstruction or in patients having gastric or pancreatic anastomosis. Use with caution in patients with hepatic or renal impairment; use not recommended in patients with severe hepatic impairment or ESRD. Use with caution is patients recently exposed to opioids; may be more sensitive to gastrointestinal adverse effects (eg, abdominal pain, diarrhea, nausea and vomiting). Contraindicated in patients who have received therapeutic opioids for >7 consecutive days immediately prior to use. **[U.S. Boxed Warning]: A trend towards an increased incidence of MI was observed in alvimopan (low dose) treated patients compared to placebo in a 12-month study in patients treated with opioids for chronic pain. Other short-term studies have not observed this trend and a causal relationship has not been found.** MI was generally observed more frequently in the initial 1-4 months of treatment. Patients of Japanese descent should be monitored closely for gastrointestinal side effects (eg, abdominal pain, cramping, diarrhea) due to possibility of greater drug exposure; discontinue use if side effects occur.

Adverse Reactions Note: Incidence reported limited to bowel resection patients only.

1% to 10%:

Endocrine & metabolic: Hypokalemia (10%)

Gastrointestinal: Dyspepsia (7%)

Genitourinary: Urinary retention (3%)

Hematologic and oncologic: Anemia (5%)

Neuromuscular & skeletal: Back pain (3%)

Drug Interactions

Metabolism/Transport Effects None known.

Avoid Concomitant Use There are no known interactions where it is recommended to avoid concomitant use.

Increased Effect/Toxicity

The levels/effects of Alvimopan may be increased by: Analgesics (Opioid)

Decreased Effect There are no known significant interactions involving a decrease in effect.

Ethanol/Nutrition/Herb Interactions Food: When administered with a high-fat meal, extent and rate of absorption may be reduced (C_{max} and AUC decreased by ~38% and 21%, respectively).

Storage/Stability Store at 25°C (77°F); excursions permitted to 15°C to 30°C (59°F to 86°F).

Mechanism of Action An opioid receptor antagonist which blocks opioid binding at the mu receptor; alvimopan has restricted ability to cross the blood-brain barrier at therapeutic doses. It selectively and competitively binds to the GI tract mu opioid receptors and antagonizes the peripheral effects of opioids on gastrointestinal motility and secretion. Does not affect opioid analgesic effects or induce opioid withdrawal symptoms.

Pharmacodynamics/Kinetics

Distribution: V_d: 20-40 L

Protein binding: Parent drug: 80%; metabolite: 94% (both primarily to albumin)

Metabolism: Hydrolyzed to an amide hydrolysis compound (active metabolite) by gut microflora; further metabolism of active metabolite to glucuronide conjugates and other minor metabolites.

Bioavailability: ~6% (range: 1% to 19%)

Half-life elimination: 10-17 hours

Time to peak, plasma: Parent drug: ~2 hours; Metabolite: 36 hours

Excretion: Urine (~35% as unchanged drug and metabolites); feces (via biliary excretion)

Dosage Note: For hospital use only

Oral: Adults:

Initial: 12 mg administered 30 minutes to 5 hours prior to surgery

Maintenance: 12 mg twice daily beginning the day after surgery for a maximum of 7 days or until discharged from hospital (maximum total treatment: 15 doses)

Dosage adjustment in renal impairment:

Mild-to-severe impairment: No adjustment needed; use caution

ESRD: Use not recommended

Dosage adjustment in hepatic impairment:

Mild-to-moderate impairment (Child-Pugh class A or B): No adjustment needed; use caution

Severe impairment (Child-Pugh class C): Use not recommended

Dietary Considerations Take with or without food; high-fat meals may decrease the rate and extent of absorption

Administration Patient must be hospitalized. Initial dose should be administered 30 minutes to 5 hours prior to surgery. May be administered with or without food.

Dosage Forms Excipient information presented when available (limited, particularly for generics); consult specific product labeling.

Capsule, Oral:

Entereg: 12 mg

◆ ALX-0600 *see* Teduglutide *on page 1995*

◆ Alyacen 1/35 *see* Ethinyl Estradiol and Norethindrone *on page 793*

◆ Alyacen 7/7/7 *see* Ethinyl Estradiol and Norethindrone *on page 793*

Amantadine (a MAN ta deen)

Brand Names: Canada Dom-Amantadine; Mylan-Amantadine; PHL-Amantadine; PMS-Amantadine

Index Terms Adamantanamine Hydrochloride; Amantadine Hydrochloride; Symmetrel

Pharmacologic Category Anti-Parkinson's Agent, Dopamine Agonist; Antiviral Agent; Antiviral Agent, Adamantane

Additional Appendix Information

Antiparkinsonian Agents *on page 2289*

Use Prophylaxis and treatment of influenza A viral infection (per manufacturer labeling; also refer to current ACIP guidelines for recommendations during current flu season); treatment of parkinsonism; treatment of drug-induced extrapyramidal symptoms

Pregnancy Risk Factor C

Pregnancy Considerations Teratogenic effects were observed in animal studies and in case reports in humans.

Influenza infection may be more severe in pregnant women. Untreated influenza infection is associated with an increased risk of adverse events to the fetus and an increased risk of complications or death to the mother. Oseltamivir and zanamivir are currently recommended for the treatment or prophylaxis influenza in pregnant women and women up to 2 weeks postpartum. Antiviral agents are currently recommended as an adjunct to vaccination and should not be used as a substitute for vaccination in pregnant women (consult current CDC guidelines).

Healthcare providers are encouraged to refer women exposed to influenza vaccine, or who have taken an antiviral medication during pregnancy to the Vaccines and Medications in Pregnancy Surveillance System (VAMPSS) by contacting The Organization of Teratology Information Specialists (OTIS) at (877) 311-8972

Breast-Feeding Considerations The CDC recommends that women infected with the influenza virus follow general precautions (eg, frequent hand washing) to decrease viral transmission to the child. Mothers with influenza-like illnesses at delivery should consider avoiding close contact with the infant until they have received 48 hours of antiviral medication, fever has resolved, and cough and secretions can be controlled. These measures may help decrease (but not eliminate) the risk of transmitting influenza to the newborn during breast-feeding. During this time, breast milk can be expressed and bottle-fed to the infant by another person who is not infected. Protective measures, such as wearing a face mask, changing into a clean gown or clothing, and strict hand hygiene should be continued by the mother for ≥7 days after the onset of symptoms or until symptom-free for 24 hours. Infant care should be performed by a noninfected person when possible (consult current CDC guidelines).

Contraindications Hypersensitivity to amantadine or any component of the formulation

Warnings/Precautions May cause CNS depression, which may impair physical or mental abilities; patients must be cautioned about performing tasks which require mental alertness (eg, operating machinery or driving). There have been reports of suicidal ideation/attempt in patients with and without a history of psychiatric illness. Use with caution in patients with liver disease, a history of recurrent and eczematoid dermatitis, uncontrolled psychosis or severe psychoneurosis, seizures and in those receiving CNS stimulant drugs; reduce dose in renal disease; when treating Parkinson's disease, do not discontinue abruptly. In many patients, the therapeutic benefits of amantadine are limited to a few months. Abrupt discontinuation may cause agitation, anxiety, delirium, delusions, depression, hallucinations, paranoia, parkinsonian crisis, slurred speech, or stupor. Upon discontinuation of amantadine therapy, gradually taper dose. Elderly patients may be more susceptible to the CNS effects (using 2 divided daily doses may minimize this effect); may require dosage reductions based on renal function. Use with caution in patients with HF, peripheral edema, or orthostatic hypotension; dosage reduction may be required. Avoid in untreated angle closure glaucoma.

Dopamine agonists have been associated with compulsive behaviors and/or loss of impulse control, which has manifested as pathological gambling, libido increases (hypersexuality), and/or binge eating. Causality has not been established, and controversy exists as to whether this phenomenon is related to the underlying disease, prior behaviors/addictions, and/or drug therapy. Dose reduction or discontinuation of therapy has been reported to reverse these behaviors in some, but not all cases. Risk for melanoma development is increased in Parkinson's disease patients; drug causation or factors contributing to risk have not been established. Patients should be monitored closely and periodic skin examinations should be performed.

Due to increased resistance, the ACIP has recommended that rimantadine and amantadine no longer be used for the treatment or prophylaxis of influenza A in the United States until susceptibility has been re-established; consult current guidelines. Safety and efficacy have not been established in children <1 year of age.

Adverse Reactions

1% to 10%:

Cardiovascular: Orthostatic hypotension, peripheral edema

Central nervous system: Agitation, anxiety, ataxia, confusion, delirium, depression, dizziness, dream abnormality, fatigue, hallucinations, headache, insomnia, irritability, lightheadedness, nervousness, somnolence

Dermatologic: Livedo reticularis

Gastrointestinal: Anorexia, constipation, diarrhea, nausea, xerostomia

Respiratory: Dry nose

<1% (Limited to important or life-threatening): Aggressive behavior, agranulocytosis, alkaline phosphatase increased, allergic reaction, ALT increased, AST increased, amnesia, anaphylaxis, arrhythmia, bilirubin increased, BUN increased, cardiac arrest, coma, CPK increased, creatinine increased, delusions, diaphoresis, dysphagia, dyspnea, eczematoid dermatitis, euphoria, GGT increased, heart failure, hyperkinesis, LDH increased, leukopenia, mania, neutropenia, neuroleptic malignant syndrome (NMS; associated with dosage reduction or abrupt withdrawal of amantadine), oculogyric episodes, paresthesia, photosensitivity, psychosis, pulmonary edema, rash, respiratory failure (acute), seizures, suicidal ideation, suicide, urinary retention, withdrawal reactions (may include delirium, hallucinations, and psychosis), visual disturbances

Reported with dopamine agonists: Impulsive/compulsive behaviors (eg, pathological gambling, hypersexuality, binge eating)

Drug Interactions

Metabolism/Transport Effects None known.

Avoid Concomitant Use

Avoid concomitant use of Amantadine with any of the following: Amisulpride

Increased Effect/Toxicity

Amantadine may increase the levels/effects of: Glycopyrrolate; Highest Risk QTc-Prolonging Agents; Moderate Risk QTc-Prolonging Agents; Trimethoprim

The levels/effects of Amantadine may be increased by: MAO Inhibitors; Methylphenidate; Mifepristone; Trimethoprim

Decreased Effect

Amantadine may decrease the levels/effects of: Amisulpride; Antipsychotics (Typical); Influenza Virus Vaccine (Live/Attenuated)

The levels/effects of Amantadine may be decreased by: Amisulpride; Antipsychotics (Atypical); Antipsychotics (Typical); Metoclopramide

Ethanol/Nutrition/Herb Interactions Ethanol: Avoid ethanol (may increase CNS adverse effects).

Storage/Stability Store at 25°C (77°F); excursions permitted to 15°C to 30°C (59°F to 86°F).

Mechanism of Action As an antiviral, blocks the uncoating of influenza A virus preventing penetration of virus into host; antiparkinsonian activity may be due to its blocking the reuptake of dopamine into presynaptic neurons or by increasing dopamine release from presynaptic fibers

Pharmacodynamics/Kinetics

Onset of action: Antidyskinetic: Within 48 hours

Absorption: Well absorbed

Distribution: V_d: Normal: 1.5-6.1 L/kg; Renal failure: 5.1 ± 0.2 L/kg; in saliva, tear film, and nasal secretions; in animals, tissue (especially lung) concentrations higher than serum concentrations; crosses blood-brain barrier

Protein binding: Normal renal function: ~67%; Hemodialysis: ~59%

Metabolism: Not appreciable; small amounts of an acetyl metabolite identified

Bioavailability: 86% to 90%

Half-life elimination: Normal renal function: 16 ± 6 hours (9-31 hours); Healthy, older (≥60 years) males: 29 hours (range: 20-41 hours); End-stage renal disease: 7-10 days

Time to peak, plasma: 2-4 hours

Excretion: Urine (80% to 90% unchanged) by glomerular filtration and tubular secretion

Dosage Oral:

Children: Influenza A treatment/prophylaxis: **Note:** Due to issues of resistance, amantadine is no longer recommended for the treatment or prophylaxis of influenza A. Please refer to the current ACIP recommendations.

Influenza A treatment:

1-9 years: 5 mg/kg/day in 2 divided doses (manufacturers range: 4.4-8.8 mg/kg/day); maximum dose: 150 mg/day

≥10 years and <40 kg: 5 mg/kg/day in 2 divided doses (CDC, 2011)

≥10 years and ≥40 kg: 100 mg twice daily (CDC, 2011)

Note: Initiate within 24-48 hours after onset of symptoms; continue for 24-48 hours after symptom resolution (duration of therapy is generally 3-5 days)

Influenza A prophylaxis: Refer to "Influenza A treatment" dosing. **Note:** Continue prophylaxis throughout the peak influenza activity in the community or throughout the entire influenza season in patients who cannot be vaccinated. Development of immunity following vaccination takes ~2 weeks; amantadine therapy should be considered for high-risk patients from the time of vaccination until immunity has developed. For children <9 years receiving influenza vaccine for the first time, amantadine prophylaxis should continue for 6 weeks (4 weeks after the first dose and 2 weeks after the second dose).

Adults:

Drug-induced extrapyramidal symptoms: 100 mg twice daily; may increase to 300 mg/day in divided doses, if needed

Parkinson's disease: Usual dose: 100 mg twice daily as monotherapy; may increase to 400 mg/day in divided doses, if needed, with close monitoring. **Note:** Patients with a serious concomitant illness or those receiving high doses of other anti-parkinson drugs should be started at 100 mg/day; may increase to 100 mg twice daily, if needed, after one to several weeks.

Influenza A treatment/prophylaxis: **Note:** Due to issues of resistance, amantadine is no longer recommended for the treatment or prophylaxis of influenza A. Please refer to the current ACIP recommendations. The following is based on the manufacturer's labeling:

Influenza A treatment: 200 mg once daily **or** 100 mg twice daily (may be preferred to reduce CNS effects); **Note:** Initiate within 24-48 hours after onset of symptoms; continue for 24-48 hours after symptom resolution (duration of therapy is generally 3-5 days).

Influenza A prophylaxis: 200 mg once daily **or** 100 mg twice daily (may be preferred to reduce CNS effects). **Note:** Continue prophylaxis throughout the peak influenza activity in the community or throughout the entire influenza season in patients who cannot be vaccinated. Development of immunity following vaccination takes ~2 weeks; amantadine therapy should be considered for high-risk patients from the time of vaccination until immunity has developed.

Elderly (≥65 years): Adjust dose based on renal function; some patients tolerate the drug better when it is given in 2 divided daily doses (to avoid adverse neurologic reactions).

Influenza A treatment/prophylaxis: 100 mg once daily

Dosage adjustment in renal impairment:

Cl_{cr} 30-50 mL/minute: Administer 200 mg on day 1, then 100 mg/day

Cl_{cr} 15-29 mL/minute: Administer 200 mg on day 1, then 100 mg on alternate days

Cl_{cr} <15 mL/minute: Administer 200 mg every 7 days

Hemodialysis: Administer 200 mg every 7 days

Peritoneal dialysis: No supplemental dose is needed

Continuous arteriovenous or venous-venous hemofiltration: No supplemental dose is needed

Dosage adjustment in hepatic impairment: No dosage adjustment provided in manufacturer's labeling; use with caution.

Monitoring Parameters Renal function, Parkinson's symptoms, mental status, influenza symptoms, blood pressure

Test Interactions May interfere with urine detection of amphetamines/methamphetamines (false-positive).

Dosage Forms Excipient information presented when available (limited, particularly for generics); consult specific product labeling.

Capsule, Oral, as hydrochloride:

Generic: 100 mg

Syrup, Oral, as hydrochloride:

Generic: 50 mg/5 mL (10 mL, 473 mL)

Tablet, Oral, as hydrochloride:

Generic: 100 mg

- ◆ Amantadine Hydrochloride *see* Amantadine *on page 92*
- ◆ Amaryl *see* Glimepiride *on page 956*
- ◆ Amatine® (Can) *see* Midodrine *on page 1363*
- ◆ Ambi 10PEH/400GFN [OTC] *see* Guaifenesin and Phenylephrine *on page 978*
- ◆ Ambien *see* Zolpidem *on page 2242*
- ◆ Ambien CR *see* Zolpidem *on page 2242*
- ◆ Ambifed DM *see* Guaifenesin, Pseudoephedrine, and Dextromethorphan *on page 979*
- ◆ Ambifed-G [OTC] *see* Guaifenesin and Pseudoephedrine *on page 978*
- ◆ Ambifed-G DM *see* Guaifenesin, Pseudoephedrine, and Dextromethorphan *on page 979*
- ◆ AmBisome *see* Amphotericin B (Liposomal) *on page 128*
- ◆ AmBisome® (Can) *see* Amphotericin B (Liposomal) *on page 128*

Ambrisentan (am bri SEN tan)

Brand Names: U.S. Letairis

Brand Names: Canada Volibris

Index Terms BSF208075

Pharmacologic Category Endothelin Receptor Antagonist; Vasodilator

Use Pulmonary arterial hypertension: Treatment of pulmonary artery hypertension (PAH) World Health Organization (WHO) Group I to improve exercise ability and delay clinical worsening

Pregnancy Risk Factor X

Pregnancy Considerations [U.S. Boxed Warning]: May cause birth defects; use in pregnancy is contraindicated. Exclude pregnancy prior to initiation of therapy and obtain pregnancy tests monthly during treatment and for 1 month after therapy is complete. Reliable contraception must be used during therapy and for 1 month after stopping treatment. Based on animal studies, ambrisentan is likely to produce major birth defects if used by pregnant women. Two reliable methods of contraception (eg, hormone method with a barrier method or 2 barrier methods) must be used throughout treatment and for 1 month after stopping treatment. Patients who have undergone a tubal ligation or the insertion of a contraceptive implant or intrauterine device (Copper T 380A or LNg 20) do not require additional contraceptive measures. A missed menses or suspected pregnancy should be reported to a healthcare provider and prompt immediate pregnancy testing. Sperm counts may be reduced in men during treatment (as observed with bosentan). In general, women with pulmonary hypertension should avoid pregnancy. (Badesch, 2007; McLaughlin, 2009)

Breast-Feeding Considerations It is not known if ambrisentan is excreted in breast milk. Due to the potential for serious adverse reactions in the nursing infant, the manufacturer recommends a decision be made whether to discontinue nursing or to discontinue the drug, taking into account the importance of treatment to the mother.

Prescribing and Access Restrictions As a requirement of the REMS program, access to this medication is restricted. Only prescribers and pharmacies registered with this program may prescribe and dispense ambrisentan. Further information may be obtained from the manufacturer, Gilead Sciences, Inc at www.letairisrems.com or 1-866-664-5327.

Medication Guide Available Yes

Contraindications Pregnancy; idiopathic pulmonary fibrosis, including idiopathic pulmonary fibrosis with pulmonary hypertension (WHO Group 3)

Canadian labeling: Additional contraindications (not in U.S. labeling): Hypersensitivity to ambrisentan or any component of the formulation

Warnings/Precautions Hazardous agent - use appropriate precautions for handling and disposal (NIOSH, 2012). **[U.S. Boxed Warning]: May cause birth defects; use in pregnancy is contraindicated. Exclude pregnancy prior to initiation of therapy and obtain pregnancy tests monthly during treatment and for 1 month after therapy is complete. Reliable contraception must be**

used during therapy and for 1 month after stopping treatment. Two reliable methods of contraception (eg, hormone method with a barrier method or 2 barrier methods) must be used throughout treatment and for 1 month after stopping treatment. Patients who have undergone a tubal ligation or the insertion of a contraceptive implant or intrauterine device (Copper T 380A or LNg 20) do not require additional contraceptive measures. A missed menses or suspected pregnancy should be reported to a healthcare provider and prompt immediate pregnancy testing. Women should also be educated on the appropriate use of emergency contraception if failure of contraceptive is known or suspected or in the event of unprotected sex.

[U.S. Boxed Warning]: Because of the high likelihood of teratogenic effects, ambrisentan is only available through the Letairis REMS restricted distribution program. Patients, prescribers, and pharmacies must be registered with and meet conditions of the program. Call 1-866-664-5327 or visit www.letairisrems.com for more information.

Use caution in patients with low hemoglobin levels. May cause decreases in hemoglobin and hematocrit (monitoring of hemoglobin is recommended. Use not recommended in patients with clinically significant anemia. Development of peripheral edema due to treatment and/or disease state (pulmonary arterial hypertension) may occur; a higher incidence is seen in elderly patients. Sperm count may be reduced in men during treatment (as observed with bosentan). No changes in sperm function or hormone levels have been noted. Fertility issues may require discussion with patient. Increases in serum liver aminotransferases have been reported during postmarketing use; however, in the majority of the cases, alternative causes of hepatotoxicity could be identified. Perform liver enzyme testing only when clinically indicated. Discontinue therapy if signs/symptoms of hepatic injury appear, if serum liver aminotransferases >5 times ULN are observed, or if aminotransferases are increased in the presence of bilirubin >2 times ULN. Hepatotoxicity has been reported with other endothelin receptor antagonists (eg, bosentan); however, ambrisentan may be tried in patients that have experienced asymptomatic increases in liver enzymes caused by another endothelin receptor antagonist after the liver enzymes have returned to normal. Use caution in patients with mild hepatic impairment; use not recommended in patients with moderate-to-severe impairment. There have also been postmarketing reports of fluid retention requiring treatment (eg, diuretics, fluid management, hospitalization). Further evaluation may be necessary to determine cause and appropriate treatment or discontinuation of therapy. Discontinue in any patient with pulmonary edema suggestive of pulmonary veno-occlusive disease (PVOD).

Adverse Reactions

>10%:

Cardiovascular: Peripheral edema (17%)

Central nervous system: Headache (15%)

1% to 10%:

Cardiovascular: Palpitation (5%), flushing (4%)

Gastrointestinal: Constipation (4%), abdominal pain (3%)

Hematologic: Hemoglobin decreased (7% to 10%)

Respiratory: Nasal congestion (6%), dyspnea (4%), nasopharyngitis (3%), sinusitis (3%)

Postmarketing and/or case reports: Anemia, angioedema, dizziness, fatigue, fluid retention, heart failure, hypersensitivity, liver enzymes increased, nausea, rash, vomiting, weakness

Drug Interactions

Metabolism/Transport Effects Substrate of CYP2C19 (minor), CYP3A4 (minor), P-glycoprotein, UGT1A3, UGT1A9, UGT2B7; **Note:** Assignment of Major/Minor substrate status based on clinically relevant drug interaction potential

Avoid Concomitant Use There are no known interactions where it is recommended to avoid concomitant use.

Increased Effect/Toxicity

The levels/effects of Ambrisentan may be increased by: CycloSPORINE (Systemic)

Decreased Effect There are no known significant interactions involving a decrease in effect.

Ethanol/Nutrition/Herb Interactions

Food: Grapefruit/grapefruit juice may increase levels/effects of ambrisentan.

Herb/Nutraceutical: Avoid St John's wort (concurrent use may decrease levels/effects of ambrisentan).

Storage/Stability Store at 25°C (77°F); excursions are permitted between 15°C and 30°C (59°F and 86°F). Store in original packaging.

Mechanism of Action Blocks endothelin receptor subtypes ET_A and ET_B on vascular endothelium and smooth muscle. Stimulation of ET_A receptors, located primarily in pulmonary vascular smooth muscle cells is associated with vasoconstriction and cellular proliferation. Stimulation of ET_B receptors, located in both pulmonary vascular endothelial cells and smooth muscle cells is associated with vasodilation, antiproliferative effects, and endothelin clearance. Although ambrisentan blocks both ET_A and ET_B receptors, the affinity is greater for the ET_A receptor (>4000 fold higher affinity).

Pharmacodynamics/Kinetics

Protein binding: 99%

Metabolism: Hepatic via CYP3A4, CYP2C19, and uridine 5'-diphosphate glucuronosyltransferases (UGTs) 1A9S, 2B7S, and 1A3S; *in vitro* studies also suggest it is a substrate of organic anion transporting polypeptides (OATP) 1B1 and 1B3 and P-glycoprotein (P-gp)

Half-life elimination: ~9 hours

Time to peak, plasma: ~2 hours

Excretion: Primarily nonrenal

Dosage Oral: Adults: Initial: 5 mg once daily; if tolerated, may increase to maximum 10 mg once daily

Coadministration with cyclosporine: Ambrisentan dose should not exceed 5 mg/day

Dosage adjustment in renal impairment:

Mild-to-moderate renal impairment: No dosage adjustment necessary.

Severe renal impairment: There is no data available for use in severe renal impairment.

Dosage adjustment in hepatic impairment:

Mild hepatic impairment: There is no data available for use in mild hepatic impairment; exposure may be increased.

Moderate-to-severe hepatic impairment: Use not recommended

Dietary Considerations Avoid grapefruit and grapefruit juice.

Administration Swallow tablet whole. Do not split, crush, or chew tablets. May be administered with or without food.

Hazardous agent; use appropriate precautions for handling and disposal (NIOSH, 2012).

Monitoring Parameters Monitor for significant peripheral edema and evaluate etiology if it occurs; liver enzyme testing when clinically appropriate

A woman of childbearing potential must have a negative pregnancy test prior to the initiation of therapy, monthly during treatment, and 1 month after stopping treatment. Hemoglobin and hematocrit should be measured at ▶

baseline, at 1 month, and periodically thereafter (generally stabilizes after the first few weeks of treatment).

Dosage Forms Excipient information presented when available (limited, particularly for generics); consult specific product labeling.

Tablet, Oral:

Letairis: 5 mg, 10 mg [contains fd&c red #40 aluminum lake]

◆ AMD3100 *see* Plerixafor *on page 1657*
◆ Amerge *see* Naratriptan *on page 1429*
◆ A-Methapred *see* MethylPREDNISolone *on page 1340*
◆ Amethia *see* Ethinyl Estradiol and Levonorgestrel *on page 787*
◆ Amethia Lo *see* Ethinyl Estradiol and Levonorgestrel *on page 787*
◆ Amethocaine Hydrochloride *see* Tetracaine (Ophthalmic) *on page 2034*
◆ Amethocaine Hydrochloride *see* Tetracaine (Systemic) *on page 2033*
◆ Amethocaine Hydrochloride *see* Tetracaine (Topical) *on page 2034*
◆ Amethopterin *see* Methotrexate *on page 1324*
◆ Amethyst *see* Ethinyl Estradiol and Levonorgestrel *on page 787*
◆ Ametop™ (Can) *see* Tetracaine (Topical) *on page 2034*
◆ Amfepramone *see* Diethylpropion *on page 604*
◆ AMG 073 *see* Cinacalcet *on page 428*
◆ AMG-162 *see* Denosumab *on page 568*
◆ AMG 531 *see* RomiPLOStim *on page 1850*
◆ Amicar *see* Aminocaproic Acid *on page 100*
◆ Amidate *see* Etomidate *on page 801*
◆ Amidate® (Can) *see* Etomidate *on page 801*

Amifostine (am i FOS teen)

Brand Names: U.S. Ethyol

Brand Names: Canada Ethyol®

Index Terms Ethiofos; Gammaphos; WR-2721; YM-08310

Pharmacologic Category Adjuvant, Chemoprotective Agent (Cytoprotective); Antidote

Use Reduce the incidence of moderate-to-severe xerostomia in patients undergoing postoperative radiation treatment for head and neck cancer, where the radiation port includes a substantial portion of the parotid glands; reduce the cumulative renal toxicity associated with repeated administration of cisplatin

Unlabeled Use Prevention of radiation proctitis in patients with rectal cancer

Pregnancy Risk Factor C

Pregnancy Considerations Animal studies have demonstrated embryotoxicity. There are no adequate and well-controlled studies in pregnant women.

Breast-Feeding Considerations Due to the potential for adverse reactions in the nursing infant, breast-feeding should be discontinued.

Contraindications Hypersensitivity to aminothiol compounds or any component of the formulation

Warnings/Precautions Patients who are hypotensive or dehydrated should not receive amifostine. Interrupt antihypertensive therapy for 24 hours before treatment; patients who cannot safely stop their antihypertensives 24 hours before, should not receive amifostine. Adequately hydrated prior to treatment and keep in a supine position during infusion. Monitor blood pressure every 5 minutes during the infusion. If hypotension requiring interruption of therapy occurs, patients should be placed in the Trendelenburg position and given an infusion of normal saline using a separate I.V. line; subsequent infusions may require a dose reduction. Infusions >15 minutes are associated with a higher incidence of adverse effects. Use caution in patients with cardiovascular and cerebrovascular disease and any other patients in whom the adverse effects of hypotension may have serious adverse events.

Serious cutaneous reactions, including erythema multiforme, Stevens-Johnson syndrome, toxic epidermal necrolysis, toxoderma and exfoliative dermatitis have been reported with amifostine. May be delayed, developing up to weeks after treatment initiation. Cutaneous reactions have been reported more frequently when used as a radioprotectant. Discontinue treatment for severe/serious cutaneous reaction, or with fever. Withhold treatment and obtain dermatologic consultation for rash involving lips or mucosa (of unknown etiology outside of radiation port) and for bullous, edematous or erythematous lesions on hands, feet, or trunk; reinitiate only after careful evaluation.

It is recommended that antiemetic medication, including dexamethasone 20 mg I.V. and a serotonin 5-HT_3 receptor antagonist be administered prior to and in conjunction with amifostine. Rare hypersensitivity reactions, including anaphylaxis and allergic reaction, have been reported; discontinue if allergic reaction occurs; do not rechallenge. Medications for the treatment of hypersensitivity reactions should be available.

Reports of clinically-relevant hypocalcemia are rare, but serum calcium levels should be monitored in patients at risk of hypocalcemia, such as those with nephrotic syndrome; may require calcium supplementation. Should not be used (in patients receiving chemotherapy for malignancies other than ovarian cancer) where chemotherapy is expected to provide significant survival benefit or in patients receiving definitive radiotherapy, unless within the context of a clinical trial. Safety and efficacy in children have not been established.

Adverse Reactions

>10%:

Cardiovascular: Hypotension (15% to 61%; grades 3/4: 3% to 8%; dose dependent)

Gastrointestinal: Nausea/vomiting (53% to 96%; grades 3/4: 8% to 30%; dose dependent)

1% to 10%: Endocrine & metabolic: Hypocalcemia (clinically significant: 1%)

<1% (Limited to important or life-threatening): Apnea, anaphylactoid reactions, anaphylaxis, arrhythmia, atrial fibrillation, atrial flutter, back pain, bradycardia, cardiac arrest, chest pain, chest tightness, chills, cutaneous eruptions, dizziness, erythema multiforme, exfoliative dermatitis, extrasystoles, dyspnea, fever, flushing, hiccups, hypersensitivity reactions (fever, rash, hypoxia, dyspnea, laryngeal edema), hypertension (transient), hypoxia, malaise, MI, myocardial ischemia, pruritus, rash (mild), renal failure, respiratory arrest, rigors, seizure, sneezing, somnolence, Stevens-Johnson syndrome, supraventricular tachycardia, syncope, tachycardia, toxic epidermal necrolysis, toxoderma, urticaria

Drug Interactions

Metabolism/Transport Effects None known.

Avoid Concomitant Use There are no known interactions where it is recommended to avoid concomitant use.

Increased Effect/Toxicity

The levels/effects of Amifostine may be increased by: Antihypertensives

Decreased Effect There are no known significant interactions involving a decrease in effect.

Preparation for Administration For I.V. infusion, reconstitute intact vials with 9.7 mL 0.9% sodium chloride injection and dilute in 0.9% sodium chloride to a final concentration of 5-40 mg/mL. For SubQ administration, reconstitute with 2.5 mL NS or SWFI.

Storage/Stability Store intact vials of lyophilized powder at room temperature of 20°C to 25°C (68°F to 77°F). Reconstituted solutions (500 mg/10 mL) and solutions for infusion are chemically stable for up to 5 hours at room temperature (25°C) or up to 24 hours under refrigeration (2°C to 8°C).

Mechanism of Action Prodrug that is dephosphorylated by alkaline phosphatase in tissues to a pharmacologically-active free thiol metabolite. The free thiol is available to bind to, and detoxify, reactive metabolites of cisplatin; and can also act as a scavenger of free radicals that may be generated (by cisplatin or radiation therapy) in tissues.

Pharmacodynamics/Kinetics

Distribution: V_d: 3.5 L

Metabolism: Hepatic dephosphorylation to two metabolites (active-free thiol and disulfide)

Half-life elimination: ~8-9 minutes

Excretion: Urine

Clearance, plasma: 2.17 L/minute

Dosage Note: Antiemetic medication, including dexamethasone 20 mg I.V. and a serotonin 5-HT_3 receptor antagonist, is recommended prior to and in conjunction with amifostine.

Adults:

Cisplatin-induced renal toxicity, reduction: I.V.: 910 mg/m^2 over 15 minutes once daily 30 minutes prior to cisplatin

For 910 mg/m^2 doses, the manufacturer suggests the following blood pressure-based adjustment schedule:

The infusion of amifostine should be interrupted if the systolic blood pressure decreases significantly from baseline, as defined below:

Decrease of 20 mm Hg if baseline systolic blood pressure <100

Decrease of 25 mm Hg if baseline systolic blood pressure 100-119

Decrease of 30 mm Hg if baseline systolic blood pressure 120-139

Decrease of 40 mm Hg if baseline systolic blood pressure 140-179

Decrease of 50 mm Hg if baseline systolic blood pressure ≥180

If blood pressure returns to normal within 5 minutes (assisted by fluid administration and postural management) and the patient is asymptomatic, the infusion may be restarted so that the full dose of amifostine may be administered. If the full dose of amifostine cannot be administered, the dose of amifostine for subsequent cycles should be 740 mg/m^2.

Xerostomia from head and neck cancer, reduction:

I.V.: 200 mg/m^2 over 3 minutes once daily 15-30 minutes prior to radiation therapy **or**

SubQ (unlabeled route): 500 mg once daily prior to radiation therapy

Prevention of radiation proctitis in rectal cancer (unlabeled use): I.V.: 340 mg/m^2 once daily prior to radiation therapy (Keefe, 2007; Peterson, 2008)

Dosage adjustment in renal impairment: No dosage adjustment provided in manufacturer's labeling.

Dosage adjustment in hepatic impairment: No dosage adjustment provided in manufacturer's labeling.

Administration I.V.: Administer over 3 minutes (prior to radiation therapy) or 15 minutes (prior to cisplatin); administration as a longer infusion is associated with a higher incidence of side effects. Patients should be kept in supine position during infusion. **Note:** SubQ administration (unlabeled) has been used.

Monitoring Parameters Blood pressure should be monitored every 5 minutes during the infusion and after administration if clinically indicated; serum calcium levels (in patients at risk for hypocalcemia). Evaluate for cutaneous reactions prior to each dose.

Additional Information Oncology Comment: The American Society of Clinical Oncology (ASCO) guidelines for the use of protectants for chemotherapy and radiation (Hensley, 2008) recommend the use of amifostine for prevention of nephrotoxicity due to cisplatin-based chemotherapy and to decrease the incidence of acute and delayed radiation therapy-induced xerostomia. The ASCO guidelines do not recommend the use of amifostine to reduce the incidence of neutropenia or thrombocytopenia associated with chemotherapy or radiation therapy, neurotoxicity or ototoxicity associated with platinum-based chemotherapy, radiation therapy-induced mucositis associated with head and neck cancer, or esophagitis due to chemotherapy in patients with nonsmall cell lung cancer. Additionally, the guidelines do not support the use of amifostine in patients with head and neck cancer receiving concurrent platinum-based chemotherapy.

Dosage Forms Excipient information presented when available (limited, particularly for generics); consult specific product labeling.

Solution Reconstituted, Intravenous:

Ethyol: 500 mg (1 ea)

Generic: 500 mg (1 ea)

Solution Reconstituted, Intravenous [preservative free]:

Generic: 500 mg (1 ea)

◆ Amigesic® (Can) *see* Salsalate *on page 1873*

Amikacin (am i KAY sin)

Brand Names: Canada Amikacin Sulfate Injection, USP; Amikin®

Index Terms Amikacin Sulfate

Pharmacologic Category Antibiotic, Aminoglycoside

Use Treatment of serious infections (bone infections, respiratory tract infections, endocarditis, and septicemia) due to organisms resistant to gentamicin and tobramycin, including *Pseudomonas*, *Proteus*, *Serratia*, and other gram-negative bacilli; documented infection of mycobacterial organisms susceptible to amikacin

Unlabeled Use Bacterial endophthalmitis; *Mycobacterium avium* complex (MAC; fibrocavitary or severe nodular/bronchiectatic disease)

Pregnancy Risk Factor D

Pregnancy Considerations Adverse events were not observed in the initial animal reproduction studies; however, renal toxicity has been reported in additional studies. Amikacin crosses the placenta, produces detectable serum levels in the fetus, and concentrates in the fetal kidneys. Because of several reports of total irreversible bilateral congenital deafness in children whose mothers received another aminoglycoside (streptomycin) during pregnancy, the manufacturer classifies amikacin as pregnancy risk factor D. Although serious side effects to the fetus have not been reported following maternal use of amikacin, a potential for harm exists.

Due to pregnancy-induced physiologic changes, some pharmacokinetic parameters of amikacin may be altered. Pregnant women have an average-to-larger volume of distribution which may result in lower peak serum levels than for the same dose in nonpregnant women. Serum half-life may also be shorter.

Breast-Feeding Considerations Amikacin is excreted into breast milk in trace amounts; however, it is not absorbed when taken orally. This limited oral absorption may minimize exposure to the nursing infant. Nondose-related effects could include modification of bowel flora. Breast-feeding is not recommended by the manufacturer.

Contraindications Hypersensitivity to amikacin sulfate or any component of the formulation; cross-sensitivity may exist with other aminoglycosides

Warnings/Precautions [U.S. Boxed Warning]: Amikacin may cause neurotoxicity, nephrotoxicity, and/or neuromuscular blockade and respiratory paralysis; usual risk factors include pre-existing renal impairment, concomitant neuro-/nephrotoxic medications, advanced age and dehydration. Dose and/or frequency of administration must be monitored and modified in patients with renal impairment. Drug should be discontinued if signs of ototoxicity, nephrotoxicity, or hypersensitivity occur. Ototoxicity is proportional to the amount of drug given and the duration of treatment. Tinnitus or vertigo may be indications of vestibular injury and impending bilateral irreversible damage. Renal damage is usually reversible. Use with caution in patients with neuromuscular disorders, hearing loss and hypocalcemia. Prolonged use may result in fungal or bacterial superinfection, including *C. difficile*-associated diarrhea (CDAD) and pseudomembranous colitis; CDAD has been observed >2 months postantibiotic treatment. Solution contains sodium metabisulfate; use caution in patients with sulfite allergy.

Adverse Reactions

1% to 10%:

Central nervous system: Neurotoxicity

Genitourinary: Nephrotoxicity

Otic: Auditory ototoxicity, vestibular ototoxicity

<1% (Limited to important or life-threatening): Dyspnea, eosinophilia, hypersensitivity reaction

Drug Interactions

Metabolism/Transport Effects None known.

Avoid Concomitant Use

Avoid concomitant use of Amikacin with any of the following: BCG; Gallium Nitrate

Increased Effect/Toxicity

Amikacin may increase the levels/effects of: AbobotulinumtoxinA; Bisphosphonate Derivatives; CARBOplatin; Colistimethate; CycloSPORINE (Systemic); Gallium Nitrate; Neuromuscular-Blocking Agents; OnabotulinumtoxinA; RimabotulinumtoxinB; Tenofovir

The levels/effects of Amikacin may be increased by: Amphotericin B; Capreomycin; Cephalosporins (2nd Generation); Cephalosporins (3rd Generation); Cephalosporins (4th Generation); CISplatin; Loop Diuretics; Nonsteroidal Anti-Inflammatory Agents; Tenofovir; Vancomycin

Decreased Effect

Amikacin may decrease the levels/effects of: BCG; Sodium Picosulfate; Typhoid Vaccine

The levels/effects of Amikacin may be decreased by: Penicillins

Storage/Stability Store at controlled room temperature. Following admixture at concentrations of 0.25-5 mg/mL, amikacin is stable for 24 hours at room temperature and 2 days at refrigeration when mixed in D_5W, NS, and LR.

Mechanism of Action Inhibits protein synthesis in susceptible bacteria by binding to 30S ribosomal subunits

Pharmacodynamics/Kinetics

Absorption:

I.M.: Rapid

Oral: Poorly absorbed

Distribution: V_d: 0.25 L/kg; primarily into extracellular fluid (highly hydrophilic); penetrates blood-brain barrier when meninges inflamed

Relative diffusion of antimicrobial agents from blood into CSF: Good only with inflammation (exceeds usual MICs)

CSF:blood level ratio: Normal meninges: 10% to 20%; Inflamed meninges: 15% to 24%

Protein-binding: 0% to 11%

Half-life elimination (renal function and age dependent):

Infants: Low birth weight (1-3 days): 7-9 hours; Full-term >7 days: 4-5 hours

Children: 1.6-2.5 hours

Adults: Normal renal function: 1.4-2.3 hours; Anuria/end-stage renal disease: 28-86 hours

Time to peak, serum: I.M.: 45-120 minutes

Excretion: Urine (94% to 98%)

Dosage Note: Individualization is critical because of the low therapeutic index

In underweight and nonobese patients, use of total body weight (TBW) instead of ideal body weight for determining the initial mg/kg/dose is widely accepted (Nicolau, 1995). Ideal body weight (IBW) also may be used to determine doses for patients who are neither underweight nor obese (Gilbert, 2009).

Initial and periodic peak and trough plasma drug levels should be determined, particularly in critically-ill patients with serious infections or in disease states known to significantly alter aminoglycoside pharmacokinetics (eg, cystic fibrosis, burns, or major surgery). Manufacturer recommends a maximum daily dose of 15 mg/kg/day (or 1.5 g/day in heavier patients). Higher doses may be warranted based on therapeutic drug monitoring or susceptibility information.

Usual dosage range:

Infants and Children: I.M., I.V.: 5-7.5 mg/kg/dose every 8 hours

Adults:

I.M., I.V.: 5-7.5 mg/kg/dose every 8 hours; **Note:** Some clinicians suggest a daily dose of 15-20 mg/kg for all patients with normal renal function. This dose is at least as efficacious with similar, if not less, toxicity than conventional dosing.

Intrathecal/intraventricular (unlabeled route): Meningitis (susceptible gram-negative organisms): 5-50 mg/day

Indication-specific dosing:

Adults:

Endophthalmitis, bacterial (unlabeled use): Intravitreal: 0.4 mg/0.1 mL NS in combination with vancomycin

Hospital-acquired pneumonia (HAP): I.V.: 20 mg/kg/day with antipseudomonal beta-lactam or carbapenem (American Thoracic Society/ATS guidelines)

Meningitis (susceptible gram-negative organisms):

I.V.: 5 mg/kg every 8 hours (administered with another bactericidal drug)

Intrathecal/intraventricular (unlabeled route): Usual dose: 30 mg/day (IDSA, 2004); Range: 5-50 mg/day (with concurrent systemic antimicrobial therapy) (Gilbert, 1986; Guardado, 2008; IDSA, 2004; Kasiakou, 2005)

***Mycobacterium avium* complex (MAC) (unlabeled use):** I.V.: Adjunct therapy (with macrolide, rifamycin, and ethambutol): 8-25 mg/kg 2-3 times weekly for first 2-3 months for severe disease (maximum single dose for age >50 years: 500 mg) (Griffith, 2007)

Mycobacterium fortuitum, M. chelonae, or M. abscessus: I.V.: 10-15 mg/kg daily for at least 2 weeks with high dose cefoxitin

Dosage adjustment in renal impairment: Some patients may require larger or more frequent doses if serum levels document the need (ie, cystic fibrosis or febrile granulocytopenic patients).

Cl_{cr} ≥60 mL/minute: Administer every 8 hours
Cl_{cr} 40-60 mL/minute: Administer every 12 hours
Cl_{cr} 20-40 mL/minute: Administer every 24 hours
Cl_{cr} <20 mL/minute: Loading dose, then monitor levels

Intermittent hemodialysis (IHD) (administer after hemodialysis on dialysis days): Dialyzable (20%; variable; dependent on filter, duration, and type of HD): 5-7.5 mg/kg every 48-72 hours. Follow levels. Redose when pre-HD concentration <10 mg/L; redose when post-HD concentration <6-8 mg/L (Heintz, 2009). **Note:** Dosing dependent on the assumption of 3 times/week, complete IHD sessions.

Peritoneal dialysis (PD): Dose as Cl_{cr} <20 mL/minute: Follow levels

Continuous renal replacement therapy (CRRT) (Heintz, 2009; Trotman, 2005): Drug clearance is highly dependent on the method of renal replacement, filter type, and flow rate. Appropriate dosing requires close monitoring of pharmacologic response, signs of adverse reactions due to drug accumulation, as well as drug concentrations in relation to target trough (if appropriate). The following are general recommendations only (based on dialysate flow/ultrafiltration rates of 1-2 L/hour and minimal residual renal function) and should not supersede clinical judgment:

CVVH/CVVHD/CVVHDF: Loading dose of 10 mg/kg followed by maintenance dose of 7.5 mg/kg every 24-48 hours

Note: For severe gram-negative rod infections, target peak concentration of 15-30 mg/L; redose when concentration <10 mg/L (Heintz, 2009).

Dosage adjustment in hepatic impairment: No dosage adjustment provided in manufacturer's labeling.

Dosing in obesity: In moderate obesity (TBW/IBW ≥1.25) or greater, (eg, morbid obesity [TBW/IBW >2]), initial dosage requirement may be estimated using a dosing weight of IBW + 0.4 (TBW - IBW) (Traynor, 1995).

Dietary Considerations Some products may contain sodium.

Administration Administer around-the-clock to promote less variation in peak and trough serum levels. Do not mix with other drugs, administer separately.

I.M.: Administer I.M. injection in large muscle mass.

I.V.: Infuse over 30-60 minutes.

Some penicillins (eg, carbenicillin, ticarcillin, and piperacillin) have been shown to inactivate *in vitro*. This has been observed to a greater extent with tobramycin and gentamicin, while amikacin has shown greater stability against inactivation. Concurrent use of these agents may pose a risk of reduced antibacterial efficacy *in vivo*, particularly in the setting of profound renal impairment. However, definitive clinical evidence is lacking. If combination penicillin/aminoglycoside therapy is desired in a patient with renal dysfunction, separation of doses (if feasible), and routine monitoring of aminoglycoside levels, CBC, and clinical response should be considered.

Intrathecal/Intraventricular (unlabeled route): Reserved solely for meningitis due to susceptible gram-negative organisms. Available formulation contains sodium metabisulfite. If possible, consider alternative therapy with gentamicin or tobramycin as both of these agents are available as preservative-free formulations.

Monitoring Parameters Urinalysis, BUN, serum creatinine, appropriately timed peak and trough concentrations, vital signs, temperature, weight, I & O, hearing parameters

Initial and periodic peak and trough plasma drug levels should be determined, particularly in critically-ill patients with serious infections or in disease states known to significantly alter aminoglycoside pharmacokinetics (eg, cystic fibrosis, burns, or major surgery). Aminoglycoside levels measured from blood taken from Silastic® central catheters can sometimes give falsely high readings (draw levels from alternate lumen or peripheral stick, if possible).

Some penicillin derivatives may accelerate the degradation of aminoglycosides *in vitro*. This may be clinically-significant for certain penicillin (ticarcillin, piperacillin, carbenicillin) and aminoglycoside (gentamicin, tobramycin) combination therapy in patients with significant renal impairment. Close monitoring of aminoglycoside levels is warranted.

Reference Range

Therapeutic levels:

Peak:

Life-threatening infections: 25-40 mcg/mL
Serious infections: 20-25 mcg/mL
Urinary tract infections: 15-20 mcg/mL

Trough: <8 mcg/mL

The American Thoracic Society (ATS) recommends trough levels of <4-5 mcg/mL for patients with hospital-acquired pneumonia.

Toxic concentration: Peak: >40 mcg/mL; Trough: >10 mcg/mL

Timing of serum samples: Draw peak 30 minutes after completion of 30-minute infusion or at 1 hour following initiation of infusion or I.M. injection; draw trough within 30 minutes prior to next dose

Test Interactions Some penicillin derivatives may accelerate the degradation of aminoglycosides *in vitro*, leading to a potential underestimation of aminoglycoside serum concentration.

Additional Information Aminoglycoside levels measured from blood taken from central venous catheters can sometimes give falsely high readings (draw levels from alternate lumen or peripheral stick, if possible).

Dosage Forms Excipient information presented when available (limited, particularly for generics); consult specific product labeling.

Solution, Injection, as sulfate:

Generic: 500 mg/2 mL (2 mL); 1 g/4 mL (4 mL)

Solution, Injection, as sulfate [preservative free]:

Generic: 500 mg/2 mL (2 mL); 1 g/4 mL (4 mL)

◆ **Amikacin Sulfate** *see* Amikacin *on page 97*

◆ **Amikacin Sulfate Injection, USP (Can)** *see* Amikacin *on page 97*

◆ **Amikin® (Can)** *see* Amikacin *on page 97*

AMILoride (a MIL oh ride)

Brand Names: Canada Apo-Amiloride®; Midamor

Index Terms Amiloride Hydrochloride

Pharmacologic Category Antihypertensive; Diuretic, Potassium-Sparing

Use Counteracts potassium loss induced by other diuretics in the treatment of hypertension or edematous conditions including CHF, hepatic cirrhosis, and hypoaldosteronism; usually used in conjunction with more potent diuretics such as thiazides or loop diuretics

Unlabeled Use Cystic fibrosis; reduction of lithium-induced polyuria; pediatric hypertension

Pregnancy Risk Factor B

Dosage Oral:

Children 1-17 years: Hypertension (unlabeled use): 0.4-0.625 mg/kg/day (maximum: 20 mg/day)

Adults: 5-10 mg/day (up to 20 mg)

Hypertension (JNC 7): 5-10 mg/day in 1-2 divided doses

Elderly: Initial: 5 mg once daily or every other day

Dosing adjustment in renal impairment:
Manufacturer's recommendations: Use of amiloride in patients with diabetes mellitus or S_{cr} >1.5 mg/dL should be done with caution and is contraindicated in patients with anuria, acute or chronic renal insufficiency, or evidence of diabetic nephropathy.
Alternate recommendations (Aronoff, 2007):
Cl_{cr} 10-50 mL/minute: Administer at 50% of normal dose.
Cl_{cr} <10 mL/minute: Avoid use.
Dosing adjustment in hepatic impairment: No dosage adjustment provided in the manufacturer's labeling; use with caution.

Additional Information Complete prescribing information should be consulted for additional detail.

Dosage Forms Excipient information presented when available (limited, particularly for generics); consult specific product labeling.
Tablet, Oral, as hydrochloride:
Generic: 5 mg

- **Amiloride Hydrochloride** *see* AMILoride *on page 99*
- **2-Amino-6-Mercaptopurine** *see* Thioguanine *on page 2045*
- **2-Amino-6-Methoxypurine Arabinoside** *see* Nelarabine *on page 1434*
- **2-Amino-6-Trifluoromethoxy-benzothiazole** *see* Riluzole *on page 1819*
- **Aminobenzylpenicillin** *see* Ampicillin *on page 130*

Aminocaproic Acid (a mee noe ka PROE ik AS id)

Brand Names: U.S. Amicar
Index Terms EACA; Epsilon Aminocaproic Acid
Pharmacologic Category Antifibrinolytic Agent; Antihemophilic Agent; Hemostatic Agent; Lysine Analog
Use To enhance hemostasis when fibrinolysis contributes to bleeding (causes may include cardiac surgery, hematologic disorders, neoplastic disorders, abruptio placentae, hepatic cirrhosis, and urinary fibrinolysis)
Unlabeled Use Treatment of traumatic hyphema; control bleeding in thrombocytopenia; control oral bleeding in congenital and acquired coagulation disorders; topical treatment (mouth rinse) of bleeding associated with dental procedures in patients on oral anticoagulant therapy; prevention of perioperative bleeding associated with cardiac surgery; prevention of bleeding associated with extracorporeal membrane oxygenation (ECMO); prevention of perioperative bleeding associated with spinal surgery (eg, idiopathic scoliosis)
Pregnancy Risk Factor C
Dosage
Acute bleeding: Adults: Oral, I.V.: Loading dose: 4-5 g during the first hour, followed by 1 g/hour (or 1.25 g/hour using oral solution) for 8 hours or until bleeding controlled (maximum daily dose: 30 g)
Control of bleeding with severe thrombocytopenia (unlabeled use) (Bartholomew, 1989; Gardner, 1980): Adults:
Initial: I.V.: 100 mg/kg (maximum dose: 5 g) over 30-60 minutes
Maintenance: Oral, I.V.: 1-4 g every 4-8 hours or 1 g/hour (maximum daily dose: 24 g)
Control of oral bleeding in congenital and acquired coagulation disorder (unlabeled use): Adults: Oral: 50-60 mg/kg every 4 hours (Mannucci, 1998)
Prevention of dental procedure bleeding in patients on oral anticoagulant therapy (unlabeled use): Adults: Oral rinse: Hold 4 g/10 mL in mouth for 2 minutes then spit out. Repeat every 6 hours for 2 days after procedure (Souto, 1996). Concentration and frequency may vary by institution and product availability.
Prevention of perioperative bleeding associated with cardiac surgery (unlabeled use): I.V.:
Children: 100 mg/kg given over 20-30 minutes after induction and prior to incision, 100 mg/kg during cardiopulmonary bypass, and 100 mg/kg after heparin reversal over 3 hours (Chauhan, 2004)
Adults: Loading dose of 75-150 mg/kg (typically 5-10 g), followed by 10-15 mg/kg/hour (typically 1 g/hour); may add 2-2.5 g/L of cardiopulmonary bypass circuit priming solution (Gravlee, 2008)
or
Loading dose of 10 g followed by 2 g/hour during surgery; no medication added to the bypass circuit (Fergusson, 2008)
or
10 g over 20-30 minutes prior to skin incision, followed by 10 g after heparin administration then 10 g at discontinuation of cardiopulmonary bypass (Vander Salm, 1996)
Prevention of bleeding associated with extracorporeal membrane oxygenation (ECMO) (unlabeled use): Children: I.V.: 100 mg/kg prior to or immediately after cannulation, followed by 25-30 mg/kg/hour for up to 72 hours (Downard, 2003; Horwitz, 1998; Wilson, 1993)
Prevention of perioperative bleeding associated with spinal surgery (eg, idiopathic scoliosis) (unlabeled use): Children and Adolescents: I.V.: 100 mg/kg given over 15-20 minutes after induction, followed by 10 mg/kg/hour for the remainder of the surgery; discontinue at time of wound closure (Florentino-Pineda, 2001; Florentino-Pineda, 2004)
Traumatic hyphema (unlabeled use): Children and Adults: Oral: 50 mg/kg/dose every 4 hours (maximum daily dose: 30 g) for 5 days (Brandt, 2001; Crouch, 1999)

Dosage adjustment in renal impairment: May accumulate in patients with decreased renal function. When used during cardiopulmonary bypass in anephric patients, a normal or slightly reduced loading dose and a continuous infusion rate of 5 mg/kg/hour has been recommended (Gravlee, 2008).
Dosage adjustment in hepatic impairment: No dosage adjustment provided in manufacturer's labeling.

Additional Information Complete prescribing information should be consulted for additional detail.

Dosage Forms Excipient information presented when available (limited, particularly for generics); consult specific product labeling.
Solution, Intravenous:
Generic: 250 mg/mL (20 mL)
Syrup, Oral:
Amicar: 25% (473 mL) [raspberry flavor]
Generic: 25% (237 mL, 473 mL)
Tablet, Oral:
Amicar: 500 mg, 1000 mg [scored]
Generic: 500 mg, 1000 mg

Aminolevulinic Acid (a MEE noh lev yoo lin ik AS id)

Brand Names: U.S. Levulan Kerastick
Brand Names: Canada Levulan® Kerastick®
Index Terms 5-ALA; 5-Aminolevulinic Acid; ALA; Amino Levulinic Acid; Aminolevulinic Acid Hydrochloride
Pharmacologic Category Photosensitizing Agent, Topical; Topical Skin Product
Use Treatment of minimally to moderately thick actinic keratoses (grade 1 or 2) of the face or scalp; to be used in conjunction with blue light illumination
Unlabeled Use Photodynamic treatment of low-risk superficial basal cell skin cancer and low-risk squamous cell skin cancer *in situ* (Bowen's disease)
Pregnancy Risk Factor C

Dosage Adults: Topical: Apply to actinic keratoses **(not** perilesional skin) followed 14-18 hours later by blue light illumination. Application/treatment may be repeated at a treatment site (once) after 8 weeks.

Additional Information Complete prescribing information should be consulted for additional detail.

Dosage Forms Excipient information presented when available (limited, particularly for generics); consult specific product labeling.

Solution Reconstituted, External, as hydrochloride:

Levulan Kerastick: 20% (1 ea) [contains alcohol, usp, isopropyl alcohol, laureth, polyethylene glycol]

◆ **Amino Levulinic Acid** *see* Aminolevulinic Acid *on page 100*

◆ **5-Aminolevulinic Acid** *see* Aminolevulinic Acid *on page 100*

◆ **Aminolevulinic Acid Hydrochloride** *see* Aminolevulinic Acid *on page 100*

◆ **4-aminopyridine** *see* Dalfampridine *on page 534*

◆ **5-Aminosalicylic Acid** *see* Mesalamine *on page 1305*

Amiodarone (a MEE oh da rone)

Brand Names: U.S. Cordarone; Nexterone; Pacerone

Brand Names: Canada Amiodarone Hydrochloride Injection; Apo-Amiodarone; Ava-Amiodarone; Cordarone; Dom-Amiodarone; Mylan-Amiodarone; PHL-Amiodarone; PMS-Amiodarone; PRO-Amiodarone; ratio-Amiodarone; Riva-Amiodarone; Sandoz-Amiodarone; Teva-Amiodarone

Index Terms Amiodarone Hydrochloride

Pharmacologic Category Antiarrhythmic Agent, Class III

Additional Appendix Information

Adult ACLS Algorithms *on page 2363*

Beers Criteria – Potentially Inappropriate Medications for Geriatrics *on page 2368*

Dosing Considerations for the Critically-Ill Patient With Morbid Obesity *on page 2379*

Pediatric ALS (PALS) Algorithms *on page 2359*

Use Management of life-threatening recurrent ventricular fibrillation (VF) or hemodynamically-unstable ventricular tachycardia (VT) refractory to other antiarrhythmic agents or in patients intolerant of other agents used for these conditions

Unlabeled Use

Atrial fibrillation (AF): Pharmacologic conversion of AF to and maintenance of normal sinus rhythm; treatment of AF in patients with heart failure [no accessory pathway] who require heart rate control (ACC/AHA/ESC Practice Guidelines) or in patients with hypertrophic cardiomyopathy (ACCF/AHA Practice Guidelines); prevention of postoperative AF associated with cardiothoracic surgery

Paroxysmal supraventricular tachycardia (SVT) (not initial drug of choice)

Ventricular tachyarrhythmias (ACLS/PALS guidelines): Cardiac arrest with persistent VT or VF if defibrillation, CPR, and vasopressor administration have failed; control of hemodynamically-stable monomorphic VT, polymorphic VT with a normal baseline QT interval, or wide-complex tachycardia of uncertain origin; control of rapid ventricular rate due to accessory pathway conduction in pre-excited atrial arrhythmias (ACLS guidelines) or stable narrow-complex tachycardia (ACLS guidelines)

Adjunct to ICD therapy to suppress symptomatic ventricular tachyarrhythmias in otherwise optimally-treated patients with heart failure (ACC/AHA/ESC Practice Guidelines)

Pregnancy Risk Factor D

Pregnancy Considerations Adverse events have been observed in some animal reproduction studies. Amiodarone crosses the placenta (~10% to 50%) and may cause fetal harm when administered to a pregnant woman, leading to congenital goiter and hypo- or hyperthyroidism. Growth retardation and premature birth have also been noted (ESG, 2011). Amiodarone should be used in pregnant women only to treat arrhythmias that are life-threatening or refractory to other treatments (Blomström-Lundqvist, 2003; ESG, 2011).

Breast-Feeding Considerations Amiodarone and its active metabolite are excreted into human milk. Breast-feeding may lead to significant infant exposure and potential toxicity. Due to the long half-life, amiodarone may be present in breast milk for several days following discontinuation of maternal therapy (Hall, 2003). The manufacturer recommends that breast-feeding be discontinued if treatment is needed.

Medication Guide Available Yes

Contraindications Hypersensitivity to amiodarone, iodine, or any component of the formulation; severe sinus-node dysfunction; second- and third-degree heart block (except in patients with a functioning artificial pacemaker); bradycardia causing syncope (except in patients with a functioning artificial pacemaker); cardiogenic shock

Warnings/Precautions **[U.S. Boxed Warning]: Only indicated for patients with life-threatening arrhythmias because of risk of toxicity. Alternative therapies should be tried first before using amiodarone. Patients should be hospitalized when amiodarone is initiated.** Currently, the 2005 ACLS guidelines recommend I.V. amiodarone as the preferred antiarrhythmic for the treatment of pulseless VT/VF, both life-threatening arrhythmias. In patients with non-life-threatening arrhythmias (eg, atrial fibrillation), amiodarone should be used only if the use of other antiarrhythmics has proven ineffective or are contraindicated.

[U.S. Boxed Warning]: Lung damage (abnormal diffusion capacity) may occur without symptoms. Monitor for pulmonary toxicity. Evaluate new respiratory symptoms; pre-existing pulmonary disease does not increase risk of developing pulmonary toxicity, but if pulmonary toxicity develops then the prognosis is worse. The lowest effective dose should be used as appropriate for the acuity/severity of the arrhythmia being treated. **[U.S. Boxed Warning]: Liver toxicity is common, but usually mild with evidence of increased liver enzymes. Severe liver toxicity can occur and has been fatal in a few cases.**

[U.S. Boxed Warning]: Amiodarone can exacerbate arrhythmias, by making them more difficult to tolerate or reverse; other types of arrhythmias have occurred, including significant heart block, sinus bradycardia new ventricular fibrillation, incessant ventricular tachycardia, increased resistance to cardioversion, and polymorphic ventricular tachycardia associated with QT_c prolongation (torsade de pointes [TdP]). Risk may be increased with concomitant use of other antiarrhythmic agents or drugs that prolong the QT_c interval. Proarrhythmic effects may be prolonged.

Monitor pacing or defibrillation thresholds in patients with implantable cardiac devices (eg, pacemakers, defibrillators). Use very cautiously and with close monitoring in patients with thyroid or liver disease. May cause hyper- or hypothyroidism. Hyperthyroidism may result in thyrotoxicosis and may aggravate or cause breakthrough arrhythmias. If any new signs of arrhythmia appear, hyperthyroidism should be considered. Thyroid function should be monitored prior to treatment and periodically thereafter.

May cause optic neuropathy and/or optic neuritis, usually resulting in visual impairment. Corneal microdeposits occur in a majority of patients, and may cause visual disturbances in some patients (blurred vision, halos); these are not generally considered a reason to discontinue treatment. Corneal refractive laser surgery is generally contraindicated in amiodarone users. Avoid excessive exposure to sunlight; may cause photosensitivity.

Amiodarone is a potent inhibitor of CYP enzymes and transport proteins (including p-glycoprotein), which may lead to increased serum concentrations/toxicity of a number of medications. Particular caution must be used when a drug with QT_c-prolonging potential relies on metabolism via these enzymes, since the effect of elevated concentrations may be additive with the effect of amiodarone. Carefully assess risk:benefit of coadministration of other drugs which may prolong QT_c interval. Patients may still be at risk for amiodarone–related drug interactions after the drug has been discontinued. The pharmacokinetics are complex (due to prolonged duration of action and half-life) and difficult to predict. Correct electrolyte disturbances, especially hypokalemia or hypomagnesemia, prior to use and throughout therapy. Use caution when initiating amiodarone in patients on warfarin. Cases of increased INR with or without bleeding have occurred in patients treated with warfarin; monitor INR closely after initiating amiodarone in these patients.

In the treatment of atrial fibrillation in older adults, avoid antiarrhythmics as first-line treatment. In older adults, data suggests rate control may provide more benefits than risks compared to rhythm control for most patients (Beers Criteria).

May cause hypotension and bradycardia (infusion-rate related). Hypotension with rapid administration has been attributed to the emulsifier polysorbate 80. Commercially-prepared premixed solutions do not contain polysorbate 80 and may have a lower incidence of hypotension. Caution in surgical patients; may enhance hemodynamic effect of anesthetics; associated with increased risk of adult respiratory distress syndrome (ARDS) postoperatively. Vials for injection contain benzyl alcohol, which has been associated with "gasping syndrome" in neonates. Commercially-prepared premixed solutions do not contain benzyl alcohol. Commercially-prepared premixed infusion contains the excipient cyclodextrin (sulfobutyl ether beta-cyclodextrin), which may accumulate in patients with renal insufficiency.

Adverse Reactions In a recent meta-analysis, adult patients taking lower doses of amiodarone (152-330 mg daily for at least 12 months) were more likely to develop thyroid, neurologic, skin, ocular, and bradycardic abnormalities than those taking placebo (Vorperian, 1997). Pulmonary toxicity was similar in both the low-dose amiodarone group and in the placebo group, but there was a trend towards increased toxicity in the amiodarone group. Gastrointestinal and hepatic events were seen to a similar extent in both the low-dose amiodarone group and placebo group. As the frequency of adverse events varies considerably across studies as a function of route and dose, a consolidation of adverse event rates is provided by Goldschlager, 2000.

>10%:

Cardiovascular: Hypotension (I.V. 16%, refractory in rare cases)

Central nervous system (3% to 40%): Abnormal gait/ataxia, dizziness, fatigue, headache, malaise, impaired memory, involuntary movement, insomnia, poor coordination, peripheral neuropathy, sleep disturbances, tremor

Dermatologic: Photosensitivity (10% to 75%)

Endocrine & Metabolic: Hypothyroidism (1% to 22%)

Gastrointestinal: Nausea, vomiting, anorexia, and constipation (10% to 33%)

Hepatic: AST or ALT level >2x normal (15% to 50%)

Ocular: Corneal microdeposits (>90%; causes visual disturbance in <10%)

1% to 10%:

Cardiovascular: CHF (3%), bradycardia (3% to 5%), AV block (5%), conduction abnormalities, SA node dysfunction (1% to 3%), cardiac arrhythmia, flushing, edema. Additional effects associated with I.V. administration include asystole, atrial fibrillation, cardiac arrest, electromechanical dissociation, pulseless electrical activity (PEA), ventricular tachycardia, and cardiogenic shock.

Dermatologic: Slate blue skin discoloration (<10%)

Endocrine & metabolic: Hyperthyroidism (3% to 10%; more common in iodine-deficient regions of the world), libido decreased

Gastrointestinal: Abdominal pain, abnormal salivation, abnormal taste (oral), diarrhea, nausea (I.V.)

Hematologic: Coagulation abnormalities

Hepatic: Hepatitis and cirrhosis (<3%)

Local: Phlebitis (I.V., with concentrations >3 mg/mL)

Ocular: Visual disturbances (2% to 9%), halo vision (<5% occurring especially at night), optic neuritis (1%)

Respiratory: Pulmonary toxicity has been estimated to occur at a frequency between 2% and 7% of patients (some reports indicate a frequency as high as 17%). Toxicity may present as hypersensitivity pneumonitis; pulmonary fibrosis (cough, fever, malaise); pulmonary inflammation; interstitial pneumonitis; or alveolar pneumonitis. ARDS has been reported in up to 2% of patients receiving amiodarone, and postoperatively in patients receiving oral amiodarone.

Miscellaneous: Abnormal smell (oral)

<1% (Limited to important or life-threatening): Acute intracranial hypertension (I.V.), acute renal failure, acute respiratory distress syndrome, agranulocytosis, alopecia, anaphylactic shock, angioedema, aplastic anemia, bone marrow granuloma, bronchiolitis obliterans organizing pneumonia (BOOP), bronchospasm, cholestatic hepatitis, confusion, delirium, demyelinating polyneuropathy, disorientation, drug rash with eosinophilia and systemic symptoms (DRESS), dyspnea, encephalopathy, eczema, eosinophilic pneumonia, epididymitis (noninfectious), erectile dysfunction, erythema multiforme, exfoliative dermatitis, fever, granuloma, hallucination, hemolytic anemia, hemoptysis, hyperglycemia, hypertriglyceridemia, hypotension (oral), hypoxia, impotence, injection site reactions, leukocytoclastic vasculitis, muscle weakness, myopathy, neutropenia, optic neuropathy, pancreatitis, pancytopenia, parkinsonian symptoms, photophobia, pleural effusion, pleuritis, proarrhythmia, pruritus, pseudotumor cerebri, pulmonary alveolar hemorrhage, pulmonary edema, pulmonary infiltrates, pulmonary mass, QT interval increased, rash, renal impairment, renal insufficiency, respiratory failure, rhabdomyolysis, SIADH, sinus arrest, skin cancer, spontaneous ecchymosis, Stevens-Johnson syndrome, thrombocytopenia, thyroid nodules, thyroid cancer, thyrotoxicosis, torsade de pointes (rare), toxic epidermal necrolysis, urticaria, vasculitis, ventricular fibrillation, wheezing

Drug Interactions

Metabolism/Transport Effects **Substrate** of CYP1A2 (minor), CYP2C19 (minor), CYP2C8 (major), CYP2D6 (minor), CYP3A4 (major), P-glycoprotein; **Note:** Assignment of Major/Minor substrate status based on clinically relevant drug interaction potential; **Inhibits** CYP1A2 (weak), CYP2A6 (moderate), CYP2B6 (weak), CYP2C9 (moderate), CYP2D6 (moderate), CYP3A4 (weak), P-glycoprotein

Avoid Concomitant Use

Avoid concomitant use of Amiodarone with any of the following: Agalsidase Alfa; Agalsidase Beta; Antiarrhythmic Agents (Class Ia); Azithromycin (Systemic); Bosutinib; Conivaptan; Fingolimod; Fusidic Acid (Systemic); Grapefruit Juice; Highest Risk QTc-Prolonging Agents; Ivabradine; Mifepristone; Moderate Risk QTc-Prolonging

Agents; Pomalidomide; Propafenone; Protease Inhibitors; Silodosin; Tegafur; Thioridazine; Topotecan; VinCRIStine (Liposomal)

Increased Effect/Toxicity

Amiodarone may increase the levels/effects of: Afatinib; Antiarrhythmic Agents (Class Ia); ARIPiprazole; Beta-Blockers; Bosentan; Bosutinib; Cardiac Glycosides; Colchicine; CycloSPORINE (Systemic); CYP2A6 Substrates; CYP2C9 Substrates; CYP2D6 Substrates; Dabigatran Etexilate; Everolimus; Fesoterodine; Flecainide; Fosphenytoin; Highest Risk QTc-Prolonging Agents; HMG-CoA Reductase Inhibitors; Lidocaine (Systemic); Lidocaine (Topical); Lomitapide; Loratadine; Metoprolol; Mipomersen; P-glycoprotein/ABCB1 Substrates; Phenytoin; Pomalidomide; Porfimer; Propafenone; Prucalopride; Rivaroxaban; Silodosin; Thioridazine; Topotecan; VinCRIStine (Liposomal); Vitamin K Antagonists

The levels/effects of Amiodarone may be increased by: Azithromycin (Systemic); Boceprevir; Calcium Channel Blockers (Nondihydropyridine); Cimetidine; Conivaptan; CYP2C8 Inhibitors (Moderate); CYP2C8 Inhibitors (Strong); CYP3A4 Inhibitors (Moderate); CYP3A4 Inhibitors (Strong); Dasatinib; Deferasirox; Fingolimod; Fosphenytoin; Fusidic Acid (Systemic); Grapefruit Juice; Ivabradine; Ivacaftor; Lidocaine (Topical); Luliconazole; Mifepristone; Moderate Risk QTc-Prolonging Agents; P-glycoprotein/ABCB1 Inhibitors; Protease Inhibitors; QTc-Prolonging Agents (Indeterminate Risk and Risk Modifying); Simeprevir; Telaprevir

Decreased Effect

Amiodarone may decrease the levels/effects of: Agalsidase Alfa; Agalsidase Beta; Clopidogrel; Codeine; Sodium Iodide I131; Tamoxifen; Tegafur; TraMADol

The levels/effects of Amiodarone may be decreased by: Bile Acid Sequestrants; Bosentan; CYP2C8 Inducers (Strong); CYP3A4 Inducers (Strong); Dabrafenib; Deferasirox; Etravirine; Fosphenytoin; Grapefruit Juice; Herbs (CYP3A4 Inducers); Mitotane; Orlistat; Peginterferon Alfa-2b; P-glycoprotein/ABCB1 Inducers; Phenytoin; Rifampin; Tocilizumab

Ethanol/Nutrition/Herb Interactions

Food: Increases the rate and extent of absorption of amiodarone. Grapefruit juice increases bioavailability of oral amiodarone by 50% and decreases the conversion of amiodarone to N-DEA (active metabolite); altered effects are possible. Management: Take consistently with regard to meals; grapefruit juice should be avoided during therapy.

Herb/Nutraceutical: St John's wort may decrease amiodarone levels or enhance photosensitization. Ephedra may worsen arrythmia. Management: Avoid St John's wort, ephedra and dong quai.

Storage/Stability

Tablets: Store at 20°C to 25°C (68°F to 77°F); excursions are permitted between 15°C and 30°C (59°F and 86°F); protect from light.

Injection: Store undiluted vials and premixed solutions (Nexterone) at 20°C to 25°C (68°F to 77°F); excursions are permitted between 15°C and 30°C (59°F and 86°F). Protect from light during storage; protect from excessive heat. There is no need to protect solutions from light during administration. When vial contents are admixed in D_5W to a final concentration of 1-6 mg/mL, amiodarone is stable for 24 hours in glass or polyolefin bottles and for 2 hours in polyvinyl chloride (PVC) bags; do not use evacuated glass containers as buffer may cause precipitation. Nexterone is available as premixed solutions. Although amiodarone adsorbs to PVC tubing, all clinical studies used PVC tubing and the recommended doses account for adsorption; in adults, PVC tubing is recommended.

Mechanism of Action Class III antiarrhythmic agent which inhibits adrenergic stimulation (alpha- and beta-blocking properties), affects sodium, potassium, and calcium channels, prolongs the action potential and refractory period in myocardial tissue; decreases AV conduction and sinus node function

Pharmacodynamics/Kinetics

Absorption: Slow and variable

Onset of action: Oral: 2 days to 3 weeks; I.V.: May be more rapid

Peak effect: 1 week to 5 months

Duration after discontinuing therapy: 7-50 days

Note: Mean onset of effect and duration after discontinuation may be shorter in children than adults

Distribution: V_d: 66 L/kg (range: 18-148 L/kg)

Protein binding: 96%

Metabolism: Hepatic via CYP2C8 and 3A4 to active N-desethylamiodarone metabolite; possible enterohepatic recirculation

Bioavailability: Oral: 35% to 65%

Half-life elimination: Terminal: 40-55 days (range: 26-107 days); shorter in children

Time to peak, serum: Oral: 3-7 hours

Excretion: Feces; urine (<1% as unchanged drug)

Dosage Note: Lower loading and maintenance doses are preferable in women and all patients with low body weight.

Oral: Adults:

Ventricular arrhythmias: 800-1600 mg daily in 1-2 doses for 1-3 weeks, then when adequate arrhythmia control is achieved, decrease to 600-800 mg daily in 1-2 doses for 1 month; maintenance: 400 mg daily. Lower doses are recommended for supraventricular arrhythmias.

Atrial fibrillation:

Pharmacologic cardioversion (unlabeled use): ACC/AHA/ESC Practice Guidelines: *Inpatient:* 1.2-1.8 g daily in divided doses until 10 g total, then 200-400 mg daily maintenance. *Outpatient:* 600-800 mg daily in divided doses until 10 g total, then 200-400 mg daily maintenance; although not supported by clinical evidence, a maintenance dose of 100 mg daily is commonly used especially for the elderly or patients with low body mass (Fuster, 2006; Zimetbaum, 2007). **Note:** Other regimens have been described and may be used clinically:

400 mg 3 times daily for 5-7 days, then 400 mg daily for 1 month, then 200 mg daily

or

10 mg/kg/day for 14 days, followed by 300 mg daily for 4 weeks, followed by maintenance dosage of 200 mg daily (Roy, 2000)

Prophylaxis following open heart surgery (unlabeled use): Starting in postop recovery: 400 mg twice daily for up to 7 days. Alternative regimen of amiodarone: 600 mg daily for 7 days prior to surgery, followed by 200 mg daily until hospital discharge, has also been shown to decrease the risk of postoperative atrial fibrillation. **Note:** A variety of regimens have been used in clinical trials.

I.V.:

Children:

Pulseless VT or VF: I.V., I.O.: 5 mg/kg (maximum: 300 mg per dose) rapid bolus; may repeat twice up to a maximum total dose of 15 mg/kg during acute treatment (PALS, 2010).

Perfusing tachycardias: I.V., I.O.: Loading dose: 5 mg/kg (maximum: 300 mg per dose) over 20-60 minutes; may repeat twice up to maximum total dose of 15 mg/kg during acute treatment (PALS, 2010).

Adults:

Atrial fibrillation:

Pharmacologic cardioversion (ACC/AHA/ESC Practice Guidelines) (unlabeled use): 5-7 mg/kg over 30-60 minutes, then 1.2-1.8 g daily continuous infusion until 10 g total. Maintenance: See oral dosing.

Prophylaxis following open heart surgery (unlabeled use): Starting at postop recovery, 1000 mg infused over 24 hours for 2 days has been shown to reduce the risk of postoperative atrial fibrillation. **Note:** A variety of regimens have been used in clinical trials.

Pulseless VT or VF (ACLS, 2010): I.V. push, I.O.: Initial: 300 mg rapid bolus; if pulseless VT or VF continues after subsequent defibrillation attempt or recurs, administer supplemental dose of 150 mg. **Note:** In this setting, administering **undiluted** is preferred (Dager, 2006; Skrifvars, 2004). *The Handbook of Emergency Cardiovascular Care* (Hazinski, 2010) and the 2010 ACLS guidelines, do not make any specific recommendations regarding dilution of amiodarone in this setting. Experience limited with I.O. administration of amiodarone. Maximum recommended total daily dose is 2.2 g (ACLS, 2010).

Upon return of spontaneous circulation, follow with an infusion of 1 mg/minute for 6 hours, then 0.5 mg/minute for 18 hours (mean daily doses >2.1 g/day have been associated with hypotension).

Stable VT or SVT (unlabeled use): First 24 hours: 1050 mg according to following regimen

Step 1: 150 mg (100 mL) over first 10 minutes (mix 3 mL in 100 mL D_5W)

Step 2: 360 mg (200 mL) over next 6 hours (mix 18 mL in 500 mL D_5W): 1 mg/minute

Step 3: 540 mg (300 mL) over next 18 hours: 0.5 mg/minute

Note: After the first 24 hours: 0.5 mg/minute utilizing concentration of 1-6 mg/mL

Breakthrough stable VT or SVT: 150 mg supplemental doses in 100 mL D_5W or NS over 10 minutes (mean daily doses >2.1 g/day have been associated with hypotension)

I.V. to oral therapy conversion: Use the following as a guide:

<1-week I.V. infusion: 800-1600 mg daily

1- to 3-week I.V. infusion: 600-800 mg daily

>3-week I.V. infusion: 400 mg daily

Note: Conversion from I.V. to oral therapy has not been formally evaluated. Some experts recommend a 1-2 day overlap when converting from I.V. to oral therapy especially when treating ventricular arrhythmias.

Recommendations for conversion to intravenous amiodarone after oral administration: During long-term amiodarone therapy (ie, ≥4 months), the mean plasma-elimination half-life of the active metabolite of amiodarone is 61 days. Replacement therapy may not be necessary in such patients if oral therapy is discontinued for a period <2 weeks, since any changes in serum amiodarone concentrations during this period may **not** be clinically significant.

Elderly: No specific guidelines available. Dose selection should be cautious, at low end of dosage range, and titration should be slower to evaluate response. Although not supported by clinical evidence, a maintenance dose of 100 mg daily is commonly used especially for the elderly or patients with low body mass (Fuster, 2006; Zimetbaum, 2007).

Dosing adjustment in renal impairment: No dosage adjustment necessary

Hemodialysis: Not dialyzable (0% to 5%); supplemental dose is not necessary.

Peritoneal dialysis: Not dialyzable (0% to 5%); supplemental dose is not necessary.

Dosing adjustment in hepatic impairment: Dosage adjustment is probably necessary in substantial hepatic impairment. No specific guidelines available. If hepatic enzymes exceed 3 times normal or double in a patient with an elevated baseline, consider decreasing the dose or discontinuing amiodarone.

Dietary Considerations Take consistently with regard to meals. Amiodarone is a potential source of large amounts of inorganic iodine; ~3 mg of inorganic iodine per 100 mg of amiodarone is released into the systemic circulation. Recommended daily allowance for iodine in adults is 150 mcg.

Grapefruit juice is not recommended.

Usual Infusion Concentrations: Pediatric Note: Premixed solutions available.

I.V. infusion: 1.8 mg/mL

Usual Infusion Concentrations: Adult Note: Premixed solutions available.

I.V. infusion: 450 mg in 250 mL (concentration: 1.8 mg/mL) of D_5W or NS

Administration

Oral: Administer consistently with regard to meals. Take in divided doses with meals if GI upset occurs or if taking large daily dose. If GI intolerance occurs with single-dose therapy, use twice daily dosing.

I.V.: For infusions >1 hour, use concentrations ≤2 mg/mL unless a central venous catheter is used; commercially-prepared premixed solutions in concentrations of 1.5 mg/mL and 1.8 mg/mL are available. Use only volumetric infusion pump; use of drop counting may lead to underdosage. Administer through an I.V. line located as centrally as possible. For continuous infusions, an in-line filter has been recommended during administration to reduce the incidence of phlebitis. During pulseless VT/VF, administering **undiluted** is preferred (Dager, 2006; Skrifvars, 2004). *The Handbook of Emergency Cardiovascular Care* (Hazinski, 2010) and the 2010 ACLS guidelines do not make any specific recommendations regarding dilution of amiodarone in this setting.

Adjust administration rate to urgency (give more slowly when perfusing arrhythmia present). Slow the infusion rate if hypotension or bradycardia develops. Infusions >2 hours must be administered in a non-PVC container (eg, glass or polyolefin). PVC tubing is recommended for administration regardless of infusion duration. **Incompatible** with heparin; flush with saline prior to and following infusion. **Note:** I.V. administration at lower flow rates (potentially associated with use in pediatrics) and higher concentrations than recommended may result in leaching of plasticizers (DEHP) from intravenous tubing. DEHP may adversely affect male reproductive tract development. Alternative means of dosing and administration (1 mg/kg aliquots) may need to be considered.

Monitoring Parameters Blood pressure, heart rate (ECG) and rhythm throughout therapy; assess patient for signs of lethargy, edema of the hands or feet, weight loss, and pulmonary toxicity (baseline pulmonary function tests and chest X-ray; continue monitoring chest X-ray annually during therapy); liver function tests (semiannually); monitor serum electrolytes, especially potassium and magnesium. Assess thyroid function tests before initiation of treatment and then periodically thereafter (some experts suggest every 3-6 months). If signs or symptoms of thyroid disease or arrhythmia breakthrough/exacerbation occur then immediate re-evaluation is necessary. Amiodarone partially inhibits the peripheral conversion of thyroxine (T_4) to triiodothyronine (T_3); serum T_4 and reverse triiodothyronine (rT_3) concentrations may be increased and serum T_3 may be decreased; most patients remain clinically euthyroid, however, clinical hypothyroidism or hyperthyroidism may occur.

Perform regular ophthalmic exams.

Patients with implantable cardiac devices: Monitor pacing or defibrillation thresholds with initiation of amiodarone and during treatment.

Consult individual institutional policies and procedures.

Reference Range Therapeutic: 0.5-2.5 mg/L (SI: 1-4 micromole/L) (parent); desethyl metabolite is active and is present in equal concentration to parent drug

Dosage Forms Excipient information presented when available (limited, particularly for generics); consult specific product labeling.

Solution, Intravenous, as hydrochloride:
- Nexterone: 150 mg/100 mL (100 mL); 360 mg/200 mL (200 mL)
- Generic: 150 mg/3 mL (3 mL); 450 mg/9 mL (9 mL); 900 mg/18 mL (18 mL)

Tablet, Oral, as hydrochloride:
- Cordarone: 200 mg [scored]
- Pacerone: 100 mg
- Pacerone: 200 mg [scored; contains fd&c red #40, fd&c yellow #6 (sunset yellow)]
- Pacerone: 400 mg [scored; contains fd&c yellow #10 aluminum lake]
- Generic: 100 mg, 200 mg, 400 mg

Extemporaneous Preparations A 5 mg/mL oral suspension may be made with tablets and either a 1:1 mixture of Ora-Sweet® and Ora-Plus® or a 1:1 mixture of Ora-Sweet® SF and Ora-Plus® adjusted to a pH between 6-7 using a sodium bicarbonate solution (5 g/100 mL of distilled water). Crush five 200 mg tablets in a mortar and reduce to a fine powder. Add small portions of the chosen vehicle and mix to a uniform paste; mix while adding the vehicle in incremental proportions to **almost** 200 mL; transfer to a calibrated bottle, rinse mortar with vehicle, and add quantity of vehicle sufficient to make 200 mL. Label "shake well" and "protect from light". Stable for 42 days at room temperature or 91 days refrigerated (preferred) (Nahata, 2004).

Nahata MC, Pai VB, and Hipple TF, *Pediatric Drug Formulations*, 5th ed, Cincinnati, OH: Harvey Whitney Books Co, 2004.

◆ Amiodarone Hydrochloride *see* Amiodarone *on page 101*

◆ Amiodarone Hydrochloride Injection (Can) *see* Amiodarone *on page 101*

◆ Amitiza *see* Lubiprostone *on page 1254*

Amitriptyline (a mee TRIP ti leen)

Brand Names: Canada Bio-Amitriptyline; Dom-Amitriptyline; Elavil; Levate®; Novo-Triptyn; PMS-Amitriptyline

Index Terms Amitriptyline Hydrochloride; Elavil

Pharmacologic Category Antidepressant, Tricyclic (Tertiary Amine)

Additional Appendix Information

Antidepressant Agents *on page 2284*

Beers Criteria – Potentially Inappropriate Medications for Geriatrics *on page 2368*

Use Relief of symptoms of depression

Unlabeled Use Analgesic for certain chronic and neuropathic pain (including diabetic neuropathy); prophylaxis against migraine headaches; treatment of depressive disorders in children; post-traumatic stress disorder (PTSD)

Pregnancy Risk Factor C

Pregnancy Considerations Adverse events have been observed in some animal reproduction studies. Amitriptyline crosses the human placenta; CNS effects, limb deformities, and developmental delay have been noted in case reports (causal relationship not established). Tricyclic antidepressants may be associated with irritability, jitteriness, and convulsions (rare) in the neonate (Yonkers, 2009).

The ACOG recommends that therapy for depression during pregnancy be individualized; treatment should incorporate the clinical expertise of the mental health clinician, obstetrician, primary healthcare provider, and pediatrician (ACOG, 2008). According to the American Psychiatric Association (APA), the risks of medication treatment should be weighed against other treatment options and untreated depression. For women who discontinue antidepressant medications during pregnancy and who may be at high risk for postpartum depression, the medications can be restarted following delivery (APA, 2010). Treatment algorithms have been developed by the ACOG and the APA for the management of depression in women prior to conception and during pregnancy (Yonkers, 2009). Although not a first-line agent, amitriptyline may be used for the treatment of post-traumatic stress disorder in pregnant women (Bandelow, 2008). Migraine prophylaxis should be avoided during pregnancy; if needed, amitriptyline may be used if other agents are ineffective or contraindicated (Pringsheim, 2012).

Breast-Feeding Considerations Amitriptyline is excreted into breast milk. Based on information from six mother/infant pairs, following maternal use of amitriptyline 75-175 mg/day, the estimated exposure to the breast-feeding infant would be 0.2% to 1.9% of the weight-adjusted maternal dose. Adverse events have not been reported in nursing infants (four cases). Infants should be monitored for signs of adverse events; routine monitoring of infant serum concentrations is not recommended (Fortinguerra, 2009). Migraine prophylaxis should be avoided in women who are nursing; if needed, amitriptyline may be used if other agents are ineffective or contraindicated (Pringsheim, 2012). Due to the potential for serious adverse reactions in the nursing infant, the manufacturer recommends a decision be made whether to discontinue nursing or to discontinue the drug, taking into account the importance of treatment to the mother.

Medication Guide Available Yes

Contraindications Hypersensitivity to amitriptyline or any component of the formulation (cross-sensitivity with other tricyclics may occur); use of MAO inhibitors within past 14 days; acute recovery phase following myocardial infarction; concurrent use of cisapride

Warnings/Precautions **[U.S. Boxed Warning]: Antidepressants increase the risk of suicidal thinking and behavior in children, adolescents, and young adults (18-24 years of age) with major depressive disorder (MDD) and other psychiatric disorders;** consider risk prior to prescribing. Short-term studies did not show an increased risk in patients >24 years of age and showed a decreased risk in patients ≥65 years. Closely monitor for clinical worsening, suicidality, or unusual changes in behavior; the patient's family or caregiver should be instructed to closely observe the patient and communicate condition with healthcare provider. Such observation would generally include at least weekly face-to-face contact with patients or their family members or caregivers during the first 4 weeks of treatment, then every other week visits for the next 4 weeks, then at 12 weeks, and as clinically indicated beyond 12 weeks. Additional contact by telephone may be appropriate between face-to-face visits. Adults treated with antidepressants should be observed similarly for clinical worsening and suicidality, especially during the initial few months of a course of drug therapy, or at times of dose changes, either increases or decreases. A medication guide should be dispensed with each prescription. **Amitriptyline is not FDA-approved for use in children <12 years of age.**

The possibility of a suicide attempt is inherent in major depression and may persist until remission occurs. Monitor for worsening of depression or suicidality, especially during initiation of therapy (generally first 1-2 months) or with dose increases or decreases. Worsening depression and severe abrupt suicidality that are not part of the presenting symptoms may require discontinuation or modification of drug therapy. The patient's family or caregiver should be alerted to monitor patients for the emergence of suicidality and associated behaviors (such as agitation, irritability, hostility, impulsivity, and hypomania) and notify healthcare provider.

May worsen psychosis in some patients or precipitate a shift to mania or hypomania in patients with bipolar disorder. Patients presenting with depressive symptoms should be screened for bipolar disorder. Monotherapy in patients with bipolar disorder should be avoided. **Amitriptyline is not FDA approved for bipolar depression.**

The degree of sedation, anticholinergic effects, orthostasis, and conduction abnormalities are high relative to other antidepressants. Amitriptyline often causes drowsiness/sedation, resulting in impaired performance of tasks requiring alertness (eg, operating machinery or driving). Sedative effects may be additive with other CNS depressants and/or ethanol. Use with caution in patients with a history of cardiovascular disease (including previous MI, stroke, tachycardia, or conduction abnormalities). Use with caution in patients with urinary retention, benign prostatic hyperplasia, narrow-angle glaucoma, xerostomia, visual problems, constipation, or a history of bowel obstruction.

TCAs may rarely cause bone marrow suppression; monitor for any signs of infection and obtain CBC if symptoms (eg, fever, sore throat) evident. May alter glucose control - use with caution in patients with diabetes. Recommended by the manufacturer to discontinue prior to elective surgery; risks exist for drug interactions with anesthesia and for cardiac arrhythmias. However, definitive drug interactions have not been widely reported in the literature and continuation of tricyclic antidepressants is generally recommended as long as precautions are taken to reduce the significance of any adverse events that may occur (Pass, 2004). May lower seizure threshold - use caution in patients with a previous seizure disorder or condition predisposing to seizures such as brain damage, alcoholism, or concurrent therapy with other drugs which lower the seizure threshold. Hyperpyrexia has been observed with TCAs in combination with anticholinergics and/or neuroleptics, particularly during hot weather. May increase the risks associated with electroconvulsive therapy. Bone fractures have been associated with antidepressant treatment. Consider the possibility of a fragility fracture if an antidepressant-treated patient presents with unexplained bone pain, point tenderness, swelling, or bruising (Rabenda, 2013; Rizzoli, 2012). Use with caution in hyperthyroid patients or those receiving thyroid supplementation. Use with caution in patients with hepatic or renal dysfunction. Avoid use in the elderly due to its potent anticholinergic and sedative properties, and potential to cause orthostatic hypotension. In addition, may cause or exacerbate syndrome of inappropriate antidiuretic hormone secretion or hyponatremia; monitor sodium closely with initiation or dosage adjustments in older adults (Beers Criteria).

Abrupt discontinuation or interruption of antidepressant therapy has been associated with a discontinuation syndrome. Symptoms arising may vary with antidepressant however commonly include nausea, vomiting, diarrhea, headaches, light-headedness, dizziness, diminished appetite, sweating, chills, tremors, paresthesias, fatigue, somnolence, and sleep disturbances (eg, vivid dreams, insomnia). Greater risks for developing a discontinuation syndrome have been associated with antidepressants with shorter half-lives, longer durations of treatment, and abrupt discontinuation. For antidepressants of short or intermediate half-lives, symptoms may emerge within 2-5 days after treatment discontinuation and last 7-14 days (APA, 2010; Fava, 2006; Haddad, 2001; Shelton, 2001; Warner, 2006).

Adverse Reactions Anticholinergic effects may be pronounced; moderate to marked sedation can occur (tolerance to these effects usually occurs).

Frequency not defined.

Cardiovascular: Orthostatic hypotension, tachycardia, ECG changes (nonspecific), AV conduction changes, cardiomyopathy (rare), MI, stroke, heart block, arrhythmia, syncope, hypertension, palpitation

Central nervous system: Restlessness, dizziness, insomnia, sedation, fatigue, anxiety, cognitive function impaired, seizure, extrapyramidal symptoms, coma, hallucinations, confusion, disorientation, coordination impaired, ataxia, headache, nightmares, hyperpyrexia

Dermatologic: Allergic rash, urticaria, photosensitivity, alopecia

Endocrine & metabolic: Syndrome of inappropriate ADH secretion

Gastrointestinal: Weight gain, xerostomia, constipation, paralytic ileus, nausea, vomiting, anorexia, stomatitis, peculiar taste, diarrhea, black tongue

Genitourinary: Urinary retention

Hematologic: Bone marrow depression, purpura, eosinophilia

Neuromuscular & skeletal: Numbness, paresthesia, peripheral neuropathy, tremor, weakness

Ocular: Blurred vision, mydriasis, ocular pressure increased

Otic: Tinnitus

Miscellaneous: Diaphoresis, withdrawal reactions (nausea, headache, malaise)

Postmarketing and/or case reports: Neuroleptic malignant syndrome (rare), serotonin syndrome (rare)

Drug Interactions

Metabolism/Transport Effects Substrate of CYP1A2 (minor), CYP2B6 (minor), CYP2C19 (minor), CYP2C9 (minor), CYP2D6 (major), CYP3A4 (minor); **Note:** Assignment of Major/Minor substrate status based on clinically relevant drug interaction potential; **Inhibits** CYP1A2 (weak), CYP2C19 (weak), CYP2C9 (weak), CYP2D6 (weak), CYP2E1 (weak)

Avoid Concomitant Use

Avoid concomitant use of Amitriptyline with any of the following: Aclidinium; Cisapride; Iobenguane I 123; Ipratropium (Oral Inhalation); Linezolid; MAO Inhibitors; Methylene Blue; Moxonidine; Tiotropium; Umeclidinium

Increased Effect/Toxicity

Amitriptyline may increase the levels/effects of: Alpha-/Beta-Agonists (Direct-Acting); Alpha1-Agonists; Amphetamines; Analgesics (Opioid); Anticholinergics; Antipsychotics; Aspirin; Beta2-Agonists; Cisapride; Citalopram; Desmopressin; Escitalopram; Highest Risk QTc-Prolonging Agents; Methylene Blue; Metoclopramide; Moderate Risk QTc-Prolonging Agents; NSAID (COX-2 Inhibitor); NSAID (Nonselective); QuiNIDine; Serotonin Modulators; Sodium Phosphates; Sulfonylureas; Tiotropium; TraMADol; Vitamin K Antagonists; Yohimbine

The levels/effects of Amitriptyline may be increased by: Abiraterone Acetate; Aclidinium; Altretamine; Antipsychotics; BuPROPion; Cimetidine; Cinacalcet; Citalopram; Cobicistat; CYP2D6 Inhibitors (Moderate); CYP2D6 Inhibitors (Strong); Dexmethylphenidate; DULoxetine; Escitalopram; FLUoxetine; FluvoxaMINE; Ipratropium (Oral Inhalation); Linezolid; Lithium; MAO Inhibitors; Methylphenidate; Metoclopramide; Metyrosine; Mifepristone; PARoxetine; Pramlintide; Protease Inhibitors; QuiNIDine; Sertraline; Terbinafine (Systemic); Thyroid

Products; TraMADol; Umeclidinium; Valproic Acid and Derivatives

Decreased Effect

Amitriptyline may decrease the levels/effects of: Acetylcholinesterase Inhibitors (Central); Alpha2-Agonists; Alpha2-Agonists (Ophthalmic); Iobenguane I 123; Moxonidine

The levels/effects of Amitriptyline may be decreased by: Acetylcholinesterase Inhibitors (Central); Barbiturates; CarBAMazepine; Peginterferon Alfa-2b; St Johns Wort

Ethanol/Nutrition/Herb Interactions

Ethanol: May increase CNS depression; monitor for increased effects with coadministration. Caution patients about effects.

Food: Grapefruit juice may inhibit the metabolism of some TCAs and clinical toxicity may result.

Herb/Nutraceutical: St John's wort may decrease amitriptyline levels. Avoid valerian, St John's wort, kava kava, gotu kola (may increase CNS depression).

Mechanism of Action Increases the synaptic concentration of serotonin and/or norepinephrine in the central nervous system by inhibition of their reuptake by the presynaptic neuronal membrane

Pharmacodynamics/Kinetics

Onset of action: Migraine prophylaxis: 6 weeks, higher dosage may be required in heavy smokers because of increased metabolism; Depression: 4-6 weeks, reduce dosage to lowest effective level

Distribution: Crosses placenta; enters breast milk

Metabolism: Hepatic to nortriptyline (active), hydroxy and conjugated derivatives; may be impaired in the elderly

Half-life elimination: Adults: 9-27 hours (average: 15 hours)

Time to peak, serum: ~4 hours

Excretion: Urine (18% as unchanged drug); feces (small amounts)

Dosage

Children:

Chronic pain management (unlabeled use): Oral: Initial: 0.1 mg/kg at bedtime, may advance as tolerated over 2-3 weeks to 0.5-2 mg/kg at bedtime

Depressive disorders (unlabeled use): Oral: Initial doses of 1 mg/kg/day given in 3 divided doses with increases to 1.5 mg/kg/day have been reported in a small number of children (n=9) 9-12 years of age; clinically, doses up to 3 mg/kg/day (5 mg/kg/day if monitored closely) have been proposed

Migraine prophylaxis (unlabeled use): Oral: Initial: 0.25 mg/kg/day, given at bedtime; increase dose by 0.25 mg/kg/day to maximum 1 mg/kg/day. Reported dosing ranges: 0.1-2 mg/kg/day; maximum suggested dose: 10 mg.

Adolescents: Depressive disorders: Oral: Initial: 25-50 mg/day; may administer in divided doses; increase gradually to 100 mg/day in divided doses

Adults:

Depression: Oral: 50-150 mg/day single dose at bedtime or in divided doses; dose may be gradually increased up to 300 mg/day

Chronic pain management (unlabeled use): Oral: Initial: 25 mg at bedtime; may increase as tolerated to 100 mg/day

Diabetic neuropathy (unlabeled use): Oral: 25-100 mg/day (Bril, 2011)

Migraine prophylaxis (unlabeled use): Oral: Initial: 10-25 mg at bedtime; usual dose: 150 mg; reported dosing ranges: 10-400 mg/day

Post-traumatic stress disorder (PTSD) (unlabeled use): Oral: 75-200 mg/day

Elderly: Depression: Oral: Initial: 10-25 mg at bedtime; dose should be increased in 10-25 mg increments every week if tolerated; dose range: 25-150 mg/day

Discontinuation of therapy: Upon discontinuation of antidepressant therapy, gradually taper the dose to minimize the incidence of withdrawal symptoms and allow for the detection of re-emerging symptoms. Evidence supporting ideal taper rates is limited. APA and NICE guidelines suggest tapering therapy over at least several weeks with consideration to the half-life of the antidepressant; antidepressants with a shorter half-life may need to be tapered more conservatively. In addition for long-term treated patients, WFSBP guidelines recommend tapering over 4-6 months. If intolerable withdrawal symptoms occur following a dose reduction, consider resuming the previously prescribed dose and/or decrease dose at a more gradual rate (APA, 2010; Bauer, 2002; Haddad, 2001; NCCMH, 2010; Schatzberg, 2006; Shelton, 2001; Warner, 2006).

MAO inhibitor recommendations:

Switching to or from an MAO inhibitor antidepressant:

Allow 14 days to elapse between discontinuing an MAO inhibitor intended to treat depression and initiation of amitriptyline.

Allow 14 days to elapse between discontinuing amitriptyline and initiation of an MAO inhibitor intended to treat depression.

Use with reversible MAO inhibitors (such as linezolid or I.V. methylene blue):

Do not initiate amitriptyline in patients receiving linezolid or I.V. methylene blue; consider other interventions for psychiatric condition.

If urgent treatment with linezolid or I.V. methylene blue is required in a patient already receiving amitriptyline and potential benefits outweigh potential risks, discontinue amitriptyline promptly and administer linezolid or I.V. methylene blue. Monitor for serotonin syndrome for 2 weeks or until 24 hours after the last dose of linezolid or I.V. methylene blue, whichever comes first. May resume amitriptyline 24 hours after the last dose of linezolid or I.V. methylene blue.

Dosage interval in hepatic impairment: Use with caution and monitor plasma levels and patient response

Hemodialysis: Nondialyzable

Monitoring Parameters Monitor blood pressure and pulse rate prior to and during initial therapy; evaluate mental status, suicide ideation (especially at the beginning of therapy or when doses are increased or decreased); ECG in older adults and patients with cardiac disease

Reference Range Therapeutic: Amitriptyline and nortriptyline 100-250 ng/mL (SI: 360-900 nmol/L); nortriptyline 50-150 ng/mL (SI: 190-570 nmol/L); Toxic: >0.5 mcg/mL; plasma levels do not always correlate with clinical effectiveness

Test Interactions May cause false-positive reaction to EMIT immunoassay for imipramine

Dosage Forms Excipient information presented when available (limited, particularly for generics); consult specific product labeling.

Tablet, Oral, as hydrochloride:

Generic: 10 mg, 25 mg, 50 mg, 75 mg, 100 mg, 150 mg

Amitriptyline and Chlordiazepoxide

(a mee TRIP ti leen & klor dye az e POKS ide)

Index Terms Chlordiazepoxide and Amitriptyline Hydrochloride; Limbitrol

Pharmacologic Category Antidepressant, Tricyclic (Tertiary Amine); Benzodiazepine

Additional Appendix Information

Beers Criteria – Potentially Inappropriate Medications for Geriatrics *on page 2368*

Use Treatment of moderate-to-severe anxiety and/or agitation and depression

Medication Guide Available Yes

Dosage Initial: 3-4 tablets in divided doses; this may be increased to 6 tablets/day as required; some patients respond to smaller doses and can be maintained on 2 tablets

Discontinuation of therapy: Upon discontinuation of antidepressant therapy, gradually taper the dose to minimize the incidence of withdrawal symptoms and allow for the detection of re-emerging symptoms. Evidence supporting ideal taper rates is limited. APA and NICE guidelines suggest tapering therapy over at least several weeks with consideration to the half-life of the antidepressant; antidepressants with a shorter half-life may need to be tapered more conservatively. In addition for long-term treated patients, WFSBP guidelines recommend tapering over 4-6 months. If intolerable withdrawal symptoms occur following a dose reduction, consider resuming the previously prescribed dose and/or decrease dose at a more gradual rate (APA, 2010; Bauer, 2002; Haddad, 2001; NCCMH, 2010; Schatzberg, 2006; Shelton, 2001; Warner, 2006).

MAO inhibitor recommendations:

Switching to or from an MAO inhibitor intended to treat psychiatric disorders:

Allow 14 days to elapse between discontinuing an MAO inhibitor intended to treat psychiatric disorders and initiation of amitriptyline/chlordiazepoxide.

Allow 14 days to elapse between discontinuing amitriptyline/chlordiazepoxide and initiation of an MAO inhibitor intended to treat psychiatric disorders.

Use with reversible MAO inhibitors (such as linezolid or I.V. methylene blue):

Do not initiate amitriptyline/chlordiazepoxide in patients receiving linezolid or I.V. methylene blue; consider other interventions for psychiatric condition.

If urgent treatment with linezolid or I.V. methylene blue is required in a patient already receiving amitriptyline/chlordiazepoxide and potential benefits outweigh potential risks, discontinue amitriptyline/chlordiazepoxide promptly and administer linezolid or I.V. methylene blue. Monitor for serotonin syndrome for 2 weeks or until 24 hours after the last dose of linezolid or I.V. methylene blue, whichever comes first. May resume amitriptyline/chlordiazepoxide 24 hours after the last dose of linezolid or I.V. methylene blue.

Dosage adjustment in renal impairment: No dosage adjustment provided in manufacturer's labeling; use with caution.

Dosage adjustment in hepatic impairment: No dosage adjustment provided in manufacturer's labeling; use with caution.

Additional Information Complete prescribing information should be consulted for additional detail.

Dosage Forms Excipient information presented when available (limited, particularly for generics); consult specific product labeling.

Tablet: 12.5/5: Amitriptyline hydrochloride 12.5 mg and chlordiazepoxide 5 mg; 25/10: Amitriptyline hydrochloride 25 mg and chlordiazepoxide 10 mg

Controlled Substance C-IV

Amitriptyline and Perphenazine

(a mee TRIP ti leen & per FEN a zeen)

Brand Names: Canada PMS-Levazine

Index Terms Perphenazine and Amitriptyline Hydrochloride

Pharmacologic Category Antidepressant, Tricyclic (Tertiary Amine); Antipsychotic Agent, Typical, Phenothiazine

Additional Appendix Information

Beers Criteria – Potentially Inappropriate Medications for Geriatrics *on page 2368*

Use Treatment of patients with moderate-to-severe anxiety and/or agitation and depression; schizophrenia with depressive symptoms

Medication Guide Available Yes

Dosage Oral: Adults:

Depression and anxiety:

Initial: One tablet (amitriptyline 25 mg/perphenazine 2 mg or amitriptyline 25 mg/perphenazine 4 mg) 3-4 times/day **or** 1 tablet (amitriptyline 50 mg/perphenazine 4 mg) 2 times/day; initial therapeutic response may be observed after several days or upwards of a few weeks or longer (maximum daily dose: amitriptyline 200 mg/perphenazine 16 mg)

Maintenance: Smallest dose necessary for symptom relief; usually 1 tablet (amitriptyline 25 mg/perphenazine 2 mg or amitriptyline 25 mg/perphenazine 4 mg) 2-4 times/day **or** 1 tablet (amitriptyline 50 mg/perphenazine 4 mg) 2 times/day

Schizophrenia and depression:

Initial: Two tablets (amitriptyline 25 mg/perphenazine 4 mg) 3 times/day; if necessary, a fourth dose may be given at bedtime; initial therapeutic response may be observed after several days or upwards of a few weeks or longer (maximum daily dose: amitriptyline 200 mg/perphenazine 16 mg) (maximum: 64 mg/day of perphenazine)

Maintenance: Smallest dose necessary for symptom relief; usually 1 tablet (amitriptyline 25 mg/perphenazine 2 mg or amitriptyline 25 mg/perphenazine 4 mg) 2-4 times/day **or** 1 tablet (amitriptyline 50 mg/perphenazine 4 mg) 2 times/day

Elderly: One tablet (amitriptyline 10 mg/perphenazine 4 mg) 3-4 times/day

Discontinuation of therapy: Upon discontinuation of antidepressant therapy, gradually taper the dose to minimize the incidence of withdrawal symptoms and allow for the detection of re-emerging symptoms. Evidence supporting ideal taper rates is limited. APA and NICE guidelines suggest tapering therapy over at least several weeks with consideration to the half-life of the antidepressant; antidepressants with a shorter half-life may need to be tapered more conservatively. In addition for long-term treated patients, WFSBP guidelines recommend tapering over 4-6 months. If intolerable withdrawal symptoms occur following a dose reduction, consider resuming the previously prescribed dose and/or decrease dose at a more gradual rate (APA, 2010; Bauer, 2002; Haddad, 2001; NCCMH, 2010; Schatzberg, 2006; Shelton, 2001; Warner, 2006).

MAO inhibitor recommendations:

Switching to or from an MAO inhibitor intended to treat psychiatric disorders:

Allow 14 days to elapse between discontinuing an MAO inhibitor intended to treat psychiatric disorders and initiation of amitriptyline/perphenazine.

Allow 14 days to elapse between discontinuing amitriptyline/perphenazine and initiation of an MAO inhibitor intended to treat psychiatric disorders.

Use with reversible MAO inhibitors (such as linezolid or I.V. methylene blue):

Do not initiate amitriptyline/perphenazine in patients receiving linezolid or I.V. methylene blue; consider other interventions for psychiatric condition.

If urgent treatment with linezolid or I.V. methylene blue is required in a patient already receiving amitriptyline/perphenazine and potential benefits outweigh potential risks, discontinue amitriptyline/perphenazine promptly and administer linezolid or I.V. methylene blue. Monitor for serotonin syndrome for 2 weeks or until 24 hours after the last dose of linezolid or I.V. methylene blue, whichever comes first. May resume amitriptyline/perphenazine 24 hours after the last dose of linezolid or I.V. methylene blue.

Dosage adjustment in renal impairment: No dosage adjustment provided in manufacturer's labeling.

Dosage adjustment in hepatic impairment: Use caution; no dosage adjustment provided in manufacturer's labeling.

Additional Information Complete prescribing information should be consulted for additional detail.

Dosage Forms Excipient information presented when available (limited, particularly for generics); consult specific product labeling.

Tablet:

2-10: Amitriptyline hydrochloride 10 mg and perphenazine 2 mg

4-10: Amitriptyline hydrochloride 10 mg and perphenazine 4 mg

2-25: Amitriptyline hydrochloride 25 mg and perphenazine 2 mg

4-25: Amitriptyline hydrochloride 25 mg and perphenazine 4 mg

4-50: Amitriptyline hydrochloride 50 mg and perphenazine 4 mg

◆ **Amitriptyline Hydrochloride** *see* Amitriptyline *on page 105*

◆ **AMJ 9701** *see* Palifermin *on page 1548*

AmLODIPine (am LOE di peen)

Brand Names: U.S. Norvasc

Brand Names: Canada Accel-Amlodipine; Amlodipine-Odan; Apo-Amlodipine®; CO Amlodipine; Dom-Amlodipine; GD-Amlodipine; JAMP-Amlodipine; Manda-Amlodipine; Mint-Amlodipine; Mylan-Amlodipine; Norvasc®; PHL-Amlodipine; PMS-Amlodipine; Q-Amlodipine; RAN™-Amlodipine; ratio-Amlodipine; Riva-Amlodipine; Sandoz Amlodipine; Septa-Amlodipine; Teva-Amlodipine; ZYM-Amlodipine

Index Terms Amlodipine Besylate

Pharmacologic Category Antianginal Agent; Antihypertensive; Calcium Channel Blocker; Calcium Channel Blocker, Dihydropyridine

Additional Appendix Information

Calcium Channel Blockers - Comparative Pharmacokinetics *on page 2296*

Use Treatment of hypertension; treatment of symptomatic chronic stable angina, vasospastic (Prinzmetal's) angina (confirmed or suspected); prevention of hospitalization due to angina with documented CAD (limited to patients without heart failure or ejection fraction <40%)

Pregnancy Risk Factor C

Pregnancy Considerations Adverse events were observed in some animal reproduction studies. Untreated chronic maternal hypertension is associated with adverse events in the fetus, infant, and mother. If treatment for hypertension during pregnancy is needed, other agents are preferred (ACOG, 2012; Chobanian, 2003).

Breast-Feeding Considerations It is not known if amlodipine is excreted into breast milk. The manufacturer recommends nursing be discontinued during treatment. Breast-fed infants of mothers taking medications for hypertension should be monitored for adverse effects (Chobanian, 2003).

Contraindications Hypersensitivity to amlodipine or any component of the formulation

Warnings/Precautions Increased angina and/or MI has occurred with initiation or dosage titration of calcium channel blockers. Symptomatic hypotension with or without syncope can rarely occur; blood pressure must be lowered at a rate appropriate for the patient's clinical condition. Use caution in severe aortic stenosis and/or hypertrophic cardiomyopathy with outflow tract obstruction. Use caution in patients with hepatic impairment; may require lower starting dose; titrate slowly with severe hepatic impairment. The most common side effect is peripheral edema; occurs within 2-3 weeks of starting therapy. Reflex tachycardia may occur with use. Peak antihypertensive effect is delayed; dosage titration should occur after 7-14 days on a given dose. Initiate at a lower dose in the elderly.

Adverse Reactions

>10%:

Cardiovascular: Peripheral edema (2% to 11% dose related; female 15%; male 6%; HF patients 27% to 28% [Packer, 1996; Packer, 2013])

Respiratory: Pulmonary edema (HF patients 7% to 15% [Packer, 1996; Packer, 2013])

1% to 10%:

Cardiovascular: Palpitations (1% to 5% dose related), flushing (1% to 3% dose related, more frequent in females)

Central nervous system: Fatigue (5%), dizziness (1% to 3% dose related), male sexual disorder (1% to 2%), drowsiness (1%)

Dermatologic: Pruritus (1% to 2%), skin rash (1% to 2%)

Gastrointestinal: Nausea (3%), abdominal pain (2%)

Neuromuscular & skeletal: Muscle cramps (1% to 2%), weakness (1% to 2%)

Respiratory: Dyspnea (1% to 2%)

<1% (Limited to important or life-threatening): Acute interstitial nephritis, angioedema, anorexia, atrial fibrillation, bradycardia, cardiac arrhythmia, cholestasis, conjunctivitis, depersonalization, depression, diarrhea, difficulty in micturition, diplopia, dysphagia, epistaxis, erythema multiforme, erythematous rash, exfoliative dermatitis, eye pain, female sexual disorder, gingival hyperplasia, gynecomastia, hepatitis, hot flash, hyperglycemia, hypersensitivity angiitis, hypersensitivity reaction, hypoesthesia, increased serum transaminases, increased thirst, insomnia, jaundice, leukopenia, maculopapular rash, myalgia, nocturia, nonthrombocytopenic purpura, orthostatic hypotension, osteoarthritis, pain, pancreatitis, paresthesia, peripheral ischemia, peripheral neuropathy, phototoxicity, purpura, rigors, Stevens-Johnson syndrome, syncope, tachycardia, thrombocytopenia, tremor, urinary frequency, vasculitis, ventricular tachycardia, weight gain, weight loss

Drug Interactions

Metabolism/Transport Effects Substrate of CYP3A4 (major); **Note:** Assignment of Major/Minor substrate status based on clinically relevant drug interaction potential; **Inhibits** CYP1A2 (weak), CYP2A6 (weak), CYP2B6 (weak), CYP2C8 (weak), CYP2C9 (weak), CYP2D6 (weak), CYP3A4 (weak)

Avoid Concomitant Use

Avoid concomitant use of AmLODIPine with any of the following: Conivaptan; Fusidic Acid (Systemic); Pimozide

Increased Effect/Toxicity

AmLODIPine may increase the levels/effects of: Amifostine; Antihypertensives; ARIPiprazole; Atosiban; Beta-Blockers; Calcium Channel Blockers (Nondihydropyridine); Dofetilide; Fosphenytoin; Hypotensive Agents; Lomitapide; Magnesium Salts; Neuromuscular-Blocking Agents (Nondepolarizing); Nitroprusside; Obinutuzumab; Phenytoin; Pimozide; QuiNIDine; RiTUXimab; Simvastatin; Tacrolimus (Systemic)

The levels/effects of AmLODIPine may be increased by: Alpha1-Blockers; Antifungal Agents (Azole Derivatives, Systemic); Brimonidine (Topical); Calcium Channel Blockers (Nondihydropyridine); Conivaptan; CycloSPORINE (Systemic); CYP3A4 Inhibitors (Moderate); CYP3A4 Inhibitors (Strong); Dasatinib; Diazoxide; Fluconazole; Fusidic Acid (Systemic); Grapefruit Juice; Herbs (Hypotensive Properties); Ivacaftor; Luliconazole; Macrolide Antibiotics; Magnesium Salts; MAO Inhibitors; Mifepristone; Pentoxifylline; Phosphodiesterase 5 Inhibitors; Prostacyclin Analogues; Protease Inhibitors; QuiNIDine; Simeprevir

Decreased Effect

AmLODIPine may decrease the levels/effects of: Clopidogrel; QuiNIDine

The levels/effects of AmLODIPine may be decreased by: Barbiturates; Bosentan; Calcium Salts; CarBAMazepine; CYP3A4 Inducers (Strong); Dabrafenib; Deferasirox; Herbs (CYP3A4 Inducers); Herbs (Hypertensive Properties); Melatonin; Methylphenidate; Mitotane; Nafcillin; Rifamycin Derivatives; Tocilizumab; Yohimbine

Ethanol/Nutrition/Herb Interactions

Food: Grapefruit juice may modestly increase amlodipine levels.

Herb/Nutraceutical: St John's wort may decrease amlodipine levels. Avoid herbs with *hypertensive* properties (bayberry, blue cohosh, cayenne, ephedra, ginger, ginseng [American], kola, licorice). Avoid herbs with *hypotensive* properties (black cohosh, California poppy, coleus, garlic, goldenseal, hawthorn, mistletoe, periwinkle, quinine, shepherd's purse).

Storage/Stability Store at room temperature of 15°C to 30°C (59°F to 86°F).

Mechanism of Action Inhibits calcium ion from entering the "slow channels" or select voltage-sensitive areas of vascular smooth muscle and myocardium during depolarization, producing a relaxation of coronary vascular smooth muscle and coronary vasodilation; increases myocardial oxygen delivery in patients with vasospastic angina. Amlodipine directly acts on vascular smooth muscle to produce peripheral arterial vasodilation reducing peripheral vascular resistance and blood pressure.

Pharmacodynamics/Kinetics

Duration of antihypertensive effect: 24 hours

Absorption: Oral: Well absorbed

Distribution: V_d: 21 L/kg

Protein binding: 93% to 98%

Metabolism: Hepatic (>90%) to inactive metabolites

Bioavailability: 64% to 90%

Half-life elimination: Terminal: 30-50 hours; increased with hepatic dysfunction

Time to peak, plasma: 6-12 hours

Excretion: Urine (10% of total dose as unchanged drug, 60% of total dose as metabolites)

Dosage Oral:

Children 6-17 years: Hypertension: 2.5-5 mg once daily

Adults:

Hypertension: Initial dose: 5 mg once daily; maximum dose: 10 mg once daily. In general, titrate in 2.5 mg increments over 7-14 days. Usual dosage range (JNC 7): 2.5-10 mg once daily.

Angina: Usual dose: 5-10 mg; most patients require 10 mg for adequate effect

Elderly: Dosing should start at the lower end of dosing range and titrated to response due to possible increased incidence of hepatic, renal, or cardiac impairment. Elderly patients also show decreased clearance of amlodipine.

Hypertension: 2.5 mg once daily

Angina: 5 mg once daily

Dosage adjustment in renal impairment: Dialysis: Hemodialysis and peritoneal dialysis do not enhance elimination. Supplemental dose is not necessary.

Dosage adjustment in hepatic impairment:

Angina: Administer 5 mg once daily.

Hypertension: Administer 2.5 mg once daily.

Dietary Considerations May be taken without regard to meals.

Administration May be administered without regard to meals.

Monitoring Parameters Heart rate, blood pressure, peripheral edema

Dosage Forms Excipient information presented when available (limited, particularly for generics); consult specific product labeling.

Tablet, Oral:

Norvasc: 2.5 mg, 5 mg, 10 mg

Generic: 2.5 mg, 5 mg, 10 mg

Extemporaneous Preparations A 1 mg/mL oral suspension may be made with tablets and either a 1:1 mixture of simple syrup and 1% methylcellulose or a 1:1 mixture of Ora-Plus® and Ora-Sweet®. Crush fifty 5 mg tablets in a mortar and reduce to a fine powder. Add small portions of the chosen vehicle and mix to a uniform paste; mix while adding the vehicle in incremental proportions to **almost** 250 mL; transfer to a calibrated bottle, rinse mortar with vehicle, and add quantity of vehicle sufficient to make 250 mL. Label "shake well" and "refrigerate". Stable for 56 days at room temperature or 91 days refrigerated.

Nahata MC, Morosco RS, and Hipple TF, "Stability of Amlodipine Besylate in Two Liquid Dosage Forms," *J Am Pharm Assoc (Wash)*, 1999, 39(3):375-7.

◆ **Amlodipine, Aliskiren, and Hydrochlorothiazide** *see* Aliskiren, Amlodipine, and Hydrochlorothiazide *on page 76*

Amlodipine and Atorvastatin

(am LOW di peen & a TORE va sta tin)

Brand Names: U.S. Caduet®

Brand Names: Canada Caduet®

Index Terms Atorvastatin and Amlodipine; Atorvastatin Calcium and Amlodipine Besylate

Pharmacologic Category Antianginal Agent; Antihypertensive; Antilipemic Agent, HMG-CoA Reductase Inhibitor; Calcium Channel Blocker; Calcium Channel Blocker, Dihydropyridine

Use For use when treatment with both amlodipine and atorvastatin is appropriate:

Amlodipine: Treatment of hypertension; treatment of chronic stable angina, vasospastic (Prinzmetal's) angina (confirmed or suspected); prevention of hospitalization or to decrease coronary revascularization procedure due to angina with documented CAD (limited to patients without heart failure or ejection fraction <40%)

Atorvastatin: Treatment of dyslipidemias or primary prevention of cardiovascular disease (atherosclerotic) as detailed here:

Primary prevention of cardiovascular disease (high-risk for CVD): To reduce the risk of MI or stroke in patients without evidence of coronary heart disease who have multiple CVD risk factors or type 2 diabetes; also reduces the risk for angina or revascularization procedures in patients with multiple CVD risk factors without evidence of coronary heart disease

Secondary prevention of cardiovascular disease: To reduce the risk of MI, stroke, revascularization procedures, angina, and hospitalization for heart failure

Treatment of dyslipidemias: To reduce elevations in total cholesterol, LDL-C, apolipoprotein B, and triglycerides in patients with elevations of one or more components, and/or to increase low HDL-C as present in heterozygous familial/nonfamilial hypercholesterolemia and mixed dyslipidemia (Fredrickson type IIa and IIb hyperlipidemias); treatment of primary dysbetalipoproteinemia (Fredrickson type III), elevated serum TG levels (Fredrickson type IV), and homozygous familial hypercholesterolemia

Treatment of heterozygous familial hypercholesterolemia (HeFH) in adolescent patients (10-17 years of age, females >1 year postmenarche) having LDL-C ≥190 mg/dL or LDL-C ≥160 mg/dL with positive family history of premature cardiovascular disease (CVD) or with two or more CVD risk factors.

Pregnancy Risk Factor X

Dosage Oral: **Note:** Dose is individualized; combination product may be used as initial therapy or substituted for individual components in patients currently maintained on both agents separately or in patients not adequately controlled with monotherapy (using one of the agents or an agent within same pharmacologic class).

Children 10-17 years (females >1 year postmenarche): Hypertension and hyperlipidemia:

Initial therapy: Amlodipine 2.5 mg and atorvastatin 10 mg once daily; dose may be titrated after 1-2 weeks (amlodipine component) and after 2-4 weeks (atorvastatin component) to a maximum daily dose: Amlodipine 5 mg; atorvastatin 20 mg

Add-on therapy/replacement therapy: Amlodipine 2.5-5 mg and atorvastatin 10-20 mg once daily; dose may be titrated after 1-2 weeks (amlodipine component) and after 2-4 weeks (atorvastatin component) to a maximum daily dose: Amlodipine 5 mg; atorvastatin 20 mg

Adults: Hypertension, angina, and hyperlipidemia:

Initial therapy: Amlodipine 5 mg and atorvastatin 10-20 mg once daily; dose may be titrated after 1-2 weeks (amlodipine component) and after 2-4 weeks (atorvastatin component) to a maximum daily dose: Amlodipine 10 mg; atorvastatin 80 mg

Add-on therapy/replacement therapy: Amlodipine 5-10 mg and atorvastatin 10-80 mg once daily; dose may be titrated after 1-2 weeks (amlodipine component) and after 2-4 weeks (atorvastatin component) to a maximum daily dose: Amlodipine 10 mg; atorvastatin 80 mg

Elderly: Consider starting amlodipine at the lower end of dosing range due to increased incidence of hepatic, renal, or cardiac impairment. Elderly patients also show decreased clearance of amlodipine.

Dosage adjustment for atorvastatin with concomitant medications:

Boceprevir, nelfinavir: Use lowest effective atorvastatin dose (not to exceed 40 mg daily)

Clarithromycin, itraconazole, fosamprenavir, ritonavir (plus darunavir, fosamprenavir, or saquinavir): Use lowest effective atorvastatin dose (not to exceed 20 mg daily)

Dosage adjustment in renal impairment: No dosage adjustment is necessary

Dosage adjustment in hepatic impairment: Contraindicated in patients with active liver disease

Additional Information Complete prescribing information should be consulted for additional detail.

Dosage Forms Excipient information presented when available (limited, particularly for generics); consult specific product labeling.

Tablet, oral: Amlodipine 2.5 mg and atorvastatin 10 mg; Amlodipine 2.5 mg and atorvastatin 20 mg; Amlodipine 2.5 mg and atorvastatin 40 mg; Amlodipine 5 mg and atorvastatin 10 mg; Amlodipine 5 mg and atorvastatin 20 mg; Amlodipine 5 mg and atorvastatin 40 mg; Amlodipine 5 mg and atorvastatin 80 mg; Amlodipine 10 mg and atorvastatin 10 mg; Amlodipine 10 mg and atorvastatin 20 mg; Amlodipine 10 mg and atorvastatin 40 mg; Amlodipine 10 mg and atorvastatin 80 mg

Caduet®:

2.5/10: Amlodipine 2.5 mg and atorvastatin 10 mg
2.5/20: Amlodipine 2.5 mg and atorvastatin 20 mg
2.5/40: Amlodipine 2.5 mg and atorvastatin 40 mg
5/10: Amlodipine 5 mg and atorvastatin 10 mg
5/20: Amlodipine 5 mg and atorvastatin 20 mg
5/40: Amlodipine 5 mg and atorvastatin 40 mg
5/80: Amlodipine 5 mg and atorvastatin 80 mg
10/10: Amlodipine 10 mg and atorvastatin 10 mg
10/20: Amlodipine 10 mg and atorvastatin 20 mg
10/40: Amlodipine 10 mg and atorvastatin 40 mg
10/80: Amlodipine 10 mg and atorvastatin 80 mg

Amlodipine and Benazepril

(am LOE di peen & ben AY ze pril)

Brand Names: U.S. Lotrel®

Index Terms Benazepril Hydrochloride and Amlodipine Besylate

Pharmacologic Category Angiotensin-Converting Enzyme (ACE) Inhibitor; Antianginal Agent; Antihypertensive; Calcium Channel Blocker; Calcium Channel Blocker, Dihydropyridine

Use Treatment of hypertension

Pregnancy Risk Factor D

Dosage Oral: **Note:** Dose is individualized; combination product may be substituted for individual components in patients currently maintained on both agents separately or in patients not adequately controlled with monotherapy (using one of the agents or an agent within same antihypertensive class).

Adults: 2.5-10 mg (amlodipine) and 10-40 mg (benazepril) once daily; maximum: Amlodipine: 10 mg/day; benazepril: 80 mg/day

Elderly: Initial dose: 2.5 mg based on amlodipine component

Dosage adjustment in renal impairment: Cl_{cr} ≤30 mL/minute: Use of combination product is not recommended.

Dosage adjustment in hepatic impairment: Initial dose: 2.5 mg based on amlodipine component

Additional Information Complete prescribing information should be consulted for additional detail.

Dosage Forms Excipient information presented when available (limited, particularly for generics); consult specific product labeling.

Capsule, oral:

2.5/10: Amlodipine 2.5 mg and benazepril hydrochloride 10 mg

5/10: Amlodipine 5 mg and benazepril hydrochloride 10 mg

5/20: Amlodipine 5 mg and benazepril hydrochloride 20 mg

5/40: Amlodipine 5 mg and benazepril hydrochloride 40 mg

10/20: Amlodipine 10 mg and benazepril hydrochloride 20 mg

10/40: Amlodipine 10 mg and benazepril hydrochloride 40 mg
Lotrel® 2.5/10: Amlodipine 2.5 mg and benazepril hydrochloride 10 mg
Lotrel® 5/10: Amlodipine 5 mg and benazepril hydrochloride 10 mg
Lotrel® 5/20: Amlodipine 5 mg and benazepril hydrochloride 20 mg
Lotrel® 5/40: Amlodipine 5 mg and benazepril hydrochloride 40 mg
Lotrel® 10/20: Amlodipine 10 mg and benazepril hydrochloride 20 mg
Lotrel® 10/40: Amlodipine 10 mg and benazepril hydrochloride 40 mg

Amlodipine and Olmesartan

(am LOE di peen & olme SAR tan)

Brand Names: U.S. Azor™

Index Terms Amlodipine Besylate and Olmesartan Medoxomil; Olmesartan and Amlodipine

Pharmacologic Category Angiotensin II Receptor Blocker; Antianginal Agent; Antihypertensive; Calcium Channel Blocker; Calcium Channel Blocker, Dihydropyridine

Use Treatment of hypertension, including initial treatment in patients who will require multiple antihypertensives for adequate control

Pregnancy Risk Factor D

Dosage Oral: Dose is individualized; combination product may be substituted for individual components in patients currently maintained on both agents separately or in patients not adequately controlled with monotherapy (using one of the agents or an agent the within same antihypertensive class). May also be used as initial therapy in patients who are likely to need >1 antihypertensive to control blood pressure.

Adults: Hypertension:

Initial therapy (antihypertensive naive): Amlodipine 5 mg/olmesartan 20 mg once daily; dose may be increased after 1-2 weeks of therapy. Maximum recommended dose: Amlodipine 10 mg/day; olmesartan 40 mg/day.

Add-on/replacement therapy: Amlodipine 5-10 mg and olmesartan 20-40 mg once daily depending upon previous doses, current control, and goals of therapy; dose may be titrated after 2 weeks of therapy. Maximum recommended doses: Amlodipine 10 mg/day; olmesartan 40 mg/day.

Elderly: Initial therapy is not recommended in patients ≥75 years of age.

Dosing adjustment in renal impairment: No specific guidelines for dosage adjustment

Dosing adjustment in hepatic impairment: Initial therapy is not recommended

Additional Information Complete prescribing information should be consulted for additional detail.

Dosage Forms Excipient information presented when available (limited, particularly for generics); consult specific product labeling.

Tablet:

Azor™ 5/20: Amlodipine 5 mg and olmesartan medoxomil 20 mg
Azor™ 5/40: Amlodipine 5 mg and olmesartan medoxomil 40 mg
Azor™ 10/20: Amlodipine 10 mg and olmesartan medoxomil 20 mg
Azor™ 10/40: Amlodipine 10 mg and olmesartan medoxomil 40 mg

◆ **Amlodipine and Telmisartan** *see* Telmisartan and Amlodipine *on page* 2004

Amlodipine and Valsartan

(am LOE di peen & val SAR tan)

Brand Names: U.S. Exforge®

Index Terms Amlodipine Besylate and Valsartan; Valsartan and Amlodipine

Pharmacologic Category Angiotensin II Receptor Blocker; Antianginal Agent; Antihypertensive; Calcium Channel Blocker; Calcium Channel Blocker, Dihydropyridine

Use Treatment of hypertension

Pregnancy Risk Factor D

Dosage Oral: Dose is individualized; combination product may be used as initial therapy or substituted for individual components in patients currently maintained on both agents separately or in patients not adequately controlled with monotherapy (using one of the agents or an agent within same antihypertensive class).

Adults: Hypertension:

Initial therapy: Amlodipine 5 mg and valsartan 160 mg once daily, dose may be titrated after 1-2 weeks of therapy. Maximum recommended doses: Amlodipine 10 mg daily; valsartan 320 mg daily

Add-on/replacement therapy: Amlodipine 5-10 mg and valsartan 160-320 mg once daily; dose may be titrated after 3-4 weeks of therapy. Maximum recommended doses: Amlodipine 10 mg daily; valsartan 320 mg daily

Elderly: Use of lower initial doses should be considered.

Dosing adjustment in renal impairment:

Cl_{cr} ≥30 mL/minute: No dosage adjustment necessary.

Cl_{cr} <30 mL/minute: No dosage adjustment provided in manufacturer's labeling; safety and efficacy has not been established.

Dosing adjustment in hepatic impairment:

Mild-to-moderate impairment: Use with caution; amlodipine elimination prolonged and valsartan exposure doubled in patients with mild-to-moderate chronic disease compared to healthy volunteers. No dosage adjustment for valsartan is necessary; however, a lower initial amlodipine dose may be required (possibly requiring use of the individual agents).

Severe impairment: No dosage adjustment provided in manufacturer's labeling; however, similar to patients with mild to moderate impairment, a lower initial amlodipine dose may be required (possibly requiring use of the individual agents); titrate slowly.

Additional Information Complete prescribing information should be consulted for additional detail.

Dosage Forms Excipient information presented when available (limited, particularly for generics); consult specific product labeling.

Tablet:

Exforge®:

5/160: Amlodipine 5 mg and valsartan 160 mg
5/320: Amlodipine 5 mg and valsartan 320 mg
10/160: Amlodipine 10 mg and valsartan 160 mg
10/320: Amlodipine 10 mg and valsartan 320 mg

◆ **Amlodipine Besylate** *see* AmLODIPine *on page* 109

◆ **Amlodipine Besylate, Aliskiren Hemifumarate, and Hydrochlorothiazide** *see* Aliskiren, Amlodipine, and Hydrochlorothiazide *on page* 76

◆ **Amlodipine Besylate and Olmesartan Medoxomil** *see* Amlodipine and Olmesartan *on page* 112

◆ **Amlodipine Besylate and Telmisartan** *see* Telmisartan and Amlodipine *on page* 2004

◆ **Amlodipine Besylate and Valsartan** *see* Amlodipine and Valsartan *on page* 112

◆ **Amlodipine Besylate, Olmesartan Medoxomil, and Hydrochlorothiazide** *see* Olmesartan, Amlodipine, and Hydrochlorothiazide *on page 1498*

◆ **Amlodipine Besylate, Valsartan, and Hydrochlorothiazide** *see* Amlodipine, Valsartan, and Hydrochlorothiazide *on page 113*

◆ **Amlodipine, Hydrochlorothiazide, and Aliskiren** *see* Aliskiren, Amlodipine, and Hydrochlorothiazide *on page 76*

◆ **Amlodipine, Hydrochlorothiazide, and Olmesartan** *see* Olmesartan, Amlodipine, and Hydrochlorothiazide *on page 1498*

◆ **Amlodipine, Hydrochlorothiazide, and Valsartan** *see* Amlodipine, Valsartan, and Hydrochlorothiazide *on page 113*

◆ **Amlodipine-Odan (Can)** *see* AmLODIPine *on page 109*

Amlodipine, Valsartan, and Hydrochlorothiazide

(am LOE di peen, val SAR tan, & hye droe klor oh THYE a zide)

Brand Names: U.S. Exforge HCT®

Index Terms Amlodipine Besylate, Valsartan, and Hydrochlorothiazide; Amlodipine, Hydrochlorothiazide, and Valsartan; Hydrochlorothiazide, Amlodipine, and Valsartan; Valsartan, Hydrochlorothiazide, and Amlodipine

Pharmacologic Category Angiotensin II Receptor Blocker; Antianginal Agent; Antihypertensive; Calcium Channel Blocker; Calcium Channel Blocker, Dihydropyridine; Diuretic, Thiazide

Use Treatment of hypertension (not for initial therapy)

Pregnancy Risk Factor D

Dosage Oral: **Note:** Not for initial therapy. Dose is individualized; combination product may be substituted for individual components in patients currently maintained on all three agents separately or in patients not adequately controlled with any two of the following antihypertensive classes: Calcium channel blockers, angiotensin II receptor blockers, and diuretics.

Adults: Hypertension: Add-on/switch/replacement therapy: Amlodipine 5-10 mg and valsartan 160-320 mg and hydrochlorothiazide 12.5-25 mg once daily; dose may be titrated after 2 weeks of therapy. Maximum recommended daily dose: Amlodipine 10 mg/valsartan 320 mg/hydrochlorothiazide 25 mg

Elderly: Use of lower initial doses should be considered.

Dosage adjustment in renal impairment:

Cl_{cr} ≥30 mL/minute: No dosage adjustment necessary.

Cl_{cr} <30 mL/minute: No dosage adjustment provided in manufacturer's labeling; safety and efficacy has not been established; hydrochlorothiazide is usually ineffective when Cl_{cr} <30 mL/minute and is contraindicated in patients who are anuric.

Dosage adjustment in hepatic impairment:

Mild-to-moderate impairment: Use with caution; amlodipine elimination prolonged and valsartan exposure doubled in patients with mild-to-moderate chronic disease compared to healthy volunteers. No dosage adjustment for valsartan is necessary; however, a lower initial amlodipine dose may be required (possibly requiring use of the individual agents).

Severe impairment: No dosage adjustment provided in manufacturer's labeling; however, similar to patients with mild to moderate impairment, a lower initial amlodipine dose may be required (possibly requiring use of the individual agents); titrate slowly.

Additional Information Complete prescribing information should be consulted for additional detail.

Dosage Forms Excipient information presented when available (limited, particularly for generics); consult specific product labeling.

Tablet, oral:

Exforge HCT®:

Amlodipine 5 mg, valsartan 160 mg, and hydrochlorothiazide 12.5 mg

Amlodipine 5 mg, valsartan 160 mg, and hydrochlorothiazide 25 mg

Amlodipine 10 mg, valsartan 160 mg, and hydrochlorothiazide 12.5 mg

Amlodipine 10 mg, valsartan 160 mg, and hydrochlorothiazide 25 mg

Amlodipine 10 mg, valsartan 320 mg, and hydrochlorothiazide 25 mg

◆ **Ammens® Original Medicated [OTC]** *see* Zinc Oxide *on page 2230*

◆ **Ammens® Shower Fresh [OTC]** *see* Zinc Oxide *on page 2230*

◆ **Ammonapse** *see* Sodium Phenylbutyrate *on page 1923*

Ammonium Chloride (a MOE nee um KLOR ide)

Pharmacologic Category Electrolyte Supplement, Parenteral

Use Treatment of hypochloremic states or metabolic alkalosis

Pregnancy Risk Factor C

Dosage Metabolic alkalosis: The following equations represent different methods of correction utilizing either the serum HCO_3^-, the serum chloride, or the base excess

Dosing of mEq NH_4 Cl via the chloride-deficit method (hypochloremia):

Dose of mEq NH_4Cl = [0.2 L/kg x body weight (kg)] x [103 - observed serum chloride]; administer 50% of dose over 12 hours, then re-evaluate

Note: 0.2 L/kg is the estimated chloride volume of distribution and 103 is the average normal serum chloride concentration (mEq/L)

Dosing of mEq NH_4 Cl via the bicarbonate-excess method (refractory hypochloremic metabolic alkalosis):

Dose of NH_4Cl = [0.5 L/kg x body weight (kg)] x (observed serum HCO_3^- - 24); administer 50% of dose over 12 hours, then re-evaluate

Note: 0.5 L/kg is the estimated bicarbonate volume of distribution and 24 is the average normal serum bicarbonate concentration (mEq/L)

These equations will yield different requirements of ammonium chloride

Dosage adjustment in renal impairment: Severe impairment: use is contraindicated.

Dosage adjustment in hepatic impairment: Severe impairment: use is contraindicated.

Additional Information Complete prescribing information should be consulted for additional detail.

Dosage Forms Excipient information presented when available (limited, particularly for generics); consult specific product labeling.

Injection, solution: Ammonium 5 mEq/mL and chloride 5 mEq/mL (20 mL) [equivalent to ammonium chloride 267.5 mg/mL]

◆ **Ammonul®** *see* Sodium Phenylacetate and Sodium Benzoate *on page 1922*

◆ **AMN107** *see* Nilotinib *on page 1458*

◆ **Amnesteem** *see* ISOtretinoin *on page 1129*

Amobarbital (am oh BAR bi tal)

Brand Names: U.S. Amytal Sodium
Brand Names: Canada Amytal®
Index Terms Amobarbital Sodium; Amylobarbitone
Pharmacologic Category Barbiturate
Additional Appendix Information
Beers Criteria – Potentially Inappropriate Medications for Geriatrics *on page 2368*
Use Hypnotic in short-term treatment of insomnia; reduce anxiety and provide sedation preoperatively
Unlabeled Use Therapeutic or diagnostic "Amytal® Interviewing"; Wada test
Pregnancy Risk Factor D
Dosage
Children:
Sedative: I.M., I.V.: 6-12 years: Manufacturer's dosing range: 65-500 mg
Hypnotic (unlabeled use): I.M.: 2-3 mg/kg (maximum: 500 mg)
Adults:
Hypnotic: I.M., I.V.: 65-200 mg at bedtime (maximum single dose: 1000 mg)
Sedative: I.M., I.V.: 30-50 mg 2-3 times/day (maximum single dose: 1000 mg)
"Amytal® interview" (unlabeled use): I.V.: 50-100 mg/minute for total dose of 200-1000 mg or until patient experiences drowsiness, impaired attention, slurred speech, or nystagmus
Wada test (unlabeled use): Intra-arterial: 100 mg over 4-5 seconds via percutaneous transfemoral catheter
Dosing adjustment in renal/hepatic impairment: Dosing should be reduced; specific recommendations not available.
Additional Information Complete prescribing information should be consulted for additional detail.
Dosage Forms Excipient information presented when available (limited, particularly for generics); consult specific product labeling.
Solution Reconstituted, Injection, as sodium:
Amytal Sodium: 500 mg (1 ea)
Controlled Substance C-II

◆ Amobarbital Sodium *see* Amobarbital *on page 114*
◆ Amoclan *see* Amoxicillin and Clavulanate *on page 119*

Amoxapine (a MOKS a peen)

Index Terms Asendin [DSC]
Pharmacologic Category Antidepressant, Tricyclic (Secondary Amine)
Additional Appendix Information
Antidepressant Agents *on page 2284*
Beers Criteria – Potentially Inappropriate Medications for Geriatrics *on page 2368*
Use Treatment of depression (including endogenous, neurotic, psychotic, and reactive depression); treatment of depression accompanied by anxiety or agitation
Pregnancy Risk Factor C
Pregnancy Considerations Adverse events were observed in some animal reproduction studies. Tricyclic antidepressants may be associated with irritability, jitteriness, and convulsions (rare) in the neonate (Yonkers, 2009).

The ACOG recommends that therapy for depression during pregnancy be individualized; treatment should incorporate the clinical expertise of the mental health clinician, obstetrician, primary healthcare provider, and pediatrician (ACOG, 2008). According to the American Psychiatric Association (APA), the risks of medication treatment should be weighed against other treatment options and untreated depression. For women who discontinue antidepressant medications during pregnancy and who may be at high risk for postpartum depression, the medications can be restarted following delivery (APA, 2010). Treatment algorithms have been developed by the ACOG and the APA for the management of depression in women prior to conception and during pregnancy (Yonkers, 2009).
Breast-Feeding Considerations Amoxapine is excreted into breast milk. A case report notes low concentrations of amoxapine and its active metabolite in the milk of a nonnursing woman who developed galactorrhea during therapy (Gelenberg, 1979). The manufacturer recommends that caution be used if administered to a nursing woman.
Medication Guide Available Yes
Contraindications Hypersensitivity to amoxapine or any component of the formulation; use with or within 14 days of MAO inhibitors; acute recovery phase following myocardial infarction
Warnings/Precautions [U.S. Boxed Warning]: Antidepressants increase the risk of suicidal thinking and behavior in children, adolescents, and young adults (18-24 years of age) with major depressive disorder (MDD) and other psychiatric disorders; consider risk prior to prescribing. Short-term studies did not show an increased risk in patients >24 years of age and showed a decreased risk in patients ≥65 years. Closely monitor for clinical worsening, suicidality, or unusual changes in behavior; the patient's family or caregiver should be instructed to closely observe the patient and communicate condition with healthcare provider. A medication guide should be dispensed with each prescription. **Amoxapine is not FDA approved for use in pediatric patients.**

The possibility of a suicide attempt is inherent in major depression and may persist until remission occurs. Monitor for worsening of depression or suicidality, especially during initiation of therapy (generally first 1-2 months) or with dose increases or decreases. Use caution in high-risk patients. Worsening depression and severe abrupt suicidality that are not part of the presenting symptoms may require discontinuation or modification of drug therapy. The patient's family or caregiver should be alerted to monitor patients for the emergence of suicidality and associated behaviors (such as agitation, irritability, hostility, impulsivity, and hypomania) and notify the healthcare provider.

May worsen psychosis in some patients or precipitate a shift to mania or hypomania in patients with bipolar disorder. Patients presenting with depressive symptoms should be screened for bipolar disorder. Monotherapy in patients with bipolar disorder should be avoided. **Amoxapine is not FDA approved for bipolar depression.** May cause extrapyramidal symptoms, including pseudoparkinsonism, acute dystonic reactions, akathisia, and tardive dyskinesia (risk of these reactions is low). The risk for tardive dyskinesia (may be irreversible) increases with long-term treatment and higher cumulative doses. Therapy should be discontinued in any patient if signs/symptoms of tardive dyskinesia appear. May be associated with neuroleptic malignant syndrome.

The degree of sedation, anticholinergic effects, orthostasis, and conduction abnormalities are moderate relative to other antidepressants. May cause drowsiness/sedation, resulting in impaired performance of tasks requiring alertness (eg, operating machinery or driving). Sedative effects may be additive with other CNS depressants and/or ethanol. Use with caution in patients with a history of cardiovascular disease (including previous MI, stroke, tachycardia, or conduction abnormalities). Use with caution in patients with urinary retention, benign prostatic hyperplasia, narrow-angle glaucoma, xerostomia, visual problems, constipation, or a history of bowel obstruction.

May lower seizure threshold - use caution in patients with a previous seizure disorder or condition predisposing to seizures such as brain damage, alcoholism, or concurrent therapy with other drugs which lower the seizure threshold. May increase the risks associated with electroconvulsive therapy. Bone fractures have been associated with antidepressant treatment. Consider the possibility of a fragility fracture if an antidepressant-treated patient presents with unexplained bone pain, point tenderness, swelling, or bruising (Rabenda, 2013; Rizzoli, 2012). Use with caution in hyperthyroid patients or those receiving thyroid supplementation.

Use caution in elderly patients; may cause or exacerbate syndrome of inappropriate antidiuretic hormone secretion or hyponatremia; monitor sodium closely with initiation or dosage adjustments in older adults. May be inappropriate in older adults depending on comorbidities (eg, dementia, delirium) due to its potent anticholinergic effects (Beers Criteria). May also have increased risk of adverse events, including tardive dyskinesia (particularly older women) and sedation.

Abrupt discontinuation or interruption of antidepressant therapy has been associated with a discontinuation syndrome. Symptoms arising may vary with antidepressant however commonly include nausea, vomiting, diarrhea, headaches, light-headedness, dizziness, diminished appetite, sweating, chills, tremors, paresthesias, fatigue, somnolence, and sleep disturbances (eg, vivid dreams, insomnia). Greater risks for developing a discontinuation syndrome have been associated with antidepressants with shorter half-lives, longer durations of treatment, and abrupt discontinuation. For antidepressants of short or intermediate half-lives, symptoms may emerge within 2-5 days after treatment discontinuation and last 7-14 days (APA, 2010; Fava, 2006; Haddad, 2001; Shelton, 2001; Warner, 2006).

Adverse Reactions

>10%:

Central nervous system: Drowsiness (14%)

Gastrointestinal: Xerostomia (14%), constipation (12%)

1% to 10%:

Cardiovascular: Palpitations

Central nervous system: Anxiety, ataxia, confusion, dizziness, EEG abnormalities, excitement, fatigue, headache, insomnia, nervousness, nightmares, restlessness

Dermatologic: Edema, skin rash

Endocrine: Prolactin levels increased

Gastrointestinal: Appetite increased, nausea

Neuromuscular & skeletal: Tremor, weakness

Ocular: Blurred vision (7%)

Miscellaneous: Diaphoresis

<1% (Limited to important or life-threatening): Agranulocytosis, allergic reactions, diarrhea, extrapyramidal symptoms, fever, galactorrhea, hepatitis, hypertension, hypomania. impotence, incoordination, intraocular pressure increased, leukopenia, menstrual irregularity, mydriasis, neuroleptic malignant syndrome, numbness, painful ejaculation, paresthesia, photosensitivity, seizure, SIADH, syncope, tardive dyskinesia, testicular edema, tinnitus, urinary retention, vasculitis, vomiting

Drug Interactions

Metabolism/Transport Effects Substrate of CYP2D6 (major); **Note:** Assignment of Major/Minor substrate status based on clinically relevant drug interaction potential

Avoid Concomitant Use

Avoid concomitant use of Amoxapine with any of the following: Aclidinium; Iobenguane I 123; Ipratropium (Oral Inhalation); Linezolid; MAO Inhibitors; Methylene Blue; Moxonidine; Tiotropium; Umeclidinium

Increased Effect/Toxicity

Amoxapine may increase the levels/effects of: Alpha-/Beta-Agonists (Direct-Acting); Alpha1-Agonists; Amphetamines; Analgesics (Opioid); Anticholinergics; Antipsychotics; Beta2-Agonists; Citalopram; Desmopressin; Escitalopram; Highest Risk QTc-Prolonging Agents; Methylene Blue; Metoclopramide; Moderate Risk QTc-Prolonging Agents; QuiNIDine; Serotonin Modulators; Sodium Phosphates; Sulfonylureas; Tiotropium; TraMADol; Vitamin K Antagonists; Yohimbine

The levels/effects of Amoxapine may be increased by: Abiraterone Acetate; Aclidinium; Altretamine; Antipsychotics; Cimetidine; Cinacalcet; Citalopram; Cobicistat; CYP2D6 Inhibitors (Moderate); CYP2D6 Inhibitors (Strong); Dexmethylphenidate; DULoxetine; Escitalopram; FLUoxetine; FluvoxaMINE; Ipratropium (Oral Inhalation); Linezolid; Lithium; MAO Inhibitors; Methylphenidate; Metoclopramide; Metyrosine; Mifepristone; PARoxetine; Pramlintide; Protease Inhibitors; QuiNIDine; Sertraline; Terbinafine (Systemic); Thyroid Products; TraMADol; Umeclidinium; Valproic Acid and Derivatives

Decreased Effect

Amoxapine may decrease the levels/effects of: Acetylcholinesterase Inhibitors (Central); Alpha2-Agonists; Alpha2-Agonists (Ophthalmic); Iobenguane I 123; Moxonidine

The levels/effects of Amoxapine may be decreased by: Acetylcholinesterase Inhibitors (Central); Barbiturates; CarBAMazepine; Peginterferon Alfa-2b; St Johns Wort

Ethanol/Nutrition/Herb Interactions

Ethanol: May increase CNS depression; monitor for increased effects with coadministration. Caution patients about effects.

Food: Grapefruit juice may inhibit the metabolism of some TCAs and clinical toxicity may result.

Herb/Nutraceutical: Avoid valerian, St John's wort, SAMe, kava kava.

Storage/Stability Store at 20°C to 25°C (68°F to 77°F).

Mechanism of Action Reduces the reuptake of serotonin and norepinephrine. The metabolite, 7-OH-amoxapine has significant dopamine receptor blocking activity similar to haloperidol.

Pharmacodynamics/Kinetics

Onset of antidepressant effect: Usually occurs after 1-2 weeks, but may require 4-6 weeks

Absorption: Rapid and well absorbed

Distribution: V_d: 0.9-1.2 L/kg

Protein binding: ~90%

Metabolism: Extensively metabolized; hepatic hydroxylation produces two active metabolites, 7-hydroxyamoxapine (7-OH-amoxapine) and 8-hydroxyamoxapine (8-OH-amoxapine); metabolites undergo conjugation to form glucuronides

Half-life elimination: 8 hours; 7-hydroxyamoxapine metabolite: 4-6 hours; 8-hydroxyamoxapine metabolite: 30 hours

Time to peak, serum: ~90 minutes

Excretion: Urine (as unchanged drug and metabolites)

Dosage Oral:

Adults:

Outpatients: Initial: 50 mg 2-3 times/day; dose may be increased to 100 mg 2-3 times/day by the end of the first week, if tolerated. Usual effective dose: 200-300 mg/day; if 300 mg daily has been reached and maintained for at least 2 weeks and no response is observed, may further increase to 400 mg/day. Once an effective dose is reached, doses ≤300 mg may be given once daily at bedtime and doses >300 mg/day should be divided.

Inpatients: Hospitalized patients refractory to antidepressant therapy (and no history of seizures) may be cautiously titrated to 600 mg/day in divided doses.

Maintenance: Outpatients and Inpatients: Once symptoms are controlled, gradually decrease to lowest dose that will maintain remission.

Elderly: Use caution or avoid in the elderly. Initial: 25 mg 2-3 times/day; dose may be increased to 50 mg 2-3 times/day by the end of the first week, if tolerated; usual effective dose: 100-150 mg/day; if dose is ineffective, may further increase cautiously to 300 mg/day; once an effective dose is reached, doses ≤300 mg may be given once daily at bedtime. Maintenance: Once symptoms are controlled, gradually decrease to the lowest dose that will maintain remission.

Discontinuation of therapy: Upon discontinuation of antidepressant therapy, gradually taper the dose to minimize the incidence of withdrawal symptoms and allow for the detection of re-emerging symptoms. Evidence supporting ideal taper rates is limited. APA and NICE guidelines suggest tapering therapy over at least several weeks with consideration to the half-life of the antidepressant; antidepressants with a shorter half-life may need to be tapered more conservatively. In addition for long-term treated patients, WFSBP guidelines recommend tapering over 4-6 months. If intolerable withdrawal symptoms occur following a dose reduction, consider resuming the previously prescribed dose and/or decrease dose at a more gradual rate (APA, 2010; Bauer, 2002; Haddad, 2001; NCCMH, 2010; Schatzberg, 2006; Shelton, 2001; Warner, 2006).

MAO inhibitor recommendations:

Switching to or from an MAO inhibitor intended to treat psychiatric disorders:

Allow 14 days to elapse between discontinuing an MAO inhibitor intended to treat psychiatric disorders and initiation of amoxapine.

Allow 14 days to elapse between discontinuing amoxapine and initiation of an MAO inhibitor intended to treat psychiatric disorders.

Use with reversible MAO inhibitors (such as linezolid or I.V. methylene blue):

Do not initiate amoxapine in patients receiving linezolid or I.V. methylene blue; consider other interventions for psychiatric condition.

If urgent treatment with linezolid or I.V. methylene blue is required in a patient already receiving amoxapine and potential benefits outweigh potential risks, discontinue amoxapine promptly and administer linezolid or I.V. methylene blue. Monitor for serotonin syndrome for 2 weeks or until 24 hours after the last dose of linezolid or I.V. methylene blue, whichever comes first. May resume amoxapine 24 hours after the last dose of linezolid or I.V. methylene blue.

Dosage adjustment in renal impairment: No dosage adjustment provided in manufacturer's labeling. However, amoxapine is primarily eliminated renally, and renal failure may develop in overdoses; use with caution.

Dosage adjustment in hepatic impairment: No dosage adjustment provided in manufacturer's labeling.

Monitoring Parameters Monitor blood pressure and pulse rate prior to and during initial therapy evaluate mental status, suicide ideation (especially at the beginning of therapy or when doses are increased or decreased); ECG in older adults and patients with cardiac disease

Additional Information Extrapyramidal reactions and tardive dyskinesia may occur.

Dosage Forms Excipient information presented when available (limited, particularly for generics); consult specific product labeling.

Tablet, Oral:

Generic: 25 mg, 50 mg, 100 mg, 150 mg

Amoxicillin (a moks i SIL in)

Brand Names: U.S. Moxatag

Brand Names: Canada Apo-Amoxi®; Mylan-Amoxicillin; Novamoxin®; NTP-Amoxicillin; Nu-Amoxi; PHL-Amoxicillin; PMS-Amoxicillin; Pro-Amox-250; Pro-Amox-500

Index Terms *p*-Hydroxyampicillin; Amoxicillin Trihydrate; Amoxil; Amoxycillin

Pharmacologic Category Antibiotic, Penicillin

Additional Appendix Information

Prevention of Infective Endocarditis *on page 2353*

Use Treatment of otitis media, sinusitis, and infections caused by susceptible organisms involving the upper and lower respiratory tract, skin, and urinary tract; prophylaxis of infective endocarditis in patients undergoing surgical or dental procedures; as part of a multidrug regimen for *H. pylori* eradication; periodontitis

Unlabeled Use Postexposure prophylaxis for anthrax exposure with documented susceptible organisms; chronic oral antimicrobial suppression of prosthetic joint infection

Pregnancy Risk Factor B

Pregnancy Considerations Adverse events have not been observed in animal reproduction studies. Maternal use of amoxicillin has generally not resulted in an increased risk of adverse fetal effects; however, an increased risk of cleft lip with cleft palate has been observed in some studies. It is the drug of choice for the treatment of chlamydial infections in pregnancy and for anthrax prophylaxis when penicillin susceptibility is documented. Amoxicillin may be used in certain situations prior to vaginal delivery in women at high risk for endocarditis.

Due to pregnancy-induced physiologic changes, oral amoxicillin clearance is increased during pregnancy resulting in lower concentrations and smaller AUCs. Oral ampicillin-class antibiotics are poorly absorbed during labor.

Breast-Feeding Considerations Very small amounts of amoxicillin are excreted in breast milk. The manufacturer recommends that caution be exercised when administering amoxicillin to nursing women. Nondose-related effects could include modification of bowel flora and allergic sensitization of the infant.

Contraindications Hypersensitivity to amoxicillin, penicillin, other beta-lactams, or any component of the formulation

Warnings/Precautions In patients with renal impairment, doses and/or frequency of administration should be modified in response to the degree of renal impairment; in addition, use of certain dosage forms (eg, extended release 775 mg tablet and immediate release 875 mg tablet) should be avoided in patients with Cl_{cr} <30 mL/minute or patients requiring hemodialysis. A high percentage of patients with infectious mononucleosis have developed rash during therapy with amoxicillin; ampicillin-class antibiotics not recommended in these patients. Serious and occasionally severe or fatal hypersensitivity (anaphylactoid) reactions have been reported in patients on penicillin therapy, especially with a history of beta-lactam hypersensitivity, history of sensitivity to multiple allergens, or previous IgE-mediated reactions (eg, anaphylaxis, angioedema, urticaria). Use with caution in asthmatic patients. Prolonged use may result in fungal or bacterial superinfection, including *C. difficile*-associated diarrhea (CDAD) and pseudomembranous colitis; CDAD has been observed >2 months postantibiotic treatment. Chewable tablets contain phenylalanine.

Adverse Reactions Frequency not defined.

Cardiovascular: Hypersensitivity angiitis

Central nervous system: Agitation, anxiety, behavioral changes, confusion, dizziness, headache, hyperactivity (reversible), insomnia, seizure

Dermatologic: Acute generalized exanthematous pustulosis, erythematous maculopapular rash, erythema multiforme, exfoliative dermatitis, Stevens-Johnson syndrome, toxic epidermal necrolysis, urticaria

Gastrointestinal: Dental discoloration (brown, yellow, or gray; rare), diarrhea, hemorrhagic colitis, melanoglossia, mucocutaneous candidiasis, nausea, pseudomembranous colitis, vomiting

Genitourinary: Crystalluria

Hematologic & oncologic: Agranulocytosis, anemia, eosinophilia, hemolytic anemia, leukopenia,thrombocytopenia, thrombocytopenia purpura

Hepatic: Cholestatic hepatitis, cholestatic jaundice, hepatitis (acute cytolytic), increased serum ALT, increased serum AST

Hypersensitivity: Anaphylaxis

Immunologic: Serum sickness-like reaction

Drug Interactions

Metabolism/Transport Effects None known.

Avoid Concomitant Use

Avoid concomitant use of Amoxicillin with any of the following: BCG

Increased Effect/Toxicity

Amoxicillin may increase the levels/effects of: Methotrexate; Vitamin K Antagonists

The levels/effects of Amoxicillin may be increased by: Allopurinol; Probenecid

Decreased Effect

Amoxicillin may decrease the levels/effects of: BCG; Mycophenolate; Sodium Picosulfate; Typhoid Vaccine

The levels/effects of Amoxicillin may be decreased by: Tetracycline Derivatives

Storage/Stability

Amoxil®: Oral suspension remains stable for 14 days at room temperature or if refrigerated (refrigeration preferred). Unit-dose antibiotic oral syringes are stable at room temperature for at least 72 hours (Tu, 1988).

Moxatag™: Store at 25°C (77°F); excursions permitted to 15°C to 30°C (59°F to 86°F).

Mechanism of Action Inhibits bacterial cell wall synthesis by binding to one or more of the penicillin-binding proteins (PBPs) which in turn inhibits the final transpeptidation step of peptidoglycan synthesis in bacterial cell walls, thus inhibiting cell wall biosynthesis. Bacteria eventually lyse due to ongoing activity of cell wall autolytic enzymes (autolysins and murein hydrolases) while cell wall assembly is arrested.

Pharmacodynamics/Kinetics

Absorption: Oral: Rapid and nearly complete; food does not interfere

Extended-release tablet: Rate of absorption is slower compared to immediate-release formulations; food decreases the rate but not extent of absorption

Distribution: Widely to most body fluids and bone; poor penetration into cells, eyes, and across normal meninges

Pleural fluids, lungs, and peritoneal fluid; high urine concentrations are attained; also into synovial fluid, liver, prostate, muscle, and gallbladder; penetrates into middle ear effusions, maxillary sinus secretions, tonsils, sputum, and bronchial secretions

CSF:blood level ratio: Normal meninges: <1%; Inflamed meninges: 8% to 90%

Protein binding: 17% to 20%

Metabolism: Partially hepatic

Half-life elimination:

Neonates, full-term: 3.7 hours

Infants and Children: 1-2 hours

Adults: Normal renal function: 0.7-1.4 hours

Cl_{cr} <10 mL/minute: 7-21 hours

Time to peak: Capsule: 2 hours; Extended-release tablet: 3.1 hours; Suspension: 1 hour

Excretion: Urine (60% as unchanged drug); lower in neonates

Note: Extended-release tablets: In healthy volunteers, serum drug concentrations were below 0.25 mcg/mL and undetectable at 16 hours following dosing.

Dosage

Usual dosage range:

Children ≤3 months: Oral: 20-30 mg/kg/day divided every 12 hours

Children >3 months and <40 kg: Oral: 20-100 mg/kg/day in divided doses every 8-12 hours

Children >3 months and ≥40 kg: Refer to adult dosing

Children ≥12 years: Oral: Extended-release tablet: 775 mg once daily

Adults: Oral: 250-500 mg every 8 hours or 500-875 mg twice daily

Extended-release tablet: 775 mg once daily

Indication-specific dosing:

Children >3 months and <40 kg: Oral: **Note:** In general, children >3 months and ≥40 kg should be dosed according to the adult recommendations except where indicated.

Acute otitis media: 80-90 mg/kg/day divided every 12 hours

Community-acquired pneumonia (CAP) (IDSA/PIDS, 2011): Note: In children ≥5 years, a macrolide antibiotic should be added if atypical pneumonia cannot be ruled out.

Empiric treatment or *S. pneumoniae* (MICs to penicillin ≤2.0 mcg/mL) (preferred): 90 mg/kg/day in 2-3 divided doses (maximum: 4 g/day). **Note:** Dividing in 3 doses is recommended for MIC = 2 mcg/mL.

Group A *Streptococcus* (moderate-to-severe) (preferred): 50-75 mg/kg/day in 2 divided doses (maximum: 4 g/day)

H. influenzae (beta-lactamase negative) mild infection (preferred): 75-100 mg/kg/day in 3 divided doses (maximum: 4 g/day)

Ear, nose, throat, genitourinary tract, or skin/skin structure infections: Note: Amoxicillin-clavulanate is preferred for first-line treatment of acute bacterial rhinosinusitis (Chow, 2012):

Mild-to-moderate: 25 mg/kg/day in divided doses every 12 hours **or** 20 mg/kg/day in divided doses every 8 hours

Severe: 45 mg/kg/day in divided doses every 12 hours **or** 40 mg/kg/day in divided doses every 8 hours

Tonsillitis and/or pharyngitis: Children ≥12 years: Extended-release tablet: 775 mg once daily

Lower respiratory tract infections: 45 mg/kg/day in divided doses every 12 hours **or** 40 mg/kg/day in divided doses every 8 hours

Lyme disease: 25-50 mg/kg/day divided every 8 hours (maximum: 500 mg)

Pharyngitis, group A streptococci (IDSA guidelines): 50 mg/kg once daily or alternatively, 25 mg/kg twice daily (maximum total daily dose: 1000 mg) for 10 days (Shulman, 2012)

Postexposure inhalational anthrax prophylaxis (ACIP recommendations): Children <40 kg: 45 mg/kg/day divided into 3 daily doses (maximum: 500 mg/dose) (ACIP, 2010). **Note:** The AAP recommends a higher dose (80 mg/kg/day divided into 3 daily doses [maximum: 500 mg/dose]) due to the lack of data on amoxicillin dosages for treating anthrax and the high mortality rate.

Note: Use **only** if isolates of the specific *B. anthracis* are sensitive to amoxicillin (MIC ≤0.125 mcg/mL). Duration of antibiotic postexposure prophylaxis (PEP) is ≥60 days in a previously-unvaccinated exposed person. Antimicrobial therapy should continue for 14 days after the third dose of PEP vaccine. Those who are partially or fully vaccinated should receive at least a 30-day course of antimicrobial PEP and continue with licensed vaccination regimen.

Unvaccinated workers, even those wearing personal protective equipment with adequate respiratory protection, should receive antimicrobial PEP. Antimicrobial PEP is not required for fully-vaccinated people (five-dose I.M. vaccination series with a yearly booster) who enter an anthrax area clothed in personal protective equipment. If respiratory protection is disrupted, a 30-day course of antimicrobial therapy is recommended (ACIP, 2010).

Prophylaxis against infective endocarditis: 50 mg/kg 1 hour before procedure. **Note:** American Heart Association (AHA) guidelines now recommend prophylaxis only in patients undergoing invasive procedures and in whom underlying cardiac conditions may predispose to a higher risk of adverse outcomes should infection occur. As of April 2007, routine prophylaxis for GI/GU procedures is no longer recommended by the AHA.

Adults: Oral:

Chlamydial infection during pregnancy (unlabeled use): 500 mg 3 times/day for 7 days (CDC, 2010)

Ear, nose, throat, genitourinary tract, or skin/skin structure infections: Note: Amoxicillin-clavulanate is preferred for first-line treatment of acute bacterial rhinosinusitis (Chow, 2012):

Mild-to-moderate: 500 mg every 12 hours **or** 250 mg every 8 hours

Severe: 875 mg every 12 hours **or** 500 mg every 8 hours

Tonsillitis and/or pharyngitis: Extended-release tablet: 775 mg once daily

***Helicobacter pylori* eradication:** 1000 mg twice daily; requires combination therapy with at least one other antibiotic and an acid-suppressing agent (proton pump inhibitor or H_2 blocker)

Lower respiratory tract infections: 875 mg every 12 hours **or** 500 mg every 8 hours

Lyme disease: 500 mg every 6-8 hours (depending on size of patient) for 21-30 days

Periodontitis (aggressive) (in combination with metronidazole) associated with presense of *Actinobacillus actinomycetemcomitans* (AA): Oral: 500 mg every 8 hours for 10 days used in addition to scaling and root planing (Varela, 2011)

Pharyngitis, group A streptococci (IDSA guidelines): 1000 mg once daily or 500 mg twice daily (maximum daily dose: 1000 mg) for 10 days (Shulman, 2012)

Postexposure inhalational anthrax prophylaxis (ACIP recommendations): 500 mg every 8 hours. **Note:** Use **only** if isolates of the specific *B. anthracis* are sensitive to amoxicillin (MIC ≤0.125 mcg/mL); may be administered to pregnant and breast-feeding women. Duration of antibiotic postexposure prophylaxis (PEP) is ≥60 days in a previously unvaccinated exposed person. Antimicrobial therapy should continue for 14 days after the third dose of PEP vaccine. Those who are partially or fully vaccinated should receive at least a 30-day course of antimicrobial PEP and continue with licensed vaccination regimen. Unvaccinated workers, even those wearing personal protective equipment with adequate respiratory protection, should receive antimicrobial PEP. Antimicrobial PEP is not required for fully vaccinated people (five-dose I.M. vaccination series with a yearly booster) who enter an anthrax area clothed in personal protective equipment. If respiratory protection is disrupted, a 30-day course of antimicrobial therapy is recommended (ACIP, 2010).

Prophylaxis against infective endocarditis: Oral: 2 g 30-60 minutes before procedure. **Note:** American Heart Association (AHA) guidelines now recommend prophylaxis only in patients undergoing invasive procedures and in whom underlying cardiac conditions may predispose to a higher risk of adverse outcomes should infection occur. As of April 2007, routine prophylaxis for GI/GU procedures is no longer recommended by the AHA.

Prophylaxis in total joint replacement patients undergoing dental procedures which produce bacteremia: 2 g 1 hour prior to procedure

Prosthetic joint infection, chronic antimicrobial suppression of prosthetic joint infection associated with beta-hemolytic streptococci, penicillin-susceptible *Enterococcus* spp, or *Propionibacterium* spp (unlabeled use): Oral: 500 mg 3 times daily (Osmon, 2013)

Dosage adjustment in renal impairment: Use of certain dosage forms (eg, extended-release 775 mg tablet and immediate-release 875 mg tablet) should be avoided in patients with Cl_{cr} <30 mL/minute or patients requiring hemodialysis.

Cl_{cr} 10-30 mL/minute: 250-500 mg every 12 hours

Cl_{cr} <10 mL/minute: 250-500 mg every 24 hours

Dialysis: Moderately dialyzable (20% to 50%) by hemo- or peritoneal dialysis; approximately 50 mg of amoxicillin per liter of filtrate is removed by continuous arteriovenous or venovenous hemofiltration; dose as per Cl_{cr} <10 mL/minute guidelines

Dosage adjustment in hepatic impairment: No dosage adjustment provided in manufacturer's labeling.

Dietary Considerations May be taken with food. Some products may contain phenylalanine.

Moxatag™: Take within 1 hour of finishing a meal.

Administration Administer around-the-clock to promote less variation in peak and trough serum levels. The appropriate amount of suspension may be mixed with formula, milk, fruit juice, water, ginger ale, or cold drinks; administer dose immediately after mixing.

Moxatag™ extended release tablet: Administer within 1 hour of finishing a meal.

Some penicillins (eg, carbenicillin, ticarcillin, and piperacillin) have been shown to inactivate aminoglycosides *in vitro*. This has been observed to a greater extent with tobramycin and gentamicin, while amikacin has shown greater stability against inactivation. Concurrent use of these agents may pose a risk of reduced antibacterial efficacy *in vivo*, particularly in the setting of profound renal impairment. However, definitive clinical evidence is lacking. If combination penicillin/aminoglycoside therapy is desired in a patient with renal dysfunction, separation of doses (if feasible), and routine monitoring of aminoglycoside levels, CBC, and clinical response should be considered.

Monitoring Parameters With prolonged therapy, monitor renal, hepatic, and hematologic function periodically; assess patient at beginning and throughout therapy for infection; monitor for signs of anaphylaxis during first dose

Test Interactions May interfere with urinary glucose tests using cupric sulfate (Benedict's solution, Clinitest®)

Some penicillin derivatives may accelerate the degradation of aminoglycosides *in vitro*, leading to a potential underestimation of aminoglycoside serum concentration.

Dosage Forms Excipient information presented when available (limited, particularly for generics); consult specific product labeling.

Capsule, Oral:

Generic: 250 mg, 500 mg

Suspension Reconstituted, Oral:

Generic: 125 mg/5 mL (80 mL, 100 mL, 150 mL); 200 mg/5 mL (50 mL, 75 mL, 100 mL); 250 mg/5 mL (80 mL, 100 mL, 150 mL); 400 mg/5 mL (50 mL, 75 mL, 100 mL)

Tablet, Oral:
Generic: 500 mg, 875 mg
Tablet Chewable, Oral:
Generic: 125 mg, 250 mg
Tablet Extended Release 24 Hour, Oral:
Moxatag: 775 mg [contains cremophor el, fd&c blue #2 aluminum lake]

Amoxicillin and Clavulanate
(a moks i SIL in & klav yoo LAN ate)

Brand Names: U.S. Amoclan; Augmentin; Augmentin ES-600; Augmentin XR

Brand Names: Canada Amoxi-Clav; Apo-Amoxi-Clav; Clavulin; Novo-Clavamoxin; ratio-Aclavulanate

Index Terms Amoxicillin and Clavulanate Potassium; Amoxicillin and Clavulanic Acid; Clavulanic Acid and Amoxicillin

Pharmacologic Category Antibiotic, Penicillin

Use Treatment of otitis media, sinusitis, and infections caused by susceptible organisms involving the lower respiratory tract, skin and skin structure, and urinary tract; spectrum same as amoxicillin with additional coverage of beta-lactamase producing *B. catarrhalis*, *H. influenzae*, *N. gonorrhoeae*, and *S. aureus* (not MRSA). The expanded coverage of this combination makes it a useful alternative when amoxicillin resistance is present and patients cannot tolerate alternative treatments.

Unlabeled Use Chronic antimicrobial suppression of prosthetic joint infection

Pregnancy Risk Factor B

Pregnancy Considerations Adverse events have not been observed in animal reproduction studies. Both amoxicillin and clavulanic acid cross the placenta. Maternal use of amoxicillin/clavulanate has generally not resulted in an increased risk of birth defects. A possible increased risk of necrotizing enterocolitis in neonates or bowel disorders in children exposed to amoxicillin/clavulanate *in utero* has been observed. In women with acute infections during pregnancy, amoxicillin/clavulanate may be given if an antibiotic is required and appropriate based on bacterial sensitivity; however, use is not recommended in the management of preterm premature rupture of membranes. Oral ampicillin-class antibiotics are poorly absorbed during labor. When used during pregnancy, pharmacokinetic changes have been observed with amoxicillin alone (refer to the Amoxicillin monograph for details).

Breast-Feeding Considerations Amoxicillin is found in breast milk. The manufacturer recommends that caution be used if administered to breast-feeding women. The use of amoxicillin/clavulanate may be safe while breast-feeding. However, the risk of adverse events in the infant may be increased when compared to the use of amoxicillin alone and the risk may be related to maternal dose. Nondose-related effects could include modification of bowel flora and allergic sensitization of the infant.

Contraindications Hypersensitivity to amoxicillin, clavulanic acid, penicillin, or any component of the formulation; history of cholestatic jaundice or hepatic dysfunction with amoxicillin/clavulanate potassium therapy; Augmentin XR: severe renal impairment (Cl_{cr} <30 mL/minute) and hemodialysis patients

Canadian labeling: Additional contraindications (not in U.S. labeling): Hypersensitivity to cephalosporins; suspected or confirmed mononucleosis

Warnings/Precautions Hypersensitivity reactions, including anaphylaxis (some fatal), have been reported. Prolonged use may result in fungal or bacterial superinfection, including *C. difficile*-associated diarrhea (CDAD) and pseudomembranous colitis; CDAD has been observed >2 months postantibiotic treatment. In patients with renal impairment, doses and/or frequency of administration should be modified in response to the degree of renal impairment. High percentage of patients with infectious mononucleosis have developed rash during therapy; ampicillin-class antibiotics not recommended in these patients. Incidence of diarrhea is higher than with amoxicillin alone. Due to differing content of clavulanic acid, not all formulations are interchangeable. Low incidence of cross-allergy with cephalosporins exists. Some products contain phenylalanine.

Adverse Reactions

>10%: Gastrointestinal: Diarrhea (3% to 34%; incidence varies upon dose and regimen used)

1% to 10%:
- Dermatologic: Diaper rash, skin rash, urticaria
- Gastrointestinal: Abdominal discomfort, loose stools, nausea, vomiting
- Genitourinary: Vaginitis, vaginal mycosis
- Miscellaneous: Moniliasis

<1% (Limited to important or life-threatening): Alkaline phosphatase increased, cholestatic jaundice, flatulence, headache, hepatic dysfunction, hepatitis, liver function tests increased, prothrombin time increased, thrombocytosis, vasculitis (hypersensitivity)

Additional adverse reactions seen with **ampicillin-class antibiotics:** Agitation, agranulocytosis, alkaline phosphatase increased, anaphylaxis, anemia, angioedema, anxiety, behavioral changes, bilirubin increased, black "hairy" tongue, confusion, convulsions, crystalluria, dizziness, enterocolitis, eosinophilia, erythema multiforme, exanthematous pustulosis, exfoliative dermatitis, gastritis, glossitis, hematuria, hemolytic anemia, hemorrhagic colitis, indigestion, insomnia, hyperactivity, interstitial nephritis, leukopenia, mucocutaneous candidiasis, pruritus, pseudomembranous colitis, serum sickness-like reaction, Stevens-Johnson syndrome, stomatitis, transaminases increased, thrombocytopenia, thrombocytopenic purpura, tooth discoloration, toxic epidermal necrolysis

Drug Interactions

Metabolism/Transport Effects None known.

Avoid Concomitant Use

Avoid concomitant use of Amoxicillin and Clavulanate with any of the following: BCG

Increased Effect/Toxicity

Amoxicillin and Clavulanate may increase the levels/effects of: Methotrexate; Vitamin K Antagonists

The levels/effects of Amoxicillin and Clavulanate may be increased by: Allopurinol; Probenecid

Decreased Effect

Amoxicillin and Clavulanate may decrease the levels/effects of: BCG; Mycophenolate; Sodium Picosulfate; Typhoid Vaccine

The levels/effects of Amoxicillin and Clavulanate may be decreased by: Tetracycline Derivatives

Preparation for Administration Reconstitute powder for oral suspension with appropriate amount of water as specified on the bottle. Shake vigorously until suspended. Discard unused suspension after 7-10 days (consult manufacturer labeling for specific recommendations).

Storage/Stability

Powder for oral suspension: Store dry powder at room temperature of 25°C (77°F). Reconstituted oral suspension should be kept in refrigerator. Unit-dose antibiotic oral syringes are stable under refrigeration for 24 hours (Tu, 1988).

Tablet: Store at room temperature of 25°C (77°F).

Mechanism of Action Clavulanic acid binds and inhibits beta-lactamases that inactivate amoxicillin resulting in amoxicillin having an expanded spectrum of activity. Amoxicillin inhibits bacterial cell wall synthesis by binding to one or more of the penicillin-binding proteins (PBPs) which in turn inhibits the final transpeptidation step of peptidoglycan synthesis in bacterial cell walls, thus inhibiting cell wall biosynthesis. Bacteria eventually lyse due to ongoing activity of cell wall autolytic enzymes (autolysins and murein hydrolases) while cell wall assembly is arrested.

Pharmacodynamics/Kinetics Amoxicillin pharmacokinetics are not affected by clavulanic acid.

Amoxicillin: See Amoxicillin monograph.

Clavulanic acid:

Protein binding: ~25%
Metabolism: Hepatic
Half-life elimination: 1 hour
Time to peak: 1 hour
Excretion: Urine (30% to 40% as unchanged drug)

Dosage Note: Dose is based on the amoxicillin component; see "Augmentin Product-Specific Considerations" table.

Usual dosage range:

Infants <3 months: Oral: 30 mg/kg/day divided every 12 hours using the 125 mg/5 mL suspension

Children ≥3 months and <40 kg: Oral: 20-90 mg/kg/day divided every 8-12 hours

Children >40 kg and Adults: Oral: 250-500 mg every 8 hours or 875 mg every 12 hours

Indication-specific dosing:

Children ≥3 months and <40 kg: Oral:

Community-acquired pneumonia (CAP) (IDSA/PIDS, 2011): Note: In children ≥5 years, a macrolide antibiotic should be added if atypical pneumonia cannot be ruled out.

Presumed bacterial (mild-to-moderate infection) (alternative to amoxicillin): 90 mg/kg/day divided every 12 hours

H. influenzae (typeable or nontypeable; beta-lactamase producing), step-down therapy or mild infection (preferred): 45 mg/kg/day divided every 8 hours **or** 90 mg/kg/day divided every 12 hours

Group A streptococci, chronic carrier treatment (IDSA guidelines): Refer to adult dosing.

Lower respiratory tract infections, severe infections, sinusitis: 45 mg/kg/day divided every 12 hours **or** 40 mg/kg/day divided every 8 hours

Mild-to-moderate infections: 25 mg/kg/day divided every 12 hours or 20 mg/kg/day divided every 8 hours

Otitis media (amoxicillin 600 mg and clavulanate potassium 42.9 mg per 5 mL): 90 mg/kg/day divided every 12 hours for 10 days in children with severe illness and when coverage for β-lactamase-positive *H. influenzae* and *M. catarrhalis* is needed.

Children <16 years: Oral:

Acute bacterial rhinosinusitis: 45 mg/kg/day divided every 12 hours (preferred) for 10-14 days. **Note:** May use high-dose therapy (90 mg/kg/day divided every 12 hours) if initial therapy fails, in areas with high endemic rates of penicillin-nonsusceptible *S. pneumoniae*, those with severe infections, daycare attendance, age <2 years, recent hospitalization, antibiotic use within the past month, or who are immunocompromised (Chow, 2012).

Children ≥16 years and Adults: Oral:

Acute bacterial rhinosinusitis: Extended release tablet: 2000 mg every 12 hours for 10 days or 500 mg every 8 hours or 875 mg every 12 hours for 5-7 days **Note:** May use high-dose therapy (extended release: 2000 mg every 12 hours) if initial therapy fails, in areas with high endemic rates of penicillin-nonsusceptible *S. pneumoniae*, those with severe infections, age >65 years, recent hospitalization, antibiotic use within the past month, or who are immunocompromised (Chow, 2012).

Bite wounds (animal/human): 875 mg every 12 hours **or** 500 mg every 8 hours

Chronic obstructive pulmonary disease: 875 mg every 12 hours **or** 500 mg every 8 hours

Diabetic foot: Extended release tablet: Two 1000 mg tablets every 12 hours for 7-14 days

Erysipelas: 875 mg every 12 hours **or** 500 mg every 8 hours

Febrile neutropenia: 875 mg every 12 hours

Group A streptococci, chronic carrier treatment (IDSA guidelines): 40 mg/kg/day divided every 8 hours (maximum: 2000 mg daily) for 10 days (Shulman, 2012)

Pneumonia:

Aspiration: 875 mg every 12 hours

Community-acquired: Extended release tablet: Two 1000 mg tablets every 12 hours for 7-10 days

Prosthetic joint infection, chronic antimicrobial suppression, oxacillin-susceptible *Staphylococci* (alternative to cephalexin or cefadroxil) (unlabeled use): 500 mg 3 times daily (Osmon, 2013)

Pyelonephritis (acute, uncomplicated): 875 mg every 12 hours **or** 500 mg every 8 hours

Skin abscess: 875 mg every 12 hours

Dosage adjustment in renal impairment:

Cl_{cr} <30 mL/minute: Do not use 875 mg tablet or extended release tablets

Cl_{cr} 10-30 mL/minute: 250-500 mg every 12 hours

Cl_{cr} <10 mL/minute: 250-500 every 24 hours

Hemodialysis: Moderately dialyzable (20% to 50%)

250-500 mg every 24 hours; administer dose during and after dialysis. Do not use extended release tablets.

Peritoneal dialysis: Moderately dialyzable (20% to 50%)

Amoxicillin: Administer 250 mg every 12 hours

Clavulanic acid: Dose for Cl_{cr} <10 mL/minute

Continuous arteriovenous or venovenous hemofiltration effects:

Amoxicillin: ~50 mg of amoxicillin/L of filtrate is removed

Clavulanic acid: Dose for Cl_{cr} <10 mL/minute

Augmentin Product-Specific Considerations

Strength	Form	Consideration
125 mg	S	q8h dosing
	S	For adults having difficulty swallowing tablets, 125 mg/5 mL suspension may be substituted for 500 mg tablet.
200 mg	CT, S	q12h dosing
	CT	Contains phenylalanine
	S	For adults having difficulty swallowing tablets, 200 mg/5 mL suspension may be substituted for 875 mg tablet.
250 mg	S, T	q8h dosing
	T	Not for use in patients <40 kg
	S	For adults having difficulty swallowing tablets, 250 mg/5 mL suspension may be substituted for 500 mg tablet.
400 mg	CT, S	q12h dosing
	CT	Contains phenylalanine
	S	For adults having difficulty swallowing tablets, 400 mg/5 mL suspension may be substituted for 875 mg tablet.
500 mg	T	q8h or q12h dosing
600 mg	S	q12h dosing
		Not for use in adults or children ≥40 kg
		600 mg/5 mL suspension is not equivalent to or interchangeable with 200 mg/5 mL or 400 mg/5 mL due to differences in clavulanic acid.
875 mg	T	q12h dosing; not for use in Cl_{cr} <30 mL/minute
1000 mg	XR	q12h dosing
		Not for use in children <16 years of age
		Not interchangeable with two 500 mg tablets
		Not for use if Cl_{cr} <30 mL/minute or hemodialysis

Legend: CT = chewable tablet, S = suspension, T = tablet, XR = extended release.

Dosage adjustment in hepatic impairment: No dosage adjustment provided in manufacturer's labeling; use with caution. Use contraindicated in patients with a history of amoxicillin and clavulanate-associated hepatic dysfunction.

Dietary Considerations May be taken with meals or on an empty stomach; take with meals to increase absorption and decrease GI upset; may mix with milk, formula, or juice. Extended release tablets should be taken with food. Some products may contain sodium. Some products contain phenylalanine; if you have phenylketonuria or PKU, avoid use. All dosage forms contain potassium.

Administration Administer around-the-clock to promote less variation in peak and trough serum levels. Administer with food to increase absorption and decrease stomach upset; shake suspension well before use. Extended release tablets should be administered with food.

Some penicillins (eg, carbenicillin, ticarcillin, and piperacillin) have been shown to inactivate aminoglycosides *in vitro*. This has been observed to a greater extent with tobramycin and gentamicin, while amikacin has shown greater stability against inactivation. Concurrent use of these agents may pose a risk of reduced antibacterial efficacy *in vivo*, particularly in the setting of profound renal impairment. However, definitive clinical evidence is lacking. If combination penicillin/aminoglycoside therapy is desired in a patient with renal dysfunction, separation of doses (if feasible), and routine monitoring of aminoglycoside levels, CBC, and clinical response should be considered.

Monitoring Parameters Assess patient at beginning and throughout therapy for infection; with prolonged therapy, monitor renal, hepatic, and hematologic function periodically; monitor for signs of anaphylaxis during first dose

Test Interactions May interfere with urinary glucose tests using cupric sulfate (Benedict's solution, Clinitest®, Fehling's solution).

Some penicillin derivatives may accelerate the degradation of aminoglycosides *in vitro*, leading to a potential underestimation of aminoglycoside serum concentration.

Additional Information Two 250 mg tablets are not equivalent to a 500 mg tablet (both tablet sizes contain equivalent clavulanate). Two 500 mg tablets are not equivalent to a single 1000 mg extended release tablet.

Dosage Forms Excipient information presented when available (limited, particularly for generics); consult specific product labeling. [DSC] = Discontinued product

Powder for suspension, oral:

Generic: 200: Amoxicillin 200 mg and clavulanate potassium 28.5 mg per 5 mL (50 mL, 75 mL, 100 mL); 250: Amoxicillin 250 mg and clavulanate potassium 62.5 mg per 5 mL (75 mL, 100 mL, 150 mL); 400: Amoxicillin 400 mg and clavulanate potassium 57 mg per 5 mL (50 mL, 75 mL, 100 mL); 600: Amoxicillin 600 mg and clavulanate potassium 42.9 mg per 5 mL (75 mL, 125 mL, 200 mL)

Amoclan:

200: Amoxicillin 200 mg and clavulanate potassium 28.5 mg per 5 mL (50 mL, 75 mL, 100 mL) [contains phenylalanine 7 mg/5 mL and potassium 0.14 mEq/5 mL; fruit flavor]

400: Amoxicillin 400 mg and clavulanate potassium 57 mg per 5 mL (50 mL, 75 mL, 100 mL) [contains phenylalanine 7 mg/5 mL and potassium 0.29 mEq/5 mL; fruit flavor]

600: Amoxicillin 600 mg and clavulanate potassium 42.9 mg per 5 mL (75 mL, 125 mL, 200 mL) [contains phenylalanine 7 mg/5 mL, potassium 0.248 mEq/5 mL; orange flavor]

Augmentin:

125: Amoxicillin 125 mg and clavulanate potassium 31.25 mg per 5 mL (75 mL, 100 mL, 150 mL) [contains potassium 0.16 mEq/5 mL; banana flavor]

200: Amoxicillin 200 mg and clavulanate potassium 28.5 mg per 5 mL (50 mL, 75 mL, 100 mL) [contains phenylalanine 7 mg/5 mL and potassium 0.14 mEq/5 mL; orange flavor] [DSC]

250: Amoxicillin 250 mg and clavulanate potassium 62.5 mg per 5 mL (75 mL, 100 mL, 150 mL) [contains potassium 0.32 mEq/5 mL; orange flavor]

400: Amoxicillin 400 mg and clavulanate potassium 57 mg per 5 mL (50 mL, 75 mL, 100 mL) [contains phenylalanine 7 mg/5 mL and potassium 0.29 mEq/5 mL; orange flavor] [DSC]

Augmentin ES-600:

600: Amoxicillin 600 mg and clavulanate potassium 42.9 mg per 5 mL (75 mL, 125 mL, 200 mL) [contains phenylalanine 7 mg/5 mL, potassium 0.23 mEq/5 mL; strawberry cream flavor]

Tablet, oral:

Generic: 250: Amoxicillin 250 mg and clavulanate potassium 125 mg; 500: Amoxicillin 500 mg and clavulanate potassium 125 mg; 875: Amoxicillin 875 mg and clavulanate potassium 125 mg

Augmentin:

250: Amoxicillin 250 mg and clavulanate potassium 125 mg [contains potassium 0.63 mEq/tablet] [DSC]

500: Amoxicillin 500 mg and clavulanate potassium 125 mg [contains potassium 0.63 mEq/tablet]

875: Amoxicillin 875 mg and clavulanate potassium 125 mg [contains potassium 0.63 mEq/tablet]

Tablet, chewable, oral:

Generic: 200: Amoxicillin 200 mg and clavulanate potassium 28.5 mg [contains phenylalanine]; 400: Amoxicillin 400 mg and clavulanate potassium 57 mg [contains phenylalanine]

Tablet, extended release, oral:

Generic: Amoxicillin 1000 mg and clavulanate acid 62.5 mg

Augmentin XR: 1000: Amoxicillin 1000 mg and clavulanate acid 62.5 mg [contains potassium 12.6 mg (0.32 mEq) and sodium 29.3 mg (1.27 mEq) per tablet; packaged in either a 7-day or 10-day package]

Dosage Forms: Canada Note: Also refer to Dosage Forms. Excipient information presented when available (limited, particularly for generics); consult specific product labeling.

Powder for suspension, oral:

Clavulin:

125: Amoxicillin 125 mg and clavulanate potassium 31.25 mg per 5 mL (100 mL) [contains aspartame]

200: Amoxicillin 200 mg and clavulanate potassium 28.5 mg per 5 mL (70 mL) [contains aspartame]

250: Amoxicillin 250 mg and clavulanate potassium 62.5 mg per 5 mL (100 mL) [contains aspartame]

400: Amoxicillin 400 mg and clavulanate potassium 57 mg per 5 mL (70 mL) [contains aspartame]

Tablet, oral:

Clavulin:

500: Amoxicillin 500 mg and clavulanate potassium 125 mg

875: Amoxicillin 875 mg and clavulanate potassium 125 mg

◆ **Amoxicillin and Clavulanate Potassium** *see* Amoxicillin and Clavulanate *on page 119*

◆ **Amoxicillin and Clavulanic Acid** *see* Amoxicillin and Clavulanate *on page 119*

◆ **Amoxicillin, Clarithromycin, and Lansoprazole** *see* Lansoprazole, Amoxicillin, and Clarithromycin *on page 1173*

- ◆ **Amoxicillin, Clarithromycin, and Omeprazole** *see* Omeprazole, Clarithromycin, and Amoxicillin *on page 1508*
- ◆ **Amoxicillin Trihydrate** *see* Amoxicillin *on page 116*
- ◆ **Amoxi-Clav (Can)** *see* Amoxicillin and Clavulanate *on page 119*
- ◆ **Amoxil** *see* Amoxicillin *on page 116*
- ◆ **Amoxycillin** *see* Amoxicillin *on page 116*
- ◆ **Amphetamine and Dextroamphetamine** *see* Dextroamphetamine and Amphetamine *on page 589*
- ◆ **Amphojel® (Can)** *see* Aluminum Hydroxide *on page 89*
- ◆ **Amphotec** *see* Amphotericin B Cholesteryl Sulfate Complex *on page 122*
- ◆ **Amphotec® (Can)** *see* Amphotericin B Cholesteryl Sulfate Complex *on page 122*

Amphotericin B Cholesteryl Sulfate Complex

(am foe TER i sin bee kole LES te ril SUL fate KOM plecks)

Brand Names: U.S. Amphotec

Brand Names: Canada Amphotec®

Index Terms ABCD; Amphotericin B Colloidal Dispersion

Pharmacologic Category Antifungal Agent, Parenteral

Use Treatment of invasive aspergillosis in patients who have failed amphotericin B deoxycholate treatment, or who have renal impairment or experience unacceptable toxicity which precludes treatment with amphotericin B deoxycholate in effective doses.

Unlabeled Use Effective in patients with serious *Candida* species infections

Pregnancy Risk Factor B

Pregnancy Considerations Adverse events were not observed in animal reproduction studies. Amphotericin crosses the placenta and enters the fetal circulation. Amphotericin B is recommended for the treatment of serious systemic fungal diseases in pregnant women; refer to current guidelines (King, 1998).

Breast-Feeding Considerations It is not known if amphotericin is excreted into breast milk. Due to its poor oral absorption, systemic exposure to the nursing infant is expected to be decreased; however, because of the potential for toxicity, breast-feeding is not recommended (Mactal-Haaf, 2001).

Contraindications Hypersensitivity to amphotericin B or any component of the formulation (unless the benefits outweigh the possible risk to the patient)

Warnings/Precautions Anaphylaxis has been reported with amphotericin B-containing drugs. If severe respiratory distress occurs, the infusion should be immediately discontinued; the patient should not receive further infusions. During the initial dosing, the drug should be administered under close clinical observation. Acute infusion reactions, sometimes severe, may occur 1-3 hours after starting infusion. These reactions are usually more common with the first few doses and generally diminish with subsequent doses. Pretreatment with antihistamines/corticosteroids and/or decreasing the rate of infusion can be used to manage reactions. Avoid rapid infusion.

Adverse Reactions

>10%:

Cardiovascular: Hypotension, tachycardia
Central nervous system: Chills, fever
Endocrine & metabolic: Hypokalemia
Gastrointestinal: Vomiting
Hepatic: Hyperbilirubinemia
Renal: Creatinine increased

5% to 10%:

Cardiovascular: Chest pain, facial edema, hypertension
Central nervous system: Abnormal thinking, headache, insomnia, somnolence, tremor
Dermatologic: Pruritus, rash, sweating
Endocrine & metabolic: Hyperglycemia, hypocalcemia, hypomagnesemia, hypophosphatemia
Gastrointestinal: Abdominal enlargement, abdominal pain, diarrhea, dry mouth, hematemesis, jaundice, nausea, stomatitis
Hematologic: Anemia, hemorrhage, thrombocytopenia
Hepatic: Alkaline phosphatase increased, liver function test abnormal
Neuromuscular & skeletal: Back pain, rigor
Respiratory: Cough increased, dyspnea, epistaxis, hypoxia, rhinitis

<5% (Limited to important or life-threatening): Acidosis, arrhythmias (both atrial and ventricular), cardiac arrest, gastrointestinal hemorrhage, heart failure, injection site pain/reaction, liver failure, oliguria, pleural effusion, renal failure, seizure, syncope

Note: Amphotericin B colloidal dispersion has an improved therapeutic index compared to conventional amphotericin B, and has been used safely in patients with amphotericin B-related nephrotoxicity; however, continued decline of renal function has occurred in some patients.

Drug Interactions

Metabolism/Transport Effects None known.

Avoid Concomitant Use

Avoid concomitant use of Amphotericin B Cholesteryl Sulfate Complex with any of the following: Gallium Nitrate

Increased Effect/Toxicity

Amphotericin B Cholesteryl Sulfate Complex may increase the levels/effects of: Aminoglycosides; Colistimethate; CycloSPORINE (Systemic); Flucytosine; Gallium Nitrate

The levels/effects of Amphotericin B Cholesteryl Sulfate Complex may be increased by: Corticosteroids (Orally Inhaled); Corticosteroids (Systemic)

Decreased Effect

Amphotericin B Cholesteryl Sulfate Complex may decrease the levels/effects of: Saccharomyces boulardii

The levels/effects of Amphotericin B Cholesteryl Sulfate Complex may be decreased by: Antifungal Agents (Azole Derivatives, Systemic)

Preparation for Administration Reconstitute 50 mg and 100 mg vials with 10 mL and 20 mL of SWI, respectively. The reconstituted vials contain 5 mg/mL of amphotericin B. Shake the vial gently by hand until all solid particles have dissolved. Further dilute amphotericin B colloidal dispersion with D_5W.

Storage/Stability Store intact vials at 15°C to 30°C (59°F to 86°F). After reconstitution, the solution should be refrigerated at 2°C to 8°C (36°F to 46°F) and used within 24 hours. Concentrations of 0.1-2 mg/mL in D_5W are stable for 24 hours at 2°C to 8°C (36°F to 46°F).

Mechanism of Action Binds to ergosterol altering cell membrane permeability in susceptible fungi and causing leakage of cell components with subsequent cell death. Proposed mechanism suggests that amphotericin causes an oxidation-dependent stimulation of macrophages (Lyman, 1992).

Pharmacodynamics/Kinetics

Distribution: V_d: Total volume increases with higher doses, reflects increasing uptake by tissues (with 4 mg/kg/day = 4 L/kg); predominantly distributed in the liver; concentrations in kidneys and other tissues are lower than observed with conventional amphotericin B

Half-life elimination: ~28 hours; prolonged with higher doses

Dosage Children and Adults: I.V.: *Usual dosage range:* 3-4 mg/kg/day. **Note:** 6 mg/kg/day has been used for treatment of life-threatening invasive aspergillosis in immunocompromised patients (Bowden, 2002).

Premedication: For patients who experience chills, fever, hypotension, nausea, or other nonanaphylactic infusion-related immediate reactions, premedicate with the following drugs 30-60 minutes prior to drug administration: A nonsteroidal with or without diphenhydramine **or** acetaminophen with diphenhydramine **or** hydrocortisone 50-100 mg with or without a nonsteroidal and diphenhydramine (Paterson, 2008).

Test dose: For patients receiving their first dose in a new treatment course, a small amount (10 mL of the final preparation, containing between 1.6-8.3 mg) infused over 15-30 minutes is recommended. The patient should then be observed for an additional 30 minutes.

Dosage adjustment in renal impairment:

Mild to moderate impairment: No dosage adjustment provided in manufacturer's labeling. However, no pharmacokinetic changes were noted in patients with mild-to-moderate impairment.

Severe impairment: No dosage adjustment provided in manufacturer's labeling (has not been studied).

Dosage adjustment in hepatic impairment: No dosage adjustment provided in manufacturer's labeling (has not been studied).

Administration Initially infuse at 1 mg/kg/hour. Rate of infusion may be increased with subsequent doses as patient tolerance allows (minimum infusion time: 2 hours). For a patient who experiences chills, fever, hypotension, nausea, or other nonanaphylactic infusion-related reactions, premedicate with the following drugs 30-60 minutes prior to drug administration: A nonsteroidal with or without diphenhydramine **or** acetaminophen with diphenhydramine **or** hydrocortisone 50-100 mg with or without a nonsteroidal and diphenhydramine (Paterson, 2008). If the patient experiences rigors during the infusion, meperidine may be administered. If severe respiratory distress occurs, the infusion should be immediately discontinued.

Monitoring Parameters Liver function tests, serum electrolytes (especially potassium and magnesium), BUN, serum creatinine, CBC, prothrombin time; temperature, I/O; signs of hypokalemia (muscle weakness, cramping, drowsiness, ECG changes)

Additional Information Controlled trials which compare the original formulation of amphotericin B to the newer liposomal formulations (ie, Amphotec®) are lacking. Thus, comparative data discussing differences among the formulations should be interpreted cautiously. Although the risk of nephrotoxicity and infusion-related adverse effects may be less with Amphotec®, the efficacy profiles of Amphotec® and the original amphotericin formulation are comparable. Consequently, Amphotec® should be restricted to those patients who cannot tolerate or fail a standard amphotericin B formulation.

Dosage Forms Excipient information presented when available (limited, particularly for generics); consult specific product labeling.

Suspension Reconstituted, Intravenous:

Amphotec: 50 mg (1 ea); 100 mg (1 ea) [contains edetate disodium, hydrochloric acid, lactose, sodium cholesteryl sulfate, tromethamine]

◆ **Amphotericin B Colloidal Dispersion** *see* Amphotericin B Cholesteryl Sulfate Complex *on page 122*

Amphotericin B (Conventional)

(am foe TER i sin bee con VEN sha nal)

Brand Names: Canada Fungizone

Index Terms Amphotericin B Deoxycholate; Amphotericin B Desoxycholate; Conventional Amphotericin B

Pharmacologic Category Antifungal Agent, Parenteral

Additional Appendix Information

Antifungal Agents *on page 2286*

Desensitization Protocols *on page 2325*

Use Treatment of severe systemic and central nervous system infections caused by susceptible fungi such as *Candida* species, *Histoplasma capsulatum*, *Cryptococcus neoformans*, *Aspergillus* species, *Blastomyces dermatitidis*, *Torulopsis glabrata*, and *Coccidioides immitis*; fungal peritonitis; irrigant for bladder fungal infections; used in fungal infection in patients with bone marrow transplantation, amebic meningoencephalitis, ocular aspergillosis (intraocular injection), candidal cystitis (bladder irrigation), chemoprophylaxis (low-dose I.V.), immunocompromised patients at risk of aspergillosis (intranasal/nebulized), refractory meningitis (intrathecal), coccidioidal arthritis (intra-articular/I.M.).

Low-dose amphotericin B has been administered after bone marrow transplantation to reduce the risk of invasive fungal disease.

Unlabeled Use Treatment of fungal endophthalmitis

Pregnancy Risk Factor B

Pregnancy Considerations Adverse events were not observed in animal reproduction studies. Amphotericin crosses the placenta and enters the fetal circulation. No teratogenic or undue systemic toxicity (electrolyte imbalance or renal dysfunction) has been reported in the mother or fetus. Toxic maternal effects are to be expected and must be monitored (Perfect, 2010). Amphotericin B is recommended for the treatment of serious systemic fungal diseases in pregnant women. Refer to current guidelines (King, 1998).

Breast-Feeding Considerations It is not known if amphotericin is excreted into breast milk. Due to its poor oral absorption, systemic exposure to the nursing infant is expected to be decreased; however, because of the potential for toxicity, breast-feeding is not recommended (Mactal-Haaf, 2001).

Contraindications Hypersensitivity to amphotericin or any component of the formulation

Warnings/Precautions Anaphylaxis has been reported with amphotericin B-containing drugs. During the initial dosing, the drug should be administered under close clinical observation. May cause nephrotoxicity; usual risk factors include underlying renal disease, concomitant nephrotoxic medications and daily and/or cumulative dose of amphotericin. Avoid use with other nephrotoxic drugs; drug-induced renal toxicity usually improves with interrupting therapy, decreasing dosage, or increasing dosing interval. However permanent impairment may occur, especially in patients receiving large cumulative dose (eg, >5 g) and in those also receiving other nephrotoxic drugs. Hydration and sodium repletion prior to administration may reduce the risk of developing nephrotoxicity. Frequent monitoring of renal function is recommended. Acute reactions (eg, fever, shaking chills, hypotension, anorexia, nausea, vomiting, headache, tachypnea) are most common 1-3 hours after starting the infusion and diminish with continued therapy. Avoid rapid infusion to prevent hypotension, hypokalemia, arrhythmias, and shock. If therapy is stopped for >7 days, restart at the lowest dose recommended and increase gradually. Leukoencephalopathy has been reported following administration of amphotericin. Total body irradiation has been reported to be a possible predisposition.

[U.S. Boxed Warning]: Should be used primarily for treatment of progressive, potentially life-threatening fungal infections, not noninvasive forms of infection. [U.S. Boxed warning]: Verify the product name and dosage if dose exceeds 1.5 mg/kg.

Adverse Reactions

Systemic:

>10%:

Cardiovascular: Hypotension, tachypnea

Central nervous system: Fever, chills, headache (less frequent with I.T.), malaise

Endocrine & metabolic: Hypokalemia, hypomagnesemia

Gastrointestinal: Anorexia, nausea (less frequent with I.T.), vomiting (less frequent with I.T.), diarrhea, heartburn, cramping epigastric pain

Hematologic: Normochromic-normocytic anemia

Local: Pain at injection site with or without phlebitis or thrombophlebitis (incidence may increase with peripheral infusion of admixtures)

Neuromuscular & skeletal: Generalized pain, including muscle and joint pains (less frequent with I.T.)

Renal: Decreased renal function and renal function abnormalities including azotemia, renal tubular acidosis, nephrocalcinosis (>0.1 mg/mL)

1% to 10%:

Cardiovascular: Hypertension, flushing

Central nervous system: Delirium, arachnoiditis, pain along lumbar nerves (especially I.T. therapy)

Genitourinary: Urinary retention

Hematologic: Leukocytosis

Neuromuscular & skeletal: Paresthesia (especially with I.T. therapy)

<1% (Limited to important or life-threatening): Acute liver failure, agranulocytosis, anuria, arrhythmias, bone marrow suppression, bronchospasm, cardiac arrest, cardiac failure, coagulation defects, convulsions, diplopia, dyspnea, eosinophilia, hearing loss, hemorrhagic gastroenteritis, hepatitis, hypersensitivity pneumonitis, increased liver function tests, jaundice, leukoencephalopathy, leukopenia, maculopapular rash, melena, nephrogenic diabetes insipidus, oliguria, peripheral neuropathy, pruritus, pulmonary edema, renal failure, renal tubular acidosis, shock, skin exfoliation, Stevens-Johnson syndrome, thrombocytopenia, tinnitus, toxic epidermal necrolysis, transient vertigo, ventricular fibrillation, vision changes, wheezing

Drug Interactions

Metabolism/Transport Effects None known.

Avoid Concomitant Use

Avoid concomitant use of Amphotericin B (Conventional) with any of the following: Gallium Nitrate

Increased Effect/Toxicity

Amphotericin B (Conventional) may increase the levels/effects of: Aminoglycosides; Colistimethate; CycloSPORINE (Systemic); Flucytosine; Gallium Nitrate

The levels/effects of Amphotericin B (Conventional) may be increased by: Corticosteroids (Orally Inhaled); Corticosteroids (Systemic)

Decreased Effect

Amphotericin B (Conventional) may decrease the levels/effects of: Saccharomyces boulardii

The levels/effects of Amphotericin B (Conventional) may be decreased by: Antifungal Agents (Azole Derivatives, Systemic)

Preparation for Administration Add 10 mL of SWFI (without a bacteriostatic agent) to each vial of amphotericin B. Further dilute with 250-500 mL D_5W; final concentration should not exceed 0.1 mg/mL (peripheral infusion) or 0.25 mg/mL (central infusion).

Storage/Stability Store intact vials under refrigeration. Protect from light. Reconstituted vials are stable, protected from light, for 24 hours at room temperature and 1 week when refrigerated. Parenteral admixtures are stable, protected from light, for 24 hours at room temperature and 2 days under refrigeration. Short-term exposure (<24 hours) to light during I.V. infusion does **not** appreciably affect potency.

Mechanism of Action Binds to ergosterol altering cell membrane permeability in susceptible fungi and causing leakage of cell components with subsequent cell death. Proposed mechanism suggests that amphotericin causes an oxidation-dependent stimulation of macrophages (Lyman, 1992).

Pharmacodynamics/Kinetics

Distribution: Minimal amounts enter the aqueous humor, bile, CSF (inflamed or noninflamed meninges), pericardial fluid, pleural fluid, and synovial fluid

Protein binding, plasma: 90%

Half-life elimination: Biphasic: Initial: 15-48 hours; Terminal: 15 days

Time to peak: Within 1 hour following a 4- to 6-hour dose

Excretion: Urine (2% to 5% as biologically active form); ~40% eliminated over a 7-day period and may be detected in urine for at least 7 weeks after discontinued use

Dosage Premedication: For patients who experience infusion-related immediate reactions, premedicate with the following drugs 30-60 minutes prior to drug administration: NSAID and/or diphenhydramine **or** acetaminophen with diphenhydramine **or** hydrocortisone. If the patient experiences rigors during the infusion, meperidine may be administered.

Usual dosage ranges:

Infants and Children:

Test dose: I.V.: 0.1 mg/kg/dose to a maximum of 1 mg; infuse over 30-60 minutes. Many clinicians believe a test dose is unnecessary.

Maintenance dose: 0.25-1 mg/kg/day given once daily; infuse over 2-6 hours. Once therapy has been established, amphotericin B can be administered on an every-other-day basis at 1-1.5 mg/kg/dose; cumulative dose: 1.5-2 g over 6-10 weeks.

Duration of therapy: Varies with nature of infection, usual duration is 4-12 weeks or cumulative dose of 1-4 g

Adults:

Test dose: 1 mg infused over 20-30 minutes. Many clinicians believe a test dose is unnecessary.

Maintenance dose: Usual: 0.3-1.5 mg/kg/day; 1-1.5 mg/kg over 4-6 hours every other day may be given once therapy is established; aspergillosis, rhinocerebral mucormycosis, often require 1-1.5 mg/kg/day; do not exceed 1.5 mg/kg/day

Indication-specific dosing:

Infants and Children:

Aspergillosis (HIV-exposed/-positive): I.V.: 1-1.5 mg/kg/day once daily (CDC, 2009)

Candidiasis (HIV-exposed/-positive):

Invasive: I.V.: 0.5-1.5 mg/kg/day once daily (CDC, 2009)

Esophageal: I.V.: 0.3-0.5 mg/kg/day once daily (CDC, 2009)

Oropharyngeal, refractory: I.V.: 0.3-0.5 mg/kg/day (CDC, 2009)

Coccidioidomycosis (HIV-exposed/-positive): I.V.: 0.5-1 mg/kg/day (CDC, 2009)

Cryptococcus, **CNS disease (HIV-exposed/-positive):** I.V.: 0.7-1 mg/kg/day plus flucytosine; **Note:** Minimum 2 week induction followed by consolidation and chronic suppressive therapy; may increase amphotericin dose to 1.5 mg/kg/day if flucytosine is not tolerated.

Cryptococcus, **disseminated (non-CNS disease) or severe pulmonary disease (HIV-exposed/-positive):** I.V.: 0.7-1 mg/kg/day once daily with or without flucytosine

Histoplasma, CNS or severe disseminated: I.V.: 1 mg/kg/day once daily (CDC, 2009)

Adults:

Aspergillosis, disseminated: I.V.: 0.6-0.7 mg/kg/day for 3-6 months

Bone marrow transplantation (prophylaxis): I.V.: Low-dose amphotericin B 0.1-0.25 mg/kg/day has been administered after bone marrow transplantation to reduce the risk of invasive fungal disease.

Candidemia (neutropenic or non-neutropenic): I.V.: 0.5-1 mg/kg/day until 14 days after first negative blood culture and resolution of signs and symptoms (Pappas, 2009)

Candidiasis, chronic, disseminated: I.V.: 0.5-0.7 mg/kg/day for 3-6 months and resolution of radiologic lesions (Pappas, 2009)

Dematiaceous fungi: I.V.: 0.7 mg/kg/day in combination with an azole

Endocarditis: I.V.: 0.6-1 mg/kg/day (with or without flucytosine) for 6 weeks after valve replacement; **Note:** If isolates susceptible and/or clearance demonstrated, guidelines recommend step-down to fluconazole; also for long-term suppression therapy if valve replacement is not possible (Pappas, 2009)

Endophthalmitis, fungal (unlabeled use):

Intravitreal: 5-12.5 mcg (with or without concomitant systemic therapy) (Brod, 1990)

I.V.: 0.7-1 mg/kg/day (with flucytosine) for at least 4-6 weeks (Pappas, 2009)

Esophageal candidiasis: I.V.: 0.3-0.7 mg/kg/day for 14-21 days after clinical improvement (Pappas, 2009)

Histoplasmosis: Chronic, severe pulmonary or disseminated: I.V.: 0.5-1 mg/kg/day for 7 days, then 0.8 mg/kg every other day (or 3 times/week) until total dose of 10-15 mg/kg; may continue itraconazole as suppressive therapy (lifelong for immunocompromised patients)

Meningitis:

Candidal: I.V.: 0.7-1 mg/kg/day (with or without flucytosine) for at least 4 weeks; **Note:** Liposomal amphotericin favored by IDSA guidelines based on decreased risk of nephrotoxicity and potentially better CNS penetration (Pappas, 2009)

Cryptococcal or Coccidioides: I.T.: Initial: 0.01-0.05 mg as single daily dose; may increase daily in increments of 0.025-0.1 mg as tolerated (maximum: 1.5 mg/day; most patients will tolerate a maximum dose of ~0.5 mg/treatment). Once titration to a maximum tolerated dose is achieved, that dose is administered daily. Once CSF improvement noted, may decrease frequency on a weekly basis (eg, 5 times/week, then 3 times/week, then 2 times/week, then once weekly, then once every other week, then once every 2 weeks, etc) until administration occurs once every 6 weeks. Typically, concurrent oral azole therapy is maintained (Stevens, 2001). **Note:** IDSA notes that the use of I.T. amphotericin for cryptococcal meningitis is generally discouraged and rarely necessary (Perfect, 2010).

Histoplasma: I.V.: 0.5-1 mg/kg/day for 7 days, then 0.8 mg/kg every other day (or 3 times/week) for 3 months total duration; follow with fluconazole suppressive therapy for up to 12 months

Meningoencephalitis, cryptococcal (Perfect, 2010): I.V.:

HIV positive: Induction: 0.7-1 mg/kg/day (plus flucytosine 100 mg/kg/day) for 2 weeks, then change to oral fluconazole for at least 8 weeks; alternatively, amphotericin (0.7-1 mg/kg/day) may be continued uninterrupted for 4-6 weeks; maintenance: amphotericin 1 mg/kg/week for ≥1 year may be considered, but inferior to use of azoles

HIV negative: Induction: 0.7-1 mg/kg/day (plus flucytosine 100 mg/kg/day) for 2 weeks (low-risk patients), ≥4 weeks (non-low-risk, but without neurologic complication, immunosuppression, underlying disease, and negative CSF culture at 2 weeks), >6 weeks (neurologic complication or patients intolerant of flucytosine) Follow with azole consolidation/maintenance treatment.

Oropharyngeal candidiasis: I.V.: 0.3 mg/kg/day for 7-14 days (Pappas, 2009)

Osteoarticular candidiasis: I.V.: 0.5-1 mg/kg/day for several weeks, followed by fluconazole for 6-12 months (osteomyelitis) or 6 weeks (septic arthritis) (Pappas, 2009)

Penicillium marneffei: I.V.: 0.6 mg/kg/day for 2 weeks

Pneumonia: Cryptococcal (mild-to-moderate): I.V.:

HIV positive: 0.5-1 mg/kg/day

HIV negative: 0.5-0.7 mg/kg/day (plus flucytosine) for 2 weeks

Sporotrichosis: Pulmonary, meningeal, osteoarticular, or disseminated: I.V.: Total dose of 1-2 g, then change to oral itraconazole or fluconazole for suppressive therapy

Urinary tract candidiasis (Pappas, 2009):

Fungus balls: I.V.: 0.5-0.7 mg/kg/day with or without flucytosine 25 mg/kg 4 times daily

Pyelonephritis: I.V.: 0.5-0.7 mg/kg/day with or without flucytosine 25 mg/kg 4 times daily for 2 weeks

Symptomatic cystitis: I.V.: 0.3-0.6 mg/kg/day for 1-7 days

Bladder irrigation: Irrigate with 50 mcg/mL solution instilled periodically or continuously for 5-10 days or until cultures are clear for fluconazole-resistant *Candida*

Dosage adjustment in renal impairment: If renal dysfunction is due to the drug, the daily total can be decreased by 50% or the dose can be given every other day; I.V. therapy may take several months

Renal replacement therapy: Poorly dialyzed; no supplemental dose or dosage adjustment necessary, including patients on intermittent hemodialysis or CRRT.

Peritoneal dialysis (PD): Administration in dialysate: 1-2 mg/L of peritoneal dialysis fluid either with or without low-dose I.V. amphotericin B (a total dose of 2-10 mg/kg given over 7-14 days). Precipitate may form in ionic dialysate solutions.

Dosage adjustment in hepatic impairment: No dosage adjustment provided in manufacturer's labeling.

Administration

I.V.: May be infused over 4-6 hours. For a patient who experiences chills, fever, hypotension, nausea, or other nonanaphylactic infusion-related reactions, premedicate with the following drugs 30-60 minutes prior to drug administration: A nonsteroidal (eg, ibuprofen, choline magnesium trisalicylate) ± diphenhydramine **or** acetaminophen with diphenhydramine **or** hydrocortisone. If the patient experiences rigors during the infusion, meperidine may be administered. Bolus infusion of normal saline immediately preceding, or immediately preceding and following amphotericin B may reduce drug-induced nephrotoxicity. Risk of nephrotoxicity increases with amphotericin B doses >1 mg/kg/day. Infusion of admixtures more concentrated than 0.25 mg/mL should be limited to patients absolutely requiring volume contraction.

Intravitreal (labeled use/route): Administer amphotericin intravitreally with a final concentration of 5 mcg/0.1 mL NS (John, 2007)

Monitoring Parameters BUN and serum creatinine levels should be determined every other day when therapy is increased and at least weekly thereafter. Renal function (monitor frequently during therapy), electrolytes (especially potassium and magnesium), liver function tests, temperature, PT/PTT, CBC; monitor input and output; monitor for signs of hypokalemia (muscle weakness, cramping, drowsiness, ECG changes, etc)

Additional Information Premedication with diphenhydramine and acetaminophen may reduce the severity of acute infusion-related reactions. Meperidine reduces the duration of amphotericin B-induced rigors and chilling. Hydrocortisone may be used in patients with severe or refractory infusion-related reactions. Bolus infusion of normal saline immediately preceding, or immediately preceding and following amphotericin B may reduce drug-induced nephrotoxicity. Risk of nephrotoxicity increases with amphotericin B doses >1 mg/kg/day. Infusion of admixtures more concentrated than 0.25 mg/mL should be limited to patients absolutely requiring volume restriction. Amphotericin B does not have a bacteriostatic constituent, subsequently admixture expiration is determined by sterility more than chemical stability.

Dosage Forms Excipient information presented when available (limited, particularly for generics); consult specific product labeling.

Solution Reconstituted, Injection, as desoxycholate:
Generic: 50 mg (1 ea)

- **Amphotericin B Deoxycholate** *see* Amphotericin B (Conventional) *on page 123*
- **Amphotericin B Desoxycholate** *see* Amphotericin B (Conventional) *on page 123*

Amphotericin B (Lipid Complex)

(am foe TER i sin bee LIP id KOM pleks)

Brand Names: U.S. Abelcet

Brand Names: Canada Abelcet®

Index Terms ABLC

Pharmacologic Category Antifungal Agent, Parenteral

Use Treatment of invasive fungal infection in patients who are refractory to or intolerant of conventional amphotericin B (amphotericin B deoxycholate) therapy

Pregnancy Risk Factor B

Pregnancy Considerations Adverse events were not observed in animal reproduction studies. Amphotericin crosses the placenta and enters the fetal circulation. Amphotericin B is recommended for the treatment of serious, systemic fungal diseases in pregnant women, refer to current guidelines (King, 1998).

Breast-Feeding Considerations It is not known if amphotericin is excreted into breast milk. Due to its poor oral absorption, systemic exposure to the nursing infant is expected to be decreased; however, because of the potential for toxicity, breast-feeding is not recommended (Mactal-Haaf, 2001).

Contraindications Hypersensitivity to amphotericin or any component of the formulation

Warnings/Precautions Anaphylaxis has been reported with amphotericin B-containing drugs. If severe respiratory distress occurs, the infusion should be immediately discontinued. During the initial dosing, the drug should be administered under close clinical observation. Acute reactions (including fever and chills) may occur 1-2 hours after starting an intravenous infusion. These reactions are usually more common with the first few doses and generally diminish with subsequent doses. Infusion has been rarely associated with hypotension, bronchospasm, arrhythmias, and shock. Acute pulmonary toxicity has been reported in patients receiving leukocyte transfusions and amphotericin B; amphotericin B lipid complex and concurrent leukocyte transfusions are not recommended. Concurrent use with antineoplastic agents may enhance the potential for renal toxicity, bronchospasm or hypotension; use with caution. Concurrent use of amphotericin B with other nephrotoxic drugs may enhance the potential for drug-induced renal toxicity.

Adverse Reactions Nephrotoxicity and infusion-related hyperpyrexia, rigor, and chilling are reduced relative to amphotericin deoxycholate.

>10%:
Central nervous system: Chills (18%), fever (14%)
Renal: Serum creatinine increased (11%)
Miscellaneous: Multiple organ failure (11%)

1% to 10%:
Cardiovascular: Hypotension (8%), cardiac arrest (6%), hypertension (5%), chest pain (3%)
Central nervous system: Headache (6%), pain (5%)
Dermatologic: Rash (4%)
Endocrine & metabolic: Hypokalemia (5%), bilirubinemia (4%)
Gastrointestinal: Nausea (9%), vomiting (8%), diarrhea (6%), gastrointestinal hemorrhage (4%), abdominal pain (4%)
Hematologic: Thrombocytopenia (5%), anemia (4%), leukopenia (4%)
Renal: Renal failure (5%)
Respiratory: Respiratory failure (8%), dyspnea (6%), respiratory disorder (4%)
Miscellaneous: Sepsis (7%), infection (5%)

<1% (Limited to important or life-threatening): Allergic reactions, anaphylactoid reactions, anuria, arrhythmias, asthma, blood dyscrasias, bronchospasm, BUN increased, cardiomyopathy, cerebral vascular accident, cholangitis, cholecystitis, coagulation abnormalities, deafness, dysuria, encephalopathy, eosinophilia, erythema multiforme, exfoliative dermatitis, extrapyramidal syndrome, hearing loss, hemoptysis, hepatic failure (acute), hepatitis, hepatomegaly, hepatotoxicity, hyper-/hypocalcemia, hyperkalemia, hypomagnesemia, injection site reaction, jaundice, leukocytosis, MI, myasthenia, oliguria, peripheral neuropathy, pleural effusion, pulmonary edema, pulmonary embolism, renal function decreased, renal tubular acidosis, seizures, shock, tachycardia, thrombophlebitis, transaminases increased, veno-occlusive liver disease, ventricular fibrillation, vertigo (transient), visual impairment

Drug Interactions

Metabolism/Transport Effects None known.

Avoid Concomitant Use

Avoid concomitant use of Amphotericin B (Lipid Complex) with any of the following: Gallium Nitrate

Increased Effect/Toxicity

Amphotericin B (Lipid Complex) may increase the levels/effects of: Aminoglycosides; Colistimethate; CycloSPORINE (Systemic); Flucytosine; Gallium Nitrate

The levels/effects of Amphotericin B (Lipid Complex) may be increased by: Corticosteroids (Orally Inhaled); Corticosteroids (Systemic)

Decreased Effect

Amphotericin B (Lipid Complex) may decrease the levels/effects of: Saccharomyces boulardii

The levels/effects of Amphotericin B (Lipid Complex) may be decreased by: Antifungal Agents (Azole Derivatives, Systemic)

Preparation for Administration Shake the vial gently until there is no evidence of any yellow sediment at the bottom. Withdraw the appropriate dose from the vial using an 18-gauge needle. Remove the 18-gauge needle and attach the provided 5-micron filter needle to filter, and dilute the dose with D_5W to a final concentration of 1 mg/mL. Limited data suggests $D_{10}W$ and $D_{15}W$ may also be used for dilution (data on file [Sigma-Tau Pharmaceuticals, 2014]). Each filter needle may be used to filter up to four 100 mg vials. A final concentration of 2 mg/mL may be used for pediatric patients and patients with cardiovascular disease.

Do not dilute with saline solutions or mix with other drugs or electrolytes - compatibility has not been established

Storage/Stability Intact vials should be stored at 2°C to 8°C (35°F to 46°F); do not freeze. Protect intact vials from exposure to light. Solutions for infusion are stable for 48 hours under refrigeration and for an additional 6 hours at room temperature.

Mechanism of Action Binds to ergosterol altering cell membrane permeability in susceptible fungi and causing leakage of cell components with subsequent cell death. Proposed mechanism suggests that amphotericin causes an oxidation-dependent stimulation of macrophages.

Pharmacodynamics/Kinetics Note: Exhibits nonlinear kinetics; volume of distribution and clearance from blood increases with increasing dose.

Distribution: V_d: Increases with higher doses (likely reflects increased uptake by tissues); 131 L/kg with 5 mg/kg/day

Half-life elimination: 173 hours following multiple doses

Excretion: 0.9% of dose excreted in urine over 24 hours; effects of hepatic and renal impairment on drug disposition are unknown

Dialysis: Amphotericin B (lipid complex) is not hemodialyzable

Dosage I.V.: **Note:** Premedication: For patients who experience infusion-related immediate reactions, premedicate with the following drugs 30-60 minutes prior to drug administration: A nonsteroidal anti-inflammatory agent ± diphenhydramine **or** acetaminophen with diphenhydramine **or** hydrocortisone. If the patient experiences rigors during the infusion, meperidine may be administered.

Children and Adults:

Usual dose: 5 mg/kg once daily

Manufacturer's labeling: Invasive fungal infections (when patients are intolerant or refractory to conventional amphotericin B): 5 mg/kg/day

Indication-specific dosing:

Infants and Children:

Aspergillosis (HIV-positive patients) (alternative to preferred therapy): 5 mg/kg/day for ≥12 weeks (CDC, [pediatric], 2009)

Candidiasis, invasive (HIV-positive patients) (alternative to preferred therapy): 5 mg/kg/day; treatment duration based on clinical response, treat until 2-3 weeks after last positive blood culture (CDC [pediatric], 2009)

***Cryptococcus neoformans*, disseminated disease (non-CNS disease) (HIV-positive patients):** 5 mg/kg/day (with or without flucytosine); treatment duration of non-CNS disease varies by clinical response and site/severity of infection (CDC [pediatric], 2009)

Adults:

Aspergillosis, invasive (HIV-positive or HIV-negative patients) (alternative to preferred therapy): 5 mg/kg/day; duration of treatment in HIV-negative patients depends on site of infection, extent of disease and level of immunosuppression; in HIV-positive patients, treat until CD4 count >200 cells/mm^3 and evidence of clinical response (CDC [adults], 2009; Walsh, 2008)

Blastomycosis, moderately-severe-to-severe (unlabeled dose): 3-5 mg/kg/day for 1-2 weeks or until improvement, followed by oral itraconazole (Chapman, 2008)

Candidiasis (unlabeled dose):

Chronic disseminated candidiasis, pericarditis or myocarditis due to Candida, suppurative thrombophlebitis: 3-5 mg/kg/day. **Note:** In chronic disseminated candidiasis, transition to fluconazole after several weeks in stable patients is preferred (Pappas, 2009)

CNS candidiasis: 3-5 mg/kg/day (with or without flucytosine) for several weeks, followed by fluconazole (Pappas, 2009)

Endocarditis due to Candida, infected pacemaker, ICD, or VAD: 3-5 mg/kg/day (with or without flucytosine); continue to treat for 4-6 weeks after device removal unless device cannot be removed then chronic suppression with fluconazole is recommended (Pappas, 2009)

Coccidioidomycosis (unlabeled dose):

Progressive, disseminated: (alternative to preferred therapy): 2-5 mg/kg/day (Galgiani, 2005)

HIV-positive patients with severe, nonmeningeal infection: 4-6 mg/kg/day until clinical improvement, then switch to fluconazole or itraconazole (CDC, 2009)

Cryptococcosis:

Cryptococcal meningoencephalitis in HIV-positive patients (as an alternative to conventional amphotericin B in patients with renal concerns): Induction therapy: 4-6 mg/kg/day (unlabeled dose; CDC [adult], 2009) or 5 mg/kg/day (Perfect, 2010) with flucytosine for at least 2 weeks, followed by oral fluconazole. **Note:** If flucytosine is not given due to intolerance, duration of amphotericin B lipid complex therapy should be 4-6 weeks (Perfect, 2010).

Cryptococcal meningoencephalitis in HIV-negative patients and nontransplant patients (as an alternative to conventional amphotericin B): Induction therapy: 5 mg/kg/day (with flucytosine if possible) for ≥4 weeks followed by oral fluconazole. **Note:** If flucytosine is not given or treatment is interrupted, consider prolonging induction therapy for an additional 2 weeks (Perfect, 2010).

Cryptococcal meningoencephalitis in transplant recipients: Induction therapy: 5 mg/kg/day (with flucytosine) for at least 2 weeks, followed by oral fluconazole **Note:** If flucytosine is not given, duration of amphotericin B lipid complex therapy should be 4-6 weeks (Perfect, 2010).

Nonmeningeal cryptococcosis: Induction therapy: 5 mg/kg/day (with flucytosine if possible) for ≥4 weeks may be used for severe pulmonary cryptococcosis or for cryptococcemia with evidence of high fungal burden, followed by oral fluconazole. **Note:** If flucytosine is not given or treatment is interrupted, consider prolonging induction therapy for an additional 2 weeks (Perfect, 2010).

Histoplasmosis:

Acute pulmonary (moderately-severe-to-severe): 5 mg/kg/day for 1-2 weeks, followed by oral itraconazole (Wheat, 2007)

Progressive disseminated (alternative to preferred therapy): 5 mg/kg/day for 1-2 weeks, followed by oral itraconazole (Wheat, 2007)

Sporotrichosis (unlabeled dose):

Meningeal: 5 mg/kg/day for 4-6 weeks, followed by oral itraconazole (Kauffman, 2007)

Pulmonary, osteoarticular, and disseminated: 3-5 mg/kg/day, followed by oral itraconazole after a favorable response is seen with amphotericin initial therapy (Kauffman, 2007)

Dosing adjustment in renal impairment:
Manufacturer's recommendations: No dosage adjustment provided in manufacturer's labeling (has not been studied).
Alternate recommendations (Aronoff, 2007):
Intermittent hemodialysis: No supplemental dosage necessary.
Peritoneal dialysis: No supplemental dosage necessary.
Continuous renal replacement therapy (CRRT): No supplemental dosage necessary.
Dosing adjustment in hepatic impairment: No dosage adjustment provided in manufacturer's labeling (has not been studied).

Dietary Considerations If on parenteral nutrition, may need to adjust the amount of lipid infused. The lipid portion of amphotericin B (lipid complex) formulation contains 0.045 kcal per 5 mg (Sacks, 1997).

Administration For patients who experience nonanaphylactic infusion-related reactions, premedicate 30-60 minutes prior to drug administration with a nonsteroidal anti-inflammatory agent ± diphenhydramine **or** acetaminophen with diphenhydramine **or** hydrocortisone. If the patient experiences rigors during the infusion, meperidine may be administered.

Administer at an infusion rate of 2.5 mg/kg/hour (eg, over 2 hours for 5 mg/kg). Invert infusion container several times prior to administration and every 2 hours during infusion if it exceeds 2 hours. **Do not use an in-line filter during administration.** Flush line with dextrose; normal saline may cause precipitate.

Monitoring Parameters BUN and serum creatinine levels should be determined every other day while therapy is increased and at least weekly thereafter. Renal function (monitor frequently during therapy), electrolytes (especially potassium and magnesium), liver function tests, temperature, PT/PTT, CBC; monitor input and output; monitor for signs of hypokalemia (muscle weakness, cramping, drowsiness, ECG changes, etc)

Additional Information As a modification of dimyristoyl phosphatidylcholine:dimyristoyl phosphatidylglycerol 7:3 (DMPC:DMPG) liposome, amphotericin B lipid-complex has a higher drug to lipid ratio and the concentration of amphotericin B is 33 M. ABLC is a ribbon-like structure, not a liposome.

Controlled trials which compare the original formulation of amphotericin B to the newer liposomal formulations (ie, Abelcet®) are lacking. Thus, comparative data discussing differences among the formulations should be interpreted cautiously. Although the risk of nephrotoxicity and infusion-related adverse effects may be less with Abelcet®, the efficacy profiles of Abelcet® and the original amphotericin formulation are comparable. Consequently, Abelcet® should be restricted to those patients who cannot tolerate or fail a standard amphotericin B formulation.

Dosage Forms Excipient information presented when available (limited, particularly for generics); consult specific product labeling.
Suspension, Intravenous:
Abelcet: 5 mg/mL (20 mL)

Amphotericin B (Liposomal)
(am foe TER i sin bee lye po SO mal)

Brand Names: U.S. AmBisome
Brand Names: Canada AmBisome®
Index Terms Amphotericin B Liposome; L-AmB
Pharmacologic Category Antifungal Agent, Parenteral
Use Empirical therapy for presumed fungal infection in febrile, neutropenic patients; treatment of patients with *Aspergillus* species, *Candida* species, and/or *Cryptococcus* species infections refractory to amphotericin B desoxycholate (conventional amphotericin), or in patients where renal impairment or unacceptable toxicity precludes the use of amphotericin B desoxycholate; treatment of cryptococcal meningitis in HIV-infected patients; treatment of visceral leishmaniasis

Unlabeled Use Treatment of systemic *Histoplasmosis* infection; empiric treatment of fungal meningitis or osteoarticular infections

Pregnancy Risk Factor B

Pregnancy Considerations Adverse events were not observed in animal reproduction studies. Amphotericin crosses the placenta and enters the fetal circulation. Amphotericin B is recommended for the treatment of serious systemic fungal diseases in pregnant women; refer to current guidelines (King, 1998).

Breast-Feeding Considerations It is not known if amphotericin is excreted into breast milk. Due to its poor oral absorption, systemic exposure to the nursing infant is expected to be decreased; however, because of the potential for toxicity, breast-feeding is not recommended (Mactal-Haaf, 2001).

Contraindications Hypersensitivity to amphotericin B deoxycholate or any component of the formulation

Warnings/Precautions Patients should be under close clinical observation during initial dosing. As with other amphotericin B-containing products, anaphylaxis has been reported. Facilities for cardiopulmonary resuscitation should be available during administration. Acute infusion reactions (including fever and chills) may occur 1-2 hours after starting infusions; reactions are more common with the first few doses and generally diminish with subsequent doses. Immediately discontinue infusion if severe respiratory distress occurs; the patient should not receive further infusions. Concurrent use of amphotericin B with other nephrotoxic drugs may enhance the potential for drug-induced renal toxicity. Concurrent use with antineoplastic agents may enhance the potential for renal toxicity, bronchospasm or hypotension. Acute pulmonary toxicity has been reported in patients receiving simultaneous leukocyte transfusions and amphotericin B. Safety and efficacy have not been established in patients <1 month of age.

Adverse Reactions Percentage of adverse reactions is dependent upon population studied and may vary with respect to premedications and underlying illness. Incidence of decreased renal function and infusion-related events are lower than rates observed with amphotericin B deoxycholate.

>10%:
Cardiovascular: Peripheral edema (15%), edema (12% to 14%), tachycardia (9% to 19%), hypotension (7% to 14%), hypertension (8% to 20%), chest pain (8% to 12%), hypervolemia (8% to 12%)
Central nervous system: Chills (29% to 48%), insomnia (17% to 22%), headache (9% to 20%), anxiety (7% to 14%), pain (14%), confusion (9% to 13%)
Dermatologic: Rash (5% to 25%), pruritus (11%)
Endocrine & metabolic: Hypokalemia (31% to 51%), hypomagnesemia (15% to 50%), hyperglycemia (8% to 23%), hypocalcemia (5% to 18%), hyponatremia (9% to 12%)
Gastrointestinal: Nausea (16% to 40%), vomiting (11% to 32%), diarrhea (11% to 30%), abdominal pain (7% to 20%), constipation (15%), anorexia (10% to 14%)
Hematologic: Anemia (27% to 48%), blood transfusion reaction (9% to 18%), leukopenia (15% to 17%), thrombocytopenia (6% to 13%)
Hepatic: Alkaline phosphatase increased (7% to 22%), bilirubinemia (≤18%), ALT increased (15%), AST increased (13%), liver function tests abnormal (not specified) (4% to 13%)
Local: Phlebitis (9% to 11%)

Neuromuscular & skeletal: Weakness (6% to 13%), back pain (12%)
Renal: Nephrotoxicity (14% to 47%), creatinine increased (18% to 40%), BUN increased (7% to 21%), hematuria (14%)
Respiratory: Dyspnea (18% to 23%), lung disorder (14% to 18%), cough (2% to 18%), epistaxis (9% to 15%), pleural effusion (13%), rhinitis (11%)
Miscellaneous: Infusion reactions (4% to 21%), sepsis (7% to 14%), infection (11% to 13%)

2% to 10%:
Cardiovascular: Arrhythmia, atrial fibrillation, bradycardia, cardiac arrest, cardiomegaly, facial swelling, flushing, orthostatic hypotension, valvular heart disease, vascular disorder, vasodilation
Central nervous system: Agitation, abnormal thinking, coma, depression, dysesthesia, dizziness (7% to 9%), hallucinations, malaise, nervousness, seizure, somnolence
Dermatologic: Alopecia, bruising, cellulitis, dry skin, maculopapular rash, petechia, purpura, skin discoloration, skin disorder, skin ulcer, urticaria, vesiculobullous rash
Endocrine & metabolic: Acidosis, fluid overload, hypernatremia (4%), hyperchloremia, hyperkalemia, hypermagnesemia, hyperphosphatemia, hypophosphatemia, hypoproteinemia, lactate dehydrogenase increased, nonprotein nitrogen increased
Gastrointestinal: Abdomen enlarged, amylase increased, dyspepsia, dysphagia, eructation, fecal incontinence, flatulence, gastrointestinal hemorrhage (10%), hematemesis, hemorrhoids, gum/oral hemorrhage, ileus, mucositis, rectal disorder, stomatitis, ulcerative stomatitis, xerostomia
Genitourinary: Vaginal hemorrhage
Hematologic: Coagulation disorder, hemorrhage, prothrombin decreased
Hepatic: Hepatocellular damage, hepatomegaly, veno-occlusive liver disease
Local: Injection site inflammation
Neuromuscular & skeletal: Arthralgia, bone pain, dystonia, myalgia, neck pain, paresthesia, rigors, tremor
Ocular: Conjunctivitis, dry eyes, eye hemorrhage
Renal: Abnormal renal function, acute renal failure, dysuria, renal failure, toxic nephropathy, urinary incontinence
Respiratory: Asthma, atelectasis, dry nose, hemoptysis, hyperventilation, pharyngitis, pneumonia, pulmonary edema, respiratory alkalosis, respiratory insufficiency, respiratory failure, sinusitis, hypoxia (6% to 8%)
Miscellaneous: Allergic reaction, cell-mediated immunological reaction, flu-like syndrome, graft-versus-host disease, herpes simplex, hiccup, procedural complication (8% to 10%), diaphoresis (7%)

Postmarketing and/or case reports: Agranulocytosis, angioedema, bronchospasm, cyanosis/hypoventilation, erythema, hemorrhagic cystitis, rhabdomyolysis

Drug Interactions

Metabolism/Transport Effects None known.

Avoid Concomitant Use

Avoid concomitant use of Amphotericin B (Liposomal) with any of the following: Gallium Nitrate

Increased Effect/Toxicity

Amphotericin B (Liposomal) may increase the levels/effects of: Aminoglycosides; Colistimethate; CycloSPORINE (Systemic); Flucytosine; Gallium Nitrate

The levels/effects of Amphotericin B (Liposomal) may be increased by: Corticosteroids (Orally Inhaled); Corticosteroids (Systemic)

Decreased Effect

Amphotericin B (Liposomal) may decrease the levels/effects of: Saccharomyces boulardii

The levels/effects of Amphotericin B (Liposomal) may be decreased by: Antifungal Agents (Azole Derivatives, Systemic)

Preparation for Administration Reconstitute with 12 mL SWFI to a concentration of 4 mg/mL. The use of any solution other than those recommended, or the presence of a bacteriostatic agent in the solution, may cause precipitation. **Shake the vial vigorously** for 30 seconds, until dispersed into a translucent yellow suspension.

Filtration and dilution: The 5-micron filter should be on the syringe used to remove the reconstituted AmBisome®. Dilute to a final concentration of 1-2 mg/mL (0.2-0.5 mg/mL for infants and small children).

Storage/Stability Store intact vials at ≤25°C (≤77°F). Reconstituted vials are stable refrigerated at 2°C to 8°C (36°F to 46°F) for 24 hours. Do not freeze. Manufacturer's labeling states infusion should begin within 6 hours of dilution with D_5W; data on file with Astellas Pharma shows extended formulation stability when admixed in D_5W at 0.2-2 mg/mL (in polyolefin or PVC bags) for up to 11 days when stored refrigerated at 2°C to 8°C (36°F to 46°F).

Mechanism of Action Binds to ergosterol altering cell membrane permeability in susceptible fungi and causing leakage of cell components with subsequent cell death. Proposed mechanism suggests that amphotericin causes an oxidation-dependent stimulation of macrophages (Lyman, 1992).

Pharmacodynamics/Kinetics Half-life elimination: 7-10 hours (following a single 24-hour dosing interval); Terminal half-life: 100-153 hours (following multiple dosing up to 49 days)

Dosage

Usual dosage range:

Children ≥1 month: I.V.: 3-6 mg/kg/day

Adults: I.V.: 3-6 mg/kg/day; **Note:** Higher doses (7.5-15 mg/kg/day) have been used clinically in special cases (CDC [parameningeal], 2012; Kauffman, 2012; Walsh, 2001)

Note: Premedication: For patients who experience nonanaphylactic infusion-related immediate reactions, premedicate with the following drugs 30-60 minutes prior to drug administration: A nonsteroidal anti-inflammatory agent ± diphenhydramine; **or** acetaminophen with diphenhydramine; **or** hydrocortisone. If the patient experiences rigors during the infusion, meperidine may be administered.

Indication-specific dosing:

Children ≥1 month: I.V.:

Empiric therapy: 3 mg/kg/day

Systemic fungal infections *(Aspergillus, Candida, Cryptococcus)*: 3-5 mg/kg/day

Systemic fungal infections (HIV-exposed/-positive [CDC, 2009; unlabeled use]):

Aspergillosis: 5 mg/kg/day once daily

Candida, invasive: 5 mg/kg/day once daily (may consider addition of oral flucytosine for severe disease)

Cryptococcal meningitis: 4-6 mg/kg/day once daily plus oral flucytosine

Cryptococcus, disseminated (non-CNS): 3-5 mg/kg/day (may consider addition of oral flucytosine)

Histoplasmosis: 3-5 mg/kg/day once daily

Visceral leishmaniasis:

Immunocompetent: 3 mg/kg/day on days 1-5, and 3 mg/kg/day on days 14 and 21; a repeat course may be given in patients who do not achieve parasitic clearance

Note: Alternate regimen of 10 mg/kg/day for 2 days has been reportedly effective.

Immunocompromised: 4 mg/kg/day on days 1-5, and 4 mg/kg/day on days 10, 17, 24, 31, and 38

Adults: I.V.:

Cryptococcal meningitis (HIV-positive): 6 mg/kg/day or 4-6 mg/kg/day in combination with addition of oral flucytosine 25 mg/kg 4 times daily (unlabeled combination; CDC, 2009)

Empiric candidiasis therapy: 3-5 mg/kg/day (Pappas, 2009)

Endocarditis: I.V.: 3-5 mg/kg/day (with or without flucytosine 25 mg/kg 4 times daily) for 6 weeks after valve replacement; **Note:** If isolates susceptible and/or clearance demonstrated, guidelines recommend step-down to fluconazole; also for long-term suppression therapy if valve replacement is not possible (Pappas, 2009)

Fungal sinusitis: Limited data in immunocompromised patients have shown efficacy with 3-10 mg/kg/day (Barron, 2005; Pagano, 2004; Rokicka, 2006). **Note:** An azole antifungal is recommended if causative organism is *Aspergillus* spp or *Pseudallescheria boydii* (*Scedosporium* sp).

Meningitis (secondary to contaminated [eg, *Exserohilum rostratum*] steroid products), severe or in patients not improving with voriconazole monotherapy (unlabeled use) (CDC [parameningeal], 2012; Kauffman, 2012): I.V.: 5-6 mg/kg/day in combination with voriconazole for ≥3 months; a higher dose (7.5 mg/kg/day) may be considered in patients who are not improving. **Note:** Consult an infectious disease specialist and current CDC guidelines for specific treatment recommendations.

Osteoarticular candidiasis: I.V.: 3-5 mg/kg/day for several weeks, followed by fluconazole for 6-12 months (osteomyelitis) or 6 weeks (septic arthritis) (Pappas, 2009)

Osteoarticular infection (secondary to contaminated [eg, *Exserohilum rostratum*] steroid products), severe or in patients with clinical instability (unlabeled use) (CDC [osteoarticular], 2012; Kauffman, 2012): I.V.: 5 mg/kg/day in combination with voriconazole for ≥3 months. **Note:** Consult an infectious disease specialist and current CDC guidelines for specific treatment recommendations.

Systemic fungal infections *(Aspergillus, Candida, Cryptococcus)* : 3-5 mg/kg/day

General invasive Candidal disease: 3-5 mg/kg/day with oral flucytosine 25 mg/kg 4 times daily (unlabeled combination; Pappas, 2009)

Candidal meningitis: 3-5 mg/kg/day with or without oral flucytosine 25 mg/kg 4 times daily (unlabeled combination; Pappas, 2009)

Histoplasmosis (unlabeled use): 3-5 mg/kg/day (CDC, 2009)

Visceral leishmaniasis:

Immunocompetent: 3 mg/kg/day on days 1-5, and 3 mg/kg/day on days 14 and 21; a repeat course may be given in patients who do not achieve parasitic clearance

Note: Alternate regimen of 2 mg/kg/day for 5 days has been reportedly effective.

Immunocompromised: 4 mg/kg/day on days 1-5, and 4 mg/kg/day on days 10, 17, 24, 31, and 38

Dosage adjustment in renal impairment: None necessary; effects of renal impairment are not currently known

Poorly dialyzed; no supplemental dose or dosage adjustment necessary, including patients on intermittent hemodialysis, peritoneal dialysis, or continuous renal replacement therapy (eg, CVVHD).

Dosage adjustment in hepatic impairment: No dosage adjustment provided in manufacturer's labeling (has not been studied).

Dietary Considerations If on parenteral nutrition, may need to adjust the amount of lipid infused. The lipid portion of amphotericin B (liposomal) formulation contains 0.27 kcal per 5 mg (Sacks, 1997).

Administration Administer via intravenous infusion, over a period of approximately 2 hours. Infusion time may be reduced to approximately 1 hour in patients in whom the treatment is well-tolerated. If the patient experiences discomfort during infusion, the duration of infusion may be increased. Administer at a rate of 2.5 mg/kg/hour. Existing intravenous line should be flushed with D_5W prior to infusion (if not feasible, administer through a separate line). An in-line membrane filter (not less than 1 micron) may be used.

For a patient who experiences chills, fever, hypotension, nausea, or other nonanaphylactic infusion-related reactions, premedicate with the following drugs, 30-60 minutes prior to drug administration: A nonsteroidal (eg, ibuprofen, choline magnesium trisalicylate) ± diphenhydramine **or** acetaminophen with diphenhydramine **or** hydrocortisone. If the patient experiences rigors during the infusion, meperidine may be administered.

Monitoring Parameters BUN and serum creatinine levels should be determined every other day while therapy is increased and at least weekly thereafter. Renal function (monitor frequently during therapy), electrolytes (especially potassium and magnesium), liver function tests, temperature, hematocrit, PT/PTT, CBC; monitor input and output; monitor for signs of hypokalemia (muscle weakness, cramping, drowsiness, ECG changes, etc); monitor cardiac function if used concurrently with corticosteroids

Test Interactions Falsely-elevated serum phosphate may occur when using the PHOSm assay.

Additional Information Amphotericin B (liposomal) is a true single bilayer liposomal drug delivery system. Liposomes are closed, spherical vesicles created by mixing specific proportions of amphophilic substances such as phospholipids and cholesterol so that they arrange themselves into multiple concentric bilayer membranes when hydrated in aqueous solutions. Single bilayer liposomes are then formed by microemulsification of multilamellar vesicles using a homogenizer. Amphotericin B (liposomal) consists of these unilamellar bilayer liposomes with amphotericin B intercalated within the membrane. Due to the nature and quantity of amphophilic substances used, and the lipophilic moiety in the amphotericin B molecule, the drug is an integral part of the overall structure of the amphotericin B liposomal liposomes. Amphotericin B (liposomal) contains true liposomes that are <100 nm in diameter.

Dosage Forms Excipient information presented when available (limited, particularly for generics); consult specific product labeling.

Suspension Reconstituted, Intravenous:

AmBisome: 50 mg (1 ea) [contains cholesterol, distearoyl phosphatidylglycerol, hydrogenated soy phosphatidylcholine, sodium succinate hexahydrate, sucrose, tocopherol, dl-alpha]

◆ **Amphotericin B Liposome** *see* Amphotericin B (Liposomal) *on page* 128

Ampicillin (am pi SIL in)

Brand Names: Canada Ampicillin for Injection; Apo-Ampi®; Novo-Ampicillin; Nu-Ampi

Index Terms Aminobenzylpenicillin; Ampicillin Sodium; Ampicillin Trihydrate

Pharmacologic Category Antibiotic, Penicillin

Additional Appendix Information

Antibiotic Treatment of Adults With Infective Endocarditis *on page 2355*

Prevention of Infective Endocarditis *on page 2353*

Use Treatment of susceptible bacterial infections (nonbeta-lactamase-producing organisms); treatment or prophylaxis of infective endocarditis; susceptible bacterial infections caused by streptococci, pneumococci, nonpenicillinase-producing staphylococci, *Listeria*, meningococci; some strains of *H. influenzae*, *Salmonella*, *Shigella*, *E. coli*, *Enterobacter*, and *Klebsiella*

Unlabeled Use Surgical (perioperative) prophylaxis in patients undergoing liver transplantation (Bratzler, 2013)

Pregnancy Risk Factor B

Pregnancy Considerations Adverse events have not been observed in animal reproduction studies. Ampicillin crosses the placenta, providing detectable concentrations in the cord serum and amniotic fluid. Maternal use of ampicillin has generally not resulted in an increased risk of birth defects. Ampicillin is recommended for use in pregnant women for the management of preterm premature rupture of membranes (PPROM) and for the prevention of early-onset group B streptococcal (GBS) disease in newborns. Ampicillin may also be used in certain situations prior to vaginal delivery in women at high risk for endocarditis.

The volume of distribution of ampicillin is increased during pregnancy and the half-life is decreased. As a result, serum concentrations in pregnant patients are approximately 50% of those in nonpregnant patients receiving the same dose. Higher doses may be needed during pregnancy. Although oral absorption is not altered during pregnancy, oral ampicillin is poorly absorbed during labor.

Breast-Feeding Considerations Ampicillin is excreted in breast milk. The manufacturer recommends that caution be exercised when administering ampicillin to nursing women. Due to the low concentrations in human milk, minimal toxicity would be expected in the nursing infant. Nondose-related effects could include modification of bowel flora and allergic sensitization.

Contraindications Hypersensitivity to ampicillin, any component of the formulation, or other penicillins

Warnings/Precautions Dosage adjustment may be necessary in patients with renal impairment. Serious and occasionally severe or fatal hypersensitivity (anaphylactoid) reactions have been reported in patients on penicillin therapy, especially with a history of beta-lactam hypersensitivity, history of sensitivity to multiple allergens, or previous IgE-mediated reactions (eg, anaphylaxis, angioedema, urticaria). Use with caution in asthmatic patients. High percentage of patients with infectious mononucleosis have developed rash during therapy with ampicillin; ampicillin-class antibiotics not recommended in these patients. Appearance of a rash should be carefully evaluated to differentiate a nonallergic ampicillin rash from a hypersensitivity reaction. Ampicillin rash occurs in 5% to 10% of children receiving ampicillin and is a generalized dull red, maculopapular rash, generally appearing 3-14 days after the start of therapy. It normally begins on the trunk and spreads over most of the body. It may be most intense at pressure areas, elbows, and knees. Prolonged use may result in fungal or bacterial superinfection, including *C. difficile*-associated diarrhea (CDAD) and pseudomembranous colitis; CDAD has been observed >2 months post-antibiotic treatment.

Adverse Reactions Frequency not defined.

Central nervous system: Fever, penicillin encephalopathy, seizure

Dermatologic: Erythema multiforme, exfoliative dermatitis, rash, urticaria

Note: Appearance of a rash should be carefully evaluated to differentiate (if possible) nonallergic ampicillin rash from hypersensitivity reaction. Incidence is higher in patients with viral infection, *Salmonella* infection, lymphocytic leukemia, or patients that have hyperuricemia.

Gastrointestinal: Black hairy tongue, diarrhea, enterocolitis, glossitis, nausea, pseudomembranous colitis, sore mouth or tongue, stomatitis, vomiting, oral candidiasis

Hematologic: Agranulocytosis, anemia, hemolytic anemia, eosinophilia, leukopenia, thrombocytopenia purpura

Hepatic: AST increased

Renal: Interstitial nephritis (rare)

Respiratory: Laryngeal stridor

Miscellaneous: Anaphylaxis, serum sickness-like reaction

Drug Interactions

Metabolism/Transport Effects None known.

Avoid Concomitant Use

Avoid concomitant use of Ampicillin with any of the following: BCG

Increased Effect/Toxicity

Ampicillin may increase the levels/effects of: Methotrexate; Vitamin K Antagonists

The levels/effects of Ampicillin may be increased by: Allopurinol; Probenecid

Decreased Effect

Ampicillin may decrease the levels/effects of: Atenolol; BCG; Mycophenolate; Sodium Picosulfate; Typhoid Vaccine

The levels/effects of Ampicillin may be decreased by: Chloroquine; Lanthanum; Tetracycline Derivatives

Ethanol/Nutrition/Herb Interactions Food: Food decreases ampicillin absorption rate; may decrease ampicillin serum concentration. Management: Take at equal intervals around-the-clock, preferably on an empty stomach (1 hour before or 2 hours after meals). Maintain adequate hydration, unless instructed to restrict fluid intake.

Preparation for Administration I.V.: Minimum volume: Concentration should not exceed 30 mg/mL due to concentration-dependent stability restrictions. Standard diluent: 500 mg/50 mL NS; 1 g/50 mL NS; 2 g/100 mL NS.

Storage/Stability

Oral: Oral suspension is stable for 7 days at room temperature or for 14 days under refrigeration.

I.V.:

Solutions for I.M. or direct I.V. should be used within 1 hour. Solutions for I.V. infusion will be inactivated by dextrose at room temperature. If dextrose-containing solutions are to be used, the resultant solution will only be stable for 2 hours versus 8 hours in the 0.9% sodium chloride injection. D_5W has limited stability.

Stability of parenteral admixture in NS at room temperature (25°C) is 8 hours.

Stability of parenteral admixture in NS at refrigeration temperature (4°C) is 2 days.

Mechanism of Action Inhibits bacterial cell wall synthesis by binding to one or more of the penicillin-binding proteins (PBPs) which in turn inhibits the final transpeptidation step of peptidoglycan synthesis in bacterial cell walls, thus inhibiting cell wall biosynthesis. Bacteria eventually lyse due to ongoing activity of cell wall autolytic enzymes (autolysins and murein hydrolases) while cell wall assembly is arrested.

Pharmacodynamics/Kinetics

Absorption: Oral: 50%

Distribution: Bile, blister, and tissue fluids; penetration into CSF occurs with inflamed meninges only, good only with inflammation (exceeds usual MICs)

Normal meninges: Nil; Inflamed meninges: 5% to 10%

Protein binding: 15% to 25%

Half-life elimination:
Children and Adults: 1-1.8 hours
Anuria/end-stage renal disease: 7-20 hours
Time to peak: Oral: Within 1-2 hours
Excretion: Urine (~90% as unchanged drug) within 24 hours

Dosage

Usual dosage range:

Infants and Children:

Oral: 50-100 mg/kg/day in doses divided every 6 hours (maximum: 2-4 g/day)

I.M., I.V.: 100-400 mg/kg/day in divided doses every 6 hours (maximum: 12 g/day)

Adults:

Oral: 250-500 mg every 6 hours

I.M., I.V.: 1-2 g every 4-6 hours or 50-250 mg/kg/day in divided doses (maximum: 12 g/day)

Indication-specific dosing:

Infants and Children:

Community-acquired pneumonia (CAP) (IDSA/PIDS, 2011): Infants >3 months and Children: I.V.: **Note:** May consider addition of vancomycin or clindamycin to empiric therapy if community-acquired MRSA suspected. In children ≥5 years, a macrolide antibiotic should be added if atypical pneumonia cannot be ruled out.

Empiric treatment or *S. pneumoniae* (moderate-to-severe; MICs to penicillin ≤2.0 mcg/mL) or *H. influenzae* (beta-lactamase negative) (preferred): 150-200 mg/kg/day divided every 6 hours

Group A *Streptococcus* (moderate-to-severe) (preferred): 200 mg/kg/day divided every 6 hours

S. pneumoniae (moderate-to-severe; MICs to penicillin ≥4.0 mcg/mL) (alternative to ceftriaxone): 300-400 mg/kg/day divided every 6 hours

Prophylaxis against infective endocarditis:

Dental, oral, or respiratory tract procedures: I.M., I.V.: 50 mg/kg within 30-60 minutes prior to procedure in patients not allergic to penicillin and unable to take oral amoxicillin. Intramuscular injections should be avoided in patients who are receiving anticoagulant therapy. In these circumstances, orally administered regimens should be given whenever possible. Intravenously administered antibiotics should be used for patients who are unable to tolerate or absorb oral medications.

Note: American Heart Association (AHA) guidelines now recommend prophylaxis only in patients undergoing invasive procedures and in whom underlying cardiac conditions may predispose to a higher risk of adverse outcomes should infection occur.

Genitourinary and gastrointestinal tract procedures: I.M., I.V.:

High-risk patients: 50 mg/kg (maximum: 2 g) within 30 minutes prior to procedure, followed by ampicillin 25 mg/kg (or amoxicillin 25 mg/kg orally) 6 hours later; must be used in combination with gentamicin. **Note:** As of April 2007, routine prophylaxis for GI/GU procedures is no longer recommended by the AHA.

Moderate-risk patients: 50 mg/kg within 30 minutes prior to procedure

Mild-to-moderate infections:

Oral: 50-100 mg/kg/day in doses divided every 6 hours (maximum: 2-4 g/day)

I.M., I.V.: 100-150 mg/kg/day in divided doses every 6 hours (maximum: 2-4 g/day)

Severe infections, meningitis: I.M., I.V.: 200-400 mg/kg/day in divided doses every 6 hours (maximum: 6-12 g/day)

Surgical (perioperative) prophylaxis in liver transplantation (unlabeled use): Children ≥1 year: I.V.: 50 mg/kg within 60 minutes prior to surgery (maximum: 2000 mg/dose) in combination with cefotaxime. Doses may be repeated in 2 hours if procedure is lengthy or if there is excessive blood loss (Bratzler, 2013).

Adults:

Cholangitis (acute): I.V.: 2 g every 4 hours with gentamicin

Diverticulitis: I.M., I.V.: 2 g every 6 hours with metronidazole

Endocarditis:

Infective: I.V.: 12 g/day via continuous infusion or divided every 4 hours

Prophylaxis: Dental, oral, or respiratory tract: I.M., I.V.: 2 g within 30-60 minutes prior to procedure in patients not allergic to penicillin and unable to take oral amoxicillin. Intramuscular injections should be avoided in patients who are receiving anticoagulant therapy. In these circumstances, orally administered regimens should be given whenever possible. Intravenously administered antibiotics should be used for patients who are unable to tolerate or absorb oral medications.

Note: American Heart Association (AHA) guidelines now recommend prophylaxis only in patients undergoing invasive procedures and in whom underlying cardiac conditions may predispose to a higher risk of adverse outcomes should infection occur.

Prophylaxis in total joint replacement patient: I.M., I.V.: 2 g 1 hour prior to the procedure

Genitourinary and gastrointestinal tract procedures:

High-risk patients: I.M., I.V.: 2 g within 30 minutes prior to procedure, followed by ampicillin 1 g (or amoxicillin 1 g orally) 6 hours later; must be used in combination with gentamicin. **Note:** As of April 2007, routine prophylaxis for GI/GU procedures is no longer recommended by the AHA.

Moderate-risk patients: I.M., I.V.: 2 g within 30 minutes prior to procedure

Group B streptococcus (neonatal prophylaxis): I.V.: 2 g initial dose, then 1 g every 4 hours until delivery (CDC, 2010)

***Listeria* infections:** I.V.: 2 g every 4 hours (consider addition of aminoglycoside)

Mild-to-moderate infections: Oral: 250-500 mg every 6 hours

Prosthetic joint infection, *Enterococcus* spp (penicillin-susceptible): I.V.: 12 g continuous infusion every 24 hours **or** 2 g every 4 hours for 4-6 weeks; consider addition of aminoglycoside (Osmon, 2013)

Sepsis/meningitis: I.M., I.V.: 150-250 mg/kg/day divided every 3-4 hours (range: 6-12 g/day)

Surgical (perioperative) prophylaxis in liver transplantation (unlabeled use): I.V.: 2 g within 60 minutes prior to surgery in combination with cefotaxime. Doses may be repeated in 2 hours if procedure is lengthy or if there is excessive blood loss (Bratzler, 2013).

Urinary tract infections (*Enterococcus* suspected): I.V.: 1-2 g every 6 hours with gentamicin

Dosage adjustment in renal impairment:

Cl_{cr} >50 mL/minute: Administer every 6 hours

Cl_{cr} 10-50 mL/minute: Administer every 6-12 hours

Cl_{cr} <10 mL/minute: Administer every 12-24 hours

Intermittent hemodialysis (IHD) (administer after hemodialysis on dialysis days): Dialyzable (20% to 50%): I.V.: 1-2 g every 12-24 hours (Heintz, 2009). **Note:** Dosing dependent on the assumption of 3 times/week, complete IHD sessions.

Peritoneal dialysis (PD): 250 mg every 12 hours

Continuous renal replacement therapy (CRRT) (Heintz, 2009): Drug clearance is highly dependent on the method of renal replacement, filter type, and flow rate. Appropriate dosing requires close monitoring of pharmacologic response, signs of adverse reactions due to drug accumulation, as well as drug concentrations in relation to target trough (if appropriate). The following are general recommendations only (based on dialysate flow/ultrafiltration rates of 1-2 L/hour and minimal residual renal function) and should not supersede clinical judgment:

CVVH: Loading dose of 2 g followed by 1-2 g every 8-12 hours

CVVHD: Loading dose of 2 g followed by 1-2 g every 8 hours

CVVHDF: Loading dose of 2 g followed by 1-2 g every 6-8 hours

Dosage adjustment in hepatic impairment: No dosage adjustment provided in manufacturer's labeling.

Dietary Considerations Take on an empty stomach 1 hour before or 2 hours after meals. Some products may contain sodium.

Administration Administer around-the-clock to promote less variation in peak and trough serum levels.

Oral: Administer on an empty stomach (ie, 1 hour prior to, or 2 hours after meals) to increase total absorption.

I.V.: Administer over 3-5 minutes (125-500 mg) or over 10-15 minutes (1-2 g). More rapid infusion may cause seizures. Ampicillin and gentamicin should not be mixed in the same I.V. tubing.

Some penicillins (eg, carbenicillin, ticarcillin, and piperacillin) have been shown to inactivate aminoglycosides *in vitro*. This has been observed to a greater extent with tobramycin and gentamicin, while amikacin has shown greater stability against inactivation. Concurrent use of these agents may pose a risk of reduced antibacterial efficacy *in vivo*, particularly in the setting of profound renal impairment. However, definitive clinical evidence is lacking. If combination penicillin/aminoglycoside therapy is desired in a patient with renal dysfunction, separation of doses (if feasible), and routine monitoring of aminoglycoside levels, CBC, and clinical response should be considered.

Monitoring Parameters With prolonged therapy, monitor renal, hepatic, and hematologic function periodically; observe signs and symptoms of anaphylaxis during first dose

Test Interactions May interfere with urinary glucose tests using cupric sulfate (Benedict's solution, Clinitest®)

Some penicillin derivatives may accelerate the degradation of aminoglycosides *in vitro*, leading to a potential underestimation of aminoglycoside serum concentration.

Dosage Forms Excipient information presented when available (limited, particularly for generics); consult specific product labeling.

Capsule, Oral:

Generic: 250 mg, 500 mg

Solution Reconstituted, Injection, as sodium [strength expressed as base]:

Generic: 125 mg (1 ea); 250 mg (1 ea); 500 mg (1 ea); 1 g (1 ea); 2 g (1 ea); 10 g (1 ea)

Solution Reconstituted, Injection, as sodium [strength expressed as base, preservative free]:

Generic: 250 mg (1 ea); 500 mg (1 ea)

Solution Reconstituted, Intravenous, as sodium [strength expressed as base]:

Generic: 1 g (1 ea); 2 g (1 ea); 10 g (1 ea)

Solution Reconstituted, Intravenous, as sodium [strength expressed as base, preservative free]:

Generic: 10 g (1 ea)

Suspension Reconstituted, Oral:

Generic: 125 mg/5 mL (100 mL, 200 mL); 250 mg/5 mL (100 mL, 200 mL)

Ampicillin and Sulbactam

(am pi SIL in & SUL bak tam)

Brand Names: U.S. Unasyn®

Brand Names: Canada Unasyn®

Index Terms Sulbactam and Ampicillin

Pharmacologic Category Antibiotic, Penicillin

Additional Appendix Information

Antibiotic Treatment of Adults With Infective Endocarditis *on page 2355*

Use Treatment of susceptible bacterial infections involved with skin and skin structure, intra-abdominal infections, gynecological infections; spectrum is that of ampicillin plus organisms producing beta-lactamases such as *S. aureus*, *H. influenzae*, *E. coli*, *Klebsiella*, *Acinetobacter*, *Enterobacter*, and anaerobes

Unlabeled Use Treatment of acute bacterial rhinosinusitis (ABRS); endocarditis; intravascular catheter-associated bloodstream infection caused by susceptible bacteria; community-acquired pneumonia; early-onset hospital-acquired pneumonia; surgical (perioperative) prophylaxis

Pregnancy Risk Factor B

Pregnancy Considerations Adverse events have not been observed in animal reproduction studies. Both ampicillin and sulbactam cross the placenta. Maternal use of penicillins has generally not resulted in an increased risk of birth defects. When used during pregnancy, pharmacokinetic changes have been observed with ampicillin alone (refer to the Ampicillin monograph for details). Ampicillin/sulbactam may be considered for prophylactic use prior to cesarean delivery (consult current guidelines).

Breast-Feeding Considerations Ampicillin and sulbactam are both excreted into breast milk in low concentrations. The manufacturer recommends that caution be used if administering to lactating women. Nondose-related effects could include modification of bowel flora and allergic sensitization of the infant. The maternal dose of sulbactam does not need altered in the postpartum period. Also refer to the Ampicillin monograph.

Contraindications Hypersensitivity to ampicillin, sulbactam, penicillins, or any component of the formulations

Warnings/Precautions Dosage adjustment may be necessary in patients with renal impairment. Serious and occasionally severe or fatal hypersensitivity (anaphylactoid) reactions have been reported in patients on penicillin therapy, especially with a history of beta-lactam hypersensitivity, history of sensitivity to multiple allergens, or previous IgE-mediated reactions (eg, anaphylaxis, angioedema, urticaria). High percentage of patients with infectious mononucleosis have developed rash during therapy with ampicillin; ampicillin-class antibiotics not recommended in these patients. Appearance of a rash should be carefully evaluated to differentiate a nonallergic ampicillin rash from a hypersensitivity reaction. Prolonged use may result in fungal or bacterial superinfection, including *C. difficile*-associated diarrhea (CDAD) and pseudomembranous colitis; CDAD has been observed >2 months postantibiotic treatment.

Adverse Reactions Also see Ampicillin.

>10%: Local: Pain at injection site (I.M.)

1% to 10%:

Dermatologic: Rash

Gastrointestinal: Diarrhea

Local: Pain at injection site (I.V.), thrombophlebitis

Miscellaneous: Allergic reaction (may include serum sickness, urticaria, bronchospasm, hypotension, etc)

<1% (Limited to important or life-threatening): Abdominal distension, agranulocytosis, anemia. atypical lymphocytosis, candidiasis, chest pain, chills, dysuria, edema, eosinophilia, epistaxis, erythema, facial swelling, fatigue, flatulence, gastritis, glossitis, hairy tongue, headache, interstitial nephritis, itching, leukopenia, liver enzymes

increased, malaise, mucosal bleeding, nausea, pseudomembranous colitis, seizure, stomatitis, substernal pain, throat tightness, thrombocytopenia, urine retention, vomiting

Drug Interactions

Metabolism/Transport Effects None known.

Avoid Concomitant Use

Avoid concomitant use of Ampicillin and Sulbactam with any of the following: BCG

Increased Effect/Toxicity

Ampicillin and Sulbactam may increase the levels/effects of: Methotrexate; Vitamin K Antagonists

The levels/effects of Ampicillin and Sulbactam may be increased by: Allopurinol; Probenecid

Decreased Effect

Ampicillin and Sulbactam may decrease the levels/effects of: Atenolol; BCG; Mycophenolate; Sodium Picosulfate; Typhoid Vaccine

The levels/effects of Ampicillin and Sulbactam may be decreased by: Chloroquine; Lanthanum; Tetracycline Derivatives

Preparation for Administration I.M. and direct I.V. administration: Use within several hours after preparation. Reconstitute with sterile water for injection or 0.5% or 2% lidocaine hydrochloride injection (I.M.). Sodium chloride 0.9% (NS) is the diluent of choice for I.V. piggyback use.

Storage/Stability Prior to reconstitution, store at controlled room temperature 20°C to 25°C (68°F to 77°F). Solutions made in NS are stable up to 72 hours when refrigerated whereas dextrose solutions (same concentration) are stable for only 4 hours. For stability related to specific concentrations and temperatures, see prescribing information.

Mechanism of Action Inhibits bacterial cell wall synthesis by binding to one or more of the penicillin-binding proteins (PBPs) which in turn inhibits the final transpeptidation step of peptidoglycan synthesis in bacterial cell walls, thus inhibiting cell wall biosynthesis. Bacteria eventually lyse due to ongoing activity of cell wall autolytic enzymes (autolysins and murein hydrolases) while cell wall assembly is arrested. The addition of sulbactam, a beta-lactamase inhibitor, to ampicillin extends the spectrum of ampicillin to include some beta-lactamase-producing organisms.

Pharmacodynamics/Kinetics

Ampicillin: See Ampicillin monograph.

Sulbactam:

Distribution: Widely distributed to bile, blister, and tissue fluids; distributed to cerebrospinal fluid in the presence of inflamed meninges

Protein binding: 38%

Half-life elimination: Normal renal function: 1-1.3 hours; **Note:** Elimination kinetics of both ampicillin and sulbactam are similarly affected in patients with renal impairment, therefore, the blood concentration ratio is expected to remain constant regardless of renal function.

Excretion: Urine (~75% to 85% as unchanged drug) within 8 hours

Dosage Note: Unasyn® (ampicillin/sulbactam) is a combination product.

Usual dosage range:

Children and Adolescents: I.V.: 100-400 mg ampicillin/kg/day divided every 6 hours (maximum: 8 g ampicillin daily, 12 g Unasyn®). **Note:** The American Academy of Pediatrics recommends a dose of up to 300 mg ampicillin/kg/day for severe infection in infants >1 month of age.

Adults: I.M., I.V.: 1000-2000 mg ampicillin (1500-3000 mg Unasyn®) every 6 hours (maximum: 8 g ampicillin daily, 12 g Unasyn®)

Indication-specific dosing:

Infants, Children, and Adolescents:

Endocarditis (unlabeled use) (Baddour, 2005): *Enterococcus organism (resistant to penicillin/susceptible to aminoglycoside and vancomycin):* I.V.: 300 mg ampicillin/kg/day in 4 divided doses with concomitant gentamicin for 6 weeks

Intravascular catheter-associated bloodstream infection (unlabeled use) (IDSA, 2009):

Infants: I.V.: 100-150 mg ampicillin/kg/day in 4 divided doses

Children and Adolescents: I.V.: 100-200 mg ampicillin/kg/day in 4 divided doses

Children and Adolescents:

Epiglottitis: I.V.: 100-200 mg ampicillin/kg/day divided in 4 doses

Mild-to-moderate infections: I.V.: 100-200 mg ampicillin/kg/day (150-300 mg Unasyn®) divided every 6 hours (maximum: 8 g ampicillin daily, 12 g Unasyn®)

Peritonsillar and retropharyngeal abscess: I.V.: 200 mg ampicillin/kg/day in 4 divided doses

Severe infections: I.V.: 200-400 mg ampicillin/kg/day divided every 6 hours (maximum: 8 g ampicillin daily, 12 g Unasyn®)

Surgical (perioperative) prophylaxis (unlabeled use): Children ≥1 year: I.V.: 50 mg ampicillin/kg within 60 minutes prior to surgical incision (maximum dose: 2000 mg ampicillin). Doses may be repeated in 2 hours if procedure is lengthy or if there is excessive blood loss (Bratzler, 2013).

Adults: Doses expressed as ampicillin/sulbactam combination:

Acute bacterial rhinosinusitis, severe infection requiring hospitalization (unlabeled use): I.V.: 1500-3000 mg every 6 hours for 5-7 days (Chow, 2012)

Amnionitis, cholangitis, diverticulitis, endomyometritis (with doxycycline), endophthalmitis, epididymitis/orchitis, liver abscess (with metronidazole), or peritonitis: I.V.: 3000 mg every 6 hours

Bite (human, canine/feline): *Pasteurella multocida:* I.V.: 1500-3000 mg every 6 hours

Endocarditis (unlabeled use) (Baddour, 2005):

Enterococcus organism (resistant to penicillin/susceptible to aminoglycoside and vancomycin): I.V.: 3000 mg every 6 hours with concomitant gentamicin for 6 weeks. **Note:** If enterococcus is gentamicin resistant, then >6 weeks of ampicillin-sulbactam therapy needed.

HACEK organism: I.V.: 3000 mg every 6 hours for 4 weeks

Intravascular catheter-associated bloodstream infection, *Acinetobacter* spp (unlabeled use) (IDSA, 2009): I.V.: 3000 mg every 6 hours

Orbital cellulitis: I.V.: 3000 mg every 6 hours

Osteomyelitis (diabetic foot) (Lipsky, 2004): I.V.: 3000 mg every 6 hours

Pelvic inflammatory disease: I.V.: 3000 mg every 6 hours with doxycycline

Peritonitis associated with CAPD: Intraperitoneal:

Intermittent: 3000 mg added to one exchange every 12 hours; allow to dwell for at least 6 hours (Blackwell, 1990; Li, 2010)

Continuous: Loading dose: 1500 mg per liter of dialysate; maintenance dose: 150 mg per liter of dialysate (Li, 2010)

Pneumonia:

Aspiration or community-acquired: I.V.: 1500-3000 mg every 6 hours

Hospital-acquired: I.V.: 3000 mg every 6 hours

Surgical (perioperative) prophylaxis (unlabeled use): I.V.: 3000 mg within 60 minutes prior to surgical incision. Doses may be repeated in 2 hours if procedure is lengthy or if there is excessive blood loss (Bratzler, 2013).

Urinary tract infections, pyelonephritis: I.V.: 3000 mg every 6 hours for 14 days

Dosage adjustment in renal impairment: Note: Estimation of renal function for the purpose of drug dosing should be done using the Cockcroft-Gault formula.

Cl_{cr} 15-29 mL/minute/1.73 m^2: 1500-3000 mg every 12 hours

Cl_{cr} 5-14 mL/minute/1.73 m^2: 1500-3000 mg every 24 hours

Intermittent hemodialysis (IHD) (administer after hemodialysis on dialysis days): 1500-3000 mg every 12-24 hours (Heintz, 2009). **Note:** Dosing dependent on the assumption of 3 times weekly, complete IHD sessions.

Peritoneal dialysis (PD): 3000 mg every 24 hours

Continuous renal replacement therapy (CRRT): Drug clearance is highly dependent on the method of renal replacement, filter type, and flow rate. Appropriate dosing requires close monitoring of pharmacologic response, signs of adverse reactions due to drug accumulation, as well as drug levels in relation to target trough (if appropriate). The following are general recommendations only (based on dialysate flow/ultrafiltration rates of 1-2 L/hour and minimal residual renal function) and should not supersede clinical judgment (Heintz, 2009; Trotman, 2005):

CVVH: Initial: 3000 mg; maintenance: 1500-3000 mg every 8-12 hours

CVVHD: Initial: 3000 mg; maintenance: 1500-3000 mg every 8 hours

CVVHDF: Initial: 3000 mg; maintenance: 1500-3000 mg every 6-8 hours

Dosage adjustment in hepatic impairment: No dosage adjustment provided in manufacturer's labeling.

Dietary Considerations Some products may contain sodium.

Administration Administer around-the-clock to promote less variation in peak and trough serum levels. Administer by slow injection over 10-15 minutes or I.V. over 15-30 minutes. Ampicillin and gentamicin should not be mixed in the same I.V. tubing.

Some penicillins (eg, ampicillin, carbenicillin, ticarcillin, and piperacillin) have been shown to inactivate aminoglycosides *in vitro*. This has been observed to a greater extent with tobramycin and gentamicin, while amikacin has shown greater stability against inactivation. Concurrent Y-site administration should be avoided.

Monitoring Parameters With prolonged therapy, monitor hematologic, renal, and hepatic function; monitor for signs of anaphylaxis during first dose

Test Interactions May interfere with urinary glucose tests using cupric sulfate (Benedict's solution, Clinitest®).

Some penicillin derivatives may accelerate the degradation of aminoglycosides *in vitro*, leading to a potential underestimation of aminoglycoside serum concentration.

Dosage Forms Excipient information presented when available (limited, particularly for generics); consult specific product labeling.

Injection, powder for reconstitution: 1.5 g: Ampicillin 1 g and sulbactam 0.5 g; 3 g: Ampicillin 2 g and sulbactam 1 g; 15 g: Ampicillin 10 g and sulbactam 5 g

Unasyn®:

1.5 g: Ampicillin 1 g and sulbactam 0.5 g [contains sodium 115 mg (5 mEq)/1.5 g)]

3 g: Ampicillin 2 g and sulbactam 1 g [contains sodium 115 mg (5 mEq)/1.5 g)]

15 g: Ampicillin 10 g and sulbactam 5 g [bulk package; contains sodium 115 mg (5 mEq)/1.5 g)]

- ◆ **Ampicillin for Injection (Can)** *see* Ampicillin *on page 130*
- ◆ **Ampicillin Sodium** *see* Ampicillin *on page 130*
- ◆ **Ampicillin Trihydrate** *see* Ampicillin *on page 130*
- ◆ **AMPT** *see* Metyrosine *on page 1355*
- ◆ **Ampyra** *see* Dalfampridine *on page 534*
- ◆ **AMR101** *see* Icosapent Ethyl *on page 1038*
- ◆ **Amrix** *see* Cyclobenzaprine *on page 502*
- ◆ **Amturnide™** *see* Aliskiren, Amlodipine, and Hydrochlorothiazide *on page 76*
- ◆ **Amvisc** *see* Hyaluronate and Derivatives *on page 1000*
- ◆ **Amvisc Plus** *see* Hyaluronate and Derivatives *on page 1000*
- ◆ **Amylase, Lipase, and Protease** *see* Pancrelipase *on page 1558*

Amyl Nitrite (AM il NYE trite)

Index Terms Isoamyl Nitrite

Pharmacologic Category Antianginal Agent; Antidote; Vasodilator

Use Coronary vasodilator in angina pectoris

Note: Given the widespread use of newer nitrate compounds, the use of amyl nitrite for patients experiencing angina pectoris has fallen out of favor.

Unlabeled Use Adjunct treatment of cyanide toxicity; produce changes in the intensity of heart murmurs; provocation of latent left ventricular outflow tract (LVOT) gradient during echocardiography in patients with hypertrophic cardiomyopathy (HCM)

Pregnancy Risk Factor C

Dosage Inhalation:

Angina: Adults: 2-6 nasal inhalations from 1 crushed ampul; may repeat in 3-5 minutes

Cyanide poisoning (unlabeled use): Children and Adults: 0.3 mL ampul crushed into a gauze pad and placed in front of the patient's mouth (or endotracheal tube if patient is intubated) to inhale over 15-30 seconds; repeat every minute until sodium nitrite can be administered. **Note:** Must separate administrations by at least 30 seconds to allow for adequate oxygenation; each ampul will last for ~3 minutes Amyl nitrite is a temporary intervention that should only be used until I.V. sodium nitrite infusion is ready for administration.

Pharmacologic provocation of latent left ventricular outflow tract (LVOT) gradient in hypertrophic cardiomyopathy (HCM) (unlabeled use): Adults: 3-4 deep inhalations from 1 crushed ampul over a 10-15 second period (Gersh, 2011; Nagueh, 2011; Reagan, 2005). **Note:** The use of more physiologic testing (eg, treadmill testing with Doppler echocardiography) may be preferred over amyl nitrite inhalation (Maron, 2003: Nagueh, 2011).

Additional Information Complete prescribing information should be consulted for additional detail.

Dosage Forms Excipient information presented when available (limited, particularly for generics); consult specific product labeling.

Liquid, for inhalation: USP: 85% to 103% (0.3 mL)

- ◆ **Amylobarbitone** *see* Amobarbital *on page 114*
- ◆ **Amytal® (Can)** *see* Amobarbital *on page 114*
- ◆ **Amytal Sodium** *see* Amobarbital *on page 114*

- **AN100226** *see* Natalizumab *on page 1431*
- **Anacaine** *see* Benzocaine *on page 240*
- **Anacin® Advanced Headache Formula [OTC]** *see* Acetaminophen, Aspirin, and Caffeine *on page 33*
- **Anadrol-50** *see* Oxymetholone *on page 1539*
- **Anafranil** *see* ClomiPRAMINE *on page 462*
- **Anafranil® (Can)** *see* ClomiPRAMINE *on page 462*

Anagrelide (an AG gre lide)

Brand Names: U.S. Agrylin

Brand Names: Canada Agrylin; Dom-Anagrelide; Mylan-Anagrelide; PMS-Anagrelide; Sandoz-Anagrelide

Index Terms Anagrelide Hydrochloride; BL4162A

Pharmacologic Category Phosphodiesterase-3 Enzyme Inhibitor; Phospholipase A_2 Inhibitor

Use Thrombocythemia: Treatment of thrombocythemia associated with myeloproliferative disorders (eg, chronic myelogenous leukemia, essential thrombocythemia, polycythemia vera, myeloid metaplasia with myelofibrosis, or other myeloproliferative disorder) to reduce the risk of thrombosis and reduce associated symptoms (including thrombohemorrhagic events)

Pregnancy Risk Factor C

Dosage Note: Maintain initial dose for ≥1 week, then adjust to the lowest effective dose to reduce and maintain platelet count <600,000/mm^3 ideally to the normal range; the dose must not be increased by >0.5 mg per day in any 1 week; maximum single dose: 2.5 mg; maximum daily dose: 10 mg

Thrombocythemia:

Children: Oral: Initial: 0.5 mg once daily (range: 0.5 mg 1-4 times daily)

Adults: Oral: Initial: 0.5 mg 4 times daily or 1 mg twice daily (most patients will experience adequate response at dose ranges of 1.5-3 mg per day)

Thrombocythemia, essential (unlabeled dosing): Adults: Oral: 0.5 mg twice daily for 1 week, then adjust dose to maintain platelet counts at normal (≤450,000/mm^3) or near normal (450,000/mm^3 to 600,000/mm^3) levels (Gisslinger, 2013).

Elderly: There are no special requirements for dosing in the elderly

Dosage adjustment in renal impairment: Renal insufficiency: No dosage adjustment necessary; monitor closely.

Dosage adjustment in hepatic impairment:

Moderate impairment: Initial: 0.5 mg once daily; maintain for at least 1 week with careful monitoring of cardiovascular status; the dose must not be increased by >0.5 mg per day in any 1 week.

Severe impairment: Use is contraindicated.

Additional Information Complete prescribing information should be consulted for additional detail.

Dosage Forms Excipient information presented when available (limited, particularly for generics); consult specific product labeling.

Capsule, Oral:

Agrylin: 0.5 mg

Generic: 0.5 mg, 1 mg

- **Anagrelide Hydrochloride** *see* Anagrelide *on page 136*

Anakinra (an a KIN ra)

Brand Names: U.S. Kineret

Brand Names: Canada Kineret®

Index Terms IL-1Ra; Interleukin-1 Receptor Antagonist

Pharmacologic Category Antirheumatic, Disease Modifying; Interleukin-1 Receptor Antagonist

Use Treatment of moderately- to severely-active rheumatoid arthritis (RA) in adult patients who have failed one or more disease-modifying antirheumatic drugs (DMARDs; may be used alone or in combination with DMARDs [other than tumor necrosis factor-blocking agents]); treatment of neonatal-onset multisystem inflammatory disease (NOMID), which is a cryopyrin-associated periodic syndrome (CAPS)

Pregnancy Risk Factor B

Pregnancy Considerations Animal reproduction studies have not revealed any evidence of impaired fertility or harm to fetus. Women exposed to anakinra during pregnancy may contact the Organization of Teratology Information Services (OTIS), Rheumatoid Arthritis and Pregnancy Study at 1-877-311-8972.

Breast-Feeding Considerations Endogenous interleukin-1 receptor antagonist can be found in breast milk; although specific excretion of anakinra is not known. Use caution if administering to a nursing woman.

Contraindications Hypersensitivity to *E. coli*-derived proteins, anakinra, or any component of the formulation

Warnings/Precautions Anakinra is associated with an increased risk of infection in rheumatoid arthritis studies. Do not initiate in patients with an active infection. Patients who develop a new infection while undergoing treatment should be monitored closely. If a patient receiving anakinra for rheumatoid arthritis develops a serious infection, therapy should be discontinued; if a patient receiving anakinra for neonatal-onset multisystem inflammatory disease (NOMID) develop a serious infection, the risk of a NOMID flare should be weighed against the risks associated with continued treatment. Safety and efficacy have not been evaluated in immunosuppressed patients or patients with chronic infections; the impact on active or chronic infections has not been determined. Immunosuppressive therapy (including anakinra) may lead to reactivation of latent tuberculosis or other atypical or opportunistic infections; test patients for latent TB prior to initiation, and treat latent TB infection prior to use.

A decrease in neutrophil count may occur during treatment; assess neutrophil count at baseline, monthly for 3 months, then every 3 months for up to 1 year; in a limited number of patients with NOMID, neutropenia resolved over time with continued anakinra administration. May affect defenses against malignancies; impact on the development and course of malignancies is not fully defined; as compared to the general population, an increased risk of lymphoma has been noted in clinical trials; however, rheumatoid arthritis has been previously associated with an increased rate of lymphoma.

Potentially significant drug-drug interactions may exist, requiring dose or frequency adjustment, additional monitoring, and/or selection of alternative therapy. Use is not recommended in combination with tumor necrosis factor antagonists. Patients should be brought up to date with all immunizations before initiating therapy; live vaccines should not be given concurrently; there is no data available concerning the effects of therapy on vaccination or secondary transmission of live vaccines in patients receiving therapy. Hypersensitivity reactions, including anaphylactic reactions and angioedema have been reported; discontinue use if severe hypersensitivity occurs. Injection site reactions commonly occur and are generally mild with a duration of 14-28 days. Use caution in patients with renal impairment; extended dosing intervals (every other day) are recommended for severe renal insufficiency (Cl_{cr} <30 mL/minute) and ESRD. Use with caution in patients with asthma; may have increased risk of serious infection. Use caution in the elderly due to the potential for higher risk of infections. The packaging (needle cover) contains latex.

Adverse Reactions

>10%:

Central nervous system: Headache (12% to 14%), fever (12%)

Gastrointestinal: Nausea (8%)

Local: Injection site reaction (RA: ≤71%; mild: 73%; moderate; 24%; severe: 3%; NOMID: 16%)

Neuromuscular & skeletal: Arthralgia (6% to 12%)

Respiratory: Nasopharyngitis (12%)

Miscellaneous: Infection (39% versus 37% in placebo; serious infection 2% to 3%)

1% to 10%:

Gastrointestinal: Diarrhea (7%)

Hematologic: Neutropenia (5% to 8%)

<1% (Limited to important or life-threatening): Cellulitis, hypersensitivity reactions (including anaphylaxis, angioedema, pruritus, rash, urticaria), leukopenia, opportunistic infection, pneumonia (bacterial), pulmonary fibrosis, secondary malignancies (including lymphoma, melanoma), thrombocytopenia

Drug Interactions

Metabolism/Transport Effects None known.

Avoid Concomitant Use

Avoid concomitant use of Anakinra with any of the following: Abatacept; Anti-TNF Agents; BCG; Canakinumab; Natalizumab; Pimecrolimus; Tacrolimus (Topical); Tofacitinib; Vaccines (Live)

Increased Effect/Toxicity

Anakinra may increase the levels/effects of: Abatacept; Canakinumab; Leflunomide; Natalizumab; Tofacitinib; Vaccines (Live)

The levels/effects of Anakinra may be increased by: Anti-TNF Agents; Denosumab; Pimecrolimus; Roflumilast; Tacrolimus (Topical); Trastuzumab

Decreased Effect

Anakinra may decrease the levels/effects of: BCG; Coccidioidin Skin Test; Sipuleucel-T; Vaccines (Inactivated); Vaccines (Live)

The levels/effects of Anakinra may be decreased by: Echinacea

Storage/Stability Store in refrigerator at 2°C to 8°C (36°F to 46°F); do not freeze. Do not shake. Protect from light.

Mechanism of Action Antagonist of the interleukin-1 (IL-1) receptor. Endogenous IL-1 is induced by inflammatory stimuli and mediates a variety of immunological responses, including degradation of cartilage (loss of proteoglycans) and stimulation of bone resorption.

Pharmacodynamics/Kinetics

Bioavailability: SubQ: 95%

Half-life elimination: Terminal: 4-6 hours; Severe renal impairment (Cl_{cr} <30 mL/minute): ~7 hours; ESRD: 9.7 hours (Yang, 2003)

Time to peak: SubQ: 3-7 hours

Dosage

Neonatal-onset multisystem inflammatory disease (NOMID): Infants, Children, Adolescents, and Adults: SubQ: Initial: 1-2 mg/kg daily in 1-2 divided doses; adjust dose in 0.5-1 mg/kg increments as needed; usual maintenance dose: 3-4 mg/kg daily (maximum: 8 mg/kg daily). **Note:** The prefilled syringe does not allow doses lower than 20 mg to be administered.

Rheumatoid arthritis (RA): Adults: SubQ: 100 mg once daily (administer at approximately the same time each day)

Dosage adjustment in renal impairment:

Cl_{cr} ≥30 mL/minute: No dosage adjustment necessary.

Cl_{cr} <30 mL/minute:

NOMID: Infants, Children, Adolescents, and Adults: No dosage adjustment necessary; however, decrease frequency of administration to every other day.

RA: Adults: 100 mg every other day

ESRD (**Note:** <2.5% of the dose is removed by hemodialysis or CAPD):

NOMID: Infants, Children, Adolescents, and Adults: No dosage adjustment necessary; however, decrease frequency of administration to every other day.

RA: Adults: 100 mg every other day

Dosage adjustment in hepatic impairment: No dosage adjustments provided in the manufacturer's labeling (has not been studied).

Administration SubQ: Inject into outer area of upper arms, abdomen (do not use within 2 inches of belly button), front of middle thighs, or upper outer buttocks. Rotate injection sites. Allow solution to warm to room temperature prior to use (30 minutes). Do not shake. Provided in single-use, preservative free syringes with 27-gauge needles; discard any unused portion. When used for the treatment of neonatal-onset multisystem inflammatory disease (NOMID), once-daily administration is preferred; however, the dose may also be divided and administered twice daily.

pH: 6.5 (solution in syringe)

Monitoring Parameters CBC with differential (baseline, then monthly for 3 months, then every 3 months for a period up to 1 year); TB test (baseline); serum creatinine; signs/symptoms of infection

Additional Information Anakinra is produced by recombinant DNA/*E. coli* technology.

Dosage Forms Excipient information presented when available (limited, particularly for generics); consult specific product labeling.

Solution, Subcutaneous [preservative free]:

Kineret: 100 mg/0.67 mL (0.67 mL) [contains disodium edta, polysorbate 80]

◆ **Analpram E™** *see* Pramoxine and Hydrocortisone *on page 1699*

◆ **Analpram HC®** *see* Pramoxine and Hydrocortisone *on page 1699*

◆ **Anandron® (Can)** *see* Nilutamide *on page 1459*

◆ **Anaprox** *see* Naproxen *on page 1425*

◆ **Anaprox DS** *see* Naproxen *on page 1425*

◆ **Anascorp** *see* *Centruroides* Immune F(ab')$_2$ (Equine) *on page 390*

◆ **Anaspaz** *see* Hyoscyamine *on page 1026*

Anastrozole (an AS troe zole)

Brand Names: U.S. Arimidex

Brand Names: Canada Apo-Anastrozole; Arimidex; Auro-Anastrozole; Bio-Anastrozole; Co-Anastrozole; JAMP-Anastrozole; Mar-Anastrozole; Med-Anastrozole; Mint-Anastrozole; Mylan-Anastrozole; PMS-Anastrozole; Riva-Anastrozole; Sandoz-Anastrozole; Taro-Anastrozole; Teva-Anastrozole; Zinda-Anastrozole

Index Terms ICI-D1033; ZD1033

Pharmacologic Category Antineoplastic Agent, Aromatase Inhibitor

Use Breast cancer:

First-line treatment of locally-advanced or metastatic breast cancer (hormone receptor-positive or unknown) in postmenopausal women

Adjuvant treatment of early hormone receptor-positive breast cancer in postmenopausal women

Treatment of advanced breast cancer in postmenopausal women with disease progression following tamoxifen therapy

Unlabeled Use Treatment of recurrent or metastatic endometrial or uterine cancers, treatment of recurrent ovarian cancer

Pregnancy Risk Factor X

Pregnancy Considerations Adverse events were observed in animal reproduction studies. Anastrozole is contraindicated in women who are or may become pregnant (may cause fetal harm if administered during pregnancy). Use in premenopausal women with breast cancer does not provide any clinical benefit.

Breast-Feeding Considerations It is not known if anastrozole is excreted in breast milk. Due to the potential for serious adverse reactions in the nursing infant, a decision should be made whether to discontinue nursing or to discontinue the drug, taking into account the importance of treatment to the mother. The Canadian labeling contraindicates use in lactating women.

Contraindications Hypersensitivity to anastrozole or any component of the formulation; use in women who are or may become pregnant

Canadian labeling: Additional contraindications (not in U.S. labeling): Lactating women

Warnings/Precautions Hazardous agent - use appropriate precautions for handling and disposal (NIOSH, 2012). Use is contraindicated in women who are or may become pregnant. Anastrozole offers no clinical benefit in premenopausal women with breast cancer. Patients with pre-existing ischemic cardiac disease have an increased risk for ischemic cardiovascular events.

Due to decreased circulating estrogen levels, anastrozole is associated with a reduction in bone mineral density (BMD); decreases (from baseline) in total hip and lumbar spine BMD have been reported. Patients with pre-existing osteopenia are at higher risk for developing osteoporosis (Eastell, 2008). When initiating anastrozole treatment, follow available guidelines for bone mineral density management in postmenopausal women with similar fracture risk; concurrent use of bisphosphonates may be useful in patients at risk for fractures.

Elevated total cholesterol levels (contributed to by LDL cholesterol increases) have been reported in patients receiving anastrozole; use with caution in patients with hyperlipidemias; cholesterol levels should be monitored/managed in accordance with current guidelines for patients with LDL elevations. Plasma concentrations in patients with stable hepatic cirrhosis were within the range of concentrations seen in normal subjects across all clinical trials; use has not been studied in patients with severe hepatic impairment. Safety and efficacy in children have not been established.

Adverse Reactions

>10%:

Cardiovascular: Vasodilatation (25% to 36%), ischemic heart disease (4%; 17% in patients with pre-existing ischemic heart disease), hypertension (2% to 13%), angina pectoris (2%; 12% in patients with pre-existing ischemic heart disease), edema (7% to 11%)

Central nervous system: Fatigue (19%), mood disorder (19%), headache (9% to 18%), pain (11% to 17%), depression (2% to 13%)

Dermatologic: Skin rash (6% to 11%)

Endocrine & metabolic: Hot flash (12% to 36%)

Gastrointestinal: Gastrointestinal distress (29% to 34%), nausea (11% to 20%), vomiting (8% to 13%)

Neuromuscular & skeletal: Weakness (13% to 19%), arthritis (17%), arthralgia (2% to 15%), back pain (10% to 12%), ostealgia (6% to 12%), osteoporosis (11%)

Respiratory: Pharyngitis (6% to 14%), dyspnea (8% to 11%), increased cough (7% to 11%)

1% to 10%:

Cardiovascular: Peripheral edema (5% to 10%), chest pain (5% to 7%), venous thrombosis (2% to 4%; including pulmonary embolism, thrombophlebitis, retinal vein thrombosis), myocardial infarction (1%)

Central nervous system: Insomnia (2% to 10%), dizziness (5% to 8%), paresthesia (5% to 7%), anxiety (2% to 6%), confusion (2% to 5%), drowsiness (2% to 5%), malaise (2% to 5%), nervousness (2% to 5%), carpal tunnel syndrome (3%), hypertonia (3%), cerebrovascular insufficiency (2%), lethargy (1%)

Dermatologic: Alopecia (2% to 5%), pruritus (2% to 5%), diaphoresis (1% to 5%)

Endocrine & metabolic: Hypercholesterolemia (9%), increased serum cholesterol (9%), weight gain (2% to 9%), increased gamma-glutamyl transferase (2% to 5%), weight loss (2% to 5%)

Gastrointestinal: Constipation (7% to 9%), diarrhea (7% to 9%), abdominal pain (6% to 9%), anorexia (5% to 8%), dyspepsia (7%), gastrointestinal disease (7%), xerostomia (4% to 6%)

Genitourinary: Mastalgia (2% to 8%), urinary tract infection (2% to 8%), pelvic pain (5% to 7%), vulvovaginitis (6%), vaginal dryness (1% to 5%), vaginal hemorrhage (1% to 5%), vaginal discharge (4%), vaginitis (4%), leukorrhea (2% to 3%)

Hematologic & oncologic: Lymphedema (10%), breast neoplasm (5%), neoplasm (5%), anemia (2% to 5%), leukopenia (2% to 5%), tumor flare (3%)

Hepatic: Increased serum alkaline phosphatase (2% to 5%), increased serum ALT (2% to 5%), increased serum AST (2% to 5%)

Infection: Infection (2% to 9%)

Neuromuscular & skeletal: Bone fracture (1% to 10%), arthrosis (7%), myalgia (2% to 6%), neck pain (2% to 5%), pathological fracture (2% to 5%)

Ophthalmic: Cataract (6%)

Respiratory: Flu-like symptoms (2% to 7%), sinusitis (2% to 6%), bronchitis (2% to 5%), rhinitis (2% to 5%)

Miscellaneous: Accidental injury (2% to 10%), cyst (5%), fever (2% to 5%)

<1% (Limited to important or life-threatening): Anaphylaxis, angioedema, cerebral infarction, cerebral ischemia, dermal ulcer, endometrial carcinoma, erythema multiforme, hepatitis, hepatomegaly, hypercalcemia, hypersensitivity angiitis (including anaphylactoid purpura [IgA vasculitis]), jaundice, joint stiffness, pulmonary embolism, retinal thrombosis, skin blister, skin lesion, Stevens-Johnson syndrome, tenosynovitis (stenosing), urticaria

Drug Interactions

Metabolism/Transport Effects Inhibits CYP1A2 (weak), CYP2C8 (weak), CYP2C9 (weak), CYP3A4 (weak)

Avoid Concomitant Use

Avoid concomitant use of Anastrozole with any of the following: Estrogen Derivatives; Pimozide

Increased Effect/Toxicity

Anastrozole may increase the levels/effects of: ARIPiprazole; Dofetilide; Lomitapide; Methadone; Pimozide; Vitamin K Antagonists

Decreased Effect

Anastrozole may decrease the levels/effects of: Cardiac Glycosides; Vitamin K Antagonists

The levels/effects of Anastrozole may be decreased by: Estrogen Derivatives; Tamoxifen

Storage/Stability Store at 20°C to 25°C (68°F to 77°F).

Mechanism of Action Potent and selective nonsteroidal aromatase inhibitor. By inhibiting aromatase, the conversion of androstenedione to estrone, and testosterone to estradiol, is prevented, thereby decreasing tumor mass or delaying progression in patients with tumors responsive to hormones. Anastrozole causes an 85% decrease in estrone sulfate levels.

Pharmacodynamics/Kinetics

Onset of estradiol reduction: 70% reduction after 24 hours; 80% after 2 weeks therapy

Duration of estradiol reduction: 6 days

Absorption: Well absorbed; extent of absorption not affected by food
Protein binding, plasma: 40%
Metabolism: Extensively hepatic (~85%) via N-dealkylation, hydroxylation, and glucuronidation; primary metabolite (triazole) inactive
Half-life elimination: ~50 hours
Time to peak, plasma: ~2 hours without food; 5 hours with food
Excretion: Feces; urine (urinary excretion accounts for ~10% of total elimination, mostly as metabolites)

Dosage Oral: Adults: Females: Postmenopausal:
Breast cancer, advanced: 1 mg once daily; continue until tumor progression
Breast cancer, early (adjuvant treatment): 1 mg once daily; optimal duration unknown, duration in clinical trial is 5 years

Dosage adjustment in renal impairment: No dosage adjustment necessary.
Dosage adjustment in hepatic impairment:
Mild to moderate impairment or stable hepatic cirrhosis: No dosage adjustment necessary.
Severe hepatic impairment: No dosage adjustment provided in manufacturer's labeling (has not been studied).

Dietary Considerations May be taken with or without food.

Administration May be administered with or without food.
Hazardous agent; use appropriate precautions for handling and disposal (NIOSH, 2012).

Monitoring Parameters Bone mineral density; total cholesterol and LDL

Additional Information Oncology Comment: The American Society of Clinical Oncology (ASCO) guidelines for adjuvant endocrine therapy in postmenopausal women with HR-positive breast cancer (Burstein, 2010) recommend considering aromatase inhibitor (AI) therapy at some point in the treatment course (primary, sequentially, or extended). Optimal duration at this time is not known; however, treatment with an AI should not exceed 5 years in primary and extended therapies, and 2-3 years if followed by tamoxifen in sequential therapy (total of 5 years). If initial therapy with AI has been discontinued before the 5 years, consideration should be taken to receive tamoxifen for a total of 5 years. The optimal time to switch to an AI is also not known, but data supports switching after 2-3 years of tamoxifen (sequential) or after 5 years of tamoxifen (extended). If patient becomes intolerant or has poor adherence, consideration should be made to switch to another AI or initiate tamoxifen.

Dosage Forms Excipient information presented when available (limited, particularly for generics); consult specific product labeling.
Tablet, Oral:
Arimidex: 1 mg
Generic: 1 mg

- **Anbesol [OTC]** *see* Benzocaine *on page* 240
- **Anbesol® Baby (Can)** *see* Benzocaine *on page* 240
- **Anbesol Cold Sore Therapy [OTC]** *see* Benzocaine *on page* 240
- **Anbesol JR [OTC]** *see* Benzocaine *on page* 240
- **Anbesol Maximum Strength [OTC]** *see* Benzocaine *on page* 240
- **Ancef** *see* CeFAZolin *on page* 362
- **Anchoic Acid** *see* Azelaic Acid *on page* 211
- **Ancobon** *see* Flucytosine *on page* 871
- **Andriol® (Can)** *see* Testosterone *on page* 2026
- **Androderm** *see* Testosterone *on page* 2026
- **Androderm® (Can)** *see* Testosterone *on page* 2026
- **AndroGel** *see* Testosterone *on page* 2026
- **AndroGel® (Can)** *see* Testosterone *on page* 2026
- **AndroGel Pump** *see* Testosterone *on page* 2026
- **Android** *see* MethylTESTOSTERone *on page* 1344
- **Andropository (Can)** *see* Testosterone *on page* 2026
- **Androxy** *see* Fluoxymesterone *on page* 889
- **AneCream [OTC]** *see* Lidocaine (Topical) *on page* 1212
- **AneCream5 [OTC]** *see* Lidocaine (Topical) *on page* 1212
- **Anectine** *see* Succinylcholine *on page* 1954
- **Aneurine Hydrochloride** *see* Thiamine *on page* 2045
- **Anexate (Can)** *see* Flumazenil *on page* 877
- **Angiomax** *see* Bivalirudin *on page* 262
- **Angiomax® (Can)** *see* Bivalirudin *on page* 262

Anidulafungin (ay nid yoo la FUN jin)

Brand Names: U.S. Eraxis
Brand Names: Canada Eraxis
Index Terms LY303366
Pharmacologic Category Antifungal Agent, Parenteral; Echinocandin
Additional Appendix Information
Antifungal Agents *on page* 2286

Use Treatment of candidemia and other forms of *Candida* infections (including those of intra-abdominal, peritoneal, and esophageal locus)

Pregnancy Risk Factor B

Pregnancy Considerations Adverse effects were observed in animal reproduction studies.

Breast-Feeding Considerations It is not known if anidulafungin is excreted in breast milk. The manufacturer recommends that caution be exercised when administering anidulafungin to nursing women.

Contraindications Hypersensitivity to anidulafungin, other echinocandins, or any component of the formulation

Warnings/Precautions Severe hypersensitivity reactions, including anaphylactic reactions and anaphylactic shock have been reported; immediate treatment for hypersensitivity reactions should be available. Discontinue treatment immediately if reactions occur. Infusion reactions (eg, bronchospasm, dyspnea, flushing, hypotension, pruritus, rash, urticaria) may occur; do not exceed rate of infusion. Elevated liver function tests, hepatitis, and hepatic failure have been reported. Monitor for progressive hepatic impairment if increased transaminase enzymes noted. Safety and efficacy have not been established in other *Candida* infections (eg, endocarditis, osteomyelitis, meningitis).

Adverse Reactions
>10%:
Cardiovascular: Hypotension (15%), hypertension (12%), peripheral edema (11%)
Central nervous system: Fever (9% to 18%), insomnia (15%)
Endocrine & metabolic: Hypokalemia (≤25%), hypomagnesemia (12%)
Gastrointestinal: Nausea (7% to 24%), diarrhea (9% to 18%), vomiting (7% to 18%)
Genitourinary: Urinary tract infection (15%)
Hepatic: Alkaline phosphatase increased (12%)
Respiratory: Dyspnea (12%)
Miscellaneous: Bacteremia (18%)
2% to 10%:
Cardiovascular: Deep vein thrombosis (10%), chest pain (5%)
Central nervous system: Confusion (8%), headache (8%), depression (6%)
Dermatologic: Decubitus ulcer (5%)

Endocrine & metabolic: Hypoglycemia (7%), dehydration (6%), hyperglycemia (6%), hyperkalemia (6%)
Gastrointestinal: Constipation (8%), dyspepsia (7%), abdominal pain (6%), oral candidiasis (5%)
Hematologic: Anemia (8% to 9%), thrombocythemia (6%), leukocytosis (5% to 8%)
Hepatic: Transaminases increased (≤5%)
Neuromuscular & skeletal: Back pain (5%)
Renal: Creatinine increased (5%)
Respiratory: Pleural effusion (10%), cough (7%), pneumonia (6%), respiratory distress (6%)
Miscellaneous: Sepsis (7%)

<2% (Limited to important or life-threatening): Amylase increased, anaphylactic shock, anaphylaxis, angioedema, atrial fibrillation, bundle branch block (right), cholestasis, clostridial infection, coagulopathy, ECG abnormality (including QT prolongation), hepatic dysfunction, hepatic necrosis, hepatitis, infusion-related reaction, prothrombin time prolonged, seizure, sinus arrhythmia, thrombocytopenia, thrombophlebitis, ventricular extrasystoles, vision blurred

Drug Interactions

Metabolism/Transport Effects None known.

Avoid Concomitant Use There are no known interactions where it is recommended to avoid concomitant use.

Increased Effect/Toxicity There are no known significant interactions involving an increase in effect.

Decreased Effect

Anidulafungin may decrease the levels/effects of: Saccharomyces boulardii

Preparation for Administration Aseptically add 15 mL (50 mg vial) or 30 mL (100 mg vial) of sterile water for injection to each vial. Further dilute 50 mg or 100 mg vials in 50 mL or 100 mL, respectively, of D_5W or NS.

Storage/Stability Store vials at 2°C to 8°C (36°F to 46°F); excursions at 25°C (77°F) are permitted for 96 hours and the vial may be returned to storage at 2°C to 8°C (36°F to 46°F). Do not freeze. The reconstituted solution can be stored for up to 24 hours at temperatures up to 25°C (77°F) prior to dilution into the infusion solution. The infusion solution may be stored for up to 48 hours at temperatures up to 25°C (77°F) or stored in the freezer for ≥72 hours prior to administration.

Mechanism of Action Noncompetitive inhibitor of 1,3-beta-D-glucan synthase resulting in reduced formation of 1,3-beta-D-glucan, an essential polysaccharide comprising 30% to 60% of *Candida* cell walls (absent in mammalian cells); decreased glucan content leads to osmotic instability and cellular lysis

Pharmacodynamics/Kinetics

Distribution: 30-50 L
Protein binding: ~99%
Metabolism: No hepatic metabolism observed; undergoes slow chemical hydrolysis to open-ring peptide-lacking antifungal activity
Half-life elimination: Terminal: 40-50 hours
Excretion: Feces (30%, 10% as unchanged drug); urine (<1%)

Dosage I.V.: Adults:

Candidemia, intra-abdominal or peritoneal candidiasis: Initial dose: 200 mg on day 1; subsequent dosing: 100 mg daily; treatment should continue until 14 days after last positive culture

Esophageal candidiasis: Initial dose: 100 mg on day 1; subsequent dosing: 50 mg daily; treatment should continue for a minimum of 14 days and for at least 7 days after symptom resolution

Dosage adjustment in renal impairment: No dosage adjustment necessary, including dialysis patients.

Dosage adjustment in hepatic impairment: No dosage adjustment necessary.

Administration For intravenous use only; infusion rate should not exceed 1.1 mg/minute (1.4 mL/minute or 84 mL/hour).

Monitoring Parameters Liver function tests

Dosage Forms Excipient information presented when available (limited, particularly for generics); consult specific product labeling.

Solution Reconstituted, Intravenous [preservative free]:
Eraxis: 50 mg (1 ea); 100 mg (1 ea) [contains polysorbate 80]

◆ Ansaid® (Can) *see* Flurbiprofen (Systemic) *on page 892*
◆ Ansamycin *see* Rifabutin *on page 1809*
◆ Antabuse *see* Disulfiram *on page 637*
◆ Antacid [OTC] *see* Calcium Carbonate *on page 318*
◆ Antacid Extra Strength [OTC] *see* Calcium Carbonate *on page 318*
◆ Antagon *see* Ganirelix *on page 940*
◆ Antara *see* Fenofibrate and Derivatives *on page 837*
◆ Anthraforte® (Can) *see* Anthralin *on page 140*

Anthralin (AN thra lin)

Brand Names: U.S. Dritho-Creme HP; Zithranol; Zithranol-RR

Brand Names: Canada Anthraforte®; Anthranol®; Anthrascalp®; Micanol®

Index Terms Dithranol

Pharmacologic Category Antipsoriatic Agent; Keratolytic Agent

Use Treatment of psoriasis (quiescent or chronic psoriasis)

Pregnancy Risk Factor C

Dosage Children (unlabeled) and Adults: Topical: Generally, apply once a day or as directed. The irritant potential of anthralin is directly related to the strength being used and each patient's individual tolerance. Always commence treatment using a short, daily contact time (5-10 minutes) for at least 1 week using the lowest strength possible. Contact time may be gradually increased (to 20-30 minutes) as tolerated.

Skin application: Apply sparingly only to psoriatic lesions and rub gently and carefully into the skin until absorbed. Avoid applying an excessive quantity which may cause unnecessary soiling and staining of the clothing or bed linen.

Scalp application: Comb hair to remove scalar debris, wet hair and, after suitably parting, rub cream well into the lesions, taking care to prevent the cream from spreading onto the forehead.

Remove by washing or showering; optimal period of contact will vary according to the strength used and the patient's response to treatment. Continue treatment until the skin is entirely clear (ie, when there is nothing to feel with the fingers and the texture is normal).

Additional Information Complete prescribing information should be consulted for additional detail.

Dosage Forms Excipient information presented when available (limited, particularly for generics); consult specific product labeling.

Cream, External:
Dritho-Creme HP: 1% (50 g) [contains methylparaben]
Zithranol-RR: 1.2% (45 g) [contains brilliant blue fcf (fd&c blue #1)]

Shampoo, External:
Zithranol: 1% (85 g) [contains brilliant blue fcf (fd&c blue #1)]

◆ Anthranol® (Can) *see* Anthralin *on page 140*
◆ Anthrascalp® (Can) *see* Anthralin *on page 140*

Anthrax Vaccine Adsorbed

(AN thraks vak SEEN ad SORBED)

Brand Names: U.S. BioThrax®

Index Terms AVA

Pharmacologic Category Vaccine, Inactivated (Bacterial)

Additional Appendix Information

Immunization Administration Recommendations *on page 2334*

Immunization Recommendations *on page 2339*

Use Immunization against *Bacillus anthracis* in persons at high risk for exposure.

The Advisory Committee on Immunization Practices (ACIP) recommends routine vaccination (pre-exposure vaccination) for the following (CDC, 2010):

- Persons who work directly with the organism in the laboratory
- Persons who handle animals or animal products only when
  - potentially infected in research settings;
  - in areas of high incidence of enzootic anthrax; or
  - where standards and restrictions are not sufficient to prevent exposure
- Military personnel deployed to areas with high risk of exposure as recommended by the Department of Defense (DoD)
- Persons engaged in environmental investigations or remediation efforts

Routine immunization for the general population is not recommended. Routine vaccination may be offered to emergency and other responders (police and fire departments, the National Guard, etc) on a voluntary basis under the direction of a comprehensive occupational health and safety program.

The ACIP recommends postexposure prophylaxis after inhalation exposure to aerosolized *Bacillus anthracis* spores for the following (in the absence of completing a pre-exposure, routine vaccination schedule):

- The general public, including pregnant and breast-feeding women
- Medical professionals
- Children ages 0-18 years as determined on an event-by-event basis
- Persons engaged in handling certain animals or animal products
- Persons who work directly with the organism in the laboratory (postexposure vaccination dependant upon pre-event vaccination status)
- Military personnel as recommended by the DoD
- Persons engaged in environmental investigations or remediation efforts (postexposure vaccination dependent upon pre-event vaccination status)
- Emergency and other responders (police and fire departments, the National Guard, etc)
- Persons working in postal facilities

Pregnancy Risk Factor D

Pregnancy Considerations Adverse events were not observed in animal developmental toxicity studies. Data from the Department of Defense suggest the vaccine may be linked with a slightly increased number of atrial septal defects when given during the first trimester of pregnancy; however, when premature infants are excluded from analysis, the association is not statistically significant. Current ACIP guidelines recommend deferring pre-exposure vaccination when possible; however, postexposure prophylaxis is recommended in pregnant women. Male fertility is not affected by vaccine administration (CDC, 2010).

Breast-Feeding Considerations There are no adequate and well-controlled studies using this vaccine in breast-feeding women; however, the administration of nonlive vaccines during breast-feeding is generally not medically contraindicated. Current ACIP guidelines recommend deferring pre-exposure vaccination when possible; however postexposure prophylaxis is recommended in breast-feeding women (CDC, 2010).

Prescribing and Access Restrictions Not commercially available in U.S.; presently, all anthrax vaccine lots are owned by the U.S. Department of Defense. The Center for Disease Control (CDC) does not currently recommend routine vaccination of the general public.

Contraindications Anaphylactic or anaphylactic-like reaction following a previous dose of anthrax vaccine or any component of the formulation

Warnings/Precautions Immediate treatment for anaphylactic/anaphylactoid reaction should be available during vaccine use. May consider deferring administration in patients with moderate or severe acute illness (with or without fever) in pre-exposure vaccination programs; may administer to patients with mild acute illness (with or without fever). When used for postexposure prophylaxis, consider the benefits versus risks in patients with moderate or severe acute illness. Vaccination is not recommended after cutaneous or gastrointestinal exposures that pose no risk of inhalational exposure to *Bacillus anthracis* spores; antimicrobial postexposure prophylaxis may be considered in these patients. Vaccination may not result in effective immunity in all patients. Response depends upon multiple factors (eg, type of vaccine, age of patient) and may be improved by administering the vaccine at the recommended dose, route, and interval. Vaccines may not be effective if administered during periods of altered immune competence (CDC, 2011). Use with caution in severely immunocompromised patients (eg, patients receiving chemo/radiation therapy or other immunosuppressive therapy (including high dose corticosteroids); may have a reduced response to vaccination. In general, household and close contacts of persons with altered immunocompetence may receive all age appropriate vaccines. Persons with a history of anthrax disease may have an increased risk for adverse reactions from the vaccine. Syncope has been reported with use of injectable vaccines and may be accompanied by transient visual disturbances, weakness, or tonic-clonic movements. Procedures should be in place to avoid injuries from falling and to restore cerebral perfusion if syncope occurs.

Use with caution in patients with a history of bleeding disorders (including thrombocytopenia) and/or patients on anticoagulant therapy; bleeding/hematoma may occur from I.M. administration. For patients at risk of hemorrhage following intramuscular injection, the vaccine can be administered SubQ. In order to maximize vaccination rates, the ACIP recommends simultaneous administration of all age-appropriate vaccines (live or inactivated) for which a person is eligible at a single clinic visit, unless contraindications exist. Packaging may contain natural latex rubber. Safety and efficacy in children <18 years of age or adults ≥65 years have not been established. Use in children <18 years is recommended by the ACIP as determined on an event-by-event basis.

Adverse Reactions All serious adverse reactions must be reported to the U.S. Department of Health and Human Services (DHHS) Vaccine Adverse Event Reporting System (VAERS) 1-800-822-7967 or online at https://vaers.hhs.gov/esub/index.

Note: Percentages reported with I.M. administration; the incidence of local reactions may be increased with SubQ administration.

>10%:

Central nervous system: Fatigue (4% to 12%)

Local: Injection site reactions: Tenderness (41% to 51%), erythema (15% to 48%), edema (5% to 30%), induration (7% to 23%), pain (13% to 20%), warmth (4% to 19%); arm motion limitation (9% to 15%)
Neuromuscular & skeletal: Muscle ache (3% to 13%)
Miscellaneous: Burning sensation (45% to 97%)

1% to 10%:
Central nervous system: Headache (4% to 9%)
Local: Injection site reactions: Itching (1% to 10%), nodule (3% to 9%), bruise (2% to 5%)
Miscellaneous: Tender/painful axillary adenopathy (≤1%)

Postmarketing and/or case reports: Allergic reactions, anaphylactoid reaction, anaphylaxis, angioedema, arthralgia, arthropathy, cellulitis, dizziness, erythema multiforme, lymphadenopathy, myalgia, pain, paresthesia, pruritus, rash, rhabdomyolysis, Stevens-Johnson syndrome, syncope, tremor, ulnar nerve neuropathy, urticaria

Drug Interactions

Metabolism/Transport Effects None known.

Avoid Concomitant Use There are no known interactions where it is recommended to avoid concomitant use.

Increased Effect/Toxicity There are no known significant interactions involving an increase in effect.

Decreased Effect

The levels/effects of Anthrax Vaccine Adsorbed may be decreased by: Belimumab; Fingolimod; Immunosuppressants

Storage/Stability Store under refrigeration at 2°C to 8°C (36°F to 46°F); do not freeze.

Mechanism of Action Active immunization against *Bacillus anthracis*. The vaccine is prepared from a cell-free filtrate of *B. anthracis*, but no dead or live bacteria. Completion of the entire vaccination series is required for full protection; annual boosters are required to maintain immunity.

Dosage

Children <18 years: Safety and efficacy have not been established. **Note:** Use in children is recommended by the ACIP as determined on an event-by-event basis; refer to adult dosing for postexposure prophylaxis.

Adults:

I.M.:

Primary immunization: Three injections of 0.5 mL each given at day 0, 1 month, and 6 months. Booster injections of 0.5 mL each should be given at 12 and 18 months after the initiation of the series.

Subsequent booster injections: 0.5 mL at 1-year intervals are recommended in persons who remain at risk

SubQ:

Primary Immunization: Four injections of 0.5 mL each given at day 0, 2 weeks, 4 weeks, and 6 months. Booster injections of 0.5 mL each should be given at 12 and 18 months.

Subsequent booster injections: 0.5 mL at 1-year intervals are recommended in persons who remain at risk.

Note: SubQ administration is only to be used for primary immunization in persons who are at risk for hematoma formation following I.M. injection.

Postexposure prophylaxis (inhalation exposure) (CDC, 2010): Three injections of 0.5 mL each given at day 0, week 2, and week 4. Administer with a 60-day course of antibiotics. (Vaccination should begin within 10 days of exposure. Refer to guidelines provided as part of emergency use authorization [EUA] or investigational new drug [IND] application at the time of the event). **Note:** Additional considerations for postexposure prophylaxis following occupational exposures:

Fully vaccinated: Personnel who have completed the primary vaccination series and booster injections do not require postexposure prophylaxis if wearing protective equipment. If respiratory protection is disrupted, a 30-day course of antimicrobial therapy is recommended.

Previously unvaccinated: Workers should receive the vaccine as directed per postexposure prophylaxis along with the 60-day course of antimicrobial therapy (antimicrobial therapy should continue for 14 days after the third dose of PEP vaccine), then switch to the licensed regimen at the 6-month dose.

Partially vaccinated: Any person who started but did not complete the primary vaccination series should receive a 30-day course of antimicrobial therapy and continue with the primary vaccination schedule.

Elderly: Safety and efficacy have not been established for patients >65 years of age

Administration Shake well before use. Do not use if discolored or contains particulate matter. Do not use the same site for more than one injection. Do not mix with other injections.

Pre-exposure (routine vaccination): For I.M. administration; do not inject I.V. or intradermally. For patients at risk of hemorrhage following intramuscular injection, the vaccine can be administered SubQ.

Postexposure prophylaxis: Administer SubQ.

Simultaneous administration of vaccines helps ensure the patients will be fully vaccinated by the appropriate age. Simultaneous administration of vaccines is defined as administering >1 vaccine on the same day at different anatomic sites. Separate vaccines should not be combined in the same syringe unless indicated by product specific labeling. Separate needles and syringes should be used for each injection. The ACIP prefers each dose of a specific vaccine in a series come from the same manufacturer when possible. Adolescents and adults should be vaccinated while seated or lying down. In general, preterm infants should be vaccinated at the same chronological age as full-term infants (CDC, 2011).

Antipyretics have not been shown to prevent febrile seizures. Antipyretics may be used to treat fever or discomfort following vaccination (CDC, 2011). One study reported that routine prophylactic administration of acetaminophen to prevent fever prior to vaccination decreased the immune response of some vaccines; the clinical significance of this reduction in immune response has not been established (Prymula, 2009).

Monitoring Parameters Monitor for local reactions, chills, fever, anaphylaxis. Monitor for syncope for 15 minutes following administration. If seizure-like activity associated with syncope occurs, maintain patient in supine or Trendelenburg position to reestablish adequate cerebral perfusion.

Additional Information U.S. federal law requires that the name of medication, date of administration, the vaccine manufacturer, lot number of vaccine, and the administering person's name, title and address be entered into the patient's permanent medical record.

Dosage Forms Excipient information presented when available (limited, particularly for generics); consult specific product labeling.

Injection, suspension:

BioThrax®: *Bacillus anthracis* proteins (5 mL) [contains aluminum, natural rubber/natural latex in packaging]

- **Anti-4 Alpha Integrin** *see* Natalizumab *on page 1431*
- **Anti-D Immunoglobulin** *see* Rh_o(D) Immune Globulin *on page 1801*
- **Antibody-Drug Conjugate SGN-35** *see* Brentuximab Vedotin *on page 278*
- **Anti-CD20 Monoclonal Antibody** *see* RiTUXimab *on page 1833*
- **Anti-CD30 ADC SGN-35** *see* Brentuximab Vedotin *on page 278*

Antihemophilic Factor (Human)

(an tee hee moe FIL ik FAK tor HYU man)

Brand Names: U.S. Hemofil M; Koāte®-DVI; Monoclate-P®

Brand Names: Canada Hemofil M

Index Terms AHF (Human); Factor VIII (Human); Kaote DVI

Pharmacologic Category Antihemophilic Agent; Blood Product Derivative

Use Prevention and treatment of hemorrhagic episodes in patients with hemophilia A (classic hemophilia); perioperative management of hemophilia A; can be of significant therapeutic value in patients with acquired factor VIII inhibitors not exceeding 10 Bethesda units/mL

Pregnancy Risk Factor C

Pregnancy Considerations Animal reproduction studies have not been conducted. Parvovirus B19 or hepatitis A, which may be present in plasma-derived products, may affect a pregnant woman more seriously than nonpregnant women.

Breast-Feeding Considerations It is not known if this product is excreted into breast milk.

Contraindications Hypersensitivity to any component of the formulation

Warnings/Precautions Risk of viral transmission is not totally eradicated. Because antihemophilic factor is prepared from pooled plasma, it may contain the causative agent of viral hepatitis and other viral diseases. Hepatitis B vaccination is recommended for all patients. Hepatitis A vaccination is also recommended for seronegative patients. Antihemophilic factor contains trace amounts of blood groups A and B isohemagglutinins and when large or frequently repeated doses are given to individuals with blood groups A, B, and AB, the patient should be monitored for signs of progressive anemia and the possibility of intravascular hemolysis should be considered. The dosage requirement will vary in patients with factor VIII inhibitors; optimal treatment should be determined by clinical response. Natural rubber latex is a component of Hemofil M packaging. Hemofil M and Monoclate-P® contain trace amounts of mouse protein. Products contain naturally-occurring von Willebrand factor for stabilization, however efficacy has not been established for the treatment of von Willebrand disease. Products vary by preparation method; final formulations contain human albumin.

Adverse Reactions <1% (Limited to important or life-threatening): Acute hemolytic anemia, AHF inhibitor development, allergic reactions (rare), anaphylaxis (rare), bleeding tendency increased, blurred vision, chest tightness, chills, fever, headache, hyperfibrinogenemia, jittery feeling, lethargy, nausea, somnolence, stinging at the infusion site, stomach discomfort, tingling, urticaria, vasomotor reactions with rapid infusion, vomiting

Drug Interactions

Metabolism/Transport Effects None known.

Avoid Concomitant Use There are no known interactions where it is recommended to avoid concomitant use.

Increased Effect/Toxicity There are no known significant interactions involving an increase in effect.

Decreased Effect There are no known significant interactions involving a decrease in effect.

Preparation for Administration If refrigerated, the dried concentrate and diluent should be warmed to room temperature before reconstitution. Gently swirl or rotate vial after adding diluent; do not shake vigorously.

Storage/Stability Store under refrigeration, 2°C to 8°C (36°F to 46°F); avoid freezing. Use within 3 hours of reconstitution. Do not refrigerate after reconstitution, precipitation may occur.

Hemofil M: May also be stored at room temperature not to exceed 30°C (86°F).

Koāte®-DVI; Monoclate-P®: May also be stored at room temperature of 25°C (77°F) for ≤6 months.

Mechanism of Action Protein (factor VIII) in normal plasma which is necessary for clot formation and maintenance of hemostasis; activates factor X in conjunction with activated factor IX; activated factor X converts prothrombin to thrombin, which converts fibrinogen to fibrin, and with factor XIII forms a stable clot

Pharmacodynamics/Kinetics Half-life elimination: Mean: 8-27 hours

Dosage Children and Adults: I.V.: Individualize dosage based on coagulation studies performed prior to treatment and at regular intervals during treatment. In general, administration of factor VIII 1 unit/kg will increase circulating factor VIII levels by ~2 units/dL. (General guidelines presented; consult individual product labeling for specific dosing recommendations.)

Dosage based on desired factor VIII increase (%):

To calculate dosage needed based on desired factor VIII increase (%):

Body weight (kg) x 0.5 units/kg x desired factor VIII increase (%) = units factor VIII required

For example:

50 kg x 0.5 units/kg x 30 (% increase) = 750 units factor VIII

Dosage based on expected factor VIII increase (%):

It is also possible to calculate the **expected** % factor VIII increase:

(# units administered x 2%/units/kg) divided by body weight (kg) = expected % factor VIII increase

For example:

(1400 units x 2%/units/kg) divided by 70 kg = 40%

General guidelines:

Minor hemorrhage: 10-20 units/kg as a single dose to achieve FVIII plasma level ~20% to 40% of normal. Mild superficial or early hemorrhages may respond to a single dose; may repeat dose every 12-24 hours for 1-3 days until bleeding is resolved or healing achieved.

Moderate hemorrhage/minor surgery: 15-25 units/kg to achieve FVIII plasma level 30% to 50% of normal. If needed, may continue with a maintenance dose of 10-15 units/kg every 8-12 hours.

Major to life-threatening hemorrhage: Initial dose 40-50 units/kg, followed by a maintenance dose of 20-25 units/kg every 8-12 hours until threat is resolved, to achieve FVIII plasma level 80% to 100% of normal.

Major surgery: 50 units/kg given preoperatively to raise factor VIII level to 100% before surgery begins. May repeat as necessary after 6-12 hours initially and for a total of 10-14 days until healing is complete. Intensity of therapy may depend on type of surgery and postoperative regimen.

Bleeding prophylaxis: May be administered on a regular basis for bleeding prophylaxis. Doses of 24-40 units/kg 3 times/week have been reported in patients with severe hemophilia to prevent joint bleeding.

If bleeding is not controlled with adequate dose, test for presence of inhibitor. It may not be possible or practical to control bleeding if inhibitor titers are >10 Bethesda units/mL.

Elderly: Response in the elderly is not expected to differ from that of younger patients; dosage should be individualized

Dosage adjustment in renal impairment: No dosage adjustment provided in manufacturer's labeling.

Dosage adjustment in hepatic impairment: No dosage adjustment provided in manufacturer's labeling.

Administration Administer I.V. over 5-10 minutes (maximum: 10 mL/minute). Infuse Monoclate-P® at 2 mL/minute.

Monitoring Parameters Heart rate and blood pressure (before and during I.V. administration); AHF levels prior to and during treatment; in patients with circulating inhibitors, the inhibitor level should be monitored; hematocrit; monitor for signs and symptoms of intravascular hemolysis; bleeding

Reference Range Classification of hemophilia; normal is defined as 1 unit/mL of factor VIII

Severe: Factor level <1% of normal

Moderate: Factor level 1% to 5% of normal

Mild: Factor level >5% to <40% of normal

Dosage Forms Excipient information presented when available (limited, particularly for generics); consult specific product labeling. [DSC] = Discontinued product

Injection, powder for reconstitution:

Hemofil M: ~250 units, ~500 units, ~1000 units, ~1700 units [contains albumin (human), mouse protein; packaging may contain natural rubber latex]. Supplied with diluent.

Koāte®-DVI: ~250 units, ~500 units, ~1000 units [contains albumin (human), aluminum, polysorbate 80]. Supplied with diluent.

Monoclate-P®: ~250 units, ~500 units, ~1000 units, ~1500 units [contains albumin (human), mouse protein]. Supplied with diluent.

Antihemophilic Factor (Recombinant)

(an tee hee moe FIL ik FAK tor ree KOM be nant)

Brand Names: U.S. Advate; Helixate FS; Kogenate FS; Kogenate FS Bio-Set; Recombinate; Xyntha; Xyntha Solofuse

Brand Names: Canada Advate; Helixate® FS; Kogenate® FS; Xyntha®

Index Terms AHF (Recombinant); Factor VIII (Recombinant); Novoeight; rAHF

Pharmacologic Category Antihemophilic Agent

Use Prevention and treatment of hemorrhagic episodes in patients with hemophilia A (classic hemophilia or congenital factor VIII deficiency); perioperative management of hemophilia A; routine prophylaxis in patients with hemophilia A to prevent bleeding episodes (Advate, Helixate® FS, Kogenate® FS)

Note: Helixate® FS and Kogenate® FS are also approved in children with hemophilia A with no pre-existing joint damage to reduce risk of joint damage. In addition, Recombinate can be of therapeutic value in patients with acquired factor VIII inhibitors ≤10 Bethesda units/mL.

Pregnancy Risk Factor C

Pregnancy Considerations Animal reproduction studies have not been conducted. Safety and efficacy in pregnant women has not been established. Use during pregnancy only if clearly needed.

Breast-Feeding Considerations It is not known if antihemophilic factor (recombinant) is excreted in breast milk. The manufacturer recommends that caution be exercised when administering antihemophilic factor (recombinant) to nursing women.

Contraindications Hypersensitivity to any component of the formulation

Warnings/Precautions Monitor for signs of formation of antibodies to factor VIII; may occur at anytime but more common in young children with severe hemophilia. The dosage requirement will vary in patients with factor VIII inhibitors; optimal treatment should be determined by clinical response. Allergic hypersensitivity reactions (including anaphylaxis) may occur; monitor. Products vary by preparation method. Recombinate is stabilized using human albumin. Helixate® FS and Kogenate® FS are stabilized with sucrose. Advate, Helixate® FS, Kogenate® FS, and Xyntha® may contain trace amounts of mouse or hamster protein. Recombinate may contain mouse, hamster or bovine protein. Some products may contain polysorbate 80. Products may contain von Willebrand factor for stabilization; however, efficacy has not been established for the treatment of von Willebrand's disease.

Adverse Reactions Actual frequency may vary by product.

>1%:

Central nervous system: Chills, dizziness, fever, headache, pain

Dermatologic: Pruritus, rash, urticaria

Gastrointestinal: Constipation, diarrhea, nausea, taste perversion, vomiting

Local: Injection/infusion site reactions

Neuromuscular & skeletal: Arthralgia, joint swelling, pain in extremity, weakness

Otic: Ear infection, ear pain

Respiratory: Cough, nasal congestion, nasopharyngitis, pharyngolaryngeal pain, rhinorrhea, sinusitis

Miscellaneous: Catheter thrombosis, catheter infection, factor VIII inhibitor formation, flu-like syndrome, influenza

≤1% (Limited to important or life-threatening): Abdominal pain, adenopathy, allergic reactions, anaphylaxis, anemia, angioedema, anorexia, arthralgia, AST increased, chest discomfort, chest pain, cyanosis, depersonalization, diaphoresis, dyspnea, edema, epistaxis, erythema, facial edema, facial flushing, factor VIII decreased, fatigue, GI hemorrhage, hematoma, hives, hot flashes, hyperhidrosis, hypersensitivity reaction, hyper-/hypotension (slight), infection, laryngeal edema, lethargy, malaise, pallor, paresthesia, restlessness, rhinitis, rigors, shortness of breath, somnolence, tachycardia, tremor, urinary tract infection, vasodilation, venous catheter access complications

Drug Interactions

Metabolism/Transport Effects None known.

Avoid Concomitant Use There are no known interactions where it is recommended to avoid concomitant use.

Increased Effect/Toxicity There are no known significant interactions involving an increase in effect.

Decreased Effect There are no known significant interactions involving a decrease in effect.

Preparation for Administration If refrigerated, the dried concentrate and diluent should be warmed to room temperature before reconstitution. Gently agitate or rotate vial after adding diluent, do not shake vigorously. Refer to product specific labeling for reconstitution instructions; recommendations vary by product.

Storage/Stability Prior to reconstitution, store refrigerated at 2°C to 8°C (36°F to 46°F); avoid freezing. Use within 3 hours of reconstitution. Do not refrigerate after reconstitution.

Advate: May also be stored at room temperature for up to 6 months.

Helixate® FS: May also be stored at room temperature (not to exceed 25°C [77°F]) up to 3 months; do not return to refrigerator. Avoid prolonged exposure to light during storage.

Kogenate® FS: May also be stored at room temperature (not to exceed 25°C [77°F]) up to 12 months; do not return to refrigerator. Avoid prolonged exposure to light during storage.

Recombinate: May also be stored at room temperature, not to exceed 30°C (86°F).

Xyntha®: May also be stored at room temperature (not to exceed 25°C [77°F]) up to 3 months; after room temperature storage, product may be returned to the refrigerator until the expiration date; however, do not store at room temperature and return to refrigerator temperature more than once. Avoid prolonged exposure to light during storage.

Xyntha® Solofuse™: May also be stored at room temperature not to exceed 25°C [77°F]) up to 3 months; do not return to refrigerator; after 3 months at room temperature, must use immediately or discard.

Mechanism of Action Factor VIII replacement, necessary for clot formation and maintenance of hemostasis. It activates factor X in conjunction with activated factor IX; activated factor X converts prothrombin to thrombin, which converts fibrinogen to fibrin, and with factor XIII forms a stable clot.

Pharmacodynamics/Kinetics

Distribution: V_{ss}: ~0.4 dL/kg

Half-life elimination: Mean: ~11-15 hours

Dosage I.V.:

Hemophilia A: Children and Adults: Individualize dosage based on coagulation studies performed prior to treatment and at regular intervals during treatment. In general, administration of factor VIII 1 unit/kg will increase circulating factor VIII levels by ~2 units/dL. (General guidelines presented; consult individual product labeling for specific dosing recommendations.)

Dosage based on desired factor VIII increase (%):

To calculate dosage needed based on desired factor VIII increase (%):

[Body weight (kg) x desired factor VIII increase (%)] divided by 2 (%/units/kg) = units factor VIII required

For example:

50 kg x 30 (% increase) divided by 2 = 750 units factor VIII

Dosage based on expected factor VIII increase (%):

It is also possible to calculate the **expected** % factor VIII increase:

[# units administered x 2 (%/units/kg)] divided by body weight (kg) = expected % factor VIII increase

For example:

[1400 units x 2] divided by 70 kg = 40%

General guidelines (consult individual product labeling for specific dosage recommendations): Note: Children <6 years may require more frequent administration.

Minor hemorrhage: 10-20 units/kg as a single dose to achieve FVIII plasma level ~20% to 40% of normal. Mild superficial or early hemorrhages may respond to a single dose; may repeat dose every 12-24 hours for 1-3 days until bleeding is resolved or healing achieved.

Moderate hemorrhage/minor surgery: 15-30 units/kg to achieve FVIII plasma level 30% to 60% of normal. May repeat 1 dose at 12-24 hours if needed. Some products suggest continuing for ≥3 days until pain and disability are resolved.

Major to life-threatening hemorrhage: Initial dose 30-50 units/kg followed by a maintenance dose of 20-50 units/kg every 8-24 hours until threat is resolved, to achieve FVIII plasma level 60% to 100% of normal.

Minor surgery (including tooth extraction): 15-50 units/kg to raise factor VIII level to ~30-100% before procedure/surgery. May repeat every 12-24 hours until bleeding is resolved.

Major surgery: 40-60 units/kg given preoperatively to raise factor VIII level to ~60% to 120% before surgery begins. May repeat as necessary after 6-24 hours until wound healing. Intensity of therapy may depend on type of surgery and postoperative regimen.

If bleeding is not controlled with adequate dose, test for presence of inhibitor. It may not be possible or practical to control bleeding if inhibitor titers >10 Bethesda units/mL.

Routine prophylaxis to prevent bleeding episodes and joint damage (Helixate® FS, Kogenate® FS): Children (without pre-existing joint damage): 25 units/kg every other day

Routine prophylaxis to prevent bleeding episodes (Advate): Children and Adults: 20-40 units/kg every other day (3-4 times weekly). Alternatively, an every-third-day dosing regimen may be used to target factor VIII trough levels of ≥1%.

Elderly: Response in the elderly is not expected to differ from that of younger patients; dosage should be individualized

Dosage adjustment in renal impairment: No dosage adjustment provided in manufacturer's labeling.

Dosage adjustment in hepatic impairment: No dosage adjustment provided in manufacturer's labeling.

Dietary Considerations Some products may contain sodium.

Administration Use administration sets/tubing provided by manufacturer (if provided).

Advate: Infuse over ≤5 minutes (maximum: 10 mL/minute)

Helixate® FS, Kogenate® FS: Infuse over 1-15 minutes; based on patient tolerability

Recombinate reconstituted with 5 mL of SWFI: Infuse at a rate of ≤5 mL/minute (maximum: 5 mL/minute)

Recombinate reconstituted with 10 mL of SWFI: Infuse at a rate of ≤10 mL/minute (maximum: 10 mL/minute)

Xyntha®, Xyntha® Solufuse™: Infuse over several minutes; adjust based on patient comfort. Do not admix or administer in same tubing as other medications.

Monitoring Parameters Heart rate and blood pressure (before and during I.V. administration); plasma factor VIII activity prior to and during treatment; development of factor VIII inhibitors; signs of bleeding; hemoglobin, hematocrit

Reference Range Classification of hemophilia; normal is defined as 1 unit/mL of factor VIII

Severe: Factor level <1% of normal

Moderate: Factor level 1% to 5% of normal

Mild: Factor level >5% to <40% of normal

Product Availability

Novoeight: FDA approved October 2013; availability anticipated in the second quarter of 2015.

Novoeight is indicated for use in children and adults with hemophilia A (congenital factor VIII deficiency or classic hemophilia) for control and prevention of bleeding episodes, perioperative management, and routine prophylaxis to prevent or reduce the frequency of bleeding episodes.

Dosage Forms Excipient information presented when available (limited, particularly for generics); consult specific product labeling.

Kit, Intravenous:

Kogenate FS: 250 units, 500 units, 1000 units

Kit, Intravenous [preservative free]:

Helixate FS: 250 units, 500 units, 1000 units, 2000 units, 3000 units [contains polysorbate 80]

Kogenate FS: 2000 units, 3000 units

Kogenate FS Bio-Set: 250 units, 500 units, 1000 units, 2000 units, 3000 units

Xyntha: 250 units, 500 units, 1000 units, 2000 units [albumin free; contains mouse protein (murine) (hamster), polysorbate 80]
Xyntha Solofuse: 250 units, 500 units, 1000 units, 2000 units, 3000 units [albumin free; contains mouse protein (murine) (hamster), polysorbate 80]
Solution Reconstituted, Intravenous:
Advate: 250 units (1 ea) [albumin free]
Advate: 250 units (1 ea) [albumin free; contains polysorbate 80]
Advate: 500 units (1 ea) [albumin free]
Advate: 500 units (1 ea) [albumin free; contains polysorbate 80]
Advate: 1000 units (1 ea) [albumin free]
Advate: 1000 units (1 ea) [albumin free; contains polysorbate 80]
Advate: 1500 units (1 ea) [albumin free]
Advate: 1500 units (1 ea) [albumin free; contains polysorbate 80]
Advate: 2000 units (1 ea); 3000 units (1 ea) [albumin free]
Solution Reconstituted, Intravenous [preservative free]:
Advate: 250 units (1 ea); 500 units (1 ea); 1000 units (1 ea); 1500 units (1 ea); 2000 units (1 ea); 3000 units (1 ea); 4000 units (1 ea) [albumin free; contains polysorbate 80]
Recombinate: 220-400 UNIT (1 ea); 401-800 UNIT (1 ea); 801-1240 UNIT (1 ea); 1241-1800 UNIT (1 ea); 1801-2400 UNIT (1 ea) [contains albumin human, polyethylene glycol, polysorbate 80]

Antihemophilic Factor/von Willebrand Factor Complex (Human)

(an tee hee moe FIL ik FAK tor von WILL le brand FAK tor KOM plex HYU man)

Brand Names: U.S. Alphanate®; Humate-P®; Wilate®
Brand Names: Canada Humate-P®
Index Terms AHF (Human); Factor VIII (Human); Factor VIII Concentrate; FVIII/vWF; von Willebrand Factor/Factor VIII Complex; VWF/FVIII Concentrate; VWF:RCo; vWF: RCof
Pharmacologic Category Antihemophilic Agent; Blood Product Derivative
Use
Factor VIII deficiency: Alphanate®, Humate-P®: Prevention and treatment of hemorrhagic episodes in patients with hemophilia A (classical hemophilia) or acquired factor VIII deficiency (Alphanate® only); **Note:** Wilate® is not approved for use in patients with hemophilia A or acquired factor VIII deficiency
von Willebrand disease (VWD):
Alphanate®: Prophylaxis with surgical and/or invasive procedures in patients with VWD when desmopressin is either ineffective or contraindicated; **Note:** Not indicated for patients with severe VWD undergoing major surgery
Humate-P®: Treatment of spontaneous or trauma-induced bleeding, as well as prevention of excessive bleeding during and after surgery in patients with severe VWD, including mild or moderate disease where use of desmopressin is known or suspected to be inadequate; **Note:** Not indicated for the prophylaxis of spontaneous bleeding episodes
Wilate®: Treatment of spontaneous and trauma-induced bleeding in patients with severe VWD, including mild or moderate disease where use of desmopressin is known or suspected to be inadequate or contraindicated; **Note:** Not indicated for prophylaxis of spontaneous bleeding or prevention of excessive bleeding during and after surgery)
Pregnancy Risk Factor C

Dosage
Factor VIII deficiency: General guidelines (consult specific product labeling for Alphanate® or Humate-P®): Children and Adults: I.V.:
Individualize dosage based on coagulation studies performed prior to treatment and at regular intervals during treatment; in general, administration of factor VIII 1 unit/kg will increase circulating factor VIII levels by ~2 units/dL.
Minor hemorrhage: Loading dose: FVIII:C 15 units/kg to achieve FVIII:C plasma level ~30% of normal. If second infusion is needed, half the loading dose may be given once or twice daily for 1-2 days.
Moderate hemorrhage: Loading dose: FVIII:C 25 units/kg to achieve FVIII:C plasma level ~50% of normal; Maintenance: FVIII:C 15 units/kg every 8-12 hours for 1-2 days in order to maintain FVIII:C plasma levels at 30% of normal. Repeat the same dose once or twice daily for up to 7 days or until adequate wound healing.
Life-threatening hemorrhage/major surgery: Loading dose: FVIII:C 40-50 units/kg; Maintenance: FVIII:C 20-25 units/kg every 8-12 hours to maintain FVIII:C plasma levels at 80% to 100% of normal for 7 days. Continue same dose once or twice daily for another 7 days in order to maintain FVIII:C levels at 30% to 50% of normal.

von Willebrand disease (VWD): Treatment:
Humate-P®: Children and Adults: I.V.: Individualize dosage based on coagulation studies performed prior to treatment and at regular intervals during treatment; in general, administration of factor VIII 1 unit/kg would be expected to raise circulating VWF:RCo ~5 units/dL
Type 1, mild VWD: Minor hemorrhage (if desmopressin is not appropriate) or major hemorrhage:
Loading dose: VWF:RCo 40-60 units/kg
Maintenance dose: VWF:RCo 40-50 units/kg every 8-12 hours for 3 days, keeping VWF:RCo nadir >50%; follow with 40-50 units/kg daily for up to 7 days
Type 1, moderate or severe VWD:
Minor hemorrhage: VWF:RCo 40-50 units/kg for 1-2 doses
Major hemorrhage:
Loading dose: VWF:RCo 50-75 units/kg
Maintenance dose: VWF:RCo 40-60 units/kg every 8-12 hours for 3 days to keep the VWF:RCo nadir >50%, then 40-60 units/kg daily for a total of up to 7 days
Types 2 and 3 VWD:
Minor hemorrhage: VWF:RCo 40-50 units/kg for 1-2 doses
Major hemorrhage:
Loading dose: VWF:RCo 60-80 units/kg
Maintenance dose: VWF:RCo 40-60 units/kg every 8-12 hours for 3 days, keeping the VWF:RCo nadir >50%; follow with 40-60 units/kg daily for a total of up to 7 days
Wilate®: Children and Adults: I.V.:
Minor hemorrhage:
Loading dose: VWF:RCo: 20-40 units/kg
Maintenance dose: 20-30 units/kg every 12-24 hours for ≤3 days, keeping the VWF:RCo nadir >30%
Major hemorrhage:
Loading dose: VWF:RCo: 40-60 units/kg
Maintenance dose: 20-40 units/kg every 12-24 hours for 5-7 days, keeping the VWF:RCo nadir >50%

von Willebrand disease (VWD): Prophylaxis:
Alphanate®: Surgery/procedure prophylaxis (except patients with type 3 undergoing major surgery):
Children: I.V.:
Preoperative dose: VWF:RCo: 75 units/kg 1 hour prior to surgery

Maintenance dose: VWF:RCo: 50-75 units/kg every 8-12 hours as clinically needed. May reduce dose after third postoperative day; continue treatment until healing is complete.

Adults: I.V.:

Preoperative dose: VWF:RCo: 60 units/kg 1 hour prior to surgery

Maintenance dose: VWF:RCo: 40-60 units/kg every 8-12 hours as clinically needed. May reduce dose after third postoperative day; continue treatment until healing is complete. For minor procedures, maintain VWF of 40% to 50% during postoperative days 1-3; for major procedures maintain VWF of 40% to 50% for ≥3-7 days.

Humate-P®: Surgery/procedure prevention of bleeding: Children and Adults: I.V.:

Emergency surgery: Administer VWF:RCo 50-60 units/kg; monitor trough coagulation factor levels for subsequent doses

Surgical management (nonemergency):

Loading dose calculation based on baseline target VWF:RCo: (Target peak VWF:RCo - Baseline VWF:RCo) x weight (in kg) / IVR = units VWF:RCo required. Administer loading dose 1-2 hours prior to surgery. **Note:** If *in vivo* recovery (IVR) not available, assume 2 units/dL per units/kg of VWF:RCo product administered.

Target concentrations for VWF:RCo following loading dose:

Major surgery: 100 units/dL

Minor surgery: 50-60 units/dL

Maintenance dose: Initial: One-half loading dose, followed by subsequent dosing determined by target trough concentrations, generally every 8-12 hours. Patients with shorter half-lives may require dosing every 6 hours.

Target maintenance trough VWF:RCo concentrations:

Major surgery: >50 units/dL for up to 3 days, followed by >30 units/dL for a minimum total treatment of 72 hours

Minor surgery: ≥30 units/dL for a minimum duration of 48 hours

Oral surgery: ≥30 units/dL for a minimum duration of 8-12 hours

Elderly: Response in the elderly is not expected to differ from that of younger patients; dosage should be individualized

Dosage adjustment in renal impairment: No dosage adjustment provided in manufacturer's labeling.

Dosage adjustment in hepatic impairment: No dosage adjustment provided in manufacturer's labeling.

Additional Information Complete prescribing information should be consulted for additional detail.

Dosage Forms Excipient information presented when available (limited, particularly for generics); consult specific product labeling. [DSC] = Discontinued product

Injection, powder for reconstitution [human derived]:

Alphanate®:

250 units [Factor VIII and VWF:RCo ratio varies by lot; contains sodium ≥10 mEq/vial, albumin and polysorbate 80; packaged with diluent]

500 units [Factor VIII and VWF:RCo ratio varies by lot; contains sodium ≥10 mEq/vial, albumin and polysorbate 80; packaged with diluent]

1000 units [Factor VIII and VWF:RCo ratio varies by lot; contains sodium ≥10 mEq/vial, albumin and polysorbate 80; packaged with diluent]

1500 units [Factor VIII and VWF:RCo ratio varies by lot; contains sodium ≥10 mEq/vial, albumin and polysorbate 80; packaged with diluent]

Humate-P®:

FVIII 250 units and VWF:RCo 600 units [contains albumin; packaged with diluent]

FVIII 500 units and VWF:RCo 1200 units [contains albumin; packaged with diluent]

FVIII 1000 units and VWF:RCo 2400 units [contains albumin; packaged with diluent]

Wilate®:

FVIII 450 units and VWF:RCo 450 units [contains polysorbate 80 (in diluent); packaged with diluent] [DSC]

FVIII 500 units and VWF:RCo 500 units [contains polysorbate 80 (in diluent); packaged with diluent]

FVIII 900 units and VWF:RCo 900 units [contains polysorbate 80 (in diluent); packaged with diluent] [DSC]

FVIII 1000 units and VWF:RCo 1000 units [contains polysorbate 80 (in diluent); packaged with diluent]

◆ **Anti-Hist [OTC]** *see* DiphenhydrAMINE (Systemic) *on page 622*

◆ **Anti-Hist Allergy [OTC]** *see* DiphenhydrAMINE (Systemic) *on page 622*

Anti-inhibitor Coagulant Complex (Human)

(an TEE in HI bi tor coe AG yoo lant KOM pleks HYU man)

Brand Names: U.S. Feiba NF; Feiba VH Immuno

Brand Names: Canada FEIBA NF

Index Terms Activated PCC; AICC; aPCC; Coagulant Complex Inhibitor; Factor Eight Inhibitor Bypassing Activity; Factor VIII Inhibitor Bypassing Activity; FEIBA VH

Pharmacologic Category Activated Prothrombin Complex Concentrate (aPCC); Antihemophilic Agent; Blood Product Derivative

Use Hemophilia A & B patients with inhibitors who are to undergo surgery or those who are bleeding

Unlabeled Use Acquired hemophilia with factor VIII or factor IX inhibitor titers >5 Bethesda units (BU); treatment of life-threatening bleeding associated with dabigatran

Pregnancy Risk Factor C

Dosage

Children and Adults: I.V.: **Note:** Considered a first-line treatment when factor VIII inhibitor titer is >5 Bethesda units (BU) (antihemophilic factor may be preferred when titer <5 BU)

General dosing guidelines: 50-100 units/kg (maximum: 200 units/kg/day). If total single dose exceeds 100 units/kg or total daily dose exceeds 200 units/kg/day, monitor closely for DIC and/or coronary ischemia.

Joint hemorrhage: 50 units/kg every 12 hours; if hemorrhage continues, may increase to 100 units/kg every 12 hours; continue until signs of clinical improvement occur (maximum: 200 units/kg/day)

Mucous membrane bleeding: 50 units/kg every 6 hours; if hemorrhage continues, may increase to 100 units/kg every 6 hours up to 2 doses only (maximum: 200 units/kg/day)

Soft tissue hemorrhage (eg, retroperitoneal bleed): 100 units/kg every 12 hours (maximum: 200 units/kg/day)

Other severe hemorrhage (eg, intracranial hemorrhage): 100 units/kg every 12 hours; may be used every 6 hours if needed; continue until clinical improvement (maximum: 200 units/kg/day unless severity of hemorrhage justifies higher doses).

Adults: I.V.:

Hemorrhage (moderate-to-severe) due to acquired hemophilia (unlabeled use): **Optimal dosing has not been established:** 50-100 units/kg every 8-12 hours until bleeding controlled has been suggested; may continue for 24-72 hours based on site, type, and severity of bleeding (maximum: 200 units/kg/day) (Huth-Kuhne, 2009; Sallah, 2004).

Life-threatening hemorrhage associated with dabigatran (unlabeled use): **Optimal dosing has not been established.** In one case study involving a patient with bleeding that occurred during cardiac ablation while on dabigatran, the use of 26 units/kg was effective in rapidly reducing the amount of bleeding. After ~30 hours later, the patient received an additional dose of 16 unit/kg for a concern of rebleeding (Dager, 2013). Others have recommended the use of 50 units/kg (Weitz, 2012; Heidbuchel, 2013). **Note:** The use of FEIBA (activated 4-factor PCC) may be associated with a higher risk of thrombosis compared to nonactivated PCCs especially with higher doses; monitor closely for arterial and venous thrombosis.

Dosage adjustment in renal impairment: No dosage adjustment provided in manufacturer's labeling.

Dosage adjustment in hepatic impairment: Use with caution in patients with a history of liver disease.

Additional Information Complete prescribing information should be consulted for additional detail.

Dosage Forms Excipient information presented when available (limited, particularly for generics); consult specific product labeling.

Solution Reconstituted, Intravenous:

Feiba NF: (1 ea)

Feiba VH Immuno: (1 ea)

Solution Reconstituted, Intravenous [preservative free]:

Feiba NF: 500 units (1 ea); 1000 units (1 ea); 2500 units (1 ea)

◆ Anti-Itch Maximum Strength [OTC] *see* Hydrocortisone (Topical) *on page* 1011

Antipyrine and Benzocaine

(an tee PYE reen & BEN zoe kane)

Brand Names: U.S. Aurodex®

Brand Names: Canada Auralgan®

Index Terms Benzocaine and Antipyrine

Pharmacologic Category Otic Agent, Analgesic; Otic Agent, Cerumenolytic

Use Temporary relief of pain and reduction of swelling associated with acute congestive and serous otitis media; facilitates ear wax removal

Pregnancy Risk Factor C

Dosage Otic: Children and Adults:

Otitis media: Fill ear canal with solution; moisten cotton pledget with antipyrine and benzocaine solution, place in external ear, repeat every 1-2 hours until pain and congestion are relieved

Ear wax removal: Instill drops 3 times/day for 2-3 days; before and after ear wax removal, moisten cotton pledget with antipyrine and benzocaine solution and place in external ear after solution instillation.

Dosage adjustment in renal impairment: No dosage adjustment provided in manufacturer's labeling.

Dosage adjustment in hepatic impairment: No dosage adjustment provided in manufacturer's labeling.

Additional Information Complete prescribing information should be consulted for additional detail.

Dosage Forms Excipient information presented when available (limited, particularly for generics); consult specific product labeling.

Solution, otic [drops]: Antipyrine 5.4% and benzocaine 1.4% (10 mL, 15 mL)

Aurodex™: Antipyrine 5.4% and benzocaine 1.4% (10 mL)

Antithrombin (an tee THROM bin)

Brand Names: U.S. ATryn; Thrombate III

Brand Names: Canada Antithrombin III NF; Thrombate III®

Index Terms Antithrombin Alfa; Antithrombin III; AT; AT-III; hpAT; rhAT; rhATIII

Pharmacologic Category Anticoagulant; Blood Product Derivative

Use Prophylaxis (ATryn®, Thrombate III®) of thromboembolic events in patients with hereditary antithrombin (AT or AT-III) deficiency undergoing surgical or obstetrical procedures (eg, childbirth); treatment (Thrombate III®) of thromboembolism in patients with hereditary AT deficiency

Pregnancy Risk Factor B (Thrombate III®); C (ATryn®)

Dosage I.V.: Adults: Antithrombin deficiency:

Atryn®: Prophylaxis of thrombosis during surgical or obstetrical procedures:

Dosing is individualized based on pretherapy antithrombin (AT) activity levels. Therapy should begin before delivery or ~24 hours prior to surgery to obtain target AT activity levels. Dosing should be targeted to keep levels between 80% to 120% of normal. Loading dose should be given as a 15-minute infusion, followed by maintenance dose as a continuous infusion. Doses may be calculated based on the following formulas:

Surgical patients (nonpregnant):

Loading dose: [(100 - baseline AT activity level) **divided** by 2.3] x body weight (kg) = units of antithrombin required

Maintenance infusion: [(100 - baseline AT activity level) **divided** by 10.2] x body weight (kg) = units of antithrombin required/hour

Pregnant patients: **Note:** Pregnant women undergoing surgical procedures (other than a Cesarean section) should also be dosed according to the formula below.

Loading dose: [(100 - baseline AT activity level) **divided** by 1.3] x body weight (kg) = units of antithrombin required

Maintenance infusion: [(100 - baseline AT activity level) **divided** by 5.4] x body weight (kg) = units of antithrombin required/hour

Dosing adjustments: Adjustments should be made based on AT activity levels to maintain levels between 80% to 120% of normal. Surgery or delivery may rapidly decrease AT levels; check AT level just after surgery or delivery. The first AT level should be obtained 2 hours after initiation and adjusted as follows:

AT activity level <80%: Increase infusion rate by 30%; recheck AT level 2 hours after adjustment. Alternatively, an additional bolus dose (using loading dose formula) may be needed to rapidly restore AT levels. Calculate the additional bolus/loading dose using the last available AT activity result. After additional loading/bolus dose given, resume maintenance infusion at the same rate prior to bolus administration.

AT activity level 80% to 120%: No dosage adjustment needed; recheck AT level in 6 hours

AT activity level >120%: Decrease infusion rate by 30%; recheck AT level 2 hours after adjustment

Thrombate III®: Prophylaxis of thrombosis during surgical or obstetrical procedures or treatment of thromboembolism:

Initial loading dose: Dosing is individualized based on pretherapy antithrombin (AT) levels. The initial dose should raise AT levels to 120% and may be calculated based on the following formula:

[(desired AT level % - baseline AT level %) x body weight (kg)] **divided** by 1.4 = units of antithrombin required

For example, if a 70 kg adult patient had a baseline AT level of 57%, the initial dose would be

[(120% - 57%) x 70] divided by 1.4 = 3150 units

Maintenance dose: In general, subsequent dosing should be targeted to keep levels between 80% to 120% which may be achieved by administering 60% of the initial loading dose every 24 hours. Adjustments may be made by adjusting dose or interval. Maintain level within normal range for 2-8 days depending on type of procedure/situation.

Dosage adjustment in renal impairment: No dosage adjustment provided in the manufacturer's labeling.

Dosage adjustment in hepatic impairment: No dosage adjustment provided in the manufacturer's labeling.

Additional Information Complete prescribing information should be consulted for additional detail.

Dosage Forms Excipient information presented when available (limited, particularly for generics); consult specific product labeling.

Solution Reconstituted, Intravenous:

Thrombate III: 500 units (1 ea); 1000 units (1 ea)

ATryn: 1750 units (1 ea)

◆ **Antithrombin III** *see* Antithrombin *on page 148*

◆ **Antithrombin III NF (Can)** *see* Antithrombin *on page 148*

◆ **Antithrombin Alfa** *see* Antithrombin *on page 148*

Antithymocyte Globulin (Equine)

(an te THY moe site GLOB yu lin, E kwine)

Brand Names: U.S. Atgam

Brand Names: Canada Atgam®

Index Terms Antithymocyte Immunoglobulin; ATG; Horse Antihuman Thymocyte Gamma Globulin; Lymphocyte Immune Globulin

Pharmacologic Category Immune Globulin; Immunosuppressant Agent; Polyclonal Antibody

Use Prevention and treatment of acute renal allograft rejection; treatment of moderate-to-severe aplastic anemia in patients not considered suitable candidates for bone marrow transplantation

Unlabeled Use Prevention and treatment of other solid organ allograft rejection; prevention or treatment of graft-versus-host disease (GVHD) following allogeneic stem cell transplantation; treatment of myelodysplastic syndrome (MDS)

Pregnancy Risk Factor C

Pregnancy Considerations Animal reproduction studies have not been conducted. Women exposed to Atgam® during pregnancy may be enrolled in the National Transplantation Pregnancy Registry (877-955-6877).

Breast-Feeding Considerations It is not known if antithymocyte globulin (equine) is excreted into breast milk. The manufacturer recommends caution be used if administered to a nursing woman.

Contraindications History of severe systemic reaction to prior administration of antithymocyte globulin or other equine gamma globulins

Warnings/Precautions For I.V. use only. Must be administered via central line due to chemical phlebitis. **[U.S. Boxed Warning]: Should only be used by physicians experienced in immunosuppressive therapy or management of solid organ or bone marrow transplant patients. Adequate laboratory and supportive medical resources must be readily available in the facility for patient management.** Hypersensitivity and anaphylactic reactions can occur; immediate treatment (including epinephrine 1:1000) should be available. Rash, dyspnea, hypotension, tachycardia, or anaphylaxis precludes further administration of the drug. Respiratory distress, hypotension, or pain (chest, flank or back) may indicate an anaphylactoid/anaphylactic reaction. Discontinue if severe and unremitting thrombocytopenia and/or leukopenia occur in transplant patients. Clinically significant hemolysis has been reported (rarely); severe and unremitting hemolysis may require treatment discontinuation; chest, flank or back pain may indicate hemolysis. Monitor closely for signs of infection; there may be an increased incidence of cytomegalovirus (CMV) infection. Dose must be administered over at least 4 hours. Patient may need to be pretreated with an antipyretic, antihistamine, and/or corticosteroid. Intradermal skin testing is recommended prior to first-dose administration. Product of equine and human plasma; may have a risk of transmitting disease, including a theoretical risk of Creutzfeldt-Jakob disease (CJD). Product potency and activity may vary from lot to lot.

Adverse Reactions

>10%:

Central nervous system: Chills, fever, headache

Dermatologic: Pruritus, rash, urticaria, wheal/flare

Hematologic: Leukopenia, thrombocytopenia

Neuromuscular & skeletal: Arthralgia

1% to 10%:

Cardiovascular: Bradycardia, cardiac irregularity, chest pain, edema, heart failure, hyper-/hypotension, myocarditis

Central nervous system: Agitation, encephalitis, lethargy, lightheadedness, listlessness, seizure, viral encephalopathy

Gastrointestinal: Diarrhea, nausea, stomatitis, vomiting

Hepatic: Hepatosplenomegaly, liver function tests abnormal

Local: Injection site reactions (pain, redness, swelling), phlebitis, thrombophlebitis, burning soles/palms

Neuromuscular & skeletal: Aches, back pain, joint stiffness, myalgia

Ocular: Periorbital edema

Renal: Proteinuria, renal function tests abnormal

Respiratory: Dyspnea, pleural effusion, respiratory distress

Miscellaneous: Anaphylactic reaction, diaphoresis, lymphadenopathy, night sweats, serum sickness, viral infection

<1% (Limited to important or life-threatening: Abdominal pain, acute renal failure, anaphylactoid reaction, anemia, aplasia, apnea, confusion, cough, deep vein thrombosis, disorientation, dizziness, eosinophilia, epigastric pain, epistaxis, erythema, faintness, flank pain, GI bleeding, GI perforation, granulocytopenia, hemolysis, hemolytic anemia, herpes simplex reactivation, hiccups, hyperglycemia, iliac vein obstruction, infection, involuntary movement, kidney enlarged/ruptured, laryngospasm, malaise, neutropenia, pancytopenia, paresthesia, pulmonary edema, renal artery thrombosis, rigidity, sore mouth/throat, tachycardia, toxic epidermal necrosis, tremor, vasculitis, viral hepatitis, weakness, wound dehiscence

Drug Interactions

Metabolism/Transport Effects None known.

Avoid Concomitant Use

Avoid concomitant use of Antithymocyte Globulin (Equine) with any of the following: BCG; Natalizumab; Pimecrolimus; Tacrolimus (Topical); Tofacitinib; Vaccines (Live)

Increased Effect/Toxicity

Antithymocyte Globulin (Equine) may increase the levels/effects of: Leflunomide; Natalizumab; Tofacitinib; Vaccines (Live)

The levels/effects of Antithymocyte Globulin (Equine) may be increased by: Denosumab; Pimecrolimus; Roflumilast; Tacrolimus (Topical); Trastuzumab

Decreased Effect

Antithymocyte Globulin (Equine) may decrease the levels/effects of: BCG; Coccidioidin Skin Test; Sipuleucel-T; Vaccines (Inactivated); Vaccines (Live)

The levels/effects of Antithymocyte Globulin (Equine) may be decreased by: Echinacea

Preparation for Administration Dilute into inverted bottle of sterile vehicle to ensure that undiluted lymphocyte immune globulin does not contact air. Gently rotate or swirl to mix; do not shake. Final concentration should be 4 mg/mL. May be diluted in NS, $D_5$1/4NS, $D_5$1/2NS **(do not use D_5W; low salt concentrations may result in precipitation)**.

Storage/Stability Refrigerate ampuls at 2°C to 8°C (36°F to 46°F); do not freeze. Diluted solution is stable for 24 hours (including infusion time) at refrigeration. Allow infusion solution to reach room temperature prior to administration.

Mechanism of Action Immunosuppressant involved in the elimination of antigen-reactive T lymphocytes (killer cells) in peripheral blood or alteration in the function of T-lymphocytes, which are involved in humoral immunity and partly in cell-mediated immunity; induces complete or partial hematologic response in aplastic anemia

Pharmacodynamics/Kinetics

Distribution: Poorly into lymphoid tissues; binds to circulating lymphocytes, granulocytes, platelets, bone marrow cells

Half-life elimination, plasma: 1.5-12 days

Excretion: Urine (~1%)

Dosage An intradermal skin test is recommended prior to administration of the initial dose of ATG; use 0.1 mL of a fresh 1:1000 dilution of ATG in normal saline; observe every 15-20 minutes for 1 hour. A positive skin reaction consists of a wheal ≥10 mm in diameter. If a positive skin test occurs, the first infusion should be administered in a controlled environment with intensive life support immediately available. A systemic reaction precludes further administration of the drug. The absence of a reaction does **not** preclude the possibility of an immediate sensitivity reaction.

Premedication with diphenhydramine, hydrocortisone, and acetaminophen is recommended prior to first dose.

Children: I.V.:

Aplastic anemia protocol: 10-20 mg/kg/day for 8-14 days; then administer every other day for 7 more doses; additional doses may be given every other day for 21 total doses in 28 days **or**

Unlabeled dosing: Children >10 kg: 40 mg/kg/day for 4 days (Rosenfeld, 1995)

Renal allograft: 5-25 mg/kg/day

Acute GVHD treatment (unlabeled use): 30 mg/kg/dose every other day for 6 doses (MacMillan, 2007) **or** 15 mg/kg/dose twice daily for 10 doses (MacMillan, 2002)

Adults: I.V.:

Aplastic anemia protocol: 10-20 mg/kg/day for 8-14 days, then administer every other day for 7 more doses, for a total of 21 doses in 28 days **or**

Unlabeled dosing: 40 mg/kg/day for 4 days (Rosenfeld, 1995)

Renal allograft:

Rejection prophylaxis: 15 mg/kg/day for 14 days, then give every other day for 7 more doses for a total of 21 doses in 28 days; the initial dose should be administered within 24 hours before or after transplantation

Rejection treatment: 10-15 mg/kg/day for 14 days, then administer every other day for 7 more doses for a total of 21 doses in 28 days

Acute GVHD treatment (unlabeled use): 30 mg/kg/dose every other day for 6 doses (MacMillan, 2007) **or** 15 mg/kg/dose twice daily for 10 doses (MacMillan, 2002)

Myelodysplastic syndrome (unlabeled use): 40 mg/kg/dose once daily for 4 days; an intradermal test dose was administered prior to treatment (Molldrem, 2002)

Dosage adjustment for toxicity:

Anaphylaxis: Stop infusion immediately; administer epinephrine. May require corticosteroids, respiration assistance, and/or other resuscitative measures. Do not resume infusion.

Hemolysis (severe and unremitting): May require discontinuation of treatment.

Administration Infuse dose over at least 4 hours. Any severe systemic reaction to the skin test, such as generalized rash, tachycardia, dyspnea, hypotension, or anaphylaxis, should preclude further therapy. Epinephrine and resuscitative equipment should be nearby. Patient may need to be pretreated with an antipyretic, antihistamine, and/or corticosteroid. Mild itching and erythema can be treated with antihistamines. May cause vein irritation (chemical phlebitis) if administered peripherally. Infuse into a vascular shunt, arterial venous fistula, or high-flow central vein through a 0.2-1 micron in-line filter.

First dose: Premedicate with diphenhydramine orally 30 minutes prior to and hydrocortisone I.V. 15 minutes prior to infusion and acetaminophen 2 hours after start of infusion.

Monitoring Parameters Lymphocyte profile, CBC with differential and platelet count, vital signs during administration

Dosage Forms Excipient information presented when available (limited, particularly for generics); consult specific product labeling.

Injectable, Intravenous:

Atgam: 50 mg/mL (5 mL) [thimerosal free]

Antithymocyte Globulin (Rabbit)

(an te THY moe site GLOB yu lin RAB bit)

Brand Names: U.S. Thymoglobulin

Brand Names: Canada Thymoglobulin

Index Terms Antithymocyte Immunoglobulin; rATG

Pharmacologic Category Immune Globulin; Immunosuppressant Agent; Polyclonal Antibody

Use Treatment of acute rejection of renal transplant; used in conjunction with concomitant immunosuppression

Unlabeled Use Induction therapy in renal transplant; treatment of myelodysplastic syndrome (MDS)

Pregnancy Risk Factor C

Pregnancy Considerations Animal reproduction studies have not been conducted. Women exposed to thymoglobulin during pregnancy may be enrolled in the National Transplantation Pregnancy Registry (877-955-6877).

Breast-Feeding Considerations This product has not been evaluated in nursing women; the manufacturer recommends that breast-feeding be discontinued if therapy is needed.

Contraindications Hypersensitivity to antithymocyte globulin, rabbit proteins, or any component of the formulation; acute or chronic infection

Warnings/Precautions [U.S. Boxed Warning]: Should only be used by physicians experienced in immunosuppressive therapy for the treatment of renal transplant patients. Medical surveillance is required during the infusion. Initial dose must be administered over at least 6 hours into a high flow vein; patient may need pretreatment with an antipyretic, antihistamine, and/or corticosteroid. Hypersensitivity and fatal anaphylactic reactions can occur; immediate treatment (including epinephrine 1:1000) should be available. An increased incidence of lymphoma, post-transplant lymphoproliferative disease (PTLD), other malignancies, or severe infections may develop following concomitant use of immunosuppressants and prolonged use or overdose of antithymocyte globulin. Appropriate antiviral, antibacterial, antiprotozoal, and/or antifungal prophylaxis is recommended. Reversible neutropenia or thrombocytopenia may result from the development of cross-reactive antibodies.

Release of cytokines by activated monocytes and lymphocytes may cause fatal cytokine release syndrome (CRS) during administration of antithymocyte globulin. Rapid infusion rates of have been associated with CRS in case reports. Symptoms range from a mild, self-limiting "flu-like reaction" to severe, life-threatening reactions. Severe or life-threatening symptoms include hypotension, acute respiratory distress syndrome, pulmonary edema, myocardial infarction, and tachycardia. Patients should not be immunized with attenuated live viral vaccines during or shortly after treatment; safety of immunization following therapy has not been studied.

Adverse Reactions

>10%:

Cardiovascular: Hypertension, peripheral edema, tachycardia

Central nervous system: Chills, fever, headache, pain, malaise

Endocrine & metabolic: Hyperkalemia

Gastrointestinal: Abdominal pain, diarrhea, nausea

Genitourinary: Urinary tract infection

Hematologic: Leukopenia, thrombocytopenia

Neuromuscular & skeletal: Weakness

Respiratory: Dyspnea

Miscellaneous: Antirabbit antibody development, cytomegalovirus infection, sepsis, systemic infection

1% to 10%:

Central nervous system: Dizziness

Gastrointestinal: Gastritis, gastrointestinal moniliasis

Miscellaneous: Herpes simplex infection, oral moniliasis

Postmarketing and/or case reports: Anaphylaxis, cytokine release syndrome, PTLD, neutropenia, serum sickness (delayed)

Drug Interactions

Metabolism/Transport Effects None known.

Avoid Concomitant Use

Avoid concomitant use of Antithymocyte Globulin (Rabbit) with any of the following: BCG; Natalizumab; Pimecrolimus; Tacrolimus (Topical); Tofacitinib; Vaccines (Live)

Increased Effect/Toxicity

Antithymocyte Globulin (Rabbit) may increase the levels/effects of: Leflunomide; Natalizumab; Tofacitinib; Vaccines (Live)

The levels/effects of Antithymocyte Globulin (Rabbit) may be increased by: Denosumab; Pimecrolimus; Roflumilast; Tacrolimus (Topical); Trastuzumab

Decreased Effect

Antithymocyte Globulin (Rabbit) may decrease the levels/effects of: BCG; Coccidioidin Skin Test; Sipuleucel-T; Vaccines (Inactivated); Vaccines (Live)

The levels/effects of Antithymocyte Globulin (Rabbit) may be decreased by: Echinacea

Preparation for Administration Allow vials to reach room temperature, then reconstitute each vial with SWFI 5 mL. Rotate vial gently until dissolved. Prior to administration, further dilute one vial in 50 mL saline or dextrose (total volume is usually 50-500 mL depending on total number of vials needed per dose). Mix by gently inverting infusion bag once or twice.

Storage/Stability Store powder under refrigeration at 2°C to 8°C (36°F to 46°F); do not freeze. Protect from light. Reconstituted product is stable for up to 24 hours at room temperature; however, since it contains no preservatives, it should be used immediately following reconstitution.

Mechanism of Action Polyclonal antibody which appears to cause immunosuppression by acting on T-cell surface antigens and depleting CD4 lymphocytes

Pharmacodynamics/Kinetics

Duration: Lymphopenia may persist ≥1 year

Half-life elimination, plasma: 2-3 days

Dosage I.V.: Children and Adults: Treatment of acute rejection: 1.5 mg/kg/day for 7-14 days

Dosage adjustment for toxicity:

WBC count 2000-3000 cells/mm^3 or platelet count 50,000-75,000 cells/mm^3: Reduce dose by 50%

WBC count <2000 cells/mm^3 or platelet count <50,000 cells/mm^3: Consider discontinuing treatment

Administration The first dose should be infused over at least 6 hours through a high-flow vein. Subsequent doses should be administered over at least 4 hours. Administer through an in-line 0.22 micron filter. Premedication with corticosteroids, acetaminophen, and/or an antihistamine may reduce infusion-related reactions.

Monitoring Parameters Lymphocyte profile, CBC with differential and platelet count; vital signs during administration; signs and symptoms of infection

Test Interactions Potential interference with rabbit antibody-based immunoassays

Dosage Forms Excipient information presented when available (limited, particularly for generics); consult specific product labeling.

Solution Reconstituted, Intravenous:

Thymoglobulin: 25 mg (1 ea) [contains glycine, mannitol, sodium chloride]

◆ **Antithymocyte Immunoglobulin** *see* Antithymocyte Globulin (Equine) *on page 149*

◆ **Antithymocyte Immunoglobulin** *see* Antithymocyte Globulin (Rabbit) *on page 150*

◆ **Antitumor Necrosis Factor Alpha (Human)** *see* Adalimumab *on page 45*

◆ **Anti-VEGF Monoclonal Antibody** *see* Bevacizumab *on page 251*

◆ **Anti-VEGF rhuMAb** *see* Bevacizumab *on page 251*

◆ **Antivenin (*Centruroides*) Immune F(ab')$_2$ (Equine)** *see Centruroides* Immune F(ab')$_2$ (Equine) *on page 390*

◆ **Antivenin Scorpion** *see Centruroides* Immune F(ab')$_2$ (Equine) *on page 390*

◆ **Antivenom (*Centruroides*) Immune F(ab')$_2$ (Equine)** *see Centruroides* Immune F(ab')$_2$ (Equine) *on page 390*

◆ **Antivenom Scorpion** *see Centruroides* Immune F(ab')$_2$ (Equine) *on page 390*

◆ **Antivert** *see* Meclizine *on page 1277*

◆ **Antizol** *see* Fomepizole *on page 910*

◆ **Anucort-HC** *see* Hydrocortisone (Topical) *on page 1011*

◆ **Anusol-HC** *see* Hydrocortisone (Topical) *on page 1011*

◆ **Anuzinc (Can)** *see* Zinc Sulfate *on page 2230*

◆ **Anzemet** *see* Dolasetron *on page 647*

◆ **4-AP** *see* Dalfampridine *on page 534*

◆ **AP24534** *see* PONATinib *on page 1676*

◆ **APAP 500 [OTC]** *see* Acetaminophen *on page 28*

◆ **APAP (abbreviation is not recommended)** *see* Acetaminophen *on page 28*

◆ **APC8015** *see* Sipuleucel-T *on page 1902*

◆ **aPCC** *see* Anti-inhibitor Coagulant Complex (Human) *on page 147*

◆ **ApexiCon** *see* Diflorasone *on page 604*

◆ **ApexiCon E** *see* Diflorasone *on page 604*

◆ **Apidra** *see* Insulin Glulisine *on page 1089*

◆ Apidra® (Can) *see* Insulin Glulisine *on page 1089*
◆ Apidra SoloStar *see* Insulin Glulisine *on page 1089*

Apixaban (a PIX a ban)

Brand Names: U.S. Eliquis
Brand Names: Canada Eliquis®
Pharmacologic Category Factor Xa Inhibitor
Additional Appendix Information

Antithrombotic Therapy in Patients With Atrial Fibrillation *on page 2366*
Oral Anticoagulant Comparison Chart *on page 2307*
Reversal of Oral Anticoagulants *on page 2308*

Use

To reduce the risk of stroke and systemic embolism in patients with nonvalvular atrial fibrillation

Canadian labeling: Additional use (not in U.S. labeling): Postoperative prophylaxis of venous thromboembolism (VTE) following elective knee or hip replacement surgery

Unlabeled Use Initial treatment of VTE; extended treatment of VTE to reduce the risk of recurrent DVT and/or PE (in patients completing 6-12 months of standard anticoagulation for venous thromboembolism)

Pregnancy Risk Factor B

Pregnancy Considerations Adverse events were not observed in animal reproduction studies. Data are insufficient to evaluate the safety of oral factor Xa inhibitors during pregnancy; use during pregnancy should be avoided (Bates, 2012).

Breast-Feeding Considerations It is not known if apixaban is excreted into breast milk. Apixaban is not recommended for use in breast-feeding women; use of alternative anticoagulants is preferred (Bates, 2012)

Medication Guide Available Yes

Contraindications

U.S. labeling: Severe hypersensitivity reaction (ie, anaphylaxis) to apixaban or any component of the formulation; active pathological bleeding

Canadian labeling: Hypersensitivity to apixaban or any component of the formulation; clinically-significant active bleeding (including gastrointestinal bleeding); lesions or conditions at increased risk of clinically-significant bleeding (eg, cerebral infarct [ischemic or hemorrhagic], active peptic ulcer disease with recent bleeding; patients with spontaneous or acquired impairment of hemostasis); hepatic disease associated with coagulopathy and clinically-relevant bleeding risk; concomitant systemic treatment with agents that are strong inhibitors of both CYP3A4 and P-glycoprotein (P-gp); concomitant treatment with any other anticoagulant including unfractionated heparin (except at doses used to maintain patency of central venous or arterial catheter), low molecular weight heparins, heparin derivatives (eg, fondaparinux), and oral anticoagulants including warfarin, dabigatran, rivaroxaban except when transitioning to or from apixaban therapy

Warnings/Precautions [U.S. Boxed Warning]: When used to prevent stroke in patients with nonvalvular atrial fibrillation, an increased risk of stroke may occur upon apixaban discontinuation if patient is not adequately anticoagulated with an alternative anticoagulant. If apixaban must be discontinued for reasons other than bleeding, consider the use of another anticoagulant to prevent stroke from occurring.

Monitor for signs and symptoms of bleeding. Discontinue therapy with severe hemorrhage and promptly evaluate for bleeding source. No specific antidote exists for apixaban reversal; apixaban is not dialyzable. Although not evaluated in clinical trials, in the event of apixaban-related hemorrhage, the use of prothrombin complex concentrate (PCC), activated prothrombin complex concentrate, or recombinant factor VIIa may be considered. The use of activated oral charcoal may be considered if ingestion occurred within 2-6 hours of presentation.

Spinal or epidural hematomas, including subsequent paralysis, may occur with neuraxial anesthesia (epidural or spinal anesthesia) or spinal puncture in patients who are anticoagulated; the risk is increased with concomitant administration of other drugs that affect hemostasis (eg, NSAIDS, platelet inhibitors, other anticoagulants), in patients with a history of traumatic or repeated epidural or spinal punctures, or a history of spinal deformity or surgery. In patients who receive both apixaban and neuraxial anesthesia, Canadian labeling recommends to avoid removal of epidural catheter for at least 24 hours following last apixaban dose; avoid apixaban administration for at least 5 hours following epidural or intrathecal catheter removal. Monitor for signs of neurologic impairment (eg, numbness/weakness of legs, bowel/bladder dysfunction); prompt diagnosis and treatment are necessary.

In a clinical trial of high-risk, post-acute coronary syndrome (ACS) patients (unlabeled use), use of apixaban in addition to standard antiplatelet therapy increased the incidence of major bleeding (including intracranial and fatal bleeding) without any significant clinical benefit (Alexander, 2011). In acutely ill patients (eg, heart failure, respiratory failure) at risk for venous thromboembolism (VTE) receiving apixaban for extended VTE prophylaxis (unlabeled use), an increased incidence of major bleeding without greater efficacy was observed with extended apixaban therapy (eg, 30 days) versus low molecular weight heparin (enoxaparin) therapy for 1-2 weeks (Goldhaber, 2011). Use in patients undergoing hip fracture surgery has not been studied; avoid use in these patients.

Use with caution in moderate impairment (Child-Pugh class B) as there is limited clinical experience in these patients; dosing recommendations cannot be provided. Use in severe hepatic impairment (Child-Pugh class C) is not recommended. Patients with ALT/AST >2 times ULN or total bilirubin ≥1.5 times ULN and undergoing major orthopedic surgery (approved use in Canada; not an approved use in U.S.) were excluded from clinical trials; use with caution in these patients. Systemic exposure increases with worsening renal function. Bleeding risk may be increased in severe renal impairment (Cl_{cr} <15-29 mL/minute); use with caution. Recommendations regarding use in patients with Cl_{cr} <15 mL/minute or receiving dialysis cannot be made (has not been evaluated). Dosage reduction is recommended for patients with nonvalvular atrial fibrillation with a serum creatinine ≥1.5 mg/dL **and** are *either* ≥80 years of age or weigh ≤60 kg. Safety and efficacy have not been established in patients with prosthetic heart valves or significant rheumatic heart disease (eg, mitral stenosis); use is not recommended. Non-valvular atrial fibrillation is defined as atrial fibrillation that occurs in the absence of rheumatic mitral valve disease, mitral valve repair, or prosthetic heart valve (Fuster, 2011).

High potential for interactions (eg, CYP3A4 inducers/inhibitors, P-gp inducers/inhibitors, antiplatelet agents); refer to Drug Interactions for in-depth discussion. Systemic exposure is increased ~32% in patients >65 years of age and may be increased by 20% to 30% in patients <50 kg and decreased by 20% to 30% in patients >120 kg; dosage reduction is recommended for patients with nonvalvular atrial fibrillation with any 2 of the following: ≥80 years of age, weight ≤60 kg or serum creatinine ≥1.5 mg/dL.

Discontinue apixaban at least 24-48 hours prior to elective surgery or invasive procedures depending on risk or location of bleeding.

Adverse Reactions Note: Includes adverse reactions from nonvalvular atrial fibrillation and hip/knee replacement surgery clinical trials.

>10%: Hematologic: Bleeding (5% to 12%; major: ≤2%; clinically-relevant non-major bleeding: 2% to 4%)

1% to 10%:

Dermatologic: Bruising (1%)

Gastrointestinal: Nausea (3%)

Hematologic: Anemia (3%), postprocedural hemorrhage (1%)

Hepatic: GGT increased (1%), transaminases increased (1%)

<1% (Limited to important or life-threatening): Alkaline phosphatase increased, allergic edema, anaphylaxis, bilirubin increased, epistaxis, GI hemorrhage, gingival bleeding, hematemesis, hematochezia, hematuria, hemoptysis, hypersensitivity, hypotension, incision site hematoma, incision site hemorrhage, intracranial hemorrhage, intraocular hemorrhage, melena, muscle hemorrhage, rash, rectal hemorrhage, syncope, thrombocytopenia, wound secretion

Drug Interactions

Metabolism/Transport Effects Substrate of BCRP, CYP1A2 (minor), CYP2C19 (minor), CYP2C8 (minor), CYP2C9 (minor), CYP3A4 (major), P-glycoprotein; **Note:** Assignment of Major/Minor substrate status based on clinically relevant drug interaction potential; **Inhibits** CYP2C19 (weak)

Avoid Concomitant Use

Avoid concomitant use of Apixaban with any of the following: Anticoagulants; CYP3A4 Inducers (Strong); CYP3A4 Inhibitors (Strong); Dabigatran Etexilate; Omacetaxine; Rivaroxaban; St Johns Wort

Increased Effect/Toxicity

Apixaban may increase the levels/effects of: Anticoagulants; Collagenase (Systemic); Deferasirox; Ibritumomab; Omacetaxine; Rivaroxaban; Tositumomab and Iodine I 131 Tositumomab

The levels/effects of Apixaban may be increased by: Agents with Antiplatelet Properties; CYP3A4 Inhibitors (Moderate); CYP3A4 Inhibitors (Strong); Dabigatran Etexilate; Dasatinib; Fusidic Acid (Systemic); Herbs (Anticoagulant/Antiplatelet Properties); Ibrutinib; Ivacaftor; Luliconazole; Mifepristone; Nonsteroidal Anti-Inflammatory Agents; Omega-3 Fatty Acids; Pentosan Polysulfate Sodium; P-glycoprotein/ABCB1 Inhibitors; Prostacyclin Analogues; Salicylates; Simeprevir; Sugammadex; Thrombolytic Agents; Tibolone; Tipranavir; Vitamin E

Decreased Effect

The levels/effects of Apixaban may be decreased by: Bosentan; CYP3A4 Inducers (Strong); Dabrafenib; Deferasirox; Estrogen Derivatives; P-glycoprotein/ABCB1 Inducers; Progestins; St Johns Wort; Tocilizumab

Ethanol/Nutrition/Herb Interactions

Food: Grapefruit juice may increase levels/effects of apixaban; use caution.

Herb/Nutraceutical: St John's wort may reduce apixaban systemic exposure; use with caution or if possible, avoid concomitant use.

Storage/Stability Store at 20°C to 25°C (68°F to 77°F); excursions permitted between 15°C to 30°C (59°F to 86°F).

Mechanism of Action Inhibits platelet activation and fibrin clot formation via direct, selective and reversible inhibition of free and clot-bound factor Xa (FXa). FXa, as part of the prothrombinase complex consisting also of factor Va, calcium ions, and phospholipid, catalyzes the conversion of prothrombin to thrombin. Thrombin both activates platelets and catalyzes the conversion of fibrinogen to fibrin.

Pharmacodynamics/Kinetics

Onset: 3-4 hours

Distribution: V_{ss}: ~21 L

Protein binding: ~87%

Metabolism: Hepatic predominantly via CYP3A4/5 and to a lesser extent via CYP1A2, 2C8, 2C9, 2C19, and 2J2 to inactive metabolites; substrate of P-glycoprotein (P-gp) and breast cancer resistant protein (BCRP)

Bioavailability: ~50%

Half-life elimination: 2.5 mg dose (repeated oral administration): ~8 hours; 5 mg single dose: ~15 hours (Frost, 2012)

Time to peak: 3-4 hours

Excretion: Urine (~27% as parent drug); feces (~25% of dose recovered as metabolites)

Dosage Oral:

Adults:

Nonvalvular atrial fibrillation (to prevent stroke and systemic embolism): 5 mg twice daily **unless** patient has any 2 of the following: Age ≥80 years, body weight ≤60 kg, or serum creatinine ≥1.5 mg/dL, then reduce dose to 2.5 mg twice daily.

Per the American Heart Association, the following apixaban doses have been recommended based on the following criteria (Furie, 2012):

Patients with ≥1 additional risk factor for stroke and ≤**1** of the following: Age ≥80 years, weight ≤60 kg, or serum creatinine ≥1.5 mg/dL (also see dosage adjustment in renal impairment): Alternative to aspirin or warfarin depending on suitability of vitamin K antagonist (VKA) therapy: 5 mg twice daily

Patients with ≥1 additional risk factor for stroke and ≥**2** of the following: Age ≥80 years, weight ≤60 kg, or serum creatinine ≥1.5 mg/dL (also see dosage adjustment in renal impairment): Alternative to aspirin or warfarin depending on suitability of vitamin K antagonist (VKA) therapy: 2.5 mg twice daily

Conversion from warfarin to apixaban: Discontinue warfarin and initiate apixaban when INR is <2.0

Conversion from apixaban to warfarin: **Note:** Apixaban affects the **INR**; measuring the INR during coadministration with warfarin therapy may not be useful for determining an appropriate dose of warfarin.

U.S. labeling: If continuous anticoagulation is necessary, discontinue apixaban and begin both a parenteral anticoagulant with warfarin when the next dose of apixaban is due; discontinue parenteral anticoagulant when INR reaches an acceptable range.

Canadian labeling: Initiate warfarin or other vitamin K antagonist (VKA) at usual starting doses and continue apixaban until INR ≥2, then discontinue apixaban. During concomitant therapy, manufacturer recommends initiating INR testing on day 3 and just prior to each dose of apixaban.

Conversion between apixaban and other non-warfarin anticoagulants: Discontinue anticoagulant being taken and begin the other at the next scheduled dose.

Postoperative venous thromboprophylaxis: Canadian labeling (not in U.S. labeling):

Hip replacement surgery: 2.5 mg twice daily beginning 12-24 hours postoperatively and after achievement of hemostasis; duration: 32-38 days

Knee replacement surgery: 2.5 mg twice daily beginning 12-24 hours postoperatively and after achievement of hemostasis; duration: 10-14 days

Venous thromboembolism (DVT or PE) treatment (unlabeled use):

Initial treatment: 10 mg twice daily for 7 days followed by 5 mg twice daily for 6 months (Agnelli, 2013b)

Extended treatment: After at least 6 months of initial standard therapy (or apixaban) administer apixaban 2.5 mg twice daily for an additional 12 months. **Note:** Patients in the extended treatment trial completed

6-12 months of initial standard anticoagulant therapy (or apixaban) and uncertainty existed about whether or not to continue anticoagulation. Patients were also randomized to a 5 mg twice daily dosage; however, slightly more non-major bleeding occurred (Agnelli, 2013a).

Elderly: Refer to adult dosing. Nonvalvular atrial fibrillation (to prevent stroke and systemic embolism): If patient is ≥80 years of age **and** *either* weighs ≤60 kg or has a serum creatinine ≥1.5 mg/dL, then reduce dose to 2.5 mg twice daily.

Dosage adjustment of apixaban with concomitant medications:

U.S. labeling: Dual strong CYP3A4 and P-glycoprotein inhibitors (eg, clarithromycin, ketoconazole, itraconazole, ritonavir): 2.5 mg twice daily; **Note:** Avoid concomitant use if patient is already taking apixaban 2.5 mg twice daily or patient meets 2 of the following criteria: Age ≥80 years, body weight ≤60 kg, or serum creatinine ≥1.5 mg/dL.

Canadian labeling: Dual CYP3A4 and P-glycoprotein inhibitors: No dosage adjustment necessary for moderate dual inhibitors. Use is contraindicated with strong dual inhibitors.

Dosage adjustment in renal impairment:

U.S. labeling: Nonvalvular atrial fibrillation (to prevent stroke and systemic embolism):

Serum creatinine ≥1.5 mg/dL **and** *either* age ≥80 years or body weight ≤60 kg: 2.5 mg twice daily

Cl_{cr} <15 mL/minute: No dosage adjustment provided in manufacturer's labeling (has not been studied). **Note:** When used to prevent stroke with nonvalvular atrial fibrillation and Cl_{cr} <25 mL/minute, the American Heart Association/American Stroke Association recommends to avoid use (Furie, 2012).

Canadian labeling: **Note:** Estimated creatinine clearance (eCl_{cr}) may be calculated using Cockcroft-Gault equation.

Nonvalvular atrial fibrillation (to prevent stroke and systemic embolism):

eCl_{cr} ≥25 mL/minute: No dosage adjustment necessary. Patients with serum creatinine ≥1.5 mg/dL and either age ≥80 years or body weight ≤60 kg: 2.5 mg twice daily

eCl_{cr} 15-24 mL/minute: No dosage adjustment provided in manufacturer's labeling (very limited data).

eCl_{cr} <15 mL/minute: Use is not recommended.

Dialysis: Use is not recommended.

Postoperative venous thromboprophylaxis:

eCl_{cr} ≥30 mL/minute): No dosage adjustment required.

eCl_{cr} 15 -29 mL/minute: No dosage adjustment provided in manufacturer's labeling; use with caution as bleeding risk may be increased.

eCl_{cr} <15 mL/minute: Use is not recommended.

Dialysis: Use is not recommended.

Dosage adjustment in hepatic impairment:

U.S. labeling:

Mild impairment (Child-Pugh class A): No dosage adjustment required.

Moderate impairment (Child-Pugh class B): No dosage adjustment provided in manufacturer's labeling; use with caution (limited clinical experience in these patients).

Severe impairment (Child-Pugh class C): Use is not recommended.

Canadian labeling:

Mild or moderate impairment (Child-Pugh class A or B): No dosage adjustment required; use with caution.

Severe impairment (Child-Pugh class C): Use is not recommended.

Note: Use is contraindicated in patients with hepatic disease associated with coagulopathy and clinically-relevant bleeding risk.

Dietary Considerations May be taken without regard to meals.

Administration May be administered without regard to meals. After hip/knee replacement (Canadian labeling), initial dose should be administered 12-24 hours postoperatively.

Monitoring Parameters Renal and hepatic function; signs of bleeding; routine monitoring of coagulation tests is not required. Although not recommended to assess effectiveness, the prothrombin time (PT), INR, and aPTT are prolonged with apixaban. Anti-FXa assay may be helpful (plasma concentrations and anti-FXa activity exhibit linear relationship) in guiding clinical decisions.

When converting from apixaban to a vitamin K antagonist (VKA), Canadian labeling recommends INR testing just prior to each dose of apixaban beginning on day 3 of concurrent therapy with the VKA.

Reference Range Predicted steady state anti-FXa activity: Peak: 1.3 units/mL; trough: 0.84 units/mL

Dosage Forms Excipient information presented when available (limited, particularly for generics); consult specific product labeling.

Tablet, Oral:

Eliquis: 2.5 mg, 5 mg

- ◆ **Aplenzin** *see* BuPROPion *on page* 296
- ◆ **Aplisol** *see* Tuberculin Tests *on page* 2134
- ◆ **Aplonidine** *see* Apraclonidine *on page* 158
- ◆ **APO-066** *see* Deferiprone *on page* 561
- ◆ **Apo-Acebutolol® (Can)** *see* Acebutolol *on page* 28
- ◆ **Apo-Acetaminophen (Can)** *see* Acetaminophen *on page* 28
- ◆ **Apo-Acyclovir (Can)** *see* Acyclovir (Systemic) *on page* 42
- ◆ **Apo-Alendronate® (Can)** *see* Alendronate *on page* 69
- ◆ **Apo-Alfuzosin® (Can)** *see* Alfuzosin *on page* 73
- ◆ **Apo-Alpraz® (Can)** *see* ALPRAZolam *on page* 81
- ◆ **Apo-Alpraz® TS (Can)** *see* ALPRAZolam *on page* 81
- ◆ **Apo-Amiloride® (Can)** *see* AMILoride *on page* 99
- ◆ **Apo-Amiodarone (Can)** *see* Amiodarone *on page* 101
- ◆ **Apo-Amlodipine® (Can)** *see* AmLODIPine *on page* 109
- ◆ **Apo-Amoxi® (Can)** *see* Amoxicillin *on page* 116
- ◆ **Apo-Amoxi-Clav (Can)** *see* Amoxicillin and Clavulanate *on page* 119
- ◆ **Apo-Ampi® (Can)** *see* Ampicillin *on page* 130
- ◆ **Apo-Anastrozole (Can)** *see* Anastrozole *on page* 137
- ◆ **Apo-Atenol® (Can)** *see* Atenolol *on page* 186
- ◆ **Apo-Atomoxetine (Can)** *see* AtoMOXetine *on page* 187
- ◆ **Apo-Atorvastatin (Can)** *see* AtorvaSTATin *on page* 190
- ◆ **Apo-Azathioprine® (Can)** *see* AzaTHIOprine *on page* 208
- ◆ **Apo-Azithromycin® (Can)** *see* Azithromycin (Systemic) *on page* 214
- ◆ **Apo-Baclofen® (Can)** *see* Baclofen *on page* 221
- ◆ **Apo-Beclomethasone® (Can)** *see* Beclomethasone (Nasal) *on page* 229
- ◆ **Apo-Benztropine® (Can)** *see* Benztropine *on page* 243
- ◆ **Apo-Bicalutamide® (Can)** *see* Bicalutamide *on page* 258
- ◆ **Apo-Bisacodyl [OTC] (Can)** *see* Bisacodyl *on page* 259
- ◆ **Apo-Bisoprolol® (Can)** *see* Bisoprolol *on page* 261

- **Apo-Nabumetone® (Can)** *see* Nabumetone *on page 1413*
- **Apo-Nadol (Can)** *see* Nadolol *on page 1415*
- **Apo-Napro-Na (Can)** *see* Naproxen *on page 1425*
- **Apo-Napro-Na DS (Can)** *see* Naproxen *on page 1425*
- **Apo-Naproxen (Can)** *see* Naproxen *on page 1425*
- **Apo-Naproxen EC (Can)** *see* Naproxen *on page 1425*
- **Apo-Naproxen SR (Can)** *see* Naproxen *on page 1425*
- **Apo-Nifed PA® (Can)** *see* NIFEdipine *on page 1455*
- **Apo-Nitrofurantoin® (Can)** *see* Nitrofurantoin *on page 1464*
- **Apo-Nizatidine® (Can)** *see* Nizatidine *on page 1470*
- **Apo-Norflox® (Can)** *see* Norfloxacin *on page 1475*
- **Apo-Nortriptyline® (Can)** *see* Nortriptyline *on page 1475*
- **Apo-Oflox® (Can)** *see* Ofloxacin (Systemic) *on page 1490*
- **Apo-Olanzapine (Can)** *see* OLANZapine *on page 1493*
- **Apo-Olanzapine ODT (Can)** *see* OLANZapine *on page 1493*
- **Apo-Omeprazole® (Can)** *see* Omeprazole *on page 1505*
- **Apo-Ondansetron® (Can)** *see* Ondansetron *on page 1510*
- **Apo-Orciprenaline® (Can)** *see* Metaproterenol *on page 1309*
- **Apo-Oxaprozin® (Can)** *see* Oxaprozin *on page 1527*
- **Apo-Oxazepam® (Can)** *see* Oxazepam *on page 1529*
- **Apo-Oxcarbazepine® (Can)** *see* OXcarbazepine *on page 1530*
- **Apo-Oxybutynin (Can)** *see* Oxybutynin *on page 1533*
- **Apo-Oxycodone/Acet (Can)** *see* Oxycodone and Acetaminophen *on page 1538*
- **Apo-Oxycodone CR (Can)** *see* OxyCODONE *on page 1535*
- **Apo-Paclitaxel® (Can)** *see* PACLitaxel *on page 1543*
- **Apo-Pantoprazole® (Can)** *see* Pantoprazole *on page 1563*
- **Apo-Paroxetine (Can)** *see* PARoxetine *on page 1575*
- **Apo-Pen VK (Can)** *see* Penicillin V Potassium *on page 1611*
- **Apo-Perphenazine® (Can)** *see* Perphenazine *on page 1624*
- **Apo-Pimozide® (Can)** *see* Pimozide *on page 1648*
- **Apo-Pindol (Can)** *see* Pindolol *on page 1649*
- **Apo-Pioglitazone® (Can)** *see* Pioglitazone *on page 1649*
- **Apo-Piroxicam® (Can)** *see* Piroxicam *on page 1656*
- **Apo-Pramipexole® (Can)** *see* Pramipexole *on page 1695*
- **Apo-Pravastatin® (Can)** *see* Pravastatin *on page 1700*
- **Apo-Prazo® (Can)** *see* Prazosin *on page 1703*
- **Apo-Prednisone® (Can)** *see* PredniSONE *on page 1707*
- **Apo-Primidone® (Can)** *see* Primidone *on page 1715*
- **Apo-Procainamide® (Can)** *see* Procainamide *on page 1718*
- **Apo-Prochlorperazine (Can)** *see* Prochlorperazine *on page 1722*
- **Apo-Propafenone® (Can)** *see* Propafenone *on page 1731*
- **Apo-Propranolol (Can)** *see* Propranolol *on page 1737*
- **Apo-Quetiapine (Can)** *see* QUEtiapine *on page 1757*
- **Apo-Quinapril (Can)** *see* Quinapril *on page 1761*
- **Apo-Quinidine® (Can)** *see* QuiNIDine *on page 1764*
- **Apo-Quinine® (Can)** *see* QuiNINE *on page 1766*
- **Apo-Rabeprazole (Can)** *see* RABEprazole *on page 1769*
- **Apo-Raloxifene® (Can)** *see* Raloxifene *on page 1774*
- **Apo-Ramipril (Can)** *see* Ramipril *on page 1778*
- **Apo-Ranitidine® (Can)** *see* Ranitidine *on page 1782*
- **Apo-Riluzole® (Can)** *see* Riluzole *on page 1819*
- **Apo-Risedronate® (Can)** *see* Risedronate *on page 1824*
- **Apo-Risperidone (Can)** *see* RisperiDONE *on page 1826*
- **Apo-Rivastigmine (Can)** *see* Rivastigmine *on page 1841*
- **Apo-Rizatriptan® (Can)** *see* Rizatriptan *on page 1844*
- **Apo-Rosuvastatin (Can)** *see* Rosuvastatin *on page 1858*
- **Apo-Salvent® (Can)** *see* Albuterol *on page 61*
- **Apo-Salvent® AEM (Can)** *see* Albuterol *on page 61*
- **Apo-Salvent® CFC Free (Can)** *see* Albuterol *on page 61*
- **Apo-Salvent® Sterules (Can)** *see* Albuterol *on page 61*
- **Apo-Selegiline (Can)** *see* Selegiline *on page 1884*
- **Apo-Sertraline (Can)** *see* Sertraline *on page 1889*
- **Apo-Sildenafil® (Can)** *see* Sildenafil *on page 1894*
- **Apo-Simvastatin (Can)** *see* Simvastatin *on page 1899*
- **Apo-Sotalol® (Can)** *see* Sotalol *on page 1942*
- **Apo-Sucralfate (Can)** *see* Sucralfate *on page 1955*
- **Apo-Sulfasalazine (Can)** *see* SulfaSALAzine *on page 1964*
- **Apo-Sulfatrim (Can)** *see* Sulfamethoxazole and Trimethoprim *on page 1959*
- **Apo-Sulfatrim DS (Can)** *see* Sulfamethoxazole and Trimethoprim *on page 1959*
- **Apo-Sulfatrim Pediatric (Can)** *see* Sulfamethoxazole and Trimethoprim *on page 1959*
- **Apo-Sulin® (Can)** *see* Sulindac *on page 1967*
- **Apo-Sumatriptan (Can)** *see* SUMAtriptan *on page 1969*
- **Apo-Tamox® (Can)** *see* Tamoxifen *on page 1987*
- **Apo-Temazepam (Can)** *see* Temazepam *on page 2005*
- **Apo-Terazosin® (Can)** *see* Terazosin *on page 2015*
- **Apo-Terbinafine (Can)** *see* Terbinafine (Systemic) *on page 2017*
- **Apo-Tetra (Can)** *see* Tetracycline *on page 2034*
- **Apo-Theo LA® (Can)** *see* Theophylline *on page 2042*
- **Apo-Ticlopidine® (Can)** *see* Ticlopidine *on page 2059*
- **Apo-Timol® (Can)** *see* Timolol (Systemic) *on page 2064*
- **Apo-Timop® (Can)** *see* Timolol (Ophthalmic) *on page 2064*
- **Apo-Tizanidine (Can)** *see* TiZANidine *on page 2074*
- **Apo-Tolbutamide® (Can)** *see* TOLBUTamide *on page 2085*
- **Apo-Topiramate (Can)** *see* Topiramate *on page 2090*
- **Apo-Tramadol/Acet® (Can)** *see* Acetaminophen and Tramadol *on page 33*
- **Apo-Trazodone® (Can)** *see* TraZODone *on page 2112*
- **Apo-Trazodone D® (Can)** *see* TraZODone *on page 2112*
- **Apo-Triazide (Can)** *see* Hydrochlorothiazide and Triamterene *on page 1006*

Apraclonidine (a pra KLOE ni deen)

Brand Names: U.S. Iopidine

Brand Names: Canada Iopidine®

Index Terms Aplonidine; Apraclonidine Hydrochloride; p-Aminoclonidine

Pharmacologic Category Alpha$_2$ Agonist, Ophthalmic

Use Prevention and treatment of postsurgical intraocular pressure (IOP) elevation; short-term, adjunctive therapy in patients who require additional reduction of IOP

Pregnancy Risk Factor C

Dosage Adults: Ophthalmic:

0.5%: Instill 1-2 drops in the affected eye(s) 3 times/day

1%: Instill 1 drop in operative eye 1 hour prior to anterior segment laser surgery, second drop in eye immediately upon completion of procedure

Dosing adjustment in renal impairment: Although the topical use of apraclonidine has not been studied in renal failure patients, structurally-related clonidine undergoes a significant increase in half-life in patients with severe renal impairment; close monitoring of cardiovascular parameters in patients with impaired renal function is advised.

Dosing adjustment in hepatic impairment: Close monitoring of cardiovascular parameters in patients with impaired liver function is advised because the systemic dosage form of clonidine is partially metabolized in the liver.

Additional Information Complete prescribing information should be consulted for additional detail.

Dosage Forms Excipient information presented when available (limited, particularly for generics); consult specific product labeling.

Solution, Ophthalmic:

Iopidine: 0.5% (5 mL, 10 mL); 1% (1 ea) [contains benzalkonium chloride]

Generic: 0.5% (5 mL, 10 mL)

Aprepitant (ap RE pi tant)

Brand Names: U.S. Emend

Brand Names: Canada Emend®

Index Terms L 754030; MK 869

Pharmacologic Category Antiemetic; Substance P/Neurokinin 1 Receptor Antagonist

Use Prevention of acute and delayed nausea and vomiting associated with moderately- and highly-emetogenic chemotherapy (in combination with other antiemetics); prevention of postoperative nausea and vomiting (PONV)

Pregnancy Risk Factor B

Pregnancy Considerations Teratogenic effects were not observed in animal reproduction studies. Use during pregnancy only if clearly needed. Efficacy of hormonal contraceptive may be reduced; alternative or additional methods of contraception should be used both during treatment with fosaprepitant or aprepitant and for at least 1 month following the last fosaprepitant/aprepitant dose.

Breast-Feeding Considerations It is not known if aprepitant is excreted in breast milk. Due to the potential for adverse reactions in the nursing infant, the decision to discontinue aprepitant or to discontinue breast-feeding should take into account the benefits of treatment to the mother.

Contraindications Hypersensitivity to aprepitant or any component of the formulation; concurrent use with cisapride or pimozide

Warnings/Precautions Potentially significant drug-drug interactions may exist, requiring dose or frequency adjustment, additional monitoring, and/or selection of alternative therapy. Use caution with severe hepatic impairment (Child-Pugh class C); has not been studied. Not studied for treatment of existing nausea and vomiting. Chronic continuous administration is not recommended.

Adverse Reactions Note: Adverse reactions reported as part of a combination chemotherapy regimen or with general anesthesia.

>10%:

Central nervous system: Fatigue (≤18%)

Gastrointestinal: Nausea (6% to 13%), constipation (9% to 10%)

Neuromuscular & skeletal: Weakness (≤18%)

Miscellaneous: Hiccups (11%)

1% to 10%:

Cardiovascular: Hypotension (≤6%), bradycardia (≤4%)

Central nervous system: Dizziness (≤7%)

Endocrine & metabolic: Dehydration (≤6%)

Gastrointestinal: Diarrhea (≤10%), dyspepsia (≤6%), abdominal pain (≤5%), epigastric discomfort (4%), gastritis (4%), stomatitis (3%)

Hepatic: ALT increased (≤6%), AST increased (3%)

Renal: Proteinuria (7%), BUN increased (5%)

>0.5% (Limited to important or life-threatening): Acid reflux, acne, albumin decreased, alkaline phosphatase increased, anaphylactic reaction, anemia, angioedema, anxiety, appetite decreased, arthralgia, back pain, bilirubin increased, candidiasis, confusion, conjunctivitis, cough, deglutition disorder, depression, diabetes mellitus, diaphoresis, disorientation, duodenal ulcer (perforating), DVT, dysarthria, dysphagia, dyspnea, dysuria, edema, enterocolitis, eructation, erythrocyturia, febrile neutropenia, flatulence, flushing, glucosuria, herpes simplex, hyperglycemia, hypersensitivity reaction, hypertension, hypoesthesia, hypokalemia, hyponatremia, hypothermia, hypovolemia, hypoxia, leukocytes increased, leukocyturia, malaise, MI, miosis, muscular weakness, musculoskeletal pain, myalgia, nasal secretion, neutropenic sepsis, obstipation, pain, palpitation, pelvic pain, peripheral neuropathy, pharyngitis, pharyngolaryngeal pain, pneumonia, pneumonitis, pruritus, pulmonary embolism, rash, renal insufficiency, respiratory infection, respiratory insufficiency, rigors, salivation increased, sensory disturbance, sensory neuropathy, septic shock, Stevens-Johnson syndrome, syncope, tachycardia, taste disturbance, thrombocytopenia, toxic

epidermal necrolysis, tremor, urinary tract infection, urticaria, visual acuity decreased, vocal disturbance, weight loss, wheezing, xerostomia

Drug Interactions

Metabolism/Transport Effects Substrate of CYP1A2 (minor), CYP2C19 (minor), CYP3A4 (major); **Note:** Assignment of Major/Minor substrate status based on clinically relevant drug interaction potential; **Inhibits** CYP2C19 (weak), CYP2C9 (weak), CYP3A4 (moderate); **Induces** CYP2C9 (strong), CYP3A4 (weak/moderate)

Avoid Concomitant Use

Avoid concomitant use of Aprepitant with any of the following: Axitinib; Bosutinib; Cisapride; Conivaptan; Fusidic Acid (Systemic); Ibrutinib; Ivabradine; Lomitapide; Pimozide; Simeprevir; Tolvaptan; Ulipristal

Increased Effect/Toxicity

Aprepitant may increase the levels/effects of: ARIPiprazole; Avanafil; Benzodiazepines (metabolized by oxidation); Bosentan; Bosutinib; Budesonide (Systemic, Oral Inhalation); Cisapride; Colchicine; Corticosteroids (Systemic); CYP3A4 Substrates; Diltiazem; Dofetilide; Eplerenone; Everolimus; FentaNYL; Halofantrine; Ibrutinib; Imatinib; Ivabradine; Ivacaftor; Lomitapide; Lurasidone; OxyCODONE; Pimecrolimus; Pimozide; Propafenone; Ranolazine; Salmeterol; Saxagliptin; Simeprevir; Tolvaptan; Ulipristal; Vilazodone; Zuclopenthixol

The levels/effects of Aprepitant may be increased by: Conivaptan; CYP3A4 Inhibitors (Moderate); CYP3A4 Inhibitors (Strong); Dasatinib; Diltiazem; Fusidic Acid (Systemic); Ivacaftor; Luliconazole; Mifepristone; Simeprevir

Decreased Effect

Aprepitant may decrease the levels/effects of: ARIPiprazole; Axitinib; Contraceptives (Estrogens); Contraceptives (Progestins); CYP2C9 Substrates; Diclofenac (Systemic); Ibrutinib; Ifosfamide; PARoxetine; Saxagliptin; Simeprevir; TOLBUTamide; Warfarin

The levels/effects of Aprepitant may be decreased by: Bosentan; CYP3A4 Inducers (Strong); Dabrafenib; Deferasirox; Herbs (CYP3A4 Inducers); Mitotane; PARoxetine; Rifampin; Tocilizumab

Ethanol/Nutrition/Herb Interactions

Food: Aprepitant serum concentration may be increased when taken with grapefruit juice; avoid concurrent use.

Herb/Nutraceutical: Avoid St John's wort (may decrease aprepitant levels).

Storage/Stability Store at room temperature of 20°C to 25°C (68°F to 77°F).

Mechanism of Action Prevents acute and delayed vomiting by inhibiting the substance P/neurokinin 1 (NK_1) receptor; augments the antiemetic activity of 5-HT_3 receptor antagonists and corticosteroids to inhibit acute and delayed phases of chemotherapy-induced emesis.

Pharmacodynamics/Kinetics

Distribution: V_d: ~70 L; crosses the blood-brain barrier

Protein binding: >95%

Metabolism: Extensively hepatic via CYP3A4 (major); CYP1A2 and CYP2C19 (minor); forms 7 metabolites (weakly active)

Bioavailability: ~60% to 65%

Half-life elimination: Terminal: ~9-13 hours

Time to peak, plasma: ~3-4 hours

Dosage

Prevention of chemotherapy-induced nausea/vomiting: Adults: Oral:

Highly-emetogenic chemotherapy: 125 mg 1 hour prior to chemotherapy on day 1, followed by 80 mg once daily on days 2 and 3 (in combination with a 5-HT_3 antagonist antiemetic on day 1 and dexamethasone on days 1-4)

Moderately-emetogenic chemotherapy: 125 mg 1 hour prior to chemotherapy on day 1, followed by 80 mg once daily on days 2 and 3 (in combination with a 5-HT_3 antagonist antiemetic and dexamethasone on day 1)

Prevention of PONV: Adults: Oral: 40 mg within 3 hours prior to induction

Dosage adjustment in renal impairment: No dosage adjustment necessary.

ESRD undergoing dialysis: No dosage adjustment necessary.

Dosage adjustment in hepatic impairment:

Mild-to-moderate impairment (Child-Pugh class A or B): No dosage adjustment necessary

Severe impairment (Child-Pugh class C): Use with caution; no data available.

Dietary Considerations May be taken with or without food.

Administration

Chemotherapy-induced nausea/vomiting: Administer with or without food. First dose should be given 1 hour prior to antineoplastic therapy; subsequent doses should be given in the morning.

PONV: Administer within 3 hours prior to induction; follow healthcare providers instructions about food/drink restrictions prior to surgery.

Dosage Forms Excipient information presented when available (limited, particularly for generics); consult specific product labeling.

Capsule, Oral:

Emend: 40 mg, 80 mg, 125 mg, 80 & 125 MG

Extemporaneous Preparations A 20 mg/mL oral aprepitant suspension may be prepared with capsules and a 1:1 combination of Ora-Sweet® and Ora-Plus® (or Ora-Blend®). Empty the contents of four 125 mg capsules into a mortar and reduce to a fine powder (process will take 10-15 minutes). Add small portions of vehicle and mix to a uniform paste. Add sufficient vehicle to form a liquid; transfer to a graduated cylinder, rinse mortar with vehicle, and add quantity of vehicle sufficient to make 25 mL. Label "shake well" and "refrigerate". Stable for 90 days refrigerated.

Dupuis LL, Lingertat-Walsh K, and Walker SE, "Stability of an Extemporaneous Oral Liquid Aprepitant Formulation," *Support Care Cancer*, 2009, 17(6):701-6.

- **Aprepitant Injection** *see* Fosaprepitant *on page* 919
- **Apresoline** *see* HydrALAZINE *on page* 1002
- **Apresoline® (Can)** *see* HydrALAZINE *on page* 1002
- **Apri** *see* Ethinyl Estradiol and Desogestrel *on page* 784
- **Apriso** *see* Mesalamine *on page* 1305
- **Aprodine [OTC]** *see* Triprolidine and Pseudoephedrine *on page* 2131

Aprotinin (a proe TYE nin)

Brand Names: U.S. Trasylol

Brand Names: Canada Trasylol®

Pharmacologic Category Blood Product Derivative; Hemostatic Agent

Use Prevention of perioperative blood loss in patients who are at increased risk for blood loss and blood transfusions in association with cardiopulmonary bypass in coronary artery bypass graft (CABG) surgery

Note: Aprotinin has been withdrawn from the worldwide market due to evidence demonstrating an increased risk of renal dysfunction, myocardial infarction, and mortality in patients undergoing cardiac surgery (Canada has lifted this suspension); use limited to investigational use in the U.S. only according to a special treatment protocol allowing for treatment in select patients at increased risk of blood loss and transfusion during CABG surgery when alternative therapies are unacceptable.

Pregnancy Risk Factor B

Prescribing and Access Restrictions Available in U.S. under an investigational new drug (IND) process. The program will provide aprotinin for the treatment of adult patients undergoing coronary artery bypass graft (CABG) surgery requiring cardiopulmonary bypass (CPB) who are at increased risk of bleeding and transfusion during CABG surgery with no acceptable therapeutic alternative. Healthcare providers using aprotinin for this situation must also ensure that the benefits outweigh the risks for their patient. Healthcare providers with patients who may qualify can access information and forms for enrollment by contacting Bayer Medical Communications at (888) 842-2937.

Dosage Adults: Test dose: **All** patients should receive a 1 mL (1.4 mg) I.V. test dose at least 10 minutes prior to the loading dose to assess the potential for allergic reactions.

Notes:

The loading dose should be given after induction of anesthesia but prior to sternotomy. In patients with previous exposure to aprotinin, administer loading dose just prior to cannulation. A constant infusion is continued until surgery is complete.

To avoid physical incompatibility with heparin when adding to pump-prime solution, each agent should be added during recirculation to assure adequate dilution.

Regimen A (standard dose):

2 million KIU (280 mg; 200 mL) loading dose I.V. over 20-30 minutes

2 million KIU (280 mg; 200 mL) into pump prime volume

500,000 KIU/hour (70 mg/hour; 50 mL/hour) I.V. during operation

Regimen B (low dose):

1 million KIU (140 mg; 100 mL) loading dose I.V. over 20-30 minutes

1 million KIU (140 mg; 100 mL) into pump prime volume

250,000 KIU/hour (35 mg/hour; 25 mL/hour) I.V. during operation

Dosage adjustment in renal impairment: No adjustment required, but increased risk of worsening renal dysfunction with use; monitor closely

Dosage adjustment in hepatic impairment: No information available

Additional Information Complete prescribing information should be consulted for additional detail.

Dosage Forms Excipient information presented when available (limited, particularly for generics); consult specific product labeling.

Solution, Intravenous:

Trasylol: 10,000 KIU/mL (100 mL, 200 mL)

◆ Aptivus *see* Tipranavir *on page 2070*

◆ Aptivus® (Can) *see* Tipranavir *on page 2070*

◆ Aquacort® (Can) *see* Hydrocortisone (Topical) *on page 1011*

◆ AquaMEPHYTON® (Can) *see* Phytonadione *on page 1644*

◆ Aquanil HC [OTC] *see* Hydrocortisone (Topical) *on page 1011*

◆ Aquaphilic/Carbamide [OTC] *see* Urea *on page 2140*

◆ Aquasol A *see* Vitamin A *on page 2201*

◆ Aquasol E [OTC] *see* Vitamin E *on page 2202*

◆ Aquavit-E [OTC] *see* Vitamin E *on page 2202*

◆ Aqueous Procaine Penicillin G *see* Penicillin G Procaine *on page 1610*

◆ Aqueous Selenium [OTC] *see* Selenium *on page 1888*

◆ Aqueous Vitamin E [OTC] *see* Vitamin E *on page 2202*

◆ Ara-C *see* Cytarabine (Conventional) *on page 517*

◆ Arabinosylcytosine *see* Cytarabine (Conventional) *on page 517*

◆ Aralen *see* Chloroquine *on page 409*

◆ Aranelle *see* Ethinyl Estradiol and Norethindrone *on page 793*

◆ Aranesp (Can) *see* Darbepoetin Alfa *on page 543*

◆ Aranesp (Albumin Free) *see* Darbepoetin Alfa *on page 543*

◆ Arava *see* Leflunomide *on page 1178*

◆ Arava® (Can) *see* Leflunomide *on page 1178*

◆ Arbinoxa *see* Carbinoxamine *on page 343*

◆ Arcalyst *see* Rilonacept *on page 1816*

◆ Arcapta Neohaler *see* Indacaterol *on page 1065*

◆ Aredia® (Can) *see* Pamidronate *on page 1555*

◆ Arestin Microspheres (Can) *see* Minocycline *on page 1373*

Arformoterol (ar for MOE ter ol)

Brand Names: U.S. Brovana

Index Terms (R,R)-Formoterol L-Tartrate; Arformoterol Tartrate

Pharmacologic Category Beta$_2$-Adrenergic Agonist; Beta$_2$-Adrenergic Agonist, Long-Acting

Use Long-term maintenance treatment of bronchoconstriction in chronic obstructive pulmonary disease (COPD), including chronic bronchitis and emphysema

Pregnancy Risk Factor C

Medication Guide Available Yes

Dosage Nebulization: Adults: COPD: 15 mcg twice daily; maximum: 30 mcg/day

Dosage adjustment in renal impairment: No adjustment required

Dosage adjustment in hepatic impairment: No dosage adjustment required, but use caution; systemic drug exposure prolonged (1.3- to 2.4-fold)

Additional Information Complete prescribing information should be consulted for additional detail.

Dosage Forms Excipient information presented when available (limited, particularly for generics); consult specific product labeling.

Nebulization Solution, Inhalation:

Brovana: 15 mcg/2 mL (2 mL)

◆ Arformoterol Tartrate *see* Arformoterol *on page 160*

Argatroban (ar GA troh ban)

Pharmacologic Category Anticoagulant, Thrombin Inhibitor

Additional Appendix Information

Dosing Considerations for the Critically-Ill Patient With Morbid Obesity *on page 2379*

Reversal of Oral Anticoagulants *on page 2308*

Use Prophylaxis or treatment of thrombosis in patients with heparin-induced thrombocytopenia (HIT); adjunct to percutaneous coronary intervention (PCI) in patients who have or are at risk of thrombosis associated with HIT

Unlabeled Use To maintain extracorporeal circuit patency (prefilter administration) of continuous renal replacement therapy (CRRT) in critically-ill patients with HIT

Pregnancy Risk Factor B

Pregnancy Considerations Adverse events were not observed in animal studies. Information related to argatroban in pregnancy is limited. Use of parenteral direct thrombin inhibitors in pregnancy should be limited to those women who have severe allergic reactions to heparin, including heparin-induced thrombocytopenia, and who cannot receive danaparoid (Guyatt, 2012).

Breast-Feeding Considerations It is not known if argatroban is excreted in human milk. Because of the serious potential of adverse effects to the nursing infant, a decision to discontinue nursing or discontinue argatroban should be considered.

Contraindications Hypersensitivity to argatroban or any component of the formulation; overt major bleeding

Warnings/Precautions Hemorrhage can occur at any site in the body. Extreme caution should be used when there is an increased danger of hemorrhage, such as severe hypertension, immediately following lumbar puncture, spinal anesthesia, major surgery (including brain, spinal cord, or eye surgery), congenital or acquired bleeding disorders, and gastrointestinal ulcers. Use caution in critically-ill patients; reduced clearance may require dosage reduction. Use caution with hepatic dysfunction. Argatroban prolongs the PT/INR. Concomitant use with warfarin will cause increased prolongation of the PT and INR greater than that of warfarin alone. If warfarin is initiated concurrently with argatroban, initial PT/INR goals while on argatroban may require modification; alternative guidelines for monitoring therapy should be followed. Safety and efficacy for use with other thrombolytic agents has not been established. Discontinue all parenteral anticoagulants prior to starting therapy. Allow reversal of heparin's effects before initiation. Patients with hepatic dysfunction may require >4 hours to achieve full reversal of argatroban's anticoagulant effect following treatment. Avoid use during PCI in patients with elevations of ALT/AST (≥3 times ULN); the use of argatroban in these patients has not been evaluated. Limited pharmacokinetic and dosing information is available from use in critically-ill children with heparin-induced thrombocytopenia.

Adverse Reactions As with all anticoagulants, bleeding is the major adverse effect of argatroban. Hemorrhage may occur at virtually any site. Risk is dependent on multiple variables, including the intensity of anticoagulation and patient susceptibility.

>10%:

Cardiovascular: Chest pain (PCI related: <1% to 15%), hypotension (7% to 11%)

Gastrointestinal: Gastrointestinal bleed (major: <1% to 3%; minor: 3% to 14%)

Genitourinary: Genitourinary bleed and hematuria (major: <1%; minor: 2% to 12%)

1% to 10%:

Cardiovascular: Vasodilation (1% to 10%), cardiac arrest (6%), ventricular tachycardia (5%), bradycardia (5%), myocardial infarction (PCI: 4%), atrial fibrillation (3%), angina (2%), CABG-related bleeding (minor, 2%), myocardial ischemia (2%), cerebrovascular disorder (<1% to 2%), thrombosis (<1% to 2%)

Central nervous system: Fever (<1% to 7%), headache (5%), pain (5%), intracranial bleeding (1% to 4%)

Dermatologic: Skin reactions (bullous eruption, rash; 1% to <10%)

Gastrointestinal: Nausea (5% to 7%), diarrhea (6%), vomiting (4% to 6%), abdominal pain (3% to 4%)

Genitourinary: Urinary tract infection (5%)

Hematologic: Hemoglobin decreased (<2 g/dL), hematocrit decreased (minor: 2% to 10%; major: <1%)

Local: Bleeding at injection or access site (minor: 2% to 5%)

Neuromuscular & skeletal: Back pain (PCI related: 8%)

Renal: Abnormal renal function (3%)

Respiratory: Dyspnea (8% to 10%), cough (3% to 10%), hemoptysis (minor: <1% to 3%), pneumonia (3%)

Miscellaneous: Sepsis (6%), infection (4%)

<1% (Limited to important or life-threatening): Allergic reactions, constipation (infants and children), GERD, hypokalemia (infants and children), limb and below-the-knee stump bleed, multisystem hemorrhage and DIC, pulmonary edema, retroperitoneal bleeding

Drug Interactions

Metabolism/Transport Effects None known.

Avoid Concomitant Use

Avoid concomitant use of Argatroban with any of the following: Apixaban; Dabigatran Etexilate; Omacetaxine; Rivaroxaban

Increased Effect/Toxicity

Argatroban may increase the levels/effects of: Anticoagulants; Collagenase (Systemic); Deferasirox; Ibritumomab; Omacetaxine; Rivaroxaban; Tositumomab and Iodine I 131 Tositumomab

The levels/effects of Argatroban may be increased by: Agents with Antiplatelet Properties; Apixaban; Dabigatran Etexilate; Dasatinib; Herbs (Anticoagulant/Antiplatelet Properties); Ibrutinib; Nonsteroidal Anti-Inflammatory Agents; Omega-3 Fatty Acids; Pentosan Polysulfate Sodium; Prostacyclin Analogues; Salicylates; Sugammadex; Thrombolytic Agents; Tibolone; Tipranavir; Vitamin E

Decreased Effect

The levels/effects of Argatroban may be decreased by: Estrogen Derivatives; Progestins

Preparation for Administration

Vials for injection, 2.5 mL (100 mg/mL) concentrate: Prior to administration, each vial must be diluted to a final concentration of 1 mg/mL. Solution may be mixed with 0.9% sodium chloride injection, 5% dextrose injection, or lactated Ringer's injection. Do not mix with other medications. To prepare solution for I.V. administration, dilute each 250 mg vial with 250 mL of diluent or dilute 500 mg per 500 mL of diluent. Mix by repeated inversion for 1 minute. A slight but brief haziness may occur prior to mixing.

Premixed vials for infusion, 50 mL or 125 mL (1 mg/mL): No further dilution is required.

Storage/Stability

Vials for injection, 2.5 mL (100 mg/mL) concentrate: Prior to use, store at 15°C to 30°C (59°F to 86°F). Protect from light. The diluted, prepared solution is stable for 24 hours at 15°C to 30°C (59°F to 86°F) in ambient indoor light. Do not expose to direct sunlight. Prepared solutions that are protected from light and kept at controlled room temperature of 20°C to 25°C (68°F to 77°F) or under refrigeration at 2°C to 8°C (36°F to 46°F) are stable for up to 96 hours.

Premixed vials for infusion, 50 mL or 125 mL (1 mg/mL): Store at controlled room temperature of 20°C to 25°C (68°F to 77°F). Keep in original container to protect from light.

Mechanism of Action A direct, highly-selective thrombin inhibitor. Reversibly binds to the active thrombin site of free and clot-associated thrombin. Inhibits fibrin formation; activation of coagulation factors V, VIII, and XIII; activation of protein C; and platelet aggregation.

Pharmacodynamics/Kinetics

Onset of action: Immediate

Distribution: 174 mL/kg

Protein binding: Albumin: 20%; α_1-acid glycoprotein: 35%

Metabolism: Hepatic via hydroxylation and aromatization. Metabolism via CYP3A4/5 to four known metabolites plays a minor role. Unchanged argatroban is the major plasma component. Plasma concentration of metabolite M1 is 0% to 20% of the parent drug and is three- to fivefold weaker.

Half-life elimination: 39-51 minutes; Hepatic impairment: ≤181 minutes

Time to peak: Steady-state: 1-3 hours

Excretion: Feces (65%); urine (22%); low quantities of metabolites M2-4 in urine

Clearance is decreased in critically-ill pediatric patients

Dosage I.V.:

Children: **Heparin-induced thrombocytopenia** (dosing based on limited data from critically-ill patients):

Initial dose: 0.75 mcg/kg/minute

Maintenance dose: Patient may not be at steady-state but measure aPTT after 2 hours; adjust dose until the steady-state aPTT is 1.5-3 times the initial baseline value, not exceeding 100 seconds; dosage may be adjusted in increments of 0.1-0.25 mcg/kg/minute. **Note:** Frequent dosage adjustments may be required to maintain desired anticoagulant activity.

Adults:

Heparin-induced thrombocytopenia:

Initial dose: 2 mcg/kg/minute

Obesity: Pharmacokinetics and pharmacodynamics have not been evaluated prospectively in obese patients; however, retrospective data suggests using actual body weight to dose and that adjustment of initial dose is unnecessary in obesity (BMI up to 51 kg/m^2) (Rice, 2007); weight range included in phase II and III clinical trials: 33-204 kg (actual body weight).

Maintenance dose: Patient may not be at steady-state but measure aPTT after 2 hours; adjust dose until the steady-state aPTT is 1.5-3 times the initial baseline value, not exceeding 100 seconds; dosage should not exceed 10 mcg/kg/minute

Note: Critically-ill patients with normal hepatic function have become excessively anticoagulated with FDA-approved or lower starting doses of argatroban. Doses between 0.15-1.3 mcg/kg/minute were required to maintain aPTTs in the target range (Reichert, 2003). In a prospective observational study of critically-ill patients with multiple organ dysfunction (MODS) and suspected or proven HIT, an initial infusion dose of 0.2 mcg/kg/minute was found to be sufficient and safe in this population (Beiderlinden, 2007). Consider reducing starting dose to 0.2 mcg/kg/minute in critically-ill patients with MODS defined as a minimum number of two organ failures. Another report of a cardiac patient with anasarca secondary to acute renal failure had a reduction in argatroban clearance similar to patients with hepatic dysfunction. Reduced clearance may have been due to reduced liver perfusion (de Denus, 2003). The American College of Chest Physicians has recommended an initial infusion rate of 0.5-1.2 mcg/kg/minute for patients with heart failure, MODS, severe anasarca, or postcardiac surgery (Linkins, 2012).

Conversion to oral anticoagulant: Because there may be a combined effect on the INR when argatroban is combined with warfarin, loading doses of warfarin should not be used. Warfarin therapy should be started at the expected daily dose.

Patients receiving ≤2 mcg/kg/minute of argatroban: Argatroban therapy can be stopped when the combined INR on warfarin and argatroban is >4; repeat INR measurement in 4-6 hours; if INR is below therapeutic level, argatroban therapy may be restarted. Repeat procedure daily until desired INR on warfarin alone is obtained.

Patients receiving >2 mcg/kg/minute of argatroban: In order to predict the INR on warfarin alone, reduce dose of argatroban to 2 mcg/kg/minute; measure INR for argatroban and warfarin 4-6 hours after dose reduction; argatroban therapy can be stopped when the combined INR on warfarin and argatroban is >4. Repeat INR measurement in 4-6 hours; if INR is below therapeutic level, argatroban therapy may be restarted. Repeat procedure daily until desired INR on warfarin alone is obtained.

Note: The American College of Chest Physicians suggests monitoring chromogenic factor X assay when transitioning from argatroban to warfarin (Garcia, 2012) or overlapping administration of warfarin for a minimum of 5 days until INR is within target range; recheck INR after anticoagulant effect of argatroban has dissipated (Guyatt, 2012). Factor X levels <45% have been associated with INR values >2 after the effects of argatroban have been eliminated (Arpino, 2005).

Prefilter administration for continuous renal replacement therapy (CRRT) in critically-ill patients with HIT (unlabeled use; Link, 2009): 0.1-1.5 mcg/kg/minute. **Note:** Loading dose of 100 mcg/kg was administered during clinical trial; however, this may be unnecessary.

Percutaneous coronary intervention (PCI):

Initial: Begin infusion of 25 mcg/kg/minute and administer bolus dose of 350 mcg/kg (over 3-5 minutes). ACT should be checked 5-10 minutes after bolus infusion; proceed with procedure if ACT >300 seconds.

Obesity: Pharmacokinetics and pharmacodynamics have not been evaluated prospectively in obese patients; however, retrospective data suggests using actual body weight to dose and that adjustment of initial dose is unnecessary in obesity (BMI up to 51 kg/m^2) (Hursting, 2008); weight range included in phase II and III clinical trials: 49-141 kg (actual body weight).

Following initial bolus:

ACT <300 seconds: Give an additional 150 mcg/kg bolus, and increase infusion rate to 30 mcg/kg/minute (recheck ACT in 5-10 minutes)

ACT >450 seconds: Decrease infusion rate to 15 mcg/kg/minute (recheck ACT in 5-10 minutes)

Once a therapeutic ACT (300-450 seconds) is achieved, infusion should be continued at this dose for the duration of the procedure.

If dissection, impending abrupt closure, thrombus formation during PCI, or inability to achieve ACT >300 seconds: An additional bolus of 150 mcg/kg, followed by an increase in infusion rate to 40 mcg/kg/minute may be administered.

Note: Post-PCI anticoagulation, if required, may be achieved by continuing infusion at a reduced dose of 2-10 mcg/kg/minute, with close monitoring of aPTT.

Elderly: No adjustment is necessary for patients with normal liver function

Dosage adjustment in renal impairment: Removal during hemodialysis and continuous venovenous hemofiltration is clinically insignificant. No dosage adjustment required.

Dosage adjustment in hepatic impairment: Decreased clearance and increased elimination half-life are seen with hepatic impairment; dose should be reduced.

Children: Initial dose: 0.2 mcg/kg/minute; adjust dose in increments of ≤0.05 mcg/kg/minute

Adults: Per manufacturer labeling, the initial dose for moderate-to-severe hepatic impairment (Child-Pugh classes B and C) is 0.5 mcg/kg/minute; monitor aPTT closely and adjust dose as necessary. However, patients with severe hepatic impairment (Child-Pugh class C) may require further reduction of the initial dose. One case report describes a dose of 0.05 mcg/kg/minute required to maintain a stable, therapeutic aPTT in a patient with severe hepatic impairment (Yarbrough, 2012). **Note:** During PCI, avoid use in patients with elevations of ALT/AST (≥3 times ULN); the use of argatroban in these patients has not been evaluated.

Usual Infusion Concentrations: Pediatric Note: Premixed solutions available.

I.V. infusion: 1000 **mcg**/mL

Usual Infusion Concentrations: Adult Note: Premixed solutions available.

I.V. infusion: 250 mg in 250 mL (concentration: 1000 **mcg**/mL) in D_5W or NS

Administration The 2.5 mL (100 mg/mL) **concentrated** vial **must be diluted to 1 mg/mL** prior to administration. The premixed 50 mL or 125 mL (1 mg/mL) vial requires no further dilution. The premixed 1 mg/mL vial may be inverted for use with an infusion set.

Monitoring Parameters Obtain baseline aPTT prior to start of therapy. Patient may not be at steady-state but check aPTT 2 hours after start of therapy to adjust dose, keeping the steady-state aPTT 1.5-3 times the initial baseline value (not exceeding 100 seconds). Monitor hemoglobin, hematocrit, signs and symptoms of bleeding.

PCI: Monitor ACT before dosing, 5-10 minutes after bolus dosing, and after any change in infusion rate and at the end of the procedure. Additional ACT assessments should be made every 20-30 minutes during extended PCI procedures.

Test Interactions Argatroban may elevate PT/INR levels in the absence of warfarin. If warfarin is started, initial PT/INR goals while on argatroban may require modification. The American College of Chest Physicians suggests monitoring chromogenic factor X assay when transitioning from argatroban to warfarin (Garcia, 2012) or overlapping administration of warfarin for a minimum of 5 days until INR is within target range; recheck INR after anticoagulant effect of argatroban has dissipated (Guyatt, 2012). Factor Xa levels <45% have been associated with INR values >2 after the effects of argatroban have been eliminated (Arpino, 2005).

Additional Information Platelet counts recovered by day 3 in 53% of patients with heparin-induced thrombocytopenia and in 58% of patients with heparin-induced thrombocytopenia with thrombosis syndrome.

Dosage Forms Excipient information presented when available (limited, particularly for generics); consult specific product labeling.

Solution, Intravenous:

Generic: 125 mg/125 mL (125 mL); 100 mg/mL (2.5 mL)

Solution, Intravenous [preservative free]:

Generic: 50 mg/50 mL (50 mL)

Arginine (AR ji neen)

Brand Names: U.S. R-Gene 10

Index Terms Arginine HCl; Arginine Hydrochloride; L-Arginine; L-Arginine Hydrochloride

Pharmacologic Category Diagnostic Agent

Use Pituitary function test (growth hormone)

Unlabeled Use Management of severe, uncompensated, metabolic alkalosis (pH ≥7.55) **after** optimizing therapy with sodium and potassium supplements

Pregnancy Risk Factor B

Dosage I.V.: Pituitary function test:

Children: 0.5 g/kg/dose administered over 30 minutes

Adults: 30 g (300 mL) administered over 30 minutes

Additional Information Complete prescribing information should be consulted for additional detail.

Dosage Forms Excipient information presented when available (limited, particularly for generics); consult specific product labeling.

Solution, Intravenous, as hydrochloride [preservative free]:

R-Gene 10: 10% (300 mL)

- ◆ **Arginine HCl** *see* Arginine *on page* 163
- ◆ **Arginine Hydrochloride** *see* Arginine *on page* 163
- ◆ **8-Arginine Vasopressin** *see* Vasopressin *on page* 2172
- ◆ **Aricept** *see* Donepezil *on page* 650
- ◆ **Aricept® (Can)** *see* Donepezil *on page* 650
- ◆ **Aricept ODT** *see* Donepezil *on page* 650
- ◆ **Aricept® RDT (Can)** *see* Donepezil *on page* 650
- ◆ **Aridol** *see* Mannitol *on page* 1266
- ◆ **Arimidex** *see* Anastrozole *on page* 137

ARIPiprazole (ay ri PIP ray zole)

Brand Names: U.S. Abilify; Abilify Discmelt; Abilify Maintena

Brand Names: Canada Abilify

Index Terms BMS 337039; OPC-14597

Pharmacologic Category Antipsychotic Agent, Atypical

Additional Appendix Information

Antipsychotic Agents *on page* 2290

Beers Criteria – Potentially Inappropriate Medications for Geriatrics *on page* 2368

Use

Oral:

Bipolar I disorder: For the acute treatment of manic and mixed episodes associated with bipolar I disorder in pediatric patients 10 to 17 years of age as monotherapy; for the acute and maintenance treatment of manic and mixed episodes associated with bipolar I disorder in adults, both as monotherapy and as an adjunct to lithium or valproate.

Irritability associated with autistic disorder: For the treatment of irritability associated with autistic disorder in pediatric patients 6 to 17 years of age.

Major depressive disorder: For use as an adjunctive treatment to antidepressants for the treatment of major depressive disorder in adults.

Schizophrenia: For the acute treatment of schizophrenia in adolescents 13 to 17 years of age; for the acute and maintenance treatment of schizophrenia in adults.

Injection:

Agitation associated with schizophrenia or bipolar mania (immediate-release injection only): For the acute treatment of agitation associated with schizophrenia or bipolar mania, manic or mixed in adults.

Schizophrenia (extended-release injection only): For the treatment of schizophrenia in adults.

Unlabeled Use Depression with psychotic features; aggression (children); conduct disorder (children); Tourette syndrome (children); pervasive developmental disorder not otherwise specified (PDD-NOS) (children); Asperger's Disorder (children); psychosis/agitation related to Alzheimer's dementia

Pregnancy Risk Factor C

Pregnancy Considerations Adverse events were observed in animal reproduction studies. Aripiprazole crosses the placenta; aripiprazole and dehydro-aripiprazole can be detected in the cord blood at delivery (Nguyen, 2011; Wantanabe, 2011). Antipsychotic use during the third trimester of pregnancy has a risk for abnormal muscle movements (extrapyramidal symptoms [EPS]) and/or withdrawal symptoms in newborns following delivery. Symptoms in the newborn may include agitation, feeding disorder, hypertonia, hypotonia, respiratory distress, somnolence, and tremor; these effects may be self-limiting or require hospitalization.

Treatment algorithms have been developed by the ACOG and the APA for the management of depression in women prior to conception and during pregnancy (Yonkers, 2009). The ACOG recommends that therapy during pregnancy be individualized; treatment with psychiatric medications during pregnancy should incorporate the clinical expertise of the mental health clinician, obstetrician, primary healthcare provider, and pediatrician. Safety data related to atypical antipsychotics during pregnancy is limited and routine use is not recommended. However, if a woman is inadvertently exposed to an atypical antipsychotic while pregnant, continuing therapy may be preferable to switching to a typical antipsychotic that the fetus has not yet been exposed to; consider risk:benefit (ACOG, 2008).

Healthcare providers are encouraged to enroll women 18-45 years of age exposed to aripiprazole during pregnancy in the Atypical Antipsychotics Pregnancy Registry (866-961-2388 or http://www.womensmentalhealth.org/pregnancyregistry).

Breast-Feeding Considerations Aripiprazole is excreted in breast milk (Schlotterbeck, 2007; Watanabe, 2011). In one case report, milk concentrations were ~20% of the maternal plasma concentration (maternal dose: 15 mg/day; ~6 months postpartum) (Schlotterbeck, 2007); however, aripiprazole was not detected in the breast milk in a second case (limit of detection 10 ng/mL; maternal dose: 15 mg/day; ~1 month postpartum) (Lutz, 2010). Aripiprazole was also detected in the neonatal blood 6 days after delivery in a breast-fed infant also exposed during pregnancy. In this case report, the authors suggest *in utero* exposure could have contributed to the findings due to the long elimination half-life of aripiprazole (Watanabe, 2011). In one report, lactation was not able to be established, possibly due to changes in maternal prolactin potentially caused by aripiprazole (Mendhekar, 2006). The manufacturer recommends a decision be made whether to discontinue nursing or to discontinue the drug, taking into account the importance of treatment to the mother.

Medication Guide Available Yes

Contraindications Known hypersensitivity (eg, anaphylaxis, pruritus, urticaria) to aripiprazole.

Warnings/Precautions [U.S. Boxed Warning]: Elderly patients with dementia-related psychosis treated with antipsychotics are at an increased risk of death compared to placebo. Most deaths appeared to be either cardiovascular (eg, heart failure, sudden death) or infectious (eg, pneumonia) in nature. In addition, an increased incidence of cerebrovascular effects (eg, transient ischemic attack, cerebrovascular accidents) has been reported in studies of placebo-controlled trials of aripiprazole in elderly patients with dementia-related psychosis. Aripiprazole is not approved for the treatment of dementia-related psychosis.

[U.S. Boxed Warning]: Antidepressants increase the risk of suicidal thinking and behavior in children, adolescents, and young adults (18-24 years of age) with major depressive disorder (MDD) and other psychiatric disorders; consider risk prior to prescribing. The possibility of a suicide attempt is inherent in major depression and may persist until remission occurs. Patients treated with antidepressants should be observed for clinical worsening and suicidality, especially during the initial few months of a course of drug therapy, or at times of dose changes, either increases or decreases. Prescriptions should be written for the smallest quantity consistent with good patient care. The patient's family or caregiver should be alerted to monitor patients for the emergence of suicidality and associated behaviors; patients should be instructed to notify their healthcare provider if any of these symptoms or worsening depression or psychosis occur.

Leukopenia, neutropenia, and agranulocytosis (sometimes fatal) have been reported in clinical trials and postmarketing reports with antipsychotic use; presence of risk factors (eg, pre-existing low WBC or history of drug-induced leuko-/neutropenia) should prompt periodic blood count assessment. Discontinue therapy at first signs of blood dyscrasias or if absolute neutrophil count <1000/mm^3.

A medication guide concerning the use of antidepressants should be dispensed with each prescription. **Aripiprazole is not FDA approved for adjunctive treatment of depression in children.**

May cause extrapyramidal symptoms (EPS), including pseudoparkinsonism, acute dystonic reactions, akathisia, and tardive dyskinesia (risk of these reactions is very low relative to typical/conventional antipsychotics, frequencies reported are similar to placebo). Risk of dystonia (and probably other EPS) may be greater with increased doses, use of conventional antipsychotics, males, and younger patients. May be associated with neuroleptic malignant syndrome (NMS).

May be sedating, use with caution in disorders where CNS depression is a feature. May cause orthostatic hypotension (although reported rates are similar to placebo); use caution in patients at risk of this effect or those who would not tolerate transient hypotensive episodes (cerebrovascular disease, cardiovascular disease, or other medications which may predispose).

Use caution in patients with Parkinson's disease; predisposition to seizures; and severe cardiac disease. May alter cardiac conduction; life-threatening arrhythmias have occurred with therapeutic doses of antipsychotics. Esophageal dysmotility and aspiration have been associated with antipsychotic use; use caution in patients at risk of pneumonia (eg, Alzheimer's disease). May alter temperature regulation.

Atypical antipsychotics have been associated with metabolic changes including loss of glucose control, lipid changes, and weight gain (risk profile varies with product). Development of hyperglycemia in some cases, may be extreme and associated with ketoacidosis, hyperosmolar coma, or death. Reports of hyperglycemia with aripiprazole therapy have been few and specific risk associated with this agent is not known. Use caution in patients with diabetes or other disorders of glucose regulation; monitor for worsening of glucose control.

Use in elderly patients with dementia is associated with an increased risk of mortality and cerebrovascular accidents; avoid antipsychotic use for behavioral problems associated with dementia unless alternative nonpharmacologic therapies have failed and patient may harm self or others. In addition, use may cause or exacerbate syndrome of inappropriate antidiuretic hormone secretion or hyponatremia; monitor sodium closely with initiation or dosage adjustments in older adults (Beers Criteria).

Tablets contain lactose; avoid use in patients with galactose intolerance or glucose-galactose malabsorption.

Abilify Discmelt®: Use caution in phenylketonuria; contains phenylalanine.

There are two formulations available for intramuscular administration: Abilify® is an immediate release short-acting formulation and Abilify Maintena™ is an extended-release formulation. These products are **not** interchangeable.

Adverse Reactions Unless otherwise noted, frequency of adverse reactions is shown as reported for adult patients receiving oral administration. Spectrum and incidence of adverse effects similar in children; exceptions noted when incidence much higher in children.

>10%:

Central nervous system: Headache (adults 27%; children 13%; injection 12%), extrapyramidal reaction (dose-related; 8% to 26%), akathisia (dose-related; adults 2% to 25%; children 6% to 10%), cognitive dysfunction (children 24%; adults 11%; injection 9%), drowsiness (children 10% to 24%; adults 11%; injection 11%), sedation (dose-related; children 8% to 24%; adults 4% to 13%; injection 3% to 9%), fatigue (dose-related; children 4% to 22%; adults 6% to 8%; injection 2%), agitation (19%), insomnia (8% to 18%), anxiety (4% to 17%), restlessness (2% to 12%)

Gastrointestinal: Nausea (8% to 15%; injection 9%), vomiting (4% to 14%; injection 3%), constipation (adults 5% to 11%; children 3%)

1% to 10%:

Cardiovascular: Chest pain (1% to 10%), tachycardia (2%; injection <1%), hypertension (≥1%), orthostatic hypotension (including injection, ≤1%), peripheral edema (≥1%)

Central nervous system: Dizziness (3% to 10%; injection 8%), drooling (children 4% to 9%), lethargy (children 2% to 5%), nervousness (3%), pain (3%), ataxia (≥1%), dystonia (children 1%), hypersomnia (children 1%)

Dermatologic: Skin rash (children ≥1% to 2%)

Endocrine & metabolic: Weight gain (≥7% body weight; 2% to 8%), weight loss (>1%), increased thirst (children 1%)

Gastrointestinal: Dyspepsia (9%), sialorrhea (dose-related; 3% to 8%), decreased appetite (children 4% to 7%), increased appetite (children 3% to 7%), diarrhea (children 5%), xerostomia (adults 2% to 5%; children 1%), toothache (4%), abdominal distress (3%), gastric distress (3%), upper abdominal pain (children 3%)

Genitourinary: Dysmenorrhea (children 2%)

Local: Injection site reaction (injection >1%)

Neuromuscular & skeletal: Increased creatine phosphokinase (1% to 10%), tremor (dose-related; 5% to 10%), weakness (1% to 10%), arthralgia (adults 4%; children 1%), limb pain (4%), stiffness (adults 4%; children 1%), myalgia (2% to 3%), muscle cramps (2%), muscle spasm (2%), dyskinesia (children 1%)

Ophthalmic: Blurred vision (3% to 8%), accommodation disturbance (3%)

Respiratory: Aspiration pneumonia (1% to 10%), dyspnea (1% to 10%), nasal congestion (1% to 10%), upper respiratory tract infection (6%), nasopharyngitis (children 3% to 6%), cough (3%), pharyngolaryngeal pain (3%), rhinorrhea (children 2%)

Miscellaneous: Fever (children 5% to 9%)

<1% (Limited to important or life-threatening): Abnormal bilirubin levels, agranulocytosis, akinesia, alopecia, amenorrhea, anaphylaxis, angina pectoris, angioedema, anorexia, anorgasmia, atrial fibrillation, atrial flutter, atrioventricular block, bradycardia, cardiorespiratory arrest, catatonia, cerebrovascular accident, choreoathetosis, cogwheel rigidity, delirium, depression, diabetes mellitus, diabetic ketoacidosis, diplopia, disruption of body temperature regulation, edema, erectile dysfunction, esophagitis, extrasystoles, gynecomastia, hepatitis, homicidal ideation, hostility, hyperglycemia, hyperlipidemia, hypersensitivity, hypertonia, hypoglycemia, hypokalemia, hypokinesia, hyponatremia, hypotension, hypothermia, hypotonia, increased blood urea nitrogen, increased creatinine clearance, increased gamma-glutamyl transferase, increased lactate dehydrogenase, increased serum prolactin, intentional injury, ischemic heart disease, jaundice, leukopenia, mastalgia, memory impairment, myocardial infarction, myoclonus, neuroleptic malignant syndrome, neutropenia, nocturia, pancreatitis, Parkinson's disease, priapism, prolonged Q-T interval on ECG, rhabdomyolysis, seizure (including injection), suicidal ideation, suicidal tendencies, supraventricular tachycardia, syncope, tardive dyskinesia, thrombocytopenia, tics, tonic-clonic seizures, uncontrolled diabetes mellitus, urinary retention, ventricular tachycardia

Drug Interactions

Metabolism/Transport Effects Substrate of CYP2D6 (major), CYP3A4 (major); **Note:** Assignment of Major/Minor substrate status based on clinically relevant drug interaction potential

Avoid Concomitant Use

Avoid concomitant use of ARIPiprazole with any of the following: Amisulpride; Azelastine (Nasal); Fusidic Acid (Systemic); Metoclopramide; Paraldehyde; Sulpiride

Increased Effect/Toxicity

ARIPiprazole may increase the levels/effects of: Alcohol (Ethyl); Amisulpride; Azelastine (Nasal); Buprenorphine; CNS Depressants; DULoxetine; FLUoxetine; Haloperidol; Highest Risk QTc-Prolonging Agents; Hydrocodone; Methylphenidate; Moderate Risk QTc-Prolonging Agents; Paraldehyde; PARoxetine; Ritonavir; Serotonin Modulators; Sulpiride; Zolpidem

The levels/effects of ARIPiprazole may be increased by: Abiraterone Acetate; Acetylcholinesterase Inhibitors (Central); Brimonidine (Topical); CYP2D6 Inhibitors (Moderate); CYP2D6 Inhibitors (Strong); CYP2D6 Inhibitors (Weak); CYP3A4 Inhibitors (Moderate); CYP3A4 Inhibitors (Strong); CYP3A4 Inhibitors (Weak); Dasatinib; Doxylamine; Droperidol; DULoxetine; FLUoxetine; Fusidic Acid (Systemic); Haloperidol; HydrOXYzine; Ivacaftor; Lithium formulations; Luliconazole; Magnesium Sulfate; Methylphenidate; Metoclopramide; Metyrosine; Mifepristone; PARoxetine; Perampanel; Ritonavir; Serotonin Modulators; Sertraline; Simeprevir; Sodium Oxybate; Tetrabenazine

Decreased Effect

ARIPiprazole may decrease the levels/effects of: Amphetamines; Anti-Parkinson's Agents (Dopamine Agonist); Haloperidol; Quinagolide

The levels/effects of ARIPiprazole may be decreased by: Bosentan; CYP3A4 Inducers; CYP3A4 Inducers (Strong); Dabrafenib; Deferasirox; Lithium formulations; Mitotane; Peginterferon Alfa-2b; Tocilizumab

Ethanol/Nutrition/Herb Interactions

Ethanol: May increase CNS depression; monitor for increased effects with coadministration. Caution patients about effects.

Food: Ingestion with a high-fat meal delays time to peak plasma level.

Herb/Nutraceutical: St John's wort may decrease aripiprazole levels. Avoid kava kava, gotu kola, valerian, St John's wort (may increase CNS depression).

Preparation for Administration

Injection, powder for reconstitution: Reconstitute using 1.5 mL sterile water for injection (SWFI) (provided) for the 300 mg vial or 1.9 mL SWFI (provided) for the 400 mg vial to a final concentration of 200 mg/mL; residual SWFI should be discarded after reconstitution. Shake vigorously for 30 seconds or until the suspension is uniform; the resulting suspension will be milky white and opaque. If the suspension is not administered immediately after reconstitution, shake vigorously for 60 seconds prior to administration.

Storage/Stability

Injection, powder for reconstitution: Store unused vials at 25°C (77°F); excursions permitted to 15°C to 30°C (59°F to 86°F). If the suspension is not administered immediately after reconstitution, store at room temperature in the vial (do not store in a syringe); shake vigorously for 60 seconds prior to administration.

Injection solution: Store at 25°C (77°F); excursions permitted to 15°C to 30°C (59°F to 86°F). Protect from light.

Oral solution: Store at 25°C (77°F); excursions permitted to 15°C to 30°C (59°F to 86°F). Use within 6 months after opening.

Tablet: Store at 25°C (77°F); excursions permitted to 15°C to 30°C (59°F to 86°F).

Mechanism of Action Aripiprazole is a quinolinone antipsychotic which exhibits high affinity for D_2, D_3, 5-HT_{1A}, and 5-HT_{2A} receptors; moderate affinity for D_4, 5-HT_{2C}, 5-HT_7, $alpha_1$ adrenergic, and H_1 receptors. It also possesses moderate affinity for the serotonin reuptake transporter; has no affinity for muscarinic (cholinergic) receptors. Aripiprazole functions as a partial agonist at the D_2 and $5\text{-}HT_{1A}$ receptors, and as an antagonist at the $5\text{-}HT_{2A}$ receptor.

Pharmacodynamics/Kinetics

Onset of action: Initial: 1-3 weeks

Absorption: Well absorbed

Distribution: V_d: 4.9 L/kg

Protein binding: ≥99%, primarily to albumin

Metabolism: Hepatic, via CYP2D6, CYP3A4 (dehydro-aripiprazole metabolite has affinity for D_2 receptors similar to the parent drug and represents 40% of the parent drug exposure in plasma)

Bioavailability: I.M.: 100%; Tablet: 87%

Half-life elimination: Aripiprazole: 75 hours; dehydro-aripiprazole: 94 hours; I.M., extended release (terminal): ~30-47 days (dose-dependent)

CYP2D6 poor metabolizers: Aripiprazole: 146 hours

Time to peak, plasma:

I.M.:

Immediate release: 1-3 hours

Extended release: 5-7 days

Tablet: 3-5 hours

With high-fat meal: Aripiprazole: Delayed by 3 hours; dehydro-aripiprazole: Delayed by 12 hours

Excretion: Feces (55%, ~18% of the total dose as unchanged drug); urine (25%, <1% of the total dose as unchanged drug)

Dosage Note: Oral solution may be substituted for the oral tablet on a mg-per-mg basis, up to 25 mg. Patients receiving 30 mg tablets should be given 25 mg oral solution. Orally disintegrating tablets (Abilify Discmelt®) are bioequivalent to the immediate release tablets (Abilify®).

Children ≥6 years: Irritability associated with autistic disorder: Oral: Initial: 2 mg once daily for 7 days, followed by an increase to 5 mg once daily; subsequent dose increases may be made in 5 mg increments at intervals of ≥1 week as needed, up to a maximum of 15 mg/day. Efficacy of continued treatment >8 weeks has not been established; the need for ongoing treatment should be assessed periodically.

Children ≥10 years (U.S. labeling): Bipolar I disorder (acute manic or mixed episodes) Oral:

Stabilization: Initial: 2 mg once daily for 2 days, followed by 5 mg once daily for 2 days with a further increase to target dose of 10 mg once daily as monotherapy or as adjunct to lithium or valproic acid; subsequent dose increases may be made in 5 mg increments, up to a maximum of 30 mg/day

Maintenance: Continue stabilization dose for up to 6 weeks; efficacy of continued treatment >6 weeks has not been established.

Adolescents ≥13 years (Canadian labeling): Bipolar I disorder (acute manic or mixed episodes): Oral: Initial: 2 mg once daily for 2 days, followed by 5 mg once daily for 2 days with a further increase to target dose of 10 mg once daily as monotherapy; subsequent dose increases may be made in 5 mg increments, up to a maximum of 30 mg/day. **Note:** Not approved for maintenance or as adjunctive therapy.

Adolescents ≥13 years (U.S. labeling) or ≥15 years (Canadian labeling): Schizophrenia: Oral: Initial: 2 mg once daily for 2 days, followed by 5 mg once daily for 2 days with a further increase to target dose of 10 mg once daily; subsequent dose increases may be made in 5 mg increments up to a maximum of 30 mg/day (30 mg/day not shown to be more efficacious than 10 mg/day)

Adults:

Acute agitation (schizophrenia/bipolar mania): I.M.: 9.75 mg as a single dose (range: 5.25-15 mg); repeated doses may be given at ≥2-hour intervals to a maximum of 30 mg/day. **Note:** If ongoing therapy with aripiprazole is necessary, transition to oral therapy as soon as possible.

Bipolar I disorder (acute manic or mixed episodes): Oral:

Stabilization:

Monotherapy: Initial: 15 mg once daily. May increase to 30 mg once daily if clinically indicated; safety of doses >30 mg/day has not been evaluated

Adjunct to lithium or valproic acid: Initial: 10-15 mg once daily. May increase to 30 mg once daily if clinically indicated; safety of doses >30 mg/day has not been evaluated.

Maintenance: Continue stabilization dose for up to 6 weeks; efficacy of continued treatment >6 weeks has not been established

Depression (adjunctive with antidepressants): Oral: Initial: 2-5 mg/day (range: 2-15 mg/day); dose adjustments of up to 5 mg/day may be made in intervals of ≥1 week. **Note:** Dosing based on patients already receiving antidepressant therapy.

Schizophrenia:

Oral: 10-15 mg once daily; may be increased to a maximum of 30 mg once daily (efficacy at dosages above 10-15 mg has not been shown to be increased). Dosage titration should not be more frequent than every 2 weeks.

I.M, extended release (Abilify Maintena™): 400 mg once monthly (doses should be separated by ≥26 days); **Note:** Tolerability should be established using oral aripiprazole prior to initiation of parenteral therapy. Continue oral aripiprazole (or other oral antipsychotic) for 14 days during initiation of parenteral therapy.

Missed doses:

Second or third doses missed:

>4 weeks but <5 weeks since last dose: Administer next dose as soon as possible

>5 weeks since last dose: Administer oral aripiprazole for 14 days with next injection

Fourth or subsequent doses missed:

>4 weeks but <6 weeks since last dose: Administer next dose as soon as possible

>6 weeks since last dose: Administer oral aripiprazole for 14 days with next injection

Dosage adjustment for adverse effects: Consider reducing dose to 300 mg once monthly

Elderly: Refer to adult dosing

Dosage adjustment with concurrent CYP450 inducer or inhibitor therapy:

Oral:

CYP3A4 inducers (eg, carbamazepine): Aripiprazole dose should be doubled; dose should be subsequently reduced if concurrent inducer agent discontinued.

Strong CYP3A4 inhibitors (eg, ketoconazole): Aripiprazole dose should be reduced to 50% of the usual dose, and proportionally increased upon discontinuation of the inhibitor agent.

Strong CYP2D6 inhibitors (eg, fluoxetine, paroxetine): Aripiprazole dose should be reduced to 50% of the usual dose, and proportionally increased upon discontinuation of the inhibitor agent. **Note:** Dose reduction does not apply to patients with major depressive disorder; follow usual dosing recommendations.

CYP3A4 and CYP2D6 inhibitors: Aripiprazole dose should be reduced to 25% of the usual dose. In patients receiving inhibitors of differing (eg, moderate 3A4/strong 2D6) or same (eg, moderate 3A4/moderate 2D6) potencies (excluding concurrent strong inhibitors), further dosage adjustments can be made to achieve the desired clinical response. In patients receiving strong CYP3A4 and 2D6 inhibitors, aripiprazole dose is proportionally increased upon discontinuation of one or both inhibitor agents.

I.M., extended release (Abilify Maintena™): **Note:** Dosage adjustments are not recommended for concomitant use of CYP3A4 inhibitors, CYP2D6 inhibitors or CYP3A4 inducers for <14 days. In patients who had their aripiprazole dose adjusted for concomitant therapy, the aripiprazole dose may need to be increased if the CYP3A4 and/ or CYP2D6 inhibitor is withdrawn.

CYP3A4 inducers: Avoid use; aripiprazole serum concentrations may fall below effective levels.

Strong CYP3A4 or CYP2D6 inhibitors:

Current aripiprazole dose of 300 mg once monthly: Reduce aripiprazole dose to 200 mg once monthly

Current aripiprazole dose of 400 mg once monthly: Reduce aripiprazole dose to 300 mg once monthly

Strong CYP3A4 inhibitors **and** CYPD2D6 inhibitors:

Current aripiprazole dose of 300 mg once monthly: Reduce aripiprazole dose to 160 mg once monthly

Current aripiprazole dose of 400 mg once monthly: Reduce aripiprazole dose to 200 mg once monthly

Dosage adjustment based on CYP2D6 metabolizer status:

Oral: Aripiprazole dose should be reduced to 50% of the usual dose in CYP2D6 poor metabolizers and to 25% of the usual dose in poor metabolizers receiving a concurrent strong CYP3A4 inhibitor; subsequently adjust dose for favorable clinical response.

I.M., extended release (Abilify Maintena™): Reduce aripiprazole dose to 300 mg once monthly in CYP2D6 poor metabolizers; reduce dose to 200 mg once monthly in CYP2D6 poor metabolizers receiving a concurrent CYP3A4 inhibitor for >14 days.

Dosage adjustment in renal impairment: No dosage adjustment necessary.

Dosage adjustment in hepatic impairment: No dosage adjustment necessary.

Dietary Considerations May be taken with or without food. Some products may contain phenylalanine.

Administration

Injection: For I.M. use only; do not administer SubQ or I.V.; **Note:** Immediate release and extended release parenteral products are **not** interchangeable.

Immediate release (Abilify®): Inject slowly into deep muscle mass

Extended release (Abilify Maintena™): Inject slowly into gluteal muscle using the provided 1.5 inch (38 mm) needle for nonobese patients or the provided 2 inch (50 mm) needle for obese patients. Do not massage muscle after administration. Rotate injection sites between the two gluteal muscles. Administer monthly (doses should be separated by ≥26 days).

Oral: May be administered with or without food. Tablet and oral solution may be interchanged on a mg-per-mg basis, up to 25 mg. Doses using 30 mg tablets should be exchanged for 25 mg oral solution. Orally disintegrating tablets (Abilify Discmelt®) are bioequivalent to the immediate release tablets (Abilify®).

Orally disintegrating tablet: Remove from foil blister by peeling back (do not push tablet through the foil). Place tablet in mouth immediately upon removal. Tablet dissolves rapidly in saliva and may be swallowed without liquid. If needed, can be taken with liquid. Do not split tablet.

Monitoring Parameters Vital signs; fasting lipid profile and fasting blood glucose/Hb A_{1c} (prior to treatment, at 3 months, then annually); CBC frequently during first few months of therapy in patients with pre-existing low WBC or a history of drug-induced leukopenia/neutropenia; BMI, personal/family history of diabetes, waist circumference, blood pressure, mental status, abnormal involuntary movement scale (AIMS), extrapyramidal symptoms (EPS). Weight should be assessed prior to treatment, at 4 weeks, 8 weeks, 12 weeks, and then at quarterly intervals. Consider titrating to a different antipsychotic agent for a weight gain ≥5% of the initial weight.

Dosage Forms Excipient information presented when available (limited, particularly for generics); consult specific product labeling.

Solution, Intramuscular:

Abilify: 9.75 mg/1.3 mL (1.3 mL)

Solution, Oral:

Abilify: 1 mg/mL (150 mL) [contains methylparaben, propylene glycol, propylparaben; orange cream flavor]

Suspension Reconstituted, Intramuscular:

Abilify Maintena: 300 mg (1 ea); 400 mg (1 ea)

Tablet, Oral:

Abilify: 2 mg, 5 mg, 10 mg, 15 mg, 20 mg, 30 mg

Tablet Dispersible, Oral:

Abilify Discmelt: 10 mg, 15 mg [contains aspartame, fd&c blue #2 aluminum lake]

◆ **Aristospan® (Can)** *see* Triamcinolone (Systemic) *on page 2121*

◆ **Aristospan Intra-Articular** *see* Triamcinolone (Systemic) *on page 2121*

◆ **Aristospan Intralesional** *see* Triamcinolone (Systemic) *on page 2121*

◆ **Arixtra** *see* Fondaparinux *on page 911*

◆ **Arixtra® (Can)** *see* Fondaparinux *on page 911*

Armodafinil (ar moe DAF i nil)

Brand Names: U.S. Nuvigil

Index Terms R-modafinil

Pharmacologic Category Central Nervous System Stimulant

Use Improve wakefulness in patients with excessive daytime sleepiness associated with narcolepsy and shift work sleep disorder (SWSD); adjunctive therapy for obstructive sleep apnea/hypopnea syndrome (OSAHS)

Pregnancy Risk Factor C

Pregnancy Considerations Adverse events have been observed in animal reproduction studies, including visceral and skeletal abnormalities and decreased fetal weight. Efficacy of steroidal contraceptives may be decreased; alternate means of contraception should be considered during therapy and for 1 month after armodafinil is discontinued. A pregnancy registry has been established for patients exposed to armodafinil; healthcare providers are encouraged to register pregnant patients or pregnant women may register themselves by calling 1-866-404-4106.

Breast-Feeding Considerations It is not known if armodafinil or its metabolite is excreted into breast milk. The manufacture recommends caution be used if administered to a nursing woman.

Medication Guide Available Yes

Contraindications Hypersensitivity to armodafinil, modafinil, or any component of the formulation

Warnings/Precautions For use following complete evaluation of sleepiness and in conjunction with other standard treatments (eg, CPAP). The degree of sleepiness should be reassessed frequently; some patients may not return to a normal level of wakefulness. Patients with excessive sleepiness should be advised to avoid driving or any other potentially dangerous activity. Use >12 weeks has not been studied; patient should be reevaluated to determine effectiveness if use exceeds 12 weeks. Use is not recommended in patients with a history of angina or myocardial infarction, left ventricular hypertrophy, or patients with mitral valve prolapse who have developed mitral valve prolapse syndrome with previous CNS stimulant use. Patients with these conditions may also experience chest pain, palpitations, dyspnea, and transient ischemic T-wave changes on ECG. Increased blood pressure monitoring may be required in patients taking armodafinil. New or additional antihypertensive therapy may be needed.

Serious and life-threatening rashes including Stevens-Johnson syndrome, toxic epidermal necrolysis, and drug rash with eosinophilia and systemic symptoms (DRESS) have been reported. In modafinil clinical trials, rashes were more likely to occur in children; serious, postmarketing reactions have occurred with modafinil in adults and children as well as with armodafinil in adults. Most cases have been reported within the first 5 weeks of initiating therapy; however, rare cases have occurred after prolonged therapy. No risk factors have been identified to predict occurrence or severity of these reactions. Patients should be advised to discontinue use at first sign of rash (unless the rash is clearly not drug-related). Rare cases of multiorgan hypersensitivity reactions (with modafinil) and cases of angioedema and anaphylactoid reactions (armodafinil) have been reported. Signs and symptoms of multiorgan hypersensitivity reactions are diverse. Patients typically present with fever and rash associated with other organ system involvement. Patients should be advised to discontinue therapy and promptly report any signs or symptoms related to these adverse effects.

Caution should be exercised when modafinil is given to patients with a history of psychosis, depression, or mania; use may worsen symptoms (eg, mania, hallucinations, suicidal thoughts) of these disease; discontinue therapy if psychiatric symptoms develop. Use may impair the ability to engage in potentially hazardous activities; patients must be cautioned about performing tasks which require mental alertness (eg, operating machinery or driving). Stimulants may unmask tics in individuals with coexisting Tourette's syndrome. Use caution with hepatic impairment; consider use of a reduced dosage in patients with hepatic impairment or elderly patients. Safety and efficacy have not been established in patients with severe renal impairment. Use with caution in patients with a history of drug abuse; potential for drug dependency exists.

Adverse Reactions

>10%: Central nervous system: Headache (14% to 23%; dose-related)

1% to 10%:

Cardiovascular: Palpitation (2%), heart rate increased (1%)

Central nervous system: Dizziness (5%), insomnia (4% to 6%; dose related), anxiety (4%), depression (1% to 3%; dose related), fatigue (2%), agitation (1%), attention disturbance (1%), depressed mood (1%), migraine (1%), nervousness (1%), pain (1%), pyrexia (1%), tremor (1%)

Dermatologic: Rash (1% to 4%; dose related), contact dermatitis (1%), hyperhidrosis (1%)

Gastrointestinal: Nausea (6% to 9%; dose related), xerostomia (2% to 7%; dose related), diarrhea (4%), abdominal pain (2%), dyspepsia (2%), anorexia (1%), appetite decreased (1%), constipation (1%), loose stools (1%), vomiting (1%)

Genitourinary: Polyuria (1%)

Hepatic: GGT increased (1%)

Neuromuscular & skeletal: Paresthesia (1%)

Respiratory: Dyspnea (1%)

Miscellaneous: Flu-like syndrome (1%), seasonal allergy (1%), thirst (1%)

Postmarketing and/or case reports: Angioedema, hypersensitivity, liver enzymes increased, nonimmunologic anaphylaxis (formerly known as anaphylactoid reaction), pancytopenia, systolic blood pressure increased

Drug Interactions

Metabolism/Transport Effects Substrate of CYP3A4 (major); **Note:** Assignment of Major/Minor substrate status based on clinically relevant drug interaction potential; **Inhibits** CYP2C19 (moderate); **Induces** CYP3A4 (weak/moderate)

Avoid Concomitant Use

Avoid concomitant use of Armodafinil with any of the following: Axitinib; Conivaptan; Fusidic Acid (Systemic); Iobenguane I 123; Simeprevir

Increased Effect/Toxicity

Armodafinil may increase the levels/effects of: Citalopram; CYP2C19 Substrates; Sympathomimetics

The levels/effects of Armodafinil may be increased by: AtoMOXetine; Cannabinoids; Conivaptan; CYP3A4 Inhibitors (Moderate); CYP3A4 Inhibitors (Strong); Dasatinib; Fusidic Acid (Systemic); Ivacaftor; Linezolid; Luliconazole; Mifepristone; Simeprevir

Decreased Effect

Armodafinil may decrease the levels/effects of: ARIPiprazole; Axitinib; Clopidogrel; Contraceptives (Estrogens); CycloSPORINE (Systemic); Ibrutinib; Iobenguane I 123; Saxagliptin; Simeprevir

The levels/effects of Armodafinil may be decreased by: Bosentan; CYP3A4 Inducers (Strong); Dabrafenib; Deferasirox; Herbs (CYP3A4 Inducers); Mitotane; Tocilizumab

Ethanol/Nutrition/Herb Interactions

Ethanol: Avoid or limit ethanol.

Food: Delays absorption, but minimal effects on bioavailability. Food may affect the onset and time course of armodafinil.

Storage/Stability Store at 20°C to 25°C (68°F to 77°F).

Mechanism of Action The exact mechanism of action of armodafinil is unknown. It is the R-enantiomer of modafinil. Armodafinil binds to the dopamine transporter and inhibits dopamine reuptake, which may result in increased extracellular dopamine levels in the brain. However, it does not appear to be a dopamine receptor agonist and also does not appear to bind to or inhibit the most common receptors or enzymes that are relevant for sleep/wake regulation.

Pharmacodynamics/Kinetics

Absorption: Readily absorbed

Distribution: V_d: 42 L

Protein binding: ~60% (based on modafinil; primarily albumin)

Metabolism: Hepatic, multiple pathways, including amine hydrolysis and CYP3A4/5; metabolites include R-modafinil acid and modafinil sulfone

Half-life elimination: 15 hours; Steady state: ~7 days

Time to peak, plasma: 2 hours (fasted)

Excretion: Urine (based on modafinil: 80% predominantly as metabolites; <10% as unchanged drug)

Dosage Oral:

Adults:

Narcolepsy: 150-250 mg once daily in the morning

Obstructive sleep apnea/hypopnea syndrome (OSAHS): 150-250 mg once daily in the morning; doses >150 mg have not been shown to have an increased benefit

Shift work sleep disorder (SWSD): 150 mg given once daily ~1 hour prior to work shift

Elderly: Consider lower initial dosage. Concentrations were almost doubled in clinical trials (based on modafinil)

Dosage adjustment in renal impairment: Safety and efficacy have not been established in severe renal impairment.

Dosage adjustment in hepatic impairment: Severe hepatic impairment: The manufacturer recommends a reduced dose; based on modafinil pharmacokinetics, a dose reduction of one-half the normal dose should be considered.

Dietary Considerations Take with or without meals.

Administration May be administered without regard to food.

Monitoring Parameters Signs of hypersensitivity, rash, psychiatric symptoms, levels of sleepiness, blood pressure, and drug abuse

Dosage Forms Excipient information presented when available (limited, particularly for generics); consult specific product labeling.

Tablet, Oral:

Nuvigil: 50 mg, 150 mg, 250 mg

Controlled Substance C-IV

- **Armour Thyroid** *see* Thyroid, Desiccated *on page 2052*
- **Aromasin** *see* Exemestane *on page 813*
- **Aromasin® (Can)** *see* Exemestane *on page 813*
- **Arranon** *see* Nelarabine *on page 1434*

Arsenic Trioxide (AR se nik tri OKS id)

Brand Names: U.S. Trisenox

Brand Names: Canada Trisenox

Index Terms As_2O_3

Pharmacologic Category Antineoplastic Agent, Miscellaneous

Use Remission induction and consolidation in patients with relapsed or refractory acute promyelocytic leukemia (APL) characterized by t(15;17) translocation or PML/RAR-alpha gene expression

Unlabeled Use Initial treatment of APL, treatment of myelodysplastic syndrome (MDS)

Pregnancy Risk Factor D

Pregnancy Considerations Increased resorptions, neural-tube defects, and ophthalmic abnormalities have been observed in animal studies. Arsenic crosses the human placenta. In studies of women exposed to high levels of arsenic from drinking water, cord blood levels were similar to maternal serum levels. Dimethylarsinic acid (DMA) was the form of arsenic found in the fetus. An increased risk of low birth weight and still births were observed in women who ingested high levels of dietary arsenic. Women of childbearing potential should avoid pregnancy. The Canadian labeling contraindicates use in pregnant women. It also recommends that women of childbearing potential avoid pregnancy, and male patients wear condoms during intercourse with women who are pregnant or of childbearing potential during therapy and for 3 months following therapy discontinuation.

Breast-Feeding Considerations Arsenic is naturally found in breast milk; concentrations range from 0.2-6 mcg/kg. In studies of women exposed to high levels of arsenic from drinking water, breast milk concentrations were low (~3.1 mcg/kg) and did not correlate with maternal serum levels. The possible effect of maternal arsenic trioxide therapy on breast milk concentrations is not known. Due to the potential for serious adverse reactions in a nursing infant, breast-feeding during therapy is not recommended. The Canadian labeling contraindicates use in nursing women and recommends avoiding nursing for 3 months after therapy discontinuation.

Contraindications

Hypersensitivity to arsenic or any component of the formulation

Canadian labeling: Additional contraindications (not in U.S. labeling): Pregnancy; breast-feeding

Warnings/Precautions Hazardous agent - use appropriate precautions for handling and disposal (NIOSH, 2012). **[U.S. Boxed Warnings]: May prolong the QT interval. May lead to torsade de pointes or complete AV block.** Risk factors for torsade de pointes include extent of prolongation, HF, a history of torsade de pointes, preexisting QT interval prolongation, patients taking medications know to prolong the QT interval or potassium-wasting diuretics, and conditions which cause hypokalemia or hypomagnesemia. If possible, discontinue all medications known to prolong the QT interval. **[U.S. Boxed Warning]: A baseline 12-lead ECG, serum electrolytes (potassium, calcium, magnesium), and creatinine should be obtained prior to treatment.** Correct electrolyte abnormalities prior to treatment and monitor potassium and magnesium levels during therapy (maintain potassium >4 mEq/dL and magnesium >1.8 mg/dL). If baseline QT_c >500 msec, correct prior to treatment. If QT_c >500 msec during treatment, reassess, correct contributing factors, and consider temporarily withholding treatment. If syncope or irregular heartbeat develop during therapy, hospitalize patient and do not reinitiate until QT_c <460 msec, electrolyte abnormalities are corrected and syncope/irregular heartbeat has resolved. Monitor ECG weekly; more frequently if clinically indicated.

[U.S. Boxed Warning]: May cause APL differentiation syndrome (formerly called retinoic-acid-APL [RA-APL] syndrome) in patients with APL, which is characterized by dyspnea, fever, weight gain, pulmonary infiltrates, and pleural or pericardial effusions. May be fatal. High-dose steroids (dexamethasone 10 mg I.V. twice daily for ≥3 days; begin at initial presentation) have been used for treatment; in general, most patients may continue arsenic trioxide during treatment of APL differentiation syndrome. May lead to the development of hyperleukocytosis (leukocytes ≥10,000/mm^3); did not correlate with baseline WBC counts and generally was not as high during consolidation as observed during induction treatment. Use with caution in patients with hepatic impairment; in patients with severe hepatic impairment, monitor closely for toxicity. Use with caution in patients with severe renal impairment; systemic exposure to metabolites may be higher; has not been studied in dialysis patients. Monitor electrolytes, CBC with differential, and coagulation parameters at least twice a week during induction and weekly during consolidation; more frequently if clinically indicated. **[U.S. Boxed Warning]: Should be administered under the supervision of a physician experienced in acute leukemia management.**

Adverse Reactions

>10%:

Cardiovascular: Tachycardia (55%), edema (40%), QT interval >500 msec (40%), chest pain (25%; grades 3/4: 5%), hypotension (25%; grades 3/4: 5%)

Central nervous system: Fatigue (63%), fever (63%), headache (60%), insomnia (43%), anxiety (30%), dizziness (23%), depression (20%), pain (15%)

Dermatologic: Dermatitis (43%), pruritus (33%), bruising (20%), dry skin (15%), erythema (13%)

Endocrine & metabolic: Hypokalemia (50%; grades 3/4: 13%), hyperglycemia (45%; grades 3/4: 13%), hypomagnesemia (45%; grades 3/4: 13%), hyperkalemia (18%; grades 3/4: 5%)

Gastrointestinal: Nausea (75%), abdominal pain (58%), vomiting (58%), diarrhea (53%), sore throat (35%), constipation (28%), anorexia (23%), appetite decreased (15%), weight gain (13%)

Genitourinary: Vaginal hemorrhage (13%)

Hematologic: Leukocytosis (50%; grades 3/4: 3%), APL differentiation syndrome (23%; grades 3/4: 8%), anemia (20%; grades 3/4: 5%), thrombocytopenia (18%; grades 3/4: 13%), febrile neutropenia (13%; grades 3/4: 8%)

Hepatic: ALT increased (20%; grades 3/4: 5%), AST increased (13%; grades 3/4: 3%)

Local: Injection site: Pain (20%), erythema (13%)

Neuromuscular & skeletal: Rigors (38%), arthralgia (33%), paresthesia (33%), myalgia (25%), bone pain (23%), back pain (18%), limb pain (13%), neck pain (13%), tremor (13%)

Respiratory: Cough (65%), dyspnea (53%; grades 3/4: 10%), epistaxis (25%), hypoxia (23%), pleural effusion (20%), sinusitis (20%), postnasal drip (13%), upper respiratory tract infection (13%), wheezing (13%)
Miscellaneous: Herpes simplex (13%), diaphoresis (13%)

1% to 10%:
Cardiovascular: Hypertension (10%), flushing (10%), pallor (10%), palpitation (10%), facial edema (8%), abnormal ECG (not QT prolongation) (8%), atrial dysrhythmia (5%), torsade de pointes (3%)
Central nervous system: Seizure (8%; grades 3/4: 5%), somnolence (8%), agitation (5%), coma (5%), confusion (5%)
Dermatologic: Hyperpigmentation (8%), petechia (8%), skin lesions (8%), urticaria (8%), local exfoliation (5%)
Endocrine & metabolic: Hypocalcemia (10%), hypoglycemia (8%), intermenstrual bleeding (8%), acidosis (5%)
Gastrointestinal: Dyspepsia (10%), loose stools (10%), abdominal distension (8%), abdominal tenderness (8%), caecitis (children: 8%), fecal incontinence (8%), gastrointestinal hemorrhage (8%), hemorrhagic diarrhea (8%), oral blistering (8%), weight loss (8%), xerostomia (8%), oral candidiasis (5%)
Genitourinary: Incontinence (5%)
Hematologic: Neutropenia (10%; grades 3/4: 10%), DIC (8%), hemorrhage (8%)
Local: Injection site edema (10%)
Neuromuscular & skeletal: Weakness (10%)
Ocular: Blurred vision (10%), eye irritation (10%), dry eye (8%), eyelid edema (5%), painful red eye (5%)
Otic: Earache (8%), tinnitus (5%)
Renal: Renal failure (8%; grades 3/4: 3%), renal impairment (8%), oliguria (5%)
Respiratory: Breath sounds decreased (10%), crepitations (10%), rales (10%), hemoptysis (8%), pulmonary edema (children: 8%), rhonchi (8%), tachypnea (8%), nasopharyngitis (5%)
Miscellaneous: Bacterial infection (8%), herpes zoster (8%), lymphadenopathy (8%), night sweats (8%), hypersensitivity (5%), sepsis (5%; grades 3/4: 5%)

<1% (Limited to important or life-threatening): Acute respiratory distress syndrome, AV block, capillary leak syndrome, CHF, heart block, hypoalbuminemia, hyponatremia, hypophosphatemia, lipase increased, mitochondrial myopathy, pancytopenia, peripheral neuropathy, pneumonitis, pulmonary infiltrate, respiratory distress, stomatitis, ventricular extrasystoles, ventricular tachycardia

Drug Interactions

Metabolism/Transport Effects None known.

Avoid Concomitant Use

Avoid concomitant use of Arsenic Trioxide with any of the following: CloZAPine; Highest Risk QTc-Prolonging Agents; Ivabradine; Mifepristone; Moderate Risk QTc-Prolonging Agents

Increased Effect/Toxicity

Arsenic Trioxide may increase the levels/effects of: CloZAPine; Highest Risk QTc-Prolonging Agents; Hypoglycemic Agents

The levels/effects of Arsenic Trioxide may be increased by: Herbs (Hypoglycemic Properties); Ivabradine; MAO Inhibitors; Mifepristone; Moderate Risk QTc-Prolonging Agents; QTc-Prolonging Agents (Indeterminate Risk and Risk Modifying); Salicylates; Selective Serotonin Reuptake Inhibitors

Decreased Effect

The levels/effects of Arsenic Trioxide may be decreased by: Loop Diuretics

Ethanol/Nutrition/Herb Interactions Herb/Nutraceutical: Avoid homeopathic products (arsenic is present in some homeopathic medications). Avoid hypoglycemic herbs, including alfalfa, aloe, bilberry, bitter melon, burdock, celery, damiana, fenugreek, garcinia, garlic, ginger, ginseng, gymnema, marshmallow, and stinging nettle (may enhance the hypoglycemic effect of arsenic trioxide).

Preparation for Administration Hazardous agent; use appropriate precautions for handling and disposal (NIOSH, 2012). Dilute in 100-250 mL D_5W or 0.9% NaCl. Discard unused portion of ampul.

Storage/Stability Store at 25°C (77°F); excursions permitted to 15°C to 30°C (59°F to 86°F); do not freeze. Following dilution, stable for 24 hours at room temperature or 48 hours when refrigerated.

Mechanism of Action Induces apoptosis in APL cells via morphological changes and DNA fragmentation; also damages or degrades the fusion protein PML-RAR alpha

Pharmacodynamics/Kinetics

Distribution: V_{dss}: As^{III}: 562 L; widely distributed throughout body tissues; orally administered arsenic trioxide distributes into the CNS
Metabolism: Arsenic trioxide is immediately hydrolyzed to the active form, arsenious acid (As^{III}) which is methylated (hepatically) to the less active pentavalent metabolites, monomethylarsonic acid (MMA^{V}) and dimethylarsinic acid (DMA^{V}) by methyltransferases; As^{III} is also oxidized to the minor metabolite, arsenic acid (As^{V})
Half-life elimination: AS^{III}: 10-14 hours; MMA^{V}: ~32 hours; DMA^{V}: ~72 hours
Time to peak: As^{III}: At the end of infusion; MMA^{V} and DMA^{V}; ~10-24 hours
Excretion: Urine (MMA^{V}, DMA^{V}, and 15% of a dose as unchanged As^{III})

Dosage I.V.:

APL, relapsed or refractory: Children ≥4 years (U.S. labeling) or ≥5 years (Canadian labeling) and Adults:
Induction: 0.15 mg/kg/day; administer daily until bone marrow remission; maximum induction: 60 doses
Consolidation: 0.15 mg/kg/day starting 3-6 weeks after completion of induction therapy; maximum consolidation: 25 doses over a period of up to 5 weeks

APL initial treatment (unlabeled use):
Children: Induction, consolidation, and maintenance (Mathews, 2006):
Induction: 0.15 mg/kg/day (maximum dose: 10 mg); administer daily until bone marrow remission; maximum induction: 60 doses
Consolidation: 0.15 mg/kg/day (maximum dose: 10 mg) for 4 weeks, starting 4 weeks after completion of induction therapy
Maintenance: 0.15 mg/kg/dose (maximum dose: 10 mg) administered 10 days per month for 6 months, starting 4 weeks after completion of consolidation therapy

Adults:
Induction, consolidation, and maintenance (Mathews, 2006):
Induction: 10 mg/day; administer daily until bone marrow remission; maximum induction: 60 doses
Consolidation: 10 mg/day for 4 weeks, starting 4 weeks after completion of induction therapy
Maintenance: 10 mg/dose administered 10 days per month for 6 months, starting 4 weeks after completion of consolidation therapy

Consolidation therapy after remission induction with tretinoin, daunorubicin and cytarabine (Powell, 2007; Powell, 2010): Two consolidation courses (2 weeks apart): 0.15 mg/kg/day 5 days/week for 5 weeks

In combination with tretinoin (Estey, 2006; Ravandi, 2009):
Induction (beginning 10 days after initiation of tretinoin): 0.15 mg/kg/day until bone marrow remission; maximum induction: 75 doses
Consolidation: 0.15 mg/kg/day Monday through Friday for 4 weeks every 8 weeks for 4 cycles (weeks 1 to 4, 9 to 12, 17 to 20, and 25 to 28)

MDS (unlabeled uses): Adults: 0.25 mg/kg/day 5 consecutive days/week for 2 weeks, followed by a 2-week rest period (Schiller, 2006)

Dosage adjustment in renal impairment:
Mild-to-moderate impairment (Cl_{cr} ≥30 mL/minute): No dosage adjustment provided in manufacturer's labeling.
Severe renal impairment (Cl_{cr} <30 mL/minute): Use with caution (systemic exposure to metabolites may be higher); may require dosage reduction; monitor closely for toxicity
Dialysis patients: Has not been studied

Dosage adjustment in hepatic impairment: No dosage adjustment provided in manufacturer's labeling; use with caution. Patients with severe impairment (Child-Pugh class C) should be monitored closely for toxicity.

Dosing in obesity: *ASCO Guidelines for appropriate chemotherapy dosing in obese adults with cancer:* Utilize patient's actual body weight (full weight) for calculation of body surface area- or weight-based dosing, particularly when the intent of therapy is curative; manage regimen-related toxicities in the same manner as for nonobese patients; if a dose reduction is utilized due to toxicity, consider resumption of full weight-based dosing with subsequent cycles, especially if cause of toxicity (eg, hepatic or renal impairment) is resolved (Griggs, 2012).
Note: The Canadian labeling recommends dosing obese pediatric patients based on ideal body weight.

Administration Administer as I.V. infusion over 1-2 hours. If acute vasomotor reactions occur, infuse over a maximum of 4 hours. Does not require administration via a central venous catheter.

Hazardous agent; use appropriate precautions for handling and disposal (NIOSH, 2012).

Monitoring Parameters Baseline then weekly 12-lead ECG; monitor electrolytes, CBC with differential, and coagulation at baseline then at least twice weekly during induction and at least weekly during consolidation; more frequent monitoring may be necessary in unstable patients

Dosage Forms Excipient information presented when available (limited, particularly for generics); consult specific product labeling.
Solution, Intravenous:
Trisenox: 10 mg/10 mL (10 mL)

◆ **Artane** *see* Trihexyphenidyl *on page 2127*

◆ **Artemether and Benflumetol** *see* Artemether and Lumefantrine *on page 171*

Artemether and Lumefantrine
(ar TEM e ther & loo me FAN treen)

Brand Names: U.S. Coartem

Index Terms Artemether and Benflumetol; Benflumetol and Artemether; Lumefantrine and Artemether

Pharmacologic Category Antimalarial Agent

Use Treatment of acute, uncomplicated malaria infections due to *Plasmodium falciparum*, including geographical regions where chloroquine resistance has been reported

Pregnancy Risk Factor C

Dosage Oral: Three-day schedule for the treatment of uncomplicated malaria (chloroquine-resistant uncomplicated *P. falciparum*):
Children 2 months to ≤16 years:
5 to <15 kg: One tablet at hour 0 and hour 8 on the first day, then 1 tablet twice daily on day 2 and day 3 (total of 6 tablets per treatment course)
15 to <25 kg: Two tablets at hour 0 and hour 8 on the first day, then 2 tablets twice daily on day 2 and day 3 (total of 12 tablets per treatment course)
25 to <35 kg: Three tablets at hour 0 and hour 8 on the first day, then 3 tablets twice daily on day 2 and day 3 (total of 18 tablets per treatment course)
≥35 kg: Four tablets at hour 0 and hour 8 on the first day, then 4 tablets twice daily on day 2 and day 3 (total of 24 tablets per treatment course)
Children >16 years and Adults:
25 to <35 kg: Three tablets at hour 0 and hour 8 on the first day, then 3 tablets twice daily on day 2 and day 3 (total of 18 tablets per treatment course)
≥35 kg: Four tablets at hour 0 and hour 8 on the first day, then 4 tablets twice daily on day 2 and day 3 (total of 24 tablets per treatment course)

Dosage adjustment in renal impairment: Dosage adjustment not recommended in mild or moderate impairment. Use caution in severe renal impairment (has not been studied).

Dosage adjustment in hepatic impairment: Dosage adjustments are not recommended in mild or moderate impairment. Use caution in severe impairment (has not been studied).

Additional Information Complete prescribing information should be consulted for additional detail.

Dosage Forms Excipient information presented when available (limited, particularly for generics); consult specific product labeling.
Tablet:
Coartem: Artemether 20 mg and lumefantrine 120 mg

◆ **Artemisinin Derivative** *see* Artesunate *on page 171*

Artesunate (ar TES oo nate)

Index Terms Artemisinin Derivative; Artesunic Acid; Dihydroartemisinin Hemisuccinate Sodium; Dihydroqinghaosu Hemisuccinate Sodium; Nuartez™; P01BE03; Qinghao Derivative; Qinghaosu Derivative; Sodium Artesunate

Pharmacologic Category Antimalarial Agent; Artemisinin Derivative

Unlabeled Use Treatment of severe malaria

Pregnancy Considerations Teratogenic effects have been observed in animal reproduction studies. Limited studies in pregnant women have not revealed an increased risk of congenital abnormalities in newborns (McGready, 1998; McGready, 2008). Malaria infection in pregnant women may be more severe than in nonpregnant women. Because *P. falciparum* malaria can cause maternal death, congenital malaria, and fetal loss, pregnant women traveling to malaria-endemic areas must use personal protection against mosquito bites.

Breast-Feeding Considerations The benefits of breast-feeding to mother and infants should be weighed against the potential risk from infant exposure to artesunate.

Prescribing and Access Restrictions Investigational agent – not approved for use in the U.S.

Artesunate is available in the U.S. for I.V. use in patients with malaria through an Investigational New Drug (IND) protocol. To obtain artesunate via the IND protocol, clinicians must contact the Centers for Disease Control (CDC) Malaria Hotline at 770-488-7788 (business hours) or 770-488-7100 (nonbusiness hours) and request to speak with a CDC Malaria Branch clinician.

Eligibility criteria under the IND protocol include (Hess, 2010):
- **Patients must have malaria:** Diagnosis by microscopy or strong clinical suspicion of *Plasmodium falciparum* or other *Plasmodium* spp. infection
- **Patients must require parenteral therapy:** Unable to take oral medications, high-density parasitemia (eg, >5%), or diagnosis of severe malaria

- **I.V. artesunate must be the preferred treatment:** I.V. artesunate is at least as readily available as I.V. quinidine or the patient has experienced quinidine failure (eg, parasitemia >10% baseline after 48 hours of quinidine therapy), quinidine intolerance, or contraindications to quinidine

For medical access to I.V. artesunate in Canada, please refer to special access information on the Public Health Agency of Canada website, http://www.phac-aspc.gc.ca/tmp-pmv/quinine/.

Contraindications Hypersensitivity to artesunate or any component of the formulation (Hess, 2010)

Warnings/Precautions Severe allergic reactions have been reported with oral administration of artesunate (Leonardi, 2001); monitor for signs of hypersensitivity and discontinue treatment in patients who develop severe hypersensitivity reactions (eg, angioedema, dyspnea, erythema, anaphylaxis). QT prolongation has been reported with other artemisinin derivatives (eg, artemether); however, one report suggests that the mean QT_c interval was unaffected by artesunate (Maude, 2010).

Adverse Reactions Frequency not defined.

Cardiovascular: Hypotension

Central nervous system: Anxiety, dizziness, headache, restlessness, slurred speech

Dermatologic: Angioedema, erythema, pruritus, rash, urticaria

Endocrine & metabolic: Hypoglycemia

Gastrointestinal: Anorexia, diarrhea, metallic taste, nausea, vomiting

Hematologic: Anemia, hemolysis, neutropenia, reticulocytopenia

Hepatic: ALT increased

Neuromuscular & skeletal: Ataxia, hyperreflexia, tremor

Renal: BUN increased

Respiratory: Dyspnea

Miscellaneous: Hypersensitivity reaction

Preparation for Administration Reconstitute vial with 11 mL of phosphate buffer diluent to a final concentration of 10 mg/mL; gently swirl for 5-6 minutes to mix.

Storage/Stability Reconstituted solutions are stable for 1 hour following reconstitution.

Mechanism of Action

Artesunate, a semisynthetic derivative of artemisinin, is a prodrug which is converted to dihydroartemisinin (DHA). DHA is an antimalarial agent active against all of the erythrocytic stages of the parasite including gametocytes; inhibits parasite metabolism and enhances the clearance of infected erythrocytes.

Antiparasitic activity is hypothesized to involve cleavage of the $Fe^{2+}$of endoperoxide bridge, thereby producing free radicals and damaging parasite proteins. DHA may also inhibit calcium adenosine triphosphatase (cATP) of the sarcoplasmic endoplasmic reticulum and impair parasite protein folding.

Pharmacodynamics/Kinetics

Distribution: V_{dss}: Adults infected with severe malaria: Artesunate: 15.2 L/kg (range: 2.2-39 L/kg); Dihydroartemisinin (DHA): 1.9 L/kg (range: 0.8-11.5 L/kg) (Newton, 2006)

Protein binding: Dihydroartemisinin (DHA): 47% to 76%

Metabolism: Artesunate (prodrug) is rapidly hydrolyzed to an active metabolite, dihydroartemisinin (DHA). DHA undergoes hepatic metabolism via CYP2B6, CYP2C19, and CYP3A4 to inactive metabolites (Hess, 2010).

Half-life elimination: Artesunate: Adults infected with severe malaria: 0.22 hours (range: 0.08-0.61 hours); Dihydroartesiminin (DHA): 0.34 hours (range: 0.14-0.87 hours) (Newton, 2006)

Time to peak: Dihyrdoartemisinin (DHA): Adults infected with severe malaria: Within 15 minutes (Newton, 2006)

Dosage I.V.: Children and Adults: 2.4 mg/kg/dose initially, followed by 2.4 mg/kg/dose at 12 hours, 24 hours, and 48 hours after the initial dose for a total of 4 doses over a period of 3 days; longer treatment duration (eg, an additional 4 days [Hess, 2010]) may be required in severely-ill patients or in patients unable to transition to oral therapy (Hess, 2010; Rosenthal, 2008). **Note:** Because of the short half-life of artesunate and a high risk of recrudescence, oral antimalarial therapy must begin ≤4 hours after the last dose of I.V. artesunate. Appropriate oral therapies include atovaquone-proguanil, doxycycline (in patients >8 years of age and nonpregnant adults), clindamycin, **or** mefloquine (CDC, 2009, Hess, 2010; Rosenthal, 2008).

Dosage adjustment in renal impairment: No dosage adjustment necessary (Rosenthal, 2008).

Dosage adjustment in hepatic impairment: No dosage adjustment necessary (Rosenthal, 2008).

Administration I.V.: Administer via I.V. bolus over 1–2 minutes through a 0.8-micron hydrophilic polyethersulfone filter (Hess, 2010)

- Artesunic Acid *see* Artesunate *on page 171*
- Arthrotec® *see* Diclofenac and Misoprostol *on page 600*
- Arzerra *see* Ofatumumab *on page 1489*
- As_2O_3 *see* Arsenic Trioxide *on page 169*
- ASA *see* Aspirin *on page 177*
- 5-ASA *see* Mesalamine *on page 1305*
- ASA and Diphenhydramine *see* Aspirin and Diphenhydramine *on page 182*
- Asacol [DSC] *see* Mesalamine *on page 1305*
- Asacol (Can) *see* Mesalamine *on page 1305*
- Asacol 800 (Can) *see* Mesalamine *on page 1305*
- Asacol HD *see* Mesalamine *on page 1305*
- Asaphen (Can) *see* Aspirin *on page 177*
- Asaphen E.C. (Can) *see* Aspirin *on page 177*
- Asclera *see* Polidocanol *on page 1666*
- Ascocid [OTC] *see* Ascorbic Acid *on page 172*
- Ascocid-ISO-pH [OTC] *see* Ascorbic Acid *on page 172*
- Ascor L 500 *see* Ascorbic Acid *on page 172*
- Ascor L NC *see* Ascorbic Acid *on page 172*

Ascorbic Acid (a SKOR bik AS id)

Brand Names: U.S. Acerola C 500 [OTC]; Asco-Tabs-1000 [OTC]; Ascocid [OTC]; Ascocid-ISO-pH [OTC]; Ascor L 500; Ascor L NC; BProtected Vitamin C [OTC]; C Complex [OTC]; C-500 [OTC]; C-Time [OTC]; Cemill SR [OTC]; Cemill [OTC]; Chew-C [OTC]; Ester-C [OTC]; Fruit C 500 [OTC]; Fruit C [OTC]; Fruity C [OTC]; Mega-C/A Plus; Vita-C [OTC]

Brand Names: Canada Proflavanol C™; Revitalose C-1000®

Index Terms Vitamin C

Pharmacologic Category Vitamin, Water Soluble

Use Prevention and treatment of scurvy; acidify the urine

Unlabeled Use In large doses, to decrease the severity of "colds"; dietary supplementation; a 20-year study was recently completed involving 730 individuals which indicates a possible decreased risk of death by stroke when ascorbic acid at doses ≥45 mg/day was administered

Pregnancy Risk Factor C

Dosage Oral, I.M., I.V., SubQ:

Recommended adequate intake (AI):

0-6 months: 40 mg

6-12 months: 50 mg

Recommended daily allowance (RDA):
1-3 years: 15 mg; upper limit of intake should not exceed 400 mg/day
4-8 years: 25 mg; upper limit of intake should not exceed 650 mg/day
9-13 years: 45 mg; upper limit of intake should not exceed 1200 mg/day
14-18 years: Upper limit of intake should not exceed 1800 mg/day
Males: 75 mg
Females: 65 mg
Adults: Upper limit of intake should not exceed 2000 mg/day
Males: 90 mg
Females: 75 mg
Pregnant females:
≤18 years: 80 mg; upper limit of intake should not exceed 1800 mg/day
19-50 years: 85 mg; upper limit of intake should not exceed 2000 mg/day
Lactating females:
≤18 years: 115 mg; upper limit of intake should not exceed 1800 mg/day
19-50 years: 120 mg; upper limit of intake should not exceed 2000 mg/day
Adult smoker: Add an additional 35 mg/day
Children:
Scurvy: 100-300 mg/day in divided doses for at least 2 weeks
Urinary acidification: 500 mg every 6-8 hours
Dietary supplement: 35-100 mg/day
Adults:
Scurvy: 100-250 mg 1-2 times/day for at least 2 weeks
Urinary acidification: 4-12 g/day in 3-4 divided doses
Prevention and treatment of colds: 1-3 g/day
Dietary supplement: 50-200 mg/day

Additional Information Complete prescribing information should be consulted for additional detail.

Dosage Forms Excipient information presented when available (limited, particularly for generics); consult specific product labeling. [DSC] = Discontinued product
Capsule Extended Release, Oral:
C-Time: 500 mg
Generic: 500 mg
Crystals, Oral:
Vita-C: (120 g, 480 g) [animal products free, gelatin free, gluten free, lactose free, no artificial color(s), no artificial flavor(s), starch free, sugar free, yeast free]
Granules, Oral:
Generic: (1 g [DSC], 100 g, 500 g, 1000 g)
Liquid, Oral:
BProtected Vitamin C: 500 mg/5 mL (236 mL) [contains propylene glycol, saccharin sodium, sodium benzoate; citrus flavor]
Generic: 500 mg/5 mL (473 mL)
Powder, Oral:
Ascocid: (227 g)
Generic: (113 g, 120 g, 480 g)
Powder Effervescent, Oral:
Ascocid-ISO-pH: (150 g) [corn free, rye free, wheat free]
Solution, Injection:
Generic: 500 mg/mL (50 mL)
Solution, Injection [preservative free]:
Ascor L 500: 500 mg/mL (50 mL)
Ascor L NC: 500 mg/mL (50 mL) [corn free]
Mega-C/A Plus: 500 mg/mL (50 mL)
Generic: 250 mg/mL (30 mL)
Syrup, Oral:
Generic: 500 mg/5 mL (118 mL, 473 mL)
Tablet, Oral:
Asco-Tabs-1000: 1000 mg [color free, starch free, sugar free]
Ester-C:
Generic: 100 mg, 250 mg, 500 mg, 1000 mg, 1000 mg
Tablet, Oral [preservative free]:
Generic: 250 mg, 500 mg
Tablet Chewable, Oral:
Chew-C: 500 mg
Fruit C 500: 500 mg [animal products free, gelatin free, gluten free, kosher certified, lactose free, no artificial color(s), no artificial flavor(s), starch free, sugar free, yeast free]
Fruit C: 100 mg [animal products free, gelatin free, gluten free, lactose free, no artificial color(s), no artificial flavor(s), starch free, sugar free, yeast free]
Fruity C: 250 mg
Generic: 100 mg, 250 mg, 500 mg
Tablet Chewable, Oral [preservative free]:
C-500: 500 mg [animal products free, gluten free, soy free, starch free, yeast free; contains fd&c yellow #6 aluminum lake; orange flavor]
Generic: 500 mg,
Tablet Extended Release, Oral:
C Complex: [contains rose hips]
Cemill: 500 mg
Cemill SR: 1000 mg
Generic: 500 mg, 1000 mg, 1500 mg
Tablet Extended Release, Oral [preservative free]:
C Complex: [corn free, no artificial color(s), no artificial flavor(s), starch free, sugar free, wheat free, yeast free]
Generic: 1000 mg
Wafer, Oral [preservative free]:
Acerola C 500: 500 mg (50 ea) [corn free, no artificial color(s), no artificial flavor(s), wheat free, yeast free; contains acerola (malpighia glabra)]

◆ **Asco-Tabs-1000 [OTC]** *see* Ascorbic Acid *on page 172*
◆ **Ascriptin® Maximum Strength [OTC]** *see* Aspirin *on page 177*
◆ **Ascriptin® Regular Strength [OTC]** *see* Aspirin *on page 177*

Asenapine (a SEN a peen)

Brand Names: U.S. Saphris
Brand Names: Canada Saphris®
Pharmacologic Category Antimanic Agent; Antipsychotic Agent, Atypical
Additional Appendix Information
Antipsychotic Agents *on page 2290*
Beers Criteria – Potentially Inappropriate Medications for Geriatrics *on page 2368*

Use Acute and maintenance treatment of schizophrenia; treatment of acute mania or mixed episodes associated with bipolar I disorder (as monotherapy or in combination with lithium or valproate)

Pregnancy Risk Factor C

Dosage Sublingual: Adults: **Note:** Safety of doses >20 mg/day has not been evaluated:
Schizophrenia:
Acute treatment: Initial: 5 mg twice daily. Daily doses >20 mg/day in clinical trials did not appear to offer any additional benefits and increased risk of adverse effects.
Maintenance treatment: Initial: 5 mg twice daily; may increase to 10 mg twice daily after 1 week based on tolerability
Bipolar disorder:
Monotherapy: Initial: 10 mg twice daily; decrease to 5 mg twice daily if dose not tolerated

Combination therapy (with lithium or valproate): 5 mg twice daily; may increase to 10 mg twice daily based on tolerability

Dosing adjustment in renal impairment: No dosage adjustment is necessary

Dosing adjustment in hepatic impairment:

Mild-to-moderate hepatic impairment (Child-Pugh class A or B): No dosage adjustment is necessary

Severe hepatic impairment (Child-Pugh class C): Use is not recommended

Additional Information Complete prescribing information should be consulted for additional detail.

Dosage Forms Excipient information presented when available (limited, particularly for generics); consult specific product labeling.

Tablet Sublingual, Sublingual:

Saphris: 5 mg

Saphris: 5 mg [black cherry flavor]

Saphris: 10 mg

Saphris: 10 mg [black cherry flavor]

◆ Asendin [DSC] *see* Amoxapine *on page 114*

◆ Asmanex 7 Metered Doses *see* Mometasone (Oral Inhalation) *on page 1392*

◆ Asmanex 14 Metered Doses *see* Mometasone (Oral Inhalation) *on page 1392*

◆ Asmanex 30 Metered Doses *see* Mometasone (Oral Inhalation) *on page 1392*

◆ Asmanex 60 Metered Doses *see* Mometasone (Oral Inhalation) *on page 1392*

◆ Asmanex 120 Metered Doses *see* Mometasone (Oral Inhalation) *on page 1392*

◆ Asmanex® Twisthaler® (Can) *see* Mometasone (Oral Inhalation) *on page 1392*

◆ ASNase *see* Asparaginase (*E. coli*) *on page 174*

◆ Asparaginase *see* Asparaginase (*E. coli*) *on page 174*

Asparaginase (*E. coli*) (a SPEAR a ji nase e ko lye)

Brand Names: U.S. Elspar

Brand Names: Canada Kidrolase

Index Terms *E. coli* Asparaginase; ASNase; Asparaginase; L-ASP; L-asparaginase (*E. coli*)

Pharmacologic Category Antineoplastic Agent, Miscellaneous; Enzyme

Use Acute lymphoblastic leukemia (ALL): Treatment (in combination with other chemotherapy) of ALL

Unlabeled Use Treatment of lymphoblastic lymphoma

Pregnancy Risk Factor C

Pregnancy Considerations Adverse events were observed in animal reproduction studies. Use during pregnancy only if clearly needed.

Breast-Feeding Considerations It is not known if asparaginase is excreted in human milk. Due to the potential for serious adverse reactions in the nursing infant, the decision to discontinue asparaginase or to discontinue breast-feeding should take into account the importance of treatment to the mother.

Contraindications History of serious allergic reaction to asparaginase (*E. coli*-derived) or any component of the formulation; history of serious thrombosis, pancreatitis, or serious hemorrhagic events with prior L-asparaginase treatment

Canadian labeling: Additional contraindications (not in U.S. labeling): Hepatic insufficiency, pregnancy, breast-feeding, recent yellow fever vaccination, concurrent administration with phenytoin

Warnings/Precautions Hazardous agent - use appropriate precautions for handling and disposal (NIOSH, 2012). Severe allergic reactions may occur; observe for 1 hour after administration (although reactions may also occur beyond 1 hour after administration); immediate treatment for hypersensitivity reactions should be available during administration. Discontinue if serious allergic reaction occurs. Prior exposure to asparaginase is a risk factor for allergic reactions; I.V. administration (compared to I.M. or SubQ administration) and younger age also may be associated with hypersensitivity reactions (Stock, 2011; Woo, 2000). Patients who have an allergic reaction to *E. coli* asparaginase may also react to asparaginase (*Erwinia*) or to pegaspargase.

Altered liver function tests (eg, increased AST, ALT, alkaline phosphatase, bilirubin, and decreased serum albumin, plasma fibrinogen) may occur with therapy; fulminant hepatic failure has also occurred. Fatty liver may be observed on biopsy. Use with caution in patients with pre-existing hepatic impairment; may alter function. Monitor liver function tests at baseline and periodically during treatment. Serious thrombosis, including sagittal sinus thrombosis may occur; discontinue with serious thrombotic events. Anticoagulaton prophylaxis during therapy may be considered in some patients (Farge, 2013). The risk for thrombosis may be higher in adult patients (Stock, 2011). Increased prothrombin time, partial thromboplastin time and hypofibrinogenemia may occur; cerebrovascular hemorrhage has been reported; monitor coagulation parameters at baseline and periodically during and after therapy; use cautiously in patients with an underlying coagulopathy.May cause hyperglycemia/glucose intolerance (possibly irreversible). Cases of diabetic ketoacidosis have been observed; monitor blood glucose as clinically necessary. May cause serious and possibly fulminant or fatal pancreatitis; promptly evaluate patients with abdominal pain; the manufacturer recommends to discontinue permanently if pancreatitis develops. May consider continuing therapy for asymptomatic chemical pancreatitis (amylase or lipase >3 times ULN) or only radiologic abnormalities; monitor closely for rising amylase and/or lipase levels (Stock, 2011). Discontinue permanently for clinical pancreatitis (eg, vomiting, severe abdominal pain) with amylase/lipase elevation >3 times ULN for >3 days and/or development of a pancreatic pseudocyst. Avoid alcohol use (Stock, 2011).

Posterior reversible encephalopathy syndrome (PRES) has been observed in patients treated with asparaginase (in combination with other chemotherapy agents). Monitor for signs/symptoms of PRES (eg, altered mental status, headache, hypertension, seizures, visual disturbances); interrupt therapy for suspected PRES. Control blood pressure and closely monitor for seizure activity. Appropriate measures must be taken to prevent tumor lysis syndrome and subsequent hyperuricemia and uric acid nephropathy; monitor, consider antihyperuricemic therapy, hydration and urinary alkalization.

Do not interchange *E. coli* asparaginase for *Erwinia* asparaginase or pegaspargase; ensure the proper formulation, route of administration, and dose prior to administration.

Adverse Reactions Note: Immediate effects: Fever, chills, nausea, and vomiting occur in 50% to 60% of patients.

>10%:

Central nervous system: Fatigue, fever, chills, depression, agitation, seizure (10% to 60%), somnolence, stupor, confusion, coma (25%)

Endocrine & metabolic: Hyperglycemia/glucose intolerance (10%)

Gastrointestinal: Nausea, vomiting (50% to 60%), anorexia, abdominal cramps (70%), acute pancreatitis (15%, may be severe in some patients)

Hematologic: Hypofibrinogenemia and depression of clotting factors V and VIII, variable decrease in factors VII and IX, severe protein C deficiency and decrease in antithrombin III (may be dose limiting or fatal)

Hepatic: Transaminases, bilirubin, and alkaline phosphatase increased (transient)

Hypersensitivity: Acute allergic reactions (fever, rash, urticaria, arthralgia, hypotension, angioedema, bronchospasm, anaphylaxis (15% to 35%); may be dose limiting in some patients, may be fatal)

Renal: Azotemia (66%)

1% to 10%:

Endocrine & metabolic: Hyperuricemia

Gastrointestinal: Stomatitis

Miscellaneous: Allergic reaction (including anaphylaxis), antibody formation/immunogenicity (~25%)

<1% (Limited to important or life-threatening) and/or frequency not defined: Acute renal failure, albumin decreased, cerebrovascular hemorrhage, cerebrovascular thrombosis, disorientation, fatty liver, fibrinogen decreased, glucosuria, hallucinations, headache, hemorrhagic pancreatitis, hyper-/hypolipidemia, hyperthermia, hypocholesterolemia, hypotension, insulin-dependent diabetes, intracranial hemorrhage, irritability, ketoacidosis, laryngospasm, malabsorption syndrome, myelosuppression (mild–to-moderate anemia, leukopenia, and thrombocytopenia; onset: 7 days; nadir: 14 days; recovery: 21 days), pancreatic pseudocyst, Parkinsonian symptoms (including tremor and increased muscle tone), partial thromboplastin time increased, peripheral edema, polyuria, proteinuria, prothrombin time increased, pruritus, rash, renal insufficiency, serum ammonia increased, serum cholesterol decreased, sagittal sinus thrombosis, stroke (hemorrhagic and thrombotic), thrombosis, urticaria, venous thrombosis

Drug Interactions

Metabolism/Transport Effects None known.

Avoid Concomitant Use There are no known interactions where it is recommended to avoid concomitant use.

Increased Effect/Toxicity

Asparaginase (E. coli) may increase the levels/effects of: Dexamethasone (Systemic)

Decreased Effect There are no known significant interactions involving a decrease in effect.

Preparation for Administration Hazardous agent; use appropriate precautions for handling and disposal (NIOSH, 2012). For I.V. administration, reconstitute lyophilized powder with 5 mL sterile water for injection or NS. For I.M. administration, the manufacturer recommends reconstitution of the lyophilized powder with 2 mL NS to a concentration of 5000 units/mL; however, some institutions reconstitute with 1 mL NS for I.M. use, resulting in a concentration of 10,000 units/mL. Shake well, but not too vigorously. A 5 micron filter may be used to remove fiber-like particles in the solution (do not use a 0.2 micron filter; has been associated with loss of potency).

Standard I.M. dilution: 5000 units/mL (10,000 units/mL has been used by some institutions)

Standard I.V. dilution: Dilute in 50-250 mL NS or D_5W

Storage/Stability Intact vials of powder should be refrigerated at 2°C to 8°C (36°F to 48°F). Reconstituted solutions are stable 1 week refrigerated at 8°C (Stecher, 1999), although the manufacturer recommends use within 8 hours. Solutions for I.V. infusion are stable for 8 hours at room temperature or under refrigeration.

Mechanism of Action In leukemic cells, asparaginase hydrolyzes L-asparagine to ammonia and L-aspartic acid, leading to depletion of asparagine. Leukemia cells, especially lymphoblasts, require exogenous asparagine; normal cells can synthesize asparagine. Asparagine depletion in leukemic cells leads to inhibition of protein synthesis and apoptosis. Asparaginase is cycle-specific for the G_1 phase.

Pharmacodynamics/Kinetics

Distribution: I.V.: Slightly higher than plasma volume; <1% CSF penetration

Metabolism: Systemically degraded

Half-life elimination: I.M.: 34-49 hours; I.V.: 8-30 hours

Time to peak, plasma: I.M.: 14-24 hours

Dosage Note: Dose, frequency, number of doses, and start date may vary by protocol and treatment phase.

Acute lymphoblastic leukemia (ALL): Manufacturer's U.S. labeling: Children and Adults: I.V., I.M.: 6000 units/m²/dose 3 times weekly

CCG 1922 protocol (unlabeled dosing): Children: I.M.: 6000 units/m²/dose 3 times weekly for 9 doses beginning either on day 2, 3, or 4 (induction phase) and 6000 units/m²/dose on Monday, Wednesday, and Friday for 6 doses beginning day 3 (delayed intensification phase) (Bostrom, 2004)

DFCI-ALL Consortium protocol 00-01 (unlabeled dosing): Children: I.M.: 25,000 units/m² for 1 dose (induction phase) and 25,000 units/m²/dose weekly for 30 weeks (intensification phase) (Vrooman, 2013)

DFCI-ALL Consortium protocol 95-01 (unlabeled dosing): Children: I.M.: 25,000 units/m² for 1 dose on day 4 (induction phase) and 25,000 units/m²/dose weekly for 20 weeks (intensification phase) (Moghrabi, 2007)

Hyper-CVAD regimen (unlabeled dosing): Adolescents ≥13 years and Adults: I.V. 20,000 units weekly for 4 doses (starting on day 2) during either months 7 and 19 or months 7 and 11 of intensification phase (Thomas, 2010)

Larson regimen (unlabeled dosing): Adults: SubQ: 6000 units/m²/dose on days 5, 8, 11, 15, 18, and 22 (induction phase) and on days 15, 18, 22, and 25 (early intensification phase) (Larson, 1995)

Linker regimen (unlabeled dosing): Adults: I.M.:

Remission induction: 6000 units/m²/dose on days 17-28; if bone marrow on day 28 is positive for residual leukemia: 6000 units/m²/dose on days 29-35 (Linker, 1991)

Consolidation (Treatment A; cycles 1, 3, 5, and 7): 12,000 units/m²/dose on days 2, 4, 7, 9, 11, and 14 (Linker, 1991)

Lymphoblastic lymphoma (unlabeled use): Adolescents >15 years and Adults: Hyper-CVAD regimen: I.V.: 20,000 units weekly for 4 doses (starting on day 2) for 2 cycles (months 7 and 11) during maintenance phase (Thomas, 2004)

Dosage adjustment for toxicity:

Allergic reaction/hypersensitivity: Discontinue for severe reactions.

Neurotoxicity (posterior reversible encephalopathy syndrome; PRES): Interrupt therapy for suspected PRES; control blood pressure and closely monitor for seizure activity.

Pancreatitis: Discontinue permanently (per manufacturer).

Thrombotic event: Discontinue for serious reactions.

Dosage adjustment in renal impairment: No dosage adjustment provided in manufacturer's labeling.

Dosage adjustment in hepatic impairment: No dosage adjustment provided in manufacturer's labeling.

Dosing in obesity: *ASCO Guidelines for appropriate chemotherapy dosing in obese adults with cancer:* Utilize patient's actual body weight (full weight) for calculation of body surface area- or weight-based dosing, particularly when the intent of therapy is curative; manage regimen-related toxicities in the same manner as for nonobese patients; if a dose reduction is utilized due to toxicity, consider resumption of full weight-based dosing with subsequent cycles, especially if cause of toxicity (eg, hepatic or renal impairment) is resolved (Griggs, 2012).

Administration May be administered I.M. or I.V.; has been administered SubQ (unlabeled route; Larson, 1995) in specific protocols. Observe patients for 1 hour after administration; have epinephrine, diphenhydramine, and hydrocortisone at the bedside. A physician should be readily accessible.

I.M.: Doses should be given as a deep intramuscular injection into a large muscle; volumes >2 mL should be divided and administered in 2 separate sites.

I.V.: Infuse over at least 30 minutes through the side arm of a NS or D_5W infusion.

Gelatinous fiber-like particles may develop on standing. Filtration through a 5-micron filter during administration will remove the particles with no loss of potency.

Hazardous agent; use appropriate precautions for handling and disposal (NIOSH, 2012).

Monitoring Parameters CBC with differential, urinalysis, amylase, liver function prior to and frequently during therapy, liver enzymes, coagulation parameters (baseline and periodic), renal function tests, urine dipstick for glucose, blood glucose, uric acid. Monitor for allergic reaction, be prepared to treat anaphylaxis at each administration; monitor for onset of abdominal pain and mental status changes. Monitor vital signs during administration.

Test Interactions Decreased thyroxine and thyroxine-binding globulin

Additional Information Some institutions recommended the following precautions for asparaginase administration: Parenteral epinephrine, diphenhydramine, and hydrocortisone available at bedside; freely running I.V. in place; physician readily accessible; monitor the patient closely for 30-60 minutes; avoid administering at night.

An asparaginase desensitization regimen has been administered for patients who react to a test dose, or are being retreated following a break in therapy. Doses are doubled and given every 10 minutes until the total daily dose for that day has been administered. One schedule begins with a total of 1 unit given I.V. and doubles the dose every 10 minutes until the total amount given is the planned dose for that day (Elspar product information, 2006).

The *E. coli* and the *Erwinia* strains of asparaginase differ slightly in their gene sequencing, and have slight differences in their enzyme characteristics. Both are highly specific for asparagine and have <10% activity for the D-isomer.

Product Availability Elspar: Manufacturing of asparaginase (*E. coli*) was discontinued by Lundbeck at the end of 2012. Elspar was acquired by Recordati Rare Diseases; availability information is currently unavailable.

Dosage Forms Excipient information presented when available (limited, particularly for generics); consult specific product labeling.

Solution Reconstituted, Injection:

Elspar: 10,000 units (1 ea)

Asparaginase (*Erwinia*)

(a SPEAR a ji nase er WIN i ah)

Brand Names: U.S. Erwinaze

Brand Names: Canada Erwinase®

Index Terms *Erwinia chrysanthemi*; Asparaginase *Erwinia chrysanthemi*; L-asparaginase (*Erwinia*)

Pharmacologic Category Antineoplastic Agent, Miscellaneous; Enzyme

Use Treatment (in combination with other chemotherapy) of acute lymphoblastic leukemia (ALL) in patients with hypersensitivity to *E. coli*-derived asparaginase

Pregnancy Risk Factor C

Pregnancy Considerations Animal reproduction studies have not been conducted. The effects on human pregnancy are unknown.

Breast-Feeding Considerations According to the manufacturer, the decision to continue or discontinue breast-feeding during therapy should take into account the risk of exposure to the infant and the benefits of treatment to the mother.

Prescribing and Access Restrictions Erwinaze™ is distributed through Accredo Health Group, Inc. (1-877-900-9223).

Contraindications History of serious hypersensitivity reactions, including anaphylaxis to asparaginase (*Erwinia*) or any component of the formulation; history of serious pancreatitis, serious thrombosis, or serious hemorrhagic event with prior asparaginase treatment

Canadian labeling: Additional contraindications (not in the U.S. labeling): Women who are or may become pregnant

Warnings/Precautions Hazardous agent - use appropriate precautions for handling and disposal (NIOSH, 2012).

Serious hypersensitivity reactions, including anaphylaxis, have occurred in 5% of patients in clinical trials. Immediate treatment for hypersensitivity reactions should be available during treatment; discontinue for serious hypersensitivity (and administer appropriate treatment for reaction).

Pancreatitis has been reported in 4% of patients in clinical trials; promptly evaluate with symptoms suggestive of pancreatitis. For mild pancreatitis, withhold treatment until signs and symptoms subside and amylase returns to normal; may resume after resolution. Discontinue for severe or hemorrhagic pancreatitis characterized by abdominal pain >72 hours and amylase ≥2 x ULN. Further use is contraindicated if severe pancreatitis is diagnosed.

Serious thrombotic events, including sagittal sinus thrombosis, have been reported with asparaginase formulations. Decreases in fibrinogen, protein C activity, protein S activity, and antithrombin III have been noted following a 2-week treatment course. Discontinue for hemorrhagic or thrombotic events; may resume treatment after resolution (contraindicated with history of serious thrombosis or hemorrhagic event with prior asparaginase treatment).

In clinical trials, 2% of patients experienced glucose intolerance; may be irreversible; monitor glucose levels (baseline and periodic) during treatment; may require insulin administration.

Adverse Reactions

>10%: Miscellaneous: Allergic reaction/hypersensitivity (17%; grades 3/4: 5% to 9%; includes anaphylaxis, urticaria)

1% to 10%:

Cardiovascular: Thrombosis (2%; grades 3/4: ≤1%)

Central nervous system: Fever (3%), headache (1%), seizure (1%)

Endocrine & metabolic: Glucose intolerance (2%), hyperglycemia (2%; grades 3/4: 2%), hyperammonemia (1%)

Gastrointestinal: Pancreatitis (4%; grades 3/4: ≤1%), nausea (2%), vomiting (2%), abdominal pain (1%), diarrhea (1%)

Hematologic: Coagulation abnormalities (3%; grades 3/4: ≤1%), hemorrhage (1%; grades 3/4: <1%)

Hepatic: Transaminases increased (3%; grades 3/4: ≤2%), hyperbilirubinemia (1%)

<1% (Limited to important or life-threatening): Acute renal failure, albumin decreased, alkaline phosphatase increased, anorexia, azotemia, bone marrow depression (rare), chills, cholesterol decreased, disseminated intravascular coagulation (DIC), hepatomegaly, injection site reactions, irritability, lipids (total) decreased/increased, malabsorption syndrome, proteinuria, transient ischemic event, weight loss

Drug Interactions

Metabolism/Transport Effects None known.

Avoid Concomitant Use There are no known interactions where it is recommended to avoid concomitant use.

Increased Effect/Toxicity

Asparaginase (Erwinia) may increase the levels/effects of: Dexamethasone (Systemic)

Decreased Effect There are no known significant interactions involving a decrease in effect.

Preparation for Administration Hazardous agent; use appropriate precautions for handling and disposal (NIOSH, 2012). Reconstitute each vial with 1 mL of preservative free sodium chloride 0.9% (NS) to obtain a concentration of 10,000 units/mL, or with 2 mL preservative free NS to obtain a concentration of 5,000 units/mL. Gently direct the NS down the wall of the vial (do not inject forcefully into or onto the powder). Dissolve by gently swirling or mixing; do not shake or invert the vial. Resulting reconstituted solution should be clear and colorless and free of visible particles or protein aggregates. Withdraw appropriate volume for dose into a polypropylene syringe.

Storage/Stability Store intact vials refrigerated at 2°C to 8°C (36°F to 48°F). Protect from light. Within 15 minutes of reconstitution, withdraw appropriate volume for dose into a polypropylene syringe. Do not freeze or refrigerate reconstituted solution; discard if not administered within 4 hours.

Mechanism of Action Asparaginase catalyzes the deamidation of asparagine to aspartic acid and ammonia, reducing circulating levels of asparagine. Leukemia cells lack asparagine synthetase and are unable to synthesize asparagine. Asparaginase reduces the exogenous asparagine source for the leukemic cells, resulting in cytotoxicity specific to leukemic cells.

Pharmacodynamics/Kinetics Half-life elimination: I.M.: ~16 hours (Asselin, 1993; Avramis, 2005)

Dosage

I.M.: Children and Adults: Acute lymphoblastic leukemia (ALL):

As a substitute for pegaspargase: 25,000 units/m^2 3 times/week (Mon, Wed, Fri) for 6 doses for each planned pegaspargase dose

As a substitute for asparaginase (E. coli): 25,000 units/m^2 for each planned asparaginase (*E. coli*) dose

Canadian labeling (not in the U.S. labeling): ALL induction:

Children <14 years: I.M.: 6000 units/m^2 3 times/week for 9 doses beginning day 4 of week 1 (in combination with vincristine, prednisone, methotrexate, and daunorubicin)

Children >14 years and Adults: SubQ: 10,000 units/m^2 days 1, 3, and 5 of week 4 and day 1 of week 5 (in combination with prednisolone, vincristine, mercaptopurine, and methotrexate) **or** 10,000 units/m^2 3 times/week (starting week 4) for 4 weeks (in combination with prednisolone, vincristine, and daunorubicin)

Dosage adjustment for toxicity:

Hemorrhagic or thrombotic event: Discontinue treatment; may resume treatment upon symptom resolution

Pancreatitis:

Mild pancreatitis: Withhold treatment until signs and symptoms subside and amylase returns to normal; may resume after resolution

Severe or hemorrhagic pancreatitis (abdominal pain >72 hours and amylase ≥2 x ULN): Discontinue treatment; further use is contraindicated.

Serious hypersensitivity: Discontinue treatment

Dosage adjustment in renal impairment: No dosage adjustment provided in the manufacturer's labeling.

Dosage adjustment in hepatic impairment: No dosage adjustment provided in the manufacturer's labeling.

Dosing in obesity: *ASCO Guidelines for appropriate chemotherapy dosing in obese adults with cancer:* Utilize patient's actual body weight (full weight) for calculation of body surface area- or weight-based dosing, particularly when the intent of therapy is curative; manage regimen-related toxicities in the same manner as for nonobese patients; if a dose reduction is utilized due to toxicity, consider resumption of full weight-based dosing with subsequent cycles, especially if cause of toxicity (eg, hepatic or renal impairment) is resolved (Griggs, 2012).

Administration

Administer I.M.; volume of each single injection site should be limited to 2 mL; use multiple injections for volumes >2 mL

Canadian labeling (additional administration routes not in the U.S. labeling): May also be administered SubQ and I.V., although I.M. and SubQ are preferred

Hazardous agent; use appropriate precautions for handling and disposal (NIOSH, 2012).

Monitoring Parameters CBC with differential, amylase, liver enzymes, blood glucose, coagulation parameters, symptoms of hypersensitivity, symptoms of pancreatitis, thrombosis, or hemorrhage

Dosage Forms Excipient information presented when available (limited, particularly for generics); consult specific product labeling.

Solution Reconstituted, Intramuscular:

Erwinaze: 10,000 units (1 ea)

◆ **Asparaginase *Erwinia chrysanthemi*** *see* Asparaginase (*Erwinia*) *on page 176*

◆ **Aspart Insulin** *see* Insulin Aspart *on page 1086*

◆ **Aspercin [OTC]** *see* Aspirin *on page 177*

◆ ***Aspergillus niger*** *see* Alpha-Galactosidase *on page 80*

◆ **Aspergum® [OTC]** *see* Aspirin *on page 177*

Aspirin (AS pir in)

Brand Names: U.S. Ascriptin® Maximum Strength [OTC]; Ascriptin® Regular Strength [OTC]; Aspercin [OTC]; Aspergum® [OTC]; Aspir-low [OTC]; Aspirtab [OTC]; Bayer® Aspirin Extra Strength [OTC]; Bayer® Aspirin Regimen Adult Low Strength [OTC]; Bayer® Aspirin Regimen Children's [OTC]; Bayer® Aspirin Regimen Regular Strength [OTC]; Bayer® Genuine Aspirin [OTC]; Bayer® Plus Extra Strength [OTC]; Bayer® Women's Low Dose Aspirin [OTC]; Buffasal [OTC]; Bufferin® Extra Strength [OTC]; Bufferin® [OTC]; Buffinol [OTC]; Ecotrin® Arthritis Strength [OTC]; Ecotrin® Low Strength [OTC]; Ecotrin® [OTC]; Halfprin® [OTC]; St Joseph® Adult Aspirin [OTC]; Tri-Buffered Aspirin [OTC]

Brand Names: Canada Asaphen; Asaphen E.C.; Entrophen®; Novasen; Praxis ASA EC 81 Mg Daily Dose

Index Terms Acetylsalicylic Acid; ASA; Baby Aspirin

Pharmacologic Category Antiplatelet Agent; Salicylate

Additional Appendix Information

Beers Criteria – Potentially Inappropriate Medications for Geriatrics *on page 2368*

Desensitization Protocols *on page 2325*

Oral Antiplatelet Comparison Chart *on page 2313*

Use Treatment of mild-to-moderate pain, inflammation, and fever; prevention and treatment of acute coronary syndromes (ST-elevation MI, non-ST-elevation MI, unstable angina), acute ischemic stroke, and transient ischemic episodes; management of rheumatoid arthritis, rheumatic fever, osteoarthritis; adjunctive therapy in revascularization procedures (coronary artery bypass graft [CABG], percutaneous transluminal coronary angioplasty [PTCA], carotid endarterectomy), stent implantation

Unlabeled Use Low doses have been used in the prevention of pre-eclampsia, complications associated with autoimmune disorders such as lupus or antiphospholipid syndrome; colorectal cancer; Kawasaki disease; alternative therapy for prevention of thromboembolism associated with atrial fibrillation in patients not candidates for warfarin; ▶

pericarditis including pericarditis associated with MI; thromboprophylaxis for aortic valve repair, Blalock-Taussig shunt placement, carotid artery stenosis, coronary artery disease, Fontan surgery, peripheral arterial occlusive disease, peripheral artery percutaneous transluminal angioplasty, peripheral artery bypass graft surgery, prosthetic valves, ventricular assist device (VAD) placement

Pregnancy Considerations Salicylates have been noted to cross the placenta and enter fetal circulation. Adverse effects reported in the fetus include mortality, intrauterine growth retardation, salicylate intoxication, bleeding abnormalities, and neonatal acidosis. Use of aspirin close to delivery may cause premature closure of the ductus arteriosus. Adverse effects reported in the mother include anemia, hemorrhage, prolonged gestation, and prolonged labor (Østensen, 1998). Aspirin has been used for the prevention of pre-eclampsia; however, the ACOG currently recommends that it not be used in low-risk women (ACOG, 2002). Low-dose aspirin is used to treat complications resulting from antiphospholipid syndrome in pregnancy (either primary or secondary to SLE) (Carp, 2004; Guyatt, 2012; Tincani, 2003). In general, low doses during pregnancy needed for the treatment of certain medical conditions have not been shown to cause fetal harm, however, discontinuing therapy prior to delivery is recommended (Østensen, 2006). Use of safer agents for routine management of pain or headache should be considered.

Breast-Feeding Considerations Low amounts of aspirin can be found in breast milk. Milk/plasma ratios ranging from 0.03-0.3 have been reported. Peak levels in breast milk are reported to be at ~9 hours after a dose. Metabolic acidosis was reported in one infant following an aspirin dose of 3.9 g/day in the mother. The WHO considers occasional doses of aspirin to be compatible with breast-feeding, but to avoid long-term therapy and consider monitoring the infant for adverse effects (WHO, 2002). Other sources suggest avoiding aspirin while breast-feeding due to the theoretical risk of Reye's syndrome (Bar-Oz, 2003; Spigset, 2000). When used for vascular indications, breast-feeding may be continued during low-dose aspirin therapy (Guyatt, 2012).

Contraindications Hypersensitivity to salicylates, other NSAIDs, or any component of the formulation; asthma; rhinitis; nasal polyps; inherited or acquired bleeding disorders (including factor VII and factor IX deficiency); do not use in children (<16 years of age) for viral infections (chickenpox or flu symptoms), with or without fever, due to a potential association with Reye's syndrome

Warnings/Precautions Use with caution in patients with platelet and bleeding disorders, renal dysfunction, dehydration, erosive gastritis, or peptic ulcer disease. Heavy ethanol use (>3 drinks/day) can increase bleeding risks. Avoid use in severe renal failure or in severe hepatic failure. Low-dose aspirin for cardioprotective effects is associated with a two- to fourfold increase in UGI events (eg, symptomatic or complicated ulcers); risks of these events increase with increasing aspirin dose; during the chronic phase of aspirin dosing, doses >81 mg are not recommended unless indicated (Bhatt, 2008). Use of safer agents for routine management of pain or headache throughout pregnancy should be considered. If possible, avoid use during the third trimester of pregnancy.

Discontinue use if tinnitus or impaired hearing occurs. Caution in mild-to-moderate renal failure (only at high dosages). Patients with sensitivity to tartrazine dyes, nasal polyps, and asthma may have an increased risk of salicylate sensitivity. In the treatment of acute ischemic stroke, avoid aspirin for 24 hours following administration of alteplase; administration within 24 hours increases the risk of hemorrhagic transformation (Jauch, 2013). Concurrent use of aspirin and clopidogrel is not recommended for secondary prevention of ischemic stroke or TIA in patients unable to take oral anticoagulants due to hemorrhagic risk (Furie, 2011). Surgical patients should avoid ASA if possible, for 1-2 weeks prior to surgery, to reduce the risk of excessive bleeding (except in patients with cardiac stents that have not completed their full course of dual antiplatelet therapy [aspirin, clopidogrel]; patient-specific situations need to be discussed with cardiologist; AHA/ACC/SCAI/ACS/ADA Science Advisory provides recommendations). When used concomitantly with ≤325 mg of aspirin, NSAIDs (including selective COX-2 inhibitors) substantially increase the risk of gastrointestinal complications (eg, ulcer); concomitant gastroprotective therapy (eg, proton pump inhibitors) is recommended (Bhatt, 2008).

Elderly: Avoid chronic use of doses >325 mg/day (unless alternative agents ineffective and patient can receive concomitant gastroprotective agent); nonselective oral NSAID use is associated with an increased risk of GI bleeding and peptic ulcer disease in older adults in high risk category (eg, >75 years or age or receiving concomitant oral/parenteral corticosteroids, anticoagulants, or antiplatelet agents) (Beers Criteria).

When used for self-medication (OTC labeling): Children and teenagers who have or are recovering from chickenpox or flu-like symptoms should not use this product. Changes in behavior (along with nausea and vomiting) may be an early sign of Reye's syndrome; patients should be instructed to contact their healthcare provider if these occur.

Adverse Reactions As with all drugs which may affect hemostasis, bleeding is associated with aspirin. Hemorrhage may occur at virtually any site. Risk is dependent on multiple variables including dosage, concurrent use of multiple agents which alter hemostasis, and patient susceptibility. Many adverse effects of aspirin are dose related, and are extremely rare at low dosages. Other serious reactions are idiosyncratic, related to allergy or individual sensitivity. Accurate estimation of frequencies is not possible.

Cardiovascular: Hypotension, tachycardia, dysrhythmias, edema

Central nervous system: Fatigue, insomnia, nervousness, agitation, confusion, dizziness, headache, lethargy, cerebral edema, hyperthermia, coma

Dermatologic: Rash, angioedema, urticaria

Endocrine & metabolic: Acidosis, hyperkalemia, dehydration, hypoglycemia (children), hyperglycemia, hypernatremia (buffered forms)

Gastrointestinal: Nausea, vomiting, dyspepsia, epigastric discomfort, heartburn, stomach pain, gastrointestinal ulceration (6% to 31%), gastric erosions, gastric erythema, duodenal ulcers

Hematologic: Anemia, disseminated intravascular coagulation (DIC), prothrombin times prolonged, coagulopathy, thrombocytopenia, hemolytic anemia, bleeding, iron-deficiency anemia

Hepatic: Hepatotoxicity, transaminases increased, hepatitis (reversible)

Neuromuscular & skeletal: Rhabdomyolysis, weakness, acetabular bone destruction (OA)

Otic: Hearing loss, tinnitus

Renal: Interstitial nephritis, papillary necrosis, proteinuria, renal failure (including cases caused by rhabdomyolysis), BUN increased, serum creatinine increased

Respiratory: Asthma, bronchospasm, dyspnea, laryngeal edema, hyperpnea, tachypnea, respiratory alkalosis, noncardiogenic pulmonary edema

Miscellaneous: Anaphylaxis, prolonged pregnancy and labor, stillbirths, low birth weight, peripartum bleeding, Reye's syndrome

Postmarketing and/or case reports: Colonic ulceration, esophageal stricture, esophagitis with esophageal ulcer, esophageal hematoma, oral mucosal ulcers (aspirin-containing chewing gum), coronary artery spasm, conduction defect and atrial fibrillation (toxicity), delirium, ischemic brain infarction, colitis, rectal stenosis (suppository), cholestatic jaundice, periorbital edema, rhinosinusitis

Drug Interactions

Metabolism/Transport Effects Substrate of CYP2C9 (minor); **Note:** Assignment of Major/Minor substrate status based on clinically relevant drug interaction potential; **Induces** CYP2C19 (weak/moderate)

Avoid Concomitant Use

Avoid concomitant use of Aspirin with any of the following: Floctafenine; Influenza Virus Vaccine (Live/Attenuated); Ketorolac (Nasal); Ketorolac (Systemic); Omacetaxine

Increased Effect/Toxicity

Aspirin may increase the levels/effects of: Alendronate; Anticoagulants; Carbonic Anhydrase Inhibitors; Carisoprodol; Collagenase (Systemic); Corticosteroids (Systemic); Dabigatran Etexilate; Heparin; Hypoglycemic Agents; Ibritumomab; Methotrexate; NSAID (COX-2 Inhibitor); Omacetaxine; PRALAtrexate; Rivaroxaban; Salicylates; Thrombolytic Agents; Ticagrelor; Tositumomab and Iodine I 131 Tositumomab; Valproic Acid and Derivatives; Varicella Virus-Containing Vaccines; Vitamin K Antagonists

The levels/effects of Aspirin may be increased by: Agents with Antiplatelet Properties; Ammonium Chloride; Antidepressants (Tricyclic, Tertiary Amine); Calcium Channel Blockers (Nondihydropyridine); Dasatinib; Floctafenine; Ginkgo Biloba; Glucosamine; Herbs (Anticoagulant/Antiplatelet Properties); Ibrutinib; Influenza Virus Vaccine (Live/Attenuated); Ketorolac (Nasal); Ketorolac (Systemic); Loop Diuretics; Multivitamins/Fluoride (with ADE); Multivitamins/Minerals (with ADEK, Folate, Iron); Multivitamins/Minerals (with AE, No Iron); NSAID (Nonselective); Omega-3 Fatty Acids; Pentosan Polysulfate Sodium; Pentoxifylline; Potassium Acid Phosphate; Prostacyclin Analogues; Selective Serotonin Reuptake Inhibitors; Serotonin/Norepinephrine Reuptake Inhibitors; Tipranavir; Treprostinil; Vitamin E

Decreased Effect

Aspirin may decrease the levels/effects of: ACE Inhibitors; Carisoprodol; Hyaluronidase; Loop Diuretics; Multivitamins/Fluoride (with ADE); Multivitamins/Minerals (with ADEK, Folate, Iron); Multivitamins/Minerals (with AE, No Iron); NSAID (Nonselective); Probenecid; Ticagrelor; Tiludronate

The levels/effects of Aspirin may be decreased by: Corticosteroids (Systemic); Floctafenine; Ketorolac (Nasal); Ketorolac (Systemic); NSAID (Nonselective)

Ethanol/Nutrition/Herb Interactions

Ethanol: Avoid ethanol (may enhance gastric mucosal damage).

Food: Food may decrease the rate but not the extent of oral absorption.

Folic acid: Hyperexcretion of folate; folic acid deficiency may result, leading to macrocytic anemia.

Iron: With chronic aspirin use and at doses of 3-4 g/day, iron-deficiency anemia may result.

Sodium: Hypernatremia resulting from buffered aspirin solutions or sodium salicylate containing high sodium content. Avoid or use with caution in CHF or any condition where hypernatremia would be detrimental.

Benedictine liqueur, prunes, raisins, tea, and gherkins: Potential salicylate accumulation.

Fresh fruits containing vitamin C: Displace drug from binding sites, resulting in increased urinary excretion of aspirin.

Herb/Nutraceutical: Avoid cat's claw, dong quai, evening primrose, feverfew, garlic, ginger, ginkgo, red clover, horse chestnut, green tea, ginseng (all have additional antiplatelet activity). Limit curry powder, paprika, licorice; may cause salicylate accumulation. These foods contain 6 mg salicylate/100 g. An ordinary American diet contains 10-200 mg/day of salicylate.

Storage/Stability Keep suppositories in refrigerator; do not freeze. Hydrolysis of aspirin occurs upon exposure to water or moist air, resulting in salicylate and acetate, which possess a vinegar-like odor. Do not use if a strong odor is present.

Mechanism of Action Irreversibly inhibits cyclooxygenase-1 and 2 (COX-1 and 2) enzymes, via acetylation, which results in decreased formation of prostaglandin precursors; irreversibly inhibits formation of prostaglandin derivative, thromboxane A_2, via acetylation of platelet cyclooxygenase, thus inhibiting platelet aggregation; has antipyretic, analgesic, and anti-inflammatory properties

Pharmacodynamics/Kinetics

Duration: 4-6 hours

Absorption: Rapid

Distribution: V_d: 10 L; readily into most body fluids and tissues

Metabolism: Hydrolyzed to salicylate (active) by esterases in GI mucosa, red blood cells, synovial fluid, and blood; metabolism of salicylate occurs primarily by hepatic conjugation; metabolic pathways are saturable

Bioavailability: 50% to 75% reaches systemic circulation

Half-life elimination: Parent drug: 15-20 minutes; Salicylates (dose dependent): 3 hours at lower doses (300-600 mg), 5-6 hours (after 1 g), 10 hours with higher doses

Time to peak, serum: ~1-2 hours

Excretion: Urine (75% as salicyluric acid, 10% as salicylic acid)

Dosage

Children:

Analgesic and antipyretic: Oral, rectal: 10-15 mg/kg/dose every 4-6 hours, up to a total of 4 g/day

Anti-inflammatory: Oral: Initial: 60-90 mg/kg/day in divided doses; usual maintenance: 80-100 mg/kg/day divided every 6-8 hours; monitor serum concentrations

Antiplatelet effects: Adequate pediatric studies have not been performed; pediatric dosage is derived from adult studies and clinical experience and is not well established. Doses are typically rounded to a convenient amount (eg, 1/2 of 81 mg tablet).

Acute ischemic stroke (AIS): Oral:

Noncardioembolic: 1-5 mg/kg/dose once daily for ≥2 years; patients with recurrent AIS or TIAs should be transitioned to clopidogrel, LMWH, or warfarin (Monagle, 2012)

Secondary to Moyamoya and non-Moyamoya vasculopathy: 1-5 mg/kg/dose once daily. **Note:** In non-Moyamoya vasculopathy, continue aspirin for 3 months, with subsequent use guided by repeat cerebrovascular imaging (Monagle, 2012).

Blalock-Taussig shunts, primary prophylaxis (unlabeled use): Oral: 1-5 mg/kg/dose once daily (Monagle, 2012)

Fontan surgery, primary prophylaxis: Oral: 5 mg/kg/dose once daily (Monagle, 2011)

Prosthetic heart valve: Oral:

Bioprosthetic aortic valve (in normal sinus rhythm): 1-5 mg/kg/dose once daily (Monagle, 2012; Guyatt, 2012)

Mechanical aortic and/or mitral valve: Low-dose aspirin (eg, 1-5 mg/kg/day) combined with vitamin K antagonist (eg, warfarin) is recommended as first-line antithrombotic therapy (Guyatt, 2012). Alternative regimens: 6-20 mg/kg/dose once daily in combination with dipyridamole (Bradley, 1985; El Makhlouf, 1987; LeBlanc, 1993; Serra, 1987; Solymar, 1991)

Ventricular assist device (VAD) placement: Oral: 1-5 mg/kg/dose once daily initiated within 72 hours of VAD placement; should be used with heparin (initiated between 8-48 hours following implantation) (Monagle, 2012)

Kawasaki disease (unlabeled use): Oral: 80-100 mg/kg/day divided every 6 hours for up to 14 days (until fever resolves for at least 48 hours); then decrease dose to 3-5 mg/kg/day once daily; in patients without coronary artery abnormalities, give lower dose (ie, 3-5 mg/kg/day) for at least 6-8 weeks. In patients with coronary artery abnormalities, low-dose aspirin should be continued indefinitely (in combination with warfarin). **Note:** Combine with I.V. immune globulin treatment within 10 days of symptom onset (Newbuger, 2004).

Adults: **Note:** For most cardiovascular uses, typical maintenance dosing of aspirin is 81 mg once daily.

Acute coronary syndrome (ST-segment elevation myocardial infarction [STEMI], unstable angina (UA)/non-ST-segment elevation myocardial infarction [NSTEMI]): Oral: Initial: 162-325 mg given on presentation (patient should chew nonenteric-coated aspirin especially if not taking before presentation); for patients unable to take oral, may use rectal suppository (300-600 mg [Antman, 2004; Maalouf, 2009]). Maintenance (secondary prevention): 75-162 mg once daily indefinitely (Anderson, 2007) or 81-325 mg once daily; 81 mg once daily preferred (O'Gara, 2013). **Note:** When aspirin is used with ticagrelor, the recommended maintenance dose of aspirin is 81 mg/day (Jneid, 2012; O'Gara, 2013).

UA/NSTEMI: Concomitant antiplatelet therapy (Jneid, 2012):

If invasive strategy chosen: Aspirin is recommended in combination with either clopidogrel, ticagrelor, (or prasugrel if at the time of PCI) or an I.V. GP IIb/IIIa inhibitor (if given before PCI, eptifibatide and tirofiban are preferred agents).

If noninvasive strategy chosen: Aspirin is recommended in combination with clopidogrel or ticagrelor.

Analgesic and antipyretic:

Oral: 325-650 mg every 4-6 hours up to 4 g/day

Rectal: 300-600 mg every 4-6 hours up to 4 g/day

Anti-inflammatory: Oral: Initial: 2.4-3.6 g/day in divided doses; usual maintenance: 3.6-5.4 g/day; monitor serum concentrations

Aortic valve repair (unlabeled use): Oral: 50-100 mg once daily (Guyatt, 2012)

Atrial fibrillation (in patients not candidates for oral anticoagulation or at low risk of ischemic stroke) (unlabeled use): Oral: 75-325 mg once daily (Furie, 2011; Fuster, 2006). **Note:** Combination therapy with clopidogrel has been suggested over aspirin alone for those patients who are unsuitable for or choose not to take oral anticoagulant for reasons other than concerns for bleeding (Guyatt, 2012).

As an alternative to adjusted-dose warfarin in patients with atrial fibrillation and mitral stenosis: 75-325 mg once daily with (preferred) or without clopidogrel (Guyatt, 2012)

CABG: Oral: 100-325 mg once daily initiated either preoperatively or within 6 hours postoperatively; continue indefinitely (Hillis, 2011)

Carotid artery stenosis (unlabeled use): Oral: 75-100 mg once daily. **Note:** When symptomatic (including recent carotid endarterectomy), the use of clopidogrel or aspirin/extended-release dipyridamole has been suggested over aspirin alone (Guyatt, 2012).

Coronary artery disease (CAD), established (unlabeled use): Oral: 75-100 mg once daily (Guyatt, 2012)

PCI: Oral:

Non-emergent PCI: Preprocedure: 81-325 mg (325 mg [nonenteric coated] in aspirin-naive patients) starting at least 2 hours (preferably 24 hours) before procedure. Postprocedure: 81 mg once daily continued indefinitely (in combination with a $P2Y_{12}$ inhibitor [eg, clopidogrel, prasugrel, ticagrelor] up to 12 months) (Levine, 2011)

Primary PCI: Preprocedure: 162-325 mg as early as possible prior to procedure; 325 mg preferred followed by a maintenance dose of 81 mg once daily even when a stent is deployed (O'Gara, 2013).

Alternatively, in patients who have undergone elective PCI with either bare metal or drug-eluting stent placement: The American College of Chest Physicians recommends the use of 75-325 mg once daily (in combination with clopidogrel) for 1 month (BMS) or 3-6 months (dependent upon DES type) followed by 75-100 mg once daily (in combination with clopidogrel) for up to12 months. For patients who underwent PCI but did not have stent placement, 75-325 mg once daily (in combination with clopidogrel) for 1 month is recommended. In either case, single antiplatelet therapy (either aspirin or clopidogrel) is recommended indefinitely (Guyatt, 2012).

Pericarditis (unlabeled use): Oral: Initial: 2.4-3.6 g daily in 3-4 divided doses; usual maintenance: 3.6-5.4 g daily in divided doses; gradually taper over 2- to 3-week period as appropriate (Imazio, 2004; Imazio, 2009). In the treatment of postmyocardial infarction pericarditis, an initial dose of 650 mg 4 times daily increased to 975 mg 4 times daily if necessary (after 24 hours) has been used (Berman, 1981; O'Gara, 2013).

Peripheral arterial disease (unlabeled use): Oral: 75-100 mg once daily (Guyatt, 2012) **or** 75-325 mg once daily; may use in conjunction with clopidogrel in those who are not at an increased risk of bleeding but are of high cardiovascular risk. **Note:** These recommendations also pertain to those with intermittent claudication or critical limb ischemia, prior lower extremity revascularization, or prior amputation for lower extremity ischemia (Rooke, 2011).

Peripheral artery percutaneous transluminal angioplasty (with or without stenting) or peripheral artery bypass graft surgery, postprocedure (unlabeled use): Oral: 75-100 mg once daily (Guyatt, 2012). **Note:** For below-knee bypass graft surgery with prosthetic grafts, combine with clopidogrel (Guyatt, 2012).

Pre-eclampsia prevention (women at risk) (unlabeled use): Oral: 75-100 mg once daily starting in the second trimester (Guyatt, 2012)

Primary prevention: Oral:

American College of Cardiology/American Heart Association: Prevention of myocardial infarction: 75-162 mg once daily. **Note:** Patients are most likely to benefit if their 10-year coronary heart disease risk is ≥6% (Antman, 2004).

American College of Chest Physicians: Prevention of myocardial infarction and stroke: Select individuals ≥50 years of age (without symptomatic cardiovascular disease): 75-100 mg once daily (Guyatt, 2012; Grade 2B, weak recommendation)

Prosthetic heart valve: Oral:

Bioprosthetic aortic valve (patient in normal sinus rhythm) (unlabeled use): 50-100 mg once daily; usual dose: 81 mg once daily. **Note:** If mitral bioprosthetic valve, oral anticoagulation with warfarin (instead of aspirin) is recommended for the first 3 months postoperatively, followed by aspirin alone (Guyatt, 2012).

Mechanical aortic or mitral valve (unlabeled use):

Low risk of bleeding: 50-100 mg once daily (in combination with warfarin) (Guyatt, 2012)

History of thromboembolism while receiving oral anticoagulants: 75-100 mg once daily (in combination with warfarin) (Furie, 2011)

Transcatheter aortic bioprosthetic valve (unlabeled use): 50-100 mg once daily (in combination with clopidogrel) (Guyatt, 2012)

Stroke/TIA: Oral:

Acute ischemic stroke/TIA: Initial: 160-325 mg within 48 hours of stroke/TIA onset, followed by 75-100 mg once daily (Guyatt, 2012). The AHA/ASA recommends an initial dose of 325 mg within 24-48 hours after stroke; do not administer aspirin within 24 hours after administration of alteplase (Jauch, 2013).

Cardioembolic, secondary prevention (oral anticoagulation unsuitable): 75-100 mg once daily (in combination with clopidogrel) (Guyatt, 2012; The ACTIVE Investigators [Connolly, 2009])

Cryptogenic with patent foramen ovale (PFO) or atrial septal aneurysm: 50-100 mg once daily (Guyatt, 2012)

Noncardioembolic, secondary prevention: 75-325 mg once daily (Smith, 2011) **or** 75-100 mg once daily (Guyatt, 2012). **Note:** Combination aspirin/extended release dipyridamole or clopidogrel is preferred over aspirin alone (Guyatt, 2012).

Women at high risk, primary prevention: 81 mg once daily **or** 100 mg every other day (Goldstein, 2010)

Dosing adjustment in renal impairment: Cl_{cr} <10 mL/minute: Avoid use.

Hemodialysis: Dialyzable (50% to 100%)

Dosing adjustment in hepatic disease: Avoid use in severe liver disease.

Dietary Considerations Take with food or large volume of water or milk to minimize GI upset.

Administration Do not crush enteric coated tablet. Administer with food or a full glass of water to minimize GI distress. For acute myocardial infarction, have patient chew tablet.

Reference Range Timing of serum samples: Peak levels usually occur 2 hours after ingestion. Salicylate serum concentrations correlate with the pharmacological actions and adverse effects observed. The serum salicylate concentration (mcg/mL) and the corresponding clinical correlations are as follows: See table.

Serum Salicylate: Clinical Correlations

Serum Salicylate Concentration (mcg/mL)	Desired Effects	Adverse Effects / Intoxication
~100	Antiplatelet Antipyresis Analgesia	GI intolerance and bleeding, hypersensitivity, hemostatic defects
150-300	Anti-inflammatory	Mild salicylism
250-400	Treatment of rheumatic fever	Nausea/vomiting, hyperventilation, salicylism, flushing, sweating, thirst, headache, diarrhea, and tachycardia
>400-500		Respiratory alkalosis, hemorrhage, excitement, confusion, asterixis, pulmonary edema, convulsions, tetany, metabolic acidosis, fever, coma, cardiovascular collapse, renal and respiratory failure

Test Interactions False-negative results for glucose oxidase urinary glucose tests (Clinistix®); false-positives using the cupric sulfate method (Clinitest®); also, interferes with Gerhardt test, VMA determination; 5-HIAA, xylose tolerance test and T_3 and T_4

Dosage Forms Excipient information presented when available (limited, particularly for generics); consult specific product labeling.

Caplet, oral: 500 mg
- Bayer® Aspirin Extra Strength: 500 mg
- Bayer® Genuine Aspirin: 325 mg
- Bayer® Women's Low Dose Aspirin: 81 mg [contains elemental calcium 300 mg]

Caplet, oral [buffered]:
- Ascriptin® Maximum Strength: 500 mg [contains aluminum hydroxide, calcium carbonate, magnesium hydroxide]
- Bayer® Plus Extra Strength: 500 mg [contains calcium carbonate]

Caplet, enteric coated, oral:
- Bayer® Aspirin Regimen Regular Strength: 325 mg

Gum, chewing, oral:
- Aspergum®: 227 mg (12s) [cherry flavor]
- Aspergum®: 227 mg (12s) [orange flavor]

Suppository, rectal: 300 mg (12s); 600 mg (12s)

Tablet, oral: 325 mg
- Aspercin: 325 mg
- Aspirtab: 325 mg
- Bayer® Genuine Aspirin: 325 mg

Tablet, oral [buffered]: 325 mg
- Ascriptin® Regular Strength: 325 mg [contains aluminum hydroxide, calcium carbonate, magnesium hydroxide]
- Buffasal: 325 mg [contains magnesium oxide]
- Bufferin®: 325 mg [contains calcium carbonate, magnesium carbonate, magnesium oxide]
- Bufferin® Extra Strength: 500 mg [contains calcium carbonate, magnesium carbonate, magnesium oxide]
- Buffinol: 324 mg [sugar free; contains magnesium oxide]
- Tri-Buffered Aspirin: 325 mg [contains calcium carbonate, magnesium carbonate, magnesium oxide]

Tablet, chewable, oral: 81 mg
- Bayer® Aspirin Regimen Children's: 81 mg [cherry flavor]
- Bayer® Aspirin Regimen Children's: 81 mg [orange flavor]
- St Joseph® Adult Aspirin: 81 mg

Tablet, enteric coated, oral: 81 mg, 325 mg, 650 mg
- Aspir-low: 81 mg
- Bayer® Aspirin Regimen Adult Low Strength: 81 mg
- Ecotrin®: 325 mg
- Ecotrin® Arthritis Strength: 500 mg
- Ecotrin® Low Strength: 81 mg
- Halfprin®: 81 mg, 162 mg
- St Joseph® Adult Aspirin: 81 mg

- **Aspirin, Acetaminophen, and Caffeine** *see* Acetaminophen, Aspirin, and Caffeine *on page 33*
- **Aspirin and Carisoprodol** *see* Carisoprodol and Aspirin *on page 352*

Aspirin and Diphenhydramine

(AS pir in & dye fen HYE dra meen)

Brand Names: U.S. Bayer® PM [OTC]

Index Terms ASA and Diphenhydramine; Aspirin and Diphenhydramine Citrate; Diphenhydramine and ASA; Diphenhydramine and Aspirin; Diphenhydramine Citrate and Aspirin

Pharmacologic Category Analgesic, Miscellaneous

Use Aid in the relief of insomnia accompanied by minor pain or headache

Dosage Oral: Children ≥12 years and Adults: Pain-associated insomnia: Two caplets (1000 mg aspirin/77 mg diphenhydramine citrate) at bedtime if needed or as directed by physician; do not exceed recommended dosage; not for use in children <12 years of age

Additional Information Complete prescribing information should be consulted for additional detail.

Dosage Forms Excipient information presented when available (limited, particularly for generics); consult specific product labeling.

Caplet, oral:

Bayer® PM: Aspirin 500 mg and diphenhydramine citrate 38.3 mg

- **Aspirin and Diphenhydramine Citrate** *see* Aspirin and Diphenhydramine *on page 182*

Aspirin and Dipyridamole

(AS pir in & dye peer ID a mole)

Brand Names: U.S. Aggrenox®

Brand Names: Canada Aggrenox®

Index Terms Aspirin and Extended-Release Dipyridamole; Dipyridamole and Aspirin

Pharmacologic Category Antiplatelet Agent

Use Reduction in the risk of stroke in patients who have had transient ischemia of the brain or ischemic stroke due to thrombosis

Unlabeled Use Hemodialysis graft patency; symptomatic carotid artery stenosis (including recent carotid endarterectomy)

Pregnancy Risk Factor D

Dosage Oral: Adults:

Stroke prevention: One capsule (dipyridamole 200 mg, aspirin 25 mg) twice daily

Alternative regimen for patients with intolerable headache: One capsule at bedtime and low-dose aspirin in the morning. Return to usual dose (1 capsule twice daily) as soon as tolerance to headache develops (usually within a week).

Carotid artery stenosis, symptomatic (including recent carotid endarterectomy) (unlabeled use): One capsule (dipyridamole 200 mg, aspirin 25 mg) twice daily (Guyatt, 2012)

Hemodialysis graft patency (unlabeled use): One capsule (dipyridamole 200 mg, aspirin 25 mg) twice daily

Dosage adjustment in renal impairment: Avoid use in patients with severe renal dysfunction (Cl_{cr} <10 mL/minute). Studies have not been done in patients with renal impairment.

Dosage adjustment in hepatic impairment: Avoid use in patients with severe hepatic impairment. Studies have not been done in patients with varying degrees of hepatic impairment.

Elderly: Plasma concentrations were 40% higher, but specific dosage adjustments have not been recommended.

Additional Information Complete prescribing information should be consulted for additional detail.

Dosage Forms Excipient information presented when available (limited, particularly for generics); consult specific product labeling.

Capsule, variable release:

Aggrenox®: Aspirin 25 mg [immediate release] and dipyridamole 200 mg [extended release] [contains lactose, sucrose]

- **Aspirin and Extended-Release Dipyridamole** *see* Aspirin and Dipyridamole *on page 182*
- **Aspirin and Oxycodone** *see* Oxycodone and Aspirin *on page 1539*
- **Aspirin, Caffeine and Acetaminophen** *see* Acetaminophen, Aspirin, and Caffeine *on page 33*
- **Aspirin, Caffeine, and Butalbital** *see* Butalbital, Aspirin, and Caffeine *on page 305*
- **Aspirin, Caffeine, and Orphenadrine** *see* Orphenadrine, Aspirin, and Caffeine *on page 1517*
- **Aspirin, Carisoprodol, and Codeine** *see* Carisoprodol, Aspirin, and Codeine *on page 352*
- **Aspirin, Dihydrocodeine, and Caffeine** *see* Dihydrocodeine, Aspirin, and Caffeine *on page 611*
- **Aspirin Free Anacin Extra Strength [OTC]** *see* Acetaminophen *on page 28*
- **Aspirin, Orphenadrine, and Caffeine** *see* Orphenadrine, Aspirin, and Caffeine *on page 1517*
- **Aspir-low [OTC]** *see* Aspirin *on page 177*
- **Aspirtab [OTC]** *see* Aspirin *on page 177*
- **Astagraf XL** *see* Tacrolimus (Systemic) *on page 1976*
- **Astelin** *see* Azelastine (Nasal) *on page 211*
- **Astepro** *see* Azelastine (Nasal) *on page 211*
- **Asthmanefrin Refill [OTC]** *see* EPINEPHrine (Systemic, Oral Inhalation) *on page 714*
- **Asthmanefrin Starter Kit [OTC]** *see* EPINEPHrine (Systemic, Oral Inhalation) *on page 714*
- **Astramorph** *see* Morphine (Systemic) *on page 1398*
- **AT** *see* Antithrombin *on page 148*
- **AT-III** *see* Antithrombin *on page 148*
- **Atacand** *see* Candesartan *on page 327*
- **Atacand HCT** *see* Candesartan and Hydrochlorothiazide *on page 329*
- **Atacand Plus (Can)** *see* Candesartan and Hydrochlorothiazide *on page 329*
- **Atarax (Can)** *see* HydrOXYzine *on page 1025*
- **Atasol (Can)** *see* Acetaminophen *on page 28*

Atazanavir (at a za NA veer)

Brand Names: U.S. Reyataz

Brand Names: Canada Reyataz

Index Terms Atazanavir Sulfate; ATV; BMS-232632

Pharmacologic Category Antiretroviral, Protease Inhibitor (Anti-HIV)

Use Treatment of HIV-1 infections in combination with at least two other antiretroviral agents

Pregnancy Risk Factor B

Pregnancy Considerations Adverse events were not observed in animal reproduction studies. Atazanavir crosses the placenta with cord blood concentrations reported as 13% to 21% of maternal serum concentrations at delivery. An increased risk of teratogenic effects has not been observed based on information collected by the antiretroviral pregnancy registry. A small increased risk of preterm birth has been associated with maternal use of protease inhibitor-based combination antiretroviral (ARV) therapy during pregnancy; however, the benefits of use generally outweigh this risk and protease inhibitors (PIs) should not be withheld if otherwise recommended. Hyperglycemia, new onset of diabetes mellitus, or diabetic ketoacidosis have been reported with PIs; it is not clear if pregnancy increases this risk. Hyperbilirubinemia or hypoglycemia may occur in neonates following *in utero* exposure to atazanavir, although data are conflicting.

The DHHS Perinatal HIV Guidelines recommend atazanavir as a preferred PI when combined with low-dose ritonavir boosting. Pharmacokinetic studies suggest that standard dosing during pregnancy may provide decreased plasma concentrations and some experts recommend increased doses during the second and third trimesters. However, the manufacturer notes that dose adjustment is not required unless using concomitant H_2-receptor blockers or tenofovir or for ARV-naive pregnant women taking efavirenz. May give as once-daily dosing.

Regardless of CD4 count or HIV RNA copy number, all HIV-infected pregnant women should receive a combination antepartum ARV drug regimen; this includes women who require therapy for their own health, as well as women who do not yet require therapy for their own health. ARV therapy should be started as soon as possible if required for the woman's health Although earlier initiation may be more effective in reducing the perinatal transmission of HIV), also consider maternal conditions (eg, nausea and vomiting) and the potential risks of first trimester fetal exposure for specific agents. Plasma HIV RNA levels should be assessed at ~34-36 weeks gestation in order to help determine mode of delivery. If ARV therapy must be interrupted for <24 hours during the peripartum period, stop then restart all medications simultaneously in order to decrease the chance of developing resistance. Long-term follow-up is recommended for all infants exposed to ARV medications.

Healthcare providers are encouraged to enroll pregnant women exposed to antiretroviral medications in the Antiretroviral Pregnancy Registry (1-800-258-4263 or www.-APRegistry.com). Healthcare providers caring for HIV-infected women and their infants may contact the National Perinatal HIV Hotline (888-448-8765) for clinical consultation (DHHS [perinatal], 2012).

Breast-Feeding Considerations Atazanavir is excreted into breast milk. Maternal or infant antiretroviral therapy does not completely eliminate the risk of postnatal HIV transmission. In addition, multiclass-resistant virus has been detected in breast-feeding infants despite maternal therapy. Therefore, in the United States, where formula is accessible, affordable, safe, and sustainable, and the risk of infant mortality due to diarrhea and respiratory infections is low, complete avoidance of breast-feeding by HIV-infected women is recommended to decrease potential transmission of HIV (DHHS [perinatal], 2012).

Contraindications Hypersensitivity (eg, Stevens-Johnson syndrome, erythema multiforme, or toxic skin eruptions) to atazanavir or any component of the formulation; concurrent therapy with alfuzosin, cisapride, ergot derivatives (dihydroergotamine, ergonovine, ergotamine, methylergonovine), indinavir, irinotecan, lovastatin, midazolam (oral), pimozide, rifampin, sildenafil (when used for pulmonary artery hypertension [eg, Revatio]), simvastatin, St John's wort, or triazolam

Canadian labeling: Additional contraindications (not in U.S. labeling): Concomitant use of quinidine or bepridil (currently not marketed in Canada)

Warnings/Precautions Atazanavir may prolong PR interval, use with caution in patients with pre-existing conduction abnormalities or with medications which prolong AV conduction (dosage adjustment required with some agents); rare cases of second-degree AV block have been reported. May cause or exacerbate pre-existing hepatic dysfunction; use caution in patients with transaminase elevations prior to therapy or underlying hepatic disease, such as hepatitis B or C or cirrhosis; monitor closely. Asymptomatic elevations in bilirubin (unconjugated) occur commonly during therapy with atazanavir; consider alternative therapy if bilirubin is >5 times ULN. Evaluate alternative etiologies if transaminase elevations also occur.

Cases of nephrolithiasis have been reported in postmarketing surveillance; temporary or permanent discontinuation of therapy should be considered if symptoms develop.

Protease inhibitors have been associated with a variety of hypersensitivity events (some severe), including rash, anaphylaxis (rare), angioedema, bronchospasm, erythema multiforme, Stevens-Johnson syndrome (rare) and/or toxic skin eruptions (including DRESS [drug rash, eosinophilia and systemic symptoms] syndrome). It is generally recommended to discontinue treatment if severe rash or moderate symptoms accompanied by other systemic symptoms occur.

Use with caution in patients with hemophilia A or B; increased bleeding during protease inhibitor therapy has been reported. Changes in glucose tolerance, hyperglycemia, exacerbation of diabetes, DKA, and new-onset diabetes mellitus have been reported in patients receiving protease inhibitors. May be associated with fat redistribution (buffalo hump, increased abdominal girth, breast engorgement, facial atrophy). Immune reconstitution syndrome may develop resulting in the occurrence of an inflammatory response to an indolent or residual opportunistic infection during initial HIV treatment or activation of autoimmune disorders (eg, Graves' disease, polymyositis, Guillain-Barré syndrome) later in therapy; further evaluation and treatment may be required. Do not use in children <3 months of age due to potential for kernicterus. Potentially significant drug-drug interactions may exist, requiring dose or frequency adjustment, additional monitoring, and/or selection of alternative therapy.

Adverse Reactions Includes data from both treatment-naive and treatment-experienced patients. Percentages listed for adults unless otherwise specified.

>10%:

- Dermatologic: Skin rash (3% to 21%; median onset: 7 weeks)
- Endocrine & metabolic: Increased serum cholesterol (≥240 mg/dL: 6% to 25%), increased amylase (≤14%)
- Gastrointestinal: Nausea (3% to 14%)
- Hepatic: Increased serum bilirubin (≥2.6 times ULN: 35% to 49%), jaundice (children 13% to 15%; adults 5% to 9%)
- Neuromuscular & skeletal: Increased creatine phosphokinase (6% to 11%)
- Respiratory: Cough (children 21%)
- Miscellaneous: Fever (children 18% to 19%; adults 2%)

2% to 10%:

- Cardiovascular: First degree atrioventricular block (6%), second degree atrioventricular block (children 2%; adults [rare])
- Central nervous system: Headache (1% to 6%; children 7%), peripheral neuropathy (<1% to 4%), insomnia (<1% to 3%), depression (2%), dizziness (<1% to 2%)
- Endocrine & metabolic: Increased serum triglycerides (<1% to 8%), hyperglycemia (≥251 mg/dL: 5%)
- Gastrointestinal: Diarrhea (children 8%; adults 1% to 3%, vomiting (children 8%; adults 3% to 4%), increased serum lipase (<1% to 5%), abdominal pain (4%)

Hematologic: Neutropenia (3% to 7%), decreased hemoglobin (<1% to 5%), thrombocytopenia (2%)
Hepatic: Increased serum ALT (>5 times ULN: 3% to 9%; 10% to 25% in patients seropositive for hepatitis B and/or C), increased serum AST (>5 times ULN: 2% to 7%; 9% to 10% in patients seropositive for hepatitis B and/or C)
Neuromuscular & skeletal: Myalgia (4%)
Respiratory: Rhinorrhea (children 6%)

<2% (Limited to important or life-threatening): Alopecia, cholecystitis, cholelithiasis, cholestasis, complete atrioventricular block (rare), diabetes mellitus, DRESS syndrome, edema, erythema multiforme, immune reconstitution syndrome, interstitial nephritis, left bundle branch block, maculopapular rash, nephrolithiasis, pancreatitis, prolongation P-R interval on ECG, prolonged Q-T interval on ECG, Stevens-Johnson syndrome, torsades de pointes

Drug Interactions

Metabolism/Transport Effects **Substrate** of CYP3A4 (major); **Note:** Assignment of Major/Minor substrate status based on clinically relevant drug interaction potential; **Inhibits** CYP1A2 (weak), CYP2C8 (weak), CYP2C9 (weak), CYP3A4 (strong), UGT1A1

Avoid Concomitant Use

Avoid concomitant use of Atazanavir with any of the following: Ado-Trastuzumab Emtansine; Alfuzosin; Amiodarone; Apixaban; Avanafil; Axitinib; Bosutinib; Buprenorphine; Cabozantinib; Cisapride; Conivaptan; Crizotinib; Dronedarone; Eplerenone; Ergot Derivatives; Etravirine; Everolimus; Fusidic Acid (Systemic); Halofantrine; Ibrutinib; Imatinib; Indinavir; Irinotecan; Ivabradine; Lapatinib; Lomitapide; Lovastatin; Lurasidone; Macitentan; Midazolam; Nevirapine; Nilotinib; Nisoldipine; Pimozide; Pomalidomide; QuiNIDine; Ranolazine; Red Yeast Rice; Regorafenib; Rifampin; Rivaroxaban; Salmeterol; Silodosin; Simeprevir; Simvastatin; St Johns Wort; Tamsulosin; Ticagrelor; Tolvaptan; Toremifene; Triazolam; Ulipristal; Vemurafenib; VinCRIStine (Liposomal); Voriconazole

Increased Effect/Toxicity

Atazanavir may increase the levels/effects of: Ado-Trastuzumab Emtansine; Alfuzosin; Almotriptan; Alosetron; ALPRAZolam; Amiodarone; Apixaban; ARIPiprazole; AtorvaSTATin; Avanafil; Axitinib; Bedaquiline; Bortezomib; Bosentan; Bosutinib; Brentuximab Vedotin; Brinzolamide; Budesonide (Nasal); Budesonide (Systemic, Oral Inhalation); Buprenorphine; Cabozantinib; Calcium Channel Blockers (Dihydropyridine); Calcium Channel Blockers (Nondihydropyridine); CarBAMazepine; Cisapride; Clarithromycin; Colchicine; Conivaptan; Contraceptives (Progestins); Corticosteroids (Orally Inhaled); Crizotinib; CycloSPORINE (Systemic); CYP3A4 Substrates; Dienogest; Digoxin; Dofetilide; Dronedarone; Dutasteride; Enfuvirtide; Enzalutamide; Eplerenone; Ergot Derivatives; Etravirine; Everolimus; FentaNYL; Fesoterodine; Fluticasone (Nasal); Fluticasone (Oral Inhalation); GuanFACINE; Halofantrine; Highest Risk QTc-Prolonging Agents; Ibrutinib; Iloperidone; Imatinib; Indinavir; Irinotecan; Ivabradine; Ivacaftor; Ixabepilone; Lacosamide; Lapatinib; Levomilnacipran; Lomitapide; Lovastatin; Lumefantrine; Lurasidone; Macitentan; Maraviroc; Meperidine; MethylPREDNISolone; Midazolam; Mifepristone; Moderate Risk QTc-Prolonging Agents; Nefazodone; Nevirapine; Nilotinib; Nisoldipine; Ospemifene; OxyCODONE; Paricalcitol; PAZOPanib; Pimecrolimus; Pimozide; Pitavastatin; Pomalidomide; PONATinib; Propafenone; Protease Inhibitors; QUEtiapine; QuiNIDine; Ranolazine; Red Yeast Rice; Regorafenib; Repaglinide; Rifabutin; Rilpivirine; Riociguat; Rivaroxaban; RomiDEPsin; Rosuvastatin; Ruxolitinib; Salmeterol; Saxagliptin; Sildenafil; Silodosin; Simeprevir; Simvastatin; SORAfenib; Tacrolimus (Systemic); Tacrolimus (Topical); Tadalafil; Tamsulosin; Temsirolimus; Tenofovir; Ticagrelor; Tofacitinib; Tolterodine; Tolvaptan; Toremifene; TraZODone; Triazolam; Tricyclic Antidepressants; Ulipristal; Vardenafil; Vemurafenib; Vilazodone; VinCRIStine (Liposomal); Voriconazole; Warfarin; Zuclopenthixol

The levels/effects of Atazanavir may be increased by: Clarithromycin; CycloSPORINE (Systemic); CYP3A4 Inhibitors (Moderate); CYP3A4 Inhibitors (Strong); Dasatinib; Delavirdine; Enfuvirtide; Fusidic Acid (Systemic); Indinavir; Luliconazole; Posaconazole; Simeprevir; Telaprevir

Decreased Effect

Atazanavir may decrease the levels/effects of: Abacavir; Boceprevir; Clarithromycin; Contraceptives (Estrogens); Delavirdine; Didanosine; Ifosfamide; Meperidine; Prasugrel; Telaprevir; Theophylline Derivatives; Ticagrelor; Valproic Acid and Derivatives; Voriconazole; Zidovudine

The levels/effects of Atazanavir may be decreased by: Antacids; Boceprevir; Bosentan; Buprenorphine; CarBAMazepine; CYP3A4 Inducers (Strong); Dabrafenib; Deferasirox; Didanosine; Efavirenz; Etravirine; Garlic; H2-Antagonists; Minocycline; Mitotane; Nevirapine; Proton Pump Inhibitors; Rifampin; St Johns Wort; Tenofovir; Tocilizumab; Voriconazole

Ethanol/Nutrition/Herb Interactions

Food: Bioavailability of atazanavir increased when taken with food. Management: Administer with food.
Herb/Nutraceutical: St John's wort decreases serum concentrations of protease inhibitors and may lead to treatment failures. Garlic may decrease the serum concentration of protease inhibitors. Management: Concurrent use of St John's wort is contraindicated. Use of garlic supplements while taking protease inhibitors is not recommended.

Storage/Stability Store at 25°C (77°F); excursions permitted to 15°C to 30°C (59°F to 86°F).

Mechanism of Action Binds to the site of HIV-1 protease activity and inhibits cleavage of viral Gag-Pol polyprotein precursors into individual functional proteins required for infectious HIV. This results in the formation of immature, noninfectious viral particles.

Pharmacodynamics/Kinetics

Absorption: Rapid; enhanced with food
Protein binding: 86%
Metabolism: Hepatic, via multiple pathways including CYP3A4; forms two metabolites (inactive)
Half-life elimination: Unboosted therapy: 7-8 hours; Boosted therapy (with ritonavir): 9-18 hours
Time to peak, plasma: 2-3 hours
Excretion: Feces (79%, 20% of total dose as unchanged drug); urine (13%, 7% of total dose as unchanged drug)

Dosage Oral:

Children 6 to <18 years:

Antiretroviral-naive patients: Note: Ritonavir-boosted atazanavir dosing regimen is preferred:

Ritonavir-unboosted regimen:

- Children 6 years to <13 years: Dose not established; use not recommended
- Children ≥13 years and <40 kg **who are not able to tolerate ritonavir**: No dosage recommendations provided in the manufacturer's labeling.
- Children ≥13 years and ≥40 kg **who are not able to tolerate ritonavir**: Atazanavir 400 mg once daily (without ritonavir)

Ritonavir-boosted regimen:

- 15 to <20 kg: Atazanavir 150 mg once daily **plus** ritonavir 100 mg once daily
- 20 to <40 kg: Atazanavir 200 mg once daily **plus** ritonavir 100 mg once daily
- ≥40 kg: Atazanavir 300 mg once daily **plus** 100 mg ritonavir once daily

Alternate recommendations (DHHS [pediatric], 2011):
15-24 kg: Atazanavir 150 mg once daily **plus** ritonavir 80 mg once daily
25-31 kg: Atazanavir 200 mg once daily **plus** ritonavir 100 mg once daily
32-38 kg: Atazanavir 250 mg once daily **plus** ritonavir 100 mg once daily
≥39 kg: Atazanavir 300 mg once daily **plus** 100 mg ritonavir once daily. **Note:** Treatment-naive patients ≥39 kg and ≥13 years of age who are unable to tolerate ritonavir, refer to adult dosing.

Antiretroviral-experienced patients: Note: Atazanavir without ritonavir is not recommended in antiretroviral-experienced patients with prior virologic failure:
Ritonavir-unboosted regimen: Use not recommended
Ritonavir-boosted regimen:
15 to <20 kg: Atazanavir 150 mg once daily **plus** ritonavir 100 mg once daily
20 to <40 kg: Atazanavir 200 mg once daily **plus** ritonavir 100 mg once daily
≥40 kg: Atazanavir 300 mg once daily **plus** 100 mg ritonavir once daily
Alternate recommendations (DHHS [pediatric], 2011):
25-31 kg: Atazanavir 200 mg once daily **plus** ritonavir 100 mg once daily
32-38 kg: Atazanavir 250 mg once daily **plus** ritonavir 100 mg once daily
≥39 kg: Atazanavir 300 mg once daily **plus** 100 mg ritonavir once daily

Dosing adjustment for concomitant therapy: Children (antiretroviral-experienced or antiretroviral-naive patients): Coadministration with H_2 antagonists, proton pump inhibitors, or tenofovir:
Children 6 to <13 years: Use not recommended.
Children ≥13 years and <40 kg: Use not recommended.
Children ≥13 years and ≥40 kg:
Ritonavir-unboosted regimen: Use not recommended.
Ritonavir-boosted regimen: Refer to adult dosing.

Adults:

Antiretroviral-naive patients: Atazanavir 300 mg once daily **plus** ritonavir 100 mg once daily **or** atazanavir 400 mg once daily in patients unable to tolerate ritonavir. **Note:** Recommended (with ritonavir) as a first-line therapy with tenofovir/emtricitabine in nonpregnant antiretroviral-naive patients (DHHS, 2013). Acceptable alternative regimens would be atazanavir plus lamivudine/zidovudine **or** atazanavir plus abacavir/lamivudine. Do not use tenofovir with unboosted atazanavir (DHHS, 2013).

Antiretroviral-experienced patients: Atazanavir 300 mg once daily **plus** ritonavir 100 mg once daily. **Note:** Atazanavir without ritonavir is not recommended in antiretroviral-experienced patients with prior virologic failure.

Pregnant patients: Atazanavir 300 mg once daily **plus** ritonavir 100 mg once daily. **Note:** Preferred regimen for pregnant patients who are antiretroviral-naive. Postpartum dosage adjustment not needed. Observe patient for adverse events, especially within 2 months after delivery. Dose adjustments required for concomitant tenofovir *or* H_2 antagonist use (insufficient information for dose adjustment if *both* tenofovir and an H_2 antagonist are used). Some experts recommend atazanavir 400 mg plus ritonavir 100 mg in all pregnant women during the second and third trimesters due to decreased plasma concentrations (DHHS [perinatal], 2012).

Dosage adjustments for concomitant therapy: Adults:

Coadministration with efavirenz:

Antiretroviral-naive patients: Atazanavir 400 mg plus ritonavir 100 mg given with efavirenz 600 mg (all once daily but administered at different times; atazanavir and ritonavir with food and efavirenz on an empty stomach).

Antiretroviral-experienced patients: Concurrent use not recommended due to decreased atazanavir exposure.

Coadministration with didanosine buffered or enteric-coated formulations: Administer atazanavir 2 hours before or 1 hour after didanosine buffered or enteric coated formulations

Coadministration with H_2 antagonists:

Antiretroviral-naive patients: Atazanavir 300 mg plus ritonavir 100 mg given simultaneously with, or at least 10 hours after an H_2 antagonist equivalent dose of ≤80 mg famotidine/day

Patients unable to tolerate ritonavir: Atazanavir 400 mg once daily given at least 2 hours before or at least 10 hours after an H_2 antagonist equivalent daily dose of ≤40 mg famotidine (single dose ≤20 mg)

Antiretroviral-experienced patients: Atazanavir 300 mg plus ritonavir 100 mg given simultaneously with, or at least 10 hours after an H_2 antagonist equivalent dose of ≤40 mg famotidine/day

Antiretroviral-experienced pregnant patients in the second or third trimester: Atazanavir 400 mg plus ritonavir 100 mg simultaneously with, or at least 10 hours after an H_2 antagonist. **Note:** Insufficient information for dose adjustment if tenofovir **and** an H_2 antagonist are used.

Coadministration with proton pump inhibitors:

U.S. labeling:

Antiretroviral-naive patients: Atazanavir 300 mg plus ritonavir 100 mg given 12 hours after a proton pump inhibitor equivalent dose of ≤20 mg omeprazole/day

Antiretroviral-experienced patients: Concurrent use not recommended. (**Note:** One study noted adequate serum concentrations when atazanavir 400 mg plus ritonavir 100 mg was given at the same time or 12 hours after omeprazole 20 mg.)

Canadian labeling: Concurrent use is not recommended; however, if unavoidable, administer atazanavir 400 mg plus ritonavir 100 mg once daily with proton pump inhibitor equivalent dose of ≤20 mg omeprazole/day. **Note:** Manufacturer labeling does not specify patient population (antiretroviral- naïve and/or experienced) to which dosing recommendation applies.

Coadministration with tenofovir:

Antiretroviral-naive patients: Atazanavir 300 mg plus ritonavir 100 mg given with tenofovir 300 mg (all as a single daily dose)

Antiretroviral-experienced patients: Atazanavir 300 mg plus ritonavir 100 mg given with tenofovir 300 mg (all as a single daily dose); if H_2 antagonist coadministered (not to exceed equivalent daily dose of ≤40 mg famotidine), increase atazanavir to 400 mg (plus ritonavir 100 mg) once daily

Antiretroviral-experienced pregnant patients in the second or third trimester: Atazanavir 400 mg plus ritonavir 100 mg. **Note:** Insufficient information for dose adjustment if tenofovir **and** an H_2 antagonist are used

Dosage adjustment in renal impairment:
Not on hemodialysis: No dosage adjustment necessary
Hemodialysis:
Antiretroviral-naive patients: Use boosted therapy of atazanavir 300 mg with ritonavir 100 mg once daily
Antiretroviral-experienced patients: Not recommended

Dosage adjustment in hepatic impairment:
Atazanavir:
Mild-to-moderate hepatic insufficiency: Use with caution; if moderate insufficiency (Child-Pugh class B) and no prior virologic failure, reduce dose to 300 mg once daily.
Severe hepatic insufficiency (Child-Pugh class C): Not recommended
Note: Patients with underlying hepatitis B or C may be at increased risk of hepatic decompensation.

Atazanavir/ritonavir: Use not recommended in hepatic impairment (has not been studied).

Dietary Considerations Must be taken with food; enhances absorption.

Administration Administer with food. Swallow capsules whole with water; do not open capsules.

Monitoring Parameters Viral load, CD4, serum glucose; liver function tests, bilirubin, drug levels (with certain concomitant medications), ECG monitoring in patients with prolonged PR interval or with concurrent AV nodal blocking drugs

Additional Information A listing of medications that should not be used concurrently is available with each bottle and patients should be provided with this information.

Dosage Forms Excipient information presented when available (limited, particularly for generics); consult specific product labeling. [DSC] = Discontinued product

Capsule, Oral, as sulfate:

Reyataz: 100 mg [DSC], 150 mg, 200 mg, 300 mg [contains fd&c blue #2 (indigotine)]

◆ Atazanavir Sulfate *see* Atazanavir *on page 182*

◆ Atelvia *see* Risedronate *on page 1824*

Atenolol (a TEN oh lole)

Brand Names: U.S. Tenormin

Brand Names: Canada Apo-Atenol®; Ava-Atenolol; CO Atenolol; Dom-Atenolol; JAMP-Atenolol; Mint-Atenolol; Mylan-Atenolol; Nu-Atenol; PMS-Atenolol; RAN™-Atenolol; ratio-Atenolol; Riva-Atenolol; Sandoz-Atenolol; Septa-Atenolol; Tenormin®; Teva-Atenolol

Pharmacologic Category Antianginal Agent; Antihypertensive; Beta-Blocker, Beta-1 Selective

Additional Appendix Information

Beta-Blockers *on page 2294*

Use Treatment of hypertension, alone or in combination with other agents; management of angina pectoris; secondary prevention postmyocardial infarction

Unlabeled Use Acute ethanol withdrawal (in combination with a benzodiazepine), supraventricular and ventricular arrhythmias, and migraine headache prophylaxis

Pregnancy Risk Factor D

Pregnancy Considerations Studies in pregnant women have demonstrated a risk to the fetus; therefore, the manufacturer classifies atenolol as pregnancy category D. Atenolol crosses the placenta and is found in cord blood. In a cohort study, an increased risk of cardiovascular defects was observed following maternal use of beta-blockers during pregnancy. Intrauterine growth restriction (IUGR), small placentas, as well as fetal/neonatal bradycardia, hypoglycemia, and/or respiratory depression have been observed following *in utero* exposure to beta-blockers as a class. Adequate facilities for monitoring infants at birth should be available. Untreated chronic maternal hypertension and pre-eclampsia are also associated with adverse events in the fetus, infant, and mother. The maternal pharmacokinetic parameters of atenolol during the second and third trimesters are within the ranges reported in nonpregnant patients. Although atenolol has shown efficacy in the treatment of hypertension in pregnancy, it is not the drug of choice due to potential IUGR in the infant.

Breast-Feeding Considerations Atenolol is excreted in breast milk and has been detected in the serum and urine of nursing infants. Peak concentrations in breast milk have been reported to occur between 2-8 hours after the maternal dose and in some cases are higher than the peak maternal serum concentration. Although most studies have not reported adverse events in nursing infants, avoiding maternal use while nursing infants with renal dysfunction or infants <44 weeks postconceptual age has been suggested. Beta-blockers with less distribution into breast milk may be preferred. The manufacturer recommends that caution be exercised when administering atenolol to nursing women.

Contraindications Hypersensitivity to atenolol or any component of the formulation; sinus bradycardia; sinus node dysfunction; heart block greater than first-degree (except in patients with a functioning artificial pacemaker); cardiogenic shock; uncompensated cardiac failure; pulmonary edema; pregnancy

Warnings/Precautions Consider pre-existing conditions such as sick sinus syndrome before initiating. Administer cautiously in compensated heart failure and monitor for a worsening of the condition (efficacy of atenolol in heart failure has not been established). **[U.S. Boxed Warning]: Beta-blocker therapy should not be withdrawn abruptly (particularly in patients with CAD), but gradually tapered to avoid acute tachycardia, hypertension, and/or ischemia.** Chronic beta-blocker therapy should not be routinely withdrawn prior to major surgery. Beta-blockers should be avoided in patients with bronchospastic disease (asthma). Atenolol, with B_1 selectivity, has been used cautiously in bronchospastic disease with close monitoring. May precipitate or aggravate symptoms of arterial insufficiency in patients with PVD and Raynaud's disease; use with caution and monitor for progression of arterial obstruction. Use cautiously in patients with diabetes - may mask hypoglycemic symptoms. May mask signs of hyperthyroidism (eg, tachycardia); use caution if hyperthyroidism is suspected, abrupt withdrawal may precipitate thyroid storm. Alterations in thyroid function tests may be observed. Use cautiously in the renally impaired (dosage adjustment required). Caution in myasthenia gravis or psychiatric disease (may cause CNS depression). Bradycardia may be observed more frequently in elderly patients (>65 years of age); dosage reductions may be necessary. Adequate alpha-blockade is required prior to use of any beta-blocker for patients with untreated pheochromocytoma. May induce or exacerbate psoriasis. Use caution with history of severe anaphylaxis to allergens; patients taking beta-blockers may become more sensitive to repeated challenges. Treatment of anaphylaxis (eg, epinephrine) in patients taking beta-blockers may be ineffective or promote undesirable effects. Use with caution in patients on concurrent digoxin, verapamil, or diltiazem; bradycardia or heart block can occur. Use with caution in patients receiving inhaled anesthetic agents known to depress myocardial contractility.

Adverse Reactions

1% to 10%:

Cardiovascular: Persistent bradycardia, hypotension, chest pain, edema, heart failure, second- or third-degree AV block, Raynaud's phenomenon

Central nervous system: Dizziness, fatigue, insomnia, lethargy, confusion, mental impairment, depression, headache, nightmares

Gastrointestinal: Constipation, diarrhea, nausea

Genitourinary: Impotence

Miscellaneous: Cold extremities

<1% (Limited to important or life-threatening): Alopecia, dyspnea (especially with large doses), hallucinations, impotence, liver enzymes increased, lupus syndrome, Peyronie's disease, positive ANA, psoriasiform rash, psychosis, thrombocytopenia, wheezing

Drug Interactions

Metabolism/Transport Effects None known.

Avoid Concomitant Use

Avoid concomitant use of Atenolol with any of the following: Floctafenine; Methacholine

Increased Effect/Toxicity

Atenolol may increase the levels/effects of: Alpha-/Beta-Agonists (Direct-Acting); Alpha1-Blockers; Alpha2-Agonists; Amifostine; Antihypertensives; Bupivacaine; Cardiac Glycosides; Cholinergic Agonists; Ergot Derivatives; Fingolimod; Hypotensive Agents; Insulin; Lidocaine (Systemic); Lidocaine (Topical); Mepivacaine; Methacholine; Midodrine; Obinutuzumab; RiTUXimab; Sulfonylureas

The levels/effects of Atenolol may be increased by: Acetylcholinesterase Inhibitors; Alpha2-Agonists; Amiodarone; Anilidopiperidine Opioids; Brimonidine (Topical); Calcium Channel Blockers (Dihydropyridine); Calcium Channel Blockers (Nondihydropyridine); Diazoxide; Dipyridamole; Disopyramide; Dronedarone; Floctafenine; Glycopyrrolate; Herbs (Hypotensive Properties); MAO Inhibitors; Pentoxifylline; Phosphodiesterase 5 Inhibitors; Prostacyclin Analogues; Regorafenib; Reserpine

Decreased Effect

Atenolol may decrease the levels/effects of: Beta2-Agonists; Theophylline Derivatives

The levels/effects of Atenolol may be decreased by: Ampicillin; Herbs (Hypertensive Properties); Methylphenidate; Nonsteroidal Anti-Inflammatory Agents; Yohimbine

Ethanol/Nutrition/Herb Interactions

Food: Atenolol serum concentrations may be decreased if taken with food.

Herb/Nutraceutical: Dong quai has estrogenic activity. Ephedra, yohimbe, and ginseng may worsen hypertension. Garlic may have increased antihypertensive effect. Management: Avoid dong quai, ephedra, yohimbe, ginseng, and garlic.

Storage/Stability Protect from light.

Mechanism of Action Competitively blocks response to beta-adrenergic stimulation, selectively blocks beta$_1$-receptors with little or no effect on beta$_2$-receptors except at high doses

Pharmacodynamics/Kinetics

Onset of action: Peak effect: Oral: 2-4 hours

Duration: Normal renal function: 12-24 hours

Absorption: Oral: Rapid, incomplete (~50%)

Distribution: Low lipophilicity; does not cross blood-brain barrier

Protein binding: 6% to 16%

Metabolism: Limited hepatic

Half-life elimination: Beta:

- Neonates: ≤35 hours; Mean: 16 hours
- Children: 4.6 hours; children >10 years may have longer half-life (>5 hours) compared to children 5-10 years (<5 hours)
- Adults: Normal renal function: 6-7 hours, prolonged with renal impairment; End-stage renal disease: 15-35 hours

Time to peak, plasma: Oral: 2-4 hours

Excretion: Feces (50%); urine (40% as unchanged drug)

Dosage Oral:

Children: Hypertension: 0.5-1 mg/kg/dose given daily; range of 0.5-1.5 mg/kg/day; maximum dose: 2 mg/kg/day up to 100 mg/day

Adults:

- Hypertension: 25-50 mg once daily, may increase to 100 mg/day. Doses >100 mg are unlikely to produce any further benefit.
- Angina pectoris: 50 mg once daily, may increase to 100 mg/day. Some patients may require 200 mg/day.
- Postmyocardial infarction: 100 mg/day or 50 mg twice daily for 6-9 days postmyocardial infarction.
- Thyrotoxicosis (unlabeled use): 25-100 mg once or twice daily (Bahn, 2011)

Elderly: Hypertension: Consider lower initial doses and titrate to response (Aronow, 2011).

Dosage adjustment in renal impairment:

- Cl_{cr} >35 mL/minute/1.73 m^2: No dosage adjustment necessary.
- Cl_{cr} 15-35 mL/minute/1.73 m^2: Maximum dose: 50 mg daily
- Cl_{cr} <15 mL/minute/1.73 m^2: Maximum dose: 25 mg daily

Hemodialysis: Moderately dialyzable (20% to 50%) via hemodialysis; administer dose postdialysis or administer 25-50 mg supplemental dose.

Peritoneal dialysis: Elimination is not enhanced; supplemental dose is not necessary.

Dosage adjustment in hepatic impairment: No dosage adjustment provided in the manufacturer's labeling; however, atenolol undergoes minimal hepatic metabolism.

Dietary Considerations May be taken without regard to meals.

Administration When administered acutely for cardiac treatment, monitor ECG and blood pressure. May be administered without regard to meals.

Monitoring Parameters Acute cardiac treatment: Monitor ECG and blood pressure

Test Interactions Increased glucose; decreased HDL

Dosage Forms Excipient information presented when available (limited, particularly for generics); consult specific product labeling.

Tablet, Oral:

- Tenormin: 25 mg
- Tenormin: 50 mg [scored]
- Tenormin: 100 mg
- Generic: 25 mg, 50 mg, 100 mg

Extemporaneous Preparations A 2 mg/mL oral suspension may be made with tablets. Crush four 50 mg tablets in a mortar and reduce to a fine powder. Add a small amount of glycerin and mix to a uniform paste. Mix while adding Ora-Sweet® SF vehicle in incremental proportions to **almost** 100 mL; transfer to a calibrated bottle, rinse mortar with vehicle, and add quantity of vehicle sufficient to make 100 mL. Label "shake well" and "refrigerate". Stable for 90 days.

Nahata MC, Pai VB, and Hipple TF, *Pediatric Drug Formulations*, 5th ed, Cincinnati, OH: Harvey Whitney Books Co, 2004.

- **ATG** *see* Antithymocyte Globulin (Equine) *on page 149*
- **Atgam** *see* Antithymocyte Globulin (Equine) *on page 149*
- **Atgam® (Can)** *see* Antithymocyte Globulin (Equine) *on page 149*
- **Athletes Foot Spray [OTC]** *see* Tolnaftate *on page 2087*
- **Ativan** *see* LORazepam *on page 1242*
- **Atlizumab** *see* Tocilizumab *on page 2080*
- **ATNAA** *see* Atropine and Pralidoxime *on page 200*

AtoMOXetine (AT oh mox e teen)

Brand Names: U.S. Strattera

Brand Names: Canada Apo-Atomoxetine; DOM-Atomoxetine; Mylan-Atomoxetine; PMS-Atomoxetine; RIVA-Atomoxetine; Sandoz-Atomoxetine; Strattera; Teva-Atomoxetine

Index Terms Atomoxetine Hydrochloride; LY139603; Methylphenoxy-Benzene Propanamine; Tomoxetine

Pharmacologic Category Norepinephrine Reuptake Inhibitor, Selective

Use Attention deficit hyperactivity disorder: Treatment of attention deficit hyperactivity disorder (ADHD)

Pregnancy Risk Factor C

Pregnancy Considerations Adverse events have been observed in animal reproduction studies. Information related to atomoxetine use in pregnancy is limited; appropriate contraception is recommended for sexually active women of childbearing potential (Heiligenstein, 2003).

Breast-Feeding Considerations It is not known if atomoxetine is excreted in breast milk. The manufacturer recommends that caution be exercised when administering atomoxetine to nursing women.

Medication Guide Available Yes

Contraindications Hypersensitivity to atomoxetine or any component of the formulation; use with or within 14 days of MAO inhibitors; narrow-angle glaucoma; current or past history of pheochromocytoma; severe cardiac or vascular disorders in which the condition would be expected to deteriorate with clinically important increases in blood pressure (eg, 15 to 20 mm Hg) or heart rate (eg, 20 beats/minute).

Canadian labeling: Additional contraindications (not in U.S. labeling): Symptomatic cardiovascular diseases, moderate-to-severe hypertension; advanced arteriosclerosis; uncontrolled hyperthyroidism

Warnings/Precautions [U.S. Boxed Warning]: Use caution in pediatric patients; may be an increased risk of suicidal ideation. Closely monitor for clinical worsening, suicidality, or unusual changes in behavior; especially during the initial few months of a course of drug therapy, or at times of dose changes, either increases or decreases. The family or caregiver should be instructed to closely observe the patient and communicate condition with healthcare provider. New or worsening symptoms of hostility or aggressive behaviors have been associated with atomoxetine, particularly with the initiation of therapy. Treatment-emergent psychotic or manic symptoms (eg, hallucinations, delusional thinking, mania) may occur in children and adolescents without a prior history of psychotic illness or mania; consider discontinuation of treatment if symptoms occur. Use caution in patients with comorbid bipolar disorder; therapy may induce mixed/manic episode. Atomoxetine is not approved for major depressive disorder. Patients presenting with depressive symptoms should be screened for bipolar disorder. Recommended to be used as part of a comprehensive treatment program for attention deficit disorders. Atomoxetine does not worsen anxiety in patients with existing anxiety disorders or tics related to Tourette's disorder.

Use caution with hepatic disease (dosage adjustments necessary in moderate and severe hepatic impairment). Use may be associated with rare but severe hepatotoxicity, including hepatic failure; discontinue and do not restart if signs or symptoms of hepatotoxic reaction (eg, jaundice, pruritus, flu-like symptoms, dark urine, right upper quadrant tenderness) or laboratory evidence of liver disease are noted. Use caution in patients who are poor metabolizers of CYP2D6 metabolized drugs ("poor metabolizers"), bioavailability increases; dosage adjustments are recommended in patients known to be CYP2D6 poor metabolizers.

Orthostasis can occur; use caution in patients predisposed to hypotension or those with abrupt changes in heart rate or blood pressure. Atomoxetine has been associated with serious cardiovascular events including sudden death in patients with pre-existing structural cardiac abnormalities or other serious heart problems (sudden death in children and adolescents; sudden death, stroke, and MI in adults). Atomoxetine should be avoided in patients with known serious structural cardiac abnormalities, cardiomyopathy, serious heart rhythm abnormalities, or other serious cardiac problems that could increase the risk of sudden death that these conditions alone carry. Patients should be carefully evaluated for cardiac disease prior to initiation of therapy. Perform a prompt cardiac evaluation in patients who develop symptoms of exertional chest pain, unexplained syncope, or other symptoms suggestive of cardiac disease during treatment. May cause increased heart rate or blood pressure; use caution with hypertension or other cardiovascular or cerebrovascular disease; CYP2D6 poor metabolizers may experience greater increases in blood pressure and heart rate effects. Use caution in patients with a history of urinary retention or bladder outlet obstruction; may cause urinary retention/hesitancy; use caution in patients with history of urinary retention or bladder outlet obstruction. Priapism has been associated with use (rarely). Allergic reactions (including anaphylactic reactions, angioneurotic edema, urticaria, and rash) may occur (rare).

Growth in pediatric patients should be monitored during treatment. Height and weight gain may be reduced during the first 9-12 months of treatment, but should recover by 3 years of therapy.

Adverse Reactions Percentages as reported in children and adults; some adverse reactions may be increased in "poor metabolizers" (CYP2D6).

>10%:
- Central nervous system: Headache (2% to 19%), insomnia (2% to 15%), drowsiness (4% to 11%)
- Gastrointestinal: Nausea (7% to 26%), xerostomia (20%), abdominal pain (7% to 18%), decreased appetite (11% to 16%), vomiting (3% to 11%)

1% to 10%:
- Cardiovascular: Systolic hypertension (4% to 5%), increased diastolic blood pressure (≤4%), palpitations (3%), syncope (1% to 3%), flushing (≥2%), tachycardia (<1% to ≥2%), orthostatic hypotension (<2%)
- Central nervous system: Fatigue (6% to 10%), dizziness (5% to 8%), depression (4% to 7%), irritability (≤6%), abnormal dreams (4%), chills (3%), disturbed sleep (3%), paresthesia (3% adults; postmarketing observation in children), agitation (2%), anxiety (2%), restlessness (2%), emotional lability (1% to 2%)
- Dermatologic: Hyperhidrosis (4%), excoriation (2% to 4%), skin rash (2%)
- Endocrine & metabolic: Weight loss (2% to 7%), decreased libido (3% to 4%), hot flash (3%), increased thirst (2%), menstrual disease (2%)
- Gastrointestinal: Constipation (1% to 9%), dyspepsia (4%), anorexia (≤3%), diarrhea (2%), dysgeusia (2%), flatulence (2%)
- Genitourinary: Erectile dysfunction (8%), urinary retention (6%), ejaculatory disorder (4%), dysmenorrhea (3%), dysuria (3%), orgasm abnormal (2%), pollakiuria (2%), prostatitis (2%), urinary frequency (2%)
- Neuromuscular & skeletal: Tremor (1% to 5%), back pain (2%), muscle spasm (2%), weakness (2%)
- Ophthalmic: Conjunctivitis (1% to 3%), mydriasis (≥2%)
- Respiratory: Sinus headache (3%), pharyngolaryngeal pain (≥2%), oropharyngeal pain (2%)
- Miscellaneous: Jitteriness (2%), therapeutic response unexpected (2%)

Limited to important or life-threatening: Aggressive behavior, allergy disorder, anaphylaxis, angioedema, cerebrovascular accident, delusions, growth suppression (children), hallucination, hepatotoxicity, hostility, hyperhidrosis, hypersensitivity reaction, hypoesthesia, hypomania, impulsivity, jaundice, mania, myocardial infarction, panic attack, pelvic pain, peripheral vascular disease, priapism, pruritus, prolonged Q-T interval on ECG, Raynaud's phenomenon, seizure (including patients with no prior history or known risk factors for seizure), severe hepatic disease, suicidal ideation, testicular pain, tics, urticaria

Drug Interactions

Metabolism/Transport Effects Substrate of CYP2C19 (minor), CYP2D6 (major); **Note:** Assignment of Major/Minor substrate status based on clinically relevant drug interaction potential; **Inhibits** CYP2D6 (weak), CYP3A4 (weak)

Avoid Concomitant Use

Avoid concomitant use of AtoMOXetine with any of the following: Iobenguane I 123; MAO Inhibitors; Pimozide

Increased Effect/Toxicity

AtoMOXetine may increase the levels/effects of: ARIPiprazole; Beta2-Agonists; Dofetilide; Lomitapide; Pimozide; Sympathomimetics

The levels/effects of AtoMOXetine may be increased by: Abiraterone Acetate; CYP2D6 Inhibitors (Moderate); CYP2D6 Inhibitors (Strong); Darunavir; MAO Inhibitors

Decreased Effect

AtoMOXetine may decrease the levels/effects of: Iobenguane I 123

The levels/effects of AtoMOXetine may be decreased by: Peginterferon Alfa-2b

Ethanol/Nutrition/Herb Interactions Ethanol: May increase CNS depression; monitor for increased effects with coadministration. Caution patients about effects.

Storage/Stability Store at 25°C (77°F); excursions are permitted between 15°C and 30°C (59°F and 86°F).

Mechanism of Action Selectively inhibits the reuptake of norepinephrine (Ki 4.5nM) with little to no activity at the other neuronal reuptake pumps or receptor sites.

Pharmacodynamics/Kinetics

Absorption: Rapid

Distribution: V_d: I.V.: 0.85 L/kg

Protein binding: 98%, primarily albumin

Metabolism: Hepatic, via CYP2D6 and CYP2C19; forms metabolites (4-hydroxyatomoxetine, active, equipotent to atomoxetine; N-desmethylatomoxetine, limited activity)

Bioavailability: 63% in extensive metabolizers; 94% in poor metabolizers

Half-life elimination: Atomoxetine: 5 hours (up to 24 hours in poor metabolizers); Active metabolites: 4-hydroxyatomoxetine: 6-8 hours; N-desmethylatomoxetine: 6-8 hours (34-40 hours in poor metabolizers)

Time to peak, plasma: 1-2 hours

Excretion: Urine (80%, as conjugated 4-hydroxy metabolite); feces (17%)

Dosage Oral: **Note:** Atomoxetine may be discontinued without the need for tapering dose.

ADHD treatment:

U.S. labeling:

Children ≥6 years and ≤70 kg:

Initial: 0.5 mg/kg/day, increase after minimum of 3 days to ~1.2 mg/kg/day; may administer as either a single daily dose or 2 evenly divided doses in morning and late afternoon/early evening. Maximum daily dose: 1.4 mg/kg or 100 mg, whichever is less.

Dosage adjustment in patients receiving strong CYP2D6 inhibitors (eg, paroxetine, fluoxetine, quinidine) or patients known to be CYP2D6 poor metabolizers: Initial: 0.5 mg/kg/day; if tolerating therapy but inadequate response, may increase after minimum of 4 weeks to 1.2 mg/kg/day.

Children ≥6 years and >70 kg and Adults:

Initial: 40 mg/day, increased after minimum of 3 days to ~80 mg/day; may administer as either a single daily dose or two evenly divided doses in morning and late afternoon/early evening. May increase to 100 mg/day in 2-4 additional weeks to achieve optimal response. Maximum daily dose: 100 mg/day.

Dosage adjustment in patients receiving strong CYP2D6 inhibitors (eg, paroxetine, fluoxetine, quinidine) or patients known to be CYP2D6 poor metabolizers: Initial: 40 mg/day; if tolerating therapy but inadequate response, may increase after minimum of 4 weeks to 80 mg/day.

Canadian labeling:

Children ≥6 years and ≤70 kg:

Initial: ~0.5 mg/kg/day for 7-14 days (Step 1); if tolerated, may increase to ~0.8 mg/kg/day for 7-14 days (Step 2), then to ~1.2 mg/kg/day (Step 3); reevaluate after ≥30 days and adjust for response if necessary. Maximum daily dose: 1.4 mg/kg or 100 mg, whichever is less. **Note:** Children should weigh at least 20 kg at the time of initiation as 10 mg is the lowest available capsule strength and capsules are to be swallowed whole.

Dosing recommendations according to weight:

Initial (Step 1):

20-29 kg: 10 mg/day

30-44 kg: 18 mg/day

45-64 kg: 25 mg/day

65-70 kg: 40 mg/day

First titration (Step 2):

20-29 kg: 18 mg/day

30-44 kg: 25 mg/day

45-64 kg: 40 mg/day

65-70 kg: 60 mg/day

Second titration (Step 3):

20-29 kg: 25 mg/day

30-44 kg: 40 mg/day

45-64 kg: 60 mg/day

65-70 kg: 80 mg/day

Dosage adjustment in patients receiving strong CYP2D6 inhibitors: Initial: 0.5 mg/kg/day; may increase to next dosage level after 14 days if previous dose is well tolerated but response is inadequate. **Note:** Canadian labeling does not include specific dosing recommendations in regards to patients who are poor CYP2D6 metabolizers although similar dose reductions would appear necessary.

Children ≥6 years and >70 kg and Adults:

Initial: 40 mg/day for 7-14 days (Step 1); if tolerated, may increase dose at 7-14 day intervals to 60 mg/day (Step 2) then to 80 mg/day (Step 3). If optimal response is not obtained after 2-4 additional weeks, may increase to a maximum dose of 100 mg/day.

Dosage adjustment in patients receiving strong CYP2D6 inhibitors: Initial: 40 mg/day; may increase to next dosage level after 14 days if previous dose is well tolerated but response is inadequate. **Note:** Canadian labeling does not include specific dosing recommendations in regards to patients who are poor CYP2D6 metabolizers although similar dose reductions would appear necessary.

Elderly: Use has not been evaluated in the elderly.

Dosage adjustment in renal impairment: No dosage adjustment necessary

Dosage adjustment in hepatic impairment:

Mild impairment (Child-Pugh class A): No dosage adjustment provided in manufacturer's labeling.

Moderate impairment (Child-Pugh class B): All doses should be reduced to 50% of normal.

Severe impairment (Child-Pugh class C): All doses should be reduced to 25% of normal.

Administration Administer with or without food as a single daily dose in the morning or as two evenly divided doses in morning and late afternoon/early evening. Swallow capsules whole; do not open capsules. If opened accidentally, do not touch eyes; wash hands immediately (product is an ocular irritant).

Monitoring Parameters Patient growth (weight/height gain in children); attention, hyperactivity, anxiety, worsening of aggressive behavior or hostility; blood pressure and pulse (baseline and following dose increases and periodically during treatment)

Family members and caregivers need to monitor patient daily for emergence of irritability, agitation, unusual changes in behavior, and suicide ideation. Pediatric patients should be monitored closely for suicidality, clinical worsening, or unusual changes in behavior, especially during the initial for months of therapy or at times of dose changes. Appearance of symptoms needs to be immediately reported to healthcare provider.

Thoroughly evaluate for cardiovascular risk. Monitor heart rate, blood pressure, and consider obtaining ECG prior to initiation (Martinez-Raga J, 2013; Vetter, 2008). Periodically reevaluate the long-term usefulness of the drug for the individual patient.

Dosage Forms Excipient information presented when available (limited, particularly for generics); consult specific product labeling.

Capsule, Oral:

Strattera: 10 mg, 18 mg, 25 mg, 40 mg, 60 mg

Strattera: 80 mg, 100 mg [contains fd&c blue #2 (indigotine)]

◆ Atomoxetine Hydrochloride *see* AtoMOXetine *on page 187*

AtorvaSTATin (a TORE va sta tin)

Brand Names: U.S. Lipitor

Brand Names: Canada Apo-Atorvastatin; Ava-Atorvastatin; CO Atorvastatin; Dom-Atorvastatin; GD-Atorvastatin; Lipitor; Mylan-Atorvastatin; Novo-Atorvastatin; PMS-Atorvastatin; RAN-Atorvastatin; ratio-Atorvastatin; Sandoz-Atorvastatin

Index Terms Atorvastatin Calcium

Pharmacologic Category Antilipemic Agent, HMG-CoA Reductase Inhibitor

Use Treatment of dyslipidemias or primary prevention of cardiovascular disease (atherosclerotic) as detailed below:

Prevention of cardiovascular disease:

Primary prevention of cardiovascular disease (high-risk for CVD): To reduce the risk of MI or stroke in patients without evidence of heart disease who have multiple CVD risk factors or type 2 diabetes. Treatment reduces the risk for angina or revascularization procedures in patients with multiple risk factors.

Secondary prevention of cardiovascular disease: To reduce the risk of nonfatal MI, nonfatal stroke, revascularization procedures, hospitalization for heart failure, and angina in patients with evidence of coronary heart disease.

Primary and secondary prevention of atherosclerotic cardiovascular disease (ASCVD) according to the American College of Cardiology/American Heart Association: To reduce the risk of ASCVD in patients with clinical ASCVD (eg, coronary heart disease, stroke/TIA, or peripheral arterial disease presumed to be of atherosclerotic origin) who are less than 75 years of age; in patients without clinical ASCVD if LDL-C is 190 mg/dL or greater; in patients without clinical ASCVD who have type 1 or type 2 diabetes and are between 40 and 75 years of age with an estimated 10-year ASCVD risk 7.5% or greater; in patients with an estimated 10-year ASCVD risk 7.5% or greater and who are between 40 and 75 years of age (Stone, 2013)

Treatment of dyslipidemias: To reduce elevations in total cholesterol (C), LDL-C, apolipoprotein B, and triglycerides in patients with elevations of one or more components, and/or to increase low HDL-C as present in Fredrickson type IIa, IIb, III, and IV hyperlipidemias, heterozygous familial and nonfamilial hypercholesterolemia, and homozygous familial hypercholesterolemia

Treatment of heterozygous familial hypercholesterolemia (HeFH) in adolescent patients (10-17 years of age, females >1 year postmenarche) having LDL-C ≥190 mg/dL or LDL-C ≥160 mg/dL with positive family history of premature cardiovascular disease (CVD) or with two or more CVD risk factors.

Unlabeled Use Secondary prevention in patients who have experienced a noncardioembolic stroke/TIA or following an ACS event regardless of baseline LDL-C using intensive lipid-lowering therapy

Pregnancy Risk Factor X

Pregnancy Considerations Adverse events were observed in animal reproductions studies. There are reports of congenital anomalies following maternal use of HMG-CoA reductase inhibitors in pregnancy; however, maternal disease, differences in specific agents used, and the low rates of exposure limit the interpretation of the available data (Godfrey, 2012; Lecarpentier, 2012). Cholesterol biosynthesis may be important in fetal development; serum cholesterol and triglycerides increase normally during pregnancy. The discontinuation of lipid lowering medications temporarily during pregnancy is not expected to have significant impact on the long term outcomes of primary hypercholesterolemia treatment.

Use of atorvastatin is contraindicated in pregnancy or those who may become pregnant. HMG-CoA reductase inhibitors should be discontinued prior to pregnancy (ADA, 2013). If treatment of dyslipidemias is needed in pregnant women or in women of reproductive age, other agents are preferred (Berglund, 2012; Stone, 2013). The manufacturer recommends administration to women of childbearing potential only when conception is highly unlikely and patients have been informed of potential hazards.

Breast-Feeding Considerations It is not known if atorvastatin is excreted into breast milk. Due to the potential for serious adverse reactions in a nursing infant, use while breast-feeding is contraindicated by the manufacturer.

Contraindications Hypersensitivity to atorvastatin or any component of the formulation; active liver disease; unexplained persistent elevations of serum transaminases; pregnancy (or those who may become pregnant); breast-feeding

Note: Telaprevir Canadian product monograph contraindicates use with atorvastatin.

Warnings/Precautions Secondary causes of hyperlipidemia should be ruled out prior to therapy. Atorvastatin has not been studied when the primary lipid abnormality is chylomicron elevation (Fredrickson types I and V). Liver function tests must be obtained prior to initiating therapy, repeat if clinically indicated thereafter. May cause hepatic dysfunction. Use with caution in patients who consume large amounts of ethanol or have a history of liver disease; monitoring is recommended. Use is contraindicated in patients with active liver disease or unexplained persistent elevations of serum transaminases; monitoring is recommended. Use high-dose atorvastatin with caution in patients with prior stroke or TIA; the risk of hemorrhagic stroke may be increased.

Rhabdomyolysis with acute renal failure has occurred. Risk is dose related and is increased with concurrent use of lipid-lowering agents which may cause rhabdomyolysis (fibric acid derivatives or niacin at doses ≥1 g/day) or during concurrent use with potent CYP3A4 inhibitors (including amiodarone, clarithromycin, erythromycin, itraconazole, ketoconazole, nefazodone, grapefruit juice in large quantities, verapamil, or protease inhibitors such as indinavir, nelfinavir, or ritonavir). Ensure patient is on the lowest effective atorvastatin dose. If concurrent use of clarithromycin or combination protease inhibitors (eg, lopinavir/ritonavir or ritonavir/saquinavir) is warranted consider dose adjustment of atorvastatin. Do not use with cyclosporine, gemfibrozil, tipranavir plus ritonavir, or telaprevir. Monitor closely if used with other drugs associated with myopathy. Weigh the risk versus benefit when combining any of these drugs with atorvastatin. Discontinue in any patient in which CPK levels are markedly elevated (>10 times ULN) or if myopathy is suspected/diagnosed. The manufacturer recommends temporary discontinuation for elective major surgery, acute medical or surgical conditions, or in any patient experiencing an acute or serious condition predisposing to renal failure (eg, sepsis, hypotension, trauma, uncontrolled seizures). However, based upon current evidence, HMG-CoA reductase inhibitor therapy should be continued in the perioperative period unless risk outweighs cardioprotective benefit. Use with caution in patients with advanced age, these patients are predisposed to myopathy. Immune-mediated necrotizing myopathy (IMNM), an autoimmune-mediated myopathy, has been reported (rarely) with HMG-CoA reductase inhibitor therapy. IMNM presents as proximal muscle weakness with elevated CPK levels, which persists despite discontinuation of HMG-CoA reductase inhibitor therapy; additionally, muscle biopsy may show necrotizing myopathy with limited inflammation; immunosuppressive therapy (eg, corticosteroids, azathioprine) may be used for treatment.

Adverse Reactions

>10%:

Gastrointestinal: Diarrhea (5% to 14%)

Neuromuscular & skeletal: Arthralgia (4% to 12%)

Respiratory: Nasopharyngitis (4% to 13%)

2% to 10%:

Central nervous system: Insomnia (1% to 5%)

Gastrointestinal: Nausea (4% to 7%), dyspepsia (3% to 6%)

Genitourinary: Urinary tract infection (4% to 8%)

Hepatic: Transaminases increased (2% to 3% with 80 mg/day dosing)

Neuromuscular & skeletal: Limb pain (3% to 9%), myalgia (3% to 8%), muscle spasms (2% to 5%), musculoskeletal pain (2% to 5%)

Respiratory: Pharyngolaryngeal pain (1% to 4%)

<2% (Limited to important or life-threatening): Alkaline phosphatase increased, alopecia, amnesia (reversible), anaphylaxis, anemia, angioneurotic edema, anorexia, biliary pain, blood glucose increased, blurred vision, bullous rash, bullous rash, bursitis, cholestasis, cholestatic jaundice, cognitive impairment (reversible), colitis, confusion (reversible), CPK increased, depression, diabetes mellitus (new onset), dizziness, duodenal ulcer, dysphagia, ecchymosis, emotional lability, epistaxis, eructation, erythema multiforme, esophagitis, fatigue, flatulence, gastritis, gastroenteritis, gingival hemorrhage, glossitis, glycosylated hemoglobin (Hb A_{1c}) increased, hematuria, hepatic failure, hepatitis, hyper-/hypoglycemia, incoordination, jaundice, joint swelling, leg cramps, malaise, melena, memory disturbance (reversible), memory impairment (reversible), metrorrhagia, migraine, muscle fatigue, myasthenia, myopathy, myositis, neck pain, neck rigidity, nephritis, nightmare, pancreatitis, paresthesia, parosmia, peripheral neuropathy, petechiae, photosensitivity, pruritus, rectal hemorrhage, rhabdomyolysis, Stevens-Johnson syndrome, stomatitis, syncope, taste loss, taste perversion, tendinous contracture, tendon rupture, tenesmus, thrombocytopenia, tinnitus, torticollis, toxic epidermal necrolysis, urticaria, vaginal hemorrhage, vomiting

Additional class-related events or case reports (not necessarily reported with atorvastatin therapy): Cataracts, cirrhosis, dermatomyositis, eosinophilia, erectile dysfunction, extraocular muscle movement impaired, fulminant hepatic necrosis, gynecomastia, hemolytic anemia, immune-mediated necrotizing myopathy (IMNM), interstitial lung disease, ophthalmoplegia, peripheral nerve palsy, polymyalgia rheumatica, positive ANA, renal failure (secondary to rhabdomyolysis), systemic lupus erythematosus-like syndrome, thyroid dysfunction, tremor, vasculitis, vertigo

Drug Interactions

Metabolism/Transport Effects **Substrate** of CYP3A4 (major), P-glycoprotein, SLCO1B1; **Note:** Assignment of Major/Minor substrate status based on clinically relevant drug interaction potential; **Inhibits** CYP3A4 (weak), P-glycoprotein

Avoid Concomitant Use

Avoid concomitant use of AtorvaSTATin with any of the following: Bosutinib; Conivaptan; CycloSPORINE (Systemic); Fusidic Acid (Systemic); Gemfibrozil; Pimozide; Pomalidomide; Posaconazole; Red Yeast Rice; Silodosin; Telaprevir; Tipranavir; Topotecan; VinCRIStine (Liposomal)

Increased Effect/Toxicity

AtorvaSTATin may increase the levels/effects of: Afatinib; Aliskiren; ARIPiprazole; Bosutinib; Cimetidine; DAPTOmycin; Digoxin; Diltiazem; Dofetilide; Everolimus; Ketoconazole (Systemic); Lomitapide; Midazolam; PAZOPanib; P-glycoprotein/ABCB1 Substrates; Pimozide; Pomalidomide; Prucalopride; Rivaroxaban; Silodosin; Spironolactone; Topotecan; Trabectedin; Verapamil; VinCRIStine (Liposomal)

The levels/effects of AtorvaSTATin may be increased by: Amiodarone; Azithromycin (Systemic); Bezafibrate; Boceprevir; Clarithromycin; Cobicistat; Colchicine; Conivaptan; CycloSPORINE (Systemic); CYP3A4 Inhibitors (Moderate); CYP3A4 Inhibitors (Strong); Cyproterone; Danazol; Dasatinib; Diltiazem; Dronedarone; Eltrombopag; Erythromycin (Systemic); Fenofibrate and Derivatives; Fluconazole; Fusidic Acid (Systemic); Gemfibrozil; Grapefruit Juice; Itraconazole; Ivacaftor; Ketoconazole (Systemic); Luliconazole; Mifepristone; Niacin; Niacinamide; P-glycoprotein/ABCB1 Inhibitors; Posaconazole; Protease Inhibitors; QuiNINE; Raltegravir; Ranolazine; Red Yeast Rice; Sildenafil; Simeprevir; Telaprevir; Telithromycin; Tipranavir; Verapamil; Voriconazole

Decreased Effect

AtorvaSTATin may decrease the levels/effects of: Dabigatran Etexilate; Lanthanum

The levels/effects of AtorvaSTATin may be decreased by: Antacids; Bexarotene (Systemic); Bile Acid Sequestrants; Bosentan; CYP3A4 Inducers (Strong); Dabrafenib; Deferasirox; Efavirenz; Etravirine; Fosphenytoin; Mitotane; P-glycoprotein/ABCB1 Inducers; Phenytoin; Rifamycin Derivatives; St Johns Wort; Tocilizumab

Ethanol/Nutrition/Herb Interactions

Ethanol: Ethanol may enhance the potential of adverse hepatic effects. Management: Avoid excessive ethanol consumption.

Food: Atorvastatin serum concentrations may be increased by grapefruit juice. Management: Avoid concurrent intake of large quantities of grapefruit juice (>1 quart/day). Red yeast rice contains an estimated 2.4 mg lovastatin per 600 mg rice.

Herb/Nutraceutical: St John's wort may decrease atorvastatin levels.

Storage/Stability Store at controlled room temperature of 20°C to 25°C (68°F to 77°F).

Mechanism of Action Inhibitor of 3-hydroxy-3-methylglutaryl coenzyme A (HMG-CoA) reductase, the rate-limiting enzyme in cholesterol synthesis (reduces the production of mevalonic acid from HMG-CoA); this then results in a compensatory increase in the expression of LDL receptors on hepatocyte membranes and a stimulation of LDL catabolism

Pharmacodynamics/Kinetics

Onset of action: Initial changes: 3-5 days; Maximal reduction in plasma cholesterol and triglycerides: 2 weeks

Absorption: Rapid

Distribution: V_d: ~381 L
Protein binding: ≥98%
Metabolism: Hepatic; forms active ortho- and parahydroxylated derivates and an inactive beta-oxidation product
Bioavailability: ~14% (parent drug); ~30% (parent drug and equipotent metabolites)
Half-life elimination: Parent drug: 14 hours; Equipotent metabolites: 20-30 hours
Time to peak, serum: 1-2 hours
Excretion: Bile; urine (<2% as unchanged drug)

Dosage Oral:

Primary prevention: Note: Doses should be individualized according to the baseline LDL-cholesterol concentrations, the recommended goal of therapy, and patient response; adjustments should be made at intervals of 2-4 weeks (4 weeks for children)

Children 10-17 years (females >1 year postmenarche):
HeFH: 10 mg once daily (maximum: 20 mg/day)

Adults:
Hypercholesterolemia (heterozygous familial and nonfamilial) and mixed hyperlipidemia (Fredrickson types IIa and IIb): Initial: 10-20 mg once daily; patients requiring >45% reduction in LDL-C may be started at 40 mg once daily; range: 10-80 mg once daily
Homozygous familial hypercholesterolemia: 10-80 mg once daily

ACC/AHA Blood Cholesterol Guideline recommendations to reduce the risk of atherosclerotic cardiovascular disease (ASCVD) (Stone, 2013): Adults ≥21 years:

Primary Prevention:
LDL-C ≥190 mg/dL: High intensity therapy: 80 mg once daily; if unable to tolerate, may reduce dose to 40 mg once daily
Type 1 or 2 diabetes and age 40-75 years: Moderate intensity therapy: 10-20 mg once daily
Type 1 or 2 diabetes, age 40-75 years, and an estimated 10-year ASCVD risk ≥7.5%: High intensity therapy: 80 mg once daily; if unable to tolerate, may reduce dose to 40 mg once daily
Age 40-75 years and an estimated 10-year ASCVD risk ≥7.5%: Moderate to high intensity therapy: 10-80 mg once daily

Secondary prevention:
Patient has clinical ASCVD (eg, coronary heart disease, stroke/TIA, or peripheral arterial disease presumed to be of atherosclerotic origin) **and:**
Age ≤75 years: High intensity therapy: 80 mg once daily; if unable to tolerate, may reduce dose to 40 mg once daily
Age >75 years or not a candidate for high intensity therapy: Moderate intensity therapy: 10-20 mg once daily

Intensive lipid-lowering after an ACS event regardless of baseline LDL (unlabeled use): Initial: 80 mg once daily; adjust based on patient tolerability and recommended goal LDL-C (Cannon, 2004; Pederson, 2005; Schwartz, 2001). **Note:** Currently, the ACC/AHA guidelines for UA/NSTEMI do not specify which statin to use (Anderson, 2013).

Noncardioembolic stroke/TIA (unlabeled use): Initial: 80 mg once daily; adjust based on patient tolerability and recommended goal LDL-C (Adams, 2008; Amarenco, 2006)

Dosage adjustment for atorvastatin with concomitant medications:
Boceprevir, nelfinavir: Use lowest effective atorvastatin dose (not to exceed 40 mg daily)
Clarithromycin, itraconazole, fosamprenavir, ritonavir (plus darunavir, fosamprenavir, or saquinavir): Use lowest effective atorvastatin dose (not to exceed 20 mg daily)
Lomitapide: Consider atorvastatin dose reduction (per lomitapide manufacturer).

Dosing adjustment for toxicity:
Severe muscle symptoms or fatigue: Promptly discontinue use; evaluate CPK, creatinine, and urinalysis for myoglobinuria (Stone, 2013).
Mild to moderate muscle symptoms: Discontinue use until symptoms can be evaluated; evaluate patient for conditions that may increase the risk for muscle symptoms (eg, hypothyroidism, reduced renal or hepatic function, rheumatologic disorders such as polymyalgia rheumatica, steroid myopathy, vitamin D deficiency, or primary muscle diseases). Upon resolution, resume the original or lower dose of atorvastatin. If muscle symptoms recur, discontinue atorvastatin use. After muscle symptom resolution, may then use a low dose of a different statin; gradually increase if tolerated. In the absence of continued statin use, if muscle symptoms or elevated CPK continues after 2 months, consider other causes of muscle symptoms. If determined to be due to another condition aside from statin use, may resume statin therapy at the original dose (Stone, 2013).

Dosage adjustment in renal impairment: No dosage adjustment necessary.

Dosage adjustment in hepatic impairment: Contraindicated in active liver disease or in patients with unexplained persistent elevations of serum transaminases.

Dietary Considerations May take with food if desired; may take without regard to time of day. Before initiation of therapy, patients should be placed on a standard cholesterol-lowering diet for 3-6 months and the diet should be continued during drug therapy. Red yeast rice contains an estimated 2.4 mg lovastatin per 600 mg rice. Atorvastatin serum concentration may be increased when taken with grapefruit juice; avoid concurrent intake of large quantities (>1 quart/day).

Administration May be administered with food if desired; may take without regard to time of day.

Monitoring Parameters

2013 ACC/AHA Blood Cholesterol Guideline recommendations (Stone, 2013):

Lipid panel (total cholesterol, HDL, LDL, triglycerides): Baseline lipid panel; fasting lipid profile within 4-12 weeks after initiation or dose adjustment and every 3-12 months (as clinically indicated) thereafter. If 2 consecutive LDL levels are <40 mg/dL, consider decreasing the dose.

Hepatic transaminase levels: Baseline measurement of hepatic transaminase levels (ie, ALT); measure hepatic function if symptoms suggest hepatotoxicity (eg, unusual fatigue or weakness, loss of appetite, abdominal pain, dark-colored urine or yellowing of skin or sclera) during therapy.

CPK: CPK should not be routinely measured. Baseline CPK measurement is reasonable for some individuals (eg, family history of statin intolerance or muscle disease, clinical presentation, concomitant drug therapy that may increase risk of myopathy). May measure CPK in any patient with symptoms suggestive of myopathy (pain, tenderness, stiffness, cramping, weakness, or generalized fatigue).

Evaluate for new-onset diabetes mellitus during therapy; if diabetes develops, continue statin therapy and encourage adherence to a heart-healthy diet, physical activity, a healthy body weight, and tobacco cessation.

If patient develops a confusional state or memory impairment, may evaluate patient for nonstatin causes (eg, exposure to other drugs), systemic and neuropsychiatric causes, and the possibility of adverse effects associated with statin therapy.

Manufacturer recommendation: Liver enzyme tests at baseline and repeated when clinically indicated. Measure CPK when myopathy is being considered or may measure CPK periodically in high risk patients (eg, drug-drug interaction). Upon initiation or titration, lipid panel should be analyzed within 2-4 weeks.

Dosage Forms Excipient information presented when available (limited, particularly for generics); consult specific product labeling.

Tablet, Oral:

Lipitor: 10 mg, 20 mg, 40 mg, 80 mg

Generic: 10 mg, 20 mg, 40 mg, 80 mg

◆ **Atorvastatin and Amlodipine** *see* Amlodipine and Atorvastatin *on page 110*

◆ **Atorvastatin and Ezetimibe** *see* Ezetimibe and Atorvastatin *on page 818*

◆ **Atorvastatin Calcium** *see* AtorvaSTATin *on page 190*

◆ **Atorvastatin Calcium and Amlodipine Besylate** *see* Amlodipine and Atorvastatin *on page 110*

Atovaquone (a TOE va kwone)

Brand Names: U.S. Mepron

Brand Names: Canada Mepron®

Pharmacologic Category Antiprotozoal

Use

Pneumocystis jirovecii pneumonia (PCP) prophylaxis: Prevention of PCP in patients who are intolerant to trimethoprim-sulfamethoxazole (TMP-SMZ)

Pneumocystis jirovecii pneumonia (PCP) treatment: Acute oral treatment of mild-to-moderate PCP in patients who are intolerant to TMP-SMZ

Unlabeled Use Treatment of babesiosis; treatment/chronic maintenance of *Toxoplasma gondii* encephalitis; primary prophylaxis of HIV-infected persons at high risk for developing *Toxoplasma gondii* encephalitis

Pregnancy Risk Factor C

Pregnancy Considerations Adverse events were observed in animal reproduction studies. Diagnosis and treatment of *Pneumocystis jirovecii* pneumonia (PCP) in pregnant women is the same as in nonpregnant women; however, information specific to the use of atovaquone in pregnancy is limited (DHHS [OI], 2013).

Breast-Feeding Considerations It is not known if atovaquone is excreted in breast milk. The manufacturer recommends that caution be exercised when administering atovaquone to nursing women.

Contraindications Patients who have or develop potentially life-threatening allergic reaction to atovaquone or any component of the formulation

Warnings/Precautions When used for *Pneumocystis jirovecii* pneumonia (PCP) treatment, has only been indicated in mild-to-moderate PCP; not studied for use in severe PCP; atovaquone has less adverse effects than trimethoprim-sulfamethoxazole (TMP-SMZ; the treatment of choice for mild-to-moderate PCP), although atovaquone is less effective than TMP-SMZ (DHHS [OI], 2013). Use with caution in elderly patients. Absorption may be decreased in patients who have diarrhea or vomiting; monitor closely and consider use of an antiemetic; if severe, consider use of an alternative antiprotozoal. Consider parenteral therapy with alternative agents in patients who have difficulty taking atovaquone with food; gastrointestinal disorders may limit absorption of oral medications; may not achieve adequate plasma levels. Use with caution in patients with severe hepatic impairment; monitor closely; rare cases of hepatitis, elevated liver function tests, and liver failure have been reported. Potentially significant drug-drug interactions may exist, requiring dose or frequency adjustment, additional monitoring, and/or selection of alternative therapy.

Adverse Reactions Note: Adverse reaction statistics have been compiled from studies including patients with advanced HIV disease. Consequently, it is difficult to distinguish reactions attributed to atovaquone from those caused by the underlying disease or a combination thereof.

>10%:

Central nervous system: Fever (14% to 40%), headache (16% to 31%), insomnia (10% to 19%), depression, pain

Dermatologic: Rash (22% to 46%), pruritus (5% to ≥10%)

Gastrointestinal: Diarrhea (19% to 42%), nausea (21% to 32%), vomiting (14% to 22%), abdominal pain (4% to 21%)

Neuromuscular & skeletal: Weakness (8% to 31%), myalgia

Respiratory: Cough (14% to 25%), rhinitis (5% to 24%), dyspnea (15% to 21%), sinusitis (7% to ≥10%)

Miscellaneous: Infection (18% to 22%), diaphoresis, flu-like syndrome

1% to 10%:

Cardiovascular: Hypotension (≤1%)

Central nervous system: Dizziness (3% to 8%), anxiety (≤7%)

Endocrine & metabolic: Hyponatremia (7% to 10%), hyperglycemia (≤9%), hypoglycemia (≤1%)

Gastrointestinal: Amylase increased (7% to 8%), anorexia (≤7%), dyspepsia (≤5%), constipation (≤3%), taste perversion (≤3%)

Hematologic: Anemia (4% to 6%), neutropenia (3% to 5%)

Hepatic: Liver enzymes increased (4% to 8%)

Renal: BUN increased (≤1%), creatinine increased (≤1%)

Respiratory: Bronchospasm (2% to 4%)

Miscellaneous: Oral moniliasis (5% to 10%)

Postmarketing and/or case reports: Acute renal failure, allergic reaction, angioedema, erythema multiforme, hepatitis (rare), hypersensitivity reactions, liver failure (rare), methemoglobinemia, pancreatitis, skin desquamation, Stevens-Johnson syndrome, throat tightness, thrombocytopenia, urticaria, vortex keratopathy

Drug Interactions

Metabolism/Transport Effects None known.

Avoid Concomitant Use

Avoid concomitant use of Atovaquone with any of the following: Efavirenz; Rifamycin Derivatives; Ritonavir

Increased Effect/Toxicity

Atovaquone may increase the levels/effects of: Etoposide; Hypoglycemic Agents

The levels/effects of Atovaquone may be increased by: Herbs (Hypoglycemic Properties); MAO Inhibitors; Salicylates; Selective Serotonin Reuptake Inhibitors

Decreased Effect

Atovaquone may decrease the levels/effects of: Indinavir

The levels/effects of Atovaquone may be decreased by: Efavirenz; Loop Diuretics; Metoclopramide; Rifamycin Derivatives; Ritonavir; Tetracycline

Ethanol/Nutrition/Herb Interactions

Food: Ingestion with a fatty meal increases absorption. Management: Administer with food, preferably high-fat meals (peanuts or ice cream).

Herb/Nutraceutical: Herbs with hypoglycemic properties may enhance the hypoglycemic effect of atovaquone. Management: Avoid alfalfa, aloe, bilberry, bitter melon, burdock, celery, damiana, fenugreek, garcinia, garlic, ginger, ginseng (American), gymnema, marshmallow, and stinging nettle.

Storage/Stability Store at 15°C to 25°C (59°F to 77°F). Do not freeze. Dispense in tight container.

▶

Mechanism of Action Inhibits electron transport in mitochondria resulting in the inhibition of key metabolic enzymes responsible for the synthesis of nucleic acids and ATP

Pharmacodynamics/Kinetics

Absorption: Significantly increased with a high-fat meal

Distribution: V_{dss}: 0.6 ± 0.17 L/kg

Protein binding: >99%

Metabolism: Undergoes enterohepatic recirculation

Bioavailability: 32% to 62%

Half-life elimination: 1.5-4 days

Excretion: Feces (>94% as unchanged drug); urine (<1%)

Dosage

Pneumocystis jirovecii pneumonia (PCP), prevention:

Infants and Children <13 years (unlabeled use; CDC, 2009): Oral:

1-3 months: 30 mg/kg once daily with food

4-24 months: 45 mg/kg once daily with food

>24 months: 30 mg/kg once daily with food

Adolescents ≥13 years and Adults: Oral: 1500 mg once daily with food

PCP, mild-to-moderate, treatment:

Infants and Children <13 years (unlabeled use; CDC, 2009): Oral:

Birth to 3 months: 30-40 mg/kg/day in 2 divided doses with food (maximum: 1500 mg daily)

3-24 months: 45 mg/kg/day in 2 divided doses with food (maximum: 1500 mg daily)

≥24 months: 30-40 mg/kg/day in 2 divided doses with food (maximum: 1500 mg daily)

Adolescents ≥13 years and Adults: Oral: 750 mg twice daily with food for 21 days

Babesiosis (unlabeled use): Oral:

Children: 40 mg/kg/day in 2 divided doses with azithromycin for 7-10 days (maximum: 1500 mg daily). **Note:** Relapsing infection may require at least 6 weeks of therapy (Vannier, 2012).

Adults: 750 mg twice daily with azithromycin for 7-10 days; **Note:** Relapsing infection may require at least 6 weeks of therapy (Vannier, 2012)

Toxoplasma gondii prophylaxis (CDC, 2009): Infants and Children <13 years (unlabeled use; either as monotherapy or with pyrimethamine plus leucovorin): Oral:

1-3 months: 30 mg/kg once daily with food

4-24 months: 45 mg/kg once daily with food

>24 months: 30 mg/kg once daily with food

Toxoplasma gondii encephalitis (unlabeled use) (DHHS [OI], 2013): Adolescents ≥13 years and Adults: Oral:

Prophylaxis: 1500 mg once daily with food (either as monotherapy or with pyrimethamine plus leucovorin)

Treatment: 1500 mg twice daily with food (either with pyrimethamine plus leucovorin, or with sulfadiazine, or as monotherapy) for at least 6 weeks (longer if extensive disease or incomplete response)

Chronic maintenance: 750-1500 mg twice daily with food (either with pyrimethamine plus leucovorin, or with sulfadiazine, or as monotherapy); may discontinue when asymptomatic and CD4 count >200/mm^3 for 6 months

Dosage adjustment in renal impairment: No dosage adjustment provided in manufacturer's labeling (has not been studied). However, atovaquone is not appreciably renally excreted.

Dosage adjustment in hepatic impairment: No dosage adjustment provided in manufacturer's labeling (has not been studied). However, atovaquone undergoes enterohepatic cycling and primarily hepatic excretion.

Dietary Considerations Must be taken with meals.

Administration Must be administered with meals. Shake suspension gently before use. Once opened, the foil pouch can be emptied on a dosing spoon, in a cup, or directly into the mouth.

Monitoring Parameters Hepatic function, CD4 count (for chronic maintenance treatment in toxoplasmosis)

Dosage Forms Excipient information presented when available (limited, particularly for generics); consult specific product labeling.

Suspension, Oral:

Mepron: 750 mg/5 mL (5 mL, 210 mL) [contains benzyl alcohol; citrus flavor]

Atovaquone and Proguanil

(a TOE va kwone & pro GWA nil)

Brand Names: U.S. Malarone®

Brand Names: Canada Malarone®; Malarone® Pediatric

Index Terms Atovaquone and Proguanil Hydrochloride; Proguanil and Atovaquone; Proguanil Hydrochloride and Atovaquone

Pharmacologic Category Antimalarial Agent

Use

Malaria prevention: Prophylaxis of *Plasmodium falciparum* malaria, including areas where chloroquine resistance has been reported

Malaria treatment: Treatment of acute, uncomplicated *P. falciparum* malaria

Pregnancy Risk Factor C

Pregnancy Considerations Teratogenic effects were not observed with the combination of atovaquone/proguanil in animal reproduction studies using concentrations similar to the estimated human exposure. The pharmacokinetics of atovaquone and proguanil are changed during pregnancy. Malaria infection in pregnant women may be more severe than in nonpregnant women. Because *P. falciparum* malaria can cause maternal death and fetal loss, pregnant women traveling to malaria-endemic areas must use personal protection against mosquito bites. Atovaquone/proguanil may be used as an alternative treatment of malaria in pregnant women; consult current CDC guidelines.

Breast-Feeding Considerations Small quantities of proguanil are found in breast milk. This combination is not recommended if nursing infants <5 kg (safety data is limited concerning therapeutic use in infants <5 kg)

Contraindications Hypersensitivity to atovaquone, proguanil, or any component of the formulation; prophylactic use in severe renal impairment (Cl_{cr} <30 mL/minute)

Warnings/Precautions Not indicated for cerebral malaria or other severe manifestations of complicated malaria. Delayed cases of *P. falciparum* malaria may occur after stopping prophylaxis; travelers returning from endemic areas who develop febrile illnesses should be evaluated for malaria. Recrudescent infections or infections following prophylaxis with this agent should be treated with alternative agent(s). Absorption of atovaquone may be decreased in patients who have diarrhea or vomiting; monitor closely and consider use of an antiemetic. If severe, consider use of an alternative antimalarial. Increased transaminase levels and hepatitis have been reported with prophylactic use; single case report of hepatic failure requiring transplantation documented. Monitor closely and use caution in patients with existing hepatic impairment. Elevations in AST/ALT may persist for up to 4 weeks following treatment (Looareesuwan, 1999). Administer with caution to patients with pre-existing renal disease. May use with caution for treatment of malaria treatment in patients with severe renal impairment (Cl_{cr} <30 mL/minute) if benefit outweighs risk. Contraindicated for prophylactic use in severe renal impairment due to the risk of pancytopenia in patients with severe renal impairment treated with proguanil. Treatment failures have been reported in patients >100 kg (case reports); follow-up monitoring is recommended (Durand, 2008).

Adverse Reactions The following adverse reactions were reported in patients being treated for malaria. When used for prophylaxis, reactions are similar to those seen with placebo.

>10%:

Gastrointestinal: Abdominal pain (17%), nausea (12%), vomiting (children 10% to 13%, adults 12%)

Hepatic: Transaminase increases (ALT 27%, AST 17%; increased LFT values typically normalized after ~4 weeks)

1% to 10%:

Central nervous system: Headache (10%), dizziness (5%)

Dermatologic: Pruritus (children 6%)

Gastrointestinal: Diarrhea (children 6%, adults 8%), anorexia (5%)

Neuromuscular & skeletal: Weakness (8%)

Postmarketing and/or case reports: Anaphylaxis (rare), anemia (rare), angioedema, cholestasis, erythema multiforme (rare), hallucinations, hepatitis (rare), hepatic failure (case report), neutropenia, pancytopenia (with severe renal impairment), photosensitivity, psychotic episodes (rare), rash, seizure (rare), Stevens-Johnson syndrome (rare), stomatitis, urticaria, vasculitis (rare)

Drug Interactions

Metabolism/Transport Effects None known.

Avoid Concomitant Use

Avoid concomitant use of Atovaquone and Proguanil with any of the following: Artemether; Efavirenz; Lumefantrine; Rifamycin Derivatives; Ritonavir

Increased Effect/Toxicity

Atovaquone and Proguanil may increase the levels/effects of: Antipsychotic Agents (Phenothiazines); Dapsone (Systemic); Dapsone (Topical); Etoposide; Hypoglycemic Agents; Lumefantrine; Warfarin

The levels/effects of Atovaquone and Proguanil may be increased by: Artemether; Dapsone (Systemic); Herbs (Hypoglycemic Properties); MAO Inhibitors; Salicylates; Selective Serotonin Reuptake Inhibitors

Decreased Effect

Atovaquone and Proguanil may decrease the levels/effects of: Indinavir

The levels/effects of Atovaquone and Proguanil may be decreased by: Efavirenz; Loop Diuretics; Metoclopramide; Rifamycin Derivatives; Ritonavir; Tetracycline

Ethanol/Nutrition/Herb Interactions

Food: Atovaquone taken with dietary fat significantly increases the rate and extent of absorption; AUC is increased 2-3 times and C_{max} is increased 5 times as compared to administration during a fasted state. Management: Administer with food or milk-based drink at the same time each day.

Herb/Nutraceutical: Herbs with hypoglycemic properties may enhance the hypoglycemic effect of atovaquone. This includes alfalfa, aloe, bilberry, bitter melon, burdock, celery, damiana, fenugreek, garcinia, garlic, ginger, ginseng (American), gymnema, marshmallow, stinging nettle. Management: Monitor for increased risk of hypoglycemia during concomitant use.

Storage/Stability Store at 25°C (77°F); excursions permitted to 15°C to 30°C (59°F to 86°F).

Mechanism of Action

Atovaquone: Selectively inhibits parasite mitochondrial electron transport.

Proguanil: The metabolite cycloguanil inhibits dihydrofolate reductase, disrupting deoxythymidylate synthesis. Together, atovaquone/cycloguanil affect the erythrocytic and exoerythrocytic stages of development.

Pharmacodynamics/Kinetics

Absorption:

Atovaquone: The rate and extent of absorption is increased when administered with dietary fat.

Proguanil: Extensive

Distribution: V_d:

Atovaquone: Children and Adults: ~8.8 L/kg

Proguanil: Children >15 years and Adults and 31-110 kg: 1617-2502 L; Pediatric patients ≤15 years and 11-56 kg: 462-966 L; concentrated in erythrocytes

Protein binding:

Atovaquone: >99%

Proguanil: 75%

Metabolism: Proguanil: Hepatic to active metabolites, cycloguanil (via CYP2C19) and 4-chlorophenylbiguanide

Bioavailability: Atovaquone/proguanil: 23% when administered with food

Half-life elimination:

Atovaquone: 2-3 days (adults), 1-2 days (children)

Proguanil: 12-21 hours

Excretion:

Atovaquone: Feces (>94% as unchanged drug); urine (<0.6%)

Proguanil: Urine (40% to 60%)

Dosage Oral:

Children and Adolescents (dosage based on body weight):

Prevention of malaria: Start 1-2 days prior to entering a malaria-endemic area, continue throughout the stay and for 7 days after returning. Take as a single dose, once daily.

5-8 kg (unlabeled dosing): Atovaquone/proguanil 31.25 mg/12.5 mg (Boggild, 2007)

9-10 kg (unlabeled dosing): Atovaquone/proguanil 46.8 mg/18.75 mg (Boggild, 2007)

11-20 kg: Atovaquone/proguanil 62.5 mg/25 mg

21-30 kg: Atovaquone/proguanil 125 mg/50 mg

31-40 kg: Atovaquone/proguanil 187.5 mg/75 mg

>40 kg: Atovaquone/proguanil 250 mg/100 mg

Treatment of acute malaria: Take as a single dose, once daily for 3 consecutive days.

5-8 kg: Atovaquone/proguanil 125 mg/50 mg

9-10 kg: Atovaquone/proguanil 187.5 mg/75 mg

11-20 kg: Atovaquone/proguanil 250 mg/100 mg

21-30 kg: Atovaquone/proguanil 500 mg/200 mg

31-40 kg: Atovaquone/proguanil 750 mg/300 mg

>40 kg: Atovaquone/proguanil 1000 mg/400 mg

Adults:

Prevention of malaria: Atovaquone/proguanil 250 mg/100 mg once daily; start 1-2 days prior to entering a malaria-endemic area, continue throughout the stay and for 7 days after returning

Treatment of acute malaria: Atovaquone/proguanil 1000 mg/400 mg as a single dose, once daily for 3 consecutive days

Elderly: Use with caution.

Dosage adjustment in renal impairment:

Cl_{cr} ≥30 mL/minute: No dosage adjustment necessary.

Cl_{cr} <30 mL/minute:

Prophylaxis: Use is contraindicated.

Treatment: No dosage adjustment necessary; however, use with extreme caution and only if the benefits outweigh the risks.

Dosage adjustment in hepatic impairment:

Mild-to-moderate impairment: No dosage adjustment necessary.

Severe impairment; No dosage adjustment provided in manufacturer's labeling (has not been studied).

Dietary Considerations Must be taken with food or milk-based drink.

Administration Administer with food or milk-based drink at the same time each day. If vomiting occurs within 1 hour of administration, repeat the dose. For patients who have difficulty swallowing tablets, tablets may be crushed and mixed with condensed milk just prior to administration.

Monitoring Parameters Liver and renal function; closely monitor response to treatment in patients with vomiting or diarrhea and in patients >100 kg (Durand, 2008)

Dosage Forms Excipient information presented when available (limited, particularly for generics); consult specific product labeling.

Tablet, oral: Atovaquone 250 mg and proguanil hydrochloride 100 mg

Malarone®: Atovaquone 250 mg and proguanil hydrochloride 100 mg

Tablet, oral [pediatric]:

Malarone®: Atovaquone 62.5 mg and proguanil hydrochloride 25 mg

◆ Atovaquone and Proguanil Hydrochloride *see* Atovaquone and Proguanil *on page 194*

◆ ATRA *see* Tretinoin (Systemic) *on page 2117*

◆ Atrac-Tain [OTC] *see* Urea *on page 2140*

Atracurium (a tra KYOO ree um)

Brand Names: Canada Atracurium Besylate Injection

Index Terms Atracurium Besylate

Pharmacologic Category Neuromuscular Blocker Agent, Nondepolarizing

Additional Appendix Information

Dosing Considerations for the Critically-Ill Patient With Morbid Obesity *on page 2379*

Use Adjunct to general anesthesia to facilitate endotracheal intubation and to relax skeletal muscles during surgery; to facilitate mechanical ventilation in ICU patients; does not relieve pain or produce sedation

Pregnancy Risk Factor C

Pregnancy Considerations Adverse events were observed in animal reproduction studies. Small amounts of atracurium have been shown to cross the placenta when given to women during cesarean section.

Breast-Feeding Considerations It is not known if atracurium is excreted in breast milk. The manufacturer recommends that caution be exercised when administering atracurium to nursing women.

Contraindications Hypersensitivity to atracurium besylate or any component of the formulation

Warnings/Precautions Reduce initial dosage and inject slowly (over 1-2 minutes) in patients in whom substantial histamine release would be potentially hazardous (eg, patients with clinically-important cardiovascular disease). Maintenance of an adequate airway and respiratory support is critical. Certain clinical conditions may result in potentiation or antagonism of neuromuscular blockade:

Potentiation: Electrolyte abnormalities, severe hyponatremia, severe hypocalcemia, severe hypokalemia, hypermagnesemia, neuromuscular diseases, acidosis, acute intermittent porphyria, renal failure, hepatic failure

Antagonism: Alkalosis, hypercalcemia, demyelinating lesions, peripheral neuropathies, diabetes mellitus

Increased sensitivity in patients with myasthenia gravis, Eaton-Lambert syndrome; resistance in burn patients (>30% of body) for period of 5-70 days postinjury; resistance in patients with muscle trauma, denervation, immobilization, infection, chronic treatment with atracurium. Cross-sensitivity with other neuromuscular-blocking agents may occur; use extreme caution in patients with previous anaphylactic reactions. Use caution in the elderly. Bradycardia may be more common with atracurium than with other neuromuscular-blocking agents since it has no clinically-significant effects on heart rate to counteract the bradycardia produced by anesthetics. Should be administered by adequately trained individuals familiar with its use. Some dosage forms may contain benzyl alcohol which has been associated with "gasping syndrome" in neonates.

Adverse Reactions Mild, rare, and generally suggestive of histamine release

1% to 10%: Cardiovascular: Flushing

<1%: Bronchial secretions, erythema, hives, itching, wheezing

Postmarketing and/or case reports: Allergic reaction, bradycardia, bronchospasm, dyspnea, hypotension, injection site reaction, seizure, acute quadriplegic myopathy syndrome (prolonged use), laryngospasm, myositis ossificans (prolonged use), tachycardia, urticaria

Causes of prolonged neuromuscular blockade: Excessive drug administration; cumulative drug effect, metabolism/excretion decreased (hepatic and/or renal impairment); accumulation of active metabolites; electrolyte imbalance (hypokalemia, hypocalcemia, hypermagnesemia, hypernatremia); hypothermia

Drug Interactions

Metabolism/Transport Effects None known.

Avoid Concomitant Use

Avoid concomitant use of Atracurium with any of the following: QuiNINE

Increased Effect/Toxicity

Atracurium may increase the levels/effects of: Cardiac Glycosides; Corticosteroids (Systemic); OnabotulinumtoxinA; RimabotulinumtoxinB

The levels/effects of Atracurium may be increased by: AbobotulinumtoxinA; Aminoglycosides; Calcium Channel Blockers; Capreomycin; Colistimethate; CycloSPORINE (Systemic); Fosphenytoin-Phenytoin; Inhalational Anesthetics; Ketorolac (Nasal); Ketorolac (Systemic); Lincosamide Antibiotics; Lithium; Loop Diuretics; Magnesium Salts; Polymyxin B; Procainamide; QuiNIDine; QuiNINE; Spironolactone; Tetracycline Derivatives; Vancomycin

Decreased Effect

The levels/effects of Atracurium may be decreased by: Acetylcholinesterase Inhibitors; Fosphenytoin-Phenytoin; Loop Diuretics

Preparation for Administration Atracurium should not be mixed with alkaline solutions.

Storage/Stability Refrigerate intact vials at 2°C to 8°C (36°F to 46°F); protect from freezing. Use vials within 14 days upon removal from the refrigerator to room temperature of 25°C (77°F). Dilutions of 0.2 mg/mL or 0.5 mg/mL in 0.9% sodium chloride, dextrose 5% in water, or 5% dextrose in sodium chloride 0.9% are stable for up to 24 hours at room temperature or under refrigeration.

Mechanism of Action Blocks neural transmission at the myoneural junction by binding with cholinergic receptor sites

Pharmacodynamics/Kinetics

Onset of action (dose dependent): 2-3 minutes

Duration: Recovery begins in 20-35 minutes following initial dose of 0.4-0.5 mg/kg under balanced anesthesia; recovery to 95% of control takes 60-70 minutes

Metabolism: Undergoes ester hydrolysis and Hofmann elimination (nonbiologic process independent of renal, hepatic, or enzymatic function); metabolites have no neuromuscular blocking properties; laudanosine, a product of Hofmann elimination, is a CNS stimulant and can accumulate with prolonged use. Laudanosine is hepatically metabolized.

Half-life elimination: Biphasic: Adults: Initial (distribution): 2 minutes; Terminal: 20 minutes

Excretion: Urine (<5%)

Dosage I.V. (not to be used I.M.): Dose to effect; doses must be individualized due to interpatient variability

Adjunct to surgical anesthesia (neuromuscular blockade):

Children 1 month to 2 years: Initial: 0.3-0.4 mg/kg followed by maintenance doses as needed to maintain neuromuscular blockade

Children >2 years, Adolescents, and Adults: 0.4-0.5 mg/kg, then 0.08-0.1 mg/kg administered 20-45 minutes after initial dose to maintain neuromuscular block; repeat dose at 15- to 25-minute intervals

Initial dose after succinylcholine for intubation (balanced anesthesia): Adults: 0.3-0.4 mg/kg

Pretreatment/priming: 10% of intubating dose (eg, 0.04-0.05 mg/kg) given 2-4 minutes before the larger second dose (Mehta, 1985; Miller, 2010). **Note:** Although priming has been advocated by some, priming may either be uncomfortable for the patient, increase the risk of aspiration and difficulty swallowing, or intubating conditions after priming may not be as good as that seen with succinylcholine (Miller, 2010).

Maintenance infusion for continued surgical relaxation during extended surgical procedures: At initial signs of recovery from bolus dose, a continuous infusion may be initiated at a rate of 9-10 **mcg**/kg/**minute** (0.54-0.6 **mg**/kg/**hour**); block usually maintained by a rate of 5-9 **mcg**/kg/**minute** (0.3-0.54 **mg**/kg/**hour**) under balanced anesthesia; range: 2-15 **mcg**/kg/**minute** (0.12-0.9 **mg**/kg/**hour**)

ICU paralysis (eg, facilitate mechanical ventilation) in selected adequately sedated patients (unlabeled dosing): Adults: Initial bolus of 0.4-0.5 mg/kg, followed by 4-20 **mcg**/kg/**minute** (0.24-1.2 **mg**/kg/**hour**) (Greenberg, 2013; Murray, 2002)

Dosage adjustment in renal impairment: No dosage adjustment necessary.

Dosage adjustment in hepatic impairment: No dosage adjustment necessary.

Dosing in obesity: Morbidly-obese patients should be dosed using ideal body weight or an adjusted body weight (ie, between IBW and total body weight [TBW]) (Erstad, 2004). In a bariatric surgical population of morbidly-obese patients who were administered an induction dose of atracurium based on TBW as compared to IBW, time to recovery of twitch response was prolonged (Kralingen, 2011).

Administration May be given undiluted as a bolus injection; not for I.M. injection due to tissue irritation; administration via infusion requires the use of an infusion pump; use infusion solutions within 24 hours of preparation

Monitoring Parameters Vital signs (heart rate, blood pressure, respiratory rate); degree of muscle relaxation (via peripheral nerve stimulator and presence of spontaneous movement); renal function (serum creatinine, BUN) and liver function when in ICU

In the ICU setting, prolonged paralysis and generalized myopathy, following discontinuation of agent, may be minimized by appropriately monitoring degree of blockade.

Additional Information Atracurium is classified as an intermediate-duration neuromuscular-blocking agent. It does not appear to have a cumulative effect on the duration of blockade. It does not relieve pain or produce sedation.

Dosage Forms Excipient information presented when available (limited, particularly for generics); consult specific product labeling.

Solution, Intravenous, as besylate:

Generic: 50 mg/5 mL (5 mL); 100 mg/10 mL (10 mL)

Solution, Intravenous, as besylate [preservative free]:

Generic: 50 mg/5 mL (5 mL)

- ◆ **Atracurium Besylate** *see* Atracurium *on page 196*
- ◆ **Atracurium Besylate Injection (Can)** *see* Atracurium *on page 196*
- ◆ **Atralin** *see* Tretinoin (Topical) *on page 2120*
- ◆ **Atriance™ (Can)** *see* Nelarabine *on page 1434*
- ◆ **Atripla** *see* Efavirenz, Emtricitabine, and Tenofovir *on page 690*
- ◆ **AtroPen** *see* Atropine *on page 197*

Atropine (A troe peen)

Brand Names: U.S. AtroPen; Atropine-Care; Isopto Atropine

Brand Names: Canada Dioptic's Atropine Solution; Isopto® Atropine

Index Terms Atropine Sulfate

Pharmacologic Category Anticholinergic Agent; Anticholinergic Agent, Ophthalmic; Antidote; Antispasmodic Agent, Gastrointestinal; Ophthalmic Agent, Mydriatic

Additional Appendix Information

Adult ACLS Algorithms *on page 2363*

Beers Criteria – Potentially Inappropriate Medications for Geriatrics *on page 2368*

Pediatric ALS (PALS) Algorithms *on page 2359*

Use

Injection: Preoperative medication to inhibit salivation and secretions; treatment of symptomatic sinus bradycardia, AV block (nodal level); antidote for anticholinesterase poisoning (carbamate insecticides, nerve agents, organophosphate insecticides); adjuvant use with anticholinesterases (eg, edrophonium, neostigmine) to decrease their side effects during reversal of neuromuscular blockade

Note: Use is no longer recommended in the management of asystole or pulseless electrical activity (PEA) (ACLS, 2010).

Ophthalmic: Produce mydriasis and cycloplegia for examination of the retina and optic disc and accurate measurement of refractive errors; produce papillary dilation in inflammatory conditions (eg, uveitis)

Pregnancy Risk Factor B/C (manufacturer specific)

Pregnancy Considerations Animal reproduction studies have not been conducted. Atropine has been found to cross the human placenta.

Breast-Feeding Considerations Trace amounts of atropine are excreted into breast milk. Anticholinergic agents may suppress lactation.

Prescribing and Access Restrictions The AtroPen® formulation is available for use primarily by the Department of Defense.

Contraindications Hypersensitivity to atropine or any component of the formulation; narrow-angle glaucoma; adhesions between the iris and lens (ophthalmic product); pyloric stenosis; prostatic hypertrophy

Note: No contraindications exist in the treatment of life-threatening organophosphate or carbamate insecticide or nerve agent poisoning.

Warnings/Precautions Heat prostration may occur in the presence of high environmental temperatures. Psychosis may occur in sensitive individuals or following use of excessive doses. Avoid use if possible in patients with obstructive uropathy or in other conditions resulting in urinary retention; use is contraindicated in patients with prostatic hypertrophy. Avoid use in patients with paralytic ileus, intestinal atony of the elderly or debilitated patient, severe ulcerative colitis, and toxic megacolon complicating ulcerative colitis. Use with caution in patients with autonomic neuropathy, hyperthyroidism, renal or hepatic impairment, myocardial ischemia, HF, tachyarrhythmias (including sinus tachycardia), hypertension, and hiatal hernia associated with reflux esophagitis. Treatment-related blood pressure increases and tachycardia may lead to ischemia, precipitate an MI, or increase arrhythmogenic potential. In heart transplant recipients, atropine will likely be ineffective in treatment of bradycardia due to lack of vagal innervation of the transplanted heart; cholinergic reinnervation may occur over time (years), so atropine may be used cautiously; however, some may experience paradoxical slowing of the heart rate and high-degree AV block upon administration (ACLS, 2010; Bernheim, 2004).

Avoid relying on atropine for effective treatment of type II second-degree or third-degree AV block (with or without a new wide QRS complex). Asystole or bradycardic pulseless electrical activity (PEA): Although no evidence exists for significant detrimental effects, routine use is unlikely to have a therapeutic benefit and is no longer recommended (ACLS, 2010).

AtroPen®: There are no absolute contraindications for the use of atropine in severe organophosphate or carbamate insecticide or nerve agent poisonings; however in mild poisonings, use caution in those patients where the use of atropine would be otherwise contraindicated. Formulation for use by trained personnel only. Clinical symptoms consistent with highly-suspected organophosphate or carbamate insecticides or nerve agent poisoning should be treated with antidote immediately; administration should not be delayed for confirmatory laboratory tests. Signs of atropinization include flushing, mydriasis, tachycardia, and dryness of the mouth or nose. Monitor effects closely when administering subsequent injections as necessary. The presence of these effects is not indicative of the success of therapy; inappropriate use of mydriasis as an indicator of successful treatment has resulted in atropine toxicity. Reversal of bronchial secretions is the preferred indicator of success. Adjunct treatment with a cholinesterase reactivator (eg, pralidoxime) may be required in patients with toxicity secondary to organophosphorus insecticides or nerve agents. Treatment should always include proper evacuation and decontamination procedures; medical personnel should protect themselves from inadvertent contamination. Antidotal administration is intended only for initial management; definitive and more extensive medical care is required following administration. Individuals should not rely solely on antidote for treatment, as other supportive measures (eg, artificial respiration) may still be required. Atropine reverses the muscarinic but not the nicotinic effects associated with anticholinesterase toxicity.

Children may be more sensitive to the anticholinergic effects of atropine; use with caution in children with spastic paralysis. May be inappropriate in older adults depending on comorbidities (eg, dementia, delirium) due to its potent anticholinergic effects (Beers Criteria).

Adverse Reactions Severity and frequency of adverse reactions are dose related and vary greatly; listed reactions are limited to significant and/or life-threatening.

Cardiovascular: Cardiac arrhythmia, flushing, hypotension, palpitations, tachycardia
Central nervous system: Ataxia, coma, delirium, disorientation, dizziness, drowsiness, excitement, hallucination, headache, insomnia, nervousness
Dermatologic: Anhidrosis, scarlatiniform rash, skin rash, urticaria
Gastrointestinal: Ageusia, bloating, constipation, delayed gastric emptying, nausea, paralytic ileus, vomiting, xerostomia
Genitourinary: Urinary hesitancy, urinary retention
Hypersensitivity: Anaphylaxis
Neuromuscular & skeletal: Laryngospasm, weakness
Ocular: Angle-closure glaucoma, blurred vision, cycloplegia, dry eye syndrome, increased intraocular pressure, mydriasis
Respiratory: Dry nose, dry throat, dyspnea, pulmonary edema
Miscellaneous: Fever

Drug Interactions

Metabolism/Transport Effects None known.

Avoid Concomitant Use

Avoid concomitant use of Atropine with any of the following: Aclidinium; Ipratropium (Oral Inhalation); Potassium Chloride; Tiotropium; Umeclidinium

Increased Effect/Toxicity

Atropine may increase the levels/effects of: AbobotulinumtoxinA; Analgesics (Opioid); Anticholinergics; Cannabinoids; Mirabegron; OnabotulinumtoxinA; Potassium Chloride; RimabotulinumtoxinB; Thiazide Diuretics; Tiotropium; Topiramate

The levels/effects of Atropine may be increased by: Aclidinium; Ipratropium (Oral Inhalation); Pramlintide; Umeclidinium

Decreased Effect

Atropine may decrease the levels/effects of: Acetylcholinesterase Inhibitors (Central); Secretin

The levels/effects of Atropine may be decreased by: Acetylcholinesterase Inhibitors (Central)

Preparation for Administration Preparation of bulk atropine solution for mass chemical terrorism: Add atropine sulfate powder to 100 mL NS in polyvinyl chloride bags to yield a final concentration of 1 mg/mL. Stable for 72 hours at 4°C to 8°C (39°F to 46°F); 20°C to 25°C (68°F to 77°F); 32°C to 36°C (90°F to 97°F) (Dix, 2003).

Storage/Stability Store injection at controlled room temperature of 15°C to 30°C (59°F to 86°F); avoid freezing. In addition, AtroPen® should be protected from light.

Mechanism of Action Blocks the action of acetylcholine at parasympathetic sites in smooth muscle, secretory glands, and the CNS; increases cardiac output, dries secretions. Atropine reverses the muscarinic effects of cholinergic poisoning due to agents with acetylcholinesterase inhibitor activity by acting as a competitive antagonist of acetylcholine at muscarinic receptors. The primary goal in cholinergic poisonings is reversal of bronchorrhea and bronchoconstriction. Atropine has no effect on the nicotinic receptors responsible for muscle weakness, fasciculations, and paralysis.

Pharmacodynamics/Kinetics

Onset of action: I.M., I.V.: Rapid
Absorption: I.M.: Rapid and well absorbed
Distribution: Widely throughout the body; crosses blood-brain barrier
Metabolism: Hepatic via enzymatic hydrolysis
Half-life elimination: 2-3 hours; Children <2 years of age: 7 hours; Elderly 65-75 years of age: 10 hours
Time to peak: I.M.: 3 minutes
Excretion: Urine (30% to 50% as unchanged drug and metabolites)

Dosage

Infants and Children: Doses <0.1 mg have been associated with paradoxical bradycardia.

Inhibit salivation and secretions (preanesthesia): I.M., I.V., SubQ:

<5 kg: 0.02 mg/kg/dose 30-60 minutes preop then every 4-6 hours as needed. Use of a minimum dosage of 0.1 mg in neonates <5 kg will result in dosages >0.02 mg/kg. There is no documented minimum dosage in this age group.

>5 kg: 0.01-0.02 mg/kg/dose to a maximum 0.4 mg/dose 30-60 minutes preop; minimum dose: 0.1 mg

Alternate dosing:

3-7 kg (7-16 lb): 0.1 mg
8-11 kg (17-24 lb): 0.15 mg
11-18 kg (24-40 lb): 0.2 mg
18-29 kg (40-65 lb): 0.3 mg
>30 kg (>65 lb): 0.4 mg

Bradycardia:

I.V., I.O.: 0.02 mg/kg, minimum dose recommended by PALS: 0.1 mg; however, use of a minimum dosage of 0.1 mg in patients <5 kg will result in dosages >0.02 mg/kg and is not recommended (Barrington, 2011); there is no documented minimum dosage in this age group; maximum single dose: 0.5 mg; may repeat once in 3-5 minutes; maximum total dose: 1 mg (PALS, 2010).

Endotracheal: 0.04-0.06 mg/kg; may repeat once if needed (PALS, 2010)

Children: Organophosphate or carbamate insecticide or nerve agent poisoning: **Note:** The dose of atropine required varies considerably with the severity of poisoning. The total amount of atropine used for carbamate poisoning is usually less than with organophosphate insecticide or nerve agent poisoning. Severely poisoned patients may exhibit significant tolerance to atropine; ≥2 times the suggested doses may be needed. Titrate to pulmonary status (decreased bronchial secretions); consider administration of atropine via continuous I.V. infusion in patients requiring large doses of atropine. Once patient is stable for a period of time, the dose/dosing frequency may be decreased. Pralidoxime is a component of the management of organophosphate insecticide and nerve agent toxicity; refer to Pralidoxime monograph for the specific route and dose.

I.V., I.M. (unlabeled dose): Initial: 0.05-0.1 mg/kg; repeat every 5-10 minutes as needed, doubling the dose if previous dose does not induce atropinization (Hegenbarth, 2008; Rotenberg, 2003). Maintain atropinization by administering repeat doses as needed for ≥2-12 hours based on recurrence of symptoms (Reigart, 1999).

I.V. infusion (unlabeled dose): Following atropinization, administer 10% to 20% of the total loading dose required to induce atropinization as a continuous I.V. infusion per hour; adjust as needed to maintain adequate atropinization without atropine toxicity (Eddleston, 2004b; Roberts, 2007).

I.M. (AtroPen®):

Mild symptoms (≥2 mild symptoms): Administer the weight-based dose listed below as soon as an exposure is known or strongly suspected. If severe symptoms develop after the first dose, 2 additional doses should be repeated in rapid succession 10 minutes after the first dose; do not administer more than 3 doses. If profound anticholinergic effects occur in the absence of excessive bronchial secretions, further doses of atropine should be withheld.

Severe symptoms (≥1 severe symptoms): Immediately administer **three** weight-based doses in rapid succession.

Weight-based dosing:

<6.8 kg (15 lb): 0.25 mg/dose
6.8-18 kg (15-40 lb): 0.5 mg/dose
18-41 kg (40-90 lb): 1 mg/dose
>41 kg (>90 lb): 2 mg/dose

Symptoms of insecticide or nerve agent poisoning, as provided by manufacturer in the AtroPen® product labeling, to guide therapy:

Mild symptoms: Blurred vision, bradycardia, breathing difficulties, chest tightness, coughing, drooling, miosis, muscular twitching, nausea, runny nose, salivation increased, stomach cramps, tachycardia, teary eyes, tremor, vomiting, or wheezing

Severe symptoms: Breathing difficulties (severe), confused/strange behavior, defecation (involuntary), muscular twitching/generalized weakness (severe), respiratory secretions (severe), seizure, unconsciousness, urination (involuntary); **Note:** Infants may become drowsy or unconscious with muscle floppiness as opposed to muscle twitching.

Endotracheal (unlabeled route): Increase the dose by 2-3 times the usual I.V. dose. Mix with 3-5 mL of normal saline and administer. Flush with 3-5 mL of NS and follow with 5 assisted manual ventilations (Rotenberg, 2003).

Adults (doses <0.5 mg have been associated with paradoxical bradycardia):

Inhibit salivation and secretions (preanesthesia): I.M., I.V., SubQ: 0.4-0.6 mg 30-60 minutes preop and repeat every 4-6 hours as needed

Bradycardia: **Note:** Atropine may be ineffective in heart transplant recipients: I.V.: 0.5 mg every 3-5 minutes, not to exceed a total of 3 mg or 0.04 mg/kg (ACLS, 2010)

Neuromuscular blockade reversal: I.V.: 25-30 mcg/kg 30-60 seconds before neostigmine or 7-10 mcg/kg 30-60 seconds before edrophonium

Organophosphate or carbamate insecticide or nerve agent poisoning: **Note:** The dose of atropine required varies considerably with the severity of poisoning. The total amount of atropine used for carbamate poisoning is usually less than with organophosphate insecticide or nerve agent poisoning. Severely poisoned patients may exhibit significant tolerance to atropine; ≥2 times the suggested doses may be needed. Titrate to pulmonary status (decreased bronchial secretions); consider administration of atropine via continuous I.V. infusion in patients requiring large doses of atropine. Once patient is stable for a period of time, the dose/dosing frequency may be decreased. Pralidoxime is a component of the management of organophosphate insecticide and nerve agent toxicity; refer to Pralidoxime monograph for the specific route and dose.

I.V., I.M. (unlabeled dose): Initial: 1-6 mg (ATSDR, 2011; Roberts, 2007); repeat every 3-5 minutes as needed, doubling the dose if previous dose did not induce atropinization (Eddleston, 2004b; Roberts, 2007). Maintain atropinization by administering repeat doses as needed for ≥2-12 hours based on recurrence of symptoms (Reigart, 1999).

I.V. Infusion (unlabeled dose): Following atropinization, administer 10% to 20% of the total loading dose required to induce atropinization as a continuous I.V. infusion per hour; adjust as needed to maintain adequate atropinization without atropine toxicity (Eddleston, 2004b; Roberts, 2007)

I.M. (AtroPen®):

Mild symptoms (≥2 mild symptoms): Administer 2 mg as soon as an exposure is known or strongly suspected. If severe symptoms develop after the first dose, 2 additional doses should be repeated in rapid succession 10 minutes after the first dose; do not administer more than 3 doses. If profound anticholinergic effects occur in the absence of excessive bronchial secretions, further doses of atropine should be withheld.

Severe symptoms (≥1 severe symptoms): Immediately administer **three** 2 mg doses in rapid succession.

Symptoms of insecticide or nerve agent poisoning, as provided by manufacturer in the AtroPen® product labeling, to guide therapy:

Mild symptoms: Blurred vision, bradycardia, breathing difficulties, chest tightness, coughing, drooling, miosis, muscular twitching, nausea, runny nose, salivation increased, stomach cramps, tachycardia, teary eyes, tremor, vomiting, or wheezing

Severe symptoms: Breathing difficulties (severe), confused/strange behavior, defecation (involuntary), muscular twitching/generalized weakness (severe), respiratory secretions (severe), seizure, unconsciousness, urination (involuntary)

Mydriasis, cycloplegia (preprocedure): Ophthalmic (1% solution): Instill 1-2 drops 1 hour before procedure.

Uveitis: Ophthalmic:

1% solution: Instill 1-2 drops up to 4 times/day

Ointment: Apply a small amount in the conjunctival sac up to 3 times/day; compress the lacrimal sac by digital pressure for 1-3 minutes after instillation

Dosage adjustment in renal impairment: No dosage adjustment provided in manufacturer's labeling.

Dosage adjustment in hepatic impairment: No dosage adjustment provided in manufacturer's labeling.

Administration

I.M.: AtroPen®: Administer to the outer thigh. Firmly grasp the autoinjector with the green tip (0.5 mg, 1 mg, and 2 mg autoinjector) or black tip (0.25 mg autoinjector) pointed down; remove the yellow safety release (0.5 mg, 1 mg, and 2 mg autoinjector) or gray safety release (0.25 autoinjector). Jab the green tip at a 90° angle against the outer thigh; may be administered through clothing as long as pockets at the injection site are empty. In thin patients or patients <6.8 kg (15 lb), bunch up the thigh prior to injection. Hold the autoinjector in place for 10 seconds following the injection; remove the autoinjector and massage the injection site. After administration, the needle will be visible; if the needle is not visible, repeat the above steps. After use, bend the needle against a hard surface (needle does not retract) to avoid accidental injury.

I.V.: Administer undiluted by rapid I.V. injection; slow injection may result in paradoxical bradycardia. In bradycardia, atropine administration should not delay treatment with external pacing.

Endotracheal: Dilute in NS or sterile water. Absorption may be greater with sterile water. Stop compressions (if using for cardiac arrest), spray the drug quickly down the tube. Follow immediately with several quick insufflations and continue chest compressions.

Monitoring Parameters Heart rate, blood pressure, pulse, mental status; intravenous administration requires a cardiac monitor

Organophosphate or carbamate insecticide or nerve agent poisoning: Heart rate, blood pressure, respiratory status, oxygenation secretions. Maintain atropinization with repeated dosing as indicated by clinical status. Crackles in lung bases, or continuation of cholinergic signs, may be signs of inadequate dosing. Pulmonary improvement may not parallel other signs of atropinization. Monitor for signs and symptoms of atropine toxicity (eg, fever, muscle fasciculations, delirium); if toxicity occurs, discontinue atropine and monitor closely.

Consult individual institutional policies and procedures.

Dosage Forms Excipient information presented when available (limited, particularly for generics); consult specific product labeling.

Device, Intramuscular, as sulfate:

AtroPen: 0.25 mg/0.3 mL (0.3 mL) [pyrogen free]

AtroPen: 0.5 mg/0.7 mL (0.7 mL); 1 mg/0.7 mL (0.7 mL); 2 mg/0.7 mL (0.7 mL) [pyrogen free; contains phenol]

Ointment, Ophthalmic, as sulfate:

Generic: 1% (3.5 g)

Solution, Injection, as sulfate:

Generic: 0.05 mg/mL (5 mL); 0.1 mg/mL (5 mL, 10 mL); 0.4 mg/mL (1 mL, 20 mL); 1 mg/mL (1 mL)

Solution, Injection, as sulfate [preservative free]:

Generic: 0.4 mg/mL (1 mL); 0.8 mg/mL (0.5 mL); 1 mg/mL (1 mL)

Solution, Ophthalmic, as sulfate:

Atropine-Care: 1% (2 mL, 5 mL, 15 mL) [contains benzalkonium chloride, edetate disodium]

Isopto Atropine: 1% (5 mL, 15 mL)

Generic: 1% (5 mL, 15 mL)

◆ **Atropine and Diphenoxylate** *see* Diphenoxylate and Atropine *on page* 625

Atropine and Pralidoxime

(A troe peen & pra li DOKS eem)

Brand Names: U.S. ATNAA; Duodote™

Index Terms Atropine and Pralidoxime Chloride; Mark 1™; NAAK; Nerve Agent Antidote Kit; Pralidoxime and Atropine

Pharmacologic Category Anticholinergic Agent; Antidote

Use

ATNAA: Treatment of poisoning in patients who have been exposed to organophosphate nerve agents (eg, tabun, sarin, soman) that have acetylcholinesterase-inhibiting activity for self- or buddy-administration by military personnel

Duodote™: Treatment of poisoning by organophosphate nerve agents (eg, tabun, sarin, soman) or organophosphate insecticides for use by trained emergency medical services personnel

Pregnancy Risk Factor C

Prescribing and Access Restrictions

ATNAA (**A**ntidote **T**reatment-**N**erve **A**gent **A**uto-Injector) is only available for use by U.S. Armed Forces military personnel. Information on distribution is available at Defense Services Supply Center-Philadelphia at 215-737-2341.

Duodote™ is only available for use by trained emergency medical services personnel to treat civilians. Distribution is limited to directly from manufacturer (Meridian Medical Technologies, Inc) to emergency medical service organizations or their suppliers.

Dosage I.M.: Adults: Organophosphate insecticide or nerve agent poisoning: **Note:** If exposure is suspected, antidotal therapy should be given immediately as soon as symptoms appear (critical to administer immediately in case of soman exposure). Definitive medical care should be sought after any injection given. One injection only may be given as self-aid. If repeat injections needed, administration must be done by another trained individual. Emergency medical personnel who have self-administered a dose must determine capacity to continue to provide care.

ATNAA:

Mild symptoms (some or all mild symptoms): Self-Aid or Buddy-Aid: 1 injection (wait 10-15 minutes for effect); if the patient is able to ambulate, and knows who and where they are, then no further injections are needed. If symptoms still present: Buddy-Aid: May repeat 1-2 more injections

Severe symptoms (if most or all): Buddy-Aid: If no self-aid given, 3 injections in rapid succession; if 1 self-aid injection given, 2 injections in rapid succession

Maximum cumulative dose: 3 injections

Symptoms of organophosphate insecticide or nerve agent poisoning, as provided by the manufacturer in the ATNAA product labeling to guide therapy:

Mild symptoms: Breathing difficulties, chest tightness, coughing, difficulty in seeing, drooling, headache, localized sweating and muscular twitching, miosis, nausea (with or without vomiting), runny nose, stomach cramps, tachycardia (followed by bradycardia), wheezing

Severe symptoms: Bradycardia, confused/strange behavior, convulsions, increased wheezing and breathing difficulties, involuntary urination/defecation, miosis (severe), muscular twitching/generalized weakness (severe), red/teary eyes, respiratory failure, unconsciousness, vomiting

Duodote™:

Mild symptoms (≥2 mild symptoms): 1 injection (wait 10-15 minutes for effect); if after 10-15 minutes no severe symptoms emerge, no further injections are indicated; if any severe symptoms emerge at any point following the initial injection, repeat dose by giving 2 additional injections in rapid succession. Transport to medical care facility.

Severe symptoms (≥1 severe symptom): 3 injections in rapid succession. Transport to medical care facility.

Maximum cumulative dose: 3 injections unless medical care support (eg, hospital, respiratory support) is available

Symptoms of organophosphate insecticide or nerve agent poisoning, as provided by manufacturer in the Duodote™ product labeling to guide therapy:

Mild symptoms: Airway secretions increased, blurred vision, bradycardia, breathing difficulties, chest tightness, drooling miosis, nausea, vomiting, runny nose, salivation, stomach cramps (acute onset), tachycardia, teary eyes, tremors/muscular twitching, wheezing/coughing

Severe symptoms: Breathing difficulties (severe), confused/strange behavior, convulsions, copious secretions from lung or airway, involuntary urination/defecation, muscular twitching/generalized weakness (severe)

Dosage adjustment in renal impairment: Use caution in renal impairment; pralidoxime is renally eliminated.

Dosage adjustment in hepatic impairment: No dosage adjustment provided in manufacturer's labeling.

Additional Information Complete prescribing information should be consulted for additional detail.

Dosage Forms Excipient information presented when available (limited, particularly for generics); consult specific product labeling.

Injection, solution:

ATNAA, Duodote™: Atropine 2.1 mg/0.7 mL and pralidoxime chloride 600 mg/2 mL [contains benzyl alcohol; prefilled autoinjector]

◆ **Atropine and Pralidoxime Chloride** *see* Atropine and Pralidoxime *on page* *200*

◆ **Atropine-Care** *see* Atropine *on page* *197*

◆ **Atropine, Hyoscyamine, Phenobarbital, and Scopolamine** *see* Hyoscyamine, Atropine, Scopolamine, and Phenobarbital *on page* *1028*

◆ **Atropine Sulfate** *see* Atropine *on page* *197*

◆ **Atropine Sulfate and Edrophonium Chloride** *see* Edrophonium and Atropine *on page* *687*

◆ **Atrovent** *see* Ipratropium (Nasal) *on page* *1112*

◆ **Atrovent® (Can)** *see* Ipratropium (Nasal) *on page* *1112*

◆ **Atrovent HFA** *see* Ipratropium (Systemic) *on page* *1111*

◆ **ATryn** *see* Antithrombin *on page* *148*

◆ **ATV** *see* Atazanavir *on page* *182*

◆ **Aubagio** *see* Teriflunomide *on page* *2021*

◆ **Aubra** *see* Ethinyl Estradiol and Levonorgestrel *on page* *787*

◆ **Augmentin** *see* Amoxicillin and Clavulanate *on page* *119*

◆ **Augmentin ES-600** *see* Amoxicillin and Clavulanate *on page* *119*

◆ **Augmentin XR** *see* Amoxicillin and Clavulanate *on page* *119*

◆ **Auralgan® (Can)** *see* Antipyrine and Benzocaine *on page* *148*

Auranofin (au RANE oh fin)

Brand Names: U.S. Ridaura

Brand Names: Canada Ridaura®

Pharmacologic Category Gold Compound

Use Management of active stage classic or definite rheumatoid arthritis in patients who do not respond to or tolerate other agents

Pregnancy Risk Factor C

Dosage Oral: Adults: 6 mg/day in 1-2 divided doses; after 6 months may be increased to 9 mg/day in 3 divided doses; discontinue therapy if no response after 3 months at 9 mg/day

Note: Signs of clinical improvement may not be evident until after 3 months of therapy.

Dosage adjustment in renal impairment: There are no dosage adjustments provided in the manufacturer's labeling. The following guidelines have been used by some clinicians (Aronoff, 2007):

Cl_{cr} 50-80 mL/minute: Reduce dose to 50%

Cl_{cr} <50 mL/minute: Avoid use

Dosage adjustment in hepatic impairment: No dosage adjustment provided in manufacturer's labeling.

Additional Information Complete prescribing information should be consulted for additional detail.

Dosage Forms Excipient information presented when available (limited, particularly for generics); consult specific product labeling.

Capsule, Oral:

Ridaura: 3 mg [contains benzyl alcohol]

◆ **Auraphene-B [OTC]** *see* Carbamide Peroxide *on page* *340*

◆ **Auro-Alendronate (Can)** *see* Alendronate *on page* *69*

◆ **Auro-Anastrozole (Can)** *see* Anastrozole *on page* *137*

◆ **Auro-Cefprozil (Can)** *see* Cefprozil *on page* *377*

◆ **Auro-Cefuroxime (Can)** *see* Cefuroxime *on page* *386*

◆ **Auro-Ciprofloxacin (Can)** *see* Ciprofloxacin (Systemic) *on page* *430*

◆ **Auro-Citalopram (Can)** *see* Citalopram *on page* *440*

◆ **Auro-Cyclobenzaprine (Can)** *see* Cyclobenzaprine *on page* *502*

◆ **Aurodex®** *see* Antipyrine and Benzocaine *on page* *148*

◆ **Auro-Gabapentin (Can)** *see* Gabapentin *on page* *933*

◆ **Auro-Irbesartan (Can)** *see* Irbesartan *on page* *1113*

◆ **Auro-Lamotrigine (Can)** *see* LamoTRIgine *on page* *1165*

◆ **Auro-Letrozole (Can)** *see* Letrozole *on page* *1185*

◆ **Auro-Levetiracetam (Can)** *see* LevETIRAcetam *on page* *1194*

◆ **Auro-Lisinopril (Can)** *see* Lisinopril *on page* *1226*

◆ **Auro-Losartan (Can)** *see* Losartan *on page* *1247*

◆ **Auro-Meloxicam (Can)** *see* Meloxicam *on page* *1284*

◆ **Auro-Mirtazapine (Can)** *see* Mirtazapine *on page* *1379*

◆ **Auro-Nevirapine (Can)** *see* Nevirapine *on page* *1444*

◆ **Auro-Paroxetine (Can)** *see* PARoxetine *on page* *1575*

◆ **Auro-Pioglitazone (Can)** *see* Pioglitazone *on page* *1649*

◆ **Auro-Quetiapine (Can)** *see* QUEtiapine *on page* *1757*

◆ **Auro-Ramipri (Can)** *see* Ramipril *on page* *1778*

◆ **Auro-Sertraline (Can)** *see* Sertraline *on page* *1889*

Avanafil (a VAN a fil)

Brand Names: U.S. Stendra

Index Terms Stendra

Pharmacologic Category Phosphodiesterase-5 Enzyme Inhibitor

Use Treatment of erectile dysfunction (ED)

Pregnancy Risk Factor C

Pregnancy Considerations Based on data from animal reproduction studies, avanafil is predicted to have a low risk for major developmental abnormalities in humans. This product is not indicated for use in women.

Breast-Feeding Considerations This product is not indicated for use in women.

Contraindications Hypersensitivity to avanafil or any component of the formulation; concurrent (regular or intermittent) use of organic nitrates in any form (eg, nitroglycerin, isosorbide dinitrate)

Warnings/Precautions There is a degree of cardiac risk associated with sexual activity; therefore, physicians may wish to consider the patient's cardiovascular status prior to initiating any treatment for erectile dysfunction. Use caution in patients with anatomical deformation of the penis (angulation, cavernosal fibrosis, or Peyronie's disease) and in patients who have conditions which may predispose them to priapism (sickle cell anemia, multiple myeloma, leukemia). Instruct patients to seek immediate medical attention if erection persists >4 hours.

Use is not recommended in patients with hypotension (<90/50 mm Hg); uncontrolled hypertension (>170/100 mm Hg); unstable angina or angina during intercourse; life-threatening arrhythmias, stroke, or MI within the last 6 months; cardiac failure or coronary artery disease causing unstable angina. Safety and efficacy have not been studied in these patients. Use caution in patients with left ventricular outflow obstruction (eg, aortic stenosis). Use caution with alpha-blockers; dosage adjustment is needed. Avoid or limit concurrent substantial alcohol consumption as this may increase the risk of symptomatic hypotension.

Rare cases of nonarteritic ischemic optic neuropathy (NAION) have been reported; risk may be increased with history of vision loss. Other risk factors for NAION include heart disease, diabetes, hypertension, smoking, age >50 years, or history of certain eye problems. Sudden decrease or loss of hearing has been reported rarely; hearing changes may be accompanied by tinnitus and dizziness.

Safety and efficacy have not been studied in patients with the following conditions, therefore, use in these patients is not recommended at this time: Severe hepatic impairment (Child-Pugh class C); severe renal impairment; end-stage renal disease requiring dialysis; retinitis pigmentosa or other degenerative retinal disorders. The safety and efficacy of avanafil with other treatments for erectile dysfunction have not been studied and are not recommended as combination therapy. Concomitant use with all forms of nitrates is contraindicated. If nitrate administration is medically necessary, at least 12 hours should elapse from time of last dose of avanafil to time of nitrate administration; administer only under close medical supervision with appropriate hemodynamic monitoring. Avoid use in patients taking strong CYP3A4 inhibitors (see Drug Interactions); dosage reduction recommended in patients taking moderate CYP3A4 inhibitors. Potential underlying causes of erectile dysfunction should be evaluated prior to treatment.

Adverse Reactions

>10%: Central nervous system: Headache (5% to 12%)

2% to 10%:

Cardiovascular: Flushing (3% to 10%), ECG abnormal (1% to 3%)

Central nervous system: Dizziness (1% to 2%)

Neuromuscular & skeletal: Back pain (1% to 3%)

Respiratory: Nasopharyngitis (1% to 5%), nasal congestion (1% to 3%), upper respiratory infection (1% to 3%)

<2% (Limited to important or life-threatening): ALT increased, angina, arthralgia, balanitis, color vision change, depression, DVT, dyspnea (exertional), gastritis, gastroesophageal reflux, hearing loss, hematuria, hyperglycemia, hypertension, hypoglycemia, hypotension, myalgia, nausea, nephrolithiasis, nonarteritic ischemic optic neuropathy (NAION), palpitations, peripheral edema, pollakiuria, priapism, rash, tinnitus, urinary tract infection, vertigo, vision loss (temporary or permanent) vomiting, wheezing

Drug Interactions

Metabolism/Transport Effects **Substrate** of CYP3A4 (major); **Note:** Assignment of Major/Minor substrate status based on clinically relevant drug interaction potential

Avoid Concomitant Use

Avoid concomitant use of Avanafil with any of the following: Alprostadil; Amyl Nitrite; CYP3A4 Inhibitors (Strong); Fusidic Acid (Systemic); Itraconazole; Ketoconazole (Systemic); Phosphodiesterase 5 Inhibitors; Posaconazole; Riociguat; Vasodilators (Organic Nitrates); Voriconazole

Increased Effect/Toxicity

Avanafil may increase the levels/effects of: Alpha1-Blockers; Alprostadil; Amyl Nitrite; Antihypertensives; Bosentan; Phosphodiesterase 5 Inhibitors; Riociguat; Vasodilators (Organic Nitrates)

The levels/effects of Avanafil may be increased by: Alcohol (Ethyl); CYP3A4 Inhibitors (Moderate); CYP3A4 Inhibitors (Strong); Dasatinib; Fluconazole; Fusidic Acid (Systemic); Itraconazole; Ivacaftor; Ketoconazole (Systemic); Lorcaserin; Luliconazole; Mifepristone; Posaconazole; Sapropterin; Simeprevir; Voriconazole

Decreased Effect

The levels/effects of Avanafil may be decreased by: Bosentan; CYP3A4 Inducers (Strong); Dabrafenib; Deferasirox; Etravirine; Herbs (CYP3A4 Inducers); Mitotane; Tocilizumab

Ethanol/Nutrition/Herb Interactions Ethanol: Substantial consumption of ethanol may increase the risk of hypotension and orthostasis. Lower ethanol consumption has not been associated with significant changes in blood pressure or increase in orthostatic symptoms. Management: Avoid or limit ethanol consumption.

Food: Avoid grapefruit juice.

Storage/Stability Store at 20°C to 25°C (68°F to 77°F); excursions permitted to 30°C (86°F). Protect from light.

Mechanism of Action Does not directly cause penile erections, but affects the response to sexual stimulation. The physiologic mechanism of erection of the penis involves release of nitric oxide (NO) in the corpus cavernosum during sexual stimulation. NO then activates the enzyme guanylate cyclase, which results in increased levels of cyclic guanosine monophosphate (cGMP), producing smooth muscle relaxation and inflow of blood to the corpus cavernosum. Avanafil enhances the effect of NO by inhibiting phosphodiesterase type 5 (PDE-5), which is responsible for degradation of cGMP in the corpus cavernosum; when sexual stimulation causes local release of NO, inhibition of PDE-5 by avanafil causes increased levels of cGMP in the corpus cavernosum, resulting in smooth muscle relaxation and inflow of blood to the corpus cavernosum; at recommended doses, it has no effect in the absence of sexual stimulation.

Pharmacodynamics/Kinetics

Absorption: Rapid

Protein binding: ~99%

Metabolism: Hepatic via CYP3A4 (major), CYP2C (minor); forms metabolites (active and inactive)

Half-life elimination: Terminal: ~5 hours

Time to peak, plasma: 30-45 minutes (fasting); 1.12-1.25 hours (high-fat meal)

Excretion: Feces (~62%); urine (~21%)

Dosage Oral: Erectile dysfunction:

Adults: Initial: 100 mg 30 minutes prior to sexual activity; to be given as one single dose and not given more than once daily; dosing range: 50-200 mg once daily

Elderly ≥65 years: Refer to adult dosing.

Dosing adjustment with concomitant medications:

Alpha-blocker (dose should be stable at time of avanafil initiation): Initial avanafil dose: 50 mg every 24 hours

Moderate CYP34A inhibitors (including aprepitant, diltiazem, erythromycin, fluconazole, fosamprenavir, verapamil): Maximum avanafil dose: 50 mg every 24 hours

Dosage adjustment in renal impairment:

Cl_{cr} ≥30 mL/minute: No dosage adjustment necessary.

Cl_{cr} <30 mL/minute: Has not been studied; use is not recommended by the manufacturer.

ESRD requiring hemodialysis: Has not been studied; use is not recommended by the manufacturer.

Dosage adjustment in hepatic impairment:

Mild-to-moderate hepatic impairment (Child-Pugh class A or B): No adjustment required

Severe hepatic impairment (Child-Pugh class C): Has not been studied; use is not recommended by the manufacturer

Dietary Considerations May take with or without food. Avoid grapefruit juice.

Administration May be administered with or without food, 30 minutes prior to sexual activity.

Monitoring Parameters Monitor for response, adverse reactions, blood pressure, and heart rate.

Product Availability Stendra: FDA approved April 2012; availability currently undetermined.

Dosage Forms Excipient information presented when available (limited, particularly for generics); consult specific product labeling.

Tablet, Oral:

Stendra: 50 mg, 100 mg, 200 mg

- ◆ **Ava-Naproxen EC (Can)** *see* Naproxen *on page 1425*
- ◆ **Avandamet** *see* Rosiglitazone and Metformin *on page 1858*
- ◆ **Avandaryl** *see* Rosiglitazone and Glimepiride *on page 1857*
- ◆ **Avandia** *see* Rosiglitazone *on page 1855*
- ◆ **Ava-Nortriptyline (Can)** *see* Nortriptyline *on page 1475*
- ◆ **Ava-Olanzapine (Can)** *see* OLANZapine *on page 1493*
- ◆ **Ava-Omeprazole (Can)** *see* Omeprazole *on page 1505*
- ◆ **Ava-Pantoprazole (Can)** *see* Pantoprazole *on page 1563*
- ◆ **Ava-Pioglitazone (Can)** *see* Pioglitazone *on page 1649*
- ◆ **Ava-Pramipexole (Can)** *see* Pramipexole *on page 1695*
- ◆ **Avapro** *see* Irbesartan *on page 1113*
- ◆ **Avapro® HCT** *see* Irbesartan and Hydrochlorothiazide *on page 1115*
- ◆ **Ava-Quetiapine (Can)** *see* QUEtiapine *on page 1757*
- ◆ **AVAR** *see* Sulfur and Sulfacetamide *on page 1966*
- ◆ **Ava-Ramipril (Can)** *see* Ramipril *on page 1778*
- ◆ **AVAR-e** *see* Sulfur and Sulfacetamide *on page 1966*
- ◆ **AVAR-e Green** *see* Sulfur and Sulfacetamide *on page 1966*

- AVAR-e LS *see* Sulfur and Sulfacetamide *on page 1966*
- Ava-Risperidone (Can) *see* RisperiDONE *on page 1826*
- AVAR LS *see* Sulfur and Sulfacetamide *on page 1966*
- Ava-Simvastatin (Can) *see* Simvastatin *on page 1899*
- Avastin *see* Bevacizumab *on page 251*
- Ava-Sumatriptan (Can) *see* SUMAtriptan *on page 1969*
- Ava-Tamsulosin CR (Can) *see* Tamsulosin *on page 1990*
- Ava-Valsartan (Can) *see* Valsartan *on page 2154*
- Ava-Valsartan/HCT (Can) *see* Valsartan and Hydrochlorothiazide *on page 2156*
- Avaxim (Can) *see* Hepatitis A Vaccine *on page 990*
- Avaxim-Pediatric (Can) *see* Hepatitis A Vaccine *on page 990*
- AVC Vaginal *see* Sulfanilamide *on page 1963*
- AVE 0005 *see* Aflibercept (Ophthalmic) *on page 56*
- Avelox *see* Moxifloxacin (Systemic) *on page 1404*
- Avelox ABC Pack *see* Moxifloxacin (Systemic) *on page 1404*
- Avelox I.V. (Can) *see* Moxifloxacin (Systemic) *on page 1404*
- Aventyl® (Can) *see* Nortriptyline *on page 1475*
- Aviane *see* Ethinyl Estradiol and Levonorgestrel *on page 787*
- Avian Influenza Virus Vaccine *see* Influenza Virus Vaccine (H5N1) *on page 1076*
- Avidoxy *see* Doxycycline *on page 668*
- AVINza *see* Morphine (Systemic) *on page 1398*
- Avita *see* Tretinoin (Topical) *on page 2120*
- Avodart *see* Dutasteride *on page 680*
- Avodart® (Can) *see* Dutasteride *on page 680*
- Avonex® *see* Interferon Beta-1a *on page 1104*
- Avonex® Pen™ *see* Interferon Beta-1a *on page 1104*
- AVP *see* Vasopressin *on page 2172*
- Axert *see* Almotriptan *on page 79*
- Axid *see* Nizatidine *on page 1470*
- Axid® (Can) *see* Nizatidine *on page 1470*
- Axid AR [OTC] *see* Nizatidine *on page 1470*
- Axiron® *see* Testosterone *on page 2026*
- Axiron *see* Testosterone *on page 2026*

Axitinib (ax I ti nib)

Brand Names: U.S. Inlyta

Brand Names: Canada Inlyta®

Index Terms AG-013736; Inlyta®

Pharmacologic Category Antineoplastic Agent, Tyrosine Kinase Inhibitor; Vascular Endothelial Growth Factor (VEGF) Inhibitor

Use Treatment of advanced renal cell cancer (RCC) after failure of one prior systemic treatment

Pregnancy Risk Factor D

Pregnancy Considerations Teratogenic, embryotoxic, and fetotoxic events were observed in animal reproduction studies when administered in doses less than the normal human dose. Based on its mechanism of action and because axitinib inhibits angiogenesis (a critical component of fetal development), adverse effects on pregnancy would be expected. Women of childbearing potential should be advised to avoid pregnancy during therapy.

Breast-Feeding Considerations The decision to discontinue axitinib or discontinue breast-feeding during therapy should take into account the benefits of treatment to the mother.

Prescribing and Access Restrictions Available from select specialty pharmacies. Further information may be obtained at 877-744-5675 or www.inlytahcp.com.

Contraindications There are no contraindications listed within the manufacturer's labeling.

Warnings/Precautions Hazardous agent - use appropriate precautions for handling and disposal (meets NIOSH, 2012 criteria). May cause hypertension; the median onset is within the first month, and has been observed as early as 4 days after treatment initiation. Hypertensive crisis has been reported. Blood pressure should be well-controlled prior to treatment initiation. Monitor blood pressure and treat with standard antihypertensive therapy. Persistent hypertension (despite antihypertensive therapy) may require dose reduction; discontinue if severe and persistent despite concomitant antihypertensives (or dose reduction), or with evidence of hypertensive crisis. Monitor for hypotension if on antihypertensive therapy and axitinib is withheld or discontinued.

Gastrointestinal perforation and fistulas (including a fatality) have been reported. Monitor for signs/symptoms throughout treatment. Has not been studied in patients with recent active gastrointestinal bleeding; use is not recommended.

Arterial thrombotic events (cerebrovascular accident, MI, retinal artery occlusion, and transient ischemic attack), with fatalities, have been reported. Venous thrombotic events, including pulmonary embolism, deep vein thrombosis, retinal vein occlusion and retinal vein thrombosis, have been observed (with some fatalities). Use with caution in patients with a history of or risks for arterial or venous thrombotic events; has not been studied in patients within 12 months of an arterial thrombotic event or within 6 months of a venous thrombotic event. Hemorrhagic events (cerebral hemorrhage, gastrointestinal hemorrhage, hematuria, hemoptysis, and melena) have been reported (with some fatalities). Temporarily interrupt treatment with any hemorrhage requiring medical intervention.

Cases of reversible posterior leukoencephalopathy syndrome (RPLS) have been reported. Symptoms of RPLS include confusion, headache, hypertension (mild-to-severe), lethargy, seizure, blindness and/or other vision, or neurologic disturbances; interrupt treatment and manage hypertension. MRI is recommended to confirm RPLS diagnosis. Discontinue axitinib if RPLS is confirmed. The safety of reinitiating axitinib in patients previously experiencing RPLS is unknown.

Hypothyroidism occurs commonly with tyrosine kinase inhibitors, including axitinib. Hyperthyroidism has also been reported. Monitor thyroid function. Thyroid disorders should be treated according to standard practice to achieve/maintain euthyroid state. Proteinuria is associated with use. Monitor for proteinuria. If moderate or severe proteinuria occurs, reduce dose or temporarily withhold treatment. Although the effect on wound healing has not been studied with axitinib, vascular endothelial growth factor (VEGF) receptor inhibitors are associated with impaired wound healing. Discontinue treatment at least 24 hours prior to scheduled surgery; treatment reinitiation should be guided by clinical judgment and wound assessment. Has not been studied in patients with evidence of untreated brain metastases; use is not recommended. Systemic exposure to axitinib is increased in patients with moderate hepatic impairment; dose reductions are recommended. Has not been studied in patients with severe hepatic impairment. Increases in ALT have been observed during treatment; monitor liver function tests.

Adverse Reactions

>10%:

Cardiovascular: Hypertension (40%; grades 3/4: 16%)

Central nervous system: Fatigue (39%), dysphonia (31%), headache (14%)

Dermatologic: Palmar-plantar erythrodysesthesia syndrome (27%; grades 3/4: 5%), rash (13%; grades 3/4: <1%)

Endocrine & metabolic: Bicarbonate decreased (44%), hypocalcemia (39%), hyperglycemia (28%), hypothyroidism (19%; grades 3/4: <1%), hypernatremia (17%), hyperkalemia (15%), hypoalbuminemia (15%), hyponatremia (13%), hypophosphatemia (13%), hypoglycemia (11%)

Gastrointestinal: Diarrhea (55%; grades 3/4: 11%), appetite decreased (34%), nausea (32%; grades 3/4: 3%), lipase increased (3% to 27%), amylase increased (25%), weight loss (25%), vomiting (24%; grades 3/4: 3%), constipation (20%), mucosal inflammation (15%), stomatitis (15%), abdominal pain (8% to 14%), taste alteration (11%)

Hematologic: Anemia (4% to 35%; grades 3/4: <1%), lymphopenia (33%; grades 3/4: 3%), hemorrhage (16%; grades 3/4 1%), thrombocytopenia (15%; grades 3/4: <1%), leukopenia (11%)

Hepatic: Alkaline phosphatase increased (30%), ALT increased (22%; grades 3/4: <1%), AST increased (20%; grades 3/4: <1%)

Neuromuscular & skeletal: Weakness (21%), arthralgia (15%), limb pain (13%)

Renal: Creatinine increased (55%), proteinuria (11%; grade 3: 3%)

Respiratory: Cough (15%), dyspnea (15%)

1% to 10%:

Cardiovascular: Venous thrombotic events (grades 3/4: 3%), arterial thrombotic events (2%; grade 3/4: 1%), deep vein thrombosis (1%), transient ischemic attack (1%)

Central nervous system: Dizziness (9%)

Dermatologic: Dry skin (10%), pruritus (7%), alopecia (4%), erythema (2%)

Endocrine & metabolic: Dehydration (6%), hyperthyroidism (1%)

Gastrointestinal: Dyspepsia (10%), hemorrhoids (4%), rectal hemorrhage (2%), fistula (1%), gastrointestinal perforation (≤1%)

Hematologic: Hemoglobin increased (9%), polycythemia (1%)

Neuromuscular & skeletal: Myalgia (7%)

Ocular: Retinal vein occlusion/thrombosis (1%)

Otic: Tinnitus (3%)

Renal: Hematuria (3%)

Respiratory: Epistaxis (6%), hemoptysis (2%), pulmonary embolism (2%)

<1% (Limited to important or life-threatening): Cerebral bleeding, cerebrovascular accident, fever, hypertensive crisis, heart failure, neutropenia, reversible posterior leukoencephalopathy syndrome (RPLS)

Drug Interactions

Metabolism/Transport Effects **Substrate** of CYP1A2 (minor), CYP2C19 (minor), CYP3A4 (major), UGT1A1; **Note:** Assignment of Major/Minor substrate status based on clinically relevant drug interaction potential

Avoid Concomitant Use

Avoid concomitant use of Axitinib with any of the following: CYP3A4 Inducers (Strong); CYP3A4 Inducers (Weakly to Moderately Effective); CYP3A4 Inhibitors (Strong); Fusidic Acid (Systemic); Grapefruit Juice; St Johns Wort

Increased Effect/Toxicity

Axitinib may increase the levels/effects of: Bisphosphonate Derivatives; Vitamin K Antagonists

The levels/effects of Axitinib may be increased by: CYP3A4 Inhibitors (Moderate); CYP3A4 Inhibitors (Strong); Dasatinib; Fusidic Acid (Systemic); Grapefruit Juice; Ivacaftor; Luliconazole; Mifepristone; Simeprevir

Decreased Effect

Axitinib may decrease the levels/effects of: Cardiac Glycosides; Vitamin K Antagonists

The levels/effects of Axitinib may be decreased by: Bosentan; CYP3A4 Inducers (Strong); CYP3A4 Inducers (Weakly to Moderately Effective); Dabrafenib; Deferasirox; St Johns Wort; Tocilizumab

Ethanol/Nutrition/Herb Interactions

Food: Axitinib serum concentrations may be increased when taken with grapefruit or grapefruit juice. Management: Avoid concurrent use.

Herb/Nutraceutical: St John's wort may decrease axitinib serum concentrations. Management: Avoid concurrent use.

Storage/Stability Store at 20°C to 25°C (68°F to 77°F); excursions permitted to 15°C to 30°C (59°F to 86°F).

Mechanism of Action Axitinib is a selective second generation tyrosine kinase inhibitor which blocks angiogenesis and tumor growth by inhibiting vascular endothelial growth factor receptors (VEGFR-1, VEGFR-2, and VEGFR-3).

Pharmacodynamics/Kinetics

Absorption: Rapid (Rugo, 2005)

Distribution: V_d: 160 L

Protein binding: >99%; to albumin (primarily) and to alpha$_1$ acid glycoprotein (AAG)

Metabolism: Hepatic; primarily via CYP3A4/5 and to a lesser extend via CYP1A2, CYP2C19 and UGT1A1

Bioavailability: 58%

Half-life elimination: 2.5-6 hours

Time to peak: 2.5-4 hours

Excretion: Feces (~41%; 12% as unchanged drug); urine (~23%; as metabolites)

Dosage Oral: Adults: Renal cell cancer, advanced: Initial: 5 mg twice daily (approximately every 12 hours)

Dose increases: If dose is tolerated (no adverse events above grade 2, blood pressure is normal and no antihypertensive use) for at least 2 consecutive weeks, may increase the dose to 7 mg twice daily, and then further increase (using the same tolerance criteria) to 10 mg twice daily.

Dose decreases: For adverse events, reduce dose from 5 mg twice daily to 3 mg twice daily; further reduce to 2 mg twice daily if adverse events persist.

Dosage adjustment for strong CYP3A4 inhibitors: Avoid concomitant administration with strong CYP3A4 inhibitors (eg, clarithromycin, itraconazole, ketoconazole, nefazodone, protease inhibitors, telithromycin, voriconazole, grapefruit juice); if concomitant administration with a strong CYP3A4 inhibitor cannot be avoided, ~50% dosage reduction is recommended; adjust dose based on individual tolerance and safety. When the strong CYP3A4 inhibitor is discontinued, resume previous axitinib dose after 3-5 half-lives of the inhibitor have passed.

Dosing adjustment for toxicity:

Adverse events: May require temporary interruption, dose decreases (reduce dose from 5 mg twice daily to 3 mg twice daily; further reduce to 2 mg twice daily) or discontinuation

Hypertension: Treat with standard antihypertensive therapy.

Persistent hypertension: May require dose reduction

Severe, persistent (despite antihypertensives and dose reduction), or evidence of hypertensive crisis: Discontinue treatment

Hemorrhage: Any bleeding requiring medical intervention: Temporarily interrupt treatment.

Proteinuria (moderate-to-severe): Reduce dose or temporarily interrupt treatment.

Dosing adjustment in renal impairment:

Mild-to-severe renal impairment (Cl_{cr} 15 to <89 mL/minute): No initial dosage adjustment necessary

End-stage renal disease: (ESRD) No dosage adjustment provided in the manufacturer's labeling

Dosing adjustment in hepatic impairment:

Mild impairment (Child-Pugh class A): No starting dosage adjustment necessary

Moderate impairment (Child-Pugh class B): Reduce starting dose by ~50%; increase or decrease based on individual tolerance

Severe impairment (Child-Pugh class C): No dosage adjustment provided in the manufacturer's labeling (has not been studied)

Dietary Considerations May be taken without regard to food. Avoid grapefruit and grapefruit juice.

Administration Oral: Swallow tablet whole with a glass of water. May be taken with or without food. If a dose is missed or vomited, do not make up; resume dosing with the next scheduled dose.

Hazardous agent; use appropriate precautions for handling and disposal (meets NIOSH, 2012 criteria).

Monitoring Parameters Hepatic function (ALT, AST, and bilirubin; baseline and periodic), thyroid function (baseline and periodic), urinalysis (for proteinuria; baseline and periodically); blood pressure, signs/symptoms of RPLS, gastrointestinal bleeding/perforation/fistula

Thyroid function testing recommendations (Hamnvik, 2011):

Pre-existing levothyroxine therapy: Obtain baseline TSH levels, then monitor every 4 weeks until levels and levothyroxine dose are stable, then monitor every 2 months

Without pre-existing thyroid hormone replacement: TSH at baseline, then monthly for 4 months, then every 2-3 months

Dosage Forms Excipient information presented when available (limited, particularly for generics); consult specific product labeling.

Tablet, Oral:

Inlyta: 1 mg, 5 mg

- AY-25650 *see* Triptorelin *on page 2131*
- Aygestin *see* Norethindrone *on page 1472*
- Ayr [OTC] *see* Sodium Chloride *on page 1914*
- Ayr Nasal Mist Allergy/Sinus [OTC] *see* Sodium Chloride *on page 1914*
- Ayr Saline Nasal [OTC] *see* Sodium Chloride *on page 1914*
- Ayr Saline Nasal Drops [OTC] *see* Sodium Chloride *on page 1914*
- Ayr Saline Nasal Gel [OTC] *see* Sodium Chloride *on page 1914*
- Ayr Saline Nasal No-Drip [OTC] *see* Sodium Chloride *on page 1914*
- AYR Saline Nasal Rinse [OTC] *see* Sodium Chloride *on page 1914*
- 5-Aza-2'-deoxycytidine *see* Decitabine *on page 556*

AzaCITIDine (ay za SYE ti deen)

Brand Names: U.S. Vidaza

Brand Names: Canada Vidaza®

Index Terms 5-Azacytidine; 5-AZC; AZA-CR; Azacytidine; Ladakamycin

Pharmacologic Category Antineoplastic Agent, DNA Methylation Inhibitor

Use Treatment of myelodysplastic syndrome (MDS)

Unlabeled Use Treatment of acute myelogenous leukemia (AML)

Pregnancy Risk Factor D

Pregnancy Considerations Embryotoxicity, fetal death, and fetal abnormalities were observed in animal studies. There are no adequate and well-controlled studies in pregnant women. Women of childbearing potential should be advised to avoid pregnancy during treatment. In addition, males should be advised to avoid fathering a child while on azacitidine therapy.

Breast-Feeding Considerations Due to the potential for serious adverse reactions in the nursing infant, breast-feeding is not recommended.

Contraindications Hypersensitivity to azacitidine, mannitol, or any component of the formulation; advanced malignant hepatic tumors

Warnings/Precautions Hazardous agent - use appropriate precautions for handling and disposal (NIOSH, 2012). Azacitidine may be hepatotoxic, use caution with hepatic impairment; use is contraindicated in patients with advanced malignant hepatic tumors. Progressive hepatic coma leading to death has been reported (rare) in patients with extensive tumor burden, especially those with a baseline albumin <30 g/L. Use caution with renal impairment; dose adjustment may be required. Serum creatinine elevations, renal tubular acidosis, and renal failure have been reported with combination chemotherapy; decrease or withhold dose for unexplained elevations in BUN or serum creatinine or reductions in serum bicarbonate to <20 mEq/L. Patients with renal and hepatic impairment were excluded from clinical studies. Neutropenia, thrombocytopenia, and anemia are common; may cause therapy delays and/or dosage reductions. Not FDA approved for use in children.

Adverse Reactions

>10%:

Cardiovascular: Peripheral edema (7% to 19%), chest pain (16%), pallor (16%), pitting edema (15%)

Central nervous system: Fever (30% to 52%), fatigue (13% to 36%), headache (22%), dizziness (19%), anxiety (5% to 13%), depression (12%), insomnia (9% to 11%), malaise (11%), pain (11%)

Dermatologic: Bruising (19% to 31%), petechiae (11% to 24%), erythema (7% to 17%), skin lesion (15%), rash (10% to 14%), pruritus (12%)

Endocrine & metabolic: Hypokalemia (6% to 13%)

Gastrointestinal: Nausea (48% to 71%), vomiting (27% to 54%), diarrhea (36%), constipation (34% to 50%), anorexia (13% to 21%), weight loss (16%), abdominal pain (11% to 16%), abdominal tenderness (12%)

Hematologic: Thrombocytopenia (66% to 70%; grades 3/4: 58%), anemia (51% to 70%; grades 3/4: 14%), neutropenia (32% to 66%; grades 3/4: 61%), leukopenia (18% to 48%; grades 3/4: 15%), febrile neutropenia (14% to 16%; grades 3/4: 13%), myelosuppression (nadir: days 10-17; recovery: days 28-31)

Local: Injection site reactions (14% to 29%): Erythema (35% to 43%; more common with I.V. administration), pain (19% to 23%; more common with I.V. administration), bruising (5% to 14%)

Neuromuscular & skeletal: Weakness (29%), rigors (26%), arthralgia (22%), limb pain (20%), back pain (19%), myalgia (16%)

Respiratory: Cough (11% to 30%), dyspnea (5% to 29%), pharyngitis (20%), epistaxis (16%), nasopharyngitis (15%), upper respiratory tract infection (9% to 13%), pneumonia (11%), crackles (11%)

Miscellaneous: Diaphoresis (11%)

5% to 10%:

Cardiovascular: Cardiac murmur (10%), hypertension (≤9%), tachycardia (9%), hypotension (7%), syncope (6%), chest wall pain (5%)

Central nervous system: Lethargy (7% to 8%), hypoesthesia (5%), postprocedural pain (5%)

Dermatologic: Cellulitis (8%), urticaria (6%), dry skin (5%), skin nodule (5%)

Gastrointestinal: Gingival bleeding (10%), oral mucosal petechiae (8%), stomatitis (8%), weight loss (≤8%), dyspepsia (6% to 7%), hemorrhoids (7%), abdominal distension (6%), loose stools (6%), dysphagia (5%), oral hemorrhage (5%), tongue ulceration (5%)

Genitourinary: Dysuria (8%), urinary tract infection (8% to 9%)

Hematologic: Hematoma (9%), postprocedural hemorrhage (6%)

Local: Injection site reactions: Pruritus (7%), hematoma (6%), rash (6%), granuloma (5%), induration (5%), pigmentation change (5%), swelling (5%)

Neuromuscular & skeletal: Muscle cramps (6%)

Renal: Hematuria (≤6%)

Respiratory: Rhinorrhea (10%), rales (9%), wheezing (9%), breath sounds decreased (8%), pharyngolaryngeal pain (6%), pleural effusion (6%), postnasal drip (6%), rhinitis (6%), rhonchi (6%), nasal congestion (6%), atelectasis (5%), sinusitis (5%)

Miscellaneous: Lymphadenopathy (10%), herpes simplex (9%), night sweats (9%), transfusion reaction (7%), mouth hemorrhage (5%)

<5% (Limited to important or life-threatening): Abscess (limb, perirectal), acute febrile neutrophilic dermatosis (Sweet's syndrome), agranulocytosis, anaphylactic shock, atrial fibrillation, azotemia, blastomycosis, bone marrow depression/failure, bone pain aggravated, cardiac failure, cardiorespiratory arrest, catheter site hemorrhage, cellulitis, cerebral hemorrhage, CHF, cholecystectomy, cholecystitis, congestive cardiomyopathy, dehydration, diverticulitis, eye hemorrhage, fibrosis (interstitial and alveolar), gastrointestinal hemorrhage, glycosuria, hemoptysis, hepatic coma, hypersensitivity reaction, hypophosphatemia, infection (bacterial), injection site infection, injection site necrosis, interstitial lung disease, intracranial hemorrhage, leukemia cutis, lung infiltration, melena, neutropenic sepsis, orthostatic hypotension, pancytopenia, pneumonitis, polyuria, pyoderma gangrenosum, renal failure, renal tubular acidosis, seizure, respiratory distress, sepsis, septic shock, serum bicarbonate levels decreased, serum creatinine increased, splenomegaly, systemic inflammatory response syndrome, toxoplasmosis, tumor lysis syndrome

Drug Interactions

Metabolism/Transport Effects None known.

Avoid Concomitant Use

Avoid concomitant use of AzaCITIDine with any of the following: BCG; CloZAPine; Natalizumab; Pimecrolimus; Tacrolimus (Topical); Tofacitinib; Vaccines (Live)

Increased Effect/Toxicity

AzaCITIDine may increase the levels/effects of: CloZAPine; Leflunomide; Natalizumab; Tofacitinib; Vaccines (Live)

The levels/effects of AzaCITIDine may be increased by: Denosumab; Pimecrolimus; Roflumilast; Tacrolimus (Topical); Trastuzumab

Decreased Effect

AzaCITIDine may decrease the levels/effects of: BCG; Coccidioidin Skin Test; Sipuleucel-T; Vaccines (Inactivated); Vaccines (Live)

The levels/effects of AzaCITIDine may be decreased by: Echinacea

Preparation for Administration Hazardous agent; use appropriate precautions for handling and disposal (NIOSH, 2012).

SubQ: To prepare a 25 mg/mL suspension, slowly add 4 mL SWFI to each vial. Vigorously shake or roll vial until a suspension is formed (suspension will be cloudy).

I.V.: Reconstitute vial with 10 mL SWFI to form a 10 mg/mL solution; vigorously shake until solution is dissolved and clear. Mix in 50-100 mL of NS or lactated Ringer's injection for infusion.

Storage/Stability Prior to reconstitution, store powder at room temperature of 25°C (77°F); excursions permitted to 15°C to 30°C (59°F to 86°F).

SubQ: Following reconstitution, suspension may be stored at room temperature for up to 1 hour, or immediately refrigerated at 2°C to 8°C (36°F to 46°F) and stored for up to 8 hours.

I.V.: **Solutions for I.V. administration have very limited stability and must be prepared immediately prior to each dose.** Administration must be completed within 1 hour of (vial) reconstitution.

Mechanism of Action Antineoplastic effects may be a result of azacitidine's ability to promote hypomethylation of DNA leading to direct toxicity of abnormal hematopoietic cells in the bone marrow.

Pharmacodynamics/Kinetics

Absorption: SubQ: Rapid and complete

Distribution: V_d: I.V.: 76 ± 26 L; does not cross blood-brain barrier

Metabolism: Hepatic; hydrolysis to several metabolites

Bioavailability: SubQ: ~89%

Half-life elimination: I.V., SubQ: ~4 hours

Time to peak, plasma: SubQ: 30 minutes

Excretion: Urine (50% to 85%); feces (minor)

Dosage

Children: I.V.: Refractory AML (unlabeled use): 250 mg/m²/dose days 4 and 5 every 4 weeks (Steuber, 1996) **or** 300 mg/m²/dose days 4 and 5 every 4 weeks (Hurwitz, 1995)

Adults:

MDS: I.V., SubQ: 75 mg/m²/day for 7 days repeated every 4 weeks. Dose may be increased to 100 mg/m²/day if no benefit is observed after 2 cycles and no toxicity other than nausea and vomiting have occurred. Treatment is recommended for at least 4 cycles; treatment may be continued as long as patient continues to benefit.

Note: Alternate (unlabeled) schedules (which have produced hematologic response) have been used for convenience in community oncology centers (Lyons, 2009):

75 mg/m²/day for 5 days (Mon-Fri), 2 days rest (Sat, Sun), then 75 mg/m²/day for 2 days (Mon, Tues); repeat cycle every 28 days **or**

50 mg/m²/day for 5 days (Mon-Fri), 2 days rest (Sat, Sun), then 50 mg/m²/day for 5 days (Mon-Fri); repeat cycle every 28 days **or**

75 mg/m²/day for 5 days (Mon-Fri), repeat cycle every 28 days

AML (unlabeled use): SubQ: 75 mg/m²/day for 7 days repeated every 4 weeks (Sudan, 2006)

Elderly: Refer to adult dosing; due to the potential for decreased renal function in the elderly, select dose carefully and closely monitor renal function

Dosage adjustment based on hematology: Adults: MDS: I.V., SubQ:

For baseline WBC ≥3.0 x 10⁹/L, ANC ≥1.5 x 10⁹/L, and platelets ≥75 x 10⁹/L:

Nadir count: ANC <0.5 x 10⁹/L or platelets <25 x 10⁹/L: Administer 50% of dose during next treatment course

Nadir count: ANC 0.5-1.5 x 10^9/L or platelets 25-50 x 10^9/L: Administer 67% of dose during next treatment course

Nadir count: ANC >1.5 x 10^9/L or platelets >50 x 10^9/L: Administer 100% of dose during next treatment course

For baseline WBC <3 x 10^9/L, ANC <1.5 x 10^9/L, or platelets <75 x 10^9/L: Adjust dose as follows based on nadir counts and bone marrow biopsy cellularity at the time of nadir, unless clear improvement in differentiation at the time of the next cycle:

WBC or platelet nadir decreased 50% to 75% from baseline and bone marrow biopsy cellularity at time of nadir 30% to 60%: Administer 100% of dose during next treatment course

WBC or platelet nadir decreased 50% to 75% from baseline and bone marrow biopsy cellularity at time of nadir 15% to 30%: Administer 50% of dose during next treatment course

WBC or platelet nadir decreased 50% to 75% from baseline and bone marrow biopsy cellularity at time of nadir <15%: Administer 33% of dose during next treatment course

WBC or platelet nadir decreased >75% from baseline and bone marrow biopsy cellularity at time of nadir 30% to 60%: Administer 75% of dose during next treatment course

WBC or platelet nadir decreased >75% from baseline and bone marrow biopsy cellularity at time of nadir 15% to 30%: Administer 50% of dose during next treatment course

WBC or platelet nadir decreased >75% from baseline and bone marrow biopsy cellularity at time of nadir <15%: Administer 33% of dose during next treatment course

Note: If a nadir defined above occurs, administer the next treatment course 28 days after the start of the preceding course as long as WBC and platelet counts are >25% above the nadir and rising. If a >25% increase above the nadir is not seen by day 28, reassess counts every 7 days. If a 25% increase is not seen by day 42, administer 50% of the scheduled dose.

Dosage adjustment based on serum electrolytes: The manufacturer recommends that if serum bicarbonate falls to <20 mEq/L (unexplained decrease): Reduce dose by 50% for next treatment course

Dosage adjustment based on renal toxicity: If increases in BUN or serum creatinine (unexplained) occur, delay next cycle until values reach baseline or normal, then reduce dose by 50% for next treatment course.

Dosage adjustment in renal impairment: Not studied in patients with renal impairment; select dose carefully (excretion is primarily renal; consider dose reduction); monitor closely for toxicity

Dosage adjustment in hepatic impairment: Not studied in patients with hepatic impairment; use caution. Contraindicated in patients with advanced malignant hepatic tumors.

Dosing in obesity: *ASCO Guidelines for appropriate chemotherapy dosing in obese adults with cancer:* Utilize patient's actual body weight (full weight) for calculation of body surface area- or weight-based dosing, particularly when the intent of therapy is curative; manage regimen-related toxicities in the same manner as for nonobese patients; if a dose reduction is utilized due to toxicity, consider resumption of full weight-based dosing with subsequent cycles, especially if cause of toxicity (eg, hepatic or renal impairment) is resolved (Griggs, 2012).

Administration

SubQ: Premedication for nausea and vomiting is recommended. The manufacturer recommends equally dividing volumes >4 mL into 2 syringes and injecting into 2 separate sites; however, policies for maximum SubQ administration volume may vary by institution; interpatient variations may also apply. Administer subsequent injections at least 1 inch from previous injection sites. Allow refrigerated suspensions to come to room temperature (up to 30 minutes) prior to administration. Resuspend by inverting the syringe 2-3 times and then rolling the syringe between the palms for 30 seconds. If azacitidine suspension comes in contact with the skin, immediately wash with soap and water.

I.V.: Premedication for nausea and vomiting is recommended. Infuse over 10-40 minutes; infusion must be completed within 1 hour of (vial) reconstitution.

Hazardous agent; use appropriate precautions for handling and disposal (NIOSH, 2012).

Monitoring Parameters Liver function tests, electrolytes, CBC with differential and platelets, renal function tests (BUN and serum creatinine) should be obtained prior to initiation of therapy. Electrolytes, renal function (BUN and creatinine), CBC should be monitored prior to each cycle and periodically as needed to monitor response and toxicity.

Additional Information Oncology Comment: Azacitidine treatment for MDS is associated with an improvement in quality of life (including a reduction in transfusion requirements), a decrease in transformation to AML, and improved survival, when compared to best supportive care. Treatment should be continued for a minimum of 4-6 cycles (NCCN MDS guidelines v.2.2009).

Dosage Forms Excipient information presented when available (limited, particularly for generics); consult specific product labeling.

Suspension Reconstituted, Injection [preservative free]:
Vidaza: 100 mg (1 ea)
Generic: 100 mg (1 ea)

- **AZA-CR** *see* AzaCITIDine *on page 206*
- **Azactam** *see* Aztreonam *on page 218*
- **Azactam in Dextrose** *see* Aztreonam *on page 218*
- **Azacytidine** *see* AzaCITIDine *on page 206*
- **5-Azacytidine** *see* AzaCITIDine *on page 206*
- **5-Aza-dCyd** *see* Decitabine *on page 556*
- **Azaepothilone B** *see* Ixabepilone *on page 1139*
- **Azasan** *see* AzaTHIOprine *on page 208*
- **AzaSite** *see* Azithromycin (Ophthalmic) *on page 217*

AzaTHIOprine (ay za THYE oh preen)

Brand Names: U.S. Azasan; Imuran

Brand Names: Canada Apo-Azathioprine®; Imuran®; Mylan-Azathioprine; Teva-Azathioprine

Index Terms Azathioprine Sodium

Pharmacologic Category Immunosuppressant Agent

Use Adjunctive therapy in prevention of rejection of kidney transplants; management of active rheumatoid arthritis (RA)

Unlabeled Use Adjunct in prevention of rejection of solid organ (nonrenal) transplants; remission maintenance or reduction of steroid use in Crohn's disease (CD) and in ulcerative colitis (UC); dermatomyositis/polymyositis; erythema multiforme; pemphigus vulgaris, lupus nephritis (maintenance), chronic refractory immune thrombocytopenia (ITP), relapsed/remitting multiple sclerosis

Pregnancy Risk Factor D

Pregnancy Considerations Azathioprine was found to be teratogenic in animal studies; temporary depression in spermatogenesis and reduction in sperm viability and sperm count were also reported in mice. Azathioprine crosses the placenta in humans; congenital anomalies, immunosuppression, hematologic toxicities (lymphopenia, pancytopenia), and intrauterine growth retardation have been reported. There are no adequate and well-controlled studies in pregnant women. Azathioprine should not be used to treat rheumatoid arthritis during pregnancy. The potential benefit to the mother versus possible risk to the fetus should be considered when treating other disease states. Women of childbearing potential should avoid becoming pregnant during treatment.

The National Transplantation Pregnancy Registry (NTPR, Temple University) is a registry for pregnant women taking immunosuppressants following any solid organ transplant. The NTPR encourages reporting of all immunosuppressant exposures during pregnancy in transplant recipients at 877-955-6877.

Breast-Feeding Considerations Due to risk of immunosuppression and serious adverse effects in the nursing infant, breast-feeding is not recommended.

Contraindications Hypersensitivity to azathioprine or any component of the formulation; pregnancy (in patients with rheumatoid arthritis); patients with rheumatoid arthritis and a history of treatment with alkylating agents (eg, cyclophosphamide, chlorambucil, melphalan) may have a prohibitive risk of neoplasia with azathioprine treatment

Warnings/Precautions Hazardous agent - use appropriate precautions for handling and disposal (NIOSH, 2012).

[U.S. Boxed Warning]: Immunosuppressive agents, including azathioprine, are associated with the development of lymphoma and other malignancies, especially of the skin. Hepatosplenic T-Cell Lymphoma (HSTCL), a rare white blood cell cancer that is usually fatal, has predominantly occurred in adolescents and young adults treated for Crohn's disease or ulcerative colitis and receiving TNF blockers (eg, adalimumab, certolizumab pegol, etanercept, golimumab), azathioprine, and/or mercaptopurine. Most cases have occurred in patients treated with a combination of immunosuppressant agents, although there have been reports of HSTCL in patients receiving azathioprine or mercaptopurine monotherapy. Renal transplant patients are also at increased risk for malignancy (eg, skin cancer, lymphoma); limit sun and ultraviolet light exposure and use appropriate sun protection. Dose-related hematologic toxicities (leukopenia, thrombocytopenia, and anemias, including macrocytic anemia, or pancytopenia) may occur; delayed toxicities may also occur. May be more severe with renal transplants undergoing rejection; dosage modification for hematologic toxicity may be necessary. Chronic immunosuppression increases the risk of serious infections; may require dosage reduction. Use with caution in patients with liver disease or renal impairment; monitor hematologic function closely. Azathioprine is metabolized to mercaptopurine; concomitant use may result in profound myelosuppression and should be avoided. Patients with genetic deficiency of thiopurine methyltransferase (TPMT) or concurrent therapy with drugs which may inhibit TPMT may be sensitive to myelosuppressive effects. Patients with intermediate TPMT activity may be at risk for increased myelosuppression; those with low or absent TPMT activity are at risk for developing severe myelotoxicity. TPMT genotyping or phenotyping may assist in identifying patients at risk for developing toxicity. Consider TPMT testing in patients with abnormally low CBC unresponsive to dose reduction. TPMT testing does not substitute for CBC monitoring. Xanthine oxidase inhibitors may increase risk for hematologic toxicity; reduce azathioprine dose when used concurrently with allopurinol; patients with low or absent TPMT activity may require further dose reductions or discontinuation.

Hepatotoxicity (transaminase, bilirubin, and alkaline phosphatase elevations) may occur, usually in renal transplant patients and generally within 6 months of transplant; normally reversible with discontinuation; monitor liver function periodically. Rarely, hepatic sinusoidal obstruction syndrome (SOS; formerly called veno-occlusive disease) has been reported; discontinue if hepatic SOS is suspected. Severe nausea, vomiting, diarrhea, rash, fever, malaise, myalgia, hypotension, and liver enzyme abnormalities may occur within the first several weeks of treatment and are generally reversible upon discontinuation. **[U.S. Boxed Warning]: Should be prescribed by physicians familiar with the risks, including hematologic toxicities and mutagenic potential.** Immune response to vaccines may be diminished.

Adverse Reactions Frequency not always defined; dependent upon dose, duration, indication, and concomitant therapy.

Central nervous system: Fever, malaise

Gastrointestinal: Nausea/vomiting (RA 12%), diarrhea

Hematologic: Leukopenia (renal transplant >50%; RA 28%), thrombocytopenia

Hepatic: Alkaline phosphatase increased, bilirubin increased, hepatotoxicity, transaminases increased

Neuromuscular & skeletal: Myalgia

Miscellaneous: Infection (renal transplant 20%; RA <1%; includes bacterial, fungal, protozoal, viral), neoplasia (renal transplant 3% [other than lymphoma], 0.5% [lymphoma])

Postmarketing and/or case reports: Abdominal pain, alopecia, anemia, arthralgia, bleeding, bone marrow suppression, fever, hepatic sinusoidal obstruction syndrome (SOS; veno-occlusive disease), hepatosplenic T-cell lymphoma, hypersensitivity, hypotension, interstitial pneumonitis, lymphoma, macrocytic anemia, negative nitrogen balance, pancreatitis, pancytopenia, rash, skin cancer, steatorrhea, Sweet's syndrome (acute febrile neutrophilic dermatosis)

Drug Interactions

Metabolism/Transport Effects None known.

Avoid Concomitant Use

Avoid concomitant use of AzaTHIOprine with any of the following: BCG; Febuxostat; Mercaptopurine; Natalizumab; Pimecrolimus; Tacrolimus (Topical); Tofacitinib

Increased Effect/Toxicity

AzaTHIOprine may increase the levels/effects of: Leflunomide; Mercaptopurine; Natalizumab; Tofacitinib; Vaccines (Live)

The levels/effects of AzaTHIOprine may be increased by: 5-ASA Derivatives; ACE Inhibitors; Allopurinol; Denosumab; Febuxostat; Pimecrolimus; Ribavirin; Roflumilast; Sulfamethoxazole; Tacrolimus (Topical); Trastuzumab; Trimethoprim

Decreased Effect

AzaTHIOprine may decrease the levels/effects of: BCG; Coccidioidin Skin Test; Sipuleucel-T; Vaccines (Inactivated); Vitamin K Antagonists

The levels/effects of AzaTHIOprine may be decreased by: Echinacea

Ethanol/Nutrition/Herb Interactions Herb/Nutraceutical: Avoid cat's claw, echinacea (have immunostimulant properties).

Preparation for Administration Hazardous agent; use appropriate precautions for handling and disposal (NIOSH, 2012).

Powder for injection: Reconstitute each vial with 10 mL sterile water for injection; may further dilute for infusion (in D_5W, $\frac{1}{2}$NS, or NS).

Storage/Stability

Tablet: Store at room temperature of 15°C to 25°C (59°F to 77°F). Protect from light and moisture.

Powder for injection: Store intact vials at room temperature of 15°C to 25°C (59°F to 77°F). Protect from light. Reconstituted solution should be used within 24 hours; solutions diluted in D_5W, ½NS, or NS for infusion are stable at room temperature or refrigerated for up to 16 days (Johnson, 1981); however, the manufacturer recommends use within 24 hours of reconstitution.

Mechanism of Action Azathioprine is an imidazolyl derivative of mercaptopurine; antagonizes purine metabolism and may inhibit synthesis of DNA, RNA, and proteins; may also interfere with cellular metabolism and inhibit mitosis. The 6-thioguanine nucleotides appear to mediate the majority of azathioprine's immunosuppressive and toxic effects.

Pharmacodynamics/Kinetics

Absorption: Oral: Well absorbed

Distribution: Crosses placenta

Protein binding: ~30%

Metabolism: Hepatic, to 6-mercaptopurine, possibly by glutathione S-transferase (GST). Further metabolism of 6-mercaptopurine (in the liver and GI tract), via three major pathways: Hypoxanthine guanine phosphoribosyltransferase (to active metabolites: 6-thioguanine-nucleotides, or 6-TGNs), xanthine oxidase (to inactive metabolite: 6-thiouric acid), and thiopurine methyltransferase (TPMT) (to inactive metabolite: 6-methylmercaptopurine)

Half-life elimination: Parent drug: 12 minutes; mercaptopurine: 0.7-3 hours; End-stage renal disease: Slightly prolonged

Time to peak, plasma: Oral: 1-2 hours (including metabolites)

Excretion: Urine (primarily as metabolites)

Dosage Note: Patients with intermediate TPMT activity may be at risk for increased myelosuppression; those with low or absent TPMT activity receiving conventional azathioprine doses are at risk for developing severe, life-threatening myelotoxicity. Dosage reductions are recommended for patients with reduced TPMT activity.

I.V. dose is equivalent to oral dose (dosing should be transitioned from I.V. to oral as soon as tolerated): Adults:

Renal transplantation (treatment usually started the day of transplant, however, has been initiated [rarely] 1-3 days prior to transplant): Oral, I.V.: Initial: 3-5 mg/kg/day usually given as a single daily dose, then 1-3 mg/kg/day maintenance

Rheumatoid arthritis: Oral:

Initial: 1 mg/kg/day (50-100 mg) given once daily or divided twice daily for 6-8 weeks; may increase by 0.5 mg/kg every 4 weeks until response or up to 2.5 mg/kg/day; an adequate trial should be a minimum of 12 weeks

Maintenance dose: Reduce dose by 0.5 mg/kg (~25 mg daily) every 4 weeks until lowest effective dose is reached; optimum duration of therapy not specified; may be discontinued abruptly

Crohn's disease, remission maintenance or reduction of steroid use (unlabeled use): Oral: 2-3 mg/kg/day (Lichtenstein, 2009)

Dermatomyositis/polymyositis, adjunctive management (unlabeled use): Oral: 50 mg/day in conjunction with prednisone; increase by 50 mg/week to total dose of 2-3 mg/kg/day (Briemberg, 2003); **Note:** Onset of beneficial effects may take 3-6 months; however, may be preferred over methotrexate in patients with pulmonary or hepatic toxicity.

Immune thrombocytopenia (ITP), chronic refractory (unlabeled use): Oral: Maintenance: 100-200 mg/day (Boruchov, 2007)

Lupus nephritis, maintenance (unlabeled use): Oral: Initial: 2 mg/kg/day; may reduce to 1.5 mg/kg/day after 1 month (if proteinuria <1 g/day and serum creatinine stable) (Moroni, 2006) **or** target dose: 2 mg/kg/day (Hahn, 2012; Houssiau, 2010)

Ulcerative colitis, remission maintenance or reduction of steroid use (unlabeled use): Oral: 1.5-2.5 mg/kg/day (Kornbluth, 2010)

Dosage adjustment for concomitant use with allopurinol: Reduce azathioprine dose to one-third or one-fourth the usual dose when used concurrently with allopurinol. Patients with low or absent TPMT activity may require further dose reductions or discontinuation.

Dosage adjustment for toxicity:

Rapid WBC count decrease, persistently low WBC count, or serious infection: Reduce dose or temporarily withhold treatment

Severe toxicity in renal transplantation: May require discontinuation

Hepatic sinusoidal obstruction syndrome (SOS; veno-occlusive disease): Permanently discontinue

Dosage adjustment in renal impairment: No dosage adjustment provided in manufacturer's labeling; however, the following adjustments have been recommended (Aronoff, 2007):

Cl_{cr} >50 mL/minute: No adjustment recommended

Cl_{cr} 10-50 mL/minute: Administer 75% of normal dose

Cl_{cr} <10 mL/minute: Administer 50% of normal dose

Hemodialysis (dialyzable; ~45% removed in 8 hours): Administer 50% of normal dose; supplement: 0.25 mg/kg

CRRT: Administer 75% of normal dose

Dosage adjustment in hepatic impairment: No dosage adjustment provided in manufacturer's labeling.

Dietary Considerations May be taken with food.

Administration

I.V.: Azathioprine can be administered IVP over 5 minutes at a concentration not to exceed 10 mg/mL **or** diluted and given as an intermittent infusion usually over 30-60 minutes or as an extended infusion over up to 8 hours.

Oral: Administering tablets after meals or in divided doses may decrease adverse GI events.

Hazardous agent; use appropriate precautions for handling and disposal (NIOSH, 2012).

Monitoring Parameters CBC with differential and platelets (weekly during first month, twice monthly for months 2 and 3, then monthly; monitor more frequently with dosage modifications), total bilirubin, liver function tests, creatinine clearance, TPMT genotyping or phenotyping (consider TPMT testing in patients with abnormally low CBC unresponsive to dose reduction); monitor for symptoms of infection

For use as immunomodulatory therapy in CD or UC, monitor CBC with differential weekly for 1 month, then biweekly for 1 month, followed by monitoring every 1-2 months throughout the course of therapy; monitor more frequently if symptomatic. LFTs should be assessed every 3 months. Monitor for signs/symptoms of malignancy (eg, splenomegaly, hepatomegaly, abdominal pain, persistent fever, night sweats, weight loss).

Test Interactions TPMT phenotyping results will not be accurate following recent blood transfusions.

Dosage Forms Excipient information presented when available (limited, particularly for generics); consult specific product labeling.

Solution Reconstituted, Injection [preservative free]:

Generic: 100 mg (1 ea)

Tablet, Oral:

Azasan: 75 mg, 100 mg [scored]

Imuran: 50 mg [scored]

Generic: 50 mg

Extemporaneous Preparations Hazardous agent: Use appropriate precautions for handling and disposal.

A 50 mg/mL oral suspension may be prepared with tablets. Crush one-hundred-twenty 50 mg tablets in a mortar and reduce to a fine powder. Add 40 mL of either cherry syrup (diluted 1:4 with Simple Syrup, USP); a 1:1 mixture of Ora-Sweet® and Ora-Plus®; or a 1:1 mixture of Ora-Sweet® SF and Ora-Plus®, and mix to a uniform paste. Mix while adding the vehicle in incremental proportions to **almost** 120 mL; transfer to a calibrated bottle, rinse mortar with vehicle, and add quantity of vehicle sufficient to make 120 mL. Label "shake well", "refrigerate", and "protect from light". Stable for 60 days refrigerated.

Allen LV Jr and Erickson MA 3rd, "Stability of Acetazolamide, Allopurinol, Azathioprine, Clonazepam, and Flucytosine in Extemporaneously Compounded Oral Liquids," *Am J Health Syst Pharm*, 1996, 53(16):1944-9.

◆ **Azathioprine Sodium** *see* AzaTHIOprine *on page* 208

◆ **5-AZC** *see* AzaCITIDine *on page* 206

◆ **AZD6140** *see* Ticagrelor *on page* 2055

◆ **AZD6474** *see* Vandetanib *on page* 2162

Azelaic Acid (a zeh LAY ik AS id)

Brand Names: U.S. Azelex; Finacea

Brand Names: Canada Finacea®

Index Terms Anchoic Acid; Lepargylic Acid

Pharmacologic Category Topical Skin Product, Acne

Use

Azelex®: Treatment of mild-to-moderate inflammatory acne vulgaris

Finacea®: Treatment of inflammatory papules and pustules of mild-to-moderate rosacea

Pregnancy Risk Factor B

Dosage Topical:

Adolescents ≥12 years and Adults: Acne vulgaris: Cream 20%: Apply a thin film to the affected area(s) twice daily, in the morning and evening; may reduce to once daily if persistent skin irritation occurs. Improvement in condition is usually seen within 4 weeks.

Adults: Rosacea: Gel 15%: Apply a thin layer to the affected area(s) of the face twice daily, in the morning and evening; reassess if no improvement after 12 weeks of therapy.

Additional Information Complete prescribing information should be consulted for additional detail.

Dosage Forms Excipient information presented when available (limited, particularly for generics); consult specific product labeling.

Cream, External:

Azelex: 20% (30 g, 50 g)

Gel, External:

Finacea: 15% (50 g) [contains benzoic acid, disodium edta, polysorbate 80, propylene glycol]

Azelastine (Nasal) (a ZEL as teen)

Brand Names: U.S. Astelin; Astepro

Brand Names: Canada Astelin

Index Terms Azelastine Hydrochloride

Pharmacologic Category Histamine H_1 Antagonist; Histamine H_1 Antagonist, Second Generation

Use Treatment of the symptoms of seasonal or perennial allergic rhinitis such as rhinorrhea, sneezing, and nasal pruritus; treatment of the symptoms of vasomotor rhinitis

Pregnancy Risk Factor C

Dosage

Perennial allergic rhinitis: Intranasal (Astepro):

Children 6 to <12 years: One spray in each nostril twice daily

Children ≥12 years, Adolescents, and Adults: Two sprays in each nostril twice daily

Seasonal allergic rhinitis: Intranasal:

Children 5 to <12 years (Astelin): One spray in each nostril twice daily

Children 6 to <12 years (Astepro): One spray in each nostril twice daily

Children ≥12 years, Adolescents, and Adults (Astelin, Astepro): 1-2 sprays in each nostril twice daily; alternatively, Astepro (azelastine 0.15%) may be administered as 2 sprays in each nostril once daily

Vasomotor rhinitis: Intranasal: Children ≥12 years, Adolescents, and Adults (Astelin): Two sprays in each nostril twice daily

Dosage adjustment in renal impairment: No dosage adjustment provided in manufacturer's labeling.

Dosage adjustment in hepatic impairment: No dosage adjustment necessary.

Additional Information Complete prescribing information should be consulted for additional detail.

Dosage Forms Considerations

Astelin and Astepro 30 mL bottles contain 200 sprays each.

Dosage Forms Excipient information presented when available (limited, particularly for generics); consult specific product labeling.

Solution, Nasal, as hydrochloride:

Astelin: 137 mcg/spray (30 mL) [contains benzalkonium chloride, edetate disodium]

Astepro: 0.15% (30 mL) [contains benzalkonium chloride, edetate disodium]

Generic: 137 mcg/spray (30 mL)

Azelastine (Ophthalmic) (a ZEL as teen)

Brand Names: U.S. Optivar

Index Terms Azelastine Hydrochloride

Pharmacologic Category Histamine H_1 Antagonist; Histamine H_1 Antagonist, Second Generation

Use Treatment of itching of the eye associated with seasonal allergic conjunctivitis

Pregnancy Risk Factor C

Dosage Ophthalmic: Children ≥3 years and Adults: Instill 1 drop into affected eye(s) twice daily.

Dosage adjustment in renal impairment: No dosage adjustment provided in manufacturer's labeling.

Dosage adjustment in hepatic impairment: No dosage adjustment provided in manufacturer's labeling.

Additional Information Complete prescribing information should be consulted for additional detail.

Dosage Forms Excipient information presented when available (limited, particularly for generics); consult specific product labeling.

Solution, Ophthalmic, as hydrochloride:

Optivar: 0.05% (6 mL) [contains benzalkonium chloride]

Generic: 0.05% (6 mL)

Azelastine and Fluticasone

(a ZEL as teen & floo TIK a sone)

Brand Names: U.S. Dymista™

Index Terms Fluticasone Propionate and Azelastine Hydrochloride

Pharmacologic Category Corticosteroid, Nasal; Histamine H_1 Antagonist, Second Generation

Use Symptomatic relief of seasonal allergic rhinitis

Pregnancy Risk Factor C

Dosage Intranasal: Seasonal allergic rhinitis: Children ≥12 years and Adults: 1 spray (137 mcg azelastine/50 mcg fluticasone) per nostril twice daily

Dosage adjustment in renal impairment: No dosage adjustment provided in manufacturer's labeling.

Dosage adjustment in hepatic impairment: No dosage adjustment necessary.

Additional Information Complete prescribing information should be consulted for additional detail.

Dosage Forms Excipient information presented when available (limited, particularly for generics); consult specific product labeling.

Suspension, intranasal [spray]:

Dymista™: Azelastine hydrochloride 0.1% [137 mcg/spray] and fluticasone propionate 0.037% [50 mcg/spray] (23 g) [contains benzalkonium chloride; 120 metered sprays]

◆ Azelastine Hydrochloride *see* Azelastine (Nasal) *on page 211*

◆ Azelastine Hydrochloride *see* Azelastine (Ophthalmic) *on page 211*

◆ Azelex *see* Azelaic Acid *on page 211*

◆ Azidothymidine *see* Zidovudine *on page 2226*

◆ Azidothymidine, Abacavir, and Lamivudine *see* Abacavir, Lamivudine, and Zidovudine *on page 20*

◆ Azilect *see* Rasagiline *on page 1786*

◆ Azilect® (Can) *see* Rasagiline *on page 1786*

Azilsartan (ay zil SAR tan)

Brand Names: U.S. Edarbi

Brand Names: Canada Edarbi™

Index Terms Azilsartan Medoxomil; AZL-M

Pharmacologic Category Angiotensin II Receptor Blocker; Antihypertensive

Additional Appendix Information

Angiotensin Agents *on page 2280*

Use Treatment of hypertension; may be used alone or in combination with other antihypertensives

Pregnancy Risk Factor D

Pregnancy Considerations [U.S. Boxed Warning]: Drugs that act on the renin-angiotensin system can cause injury and death to the developing fetus. Discontinue as soon as possible once pregnancy is detected. The use of drugs which act on the renin-angiotensin system are associated with oligohydramnios. Oligohydramnios, due to decreased fetal renal function, may lead to fetal lung hypoplasia and skeletal malformations. Use is also associated with anuria, hypotension, renal failure, skull hypoplasia, and death in the fetus/neonate. The exposed fetus should be monitored for fetal growth, amniotic fluid volume, and organ formation. Infants exposed *in utero* should be monitored for hyperkalemia, hypotension, and oliguria.

Untreated chronic maternal hypertension is also associated with adverse events in the fetus, infant, and mother. If treatment for hypertension during pregnancy is needed, other agents are preferred (ACOG, 2012; Chobanian, 2003). In women of reproductive potential, angiotensin II receptor blockers should be discontinued prior to conception or as soon as pregnancy is confirmed (Chobanian, 2003).

Breast-Feeding Considerations It is not known if azilsartan is excreted into breast milk. Due to the potential for serious adverse reactions in the nursing infant, the manufacturer recommends a decision be made whether to discontinue nursing or to discontinue the drug, taking into account the importance of treatment to the mother. Breast-fed infants of mothers taking medications for hypertension should be monitored for adverse effects (Chobanian, 2003).

Contraindications

U.S. labeling: Concomitant use with aliskiren in patients with diabetes mellitus

Canadian labeling: Hypersensitivity to azilsartan medoxomil or any component of the formulation; concomitant use with aliskiren in patients with diabetes or moderate-to-severe renal impairment (GFR <60 mL/minute/1.73 m^2).

Warnings/Precautions [U.S. Boxed Warning]: Drugs that act on the renin-angiotensin system can cause injury and death to the developing fetus. Discontinue as soon as possible once pregnancy is detected. Angiotensin II receptor blockers may cause hyperkalemia; avoid potassium supplementation unless specifically required by healthcare provider. Avoid use or use a smaller dose in patients who are volume depleted; correct depletion first. May be associated with deterioration of renal function and/or increases in serum creatinine, particularly in patients with low renal blood flow (eg, renal artery stenosis, heart failure, volume depletion) whose glomerular filtration rate (GFR) is dependent on efferent arteriolar vasoconstriction by angiotensin II. Use with caution in unstented unilateral/bilateral renal artery stenosis. When unstented bilateral renal artery stenosis is present, use is generally avoided due to the elevated risk of deterioration in renal function unless possible benefits outweigh risks. Use with caution in pre-existing renal insufficiency; significant aortic/mitral stenosis. Potentially significant drug-drug interactions may exist, requiring dose or frequency adjustment, additional monitoring, and/or selection of alternative therapy.

Angioedema has been reported rarely with some angiotensin II receptor antagonists (ARBs) and may occur at any time during treatment (especially following first dose). It may involve the head and neck (potentially compromising airway) or the intestine (presenting with abdominal pain). Patients with idiopathic or hereditary angioedema or previous angioedema associated with ACE-inhibitor therapy may be at an increased risk. Prolonged frequent monitoring may be required, especially if tongue, glottis, or larynx are involved, as they are associated with airway obstruction. Patients with a history of airway surgery may have a higher risk of airway obstruction. Discontinue therapy immediately if angioedema occurs. Aggressive early management is critical. Intramuscular (I.M.) administration of epinephrine may be necessary. Do not readminister to patients who have had angioedema with ARBs.

Adverse Reactions

Cardiovascular: Hypotension, orthostatic hypotension

Central nervous system: Dizziness, fatigue

Gastrointestinal: Diarrhea (2%), nausea

Hematologic: Hemoglobin decreased, hematocrit decreased, leukopenia (rare), RBC decreased, thrombocytopenia (rare)

Neuromuscular & skeletal: Muscle spasm, weakness

Renal: Serum creatinine increased

Respiratory: Cough

Drug Interactions

Metabolism/Transport Effects Substrate of CYP2C9 (minor); **Note:** Assignment of Major/Minor substrate status based on clinically relevant drug interaction potential

Avoid Concomitant Use There are no known interactions where it is recommended to avoid concomitant use.

Increased Effect/Toxicity

Azilsartan may increase the levels/effects of: ACE Inhibitors; Amifostine; Antihypertensives; CycloSPORINE (Systemic); Hypotensive Agents; Lithium; Nonsteroidal Anti-Inflammatory Agents; Obinutuzumab; Potassium-Sparing Diuretics; RiTUXimab; Sodium Phosphates

The levels/effects of Azilsartan may be increased by: Alfuzosin; Aliskiren; Brimonidine (Topical); Canagliflozin; Diazoxide; Eplerenone; Heparin; Heparin (Low Molecular

Weight); Herbs (Hypotensive Properties); MAO Inhibitors; Pentoxifylline; Phosphodiesterase 5 Inhibitors; Potassium Salts; Prostacyclin Analogues; Tolvaptan; Trimethoprim

Decreased Effect

The levels/effects of Azilsartan may be decreased by: Herbs (Hypertensive Properties); Methylphenidate; Nonsteroidal Anti-Inflammatory Agents; Rifamycin Derivatives; Yohimbine

Ethanol/Nutrition/Herb Interactions Herb/Nutraceutical: Avoid ephedra, yohimbe, ginseng (may worsen hypertension). Avoid garlic (may have increased antihypertensive effect).

Storage/Stability Store at 25°C (77°F); excursions permitted to 15°C to 30°C (59°F to 86°F). Protect from moisture and light. Dispense and store in original container.

Mechanism of Action Angiotensin II (which is formed by enzymatic conversion from angiotensin I) is the primary pressor agent of the renin-angiotensin system. Effects of angiotensin II include vasoconstriction, stimulation of aldosterone synthesis/release, cardiac stimulation, and renal sodium reabsorption. Azilsartan inhibits angiotensin II's vasoconstrictor and aldosterone-secreting effects by selectively blocking the binding of angiotensin II to the AT_1 receptor in vascular smooth muscle and adrenal gland tissues (azilsartan has a stronger affinity for the AT_1 receptor than the AT_2 receptor). The action is independent of the angiotensin II synthesis pathways. Azilsartan does not inhibit ACE (kininase II), therefore it does not affect the response to bradykinin (the clinical relevance of this is unknown) and does not bind to or inhibit other receptors or ion channels of importance in cardiovascular regulation.

Pharmacodynamics/Kinetics

Distribution: V_d: ~16 L

Protein binding: >99%; primarily to serum albumin

Metabolism: Gut: prodrug hydrolyzed to active metabolite; Hepatic: primarily via CYP2C9 to inactive metabolites

Bioavailability: ~60%

Half-life elimination: ~11 hours

Time to peak, serum: 1.5-3 hours

Excretion: Feces (~55%); urine (~42%, 15% as unchanged drug)

Clearance: 2.3 mL/minute

Dosage Oral: Adults:

U.S. labeling: 80 mg once daily; consider initial dose of 40 mg once daily in patients with volume depletion (eg, patients receiving high-dose diuretics)

Canadian labeling: Initial: 40 mg once daily; may increase to 80 mg once daily if necessary

Dosage adjustment in renal impairment:

U.S. labeling: No dosage adjustment necessary; however, carefully monitor the patient.

Canadian labeling:

Mild-to-moderate impairment: No dosage adjustment is necessary; however, carefully monitor the patient.

Severe impairment or end stage renal disease (ESRD): No dosage adjustment provided in manufacturer's labeling (has not been studied). Use with caution.

Dosage adjustment in hepatic impairment:

U.S. labeling:

Mild-to-moderate impairment: No dosage adjustment necessary; however, carefully monitor the patient.

Severe impairment: No dosage adjustment provided in manufacturer's labeling (has not been studied).

Canadian labeling:

Mild-to-moderate moderate impairment: There is no specific dosage adjustment provided in manufacturer's labeling; however, a reduced initial dose is recommended. Do not exceed daily dose of 80 mg.

Severe impairment: Use is not recommended.

Dietary Considerations May be taken with or without food.

Administration Administer without regard to food.

Monitoring Parameters Electrolytes, serum creatinine, BUN; blood pressure

Dosage Forms Excipient information presented when available (limited, particularly for generics); consult specific product labeling.

Tablet, Oral, as medoxomil:

Edarbi: 40 mg, 80 mg

Azilsartan and Chlorthalidone

(ay zil SAR tan & klor THAL i done)

Brand Names: U.S. Edarbyclor

Brand Names: Canada Edarbyclor™

Index Terms Azilsartan Medoxomil and Chlorthalidone; Chlorthalidone and Azilsartan

Pharmacologic Category Angiotensin II Receptor Blocker; Antihypertensive; Diuretic, Thiazide

Use Treatment of hypertension

Pregnancy Risk Factor D

Dosage Dose is individualized; combination product may be substituted for individual components in patients currently maintained on both agents separately or in patients not adequately controlled with monotherapy (using one of the agents or an agent within the same antihypertensive class). May also be used as initial therapy in patients who are likely to need >1 antihypertensive to control blood pressure.

Oral: Adults: Hypertension: *Initial therapy:* Azilsartan 40 mg/chlorthalidone 12.5 mg once daily; dose may be increased after 2-4 weeks of therapy to azilsartan 40 mg/chlorthalidone 25 mg once daily. Maximum recommended dose: Azilsartan 40 mg/day; chlorthalidone 25 mg/day

Dosage adjustment in renal impairment:

Mild-to-moderate renal impairment (eGFR 30-90 mL/minute/1.73 m^2): No dosage adjustment necessary.

Severe renal impairment (eGFR <30 mL/minute/1.73 m^2): No dosage adjustment provided in manufacturer's labeling (has not been studied); use with caution.

Dosage adjustment in hepatic impairment:

U.S. labeling:

Mild-to-moderate hepatic impairment: No initial dosage adjustment necessary; monitor patient carefully.

Severe hepatic impairment: No dosage adjustment provided in manufacturer's labeling (has not been studied); use with caution.

Canadian labeling:

Mild-to-moderate hepatic impairment: Initial dosage reduction is recommended although specific adjustments are not provided in the manufacturer labeling; monitor patient carefully.

Severe hepatic impairment: Use is not recommended (has not been studied).

Additional Information Complete prescribing information should be consulted for additional detail.

Dosage Forms Excipient information presented when available (limited, particularly for generics); consult specific product labeling.

Tablet, Oral:

Edarbyclor: 40/25: Azilsartan medoxomil 40 mg and chlorthalidone 25 mg, 40/12.5: Azilsartan medoxomil 40 mg and chlorthalidone 12.5 mg

◆ **Azilsartan Medoxomil** *see* Azilsartan *on page 212*

◆ **Azilsartan Medoxomil and Chlorthalidone** *see* Azilsartan and Chlorthalidone *on page 213*

Azithromycin (Systemic) (az ith roe MYE sin)

Brand Names: U.S. Zithromax; Zithromax Tri-Pak; Zithromax Z-Pak; Zmax

Brand Names: Canada Apo-Azithromycin®; Ava-Azithromycin; Azithromycin for Injection; CO Azithromycin; Dom-Azithromycin; GD-Azithromycin; Mylan-Azithromycin; Novo-Azithromycin; PHL-Azithromycin; PMS-Azithromycin; PRO-Azithromycin; ratio-Azithromycin; Riva-Azithromycin; Sandoz-Azithromycin; Zithromax®; Zithromax® For Intravenous Injection; Zmax SR™

Index Terms Azithromycin Dihydrate; Azithromycin Monohydrate; Z-Pak; Zithromax TRI-PAK™; Zithromax Z-PAK®

Pharmacologic Category Antibiotic, Macrolide

Additional Appendix Information

Prevention of Infective Endocarditis *on page 2353*

Use Oral, I.V.: Treatment of acute otitis media due to *H. influenzae, M. catarrhalis*, or *S. pneumoniae*; pharyngitis/tonsillitis due to *S. pyogenes*, community-acquired pneumonia due to *Chlamydia pneumonia, H. influenzae, M. pneumoniae*, or *S. pneumoniae*; pelvic inflammatory disease (PID) due to *C. trachomatis, N. gonorrhoeae*, or *M. hominis*; genital ulcer disease (in men) due to *H. ducreyi* (chancroid); acute bacterial exacerbations of chronic obstructive pulmonary disease (COPD) due to *H. influenzae, M. catarrhalis*, or *S. pneumoniae*; acute bacterial sinusitis due to *H. influenzae, M. catarrhalis*, or *S. pneumoniae*; prevention of *Mycobacterium avium* complex (MAC) (alone or in combination with rifabutin) in patients with advanced HIV infection; treatment of disseminated MAC (in combination with ethambutol) in patients with advanced HIV infection; skin and skin structure infections (uncomplicated) due to *S. aureus, S. pyogenes*, or *S. agalactiae*; urethritis and cervicitis due to *C. trachomatis* or *N. gonorrhoeae*

Unlabeled Use Treatment of babesiosis; cat scratch disease; gonococcal infections of the pharynx or rectum (combination therapy) and expedited partner therapy; granuloma inguinale (donovanosis); *Mycoplasma genitalium* infections; pertussis; prophylaxis of infective endocarditis in select patients who are allergic to penicillin and undergoing dental procedures; prevention of pulmonary exacerbations in patients with noncystic fibrosis bronchiectasis; treatment of *Shigella dysenteriae* type 1

Pregnancy Risk Factor B

Pregnancy Considerations Adverse events were not observed in animal reproduction studies. Azithromycin crosses the placenta. Fetal malformations have not been observed following maternal use of azithromycin. The maternal serum half-life of azithromycin is unchanged in early pregnancy and decreased at term; however, high concentrations of azithromycin are sustained in the myometrium and adipose tissue. Azithromycin is recommended for the treatment of several infections, including chlamydia, gonococcal infections, and *Mycobacterium avium* complex (MAC) in pregnant patients (consult current guidelines).

Breast-Feeding Considerations Azithromycin is excreted in low amounts into breast milk. The manufacturer recommends that caution be exercised when administering azithromycin to breast-feeding women. Nondose-related effects could include modification of bowel flora.

Contraindications Hypersensitivity to azithromycin, other macrolide (eg, azalide or ketolide) antibiotics, or any component of the formulation; history of cholestatic jaundice/hepatic dysfunction associated with prior azithromycin use

Note: The manufacturer does not list concurrent use of pimozide as a contraindication; however, azithromycin is listed as a contraindication in the manufacturer's labeling for pimozide.

Warnings/Precautions Use with caution in patients with pre-existing liver disease; hepatocellular and/or cholestatic hepatitis, with or without jaundice, hepatic necrosis, failure and death have occurred. Discontinue immediately if symptoms of hepatitis occur (malaise, nausea, vomiting, abdominal colic, fever). Allergic reactions have been reported (rare); reappearance of allergic reaction may occur shortly after discontinuation without further azithromycin exposure. May mask or delay symptoms of incubating gonorrhea or syphilis, so appropriate culture and susceptibility tests should be performed prior to initiating a treatment regimen. Prolonged use may result in fungal or bacterial superinfection, including *C. difficile*-associated diarrhea (CDAD); CDAD has been observed >2 months postantibiotic treatment. Use caution with renal dysfunction. Macrolides (especially erythromycin) have been associated with rare QT_c prolongation and ventricular arrhythmias, including torsade de pointes; consider avoiding use in patients with prolonged QT interval, congenital long QT syndrome, history of torsade de pointes, bradyarrhythmias, uncorrected hypokalemia or hypomagnesemia, clinically significant bradycardia, uncompensated heart failure, or concurrent use of Class IA (eg, quinidine, procainamide) or Class III (eg, amiodarone, dofetilide, sotalol) antiarrhythmic agents or other drugs known to prolong the QT interval. A recent retrospective cohort study (under FDA review) demonstrated an increased cardiac risk with azithromycin relative to amoxicillin or ciprofloxacin, and similar risk compared to levofloxacin; notably, increased cardiac mortality (an estimated 47 additional deaths per 1 million 5-day courses of treatment compared to amoxicillin) was associated with higher baseline cardiovascular risk (Ray, 2012). Use with caution in patients with myasthenia gravis.

Oral suspensions (immediate release and extended release) are not interchangeable.

Adverse Reactions

>10%: Gastrointestinal: Diarrhea (4% to 9%; high single-dose regimens 12% to 14%), nausea (≤7%; high single-dose regimens 18%)

2% to 10%:

Dermatologic: Pruritus, rash

Gastrointestinal: Abdominal pain, anorexia, cramping, vomiting (especially with high single-dose regimens)

Genitourinary: Vaginitis

Local: (with I.V. administration): Injection site pain, inflammation

≤1% (Limited to important or life-threatening): Acute renal failure, aggressive behavior agitation, allergic reaction, anaphylaxis, anemia, angioedema, anxiety, arrhythmia (including ventricular tachycardia), arthralgia, bronchospasm, candidiasis, chest pain, cholestatic jaundice, conjunctivitis (pediatric patients), constipation, cough increased, deafness, dehydration, dermatitis (fungal), diaphoresis, dizziness, dyspepsia, eczema, edema, enteritis, erythema multiforme (rare), facial edema, fatigue fever, flatulence, fungal infection, gastritis, headache, hearing disturbance, hearing loss, hepatic failure, hepatic necrosis, hepatitis, hyperactivity, hyperkinesia, hypotension, insomnia, interstitial nephritis, jaundice, leukopenia, LFTs increased, loss of smell, loss of taste, malaise, melena, mucositis, nephritis, nervousness, neutropenia (mild), oral candidiasis, oral moniliasis, pain, palpitation, pancreatitis, paresthesia, pharyngitis, photosensitivity, pleural effusion, pseudomembranous colitis, pyloric stenosis, QT_c prolongation (rare), rhinitis, seizure, smell perversion, somnolence, somnolence, Stevens-Johnson syndrome (rare), syncope, taste perversion, thrombocytopenia, tinnitus, tongue discoloration (rare), torsade de pointes (rare), toxic epidermal necrolysis (rare), urticaria, vertigo, vesiculobullous rash, weakness

Drug Interactions

Metabolism/Transport Effects Substrate of CYP3A4 (minor); **Note:** Assignment of Major/Minor substrate status based on clinically relevant drug interaction potential; **Inhibits** CYP1A2 (weak), P-glycoprotein

Avoid Concomitant Use

Avoid concomitant use of Azithromycin (Systemic) with any of the following: Amiodarone; BCG; Highest Risk QTc-Prolonging Agents; Ivabradine; Mifepristone; Pimozide; QuiNINE; Terfenadine

Increased Effect/Toxicity

Azithromycin (Systemic) may increase the levels/effects of: Amiodarone; AtorvaSTATin; Cardiac Glycosides; CycloSPORINE (Systemic); Highest Risk QTc-Prolonging Agents; Ivermectin (Systemic); Lovastatin; Moderate Risk QTc-Prolonging Agents; Pimozide; QuiNINE; Rilpivirine; Rivaroxaban; Simvastatin; Tacrolimus (Systemic); Tacrolimus (Topical); Terfenadine; Vitamin K Antagonists

The levels/effects of Azithromycin (Systemic) may be increased by: Ivabradine; Mifepristone; Nelfinavir; QTc-Prolonging Agents (Indeterminate Risk and Risk Modifying)

Decreased Effect

Azithromycin (Systemic) may decrease the levels/effects of: BCG; Sodium Picosulfate; Typhoid Vaccine

Ethanol/Nutrition/Herb Interactions Food: Rate and extent of GI absorption may be altered depending upon the formulation. Azithromycin suspension, not tablet form, has significantly increased absorption (46%) with food.

Preparation for Administration Injection (Zithromax®): Prepare initiation solution by adding 4.8 mL of sterile water for injection to the 500 mg vial (resulting concentration: 100 mg/mL). Use of a standard syringe is recommended due to the vacuum in the vial (which may draw additional solution through an automated syringe).

The initial solution should be further diluted to a concentration of 1 mg/mL (500 mL) to 2 mg/mL (250 mL) in 0.9% sodium chloride, 5% dextrose in water, or lactated Ringer's. The diluted solution is stable for 24 hours at or below room temperature (30°C or 86°F) and for 7 days if stored under refrigeration (5°C or 41°F).

Storage/Stability

Injection (Zithromax®): Store intact vials of injection at room temperature. Reconstituted solution is stable for 24 hours when stored below 30°C (86°F).

Suspension, immediate release (Zithromax®): Store dry powder below 30°C (86°F). Following reconstitution, store at 5°C to 30°C (41°F to 86°F).

Suspension, extended release (Zmax®): Store dry powder ≤30°C (86°F). Following reconstitution, store at 25°C (77°F); excursions permitted to 15°C to 30°C (59°F to 86°F); do not refrigerate or freeze. Should be consumed within 12 hours following reconstitution.

Tablet (Zithromax®): Store between 15°C to 30°C (59°F to 86°F).

Mechanism of Action Inhibits RNA-dependent protein synthesis at the chain elongation step; binds to the 50S ribosomal subunit resulting in blockage of transpeptidation

Pharmacodynamics/Kinetics

Absorption: Oral: Rapid

Distribution: Extensive tissue; distributes well into skin, lungs, sputum, tonsils, and cervix; penetration into CSF is poor; V_d: 31-33 L/kg

Protein binding (concentration dependent): Oral, I.V.: 7% to 51%

Metabolism: Hepatic

Bioavailability: Oral: 38%, decreased by 17% with extended release suspension; variable effect with food (increased with immediate or delayed release oral suspension, unchanged with tablet)

Half-life elimination: Oral, I.V.: Terminal: Immediate release: 68-72 hours; Extended release: 59 hours

Time to peak, serum: Oral: Immediate release: 2-3 hours; Extended release: 5 hours

Excretion: Oral, I.V.: Biliary (major route); urine (6%)

Dosage Note: Extended release suspension (Zmax®) is not interchangeable with immediate release formulations. Use should be limited to approved indications. All doses are expressed as immediate release azithromycin unless otherwise specified.

Usual dosage range:

Children ≥6 months: Oral: 5-12 mg/kg given once daily (maximum: 500 mg daily) **or** 30 mg/kg as a single dose (maximum: 1500 mg)

Extended release suspension (Zmax®): 60 mg/kg as a single dose; **Note:** Extended release suspension (Zmax®): Dose in mL is equal to the weight in lbs for patients <75 lbs (34 kg). Pediatric patients ≥75 lbs should receive the adult dose.

Adolescents ≥16 years and Adults:

Oral: 250-600 mg once daily **or** 1-2 g as a single dose

Extended release suspension (Zmax®): 2 g as a single dose

I.V.: 250-500 mg once daily

Indication-specific dosing:

Children:

Bacterial sinusitis: Oral: 10 mg/kg once daily for 3 days (maximum: 500 mg daily)

Cat scratch disease (unlabeled use; Bass, 1998; Stevens, 2005): Oral:

<45.5 kg: 10 mg/kg as a single dose, then 5 mg/kg once daily for 4 additional days

>45.5 kg: 500 mg as a single dose, then 250 mg once daily for 4 additional days

Community-acquired pneumonia (CAP) (IDSA/PIDS, 2011): Infants >3 months and Children: **Note:** A beta-lactam antibiotic should be added if typical bacterial pneumonia cannot be ruled out

Presumed mild infection or step-down therapy, atypical (*M. pneumoniae, C. pneumoniae, C. trachomatis*) (preferred): Oral: 10 mg/kg (maximum dose: 500 mg) as a single dose on the first day, followed by 5 mg/kg/day (maximum dose: 250 mg) on days 2 through 5.

Presumed moderate-to-severe infection, atypical (*M. pneumoniae, C. pneumoniae, C. trachomatis*): I.V.: 10 mg/kg/day on days 1 and 2, then switch to oral azithromycin therapy if possible to finish the 5-day course

Alternative regimens for community-acquired pneumonia: Oral: 10 mg/kg (maximum dose: 500 mg) once daily for 3 days (Kogan, 2003)

Extended release suspension (Zmax®):

<75 lbs (34 kg): 60 mg/kg as a single dose

≥75 lbs (34 kg): Refer to adult dosing

Disseminated *M. avium* complex disease in patients with advanced HIV infection (unlabeled use; CDC, 2009):

Treatment: 10-12 mg/kg/day (maximum: 500 mg) in combination with ethambutol; patients with severe disease should also receive rifabutin

Primary prophylaxis: 20 mg/kg (maximum: 1200 mg) once weekly (preferred) or alternatively, 5 mg/kg/day once daily (maximum: 250 mg daily)

Secondary prophylaxis: 5 mg/kg/day once daily (maximum: 250 mg daily) in combination with ethambutol, with or without rifabutin

Otitis media: Oral:

1-day regimen: 30 mg/kg as a single dose (maximum: 1500 mg)

3-day regimen: 10 mg/kg once daily for 3 days (maximum: 500 mg daily)

5-day regimen: 10 mg/kg on day 1 (maximum: 500 mg daily) followed by 5 mg/kg/day once daily on days 2-5 (maximum: 250 mg daily)

Pertussis (unlabeled use; CDC, 2005):

Children <6 months: 10 mg/kg/day for 5 days

Children ≥6 months: 10 mg/kg on day 1 (maximum: 500 mg daily) followed by 5 mg/kg/day once daily on days 2-5 (maximum: 250 mg daily)

Pharyngitis (including susceptible group A streptococci), tonsillitis (IDSA guidelines): Children ≥2 years: Oral: 12 mg/kg/day once daily for 5 days (maximum: 500 mg daily). **Note:** Recommended by the Infectious Disease Society of America (IDSA) as an alternative agent for group A streptococcal pharyngitis in penicillin-allergic patients (Shulman, 2012)

Prophylaxis against infective endocarditis (unlabeled use): 15 mg/kg 30-60 minutes before procedure (maximum: 500 mg). **Note:** American Heart Association (AHA) guidelines now recommend prophylaxis only in patients undergoing invasive procedures and in whom underlying cardiac conditions may predispose to a higher risk of adverse outcomes should infection occur. As of April 2007, routine prophylaxis for GI/GU procedures is no longer recommended by the AHA.

Shigella dysentery type 1 (unlabeled use): Oral: 6-20 mg/kg/day for 1-5 days (WHO, 2005)

Uncomplicated chlamydial urethritis or cervicitis (unlabeled use): Children ≥45 kg: 1 g as a single dose (CDC, 2010)

Adolescents ≥16 years and Adults:

Babesiosis (unlabeled use): Oral: 500-1000 mg on day 1, followed by 250 mg once daily for 7-10 days with atovaquone; higher doses may be required in immunocompromised patients (600-1000 mg daily). **Note:** Relapsing infection may require at least 6 weeks of therapy (Vannier, 2012; Wormser, 2006).

Bacterial sinusitis: Oral: 500 mg daily for a total of 3 days

Extended release suspension (Zmax®): 2 g as a single dose

Cat scratch disease (unlabeled use): Oral: >45.5 kg: 500 mg as a single dose, then 250 mg once daily for 4 additional days (Bass, 1998; Stevens, 2005)

Chancroid due to *H. ducreyi*: Oral: 1 g as a single dose (CDC, 2010)

***C. trachomatis* urethritis/cervicitis:** Oral: 1 g as a single dose

Community-acquired pneumonia:

Oral: 500 mg on day 1 followed by 250 mg once daily on days 2-5

Extended release suspension (Zmax®): 2 g as a single dose

I.V.: 500 mg as a single dose for at least 2 days, follow I.V. therapy by the oral route with a single daily dose of 500 mg to complete a 7- to 10-day course of therapy.

Disseminated *M. avium* complex disease in patients with advanced HIV infection: Oral:

Treatment: 600 mg daily in combination with ethambutol

Primary prophylaxis: 1200 mg once weekly (preferred), with or without rifabutin **or** alternatively, 600 mg twice weekly (CDC, 2009)

Secondary prophylaxis: 500-600 mg daily in combination with ethambutol (CDC, 2009)

Gonococcal infection, uncomplicated (cervix, rectum, urethra) (unlabeled regimen): Oral: 1 g as a single dose in combination with ceftriaxone (preferred) or cefixime (only if ceftriaxone unavailable); if cefixime is used, test-of-cure in 7 days is recommended (CDC, 2012). **Note:** Monotherapy with azithromycin single dose of 2 g has been associated with resistance and/or treatment failure; however, may be appropriate for treatment of a gonococcal infection in pregnant women who cannot tolerate a cephalosporin (CDC, 2010).

Patients with severe cephalosporin allergy: 2 g as a single dose and test-of-cure in 7 days (CDC, 2012)

Gonococcal infection, uncomplicated (pharynx) (unlabeled use): 1 g as a single dose in combination with ceftriaxone (CDC, 2012)

Gonococcal infection, expedited partner therapy (unlabeled use): Oral: 1 g as a single dose in combination with cefixime (CDC, 2012). **Note:** Only used if a heterosexual partner cannot be linked to evaluation and treatment in a timely manner; dose delivered to partner by patient, collaborating pharmacy, or disease investigation specialist.

Granuloma inguinale (donovanosis) (unlabeled use): Oral: 1 g once a week for at least 3 weeks (and until lesions have healed) (CDC, 2010)

Mild-to-moderate respiratory tract, skin, and soft tissue infections: Oral: 500 mg in a single loading dose on day 1 followed by 250 mg daily as a single dose on days 2-5

Alternative regimen: Bacterial exacerbation of COPD: 500 mg daily for a total of 3 days

***M. genitalium* infections (unlabeled use)** (confirmed cases in males or females or clinically significant persistent urethritis in males): Oral: 1 g as a single dose or 500 mg on day 1, followed by 250 mg daily on days 2-5 (Manhart, 2011):

Note: Follow up patients on either regimen in 3-4 weeks for test of cure; consider moxifloxacin for treatment failures (Manhart, 2011)

Pelvic inflammatory disease (PID): I.V.: 500 mg as a single dose for 1-2 days, follow I.V. therapy by the oral route with a single daily dose of 250 mg to complete a 7-day course of therapy

Pertussis (unlabeled use; CDC, 2005): Oral: 500 mg on day 1 followed by 250 mg daily on days 2-5 (maximum: 500 mg daily)

Pharyngitis, group A streptococci in penicillin-allergic patients (IDSA guidelines): Oral: 12 mg/kg once daily (maximum: 500 mg daily) for 5 days. **Note:** Recommended by the Infectious Disease Society of America (IDSA) as an alternative agent for group A streptococcal pharyngitis in penicillin-allergic patients (Shulman, 2012).

Prophylaxis against infective endocarditis (unlabeled use): Oral: 500 mg 30-60 minutes prior to the procedure. **Note:** American Heart Association (AHA) guidelines now recommend prophylaxis only in patients undergoing invasive procedures and in whom underlying cardiac conditions may predispose to a higher risk of adverse outcomes should infection occur. As of April 2007, routine prophylaxis for GI/GU procedures is no longer recommended by the AHA.

Prophylaxis against sexually-transmitted diseases following sexual assault (unlabeled use): Oral: 1 g as a single dose (in combination with a cephalosporin and metronidazole) (CDC, 2010)

Shigella dysentery type 1 (unlabeled use): Oral: 1000-1500 mg once daily for 1-5 days (WHO, 2005)

Adults:

Prevention of pulmonary exacerbations in patients with noncystic fibrosis bronchiectasis (unlabeled use): Oral: 500 mg 3 days per week. **Note:** Duration of treatment in clinical trial was 6 months; durations >6 months have not been evaluated. Trial patients had ≥1 exacerbation in the past year, no macrolide treatment for >3 months in the past 6 months, and were screened for nontuberculous mycobacterial infection prior to treatment (Wong, 2012). A more selective approach for patients with functionally mild disease has been suggested (Wilson, 2012).

Dosage adjustment in renal impairment: Use with caution in patients with GFR <10 mL/minute (AUC increased by 35% compared to patients with normal renal function); however, no dosage adjustment is provided in the manufacturer's labeling.

No supplemental dose or dosage adjustment necessary, including patients on intermittent hemodialysis, peritoneal dialysis, or continuous renal replacement therapy (eg, CVVHD) (Aronoff, 2007; Heintz, 2009).

Dosage adjustment in hepatic impairment: Azithromycin is predominantly hepatically eliminated; however, there is no dosage adjustment provided in the manufacturer's labeling, Use with caution due to potential for hepatotoxicity (rare); discontinue immediately for signs or symptoms of hepatitis.

Dietary Considerations

Some products may contain sodium and/or sucrose.

Oral suspension, immediate release, may be administered with or without food.

Oral suspension, extended release, should be taken on an empty stomach (at least 1 hour before or 2 hours following a meal).

Tablet may be administered with food to decrease GI effects.

Administration

I.V.: Infusate concentration and rate of infusion for azithromycin for injection should be either 1 mg/mL over 3 hours or 2 mg/mL over 1 hour. Other medications should not be infused simultaneously through the same I.V. line.

Oral: Immediate release suspension and tablet may be taken without regard to food; extended release suspension should be taken on an empty stomach (at least 1 hour before or 2 hours following a meal), within 12 hours of reconstitution.

Monitoring Parameters Liver function tests, CBC with differential; when used as part of alternative treatment for gonococcal infection, test-of-cure 7 days after dose (CDC, 2012)

Additional Information Zithromax® tablets and immediate release suspension may be interchanged (eg, two Zithromax® 250 mg tablets may be substituted for one Zithromax® 500 mg tablet or the tablets may be substituted with the immediate release suspension); however, the extended release suspension (Zmax®) is not bioequivalent with Zithromax® and therefore should not be interchanged.

Azithromycin is not recommended for treatment of early syphilis; the 23S rRNA mutation, which has been associated with macrolide resistance, has been documented in multiple geographic areas and in the MSM population. If a penicillin allergic patient cannot take doxycycline (preferred alternative to penicillin), azithromycin (single 2 g dose orally) may be considered but close clinical follow-up is needed (Ghanem, 2011).

Dosage Forms Excipient information presented when available (limited, particularly for generics); consult specific product labeling.

Packet, Oral, as dihydrate [strength expressed as base]:
- Zithromax: 1 g (3 ea, 10 ea) [cherry-banana flavor]
- Generic: 1 g (3 ea, 10 ea)

Solution Reconstituted, Intravenous, as dihydrate [strength expressed as base]:
- Zithromax: 500 mg (1 ea)

Solution Reconstituted, Intravenous, as hydrogencitrate [strength expressed as base]:
- Generic: 2.5 g (1 ea)

Solution Reconstituted, Intravenous, as monohydrate [strength expressed as base]:
- Generic: 500 mg (1 ea)

Solution Reconstituted, Intravenous, as monohydrate [strength expressed as base, preservative free]:
- Generic: 500 mg (1 ea)

Suspension Reconstituted, Oral, as dihydrate [strength expressed as base]:
- Zithromax: 100 mg/5 mL (15 mL) [cherry-vanilla-banana flavor]
- Zithromax: 200 mg/5 mL (15 mL, 22.5 mL, 30 mL) [cherry flavor]
- Zmax: 2 g (1 ea) [cherry-banana flavor]
- Generic: 100 mg/5 mL (15 mL); 200 mg/5 mL (15 mL, 22.5 mL, 30 mL)

Suspension Reconstituted, Oral, as monohydrate [strength expressed as base]:
- Generic: 100 mg/5 mL (15 mL); 200 mg/5 mL (15 mL, 22.5 mL, 30 mL)

Tablet, Oral, as anhydrous:
- Generic: 250 mg, 500 mg, 600 mg

Tablet, Oral, as dihydrate [strength expressed as base]:
- Zithromax: 250 mg, 500 mg, 600 mg
- Zithromax Tri-Pak: 500 mg
- Zithromax Z-Pak: 250 mg
- Generic: 250 mg, 500 mg, 600 mg

Tablet, Oral, as monohydrate [strength expressed as base]:
- Generic: 250 mg, 500 mg, 600 mg

Azithromycin (Ophthalmic) (az ith roe MYE sin)

Brand Names: U.S. AzaSite

Pharmacologic Category Antibiotic, Macrolide; Antibiotic, Ophthalmic

Use Treatment of bacterial conjunctivitis caused by susceptible microorganisms

Pregnancy Risk Factor B

Dosage Ophthalmic: **Usual dosage range:** Bacterial conjunctivitis: Children ≥1 year and Adults: Instill 1 drop into affected eye(s) twice daily (8-12 hours apart) for 2 days, then 1 drop into affected eye(s) once daily for 5 days

Additional Information Complete prescribing information should be consulted for additional detail.

Dosage Forms Excipient information presented when available (limited, particularly for generics); consult specific product labeling.

Solution, Ophthalmic:
- AzaSite: 1% (2.5 mL) [contains benzalkonium chloride, disodium edta]

- ◆ **Azithromycin Dihydrate** *see* Azithromycin (Systemic) *on page 214*
- ◆ **Azithromycin for Injection (Can)** *see* Azithromycin (Systemic) *on page 214*
- ◆ **Azithromycin Monohydrate** *see* Azithromycin (Systemic) *on page 214*
- ◆ **AZL-M** *see* Azilsartan *on page 212*
- ◆ **Azo-Gesic [OTC]** *see* Phenazopyridine *on page 1627*

◆ **Azolen Tincture [OTC]** *see* Miconazole (Topical) *on page 1358*
◆ **Azopt** *see* Brinzolamide *on page 281*
◆ **Azopt® (Can)** *see* Brinzolamide *on page 281*
◆ **Azor™** *see* Amlodipine and Olmesartan *on page 112*
◆ **AZT™ (Can)** *see* Zidovudine *on page 2226*
◆ **AZT + 3TC (error-prone abbreviation)** *see* Lamivudine and Zidovudine *on page 1164*
◆ **AZT, Abacavir, and Lamivudine** *see* Abacavir, Lamivudine, and Zidovudine *on page 20*
◆ **AZT (error-prone abbreviation)** *see* Zidovudine *on page 2226*
◆ **Azthreonam** *see* Aztreonam *on page 218*

Aztreonam (AZ tree oh nam)

Brand Names: U.S. Azactam; Azactam in Dextrose; Cayston

Brand Names: Canada Cayston

Index Terms Azthreonam

Pharmacologic Category Antibiotic, Miscellaneous

Use

Injection: Treatment of patients with urinary tract infections, lower respiratory tract infections, septicemia, skin/skin structure infections, intra-abdominal infections, and gynecological infections caused by susceptible gram-negative bacilli

Inhalation: Improve respiratory symptoms in cystic fibrosis (CF) patients with *Pseudomonas aeruginosa*

Unlabeled Use Surgical (perioperative) prophylaxis

Pregnancy Risk Factor B

Pregnancy Considerations Adverse events have not been observed in animal reproduction studies; therefore, the manufacturer classifies aztreonam as pregnancy category B. Aztreonam crosses the placenta and enters cord blood during middle and late pregnancy. Distribution to the fetus is minimal in early pregnancy. The amount of aztreonam available systemically following inhalation is significantly less in comparison to doses given by injection.

Breast-Feeding Considerations Very small amounts of aztreonam are excreted in breast milk. The poor oral absorption of aztreonam (<1%) may limit adverse effects to the infant. Nondose-related effects could include modification of bowel flora. Maternal use of aztreonam inhalation is not likely to pose a risk to breast-feeding infants.

Prescribing and Access Restrictions Cayston (aztreonam inhalation solution) is only available through a select group of specialty pharmacies and cannot be obtained through a retail pharmacy. Because Cayston® may only be used with the Altera Nebulizer System, it can only be obtained from the following specialty pharmacies: Cystic Fibrosis Services, Inc; IV Solutions; Foundation Care; and Pharmaceutical Specialties, Inc. This network of specialty pharmacies ensures proper access to both the drug and device. To obtain the medication and proper nebulizer, contact the Cayston Access Program at 1-877-7CAYSTON (1-877-722-9786) or at www.cayston.com.

Contraindications Hypersensitivity to aztreonam or any component of the formulation

Warnings/Precautions Rare cross-allergenicity to penicillins, cephalosporins, or carbapenems may occur; use with caution in patients with a history of hypersensitivity to beta-lactams. Use caution in renal impairment; dosing adjustment required for the injectable formulation. Prolonged use may result in fungal or bacterial superinfection, including *C. difficile*-associated diarrhea (CDAD) and pseudomembranous colitis; CDAD has been observed >2 months postantibiotic treatment. Use with caution in bone marrow transplant patients with multiple risk factors for toxic epidermal necrolysis (TEN) (eg, sepsis, radiation therapy, drugs known to cause TEN); rare cases of TEN in this population have been reported. Patients colonized with *Burkholderia cepacia* have not been studied. Potentially significant interactions may exist, requiring dose or frequency adjustment, additional monitoring, and/or selection of alternative therapy. Safety and efficacy has not been established in patients with FEV_1 <25% or >75% predicted. To reduce the development of resistant bacteria and maintain efficacy reserve use for CF patients with known *Pseudomonas aeruginosa*. Bronchospasm may occur occur following nebulization; administer a bronchodilator prior to treatment.

Adverse Reactions

Inhalation:

>10%:

Respiratory: Cough (54%), nasal congestion (16%), wheezing (16%), sore throat (12%)

Miscellaneous: Fever (13%; more common in children)

1% to 10%:

Cardiovascular: Chest discomfort (8%)

Dermatologic: Skin rash (2%)

Gastrointestinal: Abdominal pain (7%), vomiting (6%)

Respiratory: Bronchospasm (3%)

<1%, postmarketing, and/or case reports: Arthralgia, facial edema, hypersensitivity reaction, joint swelling, tightness in chest and throat

Injection:

>10%:

Hematologic & oncologic: Neutropenia (children 3% to 11%; adults <1%)

Hepatic: Increased serum transaminases (ALT/AST; children 4% to 6%; >3 times ULN: 15% to 20%, high dose)

Local: Pain at injection site (children 12%, adults 2%)

1% to 10%:

Dermatologic: Skin rash (children 4%, adults 1%)

Gastrointestinal: Diarrhea (1%), nausea (1%), vomiting (1%)

Hematologic & oncologic: Eosinophilia (children 6%, adults <1%), thrombocythemia (children 4%, adults <1%)

Local: Injection site reaction (1% to 3%) (erythema, induration; more common in children), inflammation at injection site (2%)

Renal: Increased serum creatinine (children 6%)

Miscellaneous: Fever (≤1%)

<1% (Limited to important or life-threatening): Anaphylaxis, anemia, angioedema, aphthous stomatitis, *Clostridium difficile* associated diarrhea, erythema multiforme, exfoliative dermatitis, gastrointestinal hemorrhage, hepatitis, leukocytosis, leukopenia, oral mucosa ulcer, pancytopenia, positive direct Coombs test, prolonged partial thromboplastin time, prolonged prothrombin time, pseudomembranous colitis, seizure, thrombocytopenia, toxic epidermal necrolysis, vaginitis, ventricular bigeminy (transient), ventricular premature contractions (transient), vulvovaginal candidiasis

Drug Interactions

Metabolism/Transport Effects None known.

Avoid Concomitant Use

Avoid concomitant use of Aztreonam with any of the following: BCG

Increased Effect/Toxicity There are no known significant interactions involving an increase in effect.

Decreased Effect

Aztreonam may decrease the levels/effects of: BCG; Sodium Picosulfate; Typhoid Vaccine

Preparation for Administration

Inhalation: Reconstitute immediately prior to use. Squeeze diluent into opened glass vial. Replace rubber stopper and gently swirl vial until contents have completely dissolved.

I.M.: Reconstitute vial with at least 3 mL SWFI, sterile bacteriostatic water for injection, NS, or bacteriostatic sodium chloride per gram of aztreonam; immediately shake vigorously.

I.V.:

Bolus injection: Reconstitute vial with 6-10 mL SWFI; immediately shake vigorously.

Infusion: Reconstitute vial with at least 3 mL SWFI per gram of aztreonam; immediately shake vigorously. Reconstituted solutions are colorless to light yellow straw and may turn pink upon standing without affecting potency. Further dilute in an appropriate solution for infusion to a final concentration ≤2% (ie, final concentration should not exceed 20 mg/mL).

Storage/Stability

Inhalation: Prior to reconstitution, store at 2°C to 8°C (36°F to 46°F). Once removed from refrigeration, aztreonam and the diluent may be stored at room temperature (up to 25°C [77°F]) for ≤28 days. Protect from light. Use immediately after reconstitution.

Vials: Prior to reconstitution, store at room temperature; avoid excessive heat. After reconstitution, solutions for infusion with a final concentration of ≤20 mg/mL should be used within 48 hours if stored at room temperature or within 7 days if refrigerated. Solutions for infusion with a final concentration of >20 mg/mL (if prepared with SWFI or NS **only**) should also be used within 48 hours if stored at room temperature or within 7 days if refrigerated; all other solutions for infusion with a final concentration >20 mg/mL must be used immediately after preparation (unless prepared with SWFI or NS).

Premixed frozen containers: Store unused container frozen at ≤ -20°C (-4°F). Frozen container can be thawed at room temperature of 25°C (77°F) or in a refrigerator, 2°C to 8°C (36°F to 46°F). Thawed solution should be used within 48 hours if stored at room temperature or within 14 days if stored under refrigeration. **Do not freeze.**

Mechanism of Action Inhibits bacterial cell wall synthesis by binding to one or more of the penicillin-binding proteins (PBPs) which in turn inhibits the final transpeptidation step of peptidoglycan synthesis in bacterial cell walls, thus inhibiting cell wall biosynthesis. Bacteria eventually lyse due to ongoing activity of cell wall autolytic enzymes (autolysins and murein hydrolases) while cell wall assembly is arrested. Monobactam structure makes cross-allergenicity with beta-lactams unlikely.

Pharmacodynamics/Kinetics

Absorption: I.M.: Well absorbed; I.M. and I.V. doses produce comparable serum concentrations; Inhalation: Low systemic absorption

Distribution: Injection: Widely to most body fluids and tissues

V_d: Children: 0.2-0.29 L/kg; Adults: 0.2 L/kg

Relative diffusion of antimicrobial agents from blood into CSF: Good only with inflammation (exceeds usual MICs)

CSF:blood level ratio: Meninges: Inflamed: 8% to 40%; Normal: ~1%

Protein binding: 56%

Metabolism: Injection: Hepatic (minor %)

Half-life elimination: Injection:

Children 2 months to 12 years: 1.7 hours

Adults: Normal renal function: 1.7-2.9 hours

End-stage renal disease: 6-8 hours

Time to peak: I.M., I.V. push: Within 60 minutes; I.V. infusion: 1.5 hours

Excretion: Injection: Urine (60% to 70% as unchanged drug); feces (~13% to 15%)

Dosage

Children ≥9 months and Adolescents: I.V.:

Mild-to-moderate infections: 30 mg/kg/dose every 8 hours; maximum: 120 mg/kg/day (8 g daily)

Moderate-to-severe infections: 30 mg/kg/dose every 6-8 hours; maximum: 120 mg/kg/day (8 g daily)

Cystic fibrosis: 50 mg/kg/dose every 6-8 hours (ie, up to 200 mg/kg/day); maximum: 8 g daily. **Note:** Higher doses (8-12 g daily) may be needed for patients with cystic fibrosis (Zobell, 2013).

Children ≥1 year: Surgical (perioperative) prophylaxis (unlabeled use): I.V.: 30 mg/kg within 60 minutes prior to surgery (maximum: 2000 mg per dose). Doses may be repeated in 4 hours if procedure is lengthy or if there is excessive blood loss (Bratzler, 2013).

Children ≥7 years, Adolescents, and Adults: Inhalation (nebulizer): Cystic fibrosis: 75 mg 3 times daily (at least 4 hours apart) for 28 days; do not repeat for 28 days after completion

Adults:

Urinary tract infection: I.M., I.V.: 500 mg to 1 g every 8-12 hours

Moderately severe systemic infections: 1 g I.V. or I.M. or 2 g I.V. every 8-12 hours. **Note:** I.V. route preferred for septicemia, intra-abdominal abscess, or peritonitis; higher doses (8-12 g daily) may be needed for patients with cystic fibrosis (Zobell, 2013) or other infections (Solomkin, 2010).

Severe systemic or life-threatening infections (eg, *Pseudomonas aeruginosa*): I.V.: 2 g every 6-8 hours; maximum: 8 g daily. **Note:** Higher doses (8-12 g daily) may be needed for patients with cystic fibrosis (Zobell, 2013) or other infections (Solomkin, 2010).

Surgical (perioperative) prophylaxis (unlabeled use): I.V.: 2 g within 60 minutes prior to surgery. Doses may be repeated in 4 hours if procedure is lengthy or if there is excessive blood loss (Bratzler, 2013).

Dosage adjustment in renal impairment:

Oral inhalation: Dosage adjustment not required for mild, moderate, or severe renal impairment

I.M., I.V.: Adults: Following initial dose, maintenance doses should be given as follows:

Cl_{cr} 10-30 mL/minute: 50% of usual dose at the usual interval

Cl_{cr} <10 mL/minute: 25% of usual dosage at the usual interval

Intermittent hemodialysis (IHD): Dialyzable (20% to 50%): Loading dose of 500 mg, 1 g, or 2 g, followed by 25% of initial dose at usual interval; for serious/life-threatening infections, administer 12.5% of initial dose after each hemodialysis session (given in addition to the maintenance doses). Alternatively, may administer 500 mg every 12 hours (Heintz, 2009). **Note:** Dosing dependent on the assumption of 3 times/week, complete IHD sessions.

Peritoneal dialysis (PD): Administer as for Cl_{cr} <10 mL/minute (Aronoff, 2007)

Continuous renal replacement therapy (CRRT) (Heintz, 2009; Trotman, 2005): Drug clearance is highly dependent on the method of renal replacement, filter type, and flow rate. Appropriate dosing requires close monitoring of pharmacologic response, signs of adverse reactions due to drug accumulation, as well as drug concentrations in relation to target trough (if appropriate). The following are general recommendations only (based on dialysate flow/ultrafiltration rates of 1-2 L/hour and minimal residual renal function) and should not supersede clinical judgment:

CVVH: Loading dose of 2 g followed by 1-2 g every 12 hours

CVVHD/CVVHDF: Loading dose of 2 g followed by either 1 g every 8 hours **or** 2 g every 12 hours (Heintz, 2009)

Dosage adjustment in hepatic impairment: No dosage adjustment provided in manufacturer's labeling. Use with caution (minor hepatic elimination occurs).

Administration

Inhalation: Administer using only an Altera nebulizer system; **administer alone; do not mix with other nebulizer medications**. Administer a bronchodilator before administration of aztreonam (short-acting: 15 minutes to 4 hours before; long-acting: 30 minutes to 12 hours before). For patients on multiple inhaled therapies, administer bronchodilator first, then mucolytic, and lastly, aztreonam. To administer Cayston, pour reconstituted solution into the handset of the nebulizer system, turn unit on. Place the mouthpiece in the patient's mouth and encourage to breath normally through the mouth. Administration time is usually 2-3 minutes. Administer doses ≥4 hours apart.

Injection: Doses >1 g should be administered I.V.

I.M.: Administer by deep injection into large muscle mass, such as upper outer quadrant of gluteus maximus or the lateral part of the thigh

I.V.: Administer by slow I.V. push over 3-5 minutes or by intermittent infusion over 20-60 minutes.

Monitoring Parameters

Injection: Periodic liver function test; monitor for signs of anaphylaxis during first dose

Inhalation: Consider measuring FEV_1 prior to initiation of therapy

Test Interactions May interfere with urine glucose tests containing cupric sulfate (Benedict's solution, Clinitest); positive Coombs' test

Additional Information Although marketed as an agent similar to aminoglycosides, aztreonam is a monobactam antimicrobial with almost pure gram-negative aerobic activity. It cannot be used for gram-positive infections.

Dosage Forms Excipient information presented when available (limited, particularly for generics); consult specific product labeling.

Solution, Intravenous:
- Azactam in Dextrose: 1 g (50 mL); 2 g (50 mL) [sodium free]

Solution Reconstituted, Inhalation [preservative free]:
- Cayston: 75 mg (84 mL) [arginine free]

Solution Reconstituted, Injection:
- Azactam: 1 g (1 ea); 2 g (1 ea) [sodium free]
- Generic: 1 g (1 ea); 2 g (1 ea)

- Azulfidine *see* SulfaSALAzine *on page 1964*
- Azulfidine EN-tabs *see* SulfaSALAzine *on page 1964*
- Azurette *see* Ethinyl Estradiol and Desogestrel *on page 784*
- B-2-400 [OTC] *see* Riboflavin *on page 1809*
- B6 *see* Pyridoxine *on page 1753*
- B1939 *see* Eribulin *on page 734*
- B2036-PEG *see* Pegvisomant *on page 1600*
- Baby Anbesol [OTC] *see* Benzocaine *on page 240*
- Baby Aspirin *see* Aspirin *on page 177*
- Baby Ayr Saline [OTC] *see* Sodium Chloride *on page 1914*
- BabyBIG® *see* Botulism Immune Globulin (Intravenous-Human) *on page 277*
- Baciguent® (Can) *see* Bacitracin *on page 220*
- BACiiM *see* Bacitracin *on page 220*
- Baciject® (Can) *see* Bacitracin *on page 220*
- Bacillus Calmette-Guérin (BCG) Live *see* BCG *on page 226*

Bacitracin (bas i TRAY sin)

Brand Names: U.S. BACiiM

Brand Names: Canada Baciguent®; Baciject®

Pharmacologic Category Antibiotic, Miscellaneous; Antibiotic, Ophthalmic; Antibiotic, Topical

Use Treatment of susceptible bacterial infections mainly (has activity against gram-positive bacilli); due to toxicity risks, systemic and irrigant uses of bacitracin should be limited to situations where less toxic alternatives would not be effective

Unlabeled Use Oral administration: Treatment of *Clostridium difficile*-associated diarrhea; has been used for enteric eradication of vancomycin-resistant enterococci (VRE)

Dosage Do not administer I.V.:

Infants: I.M.:
- ≤2.5 kg: 900 units/kg/day in 2-3 divided doses
- >2.5 kg: 1000 units/kg/day in 2-3 divided doses

Adults: Oral:
- *Clostridium difficile*-associated diarrhea (unlabeled use): 25,000 units 4 times daily for 7-10 days (Dudley 1986; Young, 1985). **Note:** May be considered when other more established regimens (eg, metronidazole or vancomycin) fail; not routinely used (Cohen, 2010).
- Enteric VRE eradication (unlabeled use): 25,000 units 4 times daily for 7-10 days (Chia, 1995; O'Donovan, 1994)

Children and Adults:
- Topical: Apply 1-3 times daily
- Ophthalmic, ointment: Instill 1/4" to 1/2" ribbon every 3-4 hours into conjunctival sac for acute infections, or 2-3 times daily for mild-to-moderate infections for 7-10 days

Additional Information Complete prescribing information should be consulted for additional detail.

Dosage Forms Excipient information presented when available (limited, particularly for generics); consult specific product labeling.

Ointment, Ophthalmic:
- Generic: 500 units/g (1 g, 3.5 g)

Ointment, External, as zinc [strength expressed as base]:
- Generic: 500 units/g (1 ea, 1 g, 14 g, 14.2 g, 15 g, 28 g, 28.35 g, 28.4 g, 30 g, 120 g, 453.9 g, 454 g)

Solution Reconstituted, Intramuscular:
- BACiiM: 50,000 units (1 ea)
- Generic: 50,000 units (1 ea)

Solution Reconstituted, Intramuscular [preservative free]:
- Generic: 50,000 units (1 ea)

Bacitracin and Polymyxin B
(bas i TRAY sin & pol i MIKS in bee)

Brand Names: U.S. AK-Poly-Bac™; Polycin™; Polysporin® [OTC]

Brand Names: Canada LID-Pack®; Optimyxin®

Index Terms Polymyxin B and Bacitracin

Pharmacologic Category Antibiotic, Ophthalmic; Antibiotic, Topical

Use Treatment of superficial infections caused by susceptible organisms

Pregnancy Risk Factor C

Dosage Children and Adults:
- Ophthalmic ointment: Instill 1/2" ribbon in the affected eye(s) every 3-4 hours for acute infections or 2-3 times/day for mild-to-moderate infections for 7-10 days
- Topical ointment/powder: Apply to affected area 1-4 times/day; may cover with sterile bandage if needed

Additional Information Complete prescribing information should be consulted for additional detail.

Dosage Forms Excipient information presented when available (limited, particularly for generics); consult specific product labeling.

Ointment, ophthalmic: Bacitracin 500 units and polymyxin B 10,000 units per g (3.5 g)
- AK-Poly-Bac™: Bacitracin 500 units and polymyxin B 10,000 units per g (3.5 g)
- Polycin™: Bacitracin 500 units and polymyxin B 10,000 units per g (3.5 g)

Ointment, topical: Bacitracin 500 units and polymyxin B 10,000 units per g (15 g, 30 g)

Polysporin®: Bacitracin 500 units and polymyxin B 10,000 units per g (0.9 g, 15 g, 30 g)

Powder, topical:

Polysporin®: Bacitracin 500 units and polymyxin B 10,000 units per g (10 g)

Bacitracin, Neomycin, and Polymyxin B

(bas i TRAY sin, nee oh MYE sin, & pol i MIKS in bee)

Brand Names: U.S. Neo-Polycin™; Neosporin® Neo To Go® [OTC]; Neosporin® Topical [OTC]

Index Terms Neomycin, Bacitracin, and Polymyxin B; Polymyxin B, Bacitracin, and Neomycin; Triple Antibiotic

Pharmacologic Category Antibiotic, Ophthalmic; Antibiotic, Topical

Use Helps prevent infection in minor cuts, scrapes, and burns; short-term treatment of superficial external ocular infections caused by susceptible organisms

Pregnancy Risk Factor C

Dosage Children and Adults:

Ophthalmic: Ointment: Instill 1/2" into the conjunctival sac every 3-4 hours for 7-10 days for acute infections

Topical: Apply 1-3 times/day to infected area; may cover with sterile bandage as needed

Additional Information Complete prescribing information should be consulted for additional detail.

Dosage Forms Excipient information presented when available (limited, particularly for generics); consult specific product labeling.

Ointment, ophthalmic: Bacitracin 400 units, neomycin 3.5 mg, and polymyxin B 10,000 units per g (3.5 g)

Neo-Polycin™: Bacitracin 400 units, neomycin 3.5 mg, and polymyxin B 10,000 units per g (3.5 g)

Ointment, topical: Bacitracin 400 units, neomycin 3.5 mg, and polymyxin B 5000 units per g (0.9 g, 15 g, 30 g, 454 g)

Neosporin®: Bacitracin 400 units, neomycin 3.5 mg, and polymyxin B 5000 units per g (15 g, 30 g)

Neosporin® Neo To Go®: Bacitracin 400 units, neomycin 3.5 mg, and polymyxin B 5000 units per g (0.9 g)

Bacitracin, Neomycin, Polymyxin B, and Hydrocortisone

(bas i TRAY sin, nee oh MYE sin, pol i MIKS in bee, & hye droe KOR ti sone)

Brand Names: U.S. Cortisporin® Ointment; Neo-Polycin™ HC

Brand Names: Canada Cortisporin® Topical Ointment

Index Terms Hydrocortisone, Bacitracin, Neomycin, and Polymyxin B; Neomycin, Bacitracin, Polymyxin B, and Hydrocortisone; Polymyxin B, Bacitracin, Neomycin, and Hydrocortisone

Pharmacologic Category Antibiotic, Ophthalmic; Antibiotic, Topical; Corticosteroid, Ophthalmic; Corticosteroid, Topical

Use Prevention and treatment of susceptible inflammatory conditions where bacterial infection (or risk of infection) is present

Pregnancy Risk Factor C

Dosage Children and Adults:

Ophthalmic: Ointment: Instill 1/2 inch ribbon to inside of lower lid every 3-4 hours until improvement occurs

Topical: Apply sparingly 2-4 times/day. Therapy should be discontinued when control is achieved; if no improvement is seen, reassessment of diagnosis may be necessary.

Additional Information Complete prescribing information should be consulted for additional detail.

Dosage Forms Excipient information presented when available (limited, particularly for generics); consult specific product labeling.

Ointment, ophthalmic: Bacitracin 400 units, neomycin 3.5 mg, polymyxin B 10,000 units, and hydrocortisone 10 mg per g (3.5 g)

Neo-Polycin™ HC: Bacitracin 400 units, neomycin 3.5 mg, polymyxin B 10,000 units, and hydrocortisone 10 mg per g (3.5 g)

Ointment, topical:

Cortisporin®: Bacitracin 400 units, neomycin 3.5 mg, polymyxin B 5000 units, and hydrocortisone 10 mg per g (15 g)

Baclofen (BAK loe fen)

Brand Names: U.S. Gablofen; Lioresal

Brand Names: Canada Apo-Baclofen®; Ava-Baclofen; Dom-Baclofen; Lioresal®; Lioresal® D.S.; Lioresal® Intrathecal; Med-Baclofen; Mylan-Baclofen; Novo-Baclofen; Nu-Baclo; PHL-Baclofen; PMS-Baclofen; ratio-Baclofen; Riva-Baclofen

Pharmacologic Category Skeletal Muscle Relaxant

Use Treatment of reversible spasticity associated with multiple sclerosis or spinal cord lesions

Orphan drug: Intrathecal: Treatment of intractable spasticity caused by spinal cord injury, multiple sclerosis, and other spinal disease (spinal ischemia or tumor, transverse myelitis, cervical spondylosis, degenerative myelopathy)

Unlabeled Use Intractable hiccups, intractable pain relief, bladder spasticity, trigeminal neuralgia, cerebral palsy, short-term treatment of spasticity in children with cerebral palsy, Huntington's chorea

Pregnancy Risk Factor C

Pregnancy Considerations Adverse events were observed in animal reproduction studies. Withdrawal symptoms in the neonate were noted in a case report following the maternal use of oral baclofen 20 mg 4 times/day throughout pregnancy (Ratnayaka, 2001). Plasma concentrations following administration of intrathecal baclofen are significantly less than those with oral doses; exposure to the fetus is expected to be limited (Morton, 2009).

Breast-Feeding Considerations Baclofen is excreted into breast milk. Very small amounts were found in the breast milk of a woman 14 days postpartum after oral use. Following a single oral dose of baclofen 20 mg, the total amount of baclofen excreted in breast milk within 26 hours was 22 mcg (Eriksson, 1981). Adverse events were not observed in a nursing infant following maternal use of intrathecal baclofen 200 mcg/day throughout pregnancy and while nursing (Morton, 2009). Due to the potential for adverse events in the nursing infant, breast-feeding is not recommended by the manufacturer.

Contraindications Hypersensitivity to baclofen or any component of the formulation

Warnings/Precautions Use with caution in patients with seizure disorder or impaired renal function. **[U.S. Boxed Warning]: Avoid abrupt withdrawal of the drug; abrupt withdrawal of intrathecal baclofen has resulted in severe sequelae (hyperpyrexia, obtundation, rebound/exaggerated spasticity, muscle rigidity, and rhabdomyolysis), leading to organ failure and some fatalities.** Risk may be higher in patients with injuries at T-6 or above, history of baclofen withdrawal, or limited ability to communicate. May cause CNS depression, which may impair physical or mental abilities; patients must be cautioned about performing tasks which require mental alertness (eg, operating machinery or driving). Elderly are more sensitive to the effects of baclofen and are more likely to experience adverse CNS effects at higher doses.

Cases (most from pharmacy compounded preparations) of intrathecal mass formation at the implanted catheter tip have been reported; may lead to loss of clinical response, pain or new/worsening neurological effects. Neurosurgical evaluation and/or an appropriate imaging study should be considered if a mass is suspected.

Adverse Reactions

>10%:

Central nervous system: Drowsiness, vertigo, dizziness, psychiatric disturbances, insomnia, slurred speech, ataxia, hypotonia

Neuromuscular & skeletal: Weakness

1% to 10%:

Cardiovascular: Hypotension

Central nervous system: Fatigue, confusion, headache

Dermatologic: Rash

Gastrointestinal: Nausea, constipation

Genitourinary: Polyuria

<1% (Limited to important or life-threatening): Chest pain, dyspnea, dysuria, enuresis, hematuria, impotence, inability to ejaculate, nocturia, palpitation, syncope, urinary retention; withdrawal reactions have occurred with abrupt discontinuation (particularly severe with intrathecal use).

Drug Interactions

Metabolism/Transport Effects None known.

Avoid Concomitant Use

Avoid concomitant use of Baclofen with any of the following: Azelastine (Nasal); Paraldehyde

Increased Effect/Toxicity

Baclofen may increase the levels/effects of: Alcohol (Ethyl); Azelastine (Nasal); Buprenorphine; CNS Depressants; Hydrocodone; Methotrimeprazine; Metyrosine; Mirtazapine; Paraldehyde; Pramipexole; ROPINIRole; Rotigotine; Selective Serotonin Reuptake Inhibitors; Zolpidem

The levels/effects of Baclofen may be increased by: Brimonidine (Topical); Doxylamine; Droperidol; HydrOXYzine; Magnesium Sulfate; Methotrimeprazine; Perampanel; Sodium Oxybate; Tapentadol

Decreased Effect There are no known significant interactions involving a decrease in effect.

Ethanol/Nutrition/Herb Interactions

Ethanol: May increase CNS depression; monitor for increased effects with coadministration. Caution patients about effects.

Herb/Nutraceutical: Avoid valerian, St John's wort, kava kava, gotu kola.

Preparation for Administration Intrathecal: For screening dosages, dilute with preservative-free sodium chloride to a final concentration of 50 mcg/mL. For maintenance infusions, concentrations of 500-2000 mcg/mL may be used.

Mechanism of Action Inhibits the transmission of both monosynaptic and polysynaptic reflexes at the spinal cord level, possibly by hyperpolarization of primary afferent fiber terminals, with resultant relief of muscle spasticity

Pharmacodynamics/Kinetics

Onset of action: 3-4 days

Peak effect: 5-10 days

Absorption (dose dependent): Oral: Rapid

Protein binding: 30%

Metabolism: Hepatic (15% of dose)

Half-life elimination: 3.5 hours

Time to peak, serum: Oral: Within 2-3 hours

Excretion: Urine and feces (85% as unchanged drug)

Dosage

Oral (avoid abrupt withdrawal of drug):

Children (unlabeled use):

Spasticity: Caution: Pediatric dosing expressed as a daily amount, and **NOT** in mg/kg. Limited published data in children; the following is a compilation of small prospective studies (Albright, 1996; Milla, 1977; Scheinberg, 2006) and one large retrospective study (Lubsch, 2006):

<2 years: 10-20 mg daily divided every 8 hours; titrate dose every 3 days in increments of 5-15 mg/day to a maximum of 40 mg daily

2-7 years: Initial: 20-30 mg daily divided every 8 hours; titrate dose every 3 days in increments of 5-15 mg/day to a maximum of 60 mg daily

≥8 years: 30-40 mg daily divided every 8 hours; titrate dose every 3 days in increments of 5-15 mg/day to a maximum of 120 mg daily

Note: Baclofen dose may need to be increased over time. One retrospective analysis (Lubsch, 2006) suggested that increased doses were needed as the time increased from spasticity onset, as age increased, and as the number of concomitant antispasticity medications increased. A small number of patients required daily doses exceeding 200 mg.

Spasticity in cerebral palsy (unlabeled use): Initial: 5-10 mg/day in 3 divided doses (Delgado, 2010)

Adults: 5 mg 3 times/day, may increase 5 mg/dose every 3 days to a maximum of 80 mg/day

Hiccups (unlabeled use): Usual effective dose: 10-20 mg 2-3 times/day

Intrathecal: Children and Adults:

Test dose: 50-100 mcg, doses >50 mcg should be given in 25 mcg increments, separated by 24 hours. A screening dose of 25 mcg may be considered in very small patients. Patients not responding to screening dose of 100 mcg should not be considered for chronic infusion/implanted pump.

Maintenance: After positive response to test dose, a maintenance intrathecal infusion can be administered via an implanted intrathecal pump. Initial dose via pump: Infusion at a 24-hour rate dosed at twice the test dose. Avoid abrupt discontinuation.

Elderly: Oral (the lowest effective dose is recommended): Initial: 5 mg 2-3 times/day, increasing gradually as needed; if benefits are not seen, withdraw the drug slowly.

Dosage adjustment in renal impairment: Oral: No dosage adjustment provided in the manufacturer's labeling. However, baclofen is primarily renally eliminated; use with caution; dosage reduction may be necessary.

Dosage adjustment in hepatic impairment: Oral: No dosage adjustment provided in the manufacturer's labeling.

Administration Intrathecal: For screening dosages, administer as a bolus injection (50 mcg/mL concentration) into the subarachnoid space, followed by maintenance infusion (500-2000 mcg/mL concentration).

Test Interactions Increased alkaline phosphatase, AST, glucose, ammonia (B); decreased bilirubin (S)

Dosage Forms Excipient information presented when available (limited, particularly for generics); consult specific product labeling.

Solution, Intrathecal:

Gablofen: 50 mcg/mL (1 mL)

Lioresal: 0.05 mg/mL (1 mL); 10 mg/20 mL (20 mL)

Solution, Intrathecal [preservative free]:
Gablofen: 10,000 mcg/20 mL (20 mL); 20,000 mcg/20 mL (20 mL); 40,000 mcg/20 mL (20 mL) [antioxidant free]
Lioresal: 10 mg/5 mL (5 mL); 40 mg/20 mL (20 mL) [antioxidant free, pyrogen free]
Tablet, Oral:
Generic: 10 mg, 20 mg

Extemporaneous Preparations A 5 mg/mL oral suspension may be made with tablets. Crush thirty 20 mg tablets in a mortar and reduce to a fine powder. Add a small amount of glycerin and mix to a uniform paste. Mix while adding Simple Syrup, NF in incremental proportions to **almost** 120 mL; transfer to a calibrated bottle, rinse mortar with vehicle, and add a sufficient quantity of vehicle to make 120 mL. Label "shake well" and "refrigerate". Stable for 35 days (Johnson, 1993).

A 10 mg/mL oral suspension may be made with tablets. Crush one-hundred-twenty 10 mg tablets in a mortar and reduce to a fine powder. Add small portions (60 mL) of a 1:1 mixture of Ora-Sweet® and Ora-Plus® and mix to a uniform paste; mix while adding the vehicle in incremental proportions to **almost** 120 mL; transfer to a calibrated bottle, rinse mortar with vehicle, and add quantity of vehicle sufficient to make 120 mL. Label "shake well" and "refrigerate". Stable for 60 days (Allen, 1996).

Allen LV Jr and Erickson MA 3rd, "Stability of Baclofen, Captopril, Diltiazem Hydrochloride, Dipyridamole, and Flecainide Acetate in Extemporaneously Compounded Oral Liquids," *Am J Health Syst Pharm*, 1996, 53(18):2179-84.

Johnson CE and Hart SM, "Stability of an Extemporaneously Compounded Baclofen Oral Liquid," *Am J Hosp Pharm*, 1993, 50 (11):2353-5.

◆ **Bactocill in Dextrose** *see* Oxacillin *on page 1523*
◆ **Bactrim** *see* Sulfamethoxazole and Trimethoprim *on page 1959*
◆ **Bactrim DS** *see* Sulfamethoxazole and Trimethoprim *on page 1959*
◆ **Bactroban** *see* Mupirocin *on page 1407*
◆ **Bactroban® (Can)** *see* Mupirocin *on page 1407*
◆ **Bactroban Nasal** *see* Mupirocin *on page 1407*
◆ **Baking Soda** *see* Sodium Bicarbonate *on page 1912*
◆ **BAL** *see* Dimercaprol *on page 617*
◆ **Bal in Oil** *see* Dimercaprol *on page 617*
◆ **Balmex® [OTC]** *see* Zinc Oxide *on page 2230*
◆ **Balminil Decongestant (Can)** *see* Pseudoephedrine *on page 1746*
◆ **Balminil DM D (Can)** *see* Pseudoephedrine and Dextromethorphan *on page 1748*
◆ **Balminil DM + Decongestant + Expectorant (Can)** *see* Guaifenesin, Pseudoephedrine, and Dextromethorphan *on page 979*
◆ **Balminil DM E (Can)** *see* Guaifenesin and Dextromethorphan *on page 976*
◆ **Balminil Expectorant (Can)** *see* GuaiFENesin *on page 974*

Balsalazide (bal SAL a zide)

Brand Names: U.S. Colazal; Giazo
Index Terms Balsalazide Disodium
Pharmacologic Category 5-Aminosalicylic Acid Derivative; Anti-inflammatory Agent
Use Treatment of mildly- to moderately-active ulcerative colitis
Giazo™: Only approved in males ≥18 years; effectiveness in females was not demonstrated
Pregnancy Risk Factor B

Pregnancy Considerations Teratogenic effects were not observed in animal reproduction studies. Mesalamine (5-aminosalicylic acid) is the active metabolite of balsalazide; mesalamine is known to cross the placenta.

Breast-Feeding Considerations Mesalamine, 5-aminosalicylic acid, is the active metabolite of balsalazide. Low levels of mesalamine enter breast milk; a case of bloody diarrhea in a breast-fed infant has been reported.

Contraindications Hypersensitivity to balsalazide or its metabolites, salicylates, or any component of the formulation

Warnings/Precautions Pyloric stenosis may prolong gastric retention of balsalazide. Renal toxicity and hepatic failure have been observed with other mesalamine (5-aminosalicylic acid) products; use with caution in patients with known renal or hepatic disease. Symptomatic worsening of ulcerative colitis may occur following initiation of treatment. May cause an acute intolerance syndrome (cramping, acute abdominal pain, bloody diarrhea; sometimes fever, headache, rash); discontinue if this occurs. May cause staining of teeth or tongue if capsule is opened and sprinkled on food.

Adverse Reactions
>10%:
Central nervous system: Headache (children 15%; adults 8%)
Gastrointestinal: Abdominal pain (children 12% to 13%; adults ≤6%)
1% to 10%:
Central nervous system: Insomnia (adults 2%), fatigue (children 4%; adults ≤2%), fever (children 6%; adults 2%)
Endocrine & metabolic: Dysmenorrhea (children 3%)
Gastrointestinal: Vomiting (children 10%; adults ≤4%), diarrhea (children 9%; adults ≤5%), ulcerative colitis exacerbation (children 6%; adults 1%), nausea (children 4%; adults 5%), hematochezia (children 4%), stomatitis (children 3%), anorexia (adults 2%), dyspepsia (adults 2%), flatulence (adults ≤2%), cramps (adults 1%), constipation (adults ≤1%), xerostomia (adults ≤1%)
Genitourinary: Urinary tract infection (adults 1% to 4%)
Hematologic: Anemia (4%)
Neuromuscular & skeletal: Arthralgia (adults ≤4%), musculoskeletal pain (adults 2%), myalgia (adults ≤1%)
Respiratory: Respiratory infection (adults ≤4%), cough (children 3%; adults 2%), pharyngitis (children 6%; adults 2%), pharyngolaryngeal pain (children 3%; adults 4%), rhinitis (adults 2%)
Miscellaneous: Flu-like syndrome (children 4%; adults 1%)
<1% (Limited to important or life-threatening): Alopecia, alveolitis, AST increased, back pain, blood pressure increased, cholestatic jaundice, cirrhosis, defecation urgency, dizziness, dyspnea, edema, erythema nodosum, facial edema, fever, gastroenteritis, gastroesophageal reflux, hard stool, heart rate increased, hepatocellular damage, hepatotoxicity, hyperbilirubinemia, hypersensitivity, interstitial nephritis, jaundice, Kawasaki-like syndrome, lethargy, liver failure, liver necrosis, liver function tests increased, malaise, myocarditis, pain, pancreatitis, pericarditis, pleural effusion, pneumonia (with and without eosinophilia), pruritus, rash, renal failure, vasculitis

Drug Interactions
Metabolism/Transport Effects None known.
Avoid Concomitant Use There are no known interactions where it is recommended to avoid concomitant use.
Increased Effect/Toxicity
Balsalazide may increase the levels/effects of: Heparin; Heparin (Low Molecular Weight); Thiopurine Analogs; Varicella Virus-Containing Vaccines

The levels/effects of Balsalazide may be increased by: Nonsteroidal Anti-Inflammatory Agents

Decreased Effect

Balsalazide may decrease the levels/effects of: Cardiac Glycosides

Storage/Stability Store at controlled room temperature of 20°C to 25°C (68°F to 77°F); excursions permitted to 15°C to 30°C (59°F to 86°F).

Mechanism of Action Balsalazide is a prodrug, converted by bacterial azoreduction to 5-aminosalicylic acid (mesalamine, active), 4-aminobenzoyl-β-alanine (inert), and their metabolites. 5-aminosalicylic acid may decrease inflammation by blocking the production of arachidonic acid metabolites topically in the colon mucosa.

Pharmacodynamics/Kinetics

Onset of action: Delayed; may require several days to weeks

Absorption: Very low and variable

Protein binding: Balsalazide: ≥99%

Metabolism: Azoreduced in the colon to 5-aminosalicylic acid (active), 4-aminobenzoyl-β-alanine (inert), and N-acetylated metabolites

Half-life elimination: Primary effect is topical (colonic mucosa); therapeutic effect appears not to be influenced by the systemic half-life of balsalazide (1.9 hours) or its metabolites (5-ASA [9.5 hours], N-Ac-5-ASA [10.4 hours])

Time to peak: Balsalazide: Capsule: 1-2 hours; Tablet: 0.5 hours

Excretion: Feces (65% as 5-aminosalicylic acid, 4-aminobenzoyl-β-alanine, and N-acetylated metabolites); urine (<16% as N-acetylated metabolites); Parent drug: Urine or feces (<1%)

Dosage Oral:

Capsule:

Children 5-17 years: 750 mg 3 times daily for up to 8 weeks **or** 2.25 g (three 750 mg capsules) 3 times daily for up to 8 weeks

Adults: 2.25 g (three 750 mg capsules) 3 times daily for up to 8-12 weeks

Tablet (Giazo™): Adults: Males: 3.3 g (three 1.1 g tablets) twice daily for up to 8 weeks

Elderly: Refer to adult dosing.

Dosage adjustment in renal impairment: No dosage adjustment provided in manufacturer's labeling. Renal toxicity has been observed with other 5-aminosalicylic acid products; use with caution.

Dosage adjustment in hepatic impairment: No dosage adjustment provided in manufacturer's labeling.

Dietary Considerations Some products may contain sodium. Take tablets with or without food.

Administration

Capsule: Should be swallowed whole or may be opened and sprinkled on applesauce. Applesauce mixture may be chewed; swallow immediately, do not store mixture for later use. When sprinkled on food, may cause staining of teeth or tongue.

Tablet: Administer with or without food.

Monitoring Parameters Improvement or worsening of symptoms; renal function (prior to initiation, then periodically); liver function tests

Additional Information Balsalazide 750 mg is equivalent to mesalamine 267 mg

Dosage Forms Excipient information presented when available (limited, particularly for generics); consult specific product labeling.

Capsule, Oral, as disodium:

Colazal: 750 mg

Generic: 750 mg

Tablet, Oral:

Giazo: 1.1 g

◆ **Balsalazide Disodium** *see* Balsalazide *on page 223*

◆ **Balsam Peru, Castor Oil, and Trypsin** *see* Trypsin, Balsam Peru, and Castor Oil *on page 2133*

◆ **Balziva** *see* Ethinyl Estradiol and Norethindrone *on page 793*

◆ **Banophen [OTC]** *see* DiphenhydrAMINE (Systemic) *on page 622*

◆ **Banzel** *see* Rufinamide *on page 1865*

◆ **Banzel™ (Can)** *see* Rufinamide *on page 1865*

◆ **Baraclude** *see* Entecavir *on page 711*

◆ **Baraclude® (Can)** *see* Entecavir *on page 711*

◆ **Baridium [OTC]** *see* Phenazopyridine *on page 1627*

◆ **Basaljel® (Can)** *see* Aluminum Hydroxide *on page 89*

◆ **Base Ointment** *see* Zinc Oxide *on page 2230*

Basiliximab (ba si LIK si mab)

Brand Names: U.S. Simulect

Brand Names: Canada Simulect®

Pharmacologic Category Immunosuppressant Agent; Monoclonal Antibody

Use Prophylaxis of acute organ rejection in renal transplantation (in combination with cyclosporine and corticosteroids)

Unlabeled Use Treatment of refractory acute graft-versus-host disease (GVHD); prevention of liver or cardiac transplant rejection

Pregnancy Risk Factor B

Pregnancy Considerations Teratogenic effects were not observed in animal studies. IL-2 receptors play an important role in the development of the immune system. Use in pregnant women only when benefit exceeds potential risk to the fetus. Women of childbearing potential should use effective contraceptive measures before beginning treatment and for 4 months after completion of therapy with this agent. The National Transplantation Pregnancy Registry (NTPR, Temple University) is a registry for pregnant women taking immunosuppressants following any solid organ transplant. The NTPR encourages reporting of all immunosuppressant exposures during pregnancy in transplant recipients at 877-955-6877.

Breast-Feeding Considerations It is not known whether basiliximab is excreted in human milk. Because many immunoglobulins are secreted in milk and the potential for serious adverse reactions exists, a decision should be made whether to discontinue nursing or discontinue the drug, taking into account the importance of the drug to the mother.

Contraindications Hypersensitivity to basiliximab or any component of the formulation

Warnings/Precautions To be used as a component of an immunosuppressive regimen which includes cyclosporine and corticosteroids. The incidence of lymphoproliferative disorders and/or opportunistic infections may be increased by immunosuppressive therapy. Severe hypersensitivity reactions, occurring within 24 hours, have been reported. Reactions, including anaphylaxis, have occurred both with the initial exposure and/or following re-exposure after several months. Use caution during re-exposure to a subsequent course of therapy in a patient who has previously received basiliximab; patients in whom concomitant immunosuppression was prematurely discontinued due to abandoned transplantation or early graft loss are at increased risk for developing a severe hypersensitivity reaction upon re-exposure. Discontinue permanently if a severe reaction occurs. Medications for the treatment of hypersensitivity reactions should be available for immediate use. Treatment may result in the development of human antimurine antibodies (HAMA); however, limited evidence suggesting the use of muromonab-CD3 or other murine products is not precluded. **[U.S. Boxed Warning]: Should be administered under the supervision of a physician experienced in immunosuppression therapy and organ transplant management.** In renal transplant patients receiving basiliximab plus prednisone, cyclosporine, and mycophenolate, new-onset diabetes, glucose intolerance, and impaired fasting glucose were observed at rates significantly higher than observed in patients receiving prednisone, cyclosporine, and mycophenolate without basiliximab (Aasebo, 2010).

Adverse Reactions Administration of basiliximab did not appear to increase the incidence or severity of adverse effects in clinical trials. Adverse events were reported in 96% of both the placebo and basiliximab groups.

>10%:

Cardiovascular: Hypertension, peripheral edema

Central nervous system: Fever, headache, insomnia, pain

Dermatologic: Acne, wound complications

Endocrine & metabolic: Hypercholesterolemia, hyperglycemia, hyper-/hypokalemia, hyperuricemia, hypophosphatemia

Gastrointestinal: Abdominal pain, constipation, diarrhea, dyspepsia, nausea, vomiting

Genitourinary: Urinary tract infection

Hematologic: Anemia

Neuromuscular & skeletal: Tremor

Respiratory: Dyspnea, infection (upper respiratory)

Miscellaneous: Viral infection

3% to 10%:

Cardiovascular: Abnormal heart sounds, angina, arrhythmia, atrial fibrillation, chest pain, generalized edema, heart failure, hypotension, tachycardia

Central nervous system: Agitation, anxiety, depression, dizziness, fatigue, hypoesthesia, malaise

Dermatologic: Cyst, hypertrichosis, pruritus, rash, skin disorder, skin ulceration

Endocrine & metabolic: Acidosis, dehydration, diabetes mellitus, fluid overload, glucocorticoids increased, hyper-/hypocalcemia, hyperlipemia, hypertriglyceridemia, hypoglycemia, hypomagnesemia, hyponatremia, hypoproteinemia

Gastrointestinal: Abdomen enlarged, esophagitis, flatulence, gastroenteritis, GI hemorrhage, gingival hyperplasia, melena, moniliasis, stomatitis (including ulcerative), weight gain

Genitourinary: Bladder disorder, dysuria, genital edema (male), impotence, ureteral disorder, urinary frequency, urinary retention

Hematologic: Hematoma, hemorrhage, leukopenia, polycythemia, purpura, thrombocytopenia, thrombosis

Neuromuscular & skeletal: Arthralgia, arthropathy, back pain, cramps, fracture, hernia, leg pain, myalgia, neuropathy, paresthesia, rigors, weakness

Ocular: Abnormal vision, cataract, conjunctivitis

Renal: Albuminuria, hematuria, nonprotein nitrogen increased, oliguria, renal function abnormal, renal tubular necrosis

Respiratory: Bronchitis, bronchospasm, cough, pharyngitis, pneumonia, pulmonary edema, rhinitis, sinusitis

Miscellaneous: Accidental trauma, cytomegalovirus (CMV) infection, herpes infection (simplex and zoster), infection, sepsis

Postmarketing and/or case reports: Anaphylaxis, capillary leak syndrome, cytokine release syndrome, diabetes (new onset), fasting glucose impaired, glucose intolerance, hypersensitivity reaction (including heart failure, hypotension, tachycardia, bronchospasm, dyspnea, pulmonary edema, respiratory failure, sneezing, pruritus, rash, urticaria), lymphoproliferative disease

Drug Interactions

Metabolism/Transport Effects None known.

Avoid Concomitant Use

Avoid concomitant use of Basiliximab with any of the following: BCG; Belimumab; Natalizumab; Pimecrolimus; Tacrolimus (Topical); Tofacitinib; Vaccines (Live)

Increased Effect/Toxicity

Basiliximab may increase the levels/effects of: Belimumab; Hypoglycemic Agents; Leflunomide; Natalizumab; Tofacitinib; Vaccines (Live)

The levels/effects of Basiliximab may be increased by: Abciximab; Denosumab; Herbs (Hypoglycemic Properties); MAO Inhibitors; Pimecrolimus; Roflumilast; Salicylates; Selective Serotonin Reuptake Inhibitors; Tacrolimus (Topical); Trastuzumab

Decreased Effect

Basiliximab may decrease the levels/effects of: BCG; Coccidioidin Skin Test; Sipuleucel-T; Vaccines (Inactivated); Vaccines (Live)

The levels/effects of Basiliximab may be decreased by: Echinacea; Loop Diuretics

Ethanol/Nutrition/Herb Interactions Herb/Nutraceutical: Echinacea may diminish the therapeutic effect of basiliximab. Avoid hypoglycemic herbs, including alfalfa, bilberry, bitter melon, burdock, celery, damiana, fenugreek, garcinia, garlic, ginger, ginseng, gymnema, marshmallow, and stinging nettle (may enhance the hypoglycemic effect of basiliximab).

Preparation for Administration Reconstitute with preservative-free sterile water for injection (reconstitute 10 mg vial with 2.5 mL, 20 mg vial with 5 mL). Shake gently to dissolve. May further dilute reconstituted solution with 25 mL (10 mg) or 50 mL (20 mg) 0.9% sodium chloride or dextrose 5% in water. When mixing the solution, gently invert the bag to avoid foaming. Do not shake solutions diluted for infusion.

Storage/Stability Store intact vials refrigerated at 2°C to 8°C (36°F to 46°F). Should be used immediately after reconstitution; however, if not used immediately, reconstituted solution may be stored at 2°C to 8°C for up to 24 hours or at room temperature for up to 4 hours. Discard the reconstituted solution if not used within 24 hours.

Mechanism of Action Chimeric (murine/human) immunosuppressant monoclonal antibody which blocks the alpha-chain of the interleukin-2 (IL-2) receptor complex; this receptor is expressed on activated T lymphocytes and is a critical pathway for activating cell-mediated allograft rejection

Pharmacodynamics/Kinetics

Duration: Mean: 36 days (determined by IL-2R alpha saturation)

Distribution: Mean: V_d: Children 1-11 years: 4.8 ± 2.1 L; Adolescents 12-16 years: 7.8 ± 5.1 L; Adults: 8.6 ± 4.1 L

Half-life elimination: Children 1-11 years: 9.5 days; Adolescents 12-16 years: 9.1 days; Adults: Mean: 7.2 days

Dosage Note: Patients previously administered basiliximab should only be re-exposed to a subsequent course of therapy with extreme caution.

I.V.:

Children <35 kg: Acute renal transplant rejection prophylaxis: 10 mg within 2 hours prior to transplant surgery, followed by a second 10 mg dose 4 days after transplantation; the second dose should be withheld if complications occur (including severe hypersensitivity reactions or graft loss)

Children ≥35 kg and Adults: Acute renal transplant rejection prophylaxis: 20 mg within 2 hours prior to transplant surgery, followed by a second 20 mg dose 4 days after transplantation; the second dose should be withheld if complications occur (including severe hypersensitivity reactions or graft loss)

Adults:

Acute cardiac transplant rejection prophylaxis (unlabeled use): 20 mg on the day of transplant, followed by a second dose 4 days after transplantation (Mehra, 2005); usually given within the first hour postoperatively

Acute liver transplant rejection prophylaxis (unlabeled use): 20 mg within 6 hours of organ reperfusion, followed by a second 20 mg dose 4 days after transplantation (Neuhaus, 2002)

Treatment of refractory acute GVHD (unlabeled use): 20 mg on days 1 and 4; may repeat for recurrent acute GVHD (Schmidt-Hieber, 2005)

Dosage adjustment in renal impairment: No dosage adjustment provided in manufacturer's labeling.

Dosage adjustment in hepatic impairment: No dosage adjustment provided in manufacturer's labeling.

Administration For intravenous administration only. Infuse as a bolus or I.V. infusion over 20-30 minutes. (Bolus dosing is associated with nausea, vomiting, and local pain at the injection site.) Administer only after assurance that patient will receive renal graft and immunosuppression. For the treatment of acute GVHD (unlabeled use), the dose was diluted in 250 mL NS and administered over 30 minutes (Schmidt-Hieber, 2005).

Monitoring Parameters Signs and symptoms of acute rejection; hypersensitivity, infection

Dosage Forms Excipient information presented when available (limited, particularly for generics); consult specific product labeling.

Solution Reconstituted, Intravenous [preservative free]:

Simulect: 10 mg (1 ea); 20 mg (1 ea)

- ◆ BAY 43-9006 *see* SORAfenib *on page 1938*
- ◆ BAY 59-7939 *see* Rivaroxaban *on page 1838*
- ◆ BAY 63-2521 *see* Riociguat *on page 1822*
- ◆ BAY 73-4506 *see* Regorafenib *on page 1793*
- ◆ Baycadron *see* Dexamethasone (Systemic) *on page 580*
- ◆ Bayer® Aspirin Extra Strength [OTC] *see* Aspirin *on page 177*
- ◆ Bayer® Aspirin Regimen Adult Low Strength [OTC] *see* Aspirin *on page 177*
- ◆ Bayer® Aspirin Regimen Children's [OTC] *see* Aspirin *on page 177*
- ◆ Bayer® Aspirin Regimen Regular Strength [OTC] *see* Aspirin *on page 177*
- ◆ Bayer® Genuine Aspirin [OTC] *see* Aspirin *on page 177*
- ◆ Bayer® Plus Extra Strength [OTC] *see* Aspirin *on page 177*
- ◆ Bayer® PM [OTC] *see* Aspirin and Diphenhydramine *on page 182*
- ◆ Bayer® Women's Low Dose Aspirin [OTC] *see* Aspirin *on page 177*
- ◆ Baza Antifungal [OTC] *see* Miconazole (Topical) *on page 1358*
- ◆ Baza® Clear [OTC] *see* Vitamin A and Vitamin D (Topical) *on page 2202*
- ◆ Bazedoxifene and Estrogens (Conjugated/Equine) *see* Estrogens (Conjugated/Equine) and Bazedoxifene *on page 765*
- ◆ B-Caro-T [OTC] *see* Beta-Carotene *on page 246*

BCG (bee see jee)

Brand Names: U.S. TheraCys; Tice BCG

Brand Names: Canada BCG Vaccine; ImmuCyst®; Oncotice™

Index Terms Bacillus Calmette-Guérin (BCG) Live; BCG Vaccine U.S.P. *(percutaneous use product)*; BCG, Live

Pharmacologic Category Biological Response Modulator; Vaccine, Live (Bacterial)

Additional Appendix Information

Immunization Administration Recommendations *on page 2334*

Immunization Recommendations *on page 2339*

Use

BCG intravesical: Treatment and prophylaxis of carcinoma *in situ* of the bladder; prophylaxis of primary or recurrent superficial or minimally invasive papillary tumors following transurethral resection

BCG vaccine: Immunization against *Mycobacterium tuberculosis* in persons not previously infected and who are at high risk for exposure

BCG vaccine is not routinely administered for the prevention of *M. tuberculosis* in the United States. The Advisory Committee on Immunization Practices (ACIP) recommends vaccination be considered for the following:

- Children with a negative tuberculin skin test who are continually exposed to (and cannot be separated from) adults who are untreated or ineffectively treated for TB disease when the child cannot be given long-term treatment for infection **or** if the adult has TB caused by strains resistant to isoniazid and rifampin.
- Healthcare workers with a high percentage of patients with *M. tuberculosis* strains resistant to both isoniazid and rifampin, if there is ongoing transmission of the resistant strains and subsequent infection is likely, or if comprehensive infection-control precautions have not been successful. In addition, healthcare workers should be counseled on the risks and benefits of vaccination and treatment of latent TB infection

Pregnancy Risk Factor C

Dosage

Immunization against tuberculosis: Percutaneous: **Note:** Initial lesion usually appears after 10-14 days consisting of small, red papule at injection site and reaches maximum diameter of 3 mm in 4-6 weeks.

Children <1 month: 0.2-0.3 mL (half-strength dilution). Administer tuberculin test (5 TU) after 2-3 months; repeat vaccination after 1 year of age for negative tuberculin test if indications persist.

Children >1 month and Adults: 0.2-0.3 mL (full strength dilution); conduct postvaccinal tuberculin test (5 TU of PPD) in 2-3 months; if test is negative, repeat vaccination.

Immunotherapy for bladder cancer: Intravesicular: Adults: **Note:** Treatment should begin 7-14 days after biopsy or TUR. The contents of one vial is used for each dose.

TheraCys®: One dose instilled into bladder (retain for 2 hours) once weekly for 6 weeks followed by 1 treatment at 3, 6, 12, 18, and 24 months after initial treatment

TICE® BCG: One dose instilled into the bladder (retain for 2 hours) once weekly for 6 weeks (may repeat cycle 1 time) followed by approximately once monthly for at least 6-12 months

Dosage adjustment in renal impairment: No dosage adjustment provided in manufacturer's labeling.

Dosage adjustment in hepatic impairment: No dosage adjustment provided in manufacturer's labeling.

Additional Information Complete prescribing information should be consulted for additional detail.

Dosage Forms Excipient information presented when available (limited, particularly for generics); consult specific product labeling.

Injectable, Injection:

Generic: 50 mg (1 ea)

Suspension Reconstituted, Intravesical:

Tice BCG: 50 mg (1 ea)

Suspension Reconstituted, Intravesical [preservative free]:
TheraCys: 81 mg (1 ea) [contains monosodium glutamate (sodium glutamate)]

- **BCG, Live** *see* BCG *on page 226*
- **BCG Vaccine (Can)** *see* BCG *on page 226*
- **BCG Vaccine U.S.P.** *(percutaneous use product) see* BCG *on page 226*
- **BCNU** *see* Carmustine *on page 352*
- **beano® [OTC]** *see* Alpha-Galactosidase *on page 80*
- **beano® Meltaways [OTC]** *see* Alpha-Galactosidase *on page 80*
- **Bebulin VH** *see* Factor IX Complex (Human) [(Factors II, IX, X)] *on page 822*

Becaplermin (be KAP ler min)

Brand Names: U.S. Regranex

Index Terms Recombinant Human Platelet-Derived Growth Factor B; rPDGF-BB

Pharmacologic Category Growth Factor, Platelet-Derived; Topical Skin Product

Use Adjunctive treatment of diabetic neuropathic ulcers occurring on the lower limbs and feet that extend into subcutaneous tissue (or beyond) and have adequate blood supply

Pregnancy Risk Factor C

Dosage Topical: Adults: Diabetic ulcers: Apply appropriate amount of gel once daily with a cotton swab or similar tool, as a coating over the ulcer. The amount of becaplermin to be applied will vary depending on the size of the ulcer area.

Note: If the ulcer does not decrease in size by ~30% after 10 weeks of treatment or complete healing has not occurred in 20 weeks, continued treatment with becaplermin gel should be reassessed.

To calculate the length of gel applied to the ulcer, measure the greatest length of the ulcer by the greatest width of the ulcer. Tube size and unit of measure will determine the formula used in the calculation. Recalculate amount of gel needed every 1-2 weeks, depending on the rate of change in ulcer area.

Centimeters:

15 g tube: [ulcer length (cm) x width (cm)] divided by 4 = length of gel (cm)

2 g tube: [ulcer length (cm) x width (cm)] divided by 2 = length of gel (cm)

Inches:

15 g tube: [length (in) x width (in)] x 0.6 = length of gel (in)

2 g tube: [length (in) x width (in)] x 1.3 = length of gel (in)

Additional Information Complete prescribing information should be consulted for additional detail.

Dosage Forms Excipient information presented when available (limited, particularly for generics); consult specific product labeling.

Gel, External:

Regranex: 0.01% (15 g) [contains metacresol, methylparaben, propylparaben]

Beclomethasone (Systemic)
(be kloe METH a sone)

Brand Names: U.S. Qvar

Brand Names: Canada QVAR®

Index Terms Vanceril

Pharmacologic Category Corticosteroid, Inhalant (Oral)

Additional Appendix Information

Inhaled Corticosteroids *on page 2298*

Use Oral inhalation: Maintenance and prophylactic treatment of asthma; includes those who require corticosteroids and those who may benefit from a dose reduction/elimination of systemically-administered corticosteroids. Not for relief of acute bronchospasm.

Pregnancy Risk Factor C

Pregnancy Considerations Adverse events were observed in some animal reproduction studies. Hypoadrenalism may occur in newborns following maternal use of corticosteroids in pregnancy. Based on available data, an overall increased risk of congenital malformations or a decrease in fetal growth has not been associated with maternal use of inhaled corticosteroids during pregnancy (Bakhireva, 2005; NAEPP, 2005; Namazy, 2004). Uncontrolled asthma is associated with adverse events in pregnancy (increased risk of perinatal mortality, pre-eclampsia, preterm birth, low birth weight infants). Inhaled corticosteroids are recommended for the treatment of asthma during pregnancy (most information available using budesonide) (ACOG, 2008; NAEPP, 2005).

Breast-Feeding Considerations Other corticosteroids have been found in breast milk; however, information for beclomethasone is not available. Due to the potential for serious adverse reactions in the nursing infant, the manufacturer recommends a decision be made whether to discontinue nursing or to discontinue the drug, taking into account the importance of treatment to the mother. Use of inhaled corticosteroids is not a contraindication to breast-feeding (NAEPP, 2005).

Contraindications Hypersensitivity to beclomethasone or any component of the formulation; status asthmaticus, or other acute asthma episodes requiring intensive measures

Canadian labeling: Additional contraindications (not in U.S. labeling): Moderate-to-severe bronchiectasis requiring intensive measures; untreated fungal, bacterial, or tubercular infections of the respiratory tract

Warnings/Precautions May cause hypercorticism or suppression of hypothalamic-pituitary-adrenal (HPA) axis, particularly in younger children or in patients receiving high doses for prolonged periods. HPA axis suppression may lead to adrenal crisis. Withdrawal and discontinuation of a corticosteroid should be done slowly and carefully. Particular care is required when patients are transferred from systemic corticosteroids to inhaled products due to possible adrenal insufficiency or withdrawal from steroids, including an increase in allergic symptoms. Patients receiving >20 mg per day of prednisone (or equivalent) may be most susceptible. Fatalities have occurred due to adrenal insufficiency in asthmatic patients during and after transfer from systemic corticosteroids to aerosol steroids; aerosol steroids do **not** provide the systemic steroid needed to treat patients having trauma, surgery, or infections.

Bronchospasm may occur with wheezing after inhalation; if this occurs, stop steroid and treat with a fast-acting bronchodilator. Supplemental steroids (oral or parenteral) may be needed during stress or severe asthma attacks. Not to be used in status asthmaticus or for the relief of acute bronchospasm. Corticosteroid use may cause psychiatric disturbances, including depression, euphoria, insomnia, mood swings, and personality changes. Pre-existing psychiatric conditions may be exacerbated by corticosteroid use. Prolonged use of corticosteroids may also increase the incidence of secondary infection, mask acute infection (including fungal infections), prolong or exacerbate viral infections, or limit response to vaccines. Avoid use in patients with ocular herpes or untreated viral, fungal, parasitic or bacterial systemic infections (Canadian labeling contraindicates use with untreated respiratory infections).

Exposure to chickenpox should be avoided. Close observation is required in patients with latent tuberculosis and/or TB reactivity; restrict use in active TB (only in conjunction with antituberculosis treatment). Prolonged treatment with corticosteroids has been associated with the development of Kaposi's sarcoma (case reports); if noted, discontinuation of therapy should be considered.

Use with caution in patients with thyroid disease, hepatic impairment, renal impairment, cardiovascular disease, diabetes, glaucoma, cataracts, myasthenia gravis, patients at risk for osteoporosis, patients at risk for seizures, or GI diseases (diverticulitis, peptic ulcer, ulcerative colitis) due to perforation risk. Use caution following acute MI (corticosteroids have been associated with myocardial rupture). Because of the risk of adverse effects, systemic corticosteroids should be used cautiously in the elderly in the smallest possible effective dose for the shortest duration.

Orally-inhaled corticosteroids may cause a reduction in growth velocity in pediatric patients (~1 centimeter per year [range: 0.3-1.8 cm per year] and related to dose and duration of exposure). To minimize the systemic effects of orally-inhaled corticosteroids, each patient should be titrated to the lowest effective dose. Growth should be routinely monitored in pediatric patients. Safety and efficacy have not been established in children <5 years of age. There have been reports of systemic corticosteroid withdrawal symptoms (eg, joint/muscle pain, lassitude, depression) when withdrawing oral inhalation therapy.

Adverse Reactions

>10%: Central nervous system: Headache (12%)

1% to 10%:

- Central nervous system: Dysphonia (1% to 3%), pain (2%)
- Endocrine & metabolic: Dysmenorrhea (1% to 3%)
- Gastrointestinal: Nausea (1%)
- Neuromuscular & skeletal: Back pain (1%)
- Respiratory: Upper respiratory tract infection (9%), pharyngitis (8%), rhinitis (6%), sinusitis (3%), cough (1% to 3%)

<1% (Limited to important or life-threatening): Anaphylactic/anaphylactoid reactions; growth velocity reduction in children/adolescents; HPA function suppression; immediate and delayed hypersensitivity reactions (angioedema, bronchospasm, rash, urticaria); psychiatric and behavioral changes (such as aggressiveness, depression, sleep disturbances, psychomotor hyperactivity, suicidal ideation; more common in children); rarely glaucoma, increased intraocular pressure, and cataracts have been reported with inhaled corticosteroids

Drug Interactions

Metabolism/Transport Effects None known.

Avoid Concomitant Use

Avoid concomitant use of Beclomethasone (Oral Inhalation) with any of the following: Aldesleukin; BCG; Natalizumab; Pimecrolimus; Tacrolimus (Topical); Tofacitinib

Increased Effect/Toxicity

Beclomethasone (Oral Inhalation) may increase the levels/effects of: Amphotericin B; Deferasirox; Leflunomide; Loop Diuretics; Natalizumab; Thiazide Diuretics; Tofacitinib

The levels/effects of Beclomethasone (Oral Inhalation) may be increased by: Denosumab; Pimecrolimus; Tacrolimus (Topical); Telaprevir; Trastuzumab

Decreased Effect

Beclomethasone (Oral Inhalation) may decrease the levels/effects of: Aldesleukin; Antidiabetic Agents; BCG; Coccidioidin Skin Test; Corticorelin; Hyaluronidase; Sipuleucel-T; Telaprevir; Vaccines (Inactivated)

The levels/effects of Beclomethasone (Oral Inhalation) may be decreased by: Echinacea

Storage/Stability Do not store near heat or open flame. Do not puncture canisters. Store at 25°C (77°F); excursions permitted between 15°C to 30°C (59°F to 86°F). Rest QVAR® on concave end of canister with actuator on top.

Mechanism of Action Controls the rate of protein synthesis; depresses the migration of polymorphonuclear leukocytes, fibroblasts; reverses capillary permeability and lysosomal stabilization at the cellular level to prevent or control inflammation

Pharmacodynamics/Kinetics

Onset of action: Therapeutic effect: 1-4 weeks

Absorption: Readily; quickly hydrolyzed by pulmonary esterases to active metabolite (beclomethasone-17-monoproprionate [17-BMP]) during absorption

Protein binding: 17-BMP: 94% to 96%

Metabolism: Pro-drug; undergoes rapid conversion to 17-BMP during absorption; followed by additional metabolism via CYP3A4 to other, less active metabolites (beclomethasone-21-monopropionate [21-BMP] and beclomethasone [BOH])

Half-life elimination: 17-BMP: 3 hours

Time to peak, plasma: Oral inhalation: BDP: 0.5 hours; 17-BMP: 0.7 hours

Excretion: Mainly in feces; urine (<10%)

Dosage Inhalation, oral: Asthma (doses should be titrated to the lowest effective dose once asthma is controlled):

U.S. labeling:

- Children 5-11 years: Initial: 40 mcg twice daily; maximum dose: 80 mcg twice daily
- Children ≥12 years and Adults:
  - Patients previously on bronchodilators only: Initial dose 40-80 mcg twice daily; maximum dose: 320 mcg twice day
  - Patients previously on inhaled corticosteroids: Initial dose 40-160 mcg twice daily; maximum dose: 320 mcg twice daily
- NIH Asthma Guidelines (NIH, 2007):
  - Children 5-11 years:
    - "Low" dose: 80-160 mcg/day
    - "Medium" dose: >160-320 mcg/day
    - "High" dose: >320 mcg/day
  - Children ≥12 years and Adults:
    - "Low" dose: 80-240 mcg/day
    - "Medium" dose: >240-480 mcg/day
    - "High" dose: >480 mcg/day

Canadian labeling:

- Children 5-11 years: Initial: 50 mcg twice daily; maximum dose: 100 mcg twice daily
- Children ≥12 years and Adults:
  - Mild asthma: 50-100 mcg twice daily; maximum dose: 100 mcg twice daily
  - Moderate asthma: 100-250 mcg twice daily; maximum dose: 250 mcg twice daily
  - Severe asthma: 300-400 mcg twice daily; maximum dose: 400 mcg twice daily

Conversion from oral systemic corticosteroid to orally inhaled corticosteroid: Initiation of oral inhalation therapy should begin in patients whose asthma is reasonably stabilized on oral corticosteroids (OCS). A gradual dose reduction of OCS should begin ~7 days after starting inhaled therapy. U.S. labeling recommends reducing prednisone dose no more rapidly than ≤2.5 mg/day (or equivalent of other OCS) every 1-2 weeks. The Canadian labeling recommends decreasing the daily dose of prednisone by 1 mg (or equivalent of other OCS) every 7 days or more in closely monitored patients. If adrenal insufficiency occurs, temporarily increase the OCS dose and follow with a more gradual withdrawal. **Note:** When transitioning from systemic to inhaled corticosteroids, supplemental systemic corticosteroid therapy may be necessary during periods of stress or during severe asthma attacks.

Administration Canister does not need shaken prior to use. Prime canister by spraying twice into the air prior to initial use or if not in use for >10 days. Avoid spraying in face or eyes. Exhale fully prior to bringing inhaler to mouth. Place inhaler in mouth, close lips around mouthpiece, and inhale slowly and deeply. Remove inhaler and hold breath for approximately 5-10 seconds. Rinse mouth and throat after use to prevent *Candida* infection. Do not wash or put inhaler in water; mouth piece may be cleaned with a dry tissue or cloth. Discard after the "discard by" date or after labeled number of doses has been used, even if container is not completely empty. Patients using a spacer should inhale immediately due to decreased amount of medication that is delivered with a delayed inspiration.

Monitoring Parameters Growth (adolescents) and signs/symptoms of HPA axis suppression/adrenal insufficiency; signs/symptoms of oral candidiasis; ocular effects (eg, cataracts, increased intraocular pressure, glaucoma)

Additional Information Effects of inhaled steroids on growth have been observed in the absence of laboratory evidence of HPA axis suppression, suggesting that growth velocity is a more sensitive indicator of systemic corticosteroid exposure in pediatric patients than some commonly used tests of HPA axis function. The long-term effects of this reduction in growth velocity associated with orally-inhaled corticosteroids, including the impact on final adult height, are unknown. The potential for "catch up" growth following discontinuation of treatment with inhaled corticosteroids has not been adequately studied.

Dosage Forms Considerations

QVAR 8.7 g canisters contain 120 inhalations.

Dosage Forms Excipient information presented when available (limited, particularly for generics); consult specific product labeling.

Aerosol Solution, Inhalation, as dipropionate:

Qvar: 40 mcg/actuation (8.7 g); 80 mcg/actuation (8.7 g)

Dosage Forms: Canada Excipient information presented when available (limited, particularly for generics); consult specific product labeling.

Aerosol, for oral inhalation, as dipropionate:

QVAR™: 50 mcg/inhalation (6.5 g) [chlorofluorocarbon free; contains ethanol; 100 metered actuations]

QVAR™: 50 mcg/inhalation (12.4 g) [chlorofluorocarbon free; contains ethanol; 200 metered actuations]

QVAR™: 100 mcg/inhalation (6.5 g) [chlorofluorocarbon free; contains ethanol; 100 metered actuations]

QVAR™: 100 mcg/inhalation (12.4 g) [chlorofluorocarbon free; contains ethanol; 200 metered actuations]

Beclomethasone (Nasal) (be kloe METH a sone)

Brand Names: U.S. Beconase AQ; Qnasl

Brand Names: Canada Apo-Beclomethasone®; Mylan-Beclo AQ; Nu-Beclomethasone; Rivanase AQ

Index Terms Beclomethasone Dipropionate

Pharmacologic Category Corticosteroid, Nasal

Additional Appendix Information

Inhaled Corticosteroids *on page 2298*

Use

Beconase AQ®: Symptomatic treatment of seasonal or perennial allergic rhinitis; nonallergic (vasomotor) rhinitis; prevent recurrence of nasal polyps following surgery

Qnasl™: Symptomatic treatment of seasonal or perennial allergic rhinitis

Unlabeled Use Adjunct to antibiotics in empiric treatment of acute bacterial rhinosinusitis (ABRS) (Chow, 2012)

Pregnancy Risk Factor C

Dosage Inhalation, nasal:

Children 6-11 years (Beconase® AQ): Rhinitis, nasal polyps (postsurgical prophylaxis): Initial: One inhalation each nostril twice daily (total dose: 168 mcg/day); if response inadequate, may increase to 2 inhalations each nostril twice daily (total dose: 336 mcg/day)

Children ≥12 years and Adults:

Beconase® AQ: Rhinitis, nasal polyps (postsurgical prophylaxis): 1-2 inhalations each nostril twice daily; total dose: 168-336 mcg/day

Qnasl™: Allergic rhinitis: Two inhalations each nostril once daily; total dose: 320 mcg/day

Dosage adjustment in renal impairment: No dosage adjustment provided in manufacturer's labeling.

Dosage adjustment in hepatic impairment: No dosage adjustment provided in manufacturer's labeling.

Additional Information Complete prescribing information should be consulted for additional detail.

Dosage Forms Considerations

Beconase AQ 25 g bottles contain 180 sprays.

Qnasl 8.7 g bottles contain 120 actuations.

Dosage Forms Excipient information presented when available (limited, particularly for generics); consult specific product labeling.

Aerosol Solution, Nasal, as dipropionate:

Qnasl: 80 mcg/actuation (8.7 g)

Suspension, Nasal, as dipropionate:

Beconase AQ: 42 mcg/spray (25 g) [contains benzalkonium chloride]

◆ **Beclomethasone Dipropionate** *see* Beclomethasone (Nasal) *on page 229*

◆ **Beconase AQ** *see* Beclomethasone (Nasal) *on page 229*

Bedaquiline (bed AK wi leen)

Brand Names: U.S. Sirturo

Index Terms AIDS222089; R207910; TMC207

Pharmacologic Category Antitubercular Agent

Use Multidrug-resistant tuberculosis: Treatment of pulmonary multidrug-resistant tuberculosis (MDR-TB) in combination therapy in adults (≥18 years of age) when other alternatives are not available

Pregnancy Risk Factor B

Pregnancy Considerations Adverse events were not observed in animal reproduction studies.

Breast-Feeding Considerations It is not known if bedaquiline is excreted into breast milk. Due to the potential for serious adverse reactions in the nursing infant, a decision should be made whether to discontinue nursing or to discontinue the drug, taking into account the importance of treatment to the mother.

Medication Guide Available Yes

Contraindications There are no contraindications listed within the manufacturer's labeling.

Warnings/Precautions [U.S. Boxed Warning]: May prolong QT_c interval. Use with drugs that prolong the QT_c interval may cause additive prolongation. Monitor ECG weekly with concurrent administration of other medications known to prolong the QT_c interval (including fluoroquinolones, macrolide antibiotics or clofazimine) or in patients with a history of torsade de pointes, congenital long QT syndrome, bradyarrhythmias, hypothyroidism, uncompensated heart failure, and low serum electrolyte levels (CDC, 2013). Baseline potassium, calcium and magnesium should be obtained and corrected, if abnormal. Also evaluate serum electrolytes if QT prolongation is detected during therapy. Discontinue therapy if patient develops confirmed QT_cF interval of >500 ms or ventricular arrhythmia and monitor ECG to confirm return to baseline. If patient experiences syncope, obtain ECG to assess potential QT_c prolongation.

Increased risk of hepatic reactions; avoid alcohol intake and other known hepatotoxic drugs, especially in patients with low hepatic reserve. Monitor AST, ALT, alkaline phosphatase, and bilirubin at baseline and monthly during therapy. Monitor more frequently if patient has underlying hepatic disease or is receiving concomitant hepatotoxic drugs (CDC, 2013). Further evaluate patients with evidence of liver dysfunction (AST/ALT and/or bilirubin elevations, and/or symptoms [eg, fatigue, nausea, anorexia, jaundice, dark urine, liver tenderness, hepatomegaly]). Discontinue use if aminotransferase elevations are accompanied by total bilirubin elevation >2 times ULN, aminotransferase elevations are >8 times ULN, or aminotransferase elevations continue for >2 weeks. May be used for 24 weeks in adults with an isolate showing genotypic or phenotypic resistance to both isoniazid and rifampin when another effective treatment regimen cannot be used. Use for >24 weeks should be evaluated on a case-by-case basis. Consider discontinuing bedaquiline 4 or 5 months before discontinuation of other drugs in the patient's regimen. Bedaquiline's long terminal half-life may predispose to acquired resistance if it is the sole antitubercular drug remaining in the patient's system. Safety and effectiveness has not been studied in children, HIV-1 infected persons, pregnant women, patients with extrapulmonary tuberculosis, or patients with comorbidities receiving other medications. When another effective treatment regimen cannot be used, bedaquiline may be evaluated for use on a case-by-case basis (CDC, 2013).

Administer by directly observed therapy (DOT) and use only in multidrug regimens (≥3 drugs) also active against *M. tuberculosis* isolate; if failure/relapse occurs, have isolate tested for bedaquiline MIC. Should not be used for latent, extrapulmonary (eg, CNS) or drug-sensitive tuberculosis, or nontuberculous mycobacteria. **[U.S. Boxed Warning]: Increased risk of death in clinical trials of bedaquiline versus placebo. Only use if no other effective treatment regimen is available.**

Adverse Reactions

>10%:

- Cardiovascular: Chest pain (11%)
- Central nervous system: Headache (28%)
- Gastrointestinal: Nausea (38%)
- Hepatic: Transaminases increased (9%; ALT increased >3 x ULN: 11%; AST increased >3 x ULN: 11%)
- Neuromuscular & skeletal: Arthralgia (33%)
- Respiratory: Hemoptysis (18%)

1% to 10%:

- Dermatologic: Rash (8%)
- Gastrointestinal: Anorexia (9%), amylase increased (3%)

Frequency not defined: QT prolongation

Drug Interactions

Metabolism/Transport Effects **Substrate** of CYP3A4 (major); **Note:** Assignment of Major/Minor substrate status based on clinically relevant drug interaction potential

Avoid Concomitant Use

Avoid concomitant use of Bedaquiline with any of the following: Alcohol (Ethyl); BCG; CYP3A4 Inducers (Strong); Highest Risk QTc-Prolonging Agents; Ivabradine; Mifepristone; St Johns Wort

Increased Effect/Toxicity

Bedaquiline may increase the levels/effects of: Highest Risk QTc-Prolonging Agents; Moderate Risk QTc-Prolonging Agents

The levels/effects of Bedaquiline may be increased by: Alcohol (Ethyl); CYP3A4 Inhibitors (Strong); Ivabradine; Mifepristone; QTc-Prolonging Agents (Indeterminate Risk and Risk Modifying)

Decreased Effect

Bedaquiline may decrease the levels/effects of: BCG; Sodium Picosulfate; Typhoid Vaccine

The levels/effects of Bedaquiline may be decreased by: Bosentan; CYP3A4 Inducers (Strong); Dabrafenib; Deferasirox; St Johns Wort; Tocilizumab

Ethanol/Nutrition/Herb Interactions

Ethanol: May increase risk of hepatic-related adverse drug reactions. Management: Avoid alcohol use during therapy.

Food: Administration with a standard meal (~22 g fat; 558 calories) increases bioavailability by approximately two-fold. Management: Administer with food.

Storage/Stability Store at 25°C (77°F); excursions permitted to 15°C to 30°C (59°F to 86°F). Dispense in original container. If tablets are dispensed outside original container, store in tight light-resistant container and give an expiration date of ≤3 months.

Mechanism of Action As a diarylquinoline antimycobacterial, inhibits the proton transfer chain of mycobacterial ATP synthase required for energy generation in *M. tuberculosis*. It is not active against human ATP synthase.

Pharmacodynamics/Kinetics

Absorption: Significantly increased with food

Distribution: V_d: ~164 L

Protein binding: ~100%

Metabolism: Hepatic via CYP3A4; forms N-monodesmethyl metabolite (M2) which has 4-6 times less antimycobacterial potency than parent drug

Half-life elimination: Terminal: 5.5 months (bedaquiline and M2 metabolite)

Time to peak, serum: Oral: 5 hours

Excretion: Feces; urine (<0.001%)

Dosage Note: Use with ≥3 drugs also active against the patient's *M. tuberculosis* isolate.

Usual dosage range: Adults: Oral: Directly observed therapy (DOT):

Weeks 1-2: 400 mg once daily. **Note:** If a dose is missed during weeks 1-2, do not make up the missed dose, and continue the usual dosing schedule.

Weeks 3-24: 200 mg 3 times weekly (total weekly dose: 600 mg). **Note:** Space doses at least 48 hours apart. If a dose is missed during weeks 3-24, administer the missed dose as soon as possible, and resume the 3-times-weekly schedule.

Dosage adjustment in renal impairment:

Mild-to-moderate renal impairment: No dosage adjustment necessary.

Severe renal impairment: No dosage adjustment provided in manufacturer's labeling; use with caution.

Intermittent hemodialysis (IHD) or peritoneal dialysis (PD): No dosage adjustment provided in manufacturer's labeling. Use with caution (CDC, 2013); bedaquiline is highly protein bound and not likely to be removed by dialysis.

Dosage adjustment in hepatic impairment:

Mild or moderate impairment (Child-Pugh class A or B): No dosage adjustment necessary.

Severe impairment (Child-Pugh class C): No dosage adjustment provided in manufacturer's labeling; use should be avoided (CDC, 2013).

Dietary Considerations Tablets should be taken with meals.

Administration Oral: Administer with food; swallow tablets whole. During weeks 3-24 of therapy, space doses at least 48 hours apart. Administer by directly observed therapy (DOT).

Monitoring Parameters ECG should be obtained at baseline and at weeks 2, 12, and 24 during therapy. Monitor ECG weekly with concurrent administration of other medications known to prolong the QT_c interval (including fluoroquinolones, macrolide antibiotics, or clofazimine) or if the patient has conditions predisposing them to QT_c prolongation (torsade de pointes, congenital long QT syndrome, hypothyroidism, uncompensated heart failure, bradyarrhythmias) (CDC, 2013). If QT_c prolongation is detected during therapy, monitor ECG frequently to confirm QT_c return to baseline. Baseline potassium, calcium, and magnesium should be obtained and corrected, if abnormal. Discontinue therapy if patient develops confirmed QT_cF interval of >500 ms or ventricular arrhythmia.

Monitor AST, ALT, alkaline phosphatase, and bilirubin at baseline, monthly during treatment, and as needed. Monitor more frequently if patient has underlying hepatic disease or is receiving concomitant hepatotoxic drugs (CDC, 2013). If AST or ALT >3 x upper limit of normal (ULN), repeat test in 48 hours, test for viral hepatitis and discontinue other hepatotoxic medications. Further evaluate patients with evidence of liver dysfunction (AST/ALT and/or bilirubin elevations, and/or symptoms [eg fatigue, nausea, anorexia, hepatomegaly]). Discontinue if AST or ALT elevations persist >2 weeks, are >8 x ULN, or if elevations also include total bilirubin >2 x ULN.

Monitor weekly for arthralgias, chest pain, headache, hemoptysis, nausea, and rash. Monitoring serum bedaquiline levels may be considered in patients with renal impairment. Sputum specimens should be evaluated monthly throughout treatment and at the end of treatment, even if cultures become negative. Specimens positive for *M. tuberculosis* (including pretreatment specimen) should be evaluated further by a laboratory (in conjunction with a state public health laboratory) that performs bedaquiline resistance testing (CDC, 2013).

Dosage Forms Excipient information presented when available (limited, particularly for generics); consult specific product labeling.

Tablet, Oral:

Sirturo: 100 mg

◆ **Behenyl Alcohol** *see* Docosanol *on page 644*

Belatacept (bel AT a sept)

Brand Names: U.S. Nulojix

Index Terms BMS-224818; LEA29Y

Pharmacologic Category Selective T-Cell Costimulation Blocker

Use Prophylaxis of organ rejection concomitantly with basiliximab induction, mycophenolate, and corticosteroids in Epstein-Barr virus (EBV) seropositive kidney transplant recipients

Pregnancy Risk Factor C

Pregnancy Considerations Teratogenic effects were not observed in animal studies. There are no adequate and well-controlled studies in pregnant women. Due to the potential risk for development of autoimmune disease in the fetus, use during pregnancy only if clearly needed. A pregnancy registry has been established to monitor outcomes of women exposed to belatacept during pregnancy (1-877-955-6877).

Breast-Feeding Considerations It is not known if belatacept is excreted in breast milk. Due to the potential for adverse reactions and possible effects on the developing immune system, breast-feeding is not recommended.

Prescribing and Access Restrictions The ENLiST registry has been created to further determine the safety of belatacept, particularly the incidence of post-transplant lymphoproliferative disorder (PTLD) and progressive multifocal leukoencephalopathy (PML), in EBV-seropositive kidney transplant patients. Transplant centers are encouraged to participate (1-800-321-1335).

Medication Guide Available Yes

Contraindications Transplant patients who are Epstein-Barr virus (EBV) seronegative or with unknown EBV status

Warnings/Precautions [U.S. Boxed Warning]: Risk of post-transplant lymphoproliferative disorder (PTLD) is increased, primarily involving the CNS, in patients receiving belatacept compared to patients receiving cyclosporine-based regimens. Degree of immunosuppression is a risk factor for PTLD developing; do not exceed recommended dosing. Patients who are Epstein-Barr virus seronegative (EBV) are at an even higher risk; use is contraindicated in patients without evidence of immunity to EBV. Therapy is only appropriate in patients who are EBV seropositive via evidence of acquired immunity, such as presence of IgG antibodies to viral capsid antigen [VCA] and EBV nuclear antigen [EBNA]. Cytomegalovirus (CMV) infection also increases the risk for PTLD; CMV prophylaxis is recommended for a minimum of 3 months following transplantation. Although CMV disease is a risk for PTLD and CMV seronegative patients are at an increased risk for CMV disease, the clinical role, if any, of determining CMV serology to determine risk of PTLD development has not been determined.

[U.S. Boxed Warning]: Risk for infection is increased. Immunosuppressive therapy may lead to opportunistic infections, sepsis, and/or fatal infections. Tuberculosis (TB) is increased; test patients for latent TB prior to initiation, and treat latent TB infection prior to use. Patients receiving immunosuppressive therapy are at an increased risk of activation of latent viral infections, including John Cunningham virus (JCV) and BK virus infection. Activation of JCV may result in progressive multifocal leukoencephalopathy (PML), a rare and potentially fatal condition affecting the CNS. Symptoms of PML include apathy, ataxia, cognitive deficiencies, confusion, and hemiparesis. Polyoma virus-associated nephropathy (PVAN), primarily from activation of BK virus, may also occur and lead to the deterioration of renal function and/or renal graft loss. Risk factors for the development of PML and PVAN include immunosuppression and treatment with immunosuppressant therapy. The onset of PML or PVAN may warrant a reduction in immunosuppressive therapy; however, in transplant recipients, the risk of reduced immunosuppression and graft rejection should be considered.

[U.S. Boxed Warning]: Risk for malignancy is increased. Malignancy, including skin malignancy and post-transplant lymphoproliferative disease, is associated with the use of immunosuppressants, including belatacept; higher than recommended doses or more frequent dosing is not recommended; patients should be advised to limit their exposure to sunlight/UV light.

[U.S. Boxed Warning]: Therapy is not recommended in liver transplant patients due to increased risk of graft loss and death. [U.S. Boxed Warning]: Should be administered under the supervision of a physician experienced in immunosuppressive therapy. Patients should not be immunized with attenuated or live viral vaccines during or shortly after treatment; safety of immunization following therapy has not been studied. An increased risk of acute rejection and graft loss has been observed with belatacept when corticosteroids were minimized to 5 mg daily between day 3 and week 6 post-transplant; corticosteroid dosing should be consistent with clinical trial experience (ie, tapered to ~15 mg daily by the first 6 weeks post-transplant and remain at ~10 mg daily for the first 6 months post-transplant). Patients should not be immunized with attenuated or live viral vaccines during or shortly after treatment; safety of immunization following therapy has not been studied.

Adverse Reactions Incidences reported occurred during clinical trials using belatacept compared to a cyclosporine control regimen. All patients also received basiliximab induction, mycophenolate mofetil, and corticosteroids, and were followed up to 3 years.

>10%:

Cardiovascular: Peripheral edema (34%), hypertension (32%), hypotension (18%)

Central nervous system: Fever (28%), headache (21%), insomnia (15%)

Endocrine & metabolic: Hypokalemia (21%), hyperkalemia (20%), hypophosphatemia (19%), lipid metabolism disorder (19%), hyperglycemia (16%), hypocalcemia (13%), hypercholesterolemia (11%)

Gastrointestinal: Diarrhea (39%), constipation (33%), nausea (24%), vomiting (22%), abdominal pain (19%)

Genitourinary: Urinary tract infection (37%), dysuria (11%)

Hematologic & oncologic: Anemia (45%), leukopenia (20%)

Infection: Increased susceptibility to infection (72% to 82%, serious infection 24% to 36%), herpes (7% to 14%), cytomegalovirus disease (11% to 13%), influenza (11%)

Neuromuscular & skeletal: Arthralgia (17%), back pain (13%)

Renal: Proteinuria (16%; up to 33% 2+ proteinuria at 1 month post-transplant), renal graft dysfunction (25%), hematuria (16%), increased serum creatinine (15%)

Respiratory: Cough (24%), upper respiratory tract infection (15%), nasopharyngitis (13%), dyspnea (12%)

1% to 10%:

Cardiovascular: Arteriovenous fistula site complication (thrombosis, <10%), atrial fibrillation (<10%)

Central nervous system: Anxiety (10%), Guillain-Barré syndrome (<10%), dizziness (9%)

Dermatologic: Alopecia (<10%), hyperhidrosis (<10%), acne vulgaris (8%)

Endocrine & metabolic: Diabetes mellitus (new onset, 5% to 8%), hypomagnesemia (7%), hyperuricemia (5%)

Gastrointestinal: Stomatitis (<10%), upper abdominal pain (9%)

Genitourinary: Urinary incontinence (<10%)

Hematologic & oncologic: Hematoma (<10%), lymphocele (<10%), neutropenia (<10%), malignant neoplasm (4%), malignant neoplasm of skin (nonmelanoma, 2%)

Immunologic: Antibody development (2%)

Infection: Polyoma virus (3% to 4%)

Neuromuscular & skeletal: Musculoskeletal pain (<10%), tremor (8%)

Renal: Acute renal failure (<10%), chronic allograft nephropathy (<10%), hydronephrosis (<10%), renal insufficiency (<10%), renal artery stenosis (<10%), renal tubular necrosis (9%), renal disease (BK virus-associated, 1%)

Respiratory: Bronchitis (10%), tuberculosis (1% to 2%)

Miscellaneous: Infusion related reaction (5%)

<1%, postmarketing, and/or case reports (Limited to important or life-threatening): Aspergillosis (cerebral; higher dosing regimen), encephalitis (Chagas, West Nile; higher dosing regimen), lymphoproliferative disorder (post-transplant; incidence is 9-fold higher in non-EBV seropositive patients), meningitis (cryptococcal), progressive multifocal leukoencephalopathy (higher dosing regimen), renal graft rejection

Drug Interactions

Metabolism/Transport Effects None known.

Avoid Concomitant Use

Avoid concomitant use of Belatacept with any of the following: BCG; Belimumab; Natalizumab; Pimecrolimus; Tacrolimus (Topical); Tofacitinib; Vaccines (Live)

Increased Effect/Toxicity

Belatacept may increase the levels/effects of: Belimumab; Leflunomide; Mycophenolate; Natalizumab; Tofacitinib; Vaccines (Live)

The levels/effects of Belatacept may be increased by: Denosumab; Pimecrolimus; Roflumilast; Tacrolimus (Topical); Trastuzumab

Decreased Effect

Belatacept may decrease the levels/effects of: BCG; Coccidioidin Skin Test; Sipuleucel-T; Vaccines (Inactivated); Vaccines (Live)

The levels/effects of Belatacept may be decreased by: Echinacea

Preparation for Administration Reconstitute each vial with 10.5 mL of diluent (SWFI, NS, or D_5W) using the provided silicone-free disposable syringe, and an 18- to 21-gauge needle. Reconstitute using **only** the silicone-free syringe provided (discard if powder is inadvertently mixed using a siliconized syringe, translucent particles may develop). Inject the diluent down the side of the vial to avoid foaming. Rotate the vial and invert with gentle swirling until completely dissolved; do **not** shake vial. The reconstituted solution should be clear to slightly opalescent and colorless to pale yellow. Immediately transfer the reconstituted solution using the same silicone-free syringe to an infusion bag or bottle with NS or D_5W (if NS or D_5W were used to reconstitute, the same fluid should be used to further dilute). The final concentration should range from 2 mg/mL and 10 mg/mL (typical infusion volume is 100 mL). Prior to adding belatacept to the infusion solution, the manufacturer recommends withdrawing a volume equal to the amount of belatacept to be added. Mix gently; do not shake.

Storage/Stability Prior to use, store refrigerated at 2°C to 8°C (36°F to 46°F). Protect from light. After dilution, the infusion solution (reconstituted solution must be further diluted immediately) may be stored refrigerated for up to 24 hours, with a maximum of 4 hours of the 24 hours at room temperature, 20°C to 25°C (68°F to 77°F), and room light. Infusion must be completed within 24 hours of reconstitution.

Mechanism of Action Fusion protein which acts as a selective T-cell (lymphocyte) costimulation blocker by binding to CD80 and CD86 receptors on antigen presenting cells (APC), blocking the required CD28 mediated interaction between APCs and T cells needed to activate T lymphocytes. T-cell stimulation results in cytokine production and proliferation, mediators in immunologic rejection associated with kidney transplantation.

Pharmacodynamics/Kinetics

Distribution: V_{ss}: 0.11 L/kg (transplant patients)

Half-life elimination: ~10 days (healthy patients and kidney transplant patients)

Dosage Note: Dosing is based on actual body weight at the time of transplantation; do not modify weight-based dosing during course of therapy unless the change in body weight is >10%. The prescribed dose must be evenly divisible by 12.5 mg to allow accurate preparation of the reconstituted solution using the required disposable syringe provided by the manufacturer. For example, the calculated dose for a 64 kg patient: 64 kg x 10 mg per kg = 640 mg. The nearest doses to 640 mg that are evenly divisible by 12.5 mg would be 637.5 mg or 650 mg; the closest dose to the calculated dose is 637.5 mg, therefore, 637.5 should be the actual prescribed dose for the patient.

Kidney transplant, prophylaxis of organ rejection: Adults: I.V.:

Initial phase: 10 mg/kg on Day 1 (day of transplant, prior to implantation) and on day 5 (~96 hours after Day 1 dose), followed by 10 mg/kg given at the end of Week 2, Week 4, Week 8, and Week 12 following transplantation

Maintenance phase: 5 mg/kg every 4 weeks (plus or minus 3 days) beginning at Week 16 following transplantation

Concomitant therapy: Belatacept should be used in combination with basiliximab induction, mycophenolate mofetil, and corticosteroids. Corticosteroids should be tapered to ~15 mg (10-20 mg) daily by the first 6 weeks and remain at ~10 mg (5-10 mg) daily for the first 6 months post-transplant.

Dosage adjustment in renal impairment: No dosage adjustment provided in manufacturer's labeling; however, renal function did not affect clearance in pharmacokinetic studies of kidney transplant patients.

Dosage adjustment in hepatic impairment: No dosage adjustment provided in manufacturer's labeling; however, hepatic function did not affect clearance in pharmacokinetic studies of kidney transplant patients.

Dietary Considerations May contain sucrose.

Administration Administer as an I.V. infusion over 30 minutes using an infusion set with a 0.2-1.2 micron low protein-binding filter. Prior to administration, inspect visually and do not use if solution is discolored or contains particulate matter.

Monitoring Parameters New-onset or worsening neurological, cognitive, or behavioral signs/symptoms; signs/symptoms of infection; TB screening prior to therapy initiation; EBV seropositive verification prior to therapy initiation

Additional Information If additional silicone-free disposable syringes are needed, contact Bristol-Myers Squibb at 1-888-NULOJIX.

Dosage Forms Excipient information presented when available (limited, particularly for generics); consult specific product labeling.

Solution Reconstituted, Intravenous:

Nulojix: 250 mg (1 ea)

Belimumab (be LIM yoo mab)

Brand Names: U.S. Benlysta

Brand Names: Canada Benlysta

Pharmacologic Category Monoclonal Antibody

Use

Systemic lupus erythematosus: Treatment of adult patients with active, autoantibody-positive systemic lupus erythematosus (SLE) who are receiving standard therapy.

Limitations of use: Use is not recommended in patients with severe active lupus nephritis, severe active CNS lupus, or in combination with other biologics, including B-cell targeted therapies or intravenous (IV) cyclophosphamide.

Pregnancy Risk Factor C

Pregnancy Considerations Adverse events were observed in some animal reproduction studies. IgG molecules are known to cross the placenta (belimumab is an engineered IgG molecule). Effective contraception should be used during and for at least 4 months following treatment in women of childbearing potential. Healthcare providers are encouraged to enroll women exposed to belimumab during pregnancy in a pregnancy registry (877-681-6296); patients may also enroll themselves.

Breast-Feeding Considerations It is not known if belimumab is excreted in breast milk. Because IgG molecules are excreted in breast milk, a decision should be made whether to discontinue nursing or to discontinue the drug, taking into account the importance of treatment to the mother.

Medication Guide Available Yes

Contraindications Hypersensitivity (anaphylaxis) to belimumab or any component of the formulation

Warnings/Precautions Deaths due to infection, cardiovascular disease, and suicide were higher in belimumab patients compared to placebo during clinical trials. Serious and potentially fatal infections may occur during treatment. Use with caution in patients with chronic infections; treatment should not be undertaken if receiving therapy for chronic infection. Consider interrupting belimumab in patients who develop new infections and initiate appropriate anti-infective treatment; monitor closely.

Acute hypersensitivity reactions including anaphylaxis (with fatalities) and infusion-related reactions (eg, bradycardia, hypotension, myalgia, headache, rash, and urticaria) have been reported, including patients who had previously tolerated infusions of belimumab; onset may occur within hours of the infusion or may be delayed. Monitor for an appropriate time following administration. Discontinue for severe reactions (anaphylaxis, angioedema); infusion may be slowed or temporarily interrupted for other infusion-related reactions. Risk for hypersensitivity reactions may be increased with history of multiple drug allergies or significant hypersensitivity. Immunosuppressants may increase risk of malignancy. May cause psychiatric adverse effects, including anxiety, insomnia, or new/worsening depression. Potentially significant drug-drug interactions may exist, requiring dose or frequency adjustment, additional monitoring, and/or selection of alternative therapy. Live vaccines should not be given within 30 days before or concurrently with belimumab. Black/African-American patients may have a lower response rate; use with caution.

Adverse Reactions

>10%:

Gastrointestinal: Nausea (15%), diarrhea (12%)

Miscellaneous: Infusion-related reaction (17%), hypersensitivity (13%)

≥3% to 10%:

Central nervous system: Fever (10%), insomnia (6% to 7%), migraine (5%), depression (5% to 6%), anxiety (4%), headache (≥3%)

Dermatologic: Skin reactions (≥3%)

Gastrointestinal: Viral gastroenteritis (3%)

Genitourinary: Urinary tract infection (site not specified >5%), cystitis (4%)

Hematologic: Leukopenia (4%)

Neuromuscular & skeletal: Pain in extremity (6%)

Respiratory: Bronchitis (9%), nasopharyngitis (9%), pharyngitis (5%), sinusitis (>5%), upper respiratory infection (>5%)

Miscellaneous: Influenza (>5%)

<3% (Limited to important or life-threatening): Anaphylaxis (including fatalities), angioedema, antibody formation, bradycardia, cellulitis, dyspnea, eyelid edema, hypotension, myalgia, pneumonia, pruritus, rash, suicide, urticaria

Drug Interactions

Metabolism/Transport Effects None known.

Avoid Concomitant Use

Avoid concomitant use of Belimumab with any of the following: Abatacept; BCG; Belatacept; Cyclophosphamide; Etanercept; Monoclonal Antibodies; Natalizumab; Pimecrolimus; Tacrolimus (Topical); Tofacitinib; Vaccines (Live)

Increased Effect/Toxicity

Belimumab may increase the levels/effects of: Cyclophosphamide; Leflunomide; Natalizumab; Tofacitinib; Vaccines (Live)

The levels/effects of Belimumab may be increased by: Abatacept; Abciximab; Belatacept; Denosumab; Etanercept; Monoclonal Antibodies; Pimecrolimus; Roflumilast; Tacrolimus (Topical); Trastuzumab

Decreased Effect

Belimumab may decrease the levels/effects of: BCG; Coccidioidin Skin Test; Sipuleucel-T; Vaccines (Inactivated); Vaccines (Live)

The levels/effects of Belimumab may be decreased by: Echinacea

Preparation for Administration To reconstitute, allow vial to reach room temperature. Reconstitute 120 mg vial with 1.5 mL of SWFI. Reconstitute 400 mg vial with 4.8 mL of SWFI. To minimize foaming, direct SWFI toward the side of the vial. Gently swirl for 60 seconds every 5 minutes until powder has dissolved (usual reconstitution time is 10-15 minutes, but may take up to 30 minutes); do not shake. If utilizing a mechanical reconstitution device, do not exceed 500 rpm or 30 minutes. Further dilute reconstituted solution in 250 mL of 0.9% sodium chloride by first removing and discarding the volume equivalent to the volume of the reconstituted solution to be added to prepare the appropriate dose; add the appropriate volume of the reconstituted solution to the infusion container and gently invert to mix solution. Protect from light. Solution may be stored refrigerated or at room temperature.

Storage/Stability Prior to reconstitution, store unused vials between 2°C to 8°C (36°F to 46°F); do not freeze. Protect from light. Prior to further dilution, the reconstituted solution must be stored under refrigeration. The diluted solution may be stored refrigerated or at room temperature. Infusion must be completed within 8 hours of reconstitution.

Mechanism of Action Belimumab is an IgG1-lambda monoclonal antibody that prevents the survival of B lymphocytes by blocking the binding of soluble human B lymphocyte stimulator protein (BLyS) to receptors on B lymphocytes. This reduces the activity of B-cell mediated immunity and the autoimmune response.

Pharmacodynamics/Kinetics

Onset of action: B cells: 8 weeks; Clinical improvement (SLE Responder Index and flare reduction): 16 weeks (Navarra, 2011)

Distribution: V_d: 5.29 L

Half-life elimination: 19.4 days

Dosage I.V.: Adults: Initial: 10 mg/kg every 2 weeks for 3 doses; Maintenance: 10 mg/kg every 4 weeks

Dosing adjustment in renal impairment: No dosage adjustment is necessary for Cl_{cr} ≥15 mL/minute; has not been studied in Cl_{cr}<15 mL/minute

Dosing adjustment in hepatic impairment: No dosage adjustment provided in manufacturer's labeling (has not been studied).

Administration Administer intravenously over 1 hour through a dedicated I.V. line. Do **NOT** administer as an I.V. push or bolus. Discontinue infusion for severe hypersensitivity reaction (eg, anaphylaxis, angioedema). The infusion may be slowed or temporarily interrupted for minor reactions. Consider premedicating with an antihistamine and antipyretic for prophylaxis against hypersensitivity or infusion reactions.

Monitoring Parameters Monitor for hypersensitivity and/or infusion reactions; infections; worsening of depression, mood changes, or suicidal thoughts

Dosage Forms Excipient information presented when available (limited, particularly for generics); consult specific product labeling.

Solution Reconstituted, Intravenous [preservative free]:

Benlysta: 120 mg (1 ea); 400 mg (1 ea) [contains polysorbate 80]

◆ **Belladonna Alkaloids With Phenobarbital** *see* Hyoscyamine, Atropine, Scopolamine, and Phenobarbital *on page 1028*

Belladonna and Opium (bel a DON a & OH pee um)

Index Terms B&O; Opium and Belladonna

Pharmacologic Category Analgesic Combination (Opioid); Antispasmodic Agent, Urinary

Additional Appendix Information

Beers Criteria – Potentially Inappropriate Medications for Geriatrics *on page 2368*

Use Relief of moderate-to-severe pain associated with ureteral spasms not responsive to nonopioid analgesics and to space intervals between injections of opioids

Pregnancy Risk Factor C

Dosage Rectal: Children >12 years and Adults: 1 suppository 1-2 times/day, up to 4 doses/day

Additional Information Complete prescribing information should be consulted for additional detail.

Dosage Forms Excipient information presented when available (limited, particularly for generics); consult specific product labeling.

Suppository: Belladonna extract 16.2 mg and opium 30 mg; belladonna extract 16.2 mg and opium 60 mg

Controlled Substance C-II

◆ **Belviq** *see* Lorcaserin *on page 1245*

◆ **Benadryl [OTC]** *see* DiphenhydrAMINE (Systemic) *on page 622*

◆ **Benadryl® (Can)** *see* DiphenhydrAMINE (Systemic) *on page 622*

◆ **Benadryl-D® Allergy & Sinus [OTC]** *see* Diphenhydramine and Phenylephrine *on page 625*

◆ **Benadryl-D® Children's Allergy & Sinus [OTC]** *see* Diphenhydramine and Phenylephrine *on page 625*

◆ **Benadryl Allergy [OTC]** *see* DiphenhydrAMINE (Systemic) *on page 622*

◆ **Benadryl Allergy Childrens [OTC]** *see* DiphenhydrAMINE (Systemic) *on page 622*

◆ **Benadryl Dye-Free Allergy [OTC]** *see* DiphenhydrAMINE (Systemic) *on page 622*

Benazepril (ben AY ze pril)

Brand Names: U.S. Lotensin

Brand Names: Canada Lotensin

Index Terms Benazepril Hydrochloride

Pharmacologic Category Angiotensin-Converting Enzyme (ACE) Inhibitor; Antihypertensive

Additional Appendix Information

Angiotensin Agents *on page 2280*

Use Treatment of hypertension, either alone or in combination with other antihypertensive agents

Pregnancy Risk Factor D

Pregnancy Considerations [U.S. Boxed Warning]: Drugs that act on the renin-angiotensin system can cause injury and death to the developing fetus. Discontinue as soon as possible once pregnancy is detected. Benazepril crosses the placenta; teratogenic effects may occur following maternal use during pregnancy. Drugs that act on the renin-angiotensin system are associated with oligohydramnios. Oligohydramnios, due to decreased fetal renal function, may lead to fetal lung hypoplasia and skeletal malformations. Their use in pregnancy is also associated with anuria, hypotension, renal failure, skull hypoplasia, and death in the fetus/neonate. Chronic maternal hypertension itself is also associated with adverse events in the fetus/infant. ACE inhibitors are not recommended during pregnancy to treat maternal hypertension or heart failure. Use of an ACE inhibitor should also be avoided in any woman of reproductive age. Women who are planning a pregnancy should be considered for other medication options if an ACE inhibitor is currently prescribed or the ACE inhibitor should be discontinued as soon as possible once pregnancy is detected. The exposed fetus should be monitored for fetal growth, amniotic fluid volume, and organ formation. Infants exposed to an ACE inhibitor *in utero* should be monitored for hyperkalemia, hypotension, and oliguria.

Breast-Feeding Considerations Small amounts of benazepril and benazeprilat are found in breast milk.

Contraindications Hypersensitivity to benazepril or any component of the formulation; patients with a history of angioedema (with or without prior ACE inhibitor therapy); concomitant use with aliskiren in patients with diabetes mellitus

Canadian labeling: Additional contraindications (not in U.S. labeling): Concomitant use with aliskiren in patients with moderate to severe renal impairment (GFR <60 mL/minute/1.73 m^2); pregnancy; breast-feeding; rare hereditary problems of galactose intolerance (eg, galactosemia, Lapp Lactase deficiency or glucose-galactose malabsorption)

Warnings/Precautions Anaphylactic reactions may occur rarely with ACE inhibitors. At any time during treatment (especially following first dose) angioedema may occur rarely with ACE inhibitors. It may involve the head and neck (potentially compromising airway) or the intestine (presenting with abdominal pain). African-Americans and patients with idiopathic or hereditary angioedema may be at an increased risk. Prolonged frequent monitoring may be required especially if tongue, glottis, or larynx are involved as they are associated with airway obstruction. Patients with a history of airway surgery may have a higher risk of airway obstruction. Aggressive early and appropriate management is critical. Contraindicated in patients with history of angioedema with or without prior ACE inhibitor therapy. Hypersensitivity reactions may be seen during hemodialysis (eg, CVVHD) with high-flux dialysis membranes (eg, AN69), and rarely, during low density lipoprotein apheresis with dextran sulfate cellulose. Rare cases of anaphylactoid reactions have been reported in patients undergoing sensitization treatment with hymenoptera (bee, wasp) venom while receiving ACE inhibitors.

Symptomatic hypotension with or without syncope can occur with ACE inhibitors (usually with the first several doses); effects are most often observed in volume depleted patients; close monitoring of patient is required especially with initial dosing and dosing increases; blood pressure must be lowered at a rate appropriate for the patient's clinical condition. Initiation of therapy in patients with ischemic heart disease or cerebrovascular disease warrants close observation due to the potential consequences posed by falling blood pressure (eg, MI, stroke). **[U.S. Boxed Warning]: Drugs that act on the renin-angiotensin system can cause injury and death to the developing fetus. Discontinue as soon as possible once pregnancy is detected.** Use with caution in hypertrophic cardiomyopathy with outflow tract obstruction, severe aortic stenosis, or before, during, or immediately after major surgery.

Hyperkalemia may occur with ACE inhibitors; risk factors include renal dysfunction, diabetes mellitus, concomitant use of potassium-sparing diuretics, potassium supplements and/or potassium-containing salts. Use cautiously, if at all, with these agents and monitor potassium periodically. Cough may occur with ACE inhibitors. Other causes of cough should be considered (eg, pulmonary congestion in patients with heart failure) and excluded prior to discontinuation. Use with caution in patients with diabetes receiving insulin or oral antidiabetic agents; may be at increased risk for episodes of hypoglycemia.

May be associated with deterioration of renal function and/or increases in serum creatinine, particularly in patients with low renal blood flow (eg, renal artery stenosis, heart failure) whose glomerular filtration rate (GFR) is dependent on efferent arteriolar vasoconstriction by angiotensin II; deterioration may result in oliguria, acute renal failure, and progressive azotemia. Small increases in serum creatinine may occur following initiation; consider discontinuation only in patients with progressive and/or significant deterioration in renal function. Use with caution in patients with unstented unilateral/bilateral renal artery stenosis. When unstented bilateral renal artery stenosis is present, use is generally avoided due to the elevated risk of deterioration in renal function unless possible benefits outweigh risks. Potentially significant drug-drug interactions may exist, requiring dose or frequency adjustment, additional monitoring, and/or selection of alternative therapy.

Rare toxicities associated with ACE inhibitors include cholestatic jaundice (which may progress to fulminant hepatic necrosis), agranulocytosis, neutropenia, or leukopenia with myeloid hypoplasia. Patients with collagen vascular diseases (especially with concomitant renal impairment) or renal impairment alone may be at increased risk for hematologic toxicity; periodically monitor CBC with differential in these patients.

Adverse Reactions

1% to 10%:

Cardiovascular: Postural dizziness (2%)

Central nervous system: Headache (6%), dizziness (4%), somnolence (2%)

Renal: Serum creatinine increased (2%), worsening of renal function may occur in patients with bilateral renal artery stenosis or hypovolemia

Respiratory: Cough (1% to 10%)

<1% (Limited to important or life-threatening): Agranulocytosis, alopecia, anaphylactoid reaction, angina, angioedema (includes head, neck and intestinal angioedema), arthralgia, arthritis, asthma, BUN increased (transient), dermatitis, dyspnea, ECG changes, eosinophilia, flushing, gastritis, hemolytic anemia, hyperbilirubinemia, hyperglycemia, hyperkalemia, hypersensitivity, hypertonia, hyponatremia, hypotension, impotence, insomnia, leukopenia, myalgia, neutropenia, orthostatic hypotension, palpitations, pancreatitis, paresthesia, pemphigus, peripheral edema, photosensitivity, proteinuria, pruritus, rash, shock, Stevens-Johnson syndrome, syncope, thrombocytopenia, transaminases increased, uric acid increased, vomiting

Eosinophilic pneumonitis, anaphylaxis, neutropenia, agranulocytosis, renal insufficiency, and renal failure have been reported with other ACE inhibitors. In addition, a syndrome including fever, myalgia, arthralgia, interstitial nephritis, vasculitis, rash, eosinophilia, and elevated ESR has been reported to be associated with ACE inhibitors.

Drug Interactions

Metabolism/Transport Effects None known.

Avoid Concomitant Use There are no known interactions where it is recommended to avoid concomitant use.

Increased Effect/Toxicity

Benazepril may increase the levels/effects of: Allopurinol; Amifostine; Antihypertensives; AzaTHIOprine; CycloSPORINE (Systemic); Ferric Gluconate; Gold Sodium Thiomalate; Hypotensive Agents; Iron Dextran Complex; Lithium; Nonsteroidal Anti-Inflammatory Agents; Obinutuzumab; RiTUXimab; Sodium Phosphates

The levels/effects of Benazepril may be increased by: Alfuzosin; Aliskiren; Angiotensin II Receptor Blockers; Brimonidine (Topical); Canagliflozin; Diazoxide; DPP-IV Inhibitors; Eplerenone; Everolimus; Heparin; Heparin (Low Molecular Weight); Herbs (Hypotensive Properties); Hydrochlorothiazide; Loop Diuretics; MAO Inhibitors; Pentoxifylline; Phosphodiesterase 5 Inhibitors; Potassium Salts; Potassium-Sparing Diuretics; Prostacyclin Analogues; Sirolimus; Temsirolimus; Thiazide Diuretics; TiZANidine; Tolvaptan; Trimethoprim

Decreased Effect

Benazepril may decrease the levels/effects of: Hydrochlorothiazide

The levels/effects of Benazepril may be decreased by: Antacids; Aprotinin; Herbs (Hypertensive Properties); Icatibant; Lanthanum; Methylphenidate; Nonsteroidal Anti-Inflammatory Agents; Salicylates; Yohimbine

Ethanol/Nutrition/Herb Interactions

Food: Potassium supplements and/or potassium-containing salts may cause or worsen hyperkalemia. Management: Consult prescriber before consuming a potassium-rich diet, potassium supplements, or salt substitutes.

Herb/Nutraceutical: Some herbal medications may worsen hypertension (eg, licorice); others may increase the antihypertensive effect of benazepril (eg, shepherd's purse). Management: Avoid bayberry, blue cohosh, cayenne, ephedra, ginger, ginseng (American), kola, licorice, and yohimbe. Avoid black cohosh, California poppy, coleus, golden seal, hawthorn, mistletoe, periwinkle, quinine, and shepherd's purse.

Storage/Stability Store at ≤30°C (86°F). Protect from moisture.

Mechanism of Action Competitive inhibition of angiotensin I being converted to angiotensin II, a potent vasoconstrictor, through the angiotensin I-converting enzyme (ACE) activity, with resultant lower levels of angiotensin II which causes an increase in plasma renin activity and a reduction in aldosterone secretion

Pharmacodynamics/Kinetics

Reduction in plasma angiotensin-converting enzyme (ACE) activity:

Onset of action: Peak effect: 1-2 hours after 2-20 mg dose

Duration: >90% inhibition for 24 hours after 5-20 mg dose

Reduction in blood pressure:

Peak effect: Single dose: 2-4 hours; Continuous therapy: 2 weeks

Absorption: Rapid (37%); food does not alter significantly; metabolite (benazeprilat) itself unsuitable for oral administration due to poor absorption

Distribution: V_d: ~8.7 L

Protein binding:

Benazepril: ~97%

Benazeprilat: ~95%

Metabolism: Rapidly and extensively hepatic to its active metabolite, benazeprilat, via enzymatic hydrolysis; extensive first-pass effect

Half-life elimination: Benazeprilat: Effective: 10-11 hours; Terminal: Children: 5 hours, Adults: 22 hours

Time to peak: Parent drug: 0.5-1 hour

Excretion:

Urine (trace amounts as benazepril; 20% as benazeprilat; 12% as other metabolites)

Clearance: Nonrenal clearance (ie, biliary, metabolic) appears to contribute to the elimination of benazeprilat (11% to 12%), particularly patients with severe renal impairment; hepatic clearance is the main elimination route of unchanged benazepril

Dialysis: ~6% of metabolite removed within 4 hours of dialysis following 10 mg of benazepril administered 2 hours prior to procedure; parent compound not found in dialysate

Dosage Oral: Hypertension:

Children ≥6 years: Initial: 0.2 mg/kg/day (up to 10 mg/day) as monotherapy; dosing range: 0.1-0.6 mg/kg/day (maximum dose: 40 mg/day)

Adults: Initial: 10 mg/day in patients not receiving a diuretic; 20-80 mg/day as a single dose or 2 divided doses; the need for twice-daily dosing should be assessed by monitoring peak (2-6 hours after dosing) and trough responses.

Note: Patients taking diuretics should have them discontinued 2-3 days prior to starting benazepril. If they cannot be discontinued, then initial dose should be 5 mg; restart after blood pressure is stabilized if needed.

Elderly: Oral: Initial: 5-10 mg/day in single or divided doses; usual range: 20-40 mg/day; adjust for renal function; also see **Note** in adult dosing.

Dosage adjustment in renal impairment: Cl_{cr} <30 mL/minute:

Children: Use is not recommended.

Adults: Administer 5 mg/day initially; maximum daily dose: 40 mg.

Hemodialysis: Moderately dialyzable (20% to 50%); administer dose postdialysis or administer 25% to 35% supplemental dose.

Peritoneal dialysis: Supplemental dose is not necessary.

Dosage adjustment in hepatic impairment: No dosage adjustment provided in manufacturer's labeling (has not been studied); use with caution.

Monitoring Parameters Blood pressure; serum creatinine and potassium; if patient has collagen vascular disease and/or renal impairment, periodically monitor CBC with differential

Dosage Forms Excipient information presented when available (limited, particularly for generics); consult specific product labeling.

Tablet, Oral, as hydrochloride:

Lotensin: 10 mg, 20 mg, 40 mg

Generic: 5 mg, 10 mg, 20 mg, 40 mg

Extemporaneous Preparations A 2 mg/mL oral suspension may be made with tablets. Mix fifteen benazepril 20 mg tablets in an amber polyethylene terephthalate bottle with Ora-Plus® 75 mL. Shake for 2 minutes, allow suspension to stand for ≥1 hour, then shake again for at least 1 additional minute. Add Ora-Sweet® 75 mL to suspension and shake to disperse. Will make 150 mL of a 2 mg/mL suspension. Label "shake well" and "refrigerate". Stable for 30 days.

Lotensin® prescribing information, Novartis Pharmaceuticals Corporation, Suffern, NY, 2009.

Benazepril and Hydrochlorothiazide

(ben AY ze pril & hye droe klor oh THYE a zide)

Brand Names: U.S. Lotensin HCT®

Index Terms Benazepril Hydrochloride and Hydrochlorothiazide; Hydrochlorothiazide and Benazepril

Pharmacologic Category Angiotensin-Converting Enzyme (ACE) Inhibitor; Antihypertensive; Diuretic, Thiazide

Use Treatment of hypertension

Pregnancy Risk Factor D

Dosage Note: Not for initial therapy; dose should be individualized.

Oral: Range: Benazepril: 5-20 mg; Hydrochlorothiazide: 6.25-25 mg/day

Add-on therapy:

Patients not adequately controlled on benazepril monotherapy: Initiate benazepril 10-20 mg/hydrochlorothiazide 12.5 mg; titrate to effect at 2- to 3-week intervals

Patients controlled on hydrochlorothiazide 25 mg/day but experience significant potassium loss with this regimen: Initiate benazepril 5 mg/hydrochlorothiazide 6.25 mg

Replacement therapy: Substitute for the individually titrated components

Dosage adjustment in renal impairment: Cl_{cr} ≤30 mL/minute: Not recommended; loop diuretics are preferred.

Dosage adjustment in hepatic impairment: No dosage adjustment provided in manufacturer's labeling (has not been studied); use with caution.

Additional Information Complete prescribing information should be consulted for additional detail.

Dosage Forms Excipient information presented when available (limited, particularly for generics); consult specific product labeling.

Tablet: 5/6.25: Benazepril hydrochloride 5 mg and hydrochlorothiazide 6.25 mg; 10/12.5: Benazepril hydrochloride 10 mg and hydrochlorothiazide 12.5 mg; 20/12.5: Benazepril hydrochloride 20 mg and hydrochlorothiazide 12.5 mg; 20/25: Benazepril hydrochloride 20 mg and hydrochlorothiazide 25 mg

Lotensin HCT® 10/12.5: Benazepril hydrochloride 10 mg and hydrochlorothiazide 12.5 mg

Lotensin HCT® 20/12.5: Benazepril hydrochloride 20 mg and hydrochlorothiazide 12.5 mg

Lotensin HCT® 20/25: Benazepril hydrochloride 20 mg and hydrochlorothiazide 25 mg

◆ **Benazepril Hydrochloride** *see* Benazepril *on page 234*

◆ **Benazepril Hydrochloride and Amlodipine Besylate** *see* Amlodipine and Benazepril *on page 111*

◆ **Benazepril Hydrochloride and Hydrochlorothiazide** *see* Benazepril and Hydrochlorothiazide *on page 236*

Bendamustine (ben da MUS teen)

Brand Names: U.S. Treanda

Brand Names: Canada Treanda

Index Terms Bendamustine Hydrochloride; Cytostasan; SDX-105

Pharmacologic Category Antineoplastic Agent; Antineoplastic Agent, Alkylating Agent; Antineoplastic Agent, Alkylating Agent (Nitrogen Mustard)

Use

Chronic lymphocytic leukemia: Treatment of chronic lymphocytic leukemia (CLL)

Non-Hodgkin lymphoma: Treatment of indolent B-cell non-Hodgkin lymphoma (NHL) which has progressed during or within 6 months of rituximab treatment or a rituximab-containing regimen

Unlabeled Use Treatment of relapsed or refractory Hodgkin lymphoma; treatment of mantle cell lymphoma; salvage therapy for relapsed multiple myeloma; first-line therapy for follicular lymphoma; treatment of Waldenström's macroglobulinemia

Pregnancy Risk Factor D

Pregnancy Considerations Teratogenic and nonteratogenic events were observed in animal reproduction studies following intraperitoneal dosing. May cause fetal harm if administered during pregnancy. For women and men of reproductive potential, the U.S. labeling recommends effective contraception during and for 3 months after treatment. The Canadian labeling recommends effective contraception beginning 2 weeks prior to treatment and for ≥1 month after treatment.

Breast-Feeding Considerations It is not known if bendamustine is excreted in breast milk. Due to the potential for serious adverse reactions in the nursing infant, the decision to discontinue bendamustine or discontinue breastfeeding should take into account the benefits of treatment to the mother.

Contraindications Hypersensitivity (eg, anaphylactic or anaphylactoid reactions) to bendamustine or any component of the formulation

Warnings/Precautions Hazardous agent - use appropriate precautions for handling and disposal (NIOSH, 2012). Myelosuppression (neutropenia, thrombocytopenia, and anemia) is a common toxicity; may require therapy delay and/or dose reduction; monitor blood counts frequently (nadirs typically occurred in the third week of treatment). Complications due to febrile neutropenia and severe thrombocytopenia have been reported (some fatal). ANC should recover to ≥1000/mm³ and platelets to ≥75,000/mm³ prior to cycle initiation. Pneumonia, sepsis, and septic shock have been reported; fatalities due to infection have occurred; patients with myelosuppression are more susceptible to infection; monitor closely.

Infusion reactions, including chills, fever, pruritus, and rash are common; rarely, anaphylactic and anaphylactoid reactions have occurred, particularly with the second or subsequent cycle(s). Patients who experienced grade 3 or higher allergic reactions should not be rechallenged. Consider premedication with antihistamines, antipyretics, and corticosteroids for patients with a history of grade 1 or 2 infusion reaction. Discontinue for severe allergic reaction or grade 4 infusion reaction; consider discontinuation with grade 3 infusion reaction. Rash, toxic skin reactions and bullous exanthema have been reported with monotherapy and in combination with other antineoplastics; may be progressive or worsen with continued treatment; discontinue bendamustine treatment for severe or progressive skin reaction; monitor closely; withhold or discontinue bendamustine treatment for severe or progressive skin reaction. The risk for severe skin toxicity is increased with concurrent use of allopurinol and other medications known to cause skin toxicity; Stevens-Johnson syndrome (SJS) and toxic epidermal necrolysis (TEN) have been reported. TEN has also been reported when used in combination with rituximab. Bendamustine is an irritant with vesicant-like properties; ensure proper needle or catheter placement prior to and during infusion; avoid extravasation; erythema, marked swelling, and pain have been reported with extravasation. Bendamustine is associated with a moderate emetic potential (Basch, 2011); antiemetics are recommended to prevent nausea and vomiting.

Tumor lysis syndrome (usually occurring in the first treatment cycle) may occur as a consequence of antineoplastic treatment, including treatment with bendamustine. May lead to life-threatening acute renal failure; vigorous hydration and prophylactic measures (eg, antihyperuricemic therapy) should be instituted prior to treatment in high-risk patients; monitor closely. **Note:** Allopurinol may increase the risk for bendamustine skin toxicity. May cause hypokalemia; monitor potassium closely during therapy, particularly in patients with cardiac disease.

Per manufacturer's labeling, use with caution in patients with mild hepatic impairment. However, a pharmacokinetic study showed only slight differences in bendamustine AUC and C_{max} in patients with mild hepatic impairment (defined in the study as total bilirubin 1-1.5 times ULN or AST greater than ULN), as compared to patients with normal hepatic function (Owen, 2010). Use is not recommended in patients with moderate (AST or ALT 2.5-10 times ULN and ▶

total bilirubin 1.5-3 times ULN) or severe (total bilirubin >3 times ULN) hepatic impairment.

Use with caution in patients with mild-to-moderate renal impairment. The U.S. and Canadian product labels do not recommend use in patients with Cl_{cr} <40 mL/minute. A pharmacokinetic study illustrated only slight differences in bendamustine AUC and C_{max} in patients with mild (Cl_{cr} >50 to ≤80 mL/minute) and moderate (Cl_{cr} >30 to ≤50 mL/minute) renal dysfunction, compared to patients with normal renal function (Owen, 2010). A retrospective safety study found no significant difference in lab toxicities between CLL patients with renal impairment (Cl_{cr} <40 mL/minute) compared to those without renal impairment, although an increase in grades 3/4 thrombocytopenia and grades 3/4 BUN increases were detected in patients with renal impairment (Nordstrom, 2012); monitor blood counts and renal function. **Note:** UK labeling (Levact prescribing information, October, 2010) recommends no dosage adjustment for patients with Cl_{cr} >10 mL/minute. Secondary malignancies (including myelodysplastic syndrome, myeloproliferative disorders, acute myeloid leukemia and bronchial cancer) and premalignant diseases have been reported in patients who have received bendamustine.

Adverse Reactions

>10%:

Cardiovascular: Peripheral edema (NHL 13%; grades 3/4: <1%)

Central nervous system: Fatigue (NHL 57% [grades 3/4: 11%]; CLL 9%), headache (21%), dizziness (14%), chills (6% to 14%), insomnia (13%)

Dermatologic: Skin rash (8% to 16%; grades 3/4: ≤3%)

Endocrine & metabolic: Weight loss (NHL 18% [grades 3/4: 2%]; CLL 7%); dehydration (14%)

Gastrointestinal: Nausea (NHL 75% [grades 3/4: 4%]; CLL 20% [grades 3/4: <1%]), vomiting (NHL 40% [grades 3/4: 3%]; CLL 16% [grades 3/4: <1%]), diarrhea (NHL 37% [grades 3/4: 3%]; CLL 9% [grades 3/4: 1%]), constipation (NHL 29%; grades 3/4: <1%), anorexia (NHL 23%; grades 3/4: 2%), stomatitis (NHL 15%; grades 3/4: <1%), decreased appetite (NHL 13%; grades 3/4: <1%), abdominal pain (NHL 5% to 13%; grades 3/4: 1%), dyspepsia (11%)

Hematologic & oncologic: Lymphocytopenia (NHL 99% [grades 3/4: 94%]; CLL 68% [grades 3/4: 47%]), bone marrow depression (grades 3/4: 98%; nadir: In week 3), leukopenia (NHL 94% [grades 3/4: 56%]; CLL 61% [grades 3/4: 28%]), decreased hemoglobin (88% to 89%; grades 3/4: 11% to 13%), decreased neutrophils (NHL 86% [grades 3/4: 60%]; CLL 75% [grades 3/4: 43%]), thrombocytopenia (77% to 86%; grades 3/4: NHL 25%; CLL 11%)

Hepatic: Increased serum bilirubin (34%; grades 3/4: 3%)

Neuromuscular & skeletal: Back pain (14%), weakness (8% to 11%)

Respiratory: Cough (NHL 22%; CLL 4%), dyspnea (16%)

Miscellaneous: Fever (NHL 34%; CLL 24%)

1% to 10%:

Cardiovascular: Tachycardia (7%), chest pain (6%), hypotension (6%), exacerbation of hypertension (≤3%)

Central nervous system: Anxiety (8%), depression (6%), pain (6%)

Dermatologic: Pruritus (5% to 6%), hyperhidrosis (5%), night sweats (5%), xeroderma (5%)

Endocrine & metabolic: Hypokalemia (9%), hyperuricemia (7%; grades 3/4: 2%), hyperglycemia (grades 3/4: 3%), hypocalcemia (grades 3/4: 2%), hyponatremia (grades 3/4: 2%)

Gastrointestinal: Gastroesophageal reflux disease (10%), xerostomia (9%), dysgeusia (7%), oral candidiasis (6%), abdominal distention (5%)

Genitourinary: Urinary tract infection (10%)

Hematologic & oncologic: Febrile neutropenia (6%)

Hepatic: Increased serum ALT (grades 3/4: 3%), increased serum AST (grades 3/4: 1%)

Hypersensitivity: Hypersensitivity (5%; grades 3/4: 1%)

Infection: Herpes zoster (10%), infection (6%; grades 3/4: 2%), herpes simplex infection (3%)

Local: Infusion site reaction (6%), catheter pain (5%)

Neuromuscular & skeletal: Arthralgia (6%), limb pain (5%), ostealgia (5%)

Renal: Increased serum creatinine (grades 3/4: 2%)

Respiratory: Upper respiratory tract infection (10%), sinusitis (9%), pharyngolaryngeal pain (8%), pneumonia (8%), nasopharyngitis (6% to 7%), nasal congestion (5%), wheezing (5%)

<1% (Limited to important or life-threatening): Acute renal failure, alopecia, anaphylaxis, bronchogenic carcinoma, bullous rash, cardiac failure, dermatitis, dermatological reaction (toxic), drowsiness, erythema, exacerbation of hepatitis B, hemolysis, infusion related reaction, mucositis, myelodysplastic syndrome, myeloid leukemia (acute), myeloproliferative disease, pneumonitis, pulmonary fibrosis, sepsis, septic shock, skin necrosis, Stevens-Johnson syndrome, toxic epidermal necrolysis, tumor lysis syndrome

Drug Interactions

Metabolism/Transport Effects **Substrate** of BCRP, CYP1A2 (minor), P-glycoprotein; **Note:** Assignment of Major/Minor substrate status based on clinically relevant drug interaction potential

Avoid Concomitant Use

Avoid concomitant use of Bendamustine with any of the following: CloZAPine

Increased Effect/Toxicity

Bendamustine may increase the levels/effects of: CloZAPine

The levels/effects of Bendamustine may be increased by: Allopurinol; CYP1A2 Inhibitors (Strong)

Decreased Effect

The levels/effects of Bendamustine may be decreased by: CYP1A2 Inducers (Strong)

Preparation for Administration Hazardous agent; use appropriate precautions for handling and disposal (NIOSH, 2012). Reconstitute 25 mg vial with 5 mL and 100 mg vial with 20 mL of sterile water for injection to a concentration of 5 mg/mL; powder usually dissolves within 5 minutes. Prior to administration, dilute appropriate dose in 500 mL NS (or $D_{2.5}$½NS) to a final concentration of 0.2-0.6 mg/mL; mix thoroughly.

Storage/Stability Prior to reconstitution, store intact vials up to 25°C (77°F); excursions permitted up to 30°C (86°F). Protect from light. The solution in the vial (reconstituted with SWFI) is stable for 30 minutes (transfer to 500 mL infusion bag within that 30 minutes). The solution diluted in 500 mL for infusion is stable for 24 hours refrigerated or 3 hours at room temperature and room light. Infusion must be completed within these time frames.

Mechanism of Action Bendamustine is an alkylating agent (nitrogen mustard derivative) with a benzimidazole ring (purine analog) which demonstrates only partial cross-resistance (*in vitro*) with other alkylating agents. It leads to cell death via single and double strand DNA cross-linking. Bendamustine is active against quiescent and dividing cells. The primary cytotoxic activity is due to bendamustine (as compared to metabolites).

Pharmacodynamics/Kinetics

Distribution: V_{ss}: ~20-25 L

Protein binding: 94% to 96%

Metabolism: Hepatic (extensive), via CYP1A2 to active (minor) metabolites gamma-hydroxy bendamustine (M3) and N-desmethyl-bendamustine (M4); also via hydrolysis to low cytotoxic metabolites, monohydroxy bendamustine (HP1) and dihydroxy bendamustine (HP2)

Half-life elimination: Bendamustine: ~40 minutes; M3: ~3 hours; M4: ~30 minutes

Time to peak, serum: At end of infusion

Excretion: Feces (~25%); urine (~50%; ~3% as active parent drug)

Dosage Note: Bendamustine is associated with a moderate emetic potential (Basch, 2011); antiemetics are recommended to prevent nausea and vomiting.

Chronic lymphocytic leukemia (CLL): Adults: I.V.: 100 mg/m^2 over 30 minutes on days 1 and 2 of a 28-day treatment cycle (as a single agent) for up to 6 cycles (Knauf, 2009; Knauf, 2012)

CLL, relapsed/refractory (unlabeled dosing): Adults: I.V.: 70 mg/m^2 on days 1 and 2 of a 28-day treatment cycle (in combination with rituximab) for up to 6 cycles (Fischer, 2011)

Non-Hodgkin lymphomas: Adults: I.V.:

Lymphoma, indolent B-cell, refractory: 120 mg/m^2 over 60 minutes on days 1 and 2 of a 21-day treatment cycle (as a single agent) for up to 8 cycles (Kahl, 2010)

Lymphoma, indolent B-cell, follicular, or mantle cell, first-line (unlabeled use): 90 mg/m^2 on days 1 and 2 of a 28-day treatment cycle (in combination with rituximab) for up to 6 cycles (Rummel, 2009)

Lymphoma, follicular, relapsed or refractory (unlabeled use): 90 mg/m^2 on days 1 and 2 of a 35-day treatment cycle (in combination with bortezomib and rituximab) for 5 cycles (Fowler, 2011)

Lymphoma, mantle cell, relapsed or refractory (unlabeled use): 90 mg/m^2 over 30 minutes on days 2 and 3 of a 28-day treatment cycle (in combination with rituximab) for up to 4 cycles (Rummel, 2005)

Hodgkin lymphoma, relapsed or refractory (unlabeled use): Adults: I.V.: 120 mg/m^2 on days 1 and 2 of a 28-day treatment cycle for up to 6 cycles (Moskowitz, 2009)

Multiple myeloma, salvage therapy (unlabeled use): Adults: I.V.: 90-100 mg/m^2 on days 1 and 2 of a 28-day treatment cycle for at least 2 cycles (Knop, 2005)

Waldenström's macroglobulinemia, refractory (unlabeled use): Adults: I.V.: 90 mg/m^2 on days 1 and 2 of a 28-day treatment cycle (in combination with rituximab) for 6 cycles (Treon, 2011) **or** 90 mg/m^2 over 30 minutes on days 2 and 3 of a 28-day treatment cycle (in combination with rituximab) for 4 cycles (Rummel, 2005)

Dosage adjustment for toxicity:

Infusion reactions:

Grade 1 or 2: Consider premedication with antihistamines, antipyretics, and corticosteroids in subsequent cycles

Grade 3: Consider discontinuing treatment

Grade 4: Discontinue treatment

Skin reaction, severe or progressive: Withhold or discontinue treatment

Treatment delay:

Hematologic toxicity ≥grade 4: Delay treatment until resolves (ANC ≥1000/mm^3, platelets ≥75,000/mm^3)

Nonhematologic toxicity ≥grade 2 (clinically significant): Delay treatment until resolves to ≤grade 1

Dose modification in CLL:

Hematologic toxicity ≥grade 3: Reduce dose to 50 mg/m^2 on days 1 and 2 of each treatment cycle. For recurrent hematologic toxicity (≥grade 3), further reduce dose to 25 mg/m^2 on days 1 and 2 of the treatment cycle. May cautiously re-escalate dose in subsequent cycles.

Nonhematologic toxicity ≥grade 3 (clinically significant): Reduce dose to 50 mg/m^2 on days 1 and 2 of the treatment cycle with discretion. May cautiously re-escalate dose in subsequent cycles.

Dose modification in NHL:

Hematologic toxicity grade 4: Reduce dose to 90 mg/m^2 on days 1 and 2 of each treatment cycle. For recurrent hematologic toxicity (grade 4), further reduce dose to 60 mg/m^2 on days 1 and 2 of each treatment cycle.

Nonhematologic toxicity ≥grade 3: Reduce dose to 90 mg/m^2 on days 1 and 2 of the treatment cycle with discretion. For recurrent toxicity ≥grade 3, further reduce dose to 60 mg/m^2 on days 1 and 2 of each treatment cycle.

Dosage adjustment in renal impairment:

Cl_{cr} <40 mL/minute: Use is not recommended in the U.S. and Canadian manufacturers' labeling.

Study data suggest minor changes in systemic exposure may occur with mild-to-moderate renal impairment. Based on a pharmacokinetic study (patients receiving 120 mg/m^2 for 2 days every 21 days), only slight differences in bendamustine AUC and C_{max} were demonstrated in patients with mild (Cl_{cr} >50 to ≤80 mL/minute) and moderate (Cl_{cr} >30 to ≤50 mL/minute) renal dysfunction, compared to patients with normal renal function (Owen, 2010). A retrospective study of bendamustine in CLL and NHL patients with renal impairment (Cl_{cr} <40 mL/minute) compared to those without (Cl_{cr} ≥60 mL/minute) found no significant difference in lab toxicities in CLL patients with renal impairment compared to those without renal impairment, although an increase in grades 3/4 thrombocytopenia was noted in NHL patients and grades 3/4 BUN increases were higher when combining data for CLL and NHL (Nordstrom, 2012).

Note: UK manufacturer's labeling (Levact [prescribing information], October, 2010) recommends no dosage adjustment for patients with Cl_{cr} >10 mL/minute.

Dosage adjustment in hepatic impairment:

Mild impairment: Per U.S. and Canadian manufacturers' labeling, use with caution. However, a pharmacokinetic study showed only slight differences in bendamustine AUC and C_{max} in patients with mild hepatic impairment (defined in the study as total bilirubin 1-1.5 times ULN or AST greater than ULN), compared to patients with normal hepatic function (Owen, 2010).

Moderate impairment (AST or ALT 2.5-10 times ULN and total bilirubin 1.5-3 times ULN): Use is not recommended.

Severe impairment (total bilirubin >3 times ULN): Use is not recommended.

Dosing in obesity: *ASCO Guidelines for appropriate chemotherapy dosing in obese adults with cancer:* Utilize patient's actual body weight (full weight) for calculation of body surface area- or weight-based dosing, particularly when the intent of therapy is curative; manage regimen-related toxicities in the same manner as for nonobese patients; if a dose reduction is utilized due to toxicity, consider resumption of full weight-based dosing with subsequent cycles, especially if cause of toxicity (eg, hepatic or renal impairment) is resolved (Griggs, 2012).

Administration Infuse over 30 minutes for the treatment of CLL and over 60 minutes for NHL; administration times for unlabeled uses/doses vary by protocol. Consider premedication with antihistamines, antipyretics, and corticosteroids for patients with a previous grade 1 or 2 infusion reaction to bendamustine. Bendamustine is associated with a moderate emetic potential (Basch, 2011); antiemetics are recommended to prevent nausea and vomiting.

Irritant with vesicant-like properties; ensure proper needle or catheter placement prior to and during infusion. Avoid extravasation; monitor I.V. site for redness, swelling, or pain.

Extravasation management: If extravasation occurs, stop infusion immediately and disconnect (leave cannula/needle in place); gently aspirate extravasated solution (do **NOT** flush the line); remove needle/cannula; elevate extremity. Apply dry cold compresses for 20 minutes 4 times daily (Perez Fildago, 2012). May be managed with sodium thiosulfate in the same manner as mechlorethamine extravasation (Schulmeister, 2011).

Sodium thiosulfate 1/6 M solution (instructions for mechlorethamine): Inject subcutaneously into extravasation area using 2 mL for each mg of drug suspected to have extravasated (Perez Fidalgo, 2012; Polovich, 2009).

Hazardous agent; use appropriate precautions for handling and disposal (NIOSH, 2012).

Monitoring Parameters CBC with differential and platelets (monitored weekly [initially] in clinical trials); serum creatinine; ALT, AST, and total bilirubin; monitor potassium and uric acid levels in patients at risk for tumor lysis syndrome; monitor for infusion reactions anaphylaxis, infection, and dermatologic toxicity; monitor I.V. site during and after infusion.

Canadian labeling also recommends periodic monitoring of blood pressure, serum glucose, and ECG (in patients with cardiac disease particularly if concomitant electrolyte disturbances).

Dosage Forms Excipient information presented when available (limited, particularly for generics); consult specific product labeling.

Solution Reconstituted, Intravenous:

Treanda: 25 mg (1 ea); 100 mg (1 ea)

◆ **Bendamustine Hydrochloride** *see* Bendamustine *on page* 237

◆ **Benefiber [OTC]** *see* Wheat Dextrin *on page* 2215

◆ **Benefiber Drink Mix [OTC]** *see* Wheat Dextrin *on page* 2215

◆ **Benefiber For Children [OTC]** *see* Wheat Dextrin *on page* 2215

◆ **Benefiber Plus Calcium [OTC]** *see* Wheat Dextrin *on page* 2215

◆ **BeneFIX** *see* Factor IX (Recombinant) *on page* 827

◆ **BeneFix (Can)** *see* Factor IX (Recombinant) *on page* 827

◆ **Benemid [DSC]** *see* Probenecid *on page* 1716

◆ **Benflumetol and Artemether** *see* Artemether and Lumefantrine *on page* 171

◆ **BenGay® [OTC]** *see* Methyl Salicylate and Menthol *on page* 1344

◆ **Benicar** *see* Olmesartan *on page* 1497

◆ **Benicar HCT** *see* Olmesartan and Hydrochlorothiazide *on page* 1499

◆ **Benlysta** *see* Belimumab *on page* 233

◆ **Benoxinate Hydrochloride and Fluorescein Sodium** *see* Fluorescein and Benoxinate *on page* 880

Bentoquatam (BEN toe kwa tam)

Brand Names: U.S. Ivy Block [OTC]

Index Terms Quaternium-18 Bentonite

Pharmacologic Category Topical Skin Product

Use Skin protectant for the prevention of poison ivy, poison oak, and poison sumac

Dosage Skin protectant: Children ≥6 years and Adults: Topical: Apply to skin 15 minutes prior to potential exposure to poison ivy, poison oak, or poison sumac; may reapply every 4 hours

Additional Information Complete prescribing information should be consulted for additional detail.

Dosage Forms Excipient information presented when available (limited, particularly for generics); consult specific product labeling.

Lotion, topical:

Ivy Block: 5% (30 mL, 120 mL) [contains benzyl alcohol, ethanol 25%]

◆ **Bentyl** *see* Dicyclomine *on page* 601

◆ **Bentylol (Can)** *see* Dicyclomine *on page* 601

◆ **Benuryl™ (Can)** *see* Probenecid *on page* 1716

◆ **Benylin® 3.3 mg-D-E (Can)** *see* Guaifenesin, Pseudoephedrine, and Codeine *on page* 979

◆ **Benylin® D for Infants (Can)** *see* Pseudoephedrine *on page* 1746

◆ **Benylin® DM-D (Can)** *see* Pseudoephedrine and Dextromethorphan *on page* 1748

◆ **Benylin® DM-D-E (Can)** *see* Guaifenesin, Pseudoephedrine, and Dextromethorphan *on page* 979

◆ **Benylin DM-E (Can)** *see* Guaifenesin and Dextromethorphan *on page* 976

◆ **Benylin® E Extra Strength (Can)** *see* GuaiFENesin *on page* 974

◆ **Benzamycin®** *see* Erythromycin and Benzoyl Peroxide *on page* 744

◆ **Benzamycin® Pak** *see* Erythromycin and Benzoyl Peroxide *on page* 744

◆ **Benzathine Benzylpenicillin** *see* Penicillin G Benzathine *on page* 1606

◆ **Benzathine Penicillin G** *see* Penicillin G Benzathine *on page* 1606

◆ **Benzene Hexachloride** *see* Lindane *on page* 1217

◆ **Benzhexol Hydrochloride** *see* Trihexyphenidyl *on page* 2127

◆ **Benzmethyzin** *see* Procarbazine *on page* 1720

Benzocaine (BEN zoe kane)

Brand Names: U.S. Anacaine; Anbesol Cold Sore Therapy [OTC]; Anbesol JR [OTC]; Anbesol Maximum Strength [OTC]; Anbesol [OTC]; Baby Anbesol [OTC]; Benz-O-Sthetic [OTC]; Benzocaine Oral Anesthetic [OTC]; Bi-Zets/Benzotroches [OTC]; Cepacol Dual Relief [OTC]; Cepacol Sensations Hydra [OTC]; Cepacol Sensations Warming [OTC]; Cepacol Sore Throat + Coating [OTC]; Cepacol Sore Throat Max Numb [OTC]; Cepacol Sore Throat [OTC]; Chiggerex [OTC]; Chiggertox [OTC]; Dent-O-Kain/20 [OTC]; Dentapaine [OTC]; Foille [OTC]; Hurri-Caine One [OTC]; Hurricaine [OTC]; Ivy-Rid [OTC]; Kank-A Mouth Pain [OTC]; Ora-film [OTC]; Oral Pain Relief Max St [OTC]; Pinnacaine Otic; Sore Throat Relief [OTC]; Topex Topical Anesthetic; Trocaine Throat [OTC]; Zilactin Baby [OTC]

Brand Names: Canada Anbesol® Baby; Zilactin Baby®; Zilactin-B®

Index Terms Ethyl Aminobenzoate

Pharmacologic Category Antihemorrhoidal Agent; Local Anesthetic

Use Temporary relief of pain associated with pruritic dermatosis, pruritus, minor burns, acute congestive, bee stings, and insect bites; mouth and gum irritations (toothache, minor sore throat pain, canker sores, dentures, orthodontia, teething, mucositis, stomatitis); sunburn; hemorrhoids; anesthetic lubricant for passage of catheters and endoscopic tubes

Pregnancy Risk Factor C

Pregnancy Considerations Reproduction studies have not been conducted.

Breast-Feeding Considerations It is not known if benzocaine is excreted in breast milk. The manufacturer recommends that caution be exercised when administering benzocaine to nursing women.

Contraindications Hypersensitivity to benzocaine, other ester-type local anesthetics, or any component of the formulation; secondary bacterial infection of area; ophthalmic use

Warnings/Precautions Methemoglobinemia has been reported following topical use, particularly with higher concentration (14% to 20%) spray formulations applied to the mouth or mucous membranes. When applied as a spray to the mouth or throat, multiple sprays (or sprays of longer than indicated duration) are not recommended. Use caution with breathing problems (asthma, bronchitis, emphysema, in smokers), inflamed/damaged mucosa, heart disease, and hemoglobin or enzyme abnormalities (glucose-6-phosphate dehydrogenase deficiency, hemoglobin-M disease, NADH-methemoglobin reductase deficiency, pyruvate-kinase deficiency). Alternatives to benzocaine sprays, such as topical lidocaine preparations, should be considered for patients at higher risk of this reaction. Due to the heightened risk of methemoglobinemia, not recommended for use in patients <2 years of age unless under the advice and supervision by a healthcare professional.

The classical clinical finding of methemoglobinemia is chocolate brown-colored arterial blood. However, suspected cases should be confirmed by co-oximetry, which yields a direct and accurate measure of methemoglobin levels. Standard pulse oximetry readings or arterial blood gas values are not reliable. Clinically significant methemoglobinemia requires immediate treatment.

When topical anesthetics are used prior to cosmetic or medical procedures, the lowest amount of anesthetic necessary for pain relief should be applied. High systemic levels and toxic effects (eg, methemoglobinemia, irregular heart beats, respiratory depression, seizures, death) have been reported in patients who (without supervision of a trained professional) have applied topical anesthetics in large amounts (or to large areas of the skin), left these products on for prolonged periods of time, or have used wraps/dressings to cover the skin following application.

When used for self-medication (OTC), notify healthcare provider if condition worsens or does not improve within the timeframe noted on the product labeling or if accompanied by additional symptoms (eg, swelling, rash, headache, nausea, vomiting, or fever). Do not use topical products on open wounds; avoid contact with the eyes.

Adverse Reactions Frequency not defined.

Hematologic: Methemoglobinemia

Local: Burning, contact dermatitis, edema, erythema, pruritus, rash, stinging, tenderness, urticaria

Miscellaneous: Hypersensitivity

Drug Interactions

Metabolism/Transport Effects None known.

Avoid Concomitant Use There are no known interactions where it is recommended to avoid concomitant use.

Increased Effect/Toxicity

Benzocaine may increase the levels/effects of: Prilocaine; Sodium Nitrite

The levels/effects of Benzocaine may be increased by: Nitric Oxide

Decreased Effect

Benzocaine may decrease the levels/effects of: Technetium Tc 99m Tilmanocept

Mechanism of Action Ester local anesthetic blocks both the initiation and conduction of nerve impulses by decreasing the neuronal membrane's permeability to sodium ions, which results in inhibition of depolarization with resultant blockade of conduction

Pharmacodynamics/Kinetics

Absorption: Topical: Poor to intact skin; well absorbed from mucous membranes and traumatized skin

Metabolism: Hepatic (to a lesser extent) and plasma via hydrolysis by cholinesterase

Excretion: Urine (as metabolites)

Dosage Note: These are general dosing guidelines; refer to specific product labeling for dosing instructions.

Children ≥4 months: Topical (oral): Teething pain: 7.5% to 10%: Apply to affected gum area up to 4 times daily

Children ≥2 years and Adults:

Topical:

Bee stings, insect bites, minor burns, sunburn: 5% to 20%: Apply to affected area 3-4 times daily as needed. In cases of bee stings, remove stinger before treatment.

Boils: 20%: Apply to affected area up to 2 times daily (maximum: 2 times/day)

Lubricant for passage of catheters and instruments: 20%: Apply evenly to exterior of instrument prior to use.

Topical (oral): Mouth and gum irritation: 10% to 20%: Apply thin layer to affected area up to 4 times daily

Children ≥5 years and Adults: Oral: Sore throat: Allow 1 lozenge (10-15 mg) to dissolve slowly in mouth; may repeat every 2 hours as needed

Children ≥6 years and Adults: Topical (oral) spray: 5%: Sore throat or mouth: One spray to affected area, then wait ≥1 minute and spit; may repeat up to 4 times daily. **Note:** Children 6-11 years should only use under adult supervision.

Children ≥12 years and Adults: Rectal: Hemorrhoids: 5% to 20%: Apply externally to affected area up to 6 times daily

Dietary Considerations Some products may contain sodium.

Administration Avoid application to large areas of broken skin, especially in children. When possible, apply to clean, dry area. When administering a spray formulation, the number of sprays administered and the length of each spray should be monitored and recorded.

Monitoring Parameters Monitor patients for signs and symptoms of methemoglobinemia such as pallor, cyanosis, nausea, muscle weakness, dizziness, confusion, agitation, dyspnea and tachycardia. The classical clinical finding of methemoglobinemia is chocolate brown-colored arterial blood. However, suspected cases should be confirmed by co-oximetry, which yields a direct and accurate measure of methemoglobin levels. Standard pulse oximetry readings or arterial blood gas values are not reliable. Clinically significant methemoglobinemia requires immediate treatment.

Dosage Forms Excipient information presented when available (limited, particularly for generics); consult specific product labeling.

Aerosol, External:

Ivy-Rid: 2% (82.5 mL)

Gel, Mouth/Throat:

Anbesol: 10% (9 g) [contains benzyl alcohol, brilliant blue fcf (fd&c blue #1), fd&c yellow #10 (quinoline yellow), fd&c yellow #6 (sunset yellow), methylparaben, propylene glycol, saccharin; cool mint flavor]

Anbesol JR: 10% (9 g) [contains methylparaben]

Anbesol Maximum Strength: 20% (9 g) [contains brilliant blue fcf (fd&c blue #1), fd&c red #40, fd&c yellow #10 (quinoline yellow), methylparaben, saccharin]

Baby Anbesol: 7.5% (9 g)

Benz-O-Sthetic: 20% (15 g) [contains benzyl alcohol, saccharin sodium]
Benz-O-Sthetic: 20% (29 g) [contains benzyl alcohol, saccharin sodium; bubble-gum flavor]
Benz-O-Sthetic: 20% (29 g) [contains benzyl alcohol, saccharin sodium; cherry flavor]
Dentapaine: 20% (11 g)
Hurricaine: 20% (5.25 g) [contains polyethylene glycol, saccharin sodium]
Hurricaine: 20% (28.4 g) [contains polyethylene glycol, saccharin sodium; mint flavor]
Hurricaine: 20% (30 g) [contains polyethylene glycol, saccharin sodium; pina colada flavor]
Hurricaine: 20% (30 g) [contains polyethylene glycol, saccharin sodium; watermelon flavor]
Hurricaine: 20% (5.25 g, 30 g) [contains polyethylene glycol, saccharin sodium; wild cherry flavor]
Oral Pain Relief Max St: 20% (14.2 g) [contains saccharin sodium]
Zilactin Baby: 10% (9.4 g) [alcohol free, dye free, saccharin free]

Liquid, External:
Chiggertox: 2.1% (30 mL)

Liquid, Mouth/Throat:
Anbesol: 10% (12 mL) [contains brilliant blue fcf (fd&c blue #1), fd&c yellow #10 (quinoline yellow), fd&c yellow #6 (sunset yellow), methylparaben, saccharin; cool mint flavor]
Anbesol Maximum Strength: 20% (12 mL) [contains benzyl alcohol, brilliant blue fcf (fd&c blue #1), fd&c red #40, fd&c yellow #10 (quinoline yellow), methylparaben, polyethylene glycol, propylene glycol, saccharin]
Benz-O-Sthetic: 20% (56 g) [contains benzyl alcohol, brilliant blue fcf (fd&c blue #1), fd&c red #40, fd&c yellow #10 (quinoline yellow), polyethylene glycol, propylene glycol, saccharin]
Cepacol Dual Relief: 5% (22.2 mL) [sugar free; cherry flavor]
Dent-O-Kain/20: 20% (9 mL) [contains benzyl alcohol, brilliant blue fcf (fd&c blue #1), d&c yellow #11 (quinoline yellow ss), fd&c red #40, propylene glycol, saccharin]
Oral Pain Relief Max St: 20% (15 mL) [contains benzyl alcohol, brilliant blue fcf (fd&c blue #1), fd&c red #40, fd&c yellow #10 (quinoline yellow), methylparaben, polyethylene glycol, propylene glycol, saccharin]

Lozenge, Mouth/Throat:
Bi-Zets/Benzotroches: 15 mg (10 ea) [orange flavor]
Cepacol Sensations Hydra: 3 mg (20 ea) [contains brilliant blue fcf (fd&c blue #1), fd&c yellow #10 (quinoline yellow)]
Cepacol Sensations Warming: 4 mg (20 ea) [contains fd&c red #40, fd&c yellow #10 (quinoline yellow)]
Cepacol Sore Throat: 15 mg (576 ea) [contains fd&c red #40; cherry flavor]
Cepacol Sore Throat: 15% (16 ea) [contains fd&c yellow #10 (quinoline yellow), fd&c yellow #6 (sunset yellow); honey-lemon flavor]
Cepacol Sore Throat: 15 mg (16 ea) [sugar free; contains fd&c red #40; cherry flavor]
Cepacol Sore Throat + Coating: 15 mg (16 ea) [sugar free; contains brilliant blue fcf (fd&c blue #1), fd&c yellow #10 (quinoline yellow); lemon-lime flavor]
Cepacol Sore Throat Max Numb: 15 mg (16 ea) [contains fd&c red #40; cherry flavor]
Cepacol Sore Throat Max Numb: 15 mg (16 ea) [sugar free; contains fd&c red #40; cherry flavor]
Sore Throat Relief: 10 mg (2 ea) [wild cherry flavor]
Trocaine Throat: 10 mg (1 ea)

Ointment, External:
Anacaine: 10% (30 g)
Anbesol Cold Sore Therapy: 20% (9 g) [contains aloe, vitamin e]
Chiggerex: 2% (52.5 g)
Foille: 5% (28 g)

Solution, Mouth/Throat:
Benz-O-Sthetic: 20% (30 mL) [contains polyethylene glycol, saccharin]
Benzocaine Oral Anesthetic: 20% (59.7 g) [contains alcohol, usp, polyethylene glycol, saccharin sodium]
Hurricaine: 20% (57 g) [contains polyethylene glycol, saccharin sodium]
Hurricaine: 20% (30 mL) [contains polyethylene glycol, saccharin sodium; pina colada flavor]
Hurricaine: 20% (57 g, 30 mL) [contains polyethylene glycol, saccharin sodium; wild cherry flavor]
HurriCaine One: 20% (2 ea, 25 ea) [contains polyethylene glycol, saccharin sodium]
Kank-A Mouth Pain: 20% (9.75 mL) [contains benzyl alcohol, propylene glycol, saccharin sodium]
Topex Topical Anesthetic: 20% (57 g) [cherry flavor]

Solution, Otic:
Pinnacaine Otic: 20% (15 mL)

Strip, Mouth/Throat:
Ora-film: 6% (12 ea) [contains brilliant blue fcf (fd&c blue #1), menthol, methylparaben, propylparaben, tartrazine (fd&c yellow #5)]

Swab, Mouth/Throat:
Benz-O-Sthetic: 20% (2 ea) [contains benzyl alcohol, polyethylene glycol, saccharin sodium]
Benz-O-Sthetic: 20% (2 ea) [contains benzyl alcohol, polyethylene glycol, saccharin sodium; cherry flavor]
Hurricaine: 20% (72 ea) [contains polyethylene glycol, saccharin sodium; wild cherry flavor]

◆ **Benzocaine and Antipyrine** *see* Antipyrine and Benzocaine *on page* 148

Benzocaine, Butamben, and Tetracaine

(BEN zoe kane, byoo TAM ben, & TET ra kane)

Brand Names: U.S. Cetacaine

Index Terms Benzocaine, Butamben, and Tetracaine Hydrochloride; Benzocaine, Butyl Aminobenzoate, and Tetracaine; Butamben, Tetracaine, and Benzocaine; Exactacain; Tetracaine, Benzocaine, and Butamben

Pharmacologic Category Local Anesthetic

Use Topical anesthetic to control pain in surgical or endoscopic procedures, or other procedures in the ear, nose, mouth, pharynx, larynx, trachea, bronchi, and esophagus (may also be used for vaginal or rectal procedure, when feasible); anesthetic for accessible mucous membranes except for the eyes; to control pain or gagging (spray only)

Dosage Topical anesthetic: **Note:** Decrease dose in the acutely-ill patient.

Children: Dose has not been established; dose reduction is suggested

Adults: Cetacaine:

Spray: Apply for ≤1 second; use of sprays >2 seconds is contraindicated. **Note:** Spray provides ~200 mg/second

Gel: Apply 200 mg (~1/4 to 1/2 inch); application of >400 mg (>1 inch) is contraindicated

Liquid: Apply 200 mg (~0.2 mL); application of >400 mg (~0.4 mL) is contraindicated

Elderly: Dose reduction is suggested

Dosage adjustment in renal impairment: No dosage adjustment provided in manufacturer's labeling.

Dosage adjustment in hepatic impairment: No dosage adjustment provided in manufacturer's labeling.

Additional Information Complete prescribing information should be consulted for additional detail.

Dosage Forms Excipient information presented when available (limited, particularly for generics); consult specific product labeling.

Aerosol, spray, topical [kit]:

Cetacaine: Benzocaine 14%, butamben 2%, and tetracaine hydrochloride 2% (56 g) [delivers benzocaine 28 mg, butamben 4 mg, and tetracaine hydrochloride 4 mg per second; contains benzalkonium chloride, chlorofluorocarbon; packaged with cannula assortment]

Aerosol, spray, topical:

Cetacaine: Benzocaine 14%, butamben 2%, and tetracaine hydrochloride 2% (56 g) [delivers benzocaine 28 mg, butamben 4 mg, and tetracaine hydrochloride 4 mg per second; contains benzalkonium chloride, chlorofluorocarbon; packaged with cannula]

Gel, topical:

Cetacaine: Benzocaine 14%, butamben 2%, and tetracaine hydrochloride 2% (29 g [DSC]) [provides benzocaine 28 mg, butamben 4 mg and tetracaine hydrochloride 4 mg per 0.5 inch (13 mm) x 3/16 inch (5 mm) application; contains benzalkonium chloride]

Cetacaine: Benzocaine 14%, butamben 2%, and tetracaine hydrochloride 2% (32 g) [delivers benzocaine 28 mg, butamben 4 mg and tetracaine hydrochloride 4 mg per pump actuation ~0.25 inch (6.5 mm) x 0.5 inch (13 mm) long application; contains benzalkonium chloride]

Liquid, topical [kit]:

Cetacaine: Benzocaine 14%, butamben 2%, and tetracaine hydrochloride 2% (14 g) [provides benzocaine 28 mg, butamben 4 mg, and tetracaine hydrochloride 4 mg per 6-7 drops (0.2 mL); contains benzalkonium chloride; packaged with syringes and applicator tips]

Liquid, topical:

Cetacaine: Benzocaine 14%, butamben 2%, and tetracaine hydrochloride 2% (14 g, 30 g) [provides benzocaine 28 mg, butamben 4 mg, and tetracaine hydrochloride 4 mg per 6-7 drops (0.2 mL); contains benzalkonium chloride]

◆ **Benzocaine, Butamben, and Tetracaine Hydrochloride** *see* Benzocaine, Butamben, and Tetracaine *on page 242*

◆ **Benzocaine, Butyl Aminobenzoate, and Tetracaine** *see* Benzocaine, Butamben, and Tetracaine *on page 242*

◆ **Benzocaine Oral Anesthetic [OTC]** *see* Benzocaine *on page 240*

◆ **Benzoic Acid, Hyoscyamine, Methenamine, Methylene Blue, and Phenyl Salicylate** *see* Methenamine, Phenyl Salicylate, Methylene Blue, Benzoic Acid, and Hyoscyamine *on page 1319*

◆ **Benzoic Acid, Methenamine, Methylene Blue, Phenyl Salicylate, and Hyoscyamine** *see* Methenamine, Phenyl Salicylate, Methylene Blue, Benzoic Acid, and Hyoscyamine *on page 1319*

Benzonatate (ben ZOE na tate)

Brand Names: U.S. Tessalon Perles; Zonatuss

Index Terms Tessalon Perles

Pharmacologic Category Antitussive

Use Symptomatic relief of nonproductive cough

Pregnancy Risk Factor C

Dosage Children >10 years and Adults: Oral: 100-200 mg 3 times/day as needed for cough; maximum dose: 600 mg/day

Dosage adjustment in renal impairment: No dosage adjustment provided in manufacturer's labeling.

Dosage adjustment in hepatic impairment: No dosage adjustment provided in manufacturer's labeling.

Additional Information Complete prescribing information should be consulted for additional detail.

Dosage Forms Excipient information presented when available (limited, particularly for generics); consult specific product labeling.

Capsule, Oral:

Tessalon Perles: 100 mg

Zonatuss: 150 mg [contains brilliant blue fcf (fd&c blue #1)]

Generic: 100 mg, 200 mg

◆ **Benz-O-Sthetic [OTC]** *see* Benzocaine *on page 240*

◆ **Benzoyl Peroxide and Adapalene** *see* Adapalene and Benzoyl Peroxide *on page 48*

◆ **Benzoyl Peroxide and Erythromycin** *see* Erythromycin and Benzoyl Peroxide *on page 744*

Benzoyl Peroxide and Hydrocortisone

(BEN zoe il peer OKS ide & hye droe KOR ti sone)

Brand Names: U.S. Vanoxide-HC®

Brand Names: Canada Vanoxide-HC®

Index Terms Hydrocortisone and Benzoyl Peroxide

Pharmacologic Category Acne Products; Topical Skin Product; Topical Skin Product, Acne

Use Treatment of acne vulgaris and oily skin

Pregnancy Risk Factor C

Dosage Adolescents ≥12 years and Adults: Topical: Apply thin film 1-3 times/day

Additional Information Complete prescribing information should be consulted for additional detail.

Dosage Forms Excipient information presented when available (limited, particularly for generics); consult specific product labeling.

Lotion, topical:

Vanoxide-HC®: Benzoyl peroxide 5% and hydrocortisone 0.5% (25 g)

Benztropine (BENZ troe peen)

Brand Names: U.S. Cogentin

Brand Names: Canada Apo-Benztropine®; Benztropine Omega; PMS-Benztropine

Index Terms Benztropine Mesylate

Pharmacologic Category Anti-Parkinson's Agent, Anticholinergic; Anticholinergic Agent

Additional Appendix Information

Antiparkinsonian Agents *on page 2289*

Beers Criteria – Potentially Inappropriate Medications for Geriatrics *on page 2368*

Use Adjunctive treatment of Parkinson's disease; aid in the treatment of drug-induced extrapyramidal symptoms (except tardive dyskinesia)

Pregnancy Considerations Animal reproduction studies have not been conducted. Paralytic ileus (which resolved rapidly) was reported in two newborns exposed to a combination of benztropine and chlorpromazine during the second and third trimesters and the last 6 weeks of pregnancy, respectively (Falterman, 1980).

Breast-Feeding Considerations It is not known if benztropine is excreted in breast milk. Anticholinergic agents may suppress lactation.

Contraindications Hypersensitivity to benztropine or any component of the formulation; children <3 years of age (due to atropine-like adverse effects)

Warnings/Precautions Use with caution in children >3 years of age due to its anticholinergic effects (dose has not been established). Use is contraindicated in children <3 years of age. Use with caution in hot weather or during exercise. May cause anhydrosis and hyperthermia, which may be severe. The risk is increased in hot environments, particularly in the elderly, alcoholics, patients with CNS disease, and those with prolonged outdoor exposure.

Use with caution in patients >65 years of age; response in elderly may be altered. Initiate at low doses in the elderly and increase as needed while monitoring for adverse events. Avoid use of oral benztropine in older adults for prevention of extrapyramidal symptoms with antipsychotics and alternative agents preferred in the treatment of Parkinson's disease. May be inappropriate in older adults depending on comorbidities (eg, dementia, delirium) due to its potent anticholinergic effects (Beers Criteria). Avoid use in patients with myasthenia gravis, may precipitate myasthenic crisis. Avoid use in angle-closure glaucoma.

Use with caution in patients with tachycardia, cardiac arrhythmias, hypertension, hypotension, glaucoma, prostatic hyperplasia (especially in the elderly), any tendency toward urinary retention, liver or kidney disorders, and obstructive disease of the GI or GU tracts. When given in large doses or to susceptible patients, may cause weakness and inability to move particular muscle groups.

May be associated with confusion, visual hallucinations, or excitement (generally at higher dosages). Intensification of symptoms or toxic psychosis may occur in patients with mental disorders. May cause CNS depression, which may impair physical or mental abilities; patients must be cautioned about performing tasks which require mental alertness (eg, operating machinery or driving). Benztropine does not relieve symptoms of tardive dyskinesia and may potentially exacerbate symptoms.

Potentially significant drug-drug interactions may exist, requiring dose or frequency adjustment, additional monitoring, and/or selection of alternative therapy.

Adverse Reactions Frequency not defined.

Cardiovascular: Tachycardia

Central nervous system: Confusion, depression, disorientation, exacerbation of pre-existing psychotic symptoms, fever, listlessness, memory impairment, nervousness, toxic psychosis, visual hallucinations

Dermatologic: Rash

Endocrine & metabolic: Heat stroke, hyperthermia

Gastrointestinal: Constipation, nausea, paralytic ileus, vomiting, xerostomia

Genitourinary: Urinary retention, dysuria

Neuromuscular & skeletal: Numbness of fingers

Ocular: Blurred vision, mydriasis

Drug Interactions

Metabolism/Transport Effects **Substrate** of CYP2D6 (minor); **Note:** Assignment of Major/Minor substrate status based on clinically relevant drug interaction potential

Avoid Concomitant Use

Avoid concomitant use of Benztropine with any of the following: Aclidinium; Ipratropium (Oral Inhalation); Potassium Chloride; Tiotropium; Umeclidinium

Increased Effect/Toxicity

Benztropine may increase the levels/effects of: AbobotulinumtoxinA; Analgesics (Opioid); Anticholinergics; Cannabinoids; Mirabegron; OnabotulinumtoxinA; Potassium Chloride; RimabotulinumtoxinB; Thiazide Diuretics; Tiotropium; Topiramate

The levels/effects of Benztropine may be increased by: Aclidinium; Ipratropium (Oral Inhalation); Pramlintide; Umeclidinium

Decreased Effect

Benztropine may decrease the levels/effects of: Acetylcholinesterase Inhibitors (Central); Ioflupane I 123; Secretin

The levels/effects of Benztropine may be decreased by: Acetylcholinesterase Inhibitors (Central); Peginterferon Alfa-2b

Ethanol/Nutrition/Herb Interactions Ethanol: Avoid ethanol (may increase CNS depression).

Mechanism of Action Possesses both anticholinergic and antihistaminic effects. *In vitro* anticholinergic activity approximates that of atropine; *in vivo* it is only about half as active as atropine. Animal data suggest its antihistaminic activity and duration of action approach that of pyrilamine maleate. May also inhibit the reuptake and storage of dopamine, thereby prolonging the action of dopamine.

Pharmacodynamics/Kinetics

Onset of action: I.M., I.V.: Within a few minutes

Metabolism: Hepatic (N-oxidation, N-dealkylation, and ring hydroxylation) (from animal studies only)

Time to peak, plasma: 7 hours

Dosage

Drug-induced extrapyramidal symptoms: Oral, I.M., I.V.:

Children >3 years (unlabeled dose): 0.02-0.05 mg/kg/dose 1-2 times daily

Adults: 1-4 mg 1-2 times daily or 1-2 mg 2-3 times daily for reactions developing soon after initiation of antipsychotic medication; usually provides relief within 1-2 days, but may continue for up to 1-2 weeks; withdraw after 1-2 weeks to reassess continued need for therapy. May reinitiate benztropine if symptoms recur.

Acute dystonia: Adults: I.M., I.V.: 1-2 mg

Parkinsonism, idiopathic or postencephalitic: Adults: Oral, I.M., I.V.: Usual dose: 1-2 mg daily; range: 0.5-6 mg daily in a single dose at bedtime or divided in 2-4 doses; titrate dose in 0.5 mg increments at 5- to 6-day intervals up to a maximum daily dose of 6 mg.

Note: Dosing should be individualized based on patient age, weight, and type of parkinsonism being treated. Lower initial doses may be appropriate for older and thinner patients. Low initial doses (0.5-1 mg) may also be appropriate for idiopathic parkinsonism and may be adequate for maintenance. Higher initial doses (2 mg daily) may be required for postencephalitic parkinsonism. Dosing schedule should also be individualized; patients may respond more favorably to either once daily bedtime dosing or 2-4 divided doses throughout the day; however, once daily bedtime dosing is often effective.

Elderly: Use caution or avoid; anticholinergics generally not tolerated in older adults. If used, start at low end of dosing range and increase only as needed and as tolerated.

Dosage adjustment in renal impairment: No dosage adjustment provided in manufacturer's labeling.

Dosage adjustment in hepatic impairment: No dosage adjustment provided in manufacturer's labeling.

Dietary Considerations Tablet may be taken with or without food.

Administration

Oral: May be given with or without food.

Injectable: May administer I.M or I.V. if oral route is unacceptable. Manufacturer's labeling states there is no difference in onset of effect after I.V. or I.M. injection and therefore there is usually no need to use the I.V. route. No specific instructions on administering benztropine I.V. are provided in the labeling. The I.V. route has been reported in the literature (slow I.V. push when reported), although specific instructions are lacking (Duncan, 2001; Lydon, 1998; Sachdev, 1993; Schramm, 2002).

Monitoring Parameters Symptoms of EPS or Parkinson's, pulse, anticholinergic effects

Dosage Forms Excipient information presented when available (limited, particularly for generics); consult specific product labeling.

Solution, Injection, as mesylate:
Cogentin: 1 mg/mL (2 mL)
Generic: 1 mg/mL (2 mL)

Tablet, Oral, as mesylate:
Generic: 0.5 mg, 1 mg, 2 mg

◆ **Benztropine Mesylate** *see* Benztropine *on page 243*

◆ **Benztropine Omega (Can)** *see* Benztropine *on page 243*

Benzyl Alcohol (BEN zill AL koe hol)

Brand Names: U.S. Ulesfia; Zilactin [OTC]

Pharmacologic Category Analgesic, Topical; Antiparasitic Agent, Topical; Pediculocide; Topical Skin Product

Use

Liquid (Zilactin®-L): Temporary relief of pain from cold sores/fever blisters

Lotion (Ulesfia™): Treatment of head lice infestation

Pregnancy Risk Factor B

Dosage Topical:

Lotion: Head lice: Children ≥6 months and Adults: Apply appropriate volume for hair length to dry hair and completely saturate the scalp; leave on for 10 minutes; rinse thoroughly with water; repeat in 7 days
Hair length 0-2 inches: 4-6 ounces
Hair length 2-4 inches: 6-8 ounces
Hair length 4-8 inches: 8-12 ounces
Hair length 8-16 inches: 12-24 ounces
Hair length 16-22 inches: 24-32 ounces
Hair length >22 inches: 32-48 ounces

Liquid (topical): Cold sores/fever blisters: Children ≥2 years and Adults: Apply to affected area up to 4 times/day

Additional Information Complete prescribing information should be consulted for additional detail.

Dosage Forms Excipient information presented when available (limited, particularly for generics); consult specific product labeling.

Gel, Mouth/Throat:
Zilactin: 10% (7.1 g) [contains propylene glycol, sd alcohol]

Lotion, External:
Ulesfia: 5% (227 g) [contains polysorbate 80, trolamine (triethanolamine)]

◆ **Benzylpenicillin Benzathine** *see* Penicillin G Benzathine *on page 1606*

◆ **Benzylpenicillin Potassium** *see* Penicillin G (Parenteral/Aqueous) *on page 1608*

◆ **Benzylpenicillin Sodium** *see* Penicillin G (Parenteral/Aqueous) *on page 1608*

Bepotastine (be poe TAS teen)

Brand Names: U.S. Bepreve

Index Terms Bepotastine Besilate

Pharmacologic Category Histamine H_1 Antagonist; Histamine H_1 Antagonist, Second Generation; Mast Cell Stabilizer

Use Treatment of itching associated with allergic conjunctivitis

Pregnancy Risk Factor C

Dosage Ophthalmic: Children ≥2 years and Adults: Allergic conjunctivitis: Instill 1 drop into the affected eye(s) twice daily

Additional Information Complete prescribing information should be consulted for additional detail.

Dosage Forms Excipient information presented when available (limited, particularly for generics); consult specific product labeling.

Solution, Ophthalmic, as besilate:
Bepreve: 1.5% (5 mL, 10 mL) [contains benzalkonium chloride]

◆ **Bepotastine Besilate** *see* Bepotastine *on page 245*

◆ **Bepreve** *see* Bepotastine *on page 245*

Beractant (ber AKT ant)

Brand Names: U.S. Survanta

Brand Names: Canada Survanta®

Index Terms Bovine Lung Surfactant; Natural Lung Surfactant

Pharmacologic Category Lung Surfactant

Use Prevention and treatment of respiratory distress syndrome (RDS) in premature infants

Prophylactic therapy: Body weight <1250 g in infants at risk for developing, or with evidence of, surfactant deficiency (administer within 15 minutes of birth)

Rescue therapy: Treatment of infants with RDS confirmed by x-ray and requiring mechanical ventilation (administer as soon as possible - within 8 hours of age)

Pregnancy Considerations Beractant is only indicated for use in premature infants.

Contraindications

There are no contraindications listed within the FDA-approved labeling

Warnings/Precautions For endotracheal administration only. Rapidly affects oxygenation and lung compliance; restrict use to a highly-supervised clinical setting with immediate availability of clinicians experienced in intubation and ventilatory management of premature infants. Transient episodes of bradycardia and decreased oxygen saturation occur. Discontinue dosing procedure and initiate measures to alleviate the condition; may reinstitute after the patient is stable. Produces rapid improvements in lung oxygenation and compliance that may require frequent adjustments to oxygen delivery and ventilator settings.

Adverse Reactions During the dosing procedure:

>10%: Cardiovascular: Transient bradycardia

1% to 10%: Respiratory: Oxygen desaturation

<1% (Limited to important or life-threatening): Apnea, endotracheal tube blockage, hypercarbia, hyper-/hypotension, post-treatment nosocomial sepsis probability increased, pulmonary air leaks, pulmonary interstitial emphysema, vasoconstriction

Drug Interactions

Metabolism/Transport Effects None known.

Avoid Concomitant Use There are no known interactions where it is recommended to avoid concomitant use.

Increased Effect/Toxicity There are no known significant interactions involving an increase in effect.

Decreased Effect There are no known significant interactions involving a decrease in effect.

Storage/Stability Refrigerate; protect from light. Prior to administration, warm by standing at room temperature for 20 minutes or held in hand for 8 minutes. **Artificial warming methods should not be used.** Unused, unopened vials warmed to room temperature may be returned to the refrigerator within 24 hours of warming only once.

Mechanism of Action Replaces deficient or ineffective endogenous lung surfactant in neonates with respiratory distress syndrome (RDS) or in neonates at risk of developing RDS. Surfactant prevents the alveoli from collapsing during expiration by lowering surface tension between air and alveolar surfaces.

Pharmacodynamics/Kinetics Excretion: Clearance: Alveolar clearance is rapid

Dosage
Endotracheal: Premature infants:
Prophylactic treatment: Administer 4 mL/kg (100 mg phospholipids/kg) as soon as possible; as many as 4 doses may be administered during the first 48 hours of life, no more frequently than 6 hours apart. The need for additional doses is determined by evidence of continuing respiratory distress; if the infant is still intubated and requiring at least 30% inspired oxygen to maintain a PaO_2 ≤80 torr.
Rescue treatment: Administer 4 mL/kg (100 mg phospholipids/kg) as soon as the diagnosis of RDS is made; may repeat if needed, no more frequently than every 6 hours to a maximum of 4 doses

Dosage adjustment in renal impairment: No dosage adjustment provided in manufacturer's labeling.
Dosage adjustment in hepatic impairment: No dosage adjustment provided in manufacturer's labeling.

Administration
For endotracheal administration only
Suction infant prior to administration. Inspect solution to verify complete mixing of the suspension (may swirl gently, but DO NOT SHAKE). Do not filter dose and avoid shaking.
Administer endotracheally by instillation through a 5-French end-hole catheter inserted into the infant's endotracheal tube.
Administer the dose in four 1 mL/kg aliquots. Each quarter-dose is instilled over 2-3 seconds followed by at least 30 seconds of manual ventilation or until stable; each quarter-dose is administered with the infant in a different position. Slightly downward inclination with head turned to the right, then repeat with head turned to the left; then slightly upward inclination with head turned to the right, then repeat with head turned to the left. Following administration of one full dose, withhold suctioning for 1 hour unless signs of significant airway obstruction.

Monitoring Parameters Continuous ECG and transcutaneous O_2 saturation should be monitored during administration; frequent arterial blood gases are necessary to prevent postdosing hyperoxia and hypocarbia

Additional Information Each mL contains 25 mg phospholipids suspended in 0.9% sodium chloride solution. Contents of 1 mL: 0.5-1.75 mg triglycerides, 1.4-3.5 mg free fatty acids, and <1 mg protein.

Dosage Forms Excipient information presented when available (limited, particularly for generics); consult specific product labeling.
Suspension, Inhalation:
Survanta: Phospholipids 25 mg/mL (4 mL, 8 mL)

◆ **Berinert** *see* C1 Inhibitor (Human) *on page* 307
◆ **Berinert® (Can)** *see* C1 Inhibitor (Human) *on page* 307
◆ **Beriplex P/N** *see* Prothrombin Complex Concentrate (Human) [(Factors II, VII, IX, X), Protein C, and Protein S] *on page* 1743

Besifloxacin (be si FLOX a sin)

Brand Names: U.S. Besivance
Brand Names: Canada Besivance™
Index Terms Besifloxacin Hydrochloride; BOL-303224-A; SS734
Pharmacologic Category Antibiotic, Fluoroquinolone; Antibiotic, Ophthalmic
Use Treatment of bacterial conjunctivitis
Pregnancy Risk Factor C
Dosage Ophthalmic: Children ≥1 year and Adults: Bacterial conjunctivitis: Instill 1 drop into affected eye(s) 3 times/day (4-12 hours apart) for 7 days
Additional Information Complete prescribing information should be consulted for additional detail.
Dosage Forms Excipient information presented when available (limited, particularly for generics); consult specific product labeling.
Suspension, Ophthalmic:
Besivance: 0.6% (5 mL) [contains benzalkonium chloride, edetate disodium dihydrate]

◆ **Besifloxacin Hydrochloride** *see* Besifloxacin *on page* 246
◆ **Besivance** *see* Besifloxacin *on page* 246
◆ **Besivance™ (Can)** *see* Besifloxacin *on page* 246
◆ **β,β-Dimethylcysteine** *see* PenicillAMINE *on page* 1603
◆ **9-Beta-D-Ribofuranosyladenine** *see* Adenosine *on page* 49
◆ **Betacaine® (Can)** *see* Lidocaine (Topical) *on page* 1212
◆ **Beta Care Betamide [OTC]** *see* Urea *on page* 2140

Beta-Carotene (BAY ta KARE oh teen)

Brand Names: U.S. A-Caro-25 [OTC]; B-Caro-T [OTC]; Caroguard [OTC]
Pharmacologic Category Vitamin, Fat Soluble
Use Prophylaxis against photosensitivity reactions in erythropoietic protoporphyria (EPP)
Dosage Oral: EPP (Lumitene™):
Children <14 years: 30-150 mg/day
Adults: 30-300 mg/day
Dosage adjustment in renal impairment: No dosage adjustment provided in manufacturer's labeling (has not been studied); use with caution.
Dosage adjustment in hepatic impairment: No dosage adjustment provided in manufacturer's labeling (has not been studied); use with caution.
Additional Information Complete prescribing information should be consulted for additional detail.
Dosage Forms Excipient information presented when available (limited, particularly for generics); consult specific product labeling.
Capsule, Oral:
A-Caro-25: 25,000 units [contains soybean lecithin, soybean oil]
Generic: 25,000 units
Capsule, Oral [preservative free]:
B-Caro-T: 15 mg [dye free]
Caroguard: 15 mg [dye free]
Generic: 25,000 units

◆ **Betaderm (Can)** *see* Betamethasone *on page* 247
◆ **Betagan** *see* Levobunolol *on page* 1196
◆ **Betagan® (Can)** *see* Levobunolol *on page* 1196
◆ **Beta HC [OTC]** *see* Hydrocortisone (Topical) *on page* 1011

Betaine (BAY ta een)

Brand Names: U.S. Cystadane
Brand Names: Canada Cystadane®
Index Terms Betaine Anhydrous
Pharmacologic Category Homocystinuria, Treatment Agent
Use Treatment of homocystinuria (eg, deficiencies or defects in cystathionine beta-synthase [CBS], 5,10-methylene tetrahydrofolate reductase [MTHFR], and cobalamin cofactor metabolism [CBL])
Pregnancy Risk Factor C
Prescribing and Access Restrictions Cystadane® may be obtained by contacting Accredo Health Group Inc at 1-888-454-8860.

Dosage Oral:

Children <3 years: Initial dose: 100 mg/kg/day administered in 2 divided doses; increase weekly by 50 mg/kg increments, as needed

Children ≥3 years and Adults: Usual dose: 6 g/day administered in divided doses of 3 g twice daily; dosages of up to 20 g/day have been necessary to control homocysteine levels in some patients

Note: Dosage in all patients can be gradually increased until plasma total homocysteine is undetectable or present only in small amounts. One study in six patients with CBS deficiency, ranging from 6-17 years of age, showed minimal benefit from exceeding a twice daily dosing schedule and a 150 mg/kg/day dosage.

Additional Information Complete prescribing information should be consulted for additional detail.

Dosage Forms Excipient information presented when available (limited, particularly for generics); consult specific product labeling.

Powder, Oral, as anhydrous:

Cystadane: 1 g/scoop (180 g)

Tablet, Oral, as anhydrous:

Generic: 300 mg

◆ **Betaine Anhydrous** *see* Betaine *on page 246*

◆ **Betaject™ (Can)** *see* Betamethasone *on page 247*

◆ **Betaloc® (Can)** *see* Metoprolol *on page 1348*

Betamethasone (bay ta METH a sone)

Brand Names: U.S. AlphaTrex; Celestone; Celestone Soluspan; Diprolene; Diprolene AF; Luxiq

Brand Names: Canada Betaderm; Betaject™; Betnesol®; Betnovate®; Celestone® Soluspan®; Diprolene®; Diprolene® Glycol; Diprosone®; Ectosone; Prevex® B; ratio-Ectosone; Ratio-Topilene; ratio-Topilene; Ratio-Topisone; ratio-Topisone; Rivasone; Rolene; Rosone; Taro-Sone; Valisone® Scalp Lotion

Index Terms Betamethasone Dipropionate; Betamethasone Dipropionate, Augmented; Betamethasone Sodium Phosphate; Betamethasone Valerate; Flubenisolone

Pharmacologic Category Corticosteroid, Systemic; Corticosteroid, Topical

Additional Appendix Information

Corticosteroids Systemic Equivalencies *on page 2297*

Topical Corticosteroids *on page 2299*

Use Inflammatory dermatoses such as seborrheic or atopic dermatitis, neurodermatitis, anogenital pruritus, psoriasis, inflammatory phase of xerosis

Unlabeled Use Accelerate fetal lung maturation in patients with preterm labor

Pregnancy Risk Factor C

Pregnancy Considerations Adverse events have been observed with corticosteroids in animal reproduction studies. Betamethasone crosses the placenta (ACOG, 2011); and is partially metabolized by placental enzymes to an inactive metabolite (Murphy, 2007). Some studies have shown an association between first trimester systemic corticosteroid use and oral clefts (Park-Wyllie, 2000; Pradat, 2003). Systemic corticosteroids may have an effect on fetal growth (decreased birth weight); however, information is conflicting (Lunghi, 2010). Hypoadrenalism may occur in newborns following maternal use of corticosteroids during pregnancy; monitor.

Due to its positive effect on stimulating fetal lung maturation, a single course of the injection is often used in patients with premature labor (24-34 weeks gestation) who are expected to deliver within 7 days (ACOG, 2011). When systemic corticosteroids are needed in pregnancy, it is generally recommended to use the lowest effective dose for the shortest duration of time, avoiding high doses during the first trimester (Leachman, 2006; Lunghi, 2010; Makol, 2011; Østensen, 2009).

Topical corticosteroids are preferred over systemic for treating conditions, such as psoriasis or atopic dermatitis in pregnant women; high potency corticosteroids are not recommended during the first trimester. Topical products are not recommended for extensive use, in large quantities, or for long periods of time in pregnant women (Bae, 2011; Koutroulis, 2011; Leachman, 2006).

Women exposed to betamethasone during pregnancy for the treatment of an autoimmune disease may contact the OTIS Autoimmune Diseases Study at 877-311-8972.

Breast-Feeding Considerations Corticosteroids are excreted in human milk. The onset of milk secretion after birth may be delayed and the volume of milk produced may be decreased by antenatal betamethasone therapy; this affect was seen when delivery occurred 3-9 days after the betamethasone dose in women between 28 and 34 weeks gestation. Antenatal betamethasone therapy did not affect milk production when birth occurred <3 days or >10 days of treatment (Henderson, 2008). It is not known if systemic absorption following topical administration results in detectable quantities in human milk. Do not apply topical corticosteroids to nipples; hypertension was noted in a nursing infant exposed to a topical corticosteroid while nursing (Leachman, 2006).

The manufacturer notes that when used systemically, maternal use of corticosteroids have the potential to cause adverse events in a nursing infant (eg, growth suppression, interfere with endogenous corticosteroid production) and therefore recommends that caution be exercised when administering betamethasone to nursing women. If there is concern about exposure to the infant, some guidelines recommend waiting 4 hours after the maternal dose of an oral systemic corticosteroid before breast-feeding in order to decrease potential exposure to the infant (based on a study using prednisolone) (Bae, 2011; Leachman, 2006; Makol, 2011; Ost, 1985).

Contraindications Hypersensitivity to betamethasone, other corticosteroids, or any component of the formulation; systemic fungal infections; I.M. administration contraindicated in idiopathic thrombocytopenia purpura

Warnings/Precautions Very high potency topical products are not for treatment of rosacea, perioral dermatitis; not for use on face, groin, or axillae; not for use in a diapered area. Avoid concurrent use of other corticosteroids.

May cause hypercorticism or suppression of hypothalamic-pituitary-adrenal (HPA) axis, particularly in younger children or in patients receiving high doses for prolonged periods. HPA axis suppression may lead to adrenal crisis. Withdrawal and discontinuation of a corticosteroid should be done slowly and carefully. Particular care is required when patients are transferred from systemic corticosteroids to inhaled products due to possible adrenal insufficiency or withdrawal from steroids, including an increase in allergic symptoms. Patients receiving >20 mg per day of prednisone (or equivalent) may be most susceptible. Fatalities have occurred due to adrenal insufficiency in asthmatic patients during and after transfer from systemic corticosteroids to aerosol steroids; aerosol steroids do not provide the systemic steroid needed to treat patients having trauma, surgery, or infections. In stressful situations, HPA axis-suppressed patients should receive adequate supplementation with natural glucocorticoids (hydrocortisone or cortisone) rather than betamethasone (due to lack of mineralocorticoid activity).

Topical corticosteroids may be absorbed percutaneously. Absorption of topical corticosteroids may cause manifestations of Cushing's syndrome, hyperglycemia, or ▶

glycosuria. Absorption is increased by the use of occlusive dressings, application to denuded skin, or application to large surface areas.

Acute myopathy has been reported with high dose corticosteroids, usually in patients with neuromuscular transmission disorders; may involve ocular and/or respiratory muscles; monitor creatine kinase; recovery may be delayed. Corticosteroid use may cause psychiatric disturbances, including depression, euphoria, insomnia, mood swings, and personality changes. Pre-existing psychiatric conditions may be exacerbated by corticosteroid use. Prolonged use of corticosteroids may also increase the incidence of secondary infection, mask acute infection (including fungal infections), prolong or exacerbate viral infections, or limit response to vaccines. Exposure to chickenpox should be avoided; corticosteroids should not be used to treat ocular herpes simplex. Corticosteroids should not be used for cerebral malaria or viral hepatitis. Close observation is required in patients with latent tuberculosis and/or TB reactivity; restrict use in active TB (only in conjunction with antituberculosis treatment). Prolonged treatment with corticosteroids has been associated with the development of Kaposi's sarcoma (case reports); if noted, discontinuation of therapy should be considered. High-dose corticosteroids should not be used to manage acute head injury.

Use with caution in patients with thyroid disease, hepatic impairment, renal impairment, cardiovascular disease, diabetes, glaucoma, cataracts, myasthenia gravis, patients at risk for osteoporosis, patients at risk for seizures, or GI diseases (diverticulitis, peptic ulcer, ulcerative colitis) due to perforation risk. Use caution following acute MI (corticosteroids have been associated with myocardial rupture). Because of the risk of adverse effects, systemic corticosteroids should be used cautiously in the elderly in the smallest possible effective dose for the shortest duration. Discontinue if skin irritation or contact dermatitis should occur; do not use in patients with decreased skin circulation. Withdraw therapy with gradual tapering of dose.

Topical use in patients ≤12 years of age is not recommended. Children may absorb proportionally larger amounts after topical application and may be more prone to systemic effects. HPA axis suppression, intracranial hypertension, and Cushing's syndrome have been reported in children receiving topical corticosteroids. Prolonged use may affect growth velocity; growth should be routinely monitored in pediatric patients.

Adverse Reactions

Systemic:

Cardiovascular: Congestive heart failure, edema, hyper-/hypotension

Central nervous system: Dizziness, headache, insomnia, intracranial pressure increased, lightheadedness, nervousness, pseudotumor cerebri, seizure, vertigo

Dermatologic: Ecchymoses, facial erythema, fragile skin, hirsutism, hyper-/hypopigmentation, perioral dermatitis (oral), petechiae, striae, wound healing impaired

Endocrine & metabolic: Amenorrhea, Cushing's syndrome, diabetes mellitus, growth suppression, hyperglycemia, hypokalemia, menstrual irregularities, pituitary-adrenal axis suppression, protein catabolism, sodium retention, water retention

Gastrointestinal: Abdominal distention, appetite increased, hiccups, indigestion, peptic ulcer, pancreatitis, ulcerative esophagitis

Local: Injection site reactions (intra-articular use), sterile abscess

Neuromuscular & skeletal: Arthralgia, muscle atrophy, fractures, muscle weakness, myopathy, osteoporosis, necrosis (femoral and humeral heads)

Ocular: Cataracts, glaucoma, intraocular pressure increased

Miscellaneous: Anaphylactoid reaction, diaphoresis, hypersensitivity, secondary infection

Topical:

Dermatologic: Acneiform eruptions, allergic dermatitis, burning, dry skin, erythema, folliculitis, hypertrichosis, irritation, miliaria, pruritus, skin atrophy, striae, vesiculation

Endocrine and metabolic effects have occasionally been reported with topical use.

Drug Interactions

Metabolism/Transport Effects None known.

Avoid Concomitant Use

Avoid concomitant use of Betamethasone with any of the following: Aldesleukin; BCG; Mifepristone; Natalizumab; Pimecrolimus; Tacrolimus (Topical); Tofacitinib

Increased Effect/Toxicity

Betamethasone may increase the levels/effects of: Acetylcholinesterase Inhibitors; Amphotericin B; Deferasirox; Leflunomide; Loop Diuretics; Natalizumab; NSAID (COX-2 Inhibitor); NSAID (Nonselective); Thiazide Diuretics; Tofacitinib; Vaccines (Live); Warfarin

The levels/effects of Betamethasone may be increased by: Antifungal Agents (Azole Derivatives, Systemic); Aprepitant; Calcium Channel Blockers (Nondihydropyridine); Denosumab; Estrogen Derivatives; Fluconazole; Fosaprepitant; Indacaterol; Macrolide Antibiotics; Mifepristone; Neuromuscular-Blocking Agents (Nondepolarizing); Pimecrolimus; Quinolone Antibiotics; Roflumilast; Salicylates; Tacrolimus (Topical); Telaprevir; Trastuzumab

Decreased Effect

Betamethasone may decrease the levels/effects of: Aldesleukin; Antidiabetic Agents; BCG; Calcitriol; Coccidioidin Skin Test; Corticorelin; Hyaluronidase; Isoniazid; Salicylates; Sipuleucel-T; Telaprevir; Urea Cycle Disorder Agents; Vaccines (Inactivated)

The levels/effects of Betamethasone may be decreased by: Aminoglutethimide; Antacids; Barbiturates; Bile Acid Sequestrants; Echinacea; Mifepristone; Mitotane; Primidone; Rifamycin Derivatives

Ethanol/Nutrition/Herb Interactions

Ethanol: Avoid ethanol (may enhance gastric mucosal irritation).

Food: Betamethasone interferes with calcium absorption.

Herb/Nutraceutical: Avoid cat's claw, echinacea (have immunostimulant properties).

Mechanism of Action Controls the rate of protein synthesis; depresses the migration of polymorphonuclear leukocytes, fibroblasts; reverses capillary permeability and lysosomal stabilization at the cellular level to prevent or control inflammation

Pharmacodynamics/Kinetics

Protein binding: 64%

Metabolism: Hepatic

Half-life elimination: 6.5 hours

Time to peak, serum: I.V.: 10-36 minutes

Excretion: Urine (<5% as unchanged drug)

Dosage Base dosage on severity of disease and patient response

Children: Use lowest dose listed as initial dose for adrenocortical insufficiency (physiologic replacement)

I.M.: ≤12 years: 0.0175-0.125 mg base/kg/day divided every 6-12 hours **or** 0.5-7.5 mg base/m^2/day divided every 6-12 hours

Oral: ≤12 years: 0.0175-0.25 mg/kg/day divided every 6-8 hours **or** 0.5-7.5 mg/m^2/day divided every 6-8 hours

Topical:

≤12 years: Use is not recommended.

≥13 years: Use minimal amount for shortest period of time to avoid HPA axis suppression

Gel, augmented formulation: Apply once or twice daily; rub in gently. **Note:** Do not exceed 2 weeks of treatment or 50 g/week.
Lotion: Apply a few drops twice daily
Augmented formulation: Apply a few drops once or twice daily; rub in gently. **Note:** Do not exceed 2 weeks of treatment or 50 mL/week.
Cream/ointment: Apply once or twice daily.
Augmented formulation: Apply once or twice daily. **Note:** Do not exceed 2 weeks of treatment or 45 g/week.

Adolescents and Adults:
Oral: 2.4-4.8 mg/day in 2-4 doses; range: 0.6-7.2 mg/day
I.M.: Betamethasone sodium phosphate and betamethasone acetate: 0.6-9 mg/day (generally, 1/3 to 1/2 of oral dose) divided every 12-24 hours

Adults:
Intrabursal, intra-articular, intradermal: 0.25-2 mL
Intralesional: Rheumatoid arthritis/osteoarthritis:
Very large joints: 1-2 mL
Large joints: 1 mL
Medium joints: 0.5-1 mL
Small joints: 0.25-0.5 mL
I.M.: Antenatal fetal maturation (unlabeled use): 12 mg every 24 hours for a total of 2 doses (ACOG, 2011). **Note:** Recommended for pregnant women with premature labor (24-34 weeks gestation) who are expected to deliver within 7 days.
Topical:
Foam: Apply to the scalp twice daily, once in the morning and once at night
Gel, augmented formulation: Apply once or twice daily; rub in gently. **Note:** Do not exceed 2 weeks of treatment or 50 g/week.
Lotion: Apply a few drops twice daily
Augmented formulation: Apply a few drops once or twice daily; rub in gently. **Note:** Do not exceed 2 weeks of treatment or 50 mL/week.
Cream/ointment: Apply once or twice daily
Augmented formulation: Apply once or twice daily. **Note:** Do not exceed 2 weeks of treatment or 45 g/week.

Dosing adjustment in hepatic impairment: Adjustments may be necessary in patients with liver failure because betamethasone is extensively metabolized in the liver

Dietary Considerations May be taken with food to decrease GI distress.

Administration

Oral: Not for alternate day therapy; once daily doses should be given in the morning. May be administered with food to decrease GI distress.

I.M.: Do **not** give injectable sodium phosphate/acetate suspension I.V.

Topical: Apply topical sparingly to areas. Not for use on broken skin or in areas of infection. Do not apply to wet skin unless directed; do not cover with occlusive dressing. Do not apply very high potency agents to face, groin, axillae, or diaper area.
Foam: Invert can and dispense a small amount onto a saucer or other cool surface. Do not dispense directly into hands. Pick up small amounts of foam and gently massage into affected areas until foam disappears. Repeat until entire affected scalp area is treated.

Monitoring Parameters Growth in children

Test Interactions May suppress the wheal and flare reactions to skin test antigens

Additional Information

Very high potency: Augmented betamethasone dipropionate ointment, lotion
High potency: Augmented betamethasone dipropionate cream, betamethasone dipropionate cream and ointment
Intermediate potency: Betamethasone dipropionate lotion, betamethasone valerate cream

Dosage Forms Excipient information presented when available (limited, particularly for generics); consult specific product labeling.

Cream, External, as dipropionate [strength expressed as base]:
Diprolene AF: 0.05% (15 g, 50 g)
Generic: 0.05% (15 g, 45 g, 50 g)
Cream, External, as valerate [strength expressed as base]:
Generic: 0.1% (15 g, 45 g)
Foam, External, as valerate:
Luxiq: 0.12% (50 g, 100 g) [contains alcohol, usp, cetyl alcohol, propylene glycol]
Generic: 0.12% (50 g, 100 g)
Gel, External, as dipropionate [strength expressed as base]:
AlphaTrex: 0.05% (15 g, 50 g)
Generic: 0.05% (15 g, 50 g)
Lotion, External, as dipropionate [strength expressed as base]:
Diprolene: 0.05% (30 mL, 60 mL) [contains isopropyl alcohol, propylene glycol]
Generic: 0.05% (30 mL, 60 mL)
Lotion, External, as valerate [strength expressed as base]:
Generic: 0.1% (60 mL)
Ointment, External, as dipropionate [strength expressed as base]:
Diprolene: 0.05% (15 g, 50 g)
Generic: 0.05% (15 g, 45 g, 50 g)
Ointment, External, as valerate:
Generic: 0.1% (15 g, 45 g)
Ointment, External, as valerate [strength expressed as base]:
Generic: 0.1% (15 g, 45 g)
Solution, Oral, as base:
Celestone: 0.6 mg/5 mL (118 mL) [cherry-orange flavor]
Suspension, Injection:
Celestone Soluspan: Betamethasone sodium phosphate 3 mg and betamethasone acetate 3 mg per 1 mL (5 mL) [contains benzalkonium chloride, edetate disodium]
Generic: Betamethasone sodium phosphate 3 mg and betamethasone acetate 3 mg per 1 mL (5 mL)

Betamethasone and Clotrimazole

(bay ta METH a sone & kloe TRIM a zole)

Brand Names: U.S. Lotrisone®

Brand Names: Canada Lotriderm®

Index Terms Clotrimazole and Betamethasone

Pharmacologic Category Antifungal Agent, Topical; Corticosteroid, Topical

Use Topical treatment of various dermal fungal infections (including tinea pedis, cruris, and corpora in patients ≥17 years of age)

Pregnancy Risk Factor C

Dosage

Children <17 years: Do not use
Children ≥17 years and Adults:
Allergic or inflammatory diseases: Topical: Apply to affected area twice daily, morning and evening
Tinea corporis, tinea cruris: Topical: Massage into affected area twice daily, morning and evening; do not use for longer than 2 weeks; re-evaluate after 1 week if no clinical improvement; do not exceed 45 g cream/week or 45 mL lotion/week
Tinea pedis: Topical: Massage into affected area twice daily, morning and evening; do not use for longer than 4 weeks; re-evaluate after 2 weeks if no clinical improvement; do not exceed 45 g cream/week or 45 mL lotion/week

Elderly: Use with caution; skin atrophy and skin ulceration (rare) have been reported in patients with thinning skin; do not use for diaper dermatitis or under occlusive dressings

Additional Information Complete prescribing information should be consulted for additional detail.

Dosage Forms Excipient information presented when available (limited, particularly for generics); consult specific product labeling.

Cream: Betamethasone dipropionate 0.05% (base) and clotrimazole 1% (15 g, 45 g)

Lotrisone®: Betamethasone dipropionate 0.05% (base) and clotrimazole 1% (15 g, 45 g) [contains benzyl alcohol]

Lotion: Betamethasone dipropionate 0.05% (base) and clotrimazole 1% (30 mL)

Lotrisone®: Betamethasone dipropionate 0.05% (base) and clotrimazole 1% (30 mL) [contains benzyl alcohol]

- ◆ **Betamethasone Dipropionate** *see* Betamethasone *on page 247*
- ◆ **Betamethasone Dipropionate and Calcipotriene Hydrate** *see* Calcipotriene and Betamethasone *on page 312*
- ◆ **Betamethasone Dipropionate, Augmented** *see* Betamethasone *on page 247*
- ◆ **Betamethasone Sodium Phosphate** *see* Betamethasone *on page 247*
- ◆ **Betamethasone Valerate** *see* Betamethasone *on page 247*
- ◆ **Betapace** *see* Sotalol *on page 1942*
- ◆ **Betapace AF** *see* Sotalol *on page 1942*
- ◆ **Betasept Surgical Scrub [OTC]** *see* Chlorhexidine Gluconate *on page 408*
- ◆ **Betaseron** *see* Interferon Beta-1b *on page 1106*
- ◆ **Betaxin® (Can)** *see* Thiamine *on page 2045*

Betaxolol (Systemic) (be TAKS oh lol)

Brand Names: U.S. Kerlone

Index Terms Betaxolol Hydrochloride

Pharmacologic Category Antihypertensive; Beta-Blocker, Beta-1 Selective

Additional Appendix Information

Beta-Blockers *on page 2294*

Use Management of hypertension

Unlabeled Use Treatment of coronary artery disease

Pregnancy Risk Factor C

Dosage Oral:

Adults: 5-10 mg/day; may increase dose to 20 mg/day after 7-14 days if desired response is not achieved.

Elderly: Refer to adult dosing; initial dose: 5 mg/day

Dosage adjustment in renal impairment: Severe impairment: Initial dose: 5 mg/day; may increase every 2 weeks up to a maximum of 20 mg/day

Hemodialysis: Initial dose: 5 mg/day; may increase every 2 weeks up to a maximum of 20 mg/day. Supplemental dose not required.

Dosage adjustment in hepatic impairment: Dosage adjustments are not routinely required.

Additional Information Complete prescribing information should be consulted for additional detail.

Dosage Forms Excipient information presented when available (limited, particularly for generics); consult specific product labeling.

Tablet, Oral, as hydrochloride:

Kerlone: 10 mg [scored]

Kerlone: 20 mg

Generic: 10 mg, 20 mg

Betaxolol (Ophthalmic) (be TAKS oh lol)

Brand Names: U.S. Betoptic-S

Brand Names: Canada Betoptic® S; Sandoz-Betaxolol

Index Terms Betaxolol Hydrochloride

Pharmacologic Category Ophthalmic Agent, Antiglaucoma

Use Treatment of chronic open-angle glaucoma or ocular hypertension

Pregnancy Risk Factor C

Dosage

Children and Adults: Ophthalmic suspension (Betoptic® S): Instill 1 drop into affected eye(s) twice daily.

Adults: Ophthalmic solution: Instill 1-2 drops into affected eye(s) twice daily.

Elderly: Ophthalmic: Refer to adult dosing.

Additional Information Complete prescribing information should be consulted for additional detail.

Dosage Forms Excipient information presented when available (limited, particularly for generics); consult specific product labeling.

Solution, Ophthalmic:

Generic: 0.5% (5 mL, 10 mL, 15 mL)

Suspension, Ophthalmic:

Betoptic-S: 0.25% (10 mL, 15 mL)

- ◆ **Betaxolol Hydrochloride** *see* Betaxolol (Ophthalmic) *on page 250*
- ◆ **Betaxolol Hydrochloride** *see* Betaxolol (Systemic) *on page 250*

Bethanechol (be THAN e kole)

Brand Names: U.S. Urecholine

Brand Names: Canada Duvoid®; PHL-Bethanechol; PMS-Bethanechol

Index Terms Bethanechol Chloride

Pharmacologic Category Cholinergic Agonist

Use Treatment of acute postoperative and postpartum nonobstructive (functional) urinary retention; treatment of neurogenic atony of the urinary bladder with retention

Unlabeled Use Gastroesophageal reflux

Pregnancy Risk Factor C

Pregnancy Considerations Reproduction studies have not been conducted.

Breast-Feeding Considerations It is not known if bethanechol is excreted in breast milk. Due to the potential for serious adverse reactions in the nursing infant, a decision should be made whether to discontinue nursing or to discontinue the drug, taking into account the importance of treatment to the mother.

Contraindications Hypersensitivity to bethanechol or any component of the formulation; mechanical obstruction of the GI or GU tract or when the strength or integrity of the GI or bladder wall is in question; hyperthyroidism, peptic ulcer disease, epilepsy, asthma, bradycardia, vasomotor instability, coronary artery disease, hypotension, or parkinsonism

Warnings/Precautions Potential for reflux infection if the sphincter fails to relax as bethanechol contracts the bladder.

Adverse Reactions Frequency not defined.

Cardiovascular: Hypotension, tachycardia, flushed skin

Central nervous system: Headache, malaise, seizure

Gastrointestinal: Abdominal cramps, belching, borborygmi, colicky pain, diarrhea, nausea, vomiting, salivation

Genitourinary: Urinary urgency

Ocular: Lacrimation, miosis

Respiratory: Asthmatic attacks, bronchial constriction

Miscellaneous: Diaphoresis

Drug Interactions

Metabolism/Transport Effects None known.

Avoid Concomitant Use There are no known interactions where it is recommended to avoid concomitant use.

Increased Effect/Toxicity

The levels/effects of Bethanechol may be increased by: Acetylcholinesterase Inhibitors; Beta-Blockers

Decreased Effect There are no known significant interactions involving a decrease in effect.

Storage/Stability Store at room temperature of 15°C to 30°C (59°F to 86°F).

Mechanism of Action Due to stimulation of the parasympathetic nervous system, bethanechol increases bladder muscle tone causing contractions which initiate urination. Bethanechol also stimulates gastric motility, increases gastric tone and may restore peristalsis.

Pharmacodynamics/Kinetics

Onset of action: 30-90 minutes

Duration: Up to 6 hours

Absorption: Variable

Dosage Oral:

Children:

Urinary retention (unlabeled use): 0.3-0.6 mg/kg/day in 3-4 divided doses

Gastroesophageal reflux (unlabeled use): 0.3-0.6 mg/kg/day in 3-4 divided doses

Adults:

Urinary retention, neurogenic bladder: Initial: 10-50 mg 3-4 times/day (some patients may require dosages of 50-100 mg 4 times/day). To determine effective dose, may initiate at a dose of 5-10 mg, with additional doses of 5-10 mg hourly until an effective cumulative dose is reached. Cholinergic effects at higher oral dosages may be cumulative.

Gastroesophageal reflux (unlabeled): 25 mg 4 times/day

Elderly: Use the lowest effective dose

Dosage adjustment in renal impairment: No dosage adjustment provided in manufacturer's labeling.

Dosage adjustment in hepatic impairment: No dosage adjustment provided in manufacturer's labeling.

Dietary Considerations Should be taken 1 hour before meals or 2 hours after meals.

Administration Should be administered 1 hour before meals or 2 hours after meals.

Monitoring Parameters Observe closely for side effects.

Test Interactions Increased lipase, amylase (S), bilirubin, aminotransferase [ALT/AST] (S)

Dosage Forms Excipient information presented when available (limited, particularly for generics); consult specific product labeling.

Tablet, Oral, as chloride:

Urecholine: 5 mg, 10 mg [scored]

Urecholine: 25 mg, 50 mg [scored; contains fd&c yellow #10 (quinoline yellow), fd&c yellow #6 (sunset yellow)]

Generic: 5 mg, 10 mg, 25 mg, 50 mg

Dosage Forms: Canada Excipient information presented when available (limited, particularly for generics); consult specific product labeling.

Tablet, as chloride:

Duvoid®: 10 mg, 25 mg, 50 mg

Extemporaneous Preparations A 1 mg/mL solution may be made with tablets. Crush twelve 10 mg tablets in a mortar and reduce to a fine powder. Add small portions of sterile water and mix to a uniform paste; mix while adding sterile water in incremental proportions to **almost** 120 mL; transfer to a calibrated bottle, rinse mortar with sterile water, and add quantity of sterile water sufficient to make 120 mL. Label "shake well" and "refrigerate". Stable for 30 days (Schlatter, 1997).

A 5 mg/mL suspension may be made with tablets and either a 1:1 mixture of Ora-Plus® and Ora-Sweet® or Ora-Plus® and Ora-Sweet® SF or 1:4 concentrated cherry syrup and simple syrup, NF mixture. Crush twelve 50 mg tablets in a mortar and reduce to a fine powder. Add small portions of chosen vehicle and mix to a uniform paste; mix while adding the vehicle in incremental proportions to **almost** 120 mL; transfer to a calibrated bottle, rinse mortar with vehicle, and add quantity of vehicle sufficient to make 120 mL. Label "shake well" and "refrigerate". Stable for 60 days refrigerated (preferred) or at room temperature (Allen, 1998; Nahata, 2004).

Allen LV Jr and Erickson MA, "Stability of Bethanechol Chloride, Pyrazinamide, Quinidine Sulfate, Rifampin, and Tetracycline Hydrochloride in Extemporaneously Compounded Oral Liquids," *Am J Health Syst Pharm*, 1998, 55(17):1804-9.

Nahata MC, Pai VB, and Hipple TF, *Pediatric Drug Formulations*, 5th ed, Cincinnati, OH: Harvey Whitney Books Co, 2004.

Schlatter JL and Saulnier JL, "Bethanechol Chloride Oral Solutions: Stability and Use in Infants," *Ann Pharmacother*, 1997, 31(3):294-6.

◆ **Bethanechol Chloride** *see* Bethanechol *on page 250*

◆ **Bethkis** *see* Tobramycin (Systemic, Oral Inhalation) *on page 2076*

◆ **Betimol** *see* Timolol (Ophthalmic) *on page 2064*

◆ **Betnesol® (Can)** *see* Betamethasone *on page 247*

◆ **Betnovate® (Can)** *see* Betamethasone *on page 247*

◆ **Betoptic-S** *see* Betaxolol (Ophthalmic) *on page 250*

◆ **Betoptic® S (Can)** *see* Betaxolol (Ophthalmic) *on page 250*

Bevacizumab (be vuh SIZ uh mab)

Brand Names: U.S. Avastin

Brand Names: Canada Avastin

Index Terms Anti-VEGF Monoclonal Antibody; Anti-VEGF rhuMAb; rhuMAb-VEGF

Pharmacologic Category Antineoplastic Agent, Monoclonal Antibody; Vascular Endothelial Growth Factor (VEGF) Inhibitor

Use

Colorectal cancer, metastatic: First-or second-line treatment of metastatic colorectal cancer (CRC) (in combination with fluorouracil-based chemotherapy); second-line treatment of metastatic CRC (in combination with fluoropyrimidine-irinotecan- or fluoropyrimidine-oxaliplatin-based chemotherapy) after progression on a first-line treatment containing bevacizumab. **Note:** Not indicated for the adjuvant treatment of CRC.

Glioblastoma: Treatment of progressive glioblastoma (as a single agent). Effectiveness is based on improvement in objective response rate.

Non-small cell lung cancer, non-squamous: First-line treatment of unresectable, locally advanced, recurrent or metastatic nonsquamous non-small cell lung cancer (NSCLC) (in combination with carboplatin and paclitaxel).

Renal cell carcinoma, metastatic: Treatment of metastatic renal cell carcinoma (RCC) (in combination with interferon alfa). **Note:** Not an approved use in Canada.

Unlabeled Use Treatment of metastatic breast cancer, recurrent/metastatic cervical cancer, recurrent endometrial cancer, recurrent advanced ovarian cancer (platinum-sensitive), soft tissue sarcomas (angiosarcoma or hemangiopericytoma/solitary fibrous tumor), age-related macular degeneration (AMD)

Pregnancy Risk Factor C

Pregnancy Considerations Teratogenic effects have been observed in animal reproduction studies. Angiogenesis is of critical importance to human fetal development, and bevacizumab inhibits angiogenesis. Adequate contraception during therapy is recommended (and for ≥6 months following last dose of bevacizumab). Patients should also be counseled regarding prolonged exposure following discontinuation of therapy due to the long half-life of bevacizumab.

Based on animal studies, bevacizumab may disrupt normal menstrual cycles and impair fertility by several effects, including reduced endometrial proliferation and follicular developmental arrest. Some parameters do not recover completely, or recover very slowly following discontinuation.

Breast-Feeding Considerations It is not known if bevacizumab is excreted in breast milk. Immunoglobulins are excreted in breast milk, and it is assumed that bevacizumab may appear in breast milk. Because of the potential for serious adverse reactions in the nursing infant, the decision to discontinue bevacizumab or to discontinue breast-feeding during therapy should take into account the benefits of treatment to the mother. The half-life of bevacizumab is up to 50 days (average 20 days), and this should be considered when decisions are made concerning breast-feeding resumption.

Note: Canadian labeling recommends to discontinue breast-feeding during treatment and to avoid breast-feeding a minimum of 6 months following discontinuation of treatment.

Contraindications

There are no contraindications listed in the manufacturer's labeling.

Canadian labeling: Hypersensitivity to bevacizumab, any component of the formulation, Chinese hamster ovary cell products or other recombinant human or humanized antibodies; untreated CNS metastases

Warnings/Precautions [U.S. Boxed Warning]: Gastrointestinal (GI) perforation (sometimes fatal) has occurred in 0.3 to 2.4% of clinical study patients receiving bevacizumab; discontinue if GI perforation occurs. Most cases occur within 50 days of treatment initiation; monitor patients for signs/symptoms (eg, fever, abdominal pain with constipation and/or nausea/vomiting). GI fistula (including enterocutaneous, esophageal, duodenal, and rectal fistulas), and intra-abdominal abscess have been reported in patients receiving bevacizumab for colorectal cancer and other cancers (not related to treatment duration). Non-GI fistula formation (including tracheoesophageal, bronchopleural, biliary, vaginal, renal, and bladder fistulas) has been observed, most commonly within the first 6 months of treatment; permanently discontinue in patients who develop internal organ fistulas. **[U.S. Boxed Warning]: The incidence of wound healing and surgical complications is increased in patients who have received bevacizumab; discontinue with wound dehiscence. Although the appropriate interval between withholding bevacizumab and elective surgery has not been defined, bevacizumab should be discontinued at least 28 days prior to surgery and should not be reinitiated for at least 28 days after surgery and until wound is fully healed.** In a retrospective review of central venous access device placements, a greater risk of wound dehiscence was observed when port placement and bevacizumab administration were separated by <14 days (Erinjeri, 2011).

[U.S. Boxed Warning]: Severe or fatal hemorrhage, including hemoptysis, gastrointestinal bleeding, central nervous system hemorrhage, epistaxis, and vaginal bleeding have been reported (up to 5 times more frequently if receiving bevacizumab). Avoid use in patients with serious hemorrhage or recent hemoptysis (≥2.5 mL blood). Serious pulmonary hemorrhage has been reported in patients receiving bevacizumab (primarily in patients with nonsmall cell lung cancer with squamous cell histology [not an FDA-approved indication]). Intracranial hemorrhage, including cases of grade 3 or 4 hemorrhage, has occurred in patients with previously treated glioblastoma. Treatment discontinuation is recommended in all patients with intracranial or other serious hemorrhage. Use with caution in patients with CNS metastases; once case of CNS hemorrhage was observed in an ongoing study of NSCLC patients with CNS metastases. Use in patients with untreated CNS metastases is contraindicated in the Canadian labeling. Use with caution in patients at risk for thrombocytopenia.

Bevacizumab is associated with an increased risk for arterial thromboembolic events (ATE), including cerebral infarction, stroke, MI, TIA, angina, and other ATEs, when used in combination with chemotherapy. History of ATE, diabetes, or ≥65 years of age may present an even greater risk. Although patients with cancer are at risk for venous thromboembolism (VTE), a meta-analysis of 15 controlled trials has demonstrated an increased risk for VTE in patients who received bevacizumab (Nalluri, 2008). Permanently discontinue therapy in patients with severe ATE or life-threatening pulmonary embolism; the safety of treatment reinitiation after ATE has not been studied.

Use with caution in patients with cardiovascular disease. Among approved and nonapproved uses evaluated thus far, the incidence of heart failure (HF) and/or left ventricular dysfunction (including LVEF decline), is higher in patients receiving bevacizumab plus chemotherapy when compared to chemotherapy alone. Bevacizumab may potentiate the cardiotoxic effects of anthracyclines. HF is more common with prior anthracycline exposure and/or left chest wall irradiation. The safety of therapy resumption or continuation in patients with cardiac dysfunction has not been studied. In studies of patients with metastatic breast cancer (an unlabeled use), the incidence of grades 3 or 4 HF was increased in patients receiving bevacizumab plus paclitaxel, compared to the control arm. Patients with metastatic breast cancer who had received prior anthracycline therapy had a higher rate of HF compared to those receiving paclitaxel alone (3.8% vs 0.6% respectively). A meta-analysis of 5 studies which enrolled patients with metastatic breast cancer who received bevacizumab suggested an association with an increased risk of heart failure; all trials included in the analysis enrolled patients who either received prior or were receiving concurrent anthracycline therapy (Choueiri, 2011).

Bevacizumab may cause and/or worsen hypertension; the incidence of severe hypertension in increased with bevacizumab. Use caution in patients with pre-existing hypertension and monitor BP closely (every 2-3 weeks during treatment; regularly after discontinuation if bevacizumab-induced hypertension occurs or worsens). Permanent discontinuation is recommended in patients who experience a hypertensive crisis or hypertensive encephalopathy. Temporarily discontinue in patients who develop uncontrolled hypertension. An increase in diastolic and systolic blood pressures were noted in a retrospective review of patients with renal insufficiency (Cl_{cr} ≤60 mL/minute) who received bevacizumab for renal cell cancer (Gupta, 2011). Cases of reversible posterior leukoencephalopathy syndrome (RPLS) have been reported. Symptoms (which include headache, seizure, confusion, lethargy, blindness and/or other vision, or neurologic disturbances) may occur from 16 hours to 1 year after treatment initiation. Resolution of symptoms usually occurs within days after discontinuation; however, neurologic sequelae may remain. RPLS may be associated with hypertension; discontinue bevacizumab and begin management of hypertension, if present. The safety of treatment reinitiation after RPLS is not known.

Infusion reactions (eg, hypertension, hypertensive crisis, wheezing, oxygen desaturation, hypersensitivity [including anaphylactic/anaphylactoid reactions], chest pain, rigors, headache, diaphoresis) may occur with the first infusion (uncommon); interrupt therapy in patients experiencing severe infusion reactions and administer appropriate therapy; there are no data to address routine premedication use or reinstitution of therapy in patients who experience severe infusion reactions. Cases of necrotizing fasciitis, including fatalities, have been reported (rarely); usually secondary to wound healing complications, GI perforation or fistula formation. Discontinue in patients who develop necrotizing fasciitis. Proteinuria and/or nephrotic syndrome have been associated with bevacizumab; risk may be increased in patients with a history of hypertension; thrombotic microangiopathy has been associated with bevacizumab-induced proteinuria. Withhold treatment for ≥2 g proteinuria/24 hours and resume when proteinuria is <2 g/24 hours; discontinue in patients with nephrotic syndrome. Elderly patients (≥65 years of age) are at higher risk for adverse events, including thromboembolic events and proteinuria; serious adverse events occurring more frequently in the elderly also include weakness, deep thrombophlebitis, sepsis, hyper-/hypotension, MI, CHF, diarrhea, constipation, anorexia, leukopenia, anemia, dehydration, hypokalemia, and hyponatremia. Potentially significant drug-drug interactions may exist, requiring dose or frequency adjustment, additional monitoring, and/or selection of alternative therapy. Microangiopathic hemolytic anemia (MAHA) has been reported when bevacizumab has been used in combination with sunitinib. Concurrent therapy with sunitinib and bevacizumab is also associated with dose-limiting hypertension in patients with metastatic renal cell cancer. The incidence of hand-foot syndrome is increased in patients treated with bevacizumab plus sorafenib in comparison to those treated with sorafenib monotherapy. When used in combination with myelosuppressive chemotherapy, increased rates of severe or febrile neutropenia and neutropenic infection were reported. Bevacizumab, in combination with chemotherapy (or biologic therapy), is associated with an increased risk of treatment-related mortality; a higher risk of fatal adverse events was identified in a meta-analysis of 16 trials in which bevacizumab was used for the treatment of various cancers (breast cancer, colorectal cancer, non small cell lung cancer, pancreatic cancer, prostate cancer, and renal cell cancer) and compared to chemotherapy alone (Ranpura, 2011). When bevacizumab is used in combination with myelosuppressive chemotherapy, increased rates of severe or febrile neutropenia and neutropenic infection have been reported. In premenopausal women receiving bevacizumab in combination with mFOLFOX (fluorouracil/oxaliplatin based chemotherapy) the incidence of ovarian failure (amenorrhea ≥3 months) was higher (34%) compared to women who received mFOLFOX alone (2%); ovarian function recovered in some patients after treatment was discontinued; premenopausal women should be informed of the potential risk of ovarian failure. Serious eye infections and vision loss due to endophthalmitis have been reported from intravitreal administration (unlabeled use/route).

Adverse Reactions Percentages reported as monotherapy and as part of combination chemotherapy regimens. Some studies only reported hematologic toxicities grades ≥4 and nonhematologic toxicities grades ≥3.

>10%:

Cardiovascular: Hypertension (12% to 34%; grades 3/4: 5% to 18%), thromboembolism (≤21%; grades 3/4: 15%; venous thromboembolism: 8%; grades 3/4: 5% to 7%; arterial thrombosis 6%; grades 3/4: 3%), hypotension (7% to 15%)

Central nervous system: Pain (8% to 62%), fatigue (≤45%; grades 3/4: 4% to 19%), headache (24% to 37%; grades 3/4: 2% to 4%), dizziness (19% to 26%), taste disorder (14% to 21%), neuropathy (sensory, grades 3/4: 1% to 17%; in combination with paclitaxel: 24%)

Dermatologic: Alopecia (6% to 32%), xeroderma (7% to 20%), exfoliative dermatitis (3% to 19%), skin discoloration (2% to 16%)

Endocrine & metabolic: Ovarian failure (34%), weight loss (15% to 20%)

Gastrointestinal: Abdominal pain (8% to 61%; grades 3/4: 8%), vomiting (47% to 52%; grades 3/4: ≤11%), anorexia (35% to 43%), constipation (4% to 40%), diarrhea (grades 3/4: 1% to 34%), stomatitis (30% to 32%), gastrointestinal hemorrhage (19% to 24%), dyspepsia (17% to 24%), flatulence (11% to 19%), nausea (grades 3/4: ≤12%)

Genitourinary: Proteinuria (4% to 36%; grades 3/4: ≤7%; median onset: 5.6 months; median time to resolution: 6.1 months)

Hematologic & oncologic: Hemorrhage (≤40%; grades 3/4: 1% to 5%), leukopenia (grades 3/4: 37%), neutropenia (grade 4: 21% to 27%)

Infection: Infection (≤55%; serious: 7% to 14%; pneumonia, catheter infection, or wound infection)

Neuromuscular & skeletal: Myalgia (8% to 19%), back pain (≤12%)

Respiratory: Upper respiratory tract infection (40% to 47%), epistaxis (19% to 35%), dyspnea (25% to 26%), rhinitis (3% to >10%)

Miscellaneous: Postoperative wound complication (including dehiscence, 1% to 15%)

1% to 10%:

Cardiovascular: Deep vein thrombosis (6% to 9%; grades 3/4: 9%), cardiac failure (grades 3/4: 1% to 4%), syncope (grades 3/4: 3%), intra-abdominal thrombosis (venous, grades 3/4: 3%), arterial thrombosis (cardio-/cerebrovascular, 2% to 4%), ventricular dysfunction (left, grades 3/4: 1%), pulmonary embolism (≤1%)

Central nervous system: Voice disorder (≤5% to 9%), neuropathy (other than sensory: grades 3/4: 1% to 5%)

Dermatologic: Dermal ulcer (≤6%), acne vulgaris (≤1%)

Endocrine & metabolic: Dehydration (grades 3/4: ≤10%), hyponatremia (grades 3/4: 4%)

Gastrointestinal: Xerostomia (4% to 7%), colitis (1% to 6%), intestinal obstruction (grades 3/4: 4% to 5%), gingival hemorrhage (minor, 2% to 4%), gastrointestinal perforation (≤4%), gastroesophageal reflux disease (≤2%), gingivitis (≤2%), oral mucosa ulcer (≤2%), fistula (1%), gastritis (≤1%), gingival pain (≤1%)

Genitourinary: Vaginal hemorrhage (4%)

Hematologic & oncologic: Febrile neutropenia (5%; grades 3/4: 4% to 5%), thrombocytopenia (5%), hemorrhage (CNS; 1% to 5%; grades 3/4: 1%)

Infection: Abscess (tooth, ≤2%; intra-abdominal, 1%)

Neuromuscular & skeletal: Weakness (10%)

Ophthalmic: Blurred vision (≤2%)

Otic: Tinnitus (≤2%), deafness (≤1%)

Respiratory: Pneumonitis (grades 3/4: 5%), hemoptysis (nonsquamous histology 2%)

Miscellaneous: Infusion related reaction (<3%)

<1% (Limited to important or life-threatening): Anaphylaxis, anastomotic ulcer, angina pectoris, antibody development (anti-bevacizumab and neutralizing), bladder fistula, bronchopleural fistula, cerebral infarction, conjunctival hemorrhage, endophthalmitis (infectious and sterile),

enterocutaneous fistula, fistula of bile duct, fulminant necrotizing fasciitis, gastrointestinal fistula (including duodenal and esophageal), gastrointestinal ulcer, hemolytic anemia (microangiopathic; when used in combination with sunitinib), hemorrhagic stroke, hypersensitivity, hypertensive crisis, hypertensive encephalopathy, increased intraocular pressure, inflammation of anterior segment of eye (toxic anterior segment syndrome), intestinal necrosis, intraocular inflammation (iritis, vitritis), mesenteric thrombosis, myocardial infarction, nasal septum perforation, nephrotic syndrome, ocular hyperemia, osteonecrosis (jaw), ovarian failure, pancytopenia, permanent vision loss, polyserositis, pulmonary hemorrhage, pulmonary hypertension, rectal fistula, renal failure, renal fistula, renal thrombotic microangiopathy, retinal detachment, retinal hemorrhage, reversible posterior leukoencephalopathy syndrome (RPLS), sepsis, subarachnoid hemorrhage, tracheoesophageal fistula, transient ischemic attacks, ureteral spasm, vaginal fistula, vitreous hemorrhage, vitreous opacity

Drug Interactions

Metabolism/Transport Effects None known.

Avoid Concomitant Use

Avoid concomitant use of Bevacizumab with any of the following: CloZAPine; SUNItinib

Increased Effect/Toxicity

Bevacizumab may increase the levels/effects of: Antineoplastic Agents (Anthracycline, Systemic); Bisphosphonate Derivatives; CloZAPine; Irinotecan; SORAfenib; SUNItinib

The levels/effects of Bevacizumab may be increased by: SUNItinib

Decreased Effect There are no known significant interactions involving a decrease in effect.

Preparation for Administration Dilute in 100 mL NS prior to infusion (the manufacturer recommends a total volume of 100 mL). Do not mix with dextrose-containing solutions.

Storage/Stability Store vials at 2°C to 8°C (36°F to 46°F); do not freeze. Protect from light; do not shake. Diluted solutions are stable for up to 8 hours under refrigeration. Discard unused portion of vial.

Mechanism of Action Bevacizumab is a recombinant, humanized monoclonal antibody which binds to, and neutralizes, vascular endothelial growth factor (VEGF), preventing its association with endothelial receptors, Flt-1 and KDR. VEGF binding initiates angiogenesis (endothelial proliferation and the formation of new blood vessels). The inhibition of microvascular growth is believed to retard the growth of all tissues (including metastatic tissue).

Pharmacodynamics/Kinetics

Distribution: V_d: 46 mL/kg

Half-life elimination: ~20 days (range: 11-50 days)

Dosage

I.V.:

Colorectal cancer, metastatic, in combination with fluorouracil-based chemotherapy: Adults: 5 mg/kg every 2 weeks (in combination with bolus-IFL) **or** 10 mg/kg every 2 weeks (in combination with FOLFOX4)

Canadian labeling: 5 mg/kg every 2 weeks (in combination with fluorouracil-based chemotherapy)

Colorectal cancer, metastatic, following first-line therapy containing bevacizumab: Adults: 5 mg/kg every 2 weeks **or** 7.5 mg/kg every 3 weeks (in combination with fluoropyrimidine-irinotecan or fluoropyrimidine-oxaliplatin based regimen)

Glioblastoma: Adults: 10 mg/kg every 2 weeks as monotherapy **or** (unlabeled dosing) 10 mg/kg every 2 weeks (in combination with irinotecan) (Vredenburgh, 2007)

Nonsmall cell lung cancer (nonsquamous cell histology): Adults: 15 mg/kg every 3 weeks (in combination with carboplatin and paclitaxel) for 4-6 cycles followed by maintenance treatment (unlabeled use) of bevacizumab 15 mg/kg every 3 weeks as monotherapy until disease progression or unacceptable toxicity (Sandler, 2006)

Renal cell cancer, metastatic: Adults: 10 mg/kg every 2 weeks (in combination with interferon alfa) **or** (unlabeled dosing) 10 mg/kg every 2 weeks as monotherapy (Yang, 2003)

Breast cancer, metastatic (unlabeled use): Adults: 10 mg/kg every 2 weeks (in combination with paclitaxel) (Miller, 2007)

Endometrial cancer, recurrent or persistent (unlabeled use): Adults: 15 mg/kg every 3 weeks (as monotherapy) until disease progression or unacceptable toxicity (Aghajanian, 2011)

Ovarian cancer, advanced recurrent (unlabeled use): Adults: 15 mg/kg every 3 weeks in combination with gemcitabine and carboplatin for 6-10 cycles, followed by 15 mg/kg as monotherapy every 3 weeks until disease progression or unacceptable toxicity (Aghajanian, 2012)

Soft tissue sarcoma, angiosarcoma, metastatic or locally advanced (unlabeled use): Adults: 15 mg/kg every 3 weeks until disease progression or unacceptable toxicity (Agulnik, 2013)

Intravitreal: Age-related macular degeneration (unlabeled use/route): Adults: 1.25 mg (0.05 mL) monthly for 3 months, then may be given scheduled (monthly) or as needed based on monthly ophthalmologic assessment (Chakravarthy, 2013; Martin, 2012)

Dosage adjustment for toxicity: I.V. administration (systemic): There are no recommended dosage reductions. Temporary suspension is recommended for severe infusion reactions, at least 4 weeks prior to (and after) elective surgery, in moderate-to-severe proteinuria (in most studies, treatment was withheld for ≥2 g proteinuria/24 hours), or in patients with severe hypertension which is not controlled with medical management. Permanent discontinuation is recommended (by the manufacturer) in patients who develop wound dehiscence and wound healing complications requiring intervention, necrotizing fasciitis, fistula (gastrointestinal and nongastrointestinal), gastrointestinal perforation, intra-abdominal abscess, hypertensive crisis, hypertensive encephalopathy, serious bleeding/hemorrhage, severe arterial thromboembolic event, nephrotic syndrome, or RPLS.

Dosage adjustment in renal impairment: No dosage adjustment provided in the manufacturer's labeling.

Dosage adjustment in hepatic impairment: No dosage adjustment provided in the manufacturer's labeling.

Administration

I.V.: Infuse the initial dose over 90 minutes. The second infusion may be shortened to 60 minutes if the initial infusion is well tolerated. The third and subsequent infusions may be shortened to 30 minutes if the 60-minute infusion is well tolerated. Monitor closely during the infusion for signs/symptoms of an infusion reaction. After tolerance at the 90-, 60-, and 30-minute infusion rates has been established, some institutions use an unlabeled 10-minute infusion rate (0.5 mg/kg/minute) for bevacizumab dosed at 5 mg/kg (Reidy, 2007). In a study evaluating the safety of the 0.5 mg/kg/minute infusion rate, proteinuria and hypertension incidences were not increased with the shorter infusion time (Shah, 2013). Do not administer I.V. push. Do not administer with dextrose solutions.

Intravitreal injection (unlabeled use/route): Adequate local anesthesia and a topical broad-spectrum antimicrobial agent should be administered prior to the procedure.

Monitoring Parameters Monitor closely during the infusion for signs/symptoms of an infusion reaction. Monitor CBC with differential; signs/symptoms of gastrointestinal perforation, fistula, or abscess (including abdominal pain, constipation, vomiting, and fever); signs/symptoms of bleeding, including hemoptysis, gastrointestinal, and/or CNS bleeding, and/or epistaxis. Monitor blood pressure every 2-3 weeks; more frequently if hypertension develops during therapy. Continue to monitor blood pressure after discontinuing due to bevacizumab-induced hypertension. Monitor for proteinuria/nephrotic syndrome with urine dipstick; collect 24-hour urine in patients with ≥2+ reading.

AMD (unlabeled use): Monitor intraocular pressure and retinal artery perfusion

Dosage Forms Excipient information presented when available (limited, particularly for generics); consult specific product labeling.

Solution, Intravenous [preservative free]:

Avastin: 100 mg/4 mL (4 mL); 400 mg/16 mL (16 mL)

Bexarotene (Systemic) (beks AIR oh teen)

Brand Names: U.S. Targretin

Pharmacologic Category Antineoplastic Agent, Miscellaneous; Retinoic Acid Derivative

Use Treatment of cutaneous manifestations of cutaneous T-cell lymphoma in patients who are refractory to at least one prior systemic therapy

Pregnancy Risk Factor X

Pregnancy Considerations **[U.S. Boxed Warning]: Bexarotene is a retinoid, a drug class associated with birth defects in humans; do not administer during pregnancy.** Bexarotene caused birth defects when administered orally to pregnant rats. It must not be given to a pregnant woman or a woman who intends to become pregnant. If a woman becomes pregnant while taking the drug, it must be stopped immediately and appropriate counseling be given. In women of childbearing potential, therapy should be started on the second or third day of a normal menstrual period. Either abstinence or two forms of reliable contraception (one should be nonhormonal) must be used for at least 1 month before initiating therapy, during therapy, and for 1 month following discontinuation of bexarotene. A negative pregnancy test (sensitivity of at least 50 mIU/mL) within 1 week prior to beginning therapy, and monthly thereafter is required for women of childbearing potential. A maximum 1 month supply is recommended so that pregnancy tests may be evaluated. Male patients must use a condom during any sexual contact with women of childbearing age during therapy, and for at least 1 month following discontinuation of bexarotene.

Breast-Feeding Considerations It is not known if bexarotene is excreted into breast milk. Due to the potential for serious adverse reactions in a nursing infant, the decision to continue or discontinue breast-feeding during therapy should take into account the risk of exposure to the infant and the benefits of treatment to the mother.

Contraindications Hypersensitivity to bexarotene or any component of the formulation; pregnancy

Warnings/Precautions Hazardous agent - use appropriate precautions for handling and disposal (NIOSH, 2012). **[U.S. Boxed Warning]: Bexarotene is a retinoid, a drug class associated with birth defects in humans; do not administer during pregnancy.** Pregnancy test needed within 1 week before initiation and every month thereafter. Effective contraception must be in place 1 month before initiation, during therapy, and for at least 1 month after discontinuation. Male patients with sexual partners who are pregnant, possibly pregnant, or who could become pregnant, must use condoms during sexual intercourse during treatment and for at least 1 month after last dose. Induces significant lipid abnormalities in a majority of patients (triglyceride, total cholesterol, and HDL); monitor lipid panel; may require dose reduction, treatment interruption, and/or concomitant antilipemic therapy; reversible on discontinuation. Pancreatitis secondary to hypertriglyceridemia has been reported. Patients with risk factors for pancreatitis (eg, prior pancreatitis, uncontrolled hyperlipidemia, excessive ethanol consumption, uncontrolled diabetes, biliary tract disease, concomitant medications causing hyperlipidemia) should generally not receive bexarotene (oral). Dose-related elevations in ALT, AST, and bilirubin have been reported; monitor for liver function test abnormalities and temporarily hold or discontinue drug if tests are >3 times the upper limit of normal (ULN) values for AST, ALT, or bilirubin. Bexarotene rapidly suppresses TSH levels by directly inhibiting TSH secretion and also affects thyroid hormone metabolism (Hamnvik, 2011). Hypothyroidism occurs in about one third to the majority of all patients; monitor free T_4 levels closely. Thyroid supplementation is usually required; in patients already receiving thyroid hormone therapy, may require increased thyroid hormone doses to achieve therapeutic levels (Hamnvik, 2011). Monitor for signs and symptoms of infection about 4-8 weeks after initiation (leukopenia may occur). Any new visual abnormalities experienced by the patient should be evaluated by an ophthalmologist (cataracts may form, or worsen, especially in the geriatric population). Retinoids are associated with photosensitivity; mild phototoxicity (sunburn, sunlight sensitivity) has occurred with bexarotene; advise patients to limit sunlight and artificial ultraviolet light during treatment. Use only with extreme caution in patients with hepatic impairment; undergoes extensive hepatic elimination. Limit additional vitamin A intake (in studies, additional vitamin A was limited to <15,000 units/day). Use caution with diabetic patients; may enhance the actions of insulin, sulfonylureas or thiazolidinediones, resulting in hypoglycemia in patients receiving these agents (hypoglycemia has not been observed with bexarotene monotherapy). Monitor blood glucose as necessary.

Adverse Reactions

>10%:

Cardiovascular: Peripheral edema (11% to 13%)

Central nervous system: Headache (30% to 42%), fever (5% to 17%), chills (10% to 13%), insomnia (5% to 11%)

Dermatologic: Rash (17% to 23%), exfoliative dermatitis (10% to 28%), dry skin (9% to 11%), alopecia (4% to 11%)

Endocrine & metabolic: Hyperlipidemia (79%), hypercholesteremia (32% to 62%), hypothyroidism (29% to 53%)

Gastrointestinal: Diarrhea (7% to 42%), anorexia (2% to 23%), nausea (8% to 16%), vomiting (4% to 13%), abdominal pain (4% to 11%)

Hematologic: Leukopenia (17% to 47%), anemia (6% to 25%), hypochromic anemia (4% to 13%)

Hepatic: LDH increased (7% to 13%)

Neuromuscular & skeletal: Weakness (20% to 45%), back pain (2% to 11%)

Miscellaneous: Infection (13% to 23%; bacterial: 1% to 13%), flu-like syndrome (4% to 13%)

<10%:

Cardiovascular: Angina pectoris, cerebrovascular accident, chest pain, heart failure (right), hypertension, syncope, tachycardia

Central nervous system: Agitation, ataxia, confusion, depression, dizziness, hyperesthesia, subdural hematoma

Dermatologic: Acne, cellulitis, cheilitis, maculopapular rash, photosensitivity, pustular rash, serous drainage, skin nodule, skin rash, skin sensitivity, sunburn, vesicular bullous rash

Endocrine & metabolic: Breast pain, hypoproteinemia, hyperglycemia

Gastrointestinal: Amylase increased, colitis, constipation, dyspepsia, flatulence, gastroenteritis, gingivitis, melena, pancreatitis, weight loss/gain, xerostomia

Genitourinary: Dysuria, hematuria, urinary incontinence, urinary tract infection, urinary urgency

Hematologic: Coagulopathy, eosinophilia, hemorrhage, lymphocytosis, thrombocythemia, thrombocytopenia

Hepatic: ALT increased, AST increased, bilirubin increased, hepatic failure

Neuromuscular & skeletal: Arthralgia, arthrosis, bone pain, myalgia, myasthenia, neuropathy

Ocular: Blepharitis, cataracts (new and worsening), conjunctivitis, corneal lesion, dry eyes, keratitis, visual field defects

Otic: Ear pain, otitis externa

Renal: Albuminuria, creatinine increased, renal function abnormal

Respiratory: Bronchitis, cough, dyspnea, hemoptysis, hypoxia, pharyngitis, pleural effusion, pneumonia, pulmonary edema, rhinitis

Miscellaneous: Monilia, sepsis

Drug Interactions

Metabolism/Transport Effects **Substrate** of CYP3A4 (minor); **Note:** Assignment of Major/Minor substrate status based on clinically relevant drug interaction potential; **Induces** CYP3A4 (weak/moderate)

Avoid Concomitant Use

Avoid concomitant use of Bexarotene (Systemic) with any of the following: Axitinib; CloZAPine; Gemfibrozil; Multivitamins/Fluoride (with ADE); Multivitamins/Minerals (with ADEK, Folate, Iron); Multivitamins/Minerals (with AE, No Iron); Simeprevir; Tetracycline Derivatives; Vitamin A

Increased Effect/Toxicity

Bexarotene (Systemic) may increase the levels/effects of: CloZAPine; Porfimer; Vitamin A

The levels/effects of Bexarotene (Systemic) may be increased by: CARBOplatin; Gemfibrozil; Multivitamins/Fluoride (with ADE); Multivitamins/Minerals (with ADEK, Folate, Iron); Multivitamins/Minerals (with AE, No Iron); PACLitaxel; Tetracycline Derivatives

Decreased Effect

Bexarotene (Systemic) may decrease the levels/effects of: ARIPiprazole; AtorvaSTATin; Axitinib; Contraceptives (Estrogens); Contraceptives (Progestins); Ibrutinib; PACLitaxel; Saxagliptin; Simeprevir; Tamoxifen

Ethanol/Nutrition/Herb Interactions

Food: Bioavailability is increased when administered with a fat-containing meal. Serum levels may be increased by grapefruit juice. Management: Administer with food. Avoid grapefruit juice.

Herb/Nutraceutical: Dong quai and St John's wort may cause photosensitization. St John's wort may decrease bexarotene levels. Additional vitamin A supplementation may lead to vitamin A toxicity (dry skin, irritation, arthralgias, myalgias, abdominal pain, hepatic changes). Management: Avoid St John's wort and dong quai. Limit the use of vitamin A supplements.

Storage/Stability Store at 2°C to 25°C (36°F to 77°F). Protect from light. Avoid humidity and high temperatures after opening bottle.

Mechanism of Action Selectively binds to and activates retinoid X receptors (RXRs). Once activated, RXRs function as transcription factors to regulate the expression of genes which control cellular differentiation and proliferation. Bexarotene inhibits the growth *in vitro* of some tumor cell lines of hematopoietic and squamous cell origin and induces tumor regression *in vivo* in some animal models.

Pharmacodynamics/Kinetics

Absorption: Improved 48% by a fat-containing meal

Protein binding: >99% to plasma proteins

Metabolism: Hepatic via CYP3A4 isoenzyme to four metabolites; further metabolized by glucuronidation

Half-life elimination: ~7 hours

Time to peak: ~2 hours

Excretion: Primarily feces; urine (<1% as unchanged drug and metabolites)

Dosage Oral: Adults:

Cutaneous T-cell lymphoma, refractory: Initial: 300 mg/m²/day taken as a single daily dose; if well tolerated, but no response after 8 weeks of therapy, may increase to 400 mg/m²/day; continue as long as clinical benefit is demonstrated.

Cutaneous T-cell lymphomas, relapsed/refractory (unlabeled dose): 150 mg daily (in combination with denileukin diftitox) (Foss, 2005)

Mycosis fungoides/Sezary syndrome, refractory/resistant (unlabeled dose): 75-150 mg daily in combination with PUVA; maximum dose: 300 mg daily (Rupoli, 2010; Singh, 2004)

Dosage adjustment for toxicity: If necessitated by toxicity, may decrease dose from 300 mg/m²/day to 200 mg/m²/day, then to 100 mg/m²/day, or temporarily hold. Upon recovery, may titrate dose upward with careful monitoring.

Hepatotoxicity: If AST, ALT, or bilirubin >3 times ULN, consider holding or discontinuing therapy.

Hypertriglyceridemia: Consider reducing dose or suspending therapy.

Dosage adjustment in renal impairment: No dosage adjustment provided in manufacturer's labeling (has not been studied); however, renal insufficiency may result in significant protein binding changes and alter pharmacokinetics of bexarotene.

Dosage adjustment in hepatic impairment: No dosage adjustment provided in manufacturer's labeling (has not been studied); however, hepatic impairment would be expected to result in decreased clearance of bexarotene due to the extensive hepatic contribution to elimination.

Dosing in obesity: *ASCO Guidelines for appropriate chemotherapy dosing in obese adults with cancer:* Utilize patient's actual body weight (full weight) for calculation of body surface area- or weight-based dosing, particularly when the intent of therapy is curative; manage regimen-related toxicities in the same manner as for nonobese patients; if a dose reduction is utilized due to toxicity, consider resumption of full weight-based dosing with subsequent cycles, especially if cause of toxicity (eg, hepatic or renal impairment) is resolved (Griggs, 2012).

Dietary Considerations Take with food. Avoid grapefruit juice.

Administration Administer with a meal. Swallow capsule whole; do not chew or dissolve (per the manufacturer).

Hazardous agent; use appropriate precautions for handling and disposal (NIOSH, 2012).

Monitoring Parameters If female, pregnancy test within 1 week before initiation then monthly while on bexarotene; lipid panel (before initiation, then weekly until lipid response established and then at 8-week intervals thereafter); liver function tests (baseline, then at 1, 2, and 4 weeks after initiation, then at 8-week intervals thereafter if stable); monitor thyroid function tests (free T_4) weekly for the first 5-7 weeks, then every 1-2 months (Hamnvik 2011); CBC with differential (baseline and periodic); blood glucose (in diabetic patients); ophthalmic exam (if visual abnormalities occur)

Test Interactions Per the manufacturer, treatment with bexarotene may interfere with CA125 assay values in patients with ovarian cancer.

Dosage Forms Excipient information presented when available (limited, particularly for generics); consult specific product labeling.

Capsule, Oral:

Targretin: 75 mg

Extemporaneous Preparations Hazardous agent: Use appropriate precautions for handling and disposal.

A 1 mg/mL oral suspension may be prepared with capsules. Cut one 75 mg capsule in half, rinse the interior contents of the capsule, and suspend with 75 mL sterile water. Administer immediately after preparation. To ensure administration of full dose, rinse empty glass with half a glass of water and administer residue.

Targretin® data on file, Eisai Inc.

Bexarotene (Topical) (beks AIR oh teen)

Brand Names: U.S. Targretin

Pharmacologic Category Antineoplastic Agent, Miscellaneous

Use Treatment of cutaneous lesions in patients with refractory cutaneous T-cell lymphoma (stage 1A and 1B) or who have not tolerated other therapies

Pregnancy Risk Factor X

Pregnancy Considerations **Bexarotene is a retinoid, a drug class associated with birth defects in humans; do not administer during pregnancy.** Bexarotene caused birth defects when administered orally to pregnant rats. It must not be given to a pregnant woman or a woman who intends to become pregnant. If a woman becomes pregnant while using the gel, it must be stopped immediately and appropriate counseling be given. In women of childbearing potential, therapy should be started on the second or third day of a normal menstrual period. Either abstinence or two forms of reliable contraception (one should be nonhormonal) must be used for at least 1 month before initiating therapy, during therapy, and for 1 month following discontinuation of bexarotene. A negative pregnancy test (sensitivity of at least 50 mIU/mL) within 1 week prior to beginning therapy, and monthly thereafter is required for women of childbearing potential. Males patients must use a condom during any sexual contact with women of childbearing age during therapy, and for 1 month following discontinuation of bexarotene

Breast-Feeding Considerations It is not known if bexarotene is excreted into breast milk. Due to the potential for serious adverse reactions in a nursing infant, the decision to continue or discontinue breast-feeding during therapy should take into account the risk of exposure to the infant and the benefits of treatment to the mother.

Contraindications Hypersensitivity to bexarotene or any component of the formulation; pregnancy

Warnings/Precautions Hazardous agent - use appropriate precautions for handling and disposal (NIOSH, 2012). **Bexarotene is a retinoid, a drug class associated with birth defects in humans; do not administer during pregnancy.** Pregnancy test needed 1 week before initiation and every month thereafter. Effective contraception must be in place 1 month before initiation, during therapy, and for at least 1 month after discontinuation. Male patients with sexual partners who are pregnant, possibly pregnant, or who could become pregnant, must use condoms during sexual intercourse during treatment and for 1 month after last dose. May induce lipid abnormalities; reversible on discontinuation. Use extreme caution in patients with underlying hypertriglyceridemia. Monitor for signs and symptoms of infection about 4-8 weeks after initiation (leukopenia may occur). May cause photosensitization. Safety and efficacy are not established in the pediatric population. Use only with extreme caution in patients with hepatic impairment. Limit additional vitamin A intake to <15,000 units/day.

Adverse Reactions

Cardiovascular: Edema (10%)

Central nervous system: Headache (14%), weakness (6%), pain (30%)

Dermatologic: Rash (14% to 72%), pruritus (6% to 40%), contact dermatitis (14%), exfoliative dermatitis (6%)

Endocrine & metabolic: Hyperlipidemia (10%)

Hematologic: Leukopenia (6%), lymphadenopathy (6%)

Neuromuscular & skeletal: Paresthesia (6%)

Respiratory: Cough (6%), pharyngitis (6%)

Miscellaneous: Diaphoresis (6%), infection (18%)

Drug Interactions

Metabolism/Transport Effects Substrate of CYP3A4 (minor); **Note:** Assignment of Major/Minor substrate status based on clinically relevant drug interaction potential; **Induces** CYP3A4 (weak/moderate)

Avoid Concomitant Use

Avoid concomitant use of Bexarotene (Topical) with any of the following: Axitinib; Multivitamins/Fluoride (with ADE); Multivitamins/Minerals (with ADEK, Folate, Iron); Multivitamins/Minerals (with AE, No Iron); Simeprevir; Tetracycline Derivatives; Vitamin A

Increased Effect/Toxicity

Bexarotene (Topical) may increase the levels/effects of: Porfimer; Vitamin A

The levels/effects of Bexarotene (Topical) may be increased by: Multivitamins/Fluoride (with ADE); Multivitamins/Minerals (with ADEK, Folate, Iron); Multivitamins/Minerals (with AE, No Iron); Tetracycline Derivatives

Decreased Effect

Bexarotene (Topical) may decrease the levels/effects of: ARIPiprazole; Axitinib; Contraceptives (Estrogens); Contraceptives (Progestins); Ibrutinib; Saxagliptin; Simeprevir

Storage/Stability Store at 2°C to 25°C (36°F to 77°F). Protect from light.

Mechanism of Action The exact mechanism is unknown. Binds and activates retinoid X receptor subtypes. Once activated, these receptors function as transcription factors that regulate the expression of genes which control cellular differentiation and proliferation.

Pharmacodynamics/Kinetics Absorption: Systemically absorbed following topical application (1% gel: <55 ng/mL)

Dosage Topical: Adults: Apply once every other day for first week, then increase on a weekly basis to once daily, 2 times/day, 3 times/day, and finally 4 times/day, according to tolerance

Dosing adjustment in renal impairment: No studies have been conducted; however, renal insufficiency may result in significant protein binding changes and alter pharmacokinetics of bexarotene

Dosing adjustment in hepatic impairment: No studies have been conducted; however, hepatic impairment would be expected to result in decreased clearance of bexarotene due to the extensive hepatic contribution to elimination

Administration Allow gel to dry before covering with clothing. Avoid application to normal skin. Use of occlusive dressings is not recommended.

Hazardous agent; use appropriate precautions for handling and disposal (NIOSH, 2012).

Monitoring Parameters If female, pregnancy test 1 week before initiation then monthly while on bexarotene; lipid panel before initiation, then weekly until lipid response established and then at 8-week intervals thereafter; baseline LFTs, repeat at 1, 2, and 4 weeks after initiation then at 8-week intervals thereafter if stable; baseline and periodic thyroid function tests; baseline CBC with periodic monitoring

Dosage Forms Excipient information presented when available (limited, particularly for generics); consult specific product labeling.

Gel, External:

Targretin: 1% (60 g) [contains alcohol, usp]

- ◆ Beyaz *see* Ethinyl Estradiol, Drospirenone, and Levomefolate *on page 797*
- ◆ BG-12 *see* Dimethyl Fumarate *on page 618*
- ◆ BI-1356 *see* Linagliptin *on page 1216*
- ◆ Biaxin *see* Clarithromycin *on page 446*
- ◆ Biaxin XL *see* Clarithromycin *on page 446*
- ◆ Biaxin XL Pac *see* Clarithromycin *on page 446*
- ◆ Biaxin BID (Can) *see* Clarithromycin *on page 446*
- ◆ BIBW 2992 *see* Afatinib *on page 54*

Bicalutamide (bye ka LOO ta mide)

Brand Names: U.S. Casodex

Brand Names: Canada Apo-Bicalutamide®; Ava-Bicalutamide; Casodex®; CO Bicalutamide; Dom-Bicalutamide; JAMP-Bicalutamide; Mylan-Bicalutamide; Novo-Bicalutamide; PHL-Bicalutamide; PMS-Bicalutamide; PRO-Bicalutamide; ratio-Bicalutamide; Sandoz-Bicalutamide

Index Terms CDX; ICI-176334

Pharmacologic Category Antineoplastic Agent, Antiandrogen

Use Treatment of metastatic prostate cancer (in combination with an LHRH agonist)

Unlabeled Use Monotherapy for locally-advanced prostate cancer

Pregnancy Risk Factor X

Pregnancy Considerations Animal studies have demonstrated teratogenicity. Bicalutamide use is contraindicated in women. Androgen receptor inhibition during pregnancy may affect fetal development.

Breast-Feeding Considerations Bicalutamide is not indicated for use in women.

Contraindications Hypersensitivity to bicalutamide or any component of the formulation; use in women, especially women who are or may become pregnant

Warnings/Precautions Hazardous agent - use appropriate precautions for handling and disposal (NIOSH, 2012). Rare cases of death or hospitalization due to hepatitis have been reported postmarketing. Use with caution in moderate-to-severe hepatic dysfunction. Hepatotoxicity generally occurs within the first 3-4 months of use; patients should be monitored for signs and symptoms of liver dysfunction. Bicalutamide should be discontinued if patients have jaundice or ALT is >2 times the upper limit of normal. Androgen-deprivation therapy may increase the risk for cardiovascular disease (Levine, 2010). May cause gynecomastia, breast pain, or lead to spermatogenesis inhibition. When used in combination with LHRH agonists, a loss of glycemic control and decrease in glucose tolerance has been reported in patients with diabetes; monitor. May cause gynecomastia or breast pain (at higher, unlabeled doses), or lead to spermatogenesis inhibition.

Adverse Reactions Adverse reaction percentages reported as part of combination regimen with an LHRH analogue unless otherwise noted.

>10%:

Cardiovascular: Peripheral edema (13%)

Central nervous system: Pain (35%)

Endocrine & metabolic: Hot flashes (53%), breast pain (6%; monotherapy [150 mg]: 39% to 85%), gynecomastia (9%; monotherapy [150 mg]: 38% to 73%)

Gastrointestinal: Constipation (22%), nausea (15%), diarrhea (12%), abdominal pain (11%)

Genitourinary: Pelvic pain (21%), hematuria (12%), nocturia (12%)

Hematologic: Anemia (11%)

Neuromuscular & skeletal: Back pain (25%), weakness (22%)

Respiratory: Dyspnea (13%)

Miscellaneous: Infection (18%)

≥2% to 10%:

Cardiovascular: Chest pain (8%), hypertension (8%), angina pectoris (2% to <5%), cardiac arrest (2% to <5%), CHF (2% to <5%), edema (2% to <5%), MI (2% to <5%), coronary artery disorder (2% to <5%), syncope (2% to <5%)

Central nervous system: Dizziness (10%), headache (7%), insomnia (7%), anxiety (5%), depression (4%), chills (2% to <5%), confusion (2% to <5%), fever (2% to <5%), nervousness (2% to <5%), somnolence (2% to <5%)

Dermatologic: Rash (9%), alopecia (2% to <5%), dry skin (2% to <5%), pruritus (2% to <5%), skin carcinoma (2% to <5%)

Endocrine & metabolic: Hyperglycemia (6%), dehydration (2% to <5%), gout (2% to <5%), hypercholesterolemia (2% to <5%), libido decreased (2% to <5%)

Gastrointestinal: Dyspepsia (7%), weight loss (7%), anorexia (6%), flatulence (6%), vomiting (6%), weight gain (5%), dysphagia (2% to <5%), gastrointestinal carcinoma (2% to <5%), melena (2% to <5%), periodontal abscess (2% to <5%), rectal hemorrhage (2% to <5%), xerostomia (2% to <5%)

Genitourinary: Urinary tract infection (9%), impotence (7%), polyuria (6%), urinary retention (5%), urinary impairment (5%), urinary incontinence (4%), dysuria (2% to <5%), urinary urgency (2% to <5%)

Hepatic: LFTs increased (7%), alkaline phosphatase increased (5%)

Neuromuscular & skeletal: Bone pain (9%), paresthesia (8%), myasthenia (7%), arthritis (5%), pathological fracture (4%), hypertonia (2% to <5%), leg cramps (2% to <5%), myalgia (2% to <5%), neck pain (2% to <5%), neuropathy (2% to <5%)

Ocular: Cataract (2% to <5%)

Renal: BUN increased (2% to <5%), creatinine increased (2% to <5%), hydronephrosis (2% to <5%)

Respiratory: Cough (8%), pharyngitis (8%), bronchitis (6%), pneumonia (4%), rhinitis (4%), asthma (2% to <5%), epistaxis (2% to <5%), sinusitis (2% to <5%)

Miscellaneous: Flu-like syndrome (7%), diaphoresis (6%), cyst (2% to <5%), hernia (2% to <5%), herpes zoster (2% to <5%), sepsis (2% to <5%)

Postmarketing and/or case reports: Bilirubin increased, glucose tolerance decreased, hemoglobin decreased, hepatitis, hepatotoxicity, hypersensitivity reactions (including angioneurotic edema and urticaria), interstitial pneumonitis, pulmonary fibrosis, WBC decreased

Drug Interactions

Metabolism/Transport Effects Inhibits CYP3A4 (moderate)

Avoid Concomitant Use

Avoid concomitant use of Bicalutamide with any of the following: Bosutinib; Ibrutinib; Ivabradine; Lomitapide; Pimozide; Simeprevir; Tolvaptan; Ulipristal

Increased Effect/Toxicity

Bicalutamide may increase the levels/effects of: ARIPiprazole; Avanafil; Bosentan; Bosutinib; Budesonide (Systemic, Oral Inhalation); Colchicine; CYP3A4 Substrates; Dofetilide; Eplerenone; Everolimus; FentaNYL; Halofantrine; Ibrutinib; Imatinib; Ivabradine; Ivacaftor; Lomitapide; Lurasidone; OxyCODONE; Pimecrolimus; Pimozide; Propafenone; Ranolazine; Salmeterol; Saxagliptin; Simeprevir; Tolvaptan; Ulipristal; Vilazodone; Vitamin K Antagonists; Zuclopenthixol

Decreased Effect
Bicalutamide may decrease the levels/effects of: Ifosfamide

Storage/Stability Store at room temperature of 20°C to 25°C (68°F to 77°F).

Mechanism of Action Androgen receptor inhibitor; pure nonsteroidal antiandrogen that binds to androgen receptors; specifically a competitive inhibitor for the binding of dihydrotestosterone and testosterone; prevents testosterone stimulation of cell growth in prostate cancer

Pharmacodynamics/Kinetics
Absorption: Rapid and complete; unaffected by food
Protein binding: 96%
Metabolism: Extensively hepatic; glucuronidation and oxidation of the R (active) enantiomer to inactive metabolites; the S enantiomer is inactive
Half-life elimination: Active enantiomer: ~6 days, ~10 days in severe liver disease
Time to peak, plasma: Active enantiomer: ~31 hours
Excretion: Urine (36%, as inactive metabolites); feces (42%, as unchanged drug and inactive metabolites)

Dosage Oral: Adults:
Prostate cancer, metastatic: 50 mg once daily (in combination with an LHRH analogue)
Prostate cancer, locally-advanced (unlabeled use): 150 mg once daily (as monotherapy) (McLeod, 2006)
Dosage adjustment in renal impairment: No adjustment required
Dosage adjustment in hepatic impairment: No adjustment required for mild, moderate, or severe hepatic impairment; use caution with moderate-to-severe impairment. Discontinue if ALT >2 times ULN or patient develops jaundice.

Dietary Considerations May be taken with or without food.

Administration Dose should be taken at the same time each day with or without food. Treatment for metastatic cancer should be started concomitantly with an LHRH analogue.

Hazardous agent; use appropriate precautions for handling and disposal (NIOSH, 2012).

Monitoring Parameters Periodically monitor CBC, ECG, echocardiograms, serum testosterone, luteinizing hormone, and prostate specific antigen (PSA). Liver function tests should be obtained at baseline and repeated regularly during the first 4 months of treatment, and periodically thereafter; monitor for signs and symptoms of liver dysfunction (discontinue if jaundice is noted or ALT is >2 times the upper limit of normal). Monitor blood glucose in patients with diabetes. If initiating bicalutamide in patients who are on warfarin, closely monitor prothrombin time.

Dosage Forms Excipient information presented when available (limited, particularly for generics); consult specific product labeling.
Tablet, Oral:
Casodex: 50 mg
Generic: 50 mg

◆ **Bicillin L-A** *see* Penicillin G Benzathine *on page 1606*
◆ **Bicillin® L-A (Can)** *see* Penicillin G Benzathine *on page 1606*
◆ **Bicillin® C-R** *see* Penicillin G Benzathine and Penicillin G Procaine *on page 1607*
◆ **Bicillin® C-R 900/300** *see* Penicillin G Benzathine and Penicillin G Procaine *on page 1607*
◆ **Bicitra** *see* Sodium Citrate and Citric Acid *on page 1917*
◆ **BiCNU** *see* Carmustine *on page 352*
◆ **BiCNU® (Can)** *see* Carmustine *on page 352*
◆ **Bidex [OTC]** *see* GuaiFENesin *on page 974*
◆ **BiDil®** *see* Isosorbide Dinitrate and Hydralazine *on page 1127*
◆ **BIG-IV** *see* Botulism Immune Globulin (Intravenous-Human) *on page 277*
◆ **Biltricide** *see* Praziquantel *on page 1702*
◆ **Biltricide® (Can)** *see* Praziquantel *on page 1702*

Bimatoprost (bi MAT oh prost)

Brand Names: U.S. Latisse; Lumigan
Brand Names: Canada Latisse®; Lumigan®; Lumigan® RC

Pharmacologic Category Ophthalmic Agent, Antiglaucoma; Prostaglandin, Ophthalmic

Use Reduction of intraocular pressure (IOP) in patients with open-angle glaucoma or ocular hypertension; hypotrichosis treatment of the eyelashes

Pregnancy Risk Factor C

Dosage Adults:
Ophthalmic: Open-angle glaucoma or ocular hypertension: Instill 1 drop into affected eye(s) once daily in the evening; do not exceed once-daily dosing (may decrease IOP-lowering effect). If used with other topical ophthalmic agents, separate administration by at least 5 minutes.
Ophthalmic, topical: Hypotrichosis of the eyelashes: Place one drop on applicator and apply evenly along the skin of the upper eyelid at base of eyelashes once daily at bedtime; repeat procedure for second eye (use a clean applicator)

Additional Information Complete prescribing information should be consulted for additional detail.

Dosage Forms Excipient information presented when available (limited, particularly for generics); consult specific product labeling.
Solution, External:
Latisse: 0.03% (3 mL, 5 mL) [contains benzalkonium chloride]
Solution, Ophthalmic:
Lumigan: 0.01% (2.5 mL, 5 mL, 7.5 mL) [contains benzalkonium chloride]

◆ **Binosto** *see* Alendronate *on page 69*
◆ **Bio-Amitriptyline (Can)** *see* Amitriptyline *on page 105*
◆ **Bio-Anastrozole (Can)** *see* Anastrozole *on page 137*
◆ **Bio-Diazepam (Can)** *see* Diazepam *on page 594*
◆ **Bio-Furosemide (Can)** *see* Furosemide *on page 931*
◆ **Bio Glo** *see* Fluorescein *on page 880*
◆ **Bio-Hydrochlorothiazide (Can)** *see* Hydrochlorothiazide *on page 1004*
◆ **Bio-Letrozole (Can)** *see* Letrozole *on page 1185*
◆ **Bionect** *see* Hyaluronate and Derivatives *on page 1000*
◆ **Bioniche Promethazine (Can)** *see* Promethazine *on page 1728*
◆ **Bio-Oxazepam (Can)** *see* Oxazepam *on page 1529*
◆ **BioQuin® Durules™ (Can)** *see* QuiNIDine *on page 1764*
◆ **Bio-Statin** *see* Nystatin (Oral) *on page 1481*
◆ **BioThrax®** *see* Anthrax Vaccine Adsorbed *on page 141*
◆ **Biphentin (Can)** *see* Methylphenidate *on page 1336*
◆ **Bird Flu Vaccine** *see* Influenza Virus Vaccine (H5N1) *on page 1076*
◆ **Bisac-Evac [OTC]** *see* Bisacodyl *on page 259*

Bisacodyl (bis a KOE dil)

Brand Names: U.S. Bisac-Evac [OTC]; Bisacodyl EC [OTC]; Bisacodyl Laxative [OTC]; Biscolax [OTC]; Correct

[OTC]; Ducodyl [OTC]; Dulcolax [OTC]; Ex-Lax Ultra [OTC]; Fleet Bisacodyl [OTC]; Fleet Laxative [OTC]; Gentle Laxative [OTC]; Laxative [OTC]; Magic Bullets [OTC]; Stimulant Laxative [OTC]; Womens Laxative [OTC]

Brand Names: Canada Apo-Bisacodyl [OTC]; Bisacodyl-Odan [OTC]; Bisacolax [OTC]; Carter's Little Pills [OTC]; Codulax [OTC]; Dulcolax [OTC]; PMS-Bisacodyl [OTC]; ratio-Bisacodyl [OTC]; Silver Bullet Suppository [OTC]; Soflax [OTC]; The Magic Bullett [OTC]; Woman's Laxative [OTC]

Pharmacologic Category Laxative, Stimulant

Additional Appendix Information

Laxatives, Classification and Properties *on page* 2304

Use Treatment of constipation; colonic evacuation prior to procedures or examination

Dosage

Children:
- Oral: >6 years: 5-10 mg (0.3 mg/kg) at bedtime or before breakfast
- Rectal suppository:
  - <2 years: 5 mg as a single dose
  - >2 years: 10 mg

Adults:
- Oral: 5-15 mg as single dose (up to 30 mg when complete evacuation of bowel is required)
- Rectal suppository: 10 mg as single dose

Dosage adjustment in renal impairment: No dosage adjustment provided in manufacturer's labeling. Use with caution in patients with impaired renal function.

Dosage adjustment in hepatic impairment: No dosage adjustment provided in manufacturer's labeling.

Additional Information Complete prescribing information should be consulted for additional detail.

Dosage Forms Excipient information presented when available (limited, particularly for generics); consult specific product labeling.

Enema, Rectal:
- Fleet Bisacodyl: 10 mg/30 mL (37 mL)

Suppository, Rectal:
- Bisac-Evac: 10 mg (1 ea, 8 ea, 12 ea, 50 ea, 100 ea, 500 ea, 1000 ea)
- Bisacodyl Laxative: 10 mg (12 ea)
- Biscolax: 10 mg (12 ea, 100 ea)
- Dulcolax: 10 mg (4 ea, 8 ea, 16 ea, 28 ea, 50 ea)
- Laxative: 10 mg (12 ea, 100 ea)
- Magic Bullets: 10 mg (12 ea, 100 ea)
- Generic: 10 mg (12 ea, 50 ea, 100 ea)

Tablet Delayed Release, Oral:
- Bisac-Evac: 5 mg [contains fd&c yellow #10 aluminum lake, fd&c yellow #6 aluminum lake]
- Bisacodyl EC: 5 mg
- Bisacodyl EC: 5 mg [contains fd&c yellow #10 (quinoline yellow), fd&c yellow #6 (sunset yellow)]
- Bisacodyl EC: 5 mg [contains fd&c yellow #10 aluminum lake, fd&c yellow #6 aluminum lake]
- Correct: 5 mg
- Ducodyl: 5 mg
- Dulcolax: 5 mg [contains fd&c yellow #10 (quinoline yellow), methylparaben, propylparaben, sodium benzoate]
- Ex-Lax Ultra: 5 mg [contains fd&c yellow #6 (sunset yellow), methylparaben]
- Fleet Laxative: 5 mg
- Gentle Laxative: 5 mg
- Stimulant Laxative: 5 mg
- Stimulant Laxative: 5 mg [contains fd&c yellow #10 aluminum lake, fd&c yellow #6 aluminum lake]
- Womens Laxative: 5 mg
- Womens Laxative: 5 mg [contains fd&c blue #1 aluminum lake, sodium benzoate, tartrazine (fd&c yellow #5)]

◆ **Bisacodyl EC [OTC]** *see* Bisacodyl *on page* 259
◆ **Bisacodyl Laxative [OTC]** *see* Bisacodyl *on page* 259
◆ **Bisacodyl-Odan [OTC] (Can)** *see* Bisacodyl *on page* 259
◆ **Bisacolax [OTC] (Can)** *see* Bisacodyl *on page* 259
◆ **bis(chloroethyl) nitrosourea** *see* Carmustine *on page* 352
◆ **bis-chloronitrosourea** *see* Carmustine *on page* 352
◆ **Biscolax [OTC]** *see* Bisacodyl *on page* 259
◆ **Bismatrol** *see* Bismuth *on page* 260
◆ **Bismatrol [OTC]** *see* Bismuth *on page* 260
◆ **Bismatrol Maximum Strength [OTC]** *see* Bismuth *on page* 260

Bismuth (BIZ muth)

Brand Names: U.S. Bismatrol Maximum Strength [OTC]; Bismatrol [OTC]; Diotame [OTC]; Kao-Tin [OTC]; Peptic Relief [OTC]; Pepto-Bismol To-Go [OTC]; Pepto-Bismol [OTC]; Pink Bismuth [OTC]; Stomach Relief Max St [OTC]; Stomach Relief Plus [OTC]; Stomach Relief [OTC]

Index Terms Bismatrol; Bismuth Subsalicylate; Pink Bismuth

Pharmacologic Category Antidiarrheal

Use Subsalicylate formulation: Symptomatic treatment of mild, nonspecific diarrhea; control of traveler's diarrhea (enterotoxigenic *Escherichia coli*); as part of a multidrug regimen for *H. pylori* eradication to reduce the risk of duodenal ulcer recurrence

Dosage Oral:
- Treatment of nonspecific diarrhea, control/relieve traveler's diarrhea: Subsalicylate: Children >12 years and Adults: 524 mg every 30 minutes to 1 hour as needed up to 8 doses/24 hours
- *Helicobacter pylori* eradication: Subsalicylate: Adults: 524 mg 4 times/day with meals and at bedtime; requires combination therapy

Dosing adjustment in renal impairment: Bismuth has been associated with nephrotoxicity in overdose (Leussnik, 2002); although there are no specific recommendations by the manufacturer, consider using with caution in patients with renal impairment.

Additional Information Complete prescribing information should be consulted for additional detail.

Dosage Forms Excipient information presented when available (limited, particularly for generics); consult specific product labeling. [DSC] = Discontinued product

Suspension, Oral, as subsalicylate:
- Bismatrol: 262 mg/15 mL (236 mL) [contains benzoic acid, d&c red #22 (eosine), saccharin sodium; wintergreen flavor]
- Bismatrol Maximum Strength: 525 mg/15 mL (236 mL) [contains benzoic acid, d&c red #22 (eosine), saccharin sodium; wintergreen flavor]
- Kao-Tin: 262 mg/15 mL (236 mL, 473 mL) [contains fd&c red #40, saccharin sodium, sodium benzoate]
- Peptic Relief: 262 mg/15 mL (237 mL) [sugar free; contains benzoic acid, d&c red #22 (eosine), saccharin sodium; mint flavor]
- Pepto-Bismol: 262 mg/15 mL (473 mL) [contains benzoic acid, d&c red #22 (eosine), saccharin sodium]
- Pink Bismuth: 262 mg/15 mL (236 mL)
- Pink Bismuth: 262 mg/15 mL (237 mL) [contains benzoic acid, d&c red #22 (eosine), saccharin sodium]
- Stomach Relief: 262 mg/15 mL (237 mL, 355 mL, 473 mL [DSC]) [contains d&c red #22 (eosine), saccharin sodium]
- Stomach Relief: 527 mg/30 mL (240 mL, 480 mL)
- Stomach Relief Max St: 525 mg/15 mL (237 mL) [contains d&c red #22 (eosine), saccharin sodium]
- Stomach Relief Plus: 525 mg/15 mL (240 mL, 480 mL)

Tablet Chewable, Oral, as subsalicylate:
Bismatrol: 262 mg [contains aspartame]
Diotame: 262 mg
Peptic Relief: 262 mg
Pepto-Bismol To-Go: 262 mg [sugar free; contains fd&c red #40 aluminum lake, saccharin sodium; cherry flavor]
Pink Bismuth: 262 mg
Pink Bismuth: 262 mg [contains saccharin sodium]
Stomach Relief: 262 mg [contains aspartame]
Generic: 262 mg

◆ **Bismuth Subsalicylate** *see* Bismuth *on page 260*

Bisoprolol (bis OH proe lol)

Brand Names: U.S. Zebeta
Brand Names: Canada Apo-Bisoprolol®; Ava-Bisoprolol; Mylan-Bisoprolol; Novo-Bisoprolol; PHL-Bisoprolol; PMS-Bisoprolol; PRO-Bisoprolol; Sandoz-Bisoprolol
Index Terms Bisoprolol Fumarate
Pharmacologic Category Antihypertensive; Beta-Blocker, Beta-1 Selective
Additional Appendix Information
Beta-Blockers *on page 2294*
Use Treatment of hypertension, alone or in combination with other agents
Unlabeled Use Chronic stable angina, supraventricular arrhythmias, PVCs, heart failure (HF)
Pregnancy Risk Factor C
Pregnancy Considerations Adverse events were observed in animal reproduction studies; therefore, the manufacturer classifies bisoprolol as pregnancy category C. In a cohort study, an increased risk of cardiovascular defects was observed following maternal use of beta-blockers during pregnancy. Intrauterine growth restriction (IUGR), small placentas, as well as fetal/neonatal bradycardia, hypoglycemia, and/or respiratory depression have been observed following *in utero* exposure to beta-blockers as a class. Adequate facilities for monitoring infants at birth should be available. Untreated chronic maternal hypertension and pre-eclampsia are also associated with adverse events in the fetus, infant, and mother. Limited information is available related to the use of bisoprolol for the treatment of hypertension in pregnancy; other agents may be more appropriate for use.
Breast-Feeding Considerations It is not known if bisoprolol is excreted into breast milk. The manufacturer recommends that caution be exercised when administering bisoprolol to nursing women.
Contraindications Cardiogenic shock; overt cardiac failure; marked sinus bradycardia or heart block greater than first-degree (except in patients with a functioning artificial pacemaker)
Warnings/Precautions Consider pre-existing conditions such as sick sinus syndrome before initiating. Use caution in patients with heart failure; use gradual and careful titration; monitor for symptoms of congestive heart failure. Use with caution in patients with myasthenia gravis, psychiatric disease (may cause CNS depression), bronchospastic disease, undergoing anesthesia; and in those with impaired hepatic function. Bradycardia may be observed more frequently in elderly patients (>65 years of age); dosage reductions may be necessary. Beta-blocker therapy should not be withdrawn abruptly (particularly in patients with CAD), but gradually tapered to avoid acute tachycardia, hypertension, and/or ischemia. Chronic beta-blocker therapy should not be routinely withdrawn prior to major surgery. Can precipitate or aggravate symptoms of arterial insufficiency in patients with PVD and Raynaud's disease; use with caution and monitor for progression of arterial obstruction. Use caution with concurrent use of digoxin, verapamil, or diltiazem; bradycardia or heart block may occur. Use with caution in patients receiving inhaled anesthetic agents known to depress myocardial contractility. Bisoprolol, with beta$_1$-selectivity, may be used cautiously in bronchospastic disease with close monitoring. Use cautiously in patients with diabetes because it can mask prominent hypoglycemic symptoms. May mask signs of hyperthyroidism (eg, tachycardia); use caution if hyperthyroidism is suspected, abrupt withdrawal may precipitate thyroid storm. Dosage adjustment is required in patients with significant hepatic or renal dysfunction. Adequate alpha-blockade is required prior to use of any beta-blocker for patients with untreated pheochromocytoma. May induce or exacerbate psoriasis. Use caution with history of severe anaphylaxis to allergens; patients taking beta-blockers may become more sensitive to repeated challenges. Treatment of anaphylaxis (eg, epinephrine) in patients taking beta-blockers may be ineffective or promote undesirable effects.
Adverse Reactions
1% to 10%:
Cardiovascular: Chest pain (1% to 2%)
Central nervous system: Fatigue (dose related; 6% to 8%), insomnia (2% to 3%), hypoesthesia (1% to 2%)
Gastrointestinal: Diarrhea (dose related; 3% to 4%), nausea (2%), vomiting (1% to 2%)
Neuromuscular & skeletal: Arthralgia (2% to 3%), weakness (dose related; ≤2%)
Respiratory: Upper respiratory infection (5%), rhinitis (3% to 4%), sinusitis (dose related; 2%), dyspnea (1% to 2%)
<1% (Limited to important or life-threatening): Abdominal pain, acne, alopecia, angioedema, anxiety, arrhythmia, asthma, back/neck pain, bradycardia (dose related), bronchitis, bronchospasm, BUN/creatinine increased, claudication, cold extremities, confusion (especially in the elderly), congestive heart failure, constipation, coughing, cutaneous vasculitis, cystitis, depression, dermatitis, dizziness, dyspepsia, dyspnea on exertion, eczema, edema, exfoliative dermatitis, flushing, gastritis, gout, hallucinations, headache, hearing decreased, hyperesthesia, hyperglycemia, hyperkalemia, hyperphosphatemia, hypertriglyceridemia, hypotension, impotence, lacrimation (abnormal), leukopenia, libido decreased, malaise, memory loss, muscle cramps, muscle/joint pain, nervousness, ocular pain/pressure, orthostatic hypotension, palpitations, paresthesia, peptic ulcer, Peyronie's disease, pharyngitis, polyuria, positive ANA titers, pruritus, psoriasis, psoriasiform eruption, purpura, rash, renal colic, restlessness, rhythm disturbances, sleep disturbances, somnolence, syncope, taste abnormality, thrombocytopenia, tinnitus, transaminases increased, tremor, twitching, uric acid increased, vasculitis, vertigo, visual disturbances, weight gain, xerostomia
Drug Interactions
Metabolism/Transport Effects Substrate of CYP2D6 (minor), CYP3A4 (major); **Note:** Assignment of Major/Minor substrate status based on clinically relevant drug interaction potential
Avoid Concomitant Use
Avoid concomitant use of Bisoprolol with any of the following: Conivaptan; Floctafenine; Fusidic Acid (Systemic); Methacholine
Increased Effect/Toxicity
Bisoprolol may increase the levels/effects of: Alpha-/Beta-Agonists (Direct-Acting); Alpha1-Blockers; Alpha2-Agonists; Amifostine; Antihypertensives; Antipsychotic Agents (Phenothiazines); Bupivacaine; Cardiac Glycosides; Cholinergic Agonists; Ergot Derivatives; Fingolimod; Hypotensive Agents; Insulin; Lidocaine (Systemic); Lidocaine (Topical); Mepivacaine; Methacholine; Midodrine; Obinutuzumab; RiTUXimab; Sulfonylureas

The levels/effects of Bisoprolol may be increased by: Acetylcholinesterase Inhibitors; Alpha2-Agonists; Aminoquinolines (Antimalarial); Amiodarone; Anilidopiperidine Opioids; Antipsychotic Agents (Phenothiazines); Brimonidine (Topical); Calcium Channel Blockers (Dihydropyridine); Calcium Channel Blockers (Nondihydropyridine); Conivaptan; CYP3A4 Inhibitors (Moderate); CYP3A4 Inhibitors (Strong); Dasatinib; Diazoxide; Dipyridamole; Disopyramide; Dronedarone; Floctafenine; Fusidic Acid (Systemic); Herbs (Hypotensive Properties); Ivacaftor; Luliconazole; MAO Inhibitors; Mifepristone; Pentoxifylline; Phosphodiesterase 5 Inhibitors; Propafenone; Prostacyclin Analogues; Regorafenib; Reserpine; Simeprevir

Decreased Effect

Bisoprolol may decrease the levels/effects of: Beta2-Agonists; Theophylline Derivatives

The levels/effects of Bisoprolol may be decreased by: Barbiturates; Bosentan; CYP3A4 Inducers (Strong); Dabrafenib; Deferasirox; Herbs (CYP3A4 Inducers); Herbs (Hypertensive Properties); Methylphenidate; Mitotane; Nonsteroidal Anti-Inflammatory Agents; Peginterferon Alfa-2b; Rifamycin Derivatives; Tocilizumab; Yohimbine

Ethanol/Nutrition/Herb Interactions Herb/Nutraceutical: Avoid dong quai if using for hypertension (has estrogenic activity). Avoid ephedra, yohimbe, ginseng (may worsen hypertension). Avoid garlic (may have increased antihypertensive effect).

Storage/Stability Store at controlled room temperature 20°C to 25°C (68°F to 77°F). Protect from moisture.

Mechanism of Action Selective inhibitor of beta$_1$-adrenergic receptors; competitively blocks beta$_1$-receptors, with little or no effect on beta$_2$-receptors at doses ≤20 mg

Pharmacodynamics/Kinetics

Onset of action: 1-2 hours

Absorption: Rapid and almost complete

Distribution: Widely; highest concentrations in heart, liver, lungs, and saliva; crosses blood-brain barrier

Protein binding: ~30%

Metabolism: Extensively hepatic; significant first-pass effect (~20%)

Bioavailability: ~80%

Half-life elimination: Normal renal function: 9-12 hours; Cl_{cr} <40 mL/minute: 27-36 hours; Hepatic cirrhosis: 8-22 hours

Time to peak: 2-4 hours

Excretion: Urine (50% as unchanged drug, remainder as inactive metabolites); feces (<2%)

Dosage Oral:

Adults:

Hypertension: Initial: 2.5-5 mg once daily; may be increased to 10 mg and then up to 20 mg once daily, if necessary; usual dose range (JNC 7): 2.5-10 mg once daily

Heart failure (unlabeled use): Initial: 1.25 mg once daily; maximum recommended dose: 10 mg once daily. **Note:** Increase dose gradually and monitor for signs and symptoms of CHF (Hunt, 2009; Lindenfeld, 2010)

Elderly: Refer to adult dosing.

Dosage adjustment in renal impairment: Cl_{cr} <40 mL/minute: Initial: 2.5 mg daily; increase cautiously.

Hemodialysis: Not dialyzable

Dosage adjustment in hepatic impairment: Hepatitis or cirrhosis: Initial: 2.5 mg daily; increase cautiously.

Dietary Considerations May be taken without regard to meals.

Administration May be administered without regard to meals.

Monitoring Parameters Blood pressure, heart rate, ECG; serum glucose regularly (in patients with diabetes)

Dosage Forms Excipient information presented when available (limited, particularly for generics); consult specific product labeling.

Tablet, Oral, as fumarate:

Zebeta: 5 mg [scored]

Zebeta: 10 mg

Generic: 5 mg, 10 mg

Bisoprolol and Hydrochlorothiazide

(bis OH proe lol & hye droe klor oh THYE a zide)

Brand Names: U.S. Ziac®

Brand Names: Canada Ziac®

Index Terms Bisoprolol Fumarate and Hydrochlorothiazide; Hydrochlorothiazide and Bisoprolol

Pharmacologic Category Antihypertensive; Beta-Blocker, Beta-1 Selective; Diuretic, Thiazide

Use Treatment of hypertension

Unlabeled Use Treatment of hypertension in the pediatric patient

Pregnancy Risk Factor C

Dosage Oral: Hypertension:

Children (unlabeled use): Initial: Bisoprolol 2.5 mg/hydrochlorothiazide 6.25 mg once daily; up to a maximum of bisoprolol 10 mg/hydrochlorothiazide 6.25 mg daily

Adults: Initial: Bisoprolol 2.5 mg and hydrochlorothiazide 6.25 mg once daily; dose may be titrated at ≥2-week intervals. Maximum dose (manufacturer recommended): Bisoprolol 20 mg/hydrochlorothiazide 12.5 mg once daily

Add-on/replacement therapy: Bisoprolol 2.5-20 mg and hydrochlorothiazide 6.25-12.5 mg once daily

Dosage adjustment in renal impairment: Caution should be used in dosing/titrating patients with renal impairment. Discontinue use with progressive renal impairment; use is contraindicated in patients with anuria.

Dosage adjustment in hepatic impairment: Caution should be used in dosing/titrating patients. Dosage adjustment necessary with severe impairment. Specific dosing recommendations are not provided in manufacturer labeling.

Additional Information Complete prescribing information should be consulted for additional detail.

Dosage Forms Excipient information presented when available (limited, particularly for generics); consult specific product labeling.

Tablet, oral: 2.5/6.25: Bisoprolol fumarate 2.5 mg and hydrochlorothiazide 6.25 mg; 5/6.25: Bisoprolol fumarate 5 mg and hydrochlorothiazide 6.25 mg; 10/6.25: Bisoprolol fumarate 10 mg and hydrochlorothiazide 6.25 mg

Ziac®: 2.5/6.25: Bisoprolol fumarate 2.5 mg and hydrochlorothiazide 6.25 mg

Ziac®: 5/6.25: Bisoprolol fumarate 5 mg and hydrochlorothiazide 6.25 mg

Ziac®: 10/6.25: Bisoprolol fumarate 10 mg and hydrochlorothiazide 6.25 mg

- **Bisoprolol Fumarate** *see* Bisoprolol *on page* 261
- **Bisoprolol Fumarate and Hydrochlorothiazide** *see* Bisoprolol and Hydrochlorothiazide *on page* 262
- **Bis-POM PMEA** *see* Adefovir *on page* 48
- **Bistropamide** *see* Tropicamide *on page* 2132
- **Bivalent Human Papillomavirus Vaccine** *see* Papillomavirus (Types 16, 18) Vaccine (Human, Recombinant) *on page* 1569

Bivalirudin

(bye VAL i roo din)

Brand Names: U.S. Angiomax

Brand Names: Canada Angiomax®

Index Terms Hirulog

Pharmacologic Category Anticoagulant, Thrombin Inhibitor

Use Anticoagulant used in conjunction with aspirin for patients with unstable angina undergoing percutaneous transluminal coronary angioplasty (PTCA) or percutaneous coronary intervention (PCI) with provisional glycoprotein IIb/IIIa inhibitor; anticoagulant used in conjunction with aspirin for patients undergoing PCI with (or at risk of) heparin-induced thrombocytopenia (HIT) / thrombosis syndrome (HITTS)

Canadian labeling: Additional uses (not in U.S. labeling): In conjunction with aspirin for treatment of patients with ST-elevation myocardial infarction (STEMI) undergoing primary PCI; anticoagulant with or without aspirin in patients undergoing cardiac surgery with (or at risk of) heparin-induced thrombocytopenia (HIT) / thrombosis syndrome (HITTS)

Unlabeled Use Heparin-induced thrombocytopenia (HIT); ST-elevation myocardial infarction (STEMI) undergoing primary PCI

Pregnancy Risk Factor B

Pregnancy Considerations Adverse events have not been observed in animal reproduction studies. Bivalirudin is used in conjunction with aspirin, which may lead to maternal or fetal adverse effects, especially during the third trimester. Use of parenteral direct thrombin inhibitors in pregnancy should be limited to those women who have severe allergic reactions to heparin, including heparin-induced thrombocytopenia, and who cannot receive danaparoid (Guyatt, 2012).

Breast-Feeding Considerations It is not known if bivalirudin is excreted in breast milk. The manufacturer recommends that caution be exercised when administering bivalirudin to nursing women.

Contraindications Hypersensitivity to bivalirudin or any component of the formulation; active major bleeding

Canadian labeling: Additional contraindications (not in U.S. labeling): Major blood clotting disorders; acute gastric or duodenal ulcer; cerebral hemorrhage; severe cerebro-spinal trauma; bacterial endocarditis; severe uncontrolled hypertension; diabetic or hemorrhagic retinopathy; proximal use of spinal/epidural anesthesia

Warnings/Precautions Not for intramuscular use. Safety and efficacy have not been established in patients with unstable angina or acute coronary syndromes who are not undergoing PTCA or PCI. Increased risk of thrombus formation (some fatal) has been reported with bivalirudin use in gamma brachytherapy. As with all anticoagulants, bleeding may occur at any site and should be considered following an unexplained fall in blood pressure or hematocrit, or any unexplained symptom. Use with caution in patients with disease states associated with increased risk of bleeding. Use with caution in patients with renal impairment; dosage reduction required.

Adverse Reactions As with all anticoagulants, bleeding is the major adverse effect of bivalirudin. Hemorrhage may occur at virtually any site. Risk is dependent on multiple variables, including the intensity of anticoagulation, concurrent use of a glycoprotein IIb/IIIa inhibitor, and patient susceptibility. Additional adverse effects are often related to idiosyncratic reactions, and the frequency is difficult to estimate. Adverse reactions reported were generally less than those seen with heparin.

>10%:

Cardiovascular: Hypotension (≤12%)
Central nervous system: Pain (≤15%), headache (≤12%)
Gastrointestinal: Nausea (≤15%)
Hematologic & oncologic: Minor hemorrhage (Protocol defined: 14%; heparin 26%; TIMI defined: 1%; heparin 3% [Lincoff, 2003])
Neuromuscular & skeletal: Back pain (9% to 42%)

1% to 10%:

Cardiovascular: Hypertension (6%), bradycardia (5%), angina pectoris (≤5%)
Central nervous system: Insomnia (7%), anxiety (6%), nervousness (5%)
Gastrointestinal: Vomiting (≤6%), abdominal pain (5%), dyspepsia (5%)
Genitourinary: Pelvic pain (6%), urinary retention (4%)
Hematologic & oncologic: Major hemorrhage (Protocol defined: 2% to 4%; heparin 4% to 9%; TIMI defined: 0.6%; heparin 0.9%; transfusion required: 1% to 2%; heparin 2% to 6% [Lincoff, 2003])
Local: Pain at injection site (≤8%)
Miscellaneous: Fever (5%)

<1% (Limited to important or life-threatening): Cerebral ischemia, confusion, facial paralysis, hemorrhage (fatal), hypersensitivity reaction (including anaphylaxis), increased susceptibility to infection, intracranial hemorrhage, oliguria, pulmonary edema, renal failure, retroperitoneal hemorrhage, sepsis, syncope, thrombocytopenia, vascular disease, venous thrombosis (during PCI, including intracoronary brachytherapy), ventricular fibrillation

Drug Interactions

Metabolism/Transport Effects None known.

Avoid Concomitant Use

Avoid concomitant use of Bivalirudin with any of the following: Apixaban; Dabigatran Etexilate; Omacetaxine; Rivaroxaban

Increased Effect/Toxicity

Bivalirudin may increase the levels/effects of: Anticoagulants; Collagenase (Systemic); Deferasirox; Ibritumomab; Omacetaxine; Rivaroxaban; Tositumomab and Iodine I 131 Tositumomab

The levels/effects of Bivalirudin may be increased by: Agents with Antiplatelet Properties; Apixaban; Dabigatran Etexilate; Dasatinib; Herbs (Anticoagulant/Antiplatelet Properties); Ibrutinib; Nonsteroidal Anti-Inflammatory Agents; Omega-3 Fatty Acids; Pentosan Polysulfate Sodium; Prostacyclin Analogues; Salicylates; Sugammadex; Thrombolytic Agents; Tibolone; Tipranavir; Vitamin E

Decreased Effect

The levels/effects of Bivalirudin may be decreased by: Estrogen Derivatives; Progestins

Preparation for Administration Reconstitute each 250 mg with 5 mL SWFI. Gently swirl to dissolve. Further dilution in D_5W or NS (50 mL to make 5 mg/mL solution **or** 500 mL to make 0.5 mg/mL solution) is required prior to infusion.

Storage/Stability Store unopened vials at 20°C to 25°C (68°F to 77°F); excursions permitted between 15°C to 30°C. Following reconstitution, vials should be stored at 2°C to 8°C for up to 24 hours. Do not freeze. Final dilutions of 0.5 mg/mL or 5 mg/mL are stable at room temperature for up to 24 hours.

Mechanism of Action Bivalirudin acts as a specific and reversible direct thrombin inhibitor; it binds to the catalytic and anionic exosite of both circulating and clot-bound thrombin. Catalytic binding site occupation functionally inhibits coagulant effects by preventing thrombin-mediated cleavage of fibrinogen to fibrin monomers, and activation of factors V, VIII, and XIII. Shows linear dose- and concentration-dependent prolongation of ACT, aPTT, PT, and TT.

Pharmacodynamics/Kinetics

Onset of action: Immediate
Duration: Coagulation times return to baseline ~1 hour following discontinuation of infusion
Distribution: 0.2 L/kg
Protein binding, plasma: Does not bind other than thrombin
Metabolism: Blood proteases

Half-life elimination: Normal renal function (Cl_{cr} ≥90 mL/minute): 25 minutes; Severe renal impairment (Cl_{cr} 10-29 mL/minute): 57 minutes; Dialysis-dependent patients (off dialysis): 3.5 hours

Excretion: Urine (20%), proteolytic cleavage

Dosage I.V.: Adults: **Note:** If clinically indicated, a glycoprotein IIb/IIIa inhibitor may be concomitantly administered during percutaneous coronary intervention (PCI). In addition to aspirin, concomitant administration of clopidogrel or prasugrel is also recommended for patients undergoing PCI (King, 2005; Kushner, 2009).

PTCA/PCI with or without HIT/HITTS: Initial: 0.75 mg/kg bolus immediately prior to procedure, followed by 1.75 mg/kg/hour for the duration of procedure and up to 4 hours postprocedure if needed; may determine ACT 5 minutes after bolus dose; may administer additional bolus of 0.3 mg/kg if necessary. If continued anticoagulation is needed after the initial 4-hour postprocedure infusion, the infusion may be continued at 0.2 mg/kg/hour for up to an additional 20 hours (U.S. labeling) or 0.25 mg/kg/hour for 4-12 hours post procedure (Canadian labeling).

Unstable angina/non-ST-elevation myocardial infarction (UA/NSTEMI) (moderate-high risk) undergoing early invasive strategy: *U.S. unlabeled dose:* Initial: 0.1 mg/kg bolus, followed by 0.25 mg/kg/hour. Once PCI is determined to be necessary, give an additional bolus of 0.5 mg/kg and increase infusion rate to 1.75 mg/kg/hour; may discontinue at end of procedure or continue for up to 4 hours postprocedure if necessary (Stone, 2006). If, after angiography, cardiac surgery is deemed necessary, discontinue bivalirudin 3 hours prior to surgery and dose with unfractionated heparin per institutional practice. If medical management is the decided treatment approach, may either discontinue bivalirudin or continue at 0.25 mg/kg/hour for up to 72 hours (Jneid, 2012).

Canadian labeling: Initial: 0.1 mg/kg bolus, followed by 0.25 mg/kg/hour for up to 72 hours if patient is medically managed. If PCI is determined to be necessary, give an additional bolus of 0.5 mg/kg and increase infusion rate to 1.75 mg/kg/hour; may resume infusion at 0.25 mg/kg/hour for 4-12 hours following PCI if necessary. If coronary artery bypass graft (CABG) surgery is deemed necessary, discontinue bivalirudin infusion 1 hour prior to CABG (on-pump) surgery and dose with unfractionated heparin or continue infusion until time of CABG (off-pump) surgery, then give 0.5 mg/kg bolus and increase infusion rate to 1.75 mg/kg/hour until end of surgery.

STEMI undergoing primary PCI: *U.S. unlabeled use:* Initial: 0.75 mg/kg bolus, followed by 1.75 mg/kg/hour for the duration of procedure; may continue postprocedure at a reduced dose if clinically indicated (Stone, 2008).

If patient received unfractionated heparin (UFH) prior to procedure and bivalirudin is the desired anticoagulant: Discontinue heparin if infusing; without measurement of ACT, may initiate bivalirudin ≥30 minutes after the last UFH bolus but before PCI occurs (Stone, 2008). Switching patients from UFH to bivalirudin has been shown to be safe compared to continuing with UFH and as needed glycoprotein IIb/IIIa inhibition; median time from prerandomization UFH bolus to bivalirudin administration within the HORIZONS-AMI trial was 64 ± 61 minutes (Dangas, 2011).

Canadian labeling: Initial: 0.75 mg/kg bolus, followed by 1.75 mg/kg/hour for the duration of procedure or for up to 4 hours postprocedure if needed; determine ACT 5 minutes after bolus dose; may administer additional bolus of 0.3 mg/kg if necessary. If continued anticoagulation is needed after the initial 4-hour postprocedure infusion, the infusion may be continued at 0.25 mg/kg/hour for 4-12 hours.

Cardiac surgery in patients with acute or subacute heparin-induced thrombocytopenia, urgent surgery required: *U.S. unlabeled use* (Linkins, 2012): Intraoperative:

Off-pump: Initial bolus: 0.75 mg/kg, followed by continuous infusion 1.75 mg/kg/hour to maintain ACT >300 seconds (Dyke, 2007). If patient needs to go on-pump, Canadian labeling recommends an additional 0.25 mg/kg bolus and increasing the infusion rate to 2.5 mg/kg/hour.

On-pump: Initial bolus: 1 mg/kg, followed by continuous infusion 2.5 mg/kg/hour; 50 mg bolus added to priming solution of cardiopulmonary bypass (CPB) circuit. Additional boluses of 0.1-0.5 mg/kg may be given to maintain ACT >2.5 times baseline ACT. **Note:** Special maneuvers needed to prevent stasis and consequent clotting within CPB circuit during or after surgery (Koster, 2007). Per Canadian labeling, after completion of CPB, provision to allow recirculation of the circuit may be done by administering 50 mg **into the circuit** followed by a continuous infusion of 50 mg/hour **into the circuit.**

Canadian labeling: Pre -and post-cardiac surgery administration: Initial bolus: 0.1 mg/kg, followed by continuous infusion 0.2 mg/kg/hour for up to 48 hours prior to surgery or for up to 14 days after surgery; maintain aPTT 1.5-2.5 times baseline aPTT.

Heparin-induced thrombocytopenia (HIT) (unlabeled use): Initial dose: 0.15-0.2 mg/kg/hour; adjust to aPTT 1.5-2.5 times baseline value (Linkins, 2012). **Note:** Although the use of bivalirudin is not a currently recommended treatment for HIT due to insufficient evidence, the American College of Chest Physicians recommends overlapping administration of warfarin for a minimum of 5 days until INR is within target range; recheck INR after the nonheparin anticoagulant effect has dissipated (Linkins, 2012).

Elderly: No dosage adjustment is needed in elderly patients with normal renal function. Puncture site hemorrhage and catheterization site hemorrhage were seen more often in patients ≥65 years of age.

Dosage adjustment in renal impairment: Infusion dose should be reduced based on degree of renal impairment; initial bolus dose remains unchanged; monitor activated coagulation time (ACT) or aPTT depending on indication.

For use in PCI:

U.S. labeling:

Cl_{cr} ≥30 mL/minute: No adjustment required.

Cl_{cr} 10-29 mL/minute: Decrease infusion rate to 1 mg/kg/hour

Dialysis-dependent patients (off dialysis during administration): Decrease infusion rate to 0.25 mg/kg/hour

Hemodialysis: Approximately 25% removed during hemodialysis

Canadian labeling: **Note:** Check ACT following dose alterations at 5 and 45 minutes in renally impaired patients. If ACT ≤250 seconds give additional bolus 0.3 mg/kg and double infusion rate to maintain ACT ~350 seconds; if ACT 250-300 seconds give additional bolus 0.3 mg/kg to maintain ACT ~350 seconds.

Cl_{cr} ≥30 mL/minute: No adjustment required.

Cl_{cr} 10-29 mL/minute: Decrease infusion rate to 1 mg/kg/hour

Dialysis-dependent patients (off dialysis during administration): Decrease infusion rate to 0.25 mg/kg/hour

For use in cardiac surgery:

Canadian labeling:

Cl_{cr} ≥30 mL/minute: No adjustment required; monitor ACT.

Cl_{cr} <30 mL/minute: No dosage adjustment provided in manufacturer's labeling; has not been studied; monitor ACT.

For use in HIT: No dosage adjustment provided in manufacturer's labeling for this population; however, the following dose ranges have been observed in small retrospective observational studies (Kiser 2006; Kiser, 2008; Tsu, 2011). Of note, critically-ill patients comprised a significant proportion of patients in these observational studies. The following dose recommendations are based on the mean dose achieving aPTT goal within these studies; overlaps may exist; **Note:** The Cockcroft-Gault equation was used in all studies to define creatinine clearance:

Cl_{cr} >60 mL/minute: 0.13 mg/kg/hour

Cl_{cr} 30-60 mL/minute: 0.08-0.1 mg/kg/hour

Cl_{cr} <30 mL/minute: 0.04-0.05 mg/kg/hour

Intermittent hemodialysis (IHD): 0.07 mg/kg/hour (Tsu, 2011)

CRRT (eg, CVVH or CVVHDF): 0.03-0.07 mg/kg/hour (Kiser, 2006; Tsu, 2011)

Sustained low-efficiency daily diafiltration (SLEDD): 0.09 mg/kg/hour (Tsu, 2011)

Dosage adjustment in hepatic impairment: No dosage adjustment is needed

Usual Infusion Concentrations: Adult I.V. infusion: 250 mg in 500 mL (concentration: 0.5 mg/mL) **or** 250 mg in 50 mL (concentration: 5 mg/mL) of D_5W or NS

Administration For I.V. administration only.

Monitoring Parameters Depends upon indication for use of bivalirudin: ACT or aPTT

Test Interactions PT/INR levels may become elevated in the absence of warfarin. If warfarin is initiated, initial PT/INR goals while on bivalirudin may require modification.

Dosage Forms Excipient information presented when available (limited, particularly for generics); consult specific product labeling.

Solution Reconstituted, Intravenous:

Angiomax: 250 mg (1 ea)

◆ **Bivigam** *see* Immune Globulin *on page 1059*

◆ **Bi-Zets/Benzotroches [OTC]** *see* Benzocaine *on page 240*

◆ **BL4162A** *see* Anagrelide *on page 136*

◆ **Blenoxane** *see* Bleomycin *on page 265*

◆ **Blenoxane® (Can)** *see* Bleomycin *on page 265*

◆ **Bleo** *see* Bleomycin *on page 265*

Bleomycin (blee oh MYE sin)

Brand Names: Canada Blenoxane®; Bleomycin Injection, USP

Index Terms Blenoxane; Bleo; Bleomycin Sulfate; BLM

Pharmacologic Category Antineoplastic Agent, Antibiotic

Use Treatment of squamous cell carcinomas of the head and neck, penis, cervix, or vulva, testicular carcinoma, Hodgkin's lymphoma, and non-Hodgkin's lymphoma; sclerosing agent for malignant pleural effusion

Unlabeled Use Treatment of ovarian germ cell tumors

Pregnancy Risk Factor D

Pregnancy Considerations Animal studies have demonstrated teratogenic and abortifacient effects. There are no adequate and well-controlled studies in pregnant women. Women of childbearing potential should avoid becoming pregnant during treatment.

Breast-Feeding Considerations Due to the potential for serious adverse reactions in the nursing infant, breast-feeding is not recommended.

Contraindications Hypersensitivity to bleomycin or any component of the formulation

Warnings/Precautions Hazardous agent - use appropriate precautions for handling and disposal (NIOSH, 2012). **[U.S. Boxed Warning]: Occurrence of pulmonary fibrosis (commonly presenting as pneumonitis; occasionally progressing to pulmonary fibrosis) is the most severe toxicity. Risk is higher in elderly patients or patients receiving >400 units total lifetime dose;** other possible risk factors include smoking and patients with prior radiation therapy or receiving concurrent oxygen (especially high inspired oxygen doses). A review of patients receiving bleomycin for the treatment of germ cell tumors suggests risk for pulmonary toxicity is increased in patients >40 years of age, with glomerular filtration rate <80 mL/minute, advanced disease, and cumulative doses >300 units (O'Sullivan, 2003). Pulmonary toxicity may include bronchiolitis obliterans and organizing pneumonia (BOOP), eosinophilic hypersensitivity, and interstitial pneumonitis, progressing to pulmonary fibrosis (Sleijfer, 2001); pulmonary toxicity may be due to a lack of the enzyme which inactivates bleomycin (bleomycin hydrolase) in the lungs (Morgan, 2011; Sleijfer, 2001). If pulmonary changes occur, withhold treatment and investigate if drug-related. In children, a younger age at treatment, cumulative dose ≥400 units/m^2 (combined with chest irradiation), and renal impairment are associated with a higher incidence of pulmonary toxicity (Huang, 2011).

A severe idiosyncratic reaction consisting of hypotension, mental confusion, fever, chills, and wheezing (similar to anaphylaxis) has been reported in 1% of lymphoma patients treated with bleomycin. Since these reactions usually occur after the first or second dose, careful monitoring is essential after these doses. Use caution when administering O_2 during surgery to patients who have received bleomycin; the risk of bleomycin-related pulmonary toxicity is increased. Use caution with renal impairment (Cl_{cr} <50 mL/minute), may require dose adjustment. May cause renal or hepatic toxicity. **[U.S. Boxed Warning]: Should be administered under the supervision of an experienced cancer chemotherapy physician.**

Adverse Reactions

>10%:

Dermatologic: Pain at the tumor site, phlebitis. About 50% of patients develop erythema, rash, striae, induration, hyperkeratosis, vesiculation, and peeling of the skin, particularly on the palmar and plantar surfaces of the hands and feet. Hyperpigmentation (50%), alopecia, nailbed changes may also occur. These effects appear dose related and reversible with discontinuation.

Gastrointestinal: Stomatitis and mucositis (30%), anorexia, weight loss

Respiratory: Tachypnea, rales, acute or chronic interstitial pneumonitis, and pulmonary fibrosis (5% to 10%); hypoxia and death (1%). Symptoms include cough, dyspnea, and bilateral pulmonary infiltrates. The pathogenesis is not certain, but may be due to damage of pulmonary, vascular, or connective tissue. Response to steroid therapy is variable and somewhat controversial.

Miscellaneous: Acute febrile reactions (25% to 50%)

1% to 10%:

Dermatologic: Skin thickening, diffuse scleroderma, onycholysis, pruritus

Miscellaneous: Anaphylactoid-like reactions (characterized by hypotension, confusion, fever, chills, and wheezing; onset may be immediate or delayed for several hours); idiosyncratic reactions (1% in lymphoma patients)

<1% (Limited to important or life-threatening): Angioedema, cerebrovascular accident, cerebral arteritis, chest pain, coronary artery disease, flagellate hyperpigmentation, hepatotoxicity, malaise, MI, myelosuppression (rare), myocardial ischemia, nausea, pericarditis,

Raynaud's phenomenon, renal toxicity, scleroderma-like skin changes, Stevens-Johnson syndrome, thrombotic microangiopathy, toxic epidermal necrolysis, vomiting

Drug Interactions

Metabolism/Transport Effects None known.

Avoid Concomitant Use

Avoid concomitant use of Bleomycin with any of the following: BCG; Brentuximab Vedotin; Natalizumab; Pimecrolimus; Tacrolimus (Topical); Tofacitinib; Vaccines (Live)

Increased Effect/Toxicity

Bleomycin may increase the levels/effects of: Leflunomide; Natalizumab; Tofacitinib; Vaccines (Live)

The levels/effects of Bleomycin may be increased by: Brentuximab Vedotin; Denosumab; Filgrastim; Gemcitabine; Pimecrolimus; Roflumilast; Sargramostim; Tacrolimus (Topical); Trastuzumab

Decreased Effect

Bleomycin may decrease the levels/effects of: BCG; Cardiac Glycosides; Coccidioidin Skin Test; Phenytoin; Sipuleucel-T; Vaccines (Inactivated); Vaccines (Live)

The levels/effects of Bleomycin may be decreased by: Echinacea

Preparation for Administration Hazardous agent; use appropriate precautions for handling and disposal (NIOSH, 2012). For I.V. use, reconstitute 15-unit vial with 5 mL with NS and the 30-unit vial with 10 mL NS; for I.M. or SubQ use, reconstitute 15-unit vial with 1-5 mL of SWFI, BWFI, or NS and the 30-unit vial with 2-10 mL of SWFI, BWFI, or NS. For intrapleural use, mix in 50-100 mL of NS.

Storage/Stability Refrigerate intact vials of powder. Intact vials are stable for up to 4 weeks at room temperature. Solutions reconstituted in NS are stable for up to 28 days refrigerated and 14 days at room temperature; however, the manufacturer recommends stability of 24 hours in NS at room temperature.

Mechanism of Action Inhibits synthesis of DNA; binds to DNA leading to single- and double-strand breaks; also inhibits (to a lesser degree) RNA and protein synthesis

Pharmacodynamics/Kinetics

Absorption: I.M. and intrapleural administration: 30% to 50% of I.V. serum concentrations; intraperitoneal and SubQ routes produce serum concentrations equal to those of I.V.

Distribution: V_d: 22 L/m^2; highest concentrations in skin, kidney, lung, heart tissues; lowest in testes and GI tract; does not cross blood-brain barrier

Protein binding: 1%

Metabolism: Via several tissues including hepatic, GI tract, skin, pulmonary, renal, and serum

Half-life elimination: Biphasic (renal function dependent):
- Normal renal function: Initial: 1.3 hours; Terminal: 9 hours
- End-stage renal disease: Initial: 2 hours; Terminal: 30 hours

Time to peak, serum: I.M.: Within 30 minutes

Excretion: Urine (50% to 70% as active drug)

Dosage Note: The risk for pulmonary toxicity increases with age >70 years and cumulative lifetime dose of >400 units; 1 unit = 1 mg. Details concerning dosage in combination regimens should also be consulted.

Children and Adults: Test dose for lymphoma patients: I.M., I.V., SubQ: Because of the possibility of an anaphylactoid reaction, the manufacturer recommends administering 1-2 units of bleomycin before the first 1-2 doses; monitor vital signs every 15 minutes; wait a minimum of 1 hour before administering remainder of dose; if no acute reaction occurs, then the regular dosage schedule may be followed. **Note:** Test doses may not be predictive of a reaction (Lam, 2005) and/or may produce false-negative results.

I.V.:

Children: Hodgkin's lymphoma (unlabeled dosing; combination regimen): ABVD: 10 units/m^2 days 1 and 15 of a 28-day treatment cycle (Hutchinson, 1998)

Adults:
- Hodgkin's lymphoma (unlabeled dosing; combination regimens):
  - ABVD: 10 units/m^2 days 1 and 15 of a 28-day treatment cycle (Straus, 2004)
  - BEACOPP: 10 units/m^2 day 8 of a 21-day treatment cycle (Dann, 2007; Diehl, 2003)
  - Stanford V: 5 units/m^2/dose in weeks 2, 4, 6, 8, 10 and 12 (Horning, 2000; Horning, 2002)
- Testicular cancer (unlabeled dosing; combination therapy): 30 units/dose days 1, 8, and 15 of a 21-day treatment cycle for 4 cycles (Culine, 2008; Nichols, 1998)
- Ovarian germ cell cancer (unlabeled use; combination therapy): 30 units/dose days 1, 8, and 15 of a 21-day treatment cycle for 3 cycles (Williams, 1994) **or** 15 units/m^2 day 1 of a 21-day treatment cycle for 4 cycles (Cushing, 2004)

Intrapleural: Adults: Malignant pleural effusion: 60 units as a single instillation; mix in 50-100 mL of NS

Elderly: Refer to adult dosing; the incidence of pulmonary toxicity is higher in patients >70 years of age.

Dosage adjustment for toxicity:

Pulmonary changes: Discontinue until determined not to be drug-related.

Pulmonary diffusion capacity for carbon monoxide (DL_{CO}) <30% to 35% of baseline: Discontinue treatment.

Dosing adjustment in renal impairment:

The U.S. labeling recommends the following adjustments (creatinine clearance should be estimated using the Cockcroft-Gault formula):
- Cl_{cr} >50 mL/minute: No dosage adjustment necessary.
- Cl_{cr} 40-50 mL/minute: Administer 70% of normal dose
- Cl_{cr} 30-40 mL/minute: Administer 60% of normal dose
- Cl_{cr} 20-30 mL/minute: Administer 55% of normal dose
- Cl_{cr} 10-20 mL/minute: Administer 45% of normal dose
- Cl_{cr} 5-10 mL/minute: Administer 40% of normal dose

The Canadian labeling recommends the following adjustment: Cl_{cr} ≤40 mL/minute: Reduce dose by 40% to 75%.

The following adjustments have also been recommended:
- Aronoff, 2007: Adults: Continuous renal replacement therapy (CRRT): Administer 75% of dose
- Kintzel, 1995: Adults:
  - Cl_{cr} 46-60 mL/minute: Administer 70% of dose
  - Cl_{cr} 31-45 mL/minute: Administer 60% of dose
  - Cl_{cr} <30 mL/minute: Consider use of alternative drug

Dosing adjustment in hepatic impairment: No dosage adjustment provided in the manufacturer's labeling (has not been studied); however, adjustment for hepatic impairment is not necessary (King, 2001).

Dosing in obesity: *ASCO Guidelines for appropriate chemotherapy dosing in obese adults with cancer:* Fixed doses (dosing which is independent of body weight or BSA), are used in some protocols (eg, testicular cancer); due to toxicity concerns, the same fixed dose should also be considered for obese patients (Griggs, 2012).

Administration

I.V. doses should be administered slowly over 10 minutes.

I.M. or SubQ: May cause pain at injection site

Intrapleural: 60 units in 50-100 mL NS; use of topical anesthetics or opioid analgesia is usually not necessary

Hazardous agent; use appropriate precautions for handling and disposal (NIOSH, 2012).

Monitoring Parameters Pulmonary function tests, including total lung volume, forced vital capacity, diffusion capacity for carbon monoxide; vital capacity, total lung capacity and pulmonary capillary blood volume may be better indicators of changes induced by bleomycin (Sleijfer, 2001); chest x-ray, renal function, liver function, temperature initially; check body weight at regular intervals

Dosage Forms Excipient information presented when available (limited, particularly for generics); consult specific product labeling.

Solution Reconstituted, Injection:
Generic: 15 units (1 ea); 30 units (1 ea)
Solution Reconstituted, Injection [preservative free]:
Generic: 15 units (1 ea); 30 units (1 ea)

- ◆ **Bleomycin Injection, USP (Can)** *see* Bleomycin *on page 265*
- ◆ **Bleomycin Sulfate** *see* Bleomycin *on page 265*
- ◆ **Bleph-10** *see* Sulfacetamide (Ophthalmic) *on page 1956*
- ◆ **Bleph 10 DPS (Can)** *see* Sulfacetamide (Ophthalmic) *on page 1956*
- ◆ **Blephamide®** *see* Sulfacetamide and Prednisolone *on page 1957*
- ◆ **BLM** *see* Bleomycin *on page 265*
- ◆ **Bloxiverz** *see* Neostigmine *on page 1441*
- ◆ **BMS-188667** *see* Abatacept *on page 20*
- ◆ **BMS 201038** *see* Lomitapide *on page 1232*
- ◆ **BMS-224818** *see* Belatacept *on page 231*
- ◆ **BMS-232632** *see* Atazanavir *on page 182*
- ◆ **BMS-247550** *see* Ixabepilone *on page 1139*
- ◆ **BMS 337039** *see* ARIPiprazole *on page 163*
- ◆ **BMS-354825** *see* Dasatinib *on page 550*
- ◆ **BMS-477118** *see* Saxagliptin *on page 1879*
- ◆ **B&O** *see* Belladonna and Opium *on page 234*

Boceprevir (boe SE pre vir)

Brand Names: U.S. Victrelis

Brand Names: Canada Victrelis®

Index Terms SCH503034

Pharmacologic Category Antiviral Agent; Protease Inhibitor

Use Treatment of chronic hepatitis C (CHC) genotype 1 (in combination with peginterferon alfa and ribavirin) in patients with compensated liver disease (including cirrhosis) who were previously untreated or have failed prior therapy with peginterferon alfa and ribavirin therapy including prior null responders, partial responders, and relapsers

Pregnancy Risk Factor B / X (in combination with ribavirin)

Pregnancy Considerations Adverse events were not observed with boceprevir in animal reproduction studies; however, boceprevir must not be used as monotherapy (must be used in combination with peginterferon alfa and ribavirin). Adverse events have been observed with ribavirin in animal reproduction studies. Use of ribavirin is contraindicated in pregnant women and males whose female partners are pregnant. A negative pregnancy test is required before initiation of therapy and pregnancy testing should be conducted monthly during treatment and for 6 months after therapy has ended. Women of childbearing potential and males must use at least 2 effective forms of contraception during treatment and continue contraceptive measures for at least 6 months after completion of therapy. One of the two forms of effective contraception may be a combined oral contraceptive product with at least 1 mg of norethindrone; oral contraceptives with <1 mg of norethindrone and other forms of hormonal contraception are contraindicated because they have not been studied. If patient or female partner becomes pregnant during treatment, she should be counseled about potential risks of exposure. If pregnancy occurs during use or within 6 months after treatment, report to the ribavirin pregnancy registry (800-593-2214).

Breast-Feeding Considerations It is not known if boceprevir is excreted into breast milk. According to the manufacturer, due to the potential for serious adverse reactions in the nursing infant, a decision should be made whether to discontinue nursing or to discontinue the drug, taking into account the importance of treatment to the mother.

Breast-feeding is not linked to the spread of hepatitis C virus; however, if nipples are cracked or bleeding, breast-feeding is not recommended (CDC, 2010).

Medication Guide Available Yes

Contraindications Hypersensitivity to boceprevir or any component of the formulation; pregnancy; male partners of pregnant women

Coadministration with CYP3A4/5 highly-dependent substrates (alfuzosin, cisapride, drospirenone, ergot derivatives, lovastatin, midazolam [oral], pimozide, sildenafil/tadalafil [when used for treatment of pulmonary arterial hypertension], simvastatin, triazolam) or strong CYP3A4/5 inducers (carbamazepine, phenobarbital, phenytoin, rifampin, St John's wort)

Refer to Peginterferon Alfa and Ribavirin monographs for individual product contraindications.

Canadian labeling: Additional contraindications (not in U.S. labeling): Autoimmune hepatitis, hepatic decompensation (Child-Pugh class B or C); coadministration with amiodarone, astemizole, propafenone, quinidine, terfenadine

Warnings/Precautions Avoid pregnancy in female patients and female partners of male patients, during therapy, and for at least 6 months after treatment; two forms of contraception should be used. Hypersensitivity reactions, angioedema and urticaria have been reported with boceprevir, peginterferon alfa, and ribavirin combination therapy. Discontinuation of combination therapy and institution of supportive measures may be necessary. Safety and efficacy have not been established in patients who have uncompensated cirrhosis, received organ transplants, or been coinfected with hepatitis B or HIV. Monotherapy is not effective for chronic hepatitis C infection. Safety and efficacy have not been established in patients documented to have less than a 2-$\log_{10}$ HCV-RNA decline by treatment week 12 with prior peginterferon alfa and ribavirin therapy. Patients who have less than 0.5-$\log_{10}$ HCV-RNA decline at treatment week 4 with peginterferon alfa and ribavirin when **initiating** boceprevir therapy are predicted to have less than a 2-$\log_{10}$ HCV-RNA decline by treatment week 12. Those poor responders treated with boceprevir will likely not have a sustained virologic response (SVR) and have a predisposition to viral resistance at treatment failure.

Anemia has been reported with peginterferon alfa and ribavirin; addition of boceprevir is associated with further hemoglobin decreases. With anemia management, average hemoglobin decrease in clinical trials was ~1 g/dL. Dose reduction of ribavirin therapy is recommended for the initial management of anemia if hemoglobin <10 g/dL; permanent discontinuation of ribavirin treatment is recommended if hemoglobin <8.5 g/dL. The addition of boceprevir to peginterferon alfa and ribavirin therapy is also associated with a higher incidence of neutropenia. Dose modifications of peginterferon alfa and ribavirin were needed more often in patients also taking boceprevir. Complete blood counts should be obtained pretreatment and at weeks 2, 4, 8, and 12, as well as other times during treatment. May be severe or life-threatening (rare);

discontinuation of therapy may be necessary. If ribavirin is permanently discontinued, boceprevir and peginterferon alfa must also be discontinued.

Adverse Reactions

>10%:

Central nervous system: Fatigue (55% to 58%), chills (33% to 34%), insomnia (30% to 34%), irritability (21% to 22%), dizziness (16% to 19%), headache

Dermatologic: Alopecia (22% to 27%), dry skin (18% to 22%), rash (16% to 17%)

Gastrointestinal: Nausea (43% to 46%), abnormal taste (35% to 44%), appetite decreased (25% to 26%), diarrhea (24% to 25%), vomiting (15% to 20%), xerostomia (11% to 15%)

Hematologic: Anemia (45% to 50%), neutropenia (14% to 31%)

Neuromuscular & skeletal: Arthralgia (19% to 23%), weakness (15% to 21%)

Respiratory: Dyspnea (8% to 11%)

1% to 10%: Hematologic: Thrombocytopenia

<1% (Limited to important or life-threatening): Angioedema, drug rash with eosinophilia and systemic symptoms (DRESS) syndrome, exfoliative dermatitis, exfoliative rash, mouth ulceration, Stevens-Johnson syndrome, stomatitis, thromboembolic events, toxic skin eruption, toxicoderma, urticaria

Drug Interactions

Metabolism/Transport Effects **Substrate** of BCRP, CYP3A4 (major), P-glycoprotein; **Note:** Assignment of Major/Minor substrate status based on clinically relevant drug interaction potential; **Inhibits** CYP3A4 (strong), P-glycoprotein

Avoid Concomitant Use

Avoid concomitant use of Boceprevir with any of the following: Ado-Trastuzumab Emtansine; Alfuzosin; Apixaban; Astemizole; Avanafil; Axitinib; Bosutinib; Cabozantinib; CarBAMazepine; Cisapride; Conivaptan; Crizotinib; CYP3A4 Inducers (Strong); Dihydroergotamine; Dronedarone; Drospirenone; Efavirenz; Eplerenone; Ergoloid Mesylates; Ergonovine; Ergotamine; Everolimus; Fosphenytoin; Halofantrine; Ibrutinib; Imatinib; Ivabradine; Lapatinib; Lomitapide; Lovastatin; Lurasidone; Macitentan; Methylergonovine; Midazolam; Nilotinib; Nisoldipine; PHENobarbital; Phenytoin; Pimozide; Pomalidomide; Primidone; Ranolazine; Red Yeast Rice; Regorafenib; Rifabutin; Rifampin; Rivaroxaban; Salmeterol; Sildenafil; Silodosin; Simeprevir; Simvastatin; St Johns Wort; Tamsulosin; Terfenadine; Ticagrelor; Tolvaptan; Toremifene; Triazolam; Ulipristal; Vemurafenib; VinCRIStine (Liposomal)

Increased Effect/Toxicity

Boceprevir may increase the levels/effects of: Ado-Trastuzumab Emtansine; Alfuzosin; Almotriptan; Alosetron; ALPRAZolam; Amiodarone; Apixaban; ARIPiprazole; Astemizole; AtorvaSTATin; Avanafil; Axitinib; Bedaquiline; Bepridil [Off Market]; Bortezomib; Bosentan; Bosutinib; Brentuximab Vedotin; Brinzolamide; Budesonide (Nasal); Budesonide (Systemic, Oral Inhalation); Buprenorphine; Cabozantinib; Cisapride; Clarithromycin; Colchicine; Conivaptan; Contraceptives (Progestins); Corticosteroids (Orally Inhaled); Crizotinib; CycloSPORINE (Systemic); CYP3A4 Substrates; Desipramine; Dienogest; Digoxin; Dihydroergotamine; Dofetilide; Dronedarone; Drospirenone; Dutasteride; Efavirenz; Enzalutamide; Eplerenone; Ergoloid Mesylates; Ergonovine; Ergotamine; Everolimus; FentaNYL; Fesoterodine; Flecainide; Fluticasone (Nasal); Fluticasone (Oral Inhalation); Fluvastatin; GuanFACINE; Halofantrine; Ibrutinib; Iloperidone; Imatinib; Itraconazole; Ivabradine; Ivacaftor; Ixabepilone; Ketoconazole (Systemic); Lacosamide; Lapatinib; Levomilnacipran; Lomitapide; Lovastatin; Lumefantrine; Lurasidone; Macitentan; Maraviroc; Methadone; Methylergonovine; MethylPREDNISolone; Midazolam; Mifepristone; Nilotinib; Nisoldipine; Ospemifene; OxyCODONE; Paricalcitol; PAZOPanib; Pimecrolimus; Pimozide; Pitavastatin; Pomalidomide; PONATinib; Posaconazole; Pravastatin; PrednisoLONE (Systemic); PredniSONE; Propafenone; QUEtiapine; QuiNIDine; Ranolazine; Red Yeast Rice; Regorafenib; Repaglinide; Rifabutin; Rilpivirine; Rivaroxaban; RomiDEPsin; Rosuvastatin; Ruxolitinib; Salmeterol; Saxagliptin; Sildenafil; Silodosin; Simeprevir; Simvastatin; Sirolimus; SORAfenib; Tacrolimus (Systemic); Tadalafil; Tamsulosin; Terfenadine; Ticagrelor; Tofacitinib; Tolterodine; Tolvaptan; Toremifene; TraZODone; Triazolam; Ulipristal; Vardenafil; Vemurafenib; Vilazodone; VinCRIStine (Liposomal); Voriconazole; Warfarin; Zuclopenthixol

The levels/effects of Boceprevir may be increased by: Clarithromycin; CycloSPORINE (Systemic); Itraconazole; Ketoconazole (Systemic); Posaconazole; Voriconazole

Decreased Effect

Boceprevir may decrease the levels/effects of: Buprenorphine; Contraceptives (Estrogens); Escitalopram; Ifosfamide; Methadone; Prasugrel; Protease Inhibitors; Ritonavir; Ticagrelor; Warfarin

The levels/effects of Boceprevir may be decreased by: Bosentan; CarBAMazepine; CYP3A4 Inducers (Strong); Dabrafenib; Deferasirox; Efavirenz; Fosphenytoin; PHENobarbital; Phenytoin; Primidone; Protease Inhibitors; Rifabutin; Rifampin; Ritonavir; St Johns Wort; Tocilizumab

Storage/Stability Store refrigerated at 2°C to 8°C (36°F to 46°F). After dispensing, may be stored at room temperature of up to 25°C (77°F) for 3 months; keep container closed tightly; avoid excessive heat.

Mechanism of Action Binds reversibly to nonstructural protein 3 (NS 3) serine protease and inhibits replication of the hepatitis C virus. Considered a direct-acting antiviral treatment for HCV, also called a specifically targeted antiviral therapy for HCV (STAT-C).

Pharmacodynamics/Kinetics

Absorption: Food (type or timing is not important) enhances absorption by up to 65%

Distribution: V_d: ~772 L

Protein binding: ~75%

Metabolism: Primarily hepatic via aldo-ketoreductase pathway to inactive metabolites. Also some oxidative CYP 3A4/5 metabolism.

Half-life elimination: Plasma: Adults: ~3 hours

Time to peak, serum: 2 hours

Excretion: Feces (79%); urine (9%)

Dosage Oral: Adults: 800 mg 3 times daily (in combination with peginterferon alfa and ribavirin). *Missed doses:* If a dose is missed, skip dose if it is <2 hours before the next dose; if ≥2 hours before next dose is due, take dose with food and resume normal dosing schedule.

Treatment-naive patients without cirrhosis (interferon-responsive [≥1-log$_{10}$ HCV-RNA decline in viral load] at week 4):

Weeks 1-4: Peginterferon alfa with concomitant ribavirin only

Weeks 5-8: Boceprevir 800 mg 3 times daily with continued peginterferon alfa and ribavirin

Weeks 9-24 (based on HCV-RNA results at week 8):

HCV-RNA **undetectable** or **detectable** at a level of <100 units/mL: Boceprevir 800 mg 3 times daily with continued peginterferon alfa and ribavirin

HCV-RNA ≥100 units/mL: Boceprevir 800 mg 3 times daily with continued peginterferon alfa and ribavirin. Recheck HCV-RNA at week 12. If HCV-RNA ≥100 units/mL at week 12 (treatment futility), discontinue treatment (boceprevir, peginterferon alfa, and ribavirin).

Weeks ≥24:

HCV-RNA **undetectable** at week 8 and week 24: Boceprevir 800 mg 3 times daily with continued peginterferon alfa and ribavirin for 4 additional weeks (through week 28)

HCV-RNA **detectable** at Week 8 and **undetectable** at week 24:

U.S. labeling: Boceprevir 800 mg 3 times daily with continued peginterferon alfa and ribavirin for 12 additional weeks (through week 36), followed by peginterferon alfa and ribavirin for additional 12 weeks (through week 48)

Canadian labeling: Boceprevir 800 mg 3 times daily with continued peginterferon alfa and ribavirin for 4 additional weeks (through week 28), followed by peginterferon alfa and ribavirin for additional 20 weeks (through week 48)

HCV-RNA **detectable** at week 24: Discontinue treatment (boceprevir, peginterferon alfa, and ribavirin)

Treatment-naive patients (interferon nonresponsive [<0.5-log_{10} HCV-RNA decline in viral load] at week 4): **Note:** Manufacturer also recommends consideration of treatment of poor responders [<1-log_{10} HCV-RNA decline in viral load at week 4] in order to maximize rate of sustained virologic response (SVR):

Weeks 1-4: Peginterferon alfa with concomitant ribavirin only

Weeks 5-48: Boceprevir 800 mg 3 times daily with continued peginterferon alfa and ribavirin

Previously-treated patients without cirrhosis (partial response or relapser): **Note:** Previously treated does not include prior treatment with boceprevir. "Partial response" includes patients with a ≥2-log_{10} HCV-RNA decrease by week 12, but a nonsustained virologic response thereafter. "Relapser" includes patients with an undetectable HCV-RNA upon completion of previous treatment, but with detectable HCV-RNA during the follow-up period.

Weeks 1-4: Peginterferon alfa with concomitant ribavirin only

Weeks 5-8: Boceprevir 800 mg 3 times daily with continued peginterferon alfa and ribavirin

Weeks 9-24 (based on HCV-RNA results at week 8):

HCV-RNA **undetectable** or <100 units/mL: Boceprevir 800 mg 3 times daily with continued peginterferon alfa and ribavirin

HCV-RNA ≥100 units/mL: Boceprevir 800 mg 3 times daily with continued peginterferon alfa and ribavirin. Recheck HCV-RNA at week 12. If HCV-RNA ≥100 units/mL at week 12, discontinue treatment (boceprevir, peginterferon alfa, and ribavirin)

Weeks ≥24:

HCV-RNA **undetectable** at week 8 and week 24: Boceprevir 800 mg 3 times daily with continued peginterferon alfa and ribavirin for 12 additional weeks (through week 36)

HCV-RNA **detectable** at Week 8 and **undetectable** at week 24: Boceprevir 800 mg 3 times daily with continued peginterferon alfa and ribavirin for 12 additional weeks (through week 36), followed by peginterferon alfa and ribavirin for additional 12 weeks (through week 48)

HCV-RNA **detectable** at week 24: Discontinue treatment (boceprevir, peginterferon alfa, and ribavirin)

Previously treated patients with <2-log_{10} HCV-RNA decline by week 12 (prior null responders):

Weeks 1-4: Peginterferon alfa with concomitant ribavirin only

Weeks 5-8: Boceprevir 800 mg 3 times daily with continued peginterferon alfa and ribavirin

Weeks 9-24 (based on HCV-RNA results at week 8):

HCV-RNA **undetectable** or <100 units/mL: Boceprevir 800 mg 3 times daily with continued peginterferon alfa and ribavirin

HCV-RNA **detectable**: Boceprevir 800 mg 3 times daily with continued peginterferon alfa and ribavirin. Recheck HCV-RNA at week 12. If HCV-RNA ≥100 units/mL at week 12, discontinue treatment (boceprevir, peginterferon alfa, and ribavirin).

Weeks ≥24:

HCV-RNA **undetectable** at week 24: Boceprevir 800 mg 3 times daily with continued peginterferon alfa and ribavirin for 24 additional weeks (through week 48)

HCV-RNA **detectable** at week 24: Discontinue treatment (boceprevir, peginterferon alfa, and ribavirin)

Cirrhosis, compensated:

Weeks 1-4: Peginterferon alfa with concomitant ribavirin only

Weeks 5-48: Boceprevir 800 mg 3 times daily with continued peginterferon alfa and ribavirin

Dosage adjustment in renal impairment:

Mild-to-severe impairment: No dosage adjustment necessary.

ESRD requiring hemodialysis: No dosage adjustment necessary. Not removed by hemodialysis.

Dosage adjustment in hepatic impairment:

Mild, moderate, or severe impairment: No dosage adjustment necessary.

Decompensated cirrhosis: No dosage adjustment provided in manufacturer's labeling (has not been studied); not approved for use in decompensated cirrhosis (safety/efficacy not established). Also refer to Peginterferon Alfa and Ribavirin individual monographs.

Dietary Considerations Take with food. The type or timing of a meal is not important as long as dose is taken with food.

Administration Administer with food. Doses should be taken approximately every 7-9 hours. Administer concurrently with peginterferon alfa and ribavirin.

Monitoring Parameters

CBC with differential at baseline, followed by CBC at weeks 2, 4, 8 and 12, then periodically (and when clinically indicated)

Serum HCV RNA at baseline, weeks 4, 8, 12 and 24, end of treatment, during treatment follow up, and when clinically indicated

Pretreatment and monthly pregnancy test up to 6 months following discontinuation of therapy for women of childbearing age

Reference Range

Treatment futility: HCV-RNA ≥100 units/mL at treatment week 12 or confirmed, detectable HCV-RNA at treatment week 24

Rapid virological response (RVR): Absence of detectable HCV RNA after 4 weeks of treatment

Early viral response (EVR): ≥2-log decrease in HCV RNA after 8-12 weeks of treatment

End of treatment response (ETR): Absence of detectable HCV RNA at end of the recommended treatment period

Sustained treatment response (STR): Absence of HCV RNA in the serum 6 months following completion of full treatment course

Sustained virologic response (SVR): Plasma HCV RNA <25 units/mL at follow up week 24

Additional Information In clinical studies of treatment-naive patients, a sustained virologic response (SVR) with peginterferon alfa, ribavirin, and boceprevir was achieved in ~68% of non-African-American patients versus 40% of controls (peginterferon alfa and ribavirin only). African-American patients had a lower rate of SVR compared to controls (42% to 53% dependent upon treatment duration versus 23% of controls). Rapid virologic response (RVR) at week 4 of lead-in treatment with peginterferon alfa and ribavirin can predict patient success after the addition of boceprevir and guide treatment duration. Patients who have marginal response during the lead-in treatment phase have a lower SVR after the addition of boceprevir; these patients may need close monitoring for regimen adherence and resistance development.

Dosage Forms Excipient information presented when available (limited, particularly for generics); consult specific product labeling.

Capsule, Oral:

Victrelis: 200 mg [contains brilliant blue fcf (fd&c blue #1), fd&c red #40, fd&c yellow #10 (quinoline yellow), fd&c yellow #6 (sunset yellow)]

◆ BOL-303224-A *see* Besifloxacin *on page 246*

◆ Boniva *see* Ibandronate *on page 1028*

◆ Boostrix® *see* Diphtheria and Tetanus Toxoids, and Acellular Pertussis Vaccine *on page 630*

Bortezomib (bore TEZ oh mib)

Brand Names: U.S. Velcade

Brand Names: Canada Velcade

Index Terms LDP-341; MLN341; PS-341

Pharmacologic Category Antineoplastic Agent; Proteasome Inhibitor

Use

Mantle cell lymphoma: Treatment of relapsed or refractory mantle cell lymphoma

Multiple myeloma: Treatment of multiple myeloma

Unlabeled Use Treatment of relapsed/refractory cutaneous T-cell lymphomas (mycosis fungoides), relapsed/refractory follicular lymphoma, relapsed/refractory peripheral T-cell lymphoma, relapsed/refractory Waldenström's macroglobulinemia, systemic light-chain amyloidosis

Pregnancy Risk Factor D

Pregnancy Considerations Adverse effects (fetal loss and decreased fetal weight) were observed in animal reproduction studies at doses less than the equivalent human dose (based on BSA). Women of reproductive potential should avoid becoming pregnant and should use effective contraception during treatment.

Breast-Feeding Considerations It is not known if bortezomib is excreted in breast milk. Due to the potential for serious adverse reactions in the nursing infant, the decision to discontinue bortezomib or to discontinue breastfeeding should take into account the benefits of treatment to the mother.

Contraindications Hypersensitivity (excluding local reactions) to bortezomib, boron, mannitol, or any component of the formulation; administration via the intrathecal route

Warnings/Precautions Hazardous agent - use appropriate precautions for handling and disposal (NIOSH, 2012). May cause or worsen peripheral neuropathy (usually sensory but may be mixed sensorimotor); risk may be increased with previous use of neurotoxic agents or pre-existing peripheral neuropathy (patients with pre-existing neuropathy should use only after risk versus benefit assessment); monitor for signs and symptoms; adjustment of dose and/or schedule may be required. The incidence of grades 2 and 3 peripheral neuropathy may be lower with SubQ route (compared to I.V.); consider subQ administration in patients with pre-existing or at high risk for peripheral neuropathy; the majority of patients with ≥grade 2 peripheral neuropathy have improvement in or resolution of symptoms with dose adjustments or discontinuation; in a study of elderly patients receiving a weekly bortezomib schedule with combination chemotherapy, the incidence of peripheral neuropathy was significantly reduced without an effect on outcome (Boccadoro, 2010; Palumbo, 2009). May cause hypotension (including postural and orthostatic); use caution with dehydration, history of syncope, or medications associated with hypotension (may require adjustment of antihypertensive medication, hydration, and mineralocorticoids and/or sympathomimetics). Has been associated with the development or exacerbation of heart failure (HF) and decreased left ventricular ejection fraction (LVEF); monitor closely in patients with risk factors for HF or existing heart disease, although HF and decreased LVEF have been observed in patients without risk factors. Has also been associated with isolated reports of QT_c prolongation.

Pulmonary disorders (some fatal) including pneumonitis, interstitial pneumonia, lung infiltrates, and acute respiratory distress syndrome (ARDS) have been reported. Pulmonary hypertension (without left heart failure or significant pulmonary disease has been reported rarely). Promptly evaluate with new or worsening cardiopulmonary symptoms; therapy interruption may be required. Tumor lysis syndrome has been reported; risk is increased in patients with high tumor burden prior to treatment. Posterior reversible leukoencephalopathy syndrome (PRES, formerly RPLS) has been reported (rarely). Promptly evaluate with new or worsening cardiopulmonary symptoms. Symptoms of PRES include confusion, headache, hypertension, lethargy, seizure, blindness and/or other vision, or neurologic disturbances; discontinue bortezomib if PRES occurs. MRI is recommended to confirm PRES diagnosis. The safety of reinitiating bortezomib in patients previously experiencing PRES is unknown. Herpes (zoster and simplex) reactivation has been reported with bortezomib; consider antiviral prophylaxis during therapy. Hematologic toxicity, including neutropenia and severe thrombocytopenia, may occur (nadirs generally occur following the last dose of a cycle and recover prior to the next cycle); risk is increased in patients with pretreatment platelet counts <75,000/µL; frequent monitoring is required throughout treatment; may require dosage or schedule adjustments; withhold treatment for platelets <30,000/µL. Hemorrhage (gastrointestinal and intracerebral) due to low platelet count has been observed. Acute liver failure has been reported (rarely) in patients receiving multiple concomitant medications and with serious underlying conditions. Hepatitis, transaminase increases, and hyperbilirubinemia have also been reported; interrupt therapy to assess reversibility. Use caution in patients with hepatic dysfunction; reduced initial doses are recommended for moderate and severe hepatic impairment (exposure is increased); closely monitor for toxicities. Hyper- and hypoglycemia may occur in diabetic patients receiving oral hypoglycemics; may require adjustment of diabetes medications. Nausea, vomiting, diarrhea or constipation may occur; may require antiemetics or antidiarrheals; ileus may occur; administer fluid and electrolytes to prevent dehydration (monitor closely); interrupt therapy for severe symptoms.

Potentially significant drug-drug/drug-food interactions may exist, requiring dose or frequency adjustment, additional monitoring, and/or selection of alternative therapy. Coadministration of strong CYP3A4 inhibitors may increase bortezomib exposure; monitor for toxicity and consider dose reduction if concurrent therapy cannot be avoided. Efficacy may be reduced when administered with strong CYP3A4 inducers; concomitant use is not recommended.

For I.V. or SubQ administration only. Intrathecal administration is contraindicated; inadvertent intrathecal administration has resulted in death. Bortezomib should **NOT** be prepared during the preparation of any intrathecal medications. After preparation, keep bortezomib in a location **away** from the separate storage location recommended for intrathecal medications. Bortezomib should **NOT** be delivered to the patient at the same time with any medications intended for central nervous system administration.

Adverse Reactions Adverse reactions and incidences reported are associated with monotherapy.

>10%:

Central nervous system: Fatigue (7% to 52%), fever (8% to 35%), headache (10% to 19%), dizziness (10% to 18%; excludes vertigo)

Dermatologic: Rash (12% to 23%)

Gastrointestinal: Diarrhea (19% to 52%), nausea (16% to 52%), constipation (25% to 30%), vomiting (9% to 29%), anorexia (14% to 21%), abdominal pain (11%), appetite decreased (11%)

Hematologic: Thrombocytopenia (30% to 34%; grade 3: 5% to 24%; grade 4: 3% to 7%; nadir: Day 11; recovery: By day 21), neutropenia (10% to 27%; grade 3: 8% to 14%; grade 4: 2% to 4%; nadir: Day 11; recovery: By day 21), anemia (19% to 23%; grade 3: 4% to 6%; grade 4: <1%), leukopenia (18% to 20%; grade 3: 5%; grade 4: 1%)

Neuromuscular & skeletal: Peripheral neuropathy (SubQ 37%; I.V. 35% to 54%; grade ≥2: 24% to 39%; grade 3: SubQ 5%; I.V. 7% to 14%; grade 4: 1%), neuralgia (23%), paresthesia (7% to 19%), weakness (7% to 16%)

Respiratory: Dyspnea (11%)

1% to 10%:

Cardiovascular: Cardiac disorder (treatment emergent; 8%), hypotension (8%; grades 3/4: 2%), heart failure (≤1%; includes acute pulmonary edema, cardiac failure, congestive cardiac failure, cardiogenic shock)

Endocrine & metabolic: Dehydration (2%)

Hematologic: Bleeding (≥grade 3: 2%)

Local: Injection site irritation (SubQ 6%; I.V. 5%)

Respiratory: Pneumonia (1%)

Miscellaneous: Herpes zoster (1% to 2%)

<1% (Limited to important or life-threatening): Acute diffuse infiltrative pulmonary disease, acute respiratory distress syndrome (ARDS), alkaline phosphatase increased, amyloidosis, anaphylaxis, angina, angina pectoris, angioedema, ascites, aspergillosis, atelectasis, atrial fibrillation exacerbation, atrial flutter, AV block, bacteremia, blindness, bone pain, bradycardia, cardiac amyloidosis, cardiac arrest, cardiac tamponade, cardiopulmonary arrest, catheter-related infection, cerebral hemorrhage, cerebrovascular accident, coma, conjunctival infection/irritation, cranial palsy, deep vein thrombosis, diplopia, disseminated intravascular coagulation (DIC), duodenitis (hemorrhagic), dysarthria, dysautonomia, dysgeusia, dyspepsia, dysphagia, edema, embolism, encephalopathy, epistaxis, fecal impaction, gastritis (hemorrhagic), gastroenteritis, gastroesophageal reflux, GGT increased, glomerular nephritis, hearing impairment, hematemesis, hematuria, hemoptysis, hemorrhagic cystitis, hepatic failure, hepatic hemorrhage, hepatitis, hepatocellular damage, herpes meningoencephalitis, hyperbilirubinemia, hyper-/hypoglycemia, hyper-/hypokalemia, hyper-/hyponatremia, hypersensitivity, hyperuricemia, hypocalcemia, hypoxia, ileus, interstitial pneumonia, intestinal perforation, intracerebral hemorrhage, ischemic colitis, ischemic stroke, laryngeal edema, left ventricular ejection fraction decreased, leukocytoclastic vasculitis, limb pain, listeriosis, lymphopenia, melena, MI, myalgia, myocardial ischemia, nasopharyngitis, neutropenic fever, ophthalmic herpes, optic neuritis, oral candidiasis, oral mucosal petechiae, pancreatitis, paralytic ileus, pericardial effusion, pericarditis, peritonitis, phlebitis, pleural effusion, pneumonitis, portal vein thrombosis, posterior reversible encephalopathy syndrome (PRES), proliferative glomerular nephritis, pruritus, psychosis, pulmonary embolism, pulmonary hypertension, pulmonary infiltrate, QT_c prolongation, renal failure, respiratory failure, respiratory insufficiency, respiratory tract infection, seizure, sepsis, septic shock, SIADH, sinus arrest, sinusitis, spinal cord compression, Stevens-Johnson syndrome, stomatitis, stroke (hemorrhagic), subarachnoid hemorrhage, subdural hematoma, suicidal ideation, Sweet's syndrome (acute febrile neutrophilic dermatosis), syncope, tachycardia, torsade de pointes, toxic epidermal necrolysis, toxoplasmosis, transaminases increased, transient ischemic attack, tumor lysis syndrome, ventricular tachycardia, weight loss

Drug Interactions

Metabolism/Transport Effects Substrate of CYP1A2 (minor), CYP2C19 (major), CYP2C9 (minor), CYP2D6 (minor), CYP3A4 (major); **Note:** Assignment of Major/Minor substrate status based on clinically relevant drug interaction potential; **Inhibits** CYP1A2 (weak), CYP2C19 (moderate), CYP2C9 (weak), CYP2D6 (weak), CYP3A4 (weak)

Avoid Concomitant Use

Avoid concomitant use of Bortezomib with any of the following: CloZAPine; CYP3A4 Inducers (Strong); Green Tea; Pimozide; St Johns Wort

Increased Effect/Toxicity

Bortezomib may increase the levels/effects of: ARIPiprazole; Citalopram; CloZAPine; CYP2C19 Substrates; Dofetilide; Highest Risk QTc-Prolonging Agents; Lomitapide; Moderate Risk QTc-Prolonging Agents; Pimozide

The levels/effects of Bortezomib may be increased by: CYP3A4 Inhibitors (Strong); Mifepristone

Decreased Effect

Bortezomib may decrease the levels/effects of: Clopidogrel

The levels/effects of Bortezomib may be decreased by: Ascorbic Acid; Bosentan; CYP2C19 Inducers (Strong); CYP3A4 Inducers (Strong); Dabrafenib; Deferasirox; Green Tea; Multivitamins/Fluoride (with ADE); Multivitamins/Minerals (with ADEK, Folate, Iron); Multivitamins/Minerals (with AE, No Iron); Peginterferon Alfa-2b; St Johns Wort; Tocilizumab

Ethanol/Nutrition/Herb Interactions

Food: Avoid grapefruit juice (may increase bortezomib levels).

Herb/Nutraceutical: Avoid St John's wort (may decrease bortezomib levels). Avoid green tea and green tea extracts (may diminish the therapeutic effect of bortezomib) (Golden, 2009). Avoid ascorbic acid supplements, including multivitamins containing ascorbic acid (may diminish bortezomib activity) during treatment, especially 12 hours before and after bortezomib treatment (Perrone, 2009).

Preparation for Administration Note: The reconstituted concentrations for I.V. and SubQ administration are different; the manufacturer provides stickers to facilitate identification of the route for reconstituted vials. The amount contained in each vial may exceed the prescribed dose; use care with dosage and volume calculations.

Hazardous agent; use appropriate precautions for handling and disposal (NIOSH, 2012). Reconstitute only with normal saline (NS). Reconstituted solutions should be clear and colorless.

I.V.: Reconstitute each 3.5 mg vial with 3.5 mL NS to a concentration of 1 mg/mL.

SubQ: Reconstitute each 3.5 mg vial with 1.4 mL NS to a concentration of 2.5 mg/mL (Moreau, 2011). If injection site reaction occurs, the more dilute 1 mg/mL concentration may be used SubQ.

Storage/Stability Prior to reconstitution, store at room temperature of 25°C (77°F); excursions permitted between 15°C to 30°C (59°F to 86°F). Once reconstituted, the manufacturer recommends use within 8 hours of reconstitution. However, stability studies have demonstrated solutions of 1 mg/mL (vial or syringe) may be stored at room temperature for up to 3 days, or under refrigeration for up to 5 days (Andre, 2005); or refrigerated in the original vial for up to 15 days (Vanderloo, 2010). Protect from light. After preparation, keep bortezomib in a location away from the separate storage location recommended for intrathecal medications.

Mechanism of Action Bortezomib inhibits proteasomes, enzyme complexes which regulate protein homeostasis within the cell. Specifically, it reversibly inhibits chymotrypsin-like activity at the 26S proteasome, leading to activation of signaling cascades, cell-cycle arrest, and apoptosis.

Pharmacodynamics/Kinetics

Distribution: 498-1884 L/m^2; distributes widely to peripheral tissues

Protein binding: ~83%

Metabolism: Hepatic primarily via CYP2C19 and 3A4 and to a lesser extent CYP1A2; forms metabolites (inactive) via deboronization followed by hydroxylation

Half-life elimination: Single dose: I.V.: 9-15 hours; multiple dosing: 1 mg/m^2: 40-193 hours; 1.3 mg/m^2: 76-108 hours

Dosage Details concerning dosing in combination regimens should also be consulted. **Note:** Consecutive doses should be separated by at least 72 hours: Adults:

Multiple myeloma (first-line therapy; in combination with melphalan and prednisone): I.V., SubQ: 1.3 mg/m^2 days 1, 4, 8, 11, 22, 25, 29, and 32 of a 42-day treatment cycle for 4 cycles, followed by 1.3 mg/m^2 days 1, 8, 22, and 29 of a 42-day treatment cycle for 5 cycles.

Alternative first-line therapy (unlabeled dosing):

CyBorD regimen: I.V.: 1.5 mg/m^2 days 1, 8, 15, and 22 of a 28-day treatment cycle for 4 cycles (may continue beyond 4 cycles) in combination with cyclophosphamide and dexamethasone (Khan, 2012)

Patients ≥65 years: I.V.: 1.3 mg/m^2 days 1, 8, 15, and 22 of a 35-day treatment cycle, in combination with **either** melphalan and prednisone or melphalan, prednisone, and thalidomide (Boccadoro, 2010; Bringhen, 2010; Palumbo, 2009)

Multiple myeloma (relapsed) and mantle cell lymphoma: I.V., SubQ: 1.3 mg/m^2 twice weekly for 2 weeks on days 1, 4, 8, and 11 of a 21-day treatment cycle. Therapy extending beyond 8 cycles may be administered by the standard schedule or may be given once weekly for 4 weeks (days 1, 8, 15, and 22), followed by a 13-day rest (days 23 through 35).

Cutaneous and peripheral T-cell lymphoma, relapsed/refractory (unlabeled use): I.V.: 1.3 mg/m^2 twice weekly for 2 weeks on days 1, 4, 8, and 11 of a 21-day treatment cycle (Zinzani, 2007)

Follicular lymphoma, relapsed/refractory (unlabeled use): I.V.: 1.3 mg/m^2 days 1, 4, 8, and 11 of a 28-day treatment cycle, in combination with bendamustine and rituximab for 6 cycles (Friedberg, 2011) **or** 1.6 mg/m^2 days 1, 8, 15, and 22 of a 35-day treatment cycle, in combination with bendamustine and rituximab for 5 cycles (Fowler, 2011)

Systemic light-chain amyloidosis (unlabeled use): I.V.: 1.3 mg/m^2 days 1, 4, 8, and 11 of a 21-day treatment cycle (with or without dexamethasone) (Kastritis, 2010)

Waldenström's macroglobulinemia, relapsed/refractory (unlabeled use): I.V.: 1.3 mg/m^2 days 1, 4, 8, and 11 of a 21-day treatment cycle (Chen, 2007) **or** 1.3 mg/m^2 days 1, 4, 8, and 11 of a 21-day treatment cycle (in combination with dexamethasone and rituximab) (Treon, 2009) **or** 1.6 mg/m^2 days 1, 8, and 15 of a 28-day treatment cycle (in combination with rituximab) (Ghobrial, 2010)

Dosage adjustment for toxicity:

Myeloma (first-line therapy):

Platelets should be ≥70,000/mm^3, ANC should be ≥1000/mm^3, and nonhematologic toxicities should resolve to grade 1 or baseline prior to therapy initiation.

Platelets ≤30,000/mm^3 or ANC ≤750/mm^3 on bortezomib day(s) (except day 1): Withhold bortezomib; if several bortezomib doses in consecutive cycles are withheld, reduce dose 1 level (1.3 mg/m^2/dose reduced to 1 mg/m^2/dose; 1 mg/m^2/dose reduced to 0.7 mg/m^2/dose)

Grade ≥3 nonhematological toxicity (other than neuropathy): Withhold bortezomib until toxicity resolves to grade 1 or baseline. May reinitiate bortezomib at 1 dose level reduction (1.3 mg/m^2/dose reduced to 1 mg/m^2/dose; 1 mg/m^2/dose reduced to 0.7 mg/m^2/dose).

Neuropathic pain and/or peripheral sensory or motor neuropathy: See "Neuropathic pain and/or peripheral sensory or motor neuropathy" toxicity adjustment guidelines below.

Relapsed multiple myeloma and mantle cell lymphoma:

Grade 3 nonhematological (excluding neuropathy) or Grade 4 hematological toxicity: Withhold until toxicity resolved; may reinitiate with a 25% dose reduction (1.3 mg/m^2/dose reduced to 1 mg/m^2/dose; 1 mg/m^2/dose reduced to 0.7 mg/m^2/dose)

Neuropathic pain and/or peripheral sensory or motor neuropathy:

Note: Consider subQ administration in patients with preexisting or at high risk for peripheral neuropathy.

Grade 1 (asymptomatic; deep tendon reflex loss or paresthesia) without pain or loss of function: No action needed

Grade 1 with pain or Grade 2 (moderate symptoms; limiting instrumental activities of daily living): Reduce dose to 1 mg/m^2

Grade 2 with pain or Grade 3 (severe symptoms; limiting self-care activities of daily living): Withhold until toxicity resolved, may reinitiate at 0.7 mg/m^2 once weekly

Grade 4 (life-threatening consequences with urgent intervention indicated): Discontinue therapy

Dosage adjustment in renal impairment: No dosage adjustment necessary. Dialysis may reduce bortezomib concentrations; administer postdialysis (Leal, 2011).

Dosage adjustment in hepatic impairment:

Mild impairment (bilirubin ≤1 times ULN and AST >UNL or bilirubin >1-1.5 times ULN): No initial dose adjustment necessary (LoRusso, 2012).

Moderate (bilirubin >1.5-3 times ULN) and severe impairment (bilirubin >3 times ULN): Reduce initial dose to 0.7 mg/m^2 in the first cycle; based on patient tolerance, may consider dose escalation to 1 mg/m^2 (LoRusso, 2012) or further dose reduction to 0.5 mg/m^2 in subsequent cycles

Dosing in obesity: *ASCO Guidelines for appropriate chemotherapy dosing in obese adults with cancer:* Utilize patient's actual body weight (full weight) for calculation of body surface area- or weight-based dosing, particularly when the intent of therapy is curative; manage regimen-related toxicities in the same manner as for nonobese patients; if a dose reduction is utilized due to toxicity, consider resumption of full weight-based dosing with subsequent cycles, especially if cause of toxicity (eg, hepatic or renal impairment) is resolved (Griggs, 2012).

Dietary Considerations Green tea and green tea extracts may diminish the therapeutic effect of bortezomib and should be avoided (Golden, 2009). Avoid grapefruit juice. Avoid additional, nondietary sources of ascorbic acid supplements, including multivitamins containing ascorbic acid (may diminish bortezomib activity) during treatment, especially 12 hours before and after bortezomib treatment (Perrone, 2009).

Administration Note: The reconstituted concentrations for I.V. and SubQ administration are different; use caution when calculating the volume for each dose. Consider SubQ administration in patients with pre-existing or at high risk for peripheral neuropathy.

I.V.: Administer via rapid I.V. push (3-5 seconds)

SubQ: Subcutaneous administration of bortezomib 1.3 mg/m² days 1, 4, 8, and 11 of a 21-day treatment cycle has been studied in a limited number of patients with relapsed multiple myeloma; doses were administered subcutaneously (concentration of 2.5 mg/mL) into the thigh or abdomen, rotating the injection site with each dose; injections at the same site within a single cycle were avoided (Moreau, 2010; Moreau, 2011). Response rates were similar to I.V. administration; decreased incidence of grade 3 or higher adverse events were observed with SubQ administration. Administer at least 1 inch from an old site and never administer to tender, bruised, erythematous, or indurated sites. If injection site reaction occurs, the more dilute 1 mg/mL concentration may be used SubQ (or I.V. administration of 1 mg/mL concentration may be considered).

For I.V. or SubQ administration only; fatalities have been reported with inadvertent intrathecal administration. Bortezomib should **NOT** be delivered to the patient at the same time with any medications intended for central nervous system administration.

Hazardous agent; use appropriate precautions for handling and disposal (NIOSH, 2012).

Monitoring Parameters CBC with differential and platelets (monitor frequently throughout therapy); liver function tests (in patients with existing hepatic impairment); signs/symptoms of peripheral neuropathy, dehydration, hypotension, or PRES; renal function, pulmonary function (with new or worsening pulmonary symptoms)

Dosage Forms Excipient information presented when available (limited, particularly for generics); consult specific product labeling.

Solution Reconstituted, Injection:

Velcade: 3.5 mg (1 ea)

Bosentan (boe SEN tan)

Brand Names: U.S. Tracleer

Brand Names: Canada CO Bosentan; Mylan-Bosentan; PMS-Bosentan; Sandoz-Bosentan; Tracleer®

Pharmacologic Category Endothelin Receptor Antagonist; Vasodilator

Use Treatment of pulmonary artery hypertension (PAH) (WHO Group I) in patients with NYHA Class II, III, or IV symptoms to improve exercise capacity and decrease the rate of clinical deterioration

Pregnancy Risk Factor X

Pregnancy Considerations **[U.S. Boxed Warning]: May cause birth defects; use in pregnancy is contraindicated. Exclude pregnancy prior to initiation of therapy and obtain pregnancy tests monthly during treatment. Reliable contraception must be used during therapy and for 1 month after stopping treatment. Hormonal contraceptives (oral, injectable, transdermal, or implantable) may not be effective and a second method of contraception (nonhormonal) is required. Patients with tubal ligation or an implanted IUD (Copper T 380A or LNg 20) do not need additional contraceptive measures.** When a hormonal or barrier contraceptive is used, one additional method of contraception is still needed if a male partner has had a vasectomy. When initiating treatment for women of reproductive potential, a negative pregnancy test should be documented within the first 5 days of a normal menstrual period and ≥11 days after the last unprotected intercourse. A missed menses or suspected pregnancy should be reported to a healthcare provider and prompt immediate pregnancy testing. Sperm counts may be reduced in men during treatment. Women of childbearing potential should avoid splitting, crushing, or handling broken tablets and exposure to the generated dust (tablet splitting is currently outside of product labeling).

Breast-Feeding Considerations Due to the potential risk of adverse events in a nursing infant, a decision should be made to discontinue nursing or discontinue therapy.

Prescribing and Access Restrictions As a requirement of the REMS program, access to this medication is restricted. Bosentan (Tracleer®) is only available through Tracleer® Access Program (T.A.P.). Only prescribers and pharmacies registered with T.A.P. may prescribe and dispense bosentan. Further information may be obtained from the manufacturer, Actelion Pharmaceuticals (1-866-228-3546 or http://www.tracleer.com/hcp/prescribing-tracleer.asp).

Medication Guide Available Yes

Contraindications Hypersensitivity to bosentan or any component of the formulation; concurrent use of cyclosporine or glyburide; pregnancy

Canadian labeling: Additional contraindications (not in U.S. labeling): Moderate-to-severe hepatic impairment and/or baseline ALT or AST >3 times the upper limit of normal (ULN), particularly when total bilirubin >2 times ULN

Warnings/Precautions Hazardous agent - use appropriate precautions for handling and disposal (NIOSH, 2012). **[U.S. Boxed Warning]: May cause hepatotoxicity; has been associated with a high incidence (~11%) of significant transaminase elevations (ALT or AST ≥3 times ULN) with or without elevations in bilirubin and rare cases of unexplained hepatic cirrhosis (after >12 months of therapy) or hepatic failure. Monitor transaminases at baseline then monthly thereafter. Adjust dosage if elevations in liver enzymes occur without symptoms of hepatic injury or elevated bilirubin. Treatment should be stopped in patients who develop elevated transaminases either in combination with symptoms of hepatic injury (unusual fatigue, jaundice, nausea, vomiting, abdominal pain, and/or fever) or elevated bilirubin (≥2 times ULN); safety of reintroduction is unknown. Avoid use in patients with baseline serum transaminases >3 times ULN or moderate-to-severe hepatic impairment.** Transaminase elevations are dose dependent, generally asymptomatic, occur both early and late in therapy, progress slowly, and are usually reversible after treatment interruption or discontinuation. Consider the benefits of treatment versus the risk of hepatotoxicity when initiating therapy in patients with WHO Class II symptoms.

[U.S. Boxed Warning]: May cause birth defects; use in pregnancy is contraindicated. Exclude pregnancy prior to initiation of therapy and obtain pregnancy tests monthly during treatment. Reliable contraception must be used during therapy and for 1 month after stopping treatment. Hormonal contraceptives (oral, injectable, transdermal, or implantable) may not be effective and a second method of contraception (nonhormonal) is required. Patients with tubal ligation or an implanted IUD (Copper T 380A or LNg 20) do not need additional contraceptive measures. (See Pregnancy Considerations.)

[U.S. Boxed Warning]: Because of the risks of hepatic impairment and the high likelihood of teratogenic effects, bosentan is only available through the T.A.P. restricted distribution program. Patients, prescribers, and pharmacies must be registered with and meet

conditions of T.A.P. Call 1-866-228-3546 or visit http://www.tracleer.com/hcp/prescribing-tracleer.asp for more information.

A reduction in hematocrit/hemoglobin may be observed within the first few weeks of therapy with subsequent stabilization of levels. Hemoglobin reductions >15% have been observed in some patients. Measure hemoglobin prior to initiating therapy, at 1 and 3 months, and every 3 months thereafter. Significant decreases in hemoglobin in the absence of other causes may warrant the discontinuation of therapy.

Development of peripheral edema due to treatment and/or disease state (pulmonary arterial hypertension) may occur. There have also been postmarketing reports of fluid retention requiring treatment (eg, diuretics, fluid management, hospitalization). Further evaluation may be necessary to determine cause and appropriate treatment or discontinuation of therapy. Bosentan should be discontinued in any patient with pulmonary edema suggestive of pulmonary veno-occlusive disease (PVOD). Bosentan may interact with many medications, resulting in potentially serious and/or life-threatening adverse events (see Drug Interactions).

Adverse Reactions

>10%:

Cardiovascular: Edema (11%)
Central nervous system: Headache (15%)
Endocrine & metabolic: Spermatogenesis inhibition (25%)
Hematologic: Hemoglobin decreased (≥1 g/dL in up to 57%; <11 g/dL: 3% to 6%; typically in first 6 weeks of therapy)
Hepatic: Transaminases increased (≥3 times ULN; up to 12%; dose-related)
Respiratory: Respiratory tract infection (22%)

1% to 10%:

Cardiovascular: Chest pain (5%), syncope (5%), flushing (4%), hypotension (4%), palpitation (4%)
Dermatologic: Pruritus (2%)
Hematologic: Anemia (3%)
Hepatic: Abnormal hepatic function (4%)
Neuromuscular & skeletal: Arthralgia (4%)
Respiratory: Sinusitis (4%)

<1% (Limited to important or life-threatening): Anaphylaxis, angioneurotic edema, heart failure (exacerbation), cirrhosis (prolonged therapy), hyperbilirubinemia, hypersensitivity, jaundice, leukocytoclastic vasculitis, leukopenia, liver failure (rare), neutropenia, peripheral edema, rash, thrombocytopenia, weight gain

Drug Interactions

Metabolism/Transport Effects **Substrate** of CYP2C9 (minor), CYP3A4 (minor), SLCO1B1; **Note:** Assignment of Major/Minor substrate status based on clinically relevant drug interaction potential; **Induces** CYP2C9 (weak/moderate), CYP3A4 (weak/moderate)

Avoid Concomitant Use

Avoid concomitant use of Bosentan with any of the following: Axitinib; CycloSPORINE (Systemic); GlyBURIDE; Simeprevir

Increased Effect/Toxicity

The levels/effects of Bosentan may be increased by: Atazanavir; Boceprevir; Cobicistat; CycloSPORINE (Systemic); CYP2C9 Inhibitors (Moderate); CYP2C9 Inhibitors (Strong); CYP3A4 Inhibitors (Moderate); CYP3A4 Inhibitors (Strong); Darunavir; Eltrombopag; Fosamprenavir; GlyBURIDE; Indinavir; Lopinavir; Nelfinavir; Phosphodiesterase 5 Inhibitors; Rifampin; Ritonavir; Saquinavir; Telaprevir; Tipranavir

Decreased Effect

Bosentan may decrease the levels/effects of: ARIPiprazole; Atazanavir; Axitinib; Boceprevir; Contraceptives (Estrogens); Contraceptives (Progestins); CycloSPORINE (Systemic); CYP3A4 Substrates; Darunavir; Fosamprenavir; GlyBURIDE; HMG-CoA Reductase Inhibitors; Ibrutinib; Indinavir; Lopinavir; Nelfinavir; Phosphodiesterase 5 Inhibitors; Saquinavir; Saxagliptin; Simeprevir; Telaprevir; Tipranavir; Vitamin K Antagonists

The levels/effects of Bosentan may be decreased by: GlyBURIDE; Rifampin

Ethanol/Nutrition/Herb Interactions

Food: Bioavailability of bosentan is not affected by food. Bosentan serum concentrations may be increased by grapefruit juice.
Herb/Nutraceutical: Avoid St John's wort (may decrease serum concentrations of bosentan).

Storage/Stability Store at 20°C to 25°C (68°F to 77°F); excursions permitted to 15°C to 30°C (59°F to 86°F).

Mechanism of Action Blocks endothelin receptors on vascular endothelium and smooth muscle. Stimulation of these receptors is associated with vasoconstriction. Although bosentan blocks both ET_A and ET_B receptors, the affinity is higher for the A subtype.

Pharmacodynamics/Kinetics

Distribution: V_d: ~18 L
Protein binding, plasma: >98% primarily to albumin
Metabolism: Hepatic via CYP2C9 and 3A4 to three primary metabolites (one contributing ~10% to 20% pharmacologic activity); autoinduction may occur with chronic dosing
Bioavailability: ~50%
Half-life elimination: 5 hours; prolonged with heart failure, possibly in PAH
Time to peak, plasma: 3-5 hours
Excretion: Feces (as metabolites); urine (<3% as unchanged drug)

Dosage Oral:

Adolescents >12 years and Adults: Pulmonary artery hypertension:
<40 kg: Initial and maintenance: 62.5 mg twice daily
≥40 kg: Initial: 62.5 mg twice daily for 4 weeks; increase to maintenance dose of 125 mg twice daily. Doses >125 mg twice daily do not appear to confer additional clinical benefit, but may increase risk of liver toxicity.
Note: When discontinuing treatment, consider a reduction in dosage to 62.5 mg twice daily for 3-7 days (to avoid clinical deterioration).

Canadian labeling (not in U.S. labeling): Children 3-18 years:
10-20 kg: Initial: 31.25 mg once daily for 4 weeks; increase to maintenance dose of 31.25 mg twice daily
>20-40 kg: Initial: 31.25 mg twice daily for 4 weeks; increase to maintenance dose of 62.5 mg twice daily
>40 kg: Initial: 62.5 mg twice daily for 4 weeks; increase to maintenance dose of 125 mg twice daily

Coadministration with protease inhibitor regimen:

Dosage adjustment for concurrent use with atazanavir/ritonavir, darunavir/ritonavir, fosamprenavir, lopinavir/ritonavir, ritonavir, saquinavir/ritonavir, tipranavir/ritonavir:
Coadministration of bosentan in patients currently receiving one of these protease inhibitor regimens for at least 10 days: Begin with bosentan 62.5 mg once daily or every other day based on tolerability
Coadministration of one of these protease inhibitor regimens in patients currently receiving bosentan: Discontinue bosentan 36 hours prior to the initiation of an above regimen. After at least 10 days of the protease inhibitor regimen, resume bosentan 62.5 mg once daily or every other day based on tolerability.

Dosage adjustment for concurrent use with indinavir or nelfinavir:
Coadministration of bosentan in patients currently receiving indinavir or nelfinavir: Begin with bosentan 62.5 mg once daily or every other day based on tolerability

Coadministration of indinavir or nelfinavir in patients currently receiving bosentan: Adjust bosentan to 62.5 mg once daily or every other day based on tolerability

Dosage adjustment in renal impairment: No dosage adjustment necessary.

Dosage adjustment in hepatic impairment:

Mild impairment (Child-Pugh class A): No dosage adjustment necessary.

Moderate-to-severe impairment (Child-Pugh class B and C) and/or baseline transaminase >3 times ULN: Use not recommended; systemic exposure significantly increased in patients with moderate impairment (not studied in patients with severe impairment).

Modification based on transaminase elevation:

If any elevation, regardless of degree, is accompanied by clinical symptoms of hepatic injury (unusual fatigue, nausea, vomiting, abdominal pain, fever, or jaundice) or a serum bilirubin ≥2 times ULN, treatment should be stopped.

AST/ALT >3 times but ≤5 times ULN: Confirm with additional test; if confirmed, reduce dose to 62.5 mg twice daily or interrupt treatment and monitor every 2 weeks. If transaminase levels return to pretreatment values, may continue or reintroduce treatment at the starting dose, as appropriate. When reintroducing treatment, recheck transaminases within 3 days and at least every 2 weeks thereafter.

AST/ALT >5 times but ≤8 times ULN: Confirm with additional test; if confirmed, stop treatment. Monitor transaminase levels at least every 2 weeks. May reintroduce treatment, as appropriate, at starting dose, following return to pretreatment values. Recheck within 3 days and at least every 2 weeks thereafter following reinitiation.

AST/ALT >8 times ULN: Stop treatment and do not reintroduce.

Dietary Considerations May be taken with or without food. Avoid grapefruit and grapefruit juice.

Administration May be administered with or without food, once in the morning and once in the evening. Women of childbearing potential should avoid excessive handling of broken tablets.

Hazardous agent; use appropriate precautions for handling and disposal (NIOSH, 2012).

Monitoring Parameters Serum transaminase (AST and ALT) and bilirubin should be determined prior to the initiation of therapy and at monthly intervals thereafter. Monitor for clinical signs and symptoms of liver injury (eg, abdominal pain, fatigue, fever, jaundice, nausea, vomiting). Hemoglobin and hematocrit should be measured at baseline, at 1 month and 3 months of treatment, and every 3 months thereafter (generally stabilizes after 4-12 weeks of treatment).

A woman of childbearing potential must have a negative pregnancy test prior to the initiation of therapy and monthly thereafter (prior to shipment of monthly refill).

Dosage Forms Excipient information presented when available (limited, particularly for generics); consult specific product labeling.

Tablet, Oral:

Tracleer: 62.5 mg, 125 mg

Extemporaneous Preparations Hazardous agent: Use appropriate precautions for handling and disposal.

Note: Tablets are not scored; a commercial pill cutter should be used to prepare a 31.25 mg dose from the 62.5 mg tablet; the half-cut 62.5 mg tablets are stable for up to 4 weeks when stored at room temperature in the high-density polyethylene plastic bottle provided by the manufacturer. Since bosentan is classified as a teratogen (Pregnancy Risk Factor X), individuals should avoid exposure to bosentan powder (dust) by taking appropriate measures (eg, using gloves and mask); women of childbearing potential should avoid exposure to dust generated from broken or split tablets.

Crushing of the tablets is not recommended; bosentan tablets will disintegrate rapidly (within 5 minutes) in 5-25 mL of water to create a suspension. An appropriate aliquot of the suspension can be used to deliver the prescribed dose. Any remaining suspension should be discarded. Bosentan should not be mixed or dissolved in liquids with a low (acidic) pH (eg, fruit juices) due to poor solubility; the drug is most soluble in solutions with a pH >8.5.

◆ **Bosulif** *see* Bosutinib *on page* 275

Bosutinib (boe SUE ti nib)

Brand Names: U.S. Bosulif

Index Terms Bosutinib Monohydrate; SKI-606

Pharmacologic Category Antineoplastic Agent, Tyrosine Kinase Inhibitor

Use Chronic myelogenous leukemia (CML): Treatment of chronic, accelerated or blast phase Philadelphia chromosome-positive (Ph+) CML in patients resistant or intolerant to prior therapy

Pregnancy Risk Factor D

Pregnancy Considerations Adverse events were observed in animal reproduction studies. Based on the mechanism of action, bosutinib may cause fetal harm if administered in pregnancy. Females of reproductive potential should use effective contraception during bosutinib treatment and for at least 30 days after completion of treatment.

Breast-Feeding Considerations It is not known if bosutinib is excreted in breast milk. Due to the potential for serious adverse reactions in the nursing infant, the decision to discontinue bosutinib or discontinue breast-feeding should take into account the benefits of treatment to the mother.

Contraindications Hypersensitivity to bosutinib or any component of the formulation

Warnings/Precautions Hazardous agent - use appropriate precautions for handling and disposal (meets NIOSH, 2012 criteria).

Diarrhea, nausea, vomiting, and abdominal pain may occur. Monitor; may require treatment interruption, dose reduction, or discontinuation. For patients experiencing diarrhea (all grades), the median time to onset was 2 days; median duration (per event) was 1 day; manage diarrhea with antidiarrheals and/or fluid replacement. Nausea and vomiting may be managed with antiemetics and/or fluid replacement.

Anemia, neutropenia, and thrombocytopenia may occur. May require treatment interruption, dose reduction, or discontinuation. Monitor blood counts weekly during first month, then monthly thereafter (or as clinically indicated). Fluid retention, manifesting as pericardial effusion, pleural effusion, pulmonary edema and/or peripheral edema may occur; may be severe. Monitor and manage appropriately; may require treatment interruption, dose reduction, or discontinuation.

Bosutinib exposure is increased in patients with hepatic impairment; dose reduction is recommended. Hepatotoxicity has been reported during treatment; dose reductions may be necessary. Monitor liver function. ALT and AST elevations may occur, usually with an onset in the first 3 months of treatment (median onset was ~30-33 days; median duration was 21 days). One case of drug-induced liver injury has been reported; full recovery occurred after discontinuation. Bosutinib exposure is increased in patients with moderate or severe renal impairment; dosage adjustment recommended in patients with severe impairment.

Potentially significant drug-drug interactions may exist, requiring dose or frequency adjustment, additional monitoring, and/or selection of alternative therapy. Avoid concurrent use with strong or moderate CYP3A4 inducers and strong or moderate CYP3A4 and/or P-gp inhibitors. Proton pump inhibitors (PPIs) may decrease bosutinib effects; consider using short acting antacids or H_2 antagonists instead of PPIs; separate administration of antacids or H_2 antagonists from bosutinib by at least 2 hours.

Adverse Reactions

>10%:

Cardiovascular: Edema (14%; grades 3/4: <1%)

Central nervous system: Fever (26%), fatigue (24%), headache (20%)

Dermatologic: Rash (35%)

Endocrine & metabolic: Bicarbonate decreased (31%), hypermagnesemia (25%; grades 3/4: 12%), hypomagnesemia (19%)

Gastrointestinal: Diarrhea (82%; grades 3/4: 8%), nausea (46%; grades 3/4: 1%), vomiting (39%; grades 3/4: 32%), abdominal pain (37%; grades 3/4: 2%), appetite decreased (13%)

Hematologic: Thrombocytopenia (41%; grades 3/4: 29% to 33%), anemia (27%; grades 3/4: 13% to 19%), neutropenia (17%; grades 3/4: 12% to 23%)

Hepatic: ALT increased (17%; grades 3/4: 7% to 9%), AST increased (14%; grades 3/4: 3% to 4%)

Neuromuscular & skeletal: Arthralgia (14%), back pain (11%), weakness (11%)

Respiratory: Cough (20%), dyspnea (12%), respiratory tract infection (12%)

1% to 10%:

Cardiovascular: Chest pain (<10%), pericardial effusion (<10%; grades 3/4: <1%)

Central nervous system: Dizziness (10%), pain (<10%)

Dermatologic: Pruritus (10%), acne (<10%), urticaria (<10%)

Endocrine & metabolic: Dehydration (<10%), hypophosphatemia (grades 3/4: 7%), uric acid increased (grades 3/4: 6%), hypocalcemia (grades 3/4: 3% to 4%)

Gastrointestinal: Abnormal taste (<10%), gastritis (<10%), lipase increased (grades 3/4: 7%)

Hematologic: Neutropenic fever (<10%), INR increased (grades 3/4: 2%)

Hepatic: Abnormal hepatic function (<10%), hepatotoxicity (<10%), bilirubin increased (grades 3/4: 1%)

Neuromuscular & skeletal: CPK increased (<10%), myalgia (<10%), bone pain (4%), muscle spasm (2%)

Otic: Tinnitus (<10%)

Renal: Creatinine increased (<10%), renal failure (<10%)

Respiratory: Nasopharyngitis (10%), bronchitis (<10%), pleural effusion (<10%; grades 3/4: <2%), pneumonia (<10%)

Miscellaneous: Hypersensitivity reactions (<10%), influenza (<10%)

<1% (Limited to important or life-threatening): Anaphylactic shock, erythema multiforme, exfoliative rash, fixed drug eruption, gastrointestinal hemorrhage, hemorrhage, pancreatitis, pericarditis, pulmonary edema, pulmonary hypertension, QT_c prolongation, respiratory failure

Drug Interactions

Metabolism/Transport Effects Substrate of CYP3A4 (major), P-glycoprotein; **Note:** Assignment of Major/Minor substrate status based on clinically relevant drug interaction potential; **Inhibits** P-glycoprotein

Avoid Concomitant Use

Avoid concomitant use of Bosutinib with any of the following: CloZAPine; CYP3A4 Inducers (Strong); CYP3A4 Inhibitors (Moderate); CYP3A4 Inhibitors (Strong); Fusidic Acid (Systemic); Modafinil; P-glycoprotein/ABCB1 Inhibitors; St Johns Wort

Increased Effect/Toxicity

Bosutinib may increase the levels/effects of: CloZAPine; Highest Risk QTc-Prolonging Agents; Moderate Risk QTc-Prolonging Agents

The levels/effects of Bosutinib may be increased by: CYP3A4 Inhibitors (Moderate); CYP3A4 Inhibitors (Strong); Dasatinib; Fusidic Acid (Systemic); Ivacaftor; Luliconazole; Mifepristone; P-glycoprotein/ABCB1 Inhibitors; Simeprevir

Decreased Effect

The levels/effects of Bosutinib may be decreased by: Antacids; Bosentan; CYP3A4 Inducers (Strong); Dabrafenib; Deferasirox; H2-Antagonists; Modafinil; P-glycoprotein/ABCB1 Inducers; Proton Pump Inhibitors; St Johns Wort; Tocilizumab

Ethanol/Nutrition/Herb Interactions

Food: Grapefruit juice may increase bosutinib plasma concentration. Management: Avoid grapefruit juice.

Herb/Nutraceutical: St John's wort may increase metabolism and decrease bosutinib plasma concentration. Management: Avoid St John's wort.

Storage/Stability Store at room temperature of 20°C to 25°C (68°F to 77°F); excursions permitted to 15°C to 30°C (59°F to 86°F).

Mechanism of Action BCR-ABL tyrosine kinase inhibitor (TKI); inhibits BCR-ABL kinase that promotes CML. Also inhibits SRC family (including SRC, LYN, and HCK). Bosutinib has minimal activity against c-KIT and platelet-derived growth factor receptor (PDGFR), which are nonspecific targets associated with toxicity in other TKIs (Cortes, 2012). Bosutinib has activity in 16 of 18 imatinib-resistant BCR-ABL mutations, with the exceptions of the T315I and V299L mutants (Cortes, 2011).

Pharmacodynamics/Kinetics

Onset:

Median time to complete hematologic response (in responders): 2 weeks (Cortes, 2011)

Median time to major cytogenetic response (in responders): 12.3 weeks (Cortes, 2011)

Median time to first complete cytogenic response: 12.9 weeks (Cortes, 2012)

Absorption: Slow (Abbas, 2012)

Distribution: V_d: 6080 ± 1230 L

Protein binding: 94% to plasma proteins

Metabolism: Hepatic via CYP3A4, primarily to inactive metabolites oxydechlorinated (M2) bosutinib and *N*-desmethylated (M5) bosutinib, also to bosutinib *N*-oxide (M6)

Half-life elimination: 22-27 hours (Cortes, 2011)

Time to peak: 4-6 hours

Excretion: Feces (91%); urine (3%)

Dosage Philadelphia chromosome-positive chronic myelogenous leukemia (Ph+CML): Adults: Oral: 500 mg once daily; continue until disease progression or unacceptable toxicity. **Note:** If complete hematologic response is not achieved by week 8 or complete cytogenetic response is not achieved by week 12, in the absence of grade 3 or higher adverse reactions, consider increasing the dose from 500 mg once daily to 600 mg once daily.

Missed doses: If a dose is missed beyond 12 hours, skip the dose and resume the usual dose the following day.

Dosage adjustment for toxicity:

Hematologic toxicity: ANC <1000/mm³ or platelets <50,000/mm³: Withhold treatment until ANC ≥1000/mm³ **and** platelets ≥50,000/mm³; if recovery occurs within 2 weeks, resume treatment at the same dose. If ANC and platelets remain low for >2 weeks, upon recovery, resume treatment with the dose reduced by 100 mg. If cytopenia recurs, withhold until recovery and resume treatment with the dose reduced by an additional 100 mg. Doses <300 mg daily have not been evaluated.

Nonhematologic toxicity:

Diarrhea: Grade 3 or 4 (≥7 stools/day increase over baseline): Withhold treatment until recovery to ≤ grade 1; may resume at 400 mg once daily.

Other clinically significant nonhematologic toxicity, moderate or severe: Withhold treatment until resolved, then consider resuming at 400 mg once daily; may re-escalate dose to 500 mg once daily if clinically appropriate.

Dosage adjustment in renal impairment:

Mild impairment (Cl_{cr} >50-80 mL/minute): No dosage adjustment provided in manufacturer's labeling, however, based on the pharmacokinetics, the need for dosage adjustment is not likely.

Moderate impairment (Cl_{cr} 30-50 mL/minute): No dosage adjustment provided in the manufacturer's labeling.

Pre-existing severe impairment (Cl_{cr} <30 mL/minute): Reduce dose to 300 mg once daily (this dose is predicted to result in an AUC similar to that of patients with normal renal function, however, there is no efficacy data for this dose in CML patients with renal impairment).

Hemodialysis: No dosage adjustment provided in the manufacturer's labeling.

Dosage adjustment in hepatic impairment:

Pre-existing impairment (mild, moderate, or severe): Reduce dose to 200 mg once daily (this dose is predicted to result in an AUC similar to that of patients with normal hepatic function, however, there is no efficacy data for this dose in CML patients with hepatic impairment).

Hepatotoxicity during treatment:

ALT or AST >5 times ULN: Withhold treatment until recovery to ≤2.5 times ULN and resume at 400 mg once daily thereafter. If recovery to ≤2.5 times ULN takes >4 weeks: Discontinue bosutinib.

ALT or AST >3 times ULN in conjunction with bilirubin elevation >2 times ULN and alkaline phosphatase <2 times ULN: Discontinue bosutinib.

Dietary Considerations Take with food.

Administration Oral: Administer with food. Swallow tablet whole; do not crush or break.

Hazardous agent; use appropriate precautions for handling and disposal (meets NIOSH, 2012 criteria).

Monitoring Parameters CBC with differential and platelets (weekly during first month, then monthly thereafter, or as clinically indicated); hepatic enzymes (monthly for first 3 months or as clinically indicated; monitor more frequently with transaminase elevations); renal function (at baseline); diarrhea episodes; fluid/edema status

Dosage Forms Excipient information presented when available (limited, particularly for generics); consult specific product labeling.

Tablet, Oral:

Bosulif: 100 mg, 500 mg

◆ **Bosutinib Monohydrate** *see* Bosutinib *on page 275*

◆ **Botox** *see* OnabotulinumtoxinA *on page 1508*

◆ **Botox Cosmetic** *see* OnabotulinumtoxinA *on page 1508*

◆ **Botulinum Toxin Type A** *see* AbobotulinumtoxinA *on page 26*

◆ **Botulinum Toxin Type A** *see* IncobotulinumtoxinA *on page 1064*

◆ **Botulinum Toxin Type A** *see* OnabotulinumtoxinA *on page 1508*

◆ **Botulinum Toxin Type B** *see* RimabotulinumtoxinB *on page 1820*

Botulism Immune Globulin (Intravenous-Human)

(BOT yoo lism i MYUN GLOB you lin, in tra VEE nus, YU man)

Brand Names: U.S. BabyBIG®

Index Terms BIG-IV

Pharmacologic Category Blood Product Derivative; Immune Globulin

Use Treatment of infant botulism caused by toxin type A or B

Pregnancy Considerations Botulism immune globulin is only indicated for use in neonates.

Prescribing and Access Restrictions Access to botulism immune globulin is restricted through the Infant Botulism Treatment and Prevention Program (IBTPP). Healthcare providers must contact the IBTPP on-call physician at (510) 231-7600 to review treatment indications and to obtain the medication. For more information, refer to http://www.infantbotulism.org or contact IBTPP@infantbotulism.org.

Contraindications Hypersensitivity to human immune globulin preparations or any component of the formulation; selective immunoglobulin A deficiency

Warnings/Precautions Hypersensitivity and anaphylactic reactions can occur; immediate treatment (including epinephrine 1:1000) should be available. Aseptic meningitis syndrome (AMS) has been reported with intravenous immune globulin administration (rare); may occur with high doses (≥2 g/kg). Immune globulin intravenous (IGIV) has been associated with antiglobulin hemolysis; monitor for signs of hemolytic anemia. Hyperproteinemia, increased serum viscosity, and hyponatremia may occur following administration of IGIV products; distinguish hyponatremia from pseudohyponatremia to prevent volume depletion, a further increase in serum viscosity, and a higher risk of thrombotic events. These adverse events have not reported with botulism immune globulin. Thrombotic events have been reported with administration of IGIV; use with caution in patients with a history of atherosclerosis or cardiovascular and/or thrombotic risk factors or patients with known/suspected hyperviscosity. Consider a baseline assessment of blood viscosity in patients at risk for hyperviscosity. Infuse at lowest practical rate in patients at risk for thrombotic events. Monitor for transfusion-related acute lung injury (TRALI); noncardiogenic pulmonary edema has been reported with IGIV use. TRALI is characterized by severe respiratory distress, pulmonary edema, hypoxemia, and fever in the presence of normal left ventricular function. Usually occurs within 1-6 hours after infusion.

Acute renal dysfunction (increased serum creatinine, oliguria, acute renal failure) can rarely occur; usually within 7 days of use (more likely with products stabilized with sucrose). Use with caution in patients with renal disease, diabetes mellitus, volume depletion, sepsis, paraproteinemia, and nephrotoxic medications due to risk of renal dysfunction. In patients at risk of renal dysfunction, the rate of infusion and concentration of solution should be minimized. Patients should not be volume depleted prior to therapy. Product of human plasma; may potentially contain infectious agents which could transmit disease. Screening of donors, as well as testing and/or inactivation or removal of certain viruses, reduces the risk. Infections thought to be transmitted by this product should be reported to the manufacturer. For I.V. infusion only; do not exceed recommended rate of administration. Not indicated for use in adults. Safety and efficacy established for infants <1 year of age; not indicated for children ≥1 year of age.

Adverse Reactions Percentages reported in open-label study except where otherwise noted; may reflect pathophysiology of infant botulism.

>10%:
- Cardiovascular: Blood pressure increased (transient, 75%), pallor (28%), edema (18%); blood pressure decreased (transient, 16%), cardiac murmur (15%)
- Central nervous system: Irritability (41%), pyrexia (17%), body temperature decreased (16%)
- Dermatologic: Contact dermatitis (24%), erythematous rash (22%, reported as 14% vs 8% in placebo-controlled study)
- Gastrointestinal: Dysphagia (65%), loose stools (25%), vomiting (20%), abdominal distension (11%)
- Otic: Otitis media (11%, reported in placebo-controlled study)
- Respiratory: Atelectasis (39%), rhonchi (34%), nasal congestion (18%), oxygen saturation decreased (17%), cough (13%), rales (13%)

1% to 10%:
- Cardiovascular: Tachycardia (7%), peripheral coldness (7%)
- Central nervous system: Agitation (10%)
- Endocrine & metabolic: Dehydration (10%), hyponatremia (6%), metabolic acidosis (5%)
- Hematologic: Hemoglobin decreased (9%), anemia (5%)
- Local: Injection site reaction (7%), injection site erythema (5%)
- Renal: Neurogenic bladder
- Respiratory: Breath sounds decreased (10%), stridor (9%), lower respiratory tract infection (8%), dyspnea (6%), tachypnea (5%)
- Miscellaneous: Oral candidiasis (8%), intubation (5%), infusion rate reactions (<5%, includes chills, back pain, fever, muscle cramps, nausea, vomiting, wheezing)

Drug Interactions

Metabolism/Transport Effects None known.

Avoid Concomitant Use There are no known interactions where it is recommended to avoid concomitant use.

Increased Effect/Toxicity There are no known significant interactions involving an increase in effect.

Decreased Effect

Botulism Immune Globulin (Intravenous-Human) may decrease the levels/effects of: Vaccines (Live)

Preparation for Administration Reconstitute with SWFI 2 mL. Swirl gently to wet powder; do not shake. Allow ~30 minutes for powder to dissolve.

Storage/Stability Prior to reconstitution, store between 2°C to 8°C (36°F to 46°F). Infusion should begin within 2 hours of reconstitution and be completed within 4 hours of reconstitution.

Mechanism of Action BIG-IV is purified immunoglobulin derived from the plasma of adults immunized with botulinum toxoid types A and B. BIG-IV provides antibodies to neutralize circulating toxins.

Pharmacodynamics/Kinetics

Duration: Protective neutralizing antibody levels: 6 months

Half-life elimination: 28 days

Dosage I.V.: Infants <1 year: Infant botulism: 50 mg/kg as a single dose as soon as diagnosis of infant botulism is made. **Note:** The recommended dose may vary with each manufactured sublot; verify dose with the prescribing information and guidance provided with each product shipment.

Dosage adjustment for toxicity: *Infusion reactions:* Slow the infusion rate or temporarily interrupt infusion for minor reaction (ie, flushing). Discontinue infusion and administer epinephrine for anaphylactic reaction or significant hypotension.

Dosage adjustment in renal impairment: Use with caution; the rate of infusion and concentration of solution should be minimized in patients with renal impairment or those at risk for renal dysfunction.

Dosage adjustment in hepatic impairment: No dosage adjustment provided in manufacturer's labeling.

Administration For I.V. infusion only. Begin infusion at 25 mg/kg/hour for the first 15 minutes; if well tolerated, may increase to a maximum rate of 50 mg/kg/hour. Infuse using low volume tubing and an infusion pump with an in-line or syringe tip 18 micron filter. Infuse through a separate I.V. line (preferred). Infusion should take 67.5 minutes at the recommended rates and should be concluded within 4 hours of reconstitution (unless infusion temporarily interrupted for adverse reaction). Do not administer if solution is turbid. Infusion should be slowed or temporarily interrupted for minor side effects; discontinue in case of hypotension or anaphylaxis. Epinephrine should be available for the treatment of acute allergic reaction.

Monitoring Parameters Renal function (BUN, serum creatinine, urinary output); vital signs (continuously during infusion); aseptic meningitis syndrome (may occur hours to days following IGIV therapy); signs of relapse (may occur up to 1 month following recovery)

Dosage Forms Excipient information presented when available (limited, particularly for generics); consult specific product labeling.

Injection, powder for reconstitution [preservative free]:

BabyBIG®: ~100 mg [contains albumin (human), sucrose; supplied with diluent]

- ◆ Boudreaux's® Butt Paste [OTC] *see* Zinc Oxide *on page 2230*
- ◆ Bovine Lung Surfactant *see* Beractant *on page 245*
- ◆ Bovine Lung Surfactant *see* Calfactant *on page 325*
- ◆ BP 8 Cough *see* Guaifenesin, Pseudoephedrine, and Dextromethorphan *on page 979*
- ◆ BP 10-1 *see* Sulfur and Sulfacetamide *on page 1966*
- ◆ BP Cleansing Wash *see* Sulfur and Sulfacetamide *on page 1966*
- ◆ BProtected Pedia Iron [OTC] *see* Ferrous Sulfate *on page 854*
- ◆ BProtected Vitamin C [OTC] *see* Ascorbic Acid *on page 172*
- ◆ BRAF(V600E) Kinase Inhibitor RO5185426 *see* Vemurafenib *on page 2176*
- ◆ Bravelle *see* Urofollitropin *on page 2141*
- ◆ Bravelle® (Can) *see* Urofollitropin *on page 2141*
- ◆ Brentuximab *see* Brentuximab Vedotin *on page 278*

Brentuximab Vedotin (bren TUX i mab ve DOE tin)

Brand Names: U.S. Adcetris

Brand Names: Canada Adcetris™

Index Terms Anti-CD30 ADC SGN-35; Anti-CD30 Antibody-Drug Conjugate SGN-35; Antibody-Drug Conjugate SGN-35; Brentuximab; SGN-35

Pharmacologic Category Antineoplastic Agent, Monoclonal Antibody

Use Treatment of Hodgkin lymphoma after failure of at least 2 prior chemotherapy regimens (in patients ineligible for transplant) or after stem cell transplant failure; treatment of systemic anaplastic large cell lymphoma (sALCL) after failure of at least 1 prior chemotherapy regimen

Pregnancy Risk Factor D

Pregnancy Considerations Embryo-fetal toxicities and fetal malformations were noted in animal reproduction studies. Based on the mechanism of action, may cause fetal harm if administered to a pregnant woman.

Breast-Feeding Considerations It is not known if brentuximab vedotin is excreted in breast milk. According to the manufacturer, the decision to continue or discontinue breast-feeding during therapy should take into account the risk of exposure to the infant and the benefits of treatment to the mother.

Contraindications U.S. labeling: Concurrent use with bleomycin

Canadian labeling: Hypersensitivity to brentuximab or any component of the formulation; concurrent use with bleomycin; patients who have or have history of progressive multifocal leukoencephalopathy

Warnings/Precautions Hazardous agent - use appropriate precautions for handling and disposal (meets NIOSH, 2012 criteria).

[U.S. Boxed Warning]: Cases of PML and death due to JC virus infection have been reported. Immunosuppression due to prior chemotherapy treatments or underlying disease may also contribute to PML development. New-onset signs/symptoms of central nervous system abnormalities (eg, changes in mood, memory, cognition, motor incoordination and/or weakness, speech and/or visual disturbances) should receive prompt evaluation with neurology consultation, brain MRI, and lumbar puncture or brain biopsy. Withhold treatment with new-onset symptoms suggestive of PML; discontinue if diagnosis of PML is confirmed.

Peripheral neuropathy is common and is generally cumulative; usually sensory neuropathy, although motor neuropathy has also been observed; neuropathy completely resolved in nearly half of patients; almost one-third had partial improvement. Monitor for symptoms of neuropathy; dose interruption, reduction or discontinuation may be recommended.

Neutropenia, thrombocytopenia and anemia may occur; neutropenia may be prolonged (≥1 week); monitor blood counts; may require dose interruption, reduction or discontinuation. Infusion reactions, including anaphylaxis have been reported; monitor during infusion. For anaphylaxis, immediately and permanently discontinue and administer appropriate medical intervention. For infusion-related reaction, interrupt infusion and administer appropriate medical intervention; premedicate for subsequent infusions (with acetaminophen, an antihistamine, and/or a corticosteroid).

Due to the risk for pulmonary injury, concurrent use with bleomycin is contraindicated. In a study comparing brentuximab combined with ABVD (doxorubicin, bleomycin, vinblastine, and dacarbazine) to brentuximab combined with AVD (doxorubicin, vinblastine, and dacarbazine), the occurrence of pulmonary toxicity was 40% in the brentuximab/ABVD group compared to a literature-based frequency of ≤25% for other bleomycin-containing regimens. There were no cases of pulmonary toxicity documented with brentuximab in combination with AVD. Pulmonary symptoms/toxicities reported with brentuximab in combination with ABVD consisted of cough, dyspnea, and interstitial infiltration/inflammation; most patients responded to corticosteroids.

Stevens-Johnson syndrome has been observed; discontinue and administer appropriate medical intervention. Tumor lysis syndrome (TLS) may occur; risk of TLS is higher in patients with a high tumor burden or with rapid tumor proliferation; monitor closely. A component of brentuximab vedotin, the microtubule-disrupting agent MMAE is excreted renally and hepatically; the impact of renal or hepatic impairment on MMAE pharmacokinetics is undetermined.

Adverse Reactions

>10%:

Cardiovascular: Peripheral edema (4% to 16%)

Central nervous system: Fatigue (41% to 49%), fever (29% to 38%), pain (7% to 28%), headache (16% to 19%), insomnia (14% to 16%), dizziness (11% to 16%), chills (12% to 13%), anxiety (7% to 11%)

Dermatologic: Rash (27% to 31%), pruritus (17% to 19%), alopecia (13% to 14%)

Gastrointestinal: Nausea (38% to 42%), diarrhea (29% to 36%), abdominal pain (9% to 25%), vomiting (17% to 22%), constipation (16% to 19%), appetite decreased (11% to 16%), weight loss (6% to 12%)

Hematologic: Neutropenia (54% to 55%; grade 4: 6% to 9%); anemia (33% to 52%; grade 4: ≤2%), thrombocytopenia (16% to 28%; grade 4: 2% to 5%)

Neuromuscular & skeletal: Peripheral sensory neuropathy (52% to 53%; grade 3: 8% to 10%), arthralgia (9% to 19%), myalgia (16% to 17%), peripheral motor neuropathy (7% to 16%; grade 3: 3% to 4%), back pain (10% to 14%)

Respiratory: Upper respiratory tract infection (12% to 47%), cough (17% to 25%), dyspnea (13% to 19%), oropharyngeal pain (9% to 11%)

Miscellaneous: Infusion reactions (grades 1/2: 12%), night sweats (9% to 12%), lymphadenopathy (10% to 11%)

1% to 10%:

Cardiovascular: Supraventricular arrhythmia

Dermatologic: Dry skin

Genitourinary: Urinary tract infection

Neuromuscular & skeletal: Limb pain, muscle spasms

Renal: Pyelonephritis

Respiratory: Pneumonitis, pneumothorax, pulmonary embolism

Miscellaneous: Antibrentuximab antibody formation, septic shock

<1% (Limited to important or life-threatening): Anaphylaxis, progressive multifocal leukoencephalopathy (PML), Stevens-Johnson syndrome, tachycardia, tumor lysis syndrome

Drug Interactions

Metabolism/Transport Effects Substrate of CYP3A4 (minor); **Note:** Assignment of Major/Minor substrate status based on clinically relevant drug interaction potential

Avoid Concomitant Use

Avoid concomitant use of Brentuximab Vedotin with any of the following: BCG; Bleomycin; Natalizumab; Pimecrolimus; Tacrolimus (Topical); Tofacitinib; Vaccines (Live)

Increased Effect/Toxicity

Brentuximab Vedotin may increase the levels/effects of: Bleomycin; Leflunomide; Natalizumab; Tofacitinib; Vaccines (Live); Vitamin K Antagonists

The levels/effects of Brentuximab Vedotin may be increased by: CYP3A4 Inhibitors (Strong); Denosumab; Pimecrolimus; Roflumilast; Tacrolimus (Topical); Trastuzumab

Decreased Effect

Brentuximab Vedotin may decrease the levels/effects of: BCG; Cardiac Glycosides; Coccidioidin Skin Test; Sipuleucel-T; Vaccines (Inactivated); Vaccines (Live); Vitamin K Antagonists

The levels/effects of Brentuximab Vedotin may be decreased by: CYP3A4 Inducers (Strong); Echinacea

Preparation for Administration Hazardous agent: Use appropriate precautions for handling and disposal (meets NIOSH, 2012 criteria). Reconstitute each 50 mg vial with 10.5 mL sterile water for injection (SWFI), resulting in a concentration of 5 mg/mL. Direct SWFI toward the vial wall; do not direct toward the cake or powder. Swirl gently to dissolve, do not shake. Reconstituted solution should be clear to slightly opalescent without visible particles. Further dilute in at least 100 mL of either NS, D_5W, or lactated Ringer's to a final concentration of 0.4 to 1.8 mg/mL; gently invert bag to mix. Do not mix with other medications. Use within 24 hours of initial reconstitution.

Storage/Stability Store intact vials refrigerated at 2°C to 8°C (36°F to 46°F) in the original carton. Protect from light. Reconstituted solution may be stored refrigerated for up to 24 hours; do not freeze. Solutions diluted for infusion may be stored for 24 hours refrigerated (do not freeze); use within 24 hours of initial reconstitution.

Mechanism of Action Brentuximab vedotin is an antibody drug conjugate (ADC) directed at CD30 consisting of 3 components: 1) a CD30-specific chimeric IgG1 antibody cAC10; 2) a microtubule-disrupting agent, monomethylauristatin E (MMAE); and 3) a protease cleavable dipeptide linker (which covalently conjugates MMAE to cAC10). The conjugate binds to cells which express CD30, and forms a complex which is internalized within the cell and releases MMAE. MMAE binds to the tubules and disrupts the cellular microtubule network, inducing cell cycle arrest (G2/M phase) and apoptosis.

Pharmacodynamics/Kinetics

Distribution: V_{dss}: ADC: 6-10 L

Metabolism: MMAE: Minimal, primarily via oxidation by CYP3A4/5

Half-life elimination: Terminal: ADC: ~4-6 days

Time to peak: ADC: At end of infusion; MMAE: ~1-3 days

Excretion: MMAE: Feces (~72%, primarily unchanged); urine

Dosage I.V.: Adults: **Note:** For patients weighing >100 kg, dose should be calculated using a weight of 100 kg.

Hodgkin lymphoma, refractory: 1.8 mg/kg (maximum dose: 180 mg) every 3 weeks, continue until disease progression, unacceptable toxicities, or a maximum of 16 cycles

Systemic anaplastic large cell lymphoma (sALCL), refractory: 1.8 mg/kg (maximum dose: 180 mg) every 3 weeks, continue until disease progression, unacceptable toxicities, or a maximum of 16 cycles

Dosage adjustment for toxicity:

Hematologic toxicity:

Grade 3 or 4 neutropenia: Withhold treatment until resolves to baseline or ≤grade 2, consider growth factor support in subsequent cycles.

Recurrent grade 4 neutropenia (despite the use of growth factor support): Consider reducing the dose to 1.2 mg/kg or discontinuing treatment

Grade 3 or 4 thrombocytopenia (Canadian labeling): Monitor closely; dose delays or platelet transfusions may be considered.

Nonhematologic toxicities:

Anaphylaxis: Discontinue immediately and permanently

Infusion reaction: Interrupt infusion and administer appropriate medical intervention. Premedicate subsequent infusions with acetaminophen, an antihistamine, and/or a corticosteroid.

Peripheral neuropathy, new or worsening grade 2 or 3: Withhold treatment until improves or returns to grade 1 or baseline; then resume with dose reduced to 1.2 mg/kg

Peripheral neuropathy, grade 4: Discontinue treatment

Progressive multifocal leukoencephalopathy (PML): Withhold treatment with new-onset symptoms suggestive of PML; discontinue if PML diagnosis confirmed

Stevens-Johnson syndrome: Discontinue and administer appropriate medical intervention

Dosage adjustment in renal impairment: No dosage adjustment provided in the manufacturer's labeling; active drug (MMAE) pharmacokinetics have not been determined in renal impairment.

Dosage adjustment in hepatic impairment: No dosage adjustment provided in the manufacturer's labeling; active drug (MMAE) pharmacokinetics have not been determined in hepatic impairment.

Administration Infuse over 30 minutes. Do not administer as I.V. push or bolus; do not mix or infuse with other medications. Hazardous agent; use appropriate precautions for handling and disposal (meets NIOSH, 2012 criteria).

Monitoring Parameters CBC with differential prior to each dose (more frequently if clinically indicated). Monitor for infusion reaction, tumor lysis syndrome, and for signs of neuropathy (hypoesthesia, hyperesthesia, paresthesia, discomfort, burning sensation, or neuropathic pain or weakness).

Dosage Forms Excipient information presented when available (limited, particularly for generics); consult specific product labeling.

Solution Reconstituted, Intravenous [preservative free]:

Adcetris: 50 mg (1 ea) [contains polysorbate 80]

◆ **Breo Ellipta** *see* Fluticasone and Vilanterol *on page 899*

◆ **Brethaire** *see* Terbutaline *on page 2019*

◆ **Brethine** *see* Terbutaline *on page 2019*

◆ **Brevibloc** *see* Esmolol *on page 748*

◆ **Brevibloc® (Can)** *see* Esmolol *on page 748*

◆ **Brevibloc in NaCl** *see* Esmolol *on page 748*

◆ **Brevibloc® Premixed (Can)** *see* Esmolol *on page 748*

◆ **Brevicon** *see* Ethinyl Estradiol and Norethindrone *on page 793*

◆ **Brevicon 0.5/35 (Can)** *see* Ethinyl Estradiol and Norethindrone *on page 793*

◆ **Brevicon 1/35 (Can)** *see* Ethinyl Estradiol and Norethindrone *on page 793*

◆ **Brevital® (Can)** *see* Methohexital *on page 1324*

◆ **Brevital Sodium** *see* Methohexital *on page 1324*

◆ **Bricanyl** *see* Terbutaline *on page 2019*

◆ **Bricanyl® Turbuhaler® (Can)** *see* Terbutaline *on page 2019*

◆ **Briellyn** *see* Ethinyl Estradiol and Norethindrone *on page 793*

◆ **Brilinta** *see* Ticagrelor *on page 2055*

◆ **Brilinta™ (Can)** *see* Ticagrelor *on page 2055*

Brimonidine (Ophthalmic) (bri MOE ni deen)

Brand Names: Canada Alphagan®; Apo-Brimonidine P®; Apo-Brimonidine®; PMS-Brimonidine Tartrate; ratio-Brimonidine; Sandoz-Brimonidine

Index Terms Brimonidine Tartrate

Pharmacologic Category $Alpha_2$ Agonist, Ophthalmic; Ophthalmic Agent, Antiglaucoma

Use Lowering of intraocular pressure (IOP) in patients with open-angle glaucoma or ocular hypertension

Pregnancy Risk Factor B

Dosage Ophthalmic: Children ≥2 years and Adults: Glaucoma, ocular hypertension: Instill 1 drop in affected eye(s) 3 times/day (approximately every 8 hours)

Additional Information Complete prescribing information should be consulted for additional detail.

Dosage Forms Excipient information presented when available (limited, particularly for generics); consult specific product labeling.

Solution, Ophthalmic, as tartrate:

Generic: 0.2% (5 mL)

Brimonidine (Topical) (bri MOE ni deen)

Brand Names: U.S. Mirvaso

Index Terms Brimonidine Tartrate

Pharmacologic Category $Alpha_2$-Adrenergic Agonist

Use Rosacea: Topical treatment of persistent (nontransient) facial erythema of rosacea in adults

Pregnancy Risk Factor B

Dosage Rosacea: Adults: Topical: Apply a pea-size amount once daily as a thin layer across the entire face covering the central forehead, each cheek, nose, and chin. Do not apply to eyes or lips.

Additional Information Complete prescribing information should be consulted for additional detail.

Dosage Forms Excipient information presented when available (limited, particularly for generics); consult specific product labeling.

Gel, External:

Mirvaso: 0.33% (30 g) [contains methylparaben, propylene glycol]

Brimonidine and Timolol

(bri MOE ni deen & TIM oh lol)

Brand Names: U.S. Combigan®

Brand Names: Canada Combigan®

Index Terms Brimonidine Tartrate and Timolol Maleate; Timolol and Brimonidine

Pharmacologic Category Alpha$_2$ Agonist, Ophthalmic; Beta-Blocker, Nonselective; Ophthalmic Agent, Antiglaucoma

Use Reduction of intraocular pressure (IOP) in patients with glaucoma or ocular hypertension

Pregnancy Risk Factor C

Dosage Ophthalmic: Children ≥2 years and Adults: Instill 1 drop into affected eye(s) twice daily

Note: In the Canadian labeling, use in children (at any age) is not recommended

Additional Information Complete prescribing information should be consulted for additional detail.

Dosage Forms Excipient information presented when available (limited, particularly for generics); consult specific product labeling.

Solution, ophthalmic [drops]:

Combigan®: Brimonidine tartrate 0.2% and timolol 0.5% (5 mL,10 mL) [contains benzalkonium chloride]

Dosage Forms: Canada Excipient information presented when available (limited, particularly for generics); consult specific product labeling.

Solution, ophthalmic [drops]:

Combigan®: Brimonidine tartrate 0.2% and timolol maleate 0.5% (2.5 mL, 5 mL,10 mL) [contains benzalkonium chloride]

◆ **Brimonidine Tartrate** *see* Brimonidine (Ophthalmic) *on page* 280

◆ **Brimonidine Tartrate** *see* Brimonidine (Topical) *on page* 280

◆ **Brimonidine Tartrate and Timolol Maleate** *see* Brimonidine and Timolol *on page* 281

◆ **Brintellix** *see* Vortioxetine *on page* 2208

Brinzolamide

(brin ZOH la mide)

Brand Names: U.S. Azopt

Brand Names: Canada Azopt®

Pharmacologic Category Carbonic Anhydrase Inhibitor (Ophthalmic); Ophthalmic Agent, Antiglaucoma

Use Treatment of elevated intraocular pressure in patients with ocular hypertension or open-angle glaucoma

Pregnancy Risk Factor C

Dosage Ophthalmic: Adults: Ocular hypertension or open-angle glaucoma: Instill 1 drop in affected eye(s) 3 times/day

Dosage adjustment in renal impairment: Severe renal impairment (Cl_{cr} <30 mL/minute): Use is not recommended (has not been studied; brinzolamide and metabolite are excreted predominately by the kidney).

Dosage adjustment in hepatic impairment: No dosage adjustment provided in manufacturer's labeling.

Additional Information Complete prescribing information should be consulted for additional detail.

Dosage Forms Excipient information presented when available (limited, particularly for generics); consult specific product labeling.

Suspension, Ophthalmic:

Azopt: 1% (10 mL, 15 mL)

◆ **Brisdelle** *see* PARoxetine *on page* 1575

◆ **British Anti-Lewisite** *see* Dimercaprol *on page* 617

◆ **BRL 43694** *see* Granisetron *on page* 972

◆ **Bromday [DSC]** *see* Bromfenac *on page* 281

Bromfenac

(BROME fen ak)

Brand Names: U.S. Bromday [DSC]; Prolensa

Index Terms Bromfenac Sodium

Pharmacologic Category Nonsteroidal Anti-inflammatory Drug (NSAID), Ophthalmic

Use Treatment of postoperative inflammation and reduction in ocular pain following cataract removal

Pregnancy Risk Factor C

Dosage Ophthalmic (Bromday®, Prolensa™): Adults: Instill 1 drop into affected eye(s) once daily beginning 1 day prior to surgery and continuing on the day of surgery and for 2 weeks postoperatively

Dosage adjustment in renal impairment: No dosage adjustment provided in manufacturer's labeling. However, dosage adjustment unlikely due to low systemic absorption.

Dosage adjustment in hepatic impairment: No dosage adjustment provided in manufacturer's labeling. However, dosage adjustment unlikely due to low systemic absorption.

Additional Information Complete prescribing information should be consulted for additional detail.

Dosage Forms Excipient information presented when available (limited, particularly for generics); consult specific product labeling. [DSC] = Discontinued product

Solution, Ophthalmic:

Bromday: 0.09% (1.7 mL [DSC]) [contains benzalkonium chloride, edetate disodium, polysorbate 80, sodium sulfite]

Prolensa: 0.07% (1.6 mL, 3 mL) [contains benzalkonium chloride, edetate disodium, sodium sulfite]

Generic: 0.09% (1.7 mL, 2.5 mL, 5 mL)

◆ **Bromfenac Sodium** *see* Bromfenac *on page* 281

Bromocriptine

(broe moe KRIP teen)

Brand Names: U.S. Cycloset; Parlodel

Brand Names: Canada Dom-Bromocriptine; PMS-Bromocriptine

Index Terms Bromocriptine Mesylate; Cycloset®

Pharmacologic Category Anti-Parkinson's Agent, Dopamine Agonist; Antidiabetic Agent, Dopamine Agonist; Ergot Derivative

Additional Appendix Information

Antiparkinsonian Agents *on page* 2289

Oral Antidiabetic Agents Comparison Table *on page* 2312

Use Treatment of hyperprolactinemia associated with amenorrhea with or without galactorrhea, infertility, or hypogonadism; treatment of prolactin-secreting adenomas; treatment of acromegaly; treatment of Parkinson's disease

Cycloset®: Management of type 2 diabetes mellitus (noninsulin dependent, NIDDM) as an adjunct to diet and exercise

Unlabeled Use Neuroleptic malignant syndrome

Pregnancy Risk Factor B

Dosage Oral:

Children: Hyperprolactinemia:

11-15 years (based on limited information): Initial: 1.25-2.5 mg daily; dosage may be increased as tolerated to achieve a therapeutic response (range: 2.5-10 mg daily).

≥16 years: Refer to adult dosing

Adults:

Acromegaly: Initial: 1.25-2.5 mg daily increasing by 1.25-2.5 mg daily as necessary every 3-7 days; usual dose: 20-30 mg/day (maximum: 100 mg/day)

Hyperprolactinemia: Initial: 1.25-2.5 mg/day; may be increased by 2.5 mg/day as tolerated every 2-7 days until optimal response (range: 2.5-15 mg/day)

Parkinsonism: 1.25 mg twice daily, increased by 2.5 mg/day in 2- to 4-week intervals as needed (maximum: 100 mg/day)

Type 2 diabetes (Cycloset®): Initial: 0.8 mg once daily; may increase at weekly intervals in 0.8 mg increments as tolerated; usual dose: 1.6-4.8 mg/day (maximum: 4.8 mg/day)

Neuroleptic malignant syndrome (unlabeled use): 2.5 mg (orally or via gastric tube) every 8-12 hours, increased to a maximum of 45 mg/day, if needed; continue therapy until NMS is controlled, then taper slowly (Gortney, 2009; Strawn, 2007)

Dosage adjustment in renal impairment: No dosage adjustment provided in manufacturer's labeling (has not been studied).

Dosage adjustment in hepatic impairment: No dosage adjustment provided in manufacturer's labeling. However, adjustment may be necessary due to extensive hepatic metabolism.

Additional Information Complete prescribing information should be consulted for additional detail.

Dosage Forms Excipient information presented when available (limited, particularly for generics); consult specific product labeling.

Capsule, Oral:

Parlodel: 5 mg

Generic: 5 mg

Tablet, Oral:

Cycloset: 0.8 mg

Parlodel: 2.5 mg [scored]

Generic: 2.5 mg

◆ **Bromocriptine Mesylate** *see* Bromocriptine *on page* 281

Brompheniramine (brome fen IR a meen)

Brand Names: U.S. J-Tan PD [OTC]; Respa-BR

Index Terms Brompheniramine Maleate; Brompheniramine Tannate

Pharmacologic Category Alkylamine Derivative; Histamine H_1 Antagonist; Histamine H_1 Antagonist, First Generation

Additional Appendix Information

Beers Criteria – Potentially Inappropriate Medications for Geriatrics *on page* 2368

Use Symptomatic relief of perennial and seasonal allergic rhinitis, vasomotor rhinitis, and other respiratory allergies

Pregnancy Risk Factor C

Dosage Oral: Allergic rhinitis, allergic symptoms, vasomotor rhinitis:

Children 2 to <6 years (J-Tan PD): 1 mg (1 mL) every 4-6 hours (maximum: 6 mg [6 mL]/24 hours)

Children 6-12 years:

J-Tan PD: 2 mg (2 mL) every 4-6 hours (maximum: 12 mg [12 mL]/24 hours)

LoHist-12: One tablet every 12 hours (maximum: 2 tablets/day)

Children >12 years (Bromax, LoHist-12): Refer to adult dosing

Adults:

Bromax: One tablet twice daily

LoHist-12: 1-2 tablets every 12 hours (maximum: 4 tablets/day)

Additional Information Complete prescribing information should be consulted for additional detail.

Dosage Forms Excipient information presented when available (limited, particularly for generics); consult specific product labeling.

Liquid, Oral, as maleate:

J-Tan PD: 1 mg/mL (30 mL) [alcohol free, dye free, sugar free; contains propylene glycol, saccharin sodium; strawberry-banana flavor]

Tablet Extended Release 12 Hour, Oral, as maleate:

Respa-BR: 11 mg [dye free]

◆ **Brompheniramine Maleate** *see* Brompheniramine *on page* 282

◆ **Brompheniramine Tannate** *see* Brompheniramine *on page* 282

◆ **Broncho Saline [OTC]** *see* Sodium Chloride *on page* 1914

◆ **Brovana** *see* Arformoterol *on page* 160

◆ **BSF208075** *see* Ambrisentan *on page* 94

◆ **BTK inhibitor PCI-32765** *see* Ibrutinib *on page* 1030

◆ **BTX-A** *see* OnabotulinumtoxinA *on page* 1508

◆ **B-type Natriuretic Peptide (Human)** *see* Nesiritide *on page* 1443

◆ **Buckleys Chest Congestion [OTC]** *see* GuaiFENesin *on page* 974

◆ **Budeprion SR** *see* BuPROPion *on page* 296

Budesonide (Systemic) (byoo DES oh nide)

Brand Names: U.S. Entocort EC; Pulmicort; Pulmicort Flexhaler; Uceris

Brand Names: Canada Entocort®; Pulmicort® Turbuhaler®

Index Terms Uceris™

Pharmacologic Category Corticosteroid, Inhalant (Oral); Corticosteroid, Systemic

Additional Appendix Information

Inhaled Corticosteroids *on page* 2298

Use

Nebulization: Maintenance and prophylactic treatment of asthma

Oral capsule: Treatment of active Crohn's disease (mild-to-moderate) involving the ileum and/or ascending colon; maintenance of remission (for up to 3 months) of Crohn's disease (mild-to-moderate) involving the ileum and/or ascending colon

Oral inhalation: Maintenance and prophylactic treatment of asthma; includes patients who require oral corticosteroids and those who may benefit from systemic dose reduction/elimination

Oral tablet: Induction of remission in patients with active ulcerative colitis (mild-to-moderate)

Pregnancy Risk Factor C (capsule, tablet)/B (inhalation)

Pregnancy Considerations Adverse events have been observed with corticosteroids in animal reproduction studies. Some studies have shown an association between first trimester systemic corticosteroid use and oral clefts (Park-Wyllie, 2000; Pradat, 2003). Systemic corticosteroids may also influence fetal growth (decreased birth weight); however, information is conflicting (Lunghi, 2010). Hypoadrenalism may occur in newborns following maternal use of corticosteroids in pregnancy; monitor. When systemic corticosteroids are needed in pregnancy, it is generally recommended to use the lowest effective dose for the shortest duration of time, avoiding high doses during the first trimester (Leachman, 2006; Lunghi, 2010). Budesonide may be used for the induction of remission in pregnant women with inflammatory bowel disease (Habal, 2012).

Based on available data, an overall increased risk of congenital malformations or a decrease in fetal growth has not been associated with maternal use of inhaled corticosteroids during pregnancy (Bakhireva, 2005; NAEPP, 2005; Namazy, 2004). In addition, studies of pregnant women specifically using inhaled budesonide have not demonstrated an increased risk of congenital abnormalities. Uncontrolled asthma is associated with adverse events on pregnancy (increased risk of perinatal mortality, pre-eclampsia, preterm birth, low birth weight infants). Inhaled corticosteroids are recommended for the treatment of asthma during pregnancy; budesonide is preferred (ACOG, 2008; NAEPP, 2005).

Breast-Feeding Considerations Following use of the powder for oral inhalation, ~0.3% to 1% of the maternal dose was found in breast milk. The maximum concentration appeared within 45 minutes of dosing. Plasma budesonide levels obtained from infants ~90 minutes after breast-feeding (~140 minutes after maternal dose) were below the limit of quantification. Concentrations of budesonide in breast milk are expected to be higher following administration of oral capsules/tablets than after an inhaled dose.

Due to the potential for serious adverse reactions in the nursing infant, the manufacturers of the oral tablets and capsules recommend a decision be made whether to discontinue nursing or to discontinue the drug, taking into account the importance of treatment to the mother. If there is concern about exposure to the infant, some guidelines recommend waiting 4 hours after the maternal dose of an oral systemic corticosteroid before breast-feeding in order to decrease potential exposure to the nursing infant (based on a study using prednisolone) (Habal, 2012; Ost, 1985).

According to the manufacturer of the product for inhalation, the decision to continue or discontinue breast-feeding during therapy should take into account the risk of minimal exposure to the infant and the benefits of breast-feeding to the mother. The use of inhaled corticosteroids is not considered a contraindication to breast-feeding (NAEPP, 2005).

Contraindications Hypersensitivity to budesonide or any component of the formulation; primary treatment of status asthmaticus, acute episodes of asthma; not for relief of acute bronchospasm

Canadian labeling: Additional contraindications (not in U.S. labeling): Moderate-to-severe bronchiectasis, pulmonary tuberculosis (active or quiescent), untreated respiratory infection (bacterial, fungal, or viral)

Warnings/Precautions May cause hypercorticism or suppression of hypothalamic-pituitary-adrenal (HPA) axis, particularly in younger children, in patients receiving high doses for prolonged periods, or with concomitant CYP3A4 inhibitor use. HPA axis suppression may lead to adrenal crisis. Withdrawal and discontinuation of a corticosteroid should be done slowly and carefully. Particular care is required when patients are transferred from systemic corticosteroids to inhaled products or corticosteroids with lower systemic effect due to possible adrenal insufficiency or withdrawal from steroids, including an increase in allergic symptoms. Patients receiving >20 mg per day of prednisone (or equivalent) may be most susceptible. Fatalities have occurred due to adrenal insufficiency in asthmatic patients during and after transfer from systemic corticosteroids to aerosol steroids; aerosol steroids do not provide the systemic steroid needed to treat patients having trauma, surgery, or infections. Do not use this product to transfer patients directly from oral corticosteroid therapy.

Bronchospasm may occur with wheezing after inhalation; if this occurs stop steroid and treat with a fast-acting bronchodilator (eg, albuterol). Supplemental steroids (oral or parenteral) may be needed during stress or severe asthma attacks. Not to be used in status asthmaticus or for the relief of acute bronchospasm. Acute myopathy has been reported with high-dose corticosteroids, usually in patients with neuromuscular transmission disorders; may involve ocular and/or respiratory muscles; monitor creatine kinase; recovery may be delayed. Corticosteroid use may cause psychiatric disturbances, including depression, euphoria, insomnia, mood swings, and personality changes. Pre-existing psychiatric conditions may be exacerbated by corticosteroid use. Prolonged use of corticosteroids may also increase the incidence of secondary infection, mask acute infection (including fungal infections), prolong or exacerbate viral infections, or limit response to vaccines. Exposure to chickenpox should be avoided; corticosteroids should not be used to treat ocular herpes simplex. Corticosteroids should not be used for viral hepatitis. Close observation is required in patients with latent tuberculosis and/or TB reactivity; restrict use in active TB (only in conjunction with antituberculosis treatment). *Candida albicans* infections may occur in the mouth and pharynx; rinsing (and spitting) with water after inhaler use may decrease risk. Prolonged treatment with corticosteroids has been associated with the development of Kaposi's sarcoma (case reports); if noted, discontinuation of therapy should be considered.

Use with caution in patients with thyroid disease, hepatic impairment, renal impairment, cardiovascular disease, diabetes, glaucoma, cataracts, myasthenia gravis, patients at risk for osteoporosis, patients at risk for seizures, or GI diseases (diverticulitis, peptic ulcer, ulcerative colitis) due to perforation risk. Use caution following acute MI (corticosteroids have been associated with myocardial rupture). Because of the risk of adverse effects, systemic corticosteroids should be used cautiously in the elderly in the smallest possible effective dose for the shortest duration.

Potentially significant interactions may exist, requiring dose or frequency adjustment, additional monitoring, and/or selection of alternative therapy. Consult drug interactions database for more detailed information.

Orally-inhaled corticosteroids may cause a reduction in growth velocity in pediatric patients (~1 centimeter per year [range: 0.3-1.8 cm per year] and related to dose and duration of exposure). To minimize the systemic effects of orally-inhaled corticosteroids, each patient should be titrated to the lowest effective dose. Growth should be routinely monitored in pediatric patients. Withdraw systemic therapy with gradual tapering of dose. There have been reports of systemic corticosteroid withdrawal symptoms (eg, joint/muscle pain, lassitude, depression) when withdrawing oral inhalation therapy. Pulmicort Flexhaler® contains lactose; very rare anaphylactic reactions have been reported in patients with severe milk protein allergy.

Adverse Reactions

Oral capsules:

>10%:

Central nervous system: Headache (21%)
Dermatologic: Bruising (5% to 15%), acne (<5% to 15%)
Gastrointestinal: Nausea (11%)
Respiratory: Respiratory infection (11%)
Miscellaneous: Fat redistribution (moon face, buffalo hump; 3% to 11%)

1% to 10%:

Cardiovascular: Edema (<5% to 7%), chest pain (<5%), facial edema (<5%), flushing (<5%), hypertension (<5%), palpitation (<5%), tachycardia (<5%)
Central nervous system: Dizziness (<5% to 7%), agitation (<5%), amnesia (<5%), confusion (<5%), fever (<5%), insomnia (<5%), malaise (<5%), nervousness (<5%), sleep disorder (<5%), somnolence (<5%), vertigo (<5%)
Dermatologic: Hirsutism (5%), alopecia (<5%), dermatitis (<5%), eczema (<5%), purpura (<5%), skin disorder (<5%), striae (2%)
Endocrine & metabolic: Hypokalemia (<5%), intermenstrual bleeding (<5%), menstrual disorder (<5%), adrenal insufficiency (≥1%)
Gastrointestinal: Diarrhea (10%), dyspepsia (6%), anus disorder (<5%), appetite increased (<5%), Crohn's disease exacerbation (<5%), enteritis (<5%), epigastric pain (<5%), gastrointestinal fistula (<5%), glossitis (<5%), hemorrhoids (<5%), intestinal obstruction (<5%), oral candidiasis (<5%), tongue edema (<5%), tooth disorder (<5%), weight gain (<5%)
Genitourinary: Dysuria (<5%), micturition frequency (<5%), nocturia (<5%), hematuria (≥1%), pyuria (≥1%), urinary tract infection (<5%)
Hematologic: Leukocytosis (<5%), anemia (≥1%), neutrophils abnormal (≥1%)
Hepatic: Alkaline phosphatase increased (≥1%)
Neuromuscular & skeletal: Arthralgia (5%), arthritis (<5%), hyperkinesia (<5%), muscle cramping (<5%), myalgia (<5%), paresthesia (<5%), tremor (<5%), weakness (<5%)
Ocular: Eye abnormality (<5%), vision abnormal (<5%)
Otic: Ear infection (<5%)
Respiratory: Sinusitis (8%), bronchitis (<5%), dyspnea (<5%), pharynx disorder (<5%), rhinitis (<5%)
Miscellaneous: Viral infection (6%), abscess (<5%), C-reactive protein increased (<5%), diaphoresis (<5%), flu-like syndrome (<5%), erythrocyte sedimentation rate increased (≥1%)

Postmarketing and/or case reports (Limited to important or life-threatening): Anaphylaxis, intracranial hypertension (benign)

Oral inhaler (Pulmicort Flexhaler®):

1% to 10%:

Cardiovascular: Syncope (1% to 3%)
Central nervous system: Fever (≥3%), headache (≥3%), pain (≥3%), insomnia (1% to 3%)
Dermatologic: Bruising (1% to 3%)
Gastrointestinal: Dyspepsia (≥5%), nausea (2% to ≥5%), abdominal pain (1% to 3%), taste perversion (1% to 3%), vomiting (1% to 3%), weight gain (1% to 3%), xerostomia (1% to 3%), gastroenteritis (viral; 2%), oral candidiasis (1%)
Neuromuscular & skeletal: Arthralgia (≥5%), weakness (≥5%), back pain (≥3%), fracture (1% to 3%), hypertonia (1% to 3%), myalgia (1% to 3%), neck pain (1% to 3%)
Otic: Otitis media (1%)
Respiratory: Nasopharyngitis (9%), cough (≥5%), rhinitis (≥5%), respiratory infection (≥3%), sinusitis (≥3%), nasal congestion (3%), pharyngitis (3%), allergic rhinitis (2%), upper respiratory tract infection (viral; 2%)
Miscellaneous: Infection (1% to 3%), voice alteration (1% to 3%)

Postmarketing and/or case reports (Limited to important or life-threatening): Aggressiveness, cataracts, depression, glaucoma, hypercorticism, hypersensitivity reactions (immediate and delayed [includes rash, contact dermatitis, angioedema, bronchospasm, urticaria]), hypocorticism, intraocular pressure increased, psychosis, wheezing (patients with severe milk allergy)

Oral tablets:

>10%: Central nervous system: Headache (11%)

1% to 10%:

Central nervous system: Mood swings (7%), fatigue (3%)
Dermatologic: Acne (2% to 5%), hirsutism (<1% to 5%)
Endocrine & metabolic: Cortisol decreased (4%)
Gastrointestinal: Nausea (5%), upper abdominal pain (4%), flatulence (3%), abdominal distension (2%), constipation (2%)
Genitourinary: Urinary tract infection (2%)
Neuromuscular & skeletal: Arthralgia (2%)

Postmarketing and/or case reports (Limited to important or life-threatening): Anaphylaxis, intracranial hypertension (benign)

Suspension for nebulization:

>10%:

Otic: Otitis media (12%)
Respiratory: Respiratory infection (38%), rhinitis (11% to 12%)

1% to 10%:

Cardiovascular: Chest pain (1% to <3%)
Central nervous system: Dysphonia (1% to <3%), fatigue (1% to <3%), mood swings (1% to <3%)
Dermatologic: Rash (4%), contact dermatitis (1% to <3%), eczema (1% to <3%), pruritus (1% to <3%), purpura (1% to <3%), pustular rash (1% to <3%)
Gastrointestinal: Gastroenteritis (5%), diarrhea (4%), vomiting (4%), abdominal pain (3%), anorexia (1% to <3%)
Hematologic: Cervical lymphadenopathy (1% to <3%)
Neuromuscular & skeletal: Fracture (1% to <3%), hyperkinesia (1% to <3%), myalgia (1% to <3%)
Ocular: Conjunctivitis (4%), eye infection (1% to <3%)
Otic: Ear infection (5%), earache (1% to <3%), otitis externa (1% to <3%)
Respiratory: Cough (8% to 9%), epistaxis (2% to 4%), stridor (1% to <3%)
Miscellaneous: Viral infection (4% to 5%), moniliasis (4% to 5%), allergic reaction (1% to <3%), flu-like syndrome (1% to <3%), herpes simplex (1% to <3%), infection (1% to <3%)

Postmarketing and/or case reports (Limited to important or life-threatening): Aggressiveness, avascular necrosis of the femoral head, bronchitis, cataracts, depression, glaucoma, growth suppression, hypercorticism, hypersensitivity reactions (immediate and delayed [includes angioedema, bronchospasm, urticaria]), hypocorticism, intraocular pressure increased, osteoporosis, psychosis

Drug Interactions

Metabolism/Transport Effects Substrate of CYP3A4 (major); **Note:** Assignment of Major/Minor substrate status based on clinically relevant drug interaction potential

Avoid Concomitant Use

Avoid concomitant use of Budesonide (Systemic, Oral Inhalation) with any of the following: Aldesleukin; BCG; Fusidic Acid (Systemic); Grapefruit Juice; Natalizumab; Pimecrolimus; Tacrolimus (Topical); Tofacitinib

Increased Effect/Toxicity

Budesonide (Systemic, Oral Inhalation) may increase the levels/effects of: Amphotericin B; Deferasirox; Leflunomide; Loop Diuretics; Natalizumab; Thiazide Diuretics; Tofacitinib

The levels/effects of Budesonide (Systemic, Oral Inhalation) may be increased by: CYP3A4 Inhibitors (Moderate); CYP3A4 Inhibitors (Strong); Dasatinib; Denosumab; Fusidic Acid (Systemic); Grapefruit Juice; Ivacaftor; Luliconazole; Mifepristone; Pimecrolimus; Simeprevir; Tacrolimus (Topical); Telaprevir; Trastuzumab

Decreased Effect

Budesonide (Systemic, Oral Inhalation) may decrease the levels/effects of: Aldesleukin; Antidiabetic Agents; BCG; Coccidioidin Skin Test; Corticorelin; Hyaluronidase; Sipuleucel-T; Vaccines (Inactivated)

The levels/effects of Budesonide (Systemic, Oral Inhalation) may be decreased by: Antacids; Bile Acid Sequestrants; Echinacea

Ethanol/Nutrition/Herb Interactions

Food: Grapefruit juice may double systemic exposure of orally administered budesonide. Administration of capsules with a high-fat meal delays peak concentration, but does not alter the extent of absorption; administration of tablets with a high-fat meal decreases peak concentration (~27%). Management: Avoid grapefruit juice when using oral capsules or tablets.

Herb/Nutraceutical: Echinacea may diminish the therapeutic effect of budesonide. Management: Avoid echinacea.

Storage/Stability

Oral capsules and tablets: Store at 25°C (77°F); excursions permitted to 15°C to 30°C (59°F to 86°F); keep container tightly closed.

Oral inhaler (Pulmicort Flexhaler®): Store at controlled room temperature of 20°C to 25°C (68°F to 77°F). Protect from moisture.

Suspension for nebulization: Store upright at 20°C to 25°C (68°F to 77°F). Protect from light. Do not refrigerate or freeze. Once aluminum package is opened, solution should be used within 2 weeks. Continue to protect from light.

Mechanism of Action Controls the rate of protein synthesis; depresses the migration of polymorphonuclear leukocytes, fibroblasts; reverses capillary permeability and lysosomal stabilization at the cellular level to prevent or control inflammation. Has potent glucocorticoid activity and weak mineralocorticoid activity.

Pharmacodynamics/Kinetics

Onset of action: Nebulization: 2-8 days; Inhalation: 24 hours

Peak effect: Nebulization: 4-6 weeks; Inhalation: 1-2 weeks

Distribution: 2.2-3.9 L/kg

Protein binding: 85% to 90%

Metabolism: Hepatic via CYP3A4 to two metabolites: 16 alpha-hydroxyprednisolone and 6 beta-hydroxybudesonide; minor activity

Bioavailability: Limited by high first-pass effect; Capsule: 9% to 21%; Nebulization: 6%; Inhalation: 6% to 13%

Half-life elimination: 2-3.6 hours

Time to peak: Capsule: 0.5-10 hours (variable in Crohn's disease); Nebulization: 10-30 minutes; Inhalation: 1-2 hours; Tablet: 7.4-19.2 hours

Excretion: Urine (60%) and feces as metabolites

Dosage

Nebulization: Asthma: Pulmicort Respules®: Children 12 months to 8 years: Titrate to lowest effective dose once patient is stable; start at 0.25 mg/day or use as follows:

Previous therapy of bronchodilators alone: 0.5 mg/day administered as a single dose or divided twice daily (maximum daily dose: 0.5 mg)

Previous therapy of inhaled corticosteroids: 0.5 mg/day administered as a single dose or divided twice daily (maximum daily dose: 1 mg)

Previous therapy of oral corticosteroids: 1 mg/day administered as a single dose or divided twice daily (maximum daily dose: 1 mg)

NIH Asthma Guidelines (NIH, 2007):

Children 0-4 years:

"Low" dose: 0.25-0.5 mg/day

"Medium" dose: >0.5-1 mg/day

"High" dose: >1 mg/day

Children 5-11 years:

"Low" dose: 0.5 mg/day

"Medium" dose: 1 mg/day

"High" dose: 2 mg/day

Oral inhalation: Asthma: Titrate to lowest effective dose once patient is stable.

U.S. labeling: Pulmicort Flexhaler®: **Note:** May increase dose after 1-2 weeks of therapy in patients who are not adequately controlled.

Children ≥6 years: Initial: 180 mcg twice daily (some patients may be initiated at 360 mcg twice daily); maximum: 360 mcg twice daily

NIH Asthma Guidelines (NIH, 2007) (administer in divided doses twice daily):

Children 5-11 years:

"Low" dose: 180-400 mcg/day

"Medium" dose: >400-800 mcg/day

"High" dose: >800 mcg/day

Children ≥12 years: Refer to adult dosing.

Adults: Initial: 360 mcg twice daily (selected patients may be initiated at 180 mcg twice daily); maximum: 720 mcg twice daily

NIH Asthma Guidelines (NIH, 2007) (administer in divided doses twice daily):

"Low" dose: 180-600 mcg/day

"Medium" dose: >600-1200 mcg/day

"High" dose: >1200 mcg/day

Canadian labeling: Pulmicort® Turbuhaler®:

Children 6-11 years:

Initial (or during periods of severe asthma or when switching from oral corticosteroid therapy): 200-400 mcg daily in 2 divided doses

Maintenance: Individualized, lowest effective dose in 2 divided doses

Children ≥12 years and Adults:

Initial (or during periods of severe asthma or when switching from oral corticosteroid therapy): 400-2400 mcg daily in 2-4 divided doses

Maintenance: 200-400 mcg twice daily (higher doses may be needed for some patients). Patients taking 400 mcg/day may take as a single daily dose.

Conversion from oral systemic corticosteroid to orally inhaled corticosteroid: Initiation of oral inhalation therapy should begin in patients whose asthma is reasonably stabilized on oral corticosteroids (OCS). A gradual dose reduction of OCS should begin ~7-10 days after starting inhaled therapy. U.S. labeling recommends reducing prednisone dose by 2.5 mg/day (or equivalent of other OCS) on a weekly basis (patients using oral inhaler) or by ≤25% every 1-2 weeks (patients using respules). The Canadian labeling recommends decreasing the daily dose of prednisone by 2.5 mg (or equivalent of other OCS) every 4 days in closely monitored patients or every 10 days if not closely monitored. If adrenal insufficiency occurs, temporarily increase the OCS dose and follow with a more gradual withdrawal. **Note:** When transitioning from systemic to inhaled corticosteroids, supplemental systemic corticosteroid therapy may be necessary during periods of stress or during severe asthma attacks.

Oral:

Capsule: Crohn's disease (active): Adults: 9 mg once daily in the morning for up to 8 weeks; recurring episodes may be treated with a repeat 8-week course of treatment

Maintenance of remission: Following treatment of active disease (control of symptoms with CDAI <150), treatment may be continued at a dosage of 6 mg once daily for up to 3 months. If symptom control is maintained for 3 months, tapering of the dosage to complete cessation is recommended. Continued dosing beyond 3 months has not been demonstrated to result in substantial benefit.

Tablet: Ulcerative colitis (active): Adults: 9 mg once daily in the morning for up to 8 weeks

Dosage adjustment in renal impairment: Inhalation, Nebulization, Oral: No dosage adjustment provided in manufacturer's labeling (has not been studied).

Dosage adjustment in hepatic impairment: Inhalation, Nebulization, Oral: No specific dosage adjustment provided in the manufacturer's labeling (has not been studied). Manufacturer labeling for oral budesonide suggests a dosage reduction may be necessary with moderate to severe impairment. Budesonide undergoes hepatic metabolism; bioavailability increased in cirrhosis; monitor closely for signs and symptoms of hypercorticism.

Dietary Considerations Oral capsules, tablets: Avoid grapefruit juice.

Administration

Oral capsule, tablet: May be administered without regard to meals. Swallow whole; do not crush, chew, or break.

Powder for inhalation:

Pulmicort Flexhaler®: Hold inhaler in upright position (mouthpiece up) to load dose. Do not shake prior to use. Unit should be primed prior to first use only. It will not need primed again, even if not used for a long time. Place mouthpiece between lips and inhale forcefully and deeply. Do not exhale through inhaler; do not use a spacer. Dose indicator does not move with every dose, usually only after 5 doses. Discard when dose indicator reads "0". Rinse mouth with water after each use to reduce incidence of candidiasis.

Pulmicort® Turbuhaler® [CAN, not available in the U.S.]: Hold inhaler in upright position (mouthpiece up) to load dose. Do not shake inhaler after dose is loaded. Unit should be primed prior to first use. Place mouthpiece between lips and inhale forcefully and deeply; mouthpiece should face up. Do not exhale through inhaler; do not use a spacer. When a red mark appears in the dose indicator window, 20 doses are left. When the red mark reaches the bottom of the window, the inhaler should be discarded. Rinse mouth with water after use to reduce incidence of candidiasis.

Suspension for nebulization: Shake well before using. Use Pulmicort Respules® with jet nebulizer connected to an air compressor; administer with mouthpiece or facemask. Do not use ultrasonic nebulizer. Do not mix with other medications in nebulizer. Rinse mouth following treatments to decrease risk of oral candidiasis (wash face if using face mask).

Monitoring Parameters Monitor growth in pediatric patients; blood pressure, serum glucose, weight with high-dose or long-term oral use; signs and symptoms of hypercorticism or adrenal suppression

Asthma: FEV_1, peak flow, and/or other pulmonary function tests

Additional Information Effects of inhaled steroids on growth have been observed in the absence of laboratory evidence of HPA axis suppression, suggesting that growth velocity is a more sensitive indicator of systemic corticosteroid exposure in pediatric patients than some commonly used tests of HPA axis function. The long-term effects of this reduction in growth velocity associated with orally-inhaled corticosteroids, including the impact on final adult height, are unknown. The potential for "catch up" growth following discontinuation of treatment with inhaled corticosteroids has not been adequately studied.

Dosage Forms Considerations

Pulmicort Flexhaler 180 mcg/actuation canisters contain 120 actuations and the 90 mcg/actuation canisters contain 60 inhalations.

Dosage Forms Excipient information presented when available (limited, particularly for generics); consult specific product labeling.

Aerosol Powder Breath Activated, Inhalation:

Pulmicort Flexhaler: 90 mcg/actuation (1 ea); 180 mcg/actuation (1 ea) [contains milk protein]

Capsule Extended Release 24 Hour, Oral:

Entocort EC: 3 mg

Generic: 3 mg

Suspension, Inhalation:

Pulmicort: 0.25 mg/2 mL (2 mL); 0.5 mg/2 mL (2 mL); 1 mg/2 mL (2 mL) [contains disodium edta, polysorbate 80]

Generic: 0.25 mg/2 mL (2 mL); 0.5 mg/2 mL (2 mL)

Tablet Extended Release 24 Hour, Oral:

Uceris: 9 mg

Dosage Forms: Canada Excipient information presented when available (limited, particularly for generics); consult specific product labeling.

Powder for oral inhalation:

Pulmicort® Turbuhaler®: 100 mcg/inhalation [delivers 200 metered actuations]; 200 mcg/inhalation [delivers 200 metered actuations]; 400 mcg/inhalation [delivers 200 metered actuations]

Budesonide (Nasal) (byoo DES oh nide)

Brand Names: U.S. Rhinocort Aqua

Brand Names: Canada Mylan-Budesonide AQ; Rhinocort® Aqua®; Rhinocort® Turbuhaler®

Pharmacologic Category Corticosteroid, Nasal

Additional Appendix Information

Inhaled Corticosteroids *on page 2298*

Use Management of symptoms of seasonal or perennial rhinitis

Canadian labeling: Additional use (not in U.S. labeling): Prevention and treatment of nasal polyps

Unlabeled Use Adjunct to antibiotics in empiric treatment of acute bacterial rhinosinusitis (ABRS) (Chow, 2012)

Pregnancy Risk Factor B

Dosage Nasal inhalation:

U.S. labeling (Rhinocort® Aqua®): Rhinitis: Children ≥6 years and Adults: 64 mcg/day as a single 32 mcg spray in each nostril. Some patients who do not achieve adequate control may benefit from increased dosage. A reduced dosage may be effective after initial control is achieved.

Maximum dose: Children <12 years: 128 mcg/day; Adults: 256 mcg/day

Canadian labeling:

Rhinocort® Aqua®: Children ≥6 years and Adults:

Nasal polyps: 256 mcg/day administered as a single 64 mcg spray in each nostril twice daily

Rhinitis: Initial: 256 mcg/day administered as two 64 mcg sprays in each nostril once daily or a single 64 mcg spray in each nostril twice daily; Maintenance: Individualize, lowest effective dose

Maximum dose: 256 mcg/day

Rhinocort® Turbuhaler®: Children ≥6 years and Adults:

Nasal polyps: 100 mcg into each nostril twice daily (maximum: 400 mcg/day)

Rhinitis: Initial: 200 mcg into each nostril once daily; Maintenance: Individualize, lowest effective dose (maximum: 400 mcg/day)

Dosage adjustment in renal impairment: No dosage adjustment provided in manufacturer's labeling (has not been studied).

Dosage adjustment in hepatic impairment: No dosage adjustment provided in manufacturer's labeling. Systemic availability of budesonide may be increased in patients with cirrhosis; monitor closely for signs and symptoms of hypercorticism; dosage reduction may be required.

Additional Information Complete prescribing information should be consulted for additional detail.

Dosage Forms Considerations
Rhinocort Aqua 8.6 g bottles contain 120 sprays.

Dosage Forms Excipient information presented when available (limited, particularly for generics); consult specific product labeling.
Suspension, Nasal:
Rhinocort Aqua: 32 mcg/actuation (8.6 g)

Dosage Forms: Canada Excipient information presented when available (limited, particularly for generics); consult specific product labeling.
Powder for nasal inhalation:
Rhinocort® Turbuhaler®: 100 mcg/inhalation [delivers 200 metered actuations]
Suspension, intranasal [spray]:
Rhinocort® Aqua®: 64 mcg/inhalation [120 metered actuations]

◆ Budesonide and Eformoterol *see* Budesonide and Formoterol *on page 287*

Budesonide and Formoterol
(byoo DES oh nide & for MOH te rol)

Brand Names: U.S. Symbicort®
Brand Names: Canada Symbicort®
Index Terms Budesonide and Eformoterol; Eformoterol and Budesonide; Formoterol and Budesonide; Formoterol Fumarate Dihydrate and Budesonide
Pharmacologic Category $Beta_2$ Agonist; $Beta_2$-Adrenergic Agonist, Long-Acting; Corticosteroid, Inhalant (Oral)
Use Treatment of asthma in patients ≥12 years of age where combination therapy is indicated; maintenance treatment of airflow obstruction associated with chronic obstructive pulmonary disease (COPD; including chronic bronchitis and emphysema)
Unlabeled Use Treatment of asthma in children 5-11 years of age where combination therapy is indicated
Pregnancy Risk Factor C
Medication Guide Available Yes
Dosage Oral inhalation:
Asthma:
Children 5-11 years (NIH Guidelines): Symbicort® 80/4.5: Two inhalations twice daily. Do not exceed 4 inhalations per day.
Children ≥12 years and Adults:
U.S. labeling: Symbicort® 80/4.5, Symbicort® 160/4.5: Two inhalations twice daily (maximum: 4 inhalations/day). Recommended starting dose combination is determined according to asthma severity. In patients not adequately controlled on the lower combination dose following 1-2 weeks of therapy, consider the higher dose combination.
Canadian labeling:
Symbicort® 100 Turbuhaler® [CAN; not available in U.S.], Symbicort® 200 Turbuhaler® [CAN; not available in U.S.]:
Initial: 1-2 inhalations twice daily until symptom control, then titrate to lowest effective dosage to maintain control
Maintenance: 1-2 inhalations once or twice daily (maximum: 8 inhalations/day as temporary treatment in periods of worsening asthma)
Symbicort® Maintenance and Reliever Therapy (Symbicort® SMART): **Note:** Not approved in the U.S.:
Maintenance: Symbicort® 100 Turbuhaler® [CAN] **or** Symbicort® 200 Turbuhaler® [CAN]: 1-2 inhalations twice daily **or** 2 inhalations once daily
Reliever therapy: Symbicort® 100 Turbuhaler [CAN] **or** Symbicort® 200 Turbuhaler® [CAN]: One additional inhalation as needed, may repeat if no relief for up to 6 inhalations total (maximum: 8 inhalations/day)
COPD: Adults:
U.S. labeling: Symbicort® 160/4.5: Two inhalations twice daily (maximum: 4 inhalations/day)
Canadian labeling: Symbicort® 200 Turbuhaler® [CAN; not available in U.S.]: Two inhalations twice daily (maximum: 4 inhalations/day)

Dosage adjustment in renal impairment: No dosage adjustment provided in the manufacturer's labeling (has not been studied).

Dosing adjustment in hepatic impairment: No dosage adjustment provided in manufacturer's labeling (has not been studied). However, close monitoring of patients with hepatic disease may be warranted due to hepatic metabolism of both agents.

Additional Information Complete prescribing information should be consulted for additional detail.

Dosage Forms Excipient information presented when available (limited, particularly for generics); consult specific product labeling.
Aerosol for oral inhalation:
Symbicort® 80/4.5: Budesonide 80 mcg and formoterol fumarate dihydrate 4.5 mcg per actuation (6.9 g) [60 metered inhalations]; budesonide 80 mcg and formoterol fumarate dihydrate 4.5 mcg per actuation (10.2 g) [120 metered inhalations]
Symbicort® 160/4.5: Budesonide 160 mcg and formoterol fumarate dihydrate 4.5 mcg per actuation (6 g) [60 metered inhalations]; budesonide 160 mcg and formoterol fumarate dihydrate 4.5 mcg per actuation (10.2 g) [120 metered inhalations]

Dosage Forms: Canada Excipient information presented when available (limited, particularly for generics); consult specific product labeling.
Powder for oral inhalation:
Symbicort® 100 Turbuhaler®: Budesonide 100 mcg and formoterol dihydrate 6 mcg per inhalation (available in 60 or 120 metered doses) [delivers ~80 mcg budesonide and 4.5 mcg formoterol per inhalation; contains lactose]
Symbicort® 200 Turbuhaler®: Budesonide 200 mcg and formoterol dihydrate 6 mcg per inhalation (available in 60 or 120 metered doses) [delivers ~160 mcg budesonide and 4.5 mcg formoterol per inhalation; contains lactose]

◆ Buffasal [OTC] *see* Aspirin *on page 177*
◆ Bufferin® [OTC] *see* Aspirin *on page 177*
◆ Bufferin® Extra Strength [OTC] *see* Aspirin *on page 177*
◆ Buffinol [OTC] *see* Aspirin *on page 177*

Bumetanide (byoo MET a nide)

Brand Names: Canada Burinex®
Index Terms Bumex
Pharmacologic Category Antihypertensive; Diuretic, Loop
Use Management of edema secondary to heart failure or hepatic or renal disease (including nephrotic syndrome)
Unlabeled Use Treatment of hypertension
Pregnancy Risk Factor C

Pregnancy Considerations Adverse events have been observed in some animal reproduction studies.

Breast-Feeding Considerations It is not known if bumetanide is excreted in breast milk. Breast-feeding is not recommended by the manufacturer.

Contraindications Hypersensitivity to bumetanide or any component of the formulation; anuria; patients with hepatic coma or in states of severe electrolyte depletion until the condition improves or is corrected

Warnings/Precautions [U.S. Boxed Warning]: Excessive amounts can lead to profound diuresis with fluid and electrolyte loss; close medical supervision and dose evaluation are required. Potassium supplementation and/or use of potassium-sparing diuretics may be necessary to prevent hypokalemia. In cirrhosis, initiate bumetanide therapy with conservative dosing and close monitoring of electrolytes; avoid sudden changes in fluid and electrolyte balance and acid/base status which may lead to hepatic encephalopathy. *In vitro* studies using pooled sera from critically-ill neonates have shown bumetanide to be a potent displacer of bilirubin; avoid use in neonates at risk for kernicterus. Coadministration of antihypertensives may increase the risk of hypotension.

Monitor fluid status and renal function in an attempt to prevent oliguria, azotemia, and reversible increases in BUN and creatinine; close medical supervision of aggressive diuresis required. Bumetanide-induced ototoxicity (usually transient) may occur with rapid I.V. administration, renal impairment, excessive doses, and concurrent use of other ototoxins (eg, aminoglycosides). Asymptomatic hyperuricemia has been reported with use.

Chemical similarities are present among sulfonamides, sulfonylureas, carbonic anhydrase inhibitors, thiazides, and loop diuretics (except ethacrynic acid); the manufacturer's labeling states that bumetanide may be used in patients allergic to furosemide. Use in patients with sulfonylurea allergy is not specifically contraindicated in product labeling; however, a risk of cross-reaction exists in patients with allergy to any of these compounds; avoid use when previous reaction has been severe. Discontinue if signs of hypersensitivity are noted.

Adverse Reactions

>10%:

Endocrine & metabolic: Hyperuricemia (18%), hypochloremia (15%), hypokalemia (15%)

Renal: Azotemia (11%)

1% to 10%:

Central nervous system: Dizziness (1%)

Endocrine & metabolic: Hyponatremia (9%), hyperglycemia (7%), phosphorus altered (5%), CO_2 content altered (4%), bicarbonate altered (3%), calcium altered (2%)

Neuromuscular & skeletal: Muscle cramps (1%)

Renal: Serum creatinine increased (7%)

Miscellaneous: LDH altered (1%)

<1% (Limited to important or life-threatening): Abdominal pain, alkaline phosphatase altered, arthritic pain, asterixis, bilirubin altered, chest pain, cholesterol altered, creatinine clearance altered, dehydration, diaphoresis, diarrhea, ear discomfort, ECG changes, encephalopathy (in patients with pre-existing liver disease), erectile dysfunction, fatigue, headache, hearing impaired, hemoglobin/hematocrit altered, hives, hyperventilation, hypotension, musculoskeletal pain, nausea, nipple tenderness, orthostatic hypotension, ototoxicity, premature ejaculation, prothrombin time altered, pruritus, rash, renal failure, Stevens-Johnson syndrome, thrombocytopenia, toxic epidermal necrolysis, transaminase altered, upset stomach, urine glucose increased, urine protein increased, vertigo, vomiting, WBC altered, weakness, xerostomia

Drug Interactions

Metabolism/Transport Effects None known.

Avoid Concomitant Use There are no known interactions where it is recommended to avoid concomitant use.

Increased Effect/Toxicity

Bumetanide may increase the levels/effects of: ACE Inhibitors; Allopurinol; Amifostine; Aminoglycosides; Antihypertensives; Cardiac Glycosides; CISplatin; Dofetilide; Hypotensive Agents; Ivabradine; Lithium; Methotrexate; Neuromuscular-Blocking Agents; Obinutuzumab; RisperiDONE; RiTUXimab; Salicylates; Sodium Phosphates; Topiramate

The levels/effects of Bumetanide may be increased by: Alfuzosin; Analgesics (Opioid); Beta2-Agonists; Brimonidine (Topical); Corticosteroids (Orally Inhaled); Corticosteroids (Systemic); CycloSPORINE (Systemic); Diazoxide; Herbs (Hypotensive Properties); Licorice; MAO Inhibitors; Methotrexate; Pentoxifylline; Phosphodiesterase 5 Inhibitors; Probenecid; Prostacyclin Analogues

Decreased Effect

Bumetanide may decrease the levels/effects of: Hypoglycemic Agents; Lithium; Neuromuscular-Blocking Agents

The levels/effects of Bumetanide may be decreased by: Bile Acid Sequestrants; Fosphenytoin; Herbs (Hypertensive Properties); Methotrexate; Methylphenidate; Nonsteroidal Anti-Inflammatory Agents; Phenytoin; Probenecid; Salicylates; Yohimbine

Ethanol/Nutrition/Herb Interactions

Food: Bumetanide serum levels may be decreased if taken with food. It has been recommended that bumetanide be administered without food (Bard, 2004).

Herb/Nutraceutical: Avoid ephedra, yohimbe, ginseng (may worsen hypertension). Avoid dong quai if using for hypertension (has estrogenic activity). Avoid garlic (may have increased antihypertensive effect).

Storage/Stability

I.V.: Store vials at 15°C to 30°C (59°F to 86°F). Infusion solutions should be used within 24 hours after preparation. Light sensitive; discoloration may occur when exposed to light.

Tablet: Store at 15°C to 30°C (59°F to 86°F).

Mechanism of Action Inhibits reabsorption of sodium and chloride in the ascending loop of Henle and proximal renal tubule, interfering with the chloride-binding cotransport system, thus causing increased excretion of water, sodium, chloride, magnesium, phosphate, and calcium; it does not appear to act on the distal tubule

Pharmacodynamics/Kinetics

Onset of action: Oral, I.M.: 0.5-1 hour; I.V.: 2-3 minutes

Peak effect: Oral: 1-2 hours; I.V.: 15-30 minutes

Duration: 4-6 hours

Distribution: V_d: Neonates and Infants: 0.26-0.39 L/kg; Adults: 9-25 L

Protein binding: 94% to 96%

Metabolism: Partially hepatic

Bioavailability: 59% to 89% (median: 80%)

Half-life elimination: Neonates: ~6 hours; Infants (1 month): ~2.4 hours; Adults: 1-1.5 hours

Excretion: Urine (81% of total dose; 45% of which is unchanged drug); feces (2% of total dose)

Dosage

Infants and Children: Oral, I.M., I.V.: 0.015-0.1 mg/kg/dose every 6-24 hours (maximum dose: 10 mg/day)

Adults:

Edema:

Oral: 0.5-2 mg/dose 1-2 times/day; if diuretic response to initial dose is not adequate, may repeat in 4-5 hours for up to 2 doses (maximum dose: 10 mg/day)

I.M., I.V.: 0.5-1 mg/dose; if diuretic response to initial dose is not adequate, may repeat in 2-3 hours for up to 2 doses (maximum dose: 10 mg/day)

Continuous I.V. infusion (unlabeled dose): Initial: 1 mg I.V. load then 0.5-2 mg/hour (Hunt, 2009)

Hypertension (unlabeled use): Oral: 0.5 mg daily (maximum dose: 5 mg/day); usual dosage range (JNC 7): 0.5-2 mg/day in 2 divided doses (Chobanian, 2003)

Dosage adjustment in renal impairment: Use is contraindicated in anuria. Use with caution in renal insufficiency due to increased risk of adverse effects.

Dosage adjustment in hepatic impairment: Use is contraindicated in hepatic coma. Use with caution in cirrhosis and ascites due to increased risk of precipitating hepatic coma; initiate with conservative doses and monitoring.

Dietary Considerations Administration with food slows the rate and reduces the extent of absorption and may reduce diuretic efficacy (Bard, 2004). May require increased intake of potassium-rich foods.

Administration

I.V.: Administer slowly, over 1-2 minutes.

Oral: An alternate-day schedule or a 3-4 daily dosing regimen with rest periods of 1-2 days in between may be the most tolerable and effective regimen for the continued control of edema.

Monitoring Parameters Blood pressure; serum electrolytes, renal function; fluid status (weight and I & O), blood pressure

Dosage Forms Excipient information presented when available (limited, particularly for generics); consult specific product labeling.

Solution, Injection:

Generic: 0.25 mg/mL (2 mL, 4 mL, 10 mL)

Tablet, Oral:

Generic: 0.5 mg, 1 mg, 2 mg

Dosage Forms: Canada Note: Solution for injection is not available in Canada. Excipient information presented when available (limited, particularly for generics); consult specific product labeling.

Tablet, Oral:

Burinex: 1 mg, 5 mg

◆ **Bumex** *see* Bumetanide *on page 287*

◆ **Buminate** *see* Albumin *on page 59*

◆ **Buminate-5% (Can)** *see* Albumin *on page 59*

◆ **Buminate-25% (Can)** *see* Albumin *on page 59*

◆ **Bupap** *see* Butalbital and Acetaminophen *on page 305*

◆ **Buphenyl** *see* Sodium Phenylbutyrate *on page 1923*

Bupivacaine (byoo PIV a kane)

Brand Names: U.S. Bupivacaine Spinal; Marcaine; Marcaine Preservative Free; Marcaine Spinal; Sensorcaine; Sensorcaine-MPF; Sensorcaine-MPF Spinal

Brand Names: Canada Marcaine®; Sensorcaine®

Index Terms Bupivacaine Hydrochloride

Pharmacologic Category Local Anesthetic

Use Local or regional anesthesia; spinal anesthesia; diagnostic and therapeutic procedures; obstetrical procedures (only 0.25% and 0.5% concentrations)

0.25%: Local infiltration, peripheral nerve block, sympathetic block, caudal or epidural block

0.5%: Peripheral nerve block, caudal and epidural block

0.75% **(not for obstetrical anesthesia)**: Retrobulbar block, epidural block. **Note:** Reserve for surgical procedures where a high degree of muscle relaxation and prolonged effect are necessary

Pregnancy Risk Factor C

Pregnancy Considerations Adverse events were observed in animal reproduction studies. Bupivacaine crosses the placenta. Bupivacaine is approved for use at term in obstetrical anesthesia or analgesia. **[U.S. Boxed Warning]: The 0.75% is not recommended for obstetrical anesthesia.** Bupivacaine 0.75% solutions have been associated with cardiac arrest following epidural anesthesia in obstetrical patients and use of this concentration is not recommended for this purpose. Use in obstetrical paracervical block anesthesia is contraindicated.

Breast-Feeding Considerations Bupivacaine is excreted in breast milk. Due to the potential for serious adverse reactions in the nursing infant, a decision should be made whether to discontinue nursing or to discontinue the drug, taking into account the importance of treatment to the mother.

Contraindications Hypersensitivity to bupivacaine hydrochloride, amide-type local anesthetics, or any component of the formulation; obstetrical paracervical block anesthesia

Note: Use as intravenous regional anesthesia (Bier block) is considered contraindicated per accepted clinical practice.

Warnings/Precautions Do not use solutions containing preservatives for caudal or epidural block. Use with caution in patients with hepatic impairment. Local anesthetics have been associated with rare occurrences of sudden respiratory arrest; convulsions due to systemic toxicity leading to cardiac arrest have also been reported, presumably following unintentional intravascular injection. Intravenous regional anesthesia (Bier block) is **not** recommended; cardiac arrest and death have occurred with this method of administration. **[U.S. Boxed Warning]: The 0.75% concentration is not recommended for obstetrical epidural anesthesia; cardiac arrest with difficult resuscitation or death has occurred.** A test dose is recommended prior to epidural administration (prior to initial dose) and all reinforcing doses with continuous catheter technique. Use caution with cardiovascular dysfunction including patients with hypotension or heart block. Bupivacaine-containing products have been associated with rare occurrences of arrhythmias, cardiac arrest, and death. Use caution in debilitated, elderly, or acutely ill patients; dose reduction may be required. Resuscitative equipment, oxygen, and other resuscitative drugs should be available for immediate use. Continuous intra-articular infusion of local anesthetics after arthroscopic or other surgical procedures is **not** an approved use; chondrolysis (primarily shoulder joint) has occurred following infusion, with some requiring arthroplasty or shoulder replacement.

Adverse Reactions Note: Incidence of adverse reactions is difficult to define. Most effects are dose related, and are often due to accelerated absorption from the injection site, unintentional intravascular injection, or slow metabolic degradation. The development of any central nervous system symptoms may be an early indication of more significant toxicity (seizure).

Cardiovascular: Hypotension, bradycardia, palpitation, heart block, ventricular arrhythmia, cardiac arrest

Central nervous system: Restlessness, anxiety, dizziness, seizure (0.1%); rare symptoms (usually associated with unintentional subarachnoid injection during high spinal anesthesia) include persistent anesthesia, paresthesia, paralysis, headache, septic meningitis, and cranial nerve palsies

Gastrointestinal: Nausea, vomiting; rare symptoms (usually associated with unintentional subarachnoid injection during high spinal anesthesia) include fecal incontinence and loss of sphincter control

Genitourinary: Rare symptoms (usually associated with unintentional subarachnoid injection during high spinal anesthesia) include urinary incontinence, loss of perineal sensation, and loss of sexual function

Neuromuscular & skeletal: Chondrolysis (continuous intra-articular administration), weakness
Ocular: Blurred vision, pupillary constriction
Otic: Tinnitus
Respiratory: Apnea, hypoventilation (usually associated with unintentional subarachnoid injection during high spinal anesthesia)
Miscellaneous: Allergic reactions (urticaria, pruritus, angioedema), anaphylactoid reactions

Drug Interactions

Metabolism/Transport Effects Substrate of CYP1A2 (minor), CYP2C19 (minor), CYP2D6 (minor), CYP3A4 (minor); **Note:** Assignment of Major/Minor substrate status based on clinically relevant drug interaction potential

Avoid Concomitant Use There are no known interactions where it is recommended to avoid concomitant use.

Increased Effect/Toxicity

The levels/effects of Bupivacaine may be increased by: Beta-Blockers; Hyaluronidase

Decreased Effect

Bupivacaine may decrease the levels/effects of: Technetium Tc 99m Tilmanocept

The levels/effects of Bupivacaine may be decreased by: Peginterferon Alfa-2b

Storage/Stability Store at controlled room temperature of 20°C to 25°C (68°F to 77°F).

Mechanism of Action Blocks both the initiation and conduction of nerve impulses by decreasing the neuronal membrane's permeability to sodium ions, which results in inhibition of depolarization with resultant blockade of conduction

Pharmacodynamics/Kinetics

Onset of action: Anesthesia (route and dose dependent): 1-17 minutes
Duration (route and dose dependent): 2-9 hours
Protein binding: ~95%
Metabolism: Hepatic; forms metabolite (pipecoloxylidine [PPX])
Half-life elimination (age dependent): Neonates: 8.1 hours; Adults: 2.7 hours
Time to peak, plasma: Caudal, epidural, or peripheral nerve block: 30-45 minutes
Excretion: Urine (~6% unchanged)

Dosage Dose varies with procedure, depth of anesthesia, vascularity of tissues, duration of anesthesia, and condition of patient. Do not use solutions containing preservatives for caudal or epidural block.

Children >12 years and Adults:
- Local anesthesia: Infiltration: 0.25% infiltrated locally; maximum: 175 mg
- Caudal block (preservative free): 15-30 mL of 0.25% or 0.5%
- Epidural block (other than caudal block; preservative free): Administer in 3-5 mL increments, allowing sufficient time to detect toxic manifestations of inadvertent I.V. or I.T. administration: 10-20 mL of 0.25% or 0.5%
  - Surgical procedures requiring a high degree of muscle relaxation and prolonged effects **only**: 10-20 mL of 0.75% (**Note:** Not to be used in obstetrical cases)
- Peripheral nerve block: 5 mL of 0.25% or 0.5%; maximum: 400 mg/day
- Sympathetic nerve block: 20-50 mL of 0.25%
- Retrobulbar anesthesia: 2-4 mL of 0.75%

Adults: Spinal anesthesia: Preservative free solution of 0.75% bupivacaine in 8.25% dextrose:
- Lower extremity and perineal procedures: 1 mL
- Lower abdominal procedures: 1.6 mL
- Normal vaginal delivery: 0.8 mL (higher doses may be required in some patients)
- Cesarean section: 1-1.4 mL

Dosage adjustment in renal impairment: No dosage adjustments provided in manufacturer's labeling; use with caution.

Dosage adjustment in hepatic impairment: No dosage adjustments provided in manufacturer's labeling; use with caution.

Administration Solutions containing preservatives should not be used for epidural or caudal blocks.

Monitoring Parameters Vital signs, state of consciousness; signs of CNS toxicity

Dosage Forms Excipient information presented when available (limited, particularly for generics); consult specific product labeling.

Solution, Injection, as hydrochloride:
- Marcaine: 0.25% (50 mL); 0.5% (50 mL) [contains methylparaben]
- Sensorcaine: 0.25% (50 mL); 0.5% (50 mL) [contains methylparaben]
- Sensorcaine-MPF: 0.25% (10 mL, 30 mL); 0.5% (10 mL, 30 mL); 0.75% (10 mL, 30 mL) [methylparaben free]
- Generic: 0.25% (10 mL, 30 mL, 50 mL); 0.5% (10 mL, 30 mL, 50 mL); 0.75% (10 mL, 30 mL)

Solution, Injection, as hydrochloride [preservative free]:
- Marcaine: 0.75% (10 mL, 30 mL)
- Marcaine Preservative Free: 0.25% (10 mL, 30 mL); 0.5% (10 mL, 30 mL)
- Generic: 0.25% (10 mL, 20 mL, 30 mL); 0.5% (10 mL, 20 mL, 30 mL); 0.75% (10 mL, 20 mL, 30 mL)

Solution, Intrathecal, as hydrochloride:
- Marcaine Spinal: 0.75% [7.5 mg/mL] (2 mL)

Solution, Intrathecal, as hydrochloride [preservative free]:
- Bupivacaine Spinal: 0.75% [7.5 mg/mL] (2 mL)
- Sensorcaine-MPF Spinal: 0.75% [7.5 mg/mL] (2 mL)

◆ **Bupivacaine Hydrochloride** *see* Bupivacaine *on page 289*

Bupivacaine (Liposomal)

(byoo PIV a kane lye po SO mal)

Brand Names: U.S. Exparel

Index Terms Bupivacaine Liposome; DepoFoam Bupivacaine; Exparel™; Liposomal Bupivacaine

Pharmacologic Category Analgesic, Nonopioid

Use Injected into the surgical site (eg, bunionectomy, hemorrhoidectomy) to provide postoperative analgesia

Pregnancy Risk Factor C

Pregnancy Considerations Adverse events were observed in animal reproduction studies. Bupivacaine crosses the placenta. Use in obstetrical paracervical block anesthesia is contraindicated; may cause fetal bradycardia and death.

Breast-Feeding Considerations Bupivacaine is excreted into breast milk. Due to the potential for serious adverse reactions in the nursing infant, the manufacturer recommends a decision be made whether to discontinue nursing or to discontinue the drug, taking into account the importance of treatment to the mother.

Contraindications Obstetrical paracervical block anesthesia

Warnings/Precautions Use with caution in patients with hepatic impairment. Local anesthetics have been associated with rare occurrences of sudden respiratory arrest; convulsions due to systemic toxicity leading to cardiac arrest have also been reported, presumably following unintentional intravascular injection. CNS effects (including stimulation and/or depression) have been reported with bupivacaine-containing products; monitor for CNS-related changes or alterations in consciousness. Additionally, use of local anesthetics have been associated with rare occurrences of localized neurological toxicity (numbness, weakness, paralysis), which may be irreversible.

Use caution with cardiovascular dysfunction including patients with hypotension or heart block. Bupivacaine-containing products have been associated with rare occurrences of arrhythmias, cardiac arrest, and death. Resuscitative equipment, oxygen, and other resuscitative drugs should be available for immediate use.

Intravascular, epidural, intrathecal, intra-articular, and regional nerve block injections should be avoided; aspiration should be performed prior to administration. Should not be used to provide presurgical anesthesia. Exparel™ and other bupivacaine products are not interchangeable due to differences in formulation and indications. Wait at least 96 hours after administration before administering other bupivacaine-containing products. Wait at least 20 minutes after administration of locally administered lidocaine before administering bupivacaine (liposomal).

Adverse Reactions

>10%: Gastrointestinal: Nausea (2% to 40%), vomiting (28%), constipation (2% to ≥10%)

1% to 10%:

Cardiovascular: Hypotension (2% to 10%), peripheral edema (2% to 10%), tachycardia (4%), bradycardia (2%), syncope (<2%), edema (<2%), hypertension (<2%), pallor (<2%), palpitation (<2%), sinus bradycardia (<2%), supraventricular extrasystoles (<2%), ventricular extrasystoles (<2%), ventricular tachycardia (<2%)

Central nervous system: Insomnia (2% to 10%), dizziness (6%), somnolence (2% to 5%), headache (4%), fever (2%), hypoesthesia (2%), agitation (<2%), anxiety (<2%), chills (<2%), confusion (<2%), depression (<2%), pain (<2%), restlessness (<2%), tremor (<2%), lethargy (1%)

Dermatologic: Pruritus (3%), erythema (<2%), hyperhidrosis (<2%), pruritic rash (<2%), urticaria (<2%)

Genitourinary: Urinary incontinence (<2%), urinary retention (<2%)

Hematologic: Anemia (hemorrhagic, postoperative; 2% to 10%)

Hepatic: AST increased (3%), ALT increased (1%)

Local: Incision site edema (2%)

Neuromuscular & skeletal: Back pain (2% to 10%), muscle spasm (2% to 10%), neck pain (<2%), paresthesia (<2%), weakness (<2%), chondrolysis (continuous intra-articular administration; develops months after surgery)

Ocular: Blurred vision (<2%)

Otic: Tinnitus (<2%)

Renal: Creatinine increased (2%)

Respiratory: Apnea (<2%), hypoxia (<2%), laryngospasm (<2%), respiratory depression/failure (<2%)

Miscellaneous: Feeling of warmth (2%), fungal infection (2%), anaphylactoid reactions (<2%), diaphoresis (<2%), hypersensitivity reactions (<2%)

Frequency not defined:

Cardiovascular: Cardiac arrest, heart block

Central nervous system: Persistent anesthesia, paralysis, seizures

Ocular: Pupillary constriction

Preparation for Administration

10 mL vial: No further dilution required

20 mL vial: For surgical procedures (eg, hemorrhoidectomy), may dilute with 10 mL of NS (total volume = 30 mL); further dilution to 0.89 mg/mL (ie, a 1:14 dilution by volume) may be considered if additional volume is necessary to cover the surgical site. Use only NS for dilution; use of water or other hypotonic agents will disrupt liposomal particles.

Storage/Stability Store at 2°C to 8°C (36°F to 46°F); do not freeze and do not heat or autoclave vials once removed from refrigerator. Unopened vials may be stored at room temperature of 20°C to 25°C (68°F to 77°F) for up to 30 days (do not re-refrigerate). Diluted vials should be used within 4 hours.

Mechanism of Action Blocks both the initiation and conduction of nerve impulses by decreasing the neuronal membrane's permeability to sodium ions, which results in inhibition of depolarization with resultant blockade of conduction.

Pharmacodynamics/Kinetics

Duration: Local: ~24 hours; Systemic: 96 hours

Protein binding: 95%

Metabolism: Hepatic via conjugation; major metabolite pipecoloxylidine (PPX; inactive)

Half-life elimination: Apparent: 24-34 hours

Time to peak, plasma: Bunionectomy: 2 hours: Hemorrhoidectomy: 30 minutes

Excretion: Urine (~6% unchanged)

Dosage Infiltration (local): Adults: Postoperative analgesia: Dose is based on surgical site and volume required to cover the area (in general, the maximum total dose is 266 mg).

Bunionectomy: 7 mL into the tissues surrounding the osteotomy and 1 mL into the subcutaneous tissue of the surgical site (total dose = 8 mL [106 mg])

Hemorrhoidectomy: 30 mL (20 mL vial diluted with 10 mL NS) divided and administered as 6 injections of 5 mL each (total dose = 30 mL [266 mg])

Dosage adjustment in renal impairment: No dosage adjustment provided in manufacturer's labeling; however, renal impairment may reduce bupivacaine elimination increasing systemic exposure and the risk of adverse effects or toxicities; use with caution.

Dosage adjustment in hepatic impairment: No dosage adjustment provided in manufacturer's labeling; however, moderate-to-severe impairment may reduce bupivacaine metabolism increasing systemic exposure and the risk of adverse effects or toxicities; use with caution.

Administration For local infiltration use only. Invert vial several times prior to withdrawing contents (resuspends particles). Administer using a ≥25 gauge needle. May administer ≥20 minutes after local lidocaine administration (if applicable). Allow topical antiseptics (eg, povidone iodine) applied to surgical site to dry prior to administration.

Bunionectomy: Infiltrate into the tissues surrounding the osteotomy and into the subcutaneous tissue.

Hemorrhoidectomy: Visualize the anal sphincter as a clock face and slowly infiltrate each aliquot (5 mL) of the diluted 20 mL vial into each of the even numbers.

Monitoring Parameters Vital signs, state of consciousness; signs of CNS toxicity, pain relief.

Dosage Forms Excipient information presented when available (limited, particularly for generics); consult specific product labeling.

Suspension, Injection:

Exparel: 1.3% (20 mL)

◆ **Bupivacaine Liposome** *see* Bupivacaine (Liposomal) *on page 290*

◆ **Bupivacaine Spinal** *see* Bupivacaine *on page 289*

◆ **Buprenex** *see* Buprenorphine *on page 291*

Buprenorphine (byoo pre NOR feen)

Brand Names: U.S. Buprenex; Butrans

Brand Names: Canada Butrans®

Index Terms Buprenorphine Hydrochloride

Pharmacologic Category Analgesic, Opioid; Analgesic, Opioid Partial Agonist

Additional Appendix Information
Opioid Conversion Table *on page 2306*

Use
Injection: Management of moderate-to-severe pain
Sublingual tablet: Treatment of opioid dependence
Transdermal patch: Management of moderate-to-severe chronic pain in patients requiring an around-the-clock opioid analgesic for an extended period of time

Unlabeled Use Injection: Management of opioid withdrawal in heroin-dependent hospitalized patients

Pregnancy Risk Factor C

Pregnancy Considerations Adverse effects have been observed in some animal reproduction studies. Buprenorphine crosses the placenta; buprenorphine and norbuprenorphine can be detected in newborn serum, urine, and meconium following in utero exposure (CSAT, 2004). Following chronic opioid therapy in pregnancy, adverse events in the newborn (including withdrawal) may occur; monitoring of the neonate is recommended. The minimum effective dose should be used if opioids are needed (Chou, 2009). The onset of withdrawal in infants of women receiving buprenorphine during pregnancy ranged from day 1 to day 8 of life, most occurring on day 1. Symptoms of withdrawal may include agitation, apnea, bradycardia, convulsions, hypertonia, myoclonus, respiratory depression, and tremor.

Buprenorphine is currently considered an alternate treatment for pregnant women who need therapy for opioid addiction (CSAT, 2004; Dow, 2012); however, use in pregnancy for this purpose is increasing (ACOG, 2012; Soyka, 2013). Buprenorphine should not be used to treat pain during labor. Women receiving buprenorphine for the treatment of addiction should be maintained on their daily dose of buprenorphine in addition to receiving the same pain management options during labor and delivery as opioid-naïve women; maintenance doses of buprenorphine will not provide adequate pain relief. Narcotic agonist-antagonists should be avoided for the treatment of labor pain in women maintained on buprenorphine due to the risk of precipitating acute withdrawal. In addition, buprenorphine should not be given to women in labor taking methadone (ACOG, 2012).

Amenorrhea may develop secondary to substance abuse; pregnancy may occur following the initiation of buprenorphine maintenance treatment. Contraception counseling is recommended to prevent unplanned pregnancies (Dow, 2012).

Breast-Feeding Considerations Buprenorphine is excreted in breast milk. Breast-feeding is not recommended by the manufacturer. Nursing infants exposed to large doses of opioids should be monitored for apnea and sedation (Montgomery, 2012).

When buprenorphine is used to treat opioid addiction in nursing women, most guidelines do not contraindicate breast-feeding as long as the infant is tolerant to the dose and other contraindications do not exist; caution should be used when nursing infants not previously exposed (ACOG, 2012; CSAT, 2004; Montgomery, 2012). If additional illicit substances are being abused, women treated with buprenorphine should pump and discard breast milk until sobriety is established (ACOG, 2012; Dow, 2012).

Prescribing and Access Restrictions Prescribing of tablets for opioid dependence is limited to physicians who have met the qualification criteria and have received a DEA number specific to prescribing this product. Tablets will be available through pharmacies and wholesalers which normally provide controlled substances.

Medication Guide Available Yes

Contraindications Hypersensitivity to buprenorphine or any component of the formulation

Transdermal patch: Additional contraindications: Significant respiratory depression; acute or severe asthma; known or suspected paralytic ileus

Warnings/Precautions An opioid-containing analgesic regimen should be tailored to each patient's needs and based upon the type of pain being treated (acute versus chronic), the route of administration, degree of tolerance for opioids (naive versus chronic user), age, weight, and medical condition. The optimal analgesic dose varies widely among patients. Doses should be titrated to pain relief/prevention.

May cause CNS depression, which may impair physical or mental abilities; patients must be cautioned about performing tasks which require mental alertness (eg, operating machinery or driving). Effects with other sedative drugs or ethanol may be potentiated. Elderly may be more sensitive to CNS depressant and constipating effects. May cause respiratory depression - use caution in patients with respiratory disease or pre-existing respiratory depression. Hypersensitivity reactions, including bronchospasm, angioneurotic edema, and anaphylactic shock, have also been reported. Potential for drug dependency exists, abrupt cessation may precipitate withdrawal. Use caution in elderly, debilitated, cachectic, pediatric patients, depression or suicidal tendencies. Tolerance, psychological and physical dependence may occur with prolonged use. Partial antagonist activity may precipitate acute opioid withdrawal in opioid-dependent individuals.

After chronic maternal exposure to opioids, neonatal withdrawal syndrome may occur in the newborn; monitor neonate closely. Signs and symptoms include irritability, hyperactivity and abnormal sleep pattern, high pitched cry, tremor, vomiting, diarrhea and failure to gain weight. Onset, duration and severity depend on the drug used, duration of use, maternal dose, and rate of drug elimination by the newborn. Opioid withdrawal syndrome in the neonate, unlike in adults, may be life-threatening and should be treated according to protocols developed by neonatology experts.

Hepatitis has been reported with buprenorphine use; hepatic events ranged from transient, asymptomatic transaminase elevations to hepatic failure; in many cases, patients had pre-existing hepatic dysfunction. Monitor liver function tests in patients at increased risk for hepatotoxicity (eg, history of alcohol abuse, pre-existing hepatic dysfunction, I.V. drug abusers) prior to and during therapy. Use with caution in patients with hepatic impairment; dosage adjustments are recommended in hepatic impairment.

Use with caution in patients with pulmonary or renal function impairment. Also use caution in patients with head injury or increased ICP, biliary tract dysfunction, pancreatitis, patients with history of hyperthyroidism, morbid obesity, adrenal insufficiency, prostatic hyperplasia, urinary stricture, toxic psychosis, pancreatitis, alcoholism, delirium tremens, or kyphoscoliosis. Avoid use in patients with CNS depression or coma as these patients are susceptible to intracranial effects of CO_2 retention. May cause hypotension; use with caution in patients with hypovolemia, cardiovascular disease (including acute MI), or drugs which may exaggerate hypotensive effects (including phenothiazines or general anesthetics). May obscure diagnosis or clinical course of patients with acute abdominal conditions. Use with caution in patients with a history of ileus or bowel obstruction; use of transdermal patch is contraindicated in patients with known or suspected paralytic ileus. Opioid therapy may lower seizure threshold; use caution in patients with a history of seizure disorders. Potentially significant drug-drug interactions may exist, requiring dose or frequency adjustment, additional monitoring, and/or selection of alternative therapy.

Transdermal patch: Indicated for the management of chronic moderate-to-severe pain when around the clock pain control is needed for an extended time period; should not be used for as-needed pain relief or for the treatment of mild pain, acute pain, or postoperative pain requiring short-term opioid analgesia. **[U.S. Boxed Warning]: May cause potentially life-threatening respiratory depression even with therapeutic use. Ensure proper dosing and titration; monitor for respiratory depression, especially within the first 24-72 hours of initiation or dose escalation. Buprenorphine transdermal patches should only be prescribed by healthcare professionals familiar with the use of potent opioids for chronic pain.** Do not exceed one 20 **mcg**/hour transdermal patch due to the risk of QTc-interval prolongation. Avoid using in patients with history of long QT syndrome or in patients with predisposing factors increasing the risk of QT abnormalities (eg, concurrent medications such as antiarrhythmics, hypokalemia, unstable heart failure, unstable atrial fibrillation). **[U.S. Boxed Warning]: Healthcare provider should be alert to problems of abuse, misuse, and diversion.** Risk of opioid abuse is increased in patients with a history or family history of alcohol or drug abuse or mental illness. **[U.S. Boxed Warning]: Proper storage, handling, and disposal of used patches are essential to prevent accidental exposures, especially in children; accidental exposure may result in a fatal overdose.** To properly dispose of Butrans® patch, fold it over on itself and flush down the toilet; alternatively, seal the used patch in the provided Patch-Disposal Unit and dispose of in the trash. Avoid exposure of application site and surrounding area to direct external heat sources. Buprenorphine release from the patch is temperature-dependent and may result in overdose. Patients who experience fever or increase in core temperature should be monitored closely. Application site reactions, including rare cases of severe reactions (eg, vesicles, discharge, "burns"), have been observed with use; onset varies from days to months after initiation; patients should be instructed to report severe reactions promptly. Therapy with the transdermal patch is not appropriate for use in the management of addictions.

Concurrent use of agonist/antagonist analgesics may precipitate withdrawal symptoms and/or reduced analgesic efficacy in patients following prolonged therapy with mu opioid agonists. Abrupt discontinuation following prolonged use may also lead to withdrawal symptoms and is not recommended; taper dose gradually when discontinuing.

Sublingual tablets, which are used for induction treatment of opioid dependence, should not be started until effects of withdrawal are evident.

Adverse Reactions

Injection:

>10%: Central nervous system: Sedation (≤66%)

1% to 10%:
- Cardiovascular: Hypotension (1% to 5%)
- Central nervous system: Dizziness/vertigo (5% to 10%), headache (1% to 5%)
- Gastrointestinal: Nausea (5% to 10%), vomiting (1% to 5%)
- Ocular: Miosis (1% to 5%)
- Respiratory: Respiratory depression (1% to 5%)
- Miscellaneous: Diaphoresis (1% to 5%)

<1%: (Limited to important or life-threatening): Amblyopia, anaphylactic shock, apnea, bradycardia, conjunctivitis, coma, cyanosis, depersonalization, depression, diplopia, euphoria, hallucinations, hypersensitivity reactions, hypertension, injection site reaction, psychosis, seizures, slurred speech, tachycardia, urinary retention, Wenckebach block

Tablet:

>10%:
- Central nervous system: Headache (30%), pain (24%), insomnia (21% to 25%), anxiety (12%), depression (11%)
- Gastrointestinal: Nausea (10% to 14%), abdominal pain (12%), constipation (8% to 11%)
- Neuromuscular & skeletal: Back pain (14%), weakness (14%)
- Respiratory: Rhinitis (11%)
- Miscellaneous: Withdrawal syndrome (18% to 22%; placebo 37%), infection (12% to 20%), diaphoresis (12% to 13%)

1% to 10%:
- Central nervous system: Chills (6%), nervousness (6%), somnolence (5%), dizziness (4%), fever (3%)
- Gastrointestinal: Vomiting (5% to 8%), diarrhea (5%), dyspepsia (3%)
- Local: Abscess formation (2%)
- Ocular: Lacrimation (5%)
- Respiratory: Cough (4%), pharyngitis (4%)
- Miscellaneous: Flu-like syndrome (6%)

<1% (Limited to important or life-threatening): Anaphylactic shock, angioedema, hepatic encephalopathy, hepatic failure, hepatic necrosis, hepatitis (including cytolytic), hepatorenal syndrome, hypersensitivity reactions, transaminases increased

Transdermal patch:

>10%:
- Central nervous system: Headache (3% to 14%), dizziness (2% to 15%), somnolence (2% to 13%)
- Gastrointestinal: Nausea (6% to 23%), constipation (3% to 13%)
- Local: Application site pruritus (4% to 15%)

1% to 10%:
- Cardiovascular: Chest pain (1% to <5%), hypertension (1% to <5%), peripheral edema (1% to <5%)
- Central nervous system: Anxiety (1% to <5%), depression (1% to <5%), fatigue (1% to 5%), fever (1% to <5%), hypoesthesia (1% to <5%), insomnia (1% to <5%), migraine (1% to <5%), pain (1% to <5%)
- Dermatologic: Hyperhydrosis (1% to <5%), pruritus (1% to <5%), rash (1% to <5%)
- Gastrointestinal: Vomiting (4% to 9%), xerostomia (6%), anorexia (1% to <5%), diarrhea (1% to <5%), dyspepsia (1% to <5%), upper abdominal pain (1% to <5%), abdominal discomfort (2%)
- Genitourinary: Urinary tract infection (1% to <5%)
- Local: Application site erythema (3% to 10%), application site irritation (1% to 6%), application site rash (3% to 8%)
- Neuromuscular & skeletal: Arthralgia (1% to <5%), back pain (1% to <5%), joint swelling (1% to <5%), muscle spasms (1% to <5%), musculoskeletal pain (1% to <5%), myalgia (1% to <5%), neck pain (1% to <5%), pain in extremity (1% to <5%), paresthesia (1% to <5%), tremor (1% to <5%), weakness (1% to <5%)
- Respiratory: Bronchitis (1% to <5%), cough (1% to <5%), dyspnea (1% to <5%), nasopharyngitis (1% to <5%), pharyngolaryngeal pain (1% to <5%), sinusitis (1% to <5%), upper respiratory tract infection (1% to <5%)
- Miscellaneous: Flu-like syndrome (1% to <5%)

<1% (Limited to important or life-threatening): ALT increased, angina, angioedema, application site dermatitis, asthma exacerbation, bradycardia, contact dermatitis, diverticulitis, hallucinations, hyper/hypoventilation, hypersensitivity reactions, hypotension, ileus, loss of consciousness, memory impairment, mental impairment, mental status changes, miosis (dose-related), orthostatic hypotension, psychoses, respiratory depression, respiratory distress, respiratory failure, syncope, tachycardia,

urinary incontinence, urinary retention, vasodilatation, visual disturbances, withdrawal syndrome

Drug Interactions

Metabolism/Transport Effects Substrate of CYP3A4 (major); **Note:** Assignment of Major/Minor substrate status based on clinically relevant drug interaction potential; **Inhibits** CYP1A2 (weak), CYP2A6 (weak), CYP2C19 (weak), CYP2D6 (weak)

Avoid Concomitant Use

Avoid concomitant use of Buprenorphine with any of the following: Atazanavir; Azelastine (Nasal); Conivaptan; Fusidic Acid (Systemic); MAO Inhibitors; Paraldehyde

Increased Effect/Toxicity

Buprenorphine may increase the levels/effects of: Alvimopan; ARIPiprazole; Azelastine (Nasal); Desmopressin; Diuretics; MAO Inhibitors; Metyrosine; Mirtazapine; Paraldehyde; Pramipexole; ROPINIRole; Rotigotine; Selective Serotonin Reuptake Inhibitors; Zolpidem

The levels/effects of Buprenorphine may be increased by: Alcohol (Ethyl); Amphetamines; Anticholinergics; Antipsychotic Agents (Phenothiazines); Atazanavir; Boceprevir; Brimonidine (Topical); Cannabinoids; CNS Depressants; Conivaptan; CYP3A4 Inhibitors (Moderate); CYP3A4 Inhibitors (Strong); Dasatinib; Doxylamine; Droperidol; Fusidic Acid (Systemic); HydrOXYzine; Ivacaftor; Luliconazole; Magnesium Sulfate; Mifepristone; Perampanel; Simeprevir; Sodium Oxybate; Succinylcholine

Decreased Effect

Buprenorphine may decrease the levels/effects of: Analgesics (Opioid); Atazanavir; Pegvisomant

The levels/effects of Buprenorphine may be decreased by: Ammonium Chloride; Boceprevir; Bosentan; CYP3A4 Inducers (Strong); Dabrafenib; Deferasirox; Efavirenz; Etravirine; Herbs (CYP3A4 Inducers); Mitotane; Mixed Agonist / Antagonist Opioids; Tocilizumab

Ethanol/Nutrition/Herb Interactions

Ethanol: May increase CNS depression; monitor for increased effects with coadministration. Caution patients about effect.

Herb/Nutraceutical: Avoid valerian, St John's wort, kava kava, gotu kola (may increase CNS depression).

Storage/Stability

Injection: Protect from excessive heat >40°C (>104°F). Protect from light.

Patch, tablet: Store at room temperature of 25°C (77°F); excursions permitted between 15°C to 30°C (59°F to 86°F).

Mechanism of Action Buprenorphine exerts its analgesic effect via high affinity binding to μ opiate receptors in the CNS; displays partial mu agonist and weak kappa antagonist activity

Pharmacodynamics/Kinetics

Onset of action: Analgesic: I.M: Within 15 minutes

Peak effect: I.M.: ~1 hour; Transdermal patch: Steady state achieved by day 3

Duration: I.M.: ≥6 hours

Absorption: I.M., SubQ: 30% to 40%

Distribution: V_d: 97-187 L/kg

Protein binding: High (~96%, primarily to alpha- and beta globulin)

Metabolism: Primarily hepatic via N-dealkylation by CYP3A4 to norbuprenorphine (active metabolite), and to a lesser extent via glucuronidation by UGT1A1 and 2B7 to buprenorphine 3-O-glucuronide; the major metabolite, norbuprenorphine, also undergoes glucuronidation via UGT1A3; extensive first-pass effect

Bioavailability (relative to I.V. administration): I.M.: 70%; Sublingual tablet: 29%; Transdermal patch: ~15%

Half-life elimination: I.V.: 2.2-3 hours; Apparent terminal half-life: Sublingual tablet: ~37 hours; Transdermal patch: ~26 hours. **Note:** Extended elimination half-life for sublingual administration may be due to depot effect (Kuhlman, 1996).

Time to peak, plasma: Sublingual: 30 minutes to 1 hour (Kuhlman, 1996)

Excretion: Feces (~70%); urine (27% to 30%)

Dosage

I.M., I.V.: Acute pain (moderate-to-severe): **Note: Long-term use is not recommended.** The following recommendations are guidelines and do not represent the maximum doses that may be required in all patients. Doses should be titrated to pain relief/prevention. In high-risk patients (eg, elderly, debilitated, presence of respiratory disease) and/or concurrent CNS depressant use, reduce dose by one-half. Buprenorphine has an analgesic ceiling.

Children 2-12 years: I.M., slow I.V.: 2-6 **mcg**/kg every 4-6 hours

Children ≥13 years and Adults:

I.M.: Initial: Opioid-naive: 0.3 mg every 6-8 hours as needed; initial dose (up to 0.3 mg) may be repeated once in 30-60 minutes after the initial dose if needed; usual dosage range: 0.15-0.6 mg every 4-8 hours as needed

Slow I.V.: Initial: Opioid-naive: 0.3 mg every 6-8 hours as needed; initial dose (up to 0.3 mg) may be repeated once in 30-60 minutes after the initial dose if needed

Adults: I.V. infusion: Opioid withdrawal in heroin-dependent hospitalized patients (unlabeled): 0.3-0.9 mg (diluted in 50-100 mL of NS) over 20-30 minutes every 6-12 hours (Welsh, 2002)

Sublingual tablet: Children ≥16 years and Adults: Opioid dependence: **Note:** The combination product, buprenorphine and naloxone, is preferred therapy over buprenorphine monotherapy for induction treatment (and stabilization/maintenance treatment) for short-acting opioid dependence (U.S. Department of Health and Human Services, 2005).

Manufacturer's labeling:

Induction: Day 1: 8 mg; Day 2 and subsequent induction days: 16 mg; usual induction dosage range: 12-16 mg/day (induction usually accomplished over 3-4 days). Treatment should begin at least 4 hours after last use of heroin or other short-acting opioids, preferably when first signs of withdrawal appear. Titrating dose to clinical effectiveness should be done as rapidly as possible to prevent undue withdrawal symptoms and patient drop-out during the induction period. There is little controlled experience with induction in patients on methadone or other long-acting opioids; consult expert physician experienced with this procedure.

Maintenance: Target dose: 16 mg daily; in some patients 12 mg daily may be effective; patients should be switched to the buprenorphine/naloxone combination product for maintenance and unsupervised therapy

Transdermal patch: Adults: Chronic pain (moderate-to-severe):

Opioid-naive patients: Initial: 5 **mcg**/hour applied once every 7 days

Opioid-experienced patients (conversion from other opioids to buprenorphine): Taper the current around-the-clock opioid for up to 7 days to ≤30 mg/day of oral morphine or equivalent before initiating therapy. Short-acting analgesics as needed may be continued until analgesia with transdermal buprenorphine is attained. There is a potential for buprenorphine to precipitate withdrawal in patients already receiving opioids.

Patients who were receiving daily dose of <30 mg of oral morphine equivalents: Initial: 5 **mcg**/hour applied once every 7 days

Patients who were receiving daily dose of 30-80 mg of oral morphine equivalents: Initial: 10 **mcg**/hour applied once every 7 days

Patient who were receiving daily dose of >80 mg of oral morphine equivalents: Buprenorphine transdermal patch, even at the maximum dose of 20 **mcg**/hour applied once every 7 days, may not provide adequate analgesia; **consider the use of an alternate analgesic.**

Dose titration (opioid-naive or opioid-experienced patients): May increase dose, based on patient's supplemental short-acting analgesic requirements, with a minimum titration interval of 72 hours (maximum dose: 20 **mcg**/hour applied once every 7 days; risk for QT_c prolongation increases with doses ≥20 **mcg**/hour patch).

Discontinuation of therapy: Taper dose gradually every 7 days to prevent withdrawal in the physically dependent patient; consider initiating immediate-release opioids, if needed.

Elderly:

I.M., slow I.V.: 0.15 mg every 6 hours; elderly patients are more likely to suffer from confusion and drowsiness compared to younger patients

Transdermal patch: Chronic pain (moderate-to-severe): No specific dosage adjustments required; use caution due to potential for increased risk of adverse events. Refer to adult dosing.

Dosage adjustment in renal impairment: Injection, sublingual, transdermal: No dosage adjustment provided in manufacturer's labeling (has not been adequately studied); use with caution.

Dosage adjustment in hepatic impairment:

Injection: No dosage adjustment provided in manufacturer's labeling; undergoes extensive hepatic metabolism; use with caution, especially in severe impairment.

Sublingual: Moderate-to-severe impairment: Dosage adjustments recommended; however, no specific recommendations are provided in the manufacturer's labeling.

Transdermal patch:

Mild-to-moderate impairment: Initial: 5 **mcg**/hour applied once every 7 days

Severe impairment: Not studied; consider alternative therapy with more flexibility for dosing adjustments.

Administration

I.M.: Administer via deep I.M. injection

I.V.: Administer slowly, over at least 2 minutes. Administration over 20-30 minutes preferred when managing opioid withdrawal in heroin-dependent hospitalized patients (Welsh, 2002).

Oral: Sublingual tablet: Tablet should be placed under the tongue until dissolved; should not be swallowed. If two or more tablets are needed per dose, all may be placed under the tongue at once, or two at a time. To ensure consistent bioavailability, subsequent doses should always be taken the same way.

Transdermal patch: Apply to patch to intact, nonirritated skin only. Apply to a hairless or nearly hairless skin site. If hairless site is not available, do not shave skin; hair at application site should be clipped. Prior to application, if the site must be cleaned, clean with clear water and allow to dry completely; do not use soaps, alcohol, lotions or abrasives due to potential for increased skin absorption. Do not use any patch that has been damaged, cut or manipulated in any way. Remove patch from protective pouch immediately before application. Remove the protective backing, and apply the sticky side of the patch to one of eight possible application sites (upper outer arm, upper chest, upper back or the side of the chest [each site on either side of the body]). Firmly press patch in place and hold for ~15 seconds. Change patch every 7 days. Rotate patch application sites; wait ≥21 days before reapplying another patch to the same skin site. Avoid exposing application site to external heat sources (eg, heating pad, electric blanket, heat lamp, hot tub). If there is difficulty with patch adhesion, the edges of the system may be taped in place with first-aid tape. If the patch falls off during the 7-day dosing interval, dispose of the patch and apply a new patch to a different skin site.

Monitoring Parameters Pain relief, respiratory and mental status, CNS depression, blood pressure; LFTs (prior to initiation and during therapy); symptoms of withdrawal; application site reactions (transdermal patch)

Dosage Forms Excipient information presented when available (limited, particularly for generics); consult specific product labeling.

Patch Weekly, Transdermal:

Butrans: 5 mcg/hr (4 ea); 10 mcg/hr (4 ea); 15 mcg/hr (4 ea); 20 mcg/hr (4 ea)

Solution, Injection:

Buprenex: 0.3 mg/mL (1 mL)

Generic: 0.3 mg/mL (1 mL)

Tablet Sublingual, Sublingual:

Generic: 2 mg, 8 mg

Controlled Substance C-III

Extemporaneous Preparations A 0.075 mg/mL solution can be made using the 0.3 mg/mL injection, 95% ethanol, and simple syrup. Add 1.26 mL of 95% ethanol to 0.3 mg buprenorphine obtained from an 0.3 mg/1 mL ampule, mix well, and add quantity of simple syrup sufficient to obtain 4 mL (final volume). Solution is stable under refrigeration and at room temperature for 30 days when stored in amber glass bottles and for 7 days when stored in oral syringes (Anagnostis, 2011; Anagnostis, 2013).

Anagnostis EA, Sadaka RE, Sailor LA, et al, "Formulation of Buprenorphine for Sublingual Use in Neonates," *J Pediatr Pharmacol Ther*, 2011, 16(4):281-4.

Anagnostis EA, personal communication, March 2013.

Buprenorphine and Naloxone

(byoo pre NOR feen & nal OKS one)

Brand Names: U.S. Suboxone; Zubsolv

Brand Names: Canada Suboxone

Index Terms Buprenorphine Hydrochloride and Naloxone Hydrochloride Dihydrate; Naloxone and Buprenorphine; Naloxone Hydrochloride Dihydrate and Buprenorphine Hydrochloride

Pharmacologic Category Analgesic, Opioid; Analgesic, Opioid Partial Agonist

Use

Opioid dependence: For the maintenance treatment of opioid dependence.

General information: Buprenorphine/naloxone should be used as part of a complete treatment plan to include counseling and psychosocial support

Pregnancy Risk Factor C

Prescribing and Access Restrictions Prescribing of tablets for opioid dependence is limited to physicians who have met the qualification criteria and have received a DEA number specific to prescribing this product. Tablets will be available through pharmacies and wholesalers which normally provide controlled substances.

Medication Guide Available Yes

Dosage Opioid dependence: Sublingual: **Note:** Buprenorphine and naloxone combination product is not recommended for use during the induction period for long-acting opioids (eg, methadone); initial treatment should begin using buprenorphine oral sublingual tablets under supervision. Patients should be switched to the combination product for maintenance and unsupervised therapy. Doses provided based on buprenorphine content.

Adolescents ≥16 years (sublingual tablet) and Adults (sublingual tablet or sublingual film [Suboxone]):

Manufacturer's labeling: Maintenance: Target dose: 16 mg daily as a single daily dose; dosage should be adjusted in increments of 2 mg or 4 mg to a level which maintains treatment and suppresses opioid withdrawal symptoms; usual range: 4-24 mg daily

Unlabeled dosing recommendations (U.S. Department of Health and Human Services, 2005):

Induction (only administer combination product for induction in patients who are dependent on **short-acting** opioids and whose last dose of opioids was >12-24 hours prior to induction):

Day 1 induction dose: Initial: 4 mg; may repeat dose after >2 hours if withdrawal symptoms not relieved; maximum daily dose on day 1: 8 mg daily

Day 2 induction dose: Previous dose from day 1 if no withdrawal symptoms present; if symptoms of withdrawal present, increase day 1 dose by 4 mg. If withdrawal symptoms not relieved after >2 hours, may administer 4 mg; maximum daily dose on day 2: 16 mg daily

Subsequent induction days: If withdrawal symptoms are not present, daily dose is established. If withdrawal symptoms are present, increase dose in increments of 2 mg or 4 mg each day as needed for symptom relief. Target daily dose by the end of the first week: 12 mg or 16 mg daily; maximum daily dose: 32 mg daily

Stabilization: Usual dose: 16-24 mg daily; maximum dose: 32 mg daily

Switching between sublingual tablets and sublingual film: Same dosage should be used as the previous administered product. **Note:** Potential for greater bioavailability with certain sublingual film strengths compared to the same strength of the sublingual tablet; monitor closely for either over- or underdosing when switching patients from one formulation to another.

Switching between sublingual film strengths: Systemic exposure may be different with various combinations of sublingual film strengths; pharmacists should not substitute one or more film strengths for another (eg, switching from three 4 mg films to a single 12 mg film, or vice-versa) without physician approval, and patients should be monitored closely for either over- or underdosing when switching between film strengths.

Adults: Sublingual tablets (Zubsolv): Maintenance: Target dose: 11.4 mg daily as a single daily dose; dosage should be adjusted in increments or decrements of 1.4 mg or 2.8 mg to a level which maintains treatment and suppresses opioid withdrawal symptoms; usual range: 2.8-17.1 mg daily. The corresponding doses going from induction with buprenorphine sublingual tablets to maintenance treatment with buprenorphine/naloxone sublingual tablets are:

Final sublingual buprenorphine dose during induction: 8 mg: Zubsolv maintenance dose: 5.7 mg buprenorphine/1.4 mg naloxone as a single daily dose

Final sublingual buprenorphine dose during induction: 12 mg: Zubsolv maintenance dose: 8.5 mg buprenorphine/2.12 mg naloxone as a single daily dose

Final sublingual buprenorphine dose during induction: 16 mg: Zubsolv maintenance dose: 11.4 mg buprenorphine/2.8 mg naloxone as a single daily dose

Switching between sublingual tablet products: Due to differences in the bioavailability of Zubsolv sublingual tablets compared to other buprenorphine/naloxone sublingual tablets, different strengths must be given to achieve equivalent doses. When switching between Zubsolv and other sublingual tablets, corresponding dosage strengths are as follows:

Zubsolv 1.4 mg/0.36 mg sublingual tablets = 2 mg/0.5 mg buprenorphine/naloxone sublingual tablets

Zubsolv 5.7 mg/1.4 mg sublingual tablets = 8 mg/2 mg buprenorphine/naloxone sublingual tablets

Dosage adjustment in renal impairment: No dosage adjustment provided in manufacturer's labeling (has not been adequately studied). Use with caution.

Dosing adjustment in hepatic impairment: Moderate-to-severe impairment: dosage adjustments recommended; however, no specific recommendations are provided in manufacturer's labeling.

Additional Information Complete prescribing information should be consulted for additional detail.

Dosage Forms Excipient information presented when available (limited, particularly for generics); consult specific product labeling.

Film, sublingual:

Suboxone: Buprenorphine 2 mg and naloxone 0.5 mg (30s); buprenorphine 4 mg and naloxone 1 mg (30s); buprenorphine 8 mg and naloxone 2 mg (30s); buprenorphine 12 mg and naloxone 3 mg (30s) [lime flavor]

Tablet, sublingual: Buprenorphine 2 mg and naloxone 0.5 mg; buprenorphine 8 mg and naloxone 2 mg

Suboxone: Buprenorphine 2 mg and naloxone 0.5 mg [DSC]; buprenorphine 8 mg and naloxone 2 mg [lemon-lime flavor] [DSC]

Zubsolv: Buprenorphine 1.4 mg and naloxone 0.36 mg; buprenorphine 5.7 mg and naloxone 1.4 mg [menthol flavor]

Controlled Substance C-III

◆ **Buprenorphine Hydrochloride** *see* Buprenorphine *on page 291*

◆ **Buprenorphine Hydrochloride and Naloxone Hydrochloride Dihydrate** *see* Buprenorphine and Naloxone *on page 295*

◆ **Buproban** *see* BuPROPion *on page 296*

BuPROPion (byoo PROE pee on)

Brand Names: U.S. Aplenzin; Budeprion SR; Buproban; Forfivo XL; Wellbutrin; Wellbutrin SR; Wellbutrin XL; Zyban

Brand Names: Canada Ava-Bupropion SR; Bupropion SR; Mylan-Bupropion XL; Novo-Bupropion SR; PMS-Bupropion SR; ratio-Bupropion SR; Sandoz-Bupropion SR; Wellbutrin SR; Wellbutrin XL; Zyban

Index Terms Bupropion Hydrobromide; Bupropion Hydrochloride

Pharmacologic Category Antidepressant, Dopamine-Reuptake Inhibitor; Smoking Cessation Aid

Additional Appendix Information

Antidepressant Agents *on page 2284*

Use Treatment of major depressive disorder, including seasonal affective disorder (SAD); adjunct in smoking cessation (Buproban®, Zyban®)

Unlabeled Use Attention-deficit/hyperactivity disorder (ADHD); depression associated with bipolar disorder

Pregnancy Risk Factor C

Pregnancy Considerations Adverse events have been observed in some animal reproduction studies. Bupropion and its metabolites were found to cross the placenta in *in vitro* studies (Earhart, 2012). An increased risk of congenital malformations has not been observed following maternal of use of bupropion during pregnancy; however, data specific to cardiovascular malformations is inconsistent. The long-term effects on development and behavior have not been studied. The ACOG recommends that antidepressant therapy during pregnancy be individualized; treatment of depression during pregnancy should incorporate the clinical expertise of the mental health clinician, obstetrician, primary healthcare provider, and pediatrician. According to the American Psychiatric Association (APA), the risks of medication treatment should be weighed against other treatment options and untreated depression. For women who discontinue antidepressant medications during pregnancy and who may be at high risk for postpartum depression, the medications can be restarted following delivery. Treatment algorithms have been developed by the ACOG and the APA for the management of depression in women prior to conception and during pregnancy (ACOG, 2008; APA, 2010; Yonkers, 2009). There is insufficient information related to the use of bupropion to recommend use in pregnancy (ACOG, 2010).

Breast-Feeding Considerations Bupropion and its metabolites are excreted into breast milk. The estimated dose to a nursing infant varies by study and has been reported as ~2% of the weight-adjusted maternal dose (range: 1.4% to 10.6%) (Davis, 2009; Haas, 2004). Adverse events have been reported with some antidepressants and a seizure was noted in one 6-month old nursing infant exposed to bupropion (a causal effect could not be confirmed) (Chaudron, 2004; Hale, 2010). Recommendations for use in nursing women vary by manufacturer labeling.

Medication Guide Available Yes

Contraindications Hypersensitivity to bupropion or any component of the formulation; seizure disorder; history of anorexia/bulimia; patients undergoing abrupt discontinuation of ethanol or sedatives, including benzodiazepines; use of MAO inhibitors or MAO inhibitors intended to treat psychiatric disorders (concurrently or within 14 days of discontinuing either bupropion or the MAO inhibitor); initiation of bupropion in a patient receiving linezolid or intravenous methylene blue; patients receiving other dosage forms of bupropion

Aplenzin™: Additional contraindications: Other conditions that increase seizure risk, including arteriovenous malformation, severe head injury, severe stroke, CNS tumor, CNS infection, or abrupt discontinuation of barbiturates or antiepileptics

Warnings/Precautions [U.S. Boxed Warning]: Use in treating psychiatric disorders: Antidepressants increase the risk of suicidal thinking and behavior in children, adolescents, and young adults (18-24 years of age) with major depressive disorder (MDD) and other psychiatric disorders; consider risk prior to prescribing. Short-term studies did not show an increased risk in patients >24 years of age and showed a decreased risk in patients ≥65 years. All patients must be closely monitored for clinical worsening, suicidality, or unusual changes in behavior, especially during the initiation of therapy (generally first 1-2 months) or following an increase or decrease in dosage. The patient's family or caregiver should be instructed to closely observe the patient and communicate condition with healthcare provider. A medication guide should be dispensed with each prescription. **Bupropion is not FDA approved for use in children.**

[U.S. Boxed Warning]: Use in smoking cessation: Serious neuropsychiatric events, including depression, suicidal thoughts, and suicide, have been reported with use; some cases may have been complicated by symptoms of nicotine withdrawal following smoking cessation. Smoking cessation (with or without treatment) is associated with nicotine withdrawal symptoms and the exacerbation of underlying psychiatric illness; however, some of the behavioral disturbances were reported in treated patients who continued to smoke. These neuropsychiatric symptoms (eg, mood disturbances, psychosis, hostility) have occurred in patients with and without pre-existing psychiatric disease; many cases resolved following therapy discontinuation although in some cases, symptoms persisted. Monitor all patients for behavioral changes and psychiatric symptoms (eg, agitation, depression, suicidal behavior, suicidal ideation); inform patients to discontinue treatment and contact their healthcare provider immediately if they experience any behavioral and/or mood changes.

The possibility of a suicide attempt is inherent in major depression and may persist until remission occurs. Use caution in high-risk patients. Worsening depression and severe abrupt suicidality that are not part of the presenting symptoms may require discontinuation or modification of drug therapy. The patient's family or caregiver should be alerted to monitor patients for the emergence of suicidality and associated behaviors (such as agitation, irritability, hostility, impulsivity, and hypomania) and notify the healthcare provider.

May worsen psychosis in some patients or precipitate a shift to mania or hypomania in patients with bipolar disorder. Patients presenting with depressive symptoms should be screened for bipolar disorder. Monotherapy in patients with bipolar disorder should be avoided. **Bupropion is not FDA approved for bipolar depression.**

May cause a dose-related risk of seizures. Use is contraindicated in patients with a history of seizures or certain conditions with high seizure risk (eg, arteriovenous malformation, severe head injury, severe stroke, CNS tumor, or CNS infection, history of anorexia/bulimia, or patients undergoing abrupt discontinuation of ethanol, benzodiazepines, barbiturates, or antiepileptic drugs). Use caution with concurrent use of antipsychotics, antidepressants, theophylline, systemic corticosteroids, stimulants (including cocaine), anorectants, or hypoglycemic agents, or with excessive use of ethanol, benzodiazepines, sedative/hypnotics, or opioids. Use with caution in seizure-potentiating metabolic disorders (hypoglycemia, hyponatremia, severe hepatic impairment, and hypoxia). The dose-dependent risk of seizures may be reduced by gradual dose increases and limiting the daily dose to bupropion hydrochloride ≤450 mg or bupropion hydrobromide ≤522 mg. Use of multiple bupropion formulations is contraindicated. Permanently discontinue if seizure occurs during therapy. Chewing, crushing, or dividing long-acting products may increase seizure risk.

May cause CNS stimulation (restlessness, anxiety, insomnia) or anorexia. May increase the risks associated with electroconvulsive therapy (ECT). Consider discontinuing, when possible, prior to ECT. May cause weight loss; use caution in patients where weight loss is not desirable. The incidence of sexual dysfunction with bupropion is generally lower than with SSRIs.

Use caution in patients with cardiovascular disease, history of hypertension, or coronary artery disease; treatment-emergent hypertension (including some severe cases) has been reported, both with bupropion alone and in combination with nicotine transdermal systems. All children diagnosed with ADHD who may be candidates for stimulant medications should have a thorough cardiovascular assessment to identify risk factors for sudden cardiac death prior to initiation of drug therapy. Use with caution in patients with hepatic or renal dysfunction and in elderly patients; reduced dose and/or frequency may be recommended. Elderly patients may be at greater risk of accumulation during chronic dosing. May cause motor or cognitive impairment in some patients; use with caution if tasks requiring alertness such as operating machinery or driving are undertaken. Anaphylactoid/anaphylactic reactions have occurred, with symptoms of pruritus, urticaria, angioedema, and dyspnea. Serious reactions have been (rarely) reported, including Stevens-Johnson syndrome and anaphylactic shock. Arthralgia, myalgia, and fever with rash and other symptoms suggestive of delayed hypersensitivity resembling serum sickness have been reported. Potentially significant interactions may exist, requiring dose or frequency adjustment, additional monitoring, and/or selection of alternative therapy.

Extended release tablet: Insoluble tablet shell may remain intact and be visible in the stool.

Adverse Reactions Frequencies, when reported, reflect highest incidence reported with sustained release product.

>10%:

Cardiovascular: Tachycardia (11%)

Central nervous system: Headache (25% to 34%), insomnia (11% to 20%), dizziness (6% to 11%)

Gastrointestinal: Xerostomia (17% to 26%), weight loss (14% to 23%), nausea (1% to 18%)

Respiratory: Pharyngitis (3% to 13%)

1% to 10%:

Cardiovascular: Palpitation (2% to 6%), arrhythmias (5%), chest pain (3% to 4%), hypertension (2% to 4%; may be severe), flushing (1% to 4%), hypotension (3%)

Central nervous system: Agitation (2% to 9%), confusion (8%), anxiety (5% to 7%), hostility (6%), nervousness (3% to 5%), sleep disturbance (4%), sensory disturbance (4%), migraine (1% to 4%), abnormal dreams (3%), irritability (2% to 3%), somnolence (2% to 3%), pain (2% to 3%), memory decreased (≤3%), fever (1% to 2%), CNS stimulation (1% to 2%), depression

Dermatologic: Rash (1% to 5%), pruritus (2% to 4%), urticaria (1% to 2%)

Endocrine & metabolic: Menstrual complaints (2% to 5%), hot flashes (1% to 3%), libido decreased (3%)

Gastrointestinal: Constipation (5% to 10%), abdominal pain (2% to 9%), diarrhea (5% to 7%), flatulence (6%), anorexia (3% to 5%), appetite increased (4%), taste perversion (2% to 4%), vomiting (2% to 4%), dyspepsia (3%), dysphagia (≤2%)

Genitourinary: Polyuria (2% to 5%), urinary urgency (≤2%), vaginal hemorrhage (≤2%), UTI (≤1%)

Neuromuscular & skeletal: Tremor (3% to 6%), myalgia (2% to 6%), weakness (2% to 4%), arthralgia (1% to 4%), arthritis (2%), akathisia (≤2%), paresthesia (1% to 2%), twitching (1% to 2%), neck pain

Ocular: Blurred vision (2% to 3%), amblyopia (2%)

Otic: Tinnitus (3% to 6%), auditory disturbance (5%)

Respiratory: Upper respiratory infection (9%), cough increased (1% to 4%), sinusitis (1% to 5%)

Miscellaneous: Infection (8% to 9%), diaphoresis (5% to 6%), allergic reaction (including anaphylaxis, pruritus, urticaria)

<1% (Limited to important or life-threatening): Accommodation abnormality, aggression, akinesia, alopecia, amnesia, anaphylactic shock, anemia, angioedema, aphasia, ataxia, atrioventricular block, bronchospasm, bruxism, colitis, coma, coordination abnormal, cystitis, deafness, delayed hypersensitivity, delirium, delusions, depersonalization, derealization, diplopia, dysarthria, dyskinesia, dyspareunia, dysphoria, dystonia, dysuria, edema, EEG abnormality, emotional lability, erythema multiforme, esophagitis, euphoria, exfoliative dermatitis, extrapyramidal syndrome, extrasystoles, facial edema, gastric reflux, gastrointestinal hemorrhage, glossitis, glycosuria, gum hemorrhage, gynecomastia, hallucinations, hepatic damage, hepatitis, hirsutism, hyper-/hypoglycemia, hyper-/hypokinesia, hypertonia, hypoesthesia, hypomania, impotence, intestinal perforation, intraocular pressure increased, jaundice, leukocytosis, leukopenia, libido increased, liver function abnormal, lymphadenopathy, manic reaction, MI, muscle weakness, musculoskeletal chest pain, mydriasis, myoclonus, neuralgia, neuropathy, orthostatic hypotension, painful erection, pancreatitis, pancytopenia, paranoia, pneumonia, photosensitivity, pulmonary embolism, rhabdomyolysis, salpingitis, sciatica, seizures (dose-related), SIADH, stomach ulcer, Stevens-Johnson syndrome, stomatitis, stroke, suicidal ideation, syncope, tardive dyskinesia, thrombocytopenia, tongue edema, urinary incontinence, urinary retention, vasodilation

Drug Interactions

Metabolism/Transport Effects Substrate of CYP1A2 (minor), CYP2A6 (minor), CYP2B6 (major), CYP2C9 (minor), CYP2D6 (minor), CYP2E1 (minor), CYP3A4 (minor); **Note:** Assignment of Major/Minor substrate status based on clinically relevant drug interaction potential; **Inhibits** CYP2D6 (strong)

Avoid Concomitant Use

Avoid concomitant use of BuPROPion with any of the following: MAO Inhibitors; Pimozide; Tamoxifen; Thioridazine

Increased Effect/Toxicity

BuPROPion may increase the levels/effects of: Alcohol (Ethyl); ARIPiprazole; AtoMOXetine; CYP2D6 Substrates; Fesoterodine; FLUoxetine; FluvoxaMINE; Iloperidone; Lorcaserin; Metoprolol; Nebivolol; PARoxetine; Pimozide; Propafenone; Tetrabenazine; Thioridazine; Tricyclic Antidepressants; Vortioxetine

The levels/effects of BuPROPion may be increased by: Alcohol (Ethyl); CYP2B6 Inhibitors (Moderate); CYP2B6 Inhibitors (Strong); MAO Inhibitors; Mifepristone; Quazepam

Decreased Effect

BuPROPion may decrease the levels/effects of: Codeine; Iloperidone; Ioflupane I 123; Tamoxifen; TraMADol

The levels/effects of BuPROPion may be decreased by: CYP2B6 Inducers (Strong); Dabrafenib; Efavirenz; Lopinavir; Peginterferon Alfa-2b; Ritonavir

Ethanol/Nutrition/Herb Interactions

Ethanol: May increase CNS depression; monitor for increased effects with coadministration. Caution patients about effects.

Herb/Nutraceutical: Avoid valerian, St John's wort, SAMe, gotu kola, kava kava (may increase CNS depression).

Storage/Stability Store at controlled room temperature of 20°C to 25°C (68°F to 77°F).

Aplenzin™, Wellbutrin XL®: Store at 15°C to 30°C (59°F to 86°F).

Mechanism of Action Aminoketone antidepressant structurally different from all other marketed antidepressants; like other antidepressants the mechanism of bupropion's activity is not fully understood. Bupropion is a relatively weak inhibitor of the neuronal uptake of norepinephrine and dopamine, and does not inhibit monoamine oxidase or the reuptake of serotonin. Metabolite inhibits the reuptake of norepinephrine. The primary mechanism of action is thought to be dopaminergic and/or noradrenergic.

Pharmacodynamics/Kinetics

Absorption: Rapid

Distribution: V_d: ~20-47 L/kg (Laizure, 1985)

Protein binding: 84%

Metabolism: Extensively hepatic via CYP2B6 to hydroxybupropion; non-CYP-mediated metabolism to erythrohydrobupropion and threohydrobupropion. Metabolite activity ranges from 20% to 50% potency of bupropion.

Half-life:

Distribution: 3-4 hours

Elimination: ~14 hours (range: 8-24 hours); Metabolites: Hydroxybupropion: 20 ± 5 hours; Erythrohydrobupropion: 33 ± 10 hours; Threohydrobupropion: 37 ± 13 hours

Extended release (Aplenzin™): 21 ± 7 hours; Metabolites: Hydroxybupropion: 24 ± 5 hours; Erythrohydrobupropion: 31 ± 8 hours; Threohydrobupropion: 51 ± 9 hours

Time to peak, serum:

Bupropion: Immediate release: Within 2 hours; Sustained release: Within 3 hours; Extended release: ~5 hours (Forfivo™ XL: 5 hours [fasting]; 12 hours [fed])

Metabolite: Hydroxybupropion: Immediate release: ~3 hours; Extended release, sustained release: ~6-7 hours

Excretion: Urine (87%, primarily as metabolites); feces (10%, primarily as metabolites)

Dosage Oral:

Children and Adolescents: ADHD (unlabeled use): Hydrochloride salt: 1.4-6 mg/kg/day (Barrickman, 1995; Conners, 1996)

Adults:

Depression: **Note:** Treatment should be periodically evaluated at appropriate intervals to ensure lowest effective dose is used.

Immediate release hydrochloride salt: Initial: 100 mg twice daily; after 3 days may increase to the usual dose of 100 mg 3 times a day; if no clinical improvement after several weeks, may increase to a maximum dose of 150 mg 3 times daily

Sustained release hydrochloride salt: Initial: 150 mg daily in the morning; if tolerated, as early as day 4, may increase to a target dose of 150 mg twice daily; if no clinical improvement after several weeks, may increase to a maximum dose of 200 mg twice daily

Extended release:

Hydrochloride salt: Initial: 150 mg once daily in the morning; if tolerated, as early as day 4, may increase to 300 mg once daily; if no clinical improvement after several weeks, may increase to a maximum dose 450 mg once daily. **Note:** Forfivo™ XL may only be used after initial dose titration with other bupropion products.

Hydrochloride salt (Forfivo™ XL): *Switching from Wellbutrin® immediate release, SR®, or XL® to Forfivo™ XL:* Patients receiving 300 mg daily of bupropion hydrochloride for at least 2 weeks and requiring a dose increase or patients already taking 450 mg daily of bupropion hydrochloride may switch to Forfivo™ XL 450 mg once daily.

Hydrobromide salt (Aplenzin™): Initial: 174 mg once daily in the morning; may increase as early as day 4 of dosing to 348 mg once daily (target dose); maximum dose: 522 mg daily. **Note:** In patients receiving 348 mg once daily, taper dose down to 174 mg once daily prior to discontinuing.

Switching from hydrochloride salt formulation (eg, Wellbutrin® immediate release, SR®, XL®, or Forfivo™ XL) to hydrobromide salt formulation (Aplenzin™):

Bupropion hydrochloride 150 mg daily is equivalent to bupropion hydrobromide 174 mg once daily

Bupropion hydrochloride 300 mg daily is equivalent to bupropion hydrobromide 348 mg once daily

Bupropion hydrochloride 450 mg daily is equivalent to bupropion hydrobromide 522 mg once daily

SAD: Initial: 150 mg once daily (Wellbutrin XL®) or 174 mg once daily (Aplenzin™) in the morning; if tolerated, may increase after 1 week to 300 mg once daily (Wellbutrin XL®) or 348 mg once daily (Aplenzin™) in the morning.

Note: Prophylactic treatment should be reserved for those patients with frequent depressive episodes and/or significant impairment. Initiate treatment in the Autumn prior to symptom onset, and discontinue in early Spring with dose tapering to 150 mg once daily for 2 weeks (Wellbutrin XL®) or 174 mg once daily (Aplenzin™), then discontinue. Doses >300 mg daily (Wellbutrin XL®) or >348 mg daily (Aplenzin™) have not been studied in SAD.

Smoking cessation (Zyban®, Buproban®): Initial: 150 mg once daily for 3 days; increase to 150 mg twice daily; treatment should continue for 7-12 weeks

Note: Therapy should begin at least 1 week before target quit date. Target quit dates are generally in the second week of treatment. If patient successfully quits smoking after 7-12 weeks, may consider ongoing maintenance therapy based on individual patient risk: benefit. Efficacy of maintenance therapy (300 mg daily) has been demonstrated for up to 6 months. Conversely, if significant progress has not been made by the seventh week of therapy, success is unlikely and treatment discontinuation should be considered.

Elderly:

Depression: Oral (hydrochloride salt): Initial: 37.5 mg of immediate release tablets twice daily or 100 mg daily of sustained release tablets; increase by 37.5-100 mg every 3-4 days as tolerated to a maximum dose of 300 mg/day (in divided doses). There is evidence that the elderly respond at 150 mg daily in divided doses, but some may require a higher dose. **Note:** Patients with Alzheimer's dementia-related depression may require a lower starting dosage of 37.5 mg once or twice daily (100 mg daily sustained release), increased as needed up to 300 mg daily in divided doses (300 mg daily for sustained release) (Rabins, 2007).

Smoking cessation: Refer to adult dosing.

Dosing conversion between hydrochloride salt immediate (Wellbutrin®), sustained (Wellbutrin SR®), and extended release (Wellbutrin XL®, Forfivo™ XL) products: Convert using same total daily dose (up to the maximum recommended dose for a given dosage form), but adjust frequency as indicated for sustained (twice daily) or extended (once daily) release products.

Discontinuation of therapy: Upon discontinuation of antidepressant therapy, gradually taper the dose to allow for the detection of re-emerging symptoms. (APA, 2010).

MAO inhibitor recommendations:

Switching to or from an MAO inhibitor antidepressant:

Allow 14 days to elapse between discontinuing an MAO inhibitor intended to treat depression and initiation of bupropion.

Allow 14 days to elapse between discontinuing bupropion and initiation of an MAO inhibitor intended to treat depression.

Use with reversible MAO inhibitors (such as linezolid or I.V. methylene blue):

Do not initiate bupropion in patients receiving linezolid or I.V. methylene blue; consider other interventions for psychiatric condition.

If urgent treatment with linezolid or I.V. methylene blue is required in a patient already receiving bupropion and potential benefits outweigh potential risks, discontinue bupropion promptly and administer linezolid or I.V. methylene blue. Monitor for increased risk of hypertensive reactions for 2 weeks or until 24 hours after the last dose of linezolid or I.V. methylene blue, whichever comes first. May resume bupropion 24 hours after the last dose of linezolid or I.V. methylene blue.

Dosing adjustment/comments in renal impairment:

Use with caution and consider a reduction in dosing frequency; limited pharmacokinetic information suggests elimination of bupropion and/or the active metabolites may be reduced.

Moderate-to-severe renal impairment: Bupropion exposure was approximately twofold higher compared to normal subjects following a 150 mg single dose administration.

End-stage renal failure: Per the manufacturer, the elimination of hydroxybupropion and threohydrobupropion are reduced in patients with end-stage renal failure.
Forfivo™ XL: Use is not recommended.

Dosing adjustment in hepatic impairment:
Note: The mean AUC increased by ~1.5-fold for hydroxybupropion and ~2.5-fold for erythro/threohydrobupropion; median T_{max} was observed 19 hours later for hydroxybupropion, 31 hours later for erythro/threohydrobupropion; mean half-life for hydroxybupropion increased fivefold, and increased twofold for erythro/threohydrobupropion in patients with severe hepatic cirrhosis compared to healthy volunteers.
Mild-to-moderate hepatic impairment: Use with caution; consider a reduced dose and/or frequency.
Forfivo™ XL: Use is not recommended.
Severe hepatic cirrhosis: Use with extreme caution; maximum dose:
Aplenzin™: 174 mg every other day
Buproban®, Zyban®: 150 mg every other day
Forfivo™ XL: Use is not recommended.
Wellbutrin®: 75 mg once daily
Wellbutrin SR®: 100 mg once daily or 150 mg every other day
Wellbutrin XL®: 150 mg every other day

Administration May be taken without regard to meals. Sustained release and extended release tablets (hydrochloride and hydrobromide salt formulations) should be swallowed whole; do not crush, chew, or divide. The insoluble shell of the extended-release tablet may remain intact during GI transit and is eliminated in the feces.

Monitoring Parameters Body weight; mental status for depression, suicidal ideation (especially at the beginning of therapy or when doses are increased or decreased), anxiety, social functioning, mania, panic attacks; blood pressure (when used in conjunction with nicotine transdermal systems)

When used for the treatment of ADHD, thoroughly evaluate for cardiovascular risk. Monitor heart rate, blood pressure, and consider obtaining ECG prior to initiation (Vetter, 2008).

Reference Range Therapeutic levels (trough, 12 hours after last dose): 50-100 ng/mL

Test Interactions May interfere with urine detection of amphetamine/methamphetamine (false-positive). Decreased prolactin levels.

Additional Information Risk of seizures: When using bupropion hydrochloride immediate release tablets, seizure risk is increased at total daily dosage >450 mg, individual dosages >150 mg, or by sudden, large increments in dose. Data for the immediate-release formulation of bupropion revealed a seizure incidence of 0.4% in patients treated at doses in the 300-450 mg/day range. The estimated seizure incidence increases almost 10-fold between 450 mg and 600 mg per day. Data for the sustained release dosage form revealed a seizure incidence of 0.1% in patients treated at a dosage range of 100-300 mg/day, and increases to ~0.4% at the maximum recommended dose of 400 mg/day.

Dosage Forms Excipient information presented when available (limited, particularly for generics); consult specific product labeling. [DSC] = Discontinued product
Tablet, Oral, as hydrochloride:
Wellbutrin: 75 mg, 100 mg
Generic: 75 mg, 100 mg
Tablet Extended Release 12 Hour, Oral:
Generic: 150 mg
Tablet Extended Release 12 Hour, Oral, as hydrochloride:
Budeprion SR: 100 mg [DSC] [contains tartrazine (fd&c yellow #5)]
Budeprion SR: 150 mg
Buproban: 150 mg
Wellbutrin SR: 100 mg, 150 mg, 200 mg
Zyban: 150 mg
Generic: 100 mg, 150 mg, 200 mg
Tablet Extended Release 24 Hour, Oral, as hydrobromide:
Aplenzin: 174 mg, 348 mg, 522 mg
Tablet Extended Release 24 Hour, Oral, as hydrochloride:
Forfivo XL: 450 mg
Wellbutrin XL: 150 mg, 300 mg
Generic: 150 mg, 300 mg

◆ **Bupropion Hydrobromide** *see* BuPROPion *on page 296*

◆ **Bupropion Hydrochloride** *see* BuPROPion *on page 296*

◆ **Bupropion SR (Can)** *see* BuPROPion *on page 296*

◆ **Burinex® (Can)** *see* Bumetanide *on page 287*

◆ **Buscopan® (Can)** *see* Scopolamine (Systemic) *on page 1881*

◆ **BuSpar** *see* BusPIRone *on page 300*

BusPIRone (byoo SPYE rone)

Brand Names: Canada Apo-Buspirone®; Bustab®; Dom-Buspirone; Novo-Buspirone; PMS-Buspirone; Riva-Buspirone

Index Terms BuSpar; Buspirone Hydrochloride

Pharmacologic Category Antianxiety Agent, Miscellaneous

Use Management of generalized anxiety disorder (GAD)

Unlabeled Use Augmentation agent for antidepressants

Pregnancy Risk Factor B

Pregnancy Considerations Adverse events have not been observed in animal reproduction studies.

Breast-Feeding Considerations It is not known if buspirone is excreted in breast milk. Breast-feeding is not recommended by the manufacturer.

Contraindications Hypersensitivity to buspirone or any component of the formulation

Warnings/Precautions Use in severe hepatic or renal impairment is not recommended. Low potential for cognitive or motor impairment; until effects on patient known, patients should be warned to use caution when performing tasks which require mental alertness (eg, operating machinery or driving). Use with MAO inhibitors may result in hypertensive reactions; concurrent use is not recommended. Restlessness syndrome has been reported in small number of patients; may be attributable to buspirone's antagonism of central dopamine receptors. Monitor for signs of any dopamine-related movement disorders (eg, dystonia, akathisia, pseudo-parkinsonism). Buspirone does not exhibit cross-tolerance with benzodiazepines or other sedative/hypnotic agents. If substituting buspirone for any of these agents, gradually withdraw the drug(s) prior to initiating buspirone.

Adverse Reactions
>10%: Central nervous system: Dizziness (12%)
1% to 10%:
Cardiovascular: Chest pain (≥1%)
Central nervous system: Drowsiness (10%), headache (6%), nervousness (5%), lightheadedness (3%), anger/hostility (2%), confusion (2%), excitement (2%), dream disturbance (≥1%)
Dermatologic: Rash (1%)
Gastrointestinal: Nausea (8%), diarrhea (2%)
Neuromuscular & skeletal: Numbness (2%), weakness (2%), incoordination (1%), musculoskeletal pain (1%), paresthesia (1%), tremor (1%)
Ocular: Blurred vision (2%)
Otic: Tinnitus (≥1%)
Respiratory: Nasal congestion (≥1%), sore throat (≥1%)
Miscellaneous: Diaphoresis (1%)

<1% (Limited to important or life-threatening): Akathisia, alcohol abuse, allergic reaction, alopecia, ALT increased, amenorrhea, angioedema, anorexia, AST increased, ataxia, bleeding disorder, bradycardia, bruising, cardiomyopathy, claustrophobia, cogwheel rigidity, conjunctivitis, CVA, dyskinesia, dystonia, edema, enuresis, eosinophilia, epistaxis, EPS, galactorrhea, hallucination, heart failure, hyper-/hypotension, hyperventilation, irritable colon, leukopenia, memory impairment, menstrual irregularity, MI, ocular pressure increased, parkinsonism, personality disorders, photophobia, PID, psychosis, rectal bleeding, restless leg syndrome, seizure, serotonin syndrome, slow reaction time, slurred speech, suicidal ideation, syncope, thrombocytopenia, thyroid abnormality, transaminase increases, visual disturbances (tunnel vision)

Drug Interactions

Metabolism/Transport Effects Substrate of CYP2D6 (minor), CYP3A4 (major); **Note:** Assignment of Major/Minor substrate status based on clinically relevant drug interaction potential

Avoid Concomitant Use

Avoid concomitant use of BusPIRone with any of the following: Azelastine (Nasal); Conivaptan; Fusidic Acid (Systemic); MAO Inhibitors; Methylene Blue; Paraldehyde

Increased Effect/Toxicity

BusPIRone may increase the levels/effects of: Alcohol (Ethyl); Antidepressants (Serotonin Reuptake Inhibitor/Antagonist); Antipsychotics; Azelastine (Nasal); Buprenorphine; CNS Depressants; Hydrocodone; MAO Inhibitors; Methylene Blue; Metoclopramide; Metyrosine; Paraldehyde; Pramipexole; ROPINIRole; Rotigotine; Selective Serotonin Reuptake Inhibitors; Serotonin Modulators; Zolpidem

The levels/effects of BusPIRone may be increased by: Antifungal Agents (Azole Derivatives, Systemic); Antipsychotics; Brimonidine (Topical); Calcium Channel Blockers (Nondihydropyridine); Conivaptan; CYP3A4 Inhibitors (Moderate); CYP3A4 Inhibitors (Strong); Dasatinib; Doxylamine; Fusidic Acid (Systemic); Grapefruit Juice; HydrOXYzine; Ivacaftor; Luliconazole; Macrolide Antibiotics; Magnesium Sulfate; Mifepristone; Perampanel; Selective Serotonin Reuptake Inhibitors; Simeprevir; Sodium Oxybate

Decreased Effect

BusPIRone may decrease the levels/effects of: Ioflupane I 123

The levels/effects of BusPIRone may be decreased by: Bosentan; CYP3A4 Inducers (Strong); Dabrafenib; Deferasirox; Mitotane; Peginterferon Alfa-2b; Rifamycin Derivatives; Tocilizumab; Yohimbine

Ethanol/Nutrition/Herb Interactions

Ethanol: Ethanol may increase CNS depression. Management: Monitor for increased effects with coadministration. Caution patients about effects.

Food: Food may decrease the absorption of buspirone, but it may also decrease the first-pass metabolism, thereby increasing the bioavailability of buspirone. Grapefruit juice may cause increased buspirone concentrations. Management: Administer with or without food, but must be consistent. Avoid intake of large quantities of grapefruit juice.

Herb/Nutraceutical: St John's wort may decrease buspirone levels or increase CNS depression. Kava kava, valerian, and gotu kola may increase CNS depression; yohimbe may diminish the therapeutic effect of buspirone. Management: Avoid St John's wort, kava kava, valerian, gotu kola, and yohimbe.

Storage/Stability Store at 25°C (77°F); excursions permitted between 15°C to 30°C (59°F to 86°F). Protect from light.

Mechanism of Action The mechanism of action of buspirone is unknown. Buspirone has a high affinity for serotonin 5-HT_{1A} and 5-HT_2 receptors, without affecting benzodiazepine-GABA receptors. Buspirone has moderate affinity for dopamine D_2 receptors.

Pharmacodynamics/Kinetics

Absorption: Rapid

Distribution: V_d: 5.3 L/kg

Protein binding: 86%

Metabolism: Hepatic oxidation, primarily via CYP3A4 to several metabolites including an active metabolite, 1-pyrimidinylpiperazine (1-PP; exhibits about 25% of the activity of buspirone); extensive first-pass effect

Half-life elimination: 2-3 hours

Time to peak, serum: 40-90 minutes

Excretion: Urine: 29% to 63% (primarily as metabolites); feces: 18% to 38%

Dosage

Generalized anxiety disorder (GAD): Adults: Oral: Initial: 7.5 mg twice daily; may increase every 2-3 days in increments of 2.5 mg twice daily to a maximum of 30 mg twice daily; a dose of 10-15 mg twice daily was most often used in clinical trials that allowed for dose titration

Augmentation agent for antidepressants (unlabeled use): Adults: Oral: Initial: 7.5 mg twice daily; may increase weekly in increments of 7.5 mg twice daily to a maximum of 30 mg twice daily (Trivedi, 2006).

Dosing adjustment in renal impairment: Patients with impaired renal function demonstrated increased plasma levels and a prolonged half-life of buspirone. Use in patients with severe renal impairment not recommended.

Dosing adjustment in hepatic impairment: Patients with impaired hepatic function demonstrated increased plasma levels and a prolonged half-life of buspirone. Use in patients with severe hepatic impairment not recommended.

Dietary Considerations May be taken with or without food, but must be consistent. Avoid large quantities of grapefruit juice.

Administration May be administered with or without food, but must be consistent.

Monitoring Parameters Mental status, symptoms of anxiety

Test Interactions The presence of buspirone may result in a false positive on a urinary assay for metanephrine/catecholamine; discontinue buspirone ≥48 hours prior to collection of urine sample for catecholamines

Additional Information Has shown little potential for abuse; needs continuous use. Because of slow onset, not appropriate for "as needed" (prn) use or for brief, situational anxiety. Ineffective for treatment of benzodiazepine or ethanol withdrawal.

Dosage Forms Excipient information presented when available (limited, particularly for generics); consult specific product labeling.

Tablet, Oral, as hydrochloride:

Generic: 5 mg, 7.5 mg, 10 mg, 15 mg, 30 mg

◆ **Buspirone Hydrochloride** *see* BusPIRone *on page* 300

◆ **Bussulfam** *see* Busulfan *on page* 301

◆ **Bustab® (Can)** *see* BusPIRone *on page* 300

Busulfan (byoo SUL fan)

Brand Names: U.S. Busulfex; Myleran

Brand Names: Canada Busulfex®; Myleran®

Index Terms Bussulfam; Busulfanum; Busulphan

Pharmacologic Category Antineoplastic Agent, Alkylating Agent

Use Palliative treatment of chronic myelogenous leukemia (CML) (oral); conditioning regimen prior to allogeneic hematopoietic progenitor cell transplantation (I.V.) for CML

Unlabeled Use Conditioning regimen prior to hematopoietic stem cell transplant (HSCT) (oral); treatment of polycythemia vera and essential thrombocytosis

Pregnancy Risk Factor D

Pregnancy Considerations Animal studies have demonstrated teratogenic effects. There are no adequate and well-controlled studies in pregnant women. May cause fetal harm if administered during pregnancy. The solvent in I.V. busulfan, DMA, is also associated with teratogenic effects and may impair fertility. Women of childbearing potential should avoid pregnancy while receiving busulfan treatment.

Breast-Feeding Considerations According to the manufacturer, the decision to continue or discontinue breastfeeding during therapy should take into account the risk of exposure to the infant and the benefits of treatment to the mother.

Contraindications Hypersensitivity to busulfan or any component of the formulation; oral busulfan is contraindicated in patients without a definitive diagnosis of CML

Warnings/Precautions Hazardous agent - use appropriate precautions for handling and disposal (NIOSH, 2012). **[U.S. Boxed Warning]: Severe bone marrow suppression is common; reduce dose or discontinue oral busulfan for unusual suppression; may require bone marrow biopsy.** May result in severe neutropenia, thrombocytopenia, anemia, bone marrow failure, and/or pancytopenia; pancytopenia may be prolonged (1 month up to 2 years) and may be reversible. Use with caution in patients with compromised bone marrow reserve (due to prior treatment or radiation therapy). Monitor closely for signs of infection (due to neutropenia) or bleeding (due to thrombocytopenia) Seizures have been reported with use; use caution in patients predisposed to seizures, history of seizures or head trauma; when using as a conditioning regimen for transplant, initiate prophylactic anticonvulsant therapy (eg, phenytoin) prior to treatment. Phenytoin increases busulfan clearance by ≥15%; busulfan kinetics and dosing recommendations for high-dose HSCT conditioning were studied with concomitant phenytoin. If alternate anticonvulsants are used, busulfan clearance may be decreased and dosing should be monitored accordingly.

Bronchopulmonary dysplasia with pulmonary fibrosis ("busulfan lung") is associated with busulfan; onset is delayed with symptoms occurring at an average of 4 years (range: 4 months to 10 years) after treatment; may be fatal. Symptoms generally include a slow onset of cough, dyspnea, and fever (low-grade), although acute symptomatic onset may also occur. Diminished diffusion capacity and decreased pulmonary compliance have been noted with pulmonary function testing. Differential diagnosis should rule out opportunistic pulmonary infection or leukemic pulmonary infiltrates; may require lung biopsy. Discontinue busulfan if toxicity develops. Pulmonary toxicity may be additive if administered with other cytotoxic agents also associated with pulmonary toxicity. Cardiac tamponade as been reported in children with thalassemia treated with high-dose oral busulfan in combination with cyclophosphamide. Busulfan has been causally related to the development of secondary malignancies (tumors and acute leukemias); chromosomal alterations may also occur. Busulfan has been associated with ovarian failure (including failure to achieve puberty).

High busulfan area under the concentration versus time curve (AUC) values (>1500 micromolar•minute) are associated with increased risk of hepatic sinusoidal obstruction syndrome (SOS; formerly called veno-occlusive disease [VOD]) due to conditioning for allogenic HSCT; patients with a history of radiation therapy, prior chemotherapy (≥3 cycles), or prior stem cell transplantation are at increased risk; monitor liver function tests periodically. Oral busulfan doses above 16 mg/kg (based on IBW) and concurrent use with alkylating agents may also increase the risk for hepatic SOS. The solvent in I.V. busulfan, DMA, may impair fertility. DMA may also be associated with hepatotoxicity, hallucinations, somnolence, lethargy, and confusion. **[U.S. Boxed Warning]: Should be administered under the supervision of an experienced cancer chemotherapy physician; for the I.V. formulation, should be experienced in management of HSCT and management of patients with severe pancytopenia; according to the manufacturer, oral busulfan should not be used until CML diagnosis has been established.** Cellular dysplasia in many organs has been observed (in addition to lung dysplasia); giant hyperchromatic nuclei have been noted in adrenal glands, liver, lymph nodes, pancreas, thyroid, and bone marrow. May obscure routine diagnostic cytologic exams (eg, cervical smear).

Adverse Reactions

I.V.:

>10%:

Cardiovascular: Tachycardia (44%), hypertension (36%; grades 3/4: 7%), edema (28% to 79%), thrombosis (33%), chest pain (26%), vasodilation (25%), hypotension (11%; grades 3/4: 3%)

Central nervous system: Insomnia (84%), fever (80%), anxiety (72% to 75%), headache (69%), chills (46%), pain (44%), dizziness (30%), depression (23%), confusion (11%)

Dermatologic: Rash (57%), pruritus (28%), alopecia (17%)

Endocrine & metabolic: Hypomagnesemia (77%), hyperglycemia (66% to 67%; grades 3/4: 15%), hypokalemia (64%), hypocalcemia (49%), hypophosphatemia (17%)

Gastrointestinal: Vomiting (43% to 100%), nausea (83% to 98%), mucositis/stomatitis (79% to 97%; grades 3/4: 26%), anorexia (85%), diarrhea (84%; grades 3/4: 5%), abdominal pain (72%), dyspepsia (44%), constipation (38%), xerostomia (26%), rectal disorder (25%), abdominal fullness (23%)

Hematologic: Myelosuppression (≤100%), neutropenia (100%; onset: 4 days; median recovery: 13 days [with G-CSF support]), thrombocytopenia (98%; median onset: 5-6 days), lymphopenia (children: 79%), anemia (69%)

Hepatic: Hyperbilirubinemia (49%; grades 3/4: 30%), ALT increased (31%; grades 3/4: 7%), hepatic sinusoidal obstruction syndrome (SOS; veno-occlusive disease) (adults: 8% to 12%; children: 21%), alkaline phosphatase increased (15%), jaundice (12%)

Local: Injection site inflammation (25%), injection site pain (15%)

Neuromuscular & skeletal: Weakness (51%), back pain (23%), myalgia (16%), arthralgia (13%)

Renal: Creatinine increased (21%), oliguria (15%)

Respiratory: Rhinitis (44%), lung disorder (34%), cough (28%), epistaxis (25%), dyspnea (25%), pneumonia (children: 21%), hiccup (18%), pharyngitis (18%)

Miscellaneous: Infection (51%; includes severe bacterial, viral [CMV], and fungal infections), allergic reaction (26%)

1% to 10%:

Cardiovascular: Arrhythmia (5%), cardiomegaly (5%), atrial fibrillation (2%), ECG abnormal (2%), heart block (2%), heart failure (grade 3/4: 2%), pericardial effusion (2%), tamponade (children with thalassemia: 2%), ventricular extrasystoles (2%), hypervolemia

Central nervous system: Lethargy (7%), hallucination (5%), agitation (2%), delirium (2%), encephalopathy (2%), seizure (2%), somnolence (2%), cerebral hemorrhage (1%)

Dermatologic: Vesicular rash (10%), vesiculobullous rash (10%), skin discoloration (8%), maculopapular rash (8%), acne (7%), exfoliative dermatitis (5%), erythema nodosum (2%)
Endocrine & metabolic: Hyponatremia (2%)
Gastrointestinal: Ileus (8%), weight gain (8%), esophagitis (grade 3: 2%), hematemesis (2%), pancreatitis (2%)
Hematologic: Prothrombin time increased (2%)
Hepatic: Hepatomegaly (6%)
Renal: Hematuria (8%), dysuria (7%), hemorrhagic cystitis (grade 3/4: 7%), BUN increased (3%; grades 3/4: 2%)
Respiratory: Asthma (8%), alveolar hemorrhage (5%), hyperventilation (5%), hemoptysis (3%), pleural effusion (3%), sinusitis (3%), atelectasis (2%), hypoxia (2%)

Oral: Frequency not defined:
Dermatologic: Hyperpigmentation of skin (5% to 10%), rash
Endocrine & metabolic: Amenorrhea, ovarian suppression
Gastrointestinal: Xerostomia
Hematologic: Myelosuppression (anemia, leukopenia, thrombocytopenia)

I.V. and/or Oral: Infrequent, postmarketing, and/or case reports: Acute leukemias, adrenal insufficiency, alopecia (permanent), aplastic anemia (may be irreversible), azoospermia, bronchopulmonary dysplasia, capillary leak syndrome, cataracts (rare), cheilosis, cholestatic jaundice, corneal thinning, dry skin, endocardial fibrosis, erythema multiforme, esophageal varices, gynecomastia, hepatic dysfunction, hepatocellular atrophy, hyperuricemia, hyperuricosuria, interstitial pulmonary fibrosis, malignant tumors, myasthenia gravis, neutropenic fever, ocular (lens) changes, ovarian failure, pancytopenia, porphyria cutanea tarda, pulmonary fibrosis, radiation myelopathy, radiation recall (skin rash), sepsis, sterility, testicular atrophy, thrombotic microangiopathy (TMA), tumor lysis syndrome, urticaria

Drug Interactions

Metabolism/Transport Effects None known.

Avoid Concomitant Use

Avoid concomitant use of Busulfan with any of the following: BCG; CloZAPine; Natalizumab; Pimecrolimus; Tacrolimus (Topical); Tofacitinib; Vaccines (Live)

Increased Effect/Toxicity

Busulfan may increase the levels/effects of: CloZAPine; Ifosfamide; Leflunomide; Natalizumab; Tofacitinib; Vaccines (Live); Vitamin K Antagonists

The levels/effects of Busulfan may be increased by: Acetaminophen; Antifungal Agents (Azole Derivatives, Systemic); Denosumab; MetroNIDAZOLE (Systemic); Pimecrolimus; Roflumilast; Tacrolimus (Topical); Trastuzumab

Decreased Effect

Busulfan may decrease the levels/effects of: BCG; Coccidioidin Skin Test; Sipuleucel-T; Vaccines (Inactivated); Vaccines (Live); Vitamin K Antagonists

The levels/effects of Busulfan may be decreased by: Echinacea; Fosphenytoin; Phenytoin

Ethanol/Nutrition/Herb Interactions

Ethanol: Avoid ethanol due to GI irritation.
Food: No clear or firm data on the effect of food on busulfan bioavailability.
Herb/Nutraceutical: Avoid St John's wort (may decrease busulfan levels).

Preparation for Administration Hazardous agent; use appropriate precautions for handling and disposal (NIOSH, 2012). Injection: Dilute NS or D_5W. The dilution volume should be 10 times the volume of busulfan injection, ensuring that the final concentration of busulfan is 0.5 mg/mL. Always add busulfan to the diluent, and not the diluent to the busulfan. Mix with several inversions. Do not use polycarbonate syringes or filters for preparation or administration.

Storage/Stability

Injection: Store intact vials under refrigeration at 2°C to 8°C (36°F to 46°F). Solutions diluted in sodium chloride (NS) injection or dextrose 5% in water (D_5W) for infusion are stable for up to 8 hours at room temperature (25°C [77°F]); the infusion must also be completed within that 8-hour timeframe. Dilution of busulfan injection in NS is stable for up to 12 hours at refrigeration (2°C to 8°C); the infusion must be completed within that 12-hour timeframe.

Tablet: Store at 25°C (77°F); excursions permitted to 15°C to 30°C (59°F to 86°F).

Mechanism of Action Busulfan is an alkylating agent which reacts with the N-7 position of guanosine and interferes with DNA replication and transcription of RNA. Busulfan has a more marked effect on myeloid cells than on lymphoid cells and is also very toxic to hematopoietic stem cells. Busulfan exhibits little immunosuppressive activity. Interferes with the normal function of DNA by alkylation and cross-linking the strands of DNA.

Pharmacodynamics/Kinetics

Absorption: Rapid and complete
Distribution: V_d: ~1 L/kg; distributes into CSF with levels equal to plasma
Protein binding: 32% to plasma proteins and 47% to red blood cells
Metabolism: Extensively hepatic (may increase with multiple doses); glutathione conjugation followed by oxidation
Bioavailability: Oral: Children ≥13 years and adults: 80% ± 20%; Children 1.5-6 years: 68% ± 31%
Half-life elimination: 2-3 hours
Time to peak, serum: Oral: ~1 hour; I.V.: Within 5 minutes
Excretion: Urine (25% to 60% predominantly as metabolites; <2% as unchanged drug)

Dosage Note: Premedicate with prophylactic anticonvulsant therapy (eg, phenytoin) prior to high-dose busulfan treatment. Prophylactic antiemetics may be necessary for high-dose (HSCT) regimens.

Children:

CML, palliation (manufacturer's labeling): Oral:
Remission induction: 60 mcg/kg/day or 1.8 mg/m²/day; titrate dose (or withhold) to maintain leukocyte counts ≥15,000/mm³ (doses >4 mg/day should be reserved for patients with the most compelling symptoms)
Maintenance: When leukocyte count ≥50,000/mm³: Resume induction dose **or** (if remission <3 months) 1-3 mg/day (to control hematologic status and prevent relapse)

HSCT conditioning regimen:
I.V.:
≤12 kg: 1.1 mg/kg/dose (actual body weight) every 6 hours for 16 doses
>12 kg: 0.8 mg/kg/dose (actual body weight) every 6 hours for 16 doses
Adjust dose to desired AUC (1125 micromolar•minute) using the following formula:
Adjusted dose (mg) = Actual dose (mg) x [target AUC (micromolar•minute)/ actual AUC (micromolar•minute)]
Reduced intensity conditioning regimen (unlabeled dosing): 0.8 mg/kg/dose for 1 dose 7-10 days prior to transplant, followed by ~0.8 mg/kg/dose (busulfan kinetics calculated after initial dose) every 6 hours for 7 doses beginning 3-6 days prior to transplant (in combination with fludarabine and antithymocyte globulin) (Pulsipher, 2009)
Oral (unlabeled use): 1 mg/kg/dose every 6 hours for 16 doses beginning 9 days prior to transplant (in combination with cyclophosphamide) (Cassileth, 1998)

Adults:

CML, palliation (manufacturer's labeling): Oral:

Remission induction: 60 mcg/kg/day or 1.8 mg/m^2/day; usual range: 4-8 mg/day; titrate dose (or withhold) to maintain leukocyte counts ≥15,000/mm^3 (doses >4 mg/day should be reserved for patients with the most compelling symptoms)

Maintenance: When leukocyte count ≥50,000/mm^3: Resume induction dose **or** (if remission <3 months) 1-3 mg/day (to control hematologic status and prevent relapse)

HSCT conditioning regimen:

I.V.: 0.8 mg/kg every 6 hours for 4 days (a total of 16 doses); **Note:** Use ideal body weight or actual body weight, (whichever is lower) for dosing.

Obesity: For obese or severely-obese patients, use of an adjusted body weight [IBW + 0.25 x (actual – IBW)] is recommended.

Reduced intensity conditioning regimen (unlabeled dosing): 0.8 mg/kg/day for 4 days starting 5 days prior to transplant (in combinations with fludarabine) (Ho, 2009)

Oral (unlabeled use): 1 mg/kg/dose every 6 hours for 16 doses (in combination with cyclophosphamide) (Socié, 2001) **or** 1 mg/kg/dose every 6 hours for 16 doses beginning 9 days prior to transplant (in combination with cyclophosphamide) (Cassileth, 1993) **or** 0.44 mg/kg/dose every 6 hours for 16 doses (in combination with cyclophosphamide) (Anderson, 1996) **or** 1 mg/kg/dose every 6 hours for 16 doses beginning 6 days prior to transplant (in combination with melphalan) (Fermand, 2005)

Polycythemia vera and essential thrombocythemia (unlabeled uses): Oral: 2-4 mg/day (Fabris, 2009; Tefferi, 2011)

Dosing adjustment in renal impairment:

I.V.: No dosage adjustment provided in the manufacturer's labeling (has not been studied).

Oral: No dosage adjustment provided in the manufacturer's labeling (elimination appears to be independent of renal function); however, some clinicians suggest adjustment is not necessary (Aronoff, 2007).

Dosing adjustment in hepatic impairment:

I.V.: No dosage adjustment provided in the manufacturer's labeling (has not been studied).

Oral: No dosage adjustment provided in the manufacturer's labeling.

Dosing in obesity: *ASCO Guidelines for appropriate chemotherapy dosing in obese adults with cancer (**Note:** Excludes HSCT dosing):* Utilize patient's actual body weight (full weight) for calculation of body surface area- or weight-based dosing, particularly when the intent of therapy is curative; manage regimen-related toxicities in the same manner as for nonobese patients; if a dose reduction is utilized due to toxicity, consider resumption of full weight-based dosing with subsequent cycles, especially if cause of toxicity (eg, hepatic or renal impairment) is resolved (Griggs, 2012).

Administration Intravenous busulfan should be infused over 2 hours via central line. Flush line before and after each infusion with 5 mL D_5W or NS. Do not use polycarbonate syringes or filters for preparation or administration

HSCT only: To facilitate ingestion of high oral doses, may insert multiple tablets into gelatin capsules.

Hazardous agent; use appropriate precautions for handling and disposal (NIOSH, 2012).

Monitoring Parameters CBC with differential and platelet count (weekly for palliative treatment; daily until engraftment for HSCT); liver function tests (evaluate transaminases, alkaline phosphatase, and bilirubin daily for at least 28 days post transplant). If conducting therapeutic drug monitoring for AUC calculations in HSCT, monitor blood samples at appropriate collections times (record collection times).

Dosage Forms Excipient information presented when available (limited, particularly for generics); consult specific product labeling.

Solution, Intravenous:

Busulfex: 6 mg/mL (10 mL)

Tablet, Oral:

Myleran: 2 mg

Extemporaneous Preparations Hazardous agent: Use appropriate precautions for handling and disposal.

A 2 mg/mL oral suspension can be prepared in a vertical flow hood with tablets and simple syrup. Crush one-hundred-twenty 2 mg tablets in a mortar and reduce to a fine powder. Add small portions of simple syrup and mix to a uniform paste; mix while adding the simple syrup in incremental proportions to **almost** 120 mL; transfer to a graduated cylinder, rinse mortar and pestle with simple syrup, and add quantity of vehicle sufficient to make 120 mL. Transfer contents of the graduated cylinder into an amber prescription bottle. Label "shake well", "refrigerate", and "caution chemotherapy". Stable for 30 days.

Allen LV, "Busulfan Oral Suspension," *US Pharm*, 1990, 15:94-5.

◆ **Busulfanum** *see* Busulfan *on page 301*

◆ **Busulfex** *see* Busulfan *on page 301*

◆ **Busulfex® (Can)** *see* Busulfan *on page 301*

◆ **Busulphan** *see* Busulfan *on page 301*

Butabarbital (byoo ta BAR bi tal)

Brand Names: U.S. Butisol Sodium

Pharmacologic Category Barbiturate

Additional Appendix Information

Beers Criteria – Potentially Inappropriate Medications for Geriatrics *on page 2368*

Use Sedative; hypnotic

Pregnancy Risk Factor D

Dosage Oral:

Children: Preoperative sedation: 2-6 mg/kg/dose (maximum: 100 mg)

Adults:

Sedative: 15-30 mg 3-4 times/day

Hypnotic: 50-100 mg at bedtime. When used for insomnia, treatment should be limited since barbiturates lose effectiveness for sleep induction and maintenance after 2 weeks.

Preop: 50-100 mg 1-1½ hours before surgery

Elderly: Use with caution; reduce dose if use is needed

Dosage adjustment in renal impairment: Reduce dose if use is needed

Dosage adjustment in hepatic impairment: Reduce dose if use is needed

Additional Information Complete prescribing information should be consulted for additional detail.

Dosage Forms Excipient information presented when available (limited, particularly for generics); consult specific product labeling.

Elixir, Oral, as sodium:

Butisol Sodium: 30 mg/5 mL (473 mL) [contains alcohol, usp, tartrazine (fd&c yellow #5); mint flavor]

Tablet, Oral, as sodium:

Butisol Sodium: 30 mg, 50 mg [scored; contains tartrazine (fd&c yellow #5)]

Controlled Substance C-III

Butalbital, Acetaminophen, and Caffeine

(byoo TAL bi tal, a seet a MIN oh fen, & KAF een)

Brand Names: U.S. Alagesic LQ; Dolgic Plus; Esgic; Esgic-Plus; Fioricet; Margesic; Orbivan [DSC]; Repan; Zebutal

Index Terms Acetaminophen, Butalbital, and Caffeine

Pharmacologic Category Barbiturate

Use Tension or muscle contraction headache: Relief of symptom complex of tension or muscle contraction headache

Pregnancy Risk Factor C

Dosage

Adults: Oral: 1-2 tablets or capsules (or 15-30 mL solution) every 4 hours; not to exceed 6 tablets or capsules (or 90 mL solution) daily

Elderly: Not recommended for use in the elderly

Dosage adjustment in renal impairment: No dosage adjustment provided in the manufacturer's labeling; use with caution, especially with severe impairment.

Dosage adjustment in hepatic impairment: No dosage adjustment provided in the manufacturer's labeling; use with caution, especially with severe impairment.

Additional Information Complete prescribing information should be consulted for additional detail.

Dosage Forms Excipient information presented when available (limited, particularly for generics); consult specific product labeling.

Capsule, oral: Butalbital 50 mg, acetaminophen 300 mg, and caffeine 40 mg

Esgic: Butalbital 50 mg, acetaminophen 325 mg, and caffeine 40 mg

Esgic-Plus: Butalbital 50 mg, acetaminophen 500 mg, and caffeine 40 mg

Fioricet: Butalbital 50 mg, acetaminophen 300 mg, and caffeine 40 mg

Margesic: Butalbital 50 mg, acetaminophen 325 mg, and caffeine 40 mg

Orbivan: Butalbital 50 mg, acetaminophen 300 mg, and caffeine 40 mg [DSC]

Zebutal: Butalbital 50 mg, acetaminophen 325 mg, and caffeine 40 mg; Butalbital 50 mg, acetaminophen 500 mg, and caffeine 40 mg

Liquid, oral:

Alagesic LQ: Butalbital 50 mg, acetaminophen 325 mg, and caffeine 40 mg per 15 mL (480 mL) [contains ethanol 7%; propylene glycol]

Tablet, oral: Butalbital 50 mg, acetaminophen 325 mg, and caffeine 40 mg; butalbital 50 mg, acetaminophen 500 mg, and caffeine 40 mg

Dolgic Plus: Butalbital 50 mg, acetaminophen 750 mg, and caffeine 40 mg

Esgic, Fioricet [DSC], Repan: Butalbital 50 mg, acetaminophen 325 mg, and caffeine 40 mg

Esgic-Plus: Butalbital 50 mg, acetaminophen 500 mg, and caffeine 40 mg

Butalbital and Acetaminophen

(byoo TAL bi tal & a seet a MIN oh fen)

Brand Names: U.S. Bupap; Orviban CF; Phrenilin Forte; Promacet

Index Terms Acetaminophen and Butalbital

Pharmacologic Category Analgesic, Miscellaneous; Barbiturate

Use Relief of the symptomatic complex of tension or muscle contraction headache

Pregnancy Risk Factor C

Dosage Oral:

Children ≥12 years and Adults:

Butalbital 50 mg and acetaminophen 300-325 mg: 1-2 tablets every 4 hours as needed (maximum: 6 tablets/24 hours)

Butalbital 50 mg and acetaminophen 650 mg: One tablet/capsule every 4 hours as needed (maximum: 6 doses/24 hours)

Elderly: Use with caution; see adult dosing

Dosage adjustment in renal impairment: No dosage adjustment provided in the manufacturer's labeling; however, use with caution; dose reduction or alternate therapy should be considered, especially with severe impairment.

Dosage adjustment in hepatic impairment: No dosage adjustment provided in the manufacturer's labeling; however, use with caution; dose reduction or alternate therapy should be considered, especially with severe impairment.

Additional Information Complete prescribing information should be consulted for additional detail.

Dosage Forms Excipient information presented when available (limited, particularly for generics); consult specific product labeling. [DSC] = Discontinued product

Tablet, oral: Butalbital 50 mg and acetaminophen 325 mg

Bupap [DSC], Promacet: Butalbital 50 mg and acetaminophen 650 mg

Bupap, Orbivan CF: Butalbital 50 mg and acetaminophen 300 mg

Capsule, oral:

PhrenilinForte: Butalbital 50 mg and acetaminophen 650 mg [may contain benzyl alcohol]

Butalbital, Aspirin, and Caffeine

(byoo TAL bi tal, AS pir in, & KAF een)

Brand Names: U.S. Fiorinal®

Brand Names: Canada Fiorinal®

Index Terms Aspirin, Caffeine, and Butalbital; Butalbital Compound

Pharmacologic Category Barbiturate

Use Relief of the symptomatic complex of tension or muscle contraction headache

Pregnancy Risk Factor C

Dosage

Oral: Adults: 1-2 tablets or capsules every 4 hours; not to exceed 6 tablets or capsules/day

Elderly: Not recommended for use in the elderly

Dosing adjustment in renal/hepatic impairment: Dosage should be reduced

Additional Information Complete prescribing information should be consulted for additional detail.

Dosage Forms Excipient information presented when available (limited, particularly for generics); consult specific product labeling.

Capsule: Butalbital 50 mg, aspirin 325 mg, and caffeine 40 mg

Fiorinal®: Butalbital 50 mg, aspirin 325 mg, and caffeine 40 mg

Tablet: Butalbital 50 mg, aspirin 325 mg, and caffeine 40 mg [DSC]

Controlled Substance C-III

◆ **Butalbital Compound** *see* Butalbital, Aspirin, and Caffeine *on page 305*

◆ **Butamben, Tetracaine, and Benzocaine** *see* Benzocaine, Butamben, and Tetracaine *on page 242*

Butenafine (byoo TEN a feen)

Brand Names: U.S. Lotrimin Ultra [OTC]; Mentax

Index Terms Butenafine Hydrochloride
Pharmacologic Category Antifungal Agent, Topical
Use Topical treatment of tinea pedis (athlete's foot), tinea cruris (jock itch), tinea corporis (ringworm), and tinea versicolor
Pregnancy Risk Factor C
Dosage Children >12 years and Adults: Topical:
Tinea corporis, tinea cruris (Lotrimin® ultra™): Apply once daily for 2 weeks to affected area and surrounding skin
Tinea versicolor (Mentax®): Apply once daily for 2 weeks to affected area and surrounding skin
Tinea pedis (Lotrimin® ultra™): Apply to affected skin between and around the toes, twice daily for 1 week, or once daily for 4 weeks
Additional Information Complete prescribing information should be consulted for additional detail.
Dosage Forms Excipient information presented when available (limited, particularly for generics); consult specific product labeling.
Cream, External, as hydrochloride:
Lotrimin Ultra: 1% (30 g) [contains benzyl alcohol, cetyl alcohol, propylene glycol, sodium benzoate]
Mentax: 1% (15 g, 30 g) [contains benzyl alcohol, sodium benzoate]

◆ Butenafine Hydrochloride *see* Butenafine *on page 305*
◆ Butisol Sodium *see* Butabarbital *on page 304*

Butoconazole (byoo toe KOE na zole)

Brand Names: U.S. Gynazole-1
Brand Names: Canada Femstat® One; Gynazole-1®
Index Terms Butoconazole Nitrate
Pharmacologic Category Antifungal Agent, Vaginal
Use Local treatment of vulvovaginal candidiasis
Pregnancy Risk Factor C
Dosage Adults: Females: Gynazole-1®: Insert 1 applicatorful (~5 g) intravaginally as a single dose
Additional Information Complete prescribing information should be consulted for additional detail.
Dosage Forms Excipient information presented when available (limited, particularly for generics); consult specific product labeling.
Cream, Vaginal, as nitrate:
Gynazole-1: 2% (5.8 g) [contains disodium edta, methylparaben, propylene glycol, propylparaben]

◆ Butoconazole Nitrate *see* Butoconazole *on page 306*

Butorphanol (byoo TOR fa nole)

Brand Names: Canada Apo-Butorphanol; PMS-Butorphanol
Index Terms Butorphanol Tartrate; Stadol
Pharmacologic Category Analgesic, Opioid; Analgesic, Opioid Partial Agonist
Additional Appendix Information
Opioid Conversion Table *on page 2306*
Use
Parenteral: Management of pain when the use of an opioid analgesic is appropriate; preoperative or preanesthetic medication; supplement to balanced anesthesia; management of pain during labor.
Nasal spray: Management of pain when the use of an opioid analgesic is appropriate.
Pregnancy Risk Factor C
Dosage Note: These are guidelines and do not represent the maximum doses that may be required in all patients. Doses should be titrated to pain relief/prevention. Butorphanol has an analgesic ceiling.

Adults:
Parenteral:
Acute pain (moderate-to-severe):
I.M.: Initial: 2 mg, may repeat every 3-4 hours as needed; usual range: 1-4 mg every 3-4 hours as needed
I.V.: Initial: 1 mg, may repeat every 3-4 hours as needed; usual range: 0.5-2 mg every 3-4 hours as needed
Preoperative medication: I.M.: 2 mg 60-90 minutes before surgery
Supplement to balanced anesthesia: I.V.: 2 mg shortly before induction and/or an incremental dose of 0.5-1 mg (up to 0.06 mg/kg), depending on previously administered sedative, analgesic, and hypnotic medications
Pain during labor (fetus >37 weeks gestation and no signs of fetal distress):
I.M., I.V.: 1-2 mg; may repeat in 4 hours
Note: Alternative analgesia should be used for pain associated with delivery or if delivery is anticipated within 4 hours

Nasal spray:
Pain: Initial: 1 spray (~1 mg per spray) in 1 nostril; if adequate pain relief is not achieved within 60-90 minutes, an additional 1 spray in 1 nostril may be given; may repeat initial dose sequence in 3-4 hours after the last dose as needed
Alternatively, an initial dose of 2 mg (1 spray in each nostril) may be used in patients who will be able to remain recumbent (in the event drowsiness or dizziness occurs); additional 2 mg doses should not be given for 3-4 hours

Elderly:
I.M., I.V.: Initial dosage should generally be 1/2 of the recommended dose; repeated dosing must be based on initial response rather than fixed intervals, but generally should be at least 6 hours apart
Nasal spray: Initial dose should not exceed 1 mg; a second dose may be given after 90-120 minutes if needed. In Canadian labeling, repeated dosing must be based on initial response rather than fixed intervals, but generally should be at least 6 hours apart.

Dosage adjustment in renal impairment:
I.M., I.V.: Initial dosage should generally be 1/2 of the recommended dose; repeated dosing must be based on initial response rather than fixed intervals, but generally should be at least 6 hours apart
Nasal spray: Initial dose should not exceed 1 mg; a second dose may be given after 90-120 minutes if needed. Repeated dosing must be based on initial response rather than fixed intervals, but generally should be at least 6 hours apart.
Canadian labeling: Cl_{cr} <30 mL/minute: Increase initial dosing interval to 6-8 hours.
Dosage adjustment in hepatic impairment:
I.M., I.V.: Initial dosage should generally be 1/2 of the recommended dose; repeated dosing must be based on initial response rather than fixed intervals, but generally should be at least 6 hours apart
Nasal spray: Initial dose should not exceed 1 mg; a second dose may be given after 90-120 minutes if needed. Repeated dosing must be based on initial response rather than fixed intervals, but generally should be at least 6 hours apart.
Canadian labeling: Increase interval of repeat dosing to 6-12 hours.
Additional Information Complete prescribing information should be consulted for additional detail.

Dosage Forms Excipient information presented when available (limited, particularly for generics); consult specific product labeling.
Solution, Injection, as tartrate:
Generic: 1 mg/mL (1 mL); 2 mg/mL (1 mL, 2 mL, 10 mL)
Solution, Injection, as tartrate [preservative free]:
Generic: 1 mg/mL (1 mL); 2 mg/mL (1 mL)
Solution, Nasal, as tartrate:
Generic: 10 mg/mL (2.5 mL)
Controlled Substance C-IV

- **Butorphanol Tartrate** *see* Butorphanol *on page* 306
- **Butrans** *see* Buprenorphine *on page* 291
- **Butrans® (Can)** *see* Buprenorphine *on page* 291
- **BW-430C** *see* LamoTRIgine *on page* 1165
- **BW524W91** *see* Emtricitabine *on page* 698
- **Bydureon** *see* Exenatide *on page* 815
- **Byetta® (Can)** *see* Exenatide *on page* 815
- **Byetta 5 MCG Pen** *see* Exenatide *on page* 815
- **Byetta 10 MCG Pen** *see* Exenatide *on page* 815
- **Bystolic** *see* Nebivolol *on page* 1433
- **Bystolic® (Can)** *see* Nebivolol *on page* 1433
- **C1 Esterase Inhibitor** *see* C1 Inhibitor (Human) *on page* 307
- **C1-INH** *see* C1 Inhibitor (Human) *on page* 307
- **C1-Inhibitor** *see* C1 Inhibitor (Human) *on page* 307
- **C1INHRP** *see* C1 Inhibitor (Human) *on page* 307
- **C2B8 Monoclonal Antibody** *see* RiTUXimab *on page* 1833
- **2C4 Antibody** *see* Pertuzumab *on page* 1625
- **C7E3** *see* Abciximab *on page* 22
- **311C90** *see* ZOLMitriptan *on page* 2240
- **C225** *see* Cetuximab *on page* 398
- **C-500 [OTC]** *see* Ascorbic Acid *on page* 172

C1 Inhibitor (Human) (cee won in HIB i ter HYU man)

Brand Names: U.S. Berinert; Cinryze
Brand Names: Canada Berinert®
Index Terms C1 Esterase Inhibitor; C1-INH; C1-Inhibitor; C1INHRP; Human C1 Inhibitor
Pharmacologic Category Blood Product Derivative
Use
Berinert®: Treatment of acute abdominal, facial, or laryngeal attacks of hereditary angioedema (HAE)
Cinryze®: Routine prophylaxis against angioedema attacks in patients with HAE
Pregnancy Risk Factor C
Prescribing and Access Restrictions Assistance with procurement and reimbursement of Cinryze® is available for healthcare providers and patients through the CINRYZE*Solutions*® program (telephone: 1-877-945-1000) or at http://www.cinryze.com/Cinryze_Solutions/Default.aspx
Dosage I.V.: Adolescents and Adults:
Routine prophylaxis against hereditary angioedema (HAE) attacks (Cinryze®): 1000 units every 3-4 days
Treatment of abdominal, facial, or laryngeal HAE attacks (Berinert®): 20 units/kg

Dosage adjustment in renal impairment: No dosage adjustment provided in manufacturer's labeling (has not been studied).
Dosage adjustment in hepatic impairment: No dosage adjustment provided in manufacturer's labeling (has not been studied).
Additional Information Complete prescribing information should be consulted for additional detail.

Dosage Forms Excipient information presented when available (limited, particularly for generics); consult specific product labeling.
Kit, Intravenous:
Berinert: 500 units
Solution Reconstituted, Intravenous [preservative free]:
Cinryze: 500 units (1 ea)

Cabazitaxel (ca baz i TAKS el)

Brand Names: U.S. Jevtana
Brand Names: Canada Jevtana
Index Terms RPR-116258A; XRP6258
Pharmacologic Category Antineoplastic Agent, Antimicrotubular; Antineoplastic Agent, Taxane Derivative
Use Treatment of hormone-refractory metastatic prostate cancer (in patients previously treated with a docetaxel-containing regimen)
Pregnancy Risk Factor D
Pregnancy Considerations Animal studies have demonstrated adverse effects (embryotoxicity, fetotoxicity and fetal loss) at doses significantly lower than human doses. There are no adequate and well-controlled studies in pregnant women. May cause fetal harm if administered during pregnancy. Pregnant women should avoid exposure to cabazitaxel.
Breast-Feeding Considerations Due to the potential for serious adverse reactions in the nursing infant, breast-feeding is not recommended.
Contraindications Hypersensitivity to cabazitaxel, polysorbate 80, or any component of the formulation; neutrophil count ≤1500/mm^3
Warnings/Precautions Hazardous agent - use appropriate precautions for handling and disposal (meets NIOSH, 2012 criteria). **[U.S. Boxed Warning]: Severe hypersensitivity reactions, including generalized rash, erythema, hypotension, and bronchospasm may occur; may require immediate discontinuation if hypersensitivity is severe. Premedicate with an I.V. antihistamine, corticosteroid and H$_2$ antagonist prior to infusion. Use in patients with history of severe hypersensitivity to cabazitaxel or polysorbate 80 is contraindicated.** Observe closely during infusion, especially during the first and second infusions; reaction may occur within minutes. Do not rechallenge after severe hypersensitivity reactions.

[U.S. Boxed Warning]: Deaths due to neutropenia have been reported. Do not administer in patients with neutrophil count ≤1500/mm^3; monitor blood counts frequently. Dose reductions are recommended following neutropenic fever or prolonged neutropenia. Administration of WBC growth factors may reduce the risk of complications due to neutropenia; consider primary WBC growth factor prophylaxis in high-risk patients (eg, >65 years of age, poor performance status, history of neutropenic fever, extensive prior radiation, poor nutrition status, or other serious comorbidities); secondary prophylaxis and therapeutic WBC growth factors should be considered in all patients with increased risk for neutropenic complications. Patients ≥65 years of age are more likely to experience certain adverse reactions, including neutropenia and neutropenic fever.

Use is not recommended in patients with hepatic impairment (total bilirubin ≥ULN or AST and/or ALT ≥1.5 times ULN). Due to extensive hepatic metabolism, cabazitaxel exposure is increased in patients with hepatic impairment. Renal failure has been reported from clinical trials; generally associated with dehydration, sepsis, or obstructive uropathy; use with caution in patients with severe renal impairment (Cl_{cr} <30 mL/minute) and end-stage renal disease. Nausea, vomiting and diarrhea may occur. Diarrhea may be severe and may result in dehydration and electrolyte imbalance. Antiemetics, antidiarrhea medication, and fluid and electrolyte replacement may be necessary. Diarrhea ≥ grade 3 may require treatment delay and or dosage reduction.

Avoid concomitant use of strong CYP3A4 inducers or inhibitors; use with moderate CYP3A4 inhibitors with caution. Strong CYP3A4 inducers (eg, carbamazepine, phenobarbital, phenytoin, rifabutin rifampin, rifapentine) may decrease the levels/effects of cabazitaxel. Strong CYP3A4 inhibitors (eg, atazanavir, clarithromycin, indinavir, itraconazole, ketoconazole, nefazodone, nelfinavir, ritonavir, saquinavir, telithromycin, voriconazole) may increase the levels/effects of cabazitaxel.

Adverse Reactions Note: Adverse reactions reported for combination therapy with prednisone.

>10%:

- Central nervous system: Fatigue (37%), fever (12%)
- Gastrointestinal: Diarrhea (47%; grades 3/4: 6%), nausea (34%), vomiting (22%), constipation (20%), abdominal pain (17%), anorexia (16%), taste alteration (11%)
- Hematologic: Anemia (98%; grades 3/4: 11%), leukopenia (96%; grades 3/4: 69%), neutropenia (94%; grades 3/4: 82%; nadir: 12 days [range: 4-17 days]), thrombocytopenia (48%; grades 3/4: 4%)
- Neuromuscular & skeletal: Weakness (20%), back pain (16%), peripheral neuropathy (13%; grades 3/4: <1%), arthralgia (11%)
- Renal: Hematuria (17%)
- Respiratory: Dyspnea (12%), cough (11%)

1% to 10%:

- Cardiovascular: Peripheral edema (9%), arrhythmia (5%), hypotension (5%)
- Central nervous system: Dizziness (8%), headache (8%), pain (5%)
- Dermatologic: Alopecia (10%)
- Endocrine & metabolic: Dehydration (5%)
- Gastrointestinal: Dyspepsia (10%), weight loss (9%), mucosal inflammation (6%)
- Genitourinary: Urinary tract infection (8%), dysuria (7%)
- Hematologic: Neutropenic fever (grades 3/4: 7%)
- Hepatic: ALT increased (grades 3/4: ≤1%), AST increased (grades 3/4: ≤1%), bilirubin increased (grades 3/4: ≤1%)
- Neuromuscular & skeletal: Muscle spasm (7%)

<1% (Limited to important or life-threatening): Hypersensitivity (eg, rash, erythema, hypotension, bronchospasm), electrolyte imbalance, renal failure, sepsis, septic shock

Drug Interactions

Metabolism/Transport Effects Substrate of CYP2C8 (minor), CYP3A4 (major); **Note:** Assignment of Major/Minor substrate status based on clinically relevant drug interaction potential

Avoid Concomitant Use

Avoid concomitant use of Cabazitaxel with any of the following: BCG; CloZAPine; Conivaptan; Fusidic Acid (Systemic); Natalizumab; Pimecrolimus; Tacrolimus (Topical); Tofacitinib; Vaccines (Live)

Increased Effect/Toxicity

Cabazitaxel may increase the levels/effects of: Antineoplastic Agents (Anthracycline, Systemic); CloZAPine; DOXOrubicin; Leflunomide; Natalizumab; Tofacitinib; Vaccines (Live); Vitamin K Antagonists

The levels/effects of Cabazitaxel may be increased by: Conivaptan; CYP3A4 Inhibitors (Moderate); CYP3A4 Inhibitors (Strong); Dasatinib; Denosumab; Fusidic Acid (Systemic); Ivacaftor; Luliconazole; Mifepristone; Pimecrolimus; Platinum Derivatives; Roflumilast; Simeprevir; Tacrolimus (Topical); Trastuzumab

Decreased Effect

Cabazitaxel may decrease the levels/effects of: BCG; Cardiac Glycosides; Coccidioidin Skin Test; Sipuleucel-T; Vaccines (Inactivated); Vaccines (Live); Vitamin K Antagonists

The levels/effects of Cabazitaxel may be decreased by: Bosentan; CYP3A4 Inducers (Strong); Dabrafenib; Deferasirox; Echinacea; Herbs (CYP3A4 Inducers); Mitotane; Tocilizumab

Ethanol/Nutrition/Herb Interactions

Food: Avoid grapefruit juice (may increase the levels/effects of cabazitaxel).

Herb/Nutraceutical: Avoid St John's wort (may increase metabolism and decrease cabazitaxel concentrations).

Preparation for Administration Hazardous agent; use appropriate precautions for handling and disposal (meets NIOSH, 2012 criteria). Do not prepare in PVC-containing infusion containers. Cabazitaxel and diluent vials contain overfill. Preparation requires 2 steps. Slowly inject the entire contents of the provided diluent into the 60 mg/1.5 mL cabazitaxel vial, directing the diluent down the vial wall. Mix gently by inverting the vial for at least 45 seconds; do not shake. Allow vial to sit so that foam dissipates and solution appears homogeneous. This results in an intermediate reconstituted concentration of 10 mg/mL. Further dilute (within 30 minutes) into a 250 mL D_5W or NS non-PVC infusion container to final concentration of 0.1-0.26 mg/mL (total doses >65 mg will require a larger infusion volume; final concentration should not exceed 0.26 mg/mL). Gently invert to mix. Do not use infusion solutions if crystals or precipitate appear; discard.

Storage/Stability Store intact vials at 25°C (77°F); excursions permitted between 15°C and 30°C (59°F and 86°F). Do not refrigerate. Do not prepare in PVC-containing infusion containers. Initial reconstituted solution (at 10 mg/mL) is stable for 30 minutes in the vial. Solutions for infusion are stable for 8 hours at room temperature or 24 hours refrigerated. Infusion should be completed within 8 hours if stored at room temperature or 24 hours if refrigerated.

Mechanism of Action Cabazitaxel is a taxane derivative which is a microtubule inhibitor; it binds to tubulin promoting assembly into microtubules and inhibiting disassembly which stabilizes microtubules. This inhibits microtubule depolymerization and cell division, arresting the cell cycle and inhibiting tumor proliferation. Unlike other taxanes, cabazitaxel has a poor affinity for multidrug resistance (MDR) proteins, therefore conferring activity in resistant tumors.

Pharmacodynamics/Kinetics

Distribution: V_{dss}: 4864 L; has greater CNS penetration than other taxanes

Protein binding: 89% to 92%; primarily to serum albumin and lipoproteins

Metabolism: Extensively hepatic; primarily via CYP3A4 and 3A5; also via CYP2C8 (minor)

Half-life elimination: Terminal: 95 hours

Excretion: Feces (76% as metabolites); Urine (~4%)

Dosage Note: Premedicate at least 30 minutes prior to each dose of cabazitaxel with an antihistamine (eg, diphenhydramine I.V. 25 mg or equivalent), a corticosteroid (eg, dexamethasone 8 mg I.V. or equivalent), and an H_2 antagonist (eg, ranitidine 50 mg I.V. or equivalent). Antiemetic prophylaxis is also recommended. Details concerning dosing in combination regimens should also be consulted.

I.V.: Adults: Prostate cancer: 25 mg/m^2/dose once every 3 weeks (in combination with prednisone)

Dosage adjustment for toxicity:
Hematologic toxicity:
Neutropenia ≥grade 3 for >1 week despite WBC growth factors: Delay treatment until ANC >1500/mm^3 and then reduce dose to 20 mg/m^2 with continued WBC growth factor secondary prophylaxis
Neutropenic fever: Delay treatment until improvement/resolution and ANC >1500/mm^3 and then reduce dose to 20 mg/m^2 with continued WBC growth factor secondary prophylaxis
Persistent hematologic toxicity (despite dosage reduction): Discontinue treatment
Nonhematologic toxicity:
Severe hypersensitivity: Discontinue immediately
Diarrhea ≥grade 3 or persistent despite appropriate medication, fluids, and electrolyte replacement: Delay treatment until improves or resolves and then reduce dose to 20 mg/m^2
Persistent diarrhea (despite dosage reduction): Discontinue treatment

Dosage adjustment in renal impairment: Severe renal impairment (Cl_{cr} <30 mL/minute) or end-stage renal disease: Use with caution
Dosage adjustment in hepatic impairment: Hepatic impairment (total bilirubin ≥ULN or AST and/or ALT ≥1.5 times ULN): Use is not recommended

Dosing in obesity: ASCO Guidelines for appropriate chemotherapy dosing in obese adults with cancer: Utilize patient's actual body weight (full weight) for calculation of body surface area- or weight-based dosing, particularly when the intent of therapy is curative; manage regimen-related toxicities in the same manner as for nonobese patients; if a dose reduction is utilized due to toxicity, consider resumption of full weight-based dosing with subsequent cycles, especially if cause of toxicity (eg, hepatic or renal impairment) is resolved (Griggs, 2012).
Dietary Considerations Avoid grapefruit juice.
Administration I.V.: Infuse over 1 hour using a 0.22 micron inline filter. Do not use polyurethane-containing infusion sets for administration. Allow to reach room temperature prior to infusion. Premedicate with an antihistamine, a corticosteroid, and an H_2 antagonist at least 30 minutes prior to infusion. Observe closely during infusion (for hypersensitivity). Antiemetic prophylaxis (oral or I.V.) is also recommended.

Hazardous agent; use appropriate precautions for handling and disposal (meets NIOSH, 2012 criteria).
Monitoring Parameters CBC with differential and platelets (weekly during first cycle, then prior to each treatment cycle); monitor for hypersensitivity
Dosage Forms Excipient information presented when available (limited, particularly for generics); consult specific product labeling.
Solution, Intravenous:
Jevtana: 60 mg/1.5 mL (1.5 mL) [contains alcohol, usp, polysorbate 80]

Cabergoline (ca BER goe leen)

Brand Names: Canada CO Cabergoline; Dostinex®
Pharmacologic Category Ergot Derivative
Additional Appendix Information
Antiparkinsonian Agents *on page 2289*
Use Treatment of hyperprolactinemic disorders, either idiopathic or due to pituitary adenomas
Canadian labeling: Additional use (not in U.S. labeling): Prevention of the onset of physiological lactation in the puerperium when clinically indicated (eg, still born baby or neonatal death, conditions that interfere with suckling, severe acute or chronic mental illness). **Note:** Not indicated for suppression of established postpartum lactation.
Pregnancy Risk Factor B
Dosage Oral: Adults:
Hyperprolactinemia:
U.S. labeling: Initial dose: 0.25 mg twice weekly; the dose may be increased by 0.25 mg twice weekly up to a maximum of 1 mg twice weekly according to the patient's serum prolactin level. Dosage increases should not occur more rapidly than every 4 weeks. Once a normal serum prolactin level is maintained for 6 months, the dose may be discontinued and prolactin levels monitored to determine if cabergoline is still required. The durability of efficacy beyond 24 months of therapy has not been established.
Canadian labeling: Initial dose: 0.5 mg once weekly or 0.25 mg twice weekly; weekly dose may be increased by 0.5 mg per week at 4 week intervals until optimal therapeutic response. Therapeutic dose: Usual: 1 mg/week (range: 0.25-2 mg/week). **Note:** May divide weekly dose into 2 or more divided doses per week (recommended for doses >1 mg/week) based on tolerability.
Lactation inhibition (Canadian labeling; not in U.S. labeling): 1 mg single dose on first day postpartum
Elderly: No dosage recommendations suggested; however, start at the low end of the dosage range

Dosage adjustment in renal impairment: No dosage adjustment required; pharmacokinetics not altered with moderate-severe renal impairment.
Dosage adjustment in hepatic impairment:
Mild-to-moderate dysfunction (Child-Pugh class B or C): No dosage adjustment required; no effect on C_{max} or AUC.
Severe dysfunction (Child-Pugh class C): There are no dosage adjustments provided in manufacturer's labeling; use caution; significant increase in AUC.
Additional Information Complete prescribing information should be consulted for additional detail.
Dosage Forms Excipient information presented when available (limited, particularly for generics); consult specific product labeling.
Tablet, Oral:
Generic: 0.5 mg

◆ **Caduet®** *see* Amlodipine and Atorvastatin *on page 110*
◆ **CaEDTA** *see* Edetate CALCIUM Disodium *on page 685*
◆ **Caelyx (Can)** *see* DOXOrubicin (Liposomal) *on page 663*
◆ **Cafcit®** *see* Caffeine *on page 309*
◆ **CAFdA** *see* Clofarabine *on page 458*

Caffeine (KAF een)

Brand Names: U.S. Cafcit®; Enerjets [OTC]; No Doz® Maximum Strength [OTC]; Vivarin® [OTC]
Index Terms Caffeine and Sodium Benzoate; Caffeine Citrate; Caffeine Sodium Benzoate; Sodium Benzoate and Caffeine
Pharmacologic Category Central Nervous System Stimulant; Phosphodiesterase Enzyme Inhibitor, Nonselective
Use
Caffeine citrate: Treatment of idiopathic apnea of prematurity
Caffeine and sodium benzoate: Treatment of acute respiratory depression (not a preferred agent)
Caffeine [OTC labeling]: Restore mental alertness or wakefulness when experiencing fatigue

Unlabeled Use Caffeine and sodium benzoate: Treatment of spinal puncture headache; CNS stimulant; diuretic; augmentation of seizure induction during electroconvulsive therapy (ECT)

Pregnancy Risk Factor C

Pregnancy Considerations Adverse events were observed in animal reproduction studies. Caffeine crosses the placenta; serum concentrations in the fetus are similar to those in the mother (Grosso, 2005). Based on current studies, usual dietary exposure to caffeine is unlikely to cause congenital malformations (Brent, 2011). However, available data shows conflicting results related to maternal caffeine use and the risk of other adverse events, such as spontaneous abortion or growth retardation (Brent, 2011; Jahanfar, 2013). The half-life of caffeine is prolonged during the second and third trimesters of pregnancy and maternal and fetal exposure is also influenced by maternal smoking or drinking (Brent, 2011; Koren, 2000). Current guidelines recommend limiting caffeine intake from all sources to ≤200 mg/day (ACOG, 2010).

Breast-Feeding Considerations Caffeine is detected in breast milk (Berlin, 1981; Hildebrant, 1983; Ryu, 1985a); concentrations may be dependent upon maternal consumption and her ability to metabolize (eg, smoker versus nonsmoker) (Brent, 2011). The ability of the breast-feeding child to metabolize caffeine is age dependant (Hildebrant, 1983). Irritability and jitteriness have been reported in the nursing infant exposed to high concentrations of caffeine in breast milk (Martin, 2007). Infant heart rates and sleep patterns were not found to be affected in normal, full-term infants exposed to lesser amounts of caffeine (Ryu, 1985b).

Contraindications Hypersensitivity to caffeine or any component of the formulation; sodium benzoate is not for use in neonates

Warnings/Precautions Use with caution in patients with a history of peptic ulcer, gastroesophageal reflux, impaired renal or hepatic function, seizure disorders, or cardiovascular disease. Avoid use in patients with symptomatic cardiac arrhythmias, agitation, anxiety, or tremor. Over-the-counter [OTC] products contain an amount of caffeine similar to one cup of coffee; limit the use of other caffeine-containing beverages or foods.

Caffeine citrate should not be interchanged with caffeine and sodium benzoate. Avoid use of products containing sodium benzoate in neonates; has been associated with a potentially fatal toxicity ("gasping syndrome"). Neonates receiving caffeine citrate should be closely monitored for the development of necrotizing enterocolitis. Caffeine serum levels should be closely monitored to optimize therapy and prevent serious toxicity.

Adverse Reactions Frequency not specified; primarily serum-concentration related.

Cardiovascular: Angina, arrhythmia (ventricular), chest pain, flushing, palpitation, sinus tachycardia, tachycardia (supraventricular), vasodilation

Central nervous system: Agitation, delirium, dizziness, hallucinations, headache, insomnia, irritability, psychosis, restlessness

Dermatologic: Urticaria

Gastrointestinal: Esophageal sphincter tone decreased, gastritis

Neuromuscular & skeletal: Fasciculations

Ocular: Intraocular pressure increased (>180 mg caffeine), miosis

Renal: Diuresis

Drug Interactions

Metabolism/Transport Effects Substrate of CYP1A2 (major), CYP2C9 (minor), CYP2D6 (minor), CYP2E1 (minor), CYP3A4 (minor); **Note:** Assignment of Major/Minor substrate status based on clinically relevant drug interaction potential; **Inhibits** CYP1A2 (weak)

Avoid Concomitant Use

Avoid concomitant use of Caffeine with any of the following: Iobenguane I 123

Increased Effect/Toxicity

Caffeine may increase the levels/effects of: Formoterol; Indacaterol; Sympathomimetics

The levels/effects of Caffeine may be increased by: Abiraterone Acetate; AtoMOXetine; Cannabinoids; Ciprofloxacin (Systemic); CYP1A2 Inhibitors (Moderate); CYP1A2 Inhibitors (Strong); Deferasirox; Linezolid; Norfloxacin; Vemurafenib

Decreased Effect

Caffeine may decrease the levels/effects of: Adenosine; Iobenguane I 123; Regadenoson

The levels/effects of Caffeine may be decreased by: Peginterferon Alfa-2b; Teriflunomide

Preparation for Administration Parenteral:

Caffeine citrate: May administer without dilution or diluted with D_5W to 10 mg caffeine citrate/mL.

Caffeine and sodium benzoate: For spinal headaches, dilute in 1000 mL NS.

Storage/Stability Store at 20°C to 25°C (68°F to 77°F).

Caffeine citrate: Injection and oral solution contain no preservatives; injection is chemically stable for at least 24 hours at room temperature when diluted to 10 mg/mL (as caffeine citrate) with D_5W, $D_{50}W$, Intralipid® 20%, and Aminosyn® 8.5%; also compatible with dopamine (600 mcg/mL), calcium gluconate 10%, heparin (1 unit/mL), and fentanyl (10 mcg/mL) at room temperature for 24 hours.

Mechanism of Action Increases levels of 3'5' cyclic AMP by inhibiting phosphodiesterase; CNS stimulant which increases medullary respiratory center sensitivity to carbon dioxide, stimulates central inspiratory drive, and improves skeletal muscle contraction (diaphragmatic contractility); prevention of apnea may occur by competitive inhibition of adenosine

Pharmacodynamics/Kinetics

Distribution: V_d:

- Neonates: 0.8-0.9 L/kg
- Children >9 months to Adults: 0.6 L/kg

Protein binding: 17% (children) to 36% (adults)

Metabolism: Hepatic, via demethylation by CYP1A2. **Note:** In neonates, interconversion between caffeine and theophylline has been reported (caffeine levels are ~25% of measured theophylline after theophylline administration and ~3% to 8% of caffeine would be expected to be converted to theophylline)

Half-life elimination:

- Neonates: 72-96 hours (range: 40-230 hours)
- Children >9 months and Adults: 5 hours

Time to peak, serum: Oral: Within 30 minutes to 2 hours

Excretion:

- Neonates ≤1 month: 86% excreted unchanged in urine
- Infants >1 month and Adults: In urine, as metabolites

Dosage

Note: Caffeine citrate should not be interchanged with the caffeine sodium benzoate formulation.

Caffeine citrate: Neonates: Apnea of prematurity: Oral, I.V.:

Loading dose: 10-20 mg/kg as caffeine citrate (5-10 mg/kg as caffeine base). If theophylline has been administered to the patient within the previous 3 days, a full or modified loading dose (50% to 75% of a loading dose) may be given.

Maintenance dose: 5 mg/kg/day as caffeine citrate (2.5 mg/kg/day as caffeine base) once daily starting 24 hours after the loading dose. Maintenance dose is adjusted based on patient's response and serum caffeine concentrations.

Caffeine and sodium benzoate:
Children: Stimulant: I.M., I.V., SubQ: 8 mg/kg every 4 hours as needed
Children ≥12 years and Adults: OTC labeling (stimulant):
Oral: 100-200 mg every 3-4 hours as needed
Adults:
Electroconvulsive therapy: I.V.: 300-2000 mg
Respiratory depression: I.M., I.V.: 250 mg as a single dose; may repeat as needed. Maximum single dose should be limited to 500 mg; maximum amount in any 24-hour period should generally be limited to 2500 mg.
Spinal puncture headache (unlabeled use):
I.V.: 500 mg in 1000 mL NS infused over 1 hour, followed by 1000 mL NS infused over 1 hour; a second course of caffeine can be given for unrelieved headache pain in 4 hours.
Oral: 300 mg as a single dose
Stimulant/diuretic (unlabeled use): I.M., I.V.: 500 mg, maximum single dose: 1 g

Dosage adjustment in renal impairment: No dosage adjustment required.

Dietary Considerations Oral formulations may be taken without regard to feedings or meals.

Administration
Oral: May be administered without regard to feedings or meals. May administer injectable formulation (caffeine citrate) orally.
Parenteral:
Caffeine citrate: Infuse loading dose over at least 30 minutes; maintenance dose may be infused over at least 10 minutes. May administer without dilution.
Caffeine and sodium benzoate: I.V. as slow direct injection. For spinal headaches, infuse diluted solution over 1 hour. Follow with 1000 mL NS; infuse over 1 hour. May administer I.M. undiluted.

Reference Range
Therapeutic: Apnea of prematurity: 8-20 mcg/mL
Potentially toxic: >20 mcg/mL
Toxic: >50 mcg/mL

Dosage Forms Excipient information presented when available (limited, particularly for generics); consult specific product labeling. [DSC] = Discontinued product
Caplet:
NoDoz® Maximum Strength: 200 mg
Injection, solution, as citrate [preservative free]: 20 mg/mL (3 mL) [equivalent to 10 mg/mL caffeine base]
Cafcit®: 20 mg/mL (3 mL) [equivalent to 10 mg/mL caffeine base]
Injection, solution [with sodium benzoate]: Caffeine 125 mg/mL and sodium benzoate 125 mg/mL (2 mL)
Lozenge:
Enerjets®: 75 mg (12s) [classic coffee, hazelnut cream, or mochamint flavor]
Solution, oral, as citrate [preservative free]: 20 mg/mL (3 mL) [equivalent to 10 mg/mL caffeine base]
Cafcit®: 20 mg/mL (3 mL) [equivalent to 10 mg/mL caffeine base]
Tablet: 200 mg
Vivarin®: 200 mg

Extemporaneous Preparations A 10 mg/mL oral solution of caffeine (as citrate) may be prepared from 10 g caffeine (anhydrous) combined with 10 g citric acid USP and dissolved in 1000 mL sterile water. Label "shake well" and "refrigerate". Stable for 3 months (Nahata, 2004).

A 20 mg/mL oral solution of caffeine (as citrate) may be made from 5 g caffeine (anhydrous) combined with 5 g citric acid USP and dissolved in 250 mL sterile water. Stir solution until completely clear, then add a 2:1 mixture of simple syrup and cherry syrup in sufficient quantity to make 500 mL. Label "shake well" and "refrigerate". Stable for 90 days (Eisenberg, 1984).

Eisenberg MG and Kang N, "Stability of Citrated Caffeine Solutions for Injectable and Enteral Use," *Am J Hosp Pharm*, 1984, 41(11):2405-6.
Nahata MC, Pai VB, and Hipple TF, *Pediatric Drug Formulations*, 5th ed, Cincinnati, OH: Harvey Whitney Books Co, 2004.

◆ **Caffeine, Acetaminophen, and Aspirin** *see* Acetaminophen, Aspirin, and Caffeine *on page 33*
◆ **Caffeine and Sodium Benzoate** *see* Caffeine *on page 309*
◆ **Caffeine, Aspirin, and Acetaminophen** *see* Acetaminophen, Aspirin, and Caffeine *on page 33*
◆ **Caffeine Citrate** *see* Caffeine *on page 309*
◆ **Caffeine, Dihydrocodeine, and Aspirin** *see* Dihydrocodeine, Aspirin, and Caffeine *on page 611*
◆ **Caffeine, Orphenadrine, and Aspirin** *see* Orphenadrine, Aspirin, and Caffeine *on page 1517*
◆ **Caffeine Sodium Benzoate** *see* Caffeine *on page 309*

Calamine (KAL a meen)

Index Terms Calamine Lotion

Pharmacologic Category Topical Skin Product

Use Employed primarily as an astringent, protectant, and soothing agent for conditions such as poison ivy, poison oak, poison sumac, sunburn, insect bites, or minor skin irritations

Dosage Topical: Children and Adults: Apply to affected area as often as needed

Additional Information Complete prescribing information should be consulted for additional detail.

Dosage Forms Excipient information presented when available (limited, particularly for generics); consult specific product labeling. [DSC] = Discontinued product
Lotion, External:
Generic: 8% (118 mL [DSC]); 8% (120 mL, 177 mL, 180 mL, 240 mL)

◆ **Calamine Lotion** *see* Calamine *on page 311*
◆ **Calan** *see* Verapamil *on page 2182*
◆ **Calan SR** *see* Verapamil *on page 2182*
◆ **Calcarb 600 [OTC]** *see* Calcium Carbonate *on page 318*
◆ **Cal-Carb Forte [OTC]** *see* Calcium Carbonate *on page 318*
◆ **Calcet Petites [OTC]** *see* Calcium and Vitamin D *on page 318*
◆ **Calci-Chew [OTC]** *see* Calcium Carbonate *on page 318*
◆ **Calcidol [OTC]** *see* Ergocalciferol *on page 733*
◆ **Calciferol [OTC]** *see* Ergocalciferol *on page 733*
◆ **Calcijex® (Can)** *see* Calcitriol *on page 314*
◆ **Calcimar (Can)** *see* Calcitonin *on page 312*
◆ **Calci-Mix [OTC]** *see* Calcium Carbonate *on page 318*
◆ **Calcio del Mar [OTC]** *see* Calcium Carbonate *on page 318*
◆ **Calcionate [OTC]** *see* Calcium Glubionate *on page 322*

Calcipotriene (kal si POE try een)

Brand Names: U.S. Calcitrene; Dovonex; Sorilux

Brand Names: Canada Dovonex®

Pharmacologic Category Topical Skin Product; Vitamin D Analog

Use Treatment of plaque psoriasis of the body (cream, foam, ointment) or of the scalp (foam, solution)

Pregnancy Risk Factor C

Dosage Plaque psoriasis: Topical: Adults:

Cream: Apply a thin film to the affected skin twice daily

Foam: Apply a thin film to the affected skin or scalp twice daily

Ointment: Apply a thin film to the affected skin once or twice daily

Solution: Apply to the affected scalp twice daily

Additional Information Complete prescribing information should be consulted for additional detail.

Dosage Forms Excipient information presented when available (limited, particularly for generics); consult specific product labeling.

Cream, External:

Dovonex: 0.005% (60 g, 120 g) [contains cetearyl alcohol, disodium edta]

Generic: 0.005% (60 g, 120 g)

Foam, External:

Sorilux: 0.005% (60 g, 120 g) [contains cetyl alcohol, edetate disodium, propylene glycol]

Ointment, External:

Calcitrene: 0.005% (60 g, 120 g) [contains disodium edta, propylene glycol]

Generic: 0.005% (60 g, 120 g)

Solution, External:

Generic: 0.005% (60 mL)

Calcipotriene and Betamethasone

(kal si POE try een & bay ta METH a sone)

Brand Names: U.S. Taclonex®

Brand Names: Canada Dovobet®; Xamiol®

Index Terms Betamethasone Dipropionate and Calcipotriene Hydrate; Calcipotriol and Betamethasone Dipropionate

Pharmacologic Category Corticosteroid, Topical; Vitamin D Analog

Use Treatment of plaque psoriasis

Unlabeled Use Treatment of corticosteroid-responsive dermatoses

Pregnancy Risk Factor C

Dosage Topical: Adults: Plaque psoriasis:

Gel (Xamiol® [CAN]): Apply to affected area of scalp once daily for up to 4 weeks (maximum recommended dose: 15 g daily or 100 g weekly). Application to >30% of body surface area is not recommended

Ointment: Apply to affected area of skin once daily for up to 4 weeks (maximum recommended dose: 100 g weekly). Application to >30% of body surface area is not recommended.

Suspension: Apply to affected area of skin or scalp once daily for up to 8 weeks (maximum recommended dose: 100 g weekly)

Dosing adjustment in renal impairment: No dosage adjustment provided in manufacturer's labeling (has not been studied in severe renal impairment).

Dosing adjustment in hepatic impairment: No dosage adjustment provided in manufacturer's labeling (has not been studied in severe hepatic impairment).

Additional Information Complete prescribing information should be consulted for additional detail.

Dosage Forms Excipient information presented when available (limited, particularly for generics); consult specific product labeling.

Ointment, topical:

Taclonex®: Calcipotriene 0.005% and betamethasone dipropionate 0.064% (60 g, 100 g)

Suspension, topical:

Taclonex®: Calcipotriene 0.005% and betamethasone dipropionate 0.064% (60 g, 120 g) [contains castor oil]

Dosage Forms: Canada Excipient information presented when available (limited, particularly for generics); consult specific product labeling.

Gel, topical:

Xamiol®: Calcipotriol 50 mcg/g and betamethasone dipropionate 0.5 mg/g (30 g, 60 g, 2 x 60 g)

Ointment, topical:

Dovobet®: Calcipotriol 50 mcg/g and betamethasone 0.5 mg/g (30 g, 60 g, 120 g)

◆ **Calcipotriol and Betamethasone Dipropionate** *see* Calcipotriene and Betamethasone *on page 312*

◆ **Calcite-500 (Can)** *see* Calcium Carbonate *on page 318*

Calcitonin (kal si TOE nin)

Brand Names: U.S. Fortical; Miacalcin

Brand Names: Canada Apo-Calcitonin; Calcimar; Caltine; Miacalcin NS; PRO-Calcitonin; Sandoz-Calcitonin

Index Terms Calcitonin (Salmon)

Pharmacologic Category Antidote; Hormone

Use

U.S. labeling: Treatment of symptomatic Paget's disease of bone (osteitis deformans); adjunctive therapy for hypercalcemia; treatment of osteoporosis in women >5 years postmenopause

Canadian labeling: Injection: Treatment of symptomatic Paget's disease of bone (osteitis deformans) in patients who are nonresponsive or intolerant to alternative therapy; adjunctive therapy for hypercalcemia; Intranasal: Treatment of osteoporosis in women >5 years postmenopause

Pregnancy Risk Factor C

Pregnancy Considerations Decreased birth weight was observed in animal reproduction studies. Calcitonin does not cross the placenta. The nasal spray formulations are not indicated for use in pregnancy.

Breast-Feeding Considerations It is not known if calcitonin is excreted in human breast milk. Calcitonin has been shown to decrease milk production in animals. Breast-feeding is not recommended by the manufacturer.

Contraindications Hypersensitivity to calcitonin salmon or any component of the formulation

Warnings/Precautions A skin test should be performed prior to initiating therapy of calcitonin salmon in patients with suspected sensitivity; have epinephrine immediately available for a possible hypersensitivity reaction. A detailed skin testing protocol is available from the manufacturers. Temporarily withdraw use of nasal spray if ulceration of nasal mucosa occurs. Discontinue for ulcerations >1.5 mm or those that penetrate below the mucosa. Patients >65 years of age may experience a higher incidence of nasal adverse events with calcitonin nasal spray.

Analyses of randomized controlled trials (in osteoporosis and osteoarthritis) have demonstrated a statistically significant increase in the risk of the development of cancer in calcitonin-treated patients (compared to placebo). The risk for malignancies is associated with long-term use of calcitonin. Definitive efficacy of calcitonin-salmon in decreasing fractures is lacking compared to other agents approved for osteoporosis treatment; consider potential benefits of therapy against risks in osteoporosis treatment, including the potential risk for malignancy with long-term use.

Adverse Reactions Unless otherwise noted, frequencies reported are with nasal spray.

>10%: Respiratory: Rhinitis (≤12%, including ulcerative)

1% to 10%:

Cardiovascular: Flushing (nasal spray: <1%; injection: 2% to 5%), angina pectoris (1% to 3%), hypertension (1% to 3%)

Central nervous system: Depression (1% to 3%), dizziness (1% to 3%), fatigue (1% to 3%)

Dermatologic: Erythematous rash (1% to 3%)

Gastrointestinal: Nausea (injection: 10%; nasal spray: 2%), abdominal pain (1% to 3%), constipation (1% to 3%), diarrhea (1% to 3%), dyspepsia (1% to 3%)

Genitourinary: Cystitis (1% to 3%)

Hematologic & oncologic: Lymphadenopathy (1% to 3%)

Infection: Increased susceptibility to infection (1% to 3%)

Local: Injection site reaction (injection: 10%)

Neuromuscular & skeletal: Back pain (5%), osteoarthritis (1% to 3%), myalgia (1% to 3%), paresthesia (1% to 3%)

Ophthalmic: Conjunctivitis (1% to 3%), abnormal lacrimation (1% to 3%)

Respiratory: Nasal mucosa ulcer (3%), bronchospasm (1% to 3%), flu-like symptoms (1% to 3%), sinusitis (1% to 3%), upper respiratory tract infection (1% to 3%)

<1% (Limited to important or life-threatening): Alopecia, altered sense of smell, anaphylactic shock, anaphylactoid reaction, anaphylaxis, anemia, anorexia, arthritis, bronchitis, bundle branch block, cerebrovascular accident, cholelithiasis, dermal ulcer, eczema, edema, gastritis, goiter, hearing loss, hematuria, hepatitis, hypersensitivity reaction, hyperthyroidism, malignant neoplasm, migraine, myocardial infarction, nephrolithiasis, neuralgia, nocturia, palpitations, parosmia, periorbital edema, pneumonia, polymyalgia rheumatica, polyuria, pyelonephritis, tachycardia, thrombophlebitis, tissue damage (nasal mucosal excoriation), vitreous opacity, weight gain

Drug Interactions

Metabolism/Transport Effects None known.

Avoid Concomitant Use There are no known interactions where it is recommended to avoid concomitant use.

Increased Effect/Toxicity There are no known significant interactions involving an increase in effect.

Decreased Effect

Calcitonin may decrease the levels/effects of: Lithium

Ethanol/Nutrition/Herb Interactions Ethanol: Avoid ethanol (may increase risk of osteoporosis).

Preparation for Administration Injection: NS has been recommended for the dilution to prepare a skin test in patients with suspected sensitivity.

Storage/Stability

Injection: Store under refrigeration at 2°C to 8°C (36°F to 46°F); protect from freezing. The following stability information has also been reported: May be stored at room temperature for up to 14 days (Cohen, 2007).

Nasal: Store unopened bottle under refrigeration at 2°C to 8°C (36°F to 46°F); do not freeze.

Fortical: After opening, store for up to 30 days at 20°C to 25°C (68°F to 77°F); excursions permitted to 15°C to 30°C (59°F to 86°F). Store in upright position.

Miacalcin: After opening, store for up to 35 days at room temperature of 15°C to 30°C (59°F to 86°F). Store in upright position.

Mechanism of Action Peptide sequence similar to human calcitonin; functionally antagonizes the effects of parathyroid hormone. Directly inhibits osteoclastic bone resorption; promotes the renal excretion of calcium, phosphate, sodium, magnesium, and potassium by decreasing tubular reabsorption; increases the jejunal secretion of water, sodium, potassium, and chloride

Pharmacodynamics/Kinetics

Onset of action:

Hypercalcemia: I.M., SubQ: ~2 hours

Paget's disease: Within a few months; may take up to 1 year for neurologic symptom improvement

Duration: Hypercalcemia: I.M., SubQ: 6-8 hours

Distribution: V_d: 0.15-0.3 L/kg

Metabolism: Metabolized in kidneys, blood and peripheral tissue

Bioavailability: I.M.: 66%; SubQ: 71%; Nasal: ~3% to 5% (relative to I.M.)

Half-life elimination (terminal): I.M. 58 minutes; SubQ 59-64 minutes; Nasal: ~18 minutes

Time to peak, plasma: SubQ ~23 minutes; Nasal: ~13 minutes

Excretion: Urine (as inactive metabolites)

Dosage Adults:

Paget's disease, symptomatic (Miacalcin): I.M., SubQ: Initial: 100 units daily; maintenance: 50 units every 1-2 days; may be preferable to maintain doses of 100 units daily for serious deformity or neurologic involvement. **Note:** Due to the risk of malignancy associated with prolonged calcitonin use, the Canadian labeling recommends limiting therapy in most patients to ≤3 months; under exceptional circumstances (eg, impending pathologic fracture), therapy may be extended to ≤6 months

Hypercalcemia (Miacalcin): Initial: I.M., SubQ: 4 units/kg every 12 hours; after 1-2 days, may increase up to 8 units/kg every 12 hours; if the response remains unsatisfactory after 2 more days, may further increase up to a maximum of 8 units/kg every 6 hours

Postmenopausal osteoporosis:

I.M., SubQ: Miacalcin: 100 units every other day

Intranasal: Fortical, Miacalcin: 200 units (1 spray) in one nostril daily

Dosage adjustment in renal impairment: No dosage adjustment provided in manufacturer's labeling.

Dosage adjustment in hepatic impairment: No dosage adjustment provided in manufacturer's labeling.

Dietary Considerations Patients with Paget's disease and hypercalcemia should follow a low calcium diet as prescribed. Recommended amounts of vitamin D and calcium intake is essential for preventing/treating osteoporosis. If dietary intake is inadequate, dietary supplementation is recommended. Women and men should consume:

Calcium: 1000 mg/day (men: 50-70 years) **or** 1200 mg/day (women ≥51 years and men ≥71 years) (IOM, 2011; NOF, 2013)

Vitamin D: 800-1000 IU/day (men and women ≥50 years) (NOF, 2013). Recommended Dietary Allowance (RDA): 600 IU/day (men and women ≤70 years) **or** 800 IU/day (men and women ≥71 years) (IOM, 2011).

Administration

Injection: May be administered I.M. or SubQ. I.M. route is preferred if the injection volume is >2 mL (use multiple injection sites if dose volume is >2 mL). SubQ route is preferred for outpatient self-administration unless the injection volume is >2 mL.

Nasal spray: Before first use, allow bottle to reach room temperature, then prime pump by releasing at least 5 sprays until full spray is produced. To administer, place nozzle into nostril with head in upright position. Alternate nostrils daily. Do not prime pump before each daily use. Discard after 30 doses.

Monitoring Parameters

Osteoporosis: Bone mineral density (BMD) should be re-evaluated every 2 years (or more frequently) after initiating therapy (NOF, 2013); annual measurements of height and weight, assessment of chronic back pain; serum calcium and 25(OH)D; consider measuring biochemical markers of bone turnover

Paget's disease: Alkaline phosphatase; pain; serum calcium and 25(OH)D

Nasal formulation: Visualization of nasal mucosa, turbinate, septum, and mucosal blood vessels (at baseline and with nasal complaints)

Reference Range

Calcium (total): Adults: 9.0-11.0 mg/dL (2.05-2.54 mmol/L), may slightly decrease with aging

Phosphorus: 2.5-4.5 mg/dL (0.81-1.45 mmol/L)

Vitamin D: There is no clear consensus on a reference range for total serum 25(OH)D concentrations or the validity of this level as it relates clinically to bone health. In addition, there is significant variability in the reporting of serum 25(OH)D levels as a result of different assay types in use; however, the following ranges have been suggested:

Adults (IOM, 2011): Sufficient levels in practically all persons: ≥20 ng/mL (50 nmol/L); concern for risk of toxicity: >50 ng/mL (125 nmol/L)

Osteoporosis patients (NOF, 2013): Recommended level to reach and maintain: ~30 ng/mL (75 nmol/L)

Dosage Forms Excipient information presented when available (limited, particularly for generics); consult specific product labeling.

Solution, Injection:

Miacalcin: 200 units/mL (2 mL)

Solution, Nasal:

Fortical: 200 units/actuation (3.7 mL)

Miacalcin: 200 units/actuation (3.7 mL)

Generic: 200 units/actuation (3.7 mL)

◆ Calcitonin (Salmon) *see* Calcitonin *on page 312*

◆ Calcitrate [OTC] *see* Calcium and Vitamin D *on page 318*

◆ Cal-Citrate [OTC] *see* Calcium Citrate *on page 321*

◆ Calcitrene *see* Calcipotriene *on page 311*

Calcitriol (kal si TRYE ole)

Brand Names: U.S. Rocaltrol; Vectical

Brand Names: Canada Calcijex®; Rocaltrol®; Silkis™

Index Terms 1,25 Dihydroxycholecalciferol

Pharmacologic Category Vitamin D Analog

Use

Management of hypocalcemia in patients on chronic renal dialysis (oral, injection); management of secondary hyperparathyroidism in patients with chronic kidney disease (CKD) (oral); management of hypocalcemia in patients with hypoparathyroidism and pseudohypoparathyroidism (oral); management of mild-to-moderate plaque psoriasis (topical)

Canadian labeling: Additional uses (not in U.S. labeling): Vitamin D-resistant rickets (oral)

Unlabeled Use Vitamin D-dependent rickets type I/pseudovitamin D deficiency rickets (PDDR)

Pregnancy Risk Factor C

Pregnancy Considerations Teratogenic effects have been observed in some animal reproduction studies. Mild hypercalcemia has been reported in a newborn following maternal use of calcitriol during pregnancy. Adverse effects on fetal development were not observed with use of calcitriol during pregnancy in women (N=9) with pseudovitamin D-dependent rickets. Doses were adjusted every 4 weeks to keep calcium concentrations within normal limits (Edouard, 2011). If calcitriol is used for the management of hypoparathyroidism in pregnancy, dose adjustments may be needed as pregnancy progresses and again following delivery. Vitamin D and calcium levels should be monitored closely and kept in the lower normal range.

Breast-Feeding Considerations Low levels are found in breast milk (~2 pg/mL)

Contraindications

U.S. labeling:

Oral, injection: Hypersensitivity to calcitriol or any component of the formulation; hypercalcemia, vitamin D toxicity

Topical: There are no contraindications listed in the manufacturer's labeling.

Canadian labeling:

Oral, injection: Hypersensitivity to calcitriol, vitamin D or its analogues or derivatives, or any component of the formulation or container; hypercalcemia, vitamin D toxicity

Topical: Ophthalmic or internal use; hypercalcemia or a history of abnormal calcium metabolism; concurrent systemic treatment of calcium homeostasis; severe renal impairment or end-stage renal disease (ESRD)

Warnings/Precautions Oral, injection: Adequate dietary (supplemental) calcium is necessary for clinical response to vitamin D. Excessive vitamin D may cause severe hypercalcemia, hypercalciuria, and hyperphosphatemia. Discontinue use immediately in patients with a calcium-phosphate product (serum calcium times phosphorus) >70 mg^2/dL^2, may resume therapy at decreased doses when levels are appropriate. Other forms of vitamin D should be withheld during therapy to avoid the potential for hypercalcemia to develop. In addition, several months may be required for ergocalciferol levels to return to baseline in patients switching from ergocalciferol therapy to calcitriol. Monitor calcium levels closely with initiation of therapy and with dose adjustments; discontinue use promptly in patients who develop hypercalcemia. Avoid abrupt dietary modifications (eg, increased intake of dairy products) which may lead to hypercalcemia; adjust calcium intake if indicated and maintain adequate hydration. Chronic hypercalcemia can result in generalized vascular and soft tissue calcification. Immobilized patients may be at a higher risk for hypercalcemia.

Use oral calcitriol with caution in patients with malabsorption syndromes (efficacy may be limited and/or response may be unpredictable). Use of calcitriol for the treatment of secondary hyperparathyroidism associated with CKD is not recommended in patients with rapidly worsening kidney function or in noncompliant patients. Increased serum phosphate levels in patients with renal failure may lead to calcification; the use of an aluminum-containing phosphate binder is recommended along with a low phosphate diet in these patients. Use with caution in patients taking cardiac glycosides; digitalis toxicity is potentiated by hypocalcemia. Concomitant use with magnesium-containing products such as antacids may lead to hypermagnesemia in patients receiving chronic renal dialysis. Products may contain coconut (capsule) or palm seed oil (oral solution). Some products may contain tartrazine.

Topical: May cause hypercalcemia; if alterations in calcium occur, discontinue treatment until levels return to normal. For external use only; not for ophthalmic, oral, or intravaginal use. Do not apply to facial skin, eyes, or lips. Absorption may be increased with occlusive dressings. Avoid or limit excessive exposure to natural or artificial sunlight, or phototherapy. The safety and effectiveness has not been evaluated in patients with erythrodermic, exfoliative, or pustular psoriasis. Canadian labeling does not recommend use in patients with hepatic or renal impairment.

Adverse Reactions

Oral, I.V.: Frequency not defined.

Cardiovascular: Cardiac arrhythmia, hypertension

Central nervous system: Apathy, headache, hyperthermia, psychosis, sensory disturbances, somnolence

Dermatologic: Erythema multiforme, erythematous skin disorders, pruritus, rash, urticaria

Endocrine & metabolic: Dehydration, growth suppression, hypercalcemia, hypercholesterolemia, libido decreased, polydipsia
Gastrointestinal: Abdominal pain, anorexia, constipation, metallic taste, nausea, pancreatitis, stomach ache, vomiting, weight loss, xerostomia
Genitourinary: Nocturia, urinary tract infection
Hepatic: ALT increased, AST increased
Local: Injection site pain (mild)
Neuromuscular & skeletal: Bone pain, myalgia, dystrophy, soft tissue calcification, weakness
Ocular: Conjunctivitis, photophobia
Renal: Albuminuria, BUN increased, creatinine increased, hypercalciuria, nephrocalcinosis, polyuria
Respiratory: Rhinorrhea
Miscellaneous: Allergic reaction, hypersensitivity reactions
<1% (Limited to important or life-threatening): Anaphylaxis

Topical:
>10%: Endocrine: Hypercalcemia (24%)
1% to 10%:
Dermatologic: Psoriasis (4%), skin discomfort (3%), pruritus (1% to 3%)
Genitourinary: Urine abnormality (4%)
Renal: Hypercalciuria (3%)
<1% (Limited to important or life-threatening): Kidney stones

Drug Interactions

Metabolism/Transport Effects Substrate of CYP3A4 (major); **Note:** Assignment of Major/Minor substrate status based on clinically relevant drug interaction potential; **Induces** CYP3A4 (weak/moderate)

Avoid Concomitant Use

Avoid concomitant use of Calcitriol with any of the following: Aluminum Hydroxide; Axitinib; Conivaptan; Fusidic Acid (Systemic); Multivitamins/Fluoride (with ADE); Multivitamins/Minerals (with ADEK, Folate, Iron); Simeprevir; Sucralfate; Sucroferric Oxyhydroxide; Vitamin D Analogs

Increased Effect/Toxicity

Calcitriol may increase the levels/effects of: Aluminum Hydroxide; Cardiac Glycosides; Magnesium Salts; Sucralfate; Vitamin D Analogs

The levels/effects of Calcitriol may be increased by: Calcium Salts; Conivaptan; CYP3A4 Inhibitors (Moderate); CYP3A4 Inhibitors (Strong); Danazol; Dasatinib; Fusidic Acid (Systemic); Ivacaftor; Luliconazole; Mifepristone; Multivitamins/Fluoride (with ADE); Multivitamins/Minerals (with ADEK, Folate, Iron); Simeprevir; Thiazide Diuretics

Decreased Effect

Calcitriol may decrease the levels/effects of: ARIPiprazole; Axitinib; Ibrutinib; Saxagliptin; Simeprevir

The levels/effects of Calcitriol may be decreased by: Bile Acid Sequestrants; Bosentan; Corticosteroids (Systemic); CYP3A4 Inducers (Strong); Dabrafenib; Deferasirox; Herbs (CYP3A4 Inducers); Mineral Oil; Mitotane; Orlistat; Sevelamer; Sucroferric Oxyhydroxide; Tocilizumab

Storage/Stability

Injection: Store at room temperature of 15°C to 30°C (59°F to 86°F). Protect from light.

Oral capsule, solution: Store at room temperature of 15°C to 30°C (59°F to 86°F). Protect from light.

Topical: Store at room temperature of 25°C (77°F); excursions permitted to 15°C to 30°C (59°F to 86°F); do not refrigerate; do not freeze.

Mechanism of Action Calcitriol, the active form of vitamin D (1,25 hydroxyvitamin D_3), binds to and activates the vitamin D receptor in kidney, parathyroid gland, intestine, and bone, stimulating intestinal calcium transport and absorption. It reduces PTH levels and improves calcium and phosphate homeostasis by stimulating bone resorption of calcium and increasing renal tubular reabsorption of calcium. Decreased renal conversion of vitamin D to its primary active metabolite (1,25 hydroxyvitamin D) in chronic renal failure leads to reduced activation of vitamin D receptor, which subsequently removes inhibitory suppression of parathyroid hormone (PTH) release; increased serum PTH (secondary hyperparathyroidism) reduces calcium excretion and enhances bone resorption.

The mechanism by which calcitriol is beneficial in the treatment of psoriasis has not been established.

Pharmacodynamics/Kinetics

Duration: Oral, I.V.: 3-5 days
Absorption: Oral: Rapid
Protein binding: 99.9%
Metabolism: Primarily to calcitroic acid and a lactone metabolite
Half-life elimination: Children ~27 hours; Healthy adults: 5-8 hours; Hemodialysis: 16-22 hours
Time to peak, serum: Oral: 3-6 hours; Hemodialysis: 8-12 hours
Excretion: Primarily feces; urine

Dosage

Hypocalcemia in patients on chronic renal dialysis:
Adults:
Oral: Initial: 0.25 mcg daily; may increase dose by 0.25 mcg daily at 4- to 8-week intervals, up to 0.5-1 mcg daily; patients with normal or mildly decreased serum calcium levels may respond to 0.25 mcg every other day
I.V.:
U.S. labeling: Initial: 1-2 mcg 3 times weekly approximately every other day. Adjust dose by 0.5-1 mcg at 2- to 4-week intervals; dosing range: 0.5-4 mcg 3 times weekly. Gradual dose reduction and discontinuation of therapy may be necessary as PTH levels decrease below target of (1.5-3 x ULN) in response to therapy.
Canadian labeling: Initial: 0.5 mcg 3 times weekly, approximately every other day. Adjust dose by 0.25-0.5 mcg at 2- to 4-week intervals; dosing range: 0.5-3 mcg 3 times weekly

Hypocalcemia in hypoparathyroidism/pseudohypoparathyroidism:
U.S. labeling: Oral:
Children 1-5 years: Usual dosage range: 0.25-0.75 mcg once daily (may adjust dose at 2- to 4-week intervals)
Children ≥6 years and Adults: Initial: 0.25 mcg daily (may adjust dose at 2- to 4-week intervals); range: 0.5-2 mcg once daily
Canadian labeling: Oral:
Children: Initial: 0.03-0.05 mcg/kg/day; evaluate response after 2 weeks and increase dose by 25% if response is inadequate. Dose may be increased or decreased by 25% every 2 weeks thereafter until therapeutic response is achieved. **Note:** May consider initial dose of 0.05 mcg/kg/day for severe hypocalcemia/ symptoms (hospitalization recommended with close monitoring and dose reduction as soon as clinically possible). Maintenance dose: 0.014-0.04 mcg/kg/day
Adults: Initial: 0.25 mcg daily; may increase dose by 0.25 mcg daily at 2- to 4-week intervals. Discontinue use immediately for hypercalcemia; may resume therapy after calcium levels normalize.

Psoriasis: Adults: Topical: Apply twice daily to affected areas (maximum: 200 g weekly); Canadian labeling recommends maximum of 30 g daily

Secondary hyperparathyroidism associated with moderate-to-severe CKD in patients not on dialysis:
U.S. labeling: Oral:
Children <3 years: Initial dose: 0.01-0.015 mcg/kg/day
Children ≥3 years and Adults: Initial: 0.25 mcg daily; may increase to 0.5 mcg daily

KDOQI guidelines for vitamin D therapy in CKD:
Children (KDOQI, 2005):
CKD stage 2, 3: Oral:
<10 kg: 0.05 mcg every other day
10-20 kg: 0.1-0.15 mcg daily
>20 kg: 0.25 mcg daily
Note: Treatment should only be started with serum 25 (OH)D >30 ng/mL, serum iPTH >70 pg/mL, serum calcium <10 mg/dL and serum phosphorus less than or equal to the age appropriate level.
CKD stage 4: Oral:
<10 kg: 0.05 mcg every other day
10-20 kg: 0.1-0.15 mcg daily
>20 kg: 0.25 mcg daily
Note: Treatment should only be started with serum 25 (OH)D >30 ng/mL, serum iPTH >110 pg/mL, serum calcium <10 mg/dL and serum phosphorus less than or equal to the age appropriate level.
CKD stage 5: Peritoneal dialysis or hemodialysis: Oral, I.V.: **Note:** The following initial doses are based on plasma PTH and serum calcium levels for patients with serum phosphorus <5.5 mg/dL in adolescents or <6.5 in infants and children, and Ca-P product <55 in adolescents or <65 in infants and children <12 years. Adjust dose based on serum phosphate, calcium and PTH levels. Administer dose with each dialysis session (3 times weekly). Intermittent I.V./oral administration is more effective than daily oral dosing.
Plasma PTH 300-500 pg/mL and serum Ca <10 mg/dL: 0.0075 mcg/kg (maximum: 0.25 mcg daily)
Plasma PTH >500-1000 pg/mL and serum Ca <10 mg/dL: 0.015 mcg/kg (maximum: 0.5 mcg daily)
Plasma PTH >1000 pg/mL and serum Ca <10.5 mg/dL: 0.025 mcg/kg (maximum: 1 mcg daily)
Adults (KDOQI, 2003):
CKD stage 3: Oral: 0.25 mcg daily. Treatment should only be started with serum 25(OH)D >30 ng/mL, serum iPTH >70 pg/mL, serum calcium <9.5 mg/dL and serum phosphorus <4.6 mg/dL
CKD stage 4: Oral: 0.25 mcg daily. Treatment should only be started with serum 25(OH)D >30 ng/mL, serum iPTH >110 pg/mL, serum calcium <9.5 mg/dL and serum phosphorus <4.6 mg/dL
CKD stage 5:
Peritoneal dialysis: Oral: Initial: 0.5-1 mcg 2-3 times weekly or 0.25 mcg daily
Hemodialysis: **Note:** The following initial doses are based on plasma PTH and serum calcium levels for patients with serum phosphorus <5.5 mg/dL and Ca-P product <55. Adjust dose based on serum phosphate, calcium, and PTH levels. Intermittent I.V. administration may be more effective than daily oral dosing. Administer per hemodialysis session.
Plasma PTH 300-600 pg/mL and serum Ca <9.5 mg/dL: Oral, I.V.: 0.5-1.5 mcg
Plasma PTH 600-1000 pg/mL and serum Ca <9.5 mg/dL:
Oral: 1-4 mcg
I.V.: 1-3 mcg
Plasma PTH >1000 pg/mL and serum Ca <10 mg/dL:
Oral: 3-7 mcg
I.V.: 3-5 mcg

Vitamin D-dependent rickets type 1/pseudovitamin D deficiency rickets (PDDR):
U.S. unlabeled use: Children and Adults: Oral: Initial: 0.5 mcg twice daily; subsequent dosing adjusted to maintain normal serum calcium and PTH levels; median dose after 2 years: 0.25 mcg daily (range: 0.1-0.5 mcg daily) (Edouard, 2011)
Canadian labeling: Children: Oral: Initial: 0.01-0.025 mcg/kg/day; evaluate response after two weeks and increase dose by 25% if response is inadequate. Dose may be increased or decreased by 25% every 2 weeks thereafter until therapeutic response is achieved. **Note:** May consider initial dose of 0.05 mcg/kg/day for severe hypocalcemia/ symptoms (hospitalization recommended with close monitoring and dose reduction as soon as clinically possible). Maintenance dose: 0.0046-0.015 mcg/kg/day.

Vitamin D-resistant rickets: *Canadian labeling (not in U.S. labeling):* Adults: Oral: Initial: 0.25 mcg daily; may increase dose by 25 mcg daily at 2- to 4-week intervals if response is inadequate; discontinue use immediately for hypercalcemia and do not resume until calcium levels normalize.

X-linked hypophosphatemic rickets: *Canadian labeling (not in U.S. labeling):* Children: Oral: Initial: 0.01-0.02 mcg/kg/day; evaluate response after 2 weeks and increase dose by 25% if response is inadequate. Dose may be increased or decreased by 25% every two weeks thereafter until therapeutic response is achieved. **Note:** May consider initial dose of 0.05 mcg/kg/day for severe hypocalcemia/ symptoms (hospitalization recommended with close monitoring and dose reduction as soon as clinically possible). Maintenance dose: 0.01-0.05 mcg/kg/day.

Elderly: Start at the lower end of the dosage range. Refer to adult dosing.

Dosage adjustment for toxicity:
Children: KDOQI guidelines (2005): CKD stages 2-4:
Serum iPTH below target range: Hold calcitriol until levels rise above target range appropriate for CKD stage, than resume treatment at half the previous dose. If the lowest dose was being used, switch to alternate day therapy.
Corrected total calcium >10.2 mg/dL: Hold calcitriol until serum calcium returns to <9.8 mg/dL then resume treatment at half the previous dose. If the lowest dose was being used, switch to alternate day therapy.
Serum phosphorus greater than the age appropriate limits: Hold calcitriol and add/increase dose of phosphate binder until levels of phosphorous decrease to age appropriate levels, then resume at half the previous dose
Adults: KDOQI guidelines (2003): CKD stage 3 and 4:
iPTH below target: Hold calcitriol until levels rise then resume treatment at half the previous dose. If the lowest dose was being used, switch to alternate day therapy.
Corrected total calcium >9.5 mg/dL: Hold calcitriol until serum calcium returns to <9.5 mg/dL, then resume treatment at half the previous dose. If the lowest dose was being used, switch to alternate day therapy.
Serum phosphorus >4.6 mg/dL: Hold calcitriol (or add/ increase dose of phosphate binder) until levels of phosphorous decrease, then resume at half the prior dose.

Dosage adjustment in renal impairment: No dosage adjustment necessary.

Dosage adjustment in hepatic impairment: No dosage adjustment provided in the manufacturer's labeling.

Dietary Considerations May be taken without regard to food. Give with meals to reduce GI problems. Adequate calcium intake should be maintained during therapy; dietary phosphorous may need to be restricted.

Administration

I.V.: May be administered as a bolus dose I.V. through the catheter at the end of hemodialysis.

Oral: May be administered without regard to food. Administer with meals to reduce GI problems.

Topical: Apply externally; not for ophthalmic, oral, or intravaginal use. Do not apply to eyes, lips, or facial skins. Rub in gently so that no medication remains visible. Limit application to only the areas of skin affected by psoriasis.

Monitoring Parameters

Manufacturer's labeling:

Oral therapy:

Dialysis patients: Serum calcium, phosphorus, magnesium, and alkaline phosphate monitored periodically

Hypoparathyroid patients: Serum calcium, phosphorus, 24 hour urinary calcium monitored periodically

Predialysis patients: Serum calcium, phosphorus, alkaline phosphatase, creatinine, and intact PTH, initially; then serum calcium, phosphorus, alkaline phosphatase, and creatinine monthly x 6 months, then periodically. Intact PTH should be monitored every 3-4 months.

During titration periods (all patients), monitor serum calcium levels at least twice weekly.

I.V. therapy: Serum calcium and phosphorus twice weekly (following initiation and during dosage adjustments) and periodically during therapy; periodic magnesium, alkaline phosphatase, 24 hour urinary calcium and phosphorous

KDOQI Guidelines: Oral and I.V. therapy: **Note:** More frequent monitoring may be necessary depending on the presence and magnitude of abnormalities, the rate of progression of CKD, and the use of treatments for CKD-mineral and bone disorders.

Children (KDOQI, 2005):

Serum calcium and phosphorous: CKD stages 2-4: At least monthly for first 3 months following initiation of therapy and at least every 3 months thereafter

CKD stage 5: At least every 2 weeks for one month following initiation of therapy and dose increases and monthly thereafter

Serum iPTH:

CKD stages 2-4: At least every 3 months

CKD stage 5: Monthly for at least 3 months following initiation of therapy or dose increases; once target levels are achieved monitor at least every 3 months thereafter

Adults (KDOQI, 2003):

Serum calcium and phosphorous:

CKD stages 3 and 4: At least monthly for first 3 months following initiation of therapy and every 3 months thereafter

CKD stage 5: At least every 2 weeks for one month following initiation of therapy or dose increases and monthly thereafter

Serum iPTH:

CKD stages 3 and 4: At least every 3 months for 6 months and every 3 months thereafter

CKD stage 5: Monthly for at least 3 months following initiation of therapy or dose increases and at least every 3 months once target levels are achieved

Reference Range

Corrected total serum calcium (KDOQI, 2003): CKD stages 3 and 4: 8.4-10.2 mg/dL (2.1-2.6 mmol/L); CKD stage 5: 8.4-9.5 mg/dL (2.1-2.37 mmol/L); KDIGO guidelines recommend maintaining normal ranges for all stages of CKD (3-5D) (KDIGO, 2009)

Phosphorus (KDOQI, 2003):

CKD stages 3 and 4: 2.7-4.6 mg/dL (0.87-1.48 mmol/L) (adults); maintain within age-appropriate limits (children)

CKD stage 5 (including those treated with dialysis): 3.5-5.5 mg/dL (1.13-1.78 mmol/L) (children >12 years and adults); 4-6 mg/dL (1.29-1.94 mmol/L) (children 1-12 years)

KDIGO guidelines recommend maintaining normal ranges for CKD stages 3-5 and lowering elevated phosphorus levels toward the normal range for CKD stage 5D (KDIGO, 2009)

Serum calcium-phosphorus product (KDOQI, 2003): CKD stage 3-5: <55 mg^2/dL^2 (children >12 years and adults); <65 mg^2/dL^2 (children ≤12 years)

PTH: Whole molecule, immunochemiluminometric assay (ICMA): 1.0-5.2 pmol/L; whole molecule, radioimmunoassay (RIA): 10.0-65.0 pg/mL; whole molecule, immunoradiometric, double antibody (IRMA): 1.0-6.0 pmol/L

Target ranges by stage of chronic kidney disease (KDIGO, 2009): CKD stage 3-5: Optimal iPTH is unknown; maintain normal range (assay-dependent); CKD stage 5D: Maintain iPTH within 2-9 times the upper limit of normal for the assay used

Dosage Forms Excipient information presented when available (limited, particularly for generics); consult specific product labeling.

Capsule, Oral:

Rocaltrol: 0.25 mcg, 0.5 mcg [contains fd&c yellow #6 (sunset yellow), methylparaben, propylparaben]

Generic: 0.25 mcg, 0.5 mcg

Ointment, External:

Vectical: 3 mcg/g (100 g)

Generic: 3 mcg/g (100 g)

Solution, Intravenous:

Generic: 1 mcg/mL (1 mL)

Solution, Oral:

Rocaltrol: 1 mcg/mL (15 mL)

Generic: 1 mcg/mL (15 mL)

Dosage Forms: Canada Excipient information presented when available (limited, particularly for generics); consult specific product labeling.

Ointment, topical:

Silkis™: 3 mcg/g (5 g, 30 g, 100 g)

◆ **Calcium 600 [OTC]** *see* Calcium Carbonate *on page 318*

Calcium Acetate (KAL see um AS e tate)

Brand Names: U.S. Calphron [OTC]; Eliphos; PhosLo; Phoslyra

Brand Names: Canada PhosLo®

Pharmacologic Category Antidote; Calcium Salt; Phosphate Binder

Use Control of hyperphosphatemia in end-stage renal failure; does not promote aluminum absorption

Pregnancy Risk Factor C

Dosage Oral: Adults, on dialysis: Initial: 1334 mg with each meal, can be increased gradually (ie, every 2-3 weeks) to bring the serum phosphate value to <6 mg/dL as long as hypercalcemia does not develop (usual dose: 2001-2668 mg calcium acetate with each meal); do not give additional calcium supplements

Dosage adjustment in renal impairment: No dosage adjustment necessary.

Dosage adjustment in hepatic impairment: No dosage adjustment provided in manufacturer's labeling.

Additional Information Complete prescribing information should be consulted for additional detail.

Dosage Forms Considerations

Calcium acetate is approximately 25% elemental calcium

Calcium acetate 667 mg = elemental calcium 169 mg = calcium 8.45 mEq = calcium 4.23 mmol

Dosage Forms Excipient information presented when available (limited, particularly for generics); consult specific product labeling.

Capsule, Oral:
PhosLo: 667 mg
Generic: 667 mg

Solution, Oral:
Phoslyra: 667 mg/5 mL (473 mL) [contains methylparaben, propylene glycol]

Tablet, Oral:
Calphron: 667 mg
Eliphos: 667 mg
Generic: 667 mg, 668 mg

◆ **Calcium Acetate and Aluminum Sulfate** *see* Aluminum Sulfate and Calcium Acetate *on page 91*

◆ **Calcium Acetylhomotaurinate** *see* Acamprosate *on page 26*

Calcium and Vitamin D

(KAL see um & VYE ta min dee)

Brand Names: U.S. Cal-CYUM [OTC]; Calcet Petites [OTC]; Calcitrate [OTC]; Caltrate 600+D [OTC]; Caltrate 600+Soy [OTC]; Caltrate ColonHealth [OTC]; Chew-Cal [OTC]; Citracal Maximum [OTC]; Citracal Petites [OTC]; Citracal Regular [OTC]; Liqua-Cal [OTC]; Os-Cal 500+D [OTC]; Oysco 500+D [OTC]; Oysco D [OTC]

Index Terms Calcium Citrate and Vitamin D; Vitamin D and Calcium Carbonate

Pharmacologic Category Calcium Salt; Electrolyte Supplement, Oral; Vitamin, Fat Soluble

Use Dietary supplement, antacid

Dosage Oral: Adults: Refer to individual monographs for dietary reference intake.

Dosage adjustment in renal impairment: Use caution in severe renal impairment

Additional Information Complete prescribing information should be consulted for additional detail.

Dosage Forms Excipient information presented when available (limited, particularly for generics); consult specific product labeling.

Caplet, oral:
Citracal Maximum: Calcium 315 mg and vitamin D 250 units [gluten free]
Os-Cal: Calcium 500 mg and vitamin D 200 units
Os-Cal Extra D: Calcium 500 mg and vitamin D 600 units

Capsule, softgel, oral: Calcium 500 mg and vitamin D 500 units; calcium 600 mg and vitamin D 100 units; calcium 600 mg and vitamin D 200 units
Liqua-Cal: Calcium 600 mg and vitamin D 200 units [contains beeswax, lecithin, and soybean oil]

Tablet, oral: Calcium 250 mg and vitamin D 125 units; calcium 315 mg and vitamin D 200 units; calcium 500 mg and vitamin D 125 units; calcium 500 mg and vitamin D 200 units; calcium 600 mg and vitamin D 125 units; calcium 600 mg and vitamin D 200 units; calcium 600 mg and vitamin D 400 units
Calcet Petites: Calcium 200 mg and vitamin D 250 units [gluten free; contains tartrazine]
Calcitrate: Calcium 315 mg and vitamin D 250 units
Caltrate 600+D: Calcium 600 mg and vitamin D 200 units [contains soybean oil]
Caltrate 600+Soy: Calcium 600 mg and vitamin D 200 units [contains soy isoflavones 25 mg]
Caltrate ColonHealth: Calcium 600 mg and vitamin D 200 units [contains soybean oil]
Citracal Petites: Calcium 200 mg and vitamin D 250 units [gluten free]
Citracal Regular: Calcium 250 mg and vitamin D 200 units [gluten free]
Oysco D: Calcium 250 mg and vitamin D 125 units
Oysco 500+D: Calcium 500 mg and vitamin D 200 units [contains tartrazine]

Tablet, chewable: Calcium 500 mg and vitamin D 100 units; calcium 500 mg and vitamin D 200 units; calcium 500 mg and vitamin D 600 units; calcium 600 mg and vitamin D 400 units
Os-Cal: Calcium 500 mg and vitamin D 600 units [sugar free; contains phenylalanine; lemon chiffon flavor]

Wafer, chewable:
Cal-CYUM: Calcium 519 mg and vitamin D 150 units (50s) [dye free; vanilla flavor]
Chew-Cal: Calcium 333 mg and vitamin D 40 units (100s, 250s)

◆ **Calcium Antacid [OTC]** *see* Calcium Carbonate *on page 318*

◆ **Calcium Antacid Extra Strength [OTC]** *see* Calcium Carbonate *on page 318*

◆ **Calcium Antacid Ultra Max St [OTC]** *see* Calcium Carbonate *on page 318*

Calcium Carbonate

(KAL see um KAR bun ate)

Brand Names: U.S. Alcalak [OTC]; Antacid Extra Strength [OTC]; Antacid [OTC]; Cal-Carb Forte [OTC]; Cal-CO3S [OTC]; Cal-Gest Antacid [OTC]; Cal-Mint [OTC]; Calcarb 600 [OTC]; Calci-Chew [OTC]; Calci-Mix [OTC]; Calcio del Mar [OTC]; Calcium 600 [OTC]; Calcium Antacid Extra Strength [OTC]; Calcium Antacid Ultra Max St [OTC]; Calcium Antacid [OTC]; Calcium High Potency [OTC]; Caltrate 600 [OTC]; Florical [OTC]; Maalox Childrens [OTC]; Maalox [OTC]; Os-Cal [OTC] [DSC]; Oysco 500 [OTC]; Titralac [OTC]; Tums E-X 750 [OTC]; Tums Freshers [OTC]; Tums Kids [OTC]; Tums Lasting Effects [OTC]; Tums Smoothies [OTC]; Tums Ultra 1000 [OTC]; Tums [OTC]

Brand Names: Canada Apo-Cal®; Calcite-500; Caltrate®; Caltrate® Select; Os-Cal®; Tums Extra Strength; Tums Smoothies; Tums® Chews Extra Strength; Tums® Regular Strength; Tums® Ultra Strength

Index Terms Oscal

Pharmacologic Category Antacid; Antidote; Calcium Salt; Electrolyte Supplement, Oral

Use As an antacid; treatment and prevention of calcium deficiency or hyperphosphatemia (eg, osteoporosis, osteomalacia, mild/moderate renal insufficiency, hypoparathyroidism, postmenopausal osteoporosis, rickets); has been used to bind phosphate

Dosage Oral (dosage is in terms of **elemental** calcium):

Dietary Reference Intake for Calcium:
1-6 months: Adequate intake: 200 mg/day
7-12 months: Adequate intake: 260 mg/day
1-3 years: RDA: 700 mg/day
4-8 years: RDA: 1000 mg/day
9-18 years: RDA:1300 mg/day
Adults, Females/Males: RDA:
19-50 years: 1000 mg/day
≥51 years, females: 1200 mg/day
51-70 years, males: 1000 mg/day
>70 years, males: 1200 mg/day
Females: Pregnancy/Lactating: RDA: Requirements are the same as in nonpregnant or nonlactating females

Hypocalcemia (dose depends on clinical condition and serum calcium level): Dose expressed in mg of **elemental calcium**
Children: 45-65 mg/kg/day in 4 divided doses
Adults: 1-2 g or more/day in 3-4 divided doses

Antacid:
Children 2-5 years (24-47 lb): Elemental calcium 161 mg as needed; maximum: 483 mg per 24 hours
Children 6-11 years (48-95 lb): Elemental calcium 322 mg as needed; maximum: 966 mg per 24 hours

Adults: Dosage based on acid-neutralizing capacity of specific product; generally, 2-4 tablets or 5-10 mL every 2 hours; maximum: 7500 mg calcium carbonate per 24 hours (equivalent to 3000 mg elemental calcium); OTC dosing recommendations may vary by product and/or manufacturer; specific product labeling should be consulted

Dietary supplementation: Adults: 500 mg to 2 g divided 2-4 times/day

Dosing adjustment in renal impairment: Cl_{cr} <25 mL/minute: Dosage adjustments may be necessary depending on the serum calcium levels

Additional Information Complete prescribing information should be consulted for additional detail.

Dosage Forms Considerations

1 g calcium carbonate = elemental calcium 400 mg = calcium 20 mEq = calcium 10 mmol

Dosage Forms Excipient information presented when available (limited, particularly for generics); consult specific product labeling. [DSC] = Discontinued product

Capsule, Oral:
- Calci-Mix: 1250 mg
- Florical: 364 mg

Capsule, Oral [preservative free]:
- Cal-CO3S: 200 mg [dye free]

Powder, Oral:
- Generic: 800 mg/2 g (480 g)

Suspension, Oral:
- Generic: 1250 mg/5 mL (5 mL, 473 mL, 500 mL)

Tablet, Oral:
- Cal-Carb Forte: 1250 mg
- Calcarb 600: 1500 mg [scored]
- Calcio del Mar: 1250 mg
- Calcium 600: 600 mg [scored]
- Calcium 600: 600 mg [contains fd&c yellow #6 aluminum lake, soy polysaccarides]
- Calcium High Potency: 600 mg
- Caltrate 600: 1500 mg [scored]
- Florical: 364 mg
- Oysco 500: 500 mg [contains brilliant blue fcf (fd&c blue #1), tartrazine (fd&c yellow #5)]
- Generic: 500 mg, 600 mg, 648 mg, 1250 mg, 1500 mg

Tablet, Oral [preservative free]:
- Calcium 600: 600 mg [lactose free, salt free, sugar free]
- Generic: 500 mg, 600 mg, 1250 mg

Tablet Chewable, Oral:
- Alcalak: 420 mg [mint flavor]
- Antacid: 420 mg [mint flavor]
- Antacid: 500 mg
- Antacid: 500 mg [assorted fruit flavor]
- Antacid: 500 mg [peppermint flavor]
- Antacid: 500 mg [contains brilliant blue fcf (fd&c blue #1), fd&c yellow #10 (quinoline yellow), fd&c yellow #6 (sunset yellow)]
- Antacid: 500 mg [contains fd&c blue #1 aluminum lake, fd&c red #40 aluminum lake, fd&c yellow #5 aluminum lake, fd&c yellow #6 aluminum lake]
- Antacid Extra Strength: 750 mg [contains brilliant blue fcf (fd&c blue #1), fd&c red #40]
- Antacid Extra Strength: 750 mg [contains fd&c red #40, fd&c yellow #6 (sunset yellow), tartrazine (fd&c yellow #5)]
- Cal-Gest Antacid: 500 mg [contains fd&c blue #1 aluminum lake, fd&c yellow #10 aluminum lake, fd&c yellow #6 aluminum lake]
- Cal-Mint: 260 mg [animal products free, gelatin free, gluten free, lactose free, no artificial color(s), no artificial flavor(s), starch free, sugar free, yeast free]
- Calci-Chew: 1250 mg [cherry flavor]
- Calcium Antacid: 500 mg
- Calcium Antacid: 500 mg [contains brilliant blue fcf (fd&c blue #1), fd&c red #40, fd&c yellow #6 (sunset yellow), soybeans (glycine max), tartrazine (fd&c yellow #5); assorted flavor]
- Calcium Antacid: 500 mg [contains fd&c blue #1 aluminum lake]
- Calcium Antacid Extra Strength: 750 mg [assorted fruit flavor]
- Calcium Antacid Extra Strength: 750 mg [contains brilliant blue fcf (fd&c blue #1), fd&c red #40, fd&c yellow #6 (sunset yellow), tartrazine (fd&c yellow #5); assorted flavor]
- Calcium Antacid Extra Strength: 750 mg [contains fd&c blue #1 aluminum lake, fd&c red #40 aluminum lake]
- Calcium Antacid Ultra Max St: 1000 mg [contains brilliant blue fcf (fd&c blue #1), fd&c red #40, fd&c yellow #6 (sunset yellow), soybeans (glycine max), tartrazine (fd&c yellow #5)]
- Maalox: 600 mg [contains aspartame; wild berry flavor]
- Maalox Childrens: 400 mg [contains aspartame; wild berry flavor]
- Os-Cal: 1250 mg [DSC]
- Titralac: 420 mg [low sodium, sugar free; contains saccharin]
- Tums: 500 mg [gluten free]
- Tums: 500 mg [gluten free; contains fd&c blue #1 aluminum lake, fd&c red #40 aluminum lake, fd&c yellow #6 aluminum lake, tartrazine (fd&c yellow #5)]
- Tums E-X 750: 750 mg
- Tums E-X 750: 750 mg [assorted flavor]
- Tums E-X 750: 750 mg [gluten free; contains fd&c blue #1 aluminum lake, fd&c red #40 aluminum lake; assorted berries flavor]
- Tums E-X 750: 750 mg [gluten free; contains fd&c blue #1 aluminum lake, fd&c red #40 aluminum lake, fd&c yellow #5 aluminum lake, fd&c yellow #6 aluminum lake; assorted fruit flavor]
- Tums E-X 750: 750 mg [sugar free]
- Tums Freshers: 500 mg [gluten free; contains brilliant blue fcf (fd&c blue #1); mint flavor]
- Tums Kids: 750 mg [scored; contains fd&c blue #1 aluminum lake, fd&c red #40 aluminum lake; cherry flavor]
- Tums Lasting Effects: 500 mg [contains fd&c red #40 aluminum lake, fd&c yellow #6 aluminum lake, tartrazine (fd&c yellow #5)]
- Tums Smoothies: 750 mg [peppermint flavor]
- Tums Smoothies: 750 mg [contains fd&c blue #1 aluminum lake, fd&c red #40 aluminum lake, fd&c yellow #6 aluminum lake, soybeans (glycine max); assorted tropical fruit flavor]
- Tums Smoothies: 750 mg [contains fd&c blue #1 aluminum lake, fd&c red #40 aluminum lake, soybeans (glycine max); berry flavor]
- Tums Smoothies: 750 mg [gluten free; contains fd&c blue #1 aluminum lake, fd&c red #40 aluminum lake, fd&c yellow #5 aluminum lake, fd&c yellow #6 aluminum lake, milk (cow)]
- Tums Ultra 1000: 1000 mg [peppermint flavor]
- Tums Ultra 1000: 1000 mg [contains fd&c blue #1 aluminum lake, fd&c red #40 aluminum lake, fd&c yellow #5 aluminum lake, fd&c yellow #6 aluminum lake; assorted berries flavor]
- Tums Ultra 1000: 1000 mg [contains fd&c red #40 aluminum lake, fd&c yellow #6 aluminum lake, tartrazine (fd&c yellow #5); assorted tropical fruit flavor]
- Tums Ultra 1000: 1000 mg [DSC] [gluten free]
- Tums Ultra 1000: 1000 mg [gluten free; contains fd&c blue #1 aluminum lake, fd&c red #40 aluminum lake, fd&c yellow #6 aluminum lake, tartrazine (fd&c yellow #5)]
- Generic: 260 mg, 500 mg

Tablet Chewable, Oral [preservative free]:
- Generic: 500 mg

Calcium Carbonate and Magnesium Hydroxide

(KAL see um KAR bun ate & mag NEE zhum hye DROKS ide)

Brand Names: U.S. Mi-Acid™ Double Strength [OTC]; Mylanta® Supreme [OTC]; Mylanta® Ultra [OTC]

Index Terms Magnesium Hydroxide and Calcium Carbonate

Pharmacologic Category Antacid

Use Hyperacidity

Dosage Adults: Oral: 2-4 tablets between meals, at bedtime, or as directed by healthcare provider

Additional Information Complete prescribing information should be consulted for additional detail.

Dosage Forms Excipient information presented when available (limited, particularly for generics); consult specific product labeling.

Liquid (Mylanta® Supreme): Calcium carbonate 400 mg and magnesium hydroxide 135 mg per 5 mL (360 mL, 720 mL) [cherry flavor]

Tablet, chewable:

Mi-Acid™ Double Strength: Calcium carbonate 700 mg and magnesium hydroxide 300 mg

Mylanta® Ultra: Calcium carbonate 700 mg and magnesium hydroxide 300 mg [cherry créme and cool mint flavors]

Calcium Chloride (KAL see um KLOR ide)

Pharmacologic Category Calcium Salt; Electrolyte Supplement, Parenteral

Use Treatment of hypocalcemia and conditions secondary to hypocalcemia (eg, tetany, seizures, arrhythmias); emergent treatment of severe hypermagnesemia

Unlabeled Use Calcium channel blocker overdose; beta-blocker overdose (refractory to glucagon and high-dose vasopressors); severe hyperkalemia ($K+ >6.5$ mEq/L with toxic ECG changes) [ACLS guidelines]; malignant arrhythmias (including cardiac arrest) associated with hypermagnesemia [ACLS guidelines]

Pregnancy Risk Factor C

Pregnancy Considerations Animal reproduction studies have not been conducted. Calcium crosses the placenta. The amount of calcium reaching the fetus is determined by maternal physiological changes. Calcium requirements are the same in pregnant and nonpregnant females (IOM, 2011). Information related to use as an antidote in pregnancy is limited. In general, medications used as antidotes should take into consideration the health and prognosis of the mother; antidotes should be administered to pregnant women if there is a clear indication for use and should not be withheld because of fears of teratogenicity (Bailey, 2003).

Breast-Feeding Considerations Calcium is excreted in breast milk. The amount of calcium in breast milk is homeostatically regulated and not altered by maternal calcium intake. Calcium requirements are the same in lactating and nonlactating females (IOM, 2011).

Contraindications Known or suspected digoxin toxicity; not recommended as routine treatment in cardiac arrest (includes asystole, ventricular fibrillation, pulseless ventricular tachycardia, or pulseless electrical activity)

Warnings/Precautions For I.V. use only; do not inject SubQ or I.M.; avoid rapid I.V. administration (do not exceed 100 mg/minute except in emergency situations). Vesicant; ensure proper catheter or needle position prior to and during infusion; avoid extravasation; extravasation may result in severe necrosis and sloughing. Monitor the I.V. site closely. Use with caution in patients with hyperphosphatemia, respiratory acidosis, renal impairment, or respiratory failure; acidifying effect of calcium chloride may potentiate acidosis. Use with caution in patients with chronic renal failure to avoid hypercalcemia; frequent monitoring of serum calcium and phosphorus is necessary. Use with caution in hypokalemic or digitalized patients since acute rises in serum calcium levels may precipitate cardiac arrhythmias; use is contraindicated with known or suspected digoxin toxicity. Hypomagnesemia is a common cause of hypocalcemia; therefore, correction of hypocalcemia may be difficult in patients with concomitant hypomagnesemia. Evaluate serum magnesium and correct hypomagnesemia (if necessary), particularly if initial treatment of hypocalcemia is refractory. Solutions may contain aluminum; toxic levels may occur following prolonged administration in premature neonates or patients with renal impairment. Avoid metabolic acidosis (ie, administer only up to 2-3 days then change to another calcium salt).

Ceftriaxone may complex with calcium causing precipitation. Fatal lung and kidney damage associated with calcium-ceftriaxone precipitates has been observed in premature and term neonates. Due to reports of precipitation reaction in neonates, do not coadminister ceftriaxone with calcium-containing solutions, even via separate infusion lines/sites or at different times in any neonate. Ceftriaxone should not be administered simultaneously with any calcium-containing solution via a Y-site in any patient. However, ceftriaxone and calcium-containing solutions may be administered sequentially of one another for use in patients **other than neonates** if infusion lines are thoroughly flushed (with a compatible fluid) between infusions.

Adverse Reactions Frequency not defined. I.V.:

Cardiovascular (following rapid I.V. injection): Arrhythmia, bradycardia, cardiac arrest, hypotension, syncope, vasodilation

Central nervous system: Sense of oppression (with rapid I.V. injection)

Endocrine & metabolic: Hypercalcemia

Gastrointestinal: Irritation, chalky taste

Hepatic: Serum amylase increased

Local (following extravasation): Tissue necrosis

Neuromuscular & skeletal: Tingling sensation (with rapid I.V. injection)

Renal: Renal calculi

Miscellaneous: Hot flashes (with rapid I.V. injection)

Postmarketing and/or case reports: Calcinosis cutis

Drug Interactions

Metabolism/Transport Effects None known.

Avoid Concomitant Use

Avoid concomitant use of Calcium Chloride with any of the following: Calcium Acetate

Increased Effect/Toxicity

Calcium Chloride may increase the levels/effects of: Calcium Acetate; CefTRIAXone; Vitamin D Analogs

The levels/effects of Calcium Chloride may be increased by: Multivitamins/Fluoride (with ADE); Multivitamins/Minerals (with ADEK, Folate, Iron); Thiazide Diuretics

Decreased Effect

Calcium Chloride may decrease the levels/effects of: Bisphosphonate Derivatives; Calcium Channel Blockers; Deferiprone; DOBUTamine; Dolutegravir; Eltrombopag; Multivitamins/Fluoride (with ADE); Phosphate Supplements; Tetracycline Derivatives; Thyroid Products; Trientine

The levels/effects of Calcium Chloride may be decreased by: Trientine

Preparation for Administration I.V.: For intermittent I.V. infusion, dilute to a maximum concentration of 20 mg/mL.

Storage/Stability Do not refrigerate solutions; I.V. infusion solutions are stable for 24 hours at room temperature.

Although calcium chloride is not routinely used in the preparation of parenteral nutrition, it is important to note that phosphate salts may precipitate when mixed with calcium salts. Solubility is improved in amino acid parenteral nutrition solutions. Check with a pharmacist to determine compatibility.

Mechanism of Action Moderates nerve and muscle performance via action potential excitation threshold regulation

Pharmacodynamics/Kinetics

Protein binding: ~40%, primarily to albumin (Wills, 1971)

Excretion: Primarily feces (80% as insoluble calcium salts); urine (20%)

Dosage Note: One gram of calcium chloride salt is equal to 270 mg of elemental calcium.

Dosages are expressed in terms of the calcium chloride salt based on a solution concentration of 100 mg/mL (10%) containing 1.4 mEq (27 mg)/mL elemental calcium.

Hypocalcemia: I.V.: **Note:** In general, I.V. calcium gluconate is preferred over I.V. calcium chloride in nonemergency settings due to the potential for extravasation with calcium chloride.

Acute, symptomatic: Manufacturer's recommendations:

Children: 2.7-5 mg/kg/dose every 4-6 hours

Adults: 200-1000 mg every 1-3 days

Severe, symptomatic (eg, seizure, tetany): Adults: 1000 mg over 10 minutes; repeat every 60 minutes until symptoms resolve (French, 2012)

Cardiac arrest or cardiotoxicity in the presence of hyperkalemia, hypocalcemia, or hypermagnesemia: **Note:** Routine use in cardiac arrest is not recommended due to the lack of improved survival (Kleinman, 2010; Neumar, 2010).

Infants and Children: I.V., I.O.: 20 mg/kg (maximum: 2000 mg/dose); may repeat as necessary (Hegenbarth, 2008; Kleinman, 2010)

Adults: I.V.: 500-1000 mg over 2-5 minutes; may repeat as necessary (Vanden Hoek, 2010)

Beta-blocker overdose, refractory to glucagon and high-dose vasopressors (unlabeled use): **Note:** Optimal dose has not been established (DeWitt, 2004)

Adults: I.V.: 20 mg/kg over 5-10 minutes followed by an infusion of 20 mg/kg/hour titrated to adequate hemodynamic response (Vanden Hoek, 2010)

Calcium channel blocker overdose (unlabeled use): **Note:** Optimal dose has not been established (DeWitt, 2004).

Infants and Children:

I.V., I.O.: Initial: 10-20 mg/kg (maximum: 2000 mg/dose) over 10-15 minutes; may repeat every 10-15 minutes (Arroyo, 2009; Kleinman, 2010); if favorable response obtained, consider I.V. infusion

I.V. infusion: 20-50 mg/kg/hour (Arroyo, 2009)

Adults:

I.V.: Initial: 1000-2000 mg over 5 minutes; may repeat every 10-20 minutes with 3-4 additional doses **or** 1000 mg every 2-3 minutes until clinical effect is achieved (DeWitt, 2004); if favorable response obtained, consider I.V. infusion

I.V. infusion: 20-40 mg/kg/hour (DeWitt, 2004; Salhanick, 2003)

Dosage adjustment in renal impairment: No initial dosage adjustment necessary; however, accumulation may occur with renal impairment and subsequent doses may require adjustment based on serum calcium concentrations.

Dosage adjustment in hepatic impairment: No initial dosage adjustment necessary; subsequent doses should be guided by serum calcium concentrations.

Administration For I.V. administration only. Not for I.M. or SubQ administration (severe necrosis and sloughing may occur). Avoid rapid administration (do not exceed 100 mg/minute except in emergency situations). For intermittent I.V. infusion, infuse diluted solution over 1 hour or no greater than 45-90 mg/kg/hour (0.6-1.2 mEq/kg/hour); administration via a central or deep vein is preferred; do not use scalp, small hand or foot veins for I.V. administration (severe necrosis and sloughing may occur). Monitor ECG if calcium is infused faster than 2.5 mEq/minute; **stop the infusion if the patient complains of pain or discomfort.** Warm solution to body temperature prior to administration. **Do not infuse calcium chloride in the same I.V. line as phosphate-containing solutions.**

Vesicant; ensure proper needle or catheter placement prior to and during I.V. infusion. Avoid extravasation.

Extravasation management: If extravasation occurs, stop infusion immediately and disconnect (leave needle/cannula in place); gently aspirate extravasated solution (do **NOT** flush the line); initiate hyaluronidase antidote; remove needle/cannula; apply dry cold compresses (Hurst, 2004); elevate extremity.

Hyaluronidase: Intradermal or SubQ: Inject a total of 1 mL (15 units/mL) as five separate 0.2 mL injections (using a 25-gauge needle) into area of extravasation at the leading edge in a clockwise manner (MacCara, 1983; Zenk, 1981).

Monitoring Parameters Monitor infusion site, ECG when appropriate; serum calcium and ionized calcium (normal: 8.5-10.2 mg/dL [total]; 4.5-5.0 mg/dL [ionized]), albumin, serum phosphate; magnesium (to facilitate calcium repletion)

Calcium channel blocker overdose, beta-blocker overdose: Hemodynamic response, serum ionized calcium concentration

Reference Range

Serum total calcium: 8.4-10.2 mg/dL (2.1-2.55 mmol/L). **Note:** Due to a poor correlation between the serum ionized calcium (free) and total serum calcium, particularly in states of low albumin or acid/base imbalances, direct measurement of ionized calcium is recommended.

In low albumin states, the corrected **total** serum calcium may be estimated by the following equation (assuming a normal albumin of 4 g/dL [40 g/L]).

Corrected total calcium (mg/dL) = measured total calcium (mg/mL) + 0.8 [4 - measured serum albumin(g/dL)]

or

Corrected total calcium (mmol/L) = measured total calcium (mmol/L) + 0.02 [40-measured serum albumin (g/L)]

Additional Information 14 mEq calcium/g (10 mL); 270 mg elemental calcium/g calcium chloride (27% elemental calcium)

Dosage Forms Considerations

1 g calcium chloride = elemental calcium 273 mg = calcium 13.6 mEq = calcium 6.8 mmol

Dosage Forms Excipient information presented when available (limited, particularly for generics); consult specific product labeling.

Solution, Intravenous:

Generic: 10% (10 mL)

Solution, Intravenous [preservative free]:

Generic: 10% (10 mL)

Calcium Citrate (KAL see um SIT rate)

Brand Names: U.S. Cal-Citrate [OTC]; Calcitrate [OTC]

Brand Names: Canada Osteocit®

Pharmacologic Category Calcium Salt

Use Dietary supplement

Dosage Oral: Dosage is in terms of **elemental** calcium

Dietary Reference Intake for Calcium:
1-6 months: Adequate intake: 200 mg/day
7-12 months: Adequate intake: 260 mg/day
1-3 years: RDA: 700 mg/day
4-8 years: RDA: 1000 mg/day
9-18 years: RDA: 1300 mg/day
Adults, Females/Males: RDA:
19-50 years: 1000 mg/day
≥51 years, females: 1200 mg/day
51-70 years, males: 1000 mg/day
>70 years, males: 1200 mg/day
Female: Pregnancy/Lactating: RDA: Requirements are the same as in nonpregnant or nonlactating females

Additional Information Complete prescribing information should be consulted for additional detail.

Dosage Forms Considerations
1 g calcium citrate = elemental calcium 211 mg = calcium 10.5 mEq = calcium 5.25 mmol

Dosage Forms Excipient information presented when available (limited, particularly for generics); consult specific product labeling.
Capsule, Oral [preservative free]:
Cal-Citrate: 150 mg [dye free]
Granules, Oral:
Generic: 760 mg/3.5 g (480 g)
Tablet, Oral:
Generic: 250 mg, 950 mg, 1040 mg
Tablet, Oral [preservative free]:
Calcitrate: 950 mg [lactose free, milk derivatives/products, no artificial color(s), no artificial flavor(s), sodium free, soy free, sugar free, wheat free, yeast free]

◆ **Calcium Citrate and Vitamin D** *see* Calcium and Vitamin D *on page* 318
◆ **Calcium Disodium Edetate** *see* Edetate CALCIUM Disodium *on page* 685
◆ **Calcium Disodiumethylenediaminetetraacetic Acid** *see* Edetate CALCIUM Disodium *on page* 685
◆ **Calcium Folinate** *see* Leucovorin Calcium *on page* 1186

Calcium Glubionate (KAL see um gloo BYE oh nate)

Brand Names: U.S. Calcionate [OTC]
Pharmacologic Category Calcium Salt
Use Dietary supplement
Dosage Dosage is in terms of **elemental** calcium
Dietary Reference Intake for Calcium: Oral:
1-6 months: Adequate intake: 200 mg/day
7-12 months: Adequate intake: 260 mg/day
1-3 years: RDA: 700 mg/day
4-8 years: RDA: 1000 mg/day
9-18 years: RDA: 1300 mg/day
Adults, Females/Males: RDA:
19-50 years: 1000 mg/day
≥51 years, females: 1200 mg/day
51-70 years, males: 1000 mg/day
>70 years, males: 1200 mg/day
Females: Pregnancy/Lactating: RDA: Requirements are the same as in nonpregnant or nonlactating females
Dietary supplement: Oral:
Infants <12 months: 5 mL 5 times/day; may mix with juice or formula
Children <4 years: 10 mL 3 times/day
Children ≥4 years and Adults: 15 mL 3 times/day

Additional Information Complete prescribing information should be consulted for additional detail.

Dosage Forms Considerations
1 g calcium glubionate = elemental calcium 63.8 mg = calcium 3.2 mEq = calcium 1.6 mmol

Dosage Forms Excipient information presented when available (limited, particularly for generics); consult specific product labeling.
Syrup, Oral:
Calcionate: 1.8 g/5 mL (473 mL) [fruit flavor]

Calcium Gluconate (KAL see um GLOO koe nate)

Brand Names: U.S. Cal-Glu [OTC]
Pharmacologic Category Calcium Salt; Electrolyte Supplement, Oral; Electrolyte Supplement, Parenteral
Use
I.V.: Treatment of hypocalcemia and conditions secondary to hypocalcemia (eg, tetany, seizures, arrhythmias); treatment of cardiac disturbances secondary to hyperkalemia; adjunctive treatment of rickets, osteomalacia, and magnesium sulfate overdose; decrease capillary permeability in allergic conditions, nonthrombocytopenic purpura, and exudative dermatoses (eg, dermatitis herpetiformis, pruritus secondary to certain drugs)
Oral: Dietary calcium supplementation

Unlabeled Use Calcium channel blocker overdose; treatment of hydrofluoric acid exposure

Pregnancy Risk Factor C

Pregnancy Considerations Animal reproduction studies have not been conducted. Calcium crosses the placenta. The amount of calcium reaching the fetus is determined by maternal physiological changes. Calcium requirements are the same in pregnant and nonpregnant females (IOM, 2011). Information related to use as an antidote in pregnancy is limited. In general, medications used as antidotes should take into consideration the health and prognosis of the mother; antidotes should be administered to pregnant women if there is a clear indication for use and should not be withheld because of fears of teratogenicity (Bailey, 2003).

Breast-Feeding Considerations Calcium is excreted in breast milk. The amount of calcium in breast milk is homeostatically regulated and not altered by maternal calcium intake. Calcium requirements are the same in lactating and nonlactating females (IOM, 2011).

Contraindications Ventricular fibrillation; hypercalcemia; concomitant use of I.V. calcium gluconate and ceftriaxone in neonates (risk of precipitation of calcium-ceftriaxone)

Warnings/Precautions Avoid too rapid I.V. administration (do not exceed 200 mg/minute except in emergency situations);may result in vasodilation, hypotension, bradycardia, arrhythmias, and cardiac arrest. Vesicant; ensure proper catheter or needle position prior to and during infusion. Avoid extravasation; may result in necrosis. Monitor the I.V. site closely. Use with caution in digitalized patients, severe hyperphosphatemia, or severe hypokalemia. Hypercalcemia may occur in patients with renal failure; frequent determination of serum calcium is necessary. Use caution with chronic renal disease. Use caution when administering calcium supplements to patients with a history of kidney stones. Hypomagnesemia is a common cause of hypocalcemia; therefore, correction of hypocalcemia may be difficult in patients with concomitant hypomagnesemia. Evaluate serum magnesium and correct hypomagnesemia (if necessary), particularly if initial treatment of hypocalcemia is refractory.

Solutions may contain aluminum; toxic levels may occur following prolonged administration in premature neonates or patients with renal dysfunction. Constipation, bloating, and gas are common with oral calcium supplements (especially carbonate salt). Taking calcium (≤500 mg) with food improves absorption. Calcium administration interferes with absorption of some minerals and drugs; use with caution. It is recommended to concomitantly administer vitamin D for optimal calcium absorption.

Ceftriaxone may complex with calcium causing precipitation. Fatal lung and kidney damage associated with calcium-ceftriaxone precipitates has been observed in premature and term neonates. Due to reports of precipitation reaction in neonates, do not coadminister ceftriaxone with calcium-containing solutions, even via separate infusion lines/sites or at different times in any neonate. Ceftriaxone should not be administered simultaneously with any calcium-containing solution via a Y-site in any patient. However, ceftriaxone and calcium-containing solutions may be administered sequentially of one another for use in patients **other than neonates** if infusion lines are thoroughly flushed (with a compatible fluid) between infusions.

Adverse Reactions Frequency not defined.

I.V.:

Cardiovascular (with rapid I.V. injection): Arrhythmia, bradycardia, cardiac arrest, hypotension, syncope, vasodilation

Central nervous system: Sense of oppression (with rapid I.V. injection)

Endocrine & metabolic: Hypercalcemia

Gastrointestinal: Chalky taste

Neuromuscular & skeletal: Tingling sensation (with rapid I.V. injection)

Miscellaneous: Heat waves (with rapid I.V. injection)

Postmarketing and/or case reports: Calcinosis cutis

Oral: Gastrointestinal: Constipation

Drug Interactions

Metabolism/Transport Effects None known.

Avoid Concomitant Use

Avoid concomitant use of Calcium Gluconate with any of the following: Calcium Acetate

Increased Effect/Toxicity

Calcium Gluconate may increase the levels/effects of: Calcium Acetate; CefTRIAXone; Vitamin D Analogs

The levels/effects of Calcium Gluconate may be increased by: Multivitamins/Fluoride (with ADE); Multivitamins/Minerals (with ADEK, Folate, Iron); Thiazide Diuretics

Decreased Effect

Calcium Gluconate may decrease the levels/effects of: Bisphosphonate Derivatives; Calcium Channel Blockers; Deferiprone; DOBUTamine; Dolutegravir; Eltrombopag; Estramustine; Multivitamins/Fluoride (with ADE); Phosphate Supplements; Quinolone Antibiotics; Strontium Ranelate; Tetracycline Derivatives; Thyroid Products; Trientine

The levels/effects of Calcium Gluconate may be decreased by: Trientine

Preparation for Administration

I.V.: Observe the vial for the presence of particulates. If particulates are observed, place vial in a 60°C to 80 °C water bath for 15-30 minutes (or until solution is clear); occasionally shake to dissolve; cool to body/room temperature before use. Do not use vial if particulates do not dissolve. **Note:** Due to the potential presence of particulates, American Regent, Inc recommends the use of a 5 micron filter when preparing calcium gluconate-containing I.V. solutions (Important Drug Administration Information, American Regent, 2013); a similar recommendation has not been noted by other manufacturers.

Inhalation: Treatment of hydrofluoric acid burns (unlabeled use): Mix 1 mL of 10% calcium gluconate solution with 4 mL NS to make a 2.5% solution.

Storage/Stability I.V.: Store at 20°C to 25°C (68°F to 77°F); excursions permitted to 15°C to 30°C (59°F to 86°F).

Usual concentrations: 1 g/100 mL D_5W or NS; 2 g/100 mL D_5W or NS.

Maximum concentration in parenteral nutrition solutions is variable depending upon concentration and solubility (consult detailed reference).

Mechanism of Action Moderates nerve and muscle performance via action potential threshold regulation.

In hydrogen fluoride exposures, calcium gluconate provides a source of calcium ions to complex free fluoride ions and prevent or reduce toxicity; administration also helps to correct fluoride-induced hypocalcemia.

Pharmacodynamics/Kinetics

Absorption: Oral: Requires vitamin D; calcium is absorbed in soluble, ionized form; solubility of calcium is increased in an acid environment

Protein binding: ~40%, primarily to albumin (Wills, 1971)

Excretion: Primarily feces (as unabsorbed calcium salts); urine (20%)

Dosage Note: One gram of calcium gluconate salt is equal to 93 mg of elemental calcium.

Dosages are expressed in terms of the calcium gluconate salt (unless otherwise specified as elemental calcium). Dosages expressed in terms of the calcium gluconate salt are based on a solution concentration of 100 mg/mL (10%) containing 0.465 mEq (9.3 mg)/mL elemental calcium, except where noted.

Dietary Reference Intake for Calcium: Oral: **Note:** Expressed in terms of elemental calcium:

1-6 months: Adequate intake: 200 mg **elemental calcium** daily

7-12 months: Adequate intake: 260 mg **elemental calcium** daily

1-3 years: RDA: 700 mg **elemental calcium** daily

4-8 years: RDA: 1000 mg **elemental calcium** daily

9-18 years: RDA: 1300 mg **elemental calcium** daily

Adults, Females/Males: RDA:

19-50 years: 1000 mg **elemental calcium** daily

≥51 years, females: 1200 mg **elemental calcium** daily

51-70 years, males: 1000 mg **elemental calcium** daily

>70 years, males: 1200 mg **elemental calcium** daily

Females: Pregnancy/Lactating: RDA: Requirements are the same as in nonpregnant or nonlactating females

Hypocalcemia: I.V.:

Infants and Children: 200-500 mg/kg/day as a continuous infusion or in 4 divided doses (maximum: 2000-3000 mg/dose)

Adults:

Mild (ionized calcium: 4-5 mg/dL [1-1.2 mmol/L]): 1000-2000 mg over 2 hours; asymptomatic patients may be given oral calcium (Ariyan, 2004; French, 2012)

Moderate-to-severe (without seizure or tetany; ionized calcium: <4 mg/dL [<1 mmol/L]): 4000 mg over 4 hours (French, 2012)

Severe symptomatic (eg, seizure, tetany): 1000-2000 mg over 10 minutes; repeat every 60 minutes until symptoms resolve (French, 2012)

Note: Repeat ionized calcium measurement 6-10 hours after completion of administration. Check for hypomagnesemia and correct if present. Consider continuous infusion if hypocalcemia is likely to recur due to ongoing losses (French, 2012).

Continuous infusion: 5-20 mg/kg/hour (Pai, 2011)

Cardiac arrest or cardiotoxicity in the presence of hyperkalemia, hypocalcemia, or hypermagnesemia: I.V.:

Infants and Children: 60-100 mg/kg/dose (maximum: 3000 mg/dose) (Hegenbarth, 2008)

Adults: 1500-3000 mg over 2-5 minutes (Vanden Hoek, 2010)

Note: Routine use in cardiac arrest is not recommended due to the lack of improved survival (Kleinman, 2010; Neumar, 2010):

Maintenance electrolyte requirements for parenteral nutrition: I.V. (Mirtallo, 2004): **Note:** Expressed in terms of **elemental calcium:**

Infants and Children (<50 kg): 0.5-4 **mEq elemental calcium**/kg/day

Adults: 10-20 **mEq elemental calcium** daily

Calcium channel blocker overdose (unlabeled use): Hypotension/conduction disturbances:

Children: I.V., I.O.: 60 mg/kg/dose administered over 30-60 minutes (Hegenbarth, 2008). **Note:** Calcium chloride may provide a more rapid increase of ionized calcium in critically-ill children. Calcium gluconate may be substituted if calcium chloride is not available.

Adults: I.V.: 60-120 mg/kg/**hour** (Salhanick, 2003) **or** 60 mg/kg/dose over 5 minutes (maximum: 3000-6000 mg/dose) every 10-20 minutes; may repeat for 3-4 additional doses (Vanden Hoek, 2010; DeWitt, 2004). In life-threatening situations, 1000 mg has been administered every 2-3 minutes until clinical effect is achieved (Buckley, 1994). In one report, 18 **g** was administered over a 3-hour period (Luscher, 1994).

Hydrofluoric acid burns, treatment (unlabeled route/use):

Children and Adults:

SubQ (unlabeled route/use): 5% to 10% solution: 0.5 **mL**/cm^2 of burned tissue (Dibbell, 1970; Hatzifotis, 2004; Kirkpatrick, 1995; Krenzelok, 1999). Infiltration should be carried 0.5 cm away from the margin of the injured tissue into the surrounding uninjured areas. Repeat if pain recurs. Local anesthesia may be required to perform procedure; pain resolution is the therapeutic endpoint and if a local anesthetic is utilized, it may be difficult to determine the success of therapy (**Note: Never** use calcium chloride for subcutaneous injection).

Intra-arterial (unlabeled route/use): Add 10 **mL** of a 10% solution to 50 mL of D_5W. Infuse over 4 hours into the artery that provides the vascular supply to the affected area (Hatzifotis, 2004; Kirkpatrick, 1995). Pain usually resolves by the end of the infusion; repeat if pain recurs. **This intervention should be used only by those accustomed to this technique. Extreme care should be taken to avoid the extravasation.** A poison information center or clinical toxicologist should be consulted prior to implementation.

Inhalation (unlabeled route/use): 2.5% nebulization solution: Mix 1 **mL** of 10% calcium gluconate solution with 4 mL NS to make a 2.5% solution and administer via nebulization (Hatzifotis, 2004).

Dosing adjustment in renal impairment: No initial dosage adjustment necessary; however, accumulation may occur with renal impairment and subsequent doses may require adjustment based on serum calcium concentrations.

Dosing adjustment in hepatic impairment: No initial dosage adjustment necessary; subsequent doses should be guided by serum calcium concentrations. In patients in the anhepatic stage of liver transplantation, equal rapid increases in ionized concentrations occur suggesting that calcium gluconate does not require hepatic metabolism for release of ionized calcium (Martin, 1990).

Administration

I.V.: Administer slowly (~1.5 mL calcium gluconate 10% per minute; not to exceed 200 mg/minute except in emergency situations) through a small needle into a large vein in order to avoid too rapid increases in the serum calcium and extravasation. **Note:** Due to the potential presence of particulates, American Regent, Inc recommends the use of a 0.22 micron inline filter for I.V. administration (1.2 micron filter if admixture contains lipids) (Important Drug Administration Information, American Regent, 2013); a similar recommendation has not been noted by other manufacturers. Not for I.M. administration.

Vesicant; ensure proper needle or catheter placement prior to and during I.V. infusion. Avoid extravasation.

Extravasation management: If extravasation occurs, stop infusion immediately and disconnect (leave needle/cannula in place); gently aspirate extravasated solution (do **NOT** flush the line); initiate hyaluronidase antidote; remove needle/cannula; apply dry cold compresses (Hurst, 2004); elevate extremity.

Hyaluronidase: Intradermal or SubQ: Inject a total of 1 mL (15 units/mL) as five separate 0.2 mL injections (using a 25-gauge needle) into area of extravasation at the leading edge in a clockwise manner (MacCara, 1983; Zenk, 1981).

Treatment of hydrofluoric acid burns (unlabeled use):

SubQ infiltration (unlabeled route): Using a 27- or 30-gauge needle, approach the wound from the distal point of injury and infiltrate directly into the affected dermis and subcutaneous tissue. The infiltration should be carried 0.5 cm away from the margin of the injured tissue into the surrounding uninjured areas (Dibbell, 1970). Avoid excessive administration as it can cause compartment syndrome and further exacerbate tissue damage. Following subungual exposure, administer to the affected area via the lateral or volar route through the fat pad (under digital nerve block); administration may also require removal of the nailbed, splitting the distal nail from the nailbed, or trimming the nail to the nailbed to reach the affected area (Kirkpatrick, 1995; Roberts, 1989).

Intra-arterial (unlabeled route): Requires radiology to place an arterial catheter in an artery supplying blood to the area of exposure; infuse over four hours (Vance, 1986). **This intervention should be used only by those accustomed to this technique. Care should be taken to avoid the extravasation.** A poison information center or clinical toxicologist should be consulted prior to implementation.

Inhalation: Dilute 10% calcium gluconate solution to a 2.5% solution and administer via nebulization.

Reference Range

Serum total calcium: 8.4-10.2 mg/dL (2.1-2.55 mmol/L). **Note:** Due to a poor correlation between the serum ionized calcium (free) and total serum calcium, particularly in states of low albumin or acid/base imbalances, direct measurement of ionized calcium is recommended.

In low albumin states, the corrected **total** serum calcium may be estimated by the following equation (assuming a normal albumin of 4 g/dL [40 g/L]).

Corrected total calcium (mg/dL) = measured total calcium (mg/mL) + 0.8 [4 - measured serum albumin(g/dL)]

or

Corrected total calcium (mmol/L) = measured total calcium (mmol/L) + 0.02 [40-measured serum albumin (g/L)]

Test Interactions I.V. administration may produce falsely decreased serum and urine magnesium concentrations

Dosage Forms Considerations

1 g calcium gluconate = elemental calcium 93 mg = calcium 4.65 mEq = calcium 2.33 mmol

Dosage Forms Excipient information presented when available (limited, particularly for generics); consult specific product labeling. [DSC] = Discontinued product

Capsule, Oral [preservative free]:

Cal-Glu: 500 mg [dye free]

Solution, Intravenous:
Generic: 10% (10 mL, 50 mL, 100 mL, 200 mL [DSC])
Solution, Intravenous [preservative free]:
Generic: 10% (100 mL)
Tablet, Oral:
Generic: 50 mg, 500 mg, 648 (60 Ca) MG [DSC]

- **Calcium High Potency [OTC]** *see* Calcium Carbonate *on page 318*
- **Calcium Leucovorin** *see* Leucovorin Calcium *on page 1186*
- **Calcium Levoleucovorin** *see* LEVOleucovorin *on page 1201*
- **Cal-CO3S [OTC]** *see* Calcium Carbonate *on page 318*
- **Cal-CYUM [OTC]** *see* Calcium and Vitamin D *on page 318*
- **Caldolor** *see* Ibuprofen *on page 1032*

Calfactant (kaf AKT ant)

Brand Names: U.S. Infasurf

Index Terms Bovine Lung Surfactant

Pharmacologic Category Lung Surfactant

Use Prevention of respiratory distress syndrome (RDS) in premature infants at high risk for RDS and for the treatment ("rescue") of premature infants who develop RDS

Prophylaxis: Therapy at birth with calfactant is indicated for premature infants <29 weeks of gestational age at significant risk for RDS. Should be administered as soon as possible, preferably within 30 minutes after birth.

Treatment: For infants ≤72 hours of age with RDS (confirmed by clinical and radiologic findings) and requiring endotracheal intubation.

Warnings/Precautions For intratracheal administration only. Rapidly affects oxygenation and lung compliance; restrict use to a highly-supervised clinical setting with immediate availability of clinicians experienced in intubation and ventilatory management of premature infants. Transient episodes of bradycardia, decreased oxygen saturation, endotracheal tube blockage or reflux of calfactant into endotracheal tube may occur. Discontinue dosing procedure and initiate measures to alleviate the condition; may reinstitute after the patient is stable. Produces rapid improvements in lung oxygenation and compliance that may require frequent adjustments to oxygen delivery and ventilator settings.

Adverse Reactions

Cardiovascular: Cyanosis (65%), bradycardia (34%)

Respiratory: Airway obstruction (39%), reflux (21%), requirement for manual ventilation (16%), reintubation (3%)

Drug Interactions

Metabolism/Transport Effects None known.

Avoid Concomitant Use There are no known interactions where it is recommended to avoid concomitant use.

Increased Effect/Toxicity There are no known significant interactions involving an increase in effect.

Decreased Effect There are no known significant interactions involving a decrease in effect.

Storage/Stability Gentle swirling or agitation of the vial of suspension is often necessary for redispersion. **Do not shake**. Visible flecks of the suspension and foaming under the surface are normal. Calfactant should be stored upright (3 mL vial) and under refrigeration at 2°C to 8°C (36°F to 46°F); protect from light; document date and time removed from refrigeration. Warming before administration is not necessary. Unopened and unused vials of calfactant that have been warmed to room temperature can be returned to refrigeration storage within 24 hours for future use. Repeated warming to room temperature should be avoided. Each single-use vial should be entered only once and the vial with any unused material should be discarded after the initial entry.

Mechanism of Action Endogenous lung surfactant is essential for effective ventilation because it modifies alveolar surface tension, thereby stabilizing the alveoli. Lung surfactant deficiency is the cause of respiratory distress syndrome (RDS) in premature infants and lung surfactant restores surface activity to the lungs of these infants.

Pharmacodynamics/Kinetics No human studies of absorption, biotransformation, or excretion have been performed

Dosage Intratracheal administration **only**: Each dose is 3 mL/kg body weight at birth; should be administered every 12 hours for a total of up to 3 doses

Dosage adjustment in renal impairment: No dosage adjustment provided in manufacturer's labeling.

Dosage adjustment in hepatic impairment: No dosage adjustment provided in manufacturer's labeling.

Administration Should be administered intratracheally through an endotracheal tube. Dose is drawn into a syringe from the single-use vial using a 20-gauge or larger needle with care taken to avoid excessive foaming. Dose should be administered in 2 or 4 equal aliquots. After each aliquot is instilled, the infant should be positioned with either the right or the left side dependent. Administration is made while ventilation is continued over 20-30 breaths for each aliquot, with small bursts timed only during the inspiratory cycles. A pause followed by evaluation of the respiratory status and repositioning should separate the aliquots. Do not dilute or sonicate.

Monitoring Parameters Following administration, patients should be carefully monitored so that oxygen therapy and ventilatory support can be modified in response to changes in respiratory status.

Additional Information Each mL = 35 mg total phospholipids (including 26 mg phosphatidylcholine, of which 16 mg is disaturated phosphatidylcholine) and 0.7 mg proteins (including 0.26 mg SP-B)

Dosage Forms Excipient information presented when available (limited, particularly for generics); consult specific product labeling.

Suspension, Inhalation:
Infasurf: 35 mg phospholipids and 0.7 mg protein per mL (3 mL, 6 mL)

- **Cal-Gest Antacid [OTC]** *see* Calcium Carbonate *on page 318*
- **Cal-Glu [OTC]** *see* Calcium Gluconate *on page 322*
- **Cal-Mint [OTC]** *see* Calcium Carbonate *on page 318*
- **Calmylin with Codeine (Can)** *see* Guaifenesin, Pseudoephedrine, and Codeine *on page 979*
- **Calphron [OTC]** *see* Calcium Acetate *on page 317*
- **Caltine (Can)** *see* Calcitonin *on page 312*
- **Caltrate® (Can)** *see* Calcium Carbonate *on page 318*
- **Caltrate 600 [OTC]** *see* Calcium Carbonate *on page 318*
- **Caltrate 600+D [OTC]** *see* Calcium and Vitamin D *on page 318*
- **Caltrate 600+Soy [OTC]** *see* Calcium and Vitamin D *on page 318*
- **Caltrate ColonHealth [OTC]** *see* Calcium and Vitamin D *on page 318*
- **Caltrate® Select (Can)** *see* Calcium Carbonate *on page 318*
- **Cambia** *see* Diclofenac (Systemic) *on page 597*
- **Camila** *see* Norethindrone *on page 1472*
- **Campath-1H** *see* Alemtuzumab *on page 66*
- **Camphorated Tincture of Opium (error-prone synonym)** *see* Paregoric *on page 1571*
- **Campral** *see* Acamprosate *on page 26*

◆ **Campral® (Can)** *see* Acamprosate *on page 26*
◆ **Camptosar** *see* Irinotecan *on page 1115*
◆ **Camptosar® (Can)** *see* Irinotecan *on page 1115*
◆ **Camptothecin-11** *see* Irinotecan *on page 1115*
◆ **camrese** *see* Ethinyl Estradiol and Levonorgestrel *on page 787*

Canakinumab (can a KIN ue mab)

Brand Names: U.S. Ilaris
Brand Names: Canada Ilaris
Index Terms ACZ885
Pharmacologic Category Interleukin-1 Beta Inhibitor; Interleukin-1 Inhibitor; Monoclonal Antibody
Use Treatment of cryopyrin-associated periodic syndromes (CAPS), including familial cold autoinflammatory syndrome (FCAS) and Muckle-Wells syndrome (MWS); systemic juvenile idiopathic arthritis (SJIA)
Pregnancy Risk Factor C
Pregnancy Considerations Adverse events were observed in animal reproduction studies. The Canadian product labeling recommends women of reproductive potential use effective contraception during treatment and for 3 months after the last dose.
Breast-Feeding Considerations It is not known if canakinumab is excreted into breast milk. The manufacturer recommends caution be used if administered to nursing women.
Medication Guide Available Yes
Contraindications Confirmed hypersensitivity to canakinumab or any component of the formulation

Canadian labeling: Additional contraindications (not in U.S. labeling): Active, severe infections
Warnings/Precautions Hypersensitivity reactions (excluding anaphylactic reactions) have been reported with use; symptoms may be similar to those that are disease-related. Use is contraindicated in patients with known hypersensitivity to canakinumab. Caution should be exercised when considering use in patients with a history of new/recurrent infections, with conditions that predispose them to infections, or with latent or localized infections. Therapy should not be initiated in patients with active or chronic infections. Patients should be evaluated for latent tuberculosis infection with a tuberculin skin test prior to starting therapy. Treat latent TB infections prior to initiating canakinumab therapy. During and following treatment, monitor for signs/symptoms of active TB. Macrophage activation syndrome (MAS may develop in patients with SJIA and should be treated aggressively. Infection or worsening SJIA may be triggers for MAS

Use may impair defenses against malignancies; impact on the development and course of malignancies is not fully defined. Tumor necrosis factor (TNF)-blocking agents should not be used in combination with canakinumab; risk of serious infection is increased. Immunizations should be up to date including pneumococcal and influenza vaccines before initiating therapy. Live vaccines should not be given concurrently. Administration of inactivated (killed) vaccines while on therapy may not be effective.
Adverse Reactions Adverse events reported in treatment of CAPS unless otherwise noted.
>10%:
Central nervous system: Headache (14%), vertigo (9% to 14%)
Gastrointestinal: Diarrhea (20%), upper abdominal pain (SJIA 7% to 16%); nausea (14%), gastroenteritis (11%), weight gain (11%)
Infection: Increased susceptibility to infection (SJIA 30% to 55%)
Local: Injection site reaction (SJIA ≤14%; CAPS 7% to 9%)
Neuromuscular and skeletal: Musculoskeletal pain (11%)
Respiratory: Nasopharyngitis (34%), rhinitis (17%), bronchitis (11%), pharyngitis (11%)
Miscellaneous: Influenza (17%)
1% to 10%:
Endocrine & metabolic: Calcium decreased (4% to 8%)
Hematologic & oncologic: Decreased white blood cell count (SJIA 10%), eosinophils increased (3% to 7%), decreased platelet count (mild, transient; SJIA 6%)
Hepatic: Bilirubin increased (3% to 7%), increased AST (3% to 6%), increased serum transaminases (SJIA 4%), increased ALT (3%)
Immunologic: Antibody development (SJIA 3%; CAPS 2%)
Renal: Creatinine clearance decreased (3% to 8%), proteinuria (4% to 8%)
<1%, postmarketing, and/or case reports: Hypersensitivity reactions, neutropenia (SJIA)
Drug Interactions
Metabolism/Transport Effects None known.
Avoid Concomitant Use
Avoid concomitant use of Canakinumab with any of the following: Anti-TNF Agents; BCG; Interleukin-1 Inhibitors; Interleukin-1 Receptor Antagonist; Natalizumab; Pimecrolimus; Tacrolimus (Topical); Tofacitinib; Vaccines (Live)
Increased Effect/Toxicity
Canakinumab may increase the levels/effects of: Leflunomide; Natalizumab; Tofacitinib; Vaccines (Live)

The levels/effects of Canakinumab may be increased by: Anti-TNF Agents; Denosumab; Interleukin-1 Inhibitors; Interleukin-1 Receptor Antagonist; Pimecrolimus; Roflumilast; Tacrolimus (Topical); Trastuzumab
Decreased Effect
Canakinumab may decrease the levels/effects of: BCG; Coccidioidin Skin Test; Sipuleucel-T; Vaccines (Inactivated); Vaccines (Live)

The levels/effects of Canakinumab may be decreased by: Echinacea
Preparation for Administration Reconstitute vial with SWFI 1 mL. After reconstituting with SWFI, swirl the vial at a 45-degree angle for ~1 minute (do not shake), then allow solution to sit for 5 minutes. Gently turn vial (without touching rubber stopper) upside down and back 10 times. Allow to sit at room temperature for ~15 minutes until solution is clear. Do not shake. Solution may have a slight brownish-yellow tint; do not use if distinctly brown in color or if particulate matter is present in the solution. Each reconstituted vial results in a final concentration of 150 mg/mL.
Storage/Stability Store powder in refrigerator at 2°C to 8°C (36°F to 46°F); do not freeze. Protect from light. After reconstitution, vials may be stored at controlled room temperature for up to 1 hour or in a refrigerator for up to 4 hours.
Mechanism of Action Canakinumab reduces inflammation by binding to interleukin-1 beta (IL-1β) (no binding to IL-1 alpha or IL-1 receptor antagonist) and preventing interaction with cell surface receptors. Cryopyrin-associated periodic syndromes (CAPS) refers to rare genetic syndromes caused by mutations in the nucleotide-binding domain, leucine rich family (NLR), pyrin domain containing 3 (NLRP-3) gene or the cold-induced autoinflammatory syndrome-1 (CIAS1) gene. Cryopyrin, a protein encoded by this gene, regulates IL-1β activation. Deficiency of cryopyrin results in excessive inflammation.
Pharmacodynamics/Kinetics
Distribution: V_d: 6 L (70 kg CAPS patient); 3.2 L (33 kg SJIA patient)
Bioavailability: Subcutaneous: 66%

Half-life elimination: 26 days

Time to peak, serum: Children: 2-7 days; Adults: ~7 days

Dosage

Cryopyrin-associated periodic syndromes (CAPS): SubQ:
Children ≥4 years and Adolescents:
15-40 kg: 2 mg/kg every 8 weeks; may increase to 3 mg/kg if response inadequate
>40 kg: 150 mg every 8 weeks
Adults >40 kg: 150 mg every 8 weeks

Systemic juvenile idiopathic arthritis (SJIA): SubQ: Children ≥2 years and ≥7.5 kg and Adolescents: 4 mg/kg every 4 weeks (maximum: 300 mg per dose)

Dosage adjustment in renal impairment: No dosage adjustment provided in manufacturer's labeling (has not been studied).

Dosage adjustment in hepatic impairment: No dosage adjustment provided in manufacturer's labeling (has not been studied).

Administration SubQ: Do not inject into scar tissue.

Monitoring Parameters CBC with differential, C-reactive protein (CRP), serum amyloid A protein A (SAA); signs of infection; latent TB screening (prior to initiating therapy); Canadian labeling also recommends blood pressure monitoring, annual lipid screening, and monitoring of neutrophil counts (at baseline, after 1-2 months and periodically thereafter)

Eye examinations for patients with CAPS (Caorsi, 2013) and symptoms of disease for patients with CAPS or SJIA (Caorsi, 2013; Lachmann, 2009; Ruperto, 2012) were also monitored in clinical trials.

Dosage Forms Excipient information presented when available (limited, particularly for generics); consult specific product labeling.

Solution Reconstituted, Subcutaneous [preservative free]:
Ilaris: 180 mg (1 ea) [contains polysorbate 80]

Dosage Forms: Canada Excipient information presented when available (limited, particularly for generics); consult specific product labeling.

Injection, powder for reconstitution:
Ilaris: 150 mg [contains polysorbate 80, sucrose]

◆ **Canasa** *see* Mesalamine *on page 1305*
◆ **Cancidas** *see* Caspofungin *on page 358*
◆ **Cancidas® (Can)** *see* Caspofungin *on page 358*

Candesartan (kan de SAR tan)

Brand Names: U.S. Atacand

Brand Names: Canada Apo-Candesartan; Atacand; CO Candesartan; DOM-Candesartan; JAMP-Candesartan; Mylan-Candesartan; PMS-Candesartan; Ran-Candesartan; Sandoz-Candesartan; Teva-Candesartan

Index Terms Candesartan Cilexetil

Pharmacologic Category Angiotensin II Receptor Blocker; Antihypertensive

Additional Appendix Information

Angiotensin Agents *on page 2280*

Use

Heart failure: Treatment of heart failure (NYHA class II-IV)

Hypertension: Alone or in combination with other antihypertensive agents in treating hypertension

Pregnancy Risk Factor D

Pregnancy Considerations [U.S. Boxed Warning]: Drugs that act on the renin-angiotensin system can cause injury and death to the developing fetus. Discontinue as soon as possible once pregnancy is detected. The use of drugs which act on the renin-angiotensin system are associated with oligohydramnios. Oligohydramnios, due to decreased fetal renal function, may lead to fetal lung hypoplasia and skeletal malformations. Use is also associated with anuria, hypotension, renal failure, skull hypoplasia, and death in the fetus/neonate. The exposed fetus should be monitored for fetal growth, amniotic fluid volume, and organ formation. Infants exposed *in utero* should be monitored for hyperkalemia, hypotension, and oliguria.

Untreated chronic maternal hypertension is also associated with adverse events in the fetus, infant, and mother. If treatment for hypertension or heart failure during pregnancy is needed, other agents are preferred (ACOG, 2012; Chobanian, 2003). In women of reproductive potential, angiotensin II receptor blockers should be discontinued prior to conception or as soon as pregnancy is confirmed (Chobanian, 2003).

Breast-Feeding Considerations It is not known if candesartan is excreted into breast milk. Due to the potential for serious adverse reactions in the nursing infant, the manufacturer recommends a decision be made whether to discontinue nursing or to discontinue the drug, taking into account the importance of treatment to the mother. Breast-fed infants of mothers taking medications for hypertension should be monitored for adverse effects (Chobanian, 2003).

Contraindications

Hypersensitivity to candesartan or any component of the formulation; concomitant use with aliskiren in patients with diabetes mellitus

Canadian labeling: Additional contraindications (not in U.S. labeling): Concomitant use with aliskiren in patients with moderate-to-severe renal impairment (GFR <60 mL/minute/1.73 m^2)

Warnings/Precautions [U.S. Boxed Warning]: Drugs that act on the renin-angiotensin system can cause injury and death to the developing fetus. Discontinue as soon as possible once pregnancy is detected. May cause hyperkalemia; avoid potassium supplementation unless specifically required by healthcare provider. Avoid use or use a smaller dose in patients who are volume depleted; correct depletion first. May be associated with deterioration of renal function and/or increases in serum creatinine, particularly in patients with low renal blood flow (eg, renal artery stenosis, heart failure) whose glomerular filtration rate (GFR) is dependent on efferent arteriolar vasoconstriction by angiotensin II; deterioration may result in oliguria, acute renal failure, and progressive azotemia. Small increases in serum creatinine may occur following initiation; consider discontinuation only in patients with progressive and/or significant deterioration in renal function. Use with caution in unstented unilateral/bilateral renal artery stenosis, pre-existing renal insufficiency, or significant aortic/mitral stenosis. Systemic exposure increases in hepatic impairment. Dosage adjustment recommended in patients with moderate hepatic impairment; pharmacokinetics have not been studied in severe hepatic impairment. Use caution when initiating in heart failure; may need to adjust dose, and/or concurrent diuretic therapy, because of candesartan-induced hypotension. Hypotension may occur during major surgery and anesthesia; use cautiously before, during, and immediately after such interventions. Potentially significant drug interactions may exist, requiring dose or frequency adjustment, additional monitoring, and/or selection of alternative therapy. Pediatric patients with a GFR <30 mL/minute/1.73 m^2 should not receive candesartan; has not been evaluated. Children <1 year of age should not receive candesartan due to potential effects on the development of immature kidneys.

Angioedema has been reported rarely with some angiotensin II receptor antagonists (ARBs) and may occur at any time during treatment (especially following first dose). It may involve the head and neck (potentially compromising airway) or the intestine (presenting with abdominal pain). Patients with idiopathic or hereditary angioedema or previous angioedema associated with ACE-inhibitor therapy may be at an increased risk. Prolonged frequent monitoring may be required, especially if tongue, glottis, or larynx are involved, as they are associated with airway obstruction. Patients with a history of airway surgery may have a higher risk of airway obstruction. Discontinue therapy immediately if angioedema occurs. Aggressive early management is critical. Intramuscular (I.M.) administration of epinephrine may be necessary. Do not readminister to patients who have had angioedema with ARBs.

Adverse Reactions Frequency not always defined.

Cardiovascular: Hypotension (heart failure 19%), angina pectoris, myocardial infarction, palpitations, tachycardia

Central nervous system: Anxiety, depression, dizziness, drowsiness, headache, paresthesia, vertigo

Dermatologic: Diaphoresis, skin rash

Endocrine & metabolic: Hyperkalemia (heart failure <1% to 6%), hyperglycemia, hypertriglyceridemia, hyperuricemia

Gastrointestinal: Dyspepsia, gastroenteritis

Genitourinary: Hematuria

Neuromuscular & skeletal: Back pain, increased creatine phosphokinase, myalgia, weakness

Renal: Increased serum creatinine (≤13% in patients with heart failure with drug discontinuation required in 6%)

Respiratory: Dyspnea, epistaxis, pharyngitis, rhinitis, upper respiratory tract infection

Miscellaneous: Fever

<1% (Limited to important or life-threatening): Agranulocytosis, anemia, angioedema, hepatic insufficiency, hepatitis, hyponatremia, leukopenia, neutropenia, thrombocytopenia

Drug Interactions

Metabolism/Transport Effects **Substrate** of CYP2C9 (minor); **Note:** Assignment of Major/Minor substrate status based on clinically relevant drug interaction potential; **Inhibits** CYP2C8 (weak), CYP2C9 (weak)

Avoid Concomitant Use There are no known interactions where it is recommended to avoid concomitant use.

Increased Effect/Toxicity

Candesartan may increase the levels/effects of: ACE Inhibitors; Amifostine; Antihypertensives; CycloSPORINE (Systemic); Hypotensive Agents; Lithium; Nonsteroidal Anti-Inflammatory Agents; Obinutuzumab; Potassium-Sparing Diuretics; RiTUXimab; Sodium Phosphates

The levels/effects of Candesartan may be increased by: Alfuzosin; Aliskiren; Brimonidine (Topical); Canagliflozin; Diazoxide; Eplerenone; Heparin; Heparin (Low Molecular Weight); Herbs (Hypotensive Properties); MAO Inhibitors; Pentoxifylline; Phosphodiesterase 5 Inhibitors; Potassium Salts; Prostacyclin Analogues; Tolvaptan; Trimethoprim

Decreased Effect

The levels/effects of Candesartan may be decreased by: Herbs (Hypertensive Properties); Methylphenidate; Nonsteroidal Anti-Inflammatory Agents; Yohimbine

Ethanol/Nutrition/Herb Interactions

Food: Potassium supplements and/or potassium-containing salts may cause or worsen hyperkalemia. Management: Consult prescriber before consuming a potassium-rich diet, potassium supplements, or salt substitutes.

Herb/Nutraceutical: Dong quai has estrogenic activity. Ephedra, yohimbe, and ginseng may worsen hypertension. Garlic may increase antihypertensive effect of candesartan. Management: Avoid dong quai if using for hypertension. Avoid ephedra, yohimbe, ginseng, and garlic.

Storage/Stability Store at 25°C (77°F); excursions permitted to 15°C to 30°C (59°F to 86°F).

Mechanism of Action Candesartan is an angiotensin receptor antagonist. Angiotensin II acts as a vasoconstrictor. In addition to causing direct vasoconstriction, angiotensin II also stimulates the release of aldosterone. Once aldosterone is released, sodium as well as water are reabsorbed. The end result is an elevation in blood pressure. Candesartan binds to the AT1 angiotensin II receptor. This binding prevents angiotensin II from binding to the receptor thereby blocking the vasoconstriction and the aldosterone secreting effects of angiotensin II.

Pharmacodynamics/Kinetics

Onset of action: 2-3 hours

Peak effect: 6-8 hours

Duration: >24 hours

Distribution: V_d: 0.13 L/kg

Protein binding: >99%

Metabolism: Parent compound bioactivated during absorption via ester hydrolysis within intestinal wall to candesartan

Bioavailability: 15%

Half-life elimination (dose dependent): 5-9 hours

Time to peak: 3-4 hours

Excretion: Urine (26%)

Dosage

Hypertension: **Note:** Antihypertensive effect usually observed within 2 weeks; maximum antihypertensive effect seen within 4-6 weeks.

Children 1 to <6 years: Oral: Initial: 0.2 mg/kg/day in 1-2 divided doses; titrate to response; usual range: 0.05-0.4 mg/kg/day; maximum daily dose: 0.4 mg/kg/day

Children ≥6 years and Adolescents <17 years: Oral:

<50 kg: Initial: 4-8 mg daily in 1-2 divided doses; titrate to response; usual range: 2-16 mg daily; maximum daily dose: 32 mg daily

>50 kg: Initial: 8-16 mg daily in 1-2 divided doses; titrate to response; usual range: 4-32 mg daily; maximum daily dose: 32 mg daily

Adults: Oral: Dosage must be individualized. Initial: 16 mg once daily; titrate to response; usual range: 8-32 mg daily in 1-2 divided doses; maximum daily dose: 32 mg daily.

Heart failure: Adults: Oral: Initial: 4 mg once daily; double the dose at 2-week intervals, as tolerated; target dose: 32 mg once daily

Note: In selected cases, concurrent therapy with an ACE inhibitor may provide additional benefit.

Elderly: No initial dosage adjustment is necessary for elderly patients (although higher concentrations (C_{max}) and AUC were observed in this population).

Dosage adjustment in renal impairment:

Children 1 to <17 years: No dosage adjustment provided in manufacturer's labeling (has not been studied). Children with GFR <30 mL/minute/1.73 m^2 should not receive candesartan.

Adults: No initial dosage adjustment necessary; however, in patients with severe renal impairment (Cl_{cr} <30 mL/minute/1.73 m^2) AUC and C_{max} were approximately doubled after repeated dosing.

Dosage adjustment in hepatic impairment:

Mild impairment (Child-Pugh class A): No initial dosage adjustment necessary.

Moderate impairment (Child-Pugh class B): Initial: 8 mg daily (AUC increased by 145%).

Severe impairment (Child-Pugh class C): No dosage adjustment provided in manufacturer's labeling (has not been studied); however, systemic exposure increases significantly in moderate impairment.

Administration Administer without regard to meals.

Monitoring Parameters Supine blood pressure, electrolytes, serum creatinine, BUN, urinalysis, symptomatic hypotension, and tachycardia; in heart failure, serum potassium during dose escalation and periodically thereafter

Additional Information May have an advantage over losartan due to minimal metabolism requirements and consequent use in mild-to-moderate hepatic impairment

Dosage Forms Excipient information presented when available (limited, particularly for generics); consult specific product labeling.

Tablet, Oral, as cilexetil:

Atacand: 4 mg, 8 mg, 16 mg, 32 mg [scored]

Generic: 4 mg, 8 mg, 16 mg, 32 mg

Extemporaneous Preparations Oral suspension may be made in concentrations ranging from 0.1-2 mg/mL; typically 1 mg/mL oral suspension suitable for majority of prescribed doses; any strength tablet may be used. A 1 mg/mL (total volume: 160 mL) oral suspension may be made with tablets and a 1:1 mixture of Ora-Plus® and Ora-Sweet SF®. Prepare the vehicle by adding 80 mL of Ora-Plus® and 80 mL of Ora-Sweet SF® or, alternatively, use 160 mL of Ora-Blend SF®. Add a small amount of vehicle to five 32 mg tablets and grind into a smooth paste using a mortar and pestle. Transfer the paste to a calibrated amber PET bottle, rinse the mortar and pestle clean using the vehicle, add this to the bottle, and then add a quantity of vehicle sufficient to make 160 mL. The suspension is stable at room temperature for 100 days unopened or 30 days after the first opening; do not freeze; label "shake well before use." (Atacand® prescribing information, 2013).

Atacand® prescribing information, AstraZeneca LP, Wilmington, DE, 2013.

Candesartan and Hydrochlorothiazide

(kan de SAR tan & hye droe klor oh THYE a zide)

Brand Names: U.S. Atacand HCT

Brand Names: Canada Apo-Candesartan HCTZ; Atacand Plus; Candesartan-HCTZ; Co-Candesartan/HCT; Mylan-Candesartan HCTZ; PMS-Candesartan HCTZ; Sandoz-Candesartan Plus; Teva-Candesartan/HCTZ

Index Terms Candesartan Cilexetil and Hydrochlorothiazide; Hydrochlorothiazide and Candesartan

Pharmacologic Category Angiotensin II Receptor Blocker; Antihypertensive; Diuretic, Thiazide

Use Hypertension: Treatment of hypertension; combination product should not be used for initial therapy

Pregnancy Risk Factor D

Dosage Hypertension, replacement therapy: Adults: Oral: Combination product can be substituted for individual agents; maximum therapeutic effect would be expected within 4 weeks

Usual dosage range:

Candesartan: 8-32 mg daily, given once daily or twice daily in divided doses

Hydrochlorothiazide: 12.5-50 mg once daily

Elderly: No initial dosage adjustment is recommended.

Dosage adjustment in renal impairment:

Cl_{cr} ≥30 mL/minute: No dosage adjustment necessary.

Cl_{cr} <30 mL/minute: No dosage adjustment provided in manufacturer's labeling (safety and efficacy not established); however, AUC and serum levels of candesartan are increased, and the half-life of hydrochlorothiazide is prolonged in severe renal impairment. Use is contraindicated in anuric patients.

Dosage adjustment in hepatic impairment:

Mild impairment (Child-Pugh class A): No dosage adjustment necessary.

Moderate-to-severe impairment (Child-Pugh classes B and C): Not recommended for initiation since an appropriate adjusted dose is not commercially available.

Additional Information Complete prescribing information should be consulted for additional detail.

Dosage Forms Excipient information presented when available (limited, particularly for generics); consult specific product labeling.

Tablet, oral: 16/12.5: Candesartan cilexetil 16 mg and hydrochlorothiazide 12.5 mg; 32/12.5: Candesartan cilexetil 32 mg and hydrochlorothiazide 12.5 mg; 32/25: Candesartan cilexetil 32 mg and hydrochlorothiazide 25 mg

Atacand HCT:

16/12.5: Candesartan cilexetil 16 mg and hydrochlorothiazide 12.5 mg

32/12.5: Candesartan cilexetil 32 mg and hydrochlorothiazide 12.5 mg

32/25: Candesartan cilexetil 32 mg and hydrochlorothiazide 25 mg

- **Candesartan Cilexetil** *see* Candesartan *on page 327*
- **Candesartan Cilexetil and Hydrochlorothiazide** *see* Candesartan and Hydrochlorothiazide *on page 329*
- **Candesartan-HCTZ (Can)** *see* Candesartan and Hydrochlorothiazide *on page 329*
- **Candistatin (Can)** *see* Nystatin (Topical) *on page 1482*
- **CanesOral® (Can)** *see* Fluconazole *on page 868*
- **Canesten® Topical (Can)** *see* Clotrimazole (Topical) *on page 476*
- **Canesten® Vaginal (Can)** *see* Clotrimazole (Topical) *on page 476*
- **CAPE** *see* Capecitabine *on page 329*

Capecitabine

(ka pe SITE a been)

Brand Names: U.S. Xeloda

Brand Names: Canada Teva-Capecitabine; Xeloda

Index Terms CAPE

Pharmacologic Category Antineoplastic Agent, Antimetabolite; Antineoplastic Agent, Antimetabolite (Pyrimidine Analog)

Use Treatment of metastatic colorectal cancer; adjuvant therapy of Dukes' C colon cancer; treatment of metastatic breast cancer

Unlabeled Use Treatment of CNS lesions from metastatic breast cancer, esophageal cancer, gastric cancer, hepatobiliary cancers (advanced), neuroendocrine (pancreatic/islet cell) tumors (metastatic or unresectable), ovarian cancer (platinum-refractory), pancreatic cancer (metastatic), unknown primary cancer

Pregnancy Risk Factor D

Pregnancy Considerations Animal reproduction studies have demonstrated teratogenicity and fetal loss. Fetal harm may occur if administered during pregnancy. Women of childbearing potential should use effective contraceptives to avoid pregnancy during treatment.

Breast-Feeding Considerations Due to the potential for serious adverse reactions in the nursing infant, the decision to discontinue capecitabine or to discontinue breastfeeding should take into account the importance of treatment to the mother.

Contraindications Hypersensitivity to capecitabine, fluorouracil, or any component of the formulation; known deficiency of dihydropyrimidine dehydrogenase (DPD); severe renal impairment (Cl_{cr} <30 mL/minute)

Warnings/Precautions Hazardous agent - use appropriate precautions for handling and disposal (NIOSH, 2012). Bone marrow suppression may occur, hematologic toxicity is more common when used in combination therapy; use with caution; dosage adjustments may be required. Product labeling recommends that patients with baseline platelets <100,000/mm^3 and/or neutrophils <1500/mm^3 not receive capecitabine therapy and also to withhold for grade 3 or 4 hematologic toxicity during treatment. Rare and unexpected severe toxicity (stomatitis, diarrhea, neutropenia, neurotoxicity) may be attributed to dihydropyrimidine dehydrogenase (DPD) deficiency.

Capecitabine may cause diarrhea (may be severe); median time to first occurrence of grade 2-4 diarrhea was 34 days; median duration of grades 3 or 4 diarrhea was 5 days. Withhold treatment for grades 2-4 diarrhea; subsequent doses should be reduced after grade 3 or 4 diarrhea or recurrence of grade 2 diarrhea. Necrotizing enterocolitis (typhlitis) has been reported. Dehydration may occur rapidly in patients with diarrhea, nausea, vomiting, anorexia, and/or weakness; adequately hydrate prior to treatment initiation. Elderly patients may be a higher risk for dehydration. **Note:** Canadian labeling recommends treatment interruption for dehydration requiring I.V. hydration lasting <24 hours and dosage reduction if I.V hydration required for ≥24 hours; correct precipitating factors and ensure rehydration prior to resuming therapy.

Hand-and-foot syndrome is characterized by numbness, dysesthesia/paresthesia, tingling, painless or painful swelling, erythema, desquamation, blistering, and severe pain; median onset is 79 days (range: 11-360 days). If grade 2 or 3 hand-and-foot syndrome occurs, interrupt administration of capecitabine until decreases to grade 1. Following grade 3 hand-and-foot syndrome, decrease subsequent doses of capecitabine. In patients with colorectal cancer, treatment with capecitabine immediately following 6 weeks of fluorouracil/leucovorin (FU/LV) therapy has been associated with an increased incidence of grade ≥3 toxicity, when compared to patients receiving the reverse sequence, capecitabine (two 3-week courses) followed by FU/LV (Hennig, 2008).

Grade 3 and 4 hyperbilirubinemia have been observed in patients with and without hepatic metastases at baseline (median onset: 64 days). Transaminase and alkaline phosphatase elevations have also been reported. If capecitabine-related grade 3 or 4 hyperbilirubinemia occurs, Interrupt treatment until bilirubin ≤3 times ULN. Use with caution in patients with mild to moderate hepatic impairment due to liver metastases; effect of severe hepatic impairment has not been studied. Use with caution in patients with mild-to-moderate renal impairment; reduce dose with moderate impairment (exposure to capecitabine and metabolites is increased) and carefully monitor and reduce subsequent dose (with any grade 2 or higher adverse effect) with mild-to-moderate impairment; use is contraindicated in severe impairment. Use with caution in patients ≥60 years of age, the incidence of treatment-related adverse events may be higher.

Cardiotoxicity has been observed with capecitabine, including myocardial infarction, ischemia, angina, dysrhythmias, cardiac arrest, cardiac failure, sudden death, ECG changes, and cardiomyopathy; may be more common in patients with a history of coronary artery disease. **[U.S. Boxed Warning]: Capecitabine may increase the anticoagulant effects of warfarin; bleeding events, including death, have occurred with concomitant use. Increases in prothrombin time (PT) and INR may occur within several days to months after capecitabine initiation, and may continue up to 1 month after capecitabine discontinuation; may occur in patients with or without liver metastases. Monitor frequently and adjust anticoagulation dosing accordingly. An increased risk of coagulopathy is correlated with a cancer diagnosis and age >60 years.** Other potentially significant drug-drug interactions may exist, requiring dose or frequency adjustment, additional monitoring, and/or selection of alternative therapy.

Adverse Reactions Frequency listed derived from monotherapy trials.

>10%:

Cardiovascular: Edema (9% to 15%)

Central nervous system: Fatigue (16% to 42%), fever (7% to 18%), pain (12%)

Dermatologic: Palmar-plantar erythrodysesthesia (hand-and-foot syndrome) (54% to 60%; grade 3: 11% to 17%; may be dose limiting), dermatitis (27% to 37%)

Gastrointestinal: Diarrhea (47% to 57%; may be dose limiting; grade 3: 12% to 13%; grade 4: 2% to 3%), nausea (34% to 53%), vomiting (15% to 37%), abdominal pain (7% to 35%), stomatitis (22% to 25%), appetite decreased (26%), anorexia (9% to 23%), constipation (9% to 15%)

Hematologic: Lymphopenia (94%; grade 4: 14%), anemia (72% to 80%; grade 4: <1% to 1%), neutropenia (2% to 26%; grade 4: 2%), thrombocytopenia (24%; grade 4: 1%)

Hepatic: Bilirubin increased (22% to 48%; grades 3/4: 11% to 23%)

Neuromuscular & skeletal: Paresthesia (21%)

Ocular: Eye irritation (13% to 15%)

Respiratory: Dyspnea (14%)

5% to 10%:

Cardiovascular: Venous thrombosis (8%), chest pain (6%)

Central nervous system: Headache (5% to 10%), lethargy (10%), dizziness (6% to 8%), insomnia (7% to 8%), mood alteration (5%), depression (5%)

Dermatologic: Nail disorder (7%), rash (7%), skin discoloration (7%), alopecia (6%), erythema (6%)

Endocrine & metabolic: Dehydration (7%)

Gastrointestinal: Motility disorder (10%), oral discomfort (10%), dyspepsia (6% to 8%), upper GI inflammatory disorders (colorectal cancer: 8%), hemorrhage (6%), ileus (6%), taste perversion (colorectal cancer: 6%)

Neuromuscular & skeletal: Back pain (10%), weakness (10%), neuropathy (10%), myalgia (9%), arthralgia (8%), limb pain (6%)

Ocular: Abnormal vision (colorectal cancer: 5%), conjunctivitis (5%)

Respiratory: Cough (7%)

Miscellaneous: Viral infection (colorectal cancer: 5%)

<5% (from monotherapy or combination therapy; limited to important or life-threatening): Abdominal distension, agranulocytosis, angina, arthritis, ascites, asthma, ataxia, atrial fibrillation, bone pain, bradycardia, bronchitis, bronchopneumonia, bronchospasm, cachexia, cardiac arrest, cardiac failure, cardiomyopathy, cerebral vascular accident, cholestatic hepatitis, coagulation disorder, colitis, confusion, deep vein thrombosis, diaphoresis, duodenitis, dysarthria, dysphagia, dysrhythmia, ecchymoses, ECG changes, encephalopathy, epistaxis, esophagitis, fibrosis, fingerprint distortion (secondary to hand-and-foot syndrome), fungal infection, gastric ulcer, gastritis, gastroenteritis, gastrointestinal perforation, hematemesis, hemoptysis, hepatic coma, hepatic failure, hepatic fibrosis, hepatitis, hepatotoxicity, hot flushes, hypokalemia, hypomagnesemia, hyper-/hypotension, hypersensitivity, hypertriglyceridemia, idiopathic thrombocytopenia purpura, ileus, infection, influenza-like illness, intestinal obstruction (~1%), jaundice, keratoconjunctivitis, lacrimal duct stenosis, laryngitis, leukopenia, loss of consciousness, lymphedema, MI, multifocal leukoencephalopathy, myocardial ischemia, myocarditis, necrotizing enterocolitis (typhlitis), neutropenic sepsis, nocturia, oral candidiasis, pancytopenia, pericardial effusion, phlebitis (venous),

photosensitivity reaction, pneumonia, proctalgia, prothrombin decreased, pruritus, pulmonary embolism, radiation recall syndrome, renal impairment, respiratory distress, sedation, sepsis, skin ulceration, sore throat, Stevens-Johnson syndrome, syncope, tachycardia, thrombocytopenic purpura, thrombophlebitis, toxic epidermal necrolysis, toxic megacolon, tremor, ventricular extrasystoles, vertigo

Drug Interactions

Metabolism/Transport Effects **Inhibits** CYP2C9 (strong)

Avoid Concomitant Use

Avoid concomitant use of Capecitabine with any of the following: BCG; CloZAPine; Gimeracil; Natalizumab; Pimecrolimus; Tacrolimus (Topical); Tofacitinib; Vaccines (Live)

Increased Effect/Toxicity

Capecitabine may increase the levels/effects of: Bosentan; Carvedilol; CloZAPine; CYP2C9 Substrates; Diclofenac (Systemic); Fosphenytoin; Lacosamide; Leflunomide; Natalizumab; Ospemifene; Phenytoin; Tofacitinib; Vaccines (Live); Vitamin K Antagonists

The levels/effects of Capecitabine may be increased by: Cimetidine; Denosumab; Gimeracil; Leucovorin Calcium-Levoleucovorin; Pimecrolimus; Roflumilast; Tacrolimus (Topical); Trastuzumab

Decreased Effect

Capecitabine may decrease the levels/effects of: BCG; Coccidioidin Skin Test; Sipuleucel-T; Vaccines (Inactivated); Vaccines (Live)

The levels/effects of Capecitabine may be decreased by: Echinacea

Ethanol/Nutrition/Herb Interactions Food: Food reduced the rate and extent of absorption of capecitabine.

Storage/Stability Store at room temperature of 25°C (77°F); excursions permitted between 15°C and 30°C (59°F and 86°F). Keep bottle tightly closed.

Mechanism of Action Capecitabine is a prodrug of fluorouracil. It undergoes hydrolysis in the liver and tissues to form fluorouracil which is the active moiety. Fluorouracil is a fluorinated pyrimidine antimetabolite that inhibits thymidylate synthetase, blocking the methylation of deoxyuridylic acid to thymidylic acid, interfering with DNA, and to a lesser degree, RNA synthesis. Fluorouracil appears to be phase specific for the G_1 and S phases of the cell cycle.

Pharmacodynamics/Kinetics

Absorption: Rapid and extensive (rate and extent reduced by food)

Protein binding: <60%; ~35% to albumin

Metabolism:

Hepatic: Inactive metabolites: 5′-deoxy-5-fluorocytidine, 5′-deoxy-5-fluorouridine

Tissue: Enzymatically metabolized to fluorouracil, which is then metabolized to active metabolites, 5-fluoroxyuridine monophosphate (F-UMP) and 5-5-fluoro-2′-deoxyuridine-5′-O-monophosphate (F-dUMP)

Half-life elimination: 0.5-1 hour

Time to peak: 1.5 hours; Fluorouracil: 2 hours

Excretion: Urine (96%, 57% as α-fluoro-β-alanine; <3% as unchanged drug); feces (<3%)

Dosage Note: Details concerning dosing in combination regimens should also be consulted. Capecitabine toxicities, particularly hand-foot syndrome, may be higher in North American populations (for the treatment of colorectal cancer); therapy initiation at doses of 1000 mg/m^2 twice daily (for 2 weeks every 21 days) may be considered (Haller, 2008; NCCN Colon Cancer Guidelines v3.2013)

Breast cancer, metastatic: Adults: Oral: 1250 mg/m^2 twice daily for 2 weeks, every 21 days (as either monotherapy or in combination with docetaxel)

Colorectal cancer, metastatic: Adults: Oral: 1250 mg/m^2 twice daily for 2 weeks, every 21 days

Dukes' C colon cancer, adjuvant therapy: Adults: Oral: 1250 mg/m^2 twice daily for 2 weeks, every 21 days, for a recommended total duration of 24 weeks (8 cycles of 2 weeks of drug administration and 1 week rest period).

Unlabeled uses:

Breast cancer, metastatic (unlabeled dosing): Adults: Oral: 1000 mg/m^2 twice daily (in combination with ixabepilone) on days 1-14 of a 3-week cycle until disease progression or unacceptable toxicity (Thomas, 2007)

Breast cancer, metastatic, HER2+ (unlabeled dosing): Adults: Oral: 1000 mg/m^2 twice daily (in combination with lapatinib) on days 1-14 of a 3-week cycle until disease progression or unacceptable toxicity (Geyer, 2006) **or** 1250 mg/m^2 twice daily (in combination with trastuzumab) on days 1-14 of a 3-week cycle (Bartsch, 2007)

Breast cancer, metastatic, HER2+ with brain metastases, first-line therapy (unlabeled dosing): Adults: Oral: 1000 mg/m^2 twice daily (in combination with lapatinib) on days 1-14 of a 3-week cycle until disease progression or unacceptable toxicity (Bachelot, 2012)

Colorectal cancer (unlabeled dosing): Adults: Oral: 1000 mg/m^2 twice daily (in combination with oxaliplatin) on days 1-14 of a 3-week cycle for 8 or 16 cycles (Cassidy, 2008; Haller, 2011; Schmoll, 2007)

Esophageal and gastric cancers (unlabeled uses): Adults: Oral:

Preoperative or definitive chemoradiation: 800 mg/m^2 twice daily (in combination with cisplatin and radiation) on days 1-5 weekly for 5 weeks (Lee, 2007; NCCN Esophageal/Esophagogastric Cancers, v2.2013; NCCN Gastric Cancer, v2.2013) **or** 625 mg/m^2 twice daily (in combination with oxaliplatin and radiation) on days 1-5 weekly for 5 weeks (Javle, 2009; NCCN Esophageal/Esophagogastric Cancers, v2.2013; NCCN Gastric Cancer, v2.2013)

Perioperative chemotherapy: 625 mg/m^2 twice daily (in combination with epirubicin and cisplatin or oxaliplatin) on days 1-21 of a 3-week cycle; 3 cycles administered both before and after surgery (NCCN Esophageal/Esophagogastric Cancers, v2.2013; NCCN Gastric Cancer, v2.2013)

Postoperative chemoradiation: 625-825 mg/m^2 twice daily on days 1-5 or days 1-7 weekly for 5 weeks (in combination with radiation) (Lee, 2006; NCCN Esophageal/Esophagogastric Cancers, v2.2013; NCCN Gastric Cancer, v2.2013)

Locally-advanced or metastatic (chemoradiation not indicated): 1000-1250 mg/m^2 twice daily (monotherapy or in combination with cisplatin with or without trastuzumab) on days 1-14 of a 3-week cycle (Bang, 2010; Hong, 2004; Kang, 2009) **or** 625 mg/m^2 twice daily (in combination with epirubicin and cisplatin or oxaliplatin) on days 1-21 of a 3-week cycle for up to 8 cycles (Cunningham, 2008; Sumpter, 2005)

Hepatobiliary cancers, advanced (unlabeled use): Adults: Oral: 650 mg/m^2 twice daily (in combination with gemcitabine) on days 1-14 of a 3-week cycle (Knox, 2005) **or** 1000 mg/m^2 twice daily (in combination with oxaliplatin) on days 1-14 of a 3-week cycle (Nehls, 2008) **or** 1250 mg/m^2 twice daily (in combination with cisplatin) on days 1-14 of a 3-week cycle (Kim, 2003); all regimens continued until disease progression or unacceptable toxicity

Neuroendocrine (pancreatic/islet cell) tumors, metastatic or unresectable: Adults: Oral: 750 mg/m² twice daily (in combination with temozolomide) on days 1-14 of a 4-week cycle (Strosberg, 2011)

Ovarian, fallopian tube, or peritoneal cancer, platinum-refractory: Adults: Oral: 1000 mg/m² twice daily on days 1-14 of a 3-week cycle until disease progression or unacceptable toxicity (Wolf, 2006)

Pancreatic cancer, metastatic (unlabeled use): Adults: Oral: 1000 mg/m² twice daily on days 1-14 of a 3-week cycle (NCCN Pancreatic Cancer v1.2013) **or** 1250 mg/m² twice daily on days 1-14 of a 3-week cycle (Cartwright, 2002) **or** 830 mg/m² twice daily (in combination with gemcitabine) on days 1-21 of a 4-week cycle until disease progression or unacceptable toxicity (Cunningham, 2009)

Unknown primary cancer (unlabeled use): Adults: Oral: 850-1000 mg/m² twice daily (in combination with oxaliplatin) on days 1-14 of a 3-week cycle for up to 6 cycles or until disease progression (Hainsworth, 2010; NCCN Occult Primary v1.2013) **or** 800 mg/m² twice daily (in combination with carboplatin and gemcitabine) on days 1-14 of a 3-week cycle for up to 8 cycles or until disease progression or unacceptable toxicity (Schneider, 2007)

Elderly: The elderly may be more sensitive to the toxic effects of fluorouracil. Insufficient data are available to provide dosage modifications.

Dosing adjustment in renal impairment:

Renal impairment at treatment initiation:

Cl_{cr} ≥51 mL/minute: Initial: No dosage adjustment necessary.

Cl_{cr} 30-50 mL/minute: Initial: Administer 75% of usual dose (Superfin, 2007).

Cl_{cr} <30 mL/minute: Use is contraindicated (Superfin, 2007).

Renal toxicity during treatment: Refer to dosage adjustment for toxicity.

Dosing adjustment in hepatic impairment:

Hepatic impairment at treatment initiation:

Mild-to-moderate impairment: No starting dose adjustment is necessary (Ecklund, 2005; Superfin, 2007); however, carefully monitor patients.

Severe hepatic impairment: No dosage adjustment provided in manufacturer's labeling (has not been studied).

Hepatotoxicity during treatment: Hyperbilirubinemia, grade 3 or 4: Interrupt treatment until bilirubin ≤3 times ULN.

Dosing in obesity: *ASCO Guidelines for appropriate chemotherapy dosing in obese adults with cancer:* Utilize patient's actual body weight (full weight) for calculation of body surface area- or weight-based dosing, particularly when the intent of therapy is curative; manage regimen-related toxicities in the same manner as for nonobese patients; if a dose reduction is utilized due to toxicity, consider resumption of full weight-based dosing with subsequent cycles, especially if cause of toxicity (eg, hepatic or renal impairment) is resolved (Griggs, 2012).

Dosage adjustment for toxicity: See table (**Note:** Capecitabine dosing recommendations apply to both monotherapy and when used in combination therapy with docetaxel).

Monitor carefully for toxicity and adjust dose as necessary. Doses reduced for toxicity should not be increased at a later time. For combination therapy, also refer to docetaxel product labeling for docetaxel dose modifications. If treatment delay is required for either capecitabine or docetaxel, withhold both agents until appropriate to resume combination treatment.

Recommended Capecitabine Dose Modifications

Toxicity Grades	During a Course of Therapy	Dose Adjustment for Next Cycle (% of starting dose)
Grade 1	Maintain dose level	Maintain dose level
Grade 2		
1st appearance	Interrupt until resolved to grade 0-1	100%
2nd appearance	Interrupt until resolved to grade 0-1	75%
3rd appearance	Interrupt until resolved to grade 0-1	50%
4th appearance	Discontinue treatment permanently	
Grade 3		
1st appearance	Interrupt until resolved to grade 0-1	75%
2nd appearance	Interrupt until resolved to grade 0-1	50%
3rd appearance	Discontinue treatment permanently	
Grade 4		
1st appearance	Discontinue permanently or If in the patient's best interest to continue, interrupt until resolved to grade 0-1	50%

Dosage adjustments for hematologic toxicity in combination therapy with ixabepilone:

Neutrophils <500/mm³ for ≥7 days or neutropenic fever: Hold for concurrent diarrhea or stomatitis until neutrophils recover to >1000/mm³, then continue at same dose

Platelets <25,000/mm³ (or <50,000/mm³ with bleeding): Hold for concurrent diarrhea or stomatitis until platelets recover to >50,000/mm³, then continue at same dose

Dietary Considerations Because current safety and efficacy data are based upon administration with food, it is recommended that capecitabine be administered with food. In all clinical trials, patients were instructed to take with water within 30 minutes after a meal.

Administration Usually administered in 2 divided doses taken 12 hours apart. Doses should be taken with water within 30 minutes after a meal. Swallow tablets whole; do not cut or crush.

Hazardous agent; use appropriate precautions for handling and disposal (NIOSH, 2012).

Monitoring Parameters Renal function should be estimated at baseline to determine initial dose. During therapy, CBC with differential, hepatic function, and renal function should be monitored. Monitor for diarrhea, hand/foot syndrome, stomatitis, and cardiotoxicity. Monitor INR closely if receiving concomitant warfarin.

Additional Information Oncology Comment: An investigational uridine prodrug, uridine triacetate (formerly called vistonuridine), has been studied in a limited number of cases of fluorouracil overdose. Of 17 patients receiving uridine triacetate beginning within 8-96 hours after fluorouracil overdose, all patients fully recovered (von Borstel, 2009). Updated data has described a total of 28 patients treated with uridine triacetate for fluorouracil overdose (including overdoses related to continuous infusions delivering fluorouracil at rates faster than prescribed), all of whom recovered fully (Bamat, 2010). An additional case report describes accidental capecitabine ingestion by a 22 month old child; uridine acetate was initiated approximately 7 hours after exposure. The patient received uridine acetate every 6 hours for a total of 20 doses through nasogastric tube administration; he was asymptomatic throughout his course and was discharged with normal laboratory values (Kanie, 2011). Refer to Uridine Triacetate monograph.

Dosage Forms Excipient information presented when available (limited, particularly for generics); consult specific product labeling.

Tablet, Oral:

Xeloda: 150 mg, 500 mg

Extemporaneous Preparations Hazardous agent: Use appropriate precautions for handling and disposal.

A 10 mg/mL oral solution may be made with tablets. Crush four 500 mg tablets in a mortar and reduce to a fine powder; add to 200 mL water. Capecitabine tablets are water soluble (data on file from Roche). Administer immediately after preparation, 30 minutes after a meal.

Judson IR, Beale PJ, Trigo JM, et al, "A Human Capecitabine Excretion Balance and Pharmacokinetic Study After Administration of a Single Oral Dose of ^{14}C-Labelled Drug," *Invest New Drugs*, 1999, 17 (1):49-56.

◆ **Capex** *see* Fluocinolone (Topical) *on page 878*

◆ **Capex® (Can)** *see* Fluocinolone (Topical) *on page 878*

◆ **Capital® and Codeine** *see* Acetaminophen and Codeine *on page 32*

◆ **Capoten® (Can)** *see* Captopril *on page 333*

◆ **Caprelsa** *see* Vandetanib *on page 2162*

Captopril (KAP toe pril)

Brand Names: Canada Apo-Capto®; Capoten®; Dom-Captopril; Mylan-Captopril; Nu-Capto; PMS-Captopril; Teva-Captopril

Index Terms ACE

Pharmacologic Category Angiotensin-Converting Enzyme (ACE) Inhibitor; Antihypertensive

Additional Appendix Information

Angiotensin Agents *on page 2280*

Use Management of hypertension; treatment of heart failure, left ventricular dysfunction after myocardial infarction, diabetic nephropathy

Unlabeled Use To delay the progression of nephropathy and reduce risks of cardiovascular events in hypertensive patients with type 1 or 2 diabetes mellitus; treatment of hypertensive crisis, rheumatoid arthritis; diagnosis of anatomic renal artery stenosis, hypertension secondary to scleroderma renal crisis; diagnosis of aldosteronism, idiopathic edema, Bartter's syndrome, postmyocardial infarction for prevention of ventricular failure; increase circulation in Raynaud's phenomenon, hypertension secondary to Takayasu's disease

Pregnancy Risk Factor D

Pregnancy Considerations **[U.S. Boxed Warning]: Drugs that act on the renin-angiotensin system can cause injury and death to the developing fetus. Discontinue as soon as possible once pregnancy is detected.** Captopril crosses the placenta; teratogenic effects may occur following maternal use during pregnancy. Drugs that act on the renin-angiotensin system are associated with oligohydramnios. Oligohydramnios, due to decreased fetal renal function, may lead to fetal lung hypoplasia and skeletal malformations. Their use in pregnancy is also associated with anuria, hypotension, renal failure, skull hypoplasia, and death in the fetus/neonate. Chronic maternal hypertension itself is also associated with adverse events in the fetus/infant. ACE inhibitors are not recommended during pregnancy to treat maternal hypertension or heart failure. Use of an ACE inhibitor should also be avoided in any woman of reproductive age. Women who are planning a pregnancy should be considered for other medication options if an ACE inhibitor is currently prescribed or the ACE inhibitor should be discontinued as soon as possible once pregnancy is detected. The exposed fetus should be monitored for fetal growth, amniotic fluid volume, and organ formation. Infants exposed to an ACE inhibitor *in utero* should be monitored for hyperkalemia, hypotension, and oliguria.

Breast-Feeding Considerations Captopril is excreted in breast milk. Breast-feeding is not recommended by the manufacturer.

Contraindications Hypersensitivity to captopril, any other ACE inhibitor, or any component of the formulation; angioedema related to previous treatment with an ACE inhibitor; concomitant use with aliskiren in patients with diabetes mellitus

Warnings/Precautions Anaphylactic reactions may occur rarely with ACE inhibitors. At any time during treatment (especially following first dose) angioedema may occur rarely with ACE inhibitors; may involve the head and neck (potentially compromising airway) or the intestine (presenting with abdominal pain). African-Americans and patients with idiopathic or hereditary angioedema may be at an increased risk. Prolonged frequent monitoring may be required especially if tongue, glottis, or larynx are involved as they are associated with airway obstruction. Patients with a history of airway surgery may have a higher risk of airway obstruction. Aggressive early and appropriate management is critical. Use in patients with previous angioedema associated with ACE inhibitor therapy is contraindicated. Severe anaphylactoid reactions may be seen during hemodialysis (eg, CVVHD) with high-flux dialysis membranes (eg, AN69), and rarely, during low density lipoprotein apheresis with dextran sulfate cellulose. Rare cases of anaphylactoid reactions have been reported in patients undergoing sensitization treatment with hymenoptera (bee, wasp) venom while receiving ACE inhibitors.

Symptomatic hypotension with or without syncope can occur with ACE inhibitors (usually with the first several doses); effects are most often observed in volume depleted patients; close monitoring of patient is required especially with initial dosing and dosing increases; blood pressure must be lowered at a rate appropriate for the patient's clinical condition. Initiation of therapy in patients with ischemic heart disease or cerebrovascular disease warrants close observation due to the potential consequences posed by falling blood pressure (eg, MI, stroke). Use with caution in hypertrophic cardiomyopathy with outflow tract obstruction, severe aortic stenosis, or before, during, or immediately after major surgery. **[U.S. Boxed Warning]: Drugs that act on the renin-angiotensin system can cause injury and death to the developing fetus. Discontinue as soon as possible once pregnancy is detected.**

Hyperkalemia may occur with ACE inhibitors; risk factors include renal dysfunction, diabetes mellitus, concomitant use of potassium-sparing diuretics, potassium supplements and/or potassium containing salts. Use cautiously, if at all, with these agents and monitor potassium closely. Cough may occur with ACE inhibitors. Other causes of cough should be considered (eg, pulmonary congestion in patients with heart failure) and excluded prior to discontinuation.

May be associated with deterioration of renal function and/or increases in serum creatinine, particularly in patients with low renal blood flow (eg, renal artery stenosis, heart failure) whose glomerular filtration rate (GFR) is dependent on efferent arteriolar vasoconstriction by angiotensin II; deterioration may result in oliguria, acute renal failure, and progressive azotemia. Small increases in serum creatinine may occur following initiation; consider discontinuation only in patients with progressive and/or significant deterioration in renal function. Use with caution in patients with unstented unilateral/bilateral renal artery stenosis. When unstented bilateral renal artery stenosis is present, use is generally avoided due to the elevated risk of deterioration in renal function unless possible benefits outweigh risks. Concomitant use of an angiotensin receptor blocker (ARB) or renin inhibitor (eg, aliskiren) is associated with an increased risk of hypotension, hyperkalemia, and renal dysfunction; concomitant use with aliskiren should be avoided in patients with GFR <60 mL/minute and is contraindicated in patients with diabetes mellitus (regardless of GFR).

Rare toxicities associated with ACE inhibitors include cholestatic jaundice (which may progress to fulminant hepatic necrosis), agranulocytosis, neutropenia, or leukopenia with myeloid hypoplasia. Patients with collagen vascular diseases (especially with concomitant renal impairment) or renal impairment alone may be at increased risk for hematologic toxicity; closely monitor CBC with differential for the first 3 months of therapy and periodically thereafter in these patients.

Adverse Reactions

Frequency not defined:

Cardiovascular: Angioedema, cardiac arrest, cerebrovascular insufficiency, rhythm disturbances, orthostatic hypotension, syncope, flushing, pallor, angina, MI, Raynaud's syndrome, CHF

Central nervous system: Ataxia, confusion, depression, nervousness, somnolence

Dermatologic: Bullous pemphigus, erythema multiforme, Stevens-Johnson syndrome, exfoliative dermatitis

Endocrine & metabolic: Alkaline phosphatase increased, bilirubin increased, gynecomastia

Gastrointestinal: Pancreatitis, glossitis, dyspepsia

Genitourinary: Urinary frequency, impotence

Hematologic: Anemia, thrombocytopenia, pancytopenia, agranulocytosis, anemia

Hepatic: Jaundice, hepatitis, hepatic necrosis (rare), cholestasis, hyponatremia (symptomatic), transaminases increased

Neuromuscular & skeletal: Asthenia, myalgia, myasthenia

Ocular: Blurred vision

Renal: Renal insufficiency, renal failure, nephrotic syndrome, polyuria, oliguria

Respiratory: Bronchospasm, eosinophilic pneumonitis, rhinitis

Miscellaneous: Anaphylactoid reactions

1% to 10%:

Cardiovascular: Hypotension (1% to 3%), tachycardia (1%), chest pain (1%), palpitation (1%)

Dermatologic: Rash (maculopapular or urticarial) (4% to 7%), pruritus (2%); in patients with rash, a positive ANA and/or eosinophilia has been noted in 7% to 10%.

Endocrine & metabolic: Hyperkalemia (1% to 11%)

Hematologic: Neutropenia may occur in up to 4% of patients with renal insufficiency or collagen-vascular disease.

Renal: Proteinuria (1%), serum creatinine increased, worsening of renal function (may occur in patients with bilateral renal artery stenosis or hypovolemia)

Respiratory: Cough (<1% to 2%)

Miscellaneous: Hypersensitivity reactions (rash, pruritus, fever, arthralgia, and eosinophilia) have occurred in 4% to 7% of patients (depending on dose and renal function); dysgeusia - loss of taste or diminished perception (2% to 4%)

<1% (Limited to important or life-threatening): Alopecia, angina, anorexia, aphthous ulcers, aplastic anemia, cholestatic jaundice, eosinophilia, erythrocyte sedimentation rate increased, exacerbations of Huntington's disease, glomerulonephritis, Guillain-Barré syndrome, hemolytic anemia, hyperthermia, insomnia, interstitial nephritis, Kaposi's sarcoma, peptic ulcer, pericarditis, psoriasis, seizure (in premature infants), systemic lupus erythematosus, vasculitis, visual hallucinations (Doane, 2013)

Drug Interactions

Metabolism/Transport Effects Substrate of CYP2D6 (major); **Note:** Assignment of Major/Minor substrate status based on clinically relevant drug interaction potential

Avoid Concomitant Use There are no known interactions where it is recommended to avoid concomitant use.

Increased Effect/Toxicity

Captopril may increase the levels/effects of: Allopurinol; Amifostine; Antihypertensives; AzaTHIOprine; CycloSPORINE (Systemic); Ferric Gluconate; Gold Sodium Thiomalate; Hypotensive Agents; Iron Dextran Complex; Lithium; Nonsteroidal Anti-Inflammatory Agents; Obinutuzumab; RiTUXimab; Sodium Phosphates

The levels/effects of Captopril may be increased by: Abiraterone Acetate; Alfuzosin; Aliskiren; Angiotensin II Receptor Blockers; Brimonidine (Topical); Canagliflozin; CYP2D6 Inhibitors (Moderate); CYP2D6 Inhibitors (Strong); Darunavir; Diazoxide; DPP-IV Inhibitors; Eplerenone; Everolimus; Heparin; Heparin (Low Molecular Weight); Herbs (Hypotensive Properties); Loop Diuretics; MAO Inhibitors; Pentoxifylline; Phosphodiesterase 5 Inhibitors; Potassium Salts; Potassium-Sparing Diuretics; Prostacyclin Analogues; Sirolimus; Temsirolimus; Thiazide Diuretics; TiZANidine; Tolvaptan; Trimethoprim

Decreased Effect

The levels/effects of Captopril may be decreased by: Antacids; Aprotinin; Herbs (Hypertensive Properties); Icatibant; Lanthanum; Methylphenidate; Nonsteroidal Anti-Inflammatory Agents; Peginterferon Alfa-2b; Salicylates; Yohimbine

Ethanol/Nutrition/Herb Interactions

Food: Captopril serum concentrations may be decreased if taken with food. Long-term use of captopril may lead to a zinc deficiency which can result in altered taste perception. Potassium supplements and/or potassium-containing salts may cause or worsen hyperkalemia. Management: Take on an empty stomach 1 hour before or 2 hours after meals. Consult prescriber before consuming a potassium-rich diet, potassium supplements, or salt substitutes.

Herb/Nutraceutical: Some herbal medications may worsen hypertension (eg, licorice); others may increase the antihypertensive effect of captopril (eg, shepherd's purse). Management: Avoid bayberry, blue cohosh, cayenne, ephedra, ginger, ginseng (American), kola, yohimbe, and licorice. Avoid black cohosh, california poppy, coleus, golden seal, hawthorn, mistletoe, periwinkle, quinine, and shepherd's purse.

Mechanism of Action Competitive inhibitor of angiotensin-converting enzyme (ACE); prevents conversion of angiotensin I to angiotensin II, a potent vasoconstrictor; results in lower levels of angiotensin II which causes an increase in plasma renin activity and a reduction in aldosterone secretion

Pharmacodynamics/Kinetics

Onset of action: Peak effect: Blood pressure reduction: 1-1.5 hours after dose

Duration: Dose related, may require several weeks of therapy before full hypotensive effect

Absorption: 60% to 75%; reduced 30% to 40% by food

Protein binding: 25% to 30%

Metabolism: 50%

Half-life elimination (renal and cardiac function dependent):

Adults, healthy volunteers: 1.9 hours; Heart failure: 2.06 hours; Anuria: 20-40 hours

Time to peak: 1 hour

Excretion: Urine (>95%) within 24 hours (40% to 50% as unchanged drug)

Dosage Note: Titrate dose according to patient's response; use lowest effective dose. Oral:

Infants: Initial: 0.15-0.3 mg/kg/dose; titrate dose upward to maximum of 6 mg/kg/day in 1-4 divided doses

Children: Initial: 0.3-0.5 mg/kg/dose; titrate upward to maximum of 6 mg/kg/day in 2-4 divided doses (NHBPEP, 2004)

Older Children: Initial: 6.25-12.5 mg/dose every 12-24 hours; titrate upward to maximum of 6 mg/kg/day

Adolescents: Initial: 12.5-25 mg/dose; titrate to a maximum of 450 mg/day

Adults:

Acute hypertension (urgency/emergency): 12.5-25 mg, may repeat as needed (may be given sublingually, but no therapeutic advantage demonstrated)

Heart failure:

Initial dose: 6.25-12.5 mg 3 times/day in conjunction with cardiac glycoside and diuretic therapy; initial dose depends upon patient's fluid/electrolyte status

Target dose: 50 mg 3 times/day

Hypertension:

Initial dose: 25 mg 2-3 times/day (a lower initial dose of 12.5 mg 3 times/day may also be considered [VA Cooperative Study Group, 1984]); may increase by 12.5-25 mg/dose at 1- to 2-week intervals up to 50 mg 3 times/day; add thiazide diuretic, unless severe renal impairment coexists then consider loop diuretic, before further dosage increases or consider other treatment options; maximum dose: 150 mg 3 times/day

Usual dose range (JNC 7): 25-100 mg/day in 2 divided doses

LV dysfunction after MI: Initial: 6.25 mg; if tolerated, follow with 12.5 mg 3 times/day; then increase to 25 mg 3 times/day during next several days and then gradually increase over next several weeks to target dose of 50 mg 3 times/day (some dose schedules are more aggressive to achieve an increased goal dose within the first few days of initiation.)

Diabetic nephropathy: Initial: 25 mg 3 times/day. May be taken with other antihypertensive therapy if required to further lower blood pressure.

Elderly: Hypertension: Consider lower initial doses and titrate to response (Aronow, 2011)

Dosage adjustment in renal impairment:

Manufacturers recommendations: Reduce initial daily dose and titrate slowly (1- to 2-week intervals) with smaller increments. Slowly back titrate to determine the minimum effective dose once the desired therapeutic effect has been reached.

Alternative recommendations (Aronoff, 2007): Adults:

Cl_{cr} 10-50 mL/minute: Administer at 75% of normal dose every 12-18 hours.

Cl_{cr} <10 mL/minute: Administer at 50% of normal dose every 24 hours.

Intermittent hemodialysis (IHD): Administer after hemodialysis on dialysis days

Peritoneal dialysis: Dose for Cl_{cr} 10-50 mL/minute; supplemental dose is not necessary

Dosage adjustment in hepatic impairment: No dosage adjustment provided in manufacturer's labeling.

Dietary Considerations Should be taken at least 1 hour before or 2 hours after eating.

Administration Unstable in aqueous solutions; to prepare solution for oral administration, mix prior to administration and use within 10 minutes.

Monitoring Parameters BUN, electrolytes, serum creatinine; blood pressure. In patients with renal impairment and/or collagen vascular disease, closely monitor CBC with differential for the first 3 months of therapy and periodically thereafter.

Test Interactions Positive Coombs' [direct]; may cause false-positive results in urine acetone determinations using sodium nitroprusside reagent

Dosage Forms Excipient information presented when available (limited, particularly for generics); consult specific product labeling.

Tablet, Oral:

Generic: 12.5 mg, 25 mg, 50 mg, 100 mg

Dosage Forms: Canada Note: Also refer to Dosage Forms. Excipient information presented when available (limited, particularly for generics); consult specific product labeling.

Tablet, Oral: 6.25 mg

Extemporaneous Preparations A 1 mg/mL oral solution may be made by allowing two 50 mg tablets to dissolve in 50 mL of distilled water. Add the contents of one 500 mg sodium ascorbate injection ampul or one 500 mg ascorbic acid tablet and allow to dissolve. Add quantity of distilled water sufficient to make 100 mL. Label "shake well" and "refrigerate". Stable for 56 days refrigerated.

Nahata MC, Pai VB, and Hipple TF, *Pediatric Drug Formulations*, 5th ed, Cincinnati, OH: Harvey Whitney Books Co, 2004.

Captopril and Hydrochlorothiazide

(KAP toe pril & hye droe klor oh THYE a zide)

Index Terms Hydrochlorothiazide and Captopril

Pharmacologic Category Angiotensin-Converting Enzyme (ACE) Inhibitor; Antihypertensive; Diuretic, Thiazide

Use Management of hypertension

Pregnancy Risk Factor C/D (2nd and 3rd trimesters)

Dosage Oral: Adults: Hypertension, CHF: May be substituted for previously titrated dosages of the individual components; alternatively, may initiate as follows:

Initial: Single tablet (captopril 25 mg/hydrochlorothiazide 15 mg) taken once daily; daily dose of captopril should not exceed 150 mg; daily dose of hydrochlorothiazide should not exceed 50 mg

Dosage adjustment in renal impairment: May respond to smaller or less frequent doses.

Dosage adjustment in hepatic impairment: No dosage adjustments provided in manufacturer's labeling; use with caution.

Additional Information Complete prescribing information should be consulted for additional detail.

Dosage Forms Excipient information presented when available (limited, particularly for generics); consult specific product labeling.

Tablet, oral: 25/15: Captopril 25 mg and hydrochlorothiazide 15 mg; 25/25: Captopril 25 mg and hydrochlorothiazide 25 mg; 50/15: Captopril 50 mg and hydrochlorothiazide 15 mg; 50/25: Captopril 50 mg and hydrochlorothiazide 25 mg

◆ **Carac** *see* Fluorouracil (Topical) *on page* 885

◆ **Carafate** *see* Sucralfate *on page* 1955

Carbachol (KAR ba kole)

Brand Names: U.S. Isopto Carbachol; Miostat

Brand Names: Canada Isopto® Carbachol; Miostat®

Index Terms Carbacholine; Carbamylcholine Chloride

Pharmacologic Category Cholinergic Agonist; Ophthalmic Agent, Antiglaucoma; Ophthalmic Agent, Miotic

Use Lowers intraocular pressure in the treatment of glaucoma; cause miosis during surgery

Pregnancy Risk Factor C

Dosage Adults:

Ophthalmic: Instill 1-2 drops up to 3 times/day

Intraocular: 0.5 mL instilled into anterior chamber before or after securing sutures

Dosage adjustment in renal impairment: No dosage adjustment provided in manufacturer's labeling.

Dosage adjustment in hepatic impairment: No dosage adjustment provided in manufacturer's labeling.

Additional Information Complete prescribing information should be consulted for additional detail.

Dosage Forms Excipient information presented when available (limited, particularly for generics); consult specific product labeling.

Solution, Intraocular:

Miostat: 0.01% (1.5 mL)

Solution, Ophthalmic:

Isopto Carbachol: 1.5% (15 mL); 3% (15 mL)

◆ Carbacholine *see* Carbachol *on page* 335

◆ Carbaglu *see* Carglumic Acid *on page* 350

CarBAMazepine (kar ba MAZ e peen)

Brand Names: U.S. Carbatrol; Epitol; Equetro; TEGretol; TEGretol-XR

Brand Names: Canada Apo-Carbamazepine®; Dom-Carbamazepine; Mapezine®; Mylan-Carbamazepine CR; Nu-Carbamazepine; PMS-Carbamazepine; Sandoz-Carbamazepine; Taro-Carbamazepine Chewable; Tegretol®; Teva-Carbamazepine

Index Terms CBZ; SPD417

Pharmacologic Category Anticonvulsant, Miscellaneous

Additional Appendix Information

Beers Criteria – Potentially Inappropriate Medications for Geriatrics *on page* 2368

Use

Carbatrol®, Tegretol®, Tegretol®-XR: Partial seizures with complex symptomatology (psychomotor, temporal lobe), generalized tonic-clonic seizures (grand mal), mixed seizure patterns, trigeminal neuralgia, glossopharyngeal neuralgia

Equetro®: Acute manic or mixed episodes associated with bipolar 1 disorder

Unlabeled Use Treatment of restless leg syndrome and post-traumatic stress disorders

Pregnancy Risk Factor D

Pregnancy Considerations Studies in pregnant women have demonstrated a risk to the fetus. Carbamazepine and its metabolites can be found in the fetus and may be associated with teratogenic effects, including spina bifida, craniofacial defects, cardiovascular malformations, and hypospadias. The risk of teratogenic effects is higher with anticonvulsant polytherapy than monotherapy.

Developmental delays have also been observed following *in utero* exposure to carbamazepine (per manufacturer); however, socioeconomic factors, maternal and paternal IQ, and polytherapy may contribute to these findings. Pregnancy may cause small decreases of carbamazepine plasma concentrations in the second and third trimesters; monitoring should be considered. When used for the treatment of bipolar disorder, use of carbamazepine should be avoided during the first trimester of pregnancy if possible. The use of a single medication for the treatment of bipolar disorder or epilepsy in pregnancy is preferred. Carbamazepine may decrease plasma concentrations of hormonal contraceptives; breakthrough bleeding or unintended pregnancy may occur and alternate or back-up methods of contraception should be considered.

Patients exposed to carbamazepine during pregnancy are encouraged to enroll themselves into the AED Pregnancy Registry by calling 1-888-233-2334. Additional information is available at www.aedpregnancyregistry.org.

Breast-Feeding Considerations Carbamazepine and its active epoxide metabolite are found in breast milk. Carbamazepine can also be detected in the serum of nursing infants. Transient hepatic dysfunction has been observed in some case reports. Nursing should be discontinued if adverse events are observed. According to the manufacturer, the decision to continue or discontinue breast-feeding during therapy should take into account the risk of exposure to the infant and the benefits of treatment to the mother. Respiratory depression, seizures, nausea, vomiting, diarrhea, and/or decreased feeding have been observed in neonates exposed to carbamazepine *in utero* and may represent a neonatal withdrawal syndrome.

Medication Guide Available Yes

Contraindications Hypersensitivity to carbamazepine, tricyclic antidepressants, or any component of the formulation; bone marrow depression; with or within 14 days of MAO inhibitor use; concurrent use of nefazodone; concomitant use of delavirdine or other non-nucleoside reverse transcriptase inhibitors

Warnings/Precautions Hazardous agent - use appropriate precautions for handling and disposal (NIOSH, 2012). **[U.S. Boxed Warning]: The risk of developing aplastic anemia or agranulocytosis is increased during treatment. Monitor CBC, platelets, and differential prior to and during therapy; discontinue if significant bone marrow suppression occurs.** A spectrum of hematologic effects has been reported with use (eg, agranulocytosis, aplastic anemia, neutropenia, leukopenia, thrombocytopenia, pancytopenia, and anemias); patients with a previous history of adverse hematologic reaction to any drug may be at increased risk. Early detection of hematologic change is important; advise patients of early signs and symptoms including fever, sore throat, mouth ulcers, infections, easy bruising, and petechial or purpuric hemorrhage.

[U.S. Boxed Warning]: Severe and sometimes fatal dermatologic reactions, including toxic epidermal necrolysis (TENS) and Stevens-Johnson syndrome (SJS), may occur during therapy. The risk is increased in patients with the variant *HLA-B*1502* allele, found almost exclusively in patients of Asian ancestry. Patients of Asian descent should be screened prior to initiating therapy. Avoid use in patients testing positive for the allele; discontinue therapy in patients who have a serious dermatologic reaction. The risk of SJS or TENS may also be increased if carbamazepine is used in combination with other antiepileptic drugs associated with these reactions. Presence of the *HLA-B*1502* allele has not been found to predict the risk of less serious dermatologic reactions such as anticonvulsant hypersensitivity syndrome or nonserious rash. The risk of developing a hypersensitivity reaction may be increased in patients with the variant *HLA-A*3101* allele. The *HLA-A*3101* allele may occur more frequently patients of African-American, Asian, European, Indian, Latin American, and Native American ancestry. Hypersensitivity has also been reported in patients experiencing reactions to other anticonvulsants; the history of hypersensitivity reactions in the patient or their immediate family members should be reviewed. Approximately 25% to 30% of patients allergic to carbamazepine will also have reactions with oxcarbazepine. Potentially serious, sometimes fatal multiorgan hypersensitivity reactions (also known as drug reaction with eosinophilia and systemic symptoms [DRESS]) have been reported with some antiepileptic drugs including carbamazepine; monitor for signs and symptoms of possible disparate manifestations associated with lymphatic, hepatic, renal, and/or hematologic organ systems; gradual discontinuation and conversion to alternate therapy may be required.

Antiepileptics are associated with an increased risk of suicidal behavior/thoughts with use (regardless of indication); patients should be monitored for signs/symptoms of depression, suicidal tendencies, and other unusual behavior changes during therapy and instructed to inform their healthcare provider immediately if symptoms occur.

Administer carbamazepine with caution to patients with history of cardiac damage, ECG abnormalities (or at risk for ECG abnormalities), hepatic or renal disease. When used to treat bipolar disorder, the smallest effective dose is suggested to reduce the risk for overdose/suicide; high-risk patients should be monitored for suicidal ideations. Prescription should be written for the smallest quantity consistent with good patient care. May activate latent psychosis and/or cause confusion or agitation; elderly patients may be at an increased risk for psychiatric effects.

Carbamazepine is not effective in absence, myoclonic, or akinetic seizures; exacerbation of certain seizure types have been seen after initiation of carbamazepine therapy in children with mixed seizure disorders. Abrupt discontinuation is not recommended in patients being treated for seizures. Dizziness or drowsiness may occur; caution should be used when performing tasks which require alertness until the effects are known. Effects with other sedative drugs or ethanol may be potentiated. Carbamazepine has a high potential for drug interactions; use caution in patients taking strong CYP3A4 inducers or inhibitors or medications significantly metabolized via CYP1A2, 2B6, 2C9, 2C19, and 3A4. Coadministration of carbamazepine and nefazodone may lead to insufficient plasma levels of nefazodone; combination is contraindicated. Coadministration yields insufficient plasma levels of delavirdine and other non-nucleoside reverse transcriptase inhibitors to achieve a therapeutic effect; concurrent use is contraindicated. Carbamazepine has mild anticholinergic activity; use with caution in patients with increased intraocular pressure, or sensitivity to anticholinergic effects. Hyponatremia caused by the syndrome of inappropriate antidiuretic hormone secretion (SIADH) may occur during therapy. Risk may be increased in the elderly or in patients also taking diuretics and may be dose-dependent. Use caution in elderly patients; may cause or exacerbate syndrome of inappropriate antidiuretic hormone secretion or hyponatremia; monitor sodium closely with initiation or dosage adjustments in older adults (Beers Criteria).

Administration of the suspension will yield higher peak and lower trough serum levels than an equal dose of the tablet form; consider a lower starting dose given more frequently (same total daily dose) when using the suspension. The suspension may contain sorbitol; avoid use in patents with hereditary fructose intolerance.

Adverse Reactions Frequency not defined, unless otherwise specified.

Cardiovascular: Hypertension (3%), atrioventricular block, cardiac arrhythmia, cardiac failure, coronary artery disease exacerbation, edema, hypotension, syncope, thromboembolism, thrombophlebitis

Central nervous system: Dizziness (44%), drowsiness (32%), headache (22%), ataxia (15%), speech disturbance (6%), abnormality in thinking (2%), paresthesia (2%), vertigo (2%), agitation, amnesia, chills, confusion, depression, fatigue, fever, hallucination, neuroleptic malignant syndrome (NMS), peripheral neuritis, slurred speech, talkativeness

Dermatologic: Pruritus (8%), skin rash (7%), abnormal thyroid function test, acute generalized exanthematous pustulosis, alopecia, dyschromia, erythema multiforme, erythema nodosum, exfoliative dermatitis, onychomadesis, purpura, skin photosensitivity, Stevens-Johnson syndrome, toxic epidermal necrolysis, urticaria

Endocrine & metabolic: Hypocalcemia, hyponatremia, SIADH, abnormal thyroid function test

Gastrointestinal: Nausea (29%), vomiting (18%), constipation (10%), xerostomia (8%), abdominal pain, anorexia, diarrhea, dry throat, gastric distress, glossitis, pancreatitis, stomatitis

Genitourinary: Impotence, urinary frequency, urinary retention

Hematologic & oncologic: Agranulocytosis, anemia, aplastic anemia, bone marrow depression, eosinophilia, leukocytosis, leukopenia, lymphadenopathy, pancytopenia, porphyria, thrombocytopenia

Hepatic: Abnormal hepatic function tests, hepatic failure, hepatitis, jaundice

Hypersensitivity: Hypersensitivity reaction, multi-organ hypersensitivity

Neuromuscular & skeletal: Weakness (8%), tremor (3%), twitching (2%), arthralgia, leg cramps, myalgia, osteoporosis, systemic lupus erythematosus exacerbation

Ophthalmic: Blurred vision (6%), cataract, conjunctivitis, diplopia, increased intraocular pressure, nystagmus, oculomotor disturbance

Otic: Hyperacusis, tinnitus

Renal: Albuminuria, azotemia, glycosuria, increased blood urea nitrogen, oliguria, renal failure

Miscellaneous: Diaphoresis

Postmarketing and/or case reports (Limited to important or life-threatening): Aseptic meningitis, defective spermatogenesis, hirsutism, lupus-like syndrome, maculopapular rash, paralysis, reduced fertility (male), suicidal ideation

Drug Interactions

Metabolism/Transport Effects Substrate of CYP2C8 (minor), CYP3A4 (major); **Note:** Assignment of Major/Minor substrate status based on clinically relevant drug interaction potential; **Induces** CYP1A2 (strong), CYP2B6 (strong), CYP2C19 (strong), CYP2C8 (strong), CYP2C9 (strong), CYP3A4 (strong), P-glycoprotein

Avoid Concomitant Use

Avoid concomitant use of CarBAMazepine with any of the following: Abiraterone Acetate; Apixaban; Artemether; Axitinib; Azelastine (Nasal); Bedaquiline; Boceprevir; Bortezomib; Bosutinib; Cabozantinib; CloZAPine; Conivaptan; Crizotinib; Dabigatran Etexilate; Dienogest; Dolutegravir; Dronedarone; Enzalutamide; Everolimus; Fusidic Acid (Systemic); Ibrutinib; Itraconazole; Ivacaftor; Lapatinib; Lumefantrine; Lurasidone; Macitentan; MAO Inhibitors; Mifepristone; Nefazodone; NIFEdipine; Nilotinib; Nisoldipine; Paraldehyde; PAZOPanib; Pirfenidone; Pomalidomide; PONATinib; Praziquantel; Ranolazine; Regorafenib; Reverse Transcriptase Inhibitors (Non-Nucleoside); Rivaroxaban; Roflumilast; RomiDEPsin; Simeprevir; Sofosbuvir; SORAfenib; Telaprevir; Ticagrelor; Tofacitinib; Tolvaptan; Toremifene; TraMADol; Ulipristal; Vandetanib; Vemurafenib; VinCRIStine (Liposomal); Voriconazole

Increased Effect/Toxicity

CarBAMazepine may increase the levels/effects of: Adenosine; Alcohol (Ethyl); Azelastine (Nasal); Buprenorphine; Clarithromycin; ClomiPRAMINE; CloZAPine; CNS Depressants; Desmopressin; Eslicarbazepine; Fosphenytoin; Hydrocodone; Ifosfamide; Lithium; MAO Inhibitors; Methotrimeprazine; Metyrosine; Mirtazapine; Paraldehyde; Phenytoin; Pramipexole; ROPINIRole; Rotigotine

The levels/effects of CarBAMazepine may be increased by: Allopurinol; Brimonidine (Topical); Calcium Channel Blockers (Nondihydropyridine); Carbonic Anhydrase Inhibitors; Cimetidine; Clarithromycin; Conivaptan; CYP3A4 Inhibitors (Moderate); CYP3A4 Inhibitors (Strong); Danazol; Darunavir; Doxylamine; Droperidol; Fluconazole; Fusidic Acid (Systemic); Grapefruit Juice; HydrOXYzine; Isoniazid; LamoTRIgine; Luliconazole; Macrolide Antibiotics; Magnesium Sulfate; Methotrimeprazine; Nefazodone; Protease Inhibitors; QuiNINE; Selective Serotonin Reuptake Inhibitors; Sodium Oxybate; Tapentadol; Telaprevir; Thiazide Diuretics; TraMADol; Zolpidem

Decreased Effect

CarBAMazepine may decrease the levels/effects of: Abiraterone Acetate; Acetaminophen; Afatinib; Apixaban; ARIPiprazole; Artemether; Axitinib; Bazedoxifene; Bedaquiline; Bendamustine; Benzodiazepines (metabolized by oxidation); Boceprevir; Bortezomib; Bosutinib; Brentuximab Vedotin; Cabozantinib; Calcium Channel Blockers (Dihydropyridine); Calcium Channel Blockers (Nondihydropyridine); Caspofungin; Clarithromycin; CloZAPine; Cobicistat; Contraceptives (Estrogens); Contraceptives (Progestins); Crizotinib; CycloSPORINE (Systemic); CYP1A2 Substrates; CYP2B6 Substrates; CYP2C19 Substrates; CYP2C8 Substrates; CYP2C9 Substrates; CYP3A4 Substrates; Dabigatran Etexilate; Dasatinib; Diclofenac (Systemic); Dienogest; Dolutegravir; Doxycycline; Dronedarone; Elvitegravir; Enzalutamide; Eslicarbazepine; Everolimus; Exemestane; Ezogabine; Felbamate; Flunarizine; Fosphenytoin; Gefitinib; GuanFACINE; Haloperidol; Ibrutinib; Imatinib; Irinotecan; Itraconazole; Ivacaftor; Ixabepilone; Lacosamide; LamoTRIgine; Lapatinib; Linagliptin; Lopinavir; Lumefantrine; Lurasidone; Macitentan; Maraviroc; Mebendazole; Methadone; MethylPREDNISolone; Mifepristone; Nefazodone; NIFEdipine; Nilotinib; Nisoldipine; OXcarbazepine; Paliperidone; PAZOPanib; Perampanel; P-glycoprotein/ABCB1 Substrates; Phenytoin; Pirfenidone; Pomalidomide; PONATinib; Praziquantel; Protease Inhibitors; QUEtiapine; QuiNINE; Ranolazine; Regorafenib; Reverse Transcriptase Inhibitors (Non-Nucleoside); RisperiDONE; Rivaroxaban; Roflumilast; RomiDEPsin; Rufinamide; Saxagliptin; Selective Serotonin Reuptake Inhibitors; Simeprevir; Sofosbuvir; SORAfenib; SUNItinib; Tadalafil; Telaprevir; Temsirolimus; Theophylline Derivatives; Thyroid Products; Ticagrelor; Tofacitinib; Tolvaptan; Topiramate; Toremifene; TraMADol; Treprostinil; Tricyclic Antidepressants; Ulipristal; Valproic Acid and Derivatives; Vandetanib; Vecuronium; Vemurafenib; VinCRIStine (Liposomal); Vitamin K Antagonists; Voriconazole; Vortioxetine; Ziprasidone; Zolpidem; Zuclopenthixol

The levels/effects of CarBAMazepine may be decreased by: Bosentan; CYP3A4 Inducers (Strong); Dabrafenib; Deferasirox; Felbamate; Fosphenytoin; Herbs (CYP3A4 Inducers); Ketorolac (Nasal); Ketorolac (Systemic); Mefloquine; Methylfolate; Mitotane; Orlistat; Phenytoin; Reverse Transcriptase Inhibitors (Non-Nucleoside); Rufinamide; Theophylline Derivatives; Tocilizumab; TraMADol; Valproic Acid and Derivatives

Ethanol/Nutrition/Herb Interactions

Ethanol: Ethanol may increase CNS depression. Management: Avoid concurrent use of ethanol.

Food: Carbamazepine serum levels may be increased if taken with food and/or grapefruit juice. Management Avoid concurrent ingestion of grapefruit juice. Maintain adequate hydration, unless instructed to restrict fluid intake.

Herb/Nutraceutical: Evening primrose may decrease seizure threshold. Valerian, St John's wort, kava kava, and gotu kola may increase CNS depression. Management: Avoid evening primrose. Avoid valerian, St John's wort, kava kava, and gotu kola.

Storage/Stability

Carbatrol®, Equetro®: Store at controlled room temperature (25°C [77°F]); excursions permitted to 15°C to 30°C (59°F to 86°F); protect from light and moisture.

Tegretol®-XR: Store at controlled room temperature, 15°C to 30°C (59°F to 86°F); protect from moisture.

Tegretol® tablets and chewable tablets: Store at ≤30°C (86°F); protect from light and moisture.

Tegretol® suspension: Store at ≤30°C (86°F); shake well before using.

Mechanism of Action In addition to anticonvulsant effects, carbamazepine has anticholinergic, antineuralgic, antidiuretic, muscle relaxant, antimanic, antidepressive, and antiarrhythmic properties; may depress activity in the nucleus ventralis of the thalamus or decrease synaptic transmission or decrease summation of temporal stimulation leading to neural discharge by limiting influx of sodium ions across cell membrane or other unknown mechanisms; stimulates the release of ADH and potentiates its action in promoting reabsorption of water; chemically related to tricyclic antidepressants

Pharmacodynamics/Kinetics

Absorption: Slow

Distribution: V_d: Neonates: 1.5 L/kg; Children: 1.9 L/kg; Adults: 0.59-2 L/kg

Protein binding: Carbamazepine: 75% to 90%, may be decreased in newborns; Epoxide metabolite: 50%

Metabolism: Hepatic via CYP3A4 to active epoxide metabolite; induces hepatic enzymes to increase metabolism

Bioavailability: 85%

Half-life elimination: **Note:** Half-life is variable because of autoinduction which is usually complete 3-5 weeks after initiation of a fixed carbamazepine regimen.

Carbamazepine: Initial: 25-65 hours; Extended release: 35-40 hours; Multiple doses: Children: 8-14 hours; Adults: 12-17 hours

Epoxide metabolite: Initial: 25-43 hours

Time to peak, serum: Unpredictable:

Immediate release: Suspension: 1.5 hour; tablet: 4-5 hours

Extended release: Carbatrol®, Equetro®: 12-26 hours (single dose), 4-8 hours (multiple doses); Tegretol®-XR: 3-12 hours

Excretion: Urine 72% (1% to 3% as unchanged drug); feces (28%)

Dosage Dosage must be adjusted according to patient's response and serum concentrations. Administer tablets (chewable or conventional) in 2-3 divided doses daily and suspension in 4 divided doses daily. Oral:

Epilepsy:

Children:

<6 years: Initial: 10-20 mg/kg/day divided twice or 3 times daily as tablets or 4 times/day as suspension; increase dose every week until optimal response and therapeutic levels are achieved

Maintenance dose: Divide into 3-4 doses daily (tablets or suspension); maximum recommended dose: 35 mg/kg/day

6-12 years: Initial: 200 mg/day in 2 divided doses (tablets or extended release tablets) or 4 divided doses (oral suspension); increase by up to 100 mg/day at weekly intervals using a twice daily regimen of extended release tablets or 3-4 times daily regimen of other formulations until optimal response and therapeutic levels are achieved

Maintenance: Usual: 400-800 mg/day; maximum recommended dose: 1000 mg/day

Note: Children <12 years who receive ≥400 mg/day of carbamazepine may be converted to extended release capsules (Carbatrol®) using the same total daily dosage divided twice daily

Children >12 years and Adults: Initial: 400 mg/day in 2 divided doses (tablets or extended release tablets) or 4 divided doses (oral suspension); increase by up to 200 mg/day at weekly intervals using a twice daily regimen of extended release tablets or capsules, or a 3-4 times/day regimen of other formulations until optimal response and therapeutic levels are achieved; usual dose: 800-1200 mg/day

Maximum recommended doses:

Children 12-15 years: 1000 mg/day

Children >15 years: 1200 mg/day

Adults: 1600 mg/day; however, some patients have required up to 1.6-2.4 g/day

Trigeminal or glossopharyngeal neuralgia: Adults: Initial: 200 mg/day in 2 divided doses (tablets, extended release tablets, or extended release capsules) or 4 divided doses (oral suspension) with food, gradually increasing in increments of 200 mg/day as needed

Maintenance: Usual: 400-800 mg daily in 2 divided doses (tablets, extended release tablets, or extended release capsules) or 4 divided doses (oral suspension); maximum dose: 1200 mg/day

Bipolar disorder: Adults: Initial: 400 mg/day in 2 divided doses (tablets, extended release tablets, or extended release capsules) or 4 divided doses (oral suspension), may adjust by 200 mg/day increments; maximum dose: 1600 mg/day.

Note: Equetro® is the only formulation specifically approved by the FDA for the management of bipolar disorder.

Neuropathic pain, critically-ill patients (unlabeled use): Initial: 50-100 mg twice daily in combination with I.V. opioids; Maintenance: 100-200 mg every 4-6 hours; maximum dose: 1200 mg daily (Barr, 2013)

Dosing adjustment in renal impairment: Dosage adjustments are not required or recommended in the manufacturer's labeling; however, the following guidelines have been used by some clinicians (Aronoff, 2007):

Children and Adults:

GFR <10 mL/minute: Administer 75% of dose

Hemodialysis, peritoneal dialysis: Administer 75% of dose (postdialysis)

Continuous renal replacement therapy (CRRT):

Children: Administer 75% of dose

Adults: No dosage adjustment recommended

Dosing adjustment in hepatic impairment: Use with caution in hepatic impairment; metabolized primarily in the liver

Dietary Considerations Drug may cause GI upset, take with large amount of water or food to decrease GI upset. May need to split doses to avoid GI upset.

Administration

Suspension: Must be given on a 3-4 times/day schedule versus tablets which can be given 2-4 times/day. Since a given dose of suspension will produce higher peak and lower trough levels than the same dose given as the tablet form, patients given the suspension should be started on lower doses given more frequently (same total daily dose) and increased slowly to avoid unwanted side effects. When carbamazepine suspension has been combined with chlorpromazine or thioridazine solutions, a precipitate forms which may result in loss of effect. Therefore, it is recommended that the carbamazepine suspension dosage form not be administered at the same time with other liquid medicinal agents or diluents. Should be administered with meals.

Extended release capsule (Carbatrol®, Equetro®): Consists of three different types of beads: Immediate release, extended-release, and enteric release. The bead types are combined in a ratio to allow twice daily dosing. May be opened and contents sprinkled over food such as a teaspoon of applesauce; may be administered with or without food; do not crush or chew.

Extended release tablet: Should be inspected for damage. Damaged extended release tablets (without release portal) should not be administered. Should be administered with meals; swallow whole, do not crush or chew.

Hazardous agent; use appropriate precautions for handling and disposal (NIOSH, 2012).

Monitoring Parameters CBC with platelet count and differential, reticulocytes, serum iron, lipid panel, liver function tests, urinalysis, BUN, serum carbamazepine levels, thyroid function tests, serum sodium; pregnancy test; ophthalmic exams (intraocular pressure, pupillary reflexes); observe patient for excessive sedation, especially when instituting or increasing therapy; signs of rash; *HLA-B*1502* genotype screening prior to therapy initiation in patients of Asian descent; suicidality (eg, suicidal thoughts, depression, behavioral changes)

Reference Range

Timing of serum samples: Absorption is slow, peak levels occur 8-65 hours after ingestion of the first dose; the half-life ranges from 8-60 hours, therefore, steady-state is achieved in 2-5 days

Epilepsy: Therapeutic levels: 4-12 mcg/mL (SI: 17-51 micromole/L)

Toxic concentration: >15 mcg/mL; patients who require higher levels of 8-12 mcg/mL (SI: 34-51 micromole/L) should be watched closely. Side effects including CNS effects occur commonly at higher dosage levels. If other anticonvulsants are given therapeutic range is 4-8 mcg/mL.

Test Interactions May cause false-positive serum TCA screen; may interact with some pregnancy tests

Dosage Forms Excipient information presented when available (limited, particularly for generics); consult specific product labeling.

Capsule Extended Release 12 Hour, Oral:

Carbatrol: 100 mg [contains fd&c blue #2 (indigotine)]

Carbatrol: 200 mg, 300 mg

Equetro: 100 mg, 200 mg, 300 mg [contains fd&c blue #2 (indigotine)]

Generic: 100 mg, 200 mg, 300 mg

Suspension, Oral:

TEGretol: 100 mg/5 mL (450 mL) [contains fd&c yellow #6 (sunset yellow), propylene glycol; citrus-vanilla flavor]

Generic: 100 mg/5 mL (450 mL)

Tablet, Oral:

Epitol: 200 mg [scored]

TEGretol: 200 mg [scored; contains fd&c red #40]

Generic: 200 mg

Tablet Chewable, Oral:

Generic: 100 mg

Tablet Extended Release 12 Hour, Oral:

TEGretol-XR: 100 mg, 200 mg, 400 mg

Generic: 200 mg, 400 mg

Extemporaneous Preparations Hazardous agent: Use appropriate precautions for handling and disposal.

Note: Commercial oral suspension is available (20 mg/mL)

A 40 mg/mL oral suspension may be made with tablets. Crush twenty 200 mg tablets in a mortar and reduce to a fine powder. Add small portions of Simple Syrup, NF and mix to a uniform paste; mix while adding the vehicle in incremental proportions to **almost** 100 mL; transfer to a calibrated bottle, rinse mortar with vehicle, and add sufficient quantity of vehicle to make 100 mL. Label "shake well" and "refrigerate". Stable for 90 days.

Nahata MC, Pai VB, and Hipple TF, *Pediatric Drug Formulations*, 5th ed, Cincinnati, OH: Harvey Whitney Books Co, 2004.

◆ Carbamide *see* Urea *on page* 2140

Carbamide Peroxide (KAR ba mide per OKS ide)

Brand Names: U.S. Auraphene-B [OTC]; Debrox [OTC]; E-R-O Ear Drops [OTC]; E-R-O Ear Wax Removal System [OTC]; Ear Drops Earwax Aid [OTC]; Ear Wax Remover [OTC]; Earwax Treatment Drops [OTC]; Gly-Oxide [OTC]; Thera-Ear [OTC]

Index Terms Urea Peroxide

Pharmacologic Category Anti-inflammatory, Locally Applied; Otic Agent, Cerumenolytic

Use Relief of minor inflammation of gums, oral mucosal surfaces, and lips including canker sores and dental irritation; emulsify and disperse ear wax

Dosage Children and Adults:

Oral: Inflammation/dental irritation: Solution (should not be used for >7 days): Oral preparation should not be used in children <2 years of age; apply several drops undiluted on affected area 4 times/day after meals and at bedtime; expectorate after 2-3 minutes **or** place 10 drops onto tongue, mix with saliva, swish for several minutes, expectorate

Otic:

Children <12 years: Tilt head sideways and individualize the dose according to patient size; 3 drops (range: 1-5 drops) twice daily for up to 4 days, tip of applicator should not enter ear canal; keep drops in ear for several minutes by keeping head tilted and placing cotton in ear

Children ≥12 years and Adults: Tilt head sideways and instill 5-10 drops twice daily up to 4 days, tip of applicator should not enter ear canal; keep drops in ear for several minutes by keeping head tilted and placing cotton in ear

Additional Information Complete prescribing information should be consulted for additional detail.

Dosage Forms Excipient information presented when available (limited, particularly for generics); consult specific product labeling.

Solution, Mouth/Throat:

Gly-Oxide: 10% (15 mL, 60 mL) [contains propylene glycol]

Solution, Otic:

Auraphene-B: 6.5% (15 mL)

Debrox: 6.5% (15 mL) [contains propylene glycol]

E-R-O Ear Drops: 6.5% (15 mL) [contains glycerin]

E-R-O Ear Wax Removal System: 6.5% (15 mL)

Ear Drops Earwax Aid: 6.5% (15 mL) [contains propylene glycol, trolamine (triethanolamine)]

Ear Wax Remover: 6.5% (15 mL) [contains propylene glycol]

Earwax Treatment Drops: 6.5% (15 mL)

Thera-Ear: 6.5% (15 mL)

◆ Carbamylcholine Chloride *see* Carbachol *on page* 335

◆ Carbatrol *see* CarBAMazepine *on page* 336

Carbidopa (kar bi DOE pa)

Brand Names: U.S. Lodosyn

Pharmacologic Category Anti-Parkinson's Agent, Decarboxylase Inhibitor

Use Given with carbidopa-levodopa in the treatment of parkinsonism to enable a lower dosage of levodopa to be used and a more rapid response to be obtained and to decrease side effects; use with carbidopa-levodopa in patients requiring additional carbidopa; has no effect without levodopa

Pregnancy Risk Factor C

Dosage Oral: Adults: **Note:** Optimal daily dosage determined by careful titration; generally if carbidopa is ≥70 mg/day, a 1:10 proportion of carbidopa:levodopa provides the most patient response.

Carbidopa augmentation in patients receiving carbidopa-levodopa:

Patients receiving Sinemet® 10/100: 25 mg carbidopa daily with first daily dose of Sinemet® 10/100; if necessary, 12.5-25 mg carbidopa may be given with each subsequent dose of Sinemet® 10/100; maximum: 200 mg carbidopa/day (including carbidopa from Sinemet®)

Patients receiving Sinemet® 25/250 or Sinemet® 25/100: 25 mg carbidopa with any dose of Sinemet® 25/250 or Sinemet® 25/100 throughout the day; maximum: 200 mg carbidopa/day (including carbidopa from Sinemet®)

Individual titration of carbidopa and levodopa: Initial: 25 mg carbidopa 3-4 times/day; administer at the same time as levodopa, initial dose of levodopa should be 20% to 25% of the previous levodopa dose in carbidopa-naive patients; first dose of carbidopa should be taken ≥12 hours after the last dose of levodopa in carbidopa-naive patients; increase or decrease dose by 1/2 or 1 tablet/day

Additional Information Complete prescribing information should be consulted for additional detail.

Dosage Forms Excipient information presented when available (limited, particularly for generics); consult specific product labeling.

Tablet, Oral:

Lodosyn: 25 mg [scored; contains fd&c yellow #6 (sunset yellow)]

Carbidopa and Levodopa
(kar bi DOE pa & lee voe DOE pa)

Brand Names: U.S. Parcopa®; Sinemet®; Sinemet® CR

Brand Names: Canada Apo-Levocarb®; Apo-Levocarb® CR; Dom-Levo-Carbidopa; Duodopa™; Levocarb CR; Nu-Levocarb; PRO-Levocarb; Sinemet®; Sinemet® CR; Teva-Levocarbidopa

Index Terms Levodopa and Carbidopa

Pharmacologic Category Anti-Parkinson's Agent, Decarboxylase Inhibitor; Anti-Parkinson's Agent, Dopamine Precursor

Additional Appendix Information

Antiparkinsonian Agents *on page* 2289

Use Idiopathic Parkinson's disease; postencephalitic parkinsonism; symptomatic parkinsonism

Duodopa™ intestinal gel: Canadian labeling (not available in U.S.): Treatment of advanced levodopa-responsive Parkinson's disease in which severe motor symptoms are not controlled by other Parkinson's agents

Unlabeled Use Restless leg syndrome

Pregnancy Risk Factor C

Pregnancy Considerations Adverse events were observed in some animal reproduction studies using this combination. Carbidopa can be detected in the umbilical cord but absorption in fetal tissue is minimal. Levodopa crosses the placenta and can be metabolized by the fetus and detected in fetal tissue (Merchant, 1995). The incidence of Parkinson's disease in pregnancy is relatively rare, and information related to the use of carbidopa/levodopa in pregnant women is limited (Ball, 1995; Cook, 1985; Golbe, 1987; Serikawa, 2011; Shulman, 2000).

Current guidelines note that the available information is insufficient to make a recommendation for the treatment of restless leg syndrome in pregnant women (Aurora, 2012).

Breast-Feeding Considerations Levodopa is excreted into breast milk. A study was done in one lactating woman at 4.5 months postpartum who had been taking carbidopa/levodopa for several years. Regardless of the formulation (sustained release or immediate release) peak levodopa concentrations in the breast milk were found ~3 hours after the maternal dose and returned to baseline ~6 hours after the dose. The highest milk concentration (3.47 nmol/L) was found following the immediate release tablet and this was 27% of the peak maternal plasma concentration (occurring 30 minutes after the dose) and ~40% of the simultaneous plasma concentration. Carbidopa was not evaluated (Thulin, 1998). The manufacturer recommends that caution be used if administered to nursing women.

Prescribing and Access Restrictions Duodopa™ intestinal gel (Canadian labeling; product not available in U.S.): In Canada, the Duodopa™ Education Program is a risk mitigation program established to provide safe and effective use of Duodopa™ in advanced Parkinson's patients. The program involves:

- Education of prescribing neurologists and other health-care providers on suitable candidates for treatment, surgical procedures (PEG tube placement), and follow-up care including infusion device education.
- Distribution of educational materials to patients and caregivers describing Duodopa™ intestinal gel and its proper use, PEG tube placement, and complications associated with the mode of administration and/or PEG tube placement.

Contraindications Hypersensitivity to levodopa, carbidopa, or any component of the formulation; narrow-angle glaucoma; use of MAO inhibitors within prior 14 days (however, may be administered concomitantly with the manufacturer's recommended dose of an MAO inhibitor with selectivity for MAO type B); history of melanoma or undiagnosed skin lesions

Canadian labeling: Additional contraindications: Clinical or laboratory evidence of uncompensated cardiovascular, cerebrovascular, endocrine, renal, hepatic, hematologic or pulmonary disease; when administration of a sympathomimetic amine (eg, epinephrine, norepinephrine or isoproterenol) is contraindicated; intestinal gel therapy in patients with any condition preventing the required placement of a PEG tube for administration.

Warnings/Precautions Use with caution in patients with history of cardiovascular disease (including myocardial infarction and arrhythmias), pulmonary diseases (such as asthma), psychosis, wide-angle glaucoma, peptic ulcer disease, seizure disorder or prone to seizures, and in severe renal and hepatic dysfunction. Use with caution when interpreting plasma/urine catecholamine levels; falsely diagnosed pheochromocytoma has been rarely reported. Severe cases or rhabdomyolysis have been reported. Sudden discontinuation of levodopa may cause a worsening of Parkinson's disease. Elderly may be more sensitive to CNS effects of levodopa. May cause or exacerbate dyskinesias. Patients have reported falling asleep while engaging in activities of daily living; this has been reported to occur without significant warning signs. May cause orthostatic hypotension; Parkinson's disease patients appear to have an impaired capacity to respond to a postural challenge; use with caution in patients at risk of hypotension (such as those receiving antihypertensive drugs) or where transient hypotensive episodes would be poorly tolerated (cardiovascular disease or cerebrovascular disease). Observe patients closely for development of depression with concomitant suicidal tendencies.

Dopamine agonists have been associated with compulsive behaviors and/or loss of impulse control, which has manifested as pathological gambling, libido increases (hypersexuality), and/or binge eating. Causality has not been established, and controversy exists as to whether this phenomenon is related to the underlying disease, prior behaviors/addictions and/or drug therapy. Dose reduction or discontinuation of therapy has been reported to reverse these behaviors in some, but not all cases. Risk for melanoma development is increased in Parkinson's disease patients; drug causation or factors contributing to risk have not been established. Patients should be monitored closely and periodic skin examinations should be performed. Dopaminergic agents have been associated with a syndrome resembling neuroleptic malignant syndrome on abrupt withdrawal or significant dosage reduction after long-term use. Protein in the diet should be distributed throughout the day to avoid fluctuations in levodopa absorption.

Intestinal gel (available in Canada, not available in U.S.): Product should be prescribed only by neurologists experienced in the treatment of Parkinson's disease and who have completed the Duodopa™ Education Program. Response to levodopa/carbidopa intestinal gel therapy should be assessed with a test period (~3 days) of administration via a temporary nasoduodenal tube prior to placement of a percutaneous endoscopic gastrostomy (PEG) tube for permanent access and administration. Sudden deterioration in therapy response with recurring motor symptoms may indicate PEG tube complications (eg, displacement) or obstruction of the infusion device. Tube or infusion device complications may require initiation of oral levodopa/carbidopa therapy until complications are resolved. Discontinue therapy 2-3 hours prior to surgical procedures requiring general anesthesia, if possible. May resume therapy postoperatively when oral fluid intake is permitted.

Adverse Reactions Frequency not defined.

Cardiovascular: Arrhythmia, chest pain, edema, flushing, hypotension, hypertension, MI, orthostatic hypotension, palpitation, phlebitis, syncope

Central nervous system: Agitation, anxiety, ataxia, confusion, delusions, dementia, depression (with or without suicidal tendencies), disorientation, dizziness, dreams abnormal, EPS, euphoria, faintness, falling, fatigue, gait abnormalities, headache, hallucinations, impulse control symptoms, insomnia, malaise, memory impairment, mental acuity decreased, nervousness, neuroleptic malignant syndrome, nightmares, on-off phenomena, paranoid ideation, pathological gambling, psychosis, seizure (causal relationship not established), somnolence

Dermatologic: Alopecia, malignant melanoma, rash

Endocrine & metabolic: Hot flashes, hyperglycemia, hypokalemia, libido increased (including hypersexuality), uric acid increased

Gastrointestinal: Abdominal pain, abdominal distress, anorexia, bruxism, constipation, diarrhea, discoloration of saliva, duodenal ulcer, dyspepsia, dysphagia, flatulence, GI bleeding, heartburn, nausea, sialorrhea, taste alterations, tongue burning sensation, weight gain/loss, vomiting, xerostomia

Genitourinary: Discoloration of urine, glycosuria, urinary frequency, priapism, proteinuria, urinary incontinence, urinary retention, urinary tract infection

Hematologic: Agranulocytosis, anemia, Coombs' test abnormal, hematocrit decreased, hemoglobin decreased, hemolytic anemia, leukopenia

Hepatic: Alkaline phosphatase abnormal, ALT abnormal, AST abnormal, bilirubin abnormal, LDH abnormal

Neuromuscular & skeletal: Back pain, dyskinesias (including choreiform, dystonic and other involuntary movements), leg pain, muscle cramps, muscle twitching, numbness, paresthesia, peripheral neuropathy, shoulder pain, tremor increased, trismus, weakness

Ocular: Blepharospasm, blurred vision, diplopia, Horner's syndrome reactivation, mydriasis, oculogyric crises (may be associated with acute dystonic reactions)

Renal: Difficult urination

Respiratory: Cough, dyspnea, hoarseness, pharyngeal pain, upper respiratory infection

Miscellaneous: Discoloration of sweat, diaphoresis increased, hiccups, hypersensitivity reactions (angioedema, pruritus, urticaria, bullous lesions [including pemphigus-like reactions], Henoch-Schönlein purpura [IgA vasculitis])

Drug Interactions

Metabolism/Transport Effects None known.

Avoid Concomitant Use

Avoid concomitant use of Carbidopa and Levodopa with any of the following: Amisulpride; Sulpiride

Increased Effect/Toxicity

Carbidopa and Levodopa may increase the levels/effects of: MAO Inhibitors

The levels/effects of Carbidopa and Levodopa may be increased by: MAO Inhibitors; Methylphenidate; Sapropterin

Decreased Effect

Carbidopa and Levodopa may decrease the levels/effects of: Amisulpride; Antipsychotics (Typical); Sulpiride

The levels/effects of Carbidopa and Levodopa may be decreased by: Amisulpride; Antipsychotics (Atypical); Antipsychotics (Typical); Fosphenytoin; Glycopyrrolate; Iron Salts; Methionine; Metoclopramide; Multivitamins/Fluoride (with ADE); Multivitamins/Minerals (with ADEK, Folate, Iron); Multivitamins/Minerals (with AE, No Iron); Phenytoin; Pyridoxine; Sulpiride

Ethanol/Nutrition/Herb Interactions

Ethanol: Avoid ethanol (due to CNS depression).

Food: Avoid high protein diets due to potential for impaired levodopa absorption; levodopa competes with certain amino acids for transport across the gut wall or across the blood-brain barrier.

Herb/Nutraceutical: Avoid kava kava (may decrease effects). Pyridoxine (vitamin B_6) in doses >10-25 mg (for levodopa alone) may decrease efficacy. Iron supplements or iron-containing multivitamins may reduce absorption of levodopa.

Storage/Stability

Tablet: Store at 20°C to 25°C (68°F to 77°F); excursions permitted between 15°C to 30°C (59°F to 86°F). Protect from light and moisture.

Intestinal gel (Canadian labeling; not available in U.S.): Store in refrigerator at 2°C to 8°C (36°F to 46°F). Keep in outer carton to protect from light. Cassettes are for single use only and should be discarded daily following infusion (up to 16 hours).

Mechanism of Action Parkinson's symptoms are due to a lack of striatal dopamine; levodopa circulates in the plasma to the blood-brain-barrier (BBB), where it crosses, to be converted by striatal enzymes to dopamine; carbidopa inhibits the peripheral plasma breakdown of levodopa by inhibiting its decarboxylation, and thereby increases available levodopa at the BBB

Pharmacodynamics/Kinetics

Distribution: Levodopa: 0.9-1.6 L/kg (in presence of carbidopa), crosses the blood-brain barrier;Carbidopa: Does not cross the blood-brain barrier

Metabolism: Levodopa: Two major pathways (decarboxylation and O-methylation) and two minor pathways (transamination and oxidation) of metabolism; Carbidopa inhibits the decarboxylation of levodopa to dopamine in the peripheral tissue to allow greater levodopa distribution into the CNS

Bioavailability:

Controlled release: Levodopa: Bioavailability is 70% to 75% relative to availability from immediate release formulation; Carbidopa: Bioavailability is ~58% relative to availability from immediate release formulation

Intestinal gel: Levodopa: Similar bioavailability relative to oral administration of tablet formulations (81% to 98%)

Half-life elimination: Immediate release: Levodopa (in presence of carbidopa): 1.5 hours; Half-life may be prolonged with controlled release formulations due to continuous absorption

Time to peak: Immediate release: 0.5 hours; Controlled release: 2 hours; Intestinal gel: therapeutic plasma levels reached 10-30 minutes following morning bolus dose

Excretion: Levodopa: Urine (as metabolites); Carbidopa: Urine (~50% of an oral dose)

Dosage

Adults:

Parkinson's disease:

Oral:

Immediate release tablet, orally-disintegrating tablet:

Initial: Carbidopa 25 mg/levodopa 100 mg 3 times/day

Dosage adjustment: Alternate tablet strengths may be substituted according to individual carbidopa/levodopa requirements. Increase by 1 tablet every 1-2 days as necessary, except when using the carbidopa 25 mg/levodopa 250 mg tablets where increases should be made using 1/2-1 tablet every 1-2 days. Use of more than 1 dosage strength or dosing 4 times/day may be required (maximum: 8 tablets of any strength/day or 200 mg of carbidopa and 2000 mg of levodopa)

Controlled release tablet:

Patients not currently receiving levodopa: Initial: Carbidopa 50 mg/levodopa 200 mg 2 times/day, at intervals not <6 hours

Patients converting from immediate release formulation to controlled release: Initial: Dosage should be substituted at an amount that provides ~10% more of levodopa/day; total calculated dosage is administered in divided doses 2-3 times/day (or ≥3 times/day for patients maintained on levodopa ≥700 mg). Intervals between doses should be 4-8 hours while awake; when divided doses are not equal, smaller doses should be given toward the end of the day. Depending on clinical response, dosage may need to be increased to provide up to 30% more levodopa/day.

Dosage adjustment: May adjust every 3 days; intervals should be between 4-8 hours during the waking day (maximum dose: 8 tablets/day)

Intestinal infusion via PEG tube: Intestinal gel (Canadian labeling; not available in U.S.): **Note:** Conversion to/from oral levodopa tablet formulations and the intestinal gel formulation can be done on a 1:1 ratio. Total daily dose (expressed in terms of levodopa) consists of a morning bolus dose, a continuous maintenance dose, and additional bolus doses when necessary. Nighttime dosing may be necessary in certain rare situations (eg, nocturnal akinesia). Dosage adjustments should be carried out over a period of a few weeks.

Morning bolus dose (based on previous morning levodopa intake and volume to fill intestinal tubing): Usual: Levodopa 100-200 mg (5-10 mL); Maximum: Levodopa 300 mg (15 mL)

Continuous maintenance dose: Adjustable in increments of 2 mg/hour (0.1 mL/hour) and based on previous daily intake of levodopa: Usual: Levodopa 40-120 mg/hour (2-6 mL/hour) infused up to 16 hours; Range: Levodopa 20-200 mg/hour (1-10 mL/hour)

Additional bolus doses: Usual: Levodopa: 10-40 mg (0.5-2 mL), if needed for daytime hypokinesia; in patients requiring >5 additional boluses/day, the maintenance dose should be increased

Restless leg syndrome (RLS) (unlabeled use; Silber, 2004): Oral:

Immediate release tablet: Carbidopa 25 mg/levodopa 100 mg (0.5-1 tablet) given in the evening, at bedtime, or upon waking during the night with RLS symptoms

Controlled release tablet: Carbidopa 25 mg/levodopa 100 mg (1 tablet) before bedtime for RLS symptoms that awaken patient during the night

Elderly: Refer to adult dosing

Dosage adjustment in renal impairment: Use with caution; manufacturer labeling makes no specific dosing recommendations

Dosage adjustment in hepatic impairment: Use with caution; manufacturer labeling makes no specific dosing recommendations

Dietary Considerations Avoid high protein diets (>2 g/kg) which may decrease the efficacy of levodopa via competition with amino acids in crossing the blood-brain barrier. Some products may contain phenylalanine.

Administration

Oral tablet formulations: Space doses evenly over the waking hours. Give with meals to decrease GI upset. Controlled release product should not be chewed or crushed. Orally-disintegrating tablets do not require water; the tablet should disintegrate on the tongue's surface before swallowing.

Intestinal gel (Canadian labeling; not available in U.S.): Gel is administered directly to the duodenum via a portable infusion pump (CADD-legacy Duodopa™ pump). Administer through a temporary nasoduodenal tube for at least 3 days to evaluate patient response and for dose optimization. Long-term administration requires placement of PEG tube for intestinal infusion. Continuous maintenance dose is infused throughout the day for up to 16 hours.

Monitoring Parameters Periodic hepatic function tests, BUN, creatinine, and CBC; periodic skin examinations; blood pressure, standing and sitting/supine; symptoms of parkinsonism, dyskinesias, mental status

Test Interactions False-positive reaction for urinary glucose with Clinitest®; false-negative reaction using Clinistix®; false-positive urine ketones with Acetest®, Ketostix®, Labstix®

Additional Information To block the peripheral conversion of levodopa to dopamine, ≥70 mg/day of carbidopa is needed. "On-off" (a clinical syndrome characterized by sudden periods of drug activity/inactivity), can be managed by giving smaller, more frequent doses of Sinemet® or adding a dopamine agonist or selegiline; when adding a new agent, doses of Sinemet® can usually be decreased. Protein in the diet should be distributed throughout the day to avoid fluctuations in levodopa absorption. Levodopa is the drug of choice when rigidity is the predominant presenting symptom.

Conversion from levodopa to carbidopa/levodopa: **Note:** Levodopa must be discontinued at least 12 hours prior to initiation of levodopa/carbidopa:

Initial dose: Levodopa portion of carbidopa/levodopa should be at least 25% of previous levodopa therapy.

Levodopa <1500 mg/day: Sinemet® or Parcopa™ (levodopa 25 mg/carbidopa 100 mg) 3-4 times/day

Levodopa ≥1500 mg/day: Sinemet® or Parcopa™ (levodopa 25 mg/carbidopa 250 mg) 3-4 times/day

Conversion from immediate release carbidopa/levodopa (Sinemet® or Parcopa™) to Sinemet® CR (50/200):

Sinemet® or Parcopa™ [total daily dose of levodopa]/Sinemet® CR:

Sinemet® or Parcopa™ (levodopa 300-400 mg/day): Sinemet® CR (50/200) 1 tablet twice daily

Sinemet® or Parcopa™ (levodopa 500-600 mg/day): Sinemet® CR (50/200) 1 1/2 tablets twice daily or 1 tablet 3 times/day

Sinemet® or Parcopa™ (levodopa 700-800 mg/day): Sinemet® CR (50/200) 4 tablets in 3 or more divided doses

Sinemet® or Parcopa™ (levodopa 900-1000 mg/day): Sinemet® CR (50/200) 5 tablets in 3 or more divided doses

Intervals between doses of Sinemet® CR should be 4-8 hours while awake; when divided doses are not equal, smaller doses should be given toward the end of the day

Dosage Forms Excipient information presented when available (limited, particularly for generics); consult specific product labeling.

Tablet: 10/100: Carbidopa 10 mg and levodopa 100 mg; 25/100: Carbidopa 25 mg and levodopa 100 mg; 25/250: Carbidopa 25 mg and levodopa 250 mg

Sinemet®:

10/100: Carbidopa 10 mg and levodopa 100 mg

25/100: Carbidopa 25 mg and levodopa 100 mg

25/250: Carbidopa 25 mg and levodopa 250 mg

Tablet, extended release: 25/100: Carbidopa 25 mg and levodopa 100 mg; 50/200: Carbidopa 50 mg and levodopa 200 mg

Tablet, orally disintegrating: 10/100: Carbidopa 10 mg and levodopa 100 mg; 25/100: Carbidopa 25 mg and levodopa 100 mg; 25/250: Carbidopa 25 mg and levodopa 250 mg

Parcopa®:

10/100: Carbidopa 10 mg and levodopa 100 mg [contains phenylalanine 3.4 mg/tablet; mint flavor]

25/100: Carbidopa 25 mg and levodopa 100 mg [contains phenylalanine 3.4 mg/tablet; mint flavor]

25/250: Carbidopa 25 mg and levodopa 250 mg [contains phenylalanine 8.4 mg/tablet; mint flavor]

Tablet, sustained release: 25/100: Carbidopa 25 mg and levodopa 100 mg; 50/200: Carbidopa 50 mg and levodopa 200 mg

Sinemet® CR:

25/100: Carbidopa 25 mg and levodopa 100 mg

50/200: Carbidopa 50 mg and levodopa 200 mg

Dosage Forms: Canada Excipient information presented when available (limited, particularly for generics); consult specific product labeling.

Intestinal gel:

Duodopa™: Carbidopa 5 mg and levodopa 20 mg/1 mL (100 mL)

Extemporaneous Preparations An oral suspension containing carbidopa 1.25 mg and levodopa 5 mg per mL may be made with tablets. Crush ten tablets each containing carbidopa 25 mg and levodopa 100 mg and reduce to a fine powder. Add small portions of a 1:1 mixture of Ora-Sweet® and Ora-Plus® and mix to a uniform paste; mix while adding the vehicle in equal proportions to **almost** 200 mL; transfer to a calibrated bottle, rinse mortar with vehicle, and add sufficient quantity of vehicle to make 200 mL. Label "shake well" and "refrigerate". Stable 42 days under refrigeration. Also stable 28 days at room temperature.

Nahata MC, Morosco RS, and Leguire LE, "Development of Two Stable Oral Suspensions of Levodopa-Carbidopa for Children With Amblyopia," *J Pediatr Ophthalmol Strabismus*, 2000, 37(6):333-7.

◆ **Carbidopa, Entacapone, and Levodopa** *see* Levodopa, Carbidopa, and Entacapone *on page 1197*

◆ **Carbidopa, Levodopa, and Entacapone** *see* Levodopa, Carbidopa, and Entacapone *on page 1197*

Carbinoxamine (kar bi NOKS a meen)

Brand Names: U.S. Arbinoxa; Palgic

Index Terms Carbinoxamine Maleate; Karbinal™ ER

Pharmacologic Category Ethanolamine Derivative; Histamine H_1 Antagonist; Histamine H_1 Antagonist, First Generation

Additional Appendix Information
Beers Criteria – Potentially Inappropriate Medications for Geriatrics *on page 2368*

Use Allergies: For the symptomatic treatment of seasonal and perennial allergic rhinitis; vasomotor rhinitis; allergic conjunctivitis caused by inhalant allergens and foods; mild, uncomplicated allergic skin manifestations of urticaria and angioedema; dermatographism; as therapy for anaphylactic reactions adjunctive to epinephrine and other standard measures after the acute manifestations have been controlled; amelioration of the severity of allergic reactions to blood or plasma.

Pregnancy Risk Factor C

Dosage Allergies: Oral:

Extended release:

Children 2 to <4 years: 3-4 mg every 12 hours

Children 4 to <6 years: 3-8 mg every 12 hours

Children 6 to <12 years: 6-12 mg every 12 hours

Children ≥12 years, Adolescents, and Adults: 6-16 mg every 12 hours

Immediate release:

Children 2 to <6 years: 0.2-0.4 mg/kg/day divided into 3-4 doses (weight-based dosing preferred) **or** 1-2 mg 3-4 times daily

Children 6 to <12 years: 2-4 mg 3-4 times daily

Children ≥12 years, Adolescents, and Adults: 4-8 mg 3-4 times daily

Dosage adjustment in renal impairment: No dosage adjustment provided in manufacturer's labeling.

Dosage adjustment in hepatic impairment: No dosage adjustment provided in manufacturer's labeling.

Additional Information Complete prescribing information should be consulted for additional detail.

Product Availability Karbinal™ ER (extended release) oral suspension: FDA approved March 2013; anticipated availability is unknown. Consult the prescribing information for additional information.

Dosage Forms Excipient information presented when available (limited, particularly for generics); consult specific product labeling.

Solution, Oral, as maleate:

Arbinoxa: 4 mg/5 mL (473 mL) [contains methylparaben, propylene glycol, propylparaben; bubble-gum flavor]

Palgic: 4 mg/5 mL (480 mL) [contains methylparaben, propylene glycol, propylparaben; bubble-gum flavor]

Generic: 4 mg/5 mL (118 mL, 473 mL)

Tablet, Oral, as maleate:

Arbinoxa: 4 mg [scored]

Palgic: 4 mg [scored]

Generic: 4 mg

- ◆ **Carbinoxamine Maleate** *see* Carbinoxamine *on page 343*
- ◆ **Carbocaine** *see* Mepivacaine *on page 1299*
- ◆ **Carbocaine® (Can)** *see* Mepivacaine *on page 1299*
- ◆ **Carbocaine Preservative-Free** *see* Mepivacaine *on page 1299*
- ◆ **Carb-O-Lac5 [OTC]** *see* Urea *on page 2140*
- ◆ **Carb-O-Lac HP [OTC]** *see* Urea *on page 2140*
- ◆ **Carbolith™ (Can)** *see* Lithium *on page 1229*

CARBOplatin (KAR boe pla tin)

Brand Names: Canada Carboplatin Injection; Carboplatin Injection - LIQ IV

Index Terms CBDCA; Paraplatin

Pharmacologic Category Antineoplastic Agent, Alkylating Agent; Antineoplastic Agent, Platinum Analog

Additional Appendix Information
Beers Criteria – Potentially Inappropriate Medications for Geriatrics *on page 2368*
Desensitization Protocols *on page 2325*

Use Initial treatment of advanced ovarian cancer in combination with other established chemotherapy agents; palliative treatment of recurrent ovarian cancer after prior chemotherapy, including cisplatin-based treatment

Unlabeled Use Treatment of bladder cancer, breast cancer (metastatic), central nervous system tumors, cervical cancer (recurrent or metastatic), endometrial cancer, esophageal cancer, head and neck cancer, Hodgkin's lymphoma (relapsed or refractory), malignant pleural mesothelioma, melanoma (advanced or metastatic), merkel cell carcinoma, neuroendocrine tumors (adrenal gland and carcinoid tumors), non-Hodgkin's lymphomas (relapsed or refractory), nonsmall cell lung cancer, retinoblastoma, sarcomas (Ewing's sarcoma and osteosarcoma), small-cell lung cancer, testicular cancer, thymic malignancies, unknown primary adenocarcinoma, and as a conditioning regimen prior to hematopoietic stem cell transplantation

Pregnancy Risk Factor D

Pregnancy Considerations Embryotoxicity and teratogenicity have been observed in animal reproduction studies. May cause fetal harm if administered during pregnancy. Women of childbearing potential should avoid becoming pregnant during treatment.

Breast-Feeding Considerations Due to the potential for toxicity in nursing infants, breast-feeding is not recommended.

Contraindications History of severe allergic reaction to carboplatin, cisplatin, other platinum-containing formulations, mannitol, or any component of the formulation; should not be used in patients with severe bone marrow depression or significant bleeding

Warnings/Precautions Hazardous agent - use appropriate precautions for handling and disposal (NIOSH, 2012). High doses have resulted in severe abnormalities of liver function tests. **[U.S. Boxed Warning]: Bone marrow suppression, which may be severe, is dose related; may result in infection (due to neutropenia) or bleeding (due to thrombocytopenia); anemia may require blood transfusion;** reduce dosage in patients with bone marrow suppression; cycles should be delayed until WBC and platelet counts have recovered. Patients who have received prior myelosuppressive therapy and patients with renal dysfunction are at increased risk for bone marrow suppression. Anemia is cumulative.

When calculating the carboplatin dose using the Calvert formula and an estimated glomerular filtration rate (GFR), the laboratory method used to measure serum creatinine may impact dosing. Compared to other methods, standardized isotope dilution mass spectrometry (IDMS) may underestimate serum creatinine values in patients with low creatinine values (eg, ≤0.7 mg/dL) and may overestimate GFR in patients with normal renal function. This may result in higher calculated carboplatin doses and increased toxicities. If using IDMS, the Food and Drug Administration (FDA) recommends that clinicians consider capping estimated GFR at a maximum of 125 mL/minute to avoid potential toxicity.

[U.S. Boxed Warning]: Anaphylactic-like reactions have been reported with carboplatin; may occur within minutes of administration. Epinephrine, corticosteroids and antihistamines have been used to treat symptoms. The risk of allergic reactions (including anaphylaxis) is increased in patients previously exposed to platinum therapy. Skin testing and desensitization protocols have been reported (Confina-Cohen, 2005; Lee, 2004; Markman, 2003). When administered as sequential infusions, taxane derivatives (docetaxel, paclitaxel) should be administered before the platinum derivatives (carboplatin, cisplatin) to limit myelosuppression and to enhance efficacy. Ototoxicity may occur when administered concomitantly with aminoglycosides. Clinically significant hearing loss has been reported to occur in pediatric patients when carboplatin was administered at higher than recommended doses in combination with other ototoxic agents (eg, aminoglycosides). In a study of children receiving carboplatin for the treatment of retinoblastoma, those <6 months of age at treatment initiation were more likely to experience ototoxicity; long-term audiology monitoring is recommended (Qaddoumi, 2012). Loss of vision (usually reversible within weeks of discontinuing) has been reported with higher than recommended doses.

Use caution in elderly patients; may cause or exacerbate syndrome of inappropriate antidiuretic hormone secretion or hyponatremia; monitor sodium closely with initiation or dosage adjustments in older adults (Beers Criteria). Peripheral neuropathy occurs infrequently, the incidence of peripheral neuropathy is increased patients >65 years of age and those who have previously received cisplatin treatment. Patients >65 years of age are more likely to develop severe thrombocytopenia.

Limited potential for nephrotoxicity unless administered concomitantly with aminoglycosides. **[U.S. Boxed Warning]: Vomiting may occur;** may be severe in patients who have received prior emetogenic therapy. **[U.S. Boxed Warning]: Should be administered under the supervision of an experienced cancer chemotherapy physician.**

Adverse Reactions Percentages reported with single-agent therapy.

>10%:

- Central nervous system: Pain (23%)
- Endocrine & metabolic: Hyponatremia (29% to 47%), hypomagnesemia (29% to 43%), hypocalcemia(22% to 31%), hypokalemia (20% to 28%)
- Gastrointestinal: Vomiting (65% to 81%), abdominal pain (17%), nausea (without vomiting: 10% to 15%)
- Hematologic: Myelosuppression (dose related and dose limiting; nadir at ~21 days with single-agent therapy), anemia (71% to 90%; grades 3/4: 21%), leukopenia (85%; grades 3/4: 15% to 26%), neutropenia (67%; grades 3/4: 16% to 21%), thrombocytopenia (62%; grades 3/4: 25% to 35%)
- Hepatic: Alkaline phosphatase increased (24% to 37%), AST increased (15% to 19%)
- Neuromuscular & skeletal: Weakness (11%)
- Renal: Creatinine clearance decreased (27%), BUN increased (14% to 22%)
- Miscellaneous: Hypersensitivity/allergic reaction (2% to 16%)

1% to 10%:

- Central nervous system: Neurotoxicity (5%)
- Dermatologic: Alopecia (2% to 3%)
- Gastrointestinal: Constipation (6%), diarrhea (6%), stomatitis/mucositis (1%), taste dysgeusia (1%)
- Hematologic: Bleeding (5%), hemorrhagic complications (5%)
- Hepatic: Bilirubin increased (5%)
- Neuromuscular & skeletal: Peripheral neuropathy (4% to 6%)
- Ocular: Visual disturbance (1%)
- Otic: Ototoxicity (1%)
- Renal: Creatinine increased (6% to 10%)
- Miscellaneous: Infection (5%)

<1% (Limited to important or life-threatening): Anaphylactic reaction, bronchospasm, cardiac failure, cerebrovascular accident, dehydration, embolism, erythema, hemolytic anemia (acute), hemolytic uremic syndrome (HUS), hyper-/hypotension, injection site reactions (pain, redness, swelling), limb ischemia (acute), necrosis (associated with extravasation), neutropenic fever, pruritus, rash, secondary malignancies, urticaria, vision loss

Drug Interactions

Metabolism/Transport Effects None known.

Avoid Concomitant Use

Avoid concomitant use of CARBOplatin with any of the following: BCG; CloZAPine; Natalizumab; Pimecrolimus; SORAfenib; Tacrolimus (Topical); Tofacitinib; Vaccines (Live)

Increased Effect/Toxicity

CARBOplatin may increase the levels/effects of: Bexarotene (Systemic); CloZAPine; Leflunomide; Natalizumab; Taxane Derivatives; Tofacitinib; Topotecan; Vaccines (Live)

The levels/effects of CARBOplatin may be increased by: Aminoglycosides; Denosumab; Pimecrolimus; Roflumilast; SORAfenib; Tacrolimus (Topical); Trastuzumab

Decreased Effect

CARBOplatin may decrease the levels/effects of: BCG; Coccidioidin Skin Test; Fosphenytoin-Phenytoin; Sipuleucel-T; Vaccines (Inactivated); Vaccines (Live)

The levels/effects of CARBOplatin may be decreased by: Echinacea

Ethanol/Nutrition/Herb Interactions Herb/Nutraceutical: Avoid black cohosh, dong quai in estrogen-dependent tumors.

Preparation for Administration

Solution for injection: Manufacturer's labeling states solution can be further diluted to concentrations as low as 0.5 mg/mL in NS or D_5W; however, most clinicians generally dilute dose in either 100 mL or 250 mL of NS or D_5W.

Concentrations used for desensitization vary based on protocol.

Hazardous agent; use appropriate precautions for handling and disposal (NIOSH, 2012). Needles or I.V. administration sets that contain aluminum should not be used in the preparation or administration of carboplatin; aluminum can react with carboplatin resulting in precipitate formation and loss of potency.

Storage/Stability Store intact vials at room temperature at 25°C (77°F); excursions permitted to 15°C to 30°C (59°F to 86°F). Protect from light. Further dilution to a concentration as low as 0.5 mg/mL is stable at room temperature (25°C) for 8 hours in NS or D_5W. Stability has also been demonstrated for dilutions in D_5W in PVC bags at room temperature for 9 days (Benaji, 1994); however, the manufacturer recommends use within 8 hours due to lack of preservative.

Mechanism of Action Carboplatin is a platinum compound alkylating agent which covalently binds to DNA; interferes with the function of DNA by producing interstrand DNA cross-links

Pharmacodynamics/Kinetics

Distribution: V_d: 16 L (based on a dose of 300-500 mg/m^2); into liver, kidney, skin, and tumor tissue

Protein binding: Carboplatin: 0%; Platinum (from carboplatin): Irreversibly binds to plasma proteins

Metabolism: Minimally hepatic to aquated and hydroxylated compounds

Half-life elimination: Cl_{cr} >60 mL/minute: Carboplatin: 2.6-5.9 hours (based on a dose of 300-500 mg/m^2); Platinum (from carboplatin): ≥5 days

Excretion: Urine (~70% as carboplatin within 24 hours; 3% to 5% as platinum within 1-4 days)

Dosage Details concerning dosing in combination regimens should also be consulted. **Note:** Doses for adults are commonly calculated by the target AUC using the Calvert formula, where **Total dose (mg) = Target AUC x (GFR + 25)**. If estimating glomerular filtration rate (GFR)

instead of a measured GFR, the Food and Drug Administration (FDA) recommends that clinicians consider capping estimated GFR at a maximum of 125 mL/minute to avoid potential toxicity.

Children: I.V.:

Glioma (unlabeled use): 175 mg/m^2 weekly for 4 weeks every 6 weeks, with a 2-week recovery period between courses (in combination with vincristine) (Packer, 1997)

Neuroblastoma, localized and unresectable (unlabeled use): Children ≥10 kg: 200 mg/m^2/day days 1, 2, and 3 every 21 days for 2 cycles (in combination with etoposide for 2 cycles then followed by cyclophosphamide, doxorubicin and vincristine) (Rubie, 1998) **or** Children <1 year: 6.6 mg/kg/day days 1, 2, and 3 (in combination with etoposide for 2 cycles, then followed by cyclophosphamide, doxorubicin, and vincristine) (Rubie, 2001)

Sarcomas: Ewing's sarcoma, osteosarcoma (unlabeled uses): 400 mg/m^2/day for 2 days every 21 days (in combination with ifosfamide and etoposide) (van Winkle, 2005)

Adults: I.V.:

Ovarian cancer, advanced: 360 mg/m^2 every 4 weeks (as a single agent) **or** 300 mg/m^2 every 4 weeks (in combination with cyclophosphamide) **or** Target AUC 4-6 (single agent; in previously-treated patients)

Unlabeled dosing: Target AUC 5-7.5 every 3 weeks (in combination with paclitaxel) (Ozols, 2003; Parmar, 2003) **or** Target AUC 5 every 3 weeks (in combination with docetaxel) (Vasey, 2004)

Bladder cancer (unlabeled use): Target AUC 5 every 3 weeks (in combination with gemcitabine and paclitaxel) (Hainsworth, 2005) **or** Target AUC 5 every 3 weeks (in combination with gemcitabine) (Bamias, 2006) **or** Target AUC 6 every 3 weeks (in combination with paclitaxel) (Vaughn, 2002)

Breast cancer, metastatic (unlabeled use): Target AUC 6 every 3 weeks (in combination with trastuzumab and paclitaxel) (Robert, 2006) **or** Target AUC 6 every 3 weeks (in combination with trastuzumab and docetaxel) (Pegram, 2004; Valero, 2011)

Cervical cancer, recurrent or metastatic (unlabeled use): Target AUC 5 every 3 weeks (in combination with paclitaxel) (Pectasides, 2009) **or** Target AUC 5-6 every 4 weeks (in combination with paclitaxel) (Tinker, 2005) **or** 400 mg/m^2 every 28 days (as a single agent) (Weiss, 1990)

Endometrial cancer (unlabeled use): Target AUC 5 every 3 weeks (in combination with paclitaxel) (Pectasides, 2008) **or** Target AUC 2 on days 1, 8, and 15 every 28 days (in combination with paclitaxel) (Secord, 2007)

Esophageal cancer (unlabeled use): Target AUC 2 on days 1, 8, 15, 22, and 29 for 1 cycle (in combination with paclitaxel) (van Meerten, 2006) **or** Target AUC 5 every 3 weeks (in combination with paclitaxel) (El-Rayes, 2004)

Head and neck cancer (unlabeled use): Target AUC 5 every 3 weeks (in combination with cetuximab) (Chan, 2005) **or** Target AUC 5 every 3 weeks (in combination with cetuximab and fluorouracil) (Vermorken, 2008) **or** 300 mg/m^2 every 4 weeks (in combination with fluorouracil) (Forastiere, 1992) **or** Target AUC 6 every 3 weeks (in combination with paclitaxel) (Clark, 2001)

Hodgkin's lymphoma, relapsed or refractory (unlabeled use): Target AUC 5 (maximum dose 800 mg) for 2 cycles (in combination with ifosfamide and etoposide) (Moskowitz, 2001)

Malignant pleural mesothelioma (unlabeled use): Target AUC 5 every 3 weeks (in combination with pemetrexed) (Castagneto, 2008; Ceresoli, 2006)

Melanoma, advanced or metastatic (unlabeled use): Target AUC 2 on days 1, 8, and 15 every 4 weeks (in combination with paclitaxel) (Rao, 2006)

Non-Hodgkin's lymphomas, relapsed or refractory (unlabeled use): Target AUC 5 (maximum dose 800 mg) per cycle for 3 cycles (in combination with rituximab, ifosfamide and etoposide) (Kewalramani, 2004)

Nonsmall cell lung cancer (unlabeled use): Target AUC 6 every 3-4 weeks (in combination with paclitaxel) (Ramalingam, 2008; Schiller, 2002; Strauss, 2008) **or** Target AUC 6 every 3 weeks (in combination with bevacizumab and paclitaxel) (Sandler, 2006) **or** Target AUC 5 every 3 weeks (in combination with pemetrexed) (Gronberg, 2009) **or** in combination with radiation therapy and paclitaxel (Belani, 2005):

Target AUC 6 every 3 weeks for 2 cycles **or**

Target AUC 6 every 3 weeks for 2 cycles; then target AUC 2 weekly for 7 weeks **or**

Target AUC 2 every week for 7 weeks; then target AUC 6 every 3 weeks for 2 cycles

Sarcomas: Ewing's sarcoma, osteosarcoma (unlabeled uses): 400 mg/m^2/day for 2 days every 21 days (in combination with ifosfamide and etoposide) (van Winkle, 2005)

Small cell lung cancer (unlabeled use): Target AUC 6 every 3 weeks (in combination with etoposide) (Skarlos, 2001) **or** Target AUC 5 every 3 weeks (in combination with irinotecan) (Hermes, 2008) **or** Target AUC 5 every 28 days (in combination with irinotecan) (Schmittel, 2006)

Testicular cancer (unlabeled use): Target AUC 7 as a one-time dose (Oliver, 2011) **or** 700 mg/m^2/day for 3 days beginning 5 days prior to peripheral stem cell infusion (in combination with etoposide) for 2 cycles (Einhorn, 2007)

Thymic malignancies (unlabeled use): Target AUC 5 every 3 weeks (in combination with paclitaxel) (Lemma, 2008)

Unknown primary adenocarcinoma (unlabeled use): Target AUC 6 every 3 weeks (in combination with paclitaxel) (Briasoulis, 2000) **or** Target AUC 6 every 3 weeks (in combination with docetaxel) (Greco, 2000) **or** Target AUC 6 every 3 weeks (in combination with paclitaxel and etoposide) (Hainsworth, 2006) **or** Target AUC 5 every 3 weeks (in combination with paclitaxel and gemcitabine) (Greco, 2002)

Elderly: The Calvert formula should be used to calculate dosing for elderly patients.

Dosage adjustment for toxicity: Platelets <50,000 cells/mm^3 or ANC <500 cells/mm^3: Administer 75% of dose

Dosing adjustment in renal impairment: Note: Dose determination with Calvert formula uses GFR and, therefore, inherently adjusts for renal dysfunction.

The manufacturer's labeling recommends the following dosage adjustment guidelines for single-agent therapy:

Adults:

Baseline Cl_{cr} 41-59 mL/minute: Initiate at 250 mg/m^2 and adjust subsequent doses based on bone marrow toxicity

Baseline Cl_{cr} 16-40 mL/minute: Initiate at 200 mg/m^2 and adjust subsequent doses based on bone marrow toxicity

Baseline Cl_{cr} ≤15 mL/minute: No dosage adjustment provided in manufacturer's labeling.

The following dosage adjustments have also been recommended:

Aronoff, 2007:

Children:

GFR <50 mL/minute: Use Calvert formula incorporating patient's GFR

Hemodialysis, peritoneal dialysis, continuous renal replacement therapy (CRRT): Use Calvert formula incorporating patient's GFR

Adults (**Note:** For dosing based on **mg/m²**):
GFR >50 mL/minute: No dosage adjustment necessary
GFR 10-50 mL/minute: Administer 50% of the dose
GFR <10 mL/minute: Administer 25% of the dose
Hemodialysis: Administer 50% of dose
Continuous ambulatory peritoneal dialysis (CAPD): Administer 25% of dose
Continuous renal replacement therapy (CRRT): 200 mg/m²

Janus, 2010: Hemodialysis: Carboplatin dose (mg) = Target AUC x 25; administer on a nondialysis day, hemodialysis should occur between 12-24 hours after carboplatin dose

Dosing adjustment in hepatic impairment: No dosage adjustment provided in manufacturer's labeling; however, carboplatin undergoes minimal hepatic metabolism therefore dosage adjustment may not be needed.

Dosing in obesity: *ASCO Guidelines for appropriate chemotherapy dosing in obese adults with cancer:* Dosing based on GFR should be considered in obese patients; GFR should not exceed 125 mL/minute (Griggs, 2012).

Administration Usually infused over 15-60 minutes, although some protocols may require infusions up to 24 hours. When administered as a part of a combination chemotherapy regimen, sequence of administration may vary by regimen; refer to specific protocol for sequence recommendation.

Needles or I.V. administration sets that contain aluminum should not be used in the preparation or administration of carboplatin; aluminum can react with carboplatin resulting in precipitate formation and loss of potency.

Hazardous agent; use appropriate precautions for handling and disposal (NIOSH, 2012).

Monitoring Parameters CBC (with differential and platelet count), serum electrolytes, serum creatinine and BUN, creatinine clearance, liver function tests; audiology evaluations (children <6 months of age)

Dosage Forms Excipient information presented when available (limited, particularly for generics); consult specific product labeling.

Solution, Intravenous:
Generic: 50 mg/5 mL (5 mL); 150 mg/15 mL (15 mL); 450 mg/45 mL (45 mL); 600 mg/60 mL (60 mL)

Solution, Intravenous [preservative free]:
Generic: 50 mg/5 mL (5 mL); 150 mg/15 mL (15 mL); 450 mg/45 mL (45 mL); 600 mg/60 mL (60 mL)

Solution Reconstituted, Intravenous:
Generic: 150 mg (1 ea)

◆ **Carboplatin Injection (Can)** *see* CARBOplatin *on page 344*
◆ **Carboplatin Injection - LIQ IV (Can)** *see* CARBOplatin *on page 344*
◆ **Carboprost** *see* Carboprost Tromethamine *on page 347*

Carboprost Tromethamine

(KAR boe prost tro METH a meen)

Brand Names: U.S. Hemabate
Brand Names: Canada Hemabate®
Index Terms Carboprost; Prostaglandin F_2 Alpha Analog; Prostaglandin F_2 Analog
Pharmacologic Category Abortifacient; Prostaglandin
Use Termination of pregnancy during the second trimester between weeks 13 and 20 of gestation; treatment of refractory postpartum hemorrhage due to uterine atony
Pregnancy Risk Factor C

Pregnancy Considerations Teratogenic effects were not observed in animal reproduction studies. When used for termination of pregnancy, carboprost tromethamine is not considered feticidal, but is used to terminate pregnancy due to its ability to stimulate uterine contractions; use is not indicated if the fetus has reached a stage of viability *in utero*. Complete termination of pregnancy may not be induced in ~20% of cases and should therefore be completed in another way.

Breast-Feeding Considerations It is not known if carboprost tromethamine is excreted in breast milk.

Contraindications Hypersensitivity to carboprost tromethamine or any component of the formulation; acute pelvic inflammatory disease; active cardiac, pulmonary, renal, or hepatic dysfunction

Warnings/Precautions [U.S. Boxed Warning] Potent oxytocic agent; use with strict adherence to recommended dosing. Carboprost should be used only by medically-trained personnel in a hospital which can provide immediate intensive care and acute surgical facilities. Transient pyrexia and increased blood pressure may be observed with treatment. Use caution with history of asthma; hypotension or hypertension; cardiovascular, adrenal, renal, or hepatic disease; anemia; jaundice; diabetes; epilepsy; or compromised uteri. Pretreatment or concomitant use of antiemetic and antidiarrheal agents is recommended to decrease incidence of GI side effects.

Adverse Reactions Frequency not defined. Effects due to increased smooth muscle contractility are most common and are generally transient and reversible upon discontinuation of therapy.

Cardiovascular: Chest pain, flushing, hypertension, syncope, palpitation, tachycardia, tightness of chest
Central nervous system: Anxiety, chills/shivering, dizziness, drowsiness, dystonia, faintness, headache, lethargy, lightheadedness, nervousness, sleep disturbance, temperature elevation (may be drug induced or due to postabortion endometritis), vasovagal syndrome, vertigo
Dermatologic: Rash
Endocrine & metabolic: Breast tenderness, dysmenorrhea-like pain, endometritis, hot flashes, thyroid storm
Gastrointestinal: Choking sensation, diarrhea (~2/3 patients), dry throat, epigastric pain, gagging/retching, hematemesis, nausea (~1/3 patients), taste alteration, thirst, throat fullness, vomiting (~2/3 patients), xerostomia
Genitourinary: Perforated uterus, posterior cervical perforation, urinary tract infection, uterine bleeding (excessive), uterine rupture, uterine sacculation
Local: Injection site pain
Neuromuscular & skeletal: Backache, leg cramps, muscular pain, paresthesia, torticollis, weakness
Ocular: Blurred vision, eye pain, eyelid twitching
Otic: Tinnitus
Respiratory: Asthma, cough, bronchospasm, dyspnea, epistaxis, hyperventilation, pulmonary edema, respiratory distress, upper respiratory tract infection, wheezing
Miscellaneous: Diaphoresis, hiccups, retained placental fragment, septic shock

Drug Interactions

Metabolism/Transport Effects None known.

Avoid Concomitant Use There are no known interactions where it is recommended to avoid concomitant use.

Increased Effect/Toxicity There are no known significant interactions involving an increase in effect.

Decreased Effect There are no known significant interactions involving a decrease in effect.

Storage/Stability Store under refrigeration at 2°C to 8°C (36°F to 46°F).

Mechanism of Action Carboprost tromethamine is a tromethamine salt analog of naturally occurring prostaglandin F_2 alpha (dinoprost) except for the addition of a methyl group at the C-15 position. This substitution produces longer duration of activity than dinoprost; carboprost stimulates uterine contractility which usually results in expulsion of the products of conception and is used to induce abortion between 13-20 weeks of pregnancy. When used postpartum, hemostasis at the placentation site is achieved through the myometrial contractions produced by carboprost.

Pharmacodynamics/Kinetics

Time to peak, serum: I.M.: 30 minutes

Excretion: Urine

Dosage I.M.: Adults:

Refractory postpartum uterine bleeding: Initial: 250 mcg; if needed, may repeat at 15- to 90-minute intervals; maximum total dose: 2 mg (8 doses)

Termination of pregnancy: Initial: 250 mcg, then 250 mcg at 1.5- to 3.5-hour intervals, depending on uterine response; a 500 mcg dose may be given if uterine response is not adequate after several 250 mcg doses; do not exceed 12 mg total dose or continuous administration for >2 days

Dosage adjustment in renal impairment: Use is contraindicated.

Dosage adjustment in hepatic impairment: Use is contraindicated.

Administration Administer deep I.M.; rotate site if repeat injections are required. Do not inject I.V.

Monitoring Parameters Termination of pregnancy: Confirmation of fetal death; cervical exam after termination of pregnancy

Dosage Forms Excipient information presented when available (limited, particularly for generics); consult specific product labeling.

Solution, Intramuscular [strength expressed as base]:

Hemabate: 250 mcg/mL (1 mL) [contains benzyl alcohol]

- Carboxypeptidase-G2 *see* Glucarpidase *on page 961*
- Cardec™ DM [OTC] *see* Chlorpheniramine, Phenylephrine, and Dextromethorphan *on page 413*
- Cardene IV *see* NiCARdipine *on page 1450*
- Cardene SR *see* NiCARdipine *on page 1450*
- Cardizem *see* Diltiazem *on page 613*
- Cardizem CD *see* Diltiazem *on page 613*
- Cardizem® CD (Can) *see* Diltiazem *on page 613*
- Cardizem LA *see* Diltiazem *on page 613*
- Cardura *see* Doxazosin *on page 656*
- Cardura-1™ (Can) *see* Doxazosin *on page 656*
- Cardura-2™ (Can) *see* Doxazosin *on page 656*
- Cardura-4™ (Can) *see* Doxazosin *on page 656*
- Cardura XL *see* Doxazosin *on page 656*

Carfilzomib (kar FILZ oh mib)

Brand Names: U.S. Kyprolis

Index Terms PR-171

Pharmacologic Category Antineoplastic Agent; Proteasome Inhibitor

Use Treatment of multiple myeloma in patients who have received at least 2 prior treatment regimens (including a proteasome inhibitor and an immunomodulator) with disease progression within 60 days after the most recent treatment

Pregnancy Risk Factor D

Pregnancy Considerations Adverse events were observed in animal reproduction studies at doses less than the recommended human dose (based on BSA). Based on the mechanism of action, adverse fetal events would be expected to occur with use in pregnant women. Females of reproductive potential are advised to avoid pregnancy during therapy.

Breast-Feeding Considerations Due to the potential for adverse reactions in nursing infants, the manufacturer recommends avoiding breast-feeding during therapy.

Contraindications There are no contraindications listed in the manufacturer's labeling.

Warnings/Precautions Hazardous agent - use appropriate precautions for handling and disposal (meets NIOSH, 2012 criteria). Thrombocytopenia (including grade 4) was observed in patients receiving carfilzomib, with platelet nadirs occurring around day 8 of each 28-day treatment cycle, and recovery to baseline by the start of the next cycle. Monitor platelets closely and adjust dose or withhold therapy if necessary. Anemia, lymphopenia, and neutropenia were also observed. Death caused by cardiac arrest has occurred within 24 hours of drug administration. Carfilzomib has been associated with the development or worsening of congestive heart failure (HF) and decreased left ventricular ejection fraction (LVEF). HF, pulmonary edema, and decreased LVEF were observed in clinical trials; monitor closely for cardiac complications; withhold therapy for grade 3 or 4 cardiac events until recovery. Patients with New York Heart Association Class III and IV heart failure, recent myocardial infarction (within 6 months), and conduction abnormalities not managed by medication were excluded from clinical trials. Pulmonary arterial hypertension (PAH) was observed (including grade 3) in studies; perform cardiac imaging or other testing as appropriate, and withhold carfilzomib until PAH is resolved or returns to baseline. Dyspnea (including 1 death) has been reported; monitor closely, and withhold carfilzomib until symptom resolution or return to baseline.

Infusion reactions such as chills, fever, arthralgia, myalgia, shortness of breath, hypotension, facial flushing, facial edema, vomiting, weakness, syncope, chest tightness, or angina may occur immediately following or within 24 hours of carfilzomib infusion. To lessen the incidence and intensity of infusion reactions, administer dexamethasone prior to drug administration. Tumor lysis syndrome (TLS) risk is increased in multiple myeloma patients with a high tumor burden. Adequately hydrate patients prior to carfilzomib therapy and monitor closely for signs and symptoms of tumor lysis syndrome. If TLS occurs, interrupt treatment until resolved.

Hepatic failure, including fatal cases, has been reported rarely (<1%). Increased transaminases and hyperbilirubinemia have also been observed. Interrupt carfilzomib therapy in patients with grade 3 or higher hepatic toxicity until resolved or recovered to baseline; monitor liver enzymes closely and for signs of toxicity.

Adverse Reactions

>10%:

Cardiovascular: Peripheral edema (24%), hypertension (14%), chest wall pain (11%)

Central nervous system: Fatigue (56%), fever (30%), headache (28%), insomnia (18%), chills (16%), dizziness (13%), hypoesthesia (12%), pain (12%)

Endocrine & metabolic: Hypokalemia (14%), hypomagnesemia (14%), hyperglycemia (12%), hypercalcemia (11%), hypophosphatemia (11%)

Gastrointestinal: Nausea (45%), diarrhea (33%), vomiting (22%), constipation (21%), anorexia (12%)

Hematologic: Anemia (47%; grade 3: 21%; grade 4: 1%), thrombocytopenia (36%; grade 3: 13%; grade 4: 10%), lymphopenia (24%; grade 3: 16%; grade 4: 2%), neutropenia (21%; grade 3: 10%; grade 4: 1%), leukopenia (14%; grade 3: 5%; grade 4:<1%)

Hepatic: AST increased (13%; grade 3: 3%; grade 4: <1%)

Neuromuscular & skeletal: Back pain (20%), arthralgia (16%), muscle spasms (14%), peripheral neuropathy (14%; grade 3: 1%), weakness (14%), limb pain (13%)

Renal: Creatinine increased (24%; grade 3: 3%; grade 4: <1%)

Respiratory: Dyspnea (35%; grade 3: 5%; grade 4: <1%), upper respiratory tract infection (28%), cough (26%), pneumonia (13%; grade 3: 10%; grade 4: <1%)

1% to 10%:

Cardiovascular: Cardiac failure (7%; includes CHF, pulmonary edema, ejection fraction decrease)

Endocrine & metabolic: Hyponatremia (10%)

Renal: Renal failure (9%)

Respiratory: Pulmonary arterial hypertension (2%)

Miscellaneous: Herpes zoster reactivation (2%)

<1% (Limited to important or life-threatening): Bilirubin increased, hepatic failure, infusion reaction, intracranial hemorrhage, multiorgan failure, myocardial ischemia, neutropenic fever, sepsis, tumor lysis syndrome

Drug Interactions

Metabolism/Transport Effects Substrate of P-glycoprotein; **Inhibits** CYP3A4 (weak), P-glycoprotein

Avoid Concomitant Use

Avoid concomitant use of Carfilzomib with any of the following: CloZAPine; Pimozide

Increased Effect/Toxicity

Carfilzomib may increase the levels/effects of: ARIPiprazole; CloZAPine; Dofetilide; Lomitapide; Pimozide

The levels/effects of Carfilzomib may be increased by: P-glycoprotein/ABCB1 Inhibitors

Decreased Effect

The levels/effects of Carfilzomib may be decreased by: P-glycoprotein/ABCB1 Inducers

Preparation for Administration Hazardous agent; use appropriate precautions for handling and disposal (meets NIOSH, 2012 criteria). Reconstitute with 29 mL sterile water for injection to a concentration of 2 mg/mL (directing solution onto the inside wall of the vial to avoid foaming). Gently invert and/or swirl vial slowly for ~1 minute to mix; do not shake. If foaming results, allow solution to sit for 2-5 minutes until foaming resolves. Reconstituted solution should be clear and colorless. May further dilute dose in 50 mL D_5W. The amount contained in each vial may exceed the prescribed dose; use care with dosage and volume calculations. Discard unused portion of the vial.

Storage/Stability Store intact vials refrigerated at 2°C to 8°C (36°F to 46°F). Do not shake; store in original carton until use to protect from light. Reconstituted drug (in the vial or in a syringe) and preparations diluted for infusion are stable for 4 hours at room temperature or for 24 hours refrigerated at 2°C to 8°C (36°F to 46°F).

Mechanism of Action Carfilzomib inhibits proteasomes, which are responsible for intracellular protein homeostasis. Specifically, it is a potent, selective, and irreversible inhibitor of chymotrypsin-like activity of the 20S proteasome, leading to cell cycle arrest and apoptosis.

Pharmacodynamics/Kinetics

Distribution: V_{dss}: 28 L

Protein binding: 97%

Metabolism: Rapid and extensive; peptidase cleavage and epoxide hydrolysis; minimal metabolism through cytochrome P450-mediated mechanisms

Half-life elimination: Doses ≥15 mg/m^2: <1 hour on day 1 of cycle 1

Dosage I.V.: Adults: **Note:** Hydrate with 250-500 mL normal saline (or other appropriate I.V. fluid) predose (recommended) and postdose (if needed) during cycle 1 (continue in subsequent cycles if necessary). Premedicate with dexamethasone (4 mg orally or I.V.) prior to all doses in cycle 1, all doses during first dose escalation cycle, and as needed with future cycles to reduce the incidence and severity of infusion reaction.

Multiple myeloma, relapsed/refractory: **Note:** Patients with a body surface area (BSA) >2.2 m^2 should be dosed based upon a maximum BSA of 2.2 m^2. Dose adjustments for weight changes of ≤20% are not necessary, per manufacturer labeling.

Cycle 1: 20 mg/m^2 on 2 consecutive days, each week for 3 weeks (days 1, 2, 8, 9, 15, and 16) of a 28-day treatment cycle

Cycle 2 and subsequent cycles (if cycle 1 is tolerated): 27 mg/m^2 on 2 consecutive days, each week for 3 weeks (days 1, 2, 8, 9, 15, and 16) of a 28-day treatment cycle. Continue until disease progression or occurrence of unacceptable toxicity.

Dosage adjustment for toxicity:

Hematologic toxicity:

ANC: Grade 3 or 4 neutropenia: Withhold dose; continue at same dose level if fully recovered before next scheduled dose. If recovered to grade 2, reduce dose by one dose level (from 27 mg/m^2 to 20 mg/m^2 or from 20 mg/m^2 to 15 mg/m^2). Consider escalating to the previous dose if reduced dose is tolerated.

Platelets: Grade 4 thrombocytopenia: Withhold dose; continue at same dose level if fully recovered before next scheduled dose. If recovered to grade 3 thrombocytopenia, reduce dose by one dose level (from 27 mg/m^2 to 20 mg/m^2 or from 20 mg/m^2 to 15 mg/m^2). Consider escalating to the previous dose if reduced dose is tolerated.

Nonhematologic toxicity:

Cardiac: Grade 3 or 4, new onset or worsening of congestive heart failure, decreased left ventricular function, or myocardial ischemia: Withhold dose until resolved or at baseline. After resolution, if appropriate to reinitiate, consider restarting at a reduced dose level (from 27 mg/m^2 to 20 mg/m^2 or from 20 mg/m^2 to 15 mg/m^2). Consider escalating to the previous dose if reduced dose is tolerated.

Hepatic: Grade 3 or 4 elevation of bilirubin, transaminases, or other liver abnormalities: Withhold dose until resolved or at baseline. After resolution, if appropriate to reinitiate, consider restarting at a reduced dose level (from 27 mg/m^2 to 20 mg/m^2 or from 20 mg/m^2 to 15 mg/m^2). Consider escalating to the previous dose if reduced dose is tolerated.

Peripheral neuropathy: Grade 3 or 4: Withhold dose until resolved or at baseline. After resolution, if appropriate to reinitiate, restart at prior dose or at a reduced dose level (from 27 mg/m^2 to 20 mg/m^2 or from 20 mg/m^2 to 15 mg/m^2). Consider escalating to the previous dose if reduced dose is tolerated.

Pulmonary toxicity

Pulmonary hypertension: Withhold dose until resolved or at baseline. After resolution, if appropriate to reinitiate, restart at prior dose or at a reduced dose level (from 27 mg/m^2 to 20 mg/m^2 or from 20 mg/m^2 to 15 mg/m^2). Consider escalating to the previous dose if reduced dose is tolerated.

Grade 3 or 4 pulmonary complications: Withhold dose until resolved or at baseline. After resolution, consider restarting (at next scheduled treatment) at a reduced dose level (from 27 mg/m^2 to 20 mg/m^2 or from 20 mg/m^2 to 15 mg/m^2). Consider escalating to the previous dose if reduced dose is tolerated.

Renal: Serum creatinine ≥2 times baseline: Withhold dose until renal function has improved to grade 1 or baseline. If renal toxicity due to carfilzomib, reduce dose at the next scheduled treatment (from 27 mg/m^2 to 20 mg/m^2 or from 20 mg/m^2 to 15 mg/m^2). Consider escalating to the previous dose if reduced dose is tolerated. If toxicity not due to carfilzomib, restart at previous dose.

Tumor lysis syndrome: Interrupt treatment until resolved.

Other grade 3 or 4 nonhematologic toxicities: Withhold dose until resolved or at baseline. After resolution, consider restarting (at next scheduled treatment) at a reduced dose level (from 27 mg/m^2 to 20 mg/m^2 or from 20 mg/m^2 to 15 mg/m^2). Consider escalating to the previous dose if reduced dose is tolerated.

Dosage adjustment in renal impairment: No dosage adjustment provided in manufacturer's labeling; however, results from a phase 2 trial in patients with renal impairment indicate that the pharmacokinetics and safety of carfilzomib were unchanged in this patient population; no dosage adjustment is necessary in patients with baseline dysfunction, including hemodialysis (Harvey, 2012; Niesvizky, 2011). **Note:** Dialysis clearance of carfilzomib has not been studied; per manufacturer labeling, administer postdialysis.

Dosage adjustment in hepatic impairment: No dosage adjustment provided in manufacturer's labeling (has not been studied; patients with ALT or AST ≥3 times ULN and bilirubin ≥2 times ULN were excluded from clinical trials).

Dosing in obesity: *ASCO Guidelines for appropriate chemotherapy dosing in obese adults with cancer:* In general, utilize patient's actual body weight (full weight) for calculation of body surface area- or weight-based dosing, particularly when the intent of therapy is curative; manage regimen-related toxicities in the same manner as for nonobese patients; if a dose reduction is utilized due to toxicity, consider resumption of full weight-based dosing with subsequent cycles, especially if cause of toxicity (eg, hepatic or renal impairment) is resolved (Griggs, 2012). **Note:** According to the manufacturer, patients with a body surface area (BSA) >2.2 m^2 should be dosed based upon a maximum BSA of 2.2 m^2; dose adjustments for weight changes of ≤20% are not necessary.

Administration I.V.: Administer over 2-10 minutes. Flush line before and after carfilzomib with NS or D_5W.

Hazardous agent; use appropriate precautions for handling and disposal (meets NIOSH, 2012 criteria).

Monitoring Parameters CBC with differential and platelets (monitor frequently throughout therapy); renal function, pulmonary function (with new or worsening pulmonary symptoms), liver function tests, serum creatinine. Signs/symptoms of infusion-related reactions, congestive heart failure, tumor lysis syndrome, and peripheral neuropathy.

Dosage Forms Excipient information presented when available (limited, particularly for generics); consult specific product labeling.

Solution Reconstituted, Intravenous:

Kyprolis: 60 mg (1 ea)

Carglumic Acid (kar GLU mik AS id)

Brand Names: U.S. Carbaglu

Index Terms N-Carbamoyl-L-Glutamic Acid; N-Carbamylglutamate

Pharmacologic Category Antidote; Metabolic Alkalosis Agent; Urea Cycle Disorder (UCD) Treatment Agent

Use Hyperammonemia: Adjunctive treatment in adult and pediatric patients of acute hyperammonemia and maintenance therapy of chronic hyperammonemia due to the deficiency of the hepatic enzyme N-acetylglutamate synthase (NAGS)

Pregnancy Risk Factor C

Pregnancy Considerations Teratogenic effects were reported in some animal reproduction studies. There are no adequate and well-controlled studies in pregnant women. However, due to the potential for irreversible fetal neurologic damage for untreated NAGS deficiency, women with this condition must remain on treatment throughout pregnancy.

Breast-Feeding Considerations It is not known if carglumic acid is excreted in breast milk. Breast-feeding is not recommended by the manufacturer.

Prescribing and Access Restrictions Carbaglu is not available through pharmaceutical wholesalers or retail pharmacies, but only through direct shipping from the Accredo specialty pharmacy. Prescribers must contact Accredo Health Group at 888-454-8860 or refer to www.-accredo.com to initiate patients on this product.

Contraindications There are no contraindications listed in the manufacturer's labeling.

Warnings/Precautions Hyperammonemia is a life-threatening emergency; management of hyperammonemia due to N-acetylglutamate synthase (NAGS) deficiency should be done in coordination with those experienced in the management of metabolic disorders. With hyperammonemia, complete protein restriction should be maintained for 24-48 hours and caloric supplementation should be maximized to reverse catabolism and nitrogen turnover.

Adverse Reactions

>10%:

Central nervous system: Fever (17%), headache (13%)
Gastrointestinal: Vomiting (26%), abdominal pain (17%), diarrhea (13%)
Hematologic: Anemia (13%)
Otic: Ear infection (13%)
Respiratory: Tonsillitis (17%), nasopharyngitis (13%)
Miscellaneous: Infections (13%)

1% to 10%:

Central nervous system: Somnolence (9%)
Dermatologic: Hyperhidrosis (9%), rash (9%)
Gastrointestinal: Anorexia (9%), dysgeusia (9%), weight loss (9%)
Neuromuscular & skeletal: Weakness (9%)
Respiratory: Pneumonia (9%)
Miscellaneous: Influenza (9%)

Drug Interactions

Metabolism/Transport Effects None known.

Avoid Concomitant Use There are no known interactions where it is recommended to avoid concomitant use.

Increased Effect/Toxicity There are no known significant interactions involving an increase in effect.

Decreased Effect There are no known significant interactions involving a decrease in effect.

Preparation for Administration

Oral: Each 200 mg tablet should be dispersed in at least 2.5 mL of water (no other foods/liquids) and taken immediately.

Oral syringe: Disperse each 200 mg tablet in 2.5 mL of water to yield a concentration of 80 mg/mL (shake gently in container). Appropriate volume of dispersion should be drawn up in an oral syringe and administered immediately (discard unused dispersion).

Nasogastric tube: Disperse each 200 mg tablet in 2.5 mL of water and shake gently. Immediately administer through a nasogastric tube, followed by flush with additional water to clear the tube.

Storage/Stability Before opening, store refrigerated at 2°C to 8°C (36°F to 46°F). After opening, do not refrigerate or store above 30°C (86°F). Protect from moisture. Discard 1 month after opening.

Mechanism of Action N-acetylglutamate synthase (NAGS) is a mitochondrial enzyme which produces N-acetylglutamate (NAG). NAG is a required allosteric activator of the hepatic mitochondrial enzyme, carbamoyl phosphate synthetase 1 (CPS 1), which converts ammonia into urea in the first step of the urea cycle. In NAGS-deficient patients, carglumic acid serves as a replacement for NAG.

Pharmacodynamics/Kinetics

Distribution: V_d: ~2657 L

Metabolism: Via intestinal flora to carbon dioxide

Half-life elimination: 5.6 hours
Time to peak: 3 hours
Excretion: Feces (60% as unchanged drug); urine (9% as unchanged drug)

Dosage Oral: Infants, Children, Adolescents, and Adults:
Acute hyperammonemia: 100-250 mg/kg/day given in 2 or 4 divided doses (rounded to the nearest 100 mg); titrate to age-appropriate plasma ammonia levels. Concomitant adjunctive ammonia-lowering therapy recommended.
Chronic hyperammonemia: Usual dose (based on limited data): <100 mg/kg/day given in 2 or 4 divided doses; titrate to age-appropriate plasma ammonia levels

Dosage adjustment in renal impairment: No dosage adjustment provided in manufacturer's labeling.
Dosage adjustment in hepatic impairment: No dosage adjustment provided in manufacturer's labeling.

Dietary Considerations Take immediately prior to meals.

Administration Administer immediately prior to meals.
Oral: Tablets should **not** be crushed or swallowed whole. Disperse each 200 mg tablet in a minimum of 2.5 mL of water immediately before use and administer orally or via a nasogastric tube. Tablets do not dissolve completely, and some particles may remain; rinse container with water and swallow rinse immediately. Follow administration via nasogastric tube by flush with additional water to clear the tube. Carglumic acid tablets should not be mixed with any other foods or liquids other than water.
Oral syringe: Disperse each 200 mg tablet in 2.5 mL of water to yield a concentration of 80 mg/mL (shake gently in container). Appropriate volume of dispersion needed for dose should be drawn up in an oral syringe and administered immediately (discard unused dispersion). After administration, oral syringe should be refilled with a minimum of 1-2 mL of water and administered immediately.

Monitoring Parameters Blood ammonia; monitor for physical signs/symptoms of hyperammonemia (eg, lethargy, ataxia, confusion, vomiting, seizures, and memory impairment)

Dosage Forms Excipient information presented when available (limited, particularly for generics); consult specific product labeling.
Tablet, Oral:
Carbaglu: 200 mg [scored]

◆ **Carimune NF** *see* Immune Globulin *on page* 1059
◆ **Caripul (Can)** *see* Epoprostenol *on page* 727
◆ **Carisoprodate** *see* Carisoprodol *on page* 351

Carisoprodol (kar eye soe PROE dole)

Brand Names: U.S. Soma
Index Terms Carisoprodate; Isobamate
Pharmacologic Category Skeletal Muscle Relaxant
Additional Appendix Information
Beers Criteria – Potentially Inappropriate Medications for Geriatrics *on page* 2368

Use Short-term (2-3 weeks) treatment of acute musculoskeletal pain

Pregnancy Risk Factor C

Pregnancy Considerations Animal data suggests that carisoprodol crosses placenta and adverse events have been observed in animal studies. Limited postmarketing data with meprobamate (the active metabolite) demonstrate a possible risk for congenital malformations. Use only if benefit outweighs the risk.

Breast-Feeding Considerations Carisoprodol and its active metabolite, meprobamate are excreted into breast milk. Carisoprodol levels in breast milk may be 2-4 times that of maternal plasma levels. The estimated dose to the infant was reported as 6.9% of the weight adjusted maternal dose in one case report (Briggs, 2008) and ~4% of the weight-adjusted maternal dose in another (Nordeng, 2001). In both cases, breast milk production was decreased requiring supplemental formula or cessation of breast-feeding. Other than slight sedation reported in one infant, no symptoms of withdrawal or other adverse events were noted in these two cases. Effects on long-term development are not known. The manufacturer recommends caution be used if carisoprodol is administered to a nursing woman.

Contraindications Hypersensitivity to carisoprodol, carbamates (eg, meprobamate), or any component of the formulation; history of acute intermittent porphyria

Warnings/Precautions Can cause CNS depression, which may impair physical or mental abilities. Concomitant use of other CNS depressants may enhance these effects. Patients must be cautioned about performing tasks which require mental alertness (eg, operating machinery or driving); postmarketing reports of motor vehicle accidents have been associated with use. Effects with other CNS-depressant drugs or ethanol may be potentiated. Use with caution in patients with hepatic/renal dysfunction. Tolerance or drug dependence may result from extended use. Limit use to 2-3 weeks; use caution in patients who may be prone to addiction. May precipitate withdrawal after abrupt cessation of prolonged use. Has been associated (rarely) with seizures in patients with and without seizure history.

Carisoprodol should be used with caution in patients who are poor CYP2C19 metabolizers; poor metabolizers have been shown to have a fourfold increase in exposure to carisoprodol and a 50% reduced exposure to the metabolite meprobamate compared to normal metabolizers. Prevalence of poor metabolizers in the Asian population is ~15% to 20% while that of Caucasians and African-Americans is ~3% to 5%. Potentially significant drug-drug interactions may exist, requiring dose or frequency adjustment, additional monitoring, and/or selection of alternative therapy. Muscle relaxants are poorly tolerated by the elderly due to potent anticholinergic effects, sedation, and risk of fracture. Efficacy is questionable at dosages tolerated by elderly patients; avoid use (Beers Criteria).

Adverse Reactions
>10%: Central nervous system: Drowsiness (13% to 17%)
1% to 10%: Central nervous system: Dizziness (7% to 8%), headache (3% to 5%)
Postmarketing and/or case reports (Limited to important or life-threatening): Abdominal cramps, agitation, allergic dermatitis, anaphylaxis, angioedema, ataxia, burning sensation of eyes, depression, drug dependence, dyspnea, epigastric pain, eosinophilia, erythema multiforme, exacerbation of asthma, fixed drug eruption, hallucination, headache, hiccups, hypersensitivity reaction, idiosyncratic reaction (symptoms may include agitation, ataxia, confusion, diplopia, disorientation, dysarthria, euphoria, extreme weakness, muscle twitching, mydriasis, temporary vision loss, and/or transient quadriplegia); insomnia, irritability, leukopenia, nausea, orthostatic hypotension, pancytopenia, paradoxical central nervous system stimulation, pruritus, psychosis, seizure, skin rash, syncope, tachycardia, transient flushing of face, tremor, urticaria, vertigo, vomiting, weakness, withdrawal syndrome (abdominal cramps, headache, insomnia, nausea, seizure)

Drug Interactions
Metabolism/Transport Effects Substrate of CYP2C19 (major); **Note:** Assignment of Major/Minor substrate status based on clinically relevant drug interaction potential
Avoid Concomitant Use
Avoid concomitant use of Carisoprodol with any of the following: Azelastine (Nasal); Paraldehyde

Increased Effect/Toxicity

Carisoprodol may increase the levels/effects of: Alcohol (Ethyl); Azelastine (Nasal); Buprenorphine; CNS Depressants; Hydrocodone; Methotrimeprazine; Metyrosine; Mirtazapine; Paraldehyde; Pramipexole; ROPINIRole; Rotigotine; Selective Serotonin Reuptake Inhibitors; Zolpidem

The levels/effects of Carisoprodol may be increased by: Aspirin; Brimonidine (Topical); CYP2C19 Inhibitors (Moderate); CYP2C19 Inhibitors (Strong); Doxylamine; Droperidol; HydrOXYzine; Luliconazole; Magnesium Sulfate; Methotrimeprazine; Perampanel; Sodium Oxybate; St Johns Wort; Tapentadol

Decreased Effect

The levels/effects of Carisoprodol may be decreased by: Aspirin; CYP2C19 Inducers (Strong); Dabrafenib; St Johns Wort

Ethanol/Nutrition/Herb Interactions

Ethanol: May increase CNS depression. Management: Instruct patients to avoid ethanol during therapy; monitor for increased effects with coadministration.

Herb/Nutraceutical: St John's wort may decrease exposure to carisoprodol and increase exposure to active metabolite (meprobamate). Kava kava, valerian, and gotu kola may increase CNS depression. Management: Avoid St John's wort, kava kava, valerian, and gotu kola.

Storage/Stability Store at 20°C to 25°C (68°F to 77°F).

Mechanism of Action Precise mechanism is not yet clear, but many effects have been ascribed to its central depressant actions. In animals, carisoprodol blocks interneuronal activity and depresses polysynaptic neuron transmission in the spinal cord and reticular formation of the brain. It is also metabolized to meprobamate, which has anxiolytic and sedative effects.

Pharmacodynamics/Kinetics

Onset of action: Rapid

Duration: 4-6 hours

Protein binding: Carisoprodol: <70%; Meprobamate: <25% (Olsen, 1994)

Metabolism: Hepatic, via CYP2C19 to active metabolite (meprobamate)

Half-life elimination: Carisoprodol: ~2 hours; Meprobamate: ~10 hours

Time to peak, plasma: 1.5-2 hours

Excretion: Urine, as metabolite

Dosage Note: Carisoprodol should only be used for short periods (2-3 weeks) due to lack of evidence of effectiveness with prolonged use.

Oral: Adolescents ≥16 years and Adults: 250-350 mg 3 times daily and at bedtime

Dosing adjustment in renal impairment: No dosage adjustment provided in manufacturer's labeling (has not been studied); carisoprodol undergoes renal excretion and should be used with caution.

Dialysis: Removed by hemo- and peritoneal dialysis

Dosing adjustment in hepatic impairment: No dosage adjustment provided in manufacturer's labeling (has not been studied); carisoprodol undergoes hepatic metabolism and should be used with caution.

Dietary Considerations May be taken with or without food.

Administration Administer with or without food.

Monitoring Parameters CNS effects (eg, mental status, excessive drowsiness); relief of pain and/or muscle spasm; signs of misuse, abuse, and addiction

Dosage Forms Excipient information presented when available (limited, particularly for generics); consult specific product labeling.

Tablet, Oral:

Soma: 250 mg, 350 mg

Generic: 250 mg, 350 mg

Controlled Substance C-IV

Carisoprodol and Aspirin

(kar eye soe PROE dole & AS pir in)

Index Terms Aspirin and Carisoprodol; Soma Compound

Pharmacologic Category Skeletal Muscle Relaxant

Use Relief of discomfort associated with acute, painful skeletal muscle conditions

Pregnancy Risk Factor C

Dosage Oral:

Children ≥16 years and Adults: Acute skeletal muscle pain: 1-2 tablets 4 times/day for 2-3 weeks (maximum: 8 tablets/24 hours)

Elderly: Avoid use in the elderly due to risk of orthostatic hypotension and CNS depression

Dosing adjustment in renal impairment: Use in renal impairment has not been studied; use with caution

Dosing adjustment in hepatic impairment: Use in hepatic impairment has not been studied; use with caution

Additional Information Complete prescribing information should be consulted for additional detail.

Dosage Forms Excipient information presented when available (limited, particularly for generics); consult specific product labeling.

Tablet: Carisoprodol 200 mg and aspirin 325 mg

Controlled Substance C-IV

Carisoprodol, Aspirin, and Codeine

(kar eye soe PROE dole, AS pir in, and KOE deen)

Index Terms Aspirin, Carisoprodol, and Codeine; Codeine, Aspirin, and Carisoprodol; Soma Compound w/Codeine

Pharmacologic Category Skeletal Muscle Relaxant

Use Skeletal muscle relaxant

Pregnancy Risk Factor C

Dosage Oral:

Adults: 1 or 2 tablets 4 times daily (maximum: 8 tablets per day); treatment should be temporary (2-3 weeks)

Elderly: Avoid or use with caution in the elderly (>65 years of age); adverse effects (eg, orthostatic hypotension and CNS depression) may be potentiated.

Dosage adjustment in renal impairment: No dosage adjustment provided in manufacturer's labeling.

Dosage adjustment in hepatic impairment: No dosage adjustment provided in manufacturer's labeling.

Additional Information Complete prescribing information should be consulted for additional detail.

Dosage Forms Excipient information presented when available (limited, particularly for generics); consult specific product labeling. [DSC] = Discontinued product

Tablet: Carisoprodol 200 mg, aspirin 325 mg, and codeine phosphate 16 mg

Controlled Substance C-III

◆ **Carmol [OTC]** *see* Urea *on page* 2140

◆ **Carmol 10 [OTC]** *see* Urea *on page* 2140

◆ **Carmol 20 [OTC]** *see* Urea *on page* 2140

◆ **Carmol-HC®** *see* Urea and Hydrocortisone *on page* 2141

Carmustine (kar MUS teen)

Brand Names: U.S. BiCNU; Gliadel Wafer

Brand Names: Canada BiCNU®; Gliadel Wafer®

Index Terms BCNU; bis(chloroethyl) nitrosourea; bis-chloronitrosourea; Carmustine Polymer Wafer; Carmustinum; WR-139021

Pharmacologic Category Antineoplastic Agent; Antineoplastic Agent, Alkylating Agent; Antineoplastic Agent, Alkylating Agent (Nitrosourea)

Use

Injection: Treatment of brain tumors (glioblastoma, brainstem glioma, medulloblastoma, astrocytoma, ependymoma, and metastatic brain tumors), multiple myeloma, Hodgkin's lymphoma (relapsed or refractory), non-Hodgkin's lymphomas (relapsed or refractory)

Wafer (implant): Adjunct to surgery in patients with recurrent glioblastoma multiforme; adjunct to surgery and radiation in patients with newly-diagnosed high-grade malignant glioma

Unlabeled Use Treatment of mycosis fungoides (topical)

Pregnancy Risk Factor D

Pregnancy Considerations Teratogenicity and embryotoxicity have been demonstrated in animal studies. Carmustine can cause fetal harm if administered to a pregnant woman. There are no adequate and well-controlled studies in pregnant women. Women of childbearing potential should avoid becoming pregnant while on treatment.

Breast-Feeding Considerations Due to the potential for serious adverse reactions in the nursing infant, breast-feeding should be discontinued.

Contraindications Hypersensitivity to carmustine or any component of the formulation

Warnings/Precautions Hazardous agent - use appropriate precautions for handling and disposal (NIOSH, 2012).

[U.S. Boxed Warning]: Injection: Bone marrow suppression (primarily thrombocytopenia and leukopenia) is the major carmustine toxicity; generally is delayed. Monitor blood counts weekly for at least 6 weeks after administration. Myelosuppression is cumulative. When given at the FDA-approved doses, treatment should not be administered less than 6 weeks apart. Consider nadir blood counts from prior dose for dosage adjustment. May cause bleeding (due to thrombocytopenia) or infections (due to neutropenia); monitor closely. Patients must have platelet counts >100,000/mm^3 and leukocytes >4000/mm^3 for a repeat dose. Anemia may occur (less common and less severe than leukopenia or thrombocytopenia). Long-term use is associated with the development of secondary malignancies (acute leukemias and bone marrow dysplasias).

[U.S. Boxed Warnings]: Injection: Dose-related pulmonary toxicity may occur; patients receiving cumulative doses >1400 mg/m^2 are at higher risk. Delayed onset of pulmonary fibrosis (may be fatal) has occurred in children up to 17 years after treatment; this occurred in ages 1-16 for the treatment of intracranial tumors; cumulative doses ranged from 770-1800 mg/m^2 (in combination with cranial radiotherapy). Pulmonary toxicity is characterized by pulmonary infiltrates and/or fibrosis and has been reported from 9 days to 43 months after nitrosourea treatment (including carmustine). Although pulmonary toxicity generally occurs in patients who have received prolonged treatment, pulmonary fibrosis has been reported with cumulative doses <1400 mg/m^2. In addition to high cumulative doses, other risk factors for pulmonary toxicity include history of lung disease and baseline predicted forced vital capacity (FVC) or carbon monoxide diffusing capacity (DL_{CO}) <70%. Baseline and periodic pulmonary function tests are recommended. For high-dose treatment (transplant; unlabeled dose), acute lung injury may occur ~1-3 months post transplant; advise patients to contact their transplant physician for dyspnea, cough, or fever; interstitial pneumonia may be managed with a course of corticosteroids. Children are at higher risk for delayed pulmonary toxicity.

Potentially significant drug-drug interactions may exist, requiring dose or frequency adjustment, additional monitoring, and/or selection of alternative therapy. Injection site burning and local tissue reactions, including swelling, pain, erythema, and necrosis have been reported. Monitor infusion site closely for infiltration or injection site reactions. Reversible increases in transaminases, bilirubin and alkaline phosphatase have been reported (rare); monitor liver function tests periodically during treatment. Renal failure, progressive azotemia, and decreased kidney size have been reported in patients who have received large cumulative doses or prolonged treatment (renal toxicity has also been reported in patients who have received lower cumulative doses); monitor renal function tests periodically during treatment. Unlabeled administration (intraarterial intracarotid route) has been associated with ocular toxicity. Consider initiating treatment at the lower end of the dose range in the elderly. Diluent contains ethanol. With wafer implantation, monitor closely for known craniotomy-related complications (seizure, intracranial infection, abnormal wound healing, brain edema); intracerebral mass effect (unresponsive to corticosteroids) has been reported; may lead to brain herniation; avoid communication between the resection cavity and the ventricular system to prevent wafer migration; communications larger than the wafer should be closed prior to implantation; wafer migration may cause obstructive hydrocephalus. **[U.S. Boxed Warning]: Injection: Should be administered under the supervision of an experienced cancer chemotherapy physician.**

Adverse Reactions

I.V.: Frequency not defined:

Cardiovascular: Arrhythmia (with high doses), chest pain, flushing (with rapid infusion), hypotension, tachycardia

Central nervous system: Ataxia, dizziness

Central nervous system: Ethanol intoxication (with high doses), headache

Dermatologic: Hyperpigmentation/skin burning (after skin contact)

Gastrointestinal: Nausea (common; dose related), vomiting (common; dose related), mucositis (with high doses), toxic enterocolitis (with high doses)

Hematologic: Leukopenia (common; onset: 5-6 weeks; recovery: after 1-2 weeks), thrombocytopenia (common: onset: ~4 weeks; recovery: after 1-2 weeks), anemia, neutropenic fever, secondary malignancies (acute leukemia, bone marrow dysplasias)

Hepatic: Alkaline phosphatase increased, bilirubin increased, hepatic sinusoidal obstruction syndrome (SOS; veno-occlusive disease; with high doses), transaminases increased

Local: Injection site reactions (burning, erythema, necrosis, pain, swelling)

Ocular: Conjunctival suffusion (with rapid infusion), neuroretinitis

Renal: Kidney size decreased, progressive azotemia, renal failure

Respiratory: Interstitial pneumonitis (with high doses), pulmonary fibrosis, pulmonary hypoplasia, pulmonary infiltrates

Miscellaneous: Allergic reaction, infection (with high doses)

Wafer:

≥4% (percentages reported only where incidence was greater compared to placebo):

Cardiovascular: Deep thrombophlebitis (10%), facial edema (6%), chest pain (5%)

Central nervous system: Brain edema (4% to 23%), confusion (10% to 23%), depression (16%), headache (15%), somnolence (14%), fever (12%), speech disorder (11%), intracranial hypertension (9%), anxiety (7%), facial paralysis (7%), pain (7%), ataxia (6%), hypesthesia (6%), hallucination (5%), seizure (grand mal 5%), meningitis (4%)

Dermatologic: Abnormal wound healing (14% to 16%), rash (5% to 12%)

Endocrine: Diabetes (5%)

Gastrointestinal: Nausea (8% to 22%), vomiting (8% to 21%), constipation (19%), abdominal pain (8%), diarrhea (5%)

Genitourinary: Urinary tract infection (21%)

Hematologic: Hemorrhage (7%)

Local: Abscess (4% to 8%)

Neuromuscular & skeletal: Weakness (22%), back pain (7%)

<4% (Limited to important or life-threatening): Abnormal thinking, allergic reaction, amnesia, aspiration pneumonia, cerebral hemorrhage, cerebral infarction, coma, cyst formation, diplopia, dizziness, dysphagia, eye pain, fecal incontinence, gastrointestinal hemorrhage, hydrocephalus, hyperglycemia, hyper-/hypotension, hypokalemia, hyponatremia, insomnia, leukocytosis, monoplegia, neck pain, paranoia, peripheral edema, sepsis, thrombocytopenia, urinary incontinence, visual field defect

Drug Interactions

Metabolism/Transport Effects None known.

Avoid Concomitant Use

Avoid concomitant use of Carmustine with any of the following: BCG; CloZAPine; Natalizumab; Pimecrolimus; Tacrolimus (Topical); Tofacitinib; Vaccines (Live)

Increased Effect/Toxicity

Carmustine may increase the levels/effects of: CloZAPine; Leflunomide; Natalizumab; Tofacitinib; Vaccines (Live)

The levels/effects of Carmustine may be increased by: Cimetidine; Denosumab; Melphalan; Pimecrolimus; Roflumilast; Tacrolimus (Topical); Trastuzumab

Decreased Effect

Carmustine may decrease the levels/effects of: BCG; Cardiac Glycosides; Coccidioidin Skin Test; Sipuleucel-T; Vaccines (Inactivated); Vaccines (Live)

The levels/effects of Carmustine may be decreased by: Echinacea

Preparation for Administration Hazardous agent; use appropriate precautions for handling and disposal (NIOSH, 2012).

Injection: Reconstitute initially with 3 mL of supplied diluent (dehydrated alcohol injection, USP); then further dilute with SWFI (27 mL), this provides a concentration of 3.3 mg/mL in ethanol 10%; protect from light; further dilute for infusion with D_5W using a non-PVC container.

Storage/Stability

Injection: Store intact vials and provided diluent under refrigeration at 2°C to 8°C (36°F to 46°F).

Reconstituted solutions are stable for 24 hours refrigerated (2°C to 8°C) and protected from light. Examine reconstituted vials for crystal formation prior to use. If crystals are observed, they may be redissolved by warming the vial to room temperature with agitation.

Solutions diluted to a concentration of 0.2 mg/mL in D_5W are stable for 8 hours at room temperature (25°C) in glass or polyolefin containers and protected from light.

Wafer: Store at or below -20°C (-4°F). Unopened foil pouches may be kept at room temperature for up to 6 hours.

Mechanism of Action Interferes with the normal function of DNA and RNA by alkylation and cross-linking the strands of DNA and RNA, and by possible protein modification; may also inhibit enzyme processes by carbamylation of amino acids in protein

Pharmacodynamics/Kinetics

Distribution: 3.3 L/kg; readily crosses blood-brain barrier producing CSF levels >50% of blood plasma levels; highly lipid soluble

Metabolism: Rapidly hepatic; forms active metabolites

Half-life elimination: Biphasic: Initial: 1.4 minutes; Secondary: 20 minutes (active metabolites: Plasma half-life of 67 hours)

Excretion: Urine (~60% to 70%) within 96 hours; lungs (6% to 10% as CO_2)

Dosage

I.V.: Adults: Brain tumors, Hodgkin's lymphoma, multiple myeloma, non-Hodgkin's lymphoma (per manufacturer labeling): 150-200 mg/m^2 every 6 weeks or 75-100 mg/m^2/day for 2 days every 6 weeks

Indication-specific dosing: I.V.:

Brain tumor, primary (unlabeled doses):

80 mg/m^2/day for 3 days every 8 weeks for 6 cycles (Brandes, 2004)

200 mg/m^2 every 8 weeks [maximum cumulative dose: 1500 mg/m^2] (Selker, 2002)

Hodgkin's lymphoma, relapsed or refractory (unlabeled dose): Mini-BEAM regimen: 60 mg/m^2 day 1 every 4-6 weeks (in combination with etoposide, cytarabine, and melphalan) (Colwill, 1995; Martin, 2001)

Multiple myeloma, relapsed, refractory (unlabeled dose): VBMCP regimen: 20 mg/m^2 day 1 every 35 days (in combination with vincristine, melphalan, cyclophosphamide, and prednisone) (Kyle, 2006; Oken, 1997)

Stem cell or bone marrow transplant, autologous (unlabeled use):

BEAM regimen: 300 mg/m^2 6 days prior to transplant (in combination with etoposide, cytarabine, and melphalan) (Chopra, 1993; Linch, 2010)

CBV regimen: 600 mg/m^2 3 days prior to transplant (in combination with cyclophosphamide and etoposide) (Reece, 1991)

Implantation (wafer): Adults: Recurrent glioblastoma multiforme, newly-diagnosed high-grade malignant glioma: 8 wafers placed in the resection cavity (total dose 61.6 mg); should the size and shape not accommodate 8 wafers, the maximum number of wafers allowed (up to 8) should be placed

Topical: Mycosis fungoides, early stage (unlabeled use; Zackheim, 2003):

Ointment (10 mg/100 grams petrolatum): Apply (with gloves) once daily to affected areas

Solution (0.2% solution in alcohol; dilute 5 mL in 60 mL water): Apply (with gloves) once daily to affected areas

Dosing adjustments for hematologic toxicity: Based on nadir counts with previous dose (manufacturer's labeling). I.V.:

If leukocytes >3000/mm^3 and platelets >75,000/mm^3: Administer 100% of dose

If leukocytes 2000-2999/mm^3 or platelets 25,000-74,999/mm^3: Administer 70% of dose

If leukocytes <2000/mm^3 or platelets <25,000/mm^3: Administer 50% of dose

Dosing adjustment in renal impairment: I.V.: The FDA-approved labeling does not contain renal dosing adjustment guidelines. The following dosage adjustments have been used by some clinicians (Kintzel, 1995):

Cl_{cr} 46-60 mL/minute: Administer 80% of dose

Cl_{cr} 31-45 mL/minute: Administer 75% of dose

Cl_{cr} ≤30 mL/minute: Consider use of alternative drug

Dosing adjustment in hepatic impairment: Dosage adjustment may be necessary; however, no specific guidelines are available.

Dosing in obesity: *ASCO Guidelines for appropriate chemotherapy dosing in obese adults with cancer (**Note:** Excludes HSCT dosing):* Utilize patient's actual body weight (full weight) for calculation of body surface area- or weight-based dosing, particularly when the intent of therapy is curative; manage regimen-related toxicities in the same manner as for nonobese patients; if a dose reduction is utilized due to toxicity, consider resumption of full weight-based dosing with subsequent cycles, especially if cause of toxicity (eg, hepatic or renal impairment) is resolved (Griggs, 2012).

Administration

Injection: Irritant (alcohol-based diluent). Significant absorption to PVC containers; should be prepared in either glass or polyolefin containers. Infuse over 2 hours (infusions <2 hours may lead to injection site pain or burning); infuse through a free-flowing saline or dextrose infusion, or administer through a central catheter to alleviate venous pain/irritation.

High-dose carmustine (transplant dose; unlabeled use): Infuse over a least 2 hours to avoid excessive flushing, agitation, and hypotension; was infused over 1 hour in some trials (Chopra, 1993). **High-dose carmustine may be fatal if not followed by stem cell rescue.** Monitor vital signs frequently during infusion; patients should be supine during infusion and may require the Trendelenburg position, fluid support, and vasopressor support.

Implant: Double glove before handling; outer gloves should be discarded as chemotherapy waste after handling wafers. Any wafer or remnant that is removed upon repeat surgery should be discarded as chemotherapy waste. The outer surface of the external foil pouch is not sterile. Open pouch gently; avoid pressure on the wafers to prevent breakage. Wafer that are broken in half may be used, however, wafers broken into more than 2 pieces should be discarded in a biohazard container. Oxidized regenerated cellulose (Surgicel®) may be placed over the wafer to secure; irrigate cavity prior to closure.

Topical (unlabeled use): Apply solution with brush or gauze pads; ointment and solution should be applied while wearing gloves to involved areas only; avoid contact with eyes or mouth (Zackheim, 2003).

Hazardous agent; use appropriate precautions for handling and disposal (NIOSH, 2012).

Monitoring Parameters CBC with differential and platelet count (weekly for at least 6 weeks after a dose), pulmonary function tests (FVC, DL_{CO}; at baseline and frequently during treatment), liver function (periodically), renal function tests (periodically); monitor blood pressure and vital signs during administration, monitor infusion site for possible infiltration

Wafer: Complications of craniotomy (seizures, intracranial infection, brain edema)

Dosage Forms Excipient information presented when available (limited, particularly for generics); consult specific product labeling.

Solution Reconstituted, Intravenous:

BiCNU: 100 mg (1 ea) [contains alcohol, usp]

Wafer, Implant:

Gliadel Wafer: 7.7 mg (8 ea) [contains polifeprosan 20]

◆ **Carmustine Polymer Wafer** *see* Carmustine *on page 352*

◆ **Carmustinum** *see* Carmustine *on page 352*

◆ **Caroguard [OTC]** *see* Beta-Carotene *on page 246*

◆ **Carrington Antifungal [OTC]** *see* Miconazole (Topical) *on page 1358*

◆ **Carter's Little Pills [OTC] (Can)** *see* Bisacodyl *on page 259*

◆ **Cartia XT** *see* Diltiazem *on page 613*

Carvedilol (KAR ve dil ole)

Brand Names: U.S. Coreg; Coreg CR

Brand Names: Canada Apo-Carvedilol®; Ava-Carvedilol; Dom-Carvedilol; JAMP-Carvedilol; Mylan-Carvedilol; Novo-Carvedilol; PMS-Carvedilol; RAN™-Carvedilol; ratio-Carvedilol; ZYM-Carvedilol

Pharmacologic Category Antihypertensive; Beta-Blocker With Alpha-Blocking Activity

Additional Appendix Information

Beta-Blockers *on page 2294*

Use Mild-to-severe heart failure of ischemic or cardiomyopathic origin (usually in addition to standard therapy); left ventricular dysfunction following myocardial infarction (MI) (clinically stable with LVEF ≤40%); management of hypertension

Unlabeled Use Angina pectoris

Pregnancy Risk Factor C

Pregnancy Considerations Because adverse events were not observed in animal reproduction studies, carvedilol is classified as pregnancy category C. In a cohort study, an increased risk of cardiovascular defects was observed following maternal use of beta-blockers during pregnancy. Intrauterine growth restriction (IUGR), small placentas, as well as fetal/neonatal bradycardia, hypoglycemia, and/or respiratory depression have been observed following *in utero* exposure to beta-blockers as a class. Adequate facilities for monitoring infants at birth should be available. Untreated chronic maternal hypertension and pre-eclampsia are also associated with adverse events in the fetus, infant, and mother. Carvedilol is not currently recommended for the initial treatment of maternal hypertension during pregnancy.

Breast-Feeding Considerations It is not known if carvedilol is excreted into human milk. The manufacturer suggests that a decision should be made to either discontinue nursing or discontinue the medication.

Contraindications Serious hypersensitivity to carvedilol or any component of the formulation; decompensated cardiac failure requiring intravenous inotropic therapy; bronchial asthma or related bronchospastic conditions; second- or third-degree AV block, sick sinus syndrome, and severe bradycardia (except in patients with a functioning artificial pacemaker); cardiogenic shock; severe hepatic impairment

Warnings/Precautions Consider pre-existing conditions such as sick sinus syndrome before initiating. Heart failure patients may experience a worsening of renal function (rare); risk factors include ischemic heart disease, diffuse vascular disease, underlying renal dysfunction, and systolic BP <100 mm Hg. Initiate cautiously and monitor for possible deterioration in patient status (eg, symptoms of HF). Worsening heart failure or fluid retention may occur during upward titration; dose reduction or temporary discontinuation may be necessary. Adjustment of other medications (ACE inhibitors and/or diuretics) may also be required. Bradycardia may be observed more frequently in elderly patients (>65 years of age); dosage reductions may be necessary.

Symptomatic hypotension with or without syncope may occur with carvedilol (usually within the first 30 days of therapy); close monitoring of patient is required especially with initial dosing and dosing increases; blood pressure must be lowered at a rate appropriate for the patient's clinical condition. Initiation with a low dose, gradual up-titration, and administration with food may help to decrease the occurrence of hypotension or syncope. Patients should be advised to avoid driving or other hazardous tasks during initiation of therapy due to the risk of syncope. Beta-blocker therapy should not be withdrawn abruptly (particularly in patients with CAD), but gradually tapered to avoid acute tachycardia, hypertension, and/or ischemia. Chronic beta-blocker therapy should not be routinely withdrawn prior to major surgery.

In general, patients with bronchospastic disease should not receive beta-blockers; if used at all, should be used cautiously with close monitoring. May precipitate or aggravate symptoms of arterial insufficiency in patients with PVD and Raynaud's disease; use with caution and monitor for progression of arterial obstruction. Use caution with concurrent use of digoxin, verapamil or diltiazem; bradycardia or heart block can occur. Use with caution in patients receiving inhaled anesthetic agents known to depress myocardial contractility. Use cautiously in patients with diabetes because it can mask prominent hypoglycemic symptoms. In patients with heart failure and diabetes, use of carvedilol may worsen hyperglycemia; may require adjustment of antidiabetic agents. May mask signs of hyperthyroidism (eg, tachycardia); if hyperthyroidism is suspected, carefully manage and monitor; abrupt withdrawal may exacerbate symptoms of hyperthyroidism or precipitate thyroid storm. May induce or exacerbate psoriasis. Use with caution in patients with myasthenia gravis or psychiatric disease (may cause CNS depression). Use with caution in patients with mild-to-moderate hepatic impairment; use is contraindicated in patients with severe impairment. Manufacturer recommends discontinuation of therapy if liver injury occurs (confirmed by laboratory testing). Adequate alpha-blockade is required prior to use of any beta-blocker for patients with untreated pheochromocytoma. Use caution with history of severe anaphylaxis to allergens; patients taking beta-blockers may become more sensitive to repeated challenges. Treatment of anaphylaxis (eg, epinephrine) in patients taking beta-blockers may be ineffective or promote undesirable effects.

Intraoperative floppy iris syndrome has been observed in cataract surgery patients who were on or were previously treated with alpha$_1$-blockers; causality has not been established and there appears to be no benefit in discontinuing alpha-blocker therapy prior to surgery. Instruct patients to inform ophthalmologist of carvedilol use when considering eye surgery.

Adverse Reactions Note: Frequency ranges include data from hypertension and heart failure trials. Higher rates of adverse reactions have generally been noted in patients with heart failure. However, the frequency of adverse effects associated with placebo is also increased in this population.

>10%:

Cardiovascular: Hypotension (9% to 20%)

Central nervous system: Dizziness (2% to 32%), fatigue (4% to 24%)

Endocrine & metabolic: Hyperglycemia (5% to 12%)

Gastrointestinal: Diarrhea (1% to 12%), weight gain (10% to 12%)

Neuromuscular & skeletal: Weakness (7% to 11%)

1% to 10%:

Cardiovascular: Bradycardia (2% to 10%), syncope (3% to 8%), peripheral edema (1% to 7%), generalized edema (5% to 6%), angina (1% to 6%), dependent edema (≤4%), AV block, cerebrovascular accident, hypertension, hyper-/hypovolemia, orthostatic hypotension, palpitation

Central nervous system: Headache (5% to 8%), depression, fever, hypoesthesia, hypotonia, insomnia, malaise, somnolence, vertigo

Endocrine & metabolic: Hypercholesterolemia (1% to 4%), hypertriglyceridemia (1%), diabetes mellitus, gout, hyperkalemia, hyperuricemia, hypoglycemia, hyponatremia

Gastrointestinal: Nausea (2% to 9%), vomiting (1% to 6%), abdominal pain, melena, periodontitis, weight loss

Genitourinary: Impotence

Hematologic: Anemia, prothrombin decreased, purpura, thrombocytopenia

Hepatic: Alkaline phosphatase increased (1% to 3%), GGT increased, transaminases increased

Neuromuscular & skeletal: Back pain (2% to 7%), arthralgia (1% to 6%), arthritis, muscle cramps, paresthesia

Ocular: Blurred vision (1% to 5%)

Renal: BUN increased (≤6%), nonprotein nitrogen increased (6%), albuminuria, creatinine increased, glycosuria, hematuria, renal insufficiency

Respiratory: Cough (5% to 8%), nasopharyngitis (4%), rales (4%), dyspnea (>3%), pulmonary edema (>3%), rhinitis (2%), nasal congestion (1%), sinus congestion (1%)

Miscellaneous: Injury (3% to 6%), allergy, flu-like syndrome, sudden death

<1% (Limited to important or life-threatening): Anaphylactoid reaction, alopecia, angioedema, aplastic anemia, amnesia, asthma, bronchospasm, bundle branch block, cholestatic jaundice, concentration decreased, diaphoresis, erythema multiforme, exfoliative dermatitis, GI hemorrhage, HDL decreased, hearing decreased, hyperbilirubinemia, hypersensitivity reaction, hypokalemia, hypokinesia, interstitial pneumonitis, leukopenia, libido decreased, migraine, myocardial ischemia, nervousness, neuralgia, nightmares, pancytopenia, paresis, peripheral ischemia, photosensitivity, pruritus, rash (erythematous, maculopapular, and psoriaform), respiratory alkalosis, seizure, Stevens-Johnson syndrome, tachycardia, tinnitus, toxic epidermal necrolysis, urinary incontinence, urticaria, xerostomia

Drug Interactions

Metabolism/Transport Effects Substrate of CYP1A2 (minor), CYP2C9 (minor), CYP2D6 (major), CYP2E1 (minor), CYP3A4 (minor), P-glycoprotein; **Note:** Assignment of Major/Minor substrate status based on clinically relevant drug interaction potential; **Inhibits** P-glycoprotein

Avoid Concomitant Use

Avoid concomitant use of Carvedilol with any of the following: Beta2-Agonists; Bosutinib; Floctafenine; Methacholine; PAZOPanib; Pomalidomide; Topotecan; VinCRIStine (Liposomal)

Increased Effect/Toxicity

Carvedilol may increase the levels/effects of: Afatinib; Alpha-/Beta-Agonists (Direct-Acting); Alpha1-Blockers; Alpha2-Agonists; Amifostine; Antihypertensives; Antipsychotic Agents (Phenothiazines); Bosutinib; Bupivacaine; Cardiac Glycosides; Cholinergic Agonists; Colchicine; CycloSPORINE (Systemic); Dabigatran Etexilate; Digoxin; Ergot Derivatives; Everolimus; Fingolimod; Hypotensive Agents; Insulin; Lidocaine (Systemic); Lidocaine (Topical); Mepivacaine; Methacholine; Midodrine; Obinutuzumab; PAZOPanib; P-glycoprotein/ABCB1 Substrates; Pomalidomide; Prucalopride; RiTUXimab; Rivaroxaban; Sulfonylureas; Topotecan; VinCRIStine (Liposomal)

The levels/effects of Carvedilol may be increased by: Abiraterone Acetate; Acetylcholinesterase Inhibitors; Alpha2-Agonists; Aminoquinolines (Antimalarial); Amiodarone; Anilidopiperidine Opioids; Antipsychotic Agents (Phenothiazines); Brimonidine (Topical); Calcium

Channel Blockers (Dihydropyridine); Calcium Channel Blockers (Nondihydropyridine); Cimetidine; CYP2C9 Inhibitors (Moderate); CYP2C9 Inhibitors (Strong); CYP2D6 Inhibitors (Moderate); CYP2D6 Inhibitors (Strong); Darunavir; Diazoxide; Digoxin; Dipyridamole; Disopyramide; Dronedarone; Floctafenine; Herbs (Hypotensive Properties); MAO Inhibitors; NiCARdipine; Pentoxifylline; P-glycoprotein/ABCB1 Inhibitors; Phosphodiesterase 5 Inhibitors; Propafenone; Prostacyclin Analogues; Regorafenib; Reserpine; Selective Serotonin Reuptake Inhibitors

Decreased Effect

Carvedilol may decrease the levels/effects of: Beta2-Agonists; Theophylline Derivatives

The levels/effects of Carvedilol may be decreased by: Barbiturates; Herbs (Hypertensive Properties); Methylphenidate; Nonsteroidal Anti-Inflammatory Agents; Peginterferon Alfa-2b; P-glycoprotein/ABCB1 Inducers; Rifamycin Derivatives; Yohimbine

Ethanol/Nutrition/Herb Interactions

Food: Food decreases rate but not extent of absorption. Administration with food minimizes risks of orthostatic hypotension.

Herb/Nutraceutical: Avoid herbs with hypertensive properties (bayberry, blue cohosh, cayenne, ephedra, ginger, ginseng [American], kola, licorice); may diminish the antihypertensive effect of carvedilol. Avoid herbs with hypotensive properties (black cohosh, California poppy, coleus, golden seal, hawthorn, mistletoe, periwinkle, quinine, shepherd's purse); may enhance the hypotensive effect of carvedilol.

Storage/Stability

Coreg®: Store at <30°C (<86°F). Protect from moisture.

Coreg CR®: Store at 25°C (77°F); excursions permitted to 15°C to 30°C (59°F to 86°F).

Mechanism of Action As a racemic mixture, carvedilol has nonselective beta-adrenoreceptor and alpha-adrenergic blocking activity. No intrinsic sympathomimetic activity has been documented. Associated effects in hypertensive patients include reduction of cardiac output, exercise- or beta-agonist-induced tachycardia, reduction of reflex orthostatic tachycardia, vasodilation, decreased peripheral vascular resistance (especially in standing position), decreased renal vascular resistance, reduced plasma renin activity, and increased levels of atrial natriuretic peptide. In CHF, associated effects include decreased pulmonary capillary wedge pressure, decreased pulmonary artery pressure, decreased heart rate, decreased systemic vascular resistance, increased stroke volume index, and decreased right arterial pressure (RAP).

Pharmacodynamics/Kinetics

Onset of action: 1-2 hours

Peak antihypertensive effect: ~1-2 hours

Absorption: Rapid and extensive

Distribution: V_d: 115 L

Protein binding: >98%, primarily to albumin

Metabolism: Extensively hepatic, via CYP2C9, 2D6, 3A4, and 2C19 (2% excreted unchanged); three active metabolites (4-hydroxyphenyl metabolite is 13 times more potent than parent drug for beta-blockade); first-pass effect; plasma concentrations in the elderly and those with cirrhotic liver disease are 50% and 4-7 times higher, respectively

Bioavailability: Immediate release: 25% to 35% (due to significant first-pass metabolism); Extended release: 85% of immediate release

Half-life elimination: 7-10 hours

Time to peak, plasma: Extended release: 5 hours

Excretion: Primarily feces

Dosage Oral: Adults: Reduce dosage if heart rate drops to <55 beats/minute.

Hypertension:

Immediate release: 6.25 mg twice daily; if tolerated, dose should be maintained for 1-2 weeks, then increased to 12.5 mg twice daily. If necessary, dosage may be increased to a maximum of 25 mg twice daily after 1-2 weeks.

Extended release: Initial: 20 mg once daily, if tolerated, dose should be maintained for 1-2 weeks then increased to 40 mg once daily if necessary; maximum dose: 80 mg once daily

Heart failure:

Immediate release: 3.125 mg twice daily for 2 weeks; if this dose is tolerated, may increase to 6.25 mg twice daily. Double the dose every 2 weeks to the highest dose tolerated by patient. (Prior to initiating therapy, other heart failure medications should be stabilized and fluid retention minimized.)

Maximum recommended dose:

Mild-to-moderate heart failure:

<85 kg: 25 mg twice daily

>85 kg: 50 mg twice daily

Severe heart failure: 25 mg twice daily

Extended release: Initial: 10 mg once daily for 2 weeks; if the dose is tolerated, increase dose to 20 mg, 40 mg, and 80 mg over successive intervals of at least 2 weeks. Maintain on lower dose if higher dose is not tolerated.

Left ventricular dysfunction following MI: **Note**: Should be initiated only after patient is hemodynamically stable and fluid retention has been minimized.

Immediate release: Initial 3.125-6.25 mg twice daily; increase dosage incrementally (ie, from 6.25-12.5 mg twice daily) at intervals of 3-10 days, based on tolerance, to a target dose of 25 mg twice daily.

Extended release: Initial: 10-20 mg once daily; increase dosage incrementally at intervals of 3-10 days, based on tolerance, to a target dose of 80 mg once daily.

Angina pectoris (unlabeled use): Immediate release: 25-50 mg twice daily

Elderly: Hypertension: Consider lower initial dose and titrate to response (Aronow, 2011)

Conversion from immediate release to extended release (Coreg CR®):

Current dose immediate release tablets 3.125 mg twice daily: Convert to extended release capsules 10 mg once daily

Current dose immediate release tablets 6.25 mg twice daily: Convert to extended release capsules 20 mg once daily

Current dose immediate release tablets 12.5 mg twice daily: Convert to extended release capsules 40 mg once daily

Current dose immediate release tablets 25 mg twice daily: Convert to extended release capsules 80 mg once daily

Dosing adjustment in renal impairment: None necessary

Dosing adjustment in hepatic impairment: Use is contraindicated in severe liver dysfunction.

Dietary Considerations Should be taken with food to minimize the risk of orthostatic hypotension.

Administration Administer with food to minimize the risk of orthostatic hypotension. Extended release capsules should not be crushed or chewed. Capsules may be opened and sprinkled on applesauce for immediate use.

Monitoring Parameters Heart rate, blood pressure (base need for dosage increase on trough blood pressure measurements and for tolerance on standing systolic pressure 1 hour after dosing); renal studies, BUN, liver function; in patient with increase risk for developing renal dysfunction, monitor during dosage titration.

Additional Information Fluid retention during therapy should be treated with an increase in diuretic dosage.

Dosage Forms Excipient information presented when available (limited, particularly for generics); consult specific product labeling.

Capsule Extended Release 24 Hour, Oral, as phosphate:
Coreg CR: 10 mg, 20 mg, 40 mg, 80 mg

Tablet, Oral:
Coreg: 3.125 mg, 6.25 mg, 12.5 mg, 25 mg
Generic: 3.125 mg, 6.25 mg, 12.5 mg, 25 mg

Dosage Forms: Canada Note: Refer to Dosage Forms. Extended-release capsules are not available in Canada.

Extemporaneous Preparations A 1.25 mg/mL carvedilol oral suspension may be made with tablets and one of two different vehicles (Ora-Blend™ or 1:1 mixture of Ora-Sweet® and Ora-Plus®). Crush five 25 mg tablets in a mortar and reduce to a fine powder; add 15 mL of purified water and mix to a uniform paste. Mix while adding chosen vehicle in incremental proportions to almost 100 mL; transfer to a calibrated amber bottle, rinse mortar with vehicle, and add quantity of vehicle sufficient to make 100 mL. Label "shake well". Stable for 84 days when stored in amber prescription bottles at room temperature (Loyd, 2006).

Carvedilol oral liquid suspensions (0.1 mg/mL and 1.67 mg/mL) made from tablets, water, Ora-Plus®, and Ora-Sweet® were stable for 12 weeks when stored in glass amber bottles at room temperature (25°C). Use one 3.125 mg tablet for the 0.1 mg/mL suspension or two 25 mg tablets for the 1.67 mg/mL suspension; grind the tablet(s) and compound a mixture with 5 mL of water, 15 mL Ora-Plus®, and 10 mL Ora-Sweet®. Final volume of each suspension: 30 mL; label "shake well" (data on file, GlaxoSmithKline, Philadelphia, PA: DOF #132 [**Note:** Manufacturer no longer disseminates this document]).

Loyd A Jr, "Carvedilol 1.25 mg/mL Oral Suspension," *Int J Pharm Compounding*, 2006, 10(3):220.

◆ Casodex *see* Bicalutamide *on page 258*

◆ Casodex® (Can) *see* Bicalutamide *on page 258*

Caspofungin (kas poe FUN jin)

Brand Names: U.S. Cancidas

Brand Names: Canada Cancidas®

Index Terms Caspofungin Acetate

Pharmacologic Category Antifungal Agent, Parenteral; Echinocandin

Additional Appendix Information

Antifungal Agents *on page 2286*

Use Treatment of invasive *Aspergillus* infections in patients who are refractory or intolerant of other therapies; treatment of candidemia and other *Candida* infections (intra-abdominal abscesses, peritonitis, pleural space); treatment of esophageal candidiasis; empirical treatment for presumed fungal infections in febrile neutropenic patients

Unlabeled Use Alternate agent in the prophylaxis against *Candida* infection in neutropenic cancer patients with substantial risk (eg, allogeneic transplant or undergoing induction therapy for acute leukemia)

Pregnancy Risk Factor C

Pregnancy Considerations Adverse events have been observed in animal reproduction studies. Caspofungin should be used during pregnancy only if potential benefit justifies the potential risk to the fetus.

Breast-Feeding Considerations It is not known if caspofungin is excreted in breast milk. The manufacturer recommends that caution be exercised when administering caspofungin to nursing women.

Contraindications Hypersensitivity to caspofungin or any component of the formulation

Warnings/Precautions Anaphylaxis and histamine-related reactions (eg, angioedema, facial swelling, bronchospasm, rash, sensation of warmth) have been reported. Discontinue if anaphylaxis occurs; consider discontinuation if histamine-related reactions occur. Administer supportive treatment if needed. Concurrent use of cyclosporine should be limited to patients for whom benefit outweighs risk, due to a high frequency of hepatic transaminase elevations observed during concurrent use. Potentially significant drug-drug interactions may exist, requiring dose or frequency adjustment, additional monitoring, and/or selection of alternative therapy. Use caution in hepatic impairment; increased transaminases and rare cases of liver impairment (including failure and hepatitis) have been reported in pediatric and adult patients. Monitor liver function tests during therapy; if tests become abnormal or worsen, consider discontinuation. Dosage reduction required in adults with moderate hepatic impairment; safety and efficacy have not been established in children with any degree of hepatic impairment and adults with severe hepatic impairment.

Adverse Reactions

>10%:

Cardiovascular: Hypotension (3% to 20%), peripheral edema (6% to 11%), tachycardia (4% to 11%)
Central nervous system: Fever (6% to 30%), chills (9% to 23%), headache (5% to 15%)
Dermatologic: Skin rash (4% to 23%)
Endocrine & metabolic: Hypokalemia (5% to 23%)
Gastrointestinal: Diarrhea (6% to 27%), vomiting (6% to 17%), nausea (4% to 15%)
Hematologic & oncologic: Decreased hemoglobin (18% to 21%), decreased hematocrit (13% to 18%), decreased white blood cell count (12%), anemia (2% to 11%)
Hepatic: Increased serum alkaline phosphatase (9% to 22%), increased serum ALT (4% to 18%), increased serum AST (2% to 16%), increased serum bilirubin (5% to 13%)
Local: Phlebitis (18%)
Renal: Increased serum creatinine (3% to 11%)
Respiratory: Respiratory failure (2% to 20%), cough (6% to 11%), pneumonia (4% to 11%)
Miscellaneous: Infusion related reaction (20% to 35%), septic shock (11% to 14%)

5% to 10%:

Cardiovascular: Hypertension (5% to 10%)
Dermatologic: Erythema (4% to 9%), pruritus (6% to 7%)
Endocrine & metabolic: Hypomagnesemia (7%), hyperglycemia (6%)
Gastrointestinal: Gastric irritation (4% to 10%), abdominal pain (4% to 9%)
Hepatic: Decreased serum albumin (7%)
Immunologic: Graft versus host disease (infants, children, and adolescents 1% to 4%)
Infection: Sepsis (5% to 7%)
Local: Catheter infection (infants, children, and adolescents 1% to 9%)
Renal: Hematuria (10%), increased blood urea nitrogen (4% to 9%)
Respiratory: Dyspnea (9%), pleural effusion (9%), respiratory distress (≤8%), rales (7%)

<5% (Limited to important or life-threatening): Abdominal distention, adult respiratory distress syndrome (ARDS), anaphylaxis, anorexia, anxiety, arthralgia, atrial fibrillation, back pain, bacteremia, blood coagulation disorder, bradycardia, cardiac arrest, cardiac arrhythmia, confusion, constipation, decreased appetite, depression, dizziness, drowsiness, dyspepsia, dystonia, edema, epistaxis, erythema multiforme, exfoliation of skin, fatigue, febrile neutropenia, flushing, hematuria, hepatic failure, hepatic necrosis, hepatitis, hepatomegaly, hepatotoxicity, hypercalcemia, hyperkalemia, hypervolemia,

hypoxia, infusion site reaction (pain/pruritus/swelling), insomnia, jaundice, limb pain, myocardial infarction, nephrotoxicity (serum creatinine ≥2 x baseline value or ≥1 mg/dL in patients with serum creatinine above ULN range), pancreatitis, petechia, pulmonary edema, pulmonary infiltrates, renal failure, renal insufficiency, seizure, skin lesion, stridor, Stevens-Johnson syndrome, tachypnea, thrombocytopenia, tremor, urinary tract infection, urticaria, weakness; histamine release (reactions include facial swelling, bronchospasm, sensation of warmth) has been reported

Drug Interactions

Metabolism/Transport Effects None known.

Avoid Concomitant Use There are no known interactions where it is recommended to avoid concomitant use.

Increased Effect/Toxicity

The levels/effects of Caspofungin may be increased by: CycloSPORINE (Systemic)

Decreased Effect

Caspofungin may decrease the levels/effects of: Saccharomyces boulardii; Tacrolimus (Systemic)

The levels/effects of Caspofungin may be decreased by: Inducers of Drug Clearance; Rifampin

Preparation for Administration Bring refrigerated vial to room temperature. Reconstitute vials using 10.8 mL 0.9% sodium chloride for injection, SWFI, or bacteriostatic water for injection, resulting in a concentration of 5 mg/mL for the 50 mg vial, and 7 mg/mL for the 70 mg vial (vials contain overfill). Mix gently to dissolve until clear solution is formed; do not use if cloudy or contains particles. Solution should be further diluted with 0.9%, 0.45%, or 0.225% sodium chloride or LR (do not exceed final concentration of 0.5 mg/mL).

Storage/Stability Store intact vials at 2°C to 8°C (36°F to 46°F). Reconstituted solution may be stored at ≤25°C (≤77°F) for 1 hour prior to preparation of infusion solution. Solutions diluted for infusion should be used within 24 hours when stored at ≤25°C (≤77°F) or within 48 hours when stored at 2°C to 8°C (36°F to 46°F).

Mechanism of Action Inhibits synthesis of β(1,3)-D-glucan, an essential component of the cell wall of susceptible fungi. Highest activity is in regions of active cell growth. Mammalian cells do not require β(1,3)-D-glucan, limiting potential toxicity.

Pharmacodynamics/Kinetics

Protein binding: ~97% to albumin

Metabolism: Slowly, via hydrolysis and *N*-acetylation as well as by spontaneous degradation, with subsequent metabolism to component amino acids. Overall metabolism is extensive.

Half-life elimination: Beta (distribution): 9-11 hours; Terminal: 40-50 hours

Excretion: Urine (41%; primarily as metabolites, ~1% of total dose as unchanged drug); feces (35%; primarily as metabolites)

Dosage Note: Duration of caspofungin treatment should be determined by patient status and clinical response.

Aspergillosis (invasive), candidemia, esophageal candidiasis, empiric therapy: Infants ≥3 months, Children, and Adolescents ≤17 years: I.V.: Initial dose: 70 mg/m² on day 1, subsequent dosing: 50 mg/m² once daily, if clinical response inadequate, may increase to 70 mg/m² once daily if tolerated, but increased efficacy not demonstrated (maximum dose: 70 mg daily). Refer to adult dosing for indication-specific recommended durations.

Aspergillosis (invasive): Adults: I.V.: Initial dose: 70 mg on day 1; subsequent dosing: 50 mg once daily. Duration of therapy should be a minimum of 6-12 weeks or throughout period of immunosuppression and until lesions have resolved (Walsh, 2008). Salvage treatment with 70 mg once daily (unlabeled dosing) has been reported (Maertens, 2006).

Candidemia: Adults: I.V.: Initial dose: 70 mg on day 1; subsequent dosing: 50 mg once daily; generally continue for at least 14 days after the last positive culture or longer if neutropenia warrants. Higher doses (150 mg once daily infused over ~2 hours) compared to the standard adult dosing regimen (50 mg once daily) have not demonstrated additional benefit or toxicity in patients with invasive candidiasis (Betts, 2009).

Esophageal candidiasis: Adults: I.V.: 50 mg once daily; continue for 7-14 days after symptom resolution. **Note:** The majority of patients studied for this indication also had oropharyngeal involvement.

Empiric therapy: Adults: I.V.: Initial dose: 70 mg on day 1; subsequent dosing: 50 mg once daily; continue until resolution of neutropenia; if fungal infection confirmed, continue for a minimum of 14 days (continue for at least 7 days after resolution of both neutropenia and clinical symptoms); if clinical response inadequate, may increase up to 70 mg once daily if tolerated, but increased efficacy not demonstrated.

Concomitant use of an enzyme inducer:

Children: Patients receiving carbamazepine, dexamethasone, efavirenz, nevirapine, phenytoin, or rifampin (and possibly other enzyme inducers): Consider 70 mg/m² once daily (maximum: 70 mg daily)

Adults:

Patients receiving rifampin: 70 mg caspofungin once daily

Patients receiving carbamazepine, dexamethasone, efavirenz, nevirapine, **or** phenytoin (and possibly other enzyme inducers): May require an increased dose of caspofungin 70 mg once daily.

Elderly: The number of patients >65 years of age in clinical studies was not sufficient to establish whether a difference in response may be anticipated.

Dosage adjustment in renal impairment: No dosage adjustment necessary.

End-stage renal disease (ESRD) requiring hemodialysis: Poorly dialyzed; no supplemental dose or dosage adjustment necessary, including patients on intermittent hemodialysis (IHD), peritoneal dialysis, or continuous renal replacement therapy (eg, CVVHD).

Dosage adjustment in hepatic impairment:

Children: Mild-to-severe insufficiency (Child-Pugh classes A, B, or C): No dosage adjustment provided in manufacturer's labeling (has not been studied).

Adults:

Mild insufficiency (Child-Pugh class A): No dosage adjustment necessary.

Moderate insufficiency (Child-Pugh class B): 70 mg on day 1 (where recommended), followed by 35 mg once daily

Severe insufficiency (Child-Pugh class C): No dosage adjustment provided in manufacturer's labeling (has not been studied).

Administration Infuse slowly, over ~1 hour. Monitor during infusion; isolated cases of possible histamine-related reactions have occurred during clinical trials (rash, flushing, pruritus, facial edema).

Monitoring Parameters Liver function; anaphylaxis or histamine-related reactions (eg, facial swelling, bronchospasm, sensation of warmth)

Dosage Forms Excipient information presented when available (limited, particularly for generics); consult specific product labeling.

Solution Reconstituted, Intravenous, as acetate:

Cancidas: 50 mg (1 ea); 70 mg (1 ea)

◆ **Caspofungin Acetate** *see* Caspofungin *on page 358*

◆ **Castor Oil, Trypsin, and Balsam Peru** *see* Trypsin, Balsam Peru, and Castor Oil *on page 2133*

Cefaclor (SEF a klor)

Brand Names: Canada Apo-Cefaclor®; Ceclor®; Novo-Cefaclor; Nu-Cefaclor; PMS-Cefaclor

Pharmacologic Category Antibiotic, Cephalosporin (Second Generation)

Use Treatment of susceptible bacterial infections including otitis media, lower respiratory tract infections, acute exacerbations of chronic bronchitis, pharyngitis and tonsillitis, urinary tract infections, skin and skin structure infections

Pregnancy Risk Factor B

Pregnancy Considerations Adverse events were not observed in animal reproduction studies. An increased risk of teratogenic effects has not been observed following maternal use of cefaclor.

Breast-Feeding Considerations Small amounts of cefaclor are excreted in breast milk. The manufacturer recommends that caution be exercised when administering cefaclor to nursing women. Nondose-related effects could include modification of bowel flora.

Contraindications Hypersensitivity to cefaclor, any component of the formulation, or other cephalosporins

Warnings/Precautions Modify dosage in patients with severe renal impairment. Prolonged use may result in fungal or bacterial superinfection, including *C. difficile*-associated diarrhea (CDAD) and pseudomembranous colitis; CDAD has been observed >2 months postantibiotic treatment. Use with caution in patients with a history of penicillin allergy, especially IgE-mediated reactions (eg, anaphylaxis, urticaria). Beta-lactamase-negative, ampicillin-resistant (BLNAR) strains of *H. influenzae* should be considered resistant to cefaclor. Extended release tablets are not approved for use in children <16 years of age.

Adverse Reactions

1% to 10%:

Dermatologic: Rash (maculopapular, erythematous, or morbilliform) (1% to 2%)
Gastrointestinal: Diarrhea (3%)
Genitourinary: Vaginitis (2%)
Hematologic: Eosinophilia (2%)
Hepatic: Transaminases increased (3%)
Miscellaneous: Moniliasis (2%)

<1% (Limited to important or life-threatening): Agitation, agranulocytosis, anaphylaxis, angioedema, aplastic anemia, arthralgia, cholestatic jaundice, CNS irritability, confusion, dizziness, hallucinations, hemolytic anemia, hepatitis, hyperactivity, insomnia, interstitial nephritis, nausea, nervousness, neutropenia, paresthesia, PT prolonged, pruritus, pseudomembranous colitis, seizure, serum-sickness, somnolence, Stevens-Johnson syndrome, thrombocytopenia, toxic epidermal necrolysis, urticaria, vomiting

Reactions reported with other cephalosporins: Abdominal pain, cholestasis, fever, hemorrhage, renal dysfunction, superinfection, toxic nephropathy

Drug Interactions

Metabolism/Transport Effects None known.

Avoid Concomitant Use

Avoid concomitant use of Cefaclor with any of the following: BCG

Increased Effect/Toxicity

Cefaclor may increase the levels/effects of: Aminoglycosides; Vitamin K Antagonists

The levels/effects of Cefaclor may be increased by: Probenecid

Decreased Effect

Cefaclor may decrease the levels/effects of: BCG; Sodium Picosulfate; Typhoid Vaccine

Ethanol/Nutrition/Herb Interactions Food: Cefaclor serum levels may be decreased slightly if taken with food. The bioavailability of cefaclor extended release tablets is decreased 23% and the maximum concentration is decreased 67% when taken on an empty stomach.

Storage/Stability Store at controlled room temperature. Refrigerate suspension after reconstitution. Discard after 14 days. Do not freeze.

Mechanism of Action Inhibits bacterial cell wall synthesis by binding to one or more of the penicillin-binding proteins (PBPs) which in turn inhibits the final transpeptidation step of peptidoglycan synthesis in bacterial cell walls, thus inhibiting cell wall biosynthesis. Bacteria eventually lyse due to ongoing activity of cell wall autolytic enzymes (autolysins and murein hydrolases) while cell wall assembly is arrested.

Pharmacodynamics/Kinetics

Absorption: Well absorbed, acid stable

Distribution: Widely throughout the body and reaches therapeutic concentration in most tissues and body fluids, including synovial, pericardial, pleural, peritoneal fluids; bile, sputum, and urine; bone, myocardium, gallbladder, skin and soft tissue

Protein binding: 25%

Metabolism: Partially hepatic

Half-life elimination: 0.5-1 hour; prolonged with renal impairment

Time to peak: Capsule: 60 minutes; Suspension: 45 minutes

Excretion: Urine (80% as unchanged drug)

Dosage

Usual dosage range:

Children >1 month: Oral: 20-40 mg/kg/day divided every 8-12 hours (maximum dose: 1 g/day)

Adults: Oral: 250-500 mg every 8 hours

Indication-specific dosing:

Children: Oral:

Otitis media: 40 mg/kg/day divided every 12 hours

Pharyngitis: 20 mg/kg/day divided every 12 hours

Dosage adjustment in renal impairment:

Cl_{cr} 10-50 mL/minute: Administer 50% to 100% of dose

Cl_{cr} <10 mL/minute: Administer 50% of dose

Hemodialysis: Moderately dialyzable (20% to 50%)

Dosage adjustment in hepatic impairment: No dosage adjustment provided in manufacturer's labeling.

Dietary Considerations Capsule and suspension may be taken with or without food.

Administration Administer around-the-clock to promote less variation in peak and trough serum levels.

Oral suspension: Shake well before using.

Monitoring Parameters Monitor renal function. Observe for signs of anaphylaxis during first dose.

Test Interactions Positive direct Coombs', false-positive urinary glucose test using cupric sulfate (Benedict's solution, Clinitest®, Fehling's solution), false-positive serum or urine creatinine with Jaffé reaction

Dosage Forms Excipient information presented when available (limited, particularly for generics); consult specific product labeling.

Capsule, Oral:

Generic: 250 mg, 500 mg

Suspension Reconstituted, Oral:

Generic: 125 mg/5 mL (150 mL); 250 mg/5 mL (150 mL); 375 mg/5 mL (100 mL)

Tablet Extended Release 12 Hour, Oral:

Generic: 500 mg

Cefadroxil (sef a DROKS il)

Brand Names: Canada Apo-Cefadroxil; PRO-Cefadroxil; Teva-Cefadroxil

Index Terms Cefadroxil Monohydrate; Duricef

Pharmacologic Category Antibiotic, Cephalosporin (First Generation)

Use

Pharyngitis and/or tonsillitis: Treatment of pharyngitis and/or tonsillitis caused by *Streptococcus pyogenes* (group A beta-hemolytic streptococci).

Skin and skin structure infections: Treatment of skin and skin structure infections caused by staphylococci and/or streptococci.

Urinary tract infection: Treatment of urinary tract infections caused by *Escherichia coli*, *Proteus mirabilis*, and *Klebsiella* species.

Unlabeled Use Chronic oral antimicrobial suppression of prosthetic joint infection with *Staphylococci* (oxacillin-susceptible) after completion of parenteral therapy

Pregnancy Risk Factor B

Pregnancy Considerations Adverse events have not been observed in animal reproduction studies. Cefadroxil crosses the placenta. Limited data is available concerning the use of cefadroxil in pregnancy; however, adverse fetal effects were not noted in a small clinical trial.

Breast-Feeding Considerations Very small amounts of cefadroxil are excreted in breast milk. The manufacturer recommends that caution be exercised when administering cefadroxil to nursing women. Nondose-related effects could include modification of bowel flora.

Contraindications Hypersensitivity to cefadroxil, any component of the formulation, or other cephalosporins

Warnings/Precautions Modify dosage in patients with renal impairment (Cl_{cr} <50 mL/minute/1.73 m^2). Use with caution in patients with a history of penicillin allergy, especially IgE-mediated reactions (eg, anaphylaxis, angioedema, urticaria). Use with caution in patients with a history of gastrointestinal disease, particularly colitis. Prolonged use may result in fungal or bacterial superinfection, including *C. difficile*-associated diarrhea (CDAD) and pseudomembranous colitis; CDAD has been observed >2 months postantibiotic treatment. Only I.M. penicillin has been shown to be effective in the prophylaxis of rheumatic fever. Cefadroxil is generally effective in the eradication of streptococci from the oropharynx; efficacy data for cefadroxil in the prophylaxis of subsequent rheumatic fever episodes are not available. Suspension may contain sulfur dioxide (sulfite); hypersensitivity reactions, including anaphylaxis and/or asthmatic exacerbations, may occur (may be life threatening).

Adverse Reactions

1% to 10%: Gastrointestinal: Diarrhea

<1% (Limited to important or life-threatening): Abdominal pain, agranulocytosis, anaphylaxis, angioedema, arthralgia, cholestasis, dyspepsia, erythema multiforme, fever, nausea, neutropenia, pruritus, pseudomembranous colitis, rash (maculopapular and erythematous), serum sickness, Stevens-Johnson syndrome, thrombocytopenia, transaminases increased, urticaria, vaginitis, vomiting

Reactions reported with other cephalosporins: Abdominal pain, aplastic anemia, BUN increased, creatinine increased, eosinophilia, hemolytic anemia, hemorrhage, pancytopenia, prothrombin time prolonged, renal dysfunction, seizure, superinfection, toxic epidermal necrolysis, toxic nephropathy

Drug Interactions

Metabolism/Transport Effects None known.

Avoid Concomitant Use

Avoid concomitant use of Cefadroxil with any of the following: BCG

Increased Effect/Toxicity

Cefadroxil may increase the levels/effects of: Vitamin K Antagonists

The levels/effects of Cefadroxil may be increased by: Probenecid

Decreased Effect

Cefadroxil may decrease the levels/effects of: BCG; Sodium Picosulfate; Typhoid Vaccine

Ethanol/Nutrition/Herb Interactions Food: Concomitant administration with food, infant formula, or cow's milk does **not** significantly affect absorption.

Preparation for Administration Powder for suspension: Refer to manufacturer's product labeling for reconstitution instructions. Shake vigorously until suspended.

Storage/Stability Store capsules, tablets and un-reconstituted oral suspension at 20°C to 25°C (68°F to 77F); excursions are permitted to 15°C to 30°C (59°F to 86°F). After reconstitution, oral suspension may be stored for 14 days under refrigeration (4°C).

Mechanism of Action Inhibits bacterial cell wall synthesis by binding to one or more of the penicillin-binding proteins (PBPs) which in turn inhibits the final transpeptidation step of peptidoglycan synthesis in bacterial cell walls, thus inhibiting cell wall biosynthesis. Bacteria eventually lyse due to ongoing activity of cell wall autolytic enzymes (autolysins and murein hydrolases) while cell wall assembly is arrested.

Pharmacodynamics/Kinetics

Absorption: Rapid and well absorbed

Excretion: Urine (>90% as unchanged drug)

Dosage

Usual dosage range: Oral:

Children: 30 mg/kg/day divided every 12 hours (maximum: 2000 mg daily)

Adults: 1-2 g daily in a single dose or 2 divided doses

Indication-specific dosing: Oral:

Pharyngitis, group A streptococci (IDSA guidelines): Children and Adults: 30 mg/kg once daily (maximum: 1 g daily) for 10 days (Shulman, 2012). **Note:** Recommended as an alternative agent in penicillin-allergic patients; however, avoid in patients with immediate type hypersensitivity to penicillin.

Prosthetic joint infection, chronic oral antimicrobial suppression, staphylococci (oxacillin-susceptible) (preferred) (unlabeled use): Adults: 500 mg every 12 hours (Osmon, 2013)

Skin and skin structure infections: Adults: 1 g daily in a single or 2 divided doses

Tonsillitis: Adults: 1 g daily in a single or 2 divided doses for 10 days

Urinary tract infections: Adults: 1 g twice daily. For uncomplicated infections: 1 or 2 g daily in a single or 2 divided doses

Dosage adjustment in renal impairment:

Cl_{cr} 25-50 mL/minute: Administer every 12 hours

Cl_{cr} 10-25 mL/minute: Administer every 24 hours

Cl_{cr} <10 mL/minute: Administer every 36 hours

Dosage adjustment in hepatic impairment: No dosage adjustment provided in manufacturer's labeling.

Administration Administer around-the-clock to promote less variation in peak and trough serum levels. Administer without regards to meals; administration with food may diminish GI complaints.

Monitoring Parameters Monitor renal function. Observe for signs and symptoms of anaphylaxis during first dose.

Test Interactions Positive direct Coombs', false-positive urinary glucose test using cupric sulfate (Benedict's solution, Clinitest®, Fehling's solution), false-positive serum or urine creatinine with Jaffé reaction

Dosage Forms Excipient information presented when available (limited, particularly for generics); consult specific product labeling.

Capsule, Oral, as monohydrate [strength expressed as base]:

Generic: 500 mg

Suspension Reconstituted, Oral, as monohydrate [strength expressed as base]:

Generic: 250 mg/5 mL (100 mL); 500 mg/5 mL (75 mL, 100 mL)

Tablet, Oral, as monohydrate [strength expressed as base]:

Generic: 1 g

◆ **Cefadroxil Monohydrate** *see* Cefadroxil *on page 361*

CeFAZolin (sef A zoe lin)

Brand Names: Canada Cefazolin For Injection; Cefazolin For Injection, USP

Index Terms Ancef; Cefazolin Sodium; Kefzol

Pharmacologic Category Antibiotic, Cephalosporin (First Generation)

Additional Appendix Information

Antibiotic Treatment of Adults With Infective Endocarditis *on page 2355*

Desensitization Protocols *on page 2325*

Dosing Considerations for the Critically-Ill Patient With Morbid Obesity *on page 2379*

Prevention of Infective Endocarditis *on page 2353*

Use Treatment of respiratory tract, skin, genital, urinary tract, biliary tract, bone and joint infections, and septicemia due to susceptible gram-positive cocci (except *Enterococcus*); some gram-negative bacilli including *E. coli, Proteus*, and *Klebsiella* may be susceptible; surgical prophylaxis

Unlabeled Use Prophylaxis against infective endocarditis

Pregnancy Risk Factor B

Pregnancy Considerations Adverse effects were not observed in animal reproduction studies. Cefazolin crosses the placenta. Adverse events have not been reported in the fetus following administration of cefazolin prior to caesarean section. Cefazolin is recommended for group B streptococcus prophylaxis in pregnant patients with a nonanaphylactic penicillin allergy. It is also one of the antibiotics recommended for prophylactic use prior to cesarean delivery and may be used in certain situations prior to vaginal delivery in women at high risk for endocarditis.

Due to pregnancy-induced physiologic changes, the pharmacokinetics of cefazolin are altered. The half-life is shorter, the AUC is smaller, and the clearance and volume of distribution are increased.

Breast-Feeding Considerations Small amounts of cefazolin are excreted in breast milk. The manufacturer recommends that caution be exercised when administering cefazolin to nursing women. Nondose-related effects could include modification of bowel flora.

Contraindications Hypersensitivity to cefazolin sodium, any component of the formulation, or other cephalosporins

Warnings/Precautions Modify dosage in patients with severe renal impairment. Use with caution in patients with a history of penicillin allergy, especially IgE-mediated reactions (eg, anaphylaxis, angioedema, urticaria). Prolonged use may result in fungal or bacterial superinfection, including *C. difficile*-associated diarrhea (CDAD) and pseudomembranous colitis; CDAD has been observed >2 months postantibiotic treatment. May be associated with increased INR, especially in nutritionally-deficient patients, prolonged treatment, hepatic or renal disease. Use with caution in patients with a history of seizure disorder; high levels, particularly in the presence of renal impairment, may increase risk of seizures. Potentially significant drug-drug interactions may exist, requiring dose or frequency adjustment, additional monitoring, and/or selection of alternative therapy.

Adverse Reactions Frequency not defined.

Cardiovascular: Localized phlebitis

Central nervous system: Seizure

Dermatologic: Pruritus, skin rash, Stevens-Johnson syndrome

Gastrointestinal: Abdominal cramps, anorexia, diarrhea, nausea, oral candidiasis, pseudomembranous colitis, vomiting

Genitourinary: Vaginitis

Hepatic: Hepatitis, increased serum transaminases

Hematologic: Eosinophilia, leukopenia, neutropenia, thrombocythemia, thrombocytopenia

Hypersensitivity: Anaphylaxis

Local: Pain at injection site

Renal: Increased blood urea nitrogen, increased serum creatinine, renal failure

Miscellaneous: Fever

Drug Interactions

Metabolism/Transport Effects None known.

Avoid Concomitant Use

Avoid concomitant use of CeFAZolin with any of the following: BCG

Increased Effect/Toxicity

CeFAZolin may increase the levels/effects of: Fosphenytoin; Phenytoin; Vitamin K Antagonists

The levels/effects of CeFAZolin may be increased by: Probenecid

Decreased Effect

CeFAZolin may decrease the levels/effects of: BCG; Sodium Picosulfate; Typhoid Vaccine

Preparation for Administration Dilute 500 mg vial with 2 mL SWFI and 1 g vial with 2.5 mL SWFI; reconstituted solution may be directly injected after further dilution with 5 mL SWFI or further diluted for I.V. administration in 50-100 mL compatible solution; 10 g vial may be diluted with 45 mL to yield 1 g/5 mL or 96 mL to yield 1 g/10 mL.

Storage/Stability Store intact vials at room temperature and protect from temperatures exceeding 40°C. Reconstituted solutions of cefazolin are light yellow to yellow. Protection from light is recommended for the powder and for the reconstituted solutions. Reconstituted solutions are stable for 24 hours at room temperature and for 10 days under refrigeration. Stability of parenteral admixture at room temperature (25°C) is 48 hours. Stability of parenteral admixture at refrigeration temperature (4°C) is 14 days.

DUPLEX: Store at 20°C to 25°C (68°F to 77°F); excursions permitted to 15°C to 30°C (59°F to 86°F) prior to activation. Following activation, stable for 24 hours at room temperature and for 7 days under refrigeration.

Mechanism of Action Inhibits bacterial cell wall synthesis by binding to one or more of the penicillin-binding proteins (PBPs) which in turn inhibits the final transpeptidation step of peptidoglycan synthesis in bacterial cell walls, thus inhibiting cell wall biosynthesis. Bacteria eventually lyse due to ongoing activity of cell wall autolytic enzymes (autolysins and murein hydrolases) while cell wall assembly is arrested.

Pharmacodynamics/Kinetics

Distribution: Widely into most body tissues and fluids including gallbladder, liver, kidneys, bone, sputum, bile, pleural, and synovial; CSF penetration is poor

Protein binding: 74% to 86%

Metabolism: Minimally hepatic

Half-life elimination: I.M. or I.V.: ~2 hours; prolonged with renal impairment

Time to peak, serum: I.M.: 0.5-2 hours

Excretion: Urine (80% to 100% as unchanged drug)

Dosage

Usual dosage range: I.M., I.V.:

Children >1 month: 25-100 mg/kg/day divided every 6-8 hours; maximum: 6 **g** daily

Adults: 250-1500 mg every 6-12 (usually 8) hours, depending on severity of infection; maximum dose: 12 **g** daily

Indication-specific dosing:

Infants and Children: I.M., I.V.:

Community-acquired pneumonia (CAP) (IDSA/PIDS, 2011), moderate-to-severe infection, *S. aureus* (methicillin-susceptible) (preferred): Infants >3 months and Children: 150 mg/kg/day divided every 8 hours

Perioperative prophylaxis (unlabeled use): Children ≥1 year: I.V.: **Note:** For most surgical procedures, joint clinical practice guidelines from the American Society of Health-System Pharmacists, Infectious Diseases Society of America, Surgical Infection Society, and Society for Healthcare Epidemiology of America (ASHP/IDSA/SIS/SHEA) recommend a dose of 30 mg/kg (maximum dose: 2000 mg) administered within 60 minutes prior to surgical incision. For procedures requiring anaerobic coverage (eg, appendectomy, small bowel surgery with intestinal obstruction, colon procedures), combine cefazolin with metronidazole as an alternative to a second generation cephalosporin with anaerobic activity (eg, cefoxitin or cefotetan). Cefazolin doses may be repeated intraoperatively in 4 hours if procedure is lengthy or if there is excessive blood loss (Bratzler, 2013)

Prophylaxis against infective endocarditis (unlabeled use): 50 mg/kg 30-60 minutes before procedure; maximum dose: 1000 mg. Intramuscular injections should be avoided in patients who are receiving anticoagulant therapy. In these circumstances, orally administered regimens should be given whenever possible. Intravenously administered antibiotics should be used for patients who are unable to tolerate or absorb oral medications.

Note: American Heart Association (AHA) guidelines now recommend prophylaxis only in patients undergoing invasive procedures and in whom underlying cardiac conditions may predispose to a higher risk of adverse outcomes should infection occur. As of April 2007, routine prophylaxis for GI/GU procedures is no longer recommended by the AHA.

Adults: I.M., I.V.:

Cholecystitis, mild-to-moderate: I.V.: 1-2 g every 8 hours for 4-7 days (provided source controlled)

Endocarditis due to MSSA (without prosthesis) (unlabeled use): I.V.: 2 g every 8 hours; **Note:** Recommended for penicillin-allergic (nonanaphylactoid) patients (Baddour, 2005)

Group B streptococcus (neonatal prophylaxis): I.V.: 2 g once, then 1 g every 8 hours until delivery (CDC, 2010)

Intra-abdominal infection, complicated, community-acquired, mild-to-moderate (in combination with metronidazole): I.V.: 1-2 g every 8 hours for 4-7 days (provided source controlled)

Prophylaxis against infective endocarditis (unlabeled use): 1 g 30-60 minutes before procedure. Intramuscular injections should be avoided in patients who are receiving anticoagulant therapy. In these circumstances, orally administered regimens should be given whenever possible. Intravenously administered antibiotics should be used for patients who are unable to tolerate or absorb oral medications.

Note: American Heart Association (AHA) guidelines now recommend prophylaxis only in patients undergoing invasive procedures and in whom underlying cardiac conditions may predispose to a higher risk of adverse outcomes should infection occur. As of April 2007, routine prophylaxis for GI/GU procedures is no longer recommended by the AHA.

Moderate-to-severe infections: I.V.: 500 mg to 1 g every 6-8 hours

Mild infection with gram-positive cocci: 250-500 mg every 8 hours

Perioperative prophylaxis:

Manufacturer's labeling: 1 g initiated 30-60 minutes prior to surgery; may repeat after 2 hours if procedure is lengthy with 500 mg to 1 g intraoperatively, followed by 500 mg to 1 g every 6-8 hours for 24 hours postoperatively.

Guideline recommendations (unlabeled): I.V.: **Note:** For most surgical procedures, joint clinical practice guidelines from the American Society of Health-System Pharmacists, Infectious Diseases Society of America, Surgical Infection Society, and Society for Healthcare Epidemiology of America (ASHP/IDSA/SIS/SHEA) recommend a dose of 2 g within 60 minutes prior to surgical incision (for nonobese patients weighing <120 kg). For procedures requiring anaerobic coverage (eg, appendectomy, small bowel surgery with intestinal obstruction, colon procedures), combine cefazolin with metronidazole as an alternative to a second generation cephalosporin with anaerobic activity (eg, cefoxitin or cefotetan). Cefazolin doses may be repeated intraoperatively in 4 hours if procedure is lengthy or if there is excessive blood loss (Bratzler, 2013).

Obesity: The ASHP/IDSA/SIS/SHEA guidelines recommend that for patients weighing ≥120 kg, a dose of 3 g within 60 minutes prior to surgical incision should be administered (Bratzler, 2013). Alternatively, for patients with BMI >40 kg/m^2, a single 2 g dose may be sufficient for common general surgical procedures lasting <5 hours; patients enrolled in this multigroup study had a BMI up to a group mean of 55.7 kg/m^2 (Ho, 2012).

Cardiothoracic surgery: I.V.: 1 g (see **"Note"**) initiated 30-60 minutes prior to surgery (usually at the time of anesthetic induction); repeat dose if the duration of operation exceeds 3 hours (Hillis, 2011). The ASHP/IDSA/SIS/SHEA guidelines recommend the use of 2 g (single dose) administered within 60 minutes prior to surgical incision (Bratzler, 2013). May either continue for ≤48 hours postoperatively or administer as a single dose preoperatively (may be preferred due to reduced cost and potential for antimicrobial resistance) (Bratzler, 2013; Bucknell, 2000; Douglas, 2011; Edwards, 2006; Hillis, 2011).

Note: For patients weighing >60 kg, the Society of Thoracic Surgeons recommends a preoperative dose of 2 g administered within 60 minutes of skin incision. If the surgical incision remains open in the operating room, follow with 1 g every 3-4 hours unless cardiopulmonary bypass is to be discontinued within 4 hours then delay administration (Engelman, 2007).

Pneumococcal pneumonia: I.V.: 500 mg every 12 hours

Prosthetic joint infection, *Staphylococci* (oxacillin-susceptible): I.V.: 1-2 g every 8 hours for 2-6 weeks (in combination with rifampin) followed by oral antibiotic treatment and suppressive regimens (Osmon, 2013)

Severe infection: I.V.: 1-1.5 g every 6 hours

UTI (uncomplicated): 1 g every 12 hours

Dosage adjustment in renal impairment:

Cl_{cr} 35-54 mL/minute: Administer full dose in intervals of ≥8 hours

Cl_{cr} 11-34 mL/minute: Administer 50% of usual dose every 12 hours

Cl_{cr} ≤10 mL/minute: Administer 50% of usual dose every 18-24 hours

Intermittent hemodialysis (IHD) (administer after hemodialysis on dialysis days): Dialyzable (20% to 50%): 500 mg to 1 g every 24 hours **or** use 1-2 g every 48-72 hours (Heintz, 2009) **or** 15-20 mg/kg (maximum dose: 2 g) after dialysis 3 times weekly (Ahern, 2003; Sowinski, 2001) **or** 2 g after dialysis if next dialysis expected in 48 hours or 3 g after dialysis if next dialysis is expected in 72 hours (Stryjewski, 2007).

Note: Dosing dependent on the assumption of 3 times weekly, complete IHD sessions.

Peritoneal dialysis (PD): 500 mg every 12 hours

Continuous renal replacement therapy (CRRT) (Heintz, 2009; Trotman, 2005): Drug clearance is highly dependent on the method of renal replacement, filter type, and flow rate. Appropriate dosing requires close monitoring of pharmacologic response, signs of adverse reactions due to drug accumulation, as well as drug concentrations in relation to target trough (if appropriate). The following are general recommendations only (based on dialysate flow/ultrafiltration rates of 1-2 L/hour and minimal residual renal function) and should not supersede clinical judgment:

CVVH: Loading dose of 2 g followed by 1-2 g every 12 hours

CVVHD/CVVHDF: Loading dose of 2 g followed by either 1 g every 8 hours **or** 2 g every 12 hours. **Note:** Dosage of 1 g every 8 hours results in similar steady-state concentrations as 2 g every 12 hours and is more cost effective (Heintz, 2009).

Dosage adjustment in hepatic impairment: No dosage adjustment provided in manufacturer's labeling.

Dietary Considerations Some products may contain sodium.

Administration

I.M.: Inject deep I.M. into large muscle mass.

I.V.: Inject direct I.V. over 5 minutes or may infuse as an intermittent infusion over 30-60 minutes.

Some penicillins (eg, carbenicillin, ticarcillin and piperacillin) have been shown to inactivate aminoglycosides *in vitro*. This has been observed to a greater extent with tobramycin and gentamicin, while amikacin has shown greater stability against inactivation. Concurrent use of these agents may pose a risk of reduced antibacterial efficacy *in vivo*, particularly in the setting of profound renal impairment. However, definitive clinical evidence is lacking. If combination penicillin/aminoglycoside therapy is desired in a patient with renal dysfunction, separation of doses (if feasible), and routine monitoring of aminoglycoside levels, CBC, and clinical response should be considered.

Monitoring Parameters Renal function periodically when used in combination with other nephrotoxic drugs, hepatic function tests, CBC; monitor for signs of anaphylaxis during first dose

Test Interactions Positive direct Coombs', false-positive urinary glucose test using cupric sulfate (Benedict's solution, Clinitest, Fehling's solution), false-positive serum or urine creatinine with Jaffé reaction.

Some penicillin derivatives may accelerate the degradation of aminoglycosides *in vitro*, leading to a potential underestimation of aminoglycoside serum concentration.

Dosage Forms Excipient information presented when available (limited, particularly for generics); consult specific product labeling.

Solution, Intravenous:
Generic: 1 g (50 mL)

Solution Reconstituted, Injection:
Generic: 500 mg (1 ea); 1 g (1 ea); 10 g (1 ea); 20 g (1 ea); 100 g (1 ea); 300 g (1 ea)

Solution Reconstituted, Injection [preservative free]:
Generic: 500 mg (1 ea); 1 g (1 ea); 10 g (1 ea); 20 g (1 ea)

Solution Reconstituted, Intravenous:
Generic: 1 g (1 ea); 2 g (1 ea)

◆ **Cefazolin For Injection (Can)** *see* CeFAZolin *on page 362*

◆ **Cefazolin For Injection, USP (Can)** *see* CeFAZolin *on page 362*

◆ **Cefazolin Sodium** *see* CeFAZolin *on page 362*

Cefdinir (SEF di ner)

Index Terms CFDN; Omnicef

Pharmacologic Category Antibiotic, Cephalosporin (Third Generation)

Use Treatment of community-acquired pneumonia, acute exacerbations of chronic bronchitis, acute bacterial otitis media, acute maxillary sinusitis, pharyngitis/tonsillitis, and uncomplicated skin and skin structure infections.

Pregnancy Risk Factor B

Pregnancy Considerations Teratogenic events have not been observed in animal reproduction studies. An increase in most types of birth defects was not found following first trimester exposure to cephalosporins.

Breast-Feeding Considerations Cefdinir is not detectable in breast milk following a single cefdinir 600 mg dose. If present in breast milk, nondose-related effects could include modification of bowel flora.

Contraindications Hypersensitivity to cefdinir, any component of the formulation, other cephalosporins, or related antibiotics

Warnings/Precautions Administer cautiously to penicillin-sensitive patients, especially IgE-mediated reactions (eg, anaphylaxis, urticaria). Prolonged use may result in fungal or bacterial superinfection, including *C. difficile*-associated diarrhea (CDAD) and pseudomembranous colitis; CDAD has been observed >2 months postantibiotic treatment. Use caution with renal dysfunction (Cl_{cr} <30 mL/minute); dose adjustment may be required.

Adverse Reactions

>10%: Gastrointestinal: Diarrhea (8% to 15%)

1% to 10%:

- Central nervous system: Headache (2%)
- Dermatologic: Rash (≤3%)
- Endocrine & metabolic: Bicarbonate decreased (≤1%), hyperglycemia (≤1%), hyperphosphatemia (≤1%)
- Gastrointestinal: Nausea (≤3%), abdominal pain (≤1%), vomiting (≤1%)
- Genitourinary: Vaginal moniliasis (≤4%), urine leukocytes increased (≤2%), urine pH increased (≤1%), urine specific gravity increased (≤1%), vaginitis (≤1%)
- Hematologic: Lymphocytes increased (≤2%), eosinophils increased (1%), lymphocytes decreased (1%), platelets increased (≤1%), PMN changes (≤1%), WBC decreased/increased (≤1%)
- Hepatic: Alkaline phosphatase increased (≤1%), ALT increased (≤1%)
- Renal: Proteinuria (1% to 2%), microhematuria (≤1%), glycosuria (≤1%)
- Miscellaneous: GGT increased (≤1%), lactate dehydrogenase increased (≤1%)

<1%, postmarketing, and/or case reports: Allergic vasculitis, amylase increased, anaphylaxis, anorexia, asthma, AST increased, bilirubin increased, bleeding tendency, bloody diarrhea, BUN increased, cardiac failure, chest pain, cholestasis, coagulation disorder, conjunctivitis, constipation, cutaneous moniliasis, disseminated intravascular coagulation (DIC), dizziness, dyspepsia, enterocolitis (acute), eosinophilic pneumonia, erythema multiforme, erythema nodosum, exfoliative dermatitis, facial edema, fever, flatulence, fulminant hepatitis, granulocytopenia, hemoglobin decreased, hemolytic anemia, hemorrhagic colitis, hepatic failure, hepatitis (acute), hyperkalemia, hyperkinesia, hypertension, hypocalcemia, hypophosphatemia, idiopathic thrombocytopenia purpura, ileus, insomnia, interstitial pneumonia (idiopathic), involuntary movement, jaundice, laryngeal edema, leukopenia, leukorrhea, loss of consciousness, maculopapular rash, melena, moniliasis, monocytes increased, myocardial infarction, nephropathy, pancytopenia, peptic ulcer, pneumonia (drug-induced), pruritus, pseudomembranous colitis, renal failure (acute), respiratory failure (acute), rhabdomyolysis, serum sickness, shock, somnolence, Stevens-Johnson syndrome, stomatitis, stools abnormal, thrombocytopenia, toxic epidermal necrolysis, upper GI bleed, urine specific gravity decreased, weakness, xerostomia

Additional reactions reported with other cephalosporins: Agranulocytosis, angioedema, aplastic anemia, asterixis, encephalopathy, hemorrhage, interstitial nephritis, neuromuscular excitability, PT prolonged, seizure, superinfection, and toxic nephropathy

Drug Interactions

Metabolism/Transport Effects None known.

Avoid Concomitant Use

Avoid concomitant use of Cefdinir with any of the following: BCG

Increased Effect/Toxicity

Cefdinir may increase the levels/effects of: Aminoglycosides; Vitamin K Antagonists

The levels/effects of Cefdinir may be increased by: Probenecid

Decreased Effect

Cefdinir may decrease the levels/effects of: BCG; Sodium Picosulfate; Typhoid Vaccine

The levels/effects of Cefdinir may be decreased by: Iron Salts; Multivitamins/Minerals (with ADEK, Folate, Iron)

Preparation for Administration Oral suspension should be mixed with 38 mL water for the 60 mL bottle and 63 mL of water for the 100 mL bottle.

Storage/Stability Capsules and unmixed powder should be stored at 25°C (77°F); excursions permitted to 15°C to 30°C (59°F to 86°F). Oral suspension should be mixed with 38 mL water for the 60 mL bottle and 63 mL of water for the 100 mL bottle. After mixing, the suspension can be stored at room temperature of 25°C (77°F) for 10 days.

Mechanism of Action Inhibits bacterial cell wall synthesis by binding to one or more of the penicillin-binding proteins (PBPs) which in turn inhibits the final transpeptidation step of peptidoglycan synthesis in bacterial cell walls, thus inhibiting cell wall biosynthesis. Bacteria eventually lyse due to ongoing activity of cell wall autolytic enzymes (autolysins and murein hydrolases) while cell wall assembly is arrested.

Pharmacodynamics/Kinetics

Distribution: V_d:

- Children 6 months to 12 years: 0.29-1.05 L/kg
- Adults: 0.06-0.64 L/kg

Protein binding: 60% to 70%

Metabolism: Minimal

Bioavailability: Capsule: 16% to 21%; suspension 25%

Half-life elimination: ~100 minutes

Time to peak, plasma: 3 hours

Excretion: Primarily urine (7% to 25% as unchanged drug)

Dosage

Usual dosage range:

Children 6 months to 12 years: Oral: 7 mg/kg/dose twice daily or 14 mg/kg/dose once daily (maximum: 600 mg/day)

Adolescents and Adults: Oral: 300 mg twice daily or 600 mg once daily

Indication-specific dosing:

Children 6 months to 12 years: Oral:

Acute bacterial otitis media, pharyngitis/tonsillitis: 7 mg/kg/dose twice daily for 5-10 days **or** 14 mg/kg/dose once daily for 10 days (maximum: 600 mg/day)

Acute maxillary sinusitis: 7 mg/kg/dose twice daily **or** 14 mg/kg/dose once daily for 10 days (maximum: 600 mg/day)

Uncomplicated skin and skin structure infections: 7 mg/kg/dose twice daily for 10 days (maximum: 600 mg/day)

Adolescents and Adults:

Acute exacerbations of chronic bronchitis, pharyngitis/tonsillitis: 300 mg twice daily for 5-10 days **or** 600 mg once daily for 10 days

Acute maxillary sinusitis: 300 mg twice daily **or** 600 mg once daily for 10 days

Community-acquired pneumonia, uncomplicated skin and skin structure infections: 300 mg twice daily for 10 days

Dosing adjustment in renal impairment: Cl_{cr} <30 mL/minute:

Children: 7 mg/kg once daily (maximum: 300 mg/day)

Adults: 300 mg once daily

Hemodialysis removes cefdinir; recommended initial dose: 300 mg (or 7 mg/kg/dose) every other day. At the conclusion of each hemodialysis session, 300 mg (or 7 mg/kg/dose) should be given. Subsequent doses (300 mg or 7 mg/kg/dose) should be administered every other day.

Dosing adjustment in hepatic impairment: No adjustment necessary.

Administration Twice daily doses should be given every 12 hours. May be administered with or without food. Manufacturer recommends administering at least 2 hours before or after antacids or iron supplements. Shake suspension well before use.

Monitoring Parameters Monitor renal function. Observe for signs and symptoms of anaphylaxis during first dose.

Test Interactions False-positive reaction for urinary ketones may occur with nitroprusside- but not nitroferricyanide-based tests. False-positive urine glucose results may occur when using Clinitest®, Benedict's solution, or Fehling's solution; glucose-oxidase-based reaction systems (eg, Clinistix®, Tes-Tape®) are recommended. May cause positive direct Coombs' test.

Dosage Forms Excipient information presented when available (limited, particularly for generics); consult specific product labeling.

Capsule, Oral:

Generic: 300 mg

Suspension Reconstituted, Oral:

Generic: 125 mg/5 mL (60 mL, 100 mL); 250 mg/5 mL (60 mL, 100 mL)

Cefditoren (sef de TOR en)

Brand Names: U.S. Spectracef

Index Terms Cefditoren Pivoxil

Pharmacologic Category Antibiotic, Cephalosporin (Third Generation)

Use Treatment of acute bacterial exacerbation of chronic bronchitis or community-acquired pneumonia (due to susceptible organisms including *Haemophilus influenzae*, *Haemophilus parainfluenzae*, *Streptococcus pneumoniae*-penicillin susceptible only, *Moraxella catarrhalis*); pharyngitis or tonsillitis (*Streptococcus pyogenes*); and uncomplicated skin and skin-structure infections (*Staphylococcus aureus* - not MRSA, *Streptococcus pyogenes*)

Pregnancy Risk Factor B

Pregnancy Considerations Adverse events have not been observed in animal reproduction studies. An increase in most types of birth defects was not found following first trimester exposure to cephalosporins.

Breast-Feeding Considerations It is not known whether cefditoren is excreted in human milk. The manufacturer recommends caution when using cefditoren during breast-feeding. If cefditoren reaches the breast milk, the limited oral absorption may minimize the effect on the nursing infant. Nondose-related effects could include modification of bowel flora.

Contraindications Hypersensitivity to cefditoren, any component of the formulation, other cephalosporins, or milk protein; carnitine deficiency

Warnings/Precautions Use with caution in patients with a history of penicillin allergy, especially IgE-mediated reactions (eg, anaphylaxis, urticaria). Prolonged use may result in fungal or bacterial superinfection, including *C. difficile*-associated diarrhea (CDAD) and pseudomembranous colitis; CDAD has been observed >2 months postantibiotic treatment. Caution in individuals with seizure disorders; high levels, particularly in the presence of renal impairment, may increase risk of seizures. Use caution in patients with renal or hepatic impairment; modify dosage in patients with severe renal impairment. Cefditoren causes renal excretion of carnitine; do not use in patients with carnitine deficiency; not for long-term therapy due to the possible development of carnitine deficiency over time. May prolong prothrombin time; use with caution in patients with a history of bleeding disorder. Cefditoren tablets contain sodium caseinate, which may cause hypersensitivity reactions in patients with milk protein hypersensitivity; this does not affect patients with lactose intolerance.

Adverse Reactions

>10%: Gastrointestinal: Diarrhea (11% to 15%)

1% to 10%:

Central nervous system: Headache (2% to 3%)

Endocrine & metabolic: Glucose increased (1% to 2%)

Gastrointestinal: Nausea (4% to 6%), abdominal pain (2%), dyspepsia (1% to 2%), vomiting (1%)

Genitourinary: Vaginal moniliasis (3% to 6%)

Hematologic: Hematocrit decreased (2%)

Renal: Hematuria (3%), urinary white blood cells increased (2%)

<1% (Limited to important or life-threatening): Acute renal failure, albumin decreased, allergic reaction, arthralgia, asthma, BUN increased, calcium decreased, eosinophilic pneumonia, coagulation time increased, erythema multiforme, fungal infection, hyperglycemia, interstitial pneumonia, leukopenia, leukorrhea, positive direct Coombs' test, potassium increased, pseudomembranous colitis, rash, sodium decreased, Stevens-Johnson syndrome, thrombocythemia, thrombocytopenia, toxic epidermal necrolysis, white blood cells increased/decreased

Reactions reported with other cephalosporins: Anaphylaxis, aplastic anemia, cholestasis, hemorrhage, hemolytic anemia, renal dysfunction, reversible hyperactivity, serum sickness-like reaction, toxic nephropathy

Drug Interactions

Metabolism/Transport Effects None known.

Avoid Concomitant Use There are no known interactions where it is recommended to avoid concomitant use.

Increased Effect/Toxicity

Cefditoren may increase the levels/effects of: Vitamin K Antagonists

The levels/effects of Cefditoren may be increased by: Probenecid

Decreased Effect

The levels/effects of Cefditoren may be decreased by: Antacids; H2-Antagonists; Proton Pump Inhibitors

Ethanol/Nutrition/Herb Interactions Food: Moderate- to high-fat meals increase bioavailability and maximum plasma concentration. Management: Take with meals. Maintain adequate hydration, unless instructed to restrict fluid intake.

Storage/Stability Store at controlled room temperature of 15°C to 30°C (59°F to 86°F). Protect from light and moisture.

Mechanism of Action Inhibits bacterial cell wall synthesis by binding to one or more of the penicillin-binding proteins (PBPs) which in turn inhibits the final transpeptidation step of peptidoglycan synthesis in bacterial cell walls, thus inhibiting cell wall biosynthesis. Bacteria eventually lyse due to ongoing activity of cell wall autolytic enzymes (autolysins and murein hydrolases) while cell wall assembly is arrested.

Pharmacodynamics/Kinetics

Distribution: 9.3 ± 1.6 L

Protein binding: 88% (*in vitro*), primarily to albumin

Metabolism: Cefditoren pivoxil is hydrolyzed to cefditoren (active) and pivalate

Bioavailability: ~14% to 16%, increased by moderate- to high-fat meal

Half-life elimination: 1.6 ± 0.4 hours

Time to peak: 1.5-3 hours

Excretion: Urine (as cefditoren and pivaloylcarnitine)

Dosage

Usual dosage range:

Children ≥12 years and Adults: Oral: 200-400 mg twice daily

Indication-specific dosing:

Children ≥12 years and Adults: Oral:

Acute bacterial exacerbation of chronic bronchitis: 400 mg twice daily for 10 days

Dental infections (unlabeled use): 400 mg twice daily for 10 days

Community-acquired pneumonia: 400 mg twice daily for 14 days

Pharyngitis, tonsillitis, uncomplicated skin and skin structure infections: 200 mg twice daily for 10 days

Dosage adjustment in renal impairment:

Cl_{cr} 30-49 mL/minute/1.73 m^2: Maximum dose: 200 mg twice daily

Cl_{cr} <30 mL/minute/1.73 m^2: Maximum dose: 200 mg once daily

End-stage renal disease: Appropriate dosing not established

Dosage adjustment in hepatic impairment:

Mild-to-moderate impairment: Adjustment not required

Severe impairment (Child-Pugh Class C): Specific guidelines not available

Dietary Considerations Cefditoren should be taken with meals. Plasma carnitine levels are decreased during therapy (39% with 200 mg dosing, 63% with 400 mg dosing); normal concentrations return within 7-10 days after treatment is discontinued.

Administration Administer with meals.

Monitoring Parameters Monitor renal function. Observe for signs and symptoms of anaphylaxis during first dose.

Test Interactions May induce a positive direct Coomb's test. May cause a false-negative ferricyanide test. Glucose oxidase or hexokinase methods recommended for blood/plasma glucose determinations. False-positive urine glucose test when using copper reduction based assays (eg, Clinitest®).

Dosage Forms Excipient information presented when available (limited, particularly for generics); consult specific product labeling.

Tablet, Oral:

Spectracef: 200 mg, 400 mg [contains sodium caseinate]

Generic: 200 mg, 400 mg

◆ **Cefditoren Pivoxil** *see* Cefditoren *on page 366*

Cefepime (SEF e pim)

Brand Names: U.S. Maxipime

Brand Names: Canada Maxipime®

Index Terms Cefepime Hydrochloride

Pharmacologic Category Antibiotic, Cephalosporin (Fourth Generation)

Use Treatment of uncomplicated and complicated urinary tract infections, including pyelonephritis caused by *Escherichia coli, Klebsiella pneumoniae*, or *Proteus mirabilis*; monotherapy for febrile neutropenia; uncomplicated skin and skin structure infections caused by *Streptococcus pyogenes* or methicillin-susceptible staphylococci; moderate-to-severe pneumonia caused by *Streptococcus pneumoniae, Pseudomonas aeruginosa, Klebsiella pneumoniae*, or *Enterobacter* species; complicated intra-abdominal infections (in combination with metronidazole) caused by *E. coli, P. aeruginosa, K. pneumoniae, Enterobacter* species, or *Bacteroides fragilis* against methicillin-susceptible staphylococci, *Enterobacter* sp, and many other gram-negative bacilli.

Children 2 months to 16 years: Empiric therapy of febrile neutropenia patients, uncomplicated skin/soft tissue infections, pneumonia, and uncomplicated/complicated urinary tract infections, including pyelonephritis.

Unlabeled Use Brain abscess (postneurosurgical prevention); malignant otitis externa; prosthetic joint infection; septic lateral/cavernous sinus thrombosis

Pregnancy Risk Factor B

Pregnancy Considerations Adverse events were not observed in animal reproduction studies. Cefepime crosses the placenta.

Breast-Feeding Considerations Small amounts of cefepime are excreted in breast milk. The manufacturer recommends that caution be exercised when administering cefepime to nursing women. Nondose-related effects could include modification of bowel flora.

Contraindications Hypersensitivity to cefepime, other cephalosporins, penicillins, other beta-lactam antibiotics, or any component of the formulation

Warnings/Precautions Severe neurological reactions (some fatal) have been reported, including encephalopathy, myoclonus, seizures, and nonconvulsive status epilepticus; risk may be increased in the presence of renal impairment (Cl_{cr} ≤60 mL/minute); ensure dose adjusted for renal function or discontinue therapy if patient develops neurotoxicity; effects are often reversible upon discontinuation of cefepime. Use with caution in patients with a history of penicillin or cephalosporin allergy, especially IgE-mediated reactions (eg, anaphylaxis, urticaria). Prolonged use may result in fungal or bacterial superinfection, including *C. difficile*-associated diarrhea (CDAD) and pseudomembranous colitis; CDAD has been observed >2 months postantibiotic treatment. Use with caution in patients with a history of gastrointestinal disease, especially colitis. May be associated with increased INR, especially in nutritionally-deficient patients, prolonged treatment, hepatic or renal disease. Use with caution in patients with a history of seizure disorder; high levels, particularly in the presence of renal impairment, may increase risk of seizures.

Adverse Reactions

>10%: Hematologic & oncologic: Positive direct Coombs test (without hemolysis; 16%)

1% to 10%:

Cardiovascular: Localized phlebitis (1%)

Central nervous system: Headache (1%)

Dermatologic: Skin rash (1% to 4%), pruritus (1%)

Endocrine & metabolic: Hypophosphatemia (3%)

Gastrointestinal: Diarrhea (≤3%), nausea (≤2%), vomiting (≤1%)

Hematologic & oncologic: Eosinophilia (2%)

Hepatic: Increased serum ALT (3%), abnormal partial thromboplastin time (2%), increased serum AST (2%), abnormal prothrombin time (1%)

Local: Local pain (1%)

Miscellaneous: Fever (1%)

<1% (Limited to important or life-threatening): Agranulocytosis, anaphylactic shock, anaphylaxis, brain disease, colitis, coma, confusion, decreased hematocrit, hallucination, hypercalcemia, hyperkalemia, hyperphosphatemia, hypocalcemia, increased blood urea nitrogen, increased serum alkaline phosphatase, increased serum

bilirubin, increased serum creatinine, leukopenia, neutropenia, oral candidiasis, pseudomembranous colitis, seizure, status epilepticus (nonconvulsive), stupor, thrombocytopenia, urticaria, vaginitis

Drug Interactions

Metabolism/Transport Effects None known.

Avoid Concomitant Use

Avoid concomitant use of Cefepime with any of the following: BCG

Increased Effect/Toxicity

Cefepime may increase the levels/effects of: Aminoglycosides; Vitamin K Antagonists

The levels/effects of Cefepime may be increased by: Probenecid

Decreased Effect

Cefepime may decrease the levels/effects of: BCG; Sodium Picosulfate; Typhoid Vaccine

Storage/Stability

Vials: Store at 20°C to 25°C (68°F to 77°F). Protect from light. After reconstitution, stable in normal saline, D_5W, and a variety of other solutions for 24 hours at room temperature and 7 days refrigerated.

Premixed solution: Store frozen at -20°C (-4°F). Thawed solution is stable for 24 hours at room temperature or 7 days under refrigeration; do not refreeze.

Mechanism of Action Inhibits bacterial cell wall synthesis by binding to one or more of the penicillin-binding proteins (PBPs) which in turn inhibits the final transpeptidation step of peptidoglycan synthesis in bacterial cell walls, thus inhibiting cell wall biosynthesis. Bacteria eventually lyse due to ongoing activity of cell wall autolytic enzymes (autolysis and murein hydrolases) while cell wall assembly is arrested.

Pharmacodynamics/Kinetics

Absorption: I.M.: Rapid and complete

Distribution: V_d: Adults: 16-20 L; penetrates into inflammatory fluid at concentrations ~80% of serum levels and into bronchial mucosa at levels ~60% of those reached in the plasma; crosses blood-brain barrier

Protein binding, plasma: ~20%

Metabolism: Minimally hepatic

Half-life elimination: 2 hours

Time to peak: I.M.: 1-2 hours; I.V.: 0.5 hours

Excretion: Urine (85% as unchanged drug)

Dosage

Usual dosage range:

Children: I.M., I.V.: 50 mg/kg/dose every 8-12 hours (not to exceed maximum adult dosing)

Adults: I.V.: 1-2 g every 8-12 hours; I.M.: 0.5-1 g every 12 hours

Indication-specific dosing:

Children ≥2 months to 16 years (<40 kg):

Febrile neutropenia: I.V.: 50 mg/kg/dose every 8 hours for 7 days or until neutropenia resolves

Skin and skin structure infections (uncomplicated) and pneumonia: I.V.: 50 mg/kg/dose every 12 hours for 10 days

Urinary tract infections, complicated and uncomplicated: I.M., I.V.: 50 mg/kg/dose every 12 hours for 7-10 days; **Note:** I.M. may be considered for mild-to-moderate infection only

Adults:

Brain abscess, postneurosurgical prevention (unlabeled use): I.V.: 2 g every 8 hours with vancomycin (Tunkel, 2004)

Febrile neutropenia, monotherapy: I.V: 2 g every 8 hours for 7 days or until the neutropenia resolves

Intra-abdominal infections, complicated, severe (in combination with metronidazole): I.V.: 2 g every 12 hours for 7-10 days. **Note:** 2010 IDSA guidelines recommend 2 g every 8-12 hours for 4-7 days (provided source controlled). Not recommended for hospital-acquired intra-abdominal infections (IAI) associated with multidrug-resistant gram negative organisms or in mild-to-moderate community-acquired IAIs due to risk of toxicity and the development of resistant organisms (Solomkin, [IDSA] 2010).

Pneumonia: I.V.:

Nosocomial (HAP/VAP): 1-2 g every 8-12 hours; **Note:** Duration of therapy may vary considerably (7-21 days); usually longer courses are required if *Pseudomonas*. In absence of *Pseudomonas*, and if appropriate empiric treatment used and patient responsive, it may be clinically appropriate to reduce duration of therapy to 7-10 days (American Thoracic Society Guidelines, 2005).

Community-acquired (including pseudomonal): 1-2 g every 12 hours for 10 days

Prosthetic joint infection, *Enterobacter spp* or *Pseudomonas aeruginosa* (unlabeled use): I.V.: 2 g every 12 hours for 4-6 weeks; **Note:** When treating *P. aeruginosa*, consider addition of an aminoglycoside (Osmon, 2013)

Skin and skin structure, uncomplicated: I.V.: 2 g every 12 hours for 10 days

Urinary tract infections, complicated and uncomplicated:

Mild-to-moderate: I.M., I.V.: 0.5-1 g every 12 hours for 7-10 days

Severe: I.V.: 2 g every 12 hours for 10 days

Dosage adjustment in renal impairment:

Children: No dosage adjustment provided in the manufacturer's labeling; however, similar dosage adjustments to adults would be anticipated based on comparable pharmacokinetics between children and adults.

Adults: Recommended maintenance schedule based on creatinine clearance (may be estimated using the Cockcroft-Gault formula), compared to normal dosing schedule: See table.

Cefepime Hydrochloride

Creatinine Clearance (mL/minute)	Recommended Maintenance Schedule			
>60 (normal recommended dosing schedule)	500 mg every 12 hours	1 g every 12 hours	2 g every 12 hours	2 g every 8 hours
30-60	500 mg every 24 hours	1 g every 24 hours	2 g every 24 hours	2 g every 12 hours
11-29	500 mg every 24 hours	500 mg every 24 hours	1 g every 24 hours	2 g every 24 hours
<11	250 mg every 24 hours	250 mg every 24 hours	500 mg every 24 hours	1 g every 24 hours

Intermittent hemodialysis (IHD) (administer after hemodialysis on dialysis days): I.V.: Initial: 1 g (single dose) on day 1. Maintenance: 0.5-1 g every 24 hours **or** 1-2 g every 48-72 hours (Heintz, 2009) **or** 2 g 3 times weekly after dialysis (Perez, 2012). **Note:** Dosing dependent on the assumption of 3 times weekly, complete IHD sessions.

Peritoneal dialysis (PD): Removed to a lesser extent than hemodialysis; administer normal recommended dose every 48 hours

Continuous renal replacement therapy (CRRT) (Heintz, 2009; Trotman, 2005): Drug clearance is highly dependent on the method of renal replacement, filter type, and flow rate. Appropriate dosing requires close monitoring of pharmacologic response, signs of adverse reactions due to drug accumulation, as well as drug concentrations in relation to target trough (if appropriate). The following are general recommendations only (based on dialysate flow/ultrafiltration rates of 1-2 L/hour and minimal residual renal function) and should not supersede clinical judgment:

CVVH: Loading dose of 2 g followed by 1-2 g every 12 hours

CVVHD/CVVHDF: Loading dose of 2 g followed by either 1 g every 8 hours **or** 2 g every 12 hours. **Note:** Dosage of 1 g every 8 hours results in similar steady-state concentrations as 2 g every 12 hours and is more cost effective (Heintz, 2009).

Note: Consider higher dosage of 4 g/day if treating *Pseudomonas* or life-threatening infections in order to maximize time above MIC (Trotman, 2005). Dosage of 2 g every 8 hours may be needed for gram-negative rods with MIC ≥4 mg/L (Heintz, 2009).

Dosage adjustment in hepatic impairment: No dosage adjustment necessary.

Administration May be administered either I.M. or I.V.

Inject deep I.M. into large muscle mass. Inject direct I.V. over 5 minutes. Infuse intermittent infusion over 30 minutes.

Monitoring Parameters Monitor renal function. Observe for signs and symptoms of anaphylaxis during first dose.

Test Interactions Positive direct Coombs', false-positive urinary glucose test using cupric sulfate (Benedict's solution, Clinitest®, Fehling's solution), false-positive serum or urine creatinine with Jaffé reaction, false-positive urinary proteins and steroids

Dosage Forms Excipient information presented when available (limited, particularly for generics); consult specific product labeling.

Solution, Intravenous, as hydrochloride:
Generic: 1 g/50 mL (50 mL); 2% (100 mL)

Solution Reconstituted, Injection, as hydrochloride:
Maxipime: 1 g (1 ea); 2 g (1 ea)
Generic: 1 g (1 ea); 2 g (1 ea)

Solution Reconstituted, Intravenous, as hydrochloride:
Maxipime: 1 g (1 ea); 2 g (1 ea)
Generic: 1 g/50 mL (1 ea); 2 g/50 mL (1 ea)

◆ **Cefepime Hydrochloride** *see* Cefepime *on page 367*

Cefixime (sef IKS eem)

Brand Names: U.S. Suprax

Brand Names: Canada Suprax®

Index Terms Cefixime Trihydrate

Pharmacologic Category Antibiotic, Cephalosporin (Third Generation)

Use Treatment of uncomplicated urinary tract infections (due to *Escherichia coli* and *Proteus mirabilis*), otitis media (due to *Haemophilus influenzae, Moraxella catarrhalis,* and *Streptococcus pyogenes*), pharyngitis and tonsillitis (due to *Streptococcus pyogenes*), acute exacerbations of chronic bronchitis (due to *Streptococcus pneumoniae* and *Haemophilus influenzae*); uncomplicated cervical/urethral gonorrhea (due to *N. gonorrhoeae* [penicillinase- and non-penicillinase-producing])

Note: Due to concerns of resistance, the CDC no longer recommends use of cefixime as a first-line regimen in the treatment of uncomplicated gonorrhea in the U.S.; ceftriaxone is the preferred cephalosporin (CDC, 2012).

Unlabeled Use Acute bacterial rhinosinusitis (ABRS) (pediatric) in combination with clindamycin; typhoid fever

Pregnancy Risk Factor B

Pregnancy Considerations Teratogenic effects were not observed in animal reproduction studies. Cefixime crosses the placenta and can be detected in the amniotic fluid. An increase in most types of birth defects was not found following first trimester exposure to cephalosporins. Cefixime may be used for the treatment of gonococcal infections in pregnant women in certain situations (refer to current guidelines).

Breast-Feeding Considerations It is not known if cefixime is excreted in breast milk. The manufacturer recommends that consideration be given to discontinuing nursing temporarily during treatment. If present in breast milk, nondose-related effects could include modification of bowel flora.

Contraindications Hypersensitivity to cefixime, any component of the formulation, or other cephalosporins

Warnings/Precautions Prolonged use may result in fungal or bacterial superinfection, including *C. difficile*-associated diarrhea (CDAD) and pseudomembranous colitis; CDAD has been observed >2 months postantibiotic treatment. Modify dosage in patients with renal impairment. Use with caution in patients with a history of penicillin allergy, especially IgE-mediated reactions (eg, anaphylaxis, urticaria). Chewable tablets contain phenylalanine.

Adverse Reactions

>10%: Gastrointestinal: Diarrhea (16%)

2% to 10%: Gastrointestinal: Abdominal pain, nausea, dyspepsia, flatulence, loose stools

<2% (Limited to important or life-threatening): Acute renal failure, anaphylactic/anaphylactoid reactions, angioedema, BUN increased, candidiasis, creatinine increased, dizziness, drug fever, eosinophilia, erythema multiforme, facial edema, fever, headache, hepatitis, hyperbilirubinemia, jaundice, leukopenia, neutropenia, pruritus, pseudomembranous colitis, PT prolonged, rash, seizure, serum sickness-like reaction, Stevens-Johnson syndrome, thrombocytopenia, toxic epidermal necrolysis, transaminases increased, urticaria, vaginitis, vomiting

Reactions reported with other cephalosporins: Agranulocytosis, aplastic anemia, colitis, hemolytic anemia, hemorrhage, interstitial nephritis, pancytopenia, superinfection

Drug Interactions

Metabolism/Transport Effects None known.

Avoid Concomitant Use

Avoid concomitant use of Cefixime with any of the following: BCG

Increased Effect/Toxicity

Cefixime may increase the levels/effects of: Aminoglycosides; Vitamin K Antagonists

The levels/effects of Cefixime may be increased by: Probenecid

Decreased Effect

Cefixime may decrease the levels/effects of: BCG; Sodium Picosulfate; Typhoid Vaccine

Ethanol/Nutrition/Herb Interactions Food: Delays cefixime absorption.

Preparation for Administration Powder for suspension: Refer to manufacturer's product labeling for reconstitution instructions.

Storage/Stability

Capsule, chewable tablet, tablet: Store at 20°C to 25°C (68°F to 77°F).

Powder for suspension: Prior to reconstitution, store at 20°C to 25°C (68°F to 77°F). After reconstitution, suspension may be stored for 14 days at room temperature or under refrigeration.

Mechanism of Action Inhibits bacterial cell wall synthesis by binding to one or more of the penicillin-binding proteins (PBPs); which in turn inhibits the final transpeptidation step of peptidoglycan synthesis in bacterial cell walls, thus inhibiting cell wall biosynthesis. Bacteria eventually lyse due to ongoing activity of cell wall autolytic enzymes (autolysins and murein hydrolases) while cell wall assembly is arrested.

Pharmacodynamics/Kinetics **Note:** Chewable tablets and oral suspension are bioequivalent. However, oral suspension and tablet (nonchewable)/capsule formulations are **not** considered bioequivalent (oral suspension AUC ~10% to 25% greater compared with tablet after doses of 100-400 mg in normal adult volunteers).

Absorption: 40% to 50%; **Note:** Capsule AUC reduced by ~15% and C_{max} by ~25% when taken with food.

Distribution: Widely throughout the body and reaches therapeutic concentration in most tissues and body fluids, including synovial, pericardial, pleural, peritoneal; bile, sputum, and urine; bone, myocardium, gallbladder, and skin and soft tissue

Protein binding: 65%

Half-life elimination: Normal renal function: 3-4 hours; Renal failure: Up to 11.5 hours

Time to peak, serum: Tablet, suspension: 2-6 hours; Capsule: 3-8 hours; Delayed with food

Excretion: Urine (50% of absorbed dose as active drug); feces (10%)

Dosage

Usual dosage range: **Note:** Otitis media should be treated using the chewable tablets or suspension **only**. Chewable tablets and suspension achieve higher peak blood levels compared to an equivalent dose using the tablet or capsule.

Children ≥6 months and ≤45 kg: Oral: 8 mg/kg/day divided every 12-24 hours (maximum: 400 mg daily)

Dosing recommendations based on body weight (doses are rounded for use of oral suspension or chewable tablet):

5 to <7.6 kg: 50 mg daily
7.6 to <10.1 kg: 80 mg daily
10.1 to <12.6 kg: 100 mg daily
12.6 to <20.6 kg: 150 mg daily
20.6 to <28.1 kg: 200 mg daily
28.1 to <33.1 kg: 250 mg daily
33.1 to <40.1 kg: 300 mg daily
40.1 to ≤45 kg: 350 mg daily

Children >45 kg or >12 years, Adolescents, and Adults: Oral: 400 mg daily divided every 12-24 hours

Indication-specific dosing:

Children: Oral:

Acute bacterial rhinosinusitis (unlabeled use): 8 mg/kg/day divided every 12 hours with concomitant clindamycin for 10-14 days. **Note:** Recommended in patients with non-type I penicillin allergy, after failure of initial therapy or in patients at risk for antibiotic resistance (eg, daycare attendance, age <2 years, recent hospitalization, antibiotic use within the past month) (Chow, 2012).

S. pyogenes **infections:**

Children ≥6 months and ≤45 kg: 8 mg/kg/day divided every 12-24 hours for ≥10 days (maximum: 400 mg daily)

Children >45 kg or >12 years and Adolescents: 400 mg daily divided every 12-24 hours for ≥10 days

Typhoid fever (unlabeled use): 15-20 mg/kg/day divided every 12 hours for 7-14 days; maximum 400 mg daily (Girgis, 1995; Stephens, 2002)

Gonococcal infection, uncomplicated: Children >45 kg: 400 mg as a single dose in combination with oral azithromycin (preferred) or oral doxycycline (CDC, 2010). **Note:** CDC no longer recommends cefixime as a first-line agent, only use as an alternative agent with test-of-cure follow up in 7 days (CDC, 2012). In Canada, due to increased antimicrobial resistance, the Public Health Agency of Canada recommends 800 mg as a single dose (unlabeled dose) for treatment of uncomplicated gonococcal infections in children ≥9 years of age.

Adults: Oral:

Gonococcal infection, uncomplicated cervical/urethral/rectal gonorrhea due to *N. gonorrhoeae:* 400 mg as a single dose in combination with oral azithromycin (preferred) or oral doxycycline (CDC, 2010). **Note:** CDC no longer recommends cefixime as a first-line agent (ceftriaxone is the preferred cephalosporin), if cefixime is used as an alternative agent, test-of-cure follow up in 7 days is recommended; in addition, cefixime is **not** an option for the treatment of uncomplicated gonorrhea of the pharynx (CDC, 2012). In Canada, due to increased antimicrobial resistance, the Public Health Agency of Canada recommends 800 mg as a single dose (unlabeled dose) for treatment of uncomplicated gonococcal infections.

Gonococcal infection, expedited partner therapy: 400 mg as a single dose in combination with oral azithromycin (CDC, 2012). **Note:** Only used if a heterosexual partner cannot be linked to evaluation and treatment in a timely manner; dose delivered to partner by patient, collaborating pharmacy, or disease investigation specialist.

S. pyogenes **infections:** 400 mg daily divided every 12-24 hours for ≥10 days

Typhoid fever (unlabeled use): 15-20 mg/kg/day in 2 divided doses for 7-14 days (Parry, 2002; WHO, 2003)

Dosage adjustment in renal impairment: Adults:

Cl_{cr} ≥60 mL/minute: No dosage adjustment necessary.
Cl_{cr} 21-59 mL/minute: 260 mg once daily
Cl_{cr} ≤20 mL/minute:
Chewable tablet, tablet: 200 mg once daily
100 mg/5 mL suspension: 172 mg once daily
200 mg/5 mL suspension: 176 mg once daily
500 mg/5 mL suspension: 180 mg once daily

Intermittent hemodialysis (not significantly removed by hemodialysis): 260 mg once daily

CAPD (not significantly removed by peritoneal dialysis):
Chewable tablet, tablet: 200 mg once daily
100 mg/5 mL suspension: 172 mg once daily
200 mg/5 mL suspension: 176 mg once daily
500 mg/5 mL suspension: 180 mg once daily

Dosage adjustment in hepatic impairment: No dosage adjustment provided in manufacturer's labeling.

Dietary Considerations Chewable tablets contain phenylalanine.

Administration May be administered with or without food. Shake oral suspension well before use. Chewable tablets must be chewed or crushed before swallowing.

Monitoring Parameters Renal function; with prolonged therapy, monitor renal and hepatic function periodically. Observe for signs and symptoms of anaphylaxis during first dose. When used as part of alternative treatment for gonococcal infection, test-of-cure 7 days after dose (CDC, 2012).

Test Interactions Positive direct Coombs', false-positive urinary glucose test using cupric sulfate (Benedict's solution, Clinitest®, Fehling's solution), may cause false-positive serum or urine creatinine with the alkaline picrate-based Jaffé reaction for measuring creatinine; false-positive urine ketones using tests with nitroprusside (but not those using nitroferricyanide).

Dosage Forms Excipient information presented when available (limited, particularly for generics); consult specific product labeling.

Capsule, Oral, as trihydrate:
Suprax: 400 mg

Suspension Reconstituted, Oral, as trihydrate:
Suprax: 100 mg/5 mL (50 mL) [strawberry flavor]

Suprax: 200 mg/5 mL (50 mL, 75 mL); 500 mg/5 mL (10 mL, 20 mL) [contains sodium benzoate; strawberry flavor]

Tablet, Oral, as trihydrate:

Suprax: 400 mg [scored]

Tablet Chewable, Oral, as trihydrate:

Suprax: 100 mg, 200 mg [contains aspartame, fd&c red #40 aluminum lake; tutti-frutti flavor]

◆ **Cefixime Trihydrate** *see* Cefixime *on page 369*
◆ **Cefotan** *see* CefoTEtan *on page 373*

Cefotaxime (sef oh TAKS eem)

Brand Names: U.S. Claforan; Claforan in D_5W

Brand Names: Canada Cefotaxime Sodium For Injection; Claforan®

Index Terms Cefotaxime Sodium

Pharmacologic Category Antibiotic, Cephalosporin (Third Generation)

Additional Appendix Information

Antibiotic Treatment of Adults With Infective Endocarditis *on page 2355*

Use Treatment of susceptible organisms in lower respiratory tract, skin and skin structure, bone and joint, urinary tract, intra-abdominal, gynecologic as well as bacteremia/ septicemia, and documented or suspected central nervous system infections (eg, meningitis). Active against most gram-negative bacilli (not *Pseudomonas* spp) and gram-positive cocci (not enterococcus). Active against many penicillin-resistant pneumococci.

Unlabeled Use Acute bacterial rhinosinusitis (ABRS); surgical (perioperative) prophylaxis

Pregnancy Risk Factor B

Pregnancy Considerations Teratogenic effects were not observed in animal reproduction studies. Cefotaxime crosses the human placenta and can be found in fetal tissue. An increase in most types of birth defects was not found following first trimester exposure to cephalosporins. During pregnancy, peak cefotaxime serum concentrations are decreased and the serum half-life is shorter. Cefotaxime is approved for use in women undergoing cesarean section (consult current guidelines for appropriate use).

Breast-Feeding Considerations Low concentrations of cefotaxime are found in breast milk. The manufacturer recommends that caution be exercised when administering cefotaxime to nursing women. Nondose-related effects could include modification of bowel flora. The pregnancy-related changes in cefotaxime pharmacokinetics continue into the early postpartum period.

Contraindications Hypersensitivity to cefotaxime, any component of the formulation, or other cephalosporins

Warnings/Precautions Modify dosage in patients with severe renal impairment. Prolonged use may result in superinfection. A potentially life-threatening arrhythmia has been reported in patients who received a rapid (<1 minute) bolus injection via central venous catheter. Granulocytopenia and more rarely agranulocytosis may develop during prolonged treatment (>10 days). Minimize tissue inflammation by changing infusion sites when needed. Use with caution in patients with a history of penicillin allergy, especially IgE-mediated reactions (eg, anaphylaxis, urticaria). Prolonged use may result in fungal or bacterial superinfection, including *C. difficile*-associated diarrhea (CDAD) and pseudomembranous colitis; CDAD has been observed >2 months postantibiotic treatment.

Adverse Reactions

1% to 10%:

Dermatologic: Pruritus, rash

Gastrointestinal: Colitis, diarrhea, nausea, vomiting

Local: Pain at injection site

<1% (Limited to important or life-threatening): Agranulocytosis, alkaline phosphatase increased, ALT increased, anaphylaxis, arrhythmia (after rapid I.V. injection via central catheter), AST increased, bilirubin increased, BUN increased, candidiasis, cholestasis, Coombs test (direct) positive, creatinine increased, encephalopathy, eosinophilia, erythema multiforme, fever, GGT increased, headache, hemolytic anemia, hepatitis, interstitial nephritis, jaundice, LDH increased, leukopenia, moniliasis, neutropenia, phlebitis, pseudomembranous colitis, Stevens-Johnson syndrome, thrombocytopenia, toxic epidermal necrolysis, transaminases increased, urticaria, vaginitis

Reactions reported with other cephalosporins: Aplastic anemia, hemorrhage, pancytopenia, renal dysfunction, seizure, superinfection, toxic nephropathy

Drug Interactions

Metabolism/Transport Effects None known.

Avoid Concomitant Use

Avoid concomitant use of Cefotaxime with any of the following: BCG

Increased Effect/Toxicity

Cefotaxime may increase the levels/effects of: Aminoglycosides; Vitamin K Antagonists

The levels/effects of Cefotaxime may be increased by: Probenecid

Decreased Effect

Cefotaxime may decrease the levels/effects of: BCG; Sodium Picosulfate; Typhoid Vaccine

Preparation for Administration Reconstituted solution is stable for 12-24 hours at room temperature and 7-10 days when refrigerated and for 13 weeks when frozen. For I.V. infusion in NS or D_5W, solution is stable for 24 hours at room temperature, 5 days when refrigerated, or 13 weeks when frozen in Viaflex® plastic containers. Thawed solutions previously of frozen premixed bags are stable for 24 hours at room temperature or 10 days when refrigerated.

Mechanism of Action Inhibits bacterial cell wall synthesis by binding to one or more of the penicillin-binding proteins (PBPs) which in turn inhibits the final transpeptidation step of peptidoglycan synthesis in bacterial cell walls, thus inhibiting cell wall biosynthesis. Bacteria eventually lyse due to ongoing activity of cell wall autolytic enzymes (autolysins and murein hydrolases) while cell wall assembly is arrested.

Pharmacodynamics/Kinetics

Distribution: Widely to body tissues and fluids including aqueous humor, ascitic and prostatic fluids, bone; penetrates CSF best when meninges are inflamed

Metabolism: Partially hepatic to active metabolite, desacetylcefotaxime

Half-life elimination:

Cefotaxime: Infants ≤1500 g: 4.6 hours; Infants >1500 g: 3.4 hours; Adults: 1-1.5 hours; prolonged with renal and/or hepatic impairment

Desacetylcefotaxime: 1.5-1.9 hours; prolonged with renal impairment

Time to peak, serum: I.M.: Within 30 minutes

Excretion: Urine (~60% as unchanged drug and metabolites)

Dosage

Usual dosage range:

Infants and Children 1 month to 12 years <50 kg: I.M., I.V.: 50-200 mg/kg/day in divided doses every 6-8 hours

Children ≥50 kg, Children >12 years, and Adults: I.M., I.V.: 1-2 g every 4-12 hours

Uncomplicated infections: I.M., I.V.: 1 g every 12 hours

Moderate-to-severe infections: I.M., I.V.: 1-2 g every 8 hours

Life-threatening infections: I.V.: 2 g every 4 hours

Indication-specific dosing:

Infants and Children:

Acute bacterial rhinosinusitis, severe infection requiring hospitalization (unlabeled use): Children: I.V.: 100-200 mg/kg/day divided every 6 hours for 10-14 days (Chow, 2012)

Community-acquired pneumonia (CAP) (IDSA/PIDS, 2011): Infants >3 months and Children: I.V.: **Note:** May consider addition of vancomycin or clindamycin to empiric therapy if community-acquired MRSA suspected. In children ≥5 years, a macrolide antibiotic should be added if atypical pneumonia cannot be ruled out.

Empiric treatment, *Haemophilus influenzae*, group A *Streptococcus*, or *S. pneumoniae* (MICs to penicillin ≤2.0 mcg/mL), patient fully immunized for *H. influenzae* type b and *S. pneumoniae*, or minimal local resistance to penicillin in invasive pneumococcal strains (alternative to ampicillin or penicillin): 50 mg/kg/dose every 8 hours

Moderate-to-severe infection, patient not fully immunized for *H. influenzae* type b and *S. pneumoniae*, or significant local resistance to penicillin in invasive pneumococcal strains (preferred): 50 mg/kg/dose every 8 hours

Moderate-to-severe infection, *H. influenzae* (beta-lactamase producing) (preferred): 50 mg/kg/dose every 8 hours

Complicated community-acquired intra-abdominal infection (in combination with metronidazole): I.V.: 150-200 mg/kg/day divided every 6-8 hours (Solomkin, 2010)

Lyme disease (as an alternative to ceftriaxone): *Cardiac or CNS manifestations:* I.V.: 150-200 mg/kg/day in divided doses every 6-8 hours for 14-28 days; maximum daily dose: 6 g/day (Halperin, 2007; Wormser, 2006)

Meningitis (in combination with vancomycin): I.V.: 225-300 mg/kg/day in divided doses every 6-8 hours (Tunkel, 2004)

Sepsis: I.V.: 150 mg/kg/day divided every 8 hours

Surgical (perioperative) prophylaxis (unlabeled use): Children ≥1 year: I.V.: 50 mg/kg within 60 minutes prior to surgery (maximum: 1000 mg per dose). Doses may be repeated in 3 hours if procedure is lengthy or if there is excessive blood loss. **Note:** preferred agent (with ampicillin) in liver transplantation (Bratzler, 2013).

Infants and Children ≤12 years:

Typhoid fever: I.M., I.V.: 150-200 mg/kg/day in 3-4 divided doses (maximum: 12 g/day); fluoroquinolone resistant: 80 mg/kg/day in 3-4 divided doses (maximum: 12 g/day)

Children ≥50 kg, Children >12 years, and Adults:

Arthritis (septic): I.V.: 1 g every 8 hours

Brain abscess, meningitis: I.V.: 2 g every 4-6 hours in combination with other antimicrobial therapy as warranted (Kowlessar, 2006; Tunkel, 2004)

Caesarean section: I.M., I.V.: 1 g as soon as the umbilical cord is clamped, then 1 g at 6- and 12-hour intervals

Lyme disease (as an alternative to ceftriaxone):

Cardiac manifestations: I.V.: 2 g every 8 hours for 14-21 days (Wormser, 2006)

CNS manifestations: I.V.: 2 g every 8 hours for 10-28 days (Halperin, 2007; Wormser, 2006)

Peritonitis (spontaneous): I.V.: 2 g every 8 hours, unless life-threatening then 2 g every 4 hours (Gilbert, 2011; Runyon, 2009)

Sepsis: I.V.: 2 g every 6-8 hours

Skin and soft tissue:

Bite wounds (animal): I.V.: 2 g every 6 hours

Mixed, necrotizing: I.V.: 2 g every 6 hours, with metronidazole or clindamycin (Stevens, 2005)

Children ≥45 kg, Adolescents ≥45 kg, and Adults:

Gonorrhea (CDC, 2010) (as an alternative to ceftriaxone):

Uncomplicated gonorrhea of the cervix, urethra, or rectum (unlabeled regimen): I.M.: 0.5 g as a single dose in combination with oral azithromycin (preferred) or oral doxycycline (alternative to preferred)

Note: May also administer 1 g as a single dose for rectal gonorrhea in adult males (per the manufacturer)

Disseminated: I.V.: 1 g every 8 hours continue for 24-48 hrs after improvement begins then switch to oral therapy. Total duration of therapy at least 7 days

Adults:

Acute bacterial rhinosinusitis, severe infection requiring hospitalization: I.V.: 2 g every 4-6 hours for 5-7 days (Chow, 2012)

Complicated community-acquired intra-abdominal infection of mild-to-moderate severity, including hepatic abscess (in combination with metronidazole): I.V.: 1-2 g every 6 -8 hours for 4-7 days (provided source controlled). **Note:** For severe infections, consider other antimicrobial agents (Bradley, 1987; Kim, 2010; Solomkin, 2010).

Surgical (perioperative) prophylaxis (unlabeled use): I.V.: 1 g within 60 minutes prior to surgical incision. Doses may be repeated in 3 hours if procedure is lengthy or if there is excessive blood loss. **Note:** preferred agent (with ampicillin) in liver transplantation (Bratzler, 2013).

Obesity: The ASHP/IDSA/SIS/SHEA guidelines recommend that for patients weighing ≥120 kg (or alternatively defined as BMI >30 kg/m^2), a dose of 2 g within 60 minutes prior to surgical incision should be administered (Bratzler, 2013).

Dosage adjustment in renal impairment:

Manufacturer's labeling: **Note:** Renal function may be estimated using Cockcroft-Gault formula for dosage adjustment purposes.

Cl_{cr} <20 mL/minute/1.73 m^2: Dose should be decreased by 50%.

Alternate recommendations:

Children: **Note:** Glomerular filtration rate (GFR) should be estimated using an acceptable pediatric method (eg, Schwartz equation, Traub-Johnson equation, or a height/weight nomogram):

The following dosage adjustments have been used by some clinicians (Aronoff, 2007):

GFR 30-50 mL/minute/1.73 m^2: 35-70 mg/kg/dose every 8-12 hours

GFR 10-29 mL/minute/1.73 m^2: 35-70 mg/kg/dose every 12 hours

GFR <10 mL/minute/1.73 m^2: 35-70 mg/kg/dose every 24 hours

Intermittent hemodialysis (IHD): 35-70 mg/kg/dose every 24 hours

Peritoneal dialysis: 35-70 mg/kg/dose every 24 hours

Continuous renal replacement therapy (CRRT): 35-70 mg/kg/dose every 12 hours

Adults: The following dosage adjustments have been used by some clinicians (Aronoff, 2007; Heintz, 2009; Trotman, 2005):

GFR >50 mL/minute: Administer every 6 hours (Aronoff, 2007)

GFR 10-50 mL/minute: Administer every 6-12 hours (Aronoff, 2007)

GFR <10 mL/minute: Administer every 24 hours **or** decrease the dose by 50% (and administer at usual intervals) (Aronoff, 2007)

Intermittent hemodialysis (IHD): Administer 1-2 g every 24 hours (on dialysis days, administer after hemodialysis). **Note:** Dosing dependent on the assumption of 3 times/week, complete IHD sessions (Heintz, 2009).

Peritoneal dialysis (PD): 1 g every 24 hours (Aronoff, 2007)

Continuous renal replacement therapy (CRRT) (Heintz, 2009; Trotman, 2005): Drug clearance is highly dependent on the method of renal replacement, filter type, and flow rate. Appropriate dosing requires close monitoring of pharmacologic response, signs of adverse reactions due to drug accumulation, as well as drug concentrations in relation to target trough (if appropriate). The following are general recommendations only (based on dialysate flow/ultrafiltration rates of 1-2 L/hour and minimal residual renal function) and should not supersede clinical judgment:

CVVH: 1-2 g every 8-12 hours
CVVHD: 1-2 g every 8 hours
CVVHDF: 1-2 g every 6-8 hours

Dosage adjustment in hepatic impairment: Dosage reduction generally not necessary unless concurrent severe renal impairment. Consider dose reduction to 0.5 g every 12 hours in patients with Cl_{cr} <5 mL/minute (Wise, 1985).

Dietary Considerations Some products may contain sodium.

Administration Can be administered IVP over at least 3-5 minutes or I.V. intermittent infusion over 15-30 minutes.

Monitoring Parameters Observe for signs and symptoms of anaphylaxis during first dose; CBC with differential (especially with long courses); renal function

Test Interactions Positive direct Coombs', false-positive urinary glucose test using cupric sulfate (Benedict's solution, Clinitest®, Fehling's solution), false-positive serum or urine creatinine with Jaffé reaction

Dosage Forms Excipient information presented when available (limited, particularly for generics); consult specific product labeling.

Solution, Intravenous:
Claforan in D_5W: 1 g/50 mL (50 mL); 2 g/50 mL (50 mL)

Solution Reconstituted, Injection:
Claforan: 500 mg (1 ea); 1 g (1 ea); 2 g (1 ea); 10 g (1 ea)
Generic: 500 mg (1 ea); 1 g (1 ea); 2 g (1 ea); 10 g (1 ea)

Solution Reconstituted, Intravenous:
Claforan: 1 g (1 ea); 2 g (1 ea)

◆ **Cefotaxime Sodium** *see* Cefotaxime *on page 371*

◆ **Cefotaxime Sodium For Injection (Can)** *see* Cefotaxime *on page 371*

CefoTEtan (SEF oh tee tan)

Index Terms Cefotan; Cefotetan Disodium

Pharmacologic Category Antibiotic, Cephalosporin (Second Generation)

Use Surgical (perioperative) prophylaxis; intra-abdominal infections and other mixed infections; respiratory tract, skin and skin structure, bone and joint, urinary tract and gynecologic infections as well as septicemia; active against gram-negative enteric bacilli including *E. coli*, *Klebsiella*, and *Proteus*; less active against staphylococci and streptococci than first generation cephalosporins, but active against anaerobes including *Bacteroides fragilis*

Pregnancy Risk Factor B

Pregnancy Considerations Adverse events have not been observed in animal reproduction studies. Cefotetan crosses the placenta and produces therapeutic concentrations in the amniotic fluid and cord serum. Cefotetan is one of the antibiotics recommended for prophylactic use prior to cesarean delivery.

Breast-Feeding Considerations Very small amounts of cefotetan are excreted in human milk. The manufacturer recommends caution when giving cefotetan to a breast-feeding mother. Nondose-related effects could include modification of bowel flora.

Contraindications Hypersensitivity to cefotetan, any component of the formulation, or other cephalosporins; previous cephalosporin-associated hemolytic anemia

Warnings/Precautions Modify dosage in patients with severe renal impairment. Although cefotetan contains the methyltetrazolethiol side chain, bleeding has not been a significant problem. Use with caution in patients with a history of penicillin allergy, especially IgE-mediated reactions (eg, anaphylaxis, urticaria). Cefotetan has been associated with a higher risk of hemolytic anemia relative to other cephalosporins (approximately threefold); monitor carefully during use and consider cephalosporin-associated immune anemia in patients who have received cefotetan within 2-3 weeks (either as treatment or prophylaxis). Prolonged use may result in fungal or bacterial superinfection, including *C. difficile*-associated diarrhea (CDAD) and pseudomembranous colitis; CDAD has been observed >2 months postantibiotic treatment. May be associated with increased INR, especially in nutritionally-deficient patients, prolonged treatment, hepatic or renal disease.

Adverse Reactions

1% to 10%:
Gastrointestinal: Diarrhea (1%)
Hepatic: Transaminases increased (1%)
Miscellaneous: Hypersensitivity reactions (1%)

<1%: Anaphylaxis, urticaria, rash, pruritus, pseudomembranous colitis, nausea, vomiting, eosinophilia, thrombocytosis, agranulocytosis, hemolytic anemia, leukopenia, thrombocytopenia, prolonged PT, bleeding, BUN increased, creatinine increased, nephrotoxicity, phlebitis, fever

Reactions reported with other cephalosporins: Seizure, Stevens-Johnson syndrome, toxic epidermal necrolysis, renal dysfunction, toxic nephropathy, cholestasis, aplastic anemia, hemolytic anemia, hemorrhage, pancytopenia, agranulocytosis, colitis, superinfection

Drug Interactions

Metabolism/Transport Effects None known.

Avoid Concomitant Use

Avoid concomitant use of CefoTEtan with any of the following: BCG

Increased Effect/Toxicity

CefoTEtan may increase the levels/effects of: Alcohol (Ethyl); Aminoglycosides; Carbocisteine; Vitamin K Antagonists

The levels/effects of CefoTEtan may be increased by: Probenecid

Decreased Effect

CefoTEtan may decrease the levels/effects of: BCG; Sodium Picosulfate; Typhoid Vaccine

Ethanol/Nutrition/Herb Interactions Ethanol: Avoid ethanol (may cause a disulfiram-like reaction).

Preparation for Administration Reconstituted solution is stable for 24 hours at room temperature and 96 hours when refrigerated. For I.V. infusion in NS or D_5W solution and after freezing, thawed solution is stable for 24 hours at room temperature or 96 hours when refrigerated. Frozen solution is stable for 12 weeks.

Mechanism of Action Inhibits bacterial cell wall synthesis by binding to one or more of the penicillin-binding proteins (PBPs) which in turn inhibits the final transpeptidation step of peptidoglycan synthesis in bacterial cell walls, thus inhibiting cell wall biosynthesis. Bacteria eventually lyse due to ongoing activity of cell wall autolytic enzymes (autolysins and murein hydrolases) while cell wall assembly is arrested.

Pharmacodynamics/Kinetics
Distribution: Widely to body tissues and fluids including bile, sputum, prostatic, peritoneal; low concentrations enter CSF
Protein binding: 76% to 90%
Half-life elimination: 3-5 hours
Time to peak, serum: I.M.: 1.5-3 hours
Excretion: Primarily urine (as unchanged drug); feces (20%)

Dosage
Usual dosage range:
Children (unlabeled use): I.M., I.V.: 20-40 mg/kg/dose every 12 hours (maximum: 6 **g** daily)
Adults: I.M., I.V.: 1-6 g daily in divided doses every 12 hours

Indication-specific dosing:
Children (unlabeled use):
Surgical (perioperative) prophylaxis: Children ≥1 year: I.V.: 40 mg/kg 30-60 minutes prior to surgery (maximum: 2000 mg/dose). Doses may be repeated in 6 hours if procedure is lengthy or if there is excessive blood loss (Bratzler, 2013).
Adolescents and Adults:
Pelvic inflammatory disease: I.V.: 2 g every 12 hours; used in combination with doxycycline (CDC, 2010)
Adults:
Orbital cellulitis, odontogenic infections: I.V.: 2 g every 12 hours (Bailey, 2007; Quayle, 1987)
Surgical (perioperative) prophylaxis:
Manufacturer recommendations: I.V.: 1-2 g 30-60 minutes prior to surgery. **Note:** When used for cesarean section, dose should be given as soon as umbilical cord is clamped.
Alternative recommendations: I.V.: 2 g within 60 minutes prior to surgery. Doses may be repeated in 6 hours if procedure is lengthy or if there is excessive blood loss (Bratzler, 2013).
Susceptible infections: I.M., I.V.: 1-6 g daily in divided doses every 12 hours; usual dose: 1-2 g every 12 hours for 5-10 days; 1-2 g may be given every 24 hours for urinary tract infection; **Note:** Due to high rates of *B. fragilis* group resistance, not recommended for the treatment of community-acquired intra-abdominal infections (Solomkin, 2010)
Urinary tract infection: I.M., I.V.: 500 mg every 12 hours or 1-2 g every 12-24 hours

Dosage adjustment in renal impairment:
Cl_{cr} 10-30 mL/minute: Administer every 24 hours
Cl_{cr} <10 mL/minute: Administer every 48 hours
Hemodialysis: Dialyzable (5% to 20%); administer 1/4 the usual dose every 24 hours on days between dialysis; administer 1/2 the usual dose on the day of dialysis.
Continuous arteriovenous or venovenous hemodiafiltration effects: Administer 750 mg every 12 hours
Dosage adjustment in hepatic impairment: No dosage adjustment provided in manufacturer's labeling.

Dietary Considerations Some products may contain sodium.

Administration
I.M.: Inject deep I.M. into large muscle mass.
I.V.: Inject direct I.V. over 3-5 minutes. Infuse intermittent infusion over 30 minutes.

Monitoring Parameters Monitor renal, hepatic, and hematologic function periodically with prolonged therapy. Monitor prothrombin time in patients at risk of prolongation during cephalosporin therapy (nutritionally-deficient, prolonged treatment, renal or hepatic disease). Monitor for signs and symptoms of hemolytic anemia, including hematologic parameters where appropriate.

Test Interactions Positive direct Coombs', false-positive urinary glucose test using cupric sulfate (Benedict's solution, Clinitest®, Fehling's solution), false-positive serum or urine creatinine with Jaffé reaction

Dosage Forms Excipient information presented when available (limited, particularly for generics); consult specific product labeling.
Solution Reconstituted, Injection:
Generic: 1 g (1 ea); 2 g (1 ea); 10 g (1 ea)
Solution Reconstituted, Intravenous:
Generic: 1 g (1 ea); 2 g (1 ea)

◆ **Cefotetan Disodium** *see* CefoTEtan *on page 373*

CefOXitin (se FOKS i tin)

Brand Names: U.S. Mefoxin
Brand Names: Canada Cefoxitin For Injection
Index Terms Cefoxitin Sodium
Pharmacologic Category Antibiotic, Cephalosporin (Second Generation)
Use Less active against staphylococci and streptococci than first generation cephalosporins, but active against anaerobes including *Bacteroides fragilis*; active against gram-negative enteric bacilli including *E. coli*, *Klebsiella*, and *Proteus*; used predominantly for respiratory tract, skin, bone and joint, urinary tract and gynecologic infections as well as septicemia; surgical (perioperative) prophylaxis; intra-abdominal infections and other mixed infections; indicated for bacterial *Eikenella corrodens* infections
Pregnancy Risk Factor B
Pregnancy Considerations Adverse events have not been observed in animal reproduction studies. Cefoxitin crosses the placenta and reaches the cord serum and amniotic fluid.

Peak serum concentrations of cefoxitin during pregnancy may be similar to or decreased compared to nonpregnant values. Maternal half-life may be shorter at term. Pregnancy-induced hypertension increases trough concentrations in the immediate postpartum period. Cefoxitin is one of the antibiotics recommended for prophylactic use prior to cesarean delivery.

Breast-Feeding Considerations Very small amounts of cefoxitin are excreted in breast milk. The manufacturer recommends that caution be exercised when administering cefoxitin to nursing women. Nondose-related effects could include modification of bowel flora. Cefoxitin pharmacokinetics may be altered immediately postpartum.
Contraindications Hypersensitivity to cefoxitin, any component of the formulation, or other cephalosporins
Warnings/Precautions Modify dosage in patients with severe renal impairment. Prolonged use may result in superinfection. Use with caution in patients with a history of penicillin allergy, especially IgE-mediated reactions (eg, anaphylaxis, urticaria). Prolonged use may result in fungal or bacterial superinfection, including *C. difficile*-associated diarrhea (CDAD) and pseudomembranous colitis; CDAD has been observed >2 months postantibiotic treatment.

Adverse Reactions
1% to 10%: Gastrointestinal: Diarrhea
<1% (Limited to important or life-threatening): Anaphylaxis, angioedema, bone marrow suppression, BUN increased, creatinine increased, dyspnea, eosinophilia, exacerbation of myasthenia gravis, exfoliative dermatitis, fever, hemolytic anemia, hypotension, interstitial nephritis, jaundice, leukopenia, nausea, nephrotoxicity (with aminoglycosides), phlebitis, prolonged PT, pruritus, pseudomembranous colitis, rash, thrombocytopenia, thrombophlebitis, toxic epidermal necrolysis, transaminases increased, urticaria, vomiting

Reactions reported with other cephalosporins: Agranulocytosis, aplastic anemia, cholestasis, colitis, erythema multiforme, hemolytic anemia, hemorrhage, pancytopenia, renal dysfunction, seizure, serum-sickness reactions, Stevens-Johnson syndrome, superinfection, toxic nephropathy, vaginitis

Drug Interactions

Metabolism/Transport Effects None known.

Avoid Concomitant Use

Avoid concomitant use of CefOXitin with any of the following: BCG

Increased Effect/Toxicity

CefOXitin may increase the levels/effects of: Aminoglycosides; Vitamin K Antagonists

The levels/effects of CefOXitin may be increased by: Probenecid

Decreased Effect

CefOXitin may decrease the levels/effects of: BCG; Sodium Picosulfate; Typhoid Vaccine

Preparation for Administration Reconstitute vials with SWFI, bacteriostatic water for injection, NS, or D_5W. For I.V. infusion, solutions may be further diluted in NS, $D_5{}^1\!/_4NS$, $D_5{}^1\!/_2NS$, D_5NS, D_5W, $D_{10}W$, LR, D_5LR, mannitol 10%, or sodium bicarbonate 5%.

Storage/Stability Reconstituted solution is stable for 6 hours at room temperature or 7 days when refrigerated; I.V. infusion in NS or D_5W solution is stable for 18 hours at room temperature or 48 hours when refrigerated. Premixed frozen solution, when thawed, is stable for 24 hours at room temperature or 21 days when refrigerated.

Mechanism of Action Inhibits bacterial cell wall synthesis by binding to one or more of the penicillin-binding proteins (PBPs) which in turn inhibits the final transpeptidation step of peptidoglycan synthesis in bacterial cell walls, thus inhibiting cell wall biosynthesis. Bacteria eventually lyse due to ongoing activity of cell wall autolytic enzymes (autolysins and murein hydrolases) while cell wall assembly is arrested.

Pharmacodynamics/Kinetics

Distribution: Widely to body tissues and fluids including pleural, synovial, ascitic, bile; poorly penetrates into CSF even with inflammation of the meninges

Protein binding: 65% to 79%

Half-life elimination: 45-60 minutes; significantly prolonged with renal impairment

Time to peak, serum: I.M.: 20-30 minutes

Excretion: Urine (85% as unchanged drug)

Dosage

Usual dosage range:

Infants >3 months and Children: I.M., I.V.: 80-160 mg/kg/day in divided doses every 4-6 hours (maximum dose: 12 g daily)

Adults: I.M., I.V.: 1-2 g every 6-8 hours (maximum dose: 12 g daily)

Note: I.M. injection is painful

Indication-specific dosing:

Infants >3 months and Children:

Mild-to-moderate infection: I.M., I.V.: 80-100 mg/kg/day in divided doses every 4-6 hours

Severe infection: I.M., I.V.: 100-160 mg/kg/day in divided doses every 4-6 hours

Surgical (perioperative) prophylaxis:

Manufacturer recommendations: I.V.: 30-40 mg/kg 30-60 minutes prior to surgical incision followed by 30-40 mg/kg/dose every 6 hours for no more than 24 hours after surgery depending on the procedure

Alternative recommendations: Children ≥1 year: I.V.: 40 mg/kg within 60 minutes prior to surgical incision (maximum: 2000 mg per dose). Doses may be repeated in 2 hours if procedure is lengthy or if there is excessive blood loss (Bratzler, 2013).

Adolescents: **Surgical (perioperative) prophylaxis:** Refer to adult dosing.

Adults:

Amnionitis, endomyometritis: I.M., I.V.: 2 g every 6-8 hours

Aspiration pneumonia, empyema, orbital cellulitis, parapharyngeal space, human bites: I.M., I.V.: 2 g every 8 hours

Intra-abdominal infection, complicated, community acquired, mild-to-moderate: I.V.: 2 g every 6 hours for 4-7 days (provided source controlled)

Liver abscess: I.V.: 1 g every 4 hours

Mycobacterium species, not MTB or MAI: I.V.: 12 g daily with amikacin

Pelvic inflammatory disease:

Inpatients: I.V.: 2 g every 6 hours **plus** doxycycline 100 mg I.V. or 100 mg orally every 12 hours until improved, followed by doxycycline 100 mg orally twice daily to complete 14 days

Outpatients: I.M.: 2 g **plus** probenecid 1 g orally as a single dose, followed by doxycycline 100 mg orally twice daily for 14 days

Surgical (perioperative) prophylaxis:

Manufacturer recommendations (procedures other than Cesarian section): I.V.: 2 g 30-60 minutes prior to surgical incision, followed by 2 g every 6 hours for no more than 24 hours after surgery depending on the procedure

Cesarean section: I.V.: 2 g as soon as umbilical cord is clamped as a single dose **or** 2 g as soon as umbilical cord is clamped followed by 2 g at 4 and 8 hours after the initial dose.

Alternative recommendations: 2 g within 60 minutes prior to surgical incision. Doses may be repeated in 2 hours if procedure is lengthy or if there is excessive blood loss (Bratzler, 2013).

Dosage adjustment in renal impairment:

Cl_{cr} 30-50 mL/minute: Administer 1-2 g every 8-12 hours

Cl_{cr} 10-29 mL/minute: Administer 1-2 g every 12-24 hours

Cl_{cr} 5-9 mL/minute: Administer 0.5-1 g every 12-24 hours

Cl_{cr} <5 mL/minute: Administer 0.5-1 g every 24-48 hours

Hemodialysis: Moderately dialyzable (20% to 50%); administer a loading dose of 1-2 g after each hemodialysis; maintenance dose as noted above based on Cl_{cr}

Continuous arteriovenous or venovenous hemodiafiltration effects: Dose as for Cl_{cr} 10-50 mL/minute

Dosage adjustment in hepatic impairment: No dosage adjustment provided in manufacturer's labeling.

Dietary Considerations Some products may contain sodium.

Administration

I.M.: Inject deep I.M. into large muscle mass.

I.V.: Can be administered IVP over 3-5 minutes at a maximum concentration of 100 mg/mL or I.V. intermittent infusion over 10-60 minutes at a final concentration for I.V. administration not to exceed 40 mg/mL

Monitoring Parameters Monitor renal function periodically when used in combination with other nephrotoxic drugs; prothrombin time. Observe for signs and symptoms of anaphylaxis during first dose.

Test Interactions Positive direct Coombs', false-positive urinary glucose test using cupric sulfate (Benedict's solution, Clinitest®, Fehling's solution), false-positive serum or urine creatinine with Jaffé reaction

Dosage Forms Excipient information presented when available (limited, particularly for generics); consult specific product labeling.

Solution, Intravenous:

Mefoxin: 1 g (50 mL); 2 g (50 mL)

Solution Reconstituted, Injection:

Generic: 10 g (1 ea)

Solution Reconstituted, Injection [preservative free]:
Generic: 10 g (1 ea)
Solution Reconstituted, Intravenous:
Generic: 1 g (1 ea); 2 g (1 ea)
Solution Reconstituted, Intravenous [preservative free]:
Generic: 1 g (1 ea); 2 g (1 ea)

◆ **Cefoxitin For Injection (Can)** *see* CefOXitin *on page 374*

◆ **Cefoxitin Sodium** *see* CefOXitin *on page 374*

Cefpodoxime (sef pode OKS eem)

Index Terms Cefpodoxime Proxetil; Vantin

Pharmacologic Category Antibiotic, Cephalosporin (Third Generation)

Use Treatment of susceptible acute, community-acquired pneumonia caused by *S. pneumoniae* or nonbeta-lactamase producing *H. influenzae*; acute uncomplicated gonorrhea caused by *N. gonorrhoeae*; uncomplicated skin and skin structure infections caused by *S. aureus* or *S. pyogenes*; acute otitis media caused by *S. pneumoniae, H. influenzae*, or *M. catarrhalis*; pharyngitis or tonsillitis; and uncomplicated urinary tract infections caused by *E. coli, Klebsiella*, and *Proteus*

Unlabeled Use Acute bacterial rhinosinusitis (ABRS) (pediatric) in combination with clindamycin

Pregnancy Risk Factor B

Pregnancy Considerations Teratogenic events were not observed in animal reproduction studies. An increase in most types of birth defects was not found following first trimester exposure to cephalosporins.

Breast-Feeding Considerations Cefpodoxime is excreted in breast milk. The manufacturer recommends discontinuing nursing or discontinuing the medication in breast-feeding women. Nondose-related effects could include modification of bowel flora.

Contraindications Hypersensitivity to cefpodoxime, any component of the formulation, or other cephalosporins

Warnings/Precautions Modify dosage in patients with severe renal impairment. Prolonged use may result in fungal or bacterial superinfection, including *C. difficile*-associated diarrhea (CDAD) and pseudomembranous colitis; CDAD has been observed >2 months postantibiotic treatment. Use with caution in patients with a history of penicillin allergy, especially IgE-mediated reactions (eg, anaphylaxis, urticaria).

Adverse Reactions

>10%:
- Dermatologic: Diaper rash (12.1%)
- Gastrointestinal: Diarrhea in infants and toddlers (15.4%)

1% to 10%:
- Central nervous system: Headache (1.1%)
- Dermatologic: Rash (1.4%)
- Gastrointestinal: Diarrhea (7.2%), nausea (3.8%), abdominal pain (1.6%), vomiting (1.1% to 2.1%)
- Genitourinary: Vaginal infection (3.1%)

<1% (Limited to important or life-threatening): Anaphylaxis, anxiety, appetite decreased, chest pain, cough, dizziness, epistaxis, eye itching, fatigue, fever, flatulence, flushing, fungal skin infection, hypotension, insomnia, malaise, nightmares, pruritus, pseudomembranous colitis, purpuric nephritis, salivation decreased, taste alteration, tinnitus, vaginal candidiasis, weakness

Reactions reported with other cephalosporins: Agranulocytosis, aplastic anemia, cholestasis, colitis, erythema multiforme, hemolytic anemia, hemorrhage, interstitial nephritis, toxic nephropathy, pancytopenia, renal dysfunction, seizure, serum-sickness reactions, Stevens-Johnson syndrome, superinfection, toxic epidermal necrolysis, urticaria, vaginitis

Drug Interactions

Metabolism/Transport Effects None known.

Avoid Concomitant Use

Avoid concomitant use of Cefpodoxime with any of the following: BCG

Increased Effect/Toxicity

Cefpodoxime may increase the levels/effects of: Aminoglycosides; Vitamin K Antagonists

The levels/effects of Cefpodoxime may be increased by: Probenecid

Decreased Effect

Cefpodoxime may decrease the levels/effects of: BCG; Sodium Picosulfate; Typhoid Vaccine

The levels/effects of Cefpodoxime may be decreased by: Antacids; H2-Antagonists

Ethanol/Nutrition/Herb Interactions Food: Food and/or low gastric pH delays absorption and may increase serum levels. Management: Take with or without food at regular intervals on an around-the-clock schedule to promote less variation in peak and trough serum levels.

Preparation for Administration Shake well before using. After mixing, keep suspension in refrigerator. Discard unused portion after 14 days.

Mechanism of Action Inhibits bacterial cell wall synthesis by binding to one or more of the penicillin-binding proteins (PBPs) which in turn inhibits the final transpeptidation step of peptidoglycan synthesis in bacterial cell walls, thus inhibiting cell wall biosynthesis. Bacteria eventually lyse due to ongoing activity of cell wall autolytic enzymes (autolysins and murein hydrolases) while cell wall assembly is arrested.

Pharmacodynamics/Kinetics

Absorption: Rapid and well absorbed (50%), acid stable; enhanced in the presence of food or low gastric pH
Distribution: Good tissue penetration, including lung and tonsils; penetrates into pleural fluid
Protein binding: 18% to 23%
Metabolism: De-esterified in GI tract to active metabolite, cefpodoxime
Half-life elimination: 2.2 hours; prolonged with renal impairment
Time to peak: Within 1 hour
Excretion: Urine (80% as unchanged drug) in 24 hours

Dosage

Usual dosage range:

Children 2 months to 12 years: Oral: 10 mg/kg/day divided every 12 hours (maximum: 200 mg/dose)
Children ≥12 years and Adults: Oral: 100-400 mg every 12 hours

Indication-specific dosing:

Children 2 months to 12 years: Oral:

Acute bacterial rhinosinusitis (unlabeled use): Children: 10 mg/kg/day divided every 12 hours (maximum: 200 mg/dose) with concomitant clindamycin for 10-14 days. **Note:** Recommended in patients with non-type I penicillin allergy, after failure of initial therapy or in patients at risk for antibiotic resistance (eg, daycare attendance, age <2 years, recent hospitalization, antibiotic use within the past month) (Chow, 2012)

Acute maxillary sinusitis: 10 mg/kg/day divided every 12 hours for 10 days (maximum: 200 mg/dose)

Acute otitis media: 10 mg/kg/day divided every 12 hours for 5 days (maximum: 200 mg/dose)

Pharyngitis/tonsillitis: 10 mg/kg/day in 2 divided doses for 5-10 days (maximum: 100 mg/dose)

Children ≥12 years and Adults: Oral:

Acute community-acquired pneumonia and bacterial exacerbations of chronic bronchitis: 200 mg every 12 hours for 14 days and 10 days, respectively

Acute maxillary sinusitis: 200 mg every 12 hours for 10 days

Pharyngitis/tonsillitis: 100 mg every 12 hours for 5-10 days

Skin and skin structure: 400 mg every 12 hours for 7-14 days

Uncomplicated gonorrhea (male and female) and rectal gonococcal infections (female): 200 mg as a single dose

Uncomplicated urinary tract infection: 100 mg every 12 hours for 7 days

Dosing adjustment in renal impairment: Cl_{cr} <30 mL/minute: Administer every 24 hours

Hemodialysis: Administer dose 3 times/week following hemodialysis

Dietary Considerations May be taken with food.

Administration Administer around-the-clock to promote less variation in peak and trough serum levels.

Monitoring Parameters Monitor renal function. Observe for signs and symptoms of anaphylaxis during first dose.

Test Interactions Positive direct Coombs', false-positive urinary glucose test using cupric sulfate (Benedict's solution, Clinitest®, Fehling's solution), false-positive serum or urine creatinine with Jaffé reaction

Dosage Forms Excipient information presented when available (limited, particularly for generics); consult specific product labeling.

Suspension Reconstituted, Oral:

Generic: 50 mg/5 mL (50 mL, 100 mL); 100 mg/5 mL (50 mL, 100 mL)

Tablet, Oral:

Generic: 100 mg, 200 mg

◆ Cefpodoxime Proxetil *see* Cefpodoxime *on page 376*

Cefprozil (sef PROE zil)

Brand Names: Canada Apo-Cefprozil®; Auro-Cefprozil; Ava-Cefprozil; Cefzil®; RAN™-Cefprozil; Sandoz-Cefprozil

Index Terms Cefzil

Pharmacologic Category Antibiotic, Cephalosporin (Second Generation)

Use Treatment of otitis media and infections involving the respiratory tract and skin and skin structure; active against methicillin-sensitive staphylococci, many streptococci, and various gram-negative bacilli including *E. coli*, some *Klebsiella*, *P. mirabilis*, *H. influenzae*, and *Moraxella*.

Pregnancy Risk Factor B

Pregnancy Considerations Adverse events were not observed in animal reproduction studies.

Breast-Feeding Considerations Small amounts of cefprozil are excreted in breast milk. The manufacturer recommends that caution be exercised when administering cefprozil to nursing women. Nondose-related effects could include modification of bowel flora.

Contraindications Hypersensitivity to cefprozil, any component of the formulation, or other cephalosporins

Warnings/Precautions Modify dosage in patients with severe renal impairment. Use with caution in patients with a history of penicillin allergy, especially IgE-mediated reactions (eg, anaphylaxis, urticaria). Prolonged use may result in fungal or bacterial superinfection, including *C. difficile*-associated diarrhea (CDAD) and pseudomembranous colitis; CDAD has been observed >2 months postantibiotic treatment. Some products may contain phenylalanine.

Adverse Reactions

1% to 10%:

Central nervous system: Dizziness (1%)

Dermatologic: Diaper rash (1.5%)

Gastrointestinal: Diarrhea (2.9%), nausea (3.5%), vomiting (1%), abdominal pain (1%)

Genitourinary: Vaginitis, genital pruritus (1.6%)

Hepatic: Transaminases increased (2%)

Miscellaneous: Superinfection

<1% (Limited to important or life-threatening): Anaphylaxis, angioedema, arthralgia, BUN increased, cholestatic jaundice, confusion, creatinine increased, eosinophilia, erythema multiforme, fever, headache, hyperactivity, insomnia, leukopenia, pseudomembranous colitis, rash, serum sickness, somnolence, Stevens-Johnson syndrome, thrombocytopenia, urticaria

Reactions reported with other cephalosporins: Agranulocytosis, aplastic anemia, colitis, hemolytic anemia, hemorrhage, interstitial nephritis, pancytopenia, renal dysfunction, seizure, superinfection, toxic epidermal necrolysis, toxic nephropathy, vaginitis

Drug Interactions

Metabolism/Transport Effects None known.

Avoid Concomitant Use

Avoid concomitant use of Cefprozil with any of the following: BCG

Increased Effect/Toxicity

Cefprozil may increase the levels/effects of: Aminoglycosides; Vitamin K Antagonists

The levels/effects of Cefprozil may be increased by: Probenecid

Decreased Effect

Cefprozil may decrease the levels/effects of: BCG; Sodium Picosulfate; Typhoid Vaccine

Ethanol/Nutrition/Herb Interactions Food: Food delays cefprozil absorption.

Mechanism of Action Inhibits bacterial cell wall synthesis by binding to one or more of the penicillin-binding proteins (PBPs) which in turn inhibits the final transpeptidation step of peptidoglycan synthesis in bacterial cell walls, thus inhibiting cell wall biosynthesis. Bacteria eventually lyse due to ongoing activity of cell wall autolytic enzymes (autolysins and murein hydrolases) while cell wall assembly is arrested.

Pharmacodynamics/Kinetics

Absorption: Well absorbed (94%)

Protein binding: 35% to 45%

Half-life elimination: Normal renal function: 1.3 hours

Time to peak, serum: Fasting: 1.5 hours

Excretion: Urine (61% as unchanged drug)

Dosage

Usual dosage range:

Infants and Children >6 months to 12 years: Oral: 7.5-15 mg/kg/day divided every 12 hours

Children >12 years and Adults: Oral: 250-500 mg every 12 hours or 500 mg every 24 hours

Indication-specific dosing:

Infants and Children >6 months to 12 years: Oral:

Otitis media: 15 mg/kg every 12 hours for 10 days

Children 2-12 years: Oral:

Pharyngitis/tonsillitis: 7.5-15 mg/kg/day divided every 12 hours for 10 days (administer for >10 days if due to *S. pyogenes*); maximum: 1 g/day

Uncomplicated skin and skin structure infections: 20 mg/kg every 24 hours for 10 days; maximum: 1 g/day

Children >12 years and Adults: Oral:

Pharyngitis/tonsillitis: 500 mg every 24 hours for 10 days

Secondary bacterial infection of acute bronchitis or acute bacterial exacerbation of chronic bronchitis: 500 mg every 12 hours for 10 days

Uncomplicated skin and skin structure infections: 250 mg every 12 hours or 500 mg every 12-24 hours for 10 days

Dosage adjustment in renal impairment: Cl_{cr} <30 mL/minute: Reduce dose by 50%

Hemodialysis: Reduced by hemodialysis; administer dose after the completion of hemodialysis

Dosage adjustment in hepatic impairment: No dosage adjustment necessary.

Dietary Considerations May be taken with food. Oral suspension may contain phenylalanine; consult product labeling.

Administration Administer around-the-clock to promote less variation in peak and trough serum levels. Chilling the reconstituted oral suspension improves flavor (do not freeze).

Monitoring Parameters Monitor renal function. Assess patient at beginning and throughout therapy for infection; monitor for signs of anaphylaxis during first dose.

Test Interactions Positive direct Coombs', false-positive urinary glucose test using cupric sulfate (Benedict's solution, Clinitest®, Fehling's solution), false-positive serum or urine creatinine with Jaffé reaction

Dosage Forms Excipient information presented when available (limited, particularly for generics); consult specific product labeling.

Suspension Reconstituted, Oral:

Generic: 125 mg/5 mL (50 mL, 75 mL, 100 mL); 250 mg/5 mL (50 mL, 75 mL, 100 mL)

Tablet, Oral:

Generic: 250 mg, 500 mg

Ceftaroline Fosamil (sef TAR oh leen FOS a mil)

Brand Names: U.S. Teflaro

Index Terms PPI-0903; PPI-0903M; T-91825; TAK-599

Pharmacologic Category Antibiotic, Cephalosporin (Fifth Generation)

Use Treatment of acute bacterial skin and skin structure infections (ABSSSI) caused by susceptible isolates of *Staphylococcus aureus* (including methicillin-susceptible and -resistant isolates), *Streptococcus pyogenes, Streptococcus agalactiae, Escherichia coli, Klebsiella pneumoniae,* and *Klebsiella oxytoca,* and community-acquired pneumonia (CAP) caused by *Streptococcus pneumoniae* (including cases with concurrent bacteremia), *Staphylococcus aureus* (methicillin-susceptible isolates only), *Haemophilus influenzae, Klebsiella pneumoniae, Klebsiella oxytoca,* and *Escherichia coli*

Pregnancy Risk Factor B

Pregnancy Considerations Adverse events have been observed in some animal reproduction studies.

Breast-Feeding Considerations It is not known if ceftaroline fosamil is excreted in breast milk. The manufacturer recommends that caution be exercised when administering ceftaroline fosamil to nursing women.

Contraindications Hypersensitivity to ceftaroline, other cephalosporins, or any component of the formulation

Warnings/Precautions Use with caution in patients with a history of penicillin cephalosporin, or carbapenem allergy, especially IgE-mediated reactions (eg, anaphylaxis, angioedema, urticaria). Seroconversion from a negative to a positive direct Coombs' test has been reported. Hemolytic anemia was not reported in clinical studies; however, if anemia develops during or after treatment, diagnostic tests should include a direct Coombs' test. If drug-induced hemolytic anemia is considered, discontinue the drug and institute supportive care as clinically indicated. Prolonged use may result in fungal or bacterial superinfection, including *C. difficile*-associated diarrhea (CDAD) and pseudomembranous colitis (including fatalities); CDAD has been observed >2 months postantibiotic treatment. Use with caution in patients with renal impairment (Cl_{cr} ≤50 mL/minute); dosage adjustments recommended. Potentially significant drug-drug interactions may exist, requiring dose or frequency adjustment, additional monitoring, and/or selection of alternative therapy.

Adverse Reactions

>10%: Hematologic: Positive Coombs' test without hemolysis (~11%)

2% to 10%:

Central nervous system: Headache (3% to 5%), insomnia (3% to 4%)

Dermatologic: Pruritus (3% to 4%), rash (3%)

Endocrine & metabolic: Hypokalemia (2%)

Gastrointestinal: Diarrhea (5%), nausea (4%), constipation (2%), vomiting (2%)

Hepatic: Transaminases increased (2%)

Local: Phlebitis (2%)

<2% (Limited to important or life-threatening): Abdominal pain, anaphylaxis, anemia, bradycardia, dizziness, *C. difficile*-associated diarrhea (CDAD), eosinophilia, fever, hepatitis, hyperglycemia, hyperkalemia, hypersensitivity, neutropenia, palpitation, seizures, renal failure, thrombocytopenia, urticaria

Drug Interactions

Metabolism/Transport Effects None known.

Avoid Concomitant Use

Avoid concomitant use of Ceftaroline Fosamil with any of the following: BCG

Increased Effect/Toxicity

Ceftaroline Fosamil may increase the levels/effects of: Vitamin K Antagonists

The levels/effects of Ceftaroline Fosamil may be increased by: Probenecid

Decreased Effect

Ceftaroline Fosamil may decrease the levels/effects of: BCG; Sodium Picosulfate; Typhoid Vaccine

Preparation for Administration Reconstitute 400 mg or 600 mg vial with 20 mL SWFI, NS, D_5W, or LR; mix gently. Reconstituted solution should be further diluted for I.V. administration in 50-250 mL of a compatible solution. Use the same solution as used for reconstitution (**Note:** If SWFI was used for reconstitution, then appropriate infusion solutions include NS, 1/2NS, D_5W, $D_{2.5}W$, or LR). Color of infusion solutions ranges from clear and light to dark yellow depending on concentration and storage conditions; potency is not affected.

Storage/Stability Store unused vials at room temperature, up to 25°C (77°F); excursions permitted to 15°C to 30°C (59°F to 86°F). Diluted solutions should be used within 6 hours when stored at room temperature or within 24 hours if refrigerated at 2°C to 8°C (36°F to 46°F).

Mechanism of Action Inhibits bacterial cell wall synthesis by binding to penicillin-binding proteins (PBPs) 1 through 3. This action blocks the final transpeptidation step of peptidoglycan synthesis in bacterial cell walls and inhibits cell wall biosynthesis. Bacteria eventually lyse due to ongoing activity of cell wall autolytic enzymes (autolysis and murein hydrolases) while cell wall assembly is arrested. Ceftaroline has a strong affinity for PBP2a, a modified PBP in MRSA, and PBP2x in *S. pneumoniae*, contributing to its spectrum of activity against these bacteria.

Pharmacodynamics/Kinetics

Distribution: V_d: 18.3-21.6 L

Protein binding: ~20%

Metabolism: Ceftaroline fosamil (inactive prodrug) undergoes rapid conversion to bioactive ceftaroline in plasma by phosphatase enzyme; ceftaroline is hydrolyzed to form inactive ceftaroline M-1 metabolite

Half-life elimination: 2.7 hours

Time to peak: 1 hour
Excretion: Urine (~88%); feces (~6%)

Dosage I.V.: Adults:

Usual dosage range: 600 mg every 12 hours

Indication-specific dosage:

Pneumonia, community-acquired: 600 mg every 12 hours for 5-7 days

Skin and skin structure, complicated: 600 mg every 12 hours for 5-14 days

Dosage adjustment in renal impairment: Note: Renal function may be estimated using the Cockcroft-Gault formula for dosage adjustment purposes.

Cl_{cr} >50 mL/minute: No dosage adjustment necessary.
Cl_{cr} >30-50 mL/minute: 400 mg every 12 hours
Cl_{cr} 15-30 mL/minute: 300 mg every 12 hours
Cl_{cr} <15 mL/minute: 200 mg every 12 hours
ESRD patients receiving hemodialysis: 200 mg every 12 hours; dose should be given after hemodialysis on dialysis days

Dosage adjustment in hepatic impairment: No dosage adjustment provided in manufacturer's labeling (has not been studied). However, ceftaroline is primarily renally eliminated.

Administration Administer by slow I.V. infusion over 60 minutes.

Monitoring Parameters Obtain specimen for culture and susceptibility prior to the first dose. Monitor for signs of anaphylaxis during first dose. Monitor renal function.

Additional Information Considered to be ineffective against *Pseudomonas aeruginosa*, *Enterococcus* species (including vancomycin-susceptible and -resistant isolates), extended-spectrum beta-lactamase (ESBL) producing or AmpC overexpressing Enterobacteriaceae.

Dosage Forms Excipient information presented when available (limited, particularly for generics); consult specific product labeling.

Solution Reconstituted, Intravenous:
Teflaro: 400 mg (1 ea); 600 mg (1 ea)

CefTAZidime (SEF tay zi deem)

Brand Names: U.S. Fortaz; Fortaz in D_5W; Tazicef

Brand Names: Canada Ceftazidime For Injection; Fortaz®

Pharmacologic Category Antibiotic, Cephalosporin (Third Generation)

Additional Appendix Information
Desensitization Protocols *on page 2325*

Use Treatment of documented susceptible *Pseudomonas aeruginosa* infection and infections due to other susceptible aerobic gram-negative organisms; empiric therapy of a febrile, granulocytopenic patient

Unlabeled Use Bacterial endophthalmitis

Pregnancy Risk Factor B

Pregnancy Considerations Teratogenic effects were not observed in animal reproduction studies. Ceftazidime crosses the placenta and reaches the cord serum and amniotic fluid. An increase in most types of birth defects was not found following first trimester exposure to cephalosporins. Maternal peak serum concentration is unchanged in the first trimester. After the first trimester, serum concentrations decrease by approximately 50% of those in nonpregnant patients. Renal clearance is increased during pregnancy.

Breast-Feeding Considerations Very small amounts of ceftazidime are excreted in breast milk. The manufacturer recommends that caution be exercised when administering ceftazidime to nursing women. Ceftazidime in not absorbed when given orally; therefore, any medication that is distributed to human milk should not result in systemic concentrations in the nursing infant. Nondose-related effects could include modification of bowel flora.

Contraindications Hypersensitivity to ceftazidime, any component of the formulation, or other cephalosporins

Warnings/Precautions Modify dosage in patients with severe renal impairment. Use with caution in patients with a history of penicillin allergy, especially IgE-mediated reactions (eg, anaphylaxis, urticaria). Prolonged use may result in fungal or bacterial superinfection, including *C. difficile*-associated diarrhea (CDAD) and pseudomembranous colitis; CDAD has been observed >2 months postantibiotic treatment. May be associated with increased INR, especially in nutritionally-deficient patients, prolonged treatment, hepatic or renal disease. Use with caution in patients with a history of seizure disorder; high levels, particularly in the presence of renal impairment, may increase risk of seizures.

Adverse Reactions

1% to 10%:

Gastrointestinal: Diarrhea (1%)
Local: Pain at injection site (1%)
Miscellaneous: Hypersensitivity reactions (2%)

<1% (Limited to important or life-threatening): Anaphylaxis, angioedema, asterixis, BUN increased, candidiasis, creatinine increased, dizziness, encephalopathy, eosinophilia, erythema multiforme, fever, headache, hemolytic anemia, hyperbilirubinemia, jaundice, leukopenia, myoclonus, nausea, neuromuscular excitability, paresthesia, phlebitis, pruritus, pseudomembranous colitis, rash, Stevens-Johnson syndrome, thrombocytosis, toxic epidermal necrolysis, transaminases increased, vaginitis, vomiting

Reactions reported with other cephalosporins: Agranulocytosis, aplastic anemia, cholestasis, colitis, hemolytic anemia, hemorrhage, interstitial nephritis, pancytopenia, prolonged PT, renal dysfunction, seizure, serum-sickness reactions, superinfection, toxic nephropathy, urticaria

Drug Interactions

Metabolism/Transport Effects None known.

Avoid Concomitant Use

Avoid concomitant use of CefTAZidime with any of the following: BCG

Increased Effect/Toxicity

CefTAZidime may increase the levels/effects of: Aminoglycosides; Vitamin K Antagonists

The levels/effects of CefTAZidime may be increased by: Probenecid

Decreased Effect

CefTAZidime may decrease the levels/effects of: BCG; Sodium Picosulfate; Typhoid Vaccine

Preparation for Administration

I.M.: Using SWFI, bacteriostatic water, lidocaine 0.5%, or lidocaine 1%, reconstitute the 500 mg vials with 1.5 mL or the 1 g vials with 3 mL; final concentration of *~280 mg/mL*

I.V.: Using SWFI, reconstitute as follows (**Note:** After reconstitution, may dilute further with a compatible solution to administer via I.V. infusion):

Fortaz®:

~100 mg/mL solution:
500 mg vial: 5.3 mL SWFI (withdraw 5 mL from the reconstituted vial to obtain a 500 mg dose)
1 g vial: 10 mL SWFI (withdraw 10 mL from the reconstituted vial to obtain a 1 g dose)
6 g vial: 56 mL SWFI (withdraw 10 mL from the reconstituted vial to obtain a 1 g dose)

~170 mg/mL solution: 2 g vial: 10 mL SWFI (withdraw 11.5 mL from the reconstituted vial to obtain a 2 g dose)

~200 mg/mL solution: 6 g vial: 26 mL SWFI (withdraw 5 mL from the reconstituted vial to obtain a 1 g dose)

Tazicef®:

~95 mg/mL solution: 1 g vial: 10 mL SWFI (withdraw 10.6 mL from the reconstituted vial to obtain a 1 g dose)

~180 mg/mL solution: 2 g vial: 10 mL SWFI (withdraw 11.2 mL from the reconstituted vial to obtain a 2 g dose)

Fortaz®, Tazicef®: ADD-Vantage® vials: Dilute in 50 or 100 mL of D_5W, NS, or 0.45% sodium chloride in an ADD-Vantage® flexible diluent container only.

Storage/Stability

Fortaz®: Store dry vials at 15°C to 30°C (59°F to 86°F). Protect from light. Reconstituted solution and solution further diluted for I.V. infusion are stable for 12 hours at room temperature, for 3 days when refrigerated, or for 12 weeks when frozen at -20°C (-4°F). After freezing, thawed solution in SWFI for I.M. administration is stable for 3 hours at room temperature or for 3 days when refrigerated; thawed solution in NS in a Viaflex® small volume container for I.V. administration is stable for 12 hours at room temperature or for 3 days when refrigerated; and thawed solution in SWFI in the original container is stable for 8 hours at room temperature or for 3 days when refrigerated.

Premixed frozen solution: Store frozen at -20°C (-4°F). Thawed solution is stable for 8 hours at room temperature or for 3 days under refrigeration; do not refreeze.

Fortaz®, Tazicef®: ADD-Vantage® vials: Following dilution, may be stored for up to 12 hours at room temperature or for 3 days under refrigeration. Freezing solutions in the ADD-Vantage® system is not recommended. Joined vials that have not been activated may be used within 14 days.

Tazicef® vials: Store dry vials at 20°C to 25°C (68°F to 77°F). Protect from light. Reconstituted vials and solution further diluted for I.V. infusion are stable for 24 hours at room temperature, for 7 days when refrigerated, or for 12 weeks when frozen at -20°C (-4°F). When thawed, solution is stable for 8 hours at room temperature and 4 days when refrigerated.

Mechanism of Action Inhibits bacterial cell wall synthesis by binding to one or more of the penicillin-binding proteins (PBPs) which in turn inhibits the final transpeptidation step of peptidoglycan synthesis in bacterial cell walls, thus inhibiting cell wall biosynthesis. Bacteria eventually lyse due to ongoing activity of cell wall autolytic enzymes (autolysins and murein hydrolases) while cell wall assembly is arrested.

Pharmacodynamics/Kinetics

Distribution: Widely throughout the body including bone, bile, skin, CSF (higher concentrations achieved when meninges are inflamed), endometrium, heart, pleural and lymphatic fluids

Protein binding: 17%

Half-life elimination: 1-2 hours, prolonged with renal impairment; Neonates <23 days: 2.2-4.7 hours

Time to peak, serum: I.M.: ~1 hour

Excretion: Urine (80% to 90% as unchanged drug)

Dosage

Usual dosage range:

Infants and Children 1 month to 12 years: I.V.: 30-50 mg/kg/dose every 8 hours (maximum dose: 6 g daily)

Adults: I.M., I.V.: 500 mg to 2 g every 8-12 hours

Indication-specific dosing:

Bacterial arthritis (gram-negative bacilli): I.V.: 1-2 g every 8 hours

Cystic fibrosis: I.V.: 30-50 mg/kg/dose every 8 hours (maximum: 6 g daily)

Endophthalmitis, bacterial (unlabeled use): Intravitreal: 2-2.25 mg/0.1 mL NS in combination with vancomycin (Jackson, 2003; Roth, 1997)

Intra-abdominal infection, severe (in combination with metronidazole): I.V.: 2 g every 8 hours for 4-7 days (provided source controlled). Not recommended for hospital-acquired intra-abdominal infections (IAI) associated with multidrug-resistant gram negative organisms or in mild-to-moderate community-acquired IAIs due to risk of toxicity and the development of resistant organisms (Solomkin, 2010).

Melioidosis: I.V.: 40 mg/kg/dose every 8 hours for 10 days, followed by oral therapy with doxycycline or TMP/SMX

Otitis externa: I.V.: 2 g every 8 hours

Peritonitis (CAPD):

Anuric, intermittent: 1-1.5 g daily

Anuric, continuous (per liter exchange): Loading dose: 250 mg; maintenance dose: 125 mg

Prosthetic joint infection, *Pseudomonas aeruginosa* (alternative to cefepime or meropenem): I.V.: 2 g every 8 hours for 4-6 weeks (consider addition of an aminoglycoside) (Osmon, 2013)

Severe infections, including meningitis, complicated pneumonia, endophthalmitis, CNS infection, osteomyelitis, gynecological, skin and soft tissue: I.V.: 2 g every 8 hours

Dosage adjustment in renal impairment:

Cl_{cr} 30-50 mL/minute: Administer every 12 hours

Cl_{cr} 10-30 mL/minute: Administer every 24 hours

Cl_{cr} <10 mL/minute: Administer every 48-72 hours

Intermittent hemodialysis (IHD) (administer after hemodialysis on dialysis days): Dialyzable (50% to 100%): 500 mg to 1 g every 24 hours **or** 1-2 g every 48-72 hours (Heintz, 2009). **Note:** Dosing dependent on the assumption of 3 times per week, complete IHD sessions.

Peritoneal dialysis (PD): Loading dose of 1 g, followed by 500 mg every 24 hours

Continuous renal replacement therapy (CRRT) (Heintz, 2009; Trotman, 2005): Drug clearance is highly dependent on the method of renal replacement, filter type, and flow rate. Appropriate dosing requires close monitoring of pharmacologic response, signs of adverse reactions due to drug accumulation, as well as drug concentrations in relation to target trough (if appropriate). The following are general recommendations only (based on dialysate flow/ultrafiltration rates of 1-2 L/hour and minimal residual renal function) and should not supersede clinical judgment:

CVVH: Loading dose of 2 g followed by 1-2 g every 12 hours

CVVHD/CVVHDF: Loading dose of 2 g followed by either 1 g every 8 hours **or** 2 g every 12 hours. **Note:** Dosage of 1 g every 8 hours results in similar steady-state concentrations as 2 g every 12 hours and is more cost effective. Dosage of 2 g every 8 hours may be needed for gram-negative rods with MIC ≥4 mg/L (Heintz, 2009).

Note: For patients receiving CVVHDF, some recommend giving a loading dose of 2 g followed by 3 g over 24 hours as a continuous I.V. infusion to maintain concentrations ≥4 times the MIC for susceptible pathogens (Heintz, 2009).

Dosage adjustment in hepatic impairment: No dosage adjustment necessary

Dietary Considerations Some products may contain sodium.

Administration Any carbon dioxide bubbles that may be present in the withdrawn solution should be expelled prior to injection. Administer around-the-clock to promote less variation in peak and trough serum levels. Ceftazidime can be administered deep I.M. into large mass muscle, IVP over 3-5 minutes, or I.V. intermittent infusion over 15-30 minutes. Do not admix with aminoglycosides in same bottle/bag. Final concentration for I.V. administration should not exceed 100 mg/mL. Ceftazidime may be administered intravitreally as 2-2.25 mg/0.1 mL NS in combination with vancomycin (separate syringes) (Jackson, 2003; Roth, 1997).

Monitoring Parameters Monitor renal function. Observe for signs and symptoms of anaphylaxis during first dose.

Test Interactions Positive direct Coombs', false-positive urinary glucose test using cupric sulfate (Benedict's solution, Clinitest®, Fehling's solution), false-positive serum or urine creatinine with Jaffé reaction

Additional Information With some organisms, resistance may develop during treatment (including *Enterobacter* spp and *Serratia* spp). Consider combination therapy or periodic susceptibility testing for organisms with inducible resistance.

Dosage Forms Excipient information presented when available (limited, particularly for generics); consult specific product labeling.

Solution, Intravenous, as sodium [strength expressed as base]:
- Fortaz in D_5W: 1 g (50 mL); 2 g (50 mL)
- Tazicef: 1 g/50 mL (50 mL)

Solution Reconstituted, Injection:
- Fortaz: 500 mg (1 ea); 1 g (1 ea); 2 g (1 ea); 6 g (1 ea)
- Tazicef: 1 g (1 ea); 2 g (1 ea); 6 g (1 ea)
- Generic: 1 g (1 ea); 2 g (1 ea); 6 g (1 ea); 100 g (1 ea)

Solution Reconstituted, Injection [preservative free]:
- Generic: 1 g (1 ea); 2 g (1 ea); 6 g (1 ea)

Solution Reconstituted, Intravenous:
- Fortaz: 1 g (1 ea); 2 g (1 ea)
- Tazicef: 1 g (1 ea); 2 g (1 ea)
- Generic: 1 g/50 mL (1 ea); 2 g/50 mL (1 ea)

◆ **Ceftazidime For Injection (Can)** *see* CefTAZidime *on page 379*

Ceftibuten (sef TYE byoo ten)

Brand Names: U.S. Cedax

Pharmacologic Category Antibiotic, Cephalosporin (Third Generation)

Use Treatment of acute exacerbations of chronic bronchitis, acute bacterial otitis media, and pharyngitis/tonsillitis

Pregnancy Risk Factor B

Pregnancy Considerations Teratogenic effects were not observed in animal reproduction studies. An increase in most types of birth defects was not found following first trimester exposure to cephalosporins.

Breast-Feeding Considerations Ceftibuten was not detectable in milk after a single 200 mg dose (limit of detection: 1 mcg/mL). It is not known if it would be detectable after a 400 mg dose or multiple doses. The manufacturer recommends that caution be exercised when administering ceftibuten to nursing women. If ceftibuten does reach the human milk, nondose-related effects could include modification of bowel flora.

Contraindications Hypersensitivity to ceftibuten, any component of the formulation, or other cephalosporins

Warnings/Precautions Modify dosage in patients with moderate-to-severe renal impairment. Prolonged use may result in fungal or bacterial superinfection, including *C. difficile*-associated diarrhea (CDAD) and pseudomembranous colitis; CDAD has been observed >2 months postantibiotic treatment. Use with caution in patients with a history of colitis and other gastrointestinal diseases. Use with caution in patients with a history of penicillin allergy, especially IgE-mediated reactions (eg, anaphylaxis, urticaria). Oral suspension formulation contains sucrose.

Adverse Reactions

1% to 10%:
- Central nervous system: Headache (≤3%), dizziness (≤1%)
- Gastrointestinal: Nausea (≤4%), diarrhea (3% to 4%), dyspepsia (≤2%), loose stools (≤2%), abdominal pain (1% to 2%), vomiting (1% to 2%)
- Hematologic: Eosinophils increased (3%), hemoglobin decreased (1% to 2%), platelets increased (≤1%)
- Hepatic: ALT increased (≤1%), bilirubin increased (≤1%)
- Renal: BUN increased (2% to 4%)

<1% (Limited to important or life-threatening): Agitation, alkaline phosphatase increased, anorexia, aphasia, AST increased, constipation, creatinine increased, dehydration, diaper rash, dyspnea, dysuria, eructation, fatigue, fever, flatulence, hematuria, hyperkinesia, insomnia, irritability, jaundice, leukopenia, melena, moniliasis, nasal congestion, paresthesia, platelets increased, pruritus, pseudomembranous colitis, psychosis, rash, rigors, serum-sickness reactions, somnolence, Stevens-Johnson syndrome, stridor, taste perversion, thrombocytopenia, toxic epidermal necrolysis, urticaria, vaginitis, xerostomia

Additional reactions reported with other cephalosporins: Allergic reaction, agranulocytosis, angioedema, aplastic anemia, anaphylaxis, asterixis, cholestasis, drug fever, encephalopathy, erythema multiforme, hemolytic anemia, hemorrhage, interstitial nephritis, neuromuscular excitability, neutropenia, pancytopenia, prolonged PT, renal dysfunction, seizure, superinfection, toxic nephropathy

Drug Interactions

Metabolism/Transport Effects None known.

Avoid Concomitant Use

Avoid concomitant use of Ceftibuten with any of the following: BCG

Increased Effect/Toxicity

Ceftibuten may increase the levels/effects of: Aminoglycosides; Vitamin K Antagonists

The levels/effects of Ceftibuten may be increased by: Probenecid

Decreased Effect

Ceftibuten may decrease the levels/effects of: BCG; Sodium Picosulfate; Typhoid Vaccine

The levels/effects of Ceftibuten may be decreased by: Multivitamins/Minerals (with ADEK, Folate, Iron); Multivitamins/Minerals (with AE, No Iron); Zinc Salts

Storage/Stability Store capsules and powder for suspension at 2°C to 25°C (36°F to 77°F). Reconstituted suspension is stable for 14 days when refrigerated at 2°C to 8°C (36°F to 46°F).

Mechanism of Action Inhibits bacterial cell wall synthesis by binding to one or more of the penicillin-binding proteins (PBPs) which in turn inhibits the final transpeptidation step of peptidoglycan synthesis in bacterial cell walls, thus inhibiting cell wall biosynthesis. Bacteria eventually lyse due to ongoing activity of cell wall autolytic enzymes (autolysins and murein hydrolases) while cell wall assembly is arrested.

Pharmacodynamics/Kinetics
- Absorption: Rapid; food decreases peak concentrations, delays T_{max}, and lowers AUC
- Distribution: V_d: Children: 0.5 L/kg; Adults: 0.21 L/kg
- Protein binding: 65%
- Half-life elimination: 2 hours; Cl_{cr} 30-49 mL/minute: 7 hours; Cl_{cr} 5-29 mL/minute: 13 hours; Cl_{cr} <5 mL/minute: 22 hours
- Time to peak: 2-3 hours
- Excretion: Urine (~56%); feces (39%)

Dosage

Usual dosage range:
- Children 6 months to <12 years: Oral: 9 mg/kg/day for 10 days (maximum dose: 400 mg/day)
- Children ≥12 years and Adults: Oral: 400 mg once daily for 10 days

Dosage adjustment in renal impairment:
Cl_{cr} ≥50 mL//minute: No adjustment needed
Cl_{cr} 30-49 mL//minute: Administer 4.5 mg/kg or 200 mg every 24 hours
Cl_{cr} 5-29 mL/minute: Administer 2.25 mg/kg or 100 mg every 24 hours.
Hemodialysis: Administer 400 mg or 9 mg/kg (maximum: 400 mg) after each hemodialysis session
Dosage adjustment in hepatic impairment: No dosage adjustment provided in manufacturer's labeling.

Dietary Considerations
Capsule: Take without regard to food.
Suspension: Take 2 hours before or 1 hour after meals.

Administration
Capsule: Administer without regard to food.
Suspension: Administer 2 hours before or 1 hour after meals. Shake well before use.

Monitoring Parameters Monitor renal, hepatic, and hematologic function periodically with prolonged therapy. Observe for signs and symptoms of anaphylaxis during first dose.

Test Interactions Positive direct Coombs', false-positive urinary glucose test using cupric sulfate (Benedict's solution, Clinitest®, Fehling's solution), false-positive serum or urine creatinine with Jaffé reaction

Dosage Forms Excipient information presented when available (limited, particularly for generics); consult specific product labeling.
Capsule, Oral:
Cedax: 400 mg [contains butylparaben, edetate calcium disodium, methylparaben, propylparaben]
Generic: 400 mg
Suspension Reconstituted, Oral:
Cedax: 90 mg/5 mL (60 mL, 90 mL, 120 mL) [contains polysorbate 80, sodium benzoate; cherry flavor]
Cedax: 180 mg/5 mL (30 mL, 60 mL) [contains sodium benzoate; cherry flavor]
Generic: 180 mg/5 mL (60 mL)

◆ Ceftin *see* Cefuroxime *on page 386*

CefTRIAXone (sef trye AKS one)

Brand Names: U.S. Rocephin

Brand Names: Canada Ceftriaxone for Injection USP; Ceftriaxone Sodium for Injection; Ceftriaxone Sodium for Injection BP

Index Terms Ceftriaxone Sodium

Pharmacologic Category Antibiotic, Cephalosporin (Third Generation)

Additional Appendix Information
Antibiotic Treatment of Adults With Infective Endocarditis *on page 2355*
Desensitization Protocols *on page 2325*
Prevention of Infective Endocarditis *on page 2353*

Use Treatment of lower respiratory tract infections, acute bacterial otitis media, skin and skin structure infections, bone and joint infections, intra-abdominal and urinary tract infections, pelvic inflammatory disease (PID), uncomplicated gonorrhea, bacterial septicemia, and meningitis; used in surgical (perioperative) prophylaxis

Unlabeled Use Treatment of chancroid, epididymitis, complicated gonococcal infections; sexually-transmitted diseases (STD); periorbital or buccal cellulitis; salmonellosis or shigellosis; atypical community-acquired pneumonia; acute bacterial rhinosinusitis (ABRS); epiglottitis, Lyme disease; used in chemoprophylaxis for high-risk contacts (close exposure to patients with invasive meningococcal disease); sexual assault; typhoid fever, Whipple's disease

Pregnancy Risk Factor B

Pregnancy Considerations Teratogenic effects have not been observed in animal reproduction studies. Ceftriaxone crosses the placenta and distributes to amniotic fluid. An increase in most types of birth defects was not found following first trimester exposure to cephalosporins. Pregnancy was found to influence the single dose pharmacokinetics of ceftriaxone when administered prior to delivery. The pharmacokinetics of ceftriaxone following multiple doses in the third trimester are similar to those of nonpregnant patients. Ceftriaxone is recommended for use in pregnant women for the treatment of gonococcal infections, Lyme disease, and may be used in certain situations prior to vaginal delivery in women at high risk for endocarditis (consult current guidelines).

Breast-Feeding Considerations Low concentrations of ceftriaxone are excreted in breast milk. The manufacturer recommends that caution be exercised when administering ceftriaxone to nursing women. Nondose-related effects could include modification of bowel flora.

Contraindications Hypersensitivity to ceftriaxone sodium, any component of the formulation, or other cephalosporins; **do not use in hyperbilirubinemic neonates**, particularly those who are premature since ceftriaxone is reported to displace bilirubin from albumin binding sites; concomitant use with intravenous calcium-containing solutions/products in neonates (≤28 days)

Warnings/Precautions Use with caution in patients with a history of penicillin allergy, especially IgE-mediated reactions (eg, anaphylaxis, urticaria). Abnormal gallbladder sonograms have been reported, possibly due to cetriaxone-calcium precipitates; discontinue in patients who develop signs and symptoms of gallbladder disease. Secondary to biliary obstruction, pancreatitis has been reported rarely. Use with caution in patients with a history of GI disease, especially colitis. Severe cases (including some fatalities) of immune-related hemolytic anemia have been reported in patients receiving cephalosporins, including ceftriaxone. Prolonged use may result in fungal or bacterial superinfection, including *C. difficile*-associated diarrhea (CDAD) and pseudomembranous colitis; CDAD has been observed >2 months postantibiotic treatment.

Potentially significant interactions may exist, requiring dose or frequency adjustment, additional monitoring, and/or selection of alternative therapy. May be associated with increased INR (rarely), especially in nutritionally-deficient patients, prolonged treatment, hepatic or renal disease. No adjustment is generally necessary in patients with renal impairment; use with caution in patients with concurrent hepatic dysfunction and significant renal disease, dosage should not exceed 2 g/day. Ceftriaxone may complex with calcium causing precipitation. Fatal lung and kidney damage associated with calcium-ceftriaxone precipitates has been observed in premature and term neonates. Do not reconstitute, admix, or coadminister with calcium-containing solutions, even via separate infusion lines/sites or at different times in any neonatal patient. Ceftriaxone should not be diluted or administered simultaneously with any calcium-containing solution via a Y-site in any patient. However, ceftriaxone and calcium-containing solution may be administered sequentially of one another for use in patients **other than neonates** if infusion lines are thoroughly flushed, with a compatible fluid, between infusions

Adverse Reactions
>10%: Local: Induration (I.M. 5% to 17%), warmth (I.M.), tightness (I.M.)
1% to 10%:
Dermatologic: Rash (2%)
Gastrointestinal: Diarrhea (3%)
Hematologic: Eosinophilia (6%), thrombocytosis (5%), leukopenia (2%)
Hepatic: Transaminases increased (3%)
Local: Tenderness at injection site (I.V. 1%), pain
Renal: BUN increased (1%)

<1% (Limited to important or life-threatening): Abdominal pain, agranulocytosis, alkaline phosphatase increased, allergic dermatitis, allergic pneumonitis, anaphylaxis, anemia, basophilia, biliary lithiasis, bilirubin increased, bronchospasm, chills, colitis, creatinine increased, diaphoresis, dizziness, dysgeusia, dyspepsia, edema, epistaxis, erythema multiforme, exanthema, fever, flatulence, flushing, gallbladder sludge, gallstones, glossitis, glycosuria, headache, hematuria, hemolytic anemia, jaundice, leukocytosis, Lyell's syndrome, lymphocytosis, lymphopenia, moniliasis, monocytosis, nausea, nephrolithiasis, neutropenia, oliguria, palpitation, pancreatitis, phlebitis, prolonged or decreased PT, pruritus, pseudomembranous colitis, renal and pulmonary ceftriaxone-calcium precipitations (neonates including some fatalities), seizure, serum sickness Stevens-Johnson syndrome, stomatitis, thrombocytopenia, toxic epidermal necrolysis, urinary casts, urticaria, vaginitis, vomiting

Reactions reported with other cephalosporins: Angioedema, allergic reaction, aplastic anemia, asterixis, cholestasis, encephalopathy, hemorrhage, hepatic dysfunction, hyperactivity (reversible), hypertonia, interstitial nephritis, LDH increased, neuromuscular excitability, pancytopenia, paresthesia, renal dysfunction, superinfection, toxic nephropathy

Drug Interactions

Metabolism/Transport Effects None known.

Avoid Concomitant Use

Avoid concomitant use of CefTRIAXone with any of the following: BCG

Increased Effect/Toxicity

CefTRIAXone may increase the levels/effects of: Aminoglycosides; Vitamin K Antagonists

The levels/effects of CefTRIAXone may be increased by: Calcium Salts (Intravenous); Probenecid; Ringer's Injection (Lactated)

Decreased Effect

CefTRIAXone may decrease the levels/effects of: BCG; Sodium Picosulfate; Typhoid Vaccine

Preparation for Administration

I.M. injection: Vials should be reconstituted with appropriate volume of diluent (including D_5W, NS, SWFI, bacteriostatic water, or 1% lidocaine) to make a final concentration of 250 mg/mL or 350 mg/mL.

Volume to add to create a **250 mg/mL** solution:
- 250 mg vial: 0.9 mL
- 500 mg vial: 1.8 mL
- 1 g vial: 3.6 mL
- 2 g vial: 7.2 mL

Volume to add to create a **350 mg/mL** solution:
- 500 mg vial: 1.0 mL
- 1 g vial: 2.1 mL
- 2 g vial: 4.2 mL

I.V. infusion: Infusion is prepared in two stages: Initial reconstitution of powder, followed by dilution to final infusion solution.

Vials: Reconstitute powder with appropriate I.V. diluent (including SWFI, D_5W, $D_{10}W$, NS) to create an initial solution of ~100 mg/mL. Recommended volume to add:
- 250 mg vial: 2.4 mL
- 500 mg vial: 4.8 mL
- 1 g vial: 9.6 mL
- 2 g vial: 19.2 mL

Note: After reconstitution of powder, further dilution into a volume of compatible solution (eg, 50-100 mL of D_5W or NS) is recommended.

Piggyback bottle: Reconstitute powder with appropriate I.V. diluent (D_5W or NS) to create a resulting solution of ~100 mg/mL. Recommended initial volume to add:
- 1 g bottle:10 mL
- 2 g bottle: 20 mL

Note: After reconstitution, to prepare the final infusion solution, further dilution to 50 mL or 100 mL volumes with the appropriate I.V. diluent (including D_5W or NS) is recommended.

Storage/Stability

Powder for injection: Prior to reconstitution, store at room temperature ≤25°C (≤77°F). Protect from light.

Premixed solution (manufacturer premixed): Store at -20°C; once thawed, solutions are stable for 3 days at room temperature of 25°C (77°F) or for 21 days refrigerated at 5°C (41°F). Do not refreeze.

Stability of reconstituted solutions:

10-40 mg/mL: Reconstituted in D_5W, $D_{10}W$, NS, or SWFI: Stable for 2 days at room temperature of 25°C (77°F) or for 10 days when refrigerated at 4°C (39°F). Stable for 26 weeks when frozen at -20°C when reconstituted with D_5W or NS. Once thawed (at room temperature), solutions are stable for 2 days at room temperature of 25°C (77°F) or for 10 days when refrigerated at 4°C (39°F); does not apply to manufacturer's premixed bags. Do not refreeze.

100 mg/mL:

Reconstituted in D_5W, SWFI, or NS: Stable for 2 days at room temperature of 25°C (77°F) or for 10 days when refrigerated at 4°C (39°F).

Reconstituted in lidocaine 1% solution or bacteriostatic water: Stable for 24 hours at room temperature of 25°C (77°F) or for 10 days when refrigerated at 4°C (39°F).

250-350 mg/mL: Reconstituted in D_5W, NS, lidocaine 1% solution, bacteriostatic water, or SWFI: Stable for 24 hours at room temperature of 25°C (77°F) or for 3 days when refrigerated at 4°C (39°F).

Mechanism of Action Inhibits bacterial cell wall synthesis by binding to one or more of the penicillin-binding proteins (PBPs) which in turn inhibits the final transpeptidation step of peptidoglycan synthesis in bacterial cell walls, thus inhibiting cell wall biosynthesis. Bacteria eventually lyse due to ongoing activity of cell wall autolytic enzymes (autolysins and murein hydrolases) while cell wall assembly is arrested.

Pharmacodynamics/Kinetics

Absorption: I.M.: Well absorbed

Distribution: V_d: 6-14 L; widely throughout the body including gallbladder, lungs, bone, bile, CSF (higher concentrations achieved when meninges are inflamed)

Protein binding: 85% to 95%

Half-life elimination: Normal renal and hepatic function: 5-9 hours; Renal impairment (mild-to-severe): 12-16 hours

Time to peak, serum: I.M.: 2-3 hours

Excretion: Urine (33% to 67% as unchanged drug); feces (as inactive drug)

Dosage

Usual dosage range:

Infants and Children: I.M., I.V.: 50-100 mg/kg/day in 1-2 divided doses (maximum: 4000 mg daily [meningitis]; 2000 mg daily [nonmeningeal infections])

Adults: I.M., I.V.: 1-2 g every 12-24 hours

Indication-specific dosing:

Infants and Children:

Acute bacterial rhinosinusitis, severe infection requiring hospitalization (unlabeled use): Children: I.V.: 50 mg/kg/day divided every 12 hours for 10-14 days (Chow, 2012)

Community-acquired pneumonia (CAP) (IDSA/PIDS, 2011): Infants >3 months and Children: I.V.: 50-100 mg/kg/day once daily or divided every 12 hours. **Note:** May consider addition of vancomycin or clindamycin to empiric therapy if community-acquired MRSA suspected. Use the higher end of the range for penicillin-resistant *S. pneumoniae*; in children ≥5 years, a macrolide antibiotic should be added if atypical pneumonia cannot be ruled out; preferred in patients not fully immunized for *H. influenzae* type b and *S. pneumoniae*, or significant local resistance to penicillin in invasive pneumococcal strains

Epiglottitis (unlabeled use): I.M., I.V.: 50-100 mg/kg once daily; reported duration of treatment ranged from 2-14 days

Gonococcal infections:

Arthritis (CDC, 2010): I.M., I.V.:

≤45 kg: 50 mg/kg/dose once daily (maximum: 1000 mg) for 7 days

>45 kg: 50 mg/kg/dose once daily (maximum: 2000 mg) for 7 days

Bacteremia (CDC, 2010): I.M., I.V.:

≤45 kg: 50 mg/kg/dose once daily (maximum: 1000 mg) for 7 days

>45 kg: 50 mg/kg/dose once daily (maximum: 2000 mg) for 7 days

Conjunctivitis, complicated (unlabeled use): I.M., I.V.:

<45 kg: 50 mg/kg in a single dose (maximum: 1000 mg)

≥45 kg: 1000 mg in a single dose

Disseminated (unlabeled use): I.M., I.V.:

Infants: 25-50 mg/kg/dose once daily for 7 days (10-14 days for meningitis) (CDC, 2010); **Note**: Use contraindicated in hyperbilirubinemic neonates.

Children <45 kg: 25-50 mg/kg/dose once daily (maximum: 1000 mg) for 7 days (CDC, 2010)

Children >45 kg: Refer to adult dosing.

Endocarditis (unlabeled use):

≤45 kg: I.M., I.V.: 50 mg/kg/day every 12 hours (maximum: 2000 mg daily) for at least 28 days

>45 kg: I.V.: 1000-2000 mg every 12 hours, for at least 28 days

Meningitis:

≤45 kg: I.V.: 50 mg/kg/day given every 12 hours (maximum: 2000 mg daily); usual duration of treatment is 10-14 days

>45 kg: I.V.: 1000-2000 mg every 12 hours; usual duration of treatment is 10-14 days

Prophylaxis (due to maternal gonococcal infection): I.M., I.V.: 25-50 mg/kg as a single dose (maximum: 125 mg) (CDC, 2010)

Uncomplicated cervicitis, pharyngitis, proctitis, urethritis, vulvovaginitis (unlabeled use) (CDC, 2010):

≤45 kg: I.M.: 125 mg as a single dose

>45 kg: Refer to adult dosing

Infective endocarditis: I.M., I.V.:

Native valve: 100 mg/kg once daily for 2-4 weeks; **Note:** If using 2-week regimen, concurrent gentamicin is recommended

Prosthetic valve: 100 mg/kg once daily for 6 weeks (with or without 2 weeks of gentamicin [dependent on penicillin MIC]); **Note:** For HACEK organisms, duration of therapy is 4 weeks

Enterococcus faecalis (resistant to penicillin, aminoglycoside, and vancomycin), native or prosthetic valve: 100 mg/kg once daily for ≥8 weeks administered concurrently with ampicillin

Prophylaxis: 50 mg/kg 30-60 minutes before procedure; maximum dose: 1000 mg. Intramuscular injections should be avoided in patients who are receiving anticoagulant therapy. In these circumstances, orally administered regimens should be given whenever possible. Intravenously administered antibiotics should be used for patients who are unable to tolerate or absorb oral medications.

Note: American Heart Association (AHA) guidelines now recommend prophylaxis only in patients undergoing invasive procedures and in whom underlying cardiac conditions may predispose to a higher risk of adverse outcomes should infection occur. As of April 2007, routine prophylaxis for GI/GU procedures is no longer recommended by the AHA.

Lyme disease, persistent arthritis (unlabeled use): I.M., I.V.: 75-100 mg/kg (maximum: 2000 mg) for 2-4 weeks

Mild-to-moderate infections: I.M., I.V.: 50-75 mg/kg/day in 1-2 divided doses every 12-24 hours (maximum: 2000 mg daily); continue until at least 2 days after signs and symptoms of infection have resolved

Meningitis (empiric treatment): I.M., I.V.: Loading dose of 100 mg/kg (maximum: 4000 mg), followed by 100 mg/kg/day divided every 12-24 hours (maximum: 4000 mg daily); usual duration of treatment is 7-14 days

Otitis media:

Acute: I.M.: 50 mg/kg in a single dose (maximum: 1000 mg)

Persistent or relapsing (unlabeled use): I.M., I.V.: 50 mg/kg once daily for 3 days

Pneumonia: I.V.: 50-75 mg/kg once daily

Prophylaxis against sexually-transmitted diseases following sexual assault (unlabeled use):

≤45 kg: I.M.: 125 mg in a single dose (in combination with azithromycin and metronidazole) (CDC, 2010)

>45 kg: Refer to adult dosing

Serious infections: I.V.: 80-100 mg/kg/day in 1-2 divided doses (maximum: 4000 mg daily)

Shigella dysentery type 1 (unlabeled dose): I.M.: 50-100 mg/kg/day for 2-5 days (WHO, 2005)

Skin/skin structure infections: I.M., I.V.: 50-75 mg/kg/day in 1-2 divided doses (maximum: 2000 mg daily)

Surgical (perioperative) prophylaxis (unlabeled dose): Children ≥1year: I.V.: 50-75 mg/kg within 60 minutes prior to surgery (maximum dose: 2000 mg) (Bratzler, 2013).

Typhoid fever (unlabeled use): I.V.: 75-80 mg/kg once daily for 5-14 days

Children >8 years (≥45 kg) and Adolescents:

Epididymitis, acute (unlabeled use): I.M.: 125 mg in a single dose

Children <15 years:

Chemoprophylaxis for high-risk contacts (close exposure to patients with invasive meningococcal disease) (unlabeled use): I.M.: 125 mg in a single dose. Children ≥15 years: Refer to adult dosing.

Adults:

Acute bacterial rhinosinusitis, severe infection requiring hospitalization (unlabeled use): I.V.: 1-2 g every 12-24 hours for 5-7 days (Chow, 2012)

Arthritis, septic (unlabeled use): I.V.: 1-2 g once daily

Brain abscess (unlabeled use): I.V.: 2 g every 12 hours with metronidazole

Cavernous sinus thrombosis (unlabeled use): I.V.: 2 g once daily with vancomycin or linezolid

Chancroid (unlabeled use): I.M.: 250 mg as single dose (CDC, 2010)

Chemoprophylaxis for high-risk contacts (close exposure to patients with invasive meningococcal disease) (unlabeled use): I.M.: 250 mg in a single dose

Cholecystitis, mild-to-moderate: 1-2 g every 12-24 hours for 4-7 days (provided source controlled)

Gonococcal infections:

Uncomplicated gonorrhea of the cervix, pharynx, urethra, or rectum (unlabeled regimen): I.M.: 250 mg in a single dose with oral azithromycin (preferred) or oral doxycycline (alternative to preferred) (CDC, 2012)

Conjunctivitis, complicated (unlabeled use): I.M.: 1 g in a single dose (CDC, 2010)

Disseminated (unlabeled use): I.M., I.V.: 1 g once daily for 24-48 hours may switch to cefixime (after improvement noted) to complete a total of 7 days of therapy (CDC, 2010)

Endocarditis (unlabeled use): I.V.: 1-2 g every 12 hours for at least 28 days (CDC, 2010)

Epididymitis, acute (unlabeled use): I.M.: 250 mg in a single dose with doxycycline (CDC, 2010)

Meningitis: I.V.: 1-2 g every 12 hours for 10-14 days (CDC, 2010)

Infective endocarditis: I.M., I.V.:

Native valve: 2 g once daily for 2-4 weeks; **Note:** If using 2-week regimen, concurrent gentamicin is recommended

Prosthetic valve: I.M., I.V.: 2 g once daily for 6 weeks (with or without 2 weeks of gentamicin [dependent on penicillin MIC]); **Note:** For HACEK organisms, duration of therapy is 4 weeks

Enterococcus faecalis (resistant to penicillin, aminoglycoside, and vancomycin), native or prosthetic valve: 2 g twice daily for ≥8 weeks administered concurrently with ampicillin

Prophylaxis: I.M., I.V.: 1 g 30-60 minutes before procedure. Intramuscular injections should be avoided in patients who are receiving anticoagulant therapy. In these circumstances, orally administered regimens should be given whenever possible. Intravenously administered antibiotics should be used for patients who are unable to tolerate or absorb oral medications.

Note: American Heart Association (AHA) guidelines now recommend prophylaxis only in patients undergoing invasive procedures and in whom underlying cardiac conditions may predispose to a higher risk of adverse outcomes should infection occur. As of April 2007, routine prophylaxis for GI/GU procedures is no longer recommended by the AHA.

Intra-abdominal infection, complicated, community-acquired, mild-to-moderate (in combination with metronidazole): 1-2 g every 12-24 hours for 4-7 days (provided source controlled)

Lyme disease (unlabeled use): I.V.: 2 g once daily for 14-28 days

Mastoiditis (hospitalized; unlabeled use): I.V.: 2 g once daily; >60 years old: 1 g once daily

Meningitis (empiric treatment): I.V.: 2 g every 12 hours for 7-14 days (longer courses may be necessary for selected organisms)

Orbital cellulitis (unlabeled use) and endophthalmitis: I.V.: 2 g once daily

Pelvic inflammatory disease: I.M.: 250 mg in a single dose plus doxycycline (with or without metronidazole) (CDC, 2010)

Pneumonia, community-acquired: I.V.: 1 g once daily, usually in combination with a macrolide; consider 2 g daily for patients at risk for more severe infection and/or resistant organisms (ICU status, age >65 years, disseminated infection)

Prophylaxis against sexually-transmitted diseases following sexual assault: I.M.: 250 mg as a single dose (in combination with azithromycin and metronidazole) (CDC, 2010)

Prosthetic joint infection: I.V.:

Staphylococci, oxacillin-susceptible: 1-2 g every 24 hours for 2-6 weeks (in combination with rifampin) followed by oral antibiotic treatment and suppressive regimens (Osmon, 2013)

Streptococci, beta-hemolytic: 2 g every 24 hours for 4-6 weeks (Osmon, 2013)

Pyelonephritis (acute, uncomplicated): Females: I.V.: 1-2 g once daily (Stamm, 1993). Many physicians administer a single parenteral dose before initiating oral therapy (Warren, 1999).

Septic/toxic shock/necrotizing fasciitis (unlabeled use): I.V.: 2 g once daily; with clindamycin for toxic shock

Surgical (perioperative) prophylaxis: I.V.: 1 g 30 minutes to 2 hours before surgery

Manufacturers recommendation: 1 g 30 minutes to 2 hours before surgery

Alternative recommendation: 1-2 g within 60 minutes prior to surgery (Bratzler, 2013).

Alternative recommendation for colorectal procedures: 2 g within 60 minutes prior to surgery with concomitant metronidazole (Bratzler, 2013).

Cholecystectomy: 1-2 g every 12-24 hours, discontinue within 24 hours unless infection outside gallbladder suspected

Syphilis (unlabeled use): I.M., I.V.: 1 g once daily for 10-14 days; **Note:** Alternative treatment for early syphilis, optimal dose, and duration have not been defined (CDC, 2010)

Typhoid fever (unlabeled use): I.V.: 2 g once daily for 14 days

Whipple's disease (unlabeled use): Initial: 2 g once daily for 10-14 days, then oral therapy for ~1 year.

Dosage adjustment in renal impairment: No dosage adjustment is generally necessary in renal impairment; **Note:** Concurrent renal and hepatic dysfunction: Maximum dose: ≤2 g daily

Poorly dialyzed; no supplemental dose or dosage adjustment necessary, including patients on intermittent hemodialysis, peritoneal dialysis, or continuous renal replacement therapy (eg, CVVHD).

Dosage adjustment in hepatic impairment: No adjustment necessary unless there is concurrent renal dysfunction (see dosage adjustment in renal impairment).

Dietary Considerations Some products may contain sodium.

Administration Do not admix with aminoglycosides in same bottle/bag. Do not reconstitute, admix, or coadminister with calcium-containing solutions. Infuse intermittent infusion over 30 minutes.

I.M.: Inject deep I.M. into large muscle mass; a concentration of 250 mg/mL or 350 mg/mL is recommended for all vial sizes except the 250 mg size (250 mg/mL is suggested); can be diluted with 1:1 water or 1% lidocaine for I.M. administration.

I.V.: Infuse as an intermittent infusion over 30 minutes. I.V. push administration over 1-4 minutes has been reported in children ≥12 years, adolescents, and adults (concentration: 100 mg/mL), primarily in patients outside the hospital setting (Baumgartner, 1983; Garrelts, 1988; Poole,1999), although a 2 g dose administered I.V. push over 5 minutes resulted in tachycardia, restlessness, diaphoresis, and palpitations in one patient (Lossos, 1994). I.V. push administration in young infants may also have been a contributing factor in risk of cardiopulmonary events occurring from interactions between ceftriaxone and calcium (Bradley, 2009).

Monitoring Parameters Prothrombin time. Observe for signs and symptoms of anaphylaxis.

Test Interactions Positive direct Coombs', false-positive urinary glucose test using cupric sulfate (Benedict's solution, Clinitest®, Fehling's solution), false-positive serum or urine creatinine with Jaffé reaction

Dosage Forms Excipient information presented when available (limited, particularly for generics); consult specific product labeling.

Solution, Intravenous:

Generic: 20 mg/mL (50 mL); 40 mg/mL (50 mL)

Solution Reconstituted, Injection:
Rocephin: 500 mg (1 ea); 1 g (1 ea)
Generic: 250 mg (1 ea); 500 mg (1 ea); 1 g (1 ea); 2 g (1 ea)
Solution Reconstituted, Intravenous:
Generic: 1 g (1 ea); 2 g (1 ea); 10 g (1 ea)

◆ **Ceftriaxone for Injection USP (Can)** *see* CefTRIAXone *on page 382*

◆ **Ceftriaxone Sodium** *see* CefTRIAXone *on page 382*

◆ **Ceftriaxone Sodium for Injection (Can)** *see* CefTRIAXone *on page 382*

◆ **Ceftriaxone Sodium for Injection BP (Can)** *see* CefTRIAXone *on page 382*

Cefuroxime (se fyoor OKS eem)

Brand Names: U.S. Ceftin; Zinacef; Zinacef in D_5W [DSC]; Zinacef in Sterile Water

Brand Names: Canada Apo-Cefuroxime; Auro-Cefuroxime; Ceftin; Cefuroxime For Injection; Cefuroxime For Injection, USP; PRO-Cefuroxime; ratio-Cefuroxime

Index Terms Cefuroxime Axetil; Cefuroxime Sodium

Pharmacologic Category Antibiotic, Cephalosporin (Second Generation)

Use Treatment of infections caused by staphylococci, group B streptococci, *H. influenzae* (type A and B), *E. coli*, *Enterobacter*, *Salmonella*, and *Klebsiella*; treatment of susceptible infections of the upper and lower respiratory tract, otitis media, urinary tract, uncomplicated skin and soft tissue, bone and joint, sepsis, uncomplicated gonorrhea, and early Lyme disease; surgical (perioperative) prophylaxis

Pregnancy Risk Factor B

Pregnancy Considerations Adverse events were not observed in animal reproduction studies. Cefuroxime crosses the placenta and reaches the cord serum and amniotic fluid. Placental transfer is decreased in the presence of oligohydramnios. Several studies have failed to identify an increased teratogenic risk to the fetus following maternal cefuroxime use.

During pregnancy, mean plasma concentrations of cefuroxime are 50% lower, the AUC is 25% lower, and the plasma half-life is shorter than nonpregnant values. At term, plasma half-life is similar to nonpregnant values and peak maternal concentrations after I.M. administration are slightly decreased. Pregnancy does not alter the volume of distribution. Cefuroxime is one of the antibiotics recommended for prophylactic use prior to cesarean delivery.

Breast-Feeding Considerations Cefuroxime is excreted in breast milk. Manufacturer recommendations vary; caution is recommended if cefuroxime I.V. is given to a nursing woman and it is recommended to consider discontinuing nursing temporarily during treatment following oral cefuroxime. Nondose-related effects could include modification of bowel flora.

Contraindications Hypersensitivity to cefuroxime, any component of the formulation, or other cephalosporins

Warnings/Precautions Modify dosage in patients with severe renal impairment. Use with caution in patients with a history of penicillin allergy, especially IgE-mediated reactions (eg, anaphylaxis, urticaria). Prolonged use may result in fungal or bacterial superinfection, including *C. difficile*-associated diarrhea (CDAD) and pseudomembranous colitis; CDAD has been observed >2 months postantibiotic treatment. May be associated with increased INR, especially in nutritionally-deficient patients, prolonged treatment, hepatic or renal disease. Tablets and oral suspension are not bioequivalent (do not substitute on a mg-per-mg basis). Some products may contain phenylalanine.

Adverse Reactions

>10%: Gastrointestinal: Diarrhea (4% to 11%, duration-dependent)

1% to 10%:
- Dermatologic: Diaper rash (3%)
- Endocrine & metabolic: Alkaline phosphatase increased (2%), lactate dehydrogenase increased (1%)
- Gastrointestinal: Nausea/vomiting (3% to 7%)
- Genitourinary: Vaginitis (≤5%)
- Hematologic: Eosinophilia (7%), hemoglobin and hematocrit decreased (10%)
- Hepatic: Transaminases increased (2% to 4%)
- Local: Thrombophlebitis (2%)

<1% (Limited to important or life-threatening): Anaphylaxis, angioedema, BUN increased, chest pain, cholestasis, colitis, creatinine increased, dyspnea, erythema multiforme, fever, GI bleeding, hemolytic anemia, hepatitis, hives, hyperbilirubinemia, hypersensitivity, interstitial nephritis, jaundice, leukopenia, neutropenia, pain at injection site, pancytopenia, positive Coombs test, prolonged PT/INR, pseudomembranous colitis, rash, renal dysfunction, seizure, Stevens-Johnson syndrome, stomach cramps, tachycardia, thrombocytopenia (rare), tongue swelling, toxic epidermal necrolysis, urticaria

Reactions reported with other cephalosporins: Agranulocytosis, aplastic anemia, asterixis, colitis, encephalopathy, hemorrhage, neuromuscular excitability, serum-sickness reactions, superinfection, toxic nephropathy

Drug Interactions

Metabolism/Transport Effects None known.

Avoid Concomitant Use

Avoid concomitant use of Cefuroxime with any of the following: BCG

Increased Effect/Toxicity

Cefuroxime may increase the levels/effects of: Aminoglycosides; Vitamin K Antagonists

The levels/effects of Cefuroxime may be increased by: Probenecid

Decreased Effect

Cefuroxime may decrease the levels/effects of: BCG; Sodium Picosulfate; Typhoid Vaccine

The levels/effects of Cefuroxime may be decreased by: Antacids; H2-Antagonists

Ethanol/Nutrition/Herb Interactions Food: Bioavailability is increased with food; cefuroxime serum levels may be increased if taken with food or dairy products.

Storage/Stability

Injection: Reconstituted solution is stable for 24 hours at room temperature and 48 hours when refrigerated. I.V. infusion in NS or D_5W solution is stable for 24 hours at room temperature, 7 days when refrigerated, or 26 weeks when frozen. After freezing, thawed solution is stable for 24 hours at room temperature or 21 days when refrigerated.

Oral suspension: Prior to reconstitution, store at 2°C to 30°C (36°F to 86°F). Reconstituted suspension is stable for 10 days at 2°C to 8°C (36°F to 46°F).

Tablet: Store at 15°C to 30°C (59°F to 86°F).

Mechanism of Action Inhibits bacterial cell wall synthesis by binding to one or more of the penicillin-binding proteins (PBPs) which in turn inhibits the final transpeptidation step of peptidoglycan synthesis in bacterial cell walls, thus inhibiting cell wall biosynthesis. Bacteria eventually lyse due to ongoing activity of cell wall autolytic enzymes (autolysins and murein hydrolases) while cell wall assembly is arrested.

Pharmacodynamics/Kinetics

Absorption: Oral (cefuroxime axetil): Increases with food

Distribution: Widely to body tissues and fluids; crosses blood-brain barrier; therapeutic concentrations achieved in CSF even when meninges are not inflamed

Protein binding: 33% to 50%

Bioavailability: Tablet: Fasting: 37%; Following food: 52%

Half-life elimination: Children 1-2 hours; Adults: 1-2 hours; prolonged with renal impairment

Time to peak, serum: I.M.: ~15-60 minutes; I.V.: 2-3 minutes; Oral: Children: 3-4 hours; Adults: 2-3 hours

Excretion: Urine (66% to 100% as unchanged drug)

Dosage Note: Cefuroxime axetil film-coated tablets and oral suspension are not bioequivalent and are not substitutable on a mg/mg basis

Usual dosage range:

Children 3 months to 12 years:

Oral: 20-30 mg/kg/day in 2 divided doses

I.M., I.V.: 75-150 mg/kg/day divided every 8 hours (maximum dose: 6 g/day)

Children ≥13 years and Adults:

Oral: 250-500 mg twice daily

I.M., I.V.: 750 mg to 1.5 g every 6-8 hours or 100-150 mg/kg/day in divided doses every 6-8 hours (maximum: 6 g/day)

Indication-specific dosing:

Children ≥1 year:

Surgical (perioperative) prophylaxis: I.V.: 50 mg/kg within 60 minutes prior to surgical incision (maximum dose: 1500 mg). Doses may be repeated in 4 hours if procedure is lengthy or if there is excessive blood loss (Bratzler, 2013).

Children ≥3 months to 12 years:

Acute bacterial maxillary sinusitis, acute otitis media, and impetigo:

Oral: Suspension: 30 mg/kg/day in 2 divided doses for 10 days (maximum dose: 1 g/day); tablet: 250 mg twice daily for 10 days

I.M., I.V.: 75-150 mg/kg/day divided every 8 hours (maximum dose: 6 g/day)

Epiglottitis: Oral: 150 mg/kg/day in 3 divided doses for 7-10 days

Pharyngitis/tonsillitis:

Oral: Suspension: 20 mg/kg/day (maximum: 500 mg/day) in 2 divided doses for 10 days; tablet: 125 mg every 12 hours for 10 days

I.M., I.V.: 75-150 mg/kg day divided every 8 hours (maximum: 6 g/day)

Adolescents: Refer to adult dosing.

Adults (all oral doses listed are for tablet formulation):

Bronchitis (acute and exacerbations of chronic bronchitis):

Oral: 250-500 mg every 12 hours for 10 days

I.V.: 500-750 mg every 8 hours (complete therapy with oral dosing)

Cellulitis, orbital: I.V.: 1.5 g every 8 hours

Cholecystitis, mild-to-moderate: I.V.: 1.5 g every 8 hours for 4-7 days (provided source controlled)

Gonorrhea:

Disseminated: I.M., I.V.: 750 mg every 8 hours

Uncomplicated:

Oral: 1 g as a single dose

I.M.: 1.5 g as single dose (administer in 2 different sites with probenecid)

Intra-abdominal infection, complicated, community-acquired, mild-to-moderate (in combination with metronidazole): I.V.: 1.5 g every 8 hours for 4-7 days (provided source controlled)

Lyme disease (early): Oral: 500 mg twice daily for 20 days

Pharyngitis/tonsillitis and sinusitis: Oral: 250 mg twice daily for 10 days

Pneumonia (uncomplicated): I.V.: 750 mg every 8 hours

Severe or complicated infections: I.M., I.V.: 1.5 g every 8 hours (up to 1.5 g every 6 hours in life-threatening infections)

Skin/skin structure infection (uncomplicated):

Oral: 250-500 mg every 12 hours for 10 days

I.M., I.V.: 750 mg every 8 hours

Surgical (perioperative) prophylaxis: I.V.:

Manufacturer's recommendation: 1.5 g 30 minutes to 1 hour prior to procedure (if procedure is prolonged can give 750 mg every 8 hours I.V. or I.M.)

Open heart: I.V.: 1.5 g every 12 hours for a total of 4 doses starting at anesthesia induction

Alternative recommendation: 1.5 g within 60 minutes prior to surgical incision. Doses may be repeated in 4 hours if procedure is lengthy or if there is excessive blood loss (Bratzler, 2013).

Urinary tract infection (uncomplicated):

Oral: 125-250 mg every 12 hours for 7-10 days

I.M., I.V.: 750 mg every 8 hours

Dosage adjustment in renal impairment:

Cl_{cr} 10-20 mL/minute: Administer every 12 hours

Cl_{cr} <10 mL/minute: Administer every 24 hours

Hemodialysis: Dialyzable (25%)

Peritoneal dialysis: Dose every 24 hours

Continuous renal replacement therapy (CRRT): 1 g every 12 hours

Dosage adjustment in hepatic impairment: No dosage adjustment provided in manufacturer's labeling.

Dietary Considerations Some products may contain phenylalanine and/or sodium.

Oral suspension: May be taken with food.

Administration

Oral suspension: Administer with food. Shake well before use.

I.M.: Inject deep I.M. into large muscle mass.

I.V.: Inject direct I.V. over 3-5 minutes. Infuse intermittent infusion over 15-30 minutes.

Monitoring Parameters Monitor renal, hepatic, and hematologic function periodically with prolonged therapy. Monitor prothrombin time in patients at risk of prolongation during cephalosporin therapy (nutritionally-deficient, prolonged treatment, renal or hepatic disease). Observe for signs and symptoms of anaphylaxis during first dose.

Test Interactions Positive direct Coombs', false-positive urinary glucose test using cupric sulfate (Benedict's solution, Clinitest®, Fehling's solution); false-negative may occur with ferricyanide test. Glucose oxidase or hexokinase-based methods should be used.

Dosage Forms Excipient information presented when available (limited, particularly for generics); consult specific product labeling. [DSC] = Discontinued product

Solution, Intravenous, as sodium [strength expressed as base]:

Zinacef in D_5W: 750 mg (50 mL [DSC])

Zinacef in Sterile Water: 1.5 g (50 mL)

Solution Reconstituted, Injection, as sodium [strength expressed as base]:

Zinacef: 750 mg (1 ea); 1.5 g (1 ea); 7.5 g (1 ea)

Generic: 750 mg (1 ea); 1.5 g (1 ea); 7.5 g (1 ea); 75 g (1 ea); 225 g (1 ea)

Solution Reconstituted, Intravenous, as sodium [strength expressed as base]:

Zinacef: 750 mg (1 ea); 1.5 g (1 ea)

Generic: 750 mg (1 ea); 1.5 g (1 ea); 7.5 g (1 ea)

Suspension Reconstituted, Oral, as axetil [strength expressed as base]:
Ceftin: 125 mg/5 mL (100 mL); 250 mg/5 mL (50 mL, 100 mL) [contains aspartame; tutti-frutti flavor]
Generic: 125 mg/5 mL (100 mL)
Tablet, Oral, as axetil [strength expressed as base]:
Ceftin: 250 mg, 500 mg
Generic: 250 mg, 500 mg

◆ Cefuroxime Axetil *see* Cefuroxime *on page 386*
◆ Cefuroxime For Injection (Can) *see* Cefuroxime *on page 386*
◆ Cefuroxime For Injection, USP (Can) *see* Cefuroxime *on page 386*
◆ Cefuroxime Sodium *see* Cefuroxime *on page 386*
◆ Cefzil *see* Cefprozil *on page 377*
◆ Cefzil® (Can) *see* Cefprozil *on page 377*
◆ CeleBREX *see* Celecoxib *on page 388*
◆ Celebrex® (Can) *see* Celecoxib *on page 388*

Celecoxib (se le KOKS ib)

Brand Names: U.S. CeleBREX

Brand Names: Canada Celebrex®

Pharmacologic Category Nonsteroidal Anti-inflammatory Drug (NSAID), COX-2 Selective

Use Relief of the signs and symptoms of osteoarthritis, ankylosing spondylitis, juvenile idiopathic arthritis (JIA), and rheumatoid arthritis; management of acute pain; treatment of primary dysmenorrhea

Pregnancy Risk Factor C (prior to 30 weeks gestation)/D (≥30 weeks gestation)

Pregnancy Considerations Teratogenic effects have been observed in some animal studies; therefore, celecoxib is classified as pregnancy category C. Celecoxib is a NSAID that primarily inhibits COX-2 whereas other currently available NSAIDs are nonselective for COX-1 and COX-2. The effects of this selective inhibition to the fetus have not been well studied and limited information is available specific to celecoxib. NSAID exposure during the first trimester is not strongly associated with congenital malformations; however, cardiovascular anomalies and cleft palate have been observed following NSAID exposure in some studies. The use of a NSAID close to conception may be associated with an increased risk of miscarriage. Nonteratogenic effects have been observed following NSAID administration during the third trimester including: Myocardial degenerative changes, prenatal constriction of the ductus arteriosus, fetal tricuspid regurgitation, failure of the ductus arteriosus to close postnatally; renal dysfunction or failure, oligohydramnios; gastrointestinal bleeding or perforation, increased risk of necrotizing enterocolitis; intracranial bleeding (including intraventricular hemorrhage), platelet dysfunction with resultant bleeding; pulmonary hypertension. Because it may cause premature closure of the ductus arteriosus, the use of celecoxib is not recommended ≥30 weeks gestation. The chronic use of NSAIDs in women of reproductive age may be associated with infertility that is reversible upon discontinuation of the medication. A registry is available for pregnant women exposed to autoimmune medications including celecoxib. For additional information contact the Organization of Teratology Information Specialists, OTIS Autoimmune Diseases Study, at 877-311-8972.

Breast-Feeding Considerations Small amounts of celecoxib are found in breast milk. The manufacturer recommends that caution be exercised when administering celecoxib to nursing women.

Medication Guide Available Yes

Contraindications Hypersensitivity to celecoxib, sulfonamides, aspirin, other NSAIDs, or any component of the formulation; perioperative pain in the setting of coronary artery bypass graft (CABG) surgery

Canadian labeling: Additional contraindications (not in U.S. labeling): Pregnancy (third trimester); women who are breast-feeding; severe, uncontrolled heart failure; active gastrointestinal ulcer (gastric, duodenal, peptic) or bleeding; inflammatory bowel disease; cerebrovascular bleeding; severe liver impairment or active hepatic disease; severe renal impairment (Cl_{cr} <30 mL/minute) or deteriorating renal disease; known hyperkalemia; use in children

Warnings/Precautions [U.S. Boxed Warning]: NSAIDs are associated with an increased risk of serious (and potentially fatal) adverse cardiovascular thrombotic events, including MI and stroke. Risk may be increased with duration of use or pre-existing cardiovascular risk factors or disease. Carefully evaluate individual cardiovascular risk profiles prior to prescribing. New-onset or exacerbation of hypertension may occur (NSAIDS may impair response to thiazide or loop diuretics); may contribute to cardiovascular events; monitor blood pressure; use with caution in patients with hypertension. May cause sodium and fluid retention; use with caution in patients with edema, cerebrovascular disease, or ischemic heart disease. Avoid use in heart failure. Long-term cardiovascular risk in children has not been evaluated.

[U.S. Boxed Warning]: Celecoxib is contraindicated for treatment of perioperative pain in the setting of coronary artery bypass graft (CABG) surgery. Risk of MI and stroke may be increased with use following CABG surgery.

[U.S. Boxed Warning]: NSAIDs may increase risk of serious gastrointestinal ulceration, bleeding, and perforation (may be fatal). These events may occur at any time during therapy and without warning. Use caution with a history of GI disease (bleeding or ulcers), concurrent therapy with aspirin, anticoagulants and/or corticosteroids, smoking, use of alcohol, the elderly or debilitated patients. When used concomitantly with ≤325 mg of aspirin, a substantial increase in the risk of gastrointestinal complications (eg, ulcer) occurs; concomitant gastroprotective therapy (eg, proton pump inhibitors) is recommended (Bhatt, 2008).

Use the lowest effective dose for the shortest duration of time, consistent with individual patient goals, to reduce risk of cardiovascular or GI adverse events. Alternate therapies should be considered for patients at high risk.

NSAIDs may cause serious skin adverse events including exfoliative dermatitis, Stevens-Johnson syndrome (SJS), and toxic epidermal necrolysis (TEN); may occur without warning and in patients without prior known sulfa allergy. Anaphylactoid reactions may occur, even without prior exposure; patients with "aspirin triad" (bronchial asthma, aspirin intolerance, rhinitis) may be at increased risk. Do not use in patients who experience bronchospasm, asthma, rhinitis, or urticaria with NSAID or aspirin therapy. Use with caution in other forms of asthma.

Use with caution in patients with decreased hepatic (dosage adjustments are recommended for moderate hepatic impairment; not recommended for patients with severe hepatic impairment) or renal function. Transaminase elevations have been reported with use; closely monitor patients with any abnormal LFT. Severe hepatic reactions (eg, fulminant hepatitis, liver failure) have occurred with NSAID use, rarely; discontinue if signs or symptoms of liver disease develop, if systemic manifestations occur, or with persistent or worsening abnormal hepatic function tests. NSAID use may compromise existing renal function; dose-dependent decreases in prostaglandin synthesis may result from NSAID use, causing a reduction in renal blood flow which may cause renal decompensation (usually reversible). Patients with impaired renal function, dehydration, heart failure, liver dysfunction, those taking diuretics, ACE inhibitors, angiotensin II receptor blockers, and the elderly are at greater risk for renal toxicity. Rehydrate patient before starting therapy; monitor renal function closely. Not recommended for use in patients with advanced renal disease or severe renal insufficiency; discontinue use with persistent or worsening abnormal renal function tests. Long-term NSAID use may result in renal papillary necrosis. Should not be considered a treatment or replacement of corticosteroid-dependent diseases.

Anaphylactoid reactions may occur, even with no prior exposure to celecoxib. Use with caution in patients with known or suspected deficiency of cytochrome P450 isoenzyme 2C9; poor metabolizers may have higher plasma levels due to reduced metabolism; consider reduced initial doses. Alternate therapies should be considered in patients with JIA who are poor metabolizers of CYP2C9.

Anemia may occur with use; monitor hemoglobin or hematocrit in patients on long-term treatment. Celecoxib does not affect PT, PTT or platelet counts; does not inhibit platelet aggregation at approved doses.

When used for juvenile idiopathic arthritis (JIA), celecoxib is not FDA-approved in children <2 years of age or in children <10 kg. Use caution with systemic onset JIA (may be at risk for disseminated intravascular coagulation). Safety and efficacy have not been established for use in children for indications other than JIA.

Adverse Reactions

≥2%

Cardiovascular: Peripheral edema

Central nervous system: Dizziness, fever, headache, insomnia

Dermatologic: Rash

Gastrointestinal: Abdominal pain, diarrhea, dyspepsia, flatulence, nausea, vomiting

Neuromuscular & skeletal: Arthralgia, back pain

Respiratory: Cough, nasopharyngitis, pharyngitis, rhinitis, sinusitis, upper respiratory tract infection

0.1% to 1.9%:

Cardiovascular: Angina, aortic valve incompetence, chest pain, coronary artery disorder, edema, facial edema, hypertension (aggravated), MI, palpitation, sinus bradycardia, tachycardia, ventricular hypertrophy

Central nervous system: Anxiety, depression, fatigue, hypoesthesia, migraine, nervousness, pain, somnolence, vertigo

Dermatologic: Alopecia, bruising, cellulitis, dermatitis, dry skin, photosensitivity, pruritus, rash (erythematous), rash (maculopapular), urticaria

Endocrine & metabolic: Hot flashes, hypercholesterolemia, hyperglycemia, hypokalemia, ovarian cyst, testosterone decreased

Gastrointestinal: Anorexia, appetite increased, constipation, diverticulitis, dysphagia, eructation, esophagitis, gastritis, gastroenteritis, gastroesophageal reflux, gastrointestinal ulcer, hemorrhoids, hiatal hernia, melena, stomatitis, tenesmus, weight gain, xerostomia

Genitourinary: Cystitis, dysuria, urinary frequency

Hematologic: Anemia, thrombocythemia

Hepatic: Alkaline phosphatase increased, transaminases increased

Neuromuscular & skeletal: Arthrosis, CPK increased, hypertonia, leg cramps, myalgia, paresthesia, synovitis, tendonitis

Ocular: Conjunctival hemorrhage, vitreous floaters

Otic: Deafness, labyrinthitis, tinnitus

Renal: Albuminuria, BUN increased, creatinine increased, hematuria, nonprotein nitrogen increased, renal calculi

Respiratory: Bronchitis, bronchospasm, dyspnea, epistaxis, laryngitis, pneumonia

Miscellaneous: Allergic reactions, allergy aggravated, cyst, diaphoresis, flu-like syndrome

<0.1% (Limited to important or life-threatening): Acute renal failure, agranulocytosis, anaphylactoid reactions, angioedema, anosmia, aplastic anemia, aseptic meningitis, cerebrovascular accident, CHF, cholelithiasis, colitis, DVT, erythema multiforme, esophageal perforation, exfoliative dermatitis, gangrene, gastrointestinal bleeding, hepatic failure, hepatic necrosis, hepatitis (including fulminant), hypoglycemia, hyponatremia, ileus, interstitial nephritis, intestinal obstruction, intestinal perforation, intracranial hemorrhage, jaundice, leukopenia, pancreatitis, pancytopenia, pulmonary embolism, renal papillary necrosis, sepsis, Stevens-Johnson syndrome, sudden death, suicide, syncope, thrombocytopenia, thrombophlebitis, toxic epidermal necrolysis, vasculitis, ventricular fibrillation

Drug Interactions

Metabolism/Transport Effects **Substrate** of CYP2C9 (major), CYP3A4 (minor); **Note:** Assignment of Major/Minor substrate status based on clinically relevant drug interaction potential; **Inhibits** CYP2C8 (moderate), CYP2D6 (moderate)

Avoid Concomitant Use

Avoid concomitant use of Celecoxib with any of the following: Floctafenine; Ketorolac (Nasal); Ketorolac (Systemic); Nonsteroidal Anti-Inflammatory Agents; NSAID (COX-2 Inhibitor); Omacetaxine; Thioridazine

Increased Effect/Toxicity

Celecoxib may increase the levels/effects of: 5-ASA Derivatives; Agents with Antiplatelet Properties; Aliskiren; Aminoglycosides; Anticoagulants; ARIPiprazole; Bisphosphonate Derivatives; CycloSPORINE (Systemic); CYP2C8 Substrates; CYP2D6 Substrates; Deferasirox; Desmopressin; Digoxin; Eplerenone; Estrogen Derivatives; Fesoterodine; Haloperidol; Lithium; Methotrexate; Metoprolol; Nebivolol; NSAID (COX-2 Inhibitor); Omacetaxine; Porfimer; Potassium-Sparing Diuretics; PRALAtrexate; Prilocaine; Quinolone Antibiotics; Sodium Nitrite; Tenofovir; Thioridazine; Thrombolytic Agents; Vancomycin; Vitamin K Antagonists

The levels/effects of Celecoxib may be increased by: ACE Inhibitors; Angiotensin II Receptor Blockers; Antidepressants (Tricyclic, Tertiary Amine); Aspirin; Corticosteroids (Systemic); CycloSPORINE (Systemic); CYP2C9 Inhibitors (Moderate); CYP2C9 Inhibitors (Strong); Floctafenine; Herbs (Anticoagulant/Antiplatelet Properties); Ketorolac (Nasal); Ketorolac (Systemic); Mifepristone; Nitric Oxide; Nonsteroidal Anti-Inflammatory Agents; Probenecid; Propafenone; Selective Serotonin Reuptake Inhibitors; Sodium Phosphates; Treprostinil

Decreased Effect

Celecoxib may decrease the levels/effects of: ACE Inhibitors; Agents with Antiplatelet Properties; Aliskiren; Angiotensin II Receptor Blockers; Beta-Blockers; Codeine; Eplerenone; HydrALAZINE; Loop Diuretics; Potassium-Sparing Diuretics; Prostaglandins (Ophthalmic); Selective Serotonin Reuptake Inhibitors; Tamoxifen; Thiazide Diuretics; TraMADol

The levels/effects of Celecoxib may be decreased by: Bile Acid Sequestrants; CYP2C9 Inducers (Strong); Dabrafenib; Peginterferon Alfa-2b

Ethanol/Nutrition/Herb Interactions

Ethanol: Avoid ethanol (increased GI irritation).

Food: Peak concentrations are delayed and AUC is increased by 10% to 20% when taken with a high-fat meal.

Herb/Nutraceutical: Avoid concomitant use with herbs possessing anticoagulation/antiplatelet properties, including alfalfa, anise, bilberry, bladderwrack, bromelain, cat's claw, celery, chamomile, coleus, cordyceps, dong quai, evening primrose, fenugreek, feverfew, garlic, ginger, ginkgo biloba, ginseng (American, Panax, Siberian), grapeseed, green tea, guggul, horse chestnuts, horseradish, licorice, prickly ash, red clover, reishi, SAMe (S-adenosylmethionine), sweet clover, turmeric, white willow.

Storage/Stability Store at 25°C (77°F); excursions permitted to 15°C to 30°C (59°F to 86°F).

Mechanism of Action Inhibits prostaglandin synthesis by decreasing the activity of the enzyme, cyclooxygenase-2 (COX-2), which results in decreased formation of prostaglandin precursors; has antipyretic, analgesic, and anti-inflammatory properties. Celecoxib does not inhibit cyclooxygenase-1 (COX-1) at therapeutic concentrations.

Pharmacodynamics/Kinetics

Distribution: V_d (apparent): ~400 L

Protein binding: ~97% primarily to albumin

Metabolism: Hepatic via CYP2C9; forms inactive metabolites

Bioavailability: Absolute: Unknown

Half-life elimination: ~11 hours (fasted)

Time to peak: ~3 hours

Excretion: Feces (~57% as metabolites, <3% as unchanged drug); urine (27% as metabolites, <3% as unchanged drug)

Dosage Note: Use the lowest effective dose for the shortest duration of time, consistent with individual patient treatment goals. Oral:

Children ≥2 years: Juvenile idiopathic arthritis (JIA):
- ≥10 kg to ≤25 kg: 50 mg twice daily
- >25 kg: 100 mg twice daily

Adults:
- Acute pain or primary dysmenorrhea: Initial dose: 400 mg, followed by an additional 200 mg if needed on day 1; maintenance dose: 200 mg twice daily as needed.
  - Canadian labeling: Recommended maximum dose for treatment of acute pain: 400 mg/day up to 7 days
- Ankylosing spondylitis: 200 mg/day as a single dose or in divided doses twice daily; if no effect after 6 weeks, may increase to 400 mg/day. If no response following 6 weeks of treatment with 400 mg/day, consider discontinuation and alternative treatment.
  - Canadian labeling: Recommended maximum dose: 200 mg/day
- Osteoarthritis: 200 mg/day as a single dose or in divided doses twice daily
- Rheumatoid arthritis: 100-200 mg twice daily

Elderly: No specific adjustment based on age is recommended. However, the AUC in elderly patients may be increased by 50% as compared to younger subjects. Initiate at the lowest recommended dose in patients weighing <50 kg.

*Dosing adjustment in poor CYP2C9 metabolizers (eg, CYP2C9*3/*3):* Consider reducing initial dose by 50%; consider alternative treatment in patients with JIA who are poor CYP2C9 metabolizers.
- Canadian labeling: Recommended maximum dose: 100 mg/day

Dosing adjustment in renal impairment:
- Advanced renal disease: Use is not recommended; however, if celecoxib treatment cannot be avoided, monitor renal function closely
- Severe renal insufficiency: Use is not recommended.
  - Canadian labeling: Cl_{cr} <30 mL/minute: Use is contraindicated.
- Abnormal renal function tests (persistent or worsening): Discontinue use

Dosing adjustment in hepatic impairment:
- Moderate hepatic impairment (Child-Pugh class B): Reduce dose by 50%
- Severe hepatic impairment (Child-Pugh class C): Use is not recommended
  - Canadian labeling: Use is contraindicated.
- Abnormal liver function tests (persistent or worsening): Discontinue use

Dietary Considerations May be taken without regard to meals.

Administration May be administered without regard to meals. Capsules may be swallowed whole or the entire contents emptied onto a teaspoon of cool or room temperature applesauce. The contents of the capsules sprinkled onto applesauce may be stored under refrigeration for up to 6 hours.

Monitoring Parameters CBC; blood chemistry profile; occult blood loss and periodic liver function tests; monitor renal function (urine output, serum BUN and creatinine; monitor response (pain, range of motion, grip strength, mobility, ADL function), inflammation; blood pressure (baseline and during treatment); observe for weight gain, edema; observe for bleeding, bruising; evaluate gastrointestinal effects (abdominal pain, bleeding, dyspepsia)

JIA: Monitor for development of abnormal coagulation tests with systemic onset JIA

Dosage Forms Excipient information presented when available (limited, particularly for generics); consult specific product labeling.

Capsule, Oral:
- CeleBREX: 50 mg, 100 mg, 200 mg, 400 mg

- Celestone *see* Betamethasone *on page 247*
- Celestone Soluspan *see* Betamethasone *on page 247*
- Celestone® Soluspan® (Can) *see* Betamethasone *on page 247*
- CeleXA *see* Citalopram *on page 440*
- Celexa® (Can) *see* Citalopram *on page 440*
- CellCept *see* Mycophenolate *on page 1407*
- CellCept Intravenous *see* Mycophenolate *on page 1407*
- Cell Culture Inactivated Influenza Vaccine, Trivalent [Flucelvax] *see* Influenza Virus Vaccine (Inactivated) *on page 1078*
- Celontin *see* Methsuximide *on page 1331*
- Celontin® (Can) *see* Methsuximide *on page 1331*
- Celsentri™ (Can) *see* Maraviroc *on page 1269*
- Cemill [OTC] *see* Ascorbic Acid *on page 172*
- Cemill SR [OTC] *see* Ascorbic Acid *on page 172*
- CEM-Urea *see* Urea *on page 2140*
- Cenestin *see* Estrogens (Conjugated A/Synthetic) *on page 765*
- Centany *see* Mupirocin *on page 1407*
- Centany AT *see* Mupirocin *on page 1407*
- *Centruroides* Immune FAB2 (Equine) *see Centruroides* Immune F(ab')$_2$ (Equine) *on page 390*

Centruroides Immune F(ab')$_2$ (Equine)

(sen tra ROY dez i MYUN fab too E kwine)

Brand Names: U.S. Anascorp

Index Terms *Centruroides* Immune FAB2 (Equine); Antivenin (*Centruroides*) Immune F(ab')$_2$ (Equine); Antivenin Scorpion; Antivenom (*Centruroides*) Immune F(ab')$_2$ (Equine); Antivenom Scorpion; Scorpion Antivenin; Scorpion Antivenom

Pharmacologic Category Antivenin

Use Treatment of scorpion envenomation

Pregnancy Risk Factor C

Pregnancy Considerations Animal reproduction studies have not been conducted. In general, medications used as antidotes should take into consideration the health and prognosis of the mother; antidotes should be administered to pregnant women if there is a clear indication for use and should not be withheld because of fears of teratogenicity (Bailey, 2003).

Breast-Feeding Considerations It is not known if this product is excreted into breast milk. The manufacturer recommends caution be used if administered to a nursing woman.

Contraindications There are no contraindications listed within the manufacturer's labeling.

Warnings/Precautions Derived from equine (horse) immune globulin F(ab')$_2$ fragments; anaphylaxis and anaphylactoid reactions are possible, especially in patients with known allergies to horse protein. Patients who have had previous treatment with *Centruroides* immune F(ab')$_2$ or other equine-derived antivenom/antitoxin may be at a higher risk for acute hypersensitivity reactions. In patients who develop an anaphylactic reaction, discontinue the infusion and administer emergency care. Immediate treatment (eg, epinephrine 1:1000, corticosteroids, diphenhydramine) should be available. In addition, delayed serum sickness may occur, usually within 2 weeks; monitor patients with follow-up visits for signs and symptoms (eg, arthralgia, fever, myalgia, rash).

Product of equine (horse) plasma; may potentially contain infectious agents (eg, viruses) which could transmit disease. May contain small amounts of cresol resulting from the manufacturing process; local reactions and myalgias may occur.

Adverse Reactions

1% to 10%:

Central nervous system: Fever (4%), fatigue (2%), headache (2%), lethargy (1%)

Dermatologic: Rash (3%), pruritus (2%)

Gastrointestinal: Vomiting (5%), nausea (2%), diarrhea (1%)

Neuromuscular & skeletal: Myalgia (2%)

Respiratory: Rhinorrhea (2%), cough (1%)

<1% (Limited to important or life-threatening): Aspiration, ataxia, chest tightness, eye edema, hypersensitivity, hypoxia, palpitation, pneumonia, respiratory distress, serum sickness (delayed)

Drug Interactions

Metabolism/Transport Effects None known.

Avoid Concomitant Use There are no known interactions where it is recommended to avoid concomitant use.

Increased Effect/Toxicity There are no known significant interactions involving an increase in effect.

Decreased Effect There are no known significant interactions involving a decrease in effect.

Preparation for Administration Reconstitute each vial with 5 mL NS; gently swirl to mix. Dilute dose (eg, 1-3 vials) with NS to a total volume of 50 mL. Inspect diluted solution; do not use if it contains particulate matter or is discolored or turbid.

Storage/Stability Store unused vials at room temperature of 25°C (77°F); excursions permitted up to 40°C (104°F); do not freeze. Discard partially used vials.

Mechanism of Action Contains venom-specific F(ab')$_2$ fragments of IgG which bind and neutralize venom toxins; thereby helping to remove the toxin from the target tissue and eliminate it from the body.

Pharmacodynamics/Kinetics

Onset: Time to resolution of symptoms: Adults: 1.91 ± 1.4 hours; Children: 1.28 ± 0.8 hours; >95% of all patients will experience resolution of symptoms within 4 hours

Distribution: V_{dss}: 13.6 L ± 5.4 L

Half-life, elimination: 159 ± 57 hours

Dosage I.V.: Children and Adults: **Note:** Initiate therapy as soon as possible after scorpion sting. Initial: 3 vials (containing ≤360 mg total protein and ≥450 LD50 [mouse] neutralizing units); may administer additional vials in 1-vial increments every 30-60 minutes as needed.

Dosing adjustment in renal impairment: There are no dosage adjustments provided in manufacturer's labeling.

Dosing adjustment in hepatic impairment: There are no dosage adjustments provided in manufacturer's labeling.

Administration I.V.: Administer over 10 minutes; monitor for return of symptoms of envenomation and repeat as needed. Medications (eg, epinephrine, corticosteroids, diphenhydramine) and equipment for resuscitation should be readily available in case of hypersensitivity reactions. Avoid I.M. since the time to peak blood concentration may be prolonged with this route of administration (Turri, 2011; Vasquez, 2010).

Monitoring Parameters Signs and symptoms of envenomation (eg, opsoclonus, involuntary muscle movement, slurred speech, paresthesias, respiratory distress, salivation, frothy sputum, vomiting); signs and symptoms of hypersensitivity reactions; follow-up visits for signs and symptoms of serum sickness (eg, arthralgia, fever, myalgia, rash)

Additional Information Each vial of *Centruroides* immune F(ab')$_2$ (equine) contains ≤120 mg total protein and ≥150 LD50 (mouse) neutralizing units.

Dosage Forms Excipient information presented when available (limited, particularly for generics); consult specific product labeling.

Solution Reconstituted, Intravenous [preservative free]:

Anascorp: (1 ea)

◆ **Cepacol Dual Relief [OTC]** *see* Benzocaine *on page 240*

◆ **Cepacol Sensations Hydra [OTC]** *see* Benzocaine *on page 240*

◆ **Cepacol Sensations Warming [OTC]** *see* Benzocaine *on page 240*

◆ **Cepacol Sore Throat [OTC]** *see* Benzocaine *on page 240*

◆ **Cepacol Sore Throat + Coating [OTC]** *see* Benzocaine *on page 240*

◆ **Cepacol Sore Throat Max Numb [OTC]** *see* Benzocaine *on page 240*

Cephalexin (sef a LEKS in)

Brand Names: U.S. Keflex

Brand Names: Canada Apo-Cephalex; Dom-Cephalexin; Keflex; Novo-Lexin; Nu-Cephalex; PMS-Cephalexin

Index Terms Cephalexin Monohydrate

Pharmacologic Category Antibiotic, Cephalosporin (First Generation)

Additional Appendix Information

Prevention of Infective Endocarditis *on page 2353*

Use Treatment of susceptible bacterial infections including respiratory tract infections, otitis media, skin and skin structure infections, bone infections, and genitourinary tract infections, including acute prostatitis; alternative therapy for acute infective endocarditis prophylaxis

Unlabeled Use Chronic antimicrobial suppression of prosthetic joint infection

Pregnancy Risk Factor B

Pregnancy Considerations Adverse events were not observed in animal reproduction studies. Cephalexin crosses the placenta and produces therapeutic concentrations in the fetal circulation and amniotic fluid. An increased risk of teratogenic effects has not been observed following maternal use of cephalexin. Peak concentrations in pregnant patients are similar to those in ▶

nonpregnant patients. Prolonged labor may decrease oral absorption.

Breast-Feeding Considerations Small amounts of cephalexin are excreted in breast milk. The manufacturer recommends that caution be exercised when administering cephalexin to nursing women. Maximum milk concentration occurs ~4 hours after a single oral dose and gradually disappears by 8 hours after administration. Nondose-related effects could include modification of bowel flora.

Contraindications Hypersensitivity to cephalexin, any component of the formulation, or other cephalosporins

Warnings/Precautions Modify dosage in patients with severe renal impairment. Use with caution in patients with a history of penicillin allergy, especially IgE-mediated reactions (eg, anaphylaxis, urticaria). Prolonged use may result in fungal or bacterial superinfection, including *C. difficile*-associated diarrhea (CDAD) and pseudomembranous colitis; CDAD has been observed >2 months postantibiotic treatment. May be associated with increased INR, especially in nutritionally-deficient patients, prolonged treatment, hepatic or renal disease.

Adverse Reactions Frequency not defined.

Central nervous system: Agitation, confusion, dizziness, fatigue, hallucinations, headache

Dermatologic: Angioedema, erythema multiforme (rare), rash, Stevens-Johnson syndrome (rare), toxic epidermal necrolysis (rare), urticaria

Gastrointestinal: Abdominal pain, diarrhea, dyspepsia, gastritis, nausea (rare), pseudomembranous colitis, vomiting (rare)

Genitourinary: Genital pruritus, genital moniliasis, vaginitis, vaginal discharge

Hematologic: Eosinophilia, hemolytic anemia, neutropenia, thrombocytopenia

Hepatic: ALT increased, AST increased, cholestatic jaundice (rare), transient hepatitis (rare)

Neuromuscular & skeletal: Arthralgia, arthritis, joint disorder

Renal: Interstitial nephritis (rare)

Miscellaneous: Allergic reactions, anaphylaxis

Drug Interactions

Metabolism/Transport Effects None known.

Avoid Concomitant Use

Avoid concomitant use of Cephalexin with any of the following: BCG

Increased Effect/Toxicity

Cephalexin may increase the levels/effects of: MetFORMIN; Vitamin K Antagonists

The levels/effects of Cephalexin may be increased by: Probenecid

Decreased Effect

Cephalexin may decrease the levels/effects of: BCG; Sodium Picosulfate; Typhoid Vaccine

The levels/effects of Cephalexin may be decreased by: Multivitamins/Minerals (with ADEK, Folate, Iron); Multivitamins/Minerals (with AE, No Iron); Zinc Salts

Ethanol/Nutrition/Herb Interactions Food: Peak antibiotic serum concentration is lowered and delayed, but total drug absorbed is not affected. Cephalexin serum levels may be decreased if taken with food.

Storage/Stability

Capsule: Store at 15°C to 30°C (59°F to 86°F).

Powder for oral suspension: Refrigerate suspension after reconstitution; discard after 14 days.

Mechanism of Action Inhibits bacterial cell wall synthesis by binding to one or more of the penicillin-binding proteins (PBPs) which in turn inhibits the final transpeptidation step of peptidoglycan synthesis in bacterial cell walls, thus inhibiting cell wall biosynthesis. Bacteria eventually lyse due to ongoing activity of cell wall autolytic enzymes (autolysins and murein hydrolases) while cell wall assembly is arrested.

Pharmacodynamics/Kinetics

Absorption: Rapid (90%); delayed in young children

Distribution: Widely into most body tissues and fluids, including gallbladder, liver, kidneys, bone, sputum, bile, and pleural and synovial fluids; CSF penetration is poor

Protein binding: 6% to 15%

Half-life elimination: Adults: 0.5-1.2 hours; prolonged with renal impairment

Time to peak, serum: ~1 hour

Excretion: Urine (80% to 100% as unchanged drug) within 8 hours

Dosage

Usual dosage range:

Children >1 year: Oral: 25-100 mg/kg/day every 6-8 hours (maximum: 4 g/day)

Adults: Oral: 250-1000 mg every 6 hours; maximum: 4 g/day

Indication-specific dosing:

Infants >3 months and Children: Oral:

Community-acquired pneumonia (CAP) (IDSA/PIDS, 2011), *S. aureus* (methicillin-susceptible), mild infection or step-down therapy (preferred): 75-100 mg/kg/day in 3-4 divided doses

Children: Oral:

Furunculosis: 25-50 mg/kg/day in 4 divided doses

Impetigo: 25 mg/kg/day in 4 divided doses

Otitis media: 75-100 mg/kg/day in 4 divided doses

Prophylaxis against infective endocarditis (dental, oral, or respiratory tract procedures): 50 mg/kg 30-60 minutes prior to procedure (maximum: 2 g). **Note:** American Heart Association (AHA) guidelines now recommend prophylaxis only in patients undergoing invasive procedures and in whom underlying cardiac conditions may predispose to a higher risk of adverse outcomes should infection occur.

Severe infections: 50-100 mg/kg/day in divided doses every 6-8 hours

Skin abscess: 50 mg/kg/day in 4 divided doses (maximum: 4 g)

Skin and skin structure infections: Children >1 year: 25-50 mg/kg/day divided every 12 hours

Streptococcal pharyngitis: Children >1 year: 25-50 mg/kg/day divided every 12 hours. **Note:** Recommended by the Infectious Disease Society of America (IDSA) as an alternative agent for group A streptococcal pharyngitis in penicillin-allergic patients (avoid in patients with immediate-type hypersensitivity to penicillin) at a dose of 40 mg/kg/day divided twice daily (maximum: 1000 mg daily) for 10 days (Shulman, 2012).

Adolescents >15 years and Adults: Oral:

Cellulitis and mastitis: 500 mg every 6 hours

Furunculosis/skin abscess: 250 mg 4 times/day

Prophylaxis against infective endocarditis (dental, oral, or respiratory tract procedures): 2 g 30-60 minutes prior to procedure. **Note:** American Heart Association (AHA) guidelines now recommend prophylaxis only in patients undergoing invasive procedures and in whom underlying cardiac conditions may predispose to a higher risk of adverse outcomes should infection occur.

Prophylaxis in total joint replacement patients undergoing dental procedures which produce bacteremia: 2 g 1 hour prior to procedure

Prosthetic joint infection, chronic oral antimicrobial suppression (unlabeled use): Oral:

Propionibacterium spp (alternative to penicillin or amoxicillin): 500 mg every 6-8 hours (Osmon, 2013)

Staphylococci, oxacillin-susceptible (preferred): 500 mg every 6-8 hours (Osmon, 2013)

Streptococci, beta-hemolytic (alternative to penicillin or amoxicillin): 500 mg every 6-8 hours (Osmon, 2013)

Skin and skin structure infections: 500 mg every 12 hours

Streptococcal pharyngitis: 500 mg every 12 hours. **Note:** Recommended by the Infectious Disease Society of America (IDSA) as an alternative agent for group A streptococcal pharyngitis in penicillin-allergic patients (avoid in patients with immediate-type hypersensitivity to penicillin) with a duration of 10 days (Shulman, 2012).

Uncomplicated cystitis: 500 mg every 12 hours for 7-14 days

Dosage adjustment in renal impairment: Adults:

Cl_{cr} 10-50 mL/minute: 500 mg every 8-12 hours

Cl_{cr} <10: 250-500 mg every 12-24 hours

Hemodialysis: 250 mg every 12-24 hours; moderately dialyzable (20% to 50%); give dose after dialysis session

Dosage adjustment in hepatic impairment: No dosage adjustment provided in manufacturer's labeling.

Dietary Considerations Take without regard to food. If GI distress, take with food.

Administration Take without regard to food. If GI distress, take with food. Give around-the-clock to promote less variation in peak and trough serum levels.

Monitoring Parameters With prolonged therapy monitor renal, hepatic, and hematologic function periodically; monitor for signs of anaphylaxis during first dose

Test Interactions Positive direct Coombs', false-positive urinary glucose test using cupric sulfate (Benedict's solution, Clinitest®, Fehling's solution), false-positive serum or urine creatinine with Jaffé reaction, false-positive urinary proteins and steroids

Dosage Forms Excipient information presented when available (limited, particularly for generics); consult specific product labeling.

Capsule, Oral:

Keflex: 250 mg, 500 mg, 750 mg [contains brilliant blue fcf (fd&c blue #1), fd&c yellow #10 (quinoline yellow), fd&c yellow #6 (sunset yellow)]

Generic: 250 mg, 500 mg, 750 mg

Suspension Reconstituted, Oral:

Generic: 125 mg/5 mL (100 mL, 200 mL); 250 mg/5 mL (100 mL, 200 mL)

Tablet, Oral:

Generic: 250 mg, 500 mg

- **Cephalexin Monohydrate** *see* Cephalexin *on page* 391
- **Ceprotin** *see* Protein C Concentrate (Human) *on page* 1743
- **Cerebyx** *see* Fosphenytoin *on page* 925
- **Cerebyx® (Can)** *see* Fosphenytoin *on page* 925
- **Cerefolin® NAC** *see* Methylfolate, Methylcobalamin, and Acetylcysteine *on page* 1335
- **Cerezyme** *see* Imiglucerase *on page* 1052
- **Cerovel** *see* Urea *on page* 2140

Certolizumab Pegol (cer to LIZ u mab PEG ol)

Brand Names: U.S. Cimzia; Cimzia Prefilled; Cimzia Starter Kit

Brand Names: Canada Cimzia®

Index Terms CDP870

Pharmacologic Category Antirheumatic, Disease Modifying; Gastrointestinal Agent, Miscellaneous; Tumor Necrosis Factor (TNF) Blocking Agent

Use

U.S. labeling:

Ankylosing spondylitis: Treatment of adults with active ankylosing spondylitis (AS)

Crohn disease: Treatment of moderately to severely active Crohn disease in patients who have inadequate response to conventional therapy

Psoriatic arthritis: Treatment of adult patients with active psoriatic arthritis

Rheumatoid arthritis: Treatment of adults with moderately to severely active rheumatoid arthritis (RA) (as monotherapy or in combination with nonbiological disease-modifying antirheumatic drugs [DMARDS])

Canadian labeling: **Rheumatoid arthritis:** Treatment of adults with moderately to severely active rheumatoid arthritis (in combination with methotrexate or as monotherapy if unable to tolerate methotrexate)

Pregnancy Risk Factor B

Pregnancy Considerations Adverse effects were not observed in animal reproduction studies. Certolizumab pegol was found to cross the human placenta. Serum concentrations in 12 infants of 10 mothers were ≥75% lower than the maternal serum at delivery (last maternal dose of 400 mg given 5-42 days prior to birth). Although placental transfer was low, infants may have a slower rate of elimination than adults. In one infant, certolizumab pegol serum concentrations decreased from 1.02 to 0.84 mcg/mL over 4 weeks. Adverse events were not reported. The safety of administering live or live-attenuated vaccines to exposed infants is not known. If a biologic agent such as certolizumab pegol is needed to treat inflammatory bowel disease during pregnancy, it is recommended to hold therapy after 30 weeks gestation (Habal, 2012).

Healthcare providers are encouraged to enroll women exposed to certolizumab pegol during pregnancy in the MotherToBaby Autoimmune Diseases Study by contacting the Organization of Teratology Information Specialists (OTIS) (877-311-8972). The Canadian labeling recommends that women of childbearing potential use reliable contraception during therapy and for at least 5 months after the last dose of certolizumab.

Breast-Feeding Considerations It is not known if certolizumab pegol is excreted in breast milk. Due to the potential for serious adverse reactions in the nursing infant, the manufacturer recommends a decision be made whether to discontinue nursing or to discontinue the drug, taking into account the importance of treatment to the mother.

Medication Guide Available Yes

Contraindications There are no contraindications listed within the manufacturer's U.S. labeling.

Canadian labeling: Hypersensitivity to certolizumab pegol or any component of the formulation; active tuberculosis or other severe infections (eg, sepsis, abscesses, opportunistic infections); moderate to severe heart failure (NYHA Class III/IV)

Warnings/Precautions [U.S. Boxed Warning]: Patients receiving certolizumab are at increased risk for serious infections which may result in hospitalization and/or fatality; infections usually developed in patients receiving concomitant immunosuppressive agents (eg, methotrexate or corticosteroids) and may present as disseminated (rather than local) disease. Active tuberculosis (or reactivation of latent tuberculosis), invasive fungal (including aspergillosis, blastomycosis, candidiasis, coccidioidomycosis, histoplasmosis, and pneumocystosis) and bacterial, viral or other opportunistic infections (including legionellosis and listeriosis) have been reported in patients receiving TNF-blocking agents, including certolizumab. Monitor closely for signs/symptoms of infection. Discontinue for serious infection or sepsis. Consider risks versus

benefits prior to use in patients with a history of chronic or recurrent infection. Consider empiric antifungal therapy in patients who are at risk for invasive fungal infection and develop severe systemic illness. Caution should be exercised when considering use in the elderly or in patients with conditions that predispose them to infections (eg, diabetes) or residence/travel from areas of endemic mycoses (blastomycosis, coccidioidomycosis, histoplasmosis), or with latent or localized infections. Do not initiate certolizumab therapy with active infection, including clinically important localized infection. Patients who develop a new infection while undergoing treatment should be monitored closely. **[U.S. Boxed Warning]: Lymphoma and other malignancies (some fatal) have been reported in children and adolescent patients receiving other TNF-blocking agents.** Approximately half of the malignancies reported in children were lymphomas (Hodgkin and non-Hodgkin) while other cases varied and included malignancies not typically observed in this population. The onset of malignancy was after a median of 30 months (range: 1-84 months) after the initiation of the TNF-blocking agent. Use of TNF blockers may affect defenses against malignancies; impact on the development and course of malignancies is not fully defined. Chronic immunosuppressant therapy use may be a predisposing factor for malignancy development; rheumatoid arthritis alone has been previously associated with an increased rate of lymphoma. Hepatosplenic T-cell lymphoma (HSTCL), a rare T-cell lymphoma, has also been associated with TNF-blocking agents, primarily reported in adolescent and young adult males with Crohn disease or ulcerative colitis, most of whom had received concurrent treatment with azathioprine and/or 6-mercaptopurine. Perform periodic skin examinations in all patients during therapy, particularly those at increased risk for skin cancer.

Tuberculosis has been reported with certolizumab treatment. **[U.S. Boxed Warnings]: Patients should be evaluated for tuberculosis risk factors and for latent tuberculosis infection (with a tuberculin skin test) prior to therapy. Treatment of latent tuberculosis should be initiated before use. Patients with initial negative tuberculin skin tests should receive continued monitoring for tuberculosis throughout treatment;** active tuberculosis has developed in this population during treatment. Use with caution in patients who have resided in regions where tuberculosis is endemic. Consider antituberculosis treatment (prior to certolizumab treatment) in patients with a history of latent or active tuberculosis if adequate treatment course cannot be confirmed, and for patients with risk factors for tuberculosis despite a negative test. Carefully consider benefits and risks of initiating certolizumab treatment in patients who have been exposed to tuberculosis.

Rare reactivation of hepatitis B virus (HBV) has occurred in chronic carriers of the virus, usually in patients receiving concomitant immunosuppressants; evaluate for HBV prior to initiation in all patients. Patients who test positive for HBV surface antigen should be referred for hepatitis B evaluation/treatment prior to certolizumab initiation. Monitor for clinical and laboratory signs of active infection during and for several months following discontinuation of treatment in HBV carriers; interrupt therapy if reactivation occurs and treat appropriately with antiviral therapy; if resumption of therapy is deemed necessary, exercise caution and monitor patient closely.

Hypersensitivity reactions, including angioedema, dyspnea, hypotension, rash, serum sickness and urticaria have been reported (rarely) with treatment; discontinue and do not resume therapy if hypersensitivity occurs. Some of these reactions have occurred after the first dose. Use with caution in patients who have experienced hypersensitivity with other TNF blockers. Use with caution in heart failure patients; worsening heart failure and new onset heart failure have been reported with TNF blockers, including certolizumab pegol; monitor closely. The Canadian labeling contraindicates use in moderate-to-severe heart failure (NYHA Class III/IV).

Rare cases of pancytopenia and other significant cytopenias, including aplastic anemia and have been reported with TNF-blocking agents. Leukopenia and thrombocytopenia have occurred with certolizumab; use with caution in patients with underlying hematologic disorders; consider discontinuing therapy with significant hematologic abnormalities. Autoantibody formation may develop; rarely resulting in autoimmune disorder, including lupus-like syndrome; monitor and discontinue if symptoms develop. A small number of patients (8%) develop antibodies to certolizumab during therapy. Antibody-positive patients may have an increased incidence of adverse events (including injection site pain/erythema, abdominal pain and erythema nodosum). Use with caution in patients with pre-existing or recent-onset CNS demyelinating disorders; rare cases of optic neuritis, seizure, peripheral neuropathy, and demyelinating disease (eg, multiple sclerosis, Guillain-Barré syndrome; new onset or exacerbation) have been reported.

Potentially significant drug-drug interactions may exist, requiring dose or frequency adjustment, additional monitoring, and/or selection of alternative therapy. Use caution when switching between biological disease modifying antirheumatic drugs (DMARDs); overlapping of biological activity may increase the risk for infection.

Patients should be up to date with all immunizations before initiating therapy; patients may receive vaccines other than live or live attenuated vaccines during therapy. There is no data available concerning the effects of therapy on vaccination or secondary transmission of live vaccines in patients receiving therapy. Use has not been studied in patients with renal impairment; however, the pharmacokinetics of the pegylated (polyethylene glycol) component may be dependent on renal function. Use with caution in the elderly, may be at higher risk for infections.

Adverse Reactions

>10%:

- Gastrointestinal: Nausea (≤11%)
- Respiratory: Upper respiratory infection (6% to 20%)
- Miscellaneous: Infection (38%; serious: 3%)

1% to 10%:

- Cardiovascular: Hypertension (≤5%)
- Central nervous system: Headache (5%), fever (3%), fatigue (≤3%)
- Dermatologic: Rash (≤9%)
- Genitourinary: Urinary tract infection (≤8%)
- Neuromuscular & skeletal: Arthralgia (6% to 7%), back pain (≤4%)
- Respiratory: Cough (≤6%), nasopharyngitis (5%), bronchitis (≤3%), pharyngitis (≤3%)
- Miscellaneous: Antibody formation (7% to 8%), positive ANA (≤4%)

<5% (Crohn's disease), <3% (RA) (limited to important or life-threatening): Alopecia, anemia, angina, anxiety, aplastic anemia, arrhythmia, atrial fibrillation, bipolar disorder, cytopenia, demyelinating disorder exacerbation, dermatitis, diarrhea, erythema nodosum, heart failure, hepatitis, hepatitis B reactivation; hypersensitivity reaction (eg, dyspnea, hot flush, hypotension, malaise, serum sickness, syncope); intestinal obstruction, leukemias, leukopenia, lupus erythematosus rash, lupus-like syndrome, lymphadenopathy, lymphomas, malignancy, MI, myocardial ischemia, nephrotic syndrome, optic neuritis, pancytopenia, pericardial effusion, pericarditis, peripheral edema, peripheral neuropathy, psoriasis, pyelonephritis,

renal failure, retinal hemorrhage, sarcoidosis, seizure, stroke, thrombocytopenia, thrombophilia, thrombophlebitis, transaminases increased, transient ischemic attack, tuberculosis, urticaria, uveitis, vasculitis

Drug Interactions

Metabolism/Transport Effects None known.

Avoid Concomitant Use

Avoid concomitant use of Certolizumab Pegol with any of the following: Abatacept; Anakinra; Anti-TNF Agents; BCG; Canakinumab; Natalizumab; Pimecrolimus; Rilonacept; RiTUXimab; Tacrolimus (Topical); Tocilizumab; Tofacitinib; Vaccines (Live)

Increased Effect/Toxicity

Certolizumab Pegol may increase the levels/effects of: Abatacept; Anakinra; Canakinumab; Leflunomide; Natalizumab; Rilonacept; Tofacitinib; Vaccines (Live)

The levels/effects of Certolizumab Pegol may be increased by: Anti-TNF Agents; Denosumab; Pimecrolimus; RiTUXimab; Roflumilast; Tacrolimus (Topical); Tocilizumab; Trastuzumab

Decreased Effect

Certolizumab Pegol may decrease the levels/effects of: BCG; Coccidioidin Skin Test; Sipuleucel-T; Vaccines (Inactivated); Vaccines (Live)

The levels/effects of Certolizumab Pegol may be decreased by: Echinacea; Pegloticase

Ethanol/Nutrition/Herb Interactions Herb/Nutraceutical: Echinacea may decrease the therapeutic effects of certolizumab. Management: Avoid concurrent use.

Preparation for Administration Vials: Allow to reach room temperature prior to reconstitution. Using aseptic technique, reconstitute each vial with 1 mL sterile water for injection (provided) to a concentration of ~200 mg/mL; the manufacturer recommends using a 20-gauge needle (provided). Gently swirl to facilitate wetting of powder; do not shake. Allow vials to set undisturbed (may take up to 30 minutes) until fully reconstituted. Reconstituted solutions should not contain visible particles or gels in the solution.

Storage/Stability

Store intact vials and syringes at 2°C to 8°C (36°F to 46°F); do not freeze. Do not separate contents of carton prior to use. Protect from light. Bring to room temperature prior to administration.

Reconstituted vials may be retained at room temperature for up to 2 hours or refrigerated (do not freeze) for up to 24 hours prior to administration. Discard unused portion of vial or syringe.

Mechanism of Action Certolizumab pegol is a pegylated humanized antibody Fab' fragment of tumor necrosis factor alpha (TNF-alpha) monoclonal antibody. Certolizumab pegol binds to and selectively neutralizes human TNF-alpha activity. (Elevated levels of TNF-alpha have a role in the inflammatory process associated with Crohn's disease and in joint destruction associated with rheumatoid arthritis.) Since it is not a complete antibody (lacks Fc region), it does not induce complement activation, antibody-dependent cell-mediated cytotoxicity, or apoptosis. Pegylation of certolizumab allows for delayed elimination and therefore an extended half-life.

Pharmacodynamics/Kinetics

Distribution: V_{ss}: 6-8 L

Bioavailability: SubQ: ~80% (range: 76% to 88%)

Half-life elimination: ~14 days

Time to peak, plasma: 54-171 hours

Dosage Note: Each 400 mg dose should be administered as 2 injections of 200 mg each

Ankylosing spondylitis: Adults: SubQ: Initial: 400 mg, repeat dose 2 and 4 weeks after initial dose; Maintenance: 200 mg every 2 weeks or 400 mg every 4 weeks

Crohn's disease: Adults: SubQ: Initial: 400 mg, repeat dose 2 and 4 weeks after initial dose; Maintenance: 400 mg every 4 weeks

Psoriatic arthritis: Adults: SubQ: Initial: 400 mg, repeat dose 2 and 4 weeks after initial dose; Maintenance: 200 mg every other week. May consider maintenance dose of 400 mg every 4 weeks.

Rheumatoid arthritis: Adults: SubQ: Initial: 400 mg, repeat dose 2 and 4 weeks after initial dose; Maintenance: 200 mg every other week. May consider maintenance dose of 400 mg every 4 weeks. May be administered alone or in combination with methotrexate.

Dosage adjustment for toxicity: Hypersensitivity, lupus-like syndrome, serious infection, sepsis, or hepatitis B reactivation: Discontinue treatment.

Dosage adjustment in renal impairment: No dosage adjustment provided in manufacturer's labeling (has not been studied); pharmacokinetics of the pegylated (polyethylene glycol) component of certolizumab pegol is expected to be dependent on renal function.

Dosage adjustment in hepatic impairment: No dosage adjustment provided in manufacturer's labeling.

Administration SubQ: Bring to room temperature prior to administration. After reconstitution (of vials), draw each vial into separate syringes (using 20-gauge needles).

Administer each syringe subcutaneously (using provided 23-gauge needle) to separate sites on abdomen or thigh. Rotate injections sites; do not administer to areas where skin is tender, bruised, red, or hard.

Monitoring Parameters Monitor improvement of symptoms and physical function assessments. Latent TB screening prior to initiating and during therapy; signs/symptoms of infection (prior to, during, and following therapy); CBC with differential; signs/symptoms/worsening of heart failure; HBV screening prior to initiating (all patients), HBV carriers (during and for several months following therapy); signs and symptoms of hypersensitivity reaction; symptoms of lupus-like syndrome; signs/symptoms of malignancy (eg, splenomegaly, hepatomegaly, abdominal pain, persistent fever, night sweats, weight loss) including periodic skin examinations.

Test Interactions Tests for latent tuberculosis may be falsely negative while on certolizumab pegol treatment. Falsely elevated aPTT assays have been reported with PTT-Lupus Anticoagulant (LA) and Standard Target Activated Partial Thromboplastin time (STA-PTT) tests from Diagnostica Stago, and with HemosiL APTT-SP liquid and HemosiL lyophilized silica tests from Instrumentation Laboratories.

Dosage Forms Excipient information presented when available (limited, particularly for generics); consult specific product labeling.

Kit, Subcutaneous:

Cimzia: 200 mg

Kit, Subcutaneous [preservative free]:

Cimzia Prefilled: 200 mg/mL

Cimzia Starter Kit: 6 X 200 mg/mL

◆ **Cerubidine** *see* DAUNOrubicin (Conventional) *on page 553*

◆ **Cerubidine® (Can)** *see* DAUNOrubicin (Conventional) *on page 553*

◆ **Cervarix®** *see* Papillomavirus (Types 16, 18) Vaccine (Human, Recombinant) *on page 1569*

◆ **Cervidil** *see* Dinoprostone *on page 619*

◆ **Cervidil® (Can)** *see* Dinoprostone *on page 619*

◆ **C.E.S.** *see* Estrogens (Conjugated/Equine, Systemic) *on page 770*

◆ **C.E.S.** *see* Estrogens (Conjugated/Equine, Topical) *on page 773*

◆ C.E.S.® (Can) *see* Estrogens (Conjugated/Equine, Systemic) *on page* 770

◆ Cetacaine *see* Benzocaine, Butamben, and Tetracaine *on page* 242

◆ Cetafen [OTC] *see* Acetaminophen *on page* 28

◆ Cetafen Extra [OTC] *see* Acetaminophen *on page* 28

Cetirizine (se TI ra zeen)

Brand Names: U.S. All Day Allergy Childrens [OTC]; All Day Allergy [OTC]; Cetirizine HCl Allergy Child [OTC]; Cetirizine HCl Childrens Alrgy [OTC]; Cetirizine HCl Childrens [OTC]; Cetirizine HCl Hives Relief [OTC]; ZyrTEC Allergy [OTC]; ZyrTEC Childrens Allergy [OTC]; ZyrTEC Childrens Hives Relief [OTC]; ZyrTEC Hives Relief [OTC]

Brand Names: Canada Aller-Relief [OTC]; Apo-Cetirizine® [OTC]; Extra Strength Allergy Relief [OTC]; PMS-Cetirizine; Reactine [OTC]; Reactine™

Index Terms Cetirizine Hydrochloride; P-071; UCB-P071

Pharmacologic Category Histamine H_1 Antagonist; Histamine H_1 Antagonist, Second Generation; Piperazine Derivative

Use Perennial and seasonal allergic rhinitis and other allergic symptoms including urticaria; chronic idiopathic urticaria

Pregnancy Considerations Maternal use of cetirizine has not been associated with an increased risk of major malformations. The use of antihistamines for the treatment of rhinitis during pregnancy is generally considered to be safe at recommended doses. Although safety data is limited, cetirizine may be a preferred second generation antihistamine for the treatment of rhinitis during pregnancy.

Breast-Feeding Considerations Cetirizine is excreted into breast milk.

Contraindications Hypersensitivity to cetirizine, hydroxyzine, or any component of the formulation

Warnings/Precautions Cetirizine should be used cautiously in patients with hepatic or renal dysfunction; dosage adjustment recommended. Use with caution in the elderly; may be more sensitive to adverse effects. May cause drowsiness; use caution performing tasks which require alertness (eg, operating machinery or driving). Effects may be potentiated when used with other sedative drugs or ethanol.

Adverse Reactions

>10%: Central nervous system: Headache (children 11% to 14%, placebo 12%), somnolence (adults 14%, children 2% to 4%)

2% to 10%:

Central nervous system: Insomnia (children 9%, adults <2%), fatigue (adults 6%), malaise (4%), dizziness (adults 2%)

Gastrointestinal: Abdominal pain (children 4% to 6%), dry mouth (adults 5%), diarrhea (children 2% to 3%), nausea (children 2% to 3%, placebo 2%), vomiting (children 2% to 3%)

Respiratory: Epistaxis (children 2% to 4%, placebo 3%), pharyngitis (children 3% to 6%, placebo 3%), bronchospasm (children 2% to 3%, placebo 2%)

<2% (Limited to important or life-threatening; as reported in adults and/or children): Aggressive reaction, anaphylaxis, angioedema, ataxia, chest pain, confusion, convulsions, depersonalization, depression, edema, fussiness, hallucinations, hemolytic anemia, hepatitis, hypertension, hypotension (severe), irritability, liver function abnormal, nervousness, ototoxicity, palpitation, paralysis, paresthesia, photosensitivity, rash, suicidal ideation, suicide, taste perversion, tongue discoloration, tongue edema, tremor, visual field defect, weakness

Drug Interactions

Metabolism/Transport Effects Substrate of CYP3A4 (minor), P-glycoprotein; **Note:** Assignment of Major/Minor substrate status based on clinically relevant drug interaction potential

Avoid Concomitant Use

Avoid concomitant use of Cetirizine with any of the following: Aclidinium; Azelastine (Nasal); Ipratropium (Oral Inhalation); Paraldehyde; Tiotropium; Umeclidinium

Increased Effect/Toxicity

Cetirizine may increase the levels/effects of: Alcohol (Ethyl); Analgesics (Opioid); Anticholinergics; Azelastine (Nasal); Buprenorphine; CNS Depressants; Hydrocodone; Methotrimeprazine; Metyrosine; Mirtazapine; Paraldehyde; Pramipexole; ROPINIRole; Rotigotine; Selective Serotonin Reuptake Inhibitors; Tiotropium; Zolpidem

The levels/effects of Cetirizine may be increased by: Aclidinium; Brimonidine (Topical); Doxylamine; Droperidol; HydrOXYzine; Ipratropium (Oral Inhalation); Magnesium Sulfate; Methotrimeprazine; Perampanel; P-glycoprotein/ABCB1 Inhibitors; Pramlintide; Sodium Oxybate; Tapentadol; Umeclidinium

Decreased Effect

Cetirizine may decrease the levels/effects of: Acetylcholinesterase Inhibitors (Central); Benzylpenicilloyl Polylysine; Betahistine; Hyaluronidase

The levels/effects of Cetirizine may be decreased by: Acetylcholinesterase Inhibitors (Central); Amphetamines; P-glycoprotein/ABCB1 Inducers

Ethanol/Nutrition/Herb Interactions Ethanol: May increase CNS depression; monitor for increased effects with coadministration. Caution patients about effects.

Storage/Stability Store at room temperature.

Syrup: Store at room temperature of 15°C to 30°C (59°F to 86°F), or under refrigeration at 2°C to 8°C (36°F to 46°F).

Mechanism of Action Competes with histamine for H_1-receptor sites on effector cells in the gastrointestinal tract, blood vessels, and respiratory tract

Pharmacodynamics/Kinetics

Onset of action: Suppression of skin wheal and flare: 0.7 hours (Simons, 1999)

Duration of action: Suppression of skin wheal and flare: ≥24 hours (Simons, 1999)

Absorption: Rapid

Distribution: 0.56 L/kg (Simons, 1999)

Protein binding, plasma: Mean: 93%

Metabolism: Limited hepatic

Half-life elimination: 8 hours

Time to peak, serum: 1 hour

Excretion: Urine (70%); feces (10%)

Dosage Oral:

Children:

6-12 months: Chronic urticaria, perennial allergic rhinitis: 2.5 mg once daily

12 months to <2 years: Chronic urticaria, perennial allergic rhinitis: 2.5 mg once daily; may increase to 2.5 mg every 12 hours if needed

2-5 years: Chronic urticaria, perennial or seasonal allergic rhinitis: Initial: 2.5 mg once daily; may be increased to 2.5 mg every 12 hours **or** 5 mg once daily

Children ≥6 years and Adults: Chronic urticaria, perennial or seasonal allergic rhinitis: 5-10 mg once daily, depending upon symptom severity

Elderly: Initial: 5 mg once daily; may increase to 10 mg/day. **Note:** Manufacturer recommends 5 mg/day in patients ≥77 years of age.

Dosage adjustment in renal/hepatic impairment:

Children <6 years: Cetirizine use not recommended

Children 6-11 years: <2.5 mg once daily

Children ≥12 and Adults:

Cl_{cr} 11-31 mL/minute, hemodialysis, or hepatic impairment: Administer 5 mg once daily

Cl_{cr} <11 mL/minute, not on dialysis: Cetirizine use not recommended

Dietary Considerations May be taken with or without food.

Administration May be administered with or without food.

Monitoring Parameters Relief of symptoms, sedation and anticholinergic effects

Test Interactions May cause false-positive serum TCA screen. May suppress the wheal and flare reactions to skin test antigens.

Dosage Forms Excipient information presented when available (limited, particularly for generics); consult specific product labeling. [DSC] = Discontinued product

Capsule, Oral, as hydrochloride:

ZyrTEC Allergy: 10 mg

Solution, Oral, as hydrochloride:

All Day Allergy Childrens: 5 mg/5 mL (118 mL) [contains methylparaben, propylene glycol, propylparaben]

All Day Allergy Childrens: 1 mg/mL (118 mL) [dye free, gluten free, sugar free; contains propylene glycol, sodium benzoate; grape flavor]

Cetirizine HCl Allergy Child: 5 mg/5 mL (120 mL) [alcohol free, dye free, gluten free, sugar free; contains methylparaben, propylene glycol, propylparaben; grape flavor]

Cetirizine HCl Allergy Child: 5 mg/5 mL (120 mL) [alcohol free, sugar free; contains methylparaben, propylene glycol, propylparaben]

Cetirizine HCl Childrens: 1 mg/mL (118 mL) [contains methylparaben, propylene glycol, propylparaben]

Cetirizine HCl Hives Relief: 5 mg/5 mL (120 mL) [alcohol free, sugar free; contains methylparaben, propylene glycol, propylparaben; grape flavor]

Syrup, Oral, as hydrochloride:

Cetirizine HCl Childrens Alrgy: 1 mg/mL (118 mL, 120 mL) [contains methylparaben, propylene glycol, propylparaben; grape flavor]

ZyrTEC Childrens Allergy: 1 mg/mL (118 mL) [contains methylparaben, propylene glycol, propylparaben; banana-grape flavor]

ZyrTEC Childrens Allergy: 1 mg/mL (118 mL) [dye free, sugar free; contains propylene glycol, sodium benzoate]

ZyrTEC Childrens Allergy: 1 mg/mL (118 mL) [dye free, sugar free; contains propylene glycol, sodium benzoate; bubble-gum flavor]

ZyrTEC Childrens Allergy: 5 mg/5 mL (5 mL, 118 mL) [dye free, sugar free; contains propylene glycol, sodium benzoate; grape flavor]

ZyrTEC Childrens Hives Relief: 1 mg/mL (118 mL) [grape flavor]

Generic: 1 mg/mL (120 mL, 480 mL); 5 mg/5 mL (5 mL, 120 mL, 473 mL)

Tablet, Oral, as hydrochloride:

All Day Allergy: 10 mg

All Day Allergy: 10 mg [contains brilliant blue fcf (fd&c blue #1)]

ZyrTEC Allergy: 10 mg

ZyrTEC Hives Relief: 10 mg

Generic: 5 mg, 10 mg

Tablet Chewable, Oral, as hydrochloride:

All Day Allergy Childrens: 5 mg, 10 mg [tutti-frutti flavor]

ZyrTEC Childrens Allergy: 5 mg [grape flavor]

ZyrTEC Childrens Allergy: 10 mg [contains fd&c blue #2 aluminum lake; grape flavor]

Generic: 5 mg, 10 mg

Tablet Dispersible, Oral, as hydrochloride:

ZyrTEC Allergy: 10 mg [DSC]

◆ **Cetirizine HCl Allergy Child [OTC]** *see* Cetirizine *on page 396*

◆ **Cetirizine HCl Childrens [OTC]** *see* Cetirizine *on page 396*

◆ **Cetirizine HCl Childrens Alrgy [OTC]** *see* Cetirizine *on page 396*

◆ **Cetirizine HCl Hives Relief [OTC]** *see* Cetirizine *on page 396*

◆ **Cetirizine Hydrochloride** *see* Cetirizine *on page 396*

◆ **Cetraxal** *see* Ciprofloxacin (Otic) *on page 435*

Cetrorelix (set roe REL iks)

Brand Names: U.S. Cetrotide

Brand Names: Canada Cetrotide®

Index Terms Cetrorelix Acetate

Pharmacologic Category Gonadotropin Releasing Hormone Antagonist

Use Inhibits premature luteinizing hormone (LH) surges in women undergoing controlled ovarian stimulation

Pregnancy Risk Factor X

Pregnancy Considerations Adverse effects, including fetal resorption and implantation loss, have been observed in animal reproduction studies. Resorption resulting in fetal loss would be expected if used in a pregnant woman; use is contraindicated during pregnancy.

Breast-Feeding Considerations It is not known if cetrorelix is excreted in breast milk. Use while breast-feeding is contraindicated by the manufacturer.

Contraindications Hypersensitivity to cetrorelix or any component of the formulation; extrinsic peptide hormones, mannitol, gonadotropin releasing hormone (GnRH) or GnRH analogs; severe renal impairment; pregnancy; breast-feeding

Warnings/Precautions Hazardous agent - use appropriate precautions for handling and disposal (NIOSH, 2012). Should only be prescribed by fertility specialists. Monitor carefully after first injection for possible hypersensitivity reactions. Use caution in women with active allergic conditions or a history of allergies; use in women with severe allergic conditions is not recommended. Pregnancy should be excluded before treatment is begun.

Adverse Reactions

1% to 10%:

Central nervous system: Headache (1%)

Endocrine & metabolic: Ovarian hyperstimulation syndrome, WHO grade II or III (4%)

Gastrointestinal: Nausea (1%)

Hepatic: ALT, AST, GGT, and alkaline phosphatase increased (1% to 2%)

Postmarketing and/or case reports: Anaphylactic reactions (cough, hypotension, rash); local injection site reactions (bruising, erythema, itching, pruritus, redness, swelling)

Drug Interactions

Metabolism/Transport Effects None known.

Avoid Concomitant Use There are no known interactions where it is recommended to avoid concomitant use.

Increased Effect/Toxicity There are no known significant interactions involving an increase in effect.

Decreased Effect There are no known significant interactions involving a decrease in effect.

Storage/Stability Store in outer carton. Once mixed, solution should be used immediately.

0.25 mg vials: Store under refrigeration at 2°C to 8°C (36°F to 46°F).

3 mg vials: Store at controlled room temperature at 25°C (77°F); excursions permitted to 15°C to 30°C (59°F to 86°F).

Mechanism of Action Competes with naturally-occurring GnRH for binding on receptors of the pituitary. This delays luteinizing hormone surge, preventing ovulation until the follicles are of adequate size.

Pharmacodynamics/Kinetics

Onset of action: 0.25 mg dose: 2 hours; 3 mg dose: 1 hour

Duration: 3 mg dose (single dose): 4 days

Absorption: Rapid

Distribution: V_d: ~1 L/kg

Protein binding: 86%

Metabolism: Transformed by peptidases; cetrorelix and peptides (1-9), (1-7), (1-6), and (1-4) are found in the bile; peptide (1-4) is the predominant metabolite

Bioavailability: 85%

Half-life elimination: 0.25 mg dose: 5 hours; 0.25 mg multiple doses: 20.6 hours; 3 mg dose: 62.8 hours

Time to peak: 0.25 mg dose: 1 hour; 3 mg dose: 1.5 hours

Excretion: Feces (5% to 10% as unchanged drug and metabolites); urine (2% to 4% as unchanged drug); within 24 hours

Dosage

Adults: Females: SubQ: Used in conjunction with controlled ovarian stimulation therapy using gonadotropins (FSH, hMG):

Single-dose regimen: 3 mg given when serum estradiol levels show appropriate stimulation response, usually stimulation day 7 (range: days 5-9). If hCG is not administered within 4 days, continue cetrorelix at 0.25 mg/day until hCG is administered.

Multiple-dose regimen: 0.25 mg morning or evening of stimulation day 5, or morning of stimulation day 6; continue until hCG is administered.

Elderly: Not intended for use in women ≥65 years of age (Phase 2 and Phase 3 studies included women 19-40 years of age)

Dosing adjustment in renal impairment:

Severe impairment: Use is contraindicated

Mild-to-moderate impairment: No dosage adjustment provided in manufacturer's labeling.

Dosing adjustment in hepatic impairment: No dosage adjustment provided in manufacturer's labeling.

Administration Cetrorelix is administered by SubQ injection following proper aseptic technique procedures. Injections should be to the lower abdomen, preferably around the navel (but staying at least 1 inch from the navel). The injection site should be rotated daily. The needle should be inserted completely into the skin at a 45-degree angle.

Hazardous agent; use appropriate precautions for handling and disposal (NIOSH, 2012).

Monitoring Parameters Ultrasound to assess follicle size

Dosage Forms Excipient information presented when available (limited, particularly for generics); consult specific product labeling.

Kit, Subcutaneous:

Cetrotide: 0.25 mg, 3 mg [contains mannitol]

◆ Cetrorelix Acetate *see* Cetrorelix *on page* 397

◆ Cetrotide *see* Cetrorelix *on page* 397

◆ Cetrotide® (Can) *see* Cetrorelix *on page* 397

Cetuximab (se TUK see mab)

Brand Names: U.S. Erbitux

Brand Names: Canada Erbitux®

Index Terms C225; IMC-C225; MOAB C225

Pharmacologic Category Antineoplastic Agent, Monoclonal Antibody; Epidermal Growth Factor Receptor (EGFR) Inhibitor

Use Treatment of *KRAS* mutation-negative (wild-type), EGFR-expressing metastatic colorectal cancer (in combination with FOLFIRI [irinotecan, fluorouracil, and leucovorin] as first-line treatment, in combination with irinotecan [in patients refractory to irinotecan-based chemotherapy], or as a single agent in patients who have failed oxaliplatin and irinotecan based chemotherapy or who are intolerant to irinotecan); treatment of squamous cell cancer of the head and neck (as a single agent for recurrent or metastatic disease after platinum-based chemotherapy failure; in combination with radiation therapy as initial treatment of locally or regionally advanced disease; in combination with platinum and fluorouracil-based chemotherapy as first-line treatment of locoregional or metastatic disease)

Note: Cetuximab is not indicated for the treatment of *KRAS* mutation-positive colorectal cancer.

Unlabeled Use Treatment of EGFR-expressing advanced nonsmall cell lung cancer (NSCLC); treatment of unresectable squamous cell skin cancer; treatment of neurological symptoms of chordoma

Pregnancy Risk Factor C

Pregnancy Considerations In pregnant cynomolgus monkeys, cetuximab was detected in the amniotic fluid and in the serum of embryos. Although teratogenic effects were not observed in animal reproduction studies, increases in embryolethality and fetal loss were noted. It is not known whether cetuximab can cause fetal harm or affect reproductive capacity. Because cetuximab inhibits epidermal growth factor (EGF), a component of fetal development, adverse effects on pregnancy would be expected. Cetuximab should only be given to a pregnant woman if the potential benefit justifies the potential risk to the fetus.

Breast-Feeding Considerations It is not known if cetuximab is excreted in breast milk. Due to the potential for serious adverse reactions in the nursing infant, the decision to discontinue cetuximab or discontinue breast-feeding should take into account the benefits of treatment to the mother. If breast-feeding is interrupted for cetuximab treatment, based on the half-life, breast-feeding should not be resumed for at least 60 days following the last cetuximab dose.

Contraindications There are no contraindications listed in the manufacturer's U.S. product labeling.

Canadian labeling: Severe hypersensitivity to cetuximab or any component of the formulation

Warnings/Precautions [U.S. Boxed Warning]: In clinical trials, serious infusion reactions have been reported in ~3% of patients; fatal outcome has been reported rarely (<1 in 1000); interrupt infusion promptly and permanently discontinue for serious infusion reactions. Reactions have included airway obstruction (bronchospasm, stridor, hoarseness), hypotension, loss of consciousness, shock, MI, and/or cardiac arrest. Premedicate with an I.V. H_1 antagonist 30-60 minutes prior to the first dose; premedication for subsequent doses is based on clinical judgement and with consideration of prior reaction to the initial infusion. The use of nebulized albuterol-based premedication to prevent infusion reaction has been reported (Tra, 2008). Approximately 90% of reactions occur with the first infusion despite the use of prophylactic antihistamines. Immediate treatment for anaphylactic/anaphylactoid reactions should be available during administration. The manufacturer recommends monitoring patients for at least 1 hour following completion of infusion, or longer if a reaction occurs. Mild-to-moderate infusion reactions are managed by slowing the infusion rate (by 50%) and administering antihistamines. Patients with pre-existing IgE antibody against cetuximab (specific for galactose-α-1,3-galactose) are reported to have a higher incidence of severe hypersensitivity reaction. Severe hypersensitivity reaction has been reported more frequently in patients living in the middle south area of the United States, including North Carolina and Tennessee (Chung, 2008; O'Neil, 2007).

[U.S. Boxed Warning]: In patients with squamous cell head and neck cancer, cardiopulmonary arrest and/or sudden death has occurred in 2% of patients receiving radiation therapy in combination with cetuximab and

in 3% of patients receiving combination chemotherapy (platinum and fluorouracil-based) with cetuximab. Closely monitor serum electrolytes (magnesium, potassium, calcium) during and after cetuximab treatment (monitor for at least 8 weeks after treatment). Use with caution in patients with history of coronary artery disease, HF, and arrhythmias; fatalities have been reported. Interstitial lung disease (ILD) has been reported; use with caution in patients with pre-existing lung disease; interrupt treatment for acute onset or worsening of pulmonary symptoms; permanently discontinue with confirmed ILD.

Acneiform rash has been reported in 76% to 88% of patients (severe in 1% to 17%), usually developing within the first 2 weeks of therapy; may require dose modification; generally resolved after discontinuation in most patients, although persisted beyond 28 days in some patients; monitor for dermatologic toxicity and corresponding infections. Acneiform rash should be treated with topical and/or oral antibiotics; topical corticosteroids are not recommended. In colorectal cancer, the presence of acneiform rash correlates with treatment response and prolonged survival (Cunningham, 2004). Other dermatologic toxicities, including dry skin, fissures, hypertrichosis, paronychial inflammation, and skin infections have been reported; related ocular toxicities (blepharitis, conjunctivitis, keratitis, ulcerative keratitis with decreased visual acuity) may also occur. Sunlight may exacerbate skin reactions (limit sun exposure). Hypomagnesemia is common (may be severe); the onset of electrolyte disturbance may occur within days to months after initiation of treatment; monitor magnesium, calcium, and potassium during treatment and for at least 8 weeks after completion; may require electrolyte replacement. Non-neutralizing anti-cetuximab antibodies were detected in 5% of evaluable patients. In a study of radiation therapy **and** cisplatin with or without cetuximab in patients with squamous cell head and neck cancer, an increase in the incidence of adverse reactions (eg, grade 3/4 mucositis, radiation recall, acneiform rash, and cardiac events including ischemia) was noted in patients receiving cetuximab, including fatal reactions; there was no improvement in the primary endpoint of progression-free survival.

In patients with colorectal cancer, cetuximab is only indicated for EGFR-expressing, *KRAS* mutation-negative metastatic colorectal cancer. Determine *KRAS* mutation status prior to treatment (the therascreen KRAS RGQ PCR Kit is approved in the U.S. to determine *KRAS* gene mutation information). Patients with a codon 12 or 13 (exon 2) *KRAS* mutation are unlikely to benefit from EGFR inhibitor therapy and should not receive cetuximab treatment; cetuximab is not effective for *KRAS* mutation-positive colorectal cancer. Cetuximab is also reported to be ineffective in patients with *BRAF* V600E mutation (Di Nicolantonio, 2008). In trials for colorectal cancer, evidence of EGFR expression was required, although the response rate did not correlate with either the percentage of cells positive for EGFR or the intensity of expression. EGFR expression has been detected in nearly all patients with head and neck cancer, therefore laboratory evidence of EGFR expression is not necessary for head and neck cancers.

Adverse Reactions Except where noted, percentages reported for studies with cetuximab monotherapy.

>10%:

Central nervous system: Fatigue (91%), pain (59%), sensory neuropathy (45%; grades 3/4: 1%), headache (38%), insomnia (27%), fever (25%), confusion (18%), anxiety (14%), chills/rigors (16%), depression (14%)

Dermatologic: Rash/desquamation (95%; grades 3/4: 16%), acneiform rash (all studies: 76% to 88%; grades 3/4: 1% to 17%; onset: ≤14 days), dry skin (57%), pruritus (47%), nail changes (31%)

Endocrine & metabolic: Hypomagnesemia (all studies: 55%; grades 3/4: 6% to 17%), dehydration (13%)

Gastrointestinal: Nausea (64%), abdominal pain (59%), constipation (53%), diarrhea (42%), vomiting (37% to 40%), stomatitis (32%), xerostomia (12%)

Neuromuscular & skeletal: Bone pain (15%), arthralgia (14%)

Respiratory: Dyspnea (48% to 49%), cough (30%)

Miscellaneous: Infection (all studies: 13% to 44%; grades 3/4: 11%), infusion reaction (all studies: 15% to 21%; grades 3/4: 2% to 5%; 90% of severe reactions occurred with first infusion)

1% to 10%:

Cardiovascular: Cardiopulmonary arrest (2%; with radiation therapy; 3% with platinum/fluorouracil-based chemotherapy)

Gastrointestinal: Taste disturbance (10%)

Renal: Renal failure (all studies: 1%)

Miscellaneous: Antibody formation (5%), sepsis (all studies: 1% to 4%)

<1% (Limited to important or life-threatening; all studies): Abscess formation, arrhythmia, aseptic meningitis, blepharitis, cardiac arrest, cellulitis, cheilitis, conjunctivitis, hypertrichosis, hypotension, interstitial lung disease (occurred between the fourth and eleventh doses), keratitis, leukopenia, loss of consciousness, MI, pulmonary embolism, radiation dermatitis, shock, skin fissure, skin infection, ulcerative keratitis

Drug Interactions

Metabolism/Transport Effects None known.

Avoid Concomitant Use There are no known interactions where it is recommended to avoid concomitant use.

Increased Effect/Toxicity There are no known significant interactions involving an increase in effect.

Decreased Effect There are no known significant interactions involving a decrease in effect.

Preparation for Administration Reconstitution is not required. Appropriate dose should be added to empty sterile container (may contain a small amount of visible white, amorphous cetuximab particles); do not shake or dilute. Discard unused portion of the vial.

Storage/Stability Store intact vials refrigerated at 2°C to 8°C (36°F to 46°F); do not freeze. Preparations in infusion containers are stable for up to 12 hours refrigerated at 2°C to 8°C (36°F to 46°F) and up to 8 hours at room temperature of 20°C to 25°C (68°F to 77°F).

Mechanism of Action Recombinant human/mouse chimeric monoclonal antibody which binds specifically to the epidermal growth factor receptor (EGFR, HER1, c-ErbB-1) and competitively inhibits the binding of epidermal growth factor (EGF) and other ligands. Binding to the EGFR blocks phosphorylation and activation of receptor-associated kinases, resulting in inhibition of cell growth, induction of apoptosis, and decreased matrix metalloproteinase and vascular endothelial growth factor production. EGFR signal transduction results in *KRAS* wild-type activation; cells with *KRAS* mutations appear to be unaffected by EGFR inhibition.

Pharmacodynamics/Kinetics

Distribution: V_d: ~2-3 L/m^2

Half-life elimination: ~112 hours (range: 63-230 hours)

Dosage Note: Premedicate with an H_1 antagonist (eg, diphenhydramine 50 mg) I.V. 30-60 minutes prior to the first dose; premedication for subsequent doses is based on clinical judgement.

Colorectal cancer, metastatic, *KRAS* mutation-negative (wild-type): Adults: I.V.:

Initial loading dose: 400 mg/m^2 infused over 120 minutes

Maintenance dose: 250 mg/m^2 infused over 60 minutes weekly until disease progression or unacceptable toxicity

Note: If given in combination with FOLFIRI (irinotecan, fluorouracil, and leucovorin), complete cetuximab infusion 1 hour prior to FOLFIRI.

Head and neck cancer (squamous cell): Adults: I.V.:

Initial loading dose: 400 mg/m² infused over 120 minutes

Maintenance dose: 250 mg/m² infused over 60 minutes weekly

Note: If given in combination with radiation therapy, administer loading dose 1 week prior to initiation of radiation course; weekly maintenance dose should be completed 1 hour prior to radiation for the duration of radiation therapy (6-7 weeks). If given in combination with chemotherapy, administer loading dose on the day of initiation of platinum and fluorouracil-based chemotherapy, cetuximab infusion should be completed 1 hour prior to initiation of chemotherapy; weekly maintenance dose should be completed 1 hour prior to chemotherapy; continue until disease progression or unacceptable toxicity. Monotherapy weekly doses should be continued until disease progression or unacceptable toxicity.

Colorectal cancer, advanced, biweekly administration (unlabeled dosing): Adults: I.V.: 500 mg/m² every 2 weeks (initial dose infused over 120 minutes, subsequent doses infused over 60 minutes) in combination with irinotecan (Pfeiffer, 2008)

Nonsmall cell lung cancer (NSCLC), EGFR-expressing, advanced (unlabeled use): Adults: I.V.: Initial loading dose: 400 mg/m², followed by maintenance dose: 250 mg/m² weekly in combination with cisplatin and vinorelbine for up to 6 cycles, then as monotherapy until disease progression or unacceptable toxicity (Pirker, 2009; Pirker, 2012)

Squamous cell skin cancer, unresectable (unlabeled use): Adults: I.V.: Initial loading dose: 400 mg/m², followed by maintenance dose: 250 mg/m² weekly until disease progression (Maubec, 2011)

Dosage adjustment for toxicity:

Infusion reactions, grade 1 or 2 and nonserious grade 3: Reduce the infusion rate by 50% and continue to use prophylactic antihistamines

Infusion reactions, severe: Immediately and permanently discontinue treatment

Pulmonary toxicity:

Acute onset or worsening pulmonary symptoms: Hold treatment

Interstitial lung disease: Permanently discontinue

Skin toxicity, mild-to-moderate: No dosage modification required

Acneiform rash, severe (grade 3 or 4):

First occurrence: Delay cetuximab infusion 1-2 weeks

If improvement, continue at 250 mg/m²

If no improvement, discontinue therapy

Second occurrence: Delay cetuximab infusion 1-2 weeks

If improvement, continue at reduced dose of 200 mg/m²

If no improvement, discontinue therapy

Third occurrence: Delay cetuximab infusion 1-2 weeks

If improvement, continue at reduced dose of 150 mg/m²

If no improvement, discontinue therapy

Fourth occurrence: Discontinue therapy

Note: Dose adjustments are not recommended for severe **radiation** dermatitis.

Dosage adjustment in renal impairment: No dosage adjustment provided in manufacturer's labeling.

Dosage adjustment in hepatic impairment: No dosage adjustment provided in manufacturer's labeling.

Administration Administer via I.V. infusion; loading dose over 2 hours, weekly maintenance dose over 1 hour. Do not administer as I.V. push or bolus. Do not shake or dilute. Administer via infusion pump or syringe pump. Following the infusion, an observation period (1 hour) is recommended; longer observation time (following an infusion reaction) may be required. Premedication with an H_1 antagonist prior to the initial dose is recommended. The maximum infusion rate is 10 mg/minute. Administer through a low protein-binding 0.22 micrometer in-line filter. Use 0.9% NaCl to flush line at the end of infusion.

For biweekly administration (unlabeled frequency and dose), the initial dose was infused over 120 minutes and subsequent doses infused over 60 minutes (Pfeiffer, 2007; Pfeiffer, 2008).

Monitoring Parameters Vital signs during infusion and observe for at least 1 hour postinfusion. Patients developing dermatologic toxicities should be monitored for the development of complications. Periodic monitoring of serum magnesium, calcium, and potassium are recommended to continue over an interval consistent with the half-life (8 weeks); monitor closely (during and after treatment) for cetuximab plus radiation therapy. *KRAS* genotyping of tumor tissue in patients with colorectal cancer (the therascreen *KRAS* RGQ PCR Kit is approved in the U.S. to determine *KRAS* gene mutation status [codon 12 or 13]).

Additional Information Oncology Comment: The National Comprehensive Cancer Network® (NCCN) guidelines for colon cancer (v.3.2013) and the American Society of Clinical Oncology (ASCO) provisional clinical opinion (Allegra, 2009) recommend genotyping tumor tissue for *KRAS* mutation in all patients with metastatic colorectal cancer (genotyping may be done on archived specimens). Patients with known codon 12 or 13 *KRAS* gene mutations are unlikely to respond to EGFR inhibitors and should not receive cetuximab. Favorable progression-free survival and overall survival has been demonstrated with cetuximab in patients with *KRAS* wild-type (Karapetis, 2008; Van Cutsem, 2008). Cetuximab is also reported to be ineffective in patients with *BRAF* V600E mutation (Di Nicolantonio, 2008). Because EGFR testing in colorectal tumors does not correlate with response, the NCCN guidelines do not recommend routine EGFR testing in colorectal cancer. Dermatologic toxicity with cetuximab is predictive for response; the presence of acneiform rash correlates with treatment response and prolonged survival (Cunningham, 2004).

Dosage Forms Excipient information presented when available (limited, particularly for generics); consult specific product labeling.

Solution, Intravenous [preservative free]:

Erbitux: 100 mg/50 mL (50 mL); 200 mg/100 mL (100 mL)

Cevimeline (se vi ME leen)

Brand Names: U.S. Evoxac

Brand Names: Canada Evoxac®

Index Terms Cevimeline Hydrochloride

Pharmacologic Category Cholinergic Agonist

Use Treatment of symptoms of dry mouth in patients with Sjögren's syndrome

Pregnancy Risk Factor C

Dosage Oral:

Adults: 30 mg 3 times/day

Elderly: No specific dosage adjustment is recommended; however, use caution when initiating due to potential for increased sensitivity

Dosage adjustment in renal impairment: No dosage adjustment provided in the manufacturer's labeling.

Dosage adjustment in hepatic impairment: No dosage adjustment provided in the manufacturer's labeling.

Additional Information Complete prescribing information should be consulted for additional detail.

Dosage Forms Excipient information presented when available (limited, particularly for generics); consult specific product labeling.

Capsule, Oral, as hydrochloride:

Evoxac: 30 mg

Generic: 30 mg

◆ **Cevimeline Hydrochloride** *see* Cevimeline *on page 400*

◆ **CFDN** *see* Cefdinir *on page 365*

◆ **CG** *see* Chorionic Gonadotropin (Human) *on page 419*

◆ **CG5503** *see* Tapentadol *on page 1992*

◆ **CGP 33101** *see* Rufinamide *on page 1865*

◆ **CGP-39393** *see* Desirudin *on page 574*

◆ **CGP-42446** *see* Zoledronic Acid *on page 2235*

◆ **CGP-57148B** *see* Imatinib *on page 1048*

◆ **CGS-20267** *see* Letrozole *on page 1185*

◆ **CGX-625** *see* Omacetaxine *on page 1501*

◆ **Champix® (Can)** *see* Varenicline *on page 2166*

◆ **Chantix** *see* Varenicline *on page 2166*

◆ **Chantix Continuing Month Pak** *see* Varenicline *on page 2166*

◆ **Chantix Starting Month Pak** *see* Varenicline *on page 2166*

◆ **Charac-25 [OTC] (Can)** *see* Charcoal, Activated *on page 401*

◆ **Charac-50 [OTC] (Can)** *see* Charcoal, Activated *on page 401*

◆ **Charactol-25 [OTC] (Can)** *see* Charcoal, Activated *on page 401*

◆ **Charactol-50 [OTC] (Can)** *see* Charcoal, Activated *on page 401*

Charcoal, Activated (CHAR kole AK tiv ay ted)

Brand Names: U.S. Actidose-Aqua [OTC]; Actidose/Sorbitol [OTC]; Char-Flo with Sorbitol [OTC]; EZ Char [OTC]; Kerr Insta-Char in Sorbitol [OTC]; Kerr Insta-Char [OTC]

Brand Names: Canada Charac-25 [OTC]; Charac-50 [OTC]; Charactol-25 [OTC]; Charactol-50 [OTC]; Charcodote Susp [OTC]; Charcodote TFS [OTC]; Charcodote-Aqueous Sus; Premium Activated Charcoal [OTC]

Index Terms Activated Carbon; Activated Charcoal; Adsorbent Charcoal; Liquid Antidote; Medicinal Carbon; Medicinal Charcoal

Pharmacologic Category Antidote

Use

Suspension: Activated charcoal is a nonabsorbable adsorbent that may be considered in the management of poisonings when gastrointestinal decontamination of drugs or chemicals is indicated (eg, presentation to a treatment facility within 1 hour of ingestion). Activated charcoal is generally an effective adsorbent of drugs and chemicals with a molecular weight range of 100-1000 daltons. Multidose activated charcoal may be considered if a patient has ingested a life-threatening amount of carbamazepine, dapsone, phenobarbital, quinine, or theophylline (Vale, 1999).

Capsules, tablets: Digestive aid

Pregnancy Considerations Activated charcoal is not absorbed systemically following oral administration. Systemic absorption would be required in order for activated charcoal to cross the placenta and reach the fetus. In general, medications used as antidotes should take into consideration the health and prognosis of the mother; antidotes should be administered to pregnant women if there is a clear indication for use and should not be withheld because of fears of teratogenicity (Bailey, 2003).

Breast-Feeding Considerations Activated charcoal is not absorbed systemically following oral administration.

Contraindications There are no absolute contraindications listed within the manufacturer's labeling.

Note: The American Academy of Clinical Toxicology (AACT) and European Association of Poisons Centres and Clinical Toxicologists (EAPCCT) consider the following to be contraindications to the use of charcoal (Chyka, 2005; Vale, 1999): Presence of intestinal obstruction or GI tract not anatomically intact; patients at risk of GI hemorrhage or perforation; patients with an unprotected airway (eg, CNS depression without intubation); if use would increase the risk and severity of aspiration

Warnings/Precautions Charcoal may cause vomiting; the risk appears to be greater when charcoal is administered with sorbitol (Chyka, 2005). I.V. antiemetics may be required to reduce the risk of vomiting or to control vomiting to facilitate administration (Vale, 1999). Due to the risk of vomiting, avoid the use of charcoal in hydrocarbon and caustic ingestions. Use caution with decreased peristalsis. Some products may contain sorbitol. Coadministration of a cathartic is **not** recommended; cathartics (eg, sorbitol, mannitol, magnesium sulfate) have not been demonstrated to change patient outcome and have no role in the management of the poisoned patient. Cathartics subject the patient to the risk of developing significant fluid and electrolyte abnormalities (AACT, 2004a). Do not use products containing sorbitol in persons with a genetic intolerance to fructose or in patients who are dehydrated; may cause excessive diarrhea. Ipecac should not be administered routinely in the management of poisoned patients (AACT, 2004b).

Not effective in the treatment of poisonings due to the ingestion of low molecular weight compounds such as cyanide, iron, ethanol, methanol, or lithium. Most effective when administered within 30-60 minutes of ingestion. Based on experimental and clinical studies, multidose activated charcoal, in most acute poisonings, has not been shown to reduce morbidity or mortality (Vale, 1999). It may be considered if a patient has ingested a life-threatening amount of carbamazepine, dapsone, phenobarbital, quinine, or theophylline, although no controlled studies have demonstrated clinical benefit.

Commercial charcoal products may contain propylene glycol. Capsules and tablets should not be used for the treatment of poisoning.

Adverse Reactions Frequency not defined.

Gastrointestinal: Abdominal distention, appendicitis, bowel obstruction, constipation, vomiting

Ocular: Corneal abrasion (with direct contact)

Respiratory: Aspiration, respiratory failure

Miscellaneous: Fecal discoloration (black)

Drug Interactions

Metabolism/Transport Effects None known.

Avoid Concomitant Use There are no known interactions where it is recommended to avoid concomitant use.

Increased Effect/Toxicity There are no known significant interactions involving an increase in effect.

Decreased Effect

Charcoal, Activated may decrease the levels/effects of: Leflunomide; Teriflunomide

Ethanol/Nutrition/Herb Interactions Food: The addition of some flavoring agents (eg, milk, ice cream, sherbet, marmalade) are known to reduce the adsorptive capacity, and therefore the efficacy, of activated charcoal and should be avoided in preference to activated charcoal-water slurries; nevertheless, these flavoring agents do not completely compromise the effectiveness of activated charcoal and may be necessary in some circumstances (eg, administration in pediatric patients) to enhance compliance (Cooney, 1995; Dagnone, 2002).

Preparation for Administration Powder: Dilute with at least 8 mL of water per 1 g of charcoal, or mix in a charcoal to water ratio of 1:4 to 1:8; mix to form a slurry (eg, mix 25 g with sufficient tap water to create a 4-ounce slurry or mix 50 g with sufficient tap water to create an 8-ounce slurry).

Storage/Stability Adsorbs gases from air, store in a closed container.

Mechanism of Action Adsorbs toxic substances, thus inhibiting GI absorption

Pharmacodynamics/Kinetics Excretion: Feces (as charcoal)

Dosage Oral, NG: **Note:** Some products may contain sorbitol; coadministration of a cathartic, including sorbitol, is **not** recommended. Some clinicians still recommend dosing activated charcoal in a 10:1 (charcoal:poison) ratio for optimal efficacy (Gude, 2009); however, the amount of poison ingested is commonly unknown, which makes this approach challenging and often impractical (Chyka, 2005).

Single dose (Chyka, 2005):

Infants <1 year: 10-25 g; **Note:** Although dosing by body weight is reported in children (0.5-1 g/kg) and published in many resources, there are no data or scientific rationale to support this recommendation.

Children 1-12 years: 25-50 g

Children >12 years and Adults: 25-100 g

Multidose:

Children: Initial dose: 25-50 g followed by multiple doses of 10-25 g every 4 hours

Adults: Initial dose: 50-100 g followed by 25-50 g every 4 hours

Administration Flavoring agents (eg, chocolate, concentrated fruit juice) or thickening agents (eg, bentonite, carboxymethylcellulose) can enhance charcoal's palatability. Check for presence of bowel sounds before administration. I.V. antiemetics may be required to reduce the risk of vomiting. The activated charcoal container should be agitated thoroughly before administration. The container should be rinsed with a small quantity of water to insure that the patient has received all of the activated charcoal (Krenzelok, 1991).

Capsules and tablets should not be used for the treatment of poisoning.

Dosage Forms Excipient information presented when available (limited, particularly for generics); consult specific product labeling.

Liquid, Oral:

Actidose-Aqua: 15 g/72 mL (72 mL); 25 g/120 mL (120 mL); 50 g/240 mL (240 mL) [sweet flavor]

Actidose/Sorbitol: 25 g/120 mL (120 mL); 50 g/240 mL (240 mL) [sweet flavor]

Kerr Insta-Char: 25 g/120 mL (120 mL); 50 g/240 mL (240 mL) [contains fd&c red #40, methylparaben sodium, propylene glycol, propylparaben sodium, sodium benzoate; cherry flavor]

Kerr Insta-Char: 50 g/240 mL (240 mL) [contains propylene glycol]

Kerr Insta-Char in Sorbitol: 25 g/120 mL (120 mL); 50 g/240 mL (240 mL) [contains fd&c red #40, methylparaben sodium, propylene glycol, propylparaben sodium, sodium benzoate; cherry flavor]

Suspension, Oral:

Char-Flo with Sorbitol: 25 g (120 mL)

Suspension Reconstituted, Oral:

EZ Char: 25 g (1 ea) [contains bentonite]

◆ **Charcodote-Aqueous Sus (Can)** *see* Charcoal, Activated *on page 401*

◆ **Charcodote Susp [OTC] (Can)** *see* Charcoal, Activated *on page 401*

◆ **Charcodote TFS [OTC] (Can)** *see* Charcoal, Activated *on page 401*

◆ **Char-Flo with Sorbitol [OTC]** *see* Charcoal, Activated *on page 401*

◆ **Chateal** *see* Ethinyl Estradiol and Levonorgestrel *on page 787*

◆ **Chemet** *see* Succimer *on page 1952*

◆ **Chenodal** *see* Chenodiol *on page 402*

◆ **Chenodeoxycholic Acid** *see* Chenodiol *on page 402*

Chenodiol (kee noe DYE ole)

Brand Names: U.S. Chenodal

Index Terms CDCA; Chenodeoxycholic Acid

Pharmacologic Category Bile Acid

Use Oral dissolution of radiolucent cholesterol gallstones in selected patients as an alternative to surgery

Unlabeled Use Cerebrotendinous xanthomatosis (CTX)

Pregnancy Risk Factor X

Prescribing and Access Restrictions Prescriptions are only dispensed by a specialty pharmacy, Centric Health Resources, which may be contacted at 866-758-7068.

Dosage Oral:

Cerebrotendinous xanthomatosis (unlabeled use): Adults: 750 mg daily in 3 divided doses (Beringer, 1984)

Gallstone dissolution (monotherapy): Adults: Initial: 250 mg twice daily for the first 2 weeks and increasing by 250 mg daily each week thereafter until the recommended or maximum tolerated dose is achieved; maintenance: 13-16 mg/kg/day in 2 divided doses. **Note:** Dosages <10 mg/kg are usually ineffective and may increase the risk of cholecystectomy.

Gallstone dissolution (combination therapy; unlabeled dose): Adults: 5-7.5 mg/kg/day once daily at bedtime, in combination with ursodeoxycholic acid, with or without adjuvant lithotripsy (Jazrawi, 1992; Pereira, 1997; Petroni, 2001)

Dosage adjustment in renal impairment: No dosage adjustment provided in manufacturer's labeling.

Dosage adjustment in hepatic impairment: Use extreme caution; contraindicated for use in presence of known hepatocyte dysfunction or bile duct abnormalities

Additional Information Complete prescribing information should be consulted for additional detail.

Dosage Forms Excipient information presented when available (limited, particularly for generics); consult specific product labeling.

Tablet, Oral:

Chenodal: 250 mg

◆ **Cheracol D [OTC]** *see* Guaifenesin and Dextromethorphan *on page 976*

◆ **Cheracol Plus [OTC]** *see* Guaifenesin and Dextromethorphan *on page 976*

◆ **Cheratussin** *see* GuaiFENesin *on page 974*

◆ **Cheratussin® DAC** *see* Guaifenesin, Pseudoephedrine, and Codeine *on page 979*

◆ **Chew-C [OTC]** *see* Ascorbic Acid *on page 172*

◆ **Chew-Cal [OTC]** *see* Calcium and Vitamin D *on page 318*

◆ **CHG** *see* Chlorhexidine Gluconate *on page 408*

◆ **Chickenpox Vaccine** *see* Varicella Virus Vaccine *on page 2168*

◆ **Chiggerex [OTC]** *see* Benzocaine *on page 240*

◆ **Chiggertox [OTC]** *see* Benzocaine *on page 240*

◆ **Childrens Advil [OTC]** *see* Ibuprofen *on page 1032*

◆ **Children's Advil® Cold (Can)** *see* Pseudoephedrine and Ibuprofen *on page 1748*

◆ **Childrens Ibuprofen [OTC]** *see* Ibuprofen *on page 1032*

- ◆ **Childrens Loratadine [OTC]** *see* Loratadine *on page 1240*
- ◆ **Childrens Motrin [OTC]** *see* Ibuprofen *on page 1032*
- ◆ **Childrens Motrin Jr Strength [OTC]** *see* Ibuprofen *on page 1032*
- ◆ **Childrens Silfedrine [OTC]** *see* Pseudoephedrine *on page 1746*
- ◆ **Children's Motion Sickness Liquid [OTC] (Can)** *see* DimenhyDRINATE *on page 616*
- ◆ **Chloditan** *see* Mitotane *on page 1385*
- ◆ **Chlodithane** *see* Mitotane *on page 1385*
- ◆ **Chloral** *see* Chloral Hydrate *on page 403*

Chloral Hydrate (KLOR al HYE drate)

Brand Names: Canada PMS-Chloral Hydrate

Index Terms Chloral; Hydrated Chloral; Trichloroacetaldehyde Monohydrate

Pharmacologic Category Hypnotic, Miscellaneous

Additional Appendix Information

Beers Criteria – Potentially Inappropriate Medications for Geriatrics *on page 2368*

Use Short-term sedative and hypnotic (<2 weeks); sedative/hypnotic for diagnostic procedures; sedative prior to EEG evaluations

Pregnancy Risk Factor C

Dosage

Children:

Sedation or anxiety: Oral, rectal: 5-15 mg/kg/dose every 8 hours (maximum: 500 mg/dose)

Prior to EEG: Oral, rectal: 20-25 mg/kg/dose, 30-60 minutes prior to EEG; may repeat in 30 minutes to maximum of 100 mg/kg or 2 g total

Hypnotic: Oral, rectal: 20-40 mg/kg/dose up to a maximum of 50 mg/kg/24 hours or 1 g/dose or 2 g/24 hours

Conscious sedation: Oral: 50-75 mg/kg/dose 30-60 minutes prior to procedure; may repeat 30 minutes after initial dose if needed, to a total maximum dose of 120 mg/kg or 1 g total

Adults: Oral:

Sedation, anxiety: 250 mg 3 times/day

Hypnotic: 500-1000 mg at bedtime or 30 minutes prior to procedure, not to exceed 2 g/24 hours

Discontinuation: Withdraw gradually over 2 weeks if patient has been maintained on high doses for prolonged period of time. Do not stop drug abruptly; sudden withdrawal may result in delirium.

Dosing adjustment/comments in renal impairment: Cl_{cr} <50 mL/minute: Avoid use

Hemodialysis: Dialyzable (50% to 100%); supplemental dose is not necessary

Dosing adjustment/comments in hepatic impairment: Avoid use in patients with severe hepatic impairment

Additional Information Complete prescribing information should be consulted for additional detail.

Controlled Substance C-IV

Chlorambucil (klor AM byoo sil)

Brand Names: U.S. Leukeran

Brand Names: Canada Leukeran®

Index Terms CB-1348; Chlorambucilum; Chloraminophene; Chlorbutinum; WR-139013

Pharmacologic Category Antineoplastic Agent, Alkylating Agent

Use

Chronic lymphocytic leukemia (CLL): Management of CLL

Lymphomas: Management of Hodgkin lymphoma and non-Hodgkin lymphomas (NHL)

Canadian labeling: Additional uses (not in U.S. labeling): Management of Waldenström's macroglobulinemia

Unlabeled Use Treatment of nephrotic syndrome (steroid sensitive) in children; treatment of Waldenström's macroglobulinemia

Pregnancy Risk Factor D

Pregnancy Considerations Animal reproduction studies have demonstrated teratogenicity. Chlorambucil crosses the human placenta. Following exposure during the first trimester, case reports have noted adverse renal effects (unilateral agenesis). Women of childbearing potential should avoid becoming pregnant while receiving treatment. **[U.S. Boxed Warning]: Affects human fertility; probably mutagenic and teratogenic as well**; chromosomal damage has been documented. Reversible and irreversible sterility (when administered to prepubertal and pubertal males), azoospermia (in adult males) and amenorrhea (in females) have been observed. Fibrosis, vasculitis and depletion of primordial follicles have been noted on autopsy of the ovaries.

Breast-Feeding Considerations It is not known if chlorambucil is excreted in breast milk. Due to the potential for serious adverse reactions in the nursing infant, the decision to discontinue chlorambucil or to discontinue breast-feeding should take into account the benefits of treatment to the mother.

Contraindications Hypersensitivity to chlorambucil or any component of the formulation; hypersensitivity to other alkylating agents (may have cross-hypersensitivity); prior (demonstrated) resistance to chlorambucil

Canadian labeling: Additional contraindications (not in U.S. labeling): Use within 4 weeks of a full course of radiation or chemotherapy

Warnings/Precautions Hazardous agent - use appropriate precautions for handling and disposal (NIOSH, 2012). Seizures have been observed; use with caution in patients with seizure disorder or head trauma; history of nephrotic syndrome and high pulse doses are at higher risk of seizures. **[U.S. Boxed Warning]: May cause severe bone marrow suppression;** neutropenia may be severe. Reduce initial dosage if patient has received myelosuppressive or radiation therapy within the previous 4 weeks, or has a depressed baseline leukocyte or platelet count. Irreversible bone marrow damage may occur with total doses approaching 6.5 mg/kg. Progressive lymphopenia may develop (recovery is generally rapid after discontinuation). Avoid administration of live vaccines to immunocompromised patients. Rare instances of severe skin reactions (eg, erythema multiforme, Stevens-Johnson syndrome, toxic epidermal necrolysis) have been reported; discontinue promptly if skin reaction occurs.

Chlorambucil is primarily metabolized in the liver. Dosage reductions should be considered in patients with hepatic impairment. **[U.S. Boxed Warning]: Affects human fertility; carcinogenic in humans and probably mutagenic and teratogenic as well;** chromosomal damage has been documented. Reversible and irreversible sterility (when administered to prepubertal and pubertal males), azoospermia (in adult males) and amenorrhea (in females) have been observed. **[U.S. Boxed Warning]: Carcinogenic;** acute myelocytic leukemia and secondary malignancies may be associated with chronic therapy. Duration of treatment and higher cumulative doses are associated with a higher risk for development of leukemia. Potentially significant drug-drug interactions may exist, requiring dose or frequency adjustment, additional monitoring, and/or selection of alternative therapy.

Adverse Reactions Frequency not always defined.

Central nervous system: Agitation (rare), ataxia (rare), confusion (rare), drug fever, fever, focal/generalized seizure (rare), hallucinations (rare)

Dermatologic: Angioneurotic edema, erythema multiforme (rare), rash, skin hypersensitivity, Stevens-Johnson syndrome (rare), toxic epidermal necrolysis (rare), urticaria

Endocrine & metabolic: Amenorrhea, infertility, SIADH (rare)

Gastrointestinal: Diarrhea (infrequent), nausea (infrequent), oral ulceration (infrequent), vomiting (infrequent)

Genitourinary: Azoospermia, cystitis (sterile)

Hematologic: Neutropenia (onset: 3 weeks; recovery: 10 days after last dose), bone marrow failure (irreversible), bone marrow suppression, anemia, leukemia (secondary), leukopenia, lymphopenia, pancytopenia, thrombocytopenia

Hepatic: Hepatotoxicity, jaundice

Neuromuscular & skeletal: Flaccid paresis (rare), muscular twitching (rare), myoclonia (rare), peripheral neuropathy, tremor (rare)

Respiratory: Interstitial pneumonia, pulmonary fibrosis

Miscellaneous: Allergic reactions, malignancies (secondary)

Drug Interactions

Metabolism/Transport Effects None known.

Avoid Concomitant Use

Avoid concomitant use of Chlorambucil with any of the following: BCG; CloZAPine; Natalizumab; Pimecrolimus; Tacrolimus (Topical); Tofacitinib; Vaccines (Live)

Increased Effect/Toxicity

Chlorambucil may increase the levels/effects of: CloZAPine; Leflunomide; Natalizumab; Tofacitinib; Vaccines (Live)

The levels/effects of Chlorambucil may be increased by: Denosumab; Pimecrolimus; Roflumilast; Tacrolimus (Topical); Trastuzumab

Decreased Effect

Chlorambucil may decrease the levels/effects of: BCG; Coccidioidin Skin Test; Sipuleucel-T; Vaccines (Inactivated); Vaccines (Live)

The levels/effects of Chlorambucil may be decreased by: Echinacea

Ethanol/Nutrition/Herb Interactions Food: Absorption is decreased when administered with food.

Storage/Stability Store in refrigerator at 2°C to 8°C (36°F to 46°F).

Mechanism of Action Alkylating agent; interferes with DNA replication and RNA transcription by alkylation and cross-linking the strands of DNA

Pharmacodynamics/Kinetics

Absorption: Rapid and complete (>70%); reduced with food

Distribution: V_d: ~0.3 L/kg

Protein binding: ~99%; primarily to albumin

Metabolism: Hepatic (extensively); primarily to active metabolite, phenylacetic acid mustard

Half-life elimination: ~1.5 hours; Phenylacetic acid mustard: ~1.8 hours

Time to peak, plasma: Within 1 hour; Phenylacetic acid mustard: 1.2-2.6 hours

Excretion: Urine (~20% to 60%, primarily as inactive metabolites, <1% as unchanged drug or phenylacetic acid mustard)

Dosage

Children: Nephrotic syndrome, steroid sensitive (unlabeled use): Oral: 0.2 mg/kg once daily for 8 weeks (Hodson, 2010)

Adults: **Note:** With bone marrow lymphocytic infiltration involvement (in CLL, Hodgkin lymphoma, or NHL), the maximum dose is 0.1 mg/kg/day. While short treatment courses are preferred, if maintenance therapy is required, the maximum dose is 0.1 mg/kg/day.

Chronic lymphocytic leukemia (CLL): Oral:

U.S. labeling: 0.1 mg/kg/day for 3-6 weeks **or** 0.4 mg/kg pulsed doses administered intermittently, biweekly, or monthly (increased by 0.1 mg/kg/dose until response/toxicity observed)

Canadian labeling: Initial: 0.15 mg/kg/day until WBC is 10,000/mm^3; interrupt treatment for 4 weeks, then may resume at 0.1 mg/kg/day until response (generally ~2 years)/toxicity observed

Unlabeled dosing for CLL: 0.4 mg/kg day 1 every 2 weeks; if tolerated may increase by 0.1 mg/kg with each treatment course to a maximum dose of 0.8 mg/kg and maximum of 24 cycles (Eichhorst, 2009) **or** 30 mg/m^2 day 1 every 2 weeks (in combination with prednisone) (Raphael, 1991) **or** 40 mg/m^2 day 1 every 4 weeks until disease progression or complete remission or response plateau for up to a maximum of 12 cycles (Rai, 2000)

Hodgkin lymphoma: Oral:

U.S. labeling: 0.2 mg/kg/day for 3-6 weeks

Canadian labeling: 0.2 mg/kg/day for 4-8 weeks

Non-Hodgkin lymphomas (NHL): Oral:

U.S. labeling: 0.1 mg/kg/day for 3-6 weeks

Canadian labeling: Initial: 0.1-0.2 mg/kg/day for 4-8 weeks; for maintenance treatment, reduce dose or administer intermittently

Waldenström's macroglobulinemia (U.S. unlabeled use): Oral: 0.1 mg/kg/day (continuously) for at least 6 months **or** 0.3 mg/kg/day for 7 days every 6 weeks for at least 6 months (Kyle, 2000)

Elderly: Refer to adult dosing; begin at the lower end of dosing range(s)

Dosage adjustment for toxicity:

Skin reactions: Discontinue treatment

Hematologic:

WBC or platelets below normal: Reduce dose

Severely depressed WBC or platelet counts: Discontinue

Persistently low neutrophil or platelet counts or peripheral lymphocytosis: May be suggestive of bone marrow infiltration; if infiltration confirmed, do not exceed 0.1 mg/kg/day.

Concurrent or within 4 weeks (before or after) of chemotherapy/radiotherapy: Initiate treatment cautiously; reduce dose; monitor closely.

Dosage adjustment in renal impairment: No dosage adjustment provided in manufacturer's labeling; however, renal elimination of unchanged chlorambucil and active metabolite (phenylacetic acid mustard) is minimal and renal impairment is not likely to affect elimination. The following adjustments have been recommended: Adults:

Aronoff, 2007:

Cl_{cr} >50 mL/minute: No adjustment necessary

Cl_{cr} 10-50 mL/minute: Administer 75% of dose

Cl_{cr} <10 mL/minute: Administer 50% of dose

Peritoneal dialysis (PD): Administer 50% of dose

Kintzel, 1995: Based on the pharmacokinetics, dosage adjustment is not indicated

Dosage adjustment in hepatic impairment: Chlorambucil undergoes extensive hepatic metabolism. Although dosage reduction should be considered in patients with hepatic impairment, no dosage adjustment is provided in the manufacturer's labeling (data is insufficient).

Dosing in obesity: *ASCO Guidelines for appropriate chemotherapy dosing in obese adults with cancer:* Utilize patient's actual body weight (full weight) for calculation of body surface area- or weight-based dosing, particularly when the intent of therapy is curative; manage regimen-related toxicities in the same manner as for nonobese patients; if a dose reduction is utilized due to toxicity, consider resumption of full weight-based dosing with subsequent cycles, especially if cause of toxicity (eg, hepatic or renal impairment) is resolved (Griggs, 2012). **Note:** The manufacturer recommends the maximum dose should not exceed 0.1 mg/kg/day if maintenance therapy is required and with bone marrow infiltration.

Administration May be administered as a single daily dose; preferably on an empty stomach.

Hazardous agent; use appropriate precautions for handling and disposal (NIOSH, 2012).

Monitoring Parameters Liver function tests, CBC with differential (weekly, with WBC monitored twice weekly during the first 3-6 weeks of treatment)

Dosage Forms Excipient information presented when available (limited, particularly for generics); consult specific product labeling.

Tablet, Oral:

Leukeran: 2 mg

Extemporaneous Preparations Hazardous agent: Use appropriate precautions for handling and disposal.

A 2 mg/mL oral suspension may be prepared with tablets. Crush sixty 2 mg tablets in a mortar and reduce to a fine powder. Add small portions of methylcellulose 1% and mix to a uniform paste (total methylcellulose: 30 mL); mix while adding simple syrup in incremental proportions to **almost** 60 mL; transfer to a graduated cylinder, rinse mortar and pestle with simple syrup, and add quantity of vehicle sufficient to make 60 mL. Transfer contents of graduated cylinder to an amber prescription bottle. Label "shake well", "refrigerate", and "protect from light". Stable for 7 days refrigerated.

Dressman JB and Poust RI, "Stability of Allopurinol and of Five Antineoplastics in Suspension," *Am J Hosp Pharm*, 1983, 40(4):616-8.

Nahata MC, Pai VB, and Hipple TF, *Pediatric Drug Formulations*, 5th ed, Cincinnati, OH: Harvey Whitney Books Co, 2004.

◆ **Chlorambucilum** *see* Chlorambucil *on page 403*

◆ **Chloraminophene** *see* Chlorambucil *on page 403*

Chloramphenicol (klor am FEN i kole)

Brand Names: Canada Chloromycetin®; Chloromycetin® Succinate; Diochloram®; Pentamycetin®

Pharmacologic Category Antibiotic, Miscellaneous

Use Treatment of serious infections due to organisms resistant to other less toxic antibiotics or when its penetrability into the site of infection is clinically superior to other antibiotics to which the organism is sensitive; useful in infections caused by *Bacteroides*, *H. influenzae*, *Neisseria meningitidis*, *Salmonella*, and *Rickettsia*; active against many vancomycin-resistant enterococci

Pregnancy Considerations Chloramphenicol crosses the placenta producing cord concentrations approaching maternal serum concentrations. An increased risk of teratogenic effects has not been associated with the use of chloramphenicol in pregnancy (Czeizel, 2000; Heinonen, 1977). "Gray Syndrome" has occurred in premature infants and newborns receiving chloramphenicol. The manufacturer recommends caution if used in a pregnant patient near term or during labor. Chloramphenicol may be used for the treatment of Rocky Mountain spotted fever in pregnant women although caution should be used when administration occurs during the third trimester (CDC, 2006).

Breast-Feeding Considerations Chloramphenicol and its inactive metabolites are excreted in breast milk. Chloramphenicol is well absorbed following oral administration; however, metabolism and excretion are highly variable in infants and children. The half-life is also significantly prolonged in low birth weight infants (Powell, 1982). Due to the potential for serious adverse reactions in the nursing infant, the manufacturer recommends that caution be exercised when administering chloramphenicol to nursing women. Other sources recommended avoiding use while breast-feeding, especially infants <34 weeks postconceptual age or when unusually large doses are needed (Atkinson, 1988; Matsuda, 1984; Plomp, 1983). Non-dose-related effects could include modification of bowel flora.

Contraindications Hypersensitivity to chloramphenicol or any component of the formulation; treatment of trivial or viral infections; bacterial prophylaxis

Warnings/Precautions Hazardous agent - use appropriate precautions for handling and disposal (NIOSH, 2012). Gray syndrome characterized by circulatory collapse, cyanosis, acidosis, abdominal distention, myocardial depression, coma, and death has occurred. Use with caution in patients with impaired renal or hepatic function and in neonates. Reduce dose with impaired liver function. Use with care in patients with glucose 6-phosphate dehydrogenase deficiency. **[U.S. Boxed Warning]: Serious and fatal blood dyscrasias (aplastic anemia, hypoplastic anemia, thrombocytopenia, and granulocytopenia) have occurred after both short-term and prolonged therapy. Monitor CBC frequently in all patients;** discontinue if evidence of myelosuppression. Irreversible bone marrow suppression may occur weeks or months after therapy. Avoid repeated courses of treatment. Should not be used for minor infections or when less potentially toxic agents are effective. Prolonged use may result in fungal or bacterial superinfection, including *C. difficile*-associated diarrhea (CDAD) and pseudomembranous colitis; CDAD has been observed >2 months postantibiotic treatment.

Adverse Reactions Frequency not defined.

Central nervous system: Confusion, delirium, depression, fever, headache

Dermatologic: Angioedema, rash, urticaria

Gastrointestinal: Diarrhea, enterocolitis, glossitis, nausea, stomatitis, vomiting

Hematologic: Aplastic anemia, bone marrow suppression, granulocytopenia, hypoplastic anemia, pancytopenia, thrombocytopenia

Ocular: Optic neuritis

Miscellaneous: Anaphylaxis, hypersensitivity reactions, Gray syndrome

Drug Interactions

Metabolism/Transport Effects Inhibits CYP2C19 (strong), CYP2C9 (weak), CYP3A4 (strong)

Avoid Concomitant Use

Avoid concomitant use of Chloramphenicol with any of the following: Ado-Trastuzumab Emtansine; Alfuzosin; Apixaban; Avanafil; Axitinib; BCG; Bosutinib; Cabozantinib; CloZAPine; Conivaptan; Crizotinib; Dronedarone; Eplerenone; Everolimus; Halofantrine; Ibrutinib; Imatinib; Ivabradine; Lapatinib; Lomitapide; Lovastatin; Lurasidone; Macitentan; Nilotinib; Nisoldipine; Pimozide; Pomalidomide; Ranolazine; Red Yeast Rice; Regorafenib; Rivaroxaban; Salmeterol; Silodosin; Simeprevir; Simvastatin; Tamsulosin; Ticagrelor; Tolvaptan; Toremifene; Ulipristal; Vemurafenib; VinCRIStine (Liposomal)

Increased Effect/Toxicity

Chloramphenicol may increase the levels/effects of: Ado-Trastuzumab Emtansine; Alfuzosin; Almotriptan; Alosetron; Anticonvulsants (Hydantoin); Apixaban; ARIPiprazole; Avanafil; Axitinib; Barbiturates; Bedaquiline; Bortezomib; Bosentan; Bosutinib; Brentuximab Vedotin; Brinzolamide; Budesonide (Nasal); Budesonide (Systemic, Oral Inhalation); Cabozantinib; Citalopram; CloZAPine; Colchicine; Conivaptan; Corticosteroids (Orally Inhaled); Crizotinib; CycloSPORINE (Systemic); CYP2C19 Substrates; CYP3A4 Substrates; Dienogest; Dofetilide; Dronedarone; Dutasteride; Enzalutamide; Eplerenone; Everolimus; FentaNYL; Fesoterodine; Fluticasone (Nasal); Fluticasone (Oral Inhalation); GuanFACINE; Halofantrine; Ibrutinib; Iloperidone; Imatinib; Ivabradine; Ivacaftor; Ixabepilone; Lacosamide;

Lapatinib; Levomilnacipran; Lomitapide; Lovastatin; Lumefantrine; Lurasidone; Macitentan; Maraviroc; MethylPREDNISolone; Mifepristone; Nilotinib; Nisoldipine; Ospemifene; OxyCODONE; Paricalcitol; PAZOPanib; Pimecrolimus; Pimozide; Pomalidomide; PONATinib; Propafenone; QUEtiapine; Ranolazine; Red Yeast Rice; Regorafenib; Repaglinide; Rilpivirine; Rivaroxaban; RomiDEPsin; Ruxolitinib; Salmeterol; Saxagliptin; Sildenafil; Silodosin; Simeprevir; Simvastatin; SORAfenib; Sulfonylureas; Tacrolimus (Systemic); Tadalafil; Tamsulosin; Ticagrelor; Tofacitinib; Tolterodine; Tolvaptan; Toremifene; Ulipristal; Vardenafil; Vemurafenib; Vilazodone; VinCRIStine (Liposomal); Vitamin K Antagonists; Voriconazole; Zuclopenthixol

Decreased Effect

Chloramphenicol may decrease the levels/effects of: BCG; Clopidogrel; Cyanocobalamin; Ifosfamide; Prasugrel; Sodium Picosulfate; Ticagrelor; Typhoid Vaccine

The levels/effects of Chloramphenicol may be decreased by: Anticonvulsants (Hydantoin); Barbiturates; Rifampin

Ethanol/Nutrition/Herb Interactions Food: May decrease intestinal absorption of vitamin B_{12} may have increased dietary need for riboflavin, pyridoxine, and vitamin B_{12}.

Storage/Stability Store at room temperature prior to reconstitution. Reconstituted solutions remain stable for 30 days. Use only clear solutions. Frozen solutions remain stable for 6 months.

Mechanism of Action Reversibly binds to 50S ribosomal subunits of susceptible organisms preventing amino acids from being transferred to growing peptide chains thus inhibiting protein synthesis

Pharmacodynamics/Kinetics

Distribution: To most tissues and body fluids
- Chloramphenicol: V_d: 0.5-1 L/kg
- Chloramphenicol succinate: V_d: 0.2-3.1 L/kg; decreased with hepatic or renal dysfunction

Protein binding: Chloramphenicol: ~60%; decreased with hepatic or renal dysfunction and in newborn infants

Metabolism:
- Chloramphenicol: Hepatic to metabolites (inactive)
- Chloramphenicol succinate: Hydrolyzed in the liver, kidney and lungs to chloramphenicol (active)

Bioavailability:
- Chloramphenicol: Oral: ~80%
- Chloramphenicol succinate: I.V.: ~70%; highly variable, dependent upon rate and extent of metabolism to chloramphenicol

Half-life elimination:
- Normal renal function:
  - Chloramphenicol: Adults: ~4 hours; Children 4-6 hours; Infants: Significantly prolonged
  - Chloramphenicol succinate: Adults: ~3 hours
- End-stage renal disease: Chloramphenicol: 3-7 hours
- Hepatic disease: Prolonged

Excretion: Urine (~30% as unchanged chloramphenicol succinate in adults, 6% to 80% in children; 5% to 15% as chloramphenicol)

Dosage

Children: Usual dosing range: I.V.: 50-100 mg/kg/day in divided doses every 6 hours; maximum daily dose: 4 g/day
- Meningitis: I.V.: Infants >30 days and Children: 75-100 mg/kg/day divided every 6 hours

Adults: 50-100 mg/kg/day in divided doses every 6 hours; maximum daily dose: 4 g/day

Dosing adjustment in renal impairment: Use with caution; monitor serum concentrations

Dosing adjustment/comments in hepatic impairment: Use with caution; monitor serum concentrations.

Dietary Considerations May have increased dietary need for riboflavin, pyridoxine, and vitamin B_{12}. Some products may contain sodium.

Administration Do not administer I.M.; can be administered IVP over at least 1 minute at a concentration of 100 mg/mL, or I.V. intermittent infusion over 15-30 minutes at a final concentration for administration of ≤20 mg/mL.

Hazardous agent; use appropriate precautions for handling and disposal (NIOSH, 2012).

Monitoring Parameters CBC with differential (baseline and every 2 days during therapy), periodic liver and renal function tests, serum drug concentration

Reference Range

Therapeutic levels:
- Meningitis:
  - Peak: 15-25 mcg/mL; toxic concentration: >40 mcg/mL
  - Trough: 5-15 mcg/mL
- Other infections:
  - Peak: 10-20 mcg/mL
  - Trough: 5-10 mcg/mL

Timing of serum samples: Draw levels 0.5-1.5 hours after completion of I.V. dose

Test Interactions May cause false-positive results in urine glucose tests when using cupric sulfate (Benedict's solution, Clinitest®).

Dosage Forms Excipient information presented when available (limited, particularly for generics); consult specific product labeling.

Solution Reconstituted, Intravenous:
- Generic: 1 g (1 ea)

◆ ChloraPrep One Step [OTC] *see* Chlorhexidine Gluconate *on page 408*

◆ Chlorbutinum *see* Chlorambucil *on page 403*

ChlordiazePOXIDE (klor dye az e POKS ide)

Index Terms Librium; Methaminodiazepoxide Hydrochloride

Pharmacologic Category Benzodiazepine

Additional Appendix Information

Beers Criteria – Potentially Inappropriate Medications for Geriatrics *on page 2368*

Benzodiazepine Comparison Table *on page 2292*

Use Management of anxiety disorder or for the short-term relief of symptoms of anxiety; withdrawal symptoms of acute alcoholism; preoperative apprehension and anxiety

Pregnancy Risk Factor D

Pregnancy Considerations Adverse events were observed in some animal reproduction studies. Chlordiazepoxide crosses the human placenta and fetal serum concentrations are similar to those in the mother. Teratogenic effects have been observed with some benzodiazepines (including chlordiazepoxide); however, additional studies are needed. The incidence of premature birth and low birth weights may be increased following maternal use of benzodiazepines; hypoglycemia and respiratory problems in the neonate may occur following exposure late in pregnancy. Neonatal withdrawal symptoms may occur within days to weeks after birth and "floppy infant syndrome" (which also includes withdrawal symptoms) has been reported with some benzodiazepines (Bergman, 1992; Iqbal, 2002; Wikner, 2007).

Breast-Feeding Considerations Chlordiazepoxide is excreted into breast milk. Drowsiness, lethargy, or weight loss in nursing infants have been observed in case reports following maternal use of some benzodiazepines (Iqbal, 2002).

Contraindications Hypersensitivity to chlordiazepoxide or any component of the formulation (cross-sensitivity with other benzodiazepines may also exist)

Warnings/Precautions Active metabolites with extended half-lives may lead to delayed accumulation and adverse effects. Use with caution in elderly or debilitated patients, pediatric patients, patients with hepatic disease (including alcoholics) or renal impairment, patients with respiratory disease or impaired gag reflex, patients with porphyria.

Causes CNS depression (dose related) resulting in sedation, dizziness, confusion, or ataxia which may impair physical and mental capabilities. Patients must be cautioned about performing tasks which require mental alertness (eg, operating machinery or driving). Use with caution in patients receiving other CNS depressants or psychoactive agents (lithium, phenothiazines). Effects with other sedative drugs or ethanol may be potentiated. Benzodiazepines have been associated with falls and traumatic injury and should be used with extreme caution in patients who are at risk of these events. In older adults, benzodiazepines increase the risk of impaired cognition, delirium, falls, fractures, and motor vehicle accidents. Due to increased sensitivity in this age group and slower metabolism of long-acting agents (such as chlordiazepoxide), avoid use for treatment of insomnia, agitation, or delirium (Beers Criteria).

Use caution in patients with depression, particularly if suicidal risk may be present. Use with caution in patients with a history of drug dependence. Benzodiazepines have been associated with dependence and acute withdrawal symptoms on discontinuation or reduction in dose. Acute withdrawal, including seizures, may be precipitated in patients after administration of flumazenil to patients receiving long-term benzodiazepine therapy.

Benzodiazepines have been associated with anterograde amnesia. Paradoxical reactions, including hyperactive or aggressive behavior have been reported with benzodiazepines, particularly in adolescent/pediatric or psychiatric patients. Does not have analgesic, antidepressant, or antipsychotic properties. Duration of use longer than 4 months has not been studied.

Adverse Reactions Frequency not defined

Cardiovascular: Edema, syncope

Central nervous system: Abnormal electroencephalogram, ataxia, confusion, drowsiness, drug-induced extrapyramidal reaction

Dermatologic: Skin rash

Endocrine & metabolic: Change in libido, menstrual disease

Gastrointestinal: Constipation, nausea

Hematologic & oncologic: Agranulocytosis, bone marrow depression

Hepatic: Hepatic insufficiency, jaundice

Miscellaneous: Paradoxical reaction

Drug Interactions

Metabolism/Transport Effects Substrate of CYP3A4 (major); **Note:** Assignment of Major/Minor substrate status based on clinically relevant drug interaction potential

Avoid Concomitant Use

Avoid concomitant use of ChlordiazePOXIDE with any of the following: Azelastine (Nasal); Conivaptan; Fusidic Acid (Systemic); OLANZapine; Paraldehyde; Sodium Oxybate

Increased Effect/Toxicity

ChlordiazePOXIDE may increase the levels/effects of: Alcohol (Ethyl); Azelastine (Nasal); Buprenorphine; CloZAPine; CNS Depressants; Fosphenytoin; Hydrocodone; Methotrimeprazine; Metyrosine; Mirtazapine; Paraldehyde; Phenytoin; Pramipexole; ROPINIRole; Rotigotine; Selective Serotonin Reuptake Inhibitors; Sodium Oxybate; Zolpidem

The levels/effects of ChlordiazePOXIDE may be increased by: Antifungal Agents (Azole Derivatives, Systemic); Aprepitant; Brimonidine (Topical); Calcium Channel Blockers (Nondihydropyridine); Cimetidine; Conivaptan; Contraceptives (Estrogens); Contraceptives (Progestins); CYP3A4 Inhibitors (Moderate); CYP3A4 Inhibitors (Strong); Dasatinib; Disulfiram; Doxylamine; Droperidol; Fosaprepitant; Fusidic Acid (Systemic); Grapefruit Juice; HydrOXYzine; Isoniazid; Ivacaftor; Luliconazole; Magnesium Sulfate; MAO Inhibitors; Methotrimeprazine; Mifepristone; OLANZapine; Perampanel; Proton Pump Inhibitors; Selective Serotonin Reuptake Inhibitors; Simeprevir; Tapentadol

Decreased Effect

The levels/effects of ChlordiazePOXIDE may be decreased by: Bosentan; CarBAMazepine; CYP3A4 Inducers (Strong); Dabrafenib; Deferasirox; Herbs (CYP3A4 Inducers); Mitotane; Rifamycin Derivatives; Theophylline Derivatives; Tocilizumab; Yohimbine

Ethanol/Nutrition/Herb Interactions

Ethanol: May increase CNS depression; monitor for increased effects with coadministration. Caution patients about effects.

Food: Serum concentrations/effects may be increased with grapefruit juice, but unlikely because of high oral bioavailability of chlordiazepoxide.

Herb/Nutraceutical: Avoid valerian, St John's wort, kava kava, gotu kola (may increase CNS depression).

Storage/Stability Store at 20°C to 25°C (68°F to 77°F). Protect from light and moisture.

Mechanism of Action Binds to stereospecific benzodiazepine receptors on the postsynaptic GABA neuron at several sites within the central nervous system, including the limbic system, reticular formation. Enhancement of the inhibitory effect of GABA on neuronal excitability results by increased neuronal membrane permeability to chloride ions. This shift in chloride ions results in hyperpolarization (a less excitable state) and stabilization.

Pharmacodynamics/Kinetics

Distribution: V_d: 3.3 L/kg (Schwartz, 1971)

Protein binding: 96% (Baskin, 1982)

Metabolism: Extensively hepatic to desmethyldiazepam (active and long-acting)

Half-life elimination: 6.6-28 hours (Schwartz, 1971)

Time to peak, serum: 0.5-2 hours (Baskin, 1982)

Excretion: Urine (minimal as unchanged drug)

Dosage Oral:

Children <6 years: Not recommended

Children ≥6 years and Adolescents: Anxiety: Usual daily dose: 5 mg 2-4 times daily. Dose may be increased to 10 mg 2-3 times daily in some patients, if necessary.

Adults:

Anxiety:

Mild-moderate anxiety: Usual daily dose: 5-10 mg 3-4 times daily

Severe anxiety: Usual daily dose: 20-25 mg 3-4 times daily

Preoperative anxiety: 5-10 mg 3-4 times daily on the days preceding surgery

Ethanol withdrawal symptoms: Initial dose: 50-100 mg; dose may be repeated as necessary to a maximum of 300 mg per 24 hours. **Note:** Frequency of repeat doses is often based on institution-specific protocols. Once agitation is under control, maintain therapy at lowest effective dose.

Elderly or debilitated patients: Usual daily dose: 5 mg 2-4 times daily. Avoid use if possible due to long-acting metabolite.

Dosage adjustment in renal impairment: Dosage adjustments are not provided in the manufacturer's labeling; however, the following guidelines have been used by some clinicians (Aronoff, 2007): Adults: Cl_{cr} <10 mL/minute: Administer 50% of dose

Peritoneal dialysis: Administer 50% of the dose (Aronoff, 2007).

Dosage adjustment/comments in hepatic impairment: There are no specific hepatic dosage adjustments provided in the manufacturer's labeling; however, chlordiazepoxide undergoes hepatic metabolism and should be used with caution.

Administration Administer orally in divided doses.

Monitoring Parameters Respiratory and cardiovascular status (including orthostasis); mental status; periodic blood counts and liver function tests; if used for ethanol withdrawal, signs/symptoms of ethanol withdrawal

Reference Range Therapeutic: 0.1-3 mcg/mL (SI: 0-10 micromole/L); Toxic: >23 mcg/mL (SI: >77 micromole/L)

Additional Information The parenteral formulation of chlordiazepoxide is no longer commercially available in the U.S. or Canada.

Dosage Forms Excipient information presented when available (limited, particularly for generics); consult specific product labeling.

Capsule, Oral, as hydrochloride:

Generic: 5 mg, 10 mg, 25 mg

Controlled Substance C-IV

◆ **Chlordiazepoxide and Amitriptyline Hydrochloride** *see* Amitriptyline and Chlordiazepoxide *on page 107*

◆ **Chlordiazepoxide and Clidinium** *see* Clidinium and Chlordiazepoxide *on page 451*

◆ **Chlorethazine** *see* Mechlorethamine (Systemic) *on page 1274*

◆ **Chlorethazine Mustard** *see* Mechlorethamine (Systemic) *on page 1274*

Chlorhexidine Gluconate

(klor HEKS i deen GLOO koe nate)

Brand Names: U.S. Betasept Surgical Scrub [OTC]; ChloraPrep One Step [OTC]; Hibiclens [OTC]; Hibistat [OTC]; Peridex; Periogard; Tegaderm CHG Dressing [OTC]

Brand Names: Canada Hibidil® 1:2000; ORO-Clense; Peridex® Oral Rinse

Index Terms 3M™ Avagard™ [OTC]; CHG

Pharmacologic Category Antibiotic, Oral Rinse; Antibiotic, Topical

Use

Topical: Skin cleanser for preoperative skin preparation, skin wound and general skin cleanser for patients; surgical scrub and antiseptic hand rinse for healthcare personnel

Oral rinse: Antibacterial dental rinse for gingivitis treatment

Periodontal chip: Adjunctive therapy to reduce pocket depth in patients with periodontitis

Unlabeled Use Oral rinse: Oropharyngeal decontamination (to reduce the risk of ventilator-associated pneumonia) in critically-ill patients with severe sepsis

Pregnancy Risk Factor B/C (manufacturer specific)

Dosage Adults:

Oral rinse: Treatment of gingivitis: Swish for 30 seconds with 15 mL (one capful) of undiluted oral rinse after toothbrushing, then expectorate; repeat twice daily (morning and evening). Therapy should be initiated immediately following a dental prophylaxis. Patient should be reevaluated and given a dental prophylaxis at intervals no longer than every 6 months.

Periodontal chip: Periodontitis: One chip is inserted into a periodontal pocket with a probing pocket depth ≥5 mm. Up to 8 chips may be inserted in a single visit. Treatment is recommended every 3 months in pockets with a remaining depth ≥5 mm. If dislodgment occurs 7 days or more after placement, the subject is considered to have had the full course of treatment. If dislodgment occurs within 48 hours, a new chip should be inserted. The chip biodegrades completely and does not need to be removed. Patients should avoid dental floss at the site of periodontal chip insertion for 10 days after placement because flossing might dislodge the chip.

Insertion of periodontal chip: Pocket should be isolated and surrounding area dried prior to chip insertion. The chip should be grasped using forceps with the rounded edges away from the forceps. The chip should be inserted into the periodontal pocket to its maximum depth. It may be maneuvered into position using the tips of the forceps or a flat instrument.

Topical: Skin cleanser for preoperative skin preparation, skin wound and general skin cleanser for patients; surgical scrub and antiseptic hand rinse for healthcare personnel:

Surgical scrub: Scrub hands and forearms for 3 minutes paying close attention to nails, cuticles, and interdigital spaces, and rinse thoroughly, wash for an additional 3 minutes, rinse, and dry thoroughly.

Surgical hand antiseptic: Lotion: Dispense 1 pumpful in palm of 1 hand; dip fingertips of opposite hand into solution and work it under nails. Spread remainder evenly over hand and just above elbow, covering all surfaces. Repeat on other hand. Dispense another pumpful in each hand and reapply to each hand up to the wrist. Allow to dry before gloving.

Healthcare personnel hand antiseptic:

Liquid or solution: Wash with ~5 mL for 15 seconds; rinse thoroughly with water and dry.

Lotion: Apply to clean, dry hands and nails. Dispense 1 pumpful (2 mL) into the palm of 1 hand; apply evenly to cover both hands up to the wrists; allow to dry without wiping.

Towelette: Rub 15 seconds paying close attention to nails and interdigital spaces; no watering or toweling necessary

Preoperative skin preparation:

Solution: Apply liberally to surgical site and swab for at least 2 minutes. Dry with sterile towel. Repeat procedure (swab for additional 2 minutes and dry with sterile towel).

Applicator (ChloraPrep®): Completely wet treatment area and use gentle back and forth strokes for 30 seconds (dry surgical sites) or 2 minutes (moist surgical sites [eg, inguinal area]); allow to completely dry (3 minutes for hairless skin; up to 1 hour in hair [avoid hairy areas]). **Note:** Do not use 26-mL applicator for head and neck surgery or an area smaller than 8.4 inches x 8.4 inches.

Preparation of skin prior to an injection: Swab: Apply swab to procedure site for 15 seconds; allow to air dry for 30 seconds (do not blot or wipe dry). **Note:** Maximum treatment area for 1 swab is ~2.5 inches x 2.5 inches.

Wound care and general skin cleansing: Rinse area with water, then apply minimum amount necessary to cover skin or wound area and wash gently. Rinse again thoroughly.

Additional Information Complete prescribing information should be consulted for additional detail.

Dosage Forms Excipient information presented when available (limited, particularly for generics); consult specific product labeling.

Liquid, External:

Betasept Surgical Scrub: 4% (118 mL, 237 mL, 473 mL, 946 mL, 3780 mL)

Hibiclens: 4% (15 mL, 118 mL, 236 mL, 473 mL, 946 mL, 3790 mL) [contains fd&c red #40, isopropyl alcohol]

Generic: 2% (118 mL); 4% (118 mL, 237 mL, 473 mL, 946 mL, 3800 mL)

Miscellaneous, External:
Hibistat: 0.5% (50 ea) [contains isopropyl alcohol]
Tegaderm CHG Dressing: (Dressing) (1 ea)
Pad, External:
Generic: 2% (2 ea, 6 ea)
Solution, External:
ChloraPrep One Step: 2% (3 mL, 10.5 mL) [latex free]
Solution, Mouth/Throat:
Peridex: 0.12% (473 mL) [contains alcohol, usp, brilliant blue fcf (fd&c blue #1), saccharin sodium]
Periogard: 0.12% (473 mL) [mint flavor]
Generic: 0.12% (15 mL, 473 mL)

◆ **Chlormeprazine** *see* Prochlorperazine *on page 1722*
◆ **2-Chlorodeoxyadenosine** *see* Cladribine *on page 444*
◆ **Chloromag** *see* Magnesium Chloride *on page 1259*
◆ **Chloromycetin® (Can)** *see* Chloramphenicol *on page 405*
◆ **Chloromycetin® Succinate (Can)** *see* Chloramphenicol *on page 405*

Chloroprocaine (klor oh PROE kane)

Brand Names: U.S. Nesacaine; Nesacaine-MPF
Brand Names: Canada Nesacaine®-CE
Index Terms Chloroprocaine Hydrochloride
Pharmacologic Category Local Anesthetic
Use Infiltration anesthesia, peripheral nerve block, epidural anesthesia
Pregnancy Risk Factor C
Dosage Dosage varies with anesthetic procedure, the area to be anesthetized, the vascularity of the tissues, depth of anesthesia required, degree of muscle relaxation required, and duration of anesthesia; range.

Children >3 years (normally developed): Maximum dose (without epinephrine): 11 mg/kg; for infiltration, concentrations of 0.5% to 1% are recommended; for nerve block, concentrations of 1% to 1.5% are recommended
Adults:
Maximum single dose (without epinephrine): 11 mg/kg; maximum dose: 800 mg
Maximum single dose (with epinephrine): 14 mg/kg; maximum dose: 1000 mg
Infiltration and peripheral nerve block:
Mandibular: 2%: 2-3 mL; total dose 40-60 mg
Infraorbital: 2%: 0.5-1 mL; total dose 10-20 mg
Brachial plexus: 2%; 30-40 mL; total dose 600-800 mg
Digital (without epinephrine): 1%; 3-4 mL; total dose: 30-40 mg
Pudendal: 2%; 10 mL each side; total dose: 400 mg
Paracervical: 1%; 3 mL per each of four sites
Caudal block: Preservative-free: 2% or 3%: 15-25 mL; may repeat at 40-60 minute intervals
Lumbar epidural block: Preservative-free: 2% or 3%: 2-2.5 mL per segment; usual total volume: 15-25 mL; may repeat with doses that are 2-6 mL less than initial dose every 40-50 minutes.

Dosage adjustment in renal impairment: No dosage adjustments provided in manufacturer's labeling. Use with caution due to increased risk of adverse effects.
Dosage adjustment in hepatic impairment: No dosage adjustments provided in manufacturer's labeling. Use with caution due to increased risk of adverse effects.
Additional Information Complete prescribing information should be consulted for additional detail.
Dosage Forms Excipient information presented when available (limited, particularly for generics); consult specific product labeling.
Solution, Injection, as hydrochloride:
Nesacaine: 1% (30 mL); 2% (30 mL) [contains disodium edta, methylparaben]
Generic: 2% (20 mL); 3% (20 mL)
Solution, Injection, as hydrochloride [preservative free]:
Nesacaine-MPF: 2% (20 mL); 3% (20 mL) [methylparaben free]

◆ **Chloroprocaine Hydrochloride** *see* Chloroprocaine *on page 409*

Chloroquine (KLOR oh kwin)

Brand Names: U.S. Aralen
Brand Names: Canada Aralen; Novo-Chloroquine
Index Terms Chloroquine Phosphate
Pharmacologic Category Aminoquinoline (Antimalarial)
Use
Malaria: Suppressive treatment and acute attacks of malaria due to *Plasmodium vivax*, *P. malariae*, *P. ovale*, and susceptible strains of *P. falciparum*.
Extraintestinal amebiasis: Treatment of extraintestinal amebiasis.
Unlabeled Use Rheumatoid arthritis; discoid lupus erythematosus
Pregnancy Considerations In animal reproduction studies, drug accumulated in fetal ocular tissues and remained for several months following drug elimination from the rest of the body. Chloroquine and its metabolites cross the placenta and can be detected in the cord blood and urine of the newborn infant (Akintonwa, 1988; Essien, 1982; Law, 2008). In one study, chloroquine and its metabolites were measurable in the cord blood 89 days (mean) after the last maternal dose (Law, 2008).

Malaria infection in pregnant women may be more severe than in nonpregnant women and has a high risk of maternal and perinatal morbidity and mortality. Therefore, pregnant women and women who are likely to become pregnant are advised to avoid travel to malaria-risk areas. Chloroquine is recommended for the treatment of pregnant women for uncomplicated malaria in chloroquine-sensitive regions; when caused by chloroquine-sensitive *P. vivax* or *P. ovale*, pregnant women should be maintained on chloroquine prophylaxis for the duration of their pregnancy (refer to current guidelines) (CDC, 2011; CDC, 2012).
Breast-Feeding Considerations Chloroquine and its metabolite can be detected in breast milk. Per product labeling, 11 lactating women with malaria were given a single oral dose of chloroquine 600 mg. The maximum daily dose to the breast-feeding infant was calculated to be 0.7% of the maternal dose. Additional information has been published and results are variable. In one study, the relative dose to the nursing infant was calculated to be 2.3% (chloroquine) and 1% (metabolite) of the weight-adjusted maternal dose with the samples obtained a median of 17 days after the last dose. Women in this study received chloroquine phosphate 750 mg daily for 3 days. This report also provides data from other studies, listing relative infant doses of chloroquine ranging from 0.9% to 9.5% of the maternal dose (Law, 2008). Due to the potential for serious adverse reactions in the nursing infant, the manufacturer recommends a decision be made whether to discontinue nursing or to discontinue the drug, taking into account the importance of treatment to the mother. Other sources consider the amount of chloroquine exposure to the nursing infant to be safe when normal maternal doses for malaria are used. However, the amount of chloroquine obtained by a nursing infant from breast milk would not provide adequate protection if therapy for malaria in the infant is needed (CDC, 2012).
Contraindications Hypersensitivity to 4-aminoquinoline compounds or any component of the formulation; the

presence of retinal or visual field changes either attributable to 4-aminoquinoline compounds or to any other etiology

Warnings/Precautions Use with caution in patients with hepatic impairment, alcoholism or in conjunction with hepatotoxic drugs. May exacerbate psoriasis or porphyria. Use caution in patients with seizure disorders. Use caution in G6PD deficiency; 4-aminoquinolines such as chloroquine has been associated with hemolysis and renal impairment. Use with caution in patients with pre-existing auditory damage; discontinue immediately if hearing defects are noted. Retinopathy, maculopathy, and macular degeneration have occurred; irreversible retinal damage has occurred with prolonged or high dose 4-aminoquinoline therapy; risk factors include age, duration of therapy, and/or high doses. Monitoring is required, especially with prolonged therapy. Discontinue immediately if signs/symptoms occur; visual changes may progress even after therapy is discontinued. Use has been associated with ECG changes, AV block, and cardiomyopathy. May cause QT prolongation and subsequent torsade de pointes; avoid use in patients with diagnosed or suspected congenital long QT syndrome. Rare hematologic reactions including agranulocytosis, aplastic anemia, neutropenia, pancytopenia, and thrombocytopenia; monitor CBC during prolonged therapy. Consider discontinuation if severe blood disorders occur that are unrelated to disease. Acute extrapyramidal disorders may occur, usually resolving after discontinuation of therapy and/or symptomatic treatment. Skeletal muscle myopathy or neuromyopathy, leading to progressive weakness and atrophy of proximal muscle groups have been reported; muscle strength (especially proximal muscles) should be assessed periodically during prolonged therapy; discontinue therapy if weakness occurs. Potentially significant drug-drug interactions may exist, requiring dose or frequency adjustment, additional monitoring, and/or selection of alternative therapy.

Certain strains of *P. falciparum* are resistant to 4-aminoquinoline compounds. Prior to initiation of therapy, it should be determined if chloroquine is appropriate for use in the region to be visited; do not use for the treatment of *P. falciparum* acquired in areas of chloroquine resistance or where chloroquine prophylaxis has failed. Patients should be treated with another antimalarial if patient is infected with a resistant strain of plasmodia. Chloroquine does not prevent relapses in patients with vivax or malariae malaria; will not prevent vivax or malariae infection when administered as a prophylactic. Also consult current CDC guidelines for treatment recommendations.

Adverse Reactions Frequency not defined.

Cardiovascular: Cardiomyopathy, ECG changes (rare; including prolonged QRS and QT_c intervals, T wave inversion or depression), hypotension (rare), torsades de pointes (rare)

Central nervous system: Agitation, anxiety, confusion, decreased deep tendon reflex, delirium, depression, extrapyramidal reaction (dystonia, dyskinesia, protrusion of the tongue, torticollis), hallucination, headache, insomnia, personality changes, polyneuropathy, psychosis, seizure

Dermatologic: Alopecia, bleaching of hair, blue gray skin pigmentation, erythema multiforme (rare), exacerbation of psoriasis, exfoliative dermatitis (rare), lichen planus, pleomorphic rash, pruritus, skin photosensitivity, Stevens-Johnson syndrome (rare), toxic epidermal necrolysis (rare), urticaria

Gastrointestinal: Abdominal cramps, anorexia, diarrhea, nausea, vomiting

Hematologic & oncologic: Agranulocytosis (rare; reversible), aplastic anemia, neutropenia, pancytopenia, thrombocytopenia

Hepatic: Hepatitis, increased liver enzymes

Hypersensitivity: Anaphylactoid reaction, anaphylaxis, angioedema

Immunologic: DRESS syndrome

Neuromuscular & skeletal: Myopathy, neuromuscular disease, proximal myopathy

Ophthalmic: Accommodation disturbances, blurred vision, corneal opacity (reversible), macular degeneration (may be irreversible), maculopathy (may be irreversible), nocturnal amblyopia, retinopathy (including irreversible changes in some patients long-term or high-dose therapy), visual field defects

Otic: Deafness (nerve), hearing loss (risk increased in patients with pre-existing auditory damage), tinnitus

Drug Interactions

Metabolism/Transport Effects **Substrate** of CYP2D6 (major), CYP3A4 (major); **Note:** Assignment of Major/Minor substrate status based on clinically relevant drug interaction potential; **Inhibits** CYP2D6 (moderate)

Avoid Concomitant Use

Avoid concomitant use of Chloroquine with any of the following: Agalsidase Alfa; Agalsidase Beta; Artemether; Conivaptan; Fusidic Acid (Systemic); Highest Risk QTc-Prolonging Agents; Ivabradine; Lumefantrine; Mefloquine; Mifepristone; Thioridazine

Increased Effect/Toxicity

Chloroquine may increase the levels/effects of: Antipsychotic Agents (Phenothiazines); ARIPiprazole; Beta-Blockers; Cardiac Glycosides; CYP2D6 Substrates; Dapsone (Systemic); Dapsone (Topical); Fesoterodine; Highest Risk QTc-Prolonging Agents; Lumefantrine; Mefloquine; Metoprolol; Moderate Risk QTc-Prolonging Agents; Prilocaine; Sodium Nitrite; Thioridazine

The levels/effects of Chloroquine may be increased by: Abiraterone Acetate; Artemether; Conivaptan; CYP2D6 Inhibitors (Moderate); CYP2D6 Inhibitors (Strong); CYP3A4 Inhibitors (Moderate); CYP3A4 Inhibitors (Strong); Dapsone (Systemic); Darunavir; Dasatinib; Fusidic Acid (Systemic); Ivabradine; Ivacaftor; Luliconazole; Mefloquine; Mifepristone; Nitric Oxide; QTc-Prolonging Agents (Indeterminate Risk and Risk Modifying); Simeprevir

Decreased Effect

Chloroquine may decrease the levels/effects of: Agalsidase Alfa; Agalsidase Beta; Ampicillin; Anthelmintics; Codeine; Rabies Vaccine; Tamoxifen; TraMADol

The levels/effects of Chloroquine may be decreased by: Antacids; Bosentan; CYP3A4 Inducers (Strong); Dabrafenib; Deferasirox; Herbs (CYP3A4 Inducers); Kaolin; Lanthanum; Mitotane; Peginterferon Alfa-2b; Tocilizumab

Ethanol/Nutrition/Herb Interactions Ethanol: Avoid ethanol (may increase GI irritation).

Storage/Stability Store at 25°C (77°F); excursions are permitted between 15°C and 30°C (59°F and 86°F).

Mechanism of Action Binds to and inhibits DNA and RNA polymerase; interferes with metabolism and hemoglobin utilization by parasites; inhibits prostaglandin effects; chloroquine concentrates within parasite acid vesicles and raises internal pH resulting in inhibition of parasite growth; may involve aggregates of ferriprotoporphyrin IX acting as chloroquine receptors causing membrane damage; may also interfere with nucleoprotein synthesis

Pharmacodynamics/Kinetics
Absorption: Rapid and almost complete
Distribution: Widely in body tissues
Protein binding: 55%
Metabolism: Partially hepatic to main metabolite, desethylchloroquine
Excretion: Urine (≥50% as unchanged drug); acidification of urine increases elimination

Dosage Oral: **Note:** Each 250 mg of chloroquine phosphate is equivalent to 150 mg of chloroquine base
Malaria chemoprophylaxis:
Children: 8.3 mg/kg/week (5 mg/kg base) on the same day each week (not to exceed 500 mg/dose [300 mg base/dose]); begin 1-2 weeks prior to exposure; continue while in endemic area and for 4 weeks after leaving endemic area (CDC, 2014)
Adults: 500 mg (300 mg base) weekly on the same day each week; begin 1-2 weeks prior to exposure; continue while in endemic area and for 4 weeks after leaving endemic area (CDC, 2014)
Malaria treatment:
Children: 16.6 mg/kg (10 mg/kg base) on day 1 (maximum: 1000 mg [600 mg base]), followed by 8.3 mg/kg (5 mg/kg base) (maximum: 500 mg [300 mg base]) 6-, 24-, and 48 hours after first dose (CDC, 2009)
Adults: 1 g (600 mg base) on day 1, followed by 500 mg (300 mg base) 6-, 24-, and 48 hours after first dose (CDC, 2009)
Extraintestinal amebiasis: Adults: 1 g (600 mg base) daily for 2 days followed by 500 mg daily (300 mg base) for at least 2-3 weeks; may be combined with an intestinal amebicide.
Lupus erythematosus (unlabeled use): Adults: 250 mg (150 mg base) once daily for ≥3 months (Bezerra, 2005; Lesiak, 2008)
Rheumatoid arthritis (unlabeled use): Adults: 250 mg (150 mg base) once daily for ≥1 year. **Note:** Not considered first-line agent. (Fowler, 1984; Freedman, 1960)

Dosage adjustment in renal impairment: The FDA-approved labeling does not contain renal dosing adjustment guidelines; the following guidelines have been used by some clinicians (Aronoff, 2007):
Cl_{cr} ≥10 mL/minute: No dosage adjustment necessary.
Cl_{cr} <10 mL/minute: Administer 50% of dose
Hemodialysis effects: Minimally removed by hemodialysis
Hemodialysis, peritoneal dialysis: Administer 50% of dose
Continuous renal replacement therapy (CRRT): No dosage adjustment necessary.

Dosage adjustment in hepatic impairment: No dosage adjustment provided in manufacturer's labeling; use with caution.

Monitoring Parameters Ophthalmic exams at baseline and periodically thereafter during prolonged therapy; visual acuity, expert slit-lamp, fundoscopic and visual field tests are recommended. Evaluate neuromuscular function periodically during prolonged therapy. Periodic CBC in patients receiving prolonged therapy

Dosage Forms Excipient information presented when available (limited, particularly for generics); consult specific product labeling.
Tablet, Oral, as phosphate:
Aralen: 500 mg [equivalent to chloroquine base 300 mg]
Generic: 250 mg [equivalent to chloroquine base 150 mg], 500 mg [equivalent to chloroquine base 300 mg]

Extemporaneous Preparations A 15 mg chloroquine phosphate/mL oral suspension (equivalent to 9 mg chloroquine base/mL) may be made from tablets and a 1:1 mixture of Ora-Sweet® and Ora-Plus®. Crush three 500 mg chloroquine phosphate tablets (equivalent to 300 mg base/tablet) in a mortar and reduce to a fine powder. Add 15 mL of the vehicle and mix to a uniform paste; mix while adding the vehicle in incremental proportions to **almost** 100 mL; transfer to a calibrated bottle, rinse mortar with vehicle, and add quantity of vehicle sufficient to make 100 mL. Label "shake well before using" and "protect from light". Stable for up to 60 days when stored in the dark at room temperature or refrigerated (preferred).

Allen LV Jr and Erickson MA 3rd, "Stability of Alprazolam, Chloroquine Phosphate, Cisapride, Enalapril Maleate, and Hydralazine Hydrochloride in Extemporaneously Compounded Oral Liquids," *Am J Health Syst Pharm*, 1998, 55(18):1915-20.

◆ **Chloroquine Phosphate** *see* Chloroquine *on page 409*

Chlorothiazide (klor oh THYE a zide)

Brand Names: U.S. Diuril; Sodium Diuril

Pharmacologic Category Antihypertensive; Diuretic, Thiazide

Use Management of hypertension; adjunctive treatment of edema

Pregnancy Risk Factor C

Dosage Note: The manufacturer states that I.V. and oral dosing are equivalent. Some clinicians may use lower I.V. doses; however, because of chlorothiazide's poor oral absorption. I.V. dosing in infants and children has not been well established.

Infants <6 months: Oral: 10-30 mg/kg/day in 2 divided doses (maximum dose: 375 mg daily)
Infants >6 months and Children: Oral: 10-20 mg/kg/day in 1-2 divided doses (maximum dose: 375 mg daily in children <2 years or 1000 mg daily in children 2-12 years)
Infants and Children: I.V. (unlabeled): 5-10 mg/kg/day in 2 divided doses (Costello, 2007)
Adults:
Hypertension: Oral: 500-2000 mg daily divided in 1-2 doses (manufacturer labeling); doses of 125-500 mg daily have also been recommended (JNC 7)
Edema: Oral, I.V.: 500-1000 mg once or twice daily; intermittent treatment (eg, therapy on alternative days) may be appropriate for some patients
ACC/AHA 2009 Heart Failure guidelines:
Oral: 250-500 mg once or twice daily (maximum daily dose: 1000 mg)
I.V.: 500-1000 mg once or twice daily plus a loop diuretic

Dosage adjustment in renal impairment: Cl_{cr} <10 mL/minute: Avoid use. Ineffective with Cl_{cr} <30 mL/minute unless in combination with a loop diuretic (Aronoff, 2007)
Note: ACC/AHA 2009 Heart Failure guidelines suggest that thiazides lose their efficacy when Cl_{cr} <40 mL/minute

Dosage adjustment in hepatic impairment: No dosage adjustments provided in manufacturer's labeling; use with caution.

Additional Information Complete prescribing information should be consulted for additional detail.

Dosage Forms Excipient information presented when available (limited, particularly for generics); consult specific product labeling.
Solution Reconstituted, Intravenous, as sodium [strength expressed as base]:
Sodium Diuril: 500 mg (1 ea)
Generic: 500 mg (1 ea)
Suspension, Oral:
Diuril: 250 mg/5 mL (237 mL) [contains alcohol, usp, benzoic acid, fd&c yellow #10 (quinoline yellow), methylparaben, propylparaben, saccharin sodium]
Tablet, Oral:
Generic: 250 mg, 500 mg

Chlorpheniramine and Acetaminophen

(klor fen IR a meen & a seet a MIN oh fen)

Brand Names: U.S. Coricidin HBP® Cold and Flu [OTC]

Index Terms Acetaminophen and Chlorpheniramine

Pharmacologic Category Alkylamine Derivative; Analgesic, Miscellaneous; Histamine H_1 Antagonist; Histamine H_1 Antagonist, First Generation

Use Symptomatic relief of congestion, headache, aches and pains of colds and flu

Dosage Adults: Oral: 2 tablets every 4 hours

Additional Information Complete prescribing information should be consulted for additional detail.

Dosage Forms Excipient information presented when available (limited, particularly for generics); consult specific product labeling.

Tablet: Chlorpheniramine maleate 2 mg and acetaminophen 325 mg

◆ **Chlorpheniramine and Dextromethorphan** *see* Dextromethorphan and Chlorpheniramine *on page 591*

Chlorpheniramine and Phenylephrine

(klor fen IR a meen & fen il EF rin)

Brand Names: U.S. Ed ChlorPed D [OTC]; Ed-A-Hist™ [OTC]; Maxichlor PEH [OTC]; nasohist™ [OTC]; NoHist LQ [OTC]; Phenagil [OTC]; Sudafed PE® Sinus + Allergy [OTC]; Triaminic® Children's Cold & Allergy [OTC]; Virdec [OTC]

Index Terms Chlorpheniramine Maleate and Phenylephrine Hydrochloride; Phenylephrine and Chlorpheniramine

Pharmacologic Category Alkylamine Derivative; Alpha-Adrenergic Agonist; Decongestant; Histamine H_1 Antagonist; Histamine H_1 Antagonist, First Generation

Use Temporary relief of upper respiratory conditions such as nasal congestion, runny nose, and sneezing due to the common cold, hay fever, or allergic or vasomotor rhinitis

Dosage Antihistamine/decongestant: Oral: **Note:** Chlorpheniramine dosing in terms of chlorpheniramine maleate; phenylephrine dosing in terms of phenylephrine hydrochloride:

Children 2-5 years:

Liquid:

Chlorpheniramine 1 mg and phenylephrine 2.5 mg per 1 mL: 1 mL every 4-6 hours (maximum: 4 mL/24 hours)

Chlorpheniramine 2 mg and phenylephrine 5 mg per 1 mL: 0.5 mL every 4 hours (maximum: 3 mL/24 hours)

Children 6-11 years:

Liquid:

Chlorpheniramine 1 mg and phenylephrine 2-2.5 mg per 1 mL: 2 mL every 4-6 hours (maximum: 8 mL/24 hours)

Chlorpheniramine 1-2 mg and phenylephrine 3.5-5 mg per 1 mL: 1 mL every 4-6 hours (maximum: 6 mL/24 hours)

Chlorpheniramine 1 mg and phenylephrine 2.5 mg per 5 mL: 10 mL every 4 hours (maximum: 60 mL/24 hours)

Chlorpheniramine 4 mg and phenylephrine 10 mg per 5 mL: 2.5 mL every 4-6 hours (maximum: 15 mL/24 hours)

Tablet: Chlorpheniramine 3-4 mg and phenylephrine 10 mg: One-half tablet every 4-6 hours (maximum: 3 tablets/24 hours)

Children ≥12 years and Adults:

Liquid: Chlorpheniramine 4 mg and phenylephrine 10 mg per 5 mL: 5 mL every 4-6 hours (maximum: 30 mL/24 hours)

Tablet: Chlorpheniramine 3-4 mg and phenylephrine 10 mg: One tablet every 4-6 hours (maximum: 6 tablets/24 hours)

Additional Information Complete prescribing information should be consulted for additional detail.

Dosage Forms Excipient information presented when available (limited, particularly for generics); consult specific product labeling.

Liquid, oral:

Ed-A-Hist™: Chlorpheniramine maleate 4 mg and phenylephrine hydrochloride 10 mg per 5 mL (473 mL) [sugar free; contains ethanol 5%, propylene glycol; grape flavor]

NoHist LQ: Chlorpheniramine maleate 4 mg and phenylephrine hydrochloride 10 mg per 5 mL (473 mL) [ethanol free, sugar free; contains propylene glycol; bubblegum flavor]

Liquid, oral [drops]:

Ed ChlorPed D: Chlorpheniramine maleate 2 mg and phenylephrine hydrochloride 5 mg per 1 mL (60 mL) [ethanol free, sugar free; contains propylene glycol; applesauce flavor]

nasohist™: Chlorpheniramine maleate 1 mg and phenylephrine hydrochloride 2 mg per 1 mL (30 mL) [dye free, ethanol free, sugar free; contains propylene glycol; orange-vanilla flavor]

Virdec: Chlorpheniramine maleate 1 mg and phenylephrine hydrochloride 3.5 mg per 1 mL (30 mL) [ethanol free, sugar free; contains propylene glycol; raspberry flavor]

Syrup, oral:

Triaminic® Children's Cold & Allergy: Chlorpheniramine maleate 1 mg and phenylephrine hydrochloride 2.5 mg per 5 mL (118 mL) [contains benzoic acid, sodium 3 mg/5 mL; orange flavor]

Tablet, oral: Chlorpheniramine maleate 4 mg and phenylephrine hydrochloride 10 mg

Ed A-Hist™: Chlorpheniramine maleate 4 mg and phenylephrine hydrochloride 10 mg [contains tartrazine; scored]

Maxichlor PEH: Chlorpheniramine maleate 4 mg and phenylephrine hydrochloride 10 mg [scored]

Phenagil: Chlorpheniramine maleate 3.5 mg and phenylephrine hydrochloride 10 mg

Chlorpheniramine and Pseudoephedrine

(klor fen IR a meen & soo doe e FED rin)

Brand Names: U.S. Dicel® Chewable [OTC]; LoHist-D [OTC]; Maxichlor PSE [OTC]; Neutrahist Pediatric [OTC]; SudoGest™ Sinus & Allergy [OTC]

Brand Names: Canada Triaminic® Cold & Allergy

Index Terms Allerest; Chlorpheniramine Maleate and Pseudoephedrine Hydrochloride; Chlorpheniramine Tannate and Pseudoephedrine Tannate; Pseudoephedrine and Chlorpheniramine

Pharmacologic Category Alkylamine Derivative; Alpha/Beta Agonist; Decongestant; Histamine H_1 Antagonist; Histamine H_1 Antagonist, First Generation

Use Relief of nasal congestion associated with the common cold, hay fever, allergic rhinitis, and other allergies

Pregnancy Risk Factor C

Dosage Rhinitis/decongestant: Oral: **Note:** All dosing is presented in terms of chlorpheniramine maleate and pseudoephedrine hydrochloride.

Children: 6-11 years:

Liquid:

Chlorpheniramine 0.8 mg and pseudoephedrine 9 mg per 1 mL: 2 mL every 4-6 hours (maximum: 8 mL/24 hours)

Chlorpheniramine 2 mg and pseudoephedrine 30 mg per 5 mL: 5 mL every 4-6 hours (maximum: 30 mL/24 hours)

Tablet:

Chlorpheniramine 2 mg and pseudoephedrine 30 mg: One tablet every 4-6 hours (maximum: 4 tablets/24 hours)

Chlorpheniramine 4 mg and pseudoephedrine 60 mg: One-half tablet every 4-6 hours (maximum: 2 tablets/24 hours)

Children ≥12 years and Adults:

Liquid: Chlorpheniramine 2 mg and pseudoephedrine 30 mg per 5 mL: 10 mL every 4-6 hours (maximum: 60 mL/24hours)

Tablet:

Chlorpheniramine 2 mg and pseudoephedrine 30 mg: Two tablets every 4-6 hours (maximum: 8 tablets/24 hours)

Chlorpheniramine 4 mg and pseudoephedrine 60 mg: One tablet every 4-6 hours (maximum: 4 tablets/24 hours)

Additional Information Complete prescribing information should be consulted for additional detail.

Dosage Forms Excipient information presented when available (limited, particularly for generics); consult specific product labeling. [DSC] = Discontinued product

Liquid, oral:

LoHist-D: Chlorpheniramine maleate 2 mg and pseudoephedrine hydrochloride 30 mg per 5 mL (473 mL) [dye free, ethanol free, sugar free; cherry flavor]

Liquid, oral [drops]:

Neutrahist Pediatric: Chlorpheniramine maleate 0.8 mg and pseudoephedrine hydrochloride 9 mg per 1 mL (30 mL) [ethanol free, sugar free; contains propylene glycol; cherry flavor]

Tablet, oral: Chlorpheniramine maleate 4 mg and pseudoephedrine hydrochloride 60 mg

Maxichlor PSE: Chlorpheniramine maleate 4 mg and pseudoephedrine hydrochloride 60 mg

SudoGest™ Sinus & Allergy: Chlorpheniramine maleate 4 mg and pseudoephedrine hydrochloride 60 mg

Tablet, chewable, oral:

Dicel® Chewables: Chlorpheniramine maleate 2 mg and pseudoephedrine hydrochloride 30 mg [ethanol free; contains sodium 17 mg/tablet, soy lecithin; strawberry-banana cream flavor]

◆ **Chlorpheniramine, Dextromethorphan, and Pseudoephedrine** *see* Chlorpheniramine, Pseudoephedrine, and Dextromethorphan *on page 414*

◆ **Chlorpheniramine Maleate and Dextromethorphan Hydrobromide** *see* Dextromethorphan and Chlorpheniramine *on page 591*

◆ **Chlorpheniramine Maleate and Hydrocodone Bitartrate** *see* Hydrocodone and Chlorpheniramine *on page 1007*

◆ **Chlorpheniramine Maleate and Phenylephrine Hydrochloride** *see* Chlorpheniramine and Phenylephrine *on page 412*

◆ **Chlorpheniramine Maleate and Pseudoephedrine Hydrochloride** *see* Chlorpheniramine and Pseudoephedrine *on page 412*

◆ **Chlorpheniramine Maleate, Dihydrocodeine Bitartrate, and Phenylephrine Hydrochloride** *see* Dihydrocodeine, Chlorpheniramine, and Phenylephrine *on page 611*

◆ **Chlorpheniramine Maleate, Pseudoephedrine Hydrochloride, and Dextromethorphan Hydrobromide** *see* Chlorpheniramine, Pseudoephedrine, and Dextromethorphan *on page 414*

Chlorpheniramine, Phenylephrine, and Dextromethorphan

(klor fen IR a meen, fen il EF rin, & deks troe meth OR fan)

Brand Names: U.S. Cardec™ DM [OTC]; Corfen-DM [OTC]; De-Chlor DM [OTC]; Ed A-Hist DM [OTC]; Father John's® Plus [OTC]; Maxichlor PEH DM [OTC] [DSC]; nasohist™ DM pediatric [OTC]; Neo DM [OTC] [DSC]; NoHist DM [OTC]; PE-Hist-DM [OTC]; Virdec DM [OTC]

Index Terms Dextromethorphan, Chlorpheniramine, and Phenylephrine; Phenylephrine, Chlorpheniramine, and Dextromethorphan

Pharmacologic Category Alkylamine Derivative; Alpha-Adrenergic Agonist; Antitussive; Decongestant; Histamine H_1 Antagonist; Histamine H_1 Antagonist, First Generation

Use Temporary relief of cough and upper respiratory symptoms associated with allergies or the common cold

Dosage Note: All dosing is presented in terms of chlorpheniramine maleate, phenylephrine hydrochloride, and dextromethorphan hydrobromide.

Oral: Relief of cough and cold symptoms:

Children: 2-5 years: Liquid: Chlorpheniramine 1 mg, phenylephrine 2.5 mg, and dextromethorphan 2.5 mg per 1 mL: 1 mL every 4-6 hours (maximum: 4 mL/24 hours)

Children: 6-11 years:

Liquid:

Chlorpheniramine 0.75 mg, phenylephrine 1.75 mg, and dextromethorphan 2.75 mg per 1 mL: 2 mL every 4-6 hours (maximum: 12 mL/24 hours)

Chlorpheniramine 1 mg, phenylephrine 2-2.5 mg, and dextromethorphan 2.5-3 mg per 1 mL: 2 mL every 4-6 hours (maximum: 8 mL/24 hours)

Chlorpheniramine 1 mg, phenylephrine 3.5 mg, and dextromethorphan 3 mg per 1 mL: 1 mL every 4-6 hours (maximum: 6 mL/24 hours)

Chlorpheniramine 2-4 mg, phenylephrine 5-10 mg, and dextromethorphan 15 mg per 5 mL: 2.5 mL every 4-6 hours (maximum: 15 mL/24 hours)

Tablet: Chlorpheniramine 4 mg, phenylephrine 10 mg, and dextromethorphan 20 mg: One-half tablet every 4-6 hours (maximum: 3 tablets/24 hours)

Children ≥12 years and Adults:

Liquid:

Chlorpheniramine 2 mg, phenylephrine 5 mg, and dextromethorphan 5 mg per 15 mL: 30 mL every 4 hours (maximum: 180 mL/24 hours)

Chlorpheniramine 2-4 mg, phenylephrine 5-10 mg, and dextromethorphan 15 mg per 5 mL: 5 mL every 4-6 hours (maximum: 30 mL/24 hours)

Tablet: Chlorpheniramine 4 mg, phenylephrine 10 mg, and dextromethorphan 20 mg: One tablet every 4-6 hours (maximum: 6 tablets/24 hours)

Additional Information Complete prescribing information should be consulted for additional detail.

Dosage Forms Excipient information presented when available (limited, particularly for generics); consult specific product labeling.

Liquid, oral:

Corfen-DM: Chlorpheniramine maleate 4 mg, phenylephrine hydrochloride 10 mg, and dextromethorphan hydrobromide 15 mg per 5 mL (473 mL) [dye free, ethanol free, sugar free; contains propylene glycol; grape flavor]

De-Chlor DM: Chlorpheniramine maleate 2 mg, phenylephrine hydrochloride 10 mg, and dextromethorphan hydrobromide 15 mg per 5 mL (473 mL) [dye free, ethanol free, sugar free; contains propylene glycol; strawberry flavor]

Ed A-Hist DM: Chlorpheniramine maleate 4 mg, phenylephrine hydrochloride 10 mg, and dextromethorphan hydrobromide 15 mg per 5 mL (473 mL) [gluten free, sugar free; contains propylene glycol; banana flavor]

Father John's® Plus: Chlorpheniramine maleate 2 mg, phenylephrine hydrochloride 5 mg, and dextromethorphan hydrobromide 5 mg per 15 mL (118 mL) [ethanol free]

NoHist DM: Chlorpheniramine maleate 4 mg, phenylephrine hydrochloride 10 mg, and dextromethorphan hydrobromide 15 mg per 5 mL (473 mL) [dye free, ethanol free, sugar free; contains propylene glycol; grape flavor]

Liquid, oral [drops]:

Cardec™ DM: Chlorpheniramine maleate 1 mg, phenylephrine hydrochloride 3.5 mg, and dextromethorphan hydrobromide 3 mg per 1 mL (30 mL) [ethanol free, gluten free, sugar free; contains propylene glycol, sodium benzoate; grape flavor]

nasohist™ DM pediatric: Chlorpheniramine maleate 1 mg, phenylephrine hydrochloride 2 mg, and dextromethorphan hydrobromide 3 mg per 1 mL (30 mL) [dye free, ethanol free, sugar free; contains propylene glycol; orange-vanilla flavor]

Neo DM: Chlorpheniramine maleate 0.75 mg, phenylephrine hydrochloride 1.75 mg, and dextromethorphan hydrobromide 2.75 mg per 1 mL (30 mL) [ethanol free, sugar free; contains propylene glycol; black cherry flavor] [DSC]

Virdec DM: Chlorpheniramine maleate 1 mg, phenylephrine hydrochloride 3.5 mg, and dextromethorphan hydrobromide 3 mg per 1 mL (30 mL) [ethanol free, gluten free, sugar free; contains propylene glycol; grape flavor]

Tablet, oral: Chlorpheniramine maleate 4 mg, phenylephrine hydrochloride 10 mg, and dextromethorphan hydrobromide 20 mg

Maxichlor PEH DM: Chlorpheniramine maleate 4 mg, phenylephrine hydrochloride 10 mg, and dextromethorphan hydrobromide 20 mg [scored] [DSC]

Chlorpheniramine, Pseudoephedrine, and Dextromethorphan

(klor fen IR a meen, soo doe e FED rin, & deks troe meth OR fan)

Brand Names: U.S. Dicel® DM Chewables [OTC]; Kidkare Children's Cough/Cold [OTC]; M-END DM [OTC]; Maxichlor PSE DM [OTC] [DSC]; Neutrahist PDX [OTC] [DSC]; Pedia Relief™ Cough-Cold [OTC]; Pediatric Cough & Cold [OTC]; Rescon DM [OTC]

Index Terms Chlorpheniramine Maleate, Pseudoephedrine Hydrochloride, and Dextromethorphan Hydrobromide; Chlorpheniramine Tannate, Pseudoephedrine Tannate, and Dextromethorphan Tannate; Chlorpheniramine, Dextromethorphan, and Pseudoephedrine; Dexchlorpheniramine Tannate, Pseudoephedrine Tannate, and Dextromethorphan Tannate; Dextromethorphan, Chlorpheniramine, and Pseudoephedrine; Pseudoephedrine, Chlorpheniramine, and Dextromethorphan

Pharmacologic Category Alkylamine Derivative; Alpha/Beta Agonist; Antitussive; Decongestant; Histamine H_1 Antagonist; Histamine H_1 Antagonist, First Generation

Use Temporarily relieves nasal congestion, runny nose, cough, and sneezing due to the common cold, hay fever, or allergic rhinitis

Dosage Relief of cold symptoms: Oral: **Note:** All dosing is presented in terms of chlorpheniramine maleate, pseudoephedrine hydrochloride, and dextromethorphan hydrobromide.

Children 6-11 years:

Liquid:

Chlorpheniramine 0.8 mg, pseudoephedrine 9 mg, and dextromethorphan 3 mg per 1 mL: 2 mL every 4-6 hours (maximum: 8 mL/24 hours)

Chlorpheniramine 1 mg, pseudoephedrine 15 mg, and dextromethorphan 5 mg per 5 mL: 10 mL every 4-6 hours (maximum: 40 mL/24 hours)

Chlorpheniramine 2 mg, pseudoephedrine 15 mg, and dextromethorphan 15 mg per 5 mL: 5 mL every 6 hours (maximum: 20 mL/24 hours)

Chlorpheniramine 2 mg, pseudoephedrine 30 mg, and dextromethorphan 10 mg per 5 mL: 5 mL every 4-6 hours (maximum: 20 mL/24 hours)

Chlorpheniramine 4 mg, pseudoephedrine 20 mg, and dextromethorphan 20 mg per 5 mL: 2.5 mL every 4-6 hours (maximum: 15 mL/24 hours)

Tablet:

Chlorpheniramine 2 mg, pseudoephedrine 30 mg, and dextromethorphan 10 mg: One tablet every 4-6 hours (maximum: 4 tablets/24 hours)

Chlorpheniramine 4 mg, pseudoephedrine 60 mg, and dextromethorphan 20 mg: One-half tablet every 4-6 hours (maximum: 2 tablets/24 hours)

Children ≥12 years and Adults:

Liquid:

Chlorpheniramine 2 mg, pseudoephedrine 15 mg, and dextromethorphan 15 mg per 5 mL: 10 mL every 6 hours (maximum: 40 mL/24 hours)

Chlorpheniramine 2 mg, pseudoephedrine 30 mg, and dextromethorphan 10 mg per 5 mL: 10 mL every 4-6 hours (maximum: 40 mL/24 hours)

Chlorpheniramine 4 mg, pseudoephedrine 20 mg, and dextromethorphan 20 mg per 5 mL: 5 mL every 4-6 hours (maximum: 30 mL/24 hours)

Tablet:

Chlorpheniramine 2 mg, pseudoephedrine 30 mg, and dextromethorphan 10 mg: Two tablets every 4-6 hours (maximum: 8 tablets/24 hours)

Chlorpheniramine 4 mg, pseudoephedrine 60 mg, and dextromethorphan 20 mg: One tablet every 4-6 hours (maximum: 4 tablets/24 hours)

Additional Information Complete prescribing information should be consulted for additional detail.

Dosage Forms Excipient information presented when available (limited, particularly for generics); consult specific product labeling.

Liquid, oral:

Kidkare Children's Cough/Cold: Chlorpheniramine maleate 1 mg, pseudoephedrine hydrochloride 15 mg, and dextromethorphan hydrobromide 5 mg per 5 mL (118 mL) [ethanol free; contains propylene glycol and sodium benzoate; cherry flavor]

Maxichlor PSE DM: Chlorpheniramine maleate 4 mg, pseudoephedrine hydrochloride 20 mg, and dextromethorphan hydrobromide 20 mg per 5 mL (473 mL) [sugar free; contains propylene glycol; vanilla flavor]

M-END DM: Chlorpheniramine maleate 2 mg, pseudoephedrine hydrochloride 15 mg, and dextromethorphan hydrobromide 15 mg per 5 mL (30 mL) [ethanol free, sugar free; contains propylene glycol; orange flavor]

Pedia Relief™ Cough-Cold: Chlorpheniramine maleate 1 mg, pseudoephedrine hydrochloride 15 mg, and dextromethorphan hydrobromide 5 mg per 5 mL (120 mL) [ethanol free; contains propylene glycol and sodium benzoate; cherry flavor]

Pediatric Cough & Cold: Chlorpheniramine maleate 1 mg, pseudoephedrine hydrochloride 15 mg, and dextromethorphan hydrobromide 5 mg per 5 mL (120 mL) [ethanol free; contains propylene glycol, sodium benzoate; wild cherry flavor]

Rescon DM: Chlorpheniramine maleate 2 mg, pseudoephedrine hydrochloride 30 mg, and dextromethorphan hydrobromide 10 mg per 5 mL (120 mL, 480 mL) [dye free, ethanol free, sugar free; cherry flavor]

Liquid, oral [drops]:

Neutrahist PDX: Chlorpheniramine maleate 0.8 mg, pseudoephedrine hydrochloride 9 mg, and dextromethorphan hydrobromide 3 mg per 1 mL (30 mL) [ethanol free, sugar free; contains propylene glycol; grape flavor] [DSC]

Tablet, oral: Chlorpheniramine maleate 4 mg, pseudoephedrine hydrochloride 60 mg, and dextromethorphan hydrobromide 20 mg

Maxichlor PSE DM: Chlorpheniramine maleate 4 mg, pseudoephedrine hydrochloride 60 mg, and dextromethorphan hydrobromide 20 mg [DSC]

Tablet, chewable, oral:

Dicel® DM Chewables: Chlorpheniramine maleate 2 mg, pseudoephedrine hydrochloride 30 mg, and dextromethorphan hydrobromide 10 mg [ethanol free; contains sodium 19 mg/tablet, soy lecithin; cotton candy flavor]

◆ **Chlorpheniramine Tannate and Pseudoephedrine Tannate** *see* Chlorpheniramine and Pseudoephedrine *on page 412*

◆ **Chlorpheniramine Tannate, Pseudoephedrine Tannate, and Dextromethorphan Tannate** *see* Chlorpheniramine, Pseudoephedrine, and Dextromethorphan *on page 414*

ChlorproMAZINE (klor PROE ma zeen)

Brand Names: Canada Chlorpromazine Hydrochloride Inj; Teva-Chlorpromazine

Index Terms Chlorpromazine Hydrochloride; CPZ; Thorazine

Pharmacologic Category Antimanic Agent; Antipsychotic Agent, Typical, Phenothiazine

Additional Appendix Information

Antipsychotic Agents *on page 2290*

Beers Criteria – Potentially Inappropriate Medications for Geriatrics *on page 2368*

Use Management of psychotic disorders (control of mania, treatment of schizophrenia); control of nausea and vomiting; relief of restlessness and apprehension before surgery; acute intermittent porphyria; adjunct in the treatment of tetanus; intractable hiccups; combativeness and/or explosive hyperexcitable behavior in children 1-12 years of age and in short-term treatment of hyperactive children

Unlabeled Use Behavioral symptoms associated with dementia (elderly); psychosis/agitation related to Alzheimer's dementia

Pregnancy Considerations Embryotoxicity was observed in animal reproduction studies. Jaundice or hyper-/hyporeflexia have been reported in newborn infants following maternal use of phenothiazines. Antipsychotic use during the third trimester of pregnancy has a risk for abnormal muscle movements (extrapyramidal symptoms [EPS]) and withdrawal symptoms in newborns following delivery. Symptoms in the newborn may include agitation, feeding disorder, hypertonia, hypotonia, respiratory distress, somnolence, and tremor; these effects may be self-limiting or require hospitalization.

Breast-Feeding Considerations Chlorpromazine and its metabolites have been detected in breast milk; concentrations in the milk do not correlate with those in the mother and may be higher than what is in the maternal plasma.

Contraindications Hypersensitivity to chlorpromazine or any component of the formulation (cross-reactivity between phenothiazines may occur); severe CNS depression; coma

Warnings/Precautions [U.S. Boxed Warning]: Elderly patients with dementia-related psychosis treated with antipsychotics are at an increased risk of death compared to placebo. Most deaths appeared to be either cardiovascular (eg, heart failure, sudden death) or infectious (eg, pneumonia) in nature. Chlorpromazine is not approved for the treatment of dementia-related psychosis. Highly sedating, use with caution in disorders where CNS depression is a feature and in patients with Parkinson's disease. Use with caution in patients with hemodynamic instability, predisposition to seizures, subcortical brain damage, severe cardiac, hepatic, or renal disease. Use caution in respiratory disease (eg, severe asthma, emphysema) due to potential for CNS effects.

Leukopenia, neutropenia, and agranulocytosis (sometimes fatal) have been reported in clinical trials and postmarketing reports with antipsychotic use; presence of risk factors (eg, pre-existing low WBC or history of drug-induced leuko/neutropenia) should prompt periodic blood count assessment. Discontinue therapy at first signs of blood dyscrasias or if absolute neutrophil count <1000/mm^3.

Esophageal dysmotility and aspiration have been associated with antipsychotic use; use with caution in patients at risk of aspiration pneumonia (ie, Alzheimer's disease). Use associated with increased prolactin levels; clinical significance of hyperprolactinemia in patients with breast cancer or other prolactin-dependent tumors is unknown. May alter temperature regulation or mask toxicity of other drugs due to antiemetic effects. May alter cardiac conduction; life-threatening arrhythmias have occurred with therapeutic doses of neuroleptics. May cause QT prolongation and subsequent torsade de pointes; avoid use in patients with diagnosed or suspected congenital long QT syndrome. Avoid concurrent use with other drugs known to prolong QT_c interval.

Use with caution in patients at risk of hypotension (orthostasis is common) or those who would tolerate transient hypotensive episodes (cerebrovascular disease, cardiovascular disease, or other medications which may predispose). Significant hypotension may occur, particularly with parenteral administration. Injection contains sulfites.

Use with caution in patients with decreased gastrointestinal motility, urinary retention, BPH, xerostomia, or visual problems (ie, narrow-angle glaucoma). Relative to other neuroleptics, chlorpromazine has a moderate potency of cholinergic blockade. May cause pigmentary retinopathy, and lenticular and corneal deposits, particularly with prolonged therapy.

May cause extrapyramidal symptoms (EPS), including pseudoparkinsonism, acute dystonic reactions, akathisia, and tardive dyskinesia. Risk of dystonia (and possibly other EPS) may be greater with increased doses, use of conventional antipsychotics, males, and younger patients. May cause neuroleptic malignant syndrome (NMS).

Use in elderly patients with dementia is associated with an increased risk of mortality and cerebrovascular accidents; avoid antipsychotic use for behavioral problems associated with dementia unless alternative nonpharmacologic therapies have failed and patient may harm self or others. In addition, may cause or exacerbate syndrome of inappropriate antidiuretic hormone secretion or hyponatremia; monitor sodium closely with initiation or dosage adjustments in older adults. May be inappropriate in older adults depending on comorbidities (eg, delirium) due to its potent anticholinergic effects (Beers Criteria). Increased risk for developing tardive dyskinesia, particularly in elderly women.

Adverse Reactions Frequency not defined.

Cardiovascular: Orthostatic hypotension, tachycardia, dizziness, nonspecific QT changes

Central nervous system: Drowsiness, dystonias, akathisia, pseudoparkinsonism, tardive dyskinesia, neuroleptic malignant syndrome, seizure

Dermatologic: Photosensitivity, dermatitis, skin pigmentation (slate gray)

Endocrine & metabolic: Lactation, breast engorgement, false-positive pregnancy test, amenorrhea, gynecomastia, hyper- or hypoglycemia

Gastrointestinal: Xerostomia, constipation, nausea

Genitourinary: Urinary retention, ejaculatory disorder, impotence

Hematologic: Agranulocytosis, eosinophilia, leukopenia, hemolytic anemia, aplastic anemia, thrombocytopenic purpura

Hepatic: Jaundice

Ocular: Blurred vision, corneal and lenticular changes, epithelial keratopathy, pigmentary retinopathy

Drug Interactions

Metabolism/Transport Effects Substrate of CYP1A2 (minor), CYP2D6 (major), CYP3A4 (minor); **Note:** Assignment of Major/Minor substrate status based on clinically relevant drug interaction potential; **Inhibits** CYP2D6 (moderate), CYP2E1 (weak)

Avoid Concomitant Use

Avoid concomitant use of ChlorproMAZINE with any of the following: Aclidinium; Amisulpride; Azelastine (Nasal); Highest Risk QTc-Prolonging Agents; Ipratropium (Oral Inhalation); Ivabradine; Metoclopramide; Mifepristone; Paraldehyde; Sulpiride; Thioridazine; Tiotropium; Umeclidinium

Increased Effect/Toxicity

ChlorproMAZINE may increase the levels/effects of: Alcohol (Ethyl); Amisulpride; Analgesics (Opioid); Anticholinergics; Antidepressants (Serotonin Reuptake Inhibitor/Antagonist); ARIPiprazole; Azelastine (Nasal); Beta-Blockers; CNS Depressants; CYP2D6 Substrates; Desmopressin; Fesoterodine; Haloperidol; Highest Risk QTc-Prolonging Agents; Methotrimeprazine; Methylphenidate; Metoprolol; Moderate Risk QTc-Prolonging Agents; Paraldehyde; Porfimer; Serotonin Modulators; Sulpiride; Thioridazine; Tiotropium; Valproic Acid and Derivatives; Zolpidem

The levels/effects of ChlorproMAZINE may be increased by: Abiraterone Acetate; Acetylcholinesterase Inhibitors (Central); Aclidinium; Antidepressants (Serotonin Reuptake Inhibitor/Antagonist); Antimalarial Agents; Beta-Blockers; Brimonidine (Topical); CYP2D6 Inhibitors (Moderate); CYP2D6 Inhibitors (Strong); Darunavir; Doxylamine; Haloperidol; HydrOXYzine; Ipratropium (Oral Inhalation); Ivabradine; Lithium formulations; Magnesium Sulfate; Methotrimeprazine; Methylphenidate; Metoclopramide; Metyrosine; Mifepristone; Perampanel; Pramlintide; QTc-Prolonging Agents (Indeterminate Risk and Risk Modifying); Serotonin Modulators; Sodium Oxybate; Tetrabenazine; Umeclidinium

Decreased Effect

ChlorproMAZINE may decrease the levels/effects of: Amphetamines; Anti-Parkinson's Agents (Dopamine Agonist); Quinagolide; Tamoxifen

The levels/effects of ChlorproMAZINE may be decreased by: Antacids; Anti-Parkinson's Agents (Dopamine Agonist); Lithium formulations; Peginterferon Alfa-2b

Ethanol/Nutrition/Herb Interactions

Ethanol: May increase CNS depression; monitor for increased effects with coadministration. Caution patients about effects.

Herb/Nutraceutical: Avoid St John's wort (may decrease chlorpromazine levels, increase photosensitization, or enhance sedative effect). Avoid dong quai (may enhance photosensitization). Avoid kava kava, gotu kola, valerian (may increase CNS depression).

Preparation for Administration Direct I.V. injection: Dilute with NS to a maximum concentration of 1 mg/mL.

I.V.: For treatment of intractable hiccups the manufacturer recommends diluting 25-50 mg of chlorpromazine in 500-1000 mL NS.

Storage/Stability Injection solution: Protect from light. A slightly yellowed solution does not indicate potency loss, but a markedly discolored solution should be discarded. Solution diluted with NS (1 mg/mL) and stored in 5 mL vials remains stable for 30 days.

Mechanism of Action Chlorpromazine is an aliphatic phenothiazine antipsychotic which blocks postsynaptic mesolimbic dopaminergic receptors in the brain; exhibits a strong alpha-adrenergic blocking effect and depresses the release of hypothalamic and hypophyseal hormones; believed to depress the reticular activating system, thus affecting basal metabolism, body temperature, wakefulness, vasomotor tone, and emesis

Pharmacodynamics/Kinetics

Onset of action: I.M.: 15 minutes; Oral: 30-60 minutes

Absorption: Rapid

Distribution: V_d: 20 L/kg

Protein binding: 92% to 97%

Metabolism: Extensively hepatic to active and inactive metabolites

Bioavailability: 20%

Half-life, biphasic: Initial: 2 hours; Terminal: 30 hours

Excretion: Urine (<1% as unchanged drug) within 24 hours

Dosage

Children ≥6 months:

Schizophrenia/psychoses:

Oral: 0.5-1 mg/kg/dose every 4-6 hours; older children may require 200 mg/day or higher

I.M., I.V.: 0.5-1 mg/kg/dose every 6-8 hours

<5 years (<22.7 kg): Maximum: 40 mg/day

5-12 years (22.7-45.5 kg): Maximum: 75 mg/day

Nausea and vomiting:

Oral: 0.5-1 mg/kg/dose every 4-6 hours as needed

I.M., I.V.: 0.5-1 mg/kg/dose every 6-8 hours

<5 years (<22.7 kg): Maximum: 40 mg/day

5-12 years (22.7-45.5 kg): Maximum: 75 mg/day

Adults:

Schizophrenia/psychoses:

Oral: Range: 30-800 mg/day in 1-4 divided doses, initiate at lower doses and titrate as needed; usual dose: 200-600 mg/day; some patients may require 1-2 g/day

I.M., I.V.: Initial: 25 mg, may repeat (25-50 mg) in 1-4 hours, gradually increase to a maximum of 400 mg/dose every 4-6 hours until patient is controlled; usual dose: 300-800 mg/day

Intractable hiccups:

Oral, I.M.: 25-50 mg 3-4 times/day

I.V. (refractory to oral or I.M. treatment): 25-50 mg via slow I.V. infusion

Nausea and vomiting:

Oral: 10-25 mg every 4-6 hours

I.M., I.V.: 25-50 mg every 4-6 hours

Elderly: Behavioral symptoms associated with dementia (unlabeled use): Initial: 10-25 mg 1-2 times/day; increase at 4- to 7-day intervals by 10-25 mg/day. Increase dose intervals (bid, tid, etc) as necessary to control behavior response or side effects; maximum daily dose: 800 mg; gradual increases (titration) may prevent some side effects or decrease their severity.

Dosing comments in renal impairment: Hemodialysis: Not dialyzable (0% to 5%)

Dosing adjustment/comments in hepatic impairment: Avoid use in severe hepatic dysfunction

Administration Do not administer SubQ (tissue damage and irritation may occur); for direct I.V. injection, administer diluted solution slow I.V. at a rate not to exceed 0.5 mg/minute in children and 1 mg/minute in adults. To reduce the risk of hypotension, patients receiving I.V. chlorpromazine must remain lying down during and for 30 minutes after the injection. **Note:** Avoid skin contact with solution; may cause contact dermatitis.

Monitoring Parameters Vital signs (especially with parenteral use); lipid profile, fasting blood glucose/Hgb A_{1c}; BMI; mental status; abnormal involuntary movement scale (AIMS); extrapyramidal symptoms (EPS); CBC in patients with risk factors for leukopenia/neutropenia

Reference Range

Therapeutic: 50-300 ng/mL (SI: 157-942 nmol/L)

Toxic: >750 ng/mL (SI: >2355 nmol/L); serum concentrations poorly correlate with expected response

Test Interactions False-positives for phenylketonuria, amylase, uroporphyrins, urobilinogen. May cause false-positive pregnancy test. May interfere with urine detection of amphetamine/methamphetamine and methadone (false-positives).

Dosage Forms Excipient information presented when available (limited, particularly for generics); consult specific product labeling.

Solution, Injection, as hydrochloride:

Generic: 25 mg/mL (1 mL, 2 mL)

Tablet, Oral, as hydrochloride:

Generic: 10 mg, 25 mg, 50 mg, 100 mg, 200 mg

◆ **Chlorpromazine Hydrochloride** *see* ChlorproMAZINE *on page 415*

◆ **Chlorpromazine Hydrochloride Inj (Can)** *see* ChlorproMAZINE *on page 415*

ChlorproPAMIDE (klor PROE pa mide)

Brand Names: Canada Apo-Chlorpropamide®

Pharmacologic Category Antidiabetic Agent, Sulfonylurea

Additional Appendix Information

Beers Criteria – Potentially Inappropriate Medications for Geriatrics *on page 2368*

Oral Antidiabetic Agents Comparison Table *on page 2312*

Use Management of blood sugar in type 2 diabetes mellitus (noninsulin dependent, NIDDM) as an adjunct to diet and exercise to lower blood glucose

Unlabeled Use Central (neurogenic) diabetes insipidus

Pregnancy Risk Factor C

Dosage Oral: The dosage of chlorpropamide is variable and should be individualized based upon the patient's response

Initial dose:

Adults: 250 mg daily in mild-to-moderate diabetes in middle-aged, stable diabetic patients

Elderly: 100-125 mg daily

Note: After 5-7 days of initiation, subsequent daily dosages may be increased or decreased by 50-125 mg at 3- to 5-day intervals (slower upward titration may be appropriate in older patients)

Maintenance dose: 100-250 mg daily; severe diabetics may require 500 mg daily; avoid doses >750 mg daily

Dosage adjustment in renal impairment: No specific dosage adjustment provided in manufacturer's labeling; conservative initial and maintenance doses are recommended.

Alternate recommendations (Aronoff, 2007):

Cl_{cr} >50 mL/minute: Reduce dose by 50%.

Cl_{cr} <50 mL/minute: Avoid use.

Hemodialysis: Avoid use.

Peritoneal dialysis: Avoid use.

Continuous renal replacement therapy (CRRT): Avoid use.

Dosage adjustment in hepatic impairment: No specific dosage adjustment provided in manufacturer's labeling; conservative initial and maintenance doses are recommended in patients with liver impairment since chlorpropamide undergoes extensive hepatic metabolism.

Additional Information Complete prescribing information should be consulted for additional detail.

Dosage Forms Excipient information presented when available (limited, particularly for generics); consult specific product labeling.

Tablet, Oral:

Generic: 100 mg, 250 mg

Chlorthalidone (klor THAL i done)

Brand Names: Canada Apo-Chlorthalidone®

Index Terms Hygroton

Pharmacologic Category Antihypertensive; Diuretic, Thiazide

Use Management of mild-to-moderate hypertension when used alone or in combination with other agents; treatment of edema associated with heart failure, renal dysfunction, hepatic cirrhosis, or corticosteroid and estrogen therapy.

Unlabeled Use Pediatric hypertension

Pregnancy Risk Factor B

Dosage Oral:

Children and Adolescents: Hypertension (unlabeled use): Initial: 0.3 mg/kg once daily, up to 2 mg/kg/day; maximum: 50 mg/day (NHBPEP, 2004; NHLBI, 2011)

Adults:

Edema: Initial: 50-100 mg once daily or 100 mg on alternate days; maximum dose: 200 mg/day

Heart failure-associated edema: Initial: 12.5-25 mg once daily; maximum dose: 100 mg/day (ACC/AHA 2009 Heart Failure Guidelines)

Hypertension: Initial: 25 mg once daily; may increase after a suitable trial to 50 mg once daily; maximum: 100 mg/day; usual dosage range (JNC 7): 12.5-25 mg/day

Elderly: Initial: 12.5-25 mg once daily or every other day; there is little advantage to using doses >25 mg/day

Dosage adjustment in renal impairment:

Cl_{cr} ≥10 mL/minute: No dosage adjustment necessary (Aronoff, 2007)

Cl_{cr} <10 mL/minute: Avoid use. Ineffective with low GFR (Aronoff, 2007)

Note: ACC/AHA 2009 Heart Failure Guidelines suggest that thiazides lose their efficacy when Cl_{cr} <40 mL/minute

Dosage adjustment in hepatic impairment: No dosage adjustment provided in manufacturer's labeling; use with caution.

Additional Information Complete prescribing information should be consulted for additional detail.

Dosage Forms Excipient information presented when available (limited, particularly for generics); consult specific product labeling.

Tablet, Oral:

Generic: 25 mg, 50 mg, 100 mg

◆ **Chlorthalidone and Azilsartan** *see* Azilsartan and Chlorthalidone *on page 213*

◆ **Chlor-Tripolon ND® (Can)** *see* Loratadine and Pseudoephedrine *on page 1242*

Chlorzoxazone (klor ZOKS a zone)

Brand Names: U.S. Lorzone; Parafon Forte DSC

Pharmacologic Category Skeletal Muscle Relaxant

Additional Appendix Information

Beers Criteria – Potentially Inappropriate Medications for Geriatrics *on page 2368*

Use Symptomatic treatment of muscle spasm and pain associated with acute musculoskeletal conditions

Dosage Muscle spasm:

Adults: Oral: 500 mg 3-4 times daily, may increase up to 750 mg 3-4 times daily. May consider dose reductions as symptoms improve.

Elderly: In general, avoid use or use cautiously at lower doses. Refer to adult dosing.

Dosage adjustment in renal impairment: No dosage adjustment provided in manufacturer's labeling.

Dosage adjustment in hepatic impairment: No dosage adjustment provided in manufacturer's labeling.

Additional Information Complete prescribing information should be consulted for additional detail.

Dosage Forms Excipient information presented when available (limited, particularly for generics); consult specific product labeling.

Tablet, Oral:

Lorzone: 375 mg [contains sodium benzoate]

Lorzone: 750 mg [scored; contains sodium benzoate]

Parafon Forte DSC: 500 mg [scored; contains brilliant blue fcf (fd&c blue #1), fd&c yellow #10 (quinoline yellow), sodium benzoate]

Generic: 500 mg

◆ **Cholecalciferol and Alendronate** *see* Alendronate and Cholecalciferol *on page 71*

Cholestyramine Resin (koe LES teer a meen REZ in)

Brand Names: U.S. Prevalite; Questran; Questran Light

Brand Names: Canada Novo-Cholamine; Novo-Cholamine Light; Olestyr; PMS-Cholestyramine; Questran; Questran Light Sugar Free; ZYM-Cholestyramine-Light; ZYM-Cholestyramine-Regular

Pharmacologic Category Antilipemic Agent, Bile Acid Sequestrant

Use Adjunct in the management of primary hypercholesterolemia; pruritus associated with elevated levels of bile acids; regression of arteriolosclerosis

Unlabeled Use Diarrhea associated with excess fecal bile acids (Westergaard, 2007); may be used to enhance elimination of digoxin when non-life-threatening toxicity occurs (Henderson, 1988)

Pregnancy Risk Factor C

Dosage Oral (dosages are expressed in terms of anhydrous resin):

Children (unlabeled use): 240 mg/kg/day in 2-3 divided doses; need to titrate dose depending on indication, response and tolerance; maximum: 8 g/day

Adults: Initial: 4 g 1-2 times/day; increase gradually over ≥1-month intervals; maintenance: 8-16 g/day divided in 2 doses; maximum: 24 g/day

Dosage adjustment in renal impairment: No dosage adjustment provided in manufacturer's labeling; however, use with caution in renal impairment; may cause hyperchloremic acidosis.

Dosage adjustment in hepatic impairment: No dosage adjustment necessary; not absorbed from the gastrointestinal tract.

Additional Information Complete prescribing information should be consulted for additional detail.

Dosage Forms Excipient information presented when available (limited, particularly for generics); consult specific product labeling. [DSC] = Discontinued product

Packet, Oral:

Prevalite: 4 g (1 ea, 42 ea, 60 ea) [contains aspartame; orange flavor]

Questran: 4 g (1 ea, 60 ea)

Questran Light: 4 g (1 ea [DSC], 60 ea [DSC]) [sugar free; contains aspartame; orange flavor]

Generic: 4 g (1 ea, 60 ea)

Powder, Oral:

Prevalite: 4 g/dose (231 g) [contains aspartame; orange flavor]

Questran: 4 g/dose (378 g)

Questran Light: 4 g/dose (210 g) [sugar free; contains aspartame]

Generic: 4 g/dose (210 g, 239.4 g, 378 g)

◆ **Choline Fenofibrate** *see* Fenofibrate and Derivatives *on page 837*

Choline Magnesium Trisalicylate

(KOE leen mag NEE zhum trye sa LIS i late)

Index Terms Tricosal; Trilisate

Pharmacologic Category Salicylate

Use Management of osteoarthritis, rheumatoid arthritis, and other arthritis; acute painful shoulder

Pregnancy Risk Factor C/D (3rd trimester)

Pregnancy Considerations Animal reproduction studies have not been conducted. Due to the known effects of other salicylates (closure of ductus arteriosus), use during late pregnancy should be avoided.

Breast-Feeding Considerations Excreted in breast milk; peak levels occur 9-12 hours after dose. Use caution if used during breast-feeding.

Contraindications Hypersensitivity to salicylates, other nonacetylated salicylates, other NSAIDs, or any component of the formulation; bleeding disorders; pregnancy (3rd trimester)

Warnings/Precautions Salicylate salts may not inhibit platelet aggregation and, therefore, should not be substituted for aspirin in the prophylaxis of thrombosis. Use with caution in patients with impaired hepatic or renal function, dehydration, erosive gastritis, asthma, or peptic ulcer. Children and teenagers who have or are recovering from chickenpox or flu-like symptoms should not use this product. Changes in behavior (along with nausea and vomiting) may be an early sign of Reye's syndrome; patients should be instructed to contact their healthcare provider if these occur.

Elderly are a high-risk population for adverse effects from NSAIDs. As many as 60% of elderly can develop peptic ulceration and/or hemorrhage asymptomatically. Use lowest effective dose for shortest period possible. Tinnitus or impaired hearing may indicate toxicity. Tinnitus may be a difficult and unreliable indication of toxicity due to age-related hearing loss or eighth cranial nerve damage. CNS adverse effects may be observed in the elderly at lower doses than younger adults.

Adverse Reactions

<20%:

Gastrointestinal: Nausea, vomiting, diarrhea, heartburn, dyspepsia, epigastric pain, constipation

Otic: Tinnitus

<2%:

Central nervous system: Headache, lightheadedness, dizziness, drowsiness, lethargy

Otic: Hearing impairment

<1%: Anorexia, asthma, BUN and creatinine increased, bruising, confusion, duodenal ulceration, dysgeusia, edema, epistaxis, erythema multiforme, esophagitis, hallucinations, hearing loss (irreversible), hepatic enzymes increased, gastric ulceration, occult bleeding, pruritus, rash, weight gain

Drug Interactions

Metabolism/Transport Effects None known.

Avoid Concomitant Use

Avoid concomitant use of Choline Magnesium Trisalicylate with any of the following: Influenza Virus Vaccine (Live/Attenuated)

Increased Effect/Toxicity

Choline Magnesium Trisalicylate may increase the levels/effects of: Anticoagulants; Carbonic Anhydrase Inhibitors; Corticosteroids (Systemic); Hypoglycemic Agents; Methotrexate; PRALAtrexate; Salicylates; Thrombolytic Agents; Valproic Acid and Derivatives; Varicella Virus-Containing Vaccines; Vitamin K Antagonists

The levels/effects of Choline Magnesium Trisalicylate may be increased by: Agents with Antiplatelet Properties; Ammonium Chloride; Calcium Channel Blockers (Nondihydropyridine); Ginkgo Biloba; Herbs (Anticoagulant/Antiplatelet Properties); Influenza Virus Vaccine (Live/Attenuated); Loop Diuretics; Potassium Acid Phosphate; Treprostinil

Decreased Effect

Choline Magnesium Trisalicylate may decrease the levels/effects of: ACE Inhibitors; Hyaluronidase; Loop Diuretics; Probenecid

The levels/effects of Choline Magnesium Trisalicylate may be decreased by: Corticosteroids (Systemic)

Ethanol/Nutrition/Herb Interactions

Ethanol: Avoid ethanol (may enhance gastric mucosal irritation).

Food: May decrease the rate but not the extent of oral absorption.

Herb/Nutraceutical: Avoid cat's claw, dong quai, evening primrose, feverfew, garlic, ginger, ginkgo, red clover, horse chestnut, green tea, ginseng (all have additional antiplatelet activity). Limit curry powder, paprika, licorice, Benedictine liqueur, prunes, raisins, tea, and gherkins; may cause salicylate accumulation. These foods contain 6 mg salicylate/100 g.

Storage/Stability Store at controlled room temperature of 15°C to 30°C (59°F to 86°F).

Mechanism of Action Weakly inhibits cyclooxygenase enzymes, which results in decreased formation of prostaglandin precursors; antipyretic, analgesic, and anti-inflammatory properties.

Other proposed mechanisms not fully elucidated (and possibly contributing to the anti-inflammatory effect to varying degrees) include inhibiting chemotaxis, altering lymphocyte activity, inhibiting neutrophil aggregation/activation, and decreasing proinflammatory cytokine levels.

Pharmacodynamics/Kinetics

Onset of action: Peak effect: ~2 hours

Absorption: Stomach and small intestines

Distribution: Readily into most body fluids and tissues; crosses placenta; enters breast milk

Half-life elimination (dose dependent): Low dose: 2-3 hours; High dose: 30 hours

Time to peak, serum: ~2 hours

Dosage Oral (based on total salicylate content):

Children <37 kg: 50 mg/kg/day given in 2 divided doses; 2250 mg/day for heavier children

Adults: 500 mg to 1.5 g 2-3 times/day **or** 3 g at bedtime; usual maintenance dose: 1-4.5 g/day

Elderly: 750 mg 3 times/day

Dosage adjustment in renal impairment: Avoid use in severe renal impairment.

Dosage adjustment in hepatic impairment: No dosage adjustment provided in manufacturer's labeling; use with caution.

Dietary Considerations Take with food or large volume of water or milk to minimize GI upset. Liquid may be mixed with fruit juice just before drinking. Hypermagnesemia resulting from magnesium salicylate; avoid or use with caution in renal insufficiency.

Administration Liquid may be mixed with fruit juice just before drinking. Do not administer with antacids.

Monitoring Parameters Serum magnesium with high dose therapy or in patients with impaired renal function; serum salicylate levels, renal function, hearing changes or tinnitus, abnormal bruising, weight gain and response (ie, pain)

Reference Range Salicylate blood levels for anti-inflammatory effect: 150-300 mcg/mL; analgesia and antipyretic effect: 30-50 mcg/mL

Test Interactions False-negative results for glucose oxidase urinary glucose tests (Clinistix®); false-positives using the cupric sulfate method (Clinitest®); also, interferes with Gerhardt test (urinary ketone analysis), VMA determination; 5-HIAA, xylose tolerance test, and T_3 and T_4; increased PBI

Dosage Forms Excipient information presented when available (limited, particularly for generics); consult specific product labeling.

Liquid, Oral:

Generic: 500 mg/5 mL (240 mL)

Tablet, Oral:

Generic: 1000 mg

◆ **Chondroitin Sulfate and Sodium Hyaluronate** *see* Sodium Chondroitin Sulfate and Sodium Hyaluronate *on page 1917*

◆ **Choriogonadotropin Alfa** *see* Chorionic Gonadotropin (Recombinant) *on page 420*

◆ **Chorionic Gonadotropin for Injection (Can)** *see* Chorionic Gonadotropin (Human) *on page 419*

Chorionic Gonadotropin (Human)

(kor ee ON ik goe NAD oh troe pin, HYU man)

Brand Names: U.S. Novarel; Pregnyl

Brand Names: Canada Chorionic Gonadotropin for Injection; Pregnyl®

Index Terms CG; hCG

Pharmacologic Category Gonadotropin; Ovulation Stimulator

Use Induces ovulation and pregnancy in anovulatory, infertile females; treatment of hypogonadotropic hypogonadism, prepubertal cryptorchidism; spermatogenesis induction with follitropin alfa

Pregnancy Risk Factor X

Pregnancy Considerations Teratogenic effects (forelimb, CNS) have been noted in animal studies at doses intended to induce superovulation (used in combination with gonadotropin). Testicular tumors in otherwise healthy men have been reported when treating secondary infertility.

Breast-Feeding Considerations It is not known if chorionic gonadotropin (human) is excreted in breast milk. The manufacturer recommends that caution be exercised when administering chorionic gonadotropin (human) to nursing women.

Contraindications Hypersensitivity to chorionic gonadotropin or any component of the formulation; precocious puberty; prostatic carcinoma or similar neoplasms; pregnancy

Warnings/Precautions Hazardous agent - use appropriate precautions for handling and disposal (NIOSH, 2012).

Use with caution in asthma, seizure disorders, migraine, cardiac or renal disease. **Not** effective in the treatment of obesity. Safety and efficacy in children <4 years of age have not been established.

Cryptorchidism: May induce precocious puberty in children being treated for cryptorchidism; discontinue if signs of precocious puberty occur.

Ovulation induction: These medications should only be used by physicians who are thoroughly familiar with infertility problems and their management. May cause ovarian hyperstimulation syndrome (OHSS); characterized by severe ovarian enlargement, abdominal pain/distention, nausea, vomiting, diarrhea, dyspnea, and oliguria, and may be accompanied by ascites, pleural effusion, hypovolemia, electrolyte imbalance, hemoperitoneum, and thromboembolic events. If severe hyperstimulation occurs, stop treatment and hospitalize patient. This syndrome ▶

develops rapidly with 24 hours to several days and generally occurs during the 7-10 days immediately following treatment. Ovarian enlargement may be accompanied by abdominal distention or abdominal pain and generally regresses without treatment within 2-3 weeks. If ovaries are abnormally enlarged on the last day of treatment, withhold hCG to reduce the risk of OHSS. In association with and separate from OHSS, thromboembolic events have been reported. May result from the use of these medications; advise patients of the potential risk of multiple births before starting the treatment.

Adverse Reactions Frequency not always defined.

Cardiovascular: Edema

Central nervous system: Depression, fatigue, headache, irritability, restlessness

Endocrine & metabolic: Gynecomastia, precocious puberty

Local: Injection site reaction, pain at injection site

Miscellaneous: Hypersensitivity reaction (local or systemic)

<1% (Limited to important or life-threatening): Arterial thrombus, ovarian cyst rupture, ovarian hyperstimulation syndrome

Drug Interactions

Metabolism/Transport Effects None known.

Avoid Concomitant Use There are no known interactions where it is recommended to avoid concomitant use.

Increased Effect/Toxicity There are no known significant interactions involving an increase in effect.

Decreased Effect There are no known significant interactions involving a decrease in effect.

Preparation for Administration Hazardous agent; use appropriate precautions for handling and disposal (NIOSH, 2012). Following reconstitution with the provided diluent, solutions are stable for 30-60 days, depending on the specific preparation, when stored at 2°C to 15°C.

Mechanism of Action Luteinizing hormone obtained from the urine of pregnant women. Stimulates production of gonadal steroid hormones by causing production of androgen by the testes; as a substitute for luteinizing hormone (LH) to stimulate ovulation

Pharmacodynamics/Kinetics

Half-life elimination: Biphasic: Initial: 11 hours; Terminal: 23 hours

Excretion: Urine

Dosage I.M.:

Children: Various regimens:

Prepubertal cryptorchidism:

4000 units 3 times/week for 3 weeks **or**

5000 units every second day for 4 injections **or**

500 units 3 times/week for 4-6 weeks **or**

15 injections of 500-1000 units given over 6 weeks

Hypogonadotropic hypogonadism: Males:

500-1000 units 3 times/week for 3 weeks, followed by the same dose twice weekly for 3 weeks **or**

4000 units 3 times/week for 6-9 months, then reduce dosage to 2000 units 3 times/week for additional 3 months

Adults:

Induction of ovulation: Females: 5000-10,000 units one day following last dose of menotropins

Spermatogenesis induction associated with hypogonadotropic hypogonadism: Males: Treatment regimens vary (range: 1000-2000 units 2-3 times a week). Administer hCG until serum testosterone levels are normal (may require 2-3 months of therapy), then may add follitropin alfa or menopausal gonadotropin if needed to induce spermatogenesis; continue hCG at the dose required to maintain testosterone levels.

Dosage adjustment in renal impairment: No dosage adjustment provided in manufacturer's labeling; use with caution.

Dosage adjustment in hepatic impairment: No dosage adjustment provided in manufacturer's labeling.

Administration I.M. administration only

Hazardous agent; use appropriate precautions for handling and disposal (NIOSH, 2012).

Monitoring Parameters

Male: Serum testosterone levels, semen analysis

Female: Ultrasound and/or estradiol levels to assess follicle development; ultrasound to assess number and size of follicles; ovulation (basal body temperature, serum progestin level, menstruation, sonography)

Reference Range Depends on application and methodology; <3 mIU/mL (SI: <3 units/L) usually normal (nonpregnant)

Test Interactions Cross-reacts with radioimmunoassay of gonadotropins, especially LH

Dosage Forms Excipient information presented when available (limited, particularly for generics); consult specific product labeling.

Solution Reconstituted, Intramuscular:

Novarel: 10,000 units (1 ea) [contains benzyl alcohol]

Pregnyl: 10,000 units (1 ea) [contains benzyl alcohol, sodium chloride]

Generic: 10,000 units (1 ea)

Chorionic Gonadotropin (Recombinant)

(kor ee ON ik goe NAD oh troe pin ree KOM be nant)

Brand Names: U.S. Ovidrel

Brand Names: Canada Ovidrel®

Index Terms Choriogonadotropin Alfa; r-hCG

Pharmacologic Category Gonadotropin; Ovulation Stimulator

Use As part of an assisted reproductive technology (ART) program, induces ovulation in infertile females who have been pretreated with follicle stimulating hormones (FSH); induces ovulation and pregnancy in infertile females when the cause of infertility is functional

Pregnancy Risk Factor X

Pregnancy Considerations Intrauterine death and impaired birth were observed in animal studies. Ectopic pregnancy, premature labor, postpartum fever, and spontaneous abortion have been reported in clinical trials. Congenital abnormalities have also been observed, however, the incidence is similar during natural conception.

Breast-Feeding Considerations It is not known if chorionic gonadotropin (recombinant) is excreted in breast milk. The manufacturer recommends that caution be exercised when administering chorionic gonadotropin (recombinant) to nursing women.

Contraindications Hypersensitivity to hCG preparations or any component of the formulation; primary ovarian failure; uncontrolled thyroid or adrenal dysfunction; uncontrolled organic intracranial lesion (ie, pituitary tumor); abnormal uterine bleeding, ovarian cyst or enlargement of undetermined origin; sex hormone dependent tumors; pregnancy

Warnings/Precautions Hazardous agent - use appropriate precautions for handling and disposal (NIOSH, 2012). Ovarian enlargement may occur; may be accompanied by abdominal distention or abdominal pain and generally regresses without treatment within 2-3 weeks. If ovaries are abnormally enlarged on the last day of treatment, withhold hCG to reduce the risk of ovarian hyperstimulation syndrome (OHSS). OHSS is characterized by severe ovarian enlargement, abdominal pain/distention, nausea, vomiting, diarrhea, dyspnea, and oliguria, and may be accompanied by ascites, pleural effusion, hypovolemia, electrolyte imbalance, hemoperitoneum, and thromboembolic events. If severe hyperstimulation occurs, stop treatment and hospitalize patient. This syndrome develops rapidly with 24 hours to several days and generally occurs during the 7-10 days immediately following treatment.

Arterial thromboembolic events have been reported in association with and separate from OHSS. These medications should only be used by healthcare providers who are thoroughly familiar with infertility problems and their management. Multiple births may result from the use of these medications; advise patients of the potential risk of multiple births before starting the treatment. Safety and efficacy have not been established in the elderly or in children.

Adverse Reactions

2% to 10%:

Endocrine & metabolic: Ovarian cyst (3%), ovarian hyperstimulation (<2% to 3%)

Gastrointestinal: Abdominal pain (3% to 4%), nausea (3%), vomiting (3%)

Local: Injection site: Pain (8%), bruising (3% to 5%), reaction (<2% to 3%), inflammation (<2% to 2%)

Miscellaneous: Postoperative pain (5%)

<2% (Limited to important or life-threatening): Abdominal enlargement, albuminuria, allergic reaction, back pain, breast pain, cardiac arrhythmia, cervical carcinoma, cervical lesion, cough, diarrhea, dizziness, dysuria, ectopic pregnancy, emotional lability, fever, flatulence, genital herpes, genital moniliasis, headache, heart murmur, hiccups, hot flashes, hyperglycemia, insomnia, intermenstrual bleeding, leukocytosis, leukorrhea, malaise, paresthesia, pharyngitis, pruritus, rash, upper respiratory tract infection, urinary incontinence, urinary tract infection, vaginal discomfort, vaginal hemorrhage, vaginitis

In addition, the following have been reported with menotropin therapy: Adnexal torsion, hemoperitoneum, mild-to-moderate ovarian enlargement, pulmonary and vascular complications. Ovarian neoplasms have also been reported (rare) with multiple drug regimens used for ovarian induction (relationship not established).

Drug Interactions

Metabolism/Transport Effects None known.

Avoid Concomitant Use There are no known interactions where it is recommended to avoid concomitant use.

Increased Effect/Toxicity There are no known significant interactions involving an increase in effect.

Decreased Effect There are no known significant interactions involving a decrease in effect.

Storage/Stability Prefilled syringe: Prior to dispensing, store at 2°C to 8°C (36°F to 46°F). Patient may store at 25°C (77°F) for up to 30 days. Protect from light.

Mechanism of Action Luteinizing hormone analogue produced by recombinant DNA techniques; stimulates late follicular maturation and intitates rupture of the ovarian follicle once follicular development has occurred

Pharmacodynamics/Kinetics

Distribution: V_d: 21.4L

Bioavailability: 40%

Half-life elimination: Initial: 4 hours; Terminal: 29 hours

Time to peak: 12-24 hours

Excretion: Urine (10% of dose)

Dosage SubQ:

Adults: Females:

Assisted reproductive technologies (ART) and ovulation induction: 250 mcg given 1 day following the last dose of follicle stimulating agent. Use only after adequate follicular development has been determined. Hold treatment when there is an excessive ovarian response.

Elderly: Safety and efficacy have not been established

Dosage adjustment in renal impairment: Safety and efficacy have not been established

Dosage adjustment in hepatic impairment: Safety and efficacy have not been established

Administration For SubQ use only; inject into stomach area.

Hazardous agent; use appropriate precautions for handling and disposal (NIOSH, 2012).

Monitoring Parameters Ultrasound and/or estradiol levels to assess follicle development; ultrasound to assess number and size of follicles; ovulation (basal body temperature, serum progestin level, menstruation, sonography)

Test Interactions May interfere with interpretation of pregnancy tests; may cross-react with radioimmunoassay of luteinizing hormone and other gonadotropins

Additional Information Clinical studies have shown r-hCG to be clinically and statistically equivalent to urinary-derived hCG products.

Dosage Forms Excipient information presented when available (limited, particularly for generics); consult specific product labeling.

Injectable, Subcutaneous:

Ovidrel: 250 mcg/0.5 mL (0.5 mL)

◆ **CI-1008** *see* Pregabalin *on page 1710*

◆ **Cialis** *see* Tadalafil *on page 1983*

Ciclesonide (Systemic) (sye KLES oh nide)

Brand Names: U.S. Alvesco

Brand Names: Canada Alvesco®

Pharmacologic Category Corticosteroid, Inhalant (Oral)

Use Prophylactic management of bronchial asthma

Pregnancy Risk Factor C

Pregnancy Considerations Adverse events were observed in some animal reproduction studies. Hypoadrenalism may occur in infants born to mothers receiving corticosteroids during pregnancy. Based on available data, an overall increased risk of congenital malformations or a decrease in fetal growth has not been associated with maternal use of inhaled corticosteroids during pregnancy (Bakhireva, 2005; NAEPP, 2005; Namazy, 2004). Uncontrolled asthma is associated with adverse events in pregnancy (increased risk of perinatal mortality, pre-eclampsia, preterm birth, low birth weight infants). Inhaled corticosteroids are recommended for the treatment of asthma during pregnancy (most information available using budesonide) (ACOG, 2008; NAEPP, 2005).

Breast-Feeding Considerations Systemic corticosteroids are excreted in human milk. It is not known if sufficient quantities of ciclesonide are absorbed following oral inhalation to produce detectable amounts in breast milk; however, oral absorption is limited (<1%). The manufacturer recommends that caution be exercised when administering ciclesonide to nursing women. The use of inhaled corticosteroids is not considered a contraindication to breast-feeding (NAEPP, 2005).

Contraindications Hypersensitivity to ciclesonide or any component of the formulation; primary treatment of acute asthma or status asthmaticus

Canadian labeling: Additional contraindications (not in U.S. labeling): Untreated fungal, bacterial, or tuberculosis infections of the respiratory tract; moderate-to-severe bronchiectasis

Warnings/Precautions May cause hypercorticism or suppression of hypothalamic-pituitary-adrenal (HPA) axis, particularly in younger children or in patients receiving high doses for prolonged periods. HPA axis suppression may lead to adrenal crisis. Withdrawal and discontinuation of a corticosteroid should be done slowly and carefully. Particular care is required when patients are transferred from systemic corticosteroids to inhaled products due to possible adrenal insufficiency or withdrawal from steroids, including an increase in allergic symptoms. Patients receiving >20 mg per day of prednisone (or equivalent) may be most susceptible. Fatalities have occurred due to adrenal insufficiency in asthmatic patients during and after transfer from systemic corticosteroids to aerosol steroids;

aerosol steroids do **not** provide the systemic steroid needed to treat patients having trauma, surgery, or infections.

Bronchospasm may occur with wheezing after inhalation; if this occurs stop steroid and treat with a fast-acting bronchodilator. Supplemental steroids (oral or parenteral) may be needed during stress or severe asthma attacks. Not to be used in status asthmaticus or for the relief of acute bronchospasm. Oropharyngeal thrush due to candida albicans infection may occur with use. Prolonged use of corticosteroids may also increase the incidence of secondary infection, mask acute infection (including fungal infections), prolong or exacerbate viral infections, or limit response to vaccines. Exposure to chickenpox and measles should be avoided; corticosteroids should not be used to treat ocular herpes simplex. Close observation is required in patients with latent tuberculosis and/or TB reactivity; restrict use in active TB (only in conjunction with antituberculosis treatment). Use in patients with TB is contraindicated in the Canadian labeling. Prolonged treatment with corticosteroids has been associated with the development of Kaposi's sarcoma (case reports); if noted, discontinuation of therapy should be considered.

Use with caution in patients with cardiovascular disease, diabetes, severe hepatic impairment, thyroid disease, psychiatric disturbances, myasthenia gravis, glaucoma, cataracts, patients at risk for osteoporosis, and patients at risk for seizures. Use in renally-impaired patients has not been studied; however, ≤20% of drug is eliminated renally. Use with caution in elderly patients.

Orally inhaled corticosteroids may cause a reduction in growth velocity in pediatric patients (~1 cm per year [range: 0.3-1.8 cm per year] and related to dose and duration of exposure). To minimize the systemic effects of orally inhaled corticosteroids, each patient should be titrated to the lowest effective dose. Growth should be routinely monitored in pediatric patients.

Adverse Reactions

>10%:
- Central nervous system: Headache (≤11%)
- Respiratory: Nasopharyngitis (≤11%)

1% to 10%:
- Cardiovascular: Facial edema (≥3%)
- Central nervous system: Dizziness (≥3%), fatigue (≥3%), dysphonia (1%)
- Dermatologic: Urticaria (≥3%)
- Gastrointestinal: Gastroenteritis (≥3%), oral candidiasis (≥3%)
- Neuromuscular & skeletal: Arthralgia (≥3%), musculoskeletal chest pain (≥3%), back pain (≥3%), extremity pain (≥3%)
- Ocular: Conjunctivitis (≥3%)
- Otic: Ear pain (2%)
- Respiratory: Upper respiratory infection (≤9%), nasal congestion (≤6%), pharyngolaryngeal pain (≤5%), hoarseness (≥3%), pneumonia (≥3%), sinusitis (≥3%), paradoxical bronchospasm (2%)
- Miscellaneous: Influenza (≥3%)

<1% (Limited to important or life-threatening): ALT increased, angioedema (with swelling of lip/pharynx/tongue), bruising, candidiasis (pharyngeal), cataract, chest discomfort, cough, dry throat, dysgeusia, dyspepsia, GGT increased, intraocular pressure increased, nausea, palpitation, pharyngitis, rash, throat irritation, weight gain, xerostomia

Drug Interactions

Metabolism/Transport Effects Substrate of CYP3A4 (minor); **Note:** Assignment of Major/Minor substrate status based on clinically relevant drug interaction potential

Avoid Concomitant Use

Avoid concomitant use of Ciclesonide (Oral Inhalation) with any of the following: Aldesleukin

Increased Effect/Toxicity

Ciclesonide (Oral Inhalation) may increase the levels/effects of: Amphotericin B; Deferasirox; Loop Diuretics; Thiazide Diuretics

The levels/effects of Ciclesonide (Oral Inhalation) may be increased by: CYP3A4 Inhibitors (Strong); Telaprevir

Decreased Effect

Ciclesonide (Oral Inhalation) may decrease the levels/effects of: Aldesleukin; Antidiabetic Agents; Corticorelin; Hyaluronidase; Telaprevir

Storage/Stability Store at 15°C to 30°C (59°F to 86°F); do not freeze.

Mechanism of Action Ciclesonide is a nonhalogenated, glucocorticoid prodrug that is hydrolyzed to the pharmacologically active metabolite des-ciclesonide following administration. Des-ciclesonide has a high affinity for the glucocorticoid receptor and exhibits anti-inflammatory activity. The mechanism of action for corticosteroids is believed to be a combination of three important properties – anti-inflammatory activity, immunosuppressive properties, and antiproliferative actions.

Pharmacodynamics/Kinetics

Absorption: 52% (lung deposition)

Protein binding: ≥99%

Metabolism: Ciclesonide hydrolyzed to its active metabolite, des-ciclesonide via esterases in nasal mucosa and lungs; des-ciclesonide undergoes further hepatic metabolism primarily via CYP3A4 and to a lesser extent via CYP2D6

Bioavailability: 63% (active metabolite)

Half-life elimination: ~6-7 hours (active metabolite)

Time to peak: ~1 hour (active metabolite)

Excretion: Feces (66%); urine (≤20% as active metabolite)

Dosage Oral inhalation (Alvesco®):

Asthma: **Note:** Titrate to the lowest effective dose once asthma stability is achieved:

U.S. labeling: Children ≥12 years and Adults:
- Prior therapy with bronchodilators alone: Initial: 80 mcg twice daily (maximum dose: 320 mcg/day)
- Prior therapy with inhaled corticosteroids: Initial: 80 mcg twice daily (maximum dose: 640 mcg/day)
- Prior therapy with oral corticosteroids: Initial: 320 mcg twice daily (maximum dose: 640 mcg/day)

Canadian labeling:
- Children 6-11 years: Initial: 100-200 mcg once daily; maintenance: 100-200 mcg/day (1-2 puffs once daily)
- Children ≥12 years and Adults: Initial: 400 mcg once daily; maintenance: 100-800 mcg/day (1-2 puffs once daily; more severe asthma may require 400 mcg twice daily)
- **Note:** Canadian Thoracic Society 2010 Asthma Management guidelines recommend dose titration in children 6-11 years who fail to achieve an adequate response in spite of adherence to therapy and/or lack of alternative factors (eg, environmental triggers) which might impair response. In children ≥12 years and adults, doses >200 mcg/day may provide minimal additional benefit while increasing risks for adverse events; add-on therapy should be considered prior to dose increases >200 mcg/day (Lougheed, 2010).

Global Strategy for Asthma Management and Prevention, 2011: Children >5 years and Adults:
- "Low" dose: 80-160 mcg/day
- "Medium" dose: >160-320 mcg/day
- "High" dose: >320 mcg/day

Conversion from oral to orally-inhaled steroid: Initiation of oral inhalation therapy should begin in patients who have previously been stabilized on oral corticosteroids (OCS). A gradual dose reduction of OCS should begin ~7-10 days after starting inhaled therapy. U.S. labeling recommends reducing prednisone dose no more rapidly than ≤2.5 mg/day on a weekly basis. The Canadian labeling recommends decreasing the daily dose of prednisone by 1 mg (or equivalent of other OCS) every 7 days in closely monitored patients, and every 10 days in patients whom close monitoring is not possible. In the presence of withdrawal symptoms, resume previous OCS dose for 1 week before attempting further dose reductions.

Dosage adjustment in renal impairment: There are no dosage adjustments provided in the manufacturer labeling (has not been studied); however, dose adjustments may not be necessary as ≤20% of drug is eliminated renally.

Dosage adjustment in hepatic impairment: Dosage adjustments are not necessary.

Administration Remove mouthpiece cover, place inhaler in mouth, close lips around mouthpiece, and inhale slowly and deeply. Press down on top of inhaler after slow inhalation has begun. Remove inhaler while holding breath for approximately 10 seconds. Breathe out slowly and replace mouthpiece on inhaler. Rinse mouth with water (and spit out) after inhalation. Do not wash or place inhaler in water. Clean mouthpiece using a dry cloth or tissue once weekly. Discard after the "discard by" date or after labeled number of doses has been used, even if container is not completely empty.

Shaking is not necessary since drug is formulated as a solution aerosol. Prime inhaler prior to initial use or if not in use for ≥7-10 days by releasing 3 puffs into the air.

Monitoring Parameters Growth (adolescents) and signs/symptoms of HPA axis suppression/adrenal insufficiency; ocular effects (eg, cataracts, increased intraocular pressure, glaucoma)

Additional Information The incidence of oral candidiasis, as well as other localized oropharyngeal effects, observed with ciclesonide use has been reported to be approximately one-half of that seen with other commonly inhaled corticosteroids such as budesonide and fluticasone. Small particle size, minimal activation, and deposition in the oropharynx may explain this decreased incidence.

Dosage Forms Considerations Alvesco 6.1 g canisters contain 60 inhalations.

Dosage Forms Excipient information presented when available (limited, particularly for generics); consult specific product labeling.

Aerosol Solution, Inhalation:

Alvesco: 80 mcg/actuation (6.1 g); 160 mcg/actuation (6.1 g)

Dosage Forms: Canada Excipient information presented when available (limited, particularly for generics); consult specific product labeling.

Aerosol for oral inhalation:

Alvesco®: 100 mcg/inhalation [30-, 60-, and 120 metered actuations]; 200 mcg/inhalation [30-, 60-, and 120 metered actuations]

Ciclesonide (Nasal) (sye KLES oh nide)

Brand Names: U.S. Omnaris; Zetonna

Brand Names: Canada Drymira; Omnaris

Pharmacologic Category Corticosteroid, Nasal

Use Management of seasonal and perennial allergic rhinitis

Unlabeled Use Adjunct to antibiotics in empiric treatment of acute bacterial rhinosinusitis (ABRS) (Chow, 2012)

Pregnancy Risk Factor C

Dosage Intranasal:

Seasonal allergic rhinitis:

Omnaris®:

U.S. labeling: Children ≥6 years and Adults: 2 sprays (50 mcg/spray) per nostril once daily; maximum: 200 mcg/day

Canadian labeling: Children ≥12 years and Adults: 2 sprays (50 mcg/spray) per nostril once daily; maximum: 200 mcg/day

Zetonna™: Children ≥12 years and Adults: 1 spray (37 mcg/spray) per nostril once daily; maximum: 74 mcg/day

Perennial allergic rhinitis: Children ≥12 years and Adults:

Omnaris®: 2 sprays (50 mcg/spray) per nostril once daily; maximum: 200 mcg/day

Zetonna™: 1 spray (37 mcg/spray) per nostril once daily; maximum: 74 mcg/day

Dosage adjustment in renal impairment: No dosage adjustment provided in manufacturer's labeling (has not been studied).

Dosage adjustment in hepatic impairment: No dosage adjustment necessary.

Additional Information Complete prescribing information should be consulted for additional detail.

Dosage Forms Considerations

Omnaris 12.5 g bottles contain 120 actuations.

Zetonna 6.1 g canisters contain 60 actuations.

Dosage Forms Excipient information presented when available (limited, particularly for generics); consult specific product labeling.

Aerosol Solution, Nasal:

Zetonna: 37 mcg/actuation (6.1 g)

Suspension, Nasal:

Omnaris: 50 mcg/actuation (12.5 g) [contains edetate sodium (tetrasodium)]

◆ Ciclodan *see* Ciclopirox *on page 423*
◆ Ciclodan Cream *see* Ciclopirox *on page 423*
◆ Ciclodan Solution *see* Ciclopirox *on page 423*

Ciclopirox (sye kloe PEER oks)

Brand Names: U.S. Ciclodan; Ciclodan Cream; Ciclodan Solution; Ciclopirox Treatment; CNL8 Nail; Loprox; Pedipirox-4 Nail; Penlac

Brand Names: Canada Apo-Ciclopirox; Loprox; Penlac; PMS-Ciclopirox; Stieprox; Taro-Ciclopirox

Index Terms Ciclopirox Olamine

Pharmacologic Category Antifungal Agent, Topical

Use

Cream/suspension: Treatment of tinea pedis (athlete's foot), tinea cruris (jock itch), tinea corporis (ringworm), cutaneous candidiasis, and tinea versicolor (pityriasis)

Gel: Treatment of tinea pedis (athlete's foot), tinea corporis (ringworm); seborrheic dermatitis of the scalp

Lacquer (solution): Topical treatment of mild-to-moderate onychomycosis of the fingernails and toenails due to *Trichophyton rubrum* (not involving the lunula) and the immediately-adjacent skin

Shampoo: Treatment of seborrheic dermatitis of the scalp

Pregnancy Risk Factor B

Dosage Topical:

Children >10 years and Adults: Tinea pedis, tinea cruris, tinea corporis, cutaneous candidiasis, and tinea versicolor: Cream/suspension: Apply twice daily, gently massage into affected areas; if no improvement after 4 weeks of treatment, re-evaluate the diagnosis.

Children ≥12 years and Adults: Onychomycosis of the fingernails and toenails: Lacquer (solution): Apply to adjacent skin and affected nails daily (as a part of a comprehensive management program for onychomycosis). Remove with alcohol every 7 days.

Children >16 years and Adults:

Tinea pedis, tinea corporis: Gel: Apply twice daily, gently massage into affected areas and surrounding skin; if no improvement after 4 weeks of treatment, re-evaluate diagnosis

Seborrheic dermatitis of the scalp:

Gel: Apply twice daily, gently massage into affected areas and surrounding skin; if no improvement after 4 weeks of treatment, re-evaluate diagnosis.

Shampoo: Apply ~5 mL to wet hair; lather, and leave in place ~3 minutes; rinse. May use up to 10 mL for longer hair. Repeat twice weekly for 4 weeks; allow a minimum of 3 days between applications; if no improvement after 4 weeks of treatment, re-evaluate diagnosis.

Dosage adjustment in renal impairment: No dosage adjustment provided in manufacturer's labeling.

Dosage adjustment in hepatic impairment: No dosage adjustment provided in manufacturer's labeling.

Additional Information Complete prescribing information should be consulted for additional detail.

Dosage Forms Excipient information presented when available (limited, particularly for generics); consult specific product labeling.

Cream, External, as olamine:

Ciclodan: 0.77% (90 g) [contains benzyl alcohol, cetyl alcohol]

Generic: 0.77% (15 g, 30 g, 90 g)

Gel, External:

Loprox: 0.77% (30 g, 45 g, 100 g) [contains isopropyl alcohol]

Generic: 0.77% (30 g, 45 g, 100 g)

Kit, External:

Ciclodan Cream: 0.77% [contains benzyl alcohol, cetyl alcohol, edetate disodium, propylene glycol]

Ciclodan Solution: 8% [contains edetate disodium, isopropyl alcohol, menthol]

Ciclopirox Treatment: 8% [contains edetate disodium, isopropyl alcohol, menthol]

CNL8 Nail: 8% [contains isopropyl alcohol]

Pedipirox-4 Nail: 8% [contains isopropyl alcohol]

Generic: 8%

Shampoo, External:

Loprox: 1% (120 mL)

Generic: 1% (120 mL)

Solution, External:

Ciclodan: 8% (6.6 mL) [contains isopropyl alcohol]

Penlac: 8% (6.6 mL) [contains ethyl acetate, isopropyl alcohol]

Generic: 8% (6.6 mL)

Suspension, External, as olamine:

Generic: 0.77% (30 mL, 60 mL)

◆ **Ciclopirox Olamine** *see* Ciclopirox *on page 423*

◆ **Ciclopirox Treatment** *see* Ciclopirox *on page 423*

◆ **Ciclosporin** *see* CycloSPORINE (Ophthalmic) *on page 515*

◆ **Ciclosporin** *see* CycloSPORINE (Systemic) *on page 508*

◆ **Cidecin** *see* DAPTOmycin *on page 541*

Cidofovir (si DOF o veer)

Brand Names: U.S. Vistide

Pharmacologic Category Antiviral Agent

Use Treatment of cytomegalovirus (CMV) retinitis in patients with acquired immunodeficiency syndrome (AIDS). **Note:** Should be administered with probenecid.

Pregnancy Risk Factor C

Pregnancy Considerations [U.S. Boxed Warning]: Possibly carcinogenic and teratogenic based on animal data. May cause hypospermia. Cidofovir was shown to be teratogenic and embryotoxic in animal studies, some at doses which also produced maternal toxicity. Reduced testes weight and hypospermia were also noted in animal studies. There are no adequate and well-controlled studies in pregnant women; use during pregnancy only if the potential benefit to the mother outweighs the possible risk to the fetus. Women of childbearing potential should use effective contraception during therapy and for 1 month following treatment. Males should use a barrier contraceptive during therapy and for 3 months following treatment.

Breast-Feeding Considerations The CDC recommends **not** to breast-feed if diagnosed with HIV to avoid postnatal transmission of the virus.

Contraindications Hypersensitivity to cidofovir; history of clinically-severe hypersensitivity to probenecid or other sulfa-containing medications; serum creatinine >1.5 mg/dL; Cl_{cr} <55 mL/minute; urine protein ≥100 mg/dL (≥2+ proteinuria); use with or within 7 days of nephrotoxic agents; direct intraocular injection

Warnings/Precautions Hazardous agent - use appropriate precautions for handling and disposal (NIOSH, 2012). **[U.S. Boxed Warning]: Dose-dependent nephrotoxicity requires dose adjustment or discontinuation if changes in renal function occur during therapy (eg, proteinuria, glycosuria, decreased serum phosphate, uric acid or bicarbonate, and elevated creatinine). Neutropenia has been reported;** monitor counts during therapy. Cases of ocular hypotony have also occurred; monitor intraocular pressure. Monitor for signs of metabolic acidosis. Safety and efficacy have not been established in children or the elderly. Administration must be accompanied by oral probenecid and intravenous saline prehydration. **[U.S. Boxed Warning]: Indicated only for CMV retinitis treatment in HIV patients; possibly carcinogenic and teratogenic based on animal data. May cause hypospermia.**

Adverse Reactions

>10%:

Central nervous system: Chills, fever, headache, pain

Dermatologic: Alopecia, rash

Gastrointestinal: Nausea, vomiting, diarrhea, anorexia

Hematologic: Anemia, neutropenia

Neuromuscular & skeletal: Weakness

Ocular: Intraocular pressure decreased, iritis, ocular hypotony, uveitis

Renal: Creatinine increased, proteinuria, renal toxicity

Respiratory: Cough, dyspnea

Miscellaneous: Infection, oral moniliasis, serum bicarbonate decreased

1% to 10%:

Renal: Fanconi syndrome

Respiratory: Pneumonia

<1%: Hepatic failure, metabolic acidosis, pancreatitis

Frequency not defined (limited to important or life-threatening reactions):

Cardiovascular: Cardiomyopathy, cardiovascular disorder, CHF, edema, orthostatic hypotension, shock, syncope, tachycardia

Central nervous system: Agitation, amnesia, anxiety, confusion, convulsion, dizziness, hallucinations, insomnia, malaise, vertigo

Dermatologic: Photosensitivity reaction, skin discoloration, urticaria

Endocrine & metabolic: Adrenal cortex insufficiency

Gastrointestinal: Abdominal pain, aphthous stomatitis, colitis, constipation, dysphagia, fecal incontinence, gastritis, GI hemorrhage, gingivitis, melena, proctitis, splenomegaly, stomatitis, tongue discoloration
Genitourinary: Urinary incontinence
Hematologic: Hypochromic anemia, leukocytosis, leukopenia, lymphadenopathy, lymphoma-like reaction, pancytopenia, thrombocytopenia, thrombocytopenic purpura
Hepatic: Hepatomegaly, hepatosplenomegaly, jaundice, liver function tests abnormal, liver damage, liver necrosis
Local: Injection site reaction
Neuromuscular & skeletal: Tremor
Ocular: Amblyopia, blindness, cataract, conjunctivitis, corneal lesion, diplopia, vision abnormal
Otic: Hearing loss
Miscellaneous: Allergic reaction, sepsis

Drug Interactions

Metabolism/Transport Effects None known.

Avoid Concomitant Use There are no known interactions where it is recommended to avoid concomitant use.

Increased Effect/Toxicity

Cidofovir may increase the levels/effects of: Tenofovir

Decreased Effect There are no known significant interactions involving a decrease in effect.

Preparation for Administration Hazardous agent; use appropriate precautions for handling and disposal (NIOSH, 2012). Dilute dose in NS 100 mL prior to infusion.

Storage/Stability Store at controlled room temperature 20°C to 25°C (68°F to 77°F). Store admixtures under refrigeration for ≤24 hours. Cidofovir infusion admixture should be administered within 24 hours of preparation at room temperature or refrigerated. Admixtures should be allowed to equilibrate to room temperature prior to use.

Mechanism of Action Cidofovir is converted to cidofovir diphosphate which is the active intracellular metabolite; cidofovir diphosphate suppresses CMV replication by selective inhibition of viral DNA synthesis. Incorporation of cidofovir into growing viral DNA chain results in reductions in the rate of viral DNA synthesis.

Pharmacodynamics/Kinetics The following pharmacokinetic data is based on a combination of cidofovir administered with probenecid:

Distribution: V_d: 0.54 L/kg; does not cross significantly into CSF
Protein binding: <6%
Metabolism: Minimal; phosphorylation occurs intracellularly
Half-life elimination, plasma: ~2.6 hours
Excretion: Urine

Dosage Adults:

Induction: 5 mg/kg I.V. over 1 hour once weekly for 2 consecutive weeks
Maintenance: 5 mg/kg over 1 hour once every other week

Note: Administer with probenecid 2 g orally 3 hours prior to each cidofovir dose and 1 g at 2 hours and 8 hours after completion of the infusion (total: 4 g)

Hydrate with at least 1 L of 0.9% NS I.V. prior to each cidofovir infusion; infuse saline over a 1- to 2-hour period immediately prior to cidofovir infusion. A second liter may be administered over a 1- to 3-hour period at the start of cidofovir infusion or immediately following infusion, if tolerated

Dosage adjustment in renal impairment:

Changes in renal function during therapy: If the creatinine increases by 0.3-0.4 mg/dL, reduce the cidofovir dose to 3 mg/kg; discontinue therapy for increases ≥0.5 mg/dL or development of ≥3+ proteinuria

Pre-existing renal impairment: Use is contraindicated with serum creatinine >1.5 mg/dL, Cl_{cr} <55 mL/minute, or urine protein ≥100 mg/dL (≥2+ proteinuria)

Dosage adjustment in hepatic impairment: No dosage adjustment provided in manufacturer's labeling.

Administration For I.V. infusion only. Infuse over 1 hour. Hydrate with 1 L of 0.9% NS I.V. prior to cidofovir infusion. A second liter may be administered over a 1- to 3-hour period immediately following infusion, if tolerated.

Hazardous agent; use appropriate precautions for handling and disposal (NIOSH, 2012).

Monitoring Parameters Serum creatinine and urine protein (within 48 hours of each dose), WBCs (prior to each dose); intraocular pressure and visual acuity, signs and symptoms of uveitis/iritis

Dosage Forms Excipient information presented when available (limited, particularly for generics); consult specific product labeling.

Solution, Intravenous:
Vistide: 75 mg/mL (5 mL)
Solution, Intravenous [preservative free]:
Generic: 75 mg/mL (5 mL)

Cilostazol (sil OH sta zol)

Brand Names: U.S. Pletal

Index Terms OPC-13013

Pharmacologic Category Antiplatelet Agent; Phosphodiesterase-3 Enzyme Inhibitor

Additional Appendix Information

Oral Antiplatelet Comparison Chart *on page 2313*

Use Symptomatic management of peripheral vascular disease, primarily intermittent claudication

Unlabeled Use Adjunct with aspirin and clopidogrel for prevention of stent thrombosis and restenosis after coronary stent placement; as an alternative agent to either aspirin or clopidogrel in a dual antiplatelet regimen when allergy or drug intolerance to either agent occurs in patients who have undergone elective PCI with bare metal or drug-eluting stent placement; secondary prevention of noncardioembolic ischemic stroke or transient ischemic attack (TIA)

Pregnancy Risk Factor C

Pregnancy Considerations Adverse events have been observed in animal reproduction studies.

Breast-Feeding Considerations It is not known if cilostazol is excreted in human milk. According to the manufacturer, the decision to continue or discontinue breastfeeding during therapy should take into account the risk of exposure to the infant and the benefits of treatment to the mother.

Contraindications Hypersensitivity to cilostazol or any component of the formulation; heart failure (HF) of any severity; hemostatic disorders or active bleeding

Warnings/Precautions [U.S. Boxed Warning]: The use of this drug is contraindicated in patients with heart failure. Use with caution in severe underlying heart disease. Use with caution in patients receiving other platelet aggregation inhibitors or in patients with thrombocytopenia. Discontinue therapy if thrombocytopenia or leukopenia occur; progression to agranulocytosis (reversible) has been reported when cilostazol was not immediately stopped. Withhold for at least 4-6 half-lives prior to elective surgical procedures. Use caution in moderate-to-severe hepatic impairment. Use cautiously in severe renal impairment (Cl_{cr} <25 mL/minute). Potentially significant drug-drug interactions may exist, requiring dose or frequency adjustment, additional monitoring, and/or selection of alternative therapy.

Adverse Reactions

>10%:

Central nervous system: Headache (27% to 34%)
Gastrointestinal: Abnormal stools (12% to 15%), diarrhea (12% to 19%)

Infection: Increased susceptibility to infection (10% to 14%)
Respiratory: Rhinitis (7% to 12%)

2% to 10%:

Cardiovascular: Peripheral edema (7% to 9%), palpitations (5% to 10%), tachycardia (4%)
Central nervous system: Dizziness (9% to 10%), vertigo (≤3%)
Gastrointestinal: Dyspepsia (6%), nausea (6% to 7%), abdominal pain (4% to 5%), flatulence (2% to 3%)
Neuromuscular & skeletal: Back pain (6% to 7%), myalgia (2% to 3%)
Respiratory: Pharyngitis (7% to 10%), cough (3% to 4%)

<2% (Limited to important or life-threatening): Agranulocytosis, anemia, aplastic anemia, asthma, atrial fibrillation, atrial flutter, blindness, blood pressure increased, bursitis, cardiac arrest, cardiac failure, cerebral hemorrhage, cerebral infarction, cerebrovascular accident, chest pain, cholelithiasis, colitis, coronary stent thrombosis, cystitis, diabetes mellitus, duodenal ulcer, duodenitis, ecchymoses, esophageal hemorrhage, esophagitis, gastrointestinal hemorrhage, gout, granulocytopenia, hematoma (extradural), hemorrhage, hemorrhage (eye), hepatic insufficiency, hot flash, hyperglycemia, hypotension, interstitial pneumonitis, intracranial hemorrhage, jaundice, leukopenia, myocardial infarction, neuralgia, nodal arrhythmia, orthostatic hypotension, pain, peptic ulcer, periodontal abscess, pneumonia, polycythemia, prolonged Q-T interval on ECG, pruritus, pulmonary hemorrhage, rectal hemorrhage, retinal hemorrhage, retroperitoneal hemorrhage, skin hypertrophy, Stevens-Johnson syndrome, subdural hematoma, supraventricular tachycardia, syncope, thrombocytopenia, thrombosis, torsades de pointes, vaginal hemorrhage, ventricular tachycardia

Drug Interactions

Metabolism/Transport Effects Substrate of CYP1A2 (minor), CYP2C19 (major), CYP2D6 (minor), CYP3A4 (major); **Note:** Assignment of Major/Minor substrate status based on clinically relevant drug interaction potential

Avoid Concomitant Use

Avoid concomitant use of Cilostazol with any of the following: Conivaptan; Fusidic Acid (Systemic); Riociguat

Increased Effect/Toxicity

Cilostazol may increase the levels/effects of: Agents with Antiplatelet Properties; Anticoagulants; Collagenase (Systemic); Dabigatran Etexilate; Ibritumomab; Riociguat; Rivaroxaban; Salicylates; Thrombolytic Agents; Tositumomab and Iodine I 131 Tositumomab

The levels/effects of Cilostazol may be increased by: Anagrelide; Antifungal Agents (Azole Derivatives, Systemic); Conivaptan; CYP2C19 Inhibitors (Moderate); CYP2C19 Inhibitors (Strong); CYP3A4 Inhibitors (Moderate); CYP3A4 Inhibitors (Strong); Dasatinib; Esomeprazole; Fusidic Acid (Systemic); Glucosamine; Herbs (Anticoagulant/Antiplatelet Properties); Ibrutinib; Ivacaftor; Luliconazole; Macrolide Antibiotics; Mifepristone; Multivitamins/Fluoride (with ADE); Multivitamins/Minerals (with ADEK, Folate, Iron); Multivitamins/Minerals (with AE, No Iron); Nonsteroidal Anti-Inflammatory Agents; Omega-3 Fatty Acids; Omeprazole; Pentosan Polysulfate Sodium; Pentoxifylline; Prostacyclin Analogues; Simeprevir; Tipranavir; Vitamin E

Decreased Effect

The levels/effects of Cilostazol may be decreased by: Bosentan; CYP3A4 Inducers (Strong); Dabrafenib; Deferasirox; Herbs (CYP3A4 Inducers); Mitotane; Nonsteroidal Anti-Inflammatory Agents; Peginterferon Alfa-2b; Tocilizumab

Ethanol/Nutrition/Herb Interactions

Food: Taking cilostazol with a high-fat meal may increase peak concentration by 90%. Grapefruit juice may increase serum levels of cilostazol and enhance toxic effects. Management: Administer cilostazol on an empty stomach 30 minutes before or 2 hours after meals. Avoid concurrent ingestion of grapefruit juice.

Herb/Nutraceutical: St John's wort may decrease the levels/effects of cilostazol. Other herbs/nutraceuticals have additional antiplatelet activity. Management: Avoid alfalfa, anise, bilberry, bladderwrack, bromelain, cat's claw, chamomile, coleus, cordyceps, dong quai, evening primrose oil, fenugreek, feverfew, garlic, ginger, ginkgo biloba, ginseng (American), ginseng (Panax), ginseng (Siberian), grapeseed, green tea, guggul, horse chestnut seed, horseradish, licorice, prickly ash, red clover, reishi, SAMe (S-adenosylmethionine), St John's wort, sweet clover, turmeric, and white willow.

Storage/Stability Store at 20°C to 25°C (68°F to 77°F); protect from light.

Mechanism of Action Cilostazol and its metabolites are inhibitors of phosphodiesterase III. As a result, cyclic AMP is increased leading to reversible inhibition of platelet aggregation, vasodilation, and inhibition of vascular smooth muscle cell proliferation.

Pharmacodynamics/Kinetics

Onset of action: 2-4 weeks; may require up to 12 weeks
Protein binding: Cilostazol 95% to 98%; active metabolites 66% to 97%
Metabolism: Hepatic via CYP3A4 (primarily), 1A2, 2C19, and 2D6; 2 active metabolites
Half-life elimination: 11-13 hours
Excretion: Urine (74%) and feces (20%) as metabolites

Dosage Adults: Oral:

Intermittent claudication: 100 mg twice daily (when refractory to exercise therapy and smoking cessation, use in combination with either aspirin or clopidogrel) (Guyatt, 2012)

PCI (following elective stent placement) (unlabeled use): 100 mg twice daily in combination with aspirin or clopidogrel. **Note:** Only recommended in patients with an allergy or intolerance to either aspirin or clopidogrel (Guyatt, 2012).

Secondary prevention of noncardioembolic stroke or TIA (unlabeled use): 100 mg twice daily. **Note:** Clopidogrel or aspirin/extended release dipyridamole recommended over the use of cilostazol (Guyatt, 2012).

Dosage adjustment for cilostazol with concomitant medications:

CYP2C19 inhibitors (eg, omeprazole): Dosage of cilostazol should be reduced to 50 mg twice daily
CYP3A4 inhibitors (eg, ketoconazole, itraconazole, erythromycin, diltiazem): Dosage of cilostazol should be reduced to 50 mg twice daily

Dosage adjustment in renal impairment: No dosage adjustment provided in the manufacturer's labeling; use with caution.

Dosage adjustment in hepatic impairment: No dosage adjustment provided in manufacturer's labeling (has not been studied in moderate-to-severe hepatic impairment); use with caution.

Dietary Considerations It is best to take cilostazol 30 minutes before or 2 hours after meals (breakfast and dinner).

Administration Administer cilostazol 30 minutes before or 2 hours after meals (breakfast and dinner).

Dosage Forms Excipient information presented when available (limited, particularly for generics); consult specific product labeling.

Tablet, Oral:
Pletal: 50 mg, 100 mg
Generic: 50 mg, 100 mg

◆ **Ciloxan** *see* Ciprofloxacin (Ophthalmic) *on page* 435

◆ **Ciloxan® (Can)** *see* Ciprofloxacin (Ophthalmic) *on page 435*

Cimetidine (sye MET i deen)

Brand Names: U.S. Cimetidine Acid Reducer [OTC]; Tagamet HB [OTC]

Brand Names: Canada Apo-Cimetidine®; Dom-Cimetidine; Mylan-Cimetidine; Novo-Cimetidine; Nu-Cimet; PMS-Cimetidine

Pharmacologic Category Histamine H_2 Antagonist

Additional Appendix Information

Contrast Media Reactions, Premedication for Prophylaxis *on page 2373*

Use Short-term treatment of active duodenal ulcers and benign gastric ulcers; maintenance therapy of duodenal ulcer; treatment of gastric hypersecretory states; treatment of gastroesophageal reflux disease (GERD)

OTC labeling: Prevention or relief of heartburn, acid indigestion, or sour stomach

Unlabeled Use Part of a multidrug regimen for *H. pylori* eradication to reduce the risk of duodenal ulcer recurrence

Pregnancy Risk Factor B

Pregnancy Considerations Teratogenic effects were not observed in animal reproduction studies; therefore, cimetidine is classified as pregnancy category B. Cimetidine crosses the placenta. An increased risk of congenital malformations or adverse events in the newborn has generally not been observed following maternal use of cimetidine during pregnancy. Histamine H_2 antagonists have been evaluated for the treatment of gastroesophageal reflux disease (GERD), as well as gastric and duodenal ulcers during pregnancy. Although if needed, cimetidine is not the agent of choice. Histamine H_2 antagonists may be used for aspiration prophylaxis prior to cesarean delivery.

Breast-Feeding Considerations Cimetidine is excreted into breast milk. The concentration of cimetidine in maternal serum in comparison to breast milk is highly variable. Breast-feeding is not recommended by the manufacturer. Consider the renal function of the breast-feeding infant.

Contraindications Hypersensitivity to cimetidine, any component of the formulation, or other H_2 antagonists

Warnings/Precautions Reversible confusional states, usually clearing within 3-4 days after discontinuation, have been linked to use. Increased age (>50 years) and renal or hepatic impairment are thought to be associated. Use caution in the elderly due to risk of confusion and other CNS effects. Dosage should be adjusted in renal/hepatic impairment or in patients receiving drugs metabolized through the P450 system.

Over the counter (OTC) cimetidine should not be taken by individuals experiencing painful swallowing, vomiting with blood, or bloody or black stools; medical attention should be sought. A physician should be consulted prior to use when pain in the stomach, shoulder, arms or neck is present; if heartburn has occurred for >3 months; or if unexplained weight loss, or nausea and vomiting occur. Frequent wheezing, shortness of breath, lightheadedness, or sweating, especially with chest pain or heartburn, should also be reported. Consultation of a healthcare provider should occur by patients if also taking theophylline, phenytoin, or warfarin; if heartburn or stomach pain continues or worsens; or if use is required for >14 days. Symptoms of GI distress may be associated with a variety of conditions; symptomatic response to H_2 antagonists does not rule out the potential for significant pathology (eg, malignancy). OTC cimetidine is not approved for use in patients <12 years of age.

Adverse Reactions

1% to 10%:

Central nervous system: Headache (2% to 4%), dizziness (1%), somnolence (1%), agitation

Endocrine & metabolic: Gynecomastia (<1% to 4%)

Gastrointestinal: Diarrhea (1%)

Frequency not defined:

Cardiovascular: AV block, bradycardia, hypotension, tachycardia, vasculitis

Central nervous system: Confusion, fever

Dermatologic: Alopecia, erythema multiforme, exfoliative dermatitis, Stevens-Johnson syndrome, toxic epidermal necrolysis, rash

Endocrine & metabolic: Edema of the breasts, sexual ability decreased

Gastrointestinal: Nausea, pancreatitis, vomiting

Hematologic: Agranulocytosis, aplastic anemia, hemolytic anemia (immune-based), neutropenia, pancytopenia, thrombocytopenia

Hepatic: ALT increased, AST increased, hepatic fibrosis (case report)

Neuromuscular & skeletal: Arthralgia, myalgia, polymyositis

Renal: Creatinine increased, interstitial nephritis

Miscellaneous: Anaphylaxis, pneumonia (causal relationship not established)

Drug Interactions

Metabolism/Transport Effects Substrate of P-glycoprotein; **Inhibits** CYP1A2 (moderate), CYP2C19 (moderate), CYP2C9 (weak), CYP2D6 (moderate), CYP2E1 (weak), CYP3A4 (moderate)

Avoid Concomitant Use

Avoid concomitant use of Cimetidine with any of the following: Dasatinib; Delavirdine; Dofetilide; EPIrubicin; Ibrutinib; Ivabradine; Lomitapide; Pimozide; Pirfenidone; PONATinib; Risedronate; Simeprevir; Thioridazine; Tolvaptan; Ulipristal

Increased Effect/Toxicity

Cimetidine may increase the levels/effects of: Agomelatine; Alfentanil; Amiodarone; Anticonvulsants (Hydantoin); ARIPiprazole; Avanafil; Benzodiazepines (metabolized by oxidation); Bosentan; Bromazepam; Budesonide (Systemic, Oral Inhalation); Calcium Channel Blockers; Capecitabine; CarBAMazepine; Carmustine; Carvedilol; Cisapride; CloZAPine; Colchicine; CYP1A2 Substrates; CYP2C19 Substrates; CYP2D6 Substrates; CYP3A4 Substrates; Dalfampridine; Dexmethylphenidate; Dofetilide; EPIrubicin; Eplerenone; Escitalopram; Everolimus; Fesoterodine; Floxuridine; Fluorouracil (Systemic); Halofantrine; Ibrutinib; Imatinib; Ivabradine; Ivacaftor; Lomitapide; Lurasidone; Mebendazole; MetFORMIN; Methylphenidate; Metoprolol; Moclobemide; Nebivolol; Nicotine; Pentoxifylline; Pimecrolimus; Pimozide; Pirfenidone; Pramipexole; Praziquantel; Procainamide; Propafenone; QuiNIDine; QuiNINE; Ranolazine; Risedronate; Roflumilast; Salmeterol; Saquinavir; Saxagliptin; Selective Serotonin Reuptake Inhibitors; Simeprevir; Sulfonylureas; Tegafur; Theophylline Derivatives; Thioridazine; Tolvaptan; Tricyclic Antidepressants; Ulipristal; Varenicline; Vitamin K Antagonists; Zaleplon; ZOLMitriptan; Zuclopenthixol

The levels/effects of Cimetidine may be increased by: AtorvaSTATin; P-glycoprotein/ABCB1 Inhibitors

Decreased Effect

Cimetidine may decrease the levels/effects of: Atazanavir; Bosutinib; Cefditoren; Cefpodoxime; Cefuroxime; Clopidogrel; Dabrafenib; Dasatinib; Delavirdine; Erlotinib; Fosamprenavir; Gefitinib; Ifosfamide; Indinavir; Iron Salts; Itraconazole; Ketoconazole (Systemic); Mesalamine; Multivitamins/Minerals (with ADEK, Folate, Iron); Nelfinavir; Nilotinib; PONATinib; Posaconazole; Rilpivirine; Tamoxifen; Vismodegib

The levels/effects of Cimetidine may be decreased by: P-glycoprotein/ABCB1 Inducers

Ethanol/Nutrition/Herb Interactions

Ethanol: Avoid ethanol (may enhance gastric mucosal irritation).

Food: Cimetidine may increase serum caffeine levels if taken with caffeine. Cimetidine peak serum levels may be decreased if taken with food.

Herb/Nutraceutical: St John's wort may decrease cimetidine levels.

Storage/Stability Tablet: Store between 15°C and 30°C (59°F to 86°F). Protect from light.

Mechanism of Action Competitive inhibition of histamine at H_2 receptors of the gastric parietal cells resulting in reduced gastric acid secretion, gastric volume and hydrogen ion concentration reduced

Pharmacodynamics/Kinetics

Onset of action: 1 hour

Duration: 80% reduction in gastric acid secretion for 4-5 hours after 300 mg dose

Absorption: Rapid

Distribution: 1.3 L/kg

Protein binding: 20%

Metabolism: Partially hepatic, forms metabolites

Bioavailability: 60% to 70%

Half-life elimination: Neonates: 3.6 hours; Children: 1.4 hours; Adults: 2 hours

Time to peak, serum: Oral: 1-2 hours

Excretion: Primarily urine (48% as unchanged drug); feces (some)

Dosage Oral:

Children: 20-40 mg/kg/day in divided doses every 6 hours

Children ≥12 years and Adults: Heartburn, acid indigestion, sour stomach (OTC labeling): 200 mg up to twice daily; may take 30 minutes prior to eating foods or beverages expected to cause heartburn or indigestion

Adults:

Short-term treatment of active ulcers: 300 mg 4 times/day or 800 mg at bedtime or 400 mg twice daily for up to 8 weeks

Note: Higher doses of 1600 mg at bedtime for 4 weeks may be beneficial for a subpopulation of patients with larger duodenal ulcers (>1 cm defined endoscopically) who are also heavy smokers (≥1 pack/day).

Duodenal ulcer prophylaxis: 400 mg at bedtime

Gastric hypersecretory conditions: 300-600 mg every 6 hours; dosage not to exceed 2.4 g/day

Gastroesophageal reflux disease: 400 mg 4 times/day or 800 mg twice daily for 12 weeks

Helicobacter pylori eradication (unlabeled use): 400 mg twice daily; requires combination therapy with antibiotics

Dosing adjustment/interval in renal impairment: Children and Adults:

Cl_{cr} 10-50 mL/minute: Administer 50% of normal dose

Cl_{cr} <10 mL/minute: Administer 25% of normal dose

Hemodialysis: Slightly dialyzable (5% to 20%); administer after dialysis

Dosing adjustment/comments in hepatic impairment: Usual dose is safe in mild liver disease but use with caution and in reduced dosage in severe liver disease; increased risk of CNS toxicity in cirrhosis suggested by enhanced penetration of CNS

Administration Administer with meals so that the drug's peak effect occurs at the proper time (peak inhibition of gastric acid secretion occurs at 1 and 3 hours after dosing in fasting subjects and approximately 2 hours in nonfasting subjects; this correlates well with the time food is no longer in the stomach offering a buffering effect)

Monitoring Parameters CBC, gastric pH, occult blood with GI bleeding; monitor renal function to correct dose.

Dosage Forms Excipient information presented when available (limited, particularly for generics); consult specific product labeling.

Solution, Oral, as hydrochloride [strength expressed as base]:

Generic: 300 mg/5 mL (237 mL, 240 mL)

Tablet, Oral:

Cimetidine Acid Reducer: 200 mg

Tagamet HB: 200 mg

Generic: 200 mg, 300 mg, 400 mg, 800 mg

Extemporaneous Preparations Note: Commercial oral solution is available (strength expressed as base: 60 mg/mL)

A 60 mg/mL oral suspension may be made with tablets. Place twenty-four 300 mg tablets in 5 mL of sterile water for ~3-5 minutes to dissolve film coating. Crush tablets in a mortar and reduce to a fine powder. Add 10 mL of glycerin and mix to a uniform paste; mix while adding Simple Syrup, NF in incremental proportions to **almost** 120 mL; transfer to a calibrated bottle, rinse mortar with vehicle, and add quantity of vehicle sufficient to make 120 mL. Label "shake well" and "refrigerate". Stable for 17 days.

Nahata MC, Pai VB, and Hipple TF, *Pediatric Drug Formulations*, 5th ed, Cincinnati, OH: Harvey Whitney Books Co, 2004.

- ◆ Cimetidine Acid Reducer [OTC] *see* Cimetidine *on page* 427
- ◆ Cimzia *see* Certolizumab Pegol *on page* 393
- ◆ Cimzia® (Can) *see* Certolizumab Pegol *on page* 393
- ◆ Cimzia Prefilled *see* Certolizumab Pegol *on page* 393
- ◆ Cimzia Starter Kit *see* Certolizumab Pegol *on page* 393

Cinacalcet (sin a KAL cet)

Brand Names: U.S. Sensipar

Brand Names: Canada Sensipar

Index Terms AMG 073; Cinacalcet Hydrochloride

Pharmacologic Category Calcimimetic

Use Treatment of secondary hyperparathyroidism in patients with chronic kidney disease (CKD) on dialysis; treatment of hypercalcemia in patients with parathyroid carcinoma; treatment of severe hypercalcemia in patients with primary hyperparathyroidism who are unable to undergo parathyroidectomy

Pregnancy Risk Factor C

Pregnancy Considerations In animal studies, there were no teratogenic effects observed, although decreased pup weights were noted. There are no adequate or well-controlled studies in pregnant women. Use in pregnancy only if potential benefit to mother justifies risk to the fetus. Women who become pregnant during cinacalcet treatment are encouraged to enroll in Amgen's Pregnancy Surveillance Program (1-800-772-6436).

Breast-Feeding Considerations Due to the potential for serious adverse effects in the nursing infant, the manufacturer recommends discontinuing nursing or discontinuing cinacalcet.

Contraindications Hypocalcemia (serum calcium lower than the lower limit of normal range)

Canadian labeling: Additional contraindications (not in U.S. labeling): Hypersensitivity to any component of the formulation

Warnings/Precautions Use is contraindicated in hypocalcemia. Monitor serum calcium and for symptoms of hypocalcemia (eg, cramps, myalgia, paresthesia, seizure, tetany); may require treatment interruption, dose reduction, or initiation (or dose increases) of calcium-based phosphate binder or vitamin D to raise serum calcium depending on calcium levels or symptoms of hypocalcemia. Use with caution in patients with a seizure disorder (seizure threshold is lowered by significant serum calcium reductions); monitor calcium levels closely. Adynamic bone disease may develop if intact parathyroid hormone (iPTH) levels are suppressed (<100 pg/mL).

Use caution in patients with moderate-to-severe hepatic impairment (Child-Pugh classes B and C); monitor serum calcium, serum phosphorus and iPTH closely. In the U.S., the long-term safety and efficacy of cinacalcet has not been evaluated in chronic kidney disease (CKD) patients with hyperparathyroidism not requiring dialysis. Not indicated for CKD patients not receiving dialysis. Although possibly related to lower baseline calcium levels, clinical studies have shown an increased incidence of hypocalcemia (<8.4 mg/dL) in patients not requiring dialysis. Monitor serum calcium and iPTH concentrations closely in patients on concurrent CYP3A4 inhibitors; dosage adjustment may be required. Cinacalcet is a strong inhibitor of CYP2D6; if on concurrent therapy with a CYP2D6 substrate, dosage adjustment of the CYP2D6 substrate may be necessary. May cause a decrease in testosterone levels (free and total); although below normal testosterone levels may occur in patients with end-stage renal disease, the clinical significance has not been determined. Use with caution in patients with cardiovascular disease; idiosyncratic hypotension, worsening of heart failure, and/or arrhythmia have been reported in patients with impaired cardiovascular function; may correlate with decreased serum calcium.

Adverse Reactions

>10%:

Central nervous system: Fatigue (12% to 21%), headache (≤21%), depression (10% to 18%)

Endocrine & metabolic: Hypocalcemia (≤66%), dehydration (≤24%), hypercalcemia (12% to 21%)

Gastrointestinal: Nausea (31% to 66%), vomiting (27% to 52%), diarrhea (≤21%), anorexia (6% to 21%), constipation (10% to 18%)

Hematologic: Anemia (6% to 17%)

Neuromuscular & skeletal: Parasthesia (14% to 29%), fracture (12% to 21%), weakness (7% to 17%), arthralgia (6% to 17%), myalgia (≤15%), limb pain (10% to 12%)

Respiratory: Upper respiratory infection (10% to 12%)

1% to 10%:

Cardiovascular: Hypertension (≤7%)

Central nervous system: Dizziness (≤10%), seizure (1%)

Endocrine & metabolic: Testosterone decreased

Neuromuscular & skeletal: Chest pain (noncardiac; ≤6%)

Postmarketing and/or case reports: Adynamic bone disease, angioedema, arrhythmia, heart failure, hypersensitivity reactions, hypotension (idiosyncratic), rash, urticaria

Drug Interactions

Metabolism/Transport Effects **Substrate** of CYP1A2 (minor), CYP2D6 (minor), CYP3A4 (major); **Note:** Assignment of Major/Minor substrate status based on clinically relevant drug interaction potential; **Inhibits** CYP2D6 (strong)

Avoid Concomitant Use

Avoid concomitant use of Cinacalcet with any of the following: Conivaptan; Fusidic Acid (Systemic); Pimozide; Tamoxifen; Thioridazine

Increased Effect/Toxicity

Cinacalcet may increase the levels/effects of: ARIPiprazole; AtoMOXetine; CYP2D6 Substrates; Fesoterodine; Iloperidone; Metoprolol; Nebivolol; Pimozide; Propafenone; Tetrabenazine; Thioridazine; Tricyclic Antidepressants; Vortioxetine

The levels/effects of Cinacalcet may be increased by: Conivaptan; CYP3A4 Inhibitors (Moderate); CYP3A4 Inhibitors (Strong); Dasatinib; Fusidic Acid (Systemic); Ivacaftor; Luliconazole; Mifepristone; Simeprevir

Decreased Effect

Cinacalcet may decrease the levels/effects of: Codeine; Iloperidone; Tacrolimus (Systemic); Tamoxifen; TraMADol

The levels/effects of Cinacalcet may be decreased by: Peginterferon Alfa-2b

Ethanol/Nutrition/Herb Interactions Food: Food increases bioavailability. Management: Administer with food or shortly after a meal.

Storage/Stability Store at 25°C (77°F); excursions permitted to 15°C to 30°C (59°F to 86°F).

Mechanism of Action Increases the sensitivity of the calcium-sensing receptor on the parathyroid gland thereby, concomitantly lowering parathyroid hormone (PTH), serum calcium, and serum phosphorus levels, preventing progressive bone disease and adverse events associated with mineral metabolism disorders.

Pharmacodynamics/Kinetics

Distribution: V_d: ~1000 L

Protein binding: ~93% to 97%

Metabolism: Hepatic (extensive) via CYP3A4, 2D6, 1A2; forms inactive metabolites

Half-life elimination: Terminal: 30-40 hours; moderate hepatic impairment: 65 hours; severe hepatic impairment: 84 hours

Time to peak, plasma: ~2-6 hours

Excretion: Urine ~80% (as metabolites); feces ~15%

Dosage Oral: Adults: **Do not titrate dose more frequently than every 2-4 weeks.** Dosage adjustment may be required in patients on concurrent CYP3A4 inhibitors.

Secondary hyperparathyroidism: Initial: 30 mg once daily (maximum daily dose: 180 mg); increase dose incrementally (60 mg, 90 mg, 120 mg, 180 mg once daily) as necessary to maintain iPTH level between 150-300 pg/mL.

Parathyroid carcinoma, primary hyperparathyroidism: Initial: 30 mg twice daily (maximum daily dose: 360 mg daily as 90 mg 4 times/day); increase dose incrementally (60 mg twice daily, 90 mg twice daily, 90 mg 3-4 times/day) as necessary to normalize serum calcium levels.

Elderly: No adjustment required; refer to adult dosing

Dosage adjustment for hypocalcemia:

If serum calcium >7.5 mg/dL but <8.4 mg/dL **or** if hypocalcemia symptoms occur: Use calcium-containing phosphate binders and/or vitamin D to raise calcium levels.

If serum calcium <7.5 mg/dL **or** if hypocalcemia symptoms persist and the dose of vitamin D cannot be increased: Withhold cinacalcet until serum calcium ≥8 mg/dL and/or symptoms of hypocalcemia resolve. Reinitiate cinacalcet at the next lowest dose.

If iPTH <150-300 pg/mL: Reduce dose or discontinue cinacalcet and/or vitamin D.

Dosage adjustment in renal impairment: No adjustment required.

Dosage adjustment in hepatic impairment: Patients with moderate-to-severe dysfunction (Child-Pugh class B or C) have an increased exposure to cinacalcet and increased half-life. Dosage adjustments may be necessary based on serum calcium, serum phosphorus, and/or iPTH.

Dietary Considerations Take with food or shortly after a meal. May be taken with vitamin D and/or phosphate binders.

Administration Administer with food or shortly after a meal. Do not break or divide tablet; should be taken whole.

Monitoring Parameters

Secondary hyperparathyroidism: Serum calcium and phosphorus levels prior to initiation and within a week of initiation or dosage adjustment; iPTH should be measured 1-4 weeks after initiation or dosage adjustment. After the maintenance dose is established, monthly calcium and phosphorus levels and iPTH every 1-3 months are required. Wait at least 12 hours after dose before drawing iPTH levels.

Parathyroid carcinoma and primary hyperparathyroidism: Serum calcium levels prior to initiation and within a week of initiation or dosage adjustment; once maintenance dose is established, obtain serum calcium every 2 months.

Reference Range

CKD K/DOQI guidelines definition of stages; chronic disease is kidney damage or GFR <60 mL/minute/1.73 m^2 for ≥3 months:

Stage 2: GFR 60-89 mL/minute/1.73 m^2 (kidney damage with mild decrease GFR)

Stage 3: GFR 30-59 mL/minute/1.73 m^2 (moderate decrease GFR)

Stage 4: GFR 15-29 mL/minute/1.73 m^2 (severe decrease GFR)

Stage 5: GFR <15 mL/minute/1.73 m^2 or dialysis (kidney failure)

Target range for iPTH: Adults:

Stage 3 CKD: 35-70 pg/mL

Stage 4 CKD: 70-110 pg/mL

Stage 5 CKD: 150-300 pg/mL

Serum phosphorus: Adults:

Stage 3 and 4 CKD: ≥2.7 to <4.6 mg/dL

Stage 5 CKD: 3.5-5.5 mg/dL

Serum calcium-phosphorus product: Adults: Stage 3-5 CKD: <55 mg^2/dL^2

Dosage Forms Excipient information presented when available (limited, particularly for generics); consult specific product labeling.

Tablet, Oral:

Sensipar: 30 mg, 60 mg, 90 mg

◆ Cinacalcet Hydrochloride *see* Cinacalcet *on page 428*

◆ Cinryze *see* C1 Inhibitor (Human) *on page 307*

◆ Cipralex® (Can) *see* Escitalopram *on page 745*

◆ Cipro *see* Ciprofloxacin (Systemic) *on page 430*

◆ Cipro XL (Can) *see* Ciprofloxacin (Systemic) *on page 430*

◆ Ciprodex® *see* Ciprofloxacin and Dexamethasone *on page 435*

Ciprofloxacin (Systemic) (sip roe FLOKS a sin)

Brand Names: U.S. Cipro; Cipro in D_5W; Cipro XR

Brand Names: Canada Apo-Ciproflox; Auro-Ciprofloxacin; Cipro; Cipro XL; CO Ciprofloxacin; Dom-Ciprofloxacin; JAMP-Ciprofloxacin; Mar-Ciprofloxacin; Mint-Ciprofloxacin; Mylan-Ciprofloxacin; Novo-Ciprofloxacin; PHL-Ciprofloxacin; PMS-Ciprofloxacin; PRO-Ciprofloxacin; RAN-Ciproflox; ratio-Ciprofloxacin; Riva-Ciprofloxacin; Sandoz-Ciprofloxacin; Taro-Ciprofloxacin

Index Terms Ciprofloxacin Hydrochloride

Pharmacologic Category Antibiotic, Fluoroquinolone

Additional Appendix Information

Antibiotic Treatment of Adults With Infective Endocarditis *on page 2355*

Desensitization Protocols *on page 2325*

Dosing Considerations for the Critically-Ill Patient With Morbid Obesity *on page 2379*

Use

Children: Complicated urinary tract infections and pyelonephritis due to *E. coli.* **Note:** Although effective, ciprofloxacin is not the drug of first choice in children.

Children and Adults: To reduce incidence or progression of disease following exposure to aerolized *Bacillus anthracis*.

Adults: Treatment of the following infections when caused by susceptible bacteria: Urinary tract infections; acute uncomplicated cystitis in females; chronic bacterial prostatitis; lower respiratory tract infections (including acute exacerbations of chronic bronchitis); acute sinusitis; skin and skin structure infections; bone and joint infections; complicated intra-abdominal infections (in combination with metronidazole); infectious diarrhea; typhoid fever due to *Salmonella typhi* (eradication of chronic typhoid carrier state has not been proven); uncomplicated cervical and urethra gonorrhea (due to *N. gonorrhoeae*); nosocomial pneumonia; empirical therapy for febrile neutropenic patients (in combination with piperacillin)

Note: As of April 2007, the CDC no longer recommends the use of fluoroquinolones for the treatment of gonococcal disease.

Unlabeled Use Acute pulmonary exacerbations in cystic fibrosis (children); cutaneous/gastrointestinal/oropharyngeal anthrax (treatment, children and adults); disseminated gonococcal infection (adults); chancroid (adults); epididymitis (adults); prophylaxis to *Neisseria meningitidis* following close contact with an infected person; empirical therapy (oral) for febrile neutropenia in low-risk cancer patients; HACEK group endocarditis; infectious diarrhea (children); periodontitis; chronic oral antimicrobial suppression of prosthetic joint infection; surgical (preoperative) prophylaxis

Pregnancy Risk Factor C

Pregnancy Considerations Adverse events have been observed in some animal reproduction studies. Ciprofloxacin crosses the placenta and produces measurable concentrations in the amniotic fluid and cord serum (Ludlam, 1997). An increased risk of teratogenic effects has not been observed in animals or humans following ciprofloxacin use during pregnancy; however, because of concerns of cartilage damage in immature animals, ciprofloxacin should only be used during pregnancy if a safer option is not available. Ciprofloxacin is recommended for prophylaxis and treatment of pregnant women exposed to anthrax (CDC, 2001a; CDC, 2001b). Serum concentrations of ciprofloxacin may be lower during pregnancy than in nonpregnant patients (Giamarellou, 1989).

Breast-Feeding Considerations Ciprofloxacin is excreted in breast milk. Due to the potential for serious adverse reactions in the nursing infant, the manufacturer recommends a decision be made whether to discontinue nursing or to discontinue the drug, taking into account the importance of treatment to the mother. However, due to the low concentrations in human milk, minimal toxicity would be expected in the nursing infant and infant serum levels were undetectable in one report (Gardner, 1992). Non-dose-related effects could include modification of bowel flora. There has been a single case report of perforated pseudomembranous colitis in a breast-feeding infant whose mother was taking ciprofloxacin (Harmon, 1992).

Medication Guide Available Yes

Contraindications Hypersensitivity to ciprofloxacin, any component of the formulation, or other quinolones; concurrent administration of tizanidine

Warnings/Precautions [U.S. Boxed Warning]: There have been reports of tendon inflammation and/or rupture with quinolone antibiotics in all ages; risk may be increased with concurrent corticosteroids, solid organ transplant recipients, and in patients >60 years of age. Rupture of the Achilles tendon sometimes requiring surgical repair has been reported most frequently; but other tendon sites (eg, rotator cuff, biceps) have also been reported. Strenuous physical activity, rheumatoid arthritis, and renal impairment may be an independent risk factor for tendonitis. Inflammation and rupture may occur bilaterally. Cases have been reported within the first 48 hours, during, and up to several months after discontinuation of therapy. Discontinue at first sign of tendon inflammation or pain.

Use with caution in patients with rheumatoid arthritis; may increase risk of tendon rupture. Use with caution in patients with a history of tendon disorders.

CNS effects may occur (tremor, restlessness, confusion, and hallucinations, increased intracranial pressure [including pseudotumor cerebri] or seizures). Reactions may occur following the first dose. Use with caution in patients with known or suspected CNS disorder or consider discontinuation if CNS effects develop. Potential for seizures, although very rare, may be increased with concomitant NSAID therapy. Use with caution in individuals at risk of seizures (CNS disorders or concurrent therapy with medications which may lower seizure threshold; status epilepticus has occurred) or if clinically appropriate, consider alternative antimicrobial therapy. Discontinue if seizures occur.

Fluoroquinolones may prolong QT_c interval; avoid use in patients with a history of or at risk for QT_c prolongation, torsade de pointes, uncorrected hypokalemia, hypomagnesemia, cardiac disease (heart failure, myocardial infarction, bradycardia) or concurrent administration of other medications known to prolong the QT interval (including Class Ia and Class III antiarrhythmics, cisapride, erythromycin, antipsychotics, and tricyclic antidepressants). Hepatocellular, cholestatic, or mixed liver injury has been reported, including hepatic necrosis, life-threatening hepatic events, and fatalities. Acute liver injury can be rapid onset (range: 1-39 days), often associated with hypersensitivity. Most fatalities occurred in patients >55 years of age. Discontinue immediately if signs/symptoms of hepatitis (abdominal tenderness, dark urine, jaundice, pruritus) occur. Additionally, temporary increases in transaminases or alkaline phosphatase or cholestatic jaundice may occur (highest risk in patients with previous liver damage).

Prolonged use may result in fungal or bacterial superinfection, including *C. difficile*-associated diarrhea (CDAD) and pseudomembranous colitis; CDAD has been observed >2 months postantibiotic treatment. Rarely crystalluria has occurred; urine alkalinity may increase the risk. Ensure adequate hydration during therapy. Adverse effects, including those related to joints and/or surrounding tissues, are increased in pediatric patients and therefore, ciprofloxacin should not be considered as drug of choice in children (exception is anthrax treatment). Peripheral neuropathy has been reported (rare); may occur soon after initiation of therapy and may be irreversible; discontinue if symptoms of sensory or sensorimotor neuropathy occur.

Fluoroquinolones have been associated with the development of serious, and sometimes fatal, hypoglycemia, most often in elderly diabetics but also in patients without diabetes. This occurred most frequently with gatifloxacin (no longer available systemically), but may occur at a lower frequency with other quinolones.

Severe hypersensitivity reactions, including anaphylaxis, have occurred with quinolone therapy. Reactions may present as typical allergic symptoms after a single dose, or may manifest as severe idiosyncratic dermatologic, vascular, pulmonary, renal, hepatic, and/or hematologic events, usually after multiple doses. Prompt discontinuation of drug should occur if skin rash or other symptoms arise. **[U.S. Boxed Warning]: Quinolones may exacerbate myasthenia gravis; avoid use (rare, potentially life-threatening weakness of respiratory muscles may occur).** Use caution in renal impairment. Avoid excessive sunlight and take precautions to limit exposure (eg, loose fitting clothing, sunscreen); may cause moderate-to-severe photosensitivity/phototoxicity reactions. Discontinue use if photosensitivity occurs. Since ciprofloxacin is ineffective in the treatment of syphilis and may mask symptoms, all patients should be tested for syphilis at the time of gonorrheal diagnosis and 3 months later. Hemolytic reactions may (rarely) occur with quinolone use in patients with latent or actual glucose-6-phosphate dehydrogenase (G6PD) deficiency.

Potentially significant interactions may exist, requiring dose or frequency adjustment, additional monitoring, and/or selection of alternative therapy. Serious and fatal reactions including seizures, status epilepticus, cardiac arrest and respiratory failure have been reported with concomitant administration of theophylline. If concurrent use is unavoidable, monitor serum theophylline levels and adjust theophylline dose as warranted.

Adverse Reactions

1% to 10%:

- Central nervous system: Neurologic events (children 2%, includes dizziness, insomnia, nervousness, somnolence); fever (children 2%); headache (I.V. administration); restlessness (I.V. administration)
- Dermatologic: Rash (children 2%, adults 1%)
- Gastrointestinal: Nausea (3%); diarrhea (children 5%, adults 2%); vomiting (children 5%, adults 1%); abdominal pain (children 3%, adults <1%); dyspepsia (children 3%)
- Hepatic: ALT increased, AST increased (adults 1%)
- Local: Injection site reactions (I.V. administration)
- Respiratory: Rhinitis (children 3%)

<1% (Limited to important or life-threatening): Abnormal gait, acute generalized exanthemous pustulosis (AGEP), acute renal failure, agitation, agranulocytosis, albuminuria, alkaline phosphatase increase, allergic reactions, anaphylactic shock, anemia, angina pectoris, angioedema, anorexia,anxiety, arthralgia, ataxia, atrial flutter, bilirubin (serum) increase, bone marrow depression (life-threatening), bronchospasm, BUN increased, candidiasis, cardiopulmonary arrest, chills, cholestatic jaundice, chromatopsia, *Clostridium difficile*-associated diarrhea (CDAD), confusion, constipation, CPK increase, crystalluria (particularly in alkaline urine), cylindruria, delirium, depression (including self-injurious behavior), dizziness, drowsiness, dyspepsia (adults), dyspnea, edema, eosinophilia, erythema multiforme/nodosum, exfoliative dermatitis, fever (adults), fixed eruption, gastrointestinal bleeding, gout flare, hallucinations, headache (oral), hematocrit decreased, hematuria, hemoglobin decreased, hemolytic anemia, hepatic failure (some fatal), hepatic necrosis, hyper-/hypoglycemia, hyper-/hypotension, hyperesthesia, hyperpigmentation, hypertonia, insomnia, interstitial nephritis, intestinal perforation, intracranial pressure increased, irritability, joint pain, laryngeal edema, LDH increased, lightheadedness, lipase increased, lymphadenopathy, malaise, manic reaction, methemoglobinemia, MI, migraine, myalgia, myasthenia gravis exacerbation, myoclonus, nephritis, nightmares, nystagmus, palpitation, pancreatitis, pancytopenia (life-threatening or fatal), paranoia, peripheral neuropathy, petechiae, photosensitivity/toxicity, pneumonitis, polyneuropathy, prolongation of PT/INR (in patients treated with vitamin K antagonists), pseudotumor cerebri, psychosis (toxic), PT decrease, pulmonary edema, renal calculi, seizure (including grand mal), serum cholesterol increased, serum creatinine increased, serum sickness-like reactions, serum triglycerides increased, status epilepticus, Stevens-Johnson syndrome, suicidal thoughts/ideation/attempts and completions, syncope, tachycardia, taste loss, tendon rupture, tendonitis, thrombocytopenia, thrombocytosis, thrombophlebitis, tinnitus, torsade de pointes, toxic epidermal necrolysis, tremor, twitching, unresponsiveness, urethral bleeding, uric acid increased, vaginitis, vasculitis, ventricular arrhythmia, visual disturbance, weakness

Drug Interactions

Metabolism/Transport Effects Substrate of P-glycoprotein; **Inhibits** CYP1A2 (strong), CYP3A4 (weak)

Avoid Concomitant Use

Avoid concomitant use of Ciprofloxacin (Systemic) with any of the following: Agomelatine; BCG; CloZAPine; Highest Risk QTc-Prolonging Agents; Ivabradine; Mifepristone; Pirfenidone; Pomalidomide; Strontium Ranelate; TiZANidine

Increased Effect/Toxicity

Ciprofloxacin (Systemic) may increase the levels/effects of: Agomelatine; ARIPiprazole; Bendamustine; Caffeine; CloZAPine; Corticosteroids (Systemic); CYP1A2 Substrates; Erlotinib; Highest Risk QTc-Prolonging Agents; Lomitapide; Methotrexate; Moderate Risk QTc-Prolonging Agents; Pentoxifylline; Pirfenidone; Pomalidomide; Porfimer; Roflumilast; ROPINIRole; Ropivacaine; Sulfonylureas; Theophylline Derivatives; TiZANidine; Varenicline; Vitamin K Antagonists

The levels/effects of Ciprofloxacin (Systemic) may be increased by: Fosphenytoin; Insulin; Ivabradine; Mifepristone; Nonsteroidal Anti-Inflammatory Agents; P-glycoprotein/ABCB1 Inhibitors; Probenecid; QTc-Prolonging Agents (Indeterminate Risk and Risk Modifying)

Decreased Effect

Ciprofloxacin (Systemic) may decrease the levels/effects of: BCG; Didanosine; Fosphenytoin; Mycophenolate; Phenytoin; Sodium Picosulfate; Sulfonylureas; Typhoid Vaccine

The levels/effects of Ciprofloxacin (Systemic) may be decreased by: Antacids; Calcium Salts; Didanosine; Iron Salts; Lanthanum; Magnesium Salts; Multivitamins/Minerals (with ADEK, Folate, Iron); Multivitamins/Minerals (with AE, No Iron); P-glycoprotein/ABCB1 Inducers; Quinapril; Sevelamer; Strontium Ranelate; Sucralfate; Zinc Salts

Ethanol/Nutrition/Herb Interactions

Food: Food decreases rate, but not extent, of absorption. Ciprofloxacin serum levels may be decreased if taken with divalent or trivalent cations. Ciprofloxacin may increase serum caffeine levels if taken concurrently. Rarely, crystalluria may occur. Enteral feedings may decrease plasma concentrations of ciprofloxacin probably by >30% inhibition of absorption. Management: May administer with food to minimize GI upset. Avoid or take ciprofloxacin 2 hours before or 6 hours after antacids, dairy products, or calcium-fortified juices alone or in a meal containing >800 mg calcium, oral multivitamins, or mineral supplements containing divalent and/or trivalent cations. Restrict caffeine intake if excessive cardiac or CNS stimulation occurs. Ensure adequate hydration during therapy. Ciprofloxacin should not be administered with enteral feedings. The feeding would need to be discontinued for 1-2 hours prior to and after ciprofloxacin administration. Nasogastric administration produces a greater loss of ciprofloxacin bioavailability than does nasoduodenal administration.

Herb/Nutraceutical: Dong quai and St John's wort may also cause photosensitization. Management: Avoid dong quai and St John's wort.

Preparation for Administration Injection, vial: May be diluted with NS, D_5W, SWFI, $D_{10}W$, $D_5{}^1/_4NS$, $D_5{}^1/_2NS$, LR.

Storage/Stability

Injection:

Premixed infusion: Store between 5°C to 25°C (41°F to 77°F); avoid freezing. Protect from light.

Vial: Store between 5°C to 30°C (41°F to 86°F); avoid freezing. Protect from light. Diluted solutions of 0.5-2 mg/mL are stable for up to 14 days refrigerated or at room temperature.

Microcapsules for oral suspension: Prior to reconstitution, store below 25°C (77°F). Protect from freezing. Following reconstitution, store below 30°C (86°F) for up to 14 days. Protect from freezing.

Tablet:

Immediate release: Store below 30°C (86°F).

Extended release: Store at room temperature of 15°C to 30°C (59°F to 86°F).

Mechanism of Action Inhibits DNA-gyrase in susceptible organisms; inhibits relaxation of supercoiled DNA and promotes breakage of double-stranded DNA

Pharmacodynamics/Kinetics

Absorption: Oral: Immediate release tablet: Rapid (~50% to 85%)

Distribution: V_d: 2.1-2.7 L/kg; tissue concentrations often exceed serum concentrations especially in kidneys, gallbladder, liver, lungs, gynecological tissue, and prostatic tissue; CSF concentrations: 10% of serum concentrations (noninflamed meninges), 14% to 37% (inflamed meninges)

Protein binding: 20% to 40%

Metabolism: Partially hepatic; forms 4 metabolites (limited activity)

Half-life elimination: Children: 2.5 hours; Adults: Normal renal function: 3-5 hours

Time to peak: Oral:

Immediate release tablet: 0.5-2 hours

Extended release tablet: Cipro XR: 1-2.5 hours

Excretion: Urine (30% to 50% as unchanged drug); feces (15% to 43%)

Dosage Note: Extended release tablets and immediate release formulations are not interchangeable. Unless otherwise specified, oral dosing reflects the use of immediate release formulations.

Usual dosage ranges:

Children (see Warnings/Precautions):

Oral: See indication-specific dosing; maximum dose: 1500 mg daily

I.V.: See indication-specific dosing; maximum dose: 800 mg daily

Adults:

Oral: 250-750 mg every 12 hours

I.V.: 200-400 mg every 12 hours

Indication-specific dosing:

Infants >3 months and Children:

Community-acquired pneumonia (CAP) (IDSA/PIDS, 2011): *H. influenzae,* moderate-to-severe infection (alternative to ampicillin, ceftriaxone, or cefotaxime): I.V.: 30 mg/kg/day divided every 12 hours

Children:

Anthrax:

Inhalational (postexposure prophylaxis):

Oral: 15 mg/kg/dose every 12 hours for 60 days; maximum: 500 mg dose

I.V.: 10 mg/kg/dose every 12 hours for 60 days; do **not** exceed 400 mg dose (800 mg daily)

Cutaneous (treatment, CDC guidelines): Oral: 10-15 mg/kg every 12 hours for 60 days (maximum: 1000 mg daily); amoxicillin 80 mg/kg/day divided every 8 hours is an option for completion of treatment after clinical improvement. **Note:** In the presence of systemic involvement, extensive edema, lesions on head/neck, refer to I.V. dosing for treatment of inhalational/gastrointestinal/oropharyngeal anthrax.

Inhalational/gastrointestinal/oropharyngeal (treatment, CDC guidelines): I.V.: Initial: 10-15 mg/kg every 12 hours for 60 days (maximum: 500 mg dose); switch to oral therapy when clinically appropriate; refer to adult dosing for notes on combined therapy and duration

Cystic fibrosis (unlabeled use):

Oral: 40 mg/kg/day divided every 12 hours administered following 1 week of I.V. therapy has been reported in a clinical trial; total duration of therapy: 10-21 days (Rubio, 1997)

I.V.: 30 mg/kg/day divided every 8 hours for 1 week, followed by oral therapy, has been reported in a clinical trial (Rubio, 1997)

Shigella dysentery type 1 (unlabeled use): Oral: 30 mg/kg/day in 2 divided doses for 3 days (WHO, 2005)

Surgical (preoperative) prophylaxis (unlabeled use): Children ≥1 year: I.V.: 10 mg/kg within 120 minutes prior to surgical incision (maximum: 400 mg) (Bratzler, 2013)

Urinary tract infection (complicated) or pyelonephritis:

Oral: 20-40 mg/kg/day in 2 divided doses (every 12 hours) for 10-21 days; maximum: 1500 mg daily. **Note:** 30-40 mg/kg/day reserved for severe infections (Red Book, 2012)

I.V.: 6-10 mg/kg every 8 hours for 10-21 days (maximum: 400 mg dose)

Adults:

Anthrax:

Inhalational (postexposure prophylaxis):

Oral: 500 mg every 12 hours for 60 days

I.V.: 400 mg every 12 hours for 60 days

Cutaneous (treatment, CDC guidelines): Oral: Immediate release formulation: 500 mg every 12 hours for 60 days. **Note:** In the presence of systemic involvement, extensive edema, lesions on head/neck, refer to I.V. dosing for treatment of inhalational/gastrointestinal/oropharyngeal anthrax

Inhalational/gastrointestinal/oropharyngeal (treatment, CDC guidelines): I.V.: 400 mg every 12 hours. **Note:** Initial treatment should include two or more agents predicted to be effective (per CDC recommendations). Continue combined therapy for 60 days.

Bone/joint infections:

Oral: 500-750 mg twice daily for ≥4-6 weeks

I.V.: Mild-to-moderate: 400 mg every 12 hours for ≥4-6 weeks; Severe/complicated: 400 mg every 8 hours for ≥4-6 weeks

Chancroid (unlabeled use): Oral: 500 mg twice daily for 3 days (CDC, 2010)

Endocarditis due to HACEK organisms (AHA guidelines, unlabeled use): Note: Not first-line option; use only if intolerant of beta-lactam therapy:

Oral: 500 mg every 12 hours for 4 weeks

I.V.: 400 mg every 12 hours for 4 weeks

Epididymitis, chlamydial (unlabeled use): Oral: 500 mg single dose (Canadian STI Guidelines, 2008)

Febrile neutropenia: I.V.: 400 mg every 8 hours for 7-14 days (combination therapy with piperacillin generally recommended)

Gonococcal infections:

Urethral/cervical gonococcal infections: Oral: 250-500 mg as a single dose (CDC recommends concomitant doxycycline or azithromycin due to possible coinfection with *Chlamydia*); **Note:** As of April 2007, the CDC no longer recommends the use of fluoroquinolones for the treatment of uncomplicated gonococcal disease.

Disseminated gonococcal infection (CDC guidelines): Oral: 500 mg twice daily to complete 7 days of therapy (initial treatment with ceftriaxone 1 g I.M./I.V. daily for 24-48 hours after improvement begins); **Note:** As of April 2007, the CDC no longer recommends the use of fluoroquinolones for the treatment of more serious gonococcal disease, unless no other options exist and susceptibility can be confirmed via culture.

Granuloma inguinale (donovanosis) (unlabeled use): Oral: 750 mg twice daily for at least 3 weeks (and until lesions have healed) (CDC, 2010)

Infectious diarrhea: Oral:

Salmonella: 500 mg twice daily for 5-7 days

Shigella (including Shigella dysentery type 1) (unlabeled regimen): 500 mg twice daily for 3 days (IDSA, 2001)

Traveler's diarrhea (unlabeled regimen): Mild: 750 mg as a single dose (CDC, 2012; de la Cabada Bauch, 2011); Severe: 500 mg twice daily for 3 days (IDSA, 2001)

Vibrio cholerae (unlabeled regimen): 1 g as a single dose (CDC, 2011)

Intra-abdominal, complicated, community-acquired (in combination with metronidazole): Note: Avoid using in settings where *E. coli* susceptibility to fluoroquinolones is <90%:

Oral: 500 mg every 12 hours for 7-14 days

I.V.: 400 mg every 12 hours for 7-14 days; **Note:** 2010 IDSA guidelines recommend treatment duration of 4-7 days (provided source controlled)

Lower respiratory tract:

Oral: 500-750 mg twice daily for 7-14 days

I.V.: Mild-to-moderate: 400 mg every 12 hours for 7-14 days; Severe/complicated: 400 mg every 8 hours for 7-14 days

Meningococcal meningitis prophylaxis (unlabeled use): Oral: 500 mg as a single dose (CDC, 2005)

Nosocomial pneumonia: I.V.: 400 mg every 8 hours for 10-14 days

Periodontitis (unlabeled use): Oral: 500 mg every 12 hours for 8-10 days (Rams, 1992)

Prostatitis (chronic, bacterial):

Oral: 500 mg every 12 hours for 28 days

I.V.: 400 mg every 12 hours for 28 days

Sinusitis (acute):

Oral: 500 mg every 12 hours for 10 days

I.V.: 400 mg every 12 hours for 10 days

Skin/skin structure infections:

Oral: 500-750 mg twice daily for 7-14 days

I.V.: Mild-to-moderate: 400 mg every 12 hours for 7-14 days; Severe/complicated: 400 mg every 8 hours for 7-14 days

Surgical (preoperative) prophylaxis (unlabeled use): I.V.: 400 mg within 120 minutes prior to surgical incision (Bratzler, 2013).

Typhoid fever: Oral: 500 mg every 12 hours for 10 days

Urinary tract infection:

Acute uncomplicated, cystitis:

Oral:

Immediate release formulation: 250 mg every 12 hours for 3 days

Extended release formulation (Cipro XR): 500 mg every 24 hours for 3 days

I.V.: 200 mg every 12 hours for 7-14 days

Complicated (including pyelonephritis):

Oral:

Immediate release formulation: 500 mg every 12 hours for 7-14 days

Extended release formulation (Cipro XR): 1000 mg every 24 hours for 7-14 days

I.V.: 400 mg every 12 hours for 7-14 days

Elderly: No adjustment needed in patients with normal renal function

Dosage adjustment in renal impairment: Adults:

Manufacturer's recommendations:

Oral, immediate release:

Cl_{cr} >50 mL/minute: No dosage adjustment necessary

Cl_{cr} 30-50 mL/minute: 250-500 mg every 12 hours

Cl_{cr} 5-29 mL/minute: 250-500 mg every 18 hours

ESRD on intermittent hemodialysis (IHD)/peritoneal dialysis (PD) (administer after dialysis on dialysis days): 250-500 mg every 24 hours

Oral, extended release:

Cl_{cr} ≥30 mL/minute: No dosage adjustment necessary

Cl_{cr} <30 mL/minute: 500 mg every 24 hours

ESRD on intermittent hemodialysis (IHD)/peritoneal dialysis (PD) (administer after dialysis on dialysis days): 500 mg every 24 hours

I.V.:

Cl_{cr} ≥30 mL/minute: No dosage adjustment necessary

Cl_{cr} 5-29 mL/minute: 200-400 mg every 18-24 hours

Alternate recommendations: Oral (immediate release), I.V.:

Cl_{cr} >50 mL/minute: No dosage adjustment necessary (Aronoff, 2007)

Cl_{cr} 10-50 mL/minute: Administer 50% to 75% of usual dose every 12 hours (Aronoff, 2007)

Cl_{cr} <10 mL/minute: Administer 50% of usual dose every 12 hours (Aronoff, 2007)

Intermittent hemodialysis (IHD) (administer after hemodialysis on dialysis days): Minimally dialyzable (<10%): Oral: 250-500 mg every 24 hours **or** I.V.: 200-400 mg every 24 hours (Heintz, 2009). **Note:** Dosing dependent on the assumption of 3 times weekly, complete IHD sessions.

Continuous renal replacement therapy (CRRT) (Heintz, 2009; Trotman, 2005): Drug clearance is highly dependent on the method of renal replacement, filter type, and flow rate. Appropriate dosing requires close monitoring of pharmacologic response, signs of adverse reactions due to drug accumulation, as well as drug concentrations in relation to target trough (if appropriate). The following are general recommendations only (based on dialysate flow/ultrafiltration rates of 1-2 L/hour and minimal residual renal function) and should not supersede clinical judgment:

CVVH/CVVHD/CVVHDF: I.V.: 200-400 mg every 12-24 hours

Dosage adjustment in hepatic impairment: No dosage adjustment provided in manufacturer's labeling (has not been studied). No pharmacokinetic changes were noted in patients with stable chronic cirrhosis, but pharmacokinetics have not been evaluated in patients with acute impairment.

Dietary Considerations Food: Drug may cause GI upset; take without regard to meals (manufacturer prefers that immediate release tablet is taken 2 hours after meals). Extended release tablet may be taken with meals that contain dairy products (calcium content <800 mg), but not with dairy products alone.

Dairy products, calcium-fortified juices, oral multivitamins, and mineral supplements: Absorption of ciprofloxacin is decreased by divalent and trivalent cations. The manufacturer states that the usual dietary intake of calcium (including meals which include dairy products) has not been shown to interfere with ciprofloxacin absorption. Immediate release ciprofloxacin and Cipro XR may be taken 2 hours before or 6 hours after any of these products.

Caffeine: Patients consuming regular large quantities of caffeinated beverages may need to restrict caffeine intake if excessive cardiac or CNS stimulation occurs.

Administration

Oral: May administer with food to minimize GI upset; avoid antacid use; maintain proper hydration and urine output. Administer immediate release ciprofloxacin and Cipro XR at least 2 hours before or 6 hours after antacids or other products containing calcium, iron, or zinc (including dairy products or calcium-fortified juices). Separate oral administration from drugs which may impair absorption (see Drug Interactions).

Oral suspension: Should not be administered through feeding tubes (suspension is oil-based and adheres to the feeding tube). Patients should avoid chewing on the microcapsules.

Nasogastric/orogastric tube: Crush immediate-release tablet and mix with water. Flush feeding tube before and after administration. Hold tube feedings at least 1 hour before and 2 hours after administration.

Tablet, extended release: Do not crush, split, or chew. May be administered with meals containing dairy products (calcium content <800 mg), but not with dairy products alone.

Parenteral: Administer by slow I.V. infusion over 60 minutes into a large vein (reduces risk of venous irritation).

Monitoring Parameters CBC, renal and hepatic function during prolonged therapy

Reference Range Therapeutic: 2.6-3 mcg/mL; Toxic: >5 mcg/mL

Test Interactions Some quinolones may produce a false-positive urine screening result for opioids using commercially-available immunoassay kits. This has been demonstrated most consistently for levofloxacin and ofloxacin, but other quinolones have shown cross-reactivity in certain assay kits. Confirmation of positive opioid screens by more specific methods should be considered.

Additional Information Although the systemic use of ciprofloxacin is only FDA-approved in children for the treatment of complicated UTI and postexposure treatment of inhalation anthrax, use of the fluoroquinolones in pediatric patients is increasing. Current recommendations by the American Academy of Pediatrics note that the systemic use of these agents in children should be restricted to infections caused by multidrug resistant pathogens with no safe or effective alternative, and when parenteral therapy is not feasible or other oral agents are not available.

Dosage Forms Excipient information presented when available (limited, particularly for generics); consult specific product labeling.

Solution, Intravenous:

Cipro in D_5W: 200 mg/100 mL (100 mL) [latex free]

Generic: 200 mg/100 mL (100 mL); 400 mg/200 mL (200 mL); 200 mg/20 mL (20 mL); 400 mg/40 mL (40 mL)

Solution, Intravenous [preservative free]:

Cipro in D_5W: 200 mg/100 mL (100 mL); 400 mg/200 mL (200 mL) [latex free]

Generic: 200 mg/100 mL (100 mL); 400 mg/200 mL (200 mL); 200 mg/20 mL (20 mL); 400 mg/40 mL (40 mL)

Suspension Reconstituted, Oral:

Cipro: 250 mg/5 mL (100 mL); 500 mg/5 mL (100 mL) [strawberry flavor]

Tablet, Oral [strength expressed as base]:

Generic: 500 mg

Tablet, Oral, as hydrochloride [strength expressed as base]:

Cipro: 250 mg, 500 mg

Generic: 100 mg, 250 mg, 500 mg, 750 mg

Tablet Extended Release 24 Hour, Oral, as base and hydrochloride [strength expressed as base]:

Cipro XR: 500 mg, 1000 mg

Generic: 500 mg, 1000 mg

Extemporaneous Preparations A 50 mg/mL oral suspension may be made using 2 different vehicles (a 1:1 mixture of Ora-Sweet and Ora-Plus or a 1:1 mixture of Methylcellulose 1% and Simple Syrup, NF). Crush twenty 500 mg tablets and reduce to a fine powder. Add a small amount of vehicle and mix to a uniform paste; mix while adding the vehicle in geometric proportions to **almost** 200 mL; transfer to a calibrated bottle, rinse mortar with vehicle, and add quantity of vehicle sufficient to make 200 mL. Label "shake well" and "refrigerate". Stable 91 days refrigerated and 70 days at room temperature. **Note:** Microcapsules for oral suspension available (50 mg/mL; 100 mg/mL); not for use in feeding tubes.

Nahata MC, Pai VB, and Hipple TF, *Pediatric Drug Formulations*, 5th ed, Cincinnati, OH: Harvey Whitney Books Co, 2004.

Ciprofloxacin (Ophthalmic) (sip roe FLOKS a sin)

Brand Names: U.S. Ciloxan

Brand Names: Canada Ciloxan®

Index Terms Ciprofloxacin Hydrochloride

Pharmacologic Category Antibiotic, Fluoroquinolone; Antibiotic, Ophthalmic

Use Treatment of superficial ocular infections (corneal ulcers, conjunctivitis) due to susceptible strains

Pregnancy Risk Factor C

Dosage Ophthalmic:

Bacterial conjunctivitis:

Ophthalmic solution: Children ≥1 year and Adults: Instill 1-2 drops into the conjunctival sac every 2 hours while awake for 2 days and 1-2 drops every 4 hours while awake for the next 5 days

Ophthalmic ointment: Children ≥2 years and Adults: Apply a 1/2 inch ribbon into the conjunctival sac 3 times/day for the first 2 days, followed by a 1/2 inch ribbon applied twice daily for the next 5 days

Corneal ulcer: Ophthalmic solution: Children ≥1 year and Adults: Instill 2 drops into affected eye every 15 minutes for the first 6 hours, then 2 drops into the affected eye every 30 minutes for the remainder of the first day. On day 2, instill 2 drops into the affected eye hourly. On days 3-14, instill 2 drops into affected eye every 4 hours. Treatment may continue after day 14 if re-epithelialization has not occurred.

Dosage adjustment in renal impairment: No dosage adjustment provided in manufacturer's labeling.

Dosage adjustment in hepatic impairment: No dosage adjustment provided in manufacturer's labeling.

Additional Information Complete prescribing information should be consulted for additional detail.

Dosage Forms Excipient information presented when available (limited, particularly for generics); consult specific product labeling.

Ointment, Ophthalmic, as hydrochloride:

Ciloxan: 0.3% (3.5 g)

Solution, Ophthalmic, as hydrochloride:

Ciloxan: 0.3% (5 mL) [contains benzalkonium chloride, edetate disodium]

Generic: 0.3% (2.5 mL, 5 mL, 10 mL)

Ciprofloxacin (Otic) (sip roe FLOKS a sin)

Brand Names: U.S. Cetraxal

Index Terms Ciprofloxacin Hydrochloride

Pharmacologic Category Antibiotic, Fluoroquinolone; Antibiotic, Otic

Use Treatment of acute otitis externa due to susceptible strains of *Pseudomonas aeruginosa* or *Staphylococcus aureus*

Pregnancy Risk Factor C

Dosage Otic: Children ≥1 year and Adults: Acute otitis externa: Instill 0.25 mL solution (contents of 1 single-dose container) into affected ear twice daily for 7 days

Additional Information Complete prescribing information should be consulted for additional detail.

Dosage Forms Excipient information presented when available (limited, particularly for generics); consult specific product labeling.

Solution, Otic, as hydrochloride [preservative free]:

Cetraxal: 0.2% (1 ea)

Generic: 0.2% (1 ea)

Ciprofloxacin and Dexamethasone

(sip roe FLOKS a sin & deks a METH a sone)

Brand Names: U.S. Ciprodex®

Brand Names: Canada Ciprodex®

Index Terms Ciprofloxacin Hydrochloride and Dexamethasone; Dexamethasone and Ciprofloxacin

Pharmacologic Category Antibiotic, Otic; Antibiotic/Corticosteroid, Otic; Corticosteroid, Otic

Use Treatment of acute otitis media in pediatric patients with tympanostomy tubes or acute otitis externa in children and adults

Pregnancy Risk Factor C

Dosage Otic:

Children: Acute otitis media in patients with tympanostomy tubes or acute otitis externa: Instill 4 drops into affected ear(s) twice daily for 7 days

Adults: Acute otitis externa: Instill 4 drops into affected ear(s) twice daily for 7 days

Dosage adjustment in renal impairment: No dosage adjustment provided in manufacturer's labeling.

Dosage adjustment in hepatic impairment: No dosage adjustment provided in manufacturer's labeling.

Additional Information Complete prescribing information should be consulted for additional detail.

Dosage Forms Excipient information presented when available (limited, particularly for generics); consult specific product labeling.

Suspension, otic:

Ciprodex®: Ciprofloxacin 0.3% and dexamethasone 0.1% (7.5 mL) [contains benzalkonium chloride]

Ciprofloxacin and Hydrocortisone

(sip roe FLOKS a sin & hye droe KOR ti sone)

Brand Names: U.S. Cipro® HC

Brand Names: Canada Cipro® HC

Index Terms Ciprofloxacin Hydrochloride and Hydrocortisone; Hydrocortisone and Ciprofloxacin

Pharmacologic Category Antibiotic/Corticosteroid, Otic

Use Treatment of acute otitis externa, sometimes known as "swimmer's ear"

Pregnancy Risk Factor C

Dosage Children >1 year of age and Adults: Otic: The recommended dosage for all patients is three drops of the suspension in the affected ear twice daily for 7 days; twice-daily dosing schedule is more convenient for patients than that of existing treatments with hydrocortisone, which are typically administered 3 or 4 times a day; a twice-daily dosage schedule may be especially helpful for parents and caregivers of young children

Dosage adjustment in renal impairment: No dosage adjustment provided in manufacturer's labeling.

Dosage adjustment in hepatic impairment: No dosage adjustment provided in manufacturer's labeling.

Additional Information Complete prescribing information should be consulted for additional detail.

Dosage Forms Excipient information presented when available (limited, particularly for generics); consult specific product labeling.

Suspension, otic:

Cipro® HC: Ciprofloxacin hydrochloride 0.2% and hydrocortisone 1% (10 mL) [contains benzyl alcohol]

- ◆ **Ciprofloxacin Hydrochloride** *see* Ciprofloxacin (Ophthalmic) *on page 435*
- ◆ **Ciprofloxacin Hydrochloride** *see* Ciprofloxacin (Otic) *on page 435*
- ◆ **Ciprofloxacin Hydrochloride** *see* Ciprofloxacin (Systemic) *on page 430*
- ◆ **Ciprofloxacin Hydrochloride and Dexamethasone** *see* Ciprofloxacin and Dexamethasone *on page 435*
- ◆ **Ciprofloxacin Hydrochloride and Hydrocortisone** *see* Ciprofloxacin and Hydrocortisone *on page 435*
- ◆ **Cipro® HC** *see* Ciprofloxacin and Hydrocortisone *on page 435*
- ◆ **Cipro in D_5W** *see* Ciprofloxacin (Systemic) *on page 430*
- ◆ **Cipro XR** *see* Ciprofloxacin (Systemic) *on page 430*

Cisatracurium (sis a tra KYOO ree um)

Brand Names: U.S. Nimbex

Brand Names: Canada Nimbex

Index Terms Cisatracurium Besylate

Pharmacologic Category Neuromuscular Blocker Agent, Nondepolarizing

Use Adjunct to general anesthesia to facilitate endotracheal intubation and to relax skeletal muscles during surgery; to facilitate mechanical ventilation in ICU patients; does not relieve pain or produce sedation

Pregnancy Risk Factor B

Pregnancy Considerations Adverse events have not been observed in animal reproduction studies.

Breast-Feeding Considerations It is not known if cisatracurium is excreted in breast milk. The manufacturer recommends that caution be exercised when administering cisatracurium to nursing women.

Contraindications Hypersensitivity to cisatracurium besylate or any component of the formulation; use of the 10 mL multiple-dose vials in premature infants (formulation contains benzyl alcohol)

Warnings/Precautions Maintenance of an adequate airway and respiratory support is critical; certain clinical conditions may result in potentiation or antagonism of neuromuscular blockade:

Potentiation: Electrolyte abnormalities, severe hyponatremia, severe hypocalcemia, severe hypokalemia, hypermagnesemia, neuromuscular diseases, acidosis, acute intermittent porphyria, renal failure, hepatic failure

Antagonism: Alkalosis, hypercalcemia, demyelinating lesions, peripheral neuropathies, diabetes mellitus

Hypothermia may slow Hoffmann elimination thereby prolonging the duration of activity (Greenberg, 2013). Increased sensitivity in patients with myasthenia gravis, Eaton-Lambert syndrome; resistance in burn patients (>30% of body) for period of 5-70 days postinjury; resistance in patients with muscle trauma, denervation, immobilization, infection. Cross-sensitivity with other neuromuscular-blocking agents may occur; use extreme caution in patients with previous anaphylactic reactions to other neuromuscular-blocking agents. Bradycardia may be more common with cisatracurium than with other neuromuscular blocking agents since it has no clinically significant effects on heart rate to counteract the bradycardia produced by anesthetics. Use caution in the elderly. Should be administered by adequately trained individuals familiar with its use. Some dosage forms may contain benzyl alcohol which has been associated with "gasping syndrome" in neonates.

Adverse Reactions <1%: Effects are minimal and transient, bradycardia and hypotension, flushing, pruritus, rash, bronchospasm, acute quadriplegic myopathy syndrome (prolonged use), myositis ossificans (prolonged use)

Drug Interactions

Metabolism/Transport Effects None known.

Avoid Concomitant Use

Avoid concomitant use of Cisatracurium with any of the following: QuiNINE

Increased Effect/Toxicity

Cisatracurium may increase the levels/effects of: Cardiac Glycosides; Corticosteroids (Systemic); OnabotulinumtoxinA; RimabotulinumtoxinB

The levels/effects of Cisatracurium may be increased by: AbobotulinumtoxinA; Aminoglycosides; Calcium Channel Blockers; Capreomycin; Colistimethate; CycloSPORINE (Systemic); Fosphenytoin-Phenytoin; Inhalational Anesthetics; Ketorolac (Nasal); Ketorolac (Systemic); Lincosamide Antibiotics; Lithium; Loop Diuretics; Magnesium Salts; Polymyxin B; Procainamide; QuiNIDine; QuiNINE; Spironolactone; Tetracycline Derivatives; Vancomycin

Decreased Effect

The levels/effects of Cisatracurium may be decreased by: Acetylcholinesterase Inhibitors; Fosphenytoin-Phenytoin; Loop Diuretics

Storage/Stability Refrigerate intact vials at 2°C to 8°C (36°F to 46°F). Use vials within 21 days upon removal from the refrigerator to room temperature of 25°C (77°F). Per the manufacturer, dilutions of 0.1 mg/mL in 0.9% sodium chloride (NS), dextrose 5% in water (D_5W), or D_5NS are stable for up to 24 hours at room temperature or under refrigeration; dilutions of 0.1-0.2 mg/mL in D_5LR are stable for up to 24 hours in the refrigerator. *Additional stability data:* Dilutions of 0.1, 2, and 5 mg/mL in D_5W or NS are stable in the refrigerator for up to 30 days; at room temperature (23°C), dilutions of 0.1 and 2 mg/mL began exhibiting substantial drug loss between 7-14 days; dilutions of 5 mg/mL in D_5W or NS are stable for up to 30 days at room temperature (23°C) (Xu, 1998). Usual concentration: 0.1-0.4 mg/mL.

Mechanism of Action Blocks neural transmission at the myoneural junction by binding with cholinergic receptor sites

Pharmacodynamics/Kinetics

Onset of action: I.V.: 2-3 minutes

Peak effect: 3-5 minutes

Duration: Recovery begins in 20-35 minutes when anesthesia is balanced; recovery is attained in 90% of patients in 25-93 minutes

Distribution: V_{dss}: 145 mL/kg (21% larger V_{dss} when receiving inhalational anesthetics)

Protein binding: Not studied due to rapid degradation at physiologic pH

Metabolism: Undergoes rapid nonenzymatic degradation in the bloodstream (Hofmann elimination) to laudanosine and inactive metabolites; laudanosine may cause CNS stimulation (association not established in humans) and has less accumulation with prolonged use than atracurium due to lower requirements for clinical effect

Half-life elimination: 22-29 minutes

Excretion: Urine (95%; <10% as unchanged drug)

Dosage I.V. (not to be used I.M.):

Operating room administration:

Infants 1-23 months: Intubating dose: 0.15 mg/kg over 5-10 seconds

Children 2-12 years: Intubating dose: 0.1-0.15 mg/kg over 5-10 seconds. (**Note:** When given during stable opioid/nitrous oxide/oxygen anesthesia, 0.1 mg/kg produces maximum neuromuscular block in an average of 2.8 minutes and clinically effective block for 28 minutes.)

Adults: Intubating dose: 0.15-0.2 mg/kg as component of propofol/nitrous oxide/oxygen induction-intubation technique. (**Note:** May produce generally good or excellent conditions for tracheal intubation in 1.5-2 minutes with clinically effective duration of action during propofol anesthesia of 55-61 minutes.) Initial dose after succinylcholine for intubation: 0.1 mg/kg; maintenance dose: 0.03 mg/kg 40-60 minutes after initial dose, then at ~20-minute intervals based on clinical criteria

Children ≥2 years and Adults: Continuous infusion: After an initial bolus, a diluted solution can be given by continuous infusion for maintenance of neuromuscular blockade during extended surgery; adjust the rate of administration according to the patient's response as determined by peripheral nerve stimulation. An initial infusion rate of 3 **mcg**/kg/**minute** (0.18 **mg**/kg/**hour**) may be required to rapidly counteract the spontaneous recovery of neuromuscular function; thereafter, a rate of 1-2 **mcg**/kg/**minute** (0.06-0.12 **mg**/kg/**hour**) should be adequate to maintain continuous neuromuscular block in the 89% to 99% range in most pediatric and adult patients. Consider reduction of the infusion rate by 30% to 40% when administering during stable isoflurane, enflurane, sevoflurane, or desflurane anesthesia. Spontaneous recovery from neuromuscular blockade following discontinuation of infusion of cisatracurium may be expected to proceed at a rate comparable to that following single bolus administration.

Intensive care unit administration:

Manufacturer's labeling: Loading dose: 0.15-0.2 mg/kg; at initial signs of recovery from bolus dose, begin the infusion at a dose of 3 **mcg**/kg/**minute** (0.18 **mg**/kg/**hour**) and adjust rate accordingly (follow the principles for infusion in the operating room); dosage ranges of 0.5-10 **mcg**/kg/**minute** (0.03-0.6 **mg**/kg/**hour**) have been reported. If patient is allowed to recover from neuromuscular blockade, readministration of a bolus dose may be necessary to quickly re-establish neuromuscular block prior to reinstituting the infusion.

or

Loading dose: 0.1 mg/kg (additional boluses of 0.05 mg/kg until train-of-four response is 3/4 or less can be used); then initiate an infusion at 2.5-3 **mcg**/kg/**minute** (0.15-0.18 **mg**/kg/**hour**) and adjust rate accordingly (Baumann, 2004; Lagneau, 2002).

or

Loading dose: 0.1 to 0.2 mg/kg; immediately following loading dose administration, begin an infusion at 1-3 **mcg**/kg/**minute** (0.06-0.18 **mg**/kg/**hour**) and adjust rate accordingly (Greenberg, 2013).

Dosing adjustment in renal impairment: Because slower times to onset of complete neuromuscular block were observed in renal dysfunction patients, extending the interval between the administration of cisatracurium and intubation attempt may be required to achieve adequate intubation conditions.

Dosage adjustment in hepatic impairment: No dosage adjustment provided in manufacturer's labeling. The time to onset of action was ~1 minute faster in patients with end-stage liver disease, but was not associated with clinically significant changes in recovery time.

Usual Infusion Concentrations: Adult I.V. infusion: 100 mg in 250 mL (total volume) (concentration: 400 **mcg**/mL) of D_5W or NS

Administration Administer I.V. only; give undiluted as bolus injection over 5-10 seconds. Continuous infusion requires the use of an infusion pump. The use of a peripheral nerve stimulator will permit the most advantageous use of cisatracurium, minimize the possibility of overdosage or underdosage and assist in the evaluation of recovery.

Do not administer I.M. (excessive tissue irritation).

Monitoring Parameters Peripheral nerve stimulator measuring twitch response (when appropriate); vital signs (heart rate, blood pressure, respiratory rate)

Additional Information Cisatracurium is classified as an intermediate-duration neuromuscular-blocking agent. It does not appear to have a cumulative effect on the duration of blockade. Neuromuscular-blocking potency is 3 times that of atracurium; maximum block is up to 2 minutes longer than for equipotent doses of atracurium.

Dosage Forms Excipient information presented when available (limited, particularly for generics); consult specific product labeling.

Solution, Intravenous:
- Nimbex: 10 mg/5 mL (5 mL)
- Nimbex: 20 mg/10 mL (10 mL) [contains benzyl alcohol]
- Nimbex: 10 mg/mL (20 mL)
- Generic: 20 mg/10 mL (10 mL)

Solution, Intravenous [preservative free]:
- Generic: 10 mg/5 mL (5 mL); 10 mg/mL (20 mL)

◆ **Cisatracurium Besylate** *see* Cisatracurium *on page 436*

◆ **cis-DDP** *see* CISplatin *on page 437*

◆ **cis-Diamminedichloroplatinum** *see* CISplatin *on page 437*

CISplatin (SIS pla tin)

Brand Names: Canada AJ-Cisplatin; Cisplatin Injection; Cisplatin Injection BP

Index Terms CDDP; cis-DDP; cis-Diamminedichloroplatinum; Platinol; Platinol-AQ

Pharmacologic Category Antineoplastic Agent, Alkylating Agent; Antineoplastic Agent, Platinum Analog

Additional Appendix Information

Beers Criteria – Potentially Inappropriate Medications for Geriatrics *on page 2368*

Use Treatment of advanced bladder cancer, metastatic testicular cancer, and metastatic ovarian cancer

Unlabeled Use Treatment of breast cancer (metastatic), central nervous system tumors, cervical cancer, endometrial cancer, esophageal cancer, gastric cancer, germ cell tumors, gestational trophoblastic disease (refractory), head and neck cancer, hepatobiliary cancer, hepatoblastoma, Hodgkin lymphoma, malignant pleural mesothelioma, melanoma (metastatic), multiple myeloma, neuroblastoma, neuroendocrine tumors, non-Hodgkin lymphoma (NHL), nonsmall cell lung cancer (NSCLC), osteosarcoma, pancreatic cancer (advanced), prostate cancer, small cell lung cancer (SCLC), soft tissue sarcomas, and unknown primary cancers

Pregnancy Risk Factor D

Pregnancy Considerations Animal reproduction studies have demonstrated teratogenicity and embryotoxicity. Women of childbearing potential should be advised to avoid pregnancy. If used in pregnancy, or if patient becomes pregnant during treatment, the patient should be apprised of potential hazard to the fetus.

Breast-Feeding Considerations Cisplatin is excreted in breast milk. Per the manufacturer, breast-feeding is not recommended.

Contraindications Hypersensitivity to cisplatin, other platinum-containing compounds, or any component of the formulation (anaphylactic-like reactions have been reported); pre-existing renal impairment; myelosuppression; hearing impairment

Warnings/Precautions Hazardous agent - use appropriate precautions for handling and disposal (NIOSH, 2012). **[U.S. Boxed Warning]: Doses >100 mg/m² once every 3-4 weeks are rarely used; verify with the prescriber. Exercise caution to avoid potential sound-alike/look-alike confusion between CISplatin and CARBOplatin.** Patients should receive adequate hydration, with or without diuretics, prior to and for 24 hours after cisplatin administration. **[U.S. Boxed Warning]: Cumulative renal toxicity may be severe.** Monitor serum creatinine, blood urea nitrogen, creatinine clearance, and serum electrolytes closely. According to the manufacturer's labeling, use is contraindicated in patients with pre-existing renal impairment and renal function must return to normal prior to administering subsequent cycles; some literature recommends reduced doses with renal impairment. Nephrotoxicity may be potentiated by aminoglycosides.

Use caution in the elderly; may cause or exacerbate syndrome of inappropriate antidiuretic hormone secretion or hyponatremia; monitor sodium closely with initiation or dosage adjustments in older adults (Beers Criteria). Elderly patients may be more susceptible to nephrotoxicity and peripheral neuropathy; select dose cautiously and monitor closely.

[U.S. Boxed Warning]: Dose-related toxicities include myelosuppression, nausea, and vomiting. Nausea and vomiting may be immediate and/or delayed; antiemetics are recommended. Diarrhea may also occur. **[U.S. Boxed Warning]: Ototoxicity, especially pronounced in children, is manifested by tinnitus or loss of high frequency hearing and occasionally, deafness; may be significant.** Pediatric patients with certain genetic variations in the thiopurine S-methyltransferase (TPMT) gene may be at increased risk of ototoxicity, even when conventional cisplatin doses are given. Ototoxicity is cumulative; audiometric testing should be performed at baseline and prior to each dose. Pediatric patients should receive audiometric testing for several years after discontinuing therapy. Severe (and possibly irreversible) neuropathies may occur with higher than recommended doses or more frequent administration; may require therapy discontinuation. Seizures, loss of motor function, loss of taste, leukoencephalopathy, and posterior reversible leukoencephalopathy syndrome (PRES [formerly RPLS]) have also been described. Serum electrolytes, particularly magnesium and potassium, should be monitored and replaced as needed during and after cisplatin therapy.

[U.S. Boxed Warning]: Anaphylactic-like reactions have been reported; may include facial edema, bronchoconstriction, tachycardia, and hypotension and may occur within minutes of administration; may be managed with epinephrine, corticosteroids, and/or antihistamines. Hyperuricemia has been reported with cisplatin use, and is more pronounced with doses >50 mg/m²; consider allopurinol therapy to reduce uric acid levels. Local infusion site reactions may occur; monitor infusion site during administration; avoid extravasation. Secondary malignancies have been reported with cisplatin in combination with other chemotherapy agents. **[U.S. Boxed Warning]: Should be administered under the supervision of an experienced cancer chemotherapy physician.** Cisplatin is a vesicant at higher concentrations, and an irritant at lower concentrations; ensure proper needle or catheter placement prior to and during infusion; avoid extravasation.

Adverse Reactions

>10%:

Central nervous system: Neurotoxicity: Peripheral neuropathy is dose- and duration-dependent.

Gastrointestinal: Nausea and vomiting (76% to 100%)

Hematologic: Anemia (≤40%), leukopenia (25% to 30%; nadir: Day 18-23; recovery: By day 39; dose related), thrombocytopenia (25% to 30%; nadir: Day 18-23; recovery: By day 39; dose related)

Hepatic: Liver enzymes increased

Renal: Nephrotoxicity (28% to 36%; acute renal failure and chronic renal insufficiency)

Otic: Ototoxicity (children 40% to 60%; adults 10% to 31%; as tinnitus, high frequency hearing loss)

1% to 10%: Local: Tissue irritation

<1% (Limited to important or life-threatening): Alopecia (mild), anaphylactic reaction, arrhythmias, arterial vasospasm (acute), autonomic neuropathy, bradycardia, bronchoconstriction, cerebral arteritis, cerebrovascular accident, dehydration, extravasation injury, heart block, heart failure, hemolytic anemia (acute), hemolytic uremic syndrome, hypercholesterolemia, hyperuricemia, hypocalcemia, hypokalemia, hypomagnesemia, hyponatremia, hypophosphatemia, hypotension, leukoencephalopathy, Lhermitte's phenomenon, limb ischemia (acute), mesenteric ischemia (acute), mouth sores, myocardial infarction, myocardial ischemia, neutropenic typhlitis, optic neuritis, orthostatic hypotension, pancreatitis, papilledema, phlebitis, reversible posterior leukoencephalopathy syndrome (RPLS), seizures, serum amylase increased, SIADH, spinal cord injury, stroke, tachycardia, tetany, thrombophlebitis, thrombotic microangiopathy, thrombotic thrombocytopenic purpura, vision loss, visual color perception changes

Drug Interactions

Metabolism/Transport Effects None known.

Avoid Concomitant Use

Avoid concomitant use of CISplatin with any of the following: BCG; CloZAPine; Natalizumab; Pimecrolimus; Tacrolimus (Topical); Tofacitinib; Vaccines (Live)

Increased Effect/Toxicity

CISplatin may increase the levels/effects of: Aminoglycosides; CloZAPine; Leflunomide; Natalizumab; Taxane Derivatives; Tofacitinib; Topotecan; Vaccines (Live); Vinorelbine

The levels/effects of CISplatin may be increased by: Denosumab; Loop Diuretics; Pimecrolimus; Roflumilast; Tacrolimus (Topical); Trastuzumab

Decreased Effect

CISplatin may decrease the levels/effects of: BCG; Coccidioidin Skin Test; Fosphenytoin-Phenytoin; Sipuleucel-T; Vaccines (Inactivated); Vaccines (Live)

The levels/effects of CISplatin may be decreased by: Echinacea

Preparation for Administration Hazardous agent; use appropriate precautions for handling and disposal (NIOSH, 2012). The infusion solution should have a final sodium chloride concentration ≥0.2%. Needles or I.V. administration sets that contain aluminum should not be used in the preparation or administration; aluminum can react with cisplatin resulting in precipitate formation and loss of potency.

Storage/Stability Store intact vials at room temperature 15°C to 25°C (59°F to 77°F). Protect from light. Do not refrigerate solution as a precipitate may form. Further dilution **stability is dependent on the chloride ion concentration** and should be mixed in solutions of NS (at least 0.3% NaCl). After initial entry into the vial, solution is stable for 28 days protected from light or for at least 7 days under fluorescent room light at room temperature.

Further dilutions in NS, D_5/0.45% NaCl or D_5/NS to a concentration of 0.05-2 mg/mL are stable for 72 hours at 4°C to 25°C. The infusion solution should have a final sodium chloride concentration ≥0.2%.

Mechanism of Action Inhibits DNA synthesis by the formation of DNA cross-links; denatures the double helix; covalently binds to DNA bases and disrupts DNA function; may also bind to proteins; the *cis*-isomer is 14 times more cytotoxic than the *trans*-isomer; both forms cross-link DNA but cis-platinum is less easily recognized by cell enzymes and, therefore, not repaired. Cisplatin can also bind two adjacent guanines on the same strand of DNA producing intrastrand cross-linking and breakage.

Pharmacodynamics/Kinetics

Distribution: I.V.: Rapidly into tissue; high concentrations in kidneys, liver, ovaries, uterus, and lungs

Protein binding: >90% (O'Dwyer, 2000)

Metabolism: Nonenzymatic; inactivated (in both cell and bloodstream) by sulfhydryl groups; covalently binds to glutathione and thiosulfate

Half-life elimination: Initial: 14-49 minutes; Beta: 0.7-4.6 hours; Gamma: 24-127 hours (O'Dwyer, 2000)

Excretion: Urine (>90%); feces (minimal)

Dosage VERIFY ANY CISPLATIN DOSE EXCEEDING 100 mg/m² PER COURSE. Pretreatment hydration with 1-2 L of I.V. fluid is recommended. Details concerning dosing in combination regimens should also be consulted.

Children: I.V.:

Germ cell tumors (unlabeled use; combination chemotherapy): 20 mg/m²/day on days 1-5 or 100 mg/m² on day 1 of a 21-day treatment cycle (Pinkerton, 1986)

Hepatoblastoma (unlabeled use; combination chemotherapy): 80 mg/m² continuous infusion over 24 hours on day 1 of a 21-day treatment cycle (Pritchard, 2000)

Medulloblastoma (unlabeled use; combination chemotherapy): 75 mg/m² on either day 0 or day 1 of each chemotherapy cycle (Packer, 2006)

Neuroblastoma, high-risk (unlabeled use; combination chemotherapy): 50 mg/m²/day on days 0-3 of a 21-day cycle (cycles 3 and 5) (Naranjo, 2011) **or** 50 mg/m²/day on days 1-4 (cycles 3, 5, and 7) (Kushner, 1994)

Osteosarcoma (unlabeled use; combination chemotherapy): 60 mg/m²/day for 2 days weeks 2, 7, 25, and 28 (neoadjuvant) or weeks 5, 10, 25, and 28 (adjuvant) (Goorin, 2003)

Adults: I.V.:

Bladder cancer, advanced: 50-70 mg/m² every 3-4 weeks; heavily pretreated patients: 50 mg/m² every 4 weeks

Ovarian cancer, metastatic:

Single agent: 100 mg/m² every 4 weeks

Combination therapy: 75-100 mg/m² every 4 weeks or (unlabeled dosing) 75 mg/m² every 3 weeks (Ozols, 2003)

Testicular cancer, metastatic: 20 mg/m²/day for 5 days repeated every 3 weeks (Cushing, 2004; Saxman, 1998)

Cervical cancer (unlabeled use): 75 mg/m² on day 1 every 3 weeks (in combination with fluorouracil and radiation) for 3 cycles (Morris, 1999) **or** 70 mg/m² on day 1 every 3 weeks for 4 cycles (in combination with fluorouracil; cycles 1 and 2 given concurrently with radiation) (Peters, 2000) **or** 50 mg/m² on day 1 every 4 weeks (in combination with radiation and fluorouracil) for 2 cycles (Whitney, 1999)

Endometrial carcinoma, recurrent, metastatic, or high-risk (unlabeled use): 50 mg/m² on day 1 every 3 weeks (in combination with doxorubicin ± paclitaxel) for 7 cycles or until disease progression or unacceptable toxicity (Fleming, 2004)

Head and neck cancer (unlabeled use):

Locally-advanced disease: 100 mg/m² every 3 weeks for 3 doses (with concurrent radiation) (Bernier, 2004; Cooper, 2004) **or** 75 mg/m² every 3 weeks (in combination with docetaxel and fluorouracil) for 4 cycles or until disease progression or unacceptable toxicity (if no disease progression after 4 cycles, chemotherapy was followed by radiation) (Vermorken, 2007) **or** 100 mg/m² every 3 weeks (in combination with docetaxel and fluorouracil) for 3 cycles or until disease progression or unacceptable toxicity (chemotherapy was followed by chemoradiation) (Posner, 2007)

Metastatic disease: 100 mg/m² every 3 weeks (in combination with fluorouracil and cetuximab) until disease progression or unacceptable toxicity or a maximum of 6 cycles (Vermorken, 2008)

Malignant pleural mesothelioma (unlabeled use): 75 mg/m² on day 1 of each 21-day cycle (in combination with pemetrexed) (Vogelzang, 2003) **or** 100 mg/m² on day 1 of a 28-day cycle (in combination with gemcitabine) (Nowak, 2002) **or** 80 mg/m² on day 1 of a 21-day cycle (in combination with gemcitabine) (van Haarst, 2002)

NSCLC (unlabeled use): **Note:** There are multiple cisplatin-containing regimens for the treatment of NSCLC. Listed below are several commonly used regimens:

100 mg/m² on day 1 every 4 weeks (in combination with etoposide) for 3-4 cycles; (Arriagada, 2007), or

100 mg/m² on day 1 every 4 weeks (in combination with vinorelbine) (Kelly, 2001; Wozniak, 1998), or

100 mg/m² on day 1 every 4 weeks (in combination with gemcitabine) (Comella, 2000), or

80 mg/m² on day 1 every 3 weeks (in combination with gemcitabine) (Ohe, 2007), or

75 mg/m² on day 1 every 3 weeks (in combination with pemetrexed) for up to 6 cycles or until disease progression or unacceptable toxicity (Scagliotti, 2008)

SCLC (unlabeled use):

Limited-stage disease: 60 mg/m² on day 1 every 3 weeks for 4 cycles (in combination with etoposide and concurrent radiation) (Turrisi, 1999)

Extensive-stage disease: 80 mg/m² on day 1 every 3 weeks (in combination with etoposide) for 4 cycles (Lara, 2009) or a maximum of 8 cycles (Ihde, 1994) **or** 60 mg/m² on day 1 every 4 weeks for 4 cycles (in combination with irinotecan) (Lara, 2009)

Testicular germ cell tumor, malignant (unlabeled use): 25 mg/m² on days 2-5 every 3 weeks (in combination with paclitaxel and ifosfamide) for 4 cycles (Kondagunta, 2005) **or** 20 mg/m² on days 1-5 every 3 weeks (in combination with bleomycin and etoposide) for 4 cycles (Nichols, 1998) **or** 20 mg/m² on days 1-5 every 3 weeks (in combination with etoposide and ifosfamide) for 4 cycles (Nichols, 1998)

Adults: Intraperitoneal: Ovarian cancer (unlabeled route): 75-100 mg/m² on day 2 of a 21-day treatment cycle (in combination with I.V. and intraperitoneal paclitaxel) for 6 cycles (Armstrong, 2006; NCCN Ovarian Cancer guidelines, v.1.2013)

Elderly: Select dose cautiously and monitor closely in the elderly; may be more susceptible to nephrotoxicity and peripheral neuropathy.

Dosage adjustment in renal impairment: Note: The manufacturer(s) recommend that repeat courses of cisplatin should not be given until serum creatinine is <1.5 mg/dL and/or BUN is <25 mg/dL and use is contraindicated in pre-existing renal impairment. The following adjustments have been recommended:

Aronoff, 2007:

Cl_{cr} 10-50 mL/minute: Administer 75% of dose

Cl_{cr} <10 mL/minute: Administer 50% of dose

Hemodialysis: Partially cleared by hemodialysis
Administer 50% of dose posthemodialysis
Continuous ambulatory peritoneal dialysis (CAPD): Administer 50% of dose
Continuous renal replacement therapy (CRRT): Administer 75% of dose
Janus, 2010: Hemodialysis: Reduce initial dose by 50%; administer post hemodialysis or on nondialysis days.
Kintzel, 1995:
Cl_{cr} 46-60 mL/minute: Administer 75% of dose
Cl_{cr} 31-45 mL/minute: Administer 50% of dose
Cl_{cr} <30 mL/minute: Consider use of alternative drug

Dosage adjustment in hepatic impairment: No dosage adjustment provided in manufacturer's labeling. However, cisplatin undergoes nonenzymatic metabolism and predominantly renal elimination; therefore, dosage adjustment is likely not necessary.

Dosing in obesity: *ASCO Guidelines for appropriate chemotherapy dosing in obese adults with cancer:* Utilize patient's actual body weight (full weight) for calculation of body surface area- or weight-based dosing, particularly when the intent of therapy is curative; manage regimen-related toxicities in the same manner as for nonobese patients; if a dose reduction is utilized due to toxicity, consider resumption of full weight-based dosing with subsequent cycles, especially if cause of toxicity (eg, hepatic or renal impairment) is resolved (Griggs, 2012).

Dietary Considerations Some products may contain sodium.

Administration Pretreatment hydration with 1-2 L of fluid is recommended prior to cisplatin administration; adequate post hydration and urinary output (>100 mL/hour) should be maintained for 24 hours after administration.

I.V.: Infuse over 6- 8 hours; has also been infused (unlabeled rates) over 30 minutes to 3 hours, at a rate of 1 mg/minute, or as a continuous infusion; infusion rate varies by protocol (refer to specific protocol for infusion details). Avoid extravasation.

Needles or I.V. administration sets that contain aluminum should not be used in the preparation or administration; aluminum may react with cisplatin resulting in precipitate formation and loss of potency.

Vesicant (at higher concentrations); ensure proper needle or catheter placement prior to and during infusion; avoid extravasation.

Extravasation management: If extravasation occurs, stop infusion immediately and disconnect (leave cannula/needle in place); gently aspirate extravasated solution (do **NOT** flush the line); initiate sodium thiosulfate antidote; elevate extremity.

Sodium thiosulfate 1/6 M solution: Inject 2 mL into existing I.V. line for each 100 mg of cisplatin extravasated; then consider also injecting 1 mL as 0.1 mL subcutaneous injections (clockwise) around the area of extravasation, may repeat subcutaneous injections several times over the next 3-4 hours (Ener, 2004).

Dimethyl sulfoxide (DMSO) may also be considered an option: Apply to a region covering twice the affected area every 8 hours for 7 days; begin within 10 minutes of extravasation; do not cover with a dressing (Perez Fidalgo, 2012).

Hazardous agent; use appropriate precautions for handling and disposal (NIOSH, 2012).

Monitoring Parameters Renal function (serum creatinine, BUN, Cl_{cr}); electrolytes (particularly magnesium, calcium, potassium [periodic]); CBC with differential and platelet count (weekly); liver function tests (periodic); audiography (baseline and prior to each subsequent dose, and following treatment in children), neurologic exam (with high dose); urine output, urinalysis

Dosage Forms Excipient information presented when available (limited, particularly for generics); consult specific product labeling.
Solution, Intravenous:
Generic: 50 mg/50 mL (50 mL); 100 mg/100 mL (100 mL)
Solution, Intravenous [preservative free]:
Generic: 50 mg/50 mL (50 mL); 100 mg/100 mL (100 mL); 200 mg/200 mL (200 mL)

◆ **Cisplatin Injection (Can)** *see* CISplatin *on page 437*
◆ **Cisplatin Injection BP (Can)** *see* CISplatin *on page 437*
◆ ***Cis*-Retinoic Acid** *see* ISOtretinoin *on page 1129*
◆ **13-*cis*-Retinoic Acid** *see* ISOtretinoin *on page 1129*
◆ **13-*cis*-Vitamin A Acid** *see* ISOtretinoin *on page 1129*

Citalopram (sye TAL oh pram)

Brand Names: U.S. CeleXA

Brand Names: Canada Apo-Citalopram®; Auro-Citalopram; Ava-Citalopram; Celexa®; Citalopram-Odan; CO Citalopram; CTP 30; Dom-Citalopram; JAMP-Citalopram; Manda-Citalopram; Mint-Citalopram; Mylan-Citalopram; PHL-Citalopram; PMS-Citalopram; Q-Citalopram; RAN™-Citalo; ratio-Citalopram; Riva-Citalopram; Sandoz-Citalopram; Septa-Citalopram; Teva-Citalopram

Index Terms Citalopram Hydrobromide; Nitalapram

Pharmacologic Category Antidepressant, Selective Serotonin Reuptake Inhibitor

Additional Appendix Information
Antidepressant Agents *on page 2284*
Selective Serotonin Reuptake Inhibitors (SSRIs) Pharmacokinetics *on page 2314*

Use Treatment of depression

Unlabeled Use Obsessive-compulsive disorder (OCD)

Pregnancy Risk Factor C

Pregnancy Considerations Adverse events have been observed in animal reproduction studies. Citalopram and its metabolites cross the human placenta. An increased risk of teratogenic effects, including cardiovascular defects, may be associated with maternal use of citalopram or other SSRIs; however, available information is conflicting. Nonteratogenic effects in the newborn following SSRI/SNRI exposure late in the third trimester include respiratory distress, cyanosis, apnea, seizures, temperature instability, feeding difficulty, vomiting, hypoglycemia, hypo- or hypertonia, hyper-reflexia, jitteriness, irritability, constant crying, and tremor. Symptoms may be due to the toxicity of the SSRIs/SNRIs or a discontinuation syndrome and may be consistent with serotonin syndrome associated with SSRI treatment. Persistent pulmonary hypertension of the newborn (PPHN) has also been reported with SSRI exposure. The long-term effects of *in utero* SSRI exposure on infant development and behavior are not known.

Due to pregnancy-induced physiologic changes, women who are pregnant may require adjusted doses of citalopram to achieve euthymia. The ACOG recommends that therapy with SSRIs or SNRIs during pregnancy be individualized; treatment of depression during pregnancy should incorporate the clinical expertise of the mental health clinician, obstetrician, primary healthcare provider, and pediatrician. According to the American Psychiatric Association (APA), the risks of medication treatment should be weighed against other treatment options and untreated depression. For women who discontinue antidepressant medications during pregnancy and who may be at high risk for postpartum depression, the medications can be restarted following delivery. Treatment algorithms have been developed by the ACOG and the APA for the management of depression in women prior to conception and during pregnancy.

Breast-Feeding Considerations Citalopram and its metabolites are excreted in breast milk. According to the manufacturer, the decision to continue or discontinue breast-feeding during therapy should take into account the risk of exposure to the infant and the benefits of treatment to the mother. Excessive somnolence, decreased feeding, colic, irritability, restlessness, and weight loss have been reported in breast-fed infants. The long-term effects on development and behavior have not been studied; therefore, citalopram should be prescribed to a mother who is breast-feeding only when the benefits outweigh the potential risks. Maternal use of an SSRI during pregnancy may cause delayed milk secretion.

Medication Guide Available Yes

Contraindications Hypersensitivity to citalopram or any component of the formulation; use of MAO inhibitors intended to treat psychiatric disorders (concurrently or within 14 days of discontinuing either citalopram or the MAO inhibitor); initiation of citalopram in a patient receiving linezolid or intravenous methylene blue; concomitant use with pimozide

Warnings/Precautions [U.S. Boxed Warning]: Antidepressants increase the risk of suicidal thinking and behavior in children, adolescents, and young adults (18-24 years of age) with major depressive disorder (MDD) and other psychiatric disorders; consider risk prior to prescribing. Short-term studies did not show an increased risk in patients >24 years of age and showed a decreased risk in patients ≥65 years. Closely monitor patients for clinical worsening, suicidality, or unusual changes in behavior, particularly during the initial 1-2 months of therapy or during periods of dosage adjustments (increases or decreases); the patient's family or caregiver should be instructed to closely observe the patient and communicate condition with healthcare provider. A medication guide concerning the use of antidepressants should be dispensed with each prescription. **Citalopram is not FDA approved for use in children.**

The possibility of a suicide attempt is inherent in major depression and may persist until remission occurs. Use caution in high-risk patients. Worsening depression and severe abrupt suicidality that are not part of the presenting symptoms may require discontinuation or modification of drug therapy. The patient's family or caregiver should be alerted to monitor patients for the emergence of suicidality and associated behaviors (such as agitation, irritability, hostility, impulsivity, and hypomania) and call healthcare provider.

May worsen psychosis in some patients or precipitate a shift to mania or hypomania in patients with bipolar disorder. Patients presenting with depressive symptoms should be screened for bipolar disorder. Monotherapy in patients with bipolar disorder should be avoided. **Citalopram is not FDA approved for the treatment of bipolar depression.**

Potentially life-threatening serotonin syndrome (SS) has occurred with serotonergic agents (eg, SSRIs, SNRIs), particularly when used in combination with other serotonergic agents (eg, triptans, TCAs, fentanyl, lithium, tramadol, buspirone, St John's wort, tryptophan) or agents that impair metabolism of serotonin (eg, MAO inhibitors intended to treat psychiatric disorders, other MAO inhibitors [ie, linezolid and intravenous methylene blue]). Discontinue treatment (and any concomitant serotonergic agent) immediately if signs/symptoms arise. May increase the risks associated with electroconvulsive therapy. Has a low potential to impair cognitive or motor performance; caution operating hazardous machinery or driving. Bone fractures have been associated with antidepressant treatment. Consider the possibility of a fragility fracture if an antidepressant-treated patient presents with unexplained bone pain, point tenderness, swelling, or bruising (Rabenda, 2013; Rizzoli, 2012).

Citalopram causes dose-dependent QT_c prolongation; torsade de pointes, ventricular tachycardia, and sudden death have been reported. Use is not recommended in patients with congenital long QT syndrome, bradycardia, recent MI, uncompensated heart failure, hypokalemia, and/or hypomagnesemia, or patients receiving concomitant medications which prolong the QT interval; if use is essential and cannot be avoided in these patients, ECG monitoring is recommended. Discontinue therapy in any patient with persistent QT_c measurements >500 msec. Serum electrolytes, particularly potassium and magnesium, should be monitored prior to initiation and periodically during therapy in any patient at increased risk for significant electrolyte disturbances; hypokalemia and/or hypomagnesemia should be corrected prior to use. Due to the QT prolongation risk, doses >40 mg/day are not recommended. Additionally, the maximum daily dose should not exceed 20 mg/day in certain populations (eg, CYP2C19 poor metabolizers, patients with hepatic impairment, elderly patients). Potentially significant interactions may exist, requiring dose or frequency adjustment, additional monitoring, and/or selection of alternative therapy. Consult drug interactions database for more detailed information.

Use with caution in patients with a previous seizure disorder or condition predisposing to seizures such as brain damage or alcoholism. May cause or exacerbate sexual dysfunction. May cause hyponatremia/SIADH (elderly at increased risk); volume depletion and diuretics may increase risk. Monitor sodium closely with initiation or dosage adjustments in older adults (Beers Criteria). Citalopram is not FDA-approved for use in children; however, if used, monitor weight and growth regularly during therapy due to the potential for decreased appetite and weight loss with SSRI use.

Abrupt discontinuation or interruption of antidepressant therapy has been associated with a discontinuation syndrome. Symptoms arising may vary with antidepressant however commonly include nausea, vomiting, diarrhea, headaches, light-headedness, dizziness, diminished appetite, sweating, chills, tremors, paresthesias, fatigue, somnolence, and sleep disturbances (eg, vivid dreams, insomnia). Greater risks for developing a discontinuation syndrome have been associated with antidepressants with shorter half-lives, longer durations of treatment, and abrupt discontinuation. For antidepressants of short or intermediate half-lives, symptoms may emerge within 2-5 days after treatment discontinuation and last 7-14 days (APA, 2010; Fava, 2006; Haddad, 2001; Shelton, 2001; Warner, 2006).

Adverse Reactions

>10%:

Central nervous system: Somnolence (18%; dose related), insomnia (15%; dose related)

Gastrointestinal: Nausea (21%), xerostomia (20%)

Miscellaneous: Diaphoresis (11%; dose related)

1% to 10%:

Cardiovascular: QT prolongation (2%), hypotension (≥1%), orthostatic hypotension (≥1%), tachycardia (≥1%), bradycardia (1%)

Central nervous system: Fatigue (5%; dose related), anxiety (4%), agitation (3%), fever (2%), yawning (2%; dose related), amnesia (≥1%), apathy (≥1%), concentration impaired (≥1%), confusion (≥1%), depression (≥1%), migraine (≥1%), suicide attempt (≥1%)

Dermatologic: Rash (≥1%), pruritus (≥1%)

Endocrine & metabolic: Libido decreased (1% to 4%), dysmenorrhea (3%), amenorrhea (≥1%)

Gastrointestinal: Diarrhea (8%), dyspepsia (5%), anorexia (4%), vomiting (4%), abdominal pain (3%), appetite increased (≥1%), flatulence (≥1%), salivation increased (≥1%), taste perversion (≥1%), weight gain/loss (≥1%)
Genitourinary: Ejaculation disorder (6%), impotence (3%; dose related), polyuria (≥1%)
Neuromuscular & skeletal: Tremor (8%), arthralgia (2%), myalgia (2%), paresthesia (≥1%)
Ocular: Abnormal accommodation (≥1%)
Respiratory: Rhinitis (5%), upper respiratory tract infection (5%), sinusitis (3%), cough (≥1%)

<1% (Limited to important or life threatening): Allergic reaction, alopecia, anaphylaxis, anemia, angina pectoris, angioedema, arthritis, asthma, atrial fibrillation, bronchitis, bundle branch block, bursitis, cardiac arrest, cardiac failure, cataracts, catatonia, cerebrovascular accident, cholelithiasis, delirium, delusions, dependence, depersonalization, diplopia, diverticulitis, duodenal ulcer, eczema, epidermal necrolysis, erythema multiforme, extrapyramidal symptoms, extrasystoles, galactorrhea, gastric ulcer, gastrointestinal hemorrhage, glaucoma, granulocytopenia, gynecomastia, hallucinations, hemolytic anemia, hepatic necrosis, hepatitis, hyperpigmentation, hypertension, hypertrichosis, hypoglycemia, hypokalemia, hyponatremia, hypothyroidism, leukocytosis, leukopenia, lymphadenopathy, lymphocytosis, lymphopenia, muscle weakness, myocardial infarction, myocardial ischemia, neuroleptic malignant syndrome, obesity, osteoporosis, pancreatitis, phlebitis, photosensitivity, pneumonia, priapism, prolactinemia, prothrombin decreased, psoriasis, psychosis, ptosis, pulmonary embolism, renal calculi, renal failure, rhabdomyolysis, seizures, serotonin syndrome, SIADH, spontaneous abortion, syncope, thrombocytopenia, thrombosis, torsade de pointes, transient ischemic attack, urinary incontinence, urinary retention, vaginal bleeding, ventricular arrhythmia, withdrawal syndrome

Drug Interactions

Metabolism/Transport Effects

Substrate of CYP2C19 (major), CYP2D6 (minor), CYP3A4 (major); **Note:** Assignment of Major/Minor substrate status based on clinically relevant drug interaction potential; **Inhibits** CYP1A2 (weak), CYP2B6 (weak), CYP2C19 (weak), CYP2D6 (weak)

Avoid Concomitant Use

Avoid concomitant use of Citalopram with any of the following: Conivaptan; Dosulepin; Fluconazole; Fusidic Acid (Systemic); Highest Risk QTc-Prolonging Agents; Iobenguane I 123; Ivabradine; Linezolid; MAO Inhibitors; Methylene Blue; Mifepristone; Moderate Risk QTc-Prolonging Agents; Pimozide; Tryptophan

Increased Effect/Toxicity

Citalopram may increase the levels/effects of: Agents with Antiplatelet Properties; Anticoagulants; Antidepressants (Serotonin Reuptake Inhibitor/Antagonist); Antipsychotics; Aspirin; BusPIRone; CarBAMazepine; CloZAPine; Collagenase (Systemic); Dabigatran Etexilate; Desmopressin; Dextromethorphan; Dosulepin; Highest Risk QTc-Prolonging Agents; Hypoglycemic Agents; Ibritumomab; Methadone; Methylene Blue; Metoclopramide; Mexiletine; NSAID (COX-2 Inhibitor); NSAID (Nonselective); Pimozide; RisperiDONE; Rivaroxaban; Salicylates; Serotonin Modulators; Thiazide Diuretics; Thrombolytic Agents; Tositumomab and Iodine I 131 Tositumomab; TraMADol; Tricyclic Antidepressants; Vitamin K Antagonists

The levels/effects of Citalopram may be increased by: Alcohol (Ethyl); Analgesics (Opioid); Antipsychotics; BusPIRone; Cimetidine; CNS Depressants; Cobicistat; Conivaptan; CYP2C19 Inhibitors (Moderate); CYP2C19 Inhibitors (Strong); CYP3A4 Inhibitors (Moderate); CYP3A4 Inhibitors (Strong); Dasatinib; Fluconazole; Fusidic Acid (Systemic); Glucosamine; Herbs (Anticoagulant/Antiplatelet Properties); Ibrutinib; Ivabradine; Ivacaftor; Linezolid; Lithium; Luliconazole; Macrolide Antibiotics; MAO Inhibitors; Metoclopramide; Metyrosine; Mifepristone; Moderate Risk QTc-Prolonging Agents; Multivitamins/Fluoride (with ADE); Multivitamins/Minerals (with ADEK, Folate, Iron); Multivitamins/Minerals (with AE, No Iron); Omega-3 Fatty Acids; Pentosan Polysulfate Sodium; Pentoxifylline; Prostacyclin Analogues; QTc-Prolonging Agents (Indeterminate Risk and Risk Modifying); Simeprevir; Tipranavir; TraMADol; Tricyclic Antidepressants; Tryptophan; Vitamin E

Decreased Effect

Citalopram may decrease the levels/effects of: Iobenguane I 123; Ioflupane I 123; Thyroid Products

The levels/effects of Citalopram may be decreased by: Bosentan; CarBAMazepine; CYP2C19 Inducers (Strong); CYP3A4 Inducers (Strong); Cyproheptadine; Dabrafenib; Deferasirox; Mitotane; NSAID (COX-2 Inhibitor); NSAID (Nonselective); Peginterferon Alfa-2b; Rifampin; Tocilizumab

Ethanol/Nutrition/Herb Interactions

Ethanol: May increase CNS depression; monitor for increased effects with coadministration. Caution patients about effects.
Herb/Nutraceutical: Avoid valerian, St John's wort, tryptophan, SAMe, kava kava, and gotu kola (may increase CNS depression).

Storage/Stability Store at 25°C (77°F); excursions permitted to 15°C to 30°C (59°F to 86°F). Protect from moisture.

Mechanism of Action A racemic bicyclic phthalane derivative, citalopram selectively inhibits serotonin reuptake in the presynaptic neurons and has minimal effects on norepinephrine or dopamine. Uptake inhibition of serotonin is primarily due to the *S*-enantiomer of citalopram. Displays little to no affinity for serotonin, dopamine, adrenergic, histamine, GABA, or muscarinic receptor subtypes.

Pharmacodynamics/Kinetics

Onset of action: Depression: The onset of action is 1-4 weeks; however, individual response varies greatly and full response may not be seen until 8-12 weeks after initiation of treatment.
Distribution: V_d: 12 L/kg
Protein binding, plasma: ~80%
Metabolism: Extensively hepatic, via CYP3A4 and 2C19 (major pathways), and 2D6 (minor pathway); metabolized to demethylcitalopram (DCT), didemethylcitalopram (DDCT), citalopram-N-oxide, and a deaminated propionic acid derivative, which are at least eight times less potent than citalopram
Bioavailability: 80%; tablets and oral solution are bioequivalent
Half-life elimination: 24-48 hours (average: 35 hours); doubled with hepatic impairment and increased by 30% (following multiple doses) to 50% (following single dose) in elderly patients (≥60 years)
Time to peak, serum: 1-6 hours, average within 4 hours
Excretion: Urine (Citalopram 10% and DCT 5%)

Note: Clearance was decreased, while half-life was significantly increased in patients with hepatic impairment. Mild-to-moderate renal impairment may reduce clearance (17%) and prolong half-life of citalopram. No pharmacokinetic information is available concerning patients with severe renal impairment. AUC and half-life were significantly increased in elderly patients (≥60 years), and in poor CYP2C19 metabolizers, steady state C_{max} and AUC was increased by 68% and 107%, respectively.

Dosage Oral:

Children and Adolescents: Obsessive-compulsive disorder (unlabeled use): 10-40 mg daily (Mukaddes, 2003; Thomsen, 1997; Thomsen, 2001)

Adults <60 years: Depression: Initial: 20 mg once daily; increase the dose by 20 mg at an interval of ≥1 week to a maximum dose of 40 mg daily. **Note:** Doses >40 mg daily are not recommended due to the risk of QT prolongation; additional efficacy with doses >40 mg daily has not been demonstrated in clinical trials.

Poor metabolizers of CYP2C19 or concurrent use of moderate-to-strong CYP2C19 inhibitors (eg, cimetidine, omeprazole): Maximum dose: 20 mg daily

Elderly ≥60 years: Depression: Initial: 20 mg once daily; maximum dose in adults ≥60 years: 20 mg daily due to increased exposure and the risk of QT prolongation. Refer to adult dosing.

Discontinuation of therapy: Upon discontinuation of antidepressant therapy, gradually taper the dose to minimize the incidence of withdrawal symptoms and allow for the detection of re-emerging symptoms. Evidence supporting ideal taper rates is limited. APA and NICE guidelines suggest tapering therapy over at least several weeks with consideration to the half-life of the antidepressant; antidepressants with a shorter half-life may need to be tapered more conservatively. In addition for long-term treated patients, WFSBP guidelines recommend tapering over 4-6 months. If intolerable withdrawal symptoms occur following a dose reduction, consider resuming the previously prescribed dose and/or decrease dose at a more gradual rate (APA, 2010; Bauer, 2002; Haddad, 2001; NCCMH, 2010; Schatzberg, 2006; Shelton, 2001; Warner, 2006).

MAO inhibitor recommendations:

Switching to or from an MAO inhibitor intended to treat psychiatric disorders:

Allow 14 days to elapse between discontinuing an MAO inhibitor intended to treat psychiatric disorders and initiation of citalopram.

Allow 14 days to elapse between discontinuing citalopram and initiation of an MAO inhibitor intended to treat psychiatric disorders.

Use with other MAO inhibitors (linezolid or I.V. methylene blue):

Do not initiate citalopram in patients receiving linezolid or I.V. methylene blue; consider other interventions for psychiatric condition.

If urgent treatment with linezolid or I.V. methylene blue is required in a patient already receiving citalopram and potential benefits outweigh potential risks, discontinue citalopram promptly and administer linezolid or I.V. methylene blue. Monitor for serotonin syndrome for 2 weeks or until 24 hours after the last dose of linezolid or I.V. methylene blue, whichever comes first. May resume citalopram 24 hours after the last dose of linezolid or I.V. methylene blue.

Dosage adjustment in renal impairment:

Mild-to-moderate impairment: No dosage adjustment necessary.

Severe impairment: Cl_{cr} <20 mL/minute: No dosage adjustment provided in manufacturer's labeling (has not been studied); use caution.

Dosage adjustment in hepatic impairment: Initial: 20 mg once daily; maximum recommended dose: 20 mg daily due to decreased clearance and the risk of QT prolongation

Dietary Considerations May be taken without regard to food.

Administration May be administered without regard to food.

Monitoring Parameters ECG (patients at increased risk for QT-prolonging effects due to certain conditions); electrolytes (potassium and magnesium concentrations [prior to initiation and periodically during therapy in patients at increased risk for electrolyte abnormalities]); signs/symptoms of arrhythmias (eg, dizziness, palpitations, syncope); liver function tests and CBC with continued therapy; monitor patient periodically for symptom resolution; signs/symptoms of serotonin syndrome; mental status for depression, suicidal ideation (especially at the beginning of therapy or when doses are increased or decreased), anxiety, social functioning, mania, panic attacks; akathisia

Dosage Forms Excipient information presented when available (limited, particularly for generics); consult specific product labeling.

Solution, Oral:

Generic: 10 mg/5 mL (240 mL)

Tablet, Oral:

CeleXA: 10 mg

CeleXA: 20 mg, 40 mg [scored]

Generic: 10 mg, 20 mg, 40 mg

◆ **Citalopram Hydrobromide** *see* Citalopram *on page 440*

◆ **Citalopram-Odan (Can)** *see* Citalopram *on page 440*

◆ **Citracal Maximum [OTC]** *see* Calcium and Vitamin D *on page 318*

◆ **Citracal Petites [OTC]** *see* Calcium and Vitamin D *on page 318*

◆ **Citracal Regular [OTC]** *see* Calcium and Vitamin D *on page 318*

◆ **Citrate of Magnesia** *see* Magnesium Citrate *on page 1260*

◆ **Citric Acid and Potassium Citrate** *see* Potassium Citrate and Citric Acid *on page 1686*

◆ **Citric Acid and Sodium Citrate** *see* Sodium Citrate and Citric Acid *on page 1917*

Citric Acid, Sodium Citrate, and Potassium Citrate

(SIT rik AS id, SOW dee um SIT rate, & poe TASS ee um SIT rate)

Brand Names: U.S. Cytra-3; Tricitrates

Index Terms Polycitra; Potassium Citrate, Citric Acid, and Sodium Citrate; Sodium Citrate, Citric Acid, and Potassium Citrate

Pharmacologic Category Alkalinizing Agent

Use Conditions where long-term maintenance of an alkaline urine is desirable as in control and dissolution of uric acid and cystine calculi of the urinary tract

Pregnancy Risk Factor Not established

Dosage Oral:

Children: 5-15 mL diluted in water after meals and at bedtime

Adults: 15-30 mL diluted in water after meals and at bedtime

Additional Information Complete prescribing information should be consulted for additional detail.

Dosage Forms Excipient information presented when available (limited, particularly for generics); consult specific product labeling. [DSC] = Discontinued product

Solution, oral:

Cytra-3: Citric acid 334 mg, sodium citrate 500 mg, and potassium citrate 550 mg per 5 mL (480 mL [DSC]) [equivalent to potassium 1 mEq, sodium 1 mEq, and bicarbonate 2 mEq per 1 mL; alcohol free, sugar free; contains sodium benzoate and propylene glycol; raspberry flavor]

Tricitrates: Citric acid 334 mg, sodium citrate 500 mg, and potassium citrate 550 mg per 5 mL (480 mL) [equivalent to potassium 1 mEq, sodium 1 mEq, and bicarbonate 2 mEq per 1 mL; alcohol free, sugar free; contains sodiuim benzoate and propylene glycol; raspberry flavor]

- ◆ Citric Acid, Sodium Picosulfate, and Magnesium Oxide *see* Sodium Picosulfate, Magnesium Oxide, and Citric Acid *on page 1925*
- ◆ Citroma [OTC] *see* Magnesium Citrate *on page 1260*
- ◆ Citro-Mag (Can) *see* Magnesium Citrate *on page 1260*
- ◆ Citrovorum Factor *see* Leucovorin Calcium *on page 1186*
- ◆ CL-118,532 *see* Triptorelin *on page 2131*
- ◆ Cl-719 *see* Gemfibrozil *on page 947*
- ◆ CL-184116 *see* Porfimer *on page 1679*
- ◆ CL-232315 *see* MitoXANtrone *on page 1386*

Cladribine (KLA dri been)

Index Terms 2-CdA; 2-Chlorodeoxyadenosine; Leustatin

Pharmacologic Category Antineoplastic Agent, Antimetabolite; Antineoplastic Agent, Antimetabolite (Purine Analog)

Use Treatment of active hairy cell leukemia

Unlabeled Use Treatment of acute myeloid leukemia (AML), chronic lymphocytic leukemia (CLL), non-Hodgkin's lymphomas (mantle cell), Waldenström's macroglobulinemia, refractory Langerhans cell histiocytosis

Pregnancy Risk Factor D

Pregnancy Considerations Teratogenic effects and fetal mortality were observed in animal reproduction studies. May cause fetal harm if administered during pregnancy. Women of reproductive potential should use highly effective contraception during treatment.

Breast-Feeding Considerations Due to the potential for serious adverse reactions in the nursing infant, the decision to discontinue cladribine or to discontinue breast-feeding should take into account the importance of treatment to the mother.

Contraindications Hypersensitivity to cladribine or any component of the formulation

Warnings/Precautions Hazardous agent - use appropriate precautions for handling and disposal (NIOSH, 2012). **[U.S. Boxed Warning]: Dose-dependent, reversible myelosuppression (neutropenia, anemia, and thrombocytopenia) is common and generally reversible;** use with caution in patients with pre-existing hematologic or immunologic abnormalities; monitor blood counts, especially during the first 4-8 weeks after treatment. **[U.S. Boxed Warning]: Serious, dose-related neurologic toxicity (including irreversible paraparesis and quadriparesis) has been reported with continuous infusions of higher doses (4-9 times the FDA-approved dose); may also occur at approved doses (rare).** Neurotoxicity may be delayed and may present as progressive, irreversible weakness; diagnostics with electromyography and nerve conduction studies were consistent with demyelinating disease. **[U.S. Boxed Warning]: Acute nephrotoxicity (eg, acidosis, anuria, increased serum creatinine), possibly requiring dialysis, has been reported with high doses (4-9 times the FDA-approved dose), particularly when administered with other nephrotoxic agents.** Use with caution in patients with renal or hepatic impairment. Fever (>100°F) may occur, with or without neutropenia, observed more commonly in the first month of treatment. Infections (bacterial, viral, and fungal) were reported more commonly in the first month after treatment (generally mild or moderate in severity, although serious infections including sepsis have been reported); the incidence is reduced in the second month; due to neutropenia and T-cell depletion, risk versus benefit of treatment should be evaluated in patients with active infections. Administration of live vaccines is not recommended during treatment with cladribine (may increase the risk of infection due to immunosuppression). Use caution in patients with high tumor burden; tumor lysis syndrome may occur (rare). **[U.S. Boxed Warning]: Should be administered under the supervision of an experienced cancer chemotherapy physician.** Diluted product may contain benzyl alcohol which has been associated with "gasping syndrome" in neonates.

Adverse Reactions

>10%:

Central nervous system: Fever (33% to 69%; ≥100°F: 67%; ≥104°F: 11%), fatigue (11% to 45%), headache (7% to 22%)

Dermatologic: Rash (10% to 27%)

Gastrointestinal: Nausea (22% to 28%), appetite decreased (8% to 17%), vomiting (9% to 13%)

Hematologic: Neutropenia (grade 4: 70%; recovery: by week 5); anemia (1% to 37%; recovery: by week 8); myelosuppression (34%; prolonged), neutropenic fever (8% to 47%; severe: 32%), thrombocytopenia (grade 4: 12%; recovery: by day 12)

Local: Injection site reactions (9% to 19%)

Respiratory: Abnormal breath sounds (4% to 11%)

Miscellaneous: Infection (month 1: 28% [serious: 6%]; month 2: 6%)

1% to 10%:

Cardiovascular: Edema (2% to 6%), tachycardia (2% to 6%), thrombosis (2%)

Central nervous system: Chills (2% to 9%), dizziness (6% to 9%), insomnia (3% to 7%), malaise (5% to 7%), pain (6%), anxiety (1%)

Dermatologic: Purpura (10%), petechiae (2% to 8%), pruritus (2% to 6%), erythema (6%), hyperhidrosis (3%), bruising (1% to 2%)

Gastrointestinal: Diarrhea (7% to 10%), constipation (4% to 9%), abdominal pain (4% to 6%), flatulence (1%)

Local: Phlebitis (2%)

Neuromuscular & skeletal: Weakness (6% to 9%), myalgia (6% to 7%), arthralgia (3% to 5%), muscle weakness (1%)

Respiratory: Cough (7% to 10%), abnormal chest sounds (9%), dyspnea (5% to 7%), epistaxis (5%), rales (1%)

Miscellaneous: Diaphoresis (9%)

<1% (Limited to important or life-threatening): Aplastic anemia, bacteremia, CD4 lymphocytopenia (nadir: 4-6 months), cellulitis, consciousness decreased, conjunctivitis, hemolytic anemia, hypereosinophilia, hypersensitivity, myelodysplastic syndrome, opportunistic infections (cytomegalovirus, fungal infections, herpes virus infections, listeriosis, Pneumocystis jirovecii), pancytopenia (prolonged), paraparesis, pneumonia, polyneuropathy (with high doses), progressive multifocal leukoencephalopathy (PML), pulmonary interstitial infiltrates, quadriparesis (reported at high doses); renal dysfunction (with high doses), renal failure, septic shock, Stevens-Johnson syndrome, stroke, toxic epidermal necrolysis, tuberculosis reactivation, tumor lysis syndrome

Drug Interactions

Metabolism/Transport Effects None known.

Avoid Concomitant Use

Avoid concomitant use of Cladribine with any of the following: BCG; CloZAPine; Natalizumab; Pimecrolimus; Tacrolimus (Topical); Tofacitinib; Vaccines (Live)

Increased Effect/Toxicity

Cladribine may increase the levels/effects of: CloZAPine; Leflunomide; Natalizumab; Tofacitinib; Vaccines (Live)

The levels/effects of Cladribine may be increased by: Denosumab; Pimecrolimus; Roflumilast; Tacrolimus (Topical); Trastuzumab

Decreased Effect

Cladribine may decrease the levels/effects of: BCG; Coccidioidin Skin Test; Sipuleucel-T; Vaccines (Inactivated); Vaccines (Live)

The levels/effects of Cladribine may be decreased by: Echinacea

Ethanol/Nutrition/Herb Interactions Ethanol: Avoid ethanol (due to GI irritation).

Preparation for Administration Hazardous agent; use appropriate precautions for handling and disposal (NIOSH, 2012).

A precipitate may develop at low temperatures and may be resolubilized at room temperature or by shaking the solution vigorously. Inadvertent freezing does not affect the solution; if freezing occurs prior to dilution, allow to thaw naturally prior to reconstitution; do not heat or microwave; do not refreeze.

To prepare a 24-hour continuous infusion: Dilute in 500 mL NS. The manufacturer recommends filtering with a 0.22 micron hydrophilic syringe filter prior to adding to infusion bag.

To prepare a 7-day continuous infusion: Dilute to a total volume of 100 mL in a CADD® medication cassette reservoir using bacteriostatic NS. Filter diluent and cladribine with a 0.22 micron hydrophilic filter prior to adding to cassette/reservoir.

Storage/Stability

Store intact vials refrigerated at 2°C to 8°C (36°F to 46°F). Protect from light. A precipitate may develop at low temperatures and may be resolubilized at room temperature or by shaking the solution vigorously. Inadvertent freezing does not affect the solution; if freezing occurs prior to dilution, allow to thaw naturally prior to reconstitution; do not heat or microwave; do not refreeze.

24-hour continuous infusion: Dilutions for infusion should be used promptly; if not used promptly, the 24-hour infusion may be stored refrigerated for up to 8 hours prior to administration.

7-day continuous infusion: Dilutions for infusion should be used promptly; if not used promptly, the 7-day infusion may be stored refrigerated for up to 8 hours prior to administration. Reconstituted solution is stable for 7 days (when diluted in bacteriostatic NS) in a CADD® medication cassette reservoir. For patients weighing >85 kg, the effectiveness of the preservative in the bacteriostatic diluent may be reduced (due to dilution).

Mechanism of Action A purine nucleoside analogue; prodrug which is activated via phosphorylation by deoxycytidine kinase to a 5'-triphosphate derivative (2-CaAMP). This active form incorporates into DNA to result in the breakage of DNA strand and shutdown of DNA synthesis and repair. This also results in a depletion of nicotinamide adenine dinucleotide and adenosine triphosphate (ATP). Cladribine is cell-cycle nonspecific.

Pharmacodynamics/Kinetics

Distribution: V_d: ~9 L/kg; penetrates CSF (CSF concentrations are ~25% of plasma concentrations)

Protein binding: ~20%

Half-life elimination: After a 2-hour infusion (with normal renal function): 5.4 hours

Excretion: Urine (18%)

Dosage

Children: I.V.:

Acute myeloid leukemia (unlabeled use): 8.9 mg/m^2/day continuous infusion for 5 days for 1 or 2 courses (Krance, 2001) **or** 9 mg/m^2/day over 30 minutes for 5 days for 1 course (in combination with cytarabine) (Crews, 2002; Rubnitz, 2009)

Langerhans cell histiocytosis, refractory (unlabeled use): 5 mg/m^2/day over 2 hours for 5 days every 21 days for up to 6 cycles (Weitzman, 2009)

Adults: Details concerning dosing in combination regimens should also be consulted.

Hairy cell leukemia: I.V.: 0.09 mg/kg/day continuous infusion for 7 days for 1 cycle **or** (unlabeled dosing) 0.1 mg/kg/day continuous infusion for 7 days for 1 cycle (Goodman, 2003; Saven, 1998)

Acute myeloid leukemia, induction (unlabeled use): I.V.: CLAG or CLAG-M regimen: 5 mg/m^2/day over 2 hours for 5 days; a second induction may be administered if needed (Robak, 2000; Wierzbowska, 2008; Wrzesień-Kuś, 2003)

Chronic lymphocytic leukemia (unlabeled use): I.V.: 0.1 mg/kg/day continuous infusion for 7 days every 4-5 weeks (Saven, 1995) **or** 0.14 mg/kg/day over 2 hours for 5 days every 28 days for 3-6 cycles (Byrd, 2003)

Mantle cell lymphoma (unlabeled use): I.V.: 5 mg/m^2/day over 2 hours for 5 days every 4 weeks for 2-6 cycles (Inwards, 2008; Rummel, 1999) **or** 5 mg/m^2/day over 2 hours for 5 days every 4 weeks for 2-6 cycles (in combination with rituximab) (Inwards, 2008)

Waldenström's macroglobulinemia (unlabeled use):

I.V.: 0.1 mg/kg/day continuous infusion for 7 days every 4 weeks for 2 cycles (Dimopoulos, 1994)

SubQ: 0.1 mg/kg/day for 5 consecutive days every month for 4 cycles (in combination with rituximab) (Laszlo, 2010)

Dosing adjustment in renal impairment: No dosage adjustment provided in the manufacturer's labeling (due to inadequate data); use with caution. The following adjustments have been used (Aronoff, 2007):

Children:

Cl_{cr} 10-50 mL/minute: Administer 50% of dose

Cl_{cr} <10 mL/minute: Administer 30% of dose

Hemodialysis: Administer 30% of dose

Continuous renal replacement therapy (CRRT): Administer 50% of dose

Adults:

Cl_{cr} 10-50 mL/minute: Administer 75% of dose

Cl_{cr} <10 mL/minute: Administer 50% of dose

Continuous ambulatory peritoneal dialysis (CAPD): Administer 50% of dose

Dosing adjustment in hepatic impairment: No dosage adjustment provided in the manufacturer's labeling (due to inadequate data); use with caution.

Dosing in obesity: ASCO Guidelines for appropriate chemotherapy dosing in obese adults with cancer: Utilize patient's actual body weight (full weight) for calculation of body surface area- or weight-based dosing, particularly when the intent of therapy is curative; manage regimen-related toxicities in the same manner as for nonobese patients; if a dose reduction is utilized due to toxicity, consider resumption of full weight-based dosing with subsequent cycles, especially if cause of toxicity (eg, hepatic or renal impairment) is resolved (Griggs, 2012).

Administration

I.V.: Administer as a continuous infusion. May also be administered over 30 minutes or over 2 hours (unlabeled administration rates) depending on indication and/or protocol.

SubQ (unlabeled route): May also be administered SubQ (Laszlo, 2010)

Hazardous agent; use appropriate precautions for handling and disposal (NIOSH, 2012).

Monitoring Parameters CBC with differential (particularly during the first 4-8 weeks post-treatment), renal and hepatic function; bone marrow biopsy (after CBC has normalized, to confirm treatment response); monitor for fever; monitor for signs/symptoms of neurotoxicity

Dosage Forms Excipient information presented when available (limited, particularly for generics); consult specific product labeling. [DSC] = Discontinued product

Solution, Intravenous:
- Generic: 1 mg/mL (10 mL [DSC])

Solution, Intravenous [preservative free]:
- Generic: 1 mg/mL (10 mL)

◆ **Claforan** *see* Cefotaxime *on page 371*

◆ **Claforan® (Can)** *see* Cefotaxime *on page 371*

◆ **Claforan in D_5W** *see* Cefotaxime *on page 371*

◆ **Claravis** *see* ISOtretinoin *on page 1129*

◆ **Clarifoam EF** *see* Sulfur and Sulfacetamide *on page 1966*

◆ **Clarinex** *see* Desloratadine *on page 575*

◆ **Clarinex-D® 12 Hour** *see* Desloratadine and Pseudoephedrine *on page 575*

◆ **Clarinex-D® 24 Hour [DSC]** *see* Desloratadine and Pseudoephedrine *on page 575*

◆ **Clarinex Reditabs** *see* Desloratadine *on page 575*

◆ **Claris** *see* Sulfur and Sulfacetamide *on page 1966*

Clarithromycin (kla RITH roe mye sin)

Brand Names: U.S. Biaxin; Biaxin XL; Biaxin XL Pac

Brand Names: Canada Accel-Clarithromycin; Apo-Clarithromycin; Ava-Clarithromycin; Biaxin; Biaxin BID; Biaxin XL; Dom-Clarithromycin; Mylan-Clarithromycin; PMS-Clarithromycin; RAN-Clarithromycin; ratio-Clarithromycin; Riva-Clarithromycin; Sandoz-Clarithromycin; Teva-Clarithromycin

Pharmacologic Category Antibiotic, Macrolide

Additional Appendix Information

Prevention of Infective Endocarditis *on page 2353*

Use

Infants and Children 6 months and older:
- Acute maxillary sinusitis due to susceptible *H. influenzae, S. pneumoniae,* or *Moraxella catarrhalis*
- Acute otitis media due to susceptible *H. influenzae, M. catarrhalis,* or *S. pneumoniae*
- Community-acquired pneumonia due to susceptible *Mycoplasma pneumoniae, S. pneumoniae,* or *Chlamydophila pneumoniae* (TWAR)
- Disseminated mycobacterial infections due to *M. avium* or *M. intracellulare*
- Pharyngitis/tonsillitis due to susceptible *S. pyogenes*
- Prevention of disseminated mycobacterial infections due to *M. avium* complex (MAC) disease in patients with advanced HIV infection (20 months of age and older)
- Uncomplicated skin/skin structure infection due to susceptible *S. aureus* or *S. pyogenes*

Adults:
- Pharyngitis/tonsillitis due to susceptible *S. pyogenes*
- Acute maxillary sinusitis due to susceptible *H. influenzae, M. catarrhalis,* or *S. pneumoniae*
- Acute exacerbation of chronic bronchitis due to susceptible *H. influenzae, H. parainfluenzae, M. catarrhalis,* or *S. pneumoniae*
- Community-acquired pneumonia due to susceptible *H. influenzae, H. parainfluenzae, M. catarrhalis, Mycoplasma pneumoniae, S. pneumoniae,* or *Chlamydophila pneumoniae* (TWAR)
- Uncomplicated skin/skin structure infections due to susceptible *S. aureus* or *S. pyogenes*
- Disseminated mycobacterial infections due to *M. avium* or *M. intracellulare*
- Prevention of disseminated mycobacterial infections due to MAC disease in patients with advanced HIV infection
- Duodenal ulcer disease due to *H. pylori* in regimens with other drugs including amoxicillin and lansoprazole or omeprazole, or in combination with omeprazole or ranitidine bismuth citrate (no longer marketed in the U.S.). **Note:** Regimens that contain clarithromycin as the single antimicrobial agent are more likely to be associated with the development of clarithromycin resistance.

Unlabeled Use Pertussis (CDC guidelines); alternate antibiotic for prophylaxis of infective endocarditis in patients who are allergic to penicillin and undergoing dental procedures (ACC/AHA guidelines); alternate antibiotic for treatment and secondary prophylaxis of bartonellosis infection in HIV-exposed/-positive infants and children (CDC guidelines) and in HIV-positive adolescents and adults (DHHS guidelines); Lyme disease (IDSA guidelines)

Pregnancy Risk Factor C

Pregnancy Considerations Adverse fetal effects have been documented in some animal reproduction studies. Clarithromycin crosses the placenta (Witt, 2003). The manufacturer recommends that clarithromycin not be used in a pregnant woman unless there are no alternative therapies. Clarithromycin is not recommended for the treatment of *Mycobacterium avium* complex (MAC) in pregnant patients (DHHS, 2013).

Breast-Feeding Considerations Clarithromycin and its active metabolite (14-hydroxy clarithromycin) are excreted into breast milk. The manufacturer recommends that caution be used if administered to nursing women.

Contraindications Hypersensitivity to clarithromycin, erythromycin, any of the macrolide antibiotics, or any component of the formulation; history of cholestatic jaundice/hepatic dysfunction associated with prior use of clarithromycin; history of QT prolongation or ventricular cardiac arrhythmia, including torsade de pointes; concomitant use with cisapride, pimozide, ergotamine, dihydroergotamine, HMG-CoA reductase inhibitors extensively metabolized by CYP3A4 (eg, lovastatin, simvastatin), astemizole or terfenadine (not available in the U.S.); concomitant use with colchicine in patients with renal or hepatic impairment

Warnings/Precautions Use has been associated with QT prolongation and infrequent cases of arrhythmias, including torsade de pointes; use is contraindicated in patients with a history of QT prolongation and ventricular arrhythmias, including torsade de pointes. Systemic exposure is increased in the elderly; may be at increased risk of torsade de pointes, particularly if concurrent severe renal impairment. Use with caution in patients at risk of prolonged cardiac repolarization. Avoid use in patients with uncorrected hypokalemia or hypomagnesemia, clinically significant bradycardia, and patients receiving Class IA (eg, quinidine, procainamide) or Class III (eg, amiodarone, dofetilide, sotalol) antiarrhythmic agents. Use caution in patients with coronary artery disease.

Elevated liver function tests and hepatitis (hepatocellular and/or cholestatic with or without jaundice) have been reported; usually reversible after discontinuation of clarithromycin. May lead to hepatic failure or death (rarely), especially in the presence of pre-existing diseases and/or concomitant use of medications. Discontinue immediately if symptoms of hepatitis occur. Dosage adjustment needed in severe renal impairment. Use with caution in patients with myasthenia gravis.

Potentially significant drug-drug interactions may exist, requiring dose or frequency adjustment, additional monitoring, and/or selection of alternative therapy. Colchicine toxicity (including fatalities) has been reported with concomitant use; concomitant use is contraindicated in patients with renal or hepatic impairment. Clarithromycin in combination with ranitidine bismuth citrate should not be used in patients with a history of acute porphyria. Prolonged use may result in fungal or bacterial superinfection, including *C. difficile*-associated diarrhea (CDAD) and pseudomembranous colitis; CDAD has been observed >2 months postantibiotic treatment. Decreased *H. pylori* eradication rates have been observed with short-term (≤7 days) combination therapy. The American College of Gastroenterology recommends 10-14 days of therapy (triple or quadruple) for eradication of *H. pylori* (Chey, 2007).

Severe acute reactions have (rarely) been reported, including anaphylaxis, Stevens-Johnson syndrome (SJS), toxic epidermal necrolysis (TEN), drug rash with eosinophilia and systemic symptoms (DRESS), and Henoch-Schönlein purpura (IgA vasculitis); discontinue therapy and initiate treatment immediately for severe acute hypersensitivity reactions. The presence of extended release tablets in the stool has been reported, particularly in patients with anatomic (eg, ileostomy, colostomy) or functional GI disorders with decreased transit times. Consider alternative dosage forms (eg, suspension) or an alternative antimicrobial for patients with tablet residue in the stool and no signs of clinical improvement.

Adverse Reactions

1% to 10%:

Central nervous system: Headache (2%)
Dermatologic: Rash (children 3%)
Gastrointestinal: Abnormal taste (adults 3% to 7%), diarrhea (adults 3% to 6%; children 6%), vomiting (children 6%), nausea (adults 3%), abdominal pain (adults 2%; children 3%), dyspepsia (adults 2%)
Hepatic: Prothrombin time increased (adults 1%)
Renal: BUN increased (4%)

<1% (Limited to important or life-threatening): Alkaline phosphatase increased, ALT increased, anaphylaxis, anorexia, anxiety, AST increased, behavioral changes, bilirubin increased, cholestatic hepatitis, *Clostridium difficile* colitis, confusion, depersonalization, depression, disorientation, dizziness, drug rash with eosinophilia and systemic symptoms (DRESS), GGT increased, glossitis, hallucinations, hearing loss (reversible), hemorrhage, Henoch-Schönlein purpura (IgA vasculitis), hepatic dysfunction, hepatic failure, hepatitis, hypoglycemia, insomnia, interstitial nephritis, jaundice, leukopenia, LDH increased, manic behavior, myalgia, neutropenia, nightmares, oral moniliasis, pancreatitis, psychosis, QT prolongation, rhabdomyolysis, seizure, serum creatinine increased, smell loss, Stevens-Johnson syndrome, stomatitis, taste loss, thrombocytopenia, tinnitus, tongue discoloration, tooth discoloration (reversible with dental cleaning), torsade de pointes, toxic epidermal necrolysis, tremor, urticaria, ventricular tachycardia, ventricular arrhythmia, vertigo, white blood cell count decreased

Drug Interactions

Metabolism/Transport Effects **Substrate** of CYP3A4 (major); **Note:** Assignment of Major/Minor substrate status based on clinically relevant drug interaction potential; **Inhibits** CYP1A2 (weak), CYP3A4 (strong), P-glycoprotein

Avoid Concomitant Use

Avoid concomitant use of Clarithromycin with any of the following: Ado-Trastuzumab Emtansine; Alfuzosin; Apixaban; Avanafil; Axitinib; BCG; Bosutinib; Cabozantinib; Cisapride; Conivaptan; Crizotinib; Dihydroergotamine; Disopyramide; Dronedarone; Eplerenone; Ergotamine; Everolimus; Fusidic Acid (Systemic); Halofantrine; Highest Risk QTc-Prolonging Agents; Ibrutinib; Imatinib; Ivabradine; Lapatinib; Lomitapide; Lovastatin; Lurasidone; Macitentan; Mifepristone; Nilotinib; Nisoldipine; Pimozide; Pomalidomide; QuiNIDine; QuiNINE; Ranolazine; Red Yeast Rice; Regorafenib; Salmeterol; Silodosin; Simeprevir; Simvastatin; Tamsulosin; Terfenadine; Ticagrelor; Tolvaptan; Topotecan; Toremifene; Ulipristal; Vemurafenib; VinCRIStine (Liposomal)

Increased Effect/Toxicity

Clarithromycin may increase the levels/effects of: Ado-Trastuzumab Emtansine; Afatinib; Alfentanil; Alfuzosin; Almotriptan; Alosetron; ALPRAZolam; Antifungal Agents (Azole Derivatives, Systemic); Antineoplastic Agents (Vinca Alkaloids); Apixaban; ARIPiprazole; AtorvaSTATin; Avanafil; Axitinib; Bedaquiline; Boceprevir; Bortezomib; Bosentan; Bosutinib; Brentuximab Vedotin; Brinzolamide; Budesonide (Nasal); Budesonide (Systemic, Oral Inhalation); BusPIRone; Cabozantinib; Calcium Channel Blockers; CarBAMazepine; Cardiac Glycosides; Cilostazol; Cisapride; CloZAPine; Cobicistat; Colchicine; Conivaptan; Corticosteroids (Orally Inhaled); Corticosteroids (Systemic); Crizotinib; CycloSPORINE (Systemic); CYP3A4 Inducers (Strong); CYP3A4 Substrates; Dabigatran Etexilate; Dienogest; Dihydroergotamine; Disopyramide; Dofetilide; Dronedarone; Dutasteride; Eletriptan; Enzalutamide; Eplerenone; Ergot Derivatives; Ergotamine; Estazolam; Everolimus; FentaNYL; Fesoterodine; Fluticasone (Nasal); Fluticasone (Oral Inhalation); GlipiZIDE; GlyBURIDE; GuanFACINE; Halofantrine; Highest Risk QTc-Prolonging Agents; Ibrutinib; Iloperidone; Imatinib; Ivabradine; Ivacaftor; Ixabepilone; Lacosamide; Lapatinib; Levomilnacipran; Lomitapide; Lovastatin; Lumefantrine; Lurasidone; Macitentan; Maraviroc; MethylPREDNISolone; Midazolam; Mifepristone; Moderate Risk QTc-Prolonging Agents; Nilotinib; Nisoldipine; Ospemifene; OxyCODONE; Paricalcitol; PAZOPanib; P-glycoprotein/ABCB1 Substrates; Pimecrolimus; Pimozide; Pitavastatin; Pomalidomide; PONATinib; Pravastatin; Propafenone; Protease Inhibitors; Prucalopride; QUEtiapine; QuiNIDine; QuiNINE; Ranolazine; Red Yeast Rice; Regorafenib; Repaglinide; Rifamycin Derivatives; Rilpivirine; Rivaroxaban; RomiDEPsin; Ruxolitinib; Salmeterol; Saxagliptin; Selective Serotonin Reuptake Inhibitors; Sildenafil; Silodosin; Simeprevir; Simvastatin; Sirolimus; SORAfenib; Tacrolimus (Systemic); Tacrolimus (Topical); Tadalafil; Tamsulosin; Telaprevir; Temsirolimus; Terfenadine; Theophylline Derivatives; Ticagrelor; Tofacitinib; Tolterodine; Tolvaptan; Topotecan; Toremifene; Triazolam; Ulipristal; Vardenafil; Vemurafenib; Vilazodone; VinCRIStine (Liposomal); Vitamin K Antagonists; Zidovudine; Zopiclone; Zuclopenthixol

The levels/effects of Clarithromycin may be increased by: Antifungal Agents (Azole Derivatives, Systemic); Boceprevir; Cobicistat; CYP3A4 Inducers (Strong); CYP3A4 Inhibitors (Moderate); CYP3A4 Inhibitors (Strong); Dasatinib; Fusidic Acid (Systemic); Ivabradine; Luliconazole; Mifepristone; Protease Inhibitors; QTc-Prolonging Agents (Indeterminate Risk and Risk Modifying); Telaprevir

Decreased Effect

Clarithromycin may decrease the levels/effects of: BCG; Clopidogrel; Ifosfamide; Prasugrel; Sodium Picosulfate; Ticagrelor; Typhoid Vaccine; Zidovudine

The levels/effects of Clarithromycin may be decreased by: CYP3A4 Inducers (Strong); Dabrafenib; Deferasirox; Etravirine; Herbs (CYP3A4 Inducers); Protease Inhibitors; Tocilizumab

Ethanol/Nutrition/Herb Interactions

Food: Immediate release: Food delays rate, but not extent of absorption; Extended release: Food increases clarithromycin AUC by ~30% relative to fasting conditions.

Herb/Nutraceutical: St John's wort may decrease clarithromycin levels; Management: Advise patient to avoid the use of St John's wort during clarithromycin therapy.

Storage/Stability

Extended release tablets: Store at 20°C to 25°C (68°F to 77°F); excursions are permitted between 15°C and 30°C (59°F and 86°F).

Immediate release tablets:

250 mg: Store at 15°C to 30°C (59°F to 86°F). Protect from light.

500 mg: Store at 20°C to 25°C (68°F to 77°F).

Granules for suspension: Store at 15°C to 30°C (59°F to 86°F) prior to and following reconstitution. Do not refrigerate. Use within 14 days of reconstitution.

Mechanism of Action Exerts its antibacterial action by binding to 50S ribosomal subunit resulting in inhibition of protein synthesis. The 14-OH metabolite of clarithromycin is twice as active as the parent compound against certain organisms.

Pharmacodynamics/Kinetics

Absorption:

Immediate release: Rapid; food delays rate, but not extent of absorption

Extended-release: Fasting is associated with ~30% lower AUC relative to administration with food

Distribution: Widely into most body tissues; manufacturer reports no data in regards to CNS penetration

Protein binding: 42% to 70% (Peters, 1992)

Metabolism: Partially hepatic via CYP3A4; converted to 14-OH clarithromycin (active metabolite)

Bioavailability: ~50%

Half-life elimination: Immediate release: Clarithromycin: 3-7 hours; 14-OH-clarithromycin: 5-9 hours

Time to peak: Immediate release: 2-3 hours; Extended release: 5-8 hours

Excretion: Urine (20% to 40% as unchanged drug; additional 10% to 15% as metabolite); feces (29% to 40% mostly as metabolites) (Ferrero, 1990)

Clearance: Approximates normal GFR

Dosage

Usual dosage range: Note: All pediatric dosing recommendations based on immediate release product formulations (tablet and oral suspension):

Infants ≥6 months, Children, and Adolescents: Oral: 7.5 mg/kg every 12 hours (maximum: 500 mg/dose) for 10 days

Adults: Oral: 250-500 mg every 12 hours **or** 1000 mg (two 500 mg extended release tablets) once daily for 7-14 days

Indication-specific dosing:

Children: Oral:

Acute otitis media: Infants ≥6 months, Children, and Adolescents: 7.5 mg/kg/dose (maximum: 500 mg/dose) every 12 hours for 10 days. **Note:** Due to increased *S. pneumoniae* and *H. influenzae* resistance, macrolides are not routinely recommended as a treatment option (Lieberthal, 2013).

Bartonellosis, treatment and secondary prophylaxis (excluding CNS infections and endocarditis) (unlabeled use): Adolescents (HIV-positive): 500 mg twice daily for at least 3 months (recommended as alternative therapy; DHHS, 2013)

Community-acquired pneumonia (CAP): Infants >3 months and Children: **Note:** A beta-lactam antibiotic should be added if typical bacterial pneumonia cannot be ruled out.

Presumed atypical *(M. pneumoniae, C. pneumoniae, C. trachomatis)* infection, mild-to-severe atypical infection or step-down therapy (alternative to azithromycin): 7.5 mg/kg/dose (maximum: 500 mg) every 12 hours (Bradley, 2011)

Lyme disease (unlabeled use): Children: 7.5 mg/kg/dose (maximum dose: 500 mg) twice daily for 14-21 days (Wormser, 2006)

Mycobacterial infection (prevention and treatment):

Manufacturer's recommendation: 7.5 mg/kg/dose (maximum: 500 mg/dose) twice daily; use in combination with other antimycobacterial agents for the treatment of disseminated MAC. **Note:** Safety of clarithromycin for MAC not studied in children <20 months.

Alternative recommendations:

HIV-exposed/-positive infants and children (CDC, 2009):

Primary prophylaxis: 7.5 mg/kg/dose (maximum: 500 mg/dose) twice daily

Secondary prophylaxis: 7.5 mg/kg/dose (maximum: 500 mg/dose) twice daily, plus ethambutol, with or without rifabutin

Treatment: 7.5-15 mg/kg/dose (maximum: 500 mg/dose) twice daily plus ethambutol, plus rifabutin (for severe disease)

HIV-positive adolescents (DHHS, 2013):

Primary prophylaxis: 500 mg twice daily (maximum: 1000 mg daily)

Secondary prophylaxis and treatment: 500 mg twice daily (maximum: 1000 mg daily) plus ethambutol; consider additional agents (eg, rifabutin, aminoglycoside, fluoroquinolone) for CD4 <50 cells/mm^3, high mycobacterial load, or ineffective antiretroviral therapy

Pertussis (unlabeled use): Infants ≥1 month, Children, and Adolescents: Oral: 7.5 mg/kg/dose (maximum: 500 mg/dose) every 12 hours for 7 days (CDC, 2005)

Pharyngitis/tonsillitis: 7.5 mg/kg/dose (maximum: 250 mg/dose) every 12 hours for 10 days. **Note:** Recommended by the Infectious Disease Society of America (IDSA) as an alternative agent for group A streptococcal pharyngitis in penicillin-allergic patients (Shulman, 2012).

Prophylaxis against infective endocarditis (unlabeled use): Children and Adolescents: Oral: 15 mg/kg/dose (maximum: 500 mg/dose) 30-60 minutes before procedure. **Note:** American Heart Association (AHA) guidelines now recommend prophylaxis only in patients undergoing invasive procedures and in whom underlying cardiac conditions may predispose to a higher risk of adverse outcomes should infection occur. As of April 2007, routine prophylaxis for GI/GU procedures is no longer recommended by the AHA (Wilson, 2007).

Sinusitis: Infants ≥6 months, Children, and Adolescents: 7.5 mg/kg/dose (maximum: 500 mg/dose) every 12 hours for 10 days

Skin/skin structure infections, uncomplicated: Infants ≥6 months, Children, and Adolescents: 7.5 mg/kg/dose (maximum: 250 mg dose) every 12 hours for 10 days

Adults: Oral:

Acute exacerbation of chronic bronchitis:

M. catarrhalis and *S. pneumoniae*: 250 mg every 12 hours for 7-14 days **or** 1000 mg (two 500 mg extended release tablets) once daily for 7 days

H. influenzae: 500 mg every 12 hours for 7-14 days **or** 1000 mg (two 500 mg extended release tablets) once daily for 7 days

H. parainfluenzae: 500 mg every 12 hours for 7 days **or** 1000 mg (two 500 mg extended release tablets) once daily for 7 days

Acute maxillary sinusitis: 500 mg every 12 hours for 14 days **or** 1000 mg (two 500 mg extended release tablets) once daily for 14 days

Bartonellosis, treatment and secondary prophylaxis in HIV-infected patients (excluding CNS infections and endocarditis) (unlabeled use): 500 mg twice daily for at least 3 months (DHHS, 2013)

Lyme disease (unlabeled use): 500 mg twice daily for 14-21 days (Wormser, 2006)

Mycobacterial infection (prevention and treatment): Manufacturer recommendations: 500 mg twice daily (use with other antimycobacterial drugs, eg, ethambutol or rifampin). Continue therapy if clinical response is observed; may discontinue when patient is considered at low risk of disseminated infection.

Alternative recommendations: (DHHS, 2013):

Primary prophylaxis: 500 mg twice daily (maximum: 1 g daily)

Secondary prophylaxis and treatment: 500 mg twice daily (maximum: 1 g daily) plus ethambutol; consider additional agents (eg, rifabutin, aminoglycoside, fluoroquinolone) for CD4 <50 cells/mm^3, high mycobacterial load, or ineffective antiretroviral therapy.

Peptic ulcer disease: Eradication of *Helicobacter pylori*: Dual or triple combination regimens with bismuth subsalicylate, amoxicillin, an H_2-receptor antagonist, or proton-pump inhibitor: 500 mg every 8-12 hours for 10-14 days

Pertussis (unlabeled use): 500 mg twice daily for 7 days (CDC, 2005)

Pharyngitis, tonsillitis: 250 mg every 12 hours for 10 days. **Note:** Recommended by the Infectious Disease Society of America (IDSA) as an alternative agent for group A streptococcal pharyngitis in penicillin-allergic patients (Shulman, 2012).

Pneumonia:

C. pneumoniae, *M. pneumoniae*, and *S. pneumoniae*: 250 mg every 12 hours for 7-14 days **or** 1000 mg (two 500 mg extended release tablets) once daily for 7 days

H. influenzae: 250 mg every 12 hours for 7 days **or** 1000 mg (two 500 mg extended release tablets) once daily for 7 days

H. parainfluenzae and *M. catarrhalis*: 1000 mg (two 500 mg extended release tablets) once daily for 7 days

Prophylaxis against infective endocarditis (unlabeled use): 500 mg 30-60 minutes prior to procedure. **Note:** American Heart Association (AHA) guidelines now recommend prophylaxis only in patients undergoing invasive procedures and in whom underlying cardiac conditions may predispose to a higher risk of adverse outcomes should infection occur. As of April 2007, routine prophylaxis for GI/GU procedures is no longer recommended by the AHA (Wilson, 2007).

Skin and skin structure infection, uncomplicated: 250 mg every 12 hours for 7-14 days

Elderly: May have age-related reductions in renal function; monitor and adjust dose if necessary

Dosing adjustment in renal impairment:

Cl_{cr} <30 mL/minute: Decrease clarithromycin dose by 50%

Hemodialysis: Administer after HD session is completed (Aronoff, 2007).

In combination with atazanavir or ritonavir:

Cl_{cr} 30-60 mL/minute: Decrease clarithromycin dose by 50%

Cl_{cr} <30 mL/minute: Decrease clarithromycin dose by 75%

Dosing adjustment in hepatic impairment: No dosing adjustment is needed as long as renal function is normal

Dietary Considerations Extended release tablets should be taken with food.

Administration Immediate release tablets and granules for suspension: Administer with or without meals. Administer every 12 hours rather than twice daily to avoid peak and trough variation. Shake suspension well before each use.

Extended release tablets: Administer with food. Do not crush or chew.

Monitoring Parameters CBC with differential, BUN, creatinine; perform culture and sensitivity studies prior to initiating drug therapy as appropriate

Dosage Forms Excipient information presented when available (limited, particularly for generics); consult specific product labeling.

Suspension Reconstituted, Oral:

Biaxin: 250 mg/5 mL (50 mL, 100 mL) [fruit punch flavor]

Generic: 125 mg/5 mL (50 mL, 100 mL); 250 mg/5 mL (50 mL, 100 mL)

Tablet, Oral:

Biaxin: 250 mg [contains brilliant blue fcf (fd&c blue #1), fd&c yellow #10 (quinoline yellow)]

Biaxin: 500 mg [contains fd&c yellow #10 (quinoline yellow)]

Generic: 250 mg, 500 mg

Tablet Extended Release 24 Hour, Oral:

Biaxin XL: 500 mg [contains fd&c yellow #10 (quinoline yellow)]

Biaxin XL Pac: 500 mg [contains fd&c yellow #10 (quinoline yellow)]

Generic: 500 mg

- **Clarithromycin, Amoxicillin, and Omeprazole** *see* Omeprazole, Clarithromycin, and Amoxicillin *on page 1508*
- **Clarithromycin, Lansoprazole, and Amoxicillin** *see* Lansoprazole, Amoxicillin, and Clarithromycin *on page 1173*
- **Claritin [OTC]** *see* Loratadine *on page 1240*
- **Claritin® (Can)** *see* Loratadine *on page 1240*
- **Claritin-D® 12 Hour Allergy & Congestion [OTC]** *see* Loratadine and Pseudoephedrine *on page 1242*
- **Claritin-D® 24 Hour Allergy & Congestion [OTC]** *see* Loratadine and Pseudoephedrine *on page 1242*
- **Claritin® Extra (Can)** *see* Loratadine and Pseudoephedrine *on page 1242*
- **Claritin Eye [OTC]** *see* Ketotifen (Ophthalmic) *on page 1156*
- **Claritin® Kids (Can)** *see* Loratadine *on page 1240*
- **Claritin® Liberator (Can)** *see* Loratadine and Pseudoephedrine *on page 1242*
- **Claritin Reditabs [OTC]** *see* Loratadine *on page 1240*
- **Clarus™ (Can)** *see* ISOtretinoin *on page 1129*
- **Clavulanic Acid and Amoxicillin** *see* Amoxicillin and Clavulanate *on page 119*
- **Clavulin (Can)** *see* Amoxicillin and Clavulanate *on page 119*
- **Clear Eyes Redness Relief [OTC]** *see* Naphazoline (Ophthalmic) *on page 1425*

Clemastine (KLEM as teen)

Brand Names: U.S. Dayhist Allergy 12 Hour Relief [OTC]; Tavist Allergy [OTC]

Index Terms Clemastine Fumarate

Pharmacologic Category Ethanolamine Derivative; Histamine H_1 Antagonist; Histamine H_1 Antagonist, First Generation

Additional Appendix Information

Beers Criteria – Potentially Inappropriate Medications for Geriatrics *on page 2368*

Use Perennial and seasonal allergic rhinitis and other allergic symptoms including urticaria

Pregnancy Risk Factor B

Dosage Oral:
Infants and Children <6 years: 0.05 mg/kg/day as **clemastine base** or 0.335-0.67 mg/day clemastine fumarate (0.25-0.5 mg base/day) divided into 2 or 3 doses; maximum daily dosage: 1.34 mg (1 mg base)
Children 6-12 years: 0.67-1.34 mg clemastine fumarate (0.5-1 mg base) twice daily; do not exceed 4.02 mg/day (3 mg/day base)
Children ≥12 years and Adults:
1.34 mg clemastine fumarate (1 mg base) twice daily to 2.68 mg (2 mg base) 3 times/day; do not exceed 8.04 mg/day (6 mg base)
OTC labeling: 1.34 mg clemastine fumarate (1 mg base) twice daily; do not exceed 2 mg base/24 hours
Elderly: Lower doses should be considered in patients >60 years

Additional Information Complete prescribing information should be consulted for additional detail.

Dosage Forms Excipient information presented when available (limited, particularly for generics); consult specific product labeling.
Syrup, Oral, as fumarate:
Generic: 0.67 mg/5 mL (120 mL)
Tablet, Oral, as fumarate:
Dayhist Allergy 12 Hour Relief: 1.34 mg [scored; sodium free]
Tavist Allergy: 1.34 mg [scored; sodium free]
Generic: 1.34 mg, 2.68 mg

◆ Clemastine Fumarate *see* Clemastine *on page 449*
◆ Clenia [DSC] *see* Sulfur and Sulfacetamide *on page 1966*
◆ Cleocin *see* Clindamycin (Systemic) *on page 451*
◆ Cleocin *see* Clindamycin (Topical) *on page 454*
◆ Cleocin in D_5W *see* Clindamycin (Systemic) *on page 451*
◆ Cleocin Phosphate *see* Clindamycin (Systemic) *on page 451*
◆ Cleocin-T *see* Clindamycin (Topical) *on page 454*

Clevidipine (klev ID i peen)

Brand Names: U.S. Cleviprex

Index Terms Clevidipine Butyrate

Pharmacologic Category Antihypertensive; Calcium Channel Blocker; Calcium Channel Blocker, Dihydropyridine

Additional Appendix Information
Calcium Channel Blockers – Comparative Pharmacokinetics *on page 2296*

Use Management of hypertension

Pregnancy Risk Factor C

Pregnancy Considerations Adverse events were observed in animal reproduction studies. Untreated chronic maternal hypertension is associated with adverse events in the fetus, infant, and mother. If treatment for hypertension during pregnancy is needed, other agents are preferred (ACOG, 2012; Chobanian, 2003).

Breast-Feeding Considerations It is not known if clevidipine is excreted into breast milk. Per the manufacturer, the possibility of infant exposure should be considered. Breast-fed infants of mothers taking medications for hypertension should be monitored for adverse effects (Chobanian, 2003).

Contraindications Hypersensitivity to clevidipine or any component of the formulation (soybeans, soy products, eggs, egg products); hypertriglyceridemia or complications of hypertriglyceridemia (eg, acute pancreatitis); lipoid nephrosis; severe aortic stenosis

Warnings/Precautions Symptomatic hypotension with or without syncope and reflex tachycardia may rarely occur. Blood pressure must be lowered at a rate appropriate for the patient's clinical condition; dosage reductions may be necessary. Treatment of clevidipine-induced tachycardia with beta-blockers is **not** recommended. After prolonged use, discontinuation may cause rebound hypertension; monitor closely for ≥8 hours after discontinuation. Use with caution in patients with heart failure (may worsen symptoms). Clevidipine is formulated within a 20% fat emulsion (0.2 g/mL); hypertriglyceridemia is an expected side effect with high-dose or extended treatment periods; median infusion duration in clinical trials was approximately 6.5 hours (Aronson, 2008). Patients who develop hypertriglyceridemia (eg, >500 mg/dL) are at risk of developing pancreatitis. A reduction in the quantity of concurrently administered lipids may be necessary. Use is contraindicated in patients with hypertriglyceridemia or complications associated with hypertriglyceridemia (eg, acute pancreatitis) and lipoid nephrosis. Withdrawal from concomitant beta-blocker therapy should be done gradually. Initiate therapy at the low end of the dosage range in the elderly, with careful upward titration if needed. Use within 12 hours of puncturing vial; maintain aseptic technique while handling.

Adverse Reactions
>10%:
Cardiovascular: Atrial fibrillation (21%)
Central nervous system: Fever (19%), insomnia (12%)
Gastrointestinal: Nausea (5% to 21%)
1% to 10%:
Central nervous system: Headache (6%)
Gastrointestinal: Vomiting (3%)
Hematologic: Postprocedural hemorrhage (3%)
Renal: Acute renal failure (9%)
Respiratory: Pneumonia (3%), respiratory failure (3%)
<1%, postmarketing, and/or case reports (Limited to important or life-threatening): Cardiac arrest, hypersensitivity, hypotension, ileus, MI, reflex tachycardia, syncope, thrombophlebitis

Drug Interactions

Metabolism/Transport Effects None known.

Avoid Concomitant Use There are no known interactions where it is recommended to avoid concomitant use.

Increased Effect/Toxicity
Clevidipine may increase the levels/effects of: Amifostine; Antihypertensives; Atosiban; Beta-Blockers; Calcium Channel Blockers (Nondihydropyridine); Hypotensive Agents; Magnesium Salts; Neuromuscular-Blocking Agents (Nondepolarizing); Nitroprusside; Obinutuzumab; QuiNIDine; RiTUXimab

The levels/effects of Clevidipine may be increased by: Alpha1-Blockers; Brimonidine (Topical); Calcium Channel Blockers (Nondihydropyridine); Diazoxide; Herbs (Hypotensive Properties); Magnesium Salts; MAO Inhibitors; Pentoxifylline; Phosphodiesterase 5 Inhibitors; Prostacyclin Analogues; QuiNIDine

Decreased Effect
Clevidipine may decrease the levels/effects of: QuiNIDine

The levels/effects of Clevidipine may be decreased by: Calcium Salts; Herbs (Hypertensive Properties); Melatonin; Methylphenidate; Yohimbine

Ethanol/Nutrition/Herb Interactions Herb/Nutraceutical: Avoid bayberry, blue cohosh, cayenne, ephedra, ginger, ginseng (American), kola, licorice (may worsen hypertension). Avoid black cohosh, California poppy, coleus, golden seal, hawthorn, mistletoe, periwinkle, quinine, shepherd's purse (may have increased antihypertensive effect).

Storage/Stability Store in refrigerator at 2°C to 8°C (36°F to 46°F). Unopened vials are stable for 2 months at room temperature. Vials are stable for 12 hours once opened. Protect from light during storage. Do not freeze.

Mechanism of Action Dihydropyridine calcium channel blocker with potent arterial vasodilating activity. Inhibits calcium ion influx through the L-type calcium channels during depolarization in arterial smooth muscle, producing a decrease in mean arterial pressure (MAP) by reducing systemic vascular resistance.

Pharmacodynamics/Kinetics

Onset of action: 2-4 minutes after start of infusion

Duration: I.V.: 5-15 minutes

Distribution: V_{dss}: 0.17 L/kg

Protein binding: >99.5%

Metabolism: Rapid hydrolysis primarily by esterases in blood and extravascular tissues to an inactive carboxylic acid metabolite and formaldehyde

Half-life elimination: Biphasic: Initial: 1 minute (predominant); Terminal: 15 minutes

Excretion: Urine (63% to 74% as metabolites); feces (7% to 22% as metabolites)

Dosage I.V.:

Adults: Initial: 1-2 mg/hour

Titration: Initial: dose may be doubled at 90-second intervals toward blood pressure goal. As blood pressure approaches goal, dose may be increased by less than double every 5-10 minutes. **Note:** For every 1-2 mg/hour increase in dose, an approximate reduction of 2-4 mm Hg in systolic blood pressure may occur.

Usual maintenance: 4-6 mg/hour; maximum: 21 mg/hour (1000 mL within a 24-hour period due to lipid load restriction). There is limited short-term experience with doses up to 32 mg/hour. Data is limited beyond 72 hours.

Elderly: Initiate at the low end of the dosage range.

Dosing adjustment in renal impairment: No adjustment required with initial infusion rate

Dosing adjustment in hepatic impairment: No adjustment required with initial infusion rate

Dietary Considerations Clevidipine is formulated in an oil-in-water emulsion containing 200 mg/mL of lipid (2 kcal/mL). If on parenteral nutrition, may need to adjust the amount of lipid infused. Emulsion contains soybean oil, egg yolk phospholipids, and glycerin.

Administration I.V.: Maintain aseptic technique. Do not use if contamination is suspected. Do not dilute. Invert vial gently several times to ensure uniformity of emulsion prior to administration. Administer as a slow continuous infusion via central or peripheral line, using infusion device allowing for calibrated infusion rates. Use within 12 hours of puncturing vial; discard any tubing and unused portion, including that currently being infused.

Monitoring Parameters Blood pressure, heart rate; patients who receive prolonged infusions of clevidipine and are not transitioned to other antihypertensive therapy should be monitored for at least 8 hours after discontinuation

Dosage Forms Excipient information presented when available (limited, particularly for generics); consult specific product labeling.

Emulsion, Intravenous:

Cleviprex: 0.5 mg/mL (50 mL, 100 mL) [contains edetate disodium, egg yolk phospholipids, soybean oil]

◆ **Clevidipine Butyrate** *see* Clevidipine *on page 450*

◆ **Cleviprex** *see* Clevidipine *on page 450*

Clidinium and Chlordiazepoxide

(kli DI nee um & klor dye az e POKS ide)

Brand Names: U.S. Librax®

Brand Names: Canada Apo-Chlorax®; Librax®

Index Terms Chlordiazepoxide and Clidinium

Pharmacologic Category Antispasmodic Agent, Gastrointestinal; Benzodiazepine

Additional Appendix Information

Beers Criteria – Potentially Inappropriate Medications for Geriatrics *on page 2368*

Use Adjunct treatment of peptic ulcer; treatment of irritable bowel syndrome

Dosage Oral: 1-2 capsules 3-4 times/day, before meals or food and at bedtime

Caution: Do not abruptly discontinue after prolonged use; taper dose gradually.

Dosage adjustment in renal impairment: No dosage adjustment provided in manufacturer's labeling.

Dosage adjustment in hepatic impairment: No dosage adjustment provided in manufacturer's labeling.

Additional Information Complete prescribing information should be consulted for additional detail.

Dosage Forms Excipient information presented when available (limited, particularly for generics); consult specific product labeling.

Capsule: Clidinium bromide 2.5 mg and chlordiazepoxide hydrochloride 5 mg

Librax®: Clidinium bromide 2.5 mg and chlordiazepoxide hydrochloride 5 mg

◆ **Climara** *see* Estradiol (Systemic) *on page 754*

◆ **ClimaraPro** *see* Estradiol and Levonorgestrel *on page 762*

◆ **Clindacin ETZ** *see* Clindamycin (Topical) *on page 454*

◆ **Clindacin-P** *see* Clindamycin (Topical) *on page 454*

◆ **Clindacin Pac** *see* Clindamycin (Topical) *on page 454*

◆ **Clindagel** *see* Clindamycin (Topical) *on page 454*

◆ **ClindaMax** *see* Clindamycin (Topical) *on page 454*

Clindamycin (Systemic) (klin da MYE sin)

Brand Names: U.S. Cleocin; Cleocin in D_5W; Cleocin Phosphate

Brand Names: Canada Apo-Clindamycin®; Ava-Clindamycin; Clindamycin Injection, USP; Clindamycine; Dalacin™ C; Mylan-Clindamycin; PMS-Clindamycin; Riva-Clindamycin; Teva-Clindamycin

Index Terms Clindamycin Hydrochloride; Clindamycin Palmitate

Pharmacologic Category Antibiotic, Lincosamide

Additional Appendix Information

Prevention of Infective Endocarditis *on page 2353*

Use Treatment of susceptible bacterial infections, mainly those caused by anaerobes, streptococci, pneumococci, and staphylococci; pelvic inflammatory disease (I.V.)

Unlabeled Use May be useful in PCP; alternate treatment for toxoplasmosis; bacterial vaginosis (oral); alternate treatment for MRSA infections; alternate antibiotic for prophylaxis of infective endocarditis in patients who are allergic to penicillin and undergoing surgical or dental procedures (ACC/AHA guidelines); group B streptococcus (GBS) infection (maternal use for neonatal prophylaxis); treatment of severe or uncomplicated malaria; treatment of babesiosis; treatment of acute bacterial rhinosinusitis (ABRS) (pediatric) (in combination with a third-generation cephalosporin); chronic oral antimicrobial suppression of prosthetic joint infection

Pregnancy Risk Factor B

Pregnancy Considerations Adverse events were not observed in animal reproduction studies. Clindamycin crosses the placenta throughout pregnancy and at term, but use during pregnancy has not been shown to cause adverse fetal effects. Clindamycin pharmacokinetics are not affected by pregnancy. Clindamycin therapy is recommended in certain pregnant patients for prophylaxis of group B streptococcal disease in newborns, prophylaxis and treatment of *Toxoplasma gondii* encephalitis, or for the treatment of *Pneumocystis* pneumonia (PCP), bacterial vaginosis, or malaria.

Breast-Feeding Considerations Small amounts of clindamycin transfer to human milk. The manufacturer does not recommend the use of clindamycin during breast-feeding. Nondose-related effects could include modification of bowel flora. One case of bloody stools in an infant occurred after a mother received clindamycin while breast-feeding; however, a casual relationship was not confirmed.

Contraindications Hypersensitivity to clindamycin, lincomycin, or any component of the formulation

Warnings/Precautions Dosage adjustment may be necessary in patients with severe hepatic dysfunction. **[U.S. Boxed Warning]: Can cause severe and possibly fatal colitis.** Prolonged use may result in fungal or bacterial superinfection, including *C. difficile*-associated diarrhea (CDAD) and pseudomembranous colitis; CDAD has been observed >2 months postantibiotic treatment. Use with caution in patients with a history of gastrointestinal disease. Discontinue drug if significant diarrhea, abdominal cramps, or passage of blood and mucus occurs. Some dosage forms contain benzyl alcohol or tartrazine. Use caution in atopic patients. Not appropriate for use in the treatment of meningitis due to inadequate penetration into the CSF.

Adverse Reactions Frequency not defined.

Cardiovascular: Cardiac arrest (rare; I.V. administration), hypotension (rare; I.V. administration)

Dermatologic: Erythema multiforme (rare), exfoliative dermatitis (rare), pruritus, rash, Stevens-Johnson syndrome (rare), urticaria

Gastrointestinal: Abdominal pain, diarrhea, esophagitis, nausea, pseudomembranous colitis, vomiting

Genitourinary: Vaginitis

Hematologic: Agranulocytosis, eosinophilia (transient), neutropenia (transient), thrombocytopenia

Hepatic: Jaundice, liver function test abnormalities

Local: Induration/pain/sterile abscess (I.M.), thrombophlebitis (I.V.)

Neuromuscular & skeletal: Polyarthritis (rare)

Renal: Renal dysfunction (rare)

Miscellaneous: Anaphylactoid reactions (rare)

Drug Interactions

Metabolism/Transport Effects Substrate of CYP3A4 (minor); **Note:** Assignment of Major/Minor substrate status based on clinically relevant drug interaction potential

Avoid Concomitant Use

Avoid concomitant use of Clindamycin (Systemic) with any of the following: BCG; Erythromycin (Systemic)

Increased Effect/Toxicity

Clindamycin (Systemic) may increase the levels/effects of: Neuromuscular-Blocking Agents

Decreased Effect

Clindamycin (Systemic) may decrease the levels/effects of: BCG; Erythromycin (Systemic); Sodium Picosulfate; Typhoid Vaccine

The levels/effects of Clindamycin (Systemic) may be decreased by: Kaolin

Ethanol/Nutrition/Herb Interactions

Food: Peak concentrations may be delayed with food.

Herb/Nutraceutical: St John's wort may decrease clindamycin levels.

Storage/Stability

Capsule: Store at room temperature of 20°C to 25°C (68°F to 77°F).

I.V.: Infusion solution in NS or D_5W solution is stable for 16 days at room temperature, 32 days refrigerated, or 8 weeks frozen. Prior to use, store vials and premixed bags at controlled room temperature 20°C to 25°C (68°F to 77°F). After initial use, discard any unused portion of vial after 24 hours.

Oral solution: Do not refrigerate reconstituted oral solution (it will thicken). Following reconstitution, oral solution is stable for 2 weeks at room temperature of 20°C to 25°C (68°F to 77°F).

Mechanism of Action Reversibly binds to 50S ribosomal subunits preventing peptide bond formation thus inhibiting bacterial protein synthesis; bacteriostatic or bactericidal depending on drug concentration, infection site, and organism

Pharmacodynamics/Kinetics

Absorption: Oral, hydrochloride: Rapid (90%)

Distribution: High concentrations in bone and urine; no significant levels in CSF, even with inflamed meninges

V_d: ~2 L/kg

Metabolism: Hepatic; forms metabolites (variable activity); Clindamycin phosphate is converted to clindamycin HCl (active)

Half-life elimination: Neonates: Premature: 8.7 hours; Full-term: 3.6 hours; Children: ~2 hours; Adults: ~2-3 hours; Elderly 4 hours (range: 3.4-5.1 hours)

Time to peak, serum: Oral: Within 60 minutes; I.M.: 1-3 hours

Excretion: Urine (10%) and feces (~4%) as active drug and metabolites

Dosage

Usual dosage ranges:

Infants and Children:

Oral: 8-40 mg/kg/day in 3-4 divided doses; Manufacturer's labeling: 8-20 mg/kg/day (as hydrochloride) or 8-25 mg/kg/day (as palmitate) in 3-4 divided doses; minimum dose of palmitate: 37.5 mg 3 times daily

I.M., I.V.: Manufacturer's labeling: 20-40 mg/kg/day in 3-4 divided doses

Adults:

Oral: 150-450 mg/dose every 6-8 hours; maximum dose: 1800 mg daily

I.M., I.V.: 1200-2700 mg daily in 2-4 divided doses; maximum dose: 4800 mg daily

Indication-specific dosing:

Infants >3 months and Children:

Community-acquired pneumonia (CAP) (IDSA/PIDS, 2011): Note: In children ≥5 years, a macrolide antibiotic should be added if atypical pneumonia cannot be ruled out.

Group A *Streptococcus:*

Moderate-to-severe infection (alternative to ampicillin/penicillin): I.V.: 40 mg/kg/day divided every 6-8 hours

Mild infection, step-down therapy (alternative to amoxicillin/penicillin): Oral: 40 mg/kg/day divided every 8 hours

Presumed bacterial (in addition to recommended antibiotic therapy), *S. pneumoniae* moderate-to-severe (MICs to penicillin ≤2.0 mcg/mL) (alternative to ampicillin/penicillin): I.V.: 40 mg/kg/day divided every 6-8 hours

S. pneumoniae:

Moderate-to-severe infection (MICs to penicillin ≥4.0 mcg/mL) (alternative to ceftriaxone): I.V.: 40 mg/kg/day divided every 6-8 hours

Mild infection, step-down therapy (MICs to penicillin ≥4.0 mcg/mL) (alternative to levofloxacin or linezolid): Oral: 30-40 mg/kg/day divided every 8 hours

S. aureus (methicillin-susceptible):

Moderate-to-severe infection (alternative to cefazolin or oxacillin): I.V.:40 mg/kg/day divided every 6-8 hours

Mild infection, step-down therapy (alternative to cephalexin): Oral: 30-40 mg/kg/day divided every 6-8 hours

S. aureus (methicillin-resistant/clindamycin-susceptible):

Moderate-to-severe infection (preferred): I.V.: 40 mg/kg/day divided every 6-8 hours; recommended duration: 7-21 days (Liu, 2011)

Mild infection, step-down therapy (preferred): Oral: 30-40 mg/kg/day divided every 6-8 hours; recommended duration: 7-21 days (Liu, 2011)

Children:

Acute bacterial rhinosinusitis (unlabeled use): Oral: 30-40 mg/kg/day divided every 8 hours with concomitant cefixime or cefpodoxime for 10-14 days. **Note:** Recommended in patients with non-type I penicillin allergy, after failure of initial therapy or in patients at risk for antibiotic resistance (eg, daycare attendance, age <2 years, recent hospitalization, antibiotic use within the past month) (Chow, 2012).

Anthrax (unlabeled dose): Note: For inhalational anthrax, combine with penicillin G (WHO, 2008):

Oral: 8-25 mg/kg/day divided every 6-8 hours

I.V.: 15-40 mg/kg/day divided every 6-8 hours

Babesiosis (unlabeled use): Oral: 20-40 mg/kg/day divided every 8 hours for 7-10 days *plus* quinine (*Medical Letter*, 2007)

Cellulitis due to MRSA (unlabeled use): Oral: 10-13 mg/kg/dose every 6-8 hours for 5-10 days (maximum: 40 mg/kg/day) (Liu, 2011)

Complicated skin/soft tissue infection due to MRSA (unlabeled use): Oral, I.V.: 10-13 mg/kg/dose every 6-8 hours for 7-14 days (maximum: 40 mg/kg/day) (Liu, 2011)

Healthcare-associated pneumonia (HAP) (methicillin-resistant/clindamycin-susceptible): Oral, I.V.: 30-40 mg/kg/day divided every 6-8 hours for 7-21 days (Liu, 2011)

Malaria, severe (unlabeled use): I.V.: Load: 10 mg/kg followed by 15 mg/kg/day divided every 8 hours *plus* I.V. quinidine gluconate; switch to oral therapy (clindamycin *plus* quinine) when able for total clindamycin treatment duration of 7 days (**Note:** Quinine duration is region specific, consult CDC for current recommendations) (CDC, 2009)

Malaria, uncomplicated treatment (unlabeled use): Oral: 20 mg/kg/day divided every 8 hours for 7 days *plus* quinine (CDC, 2009)

Osteomyelitis due to MRSA (unlabeled use): Oral, I.V.: 10-13 mg/kg/dose every 6-8 hours for a minimum of 4-6 weeks (maximum: 40 mg/kg/day) (Liu, 2011)

Pharyngitis, group A streptococci (IDSA recommendations): Oral:

Acute treatment in penicillin-allergic patients: 21 mg/kg/day divided every 8 hours (maximum: 300 mg per dose) for 10 days (Shulman, 2012).

Chronic carrier treatment: 20-30 mg/kg/day divided every 8 hours (maximum: 300 mg per dose) for 10 days (Shulman, 2012).

Prophylaxis against infective endocarditis (unlabeled use):

Oral: 20 mg/kg 30-60 minutes before procedure (Wilson, 2007)

I.M., I.V.: 20 mg/kg 30-60 minutes before procedure. Intramuscular injections should be avoided in patients who are receiving anticoagulant therapy. In these circumstances, orally administered regimens should be given whenever possible. Intravenously administered antibiotics should be used for patients who are unable to tolerate or absorb oral medications. (Wilson, 2007)

Note: American Heart Association (AHA) guidelines now recommend prophylaxis only in patients undergoing invasive procedures and in whom underlying cardiac conditions may predispose to a higher risk of adverse outcomes should infection occur. As of April 2007, routine prophylaxis for GI/GU procedures is no longer recommended by the AHA.

Septic arthritis due to MRSA (unlabeled use): Oral, I.V.: 10-13 mg/kg/dose every 6-8 hours for minimum of 3-4 weeks (maximum: 40 mg/kg/day) (Liu, 2011)

Toxoplasmosis (HIV-exposed/-positive; secondary prevention [unlabeled use]): Oral: 20-30 mg/kg/day divided every 6-8 hours (*plus* pyrimethamine and leucovorin calcium) (CDC, 2009)

Adults:

Amnionitis: I.V.: 450-900 mg every 8 hours

Anthrax (unlabeled dose):

Oral: 150-300 mg every 6 hours. **Note:** For inhalational anthrax, combine with penicillin (WHO, 2008).

I.V.:

Nonspecified disease: 600-900 mg every 6-8 hours. **Note:** For inhalational anthrax, combine with penicillin G (WHO, 2008)

Alternative regimens:

Inhalational, gastrointestinal, or complicated cutaneous disease with systemic involvement: 600 mg every 8 hours in combination with ciprofloxacin or doxycycline (Hicks, 2012)

Injectional: 600 mg every 8 hours in combination with ciprofloxacin and other antibiotics (eg, a 5-drug combination) (Hicks, 2012)

Babesiosis (unlabeled use):

Oral: 600 mg 3 times daily for 7-10 days with quinine (Vannier, 2012; Wormser, 2006)

I.V.: 300-600 mg every 6 hours for 7-10 days with quinine (Vannier, 2012; Wormser, 2006)

Note: Relapsing infection may require at least 6 weeks of therapy (Vannier, 2012)

Bacterial vaginosis (unlabeled use): Oral: 300 mg twice daily for 7 days (CDC, 2010)

Bite wounds (canine): Oral: 300 mg 4 times daily with a fluoroquinolone

Cellulitis due to MRSA (unlabeled use): Oral: 300-450 mg 3 times daily for 5-10 days (Liu, 2011)

Complicated skin/soft tissue infection due to MRSA (unlabeled use): I.V., Oral: 600 mg 3 times daily for 7-14 days (Liu, 2011)

Gangrenous pyomyositis: I.V.: 900 mg every 8 hours with penicillin G

Group B streptococcus (neonatal prophylaxis) (unlabeled use): I.V.: 900 mg every 8 hours until delivery (CDC, 2010)

Malaria, severe (unlabeled use): I.V.: Load: 10 mg/kg followed by 15 mg/kg/day divided every 8 hours *plus* I.V. quinidine gluconate; switch to oral therapy (clindamycin *plus* quinine) when able for total clindamycin treatment duration of 7 days (**Note:** Quinine duration is region specific, consult CDC for current recommendations) (CDC, 2009)

Malaria, uncomplicated treatment (unlabeled use): Oral: 20 mg/kg/day divided every 8 hours for 7 days *plus* quinine (CDC, 2009)

Orofacial/parapharyngeal space infections:

Oral: 150-450 mg every 6 hours for 7 days, maximum 1800 mg daily

I.V.: 600-900 mg every 8 hours

Osteomyelitis due to MRSA (unlabeled use): I.V., Oral: 600 mg 3 times daily for a minimum of 8 weeks (some experts combine with rifampin) (Liu, 2011)

Pelvic inflammatory disease: I.V.: 900 mg every 8 hours with gentamicin (conventional or single daily dosing); 24 hours after clinical improvement may convert to oral doxycycline 100 mg twice daily **or** clindamycin 450 mg 4 times daily to complete 14 days of total therapy. Avoid doxycycline if tubo-ovarian abscess is present (CDC, 2010).

Pharyngitis, group A streptococci (IDSA recommendations):
Acute treatment in penicillin-allergic patients: 21 mg/kg/day divided every 8 hours (maximum: 300 mg per dose) for 10 days (Shulman, 2012)
Chronic carrier treatment: 20-30 mg/kg/day divided every 8 hours (maximum: 300 mg per dose) for 10 days (Shulman, 2012)
***Pneumocystis jirovecii* pneumonia (unlabeled use):**
I.V.: 600-900 mg every 6-8 hours with primaquine for 21 days (CDC, 2009)
Oral: 300-450 mg every 6-8 hours with primaquine for 21 days (CDC, 2009)
Pneumonia due to MRSA (unlabeled use): I.V., Oral: 600 mg 3 times daily for 7-21 days (Liu, 2011)
Prophylaxis against infective endocarditis (unlabeled use):
Oral: 600 mg 30-60 minutes before procedure (Wilson, 2007)
I.M., I.V.: 600 mg 30-60 minutes before procedure. Intramuscular injections should be avoided in patients who are receiving anticoagulant therapy. In these circumstances, orally administered regimens should be given whenever possible. Intravenously administered antibiotics should be used for patients who are unable to tolerate or absorb oral medications (Wilson, 2007).
Note: American Heart Association (AHA) guidelines now recommend prophylaxis only in patients undergoing invasive procedures and in whom underlying cardiac conditions may predispose to a higher risk of adverse outcomes should infection occur. As of April 2007, routine prophylaxis for GI/GU procedures is no longer recommended by the AHA.
Prophylaxis in total joint replacement patients undergoing dental procedures which produce bacteremia (unlabeled use):
Oral: 600 mg 1 hour prior to procedure (ADA, 2003)
I.V.: 600 mg 1 hour prior to procedure (for patients unable to take oral medication) (ADA, 2003)
Prosthetic joint infection:
Chronic antimicrobial suppression, Staphylococci (oxacillin-susceptible) (alternative to cephalexin or cefadroxil) (unlabeled use): Oral: 300 mg every 6 hours (Osmon, 2013)
Propionibacterium acnes, treatment (alternative to penicillin G or ceftriaxone):
Oral: 300-450 mg every 6 hours for 4-6 weeks (Osmon, 2013)
I.V.: 600-900 mg every 8 hours for 4-6 weeks (Osmon, 2013)
Septic arthritis due to MRSA (unlabeled use): I.V., Oral: 600 mg 3 times daily for 3-4 weeks (Liu, 2011)
Toxic shock syndrome: I.V.: 900 mg every 8 hours with penicillin G or ceftriaxone
Toxoplasmosis (HIV-exposed/positive; secondary prevention [unlabeled use]): Oral: 600 mg every 8 hours (with pyrimethamine and leucovorin calcium) (CDC, 2009)

Dosing adjustment in renal impairment: No dosage adjustment required in renal impairment.
Poorly dialyzed; no supplemental dose or dosage adjustment necessary, including patients on intermittent hemodialysis, peritoneal dialysis, or continuous renal replacement therapy (eg, CVVHD).
Dosing adjustment in hepatic impairment: No adjustment required. Use caution with severe hepatic impairment.

Dietary Considerations May be taken with food.

Administration
I.M.: Deep I.M. sites, rotate sites; do not exceed 600 mg in a single injection.
I.V.: **Never administer as bolus**; administer by I.V. intermittent infusion over at least 10-60 minutes, at a rate **not** to exceed 30 mg/minute (do not exceed 1200 mg/hour); final concentration for administration should not exceed 18 mg/mL.
Oral: Administer with a full glass of water to minimize esophageal ulceration; give around-the-clock to promote less variation in peak and trough serum levels.

Monitoring Parameters Observe for changes in bowel frequency. Monitor for colitis and resolution of symptoms. During prolonged therapy monitor CBC, liver and renal function tests periodically.

Additional Information *In vitro* susceptibility rates to clindamycin are higher in community acquired versus hospital acquired MRSA, although this may vary by geographic region. The D-zone test is recommended for detection of inducible resistance to clindamycin in erythromycin-resistant but clindamycin-susceptible isolates (Liu, 2011).

Dosage Forms Excipient information presented when available (limited, particularly for generics); consult specific product labeling.
Capsule, Oral, as hydrochloride [strength expressed as base]:
Cleocin: 75 mg, 150 mg [contains brilliant blue fcf (fd&c blue #1), tartrazine (fd&c yellow #5)]
Cleocin: 300 mg [contains brilliant blue fcf (fd&c blue #1)]
Generic: 75 mg, 150 mg, 300 mg
Solution, Injection, as phosphate [strength expressed as base]:
Cleocin Phosphate: 300 mg/2 mL (2 mL) [contains benzyl alcohol]
Cleocin Phosphate: 600 mg/4 mL (4 mL) [contains benzyl alcohol, edetate disodium]
Cleocin Phosphate: 900 mg/6 mL (6 mL) [contains benzyl alcohol]
Cleocin Phosphate: 9 g/60 mL (60 mL) [contains benzyl alcohol, edetate disodium]
Generic: 300 mg/2 mL (2 mL); 600 mg/4 mL (4 mL); 900 mg/6 mL (6 mL); 9000 mg/60 mL (60 mL); 9 g/60 mL (60 mL)
Solution, Intravenous, as phosphate [strength expressed as base]:
Cleocin in D_5W: 300 mg/50 mL (50 mL); 600 mg/50 mL (50 mL); 900 mg/50 mL (50 mL) [contains edetate disodium]
Cleocin Phosphate: 600 mg/4 mL (4 mL) [contains benzyl alcohol, edetate disodium]
Cleocin Phosphate: 900 mg/6 mL (6 mL) [contains benzyl alcohol]
Generic: 300 mg/50 mL (50 mL); 600 mg/50 mL (50 mL); 900 mg/50 mL (50 mL); 300 mg/2 mL (2 mL); 600 mg/4 mL (4 mL); 900 mg/6 mL (6 mL)
Solution Reconstituted, Oral, as palmitate hydrochloride [strength expressed as base]:
Cleocin: 75 mg/5 mL (100 mL) [contains ethylparaben]
Generic: 75 mg/5 mL (100 mL)

Clindamycin (Topical) (klin da MYE sin)

Brand Names: U.S. Cleocin; Cleocin-T; Clindacin ETZ; Clindacin Pac; Clindacin-P; Clindagel; ClindaMax; Clindesse; Evoclin

Brand Names: Canada Clinda-T; Clindasol; Clindets; Dalacin T; Dalacin Vaginal; Taro-Clindamycin

Index Terms Clindamycin Phosphate

Pharmacologic Category Antibiotic, Lincosamide; Topical Skin Product, Acne

Use Treatment of bacterial vaginosis (vaginal cream, vaginal suppository); topically in treatment of severe acne

Pregnancy Risk Factor B

Dosage Indication-specific dosing:
Children ≥12 years and Adults: **Acne vulgaris:** Topical:
Gel (Cleocin T®, ClindaMax®), pledget, lotion, solution: Apply a thin film twice daily
Gel (Clindagel®), foam (Evoclin®): Apply once daily
Adults: **Bacterial vaginosis:** Intravaginal:
Suppositories: Insert one ovule (100 mg clindamycin) daily into vagina at bedtime for 3 days
Cream:
Cleocin®: One full applicator inserted intravaginally once daily before bedtime for 3 or 7 consecutive days in nonpregnant patients or for 7 consecutive days in pregnant patients
Clindesse®: One full applicator inserted intravaginally as a single dose at anytime during the day in nonpregnant patients

Additional Information Complete prescribing information should be consulted for additional detail.

Dosage Forms Excipient information presented when available (limited, particularly for generics); consult specific product labeling. [DSC] = Discontinued product
Cream, Vaginal, as phosphate [strength expressed as base]:
Cleocin: 2% (40 g) [contains benzyl alcohol]
Clindesse: 2% (5.8 g) [contains methylparaben, propylparaben]
Generic: 2% (40 g)
Foam, External, as phosphate [strength expressed as base]:
Evoclin: 1% (50 g, 100 g) [contains cetyl alcohol, propylene glycol]
Generic: 1% (50 g, 100 g)
Gel, External, as phosphate [strength expressed as base]:
Cleocin-T: 1% (30 g, 60 g) [contains methylparaben, propylene glycol]
Clindagel: 1% (40 mL [DSC], 75 mL) [contains methylparaben, polyethylene glycol, propylene glycol]
ClindaMax: 1% (30 g, 60 g)
Generic: 1% (30 g, 60 g)
Kit, External, as phosphate [strength expressed as base]:
Clindacin ETZ: 1% [contains cetyl alcohol, isopropyl alcohol, propylene glycol]
Clindacin Pac: 1% [contains cetyl alcohol, isopropyl alcohol, propylene glycol]
Lotion, External, as phosphate [strength expressed as base]:
Cleocin-T: 1% (60 mL) [contains cetostearyl alcohol, methylparaben]
ClindaMax: 1% (60 mL)
Generic: 1% (60 mL)
Solution, External, as phosphate [strength expressed as base]:
Cleocin-T: 1% (30 mL, 60 mL) [contains isopropyl alcohol, propylene glycol]
Generic: 1% (30 mL, 60 mL)
Suppository, Vaginal, as phosphate [strength expressed as base]:
Cleocin: 100 mg (3 ea)
Swab, External, as phosphate [strength expressed as base]:
Cleocin-T: 1% (60 ea) [contains isopropyl alcohol, propylene glycol]
Clindacin ETZ: 1% (60 ea) [contains isopropyl alcohol, propylene glycol]
Clindacin-P: 1% (69 ea) [contains isopropyl alcohol, propylene glycol]
Generic: 1% (60 ea)

Clindamycin and Tretinoin

(klin da MYE sin & TRET i noyn)

Brand Names: U.S. Veltin™; Ziana®

Index Terms Clindamycin Phosphate and Tretinoin; Tretinoin and Clindamycin; Veltin™

Pharmacologic Category Acne Products; Retinoic Acid Derivative; Topical Skin Product; Topical Skin Product, Acne

Use Treatment of acne vulgaris

Pregnancy Risk Factor C

Dosage Topical: Children ≥12 years and Adults: Apply once daily

Additional Information Complete prescribing information should be consulted for additional detail.

Dosage Forms Excipient information presented when available (limited, particularly for generics); consult specific product labeling.
Gel, topical:
Veltin™: Clindamycin phosphate 1.2% and tretinoin 0.025% (30 g, 60 g)
Ziana®: Clindamycin phosphate 1.2% and tretinoin 0.025% (30 g, 60 g)

◆ **Clindamycine (Can)** *see* Clindamycin (Systemic) *on page 451*
◆ **Clindamycin Hydrochloride** *see* Clindamycin (Systemic) *on page 451*
◆ **Clindamycin Injection, USP (Can)** *see* Clindamycin (Systemic) *on page 451*
◆ **Clindamycin Palmitate** *see* Clindamycin (Systemic) *on page 451*
◆ **Clindamycin Phosphate** *see* Clindamycin (Topical) *on page 454*
◆ **Clindamycin Phosphate and Tretinoin** *see* Clindamycin and Tretinoin *on page 455*
◆ **Clindasol (Can)** *see* Clindamycin (Topical) *on page 454*
◆ **Clinda-T (Can)** *see* Clindamycin (Topical) *on page 454*
◆ **Clindesse** *see* Clindamycin (Topical) *on page 454*
◆ **Clindets (Can)** *see* Clindamycin (Topical) *on page 454*
◆ **Clinolipid** *see* Fat Emulsion (Plant Based) *on page 834*
◆ **Clinpro™ 5000** *see* Fluoride *on page 880*

CloBAZam (KLOE ba zam)

Brand Names: U.S. Onfi

Brand Names: Canada Apo-Clobazam; Clobazam-10; Dom-Clobazam; Frisium; Novo-Clobazam; PMS-Clobazam

Pharmacologic Category Benzodiazepine

Use Adjunctive treatment of seizures associated with Lennox-Gastaut syndrome
Canadian labeling: Adjunctive treatment of epilepsy

Unlabeled Use Catamenial epilepsy; epilepsy (monotherapy)

Pregnancy Considerations Adverse events were observed in some animal reproduction studies. Clobazam crosses the placenta. An increased risk of fetal malformations may be associated with first trimester exposure. The Canadian labeling contraindicates use in the first trimester. The incidence of premature birth and low birth weights may be increased following maternal use of benzodiazepines; hypoglycemia and respiratory problems in the neonate may occur following exposure late in pregnancy. Neonatal withdrawal symptoms may occur within days to weeks after birth and "floppy infant syndrome" (which also includes withdrawal symptoms) has been reported with some benzodiazepines (Bergman, 1992; Iqbal, 2002; Wikner, 2007). A combination of factors influences the potential teratogenicity of anticonvulsant therapy. When treating women with epilepsy, monotherapy with the lowest effective dose and avoidance medications known to have a high incidence of teratogenic effects is recommended (Harden, 2009; Wlodarczyk, 2012).

Patients exposed to clobazam during pregnancy are encouraged to enroll themselves into the AED Pregnancy Registry by calling 1-888-233-2334. Additional information is available at www.aedpregnancyregistry.org.

Breast-Feeding Considerations Clobazam is excreted into breast milk. Use in nursing women is contraindicated in the Canadian labeling. Drowsiness, lethargy, or weight loss in nursing infants have been observed in case reports following maternal use of some benzodiazepines (Iqbal, 2002).

Medication Guide Available Yes

Contraindications There are no contraindications in the manufacturer's labeling.

Canadian labeling (not in U.S. labeling): Hypersensitivity to clobazam or any component of the formulation (cross sensitivity with other benzodiazepines may exist); myasthenia gravis; narrow-angle glaucoma; severe hepatic or respiratory disease; sleep apnea; history of substance abuse; use in the first trimester of pregnancy; breast-feeding

Warnings/Precautions Serious reactions, including Stevens-Johnson syndrome (SJS) and toxic epidermal necrolysis (TEN), have been reported. Monitor patients closely for signs and symptoms especially during the first 8 weeks or when reintroducing therapy. Permanently discontinue if SJS/TEN suspected.

Rebound or withdrawal symptoms may occur following abrupt discontinuation or large decreases in dose (more common with prolonged treatment). Cautiously taper dose if drug discontinuation is required. Use with caution in elderly or debilitated patients, patients with mild-to-moderate hepatic impairment or with pre-existing muscle weakness or ataxia (may cause muscle weakness).

Causes CNS depression (dose related) resulting in sedation, dizziness, confusion, or ataxia which may impair physical and mental capabilities. Patients must be cautioned about performing tasks which require mental alertness (eg, operating machinery or driving). Use with caution in patients receiving other CNS depressants or psychoactive agents. Effects with other sedative drugs or ethanol may be potentiated. Use with caution in patients with an impaired gag reflex or respiratory disease.

Tolerance, psychological and physical dependence may occur with prolonged use. Where possible, avoid use in patients with drug abuse, alcoholism, or psychiatric disease (eg, depression, psychosis). May increase risk of suicidal thoughts/behavior.

Acute withdrawal, including seizures, may be precipitated in patients after administration of flumazenil to patients receiving long-term benzodiazepine therapy.

Benzodiazepines have been associated with anterograde amnesia. Paradoxical reactions, including hyperactive or aggressive behavior, have been reported with benzodiazepines, particularly in adolescent/pediatric or psychiatric patients. Does not have analgesic, antidepressant, or antipsychotic properties.

Adverse Reactions

>10%:

Central nervous system: Somnolence (22%), fever (13%), lethargy (10%)

Respiratory: Upper respiratory tract infection (12%)

1% to 10%:

Central nervous system: Aggressiveness (8%), irritability (7%), ataxia (5%), fatigue (5%), insomnia (5%), sedation (5%), psychomotor hyperactivity (4%)

Gastrointestinal: Salivation increased (9%), vomiting (7%), constipation (5%), appetite increased (3%), dysphagia (2%)

Genitourinary: Urinary tract infection (4%)

Neuromuscular & skeletal: Dysarthria (3%)

Respiratory: Cough (5%), pneumonia (4%), bronchitis (2%)

Postmarketing and/or case reports (Limited to important or life-threatening): Aspiration, behavior changes, blurred vision, confusion, delirium, delusions, depression, diplopia, eosinophilia, hallucinations, leukopenia, mood changes, respiratory depression, Stevens-Johnson syndrome, suicidal ideation, suicide attempts, thrombocytopenia, toxic epidermal necrolysis

Drug Interactions

Metabolism/Transport Effects Substrate of CYP2B6 (minor), CYP2C19 (major), CYP3A4 (minor), P-glycoprotein; **Note:** Assignment of Major/Minor substrate status based on clinically relevant drug interaction potential; **Inhibits** CYP2C9 (weak), CYP2D6 (moderate), UGT1A4, UGT1A6, UGT2B4; **Induces** CYP3A4 (weak/moderate)

Avoid Concomitant Use

Avoid concomitant use of CloBAZam with any of the following: Axitinib; Azelastine (Nasal); OLANZapine; Paraldehyde; Simeprevir; Sodium Oxybate; Thioridazine

Increased Effect/Toxicity

CloBAZam may increase the levels/effects of: ARIPiprazole; Azelastine (Nasal); Buprenorphine; CloZAPine; CNS Depressants; CYP2D6 Substrates; Deferiprone; Fesoterodine; Fosphenytoin; Hydrocodone; Methotrimeprazine; Metoprolol; Metyrosine; Mirtazapine; Nebivolol; Paraldehyde; Phenytoin; Pramipexole; ROPINIRole; Rotigotine; Selective Serotonin Reuptake Inhibitors; Sodium Oxybate; Thioridazine; Zolpidem

The levels/effects of CloBAZam may be increased by: Alcohol (Ethyl); Antifungal Agents (Azole Derivatives, Systemic); Aprepitant; Brimonidine (Topical); Calcium Channel Blockers (Nondihydropyridine); Cimetidine; Contraceptives (Estrogens); Contraceptives (Progestins); CYP2C19 Inhibitors (Moderate); CYP2C19 Inhibitors (Strong); Doxylamine; Droperidol; Fosaprepitant; Grapefruit Juice; HydrOXYzine; Isoniazid; Luliconazole; Magnesium Sulfate; Methotrimeprazine; OLANZapine; Perampanel; Propafenone; Proton Pump Inhibitors; Selective Serotonin Reuptake Inhibitors; Tapentadol

Decreased Effect

CloBAZam may decrease the levels/effects of: ARIPiprazole; Axitinib; Codeine; Contraceptives (Estrogens); Contraceptives (Progestins); Ibrutinib; Saxagliptin; Simeprevir; Tamoxifen; TraMADol

The levels/effects of CloBAZam may be decreased by: CarBAMazepine; CYP2C19 Inducers (Strong); Dabrafenib; Rifamycin Derivatives; Theophylline Derivatives; Yohimbine

Ethanol/Nutrition/Herb Interactions

Ethanol: Concomitant administration may increase bioavailability of clobazam by 50%. Ethanol may also increase CNS depression; monitor for increased effects with coadministration. Caution patients about effects.

Food: Serum concentrations may be increased by grapefruit juice.

Herb/Nutraceutical: St John's wort may decrease benzodiazepine levels. Avoid valerian, St John's wort, kava kava, gotu kola (may increase CNS depression).

Storage/Stability Store at 20°C to 25°C (68°F to 77°F).

Mechanism of Action Clobazam is a 1,5 benzodiazepine which binds to stereospecific benzodiazepine receptors on the postsynaptic GABA neuron at several sites within the central nervous system, including the limbic system, reticular formation. Enhancement of the inhibitory effect of GABA on neuronal excitability results by increased neuronal membrane permeability to chloride ions. This shift in chloride ions results in hyperpolarization (a less excitable state) and stabilization.

Pharmacodynamics/Kinetics

Absorption: Rapid; ~87%

Protein binding: 80% to 90%

Metabolism: Hepatic via CYP3A4 and to a lesser extent via CYP2C19 and 2B6 (N-demethylation to active metabolite [N-desmethyl] with ~20% activity of clobazam). CYP2C19 primarily mediates subsequent hydroxylation of the N-desmethyl metabolite.

Half-life elimination: Clobazam: 36-42 hours; N-desmethyl (active): 71-82 hours

Time to peak: 30 minutes to 4 hours

Excretion: Urine (~94%), as metabolites

Dosage Oral:

Children:

- Lennox-Gastaut (adjunctive): U.S. labeling: ≥2 years: Refer to adult dosing.
- Epilepsy (adjunctive): Canadian labeling (not in U.S. labeling):
  - <2 years: Initial 0.5-1 mg/kg/day
  - 2-16 years: Initial: 5 mg daily; may be increased (no more frequently than every 5 days) to a maximum of 40 mg daily
- Epilepsy (monotherapy) (unlabeled use): 2-16 years: Initial: Titrate slowly over 1-3 weeks to target dose of ~0.5 mg/kg/day in 2 divided doses (Canadian Study Group, 1998)

Adults:

- Lennox-Gastaut (adjunctive): U.S. labeling: **Note:** Dose should be titrated according to patient tolerability and response.
  - ≤30 kg: Initial: 5 mg once daily for ≥1 week, then increase to 5 mg twice daily for ≥1 week, then increase to 10 mg twice daily thereafter
  - >30 kg: Initial: 5 mg twice daily for ≥1 week, then increase to 10 mg twice daily for ≥1 week, then increase to 20 mg twice daily thereafter
  - *CYP2C19 poor metabolizers:*
    - ≤30 kg: Initial: 5 mg once daily for ≥2 weeks, then increase to 5 mg twice daily; after ≥1 week may increase to 10 mg twice daily
    - >30 kg: Initial: 5 mg once daily for ≥1 week, then increase to 5 mg twice daily for ≥1 week, then increase to 10 mg twice daily; after ≥1 week may increase to 20 mg twice daily
- Epilepsy (adjunctive): Canadian labeling (not in U.S. labeling): Initial: 5-15 mg/day; dosage may be gradually adjusted (based on tolerance and seizure control) to a maximum of 80 mg/day. **Note:** Daily doses of up to 30 mg may be taken as a single dose at bedtime; higher doses should be divided.
- Catamenial epilepsy (unlabeled use): 20-30 mg daily for 10 days during the perimenstrual period (Feely, 1984)

Elderly: Lennox-Gastaut (adjunctive):

- ≤30 kg: Initial: 5 mg once daily for ≥2 weeks, then increase to 5 mg twice daily; after ≥1 week may increase to 10 mg twice daily based on patient tolerability and response
- >30 kg: Initial: 5 mg once daily for ≥1 week, then increase to 5 mg twice daily for ≥1 week, then increase to 10 mg twice daily; after ≥1 week may increase to 20 mg twice daily based on patient tolerability and response

Dosage adjustment in renal impairment:

U.S. labeling:

- Cl_{cr} ≥30 mL/minute: No dosage adjustment necessary.
- Cl_{cr} <30 mL/minute: No dosage adjustment provided in manufacturer's labeling (has not been studied); use with caution.

Canadian labeling: No dosage adjustment provided in manufacturer's labeling; however, a reduced dosage is recommended.

Dosage adjustment in hepatic impairment:

U.S. labeling:

- Mild-to-moderate impairment:
  - ≤30 kg: Initial: 5 mg once daily for ≥2 weeks, then increase to 5 mg twice daily; after ≥1 week may increase to 10 mg twice daily based on patient tolerability and response
  - >30 kg: Initial: 5 mg once daily for ≥1 week, then increase to 5 mg twice daily for ≥1 week, then increase to 10 mg twice daily; after ≥1 week may increase to 20 mg twice daily based on patient tolerability and response
- Severe impairment: No dosage adjustment provided in manufacturer's labeling (has not been studied). Use with caution; undergoes extensive hepatic metabolism.

Canadian labeling:

- Mild-to-moderate impairment: No dosage adjustment provided in manufacturer's labeling; however, a reduced dosage is recommended.
- Severe impairment: Use is contraindicated.

Dietary Considerations May be taken with or without food.

Administration May be administered with or without food. Tablets can be crushed and mixed in applesauce. Shake suspension well before using; only use the oral dosing syringe supplied with the suspension.

Monitoring Parameters Respiratory and mental status/suicidality (eg, suicidal thoughts, depression, behavioral changes). The Canadian labeling recommends periodic CBC, liver function, renal function and thyroid function tests.

Dosage Forms Excipient information presented when available (limited, particularly for generics); consult specific product labeling.

Suspension, Oral:

Onfi: 2.5 mg/mL (120 mL) [contains methylparaben, polysorbate 80, propylene glycol, propylparaben; berry flavor]

Tablet, Oral:

Onfi: 5 mg

Onfi: 10 mg, 20 mg [scored]

Dosage Forms: Canada Excipient information presented when available (limited, particularly for generics); consult specific product labeling.

Tablet:

Alti-Clobazam, Apo-Clobazam, Clobazam-10, Dom-Clobazam, Frisium, Novo-Clobazam, PMS-Clobazam, ratio-Clobazam: 10 mg

Controlled Substance C-IV

◆ **Clobazam-10 (Can)** *see* CloBAZam *on page 455*

Clobetasol (kloe BAY ta sol)

Brand Names: U.S. Clobetasol Propionate E; Clobex; Clobex Spray; Cormax Scalp Application; Olux; Olux-E; Temovate; Temovate E

Brand Names: Canada Clobex®; Dermovate®; Mylan-Clobetasol Cream; Mylan-Clobetasol Ointment; Mylan-Clobetasol Scalp Application; Novo-Clobetasol; PMS-Clobetasol; ratio-Clobetasol; Taro-Clobetasol

Index Terms Clobetasol Propionate

Pharmacologic Category Corticosteroid, Topical

Additional Appendix Information
Topical Corticosteroids *on page 2299*

Use Short-term relief of inflammation of moderate-to-severe corticosteroid-responsive dermatoses (very high potency topical corticosteroid)

Pregnancy Risk Factor C

Dosage Topical: Discontinue when control achieved; if improvement not seen within 2 weeks, reassessment of diagnosis may be necessary.

Children <12 years: Use is not recommended
Children ≥12 years and Adults:
Oral mucosal inflammation, dental (unlabeled use):
Cream: Apply twice daily for up to 2 weeks (maximum dose: 50 g/week); discontinue application when control is achieved; if no improvement is seen, reassessment of diagnosis may be necessary
Steroid-responsive dermatoses:
Cream, emollient cream, gel, ointment: Apply twice daily for up to 2 weeks (maximum dose: 50 g/week)
Foam (Olux-E™): Apply to affected area twice daily for up to 2 weeks (maximum dose: 50 g/week); do not apply to face or intertriginous areas
Steroid-responsive dermatoses: Foam (Olux®), solution: Apply to affected scalp twice daily for up to 2 weeks (maximum dose: 50 g/week or 50 mL/week)
Mild-to-moderate plaque-type psoriasis of nonscalp areas: Foam (Olux®): Apply to affected area twice daily for up to 2 weeks (maximum dose: 50 g/week); do not apply to face or intertriginous areas
Children ≥16 years and Adults: Moderate-to-severe plaque-type psoriasis: Emollient cream, lotion: Apply twice daily for up to 2 weeks, has been used for up to 4 weeks when application is <10% of body surface area; use with caution (maximum dose: 50 g/week)
Children ≥18 years and Adults:
Moderate-to-severe plaque-type psoriasis: Spray: Apply by spraying directly onto affected area twice daily; should be gently rubbed into skin. Should be used for not longer than 4 weeks; treatment beyond 2 weeks should be limited to localized lesions which have not improved sufficiently. Total dose should not exceed 50 g/week or 59 mL/week.
Scalp psoriasis: Shampoo: Apply thin film to dry scalp once daily; leave in place for 15 minutes, then add water, lather; rinse thoroughly
Steroid-responsive dermatoses: Lotion: Apply twice daily for up to 2 weeks (maximum dose: 50 g/week)

Additional Information Complete prescribing information should be consulted for additional detail.

Dosage Forms Excipient information presented when available (limited, particularly for generics); consult specific product labeling.
Cream, External, as propionate:
Clobetasol Propionate E: 0.05% (15 g, 30 g, 60 g) [contains cetostearyl alcohol, propylene glycol]
Clobetasol Propionate E: 0.05% (15 g, 30 g, 60 g) [contains propylene glycol]
Temovate: 0.05% (30 g, 60 g) [contains cetostearyl alcohol, chlorocresol (chloro-m-cresol), propylene glycol]
Temovate E: 0.05% (60 g)
Generic: 0.05% (15 g, 30 g, 45 g, 60 g)
Foam, External, as propionate:
Olux: 0.05% (50 g, 100 g) [contains cetyl alcohol, propylene glycol]
Olux-E: 0.05% (50 g, 100 g)
Generic: 0.05% (50 g, 100 g)
Gel, External, as propionate:
Temovate: 0.05% (60 g) [contains propylene glycol]
Generic: 0.05% (15 g, 30 g, 60 g)
Liquid, External, as propionate:
Clobex Spray: 0.05% (59 mL, 125 mL) [contains alcohol, usp]
Lotion, External, as propionate:
Clobex: 0.05% (59 mL, 118 mL)
Generic: 0.05% (59 mL, 118 mL)
Ointment, External, as propionate:
Temovate: 0.05% (15 g, 30 g) [contains propylene glycol]
Generic: 0.05% (15 g, 30 g, 45 g, 60 g)
Shampoo, External, as propionate:
Clobex: 0.05% (118 mL) [contains alcohol, usp]
Generic: 0.05% (118 mL)
Solution, External, as propionate:
Cormax Scalp Application: 0.05% (50 mL) [contains isopropyl alcohol]
Temovate: 0.05% (50 mL)
Generic: 0.05% (25 mL, 50 mL)

◆ **Clobetasol Propionate** *see* Clobetasol *on page 457*
◆ **Clobetasol Propionate E** *see* Clobetasol *on page 457*
◆ **Clobex** *see* Clobetasol *on page 457*
◆ **Clobex® (Can)** *see* Clobetasol *on page 457*
◆ **Clobex Spray** *see* Clobetasol *on page 457*

Clocortolone (kloe KOR toe lone)

Brand Names: U.S. Cloderm; Cloderm Pump

Brand Names: Canada Cloderm®

Index Terms Clocortolone Pivalate

Pharmacologic Category Corticosteroid, Topical

Additional Appendix Information
Topical Corticosteroids *on page 2299*

Use Inflammation of corticosteroid-responsive dermatoses (intermediate-potency topical corticosteroid)

Pregnancy Risk Factor C

Dosage Adults: Apply sparingly and gently; rub into affected area from 1-4 times/day. Therapy should be discontinued when control is achieved; if no improvement is seen, reassessment of diagnosis may be necessary.

Additional Information Complete prescribing information should be consulted for additional detail.

Dosage Forms Excipient information presented when available (limited, particularly for generics); consult specific product labeling.
Cream, External, as pivalate:
Cloderm: 0.1% (45 g, 90 g) [contains edetate disodium, methylparaben, propylparaben]
Cloderm Pump: 0.1% (30 g, 75 g) [contains edetate disodium, methylparaben, propylparaben]

◆ **Clocortolone Pivalate** *see* Clocortolone *on page 458*
◆ **Cloderm** *see* Clocortolone *on page 458*
◆ **Cloderm® (Can)** *see* Clocortolone *on page 458*
◆ **Cloderm Pump** *see* Clocortolone *on page 458*

Clofarabine (klo FARE a been)

Brand Names: U.S. Clolar

Brand Names: Canada Clolar®

Index Terms CAFdA; Clofarex

Pharmacologic Category Antineoplastic Agent, Antimetabolite (Purine Analog)

Use Treatment of acute lymphoblastic leukemia (ALL) in children (ages 1-21 years)

Unlabeled Use Treatment of relapsed/refractory acute lymphoblastic leukemia (ALL) in adults; treatment of acute myeloid leukemia (AML) in adults ≥60 years of age

Pregnancy Risk Factor D

Pregnancy Considerations Teratogenic effects and resorptions were observed in animal reproduction studies. May cause fetal harm if administered to a pregnant woman. Women of childbearing potential should be advised to use effective contraception and avoid becoming pregnant during therapy.

Breast-Feeding Considerations Due to the potential for serious adverse reactions in the nursing infant, breast-feeding should be avoided during clofarabine treatment.

Contraindications There are no contraindications listed within the U.S. product labeling.

Canadian labeling: Hypersensitivity to clofarabine or any component of the formulation; symptomatic CNS involvement; history of serious heart, liver, kidney, or pancreas disease; severe hepatic impairment (AST and/or ALT >5 x ULN, and/or bilirubin >3 x ULN); severe renal impairment (Cl_{cr} <30 mL/minute)

Warnings/Precautions Hazardous agent - use appropriate precautions for handling and disposal (NIOSH, 2012). Cytokine release syndrome (eg, tachypnea, tachycardia, hypotension, pulmonary edema) may develop into capillary leak syndrome, systemic inflammatory response syndrome (SIRS), and organ dysfunction; discontinue with signs/symptoms of SIRS or capillary leak syndrome (rapid onset respiratory distress, hypotension, pleural/pericardial effusion, and multiorgan failure) and consider supportive treatment with diuretics, corticosteroids, and/or albumin. Prophylactic corticosteroids may prevent or diminish the signs/symptoms of cytokine release. Monitor blood pressure during 5 days of treatment; discontinue if hypotension develops. Monitor if on concurrent medications known to affect blood pressure. Dose-dependent, reversible myelosuppression (neutropenia, thrombocytopenia, and anemia) is common; may be severe and prolonged. Monitor blood counts and platelets daily during treatment, then 1-2 times weekly or as necessary. May be at increased risk for infection due to neutropenia; opportunistic infection is increased due to prolonged neutropenia and immunocompromised state; monitor for signs and symptoms of infection and treat promptly if infection develops. May require therapy discontinuation.

Has not been studied in patients with hepatic impairment; use with caution (per manufacturer's labeling). Canadian labeling contraindicates use in severe impairment or in patients with a history of serious hepatic disease. Transaminases and bilirubin may be increased during treatment; transaminase elevations generally occur within 10 days of administration and persist for ≤15 days. In some cases, hepatotoxicity was severe and fatal. The risk for hepatotoxicity, including hepatic sinusoidal obstruction syndrome (SOS; formerly called veno-occlusive disease), is increased in patients who have previously undergone a hematopoietic stem cell transplant. Monitor liver function closely; may require therapy interruption or discontinuation; discontinue if SOS is suspected. Elevated creatinine, acute renal failure, and hematuria were observed in clinical studies. Monitor renal function closely; may require dosage reduction or therapy discontinuation. A pharmacokinetic study demonstrated that systemic exposure increases as creatinine clearance decreases (Cl_{cr} <60 mL/minute) (Bonate, 2011). Dosage reduction required for moderate renal impairment (Cl_{cr} 30-60 mL/minute); use with caution in patients with Cl_{cr} <30 mL/minute (has not been studied). Canadian labeling contraindicates use in severe impairment or in patients with a history of serious kidney disease. Minimize the use of drugs known to cause renal toxicity during the 5-day treatment period; avoid concomitant hepatotoxic medications. Tumor lysis syndrome/hyperuricemia may occur as a consequence of leukemia treatment, including treatment with clofarabine, usually occurring in the first treatment cycle. May lead to life-threatening acute renal failure; adequate hydration and prophylactic antihyperuricemic therapy throughout treatment will reduce the risk/effects of tumor lysis syndrome; monitor closely. Potentially significant drug-drug interactions may exist, requiring dose or frequency adjustment, additional monitoring, and/or selection of alternative therapy.

Adverse Reactions

>10%:

Cardiovascular: Tachycardia (35%), hypotension (29%; grade 3: 11%; grade 4: 8%), flushing (19%), hypertension (13%), edema (12%)

Central nervous system: Headache (43%), fever (39%), chills (34%), fatigue (34%), anxiety (21%), pain (15%)

Dermatologic: Pruritus (43%), rash (38%), petechiae (26%), palmar-plantar erythrodysesthesia syndrome (16%), erythema (11%)

Gastrointestinal: Vomiting (78%; grades 3/4: 9%), nausea (73%; grades 3/4: 15%), diarrhea (56%), abdominal pain (8% to 35%), anorexia (30%), gingival bleeding (17%), mucosal inflammation (16%), oral candidiasis (11%)

Hematologic: Leukopenia (grades 3/4: 88%), anemia (83%; grades 3/4: 75%), lymphopenia (grades 3/4: 82%), thrombocytopenia (81%; grades 3/4: 80%), neutropenia (grades 3/4: 10% to 64%), febrile neutropenia (55%; grade 4: 3%)

Hepatic: ALT increased (81%; grades 3/4: 43% to 44%), AST increased (74%; grades 3/4: 36%), bilirubin increased (45%; grades 3/4: 13%)

Neuromuscular & skeletal: Limb pain (30%), myalgia (14%)

Renal: Creatinine increased (50%; grades 3/4: 8%), hematuria (13%)

Respiratory: Epistaxis (27%), dyspnea (13%), pleural effusion (12%)

Miscellaneous: Infection (83%; includes bacterial, fungal, and viral), sepsis/septic shock (17%), catheter-related infection (12%)

1% to 10%:

Cardiovascular: Pericardial effusion (8%)

Central nervous system: Irritability (10%), lethargy (10%), somnolence (10%), agitation (5%), mental status change (1% to 4%)

Dermatologic: Cellulitis (8%), pruritic rash (8%)

Gastrointestinal: Proctalgia (8%), clostridium colitis (7%), stomatitis (7%), oral mucosal petechiae (5%), cecitis (1% to 4%), pancreatitis (1% to 4%)

Hepatic: Jaundice (8%)

Neuromuscular & skeletal: Back pain (10%), bone pain (10%), weakness (10%), arthralgia (9%)

Respiratory: Pneumonia (10%), respiratory distress (10%), tachypnea (9%), upper respiratory tract infection (5%), pulmonary edema (1% to 4%)

Miscellaneous: Herpes simplex (10%), bacteremia (9%), candidiasis (7%), herpes zoster (7%), staphylococcus bacteremia (6%), tumor lysis syndrome (grade 3: 6%), capillary leak syndrome (4%), hypersensitivity (1% to 4%), SIRS (2%)

<1% (Limited to important or life-threatening): Bone marrow failure, dermatitis, gastrointestinal hemorrhage, hallucination, hepatic sinusoidal obstruction syndrome (SOS; veno-occlusive disease), hepatomegaly, hypokalemia, hypophosphatemia, left ventricular systolic function decreased, right ventricular pressure increased, Stevens-Johnson syndrome, toxic epidermal necrolysis

Drug Interactions

Metabolism/Transport Effects None known.

Avoid Concomitant Use

Avoid concomitant use of Clofarabine with any of the following: BCG; CloZAPine; Natalizumab; Pimecrolimus; Tacrolimus (Topical); Tofacitinib; Vaccines (Live)

Increased Effect/Toxicity

Clofarabine may increase the levels/effects of: CloZAPine; Leflunomide; Natalizumab; Tofacitinib; Vaccines (Live); Vitamin K Antagonists

The levels/effects of Clofarabine may be increased by: Denosumab; Pimecrolimus; Roflumilast; Tacrolimus (Topical); Trastuzumab

Decreased Effect

Clofarabine may decrease the levels/effects of: BCG; Cardiac Glycosides; Coccidioidin Skin Test; Sipuleucel-T; Vaccines (Inactivated); Vaccines (Live); Vitamin K Antagonists

The levels/effects of Clofarabine may be decreased by: Echinacea

Preparation for Administration Hazardous agent; use appropriate precautions for handling and disposal (NIOSH, 2012). Clofarabine should be diluted with NS or D_5W to a final concentration of 0.15-0.4 mg/mL. Manufacturer recommends the product be filtered through a 0.2 micron filter prior to dilution.

Storage/Stability Store intact vials at room temperature of 25°C (77°F); excursions permitted to 15°C to 30°C (59°F to 86°F). Solutions diluted for infusion in D_5W or NS are stable for 24 hours at room temperature.

Mechanism of Action Clofarabine, a purine (deoxyadenosine) nucleoside analog, is metabolized to clofarabine 5'-triphosphate. Clofarabine 5'-triphosphate decreases cell replication and repair as well as causing cell death. To decrease cell replication and repair, clofarabine 5'-triphosphate competes with deoxyadenosine triphosphate for the enzymes ribonucleotide reductase and DNA polymerase. Cell replication is decreased when clofarabine 5'-triphosphate inhibits ribonucleotide reductase from reacting with deoxyadenosine triphosphate to produce deoxynucleotide triphosphate which is needed for DNA synthesis. Cell replication is also decreased when clofarabine 5'-triphosphate competes with DNA polymerase for incorporation into the DNA chain; when done during the repair process, cell repair is affected. To cause cell death, clofarabine 5'-triphosphate alters the mitochondrial membrane by releasing proteins, an inducing factor and cytochrome C.

Pharmacodynamics/Kinetics

Distribution: V_d: Children: 172 L/m^2 or 5.8 L/kg (Bonate, 2011); Elderly: 268 L/kg (Bonate, 2011)

Protein binding: 47%, primarily to albumin

Metabolism: Intracellulary by deoxycytidine kinase and mono- and diphosphokinases to active metabolite clofarabine 5'-triphosphate; limited hepatic metabolism (0.2%)

Half-life elimination: Children: ~5 hours; Children and Adults: 7 hours (Bonate, 2011); half-life may be increased in elderly and in patients with renal impairment (Bonate, 2011)

Excretion: Urine (49% to 60%, as unchanged drug)

Dosage Consider prophylactic corticosteroids (hydrocortisone 100 mg/m^2 on days 1-3) to prevent signs/symptoms of capillary leak syndrome or systemic inflammatory response syndrome (SIRS), hydration and antihyperuricemic therapy (to reduce the risk of tumor lysis syndrome/hyperuricemia), and prophylactic antiemetics.

Acute lymphoblastic leukemia (ALL): Children ≥1 year and Adults ≤21 years: I.V.: 52 mg/m^2/day days 1 through 5; repeat every 2-6 weeks; subsequent cycles should begin no sooner than 14 days from day 1 of the previous cycle (subsequent cycles may be administered when ANC ≥750/mm^3)

Acute lymphoblastic leukemia, relapsed/refractory (ALL; unlabeled use): Adults: I.V.:

Monotherapy: Induction: 40 mg/m^2/day for 5 days; may repeat induction cycle once in 3-6 weeks (depending on marrow response and recovery) (Kantarjian, 2003)

Combination therapy:

Induction: 40 mg/m^2/day for 5 days (in combination with cytarabine); may repeat one time after day 28 (if needed) (Advani, 2010) **or** 30 mg/m^2/day for 5 days (in combination with conventional chemotherapy) (Pigneux, 2011)

Consolidation: 40 mg/m^2/day for 4 days (in combination with cytarabine) for one cycle (Advani, 2010)

Acute myelocytic leukemia (AML) (unlabeled use): Adults ≥60 years: I.V.:

Monotherapy (Kantarjian, 2010):

Induction: 30 mg/m^2/day for 5 days; may repeat one time after day 28 (if needed) with 20 mg/m^2/day for 5 days

Consolidation: 20 mg/m^2/day for 5 days for up to a maximum total 6 cycles, including induction cycles

Combination therapy with cytarabine (Faderl, 2008):

Induction: 30 mg/m^2/day for 5 days; may repeat one time if needed

Consolidation: 30 mg/m^2/day for 3 days every 4-7 weeks for up to a total of 12 consolidation cycles

Dosage adjustment for toxicity:

Hematologic toxicity: ANC <500/mm^3 lasting ≥4 weeks: Reduce dose by 25% for next cycle

Nonhematologic toxicity:

Clinically significant infection: Withhold treatment until infection is under control, then restart at full dose

Grade 3 toxicity (excluding infection, nausea and vomiting, and transient elevations in transaminases and bilirubin): Withhold treatment; may reinitiate with a 25% dose-reduction with resolution or return to baseline

Grade ≥3 increase in creatinine or bilirubin: Discontinue clofarabine; may reinitiate with 25% dosage reduction when creatinine or bilirubin return to baseline and patient is stable; administer antihyperuricemic therapy for elevated uric acid.

Grade 4 toxicity (noninfectious): Discontinue treatment

Capillary leak or SIRS early signs/symptoms (eg, hypotension, tachycardia, tachypnea, pulmonary edema): Discontinue clofarabine; institute supportive measures. May consider reinitiating with a 25% dose-reduction after patient is stable and organ function recovers to baseline.

Hypotension due to any cause (Canadian labeling): Discontinue clofarabine; if hypotension resolves without pharmacologic intervention, may reinitiate with 25% dosage reduction.

Dosage adjustment in renal impairment: Clofarabine undergoes renal elimination and exposure is increased as creatinine clearance decreases (Bonate, 2011).

U.S. labeling:

Cl_{cr} 30-60 mL/minute: Reduce dose by 50%

Cl_{cr} <30 mL/minute: No dosage adjustment provided in manufacturer's labeling; use with caution (has not been studied).

Canadian labeling:

Cl_{cr} ≥30 mL/minute: No dosage adjustment provided in manufacturer's labeling; use with caution (has not been studied).

Cl_{cr} <30 mL/minute: Use is contraindicated.

NCCN AML guidelines (v.2.2012): Adults >60 years with creatinine clearance <60 mL/minute: Use is not recommended

Dosage adjustment in hepatic impairment: No dosage adjustment provided in manufacturer's labeling; use with caution (has not been studied). Canadian labeling contraindicates use in severe impairment.

Dosing in obesity: *ASCO Guidelines for appropriate chemotherapy dosing in obese adults with cancer:* Utilize patient's actual body weight (full weight) for calculation of body surface area- or weight-based dosing, particularly when the intent of therapy is curative; manage regimen-related toxicities in the same manner as for nonobese patients; if a dose reduction is utilized due to toxicity, consider resumption of full weight-based dosing with subsequent cycles, especially if cause of toxicity (eg, hepatic or renal impairment) is resolved (Griggs, 2012).

Administration

I.V. infusion: Over 1-2 hours (Faderl, 2008; Kantarjian, 2003; Kantarjian, 2010). Continuous I.V. fluids are encouraged to decrease adverse events and tumor lysis effects. Hypotension may be a sign of capillary leak syndrome or systemic inflammatory response syndrome (SIRS). Discontinue if the patient becomes hypotensive during administration; may consider therapy reinitiation with a 25% dose reduction after return to baseline. Do not administer any other medications through the same intravenous line.

Hazardous agent; use appropriate precautions for handling and disposal (NIOSH, 2012).

Monitoring Parameters CBC with differential and platelets (daily during treatment, then 1-2 times weekly or as necessary); liver and kidney function (during 5 days of clofarabine administration); blood pressure, cardiac function, and respiratory status during infusion; signs and symptoms of tumor lysis syndrome, infection, and cytokine release syndrome (tachypnea, tachycardia, hypotension, pulmonary edema); hydration status

Dosage Forms Excipient information presented when available (limited, particularly for generics); consult specific product labeling.

Solution, Intravenous [preservative free]:

Clolar: 1 mg/mL (20 mL)

◆ **Clofarex** *see* Clofarabine *on page 458*

◆ **Clolar** *see* Clofarabine *on page 458*

◆ **Clolar® (Can)** *see* Clofarabine *on page 458*

◆ **Clomid** *see* ClomiPHENE *on page 461*

◆ **Clomid® (Can)** *see* ClomiPHENE *on page 461*

ClomiPHENE (KLOE mi feen)

Brand Names: U.S. Clomid; Serophene

Brand Names: Canada Clomid®; Serophene®

Index Terms Clomiphene Citrate

Pharmacologic Category Ovulation Stimulator; Selective Estrogen Receptor Modulator (SERM)

Use Treatment of ovulatory dysfunction in patients desiring pregnancy

Pregnancy Risk Factor X

Pregnancy Considerations Embryofetal and structural malformations were observed in animal reproduction studies. The incidence of adverse fetal effects following maternal use of clomiphene for ovulation induction is similar to those seen in the general population. Clomiphene is not indicated for use in women who are already pregnant.

Breast-Feeding Considerations Clomiphene may decrease lactation.

Contraindications Hypersensitivity to clomiphene citrate or any of its components; liver disease; abnormal uterine bleeding; enlargement or development of ovarian cyst (not due to polycystic ovarian syndrome); uncontrolled thyroid or adrenal dysfunction; presence of an organic intracranial lesion such as pituitary tumor; pregnancy

Warnings/Precautions Ovarian enlargement may occur with use; may be accompanied by abdominal distention or abdominal pain and generally regresses without treatment within 2-3 weeks. If ovaries are abnormally enlarged, withhold hCG to reduce the risk of ovarian hyperstimulation syndrome (OHSS). OHSS is characterized by severe ovarian enlargement, abdominal pain/distention, nausea, vomiting, diarrhea, dyspnea, and oliguria, and may be accompanied by ascites, pleural effusion, hypovolemia, electrolyte imbalance, hemoperitoneum, and thromboembolic events. If severe hyperstimulation occurs, stop treatment and hospitalize patient. This syndrome develops rapidly within 24 hours to several days and generally occurs during the 7-10 days immediately following treatment. Use with caution in patients unusually sensitive to pituitary gonadotropins (eg, PCOS); a lower dose may be necessary. Blurring or other visual symptoms can occur; symptoms may increase with higher doses or duration of therapy; patients with visual disturbances should discontinue therapy and have an eye exam. Prolonged use may increase the risk of borderline or invasive ovarian cancer. Use caution in patients with uterine fibroids, may cause further enlargement. Multiple births may result from the use of these medications; advise patient of the potential risk of multiple births before starting the treatment. To minimize risks, use only at the lowest effective dose for the shortest duration of therapy (especially for the first course of therapy). Use should be supervised by physicians who are thoroughly familiar with infertility problems and their management.

Adverse Reactions

>10%: Endocrine & metabolic: Ovarian enlargement (14%)

1% to 10%:

Central nervous system: Headache (1%)

Endocrine & metabolic: Hot flashes (10%), breast discomfort (2%), abnormal uterine bleeding (1%)

Gastrointestinal: Distention/bloating/discomfort (6%), nausea (2%), vomiting (2%)

Ocular: Visual symptoms (2%, includes blurred vision, diplopia, floaters, lights, phosphenes, photophobia, scotomata, waves)

<1% (Limited to important or life-threatening): Abnormal accommodation, acne, allergic reaction, arrhythmia, chest pain, depression, dizziness, dyspnea, edema, endometriosis, erythema multiforme, erythema nodosum, eye pain, fatigue, fever, hepatitis, hypertension, hypertrichosis, leukocytosis, macular edema, migraine, mood changes, neoplasms, optic neuritis, ovarian cyst, ovarian hemorrhage, palpitation, PE, phlebitis, posterior vitreous detachment, pruritus, psychosis, retinal hemorrhage, retinal thrombosis, retinal vascular spasm, seizure, stroke, syncope, tachycardia, thrombophlebitis, thyroid disorder, tinnitus, transaminase increased, tubal pregnancy, uterine hemorrhage, vision loss (temporary/prolonged)

Drug Interactions

Metabolism/Transport Effects None known.

Avoid Concomitant Use

Avoid concomitant use of ClomiPHENE with any of the following: Ospemifene

Increased Effect/Toxicity

ClomiPHENE may increase the levels/effects of: Ospemifene

Decreased Effect

ClomiPHENE may decrease the levels/effects of: Ospemifene

Storage/Stability Store at room temperature of 15°C to 30°C (59°F to 86°F). Protect from light, heat, and excessive humidity.

Mechanism of Action Clomiphene is a racemic mixture consisting of zuclomiphene (~38%) and enclomiphene (~62%), each with distinct pharmacologic properties. Enclomiphene is much less potent in inducing ovulation; however, it is more rapidly absorbed and metabolized, allowing the more potent activity of zuclomiphene to predominate. Zuclomiphene acts at the level of the hypothalamus, occupying cell surface and intracellular estrogen receptors (ERs) for longer durations than estrogen. This interferes with receptor recycling, effectively depleting hypothalamic ERs and inhibiting normal estrogenic negative feedback. Impairment of the feedback signal results in increased pulsatile GnRH secretion from the hypothalamus and subsequent pituitary gonadotropin (FSH, LH) release, causing growth of the ovarian follicle, followed by follicular rupture.

Pharmacodynamics/Kinetics

Onset of action: Ovulation: 5-10 days following course of treatment

Duration: Effects are cumulative; ovulation may occur in the cycle following the last treatment

Absorption: Readily absorbed

Metabolism: Hepatic; undergoes enterohepatic recirculation

Half-life elimination: 5 days

Time to peak, plasma: ~6 hours

Excretion: Primarily feces; urine (small amounts)

Dosage Oral: Adults: Ovulation induction: Females: **Note:** Intercourse should be timed to coincide with the expected time of ovulation (usually 5-10 days after a clomiphene course).

Initial course: 50 mg once daily for 5 days. Begin on or about the fifth day of cycle if progestin-induced bleeding is scheduled or spontaneous uterine bleeding occurs prior to therapy. Therapy may be initiated at anytime in patients with no recent uterine bleeding.

Dose adjustment: Subsequent doses may be increased to 100 mg once daily for 5 days only if ovulation does not occur at the initial dose. Lower doses (12.5-25 mg daily) may be used in women sensitive to clomiphene or who consistently develop large ovarian cysts (ASRM, 2006).

Repeat courses: If needed, the 5-day cycle may be repeated as early as 30 days after the previous one. Exclude the presence of pregnancy. The lowest effective dose should be used (ASRM, 2006).

Maximum dose: 100 mg once daily for 5 days for up to 6 cycles. Discontinue if ovulation does not occur after 3 courses of treatment; or if 3 ovulatory responses occur but pregnancy is not achieved. Long-term therapy (>6 cycles) is not recommended. Re-evaluate if menses does not occur following ovulatory response. Doses have ranged from 50-250 mg daily, although doses >100 mg daily are not as successful (ASRM, 2006). The maximum recommended dose in women with PCOS is 150 mg daily (ASRM, 2008).

Dosage adjustment in renal impairment: No dosage adjustment provided in manufacturer's labeling.

Dosage adjustment in hepatic impairment: Use is contraindicated in patients with a history of liver disease or dysfunction.

Administration The total daily dose should be taken at one time to maximize effectiveness.

Monitoring Parameters Pelvic exam prior to each course of therapy; basal body temperature, serum progesterone, urinary luteinizing hormone; follicular growth and endometrial thickness may be useful in some cases; pregnancy test prior to repeat courses

Reference Range Serum progesterone: Ovulation generally occurs with levels ≥3 ng/mL; best results with levels >10 ng/mL

Test Interactions Clomiphene may increase levels of serum thyroxine and thyroxine-binding globulin (TBG)

Dosage Forms Excipient information presented when available (limited, particularly for generics); consult specific product labeling.

Tablet, Oral, as citrate:

Clomid: 50 mg [scored]

Serophene: 50 mg [scored]

Generic: 50 mg

◆ **Clomiphene Citrate** *see* ClomiPHENE *on page 461*

ClomiPRAMINE (kloe MI pra meen)

Brand Names: U.S. Anafranil

Brand Names: Canada Anafranil®; Apo-Clomipramine®; CO Clomipramine; Dom-Clomipramine; Novo-Clomipramine

Index Terms Clomipramine Hydrochloride

Pharmacologic Category Antidepressant, Tricyclic (Tertiary Amine)

Additional Appendix Information

Antidepressant Agents *on page 2284*

Beers Criteria – Potentially Inappropriate Medications for Geriatrics *on page 2368*

Use Treatment of obsessive-compulsive disorder (OCD)

Unlabeled Use Depression, panic attacks

Pregnancy Risk Factor C

Pregnancy Considerations Adverse events were observed in some animal reproduction studies. Clomipramine and its metabolite desmethylclomipramine cross the placenta and can be detected in cord blood and neonatal serum at birth (Loughhead, 2006; ter Horst, 2011). Data from five newborns found the half-life for clomipramine in the neonate to be 42 ± 16 hours following *in utero* exposure. Serum concentrations were not found to correlate to withdrawal symptoms (ter Horst, 2011). Withdrawal symptoms (including jitteriness, tremor, and seizures) have been observed in neonates whose mothers took clomipramine up to delivery.

The ACOG recommends that therapy for depression during pregnancy be individualized; treatment should incorporate the clinical expertise of the mental health clinician, obstetrician, primary healthcare provider, and pediatrician (ACOG, 2008). According to the American Psychiatric Association (APA), the risks of medication treatment should be weighed against other treatment options and untreated depression. For women who discontinue antidepressant medications during pregnancy and who may be at high risk for postpartum depression, the medications can be restarted following delivery (APA, 2010). Treatment algorithms have been developed by the ACOG and the APA for the management of depression in women prior to conception and during pregnancy (Yonkers, 2009).

Breast-Feeding Considerations Clomipramine is excreted in breast milk. Based on information from three mother-infant pairs, following maternal use of clomipramine 75-150 mg/day, the estimated exposure to the breast-feeding infant would be 0.4% to 4% of the weight-adjusted maternal dose. Adverse events have not been reported in nursing infants (information from seven cases). Infants should be monitored for signs of adverse events; routine monitoring of infant serum concentrations is not recommended (Fortinguerra, 2009). Due to the potential for serious adverse reactions in the nursing infant, the decision to continue or discontinue breast-feeding during therapy should take into account the risk of exposure to the infant and the benefits of treatment to the mother.

Medication Guide Available Yes

Contraindications Hypersensitivity to clomipramine, other tricyclic agents, or any component of the formulation; use of MAO inhibitors intended to treat psychiatric disorders (concurrently or within 14 days of discontinuing either clomipramine or the MAO inhibitor); initiation of clomipramine in a patient receiving linezolid or intravenous methylene blue; use in a patient during the acute recovery phase of MI

Warnings/Precautions [U.S. Boxed Warning]: Antidepressants increase the risk of suicidal thinking and behavior in children, adolescents, and young adults (18-24 years of age) with major depressive disorder (MDD) and other psychiatric disorders; consider risk prior to prescribing. Short-term studies did not show an increased risk in patients >24 years of age and showed a decreased risk in patients ≥65 years. Closely monitor for clinical worsening, suicidality, or unusual changes in behavior; the patient's family or caregiver should be instructed to closely observe the patient and communicate condition with healthcare provider. A medication guide should be dispensed with each prescription. **Clomipramine is FDA approved for the treatment of OCD in children ≥10 years of age.**

The possibility of a suicide attempt is inherent in major depression and may persist until remission occurs. Monitor for worsening of depression or suicidality, especially during initiation of therapy (generally first 1-2 months) or with dose increases or decreases. Use caution in high-risk patients. Worsening depression and severe abrupt suicidality that are not part of the presenting symptoms may require discontinuation or modification of drug therapy. The patient's family or caregiver should be alerted to monitor patients for the emergence of suicidality and associated behaviors (such as agitation, irritability, hostility, impulsivity, and hypomania) and notify the healthcare provider.

May worsen psychosis in some patients or precipitate a shift to mania or hypomania in patients with bipolar disorder. Patients presenting with depressive symptoms should be screened for bipolar disorder. Monotherapy in patients with bipolar disorder should be avoided. **Clomipramine is not FDA approved for bipolar depression.**

Potentially life-threatening serotonin syndrome (SS) has occurred with serotonergic agents (eg, SSRIs, SNRIs), particularly when used in combination with other serotonergic agents (eg, triptans, TCAs, fentanyl, lithium, tramadol, buspirone, St John's wort, tryptophan) or agents that impair metabolism of serotonin (eg, MAO inhibitors intended to treat psychiatric disorders, other MAO inhibitors [ie, linezolid and intravenous methylene blue]). Discontinue treatment (and any concomitant serotonergic agent) immediately if signs/symptoms arise. TCAs may rarely cause bone marrow suppression; monitor for any signs of infection and obtain CBC if symptoms (eg, fever, sore throat) evident. May cause seizures (relationship to dose and/or duration of therapy) - do not exceed maximum doses. Use caution in patients with a previous seizure disorder or condition predisposing to seizures such as brain damage, alcoholism, or concurrent therapy with other drugs which lower the seizure threshold. May increase the risks associated with electroconvulsive therapy. Bone fractures have been associated with antidepressant treatment. Consider the possibility of a fragility fracture if an antidepressant-treated patient presents with unexplained bone pain, point tenderness, swelling, or bruising (Rabenda, 2013; Rizzoli, 2012). Use with caution in patients with tumors of the adrenal medulla (eg, pheochromocytoma, neuroblastoma); may cause hypertensive crises. Has been associated with a high incidence of sexual dysfunction. Weight gain may occur.

The degree of sedation, anticholinergic effects, and conduction abnormalities are high relative to other antidepressants. Clomipramine often causes drowsiness/sedation, resulting in impaired performance of tasks requiring alertness (eg, operating machinery or driving). The risk of orthostasis is moderate to high relative to other antidepressants. Use with caution in patients with a history of cardiovascular disease (including previous MI, stroke, tachycardia, or conduction abnormalities). Use with caution in patients with urinary retention, benign prostatic hyperplasia, narrow-angle glaucoma, xerostomia, visual problems, constipation, or a history of bowel obstruction. Potentially significant drug-drug interactions may exist, requiring dose or frequency adjustment, additional monitoring, and/or selection of alternative therapy.

Recommended by the manufacturer to discontinue prior to elective surgery; risks exist for drug interactions with anesthesia and for cardiac arrhythmias. However, definitive drug interactions have not been widely reported in the literature and continuation of tricyclic antidepressants is generally recommended as long as precautions are taken to reduce the significance of any adverse events that may occur (Pass, 2004). Use with caution in hyperthyroid patients or those receiving thyroid supplementation. Use with caution in patients with hepatic impairment; increases in ALT/AST have occurred, including rare reports of severe hepatic injury (some fatal); monitor hepatic transaminases periodically in patients with hepatic impairment. Use with caution in patients with renal dysfunction. Avoid use in the elderly due to its potent anticholinergic and sedative properties, and potential to cause orthostatic hypotension. In addition, may also cause or exacerbate syndrome of inappropriate antidiuretic hormone secretion or hyponatremia; monitor sodium closely with initiation or dosage adjustments in older adults (Beers Criteria).

Abrupt discontinuation or interruption of antidepressant therapy has been associated with a discontinuation syndrome. Symptoms arising may vary with antidepressant however commonly include nausea, vomiting, diarrhea, headaches, light-headedness, dizziness, diminished appetite, sweating, chills, tremors, paresthesias, fatigue, somnolence, and sleep disturbances (eg, vivid dreams, insomnia). Greater risks for developing a discontinuation syndrome have been associated with antidepressants with shorter half-lives, longer durations of treatment, and abrupt discontinuation. For antidepressants of short or intermediate half-lives, symptoms may emerge within 2-5 days after treatment discontinuation and last 7-14 days (APA, 2010; Fava, 2006; Haddad, 2001; Shelton, 2001; Warner, 2006).

Adverse Reactions Data shown for children reflects both children and adolescents studied in clinical trials.

>10%:

Cardiovascular: Orthostatic hypotension (4% to 20%), tachycardia (2% to 20%)

Central nervous system: Somnolence (46% to 54%), dizziness (adults 54%; children 41%), headache (adults 52%; children 28%), fatigue (35% to 39%), insomnia (adults 25%; children 11%), nervousness (adults 18%; children 4%)

Endocrine & metabolic: Libido changes (adults 21%)

Gastrointestinal: Xerostomia (adults 84%, children 63%), constipation (adults 47%; children 22%), nausea (adults 33%; children 9%), dyspepsia (13% to 22%), anorexia (12% to 22%), weight gain (adults 18%; children 2%), diarrhea (7% to 13%), abdominal pain (11%), appetite increased (11%)

Genitourinary: Ejaculation failure (adults 42%, children 6%), impotence (adults 20%), micturition disorder (adults 14%; children 4%)

Neuromuscular & skeletal: Tremor (adults 54%; children 33%), myoclonus (adults 13%; children 2%), myalgia (adults 13%)

Ophthalmic: Abnormal vision (adults 18%; children 7%)

Respiratory: Pharyngitis (adults 14%), rhinitis (adults 12%)

Miscellaneous: Diaphoresis increased (adults 29%; children 9%)

1% to 10%:

Cardiovascular: Flushing (7% to 8%), chest pain (children 7%), palpitation (4%), ECG abnormality (2%), syncope (children 2%)

Central nervous system: Anxiety (adults 9%; children 2%), memory impairment (7% to 9%), sleep disorder (4% to 9%), twitching (adults 7%), concentration impaired (adults 5%), depression (adults 5%), fever (adults 4%), pain (3% to 4%), hypertonia (2% to 4%), abnormal dreaming (adults 3%), agitation (adults 3%), migraine (adults 3%), psychosomatic disorder (adults 3%), speech disorder (adults 3%), yawning (adults 3%), aggressiveness (children 2%), chills (adults 2%), depersonalization (2%), emotional lability (adults 2%), irritability (children 2%), myasthenia (1% to 2%), panic reaction (1% to 2%), abnormal thinking, vertigo

Dermatologic: Rash (4% to 8%), pruritus (adults 6%), purpura (adults 3%), body odor (children 2%), dermatitis (adults 2%), dry skin (adults 2%), urticaria (adults 1%)

Endocrine & metabolic: Hot flashes (2% to 5%), lactation (nonpuerperal; adults 4%), menstrual disorder (adults 4%), breast enlargement (adults 2%), amenorrhea (adults 1%), breast pain (adults 1%)

Gastrointestinal: Taste disturbance (4% to 8%), vomiting (7%), weight loss (children 7%), flatulence (adults 6%), tooth disorder (adults 5%), dysphagia (adults 2%), gastrointestinal disturbance (adults 2%), halitosis (children 2%), ulcerative stomatitis (children 2%), esophagitis (adults 1%)

Genitourinary: Urinary retention (children 7%; adults 2%), UTI (adults 6%), micturition frequency (adults 5%), cystitis (adults 2%), leukorrhea (adults 2%), vaginitis (adults 2%)

Hepatic: Increased serum ALT (>3 x ULN: 3%), increased serum AST (>3 x ULN: 1%)

Hypersensitivity: Hypersensitivity reaction (children 7%)

Neuromuscular & skeletal: Paresthesia (adults 9%; children 2%), paresis (children 2%), weakness (children 1%)

Ophthalmic: Lacrimation abnormal (adults 3%), anisocoria (children 2%), blepharospasm (children 2%), mydriasis (adults 2%), ocular allergy (children 2%), conjunctivitis (adults 1%)

Otic: Tinnitus (4% to 6%)

Respiratory: Bronchospasm (children 7%; adults 2%), sinusitis (adults 6%), dyspnea (children 2%), epistaxis (adults 2%), laryngitis (children 2%)

<1% (Limited to important or life-threatening): Accommodation abnormal, agranulocytosis, albuminuria, alopecia, anemia, aneurysm, anticholinergic syndrome, apathy, aphasia, apraxia, arrhythmia, ataxia, atrial flutter, blepharitis, blood in stool, bradycardia, breast fibroadenosis, bronchitis, bundle branch block, cardiac arrest, cardiac failure, catalepsy, cellulitis, cerebral hemorrhage, cervical dysplasia, cheilitis, chloasma, cholinergic syndrome, choreoathetosis, chromatopsia, chronic enteritis, colitis, coma, conjunctival hemorrhage, cyanosis, deafness, dehydration, delirium, delusion, diabetes mellitus, diplopia, duodenitis, dyskinesia, dysphonia, dystonia, eczema, edema, EEG abnormal, encephalopathy, endometrial hyperplasia, endometriosis, epididymitis, erythematous rash, exophthalmos, exostosis, extrapyramidal disorder, extrasystoles, gastric dilatation, gastric ulcer, gastroesophageal reflux disease, generalized spasm, glaucoma, glycosuria, goiter, gout, gynecomastia, hallucinations, heart block, hematuria, hemiparesis, hemoptysis, hepatitis, hostility, hyperacusis, hypercholesterolemia, hyper-/hypoesthesia, hyperglycemia, hyper-/hypokinesia, hyper-reflexia, hyperthermia, hyper-/hypothyroidism, hyperuricemia, hyper-/hypoventilation, hypnagogic hallucination, hypokalemia, ideation, intestinal obstruction, irritable bowel syndrome, keratitis, laryngismus, leukemoid reaction, leukopenia, liver injury (severe), lupus erythematosus rash, lymphadenopathy, lymphoma-like disorder, maculopapular rash, manic reaction, marrow depression, mutism, myocardial infarction, myocardial ischemia, myopathy, myositis, neuralgia, neuropathy, night blindness, oculogyric crisis, oculomotor nerve paralysis, oral/pharyngeal edema, ovarian cyst, pancytopenia, paralytic ileus, paranoia, parosmia, peptic ulcer, peripheral ischemia, phobic disorder, photophobia, photosensitivity reaction, pneumonia, polyarteritis nodosa, premature ejaculation, psoriasis, psychosis, pyelonephritis, pyuria, rectal hemorrhage, renal calculus, renal cyst, salivary gland enlargement, schizophrenic reaction, scleritis, seizure, sensory disturbance, serotonin syndrome, skin hypertrophy, skin ulceration, somnambulism, strabismus, stupor, suicidal ideation, suicide, suicide attempt, thrombocytopenia, thrombophlebitis, tongue ulceration, torticollis, urinary incontinence, uterine hemorrhage, uterine inflammation, vaginal hemorrhage, vasospasm, ventricular tachycardia, visual field defect, withdrawal syndrome

Drug Interactions

Metabolism/Transport Effects Substrate of CYP1A2 (major), CYP2C19 (major), CYP2D6 (major), CYP3A4 (minor); **Note:** Assignment of Major/Minor substrate status based on clinically relevant drug interaction potential; **Inhibits** CYP2D6 (moderate)

Avoid Concomitant Use

Avoid concomitant use of ClomiPRAMINE with any of the following: Aclidinium; Iobenguane I 123; Ipratropium (Oral Inhalation); Linezolid; MAO Inhibitors; Methylene Blue; Moxonidine; Thioridazine; Tiotropium; Umeclidinium

Increased Effect/Toxicity

ClomiPRAMINE may increase the levels/effects of: Alpha-/Beta-Agonists (Direct-Acting); Alpha1-Agonists; Amphetamines; Analgesics (Opioid); Anticholinergics; Antipsychotics; Aspirin; Beta2-Agonists; Citalopram; CYP2D6 Substrates; Desmopressin; Escitalopram; Fesoterodine; Highest Risk QTc-Prolonging Agents; Methylene Blue; Metoclopramide; Metoprolol; Milnacipran; Moderate Risk QTc-Prolonging Agents; Nebivolol; NSAID (COX-2 Inhibitor); NSAID (Nonselective); QuiNIDine; Serotonin Modulators; Sodium Phosphates; Sulfonylureas; Thioridazine; Tiotropium; TraMADol; Vitamin K Antagonists; Yohimbine

The levels/effects of ClomiPRAMINE may be increased by: Abiraterone Acetate; Aclidinium; Altretamine; Antipsychotics; BuPROPion; CarBAMazepine; Cimetidine; Cinacalcet; Citalopram; Cobicistat; CYP1A2 Inhibitors (Moderate); CYP1A2 Inhibitors (Strong); CYP2C19 Inhibitors (Moderate); CYP2C19 Inhibitors (Strong); CYP2D6 Inhibitors (Moderate); CYP2D6 Inhibitors (Strong); Deferasirox; Dexmethylphenidate; DULoxetine; Escitalopram; FLUoxetine; FluvoxaMINE; Grapefruit Juice; Ipratropium (Oral Inhalation); Linezolid; Lithium; Luliconazole; MAO Inhibitors; Methylphenidate; Metoclopramide; Metyrosine; Mifepristone; PARoxetine; Pramlintide; Propafenone; Protease Inhibitors; QuiNIDine; Sertraline; Terbinafine (Systemic); Thyroid Products; TraMADol; Umeclidinium; Valproic Acid and Derivatives; Vemurafenib

Decreased Effect

ClomiPRAMINE may decrease the levels/effects of: Acetylcholinesterase Inhibitors (Central); Alpha2-Agonists; Alpha2-Agonists (Ophthalmic); Codeine; Iobenguane I 123; Moxonidine; Tamoxifen

The levels/effects of ClomiPRAMINE may be decreased by: Acetylcholinesterase Inhibitors (Central); Barbiturates; CYP1A2 Inducers (Strong); CYP2C19 Inducers (Strong); Cyproterone; Dabrafenib; Peginterferon Alfa-2b; St Johns Wort

Ethanol/Nutrition/Herb Interactions

Ethanol: Ethanol may increase CNS depression. Management: Avoid ethanol.

Food: Serum concentrations/toxicity may be increased by grapefruit juice. Management: Avoid grapefruit juice.

Herb/Nutraceutical: St John's wort and tryptophan may increase the serotonergic effect of clomipramine, thus increasing the risk of serotonin syndrome. Clomipramine may increase the serum concentration of yohimbe. Management: Avoid valerian, St John's wort, tryptophan, SAMe, kava kava, and yohimbe.

Mechanism of Action Clomipramine appears to affect serotonin uptake while its active metabolite, desmethylclomipramine, affects norepinephrine uptake

Pharmacodynamics/Kinetics

Absorption: Rapid

Protein binding: 97%, primarily to albumin

Metabolism: Hepatic to desmethylclomipramine (DMI; active); extensive first-pass effect

Half-life elimination: Clomipramine: Mean 32 hours (range: 19-37 hours); DMI: Mean 69 hours (range: 54-77 hours)

Time to peak, plasma: 2-6 hours

Excretion: Urine and feces

Dosage

Obsessive-compulsive disorder (OCD), treatment:

Children ≥10 years and Adolescents: Oral:

Initial: 25 mg daily; gradually increase as tolerated over the first 2 weeks to 3 mg/kg/day or 100 mg daily (whichever is less) in divided doses

Maintenance: May further increase over next several weeks up to maximum of 3 mg/kg/day or 200 mg daily (whichever is less); after titration, may give as a single once daily dose at bedtime

Adults: Oral:

Initial: 25 mg daily; may gradually increase as tolerated over the first 2 weeks to ~100 mg daily in divided doses

Maintenance: May further increase over next several weeks up to a maximum of 250 mg daily; after titration, may give as a single once daily dose at bedtime

Panic attacks (unlabeled use): Adults: Oral: Initial: 10-25 mg daily; titrate gradually (usually weekly) to an effective dose (usual dosage range: 50-150 mg daily); in some studies dose was titrated up to a maximum dose of 200-250 mg daily, if needed (Bakker, 1999; Cassano, 1988; McTavish, 1990; Modigh 1992; Stein, 2010)

Discontinuation of therapy: Upon discontinuation of antidepressant therapy, gradually taper the dose to minimize the incidence of withdrawal symptoms and allow for the detection of re-emerging symptoms. Evidence supporting ideal taper rates is limited. APA and NICE guidelines suggest tapering therapy over at least several weeks with consideration to the half-life of the antidepressant; antidepressants with a shorter half-life may need to be tapered more conservatively. In addition for long-term treated patients, WFSBP guidelines recommend tapering over 4-6 months. If intolerable withdrawal symptoms occur following a dose reduction, consider resuming the previously prescribed dose and/or decrease dose at a more gradual rate (APA, 2007; APA, 2010; Bauer, 2002; Haddad, 2001; NCCMH, 2010; Schatzberg, 2006; Shelton, 2001; Warner, 2006).

MAO inhibitor recommendations:

Switching to or from an MAO inhibitor intended to treat psychiatric disorders:

Allow 14 days to elapse between discontinuing an MAO inhibitor intended to treat psychiatric disorders and initiation of clomipramine.

Allow 14 days to elapse between discontinuing clomipramine and initiation of an MAO inhibitor intended to treat psychiatric disorders.

Use with other MAO inhibitors (linezolid or I.V. methylene blue):

Do not initiate clomipramine in patients receiving linezolid or I.V. methylene blue; consider other interventions for psychiatric condition.

If urgent treatment with linezolid or I.V. methylene blue is required in a patient already receiving clomipramine and potential benefits outweigh potential risks, discontinue clomipramine promptly and administer linezolid or I.V. methylene blue. Monitor for serotonin syndrome for 2 weeks or until 24 hours after the last dose of linezolid or I.V. methylene blue, whichever comes first. May resume clomipramine 24 hours after the last dose of linezolid or I.V. methylene blue.

Dosage adjustment in renal impairment: No dosage adjustment provided in manufacturer's labeling (has not been studied). Use with caution in patients with significantly impaired renal function.

Dosage adjustment in hepatic impairment: No dosage adjustment provided in manufacturer's labeling (has not been studied). Use with caution in patients with hepatic impairment.

Administration During titration, may divide doses and administer with meals to decrease gastrointestinal side effects. After titration, may administer total daily dose at bedtime to decrease daytime sedation.

Monitoring Parameters Pulse rate and blood pressure prior to and during therapy; ECG/cardiac status in older adults and patients with cardiac disease; suicidal ideation (especially at the beginning of therapy, after initiation, or when doses are increased or decreased); signs/symptoms of serotonin syndrome; hepatic transaminases (periodically during therapy in patients with pre-existing hepatic impairment)

Test Interactions Increased glucose; may interfere with urine detection of methadone (false-positive)

Dosage Forms Excipient information presented when available (limited, particularly for generics); consult specific product labeling.

Capsule, Oral, as hydrochloride:

Anafranil: 25 mg, 50 mg, 75 mg

Generic: 25 mg, 50 mg, 75 mg

◆ **Clomipramine Hydrochloride** *see* ClomiPRAMINE *on page 462*

◆ **Clonapam (Can)** *see* ClonazePAM *on page 465*

ClonazePAM (kloe NA ze pam)

Brand Names: U.S. KlonoPIN

Brand Names: Canada Apo-Clonazepam; Clonapam; Clonazepam-R; CO Clonazepam; Dom-Clonazepam; Dom-Clonazepam-R; Mylan-Clonazepam; PHL-Clonazepam; PHL-Clonazepam-R; PMS-Clonazepam; PMS-Clonazepam-R; PRO-Clonazepam; ratio-Clonazepam; Riva-Clonazepam; Rivotril; Sandoz-Clonazepam; Teva-Clonazepam; ZYM-Clonazepam

Pharmacologic Category Benzodiazepine

Additional Appendix Information

Beers Criteria – Potentially Inappropriate Medications for Geriatrics *on page 2368*

Benzodiazepine Comparison Table *on page 2292*

Use Alone or as an adjunct in the treatment of petit mal variant (Lennox-Gastaut), akinetic, and myoclonic seizures; petit mal (absence) seizures unresponsive to succimides; panic disorder with or without agoraphobia

Unlabeled Use Restless legs syndrome; neuralgia; multifocal tic disorder; parkinsonian dysarthria; bipolar disorder; adjunct therapy for schizophrenia; burning mouth syndrome; essential tremor

Pregnancy Risk Factor D

Pregnancy Considerations Adverse events were observed in some animal reproduction studies. Clonazepam crosses the placenta. Teratogenic effects have been observed with some benzodiazepines; however, additional studies are needed. The incidence of premature birth and low birth weights may be increased following maternal use of benzodiazepines; hypoglycemia and respiratory problems in the neonate may occur following exposure late in pregnancy. Neonatal withdrawal symptoms may occur within days to weeks after birth and "floppy infant syndrome" (which also includes withdrawal symptoms) has been reported with some benzodiazepines, including clonazepam (Bergman, 1992; Iqbal, 2002; Wikner, 2007). A combination of factors influences the potential teratogenicity of anticonvulsant therapy. When treating women with epilepsy, monotherapy with the lowest effective dose and avoidance medications known to have a high incidence of teratogenic effects is recommended (Harden, 2009; Wlodarczyk, 2012).

Patients exposed to clonazepam during pregnancy are encouraged to enroll themselves into the AED Pregnancy Registry by calling 1-888-233-2334. Additional information is available at www.aedpregnancyregistry.org.

Breast-Feeding Considerations Clonazepam enters breast milk. Drowsiness, lethargy, or weight loss in nursing infants have been observed in case reports following maternal use of some benzodiazepines (Iqbal, 2002). The manufacturer states that women taking clonazepam should not breast-feed their infants.

Medication Guide Available Yes

Contraindications Hypersensitivity to clonazepam or any component of the formulation (cross-sensitivity with other benzodiazepines may exist); significant liver disease; acute narrow-angle glaucoma

Warnings/Precautions Hazardous agent - use appropriate precautions for handling and disposal (NIOSH, 2012). Antiepileptics are associated with an increased risk of suicidal behavior/thoughts with use (regardless of indication); patients should be monitored for signs/symptoms of depression, suicidal tendencies, and other unusual behavior changes during therapy and instructed to inform their healthcare provider immediately if symptoms occur.

Use with caution in elderly or debilitated patients, patients with hepatic disease (including alcoholics), or renal impairment. Use with caution in patients with respiratory disease or impaired gag reflex or ability to protect the airway from secretions (salivation may be increased). Worsening of seizures may occur when added to patients with multiple seizure types. Concurrent use with valproic acid may result in absence status. Monitoring of CBC and liver function tests has been recommended during prolonged therapy.

Causes CNS depression (dose related) resulting in sedation, dizziness, confusion, or ataxia which may impair physical and mental capabilities. Patients must be cautioned about performing tasks which require mental alertness (eg, operating machinery or driving). Use with caution in patients receiving other CNS depressants or psychoactive agents. Effects with other sedative drugs or ethanol may be potentiated. Benzodiazepines have been associated with falls and traumatic injury and should be used with extreme caution in patients who are at risk of these events.

Use caution in patients with depression, particularly if suicidal risk may be present. Use with caution in patients with a history of drug dependence. Benzodiazepines have been associated with dependence and acute withdrawal symptoms, including seizures, on discontinuation or reduction in dose. Acute withdrawal, including seizures, may be precipitated in patients after administration of flumazenil to patients receiving long-term benzodiazepine therapy.

Benzodiazepines have been associated with anterograde amnesia. Paradoxical reactions, including hyperactive or aggressive behavior, have been reported with benzodiazepines, particularly in adolescent/pediatric or psychiatric patients. Does not have analgesic, antidepressant, or antipsychotic properties.

In older adults, benzodiazepines increase the risk of impaired cognition, delirium, falls, fractures, and motor vehicle accidents. Due to increased sensitivity in this age group and slower metabolism of long-acting agents (such as clonazepam), avoid use for treatment of insomnia, agitation, or delirium (Beers Criteria).

Adverse Reactions Reactions reported in patients with seizure and/or panic disorder. Frequency not always defined.

Cardiovascular: Edema (ankle or facial), palpitation

Central nervous system: Amnesia, ataxia (seizure disorder ~30%; panic disorder 5%), behavior problems (seizure disorder ~25%), coma, confusion, coordination impaired, depression, dizziness, drowsiness (seizure disorder ~50%), emotional lability, fatigue, fever, hallucinations, headache, hysteria, insomnia, intellectual ability reduced, memory disturbance, nervousness; paradoxical reactions (including aggressive behavior, agitation, anxiety, excitability, hostility, irritability, nervousness, nightmares, sleep disturbance, vivid dreams); psychosis, slurred speech, somnolence (panic disorder 37%), vertigo

Dermatologic: Hair loss, hirsutism, skin rash

Endocrine & metabolic: Dysmenorrhea, libido increased/decreased

Gastrointestinal: Abdominal pain, anorexia, appetite increased/decreased, coated tongue, constipation, dehydration, diarrhea, encopresis, gastritis, gum soreness, nausea, weight changes (loss/gain), xerostomia

Genitourinary: Colpitis, dysuria, ejaculation delayed, enuresis, impotence, micturition frequency, nocturia, urinary retention, urinary tract infection

Hematologic: Anemia, eosinophilia, leukopenia, thrombocytopenia

Hepatic: Alkaline phosphatase increased (transient), hepatomegaly, transaminases increased (transient)

Neuromuscular & skeletal: Choreiform movements, coordination abnormal, dysarthria, hypotonia, muscle pain, muscle weakness, myalgia, tremor

Ocular: Blurred vision, eye movements abnormal, diplopia, nystagmus

Respiratory: Bronchitis, chest congestion, cough, hypersecretions, pharyngitis, respiratory depression, respiratory tract infection, rhinitis, rhinorrhea, shortness of breath, sinusitis

Miscellaneous: Allergic reaction, aphonia, dysdiadochokinesis, "glassy-eyed" appearance, hemiparesis, flu-like syndrome, lymphadenopathy

<1% (Limited to important or life-threatening): Apathy, burning skin, chest pain, depersonalization, dyspnea, excessive dreaming, hyperactivity, hypoesthesia, hypotension postural, infection, migraine, organic disinhibition, pain, paresthesia, paresis, periorbital edema, polyuria, suicidal attempt, suicide ideation, thick tongue, twitching, visual disturbance, xerophthalmia

Drug Interactions

Metabolism/Transport Effects Substrate of CYP3A4 (major); **Note:** Assignment of Major/Minor substrate status based on clinically relevant drug interaction potential

Avoid Concomitant Use

Avoid concomitant use of ClonazePAM with any of the following: Azelastine (Nasal); Conivaptan; Fusidic Acid (Systemic); OLANZapine; Paraldehyde; Sodium Oxybate

Increased Effect/Toxicity

ClonazePAM may increase the levels/effects of: Alcohol (Ethyl); Azelastine (Nasal); Buprenorphine; CloZAPine; CNS Depressants; Fosphenytoin; Hydrocodone; Methotrimeprazine; Metyrosine; Mirtazapine; Paraldehyde; Phenytoin; Pramipexole; ROPINIRole; Rotigotine; Selective Serotonin Reuptake Inhibitors; Sodium Oxybate; Zolpidem

The levels/effects of ClonazePAM may be increased by: Antifungal Agents (Azole Derivatives, Systemic); Aprepitant; Brimonidine (Topical); Calcium Channel Blockers (Nondihydropyridine); Cimetidine; Cobicistat; Conivaptan; Contraceptives (Estrogens); Contraceptives (Progestins); Cosyntropin; CYP3A4 Inhibitors (Moderate); CYP3A4 Inhibitors (Strong); Dasatinib; Doxylamine; Droperidol; Fosaprepitant; Fusidic Acid (Systemic);

Grapefruit Juice; HydrOXYzine; Isoniazid; Ivacaftor; Luliconazole; Magnesium Sulfate; Methotrimeprazine; Mifepristone; OLANZapine; Perampanel; Proton Pump Inhibitors; Selective Serotonin Reuptake Inhibitors; Simeprevir; Tapentadol; Vigabatrin

Decreased Effect

The levels/effects of ClonazePAM may be decreased by: Bosentan; CarBAMazepine; CYP3A4 Inducers (Strong); Dabrafenib; Deferasirox; Herbs (CYP3A4 Inducers); Mitotane; Rifamycin Derivatives; Theophylline Derivatives; Tocilizumab; Yohimbine

Ethanol/Nutrition/Herb Interactions

Ethanol: May increase CNS depression; monitor for increased effects with coadministration. Caution patients about effects.

Food: Clonazepam serum concentration is unlikely to be increased by grapefruit juice because of clonazepam's high oral bioavailability.

Herb/Nutraceutical: St John's wort may decrease clonazepam levels. Avoid valerian, St John's wort, kava kava, gotu kola (may increase CNS depression).

Storage/Stability Store at 25°C (77°F); excursions permitted to 15°C to 30°C (59°F to 80°F)

Mechanism of Action The exact mechanism is unknown, but believed to be related to its ability to enhance the activity of GABA; suppresses the spike-and-wave discharge in absence seizures by depressing nerve transmission in the motor cortex

Pharmacodynamics/Kinetics

Onset of action: ~20-40 minutes (Hanson, 1972)

Duration: Infants and young children: 6-8 hours (Hanson, 1972); Adults: ≤12 hours (Hanson, 1972)

Absorption: Rapidly and completely absorbed

Distribution: Children: V_d: 1.5-3 L/kg (Walson, 1996); Adults: V_d: 1.5-64.4 L/kg (Walson, 1996)

Protein binding: ~85%

Metabolism: Extensively hepatic via glucuronide and sulfate conjugation

Bioavailability: 90%

Half-life elimination: Children: 22-33 hours (Walson, 1996); Adults: 17-60 hours (Walson, 1996)

Time to peak, serum: 1-4 hours

Excretion: Urine (<2% as unchanged drug); metabolites excreted as glucuronide or sulfate conjugates

Dosage

Children <10 years or <30 kg: Seizure disorders: Oral:

Initial daily dose: 0.01-0.03 mg/kg/day (maximum: 0.05 mg/kg/day) given in 2-3 divided doses; increase by no more than 0.25-0.5 mg every third day until seizures are controlled or adverse effects seen

Usual maintenance dose: 0.1-0.2 mg/kg/day divided 3 times daily, not to exceed 0.2 mg/kg/day

Children >10 years or ≥30 kg, Adolescents, and Adults:

Seizure disorders: Oral:

Initial daily dose not to exceed 1.5 mg given in 3 divided doses; may increase by 0.5-1 mg every third day until seizures are controlled or adverse effects seen (maximum: 20 mg daily)

Usual maintenance dose: 2-8 mg daily in 1-2 divided doses (Brodie, 1997); do not exceed 20 mg daily

Adults:

Panic disorder: Oral: 0.25 mg twice daily; increase in increments of 0.125-0.25 mg twice daily every 3 days; target dose: 1 mg daily (maximum: 4 mg daily)

Discontinuation of treatment: To discontinue, treatment should be withdrawn gradually. Decrease dose by 0.125 mg twice daily every 3 days until medication is completely withdrawn.

Burning mouth syndrome (unlabeled use):

Oral: Initial: 0.25 at bedtime for 1 week; increase dose by ≤0.25 mg every week; maximum dose: 3 mg daily in 3 divided doses. **Note:** Use should be limited (Buchanan, 2008; Grushka, 1998).

Topical: May administer topically with 1 mg 3 times daily (after each meal). **Note:** Patient should be instructed to suck on the tablet, retain saliva in mouth near the pain sites without swallowing for 3 minutes, and then expectorate saliva (Gremeau-Richard, 2004).

Essential tremor (unlabeled use): Oral: Initial: 0.5 mg at bedtime; increase dose by 0.5 mg every 3-4 days; maximum dose: 6 mg daily (Biary, 1987; Thompson, 1984; Zesiewicz, 2005; Zesiewicz, 2011).

REM sleep behavior disorder (unlabeled use): 0.25-2 mg 30 minutes prior to bedtime (maximum: 4 mg 30 minutes prior to bedtime). **Note:** Use with caution in patients with dementia, gait disorders, or obstructive sleep apnea (Aurora, 2010).

Elderly: Initiate with low doses and observe closely

Dosage adjustment in renal impairment: No dosage adjustment provided in manufacturer's labeling; use with caution. Clonazepam metabolites may accumulate in patients with renal impairment.

Dosage adjustment in hepatic impairment: No dosage adjustment provided in manufacturer's labeling; use with caution.

Administration

Orally-disintegrating tablet: Open pouch and peel back foil on the blister; do not push tablet through foil. Use dry hands to remove tablet and place in mouth. May be swallowed with or without water. Use immediately after removing from package.

Tablet: Swallow whole with water.

Hazardous agent; use appropriate precautions for handling and disposal (NIOSH, 2012).

Monitoring Parameters CBC, liver and renal function tests; observe patient for excess sedation, respiratory depression; suicidality (eg, suicidal thoughts, depression, behavioral changes)

Reference Range Relationship between serum concentration and seizure control is not well established

Timing of serum samples: Peak serum levels occur 1-3 hours after oral ingestion; the half-life is 20-40 hours; therefore, steady-state occurs in 5-7 days

Therapeutic levels: 20-80 ng/mL; Toxic concentration: >80 ng/mL

Additional Information Ethosuximide or valproic acid may be preferred for treatment of absence (petit mal) seizures. Clonazepam-induced behavioral disturbances may be more frequent in mentally handicapped patients. Abrupt discontinuation after sustained use (generally >10 days) may cause withdrawal symptoms. Flumazenil, a competitive benzodiazepine antagonist at the CNS receptor site, reverses benzodiazepine-induced CNS depression.

Dosage Forms Excipient information presented when available (limited, particularly for generics); consult specific product labeling.

Tablet, Oral:

KlonoPIN: 0.5 mg [scored]

KlonoPIN: 1 mg, 2 mg

Generic: 0.5 mg, 1 mg, 2 mg

Tablet Dispersible, Oral:

Generic: 0.125 mg, 0.25 mg, 0.5 mg, 1 mg, 2 mg

Controlled Substance C-IV

Extemporaneous Preparations Hazardous agent: Use appropriate precautions for handling and disposal.

A 0.1 mg/mL oral suspension may be made with tablets and one of three different vehicles (cherry syrup; a 1:1 mixture of Ora-Sweet® and Ora-Plus®; or a 1:1 mixture of Ora-Sweet® SF and Ora-Plus®). Crush six 2 mg tablets in a mortar and reduce to a fine powder. Add 10 mL of the chosen vehicle and mix to a uniform paste; mix while adding the vehicle in incremental proportions to **almost** 120 mL; transfer to a calibrated bottle, rinse mortar with vehicle, and add quantity of vehicle sufficient to make 120 mL. Label "shake well" and "protect from light". Stable for 60 days when stored in amber prescription bottles in the dark at room temperature or refrigerated.

Allen LV Jr and Erickson MA 3rd, "Stability of Acetazolamide, Allopurinol, Azathioprine, Clonazepam, and Flucytosine in Extemporaneously Compounded Oral Liquids," Am *J Health Syst Pharm*, 1996, 53(16):1944-9.

◆ Clonazepam-R (Can) *see* ClonazePAM *on page 465*

CloNIDine (KLON i deen)

Brand Names: U.S. Catapres; Catapres-TTS-1; Catapres-TTS-2; Catapres-TTS-3; Duraclon; Kapvay

Brand Names: Canada Apo-Clonidine®; Catapres®; Dixarit®; Dom-Clonidine; Novo-Clonidine

Index Terms Clonidine Hydrochloride

Pharmacologic Category Alpha$_2$-Adrenergic Agonist; Antihypertensive

Additional Appendix Information

Beers Criteria – Potentially Inappropriate Medications for Geriatrics *on page 2368*

Use

Oral:

Immediate release: Management of hypertension (monotherapy or as adjunctive therapy)

Extended release (Kapvay™): Treatment of attention-deficit/hyperactivity disorder (ADHD) (monotherapy or as adjunctive therapy)

Epidural (Duraclon®): For continuous epidural administration as adjunctive therapy with opioids for treatment of severe cancer pain in patients tolerant to or unresponsive to opioids alone; epidural clonidine is generally more effective for neuropathic pain and less effective (or possibly ineffective) for somatic or visceral pain

Transdermal patch: Management of hypertension (monotherapy or as adjunctive therapy)

Unlabeled Use Heroin or nicotine withdrawal; severe pain; dysmenorrhea; vasomotor symptoms associated with menopause; ethanol dependence; prophylaxis of migraines; glaucoma; diabetes-associated diarrhea; impulse control disorder, clozapine-induced sialorrhea; aid in the diagnosis of growth hormone deficiency; attention-deficit/hyperactivity disorder (ADHD) and associated insomnia in children; Tourette's syndrome in children; aggression associated with conduct disorder

Pregnancy Risk Factor C

Pregnancy Considerations Adverse events have been observed in some animal reproduction studies. Clonidine crosses the placenta; concentrations in the umbilical cord plasma are similar to those in the maternal serum and concentrations in the amniotic fluid may be 4 times those in the maternal serum. The pharmacokinetics of clonidine may be altered during pregnancy (Buchanan, 2009). Untreated chronic maternal hypertension is associated with adverse events in the fetus, infant, and mother. If treatment for hypertension during pregnancy is needed, other agents are preferred (ACOG, 2012; Chobanian, 2003). **[U.S. Boxed Warning]: Epidural clonidine is not recommended for obstetrical or postpartum pain** due to risk of hemodynamic instability.

Breast-Feeding Considerations Clonidine is excreted in breast milk. Concentrations have been noted as ~7% to 8% of those in the maternal plasma following oral dosing (Atkinson, 1988; Bunjes, 1993) and twice those in the maternal serum following epidural administration. The manufacturer recommends caution be used if administered to nursing women. Another source recommends avoiding use when nursing infants born <34 weeks gestation or when large maternal doses are needed (Atkinson, 1988). Breast-fed infants of mothers taking medications for hypertension should be monitored for adverse effects (Chobanian, 2003).

Contraindications Hypersensitivity to clonidine hydrochloride or any component of the formulation

Epidural administration: Injection site infection; concurrent anticoagulant therapy; bleeding diathesis; administration above the C4 dermatome

Warnings/Precautions May cause CNS depression, which may impair physical or mental abilities; patients must be cautioned about performing tasks which require mental alertness (eg, operating machinery or driving). Sedating effects may be potentiated when used with other CNS-depressant drugs or ethanol. Use with caution in patients with severe coronary insufficiency; conduction disturbances; recent MI, CVA, or chronic renal insufficiency. May cause dose dependent reductions in heart rate; use with caution in patients with pre-existing bradycardia or those predisposed to developing bradycardia. Caution in sinus node dysfunction. Use with caution in patients concurrently receiving agents known to reduce SA node function and/or AV nodal conduction (eg, digoxin, diltiazem, metoprolol, verapamil). May cause significant xerostomia. Clonidine may cause eye dryness in patients who wear contact lenses.

[U.S. Boxed Warning]: Must dilute concentrated epidural injectable (500 mcg/mL) solution prior to use. Epidural clonidine is not recommended for perioperative, obstetrical, or postpartum pain due to risk of hemodynamic instability. Clonidine injection should be administered via a continuous epidural infusion device. Monitor closely for catheter-related infection such as meningitis or epidural abscess. Epidural clonidine is not recommended for use in patients with severe cardiovascular disease or hemodynamic instability; may lead to cardiovascular instability (hypotension, bradycardia). Symptomatic hypotension may occur with use; in all patients, use epidural clonidine with caution due to the potential for severe hypotension especially in women and those of low body weight. Most hypotensive episodes occur within the first 4 days of initiation; however, episodes may occur throughout the duration of therapy.

Gradual withdrawal is needed (taper oral immediate release or epidural dose gradually over 2-4 days to avoid rebound hypertension) if drug needs to be stopped. Patients should be instructed about abrupt discontinuation (causes rapid increase in BP and symptoms of sympathetic overactivity). In patients on both a beta-blocker and clonidine where withdrawal of clonidine is necessary, withdraw the beta-blocker first and several days before clonidine withdrawal, then slowly decrease clonidine. In children and adolescents, extended release formulation (Kapvay™) should be tapered in decrements of no more than 0.1 mg every 3-7 days. Discontinue oral immediate release formulations within 4 hours of surgery then restart as soon as possible afterwards. Discontinue oral extended release formulations up to 28 hours prior to surgery, then restart the following day.

Oral formulations of clonidine (immediate release versus extended release) are not interchangeable on a mg:mg basis due to different pharmacokinetic profiles.

Transdermal patch may contain conducting metal (eg, aluminum); remove patch prior to MRI. Due to the potential for altered electrical conductivity, remove transdermal patch before cardioversion or defibrillation. Localized contact sensitization to the transdermal system has been reported; in these patients, allergic reactions (eg, generalized rash, urticaria, angioedema) have also occurred following subsequent substitution of oral therapy.

In the elderly, avoid use as first-line antihypertensive due to high risk of CNS adverse effects; may also cause orthostatic hypotension and bradycardia (Beers Criteria). In pediatric patients, epidural clonidine should be reserved for cancer patients with severe intractable pain, unresponsive to other analgesics or epidural or spinal opioids. Use oral formulations with caution in pediatric patients since children commonly have gastrointestinal illnesses with vomiting and are susceptible to hypertensive episodes due to abrupt inability to take oral medication.

Adverse Reactions Frequency not always defined.

Oral, Transdermal: Incidence of adverse events may be less with transdermal compared to oral due to the lower peak/trough ratio.

Cardiovascular: Bradycardia (≤4%), palpitation (1%), tachycardia (1%), arrhythmia, atrioventricular block, chest pain, CHF, ECG abnormalities, flushing, orthostatic hypotension, pallor, Raynaud's phenomenon, syncope

Central nervous system: Drowsiness (12% to 38%), headache (1% to 29%), fatigue (4% to 16%), dizziness (2% to 16%), sedation (3% to 10%), insomnia (≤6%), lethargy (3%), nervousness (1% to 3%), mental depression (1%), aggression, agitation, anxiety, behavioral changes, CVA, delirium, delusional perception, fever, hallucinations (visual and auditory), irritability, malaise, nightmares, restlessness, vivid dreams

Dermatologic: Transient localized skin reactions characterized by pruritus and erythema (transdermal 15% to 50%), contact dermatitis (transdermal 8% to 34%), vesiculation (transdermal 7%), allergic contact sensitization (transdermal 5%), hyperpigmentation (transdermal 5%), burning (transdermal 3%), edema (3%), excoriation (transdermal 3%) blanching (transdermal 1%), generalized macular rash (1%), papules (transdermal 1%), throbbing (transdermal 1%), alopecia, angioedema, hives, localized hypopigmentation (transdermal), rash, urticaria

Endocrine & metabolic: Sexual dysfunction (3%), gynecomastia (1%), creatine phosphokinase increased (transient; oral), hyperglycemia (transient; oral), libido decreased

Gastrointestinal: Xerostomia (≤40%), constipation (2% to 10%), anorexia (1%), taste perversion (1%), weight gain (<1%), abdominal pain (oral), diarrhea, nausea, parotid gland pain (oral), parotitis (oral), pseudo-obstruction (oral), throat pain, vomiting

Genitourinary: Erectile dysfunction (2% to 3%), nocturia (1%), dysuria, enuresis, urinary retention

Hematologic: Thrombocytopenia (oral)

Hepatic: Liver function test (mild transient abnormalities; ≤1%), hepatitis

Neuromuscular & skeletal: Weakness (10%), arthralgia (1%), myalgia (1%), leg cramps (<1%), numbness (localized, transdermal), pain in extremities, paresthesia, tremor

Ocular: Accommodation disorder, blurred vision, burning eyes, dry eyes, lacrimation decreased, lacrimation increased

Otic: Ear pain, otitis media

Renal: Pollakiuria

Respiratory: Asthma, epistaxis, nasal congestion, nasal dryness, nasopharyngitis, respiratory tract infection, rhinorrhea

Miscellaneous: Withdrawal syndrome (1%), flu-like syndrome, thirst

Epidural: Note: The following adverse events occurred more often than placebo in cancer patients with intractable pain being treated with concurrent epidural morphine.

>10%:

Cardiovascular: Hypotension (45%), orthostatic hypotension (32%)

Central nervous system: Confusion (13%), dizziness (13%)

Gastrointestinal: Xerostomia (13%)

1% to 10%:

Cardiovascular: Chest pain (5%)

Central nervous system: Hallucinations (5%)

Gastrointestinal: Nausea/vomiting (8%)

Otic: Tinnitus (5%)

Miscellaneous: Diaphoresis (5%)

Drug Interactions

Metabolism/Transport Effects None known.

Avoid Concomitant Use

Avoid concomitant use of CloNIDine with any of the following: Azelastine (Nasal); Iobenguane I 123; Paraldehyde

Increased Effect/Toxicity

CloNIDine may increase the levels/effects of: Alcohol (Ethyl); Amifostine; Antihypertensives; Azelastine (Nasal); Beta-Blockers; Buprenorphine; Calcium Channel Blockers (Nondihydropyridine); Cardiac Glycosides; CNS Depressants; Hydrocodone; Hypotensive Agents; Methotrimeprazine; Metyrosine; Obinutuzumab; Paraldehyde; Pramipexole; RiTUXimab; ROPINIRole; Rotigotine; Selective Serotonin Reuptake Inhibitors; Zolpidem

The levels/effects of CloNIDine may be increased by: Alfuzosin; Beta-Blockers; Brimonidine (Topical); Diazoxide; Doxylamine; Droperidol; Herbs (Hypotensive Properties); HydrOXYzine; Magnesium Sulfate; MAO Inhibitors; Methotrimeprazine; Methylphenidate; Pentoxifylline; Perampanel; Phosphodiesterase 5 Inhibitors; Prostacyclin Analogues; Sodium Oxybate; Tapentadol

Decreased Effect

CloNIDine may decrease the levels/effects of: Iobenguane I 123

The levels/effects of CloNIDine may be decreased by: Antidepressants (Alpha2-Antagonist); Herbs (Hypertensive Properties); Serotonin/Norepinephrine Reuptake Inhibitors; Tricyclic Antidepressants; Yohimbine

Ethanol/Nutrition/Herb Interactions

Ethanol: Avoid ethanol (may increase CNS depression).

Herb/Nutraceutical: Avoid dong quai if using for hypertension (has estrogenic activity). Avoid ephedra, yohimbe, ginseng (may worsen hypertension). Avoid valerian, St John's wort, kava kava, gotu kola (may increase CNS depression).

Preparation for Administration Epidural formulation: Prior to administration, the 500 mcg/mL concentration must be diluted in 0.9% sodium chloride for injection (preservative-free) to a final concentration of 100 mcg/mL.

Storage/Stability

Epidural formulation: Store at 25°C (77°F); excursions permitted to 15°C to 30°C (59°F to 86°F). **Preservative free;** discard unused portion.

Tablets: Store at 25°C (77°F); excursions permitted to 15°C to 30°C (59°F to 86°F). Protect from light.

Extended release tablets: Store at 20°C to 25°C (68°F to 77°F). Protect from light.

Transdermal patches: Store below 30°C (86°F).

Mechanism of Action Stimulates $alpha_2$-adrenoceptors in the brain stem, thus activating an inhibitory neuron, resulting in reduced sympathetic outflow from the CNS, producing a decrease in peripheral resistance, renal vascular resistance, heart rate, and blood pressure; epidural clonidine may produce pain relief at spinal presynaptic and postjunctional $alpha_2$-adrenoceptors by preventing pain signal transmission; pain relief occurs only for the body regions innervated by the spinal segments where analgesic concentrations of clonidine exist. For the treatment of ADHD, the mechanism of action is unknown; it has been proposed that postsynaptic alpha$_2$-agonist stimulation regulates subcortical activity in the prefrontal cortex, the area of the brain responsible for emotions, attentions, and behaviors and causes reduced hyperactivity, impulsiveness, and distractibility.

Pharmacodynamics/Kinetics

Onset of action: Oral: Immediate release: 0.5-1 hour (maximum reduction in blood pressure: 2-4 hours); Transdermal: Initial application: 2-3 days

Duration: Oral: Immediate release: 6-10 hours

Absorption: Oral: Extended release tablets (Kapvay™) are not bioequivalent with immediate release formulations; peak plasma concentrations are 50% lower compared to immediate release formulations

Distribution: V_d: Adults: 2.9 L/kg; highly lipid soluble; distributes readily into extravascular sites

Note: Epidurally administered clonidine readily distributes into plasma via the epidural veins and attains clinically significant systemic concentrations.

Protein binding: 20% to 40%

Metabolism: Extensively hepatic to inactive metabolites; undergoes enterohepatic recirculation

Bioavailability: Oral: Immediate release: 70% to 80%; Extended release (Kapvay™): ~89% (relative to immediate release formulation); Transdermal: ~60%

Half-life elimination: Adults: Normal renal function: 12-16 hours; Renal impairment: Up to 41 hours

Epidural administration: CSF half-life elimination: 0.8-1.8 hours

Transdermal: Half-life elimination (after patch removal): ~20 hours (due to skin depot effect; increase in plasma clonidine concentrations may occur after patch removal [MacGregor, 1985])

Time to peak, plasma: Oral: Immediate release: 1-3 hours; Extended release: 7-8 hours

Excretion: Urine (40% to 60% as unchanged drug)

Dosage Note: Dosing is expressed as the salt (clonidine hydrochloride) unless otherwise noted. Formulations of clonidine (immediate release versus extended release) are not interchangeable on a mg:mg basis due to different pharmacokinetic profiles.

Children:

Oral:

Hypertension (unlabeled use): Children ≥12 years: Immediate release: Initial: 0.2 mg/day in 2 divided doses; increase gradually, if needed, in 0.1 mg/day increments at weekly intervals; maximum: 2.4 mg/day (rarely required) (NHBPEP, Fourth Report)

Severe hypertension (unlabeled use): Children: Immediate release: 0.05-0.1 mg/dose; may repeat up to a maximum total dose of 0.8 mg (NHBPEP, Fourth Report)

Clonidine tolerance test (test of growth hormone release from pituitary) (unlabeled use):

0.15 mg/m^2 as a single dose (Lanes, 1982)

or

5 mcg/kg as a single dose; maximum dose: 250 mcg (Richmond, 2008)

ADHD: **Note:** May be used alone or as an adjunct to stimulants.

Immediate release (unlabeled indication; Pliszka, 2007):

Children ≤45 kg: Initial: 0.05 mg at bedtime; sequentially increase every 3-7 days by 0.05 mg increments as twice daily, then 3 times daily, then 4 times daily; maximum daily dose: 0.2 mg/day for patients weighing 27-40.5 kg; 0.3 mg/day for patients weighing 40.5-45 kg. When discontinuing therapy, taper gradually over 1-2 weeks.

Children >45 kg: Initial: 0.1 mg at bedtime; sequentially increase every 3-7 days by 0.1 mg increments as twice daily, then 3 times daily, then 4 times daily; maximum daily dose: 0.4 mg/day. When discontinuing therapy, taper gradually over 1-2 weeks.

Extended release (Kapvay™): Children ≥6 years: Initial: 0.1 mg at bedtime; increase in 0.1 mg/day increments every 7 days until desired response, doses should be administered twice daily (either split equally or with the higher split dosage given at bedtime); maximum: 0.4 mg/day. **Note:** Maintenance treatment for >5 weeks has not been evaluated. When discontinuing therapy, taper daily dose by ≤0.1 mg every 3-7 days.

Epidural infusion: Pain management: Reserved for cancer patients with severe intractable pain, unresponsive to other opioid analgesics: Initial: 0.5 mcg/kg/**hour**; adjust with caution, based on clinical effect

Adults:

Oral:

Hypertension: Immediate release: Initial dose: 0.1 mg twice daily (maximum recommended dose: 2.4 mg/day); usual dose range (JNC 7): 0.1-0.8 mg/day in 2 divided doses

Acute hypertension (urgency) (unlabeled use): Initial 0.1-0.2 mg; may be followed by additional doses of 0.1 mg every hour, if necessary, to a maximum total dose of 0.7 mg (Atkin, 1992; Jaker, 1989)

Unlabeled route of administration: Sublingual: Initial: 0.1-0.2 mg; followed by 0.05-0.1 mg every hour until blood pressure controlled or a cumulative dose of 0.7 mg is reached (Cunningham, 1994; Matuschka, 1999)

Nicotine withdrawal symptoms (unlabeled use): Initial: 0.1 mg twice daily; titrate by 0.1 mg/day every 7 days if needed; dosage range used in clinical trials: 0.15-0.75 mg/day; duration of therapy ranged from 3-10 weeks in clinical trials (Fiore, 2008)

Transdermal:

Hypertension: Initial: 0.1 mg/24 hour patch applied once every 7 days and increase by 0.1 mg at 1- to 2-week intervals (dosages >0.6 mg/24 hours do not improve efficacy); usual dose range (JNC 7): 0.1-0.3 mg/24 hour patch applied once every 7 days

Nicotine withdrawal symptoms (unlabeled use): Initial: 0.1 mg/24 hour patch applied once every 7 days and increase by 0.1 mg at 1-week intervals if necessary; dosage range used in clinical trials: 0.1-0.2 mg/24 hour patch applied once every 7 days; duration of therapy ranged from 3-10 weeks in clinical trials (Fiore, 2008)

Epidural infusion: Pain management: Reserved for cancer patients with severe intractable pain, unresponsive to other opioid analgesics: Starting dose: 30 mcg/hour; titrate as required for relief of pain or presence of side effects; experience with doses >40 mcg/hour is limited; should be considered an adjunct to opioid therapy

Conversion from oral to transdermal: **Note:** If transitioning from oral to transdermal therapy, overlap oral regimen for 1-2 days; transdermal route takes 2-3 days to achieve therapeutic effects. An example transition is below:

Day 1: Place Catapres-TTS® 1; administer 100% of oral dose.

Day 2: Administer 50% of oral dose.

Day 3: Administer 25% of oral dose.

Day 4: Patch remains, no further oral supplement necessary.

Conversion from transdermal to oral: After transdermal patch removal, therapeutic clonidine levels persist for ~8 hours and then slowly decrease over several days. Consider starting oral clonidine no sooner than 8 hours after patch removal.

Elderly: Oral: Immediate release: Hypertension: Initial: 0.1 mg once daily at bedtime, increase gradually as needed

Dosage adjustment in renal impairment:

Children: Oral (extended release), epidural: The manufacturer recommends dosage adjustment according to degree of renal impairment; however, no specific dosage adjustment provided (has not been studied).

Adults: Oral (immediate release), transdermal, epidural: The manufacturer recommends dosage adjustment according to degree of renal impairment; however, no specific dosage adjustment provided in manufacturer's labeling. Bradycardia, sedation, and hypotension may be more likely to occur in patients with renal failure; half-life significantly prolonged in patients with severe renal failure; consider use of lower initial doses and monitor closely.

Hemodialysis: Not dialyzable (0% to 5%); supplemental dose is not necessary. Oral antihypertensive drugs given preferentially at night may reduce the nocturnal surge of blood pressure and minimize the intradialytic hypotension that may occur when taken the morning before a dialysis session (K/DOQI, 2005).

Dosage adjustment in hepatic impairment: No dosage adjustment provided in manufacturer's labeling.

Administration

Epidural: Specialized techniques are required for continuous epidural administration; administration via this route should only be performed by qualified individuals familiar with the techniques of epidural administration and patient management problems associated with this route. Familiarization of the epidural infusion device is essential. Do not discontinue clonidine abruptly; if needed, gradually reduce dose over 2-4 days to avoid withdrawal symptoms.

Oral: May be taken with or without food. Do not discontinue clonidine abruptly. If needed, gradually reduce dose over 2-4 days to avoid rebound hypertension.

Extended release tablet: Kapvay™: Swallow whole; do not crush, split, or chew.

Transdermal patch: Patches should be applied weekly at a consistent time to a clean, hairless area of the upper outer arm or chest. Rotate patch sites weekly. Redness under patch may be reduced if a topical corticosteroid spray is applied to the area before placement of the patch (Tom, 1994).

Monitoring Parameters Blood pressure, standing and sitting/supine, mental status, heart rate

When used for the treatment of ADHD, thoroughly evaluate for cardiovascular risk. Monitor heart rate, blood pressure (when started and weaned), and consider obtaining ECG prior to initiation (Vetter, 2008).

Clonidine tolerance test: In addition to growth hormone concentrations, monitor blood pressure and blood glucose (Huang, 2001).

Epidural: Carefully monitor infusion pump; inspect catheter tubing for obstruction or dislodgement to reduce risk of inadvertent abrupt withdrawal of infusion. Monitor closely for catheter-related infection (eg, meningitis or epidural abscess).

Test Interactions Positive Coombs' test

Additional Information Each 0.1 mg of clonidine hydrochloride (salt form) is equivalent to 0.087 mg of the free base.

Transdermal clonidine should only be used in patients unable to take oral medication. The transdermal product is much more expensive than oral clonidine and produces no better therapeutic effects.

When used for ADHD treatment, clonidine is recommended to be used as part of a comprehensive treatment program (eg, psychological, educational, and social) for attention-deficit disorder.

Dosage Forms Excipient information presented when available (limited, particularly for generics); consult specific product labeling. [DSC] = Discontinued product

Miscellaneous, Oral, as hydrochloride:
- Kapvay: 0.1 mg AM dose, 0.2 mg PM dose (60 ea [DSC])

Patch Weekly, Transdermal:
- Catapres-TTS-1: 0.1 mg/24 hr (4 ea)
- Catapres-TTS-2: 0.2 mg/24 hr (4 ea)
- Catapres-TTS-3: 0.3 mg/24 hr (4 ea)
- Generic: 0.1 mg/24 hr (4 ea); 0.2 mg/24 hr (4 ea); 0.3 mg/24 hr (4 ea)

Solution, Epidural, as hydrochloride:
- Duraclon: 100 mcg/mL (10 mL)

Solution, Epidural, as hydrochloride [preservative free]:
- Duraclon: 100 mcg/mL (10 mL)
- Duraclon: 500 mcg/mL (10 mL) [pyrogen free]
- Generic: 100 mcg/mL (10 mL); 500 mcg/mL (10 mL)

Tablet, Oral, as hydrochloride:
- Catapres: 0.1 mg [scored; contains brilliant blue fcf (fd&c blue #1), fd&c yellow #6 (sunset yellow)]
- Catapres: 0.2 mg, 0.3 mg [scored; contains fd&c yellow #6 (sunset yellow)]
- Generic: 0.1 mg, 0.2 mg, 0.3 mg

Tablet Extended Release 12 Hour, Oral, as hydrochloride:
- Kapvay: 0.1 mg
- Generic: 0.1 mg

Dosage Forms: Canada Note: Also refer to Dosage Forms. Epidural solution and extended-release tablets are not available in Canada.

Excipient information presented when available (limited, particularly for generics); consult specific product labeling.

Tablet, Oral, as hydrochloride: 0.025 mg

Extemporaneous Preparations

A 0.1 mg/mL oral suspension may be made from tablets. Crush thirty 0.2 mg tablets in a glass mortar and reduce to a fine powder. Slowly add 2 mL Purified Water USP and mix to a uniform paste. Slowly add Simple Syrup, NF in 15 mL increments; transfer to a calibrated bottle, rinse mortar with vehicle, and add quantity of vehicle sufficient to make 60 mL. Label "shake well" and "refrigerate". Stable for 28 days when stored in amber glass bottles and refrigerated.

Levinson ML and Johnson CE, "Stability of an Extemporaneously Compounded Clonidine Hydrochloride Oral Liquid," Am J Hosp Pharm, 1992, 49(1):122-5.

◆ **Clonidine Hydrochloride** *see* CloNIDine *on page 468*

Clopidogrel (kloh PID oh grel)

Brand Names: U.S. Plavix

Brand Names: Canada Apo-Clopidogrel; CO Clopidogrel; Dom-Clopidogrel; Mylan-Clopidogrel; Plavix; PMS-Clopidogrel; RAN-Clopidogrel; Sandoz-Clopidogrel; Teva-Clopidogrel

Index Terms Clopidogrel Bisulfate

Pharmacologic Category Antiplatelet Agent; Antiplatelet Agent, Thienopyridine

Additional Appendix Information

Desensitization Protocols *on page 2325*

Oral Antiplatelet Comparison Chart *on page 2313*

Use

Unstable angina/non-ST-segment elevation myocardial infarction: To decrease the rate of a combined end point of cardiovascular death, MI, or stroke, as well as the rate of a combined end point of cardiovascular death, MI, stroke, or refractory ischemia in patients with non-ST-segment elevation acute coronary syndrome (unstable angina/non-ST-elevation myocardial infarction [UA/NSTEMI]), including patients who are to be managed medically and those who are to be managed with coronary revascularization.

ST-segment elevation acute myocardial infarction: To reduce the rate of death from any cause and the rate of a combined end point of death, reinfarction, or stroke in patients with ST-elevation MI (STEMI).

Recent myocardial infarction, recent stroke, or established peripheral arterial disease: To reduce the rate of a combined end point of new ischemic stroke (fatal or nonfatal), new MI (fatal or nonfatal), and other vascular death in patients with a history of recent MI, recent stroke, or established peripheral arterial disease.

Canadian labeling: Additional use (not in U.S. labeling): Prevention of atherothrombotic and thromboembolic events, including stroke, in patients with atrial fibrillation with at least 1 risk factor for vascular events who are not suitable for treatment with an anticoagulant and are at a low risk for bleeding.

Unlabeled Use In patients with allergy or major gastrointestinal intolerance to aspirin, initial treatment of acute coronary syndromes (ACS) or prevention of coronary artery bypass graft closure (saphenous vein); stable coronary artery disease (in combination with aspirin); adjunctive therapy to support reperfusion with primary percutaneous coronary intervention (PCI); in patients having undergone peripheral artery percutaneous transluminal angioplasty; symptomatic carotid artery stenosis (including recent carotid endarterectomy)

Pregnancy Risk Factor B

Pregnancy Considerations Adverse events were not observed in animal reproduction studies. Information related to use during pregnancy is limited (Bauer, 2012; DeSantis, 2011; Myers, 2011).

Breast-Feeding Considerations It is not known if clopidogrel is excreted into breast milk. Due to the potential for serious adverse reactions in the nursing infant, the manufacturer recommends a decision be made whether to discontinue nursing or to discontinue the drug, taking into account the importance of treatment to the mother.

Medication Guide Available Yes

Contraindications Hypersensitivity to clopidogrel or any component of the formulation; active pathological bleeding such as peptic ulcer or intracranial hemorrhage

Canadian labeling: Additional contraindications (not in U.S. labeling): Significant liver impairment or cholestatic jaundice

Warnings/Precautions [U.S. Boxed Warning]: Patients with one or more copies of the variant *CYP2C19*2* and/or *CYP2C19*3* alleles (and potentially other reduced-function variants) may have reduced conversion of clopidogrel to its active thiol metabolite. Lower active metabolite exposure may result in reduced platelet inhibition and, thus, a higher rate of cardiovascular events following MI or stent thrombosis following PCI. Although evidence is insufficient to recommend routine genetic testing, tests are available to determine CYP2C19 genotype and may be used to determine therapeutic strategy; alternative treatment or treatment strategies may be considered if patient is identified as a CYP2C19 poor metabolizer. Genetic testing may be considered prior to initiating clopidogrel in patients at moderate or high risk for poor outcomes (eg, PCI in patients with extensive and/or very complex disease). The optimal dose for CYP2C19 poor metabolizers has yet to be determined. After initiation of clopidogrel, functional testing (eg, VerifyNow® P2Y12 assay) may also be done to determine clopidogrel responsiveness (Holmes, 2010).

Use with caution in patients who may be at risk of increased bleeding, including patients with PUD, trauma, or surgery. In patients with coronary stents, premature interruption of therapy may result in stent thrombosis with subsequent fatal and nonfatal MI. Duration of therapy, in general, is determined by the type of stent placed (bare metal or drug eluting) and whether an ACS event was ongoing at the time of placement. Consider discontinuing 5 days before elective surgery (except in patients with cardiac stents that have not completed their full course of dual antiplatelet therapy; patient-specific situations need to be discussed with cardiologist; AHA/ACC/SCAI/ACS/ADA Science Advisory provides recommendations). Discontinue at least 5 days before elective CABG; when urgent CABG is necessary, the ACCF/AHA CABG guidelines recommend discontinuation for at least 24 hours prior to surgery (Hillis, 2011). The ACCF/AHA STEMI guidelines recommend discontinuation for at least 24 hours prior to *on-pump* CABG; *off-pump* CABG may be performed within 24 hours of clopidogrel administration if the benefits of prompt revascularization outweigh the risks of bleeding (O'Gara, 2013).

Because of structural similarities, cross-reactivity is possible among the thienopyridines (clopidogrel, prasugrel, and ticlopidine); use with caution or avoid in patients with previous thienopyridine hypersensitivity. Use of clopidogrel is contraindicated in patients with hypersensitivity to clopidogrel, although desensitization may be considered for mild-to-moderate hypersensitivity.

Use caution in concurrent treatment with anticoagulants (eg, heparin, warfarin) or other antiplatelet drugs; bleeding risk is increased. Concurrent use with drugs known to inhibit CYP2C19 (eg, proton pump inhibitors) may reduce levels of active metabolite and subsequently reduce clinical efficacy and increase the risk of cardiovascular events; if possible, avoid concurrent use of moderate-to-strong CYP2C19 inhibitors. In patients requiring antacid therapy, consider use of an acid-reducing agent lacking (eg, ranitidine/famotidine) or with less CYP2C19 inhibition. According to the manufacturer, avoid concurrent use of omeprazole (even when scheduled 12 hours apart) or esomeprazole; if a PPI is necessary, the use of an agent with comparatively less effect on the antiplatelet activity of clopidogrel is recommended. Of the PPIs, pantoprazole has the lowest degree of CYP2C19 inhibition *in vitro* (Li, 2004) and has been shown to have has less effect on conversion of clopidogrel to its active metabolite compared to omeprazole (Angiolillo, 2011). Although lansoprazole exhibits the most potent CYP2C19 inhibition *in vitro* (Li, 2004; Ogilvie, 2012), an *in vivo* study of extensive CYP2C19 metabolizers showed less reduction of the active metabolite of clopidogrel by lansoprazole/dexlansoprazole compared to esomeprazole/omeprazole (Frelinger, 2012). Avoidance of rabeprazole appears prudent due to potent *in vitro* CYP2C19 inhibition and lack of sufficient comparative *in vivo* studies with other PPIs. In contrast to these warnings, others have recommended the continued use of PPIs, regardless of the degree of inhibition, in patients with multiple risk factors for GI bleeding who are also receiving clopidogrel since no evidence has established clinically meaningful differences in outcome; however, a clinically-significant interaction cannot be excluded in those who are poor metabolizers of clopidogrel. Staggering PPIs with clopidogrel is not recommended until further evidence is available (Abraham, 2010). Concurrent use of aspirin and clopidogrel is not recommended for secondary prevention of ischemic stroke or TIA in patients unable to take oral anticoagulants due to hemorrhagic risk (Furie, 2011).

Use with caution in patients with severe liver or renal disease (experience is limited). Cases of TTP (usually occurring within the first 2 weeks of therapy), resulting in some fatalities, have been reported; urgent plasmapheresis is required. Use in patients with severe hepatic impairment or cholestatic jaundice is contraindicated in the Canadian labeling. Cases of TTP (usually occurring within the first 2 weeks of therapy), resulting in some fatalities, have been reported; urgent plasmapheresis is required. In patients with recent lacunar stroke (within 180 days), the use of clopidogrel in addition to aspirin did not significantly reduce the incidence of the primary outcome of stroke recurrence (any ischemic stroke or intracranial hemorrhage) compared to aspirin alone; the use of clopidogrel in addition to aspirin did however increase the risk of major hemorrhage and the rate of all-cause mortality (SPS3 Investigators, 2012).

Assess bleeding risk carefully prior to initiating therapy in patients with atrial fibrillation (Canadian labeling; not an approved use in U.S. labeling); in clinical trials, a significant increase in major bleeding events (including intracranial hemorrhage and fatal bleeding events) were observed in patients receiving clopidogrel plus aspirin versus aspirin alone. Vitamin K antagonist (VKA) therapy (in suitable patients) has demonstrated a greater benefit in stroke reduction than aspirin (with or without clopidogrel).

Adverse Reactions As with all drugs which may affect hemostasis, bleeding is associated with clopidogrel. Hemorrhage may occur at virtually any site. Risk is dependent on multiple variables, including the concurrent use of multiple agents which alter hemostasis and patient susceptibility.

3% to 10%:

Dermatologic: Rash (4%), pruritus (3%)

Hematologic: Bleeding (major 4%; minor 5%), purpura/bruising (5%), epistaxis (3%)

1% to 3%:

Gastrointestinal: GI hemorrhage (2%)

Hematologic: Hematoma

<1% (Limited to important or life-threatening): Acute liver failure, agranulocytosis, anaphylactoid reaction, angioedema, aplastic anemia, arthralgia, arthritis, bronchospasm, bullous eruption, colitis (including ulcerative or lymphocytic), confusion, creatinine increased, eczema, erythema multiforme, fever, glomerulopathy, hallucination, hemorrhagic stroke (≤0.2%), hepatitis, hypersensitivity reaction, hypotension, interstitial pneumonitis, intracranial hemorrhage (≤0.4%), lichen planus, liver function tests (abnormal), musculoskeletal bleeding, myalgia, ocular bleeding (including conjunctival and retinal), pancreatitis, pancytopenia, pulmonary hemorrhage, rash (erythematous or maculopapular), retroperitoneal hemorrhage, serum sickness, Stevens-Johnson syndrome, stomatitis, taste disorder, thrombotic thrombocytopenic purpura (TTP), toxic epidermal necrolysis, vasculitis, wound hemorrhage

Drug Interactions

Metabolism/Transport Effects Substrate of CYP2C19 (major), CYP3A4 (minor); **Note:** Assignment of Major/Minor substrate status based on clinically relevant drug interaction potential; **Inhibits** CYP2B6 (moderate), CYP2C9 (weak)

Avoid Concomitant Use

Avoid concomitant use of Clopidogrel with any of the following: Esomeprazole; Omeprazole

Increased Effect/Toxicity

Clopidogrel may increase the levels/effects of: Agents with Antiplatelet Properties; Anticoagulants; Collagenase (Systemic); CYP2B6 Substrates; Dabigatran Etexilate; Ibritumomab; Rivaroxaban; Salicylates; Thrombolytic Agents; Tositumomab and Iodine I 131 Tositumomab; Warfarin

The levels/effects of Clopidogrel may be increased by: Dasatinib; Glucosamine; Herbs (Anticoagulant/Antiplatelet Properties); Ibrutinib; Luliconazole; Multivitamins/Fluoride (with ADE); Multivitamins/Minerals (with ADEK, Folate, Iron); Multivitamins/Minerals (with AE, No Iron); Nonsteroidal Anti-Inflammatory Agents; Omega-3 Fatty Acids; Pentosan Polysulfate Sodium; Pentoxifylline; Prostacyclin Analogues; Rifamycin Derivatives; Tipranavir; Vitamin E

Decreased Effect

The levels/effects of Clopidogrel may be decreased by: Amiodarone; Calcium Channel Blockers; CYP2C19 Inhibitors (Moderate); CYP2C19 Inhibitors (Strong); Dexlansoprazole; Esomeprazole; Grapefruit Juice; Lansoprazole; Macrolide Antibiotics; Morphine (Liposomal); Morphine (Systemic); Nonsteroidal Anti-Inflammatory Agents; Omeprazole; Pantoprazole; RABEprazole

Ethanol/Nutrition/Herb Interactions

Food: Consumption of three 200 mL glasses of grapefruit juice a day may substantially reduce clopidogrel antiplatelet effects. Management: Avoid or minimize the consumption of grapefruit or grapefruit juice (Holmberg, 2013).

Herb/Nutraceutical: Avoid alfalfa, anise, bilberry, bladderwrack, bromelain, cat's claw, chamomile, coleus, cordyceps, dong quai, evening primrose oil, fenugreek, feverfew, garlic, ginger, ginkgo biloba, ginseng (American), ginseng (Panax), ginseng (Siberian), grape seed, green tea, guggul, horse chestnut seed, horseradish, licorice, prickly ash, red clover, reishi, SAMe (S-adenosylmethionine), sweet clover, turmeric, white willow (all have additional antiplatelet activity).

Storage/Stability Store at 25°C (77°F); excursions permitted to 15°C to 30°C (59°F to 86°F).

Mechanism of Action Clopidogrel requires *in vivo* biotransformation to an active thiol metabolite. The active metabolite irreversibly blocks the $P2Y_{12}$ component of ADP receptors on the platelet surface, which prevents activation of the GPIIb/IIIa receptor complex, thereby reducing platelet aggregation. Platelets blocked by clopidogrel are affected for the remainder of their lifespan (~7-10 days).

Pharmacodynamics/Kinetics

Onset of action: Inhibition of platelet aggregation (IPA): Dose-dependent:

300-600 mg loading dose: Detected within 2 hours

50-100 mg/day: Detected by the second day of treatment

Peak effect: Time to maximal IPA: Dose-dependent: **Note:** Degree of IPA based on adenosine diphosphate (ADP) concentration used during light aggregometry:

300-600 mg loading dose:

ADP 5 micromole/L: 20% to 30% IPA at 6 hours post administration (Montelescot, 2006)

ADP 20 micromole/L: 30% to 37% IPA at 6 hours post administration (Montelescot, 2006)

50-100 mg/day: ADP 5 micromole/L: 50% to 60% IPA at 5-7 days (Herbert, 1993)

Absorption: Well absorbed

Protein binding: Parent drug: 98%; Inactive metabolite: 94%

Metabolism: Extensively hepatic via esterase-mediated hydrolysis to a carboxylic acid derivative (inactive) and via CYP450-mediated (CYP2C19 primarily) oxidation to a thiol metabolite (active)

Half-life elimination: Parent drug: ~6 hours; Active metabolite: ~30 minutes

Time to peak, serum: ~0.75 hours

Excretion: Following administration of a single ^{14}C-labeled clopidogrel oral dose; radioactivity measured over 5 days: Urine (50%); feces (46%)

Dosage Oral: Adults:

Recent MI, recent stroke, or established peripheral arterial disease (PAD): 75 mg once daily. **Note:** The ACCF/AHA guidelines for PAD recommend clopidogrel as an alternative to aspirin (Class Ib recommendation) or in conjunction with aspirin for those who are not at an increased risk of bleeding but are of high cardiovascular risk (Class IIb recommendation). These recommendations also pertain to those with intermittent claudication or critical limb ischemia, prior lower extremity revascularization, or prior amputation for lower extremity ischemia (Rooke, 2011).

Acute coronary syndrome (ACS):

Unstable angina, non-ST-segment elevation myocardial infarction (UA/NSTEMI): Initial: 300 mg loading dose, followed by 75 mg once daily for up to 12 months (in combination with aspirin indefinitely) (Anderson, 2013). The American College of Chest Physicians recommends combination aspirin dose of 75-100 mg (Guyatt, 2012).

ST-segment elevation myocardial infarction (STEMI) receiving fibrinolytic therapy (in combination with aspirin and appropriate anticoagulant) (O'Gara, 2013): **Note**: If patient is to undergo primary PCI, see *Percutaneous coronary intervention (PCI) for acute coronary syndrome* dosing.

Age ≤75 years: Loading dose of 300 mg followed by 75 mg once daily for at least 14 days up to 1 year (in the absence of bleeding)

Age >75 years: 75 mg once daily (no loading dose) for at least 14 days up to 1 year (in the absence of bleeding)

Percutaneous coronary intervention (PCI) for acute coronary syndrome (eg, UA/NSTEMI or STEMI) (unlabeled use): 600 mg (loading dose) given as early as possible before or at the time of PCI, followed by 75 mg once daily for at least 12 months (in combination with aspirin 81 mg/day) (Anderson, 2013; Levine, 2011; O'Gara, 2013).

PCI after fibrinolytic therapy (O'Gara, 2013):

Fibrinolytic administered **with** a loading dose of clopidogrel: Continue 75 mg once daily and do not administer an additional loading dose.

Fibrinolytic administered within previous 24 hours **without** a loading dose of clopidogrel: Administer 300 mg loading dose before or at the time of PCI.

Fibrinolytic administered more than 24 hours ago without a loading dose of clopidogrel: Administer 600 mg loading dose before or at the time of PCI.

Higher versus standard maintenance dosing: May consider a maintenance dose of 150 mg once daily for 6 days, then 75 mg once daily thereafter in patients not at high risk for bleeding (Anderson, 2013; CURRENT-OASIS 7 Investigators, 2010); however, in another study, in patients with high on-treatment platelet reactivity, the use of 150 mg once daily for 6 months did not demonstrate a difference in 6-month incidence of death from cardiovascular causes, nonfatal MI, or stent thrombosis compared to standard dose therapy (Price, 2011).

Duration of clopidogrel (in combination with aspirin) after stent placement for ACS and non-ACS indications: **Premature interruption of therapy may result in stent thrombosis with subsequent fatal and nonfatal MI.** At least 12 months of clopidogrel is recommended for those with ACS receiving either stent type (bare metal [BMS] or drug eluting stent [DES]) or those receiving a DES for a non-ACS indication. Those receiving a BMS for a non-ACS indication (ie, elective PCI) should be given at least 1 month and ideally up to 12 months; if patient is at increased risk of bleeding, give for a minimum of 2 weeks (Levine, 2011). A duration >12 months, regardless of indication, may be considered in patients with DES placement (Anderson, 2013; Levine, 2011; O'Gara, 2013).

CYP2C19 poor metabolizers (ie, *CYP2C19*2* or **3* carriers): Although routine genetic testing is not recommended in patients treated with clopidogrel undergoing PCI, testing may be considered to identify poor metabolizers who would be at risk for poor outcomes while receiving clopidogrel; if identified, these patients may be considered for an alternative $P2Y_{12}$ inhibitor (Levine, 2011). An appropriate regimen for this patient population has not been established in clinical outcome trials. Although a 600 mg loading dose, followed by 150 mg once daily produced greater active metabolite exposure and antiplatelet response compared to the 300 mg/75 mg regimen, it does not appear that this dosing strategy improves outcomes for this patient population (Price, 2011; Simon, 2011).

Atrial fibrillation (in patients not candidates for warfarin and at a low risk of bleeding) (Canadian labeling; ACTIVE Investigators, 2009; unlabeled use in U.S.): 75 mg once daily (in combination with aspirin 75-100 mg once daily). **Note:** Combination may also be used as an alternative for patients with atrial fibrillation and mitral stenosis (Guyatt, 2012).

Carotid artery stenosis, symptomatic (including recent carotid endarterectomy) (unlabeled use): 75 mg once daily (Guyatt, 2012)

Coronary artery disease (CAD), established (unlabeled use): 75 mg once daily. **Note:** Established CAD defined as patients 1-year post ACS, with prior revascularization, coronary stenosis >50% by angiogram, and/or evidence for cardiac ischemia on diagnostic testing (includes patients after the first year post-ACS and/or with prior CABG surgery) (Guyatt, 2012).

Peripheral artery percutaneous transluminal angioplasty (with or without stenting) or peripheral artery bypass graft surgery, postprocedure (unlabeled use): 75 mg once daily. **Note:** For below-knee bypass graft surgery with prosthetic grafts, combine with aspirin 75-100 mg/day (Guyatt, 2012).

Prevention of coronary artery bypass graft closure (saphenous vein) and postoperative adverse cardiovascular events (unlabeled use): Aspirin-allergic patients: 75 mg once daily (Hillis, 2011)

Secondary prevention of cardioembolic stroke (patient not candidate for oral anticoagulation) (unlabeled use): 75 mg once daily (in combination with aspirin) (Guyatt, 2012).

Dosing adjustment in renal impairment: No dosage adjustment necessary (Basra, 2011). **Note:** GFR stage 5 (ie, ESRD or an eGFR <15 mL/minute) is associated with higher residual platelet reactivity with maintenance dosing (Muller, 2012).

Dosing adjustment in hepatic impairment: Use with caution; experience is limited. **Note:** Inhibition of ADP-induced platelet aggregation and mean bleeding time prolongation were similar in patients with severe hepatic impairment compared to healthy subjects after repeated doses of 75 mg once daily for 10 days.

Dietary Considerations May be taken without regard to meals. Avoid grapefruit juice (Holmberg, 2013).

Administration May be administered without regard to meals.

Monitoring Parameters Signs of bleeding; hemoglobin and hematocrit periodically. May consider platelet function testing to determine platelet inhibitory response or genotyping for CYP2C19 loss of function variant if results of testing may alter management (Anderson, 2013).

Dosage Forms Excipient information presented when available (limited, particularly for generics); consult specific product labeling.

Tablet, Oral:

Plavix: 75 mg, 300 mg

Generic: 75 mg, 300 mg

Extemporaneous Preparations A 5 mg/mL oral suspension may be made using tablets. Crush four 75 mg tablets and reduce to a fine powder. Add a small amount of a 1:1 mixture of Ora-Sweet® and Ora-Plus® and mix to a uniform paste; mix while adding the vehicle in geometric proportions to **almost** 60 mL; transfer to a calibrated bottle, rinse mortar with vehicle, and add quantity of vehicle sufficient to make 60 mL. Label "shake well". Stable 60 days at room temperature or under refrigeration.

Skillman KL, Caruthers RL, and Johnson CE, "Stability of an Extemporaneously Prepared Clopidogrel Oral Suspension," *Am J Health Syst Pharm*, 2010, 67(7):559-61.

◆ **Clopidogrel Bisulfate** *see* Clopidogrel *on page 471*

Clorazepate (klor AZ e pate)

Brand Names: U.S. Tranxene-T

Brand Names: Canada Apo-Clorazepate®; Novo-Clopate

Index Terms Clorazepate Dipotassium; Tranxene T-Tab

Pharmacologic Category Benzodiazepine

Additional Appendix Information

Benzodiazepine Comparison Table *on page 2292*

Use Treatment of generalized anxiety disorder; management of ethanol withdrawal; adjunct anticonvulsant in management of partial seizures

Pregnancy Considerations Nordiazepam, the active metabolite of clorazepate, crosses the placenta and is measurable in cord blood and amniotic fluid. Teratogenic effects have been observed with some benzodiazepines (including clorazepate); however, additional studies are needed. The incidence of premature birth and low birth weights may be increased following maternal use of benzodiazepines; hypoglycemia and respiratory problems in the neonate may occur following exposure late in pregnancy. Neonatal withdrawal symptoms may occur within days to weeks after birth and "floppy infant syndrome" (which also includes withdrawal symptoms) has been reported with some benzodiazepines (Bergman, 1992; Iqbal, 2002; Patel,1980; Rey, 1979; Wikner, 2007). A combination of factors influences the potential teratogenicity of anticonvulsant therapy. When treating women with epilepsy, monotherapy with the lowest effective dose and avoidance medications known to have a high incidence of teratogenic effects is recommended (Harden, 2009; Wlodarczyk, 2012).

Patients exposed to clorazepate during pregnancy are encouraged to enroll themselves into the AED Pregnancy Registry by calling 1-888-233-2334. Additional information is available at www.aedpregnancyregistry.org.

Breast-Feeding Considerations Nordiazepam, the active metabolite of clorazepate, is found in breast milk and is measurable in the serum of breast-feeding infants. Drowsiness, lethargy, or weight loss in nursing infants have been observed in case reports following maternal use of some benzodiazepines (Iqbal, 2002; Rey, 1979). The manufacturer states that women taking clorazepate should not breast-feed their infants.

Medication Guide Available Yes

Contraindications Hypersensitivity to clorazepate or any component of the formulation (cross-sensitivity with other benzodiazepines may exist); narrow-angle glaucoma

Warnings/Precautions Antiepileptics are associated with an increased risk of suicidal behavior/thoughts with use (regardless of indication); patients should be monitored for signs/symptoms of depression, suicidal tendencies, and other unusual behavior changes during therapy and instructed to inform their healthcare provider immediately if symptoms occur. Not recommended for use in patients <9 years of age or patients with depressive or psychotic disorders. Use with caution in elderly or debilitated patients, patients with hepatic disease (including alcoholics), or renal impairment. Active metabolites with extended half-lives may lead to delayed accumulation and adverse effects. Use with caution in patients with respiratory disease or impaired gag reflex. Avoid use in patients with sleep apnea.

Causes CNS depression (dose related) resulting in sedation, dizziness, confusion, or ataxia which may impair physical and mental capabilities. Patients must be cautioned about performing tasks which require mental alertness (eg, operating machinery or driving). Use with caution in patients receiving other CNS depressants or psychoactive agents. Effects with other sedative drugs or ethanol may be potentiated. Benzodiazepines have been associated with falls and traumatic injury and should be used with extreme caution in patients who are at risk of these events. In older adults, benzodiazepines increase the risk of impaired cognition, delirium, falls, fractures, and motor vehicle accidents. Due to increased sensitivity in this age group and slower metabolism of long-acting agents (such as clorazepate), avoid use for treatment of insomnia, agitation, or delirium (Beers Criteria).

Use caution in patients with depression, particularly if suicidal risk may be present. Use with caution in patients with a history of drug dependence. Benzodiazepines have been associated with dependence and acute withdrawal symptoms on discontinuation or reduction in dose. Acute withdrawal, including seizures, may be precipitated in patients after administration of flumazenil to patients receiving long-term benzodiazepine therapy.

Benzodiazepines have been associated with anterograde amnesia. Paradoxical reactions, including hyperactive or aggressive behavior, have been reported with benzodiazepines, particularly in adolescent/pediatric or psychiatric patients. Does not have analgesic, antidepressant, or antipsychotic properties.

Adverse Reactions Frequency not defined.

Cardiovascular: Hypotension

Central nervous system: Drowsiness, fatigue, ataxia, lightheadedness, memory impairment, insomnia, anxiety, headache, depression, slurred speech, confusion, nervousness, dizziness, irritability

Dermatologic: Rash

Endocrine & metabolic: Libido decreased

Gastrointestinal: Xerostomia, constipation, diarrhea, salivation decreased, nausea, vomiting, appetite increased or decreased

Hepatic: Jaundice, transaminase increased

Neuromuscular & skeletal: Dysarthria, tremor

Ocular: Blurred vision, diplopia

Drug Interactions

Metabolism/Transport Effects Substrate of CYP3A4 (major); **Note:** Assignment of Major/Minor substrate status based on clinically relevant drug interaction potential

Avoid Concomitant Use

Avoid concomitant use of Clorazepate with any of the following: Azelastine (Nasal); Conivaptan; Fusidic Acid (Systemic); OLANZapine; Paraldehyde; Sodium Oxybate

Increased Effect/Toxicity

Clorazepate may increase the levels/effects of: Alcohol (Ethyl); Azelastine (Nasal); Buprenorphine; CloZAPine; CNS Depressants; Fosphenytoin; Hydrocodone; Methotrimeprazine; Metyrosine; Mirtazapine; Paraldehyde; Phenytoin; Pramipexole; ROPINIRole; Rotigotine; Selective Serotonin Reuptake Inhibitors; Sodium Oxybate; Zolpidem

The levels/effects of Clorazepate may be increased by: Antifungal Agents (Azole Derivatives, Systemic); Aprepitant; Brimonidine (Topical); Calcium Channel Blockers (Nondihydropyridine); Cimetidine; Conivaptan; Contraceptives (Estrogens); Contraceptives (Progestins); CYP3A4 Inhibitors (Moderate); CYP3A4 Inhibitors (Strong); Dasatinib; Doxylamine; Droperidol; Fosamprenavir; Fosaprepitant; Fusidic Acid (Systemic); Grapefruit Juice; HydrOXYzine; Isoniazid; Ivacaftor; Luliconazole; Magnesium Sulfate; MAO Inhibitors; Methotrimeprazine; Mifepristone; OLANZapine; Perampanel; Proton Pump Inhibitors; Ritonavir; Saquinavir; Selective Serotonin Reuptake Inhibitors; Simeprevir; Tapentadol

Decreased Effect

The levels/effects of Clorazepate may be decreased by: Bosentan; CarBAMazepine; CYP3A4 Inducers (Strong); Dabrafenib; Deferasirox; Herbs (CYP3A4 Inducers); Mitotane; Rifamycin Derivatives; Theophylline Derivatives; Tocilizumab; Yohimbine

Ethanol/Nutrition/Herb Interactions

Ethanol: May increase CNS depression; monitor for increased effects with coadministration. Caution patients about effects.

Food: Serum concentrations/toxicity may be increased by grapefruit juice.

Herb/Nutraceutical: Avoid valerian, St John's wort, kava kava, gotu kola (may increase CNS depression).

Storage/Stability Store at controlled room temperature at 20°C to 25°C (68°F to 77°F). Protect from moisture; keep bottle tightly closed; dispense in tightly closed, light-resistant container.

Mechanism of Action Binds to stereospecific benzodiazepine receptors on the postsynaptic GABA neuron at several sites within the central nervous system, including the limbic system, reticular formation. Enhancement of the inhibitory effect of GABA on neuronal excitability results by increased neuronal membrane permeability to chloride ions. This shift in chloride ions results in hyperpolarization (a less excitable state) and stabilization.

Pharmacodynamics/Kinetics

Onset of action: 1-2 hours

Duration: Variable, 8-24 hours

Distribution: Appears in urine

Protein binding: Nordiazepam 97% to 98%

Metabolism: Rapidly decarboxylated to nordiazepam (active) in acidic stomach prior to absorption; hepatically to oxazepam (active)

Half-life elimination: Adults: Nordiazepam: 40-50 hours; Oxazepam: 6-8 hours

Time to peak, serum: ~1 hour

Excretion: Primarily urine

Dosage Oral:

Children 9-12 years: Anticonvulsant: Initial: 3.75-7.5 mg/dose twice daily; increase dose by 3.75 mg at weekly intervals, not to exceed 60 mg/day in 2-3 divided doses

Children >12 years and Adults: Anticonvulsant: Initial: Up to 7.5 mg/dose 2-3 times/day; increase dose by 7.5 mg at weekly intervals, not to exceed 90 mg/day

Adults:

Anxiety: 7.5-15 mg 2-4 times/day

Ethanol withdrawal: Initial: 30 mg, then 15 mg 2-4 times/day on first day; maximum daily dose: 90 mg; gradually decrease dose over subsequent days

Dosage adjustment in renal impairment: No dosage adjustment provided in manufacturer's labeling; use with caution.

Dosage adjustment in hepatic impairment: No dosage adjustment provided in manufacturer's labeling; use with caution.

Monitoring Parameters Respiratory and cardiovascular status, excess CNS depression; suicidality (eg, suicidal thoughts, depression, behavioral changes)

Reference Range Therapeutic: 0.12-1 mcg/mL (SI: 0.36-3.01 micromole/L)

Test Interactions Decreased hematocrit; abnormal liver and renal function tests

Additional Information Abrupt discontinuation after sustained use (generally >10 days) may cause withdrawal symptoms.

Dosage Forms Excipient information presented when available (limited, particularly for generics); consult specific product labeling.

Tablet, Oral, as dipotassium:

Tranxene-T: 3.75 mg [scored; contains fd&c blue #2 (indigotine)]

Tranxene-T: 7.5 mg [scored; contains fd&c yellow #6 (sunset yellow)]

Tranxene-T: 15 mg [scored]

Generic: 3.75 mg, 7.5 mg, 15 mg

Controlled Substance C-IV

◆ Clorazepate Dipotassium *see* Clorazepate *on page 475*

◆ Clotrimaderm (Can) *see* Clotrimazole (Topical) *on page 476*

◆ Clotrimazole 3 Day [OTC] *see* Clotrimazole (Topical) *on page 476*

Clotrimazole (Oral) (kloe TRIM a zole)

Index Terms Mycelex

Pharmacologic Category Antifungal Agent, Oral Nonabsorbed

Use Treatment of susceptible fungal infections, including oropharyngeal candidiasis; limited data suggest that clotrimazole troches may be effective for prophylaxis against oropharyngeal candidiasis in neutropenic patients

Pregnancy Risk Factor C

Dosage Oral: Children >3 years and Adults:

Prophylaxis: 10 mg troche dissolved 3 times/day for the duration of chemotherapy or until steroids are reduced to maintenance levels

Treatment: 10 mg troche dissolved slowly 5 times/day for 14 consecutive days

Additional Information Complete prescribing information should be consulted for additional detail.

Dosage Forms Excipient information presented when available (limited, particularly for generics); consult specific product labeling.

Lozenge, Mouth/Throat:

Generic: 10 mg (70 ea, 140 ea)

Troche, Mouth/Throat:

Generic: 10 mg

Clotrimazole (Topical) (kloe TRIM a zole)

Brand Names: U.S. Clotrimazole 3 Day [OTC]; Clotrimazole Anti-Fungal [OTC]; Desenex [OTC]; Gyne-Lotrimin 3 [OTC]; Gyne-Lotrimin [OTC]; Lotrimin AF For Her [OTC]; Lotrimin AF [OTC]

Brand Names: Canada Canesten® Topical; Canesten® Vaginal; Clotrimaderm; Trivagizole-3®

Pharmacologic Category Antifungal Agent, Topical; Antifungal Agent, Vaginal

Use Treatment of susceptible fungal infections, including dermatophytoses, superficial mycoses, and cutaneous candidiasis, as well as vulvovaginal candidiasis

Dosage

Children >3 years and Adults: Topical (cream, solution): Apply twice daily; if no improvement occurs after 4 weeks of therapy, re-evaluate diagnosis

Children >12 years and Adults:
Vaginal: Cream:
1%: Insert 1 applicatorful vaginal cream daily (preferably at bedtime) for 7 consecutive days
2%: Insert 1 applicatorful vaginal cream daily (preferably at bedtime) for 3 consecutive days
Topical (cream, solution): Apply to affected area twice daily (morning and evening) for 7 consecutive days

Additional Information Complete prescribing information should be consulted for additional detail.

Dosage Forms Excipient information presented when available (limited, particularly for generics); consult specific product labeling.

Cream, External:
Clotrimazole Anti-Fungal: 1% (15 g, 28.35 g) [contains benzyl alcohol]
Desenex: 1% (15 g, 30 g)
Lotrimin AF: 1% (12 g, 24 g)
Lotrimin AF For Her: 1% (24 g)
Generic: 1% (15 g, 30 g, 45 g)

Cream, Vaginal:
Clotrimazole 3 Day: 2% (22.2 g)
Gyne-Lotrimin: 1% (45 g) [contains benzyl alcohol]
Gyne-Lotrimin 3: 2% (21 g) [contains benzyl alcohol, cetyl alcohol]
Generic: 1% (45 g)

Solution, External:
Generic: 1% (10 mL, 30 mL)

◆ **Clotrimazole and Betamethasone** *see* Betamethasone and Clotrimazole *on page 249*

◆ **Clotrimazole Anti-Fungal [OTC]** *see* Clotrimazole (Topical) *on page 476*

CloZAPine (KLOE za peen)

Brand Names: U.S. Clozaril; FazaClo; Versacloz

Brand Names: Canada Apo-Clozapine; Clozaril; Gen-Clozapine

Pharmacologic Category Antipsychotic Agent, Atypical

Additional Appendix Information

Antipsychotic Agents *on page 2290*

Beers Criteria − Potentially Inappropriate Medications for Geriatrics *on page 2368*

Use

Schizophrenia, treatment resistant: Treatment of severely ill patients with schizophrenia who fail to respond adequately to antipsychotic treatment

Suicidal behavior in schizophrenia or schizoaffective disorder: To reduce the risk of suicidal behavior in patients with schizophrenia or schizoaffective disorder

Unlabeled Use Treatment resistant schizophrenia in children and adolescents, schizoaffective disorder; treatment resistant bipolar disorder in adults and adolescents; treatment resistant psychosis/agitation related to Alzheimer dementia and Lewy body disease

Pregnancy Risk Factor B

Pregnancy Considerations Adverse events were not observed in animal reproduction studies. Clozapine crosses the placenta and can be detected in the fetal blood and amniotic fluid (Barnas, 1994). Antipsychotic use during the third trimester of pregnancy has a risk for abnormal muscle movements (extrapyramidal symptoms [EPS]) and/or withdrawal symptoms in newborns following delivery. Symptoms in the newborn may include agitation, feeding disorder, hypertonia, hypotonia, respiratory distress, somnolence, and tremor; these effects may be self-limiting or require hospitalization.

Clozapine may theoretically cause agranulocytosis in the fetus and should not routinely be used in pregnancy (NICE, 2007). The ACOG recommends that therapy during pregnancy be individualized; treatment with psychiatric medications during pregnancy should incorporate the clinical expertise of the mental health clinician, obstetrician, primary healthcare provider, and pediatrician. Safety data related to atypical antipsychotics during pregnancy is limited and routine use is not recommended. However, if a woman is inadvertently exposed to an atypical antipsychotic while pregnant, continuing therapy may be preferable to switching to a typical antipsychotic that the fetus has not yet been exposed to; consider risk:benefit (ACOG, 2008). An increased risk of exacerbation of psychosis should be considered when discontinuing or changing treatment during pregnancy and postpartum.

Healthcare providers are encouraged to enroll women 18-45 years of age exposed to clozapine during pregnancy in the Atypical Antipsychotics Pregnancy Registry (1-866-961-2388 or http://www.womensmentalhealth.org/pregnancyregistry).

Women with amenorrhea associated with use of other antipsychotic agents may return to normal menstruation when switching to clozapine therapy. Reliable contraceptive measures should be employed by women of childbearing potential switching to clozapine therapy.

Breast-Feeding Considerations Clozapine was found to accumulate in breast milk in concentrations higher than the maternal plasma (Barnas, 1994). Breast-feeding is not recommended by the manufacturer. Clozapine may theoretically cause agranulocytosis in the nursing infant and should not routinely be used in women who are breast-feeding (NICE, 2007).

Prescribing and Access Restrictions

U.S.: Versacloz has a REMS program; Clozaril is deemed to have a REMS program (approval pending from FDA). As a requirement of the REMS program, access to this medication is restricted. Patient-specific registration is required to dispense clozapine. Information specific to each monitoring program is available from the individual manufacturers. If a patient is switched from one brand/manufacturer of clozapine to another, the patient must be entered into a new registry (must be completed by the prescriber and delivered to the dispensing pharmacy). Healthcare providers, including pharmacists dispensing clozapine, should verify the patient's hematological status and qualification to receive clozapine with all existing registries. The manufacturers of clozapine request that health care providers submit all WBC/ANC values following discontinuation of therapy to the registry for all non-rechallengable patients until WBC is ≥3500/mm^3 and ANC is ≥2000/mm^3. Further information is available at 1-877-329-2256 or at the following websites:
Clozaril: http://www.clozarilregistry.com
Fazaclo: https://www.fazacloregistry.com
Versacloz: http://www.versaclozregistry.com

Canada: Currently, there are multiple manufacturers that distribute clozapine and each manufacturer has its own registry and distribution system. Patients must be registered in a database that includes their location, prescribing physician, testing laboratory, and dispensing pharmacist before using clozapine. Information specific to each monitoring program is available from the individual manufacturers.

Contraindications Hypersensitivity to clozapine or any component of the formulation (eg, photosensitivity, vasculitis, erythema multiforme, or Stevens-Johnson syndrome [SJS]); history of clozapine-induced agranulocytosis or severe granulocytopenia

Canadian labeling: Additional contraindications (not in U.S. labeling): Active hepatic disease associated with nausea, anorexia, or jaundice; progressive hepatic disease or hepatic failure; severe renal impairment; severe cardiac disease (eg, myocarditis); patients unable to undergo blood testing

Warnings/Precautions [U.S. Boxed Warning]: Significant risk of potentially life-threatening agranulocytosis, defined as an ANC <500/mm³. Monitor ANC and WBC prior to and during treatment. ANC must be ≥2000/mm³ and WBC must be ≥3500/mm³ to begin treatment. Discontinue clozapine and do not rechallenge if ANC <1000/mm³ or WBC is <2000/mm³. Monitor for symptoms of agranulocytosis and infection (eg, fever, lethargy, or sore throat). Clozapine is only available through a restricted program requiring enrollment of prescribers, patients, and pharmacies to the Registry. Do not initiate in patients with a history of clozapine-induced agranulocytosis or granulocytopenia. Initial episodes of moderate leukopenia or granulopoietic suppression confer up to a 12-fold increased risk for subsequent episodes of agranulocytosis. Concurrent use with bone marrow suppressive agents or treatments also leads to an increased risk. WBCs must be monitored weekly for at least 4 weeks after therapy discontinuation or until WBC is ≥3500/mm³ and ANC is ≥2000/mm³. The restricted distribution system ensures appropriate WBC and ANC monitoring. Eosinophilia, defined as a blood eosinophil count of >700/mm³, has been reported to occur with clozapine and usually occurs within the first month of treatment. If eosinophilia develops, evaluate for signs or symptoms of systemic reactions (eg, rash or other allergic symptoms), myocarditis, or organ-specific disease. If systemic disease is suspected, discontinue clozapine immediately. If an eosinophilia cause unrelated to clozapine is identified treat the underlying cause and continue clozapine. In the absence of organ involvement continue clozapine under careful monitoring. If the total eosinophil count continues to increase over several weeks in the absence of systemic disease, base interruption of treatment and rechallenge (after eosinophil count decreases) on overall clinical assessment and consultation with internist or hematologist (**Note:** The Canadian labeling recommends discontinuing therapy for eosinophil count >3000/mm³; may resume therapy when eosinophil count <1000/mm³).

[U.S. Boxed Warning]: Elderly patients with dementia-related psychosis treated with antipsychotics are at an increased risk of death compared to placebo. Most deaths appeared to be either cardiovascular (eg, heart failure, sudden death) or infectious (eg, pneumonia) in nature. Clozapine is not approved for the treatment of dementia-related psychosis. Avoid antipsychotic use for behavioral problems associated with dementia unless alternative nonpharmacologic therapies have failed and patient may harm self or others. May also be inappropriate in older adults depending on comorbidities (eg, dementia, delirium) due to its potent anticholinergic effects (Beers Criteria). The elderly are more susceptible to adverse effects (including agranulocytosis, cardiovascular, anticholinergic, and tardive dyskinesia). An increased incidence of cerebrovascular effects (eg, transient ischemic attack, stroke), including fatalities, has been reported in placebo-controlled trials of atypical antipsychotics in elderly patients with dementia-related psychosis.

Cognitive and/or motor impairment (sedation) is common with clozapine, resulting in impaired performance of tasks requiring alertness (eg, operating machinery or driving); use caution in patients receiving general anesthesia. **[U.S. Boxed Warning]: Seizures have been associated with clozapine use in a dose-dependent manner. Initiate treatment with no more than 12.5 mg, titrate gradually using divided dosing. Use with caution in patients at risk of seizures, including those with a history of seizures, head trauma, brain damage, alcoholism, or concurrent therapy with medications which may lower seizure threshold. Patients should be warned that a sudden loss of consciousness may occur with seizures.** Benign transient temperature elevation (>100.4°F) may occur; peaking within the first 3 weeks of treatment. May be associated with an increase or decrease in WBC count. Rule out infection, agranulocytosis, and neuroleptic malignant syndrome (NMS) in patients presenting with fever. However, clozapine may also be associated with severe febrile reactions, including neuroleptic malignant syndrome (NMS). Clozapine's potential for extrapyramidal symptoms (including tardive dyskinesia) appears to be extremely low. Risk of dystonia (and probably other EPS) may be greater with increased doses, use of conventional antipsychotics, males, and younger patients.

[U.S. Boxed Warning]: Fatalities due to myocarditis and cardiomyopathy have been reported. Upon suspicion of these reactions discontinue clozapine and obtain a cardiac evaluation. Symptoms may include chest pain, tachycardia, palpitations, dyspenia, fever, flu-like symptoms, hypotension, or ECG changes. Patients with clozaril-related myocarditis or cardiomyopathy should generally not be rechallenged with clozapine. Myocarditis and cardiomyopathy may occur at any period during clozapine treatment, however, typically myocarditis presents within the first 2 months and cardiomyopathy after 8 weeks of treatment. Rare cases of thromboembolism, including pulmonary embolism and stroke resulting in fatalities, have been associated with clozapine. Clozapine is associated with QT prolongation and ventricular arrhythmias including torsade de pointes; cardiac arrest and sudden death may occur. Use caution in patients with a history of long QT syndrome, conditions which may increase the risk of QT prolongation (cardiovascular disease, recent MI, uncompensated heart failure, clinically significant arrhythmias, family history of long QT syndrome), concomitant use of medications known to prolong the QT interval, or treatment with medications that inhibit the metabolism of clozapine. Hypokalemia and/or hypomagnesemia may increase the risk. Consider obtaining a baseline ECG and serum chemistry panel. Correct electrolyte abnormalities prior to initiating therapy. Discontinue clozapine if QT_c interval >500 msec. Undesirable changes in lipids have been observed with antipsychotic therapy; incidence varies with product. Periodically monitor total serum cholesterol, triglycerides, LDL, and HDL concentrations.

Potentially significant drug-drug interactions may exist, requiring dose or frequency adjustment, additional monitoring, and/or selection of alternative therapy.

May cause anticholinergic effects; use with caution in patients with urinary retention, benign prostatic hyperplasia, narrow-angle glaucoma, xerostomia, visual problems, constipation, or history of bowel obstruction. Because of its potential to significantly decreased GI motility, use is associated with increased risk of paralytic ileus, bowel obstruction, fecal impaction, bowel perforation, and in rare cases death. Bowel regimens and monitoring are recommended. May cause hyperglycemia; in some cases may be extreme and associated with ketoacidosis, hyperosmolar coma, or death. Monitor for symptoms of hyperglycemia including polydipsia, polyuria, polyphagia, and weakness. Use with caution in patients with diabetes or other disorders of glucose regulation; monitor for worsening of glucose control. Antipsychotic use has been associated with esophageal dysmotility and aspiration; use with caution in patients at risk of aspiration pneumonia (eg, Alzheimer disease). Use with caution in patients with hepatic disease or impairment; monitor hepatic function regularly. Hepatitis has been reported as a consequence of therapy. Discontinuation of therapy may be necessary with significant elevations in liver function tests; may reinitiate with close monitoring and if values return to normal. Use with caution in patients with renal disease.

Use caution with cardiovascular or pulmonary disease; gradually increase dose. **[U.S. Boxed Warning]: Orthostatic hypotension, bradycardia, syncope, and cardiac arrest have been reported with clozapine treatment. Risk is highest during the initial titration period and with rapid dose increases. Symptoms can develop with the first dose and with doses as low as 12.5 mg per day. Initiate treatment with no more than 12.5 mg once daily or twice daily, titrate slowly, and use divided doses. Use with caution in patients at risk for these effects (eg, cerebrovascular disease, cardiovascular disease) or with predisposing conditions for hypotensive episodes (eg, hypovolemia, concurrent antihypertensive medication);** reactions can be fatal. Consider dose reduction if hypotension occurs. May cause tachycardia (including sustained); sustained tachycardia is not limited to a reflex response to orthostatic hypotension, and is present in all positions.

The possibility of a suicide attempt is inherent in psychotic illness or bipolar disorder; use caution in high-risk patients during initiation of therapy. Prescriptions should be written for the smallest quantity consistent with good patient care. Medication should not be stopped abruptly; taper off over 1-2 weeks. If conditions warrant abrupt discontinuation (eg, leukopenia, myocarditis, cardiomyopathy), monitor patient for psychosis and cholinergic rebound (eg, headache, nausea, vomiting, diarrhea, profuse diaphoresis). Significant weight gain has been observed with antipsychotic therapy; incidence varies with product. Monitor waist circumference and BMI. Clozapine levels may be lower in patients who smoke. Smoking cessation may cause toxicity in a patient stabilized on clozapine. Monitor change in smoking. Clozapine concentrations may be increased in CYP2D6 poor metabolizers; dose reduction may be necessary. FazaClo oral disintegrating tablets contain phenylalanine.

Adverse Reactions

>10%:

- Cardiovascular: Tachycardia (25%)
- Central nervous system: Drowsiness (39% to 46%), dizziness (19% to 27%), insomnia (2% to 20%)
- Gastrointestinal: Sialorrhea (31% to 48%), weight gain (4% to 31%), constipation (14% to 25%),nausea/vomiting (3% to 17%), abdominal discomfort/heartburn (4% to 14%)

1% to 10%:

- Cardiovascular: Hypotension (9%), syncope (6%), hypertension (4%), angina (1%), ECG changes (1%)
- Central nervous system: Headache (7%), fever (5%), agitation (4%), akinesia (4%), nightmares (4%), restlessness (4%), akathisia (3%), confusion (3%), seizure (3%), fatigue (2%), anxiety (1%), ataxia (1%), depression (1%), lethargy (1%), myoclonic jerks (1%), slurred speech (1%)
- Dermatologic: Rash (2%)
- Gastrointestinal: Xerostomia (6%), diarrhea (2%), anorexia (1%), throat discomfort (1%)
- Genitourinary: Urinary abnormalities (eg, abnormal ejaculation, retention, urgency, incontinence; 1% to 2%)
- Hematologic: Leukopenia (3%), agranulocytosis (1%), eosinophilia (1%)
- Hepatic: Liver function tests abnormal (1%)
- Neuromuscular & skeletal: Tremor (6%), hypokinesia (4%), rigidity (3%), hyperkinesia (1%), weakness (1%), pain (1%), spasm (1%)
- Ocular: Visual disturbances (5%)
- Respiratory: Dyspnea (1%), nasal congestion (1%)
- Miscellaneous: Diaphoresis (6%), tongue numbness (1%)

<1%, postmarketing, and/or case reports (limited to important or life-threatening): Amentia, amnesia, anemia, arrhythmia (atrial or ventricular), aspiration, blurred vision, bradycardia, bronchitis, cardiomyopathy (usually dilated), cataplexy, CHF, cholestasis, CPK increased, cyanosis, delirium, delusions, dermatitis, diabetes mellitus, difficult urination, DVT, dysphagia, eczema, edema, EEG abnormal, erythema multiforme, ESR increased, fecal impaction, gastric ulcer, gastroenteritis, granulocytopenia, hallucinations, hematemesis, hepatitis, hypercholesterolemia (rare), hyperglycemia, hypersensitivity reaction, hypertriglyceridemia (rare), hyperuricemia, hyponatremia, hyperosmolar coma, hypothermia, impotence, interstitial nephritis (acute), intestinal obstruction, jaundice, ketoacidosis, loss of speech, metabolic syndrome (Lamberti, 2006), MI, mitral valve insufficiency, myasthenia syndrome, mydriasis, myocarditis, narrow-angle glaucoma, neuroleptic malignant syndrome, obsessive compulsive symptoms, palpitations, pancreatitis (acute), paralytic ileus, paresthesia, Parkinsonism, pericardial effusion, pericarditis, periorbital edema, phlebitis, photosensitivity, pleural effusion, pneumonia, priapism, pruritus, psychosis exacerbated, pulmonary embolism, rectal bleeding, respiratory arrest, rhabdomyolysis, salivary gland swelling, sepsis, status epilepticus, stroke, Stevens-Johnson syndrome, tardive dyskinesia, thrombocytopenia, thrombocytosis, thromboembolism, thrombophlebitis, torsade de pointes, urticaria, vasculitis, weight loss, wheezing

Drug Interactions

Metabolism/Transport Effects

Substrate of CYP1A2 (major), CYP2A6 (minor), CYP2C19 (minor), CYP2C9 (minor), CYP2D6 (minor), CYP3A4 (minor); **Note:** Assignment of Major/Minor substrate status based on clinically relevant drug interaction potential; **Inhibits** CYP1A2 (weak), CYP2C19 (weak), CYP2C9 (weak), CYP2D6 (moderate), CYP2E1 (weak), CYP3A4 (weak)

Avoid Concomitant Use

Avoid concomitant use of CloZAPine with any of the following: Aclidinium; Amisulpride; Azelastine (Nasal); CarBAMazepine; Ciprofloxacin (Systemic); CYP3A4 Inducers (Strong); Highest Risk QTc-Prolonging Agents; Ipratropium (Oral Inhalation); Ivabradine; Metoclopramide; Mifepristone; Myelosuppressive Agents; Paraldehyde; Sulpiride; Thioridazine; Tiotropium; Umeclidinium

Increased Effect/Toxicity

CloZAPine may increase the levels/effects of: Alcohol (Ethyl); Amisulpride; Analgesics (Opioid); Anticholinergics; ARIPiprazole; Azelastine (Nasal); Buprenorphine; CNS Depressants; CYP2D6 Substrates; Fesoterodine; Highest Risk QTc-Prolonging Agents; Hydrocodone; Lomitapide; Methotrimeprazine; Methylphenidate; Metoprolol; Moderate Risk QTc-Prolonging Agents; Nebivolol; Paraldehyde; Serotonin Modulators; Sulpiride; Thioridazine; Tiotropium; Zolpidem

The levels/effects of CloZAPine may be increased by: Abiraterone Acetate; Acetylcholinesterase Inhibitors (Central); Aclidinium; Benzodiazepines; Brimonidine (Topical); CarBAMazepine; Cimetidine; Ciprofloxacin (Systemic); CYP1A2 Inhibitors (Moderate); CYP1A2 Inhibitors (Strong); Deferasirox; Doxylamine; HydrOXYzine; Ipratropium (Oral Inhalation); Ivabradine; Lithium formulations; Macrolide Antibiotics; Magnesium Sulfate; MAO Inhibitors; Methotrimeprazine; Methylphenidate; Metoclopramide; Metyrosine; Mifepristone; Myelosuppressive Agents; Nefazodone; Omeprazole; Perampanel; Pramlintide; QTc-Prolonging Agents (Indeterminate Risk and Risk Modifying); Selective Serotonin Reuptake Inhibitors; Serotonin Modulators; Sodium Oxybate; Tetrabenazine; Umeclidinium

Decreased Effect

CloZAPine may decrease the levels/effects of: Amphetamines; Anti-Parkinson's Agents (Dopamine Agonist); Codeine; Quinagolide; Tamoxifen

The levels/effects of CloZAPine may be decreased by: CarBAMazepine; CYP3A4 Inducers (Strong); Cyproterone; Lithium formulations; Omeprazole

Ethanol/Nutrition/Herb Interactions

Ethanol: May increase CNS depression; monitor for increased effects with coadministration. Caution patients about effects.

Herb/Nutraceutical: St John's wort may decrease clozapine levels. Avoid kava kava, gotu kola, valerian, St John's wort (may increase CNS depression).

Storage/Stability

Suspension: Store at ≤25°C (77°F). Protect from light. Do not refrigerate or freeze. Suspension is stable for 100 days after initial bottle opening.

Tablet: Store at ≤30°C (86°F).

Tablet, dispersible: Store at 20°C to 25°C (68°F to 77°F); excursions permitted to 15°C to 30°C (59°F to 86°F). Protect from moisture; do not remove from package until ready to use.

Mechanism of Action The therapeutic efficacy of clozapine (dibenzodiazepine antipsychotic) is proposed to be mediated through antagonism of the dopamine type 2 (D_2) and serotonin type 2A ($5\text{-}HT_{2A}$) receptors. In addition, it acts as an antagonist at alpha-adrenergic, histamine H_1, cholinergic, and other dopaminergic and serotonergic receptors.

Pharmacodynamics/Kinetics

Protein binding: 97% to serum proteins

Metabolism: Extensively hepatic; forms metabolites with limited or no activity

Bioavailability: 50% to 60% (not affected by food)

Half-life elimination: Steady state: 12 hours (range: 4-66 hours)

Time to peak: Suspension: 2.2 hours (range: 1-3.5 hours); Tablets: 2.5 hours (range: 1-6 hours)

Excretion: Urine (~50%) and feces (30%) with trace amounts of unchanged drug

Dosage Note: When converting a patient from other antipsychotics to clozapine therapy, the dosage of the other antipsychotics should be reduced or discontinued (based on clinical circumstances) by gradual tapering downwards before initiating clozapine. Combination use with other antipsychotics is not generally recommended.

Schizophrenia: Oral:

Adults: Initial: 12.5 mg once or twice daily; increased, as tolerated, in increments of 25-50 mg daily to a target dose of 300-450 mg daily (administered in divided doses) by the end of 2 weeks; may further titrate in increments not exceeding 100 mg and no more frequently than once or twice weekly. Maximum total daily dose: 900 mg. **Note:** In some efficacy studies, total daily dosage was administered in 3 divided doses.

Elderly: Experience in the elderly is limited; may initiate with 12.5 once daily for 3 days, then increase to 25 mg once daily for 3 days as tolerated; may further increase, as tolerated, in increments of 12.5-25 mg daily every 3 days to desired response; maximum total daily dosage: 300 mg (Howanitz, 1999). Mean recommended dosage range: 25-150 mg (in divided doses) (De Fazio, 2003).

Suicidal behavior in schizophrenia or schizoaffective disorder: Adults: Oral: Initial: 12.5 mg once or twice daily; increased, as tolerated, in increments of 25-50 mg daily to a target dose of 300-450 mg daily (administered in divided doses) by the end of 2 weeks; mean dose is ~300 mg daily (some patients may require up to 900 mg daily in 3 divided doses). **Note:** If no longer a suicide risk, may resume prior antipsychotic therapy after gradually tapering off clozapine over 1-2 weeks (Meltzer 2003; Wagstaff 2003).

Bipolar disorder (unlabeled use): Adults: Oral: Initial: 25 mg daily; increased, as tolerated in increments of 25 mg daily to a maximum dose of 550 mg daily. Average daily dose ~300 mg daily (Green, 2000).

Psychosis/agitation related to Alzheimer's dementia (unlabeled use): Elderly: Oral: Initial: 12.5 mg once daily; if necessary, gradually increase as tolerated not to exceed 75-100 mg daily (Rabins, 2007). Bipolar disorder (unlabeled use): Adults: Oral: Initial: 25 mg daily; increased, as tolerated in increments of 25 mg daily to a maximum dose of 550 mg daily. Average daily dose ~300 mg daily (Green, 2000).

Schizoaffective disorder (unlabeled use): Adults: Oral: Initial: 25 mg daily; increased, as tolerated to a maximum dose of 600 mg daily. Average daily dose: ~200 mg daily (Ciapparelli, 2003).

Reinitiation of therapy: If dosing is interrupted for ≥48 hours, therapy must be reinitiated at 12.5-25 mg daily; may be increased more rapidly than with initial titration, unless cardiopulmonary arrest occurred during initial titration, then retitrate with extreme caution.

Termination of therapy: In the event of planned termination of clozapine, gradual reduction in dose over a 1- to 2-week period is recommended. If conditions warrant abrupt discontinuation (eg, leukopenia), monitor patient for psychosis and cholinergic rebound (eg, headache, nausea, vomiting, diarrhea, profuse diaphoresis).

Dosage adjustment for toxicity:

Hematologic toxicity:

Eosinophilia: Canadian labeling: Interrupt therapy for eosinophil count >3000/mm^3; may resume therapy when eosinophil count <1000/mm^3

Leukopenia/granulocytopenia:

Mild (WBC 3000-3500/mm^3 and/or ANC 1500-2000/mm^3): Continue treatment; monitor WBC and ANC twice weekly until WBC >3500/mm^3 and ANC >2000/mm^3 then return to previous monitoring schedule.

Moderate (WBC 2000-3000/mm^3 and/or ANC 1000-1500/mm^3): Interrupt therapy and begin daily WBC/ANC monitoring until WBC >3000/mm^3 and ANC >1500/mm^3 followed by twice weekly monitoring until WBC >3500/mm^3 and ANC >2000/mm^3, then may consider restarting therapy; weekly WBC/ANC monitoring is required for 12 months in patients restarted on clozapine treatment. **Note:** Patient is at greater risk for developing agranulocytosis.

Severe (WBC <2000/mm^3 and/or ANC <1000/mm^3 [U.S. labeling] or ANC <1500/mm^3 [Canadian labeling]) or agranulocytosis (ANC <500/mm^3): Discontinue treatment and do not rechallenge patient; continue to monitor WBC/ANC daily for at least 4 weeks from day of discontinuation and until WBC >3000/mm^3 and ANC >1500/mm^3, then twice weekly until WBC >3500/mm^3 and ANC >2000/mm^3, then weekly after WBC >3500/mm^3.

Thrombocytopenia: Platelets <50,000/mm^3: Canadian labeling recommends discontinuing therapy.

Nonhematologic toxicity:

QT_c interval >500 msec, cardiomyopathy/myocarditis, hepatotoxicity (clinically relevant transaminase elevations or jaundice symptoms), or neuroleptic malignant syndrome: Discontinue use. Patients who develop cardiomyopathy may continue use if the benefit outweighs the risk. Do not rechallenge if patient develops myocarditis. If antipsychotic therapy is required following neuroleptic malignant syndrome, use with caution as symptoms can recur.

Note: If therapy is interrupted for reasons other than leukopenia/granulocytopenia and rechallenge is considered, the 6-month time period for initiation of biweekly WBCs may need to be reset. This determination depends upon the treatment duration, the length of the break in therapy, and whether or not an abnormal blood event occurred.

Dosage adjustment in renal impairment: No dosage adjustment provided in manufacturer's labeling (has not been studied); use with caution.

Dosage adjustment in hepatic impairment: No dosage adjustment provided in manufacturer's labeling; use with caution.

Dietary Considerations May be taken without regard to food. Some products may contain phenylalanine.

Administration May be taken without regard to food. Total daily dose may be divided into uneven doses with larger dose administered at bedtime.

Canadian labeling: Maintenance dosing ≤200 mg daily may be administered as single dose in the evening.

Orally-disintegrating tablet: Should be removed from foil blister by peeling apart (do not push tablet through the foil). Remove immediately prior to use. Place tablet in mouth and chew or allow to dissolve; swallow with saliva. If dosing requires splitting tablet, throw unused portion away.

Suspension: Shake bottle prior to use. Using syringe adaptor and oral syringe provided withdrawal dose from bottle. Administer immediately after preparation using the oral syringe provided.

Monitoring Parameters Note: The Canadian labeling recommends initiating treatment in an inpatient setting or an outpatient setting with medical supervision and monitoring of vital signs for at least 6-8 hours after the first few doses.

Mental status, ECG, WBC (see below), vital signs, fasting lipid profile and fasting blood glucose/Hgb A_{1c} (prior to treatment, at 3 months, then annually; liver function tests; electrolytes (baseline, then periodic); BMI, personal/family history of obesity; waist circumference (weight should be assessed prior to treatment, at 4 weeks, 8 weeks, 12 weeks, and then at quarterly intervals. Consider titrating to a different antipsychotic agent for a weight gain ≥5% of the initial weight); blood pressure; abnormal involuntary movement scale (AIMS). If tachycardia develops, monitor for signs of myocarditis; signs and symptoms of neuroleptic malignant syndrome.

WBC and ANC should be obtained at baseline and at least weekly for the first 6 months (26 weeks) of continuous treatment. If counts remain acceptable (WBC ≥3500/mm^3, ANC ≥2000/mm^3) during this time period, then they may be monitored every other week for the next 6 months (26 weeks). If WBC/ANC continue to remain within these acceptable limits after the second 6 months (26 weeks) of therapy, monitoring can be decreased to every 4 weeks. If clozapine is discontinued, a weekly WBC should be conducted for an additional 4 weeks or until WBC is ≥3500/mm^3 and ANC is ≥2000/mm^3. **Note:** When therapy is interrupted for >3 days, the Canadian labeling recommends weekly hematologic testing for an additional 6 weeks.

Monitoring for hematologic toxicity:

Mild leukopenia/granulocytopenia (WBC 3000-3500/mm^3 and/or ANC 1500-2000/mm^3): Monitor WBC and ANC twice weekly until WBC >3500/mm^3 and ANC >2000/mm^3 then return to previous monitoring schedule.

Moderate leukopenia/granulocytopenia (WBC 2000-3000/mm^3 and/or ANC 1000-1500/mm^3): Begin daily WBC/ANC monitoring until WBC >3000/mm^3 and ANC >1500/mm^3, followed by twice weekly monitoring until WBC >3500/mm^3 and ANC >2000/mm^3, after restarting therapy, weekly WBC/ANC monitoring is required for 12 months. **Note:** Patient is at greater risk for developing agranulocytosis.

Severe leukopenia/granulocytopenia (WBC <2000/mm^3 and/or ANC <1000/mm^3 [U.S. labeling] or ANC <1500/mm^3 [Canadian labeling]) or agranulocytosis (ANC <500/mm^3): Discontinue treatment and do not rechallenge patient; continue to monitor WBC/ANC daily for at least 4 weeks from day of discontinuation and until WBC >3000/mm^3 and ANC >1500/mm^3, then twice weekly until WBC >3500/mm^3 and ANC >2000/mm^3, then weekly after WBC >3500/mm^3.

Monitoring for nonhematologic toxicity: If therapy is interrupted for reasons other than leukopenia/granulocytopenia and rechallenge is considered, the 6-month time period for initiation of biweekly WBCs may need to be reset. This determination depends upon the treatment duration, the length of the break in therapy, and whether or not an abnormal blood event occurred.

Reference Range Clozapine levels >350 ng/mL may be associated with an increased likelihood of clinical response. However, increases of serum concentrations above this have not been shown to confer greater improvements and may increase the risk of adverse events (Remington 2013).

Product Availability Versacloz oral suspension: FDA approved February 2013; anticipated availability in Fall 2013. Consult prescribing information for additional information.

Dosage Forms Excipient information presented when available (limited, particularly for generics); consult specific product labeling.

Suspension, Oral:
- Versacloz: 50 mg/mL (100 mL) [contains methylparaben sodium, propylparaben sodium]

Tablet, Oral:
- Clozaril: 25 mg, 100 mg [scored]
- Generic: 25 mg, 50 mg, 100 mg, 200 mg

Tablet Dispersible, Oral:
- FazaClo: 12.5 mg, 25 mg, 100 mg, 150 mg, 200 mg [contains aspartame]
- Generic: 12.5 mg, 25 mg, 100 mg

- ◆ **Clozaril** *see* CloZAPine *on page* *477*
- ◆ **CMA-676** *see* Gemtuzumab Ozogamicin *on page* *950*
- ◆ **C-Met/Hepatocyte Growth Factor Receptor Tyrosine Kinase Inhibitor PF-02341066** *see* Crizotinib *on page* *497*
- ◆ **C-Met/HGFR Tyrosine Kinase Inhibitor PF-02341066** *see* Crizotinib *on page* *497*
- ◆ **CMV Hyperimmune Globulin** *see* Cytomegalovirus Immune Globulin (Intravenous-Human) *on page* *523*
- ◆ **CMV-IGIV** *see* Cytomegalovirus Immune Globulin (Intravenous-Human) *on page* *523*
- ◆ **CNJ-016®** *see* Vaccinia Immune Globulin (Intravenous) *on page* *2143*
- ◆ **CNL8 Nail** *see* Ciclopirox *on page* *423*
- ◆ **CNTO-148** *see* Golimumab *on page* *968*
- ◆ **CNTO 1275** *see* Ustekinumab *on page* *2142*
- ◆ **Coagulant Complex Inhibitor** *see* Anti-inhibitor Coagulant Complex (Human) *on page* *147*
- ◆ **Coagulation Factor I** *see* Fibrinogen Concentrate (Human) *on page* *858*
- ◆ **Coagulation Factor VIIa** *see* Factor VIIa (Recombinant) *on page* *821*
- ◆ **CO Alendronate (Can)** *see* Alendronate *on page* *69*
- ◆ **CO Amlodipine (Can)** *see* AmLODIPine *on page* *109*
- ◆ **Co-Anastrozole (Can)** *see* Anastrozole *on page* *137*
- ◆ **Coartem** *see* Artemether and Lumefantrine *on page* *171*
- ◆ **CO Atenolol (Can)** *see* Atenolol *on page* *186*
- ◆ **CO Atorvastatin (Can)** *see* AtorvaSTATin *on page* *190*

◆ **CO Azithromycin (Can)** *see* Azithromycin (Systemic) *on page 214*

◆ **CO Bicalutamide (Can)** *see* Bicalutamide *on page 258*

◆ **Cobicistat, Emtricitabine, Tenofovir, and Elvitegravir** *see* Elvitegravir, Cobicistat, Emtricitabine, and Tenofovir *on page 696*

◆ **CO Bosentan (Can)** *see* Bosentan *on page 273*

◆ **CO Cabergoline (Can)** *see* Cabergoline *on page 309*

Cocaine (koe KANE)

Index Terms Cocaine Hydrochloride

Pharmacologic Category Local Anesthetic

Use Topical anesthesia (and vasoconstriction) for mucous membranes

Pregnancy Risk Factor C

Dosage Topical application (ear, nose, throat, bronchoscopy): Dosage depends on the area to be anesthetized, tissue vascularity, technique of anesthesia, and individual patient tolerance; the lowest dose necessary to produce adequate anesthesia should be used; concentrations of 1% to 10% may be used, with 4% being the most frequently used concentration (maximum total dose: 3 mg/kg **or** 200 mg) (Liao, 1999). Lasts for 30 minutes or longer depending on concentration and vascularity of anesthetized tissue. Use reduced dosages for children, elderly, or debilitated patients.

Additional Information Complete prescribing information should be consulted for additional detail.

Dosage Forms Excipient information presented when available (limited, particularly for generics); consult specific product labeling.

Solution, External, as hydrochloride:

Generic: 4% (4 mL, 10 mL); 10% (4 mL)

Controlled Substance C-II

◆ **Cocaine Hydrochloride** *see* Cocaine *on page 482*

◆ **CO Candesartan (Can)** *see* Candesartan *on page 327*

◆ **Co-Candesartan/HCT (Can)** *see* Candesartan and Hydrochlorothiazide *on page 329*

◆ **CO Ciprofloxacin (Can)** *see* Ciprofloxacin (Systemic) *on page 430*

◆ **CO Citalopram (Can)** *see* Citalopram *on page 440*

◆ **CO Clomipramine (Can)** *see* ClomiPRAMINE *on page 462*

◆ **CO Clonazepam (Can)** *see* ClonazePAM *on page 465*

◆ **CO Clopidogrel (Can)** *see* Clopidogrel *on page 471*

◆ **Codar® GF** *see* Guaifenesin and Codeine *on page 976*

Codeine (KOE deen)

Brand Names: Canada Codeine Contin®; PMS-Codeine; ratio-Codeine

Index Terms Codeine Phosphate; Codeine Sulfate; Methylmorphine

Pharmacologic Category Analgesic, Opioid; Antitussive

Use Management of mild-to-moderately-severe pain

Unlabeled Use Short-term relief of cough in select patients

Pregnancy Risk Factor C

Pregnancy Considerations Adverse events have been observed in animal reproduction studies. Opioid analgesics cross the placenta. In humans, birth defects (including some heart defects) have been associated with maternal use of codeine during the first trimester of pregnancy (Broussard, 2011). If chronic opioid exposure occurs in pregnancy, adverse events in the newborn (including withdrawal) may occur; monitoring of the neonate is recommended. The minimum effective dose should be used if opioids are needed (Chou, 2009). Neonatal abstinence syndrome following opioid exposure may present with autonomic (eg, fever, temperature instability), gastrointestinal (eg, diarrhea, vomiting, poor feeding/weight gain), or neurologic (eg, high pitched crying, increased muscle tone, irritability, seizure, tremor) symptoms (Dow, 2012; Hudak, 2012).

Breast-Feeding Considerations Codeine and its metabolite (morphine) are found in breast milk and can be detected in the serum of nursing infants. The relative dose to a nursing infant has been calculated to be ~1% of the weight-adjusted maternal dose (Spigset, 2000). Higher levels of morphine may be found in the breast milk of lactating mothers who are "ultrarapid metabolizers" of codeine; patients with two or more copies of the variant CYP2D6*2 allele may have extensive conversion to morphine and thus increased opioid-mediated effects. In one case, excessively high serum concentrations of morphine were reported in a breast-fed infant following maternal use of acetaminophen with codeine. The mother was later found to be an "ultrarapid metabolizer" of codeine; symptoms in the infant included feeding difficulty and lethargy, followed by death. Caution should be used since most persons are not aware if they have the genotype resulting in "ultra-rapid metabolizer" status. When codeine is used in breast-feeding women, it is recommended to use the lowest dose for the shortest duration of time and observe the infant for increased sleepiness, difficulty in feeding or breathing, or limpness (FDA, 2007; Koren, 2006). The manufacturer recommends that caution be used if administered to a nursing woman. According to other guidelines, when treatment is needed for pain in nursing women, other agents should be used; if codeine cannot be avoided it should not be used for >4 days (Kahan, 2011; Wong, 2011).

Medication Guide Available Yes

Contraindications Hypersensitivity to codeine or any component of the formulation; respiratory depression in the absence of resuscitative equipment; acute or severe bronchial asthma or hypercarbia; presence or suspicion of paralytic ileus; postoperative pain management in children who have undergone tonsillectomy and/or adenoidectomy

Canadian labeling: Additional contraindications (not in U.S. labeling): Hypersensitivity to other opioid analgesics; cor pulmonale; acute alcoholism; delirium tremens; severe CNS depression; convulsive disorders; increased cerebrospinal or intracranial pressure; head injury; suspected surgical abdomen; use with or within 14 days of MAO inhibitors.

Warnings/Precautions [U.S. Boxed Warning]: Respiratory depression and death have occurred in children who received codeine following tonsillectomy and/or adenoidectomy and were found to have evidence of being ultra-rapid metabolizers of codeine due to a CYP2D6 polymorphism. Deaths have also occurred in nursing infants after being exposed to high concentrations of morphine because the mothers were ultra-rapid metabolizers. Use is contraindicated in the postoperative pain management of children who have undergone tonsillectomy and/or adenoidectomy. Use caution in patients with two or more copies of the variant CYP2D6*2 allele; may have extensive conversion to morphine and thus increased opioid-mediated effects. Avoid the use of codeine in these patients; consider alternative analgesics such as morphine or a nonopioid agent (Crews, 2012). The occurrence of this phenotype is seen in 0.5% to 1% of Chinese and Japanese, 0.5% to 1% of Hispanics, 1% to 10% of Caucasians, 3% of African-Americans, and 1% to 28% of North Africans, Ethiopians, and Arabs.

May cause dose-related respiratory depression. The risk is increased in elderly patients, debilitated patients, and patients with conditions associated with hypoxia, hypercapnia, or upper airway obstruction. Use with caution in patients with pre-existing respiratory compromise (hypoxia and/or hypercapnia), COPD or other obstructive pulmonary disease, and kyphoscoliosis or other skeletal disorder which may alter respiratory function; critical respiratory depression may occur, even at therapeutic dosages.

After chronic maternal exposure to opioids, neonatal withdrawal syndrome may occur in the newborn; monitor neonate closely. Signs and symptoms include irritability, hyperactivity and abnormal sleep pattern, high pitched cry, tremor, vomiting, diarrhea and failure to gain weight. Onset, duration and severity depend on the drug used, duration of use, maternal dose, and rate of drug elimination by the newborn. Opioid withdrawal syndrome in the neonate, unlike in adults, may be life-threatening and should be treated according to protocols developed by neonatology experts.

Use may cause or aggravate constipation; chronic use may result in obstructive bowel disease, particularly in those with underlying intestinal motility disorders. Avoid use in patients with gastrointestinal obstruction, particularly paralytic ileus. May cause hypotension; use with caution in patients with hypovolemia, cardiovascular disease (including acute MI), or drugs which may exaggerate hypotensive effects (including phenothiazines or general anesthetics). May cause CNS depression, which may impair physical or mental abilities; patients must be cautioned about performing tasks which require mental alertness (eg, operating machinery or driving).

Use with extreme caution in patients with head injury, intracranial lesions, or elevated intracranial pressure; exaggerated elevation of ICP may occur. Use with caution in patients with hypersensitivity reactions to other phenanthrene-derivative opioid agonists (hydrocodone, hydromorphone, levorphanol, oxycodone, oxymorphone), adrenal insufficiency (including Addison's disease), biliary tract dysfunction, pancreatitis, thyroid dysfunction, morbid obesity, prostatic hyperplasia and/or urinary stricture, or severe hepatic or renal impairment. Use may obscure diagnosis or clinical course of patients with acute abdominal conditions. May induce or aggravate seizures; use with caution in patients with seizure disorders. Avoid use in patients with CNS depression or coma as these patients are susceptible to intracranial effects of CO_2 retention.

Use with caution in patients with a history of drug abuse or acute alcoholism; potential for drug dependency exists. Tolerance, psychological and physical dependence may occur with prolonged use. Potentially significant drug interactions may exist, requiring dose or frequency adjustment, additional monitoring, and/or selection of alternative therapy. Effects may be potentiated when used with other sedative drugs or ethanol. Concurrent use of agonist/antagonist analgesics may precipitate withdrawal symptoms and/or reduced analgesic efficacy in patients following prolonged therapy with mu opioid agonists. Abrupt discontinuation following prolonged use may also lead to withdrawal symptoms.

Some preparations contain sulfites which may cause allergic reactions. Healthcare provider should be alert to the potential for abuse, misuse, and diversion.

Adverse Reactions Frequency not defined.

Cardiovascular: Bradycardia, cardiac arrest, circulatory depression, flushing, hyper-/hypotension, palpitation, shock, syncope, tachycardia

Central nervous system: Abnormal dreams, agitation, anxiety, apprehension, chills, coordination impaired, depression, disorientation, dizziness, drowsiness, dysphoria, euphoria, faintness, fatigue, hallucinations, headache, insomnia, intracranial pressure increased, lightheadedness, nervousness, sedation, shakiness, somnolence, vertigo

Dermatologic: Pruritus, rash, urticaria

Gastrointestinal: Abdominal cramps/pain, anorexia, biliary tract spasm, constipation, diarrhea, nausea, pancreatitis, taste disturbance, vomiting, xerostomia

Genitourinary: Urinary hesitancy/retention

Neuromuscular & skeletal: Paresthesia, rigidity, tremor, weakness

Ocular: Blurred vision, diplopia, miosis, nystagmus, visual disturbances

Respiratory: Bronchospasm, dyspnea, laryngospasm, respiratory arrest, respiratory depression

Miscellaneous: Allergic reaction, diaphoresis

Drug Interactions

Metabolism/Transport Effects **Substrate** of CYP2D6 (major); **Note:** Assignment of Major/Minor substrate status based on clinically relevant drug interaction potential

Avoid Concomitant Use

Avoid concomitant use of Codeine with any of the following: Azelastine (Nasal); Paraldehyde

Increased Effect/Toxicity

Codeine may increase the levels/effects of: Alcohol (Ethyl); Alvimopan; Azelastine (Nasal); CNS Depressants; Desmopressin; Diuretics; Hydrocodone; Metyrosine; Mirtazapine; Paraldehyde; Pramipexole; ROPINIRole; Rotigotine; Selective Serotonin Reuptake Inhibitors; Zolpidem

The levels/effects of Codeine may be increased by: Amphetamines; Anticholinergics; Antipsychotic Agents (Phenothiazines); Brimonidine (Topical); Cannabinoids; Doxylamine; Droperidol; HydrOXYzine; Magnesium Sulfate; Perampanel; Sodium Oxybate; Somatostatin Analogs; Succinylcholine; Tapentadol

Decreased Effect

Codeine may decrease the levels/effects of: Pegvisomant

The levels/effects of Codeine may be decreased by: Ammonium Chloride; CYP2D6 Inhibitors (Moderate); CYP2D6 Inhibitors (Strong); Mixed Agonist / Antagonist Opioids

Ethanol/Nutrition/Herb Interactions

Ethanol: May increase CNS depression; monitor for increased effects with coadministration. Caution patients about effects.

Herb/Nutraceutical: St John's wort may decrease codeine levels. Avoid valerian, St John's wort, kava kava, gotu kola (may increase CNS depression).

Storage/Stability Oral solution, tablet: Store at controlled room temperature.

Mechanism of Action Binds to opioid receptors in the CNS, causing inhibition of ascending pain pathways, altering the perception of and response to pain; causes cough suppression by direct central action in the medulla; produces generalized CNS depression

Pharmacodynamics/Kinetics

Onset of action: Oral: Immediate release: 0.5-1 hour

Peak effect: Oral: Immediate release: 1-1.5 hours

Duration: Immediate release: 4-6 hours

Distribution: ~3-6 L/kg

Protein binding: ~7% to 25%

Metabolism: Hepatic via UGT2B7 and UGT2B4 to codeine-6-glucuronide, via CYP2D6 to morphine (active), and via CYP3A4 to norcodeine. Morphine is further metabolized via glucuronidation to morphine-3-glucuronide and morphine-6-glucuronide (active).

Bioavailability: 53%

Half-life elimination: ~3 hours

Time to peak, plasma: Immediate release: 1 hour; Controlled release (Canadian availability; not available in the U.S.): 3.3 hours

Excretion: Urine (~90%, ~10% of the total dose as unchanged drug); feces

Dosage Oral:

Pain management (analgesic): **Note:** These are guidelines and do not represent the maximum doses that may be required in all patients. Doses should be titrated to pain relief/prevention.

Children (unlabeled use): Immediate release (tablet, oral solution): Initial: 0.5-1 mg/kg/dose every 4 hours as needed; maximum: 60 mg/dose (American Pain Society, 2008)

Adults:

Immediate release (tablet, oral solution): Initial: 15-60 mg every 4 hours as needed; maximum total daily dose: 360 mg/day; patients with prior opioid exposure may require higher initial doses. **Note:** The American Pain Society recommends an initial dose of 30-60 mg for adults with moderate pain (American Pain Society, 2008).

Controlled release: Codeine Contin® (Canadian availability; not available in U.S.): **Note:** Titrate at intervals of ≥48 hours until adequate analgesia has been achieved. Daily doses >600 mg/day should not be used; patients requiring higher doses should be switched to an opioid approved for use in severe pain. In patients who receive both Codeine Contin® and an immediate release or combination codeine product for breakthrough pain, the rescue dose of the immediate release codeine product should be ≤12.5% of the total daily Codeine Contin® dose.

Opioid-naive patients: Initial: 50 mg every 12 hours

Conversion from immediate release codeine preparations: Immediate release codeine preparations contain ~75% codeine base. Therefore, patients who are switching from immediate release codeine preparations may be transferred to a ~25% lower total daily dose of Codeine Contin®, equally divided into 2 daily doses.

*Conversion from a combination codeine product (eg, codeine with acetaminophen **or** aspirin):* See table:

Number of 30 mg Codeine Combination Tablets Daily	Initial Dose of Codeine Contin®	Maintenance Dose of Codeine Contin®
≤6	50 mg every 12 h	100 mg every 12 h
7-9	100 mg every 12 h	150 mg every 12 h
10-12	150 mg every 12 h	200 mg every 12 h
>12	200 mg every 12 h	200-300 every 12 h (maximum: 300 mg every 12 h)

Conversion from another opioid analgesic: Using the patient's current opioid dose, calculate an equivalent daily dose of immediate release codeine. A ~25% lower dose of Codeine Contin® should then be initiated, equally divided into 2 daily doses.

Discontinuation of therapy: **Note:** Gradual dose reduction is recommended if clinically appropriate. Initially reduce the total daily dose by 50% and administer equally divided into 2 daily doses for 2 days followed by a 25% reduction every 2 days thereafter.

Treatment of cough (unlabeled use): Adults: Reported doses vary; range: 7.5-120 mg/day as a single dose or in divided doses (Bolser, 2006; Smith, 2010); **Note:** The American College of Chest Physicians does not recommend the routine use of codeine as an antitussive in patients with upper respiratory infections (Bolser, 2006).

Dosing adjustment in renal impairment:

Manufacturer's recommendations: Clearance may be reduced; active metabolites may accumulate. Initiate at lower doses or longer dosing intervals followed by careful titration.

Alternate recommendations: The following guidelines have been used by some clinicians (Aronoff, 2007):

Cl_{cr} 10-50 mL/minute: Administer 75% of dose

Cl_{cr} <10 mL/minute: Administer 50% of dose

Dosing adjustment in hepatic impairment: No dosage adjustment provided in manufacturer's labeling (has not been studied); however, initial lower doses or longer dosing intervals followed by careful titration are recommended.

Administration May administer without regard to meals. Take with food or milk to decrease adverse GI effects.

Controlled release tablets: Codeine Contin® (Canadian availability; not available in U.S.): Tablets should be swallowed whole; do not chew, dissolve, or crush. All strengths may be halved, **except** the 50 mg tablets; half tablets should also be swallowed intact.

Monitoring Parameters Pain relief, respiratory and mental status, blood pressure, heart rate

Reference Range Therapeutic: Not established

Test Interactions Some quinolones may produce a false-positive urine screening result for opioids using commercially-available immunoassay kits. This has been demonstrated most consistently for levofloxacin and ofloxacin, but other quinolones have shown cross-reactivity in certain assay kits. Confirmation of positive opioid screens by more specific methods should be considered.

Dosage Forms Excipient information presented when available (limited, particularly for generics); consult specific product labeling.

Solution, Oral, as phosphate:

Generic: 30 mg/5 mL (500 mL)

Tablet, Oral, as sulfate:

Generic: 15 mg, 30 mg, 60 mg

Dosage Forms: Canada Excipient information presented when available (limited, particularly for generics); consult specific product labeling.

Tablet, controlled release:

Codeine Contin®: 50 mg, 100 mg, 150 mg, 200 mg

Controlled Substance C-II

Extemporaneous Preparations A 3 mg/mL oral suspension may be made with codeine phosphate powder, USP. Add 600 mg of powder to a 400 mL beaker. Add 2.5 mL of Sterile Water for Irrigation, USP, and stir to dissolve the powder. Mix for 10 minutes while adding Ora-Sweet® to make 200 mL; transfer to a calibrated bottle. Stable 98 days at room temperature.

Dentinger PJ and Swenson CF, "Stability of Codeine Phosphate in an Extemporaneously Compounded Syrup," *Am J Health Syst Pharm*, 2007, 64(24):2569-73.

- ◆ **Codeine and Acetaminophen** *see* Acetaminophen and Codeine *on page* *32*
- ◆ **Codeine and Guaifenesin** *see* Guaifenesin and Codeine *on page* *976*
- ◆ **Codeine and Promethazine** *see* Promethazine and Codeine *on page* *1730*
- ◆ **Codeine, Aspirin, and Carisoprodol** *see* Carisoprodol, Aspirin, and Codeine *on page* *352*
- ◆ **Codeine Contin® (Can)** *see* Codeine *on page* *482*
- ◆ **Codeine, Guaifenesin, and Pseudoephedrine** *see* Guaifenesin, Pseudoephedrine, and Codeine *on page* *979*
- ◆ **Codeine Phosphate** *see* Codeine *on page* *482*
- ◆ **Codeine Sulfate** *see* Codeine *on page* *482*
- ◆ **CO Diltiazem CD (Can)** *see* Diltiazem *on page* *613*
- ◆ **CO Diltiazem T (Can)** *see* Diltiazem *on page* *613*
- ◆ **Cod Liver Oil** *see* Vitamin A and Vitamin D (Systemic) *on page* *2202*
- ◆ **Cod Liver Oil** *see* Vitamin A and Vitamin D (Topical) *on page* *2202*

- ◆ **Codulax [OTC] (Can)** *see* Bisacodyl *on page 259*
- ◆ **CO Enalapril (Can)** *see* Enalapril *on page 701*
- ◆ **Co-Etidronate (Can)** *see* Etidronate *on page 798*
- ◆ **CO Exemestane (Can)** *see* Exemestane *on page 813*
- ◆ **CO Famciclovir (Can)** *see* Famciclovir *on page 830*
- ◆ **CO Finasteride (Can)** *see* Finasteride *on page 862*
- ◆ **CO Fluconazole (Can)** *see* Fluconazole *on page 868*
- ◆ **CO Fluoxetine (Can)** *see* FLUoxetine *on page 885*
- ◆ **CO Fluvoxamine (Can)** *see* FluvoxaMINE *on page 903*
- ◆ **CO Gabapentin (Can)** *see* Gabapentin *on page 933*
- ◆ **Cogentin** *see* Benztropine *on page 243*
- ◆ **CO Ipra-Sal (Can)** *see* Ipratropium and Albuterol *on page 1113*
- ◆ **CO Irbesartan (Can)** *see* Irbesartan *on page 1113*
- ◆ **CO Irbesartan HCT (Can)** *see* Irbesartan and Hydrochlorothiazide *on page 1115*
- ◆ **Colace [OTC]** *see* Docusate *on page 644*
- ◆ **Colace® (Can)** *see* Docusate *on page 644*
- ◆ **CO Latanoprost (Can)** *see* Latanoprost *on page 1178*
- ◆ **Colax-C® (Can)** *see* Docusate *on page 644*
- ◆ **Colazal** *see* Balsalazide *on page 223*
- ◆ **ColBenemid** *see* Colchicine and Probenecid *on page 487*

Colchicine (KOL chi seen)

Brand Names: U.S. Colcrys

Brand Names: Canada Jamp-Colchicine

Pharmacologic Category Antigout Agent

Use Prevention and treatment of acute gout flares; treatment of familial Mediterranean fever (FMF)

Unlabeled Use Primary biliary cirrhosis; pericarditis

Pregnancy Risk Factor C

Pregnancy Considerations Adverse events were observed in animal reproduction studies. Colchicine crosses the human placenta. Use during pregnancy in the treatment of familial Mediterranean fever has not shown an increase in miscarriage, stillbirth, or teratogenic effects (limited data).

Breast-Feeding Considerations Colchicine enters breast milk; exclusively breast-fed infants are expected to receive <10% of the weight-adjusted maternal dose (limited data). The manufacturer recommends that caution be used if administered to a nursing woman.

Medication Guide Available Yes

Contraindications Concomitant use of a P-glycoprotein (P-gp) or strong CYP3A4 inhibitor in presence of renal or hepatic impairment

Canadian labeling: Additional contraindications (not in U.S. labeling): Hypersensitivity to colchicine; serious gastrointestinal, hepatic, renal, and cardiac disease

Warnings/Precautions Hazardous agent - use appropriate precautions for handling and disposal (NIOSH, 2012). Myelosuppression (eg, thrombocytopenia, leukopenia, granulocytopenia, pancytopenia) and aplastic anemia have been reported in patients receiving therapeutic doses. Neuromuscular toxicity (including rhabdomyolysis) has been reported in patients receiving therapeutic doses; patients with renal dysfunction and elderly patients are at increased risk. Concomitant use of cyclosporine, diltiazem, verapamil, fibrates, and statins may increase the risk of myopathy. Clearance is decreased in renal or hepatic impairment; monitor closely for adverse effects/toxicity. Dosage adjustments may be required depending on degree of impairment or indication, and may be affected by the use of concurrent medication (CYP3A4 or P-gp inhibitors). Concurrent use of P-gp or strong CYP3A4 inhibitors is contraindicated in renal impairment; fatal toxicity has been reported. Colchicine does not have analgesic activity and should not be used to treat pain from other causes. Colchicine requires dosage adjustment when used concurrently with protease inhibitor regimens. Colchicine does not have analgesic activity and should not be used to treat pain from other causes. Canadian labeling does not include recommendations for use in children.

Adverse Reactions Frequency not always defined.

>10%: Gastrointestinal: Gastrointestinal disease (26% to 77%), diarrhea (23% to 77%), vomiting (17%), nausea (4% to 17%)

1% to 10%:

Central nervous system: Fatigue (1% to 4%), headache (1% to 2%)

Endocrine & metabolic: Gout (4%)

Gastrointestinal: Abdominal cramps, abdominal pain

Respiratory: Pharyngolaryngeal pain (3%)

<1% (Limited to important or life-threatening): Alopecia, aplastic anemia, azoospermia, bone marrow depression, generalized dermatosis, granulocytopenia, hepatotoxicity, hypersensitivity reaction, increased creatine phosphokinase, increased serum ALT, increased serum AST, lactose intolerance, leukopenia, maculopapular rash, myalgia, myasthenia, myopathy, myotonia, neuropathy, oligospermia, pancytopenia, peripheral neuritis, purpura, rhabdomyolysis, skin rash, thrombocytopenia

Drug Interactions

Metabolism/Transport Effects Substrate of CYP3A4 (major), P-glycoprotein; **Note:** Assignment of Major/Minor substrate status based on clinically relevant drug interaction potential; **Induces** CYP2C9 (weak/moderate), CYP2E1 (weak/moderate), CYP3A4 (weak/moderate)

Avoid Concomitant Use

Avoid concomitant use of Colchicine with any of the following: Axitinib; Fusidic Acid (Systemic); Simeprevir

Increased Effect/Toxicity

Colchicine may increase the levels/effects of: HMG-CoA Reductase Inhibitors

The levels/effects of Colchicine may be increased by: Cobicistat; CYP3A4 Inhibitors (Moderate); CYP3A4 Inhibitors (Strong); Dasatinib; Digoxin; Fibric Acid Derivatives; Fosamprenavir; Fusidic Acid (Systemic); Ivacaftor; Luliconazole; Mifepristone; P-glycoprotein/ABCB1 Inhibitors; Simeprevir; Telaprevir

Decreased Effect

Colchicine may decrease the levels/effects of: ARIPiprazole; Axitinib; Cyanocobalamin; Ibrutinib; Multivitamins/Fluoride (with ADE); Multivitamins/Minerals (with ADEK, Folate, Iron); Multivitamins/Minerals (with AE, No Iron); Saxagliptin; Simeprevir

The levels/effects of Colchicine may be decreased by: P-glycoprotein/ABCB1 Inducers

Ethanol/Nutrition/Herb Interactions

Ethanol: Management: Avoid ethanol.

Food: Grapefruit juice may increase colchicine serum concentrations. Management: Administer orally with water and maintain adequate fluid intake. Dose adjustment may be required based on indication if ingesting grapefruit juice. Avoid grapefruit juice with hepatic or renal impairment.

Herb/Nutraceutical: Cyanocobalamin (vitamin B_{12}) absorption may be decreased by colchicine and result in macrocytic anemia or neurologic dysfunction. Management: Consider supplementing with vitamin B_{12}.

Storage/Stability Store at 20°C to 25°C (68°F to 77°F). Protect from light.

Mechanism of Action Disrupts cytoskeletal functions by inhibiting β-tubulin polymerization into microtubules, preventing activation, degranulation, and migration of neutrophils associated with mediating some gout symptoms. In ▶

familial Mediterranean fever, may interfere with intracellular assembly of the inflammasome complex present in neutrophils and monocytes that mediate activation of interleukin-1β.

Pharmacodynamics/Kinetics

Onset of action: Oral: Pain relief: ~18-24 hours

Distribution: Concentrates in leukocytes, kidney, spleen, and liver; does not distribute in heart, skeletal muscle, and brain

V_d: 5-8 L/kg

Protein binding: ~39%

Metabolism: Hepatic via CYP3A4; 3 metabolites (2 primary, 1 minor)

Bioavailability: ~45%

Half-life elimination: 27-31 hours (multiple oral doses; young, healthy volunteers)

Time to peak, serum: Oral: 0.5-3 hours

Excretion: Urine (40% to 65% as unchanged drug); enterohepatic recirculation and biliary excretion also possible

Dosage Oral:

Familial Mediterranean fever (FMF):

U.S. labeling:

Children:

4-6 years: 0.3-1.8 mg/day in 1-2 divided doses

6-12 years: 0.9-1.8 mg/day in 1-2 divided doses

Children >12 years and Adults: 1.2-2.4 mg/day in 1-2 divided doses. Titration: Increase or decrease dose in 0.3 mg/day increments based on efficacy or adverse effects; maximum: 2.4 mg/day

Canadian labeling: Adults:1.2-2.4 mg/day in 1-2 divided doses. Titration: Increase or decrease dose in 0.3 mg/day increments based on efficacy or adverse effects; maximum: 2.4 mg/day

Gout:

U.S. labeling: Children >16 years and Adults:

Flare treatment: Initial: 1.2 mg at the first sign of flare, followed in 1 hour with a single dose of 0.6 mg (maximum: 1.8 mg within 1 hour). Patients receiving prophylaxis therapy may receive treatment dosing; wait 12 hours before resuming prophylaxis dose. **Note:** Current FDA-approved dose for gout flare is substantially lower than what has been historically used clinically. Doses larger than the currently recommended dosage for gout flare have not been proven to be more effective.

Prophylaxis: 0.6 mg once or twice daily; maximum: 1.2 mg/day

Canadian labeling: Adults:

Flare treatment: Initial: 1-1.2 mg at the first sign of flare, followed by 0.5-0.6 mg dose every 2 hours until pain relief; maximum: 3 mg/24 hours

Prophylaxis: 0.5-0.6 mg 1-4 times/week (mild-moderate cases) or 0.5-0.6 mg once or twice daily (severe cases); maximum: 1.2 mg/24 hours

Pericarditis post-STEMI (unlabeled use): Adults: 0.6 mg twice daily (Antman, 2004)

Recurrent pericarditis due to previous autoimmune or idiopathic cause (unlabeled use): Note: Dosage strength not available in the U.S.: Oral: 0.5-1 mg every 12 hours for 1 day, followed by 0.25-0.5 mg every 12 hours for 6 months (in combination with high-dose aspirin or ibuprofen) (Imazio, 2011)

Patients <70 kg or unable to tolerate higher dosing regimen: 0.5 mg every 12 hours for 1 day followed by 0.5 mg once daily.

Primary biliary cirrhosis (unlabeled use): Adults: 0.6 mg twice daily (Kaplan, 2005); **Note:** Use reserved for patients refractory to ursodiol.

Elderly: Use caution; reduce prophylactic daily dose by 50% in individuals >70 years (Terkeltaub, 2009)

Dosage adjustment for concomitant therapy with CYP3A4 or P-glycoprotein (P-gp) inhibitors: Note: Dosage adjustment also required in patients receiving CYP3A4 or P-gp inhibitors up to 14 days prior to initiation of colchicine. Treatment of gout flare with colchicine is not recommended in patients receiving prophylactic colchicine and CYP3A4 inhibitors.

Coadministration of **strong** CYP3A4 inhibitor (eg, atazanavir, clarithromycin, darunavir, indinavir, itraconazole, ketoconazole, lopinavir/ritonavir, nefazodone, nelfinavir, ritonavir, saquinavir, telithromycin, tipranavir):

FMF: Maximum dose: 0.6 mg/day (0.3 mg twice daily)

Gout prophylaxis:

If original dose is 0.6 mg twice daily, adjust dose to 0.3 mg once daily

If original dose is 0.6 mg once daily, adjust dose to 0.3 mg every other day

Gout flare treatment: Initial: 0.6 mg, followed in 1 hour by a single dose of 0.3 mg; do not repeat for at least 3 days

Coadministration of **moderate** CYP3A4 inhibitor (eg, aprepitant, diltiazem, erythromycin, fluconazole, fosamprenavir, grapefruit juice, verapamil):

FMF: Maximum dose: 1.2 mg/day (0.6 mg twice daily)

Gout prophylaxis:

If original dose is 0.6 mg twice daily, adjust dose to 0.3 mg twice daily **or** 0.6 mg once daily

If original dose is 0.6 mg once daily, adjust dose to 0.3 mg once daily

Gout flare treatment: 1.2 mg as a single dose; do not repeat for at least 3 days

Coadministration of P-gp inhibitor (eg, cyclosporine, ranolazine):

FMF: Maximum dose: 0.6 mg/day (0.3 mg twice daily)

Gout prophylaxis:

If original dose is 0.6 mg twice daily, adjust dose to 0.3 mg once daily

If original dose is 0.6 mg once daily, adjust dose to 0.3 mg every other day

Gout flare treatment: Initial: 0.6 mg as a single dose; do not repeat for at least 3 days

Dosing adjustment in renal impairment: Concurrent use of colchicine and P-gp or strong CYP3A4 inhibitors is **contraindicated** in renal impairment. Fatal toxicity has been reported. Use of colchicine to treat gout flares is not recommended in patients with renal impairment receiving prophylactic colchicine.

FMF:

Cl_{cr} 30-80 mL/minute: Monitor closely for adverse effects; dose reduction may be necessary

Cl_{cr} <30 mL/minute: Initial dose: 0.3 mg/day; use caution if dose titrated; monitor for adverse effects

Dialysis: 0.3 mg as a single dose; use caution if dose titrated; dosing can be increased with close monitoring; monitor for adverse effects. Not removed by dialysis.

Gout prophylaxis:

Cl_{cr} 30-80 mL/minute: Dosage adjustment not required; monitor closely for adverse effects

Cl_{cr} <30 mL/minute: Initial dose: 0.3 mg/day; use caution if dose titrated; monitor for adverse effects

Dialysis: 0.3 mg twice weekly; monitor closely for adverse effects

Gout flare treatment:

Cl_{cr} 30-80 mL/minute: Dosage adjustment not required; monitor closely for adverse effects

Cl_{cr} <30 mL/minute: Dosage reduction not required but may be considered; treatment course should not be repeated more frequently than every 14 days

Dialysis: 0.6 mg as a single dose; treatment course should not be repeated more frequently than every 14 days. Not removed by dialysis.

Hemodialysis: Avoid chronic use of colchicine.

Dosage adjustment in hepatic impairment: Concurrent use of colchicine and P-gp or strong CYP3A4 inhibitors is **contraindicated** in hepatic impairment. Fatal toxicity has been reported. Treatment of gout flare with colchicine is not recommended in patients with hepatic impairment receiving prophylactic colchicine.

FMF:

Mild-to-moderate impairment: Use caution; monitor closely for adverse effects

Severe impairment: Consider dosage reduction

Gout prophylaxis:

Mild-to-moderate impairment: Dosage adjustment not required; monitor closely for adverse effects

Severe impairment: Dosage adjustment should be considered

Gout flare treatment:

Mild-to-moderate impairment: Dosage adjustment not required; monitor closely for adverse effects

Severe impairment: Dosage reduction not required but may be considered; treatment course should not be repeated more frequently than every 14 days

Dietary Considerations May be taken without regard to meals. May need to supplement with vitamin B_{12}. Avoid grapefruit juice.

Administration Administer orally with water and maintain adequate fluid intake. May be administered without regard to meals.

Hazardous agent; use appropriate precautions for handling and disposal (NIOSH, 2012).

Monitoring Parameters CBC, renal and hepatic function tests

Test Interactions May cause false-positive results in urine tests for erythrocytes or hemoglobin

Additional Information Oral colchicine had been available as an unapproved medication without FDA-approved prescribing information. In August 2009, the FDA approved prescribing information for a brand name colchicine product. The currently approved prescribing information recommends a lower than historically used dosage for the treatment of acute gout. This recommendation is based on data from the AGREE trial. In this trial, low-dose colchicine (1.8 mg total) had similar efficacy to high dose colchicine (4.8 mg total). Additionally, the low dosage regimen was associated with a lower incidence (26% vs 77%) of GI adverse events. Parenteral formulation of colchicine is no longer available in the U.S.; serious life-threatening complications (eg, neutropenia, acute renal failure, thrombocytopenia, heart failure) associated with intravenous colchicine have occurred prior to market withdrawal. The risks associated with oral colchicine are believed to be lower compared to intravenous use.

Dosage Forms Excipient information presented when available (limited, particularly for generics); consult specific product labeling.

Tablet, Oral:

Colcrys: 0.6 mg [scored; contains fd&c blue #2 (indigotine), fd&c red #40]

Dosage Forms: Canada Excipient information presented when available (limited, particularly for generics); consult specific product labeling.

Tablet, oral: 1 mg [scored]

Colchicine and Probenecid

(KOL chi seen & proe BEN e sid)

Index Terms ColBenemid; Probenecid and Colchicine

Pharmacologic Category Anti-inflammatory Agent; Antigout Agent; Uricosuric Agent

Use Treatment of chronic gouty arthritis when complicated by frequent, recurrent acute attacks of gout

Dosage Oral: Adults: One tablet daily for 1 week, then 1 tablet twice daily thereafter

Note: Current prescribing information states a maximum dose of 4 tablets per day; however this exceeds the usual maximum dose of colchicine for gout prophylaxis (1.2 mg per day).

Dosage adjustment in renal impairment: Cl_{cr} <30 mL/minute: Probenecid may not be effective in patients with chronic renal insufficiency.

Dosage adjustment in hepatic impairment: No dosage adjustment provided in manufacturer's labeling; use with caution.

Additional Information Complete prescribing information should be consulted for additional detail.

Dosage Forms Excipient information presented when available (limited, particularly for generics); consult specific product labeling.

Tablet: Colchicine 0.5 mg and probenecid 0.5 g

◆ **Colcrys** *see* Colchicine *on page 485*

◆ **Coldcough PD** *see* Dihydrocodeine, Chlorpheniramine, and Phenylephrine *on page 611*

Colesevelam (koh le SEV a lam)

Brand Names: U.S. Welchol

Brand Names: Canada Lodalis

Pharmacologic Category Antilipemic Agent, Bile Acid Sequestrant

Additional Appendix Information

Oral Antidiabetic Agents Comparison Table *on page 2312*

Use

Hypercholesterolemia:

U.S. labeling: Management of elevated LDL in primary hypercholesterolemia (Fredrickson type IIa) when used alone or in combination with an HMG-CoA reductase inhibitor; management of heterozygous familial hypercholesterolemia (heFH) in adolescent patients (males and postmenarcheal females 10-17 years of age) used alone or in combination with an HMG-CoA reductase inhibitor when after an adequate trial of dietary therapy patient continues to have LDL-C ≥190 mg/dL or LDL-C ≥160 mg/dL with positive family history of premature cardiovascular disease (CVD) or with two or more CVD risk factors

Canadian labeling (Lodalis): Adjunct to diet and lifestyle modifications in the management of primary hypercholesterolemia (Fredrickson type IIa) as monotherapy or in combination with an HMG-CoA reductase inhibitor

Diabetes mellitus, type 2:

U.S. labeling: Improve glycemic control in type 2 diabetes mellitus (noninsulin dependent, NIDDM) in conjunction with diet, exercise, and insulin or oral antidiabetic agents

Pregnancy Risk Factor B

Dosage Oral:

Children 10-17 years (males and postmenarchal females):

Dyslipidemia (heterozygous familial hypercholesterolemia):

Once-daily dosing: 3.75 g (oral suspension or 6 tablets)

Twice-daily dosing: 1.875 g (3 tablets)

Note: Due to large tablet size, oral suspension is recommended in pediatric patients.

Adults:

U.S. labeling: Dyslipidemia, type 2 diabetes (combination therapy with insulin or oral antidiabetic agents):

Once-daily dosing: 3.75 g (oral suspension or 6 tablets)

Twice-daily dosing: 1.875 g (3 tablets)

Canadian labeling: Dyslipidemia:

Combination therapy: 2.5-3.75 g (4-6 tablets) daily; maximum dose: 3.75 g (6 tablets) given once daily or 1.875 g (3 tablets) given twice daily

Monotherapy: Initial: 1.875 g (3 tablets) twice daily or 3.75 g (6 tablets) once daily; maximum dose: 4.375 g (7 tablets) daily

Elderly: Refer to adult dosing.

Dosage adjustment in renal impairment: No dosage adjustment necessary; not absorbed from the gastrointestinal tract.

Dosage adjustment in hepatic impairment: No dosage adjustment necessary; not absorbed from the gastrointestinal tract.

Additional Information Complete prescribing information should be consulted for additional detail.

Dosage Forms Excipient information presented when available (limited, particularly for generics); consult specific product labeling.

Packet, Oral, as hydrochloride:

Welchol: 3.75 g (30 ea) [sugar free; contains aspartame]

Tablet, Oral, as hydrochloride:

Welchol: 625 mg

Dosage Forms: Canada Excipient information presented when available (limited, particularly for generics); consult specific product labeling.

Tablet, oral, as hydrochloride:

Lodalis: 625 mg

◆ Colestid *see* Colestipol *on page 488*

◆ Colestid Flavored *see* Colestipol *on page 488*

Colestipol (koe LES ti pole)

Brand Names: U.S. Colestid; Colestid Flavored; Micronized Colestipol HCl

Brand Names: Canada Colestid

Index Terms Colestipol Hydrochloride

Pharmacologic Category Antilipemic Agent, Bile Acid Sequestrant

Use Adjunct in management of primary hypercholesterolemia

Unlabeled Use Diarrhea associated with excess fecal bile acids (Westergaard, 2007); relief of pruritus associated with elevated levels of bile acids (Datta, 1963; Scaldaferri, 2011)

Dosage Adults: Oral:

Granules: Initial: 5 g 1-2 times/day; maintenance: 5-30 g/day given once or in divided doses; increase by 5 g/day at 1- to 2-month intervals

Tablets: Initial: 2 g 1-2 times/day; maintenance: 2-16 g/day given once or in divided doses; increase by 2 g once or twice daily at 1- to 2-month intervals

Dosage adjustment in renal impairment: No dosage adjustment necessary; not absorbed from the gastrointestinal tract.

Dosage adjustment in hepatic impairment: No dosage adjustment necessary; not absorbed from the gastrointestinal tract.

Additional Information Complete prescribing information should be consulted for additional detail.

Dosage Forms Considerations

Colestid tablets contain micronized colestipol. Generic tablets are available in micronized and non-micronized formulations.

Dosage Forms Excipient information presented when available (limited, particularly for generics); consult specific product labeling.

Granules, Oral, as hydrochloride:

Colestid: 5 g (300 g, 500 g) [unflavored flavor]

Colestid Flavored: 5 g (450 g) [contains aspartame; orange flavor]

Generic: 5 g (500 g)

Packet, Oral, as hydrochloride:

Colestid: 5 g (30 ea, 90 ea) [unflavored flavor]

Colestid Flavored: 5 g (60 ea) [contains aspartame; orange flavor]

Generic: 5 g (30 ea, 90 ea)

Tablet, Oral, as hydrochloride:

Colestid: 1 g

Micronized Colestipol HCl: 1 g

Generic: 1 g

◆ Colestipol Hydrochloride *see* Colestipol *on page 488*

◆ CO Levetiracetam (Can) *see* LevETIRAcetam *on page 1194*

◆ CO Levofloxacin (Can) *see* Levofloxacin (Systemic) *on page 1198*

◆ CO Lisinopril (Can) *see* Lisinopril *on page 1226*

Colistimethate (koe lis ti METH ate)

Brand Names: U.S. Coly-Mycin M

Brand Names: Canada Coly-Mycin® M

Index Terms Colistimethate Sodium; Colistin Methanesulfonate; Colistin Sulfomethate; Pentasodium Colistin Methanesulfonate; Polymyxin E

Pharmacologic Category Antibiotic, Miscellaneous

Use Treatment of acute or chronic infections due to sensitive strains of certain gram-negative bacilli (particularly *Pseudomonas aeruginosa*) which are resistant to other antibacterials or in patients allergic to other antibacterials

Unlabeled Use Used as nebulized inhalation in the prevention of *Pseudomonas aeruginosa* respiratory tract infections in immunocompromised patients; used as nebulized inhalation adjunct agent for the treatment of *P. aeruginosa* infections in patients with cystic fibrosis and other seriously ill or chronically ill patients; used as nebulized inhalation in the treatment of ventilator-associated pneumonia (VAP) due to multidrug-resistant *P. aeruginosa* or *Acinetobacter baumannii*

Pregnancy Risk Factor C

Pregnancy Considerations Adverse events have been observed in animal reproduction studies. Colistimethate crosses the placenta in humans.

Breast-Feeding Considerations Colistin (the active form of colistimethate sodium) and colistin sulphate (another form of colistin) are excreted in human milk. The manufacturer recommends caution if giving colistimethate sodium to a breast-feeding woman. Nondose-related effects could include modification of bowel flora.

Contraindications Hypersensitivity to colistimethate, colistin, or any component of the formulation

Warnings/Precautions Use only to prevent or treat infections strongly suspected or proven to be caused by susceptible bacteria to minimize development of bacterial drug resistance. Nephrotoxicity has been reported; use with caution in patients with pre-existing renal disease; dosage adjustments may be required. Withhold treatment if signs of renal impairment occur during treatment. Respiratory arrest has been reported with use; impaired renal function may increase the risk for neuromuscular blockade and apnea. Transient, reversible neurological disturbances (eg, dizziness, numbness, paresthesia, generalized pruritus, slurred speech, tingling, vertigo) may occur. Patients must be cautioned about performing tasks which require mental alertness (eg, operating machinery or driving).

Dose reduction may reduce neurologic symptoms; monitor closely. Use of inhaled colistimethate cause bronchoconstriction. Use with caution in patients with hyperactive airways; consider administration of a bronchodilator 15 minutes prior to administration. Colistimethate solutions change to bioactive colistin, a component of which may result in severe pulmonary toxicity. Solutions for inhalation must be mixed immediately prior to administration and used within 24 hours.

Prolonged use may result in fungal or bacterial superinfection, including *C. difficile*-associated diarrhea (CDAD) and pseudomembranous colitis; CDAD has been observed >2 months postantibiotic treatment.

Potentially significant drug-drug interactions may exist, requiring dose or frequency adjustment, additional monitoring, and/or selection of alternative therapy. Use caution when prescribing or dispensing; potential for dosing errors due to lack of standardization in literature when referring to product and dose; colistimethate (inactive prodrug) and colistin base strengths are not interchangeable; verify prescribed dose is expressed in terms of colistin base prior to dispensing.

Adverse Reactions Frequency not defined.

Central nervous system: Dizziness, fever, headache, slurred speech, vertigo

Dermatologic: Pruritus, rash, urticaria

Gastrointestinal: GI upset

Neuromuscular & skeletal: Paresthesia (extremities, oral); weakness (lower limb)

Renal: BUN increased, creatinine increased, nephrotoxicity, proteinuria, urine output decreased

Respiratory: Apnea, respiratory distress

Postmarketing, and/or case reports: Lung toxicity (bronchoconstriction, bronchospasm, chest tightness, respiratory distress, acute respiratory failure following inhalation)

Drug Interactions

Metabolism/Transport Effects None known.

Avoid Concomitant Use

Avoid concomitant use of Colistimethate with any of the following: BCG

Increased Effect/Toxicity

Colistimethate may increase the levels/effects of: Neuromuscular-Blocking Agents

The levels/effects of Colistimethate may be increased by: Aminoglycosides; Amphotericin B; Capreomycin; Polymyxin B; Vancomycin

Decreased Effect

Colistimethate may decrease the levels/effects of: BCG; Sodium Picosulfate; Typhoid Vaccine

Preparation for Administration

I.V. or I.M. use: Reconstitute each vial containing 150 mg of colistin base activity with 2 mL of SWFI resulting in a concentration of 75 mg colistin base/mL; swirl gently to avoid frothing. May further dilute in D_5W or NS for I.V. infusion.

Intrathecal/intraventricular use (unlabeled route): Reconstitute with preservative-free diluent (SWFI or NS) only; use promptly after preparation; discard unused portion of vial (Quinn, 2005).

Nebulized inhalation (unlabeled route): Reconstitute vial containing 150 mg of colistin base activity with 2 mL SWFI resulting in a concentration of 75 mg colistin base activity/mL; further dilute dose to a total volume of 3-4 mL in NS; should be used promptly after preparation; do not use after 24 hours (Wallace, 2008). May also further dilute 150 mg colistin base to a total volume of 10 mL in SWFI (concentration: 15 mg colistin base activity/mL); use promptly after preparation (Lu, 2012).

Storage/Stability Store intact vials (prior to reconstitution) at 20°C to 25°C (68°F to 77°F); excursions permitted to 15°C to 30°C (59°F to 86°F). Reconstituted vials may be refrigerated at 2°C to 8°C (36°F to 46°F) or stored at 20°C to 25°C (68°F to 77°F) for up to 7 days. Solutions for infusion should be freshly prepared; do not use beyond 24 hours.

Mechanism of Action Colistimethate (or the sodium salt [colistimethate sodium]) is the inactive prodrug which is hydrolyzed to colistin, which acts as a cationic detergent and damages the bacterial cytoplasmic membrane causing leaking of intracellular substances and cell death

Pharmacodynamics/Kinetics

Distribution: Widely, except for CNS, synovial, pleural, and pericardial fluids

Metabolism: Colistimethate sodium (inactive prodrug) is hydrolyzed to colistin (active form)

Half-life elimination: I.M., I.V.: 2-3 hours; Anuria: ≤2-3 days

Time to peak: I.V.: 10 minutes

Excretion: Primarily urine (as unchanged drug)

Dosage Note: Dosage expressed in terms of **colistin base**.

Susceptible infections: Children and Adults: I.M., I.V.: 2.5-5 mg/kg/day in 2-4 divided doses; maximum: 5 mg/kg/day

Cystic fibrosis: Adults: I.V.: 3 mg/kg/day in 3 divided doses (Young, 2013)

Bronchiectasis, pulmonary colonization/infection with susceptible organisms in patients with cystic fibrosis and noncystic fibrosis (unlabeled use/route): Adults: Inhalation: 30-150 mg in NS (3-4 mL total) via nebulizer 1-3 times daily (maximum dose: 150 mg 2 times daily) (Le, 2010; Sabuda, 2008; Steinfort, 2007). **Note:** Lower doses have been used in noncystic fibrosis patients with bronchiectasis (Steinfort, 2007); the most commonly used dose is 150 mg twice daily (Le, 2010).

Meningitis (susceptible gram-negative organisms): Adults: Intrathecal/Intraventricular (unlabeled route): 10 mg/day (IDSA, 2004); **Note:** Dosage in clinical reports has ranged from 1.6-20 mg/day in 1 or 2 divided doses (maximum single dose: 10 mg) (administered with concomitant systemic antimicrobial therapy) (Guardado, 2008; Kasiakou, 2005; Katragkou, 2005)

Ventilator-associated pneumonia due to multidrug-resistant *Pseudomonas aeruginosa* or *Acinetobacter baumannii* (unlabeled use/route): Adults: Nebulization (via ventilator circuit): 150 mg every 8 hours delivered over 60 minutes for 14 days or until successful wean from mechanical ventilation (treatment duration range: 7-19 days) (Lu, 2012).

Dosage adjustment for toxicity:

CNS toxicity: Dose reduction may reduce neurologic symptoms.

Nephrotoxicity: Withhold treatment if signs of renal impairment occur during treatment.

Dosage adjustment in obesity: Doses should be based on ideal body weight in obese patients.

Dosage adjustment in renal impairment: I.M., I.V.: Adults:

Cl_{cr} ≥80 mL/minute: No dosage adjustment necessary; maximum: 5 mg/kg/day

Cl_{cr} 50-79 mL/minute: 2.5-3.8 mg/kg/day in 2 divided doses

Cl_{cr} 30-49 mL/minute: 2.5 mg/kg/day once daily or in 2 divided doses

Cl_{cr} 10-29 mL/minute: 1.5 mg/kg every 36 hours

Intermittent hemodialysis (IHD) (administer after hemodialysis on dialysis days): 1.5 mg/kg every 24-48 hours (Heintz, 2009). **Note:** Dosing dependent on the assumption of 3 times/week, complete IHD sessions.

Continuous renal replacement therapy (CRRT) (Heintz, 2009; Trotman, 2005): Drug clearance is highly dependent on the method of renal replacement, filter type, and flow rate. Appropriate dosing requires close monitoring of pharmacologic response, signs of adverse reactions due to drug accumulation, as well as drug concentrations in relation to target trough (if appropriate). The following are general recommendations only (based on dialysate flow/ultrafiltration rates of 1-2 L/hour and minimal residual renal function) and should not supersede clinical judgment:

CVVH/CVVHD/CVVHDF: 2.5 mg/kg every 24-48 hours (frequency dependent upon site or severity of infection or susceptibility of pathogen)

Note: A single case report has demonstrated that the use of 2.5 mg/kg every 48 hours with a dialysate flow rate of 1 L/hour may be inadequate and that dosing every 24 hours was well-tolerated. Based on pharmacokinetic analysis, the authors recommend dosing as frequent as every 12 hours in patients receiving CVVHDF (Li, 2005).

Dosage adjustment in hepatic impairment: No dosage adjustment provided in manufacturer's labeling.

Dosing in obesity: Doses should be based on ideal body weight in obese patients.

Administration

Parenteral: Administer by I.M., direct I.V. injection over 3-5 minutes, intermittent infusion over 30 minutes (Conway, 1997; Beringer, 2001), or by continuous I.V. infusion. For continuous I.V. infusion, one-half of the total daily dose is administered by direct I.V. injection over 3-5 minutes followed 1-2 hours later by the remaining one-half of the total daily dose diluted in a compatible I.V. solution infused over 22-23 hours. The final concentration for continuous infusion administration should be based on the patient's fluid needs; infusion should be completed within 24 hours of preparation.

Inhalation (unlabeled route): Administer solution via nebulizer promptly following preparation to decrease possibility of high concentrations of colistin from forming which may lead to potentially life-threatening lung toxicity. Consider use of a bronchodilator (eg, albuterol) within 15 minutes prior to administration (Le, 2010). If patient is on a ventilator, place medicine in a T-piece at the midinspiratory circuit of the ventilator. One study in adult patients with VAP administered colistimethate (150 mg colistin base/10 mL SWFI) over 60 minutes (Lu, 2012).

Intrathecal/intraventricular (unlabeled route): Administer only preservative-free solutions via intrathecal/intraventricular routes. Administer promptly after preparation. Discard unused portion of vial.

Monitoring Parameters Serum creatinine, BUN; urine output; signs of neurotoxicity; signs of bronchospasm (inhalation [unlabeled route])

Additional Information

Colistimethate sodium 1 mg is equivalent to ~12,500 units of **colistimethate sodium**

Colistimethate sodium ~2.67 mg is equivalent to 1 mg of **colistin base**

Dosage Forms Excipient information presented when available (limited, particularly for generics); consult specific product labeling.

Solution Reconstituted, Injection [strength expressed as base]:

Coly-Mycin M: 150 mg (1 ea)

Generic: 150 mg (1 ea)

◆ **Colistimethate Sodium** *see* Colistimethate *on page 488*

◆ **Colistin, Hydrocortisone, Neomycin, and Thonzonium** *see* Neomycin, Colistin, Hydrocortisone, and Thonzonium *on page 1439*

◆ **Colistin Methanesulfonate** *see* Colistimethate *on page 488*

◆ **Colistin Sulfomethate** *see* Colistimethate *on page 488*

Collagenase (Systemic) (KOL la je nase)

Brand Names: U.S. Xiaflex

Index Terms Collagenase Clostridium Histolyticum

Pharmacologic Category Enzyme

Use Treatment of Dupuytren's contracture with a palpable cord

Pregnancy Risk Factor B

Medication Guide Available Yes

Dosage Intralesional: Adults: Dupuytren's contracture: Inject 0.58 mg per cord affecting a metacarpophalangeal (MP) joint or a proximal interphalangeal (PIP) joint. If contracture persists, finger extension procedure should be performed 24 hours following injection to facilitate cord disruption. If MP or PIP contracture remains, may reinject cord 4 weeks following initial injection; injections and finger extension procedures may be administered up to 3 times per cord separated by ~4 week intervals. **Note:** Only one cord should be injected at a time; if other palpable cords exist, inject in a sequential order.

Dosage adjustment in renal impairment: No adjustment necessary

Dosage adjustment in hepatic impairment: No adjustment necessary

Additional Information Complete prescribing information should be consulted for additional detail.

Dosage Forms Excipient information presented when available (limited, particularly for generics); consult specific product labeling.

Solution Reconstituted, Injection:

Xiaflex: 0.9 mg (1 ea)

Collagenase (Topical) (KOL la je nase)

Brand Names: U.S. Santyl

Brand Names: Canada Santyl®

Pharmacologic Category Enzyme, Topical Debridement

Use Promotes debridement of necrotic tissue in dermal ulcers and severe burns

Dosage Topical: Apply once daily (or more frequently if the dressing becomes soiled)

Additional Information Complete prescribing information should be consulted for additional detail.

Dosage Forms Excipient information presented when available (limited, particularly for generics); consult specific product labeling.

Ointment, External:

Santyl: 250 units/g (30 g)

◆ **Collagenase Clostridium Histolyticum** *see* Collagenase (Systemic) *on page 490*

◆ **Colocort** *see* Hydrocortisone (Topical) *on page 1011*

◆ **CO Losartan (Can)** *see* Losartan *on page 1247*

◆ **CO Losartan/HCT (Can)** *see* Losartan and Hydrochlorothiazide *on page 1249*

◆ **CO Lovastatin (Can)** *see* Lovastatin *on page 1250*

◆ **Coly-Mycin M** *see* Colistimethate *on page 488*

◆ **Coly-Mycin® M (Can)** *see* Colistimethate *on page 488*

◆ **Coly-Mycin® S** *see* Neomycin, Colistin, Hydrocortisone, and Thonzonium *on page 1439*

◆ **Colyte** *see* Polyethylene Glycol-Electrolyte Solution *on page 1669*

◆ **Combantrin™ (Can)** *see* Pyrantel Pamoate *on page 1750*

Conivaptan (koe NYE vap tan)

Brand Names: U.S. Vaprisol

Index Terms Conivaptan Hydrochloride; YM087

Pharmacologic Category Vasopressin Antagonist

Use Treatment of euvolemic and hypervolemic hyponatremia in hospitalized patients

Pregnancy Risk Factor C

Pregnancy Considerations Adverse events were observed in animal reproduction studies.

Breast-Feeding Considerations It is not known if conivaptan is excreted in breast milk. Due to the potential for serious adverse reactions in the nursing infant, a decision should be made whether to discontinue nursing or to discontinue the drug, taking into account the importance of treatment to the mother.

Contraindications Hypersensitivity to conivaptan, corn or corn products, or any component of the formulation; use in hypovolemic hyponatremia; concurrent use with strong CYP3A4 inhibitors (eg, ketoconazole, itraconazole, ritonavir, indinavir, and clarithromycin); anuria

Warnings/Precautions Monitor closely for rate of serum sodium increase and neurological status; overly rapid serum sodium correction (>12 mEq/L/24 hours) can lead to seizures, permanent neurological damage, coma, or death. Discontinue use if rate of serum sodium increase is undesirable; may reinitiate infusion (at reduced dose) if hyponatremia persists in the absence of neurological symptoms typically associated with rapid sodium rise. Of note, raising serum sodium concentrations with conivaptan has not demonstrated symptomatic benefit. Discontinue if hypovolemia or hypotension occurs. Safety and efficacy in patients with hypervolemic hyponatremia associated with heart failure have not been established. Use in small numbers of hypervolemic, hyponatremic heart failure patients led to increased adverse events. In other heart failure studies, conivaptan did not show significant improvements in outcomes over placebo. Coadministration with digoxin may increase digoxin concentrations; monitor digoxin concentrations. Use with caution in patients with hepatic impairment; dosage adjustment may be required. May cause injection-site reactions.

Adverse Reactions

>10%:

Cardiovascular: Orthostatic hypotension (6% to 14%)
Central nervous system: Fever (5% to 11%)
Endocrine & metabolic: Hypokalemia (10% to 22%)
Local: Injection site reactions including pain, erythema, phlebitis, swelling (63% to 73%)

1% to 10%:

Cardiovascular: Hypertension (6% to 8%), hypotension (5% to 8%), peripheral edema (3% to 8%), phlebitis (5%), atrial fibrillation (2% to 5%), ECG abnormality (≤5%)
Central nervous system: Headache (8% to 10%), insomnia (4% to 5%), confusion (≤5%), pain (2%)
Dermatologic: Pruritus (1% to 5%), erythema (3%)
Endocrine & metabolic: Hyponatremia (6% to 8%), hypomagnesemia (2% to 5%), hyper-/hypoglycemia (3%)
Gastrointestinal: Constipation (6% to 8%), vomiting (5% to 7%), diarrhea (≤7%), nausea (3% to 5%), dry mouth (4%), dehydration (2%), oral candidiasis (2%)
Genitourinary: Urinary tract infection (4% to 5%)
Hematologic: Anemia (5% to 6%)
Renal: Polyuria (5% to 6%), hematuria (2%)
Respiratory: Pneumonia (2% to 5%), pharyngolaryngeal pain (1% to 5%)
Miscellaneous: Thirst (3% to 6%)

<1%, postmarketing, and/or case reports (limited to important or life-threatening): Atrial arrhythmias, sepsis

Drug Interactions

Metabolism/Transport Effects Substrate of CYP3A4 (major); **Note:** Assignment of Major/Minor substrate status based on clinically relevant drug interaction potential; **Inhibits** CYP3A4 (strong)

Avoid Concomitant Use

Avoid concomitant use of Conivaptan with any of the following: Ado-Trastuzumab Emtansine; Alfuzosin; Antifungal Agents (Azole Derivatives, Systemic); Apixaban; Avanafil; Axitinib; Bosutinib; Cabozantinib; Crizotinib; CYP3A4 Inhibitors (Strong); CYP3A4 Substrates; Dronedarone; Eplerenone; Everolimus; Fusidic Acid (Systemic); Halofantrine; Ibrutinib; Imatinib; Ivabradine; Lapatinib; Lomitapide; Lovastatin; Lurasidone; Macitentan; Nilotinib; Nisoldipine; Pimozide; Pomalidomide; Ranolazine; Red Yeast Rice; Regorafenib; Rivaroxaban; Salmeterol; Silodosin; Simeprevir; Simvastatin; Tamsulosin; Ticagrelor; Tolvaptan; Toremifene; Ulipristal; Vemurafenib; VinCRIStine (Liposomal)

Increased Effect/Toxicity

Conivaptan may increase the levels/effects of: Ado-Trastuzumab Emtansine; Alfuzosin; Almotriptan; Alosetron; Apixaban; ARIPiprazole; Avanafil; Axitinib; Bedaquiline; Bortezomib; Bosentan; Bosutinib; Brentuximab Vedotin; Brinzolamide; Budesonide (Nasal); Budesonide (Systemic, Oral Inhalation); Cabozantinib; Colchicine; Corticosteroids (Orally Inhaled); Crizotinib; CYP3A4 Substrates; Dienogest; Digoxin; Dofetilide; Dronedarone; Dutasteride; Enzalutamide; Eplerenone; Everolimus; FentaNYL; Fesoterodine; Fluticasone (Nasal); Fluticasone (Oral Inhalation); GuanFACINE; Halofantrine; Ibrutinib; Iloperidone; Imatinib; Ivabradine; Ivacaftor; Ixabepilone; Lacosamide; Lapatinib; Levomilnacipran; Lomitapide; Lovastatin; Lumefantrine; Lurasidone; Macitentan; Maraviroc; MethylPREDNISolone; Mifepristone; Nilotinib; Nisoldipine; Ospemifene; OxyCODONE; Paricalcitol; PAZOPanib; Pimecrolimus; Pimozide; Pomalidomide; PONATinib; Propafenone; QUEtiapine; Ranolazine; Red Yeast Rice; Regorafenib; Repaglinide; Rilpivirine; Rivaroxaban; RomiDEPsin; Ruxolitinib; Salmeterol; Saxagliptin; Sildenafil; Silodosin; Simeprevir; Simvastatin; SORAfenib; Tadalafil; Tamsulosin; Ticagrelor; Tofacitinib; Tolterodine; Tolvaptan; Toremifene; Ulipristal; Vardenafil; Vemurafenib; Vilazodone; VinCRIStine (Liposomal); Zuclopenthixol

The levels/effects of Conivaptan may be increased by: Antifungal Agents (Azole Derivatives, Systemic); CYP3A4 Inhibitors (Moderate); CYP3A4 Inhibitors (Strong); Dasatinib; Fusidic Acid (Systemic); Luliconazole

Decreased Effect

Conivaptan may decrease the levels/effects of: Ifosfamide; Prasugrel; Ticagrelor

The levels/effects of Conivaptan may be decreased by: CYP3A4 Inducers (Strong); Dabrafenib; Deferasirox; Herbs (CYP3A4 Inducers); Mitotane; Tocilizumab

Ethanol/Nutrition/Herb Interactions Herb/Nutraceutical: St John's wort may decrease the levels/effects of conivaptan.

Storage/Stability Store at 25°C (77°F); brief excursions permitted up to 40°C (104°F). Protect from light and freezing. Do not remove protective overwrap until ready for use.

Mechanism of Action Conivaptan is an arginine vasopressin (AVP) receptor antagonist with affinity for AVP receptor subtypes V_{1A} and V_2. The antidiuretic action of AVP is mediated through activation of the V_2 receptor, which functions to regulate water and electrolyte balance at the level of the collecting ducts in the kidney. Serum levels of AVP are commonly elevated in euvolemic or hypervolemic hyponatremia, which results in the dilution of serum sodium and the relative hyponatremic state. Antagonism of the V_2 receptor by conivaptan promotes the excretion of free water (without loss of serum electrolytes) resulting in net fluid loss, increased urine output, decreased urine osmolality, and subsequent restoration of normal serum sodium concentrations.

Pharmacodynamics/Kinetics

Protein binding: 99%

Metabolism: Hepatic via CYP3A4 to four minimally-active metabolites

Half-life elimination: ~5-8 hours

Excretion: Feces (83%); urine (12%, primarily as metabolites)

Dosage I.V.: Adults: 20 mg infused over 30 minutes as a loading dose, followed by a continuous infusion of 20 mg over 24 hours (0.83 mg/hour) for 2-4 days; may increase to a maximum dose of 40 mg over 24 hours (1.7 mg/hour) if serum sodium not rising sufficiently; total duration of therapy not to exceed 4 days. **Note:** If patient requires 40 mg/24 hours, may administer two consecutive 20 mg/100 mL premixed solutions over 24 hours (ie, 20 mg over 12 hours followed by 20 mg over 12 hours).

Dosing adjustment in renal impairment:

Cl_{cr} ≥30 mL/minute: No dosage adjustment necessary.

Cl_{cr} <30 mL/minute: Use not recommended; clinical response reduced; contraindicated in anuria (no benefit expected).

Dosing adjustment in hepatic impairment:

Mild impairment: No dosage adjustment necessary.

Moderate impairment: 10 mg infused over 30 minutes as a loading dose, followed by a continuous infusion of 10 mg over 24 hours (0.42 mg/hour) for 2-4 days; may increase to a maximum dose of 20 mg over 24 hours (0.83 mg/hour) if serum sodium not rising sufficiently; total duration of therapy not to exceed 4 days.

Severe impairment: Use not recommended (not studied).

Usual Infusion Concentrations: Adult Note: Premixed solutions available.

I.V. infusion: 20 mg in 100 mL (concentration: 0.2 mg/mL) of D_5W

Administration For intravenous use only; infuse into large veins and change infusion site every 24 hours to minimize vascular irritation. Do not administer with any other product in the same intravenous line or container.

Monitoring Parameters Rate of serum sodium increase, blood pressure, volume status, urine output

Dosage Forms Excipient information presented when available (limited, particularly for generics); consult specific product labeling.

Solution, Intravenous, as hydrochloride:

Vaprisol: 20 mg (100 mL)

- ◆ Conivaptan Hydrochloride *see* Conivaptan *on page 491*
- ◆ Conjugated Estrogen *see* Estrogens (Conjugated/Equine, Systemic) *on page 770*
- ◆ Conjugated Estrogen *see* Estrogens (Conjugated/Equine, Topical) *on page 773*
- ◆ CO Norfloxacin (Can) *see* Norfloxacin *on page 1475*
- ◆ Constulose *see* Lactulose *on page 1161*
- ◆ Contac® Cold 12 Hour Relief Non Drowsy (Can) *see* Pseudoephedrine *on page 1746*
- ◆ Contac® Cold and Sore Throat, Non Drowsy, Extra Strength (Can) *see* Acetaminophen and Pseudoephedrine *on page 33*
- ◆ Contac® Cold-Chest Congestion, Non Drowsy, Regular Strength (Can) *see* Guaifenesin and Pseudoephedrine *on page 978*
- ◆ Continuous Renal Replacement Therapy *see* Electrolyte Solution, Renal Replacement *on page 691*
- ◆ ControlRx™ *see* Fluoride *on page 880*
- ◆ ControlRx™ Multi *see* Fluoride *on page 880*
- ◆ Conventional Amphotericin B *see* Amphotericin B (Conventional) *on page 123*
- ◆ Conventional Cytarabine *see* Cytarabine (Conventional) *on page 517*
- ◆ Conventional Daunomycin *see* DAUNOrubicin (Conventional) *on page 553*
- ◆ Conventional Doxorubicin *see* DOXOrubicin *on page 661*
- ◆ Conventional Paclitaxel *see* PACLitaxel *on page 1543*
- ◆ Conventional Trastuzumab *see* Trastuzumab *on page 2109*
- ◆ Conventional Vincristine *see* VinCRIStine *on page 2191*
- ◆ ConZip *see* TraMADol *on page 2099*

◆ **CO Olanzapine (Can)** *see* OLANZapine *on page 1493*
◆ **CO Olanzapine ODT (Can)** *see* OLANZapine *on page 1493*
◆ **CO Ondansetron (Can)** *see* Ondansetron *on page 1510*
◆ **CO Oxycodone CR (Can)** *see* OxyCODONE *on page 1535*
◆ **CO Pantoprazole (Can)** *see* Pantoprazole *on page 1563*
◆ **CO Paroxetine (Can)** *see* PARoxetine *on page 1575*
◆ **Copaxone** *see* Glatiramer Acetate *on page 955*
◆ **Copaxone® (Can)** *see* Glatiramer Acetate *on page 955*
◆ **Copegus** *see* Ribavirin *on page 1804*
◆ **CO Pioglitazone (Can)** *see* Pioglitazone *on page 1649*
◆ **Copolymer-1** *see* Glatiramer Acetate *on page 955*

Copper (KOP er)

Brand Names: U.S. Coppermin [OTC]; Cu-5 [OTC]
Index Terms Cupric Chloride; Cupric Chloride Dihydrate
Pharmacologic Category Trace Element, Parenteral
Use Supplement to intravenous solutions given for total parenteral nutrition (TPN) to maintain copper serum levels and to prevent depletion of endogenous stores and subsequent deficiency symptoms
Pregnancy Risk Factor C
Dosage I.V. (incorporated into parenteral nutrition):
Infants and Children: 20 mcg/kg/day
Adults: 0.3-0.5 mg/day (ASPEN, 2002); 0.5-1.5 mg/day (manufacturer's product labeling)
High output intestinal fistula: Some clinicians may use twice the recommended daily allowance (ASPEN, 2002)
Elderly: Use caution. Start at the low end of dosing range.

Dosage adjustment in renal impairment: Use caution; contains aluminum
Dosage adjustment in hepatic impairment: Use caution; dosage reduction may be required

Additional Information Complete prescribing information should be consulted for additional detail.
Dosage Forms Excipient information presented when available (limited, particularly for generics); consult specific product labeling.
Capsule, Oral [preservative free]:
Cu-5: 5 mg [dye free]
Solution, Intravenous:
Generic: 0.4 mg/mL (10 mL)
Tablet, Oral:
Coppermin: 5 mg [corn free, rye free, wheat free]

◆ **Coppermin [OTC]** *see* Copper *on page 493*
◆ **CO Pramipexole (Can)** *see* Pramipexole *on page 1695*
◆ **CO Pravastatin (Can)** *see* Pravastatin *on page 1700*
◆ **CO Quetiapine (Can)** *see* QUEtiapine *on page 1757*
◆ **CO Ramipril (Can)** *see* Ramipril *on page 1778*
◆ **CO Ranitidine (Can)** *see* Ranitidine *on page 1782*
◆ **Cordarone** *see* Amiodarone *on page 101*
◆ **Cordran** *see* Flurandrenolide *on page 891*
◆ **Cordran SP** *see* Flurandrenolide *on page 891*
◆ **Coreg** *see* Carvedilol *on page 355*
◆ **Coreg CR** *see* Carvedilol *on page 355*
◆ **CO-Repaglinide (Can)** *see* Repaglinide *on page 1797*
◆ **Corfen-DM [OTC]** *see* Chlorpheniramine, Phenylephrine, and Dextromethorphan *on page 413*
◆ **Corgard** *see* Nadolol *on page 1415*
◆ **Coricidin HBP Chest Congestion and Cough [OTC]** *see* Guaifenesin and Dextromethorphan *on page 976*
◆ **Coricidin HBP® Cold and Flu [OTC]** *see* Chlorpheniramine and Acetaminophen *on page 412*
◆ **Coricidin® HBP Cough & Cold [OTC]** *see* Dextromethorphan and Chlorpheniramine *on page 591*
◆ **Corifact®** *see* Factor XIII Concentrate (Human) *on page 829*
◆ **Corifact** *see* Factor XIII Concentrate (Human) *on page 829*
◆ **CO Risperidone (Can)** *see* RisperiDONE *on page 1826*
◆ **CO Rizatriptan (Can)** *see* Rizatriptan *on page 1844*
◆ **CO Rizatriptan ODT (Can)** *see* Rizatriptan *on page 1844*
◆ **Corlopam** *see* Fenoldopam *on page 841*
◆ **Cormax Scalp Application** *see* Clobetasol *on page 457*
◆ **CO Ropinirole (Can)** *see* ROPINIRole *on page 1851*
◆ **CO Rosuvastatin (Can)** *see* Rosuvastatin *on page 1858*
◆ **Correct [OTC]** *see* Bisacodyl *on page 259*
◆ **CortAlo** *see* Hydrocortisone (Topical) *on page 1011*
◆ **Cortamed® (Can)** *see* Hydrocortisone (Topical) *on page 1011*
◆ **Cortef** *see* Hydrocortisone (Systemic) *on page 1008*
◆ **Cortef® (Can)** *see* Hydrocortisone (Systemic) *on page 1008*
◆ **Cortenema** *see* Hydrocortisone (Topical) *on page 1011*
◆ **Cortenema® (Can)** *see* Hydrocortisone (Topical) *on page 1011*
◆ **Corticool [OTC]** *see* Hydrocortisone (Topical) *on page 1011*

Corticorelin (kor ti koe REL in)

Brand Names: U.S. Acthrel
Index Terms Corticorelin Ovine Triflutate; Human Corticotrophin-Releasing Hormone, Analogue; Ovine Corticotrophin-Releasing Hormone (oCRH)
Pharmacologic Category Diagnostic Agent
Use Diagnostic test used in adrenocorticotropic hormone (ACTH)-dependent Cushing's syndrome to differentiate between pituitary and ectopic production of ACTH
Pregnancy Risk Factor C
Dosage I.V.: Adults: Testing pituitary corticotrophin function: 1 mcg/kg; dosages >1 mcg/kg or >100 mcg have been associated with an increase in adverse effects and are not recommended.

Note: Venous blood samples should be drawn 15 minutes before and immediately prior to corticorelin administration to determine baseline ACTH and cortisol (baseline ACTH value is the average of the 2 samples). At 15-, 30-, and 60 minutes after administration, venous blood samples should be drawn again to determine response. **Basal and peak responses differ depending on AM or PM administration; therefore, any repeat evaluations on the same patient are recommended to be done at the same time of day as the initial testing.**

Dosage adjustment in renal impairment: No dosage adjustment provided in manufacturer's labeling.
Dosage adjustment in hepatic impairment: No dosage adjustment provided in manufacturer's labeling.

Additional Information Complete prescribing information should be consulted for additional detail.
Dosage Forms Excipient information presented when available (limited, particularly for generics); consult specific product labeling.
Solution Reconstituted, Intravenous, as trifluoroacetate:
Acthrel: 100 mcg (1 ea)

◆ **Corticorelin Ovine Triflutate** *see* Corticorelin *on page 493*

◆ **Cortifoam** *see* Hydrocortisone (Topical) *on page 1011*
◆ **Cortifoam™ (Can)** *see* Hydrocortisone (Topical) *on page 1011*
◆ **Cortimyxin® (Can)** *see* Neomycin, Polymyxin B, and Hydrocortisone *on page 1440*
◆ **Cortisol** *see* Hydrocortisone (Systemic) *on page 1008*
◆ **Cortisol** *see* Hydrocortisone (Topical) *on page 1011*

Cortisone (KOR ti sone)

Index Terms Compound E; Cortisone Acetate

Pharmacologic Category Corticosteroid, Systemic

Additional Appendix Information

Corticosteroids Systemic Equivalencies *on page 2297*

Use Management of adrenocortical insufficiency

Pregnancy Considerations Adequate reproduction studies have not been conducted. Cortisone crosses the placenta (Migeon, 1957). Some studies have shown an association between first trimester systemic corticosteroid use and oral clefts (Park-Wyllie, 2000; Pradat, 2003). Systemic corticosteroids may also influence fetal growth (decreased birth weight); however, information is conflicting (Lunghi, 2010). Hypoadrenalism may occur in newborns following maternal use of corticosteroids in pregnancy; monitor. When systemic corticosteroids are needed in pregnancy, it is generally recommended to use the lowest effective dose for the shortest duration of time, avoiding high doses during the first trimester (Leachman, 2006; Lunghi, 2010; Makol, 2011; Østensen, 2009).

Women exposed to cortisone during pregnancy for the treatment of an autoimmune disease may contact the OTIS Autoimmune Diseases Study at 877-311-8972.

Breast-Feeding Considerations Corticosteroids are excreted in human milk. The manufacturer notes that when used systemically, maternal use of corticosteroids have the potential to cause adverse events in a nursing infant (eg, growth suppression, interfere with endogenous corticosteroid production). Breast-feeding is not recommended by the manufacturer in women taking pharmacologic doses. If there is concern about exposure to the infant, some guidelines recommend waiting 4 hours after the maternal dose of an oral systemic corticosteroid before breast-feeding in order to decrease potential exposure to the nursing infant (based on a study using prednisolone) (Bae, 2011; Leachman, 2006; Makol, 2011; Ost, 1985).

Contraindications Hypersensitivity to cortisone acetate or any component of the formulation; serious infections, except septic shock or tuberculous meningitis; administration of live virus vaccines

Warnings/Precautions Use with caution in patients with thyroid disease, hepatic impairment, renal impairment, cardiovascular disease, diabetes, glaucoma, cataracts, myasthenia gravis, patients at risk for osteoporosis, patients at risk for seizures, or GI diseases (diverticulitis, peptic ulcer, ulcerative colitis) due to perforation risk. Use caution following acute MI (corticosteroids have been associated with myocardial rupture). Because of the risk of adverse effects, systemic corticosteroids should be used cautiously in the elderly in the smallest possible effective dose for the shortest duration. May affect growth velocity; growth should be routinely monitored in pediatric patients. Withdraw therapy with gradual tapering of dose.

May cause hypercorticism or suppression of hypothalamic-pituitary-adrenal (HPA) axis, particularly in younger children or in patients receiving high doses for prolonged periods. HPA axis suppression may lead to adrenal crisis. Withdrawal and discontinuation of a corticosteroid should be done slowly and carefully. Particular care is required when patients are transferred from systemic corticosteroids to inhaled products due to possible adrenal insufficiency or withdrawal from steroids, including an increase in allergic symptoms. Patients receiving >20 mg per day of prednisone (or equivalent) may be most susceptible. Fatalities have occurred due to adrenal insufficiency in asthmatic patients during and after transfer from systemic corticosteroids to aerosol steroids; aerosol steroids do not provide the systemic steroid needed to treat patients having trauma, surgery, or infections.

Acute myopathy has been reported with high dose corticosteroids, usually in patients with neuromuscular transmission disorders; may involve ocular and/or respiratory muscles; monitor creatine kinase; recovery may be delayed. Corticosteroid use may cause psychiatric disturbances, including depression, euphoria, insomnia, mood swings, and personality changes. Pre-existing psychiatric conditions may be exacerbated by corticosteroid use. Prolonged use of corticosteroids may also increase the incidence of secondary infection, mask acute infection (including fungal infections), prolong or exacerbate viral infections, or limit response to vaccines. Exposure to chickenpox should be avoided; corticosteroids should not be used to treat ocular herpes simplex. Corticosteroids should not be used for cerebral malaria or viral hepatitis. Close observation is required in patients with latent tuberculosis and/or TB reactivity; restrict use in active TB (only in conjunction with antituberculosis treatment). Prolonged treatment with corticosteroids has been associated with the development of Kaposi's sarcoma (case reports); if noted, discontinuation of therapy should be considered.

Adverse Reactions

>10%:

Central nervous system: Insomnia, nervousness
Gastrointestinal: Increased appetite, indigestion

1% to 10%:

Dermatologic: Hirsutism
Endocrine & metabolic: Diabetes mellitus
Neuromuscular & skeletal: Arthralgia
Ocular: Cataracts, glaucoma
Respiratory: Epistaxis

<1% (Limited to important or life-threatening): Alkalosis, Cushing's syndrome, delirium, edema, euphoria, fractures, hallucinations, hypersensitivity reactions, hypertension, hypokalemia, muscle wasting, myalgia, osteoporosis, pancreatitis, peptic ulcer, pituitary-adrenal axis suppression, pseudotumor cerebri, psychoses, seizure, skin atrophy, ulcerative esophagitis

Drug Interactions

Metabolism/Transport Effects None known.

Avoid Concomitant Use

Avoid concomitant use of Cortisone with any of the following: Aldesleukin; BCG; Mifepristone; Natalizumab; Pimecrolimus; Tacrolimus (Topical); Tofacitinib

Increased Effect/Toxicity

Cortisone may increase the levels/effects of: Acetylcholinesterase Inhibitors; Amphotericin B; Deferasirox; Leflunomide; Loop Diuretics; Natalizumab; NSAID (COX-2 Inhibitor); NSAID (Nonselective); Thiazide Diuretics; Tofacitinib; Vaccines (Live); Warfarin

The levels/effects of Cortisone may be increased by: Antifungal Agents (Azole Derivatives, Systemic); Aprepitant; Calcium Channel Blockers (Nondihydropyridine); Denosumab; Estrogen Derivatives; Fluconazole; Fosaprepitant; Indacaterol; Macrolide Antibiotics; Mifepristone; Neuromuscular-Blocking Agents (Nondepolarizing); Pimecrolimus; Quinolone Antibiotics; Roflumilast; Salicylates; Tacrolimus (Topical); Telaprevir; Trastuzumab

Decreased Effect

Cortisone may decrease the levels/effects of: Aldesleukin; Antidiabetic Agents; BCG; Calcitriol; Coccidioidin Skin Test; Corticorelin; Hyaluronidase; Isoniazid; Salicylates; Sipuleucel-T; Telaprevir; Urea Cycle Disorder Agents; Vaccines (Inactivated)

The levels/effects of Cortisone may be decreased by: Aminoglutethimide; Antacids; Barbiturates; Bile Acid Sequestrants; Echinacea; Mifepristone; Mitotane; Primidone; Rifamycin Derivatives; Somatropin; Tesamorelin

Ethanol/Nutrition/Herb Interactions Food: Limit caffeine intake.

Mechanism of Action Decreases inflammation by suppression of migration of polymorphonuclear leukocytes and reversal of increased capillary permeability

Pharmacodynamics/Kinetics

Onset of action: Peak effect: Oral: ~2 hours; I.M.: 20-48 hours

Duration: 30-36 hours

Absorption: Slow

Distribution: Muscles, liver, skin, intestines, and kidneys

Metabolism: Hepatic to inactive metabolites

Half-life elimination: 0.5-2 hours; End-stage renal disease: 3.5 hours

Excretion: Urine and feces

Dosage If possible, administer glucocorticoids before 9 AM to minimize adrenocortical suppression; dosing depends upon the condition being treated and the response of the patient. **Note:** Supplemental doses may be warranted during times of stress in the course of withdrawing therapy.

Children:

Anti-inflammatory or immunosuppressive: Oral: 2.5-10 mg/kg/day **or** 20-300 mg/m^2/day in divided doses every 6-8 hours

Physiologic replacement: Oral: 0.5-0.75 mg/kg/day **or** 20-25 mg/m^2/day in divided doses every 8 hours

Adults:

Anti-inflammatory or immunosuppressive: Oral: 25-300 mg/day in divided doses every 12-24 hours

Physiologic replacement: Oral: 25-35 mg/day

Hemodialysis: Supplemental dose is not necessary

Peritoneal dialysis: Supplemental dose is not necessary

Dietary Considerations May need diet with increased potassium, pyridoxine, vitamin C, vitamin D, folate, calcium, and phosphorus and decreased sodium; may be taken with food to decrease GI distress.

Administration Insoluble in water.

Test Interactions May suppress the wheal and flare reactions to skin test antigens

Dosage Forms Excipient information presented when available (limited, particularly for generics); consult specific product labeling.

Tablet, Oral, as acetate:

Generic: 25 mg

- ◆ **Cortisone Acetate** *see* Cortisone *on page 494*
- ◆ **Cortisporin®** *see* Neomycin, Polymyxin B, and Hydrocortisone *on page 1440*
- ◆ **Cortisporin® Ointment** *see* Bacitracin, Neomycin, Polymyxin B, and Hydrocortisone *on page 221*
- ◆ **Cortisporin® Otic (Can)** *see* Neomycin, Polymyxin B, and Hydrocortisone *on page 1440*
- ◆ **Cortisporin®-TC** *see* Neomycin, Colistin, Hydrocortisone, and Thonzonium *on page 1439*
- ◆ **Cortisporin® Topical Ointment (Can)** *see* Bacitracin, Neomycin, Polymyxin B, and Hydrocortisone *on page 221*
- ◆ **Cortomycin** *see* Neomycin, Polymyxin B, and Hydrocortisone *on page 1440*
- ◆ **Cortrosyn** *see* Cosyntropin *on page 495*
- ◆ **Cortrosyn™ (Can)** *see* Cosyntropin *on page 495*
- ◆ **Corvert** *see* Ibutilide *on page 1037*
- ◆ **CO Sertraline (Can)** *see* Sertraline *on page 1889*
- ◆ **CO Sildenafil (Can)** *see* Sildenafil *on page 1894*
- ◆ **CO Simvastatin (Can)** *see* Simvastatin *on page 1899*
- ◆ **Cosmegen** *see* DACTINomycin *on page 531*
- ◆ **Cosopt®** *see* Dorzolamide and Timolol *on page 655*
- ◆ **Cosopt® PF** *see* Dorzolamide and Timolol *on page 655*
- ◆ **Cosopt® Preservative Free (Can)** *see* Dorzolamide and Timolol *on page 655*
- ◆ **CO Sotalol (Can)** *see* Sotalol *on page 1942*
- ◆ **CO Sumatriptan (Can)** *see* SUMAtriptan *on page 1969*

Cosyntropin (koe sin TROE pin)

Brand Names: U.S. Cortrosyn

Brand Names: Canada Cortrosyn™; Synacthen® Depot

Index Terms Synacthen; Tetracosactide

Pharmacologic Category Corticosteroid, Systemic; Diagnostic Agent

Use Diagnostic test to differentiate primary adrenal from secondary (pituitary) adrenocortical insufficiency

Synacthen® Depot (Canadian availability): Additional indications: Treatment of various disease states (eg, collagen, dermatologic, endocrine, ocular, hemolytic). Consult manufacturer labeling for detailed list.

Pregnancy Risk Factor C

Pregnancy Considerations Animal reproduction studies have not been conducted with cosyntropin; adverse events have been observed with corticosteroids in animal reproduction studies. Some studies have shown an association between first trimester systemic corticosteroid use and oral clefts (Park-Wyllie, 2000; Pradat, 2003). Systemic corticosteroids may also influence fetal growth (decreased birth weight); however, information is conflicting (Lunghi, 2010). When systemic corticosteroids are needed in pregnancy, it is generally recommended to use the lowest effective dose for the shortest duration of time, avoiding high doses during the first trimester (Leachman, 2006; Lunghi, 2010; Makol, 2011; Østensen, 2009).

Breast-Feeding Considerations It is not known if cosyntropin is excreted into breast milk. The manufacturer recommends that caution be exercised when administering cosyntropin to nursing women.

Contraindications Hypersensitivity to cosyntropin or any component of the formulation

Synacthen® Depot (Canadian availability):Additional contraindications: Treatment of asthma or other allergic conditions (increased risk of anaphylactic reactions); use in premature babies and neonates <1 month; acute psychosis; untreated bacterial, fungal, and viral infections; active or latent peptic ulcer; refractory heart failure; Cushing's syndrome; treatment of primary adrenocortical insufficiency; adrenogenital syndrome

Warnings/Precautions

Cortrosyn™: Use with caution in patients with pre-existing allergic disease or a history of allergic reactions to corticotropin.

Synacthen® Depot (Canadian availability): Use is contraindicated in patients with allergic conditions. Hypersensitivity reactions (including severe reactions) may occur particularly in patients with asthma or other allergies and often within 30 minutes of administration; monitor for hypersensitivity for ~1 hour after administration. Prolonged use may increase the risk of allergic reactions; contains benzyl alcohol; avoid use in infants and children <3 years of age; contraindicated in neonates. Use caution in patients with hypertension or thromboembolic disease, nonspecific ulcerative colitis, diverticulitis, or recent intestinal anastomosis, hepatic disease, renal disease, myasthenia gravis, osteoporosis, psychiatric disturbances, thyroid disease, and/or ocular disease (cataracts, glaucoma). Avoid use in optic neuritis. Consider routine eye exams in chronic users. Use caution in patients with acute or chronic infections (especially varicella or vaccinia) or exanthematous and fungal diseases. Use with caution in patients with latent tuberculosis; treatment may reactivate latent tuberculosis. Rule out amebiasis prior to initiating therapy; may activate latent amebiasis. Live vaccines should not be given concurrently. Augmentation or resumption of therapy may be necessary in patients undergoing surgery or subjected to trauma during or within 1 year of therapy discontinuation; adjunctive rapid acting corticosteroids may be necessary during periods of stress.

Adverse Reactions Frequency not defined. **Note:** Adverse events associated with other corticosteroids may be observed when Synacthen® Depot (Canadian availability) is used for therapeutic purposes. Refer to corticosteroid monographs for comprehensive lists.

Cardiovascular: Bradycardia, hypertension, peripheral edema, tachycardia

Dermatologic: Rash

Local: Whealing with redness at the injection site

Miscellaneous: Anaphylaxis, hypersensitivity reaction

Postmarketing and/or case reports: Synacthen® Depot (Canadian availability): Adrenal hemorrhage

Drug Interactions

Metabolism/Transport Effects None known.

Avoid Concomitant Use

Avoid concomitant use of Cosyntropin with any of the following: Valproic Acid and Derivatives

Increased Effect/Toxicity

Cosyntropin may increase the levels/effects of: ClonazePAM; Diazepam; Nitrazepam; PHENobarbital; Phenytoin; Primidone; Valproic Acid and Derivatives

Decreased Effect There are no known significant interactions involving a decrease in effect.

Preparation for Administration

Powder for injection:

I.M.: Reconstitute 0.25 mg with NS 1 mL.

I.V. push: Reconstitute 0.25 mg with NS 2-5 mL.

I.V. infusion: Mix in NS or D_5W.

Solution for injection:

I.V. push: Reconstitute 0.25 mg with NS 2-5 mL.

I.V. infusion: Mix in NS or D_5W.

Storage/Stability

Powder for injection: Store at controlled room temperature of 15°C to 30°C (59°F to 86°F).

I.V. infusion: Stable for 12 hours at room temperature.

Solution for injection: Store refrigerated between 2°C to 8°C (36°F to 46°F). Protect from light and freezing.

I.V. infusion: Stable for 12 hours at room temperature.

Suspension for injection: Synacthen® Depot (Canadian availability): Store refrigerated between 2°C to 8°C (36°F to 46°F). Protect from light.

Mechanism of Action Stimulates the adrenal cortex to secrete adrenal steroids (including hydrocortisone, cortisone), androgenic substances, and a small amount of aldosterone

Pharmacodynamics/Kinetics

Duration of action: Synacthen® Depot (Canadian availability): I.M.: Plasma concentrations of 200-300 pg/mL maintained for 12 hours

Absorption: Synacthen® Depot (Canadian availability): I.M.: Rapid

Distribution: Synacthen® Depot (Canadian availability): V_d: ~43% of body weight

Half-life elimination: Synacthen® Depot (Canadian availability): 7 minutes

Time to peak, serum: I.M., I.V. push: ~1 hour; plasma cortisol levels rise in healthy individuals within 5 minutes

Excretion: Urine

Dosage

Diagnostic use: Screening of adrenocortical insufficiency:

Cosyntropin **powder** for injection (I.M., I.V.) **or** cosyntropin **solution** for injection (I.V. only [manufacturer labeling does not recommend I.M. administration of solution for injection]):

Children ≤2 years: 0.125 mg

Children >2 years and Adults:

Conventional dose: 0.25 mg; **Note:** Doses in the range of 0.25-0.75 mg have been used in clinical studies; however, maximal response is seen with 0.25 mg dose. When greater cortisol stimulation is needed, an I.V. infusion may be used: 0.25 mg administered at 0.04 mg/hour over 6 hours

Low-dose protocol (unlabeled dose): 1 mcg (Abdu, 1999); **Note:** The use of the low-dose protocol has been advocated by some clinicians, particularly in mild or secondary adrenal insufficiency. The low-dose protocol is not recommended in critically-ill patients (Marik, 2008).

Synacthen® Depot (Canadian availability): I.M.: Children >3 years and Adults: 1 mg administered as a single dose or once daily for 3 or 4 days (depending on method of testing; refer to manufacturer labeling for detailed information). **Note:** For patients with severe adrenal insufficiency, some clinicians administer dexamethasone on days that Synacthen® Depot is administered to provide steroid coverage.

Therapeutic use: Synacthen® Depot (Canadian availability): I.M.: **Note:** Titrate to lowest effective dose at the longest effective dosing interval.

Children 3-6 years: Initial: 0.25-0.5 mg daily; maintenance: 0.25-0.5 mg every 2-8 days

Children 7-15 years: Initial: 0.25-1 mg daily; maintenance: 0.25-1 mg every 2-8 days

Children ≥16 years and Adults: Initial for acute treatment: 1 mg daily for 3 days; maintenance dose is individualized: 0.5-1 mg every 2-3 days or twice weekly or 2 mg once weekly or less frequently

Transferring from corticosteroids: Synacthen® Depot (Canadian availability): Children >3 years and Adults: I.M.: Initial: 1 mg daily; gradually reduce steroid by 25% of original dose on successive days. Upon withdrawal from steroid adjust Synacthen® Depot dose as needed.

Transferring from animal-derived ACTH: Synacthen® Depot (Canadian availability): Children >3 years and Adults: I.M.: Conversion varies depending on product previously used. Manufacturer suggests that patients previously receiving ACTH gel 40 units daily should receive Synacthen® Depot 0.5 mg every other day; adjust dose based on response, preferably by extending the dosing interval.

Elderly: Refer to adult dosing.

Dosage adjustment in renal impairment: No dosage adjustment provided in manufacturer's labeling (has not been studied).

Dosage adjustment in hepatic impairment: No dosage adjustment provided in manufacturer's labeling (has not been studied).

Administration

I.V.: May administer by I.V. injection over 2 minutes or as an I.V. infusion over 4-8 hours. Synacthen® Depot (Canadian availability) should **not** be administered intravenously.

I.M.: May administer I.M. (reconstituted powder for injection only); cosyntropin injection **solution** is not recommended for I.M. administration (manufacturer recommendation).

Synacthen® Depot (Canadian availability): Shake ampul until uniform appearance; administer by I.M. injection in the buttocks. Self-administration by patient is not recommended.

Monitoring Parameters Synacthen® Depot (Canadian availability): Observe patient for ~1 hour after administration for signs/symptoms of hypersensitivity; for diagnosis of adrenocortical Insufficiency measure plasma cortisol prior to and 4-6 hours after injection; with prolonged use monitor blood pressure, weight, urinalysis, glucose, electrolytes, signs and symptoms of infection, cataract formation, intraocular pressure, bone mass density and growth in children, ECG (in children)

Reference Range Normal baseline cortisol >5 mcg/dL; normal response 30 minutes after cosyntropin injection: increase in serum cortisol concentration of >7 mcg/dL or peak response >18 mcg/dL; plasma cortisol concentrations should be measured immediately before and exactly 30 minutes after a dose. If increase in plasma cortisol levels at 30 minutes is equivocal, consider repeat cortisol sampling at 60 and/or 90 minutes.

Synacthen® Depot (Canadian availability): 5-hour test: Plasma cortisol levels double in first hour then increase more gradually; normal values at 5 hours: 37-66 mcg/dL; 3-day test (control phase days 1 and 2, dosing on days 3-5): compared to control phase, urinary cortisol excretion at least doubles on day 3 and further increases on days 4 and 5

Test Interactions Concurrent or recent use of spironolactone, hydrocortisone, cortisone, etomidate, estrogens

Additional Information Each 0.25 mg of cosyntropin is equivalent to 25 units of corticotropin.

Patient should not receive corticosteroids or spironolactone the day of the test. Some clinicians administer dexamethasone on days that Synacthen® Depot (Canadian availability) is administered to provide steroid coverage.

Dosage Forms Excipient information presented when available (limited, particularly for generics); consult specific product labeling.

Solution, Intravenous:
- Generic: 0.25 mg/mL (1 mL)

Solution Reconstituted, Injection:
- Cortrosyn: 0.25 mg (1 ea)
- Generic: 0.25 mg (1 ea)

Solution Reconstituted, Injection [preservative free]:
- Generic: 0.25 mg (1 ea)

Dosage Forms: Canada Excipient information presented when available (limited, particularly for generics); consult specific product labeling.

Injection, suspension:
- Synacthen® Depot: 1 mg/mL (1 mL) [contains benzyl alcohol]

- ◆ **Cotazym (Can)** *see* Pancrelipase *on page 1558*
- ◆ **CO Telmisartan (Can)** *see* Telmisartan *on page 2002*
- ◆ **CO Telmisartan HCT (Can)** *see* Telmisartan and Hydrochlorothiazide *on page 2004*
- ◆ **CO Temazepam (Can)** *see* Temazepam *on page 2005*
- ◆ **Co-Temozolomide (Can)** *see* Temozolomide *on page 2005*
- ◆ **CO Terbinafine (Can)** *see* Terbinafine (Systemic) *on page 2017*
- ◆ **CO Topiramate (Can)** *see* Topiramate *on page 2090*
- ◆ **CO Tramadol/Acet (Can)** *see* Acetaminophen and Tramadol *on page 33*
- ◆ **Co-Trimoxazole** *see* Sulfamethoxazole and Trimethoprim *on page 1959*
- ◆ **Cough Syrup [OTC]** *see* GuaiFENesin *on page 974*
- ◆ **Coumadin** *see* Warfarin *on page 2211*
- ◆ **Coumadin® (Can)** *see* Warfarin *on page 2211*
- ◆ **CO Valacyclovir (Can)** *see* ValACYclovir *on page 2145*
- ◆ **CO Valsartan (Can)** *see* Valsartan *on page 2154*
- ◆ **CO Venlafaxine XR (Can)** *see* Venlafaxine *on page 2178*
- ◆ **Covera® (Can)** *see* Verapamil *on page 2182*
- ◆ **Covera-HS® (Can)** *see* Verapamil *on page 2182*
- ◆ **Coversyl (Can)** *see* Perindopril Erbumine *on page 1622*
- ◆ **Co-Vidarabine** *see* Pentostatin *on page 1617*
- ◆ **Coviracil** *see* Emtricitabine *on page 698*
- ◆ **Cozaar** *see* Losartan *on page 1247*
- ◆ **CP-690, 550** *see* Tofacitinib *on page 2082*
- ◆ **CP358774** *see* Erlotinib *on page 735*
- ◆ **CPDG2** *see* Glucarpidase *on page 961*
- ◆ **CPG2** *see* Glucarpidase *on page 961*
- ◆ **CPM** *see* Cyclophosphamide *on page 504*
- ◆ **CPT-11** *see* Irinotecan *on page 1115*
- ◆ **CPZ** *see* ChlorproMAZINE *on page 415*
- ◆ **13-CRA** *see* ISOtretinoin *on page 1129*
- ◆ **CRA-032765** *see* Ibrutinib *on page 1030*
- ◆ **Creon** *see* Pancrelipase *on page 1558*
- ◆ **Crestor** *see* Rosuvastatin *on page 1858*
- ◆ **Crinone** *see* Progesterone *on page 1725*
- ◆ **Critic-Aid Clear AF [OTC]** *see* Miconazole (Topical) *on page 1358*
- ◆ **Critic-Aid Skin Care® [OTC]** *see* Zinc Oxide *on page 2230*
- ◆ **Crixivan** *see* Indinavir *on page 1068*
- ◆ **Crixivan® (Can)** *see* Indinavir *on page 1068*

Crizotinib (kriz OH ti nib)

Brand Names: U.S. Xalkori

Brand Names: Canada Xalkori

Index Terms C-Met/Hepatocyte Growth Factor Receptor Tyrosine Kinase Inhibitor PF-02341066; C-Met/HGFR Tyrosine Kinase Inhibitor PF-02341066; MET Tyrosine Kinase Inhibitor PF-02341066; PF-02341066

Pharmacologic Category Antineoplastic Agent, Anaplastic Lymphoma Kinase Inhibitor; Antineoplastic Agent, Tyrosine Kinase Inhibitor

Use Nonsmall cell lung cancer: Treatment of patients with metastatic nonsmall cell lung cancer (NSCLC) whose tumors are anaplastic lymphoma kinase (ALK)-positive (as detected by an approved test)

Pregnancy Risk Factor D

Pregnancy Considerations Adverse events have been observed in animal reproduction studies. Based on the mechanism of action, crizotinib may cause fetal harm if administered during pregnancy. Women of childbearing potential and men of reproductive potential should use adequate contraception methods during and for at least 90 days after treatment.

Breast-Feeding Considerations It is not known if crizotinib is excreted in breast milk. Due to the potential for serious adverse reactions in the nursing infant, the decision to discontinue crizotinib or to discontinue breast-feeding should take into account the benefits of treatment to the mother.

Prescribing and Access Restrictions Available through specialty pharmacies. Further information may be obtained from the manufacturer, Pfizer, at 1-877-744-5675, or at http://www.pfizerpro.com

Contraindications

U.S. labeling: There are no contraindications listed in the manufacturer's labeling.

Canadian labeling: Hypersensitivity to crizotinib or any component of the formulation; congenital long QT syndrome or with persistent Fridericia-corrected QT interval (QTcF) ≥500 msec

Warnings/Precautions Hazardous agent - use appropriate precautions for handling and disposal (meets NIOSH, 2012 criteria). Approved for use only in patients with metastatic nonsmall cell lung cancer (NSCLC) who test positive for the abnormal anaplastic lymphoma kinase (ALK) gene. The Vysis ALK break-apart FISH probe kit is approved to test for the gene abnormality.

Fatalities due to crizotinib-induced hepatotoxicity have occurred. Grade 3 or 4 ALT increases (usually asymptomatic and reversible) have been observed in clinical trials. May require dosage interruption and/or reduction; permanent discontinuation was necessary in some cases; elevations in ALT >5 x ULN were observed; concurrent ALT elevations >3 x ULN and total bilirubin elevations >2 x ULN (without alkaline phosphatase elevations) were observed rarely. Monitor liver function tests, including ALT and total bilirubin every 2 weeks during the first 2 months of therapy, then monthly and as clinically necessary. Transaminase elevation onset was within 2 months of treatment initiation. Use with caution in patients with hepatic impairment (has not been studied); crizotinib is extensively metabolized in the liver and liver impairment is likely to increase crizotinib levels.

Severe, life-threatening, and potentially fatal interstitial lung disease (ILD)/pneumonitis has been associated with crizotinib. Onset was generally within 2 months of treatment initiation. Monitor for pulmonary symptoms which may indicate ILD/pneumonitis; exclude other potential causes (eg, disease progression, infection, other pulmonary disease, or radiation therapy). Permanently discontinue if treatment-related ILD/pneumonitis is confirmed.

Symptomatic bradycardia may occur; heart rate <50 beats/minute has occurred. If possible, avoid concurrent use with other agents known to cause bradycardia (eg, beta blockers, nondihydropyridine calcium channel blockers, clonidine, digoxin). Monitor heart rate and blood pressure regularly. If symptomatic bradycardia (not life-threatening) occurs, withhold treatment until recovery to asymptomatic bradycardia or to a heart rate of ≥60 beats/minute, evaluate concurrent medications, and reduce crizotinib dose. Permanently discontinue for life-threatening bradycardia due to crizotinib; if life-threatening bradycardia occurs and concurrent medications associated with bradycardia can be discontinued, restart crizotinib at a reduced dose (with frequent monitoring). QT_c prolongation has been observed; consider periodic monitoring of ECG and electrolytes in patients with heart failure, bradyarrhythmias, electrolyte abnormalities, or who are taking medications known to prolong the QT interval. May require treatment interruption, dosage reduction, or discontinuation. Avoid use in patients with congenital long QT syndrome. Canadian labeling contraindicates use in patients with congenital long QT syndrome or persistent QTcF ≥500 msec.

Ocular toxicities (eg, blurred vision, diplopia, photophobia, photopsia, visual acuity decreased, visual brightness, visual field defect, visual impairment, and/or vitreous floaters) commonly occur. Onset is generally within 2 weeks of treatment initiation; consider ophthalmology exam, especially if photopsia or vitreous floaters occur. Severe or worsening vitreous floaters or photopsia could be a sign of retinal hole or impending detachment. Reduce initial dose in patients with severe renal impairment not requiring dialysis. Potentially significant drug-drug and drug-food interactions may exist, requiring dose or frequency adjustment, additional monitoring, and/or selection of alternative therapy. Avoid concomitant use with strong CYP3A4 inhibitors and inducers and with CYP3A4 substrates. Crizotinib is associated with a moderate emetic potential; antiemetics may be needed to prevent nausea and vomiting.

Adverse Reactions

>10%:

Cardiovascular: Edema (28%)

Central nervous system: Fatigue (20%), dizziness (16%)

Gastrointestinal: Nausea (53%), diarrhea (43%), vomiting (40%), constipation (27%), appetite decreased (19%), taste alteration (12%), esophageal disorder (11%; includes dyspepsia, dysphagia, epigastric burning/discomfort/pain, esophageal obstruction/pain/spasm/ulcer, esophagitis, gastroesophageal reflux, odynophagia, reflux esophagitis)

Hematologic: Lymphopenia (grades 3/4: 11%)

Hepatic: ALT increased (13%; grades 3/4: 5%)

Neuromuscular & skeletal: Neuropathy (13%; grades 3/4: <1%)

Ocular: Vision disorder (62%; onset: <2 weeks; includes blurred vision, diplopia, photophobia, photopsia, visual acuity decreased, visual brightness, visual field defect, visual impairment, vitreous floaters)

1% to 10%:

Cardiovascular: Bradycardia (5%), chest pain (1%)

Central nervous system: Headache (4%), insomnia (3%)

Dermatologic: Rash (10%)

Gastrointestinal: Abdominal pain (8%), stomatitis (6%)

Hematologic: Neutropenia (grades 3/4: 5%)

Hepatic: AST increased (9%; grades 3/4: 2%)

Neuromuscular & skeletal: Arthralgia (2%)

Renal: Renal cysts (1%)

Respiratory: Cough (4%), dyspnea (2%), pneumonitis (2%), upper respiratory infection (2%)

<1% (Limited to important or life-threatening): Back pain, fever, QT_c prolongation, thrombocytopenia

Drug Interactions

Metabolism/Transport Effects Substrate of CYP3A4 (major), P-glycoprotein; **Note:** Assignment of Major/Minor substrate status based on clinically relevant drug interaction potential; **Inhibits** CYP2B6 (moderate), CYP3A4 (moderate), P-glycoprotein

Avoid Concomitant Use

Avoid concomitant use of Crizotinib with any of the following: Alfentanil; Bosutinib; CycloSPORINE (Systemic); CYP3A4 Inducers (Strong); CYP3A4 Inhibitors (Strong); Dihydroergotamine; Ergotamine; FentaNYL; Fusidic Acid (Systemic); Grapefruit Juice; Highest Risk QTc-Prolonging Agents; Ibrutinib; Ivabradine; Lomitapide; Mifepristone; Pimozide; Pomalidomide; QuiNIDine; Silodosin; Simeprevir; Sirolimus; St Johns Wort; Tacrolimus (Systemic); Tolvaptan; Topotecan; Ulipristal; VinCRIStine (Liposomal)

Increased Effect/Toxicity

Crizotinib may increase the levels/effects of: Afatinib; Alfentanil; ARIPiprazole; Avanafil; Bosentan; Bosutinib; Budesonide (Systemic, Oral Inhalation); Colchicine; CycloSPORINE (Systemic); CYP2B6 Substrates; CYP3A4 Substrates; Dabigatran Etexilate; Dihydroergotamine; Eplerenone; Ergotamine; Everolimus; FentaNYL; Highest Risk QTc-Prolonging Agents; Ibrutinib; Imatinib; Ivacaftor; Lomitapide; Lurasidone; Moderate Risk QTc-Prolonging Agents; OxyCODONE; P-glycoprotein/ABCB1 Substrates; Pimecrolimus; Pimozide; Pomalidomide; Prucalopride; QuiNIDine; Rivaroxaban; Salmeterol; Saxagliptin; Silodosin; Simeprevir; Sirolimus; Tacrolimus (Systemic); Tolvaptan; Topotecan; Ulipristal; Vilazodone; VinCRIStine (Liposomal); Vitamin K Antagonists

The levels/effects of Crizotinib may be increased by: CYP3A4 Inhibitors (Moderate); CYP3A4 Inhibitors (Strong); Dasatinib; Fusidic Acid (Systemic); Grapefruit Juice; Ivabradine; Ivacaftor; Luliconazole; Mifepristone; P-glycoprotein/ABCB1 Inhibitors; QTc-Prolonging Agents (Indeterminate Risk and Risk Modifying); Simeprevir

Decreased Effect

Crizotinib may decrease the levels/effects of: Cardiac Glycosides; Ifosfamide; Vitamin K Antagonists

The levels/effects of Crizotinib may be decreased by: Bosentan; CYP3A4 Inducers (Strong); Dabrafenib; Deferasirox; P-glycoprotein/ABCB1 Inducers; St Johns Wort; Tocilizumab

Ethanol/Nutrition/Herb Interactions

Food: Grapefruit juice may increase serum crizotinib levels. Management: Avoid grapefruit and grapefruit juice.

Herb/Nutraceutical: St John's wort may decrease the serum concentration of crizotinib. Management: Avoid St John's wort.

Storage/Stability Store between 20°C and 25°C (68°F and 77°F); excursions are permitted between 15°C and 30°C (59°F and 86°F).

Mechanism of Action Tyrosine kinase receptor inhibitor, which inhibits anaplastic lymphoma kinase (ALK), Hepatocyte Growth Factor Receptor (HGFR, c-MET), and Recepteur d'Origine Nantais (RON). ALK gene abnormalities due to mutations or translocations may result in expression of oncogenic fusion proteins (eg, ALK fusion protein) which alter signaling and expression and result in increased cellular proliferation and survival in tumors which express these fusion proteins. Approximately 2% to 7% of patients with NSCLC have the abnormal echinoderm microtubule-associated protein-like 4, or EML4-ALK gene (which has a higher prevalence in never smokers or light smokers and in patients with adenocarcinoma). Crizotinib selectively inhibits ALK tyrosine kinase, which reduces proliferation of cells expressing the genetic alteration.

Pharmacodynamics/Kinetics

Distribution: V_{ss}: 1772 L

Protein binding: 91%

Metabolism: Hepatic, via CYP3A4/5

Bioavailability: 43% (range: 32% to 66%); bioavailability is reduced 14% with a high-fat meal

Half-life elimination: Terminal: 42 hours

Time to peak: 4-6 hours

Excretion: Feces (63%; 53% as unchanged drug); urine (22%; 2% as unchanged drug)

Dosage Nonsmall cell lung cancer (NSCLC), metastatic (ALK-positive): Adults: Oral: 250 mg twice daily, continue treatment until disease progression or unacceptable toxicity

Missed doses: If a dose is missed, take as soon as remembered unless it is <6 hours prior to the next scheduled dose (skip the dose if <6 hours before the next dose); do not take 2 doses at the same time to make up for a missed dose. If vomiting occurs after dose, administer the next dose at the regularly scheduled time.

Dosage adjustment for toxicity: Note: If dose reduction is necessary, reduce dose to 200 mg twice daily; if necessary, further reduce to 250 mg once daily. If unable to tolerate 250 mg once daily, permanently discontinue therapy.

Hematologic toxicity (except lymphopenia, unless lymphopenia is associated with clinical events such as opportunistic infection):

Grade 3 toxicity (WBC 1000-2000/mm³, ANC 500-1000/mm³, platelets 25,000-50,000/mm³), grade 3 anemia: Withhold treatment until recovery to ≤ grade 2, then resume at the same dose and schedule

Grade 4 toxicity (WBC <1000/mm³, ANC <500/mm³, platelets <25,000/mm³), grade 4 anemia: Withhold treatment until recovery to ≤ grade 2, then resume at 200 mg twice daily

Recurrent grade 4 toxicity on 200 mg twice daily: Withhold treatment until recovery to ≤ grade 2, then resume at 250 mg once daily

Recurrent grade 4 toxicity on 250 mg once daily: Permanently discontinue

Nonhematologic toxicities:

Cardiovascular toxicities:

QT_c prolongation:

Grade 3 QT_c prolongation (QTc >500 msec without life-threatening signs or symptoms) on at least 2 separate ECGs: Withhold treatment until recovery to baseline or to ≤ grade 1 (QT_c ≤480 msec), then resume at 200 mg twice daily.

Recurrent grade 3 QT_c prolongation at 200 mg twice daily: Withhold treatment until recovery to baseline or to ≤ grade 1, then resume at 250 mg once daily.

Recurrent grade 3 QT_c prolongation at 250 mg once daily: Permanently discontinue.

Grade 4 QT_c prolongation (QT_c >500 msec or ≥60 msec change from baseline with life-threatening symptoms): Permanently discontinue.

Bradycardia:

Grade 2 bradycardia (symptomatic with medical intervention indicated) or grade 3 bradycardia (severe/ medically significant with intervention indicated): Withhold until recovery to asymptomatic bradycardia or to a heart rate of ≥60 beats/minute, evaluate concomitant medications, then resume at 200 mg twice daily.

Grade 4 bradycardia due to crizotinib (life-threatening with urgent intervention indicated): Permanently discontinue.

Grade 4 bradycardia associated with concurrent medications known to cause bradycardia or hypotension (life-threatening with urgent intervention indicated): Withhold until recovery to asymptomatic bradycardia or to a heart rate of ≥60 beats/minute, and if concurrent medication can be discontinued, resume at 250 mg once daily with frequent monitoring.

Hepatotoxicity: Refer to dosage adjustment in hepatic impairment.

Pulmonary toxicity: Interstitial lung disease (ILD)/pneumonitis (any grade; not attributable to disease progression, infection, other pulmonary disease or radiation therapy): Permanently discontinue.

Dosage adjustment in renal impairment:

Mild to moderate impairment (Cl_{cr} 30-89 mL/minute): No dosage adjustment necessary.

Severe impairment (Cl_{cr} <30 mL/minute) not requiring dialysis: Initial: 250 mg once daily

Dosage adjustment in hepatic impairment:

Hepatotoxicity **prior to** treatment: No dosage adjustment provided in manufacturer's labeling (has not been studied); crizotinib undergoes extensive hepatic metabolism and systemic exposure may be increased with impairment; use with caution.

Hepatotoxicity **during** treatment:

Grade 3 or 4 ALT or AST elevation (ALT or AST >5 x ULN) with ≤ grade 1 total bilirubin elevation (total bilirubin ≤1.5 x ULN): Withhold treatment until recovery to ≤ grade 1 (<3 x ULN) or baseline, then resume at 200 mg twice daily.

Recurrent grade 3 or 4 ALT or AST elevation with ≤ grade 1 total bilirubin elevation: Withhold treatment until recovery to ≤ grade 1, then resume at 250 mg once daily.

Recurrent grade 3 or 4 ALT or AST elevation on 250 mg once daily: Permanently discontinue.

Grade 2, 3, or 4 ALT or AST elevation (ALT or AST >3 x ULN) with concurrent grade 2, 3, or 4 total bilirubin elevation (>1.5 x ULN) in the absence of cholestasis or hemolysis: Permanently discontinue.

Dietary Considerations Avoid grapefruit and grapefruit juice.

Administration Swallow capsules whole (do not crush, dissolve, or open capsules). Administer with or without food. Crizotinib is associated with a moderate emetic potential; antiemetics may be needed to prevent nausea and vomiting. If vomiting occurs after dose, administer the next dose at the regularly scheduled time.

Hazardous agent; use appropriate precautions for handling and disposal (meets NIOSH, 2012 criteria).

Monitoring Parameters ALK positivity; CBC with differential monthly and as clinically appropriate (monitor more frequently if grades 3 or 4 abnormalities observed or with fever or infection), liver function tests monthly and as clinically appropriate (monitor more frequently if grades 2, 3, or 4 abnormalities observed). Monitor pulmonary symptoms (for interstitial lung disease [ILD]/pneumonitis). Consider monitoring ECG and electrolytes in patients with heart failure, bradycardia, bradyarrhythmias, electrolyte abnormalities, or who are taking medications known to prolong the QT interval. Consider ophthalmic evaluation, especially if photopsia or vitreous floaters occur.

Dosage Forms Excipient information presented when available (limited, particularly for generics); consult specific product labeling.

Capsule, Oral:

Xalkori: 200 mg, 250 mg

Crofelemer (kroe FEL e mer)

Brand Names: U.S. Fulyzaq

Index Terms *Croton lechleri*; Provir; SP-303

Pharmacologic Category Antidiarrheal

Use Symptomatic relief of noninfectious diarrhea in patients with HIV/AIDS on antiretroviral therapy

Pregnancy Risk Factor C

Pregnancy Considerations Adverse events were observed in some animal reproduction studies; however, maternal toxicity was also present. Systemic absorption following oral administration is limited.

Breast-Feeding Considerations It is not known if crofelemer is excreted in breast milk; however, systemic absorption following oral administration is limited. According to the manufacturer, the decision to continue or discontinue breast-feeding during therapy should take into account the risk of exposure to the infant and the benefits of treatment to the mother.

Crofelemer is approved for use in HIV-infected persons. In the United States, where formula is accessible, affordable, safe, and sustainable, and the risk of infant mortality due to diarrhea and respiratory infections is low, complete avoidance of breast-feeding by HIV-infected women is recommended to decrease potential transmission of HIV (DHHS [perinatal], 2012).

Contraindications There are no contraindications listed in the manufacturer's labeling.

Warnings/Precautions Crofelemer is not indicated for infectious diarrhea; there is a risk of inadequate or delayed treatment if used when infectious diarrhea is present. Rule out infectious causes for diarrhea prior to initiating treatment. CD4 cell count and viral load do not have a clinical impact on crofelemer treatment; no adjustments are necessary based on CD4 cell count or viral load.

Adverse Reactions 1% to 10%:

Central nervous system: Anxiety (2%), depression (1% to 2%), dizziness (1% to 2%)

Dermatologic: Acne (1% to 2%), dermatitis (1% to 2%)

Gastrointestinal: Flatulence (3%), nausea (3%), abdominal distention (2%), giardiasis (2%), hemorrhoids (2%), abdominal pain (1% to 2%), constipation (1% to 2%), dyspepsia (1% to 2%), gastroenteritis (1% to 2%), xerostomia (1% to 2%)

Genitourinary: Urinary tract infection (2%), pollakiuria (1% to 2%)

Hematologic: Leukopenia (1% to 2%)

Hepatic: Hyperbilirubinemia (1% to 3%), ALT increased (2%), AST increased (1% to 2%)

Neuromuscular & skeletal: Arthralgia (3%), back pain (3%), musculoskeletal pain (2%), limb pain (1% to 2%)

Renal: Nephrolithiasis (1% to 2%)

Respiratory: Upper respiratory tract infection (6%), bronchitis (4%), cough (4%), nasopharyngitis (2%), sinusitis (1% to 2%)

Miscellaneous: Herpes zoster (1% to 2%), seasonal allergy (1% to 2%)

Drug Interactions

Metabolism/Transport Effects **Inhibits** CYP3A4 (weak)

Avoid Concomitant Use

Avoid concomitant use of Crofelemer with any of the following: Pimozide

Increased Effect/Toxicity

Crofelemer may increase the levels/effects of: ARIPiprazole; Dofetilide; Lomitapide; Pimozide

Decreased Effect There are no known significant interactions involving a decrease in effect.

Storage/Stability Store at 20°C to 25°C (68°F to 77°F); excursions permitted to 15°C to 30°C (59°F to 86°F).

Mechanism of Action Inhibits cyclic adenosine monophosphate (cAMP)-stimulated cystic fibrosis transmembrane conductance regulator (CFTR) chloride ion channel and calcium activated chloride ion channels at the enterocyte luminal membrane. This regulates fluid secretion and water loss (high volume) due to diarrhea, normalizing chloride ion and water flow in the GI tract.

Pharmacodynamics/Kinetics Absorption: Minimal systemic absorption

Dosage Diarrhea, noninfectious (associated with antiretroviral therapy for HIV/AIDS): Adults: Oral: 125 mg twice daily

Dosage adjustment in renal impairment: No dosage adjustment provided in the manufacturer's labeling.

Dosage adjustment in hepatic impairment: No dosage adjustment provided in the manufacturer's labeling.

Dietary Considerations May be taken with or without food.

Administration May be administered orally with or without food. Swallow whole; do not crush or chew.

Dosage Forms Excipient information presented when available (limited, particularly for generics); consult specific product labeling.

Tablet Delayed Release, Oral:

Fulyzaq: 125 mg [contains methylparaben, propylparaben]

- Crolom *see* Cromolyn (Ophthalmic) *on page 501*
- Cromoglycic Acid *see* Cromolyn (Nasal) *on page 500*
- Cromoglycic Acid *see* Cromolyn (Ophthalmic) *on page 501*

Cromolyn (Nasal) (KROE moe lin)

Brand Names: U.S. NasalCrom [OTC]

Brand Names: Canada Apo-Cromolyn Nasal Spray® [OTC]; Rhinaris-CS Anti-Allergic Nasal Mist

Index Terms Cromoglycic Acid; Cromolyn Sodium; Disodium Cromoglycate; DSCG

Pharmacologic Category Mast Cell Stabilizer

Use Prevention and treatment of seasonal and perennial allergic rhinitis

Dosage Intranasal: Allergic rhinitis (treatment and prophylaxis): Children ≥2 years and Adults: 1 spray into each nostril 3-4 times/day; may be increased to 6 times/day (symptomatic relief may require 2-4 weeks)

Dosage adjustment in renal impairment: No dosage adjustment provided in manufacturer's labeling.

Dosage adjustment in hepatic impairment: No dosage adjustment provided in manufacturer's labeling.

Additional Information Complete prescribing information should be consulted for additional detail.

Dosage Forms Excipient information presented when available (limited, particularly for generics); consult specific product labeling.

Aerosol Solution, Nasal, as sodium:

NasalCrom: 5.2 mg/actuation (13 mL, 26 mL) [contains benzalkonium chloride, edetate disodium]

Generic: 5.2 mg/actuation (26 mL)

Cromolyn (Ophthalmic) (KROE moe lin)

Brand Names: Canada Opticrom®

Index Terms Crolom; Cromoglycic Acid; Cromolyn Sodium; Disodium Cromoglycate; DSCG

Pharmacologic Category Mast Cell Stabilizer

Use Treatment of vernal keratoconjunctivitis, vernal conjunctivitis, and vernal keratitis

Pregnancy Risk Factor B

Dosage Ophthalmic: Children >4 years and Adults: 1-2 drops in each eye 4-6 times/day

Dosage adjustment in renal impairment: No dosage adjustment provided in manufacturer's labeling. However, dosage adjustment unlikely due to low systemic absorption.

Dosage adjustment in hepatic impairment: No dosage adjustment provided in manufacturer's labeling. However, dosage adjustment unlikely due to low systemic absorption.

Additional Information Complete prescribing information should be consulted for additional detail.

Dosage Forms Excipient information presented when available (limited, particularly for generics); consult specific product labeling.

Solution, Ophthalmic, as sodium:

Generic: 4% (10 mL)

- **Cromolyn Sodium** *see* Cromolyn (Nasal) *on page 500*
- **Cromolyn Sodium** *see* Cromolyn (Ophthalmic) *on page 501*

Crotamiton (kroe TAM i tonn)

Brand Names: U.S. Eurax

Brand Names: Canada Eurax Cream

Pharmacologic Category Scabicidal Agent

Use Treatment of scabies (*Sarcoptes scabiei*) and symptomatic treatment of pruritus

Pregnancy Risk Factor C

Dosage Topical:

Scabicide: Children and Adults: Wash thoroughly and scrub away loose scales, then towel dry; apply a thin layer and massage drug onto skin of the entire body from the neck to the toes (with special attention to skin folds, creases, and interdigital spaces). Repeat application in 24 hours. Take a cleansing bath 48 hours after the final application. Treatment may be repeated after 7-10 days if live mites are still present.

Pruritus: Massage into affected areas until medication is completely absorbed; repeat as necessary

Additional Information Complete prescribing information should be consulted for additional detail.

Dosage Forms Excipient information presented when available (limited, particularly for generics); consult specific product labeling.

Cream, External:

Eurax: 10% (60 g)

Lotion, External:

Eurax: 10% (60 g, 454 g)

- ***Croton lechleri*** *see* Crofelemer *on page 500*
- **CRRT** *see* Electrolyte Solution, Renal Replacement *on page 691*
- **Cruex Prescription Strength [OTC]** *see* Miconazole (Topical) *on page 1358*
- **Cryselle 28** *see* Ethinyl Estradiol and Norgestrel *on page 797*
- **Crystalline Penicillin** *see* Penicillin G (Parenteral/Aqueous) *on page 1608*
- **Crystal Violet** *see* Gentian Violet *on page 954*
- **Crystapen® (Can)** *see* Penicillin G (Parenteral/Aqueous) *on page 1608*
- **CS-747** *see* Prasugrel *on page 1699*
- **CsA** *see* CycloSPORINE (Ophthalmic) *on page 515*
- **CsA** *see* CycloSPORINE (Systemic) *on page 508*
- **C-Time [OTC]** *see* Ascorbic Acid *on page 172*
- **CTLA-4Ig** *see* Abatacept *on page 20*
- **CTP 30 (Can)** *see* Citalopram *on page 440*
- **CTX** *see* Cyclophosphamide *on page 504*
- **Cu-5 [OTC]** *see* Copper *on page 493*
- **Cubicin** *see* DAPTOmycin *on page 541*
- **Cubicin® (Can)** *see* DAPTOmycin *on page 541*
- **Cupric Chloride** *see* Copper *on page 493*
- **Cupric Chloride Dihydrate** *see* Copper *on page 493*
- **Cuprimine** *see* PenicillAMINE *on page 1603*
- **Cuprimine® (Can)** *see* PenicillAMINE *on page 1603*
- **Cutivate** *see* Fluticasone (Topical) *on page 896*
- **Cutivate™ (Can)** *see* Fluticasone (Topical) *on page 896*
- **Cuvposa** *see* Glycopyrrolate *on page 965*
- **CyA** *see* CycloSPORINE (Ophthalmic) *on page 515*
- **CyA** *see* CycloSPORINE (Systemic) *on page 508*

Cyanocobalamin (sye an oh koe BAL a min)

Brand Names: U.S. Nascobal; Physicians EZ Use B-12

Index Terms Vitamin B_{12}

Pharmacologic Category Vitamin, Water Soluble

Use Treatment of pernicious anemia; vitamin B_{12} deficiency due to dietary deficiencies or malabsorption diseases, inadequate secretion of intrinsic factor, and inadequate utilization of B_{12} (eg, during neoplastic treatment); increased B_{12} requirements due to pregnancy, thyrotoxicosis, hemorrhage, malignancy, liver or kidney disease

Dosage

Adequate intake (IOM, 1998):

Children:

0-6 months: 0.4 mcg daily

7-12 months: 0.5 mcg daily

Recommended intake (IOM, 1998):

Children:

1-3 years: 0.9 mcg daily

4-8 years: 1.2 mcg daily

9-13 years: 1.8 mcg daily

Adolescents >14 years and Adults: 2.4 mcg daily

Pregnancy: 2.6 mcg daily

Lactation: 2.8 mcg daily

Vitamin B_{12} deficiency:
I.M., deep SubQ:
Children (dosage not well established): 0.2 mcg/kg for 2 days, followed by 1000 mcg daily for 2-7 days, followed by 100 mcg weekly for 1 month; for malabsorptive causes of B_{12} deficiency, monthly maintenance doses of 100 mcg have been recommended or as an alternative 100 mcg daily for 10-15 days, then once or twice weekly for several months (Rasmussen, 2001)
Adults: May use initial treatment similar to that for pernicious anemia depending on severity of deficiency: 100 mcg daily for 6-7 days; if improvement, administer same dose on alternate days for 7 doses, then every 3-4 days for 2-3 weeks; once hematologic values have returned to normal, maintenance dosage: 100 mcg monthly.
Note: Given the lack of toxicity associated with cyanocobalamin, higher doses may be preferred, especially in cases of severe deficiency. Alternate dosing regimens exist with initial doses ranging from 100-1000 mcg every day or every other day for 1-2 weeks and maintenance doses of 100-1000 mcg every 1-3 months (Oh, 2003).
Intranasal: Adults (Nascobal): 500 mcg in one nostril once weekly
Oral: Adults: 1000-2000 mcg daily for 1-2 weeks; maintenance: 1000 mcg daily (Langan, 2011; Oh, 2003)

Pernicious anemia: I.M., deep SubQ (administer concomitantly with folic acid if needed, 1 mg daily for 1 month):
Children: 30-50 mcg daily for 2 or more weeks (to a total dose of 1000-5000 mcg), then follow with 100 mcg monthly as maintenance dosage
Adults: 100 mcg daily for 6-7 days; if improvement, administer same dose on alternate days for 7 doses, then every 3-4 days for 2-3 weeks; once hematologic values have returned to normal, maintenance dosage: 100 mcg monthly.
Note: Given the lack of toxicity associated with cyanocobalamin, higher doses may be preferred, especially in cases of severe deficiency. Alternate dosing regimens exist with initial doses ranging from 100-1000 mcg every day or every other day for 1-2 weeks and maintenance doses of 100-1000 mcg every 1-3 months (Oh, 2003).
Hematologic remission (without evidence of nervous system involvement): Adults:
Intranasal (Nascobal): 500 mcg in one nostril once weekly
Oral: 1000-2000 mcg daily
I.M., SubQ: 100-1000 mcg monthly

Dosage adjustment in renal impairment: No dosage adjustment provided in manufacturer's labeling. Use with caution; some formulations may also contain aluminum, which may accumulate in renal impairment.

Dosage adjustment in hepatic impairment: No dosage adjustment provided in manufacturer's labeling.

Additional Information Complete prescribing information should be consulted for additional detail.

Dosage Forms Excipient information presented when available (limited, particularly for generics); consult specific product labeling.
Kit, Injection:
Physicians EZ Use B-12: 1000 mcg/mL [contains benzyl alcohol]
Liquid, Sublingual:
Generic: 3000 mcg/mL (52 mL)
Lozenge, Oral:
Generic: 50 mcg (100 ea); 100 mcg (100 ea); 250 mcg (100 ea, 250 ea); 500 mcg (100 ea, 250 ea)
Solution, Injection:
Generic: 1000 mcg/mL (1 mL, 10 mL, 30 mL)
Solution, Nasal:
Nascobal: 500 mcg/0.1 mL (1.3 mL) [contains benzalkonium chloride]
Tablet, Oral:
Generic: 100 mcg, 250 mcg, 500 mcg, 1000 mcg
Tablet, Oral [preservative free]:
Generic: 100 mcg, 500 mcg, 1000 mcg
Tablet Extended Release, Oral:
Generic: 1000 mcg
Tablet Sublingual, Sublingual:
Generic: 2500 mcg
Tablet Sublingual, Sublingual [preservative free]:
Generic: 2500 mcg

- ◆ **Cyanocobalamin, Folic Acid, and Pyridoxine** *see* Folic Acid, Cyanocobalamin, and Pyridoxine *on page 908*
- ◆ **Cyanokit** *see* Hydroxocobalamin *on page 1017*
- ◆ **Cyclafem 1/35** *see* Ethinyl Estradiol and Norethindrone *on page 793*
- ◆ **Cyclafem 7/7/7** *see* Ethinyl Estradiol and Norethindrone *on page 793*
- ◆ **Cyclen (Can)** *see* Ethinyl Estradiol and Norgestimate *on page 795*
- ◆ **Cyclessa** *see* Ethinyl Estradiol and Desogestrel *on page 784*

Cyclobenzaprine (sye kloe BEN za preen)

Brand Names: U.S. Amrix; Fexmid; Flexeril [DSC]

Brand Names: Canada Apo-Cyclobenzaprine; Auro-Cyclobenzaprine; Ava-Cyclobenzaprine; Dom-Cyclobenzaprine; JAMP-Cyclobenzaprine; Mylan-Cyclobenzaprine; Novo-Cycloprine; PHL-Cyclobenzaprine; PMS-Cyclobenzaprine; Q-Cyclobenzaprine; ratio-Cyclobenzaprine; Riva-Cycloprine; ZYM-Cyclobenzaprine

Index Terms Cyclobenzaprine Hydrochloride

Pharmacologic Category Skeletal Muscle Relaxant

Additional Appendix Information
Beers Criteria – Potentially Inappropriate Medications for Geriatrics *on page 2368*

Use Short-term (2-3 weeks) treatment of muscle spasm associated with acute, painful musculoskeletal conditions

Unlabeled Use Treatment of muscle spasm associated with acute temporomandibular joint pain (TMJ)

Pregnancy Risk Factor B

Pregnancy Considerations Adverse events have not been observed in animal reproduction studies. The manufacturer recommends avoiding use during pregnancy unless clearly needed.

Breast-Feeding Considerations It is not known if cyclobenzaprine is excreted in breast milk. The manufacturer recommends that caution be exercised when administering cyclobenzaprine to nursing women.

Contraindications Hypersensitivity to cyclobenzaprine or any component of the formulation; during or within 14 days of MAO inhibitors; hyperthyroidism; congestive heart failure; arrhythmias; heart block or conduction disturbances; acute recovery phase of MI

Warnings/Precautions May cause CNS depression, which may impair physical or mental abilities; ethanol and/or other CNS depressants may enhance these effects. Patients must be cautioned about performing tasks which require mental alertness (eg, operating machinery or driving). Cyclobenzaprine shares the toxic potentials of the tricyclic antidepressants (including arrhythmias, tachycardia, and conduction time prolongation) and the usual precautions of tricyclic antidepressant therapy should be observed; use with caution in patients with urinary hesitancy or retention, angle-closure glaucoma or increased intraocular pressure, hepatic impairment, or in the elderly.

Potentially life-threatening serotonin syndrome has occurred with cyclobenzaprine when used in combination with other serotonergic agents (eg, SSRIs, SNRIs, TCAs, meperidine, tramadol, buspirone, MAO inhibitors), bupropion, and verapamil. Monitor patients closely especially during initiation/dose titration for signs/symptoms of serotonin syndrome such as mental status changes (eg, agitation, hallucinations); autonomic instability (eg, tachycardia, labile blood pressure, diaphoresis); neuromuscular changes (eg, tremor, rigidity, myoclonus); GI symptoms (eg, nausea, vomiting, diarrhea); and/or seizures. Discontinue cyclobenzaprine and any concomitant serotonergic agent immediately if signs/symptoms arise. Concomitant use or use within 14 days of discontinuing an MAO inhibitor is contraindicated.

Muscle relaxants are poorly tolerated by the elderly due to potent anticholinergic effects, sedation, and risk of fracture. Efficacy is questionable at dosages tolerated by elderly patients; avoid use (Beers Criteria). Extended release capsules not recommended for use in mild-to-severe hepatic impairment or in the elderly. Potentially significant drug-drug interactions may exist, requiring dose or frequency adjustment, additional monitoring, and/or selection of alternative therapy. Effects may be potentiated when used with other CNS depressants or ethanol.

Adverse Reactions

>10%:

Central nervous system: Drowsiness (1% to 39%), dizziness (1% to 11%)

Gastrointestinal: Xerostomia (6% to 32%)

1% to 10%:

Central nervous system: Fatigue (1% to 6%), headache (1% to 5%), confusion (1% to 3%), decreased mental acuity (1% to 3%), irritability (1% to 3%), nervousness (1% to 3%)

Gastrointestinal: Dyspepsia (≤4%), abdominal pain (1% to 3%), acid regurgitation (1% to 3%), constipation (1% to 3%), diarrhea (1% to 3%), nausea (1% to 3%), unpleasant taste (1% to 3%)

Neuromuscular & skeletal: Weakness (1% to 3%)

Ophthalmic: Blurred vision (1% to 3%)

Respiratory: Pharyngitis (1% to 3%), upper respiratory tract infection (1% to 3%)

<1% (Limited to important or life-threatening): Anaphylaxis, angioedema, cardiac arrhythmia, convulsions, hepatitis (rare), hypertonia, hypotension, paresthesia, psychosis, seizure, serotonin syndrome, skin rash, syncope, tachycardia

Drug Interactions

Metabolism/Transport Effects **Substrate** of CYP1A2 (major), CYP2D6 (minor), CYP3A4 (minor); **Note:** Assignment of Major/Minor substrate status based on clinically relevant drug interaction potential

Avoid Concomitant Use

Avoid concomitant use of Cyclobenzaprine with any of the following: Aclidinium; Azelastine (Nasal); Ipratropium (Oral Inhalation); MAO Inhibitors; Paraldehyde; Tiotropium; Umeclidinium

Increased Effect/Toxicity

Cyclobenzaprine may increase the levels/effects of: Alcohol (Ethyl); Analgesics (Opioid); Anticholinergics; Antipsychotics; Azelastine (Nasal); Buprenorphine; CNS Depressants; Hydrocodone; MAO Inhibitors; Metoclopramide; Metyrosine; Paraldehyde; Pramipexole; ROPINIRole; Rotigotine; Serotonin Modulators; Tiotropium; TraMADol; Zolpidem

The levels/effects of Cyclobenzaprine may be increased by: Abiraterone Acetate; Aclidinium; Antipsychotics; Brimonidine (Topical); CYP1A2 Inhibitors (Moderate); CYP1A2 Inhibitors (Strong); Deferasirox; Doxylamine; HydrOXYzine; Ipratropium (Oral Inhalation); Magnesium Sulfate; Perampanel; Pramlintide; Sodium Oxybate; Umeclidinium; Vemurafenib

Decreased Effect

Cyclobenzaprine may decrease the levels/effects of: Acetylcholinesterase Inhibitors (Central)

The levels/effects of Cyclobenzaprine may be decreased by: Acetylcholinesterase Inhibitors (Central); Peginterferon Alfa-2b

Ethanol/Nutrition/Herb Interactions

Ethanol: May increase CNS depression. Management: Avoid ethanol during cyclobenzaprine therapy; monitor for increased effects with coadministration.

Food: Food increases bioavailability (peak plasma concentrations increased by 35% and area under the curve by 20%) of the extended release capsule. Management: Monitor for increased effects if taken with food.

Herb/Nutraceutical: Valerian, kava kava, gotu kola may increase CNS depression. Management: Avoid use during cyclobenzaprine therapy.

Storage/Stability

Amrix, Flexeril: Store at 25°C (77°F); excursions permitted to 15°C to 30°C (59°F to 86°F). Protect from light.

Fexmid: Store at 20°C to 25°C (68°F to 77°F).

Mechanism of Action Centrally-acting skeletal muscle relaxant pharmacologically related to tricyclic antidepressants; reduces tonic somatic motor activity influencing both alpha and gamma motor neurons

Pharmacodynamics/Kinetics

Metabolism: Hepatic via CYP3A4, 1A2, and 2D6; may undergo enterohepatic recirculation

Bioavailability: 33% to 55%

Half-life elimination: Immediate release tablet: 18 hours (range: 8-37 hours); Extended release capsule: 32-33 hours

Time to peak, serum: Extended release capsule: 7-8 hours

Excretion: Urine (primarily as glucuronide metabolites); feces (as unchanged drug; Hucker, 1978)

Dosage Oral: Muscle spasm: **Note:** Do not use longer than 2-3 weeks

Capsule, extended release:

Adults: Usual: 15 mg once daily; some patients may require up to 30 mg once daily

Elderly: Use not recommended

Tablet, immediate release:

Children ≥15 years and Adults: Initial: 5 mg 3 times daily; may increase up to 10 mg 3 times daily if needed

Elderly: Initial: 5 mg; titrate dose slowly and consider less frequent dosing

Dosage adjustment in renal impairment: No dosage adjustment provided in manufacturer's labeling.

Dosage adjustment in hepatic impairment:

Capsule, extended release: Mild-to-severe impairment: Use not recommended.

Tablet, immediate release:

Mild impairment: Initial: 5 mg; use with caution; titrate slowly and consider less frequent dosing

Moderate-to-severe impairment: Use not recommended

Administration Oral: Extended release capsules: Administer at the same time each day. Do not crush or chew.

Monitoring Parameters Signs/symptoms of serotonin syndrome (patients receiving other serotonergic drugs)

Test Interactions May cause false-positive serum TCA screen (Wong, 1995)

Dosage Forms Excipient information presented when available (limited, particularly for generics); consult specific product labeling. [DSC] = Discontinued product

Capsule Extended Release 24 Hour, Oral, as hydrochloride:

Amrix: 15 mg

Amrix: 30 mg [contains brilliant blue fcf (fd&c blue #1), fd&c blue #2 (indigotine), fd&c red #40, fd&c yellow #6 (sunset yellow)]

Tablet, Oral, as hydrochloride:

Fexmid: 7.5 mg

Flexeril: 5 mg [DSC], 10 mg [DSC]

Generic: 5 mg, 7.5 mg, 10 mg

◆ **Cyclobenzaprine Hydrochloride** *see* Cyclobenzaprine *on page 502*

◆ **Cyclogyl** *see* Cyclopentolate *on page 504*

◆ **Cyclogyl® (Can)** *see* Cyclopentolate *on page 504*

◆ **Cyclomen® (Can)** *see* Danazol *on page 537*

◆ **Cyclomydril®** *see* Cyclopentolate and Phenylephrine *on page 504*

Cyclopentolate (sye kloe PEN toe late)

Brand Names: U.S. Cyclogyl

Brand Names: Canada AK Pentolate Oph Soln; Cyclogyl®; Diopentolate®; Minims Cyclopentolate; PMS-Cyclopentolate

Index Terms Cyclopentolate Hydrochloride

Pharmacologic Category Anticholinergic Agent, Ophthalmic

Use Diagnostic procedures requiring mydriasis and cycloplegia

Pregnancy Risk Factor C

Dosage Ophthalmic:

Infants: **Note:** Cyclopentolate and phenylephrine combination formulation is the preferred agent for use in infants due to lower cyclopentolate concentration and reduced risk for systemic reactions

Children: Instill 1 drop of 0.5%, 1%, or 2% in eye followed by 1 drop of 0.5% or 1% in 5 minutes, if necessary

Adults: Instill 1 drop of 1% followed by another drop in 5 minutes; 2% solution in heavily pigmented iris

Dosage adjustment in renal impairment: No dosage adjustment provided in manufacturer's labeling.

Dosage adjustment in hepatic impairment: No dosage adjustment provided in manufacturer's labeling.

Additional Information Complete prescribing information should be consulted for additional detail.

Dosage Forms Excipient information presented when available (limited, particularly for generics); consult specific product labeling.

Solution, Ophthalmic, as hydrochloride:

Cyclogyl: 0.5% (15 mL); 1% (2 mL, 5 mL, 15 mL); 2% (2 mL, 5 mL, 15 mL)

Generic: 1% (2 mL, 15 mL); 2% (2 mL, 5 mL, 15 mL)

Cyclopentolate and Phenylephrine
(sye kloe PEN toe late & fen il EF rin)

Brand Names: U.S. Cyclomydril®

Index Terms Phenylephrine and Cyclopentolate

Pharmacologic Category Ophthalmic Agent, Antiglaucoma

Use Induce mydriasis greater than that produced with cyclopentolate HCl alone

Pregnancy Risk Factor C

Dosage Ophthalmic: Infants, Children, and Adults: Instill 1 drop into the eye every 5-10 minutes, for up to 3 doses, approximately 40-50 minutes before the examination

Additional Information Complete prescribing information should be consulted for additional detail.

Dosage Forms Excipient information presented when available (limited, particularly for generics); consult specific product labeling.

Solution, ophthalmic:

Cyclomydril®: Cyclopentolate hydrochloride 0.2% and phenylephrine hydrochloride 1% (2 mL, 5 mL) [contains benzalkonium chloride]

◆ **Cyclopentolate Hydrochloride** *see* Cyclopentolate *on page 504*

Cyclophosphamide (sye kloe FOS fa mide)

Brand Names: Canada Procytox®

Index Terms CPM; CTX; CYT; Cytoxan; Neosar

Pharmacologic Category Antineoplastic Agent, Alkylating Agent; Antirheumatic Miscellaneous; Immunosuppressant Agent

Use

Oncology-related uses: Treatment of Hodgkin lymphoma, non-Hodgkin lymphomas (including Burkitt lymphoma), chronic lymphocytic leukemia (CLL), chronic myelocytic leukemia (CML), acute myelocytic leukemia (AML), acute lymphoblastic leukemia (ALL), mycosis fungoides, multiple myeloma, neuroblastoma, retinoblastoma; breast cancer; ovarian adenocarcinoma

Canadian labeling: Additional use (not in U.S. labeling): Treatment of lung cancer

Nononcology uses: Treatment of refractory nephrotic syndrome in children who are unresponsive or intolerant to corticosteroid therapy

Unlabeled Use

Oncology-related uses: Ewing's sarcoma, rhabdomyosarcoma, Wilms tumor, ovarian germ cell tumors, gestational trophoblastic tumors (high-risk), small cell lung cancer, testicular cancer, pheochromocytoma, hematopoietic stem cell transplant (HSCT) conditioning regimen

Nononcology uses: Severe rheumatoid disorders, granulomatosis with polyangiitis (GPA; Wegener's granulomatosis), myasthenia gravis, multiple sclerosis, lupus nephritis, autoimmune hemolytic anemia, idiopathic thrombocytic purpura (ITP), antibody-induced pure red cell aplasia

Pregnancy Risk Factor D

Pregnancy Considerations Cyclophosphamide crosses the placenta and can be detected in amniotic fluid (D'Incalci, 1982). Adverse events (including ectrodactylia) were observed in human studies following exposure to cyclophosphamide. Women of childbearing potential should avoid pregnancy while receiving cyclophosphamide treatment. Cyclophosphamide may also cause sterility in males and females (reversible in some cases) and amenorrhea in females. When treatment is needed for lupus nephritis, cyclophosphamide should be avoided in women who are pregnant or those who wish to preserve their fertility (Hahn, 2012). Chemotherapy, if indicated, may be administered to pregnant women with breast cancer as part of a combination chemotherapy regimen (common regimens administered during pregnancy include doxorubicin (or epirubicin), cyclophosphamide, and fluorouracil); chemotherapy should not be administered during the first trimester, after 35 weeks gestation, or within 3 weeks of planned delivery (Amant, 2010; Loibl, 2006).

Breast-Feeding Considerations Cyclophosphamide is excreted into breast milk. Leukopenia and thrombocytopenia were noted in an infant exposed to cyclophosphamide while nursing. The mother was treated with one course of cyclophosphamide 6 weeks prior to delivery then cyclophosphamide I.V. 6 mg/kg (300 mg) once daily for 3 days beginning 20 days postpartum. Complete blood counts were obtained in the breast-feeding infant on each day of therapy; WBC and platelets decreased by day 3 (Durodola, 1979). Due to the potential for adverse effects and tumorigenicity, the manufacturer recommends that the decision to discontinue cyclophosphamide or to discontinue breast-feeding should take into account the benefits of treatment to the mother.

Contraindications

U.S. labeling: Hypersensitivity to cyclophosphamide or any component of the formulation; severely depressed bone marrow function

Canadian labeling: Hypersensitivity to cyclophosphamide or its metabolites, urinary outflow obstructions, severe myelosuppression, severe renal or hepatic impairment, active infection (especially varicella zoster), severe immunosuppression

Warnings/Precautions Hazardous agent - use appropriate precautions for handling and disposal (NIOSH, 2012).

Cyclophosphamide is associated with the development of hemorrhagic cystitis; may rarely be severe and even fatal. Discontinue cyclophosphamide with severe hemorrhagic cystitis. Bladder injury is due to excretion of cyclophosphamide metabolites in the urine and appears to be dose- and treatment duration-dependent. Bladder fibrosis may also occur, either with or without cystitis. Increased hydration and frequent voiding is recommended to help prevent cystitis; some protocols utilize mesna to protect against hemorrhagic cystitis. Monitor urinalysis for hematuria. Severe or prolonged hemorrhagic cystitis may require medical or surgical treatment. Hematuria generally resolves within a few days after treatment is withheld, although it may persist. Cyclophosphamide may potentiate the cardiotoxicity of anthracyclines.

Cardiotoxicity has been reported, usually with high doses associated with transplant conditioning regimens, although may rarely occur with lower doses. Cardiac abnormalities do not appear to persist. Cardiotoxicities reported have included arrhythmia, congestive heart failure, heart block, hemorrhagic myocarditis, hemopericardium (secondary to hemorrhagic myocarditis and myocardial necrosis), pericarditis, and tachyarrhythmias. Cardiotoxicity is related to endothelial capillary damage; symptoms may be managed with diuretics, ACE inhibitors, beta blockers, or inotropics (Floyd, 2005). Use with caution in patients with pre-existing cardiovascular disease. For patients with multiple cardiac risk factors, considering monitoring during treatment (Floyd, 2005).

Pulmonary toxicities, including pneumonitis and acute respiratory distress syndrome, have been reported. Consider pulmonary function testing to assess the severity of pneumonitis (Morgan, 2011). Cyclophosphamide-induced pneumonitis is rare and may present as early (within 1-6 months) or late onset (several months to years); early onset has been reversible with discontinuation; late onset is associated with pleural thickening and may persist chronically (Malik, 1996).

Dose-related neutropenia is common; thrombocytopenia and anemia may also occur. Monitor for infections; immunosuppression and serious infections may occur; infections may require dose reduction, or interruption or discontinuation of treatment. Nausea and vomiting commonly occur; premedication with antiemetics is recommended. Stomatitis/mucositis may also occur. Anaphylactic reactions have been reported; cross-sensitivity with other alkylating agents may occur. May interfere with wound healing. Secondary malignancies (bladder cancer, myeloproliferative, and lymphoproliferative malignancies) have been reported with both single-agent and with combination chemotherapy regimens; onset may be delayed (up to several years after treatment); bladder malignancy usually occurs in patients previously experiencing hemorrhagic cystitis. May impair fertility; interferes with oogenesis and spermatogenesis; effect on fertility is generally dependent on dose and duration of treatment and may be irreversible. The age at treatment initiation and cumulative dose were determined to be risk factors for ovarian failure in cyclophosphamide use for the treatment of systemic lupus erythematosus (SLE) (Mok, 1998). Use with caution in patients with renal and hepatic impairment; dosage adjustment may be needed (use is contraindicated in severe impairment in the Canadian labeling).

Adverse Reactions Frequency not defined.

Dermatologic: Alopecia (reversible; onset: 3-6 weeks after start of treatment)

Endocrine & metabolic: Amenorrhea, azoospermia, gonadal suppression, oligospermia, oogenesis impaired, sterility

Gastrointestinal: Abdominal pain, anorexia, diarrhea, mucositis, nausea/vomiting (dose-related), stomatitis

Genitourinary: Hemorrhagic cystitis

Hematologic: Anemia, leukopenia (dose-related; recovery: 7-10 days after cessation), myelosuppression, neutropenia, neutropenic fever, thrombocytopenia

Postmarketing and/or case reports: Acute respiratory distress syndrome, anaphylactic reactions, anaphylaxis, arrhythmias (with high-dose [HSCT] therapy), bladder/urinary fibrosis, blurred vision, cardiac tamponade (with high-dose [HSCT] therapy), cardiotoxicity, confusion, dyspnea, ejection fraction decreased, erythema multiforme, gastrointestinal hemorrhage, hearing disorders, heart block, heart failure (with high-dose [HSCT] therapy), hematuria, hemopericardium, hemorrhagic colitis, hemorrhagic myocarditis (with high-dose [HSCT] therapy), hemorrhagic ureteritis, hepatic sinusoidal obstruction syndrome (SOS; formerly called veno-occlusive liver disease), hepatitis, hepatotoxicity, hypersensitivity reactions, hyperuricemia, hypokalemia, hyponatremia, interstitial pneumonitis, interstitial pulmonary fibrosis (with high doses), jaundice, latent infection reactivation, mesenteric ischemia (acute), methemoglobinemia (with high-dose [HSCT] therapy), multiorgan failure, myocardial necrosis (with high-dose [HSCT] therapy), neurotoxicity, neutrophilic eccrine hidradenitis, ovarian fibrosis, pancreatitis, pericarditis, pigmentation changes (skin/fingernails), pneumonia, pulmonary hypertension, pulmonary infiltrates, pulmonary veno-occlusive disease, pyelonephritis, radiation recall, renal tubular necrosis, reversible posterior leukoencephalopathy syndrome (RPLS), rhabdomyolysis, secondary malignancy, septic shock, sepsis, SIADH, Stevens-Johnson syndrome, testicular atrophy, thrombocytopenia (immune mediated), thrombotic disorders (arterial and venous), toxic epidermal necrolysis, toxic megacolon, tumor lysis syndrome, wound healing impaired

Drug Interactions

Metabolism/Transport Effects **Substrate** of CYP2A6 (minor), CYP2B6 (major), CYP2C19 (minor), CYP2C9 (minor), CYP3A4 (minor); **Note:** Assignment of Major/Minor substrate status based on clinically relevant drug interaction potential; **Inhibits** CYP3A4 (weak); **Induces** CYP2B6 (weak/moderate), CYP2C9 (weak/moderate)

Avoid Concomitant Use

Avoid concomitant use of Cyclophosphamide with any of the following: BCG; Belimumab; CloZAPine; Etanercept; Natalizumab; Pimecrolimus; Pimozide; Tacrolimus (Topical); Tofacitinib; Vaccines (Live)

Increased Effect/Toxicity

Cyclophosphamide may increase the levels/effects of: Antineoplastic Agents (Anthracycline, Systemic); ARIPiprazole; CloZAPine; Dofetilide; Leflunomide; Lomitapide; Natalizumab; Pimozide; Succinylcholine; Tofacitinib; Vaccines (Live); Vitamin K Antagonists

The levels/effects of Cyclophosphamide may be increased by: Allopurinol; Belimumab; CYP2B6 Inhibitors (Moderate); CYP2B6 Inhibitors (Strong); Denosumab; Etanercept; Pentostatin; Pimecrolimus; Quazepam; Roflumilast; Tacrolimus (Topical); Trastuzumab

Decreased Effect

Cyclophosphamide may decrease the levels/effects of: BCG; Cardiac Glycosides; Coccidioidin Skin Test; Sipuleucel-T; Vaccines (Inactivated); Vaccines (Live); Vitamin K Antagonists

The levels/effects of Cyclophosphamide may be decreased by: CYP2B6 Inducers (Strong); Dabrafenib; Echinacea

Ethanol/Nutrition/Herb Interactions Herb/Nutraceutical: Avoid black cohosh, dong quai in estrogen-dependent tumors.

Preparation for Administration Hazardous agent; use appropriate precautions for handling and disposal (NIOSH, 2012).

Injection powder for reconstitution: Store intact vials of powder at room temperature of 25°C (77°F). For I.V. push, reconstitute with normal saline (NS) to a concentration of 20 mg/mL. For I.V. infusion, reconstitute with sterile water or NS to a concentration of 20 mg/mL; further dilute for infusion in D_5W, 1/2NS or D_5NS.

Storage/Stability Hazardous agent; use appropriate precautions for handling and disposal (NIOSH, 2012).

Injection powder for reconstitution: Store intact vials of powder at room temperature of 25°C (77°F). Reconstituted solutions in normal saline (NS) are stable for 24 hours at room temperature and for 6 days refrigerated at 2°C to 8°C (36°F to 46°F). Solutions diluted for infusion in 1/2NS are stable for 24 hours at room temperature and for 6 days refrigerated; solutions diluted in D_5W or D_5NS are stable for 24 hours at room temperature and for 36 hours refrigerated.

Tablets: Store tablets at room temperature of 25°C (77°F); excursions permitted to 15°C to 30°C (59°F to 86°F).

Mechanism of Action Cyclophosphamide is an alkylating agent that prevents cell division by cross-linking DNA strands and decreasing DNA synthesis. It is a cell cycle phase nonspecific agent. Cyclophosphamide also possesses potent immunosuppressive activity. Cyclophosphamide is a prodrug that must be metabolized to active metabolites in the liver.

Pharmacodynamics/Kinetics

Absorption: Oral: Well absorbed

Distribution: V_d: 0.48-0.71 L/kg; crosses into CSF (not in high enough concentrations to treat meningeal leukemia)

Protein binding: 10% to 60%

Metabolism: Hepatic to active metabolites acrolein, 4-aldophosphamide, 4-hydroperoxycyclophosphamide, and nor-nitrogen mustard

Bioavailability: >75%

Half-life elimination: 3-12 hours

Time to peak, serum: Oral: ~1 hour; I.V.: Metabolites: 2-3 hours

Excretion: Urine (<30% as unchanged drug, 85% to 90% as metabolites)

Dosage Details concerning dosing in combination regimens should also be consulted. Antiemetics may be recommended (emetogenic potential varies by dose and combination therapy).

Children:

U.S. labeling:

Malignancy, solid tumor (single agent):

I.V.: 40-50 mg/kg in divided doses over 2-5 days **or** 10-15 mg/kg every 7-10 days **or** 3-5 mg/kg twice weekly

Oral: 1-5 mg/kg/day (initial and maintenance dosing)

Nephrotic syndrome, corticosteroid refractory or intolerant: Oral: 2.5-3 mg/kg/day every day for 60-90 days

Canadian labeling:

I.V.: Initial: 2-8 mg/kg (60-250 mg/m^2) in divided doses for 6 or more days; Maintenance: 10-15 mg/kg every 7-10 days or 30 mg/kg every 3-4 weeks or when bone marrow function recovers

Oral: Initial: 2-8 mg/kg (60-250 mg/m^2) in divided doses for 6 or more days; Maintenance: 2-5 mg/kg (50-150 mg/m^2) twice weekly

Indication specific and/or unlabeled uses/dosing:

Ewing's sarcoma (unlabeled use): I.V.: VAC/IE regimen: VAC: 1200 mg/m^2 (plus mesna) on day 1 of a 21-day treatment cycle (in combination with vincristine and doxorubicin [then dactinomycin when maximum doxorubicin dose reached]), alternates with IE (ifosfamide and etoposide) for a total of 17 cycles (Grier, 2003)

Hodgkin lymphoma (unlabeled dosing): I.V.: BEACOPP escalated regimen: 1200 mg/m^2 on day 0 of a 21-day treatment cycle (in combination with bleomycin, etoposide, doxorubicin, vincristine, prednisone, and procarbazine) for 4 cycles (Kelly, 2011)

Lupus nephritis (unlabeled use): I.V.: 500-1000 mg/m^2 every month for 6 months, then every 3 months for a total of 2.5-3 years (Austin, 1986; Gourley, 1996; Lehman, 2000)

Neuroblastoma (unlabeled dosing): I.V.: CE-CAdO regimen, courses 3 and 4: 300 mg/m^2 days 1-5 every 21 days for 2 cycles (Rubie, 1998) **or** 10 mg/kg days 1-5 every 21 days for 2 cycles (Rubie, 2001). **Note:** Decreased doses may be recommended for newborns or children <10 kg.

Transplant conditioning (unlabeled use): Myeloablative transplant: I.V.: 50 mg/kg/day for 4 days beginning 5 days before transplant (with or without antithymocyte globulin [equine]) (Champlin, 2007)

Adults:

U.S. labeling:

Single agent for solid tumors:

I.V.: 40-50 mg/kg in divided doses over 2-5 days **or** 10-15 mg/kg every 7-10 days **or** 3-5 mg/kg twice weekly

Oral: 1-5 mg/kg/day (initial and maintenance dosing)

Canadian labeling:

I.V.: Initial: 40-50 mg/kg (1500-1800 mg/m^2) administered as 10-20 mg/kg/day over 2-5 days; Maintenance: 10-15 mg/kg (350-550 mg/m^2) every 7-10 days **or** 3-5 mg/kg (110-185 mg/m^2) twice weekly

Oral: Initial 1-5 mg/kg/day (depending on tolerance); Maintenance: 1-5 mg/kg/day

Indication specific and/or unlabeled uses/dosing:

Acute lymphoblastic leukemia (unlabeled dosing): Multiple-agent regimens:

Hyper-CVAD regimen: I.V.: 300 mg/m^2 over 3 hours (with mesna) every 12 hours for 6 doses on days 1, 2, and 3 during odd-numbered cycles (cycles 1, 3, 5, 7) of an 8-cycle phase (Kantarjian, 2004)

Larson (CALGB8811) regimen: I.V.:

Adults <60 years: Induction phase: 1200 mg/m^2 on day 1 of a 4-week cycle; Early intensification phase: 1000 mg/m^2 on day 1 of a 4-week cycle (repeat once); Late intensification phase: 1000 mg/m^2 on day 29 of an 8-week cycle (Larson, 1995)

Adults ≥60 years: Induction phase: 800 mg/m^2 on day 1 of a 4-week cycle; Early intensification phase: 1000 mg/m^2 on day 1 of a 4-week cycle (repeat once); Late intensification phase: 1000 mg/m^2 on day 29 of an 8-week cycle (Larson, 1995)

Breast cancer (unlabeled dosing):

AC regimen: I.V.: 600 mg/m^2 on day 1 every 21 days (in combination with doxorubicin) for 4 cycles (Fisher, 1990)

CEF regimen: Oral: 75 mg/m^2/day days 1-14 every 28 days (in combination with epirubicin and fluorouracil) for 6 cycles (Levine, 1998)

CMF regimen: Oral: 100 mg/m^2/day days 1-14 every 28 days (in combination with methotrexate and fluorouracil) for 6 cycles (Levine, 1998) **or** I.V.: 600 mg/m^2 on day 1 every 21 days (in combination with methotrexate and fluorouracil); Goldhirsch, 1998)

Chronic lymphocytic leukemia (unlabeled dosing): I.V.: R-FC regimen: 250 mg/m^2/day for 3 days every 28 days (in combination with rituximab and fludarabine) for 6 cycles (Robak, 2010)

Ewing's sarcoma (unlabeled use): I.V.: VAC/IE regimen: VAC: 1200 mg/m^2 (plus mesna) on day 1 of a 21-day treatment cycle (in combination with vincristine and doxorubicin [then dactinomycin when maximum doxorubicin dose reached]), alternates with IE (ifosfamide and etoposide) for a total of 17 cycles (Grier, 2003)

Gestational trophoblastic tumors, high-risk (unlabeled use): I.V.: EMA/CO regimen: 600 mg/m^2 on day 8 of 2-week treatment cycle (in combination with etoposide, methotrexate, dactinomycin, and vincristine), continue for at least 2 treatment cycles after a normal hCG level (Escobar, 2003)

Granulomatosis with polyangiitis (GPA; Wegener's granulomatosis) (unlabeled use; in combination with glucocorticoids):

Low-dose: Oral: 1.5-2 mg/kg/day (Jayne, 2003; Stone, 2010) or 2 mg/kg/day until remission, followed by 1.5 mg/kg/day for 3 additional months (de Groot, 2009; Harper, 2012)

Pulse: I.V.: 15 mg/kg (maximum dose: 1200 mg) every 2 weeks for 3 doses, followed by maintenance pulses of either 15 mg/kg I.V. (maximum dose: 1200 mg) every 3 weeks or 2.5-5 mg/kg/day orally on days 1, 2, and 3 every 3 weeks for 3 months after remission achieved (de Groot, 2009; Harper, 2012)

Hodgkin lymphoma (unlabeled dosing): I.V.:

BEACOPP regimen: 650 mg/m^2 on day 1 every 3 weeks (in combination with bleomycin, etoposide, doxorubicin, vincristine, procarbazine, and prednisone) for 8 cycles (Diehl, 2003)

BEACOPP escalated regimen: 1200 mg/m^2 on day 1 every 3 weeks (in combination with bleomycin, etoposide, doxorubicin, vincristine, procarbazine, and prednisone) for 8 cycles (Diehl, 2003)

Multiple myeloma (unlabeled dosing): Oral: CyBorD regimen: 300 mg/m^2 on days 1, 8, 15, and 22 every 4 weeks (in combination with bortezomib and dexamethasone) for 4 cycles; may continue beyond 4 cycles (Khan, 2012)

Non-Hodgkin lymphoma (unlabeled dosing): I.V.:

R-CHOP regimen: 750 mg/m^2 on day 1 every 3 weeks (in combination with rituximab, doxorubicin, vincristine, and prednisone) for 8 cycles (Coiffier, 2002)

R-EPOCH (dose adjusted) regimen: 750 mg/m^2 on day 5 every 3 weeks (in combination with rituximab, etoposide, prednisone, vincristine, and doxorubicin) for 6-8 cycles (Garcia-Suarez, 2007)

CODOX-M/IVAC (Burkitt's lymphoma): Cycles 1 and 3 (CODOX-M): 800 mg/m^2 on day 1, followed by 200 mg/m^2 on days 2-5 (in combination with vincristine, doxorubicin, and methotrexate); CODOX-M alternates with IVAC (etoposide, ifosfamide, and cytarabine) for a total of 4 cycles (Magrath, 1996)

Lupus nephritis (unlabeled use): I.V.: 500 mg once every 2 weeks for 6 doses or 500-1000 mg/m^2 once every month for 6 doses (Hahn, 2012) **or** 500-1000 mg/m^2 every month for 6 months, then every 3 months for a total of at least 2.5 years (Austin, 1986; Gourley, 1996)

Transplant conditioning (unlabeled use): I.V.:

Nonmyeloablative transplant (allogeneic): 750 mg/m^2/day for 3 days beginning 5 days prior to transplant (in combination with fludarabine) (Khouri, 2008)

Myeloablative transplant:

100 mg/kg (based on IBW, unless actual weight <95% of IBW) as a single dose 2 days prior to transplant (in combination with total body irradiation and etoposide) (Thompson, 2008)

50 mg/kg/day for 4 days beginning 5 days before transplant (with or without antithymocyte globulin [equine]) (Champlin, 2007)

50 mg/kg/day for 4 days beginning 5 days prior to transplant (in combination with busulfan) (Cassileth, 1993)

60 mg/kg/day for 2 days (in combination with busulfan and total body irradiation) (Anderson, 1996)

1800 mg/m^2/day for 4 days beginning 7 days prior to transplant (in combination with etoposide and carmustine) (Reece, 1991)

Elderly: Refer to adult dosing. Adjust dosing for renal clearance.

Dosage adjustment for toxicity:

Hematologic toxicity: May require dose reduction or treatment interruption; Canadian labeling recommends reducing initial dose by 30% to 50% if bone marrow function compromised (due to prior radiation therapy, prior chemotherapy, or tumor infiltration)

Hemorrhagic cystitis, severe: Discontinue treatment.

Dosage adjustment in renal impairment:

U.S. labeling: No adjustment provided in the manufacturer's labeling (use with caution; elevated levels of metabolites may occur).

Canadian labeling:

Mild impairment: No dosage adjustment provided in manufacturer's labeling

Moderate impairment: Dose reduction may be necessary; manufacturer's labeling does not provide specific dosing recommendations

Severe impairment: Use is contraindicated.

The following adjustments have also been recommended:

Aronoff, 2007: Children and Adults:

Cl_{cr} ≥10 mL/minute: No dosage adjustment required.

Cl_{cr} <10 mL/minute: Administer 75% of normal dose.

Hemodialysis: Moderately dialyzable (20% to 50%); administer 50% of normal dose; administer after hemodialysis

Continuous ambulatory peritoneal dialysis (CAPD): Administer 75% of normal dose.

Continuous renal replacement therapy (CRRT): Administer 100% of normal dose.

Janus, 2010: Hemodialysis: Administer 75% of normal dose; administer after hemodialysis

Dosage adjustment in hepatic impairment: The pharmacokinetics of cyclophosphamide are not significantly altered in the presence of hepatic insufficiency.

U.S. labeling: No dosage adjustment provided in the manufacturer's labeling.

Canadian labeling:

Mild-to-moderate impairment: No dosage adjustment provided in the manufacturer's labeling.

Severe impairment: Use is contraindicated.

The following adjustments have been recommended (Floyd, 2006):

Serum bilirubin 3.1-5 mg/dL or transaminases >3 times ULN: Administer 75% of dose.

Serum bilirubin >5 mg/mL: Avoid use.

Dosing in obesity: *ASCO Guidelines for appropriate chemotherapy dosing in obese adults with cancer (**Note:** Excludes HSCT dosing):* Utilize patient's actual body weight (full weight) for calculation of body surface area- or weight-based dosing, particularly when the intent of therapy is curative; manage regimen-related toxicities in the same manner as for nonobese patients; if a dose reduction is utilized due to toxicity, consider resumption of full weight-based dosing with subsequent cycles, especially if cause of toxicity (eg, hepatic or renal impairment) is resolved (Griggs, 2012).

Dietary Considerations Tablets should be administered during or after meals.

Administration

I.V.: Infusion rate may vary based on protocol (refer to specific protocol for infusion rate). Administer by direct I.V. injection (if reconstituted in NS), IVPB, or continuous I.V. infusion

Bladder toxicity: To minimize bladder toxicity, increase normal fluid intake during and for 1-2 days after cyclophosphamide dose. Most adult patients will require a fluid intake of at least 2 L/day. High-dose regimens should be accompanied by vigorous hydration with or without mesna therapy.

Hematopoietic stem cell transplant: Approaches to reduction of hemorrhagic cystitis include infusion of 0.9% NaCl 3 L/m^2/24 hours, infusion of 0.9% NaCl 3 L/m^2/24 hours with continuous 0.9% NaCl bladder irrigation 300-1000 mL/hour, and infusion of 0.9% NaCl 1.5-3 L/m^2/24 hours with intravenous mesna. Hydration should begin at least 4 hours before cyclophosphamide and continue at least 24 hours after completion of cyclophosphamide. The dose of daily mesna used may be 67% to 100% of the daily dose of cyclophosphamide. Mesna can be administered as a continuous 24-hour intravenous infusion or be given in divided doses every 4 hours. Mesna should begin at the start of treatment, and continue at least 24 hours following the last dose of cyclophosphamide.

Oral: Tablets are not scored and should not be cut or crushed. To minimize the risk of bladder irritation, do not administer tablets at bedtime.

Hazardous agent; use appropriate precautions for handling and disposal (NIOSH, 2012).

Monitoring Parameters CBC with differential and platelets, BUN, UA, serum electrolytes, serum creatinine; monitor for signs/symptoms of hemorrhagic cystitis

Additional Information In patients with CYP2B6 G516T variant allele, cyclophosphamide metabolism is markedly increased; metabolism is not influenced by CYP2C9 and CYP2C19 isotypes.

Product Availability Cyclophosphamide capsules: FDA approved September 2013; anticipated availability is currently unknown. Refer to the prescribing information for additional information.

Dosage Forms Excipient information presented when available (limited, particularly for generics); consult specific product labeling.

Solution Reconstituted, Injection:

Generic: 500 mg (1 ea); 1 g (1 ea); 2 g (1 ea)

Tablet, Oral:

Generic: 25 mg, 50 mg

Dosage Forms: Canada

Additional dosage forms available in Canada. Excipient information presented when available (limited, particularly for generics); consult specific product labeling.

Injection, powder for reconstitution: 200 mg

Extemporaneous Preparations Hazardous agent: Use appropriate precautions for handling and disposal.

Liquid solutions or oral administration may be prepared by dissolving cyclophosphamide injection in Aromatic Elixir, N.F. Store refrigerated (in glass container) for up to 14 days.

Cyclophosphamide Prescribing Information, Baxter Healthcare Corporation, Deerfield, Il, April, 2012.

A 10 mg/mL oral suspension may be prepared by reconstituting one 2 g vial for injection with 100 mL of NaCl 0.9%, providing an initial concentration of 20 mg/mL. Mix this solution in a 1:1 ratio with either Simple Syrup, NF or Ora-Plus® to obtain a final concentration of 10 mg/mL. Label "shake well" and "refrigerate". Stable for 56 days refrigerated.

Kennedy R, Groepper D, Tagen M, et al, "Stability of Cyclophosphamide in Extemporaneous Oral Suspensions," *Ann Pharmacother*, 2010, 44(2):295-301.

◆ Cycloset® *see* Bromocriptine *on page 281*

◆ Cycloset *see* Bromocriptine *on page 281*

◆ Cyclosporin A *see* CycloSPORINE (Ophthalmic) *on page 515*

◆ Cyclosporin A *see* CycloSPORINE (Systemic) *on page 508*

CycloSPORINE (Systemic) (SYE kloe spor een)

Brand Names: U.S. Gengraf; Neoral; SandIMMUNE

Brand Names: Canada Apo-Cyclosporine; Neoral; Sandimmune I.V.; Sandoz-Cyclosporine

Index Terms Ciclosporin; CsA; CyA; Cyclosporin A

Pharmacologic Category Calcineurin Inhibitor; Immunosuppressant Agent

Use

Cyclosporine modified:

Transplant rejection prophylaxis: Prophylaxis of organ rejection in kidney, liver, and heart transplants (has been used with azathioprine and/or corticosteroids)

Rheumatoid arthritis: Treatment of severe, active rheumatoid arthritis (RA) not responsive to methotrexate alone

Psoriasis: Treatment of severe, recalcitrant plaque psoriasis in nonimmunocompromised adults unresponsive to or unable to tolerate other systemic therapy

Cyclosporine non-modified: Transplant rejection (prophylaxis/treatment): Prophylaxis of organ rejection in kidney, liver, and heart transplants (has been used with azathioprine and/or corticosteroids; treatment of chronic organ rejection)

Canadian labeling: Additional uses (not in U.S. labeling):

Cyclosporine modified: Nephrotic syndrome: Induction and maintenance of remission in steroid dependent/resistant nephrotic syndrome due to glomerular disease (eg, minimal change nephropathy, membranous glomerulonephritis, focal and segmental glomerulosclerosis); maintenance of steroid induced remission allowing for steroid dose reduction or withdrawal.

Cyclosporine modified/non-modified: Bone marrow transplant rejection (prophylaxis/treatment): Prophylaxis of graft rejection following bone marrow transplantation; prophylaxis or treatment of graft-versus-host disease (GVHD)

Unlabeled Use Prevention and treatment of acute graft-versus-host disease (GVHD) in allogeneic stem cell transplantation; treatment of chronic GVHD in allogeneic stem cell transplant; treatment of lupus nephritis; treatment of focal segmental glomerulosclerosis; treatment of severe refractory ulcerative colitis

Pregnancy Risk Factor C

Pregnancy Considerations Adverse events were not observed following the use of oral cyclosporine in animal reproduction studies (using doses that were not maternally toxic). In humans, cyclosporine crosses the placenta; maternal concentrations do not correlate with those found in the umbilical cord. Cyclosporine may be detected in the serum of newborns for several days after birth (Claris, 1993). Based on clinical use, premature births and low birth weight were consistently observed in pregnant transplant patients (additional pregnancy complications also present). Formulations may contain alcohol; the alcohol content should be taken into consideration in pregnant women.

The pharmacokinetics of cyclosporine may be influenced by pregnancy (Grimer, 2007). Cyclosporine may be used in pregnant renal, liver, or heart transplant patients (Cowan, 2012; EBPG Expert Group on Renal Transplantation, 2002; McGuire, 2009; Parhar 2012). If therapy is needed for psoriasis, other agents are preferred; however, cyclosporine may be used as an alternative agent along with close clinical monitoring; use should be avoided during the first trimester if possible (Bae, 2012). If treatment is needed for lupus nephritis, other agents are recommended to be used in pregnant women (Hahn, 2012).

Following transplant, normal menstruation and fertility may be restored within months; however, appropriate contraception is recommended to prevent pregnancy until 1-2 years following the transplant to improve pregnancy outcomes (Cowan, 2012; EBPG Expert Group on Renal Transplantation, 2002; McGuire, 2009; Parhar 2012).

A pregnancy registry has been established for pregnant women taking immunosuppressants following any solid organ transplant (National Transplantation Pregnancy Registry, Temple University, 877-955-6877).

A pregnancy registry has also been established for pregnant women taking Neoral for psoriasis or rheumatoid arthritis (Neoral Pregnancy Registry for Psoriasis and Rheumatoid Arthritis, Thomas Jefferson University, 888-522-5581).

Breast-Feeding Considerations Cyclosporine is excreted in breast milk. Concentrations of cyclosporine in milk vary widely and breast-feeding during therapy is generally not recommended (Bae, 2012; Cowan, 2012). Due to the potential for serious adverse in the nursing infant, the decision to discontinue cyclosporine or to discontinue breast-feeding should take into account the importance of treatment to the mother. Formulations may contain alcohol which may be present in breast milk and could be absorbed orally by the nursing infant.

Contraindications

Hypersensitivity to cyclosporine or any component of the formulation. I.V. cyclosporine is contraindicated in hypersensitivity to polyoxyethylated castor oil (Cremophor EL).

Rheumatoid arthritis and psoriasis: Abnormal renal function, uncontrolled hypertension, malignancies. Concomitant treatment with PUVA or UVB therapy, methotrexate, other immunosuppressive agents, coal tar, or radiation therapy are also contraindications for use in patients with psoriasis.

Canadian labeling: Additional contraindications (not in U.S. labeling): Primary or secondary immunodeficiency excluding autoimmune disease; uncontrolled infection.

Warnings/Precautions Hazardous agent - use appropriate precautions for handling and disposal (NIOSH, 2012).

[U.S. Boxed Warning]: Increased risk of lymphomas and other malignancies (including fatal outcomes), **particularly skin cancers;** risk is related to intensity/duration of therapy and the use of more than one immunosuppressive agent; all patients should avoid excessive sun/UV light exposure. **[U.S. Boxed Warning]: May cause hypertension; risk is increased with increasing doses/duration.** Use caution when changing dosage forms.

[U.S. Boxed Warning]: Renal impairment, including structural kidney damage has occurred (when used at high doses); risk is increased with increasing doses/duration; monitor renal function closely. Elevations in serum creatinine and BUN generally respond to dosage reductions. Use caution with other potentially nephrotoxic drugs (eg, acyclovir, aminoglycoside antibiotics, amphotericin B, ciprofloxacin). Elevations in serum creatinine and BUN associated with nephrotoxicity generally respond to dosage reductions. In renal transplant patients with rapidly rising BUN and creatinine, carefully evaluate to differentiate between cyclosporine-associated nephrotoxicity and renal rejection episodes. In cases of severe rejection that fail to respond to pulse steroids and monoclonal antibodies, switching to an alternative immunosuppressant agent may be preferred to increasing cyclosporine to an excessive dosage.

[U.S. Boxed Warning]: Increased risk of infection with use; serious and fatal infections have been reported. Bacterial, viral, fungal, and protozoal infections (including opportunistic infections) have occurred. Polyoma virus infections, such as the JC virus and BK virus, may result in serious and sometimes fatal outcomes. The JC virus is associated with progressive multifocal leukoencephalopathy (PML), and PML has been reported in patients receiving cyclosporine. PML may be fatal and presents with hemiparesis, apathy, confusion, cognitive deficiencies, and ataxia; consider neurologic consultation as indicated. The BK virus is associated with nephropathy, and polyoma virus-associated nephropathy (PVAN) has been reported in patients receiving cyclosporine. PVAN is associated with serious adverse effects including renal dysfunction and renal graft loss. If PML or PVAN occur in transplant patients, consider reducing immunosuppression therapy as well as the risk that reduced immunosuppression poses to grafts.

Liver injury, including cholestasis, jaundice, hepatitis, and liver failure, has been reported. These events were mainly in patients with confounding factors including infections, coadministration with other potentially hepatotoxic medications, underlying conditions, and significant comorbidities. Fatalities have also been reported rarely, primarily in transplant patients. Increased hepatic enzymes and bilirubin have occurred (when used at high doses); improvement usually seen with dosage reduction.

Should be used initially with corticosteroids in transplant patients. Significant hyperkalemia (with or without hyperchloremic metabolic acidosis) and hyperuricemia have occurred with therapy. Syndromes of microangiopathic hemolytic anemia and thrombocytopenia have occurred and may result in graft failure; it is accompanied by platelet consumption within the graft. Syndrome may occur without graft rejection. Although management of the syndrome is unclear, discontinuation or reduction of cyclosporine, in addition to streptokinase and heparin administration or plasmapheresis, has been associated with syndrome resolution. However, resolution seems to be dependent upon early detection of the syndrome via indium 111 labeled platelet scans.

May cause seizures, particularly if used with high-dose corticosteroids. Encephalopathy (including posterior reversible encephalopathy syndrome [PRES]) has also been reported; predisposing factors include hypertension, hypomagnesemia, hypocholesterolemia, high-dose corticosteroids, high cyclosporine serum concentration, and graft-versus-host disease (GVHD). Encephalopathy may be more common in patients with liver transplant compared to kidney transplant. Other neurotoxic events, such as optic disc edema (including papilloedema and potential visual impairment), have been rarely reported primarily in transplant patients.

[U.S. Boxed Warning]: The modified/non-modified formulations are not bioequivalent; cyclosporine (modified) has increased bioavailability as compared to cyclosporine (non-modified) and the products cannot be used interchangeably without close monitoring. Cyclosporine (modified) refers to the oral solution and capsule dosage formulations of cyclosporine in an aqueous dispersion (previously referred to as "microemulsion"). Potentially significant drug-drug/drug-food interactions may exist, requiring dose or frequency adjustment, additional monitoring, and/or selection of alternative therapy. Gingival hyperplasia may occur; avoid concomitant nifedipine in patients who develop gingival hyperplasia (may increase frequency of hyperplasia). Monitor cyclosporine concentrations closely following the addition, modification, or deletion of other medication. Live, attenuated vaccines may be less effective; vaccination should be avoided. Make dose adjustments based on cyclosporine blood concentrations. **[U.S. Boxed Warning]: Cyclosporine non-modified absorption is erratic; monitor blood concentrations closely. [U.S. Boxed Warning]: Prescribing and dosage adjustment should only be under the direct supervision of an experienced physician. Adequate laboratory/medical resources and follow-up are necessary.** Anaphylaxis has been reported with I.V. use; reserve for patients who cannot take oral form. **[U.S. Boxed Warning]: Risk of skin cancer may be increased in transplant patients.** Due to the increased risk for nephrotoxicity in renal transplantation, avoid using standard doses of cyclosporine in combination with everolimus; reduced cyclosporine doses are recommended; monitor cyclosporine concentrations closely. Cyclosporine and everolimus combination therapy may increase the risk for proteinuria. Cyclosporine combined with either everolimus or sirolimus may increase the risk for thrombotic microangiopathy/thrombotic thrombocytopenic purpura/hemolytic uremic syndrome (TMA/TTP/HUS). Cyclosporine has extensive hepatic metabolism and exposure is increased in patients with severe hepatic impairment; may require dose reduction.

Patients with psoriasis should avoid excessive sun exposure. **[U.S. Boxed Warning]: Risk of skin cancer may be increased with a history of PUVA and possibly methotrexate or other immunosuppressants, UVB, coal tar, or radiation.**

Rheumatoid arthritis: If receiving other immunosuppressive agents, radiation or UV therapy, concurrent use of cyclosporine is not recommended.

Products may contain corn oil, ethanol (consider alcohol content in certain patient populations, including pregnant or breast feeding women, patients with liver disease, seizure disorders, alcohol dependency, or pediatrics), or propylene glycol; injection also contains the vehicle Cremophor EL (polyoxyethylated castor oil), which has been associated with hypersensitivity (anaphylactic) reactions.

Adverse Reactions Adverse reactions reported with systemic use, including rheumatoid arthritis, psoriasis, and transplantation (kidney, liver, and heart). Percentages noted include the highest frequency regardless of indication/dosage. Frequencies may vary for specific conditions or formulation.

>10%:

Cardiovascular: Hypertension (8% to 53%), edema (5% to 14%)

Central nervous system: Headache (2% to 25%), paresthesia (1% to 11%)

Dermatologic: Hypertrichosis (5% to 19%)

Endocrine & metabolic: Hirsutism (21% to 45%), increased serum triglycerides (15%), female genital tract disease (9% to 11%)

Gastrointestinal: Nausea (2% to 23%), diarrhea (3% to 13%), gingival hyperplasia (2% to 16%), abdominal distress (<1% to 15%), dyspepsia (2% to 12%)

Genitourinary: Urinary tract infection (kidney transplant: 21%)

Infection: Increased susceptibility to infection (3% to 25%), viral infection (kidney transplant: 16%)

Neuromuscular & skeletal: Tremor (7% to 55%), leg cramps (2% to 12%)

Renal: Increased serum creatinine (16% to ≥50%), renal insufficiency (10% to 38%)

Respiratory: Upper respiratory tract infection (1% to 14%)

Kidney, liver, and heart transplant only (≤2% unless otherwise noted):

Cardiovascular: Chest pain (≤4%), flushing (<1% to 4%), glomerular capillary thrombosis, myocardial infarction

Central nervous system: Convulsions (1% to 5%), anxiety, confusion, lethargy, tingling sensation

Dermatologic: Skin infection (7%), acne vulgaris (1% to 6%), nail disease (brittle fingernails), hair breakage, night sweats, pruritus

Endocrine & metabolic: Gynecomastia (<1% to 4%), hyperglycemia, hypomagnesemia, weight loss

Gastrointestinal: Vomiting (2% to 10%), anorexia, aphthous stomatitis, constipation, dysphagia, gastritis, hiccups, pancreatitis

Genitourinary: Hematuria

Hematologic & oncologic: Leukopenia (<1% to 6%), lymphoma (<1% to 6%), anemia, thrombocytopenia, upper gastrointestinal hemorrhage

Hepatic: Hepatotoxicity (<1% to 7%)

Infection: Localized fungal infection (8%), cytomegalovirus disease (5%), septicemia (5%), abscess (4%), fungal infection (systemic: 2%)

Neuromuscular & skeletal: Arthralgia, myalgia, weakness

Ophthalmic: Conjunctivitis, visual disturbance

Otic: Hearing loss, tinnitus

Respiratory: Sinusitis (<1% to 7%), pneumonia (6%)

Miscellaneous: Fever

Rheumatoid arthritis only (1% to <3% unless otherwise noted):

Cardiovascular: Chest pain (4%), cardiac arrhythmia (2%), abnormal heart sounds, cardiac failure, myocardial infarction, peripheral ischemia

Central nervous system: Dizziness (8%), pain (6%), insomnia (4%), depression (3%), migraine (2% to 3%), anxiety, drowsiness, emotional lability, hypoesthesia, lack of concentration, malaise, neuropathy, nervousness, paranoia, vertigo

Dermatologic: Cellulitis, dermatological reaction, dermatitis, diaphoresis, dyschromia, eczema, enanthema, folliculitis, nail disease, pruritus, urticaria, xeroderma

Endocrine & metabolic: Menstrual disease (3%), decreased libido, diabetes mellitus, goiter, hot flash, hyperkalemia, hyperuricemia, hypoglycemia, increased libido, weight gain, weight loss

Gastrointestinal: Vomiting (9%), flatulence (5%), gingivitis (4%), constipation, dysgeusia, dysphagia, enlargement of salivary glands, eructation, esophagitis, gastric ulcer, gastritis, gastroenteritis, gingival hemorrhage, glossitis, peptic ulcer, tongue disease, xerostomia

Genitourinary: Leukorrhea (1%), breast fibroadenosis, hematuria, mastalgia, nocturia, urine abnormality, urinary incontinence, urinary urgency, uterine hemorrhage

Hematologic & oncologic: Purpura (3% to 4%), anemia, carcinoma, leukopenia, lymphadenopathy

Hepatic: Hyperbilirubinemia

Infection: Abscess (including renal), bacterial infection, candidiasis, fungal infection, herpes simplex infection, herpes zoster, viral infection
Neuromuscular & skeletal: Arthralgia, bone fracture, dislocation, myalgia, stiffness, synovial cyst, tendon disease, weakness
Ophthalmic: Cataract, conjunctivitis, eye pain, visual disturbance
Otic: Tinnitus, deafness, vestibular disturbance
Renal: Abscess (renal), increased blood urea nitrogen, polyuria, pyelonephritis
Respiratory: Cough (5%), dyspnea (5%), sinusitis (4%), abnormal breath sounds, bronchospasm, epistaxis, tonsillitis

Psoriasis only (1% to <3% unless otherwise noted):
Cardiovascular: Chest pain, flushing
Central nervous system: Psychiatric disturbance (4% to 5%), pain (3% to 4%), dizziness, insomnia, nervousness, vertigo
Dermatologic: Acne vulgaris, folliculitis, hyperkeratosis, pruritus, skin rash, xeroderma
Endocrine & metabolic: Hot flash
Gastrointestinal: Abdominal distention, constipation, gingival hemorrhage, increased appetite
Genitourinary: Urinary frequency
Hematologic & oncologic: Abnormal erythrocytes, altered platelet function, blood coagulation disorder, carcinoma, hemorrhagic diathesis
Hepatic: Hyperbilirubinemia
Neuromuscular & skeletal: Arthralgia (1% to 6%)
Ophthalmic: Visual disturbance
Respiratory: Flu-like symptoms (8% to 10%), bronchospasm (5%), cough (5%), dyspnea (5%), rhinitis (5%), respiratory tract infection
Miscellaneous: Fever

Postmarketing and/or case reports (Limited to important or life-threatening; any indication): Anaphylaxis/anaphylactoid reaction (possibly associated with Cremophor EL vehicle in injection formulation), brain disease, central nervous system toxicity, cholesterol increased, exacerbation of psoriasis (transformation to erythrodermic or pustular psoriasis), gout, hyperbilirubinemia, hyperkalemia, impaired consciousness, increased susceptibility to infection (including JC virus and BK virus), malignant lymphoma, migraine, papilledema, progressive multifocal leukoencephalopathy, pseudotumor cerebri, pulmonary edema (noncardiogenic), renal disease (polyoma virus-associated), reversible posterior leukoencephalopathy syndrome, thrombotic microangiopathy

Drug Interactions

Metabolism/Transport Effects Substrate of CYP3A4 (major), P-glycoprotein; **Note:** Assignment of Major/Minor substrate status based on clinically relevant drug interaction potential; **Inhibits** CYP2C9 (weak), CYP3A4 (moderate), P-glycoprotein

Avoid Concomitant Use

Avoid concomitant use of CycloSPORINE (Systemic) with any of the following: Aliskiren; AtorvaSTATin; BCG; Bosentan; Bosutinib; Conivaptan; Crizotinib; Dronedarone; Enzalutamide; Eplerenone; Fusidic Acid (Systemic); Ibrutinib; Ivabradine; Lomitapide; Lovastatin; Mifepristone; Natalizumab; PAZOPanib; Pimecrolimus; Pimozide; Pitavastatin; Pomalidomide; Potassium-Sparing Diuretics; Silodosin; Simvastatin; Sitaxentan; Tacrolimus (Systemic); Tacrolimus (Topical); Tofacitinib; Tolvaptan; Topotecan; Ulipristal; Vaccines (Live); VinCRIStine (Liposomal)

Increased Effect/Toxicity

CycloSPORINE (Systemic) may increase the levels/effects of: Afatinib; Aliskiren; Ambrisentan; ARIPiprazole; AtorvaSTATin; Avanafil; Boceprevir; Bosentan; Bosutinib; Budesonide (Systemic, Oral Inhalation); Calcium Channel Blockers (Dihydropyridine); Calcium Channel Blockers (Nondihydropyridine); Cardiac Glycosides; Caspofungin; Colchicine; CYP3A4 Substrates; Dabigatran Etexilate; Dexamethasone (Systemic); Dofetilide; DOXOrubicin; Dronedarone; Etoposide; Etoposide Phosphate; Everolimus; Ezetimibe; FentaNYL; Fibric Acid Derivatives; Fluvastatin; Halofantrine; Ibrutinib; Imipenem; Ivabradine; Ivacaftor; Leflunomide; Lomitapide; Loop Diuretics; Lovastatin; Lurasidone; Methotrexate; MethylPREDNISolone; Minoxidil (Systemic); Minoxidil (Topical); MitoXANtrone; Natalizumab; Neuromuscular-Blocking Agents; Nonsteroidal Anti-Inflammatory Agents; OxyCODONE; PAZOPanib; P-glycoprotein/ABCB1 Substrates; Pimozide; Pitavastatin; Pomalidomide; Pravastatin; PrednisoLONE (Systemic); PredniSONE; Propafenone; Protease Inhibitors; Prucalopride; Ranolazine; Repaglinide; Rivaroxaban; Rosuvastatin; Salmeterol; Saxagliptin; Silodosin; Simvastatin; Sirolimus; Sitaxentan; Tacrolimus (Systemic); Tacrolimus (Topical); Ticagrelor; Tofacitinib; Tolvaptan; Topotecan; Ulipristal; Vaccines (Live); Vilazodone; VinCRIStine (Liposomal); Zuclopenthixol

The levels/effects of CycloSPORINE (Systemic) may be increased by: ACE Inhibitors; AcetaZOLAMIDE; Aminoglycosides; Amiodarone; Amphotericin B; Androgens; Angiotensin II Receptor Blockers; Antifungal Agents (Azole Derivatives, Systemic); Boceprevir; Bromocriptine; Calcium Channel Blockers (Nondihydropyridine); Carvedilol; Chloramphenicol; Conivaptan; Crizotinib; CYP3A4 Inhibitors (Moderate); CYP3A4 Inhibitors (Strong); Dasatinib; Denosumab; Dexamethasone (Systemic); Eplerenone; Ezetimibe; Fluconazole; Fusidic Acid (Systemic); GlyBURIDE; Grapefruit Juice; Imatinib; Imipenem; Ivacaftor; Luliconazole; Macrolide Antibiotics; Melphalan; Methotrexate; MethylPREDNISolone; Metoclopramide; MetroNIDAZOLE (Systemic); Mifepristone; Nonsteroidal Anti-Inflammatory Agents; Norfloxacin; Omeprazole; P-glycoprotein/ABCB1 Inhibitors; Pimecrolimus; Potassium-Sparing Diuretics; Pravastatin; PrednisoLONE (Systemic); PredniSONE; Protease Inhibitors; Pyrazinamide; Quinupristin; Roflumilast; Sirolimus; Sulfonamide Derivatives; Tacrolimus (Systemic); Tacrolimus (Topical); Telaprevir; Temsirolimus; Ticagrelor; Trastuzumab

Decreased Effect

CycloSPORINE (Systemic) may decrease the levels/effects of: BCG; Coccidioidin Skin Test; GlyBURIDE; Ifosfamide; Mycophenolate; Sipuleucel-T; Vaccines (Inactivated); Vaccines (Live)

The levels/effects of CycloSPORINE (Systemic) may be decreased by: Adalimumab; Armodafinil; Ascorbic Acid; Barbiturates; Bosentan; CarBAMazepine; Colesevelam; CYP3A4 Inducers (Strong); Dabrafenib; Deferasirox; Dexamethasone (Systemic); Echinacea; Efavirenz; Enzalutamide; Fibric Acid Derivatives; Fosphenytoin; Griseofulvin; Imipenem; MethylPREDNISolone; Mitotane; Modafinil; Multivitamins/Fluoride (with ADE); Multivitamins/Minerals (with ADEK, Folate, Iron); Multivitamins/Minerals (with AE, No Iron); Nafcillin; Orlistat; P-glycoprotein/ABCB1 Inducers; Phenytoin; PrednisoLONE (Systemic); PredniSONE; Rifamycin Derivatives; Somatostatin Analogs; St Johns Wort; Sulfinpyrazone [Off Market]; Sulfonamide Derivatives; Tocilizumab; Vitamin E

Ethanol/Nutrition/Herb Interactions

Food: Grapefruit juice increases cyclosporine serum concentrations. Management: Avoid grapefruit juice.
Herb/Nutraceutical: St John's wort may increase the metabolism of and decrease plasma levels of cyclosporine; organ rejection and graft loss have been reported. Cat's claw and echinacea have immunostimulant properties. Management: Avoid St John's wort, cat's claw, and echinacea.

Preparation for Administration Hazardous agent - use appropriate precautions for handling and disposal (NIOSH, 2012).

Injection: To minimize leaching of DEHP, non-PVC containers and sets should be used for preparation and administration.

Sandimmune injection: Injection should be further diluted (1 mL [50 mg] of concentrate in 20-100 mL of D_5W or NS) for administration by intravenous infusion.

Storage/Stability

Capsule: Store at controlled room temperature.

Injection: Store at controlled room temperature; do not refrigerate. Ampuls and vials should be protected from light. Stability of injection of parenteral admixture at room temperature (25°C) is 6 hours in PVC; 12-24 hours in Excel, PAB containers, or glass.

Oral solution: Store at controlled room temperature; do not refrigerate. Use within 2 months after opening; should be mixed in glass containers.

Mechanism of Action Inhibition of production and release of interleukin II and inhibits interleukin II-induced activation of resting T-lymphocytes.

Pharmacodynamics/Kinetics

Absorption: Oral:

Cyclosporine (non-modified): Erratic and incomplete; dependent on presence of food, bile acids, and GI motility; larger oral doses are needed in pediatrics due to shorter bowel length and limited intestinal absorption

Cyclosporine (modified): Erratic and incomplete; increased absorption, up to 30% when compared to cyclosporine (non-modified); less dependent on food, bile acids, or GI motility when compared to cyclosporine (non-modified)

Distribution: Widely in tissues and body fluids including the liver, pancreas, and lungs

V_{dss}: 4-6 L/kg in renal, liver, and marrow transplant recipients (slightly lower values in cardiac transplant patients; children <10 years have higher values); ESRD: 3.49 L/kg

Protein binding: 90% to 98% to lipoproteins

Metabolism: Extensively hepatic via CYP3A4; forms at least 25 metabolites; extensive first-pass effect following oral administration

Bioavailability: Oral:

Cyclosporine (non-modified): Dependent on patient population and transplant type (<10% in adult liver transplant patients and as high as 89% in renal transplant patients); bioavailability of Sandimmune capsules and oral solution are equivalent; bioavailability of oral solution is ~30% of the I.V. solution

Children: 28% (range: 17% to 42%); gut dysfunction common in BMT patients and oral bioavailability is further reduced

Cyclosporine (modified): Bioavailability of Neoral capsules and oral solution are equivalent:

Children: 43% (range: 30% to 68%)

Adults: 23% greater than with cyclosporine (non-modified) in renal transplant patients; 50% greater in liver transplant patients

Half-life elimination: Oral: May be prolonged in patients with hepatic impairment and shorter in pediatric patients due to the higher metabolism rate

Cyclosporine (non-modified): Biphasic: Alpha: 1.4 hours; Terminal: 19 hours (range: 10-27 hours)

Cyclosporine (modified): Biphasic: Terminal: 8.4 hours (range: 5-18 hours)

Time to peak, serum: Oral:

Cyclosporine (non-modified): 2-6 hours; some patients have a second peak at 5-6 hours

Cyclosporine (modified): Renal transplant: 1.5-2 hours

Excretion: Primarily feces; urine (6%, 0.1% as unchanged drug and metabolites)

Dosage Neoral/Gengraf and Sandimmune are not bioequivalent and cannot be used interchangeably.

Children:

Bone marrow transplantation *(Canadian labeling)*:

Note: I.V. administration is preferred for initial therapy.

Oral: Cyclosporine (modified): Initial: 12.5-15 mg/kg daily in 2 divided doses beginning 1 day prior to transplant; Maintenance: ~12.5 mg/kg daily in 2 divided doses every 12 hours for at least 3-6 months; decrease dose gradually to zero by 1 year following transplant. Patients who develop graft versus host disease (GVHD) after discontinuation of cyclosporine may be reinitiated on therapy with a loading dose of 10-12.5 mg/kg followed by the previously established maintenance dose. Patients with mild, chronic GVHD should be treated with lowest effective dose.

I.V. Cyclosporine (non-modified): Initial: 3-5 mg/kg daily or one-third of the oral dose as a single dose (infused over 2-6 hours) beginning 1 day prior to transplant; Maintenance: may continue initial dose for up to 2 weeks; however, patients should be switched to an oral dosage form as soon as possible.

Nephrotic syndrome *(Canadian labeling)*: Oral: Cyclosporine (modified):

Initial: 4.2 mg/kg daily in 2 divided doses every 12 hours; titrate for induction of remission and renal function. Adjunct therapy with low-dose oral corticosteroids is recommended for patients with an inadequate response to cyclosporine (particularly if steroid-resistant).

Maintenance: Dose is individualized based on proteinuria, serum creatinine, and tolerability but should be maintained at lowest effective dose; maximum dose: 6 mg /kg daily. Discontinue if no improvement is observed after 3 months.

Solid organ transplant: Refer to adult dosing; children may require, and are able to tolerate, larger doses than adults.

Adults:

Psoriasis: Oral: Cyclosporine (modified): Initial dose: 2.5 mg/kg daily, divided twice daily

Titration:

U.S. labeling: Increase by 0.5 mg/kg daily if insufficient response is seen after 4 weeks of treatment. Additional dosage increases may be made every 2 weeks if needed (maximum dose: 4 mg/kg daily).

Canadian labeling: Increase by 0.5-1 mg/kg daily if insufficient response is seen after 4 weeks of treatment. Additional dosage increases may be made every 4 weeks if needed (maximum dose: 5 mg/kg daily).

Discontinue if no benefit is seen by 6 weeks of therapy at the maximum dose. Once patients are adequately controlled, the dose should be decreased to the lowest effective dose. Doses lower than 2.5 mg/kg daily may be effective. The Canadian labeling recommends attempting to wean patients off therapy if no relapse occurs within 6 months of achieving remission. Treatment longer than 1 year is not recommended.

Note: Increase the frequency of blood pressure monitoring after each alteration in dosage of cyclosporine. Cyclosporine dosage should be decreased by 25% to 50% in patients with no history of hypertension who develop sustained hypertension during therapy and, if hypertension persists, treatment with cyclosporine should be discontinued.

Rheumatoid arthritis: Oral: Cyclosporine (modified): Initial dose: 2.5 mg/kg daily, divided twice daily; salicylates, NSAIDs, and oral glucocorticoids may be continued (refer to Drug Interactions)

Titration:

U.S. labeling: Dose may be increased by 0.5-0.75 mg/kg daily if insufficient response is seen after 8 weeks of treatment; additional dosage increases may be made again at 12 weeks (maximum dose: 4 mg/kg daily). Discontinue if no benefit is seen by 16 weeks of therapy.

Canadian labeling: If insufficient response to initial dose after 6 weeks, may increase dose gradually as tolerated (maximum dose: 5 mg/kg daily); maintenance therapy should be individualized to the lowest effective and tolerable dose; may take up to 12 weeks before full effect is achieved.

Note: Increase the frequency of blood pressure monitoring after each alteration in dosage of cyclosporine. Cyclosporine dosage should be decreased by 25% to 50% in patients with no history of hypertension who develop sustained hypertension during therapy and, if hypertension persists, treatment with cyclosporine should be discontinued.

Solid organ transplant (newly-transplanted patients): Adjunct therapy with corticosteroids is recommended. Initial dose should be given 4-12 hours prior to transplant or may be given postoperatively; adjust initial dose to achieve desired plasma concentration

Oral: Dose is dependent upon type of transplant and formulation:

Cyclosporine (modified):

Renal: 9 ± 3 mg/kg daily, in 2 divided doses

Liver: 8 ± 4 mg/kg daily, in 2 divided doses

Heart: 7 ± 3 mg/kg daily, in 2 divided doses

Cyclosporine (non-modified): Initial doses of 10-14 mg/kg daily have been used for renal transplants (the manufacturer's labeling includes dosing from initial clinical trials of 15 mg/kg daily [range: 14-18 mg/kg daily]; however, this higher dosing level is rarely used any longer). Continue initial dose daily for 1-2 weeks; taper by 5% per week to a maintenance dose of 5-10 mg/kg daily; some renal transplant patients may be dosed as low as 3 mg/kg daily

Note: When using the non-modified formulation, cyclosporine levels may increase in liver transplant patients when the T-tube is closed; dose may need decreased

I.V.: Cyclosporine (non-modified): Manufacturer's labeling: Initial dose: 5-6 mg/kg daily or one-third of the oral dose as a single dose, infused over 2-6 hours; use should be limited to patients unable to take capsules or oral solution; patients should be switched to an oral dosage form as soon as possible

Note: Many transplant centers administer cyclosporine as "divided dose" infusions (in 2-3 doses daily) or as a continuous (24-hour) infusion; dosages range from 3-7.5 mg/kg daily. Specific institutional protocols should be consulted.

Conversion to cyclosporine (modified) from cyclosporine (non-modified): Start with daily dose previously used and adjust to obtain preconversion cyclosporine trough concentration. Plasma concentrations should be monitored every 4-7 days and dose adjusted as necessary, until desired trough level is obtained. When transferring patients with previously poor absorption of cyclosporine (non-modified), monitor trough levels at least twice weekly (especially if initial dose exceeds 10 mg/kg daily); high plasma levels are likely to occur.

Acute graft versus host disease (GVHD), prevention (unlabeled use in the U.S.): Adults: I.V. followed by oral: Initial: I.V.: 3 mg/kg daily 1 day prior to transplant; may convert to oral therapy when tolerated; titrate dose to appropriate cyclosporine trough concentration (in combination with methotrexate); taper per protocol (refer to specific references for tapering and target trough details); discontinue 6 months post transplant in the absence of acute GVHD (Ratanatharathorn, 1998; Ruutu, 2013; Storb, 1986a; Storb, 1986b)

or

Initial: I.V.: 5 mg/kg (continuous infusion over 20 hours) each day for 6 days (loading dose) starting 2 days prior to transplant, then 3 mg/kg over 20 hours each day for 11 days starting on post transplant day 4, then 3.75 mg/kg over 20 hours each day for 21 days starting on day 15, then **oral** (in 2 divided daily doses): 10 mg/kg daily days 36 to 83, then 8 mg/kg daily days 84 to 97, then 6 mg/kg/day days 98 to 119, then 4 mg/kg/day days 120 to 180, then discontinue (in combination with methotrexate +/- corticosteroid) (Chao, 1993; Chao, 2000)

Bone marrow transplantation *(Canadian labeling):* **Note:** I.V. administration is preferred for initial therapy.

Oral: Cyclosporine (modified): Initial: 12.5-15 mg/kg daily in 2 divided doses beginning 1 day prior to transplant. Maintenance: ~12.5 mg/kg daily in 2 divided doses every 12 hours for at least 3-6 months; decrease dose gradually to zero by 1 year following transplant. Patients who develop GVHD after discontinuation of cyclosporine may be reinitiated on therapy with a loading dose of 10-12.5 mg/kg followed by the previously established maintenance dose. Patients with mild, chronic GVHD should be treated with lowest effective dose.

I.V. Cyclosporine (non-modified): Initial: 3-5 mg/kg daily or one-third of the oral dose as a single dose (infused over 2-6 hours) beginning 1 day prior to transplant; Maintenance: May continue initial dose for up to 2 weeks; however, patients should be switched to an oral dosage form as soon as possible.

Focal segmental glomerulosclerosis (unlabeled use in U.S.): Oral: Initial: 3.5-5 mg/kg/day divided every 12 hours (in combination with oral prednisone) (Braun, 2008; Cattran, 1999)

Nephrotic syndrome *(Canadian labeling):* Oral: Cyclosporine (modified):

Initial: 3.5 mg/kg daily in 2 divided doses every 12 hours; titrate for induction of remission and renal function. Adjunct therapy with low-dose oral corticosteroids is recommended for patients with an inadequate response to cyclosporine (particularly if steroid-resistant).

Maintenance: Dose is individualized based on proteinuria, serum creatinine, and tolerability but should be maintained at lowest effective dose; maximum dose: 5 mg /kg daily. Discontinue if no improvement is observed after 3 months.

Lupus nephritis (unlabeled use): Oral: Cyclosporine (modified): Initial: 4 mg/kg daily for 1 month (reduce dose if trough concentrations >200 ng/mL); reduce dose by 0.5 mg/kg every 2 weeks to a maintenance dose of 2.5-3 mg/kg daily (Moroni, 2006)

Ulcerative colitis, severe (steroid-refractory) (unlabeled use):

I.V.: Cyclosporine (non-modified): 2-4 mg/kg daily, infused continuously over 24 hours (Lichtiger, 1994; Van Assche, 2003). **Note:** Some studies suggest no therapeutic difference between low-dose (2 mg/kg) and high-dose (4 mg/kg) cyclosporine regimens (Van Assche, 2003).

Oral: Cyclosporine (modified): 2.3-3 mg/kg every 12 hours (De Saussure, 2005; Weber, 2006)

Note: Patients responsive to I.V. therapy should be switched to oral therapy when possible.

Dosage adjustment in renal impairment:

Nephrotic syndrome: *Canadian labeling:* Initial: 2.5 mg/kg daily.

Serum creatinine levels >30% above pretreatment levels: Take another sample within 2 weeks; if the level remains >30% above pretreatment levels, decrease dosage of cyclosporine (modified) by 25% to 50%.

Psoriasis (severe):

U.S. labeling:

Serum creatinine levels ≥25% above pretreatment levels: Take another sample within 2 weeks; if the level remains ≥25% above pretreatment levels, decrease dosage of cyclosporine (modified) by 25% to 50%. If two dosage adjustments do not reverse the increase in serum creatinine levels, treatment should be discontinued.

Serum creatinine levels ≥50% above pretreatment levels: Decrease cyclosporine dosage by 25% to 50%. If two dosage adjustments do not reverse the increase in serum creatinine levels, treatment should be discontinued.

Canadian labeling: Serum creatinine levels >30% above pretreatment levels: Decrease dosage of cyclosporine (modified) by 25% to 50%. If dosage adjustment does not reverse the increase in serum creatinine levels within 30 days, discontinue treatment.

Rheumatoid arthritis: *Canadian labeling:*

Serum creatinine levels >30% above pretreatment levels: Take another sample within 2 weeks; if the level remains ≥30% above pretreatment levels, manufacturer labeling recommends reducing dose but does not provide specific dosing recommendation. If dosage adjustment does not reverse the increase in serum creatinine levels within 30 days, discontinue treatment.

Serum creatinine levels >50% above pretreatment levels: Reduce dose by 50%; if dosage adjustment does not reverse the increase in serum creatinine levels within 30 days, discontinue treatment.

Hemodialysis: Supplemental dose is not necessary.

Peritoneal dialysis: Supplemental dose is not necessary.

Dosage adjustment in hepatic impairment:

Mild-to-moderate impairment: No dosage adjustment provided in the manufacturer's labeling; monitor blood concentrations.

Severe impairment: No dosage adjustment provided in the manufacturer's labeling; however, metabolism is extensively hepatic (exposure is increased). Monitor blood concentrations; may require dose reduction.

Dietary Considerations Administer this medication consistently with relation to time of day and meals. Avoid grapefruit juice with oral cyclosporine use.

Administration

Oral solution: Do not administer liquid from plastic or styrofoam cup. May dilute Neoral oral solution with orange juice or apple juice. May dilute Sandimmune oral solution with milk, chocolate milk, or orange juice. Avoid changing diluents frequently. Mix thoroughly and drink at once. Use syringe provided to measure dose. Mix in a glass container and rinse container with more diluent to ensure total dose is taken. Do not rinse syringe before or after use (may cause dose variation).

Combination therapy with renal transplantation:

Everolimus: Administer cyclosporine at the same time as everolimus

Sirolimus: Administer cyclosporine 4 hours prior to sirolimus

I.V.: The manufacturer recommends that following dilution, intravenous admixture be administered over 2-6 hours. However, many transplant centers administer as divided doses (2-3 doses/day) or as a 24-hour continuous infusion. Discard solution after 24 hours. Anaphylaxis has been reported with I.V. use; reserve for patients who cannot take oral form. Patients should be under continuous observation for at least the first 30 minutes of the infusion, and should be monitored frequently thereafter. Maintain patent airway; other supportive measures and agents for treating anaphylaxis should be present when I.V. drug is given. To minimize leaching of DEHP, non-PVC sets should be used for administration.

Hazardous agent - use appropriate precautions for handling and disposal (NIOSH, 2012).

Monitoring Parameters Monitor blood pressure and serum creatinine after any cyclosporine dosage changes or addition, modification, or deletion of other medications. Monitor plasma concentrations periodically.

Nephrotic syndrome (Canadian labeling): Baseline blood pressure (2 readings within 2 weeks), fasting serum creatinine (at least 3 levels within 2 weeks), creatinine clearance, urinalysis, CBC, liver function, serum uric acid, serum potassium, and malignancy screening (eg, skin, mouth, lymph nodes). Biweekly monitoring of blood pressure for initial 3 months and then monthly thereafter, frequent monitoring of renal function and periodic cyclosporine trough levels are recommended during therapy. Consider renal biopsy in patients with steroid-dependent minimal change neuropathy who have been maintained on therapy >1 year.

Transplant patients: Cyclosporine trough levels, serum electrolytes, renal function, hepatic function, blood pressure, lipid profile

Psoriasis therapy: Baseline blood pressure, serum creatinine (2 levels each), BUN, CBC, serum magnesium, potassium, uric acid, lipid profile. Biweekly monitoring of blood pressure, complete blood count, serum creatinine, and levels of BUN, uric acid, potassium, lipids, and magnesium during the first 3 months of treatment for psoriasis. Monthly monitoring is recommended after this initial period. (**Note:** The Canadian labeling recommends bimonthly monitoring of serum creatinine after the initial period if serum creatinine remains stable and cyclosporine dose is ≤2.5 mg/kg daily, and monthly monitoring for higher doses). Also evaluate any atypical skin lesions prior to therapy. Increase the frequency of blood pressure monitoring after each alteration in dosage of cyclosporine.

Rheumatoid arthritis: Baseline blood pressure, and serum creatinine (2 levels each); serum creatinine every 2 weeks for first 3 months, then monthly if patient is stable. Increase the frequency of blood pressure monitoring after each alteration in dosage of cyclosporine. Additional Canadian labeling recommendations include CBC, hepatic function, urinalysis, serum potassium and uric acid (baseline and periodic thereafter).

Reference Range Reference ranges are method dependent and specimen dependent; use the same analytical method consistently

Method-dependent and specimen-dependent: Trough levels should be obtained:

Oral: 12-18 hours after dose (chronic usage)

I.V.: 12 hours after dose **or** immediately prior to next dose

Therapeutic range: Not absolutely defined, dependent on organ transplanted, time after transplant, organ function and CsA toxicity:

General range of 100-400 ng/mL

Toxic level: Not well defined, nephrotoxicity may occur at any level

Recommended cyclosporine therapeutic ranges when administered in combination with everolimus for renal transplant (Zortress product labeling, 2013):

Month 1 post-transplant: 100-200 ng/mL

Months 2 and 3 post-transplant: 75-150 ng/mL

Months 4 and 5 post-transplant: 50-100 ng/mL

Months 6-12 post-transplant: 25-50 ng/mL

Test Interactions Specific whole blood assay for cyclosporine may be falsely elevated if sample is drawn from the same central venous line through which dose was administered (even if flush has been administered and/or dose was given hours before); cyclosporine metabolites cross-react with radioimmunoassay and fluorescence polarization immunoassay

Additional Information Cyclosporine (modified): Refers to the capsule dosage formulation of cyclosporine in an aqueous dispersion (previously referred to as "microemulsion"). Cyclosporine (modified) has increased bioavailability as compared to cyclosporine (non-modified) and cannot be used interchangeably without close monitoring.

Dosage Forms Considerations

Cyclosporine (modified): Gengraf and Neoral
Cyclosporine (non-modified): SandIMMUNE

Dosage Forms Excipient information presented when available (limited, particularly for generics); consult specific product labeling.

Capsule, Oral:
- Gengraf: 25 mg, 100 mg [contains cremophor el, fd&c blue #2 (indigotine)]
- Neoral: 25 mg, 100 mg [contains alcohol, usp]
- SandIMMUNE: 25 mg [contains alcohol, usp]
- SandIMMUNE: 100 mg
- Generic: 25 mg, 50 mg, 100 mg

Solution, Intravenous:
- SandIMMUNE: 50 mg/mL (5 mL) [contains alcohol, usp, cremophor el]
- Generic: 50 mg/mL (5 mL)

Solution, Oral:
- Gengraf: 100 mg/mL (50 mL) [contains propylene glycol]
- Neoral: 100 mg/mL (50 mL) [contains alcohol, usp]
- SandIMMUNE: 100 mg/mL (50 mL) [contains alcohol, usp]
- Generic: 100 mg/mL (50 mL)

Dosage Forms: Canada

Excipient information presented when available (limited, particularly for generics); consult specific product labeling.

Capsule, Oral:
- Neoral: 10 mg, 25 mg, 50 mg, 100 mg [contains alcohol]

Solution, Intravenous:
- SandIMMUNE I.V.: 50 mg/mL (1 mL, 5 mL) [contains alcohol, cremophor el]

Solution, Oral:
- Neoral: 100 mg/mL (50 mL) [contains alcohol, propylene glycol]

CycloSPORINE (Ophthalmic)
(SYE kloe spor een)

Brand Names: U.S. Restasis

Brand Names: Canada Restasis®

Index Terms Ciclosporin; CsA; CyA; Cyclosporin A

Pharmacologic Category Calcineurin Inhibitor; Immunosuppressant Agent

Use Increase tear production when suppressed tear production is presumed to be due to keratoconjunctivitis sicca-associated ocular inflammation (in patients not already using topical anti-inflammatory drugs or punctal plugs)

Pregnancy Risk Factor C

Dosage Ophthalmic: Adolescents ≥16 years and Adults: Keratoconjunctivitis sicca: Instill 1 drop in each eye every 12 hours

Dosage adjustment in renal impairment: No dosage adjustment provided in manufacturer's labeling. However, dosage adjustment unlikely due to low systemic absorption.

Dosage adjustment in hepatic impairment: No dosage adjustment provided in manufacturer's labeling. However, dosage adjustment unlikely due to low systemic absorption.

Additional Information Complete prescribing information should be consulted for additional detail.

Dosage Forms Excipient information presented when available (limited, particularly for generics); consult specific product labeling.

Emulsion, Ophthalmic [preservative free]:
- Restasis: 0.05% (1 ea) [contains polysorbate 80]

- ◆ **Cyklokapron** *see* Tranexamic Acid *on page 2104*
- ◆ **Cymbalta** *see* DULoxetine *on page 677*
- ◆ **Cymbalta® (Can)** *see* DULoxetine *on page 677*

Cyproheptadine (si proe HEP ta deen)

Brand Names: Canada Euro-Cyproheptadine; PMS-Cyproheptadine

Index Terms Cyproheptadine Hydrochloride; Periactin

Pharmacologic Category Histamine H_1 Antagonist; Histamine H_1 Antagonist, First Generation; Piperidine Derivative

Additional Appendix Information

Beers Criteria – Potentially Inappropriate Medications for Geriatrics *on page 2368*

Use Perennial and seasonal allergic rhinitis and other allergic symptoms including urticaria

Unlabeled Use Migraine headache prophylaxis, pruritus, serotonin syndrome, spasticity associated with spinal cord damage

Pregnancy Risk Factor B

Pregnancy Considerations Adverse events have been observed in some animal reproduction studies. Maternal antihistamine use has generally not resulted in an increased risk of birth defects; however, information specific to cyproheptadine is limited. Antihistamines are recommended for the treatment of rhinitis, urticaria, and pruritus with rash in pregnant women (although second generation antihistamines may be preferred). Antihistamines are not recommended for treatment of pruritus associated with intrahepatic cholestasis in pregnancy.

Breast-Feeding Considerations It is not known if cyproheptadine is excreted into breast milk. Premature infants and newborns have a higher risk of intolerance to antihistamines. Use while breast-feeding is contraindicated by the manufacturer. Antihistamines may decrease maternal serum prolactin concentrations when administered prior to the establishment of nursing.

Contraindications Hypersensitivity to cyproheptadine or any component of the formulation; narrow-angle glaucoma; bladder neck obstruction; pyloroduodenal obstruction; symptomatic prostatic hyperplasia; stenosing peptic ulcer; concurrent use of MAO inhibitors; use in debilitated elderly patients; use in premature and term newborns due to potential association with SIDS; breast-feeding

Warnings/Precautions May cause CNS depression, which may impair physical or mental abilities; patients must be cautioned about performing tasks which require mental alertness (eg, operating machinery or driving). Effects may be potentiated when used with other sedative drugs or ethanol. Use with caution in patients with cardiovascular disease; increased intraocular pressure; respiratory disease; or thyroid dysfunction. In the elderly, avoid use of this potent anticholinergic agent due to increased risk of confusion, dry mouth, constipation, and other anticholinergic effects; clearance decreases in patients of advanced age (Beers Criteria). Antihistamines may cause excitation in young children.

Adverse Reactions Frequency not defined.

Cardiovascular: Extrasystoles, hypotension, palpitation, tachycardia

Central nervous system: Confusion, coordination disturbed, dizziness, excitation, euphoria, faintness, hallucinations, headache, hysteria, insomnia, irritability, nervousness, neuritis, restlessness, sedation, seizure, sleepiness, tremor, vertigo

Dermatologic: Angioedema, photosensitivity, rash, urticaria

Gastrointestinal: Abdominal pain, anorexia, appetite increased, constipation, diarrhea, nausea, vomiting, xerostomia

Genitourinary: Difficult urination, urinary frequency, urinary retention
Hematologic: Agranulocytosis, hemolytic anemia, leukopenia, thrombocytopenia
Hepatic: Cholestasis, hepatic failure, hepatitis, jaundice
Neuromuscular & skeletal: Paresthesia
Ocular: Blurred vision, diplopia
Otic: Labyrinthitis (acute), tinnitus
Respiratory: Bronchial secretions (thickening), nasal congestion, pharyngitis
Miscellaneous: Allergic reactions, anaphylactic shock, chills, diaphoresis, fatigue

Drug Interactions

Metabolism/Transport Effects None known.

Avoid Concomitant Use

Avoid concomitant use of Cyproheptadine with any of the following: Aclidinium; Azelastine (Nasal); Ipratropium (Oral Inhalation); Paraldehyde; Tiotropium; Umeclidinium

Increased Effect/Toxicity

Cyproheptadine may increase the levels/effects of: Alcohol (Ethyl); Analgesics (Opioid); Anticholinergics; Azelastine (Nasal); Buprenorphine; CNS Depressants; Hydrocodone; Methotrimeprazine; Metyrosine; Mirtazapine; Paraldehyde; Pramipexole; ROPINIRole; Rotigotine; Tiotropium; Zolpidem

The levels/effects of Cyproheptadine may be increased by: Aclidinium; Brimonidine (Topical); Doxylamine; Droperidol; HydrOXYzine; Ipratropium (Oral Inhalation); Magnesium Sulfate; Methotrimeprazine; Perampanel; Pramlintide; Sodium Oxybate; Tapentadol; Umeclidinium

Decreased Effect

Cyproheptadine may decrease the levels/effects of: Acetylcholinesterase Inhibitors (Central); Benzylpenicilloyl Polylysine; Betahistine; Hyaluronidase; Selective Serotonin Reuptake Inhibitors

The levels/effects of Cyproheptadine may be decreased by: Acetylcholinesterase Inhibitors (Central); Amphetamines

Ethanol/Nutrition/Herb Interactions Ethanol: May increase CNS depression; monitor for increased effects with coadministration. Caution patients about effects.

Mechanism of Action A potent antihistamine and serotonin antagonist, competes with histamine for H_1-receptor sites on effector cells in the gastrointestinal tract, blood vessels, and respiratory tract

Pharmacodynamics/Kinetics

Metabolism: Primarily by hepatic glucuronidation via UGT1A (Walker, 1996)
Half-life elimination: Metabolites: ~16 hours (Paton, 1985)
Time to peak, plasma: 6-9 hours (Paton, 1985)
Excretion: Urine (~40% primarily as metabolites); feces (2% to 20%)

Dosage

Allergic conditions: Oral:
Children: 0.25 mg/kg/day or 8 mg/m^2/day in 2-3 divided doses **or**
2-6 years: 2 mg every 8-12 hours (not to exceed 12 mg daily)
7-14 years: 4 mg every 8-12 hours (not to exceed 16 mg daily)
Adults: 4-20 mg daily divided every 8 hours (not to exceed 0.5 mg/kg/day); some patients may require up to 32 mg daily for adequate control of symptoms

Migraine headache prophylaxis (unlabeled use): Oral:
Children: 4 mg every 8-12 hours
Adults: 2 mg every 12 hours (with or without propranolol) (Holland, 2012; Rao, 2000)

Serotonin syndrome (unlabeled use): Adults: Oral: Initial: 12 mg followed by 2 mg every 2 hours or 4-8 mg every 6 hours as needed for symptom control (Boyer, 2005; Sun-Edelstein, 2008)

Spasticity associated with spinal cord damage (unlabeled use): Adults: Oral: Initial: 2-4 mg every 8 hours; maximum: 8 mg every 8 hours (Barbeau, 1982; Wainberg, 1990)

Elderly: Initiate therapy at the lower end of the dosage range

Dosage adjustment in renal impairment: No dosage adjustment provided in manufacturer's labeling. However, elimination is diminished in renal insufficiency.

Dosage adjustment in hepatic impairment: No dosage adjustment provided in manufacturer's labeling.

Test Interactions Diagnostic antigen skin test results may be suppressed; false positive serum TCA screen

Dosage Forms Excipient information presented when available (limited, particularly for generics); consult specific product labeling.

Syrup, Oral, as hydrochloride:
Generic: 2 mg/5 mL (10 mL, 473 mL)
Tablet, Oral, as hydrochloride:
Generic: 4 mg

◆ Cyproheptadine Hydrochloride *see* Cyproheptadine *on page 515*
◆ Cystadane *see* Betaine *on page 246*
◆ Cystadane® (Can) *see* Betaine *on page 246*
◆ Cystagon *see* Cysteamine (Systemic) *on page 516*
◆ Cystaran *see* Cysteamine (Ophthalmic) *on page 517*

Cysteamine (Systemic) (sis TEE a meen)

Brand Names: U.S. Cystagon; Procysbi

Index Terms Cysteamine Bitartrate; Procysbi™

Pharmacologic Category Anticystine Agent; Urinary Tract Product

Use Treatment of nephropathic cystinosis

Pregnancy Risk Factor C

Dosage Oral:

Initial: Begin therapy as soon as the diagnosis of nephropathic cystinosis has been confirmed. Initiate therapy with $^1/_6$ to $^1/_4$ of maintenance dose; titrate slowly upward over 4-6 weeks.

Maintenance dose: Dosage adjustments should be made based on target WBC cystine levels (<1 nmol half-cystine/mg protein) and/or plasma cysteamine concentrations (>0.1 mg/L). If the patient is tolerating therapy, the target WBC cystine level should be <1 nmol half-cystine/mg protein; patients with poorer tolerability may still receive benefit when WBC cystine levels are kept at <2 nmol half-cystine/mg protein. If the WBC cystine level is >1 nmol half-cystine/mg protein but plasma cysteamine is >0.1 mg/L, confirm that the patient is compliant with regard to administration (including proper dosing interval and relationship between administration of medication and food).

Immediate release:

Children and Adolescents weighing ≤50 kg: 1.3 g/m^2/day or 60 mg/kg/day (unlabeled dose; Gahl, 2002) divided into 4 doses; maximum dose: 1.95 g/m^2/day or 90 mg/kg/day (unlabeled dose; Gahl, 2002).

Adolescents and Adults weighing >50 kg: 2 g daily in 4 divided doses; maximum dose: 1.95 g/m^2/day or 90 mg/kg/day (unlabeled dose; Gahl, 2002).

Missed doses: Administer missed dose as soon as possible. If the next scheduled dose is due in <2 hours, skip the missed dose and resume the regular dosing schedule. Do not double the dose.

Switching from cysteamine hydrochloride or phosphocysteamine solutions: Initiate immediate release cysteamine bitartrate at an equimolar dose to the cysteamine hydrochloride or phosphocysteamine dose; monitor WBC cystine levels 2 weeks after the switch, then every 3 months thereafter.

Delayed release:

Children ≥6 years, Adolescents, and Adults: 1.3 g/m²/day divided every 12 hours; may increase as needed in 10% increments to a maximum dose of 1.95 g/m²/day.

Missed doses: Administer missed dose as soon as possible. If the next scheduled dose is due in <4 hours, skip the missed dose and resume the regular dosing schedule. Do not double the dose.

Switching from immediate release cysteamine bitartrate to delayed release cysteamine bitartrate: Initiate delayed release cysteamine bitartrate at a total daily dose equal to the total daily dose of the immediate release formulation; monitor WBC cystine levels and/or plasma cysteamine concentration 2 weeks after the switch, then quarterly for 6 months, then two times annually thereafter.

Dosage adjustment for toxicity:

Gastrointestinal symptoms, transient skin rashes, CNS symptoms (eg, seizures, lethargy, somnolence, depression, encephalopathy):

Immediate release: Temporarily discontinue therapy. Reinitiate at a lower dose; titrate slowly.

Delayed release: Decrease dose by 10%. May temporarily discontinue therapy and reinitiate at a lower dose; titrate slowly.

Severe skin rashes (eg, erythema multiforme bullosa, toxic epidermal necrolysis): Permanently discontinue therapy.

Dosage adjustment in renal impairment: No dosage adjustment provided in manufacturer's labeling.

Dosage adjustment in hepatic impairment: No dosage adjustment provided in manufacturer's labeling.

Additional Information Complete prescribing information should be consulted for additional detail.

Dosage Forms Excipient information presented when available (limited, particularly for generics); consult specific product labeling.

Capsule, Oral:

Cystagon: 50 mg, 150 mg

Capsule Delayed Release, Oral:

Procysbi: 25 mg, 75 mg

Cysteamine (Ophthalmic) (sis TEE a meen)

Brand Names: U.S. Cystaran

Index Terms Cysteamine Hydrochloride

Pharmacologic Category Anticystine Agent; Ophthalmic Agent

Use Treatment of corneal cystine crystal accumulation in patients with cystinosis

Pregnancy Risk Factor C

Dosage Ocular cystinosis: Adults: Ophthalmic: Instill 1 drop in each eye every hour while awake

Dosage adjustment in renal impairment: No dosage adjustment provided in manufacturer's labeling. However, dosage adjustment unlikely due to low systemic absorption.

Dosage adjustment in hepatic impairment: No dosage adjustment provided in manufacturer's labeling. However, dosage adjustment unlikely due to low systemic absorption.

Additional Information Complete prescribing information should be consulted for additional detail.

Dosage Forms Excipient information presented when available (limited, particularly for generics); consult specific product labeling.

Solution, Ophthalmic:

Cystaran: 0.44% (15 mL) [contains benzalkonium chloride]

◆ **Cysteamine Bitartrate** *see* Cysteamine (Systemic) *on page 516*

◆ **Cysteamine Hydrochloride** *see* Cysteamine (Ophthalmic) *on page 517*

◆ **Cystistat (Can)** *see* Hyaluronate and Derivatives *on page 1000*

◆ **CYT** *see* Cyclophosphamide *on page 504*

◆ **Cytarabine** *see* Cytarabine (Conventional) *on page 517*

Cytarabine (Conventional)

(sye TARE a been con VEN sha nal)

Brand Names: Canada Cytarabine Injection; Cytosar®

Index Terms Ara-C; Arabinosylcytosine; Conventional Cytarabine; Cytarabine; Cytarabine Hydrochloride; Cytosar-U; Cytosine Arabinosine Hydrochloride

Pharmacologic Category Antineoplastic Agent, Antimetabolite; Antineoplastic Agent, Antimetabolite (Pyrimidine Analog)

Use Remission induction in acute myeloid leukemia (AML), treatment of acute lymphocytic leukemia (ALL) and chronic myelocytic leukemia (CML; blast phase); prophylaxis and treatment of meningeal leukemia

Unlabeled Use AML consolidation treatment, AML salvage treatment; acute promyelocytic leukemia (APL) consolidation treatment; treatment of primary central nervous system (CNS) lymphoma; treatment of chronic lymphocytic leukemia (CLL); treatment of relapsed or refractory Hodgkin lymphoma; treatment of non-Hodgkin's lymphomas (NHL)

Pregnancy Risk Factor D

Pregnancy Considerations Teratogenic effects were demonstrated in animal studies; limb and ear defects have been noted in case reports of cytarabine exposure during the first trimester of pregnancy. The following have also been noted in the neonate: Pancytopenia, WBC depression, electrolyte abnormalities, prematurity, low birth weight, decreased hematocrit or platelets. Risk to the fetus is decreased if treatment can be avoided during the first trimester; however, women of childbearing potential should be advised of the potential risks.

Breast-Feeding Considerations Due to the potential for serious adverse reactions in the nursing infant, breast-feeding is not recommended.

Contraindications Hypersensitivity to cytarabine or any component of the formulation

Warnings/Precautions Hazardous agent - use appropriate precautions for handling and disposal (NIOSH, 2012). **[U.S. Boxed Warning]: Myelosuppression (leukopenia, thrombocytopenia and anemia) is the major toxicity of cytarabine.** Use with caution in patients with prior drug-induced bone marrow suppression. Monitor blood counts frequently; once blasts are no longer apparent in the peripheral blood, bone marrow should be monitored frequently. Monitor for signs of infection or neutropenic fever due to neutropenia or bleeding due to thrombocytopenia.

High-dose regimens are associated with CNS, gastrointestinal, ocular (reversible corneal toxicity and hemorrhagic conjunctivitis; prophylaxis with ophthalmic corticosteroid drops is recommended), pulmonary toxicities and cardiomyopathy. Neurotoxicity associated with high-dose treatment may present as acute cerebellar toxicity (with or without cerebral impairment), personality changes, or may be severe with seizure and/or coma; may be delayed, ▶

occurring up to 3-8 days after treatment has begun. Risk factors for neurotoxicity include cumulative cytarabine dose, prior CNS disease and renal impairment; high-dose therapy (>18 g/m^2 per cycle) and age >50 years also increase the risk for cerebellar toxicity (Herzig, 1987). Tumor lysis syndrome and subsequent hyperuricemia may occur with high dose cytarabine; monitor, consider allopurinol and hydrate accordingly. There have been case reports of fatal cardiomyopathy when high dose cytarabine was used in combination with cyclophosphamide as a preparation regimen for transplantation.

Use with caution in patients with impaired renal and hepatic function; may be at higher risk for CNS toxicities; dosage adjustments may be necessary. A sudden respiratory arrest syndrome is characterized by fever, myalgia, bone pain, chest pain, maculopapular rash, conjunctivitis, and malaise, and may occur 6-12 hours following administration; may be managed with corticosteroids. Anaphylaxis resulting in acute cardiopulmonary arrest has been reported (rare). There have been reports of acute pancreatitis in patients receiving continuous infusion and in patients previously treated with L-asparaginase. **[U.S. Boxed Warning]: Should be administered under the supervision of an experienced cancer chemotherapy physician. Due to the potential toxicities, induction treatment with cytarabine should be in a facility with sufficient laboratory and supportive resources.** Some products may contain benzyl alcohol; do not use products containing benzyl alcohol or products reconstituted with bacteriostatic diluent intrathecally or for high-dose cytarabine regimens. When used for intrathecal administration, should not be prepared during the preparation of any other agents; after preparation, store intrathecal medications in an isolated location or container clearly marked with a label identifying as "intrathecal" use only; delivery of intrathecal medications to the patient should only be with other medications also intended for administration into the central nervous system (Jacobson, 2009).

Adverse Reactions

Frequent:

Central nervous system: Fever
Dermatologic: Rash
Gastrointestinal: Anal inflammation, anal ulceration, anorexia, diarrhea, mucositis, nausea, vomiting
Hematologic: Myelosuppression, neutropenia (onset: 1-7 days; nadir [biphasic]: 7-9 days and at 15-24 days; recovery [biphasic]: 9-12 days and at 24-34 days), thrombocytopenia (onset: 5 days; nadir: 12-15 days; recovery 15-25 days), anemia, bleeding, leukopenia, megaloblastosis, reticulocytes decreased
Hepatic: Hepatic dysfunction, transaminases increased (acute)
Local: Thrombophlebitis

Less frequent:

Cardiovascular: Chest pain, pericarditis
Central nervous system: Dizziness, headache, neural toxicity, neuritis
Dermatologic: Alopecia, pruritus, skin freckling, skin ulceration, urticaria
Gastrointestinal: Abdominal pain, bowel necrosis, esophageal ulceration, esophagitis, pancreatitis, sore throat
Genitourinary: Urinary retention
Hepatic: Jaundice
Local: Injection site cellulitis
Ocular: Conjunctivitis
Renal: Renal dysfunction
Respiratory: Dyspnea
Miscellaneous: Allergic edema, anaphylaxis, sepsis

Infrequent and/or case reports: Acute respiratory distress syndrome, amylase increased, angina, aseptic meningitis, cardiopulmonary arrest (acute), cerebral dysfunction, cytarabine syndrome (bone pain, chest pain, conjunctivitis, fever, maculopapular rash, malaise, myalgia); exanthematous pustulosis, hepatic sinusoidal obstruction syndrome (SOS; veno-occlussive disease), hyperuricemia, injection site inflammation (SubQ injection), injection site pain (SubQ injection), interstitial pneumonitis, lipase increased, paralysis (intrathecal and I.V. combination therapy), reversible posterior leukoencephalopathy syndrome (RPLS), rhabdomyolysis, toxic megacolon

Adverse events associated with high-dose cytarabine (CNS, gastrointestinal, ocular, and pulmonary toxicities are more common with high-dose regimens):

Cardiovascular: Cardiomegaly, cardiomyopathy (in combination with cyclophosphamide)
Central nervous system: Cerebellar toxicity, coma, neurotoxicity (up to 55% in patients with renal impairment), personality change, somnolence
Dermatologic: Alopecia (complete), desquamation, rash (severe)
Gastrointestinal: Gastrointestinal ulcer, pancreatitis, peritonitis, pneumatosis cystoides intestinalis
Hepatic: Hyperbilirubinemia, liver abscess, liver damage, necrotizing colitis
Neuromuscular & skeletal: Peripheral neuropathy (motor and sensory)
Ocular: Corneal toxicity, hemorrhagic conjunctivitis
Respiratory: Pulmonary edema, syndrome of sudden respiratory distress
Miscellaneous: Sepsis

Adverse events associated with intrathecal cytarabine administration:

Central nervous system: Accessory nerve paralysis, fever, necrotizing leukoencephalopathy (with concurrent cranial irradiation, I.T. methotrexate, and I.T. hydrocortisone), neurotoxicity, paraplegia
Gastrointestinal: Dysphagia, nausea, vomiting
Ocular: Blindness (with concurrent systemic chemotherapy and cranial irradiation), diplopia
Respiratory: Cough, hoarseness
Miscellaneous: Aphonia

Drug Interactions

Metabolism/Transport Effects None known.

Avoid Concomitant Use

Avoid concomitant use of Cytarabine (Conventional) with any of the following: BCG; CloZAPine; Natalizumab; Pimecrolimus; Tacrolimus (Topical); Tofacitinib; Vaccines (Live)

Increased Effect/Toxicity

Cytarabine (Conventional) may increase the levels/effects of: CloZAPine; Leflunomide; Natalizumab; Tofacitinib; Vaccines (Live)

The levels/effects of Cytarabine (Conventional) may be increased by: Denosumab; Pimecrolimus; Roflumilast; Tacrolimus (Topical); Trastuzumab

Decreased Effect

Cytarabine (Conventional) may decrease the levels/effects of: BCG; Cardiac Glycosides; Coccidioidin Skin Test; Flucytosine; Sipuleucel-T; Vaccines (Inactivated); Vaccines (Live)

The levels/effects of Cytarabine (Conventional) may be decreased by: Echinacea

Preparation for Administration Hazardous agent; use appropriate precautions for handling and disposal (NIOSH, 2012). **Note:** Solutions containing bacteriostatic agents may be used for SubQ and standard-dose (100-200 mg/m^2) I.V. cytarabine preparations, but should not be used for the preparation of either intrathecal doses or high-dose I.V. therapies.

I.V.:

Powder for reconstitution: Reconstitute with bacteriostatic water for injection (for standard-dose).

For I.V. infusion: Further dilute in 250-1000 mL 0.9% NaCl or D_5W.

Intrathecal: Powder for reconstitution: Reconstitute with preservative free sodium chloride 0.9%; may further dilute to preferred final volume (volume generally based on institution or practitioner preference; may be up to 12 mL) with Elliott's B solution, sodium chloride 0.9% or lactated Ringer's. Intrathecal medications should not be prepared during the preparation of any other agents.

Triple intrathecal therapy (TIT): Cytarabine 30-50 mg with hydrocortisone sodium succinate 15-25 mg and methotrexate 12 mg; compatible together for up to 24 hours in a syringe; however, should be administered administer as soon as possible after preparation because intrathecal preparations are preservative free

Storage/Stability Store intact vials of powder for injection at room temperature of 20°C to 25°C (68°F to 77°F); store intact vials of solution at room temperature of 15°C to 30°C (59°F to 86°F).

I.V.:

Powder for reconstitution: Reconstituted solutions should be stored at room temperature and used within 48 hours.

For I.V. infusion: Solutions for I.V. infusion diluted in D_5W or NS are stable for 7 days at room temperature, although the manufacturer recommends administration as soon as possible after preparation.

Intrathecal: Administer as soon as possible after preparation. After preparation, store intrathecal medications in an isolated location or container clearly marked with a label identifying as "intrathecal" use only.

Mechanism of Action Inhibits DNA synthesis. Cytosine gains entry into cells by a carrier process, and then must be converted to its active compound, aracytidine triphosphate. Cytosine is a pyrimidine analog and is incorporated into DNA; however, the primary action is inhibition of DNA polymerase resulting in decreased DNA synthesis and repair. The degree of cytotoxicity correlates linearly with incorporation into DNA; therefore, incorporation into the DNA is responsible for drug activity and toxicity. Cytarabine is specific for the S phase of the cell cycle (blocks progression from the G_1 to the S phase).

Pharmacodynamics/Kinetics

Distribution: V_d: Total body water; widely and rapidly since it enters the cells readily; crosses blood-brain barrier with CSF levels of 40% to 50% of plasma level

Metabolism: Primarily hepatic; metabolized by deoxycytidine kinase and other nucleotide kinases to aracytidine triphosphate (active); about 86% to 96% of dose is metabolized to inactive uracil arabinoside (ARA-U); intrathecal administration results in little conversion to ARA-U due to the low levels of deaminase in the cerebral spinal fluid

Half-life elimination: I.V.: Initial: 7-20 minutes; Terminal: 1-3 hours; I.T.: 2-6 hours

Time to peak, plasma: SubQ: 20-60 minutes

Excretion: Urine (~80%; 90% as metabolite ARA-U) within 24 hours

Dosage Details concerning dosing in combination regimens should also be consulted.

Acute myeloid leukemia (AML) remission induction: I.V.: Children and Adults: Standard-dose (provided in the FDA-approved labeling): 100 mg/m²/day continuous infusion for 7 days **or** 200 mg/m²/day continuous infusion (as 100 mg/m² over 12 hours every 12 hours) for 7 days

Pediatric indication-specific dosing:

AML induction: *7 + 3 regimen:* I.V.:

Children <3 years (unlabeled dosing): 3.3 mg/kg/day continuous infusion for 7 days; minimum of 2 courses (in combination with daunorubicin) (Woods, 1990)

Children ≥3 years: 100 mg/m²/day continuous infusion for 7 days; minimum of 2 courses (in combination with daunorubicin) (Woods, 1990)

AML consolidation (unlabeled use): *5 + 2 + 5 regimen:* I.V.: Children ≥15 years: 100 mg/m²/day continuous infusion for 5 days for 2 consolidation courses (in combination with daunorubicin and etoposide) (Bishop, 1996)

AML salvage treatment (unlabeled use):

FLAG regimen: I.V.: Children ≥11 years: 2000 mg/m²/day over 4 hours for 5 days (in combination with fludarabine and G-CSF); may repeat once if needed (Montillo, 1998)

MEC regimen: I.V.: Children ≥5 years: 1000 mg/m²/day over 6 hours for 6 days (in combination with etoposide and mitoxantrone) (Amadori, 1991)

Acute lymphocytic leukemia (ALL; unlabeled dosing): *POG 8602/PVA regimen, intensification phase:* I.V.: Children ≥1 year: 1000 mg/m² continuous infusion over 24 hours day 1 (beginning 12 hours after start of methotrexate) every 3 weeks or every 12 weeks for 6 cycles (Land, 1994)

Chronic myeloid leukemia (CML; unlabeled dosing): SubQ: Children ≥7 years: 20 mg/m² once daily days 15 to 24 every month (in combination with interferon alfa-2b) (Guilhot, 1997)

Non-Hodgkin's lymphomas (unlabeled use): *CODOX-M/IVAC regimen:* I.V.: Children ≥3 years: Cycles 2 and 4 (IVAC): 2000 mg/m² every 12 hours days 1 and 2 (total of 4 doses/cycle) (IVAC is combination with ifosfamide, mesna and etoposide; IVAC alternates with CODOX-M) (Magrath, 1996)

Adult indication-specific dosing:

AML induction: I.V.:

7 + 3 regimens (a second induction may be administered if needed; refer to specific references): 100 mg/m²/day continuous infusion for 7 days (in combination with daunorubicin **or** idarubicin **or** mitoxantrone) (Arlin, 1990; Dillman, 1991; Fernandez, 2009; Wiernick, 1992) **or** (Adults <60 years) 200 mg/m²/day continuous infusion for 7 days (in combination with daunorubicin) (Dillman, 1991)

Low intensity therapy (unlabeled dosing): Adults ≥65 years: SubQ: 20 mg/m²/day for 14 days out of every 28-day cycle for at least 4 cycles (Fenaux, 2010) **or** 10 mg/m² every 12 hours for 21 days; if complete response not achieved, may repeat a second course after 15 days (Tilly, 1990)

AML consolidation (unlabeled use): I.V.:

5 + 2 regimens: 100 mg/m²/day continuous infusion for 5 days (in combination with daunorubicin **or** idarubicin **or** mitoxantrone) (Arlin, 1990; Wiernick, 1992)

5 + 2 + 5 regimen: 100 mg/m²/day continuous infusion for 5 days (in combination with daunorubicin **and** etoposide) (Bishop, 1996)

Single-agent: Adults ≤60 years: 3000 mg/m² over 3 hours every 12 hours on days 1, 3, and 5 (total of 6 doses); repeat every 28-35 days for 4 courses (Mayer, 1994)

AML salvage treatment (unlabeled use): I.V.:

ADE regimen: Course 1: 100 mg/m² I.V push every 12 hours for 10 days (in combination with daunorubicin and etoposide) followed by Course 2: 100 mg/m² I.V push every 12 hours for 8 days (Milligan, 2006)

CLAG regimen: 2000 mg/m²/day over 4 hours for 5 days (in combination with cladribine and G-CSF); may repeat once if needed (Wrzesień -Kuś, 2003)

CLAG-M regimen: 2000 mg/m²/day over 4 hours for 5 days (in combination with cladribine, G-CSF, and mitoxantrone); may repeat once if needed (Wierzbowska, 2008)

FLAG regimen: 2000 mg/m^2/day over 4 hours for 5 days (in combination with fludarabine and G-CSF); may repeat once if needed (Montillo, 1998)

HiDAC (high-dose cytarabine) ± an anthracycline: 3000 mg/m^2 over 1 hour every 12 hours for 12 doses (Herzig, 1985)

MEC regimen: 1000 mg/m^2/day over 6 hours for 6 days (in combination with mitoxantrone and etoposide) (Amadori, 1991) **or**

Adults <60 years: 500 mg/m^2/day continuous infusion days 1, 2, and 3 and days 8, 9, and 10 (in combination with mitoxantrone and etoposide); may administer a second course if needed (Archimbaud, 1991; Archimbaud, 1995)

Acute promyelocytic leukemia (APL) induction (unlabeled dosing): I.V.: 200 mg/m^2/day continuous infusion for 7 days beginning on day 3 of treatment (in combination with tretinoin and daunorubicin) (Ades, 2006; Powell, 2010)

APL consolidation (unlabeled use): I.V.:

In combination with idarubicin and tretinoin: High-risk patients (WBC ≥10,000/mm^3) (Sanz, 2010): Adults ≤60 years:

First consolidation course: 1000 mg/m^2/day for 4 days

Third consolidation course: 150 mg/m^2 every 8 hours for 4 days

In combination with idarubicin, tretinoin, and thioguanine: High-risk patients (WBC >10,000/mm^3) (Lo Coco, 2010): Adults ≤61 years:

First consolidation course: 1000 mg/m^2/day for 4 days

Third consolidation course: 150 mg/m^2 every 8 hours for 5 days

In combination with daunorubicin (Ades, 2006; Ades, 2008):

First consolidation course: 200 mg/m^2/day for 7 days

Second consolidation course:

Age ≤60 years and low risk (WBC <10,000/mm^3): 1000 mg/m^2 every 12 hours for 4 days (8 doses)

Age <50 years and high risk (WBC ≥10,000/mm^3): 2000 mg/m^2 every 12 hours for 5 days (10 doses)

Age 50-60 years and high risk (WBC ≥10,000/mm^3): 1500 mg/m^2 every 12 hours for 5 days (10 doses) (Ades, 2008)

Age >60 years and high risk (WBC ≥10,000/mm^3): 1000 mg/m^2 every 12 hours for 4 days (8 doses)

Acute lymphocytic leukemia (ALL; unlabeled dosing):

Induction regimen, relapsed or refractory: I.V.: 3000 mg/m^2 over 3 hours daily for 5 days (in combination with idarubicin [day 3]) (Weiss, 2002)

Dose-intensive regimen: I.V.: 3000 mg/m^2 over 2 hours every 12 hours days 2 and 3 (4 doses/cycle) of even numbered cycles (in combination with methotrexate; alternates with Hyper-CVAD) (Kantarjian, 2000)

Larson regimen (Larson, 1995): SubQ:

Early intensification phase: 75 mg/m^2/dose days 1 to 4 and 8 to 11 (4-week cycle; repeat once)

Late intensification phase: 75 mg/m^2/dose days 29 to 32 and 36 to 39

Linker protocol: I.V.: 300 mg/m^2/day days 1, 4, 8, and 11 of even numbered consolidation cycles (in combination with teniposide) (Linker, 1991)

Chronic lymphocytic leukemia (CLL; unlabeled use):

OFAR regimen: I.V.: 1000 mg/m^2/dose over 2 hours days 2 and 3 every 4 weeks for up to 6 cycles (in combination with oxaliplatin, fludarabine, and rituximab) (Tsimberidou, 2008)

Chronic myeloid leukemia (CML; unlabeled dosing): SubQ: 20 mg/m^2 once daily days 15 to 24 every month (in combination with interferon alfa-2b) (Guilhot, 1997)

CNS lymphoma, primary (unlabeled use): I.V.: 2000 mg/m^2 over 1 hour every 12 hours days 2 and 3 (total of 4 doses) every 3 weeks (in combination with methotrexate and followed by whole brain irradiation) for a total of 4 courses (Ferreri, 2009)

Hodgkin lymphoma, relapsed or refractory (unlabeled use): I.V.:

DHAP regimen: 2000 mg/m^2 over 3 hours every 12 hours day 2 (total of 2 doses/cycle) for 2 cycles (in combination with dexamethasone and cisplatin) (Josting, 2002)

ESHAP regimen: 2000 mg/m^2 day 5 (in combination with etoposide, methylprednisolone, and cisplatin) every 3 to 4 weeks for 3 or 6 cycles (Aparicio, 1999)

Mini-BEAM regimen: 100 mg/m^2 every 12 hours days 2 through 5 (total of 8 doses) every 4-6 weeks (in combination with carmustine, etoposide, and melphalan) (Colwill, 1995; Martin, 2001)

BEAM regimen (transplant preparative regimen): 200 mg/m^2 twice daily for 4 days beginning 5 days prior to transplant (in combination with carmustine, etoposide, and melphalan) (Chopra, 1993)

Non-Hodgkin's lymphomas (unlabeled use): I.V.:

CALGB 9251 regimen: Cycles 2, 4, and 6: 150 mg/m^2/day continuous infusion days 4 and 5 (Lee, 2001; Rizzieri, 2004)

CODOX-M/IVAC regimen:

Adults ≤60 years: Cycles 2 and 4 (IVAC): 2000 mg/m^2 every 12 hours days 1 and 2 (total of 4 doses/cycle) (IVAC is combination with ifosfamide, mesna, and etoposide; IVAC alternates with CODOX-M) (Magrath, 1996)

Adults ≤65 years: Cycles 2 and 4 (IVAC): 2000 mg/m^2 over 3 hours every 12 hours days 1 and 2 (total of 4 doses/cycle) (IVAC is combination with ifosfamide, mesna, and etoposide; IVAC alternates with CODOX-M) (Mead, 2008)

Adults >65 years: Cycles 2 and 4 (IVAC): 1000 mg/m^2 over 3 hours every 12 hours days 1 and 2 (total of 4 doses/cycle) (IVAC is combination with ifosfamide, mesna, and etoposide; IVAC alternates with CODOX-M) (Mead, 2008)

DHAP regimen:

Adults ≤70 years: 2000 mg/m^2 over 3 hours every 12 hours day 2 (total of 2 doses/cycle) every 3-4 weeks for 6-10 cycles (in combination with dexamethasone and cisplatin) (Velasquez, 1988)

Adults >70 years: 1000 mg/m^2 over 3 hours every 12 hours day 2 (total of 2 doses/cycle) every 3-4 weeks for 6-10 cycles (in combination with dexamethasone and cisplatin) (Velasquez, 1988)

ESHAP regimen: 2000 mg/m^2 over 2 hours day 5 every 3 to 4 weeks for 6-8 cycles (in combination with etoposide, methylprednisolone, and cisplatin) (Velasquez, 1994)

BEAM regimen (transplant preparative regimen): 200 mg/m^2 twice daily for 3 days beginning 4 days prior to transplant (in combination with carmustine, etoposide, and melphalan) (Linch 2010) **or** 100 mg/m^2 over 1 hour every 12 hours for 4 days beginning 5 days prior to transplant (in combination with carmustine, etoposide, and melphalan) (van Imhoff, 2005)

Intrathecal (I.T.):

Meningeal leukemia: Note: Optimal intrathecal chemotherapy dosing should be based on age rather than on body surface area (BSA); CSF volume correlates with age and not to BSA (Bleyer, 1983; Kerr, 2001). Dosing provided in the FDA-approved labeling is BSA-based (usual dose 30 mg/m^2 every 4 days; range: 5-75 mg/m^2 once daily for 4 days or once every 4 days until CNS findings normalize, followed by 1 additional treatment).

Children: Age-based intrathecal dosing (unlabeled):

CNS prophylaxis:

<1 year: 20 mg per dose

1 to 1.99 years: 30 mg per dose

2 to 2.99 years: 50 mg per dose

≥3 years: 70 mg per dose

ALL CNS prophylaxis, age-specific doses from literature:

Administer on day 0 of induction therapy (Gaynon, 1993):

1 to <2 years: 30 mg per dose

2 to <3 years: 50 mg per dose

≥3 years: 70 mg per dose

Administer as part of triple intrathecal therapy (TIT) on days 1 and 15 of induction therapy; days 1, 15, 50, and 64 (standard risk patients) or days 1, 15, 29, and 43 (high-risk patients) during consolidation therapy; day 1 of reinduction therapy, and during maintenance therapy (very high-risk patients receive on days 1, 22, 45, and 59 of induction, days 8, 22, 36, and 50 of consolidation therapy, days 8 and 38 of reinduction therapy, and during maintenance) (Lin, 2007):

<1 year: 18 mg per dose

1-2 years: 24 mg per dose

2-3 years: 30 mg per dose

≥3 years: 36 mg per dose

Administer on day 0 of induction therapy, then as part of TIT on days 7, 14, and 21 during consolidation therapy; as part of TIT on days 0, 28, and 35 for 2 cycles of delayed intensification therapy, and then maintenance treatment as part of TIT on day 0 every 12 weeks for 38 months (boys) or 26 months (girls) from initial induction treatment (Matloub, 2006):

1 to <2 years: 16 mg per dose

2 to <3 years: 20 mg per dose

≥3 years: 24-30 mg per dose

Administer on day 15 of induction therapy, days 1 and 15 of reinduction phase; and day 1 of cycle 2 of maintenance 1A phase (Pieters, 2007):

<1 year: 15 mg per dose

≥1 year: 20 mg per dose

Treatment, CNS leukemia (ALL): Children: Administer as part of TIT weekly until CSF remission, then every 4 weeks throughout continuation treatment (Lin, 2007):

<1 year: 18 mg per dose

1-2 years: 24 mg per dose

2-3 years: 30 mg per dose

≥3 years: 36 mg per dose

Adult unlabeled uses or doses for intrathecal therapy:

CNS prophylaxis (ALL): 100 mg weekly for 8 doses, then every 2 weeks for 8 doses, then monthly for 6 doses (high-risk patients) **or** 100 mg on day 7 or 8 with each chemotherapy cycle for 4 doses (low risk patients) **or** 16 doses (high-risk patients) (Cortes, 1995)

or as part of TIT: 40 mg days 0 and 14 during induction, days 1, 4, 8, and 11 during CNS therapy phase, every 18 weeks during intensification and maintenance phases (Storring, 2009)

CNS prophylaxis (APL, as part of TIT): 50 mg per dose; administer 1 dose prior to consolidation and 2 doses during each of 2 consolidation phases (total of 5 doses) (Ades, 2006; Ades, 2008)

CNS leukemia treatment (ALL, as part of TIT): 40 mg twice weekly until CSF cleared (Storring, 2009)

CNS lymphoma treatment: 50 mg twice a week for 4 weeks, then weekly for 4-8 weeks, then every other week for 4 weeks, then every 4 weeks for 4 doses (Glantz, 1999)

Leptomeningeal metastases treatment: 50 mg twice a week for 4 weeks, then weekly for 4 weeks then monthly for 4 doses (NCCN CNS cancer guidelines v.1.2010) **or** 40-60 mg per dose (DeAngelis, 2005)

Dosage adjustment in renal impairment: The FDA-approved labeling does not contain renal dosing adjustment guidelines; the following guidelines have been used by some clinicians:

Aronoff, 2007 (Cytarabine 100-200 mg/m^2): Children and Adults: No adjustment necessary

Kintzel, 1995 (High-dose cytarabine 1-3 g/m^2):

Cl_{cr} 46-60 mL/minute: Administer 60% of dose

Cl_{cr} 31-45 mL/minute: Administer 50% of dose

Cl_{cr} <30 mL/minute: Consider use of alternative drug

Smith, 1997 (High-dose cytarabine; ≥2 g/m^2/dose):

Serum creatinine 1.5-1.9 mg/dL or increase (from baseline) of 0.5-1.2 mg/dL: Reduce dose to 1 g/m^2/dose

Serum creatinine ≥2 mg/dL or increase (from baseline) of >1.2 mg/dL: Reduce dose to 0.1 g/m^2/day as a continuous infusion

Hemodialysis: In 4 hour dialysis sessions (with high flow polysulfone membrane) 6 hours after cytarabine 1 g/m^2 over 2 hours, 63% of the metabolite ARA-U was extracted from plasma (based on a single adult case report) (based on a single adult case report) (Radeski, 2011)

Dosage adjustment in hepatic impairment: Dose may need to be adjusted in patients with liver failure since cytarabine is partially detoxified in the liver. The FDA-approved labeling does not contain hepatic dosing adjustment guidelines; the following guideline has been used by some clinicians:

Floyd, 2006: Transaminases (any elevation): Administer 50% of dose; may increase subsequent doses in the absence of toxicities

Koren, 1992 (dose level not specified): Bilirubin >2 mg/dL: Administer 50% of dose; may increase subsequent doses in the absence of toxicities

Dosing in obesity: *ASCO Guidelines for appropriate chemotherapy dosing in obese adults with cancer:* Utilize patient's actual body weight (full weight) for calculation of body surface area- or weight-based dosing, particularly when the intent of therapy is curative; manage regimen-related toxicities in the same manner as for nonobese patients; if a dose reduction is utilized due to toxicity, consider resumption of full weight-based dosing with subsequent cycles, especially if cause of toxicity (eg, hepatic or renal impairment) is resolved (Griggs, 2012).

Administration

I.V.: Infuse standard dose therapy for AML (100-200 mg/m^2/day) as a continuous infusion. Infuse high-dose therapy (unlabeled) over 1-3 hours (usually). Other rates have been used, refer to specific reference.

I.T.: Intrathecal doses should be administered as soon as possible after preparation.

May also be administered SubQ.

Hazardous agent; use appropriate precautions for handling and disposal (NIOSH, 2012).

Monitoring Parameters Liver function tests, CBC with differential and platelet count, serum creatinine, BUN, serum uric acid

Additional Information I.V. doses ≥1.5 g/m^2 may produce conjunctivitis which can be ameliorated with prophylactic use of corticosteroid (0.1% dexamethasone) eye drops. Dexamethasone eye drops should be administered at 1-2 drops every 6 hours during and for 2-7 days after completion of cytarabine.

Dosage Forms Excipient information presented when available (limited, particularly for generics); consult specific product labeling.

Solution, Injection:
Generic: 20 mg/mL (25 mL); 100 mg/mL (20 mL)
Solution, Injection [preservative free]:
Generic: 20 mg/mL (5 mL, 50 mL); 100 mg/mL (20 mL)
Solution Reconstituted, Injection:
Generic: 100 mg (1 ea); 500 mg (1 ea); 1 g (1 ea)

◆ **Cytarabine Hydrochloride** *see* Cytarabine (Conventional) *on page 517*

◆ **Cytarabine Injection (Can)** *see* Cytarabine (Conventional) *on page 517*

◆ **Cytarabine Lipid Complex** *see* Cytarabine (Liposomal) *on page 522*

Cytarabine (Liposomal)

(sye TARE a been lye po SO mal)

Brand Names: U.S. DepoCyt

Brand Names: Canada DepoCyt®

Index Terms Cytarabine Lipid Complex; Cytarabine Liposome; DepoFoam-Encapsulated Cytarabine; DTC 101; Liposomal Cytarabine

Pharmacologic Category Antineoplastic Agent, Antimetabolite; Antineoplastic Agent, Antimetabolite (Pyrimidine Analog)

Use Treatment of lymphomatous meningitis

Pregnancy Risk Factor D

Pregnancy Considerations Reproductive studies have not been conducted with cytarabine liposomal. Cytarabine, the active component, has been associated with fetal malformations when given as a component of systemic combination chemotherapy during the first trimester. Systemic exposure following intrathecal administration of cytarabine liposomal is negligible; however, women of childbearing potential should avoid becoming pregnant during treatment.

Breast-Feeding Considerations Although the systemic exposure following intrathecal administration of cytarabine liposomal is negligible, breast-feeding is not recommended due to the potential for serious adverse reactions in the nursing infant.

Contraindications Hypersensitivity to cytarabine or any component of the formulation; active meningeal infection

Warnings/Precautions Hazardous agent - use appropriate precautions for handling and disposal (NIOSH, 2012). **[U.S. Boxed Warning]: Chemical arachnoiditis (nausea, vomiting, headache, fever) occurs commonly; may be fatal if untreated. The incidence and severity of chemical arachnoiditis is reduced by coadministration with dexamethasone; dexamethasone should be administered concomitantly with cytarabine (liposomal) to diminish chemical arachnoid symptoms.** Hydrocephalus has been reported and may be precipitated by chemical arachnoiditis. May cause neurotoxicity (including myelopathy), which may lead to permanent neurologic deficit (rare); monitor for neurotoxicity; reduce subsequent doses; discontinue with persistent neurotoxicity. The risk of neurotoxicity is increased with concurrent radiation therapy or systemic chemotherapy. The risk for neurotoxicity is increased when administered with other antineoplastic agents or with cranial/spinal irradiation. Persistent (extreme) somnolence, hemiplegia, visual disturbances (including blindness; may be permanent), deafness, cranial nerve palsies, peripheral neuropathy, and even combined neurologic features (cauda equina syndrome) have been reported. CSF flow blockage may lead to increased free cytarabine concentrations in the CSF and increase the risk for neurotoxicity; assess CSF flow prior to administration. Infectious meningitis may be associated with intrathecal administration. **[U.S. Boxed Warning]: Should be administered under the supervision of an experienced cancer chemotherapy physician; facilities appropriate for diagnosis and management of complications should be readily available.** For intrathecal use only. Intrathecal medications should not be prepared during the preparation of any other agents; after preparation, store intrathecal medications in an isolated location or container clearly marked with a label identifying as "intrathecal" use only; delivery of intrathecal medications to the patient should only be with other medications intended for administration into the central nervous system (Jacobson, 2009).

Adverse Reactions

>10%:

Cardiovascular: Peripheral edema (11%)

Central nervous system: Chemical arachnoiditis (without dexamethasone premedication: 100%; with dexamethasone premedication: 33% to 42%; grade 4: 19% to 30%; onset: ≤5 days); headache (56%), confusion (33%), fever (32%), fatigue (25%), seizure (20% to 22%), dizziness (18%), lethargy (16%), insomnia (14%), memory impairment (14%), pain (14%)

Endocrine & metabolic: Dehydration (13%)

Gastrointestinal: Nausea (46%), vomiting (44%), constipation (25%), diarrhea (12%), appetite decreased (11%)

Genitourinary: Urinary tract infection (14%)

Hematologic: Anemia (12%), thrombocytopenia (3% to 11%)

Neuromuscular & skeletal: Weakness (40%), back pain (24%), abnormal gait (23%), limb pain (15%), neck pain (14%), arthralgia (11%), neck stiffness (11%)

Ocular: Blurred vision (11%)

1% to 10%:

Cardiovascular: Tachycardia (9%), hypotension (8%), hypertension (6%), syncope (3%), edema (2%)

Central nervous system: Agitation (10%), hypoesthesia (10%), depression (8%), anxiety (7%), sensory neuropathy (3%)

Dermatologic: Pruritus (2%)

Endocrine & metabolic: Hypokalemia (7%), hyponatremia (7%), hyperglycemia (6%)

Gastrointestinal: Abdominal pain (9%), dysphagia (8%), anorexia (5%), hemorrhoids (3%), mucosal inflammation (3%)

Genitourinary: Incontinence (7%), urinary retention (5%)

Hematologic: Neutropenia (10%), contusion (2%)

Neuromuscular & skeletal: Muscle weakness (10%), tremor (9%), peripheral neuropathy (3% to 4%), abnormal reflexes (3%)

Otic: Hypoacusis (6%)

Respiratory: Dyspnea (10%), cough (7%), pneumonia (6%)

Miscellaneous: Diaphoresis (2%)

1% (Limited to important or life-threatening): Anaphylaxis, bladder control impaired, blindness, bowel control impaired, cauda equine syndrome, cranial nerve palsies, CSF protein increased, CSF WBC increased, deafness, encephalopathy, hemiplegia, hydrocephalus, infectious meningitis, intracranial pressure increased, myelopathy, neurologic deficit, numbness, papilledema, somnolence, visual disturbance

Drug Interactions

Metabolism/Transport Effects None known.

Avoid Concomitant Use

Avoid concomitant use of Cytarabine (Liposomal) with any of the following: Tofacitinib

Increased Effect/Toxicity

Cytarabine (Liposomal) may increase the levels/effects of: Tofacitinib

Decreased Effect There are no known significant interactions involving a decrease in effect.

Preparation for Administration Hazardous agent; use appropriate precautions for handling and disposal (NIOSH, 2012). Allow vial to warm to room temperature prior to withdrawal from vial. Particles may settle in diluent over time, and may be resuspended with gentle agitation or inversion immediately prior to withdrawing from the vial. Do not further dilute or mix with any other medications. Further reconstitution or dilution is not required. Intrathecal medications should not be prepared during the preparation of any other agents.

Storage/Stability Store under refrigeration at 2°C to 8°C (36°F to 46°F); protect from freezing. Avoid aggressive agitation. Withdraw from the vial immediately prior to administration; solutions should be used within 4 hours of withdrawal from the vial.

After preparation, store intrathecal medications in an isolated location or container clearly marked with a label identifying as "intrathecal" use only.

Mechanism of Action Cytarabine liposomal is a sustained-release formulation of the active ingredient cytarabine, an antimetabolite which acts through inhibition of DNA synthesis and is cell cycle-specific for the S phase of cell division. Cytarabine is converted intracellularly to its active metabolite cytarabine-5'-triphosphate (ara-CTP). Ara-CTP also appears to be incorporated into DNA and RNA; however, the primary action is inhibition of DNA polymerase, resulting in decreased DNA synthesis and repair. The liposomal formulation allows for gradual release, resulting in prolonged exposure.

Pharmacodynamics/Kinetics

Absorption: Systemic exposure following intrathecal administration is negligible since transfer rate from CSF to plasma is slow

Half-life elimination, CSF: 6-82 hours

Time to peak, CSF: Intrathecal: <1 hour

Dosage Note: Initiate dexamethasone 4 mg twice daily (oral or I.V.) for 5 days, beginning on the day of cytarabine liposomal administration.

Intrathecal: Adults:

Induction: 50 mg every 14 days for a total of 2 doses (weeks 1 and 3)

Consolidation: 50 mg every 14 days for 3 doses (weeks 5, 7, and 9), followed by an additional dose at week 13

Maintenance: 50 mg every 28 days for 4 doses (weeks 17, 21, 25, and 29)

Dosage reduction for toxicity: If drug-related neurotoxicity develops, reduce dose to 25 mg. If toxicity persists, discontinue treatment.

Dosage adjustment in renal impairment: No dosage adjustment provided in manufacturer's labeling (has not been studied).

Dosage adjustment in hepatic impairment: No dosage adjustment provided in manufacturer's labeling (has not been studied).

Administration For intrathecal use only. Dose should be removed from vial immediately before administration (must be administered within 4 hours of removal). An in-line filter should **NOT** be used. Administer directly into the CSF via an intraventricular reservoir or by direct injection into the lumbar sac. Injection should be made slowly (over 1-5 minutes). Patients should lie flat for 1 hour after lumbar puncture.

Hazardous agent; use appropriate precautions for handling and disposal (NIOSH, 2012).

Monitoring Parameters Monitor closely for signs of an immediate reaction; neurotoxicity

Test Interactions Since cytarabine liposomes are similar in appearance to WBCs, care must be taken in interpreting CSF examinations in patients receiving cytarabine liposomal.

Dosage Forms Excipient information presented when available (limited, particularly for generics); consult specific product labeling.

Suspension, Intrathecal:

DepoCyt: 50 mg/5 mL (5 mL) [contains cholesterol, dioleoylphosphatidylcholine (dopc), dipalmitoylphosphatidylglycerol (dppg), triolein]

◆ **Cytarabine Liposome** *see* Cytarabine (Liposomal) *on page 522*

◆ **CytoGam®** *see* Cytomegalovirus Immune Globulin (Intravenous-Human) *on page 523*

Cytomegalovirus Immune Globulin (Intravenous-Human)

(sye toe meg a low VYE rus i MYUN GLOB yoo lin in tra VEE nus HYU man)

Brand Names: U.S. CytoGam®

Brand Names: Canada CytoGam®

Index Terms CMV Hyperimmune Globulin; CMV-IGIV

Pharmacologic Category Blood Product Derivative; Immune Globulin

Additional Appendix Information

Immunization Administration Recommendations *on page 2334*

Immunization Recommendations *on page 2339*

Use Prophylaxis of cytomegalovirus (CMV) disease associated with kidney, lung, liver, pancreas, and heart transplants; concomitant use with ganciclovir should be considered in organ transplants (other than kidney) from CMV seropositive donors to CMV seronegative recipients

Unlabeled Use Adjunctive therapy in the treatment of CMV pneumonitis in solid organ transplant and in hematopoietic stem cell transplant

Pregnancy Risk Factor C

Pregnancy Considerations Animal reproduction studies have not been conducted.

Contraindications Hypersensitivity to cytomegalovirus immune globulin (CMV-IGIV), other immunoglobulin preparations, or any component of the formulation; selective immunoglobulin A deficiency

Warnings/Precautions Hypersensitivity and anaphylactic reactions can occur; monitor vital signs during infusion; discontinue immediately for hypotension or anaphylaxis; immediate treatment (including epinephrine 1:1000) should be available. Systemic allergic reactions are rare; may be treated with epinephrine and diphenhydramine. Aseptic meningitis syndrome (AMS) has been reported with intravenous immune globulin administration (rare); may occur with high doses (≥2 g/kg). Symptoms include severe headache, nuchal rigidity, drowsiness, fever, photophobia, painful eye movements and nausea and vomiting. Syndrome usually appears within several hours to 2 days following treatment; usually resolves within several days after discontinuation. Intravenous immune globulin has been associated with antiglobulin hemolysis; monitor for signs of hemolytic anemia. Monitor for adverse pulmonary events including transfusion-related acute lung injury (TRALI); noncardiogenic pulmonary edema has been reported with intravenous immune globulin use. TRALI is characterized by severe respiratory distress, pulmonary edema, hypoxemia, and fever in the presence of normal left ventricular function and usually occurs within 1-6 hours after infusion; may be managed with oxygen and respiratory support.

Acute renal dysfunction (increased serum creatinine, oliguria, osmotic nephrosis, acute renal failure) can rarely occur; usually within 7 days of use (more likely with products stabilized with sucrose). Patients at risk for renal failure include the elderly, patients with pre-existing renal disease, diabetes mellitus, volume depletion, sepsis, paraproteinemia, and nephrotoxic medications due to risk of renal dysfunction. In patients at risk of renal dysfunction, the rate of infusion and concentration of solution should be minimized. Discontinue if renal function deteriorates. Patients should not be volume depleted prior to therapy. Thrombotic events have been reported with administration of intravenous immune globulin; patients at risk include those with advanced age or a history of atherosclerosis, cardiovascular and/or thrombotic risk factors, or known/suspected hyperviscosity. Consider a baseline assessment of blood viscosity in patients at risk for hyperviscosity. Use with caution in patients >65 years of age. Product is stabilized with albumin. Product of human plasma; may potentially contain infectious agents which could transmit disease. Screening of donors, as well as testing and/or inactivation or removal of certain viruses, reduces the risk. Infections thought to be transmitted by this product should be reported to the manufacturer. Product is stabilized with sucrose.

Adverse Reactions

<6%:

Cardiovascular: Flushing

Central nervous system: Chills, fever

Gastrointestinal: Nausea, vomiting

Neuromuscular & skeletal: Arthralgia, back pain, muscle cramps

Respiratory: Wheezing

<1% (Limited to important or life-threatening): Abdominal pain, acute renal failure, acute respiratory distress syndrome (ARDS), acute tubular necrosis, allergic reactions (systemic), anaphylactic shock, angioneurotic edema, anuria, apnea, aseptic meningitis syndrome (AMS), blood pressure decreased, bronchospasm, bullous dermatitis, BUN increased, cardiac arrest, coma, Coomb's test positive, cyanosis, dyspnea, epidermolysis, erythema multiforme, hemolysis, hypotension, hypoxemia, leukopenia, liver dysfunction, loss of consciousness, oliguria, osmotic nephrosis, pancytopenia, proximal tubular nephropathy, pulmonary edema, renal dysfunction, rigors, seizure, serum creatinine increased, Stevens-Johnson syndrome, thromboembolism, transfusion-related acute lung injury (TRALI), tremor, vascular collapse

Drug Interactions

Metabolism/Transport Effects None known.

Avoid Concomitant Use There are no known interactions where it is recommended to avoid concomitant use.

Increased Effect/Toxicity There are no known significant interactions involving an increase in effect.

Decreased Effect

Cytomegalovirus Immune Globulin (Intravenous-Human) may decrease the levels/effects of: Vaccines (Live)

Preparation for Administration Do not admix with other medications; do not use if turbid. Do not shake vials; avoid foaming. Dilution is not recommended.

Storage/Stability Store refrigerated between 2°C and 8°C (36°F and 46°F). Infusion should begin within 6 hours after entering the vial.

Mechanism of Action CMV-IGIV is a preparation of immunoglobulin G (and trace amounts of IgA and IgM) derived from pooled healthy blood donors and contains a high titer of CMV antibodies; administration provides a passive source of antibodies against cytomegalovirus to attenuate or reduce the incidence of serious CMV disease

Dosage I.V.: Children Adolescents, and Adults:

Prophylaxis of CMV disease in kidney transplant:

Initial dose (within 72 hours of transplant): 150 mg/kg/dose

2-, 4-, 6-, and 8 weeks after transplant: 100 mg/kg/dose

12 and 16 weeks after transplant: 50 mg/kg/dose

Prophylaxis of CMV disease in liver, lung, pancreas, or heart transplant:

Initial dose (within 72 hours of transplant): 150 mg/kg/dose

2-, 4-, 6-, and 8 weeks after transplant: 150 mg/kg/dose

12 and 16 weeks after transplant: 100 mg/kg/dose

Treatment of severe CMV pneumonitis in hematopoietic stem cell transplant (unlabeled use; in combination with ganciclovir): 400 mg/kg on days 1, 2, and 7, followed by 200 mg/kg on day 14; if still symptomatic, may administer an additional 200 mg/kg on day 21 (Reed, 1988) **or** 150 mg/kg twice weekly (Alexander, 2010)

Elderly: Refer to adult dosing.

Dosage adjustment in renal impairment: No dosage adjustment provided in manufacturer's labeling; use with caution. Infuse at minimum rate possible.

Dosage adjustment in hepatic impairment: No dosage adjustment provided in manufacturer's labeling.

Dietary Considerations May contain sodium.

Administration I.V.: Administer through an I.V. line containing an in-line 15 micron filter (a 0.2 micron filter is also acceptable) using an infusion pump. Do not mix with other infusions; do not use if turbid. Begin infusion within 6 hours of entering vial, complete infusion within 12 hours of vial entry.

Initial dose: Infuse at 15 mg/kg/hour. If no adverse reactions occur within 30 minutes, may increase rate to 30 mg/kg/hour. If no adverse reactions occur within the second 30 minutes, may increase rate to 60 mg/kg/hour; maximum rate of infusion: 75 mL/hour. Monitor closely after each rate change. If patient develops nausea, back pain, or flushing during infusion, slow the rate or temporarily stop the infusion. Discontinue if blood pressure drops or in case of anaphylactic reaction.

Subsequent doses: Infuse at 15 mg/kg/hour for 15 minutes; if no adverse reactions occur, may increase rate to 30 mg/kg/hour for 15 minutes; if no adverse reactions occur, may increase rate to 60 mg/kg/hour; maximum rate of infusion: 75 mL/hour.

Monitoring Parameters Renal function (BUN, serum creatinine prior to initial infusion and periodically thereafter); urine output; vital signs, including blood pressure (throughout infusion); signs/symptoms of infusion-related adverse reactions, anaphylaxis; signs and symptoms of hemolytic anemia; blood viscosity (baseline; in patients at risk for hyperviscosity); presence of antineutrophil antibodies (if TRALI is suspected); volume status; weight gain, clinical response

Dosage Forms Excipient information presented when available (limited, particularly for generics); consult specific product labeling.

Injection, solution [preservative free]:

CytoGam®: 50 mg (± 10 mg)/mL (50 mL) [contains sodium 20-30 mEq/L, human albumin, and sucrose 50 mg/mL]

- Cytomel *see* Liothyronine *on page 1222*
- Cytomel® (Can) *see* Liothyronine *on page 1222*
- Cytosar® (Can) *see* Cytarabine (Conventional) *on page 517*
- Cytosar-U *see* Cytarabine (Conventional) *on page 517*
- Cytosine Arabinosine Hydrochloride *see* Cytarabine (Conventional) *on page 517*
- Cytostasan *see* Bendamustine *on page 237*
- Cytotec *see* Misoprostol *on page 1382*
- Cytovene *see* Ganciclovir (Systemic) *on page 939*
- Cytovene® (Can) *see* Ganciclovir (Systemic) *on page 939*
- Cytoxan *see* Cyclophosphamide *on page 504*
- Cytra-2 *see* Sodium Citrate and Citric Acid *on page 1917*

◆ **Cytra-3** *see* Citric Acid, Sodium Citrate, and Potassium Citrate *on page 443*

◆ **Cytra-K** *see* Potassium Citrate and Citric Acid *on page 1686*

◆ **D2** *see* Ergocalciferol *on page 733*

◆ **D2E7** *see* Adalimumab *on page 45*

◆ **D-3-Mercaptovaline** *see* PenicillAMINE *on page 1603*

◆ **d4T** *see* Stavudine *on page 1949*

◆ **D-23129** *see* Ezogabine *on page 819*

◆ **DA-1773** *see* Sodium Picosulfate, Magnesium Oxide, and Citric Acid *on page 1925*

Dabigatran Etexilate (da BIG a tran ett EX ill ate)

Brand Names: U.S. Pradaxa

Brand Names: Canada Pradaxa®

Index Terms Dabigatran Etexilate Mesylate

Pharmacologic Category Anticoagulant, Thrombin Inhibitor

Additional Appendix Information

Antithrombotic Therapy in Patients With Atrial Fibrillation *on page 2366*

Beers Criteria – Potentially Inappropriate Medications for Geriatrics *on page 2368*

Oral Anticoagulant Comparison Chart *on page 2307*

Reversal of Oral Anticoagulants *on page 2308*

Use Prevention of stroke and systemic embolism in patients with nonvalvular atrial fibrillation

2011 ACCF/AHA/HRS atrial fibrillation guidelines: Not recommended for patients with coexisting prosthetic heart valve or hemodynamically significant valve disease, severe renal failure (Cl_{cr} <15 mL/minute), or advanced liver disease (impaired baseline clotting function)

Canadian labeling: Additional uses (not in U.S. labeling): Postoperative thromboprophylaxis in patients who have undergone total hip or knee replacement procedures

Pregnancy Risk Factor C

Pregnancy Considerations Adverse events were observed in some animal reproduction studies. Data are insufficient to evaluate the safety of direct thrombin inhibitors during pregnancy; use of oral agents during pregnancy should be avoided (Guyatt, 2012). Consider the risks of bleeding and stroke if used during pregnancy.

Breast-Feeding Considerations It is not known if dabigatran etexilate is excreted into breast milk. The manufacturer recommends caution be used if administered to nursing women. The use of alternative anticoagulants is preferred (Guyatt, 2012).

Medication Guide Available Yes

Contraindications Serious hypersensitivity (eg, anaphylaxis) to dabigatran or any component of the formulation; active pathological bleeding; patients with mechanical prosthetic heart valve(s)

Canadian labeling: Additional contraindications (not in U.S. labeling): Severe renal impairment (Cl_{cr} <30 mL/minute); bleeding diathesis or patients with spontaneous or pharmacological hemostatic impairment; lesions at risk of clinically significant bleeding (eg, hemorrhagic or ischemic cerebral infarction) within previous 6 months; concomitant therapy with oral ketoconazole; concomitant use with other anticoagulants including unfractionated heparin (except when used to maintain central venous or arterial catheter patency), low molecular weight heparins, heparin derivatives (eg, fondaparinux), anti-thrombin agents (eg, bivalirudin), and oral anticoagulants (eg, warfarin, rivaroxaban, apixaban) except during transitioning of therapy from or to dabigatran

Warnings/Precautions [U.S. Boxed Warning]: Upon discontinuation, the risk of thrombotic events, especially stroke, is increased. If dabigatran must be discontinued for a reason other than pathological bleeding, consider the use of another anticoagulant during the time of interruption. If possible, discontinue dabigatran 1-2 days (Cl_{cr} ≥50 mL/minute) or 3-5 days (Cl_{cr} <50 mL/minute) before invasive or surgical procedures due to the risk of bleeding; consider longer times for patients undergoing major surgery, spinal puncture, or insertion of a spinal or epidural catheter or port. If surgery cannot be delayed, the risk of bleeding is elevated; weigh risk of bleeding with urgency of procedure. Bleeding risk can be assessed by the ecarin clotting time (ECT) if available; if ECT is not available, use of aPTT may provide an approximation of dabigatran's anticoagulant activity.

The most common complication is bleeding, and sometimes fatal bleeding. Risk factors for bleeding include concurrent use of drugs that increase the risk of bleeding (eg, antiplatelet agents, heparin), renal impairment, impairment, and elderly patients (especially if low body weight). Monitor for signs and symptoms of bleeding; discontinue in patients with active pathological bleeding. **Important:** No specific antidote exists for dabigatran reversal. Therapy for severe hemorrhage may include transfusions of fresh frozen plasma, packed red blood cells, or surgical intervention when appropriate (Wann, 2011). The use of a PCC (Cofact ®, not available in the U.S.) has been shown to be **ineffective** for dabigatran reversal (Eerenberg, 2011); however, the manufacturer does suggest that activated PCC (eg, FEIBA NF), recombinant factor VIIa, or concentrates of factors II, IX, or X may be considered, although their use has not been evaluated in clinical trials. FEIBA NF was reported to have been effective in rapidly reversing the anticoagulant effects of dabigatran in one case study (Dager, 2013). Platelet concentrates should be considered when thrombocytopenia is present or long-acting antiplatelet drugs have been used. Use in patients with moderate hepatic impairment (Child-Pugh class B) demonstrated large inter-subject variability; however no consistent change in exposure or pharmacodynamics was seen. Use in patients with advanced liver disease (impaired baseline clotting function) is not recommended (Wann, 2011). Use is not recommended in patients with bioprosthetic heart valves; use is contraindicated in patients with mechanical prosthetic heart valves. Use in patients with atrial fibrillation in the setting of other forms of valvular heart disease, including presence of a bioprosthetic heart valve is not recommended (has not been evaluated).

Due to an increased risk of bleeding, avoid use, if possible, with other direct thrombin inhibitors (eg, bivalirudin), unfractionated heparin or heparin derivatives, low molecular weight heparins (eg, enoxaparin), fondaparinux, thienopyridines (eg, clopidogrel), GPIIb/IIIa antagonists (eg, eptifibatide), aspirin, coumarin derivatives, sulfinpyrazone, and ticagrelor. NSAIDs should be used cautiously. Appropriate doses of unfractionated heparin may be used to maintain catheter patency. The concomitant use of P-gp inducers (eg, rifampin) may reduce dabigatran bioavailability and should be avoided. Recommendations regarding concomitant use with P-gp inhibitors (eg, ketoconazole, dronedarone) may vary (see Drug Interactions). Concomitant use with any P-gp inhibitor should be avoided for Cl_{cr} <30 mL/minute.

Evaluate renal function prior to and during therapy, particularly if used in patients with any degree of pre-existing renal impairment or in any condition that may result in a decline in renal function (eg, hypovolemia, dehydration, concomitant use of medications with a potential to affect renal function); dabigatran concentrations may increase in any degree of renal impairment and increase the risk of bleeding. In moderate impairment, serum concentrations may increase 3 times higher than normal compared to concentrations in patients with normal renal function. However, U.S. labeling only requires dosage reduction in patients with severe renal impairment (Cl_{cr} 15-30 mL/minute) and recommends avoiding use in patients with Cl_{cr} <15 mL/minute due to insufficient evidence. Per the American College of Chest Physicians, dabigatran is considered contraindicated in patients with severe renal impairment (Cl_{cr} ≤30 mL/minute) (Guyatt, 2012). The Canadian labeling also contraindicates use in severe renal impairment (Cl_{cr} <30 mL/minute) and recommends indication-specific dose reductions in patients with moderate impairment (Cl_{cr} 30-50 mL/minute). Discontinue therapy in any patient who develops acute renal failure.

In the elderly, use with extreme caution or consider other treatment options. No dosage adjustment is recommended in the U.S. labeling based on age alone (unless renal impairment coexists); however, numerous case reports of hemorrhage, including hemorrhagic stroke, have been reported in elderly patients (median age: 80 years), with a quarter of these reports occurring in patients ≥84 years of age. Some reports have resulted in fatality, particularly in those with low body weight and mild-to-moderate renal impairment; the risk is expected to be higher in patients receiving interacting drugs (eg, amiodarone) (Legrand, 2011). The RE-LY trial, although not powered to assess safety in the elderly, employed 110 mg and 150 mg twice daily regiments. The 110 mg twice daily regimen was not approved for use in the United States. The Canadian labeling recommends a dose reduction for patients ≥80 years of age with atrial fibrillation and suggests that dose reductions be considered in patients >75 years of age receiving therapy for atrial fibrillation or postoperative thromboprophylaxis. In addition, due to the frequency of renal impairment in older adults, the Canadian labeling recommends monitoring renal function at a minimum of once per year in any patient >75 years of age; use of dabigatran is contraindicated in patients with Cl_{cr} <30 mL/minute. Per the Beers Criteria, there is a greater risk of bleeding in older adults aged ≥75 years (exceeds warfarin bleeding risk) and therapy should be used with caution in patients ≥75 years of age or in patients with Cl_{cr} <30 mL/minute (Beers Criteria).

Adverse Reactions Adverse reactions listed below are reflective of both the U.S. and Canadian product information. **Important:** No specific antidote exists for dabigatran reversal; protamine and vitamin K do not reverse or impact anticoagulant effects of dabigatran. Dabigatran is dialyzable (~60% removed over 2-3 hours); however, supporting data are limited for utilizing this method. Therapy for severe hemorrhage may include transfusions of fresh frozen plasma, packed red blood cells, or surgical intervention when appropriate (Wann, 2011). The use of a PCC (Cofact®, not available in the U.S.) has been shown to be **ineffective** for dabigatran reversal (Eerenberg, 2011); however, the manufacturer does suggest that activated PCC (eg, FEIBA NF), recombinant factor VIIa, or concentrates of factors II, IX, or X may be considered, although their use has not been evaluated in clinical trials. FEIBA NF was reported to have been effective in rapidly reversing the anticoagulant effects of dabigatran in one case study (Dager, 2013). Platelet concentrates should be considered when thrombocytopenia is present or long-acting antiplatelet drugs have been used.

>10%:

Gastrointestinal: Dyspepsia (11%; includes abdominal discomfort/pain, epigastric discomfort)

Hematologic: Bleeding (8% to 33%; major: ≤6%)

1% to 10%:

Gastrointestinal: GI hemorrhage (≤6%), gastritis-like symptoms (eg, GERD, esophagitis, erosive gastritis, GI ulcer)

Hematologic: Anemia (1% to 4%), hematoma (1% to 2%), hemoglobin decreased (1% to 2%), hemorrhage (post-procedural or wound: 1% to 2%)

Hepatic: ALT increased (≥3 x ULN: 2% to 3%)

Renal: Hematuria (1%)

Miscellaneous: Wound secretion (5%), postprocedural discharge (1%)

<1% (Limited to important or life-threatening): Allergic edema, anaphylactic shock, anaphylaxis, AST increased, bloody discharge, ecchymosis, epistaxis, esophageal ulcer, hemarthrosis, hematocrit decreased, hemorrhage (catheter site, hemorrhoidal, incision site, rectal), hepatic function abnormal, occult blood positive, pruritus, rash, thrombocytopenia, urticaria

Drug Interactions

Metabolism/Transport Effects **Substrate** of P-glycoprotein

Avoid Concomitant Use

Avoid concomitant use of Dabigatran Etexilate with any of the following: Anticoagulants; Apixaban; Omacetaxine; P-glycoprotein/ABCB1 Inducers; Rivaroxaban; Sulfinpyrazone [Off Market]

Increased Effect/Toxicity

Dabigatran Etexilate may increase the levels/effects of: Anticoagulants; Collagenase (Systemic); Deferasirox; Ibritumomab; Omacetaxine; Rivaroxaban; Tositumomab and Iodine I 131 Tositumomab

The levels/effects of Dabigatran Etexilate may be increased by: Agents with Antiplatelet Properties; Amiodarone; Apixaban; Dasatinib; Dronedarone; Herbs (Anticoagulant/Antiplatelet Properties); Ibrutinib; Ketoconazole (Systemic); Nonsteroidal Anti-Inflammatory Agents; Omega-3 Fatty Acids; Pentosan Polysulfate Sodium; P-glycoprotein/ABCB1 Inhibitors; Prostacyclin Analogues; QuiNIDine; Salicylates; Sugammadex; Sulfinpyrazone [Off Market]; Thrombolytic Agents; Tibolone; Tipranavir; Verapamil; Vitamin E

Decreased Effect

The levels/effects of Dabigatran Etexilate may be decreased by: Antacids; AtorvaSTATin; Estrogen Derivatives; P-glycoprotein/ABCB1 Inducers; Progestins; Proton Pump Inhibitors

Ethanol/Nutrition/Herb Interactions

Food: Food has no affect on the bioavailability of dabigatran, but delays the time to peak plasma concentrations by 2 hours.

Herb/Nutraceutical: St John's wort may decrease levels/effects of dabigatran (concomitant use is not recommended). Concomitant use of dabigatran with herbs possessing anticoagulant/antiplatelet properties may increase the risk for bleeding.

Storage/Stability

Blister: Store at 25°C (77°F); excursions permitted between 15°C to 30°C (59°F to 86°F). Protect from moisture.

Bottle: Store at 25°C (77°F); excursions permitted between 15°C to 30°C (59°F to 86°F). Dispense and store in original manufacturer's bottle to protect from moisture; discard 4 months after opening original container.

Mechanism of Action Prodrug lacking anticoagulant activity that is converted *in vivo* to the active dabigatran, a specific, reversible, direct thrombin inhibitor that inhibits both free and fibrin-bound thrombin. Inhibits coagulation by preventing thrombin-mediated effects, including cleavage of fibrinogen to fibrin monomers, activation of factors V, VIII, XI, and XIII, and inhibition of thrombin-induced platelet aggregation.

Pharmacodynamics/Kinetics

Absorption: Rapid; initially slow postoperatively

Distribution: V_d: 50-70 L

Protein binding: 35%

Metabolism: Hepatic; dabigatran etexilate is rapidly and completely hydrolyzed to dabigatran (active form) by plasma and hepatic esterases; dabigatran undergoes hepatic glucuronidation to active acylglucuronide isomers (similar activity to parent compound; accounts for <10% of total dabigatran in plasma)

Bioavailability: 3% to 7%

Half-life elimination: 12-17 hours; Elderly: 14-17 hours; Mild-to-moderate renal impairment: 15-18 hours; Severe renal impairment: 28 hours (Stangier, 2010)

Time to peak, plasma: Dabigatran: 1 hour; delayed 2 hours by food (no effect on bioavailability)

Excretion: Urine (80%)

Dosage Oral:

Adults:

Nonvalvular atrial fibrillation (to prevent stroke and systemic embolism): 150 mg twice daily. **Note:** The American Heart Association/American Stroke Association recommends dabigatran as a reasonable alternative to warfarin in patients who have ≥1 additional risk factor for stroke and Cl_{cr} >30 mL/minute (Furie, 2012). The American College of Chest Physicians (ACCP) suggests dabigatran over warfarin for primary and secondary prevention of nonvalvular atrial fibrillation-induced cardioembolic stroke or TIA. For secondary prevention, initiate therapy within 1-2 weeks after stroke onset or earlier in patients at low bleeding risk (Guyatt, 2012).

Conversion from a parenteral anticoagulant: Initiate dabigatran ≤2 hours prior to the time of the next scheduled dose of the parenteral anticoagulant (eg, enoxaparin) or at the time of discontinuation for a continuously administered parenteral drug (eg, I.V. heparin); discontinue parenteral anticoagulant at the time of dabigatran initiation.

Conversion to a parenteral anticoagulant:

U.S. labeling: Wait 12 hours (Cl_{cr} ≥30 mL/minute) or 24 hours (Cl_{cr} <30 mL/minute) after the last dose of dabigatran before initiating a parenteral anticoagulant.

Canadian labeling: Wait 12 hours after the last dose of dabigatran before initiating a parenteral anticoagulant.

Conversion from warfarin: Discontinue warfarin and initiate dabigatran when INR <2.0

Conversion to warfarin: Start time must be adjusted based on Cl_{cr}:

Cl_{cr} >50 mL/minute: Initiate warfarin 3 days before discontinuation of dabigatran

Cl_{cr} 31-50 mL/minute: Initiate warfarin 2 days before discontinuation of dabigatran

Cl_{cr} 15-30 mL/minute: Initiate warfarin 1 day before discontinuation of dabigatran (dabigatran use is contraindicated in Canadian labeling when Cl_{cr} <30 mL/minute).

Cl_{cr} <15 mL/minute: No recommendations provided in the U.S. manufacturer's labeling.

Note: Since dabigatran contributes to INR elevation, warfarin's effect on the INR will be better reflected only after dabigatran has been stopped for ≥2 days

Postoperative thromboprophylaxis (Canadian labeling):

Knee replacement: Initial: 110 mg given 1-4 hours after completion of surgery and establishment of hemostasis **OR** 220 mg as 1 dose in postoperative patients in whom therapy is not initiated on day of surgery regardless of reason; maintenance: 220 mg once daily (total duration of therapy: 10 days; ACCP recommendation [Guyatt, 2012]: Minimum of 10-14 days; extended duration of up to 35 days suggested)

Hip replacement: Initial: 110 mg given 1-4 hours after completion of surgery and establishment of hemostasis **OR** 220 mg as 1 dose in postoperative patients in whom therapy is not initiated on day of surgery regardless of reason; maintenance: 220 mg once daily (total duration of therapy: 28-35 days; ACCP recommendation [Guyatt, 2012]: Minimum of 10-14 days; extended duration of up to 35 days suggested)

Conversion information (Canadian labeling): When transitioning from parenteral anticoagulation therapy, initiate oral dabigatran therapy ≤2 hours prior to the time of next regularly scheduled dose of intermittent parenteral anticoagulant or at the time of discontinuation for continuously administered parenteral anticoagulation therapy. When transitioning from dabigatran to I.V. anticoagulation therapy following hip- or knee-replacement surgery, allow 24 hours after the last dabigatran dose before initiating I.V. anticoagulation therapy. When transitioning from warfarin, discontinue warfarin and initiate dabigatran when INR <2.0.

Dosing adjustment with concomitant medications:

U.S. labeling: Nonvalvular atrial fibrillation (to prevent stroke and systemic embolism):

Dronedarone or ketoconazole (oral) with Cl_{cr} 30-50 mL/minute: Consider dabigatran dose reduction to 75 mg twice daily.

Any P-glycoprotein inhibitor (including dronedarone and oral ketoconazole) with Cl_{cr} <30 mL/minute: Avoid concurrent use.

Canadian labeling: Postoperative thromboprophylaxis: *Strong P-gp inhibitors (eg, amiodarone, quinidine, verapamil):* Use caution and reduce dabigatran to 150 mg once daily. In patients with Cl_{cr} 30-50 mL/minute and receiving verapamil, consider dabigatran dose reduction to 75 mg once daily. Use with the strong P-gp inhibitor ketoconazole (oral) is contraindicated.

Elderly:

Nonvalvular atrial fibrillation (to prevent stroke and systemic embolism):

U.S. labeling:

Patients >65 years: Refer to adult dosing. No dosage adjustment required unless renal impairment exists; however, increased risk of bleeding has been observed, particularly in elderly patients with low body weight and/or concomitant renal impairment.

Patients ≥80 years: **Use with extreme caution or consider other treatment options;** no dosage adjustment provided in manufacturer's labeling; however, numerous cases of hemorrhage, including hemorrhagic stroke, have been reported postmarketing, particularly in this age group of octogenarians. Due to a lack of available dosing options available in the U.S., consider avoiding use of dabigatran in this population.

Canadian labeling:

Patients <80 years: 150 mg twice daily; **Note:** The manufacturer labeling suggests that a dose reduction to 110 mg twice daily may be considered in patients >75 years with at least one other risk factor for bleeding (eg, moderate renal impairment [Cl_{cr} 30-50 mL/minute], concomitant treatment with strong P-gp inhibitors, or previous GI bleed); however, efficacy in stroke prevention may be lessened with this dose reduction.

Patients ≥80 years: 110 mg twice daily

Postoperative thromboprophylaxis (Canadian labeling): Patients >75 years: Use with caution; consider a dose of 150 mg once daily.

Dosing adjustment in renal impairment: Note: Clinical trial evaluating safety and efficacy utilized the Cockcroft-Gault formula with the use of actual body weight (data on file; Boehringer Ingelheim Pharmaceuticals Inc, 2012).

Nonvalvular atrial fibrillation (to prevent stroke and systemic embolism):

U.S. labeling:

Cl_{cr} >50 mL/minute: No dosage adjustment necessary. Use with caution in mild renal impairment (Cl_{cr} 50-80 mL/minute) due to risk for increased dabigatran exposure (area under the curve may be increased 1.5 times higher than normal).

Cl_{cr} 30-50 mL/minute: No dosage adjustment necessary **unless** patient receiving concomitant dronedarone or oral ketoconazole, then consider reducing dabigatran to 75 mg twice daily. Use with caution in moderate renal impairment due to risk for increased dabigatran exposure (area under the curve may be increased 3 times higher than normal), particularly if patient is also of advanced age.

Cl_{cr} 15-30 mL/minute: 75 mg twice daily **unless** patient receiving concomitant P-gp inhibitor (including dronedarone or oral ketoconazole), then avoid concurrent use. **Note:** Patients with Cl_{cr} <30 mL/minute were excluded from the RE-LY trial (Connolly, 2009). Dose based on pharmacokinetic data; safety and efficacy has not been established. Per the American College of Chest Physicians, dabigatran is considered contraindicated in patients with severe renal impairment (Cl_{cr} ≤30 mL/minute) (Guyatt, 2012).

Cl_{cr} <15 mL/minute: Use not recommended (has not been studied). Per the American College of Chest Physicians, dabigatran is considered contraindicated in patients with severe renal impairment (Cl_{cr} ≤30 mL/minute) (Guyatt, 2012).

ESRD requiring hemodialysis: Use not recommended (has not been studied); **Note:** Hemodialysis removes ~60% over 2-3 hours

Canadian labeling:

Cl_{cr} >50 mL/minute: No dosage adjustment necessary.

Cl_{cr} 30-50 mL/minute: No dosage adjustment necessary. **Note:** Patients with moderate renal impairment (Cl_{cr} 30-50 mL/minute) are at an increased risk for bleeding; routine assessment of renal status is recommended; use recommended unadjusted dosage of 150 mg twice daily with caution in these patients. A dosage reduction to 110 mg twice daily may be considered for patients ≥75 years and/or those with other bleeding risk factors; however, efficacy in stroke prevention may be lessened with this dose.

Cl_{cr} <30 mL/minute: Use is contraindicated.

Postoperative thromboprophylaxis: Canadian labeling:

Cl_{cr} >50 mL/minute: No dosage adjustment necessary.

Cl_{cr} 30-50 mL/minute: Initial: 75 mg given 1-4 hours after completion of surgery and establishment of hemostasis; Maintenance: 150 mg once daily **unless** patient receiving concomitant verapamil, then consider reducing dabigatran to 75 mg once daily.

Cl_{cr} <30 mL/minute: Use is contraindicated.

Dosing adjustment in hepatic impairment:

U.S. labeling: No dosage adjustment provided in manufacturer's labeling; consistent changes in exposure or pharmacodynamics were not observed in a study of patients with moderate impairment.

Canadian labeling: Use is not recommended if hepatic enzymes >3 x ULN.

Dietary Considerations May be taken without regard to meals.

Administration Do not break, chew, or open capsules, as this will lead to 75% increase in absorption and potentially serious adverse reactions. Administer with a full glass of water. May be taken without regard to meals.

Monitoring Parameters Routine monitoring of coagulation tests not required. However, the measurement of activated partial thromboplastin time (aPTT) (values >2.5 x control may indicate overanticoagulation), ecarin clotting test (ECT) if available, or thrombin time (TT; most sensitive) may be useful to determine presence of dabigatran and level of coagulopathy; CBC with differential; renal function (prior to initiation and periodically as clinically indicated [ie, situations associated with a decline in renal function]); **Note:** Canadian labeling specifically recommends renal function be routinely assessed at least once per year in elderly patients (>75 years of age) or patients with moderate renal impairment (Cl_{cr} 30-50 mL/minute)

Reference Range

At therapeutic dabigatran doses, aPTT, ECT (ecarin clotting time), and TT (thrombin time) are prolonged. A median peak aPTT of ~2 x control and a median trough aPTT of 1.5 x control were observed in subjects taking dabigatran 150 mg twice daily in the RE-LY trial

A therapeutic range has not been established for aPTT or for other tests of anticoagulant activity

Dosage Forms Excipient information presented when available (limited, particularly for generics); consult specific product labeling.

Capsule, Oral:

Pradaxa: 75 mg [contains fd&c yellow #6 (sunset yellow)]

Pradaxa: 150 mg [contains fd&c blue #2 (indigotine), fd&c yellow #6 (sunset yellow)]

Dosage Forms: Canada Excipient information presented when available (limited, particularly for generics); consult specific product labeling.

Capsule, oral:

Pradax™: 75 mg, 110 mg, 150 mg

◆ **Dabigatran Etexilate Mesylate** *see* Dabigatran Etexilate *on page 525*

Dabrafenib (da BRAF e nib)

Brand Names: U.S. Tafinlar

Brand Names: Canada Tafinlar

Index Terms GSK2118436

Pharmacologic Category Antineoplastic Agent, BRAF Kinase Inhibitor

Use Melanoma, metastatic:

U.S. labeling: Treatment of unresectable or metastatic melanoma in patients with a $BRAF^{V600E}$ mutation (as detected by an approved test).

Canadian labeling: Treatment of unresectable or metastatic melanoma in patients with a $BRAF^{V600}$ mutation (as detected by a validated test).

Note: Not recommended in patients with wild-type BRAF melanoma.

Pregnancy Risk Factor D

Pregnancy Considerations Adverse effects were observed in animal reproduction studies. Based on its mechanism of action, dabrafenib would be expected to cause fetal harm if administered to a pregnant woman. Females of reproductive potential should use a highly effective nonhormonal contraceptive during therapy and for 4 weeks after treatment is complete; hormonal contraceptives may not be effective. Spermatogenesis may be impaired in males (observed in animal studies); family planning and fertility counseling should be considered prior to therapy.

Breast-Feeding Considerations It is not known if dabrafenib is excreted into breast milk. Due to the potential for serious adverse reactions in the nursing infant, the manufacturer recommends a decision be made whether to discontinue nursing or to discontinue the drug, taking into account the importance of treatment to the mother.

Medication Guide Available Yes

Contraindications There are no contraindications listed in the manufacturer's U.S. labeling.

Canadian labeling: Hypersensitivity to dabrafenib or any component of the formulation.

Warnings/Precautions Hazardous agent – use appropriate precautions for handling and disposal (meets NIOSH, 2012 criteria). Serious febrile drug reactions (eg, serious cases of fever or fever of any severity complicated by hypotension, rigors or chills, dehydration, or renal failure in the absence of a detectable cause) were observed in dabrafenib-treated patients. The median time to initial fever was 11 days (range: 1-202 days); median duration was 3 days (range: 1-129 days). Interrupt therapy for fever ≥38.5°C (101.3°F) or for any other serious febrile reaction; evaluate promptly for signs/symptoms of infection. Dosage reduction may be required; when resuming therapy after a febrile reaction, consider prophylactic administration of antipyretics. Hyperglycemia may occur while on therapy; may require initiation of insulin or oral hypoglycemic agent therapy (or an increased dose if already taking). Monitor serum glucose as clinically necessary, particularly in patients with pre-existing diabetes or hyperglycemia. Instruct patients to report symptoms of severe hyperglycemia (eg, polydipsia, polyuria).

Cutaneous squamous cell carcinoma and keratoacanthoma (cuSCC) and melanoma were observed at an increased incidence as compared to control therapy in clinical trials. The median time to the first occurrence of cuSCC was 9 weeks (range: 1-53 weeks); approximately one-third of patients who developed cuSCC had more than one occurrence (with continued treatment). The median time between diagnosis of the first and second lesions was 6 weeks. Dermatologic evaluations should be performed prior to initiating therapy, every 2 months during therapy, and for up to 6 months post discontinuation. Uveitis (including iritis) occurred in dabrafenib-treated patients (rare). Monitor for signs/symptoms of uveitis (eg, eye pain, photophobia, and vision changes).

When administered at recommended doses for 15 days, a mean increase of ~12 msec in QTc interval from baseline has been observed. Use with caution in patients who may be at increased risk for arrhythmias (eg, torsade de pointes). Potentially significant drug-drug interactions may exist, requiring dose or frequency adjustment, additional monitoring, and/or selection of alternative therapy. Drugs affecting gastric pH (eg, proton pump inhibitors, H_2-receptor antagonists, antacids) may alter dabrafenib solubility, resulting in decreased bioavailability. Clinical trials have not been performed to evaluate concomitant administration and its effect on dabrafenib efficacy. Patients with glucose-6-phosphate dehydrogenase (G6PD) deficiency may be at risk for hemolytic anemia when administered dabrafenib; use with caution and closely observe for signs/symptoms of hemolytic anemia. Not indicated for treatment of patients with wild-type BRAF melanoma. Exposing wild-type cells to BRAF inhibitors such as dabrafenib may result in paradoxical activation of MAP-kinase signaling and increased cell proliferation. Prior to initiating therapy, confirm $BRAF^{V600E}$ mutation (U.S. labeling) or $BRAF^{V600}$ mutations (Canadian labeling) status with an approved test. Data regarding use in patients with $BRAF^{V600K}$ mutation is limited; compared to $BRAF^{V600E}$ mutation, lower response rates have been observed with $BRAF^{V600K}$ mutation. Data regarding other less common BRAF V600 mutations is lacking.

Adverse Reactions

>10%:

Central nervous system: Headache (32%)

Dermatologic: Hyperkeratosis (37%), alopecia (22%), palmar-plantar erythrodysesthesia (20%), skin rash (17%)

Endocrine & metabolic: Hyperglycemia (50%; grades 3/4: 6%), hypophosphatemia (37%)

Gastrointestinal: Constipation (11%)

Hematologic & oncologic: Papilloma (27%), keratoacanthoma and squamous cell carcinoma (7% to 11%; grades 3/4: 4%)

Hepatic: Increased serum alkaline phosphatase (19%)

Neuromuscular & skeletal: Arthralgia (27%), back pain (12%), myalgia (11%)

Respiratory: Cough (12%)

Miscellaneous: Fever (28%; grades 3/4: 3%)

1% to 10%:

Endocrine & metabolic: Hyponatremia (8%)

Gastrointestinal: Pancreatitis (<10%)

Hematologic & oncologic: Malignant melanoma (2%)

Hypersensitivity: Hypersensitivity (bullous rash, <10%)

Ophthalmic: Uveitis (including iritis, 1%)

Renal: Interstitial nephritis (<10%)

Respiratory: Nasopharyngitis (10%)

Drug Interactions

Metabolism/Transport Effects **Substrate** of BCRP, CYP2C8 (major), CYP3A4 (major), P-glycoprotein; **Note:** Assignment of Major/Minor substrate status based on clinically relevant drug interaction potential; **Inhibits** BCRP, SLCO1B1; **Induces** CYP2B6 (weak/moderate), CYP2C19 (weak/moderate), CYP2C8 (weak/moderate), CYP2C9 (weak/moderate), CYP3A4 (weak/moderate)

Avoid Concomitant Use

Avoid concomitant use of Dabrafenib with any of the following: Axitinib; Conivaptan; Fusidic Acid (Systemic); PAZOPanib; Simeprevir

Increased Effect/Toxicity

Dabrafenib may increase the levels/effects of: Highest Risk QTc-Prolonging Agents; Moderate Risk QTc-Prolonging Agents; PAZOPanib; Topotecan; Vitamin K Antagonists

The levels/effects of Dabrafenib may be increased by: Conivaptan; CYP2C8 Inhibitors (Moderate); CYP2C8 Inhibitors (Strong); CYP3A4 Inhibitors (Moderate); CYP3A4 Inhibitors (Strong); Dasatinib; Deferasirox; Fusidic Acid (Systemic); Ivacaftor; Luliconazole; Mifepristone; Simeprevir

Decreased Effect

Dabrafenib may decrease the levels/effects of: ARIPiprazole; Axitinib; Cardiac Glycosides; Contraceptives (Estrogens); Contraceptives (Progestins); CYP2B6 Substrates; CYP2C19 Substrates; CYP2C8 Substrates; CYP2C9 Substrates; CYP3A4 Substrates; Ibrutinib; Proton Pump Inhibitors; Saxagliptin; Simeprevir; Vitamin K Antagonists

The levels/effects of Dabrafenib may be decreased by: Antacids; CYP2C8 Inducers (Strong); H2-Antagonists; Proton Pump Inhibitors; St Johns Wort

Ethanol/Nutrition/Herb Interactions Food: Administration with a high-fat meal decreased C_{max} and AUC by 51% and 31%, respectively, and delayed median T_{max} by ~4 hours. Management: Administer 1 hour before or 2 hours after a meal.

Storage/Stability Store at 25°C (77°F); excursions permitted to 15°C to 30°C (59°F to 86°F).

Mechanism of Action Selectively inhibits some mutated forms of the protein kinase B-raf (BRAF). $BRAF^{V600}$ mutations result in constitutive activation of the BRAF pathway; through BRAF inhibition, dabrafenib inhibits tumor cell growth.

Pharmacodynamics/Kinetics

Absorption: Decreased with a high-fat meal

Distribution: 70.3 L

Protein binding: 99.7% to plasma proteins

Metabolism: Hepatic via CYP2C8 and CYP3A4 to hydroxy-dabrafenib (active) which is further metabolized via CYP3A4 oxidation to desmethyl-dabrafenib (active)

Bioavailability: 95%

Half-life elimination: Parent drug: 8 hours; Hydroxy-dabrafenib (active metabolite): 10 hours; Desmethyl-dabrafenib (active metabolite): 21-22 hours
Time to peak: 2 hours; delayed with a high-fat meal
Excretion: Feces (71%); urine (23%; metabolites only)

Dosage

U.S. labeling: Melanoma, metastatic or unresectable (with $BRAF^{V600E}$ mutation): Adults: Oral: 150 mg twice daily (approximately every 12 hours) until disease progression or unacceptable toxicity

Canadian labeling: Melanoma, metastatic or unresectable (with $BRAF^{V600}$ mutation): Adults: Oral: 150 mg twice daily (approximately every 12 hours) until disease progression or unacceptable toxicity

Missed doses: A missed dose may be administered up to 6 hours prior to the next dose; do not administer if <6 hours until the next dose.

Dosage adjustment for toxicity:

Recommended dose reductions for toxicity:
First dose reduction: 100 mg twice daily
Second dose reduction: 75 mg twice daily
Third dose reduction: 50 mg twice daily
If unable to tolerate 50 mg twice daily: Discontinue.

Febrile drug reaction:
Fever of 38.5°C to 40°C (101.3°F to 104°F): Interrupt therapy until temperature normalizes. Resume at the same or reduced dose.
Fever >40°C (104°F) and/or fever complicated by rigors, hypotension, dehydration, or renal failure: Interrupt therapy until temperature normalizes. Consider resuming at a reduced dose or permanently discontinue.

New primary cutaneous malignancy: No dosage modifications recommended.

Other toxicity:
Intolerable Grade 2 or any Grade 3 toxicity: Interrupt therapy until resolution to ≤ Grade 1; resume at a reduced dose.
Grade 4 toxicity (first occurrence): Interrupt therapy until resolution to ≤ Grade 1; consider resuming at a reduced dose or permanently discontinue.
Grade 4 toxicity (recurrent after dosage reduction): Permanently discontinue.
Intolerable Grade 2 or any Grade 3-4 toxicity on 50 mg twice daily: Permanently discontinue.

Dosage adjustment for renal impairment:
Mild-to-moderate impairment (GFR 30-89 mL/minute/1.73 m^2): No dosage adjustment necessary.
Severe impairment (GFR <30 mL/minute/1.73 m^2): No dosage adjustment provided in manufacturer's labeling (has not been studied)

Dosage adjustment for hepatic impairment:
Mild impairment: No dosage adjustment necessary.
Moderate-to-severe impairment: No dosage adjustment provided in manufacturer's labeling (has not been studied); however, metabolism is primarily hepatic and exposure may be increased in patients with moderate-to-severe impairment.

Dietary Considerations Take at least 1 hour before or 2 hours after a meal.

Administration

Administer orally at least 1 hour before or 2 hours after a meal; doses should be ~12 hours apart. Do not open, crush, or break capsules. A missed dose may be administered up to 6 hours prior to the next dose.

Hazardous agent; use appropriate precautions for handling and disposal (meets NIOSH, 2012 criteria).

Monitoring Parameters Serum glucose (particularly in patients with pre-existing diabetes mellitus or hyperglycemia); dermatologic evaluations prior to initiation, every 2 months during therapy, and for up to 6 months following discontinuation to assess for new cutaneous malignancies; monitor for febrile drug reactions and signs/symptoms of infections; signs/symptoms of uveitis (eg, eye pain, photophobia, and vision changes); monitor for signs/symptoms of hemolytic anemia

Dosage Forms Excipient information presented when available (limited, particularly for generics); consult specific product labeling.
Capsule, Oral:
Tafinlar: 50 mg, 75 mg

Dacarbazine (da KAR ba zeen)

Brand Names: Canada Dacarbazine for Injection

Index Terms DIC; Dimethyl Triazeno Imidazole Carboxamide; DTIC; DTIC-Dome; Imidazole Carboxamide; Imidazole Carboxamide Dimethyltriazene; WR-139007

Pharmacologic Category Antineoplastic Agent, Alkylating Agent (Triazene)

Use Treatment of malignant melanoma, Hodgkin's disease

Unlabeled Use Treatment of soft-tissue sarcomas, islet cell tumors, pheochromocytoma, medullary carcinoma of the thyroid

Pregnancy Risk Factor C

Pregnancy Considerations **[U.S. Boxed Warning]: This agent is carcinogenic and/or teratogenic when used in animals;** adverse effects have been observed in animal studies. There are no adequate and well-controlled trials in pregnant women; use in pregnancy only if the potential benefit outweighs the potential risk to the fetus.

Breast-Feeding Considerations Due to the potential for serious adverse reactions in the nursing infant, breast-feeding is not recommended.

Contraindications Hypersensitivity to dacarbazine or any component of the formulation

Warnings/Precautions Hazardous agent - use appropriate precautions for handling and disposal (NIOSH, 2012). **[U.S. Boxed Warnings]: Bone marrow suppression is a common toxicity;** leukopenia and thrombocytopenia may be severe; may result in treatment delays or discontinuation; monitor closely. **Hepatotoxicity with hepatocellular necrosis and hepatic vein thrombosis has been reported (rare),** usually with combination chemotherapy, but may occur with dacarbazine alone. The half-life is increased in patients with renal and/or hepatic impairment; use caution, monitor for toxicity and consider dosage reduction. Anaphylaxis may occur following dacarbazine administration. Extravasation may result in tissue damage and severe pain. **[U.S. Boxed Warnings]: May be carcinogenic and/or teratogenic. Should be administered under the supervision of an experienced cancer chemotherapy physician.** Carefully evaluate the potential benefits of therapy against the risk for toxicity.

Adverse Reactions Frequency not always defined.
Dermatologic: Alopecia
Gastrointestinal: Nausea and vomiting (>90%), anorexia
Hematologic: Myelosuppression (onset: 5-7 days; nadir: 7-10 days; recovery: 21-28 days), leukopenia, thrombocytopenia
Local: Pain on infusion
Infrequent, postmarketing, and/or case reports: Anaphylactic reactions, anemia, diarrhea, eosinophilia, erythema, facial flushing, facial paresthesia, flu-like syndrome (fever, myalgia, malaise), hepatic necrosis, hepatic vein occlusion, liver enzymes increased (transient), paresthesia, photosensitivity, rash, renal functions test abnormalities, taste alteration, urticaria

Drug Interactions

Metabolism/Transport Effects **Substrate** of CYP1A2 (major), CYP2E1 (major); **Note:** Assignment of Major/Minor substrate status based on clinically relevant drug interaction potential

Avoid Concomitant Use

Avoid concomitant use of Dacarbazine with any of the following: BCG; CloZAPine; Natalizumab; Pimecrolimus; Tacrolimus (Topical); Tofacitinib; Vaccines (Live)

Increased Effect/Toxicity

Dacarbazine may increase the levels/effects of: CloZAPine; Leflunomide; Natalizumab; Tofacitinib; Vaccines (Live)

The levels/effects of Dacarbazine may be increased by: Abiraterone Acetate; CYP1A2 Inhibitors (Moderate); CYP1A2 Inhibitors (Strong); CYP2E1 Inhibitors (Moderate); CYP2E1 Inhibitors (Strong); Deferasirox; Denosumab; MAO Inhibitors; Pimecrolimus; Roflumilast; Tacrolimus (Topical); Trastuzumab; Vemurafenib

Decreased Effect

Dacarbazine may decrease the levels/effects of: BCG; Coccidioidin Skin Test; Sipuleucel-T; Vaccines (Inactivated); Vaccines (Live)

The levels/effects of Dacarbazine may be decreased by: CYP1A2 Inducers (Strong); Cyproterone; Echinacea; SORAfenib

Ethanol/Nutrition/Herb Interactions

Ethanol: Avoid ethanol (due to GI irritation).

Herb/Nutraceutical: Avoid dong quai, St John's wort (may also cause photosensitization).

Preparation for Administration Hazardous agent; use appropriate precautions for handling and disposal (NIOSH, 2012). The manufacturer recommends reconstituting 100 mg and 200 mg vials with 9.9 mL and 19.7 mL SWFI, respectively, to a concentration of 10 mg/mL; some institutions use different standard dilutions (eg, 20 mg/mL).

Standard I.V. dilution: Dilute in 250-1000 mL D_5W or NS.

Storage/Stability Store intact vials under refrigeration (2°C to 8°C). Protect from light. The following stability information has also been reported: Intact vials are stable for 3 months at room temperature (Cohen, 2007). Reconstituted solution is stable for 24 hours at room temperature (20°C) and 96 hours under refrigeration (4°C) when protected from light, although the manufacturer recommends use within 72 hours if refrigerated and 8 hours at room temperature. Solutions for infusion (in D_5W or NS) are stable for 24 hours at room temperature if protected from light. Decomposed drug turns pink.

Mechanism of Action Alkylating agent which is converted to the active alkylating metabolite MTIC [(methyl-triazene-1-yl)-imidazole-4-carboxamide] via the cytochrome P450 system. The cytotoxic effects of MTIC are manifested through alkylation (methylation) of DNA at the O^6, N^7 guanine positions which lead to DNA double strand breaks and apoptosis. Non-cell cycle specific.

Pharmacodynamics/Kinetics

Distribution: V_d: 0.6 L/kg, exceeding total body water; suggesting binding to some tissue (probably liver)

Protein binding: ~5%

Metabolism: Extensively hepatic to the active metabolite MTIC [(methyl-triazene-1-yl)-imidazole-4-carboxamide]

Half-life elimination: Biphasic: Initial: 20-40 minutes, Terminal: 5 hours; Patients with renal and hepatic dysfunction: Initial: 55 minutes, Terminal: 7.2 hours

Excretion: Urine (~40% as unchanged drug)

Dosage Details concerning dosing in combination regimens should also be consulted. I.V.:

Children: Hodgkin's disease (combination chemotherapy): 375 mg/m²/dose days 1 and 15 every 4 weeks (ABVD regimen; Hutchinson, 1998)

Adults:

Hodgkin's disease (combination chemotherapy): 375 mg/m²/dose days 1 and 15 every 4 weeks (ABVD regimen)

Metastatic melanoma: 250 mg/m²/dose days 1-5 every 3 weeks

Metastatic melanoma (unlabeled dosing; in combination with cisplatin and vinblastine): 800 mg/m² on day 1 every 3 weeks (Atkins, 2008; Eton, 2002)

Soft tissue sarcoma (unlabeled use; MAID regimen): 250 mg/m²/day continuous infusion for 4 days every 3 weeks (total of 1000 mg/m²/cycle) (Antman, 1993; Antman, 1998)

Dosage adjustment in renal impairment: The FDA-approved labeling does not contain dosage adjustment guidelines. The following guidelines have been used by some clinicians (Kintzel, 1995):

Cl_{cr} 46-60 mL/minute: Administer 80% of dose

Cl_{cr} 31-45 mL/minute: Administer 75% of dose

Cl_{cr} <30 mL/minute: Administer 70% of dose

Dosage adjustment in hepatic impairment: The FDA-approved labeling does not contain adjustment guidelines. May cause hepatotoxicity; monitor closely for signs of toxicity.

Dosing in obesity: *ASCO Guidelines for appropriate chemotherapy dosing in obese adults with cancer:* Utilize patient's actual body weight (full weight) for calculation of body surface area- or weight-based dosing, particularly when the intent of therapy is curative; manage regimen-related toxicities in the same manner as for nonobese patients; if a dose reduction is utilized due to toxicity, consider resumption of full weight-based dosing with subsequent cycles, especially if cause of toxicity (eg, hepatic or renal impairment) is resolved (Griggs, 2012).

Administration Infuse over 30-60 minutes; rapid infusion may cause severe venous irritation. May also be administered as a continuous infusion (unlabeled administration rate) depending on the protocol.

Extravasation management: Local pain, burning sensation, and irritation at the injection site may be relieved by local application of hot packs. If extravasation occurs, apply cold packs. Protect exposed tissue from light following extravasation.

Hazardous agent; use appropriate precautions for handling and disposal (NIOSH, 2012).

Monitoring Parameters CBC with differential, liver function

Dosage Forms Excipient information presented when available (limited, particularly for generics); consult specific product labeling.

Solution Reconstituted, Intravenous:

Generic: 100 mg (1 ea); 200 mg (1 ea)

Solution Reconstituted, Intravenous [preservative free]:

Generic: 200 mg (1 ea)

◆ **Dacarbazine for Injection (Can)** *see* Dacarbazine *on page 530*

◆ **Dacogen** *see* Decitabine *on page 556*

◆ **DACT** *see* DACTINomycin *on page 531*

DACTINomycin (dak ti noe MYE sin)

Brand Names: U.S. Cosmegen

Brand Names: Canada Cosmegen

Index Terms ACT-D; Actinomycin; Actinomycin CI; Actinomycin D; DACT

Pharmacologic Category Antineoplastic Agent, Antibiotic

Use Treatment of Wilms' tumor, childhood rhabdomyosarcoma, Ewing's sarcoma, metastatic testicular tumors (nonseminomatous), gestational trophoblastic neoplasm; regional perfusion (palliative or adjunctive) of locally recurrent or locoregional solid tumors (sarcomas, carcinomas and adenocarcinomas)

Unlabeled Use Treatment of ovarian cancer (germ cell or stromal tumors), osteosarcoma, soft tissue sarcoma (other than rhabdomyosarcoma)

Pregnancy Risk Factor D

Pregnancy Considerations Animal reproduction studies have demonstrated teratogenic effects and fetal loss. Women of childbearing potential are advised not to become pregnant. Use only when potential benefit justifies potential risk to the fetus. **[U.S. Boxed Warning]: Avoid exposure during pregnancy.**

Breast-Feeding Considerations It is not known if dactinomycin is excreted in human breast milk. According to the manufacturer labeling, due to the potential for serious adverse reactions in the nursing infant, the decision to continue or discontinue breast-feeding during therapy should take into account the risk of exposure to the infant and the benefits of treatment to the mother.

Contraindications Hypersensitivity to dactinomycin or any component of the formulation; patients with concurrent or recent chickenpox or herpes zoster

Warnings/Precautions [U.S. Boxed Warning]: Hazardous agent - use appropriate precautions for handling and disposal (NIOSH, 2012). If accidental exposure occurs, immediately irrigate copiously for at least 15 minutes with water, saline, or balanced ophthalmic irrigation solution (eye exposure) and at least 15 minutes with water (skin exposure); prompt ophthalmic or medical consultation is also recommended. Contaminated clothing should be destroyed and shoes thoroughly cleaned prior to reuse.

Vesicant; ensure proper needle or catheter placement prior to and during infusion; avoid extravasation. **[U.S. Boxed Warning]: Extremely irritating to tissues; if extravasation occurs during I.V. use, severe damage to soft tissues will occur; has led to contracture of the arm (rare). Avoid inhalation of vapors or contact with skin, mucous membrane, or eyes; avoid exposure during pregnancy.** Recommended for I.V. administration only. The manufacturer recommends intermittent ice (15 minutes 4 times/day) for suspected extravasation.

May cause hepatic sinusoidal obstruction syndrome (SOS; formerly called veno-occlusive liver disease); use with caution in hepatobiliary dysfunction. Monitor for signs or symptoms of hepatic SOS, including bilirubin >1.4 mg/dL, unexplained weight gain, ascites, hepatomegaly, or unexplained right upper quadrant pain (Arndt, 2004). The risk of fatal SOS is increased in children <4 years of age.

Dactinomycin potentiates the effects of radiation therapy; use with caution in patients who have received radiation therapy; reduce dosages in patients who are receiving dactinomycin and radiation therapy simultaneously; combination with radiation therapy may result in increased toxicity (eg, GI toxicity, myelosuppression, severe oropharyngeal mucositis). Avoid dactinomycin use within 2 months of radiation treatment for right-sided Wilms' tumor, may increase the risk of hepatotoxicity.

Toxic effects may be delayed in onset (2-4 days following a course of treatment) and may require 1-2 weeks to reach maximum severity. Discontinue treatment with severe myelosuppression, diarrhea, or stomatitis. Long-term observation of cancer survivors is recommended due to the increased risk of second primary tumors following treatment with radiation and antineoplastic agents. Regional perfusion therapy may result in local limb edema, soft tissue damage, and possible venous thrombosis; leakage of dactinomycin into systemic circulation may result in hematologic toxicity, infection, impaired wound healing, and mucositis. Dosage is usually expressed in **MICRO**grams and should be calculated on the basis of body surface area (BSA) in obese or edematous adult patients (to relate dose to lean body mass). Avoid administration of live vaccines during dactinomycin treatment. Avoid use in infants <6 months of age (toxic effects may occur more frequently). May be associated with an increased risk of myelosuppression in the elderly; use with caution. **[U.S. Boxed Warning]: Should be administered under the supervision of an experienced cancer chemotherapy physician.**

Adverse Reactions Frequency not defined.

Central nervous system: Fatigue, fever, lethargy, malaise

Dermatologic: Acne, alopecia (reversible), cheilitis, erythema multiforme, increased pigmentation, sloughing, or erythema of previously irradiated skin; skin eruptions, Stevens-Johnson syndrome, toxic epidermal necrolysis

Endocrine & metabolic: Growth retardation, hyperuricemia, hypocalcemia

Gastrointestinal: Abdominal pain, anorexia, diarrhea, dysphagia, esophagitis, GI ulceration, mucositis, nausea, pharyngitis, proctitis, stomatitis, vomiting

Hematologic: Agranulocytosis, anemia, aplastic anemia, febrile neutropenia, leukopenia, myelosuppression (onset: 7 days, nadir: 14-21 days, recovery: 21-28 days), neutropenia, pancytopenia, reticulocytopenia, thrombocytopenia, thrombocytopenia (immune mediated)

Hepatic: Ascites, bilirubin increased, hepatic failure, hepatitis, hepatomegaly, hepatopathy thrombocytopenia syndrome, hepatotoxicity, liver function test abnormality, hepatic sinusoidal obstruction syndrome (SOS; veno-occlusive liver disease)

Local: Erythema, edema, epidermolysis, pain, tissue necrosis, and ulceration (following extravasation)

Neuromuscular & skeletal: Myalgia

Renal: Renal function abnormality

Respiratory: Pneumonitis

Miscellaneous: Anaphylactoid reaction, infection, sepsis (including neutropenic sepsis)

Drug Interactions

Metabolism/Transport Effects None known.

Avoid Concomitant Use

Avoid concomitant use of DACTINomycin with any of the following: BCG; CloZAPine; Natalizumab; Pimecrolimus; Tacrolimus (Topical); Tofacitinib; Vaccines (Live)

Increased Effect/Toxicity

DACTINomycin may increase the levels/effects of: CloZAPine; Leflunomide; Natalizumab; Tofacitinib; Vaccines (Live)

The levels/effects of DACTINomycin may be increased by: Denosumab; Pimecrolimus; Roflumilast; Tacrolimus (Topical); Trastuzumab

Decreased Effect

DACTINomycin may decrease the levels/effects of: BCG; Coccidioidin Skin Test; Sipuleucel-T; Vaccines (Inactivated); Vaccines (Live)

The levels/effects of DACTINomycin may be decreased by: Echinacea

Preparation for Administration Hazardous agent; use appropriate precautions for handling and disposal (NIOSH, 2012). Reconstitute initially with 1.1 mL of preservative-free SWFI to yield a concentration of 500 mcg/mL (diluent containing preservatives will cause precipitation). May further dilute in D_5W or NS in glass or polyvinyl chloride (PVC) containers to a recommended concentration of ≥10 mcg/mL; final concentrations <10 mcg/mL are not recommended. Cellulose ester membrane filters may partially remove dactinomycin from solution and should not be used during preparation or administration.

Storage/Stability Store at controlled room temperature of 20°C to 25°C (68°F to 77°F). Protect from light and humidity. According to the manufacturer's labeling, recommended final concentrations (≥10 mcg/mL) are stable for 10 hours at room temperature but should be administered within 4 hours due to the lack of preservative.

Mechanism of Action Binds to the guanine portion of DNA intercalating between guanine and cytosine base pairs inhibiting DNA and RNA synthesis and protein synthesis

Pharmacodynamics/Kinetics

Distribution: Children: Extensive extravascular distribution (59-714 L) (Veal, 2005); does not penetrate blood-brain barrier

Metabolism: Minimal

Half-life elimination: ~36 hours; Children: Range: 14-43 hours (Veal, 2005)

Excretion: ~30% in urine and feces within 1week

Dosage Details concerning dosing in combination regimens should also be consulted. **Note: Medication orders for dactinomycin are commonly written in MICROgrams (eg, 150 mcg) although many regimens list the dose in MILLIgrams (eg, mg/kg or mg/m²).** The dose intensity per 2-week cycle should not exceed 15 mcg/kg/day for 5 days or 400-600 mcg/m²/day for 5 days.

Children >6 months: **Wilms' tumor, rhabdomyosarcoma, Ewing's sarcoma:** I.V.: 15 mcg/kg/day for 5 days (in various combination regimens and schedules)

Unlabeled dosing:

Rhabdomyosarcoma: I.V.:

VAC regimen:

Children <1 year: 25 mcg/kg every 3 weeks, weeks 0 to 45 (in combination with vincristine and cyclophosphamide, and mesna); dose omission required following radiation therapy (Raney, 2011)

Children ≥1 year: 45 mcg/kg (maximum dose: 2500 mcg) every 3 weeks, weeks 0 to 45 (in combination with vincristine and cyclophosphamide, and mesna); dose omission required following radiation therapy (Raney, 2011)

Wilms' tumor: I.V.:

DD-4A regimen: 45 mcg/kg on day 1 every 6 weeks for 54 weeks (in combination with doxorubicin and vincristine) (Green, 1998)

EE-4A regimen: 45 mcg/kg on day 1 every 3 weeks for 18 weeks (in combination with vincristine) (Green, 1998)

VAD regimen:

Children <1 year: 750 mcg/m² every 6 weeks for 1 year (stage III disease) (in combination with vincristine and doxorubicin) (Pritchard, 1995)

Children ≥1 year: 1500 mcg/m² every 6 weeks for 1 year (stage III disease) (in combination with vincristine and doxorubicin) (Pritchard, 1995)

Osteosarcoma (unlabeled use): I.V.: 600 mcg/m²/dose days 1, 2, and 3 of weeks 15, 31, 34, 39, and 42 (as part of a combination chemotherapy regimen) (Goorin, 2003)

Adults: **Note:** Some practitioners recommend calculation of the dosage for obese or edematous adult patients on the basis of body surface area in an effort to relate dosage to lean body mass.

Testicular cancer: I.V.: 1000 mcg/m² on day 1 (as part of a combination chemotherapy regimen)

Gestational trophoblastic neoplasm: I.V.: 12 mcg/kg/day for 5 days (monotherapy) **or** 500 mcg/dose days 1 and 2 (as part of a combination chemotherapy regimen)

Wilms' tumor, Ewing's sarcoma, rhabdomyosarcoma: I.V.: 15 mcg/kg/day for 5 days (in various combination regimens and schedules)

Osteosarcoma (unlabeled use): I.V.: 600 mcg/m²/dose days 1, 2, and 3 of weeks 15, 31, 34, 39, and 42 (as part of a combination chemotherapy regimen) (Goorin, 2003)

Ovarian (germ cell) tumor (unlabeled use): I.V.: 500 mcg/day for 5 days every 4 weeks (in combination with vincristine and cyclophosphamide) (Gershenson, 1985) **or** 300 mcg/m²/day for 5 days every 4 weeks (in combination with vincristine and cyclophosphamide) (Slayton, 1985)

Regional perfusion: Adults (dosages and techniques may vary by institution; obese patients and patients with prior chemotherapy or radiation therapy may require lower doses): Lower extremity or pelvis: 50 mcg/kg; Upper extremity: 35 mcg/kg

Elderly: Elderly patients are at increased risk of myelosuppression; dosing should begin at the low end of the dosing range.

Dosage adjustment in renal impairment: No dosage adjustment provided in the manufacturer's labeling; however, based on the amount of urinary excretion, dosage adjustments may not be necessary.

Dosage adjustment in hepatic impairment:

U.S. labeling: No dosage adjustment provided in manufacturer's labeling.

Canadian labeling:

Mild impairment: No dosage adjustment provided.

Moderate-severe impairment: Dose reduction may be considered; 33% to 50% dose reductions for patients with hyperbilirubinemia have been recommended by some clinicians.

Unlabeled dosing: Any transaminase increase: Reduce dose by 50%; may increase by monitoring toxicities (Floyd, 2006)

Dosing in obesity: *ASCO Guidelines for appropriate chemotherapy dosing in obese adults with cancer:* Utilize patient's actual body weight (full weight) for calculation of body surface area- or weight-based dosing, particularly when the intent of therapy is curative; manage regimen-related toxicities in the same manner as for nonobese patients; if a dose reduction is utilized due to toxicity, consider resumption of full weight-based dosing with subsequent cycles, especially if cause of toxicity (eg, hepatic or renal impairment) is resolved (Griggs, 2012).

Administration I.V.: Administer by slow I.V. push or infuse over 10-15 minutes. Do not filter with cellulose ester membrane filters. Do not administer I.M. or SubQ.

Vesicant; ensure proper needle or catheter placement prior to and during infusion; avoid extravasation.

Extravasation management: If extravasation occurs, stop infusion immediately and disconnect (leave cannula/needle in place); gently aspirate extravasated solution (do **NOT** flush the line); remove needle/cannula; elevate extremity. Apply dry cold compresses for 20 minutes 4 times a day for 1-2 days (Perez Fildago, 2012).

Hazardous agent; use appropriate precautions for handling and disposal (NIOSH, 2012).

Monitoring Parameters CBC with differential and platelet count, liver function tests, and renal function tests; monitor for signs/symptoms of hepatic SOS, including unexplained weight gain, ascites, hepatomegaly, or unexplained right upper quadrant pain (Arndt, 2004)

Test Interactions May interfere with bioassays of antibacterial drug levels

Dosage Forms Excipient information presented when available (limited, particularly for generics); consult specific product labeling.

Solution Reconstituted, Intravenous:

Cosmegen: 0.5 mg (1 ea)

Generic: 0.5 mg (1 ea)

◆ **Dalacin™ C (Can)** *see* Clindamycin (Systemic) *on page 451*

◆ Dalacin T (Can) *see* Clindamycin (Topical) *on page 454*

◆ Dalacin Vaginal (Can) *see* Clindamycin (Topical) *on page 454*

Dalfampridine (dal FAM pri deen)

Brand Names: U.S. Ampyra

Brand Names: Canada Fampyra™

Index Terms 4-aminopyridine; 4-AP; EL-970; Fampridine; Fampridine-SR

Pharmacologic Category Potassium Channel Blocker

Use Treatment to improve walking in patients with multiple sclerosis (MS)

Pregnancy Risk Factor C

Medication Guide Available Yes

Dosage Multiple sclerosis: Adults: Oral: 10 mg every 12 hours (maximum daily dose: 20 mg); no additional benefit seen with doses >20 mg daily

Missed doses: Do not administer double or extra doses if a dose is missed.

Dosing adjustment in renal impairment: Note: Creatinine clearance is estimated with Cockcroft-Gault formula.

U.S. labeling:

Mild renal impairment (Cl_{cr} 51-80 mL/minute): No dosage adjustment recommended by the manufacturer; however, use with extreme caution as risk of seizure may be increased secondary to reduced clearance.

Moderate-to-severe renal impairment (Cl_{cr} ≤50 mL/minute): Use is contraindicated.

Canadian labeling:

Mild-to-severe impairment (Cl_{cr} ≤80 mL/minute): Use is contraindicated.

Dosing adjustment in hepatic impairment: No dosage adjustment required; drug undergoes minimal metabolism and is primarily excreted unchanged in the urine.

Additional Information Complete prescribing information should be consulted for additional detail.

Dosage Forms Excipient information presented when available (limited, particularly for generics); consult specific product labeling.

Tablet Extended Release 12 Hour, Oral:

Ampyra: 10 mg

Dosage Forms: Canada Excipient information presented when available (limited, particularly for generics); consult specific product labeling.

Tablet, extended release, oral:

Fampyra™: 10 mg

◆ Dalfopristin and Quinupristin *see* Quinupristin and Dalfopristin *on page 1768*

◆ Daliresp *see* Roflumilast *on page 1847*

◆ Dalmane® (Can) *see* Flurazepam *on page 892*

◆ *d*-Alpha Tocopherol *see* Vitamin E *on page 2202*

Dalteparin (dal TE pa rin)

Brand Names: U.S. Fragmin

Brand Names: Canada Fragmin®

Index Terms Dalteparin Sodium

Pharmacologic Category Low Molecular Weight Heparin

Use Prevention of deep vein thrombosis (DVT) which may lead to pulmonary embolism, in patients requiring abdominal surgery who are at risk for thromboembolism complications (eg, patients >40 years of age, obesity, patients with malignancy, history of DVT or pulmonary embolism, and surgical procedures requiring general anesthesia and lasting >30 minutes); prevention of DVT in patients undergoing hip-replacement surgery; patients immobile during an acute illness; prevention of ischemic complications in patients with unstable angina or non-Q-wave myocardial infarction on concurrent aspirin therapy; in patients with cancer, extended treatment (6 months) of acute symptomatic venous thromboembolism (DVT and/or PE) to reduce the recurrence of venous thromboembolism

Canadian labeling: Additional use (unlabeled use in U.S.): Treatment of acute DVT; prevention of venous thromboembolism (VTE) in patients at risk of VTE undergoing general surgery; anticoagulant in extracorporeal circuit during hemodialysis and hemofiltration

Unlabeled Use Active treatment of deep vein thrombosis (noncancer patients)

Pregnancy Risk Factor B

Pregnancy Considerations Adverse effects were not observed in animal reproduction studies. Low molecular weight heparin (LMWH) does not cross the placenta; increased risks of fetal bleeding or teratogenic effects have not been reported.

LMWH is recommended over unfractionated heparin for the treatment of acute venous thromboembolism (VTE) in pregnant women. LMWH is also recommended over unfractionated heparin for VTE prophylaxis in pregnant women with certain risk factors. LMWH should be discontinued at least 24 hours prior to induction of labor or a planned cesarean delivery. For women undergoing cesarean section and who have additional risk factors for developing VTE, the prophylactic use of LMWH may be considered. For women who require long-term anticoagulation with warfarin and who are considering pregnancy, LMWH substitution should be done prior to conception when possible. When choosing therapy, fetal outcomes (ie, pregnancy loss, malformations), maternal outcomes (ie, VTE, hemorrhage), burden of therapy, and maternal preference should be considered (Guyatt, 2012). Multiple-dose vials contain benzyl alcohol (avoid in pregnant women due to association with gasping syndrome in premature infants); use of preservative-free formulation is recommended.

Breast-Feeding Considerations In lactating women receiving prophylactic doses of dalteparin, small amounts of anti-xa activity was noted in breast milk. The milk/plasma ratio was <0.025 to 0.224. Oral absorption of low molecular weight heparin is extremely low, and is therefore unlikely to cause adverse events in a nursing infant. Use of LMWH may be continued in breast-feeding women (Guyatt, 2012).

Contraindications Hypersensitivity to dalteparin (eg, pruritus, rash, anaphylactic reactions) or any component of the formulation; history of heparin-induced thrombocytopenia (HIT) or HIT with thrombosis; hypersensitivity to heparin or pork products; active major bleeding; patients with unstable angina, non-Q-wave MI, or prolonged venous thromboembolism prophylaxis undergoing epidural/neuraxial anesthesia

Note: Use of dalteparin in patients with current HIT or HIT with thrombosis is **not** recommended and considered contraindicated due to high cross-reactivity to heparin-platelet factor-4 antibody (Guyatt [ACCP], 2012; Warkentin, 1999).

Canadian labeling: Additional contraindications (not in U.S. labeling): Septic endocarditis, major blood clotting disorders; acute gastroduodenal ulcer; cerebral hemorrhage; severe uncontrolled hypertension; diabetic or hemorrhagic retinopathy; other diseases that increase risk of hemorrhage; injuries to and operations on the CNS, eyes, and ears

Warnings/Precautions [U.S. Boxed Warning]: Spinal or epidural hematomas, including subsequent paralysis, may occur with recent or anticipated neuraxial anesthesia (epidural or spinal) or spinal puncture in patients anticoagulated with LMWH or heparinoids. Consider risk versus benefit prior to spinal procedures;

risk is increased by the use of concomitant agents which may alter hemostasis, the use of indwelling epidural catheters for analgesia, a history of spinal deformity or spinal surgery, as well as traumatic or repeated epidural or spinal punctures. Use of dalteparin is contraindicated in patients undergoing epidural/neuraxial anesthesia. Patient should be observed closely for bleeding if enoxaparin is administered during or immediately following diagnostic lumbar puncture, epidural anesthesia, or spinal anesthesia.

Use with caution in patients with pre-existing thrombocytopenia, recent childbirth, subacute bacterial endocarditis, peptic ulcer disease, pericarditis or pericardial effusion, liver or renal function impairment, recent lumbar puncture, vasculitis, concurrent use of aspirin (increased bleeding risk), previous hypersensitivity to heparin, heparin-associated thrombocytopenia. Monitor platelet count closely. Cases of dalteparin-induced thrombocytopenia and thrombosis (similar to heparin-induced thrombocytopenia [HIT]), some complicated by organ infarction, limb ischemia, or death, have been observed. In patients with a history of HIT or HIT with thrombosis, dalteparin is contraindicated. Consider discontinuation of therapy in any patient developing significant thrombocytopenia (eg, <100,000/mm^3) and/or thrombosis related to initiation of dalteparin especially when associated with a positive *in vitro* test for antiplatelet antibodies. Use caution in patients with congenital or drug-induced thrombocytopenia or platelet defects.

Monitor patient closely for signs or symptoms of bleeding. Certain patients are at increased risk of bleeding. Risk factors include bacterial endocarditis; congenital or acquired bleeding disorders; active ulcerative or angiodysplastic GI diseases; severe uncontrolled hypertension; hemorrhagic stroke; or use shortly after brain, spinal, or ophthalmology surgery; in patients treated concomitantly with platelet inhibitors; recent GI bleeding; thrombocytopenia or platelet defects; severe liver disease; hypertensive or diabetic retinopathy; or in patients undergoing invasive procedures.

Use with caution in patients with severe renal impairment; accumulation may occur with repeated dosing increasing the risk for bleeding. Multidose vials contain benzyl alcohol and should not be used in pregnant women. In neonates, large amounts of benzyl alcohol (>100 mg/kg/day) have been associated with fatal toxicity (gasping syndrome). Heparin can cause hyperkalemia by affecting aldosterone. Similar reactions could occur with dalteparin. Monitor for hyperkalemia. Do **not** administer intramuscularly. Not to be used interchangeably (unit for unit) with heparin or any other low molecular weight heparins.

There is no consensus for adjusting/correcting the weight-based dosage of LMWH for patients who are morbidly obese (BMI ≥40 kg/m^2). The American College of Chest Physicians Practice Guidelines suggest consulting with a pharmacist regarding dosing in bariatric surgery patients and other obese patients who may require higher doses of LMWH (Gould, 2012).

Adverse Reactions

Note: As with all anticoagulants, bleeding is the major adverse effect of dalteparin. Hemorrhage may occur at virtually any site. Risk is dependent on multiple variables.

>10%: Hematologic: Bleeding (3% to 14%), thrombocytopenia (including heparin-induced thrombocytopenia, <1%; cancer clinical trials: ~11%)

1% to 10%:

Hematologic: Major bleeding (up to 6%), wound hematoma (up to 3%)

Hepatic: AST >3 times upper limit of normal (5% to 9%), ALT >3 times upper limit of normal (4% to 10%)

Local: Pain at injection site (up to 12%), injection site hematoma (up to 7%)

<1% (Limited to important or life-threatening): Allergic reaction (fever, pruritus, rash, injections site reaction, bullous eruption), alopecia, anaphylactoid reaction, gastrointestinal bleeding, hemoptysis, operative site bleeding, skin necrosis, subdural hematoma, thrombosis (associated with heparin-induced thrombocytopenia). Spinal or epidural hematomas can occur following neuraxial anesthesia or spinal puncture, resulting in paralysis.

Drug Interactions

Metabolism/Transport Effects None known.

Avoid Concomitant Use

Avoid concomitant use of Dalteparin with any of the following: Apixaban; Dabigatran Etexilate; Omacetaxine; Rivaroxaban

Increased Effect/Toxicity

Dalteparin may increase the levels/effects of: ACE Inhibitors; Aliskiren; Angiotensin II Receptor Blockers; Anticoagulants; Canagliflozin; Collagenase (Systemic); Deferasirox; Eplerenone; Ibritumomab; Omacetaxine; Palifermin; Potassium Salts; Potassium-Sparing Diuretics; Rivaroxaban; Tositumomab and Iodine I 131 Tositumomab

The levels/effects of Dalteparin may be increased by: 5-ASA Derivatives; Agents with Antiplatelet Properties; Apixaban; Dabigatran Etexilate; Dasatinib; Herbs (Anticoagulant/Antiplatelet Properties); Ibrutinib; Nonsteroidal Anti-Inflammatory Agents; Omega-3 Fatty Acids; Pentosan Polysulfate Sodium; Pentoxifylline; Prostacyclin Analogues; Salicylates; Sugammadex; Thrombolytic Agents; Tibolone; Tipranavir; Vitamin E

Decreased Effect

The levels/effects of Dalteparin may be decreased by: Estrogen Derivatives; Progestins

Ethanol/Nutrition/Herb Interactions Herb/Nutraceutical: Alfalfa, anise, bilberry, bladderwrack, bromelain, cat's claw, celery, chamomile, coleus, cordyceps, dong quai, evening primrose oil, fenugreek, feverfew, garlic, ginger, ginkgo biloba, ginseng (American), ginseng (panax), ginseng (Siberian), grapeseed, green tea, guggul, horse chestnut seed, horseradish, licorice, prickly ash, red clover, reishi, SAMe (s-adenosylmethionine), sweet clover, turmeric, white willow (all have additional antiplatelet/anticoagulant activity)

Preparation for Administration Canadian labeling: If necessary, may dilute in isotonic sodium chloride or dextrose solutions to a concentration of 20 units/mL. Use within 24 hours of mixing.

Storage/Stability Store at temperatures of 20°C to 25°C (68°F to 77°F). Multidose vials may be stored for up to 2 weeks at room temperature after entering.

Mechanism of Action Low molecular weight heparin analog with a molecular weight of 4000-6000 daltons; the commercial product contains 3% to 15% heparin with a molecular weight <3000 daltons, 65% to 78% with a molecular weight of 3000-8000 daltons and 14% to 26% with a molecular weight >8000 daltons; while dalteparin has been shown to inhibit both factor Xa and factor IIa (thrombin), the antithrombotic effect of dalteparin is characterized by a higher ratio of antifactor Xa to antifactor IIa activity (ratio = 4)

Pharmacodynamics/Kinetics

Onset of action: Anti-Xa activity: Within 1-2 hours

Duration: >12 hours

Distribution: V_d: 40-60 mL/kg

Protein binding: Low affinity for plasma proteins (Howard, 1997)

Bioavailability: SubQ: 81% to 93%

Half-life elimination (route dependent): Anti-Xa activity: 2-5 hours; prolonged in chronic renal insufficiency: 3.7-7.7 hours (following a single 5000 unit dose)
Time to peak, serum: Anti-Xa activity: ~4 hours
Excretion: Primarily renal (Howard, 1997)

Dosage Adults:

I.V.: Canadian labeling (not in U.S. labeling): Anticoagulant for hemodialysis and hemofiltration:
Chronic renal failure with no other bleeding risks:
Hemodialysis/filtration ≤4 hours: I.V. bolus: 5,000 units
Hemodialysis/filtration >4 hours: I.V. bolus: 30-40 units/kg, followed by an infusion of 10-15 units/kg/hour (typically produces plasma concentrations of 0.5-1 units anti-Xa/mL)
Acute renal failure and high bleeding risk: I.V. bolus: 5-10 units/kg, followed by an infusion of 4-5 units/kg/hour (typically produces plasma concentrations of 0.2-0.4 units anti-Xa/mL)

SubQ: **Note:** Each 2500 units of anti-Xa activity is equal to 16 mg of dalteparin.
DVT prophylaxis: **Note:** In morbidly obese patients (BMI ≥40 kg/m^2), increasing the prophylactic dose by 30% may be appropriate (Nutescu, 2009):
Abdominal surgery:
Low-to-moderate DVT risk: 2500 units 1-2 hours prior to surgery, then once daily for 5-10 days postoperatively
High DVT risk: 5000 units the evening prior to surgery and then once daily for 5-10 days postoperatively. Alternatively in patients with malignancy: 2500 units 1-2 hours prior to surgery, 2500 units 12 hours later, then 5000 units once daily for 5-10 days postoperatively.
General surgery with risk factors for VTE: Canadian labeling (not in U.S. labeling): 2500 units 1-2 hours preoperatively followed by 2500-5000 units every morning (may administer 2500 units no sooner than 4 hours after surgery and 8 hours after previous dose provided hemostasis has been achieved) or if other risk factors are present (eg, malignancy, heart failure), then may administer 5000 units the evening prior to surgery followed by 5000 units every evening postoperatively; continue treatment until patient is mobilized (approximately ≥5-7 days).
Total hip replacement surgery: **Note:** Three treatment options are currently available. Dose is given for 5-10 days, although up to 14 days of treatment have been tolerated in clinical trials. The American College of Chest Physicians (ACCP) recommends a minimum duration of at least 10-14 days; extended duration of up to 35 days is suggested (Guyatt, 2012).
Postoperative regimen:
Initial: 2500 units 4-8 hours after surgery (or later if hemostasis not achieved). The ACCP recommends initiation ≥12 hours after surgery if postoperative regimen chosen (Guyatt, 2012).
Maintenance: 5000 units once daily; allow at least 6 hours to elapse after initial postsurgical dose (adjust administration time accordingly)
Preoperative regimen (starting day of surgery):
Initial: 2500 units within 2 hours **before** surgery. The ACCP recommends initiation ≥12 hours before surgery if preoperative regimen chosen (Guyatt, 2012). At 4-8 hours **after** surgery (or later if hemostasis not achieved), administer 2500 units
Maintenance: 5000 units once daily; allow at least 6 hours to elapse after initial postsurgical dose (adjust administration time accordingly)
Preoperative regimen (starting evening prior to surgery):
Initial: 5000 units 10-14 hours **before** surgery. The ACCP recommends initiation ≥12 hours before surgery if preoperative regimen chosen (Guyatt, 2012). At 4-8 hours **after** surgery (or later if hemostasis not achieved), administer 5000 units
Maintenance: 5000 units once daily, allowing 24 hours between doses
Immobility during acute illness: 5000 units once daily

Unstable angina or non-Q-wave myocardial infarction: 120 units/kg body weight (maximum dose: 10,000 units) every 12 hours for up to 5-8 days with concurrent aspirin therapy. Discontinue dalteparin once patient is clinically stable.
Obesity: Use actual body weight to calculate dose; dose capping at 10,000 units recommended (Nutescu, 2009)

Venous thromboembolism, extended treatment in cancer patients:
Initial (month 1): 200 units/kg (maximum dose: 18,000 units) once daily for 30 days
Maintenance (months 2-6): ~150 units/kg (maximum dose: 18,000 units) once daily. If platelet count between 50,000-100,000/mm^3, reduce dose by 2,500 units until platelet count recovers to ≥100,000/mm^3. If platelet count <50,000/mm^3, discontinue dalteparin until platelet count recover to >50,000/mm^3.
Obesity: Use actual body weight to calculate dose; dose capping is not recommended (Nutescu, 2009). However, the manufacturer recommends a maximum dose of 18,000 units per day for the treatment of VTE in cancer patients.

DVT (with or without PE) treatment in noncancer patients (unlabeled use in U.S.): SubQ: 200 units/kg once daily (Feissinger, 1996; Jaff, 2011; Wells, 2005) **or** 100 units/kg twice daily (Jaff, 2011).
Canadian labeling: SubQ: 200 units/kg once daily (maximum dose: 18,000 units/day) **or** alternatively, may adapt dose as follows (SubQ):
46-56 kg: 10,000 units once daily
57-68 kg: 12,500 units once daily
69-82 kg: 15,000 units once daily
≥83 kg: 18,000 units once daily
Note: If increased bleeding risk, may give 100 units/kg SubQ twice daily. Concomitant treatment with a vitamin-K antagonist is usually initiated immediately.
Obesity: Use actual body weight to calculate dose; dose capping is not recommended (Nutescu, 2009). One study demonstrated similar anti-Xa levels after 3 days of therapy in obese patients (>40% above IBW; range: 82-190 kg) compared to those ≤20% above IBW or between 20% to 40% above IBW (Wilson, 2001).
Pregnant women: 200 units/kg/dose once daily or 100 units/kg/dose every 12 hours. Discontinue ≥24 hours prior to the induction of labor or cesarean section. Dalteparin therapy may be substituted with heparin near term. Continue anticoagulation therapy for ≥6 weeks postpartum (minimum duration of therapy: 3 months). LMWH or heparin therapy is preferred over warfarin during pregnancy (Bates, 2012).

Prevention of recurrent venous thromboembolism in pregnancy (unlabeled use): 5000 units once daily. Therapy should continue for 6 weeks postpartum in high-risk women (Bates, 2012).

Dosing adjustment in renal impairment: Half-life is increased in patients with chronic renal failure, use with caution, accumulation can be expected; specific dosage adjustments have not been recommended. Accumulation was not observed in critically ill patients with severe renal insufficiency (Cl_{cr} <30 mL/minute) receiving prophylactic doses (5000 units) for a median of 7 days (Douketis, 2008). In cancer patients, receiving treatment for venous thromboembolism, if Cl_{cr} <30 mL/minute, manufacturer recommends monitoring anti-Xa levels to determine appropriate dose.

Dosing adjustment in hepatic impairment: No dosage adjustment provided in manufacturer's labeling; use with caution.

Administration

For deep SubQ injection; may be injected in a U-shape to the area surrounding the navel, the upper outer side of the thigh, or the upper outer quadrangle of the buttock. Use thumb and forefinger to lift a fold of skin when injecting dalteparin to the navel area or thigh. Insert needle at a 45- to 90-degree angle. The entire length of needle should be inserted. Do not expel air bubble from fixed-dose syringe prior to injection. Air bubble (and extra solution, if applicable) may be expelled from graduated syringes. In order to minimize bruising, do not rub injection site.

To convert from I.V. unfractionated heparin (UFH) infusion to SubQ dalteparin (Nutescu, 2007): Calculate specific dose for dalteparin based on indication, discontinue UFH and begin dalteparin within 1 hour

To convert from SubQ dalteparin to I.V. UFH infusion (Nutescu, 2007): Discontinue dalteparin; calculate specific dose for I.V. UFH infusion based on indication; omit heparin bolus/loading dose

Converting from SubQ dalteparin dosed every 12 hours: Start I.V. UFH infusion 10-11 hours after last dose of dalteparin

Converting from SubQ dalteparin dosed every 24 hours: Start I.V. UFH infusion 22-23 hours after last dose of dalteparin

I.V. (Canadian labeling; not an approved route in U.S. labeling): Administer as bolus I.V. injection or as continuous infusion. Recommended concentration for infusion: 20 units/mL.

Monitoring Parameters Periodic CBC including platelet count; stool occult blood tests; monitoring of PT and PTT is not necessary. Once patient has received 3-4 doses, anti-Xa levels, drawn 4-6 hours after dalteparin administration, may be used to monitor effect in patients with severe renal dysfunction or if abnormal coagulation parameters or bleeding should occur. For patients >190 kg, if anti-Xa monitoring is available, adjusting dose based on anti-Xa levels is recommended; if anti-Xa monitoring is unavailable, reduce dose if bleeding occurs (Nutescu, 2009).

Reference Range

Recurrent VTE prophylaxis in pregnant women: Peak anti-Xa concentrations: 0.2-0.6 units/mL (Bates, 2012)

Treatment of venous thromboembolism: Peak anti-Xa concentration target (measured 4 hours after administration): *Once-daily dosing:* 1.05 anti-Xa units/mL (Garcia, 2012); per the manufacturer, target anti-Xa range is 0.5-1.5 units/mL (measured 4-6 hours after administration and after patient received 3-4 doses)

Additional Information Neutralization of dalteparin (in overdose) with protamine 1% solution: Manufacturer's recommendations: 1 mg protamine for each 100 anti-Xa units of dalteparin; if PTT prolonged 2-4 hours after first dose (or if bleeding continues), consider additional dose of 0.5 mg for each 100 anti-Xa units of dalteparin.

Dosage Forms Excipient information presented when available (limited, particularly for generics); consult specific product labeling.

Solution, Subcutaneous:

Fragmin: 25,000 units/mL (3.8 mL) [contains benzyl alcohol]

Solution, Subcutaneous [preservative free]:

Fragmin: 10,000 units/mL (1 mL); 2500 units/0.2 mL (0.2 mL); 5000 units/0.2 mL (0.2 mL); 7500 units/0.3 mL (0.3 mL); 12,500 units/0.5 mL (0.5 mL); 15,000 units/0.6 mL (0.6 mL); 18,000 units/0.72 mL (0.72 mL)

◆ **Dalteparin Sodium** *see* Dalteparin *on page 534*

Danazol (DA na zole)

Brand Names: Canada Cyclomen®

Index Terms Danocrine

Pharmacologic Category Androgen

Use Treatment of endometriosis, fibrocystic breast disease, and hereditary angioedema

Pregnancy Risk Factor X

Dosage Adults: Oral:

Females: Endometriosis:

Mild disease: Initial: 200-400 mg/day in 2 divided doses

Moderate-to-severe disease: Initial: 800 mg/day in 2 divided doses

Maintenance: Mild-severe disease: Dosage should be individualized. Continue therapy uninterrupted for 3-6 months (up to 9 months).

Females: Fibrocystic breast disease: Range: 100-400 mg/day in 2 divided doses. Pain and tenderness may be eliminated in 2-3 months; elimination of nodularity may require therapy for 4-6 months.

Males/Females: Hereditary angioedema: Initial: 200 mg 2-3 times/day; after favorable response, decrease the dosage by 50% or less at intervals of 1-3 months or longer if the frequency of attacks dictates. If an attack occurs, increase the dosage by up to 200 mg/day.

Dosage adjustment in renal impairment: Use is contraindicated in patients with markedly impaired renal function.

Dosage adjustment in hepatic impairment: Use is contraindicated in patients with markedly impaired hepatic function.

Additional Information Complete prescribing information should be consulted for additional detail.

Dosage Forms Excipient information presented when available (limited, particularly for generics); consult specific product labeling.

Capsule, Oral:

Generic: 50 mg, 100 mg, 200 mg

◆ **Dandrex [OTC]** *see* Selenium Sulfide *on page 1888*

◆ **Danocrine** *see* Danazol *on page 537*

◆ **Dantrium** *see* Dantrolene *on page 537*

◆ **Dantrium® (Can)** *see* Dantrolene *on page 537*

Dantrolene (DAN troe leen)

Brand Names: U.S. Dantrium; Revonto

Brand Names: Canada Dantrium®

Index Terms Dantrolene Sodium

Pharmacologic Category Skeletal Muscle Relaxant

Use Treatment of spasticity associated with upper motor neuron disorders (eg, spinal cord injury, stroke, cerebral palsy, or multiple sclerosis); management of malignant hyperthermia (MH); prevention of malignant hyperthermia in susceptible individuals (preoperative/postoperative administration)

Note: Dantrolene prophylaxis is not recommended for most MH-susceptible patients, provided nontriggering anesthetics are used and an adequate supply of dantrolene is available.

Unlabeled Use Neuroleptic malignant syndrome (NMS)

Pregnancy Risk Factor C

Pregnancy Considerations Adverse events were observed in animal reproduction studies. Dantrolene crosses the human placenta. Cord blood concentrations are similar to those in the maternal plasma at term. and dantrolene can be detected in the newborn serum at delivery. Adverse events were not observed in the newborn following maternal doses of 100 mg/day administered orally prior to delivery (Shime, 1988). Uterine atony has been reported following dantrolene injection after delivery; however, this may be due in part to the mannitol contained in the I.V. preparation (Shin, 1995; Weingarten, 1987). Prophylactic use of dantrolene is not routinely recommended in pregnant women susceptible to MH prior to obstetric surgery, if use is needed, close monitoring of the mother and newborn is recommended (Krause, 2004; Norman, 1995).

Breast-Feeding Considerations Low amounts of dantrolene are excreted into breast milk. Due to the potential for serious adverse reactions in the nursing infant, the manufacturer recommends that a decision be made whether to discontinue nursing or to discontinue the drug, taking into account the importance of treatment to the mother. In a case report, the half-life of dantrolene in breast milk was calculated to be 9 hours; the highest milk concentration was 1.2 mcg/mL following a maternal I.V. dose; however, the maternal serum concentrations were not reported (Fricker, 1998).

Contraindications

I.V.: There are no contraindications listed within the manufacturer's labeling.

Oral: Active hepatic disease; should not be used when spasticity is used to maintain posture/balance during locomotion or to obtain/maintain increased function

Warnings/Precautions [U.S. Boxed Warning]: Oral: Has potential for hepatotoxicity. Higher doses (ie, ≥800 mg/day), even sporadic short courses, may increase the risk of severe hepatic injury although hepatic injury may occur at doses <400 mg/day. Overt hepatitis has been most frequently observed between the third and twelfth month of therapy. Hepatic injury appears to be greater in females, in patients >35 years of age, and those taking concurrent medications. A higher incidence of fatal hepatic events have been reported in the elderly, although concurrent disease states and concurrent use of hepatotoxic drugs may have contributed. Idiosyncratic and hypersensitivity reactions (sometimes fatal) of the liver have also occurred. Monitor hepatic function at baseline and as clinically indicated during treatment. Discontinue therapy if abnormal liver function tests occur or benefits are not observed within 45 days when utilized for chronic spasticity.

Use oral therapy with caution in patients with impaired cardiac, hepatic, or pulmonary function (particularly in obstructive pulmonary disease). May cause photosensitivity. Patients should be cautioned about performing tasks which require mental alertness (eg, operating machinery or driving). The combination of I.V. dantrolene and calcium channel blockers is not recommended. Injection contains mannitol 3 g/vial for isotonicity; the patient will receive 0.375 g/kg of mannitol with the initial I.V. dantrolene dose of 2.5 mg/kg. In addition to I.V. dantrolene, supportive measures must also be utilized for management of malignant hyperthermia. Alkaline solution; may cause tissue necrosis if extravasated (vesicant); ensure proper needle or catheter placement prior to and during infusion; avoid extravasation.

Adverse Reactions Frequency not defined.

Cardiovascular: Blood pressure (altered), heart failure, tachycardia

Central nervous system: Chills, confusion, dizziness, drowsiness, fatigue, fever, headache, insomnia, lightheadedness, malaise, mental depression, nervousness, seizure, speech disturbance

Dermatologic: Eczematoid eruption, hair growth (abnormal), pruritus, rash, urticaria

Gastrointestinal: Abdominal cramps, anorexia, constipation, diarrhea, dysphagia, gastric irritation, gastrointestinal hemorrhage, nausea, taste change, vomiting

Genitourinary: Crystalluria, difficult erection, difficult urination, nocturia, polyuria, urinary incontinence, urinary retention

Hematologic: Anemia, aplastic anemia, leukopenia, thrombocytopenia

Hepatic: Hepatitis

Local: Injection site reaction (pain, erythema, swelling), thrombophlebitis, tissue necrosis

Neuromuscular & skeletal: Back pain, muscle weakness, myalgia

Ocular: Blurred vision, diplopia, tearing (excessive)

Renal: Hematuria

Respiratory: Feeling of suffocation, pleural effusion (associated with pericarditis), pulmonary edema, respiratory depression

Miscellaneous: Anaphylaxis, diaphoresis, lymphocytic lymphoma, sialorrhea

Drug Interactions

Metabolism/Transport Effects Substrate of CYP3A4 (major); **Note:** Assignment of Major/Minor substrate status based on clinically relevant drug interaction potential

Avoid Concomitant Use

Avoid concomitant use of Dantrolene with any of the following: Azelastine (Nasal); Calcium Channel Blockers (Nondihydropyridine); Conivaptan; Fusidic Acid (Systemic); Paraldehyde

Increased Effect/Toxicity

Dantrolene may increase the levels/effects of: Alcohol (Ethyl); Azelastine (Nasal); Buprenorphine; Calcium Channel Blockers (Nondihydropyridine); CNS Depressants; Hydrocodone; Methotrimeprazine; Metyrosine; Mirtazapine; Paraldehyde; Pramipexole; ROPINIRole; Rotigotine; Selective Serotonin Reuptake Inhibitors; Vecuronium; Zolpidem

The levels/effects of Dantrolene may be increased by: Brimonidine (Topical); Conivaptan; CYP3A4 Inhibitors (Moderate); CYP3A4 Inhibitors (Strong); Dasatinib; Doxylamine; Droperidol; Fusidic Acid (Systemic); HydrOXYzine; Ivacaftor; Luliconazole; Magnesium Sulfate; Methotrimeprazine; Mifepristone; Perampanel; Simeprevir; Sodium Oxybate; Tapentadol

Decreased Effect

The levels/effects of Dantrolene may be decreased by: Bosentan; CYP3A4 Inducers (Strong); Dabrafenib; Deferasirox; Herbs (CYP3A4 Inducers); Mitotane; Tocilizumab

Ethanol/Nutrition/Herb Interactions

Ethanol: May increase CNS depression; monitor for increased effects with coadministration. Caution patients about effects.

Herb/Nutraceutical: Avoid valerian, St John's wort, kava kava, gotu kola (may increase CNS depression).

Preparation for Administration Injection, powder for reconstitution: Reconstitute vial by adding 60 mL of sterile water for injection USP (**not bacteriostatic water for injection**); incompatible with D_5W, NS, and other acidic solutions; avoid glass bottles for I.V. infusion due to potential for precipitate formation. Time for dissolution for both Dantrium® IV and Revonto® is ~20 seconds.

Storage/Stability

Capsules: Store below 40°C (104°F).

Injection, powder for reconstitution: Protect from light. Use reconstituted solution within 6 hours; avoid glass bottles for I.V. infusion due to potential for precipitate formation.

Dantrium®: Store unreconstituted vials and reconstituted solutions at controlled room temperature of 15°C to 30°C (59°F to 86°F).

Revonto®: Store unreconstituted vials and reconstituted solutions at controlled room temperature of 20°C to 25°C (68°F to 77°F).

Mechanism of Action Acts directly on skeletal muscle by interfering with release of calcium ion from the sarcoplasmic reticulum; prevents or reduces the increase in myoplasmic calcium ion concentration that activates the acute catabolic processes associated with malignant hyperthermia

Pharmacodynamics/Kinetics

Absorption: Oral: Slow and incomplete

Metabolism: Hepatic

Half-life elimination: 4-8 hours

Excretion: Feces (45% to 50%); urine (25% as unchanged drug and metabolites)

Dosage

Spasticity: Oral: **Note:** Dose should be titrated and individualized for maximum effect; use the lowest dose compatible with optimal response. Some patients may not respond until a higher daily dosage is achieved; each dose level should be maintained for 7 days to determine patient response. If no further benefit observed with the higher dose level, then decrease dosage to previous dose level. Because of the potential for hepatotoxicity, stop therapy if benefits are not evident within 45 days.

Children: Initial: 0.5 mg/kg/dose once daily for 7 days; increase to 0.5 mg/kg/dose 3 times daily for 7 days, increase to 1 mg/kg/dose 3 times daily for 7 days, and then increase to 2 mg/kg/dose 3 times daily; some patients may require 2 mg/kg/dose 4 times daily; maximum dose: 400 mg daily

Adults: Initial: 25 mg once daily for 7 days; increase to 25 mg 3 times daily for 7 days, increase to 50 mg 3 times daily for 7 days, and then increase to 100 mg 3 times daily; some patients may require 100 mg 4 times daily; maximum dose: 400 mg daily

Malignant hyperthermia (MH): Children and Adults:

Preoperative prophylaxis: **Note:** Dantrolene prophylaxis is not recommended for most MH-susceptible patients, provided nontriggering anesthetics are used and an adequate supply of dantrolene is available.

Oral: 4-8 mg/kg/day in 3-4 divided doses, begin 1-2 days prior to surgery with last dose 3-4 hours prior to surgery

I.V.: 2.5 mg/kg ~1¼ hours prior to anesthesia and infused over 1 hour with additional doses as needed and individualized

Crisis: I.V.: 2.5 mg/kg (MHAUS recommendation, available at www.mhaus.org); continuously repeat dose until symptoms subside or a cumulative dose of 10 mg/kg is reached (rarely, some patients may require up to 30 mg/kg for initial treatment). **Note:** Manufacturer's labeling suggests an initial dose of 1 mg/kg.

24-hour MH Hotline (for emergencies only):

United States: 1-800-644-9737

Outside the U.S.: 00-1-209-417-3722

Postcrisis follow-up:

MHAUS protocol suggestion: 1 mg/kg every 4-6 hours (route not specified) **or** a continuous I.V. infusion of 0.25 mg/kg/hour for at least 24 hours; further doses may be indicated

Manufacturer's recommendation: Oral: 4-8 mg/kg/day in 4 divided doses for 1-3 days; I.V. dantrolene may be used to prevent or attenuate recurrence of MH signs when oral therapy is not practical; individualize dosage beginning with 1 mg/kg or more as the clinical situation dictates

Neuroleptic malignant syndrome (unlabeled use): I.V.: 1-2.5 mg/kg, may repeat dose up to maximum cumulative dose of 10 mg/kg/day, then switch to oral dosage (Strawn, 2007; Susman, 2001)

Dosage adjustment in renal impairment: No dosage adjustment provided in manufacturer's labeling.

Dosage adjustment in hepatic impairment: No dosage adjustment provided in manufacturer's labeling; use of oral dantrolene in patients with active liver disease (eg, hepatitis and cirrhosis) is contraindicated.

Administration I.V.: Therapeutic or emergency dose can be administered with rapid continuous I.V. push. Follow-up doses should be administered over at least 1 hour.

Vesicant; ensure proper needle or catheter placement prior to and during infusion; avoid extravasation.

Extravasation management: If extravasation occurs, stop infusion immediately and disconnect (leave cannula/needle in place); gently aspirate extravasated solution (do **NOT** flush the line); remove needle/cannula; elevate extremity.

Monitoring Parameters Motor performance should be monitored for therapeutic outcomes; nausea, vomiting, and liver function tests (baseline and at appropriate intervals thereafter) should be monitored for potential hepatotoxicity; intravenous administration requires cardiac monitor and blood pressure monitor

Malignant hyperthermia: During and post-acute phase: Per MHAUS protocol, patient should be observed in an ICU for at least 24 hours since recrudescence may occur; monitor for arrhythmias; monitor vital signs (including core temperature), electrolytes, ABG, CK, end tidal CO_2 ($EtCO_2$)/capnography, urine output, urine myoglobin

Dosage Forms Excipient information presented when available (limited, particularly for generics); consult specific product labeling.

Capsule, Oral, as sodium:

Dantrium: 25 mg, 50 mg, 100 mg [contains fd&c yellow #6 (sunset yellow)]

Generic: 25 mg, 50 mg, 100 mg

Solution Reconstituted, Intravenous, as sodium:

Dantrium: 20 mg (1 ea)

Revonto: 20 mg (1 ea)

Extemporaneous Preparations A 5 mg/mL oral suspension may be made with dantrolene capsules, a citric acid solution, and either simple syrup or syrup BP (containing 0.15% w/v methylhydroxybenzoate). Add the contents of five 100 mg dantrolene capsules to a citric acid solution (150 mg citric acid powder in 10 mL water); mix while adding the chosen vehicle in incremental proportions to **almost** 100 mL. Transfer to a calibrated bottle and add quantity of vehicle sufficient to make 100 mL. Label "shake well" and "refrigerate". Simple syrup suspension is stable for 2 days refrigerated; syrup BP suspension is stable for 30 days refrigerated.

Nahata MC, Pai VB, and Hipple TF, *Pediatric Drug Formulations*, 5th ed, Cincinnati, OH: Harvey Whitney Books Co, 2004.

◆ **Dantrolene Sodium** *see* Dantrolene *on page 537*

◆ **Dapcin** *see* DAPTOmycin *on page 541*

Dapsone (Systemic) (DAP sone)

Index Terms Diaminodiphenylsulfone

Pharmacologic Category Antibiotic, Miscellaneous

Use Treatment of leprosy (due to susceptible strains of *Mycobacterium leprae*) and dermatitis herpetiformis

Unlabeled Use Prophylaxis of toxoplasmosis in severely-immunocompromised patients; alternative agent for *Pneumocystis jirovecii* pneumonia (PCP) prophylaxis (monotherapy) and treatment (in combination with trimethoprim); pemphigus vulgaris (oral), aphthous ulcers (severe), bullous systemic lupus erythematosus; all in consultation with patient's physician as significant monitoring required

Pregnancy Risk Factor C

Pregnancy Considerations Because of adverse events observed in some animal studies, dapsone is classified as pregnancy category C. Per the manufacturer, dapsone has not shown an increased risk of congenital anomalies when given during all trimesters of pregnancy. Several reports have described adverse effects in the newborn after *in utero* exposure to dapsone, including neonatal hemolytic disease, methemoglobinemia, and hyperbilirubinemia. Dapsone is an alternative for prophylaxis and treatment of *Pneumocystis jirovecii* pneumonia (PCP) in pregnant, HIV-infected patients. Dapsone is also recommended for pregnant women requiring maintenance therapy of either leprosy or dermatitis herpetiformis

Breast-Feeding Considerations Dapsone is excreted in breast milk and can be detected in the serum of nursing infants. Hemolytic anemia has been reported in a breast-fed infant. Breast-feeding is not recommended by the manufacturer due to the potential for carcinogenicity observed in animal studies and the potential for hemolysis in the neonate, especially if there is a family history of G6PD deficiency.

Contraindications Hypersensitivity to dapsone or any component of the formulation

Warnings/Precautions Use with caution in patients with severe anemia, G6PD, methemoglobin reductase deficiency or hemoglobin M deficiency; hypersensitivity to other sulfonamides; aplastic anemia, agranulocytosis and other severe blood dyscrasias have resulted in death; monitor carefully; serious dermatologic reactions (including toxic epidermal necrolysis) are rare but potential occurrences; sulfone reactions may also occur as potentially fatal hypersensitivity reactions; these, but not leprosy reactional states, require drug discontinuation. Motor loss and muscle weakness have been reported with use. Prolonged use may result in fungal or bacterial superinfection, including *C. difficile*-associated diarrhea and pseudomembranous colitis.

Adverse Reactions Frequency not always defined.

>10%: Hematologic: Reticulocyte increase (2% to 12%), hemolysis (>10%; dose related; seen in patients with and without G6PD deficiency), hemoglobin decrease (>10%; 1-2 g/dL; almost all patients), methemoglobinemia (>10%), red cell life span shortened (>10%), Agranulocytosis, anemia, leukopenia, pure red cell aplasia (case report)

Cardiovascular: Tachycardia

Central nervous system: Fever, headache, insomnia, psychosis, vertigo

Dermatologic: Bullous and exfoliative dermatitis, erythema nodosum, exfoliative dermatitis, morbilliform and scarlatiniform reactions, phototoxicity, Stevens-Johnson syndrome, toxic epidural necrolysis, urticaria

Endocrine & metabolic: Hypoalbuminemia (without proteinuria), male infertility

Gastrointestinal: Abdominal pain, nausea, pancreatitis, vomiting

Hepatic: Cholestatic jaundice, hepatitis

Neuromuscular & skeletal: Drug-induced lupus erythematosus, lower motor neuron toxicity (prolonged therapy), peripheral neuropathy (rare, nonleprosy patients)

Ocular: Blurred vision

Otic: Tinnitus

Renal: Albuminuria, nephrotic syndrome, renal papillary necrosis

Respiratory: Interstitial pneumonitis, pulmonary eosinophilia

Miscellaneous: Infectious mononucleosis-like syndrome (rash, fever, lymphadenopathy, hepatic dysfunction)

Drug Interactions

Metabolism/Transport Effects Substrate of CYP2C19 (minor), CYP2C8 (minor), CYP2C9 (major), CYP2E1 (minor), CYP3A4 (major); **Note:** Assignment of Major/Minor substrate status based on clinically relevant drug interaction potential

Avoid Concomitant Use

Avoid concomitant use of Dapsone (Systemic) with any of the following: BCG; Conivaptan; Fusidic Acid (Systemic)

Increased Effect/Toxicity

Dapsone (Systemic) may increase the levels/effects of: Antimalarial Agents; Prilocaine; Sodium Nitrite; Trimethoprim

The levels/effects of Dapsone (Systemic) may be increased by: Antimalarial Agents; Conivaptan; CYP2C9 Inhibitors (Moderate); CYP2C9 Inhibitors (Strong); CYP3A4 Inhibitors (Moderate); CYP3A4 Inhibitors (Strong); Dasatinib; Fusidic Acid (Systemic); Ivacaftor; Luliconazole; Mifepristone; Nitric Oxide; Probenecid; Simeprevir; Trimethoprim

Decreased Effect

Dapsone (Systemic) may decrease the levels/effects of: BCG; Sodium Picosulfate; Typhoid Vaccine

The levels/effects of Dapsone (Systemic) may be decreased by: Bosentan; CYP2C9 Inducers (Strong); CYP3A4 Inducers (Strong); Dabrafenib; Deferasirox; Herbs (CYP3A4 Inducers); Mitotane; Peginterferon Alfa-2b; Rifamycin Derivatives; Tocilizumab

Ethanol/Nutrition/Herb Interactions Herb/Nutraceutical: St John's wort may decrease dapsone levels.

Storage/Stability Store at 20°C to 25°C (68°F to 76°F). Protect from light.

Mechanism of Action Competitive antagonist of para-aminobenzoic acid (PABA) and prevents normal bacterial utilization of PABA for the synthesis of folic acid

Pharmacodynamics/Kinetics

Absorption: Well-absorbed

Protein binding: Dapsone: 70% to 90%; Metabolite: ~99%

Distribution: V_d: 1.5 L/kg; throughout total body water and present in all tissues, especially liver and kidney

Metabolism: Hepatic (acetylation and hydroxylation); forms multiple metabolites

Half-life elimination: 30 hours (range: 10-50 hours)

Excretion: Urine (~85%)

Dosage

Leprosy: Oral:

Children: 1-2 mg/kg/24 hours, up to a maximum of 100 mg daily, in combination with other antileprosy agents; duration of therapy is variable

Adults: 100 mg daily, in combination with other antileprosy agents; duration of therapy is variable

Dermatitis herpetiformis: Adults: Oral: Start at 50 mg daily, increase to 300 mg daily, or higher to achieve full control, reduce dosage to minimum level as soon as possible

Aphthous ulcers, severe (unlabeled use): Adults: Oral:

Initial: 25 mg daily for 3 days; increase dose in increments of 25 mg daily every 3 days up to 100 mg daily for 3 days, then increase by 25 mg daily every 7 days up to 150 mg daily. Administer in 2 divided doses (75 mg dose is administered in 3 divided doses).

Maintenance: 100-150 mg daily in 2 divided doses with or without concomitant colchicine (Rogers, 1982; Lynde 2009)

Bullous systemic lupus erythematosus (unlabeled use): Adults: Oral: 100 mg once daily with or without prednisone (Fabbri, 2003).

Pemphigus vulgaris (unlabeled use): Adults: Oral: 25 mg daily for 7 days, then increase dose in increments of 25 mg daily every 7 days up to 100 mg daily for 7 days (4 weeks total therapy) with concomitant prednisone. Administer in 2 divided doses (a 75 mg dose is administered in 3 divided doses) (Azizi, 2008). **Note:** If patient becomes lesion free, taper and discontinue gradually by decreasing dose 25 mg daily over 7 days. If no new lesions are seen, gradual taper is continued. If lesions recur, dose is increased by 25 mg daily at 7-day intervals until the patient develops no new lesions. Taper is usually ~4 weeks total.

Pneumocystis jirovecii pneumonia, alternative therapy (unlabeled use): Oral:

Prophylaxis (primary or secondary):

Infants and Children: 2 mg/kg/day once daily (maximum dose: 100 mg daily) or 4 mg/kg/dose once weekly (maximum dose: 200 mg) (CDC, 2009)

Adolescents and Adults: 100 mg daily once daily or in 2 divided doses as monotherapy or 50 mg daily in combination with weekly pyrimethamine and leucovorin **or** 200 mg weekly in combination with weekly pyrimethamine and leucovorin (DHHS, 2013)

Treatment:

Infants and Children: 2 mg/kg/day once daily (maximum dose: 100 mg daily) in combination with trimethoprim for 21 days (CDC, 2009)

Adolescents and Adults (mild-to-moderate disease): 100 mg daily once daily in combination with trimethoprim for 21 days (DHHS, 2013)

Toxoplasmosis in severely-immunocompromised patients (alternative treatment) (unlabeled use): Oral: Prophylaxis:

Infants and Children: 2 mg/kg or 15 mg/m^2 up to a maximum of 25 mg once daily, in combination with pyrimethamine and leucovorin (CDC, 2009)

Adolescents and Adults: Oral: 50 mg daily, in combination with pyrimethamine and leucovorin **or** 200 mg weekly in combination with pyrimethamine and leucovorin. (DHHS, 2013)

Dosing adjustment in renal impairment: No specific guidelines are available

Dietary Considerations Do not give with antacids, alkaline foods, or drugs.

Administration May administer with meals if GI upset occurs.

Monitoring Parameters Check G6PD levels (prior to initiation); CBC (weekly for first month, monthly for 6 months and semiannually thereafter); reticulocyte counts; liver function tests. Monitor patients for signs of jaundice and hemolysis.

Dosage Forms Excipient information presented when available (limited, particularly for generics); consult specific product labeling.

Tablet, Oral:

Generic: 25 mg, 100 mg

Extemporaneous Preparations A 2 mg/mL oral suspension may be made with tablets and a 1:1 mixture of Ora-Sweet® and Ora-Plus®. Crush eight 25 mg tablets in a mortar and reduce to a fine powder. Add small portions of vehicle and mix to a uniform paste; mix while adding the vehicle in incremental proportions to **almost** 100 mL; transfer to a calibrated bottle, rinse mortar with vehicle, and add quantity of vehicle sufficient to make 100 mL. Label "shake well". Stable for 90 days at room temperature or refrigerated.

Jacobus Pharmaceutical Company makes a 2 mg/mL proprietary liquid formulation available under an IND for the prophylaxis of *Pneumocystis jirovecii* pneumonia.

Nahata MC, Morosco RS, and Trowbridge JM, "Stability of Dapsone in Two Oral Liquid Dosage Forms," *Ann Pharmacother*, 2000, 34 (7-8):848-50.

◆ **Daptacel®** *see* Diphtheria and Tetanus Toxoids, and Acellular Pertussis Vaccine *on page 630*

DAPTOmycin (DAP toe mye sin)

Brand Names: U.S. Cubicin

Brand Names: Canada Cubicin®

Index Terms Cidecin; Dapcin; LY146032

Pharmacologic Category Antibiotic, Cyclic Lipopeptide

Additional Appendix Information

Dosing Considerations for the Critically-Ill Patient With Morbid Obesity *on page 2379*

Use Treatment of complicated skin and skin structure infections caused by susceptible aerobic gram-positive organisms; *Staphylococcus aureus* bacteremia, including right-sided native valve infective endocarditis caused by MSSA or MRSA

Unlabeled Use Treatment of severe infections caused by MRSA or VRE; treatment of prosthetic joint infection caused by staphylococci (oxacillin-susceptible or -resistant) or *Enterococcus* (penicillin-susceptible or -resistant)

Pregnancy Risk Factor B

Pregnancy Considerations Adverse events were not observed in animal reproduction studies. Successful use of daptomycin during the second and third trimesters of pregnancy has been described; however, only limited information is available from case reports.

Breast-Feeding Considerations Low concentrations of daptomycin have been detected in breast milk; however, daptomycin is poorly absorbed orally. The manufacturer recommends caution if daptomycin is used during breast-feeding. Per the Canadian product labeling, daptomycin should be discontinued while breast-feeding. Nondose-related effects could include modification of bowel flora.

Contraindications Hypersensitivity to daptomycin or any component of the formulation

Warnings/Precautions May be associated with an increased incidence of myopathy; discontinue in patients with signs and symptoms of myopathy in conjunction with an increase in CPK (>5 times ULN or 1000 units/L) or in asymptomatic patients with a CPK ≥10 times ULN. Myopathy may occur more frequently at dose and/or frequency in excess of recommended dosages. Use caution in patients receiving other drugs associated with myopathy (eg, HMG-CoA reductase inhibitors). Not indicated for the treatment of pneumonia (inactivation by pulmonary surfactant). Use caution in renal impairment (dosage adjustment required severe renal impairment [Cl_{cr} <30 mL/minute]). Limited data (eg, subgroup analysis) from cSSSI and endocarditis trials suggest possibly reduced clinical efficacy (relative to comparators) in patients with baseline moderate renal impairment (<50 mL/minute). Symptoms suggestive of peripheral neuropathy have been observed with treatment; monitor for new-onset or worsening neuropathy. Prolonged use may result in fungal or bacterial superinfection, including *C. difficile*-associated diarrhea and pseudomembranous colitis. Hypersensitivity reactions and anaphylaxis have been reported with use; discontinue use immediately with signs/symptoms of hypersensitivity and initiate appropriate treatment. Use has been associated with eosinophilic pneumonia; generally develops 2-4 weeks after therapy initiation. Monitor for signs/symptoms of eosinophilic pneumonia, including new onset or worsening fever, dyspnea, difficulty breathing, new infiltrates on chest imaging studies, and/or >25% eosinophils present in bronchoalveolar lavage. Discontinue use immediately with signs/symptoms of eosinophilic pneumonia and initiate appropriate treatment (ie, corticosteroids). May reoccur with re-exposure.

Adverse Reactions

>10%:

Gastrointestinal: Diarrhea (5% to 12%), vomiting (3% to 12%), constipation (6% to 11%)

Hematologic & oncologic: Anemia (2% to 13%)

1% to 10%:

Cardiovascular: Peripheral edema (7%), chest pain (7%), hypertension (1% to 6%), hypotension (2% to 5%)

Central nervous system: Insomnia (5% to 9%), headache (5% to7%), fever (2% to 7%), dizziness (2% to 6%), anxiety (5%)

Dermatologic: Skin rash (4% to 7%), pruritus (3% to 6%), diaphoresis (5%), erythema (5%)

Endocrine & metabolic: Hypokalemia (9%), hyperkalemia (5%), hyperphosphatemia (3%)

Gastrointestinal: Nausea (6% to 10%), abdominal pain (6%), dyspepsia (1% to 4%), loose stools (4%), gastrointestinal hemorrhage (2%)

Genitourinary: Urinary tract infection (2% to 7%)

Hematologic & oncologic: Eosinophilia (2%), increased INR (2%)

Hepatic: Increased serum transaminases (2% to 3%), increased serum alkaline phosphatase (2%)

Infection: Bacteremia (5%), sepsis (5%), fungal infection (2% to 3%)

Local: Injection site reaction (3% to 6%)

Neuromuscular & skeletal: Increased creatine phosphokinase (3% to 9%), limb pain (2% to 9%), back pain (7%), osteomyelitis (6%), weakness (5%), arthralgia (1% to 3%)

Renal: Renal failure (2% to 3%)

Respiratory: Pharyngolaryngeal pain (8%), pleural effusion (6%), cough (3%), pneumonia (3%), dyspnea (2% to 3%)

<1% (Limited to important or life-threatening): Anaphylaxis, atrial fibrillation, atrial flutter, candidiasis, cardiac arrest, *Clostridium difficile*-associated diarrhea (CDAD), coma (post anaesthesia/surgery), eczema, eosinophilic pneumonitis, hallucination, hypomagnesemia, hypersensitivity, hypoesthesia (including oral), jaundice, increased lactate dehydrogenase, lymphadenopathy, mental status changes, neutropenia (Knoll, 2013), oral candidiasis, peripheral neuropathy, proteinuria, prolonged prothrombin time, renal insufficiency, rhabdomyolysis, increased serum bicarbonate, Stevens-Johnson syndrome, stomatitis, supraventricular cardiac arrhythmia, thrombocytopenia, thrombocythemia, vertigo, vesiculobullous dermatitis, vulvovaginal candidiasis

Drug Interactions

Metabolism/Transport Effects None known.

Avoid Concomitant Use There are no known interactions where it is recommended to avoid concomitant use.

Increased Effect/Toxicity

The levels/effects of DAPTOmycin may be increased by: HMG-CoA Reductase Inhibitors

Decreased Effect There are no known significant interactions involving a decrease in effect.

Preparation for Administration Reconstitute vial with 10 mL NS. Add NS to vial and rotate gently to wet powder. Allow to stand for 10 minutes, then gently swirl to obtain completely reconstituted solution. Do not shake or agitate vial vigorously. If administering via IVPB, further dilute following reconstitution in an appropriate volume of NS. Incompatible with ReadyMED® elastomeric infusion pumps (Cardinal Health, Inc) due to an impurity (2-mercaptobenzothiazole) leaching from the pump system into the daptomycin solution.

Storage/Stability Store under refrigeration at 2°C to 8°C (36°F to 46°F). Intact vials may be stored at room temperature for up to 12 months (data on file [Cubist Pharmaceuticals, 2011]). However, the manufacturer recommends storage under refrigeration. Room temperature stability information should only be utilized in situations where the drug has been inadvertently exposed to prolonged room temperature.

Reconstituted solution (either in vial or in infusion bag) is stable for a cumulative time of 12 hours at room temperature and 48 hours if refrigerated (2°C to 8°C).

Mechanism of Action Daptomycin binds to components of the cell membrane of susceptible organisms and causes rapid depolarization, inhibiting intracellular synthesis of DNA, RNA, and protein. Daptomycin is bactericidal in a concentration-dependent manner.

Pharmacodynamics/Kinetics

Distribution: V_{ss}: 0.1 L/kg; Critically-ill patients: V_{ss}: 0.23 ± 0.14 L/kg (Vilay, 2010)

Protein binding: 90% to 93%; 84% to 88% in patients with Cl_{cr}<30 mL/minute

Half-life elimination: 8-9 hours (up to 28 hours in renal impairment)

Excretion: Urine (78%; primarily as unchanged drug); feces (6%)

Dosage I.V.: Adults:

Skin and soft tissue: 4 mg/kg once daily for 7-14 days

Bacteremia, right-sided native valve endocarditis caused by MSSA or MRSA: 6 mg/kg once daily for 2-6 weeks (some experts recommend 8-10 mg/kg once daily for complicated bacteremia or infective endocarditis [Liu, 2011])

Osteomyelitis (unlabeled use): 6 mg/kg once daily for a minimum of 8 weeks (some experts combine with rifampin) (Liu, 2011)

Prosthetic joint infection (unlabeled use):

Enterococcus spp (penicillin-susceptible or -resistant) (alternative treatment): 6 mg/kg every 24 hours for 4-6 weeks (consider adding an aminoglycoside) followed by an oral antibiotic suppressive regimen (Osmon, 2013)

Staphylococci (oxacillin-sensitive or -resistant) (alternative treatment): 6 mg/kg every 24 hours for 2-6 weeks used in combination with rifampin followed by oral antibiotic treatment and suppressive regimens (Osmon, 2013)

Septic arthritis (unlabeled use): 6 mg/kg once daily for 3-4 weeks (Liu, 2011)

Dosage adjustment in renal impairment: Cl_{cr} <30 mL/minute:

Skin and soft tissue infections: 4 mg/kg every 48 hours

Staphylococcal bacteremia: 6 mg/kg every 48 hours

Intermittent hemodialysis or peritoneal dialysis (PD): Dose as in Cl_{cr} <30 mL/minute (administer after hemodialysis on dialysis days) or (unlabeled dosing) may administer 6 mg/kg after hemodialysis 3 times weekly (Salama, 2010)

Note: High permeability intermittent hemodialysis removes ~50% during a 4-hour session (Salama, 2010).

Continuous renal replacement therapy (CRRT) (Heintz, 2009; Trotman, 2005): Drug clearance is highly dependent on the method of renal replacement, filter type, and flow rate. Appropriate dosing requires close monitoring of pharmacologic response, signs of adverse reactions due to drug accumulation, as well as drug concentrations in relation to target trough (if appropriate). The following are general recommendations only (based on dialysate flow/ultrafiltration rates of 1-2 L/hour and minimal residual renal function) and should not supersede clinical judgment:

Continuous veno-venous hemodialysis (CVVHD): 8 mg/kg every 48 hours (Vilay, 2010)

Note: For other forms of CRRT (eg, CVVH or CVVHDF), dosing as with Cl_{cr}<30 mL/minute may result in low C_{max}. May consider 4-6 mg/kg every 24 hours (or 8 mg/kg every 48 hours) depending on site or severity of infection or if not responding to standard dosing;

therapeutic drug monitoring and/or more frequent serum CPK levels may be necessary (Heintz, 2009).

Slow extended daily dialysis (or extended dialysis): 6 mg/kg every 24 hours (Kielstein, 2010); **Note:** Dialysis should be initiated within 8 hours of administering daptomycin dose to avoid dose accumulation.

Dosage adjustment in hepatic impairment: No adjustment required for mild-to-moderate impairment (Child-Pugh class A or B); not evaluated in severe hepatic impairment (Child-Pugh class C)

Administration May administer I.V. push over 2 minutes or infuse IVPB over 30 minutes. Do not use in conjunction with ReadyMED® elastomeric infusion pumps (Cardinal Health, Inc) due to an impurity (2-mercaptobenzothiazole) leaching from the pump system into the daptomycin solution.

Monitoring Parameters Monitor signs and symptoms of infection. CPK should be monitored at least weekly during therapy; more frequent monitoring if current or prior statin therapy, unexplained CPK increases, and/or renal impairment. Monitor for muscle pain or weakness, especially if noted in distal extremities. Canadian labeling recommends CPK monitoring every 48 hours with unexplained muscle pain, tenderness, weakness or cramps. Monitor for signs/symptoms of eosinophilic pneumonia.

Reference Range

Trough concentrations at steady-state:

4 mg/kg once daily: 5.9 ± 1.6 mcg/mL

6 mg/kg once daily: 6.7 ± 1.6 mcg/mL

Note: Trough concentrations are not predictive of efficacy/toxicity. Drug exhibits concentration-dependent bactericidal activity, so C_{max}:MIC ratios may be a more useful parameter.

Test Interactions Daptomycin may cause false prolongation of the PT and increase of INR with certain recombinant thromboplastin reagents. This appears to be a dose-dependent phenomenon. If PT/INR is elevated, repeat PT/INR immediately prior to next daptomycin dose (eg, trough). If PT/INR remains elevated, repeat PT/INR using alternate reagents (if available) and evaluate for other causes of elevated PT/INR.

Dosage Forms Excipient information presented when available (limited, particularly for generics); consult specific product labeling.

Solution Reconstituted, Intravenous [preservative free]:

Cubicin: 500 mg (1 ea)

◆ **Daraprim** *see* Pyrimethamine *on page 1755*

◆ **Daraprim® (Can)** *see* Pyrimethamine *on page 1755*

Darbepoetin Alfa (dar be POE e tin AL fa)

Brand Names: U.S. Aranesp (Albumin Free)

Brand Names: Canada Aranesp

Index Terms Erythropoiesis-Stimulating Agent (ESA); Erythropoiesis-Stimulating Protein; NESP; Novel Erythropoiesis-Stimulating Protein

Pharmacologic Category Colony Stimulating Factor; Erythropoiesis-Stimulating Agent (ESA); Growth Factor; Recombinant Human Erythropoietin

Use Anemia: Treatment of anemia due to concurrent myelosuppressive chemotherapy in patients with cancer (nonmyeloid malignancies) receiving chemotherapy (palliative intent) for a planned minimum of 2 additional months of chemotherapy; treatment of anemia due to chronic kidney disease (including patients on dialysis and not on dialysis)

Note: Darbepoetin is **not** indicated for use under the following conditions:

- Cancer patients receiving hormonal therapy, therapeutic biologic products, or radiation therapy unless also receiving concurrent myelosuppressive chemotherapy
- Cancer patients receiving myelosuppressive chemotherapy when the expected outcome is curative
- As a substitute for RBC transfusion in patients requiring immediate correction of anemia

Note: In clinical trials, darbepoetin has not demonstrated improved quality of life, fatigue, or well-being.

Unlabeled Use Treatment of symptomatic anemia in myelodysplastic syndrome (MDS)

Pregnancy Risk Factor C

Pregnancy Considerations Adverse events were observed in animal reproduction studies. Women who become pregnant during treatment with darbepoetin are encouraged to enroll in Amgen's Pregnancy Surveillance Program (800-772-6436).

Breast-Feeding Considerations It is not known if darbepoetin alfa is excreted in breast milk. The manufacturer recommends that caution be exercised when administering darbepoetin alfa to nursing women.

Prescribing and Access Restrictions As a requirement of the REMS program, access to this medication is restricted. Healthcare providers and hospitals must be enrolled in the ESA APPRISE (Assisting Providers and Cancer Patients with Risk Information for the Safe use of ESAs) Oncology Program (866-284-8089; http://www.esa-apprise.com) to prescribe or dispense ESAs (ie, darbepoetin alfa, epoetin alfa) to patients with cancer.

Medication Guide Available Yes

Contraindications Hypersensitivity to darbepoetin or any component of the formulation; uncontrolled hypertension; pure red cell aplasia (due to darbepoetin or other erythropoietin protein drugs)

Warnings/Precautions [U.S. Boxed Warning]: Erythropoiesis-stimulating agents (ESAs) increased the risk of serious cardiovascular events, thromboembolic events, stroke, and/or tumor progression in clinical studies when administered to target hemoglobin levels >11 g/dL (and provide no additional benefit); a rapid rise in hemoglobin (>1 g/dL over 2 weeks) may also contribute to these risks. **[U.S. Boxed Warning]: A shortened overall survival and/or increased risk of tumor progression or recurrence has been reported in studies with breast, cervical, head and neck, lymphoid, and nonsmall cell lung cancer patients.** It is of note that in these studies, patients received ESAs to a target hemoglobin of ≥12 g/dL; although risk has not been excluded when dosed to achieve a target hemoglobin of <12 g/dL. **[U.S. Boxed Warnings]: To decrease these risks, and risk of cardio- and thrombovascular events, use ESAs in cancer patients only for the treatment of anemia related to concurrent myelosuppressive chemotherapy and use the lowest dose needed to avoid red blood cell transfusions. Discontinue ESA following completion of the chemotherapy course. ESAs are <u>not</u> indicated for patients receiving myelosuppressive therapy when the anticipated outcome is curative.** A dosage modification is appropriate if hemoglobin levels rise >1 g/dL per 2-week time period during treatment (Rizzo, 2010). Use of ESAs has been associated with an increased risk of venous thromboembolism (VTE) without a reduction in transfusions in patients >65 years of age with cancer (Hershman, 2009). Improved anemia symptoms, quality of life, fatigue, or well-being have not been demonstrated in controlled clinical trials. **[U.S. Boxed Warning]: Because of the risks of decreased survival and increased risk of tumor growth or progression, all healthcare providers and hospitals are required to enroll and comply with the ESA APPRISE (Assisting Providers and Cancer Patients with Risk Information for the Safe use of ESAs) Oncology Program prior to prescribing or dispensing ESAs to cancer patients.** Prescribers and patients will have to provide written documentation of discussed risks prior to each course. ▶

[U.S. Boxed Warning]: An increased risk of death, serious cardiovascular events, and stroke was reported in patients with chronic kidney disease (CKD) administered ESAs to target hemoglobin levels ≥11 g/dL; use the lowest dose sufficient to reduce the need for RBC transfusions. An optimal target hemoglobin level, dose or dosing strategy to reduce these risks has not been identified in clinical trials. Hemoglobin rising >1 g/dL in a 2-week period may contribute to the risk (dosage reduction recommended). The American College of Physicians recommends against the use of ESAs in patients with mild to moderate anemia and heart failure or coronary heart disease (ACP [Qaseem, 2013]).

CKD patients who exhibit an inadequate hemoglobin response to ESA therapy may be at a higher risk for cardiovascular events and mortality compared to other patients. ESA therapy may reduce dialysis efficacy (due to increase in red blood cells and decrease in plasma volume); adjustments in dialysis parameters may be needed. Patients treated with epoetin may require increased heparinization during dialysis to prevent clotting of the extracorporeal circuit. CKD patients not requiring dialysis may have a better response to darbepoetin and may require lower doses. An increased risk of DVT has been observed in patients treated with epoetin undergoing surgical orthopedic procedures. Darbepoetin is **not** approved for reduction in allogeneic red blood cell transfusions in patients scheduled for surgical procedures. The risk for seizures is increased with darbepoetin use in patients with CKD; use with caution in patients with a history of seizures. Monitor closely for neurologic symptoms during the first several months of therapy. Use with caution in patients with hypertension; hypertensive encephalopathy has been reported. Use is contraindicated in patients with uncontrolled hypertension. If hypertension is difficult to control, reduce or hold darbepoetin alfa. Due to the delayed onset of erythropoiesis, darbepoetin alfa is **not** recommended for acute correction of severe anemia or as a substitute for emergency transfusion. Consider discontinuing in patients who receive a renal transplant.

Prior to treatment, correct or exclude deficiencies of iron, vitamin B_{12}, and/or folate, as well as other factors which may impair erythropoiesis (inflammatory conditions, infections, bleeding). Prior to and during therapy, iron stores must be evaluated. Supplemental iron is recommended if serum ferritin <100 mcg/L or serum transferrin saturation <20%; most patients with CKD will require iron supplementation. Poor response should prompt evaluation of these potential factors, as well as possible malignant processes and hematologic disease (thalassemia, refractory anemia, myelodysplastic disorder), occult blood loss, hemolysis, osteitis fibrosa cystic, and/or bone marrow fibrosis. Severe anemia and pure red cell aplasia (PRCA) with associated neutralizing antibodies to erythropoietin has been reported, predominantly in patients with CKD receiving SubQ darbepoetin (the I.V. route is preferred for hemodialysis patients). Cases have also been reported in patients with hepatitis C who were receiving ESAs, interferon, and ribavirin. Patients with a sudden loss of response to darbepoetin (with severe anemia and a low reticulocyte count) should be evaluated for PRCA with associated neutralizing antibodies to erythropoietin; discontinue treatment (permanently) in patients with PRCA secondary to neutralizing antibodies to erythropoietin. Antibodies may cross-react; do not switch to another ESA in patients who develop antibody-mediated anemia.

Potentially serious allergic reactions have been reported (rarely). Discontinue immediately (and permanently) in patients who experience serious allergic/anaphylactic reactions. Some products may contain albumin and the packaging of some formulations may contain latex.

Adverse Reactions

>10%:

- Cardiovascular: Hypertension (31%), peripheral edema (17%), edema (6% to 13%)
- Gastrointestinal: Abdominal pain (10% to 13%)
- Respiratory: Dyspnea (17%), cough (12%)

1% to 10%:

- Cardiovascular: Angina, fluid overload, hypotension, MI, thromboembolic events
- Central nervous system: Cerebrovascular disorder
- Dermatologic: Rash/erythema
- Local: AV graft thrombosis, vascular access complications
- Respiratory: Pulmonary embolism

<1% (Limited to important or life-threatening): Allergic reaction, anaphylactic reactions, anemia associated with neutralizing antibodies (severe; with or without other cytopenias), angioedema, bronchospasm, hypertensive encephalopathy, pure red cell aplasia (PRCA), seizure, stroke, tumor progression/recurrence (cancer patients), urticaria

Drug Interactions

Metabolism/Transport Effects None known.

Avoid Concomitant Use There are no known interactions where it is recommended to avoid concomitant use.

Increased Effect/Toxicity There are no known significant interactions involving an increase in effect.

Decreased Effect There are no known significant interactions involving a decrease in effect.

Ethanol/Nutrition/Herb Interactions Ethanol: Should be avoided due to adverse effects on erythropoiesis.

Storage/Stability Store at 2°C to 8°C (36°F to 46°F); do not freeze. Do not shake. Protect from light. Store in original carton until use. The following stability information has also been reported: May be stored at room temperature for up to 7 days (Cohen, 2007).

Mechanism of Action Induces erythropoiesis by stimulating the division and differentiation of committed erythroid progenitor cells; induces the release of reticulocytes from the bone marrow into the bloodstream, where they mature to erythrocytes. There is a dose response relationship with this effect. This results in an increase in reticulocyte counts followed by a rise in hematocrit and hemoglobin levels. When administered SubQ or I.V., darbepoetin's half-life is ~3 times that of epoetin alfa concentrations.

Pharmacodynamics/Kinetics

Onset of action: Increased hemoglobin levels not generally observed until 2-6 weeks after initiating treatment

Absorption: SubQ: Slow

Distribution: V_d: 0.06 L/kg

Bioavailability: CKD: SubQ: Adults: ~37% (range: 30% to 50%); Children: 54% (range: 32% to 70%)

Half-life elimination:

- CKD: Adults:
  - I.V.: 21 hours
  - SubQ: Nondialysis patients: 70 hours (range: 35-139 hours); Dialysis patients: 46 hours (range: 12-89 hours)
- Cancer: Adults: SubQ: 74 hours (range: 24-144 hours); Children: 49 hours
- **Note:** Darbepoetin half-life is approximately threefold longer than epoetin alfa following I.V. administration

Time to peak: SubQ:

- CKD: Adults: 48 hours (range: 12-72 hours; independent of dialysis); Children: 36 hours (range: 10-58 hours)
- Cancer: Adults: 71-90 hours (range: 28-123 hours); Children: 71 hours (range: 21-143 hours)

Dosage

Anemia associated with chronic kidney disease: Individualize dosing and use the lowest dose necessary to reduce the need for RBC transfusions.

Chronic kidney disease patients ***ON dialysis*** (I.V. route is preferred for hemodialysis patients; initiate treatment when hemoglobin is <10 g/dL; reduce dose or interrupt treatment if hemoglobin approaches or exceeds 11 g/dL):

Children ≥1 year: Conversion from epoetin alfa: I.V., SubQ: Initial dose: Epoetin alfa doses of 1500 to ≥90,000 units per week may be converted to doses ranging from 6.25-200 mcg darbepoetin alfa per week (see pediatric column in conversion table).

Adults: I.V., SubQ: Initial: 0.45 mcg/kg once weekly **or** 0.75 mcg/kg once every 2 weeks **or** epoetin alfa doses of <1500 to ≥90,000 units per week may be converted to doses ranging from 6.25-200 mcg darbepoetin alfa per week (see adult column in conversion table).

Chronic kidney disease patients ***NOT on dialysis*** (consider initiating treatment when hemoglobin is <10 g/dL; use only if rate of hemoglobin decline would likely result in RBC transfusion and desire is to reduce risk of alloimmunization or other RBC transfusion-related risks; reduce dose or interrupt treatment if hemoglobin exceeds 10 g/dL):

Adults: I.V., SubQ: Initial: 0.45 mcg/kg once every 4 weeks

Dosage adjustments for chronic kidney disease patients (either on dialysis or not on dialysis): Do not increase dose more frequently than every 4 weeks (dose decreases may occur more frequently).

If hemoglobin increases >1 g/dL in any 2-week period: Decrease dose by ≥25%

If hemoglobin does not increase by >1 g/dL after 4 weeks: Increase dose by 25%

Inadequate or lack of response: If adequate response is not achieved over 12 weeks, further increases are unlikely to be of benefit and may increase the risk for adverse events; use the minimum effective dose that will maintain a hemoglobin level sufficient to avoid red blood cell transfusions **and** evaluate patient for other causes of anemia; discontinue treatment if responsiveness does not improve

Anemia due to chemotherapy in cancer patients: Initiate treatment only if hemoglobin <10 g/dL and anticipated duration of myelosuppressive chemotherapy is ≥2 months. Titrate dosage to use the minimum effective dose that will maintain a hemoglobin level sufficient to avoid red blood cell transfusions. Discontinue darbepoetin following completion of chemotherapy. SubQ:

Adults: Initial: 2.25 mcg/kg once weekly **or** 500 mcg once every 3 weeks until completion of chemotherapy

Dosage adjustments:

Increase dose: If hemoglobin does not increase by 1 g/dL **and** remains below 10 g/dL after initial 6 weeks (for patients receiving weekly therapy only), increase dose to 4.5 mcg/kg once weekly (no dosage adjustment if using every 3 week dosing).

Reduce dose by 40% if hemoglobin increases >1 g/dL in any 2-week period **or** hemoglobin reaches a level sufficient to avoid red blood cell transfusion.

Withhold dose if hemoglobin exceeds a level needed to avoid red blood cell transfusion. Resume treatment with a 40% dose reduction when hemoglobin approaches a level where transfusions may be required.

Discontinue: On completion of chemotherapy or if after 8 weeks of therapy there is no hemoglobin response or RBC transfusions still required

Symptomatic anemia associated with MDS (unlabeled use): Adults: SubQ: 150-300 mcg once weekly (NCCN MDS guidelines v.2.2011)

Conversion from epoetin alfa to darbepoetin alfa: See table.

Conversion From Epoetin Alfa to Darbepoetin Alfa (Initial Dose)

Previous Dosage of Epoetin Alfa (units/week)	Children Darbepoetin Alfa Dosage (mcg/week)	Adults Darbepoetin Alfa Dosage (mcg/week)
<1500	Not established	6.25
1500-2499	6.25	6.25
2500-4999	10	12.5
5000-10,999	20	25
11,000-17,999	40	40
18,000-33,999	60	60
34,000-89,999	100	100
≥90,000	200	200

Note: In patients receiving epoetin alfa 2-3 times per week, darbepoetin alfa is administered once weekly. In patients receiving epoetin alfa once weekly, darbepoetin alfa is administered once every 2 weeks. The darbepoetin dose to be administered every 2 weeks is derived by adding together 2 weekly epoetin alfa doses and then converting to the appropriate darbepoetin dose. Titrate dose to hemoglobin response thereafter.

Dosage adjustment in renal impairment: No dosage adjustment necessary.

Dosage adjustment in hepatic impairment: No dosage adjustment provided in manufacturer's labeling.

Dietary Considerations Supplemental iron intake may be required in patients with low iron stores.

Administration May be administered by SubQ or I.V. injection. The I.V. route is recommended in hemodialysis patients. Do not shake; vigorous shaking may denature darbepoetin alfa, rendering it biologically inactive. Do not dilute or administer in conjunction with other drug solutions. Discard any unused portion of the vial; do not pool unused portions.

Monitoring Parameters Hemoglobin (at least once per week until maintenance dose established and after dosage changes; monitor less frequently once hemoglobin is stabilized); CKD patients should be also be monitored at least monthly following hemoglobin stability); iron stores (transferrin saturation and ferritin) prior to and during therapy; serum chemistry (CKD patients); blood pressure; fluid balance (CKD patients); seizures (CKD patients following initiation for first few months, includes new-onset or change in seizure frequency or premonitory symptoms)

Cancer patients: Examinations recommended by the ASCO/ASH guidelines (Rizzo, 2010) prior to treatment include peripheral blood smear (in some situations a bone marrow exam may be necessary), assessment for iron, folate, or vitamin B_{12} deficiency, reticulocyte count, renal function status, and occult blood loss; during ESA treatment, assess baseline and periodic iron, total iron-binding capacity, and transferrin saturation or ferritin levels.

Additional Information Oncology Comment: The American Society of Clinical Oncology (ASCO) and American Society of Hematology (ASH) 2010 updates to the clinical practice guidelines for the use of erythropoiesis-stimulating agents (ESAs) in patients with cancer indicate that ESAs are appropriate when used according to the parameters identified within the Food and Drug Administration (FDA) approved labeling for epoetin and darbepoetin (Rizzo, 2010). ESAs are an option for chemotherapy associated anemia when the hemoglobin has fallen to <10 g/dL to decrease the need for RBC transfusions. ESAs should only be used in conjunction with concurrent chemotherapy. Although the FDA label now limits ESA use to the palliative setting, the ASCO/ASH guidelines suggest using clinical judgment in weighing risks versus benefits as formal outcomes studies of ESA use defined by intent of chemotherapy treatment have not been conducted.

The ASCO/ASH guidelines continue to recommend following the FDA approved dosing (and dosing adjustment) guidelines as alternate dosing and schedules have not demonstrated consistent differences in effectiveness with regard to hemoglobin response. In patients who do not have a response within 6-8 weeks (hemoglobin rise <1-2 g/dL or no reduction in transfusions) ESA therapy should be discontinued.

Prior to the initiation of ESAs, other sources of anemia (in addition to chemotherapy or underlying hematologic malignancy) should be investigated. Examinations recommended prior to treatment include peripheral blood smear (in some situations a bone marrow exam may be necessary), assessment for iron, folate, or vitamin B_{12} deficiency, reticulocyte count, renal function status, and occult blood loss. During ESA treatment, assess baseline and periodic iron, total iron-binding capacity, and transferrin saturation or ferritin levels. Iron supplementation may be necessary.

The guidelines note that patients with an increased risk of thromboembolism (generally includes previous history of thrombosis, surgery, and/or prolonged periods of immobilization) and patients receiving concomitant medications that may increase thromboembolic risk, should begin ESA therapy only after careful consideration. With the exception of low-risk myelodysplasia-associated anemia (which has evidence supporting the use of ESAs without concurrent chemotherapy), the guidelines do not support the use of ESAs in the absence of concurrent chemotherapy.

Dosage Forms Excipient information presented when available (limited, particularly for generics); consult specific product labeling.

Solution, Injection [preservative free]:

Aranesp (Albumin Free): 25 mcg/mL (1 mL); 40 mcg/mL (1 mL); 25 mcg/0.42 mL (0.42 mL); 60 mcg/mL (1 mL); 40 mcg/0.4 mL (0.4 mL); 100 mcg/mL (1 mL); 60 mcg/0.3 mL (0.3 mL); 100 mcg/0.5 mL (0.5 mL); 150 mcg/0.75 mL (0.75 mL); 200 mcg/mL (1 mL); 300 mcg/mL (1 mL); 200 mcg/0.4 mL (0.4 mL); 300 mcg/0.6 mL (0.6 mL) [albumin free; contains polysorbate 80]

Aranesp (Albumin Free): 150 mcg/0.3 mL (0.3 mL); 500 mcg/mL (1 mL) [contains polysorbate 80]

Darifenacin (dar i FEN a sin)

Brand Names: U.S. Enablex

Brand Names: Canada Enablex®

Index Terms Darifenacin Hydrobromide; UK-88,525

Pharmacologic Category Anticholinergic Agent

Additional Appendix Information

Beers Criteria - Potentially Inappropriate Medications for Geriatrics *on page 2368*

Use Management of symptoms of bladder overactivity (urge incontinence, urgency, and frequency)

Pregnancy Risk Factor C

Pregnancy Considerations Teratogenic effects and developmental delay were observed in some animal studies. There are no adequate and well-controlled studies in pregnant women; should be used only if potential benefit outweighs possible risk to the fetus.

Breast-Feeding Considerations Although human data are not available, darifenacin is excreted in the breast milk in animals.

Contraindications Hypersensitivity to darifenacin or any component of the formulation; uncontrolled narrow-angle glaucoma; urinary retention, paralytic ileus, GI or GU obstruction

Warnings/Precautions Cases of angioedema involving the face, lips, tongue, and/or larynx have been reported during treatment; some cases have occurred after the first dose. May be life-threatening. Immediately discontinue and institute supportive care if tongue, hypopharynx, or larynx is involved. Central nervous system effects have been reported (eg, headache, confusion, hallucinations, somnolence); monitor, particularly at treatment initiation or dose increase, reduce dose or discontinue if necessary. May cause drowsiness and/or blurred vision, which may impair physical or mental abilities; patients must be cautioned about performing tasks which require mental alertness (eg, operating machinery or driving). May occur in the presence of increased environmental temperature; use caution in hot weather and/or exercise. Use with caution with hepatic impairment; dosage limitation is required in moderate hepatic impairment (Child-Pugh class B). Not recommended for use in severe hepatic impairment (Child-Pugh class C). Use with caution in patients with clinically-significant bladder outlet obstruction or prostatic hyperplasia (nonobstructive). Use caution in patients with decreased GI motility, constipation, hiatal hernia, reflux esophagitis, and ulcerative colitis. Use caution in patients with myasthenia gravis. In patients with controlled narrow-angle glaucoma, darifenacin should be used with extreme caution and only when the potential benefit outweighs risks of treatment. Use with caution in patients taking strong CYP3A4 inhibitors (see Drug Interactions); dosage limitation of darifenacin is required. This medication is associated with potent anticholinergic properties which may be inappropriate in older adults depending on comorbidities (eg, dementia, delirium) (Beers Criteria).

Adverse Reactions

>10%: Gastrointestinal: Xerostomia (19% to 35%), constipation (15% to 21%)

1% to 10%:

Cardiovascular: Hypertension (≥1%), peripheral edema (≥1%)

Central nervous system: Headache (7%), dizziness (<2%), pain (≥1%)

Dermatological: Dry skin (≥1%), pruritus (≥1%), rash (≥1%)

Gastrointestinal: Dyspepsia (3% to 8%), abdominal pain (2% to 4%), nausea (2% to 4%), vomiting (≥1%), weight gain (≥1%)

Genitourinary: Urinary tract infection (4% to 5%), vaginitis (≥1%), urinary retention (acute)

Neuromuscular & skeletal: Weakness (<3%), arthralgia (≥1%), back pain (≥1%)

Ocular: Dry eyes (2%), abnormal vision (≥1%)

Respiratory: Bronchitis (≥1%), pharyngitis (≥1%), rhinitis (≥1%), sinusitis (≥1%)

Miscellaneous: Flu-like syndrome (1% to 3%)

Postmarketing and/or case reports: Anaphylaxis, angioedema, confusion, erythema multiforme, granuloma annulare, hallucinations, hypersensitivity reactions

Drug Interactions

Metabolism/Transport Effects Substrate of CYP2D6 (minor), CYP3A4 (major); **Note:** Assignment of Major/Minor substrate status based on clinically relevant drug interaction potential; **Inhibits** CYP2D6 (moderate), CYP3A4 (weak)

Avoid Concomitant Use

Avoid concomitant use of Darifenacin with any of the following: Aclidinium; Conivaptan; Fusidic Acid (Systemic); Ipratropium (Oral Inhalation); Pimozide; Potassium Chloride; Thioridazine; Tiotropium; Umeclidinium

Increased Effect/Toxicity

Darifenacin may increase the levels/effects of: AbobotulinumtoxinA; Analgesics (Opioid); Anticholinergics; ARIPiprazole; Cannabinoids; CYP2D6 Substrates; Dofetilide; Fesoterodine; Lomitapide; Metoprolol; Mirabegron; Nebivolol; OnabotulinumtoxinA; Pimozide; Potassium Chloride; RimabotulinumtoxinB; Thiazide Diuretics; Thioridazine; Tiotropium; Topiramate

The levels/effects of Darifenacin may be increased by: Aclidinium; Conivaptan; CYP3A4 Inhibitors (Moderate); CYP3A4 Inhibitors (Strong); Dasatinib; Fusidic Acid (Systemic); Ipratropium (Oral Inhalation); Ivacaftor; Luliconazole; Mifepristone; Pramlintide; Propafenone; Simeprevir; Umeclidinium

Decreased Effect

Darifenacin may decrease the levels/effects of: Acetylcholinesterase Inhibitors (Central); Codeine; Secretin; Tamoxifen; TraMADol

The levels/effects of Darifenacin may be decreased by: Acetylcholinesterase Inhibitors (Central); Bosentan; CYP3A4 Inducers (Strong); Dabrafenib; Deferasirox; Herbs (CYP3A4 Inducers); Mitotane; Peginterferon Alfa-2b; Tocilizumab

Ethanol/Nutrition/Herb Interactions Herb/Nutraceutical: Darifenacin serum concentration may be decreased by St John's wort (avoid concurrent use.)

Storage/Stability Store at 25°C (77°F); excursions permitted to 15°C to 30°C (59°F to 86°F). Protect from light.

Mechanism of Action Selective antagonist of the M3 muscarinic (cholinergic) receptor subtype. Blockade of the receptor limits bladder contractions, reducing the symptoms of bladder irritability/overactivity (urge incontinence, urgency and frequency).

Pharmacodynamics/Kinetics

Distribution: V_{dss}: ~163 L

Protein binding: ~98% (primarily alpha$_1$-acid glycoprotein)

Metabolism: Hepatic, via CYP3A4 (major) and CYP2D6 (minor)

Bioavailability: 15% to 19%

Half-life elimination: ~13-19 hours

Time to peak, plasma: ~7 hours

Excretion: As metabolites (inactive); urine (60%), feces (40%)

Dosage Oral: Adults: Initial: 7.5 mg once daily. If response is not adequate after a minimum of 2 weeks, dosage may be increased to 15 mg once daily.

Dosage adjustment with concomitant potent CYP3A4 inhibitors (eg, azole antifungals, erythromycin, isoniazid, protease inhibitors): Daily dosage should not exceed 7.5 mg/day

Dosage adjustment in renal impairment: No adjustment required.

Dosage adjustment in hepatic impairment:

Moderate impairment (Child-Pugh class B): Daily dosage should not exceed 7.5 mg/day

Severe impairment (Child-Pugh class C): Has not been evaluated; use is not recommended

Dietary Considerations May be taken without regard to meals, with or without food.

Administration Tablet should be taken with liquid and swallowed whole; do not chew, crush, or split tablet. May be taken without regard to food.

Dosage Forms Excipient information presented when available (limited, particularly for generics); consult specific product labeling.

Tablet Extended Release 24 Hour, Oral:

Enablex: 7.5 mg, 15 mg

◆ **Darifenacin Hydrobromide** *see* Darifenacin *on page 546*

Darunavir (dar OO na veer)

Brand Names: U.S. Prezista

Brand Names: Canada Prezista®

Index Terms Darunavir Ethanolate; DRV; TMC-114

Pharmacologic Category Antiretroviral, Protease Inhibitor (Anti-HIV)

Use Treatment of HIV-1 infections in combination with ritonavir and other antiretroviral agents

Pregnancy Risk Factor C

Pregnancy Considerations Teratogenic effects have not been observed in animal reproduction studies. Darunavir crosses the placenta. Safety and pharmacokinetic data are limited in pregnancy. Serum concentrations may be low with once-daily dosing; therefore, some experts recommend twice-daily dosing during pregnancy (studies are ongoing). The DHHS Perinatal HIV Guidelines consider darunavir to be an alternative protease inhibitor (PI) when combined with low-dose ritonavir boosting. A small increased risk of preterm birth has been associated with maternal use of protease inhibitor-based combination antiretroviral (ARV) therapy during pregnancy; however, the benefits of use generally outweigh this risk and PIs should not be withheld if otherwise recommended. Hyperglycemia, new onset of diabetes mellitus, or diabetic ketoacidosis have been reported with PIs; it is not clear if pregnancy increases this risk.

Regardless of CD4 count or HIV RNA copy number, all HIV-infected pregnant women should receive a combination antepartum ARV drug regimen; this includes women who require therapy for their own health, as well as women who do not yet require therapy for their own health. ARV therapy should be started as soon as possible if required for the woman's health. Although earlier initiation may be more effective in reducing the perinatal transmission of HIV), also consider maternal conditions (eg, nausea and vomiting) and the potential risks of first trimester fetal exposure for specific agents. Plasma HIV RNA levels should be assessed at ~34-36 weeks gestation in order to help determine mode of delivery. If ARV therapy must be interrupted for <24 hours during the peripartum period, stop then restart all medications simultaneously in order to decrease the chance of developing resistance. Long-term follow-up is recommended for all infants exposed to ARV medications.

Healthcare providers are encouraged to enroll pregnant women exposed to antiretroviral medications in the Antiretroviral Pregnancy Registry (1-800-258-4263 or www.APRegistry.com). Healthcare providers caring for HIV-infected women and their infants may contact the National Perinatal HIV Hotline (888-448-8765) for clinical consultation (DHHS [perinatal], 2012).

Breast-Feeding Considerations Maternal or infant antiretroviral therapy does not completely eliminate the risk of postnatal HIV transmission. In addition, multiclass-resistant virus has been detected in breast-feeding infants despite maternal therapy. Therefore, in the United States, where formula is accessible, affordable, safe, and sustainable, and the risk of infant mortality due to diarrhea and respiratory infections is low, complete avoidance of breast-feeding by HIV-infected women is recommended to decrease potential transmission of HIV (DHHS [perinatal], 2012).

Contraindications Coadministration with medications highly dependent upon CYP3A4 for clearance and for which increased levels are associated with serious and/or life-threatening events (includes alfuzosin, cisapride, ergot alkaloids [eg, dihydroergotamine, ergonovine, ergotamine, methylergonovine], lovastatin, midazolam [oral], pimozide, rifampin, sildenafil (when used for pulmonary artery hypertension [eg, Revatio®]), simvastatin, St John's wort, triazolam

Canadian labeling: Additional contraindications: Hypersensitivity to darunavir or any component of the formulation; coadministration with amiodarone, lidocaine (systemic), quinidine; severe (Child-Pugh class C) hepatic impairment

Warnings/Precautions Darunavir has a high potential for drug interactions requiring dose or frequency adjustment, additional monitoring, and/or selection of alternative therapy.

Use with caution in patients with hepatic impairment, including active chronic hepatitis; consider interruption or discontinuation with worsening hepatic function. Not recommended in severe hepatic impairment (contraindicated in Canadian labeling). Infrequent cases of drug-induced hepatitis (including acute and cytolytic) have been reported. Liver injury has been reported with use (including some fatalities), though generally in patients on multiple medications, with advanced HIV disease, hepatitis B/C coinfection, and/or immune reconstitution syndrome. Monitor patients closely; consider interrupting or discontinuing therapy if signs/symptoms of liver impairment occur.

May cause fat redistribution (buffalo hump, increased abdominal girth, breast engorgement, facial atrophy). Patients may develop immune reconstitution syndrome resulting in the occurrence of an inflammatory response to an indolent or residual opportunistic infection during initial HIV treatment or activation of autoimmune disorders (eg, Graves' disease, polymyositis, Guillain-Barré syndrome) later in therapy; further evaluation and treatment may be required. May increase cholesterol and/or triglycerides. Pancreatitis has been observed with use. Risk for pancreatitis may be increased in patients with elevated triglycerides, advanced HIV disease, or history of pancreatitis. Protease inhibitors have been associated with glucose dysregulation; use caution in patients with diabetes. Initiation or dose adjustments of antidiabetic agents may be required. Use with caution in patients with sulfonamide allergy (contains sulfa moiety) or hemophilia. Protease inhibitors have been associated with a variety of hypersensitivity events (some severe), including rash, anaphylaxis (rare), angioedema, bronchospasm, erythema multiforme, Stevens-Johnson syndrome (rare), acute generalized exanthematous pustulosis, and/or toxic epidermal necrolysis. Discontinue treatment if severe skin reactions develop. Severe skin reactions may be accompanied by fever, malaise, fatigue, arthralgias, hepatitis, oral lesion, blisters, conjunctivitis, and/or eosinophilia. Mild-to-moderate rash may occur early in treatment and resolve with continued therapy. Treatment history and resistance data should guide use of darunavir with ritonavir.

Adverse Reactions As a class, protease inhibitors potentially cause dyslipidemias which includes elevated cholesterol and triglycerides and a redistribution of body fat centrally to cause increased abdominal girth, buffalo hump, facial atrophy, and breast enlargement. These agents also cause hyperglycemia. Frequency of adverse events is reported for darunavir/ritonavir. See also Ritonavir monograph.

>10%:

Endocrine & metabolic: Hypercholesterolemia (children: grade 3: 1%; adults: grade 2: 16% to 25%; grade 3: 1% to 10%), increased LDL cholesterol (children: grade 3: 3%; adults: grade 2: 14%; grade 3: 5% to 8%)

Gastrointestinal: Vomiting (children: 13% to 33%; adults 2% to 5%), nausea (4% to 25%), diarrhea (children: 11% to 24%; adults: 8% to 14%)

2% to 10%:

Central nervous system: Headache (children: 9%; adults: 3% to 6%), fatigue (children: 3%; adults: ≤2%)

Dermatologic: Skin rash (children: 5% to 10%; adults: 6% to 7%), pruritus (children: 8%)

Endocrine & metabolic: Hyperglycemia (grade 2: 7% to 10%; grade 3: ≤1%; grade 4: <1%), increased serum triglycerides (grade 2: 3% to 10%; grade 3: 1% to 7%; grade 4: ≤3%), increased amylase (children: grade 3: 4%, grade 4: 1%; adults: grade 2: 5% to 6%, grade 3: 3% to 7%), diabetes mellitus (2%)

Gastrointestinal: Abdominal pain (children: 8% to 10%; adults: 5% to 6%), decreased appetite (children: 8%; adults: 2%), increased serum lipase (children: grade 3: 1%; adults: grade 2: 2% to 3%, grade 3; ≤2%; grade 4: <1%), abdominal distention (2%), anorexia (2%), dyspepsia (2%)

Hepatic: Increased serum ALT (children: grade 3: 3%; grade 4: 1%; adults: grade 2: 7%, grade 3: 2% to 3%; grade 4: ≤1%), increased serum AST (children: grade 3: 1%; adults: grade 2: 6%; grade 3: 2% to 4%; grade 4: <1%), increased serum alkaline phosphatase (grade 2: ≤2%; grade 3: <1%)

Neuromuscular & skeletal: Weakness (≤3%)

<2% (Limited to important or life-threatening): Acute generalized exanthematous pustulosis, acute renal failure, acute respiratory distress, allergic dermatitis, alopecia, anemia, angioedema, biliary obstruction, bradycardia, cerebrovascular accident, dermatitis (including dermatitis medicamentosa), erythema multiforme, folliculitis, gynecomastia, hematuria, hepatic cirrhosis, hepatic failure, hepatic neoplasm (malignant), hepatitis (acute and cytolytic), hepatotoxicity, hyperbilirubinemia, hyperkalemia, hyperlipidemia, hypersensitivity, hypertension, hyperthermia, immune reconstitution syndrome, increased susceptibility to infection (including clostridium infection, parasitic infection [cryptosporidiosis], cytomegalovirus disease [encephalitis], hepatitis B, esophageal candidiasis), lipoatrophy, maculopapular rash, malignant lymphoma, metabolic acidosis, myocardial infarction, myocarditis, neoplasm (diffuse large B-cell), nephrolithiasis, neuromyopathy, obesity, oropharyngeal ulcer, osteonecrosis, osteopenia, osteoporosis, pancreatitis, pancytopenia, peripheral neuropathy, pneumothorax, progressive multifocal leukoencephalopathy, rectal hemorrhage, renal insufficiency, renal tubular necrosis, redistribution of body fat (eg, buffalo hump, increased abdominal girth, breast engorgement, facial atrophy), rhabdomyolysis (coadministration with HMG-CoA reductase inhibitors), respiratory failure, seizure, sepsis, skin rash (toxic), Stevens-Johnson syndrome, tachycardia, toxic epidermal necrolysis, transient ischemic attacks

Drug Interactions

Metabolism/Transport Effects Substrate of CYP3A4 (major); **Note:** Assignment of Major/Minor substrate status based on clinically relevant drug interaction potential; **Inhibits** CYP2D6 (weak), CYP3A4 (strong), P-glycoprotein

Avoid Concomitant Use

Avoid concomitant use of Darunavir with any of the following: Ado-Trastuzumab Emtansine; Alfuzosin; Amiodarone; Apixaban; Avanafil; Axitinib; Bosutinib; Cabozantinib; Cisapride; Conivaptan; Crizotinib; Dronedarone; Eplerenone; Ergot Derivatives; Everolimus; Fosphenytoin; Fusidic Acid (Systemic); Halofantrine; Ibrutinib; Imatinib; Ivabradine; Lapatinib; Lomitapide; Lopinavir; Lovastatin; Lurasidone; Macitentan; Midazolam; Nilotinib; Nisoldipine; PHENobarbital; Phenytoin; Pimozide; Pomalidomide; QuiNIDine; Ranolazine; Red Yeast Rice; Regorafenib; Rifampin; Rivaroxaban; Salmeterol; Saquinavir; Silodosin; Simeprevir; Simvastatin; St Johns Wort; Tamsulosin; Telaprevir; Ticagrelor; Tolvaptan; Topotecan; Toremifene; Triazolam; Ulipristal; Vemurafenib; VinCRIStine (Liposomal); Voriconazole

Increased Effect/Toxicity

Darunavir may increase the levels/effects of: Ado-Trastuzumab Emtansine; Afatinib; Alfuzosin; Almotriptan; Alosetron; ALPRAZolam; Amiodarone; Apixaban; ARIPiprazole; AtorvaSTATin; Avanafil; Axitinib; Bedaquiline; Bortezomib; Bosentan; Bosutinib; Brentuximab Vedotin; Brinzolamide; Budesonide (Nasal); Budesonide (Systemic, Oral Inhalation); Cabozantinib; Calcium Channel Blockers (Dihydropyridine); Calcium Channel Blockers (Nondihydropyridine); CarBAMazepine; Cisapride; Clarithromycin; Colchicine; Conivaptan; Corticosteroids (Orally Inhaled); Crizotinib; CycloSPORINE (Systemic); CYP2D6 Substrates; CYP3A4 Substrates; Dabigatran Etexilate; Dienogest; Digoxin; Dofetilide; Dronedarone; Dutasteride; Efavirenz; Enfuvirtide; Enzalutamide; Eplerenone; Ergot Derivatives; Everolimus; FentaNYL; Fesoterodine; Fluticasone (Nasal); Fluticasone (Oral Inhalation); GuanFACINE; Halofantrine; Ibrutinib; Iloperidone; Imatinib; Itraconazole; Ivabradine; Ivacaftor; Ixabepilone; Ketoconazole (Systemic); Lacosamide; Lapatinib; Levomilnacipran; Lomitapide; Lovastatin; Lumefantrine; Lurasidone; Macitentan; Maraviroc; Meperidine; MethylPREDNISolone; Midazolam; Mifepristone; Nefazodone; Nilotinib; Nisoldipine; Ospemifene; OxyCODONE; Paricalcitol; PAZOPanib; P-glycoprotein/ABCB1 Substrates; Pimecrolimus; Pimozide; Pomalidomide; PONATinib; Pravastatin; Propafenone; Protease Inhibitors; Prucalopride; QUEtiapine; QuiNIDine; Ranolazine; Red Yeast Rice; Regorafenib; Repaglinide; Rifabutin; Rilpivirine; Riociguat; Rivaroxaban; RomiDEPsin; Rosuvastatin; Ruxolitinib; Salmeterol; Saxagliptin; Sildenafil; Silodosin; Simeprevir; Simvastatin; SORAfenib; Tacrolimus (Systemic); Tacrolimus (Topical); Tadalafil; Tamsulosin; Temsirolimus; Tenofovir; Ticagrelor; Tofacitinib; Tolterodine; Tolvaptan; Topotecan; Toremifene; TraZODone; Triazolam; Tricyclic Antidepressants; Ulipristal; Vardenafil; Vemurafenib; Vilazodone; VinCRIStine (Liposomal); Zuclopenthixol

The levels/effects of Darunavir may be increased by: Clarithromycin; CycloSPORINE (Systemic); CYP3A4 Inhibitors (Moderate); CYP3A4 Inhibitors (Strong); Dasatinib; Delavirdine; Enfuvirtide; Etravirine; Fusidic Acid (Systemic); Itraconazole; Ketoconazole (Systemic); Luliconazole; Rifabutin; Simeprevir; Tenofovir

Decreased Effect

Darunavir may decrease the levels/effects of: Abacavir; Boceprevir; Clarithromycin; Contraceptives (Estrogens); Delavirdine; Didanosine; Etravirine; Ifosfamide; Meperidine; Methadone; Norethindrone; PARoxetine; Prasugrel; Sertraline; Telaprevir; Theophylline Derivatives; Ticagrelor; Valproic Acid and Derivatives; Voriconazole; Warfarin; Zidovudine

The levels/effects of Darunavir may be decreased by: Boceprevir; Bosentan; CYP3A4 Inducers (Strong); Dabrafenib; Deferasirox; Efavirenz; Fosphenytoin; Garlic; Lopinavir; Mitotane; PHENobarbital; Phenytoin; Rifampin; Saquinavir; St Johns Wort; Telaprevir; Tocilizumab

Ethanol/Nutrition/Herb Interactions

Food: Absorption and bioavailability are increased when administered with food. Management: Take with meals.

Herb/Nutraceutical: St John's wort may decrease the plasma levels of darunavir. Garlic may decrease the serum concentration of darunavir. Management: Taking St John's wort concomitantly with darunavir is contraindicated. Use of garlic supplements with darunavir is not recommended.

Storage/Stability Store at 25°C (77°F); excursions permitted to 15°C to 30°C (59°F to 86°F).

Mechanism of Action Binds to the site of HIV-1 protease activity and inhibits cleavage of viral Gag-Pol polyprotein precursors into individual functional proteins required for infectious HIV. This results in the formation of immature, noninfectious viral particles.

Pharmacodynamics/Kinetics All kinetic parameters derived in the presence of ritonavir coadministration.

Absorption: Increased 30% with food

Protein binding: ~95%; primarily to alpha$_1$ acid glycoprotein (AAG)

Metabolism: Hepatic, via CYP3A4 to minimally-active metabolites

Bioavailability: 82%

Half-life elimination: ~15 hours

Time to peak, plasma: 2.5-4 hours

Excretion: Feces (~80%, 41% as unchanged drug); urine (~14%, 8% as unchanged drug)

Dosage Oral:

Children ≥3 years and Adolescents: **Note:** Coadministration with ritonavir is required; do not exceed the maximum recommended darunavir adult dose (800 mg to 1200 mg daily depending upon indication). Genotypic testing is recommended in therapy-experienced patients.

Treatment-naive patients or treatment-experienced with no darunavir resistance-associated substitutions:

Dosing recommendations based on body weight using the oral suspension:

≥10 kg to <11 kg: 350 mg once daily with ritonavir 64 mg once daily

≥11 kg to <12 kg: 385 mg once daily with ritonavir 64 mg once daily

≥12 kg to <13 kg: 420 mg once daily with ritonavir 80 mg once daily

≥13 kg to <14 kg: 455 mg once daily with ritonavir 80 mg once daily

≥14 kg to <15 kg: 490 mg once daily with ritonavir 96 mg once daily

Dosing recommendations based on body weight using the oral solution or tablets:

≥15 kg to <30 kg: 600 mg once daily with ritonavir 100 mg once daily

≥30 kg to <40 kg: 675 mg once daily with ritonavir 100 mg once daily

≥40 kg: 800 mg once daily with ritonavir 100 mg once daily

Treatment-experienced patients with at ≥1 darunavir resistance-associated substitution:

Dosing recommendations based on body weight using the oral suspension:

≥10 kg to <11 kg: 200 mg twice daily with ritonavir 32 mg twice daily

≥11 kg to <12 kg: 220 mg twice daily with ritonavir 32 mg twice daily

≥12 kg to <13 kg: 240 mg twice daily with ritonavir 40 mg twice daily

≥13 kg to <14 kg: 260 mg twice daily with ritonavir 40 mg twice daily

≥14 kg to <15 kg: 280 mg twice daily with ritonavir 48 mg twice daily

Dosing recommendations based on body weight using the oral solution or tablets:

≥15 kg to <30 kg: 375 mg twice daily with ritonavir 48 mg twice daily

≥30 kg to <40 kg: 450 mg twice daily with ritonavir 60 mg twice daily

≥40 kg: 600 mg twice daily with ritonavir 100 mg twice daily

Adults:

Therapy-naive: 800 mg once daily; coadministration with ritonavir 100 mg once daily is required. **Note:** Recommended (with ritonavir) as a first-line therapy with tenofovir/emtricitabine in antiretroviral naïve patients (DHHS, 2013).

Therapy-experienced: **Note:** Genotypic testing is recommended in therapy experienced patients.

With no darunavir resistance-associated substitutions: 800 mg once daily; coadministration with ritonavir 100 mg once daily is required

With ≥1 darunavir resistance-associated substitution: 600 mg twice daily; coadministration with ritonavir 100 mg twice daily is required

If genotypic testing is not possible: 600 mg twice daily, coadministered with ritonavir 100 mg twice daily

Dosage adjustment for toxicity:

Severe rash: Discontinue treatment

New or worsening liver dysfunction: Consider interrupting or discontinuing treatment

Dosage adjustment in renal impairment:

Cl_{cr} ≥30 mL/minute: No dosage adjustment provided in manufacturer's labeling; however, need for adjustment not expected based on pharmacokinetic data.

Cl_{cr} <30 mL/minute: No dosage adjustment provided in manufacturer's labeling (has not been studied).

Dosage adjustment in hepatic impairment:

Mild-to-moderate impairment (Child-Pugh class A or B): No dosage adjustment necessary

Severe impairment (Child-Pugh class C): Use not recommended (contraindicated in Canadian labeling).

Dietary Considerations Absorption increased with food. Take with meals.

Administration Coadministration with ritonavir and food is required (bioavailability is increased). Shake suspension prior to each dose; use provided oral dosing syringe to measure dose.

Monitoring Parameters Viral load, CD4, serum glucose; transaminase levels prior to and during therapy (increase monitoring in patients at risk for liver impairment), cholesterol, triglycerides

Dosage Forms Excipient information presented when available (limited, particularly for generics); consult specific product labeling.

Suspension, Oral:

Prezista: 100 mg/mL (200 mL) [contains methylparaben sodium; strawberry cream flavor]

Tablet, Oral:

Prezista: 75 mg, 150 mg

Prezista: 400 mg, 600 mg [contains fd&c yellow #6 (sunset yellow)]

Prezista: 800 mg

◆ **Darunavir Ethanolate** *see* Darunavir *on page 547*

Dasatinib (da SA ti nib)

Brand Names: U.S. Sprycel

Brand Names: Canada Sprycel®

Index Terms BMS-354825

Pharmacologic Category Antineoplastic Agent, Tyrosine Kinase Inhibitor

Use Treatment of chronic myelogenous leukemia (CML) in chronic, accelerated or blast (myeloid or lymphoid) phase resistant or intolerant to prior therapy (including imatinib); treatment of newly-diagnosed Philadelphia chromosome-positive (Ph+) CML in chronic phase; treatment of Philadelphia chromosome-positive (Ph+) acute lymphoblastic leukemia (ALL) resistant or intolerant to prior therapy

Unlabeled Use Post-stem cell transplant (allogeneic) follow-up treatment of CML; treatment of gastrointestinal stromal tumor (GIST)

Pregnancy Risk Factor D

Pregnancy Considerations Animal reproduction studies have demonstrated fetal abnormalities (skeletal malformations, reduced ossification, edema, microhepatia) and fetal death. May cause fetal harm if administered to a pregnant woman. Not recommended for use during pregnancy or if contemplating pregnancy. Effective contraception is recommended for men and women of childbearing potential. Pregnant women are advised to avoid contact with crushed or broken tablets.

Breast-Feeding Considerations Due to the potential for serious adverse reactions in the nursing infant, the decision to discontinue dasatinib or to discontinue breast-feeding should take into account the benefits of treatment to the mother.

Contraindications There are no contraindications listed within the FDA-approved manufacturer's labeling.

Canadian labeling: Hypersensitivity to dasatinib or any other component of the formulation

Warnings/Precautions Hazardous agent - use appropriate precautions for handling and disposal (NIOSH, 2012). Severe dose-related bone marrow suppression (thrombocytopenia, neutropenia, anemia) is associated with treatment; dosage adjustment or temporary interruption may be required for severe myelosuppression; the incidence of myelosuppression is higher in patients with advanced CML and Ph+ ALL. Fatal intracranial hemorrhage has been reported in association with dasatinib use; monitor blood counts. Severe hemorrhage (including CNS, GI) may occur due to thrombocytopenia; in addition to thrombocytopenia, dasatinib may also cause platelet dysfunction. Use caution with patients taking anticoagulants or medications interfering with platelet function; not studied in clinical trials. Avoid concomitant use with CYP3A4 inducers and inhibitors; if concomitant use cannot be avoided, consider dasatinib dosage adjustments.

Cardiomyopathy, diastolic dysfunction, heart failure (congestive), left ventricular dysfunction, and MI have been reported; monitor for signs and symptoms of cardiac dysfunction. Fluid retention, including pleural and pericardial effusions, severe ascites, severe pulmonary edema, and generalized edema were reported; may be dose-related. A chest x-ray is recommended for symptoms suggestive of effusion (dyspnea or dry cough). Utilizing once-daily dosing is associated with a decreased frequency of fluid retention. The risk for pleural effusion is increased in patients with hypertension, prior cardiac history and a twice a day administration schedule; interrupt treatment for grade ≥2 effusion; may consider reinitiating at a reduced dose after resolution (Quintás-Cardama, 2007). Use caution in patients where fluid accumulation may be poorly tolerated, such as in cardiovascular disease (HF or hypertension) and pulmonary disease. Elderly may be more likely to experience dyspnea and fluid retention. Pulmonary arterial hypertension (PAH) has been reported with use, sometimes after >12 months of therapy. Evaluate for underlying cardiopulmonary disease prior to therapy initiation and during therapy; evaluate and rule out alternative etiologies in patients with symptoms suggestive of PAH (eg, dyspnea, fatigue) and interrupt therapy if symptoms are severe. Discontinue permanently with confirmed PAH diagnosis.

May prolong QT interval; use caution in patients at risk for QT prolongation, including patients with long QT syndrome; patients taking antiarrhythmic medications or other medications that lead to QT prolongation or potassium-wasting diuretics; patients with cumulative high-dose anthracycline therapy, and conditions which cause hypokalemia or hypomagnesemia. Correct hypokalemia and hypomagnesemia prior to initiation of therapy. Use caution with hepatic impairment due to extensive hepatic metabolism; patients with ALT or AST >2.5 times the upper limit of normal (ULN) or total bilirubin >2 times the ULN were excluded from clinical trials.

Adverse Reactions

≥10%:

Central nervous system: Headache (12% to 33%), fatigue (8% to 26%)

Dermatologic: Skin rash (11% to 21%; includes drug eruption, erythema, erythema multiforme, erythematous rash, erythrosis, exfoliative rash, follicular rash, heat rash, macular rash, maculopapular rash, milia, papular rash, pruritic rash, pustular rash, skin exfoliation, skin irritation, urticaria vesiculosa, vesicular rash)

Endocrine & metabolic: Fluid retention (21% to 42%; grades 3/4: 1% to 8%), hypophosphatemia (grades 3/4: 5% to 18%), hypokalemia (grades 3/4: ≤15%), hypocalcemia (grades 3/4: <1% to 12%)

Gastrointestinal: Diarrhea (18% to 31%; grades 3/4: ≤5%), nausea (9% to 24%), vomiting (5% to 16%), abdominal pain (3% to 12%)

Hematologic & oncologic: Thrombocytopenia (grades 3/4: 19% to 85%), neutropenia (grades 3/4: 22% to 79%), anemia (grades 3/4: 11% to 74%), hemorrhage (6% to 26%; grades 3/4: 1% to 9%), febrile neutropenia (4% to 12%; grades 3/4: 1% to 12%)

Infection: Increased susceptibility to infection (9% to 14%; includes bacterial, fungal, viral)

Local: Localized edema (superficial; 3% to 21%; grades 3/4: ≤1%)

Neuromuscular & skeletal: Musculoskeletal pain (≤22%), myalgia (3% to 13%), arthralgia (≤12%)

Respiratory: Pleural effusion (12% to 24%; grades 3/4: ≤11%), dyspnea (3% to 24%; grades 3/4: 2% to 3%), cough (≥10%)

Miscellaneous: Fever (5% to 18%)

1% to <10%:

Cardiovascular: Cardiac disease (≤4%; includes cardiac failure, cardiomyopathy, diastolic dysfunction, ejection fraction decreased, left ventricular dysfunction, ventricular failure), edema (generalized; ≤4%), pericardial effusion (≤3%; grades 3/4: ≤1%), prolonged Q-T interval on ECG (1%), cardiac arrhythmia, chest pain, flushing, hypertension, palpitations, tachycardia

Central nervous system: Central nervous system toxicity (bleeding; ≤3%; grades 3/4: ≤3%), chills, depression, dizziness, drowsiness, insomnia, myasthenia, neuropathy, pain, peripheral neuropathy

Dermatologic: Acne vulgaris, alopecia, dermatitis, eczema, hyperhidrosis, pruritus, urticaria, xeroderma

Endocrine & metabolic: Weight gain, weight loss

Gastrointestinal: Gastrointestinal hemorrhage (2% to 9%; grades 3/4: 1% to 7%), abdominal distention, anorexia, change in appetite, colitis (including neutropenic colitis), constipation, dysgeusia, dyspepsia, enterocolitis, gastritis, mucositis, stomatitis

Hematologic & oncologic: Bruise, pancytopenia

Hepatic: Increased serum bilirubin (grades 3/4: ≤6%), increased serum ALT (grades 3/4: ≤5%), increased serum AST (grades 3/4: ≤4%), ascites (≤1%)

Infection: Herpes virus infection, sepsis

Neuromuscular & skeletal: Muscle spasm (5%), myositis (4%), stiffness, weakness

Ophthalmic: Blurred vision, decreased visual acuity, dry eye syndrome, visual disturbance

Otic: Tinnitus

Renal: Increased serum creatinine (grades 3/4: ≤8%), hyperuricemia

Respiratory: Pulmonary edema (≤4%; grades 3/4: ≤3%), pulmonary hypertension (2%; grades 3/4: <1%), pneumonia (bacterial, viral, or fungal), pneumonitis, pulmonary infiltrates, upper respiratory tract infection

Miscellaneous: Soft tissue injury (oral)

<1% (Limited to important or life-threatening): Abnormal platelet aggregation, acute coronary syndrome, acute respiratory distress, amnesia, anal fissure, angina pectoris, asthma, atrial fibrillation, atrial flutter, bullous skin disease, cardiomegaly, cerebrovascular accident, cholecystitis, cholestasis, conjunctivitis, cor pulmonale, cranial nerve palsy (facial), decreased libido, deep vein thrombosis, dermal ulcer, dyschromia, dysphagia, embolism, erythema nodosum, esophagitis, gynecomastia, hematoma, hematuria, hemorrhage (ocular), hepatitis, hypersensitivity, hypoalbuminemia, hypotension, increased pulmonary artery pressure, inflammation (panniculitis), interstitial pulmonary disease, intestinal obstruction, intolerance to temperature, livedo reticularis, myocardial infarction, myocarditis, optic neuritis, palmar-plantar erythrodysesthesia, pancreatitis, pericarditis, polyuria, proteinuria, pulmonary embolism, pure red cell aplasia, renal failure, rhabdomyolysis, seizure, skin photosensitivity, Sweet's syndrome, syncope, tendonitis, thrombophlebitis, thrombosis, transient ischemic attacks, tumor lysis syndrome, upper gastrointestinal tract ulcer, ventricular arrhythmia, ventricular tachycardia

Drug Interactions

Metabolism/Transport Effects **Substrate** of CYP3A4 (major); **Note:** Assignment of Major/Minor substrate status based on clinically relevant drug interaction potential; **Inhibits** CYP3A4 (weak)

Avoid Concomitant Use

Avoid concomitant use of Dasatinib with any of the following: BCG; CloZAPine; Conivaptan; Fusidic Acid (Systemic); H2-Antagonists; Natalizumab; Pimecrolimus; Pimozide; Proton Pump Inhibitors; St Johns Wort; Tacrolimus (Topical); Tofacitinib; Vaccines (Live)

Increased Effect/Toxicity

Dasatinib may increase the levels/effects of: Acetaminophen; Agents with Antiplatelet Properties; Anticoagulants; ARIPiprazole; CloZAPine; CYP3A4 Substrates; Dofetilide; Highest Risk QTc-Prolonging Agents; Leflunomide; Lomitapide; Moderate Risk QTc-Prolonging Agents; Natalizumab; Pimozide; Tofacitinib; Vaccines (Live); Vitamin K Antagonists

The levels/effects of Dasatinib may be increased by: Acetaminophen; Conivaptan; CYP3A4 Inhibitors (Moderate); CYP3A4 Inhibitors (Strong); Denosumab; Fusidic Acid (Systemic); Ivacaftor; Luliconazole; Mifepristone; Pimecrolimus; Roflumilast; Simeprevir; Tacrolimus (Topical); Trastuzumab

Decreased Effect

Dasatinib may decrease the levels/effects of: BCG; Cardiac Glycosides; Coccidioidin Skin Test; Sipuleucel-T; Vaccines (Inactivated); Vaccines (Live); Vitamin K Antagonists

The levels/effects of Dasatinib may be decreased by: Antacids; Bosentan; CYP3A4 Inducers (Strong); Dabrafenib; Deferasirox; Echinacea; H2-Antagonists; Proton Pump Inhibitors; St Johns Wort; Tocilizumab

Ethanol/Nutrition/Herb Interactions

Food: Dasatinib serum concentrations may be increased when taken with grapefruit or grapefruit juice. Management: Avoid concurrent use.

Herb/Nutraceutical: Avoid St John's wort (may increase metabolism and decrease dasatinib plasma concentration).

Storage/Stability Store at 25°C (77°F); excursions permitted to 15°C to 30°C (59°F to 86°F).

Mechanism of Action BCR-ABL tyrosine kinase inhibitor; targets most imatinib-resistant BCR-ABL mutations (except the T315I and F317V mutants) by distinctly binding to active and inactive ABL-kinase. Kinase inhibition halts proliferation of leukemia cells. Also inhibits SRC family (including SRC, LKC, YES, FYN); c-KIT, EPHA2 and platelet derived growth factor receptor (PDGFRβ)

Pharmacodynamics/Kinetics

Distribution: 2505 L

Protein binding: Dasatinib: 96%; metabolite (active): 93%

Metabolism: Hepatic (extensive); metabolized by CYP3A4 (primarily), flavin-containing mono-oxygenase-3 (FOM-3) and uridine diphosphate-glucuronosyltransferase (UGT) to an active metabolite and other inactive metabolites (the active metabolite plays only a minor role in the pharmacology of dasatinib)

Half-life elimination: Terminal: 3-5 hours

Time to peak, plasma: 0.5-6 hours

Excretion: Feces (~85%, 19% as unchanged drug); urine (~4%, 0.1% as unchanged drug)

Dosage Oral: Adults: **Note:** The effect of discontinuation after complete cytogenetic remission is achieved has not been studied.

Chronic myelogenous leukemia (CML), Philadelphia chromosome-positive (Ph+), newly-diagnosed in chronic phase: 100 mg once daily until disease progression or unacceptable toxicity. In clinical studies, a dose escalation to 140 mg once daily was allowed in patients not achieving hematologic or cytogenetic response at recommended initial dosage.

CML, Ph+, resistant or intolerant:

Chronic phase: 100 mg once daily until disease progression or unacceptable toxicity. In clinical studies, a dose escalation to 140 mg once daily was allowed in patients not achieving hematologic or cytogenetic response at recommended initial dosage.

Accelerated or blast phase: 140 mg once daily until disease progression or unacceptable toxicity. In clinical studies, a dose escalation to 180 mg once daily was allowed in patients not achieving hematologic or cytogenetic response at recommended initial dosage.

Acute lymphoblastic lymphoma (ALL), Ph+: 140 mg once daily until disease progression or unacceptable toxicity. In clinical studies, a dose escalation to 180 mg once daily was allowed in patients not achieving hematologic or cytogenetic response at recommended initial dosage.

Dosage adjustment for concomitant CYP3A4 inhibitors: Avoid concomitant administration with strong CYP3A4 inhibitors (eg, clarithromycin, itraconazole, ketoconazole, nefazodone, protease inhibitors, telithromycin, voriconazole, grapefruit juice); if concomitant administration with a strong CYP3A4 inhibitor cannot be avoided, consider reducing dasatinib from 100 mg once daily to 20 mg once daily **or** from 140 mg once daily to 40 mg once daily, with careful monitoring. If reduced dose is not tolerated, the strong CYP3A4 inhibitor must be discontinued or dasatinib therapy temporarily held until concomitant inhibitor use has ceased. When a strong CYP3A4 inhibitor is discontinued, allow a washout period (~1 week) prior to adjusting dasatinib dose upward.

Dosage adjustment for concomitant CYP3A4 inducers: Avoid concomitant administration with strong CYP3A4 inducers (eg, carbamazepine, dexamethasone, phenobarbital, phenytoin, rifampin, St John's wort); if concomitant administration with a strong CYP3A4 inducer cannot be avoided, consider increasing the dasatinib dose with careful monitoring.

Dosage adjustment for toxicity:

Hematologic toxicity:

Chronic phase CML (100 mg daily starting dose): For ANC <500/mm^3 or platelets <50,000/mm^3, withhold treatment until ANC ≥1000/mm^3 and platelets ≥50,000/mm^3; then resume treatment at the original starting dose if recovery occurs in ≤7 days. If platelets <25,000/mm^3 or recurrence of ANC <500/mm^3 for >7 days, withhold treatment until ANC ≥1000/mm^3 and platelets ≥50,000/mm^3; then resume treatment at 80 mg once daily (second episode). For third episode, further reduce dose to 50 mg once daily (for newly-diagnosed patients) or discontinue (for patients resistant or intolerant to prior therapy)

Accelerated or blast phase CML and Ph+ ALL (140 mg once daily starting dose): For ANC <500/mm^3 or platelets <10,000/mm^3, if cytopenia unrelated to leukemia, withhold treatment until ANC ≥1000/mm^3 and platelets ≥20,000/mm^3; then resume treatment at the original starting dose. If cytopenia recurs, withhold treatment until ANC ≥1000/mm^3 and platelets ≥20,000/mm^3; then resume treatment at 100 mg once daily (second episode) or 80 mg once daily (third episode). For cytopenias related to leukemia (confirm with marrow aspirate or biopsy), consider dose escalation to 180 mg once daily.

Nonhematologic toxicity: Withhold treatment until toxicity improvement or resolution; if appropriate, resume treatment at a reduced dose based on the event severity. Fluid retention is managed with diuretics and supportive care. Effusions may require diuretics and/or dose interruption. Corticosteroids (eg, prednisone 20 mg/day for 3 days) may be considered for pleural or pericardial effusion with significant symptoms (hold dasatinib and reinitiate at a decreased dose when effusion resolves). Rash may be managed with steroids (topical or systemic), treatment interruption, dose reduction, or discontinuation (NCCN CML guidelines v.2.2013). Discontinue with confirmed pulmonary arterial hypertension.

Dosage adjustment for renal impairment: No dosage adjustment provided in the manufacturer's labeling. However, <4% of dasatinib and metabolites are renally excreted.

Dosage adjustment for hepatic impairment: No dosage adjustment necessary; use with caution.

Dietary Considerations May be taken without regard to food. Avoid grapefruit juice.

Administration Administer once daily (morning or evening). May be taken without regard to food. Swallow whole; do not break, crush, or chew tablets. Take with a meal or with a large glass of water if GI upset occurs.

Hazardous agent; use appropriate precautions for handling and disposal (NIOSH, 2012).

Monitoring Parameters CBC with differential (weekly for 2 months, then monthly or as clinically necessary); bone marrow biopsy; liver function tests, electrolytes including calcium, phosphorus, magnesium; monitor for fluid retention; ECG monitoring if at risk for QT_c prolongation; chest x-ray is recommended for symptoms suggestive of pleural effusion (eg, cough, dyspnea)

Thyroid function testing recommendations (Hamnvik, 2011):

Pre-existing levothyroxine therapy: Obtain baseline TSH levels, then monitor every 4 weeks until levels and levothyroxine dose are stable, then monitor every 2 months

Without pre-existing thyroid hormone replacement: TSH at baseline, then monthly for 4 months, then every 2-3 months

Additional Information Oncology Comment: In a dose finding study in chronic-phase CML, dasatinib 100 mg once daily provided comparable efficacy to the original FDA-approved dose of 70 mg twice daily. The 100 mg once daily dose was better tolerated (lower rates of pleural effusion and grades 3/4 thrombocytopenia), required fewer dose reductions, and fewer dosing interruptions or discontinuations (Shah, 2008).

Dosage Forms Excipient information presented when available (limited, particularly for generics); consult specific product labeling.

Tablet, Oral:

Sprycel: 20 mg, 50 mg, 70 mg, 80 mg, 100 mg, 140 mg

Extemporaneous Preparations Hazardous agent: Use appropriate precautions for handling and disposal.

An oral suspension may be prepared by dissolving dasatinib tablet(s) for one dose in 30 mL chilled orange or apple juice (without preservatives). After 5 minutes, swirl the contents for 3 seconds and repeat the process every 5 minutes for a total of 20 minutes following addition of tablet(s). Minimize time between end of 20 minutes and administration since suspension will taste more bitter if allowed to stand longer. Swirl contents of container one last time, then administer immediately. To ensure the full dose is administered, rinse container with 15 mL juice and administer residue. May be administered orally (or by nasogastric tube). Discard any unused portion after 60 minutes.

Sprycel® data on file, Bristol-Myers Squibb

- **Dasetta 1/35** *see* Ethinyl Estradiol and Norethindrone *on page 793*
- **Dasetta 7/7/7** *see* Ethinyl Estradiol and Norethindrone *on page 793*
- **Daunomycin** *see* DAUNOrubicin (Conventional) *on page 553*
- **DAUNOrubicin Citrate** *see* DAUNOrubicin (Liposomal) *on page 555*
- **DAUNOrubicin Citrate (Liposomal)** *see* DAUNOrubicin (Liposomal) *on page 555*
- **DAUNOrubicin Citrate Liposome** *see* DAUNOrubicin (Liposomal) *on page 555*

DAUNOrubicin (Conventional)

(daw noe ROO bi sin con VEN sha nal)

Brand Names: U.S. Cerubidine

Brand Names: Canada Cerubidine®

Index Terms Conventional Daunomycin; Daunomycin; DAUNOrubicin Hydrochloride; Rubidomycin Hydrochloride

Pharmacologic Category Antineoplastic Agent, Anthracycline

Use Treatment of acute lymphocytic leukemia (ALL) and acute myeloid leukemia (AML)

Pregnancy Risk Factor D

Pregnancy Considerations Adverse events have been observed in animal reproduction studies. Daunorubicin crosses the placenta. Women of reproductive potential should avoid pregnancy.

Breast-Feeding Considerations It is not known if daunorubicin is excreted into breast milk. Due to the potential for serious adverse reactions in the nursing infant, the manufacturer recommends a decision be made whether to discontinue nursing or to discontinue the drug, taking into account the importance of treatment to the mother.

Contraindications Hypersensitivity to daunorubicin or any component of the formulation

Warnings/Precautions Hazardous agent - use appropriate precautions for handling and disposal (NIOSH, 2012). **[U.S. Boxed Warning]: Potent vesicant; if extravasation occurs, severe local tissue damage leading to ulceration and necrosis, and pain may occur. For I.V. administration only. NOT for I.M. or SubQ administration. Administer through a rapidly flowing I.V. line.** Ensure proper needle or catheter placement prior to and during infusion. Avoid extravasation. **[U.S. Boxed Warning]: Severe bone marrow suppression may occur; may lead to infection or hemorrhage.**

[U.S. Boxed Warning]: May cause cumulative, dose-related myocardial toxicity; may lead to heart failure. The incidence of irreversible myocardial toxicity increases as the total cumulative (lifetime) dosages approach 550 mg/m^2 in adults, 400 mg/m^2 in adults receiving chest radiation, 300 mg/m^2 in children >2 years of age, or 10 mg/kg in children <2 years of age. Total cumulative dose should take into account previous or concomitant treatment with cardiotoxic agents or irradiation of chest. Although the risk increases with cumulative dose, irreversible cardiotoxicity may occur at any dose level. Cardiotoxicity may be delayed. Patients with preexisting heart disease, hypertension, concurrent administration of other antineoplastic agents, prior or concurrent chest irradiation, advanced age; and infants and children are at increased risk. Monitor left ventricular (LV) function (baseline and periodic) with ECHO or MUGA scan; monitor ECG.

[U.S. Boxed Warning]: Dosage reductions are recommended in patients with renal or hepatic impairment; significant impairment may result in increased toxicities. Use with caution in patients who have received radiation therapy; reduce dosage in patients who are receiving radiation therapy simultaneously. Secondary leukemias may occur when used with combination chemotherapy or radiation therapy. **[U.S. Boxed Warning]: Should be administered under the supervision of an experienced cancer chemotherapy physician.**

Adverse Reactions

>10%:

Cardiovascular: Transient ECG abnormalities (supraventricular tachycardia, S-T wave changes, atrial or ventricular extrasystoles); generally asymptomatic and self-limiting. CHF, dose related, may be delayed for 7-8 years after treatment.

Dermatologic: Alopecia (reversible), radiation recall

Gastrointestinal: Mild nausea or vomiting, stomatitis

Genitourinary: Discoloration of urine (red)

Hematologic: Myelosuppression (onset: 7 days; nadir: 10-14 days; recovery: 21-28 days), primarily leukopenia; thrombocytopenia and anemia

1% to 10%:

Dermatologic: Skin "flare" at injection site; discoloration of saliva, sweat, or tears

Endocrine & metabolic: Hyperuricemia

Gastrointestinal: Abdominal pain, GI ulceration, diarrhea

<1% (Limited to important or life-threatening): Anaphylactoid reaction, arrhythmia, bilirubin increased, cardiomyopathy, hepatitis, infertility; local (cellulitis, pain, thrombophlebitis at injection site); MI, myocarditis, neutropenic typhlitis, pericarditis, secondary leukemia, skin rash, sterility, systemic hypersensitivity (including urticaria, pruritus, angioedema, dysphagia, dyspnea); transaminases increased

Drug Interactions

Metabolism/Transport Effects Substrate of P-glycoprotein

Avoid Concomitant Use

Avoid concomitant use of DAUNOrubicin (Conventional) with any of the following: BCG; CloZAPine; Natalizumab; Pimecrolimus; Tacrolimus (Topical); Tofacitinib; Vaccines (Live)

Increased Effect/Toxicity

DAUNOrubicin (Conventional) may increase the levels/effects of: CloZAPine; Leflunomide; Natalizumab; Tofacitinib; Vaccines (Live)

The levels/effects of DAUNOrubicin (Conventional) may be increased by: Bevacizumab; Cyclophosphamide; Denosumab; P-glycoprotein/ABCB1 Inhibitors; Pimecrolimus; Roflumilast; Tacrolimus (Topical); Taxane Derivatives; Trastuzumab

Decreased Effect

DAUNOrubicin (Conventional) may decrease the levels/effects of: BCG; Cardiac Glycosides; Coccidioidin Skin Test; Sipuleucel-T; Vaccines (Inactivated); Vaccines (Live)

The levels/effects of DAUNOrubicin (Conventional) may be decreased by: Cardiac Glycosides; Echinacea; P-glycoprotein/ABCB1 Inducers

Ethanol/Nutrition/Herb Interactions Ethanol: Avoid ethanol (due to GI irritation).

Preparation for Administration Hazardous agent; use appropriate precautions for handling and disposal (NIOSH, 2012). Dilute vials of powder for injection with 4 mL SWFI for a final concentration of 5 mg/mL. May further dilute in 100 mL D_5W or NS.

Storage/Stability Store intact vials of powder for injection at room temperature of 15°C to 30°C (59°F to 86°F); intact vials of solution for injection should be refrigerated at 2°C to 8°C (36°F to 46°F). Protect from light. Reconstituted solution is stable for 4 days at 15°C to 25°C. Further dilution in D_5W, LR, or NS is stable at room temperature (25°C) for up to 4 weeks if protected from light.

Mechanism of Action Inhibition of DNA and RNA synthesis by intercalation between DNA base pairs and by steric obstruction. Daunomycin intercalates at points of local uncoiling of the double helix. Although the exact mechanism is unclear, it appears that direct binding to DNA (intercalation) and inhibition of DNA repair (topoisomerase II inhibition) result in blockade of DNA and RNA synthesis and fragmentation of DNA.

Pharmacodynamics/Kinetics

Distribution: Many body tissues, particularly the liver, kidneys, lung, spleen, and heart; not into CNS; V_d: 40 L/kg

Metabolism: Primarily hepatic to daunorubicinol (active), then to inactive aglycones, conjugated sulfates, and glucuronides

Half-life elimination: Distribution: 2 minutes; Elimination: 14-20 hours; Terminal: 18.5 hours; Daunorubicinol plasma half-life: 24-48 hours

Excretion: Feces (40%); urine (~25% as unchanged drug and metabolites)

Dosage I.V. (refer to individual protocols):

Children: **Note:** Cumulative dose should not exceed 300 mg/m^2 in children >2 years or 10 mg/kg in children <2 years of age; maximum cumulative doses for younger children are unknown.

- Children <2 years or BSA <0.5 m^2: ALL combination therapy: 1 mg/kg/dose per protocol, with frequency dependent on regimen employed
- Children ≥2 years and BSA ≥0.5 m^2:
  - ALL combination therapy: Remission induction: 25 mg/m^2 on day 1 every week for up to 4-6 cycles
  - AML combination therapy: Induction: I.V. continuous infusion: 30-60 mg/m^2/day on days 1-3 of cycle

Adults: **Note:** Cumulative dose should not exceed 550 mg/m^2 in adults without risk factors for cardiotoxicity and should not exceed 400 mg/m^2 in adults receiving chest irradiation.

- Range: 30-60 mg/m^2/day for 3 days, repeat dose in 3-4 weeks
- ALL combination therapy: 45 mg/m^2/day for 3 days
- AML combination therapy:
  - Adults <60 years: Induction: 45 mg/m^2/day for 3 days of the first course of induction therapy; subsequent courses: 45 mg/m^2/day for 2 days
  - Adults ≥60 years: Induction: 30 mg/m^2/day for 3 days of the first course of induction therapy; subsequent courses: 30 mg/m^2/day for 2 days

Dosing adjustment in renal impairment:

The FDA-approved labeling recommends the following adjustment: S_{cr} >3 mg/dL: Administer 50% of normal dose

The following guidelines have been used by some clinicians (Aronoff, 2007):

- Children:
  - Cl_{cr} <30 mL/minute: Administer 50% of dose
  - Hemodialysis/continuous ambulatory peritoneal dialysis (CAPD): Administer 50% of dose
- Adults: No adjustment recommended

Dosing adjustment in hepatic impairment:

The FDA-approved labeling recommends the following adjustments:

- Serum bilirubin 1.2-3 mg/dL: Administer 75% of dose
- Serum bilirubin >3 mg/dL: Administer 50% of dose

The following guidelines have been used by some clinicians (Floyd, 2006):

- Serum bilirubin 1.2-3 mg/dL: Administer 75% of dose
- Serum bilirubin 3.1-5 mg/dL: Administer 50% of dose
- Serum bilirubin >5 mg/dL: Avoid use

Dosing in obesity: *ASCO Guidelines for appropriate chemotherapy dosing in obese adults with cancer:* Utilize patient's actual body weight (full weight) for calculation of body surface area- or weight-based dosing, particularly when the intent of therapy is curative; manage regimen-related toxicities in the same manner as for nonobese patients; if a dose reduction is utilized due to toxicity, consider resumption of full weight-based dosing with subsequent cycles, especially if cause of toxicity (eg, hepatic or renal impairment) is resolved (Griggs, 2012).

Administration For I.V. administration only. Do not administer I.M. or SubQ. Administer as slow I.V. push over 1-5 minutes into the tubing of a rapidly infusing I.V. solution of D_5W or NS or may dilute further and infuse over 15-30 minutes.

Vesicant; ensure proper needle or catheter placement prior to and during infusion; avoid extravasation.

Extravasation management: If extravasation occurs, stop infusion immediately and disconnect (leave cannula/needle in place); gently aspirate extravasated solution (do **NOT** flush the line); remove needle/cannula; elevate extremity. Initiate antidote (dexrazoxane or dimethyl sulfate [DMSO]). Apply dry cold compresses for 20 minutes 4 times daily for 1-2 days (Perez Fidalgo, 2012); withhold cooling beginning 15 minutes before dexrazoxane infusion; continue withholding cooling until 15 minutes after infusion is completed. Topical DMSO should not be administered in combination with dexrazoxane; may lessen dexrazoxane efficacy.

Dexrazoxane: Adults: 1000 mg/m^2 (maximum dose: 2000 mg) I.V. (administer in a large vein remote from site of extravasation) over 1-2 hours days 1 and 2, then 500 mg/m^2 (maximum dose: 1000 mg) I.V. over 1-2 hours day 3; begin within 6 hours of extravasation. Day 2 and day 3 doses should be administered at approximately the same time (± 3 hours) as the dose on day 1 (Mouridsen, 2007; Perez Fidalgo, 2012). **Note:** Reduce dexrazoxane dose by 50% in patients with moderate to severe renal impairment (Cl_{cr} <40 mL/minute).

DMSO: Children and Adults: Apply topically to a region covering twice the affected area every 8 hours for 7 days; begin within 10 minutes of extravasation; do not cover with a dressing (Perez Fidalgo, 2012).

Hazardous agent; use appropriate precautions for handling and disposal (NIOSH, 2012).

Monitoring Parameters CBC with differential and platelet count, liver function test, ECG, left ventricular ejection function (echocardiography [ECHO] or multigated radionuclide angiography [MUGA] scan), renal function test

Dosage Forms Excipient information presented when available (limited, particularly for generics); consult specific product labeling.

Injectable, Intravenous:
- Generic: 5 mg/mL (4 mL, 10 mL)

Injectable, Intravenous [preservative free]:
- Generic: 5 mg/mL (4 mL)

Solution Reconstituted, Intravenous:
- Cerubidine: 20 mg (1 ea)
- Generic: 20 mg (1 ea)

◆ **DAUNOrubicin Hydrochloride** *see* DAUNOrubicin (Conventional) *on page 553*

DAUNOrubicin (Liposomal)

(daw noe ROO bi sin lye po SO mal)

Brand Names: U.S. DaunoXome

Index Terms DAUNOrubicin Citrate; DAUNOrubicin Citrate (Liposomal); DAUNOrubicin Citrate Liposome; Liposomal DAUNOrubicin

Pharmacologic Category Antineoplastic Agent, Anthracycline

Use First-line treatment of advanced HIV-associated Kaposi's sarcoma (KS)

Pregnancy Risk Factor D

Pregnancy Considerations Adverse events were observed in animal reproduction studies. Women of childbearing potential should avoid becoming pregnant while receiving treatment.

Breast-Feeding Considerations Based on information from daunorubicin (conventional), it is not known if daunorubicin (liposomal) is excreted into breast milk. Daunorubicin (liposomal) is indicated for advanced HIV-associated Kaposi's sarcoma. In the United States, where formula is accessible, affordable, safe, and sustainable, and the risk of infant mortality due to diarrhea and respiratory infections is low, complete avoidance of breast-feeding by HIV-infected women is recommended to decrease potential transmission of HIV (DHHS [perinatal], 2012).

Contraindications Hypersensitivity to daunorubicin citrate (liposomal), daunorubicin, or any component of the formulation

Warnings/Precautions Hazardous agent - use appropriate precautions for handling and disposal (NIOSH, 2012). **[U.S. Boxed Warning]: Monitor cardiac function regularly; especially in patients with previous therapy with high cumulative doses of anthracyclines, cyclophosphamide, or thoracic radiation, or who have pre-existing cardiac disease.** Although the risk increases with cumulative dose, irreversible cardiotoxicity may occur with anthracycline treatment at any dose level. Patients with pre-existing heart disease, hypertension, concurrent administration of other antineoplastic agents, prior or concurrent chest irradiation, and advanced age are at increased risk. Evaluate left ventricular ejection fraction (LVEF) prior to treatment and periodically during treatment.

[U.S. Boxed Warning]: May cause bone marrow suppression, particularly neutropenia; monitor closely for infections. **[U.S. Boxed Warning]: Use caution with hepatic impairment;** dosage reduction is recommended. Use caution with renal impairment; may require dose adjustment. **[U.S. Boxed Warning]: The lipid component is associated with infusion-related reactions (back pain, flushing, chest tightness) usually within the first 5 minutes of infusion;** monitor, interrupt infusion, and resume at reduced infusion rate. Safety and efficacy in children and the elderly have not been established. **[U.S. Boxed Warning]: Should be administered under the supervision of an experienced cancer chemotherapy physician.**

Adverse Reactions

>10%:

Cardiovascular: Edema (11%)

Central nervous system: Fatigue (49%), fever (47%), headache (25%), neutropenic fever (17%)

Gastrointestinal: Nausea (54%), diarrhea (38%), abdominal pain (23%), anorexia (23%), vomiting (23%)

Hematologic: Myelosuppression (onset: 7 days; nadir: 14 days; recovery 21 days), neutropenia (up to 55%; grade 4: 15%), anemia (up to 55%; grade 4: 2%), thrombocytopenia (up to 12%; grade 4: 1%)

Neuromuscular & skeletal: Rigors (19%), back pain (16%), neuropathy (13%)

Respiratory: Cough (28%), dyspnea (26%), rhinitis (12%)

Miscellaneous: Opportunistic infections (40%), allergic reactions (24%), diaphoresis (14%), infusion-related reactions (14%; includes back pain, flushing, chest tightness)

1% to 10%:

Cardiovascular: Chest pain (10%), hypertension (≤5%), palpitation (≤5%), syncope (≤5%), tachycardia (≤5%), LVEF decreased (3%), CHF/cardiomyopathy

Central nervous system: Depression (10%), malaise (10%), dizziness (8%), insomnia (6%), abnormal thinking (≤5%), amnesia (≤5%), anxiety (≤5%), ataxia (≤5%), confusion (≤5%), emotional lability (≤5%), hallucination (≤5%), meningitis (≤5%), seizure (≤5%), somnolence (≤5%)

Dermatologic: Alopecia (8%), pruritus (7%), dry skin (≤5%), folliculitis (≤5%), seborrhea (≤5%)

Endocrine & metabolic: Dehydration (≤5%), hot flashes (≤5%)

Gastrointestinal: Stomatitis (10%), constipation (7%), tenesmus (5%), appetite increased (≤5%), dental caries (≤5%), dysphagia (≤5%), gastrointestinal hemorrhage (≤5%), gastritis (≤5%), gingival bleeding (≤5%), hemorrhoids (≤5%), melena (≤5%), splenomegaly (≤5%), taste perversion (≤5%), xerostomia (≤5%)

Genitourinary: Dysuria (≤5%), nocturia (≤5%), polyuria (≤5%)

Hepatic: Hepatomegaly (≤5%)

Local: Injection site inflammation (≤5%)

Neuromuscular & skeletal: Arthralgia (7%), myalgia (7%), gait abnormal (≤5%), hyperkinesia (≤5%), hypertonia (≤5%), tremor (≤5%)

Ocular: Abnormal vision (5%) conjunctivitis (≤5%), eye pain (≤5%)

Otic: Deafness (≤5%), earache (≤5%), tinnitus (≤5%)

Respiratory: Sinusitis (8%), hemoptysis (≤5%), pulmonary infiltrate (≤5%), sputum increased (≤5%)

Miscellaneous: Flu-like syndrome (5%), hiccups (≤5%), lymphadenopathy (≤5%), thirst (≤5%)

Postmarketing and/or case reports: Angina, atrial fibrillation, cardiac arrest, MI, pericardial effusion, pericardial tamponade, pulmonary hypertension, supraventricular tachycardia, ventricular extrasystoles

Drug Interactions

Metabolism/Transport Effects Substrate of P-glycoprotein

Avoid Concomitant Use

Avoid concomitant use of DAUNOrubicin (Liposomal) with any of the following: BCG; CloZAPine; Natalizumab; Pimecrolimus; Tacrolimus (Topical); Tofacitinib; Vaccines (Live)

Increased Effect/Toxicity

DAUNOrubicin (Liposomal) may increase the levels/effects of: CloZAPine; Leflunomide; Natalizumab; Tofacitinib; Vaccines (Live)

The levels/effects of DAUNOrubicin (Liposomal) may be increased by: Bevacizumab; Cyclophosphamide; Denosumab; P-glycoprotein/ABCB1 Inhibitors; Pimecrolimus; Roflumilast; Tacrolimus (Topical); Taxane Derivatives; Trastuzumab

Decreased Effect

DAUNOrubicin (Liposomal) may decrease the levels/effects of: BCG; Cardiac Glycosides; Coccidioidin Skin Test; Sipuleucel-T; Vaccines (Inactivated); Vaccines (Live)

The levels/effects of DAUNOrubicin (Liposomal) may be decreased by: Cardiac Glycosides; Echinacea; P-glycoprotein/ABCB1 Inducers

Preparation for Administration Hazardous agent; use appropriate precautions for handling and disposal (NIOSH, 2012). Only fluid which may be mixed with DaunoXome® is D_5W. Dilute to a 1:1 solution (1 mg daunorubicin liposomal/mL D_5W). Must **not** be mixed with saline, bacteriostatic agents (such as benzyl alcohol), or any other solution.

Storage/Stability Store intact vials of solution under refrigeration at 2°C to 8°C (36°F to 46°F); do not freeze. Protect from light. Diluted daunorubicin liposomal for infusion may be refrigerated at 2°C to 8°C (36°F to 46°F) for a maximum of 6 hours. Do not use with in-line filters.

Mechanism of Action Liposomes have been shown to penetrate solid tumors more effectively, possibly because of their small size and longer circulation time. Once in tissues, daunorubicin is released. Daunorubicin inhibits DNA and RNA synthesis by intercalation between DNA base pairs and by steric obstruction; and intercalates at points of local uncoiling of the double helix. Although the exact mechanism is unclear, it appears that direct binding to DNA (intercalation) and inhibition of DNA repair (topoisomerase II inhibition) result in blockade of DNA and RNA synthesis and fragmentation of DNA.

Pharmacodynamics/Kinetics

Distribution: V_d: 5-8 L

Metabolism: Similar to daunorubicin, but metabolite plasma levels are low

Half-life elimination: Distribution: 4.4 hours; Terminal: 3-5 hours

Excretion: Primarily feces; some urine

Clearance, plasma: 17.3 mL/minute

Dosage Refer to individual protocols. I.V.:

Adults: HIV-associated KS: 40 mg/m^2 every 2 weeks

Elderly: Use with caution.

Dosage adjustment for toxicity: Withhold treatment for ANC <750/mm^3

Elderly: Use with caution.

Dosing adjustment in renal impairment: Serum creatinine >3 mg/dL: Administer 50% of normal dose

Dosing adjustment in hepatic impairment:

Bilirubin 1.2-3 mg/dL: Administer 75% of normal dose

Bilirubin >3 mg/dL: Administer 50% of normal dose

Dosing in obesity: *ASCO Guidelines for appropriate chemotherapy dosing in obese adults with cancer:* Utilize patient's actual body weight (full weight) for calculation of body surface area- or weight-based dosing, particularly when the intent of therapy is curative; manage regimen-related toxicities in the same manner as for nonobese patients; if a dose reduction is utilized due to toxicity, consider resumption of full weight-based dosing with subsequent cycles, especially if cause of toxicity (eg, hepatic or renal impairment) is resolved (Griggs, 2012).

Administration Infuse over 1 hour; do not mix with other drugs. Avoid extravasation.

Hazardous agent; use appropriate precautions for handling and disposal (NIOSH, 2012).

Monitoring Parameters CBC with differential and platelets (prior to each dose), liver function tests, renal function tests; evaluate cardiac function (baseline left ventricular ejection fraction [LVEF] prior to treatment initiation; repeat LVEF at total cumulative doses of 320 mg/m^2, and every 160 mg/m^2 thereafter; patients with pre-existing cardiac disease, history of prior chest irradiation, or history of prior anthracycline treatment should have baseline LVEF and every 160 mg/m^2 thereafter); signs and symptoms of infection or disease progression; monitor closely for infusion reactions

Dosage Forms Excipient information presented when available (limited, particularly for generics); consult specific product labeling.

Injectable, Intravenous [preservative free]:

DaunoXome: 2 mg/mL (25 mL) [pyrogen free]

- DaunoXome *see* DAUNOrubicin (Liposomal) *on page 555*
- Daxas™ (Can) *see* Roflumilast *on page 1847*
- Dayhist Allergy 12 Hour Relief [OTC] *see* Clemastine *on page 449*
- Daypro *see* Oxaprozin *on page 1527*
- Daypro® (Can) *see* Oxaprozin *on page 1527*
- Daysee *see* Ethinyl Estradiol and Levonorgestrel *on page 787*
- Daytrana *see* Methylphenidate *on page 1336*
- dCF *see* Pentostatin *on page 1617*
- DDAVP *see* Desmopressin *on page 575*
- DDAVP® (Can) *see* Desmopressin *on page 575*
- DDAVP® Melt (Can) *see* Desmopressin *on page 575*
- DDAVP Rhinal Tube *see* Desmopressin *on page 575*
- ddI *see* Didanosine *on page 602*
- 1-Deamino-8-D-Arginine Vasopressin *see* Desmopressin *on page 575*
- Debrox [OTC] *see* Carbamide Peroxide *on page 340*
- Decadron *see* Dexamethasone (Systemic) *on page 580*
- Decapeptyl® (Can) *see* Triptorelin *on page 2131*
- De-Chlor DM [OTC] *see* Chlorpheniramine, Phenylephrine, and Dextromethorphan *on page 413*

Decitabine (de SYE ta been)

Brand Names: U.S. Dacogen

Index Terms 5-Aza-2'-deoxycytidine; 5-Aza-dCyd; Deoxyazacytidine; Dezocitidine

Pharmacologic Category Antineoplastic Agent, DNA Methylation Inhibitor

Use Treatment of myelodysplastic syndrome (MDS)

Unlabeled Use Treatment of acute myelogenous leukemia (AML), sickle cell anemia

Pregnancy Risk Factor D

Pregnancy Considerations Teratogenic effects, decreased fetal weight, and increased fetal deaths were observed in animal studies. There are no adequate and well-controlled studies in pregnant women. Women of childbearing potential should be advised to avoid pregnancy during treatment and for 1 month after treatment. In addition, males should be advised to avoid fathering a child while on decitabine therapy and for 2 months after treatment.

Breast-Feeding Considerations Due to the potential for serious adverse reactions in the nursing infant, breast-feeding is not recommended.

Contraindications There are no contraindications listed within the manufacturer's labeling.

Warnings/Precautions Hazardous agent - use appropriate precautions for handling and disposal (NIOSH, 2012). The dose-limiting toxicity is bone marrow suppression; worsening neutropenia is common in first two treatment cycles and may not correlate with progression of underlying MDS; may require dosage adjustment (after the first cycle), growth factor support and/or antimicrobial agents; monitor for infection. Not studied in hepatic and renal disease; use caution.

Adverse Reactions

>10%:

Cardiovascular: Peripheral edema (25% to 27%), pallor (23%), edema (5% to 18%), cardiac murmur (16%), hypotension (6% to 11%)

Central nervous system: Fever (6% to 53%), fatigue (46%), headache (23% to 28%), insomnia (14% to 28%), dizziness (18% to 21%), chills (16%), pain (5% to 13%), confusion (8% to 12%), lethargy (12%), anxiety (9% to 11%), hypoesthesia (11%)

Dermatologic: Petechiae (12% to 39%), bruising (9% to 22%), rash (11% to 19%), erythema (5% to 14%), cellulitis (9% to 12%), lesions (5% to 11%), pruritus (9% to 11%)

Endocrine & metabolic: Hyperglycemia (6% to 33%), hypoalbuminemia (7% to 24%), hypomagnesemia (5% to 24%), hypokalemia (12% to 22%), hyperkalemia (13%), hyponatremia (19%)

Gastrointestinal: Nausea (40% to 42%), constipation (30% to 35%), diarrhea (28% to 34%), vomiting (16% to 25%), anorexia/appetite decreased (8% to 23%), abdominal pain (5% to 14%), oral mucosal petechiae (13%), stomatitis (11% to 12%), dyspepsia (10% to 12%)

Hematologic: Neutropenia (38% to 90%; grades 3/4: 37% to 87%; recovery 28-50 days), thrombocytopenia (27% to 89%; grades 3/4: 24% to 85%), anemia (31% to 82%; grades 3/4: 22%), febrile neutropenia (20% to 29%; grades 3/4: 23%), leukopenia (6% to 28%; grades 3/4: 22%), lymphadenopathy (12%)

Hepatic: Hyperbilirubinemia (6% to 14%), alkaline phosphatase increased (11%)

Local: Tenderness (11%)

Neuromuscular & skeletal: Rigors (22%), arthralgia (17% to 20%), limb pain (18% to 19%), back pain (17% to 18%), weakness (15%)

Respiratory: Cough (27% to 40%), dyspnea (29%), pneumonia (20% to 22%), pharyngitis (16%), lung crackles (14%), epistaxis (13%)

5% to 10%:

Cardiovascular: Tachycardia (8%), chest pain/discomfort (6% to 7%), facial edema (6%), hypertension (6%), heart failure (5%)

Central nervous system: Depression (9%), malaise (5%)

Dermatologic: Alopecia (8%), dry skin (8%), urticaria (6%)

Endocrine & metabolic: Hyperuricemia (10%), LDH increased (8%), bicarbonate increased (6%), dehydration (6% to 8%), hypochloremia (6%), bicarbonate decreased (5%), hypoproteinemia (5%)

Gastrointestinal: Mucosal inflammation (9%), weight loss (9%), gingival bleeding (8%), hemorrhoids (8%), loose stools (7%), tongue ulceration (7%), dysphagia (5% to 6%), oral candidiasis (6%), toothache (6%), abdominal distension (5%), gastroesophageal reflux (5%), glossodynia (5%), lip ulceration (5%), oral pain (5%), tooth abscess (5%)

Genitourinary: Urinary tract infection (7%), dysuria (6%), polyuria (5%)

Hematologic: Bacteremia (5% to 8%), hematoma (5%), pancytopenia (5%), thrombocythemia (5%)

Hepatic: Ascites (10%), AST increased (10%), hypobilirubinemia (5%)

Local: Catheter infection (8%), catheter site erythema (5%), catheter site pain (5%), injection site swelling (5%)

Neuromuscular & skeletal: Myalgia (5% to 9%), falling (8%), chest wall pain (7%), muscle spasm (7%), bone pain (6%), musculoskeletal pain/discomfort (5% to 6%), crepitation (5%)

Ocular: Blurred vision (6%)

Otic: Ear pain (6%)

Respiratory: Breath sounds abnormal (5% to 10%), hypoxia (10%), upper respiratory tract infection (10%), pharyngolaryngeal pain (8%), rales (8%), pulmonary edema (6%), sinusitis (5% to 6%), pleural effusion (5%), postnasal drip (5%), sinus congestion (5%)

Miscellaneous: Candidal infection (10%), staphylococcal infection (7%), transfusion reaction (7%), night sweats (5%)

<5% (Limited to important or life-threatening): Anaphylactic reaction, atrial fibrillation, bronchopulmonary aspergillosis, cardiomyopathy, cardiorespiratory arrest/failure, catheter site hemorrhage, cholecystitis, fungal infection, gastrointestinal hemorrhage, gingival pain, hemoptysis, hypersensitivity, intracranial hemorrhage, mental status change, MI, mycobacterium avium complex infection, peridiverticular abscess, pseudomonal lung infection, pulmonary embolism, pulmonary infiltrates, pulmonary mass, renal failure, respiratory arrest, sepsis, splenomegaly, supraventricular tachycardia, Sweet's syndrome (acute febrile neutrophilic dermatosis), urethral hemorrhage

Drug Interactions

Metabolism/Transport Effects None known.

Avoid Concomitant Use

Avoid concomitant use of Decitabine with any of the following: CloZAPine

Increased Effect/Toxicity

Decitabine may increase the levels/effects of: CloZAPine

Decreased Effect There are no known significant interactions involving a decrease in effect.

Preparation for Administration Hazardous agent; use appropriate precautions for handling and disposal (NIOSH, 2012). Vials should be reconstituted with 10 mL SWFI to a concentration of 5 mg/mL. Immediately further dilute with 50-250 mL NS, D_5W, or lactated Ringer's to a final concentration of 0.1-1 mg/mL. Use appropriate precautions for handling and disposal. Solutions not administered within 15 minutes of preparation should be prepared with cold (2°C to 8°C [36°F to 46°F]) infusion solutions.

Storage/Stability Store vials at 25°C (77°F); excursions permitted to 15°C to 30°C (59°F to 86°F). Solutions diluted for infusion may be stored for up to 7 hours under refrigeration at 2°C to 8°C (36°F to 46°F) if prepared with cold infusion fluids.

Mechanism of Action After phosphorylation, decitabine is incorporated into DNA and inhibits DNA methyltransferase causing hypomethylation and subsequent cell death (within the S-phase of the cell cycle).

Pharmacodynamics/Kinetics

Distribution: 63-89 L/m^2

Protein binding: <1%

Metabolism: Possibly via deamination by cytidine deaminase

Half-life elimination: ~30-35 minutes

Time to peak: At end of infusion

Dosage I.V.: Adults:

MDS:

15 mg/m^2 over 3 hours every 8 hours (45 mg/m^2/day) for 3 days (135 mg/m^2/cycle) every 6 weeks (treatment is recommended for at least 4 cycles and may continue until the patient no longer continues to benefit)

Adjustment for prolonged hematologic toxicity (ANC <1000/mm^3 and platelets <50,000/mm^3):

>6 weeks but <8 weeks: Delay dose for up to 2 weeks and temporarily reduce dose to 11 mg/m^2 every 8 hours (33 mg/m^2/day) for 3 days

>8 weeks but <10 weeks: Assess for disease progression; if no disease progression, delay dose for up to 2 weeks and reduce dose to 11 mg/m^2 every 8 hours (33 mg/m^2/day) for 3 days; maintain or increase dose with subsequent cycles if clinically indicated

or

20 mg/m^2 over 1 hour daily for 5 days every 28 days (delay subsequent treatment cycles until hematologic recovery (ANC ≥1000/mm^3 and platelets ≥50,000/mm^3)

AML (unlabeled use): 20 mg/m^2 over 1 hour daily for 5 days every 28 days (Cashen, 2010)

Dosage adjustment for toxicity:

Hematologic toxicity (ANC <1000/mm^3 and platelets <50,000/mm^3): Delay and/or reduce dose; see recommendations specific to each MDS dosing regimen above

Nonhematologic toxicity: Temporarily hold treatment until resolution for any of the following toxicities:

Serum creatinine ≥2 mg/dL

ALT, bilirubin ≥2 times ULN

Active or uncontrolled infection

Dosage adjustment in renal impairment: No dosage adjustment provided in manufacturer's labeling (has not been studied); use with caution.

Dosage adjustment in hepatic impairment: No dosage adjustment provided in manufacturer's labeling (has not been studied); use with caution.

Dosing in obesity: *ASCO Guidelines for appropriate chemotherapy dosing in obese adults with cancer:* Utilize patient's actual body weight (full weight) for calculation of body surface area- or weight-based dosing, particularly when the intent of therapy is curative; manage regimen-related toxicities in the same manner as for nonobese patients; if a dose reduction is utilized due to toxicity, consider resumption of full weight-based dosing with subsequent cycles, especially if cause of toxicity (eg, hepatic or renal impairment) is resolved (Griggs, 2012).

Administration Infuse over 1-3 hours. Premedication with antiemetics is recommended.

Hazardous agent; use appropriate precautions for handling and disposal (NIOSH, 2012).

Monitoring Parameters CBC with differential and platelets with each cycle, more frequently if needed; liver enzymes; serum creatinine

Dosage Forms Excipient information presented when available (limited, particularly for generics); consult specific product labeling.

Solution Reconstituted, Intravenous:

Dacogen: 50 mg (1 ea)

Generic: 50 mg (1 ea)

◆ Declomycin *see* Demeclocycline *on page 567*

◆ Decongestant [OTC] *see* Pseudoephedrine *on page 1746*

◆ Decongestant 12Hour Max St [OTC] *see* Pseudoephedrine *on page 1746*

◆ Deep Sea Nasal Spray [OTC] *see* Sodium Chloride *on page 1914*

Deferasirox (de FER a sir ox)

Brand Names: U.S. Exjade

Brand Names: Canada Exjade

Index Terms ICL670

Pharmacologic Category Chelating Agent

Use Chronic iron overload: Treatment of chronic iron overload due to blood transfusions (transfusional hemosiderosis) or due to non-transfusion-dependent thalassemia syndromes and with a liver iron concentration (LIC) of at least 5 mg iron per gram of liver dry weight (mg Fe/g dw) and serum ferritin >300 mcg/L.

Pregnancy Risk Factor C

Pregnancy Considerations Teratogenic effects were observed in animal reproduction studies. Use during pregnancy only if the potential benefit justifies the potential risk to the fetus.

Breast-Feeding Considerations It is not known if deferasirox is excreted in breast milk. The decision to discontinue deferasirox or to discontinue breast-feeding during therapy should take into account the benefits of treatment to the mother.

Prescribing and Access Restrictions Deferasirox (Exjade) is only available through a restricted distribution program called EPASS Complete Care. Prescribers must enroll patients in this program in order to obtain the medication. For patient enrollment, contact 1-888-90-EPASS (1-888-903-7277).

Contraindications Hypersensitivity to deferasirox or any component of the formulation; platelet counts <50,000/mm^3; poor performance status; high-risk myelodysplastic syndromes; advanced malignancies; creatinine clearance <40 mL/minute or serum creatinine >2 x age-appropriate ULN

Canadian labeling: Additional contraindications (not in U.S. labeling): Cl_{cr} <60 mL/minute

Warnings/Precautions [U.S. Boxed Warning]: Acute renal failure (including fatalities and cases requiring dialysis) may occur; observed more frequently in patients with comorbid conditions and advanced hematologic malignancies. Obtain serum creatinine and calculate creatinine clearance in duplicate at baseline prior to initiation, and monitor at least monthly thereafter; in patients with underlying renal dysfunction or at risk for acute renal failure, monitor creatinine weekly during the first month then at least monthly thereafter. Dose reduction, interruption, or discontinuation should be considered for serum creatinine elevations. Monitor serum creatinine and/or creatinine clearance more frequently if creatinine levels are increasing. Use with caution in renal impairment; dosage modification or treatment discontinuation may be required; reductions in initial dose are recommended for patients with Cl_{cr} 40-60 mL/minute; use is contraindicated in patients with Cl_{cr} <40 mL/minute or serum creatinine >2 times age-appropriate ULN. May cause proteinuria; monitor monthly. Renal tubular damage, including Fanconi's syndrome, has also been reported, primarily in pediatric/adolescent patients with β-thalassemia and serum ferritin levels <1500 mcg/L.

[U.S. Boxed Warning]: Hepatic injury and failure (including fatalities) may occur. Monitor transaminases and bilirubin at baseline, every 2 weeks for 1 month, then at least monthly thereafter. Hepatitis and elevated transaminases have also been reported. Hepatotoxicity is more common in patients >55 years of age and in patients with significant comorbidities (eg, cirrhosis, multiorgan failure). Reduce dose or temporarily interrupt treatment for severe or persistent increases in transaminases/bilirubin. **[U.S. Boxed Warning]: Avoid use in patients with severe (Child-Pugh class C) hepatic impairment; a dose reduction is required in patients with moderate (Child-Pugh class B) hepatic impairment.** Monitor patients with mild (Child-Pugh class A) or moderate (Child-Pugh class B) impairment closely for efficacy and for adverse reactions requiring dosage reduction.

[U.S. Boxed Warning]: Gastrointestinal (GI) hemorrhage (including fatalities) may occur; observed more frequently in elderly patients with advanced hematologic malignancies and/or low platelet counts;

discontinue treatment for suspected GI hemorrhage or ulceration. Other GI effects including irritation and ulceration have been reported. Use caution with concurrent medications that may increase risk of adverse GI effects (eg, NSAIDs, corticosteroids, anticoagulants, oral bisphosphonates). Monitor patients closely for signs/symptoms of GI ulceration/bleeding.

May cause skin rash (dose-related), including erythema multiforme; mild-to-moderate rashes may resolve without treatment interruption; for severe rash, interrupt and consider restarting at a lower dose with dose escalation and oral steroids; discontinue if erythema multiforme is suspected. Severe skin reactions, including Stevens-Johnson syndrome (SJS) and erythema multiforme, have also been reported; discontinue and evaluate if suspected. Hypersensitivity reactions, including severe reactions (anaphylaxis and angioedema) have been reported, onset is usually within the first month of treatment; discontinue if severe. Auditory (decreased hearing and high frequency hearing loss) or ocular disturbances (lens opacities, cataracts, intraocular pressure elevation, and retinal disorders) have been reported (rare); monitor and consider dose reduction or treatment interruption. Bone marrow suppression (including agranulocytosis, neutropenia, thrombocytopenia, and worsening anemia) has been reported, risk may be increased in patients with pre-existing hematologic disorders; monitor blood counts regularly; interrupt treatment in patients who develop cytopenias; may reinitiate once cause of cytopenia has been determined; use contraindicated if platelet count <50,000/mm^3. Potentially significant drug-drug interactions may exist, requiring dose or frequency adjustment, additional monitoring, and/or selection of alternative therapy. Potent UGT inducers (eg, rifampin) or bile acid sequestrants (eg, cholestyramine) may decrease the efficacy of deferasirox; avoid concomitant use. If coadministration necessary, dosage modifications may be needed; monitor serum ferritin and clinical response. Not approved for use in combination with other iron chelation therapies; safety of combinations has not been established. For transfusion-related iron overload, treatment should be initiated with evidence of chronic iron overload (ie, transfusion of ≥100 mL/kg of packed RBCs [eg, ≥20 units for a 40 kg individual] and serum ferritin consistently >1000 mcg/L). For non-transfusion-dependent iron overload, initiate with liver iron concentration ≥5 mg Fe/g dry liver weight and serum ferritin >300 mcg/L. Prior to use, consider risk versus anticipated benefit with respect to individual patient's life expectancy and prognosis. Use with caution in the elderly due to the higher incidence of toxicity (eg, hepatotoxicity) and fatal events during use. Overchelation of iron may increase development of toxicity; consider temporary interruption of treatment in transfusional iron overload when serum ferritin <500 mcg/L; in non-transfusion-dependent thalassemia when serum ferritin <300 mcg/L or hepatic iron concentration <3 mg Fe/g dry weight. May contain lactose; Canadian product labeling recommends avoiding use in patients with galactose intolerance, Lapp lactase deficiency, or glucose-galactose malabsorption syndromes. Controlled studies in myelodysplastic syndromes (MDS) and chronic iron overload due to blood transfusions have not been conducted.

Adverse Reactions

>10%:

Central nervous system: Fever (19%), headache (16%)
Dermatologic: Rash (dose related; 2% to 11%)
Gastrointestinal: Abdominal pain (dose related; 21% to 28%), nausea (dose related; 2% to 23%), vomiting (dose related; 10% to 21%), diarrhea (dose related; 5% to 20%)
Renal: Serum creatinine increased (dose related; 2% to 38%), proteinuria (19%)
Respiratory: Cough (14%), nasopharyngitis (13%), pharyngolaryngeal pain (11%)
Miscellaneous: Influenza (11%)

1% to 10%:

Central nervous system: Fatigue (6%)
Dermatologic: Urticaria (4%)
Hepatic: ALT increased (1% to 8%), transaminitis (4%)
Neuromuscular & skeletal: Arthralgia (7%), back pain (6%)
Otic: Ear infection (5%)
Respiratory: Respiratory tract infection (10%), bronchitis (9%), pharyngitis (8%), acute tonsillitis (6%), rhinitis (6%)

<1% (Limited to important or life-threatening): Acute renal failure, agranulocytosis, anaphylaxis, anemia (worsening), angioedema, anxiety, ascites, bilirubin increased, cataract, cholecystitis, cholelithiasis, constipation, cytopenias, dizziness, drug fever, duodenal ulcer, edema, erythema multiforme, esophagitis, Fanconi's syndrome, gastric ulcer, gastritis, gastrointestinal bleeding, gastrointestinal hemorrhage, glomerulonephritis, glucosuria, hearing loss (including high frequency), hematuria, Henoch-Schönlein purpura (IgA vasculitis), hepatic dysfunction, hepatic encephalopathy, hepatic failure, hepatic transaminases increased, hepatitis, hyperactivity, hypersensitivity reaction, hypocalcemia, insomnia, intraocular pressure increased, jaundice, lens opacities, leukocytoclastic vasculitis, maculopathy, neutropenia, optic neuritis, pigment disorder, purpura, renal tubular necrosis, renal tubulopathy, retinal disorder, sleep disorder, thrombocytopenia, tubulointerstitial nephritis, visual disturbance

Drug Interactions

Metabolism/Transport Effects Substrate of UGT1A1; **Inhibits** CYP1A2 (moderate), CYP2C8 (moderate); **Induces** CYP3A4 (weak/moderate)

Avoid Concomitant Use

Avoid concomitant use of Deferasirox with any of the following: Aluminum Hydroxide; Axitinib; Bile Acid Sequestrants; Pirfenidone; Simeprevir; Theophylline

Increased Effect/Toxicity

Deferasirox may increase the levels/effects of: Agomelatine; CYP1A2 Substrates; CYP2C8 Substrates; Pirfenidone; Repaglinide; Theophylline

The levels/effects of Deferasirox may be increased by: Anticoagulants; Bisphosphonate Derivatives; Corticosteroids; Corticosteroids (Systemic); Nonsteroidal Anti-Inflammatory Agents

Decreased Effect

Deferasirox may decrease the levels/effects of: ARIPiprazole; Axitinib; CYP3A4 Substrates; Ibrutinib; Saxagliptin; Simeprevir

The levels/effects of Deferasirox may be decreased by: Aluminum Hydroxide; Bile Acid Sequestrants; Fosphenytoin; PHENobarbital; Phenytoin; Rifampin; Ritonavir

Ethanol/Nutrition/Herb Interactions Food: Bioavailability is increased variably when taken with food. Management: Take on an empty stomach at the same time each day at least 30 minutes before food. Maintain adequate hydration, unless instructed to restrict fluid intake.

Storage/Stability Store at room temperature of 25°C (77°F); excursions permitted to 15°C and 30°C (59°F and 86°F). Protect from moisture.

Mechanism of Action Selectively binds iron, forming a complex which is excreted primarily through the feces.

Pharmacodynamics/Kinetics

Distribution: Adults: 14.4 ± 2.7L
Protein binding: ~99% to serum albumin
Metabolism: Hepatic via glucuronidation by UGT1A1(primarily) and UGT1A3; minor oxidation by CYP450; undergoes enterohepatic recirculation
Bioavailability: 70%

Half-life elimination: 8-16 hours
Time to peak, plasma: ~1.5-4 hours
Excretion: Feces (84%); urine (8%)

Dosage Note: Calculate dose to the nearest whole tablet size.

Chronic iron overload due to blood transfusion: Note: Treatment should only be initiated with evidence of chronic iron overload (ie, transfusion of ≥100 mL/kg of packed red blood cells [eg, ≥20 units for a 40 kg individual] and serum ferritin consistently >1000 mcg/L).

Children ≥2 years, Adolescents, and Adults: Oral:

U.S. labeling: Initial: 20 mg/kg once daily

Canadian labeling: Dosing based on treatment goal and patient's individual transfusion rate:

Treatment goal: Maintenance of acceptable body iron levels:

Initial: 10 mg/kg once daily if transfused packed red blood cells (pRBCs) <7 mL/kg/month (approximately <2 units per month for an adult)

Initial: 20 mg/kg once daily if transfused pRBCs ≥7 mL/kg/month (approximately >2 units per month for an adult)

Treatment goal: Iron overload reduction:

Initial: 20 mg/kg once daily if transfused pRBCs <14 mL/kg/month (approximately <4 units per month for an adult)

Initial: 30 mg/kg once daily if transfused pRBCs ≥14 mL/kg/month (approximately >4 units per month for an adult)

Maintenance: Adjust dose every 3-6 months based on serum ferritin trends; adjust by 5 or 10 mg/kg/day; titrate to individual response and treatment goals. Usual range: 20-30 mg/kg/day; doses up to 40 mg/kg/day may be considered for serum ferritin levels persistently >2500 mcg/L (doses above 40 mg/kg/day are not recommended). **Note:** Consider interrupting therapy for serum ferritin <500 mcg/L (risk of toxicity may be increased).

Chronic iron overload in non-transfusion-dependent thalassemia syndromes: Children ≥10 years, Adolescents, and Adults: Oral:

U.S. labeling: **Note:** Treatment should only be initiated with evidence of chronic iron overload (hepatic iron concentration ≥5 mg Fe/g dry weight and serum ferritin >300 mcg/L).

Initial: 10 mg/kg once daily. Consider increasing to 20 mg/kg once daily after 4 weeks if baseline hepatic iron concentration is >15 mg Fe/g dry weight.

Maintenance: Monitor serum ferritin monthly; if serum ferritin is <300 mcg/L, interrupt therapy and obtain hepatic iron concentration. Monitor hepatic iron concentration every 6 months; interrupt therapy when hepatic iron concentration <3 mg Fe/g dry weight. After 6 months of therapy, consider dose adjustment to 20 mg/kg/day if hepatic iron concentration >7 mg Fe/g dry weight. Reduce dose to ≤10 mg/kg when hepatic iron concentration is 3-7 mg Fe/g dry weight. Doses above 20 mg/kg/day are not recommended. After interruption, resume treatment when hepatic iron concentration >5 mg Fe/g dry weight.

Canadian labeling: **Note:** Treatment should only be initiated with evidence of chronic iron overload (hepatic iron concentration ≥5 mg Fe/g dry weight or serum ferritin consistently >800 mcg/L).

Initial: 10 mg/kg/day

Maintenance: Do not exceed 10 mg/kg/day in patients whose hepatic iron concentration was not evaluated and if serum ferritin ≤2000 mcg/L. Monitor serum ferritin monthly; consider dose adjustment by 5 or 10 mg/kg/day every 3-6 months if hepatic iron concentration ≥7 mg Fe/g dry weight or serum transferrin levels consistently >2000 mcg/L. Patients receiving >10 mg/kg should have their dose reduced to ≤10 mg/kg when hepatic iron concentration <7 mg Fe/g dry weight or serum ferritin <2000 mcg/L. Interrupt therapy when hepatic iron concentration <3 mg Fe/g dry weight or serum ferritin <300 mcg/L. Doses above 20 mg/kg/day are not recommended.

Dosage adjustment with concomitant bile acid sequestrants (eg,cholestyramine, colesevelam, colestipol) or potent UGT inducers (eg, rifampin, phenytoin, phenobarbital, ritonavir): Avoid concomitant use; if coadministration necessary, consider increasing the initial dose of deferasirox dose by 50%; monitor serum ferritin and clinical response.

Dosage adjustment for toxicity:

Bone marrow suppression: Interrupt treatment; may reinitiate once cause of cytopenia has been determined; use contraindicated if platelet count <50,000/mm^3

Dermatologic toxicity:

Rash (severe): Interrupt treatment; may reintroduce at a lower dose (with future dose escalation) and short-term oral corticosteroids

Severe skin reaction (Stevens-Johnson syndrome, erythema multiforme): Discontinue and evaluate.

Gastrointestinal: Discontinue treatment for suspected GI ulceration or hemorrhage.

Hearing loss or visual disturbance: Consider dose reduction or treatment interruption

Dosage adjustment in renal impairment: Creatinine clearance should be estimated using the Cockcroft-Gault formula.

Renal impairment at treatment initiation:

Cl_{cr} >60 mL/minute: No dosage adjustment necessary.

Cl_{cr} 40-60 mL/minute: Reduce initial dose by 50%.

Cl_{cr} <40 mL/minute or serum creatinine >2 times age-appropriate ULN: Use is contraindicated.

Renal toxicity during treatment:

U.S. labeling:

Transfusional iron overload:

Children ≥2 years and Adolescents <16 years: For increase in serum creatinine >33% above the average baseline level and above the age-appropriate ULN: Reduce daily dose by 10 mg/kg

Adolescents ≥16 years and Adults: For increase in serum creatinine ≥33% above the average baseline, repeat within 1 week; if still elevated by ≥33%: Reduce daily dose by 10 mg/kg

All patients: Cl_{cr} <40 mL/minute or serum creatinine >2 times age-appropriate ULN: Discontinue treatment.

Non-transfusion-dependent thalassemia syndromes:

Children ≥10 years and Adolescents <16 years: For increase in serum creatinine >33% above the average baseline level and above the age-appropriate ULN: Reduce daily dose by 5 mg/kg

Adolescents ≥16 years and Adults: For increase in serum creatinine ≥33% above the average baseline, repeat within 1 week; if still elevated by ≥33%: Interrupt therapy if the dose is 5 mg/kg; reduce dose by 50% if the dose is 10-20 mg/kg

All patients: Cl_{cr} <40 mL/minute or serum creatinine >2 times age-appropriate ULN: Discontinue treatment.

Canadian labeling:

Children ≥2 years and Adolescents <16 years: For increase in serum creatinine above the age-appropriate ULN for 2 consecutive levels, reduce daily dose by 10 mg/kg.

Adolescents ≥16 years and Adults: For increase in serum creatinine >33% above the average pretreatment level for 2 consecutive weekly levels, reduce daily dose by 10 mg/kg.

All patients: Progressive increase serum creatinine beyond ULN: Withhold treatment.

Dosage adjustment in hepatic impairment:

Hepatic impairment at treatment initiation:

Mild impairment (Child-Pugh class A): No dosage adjustment necessary; monitor closely for efficacy and for adverse reactions requiring dosage reduction.

Moderate impairment (Child-Pugh class B): Initial: Reduce dose by 50%; monitor closely for efficacy and for adverse reactions requiring dosage reduction.

Severe impairment (Child-Pugh class C): Avoid use.

Hepatic toxicity during treatment: Severe or persistent increases in transaminases/bilirubin: Reduce dose or temporarily interrupt treatment.

Dietary Considerations Bioavailability increased variably when taken with food; take on empty stomach 30 minutes before a meal.

Administration Oral: Administer tablets by making an oral suspension; **do not chew or swallow tablets whole.** Completely disperse tablets in water, orange juice, or apple juice (use 3.5 ounces for total doses <1 g; 7 ounces for doses ≥1 g); stir to form a fine suspension and drink entire contents. Rinse remaining residue with more fluid; drink. Avoid dispersion of tablets in milk (due to slowed dissolution) or carbonated drinks (due to foaming) (Séchaud, 2008). Administer at same time each day on an empty stomach, at least 30 minutes before food. Do not take simultaneously with aluminum-containing antacids.

Monitoring Parameters Serum ferritin (baseline, monthly thereafter), iron levels (baseline), CBC with differential, serum creatinine and creatinine clearance (2 baseline assessments then monthly thereafter; in patients who are at increased risk of complications [eg, pre-existing renal conditions, elderly, comorbid conditions, or receiving other potentially nephrotoxic medications]: weekly for the first month then at least monthly thereafter); liver iron concentration (non-transfusion-dependent thalassemia; baseline, every 6 months); urine protein (monthly); monitor serum creatinine and/or creatinine clearance more frequently if creatinine levels are increasing; serum transaminases (ALT/AST) and bilirubin (baseline, every 2 weeks for the first month, then monthly); baseline and annual auditory and ophthalmic function (including slit lamp examinations and dilated fundoscopy); performance status (in patients with hematologic malignancies); signs and symptoms of GI ulcers or hemorrhage; cumulative number of RBC units received

Canadian labeling also recommends monitoring growth and body weight every 12 months in pediatric patients.

Additional Information Deferasirox has a low affinity for binding with zinc and copper, may cause variable decreases in the serum concentration of these trace minerals.

Dosage Forms Excipient information presented when available (limited, particularly for generics); consult specific product labeling.

Tablet Soluble, Oral:

Exjade: 125 mg, 250 mg, 500 mg

Deferiprone (de FER i prone)

Brand Names: U.S. Ferriprox

Index Terms APO-066; Ferriprox®

Pharmacologic Category Chelating Agent

Use Treatment of transfusional iron overload due to thalassemia syndromes with inadequate response to other chelation therapy

Pregnancy Risk Factor D

Medication Guide Available Yes

Dosage Oral: **Note:** Round dose to the nearest 250 mg (or 1/2 tablet). If serum ferritin falls consistently below 500 mcg/L, consider temporary treatment interruption.

Adults: Transfusional iron overload: Initial: 25 mg/kg 3 times/day (75 mg/kg/day); individualize dose based on response and therapeutic goal; maximum dose: 33 mg/kg 3 times/day (99 mg/kg/day)

Elderly: Begin at the low end of dosing range

Dosage adjustment for toxicity:

ANC <1500/mm^3: Interrupt treatment

ANC <500/mm^3: In addition to treatment interruption, consider hospitalization (and other clinically-appropriate management); do not resume or rechallenge unless the potential benefits outweigh potential risks

Infection: Interrupt treatment; monitor ANC more frequently

Dosage adjustment in renal impairment: No dosage adjustments are provided in the manufacturer's labeling (has not been studied).

Dosage adjustment in hepatic impairment: No dosage adjustments are provided in the manufacturer's labeling (has not been studied).

Additional Information Complete prescribing information should be consulted for additional detail.

Dosage Forms Excipient information presented when available (limited, particularly for generics); consult specific product labeling.

Tablet, Oral:

Ferriprox: 500 mg [scored]

Deferoxamine (de fer OKS a meen)

Brand Names: U.S. Desferal

Brand Names: Canada Desferal®; PMS-Deferoxamine

Index Terms Deferoxamine Mesylate; Desferrioxamine; DFM

Pharmacologic Category Antidote; Chelating Agent

Use Adjunct in the treatment of acute iron intoxication; treatment of chronic iron overload secondary to multiple transfusions

Canadian labeling (unlabeled use in the U.S.): Diagnosis of aluminum overload; treatment of chronic aluminum overload in patients with end-stage renal failure undergoing maintenance dialysis

Unlabeled Use Diagnosis or treatment of aluminum induced toxicity associated with chronic kidney disease (CKD)

Pregnancy Risk Factor C

Pregnancy Considerations Skeletal anomalies and delayed ossification were observed in some but not all animal reproduction studies. Toxic amounts of iron or deferoxamine have not been noted to cross the placenta. In case of acute iron toxicity, treatment during pregnancy should not be withheld.

Breast-Feeding Considerations It is not known if deferoxamine is excreted in human milk; the manufacturer recommends that caution be used if administered to a breast-feeding woman.

Contraindications Hypersensitivity to deferoxamine or any component of the formulation; patients with severe renal disease or anuria

Note: Canadian labeling does not include severe renal disease or anuria as contraindications.

Warnings/Precautions Flushing of the skin, hypotension, urticaria and shock are associated with rapid I.V. infusion; administer I.M., by slow subcutaneous or slow I.V. infusion only. Auditory disturbances (tinnitus and high frequency hearing loss) have been reported following prolonged administration, at high doses, or in patients with low ferritin levels; generally reversible with early detection and immediate discontinuation. Elderly patients are at increased risk for hearing loss. Audiology exams are recommended with long-term treatment. Ocular disturbances (blurred vision, cataracts, corneal opacities, decreased visual acuity, impaired peripheral, color, and night vision, optic neuritis, retinal pigment abnormalities, scotoma, visual loss/defect) have been reported following prolonged administration, at high doses, or in patients with low ferritin levels; generally reversible with early detection and immediate discontinuation. Elderly patients are at increased risk for ocular disorders. Periodic ophthalmic exams are recommended with long-term treatment.

Deferoxamine has been associated with acute respiratory distress syndrome following excessively high-dose I.V. treatment of acute iron intoxication or thalassemia (has been reported in children and adults). High deferoxamine doses and concurrent low ferritin levels are also associated with growth retardation. Growth velocity may partially resume to pretreatment velocity rates after deferoxamine dose reduction. Patients with iron overload are at increased susceptibility to infection with *Yersinia enterocolitica* and *Yersinia pseudotuberculosis*; treatment with deferoxamine may enhance this risk; if infection develops, discontinue therapy until resolved. Rare and serious cases of mucormycosis have been reported with use; withhold treatment with signs and symptoms of mucormycosis.

Increases in serum creatinine, acute renal failure and renal tubular disorders have been reported; monitor for changes in renal function. When iron is chelated with deferoxamine, the chelate is excreted renally. Deferoxamine is readily dialyzable. Treatment with deferoxamine in patients with aluminum toxicity may cause hypocalcemia and aggravate hyperparathyroidism. Deferoxamine may cause neurological symptoms (including seizure) in patients with aluminum-related encephalopathy receiving dialysis and may precipitate dialysis dementia onset.

Deferoxamine is **not** indicated for the treatment of primary hemochromatosis (treatment of choice is phlebotomy). Patients should be informed that urine may have a reddish color. Combination treatment with ascorbic acid (>500 mg/day in adults) and deferoxamine may impair cardiac function (rare), reversible upon discontinuation of ascorbic acid. If combination treatment is warranted, initiate ascorbic acid only after one month of regular deferoxamine treatment, do not exceed ascorbic acid dose of 200 mg/day for adults (in divided doses), 100 mg/day for children ≥10 years of age, or 50 mg/day in children <10 years of age; monitor cardiac function. Do not administer deferoxamine in combination with ascorbic acid in patients with pre-existing cardiac failure.

Adverse Reactions Frequency not defined.

Cardiovascular: Flushing, hypotension, shock, tachycardia

Central nervous system: Dizziness, encephalopathy (aluminum toxicity/dialysis-related), fever, headache, seizure

Dermatologic: Angioedema, rash, urticaria

Endocrine & metabolic: Growth retardation (children), hyperparathyroidism (aggravated), hypocalcemia

Gastrointestinal: Abdominal discomfort, abdominal pain, diarrhea, nausea, vomiting

Genitourinary: Dysuria, urine discoloration (reddish color)

Hematologic: Leukopenia, thrombocytopenia

Hepatic: Hepatic dysfunction, transaminases increased

Local: Injection site: Burning, crust, edema, erythema, eschar, induration, infiltration, irritation, pain, pruritus, swelling, vesicles, wheal formation

Neuromuscular & skeletal: Arthralgia, metaphyseal dysplasia (children <3 years; dose related), muscle spasms, myalgia, neuropathy (peripheral, sensory, motor, or mixed), paresthesia

Ocular: Blurred vision, cataract, corneal opacities, dyschromatopsia, loss of vision, night blindness, optic neuritis, peripheral vision impaired, retinal pigment abnormalities, scotoma, visual acuity decreased, visual field defects

Otic: Hearing loss, tinnitus

Renal: Acute renal failure, renal tubular disorders, serum creatinine increased

Respiratory: Acute respiratory distress syndrome (dyspnea, cyanosis, and/or interstitial infiltrates), asthma

Miscellaneous: Anaphylaxis (with or without shock), hypersensitivity reaction, infections (*Yersinia*, mucormycosis)

Drug Interactions

Metabolism/Transport Effects None known.

Avoid Concomitant Use There are no known interactions where it is recommended to avoid concomitant use.

Increased Effect/Toxicity

Deferoxamine may increase the levels/effects of: Prochlorperazine

The levels/effects of Deferoxamine may be increased by: Ascorbic Acid; Multivitamins/Fluoride (with ADE); Multivitamins/Minerals (with ADEK, Folate, Iron); Multivitamins/Minerals (with AE, No Iron)

Decreased Effect There are no known significant interactions involving a decrease in effect.

Preparation for Administration

I.M.: Reconstitute with sterile water for injection (500 mg vial with 2 mL SWFI; 2000 mg vial with 8 mL SWFI) to a final concentration of 213 mg/mL

I.V.: Reconstitute with sterile water for injection (500 mg vial with 5 mL SWFI; 2000 mg vial with 20 mL SWFI) to a final concentration of 95 mg/mL; further dilute for infusion in sodium chloride 0.9%, sodium chloride 0.45%, D_5W, or LR.

SubQ: Reconstitute with sterile water for injection (500 mg vial with 5 mL SWFI; 2000 mg vial with 20 mL SWFI) to a final concentration of 95 mg/mL

Storage/Stability Prior to reconstitution, store at ≤25°C (≤77°F). Following reconstitution, may be stored at room temperature for 24 hours, although the manufacturer recommends use begin within 3 hours of reconstitution. Do not refrigerate reconstituted solution. When stored at 30°C in polypropylene infusion pump syringes, deferoxamine 250 mg/mL in sterile water for injection retained 95% of initial concentration for 14 days (Stiles, 1996).

Mechanism of Action Complexes with trivalent ions (ferric ions) to form ferrioxamine, which is removed by the kidneys, slows accumulation of hepatic iron and retards or eliminates progression of hepatic fibrosis. Also known to inhibit DNA synthesis *in vitro*.

Pharmacodynamics/Kinetics

Absorption: I.M., SubQ: Well absorbed

Distribution: Distributed throughout body fluids

Protein binding: <10%

Metabolism: Plasma enzymes; binds with iron to form ferrioxamine (iron complex)

Half-life elimination: 14 hours (plasma half-life: 20-30 minutes)

Excretion: Primarily urine (as unchanged drug and ferrioxamine); feces (via bile)

Dosage

Acute iron toxicity: **Note:** The I.V. route is used when severe toxicity is evidenced by cardiovascular collapse or systemic symptoms (coma, shock, metabolic acidosis, or gastrointestinal bleeding) or potentially severe intoxications (peak serum iron level >500 mcg/dL) (Perrone, 2011). When severe symptoms are not present, the I.M. route may be used (per the manufacturer).

Children ≥3 years:

I.M.: 90 mg/kg/dose every 8 hours (maximum: 6000 mg/24 hours)

I.V.: 15 mg/kg/hour (maximum: 6000 mg/24 hours)

Canadian labeling:

I.M.: Initial: 90 mg/kg/dose (maximum/dose: 1000 mg) followed by 45 mg/kg every 4-12 hours as needed (maximum: 6000 mg/24 hours)

I.V.: 15 mg/kg/hour up to a maximum of 80 mg/kg/dose or maximum of 6000 mg/24 hours

Adults: I.M., I.V.: Initial: 1000 mg, may be followed by 500 mg every 4 hours for 2 doses; subsequent doses of 500 mg have been administered every 4-12 hours based on clinical response (maximum recommended dose: 6000 mg/day [per manufacturer])

Canadian labeling:

I.M.: Initial: 90 mg/kg/dose (maximum/dose: 2000 mg) followed by 45 mg/kg every 4-12 hours as needed (maximum: 6000 mg/24 hours)

I.V.: 15 mg/kg/hour up to a maximum of 80 mg/kg/dose or maximum of 6000 mg/24 hours

Chronic iron overload:

Children ≥3 years:

I.V.: 20-40 mg/kg/day over 8-12 hours for 5-7 days per week; dose should not exceed 40 mg/kg/day until growth has ceased

SubQ: 20-40 mg/kg/day over 8-12 hours (maximum: 1000-2000 mg/day)

Unlabeled dosing: I.V., SubQ: 25-30 mg/kg over 8-10 hours 5-7 days per week (Brittenham, 2011)

Adults:

I.M.: 500-1000 mg/day (maximum: 1000 mg/day)

I.V.: 40-50 mg/kg/day (maximum: 60 mg/kg/day) over 8-12 hours for 5-7 days per week

SubQ: 1000-2000 mg/day or 20-40 mg/kg/day over 8-24 hours

Unlabeled dosing: I.V., SubQ: 25-50 mg/kg over 8-10 hours 5-7 days per week (Brittenham, 2011)

Canadian labeling: I.V., SubQ: 1000-4000 mg/day (20-60 mg/kg/day) over ~12 hours (may further increase iron excretion with infusion at the same dose over 24 hours). SubQ infusions are administered 4-7 days per week based on the degree of iron overload.

Diagnosis of aluminum-induced toxicity with CKD (unlabeled use; K/DOQI guidelines, 2003): Children and Adults: I.V.: Test dose: 5 mg/kg during the last hour of dialysis if serum aluminum levels are 60-200 mcg/L, or clinical signs/symptoms of toxicity, or aluminum exposure prior to parathyroid surgery. Measure aluminum just prior to deferoxamine; remeasure 2 days later (test is positive if serum aluminum is ≥50 mcg/L). Do not use if aluminum serum levels are >200 mcg/L.

Canadian labeling: **Note:** Measure serum aluminum levels prior to and after administration of deferoxamine.

Adults: I.V.: Test dose: 5 mg/kg/dose (infusion rate not to exceed 15 mg/kg/hour) following hemodialysis (preferred) or during the last hour of dialysis if serum aluminum levels are >60 mcg/L in association with serum ferritin levels >100 mcg/L; continuous rise in serum aluminum over the next 24-48 hours suggests overload. Remeasure serum aluminum levels prior to next hemodialysis, test is considered positive if serum aluminum levels increase >150 mcg/L above baseline.

Treatment of aluminum toxicity with CKD (unlabeled use; K/DOQI guidelines, 2003): Children and Adults: I.V.:

Administer after diagnostic deferoxamine test dose. **Note:** The risk for deferoxamine-associated neurotoxicity is increased if aluminum serum levels are >200 mcg/L; withhold deferoxamine and administer intensive dialysis until <200 mcg/L.

Aluminum rise ≥300 mcg/L: 5 mg/kg once a week 5 hours before dialysis for 4 months

Aluminum rise <300 mcg/L: 5 mg/kg once a week during the last hour of dialysis for 2 months

Canadian labeling: Adults: Treatment should be considered for symptomatic patients with serum aluminum levels >60 mcg/L and a positive deferoxamine test dose.

Hemodialysis: I.V.: 5 mg/kg/dose (infusion rate not to exceed 15 mg/kg/hour) once weekly for 3 months following hemodialysis (preferred) or during the last hour of dialysis administered. Withhold treatment for 1 month then perform deferoxamine test. Further treatment is not recommended if 2 consecutive tests (performed 1 month apart) yield an increase in serum aluminum levels <75 mcg/L.

Continuous ambulatory or cyclic peritoneal dialysis: Intraperitoneal (preferred), I.M., SubQ infusion (slow), or I.V. infusion (slow): 5 mg/kg/dose once weekly prior to final daily exchange

Dosing adjustment in renal impairment: Severe renal disease or anuria: Use is contraindicated in the manufacturer's U.S. labeling.

The following adjustments have been used by some clinicians (Aronoff, 2007): Adults:

Cl_{cr} >50 mL/minute: No adjustment required

Cl_{cr} 10-50 mL/minute, CRRT: Administer 25% to 50% of normal dose

Cl_{cr}<10 mL/minute, hemodialysis, peritoneal dialysis: Avoid use

Dosage adjustment in hepatic impairment: There are no dosage adjustments provided in the manufacturer's labeling (has not been studied).

Dietary Considerations Vitamin C supplements may need to be limited. The manufacturer recommends a maximum ascorbic acid dose of 200 mg/day in adults (given in divided doses), 100 mg/day in children ≥10 years of age, or 50 mg/day in children <10 years of age. Avoid concurrent use with ascorbic acid in patients with heart failure.

Administration

I.V.: Urticaria, flushing of the skin, hypotension, and shock have occurred following rapid I.V. administration; limiting infusion rate to 15mg/kg/hour may help avoid infusion-related adverse effects.

Acute iron toxicity: The manufacturer states that the I.M. route is preferred; however, the I.V. route is generally preferred in patients with severe toxicity (ie, patients in shock). For the first 1000 mg, infuse at 15 mg/kg/hour. Subsequent doses may be given over 4-12 hours at a rate not to exceed 125 mg/hour.

Chronic iron overload: Administer over 8-12 hours for 5-7 days per week; rate not to exceed 15 mg/kg/hour. In patients with poor compliance, deferoxamine may be administered on the same day of blood transfusion, either prior to or following transfusion; do not administer concurrently with transfusion. Longer infusion times (24 hours) and I.V. administration may be required in patients with severe cardiac iron deposition (Brittenham, 2011).

Diagnosis or treatment of aluminum-induced toxicity with CKD: Administer dose over 1 hour, during the last hour of dialysis (K/DOQI guidelines, 2003).

SubQ: When administered for chronic iron overload, administration over 8-12 hours using a portable infusion pump is generally recommended; however, longer infusion times (24 hours) may also be used. Topical anesthetic or glucocorticoid creams may be used for induration or erythema (Brittenham, 2011).

I.M.: I.M. administration may be used for patients with acute iron toxicity that do not exhibit severe symptoms (per the manufacturer); may also be used in the treatment of chronic iron toxicity.

Monitoring Parameters Serum iron, ferritin, total iron-binding capacity, CBC with differential, renal function tests (serum creatinine), liver function tests, serum chemistries; ophthalmologic exam (visual acuity tests, fundoscopy, slit-lamp exam) and audiometry with long-term treatment; growth and body weight in children (every 3 months)

Dialysis patients: Serum aluminum (yearly; every 3 months in patients on aluminum-containing medications)

Aluminum-induced bone disease: Serum aluminum 2 days following test dose; test is considered positive if serum aluminum increases ≥50 mcg/L

Reference Range

Iron, serum: Normal: 50-160 mcg/dL; peak levels >500 mcg/dL associated with toxicity. Consider treatment in symptomatic patients with levels ≥350 mcg/dL; toxicity cannot be excluded with serum iron levels <350 mcg/dL

Aluminum, serum: <20 mcg/L recommended baseline level in dialysis patients (K/DOQI, 2003)

Test Interactions TIBC may be falsely elevated with high serum iron concentrations or deferoxamine therapy. Imaging results may be distorted due to rapid urinary excretion of deferoxamine-bound gallium-67; discontinue deferoxamine 48 hours prior to scintigraphy.

Additional Information Oncology Comment: The National Comprehensive Cancer Network (NCCN) guidelines for myelodysplastic syndromes (MDS) recommend considering iron chelation therapy in low- or intermediate-risk MDS patients to decrease iron overload due to multiple transfusions (v.1.2012). Treatment (subcutaneous deferoxamine or oral deferasirox) is generally recommended in MDS patients who have received >20-30 RBC transfusions. For those with serum ferritin levels >2500 mcg/L, the goal to decrease ferritin levels to <1000 mcg/L.

Dosage Forms Excipient information presented when available (limited, particularly for generics); consult specific product labeling.

Solution Reconstituted, Injection, as mesylate:

Desferal: 500 mg (1 ea); 2 g (1 ea)

Generic: 500 mg (1 ea); 2 g (1 ea)

◆ **Deferoxamine Mesylate** *see* Deferoxamine *on page 561*

Degarelix (deg a REL ix)

Brand Names: U.S. Firmagon

Brand Names: Canada Firmagon®

Index Terms Degarelix Acetate; FE200486

Pharmacologic Category Antineoplastic Agent, Gonadotropin-Releasing Hormone Antagonist; Gonadotropin Releasing Hormone Antagonist

Use Treatment of advanced prostate cancer

Pregnancy Risk Factor X

Pregnancy Considerations Adverse events were observed in animal reproduction studies. Use is contraindicated in women who are or may become pregnant.

Breast-Feeding Considerations It is not known if degarelix is excreted in breast milk. This product is not indicated for use in women.

Contraindications Hypersensitivity to degarelix or any component of the formulation; pregnancy (or potential to become pregnant)

Warnings/Precautions Hazardous agent - use appropriate precautions for handling and disposal (NIOSH, 2012). Hypersensitivity reactions (including anaphylaxis, urticaria, and angioedema) have been reported. Discontinue for serious hypersensitivity reaction (immediately if dose not fully injected); manage hypersensitivity as clinically indicated. Do not rechallenge after serious hypersensitivity reaction.

Long-term androgen deprivation therapy may prolong the QT interval; use with caution in patients with a known history of QT prolongation or other risk factors for QT prolongation (eg, concomitant use of medications known to prolong QT interval, heart failure, and/or electrolyte abnormalities). Androgen-deprivation therapy may increase the risk for cardiovascular disease (Levine, 2010) and decreased bone mineral density. Androgen deprivation therapy may cause obesity and insulin resistance; the risk for diabetes is increased.

Degarelix exposure is decreased in patients with hepatic impairment, dosage adjustment is not recommended in patients with mild-to-moderate hepatic impairment, although testosterone levels should be monitored. Has not been studied in patients with severe hepatic impairment; use with caution. Data for use in patients with moderate-to-severe renal impairment (Cl_{cr} <50 mL/minute) is limited; use with caution. Potentially significant drug-drug interactions may exist, requiring dose or frequency adjustment, additional monitoring, and/or selection of alternative therapy.

Adverse Reactions

>10%:

Central nervous system: Fatigue (3% to ≥10%)

Endocrine & metabolic: Hot flash (26%), increased gamma-glutamyl transferase (≥10%), weight loss (≥10%), weight gain (9% to ≥10%)

Hepatic: Increased serum transaminases (47%)

Local: Injection site reactions (35%, grade 3: ≤2%; pain at injection site [28%], erythema at injection site [17%], swelling at injection site [6%], induration at injection site [4%], injection site nodule [3%], injection site infection [including abscess, 1%])

Miscellaneous: Fever (1% to ≥10%)

1% to 10%:

Cardiovascular: Hypertension (6%)

Central nervous system: Chills (5%), dizziness (1% to 5%), headache (1% to 5%), insomnia (1% to 5%)

Dermatologic: Diaphoresis

Endocrine & metabolic: Hypercholesterolemia (3%), gynecomastia

Gastrointestinal: Constipation (5%), nausea (1% to 5%), diarrhea

Genitourinary: Urinary tract infection (5%), erectile dysfunction, testicular atrophy

Hepatic: Increased serum ALT (10%; grade 3: <1%), increased serum AST (5%; grade 3: <1%)

Immunologic: Antibody development (antidegarelix: 10%)

Neuromuscular & skeletal: Back pain (6%), arthralgia (5%), weakness (1% to 5%)

Miscellaneous: Night sweats (1% to 5%)

<1% (Limited to important or life-threatening): Bone metastases (worsening), cerebrovascular accident, depression, hypersensitivity reaction (including anaphylaxis, urticaria, and angioedema), malignant lymphoma, mental status changes, myocardial infarction, osteoarthritis, prolonged Q-T interval on ECG, squamous cell carcinoma, unstable angina pectoris

Drug Interactions

Metabolism/Transport Effects None known.

Avoid Concomitant Use

Avoid concomitant use of Degarelix with any of the following: Highest Risk QTc-Prolonging Agents; Ivabradine; Mifepristone

Increased Effect/Toxicity

Degarelix may increase the levels/effects of: Highest Risk QTc-Prolonging Agents; Moderate Risk QTc-Prolonging Agents

The levels/effects of Degarelix may be increased by: Ivabradine; Mifepristone; QTc-Prolonging Agents (Indeterminate Risk and Risk Modifying)

Decreased Effect There are no known significant interactions involving a decrease in effect.

Preparation for Administration Hazardous agent; use appropriate precautions for handling and disposal (NIOSH, 2012); wear gloves for preparation and administration. Reconstitute with provided preservative free sterile water for injection (reconstitute each 120 mg vial with 3 mL; reconstitute the 80 mg vial with 4.2 mL). Swirl gently; do not shake (to prevent foaming). Dissolution usually takes a few minutes, although may take up to 15 minutes. Keep vial upright at all times. Tilt vial slightly, keeping needle in lowest section of vial to withdraw for administration. Administer within 1 hour of reconstitution. Use of concentrations other than those described in the manufacturer's labeling is not recommended.

Storage/Stability Store at 25°C (77°F); excursions permitted to 15°C to 30°C (59°F to 86°F). Use within 1 hour of reconstitution.

Mechanism of Action Gonadotropin-releasing hormone (GnRH) antagonist which reversibly binds to GnRH receptors in the anterior pituitary gland, blocking the receptor and decreasing secretion of luteinizing hormone (LH) and follicle stimulation hormone (FSH), resulting in rapid androgen deprivation by decreasing testosterone production, thereby decreasing testosterone levels. Testosterone levels do not exhibit an initial surge, or flare, as is typical with GnRH agonists.

Pharmacodynamics/Kinetics

Onset of action: Rapid; ~96% of patients had testosterone levels ≤50 ng/dL within 3 days (Klotz, 2008)

Distribution: V_d: >1000 L

Protein binding: ~90%

Metabolism: Hepatobiliary, via peptide hydrolysis

Bioavailability: Biphasic release: Rapid release initially, then slow release from depot formed after subcutaneous injection administration (Tornoe, 2007). Bioavailability is decreased in patients with mild-to-moderate hepatic impairment.

Half-life elimination: Loading dose: SubQ: ~53 days

Time to peak, plasma: Loading dose: SubQ: Within 2 days

Excretion: Feces (~70% to 80%, primarily as peptide fragments); urine (~20% to 30%)

Dosage

Prostate cancer, advanced: Adults: SubQ:

Loading dose: 240 mg administered as two 120 mg (3 mL) injections

Maintenance dose: 80 mg administered as one 4 mL injection every 28 days (beginning 28 days after initial loading dose)

Dosage adjustment in renal impairment:

Cl_{cr} 50-80 mL/minute: No dosage adjustment necessary.

Cl_{cr} <50 mL/minute: No dosage adjustment provided in manufacturer's labeling; use with caution.

Dosage adjustment in hepatic impairment:

Mild-to-moderate hepatic impairment: No dosage adjustment necessary; monitor serum testosterone levels

Severe hepatic impairment: No dosage adjustment provided in manufacturer's labeling (has not been studied); use with caution.

Dietary Considerations Supplementation with 500 mg calcium and 400 units of vitamin D is recommended (due to increased risk for osteoporosis with androgen deprivation therapy).

Administration Administer (deep) SubQ in the abdominal area by pinching skin and elevating SubQ tissue; insert needle deeply at a 45 degree angle. Avoid pressure exposed areas (eg, waistband, belt, or near ribs). Rotate injection site. Inject loading dose as two 3 mL injections (40 mg/mL) in different sites; maintenance dose should be administered as a single 4 mL injection (20 mg/mL); begin maintenance dose 28 days after initial loading dose. Not for I.V. use; do not inject into a vein or into muscle.

Hazardous agent; use appropriate precautions for handling and disposal (NIOSH, 2012).

Monitoring Parameters Prostate-specific antigen (PSA) periodically, serum testosterone levels (if PSA increases; in patients with hepatic impairment: monitor testosterone levels monthly until achieve castration levels, then consider monitoring every other month), liver function tests (at baseline), serum electrolytes (calcium, magnesium, potassium, sodium); bone mineral density

Screen for diabetes and cardiovascular risk prior to initiating treatment.

Test Interactions Suppression of pituitary-gonadal function may affect diagnostic tests of pituitary gonadotropic and gonadal functions.

Dosage Forms Excipient information presented when available (limited, particularly for generics); consult specific product labeling.

Solution Reconstituted, Subcutaneous, as acetate:

Firmagon: 80 mg (1 ea); 120 mg (1 ea)

◆ **Degarelix Acetate** *see* Degarelix *on page 564*

◆ **Dehydral® (Can)** *see* Methenamine *on page 1319*

◆ **Dehydrobenzperidol** *see* Droperidol *on page 675*

◆ **Delatestryl** *see* Testosterone *on page 2026*

◆ **Delatestryl® (Can)** *see* Testosterone *on page 2026*

Delavirdine (de la VIR deen)

Brand Names: U.S. Rescriptor

Brand Names: Canada Rescriptor®

Index Terms DLV; U-90152S

Pharmacologic Category Antiretroviral, Reverse Transcriptase Inhibitor, Non-nucleoside (Anti-HIV)

Use Treatment of HIV-1 infection in combination with at least two additional antiretroviral agents

Pregnancy Risk Factor C

Pregnancy Considerations Adverse events were observed in some animal reproduction studies. Hypersensitivity reactions (including hepatic toxicity and rash) are more common in women on NNRTI therapy; it is not known if pregnancy increases this risk.

Regardless of CD4 count or HIV RNA copy number, all HIV-infected pregnant women should receive a combination antepartum antiretroviral (ARV) drug regimen; this includes women who require therapy for their own health, as well as women who do not yet require therapy for their own health. ARV therapy should be started as soon as possible if required for the woman's health. Although earlier initiation may be more effective in reducing the perinatal transmission of HIV), also consider maternal conditions (eg, nausea and vomiting) and the potential risks of first trimester fetal exposure for specific agents. Plasma HIV RNA levels should be assessed at ~34-36 weeks gestation in order to help determine mode of delivery. If ARV therapy must be interrupted for <24 hours during the peripartum period, stop then restart all medications simultaneously in order to decrease the chance of developing resistance. Long-term follow-up is recommended for all infants exposed to ARV medications.

Healthcare providers are encouraged to enroll pregnant women exposed to antiretroviral medications in the Antiretroviral Pregnancy Registry (1-800-258-4263 or www.-APRegistry.com). Healthcare providers caring for HIV-infected women and their infants may contact the National Perinatal HIV Hotline (888-448-8765) for clinical consultation (DHHS [perinatal], 2012).

Breast-Feeding Considerations Maternal or infant antiretroviral therapy does not completely eliminate the risk of postnatal HIV transmission. In addition, multiclass-resistant virus has been detected in breast-feeding infants despite maternal therapy. Therefore, in the United States, where formula is accessible, affordable, safe, and sustainable, and the risk of infant mortality due to diarrhea and respiratory infections is low, complete avoidance of breast-feeding by HIV-infected women is recommended to decrease potential transmission of HIV (DHHS [perinatal], 2012).

Contraindications Hypersensitivity to delavirdine or any component of the formulation; concurrent use of alprazolam, astemizole, cisapride, ergot alkaloids, midazolam, pimozide, rifampin, terfenadine, or triazolam

Warnings/Precautions Use with caution in patients with hepatic or renal dysfunction; due to rapid emergence of resistance, delavirdine should not be used as monotherapy or as a component of an initial antiretroviral regimen; cross-resistance may be conferred to other non-nucleoside reverse transcriptase inhibitors, although potential for cross-resistance with protease inhibitors is low. Long-term effects of delavirdine are not known. May cause redistribution of fat (eg, buffalo hump, peripheral wasting with increased abdominal girth, cushingoid appearance). Patients may develop immune reconstitution syndrome resulting in the occurrence of an inflammatory response to an indolent or residual opportunistic infection during initial HIV treatment or activation of autoimmune disorders (eg, Graves' disease, polymyositis, Guillain-Barré syndrome) later in therapy; further evaluation and treatment may be required. Safety and efficacy have not been established in children. Rash, which occurs frequently, may require discontinuation of therapy; usually occurs within 1-3 weeks and lasts <2 weeks. Most patients may resume therapy following a treatment interruption. Use with caution in patients taking strong CYP3A4 inhibitors, moderate or strong CYP3A4 inducers and major CYP3A4 substrates (see Drug Interactions); consider alternative agents that avoid or lessen the potential for CYP-mediated interactions.

Adverse Reactions

Frequency of adverse reactions reported from occurrence in clinical trials with delavirdine when used as part of combination antiretroviral therapy.

>10%:

Central nervous system: Headache (19% to 20%), depressive symptoms (10% to 15%), fever (4% to 12%)
Dermatologic: Rash (16% to 32%)
Gastrointestinal: Nausea (20% to 25%), vomiting (3% to 11%)

1% to 10%:

Central nervous system: Anxiety (6% to 8%)
Endocrine & metabolic: Transaminases increased (2% to 5%), amylase increased (3%), bilirubin increased (2%)
Gastrointestinal: Diarrhea, vomiting, abdominal pain (4% to 6%)
Hematologic: Prothrombin time increased (2%), hemoglobin decreased (1% to 3%)
Respiratory: Bronchitis (6% to 8%)

Frequency not defined (limited to important or life threatening): Abscess, adenopathy, alkaline phosphatase increased, allergic reaction, angioedema, anorexia, arrhythmia, bloody stool, bone pain, bruising, cardiac insufficiency, cardiac rate abnormal, cardiomyopathy, chest congestion, cognitive impairment, colitis, confusion, conjunctivitis, dermal leukocytoclastic vasculitis, desquamation, diverticulitis, dyspnea, emotional lability, eosinophilia, erythema multiforme, fecal incontinence, fungal dermatitis, gamma glutamyl transpeptidase increased, gastroenteritis, gastrointestinal bleeding, granulocytosis, gum hemorrhage, hallucination, hematuria, hepatomegaly, hyperglycemia, hyperkalemia, hypertension, hypertriglyceridemia, hyperuricemia, hypocalcemia, hyponatremia, hypophosphatemia, infection, jaundice, kidney pain, leukopenia, lipase increased, menstrual irregularities, moniliasis (oral/vaginal), orthostatic hypotension, pancreatitis, pancytopenia, paralysis, peripheral vascular disorder, pneumonia, purpura, redistribution of body fat, renal calculi, serum creatinine increased, spleen disorder, Stevens-Johnson syndrome, tetany, thrombocytopenia, urinary tract infection, vertigo

Postmarketing and/or case reports: Acute renal failure, hemolytic anemia, hepatic failure, immune reconstitution syndrome, rhabdomyolysis

Drug Interactions

Metabolism/Transport Effects Substrate of CYP2D6 (minor), CYP3A4 (major); **Note:** Assignment of Major/Minor substrate status based on clinically relevant drug interaction potential; **Inhibits** CYP1A2 (weak), CYP2C19 (strong), CYP2C9 (strong), CYP2D6 (strong), CYP3A4 (strong)

Avoid Concomitant Use

Avoid concomitant use of Delavirdine with any of the following: Ado-Trastuzumab Emtansine; Alfuzosin; Apixaban; Astemizole; Avanafil; Axitinib; Bosutinib; Cabozantinib; CarBAMazepine; Conivaptan; Crizotinib; Dronedarone; Eplerenone; Etravirine; Everolimus; Fosamprenavir; Fosphenytoin; H2-Antagonists; Halofantrine; Ibrutinib; Imatinib; Ivabradine; Lapatinib; Lomitapide; Lovastatin; Lurasidone; Macitentan; Nilotinib; Nisoldipine; Phenytoin; Pimozide; Pomalidomide; Proton Pump Inhibitors; Ranolazine; Red Yeast Rice; Regorafenib; Rilpivirine; Rivaroxaban; Salmeterol; Silodosin; Simeprevir; Simvastatin; St Johns Wort; Tamoxifen; Tamsulosin; Terfenadine; Thioridazine; Ticagrelor; Tolvaptan; Toremifene; Ulipristal; Vemurafenib; VinCRIStine (Liposomal)

Increased Effect/Toxicity

Delavirdine may increase the levels/effects of: Ado-Trastuzumab Emtansine; Alfuzosin; Almotriptan; Alosetron; Apixaban; ARIPiprazole; Astemizole; AtoMOXetine; Avanafil; Axitinib; Bedaquiline; Bortezomib; Bosentan; Bosutinib; Brentuximab Vedotin; Brinzolamide; Budesonide (Nasal); Budesonide (Systemic, Oral Inhalation); Cabozantinib; Carvedilol; Citalopram; Colchicine; Conivaptan; Corticosteroids (Orally Inhaled); Crizotinib; CYP2C19 Substrates; CYP2C9 Substrates; CYP2D6 Substrates; CYP3A4 Substrates; Diclofenac (Systemic); Dienogest; Dofetilide; Dronedarone; Dutasteride; Enzalutamide; Eplerenone; Etravirine; Everolimus; FentaNYL; Fesoterodine; Fluticasone (Nasal); Fluticasone (Oral Inhalation); Fosamprenavir; Fosphenytoin; GuanFACINE; Halofantrine; Ibrutinib; Iloperidone; Imatinib; Ivabradine; Ivacaftor; Ixabepilone; Lacosamide; Lapatinib; Levomilnacipran; Lomitapide; Lovastatin; Lumefantrine; Lurasidone; Macitentan; Maraviroc; MethylPREDNISolone; Metoprolol; Mifepristone; Nebivolol; Nilotinib; Nisoldipine; Ospemifene; OxyCODONE; Paricalcitol; PAZOPanib; Phenytoin; Pimecrolimus; Pimozide; Pomalidomide; PONATinib; Propafenone; Protease Inhibitors; QUEtiapine; Ranolazine; Red Yeast Rice; Regorafenib; Repaglinide; Rifamycin Derivatives; Rilpivirine; Rivaroxaban; RomiDEPsin; Ruxolitinib; Salmeterol; Saxagliptin; Sildenafil; Silodosin; Simeprevir; Simvastatin; SORAfenib; Tadalafil; Tamsulosin; Terfenadine; Tetrabenazine; Thioridazine; Ticagrelor; Tofacitinib; Tolterodine; Tolvaptan; Toremifene; Ulipristal; Vardenafil; Vemurafenib; Vilazodone; VinCRIStine (Liposomal); Vortioxetine; Zuclopenthixol

Decreased Effect

Delavirdine may decrease the levels/effects of: CarBAMazepine; Clopidogrel; Codeine; Etravirine; Ifosfamide; Iloperidone; Prasugrel; Rilpivirine; Tamoxifen; Ticagrelor; TraMADol

The levels/effects of Delavirdine may be decreased by: Antacids; CarBAMazepine; CYP3A4 Inducers (Strong); Dabrafenib; Deferasirox; Fosamprenavir; Fosphenytoin; H2-Antagonists; Mitotane; Peginterferon Alfa-2b; Phenytoin; Protease Inhibitors; Proton Pump Inhibitors; Rifamycin Derivatives; St Johns Wort; Tocilizumab

Ethanol/Nutrition/Herb Interactions Herb/Nutraceutical: Delavirdine serum concentration may be decreased by St John's wort; avoid concurrent use.

Storage/Stability Store at 20°C to 25°C (68°F to 77°F). Protect from humidity.

Mechanism of Action Delavirdine binds directly to reverse transcriptase, blocking RNA-dependent and DNA-dependent DNA polymerase activities

Pharmacodynamics/Kinetics

Absorption: Rapid

Distribution: Low concentration in saliva and semen; CSF 0.4% concurrent plasma concentration

Protein binding: ~98%, primarily albumin

Metabolism: Hepatic via CYP3A4 and 2D6 (**Note:** May reduce CYP3A activity and inhibit its own metabolism.)

Bioavailability: Tablet: 85% as tablet; ~100% as oral slurry

Half-life elimination: 5.8 hours (range: 2-11 hours)

Time to peak, plasma: 1 hour

Excretion: Urine (51%, <5% as unchanged drug); feces (44%); nonlinear kinetics exhibited

Dosage Adolescents ≥16 years and Adults: Oral: 400 mg 3 times/day

Note: Only a single delavirdine mutation causes resistance; use is not recommended in initial antiretroviral regimens (DHHS, 2013).

Dosage adjustment in renal impairment: No dosage adjustment provided in manufacturer's labeling (has not been studied).

Dosage adjustment in hepatic impairment: No dosage adjustment provided in manufacturer's labeling (has not been studied). However, delavirdine is primarily metabolized by the liver, use with caution.

Dietary Considerations May be taken without regard to meals.

Administration Patients with achlorhydria should take the drug with an acidic beverage; antacids and delavirdine should be separated by 1 hour. A dispersion of delavirdine may be prepared by adding four 100 mg tablets to at least 3 oz of water. Allow to stand for a few minutes and stir until uniform dispersion. Drink immediately. Rinse glass and mouth, then swallow the rinse to ensure total dose administered. The 200 mg tablets should be taken intact.

Monitoring Parameters Liver function tests if administered with saquinavir

Additional Information Potential compliance problems, frequency of administration, and adverse effects should be discussed with patients before initiating therapy to help prevent the emergence of resistance.

Dosage Forms Excipient information presented when available (limited, particularly for generics); consult specific product labeling.

Tablet, Oral, as mesylate:

Rescriptor: 100 mg, 200 mg

Extemporaneous Preparations A dispersion of delavirdine may be made with tablets. Add four 100 mg tablets to at least 3 oz of water; allow to stand for a few minutes and stir until uniform dispersion. Administer immediately. To ensure full dose is administered, rinse glass and drink liquid; also rinse mouth and swallow following ingestion.

◆ **Delestrogen** *see* Estradiol (Systemic) *on page 754*

◆ **Delta-9-tetrahydro-cannabinol** *see* Dronabinol *on page 674*

◆ **Delta-9 THC** *see* Dronabinol *on page 674*

◆ **Deltacortisone** *see* PredniSONE *on page 1707*

◆ **Deltadehydrocortisone** *see* PredniSONE *on page 1707*

◆ **Delzicol** *see* Mesalamine *on page 1305*

◆ **Demadex** *see* Torsemide *on page 2097*

Demeclocycline (dem e kloe SYE kleen)

Index Terms Declomycin; Demeclocycline Hydrochloride; Demethylchlortetracycline

Pharmacologic Category Antibiotic, Tetracycline Derivative

Use Treatment of susceptible bacterial infections (eg, acne, urinary tract infections, respiratory infections) caused by both gram-negative and gram-positive organisms

Note: Use of demeclocycline as an antibacterial agent is uncommon; alternative tetracycline agents (eg, doxycycline, minocycline, tetracycline) are generally preferred.

Unlabeled Use Treatment of chronic syndrome of inappropriate secretion of antidiuretic hormone (SIADH)

Pregnancy Risk Factor D

Pregnancy Considerations Tetracyclines, including demeclocycline, cross the placenta and accumulate in developing teeth and long tubular bones. Tetracyclines may discolor fetal teeth following maternal use during pregnancy; the specific teeth involved and the portion of the tooth affected depends on the timing and duration of exposure relative to tooth calcification. As a class, tetracyclines are generally considered second-line antibiotics in pregnant women and their use should be avoided (Gibbons, 1960; Mylonas, 2011).

Breast-Feeding Considerations Tetracyclines are excreted into breast milk. According to the manufacturer, the decision to continue or discontinue breast-feeding during therapy should take into account the risk of exposure to the infant and the benefits of treatment to the mother.

Tetracyclines, including demeclocycline, bind to calcium (Mitrano, 2009). The calcium in maternal milk will significantly decrease the amount of demeclocycline absorbed by the breast-feeding infant. Nondose-related effects could include modification of bowel flora.

Contraindications Hypersensitivity to demeclocycline, tetracyclines, or any component of the formulation

Warnings/Precautions Photosensitivity reactions occur frequently with this drug; avoid prolonged exposure to sunlight and do not use tanning equipment. Use caution in patients with hepatic impairment; dose adjustment and/or adjustment to interval frequency recommended. Hepatotoxicity and hepatic failure have been reported rarely with use. Use with caution in patients with renal impairment; dosage modification required in patients with renal impairment. Nephrotoxicity has also been reported with use, particularly in the setting of cirrhosis. May act as an antianabolic agent and increase BUN. Dose-dependent nephrogenic diabetes insipidus is common with use; however, this adverse event of demeclocycline has been used as a therapeutic advantage in the off-label use of hyponatremia associated with SIADH. Pseudotumor cerebri has been reported with tetracycline use (usually resolves with discontinuation). Prolonged use may result in fungal or bacterial superinfection, including *C. difficile*-associated diarrhea (CDAD) and pseudomembranous colitis; CDAD has been observed >2 months postantibiotic treatment. May cause tissue hyperpigmentation, enamel hypoplasia, or permanent tooth discoloration; use of tetracyclines should be avoided during tooth development (children <8 years of age) unless other drugs are not likely to be effective or are contraindicated. Do not use during pregnancy. In addition to affecting tooth development, tetracycline use has been associated with retardation of skeletal development and reduced bone growth. Concurrent use of tetracyclines and methoxyflurane (not available in the U.S.) is not recommended; fatal renal toxicity has been reported with concurrent use.

Adverse Reactions Frequency not defined.

Cardiovascular: Pericarditis

Central nervous system: Bulging fontanels (infants), dizziness, headache, pseudotumor cerebri (adults)

Dermatologic: Angioedema, anogenital inflammatory lesions (with monilial overgrowth), erythema multiforme, erythematous rash, exfoliative dermatitis (rare), maculopapular rash, photosensitivity, pigmentation of skin, Stevens-Johnson syndrome (rare), urticaria
Endocrine & metabolic: Microscopic discoloration of thyroid gland (brown/black), nephrogenic diabetes insipidus, thyroid dysfunction (rare)
Gastrointestinal: Anorexia, diarrhea, dysphagia, enterocolitis, esophageal ulcerations, glossitis, nausea, pancreatitis, vomiting
Genitourinary: Balanitis
Hematologic: Eosinophilia, neutropenia, hemolytic anemia, thrombocytopenia
Hepatic: Hepatitis (rare), hepatotoxicity (rare), liver enzymes increased, liver failure (rare)
Neuromuscular & skeletal: Myasthenic syndrome, polyarthralgia, tooth discoloration (children <8 years, rarely in adults)
Ocular: Visual disturbances
Otic: Tinnitus
Renal: Acute renal failure, BUN increased
Respiratory: Pulmonary infiltrates
Miscellaneous: Anaphylaxis, anaphylactoid purpura, fixed drug eruptions (rare), lupus-like syndrome, superinfection, systemic lupus erythematosus exacerbation

Drug Interactions

Metabolism/Transport Effects None known.

Avoid Concomitant Use

Avoid concomitant use of Demeclocycline with any of the following: BCG; Retinoic Acid Derivatives; Strontium Ranelate

Increased Effect/Toxicity

Demeclocycline may increase the levels/effects of: Mipomersen; Neuromuscular-Blocking Agents; Porfimer; Retinoic Acid Derivatives; Vitamin K Antagonists

Decreased Effect

Demeclocycline may decrease the levels/effects of: BCG; Desmopressin; Penicillins; Sodium Picosulfate; Typhoid Vaccine

The levels/effects of Demeclocycline may be decreased by: Antacids; Bile Acid Sequestrants; Bismuth; Bismuth Subsalicylate; Calcium Salts; Iron Salts; Lanthanum; Magnesium Salts; Multivitamins/Minerals (with ADEK, Folate, Iron); Multivitamins/Minerals (with AE, No Iron); Quinapril; Strontium Ranelate; Sucralfate; Sucroferric Oxyhydroxide; Zinc Salts

Ethanol/Nutrition/Herb Interactions

Food: Demeclocycline serum levels may be decreased if taken with food, milk, or dairy products. Management: Administer 1 hour before or 2 hours after food, milk, or dairy products.
Herb/Nutraceutical: Some herbal medications may cause photosensitization. Management: Avoid dong quai and St John's wort.

Storage/Stability Store at controlled room temperature at 20°C to 25°C (68°F to 77°F).

Mechanism of Action Inhibits protein synthesis by binding with the 30S and possibly the 50S ribosomal subunit(s) of susceptible bacteria; may also cause alterations in the cytoplasmic membrane; inhibits the action of ADH in patients with chronic SIADH

Pharmacodynamics/Kinetics

Onset of action: SIADH: 2-5 days
Absorption: 66%; extent of absorption is reduced by food and by certain antacids and dairy products containing aluminum, calcium, magnesium, or iron
Distribution: 1.7 L/kg
Protein binding: 40% to 90%
Metabolism: None
Half-life elimination: 10-16 hours
Time to peak, serum: ~4 hours
Excretion: Urine (44% as unchanged drug); feces (13% to 46% as unchanged drug)

Dosage

Susceptible infections: Manufacturer's labeling:
Children >8 years: Oral: 7-13 mg/kg/day (maximum: 600 mg/day) divided every 6-12 hours
Adults: Oral: 150 mg 4 times/day or 300 mg twice daily
SIADH (unlabeled use): Adults: Oral: 600-1200 mg/day (Goh, 2004; Gross, 2008)

Dosing adjustment in renal impairment: Use with caution; dosage adjustment and/or increase in time interval between doses recommended in manufacturer's labeling; no specific adjustment recommendations provided.

Dosing adjustment in hepatic impairment: Use with caution; dosage adjustment and/or increase in time interval between doses recommended in manufacturer's labeling; no specific adjustment recommendations provided.

Dietary Considerations Due to potential for decreased absorption, administer 1 hour before or 2 hours after food or milk.

Administration Administer 1 hour before or 2 hours after food or milk. Administer with adequate amounts of fluid to decrease the risk of esophageal irritation and ulceration.

Monitoring Parameters CBC, renal and hepatic function

Dosage Forms Excipient information presented when available (limited, particularly for generics); consult specific product labeling.

Tablet, Oral, as hydrochloride:
Generic: 150 mg, 300 mg

- ◆ **Demeclocycline Hydrochloride** *see* Demeclocycline *on page 567*
- ◆ **Demerol** *see* Meperidine *on page 1297*
- ◆ **Demerol® (Can)** *see* Meperidine *on page 1297*
- ◆ **4-Demethoxydaunorubicin** *see* IDArubicin *on page 1039*
- ◆ **Demethylchlortetracycline** *see* Demeclocycline *on page 567*
- ◆ **Demser** *see* Metyrosine *on page 1355*
- ◆ **Demulen® 30 (Can)** *see* Ethinyl Estradiol and Ethynodiol Diacetate *on page 786*
- ◆ **Denavir** *see* Penciclovir *on page 1603*

Denosumab (den OH sue mab)

Brand Names: U.S. Prolia; Xgeva

Brand Names: Canada Prolia; Xgeva

Index Terms AMG-162

Pharmacologic Category Bone-Modifying Agent; Monoclonal Antibody

Use

Osteoporosis/bone loss (Prolia): Treatment of osteoporosis in postmenopausal women at high risk of fracture; treatment of osteoporosis (to increase bone mass) in men at high risk of fracture; treatment of bone loss in men receiving androgen-deprivation therapy (ADT) for nonmetastatic prostate cancer; treatment of bone loss in women receiving aromatase inhibitor (AI) therapy for breast cancer

Tumors (Xgeva): Prevention of skeletal-related events (eg, fracture, spinal cord compression, bone pain requiring surgery/radiation therapy) in patients with bone metastases from solid tumors; treatment of giant cell tumor of the bone in adults and skeletally mature adolescents that is unresectable or where surgical resection is likely to result in severe morbidity

Note: NOT indicated for prevention of skeletal-related events in patients with multiple myeloma

Unlabeled Use Treatment of bone destruction caused by rheumatoid arthritis

Pregnancy Risk Factor D (Xgeva)/X (Prolia)

Pregnancy Considerations Adverse events were observed in animal reproduction studies. Specifically, increased fetal loss, stillbirths, postnatal mortality, absent lymph nodes, abnormal bone growth, and decreased neonatal growth was observed in cynomolgus monkeys exposed to denosumab throughout pregnancy. Denosumab was measurable in the offspring at one month of age. Fetal exposure to monoclonal antibodies is expected to increase as pregnancy progresses. Women of reproductive potential should be advised to use effective contraception during denosumab treatment and for at least 5 months following the last dose. If a pregnant woman is exposed, patients or their prescribers may contact the Amgen Pregnancy Surveillance Program (800-772-6436). In addition, there is potential for a fetus to be exposed to denosumab when a pregnant woman has unprotected sex with a man treated with denosumab. It is unknown the extent that denosumab is present in seminal fluid; however, the risk of harm to the fetus is expected to be low. Men receiving denosumab who have pregnant partners should be counseled regarding this potential risk.

Breast-Feeding Considerations It is not known if denosumab is excreted in breast milk. According to the manufacturer, the decision to discontinue denosumab or discontinue breast-feeding should take into account the benefits of treatment to the mother. In some animal studies, mammary gland development was impaired following exposure to denosumab during pregnancy, resulting in impaired lactation postpartum.

Medication Guide Available Yes

Contraindications Hypersensitivity to denosumab or any component of the formulation; pre-existing hypocalcemia; pregnancy (Prolia)

Warnings/Precautions Clinically significant hypersensitivity (including anaphylaxis) has been reported. May include throat tightness, facial edema, upper airway edema, dyspnea, pruritus, rash, urticaria, and hypotension. If anaphylaxis or clinically significant hypersensitivity occurs, initiate appropriate management and permanently discontinue. Denosumab may cause or exacerbate hypocalcemia; severe symptomatic cases (including fatalities) have been reported. Monitor calcium levels; correct pre-existing hypocalcemia prior to therapy. Use caution in patients with a history of hypoparathyroidism, thyroid surgery, parathyroid surgery, malabsorption syndromes, excision of small intestine, severe renal impairment/dialysis or other conditions which would predispose the patient to hypocalcemia; monitor calcium, phosphorus, and magnesium closely during therapy. Ensure adequate calcium and vitamin D intake; supplement with calcium and vitamin D; magnesium supplementation may also be necessary. Incidence of infections may be increased, including serious skin infections, abdominal, urinary, ear, or periodontal infections. Endocarditis has also been reported following use. Patients should be advised to contact their healthcare provider if signs or symptoms of severe infection or cellulitis develop. Use with caution in patients with impaired immune systems or using concomitant immunosuppressive therapy; may be at increased risk for serious infections. Evaluate the need for continued treatment with serious infection.

Atypical femur fractures have been reported in patients receiving denosumab. The fractures may occur anywhere along the femoral shaft (may be bilateral) and commonly occur with minimal to no trauma to the area. Some patients experience prodromal pain weeks or months before the fracture occurs. Because these fractures also occur in osteoporosis patients not treated with denosumab, it is unclear if denosumab therapy is the cause for the fractures; concomitant glucocorticoids may contribute to fracture risk. Advise patients to report new/unusual hip, thigh, or groin pain; and if so, evaluate for atypical/incomplete fracture. Contralateral limb should be assessed if atypical fracture occurs. Consider interrupting therapy in patients who develop an atypical femoral fracture. Osteonecrosis of the jaw (ONJ) has been reported in patients receiving denosumab. ONJ may manifest as jaw pain, osteomyelitis, osteitis, bone erosion, tooth/periodontal infection, toothache, gingival ulceration/erosion. Risk factors include invasive dental procedures (eg, tooth extraction, dental implants, boney surgery); a diagnosis of cancer, concomitant chemotherapy or corticosteroids, poor oral hygiene, ill-fitting dentures; and comorbid disorders (anemia, coagulopathy, infection, pre-existing dental disease). In studies of patients with osseous metastasis, a longer duration of denosumab exposure was associated with a higher incidence of ONJ. Patients should maintain good oral hygiene during treatment. A dental exam and preventative dentistry should be performed prior to therapy. The benefit/risk must be assessed by the treating physician and/or dentist/surgeon prior to any invasive dental procedure; avoid invasive procedures in patients with bone metastases receiving therapy for prevention of skeletal-related events. Patients developing ONJ while on denosumab therapy should receive care by a dentist or oral surgeon; extensive dental surgery to treat ONJ may exacerbate ONJ; evaluate individually and consider discontinuing if extensive dental surgery is necessary.

Postmenopausal osteoporosis: For use in women at high risk for fracture which is defined as a history of osteoporotic fracture or multiple risk factors for fracture. May also be used in women who failed or did not tolerate other therapies.

Bone metastases: Denosumab is not indicated for the prevention of skeletal-related events in patients with multiple myeloma. In trials of with multiple myeloma patients, denosumab was noninferior to zoledronic acid in delaying time to first skeletal-related event and mortality was increased in a subset of the denosumab-treated group.

Denosumab therapy results in significant suppression of bone turnover; the long term effects of treatment are not known but may contribute to adverse outcomes such as ONJ, atypical fractures, or delayed fracture healing; monitor. Use with caution in patients with renal impairment (Cl_{cr} <30 mL/minute) or patients on dialysis; risk of hypocalcemia is increased. Dose adjustment is not needed when administered at 60 mg every 6 months (Prolia); once-monthly dosing has not been evaluated in patients with renal impairment (Xgeva). Dermatitis, eczema, and rash (which are not necessarily specific to the injection site) have been reported; consider discontinuing if severe symptoms occur. Packaging may contain natural latex rubber. May impair bone growth in children with open growth plates or inhibit eruption of dentition. In pediatrics, indicated only for the treatment of giant cell tumor of the bone in adolescents who are skeletally mature. Do not administer Prolia and Xgeva to the same patient for different indications.

Adverse Reactions A postmarketing safety program for Prolia is available to collect information on adverse events; more information is available at http://www.proliasafety.com. To report adverse events for either Prolia or Xgeva, prescribers may also call Amgen at 800-772-6436 or FDA at 800-332-1088.

Percentages noted with Prolia (60 mg every 6 months) unless specified as Xgeva (120 mg every 4 weeks):

>10%:

Central nervous system: Fatigue (Xgeva: 45%), headache (Xgeva: 13%)

Dermatologic: Dermatitis (4% to 11%), eczema (4% to 11%), skin rash (3% to 11%)

Endocrine & metabolic: Hypophosphatemia (Xgeva: 32%; grade 3: 10% to 15%), hypocalcemia (2%; Xgeva: 3% to 18%; grade 3: 3%)

Gastrointestinal: Nausea (Xgeva: 31%), diarrhea (Xgeva: 20%)

Neuromuscular & skeletal: Weakness (Xgeva: 45%), arthralgia (7% to 14%), limb pain (10% to 12%), back pain (8% to 12%)

Respiratory: Dyspnea (Xgeva: 21%), cough (Xgeva: 15%)

1% to 10%:

Cardiovascular: Peripheral edema (5%), angina pectoris (3%)

Central nervous system: Sciatica (5%)

Endocrine & metabolic: Hypercholesterolemia (7%)

Gastrointestinal: Flatulence (2%)

Hematologic & oncologic: Malignant neoplasm (new; 3% to 5%)

Infection: Serious infection (nonfatal; 4%)

Neuromuscular & skeletal: Musculoskeletal pain (6%), bone pain (4%), myalgia (3%), osteonecrosis (jaw; ≤2%; Xgeva ≤2%)

Ophthalmic: Cataract (≤5%)

Respiratory: Nasopharyngitis (7%), upper respiratory tract infection (5%)

<1% (Limited to important or life-threatening): Anaphylaxis (both formulations), antibody development (both formulations), cystitis, femur fracture (both formulations; diaphyseal, subtrochanteric), endocarditis, gastroesophageal reflux disease, hypersensitivity (both formulations), hypertension, influenza, pancreatitis, severe hypocalcemia (symptomatic; both formulations)

Drug Interactions

Metabolism/Transport Effects None known.

Avoid Concomitant Use There are no known interactions where it is recommended to avoid concomitant use.

Increased Effect/Toxicity

Denosumab may increase the levels/effects of: Immunosuppressants

Decreased Effect There are no known significant interactions involving a decrease in effect.

Ethanol/Nutrition/Herb Interactions Ethanol: Ethanol may increase risk of osteoporosis. Management: Avoid ethanol.

Storage/Stability Prior to use, store in original carton under refrigeration, 2°C to 8°C (36°F to 46°F). Do not freeze. Prior to use, bring to room temperature of 25°C (77°F) in original container (usually takes 15-30 minutes); do not use any other methods for warming. Use within 14 days once at room temperature. Protect from direct heat and light; do not expose to temperatures >25°C (77°F). Avoid vigorous shaking.

Mechanism of Action Denosumab is a monoclonal antibody with affinity for nuclear factor-kappa ligand (RANKL). Osteoblasts secrete RANKL; RANKL activates osteoclast precursors and subsequent osteolysis which promotes release of bone-derived growth factors, such as insulin-like growth factor-1 (IGF1) and transforming growth factor-beta (TGF-beta), and increases serum calcium levels. Denosumab binds to RANKL, blocks the interaction between RANKL and RANK (a receptor located on osteoclast surfaces), and prevents osteoclast formation, leading to decreased bone resorption and increased bone mass in osteoporosis. In solid tumors with bony metastases, RANKL inhibition decreases osteoclastic activity leading to decreased skeletal related events and tumor-induced bone destruction. In giant cell tumors of the bone (which express RANK and RANKL), denosumab inhibits tumor growth by preventing RANKL from activating its receptor (RANK) on the osteoclast surface, osteoclast precursors, and osteoclast-like giant cells.

Pharmacodynamics/Kinetics

Onset of action: Decreases markers of bone resorption by ~85% within 3 days; maximal reductions observed within 1 month

Duration: Markers of bone resorption return to baseline within 12 months of discontinuing therapy

Bioavailability: SubQ: 62%

Half-life elimination: ~25-28 days

Time to peak, serum: 10 days (range: 3-21 days)

Dosage Note: Administer calcium and vitamin D as necessary to prevent or treat hypocalcemia

Prevention of skeletal-related events in bone metastases from solid tumors (Xgeva): Adults: SubQ: 120 mg every 4 weeks (Fizazi, 2011; Henry, 2011; Stopeck, 2010)

Treatment of androgen deprivation-induced bone loss in men with prostate cancer (Prolia): Adults: SubQ: 60 mg as a single dose, once every 6 months (Smith, 2009)

Treatment of aromatase inhibitor-induced bone loss in women with breast cancer (Prolia): Adults: SubQ: 60 mg as a single dose, once every 6 months (Ellis, 2008)

Treatment of giant cell tumor of the bone (Xgeva): Adolescents (skeletally mature) 13-17 years and Adults: SubQ: 120 mg once every 4 weeks; during the first month, give an additional 120 mg on days 8 and 15 (Blay, 2011; Thomas, 2010)

Treatment of osteoporosis in men or postmenopausal women (Prolia): Adults: SubQ: 60 mg as a single dose, once every 6 months

Dosage adjustment in renal impairment: Cl_{cr} <30 mL/minute (including dialysis-dependent): No adjustment necessary when administered every 6 months (Prolia); once-monthly dosing has not been evaluated in patients with Cl_{cr} <30 mL/minute or on dialysis (Xgeva). Monitor patients with severe impairment (Cl_{cr} <30 mL/minute or on dialysis) due to increased risk of hypocalcemia.

Dosage adjustment in hepatic impairment: No dosage adjustment provided in manufacturer's labeling (has not been studied).

Dietary Considerations Ensure adequate calcium and vitamin D intake to prevent or treat hypocalcemia. Calcium 1000 mg/day and vitamin D ≥400 units/day is recommended in product labeling (Prolia). If dietary intake is inadequate, dietary supplementation is recommended. Women and men should consume:

Calcium: 1000 mg/day (men: 50-70 years) **or** 1200 mg/day (women ≥51 years and men ≥71 years) (IOM, 2011; NOF, 2013)

Vitamin D: 800-1000 IU/day (men and women ≥50 years) (NOF, 2013). Recommended Dietary Allowance (RDA): 600 IU/day (men and women ≤70 years) **or** 800 IU/day (men and women ≥71 years) (IOM, 2011).

Administration SubQ: Prior to administration, bring to room temperature in original container (allow to stand ~15-30 minutes); do not warm by any other method. Solution may contain trace amounts of translucent to white protein particles; do not use if cloudy, discolored (normal solution should be clear and colorless to pale yellow), or contains excessive particles or foreign matter. Avoid vigorous shaking. Administer via SubQ injection in the upper arm, upper thigh, or abdomen.

Prolia: If a dose is missed, administer as soon as possible, then continue dosing every 6 months from the date of the last injection.

Monitoring Parameters Recommend monitoring of serum creatinine, serum calcium, phosphorus and magnesium, signs and symptoms of hypocalcemia, especially in patients predisposed to hypocalcemia (severe renal impairment, thyroid/parathyroid surgery, malabsorption syndromes, hypoparathyroidism); infection, or dermatologic reactions; routine oral exam (prior to treatment);

dental exam if risk factors for ONJ; monitor for sings/symptoms of hypersensitivity

Osteoporosis: Bone mineral density (BMD) should be re-evaluated every 2 years (or more frequently) after initiating therapy (NOF, 2013); annual measurements of height and weight, assessment of chronic back pain; serum calcium and 25(OH)D; may consider monitoring biochemical markers of bone turnover

Reference Range

Calcium (total): Adults: 9.0-11.0 mg/dL (2.05-2.54 mmol/L), may slightly decrease with aging

Phosphorus: 2.5-4.5 mg/dL (0.81-1.45 mmol/L)

Vitamin D: There is no clear consensus on a reference range for total serum 25(OH)D concentrations or the validity of this level as it relates clinically to bone health. In addition, there is significant variability in the reporting of serum 25(OH)D levels as a result of different assay types in use; however, the following ranges have been suggested:

Adults (IOM, 2011): Sufficient levels in practically all persons: ≥20 ng/mL (50 nmol/L); concern for risk of toxicity: >50 ng/mL (125 nmol/L)

Osteoporosis patients (NOF, 2013): Recommended level to reach and maintain: ~30 ng/mL (75 nmol/L)

Additional Information Oncology Comment: Metastatic breast cancer: The American Society of Clinical Oncology (ASCO) updated guidelines on the role of bone-modifying agents (BMAs) in the prevention and treatment of skeletal-related events for metastatic breast cancer patients (Van Poznak, 2011). The guidelines recommend initiating a BMA (denosumab, pamidronate, zoledronic acid) in patients with metastatic breast cancer to the bone. There is currently no literature indicating the superiority of one particular BMA. Optimal duration is not defined; however, the guidelines recommend continuing therapy until substantial decline in patient's performance status. In patients with normal creatinine clearance (Cl_{cr} >60 mL/minute), no dosage/interval/infusion rate changes for pamidronate or zoledronic acid are necessary. For patients with Cl_{cr} <30 mL/minute, pamidronate and zoledronic acid are not recommended. While no renal dose adjustments are recommended for denosumab, close monitoring is advised for risk of hypocalcemia in patients with Cl_{cr} <30 mL/minute or on dialysis. The ASCO guidelines are in alignment with package insert guidelines for dosing, renal dose adjustments, infusion times, prevention and management of osteonecrosis of the jaw, and monitoring of laboratory parameter recommendations. BMAs are not the first-line therapy for pain. BMAs are to be used as adjunctive therapy for cancer-related bone pain associated with bone metastasis, demonstrating a modest pain control benefit. BMAs should be used in conjunction with agents such as NSAIDs, opioid and nonopioid analgesics, corticosteroids, radiation/surgery, and interventional procedures.

Dosage Forms Excipient information presented when available (limited, particularly for generics); consult specific product labeling.

Solution, Subcutaneous [preservative free]:

Prolia: 60 mg/mL (1 mL) [contains mouse protein (murine) (hamster)]

Xgeva: 120 mg/1.7 mL (1.7 mL)

- **Denta 5000 Plus™** *see* Fluoride *on page* 880
- **DentaGel™** *see* Fluoride *on page* 880
- **Dentapaine [OTC]** *see* Benzocaine *on page* 240
- **Dent-O-Kain/20 [OTC]** *see* Benzocaine *on page* 240
- **Deodorized Tincture of Opium (error-prone synonym)** *see* Opium Tincture *on page* 1513
- **Deoxyazacytidine** *see* Decitabine *on page* 556
- **Deoxycoformycin** *see* Pentostatin *on page* 1617
- **2'-Deoxycoformycin** *see* Pentostatin *on page* 1617
- **Depacon** *see* Valproic Acid and Derivatives *on page* 2149
- **Depakene** *see* Valproic Acid and Derivatives *on page* 2149
- **Depakote** *see* Valproic Acid and Derivatives *on page* 2149
- **Depakote ER** *see* Valproic Acid and Derivatives *on page* 2149
- **Depakote Sprinkles** *see* Valproic Acid and Derivatives *on page* 2149
- **Depen Titratabs** *see* PenicillAMINE *on page* 1603
- **DepoCyt** *see* Cytarabine (Liposomal) *on page* 522
- **DepoCyt® (Can)** *see* Cytarabine (Liposomal) *on page* 522
- **DepoDur** *see* Morphine (Liposomal) *on page* 1403
- **Depo-Estradiol** *see* Estradiol (Systemic) *on page* 754
- **DepoFoam Bupivacaine** *see* Bupivacaine (Liposomal) *on page* 290
- **DepoFoam-Encapsulated Cytarabine** *see* Cytarabine (Liposomal) *on page* 522
- **Depo-Medrol** *see* MethylPREDNISolone *on page* 1340
- **Depo-Medrol® (Can)** *see* MethylPREDNISolone *on page* 1340
- **Depo-Prevera® (Can)** *see* MedroxyPROGESTERone *on page* 1278
- **Depo-Provera** *see* MedroxyPROGESTERone *on page* 1278
- **Depo-Provera® (Can)** *see* MedroxyPROGESTERone *on page* 1278
- **Depo-SubQ Provera 104** *see* MedroxyPROGESTERone *on page* 1278
- **Depotest® 100 (Can)** *see* Testosterone *on page* 2026
- **Depo-Testosterone** *see* Testosterone *on page* 2026
- **Deprenyl** *see* Selegiline *on page* 1884
- **Depsipeptide** *see* RomiDEPsin *on page* 1848
- **DermaFungal [OTC]** *see* Miconazole (Topical) *on page* 1358
- **Dermal Therapy Finger Care [OTC]** *see* Urea *on page* 2140
- **DermaMed [OTC]** *see* Aluminum Hydroxide *on page* 89
- **Derma-Smoothe/FS® (Can)** *see* Fluocinolone (Topical) *on page* 878
- **Derma-Smoothe/FS Body** *see* Fluocinolone (Topical) *on page* 878
- **Derma-Smoothe/FS Scalp** *see* Fluocinolone (Topical) *on page* 878
- **Dermasorb HC** *see* Hydrocortisone (Topical) *on page* 1011
- **Dermasorb TA** *see* Triamcinolone (Topical) *on page* 2123
- **Dermasorb XM** *see* Urea *on page* 2140
- **Dermatop** *see* Prednicarbate *on page* 1704
- **Dermatop® (Can)** *see* Prednicarbate *on page* 1704
- **Dermazene** *see* Iodoquinol and Hydrocortisone *on page* 1109
- **Dermazole (Can)** *see* Miconazole (Topical) *on page* 1358
- **Dermovate® (Can)** *see* Clobetasol *on page* 457
- **Desenex [OTC]** *see* Clotrimazole (Topical) *on page* 476
- **Desenex [OTC]** *see* Miconazole (Topical) *on page* 1358
- **Desenex Jock Itch [OTC]** *see* Miconazole (Topical) *on page* 1358

- **Desenex Spray [OTC]** *see* Miconazole (Topical) *on page 1358*
- **Desferal** *see* Deferoxamine *on page 561*
- **Desferal® (Can)** *see* Deferoxamine *on page 561*
- **Desferrioxamine** *see* Deferoxamine *on page 561*
- **Desiccated Thyroid** *see* Thyroid, Desiccated *on page 2052*

Desipramine (des IP ra meen)

Brand Names: U.S. Norpramin

Brand Names: Canada Dom-Desipramine; Novo-Desipramine; Nu-Desipramine; PMS-Desipramine

Index Terms Desipramine Hydrochloride; Desmethylimipramine Hydrochloride

Pharmacologic Category Antidepressant, Tricyclic (Secondary Amine)

Additional Appendix Information

Antidepressant Agents *on page 2284*

Beers Criteria – Potentially Inappropriate Medications for Geriatrics *on page 2368*

Use Treatment of depression

Unlabeled Use Analgesic adjunct in chronic pain; peripheral neuropathies (including diabetic neuropathy); attention-deficit/hyperactivity disorder (ADHD); depression in children ≤12 years of age

Pregnancy Considerations Animal reproduction studies are inconclusive. Tricyclic antidepressants may be associated with irritability, jitteriness, and convulsions (rare) in the neonate (Yonkers, 2009).

The ACOG recommends that therapy for depression during pregnancy be individualized; treatment should incorporate the clinical expertise of the mental health clinician, obstetrician, primary healthcare provider, and pediatrician (ACOG, 2008). According to the American Psychiatric Association (APA), the risks of medication treatment should be weighed against other treatment options and untreated depression. For women who discontinue antidepressant medications during pregnancy and who may be at high risk for postpartum depression, the medications can be restarted following delivery (APA, 2010). Treatment algorithms have been developed by the ACOG and the APA for the management of depression in women prior to conception and during pregnancy (Yonkers, 2009).

Breast-Feeding Considerations Desipramine is excreted into breast milk. Based on information from one mother-infant pair, following maternal use of desipramine 300 mg/day, the estimated exposure to the breast-feeding infant would be 2% of the weight-adjusted maternal dose. Adverse events were not reported. Infants should be monitored for signs of adverse events; routine monitoring of infant serum concentrations is not recommended (Fortinguerra, 2009).

Medication Guide Available Yes

Contraindications Hypersensitivity to desipramine, drugs of similar chemical class, or any component of the formulation; use of MAO inhibitors intended to treat psychiatric disorders (concurrently or within 14 days of discontinuing either desipramine or the MAO inhibitor); initiation of desipramine in a patient receiving linezolid or intravenous methylene blue; use in a patient during the acute recovery phase of MI

Warnings/Precautions [U.S. Boxed Warning]: Antidepressants increase the risk of suicidal thinking and behavior in children, adolescents, and young adults (18-24 years of age) with major depressive disorder (MDD) and other psychiatric disorders; consider risk prior to prescribing. Short-term studies did not show an increased risk in patients >24 years of age and showed a decreased risk in patients ≥65 years. Closely monitor for clinical worsening, suicidality, or unusual changes in behavior; the patient's family or caregiver should be instructed to closely observe the patient and communicate condition with healthcare provider. A medication guide should be dispensed with each prescription. **Desipramine is FDA approved for the treatment of depression in adolescents.**

The possibility of a suicide attempt is inherent in major depression and may persist until remission occurs. Monitor for worsening of depression or suicidality, especially during initiation of therapy (generally first 1-2 months) or with dose increases or decreases. Use caution in high-risk patients. Worsening depression and severe abrupt suicidality that are not part of the presenting symptoms may require discontinuation or modification of drug therapy. The patient's family or caregiver should be alerted to monitor patients for the emergence of suicidality and associated behaviors (such as agitation, irritability, hostility, impulsivity, and hypomania) and notify healthcare provider.

May worsen psychosis in some patients or precipitate a shift to mania or hypomania in patients with bipolar disorder. Patients presenting with depressive symptoms should be screened for bipolar disorder. Monotherapy in patients with bipolar disorder should be avoided. **Desipramine is not FDA approved for the treatment of bipolar depression.**

Potentially life-threatening serotonin syndrome (SS) has occurred with serotonergic agents (eg, SSRIs, SNRIs), particularly when used in combination with other serotonergic agents (eg, triptans, TCAs, fentanyl, lithium, tramadol, buspirone, St John's wort, tryptophan) or agents that impair metabolism of serotonin (eg, MAO inhibitors intended to treat psychiatric disorders, other MAO inhibitors [ie, linezolid and intravenous methylene blue]). Discontinue treatment (and any concomitant serotonergic agent) immediately if signs/symptoms arise. TCAs may rarely cause bone marrow suppression; monitor for any signs of infection and obtain CBC if symptoms (eg, fever, sore throat) evident. The degree of anticholinergic blockade produced by this agent is low relative to other cyclic antidepressants; however, extreme caution should be used in patients with urinary retention, benign prostatic hyperplasia, narrow-angle glaucoma, xerostomia, visual problems, constipation, or a history of bowel obstruction. The degree of sedation with desipramine are low relative to other antidepressants. However, desipramine may cause drowsiness/sedation, resulting in impaired performance of tasks requiring alertness (eg, operating machinery or driving). The risk of orthostasis is moderate relative to other antidepressants. Due to risk of conduction abnormalities, use with extreme caution in patients with a history of cardiovascular disease (including previous MI, stroke, tachycardia, or conduction abnormalities) or in patients with a family history of sudden death, dysrhythmias, or conduction abnormalities. Use with caution in patients with diabetes mellitus; may alter glucose regulation.

Recommended by the manufacturer to discontinue prior to elective surgery; risks exist for drug interactions with anesthesia and for cardiac arrhythmias. However, definitive drug interactions have not been widely reported in the literature and continuation of tricyclic antidepressants is generally recommended as long as precautions are taken to reduce the significance of any adverse events that may occur (Pass, 2004). May lower seizure threshold - use extreme caution in patients with a previous seizure disorder or condition predisposing to seizures such as brain damage, alcoholism, or concurrent therapy with other drugs which lower the seizure threshold. In some patients, seizures may precede cardiac dysrhythmias and death. May increase the risks associated with electroconvulsive therapy. Bone fractures have been associated with antidepressant treatment. Consider the possibility of a fragility fracture if an antidepressant-treated patient presents with unexplained bone pain, point tenderness, swelling, or bruising (Rabenda, 2013; Rizzoli, 2012). Use with extreme caution in hyperthyroid patients or those receiving thyroid supplementation. Use with caution in patients with glaucoma, hepatic or renal dysfunction. Potentially significant interactions may exist, requiring dose or frequency adjustment, additional monitoring, and/or selection of alternative therapy. Consult drug interactions database for more detailed information.

Use caution in elderly patients; may cause or exacerbate syndrome of inappropriate antidiuretic hormone secretion or hyponatremia; monitor sodium closely with initiation or dosage adjustments in older adults. May be inappropriate in older adults depending on comorbidities (eg, dementia, delirium) due to its potent anticholinergic effects (Beers Criteria). May also increase risk of falling or confusional states.

Abrupt discontinuation or interruption of antidepressant therapy has been associated with a discontinuation syndrome. Symptoms arising may vary with antidepressant however commonly include nausea, vomiting, diarrhea, headaches, light-headedness, dizziness, diminished appetite, sweating, chills, tremors, paresthesias, fatigue, somnolence, and sleep disturbances (eg, vivid dreams, insomnia). Greater risks for developing a discontinuation syndrome have been associated with antidepressants with shorter half-lives, longer durations of treatment, and abrupt discontinuation. For antidepressants of short or intermediate half-lives, symptoms may emerge within 2-5 days after treatment discontinuation and last 7-14 days (APA, 2010; Fava, 2006; Haddad, 2001; Shelton, 2001; Warner, 2006).

Adverse Reactions Frequency not defined.

Cardiovascular: Arrhythmias, edema, flushing, heart block, hyper-/hypotension, MI, palpitation, stroke, tachycardia

Central nervous system: Agitation, anxiety, ataxia, confusion, delusions, disorientation, dizziness, drowsiness, EEG alterations, exacerbation of psychosis, extrapyramidal symptoms, fatigue, fever, hallucinations, headache, hypomania, incoordination, insomnia, neuroleptic malignant syndrome, nightmares, restlessness, seizure, suicidal thinking and behavior

Dermatologic: Alopecia, itching, petechiae, photosensitivity, skin rash, urticaria

Endocrine & metabolic: Breast enlargement, galactorrhea, gynecomastia, hyper-/hypoglycemia, impotence, libido changes, SIADH

Gastrointestinal: Abdominal cramps, anorexia, black tongue, constipation, diarrhea, epigastric distress, nausea, parotid edema, paralytic ileus, stomatitis, sublingual adenitis, unpleasant taste, vomiting, weight gain/loss, xerostomia

Genitourinary: Micturition delayed, nocturia, painful ejaculation, polyuria, testicular edema, urinary retention

Hematologic: Agranulocytosis, eosinophilia, purpura, thrombocytopenia

Hepatic: Alkaline phosphatase increased, cholestatic jaundice, hepatitis, liver enzymes increased

Neuromuscular & skeletal: Falling, numbness, paresthesia of extremities, peripheral neuropathy, tingling, tremor, weakness

Ocular: Blurred vision, disturbances of accommodation, intraocular pressure increased, mydriasis

Otic: Tinnitus

Miscellaneous: Allergic reaction, diaphoresis (excessive), withdrawal symptoms

Drug Interactions

Metabolism/Transport Effects **Substrate** of CYP1A2 (minor), CYP2D6 (major); **Note:** Assignment of Major/Minor substrate status based on clinically relevant drug interaction potential; **Inhibits** CYP2A6 (moderate), CYP2B6 (moderate), CYP2D6 (moderate), CYP2E1 (weak), CYP3A4 (moderate)

Avoid Concomitant Use

Avoid concomitant use of Desipramine with any of the following: Aclidinium; Bosutinib; Ibrutinib; Iobenguane I 123; Ipratropium (Oral Inhalation); Ivabradine; Linezolid; Lomitapide; MAO Inhibitors; Methylene Blue; Moxonidine; Simeprevir; Tegafur; Thioridazine; Tiotropium; Tolvaptan; Ulipristal; Umeclidinium

Increased Effect/Toxicity

Desipramine may increase the levels/effects of: Alpha-/Beta-Agonists (Direct-Acting); Alpha1-Agonists; Amphetamines; Analgesics (Opioid); Anticholinergics; Antipsychotics; Avanafil; Beta2-Agonists; Bosentan; Bosutinib; Budesonide (Systemic, Oral Inhalation); Citalopram; Colchicine; CYP2B6 Substrates; CYP2D6 Substrates; CYP3A4 Substrates; Desmopressin; Dofetilide; Eplerenone; Escitalopram; Everolimus; FentaNYL; Fesoterodine; Halofantrine; Highest Risk QTc-Prolonging Agents; Ibrutinib; Imatinib; Ivabradine; Ivacaftor; Lomitapide; Methylene Blue; Metoclopramide; Metoprolol; Moderate Risk QTc-Prolonging Agents; Nebivolol; OxyCODONE; Pimecrolimus; Propafenone; QuiNIDine; Ranolazine; Saxagliptin; Serotonin Modulators; Simeprevir; Sodium Phosphates; Sulfonylureas; Thioridazine; Tiotropium; Tolvaptan; TraMADol; Ulipristal; Vitamin K Antagonists; Yohimbine

The levels/effects of Desipramine may be increased by: Abiraterone Acetate; Aclidinium; Altretamine; Antipsychotics; Boceprevir; BuPROPion; Cimetidine; Cinacalcet; Citalopram; Cobicistat; CYP2D6 Inhibitors (Moderate); CYP2D6 Inhibitors (Strong); Dexmethylphenidate; DULoxetine; Escitalopram; FLUoxetine; FluvoxaMINE; Ipratropium (Oral Inhalation); Linezolid; Lithium; MAO Inhibitors; Methylphenidate; Metoclopramide; Metyrosine; Mifepristone; Mirabegron; PARoxetine; Pramlintide; Propafenone; Protease Inhibitors; QuiNIDine; Sertraline; Terbinafine (Systemic); Thyroid Products; TraMADol; Umeclidinium; Valproic Acid and Derivatives

Decreased Effect

Desipramine may decrease the levels/effects of: Acetylcholinesterase Inhibitors (Central); Alpha2-Agonists; Alpha2-Agonists (Ophthalmic); Codeine; Ifosfamide; Iobenguane I 123; Moxonidine; Tamoxifen; Tegafur

The levels/effects of Desipramine may be decreased by: Acetylcholinesterase Inhibitors (Central); Barbiturates; CarBAMazepine; Peginterferon Alfa-2b; St Johns Wort

Ethanol/Nutrition/Herb Interactions

Ethanol: May increase CNS depression; monitor for increased effects with coadministration. Caution patients about effects.

Food: Grapefruit juice may inhibit the metabolism of some TCAs and clinical toxicity may result.

Herb/Nutraceutical: Avoid valerian, St John's wort, SAMe, kava kava (may increase risk of serotonin syndrome and/or excessive sedation).

Storage/Stability Store at 20°C to 25°C (68°F to 77°F).

Mechanism of Action Traditionally believed to increase the synaptic concentration of norepinephrine (and to a lesser extent, serotonin) in the central nervous system by inhibition of its reuptake by the presynaptic neuronal membrane. However, additional receptor effects have been found including desensitization of adenyl cyclase, down regulation of beta-adrenergic receptors, and down regulation of serotonin receptors.

Pharmacodynamics/Kinetics

Onset of action: Earliest therapeutic effects: 2-5 days; Maximum antidepressant effect: >2 weeks

Metabolism: Hepatic

Half-life elimination: Adults: 15-24 hours (Weiner, 1981)

Time to peak, plasma: ~6 hours (Weiner, 1981)

Excretion: Urine (~70%)

Dosage Note: Not FDA approved for use in pediatric patients; controlled clinical trials have not shown tricyclic antidepressants to be superior to placebo for the treatment of depression in children and adolescents (Dopheide, 2006; Wagner, 2005).

Oral:

Children 6-12 years: Depression (unlabeled use): 1-3 mg/kg/day in divided doses; monitor carefully with doses >3 mg/kg/day; maximum dose: 5 mg/kg/day.

Adolescents: Depression: Initial dose: Start at the lower range and increase based on tolerance and response to 100 mg/day in divided or single dose; usual maintenance dose: 25-100 mg/day, but doses up to 150 mg/day may be necessary in severely depressed patients

Adults:

Depression: Initial dose: Start at the lower range and increase based on tolerance and response; usual maintenance dose: 100-200 mg/day, but doses up to 300 mg/day may be necessary in severely depressed patients

Neuropathic pain (unlabeled use): Initial: 10-25 mg/day; increase dose every 3 days as necessary until the desired effect is obtained; usual effective dose: 50-150 mg/day (maximum dose: 150 mg/day)

Elderly: Depression: Initial dose: Start at the lower range and increase based on tolerance and response to 100 mg/day in as single or divided doses; usual maintenance dose: 25-100 mg/day, but doses up to 150 mg/day may be necessary in severely depressed patients

Discontinuation of therapy: Upon discontinuation of antidepressant therapy, gradually taper the dose to minimize the incidence of withdrawal symptoms and allow for the detection of re-emerging symptoms. Evidence supporting ideal taper rates is limited. APA and NICE guidelines suggest tapering therapy over at least several weeks with consideration to the half-life of the antidepressant; antidepressants with a shorter half-life may need to be tapered more conservatively. In addition for long-term treated patients, WFSBP guidelines recommend tapering over 4-6 months. If intolerable withdrawal symptoms occur following a dose reduction, consider resuming the previously prescribed dose and/or decrease dose at a more gradual rate (APA, 2010; Bauer, 2002; Haddad, 2001; NCCMH, 2010; Schatzberg, 2006; Shelton, 2001; Warner, 2006).

MAO inhibitor recommendations:

Switching to or from an MAO inhibitor intended to treat psychiatric disorders:

Allow 14 days to elapse between discontinuing an MAO inhibitor intended to treat psychiatric disorders and initiation of desipramine.

Allow 14 days to elapse between discontinuing desipramine and initiation of an MAO inhibitor intended to treat psychiatric disorders.

Use with other MAO inhibitors (linezolid or I.V. methylene blue):

Do not initiate desipramine in patients receiving linezolid or I.V. methylene blue; consider other interventions for psychiatric condition.

If urgent treatment with linezolid or I.V. methylene blue is required in a patient already receiving desipramine and potential benefits outweigh potential risks, discontinue desipramine promptly and administer linezolid or I.V. methylene blue. Monitor for serotonin syndrome for 2 weeks or until 24 hours after the last dose of linezolid or I.V. methylene blue, whichever comes first. May resume desipramine 24 hours after the last dose of linezolid or I.V. methylene blue.

Dosage adjustment in renal impairment: No dosage adjustment provided in manufacturer's labeling; use with caution. Hemodialysis/peritoneal dialysis: Supplemental dose is not necessary.

Dosage adjustment in hepatic impairment: No dosage adjustment provided in manufacturer's labeling.

Monitoring Parameters Monitor blood pressure and pulse rate prior to and during initial therapy; evaluate mental status, suicide ideation (especially at the beginning of therapy or when doses are increased or decreased); monitor weight; ECG in older adults and those patients with cardiac disease; signs/symptoms of serotonin syndrome

When used for the treatment of ADHD, thoroughly evaluate for cardiovascular risk. Monitor heart rate, blood pressure, and consider obtaining ECG prior to initiation (Vetter, 2008); ensure PR interval ≤200 ms, QRS duration ≤120 ms, and QT_c ≤460 ms.

Test Interactions Increased glucose; decreased glucose has also been reported. May interfere with urine detection of amphetamines/methamphetamines (false-positive).

Dosage Forms Excipient information presented when available (limited, particularly for generics); consult specific product labeling.

Tablet, Oral, as hydrochloride:

Norpramin: 10 mg, 25 mg, 50 mg, 75 mg, 100 mg, 150 mg

Generic: 10 mg, 25 mg, 50 mg, 75 mg, 100 mg, 150 mg

◆ **Desipramine Hydrochloride** *see* Desipramine *on page 572*

Desirudin (des i ROO din)

Brand Names: U.S. Iprivask

Index Terms CGP-39393; Desulfato-Hirudin; Desulfatohirudin; Desulphatohirudin; r-Hirudin; Recombinant Desulfatohirudin; Recombinant Hirudin

Pharmacologic Category Anticoagulant, Thrombin Inhibitor

Use Prophylaxis of deep vein thrombosis (DVT) in patients undergoing surgery for hip replacement

Pregnancy Risk Factor C

Dosage SubQ: Adults: DVT prophylaxis: 15 mg every 12 hours; initial dose may be given up to 5-15 minutes prior to surgery (after induction of regional anesthesia, if used); has been administered for up to 12 days (average: 9-12 days) in clinical trials

Dosage adjustment in renal impairment:

Moderate renal impairment (Cl_{cr} ≥31-60 mL/minute/1.73 m^2): 5 mg every 12 hours

Severe renal impairment (Cl_{cr} <31 mL/minute/1.73 m^2): 1.7 mg every 12 hours

Dosage adjustment in hepatic impairment: No dosage adjustment provided in manufacturer's labeling (has not been studied); use with caution.

Additional Information Complete prescribing information should be consulted for additional detail.

Dosage Forms Excipient information presented when available (limited, particularly for generics); consult specific product labeling.

Solution Reconstituted, Subcutaneous:

Iprivask: 15 mg (1 ea)

◆ **Desitin® [OTC]** *see* Zinc Oxide *on page 2230*

◆ **Desitin® Creamy [OTC]** *see* Zinc Oxide *on page 2230*

Desloratadine (des lor AT a deen)

Brand Names: U.S. Clarinex; Clarinex Reditabs

Brand Names: Canada Aerius®; Aerius® Kids; Desloratadine Allergy Control

Pharmacologic Category Histamine H_1 Antagonist; Histamine H_1 Antagonist, Second Generation; Piperidine Derivative

Use Relief of nasal and non-nasal symptoms of seasonal allergic rhinitis (SAR) and perennial allergic rhinitis (PAR); treatment of chronic idiopathic urticaria (CIU)

Pregnancy Risk Factor C

Dosage Oral:

Children:

6-11 months: 1 mg once daily

12 months to 5 years: 1.25 mg once daily

6-11 years: 2.5 mg once daily

Children ≥12 years and Adults: 5 mg once daily

Dosage adjustment in renal impairment:

Children: No dosage adjustment provided in manufacturer's labeling (has not been studied).

Adults: Mild-to-severe impairment: 5 mg every other day.

Dosage adjustment in hepatic impairment:

Children: No dosage adjustment provided in manufacturer's labeling (has not been studied).

Adults: Mild-to-severe impairment: 5 mg every other day.

Additional Information Complete prescribing information should be consulted for additional detail.

Dosage Forms Excipient information presented when available (limited, particularly for generics); consult specific product labeling.

Syrup, Oral:

Clarinex: 0.5 mg/mL (473 mL) [contains edetate disodium, fd&c yellow #6 (sunset yellow), propylene glycol, sodium benzoate; bubble-gum flavor]

Tablet, Oral:

Clarinex: 5 mg [contains fd&c blue #2 aluminum lake]

Generic: 5 mg

Tablet Dispersible, Oral:

Clarinex Reditabs: 2.5 mg, 5 mg [contains aspartame; tutti-frutti flavor]

Generic: 2.5 mg, 5 mg

◆ **Desloratadine Allergy Control (Can)** *see* Desloratadine *on page 575*

Desloratadine and Pseudoephedrine

(des lor AT a deen & soo doe e FED rin)

Brand Names: U.S. Clarinex-D® 12 Hour; Clarinex-D® 24 Hour [DSC]

Index Terms Pseudoephedrine and Desloratadine

Pharmacologic Category Alpha/Beta Agonist; Decongestant; Histamine H_1 Antagonist; Histamine H_1 Antagonist, Second Generation; Piperidine Derivative

Use Relief of nasal and non-nasal symptoms of seasonal allergic rhinitis

Pregnancy Risk Factor C

Dosage Oral: Children ≥12 years and Adults:

Clarinex-D® 12 Hour: One tablet twice daily

Clarinex-D® 24 Hour: One tablet daily

Dosage adjustment in renal impairment: Use is not recommended.

Dosage adjustment in hepatic impairment: Use is not recommended.

Additional Information Complete prescribing information should be consulted for additional detail.

Dosage Forms Excipient information presented when available (limited, particularly for generics); consult specific product labeling. [DSC] = Discontinued product

Tablet, variable release:

Clarinex-D® 12 Hour: Desloratadine 2.5 mg [immediate release] and pseudoephedrine sulfate120 mg [extended release]

Clarinex-D® 24 Hour: Desloratadine 5 mg [immediate release] and pseudoephedrine sulfate 240 mg [extended release] [DSC]

◆ **Desmethylimipramine Hydrochloride** *see* Desipramine *on page 572*

Desmopressin (des moe PRES in)

Brand Names: U.S. DDAVP; DDAVP Rhinal Tube; Stimate

Brand Names: Canada Apo-Desmopressin®; DDAVP®; DDAVP® Melt; Minirin®; Novo-Desmopressin; Octostim®; PMS-Desmopressin

Index Terms 1-Deamino-8-D-Arginine Vasopressin; Desmopressin Acetate

Pharmacologic Category Antihemophilic Agent; Hemostatic Agent; Vasopressin Analog, Synthetic

Use

Injection: Treatment of diabetes insipidus; maintenance of hemostasis and control of bleeding in hemophilia A with factor VIII coagulant activity levels >5% and mild-to-moderate classic von Willebrand's disease (type 1) with factor VIII coagulant activity levels >5%

Nasal solutions (DDAVP® Nasal Spray and DDAVP® Rhinal Tube): Treatment of central diabetes insipidus

Nasal spray (Stimate®): Maintenance of hemostasis and control of bleeding in hemophilia A with factor VIII coagulant activity levels >5% and mild-to-moderate classic von Willebrand's disease (type 1) with factor VIII coagulant activity levels >5%

Tablet: Treatment of central diabetes insipidus, temporary polyuria and polydipsia following pituitary surgery or head trauma, primary nocturnal enuresis

Unlabeled Use Uremic bleeding associated with acute or chronic renal failure; prevention of surgical bleeding in patients with uremia

Pregnancy Risk Factor B

Pregnancy Considerations Adverse events were not observed in animal reproduction studies. Anecdotal reports suggest congenital anomalies and low birth weight. However, causal relationship has not been established. Desmopressin has been used safely throughout pregnancy for the treatment of diabetes insipidus (Brewster, 2005; Schrier, 2010). The use of desmopressin is limited for the treatment of von Willebrand disease in pregnant women (NHLBI, 2007).

Breast-Feeding Considerations It is not known if desmopressin is excreted in breast milk. The manufacturer recommends that caution be exercised when administering desmopressin to nursing women.

Contraindications Hypersensitivity to desmopressin or any component of the formulation; hyponatremia or a history of hyponatremia; moderate-to-severe renal impairment (Cl_{cr} <50 mL/minute)

Canadian labeling: Additional contraindications (not in U.S. labeling): Type 2B or platelet-type (pseudo) von Willebrand's disease (injection, intranasal, oral, sublingual); known hyponatremia, habitual or psychogenic polydipsia, cardiac insufficiency or other conditions requiring diuretic therapy (intranasal, sublingual); nephrosis, severe hepatic dysfunction (sublingual); primary nocturnal enuresis (intranasal)

Warnings/Precautions Allergic reactions and anaphylaxis have been reported rarely with both the I.V. and intranasal formulations. Fluid intake should be adjusted downward in the elderly and very young patients to decrease the possibility of water intoxication and hyponatremia. Use may rarely lead to extreme decreases in plasma osmolality, resulting in seizures, coma, and death. Use caution with cystic fibrosis, heart failure, renal dysfunction, polydipsia (habitual or psychogenic [contraindicated in Canadian labeling]), or other conditions associated with fluid and electrolyte imbalance due to potential hyponatremia. Use caution with coronary artery insufficiency or hypertensive cardiovascular disease; may increase or decrease blood pressure leading to changes in heart rate. Consider switching from nasal to intravenous solution if changes in the nasal mucosa (scarring, edema) occur leading to unreliable absorption. Use caution in patients predisposed to thrombus formation; thrombotic events (acute cerebrovascular thrombosis, acute myocardial infarction) have occurred (rare).

Desmopressin (intranasal and I.V.), when used for hemostasis in hemophilia, is not for use in hemophilia B, type 2B von Willebrand disease, severe classic von Willebrand disease (type 1), or in patients with factor VIII antibodies. In general, desmopressin is also not recommended for use in patients with ≤5% factor VIII activity level, although it may be considered in selected patients with activity levels between 2% and 5%.

Consider switching from nasal to intravenous administration if changes in the nasal mucosa (scarring, edema) occur leading to unreliable absorption. Consider alternative rout of administration (I.V. or intranasal) with inadequate therapeutic response at maximum recommended oral doses. Therapy should be interrupted if patient experiences an acute illness (eg, fever, recurrent vomiting or diarrhea), vigorous exercise, or any condition associated with an increase in water consumption. Some patients may demonstrate a change in response after long-term therapy (>6 months) characterized as decreased response or a shorter duration of response.

Adverse Reactions Frequency may not be defined (may be dose or route related).

Cardiovascular: Blood pressure increased/decreased (I.V.), facial flushing

Central nervous system: Headache (2% to 5%), dizziness (intranasal; ≤3%), chills (intranasal; 2%)

Dermatologic: Rash

Endocrine & metabolic: Hyponatremia, water intoxication

Gastrointestinal: Abdominal pain (intranasal; 2%), gastrointestinal disorder (intranasal; ≤2%), nausea (intranasal; ≤2%), abdominal cramps, sore throat

Hepatic: Transient increases in liver transaminases (associated primarily with tablets)

Local: Injection: Burning pain, erythema, and swelling at the injection site

Neuromuscular & Skeletal: Weakness (intranasal; ≤2%)

Ocular: Conjunctivitis (intranasal; ≤2%), eye edema (intranasal; ≤2%), lacrimation disorder (intranasal; ≤2%)

Respiratory: Rhinitis (intranasal; 3% to 8%), epistaxis (intranasal; ≤3%), nostril pain (intranasal; ≤2%), cough, nasal congestion, upper respiratory infection

<1% (Limited to important or life-threatening): Acute cerebrovascular thrombosis (I.V.), acute MI (I.V.), agitation, allergic reactions (rare), anaphylaxis (rare), balanitis, chest pain, coma, diarrhea, dyspepsia, edema, insomnia, itching eyes, light-sensitive eyes, pain, palpitation, seizure, somnolence, tachycardia, thinking abnormal, vomiting, vulval pain, warmth

Drug Interactions

Metabolism/Transport Effects None known.

Avoid Concomitant Use There are no known interactions where it is recommended to avoid concomitant use.

Increased Effect/Toxicity

Desmopressin may increase the levels/effects of: Lithium

The levels/effects of Desmopressin may be increased by: Analgesics (Opioid); CarBAMazepine; ChlorproMAZINE; LamoTRIgine; Nonsteroidal Anti-Inflammatory Agents; Selective Serotonin Reuptake Inhibitors; Tricyclic Antidepressants

Decreased Effect

The levels/effects of Desmopressin may be decreased by: Demeclocycline; Lithium

Ethanol/Nutrition/Herb Interactions Ethanol: Avoid ethanol (may decrease antidiuretic effect).

Preparation for Administration DDAVP®: Dilute solution for injection in 10-50 mL NS for I.V. infusion (10 mL for children ≤10 kg: 50 mL for adults and children >10 kg).

Storage/Stability

DDAVP®:

Nasal spray: Store at controlled room temperature of 20°C to 25°C (68°F to 77°F). Keep nasal spray in upright position.

Rhinal Tube solution: Store refrigerated at 2°C to 8°C (36°F to 46°F). May store at controlled room temperature of 20°C to 25°C (68°F to 77°F) for up to 3 weeks.

Solution for injection: Store refrigerated at 2°C to 8°C (36°F to 46°F).

Tablet: Store at controlled room temperature of 20°C to 25°C (68°F to 77°F).

DDAVP® Melt (CAN; not available in U.S.): Store at 15°C to 25°C (59°F to 77°F) in original container. Protect from moisture.

Stimate® nasal spray: Store at room temperature not to exceed 25°C (77°F). Discard 6 months after opening bottle.

Mechanism of Action In a dose dependent manner, desmopressin increases cyclic adenosine monophosphate (cAMP) in renal tubular cells which increases water permeability resulting in decreased urine volume and increased urine osmolality; increases plasma levels of von Willebrand factor, factor VIII, and t-PA contributing to a shortened activated partial thromboplastin time (aPTT) and bleeding time.

Pharmacodynamics/Kinetics

Onset of action:

Intranasal: Antidiuretic: 15-30 minutes; Increased factor VIII and von Willebrand factor (vWF) activity (dose related): 30 minutes

Peak effect: Antidiuretic: 1 hour; Increased factor VIII and vWF activity: 1.5 hours

I.V. infusion: Increased factor VIII and vWF activity: 30 minutes (dose related)

Peak effect: 1.5-2 hours

Oral tablet: Antidiuretic: ~1 hour

Peak effect: 4-7 hours

Duration: Intranasal, I.V. infusion, Oral tablet: ~6-14 hours

Absorption: Sublingual: Rapid

Bioavailability: Intranasal: ~3.5%; Oral tablet: 5% compared to intranasal, 0.16% compared to I.V.

Half-life elimination: Intranasal: ~3.5 hours; I.V. infusion: 3 hours; Oral tablet: 2-3 hours

Renal impairment: ≤9 hours

Excretion: Urine

Dosage

Children:

Diabetes insipidus:

I.M., I.V., SubQ: Canadian labeling (not in U.S. labeling): Infants and Children ≥3 months: 0.4 mcg (0.1 mL) once daily or one-tenth (1/10) of the maintenance intranasal dose. Fluid restriction should be observed.

I.V., SubQ: Children <12 years: No definitive dosing available. Adult dosing should **not** be used in this age group; adverse events such as hyponatremia-induced seizures may occur. Dose should be reduced. Some have suggested an initial dosage range of 0.1-1 mcg in 1 or 2 divided doses (Cheetham, 2002). Initiate at low dose and increase as necessary. Closely monitor serum sodium levels and urine output; fluid restriction is recommended.

Intranasal (using 100 mcg/mL nasal solution): Infants and Children 3 months to 12 years: Initial: 5 mcg/day (0.05 mL/day) divided 1-2 times/day; range: 5-30 mcg/day (0.05-0.3 mL/day) divided 1-2 times/day; adjust morning and evening doses separately for an adequate diurnal rhythm of water turnover. **Note:** The nasal spray pump can only deliver doses of 10 mcg (0.1 mL) or multiples of 10 mcg (0.1 mL); if doses other than this are needed, the rhinal tube delivery system is preferred. Fluid restriction should be observed.

Oral:

U.S. labeling: Children ≥4 years: Initial: 0.05 mg twice daily; total daily dose should be increased or decreased as needed to obtain adequate antidiuresis (range: 0.1-1.2 mg divided 2-3 times/day). Fluid restriction should be observed.

Canadian labeling (not in U.S. labeling): Children ≥5 years: Initial: 0.1 mg 3 times/day; total daily dose should be increased or decreased as needed to obtain adequate antidiuresis (range: 0.3-1.2 mg divided 3 times/day). Divide daily doses so that the evening dose is 2 times higher than the morning or afternoon dose to ensure adequate antidiuresis during the night. Fluid restriction should be observed.

Sublingual formulation: Canadian labeling (not in U.S. labeling): Infants and Children ≥3 months: Initial: 60 mcg 3 times/day; total daily dose should be increased or decreased as needed to obtain adequate antidiuresis. Usual maintenance: 60-120 mcg 3 times/day (range: 120-720 mcg divided 2-3 times/day); divide daily doses so that the evening dose is 2 times higher than the morning or afternoon dose to ensure adequate antidiuresis during the night. Fluid restriction should be observed.

Hemophilia A and von Willebrand disease (type 1):

I.V.: Infants and Children ≥3 months: 0.3 mcg/kg by slow infusion; may repeat dose if needed; if used preoperatively, administer 30 minutes before procedure

Canadian labeling (not in U.S. labeling): Maximum I.V. dose: 20 mcg

Note: Adverse events such as hyponatremia-induced seizures have been reported especially in young children using this dosing regimen (Das, 2005; Molnar, 2005; Smith, 1989; Thumfart, 2005; Weinstein, 1989). Fluid restriction and careful monitoring of serum sodium levels and urine output are necessary.

Intranasal (using high concentration spray [1.5 mg/mL]): Infants and Children ≥11 months: Refer to adult dosing.

Nocturnal enuresis:

Oral: Children ≥6 years: 0.2 mg at bedtime; dose may be titrated up to 0.6 mg to achieve desired response. Fluid intake should be limited 1 hour prior to dose until the next morning, or at least 8 hours after administration. **Note:** In the Canadian labeling, use is approved for patients ≥5 years.

Sublingual formulation: Canadian labeling (not in U.S. labeling): Children ≥5 years: Initial: 120 mcg at bedtime; dose may be titrated up to 360 mcg to achieve desired response. Fluid intake should be limited 1 hour prior to dose until the next morning, or at least 8 hours after administration.

Children ≥12 years and Adults:

Diabetes insipidus:

I.V., SubQ: 2-4 mcg/day (0.5-1 mL) in 2 divided doses or one-tenth (1/10) of the maintenance intranasal dose. Fluid restriction should be observed.

Intranasal (using 100 mcg/mL nasal solution): 10-40 mcg/day (0.1-0.4 mL) divided 1-3 times/day; adjust morning and evening doses separately for an adequate diurnal rhythm of water turnover. **Note:** The nasal spray pump can only deliver doses of 10 mcg (0.1 mL) or multiples of 10 mcg (0.1 mL); if doses other than this are needed, the rhinal tube delivery system is preferred. Fluid restriction should be observed.

Oral:

U.S. labeling: Initial: 0.05 mg twice daily; total daily dose should be increased or decreased as needed to obtain adequate antidiuresis (range: 0.1-1.2 mg divided 2-3 times/day). Fluid restriction should be observed.

Canadian labeling (not in U.S. labeling): Initial: 0.1 mg 3 times/day; total daily dose should be increased or decreased as needed to obtain adequate antidiuresis (range: 0.3-1.2 mg divided 3 times/day). Fluid restriction should be observed.

Sublingual formulation: Canadian labeling (not in U.S. labeling): Initial: 60 mcg 3 times/day; total daily dose should be increased or decreased as needed to obtain adequate antidiuresis. Usual maintenance: 60-120 mcg 3 times/day (range: 120-720 mcg divided 2-3 times/day). Fluid restriction should be observed.

Hemophilia A and mild-to-moderate von Willebrand disease (type 1):

I.V.: 0.3 mcg/kg by slow infusion; if used preoperatively, administer 30 minutes before procedure

Canadian labeling (not in U.S. labeling): Maximum I.V. dose: 20 mcg

Intranasal (using high concentration spray [1.5 mg/mL]): <50 kg: 150 mcg (1 spray); >50 kg: 300 mcg (1 spray each nostril); repeat use is determined by the patient's clinical condition and laboratory work; if using preoperatively, administer 2 hours before surgery

Adults:

Diabetes insipidus: I.M., I.V., SubQ: Canadian labeling (not in U.S. labeling): 1-4 mcg (0.25-1 mL) once daily or one-tenth (1/10) of the maintenance intranasal dose. Fluid restriction should be observed.

Uremic bleeding associated with acute or chronic renal failure (unlabeled use) (Watson, 1984): I.V.: 0.4 mcg/kg over 10 minutes

Prevention of surgical bleeding in patients with uremia (unlabeled use) (Mannucci, 1983): I.V.: 0.3 mcg/kg over 30 minutes

Dosage adjustment in renal impairment: Cl_{cr} <50 mL/minute: Use is contraindicated according to the manufacturer; however, has been used in acute and chronic renal failure patients experiencing uremic bleeding or for prevention of surgical bleeding (unlabeled uses) (Mannucci, 1983; Watson, 1984)

Dosage adjustment in hepatic impairment: No dosage adjustment provided in manufacturer's labeling.

Administration

I.M., I.V. push, SubQ injection: Central diabetes insipidus: Withdraw dose from ampul into appropriate syringe size (eg, insulin syringe). Further dilution is not required. Administer as direct injection.

I.V. infusion:

Hemophilia A, von Willebrand disease (type 1), and prevention of surgical bleeding in patients with uremia (unlabeled) (Mannucci, 1983): Infuse over 15-30 minutes

Acute uremic bleeding (unlabeled) (Watson, 1984): May infuse over 10 minutes

Intranasal:

DDAVP®: Nasal pump spray: Delivers 0.1 mL (10 mcg); for doses <10 mcg or for other doses which are not multiples, use rhinal tube. DDAVP® Nasal spray delivers fifty 10 mcg doses. For 10 mcg dose, administer in one nostril. Any solution remaining after 50 doses should be discarded. Pump must be primed prior to first use.

DDAVP® Rhinal tube: Insert top of dropper into tube (arrow marked end) in downward position. Squeeze dropper until solution reaches desired calibration mark. Disconnect dropper. Grasp the tube 3/4 inch from the end and insert tube into nostril until the fingertips reach the nostril. Place opposite end of tube into the mouth (holding breath). Tilt head back and blow with a strong, short puff into the nostril (for very young patients, an adult should blow solution into the child's nose). Reseal dropper after use.

Monitoring Parameters Blood pressure and pulse should be monitored during I.V. infusion

Note: For all indications, fluid intake, urine volume, and signs and symptoms of hyponatremia should be closely monitored especially in high-risk patient subgroups (eg, young children, elderly, patients with heart failure).

Diabetes insipidus: Urine specific gravity, plasma and urine osmolality, serum electrolytes

Hemophilia A: Factor VIII coagulant activity, factor VIII ristocetin cofactor activity, and factor VIII antigen levels, aPTT

von Willebrand disease: Factor VIII coagulant activity, factor VIII ristocetin cofactor activity, and factor VIII von Willebrand antigen levels, bleeding time

Nocturnal enuresis: Serum electrolytes if used for >7 days

Additional Information 10 mcg of desmopressin acetate is equivalent to 40 units

Dosage Forms Considerations

DDAVP and Minirin 5 mL bottles contain 50 sprays.

Stimate 2.5 mL bottles contain 25 sprays.

Dosage Forms Excipient information presented when available (limited, particularly for generics); consult specific product labeling.

Solution, Injection, as acetate:
- DDAVP: 4 mcg/mL (1 mL, 10 mL)
- Generic: 4 mcg/mL (1 mL, 10 mL)

Solution, Nasal, as acetate:
- DDAVP: 0.01% (5 mL)
- DDAVP Rhinal Tube: 0.01% (2.5 mL)
- Stimate: 1.5 mg/mL (2.5 mL) [contains benzalkonium chloride]
- Generic: 0.01% (2.5 mL, 5 mL)

Tablet, Oral, as acetate:
- DDAVP: 0.1 mg, 0.2 mg [scored]
- Generic: 0.1 mg, 0.2 mg

Dosage Forms: Canada Excipient information presented when available (limited, particularly for generics); consult specific product labeling.

Tablet, as acetate, sublingual:
- DDAVP® Melt: 60 mcg, 120 mcg, 240 mcg

◆ **Desmopressin Acetate** *see* Desmopressin *on page 575*

◆ **Desocort® (Can)** *see* Desonide *on page 578*

◆ **Desogen** *see* Ethinyl Estradiol and Desogestrel *on page 784*

◆ **Desogestrel and Ethinyl Estradiol** *see* Ethinyl Estradiol and Desogestrel *on page 784*

◆ **Desonate** *see* Desonide *on page 578*

Desonide (DES oh nide)

Brand Names: U.S. Desonate; DesOwen; DesOwen Cream w/Cetaphil Lot; DesOwen Lot w/Cetaphil Cream; DesOwen Oint w/Cetaphil Lot; LoKara; Verdeso

Brand Names: Canada Desocort®; PMS-Desonide; Tridesilon; Verdeso™

Pharmacologic Category Corticosteroid, Topical

Additional Appendix Information

Topical Corticosteroids *on page 2299*

Use Treatment of inflammatory and pruritic manifestations of corticosteroid responsive dermatosis (low-to-medium potency corticosteroid); mild-to-moderate atopic dermatitis

Pregnancy Risk Factor C

Dosage Topical:

Corticosteroid responsive dermatoses: Adults: Cream, ointment, lotion: Apply 2-3 times/day sparingly. Therapy should be discontinued when control is achieved. If no improvement is seen within 2 weeks, reassessment of diagnosis may be necessary.

Atopic dermatitis: Children ≥3 months and Adults: Foam, gel: Apply 2 times/day sparingly. Therapy should be discontinued when control is achieved. If no improvement is seen within 4 weeks, reassessment of diagnosis may be necessary.

Additional Information Complete prescribing information should be consulted for additional detail.

Dosage Forms Excipient information presented when available (limited, particularly for generics); consult specific product labeling. [DSC] = Discontinued product

Cream, External:
- DesOwen: 0.05% (60 g)
- Generic: 0.05% (15 g, 60 g)

Foam, External:
- Verdeso: 0.05% (50 g [DSC], 100 g) [contains cetyl alcohol, propylene glycol]

Gel, External:
- Desonate: 0.05% (60 g) [contains edetate disodium dihydrate, methylparaben, propylene glycol, propylparaben]

Kit, External:
- DesOwen Cream w/Cetaphil Lot: 0.05% [contains benzyl alcohol, propylene glycol]
- DesOwen Lot w/Cetaphil Cream: 0.05% [contains benzyl alcohol, cetyl alcohol, edetate sodium (tetrasodium), methylparaben, peg-30 glyceryl stearate, propylene glycol, propylparaben]
- DesOwen Oint w/Cetaphil Lot: 0.05% [contains benzyl alcohol]

Lotion, External:
- DesOwen: 0.05% (59 mL, 118 mL) [contains cetyl alcohol, edetate disodium, methylparaben, propylene glycol, propylparaben]
- LoKara: 0.05% (59 mL, 118 mL)
- Generic: 0.05% (59 mL, 118 mL)

Ointment, External:
- DesOwen: 0.05% (60 g)
- Generic: 0.05% (15 g, 60 g)

◆ **DesOwen** *see* Desonide *on page 578*

◆ **DesOwen Cream w/Cetaphil Lot** *see* Desonide *on page 578*

◆ **DesOwen Lot w/Cetaphil Cream** *see* Desonide *on page 578*

◆ **DesOwen Oint w/Cetaphil Lot** *see* Desonide *on page 578*

◆ **Desoxicream (Can)** *see* Desoximetasone *on page 579*

Desoximetasone (des oks i MET a sone)

Brand Names: U.S. Topicort; Topicort Spray

Brand Names: Canada Desoxicream; Topicort®; Topicort® Gel; Topicort® Mild; Topicort® Ointment

Pharmacologic Category Corticosteroid, Topical

Additional Appendix Information

Topical Corticosteroids *on page 2299*

Use

Cream, gel, ointment: Relief of inflammation and pruritic symptoms of corticosteroid-responsive dermatosis

Spray: Plaque psoriasis treatment

Pregnancy Risk Factor C

Dosage Note: Therapy should be discontinued when control is achieved; if no improvement is seen within 4 weeks, reassessment of diagnosis may be necessary.

Corticosteroid-responsive dermatoses: Children, Adolescents, and Adults: Topical: Cream, gel, ointment: Apply a thin film to affected area twice daily

Plaque psoriasis treatment: Adults: Topical: Spray: Apply a thin film to affected area twice daily

Dosage adjustment in renal impairment: No dosage adjustment provided in manufacturer's labeling.

Dosage adjustment in hepatic impairment: No dosage adjustment provided in manufacturer's labeling; use caution.

Additional Information Complete prescribing information should be consulted for additional detail.

Dosage Forms Excipient information presented when available (limited, particularly for generics); consult specific product labeling.

Cream, External:

Topicort: 0.05% (15 g, 60 g, 100 g) [contains cetostearyl alcohol, edetate disodium]

Topicort: 0.25% (15 g, 60 g, 100 g) [contains cetostearyl alcohol]

Generic: 0.05% (15 g, 60 g, 100 g); 0.25% (15 g, 60 g, 100 g)

Gel, External:

Topicort: 0.05% (15 g, 60 g) [contains alcohol, usp, edetate disodium, trolamine (triethanolamine)]

Generic: 0.05% (15 g, 60 g)

Liquid, External:

Topicort Spray: 0.25% (100 mL) [contains isopropyl alcohol, levomenthol]

Ointment, External:

Topicort: 0.05% (15 g, 60 g, 100 g); 0.25% (15 g, 60 g, 100 g)

Generic: 0.05% (60 g, 100 g); 0.25% (15 g, 60 g, 100 g)

◆ **Desoxyephedrine Hydrochloride** *see* Methamphetamine *on page 1317*

◆ **Desoxyn** *see* Methamphetamine *on page 1317*

◆ **Desoxyphenobarbital** *see* Primidone *on page 1715*

◆ **Desulfato-Hirudin** *see* Desirudin *on page 574*

◆ **Desulphatohirudin** *see* Desirudin *on page 574*

Desvenlafaxine (des ven la FAX een)

Brand Names: U.S. Khedezla; Pristiq

Brand Names: Canada Pristiq

Index Terms O-desmethylvenlafaxine; ODV

Pharmacologic Category Antidepressant, Serotonin/Norepinephrine Reuptake Inhibitor

Additional Appendix Information

Antidepressant Agents *on page 2284*

Use Treatment of major depressive disorder (acute and maintenance)

Pregnancy Risk Factor C

Medication Guide Available Yes

Dosage Oral: Adults: Depression: 50 mg once daily; doses up to 400 mg once daily have been studied; however, the manufacturer states there is no evidence that doses >50 mg daily confer any additional benefit. A flat dose response curve for efficacy between 50-400 mg daily has been noted as well as an increase in adverse events.

Discontinuation of therapy: Upon discontinuation of antidepressant therapy, gradually taper the dose to minimize the incidence of withdrawal symptoms and allow for the detection of re-emerging symptoms. Evidence supporting ideal taper rates is limited. APA and NICE guidelines suggest tapering therapy over at least several weeks with consideration to the half-life of the antidepressant; antidepressants with a shorter half-life may need to be tapered more conservatively. In addition for long-term treated patients, WFSBP guidelines recommend tapering over 4-6 months. If intolerable withdrawal symptoms occur following a dose reduction, consider resuming the previously prescribed dose and/or decrease dose at a more gradual rate (APA, 2010; Bauer, 2002; Haddad, 2001; NCCMH, 2010; Schatzberg, 2006; Shelton, 2001; Warner, 2006).

MAO inhibitor recommendations:

Switching to or from an MAO inhibitor intended to treat psychiatric disorders:

Allow 14 days to elapse between discontinuing an MAO inhibitor intended to treat psychiatric disorders and initiation of desvenlafaxine.

Allow 7 days to elapse between discontinuing desvenlafaxine and initiation of an MAO inhibitor intended to treat psychiatric disorders.

Use with other MAO inhibitors (linezolid or I.V. methylene blue):

Do not initiate desvenlafaxine in patients receiving linezolid or I.V. methylene blue; consider other interventions for psychiatric condition.

If urgent treatment with linezolid or I.V. methylene blue is required in a patient already receiving desvenlafaxine and potential benefits outweigh potential risks, discontinue desvenlafaxine promptly and administer linezolid or I.V. methylene blue. Monitor for serotonin syndrome for 7 days or until 24 hours after the last dose of linezolid or I.V. methylene blue, whichever comes first. May resume desvenlafaxine 24 hours after the last dose of linezolid or I.V. methylene blue.

Dosing adjustment in renal impairment:

Cl_{cr} >50 mL/minute: No dosage adjustment necessary.

Cl_{cr} 30-50 mL/minute: 50 mg once daily (maximum)

Cl_{cr} <30 mL/minute: 50 mg every other day (maximum)

End-stage renal disease (ESRD) requiring hemodialysis (HD): 50 mg every other day (maximum). Supplemental doses should not be given after HD.

Dosing adjustment in hepatic impairment:

Mild impairment: No dosage adjustment necessary.

Moderate-to-severe impairment: Initial: 50 mg once daily; maximum dose: 100 mg daily

Additional Information Complete prescribing information should be consulted for additional detail.

Dosage Forms Excipient information presented when available (limited, particularly for generics); consult specific product labeling.

Tablet Extended Release 24 Hour, Oral:

Khedezla: 50 mg

Khedezla: 100 mg [contains fd&c yellow #6 (sunset yellow)]

Pristiq: 50 mg, 100 mg

Generic: 50 mg, 100 mg

◆ Desyrel *see* TraZODone *on page 2112*

◆ Detemir Insulin *see* Insulin Detemir *on page 1088*

◆ Detrol *see* Tolterodine *on page 2088*

◆ Detrol® (Can) *see* Tolterodine *on page 2088*

◆ Detrol LA *see* Tolterodine *on page 2088*

◆ Detrol® LA (Can) *see* Tolterodine *on page 2088*

◆ Detryptoreline *see* Triptorelin *on page 2131*

Dexamethasone (Systemic)

(deks a METH a sone)

Brand Names: U.S. Baycadron; Dexamethasone Intensol; DexPak 10 Day; DexPak 13 Day; DexPak 6 Day

Brand Names: Canada Apo-Dexamethasone; Dexasone; Dom-Dexamethasone; PHL-Dexamethasone; PMS-Dexamethasone; PRO-Dexamethasone; ratio-Dexamethasone

Index Terms Decadron; Dexamethasone Sodium Phosphate

Pharmacologic Category Anti-inflammatory Agent; Antiemetic; Corticosteroid, Systemic

Additional Appendix Information

Contrast Media Reactions, Premedication for Prophylaxis *on page 2373*

Corticosteroids Systemic Equivalencies *on page 2297*

Use Primarily as an anti-inflammatory or immunosuppressant agent in the treatment of a variety of diseases including those of allergic, dermatologic, endocrine, hematologic, inflammatory, neoplastic, nervous system, renal, respiratory, rheumatic, and autoimmune origin; may be used in management of cerebral edema, chronic swelling, as a diagnostic agent, diagnosis of Cushing's syndrome, antiemetic

Unlabeled Use Dexamethasone suppression test as an indicator of depression and/or risk of suicide; prevention and treatment of acute mountain sickness and high altitude cerebral edema; accelerate fetal lung maturation in patients with preterm labor

Pregnancy Risk Factor C

Pregnancy Considerations Adverse events have been observed with corticosteroids in animal reproduction studies. Dexamethasone crosses the placenta (ACOG, 2011); and is partially metabolized to an inactive metabolite by placental enzymes (Murphy, 2007). Some studies have shown an association between first trimester systemic corticosteroid use and oral clefts (Park-Wyllie, 2000; Pradat, 2003). Systemic corticosteroids may also influence fetal growth (decreased birth weight); however, information is conflicting (Lunghi, 2010). Hypoadrenalism may occur in newborns following maternal use of corticosteroids in pregnancy; monitor.

Due to its positive effect on stimulating fetal lung maturation, the injection is often used in patients with premature labor (24-34 weeks gestation) (ACOG, 2011). When systemic corticosteroids are needed in pregnancy, it is generally recommended to use the lowest effective dose for the shortest duration of time, avoiding high doses during the first trimester (Leachman, 2006; Lunghi, 2010; Makol, 2011; Østensen, 2009).

Women exposed to dexamethasone during pregnancy for the treatment of an autoimmune disease may contact the OTIS Autoimmune Diseases Study at 877-311-8972.

Breast-Feeding Considerations Corticosteroids are excreted in human milk; information specific to dexamethasone has not been located. The manufacturer notes that when used systemically, maternal use of corticosteroids have the potential to cause adverse events in a nursing infant (eg, growth suppression, interfere with endogenous corticosteroid production). Due to the potential for serious adverse reactions in the nursing infant, the manufacturer recommends a decision be made whether to discontinue nursing or to discontinue the drug, taking into account the importance of treatment to the mother. If there is concern about exposure to the infant, some guidelines recommend waiting 4 hours after the maternal dose of an oral systemic corticosteroid before breast feeding in order to decrease potential exposure to the nursing infant (based on a study using prednisolone) (Bae, 2011; Leachman, 2006; Makol, 2011; Ost, 1985).

Contraindications Hypersensitivity to dexamethasone or any component of the formulation; systemic fungal infections, cerebral malaria

Warnings/Precautions Use with caution in patients with thyroid disease, hepatic impairment, renal impairment, cardiovascular disease, diabetes, glaucoma, cataracts, myasthenia gravis, patients at risk for osteoporosis, patients at risk for seizures, or GI diseases (diverticulitis, peptic ulcer, ulcerative colitis) due to perforation risk. Use caution following acute MI (corticosteroids have been associated with myocardial rupture). Because of the risk of adverse effects, systemic corticosteroids should be used cautiously in the elderly in the smallest possible effective dose for the shortest duration. May affect growth velocity; growth should be routinely monitored in pediatric patients. Withdraw therapy with gradual tapering of dose.

May cause hypercorticism or suppression of hypothalamic-pituitary-adrenal (HPA) axis, particularly in younger children or in patients receiving high doses for prolonged periods. HPA axis suppression may lead to adrenal crisis. Withdrawal and discontinuation of a corticosteroid should be done slowly and carefully. Particular care is required when patients are transferred from systemic corticosteroids to inhaled products due to possible adrenal insufficiency or withdrawal from steroids, including an increase in allergic symptoms. Patients receiving >20 mg per day of prednisone (or equivalent) may be most susceptible. Fatalities have occurred due to adrenal insufficiency in asthmatic patients during and after transfer from systemic corticosteroids to aerosol steroids; aerosol steroids do not provide the systemic steroid needed to treat patients having trauma, surgery, or infections. Dexamethasone does not provide adequate mineralocorticoid activity in adrenal insufficiency (may be employed as a single dose while cortisol assays are performed). The lowest possible dose should be used during treatment; discontinuation and/or dose reductions should be gradual.

Acute myopathy has been reported with high dose corticosteroids, usually in patients with neuromuscular transmission disorders; may involve ocular and/or respiratory muscles; monitor creatine kinase; recovery may be delayed. Corticosteroid use may cause psychiatric disturbances, including depression, euphoria, insomnia, mood swings, and personality changes. Pre-existing psychiatric conditions may be exacerbated by corticosteroid use. Prolonged use of corticosteroids may also increase the incidence of secondary infection, mask acute infection (including fungal infections), prolong or exacerbate viral infections, or limit response to vaccines. Exposure to chickenpox should be avoided; corticosteroids should not be used to treat ocular herpes simplex. Corticosteroids should not be used for cerebral malaria or viral hepatitis.

Close observation is required in patients with latent tuberculosis and/or TB reactivity; restrict use in active TB (only in conjunction with antituberculosis treatment). Prolonged treatment with corticosteroids has been associated with the development of Kaposi's sarcoma (case reports); if noted, discontinuation of therapy should be considered. High-dose corticosteroids should not be used to manage acute head injury.

Adverse Reactions Frequency not defined.

Cardiovascular: Arrhythmia, bradycardia, cardiac arrest, cardiomyopathy, CHF, circulatory collapse, edema, hypertension, myocardial rupture (post-MI), syncope, thromboembolism, vasculitis

Central nervous system: Depression, emotional instability, euphoria, headache, intracranial pressure increased, insomnia, malaise, mood swings, neuritis, personality changes, pseudotumor cerebri (usually following discontinuation), psychic disorders, seizure, vertigo

Dermatologic: Acne, allergic dermatitis, alopecia, angioedema, bruising, dry skin, erythema, fragile skin, hirsutism, hyper-/hypopigmentation, hypertrichosis, perianal pruritus (following I.V. injection), petechiae, rash, skin atrophy, skin test reaction impaired, striae, urticaria, wound healing impaired

Endocrine & metabolic: Adrenal suppression, carbohydrate tolerance decreased, Cushing's syndrome, diabetes mellitus, glucose intolerance decreased, growth suppression (children), hyperglycemia, hypokalemic alkalosis, menstrual irregularities, negative nitrogen balance, pituitary-adrenal axis suppression, protein catabolism, sodium retention

Gastrointestinal: Abdominal distention, appetite increased, gastrointestinal hemorrhage, gastrointestinal perforation, nausea, pancreatitis, peptic ulcer, ulcerative esophagitis, weight gain

Genitourinary: Altered (increased or decreased) spermatogenesis

Hepatic: Hepatomegaly, transaminases increased

Local: Postinjection flare (intra-articular use), thrombophlebitis

Neuromuscular & skeletal: Arthropathy, aseptic necrosis (femoral and humoral heads), fractures, muscle mass loss, myopathy (particularly in conjunction with neuromuscular disease or neuromuscular-blocking agents), neuropathy, osteoporosis, parasthesia, tendon rupture, vertebral compression fractures, weakness

Ocular: Cataracts, exophthalmos, glaucoma, intraocular pressure increased

Renal: Glucosuria

Respiratory: Pulmonary edema

Miscellaneous: Abnormal fat deposition, anaphylactoid reaction, anaphylaxis, avascular necrosis, diaphoresis, hiccups, hypersensitivity, impaired wound healing, infections, Kaposi's sarcoma, moon face, secondary malignancy

Drug Interactions

Metabolism/Transport Effects **Substrate** of CYP3A4 (major), P-glycoprotein; **Note:** Assignment of Major/Minor substrate status based on clinically relevant drug interaction potential; **Inhibits** P-glycoprotein; **Induces** CYP2A6 (weak/moderate), CYP2B6 (weak/moderate), CYP2C9 (weak/moderate), CYP3A4 (strong), P-glycoprotein

Avoid Concomitant Use

Avoid concomitant use of Dexamethasone (Systemic) with any of the following: Abiraterone Acetate; Aldesleukin; Apixaban; Artemether; Axitinib; BCG; Bedaquiline; Boceprevir; Bosutinib; Cabozantinib; CloZAPine; Conivaptan; Crizotinib; Dabigatran Etexilate; Dienogest; Dronedarone; Enzalutamide; Everolimus; Fusidic Acid (Systemic); Ibrutinib; Itraconazole; Ivacaftor; Lapatinib; Lumefantrine; Lurasidone; Macitentan; Mifepristone; Natalizumab; NIFEdipine; Nilotinib; Nisoldipine; PAZOPanib; Perampanel; Pimecrolimus; Pomalidomide; PONATinib; Praziquantel; Ranolazine; Regorafenib; Rilpivirine; Rivaroxaban; Roflumilast; RomiDEPsin; Simeprevir; Sofosbuvir; SORAfenib; Tacrolimus (Topical); Telaprevir; Ticagrelor; Tofacitinib; Tolvaptan; Toremifene; Ulipristal; Vandetanib; Vemurafenib; VinCRIStine (Liposomal)

Increased Effect/Toxicity

Dexamethasone (Systemic) may increase the levels/effects of: Acetylcholinesterase Inhibitors; Amphotericin B; Clarithromycin; CycloSPORINE (Systemic); Deferasirox; Ifosfamide; Leflunomide; Lenalidomide; Loop Diuretics; Natalizumab; NSAID (COX-2 Inhibitor); NSAID (Nonselective); Thalidomide; Thiazide Diuretics; Tofacitinib; Vaccines (Live); Warfarin

The levels/effects of Dexamethasone (Systemic) may be increased by: Antifungal Agents (Azole Derivatives, Systemic); Aprepitant; Asparaginase (E. coli); Asparaginase (Erwinia); Calcium Channel Blockers (Nondihydropyridine); Clarithromycin; Conivaptan; CycloSPORINE (Systemic); CYP3A4 Inhibitors (Moderate); CYP3A4 Inhibitors (Strong); Denosumab; Estrogen Derivatives; Fluconazole; Fosaprepitant; Fusidic Acid (Systemic); Indacaterol; Luliconazole; Macrolide Antibiotics; Mifepristone; Neuromuscular-Blocking Agents (Nondepolarizing); P-glycoprotein/ABCB1 Inhibitors; Pimecrolimus; Quinolone Antibiotics; Roflumilast; Salicylates; Tacrolimus (Topical); Telaprevir; Trastuzumab

Decreased Effect

Dexamethasone (Systemic) may decrease the levels/effects of: Abiraterone Acetate; Afatinib; Aldesleukin; Antidiabetic Agents; Apixaban; ARIPiprazole; Artemether; Axitinib; BCG; Bedaquiline; Boceprevir; Bosutinib; Brentuximab Vedotin; Cabozantinib; Calcitriol; Caspofungin; Clarithromycin; CloZAPine; Cobicistat; Coccidioidin Skin Test; Corticorelin; Crizotinib; CycloSPORINE (Systemic); CYP3A4 Substrates; Dabigatran Etexilate; Dasatinib; Dienogest; Dronedarone; Elvitegravir; Enzalutamide; Everolimus; Exemestane; Gefitinib; GuanFACINE; Hyaluronidase; Ibrutinib; Imatinib; Isoniazid; Itraconazole; Ivacaftor; Ixabepilone; Lapatinib; Linagliptin; Lumefantrine; Lurasidone; Macitentan; Maraviroc; Mifepristone; NIFEdipine; Nilotinib; Nisoldipine; PAZOPanib; Perampanel; P-glycoprotein/ABCB1 Substrates; Pomalidomide; PONATinib; Praziquantel; QUEtiapine; Ranolazine; Regorafenib; Rilpivirine; Rivaroxaban; Roflumilast; RomiDEPsin; Salicylates; Simeprevir; Sipuleucel-T; Sofosbuvir; SORAfenib; SUNItinib; Tadalafil; Telaprevir; Ticagrelor; Tofacitinib; Tolvaptan; Toremifene; Triazolam; Ulipristal; Urea Cycle Disorder Agents; Vaccines (Inactivated); Vandetanib; Vemurafenib; VinCRIStine (Liposomal); Vortioxetine; Zuclopenthixol

The levels/effects of Dexamethasone (Systemic) may be decreased by: Aminoglutethimide; Antacids; Barbiturates; Bile Acid Sequestrants; Bosentan; CYP3A4 Inducers (Strong); Dabrafenib; Echinacea; Herbs (CYP3A4 Inducers); Mifepristone; Mitotane; P-glycoprotein/ABCB1 Inducers; Primidone; Rifamycin Derivatives; Tocilizumab

Ethanol/Nutrition/Herb Interactions

Ethanol: Avoid ethanol (may enhance gastric mucosal irritation).

Food: Dexamethasone interferes with calcium absorption. Limit caffeine.

Herb/Nutraceutical: Avoid cat's claw, echinacea (have immunostimulant properties).

Preparation for Administration

Oral: Oral administration of dexamethasone for croup may be prepared using a parenteral dexamethasone formulation and mixing it with an oral flavored syrup (Bjornson, 2004).

I.V.: May be given undiluted or further diluted in NS or D_5W. Use preservative-free product when used in neonates, especially premature infants.

Storage/Stability Injection: Store intact vials at 20°C to 25°C (68°F to 77°F). Protect from light, heat, or freezing. Diluted solutions should be used within 24 hours.

Mechanism of Action Decreases inflammation by suppression of neutrophil migration, decreased production of inflammatory mediators, and reversal of increased capillary permeability; suppresses normal immune response. Dexamethasone's mechanism of antiemetic activity is unknown.

Pharmacodynamics/Kinetics

Onset of action: Acetate: Prompt

Duration of metabolic effect: 72 hours; acetate is a long-acting repository preparation

Metabolism: Hepatic

Half-life elimination: Normal renal function: 1.8-3.5 hours; Biological half-life: 36-54 hours

Time to peak, serum: Oral: 1-2 hours; I.M.: ~8 hours

Excretion: Urine and feces

Dosage Refer to individual protocols.

Children:

Antiemetic (prior to chemotherapy): Refer to individual protocols and emetogenic potential: I.V.: 10 mg/m²/dose every 12-24 hours on days of chemotherapy for severely emetogenic chemotherapy courses

Anti-inflammatory immunosuppressant: Oral, I.M., I.V.: 0.08-0.3 mg/kg/day **or** 2.5-10 mg/m²/day in divided doses every 6-12 hours

Extubation or airway edema: Oral, I.M., I.V.: 0.5-2 mg/kg/day in divided doses every 6 hours beginning 24 hours prior to extubation and continuing for 4-6 doses afterwards

Cerebral edema: I.V.: Loading dose: 1-2 mg/kg/dose as a single dose; maintenance: 1-1.5 mg/kg/day (maximum: 16 mg/day) in divided doses every 4-6 hours, taper off over 1-6 weeks

Croup (laryngotracheobronchitis): Oral, I.M., I.V.: 0.6 mg/kg once; usual maximum dose: 16 mg (doses as high as 20 mg have been used) (Bjornson, 2004; Hegenbarth, 2008; Rittichier, 2000); a single oral dose of 0.15 mg/kg has been shown effective in children with mild-to-moderate croup (Russell, 2004; Sparrow, 2006)

Bacterial meningitis: Infants and Children >6 weeks: I.V.: 0.15 mg/kg/dose every 6 hours for the first 2-4 days of antibiotic treatment; start dexamethasone 10-20 minutes before or with the first dose of antibiotic

Physiologic replacement: Oral, I.M., I.V.: 0.03-0.15 mg/kg/day **or** 0.6-0.75 mg/m²/day in divided doses every 6-12 hours

Acute mountain sickness (AMS)/high altitude cerebral edema (HACE) (unlabeled use): Oral, I.M., I.V.: 0.15 mg/kg/dose every 6 hours; consider using for high altitude pulmonary edema because of associated HACE with this condition (Luks, 2010; Pollard, 2001)

Adults:

Antiemetic:

Prophylaxis: Oral, I.V.: 10-20 mg 15-30 minutes before treatment on each treatment day

Continuous infusion regimen: Oral or I.V.: 10 mg every 12 hours on each treatment day

Mildly emetogenic therapy: Oral, I.M., I.V.: 4 mg every 4-6 hours

Delayed nausea/vomiting: Oral: 4-10 mg 1-2 times/day for 2-4 days **or**
8 mg every 12 hours for 2 days; then
4 mg every 12 hours for 2 days **or**
20 mg 1 hour before chemotherapy; then
10 mg 12 hours after chemotherapy; then
8 mg every 12 hours for 4 doses; then
4 mg every 12 hours for 4 doses

Anti-inflammatory:

Oral, I.M., I.V. (injections should be given as sodium phosphate): 0.75-9 mg/day in divided doses every 6-12 hours

Intra-articular, intralesional, or soft tissue (as sodium phosphate): 0.4-6 mg/day

Multiple myeloma: Oral, I.V.: 40 mg/day, days 1 to 4, 9 to 12, and 17 to 20, repeated every 4 weeks (alone or as part of a regimen)

Cerebral edema: I.V. 10 mg stat, 4 mg I.M./I.V. every 6 hours until response is maximized, then switch to oral regimen, then taper off if appropriate; dosage may be reduced after 2-4 days and gradually discontinued over 5-7 days

Extubation or airway edema: Oral, I.M., I.V. (injections should be given as sodium phosphate): 0.5-2 mg/kg/day in divided doses every 6 hours beginning 24 hours prior to extubation and continuing for 4-6 doses afterwards

Dexamethasone suppression test (depression/suicide indicator) (unlabeled use): Oral: 1 mg at 11 PM, draw blood at 8 AM the following day for plasma cortisol determination

Cushing's syndrome, diagnostic: Oral: 1 mg at 11 PM, draw blood at 8 AM; greater accuracy for Cushing's syndrome may be achieved by the following:

Dexamethasone 0.5 mg by mouth every 6 hours for 48 hours (with 24-hour urine collection for 17-hydroxycorticosteroid excretion)

Differentiation of Cushing's syndrome due to ACTH excess from Cushing's due to other causes: Oral: Dexamethasone 2 mg every 6 hours for 48 hours (with 24-hour urine collection for 17-hydroxycorticosteroid excretion)

Multiple sclerosis (acute exacerbation): 30 mg/day for 1 week, followed by 4-12 mg/day for 1 month

Physiological replacement: Oral, I.M., I.V. (should be given as sodium phosphate): 0.03-0.15 mg/kg/day **or** 0.6-0.75 mg/m²/day in divided doses every 6-12 hours

Treatment of shock:

Addisonian crisis/shock (ie, adrenal insufficiency/responsive to steroid therapy): I.V. (given as sodium phosphate): 4-10 mg as a single dose, which may be repeated if necessary

Unresponsive shock (ie, unresponsive to steroid therapy): I.V. (given as sodium phosphate): 1-6 mg/kg as a single I.V. dose or up to 40 mg initially followed by repeat doses every 2-6 hours while shock persists

Acute mountain sickness (AMS)/high altitude cerebral edema (HACE) (unlabeled use):

Prevention: Oral: 2 mg every 6 hours **or** 4 mg every 12 hours starting on the day of ascent; may be discontinued after staying at the same elevation for 2-3 days or if descent is initiated; do not exceed a 10 day duration (Luks, 2010). **Note:** In situations of rapid ascent to altitudes >3500 meters (such as rescue or military operations), 4 mg every 6 hours may be considered (Luks, 2010).

Treatment: Oral, I.M., I.V.:

AMS: 4 mg every 6 hours (Luks, 2010)

HACE: Initial: 8 mg as a single dose; Maintenance: 4 mg every 6 hours until symptoms resolve (Luks, 2010)

Antenatal fetal maturation (unlabeled use): I.M.: 6 mg every 12 hours for a total of 4 doses (ACOG, 2011). **Note:** Recommended for pregnant women with premature labor (24-34 weeks gestation) who are expected to deliver within 7 days.

Dosage adjustment in renal impairment: No dosage adjustment provided in manufacturer's labeling; use with caution.

Hemodialysis: Supplemental dose is not necessary

Peritoneal dialysis: Supplemental dose is not necessary

Dosage adjustment in hepatic impairment: No dosage adjustment provided in manufacturer's labeling.

Dietary Considerations May be taken with meals to decrease GI upset. May need diet with increased potassium, pyridoxine, vitamin C, vitamin D, folate, calcium, and phosphorus.

Administration

Oral: Administer with meals to decrease GI upset.

I.V.: Administer the 4 mg/mL or 10 mg/mL concentration intravenously as an undiluted or diluted solution.

I.M.: Administer the 4 mg/mL or 10 mg/mL concentration deep IM.

Intra-articular: Administer into affected joint using the 4 mg/mL concentration only.

Intralesional injection: Administer into affected area using the 4 mg/mL concentration only.

Soft tissue injection: Administer into affected tissue using the 4 mg/mL concentration only.

Topical: For external use only. Do not use on open wounds.

Monitoring Parameters Hemoglobin, occult blood loss, serum potassium, glucose, growth in children

Reference Range Dexamethasone suppression test, overnight: 8 AM cortisol <6 mcg/100 mL (dexamethasone 1 mg); plasma cortisol determination should be made on the day after giving dose

Test Interactions May suppress the wheal and flare reactions to skin test antigens

Additional Information Effects of inhaled/intranasal steroids on growth have been observed in the absence of laboratory evidence of HPA axis suppression, suggesting that growth velocity is a more sensitive indicator of systemic corticosteroid exposure in pediatric patients than some commonly used tests of HPA axis function. The long-term effects of this reduction in growth velocity associated with orally-inhaled and intranasal corticosteroids, including the impact on final adult height, are unknown. The potential for "catch up" growth following discontinuation of treatment with inhaled corticosteroids has not been adequately studied.

Withdrawal/tapering of therapy: Corticosteroid tapering following short-term use is limited primarily by the need to control the underlying disease state; tapering may be accomplished over a period of days. Following longer-term use, tapering over weeks to months may be necessary to avoid signs and symptoms of adrenal insufficiency and to allow recovery of the HPA axis. Testing of HPA axis responsiveness may be of value in selected patients. Subtle deficits in HPA response may persist for months after discontinuation of therapy, and may require supplemental dosing during periods of acute illness or surgical stress.

Dosage Forms Excipient information presented when available (limited, particularly for generics); consult specific product labeling.

Concentrate, Oral:

Dexamethasone Intensol: 1 mg/mL (30 mL) [contains alcohol, usp; unflavored flavor]

Elixir, Oral:

Baycadron: 0.5 mg/5 mL (237 mL) [contains alcohol, usp, benzoic acid, fd&c red #40, propylene glycol; raspberry flavor]

Generic: 0.5 mg/5 mL (237 mL)

Solution, Oral:

Generic: 0.5 mg/5 mL (240 mL, 500 mL)

Solution, Injection, as sodium phosphate:

Generic: 4 mg/mL (1 mL, 5 mL, 30 mL); 10 mg/mL (1 mL, 10 mL)

Solution, Injection, as sodium phosphate [preservative free]:

Generic: 10 mg/mL (1 mL)

Tablet, Oral:

DexPak 10 Day: 1.5 mg [scored; contains fd&c red #40 aluminum lake]

DexPak 13 Day: 1.5 mg [scored; contains fd&c red #40 aluminum lake]

DexPak 6 Day: 1.5 mg [scored; contains fd&c red #40 aluminum lake]

Generic: 0.5 mg, 0.75 mg, 1 mg, 1.5 mg, 2 mg, 4 mg, 6 mg

Dexamethasone (Ophthalmic)

(deks a METH a sone)

Brand Names: U.S. Maxidex; Ozurdex

Brand Names: Canada Diodex®; Maxidex®; Ozurdex®

Index Terms Dexamethasone Sodium Phosphate

Pharmacologic Category Anti-inflammatory Agent, Ophthalmic; Corticosteroid, Ophthalmic; Corticosteroid, Otic

Use Management of steroid-responsive inflammatory conditions such as allergic conjunctivitis, iritis, or cyclitis; symptomatic treatment of corneal injury from chemical, radiation, or thermal burns, or penetration of foreign bodies. The ophthalmic solution is also indicated for otic use to treat steroid-responsive inflammatory conditions of the external auditory meatus.

Ophthalmic intravitreal implant (Ozurdex®): Treatment of macular edema following branch retinal vein occlusion (BRVO) or central retinal vein occlusion (CRVO); treatment of noninfective uveitis

Pregnancy Risk Factor C

Dosage Adults:

Ophthalmic:

Anti-inflammatory:

Solution: Instill 1-2 drops into conjunctival sac every hour during the day and every other hour during the night; gradually reduce dose to 1 drop every 4 hours, then to 3-4 times/day

Suspension: Instill 1-2 drops into conjunctival sac up to 4-6 times/day; may use hourly in severe disease; taper prior to discontinuation

Macular edema (following BRVO or CRVO): Ocular implant (Ozurdex®): Intravitreal injection: 0.7 mg implant injected in affected eye

Noninfective uveitis: Ocular implant (Ozurdex®): Intravitreal injection: 0.7 mg implant injected in affected eye

Otic: Anti-inflammatory: Solution: Initial: Instill 3-4 drops into the aural canal 2-3 times a day; reduce dose gradually once a favorable response is obtained. Alternately, may pack the aural canal with a gauze wick saturated with the solution; remove from the ear after 12-24 hours. Repeat as necessary.

Dosage adjustment in renal impairment: No dosage adjustment provided in manufacturer's labeling.

Dosage adjustment in hepatic impairment: No dosage adjustment provided in manufacturer's labeling.

Additional Information Complete prescribing information should be consulted for additional detail.

Dosage Forms Excipient information presented when available (limited, particularly for generics); consult specific product labeling.

Implant, Intraocular [preservative free]:

Ozurdex: 0.7 mg (1 ea)

Solution, Ophthalmic, as phosphate:

Generic: 0.1% (5 mL)

Suspension, Ophthalmic:

Maxidex: 0.1% (5 mL)

◆ **Dexamethasone and Ciprofloxacin** *see* Ciprofloxacin and Dexamethasone *on page* 435

◆ **Dexamethasone and Tobramycin** *see* Tobramycin and Dexamethasone *on page* 2079

◆ **Dexamethasone Intensol** *see* Dexamethasone (Systemic) *on page 580*

◆ **Dexamethasone, Neomycin, and Polymyxin B** *see* Neomycin, Polymyxin B, and Dexamethasone *on page 1439*

◆ **Dexamethasone Sodium Phosphate** *see* Dexamethasone (Ophthalmic) *on page 583*

◆ **Dexamethasone Sodium Phosphate** *see* Dexamethasone (Systemic) *on page 580*

◆ **Dexasone (Can)** *see* Dexamethasone (Systemic) *on page 580*

Dexchlorpheniramine (deks klor fen EER a meen)

Index Terms Dexchlorpheniramine Maleate

Pharmacologic Category Alkylamine Derivative; Histamine H_1 Antagonist; Histamine H_1 Antagonist, First Generation

Additional Appendix Information

Beers Criteria – Potentially Inappropriate Medications for Geriatrics *on page 2368*

Use Perennial and seasonal allergic rhinitis and other allergic symptoms including urticaria

Dosage Oral:

Children:

2-5 years: 0.5 mg every 4-6 hours (do not use timed release)

6-11 years: 1 mg every 4-6 hours or 4 mg timed release at bedtime

Adults: 2 mg every 4-6 hours or 4-6 mg timed release at bedtime or every 8-10 hours

Dosage adjustment in renal impairment: No dosage adjustment provided in manufacturer's labeling.

Dosage adjustment in hepatic impairment: No dosage adjustment provided in manufacturer's labeling.

Additional Information Complete prescribing information should be consulted for additional detail.

Dosage Forms Excipient information presented when available (limited, particularly for generics); consult specific product labeling.

Syrup, Oral, as maleate:

Generic: 2 mg/5 mL (473 mL)

◆ **Dexchlorpheniramine Maleate** *see* Dexchlorpheniramine *on page 584*

◆ **Dexchlorpheniramine Tannate, Pseudoephedrine Tannate, and Dextromethorphan Tannate** *see* Chlorpheniramine, Pseudoephedrine, and Dextromethorphan *on page 414*

◆ **Dexedrine** *see* Dextroamphetamine *on page 588*

◆ **Dexedrine® (Can)** *see* Dextroamphetamine *on page 588*

◆ **Dexferrum** *see* Iron Dextran Complex *on page 1119*

◆ **Dexilant** *see* Dexlansoprazole *on page 584*

◆ **Dexiron (Can)** *see* Iron Dextran Complex *on page 1119*

Dexlansoprazole (deks lan SOE pra zole)

Brand Names: U.S. Dexilant

Brand Names: Canada Dexilant

Index Terms Kapidex; TAK-390MR

Pharmacologic Category Proton Pump Inhibitor; Substituted Benzimidazole

Use

Erosive esophagitis: For healing of all grades of erosive esophagitis for up to 8 weeks; to maintain healing of erosive esophagitis and relief of heartburn for up to 6 months.

Gastroesophageal reflux disease: For the treatment of heartburn associated with symptomatic nonerosive gastroesophageal reflux disease (GERD) for 4 weeks.

Pregnancy Risk Factor B

Medication Guide Available Yes

Dosage Oral: Adults:

Erosive esophagitis (EE): Short-term treatment: 60 mg once daily for up to 8 weeks; maintenance of healed EE and symptomatic relief of heartburn: 30 mg once daily for up to 6 months. **Note:** Doses >30 mg do not provide additional benefit during maintenance phase.

Symptomatic GERD: Short-term treatment: 30 mg once daily for 4 weeks. **Note:** Doses >30 mg do not provide additional benefit during maintenance phase.

Dosage adjustment in renal impairment: No dosage adjustment necessary

Dosage adjustment in hepatic impairment:

Mild hepatic impairment (Child-Pugh class A): No dosage adjustment necessary

Moderate hepatic impairment (Child-Pugh class B): Consider a maximum dose of 30 mg once daily

Severe hepatic impairment (Child-Pugh class C): No dosage adjustment provided in manufacturer's labeling (has not been studied).

Additional Information Complete prescribing information should be consulted for additional detail.

Dosage Forms Excipient information presented when available (limited, particularly for generics); consult specific product labeling.

Capsule Delayed Release, Oral:

Dexilant: 30 mg, 60 mg [contains fd&c blue #2 aluminum lake]

Dexmedetomidine (deks MED e toe mi deen)

Brand Names: U.S. Precedex

Brand Names: Canada Precedex

Index Terms Dexmedetomidine Hydrochloride

Pharmacologic Category $Alpha_2$-Adrenergic Agonist; Sedative

Use Sedation of initially-intubated and mechanically-ventilated patients during treatment in an intensive care setting; procedural sedation prior to and/or during awake fiberoptic intubation; sedation prior to and/or during surgical or other procedures of nonintubated patients

Unlabeled Use Awake craniotomy; procedural sedation in children (MRI, CT, EEG; with or without ketamine); treatment of shivering

Pregnancy Risk Factor C

Pregnancy Considerations Adverse effects were observed in some animal reproduction studies. Dexmedetomidine is expected to cross the placenta. Information related to use during pregnancy is limited (El-Tahan, 2012).

Breast-Feeding Considerations It is not known if dexmedetomidine is excreted in breast milk. The manufacturer recommends that caution be exercised when administering dexmedetomidine to nursing women.

Contraindications There are no contraindications listed in the manufacturer's labeling.

Warnings/Precautions Should be administered only by persons skilled in management of patients in intensive care setting or operating room. Patients should be continuously monitored. Episodes of bradycardia, hypotension, and sinus arrest have been associated with dexmedetomidine. Use caution in patients with heart block, severe ventricular dysfunction, hypovolemia, diabetes, chronic hypertension, and elderly. Use with caution in patients with hepatic impairment; dosage reductions recommended. Use with caution in patients receiving vasodilators or drugs which decrease heart rate. If medical intervention is required, treatment may include stopping or decreasing the infusion; increasing the rate of I.V. fluid administration, use of pressor agents, and elevation of the lower extremities. Transient hypertension has been primarily observed during the loading dose administration and is associated with the initial peripheral vasoconstrictive effects of dexmedetomidine. Treatment is generally unnecessary; however, reduction of infusion rate may be required. Patients may be arousable and alert when stimulated. This alone should not be considered as lack of efficacy in the absence of other clinical signs/symptoms. When withdrawn abruptly in patients who have received >24 hours of therapy, withdrawal symptoms similar to clonidine withdrawal may result (eg, hypertension, tachycardia, nervousness, nausea, vomiting, agitation, headaches). Use for >24 hours is not recommended by the manufacturer. Use of infusions >24 hours has been associated with tolerance and tachyphylaxis and dose-related increase in adverse reactions.

Adverse Reactions Frequency dependent upon dose, duration, and indication.

>10%:

Cardiovascular: Hypotension (24% to 56%), bradycardia (5% to 42%), systolic hypertension (28%), tachycardia (25%), hypertension (diastolic; 12%), hypertension (11%)

Central nervous system: Agitation (5% to 14%)

Gastrointestinal: Constipation (6% to 14%), nausea (3% to 11%)

Respiratory: Respiratory depression (37%; placebo 32%)

1% to 10%:

Cardiovascular: Atrial fibrillation (2% to 9%), peripheral edema (3% to 7%), hypovolemia (3%), edema (2%)

Central nervous system: Anxiety (5% to 9%)

Endocrine & metabolic: Hypokalemia (9%), hyperglycemia (7%), hypoglycemia (5%), increased thirst (2%), hypocalcemia (1%), hypomagnesemia (1%)

Gastrointestinal: Xerostomia (3% to 4%)

Genitourinary: Oliguria (2%)

Hematologic & oncologic: Anemia (3%)

Renal: Acute renal failure (2% to 3%), decreased urine output (1%)

Respiratory: Respiratory failure (2% to 10%), adult respiratory distress syndrome (1% to 9%), pleural effusion (2%), wheezing (≤1%)

Miscellaneous: Fever (5% to 7%), withdrawal syndrome (ICU sedation; 3% to 5%)

Postmarketing and/or case reports (Limited to important or life-threatening): Acidosis, apnea, atrioventricular block, bronchospasm, cardiac arrest, cardiac arrhythmia, confusion, delirium, diaphoresis, drug tolerance (use >24 hours), extrasystoles, hallucination, heart block, hemorrhage, hepatic insufficiency, hyperbilirubinemia, hypercapnia, hyperkalemia, hyperpyrexia, hypoventilation, hypoxia, illusion, increased blood urea nitrogen, increased gamma-glutamyl transferase, increased serum alkaline phosphatase, increased serum ALT, increased serum AST, inversion T wave on ECG, myocardial infarction, neuralgia, neuritis, oliguria, photopsia, pulmonary congestion, respiratory acidosis, rigors, seizure, sinoatrial arrest, speech disturbance, supraventricular tachycardia, tachyphylaxis (use >24 hours), ventricular arrhythmia, ventricular tachycardia, visual disturbance

Drug Interactions

Metabolism/Transport Effects Substrate of CYP2A6 (major); **Note:** Assignment of Major/Minor substrate status based on clinically relevant drug interaction potential; **Inhibits** CYP1A2 (weak), CYP2C9 (weak), CYP3A4 (weak)

Avoid Concomitant Use

Avoid concomitant use of Dexmedetomidine with any of the following: Iobenguane I 123; Pimozide

Increased Effect/Toxicity

Dexmedetomidine may increase the levels/effects of: ARIPiprazole; Beta-Blockers; Dofetilide; Hypotensive Agents; Lomitapide; Pimozide

The levels/effects of Dexmedetomidine may be increased by: Beta-Blockers; CYP2A6 Inhibitors (Moderate); CYP2A6 Inhibitors (Strong); MAO Inhibitors

Decreased Effect

Dexmedetomidine may decrease the levels/effects of: Iobenguane I 123

The levels/effects of Dexmedetomidine may be decreased by: Antidepressants (Alpha2-Antagonist); Serotonin/Norepinephrine Reuptake Inhibitors; Tricyclic Antidepressants

Preparation for Administration Dexmedetomidine injection concentrate (100 mcg/mL) must be diluted in 0.9% sodium chloride solution to achieve the required concentration (4 mcg/mL) prior to administration. Add 2 mL (200 mcg) of dexmedetomidine to 48 mL of 0.9% sodium chloride for a total volume of 50 mL (4 mcg/mL). Shake gently to mix.

Storage/Stability Store at controlled room temperature of 25°C (77°F); excursions permitted to 15°C to 30°C (59°F to 86°F).

Mechanism of Action Selective $alpha_2$-adrenoceptor agonist with anesthetic and sedative properties thought to be due to activation of G-proteins by $alpha_{2a}$-adrenoceptors in the brainstem resulting in inhibition of norepinephrine release; peripheral $alpha_{2b}$-adrenoceptors are activated at high doses or with rapid I.V. administration resulting in vasoconstriction.

Pharmacodynamics/Kinetics

Onset of action: I.V. Bolus: 5-10 minutes

Peak effect: 15-30 minutes

Duration (dose dependent): 60-120 minutes

Distribution: V_{ss}: ~118 L; rapid

Protein binding: ~94%

Metabolism: Hepatic via N-glucuronidation, N-methylation, and CYP2A6

Half-life elimination: Distribution: ~6 minutes; Terminal: ~up to 3 hours (Venn, 2002); significantly prolonged in patients with severe hepatic impairment (Cunningham, 1999)

Excretion: Urine (95%); feces (4%)

Dosage Note: Errors have occurred due to misinterpretation of dosing information. Maintenance dose expressed as mcg/kg/**hour**.

Individualized and titrated to desired clinical effect. Manufacturer recommends duration of infusion should not exceed 24 hours; however, randomized clinical trials have demonstrated efficacy and safety comparable to lorazepam and midazolam with longer-term infusions of up to ~5 days (Pandharipande, 2007; Riker, 2009).

ICU sedation:

Adults: I.V.: Initial: Loading infusion (optional; see **"Note"** below) of 1 mcg/kg over 10 minutes, followed by a maintenance infusion of 0.2-0.7 mcg/kg/**hour**; adjust rate to desired level of sedation; titration no more frequently than every 30 minutes may reduce the incidence of hypotension (Gerlach, 2009)

Note: *Loading infusion:* The loading dose may be omitted for this indication if patient is either being converted from another sedative and patient is adequately sedated or there are concerns for hemodynamic compromise. *Maintenance infusion:* Dosing ranges between 0.2-1.4 mcg/kg/**hour** have been reported during randomized controlled clinical trials (Pandharipande, 2007; Riker, 2009). Although infusion rates as high as 2.5 mcg/kg/**hour** have been used, it is thought that doses >1.5 mcg/kg/**hour** do not add to clinical efficacy (Venn, 2003).

Elderly (>65 years of age): Consider dosage reduction. No specific guidelines available. Dose selections should be cautious, at the low end of dosage range; titration should be slower, allowing adequate time to evaluate response.

Procedural sedation:

Adults: I.V.: Initial: Loading infusion of 1 mcg/kg over 10 minutes, followed by a maintenance infusion of 0.6 mcg/kg/**hour**, titrate to desired effect; usual range: 0.2-1 mcg/kg/**hour**

Fiberoptic intubation (awake): I.V. Initial: Loading infusion of 1 mcg/kg over 10 minutes, followed by a maintenance infusion of 0.7 mcg/kg/**hour** until endotracheal tube is secured (Bergese, 2010).

Elderly (>65 years of age): I.V.: Initial: Loading infusion of 0.5 mcg/kg over 10 minutes; Maintenance infusion: Dosage reduction should be considered.

Craniotomy (awake) (unlabeled use): I.V.: Initial: Loading infusion of 1 mcg/kg over 10 minutes, followed by a maintenance infusion of 0.5 mcg/kg/**hour**, titrate to desired effect (Bekker, 2008); usual range: 0.1-0.7 mcg/kg/**hour** (Piccioni, 2008)

Dosage adjustment in renal impairment: No specific guidelines available; however, dexmedetomidine pharmacokinetics were not different in patients with severe renal impairment compared to those with normal renal function.

Dosage adjustment in hepatic impairment: Consider dosage reduction. No specific guidelines available.

Usual Infusion Concentrations: Pediatric I.V. infusion: 4 mcg/mL

Usual Infusion Concentrations: Adult I.V. infusion: 200 mcg in 50 mL (concentration: 4 mcg/mL) of NS

Administration Administer using a controlled infusion device. Advisable to use administration components made with synthetic or coated natural rubber gaskets. Parenteral products should be inspected visually for particulate matter and discoloration prior to administration. If loading dose used, administer over 10 minutes; may extend to 20 minutes to further reduce vasoconstrictive effects. Titration no more frequently than every 30 minutes may reduce the incidence of hypotension when used for ICU sedation (Gerlach, 2009).

Monitoring Parameters Level of sedation; heart rate, respiration, rhythm, blood pressure; pain control

Critically-ill mechanically ventilated patients: Monitor depth of sedation with either the Richmond Agitation-Sedation Scale (RASS) or Sedation-Agitation Scale (SAS) (Barr, 2013)

Dosage Forms Excipient information presented when available (limited, particularly for generics); consult specific product labeling.

Solution, Intravenous [preservative free]:

Precedex: 200 mcg/2 mL (2 mL) [additive free]

Precedex: 200 mcg/50 mL (50 mL); 400 mcg/100 mL (100 mL) [latex free]

◆ **Dexmedetomidine Hydrochloride** *see* Dexmedetomidine *on page 584*

Dexmethylphenidate (dex meth il FEN i date)

Brand Names: U.S. Focalin; Focalin XR

Index Terms Dexmethylphenidate Hydrochloride

Pharmacologic Category Central Nervous System Stimulant

Use Treatment of attention-deficit/hyperactivity disorder (ADHD)

Pregnancy Risk Factor C

Medication Guide Available Yes

Dosage Treatment of ADHD: Oral:

Children ≥6 years: Patients not currently taking methylphenidate:

Immediate release: Initial: 2.5 mg twice daily; dosage may be adjusted in increments of 2.5-5 mg at weekly intervals (maximum dose: 20 mg/day); doses should be taken at least 4 hours apart

Extended release: Initial: 5 mg once daily; dosage may be adjusted in increments of 5 mg/day at weekly intervals (maximum dose: 30 mg/day)

Conversion to dexmethylphenidate from methylphenidate:

Immediate release: Initial: Half the total daily dose of racemic methylphenidate (maximum dexmethylphenidate dose: 20 mg/day)

Extended release: Initial: Half the total daily dose of racemic methylphenidate (maximum dexmethylphenidate dose: 30 mg/day)

Conversion from dexmethylphenidate immediate release to dexmethylphenidate extended release: When changing from Focalin® tablets to Focalin® XR capsules, patients may be switched to the same daily dose using Focalin® XR (maximum dose: 30 mg/day)

Adults: Patients not currently taking methylphenidate:

Immediate release: Initial: 2.5 mg twice daily; dosage may be adjusted in increments of 2.5-5 mg at weekly intervals (maximum dose: 20 mg/day); doses should be taken at least 4 hours apart

Extended release: Initial: 10 mg once daily; dosage may be adjusted in increments of 10 mg/day at weekly intervals (maximum dose: 40 mg/day)

Conversion to dexmethylphenidate from methylphenidate:

Immediate release: Initial: Half the total daily dose of racemic methylphenidate (maximum dexmethylphenidate dose: 20 mg/day)

Extended release: Initial: Half the total daily dose of racemic methylphenidate (maximum dexmethylphenidate dose: 40 mg/day)

Conversion from dexmethylphenidate immediate release to dexmethylphenidate extended release: When changing from Focalin® tablets to Focalin® XR capsules, patients may be switched to the same daily dose using Focalin® XR (maximum dose: 40 mg/day)

Dose reductions and discontinuation: Children ≥6 years and Adults: Reduce dose or discontinue in patients with paradoxical aggravation of symptoms. Discontinue if no improvement is seen after one month of treatment.

Dosage adjustment in renal impairment: No data available. However, considering extensive metabolism to inactive compounds, renal insufficiency expected to have minimal effect on kinetics of dexmethylphenidate.

Dosage adjustment in hepatic impairment: No data available.

Additional Information Complete prescribing information should be consulted for additional detail.

Dosage Forms Excipient information presented when available (limited, particularly for generics); consult specific product labeling.

Capsule Extended Release 24 Hour, Oral:

Generic: 30 mg

Capsule Extended Release 24 Hour, Oral, as hydrochloride:

Focalin XR: 5 mg [contains fd&c blue #2 (indigotine)]

Focalin XR: 10 mg

Focalin XR: 15 mg [contains fd&c blue #2 (indigotine)]

Focalin XR: 20 mg

Focalin XR: 25 mg [contains fd&c blue #2 (indigotine)]

Focalin XR: 30 mg

Focalin XR: 35 mg, 40 mg [contains fd&c blue #2 (indigotine)]
Generic: 15 mg, 30 mg, 40 mg
Tablet, Oral, as hydrochloride:
Focalin: 2.5 mg, 5 mg, 10 mg
Generic: 2.5 mg, 5 mg, 10 mg

Controlled Substance C-II

◆ **Dexmethylphenidate Hydrochloride** *see* Dexmethylphenidate *on page 586*

◆ **DexPak 6 Day** *see* Dexamethasone (Systemic) *on page 580*

◆ **DexPak 10 Day** *see* Dexamethasone (Systemic) *on page 580*

◆ **DexPak 13 Day** *see* Dexamethasone (Systemic) *on page 580*

Dexpanthenol (deks PAN the nole)

Index Terms Pantothenyl Alcohol

Pharmacologic Category Gastrointestinal Agent, Stimulant; Topical Skin Product

Use Prophylactic use to minimize paralytic ileus; treatment of postoperative distention; topical to relieve itching and to aid healing of minor dermatoses

Pregnancy Risk Factor C

Dosage I.M.: Adults:
Prevention of postoperative ileus: 250-500 mg stat, repeat in 2 hours, followed by doses every 6 hours until danger passes
Paralytic ileus: 500 mg stat, repeat in 2 hours, followed by doses every 6 hours, if needed

Dosage adjustment in renal impairment: No dosage adjustment provided in manufacturer's labeling.

Dosage adjustment in hepatic impairment: No dosage adjustment provided in manufacturer's labeling.

Additional Information Complete prescribing information should be consulted for additional detail.

Dosage Forms Excipient information presented when available (limited, particularly for generics); consult specific product labeling.
Solution, Injection:
Generic: 250 mg/mL (2 mL)

Dexrazoxane (deks ray ZOKS ane)

Brand Names: U.S. Totect; Zinecard

Brand Names: Canada Zinecard

Index Terms ICRF-187

Pharmacologic Category Antidote; Antidote, Extravasation; Cardioprotectant

Use
Anthracycline extravasation (Totect): Treatment of anthracycline-induced extravasation
Cardioprotectant (Zinecard): Used to reduce the incidence and severity of cardiomyopathy associated with doxorubicin administration in women with metastatic breast cancer who have received a cumulative doxorubicin dose of 300 mg/m^2 and who would benefit from continuing therapy with doxorubicin. (Not recommended for use with initial doxorubicin therapy.)

Unlabeled Use Reduction of the incidence and severity of cardiomyopathy associated with doxorubicin administration (cumulative doses >300 mg/m^2) in patients with malignancies other than metastatic breast cancer who would benefit from continuing therapy with doxorubicin; reduction of the incidence and severity of cardiomyopathy associated with continued epirubicin administration for advanced breast cancer; prevention of doxorubicin cardiomyopathy associated with acute lymphoblastic leukemia treatment in children

Pregnancy Risk Factor D

Dosage
Children: I.V.: Prevention of doxorubicin cardiomyopathy associated with acute lymphoblastic leukemia treatment (high-risk patients; unlabeled use): A 10:1 ratio of dexrazoxane:doxorubicin (eg, dexrazoxane 300 mg/m^2:doxorubicin 30 mg/m^2) was used in patients with high-risk acute lymphoblastic leukemia (Lipshultz, 2010; Moghrabi, 2007; Silverman, 2010).
Adults: I.V.:
Prevention of doxorubicin cardiomyopathy: A 10:1 ratio of dexrazoxane:doxorubicin (dexrazoxane 500 mg/m^2: doxorubicin 50 mg/m^2). **Note:** Cardiac monitoring should continue during dexrazoxane therapy; doxorubicin/dexrazoxane should be discontinued in patients who develop a decline in LVEF or clinical CHF.
Treatment of anthracycline extravasation: 1000 mg/m^2 on days 1 and 2 (maximum dose: 2000 mg), followed by 500 mg/m^2 on day 3 (maximum dose: 1000 mg); begin treatment as soon as possible, within 6 hours of extravasation

Dosage adjustment in renal impairment: Note: Renal function may be estimated using the Cockcroft-Gault formula.
Mild (Cl_{cr} ≥40 mL/minute): No dosage adjustment necessary.
Moderate-to-severe (Cl_{cr} <40 mL/minute):
Prevention of cardiomyopathy: Reduce dose by 50%, using a 5:1 dexrazoxane:doxorubicin ratio (dexrazoxane 250 mg/m^2:doxorubicin 50 mg/m^2)
Anthracycline-induced extravasation: Reduce dose by 50%

Dosage adjustment in hepatic impairment:
Prevention of cardiomyopathy: Since doxorubicin dosage is reduced in hyperbilirubinemia, a proportional reduction in dexrazoxane dosage is recommended (maintain a 10:1 ratio of dexrazoxane:doxorubicin)
Anthracycline-induced extravasation: No dosage adjustment provided in manufacturer's labeling (has not been studied).

Additional Information Complete prescribing information should be consulted for additional detail.

Dosage Forms Excipient information presented when available (limited, particularly for generics); consult specific product labeling.
Solution Reconstituted, Intravenous:
Totect: 500 mg (1 ea) [pyrogen free]
Zinecard: 250 mg (1 ea); 500 mg (1 ea) [pyrogen free]
Generic: 250 mg (1 ea); 500 mg (1 ea)

Dextran (DEKS tran)

Brand Names: U.S. LMD in D_5W; LMD in NaCl

Index Terms 10% LMD; Dextran 40; Dextran, Low Molecular Weight

Pharmacologic Category Plasma Volume Expander, Colloid

Use Blood volume expander used in treatment of shock or impending shock when blood or blood products are not available; also used as a priming fluid in pump oxygenators during cardiopulmonary bypass and for prophylaxis of venous thrombosis and pulmonary embolism in surgical procedures associated with a high risk of thromboembolic complications

Pregnancy Risk Factor C

Dosage I.V.: Dose and infusion rate are dependent upon the patient's fluid status and must be individualized:
Volume expansion/shock:
Children (Dextran 40): Infuse 10 mL/kg as rapidly as possible (maximum: 20 mL/kg/day for the first 24 hours; 10 mL/kg/day thereafter); therapy should not be continued beyond 5 days

Adults (Dextran 40): Infuse 500-1000 mL (~10 mL/kg) as rapidly as possible (maximum: 20 mL/kg/day for first 24 hours; 10 mL/kg/day thereafter); therapy should not be continued beyond 5 days

Pump prime (Dextran 40): Varies with the volume of the pump oxygenator; generally, the solution is added in a dose of 10-20 mL/kg (or 1-2 g/kg); usual maximum total dose: 20 mL/kg (or 2 g/kg)

Postoperative prophylaxis of venous thrombosis/pulmonary embolism (Dextran 40): Begin during surgical procedure and give 500-1000 mL (~10 mL/kg); an additional 50 g (500 mL) should be administered every 2-3 days during the period of risk (up to 2 weeks postoperatively); usual maximum infusion rate for nonemergency use: 4 mL/minute

Dosing in renal and/or hepatic impairment: Use with extreme caution

Additional Information Complete prescribing information should be consulted for additional detail.

Dosage Forms Excipient information presented when available (limited, particularly for generics); consult specific product labeling.

Solution, Intravenous:

LMD in D_5W: 10% Dextran 40 (500 mL) [latex free]

LMD in NaCl: 10% Dextran 40 (500 mL) [latex free]

◆ Dextran 40 *see* Dextran *on page* 587

◆ Dextran, Low Molecular Weight *see* Dextran *on page* 587

◆ Dextrin *see* Wheat Dextrin *on page* 2215

Dextroamphetamine (deks troe am FET a meen)

Brand Names: U.S. Dexedrine; ProCentra; Zenzedi

Brand Names: Canada Dexedrine®

Index Terms Dextroamphetamine Sulfate

Pharmacologic Category Central Nervous System Stimulant

Use Narcolepsy; attention-deficit/hyperactivity disorder (ADHD)

Pregnancy Risk Factor C

Pregnancy Considerations Adverse effects have been observed in animal reproduction studies. The majority of human data is based on illicit amphetamine/methamphetamine exposure and not from therapeutic maternal use (Golub, 2005). Use of amphetamines during pregnancy may lead to an increased risk of premature birth and low birth weight; newborns may experience symptoms of withdrawal. Behavioral problems may also occur later in childhood (LaGasse, 2012).

Breast-Feeding Considerations The majority of human data is based on illicit amphetamine/methamphetamine exposure and not from therapeutic maternal use (Golub, 2005). Amphetamines are excreted into breast milk and use may decrease milk production. Increased irritability, agitation, and crying have been reported in nursing infants (ACOG, 2011). The manufacturer recommends that mothers taking dextroamphetamine refrain from nursing.

Medication Guide Available Yes

Contraindications Hypersensitivity or idiosyncrasy to dextroamphetamine, other sympathomimetic amines, or any component of the formulation; advanced arteriosclerosis, symptomatic cardiovascular disease, moderate-to-severe hypertension; hyperthyroidism; glaucoma; agitated states; patients with a history of drug abuse; during or within 14 days following MAO inhibitor therapy

Warnings/Precautions [U.S. Boxed Warning]: Use has been associated with serious cardiovascular events including sudden death in patients with pre-existing structural cardiac abnormalities or other serious heart problems (sudden death in children and adolescents; sudden death, stroke and MI in adults. These products should be avoided in the patients with known serious structural cardiac abnormalities, cardiomyopathy, serious heart rhythm abnormalities, or other serious cardiac problems that could increase the risk of sudden death that these conditions alone carry. Patients should be carefully evaluated for cardiac disease prior to initiation of therapy. Use with caution in patients with hypertension and other cardiovascular conditions that might be exacerbated by increases in blood pressure or heart rate. Amphetamines may impair the ability to engage in potentially hazardous activities. May cause visual disturbances. Stimulants are associated with peripheral vasculopathy, including Raynaud's phenomenon; signs/symptoms are usually mild and intermittent, and generally improve with dose reduction or discontinuation. Digital ulceration and/or soft tissue breakdown have been observed rarely; monitor for digital changes during therapy and seek further evaluation (eg, rheumatology) if necessary.

Use with caution in patients with psychiatric or seizure disorders. May exacerbate symptoms of behavior and thought disorder in psychotic patients. Stimulants may unmask tics in individuals with coexisting Tourette's syndrome. **[U.S. Boxed Warning]: Potential for drug dependency exists; prolonged use may lead to drug dependency.** Use is contraindicated in patients with history of ethanol or drug abuse. Prescriptions should be written for the smallest quantity consistent with good patient care to minimize possibility of overdose. Abrupt discontinuation following high doses or for prolonged periods may result in symptoms for withdrawal.

Use caution in the elderly due to CNS stimulant adverse effects. Appetite suppression may occur; monitor weight during therapy, particularly in children. Use of stimulants has been associated with suppression of growth; monitor growth rate during treatment.

Adverse Reactions Frequency not defined.

Cardiovascular: Cardiomyopathy, hypertension, palpitation, tachycardia

Central nervous system: Aggression, dizziness, dyskinesia, dysphoria, euphoria, exacerbation of motor and phonic tics, headache, insomnia, mania, overstimulation, psychosis, restlessness, Tourette's syndrome

Dermatologic: Urticaria

Endocrine & metabolic: Libido changes

Gastrointestinal: Anorexia, constipation, diarrhea, unpleasant taste, weight loss, xerostomia

Genitourinary: Impotence

Neuromuscular & skeletal: Tremor

Ocular: Accommodation abnormalities, blurred vision

Drug Interactions

Metabolism/Transport Effects Substrate of CYP2D6 (minor); **Note:** Assignment of Major/Minor substrate status based on clinically relevant drug interaction potential

Avoid Concomitant Use

Avoid concomitant use of Dextroamphetamine with any of the following: Iobenguane I 123; MAO Inhibitors

Increased Effect/Toxicity

Dextroamphetamine may increase the levels/effects of: Analgesics (Opioid); Sympathomimetics

The levels/effects of Dextroamphetamine may be increased by: Alkalinizing Agents; Antacids; AtoMOXetine; Cannabinoids; Carbonic Anhydrase Inhibitors; MAO Inhibitors; Proton Pump Inhibitors; Tricyclic Antidepressants

Decreased Effect

Dextroamphetamine may decrease the levels/effects of: Antihistamines; Ethosuximide; Iobenguane I 123; Ioflupane I 123; PHENobarbital; Phenytoin

The levels/effects of Dextroamphetamine may be decreased by: Ammonium Chloride; Antipsychotics; Ascorbic Acid; Gastrointestinal Acidifying Agents;

Lithium; Methenamine; Multivitamins/Fluoride (with ADE); Multivitamins/Minerals (with ADEK, Folate, Iron); Multivitamins/Minerals (with AE, No Iron); Peginterferon Alfa-2b; Urinary Acidifying Agents

Ethanol/Nutrition/Herb Interactions

Ethanol: Potential for drug dependency may increase with prolonged use. Ethanol may increase CNS depression. Management: Avoid ethanol. Use is contraindicated in patients with history of ethanol or drug abuse.

Food: Dextroamphetamine serum levels may be altered if taken with acidic food, juices, or vitamin C. Management: Avoid caffeine. Take 30 minutes before meals.

Herb/Nutraceutical: Ephedra may cause hypertension or arrhythmias. Management: Avoid ephedra.

Storage/Stability Store at controlled room temperature of 20°C to 25°C (68°F to 77°F). Protect from light.

Mechanism of Action Amphetamines are noncatecholamine, sympathomimetic amines that promote release of catecholamines (primarily dopamine and norepinephrine) from their storage sites in the presynaptic nerve terminals. A less significant mechanism may include their ability to block the reuptake of catecholamines by competitive inhibition.

Pharmacodynamics/Kinetics

Onset of action: 1-1.5 hours

Distribution: V_d: Adults: 3.5-4.6 L/kg; distributes into CNS; mean CSF concentrations are 80% of plasma

Metabolism: Hepatic via CYP monooxygenase and glucuronidation

Half-life elimination: Adults: 10-13 hours

Time to peak, serum: Immediate release: ~3 hours; sustained release: ~8 hours

Excretion: Urine (as unchanged drug and inactive metabolites)

Dosage Oral:

Children:

Narcolepsy: 6-12 years: Initial: 5 mg/day; may increase at 5 mg/day increments in weekly intervals until side effects appear (maximum dose: 60 mg/day)

ADHD:

3-5 years: Immediate release tablets or oral solution: Initial: 2.5 mg/day; may increase at 2.5 mg/day increments in weekly intervals until optimal response is obtained; usual range: 0.1-0.5 mg/kg/dose (maximum dose: 40 mg/day)

≥6 years: Initial: 5 mg once or twice daily; may increase at 5 mg/day increments in weekly intervals until optimal response is obtained; usual range: 0.1-0.5 mg/kg/dose (5-20 mg/day) (maximum dose: 40 mg/day)

Children >12 years and Adults: Narcolepsy: 10 mg/day, may increase at 10 mg/day increments in weekly intervals until side effects appear (maximum dose: 60 mg/day)

Dosage adjustment in renal impairment: No dosage adjustment provided in manufacturer's labeling.

Dosage adjustment in hepatic impairment: No dosage adjustment provided in manufacturer's labeling.

Administration Administer initial dose upon awakening; do not administer doses late in the evening due to potential for insomnia.

Immediate release tablets and oral solution: If needed, 1-2 additional doses may be administered at intervals of 4-6 hours.

Extended release or sustained release capsules: Do not crush sustained release drug products. Formulations may be used for once-daily administration, if appropriate.

Monitoring Parameters Cardiac evaluation should be completed on any patient who develops chest pain, unexplained syncope, and any symptom of cardiac disease during treatment with stimulants; signs of peripheral vasculopathy (eg, digital changes); growth in children and CNS activity in all

When used for the treatment of ADHD, thoroughly evaluate for cardiovascular risk. Monitor heart rate, blood pressure, and consider obtaining ECG prior to initiation (Vetter, 2008).

Test Interactions Amphetamines may elevate plasma corticosteroid levels; may interfere with urinary steroid determinations.

Dosage Forms Excipient information presented when available (limited, particularly for generics); consult specific product labeling.

Capsule Extended Release 24 Hour, Oral, as sulfate:

Dexedrine: 5 mg, 10 mg, 15 mg [contains brilliant blue fcf (fd&c blue #1), fd&c blue #1 aluminum lake, fd&c red #40, fd&c yellow #10 (quinoline yellow), fd&c yellow #6 (sunset yellow)]

Generic: 5 mg, 10 mg, 15 mg

Solution, Oral, as sulfate:

ProCentra: 5 mg/5 mL (473 mL) [contains benzoic acid, saccharin sodium; bubble-gum flavor]

Generic: 5 mg/5 mL (473 mL)

Tablet, Oral, as sulfate:

Zenzedi: 2.5 mg

Zenzedi: 5 mg [scored; contains fd&c yellow #6 (sunset yellow)]

Zenzedi: 7.5 mg [contains brilliant blue fcf (fd&c blue #1), fd&c yellow #10 (quinoline yellow)]

Zenzedi: 10 mg [scored; contains fd&c blue #2 (indigotine), fd&c red #40, fd&c yellow #6 (sunset yellow)]

Generic: 5 mg, 10 mg

Controlled Substance C-II

Dextroamphetamine and Amphetamine

(deks troe am FET a meen & am FET a meen)

Brand Names: U.S. Adderall; Adderall XR

Brand Names: Canada Adderall XR

Index Terms Amphetamine and Dextroamphetamine

Pharmacologic Category Central Nervous System Stimulant

Use Attention-deficit/hyperactivity disorder (ADHD); narcolepsy

Pregnancy Risk Factor C

Medication Guide Available Yes

Dosage Oral: **Note:** Use lowest effective individualized dose; administer first dose as soon as awake.

ADHD:

Children: <3 years: Not recommended

Children: 3-5 years (Adderall): Initial 2.5 mg once daily given every morning; increase daily dose in 2.5 mg increments at weekly intervals until optimal response is obtained (maximum dose: 40 mg daily given in 1-3 divided doses); use intervals of 4-6 hours between additional doses.

Children: 6-12 years:

Adderall: Initial: 5 mg once or twice daily; increase daily dose in 5 mg increments at weekly intervals until optimal response is obtained (usual maximum dose: 40 mg daily given in 1-3 divided doses); use intervals of 4-6 hours between additional doses

Adderall XR: 5-10 mg once daily in the morning; if needed, may increase daily dose in 5-10 mg increments at weekly intervals (maximum dose: 30 mg daily)

Conversion from immediate release to extended release formulation: Patients may be switched from the immediate release formulation to the extended release formulation using the same total daily dose once daily.

Adolescents 13-17 years:

Adderall: Initial: 5 mg once or twice daily; increase daily dose in 5 mg increments at weekly intervals until optimal response is obtained (usual maximum dose: 40 mg daily given in 1-3 divided doses); use intervals of 4-6 hours between additional doses.

Adderall XR: 10 mg once daily in the morning; maybe increased to 20 mg daily after 1 week if symptoms are not controlled; higher doses (up to 60 mg daily) have been evaluated; however, there is not adequate evidence that higher doses afford additional benefit.

Canadian labeling: Maximum dose: 30 mg daily.

Conversion from immediate release to extended release formulation: Patients may be switched from the immediate release formulation to the extended release formulation using the same total daily dose once daily.

Adults:

Adderall: Initial: 5 mg once or twice daily; increase daily dose in 5 mg increments at weekly intervals until optimal response is obtained; usual maximum dose: 40 mg daily given in 1-3 divided doses per day. Use intervals of 4-6 hours between additional doses.

Adderall XR: Initial: 20 mg once daily in the morning; higher doses (up to 60 mg once daily) have been evaluated; however, there is not adequate evidence that higher doses afforded additional benefit.

Canadian labeling: Maximum dose: 30 mg daily.

Conversion from immediate release to extended release formulation: Patients may be switched from the immediate release formulation to the extended release formulation using the same total daily dose once daily.

Narcolepsy (Adderall):

Children: 6-12 years: Initial: 5 mg daily; increase daily dose in 5 mg at weekly intervals until optimal response is obtained (maximum dose: 60 mg daily given in 1-3 divided doses with intervals of 4-6 hours between doses)

Children >12 years and Adults: Initial: 10 mg daily; increase daily dose in 10 mg increments at weekly intervals until optimal response is obtained (maximum dose: 60 mg daily given in 1-3 divided doses with intervals of 4-6 hours between doses)

Dosage adjustment in renal impairment: No dosage adjustment provided in manufacturer's labeling.

Dosage adjustment in hepatic impairment: No dosage adjustment provided in manufacturer's labeling.

Additional Information Complete prescribing information should be consulted for additional detail.

Dosage Forms Excipient information presented when available (limited, particularly for generics); consult specific product labeling.

Capsule, extended release, oral:

5 mg [dextroamphetamine sulfate 1.25 mg, dextroamphetamine saccharate 1.25 mg, amphetamine aspartate monohydrate 1.25 mg, amphetamine sulfate 1.25 mg (equivalent to amphetamine base 3.1 mg)]

10 mg [dextroamphetamine sulfate 2.5 mg, dextroamphetamine saccharate 2.5 mg, amphetamine aspartate monohydrate 2.5 mg, amphetamine sulfate 2.5 mg (equivalent to amphetamine base 6.3 mg)]

15 mg [dextroamphetamine sulfate 3.75 mg, dextroamphetamine saccharate 3.75 mg, amphetamine aspartate monohydrate 3.75 mg, amphetamine sulfate 3.75 mg (equivalent to amphetamine base 9.4 mg)]

20 mg [dextroamphetamine sulfate 5 mg, dextroamphetamine saccharate 5 mg, amphetamine aspartate monohydrate 5 mg, amphetamine sulfate 5 mg (equivalent to amphetamine base 12.5 mg)]

25 mg [dextroamphetamine sulfate 6.25 mg, dextroamphetamine saccharate 6.25 mg, amphetamine aspartate monohydrate 6.25 mg, amphetamine sulfate 6.25 mg (equivalent to amphetamine base 15.6 mg)]

30 mg [dextroamphetamine sulfate 7.5 mg, dextroamphetamine saccharate 7.5 mg, amphetamine aspartate monohydrate 7.5 mg, amphetamine sulfate 7.5 mg (equivalent to amphetamine base 18.8 mg)]

Adderall XR

5 mg [dextroamphetamine sulfate 1.25 mg, dextroamphetamine saccharate 1.25 mg, amphetamine aspartate monohydrate 1.25 mg, amphetamine sulfate 1.25 mg (equivalent to amphetamine base 3.1 mg)]

10 mg [dextroamphetamine sulfate 2.5 mg, dextroamphetamine saccharate 2.5 mg, amphetamine aspartate monohydrate 2.5 mg, amphetamine sulfate 2.5 mg (equivalent to amphetamine base 6.3 mg)]

15 mg [dextroamphetamine sulfate 3.75 mg, dextroamphetamine saccharate 3.75 mg, amphetamine aspartate monohydrate 3.75 mg, amphetamine sulfate 3.75 mg (equivalent to amphetamine base 9.4 mg)]

20 mg [dextroamphetamine sulfate 5 mg, dextroamphetamine saccharate 5 mg, amphetamine aspartate monohydrate 5 mg, amphetamine sulfate 5 mg (equivalent to amphetamine base 12.5 mg)]

25 mg [dextroamphetamine sulfate 6.25 mg, dextroamphetamine saccharate 6.25 mg, amphetamine aspartate monohydrate 6.25 mg, amphetamine sulfate 6.25 mg (equivalent to amphetamine base 15.6 mg)]

30 mg [dextroamphetamine sulfate 7.5 mg, dextroamphetamine saccharate 7.5 mg, amphetamine aspartate monohydrate 7.5 mg, amphetamine sulfate 7.5 mg (equivalent to amphetamine base 18.8 mg)]

Tablet, oral:

5 mg [dextroamphetamine sulfate 1.25 mg, dextroamphetamine saccharate 1.25 mg, amphetamine aspartate monohydrate 1.25 mg, amphetamine sulfate 1.25 mg (equivalent to amphetamine base 3.13 mg)]

7.5 mg [dextroamphetamine 1.875 mg, dextroamphetamine saccharate 1.875 mg, amphetamine aspartate monohydrate 1.875 mg, amphetamine sulfate 1.875 mg (equivalent to amphetamine base 4.7 mg)]

10 mg [dextroamphetamine sulfate 2.5 mg, dextroamphetamine saccharate 2.5 mg, amphetamine aspartate monohydrate 2.5 mg, amphetamine sulfate 2.5 mg (equivalent to amphetamine base 6.3 mg)]

12.5 mg [dextroamphetamine sulfate 3.125 mg, dextroamphetamine saccharate 3.125 mg, amphetamine aspartate monohydrate 3.125 mg, amphetamine sulfate 3.125 mg (equivalent to amphetamine base 7.8 mg)]

15 mg [dextroamphetamine sulfate 3.75 mg, dextroamphetamine saccharate 3.75 mg, amphetamine aspartate monohydrate 3.75 mg, amphetamine sulfate 3.75 mg (equivalent to amphetamine base 9.4 mg)]

20 mg [dextroamphetamine sulfate 5 mg, dextroamphetamine saccharate 5 mg, amphetamine aspartate monohydrate 5 mg, amphetamine sulfate 5 mg (equivalent to amphetamine base 12.6 mg)]

30 mg [dextroamphetamine sulfate 7.5 mg, dextroamphetamine saccharate 7.5 mg, amphetamine aspartate monohydrate 7.5 mg, amphetamine sulfate 7.5 mg (equivalent to amphetamine base 18.8 mg)]

Adderall:

5 mg [dextroamphetamine sulfate 1.25 mg, dextroamphetamine saccharate 1.25 mg, amphetamine aspartate monohydrate 1.25 mg, amphetamine sulfate 1.25 mg (equivalent to amphetamine base 3.13 mg)]

7.5 mg [dextroamphetamine sulfate 1.875 mg, dextroamphetamine saccharate 1.875 mg, amphetamine aspartate monohydrate 1.875 mg, amphetamine sulfate 1.875 mg (equivalent to amphetamine base 4.7 mg)]

10 mg [dextroamphetamine sulfate 2.5 mg, dextroamphetamine saccharate 2.5 mg, amphetamine aspartate monohydrate 2.5 mg, amphetamine sulfate 2.5 mg (equivalent to amphetamine base 6.3 mg)]
12.5 mg [dextroamphetamine sulfate 3.125 mg, dextroamphetamine saccharate 3.125 mg, amphetamine aspartate monohydrate 3.125 mg, amphetamine sulfate 3.125 mg (equivalent to amphetamine base 7.8 mg)]
15 mg [dextroamphetamine sulfate 3.75 mg, dextroamphetamine saccharate 3.75 mg, amphetamine aspartate monohydrate 3.75 mg, amphetamine sulfate 3.75 mg (equivalent to amphetamine base 9.4 mg)]
20 mg [dextroamphetamine sulfate 5 mg, dextroamphetamine saccharate 5 mg, amphetamine aspartate monohydrate 5 mg, amphetamine sulfate 5 mg (equivalent to amphetamine base 12.6 mg)]
30 mg [dextroamphetamine sulfate 7.5 mg, dextroamphetamine saccharate 7.5 mg, amphetamine aspartate monohydrate 7.5 mg, amphetamine sulfate 7.5 mg (equivalent to amphetamine base 18.8 mg)]

Controlled Substance C-II

◆ **Dextroamphetamine Sulfate** *see* Dextroamphetamine *on page 588*

Dextromethorphan and Chlorpheniramine

(deks troe meth OR fan & klor fen IR a meen)

Brand Names: U.S. Coricidin® HBP Cough & Cold [OTC]; Dimetapp® Children's Long Acting Cough Plus Cold [OTC]; Robitussin® Children's Cough & Cold Long-Acting [OTC]; Scot-Tussin® DM Maximum Strength [OTC]; Triaminic® Children's Softchews® Cough & Runny Nose [OTC]

Index Terms Chlorpheniramine and Dextromethorphan; Chlorpheniramine Maleate and Dextromethorphan Hydrobromide; Dextromethorphan Hydrobromide and Chlorpheniramine Maleate

Pharmacologic Category Alkylamine Derivative; Antitussive; Histamine H_1 Antagonist; Histamine H_1 Antagonist, First Generation

Use Symptomatic relief of runny nose, sneezing, itchy/watery eyes, cough, and other upper respiratory symptoms associated with hay fever, common cold, or upper respiratory allergies

Dosage General dosing guidelines; consult specific product labeling.

Antitussive/antihistamine: Oral:
Children: 6-11 years:
Liquid: Dextromethorphan 15 mg and chlorpheniramine 2 mg every 6 hours as needed (maximum: 60 mg dextromethorphan and 8 mg chlorpheniramine/24 hours)
Chewable tablet: Dextromethorphan 10 mg and chlorpheniramine 2 mg every 4-6 hours as needed (maximum: 50 mg dextromethorphan and 10 mg chlorpheniramine/24 hours)
Children ≥12 years and Adults: Dextromethorphan 30 mg and chlorpheniramine 4 mg every 6 hours as needed (maximum: 120 mg dextromethorphan and 16 mg chlorpheniramine/24 hours)

Additional Information Complete prescribing information should be consulted for additional detail.

Dosage Forms Excipient information presented when available (limited, particularly for generics); consult specific product labeling.

Syrup, oral:
Dimetapp® Children's Long Acting Cough Plus Cold: Dextromethorphan hydrobromide 7.5 mg and chlorpheniramine maleate 1 mg per 5 mL (118 mL) [ethanol free, sugar free; contains sodium 3 mg/5 mL, sodium benzoate, propylene glycol; grape flavor]
Robitussin® Children's Cough and Cold Long-Acting: Dextromethorphan hydrobromide 15 mg and chlorpheniramine maleate 2 mg per 5 mL (118 mL) [ethanol free; contains sodium 3 mg/5 mL, sodium benzoate, propylene glycol; fruit punch flavor]
Scot-Tussin® DM Maximum Strength: Dextromethorphan hydrobromide 15 mg and chlorpheniramine maleate 2 mg per 5 mL (118 mL) [ethanol free, dye free, sugar free; cherry-strawberry flavor]

Tablet, oral:
Coricidin® HBP Cough and Cold: Dextromethorphan hydrobromide 30 mg and chlorpheniramine maleate 4 mg

Tablet, softchew, oral:
Triaminic® Children's Softchews® Cough & Runny Nose: Dextromethorphan hydrobromide 5 mg and chlorpheniramine maleate 1 mg [contains coconut oil, phenylalanine 17.6 mg/softchew, sodium 5 mg/softchew; cherry flavor]

◆ **Dextromethorphan and Guaifenesin** *see* Guaifenesin and Dextromethorphan *on page 976*

Dextromethorphan and Phenylephrine

(deks troe meth OR fan & fen il EF rin)

Brand Names: U.S. PediaCare® Children's Multi-Symptom Cold [OTC]; Safetussin® CD [OTC]; Sudafed PE® Children's Cold & Cough [OTC]; Triaminic® Day Time Cold & Cough [OTC]

Index Terms Dextromethorphan Hydrobromide and Phenylephrine Hydrochloride; Phenylephrine and Dextromethorphan

Pharmacologic Category Antitussive; Decongestant

Use Temporary relief of symptoms of hay fever, the common cold, and upper respiratory allergies including sinus/nasal congestion, minor bronchial/throat irritation, and cough

Dosage Oral: Relief of nasal/sinus congestion and cough:
Children 4-6 years: PediaCare® Children's Multi-Symptom Cold, Sudafed PE® Children's Cold & Cough, Triaminic® Day Time Cold & Cough: 5 mL every 4 hours as needed (maximum: 30 mL/24 hours)
Children 6-12 years:
PediaCare® Children's Multi-Symptom Cold, Sudafed PE® Children's Cold & Cough, Triaminic® Day Time Cold & Cough: 10 mL every 4 hours as needed (maximum: 60 mL/24 hours)
Safetussin® CD: 5 mL every 6 hours as needed (maximum: 20 mL/24 hours)
Children ≥12 years and Adults: Safetussin® CD: 10 mL every 6 hours as needed (maximum: 40 mL/24 hours)

Additional Information Complete prescribing information should be consulted for additional detail.

Dosage Forms Excipient information presented when available (limited, particularly for generics); consult specific product labeling.

Liquid, oral:
Sudafed PE® Children's Cold & Cough: Dextromethorphan hydrobromide 5 mg and phenylephrine hydrochloride 2.5 mg per 5 mL (118 mL) [ethanol free, sugar free; contains sodium 15 mg/5 mL, sodium benzoate; grape flavor]

Syrup:

PediaCare® Children's Multi-Symptom Cold: Dextromethorphan hydrobromide 5 mg and phenylephrine hydrochloride 2.5 mg per 5 mL (118 mL) [contains sodium 15 mg/5 mL; sodium benzoate; grape flavor]

Safetussin® CD: Dextromethorphan hydrobromide 15 mg and phenylephrine hydrochloride 2.5 mg per 5 mL (120 mL), [alcohol free; sugar free; contains menthol, propylene glycol; orange flavor]

Triaminic® Day Time Cold & Cough: Dextromethorphan hydrobromide 5 mg and phenylephrine hydrochloride 2.5 mg per 5 mL (120 mL, 240 mL) [contains benzoic acid; sodium 2 mg/5 mL; propylene glycol; cherry flavor]

◆ **Dextromethorphan and Promethazine** *see* Promethazine and Dextromethorphan *on page 1731*

◆ **Dextromethorphan and Pseudoephedrine** *see* Pseudoephedrine and Dextromethorphan *on page 1748*

Dextromethorphan and Quinidine

(deks troe meth OR fan & KWIN i deen)

Brand Names: U.S. Nuedexta™

Brand Names: Canada Nuedexta™

Index Terms Dextromethorphan Hydrobromide and Quinidine Sulfate; Quinidine and Dextromethorphan

Pharmacologic Category N-Methyl-D-Aspartate Receptor Antagonist

Use Treatment of pseudobulbar affect (PBA)

Pregnancy Risk Factor C

Pregnancy Considerations Adverse events were observed in animal reproduction studies using this combination.

Breast-Feeding Considerations Quinidine is excreted in breast milk; excretion of dextromethorphan is not known

Contraindications Hypersensitivity to dextromethorphan, quinidine, quinine, mefloquine, or any component of the formulation; concomitant use with quinidine or other medications containing quinidine, quinine, or mefloquine; history of quinine-, mefloquine-, or quinidine-induced thrombocytopenia; hepatitis; bone marrow depression; or lupus-like syndrome; concurrent administration with or within 2 weeks of discontinuing an MAO inhibitor; patients with prolonged QT interval, congenital QT syndrome, or history of torsade de pointes; patients with heart failure; concurrent use of drugs that prolong the QT interval and are metabolized by CYP2D6 (eg, pimozide, thioridazine); patients with complete AV block without an implanted pacemaker or patients at high risk of complete AV block

Warnings/Precautions Immune-mediated thrombocytopenia (severe or fatal) may be associated with quinidine use. Unless clearly not drug related, discontinue immediately; continued use may be associated with an increase in fatal hemorrhage. Thrombocytopenia generally resolves within a few days of discontinuation. Therapy should not be restarted in sensitized patients. Agranulocytosis, angioedema, bronchospasm, lupus-like syndrome, rash or other hypersensitivity reactions may be associated with use. Quinidine has also been associated with severe hepatotoxic reactions including granulomatous hepatitis. Use is contraindicated in patients with prior history of immune-mediated thrombocytopenia associated with structurally related drugs (eg, quinine, mefloquine) and in patients with quinidine-, quinine-, or mefloquine-induced lupus-like syndrome.

Concomitant use of moderate or strong CYP3A4 inhibitors may increase quinidine levels and prolong the QT_c interval. Quinidine inhibits CYP2D6; concomitant use with CYP2D6 substrates may cause an accumulation of concomitantly administered drug and/or reduce active metabolite formation, decreasing their safety and/or efficacy. Use with caution in patients who are poor metabolizers of CYP2D6 metabolized drugs. Quinidine in this combination product is used to inhibit CYP2D6 in order to increase plasma concentrations of dextromethorphan. In patients who are poor metabolizers, this effect would not be significant; however, adverse events related to quinidine may still be observed. Genotyping should be considered in patients considered to be at risk of quinidine toxicity prior to therapy. Symptoms associated with serotonin syndrome such as agitation, confusion, hallucinations, hyper-reflexia, myoclonus, shivering, and tachycardia may occur with concomitant proserotonergic drugs (ie, SSRIs/SNRIs or triptans); especially with higher dextromethorphan doses.

Use caution in patients with left ventricular hypertrophy or left ventricular dysfunction which are more common in patients with chronic hypertension, coronary artery disease or history of stroke; risk of QT_c prolongation may be increased. Use is contraindicated in patients with prolonged QT interval, congenital QT syndrome, or history of torsade de pointes, patients with heart failure, complete AV block without an implanted pacemaker or patients at high risk of complete AV block. Correct hypokalemia or hypomagnesemia prior to therapy. Use caution with medications which may further prolong the QT interval or cause cardiac arrhythmias. Dose dependent QT_c prolongation may occur. Monitor patients at risk following the first dose. Discontinue if arrhythmia occurs.

May cause anticholinergic effects; use caution in patients with myasthenia gravis or other conditions which may be affected. May cause dizziness; use caution in patients with motor impairment or history of falls. Safety and efficacy have not been established with severe hepatic or renal impairment; increased serum concentrations may occur. Has not shown to be safe or effective in other types of commonly occurring emotional labilities (eg, Alzheimer's disease and other dementias). Patients with a history of drug abuse should be monitored closely for signs of abuse/misuse of Nuedexta™ (eg, development of tolerance, increase in dose, or drug-seeking behavior). Abuse of dextromethorphan may cause brain damage, cardiac arrhythmia, loss of consciousness, or death. Periodically reassess the need for treatment; spontaneous improvement of PBA may occur.

Adverse Reactions Also see individual agents.

>10%: Gastrointestinal: Diarrhea (13%)

1% to 10%:

Cardiovascular: Peripheral edema (5%)
Central nervous system: Dizziness (10%)
Gastrointestinal: Vomiting (5%), flatulence (3%)
Genitourinary: Urinary tract infection (4%)
Hepatic: GGT increased (3%)
Neuromuscular & skeletal: Weakness (5%)
Respiratory: Cough (5%)
Miscellaneous: Influenza (4%)

Drug Interactions

Metabolism/Transport Effects Refer to individual components.

Avoid Concomitant Use

Avoid concomitant use of Dextromethorphan and Quinidine with any of the following: Amiodarone; Antifungal Agents (Azole Derivatives, Systemic); Bosutinib; Conivaptan; Crizotinib; Enzalutamide; Fingolimod; Fusidic Acid (Systemic); Haloperidol; Highest Risk QTc-Prolonging Agents; Ivabradine; Macrolide Antibiotics; MAO Inhibitors; Mefloquine; Mifepristone; Moderate Risk QTc-Prolonging Agents; Pimozide; Pomalidomide; Propafenone; Protease Inhibitors; Silodosin; Tamoxifen; Thioridazine; Topotecan; VinCRIStine (Liposomal)

Increased Effect/Toxicity

Dextromethorphan and Quinidine may increase the levels/effects of: Afatinib; Antipsychotics; ARIPiprazole; AtoMOXetine; Bosutinib; Calcium Channel Blockers (Dihydropyridine); Cardiac Glycosides; Colchicine;

CYP2D6 Substrates; Dabigatran Etexilate; Dalfampridine; Dextromethorphan; Everolimus; Fesoterodine; Haloperidol; Highest Risk QTc-Prolonging Agents; Iloperidone; Lomitapide; Mefloquine; Metoclopramide; Metoprolol; Nebivolol; Neuromuscular-Blocking Agents; P-glycoprotein/ABCB1 Substrates; Pimozide; Pomalidomide; Propafenone; Propranolol; Prucalopride; Rivaroxaban; Serotonin Modulators; Silodosin; Tetrabenazine; Thioridazine; Topotecan; Tricyclic Antidepressants; Verapamil; VinCRIStine (Liposomal); Vitamin K Antagonists; Vortioxetine

The levels/effects of Dextromethorphan and Quinidine may be increased by: Abiraterone Acetate; Amiodarone; Antacids; Antifungal Agents (Azole Derivatives, Systemic); Antipsychotics; Boceprevir; Calcium Channel Blockers (Dihydropyridine); Carbonic Anhydrase Inhibitors; Cimetidine; Conivaptan; Crizotinib; CYP2D6 Inhibitors (Moderate); CYP2D6 Inhibitors (Strong); CYP3A4 Inhibitors (Moderate); CYP3A4 Inhibitors (Strong); Dasatinib; Diltiazem; Fingolimod; Fosphenytoin; Fusidic Acid (Systemic); Haloperidol; Ivabradine; Ivacaftor; Luliconazole; Lurasidone; Macrolide Antibiotics; MAO Inhibitors; Mifepristone; Moderate Risk QTc-Prolonging Agents; P-glycoprotein/ABCB1 Inhibitors; PHENobarbital; Protease Inhibitors; QTc-Prolonging Agents (Indeterminate Risk and Risk Modifying); QuiNIDine; Reserpine; Selective Serotonin Reuptake Inhibitors; Simeprevir; Telaprevir; Tricyclic Antidepressants; Verapamil

Decreased Effect

Dextromethorphan and Quinidine may decrease the levels/effects of: Codeine; Dihydrocodeine; Hydrocodone; Iloperidone; Tamoxifen; TraMADol

The levels/effects of Dextromethorphan and Quinidine may be decreased by: Bosentan; Calcium Channel Blockers (Dihydropyridine); CYP3A4 Inducers (Strong); Dabrafenib; Deferasirox; Enzalutamide; Etravirine; Fosphenytoin; Kaolin; Mitotane; Peginterferon Alfa-2b; P-glycoprotein/ABCB1 Inducers; PHENobarbital; Phenytoin; Potassium-Sparing Diuretics; Primidone; Rifamycin Derivatives; Sucralfate; Tocilizumab

Ethanol/Nutrition/Herb Interactions

Ethanol: Use caution with ethanol as CNS effects may be enhanced.

Food: Avoid grapefruit juice (may increase levels of quinidine). Avoid tonic water (contains quinine).

Storage/Stability Store at controlled room temperature at 25°C (77°F); excursions permitted to 15°C to 30°C (59°F to 86°F).

Mechanism of Action Dextromethorphan may relieve the symptoms of PBA by binding to sigma-1 receptors in the brain which may be involved in behavior, however the exact mechanism of action is not known. Quinidine is used to block the rapid metabolism of dextromethorphan, thereby increasing serum concentrations. The dose of quinidine in this combination product provides serum concentrations 1% to 3% of those needed to treat cardiac arrhythmias.

Pharmacodynamics/Kinetics

Absorption: Bioavailability of dextromethorphan increased ~20-fold when administered with quinidine.

Protein binding: Dextromethorphan: 60% to 70%; Quinidine: 80% to 89%

Metabolism: Dextromethorphan: Hepatic via CYP2D6 to dextrorphan (active); Quinidine: Hepatic via CYP3A4 to 3-hydroxyquinidine (active) and other metabolites

Half-life elimination: Dextromethorphan: 13 hours in extensive metabolizers; Quinidine: 7 hours in extensive metabolizers

Time to peak: Dextromethorphan: 3-4 hours; Quinidine: 1-2 hours

Excretion: Urine

Dosage Oral: Adults: Pseudobulbar affect: One capsule once daily for 7 days, then increase to 1 capsule twice daily; reassess patient periodically to determine if continued use is necessary

Dosage adjustment in renal impairment: Dose adjustment not required for mild or moderate renal impairment; not studied with severe impairment

Dosage adjustment in hepatic impairment: Dose adjustment not required for mild or moderate hepatic impairment; however, an increase in adverse reactions is observed with moderate hepatic dysfunction; not studied with severe impairment

Dietary Considerations May be taken with or without food. Avoid grapefruit juice.

Administration May be administered with or without food. Administer twice-daily doses every 12 hours.

Monitoring Parameters QT interval 3-4 hours after the first dose in patients at risk for QTc prolongation; potassium and magnesium prior to and during therapy; CBC, liver and renal function tests; periodically assess risk factors for arrhythmias during treatment; periodically reassess the need for treatment (spontaneous improvement of PBA may occur)

Test Interactions See individual agents.

Dosage Forms Excipient information presented when available (limited, particularly for generics); consult specific product labeling.

Capsule, oral:

Nuedexta™: Dextromethorphan hydrobromide 20 mg and quinidine sulfate 10 mg

◆ **Dextromethorphan, Chlorpheniramine, and Phenylephrine** *see* Chlorpheniramine, Phenylephrine, and Dextromethorphan *on page 413*

◆ **Dextromethorphan, Chlorpheniramine, and Pseudoephedrine** *see* Chlorpheniramine, Pseudoephedrine, and Dextromethorphan *on page 414*

◆ **Dextromethorphan, Guaifenesin, and Pseudoephedrine** *see* Guaifenesin, Pseudoephedrine, and Dextromethorphan *on page 979*

◆ **Dextromethorphan Hydrobromide and Chlorpheniramine Maleate** *see* Dextromethorphan and Chlorpheniramine *on page 591*

◆ **Dextromethorphan Hydrobromide and Phenylephrine Hydrochloride** *see* Dextromethorphan and Phenylephrine *on page 591*

◆ **Dextromethorphan Hydrobromide and Quinidine Sulfate** *see* Dextromethorphan and Quinidine *on page 592*

◆ **Dex-Tuss** *see* Guaifenesin and Codeine *on page 976*

◆ **Dezocitidine** *see* Decitabine *on page 556*

◆ **dFdC** *see* Gemcitabine *on page 943*

◆ **dFdCyd** *see* Gemcitabine *on page 943*

◆ **DFM** *see* Deferoxamine *on page 561*

◆ **DFMO** *see* Eflornithine *on page 691*

◆ **DHAD** *see* MitoXANtrone *on page 1386*

◆ **DHAQ** *see* MitoXANtrone *on page 1386*

◆ **DHE** *see* Dihydroergotamine *on page 611*

◆ **D.H.E. 45** *see* Dihydroergotamine *on page 611*

◆ **DHPG Sodium** *see* Ganciclovir (Systemic) *on page 939*

◆ **Diabeta** *see* GlyBURIDE *on page 963*

◆ **DiaBeta® (Can)** *see* GlyBURIDE *on page 963*

◆ **Diabetic Siltussin DAS-Na [OTC]** *see* GuaiFENesin *on page 974*

◆ **Diabetic Siltussin-DM DAS-Na [OTC]** *see* Guaifenesin and Dextromethorphan *on page 976*

Diazepam (dye AZ e pam)

Brand Names: U.S. Diastat AcuDial; Diastat Pediatric; Diazepam Intensol; Valium

Brand Names: Canada Apo-Diazepam®; Bio-Diazepam; Diastat®; Diazemuls®; Diazepam Auto Injector; Diazepam Injection USP; Novo-Dipam; PMS-Diazepam; Valium®

Pharmacologic Category Benzodiazepine

Additional Appendix Information

Beers Criteria – Potentially Inappropriate Medications for Geriatrics *on page 2368*
Benzodiazepine Comparison Table *on page 2292*
Patient Information for Disposal of Unused Medications *on page 2393*
Status Epilepticus *on page 2375*

Use Management of anxiety disorders, ethanol withdrawal symptoms; skeletal muscle relaxant; treatment of convulsive disorders; preoperative or preprocedural sedation and amnesia

Rectal gel: Management of selected, refractory epilepsy patients on stable regimens of antiepileptic drugs requiring intermittent use of diazepam to control episodes of increased seizure activity

Unlabeled Use Panic disorders; short-term treatment of spasticity in children with cerebral palsy; sedation for mechanically-ventilated patients in the intensive care unit

Pregnancy Risk Factor D

Pregnancy Considerations Teratogenic effects have been reported in animal reproduction studies. In humans, diazepam and its metabolites (N-desmethyldiazepam, temazepam, and oxazepam) cross the placenta. Teratogenic effects have been observed with diazepam; however, additional studies are needed. The incidence of premature birth and low birth weights may be increased following maternal use of benzodiazepines; hypoglycemia and respiratory problems in the neonate may occur following exposure late in pregnancy. Neonatal withdrawal symptoms may occur within days to weeks after birth and "floppy infant syndrome" (which also includes withdrawal symptoms) has been reported with some benzodiazepines (including diazepam) (Bergman, 1992; Iqbal, 2002; Wikner, 2007). A combination of factors influences the potential teratogenicity of anticonvulsant therapy. When treating women with epilepsy, monotherapy with the lowest effective dose and avoidance of medications known to have a high incidence of teratogenic effects is recommended (Harden, 2009; Wlodarczyk, 2012).

Breast-Feeding Considerations Diazepam and N-desmethyldiazepam can be found in breast milk; the oxazepam metabolite has also been detected in the urine of a nursing infant. Drowsiness, lethargy, or weight loss in nursing infants have been observed in case reports following maternal use of some benzodiazepines, including diazepam (Iqbal, 2002). Because diazepam and its metabolites may be present in breast milk for prolonged periods following administration, one manufacturer recommends discontinuing breast-feeding for an appropriate period of time.

Contraindications Hypersensitivity to diazepam or any component of the formulation (cross-sensitivity with other benzodiazepines may exist); myasthenia gravis; severe respiratory insufficiency; severe hepatic insufficiency; sleep apnea syndrome; acute narrow-angle glaucoma; not for use in children <6 months of age (oral)

Warnings/Precautions Withdrawal has also been associated with an increase in the seizure frequency. Use with caution with drugs which may decrease diazepam metabolism. Use with caution in debilitated patients, obese patients, patients with hepatic disease (including alcoholics), or renal impairment. Active metabolites with extended half-lives may lead to delayed accumulation and adverse effects. Use with caution in patients with respiratory disease or impaired gag reflex.

Acute hypotension, muscle weakness, apnea, and cardiac arrest have occurred with parenteral administration. Acute effects may be more prevalent in patients receiving concurrent barbiturates, opioids, or ethanol. Appropriate resuscitative equipment and qualified personnel should be available during administration and monitoring. Avoid use of the injection in patients with shock, coma, or acute ethanol intoxication. Intra-arterial injection or extravasation of the parenteral formulation should be avoided. Parenteral formulation contains propylene glycol, which has been associated with toxicity when administered in high dosages. Administration of rectal gel should only be performed by individuals trained to recognize characteristic seizure activity and monitor response.

Causes CNS depression (dose-related) resulting in sedation, dizziness, confusion, or ataxia which may impair physical and mental capabilities. Patients must be cautioned about performing tasks which require mental alertness (eg, operating machinery or driving). Use with caution in patients receiving other CNS depressants or psychoactive agents. Effects with other sedative drugs or ethanol may be potentiated. The dosage of opioids should be reduced by approximately one-third when diazepam is added. Benzodiazepines have been associated with falls and traumatic injury and should be used with extreme caution in patients who are at risk of these events. Benzodiazepines with long half-lives may produce prolonged sedation and increase the risk of falls and fracture. In older adults, benzodiazepines increase the risk of impaired cognition, delirium, falls, fractures, and motor vehicle accidents. Due to increased sensitivity in this age group and slower metabolism of long-acting agents (such as diazepam), avoid use for treatment of insomnia, agitation, or delirium (Beers Criteria).

Use with caution in patients taking strong CYP3A4 inhibitors, moderate or strong CYP3A4 and CYP2C19 inducers and major CYP3A4 substrates.

Use caution in patients with depression or anxiety associated with depression, particularly if suicidal risk may be present. Use with caution in patients with a history of drug dependence. Benzodiazepines have been associated with dependence and acute withdrawal symptoms on discontinuation or reduction in dose. Acute withdrawal, including seizures, may be precipitated in patients after administration of flumazenil to patients receiving long-term benzodiazepine therapy.

Diazepam has been associated with anterograde amnesia. Psychiatric and paradoxical reactions, including hyperactive or aggressive behavior, have been reported with benzodiazepines, particularly in adolescent/pediatric or elderly patients. Does not have analgesic, antidepressant, or antipsychotic properties.

Rectal gel: Safety and efficacy have not been established in children <2 years of age.

Oral: Safety and efficacy have not been established in children <6 months of age.

Injection: Safety and efficacy have not been established in children <30 days of age. Solution for injection may contain sodium benzoate, benzyl alcohol, or benzoic acid. Large amounts have been associated with "gasping syndrome" in neonates. I.V. administration: Vesicant; ensure proper needle or catheter placement prior to and during administration; avoid extravasation.

Adverse Reactions Frequency not defined. Adverse reactions may vary by route of administration.

Cardiovascular: Hypotension, vasodilatation

Central nervous system: Amnesia, ataxia, confusion, depression, drowsiness, fatigue, headache, slurred speech, paradoxical reactions (eg, aggressiveness, agitation, anxiety, delusions, hallucinations, inappropriate behavior, increased muscle spasms, insomnia, irritability, psychoses, rage, restlessness, sleep disturbances, stimulation), vertigo

Dermatologic: Rash

Endocrine & metabolic: Libido changes

Gastrointestinal: Constipation, diarrhea, nausea, salivation changes (dry mouth or hypersalivation)

Genitourinary: Incontinence, urinary retention

Hepatic: Jaundice

Local: Phlebitis, pain with injection

Neuromuscular & skeletal: Dysarthria, tremor, weakness

Ocular: Blurred vision, diplopia

Respiratory: Apnea, asthma, respiratory rate decreased

Drug Interactions

Metabolism/Transport Effects Substrate of CYP1A2 (minor), CYP2B6 (minor), CYP2C19 (major), CYP2C9 (minor), CYP3A4 (major); **Note:** Assignment of Major/Minor substrate status based on clinically relevant drug interaction potential; **Inhibits** CYP2C19 (weak), CYP3A4 (weak)

Avoid Concomitant Use

Avoid concomitant use of Diazepam with any of the following: Azelastine (Nasal); Conivaptan; Fusidic Acid (Systemic); OLANZapine; Paraldehyde; Pimozide; Sodium Oxybate

Increased Effect/Toxicity

Diazepam may increase the levels/effects of: Alcohol (Ethyl); ARIPiprazole; Azelastine (Nasal); Buprenorphine; CloZAPine; CNS Depressants; Dofetilide; Fosphenytoin; Hydrocodone; Lomitapide; Methotrimeprazine; Metyrosine; Mirtazapine; Paraldehyde; Phenytoin; Pimozide; Pramipexole; ROPINIRole; Rotigotine; Selective Serotonin Reuptake Inhibitors; Sodium Oxybate; Zolpidem

The levels/effects of Diazepam may be increased by: Antifungal Agents (Azole Derivatives, Systemic); Aprepitant; Brimonidine (Topical); Calcium Channel Blockers (Nondihydropyridine); Cimetidine; Conivaptan; Contraceptives (Estrogens); Contraceptives (Progestins); Cosyntropin; CYP2C19 Inhibitors (Moderate); CYP2C19 Inhibitors (Strong); CYP3A4 Inhibitors (Moderate); CYP3A4 Inhibitors (Strong); Dasatinib; Disulfiram; Doxylamine; Droperidol; Etravirine; Fosamprenavir; Fosaprepitant; Fusidic Acid (Systemic); Grapefruit Juice; HydrOXYzine; Isoniazid; Ivacaftor; Luliconazole; Magnesium Sulfate; Methotrimeprazine; Mifepristone; OLANZapine; Perampanel; Proton Pump Inhibitors; Ritonavir; Saquinavir; Selective Serotonin Reuptake Inhibitors; Simeprevir; Tapentadol

Decreased Effect

The levels/effects of Diazepam may be decreased by: Bosentan; CarBAMazepine; CYP2C19 Inducers (Strong); CYP3A4 Inducers (Strong); Dabrafenib; Deferasirox; Etravirine; Herbs (CYP3A4 Inducers); Mitotane; Rifamycin Derivatives; Theophylline Derivatives; Tocilizumab; Yohimbine

Ethanol/Nutrition/Herb Interactions

Ethanol: Ethanol may increase CNS depression. Potential for drug dependency exists. Management: Avoid ethanol.

Food: Diazepam serum concentrations may be decreased if taken with food. Grapefruit juice may increase diazepam serum concentrations. Management: Avoid concurrent use of grapefruit juice. Maintain adequate hydration, unless instructed to restrict fluid intake.

Herb/Nutraceutical: St John's wort may decrease diazepam levels. Yohimbe may decrease the effectiveness of diazepam. Kava kava, valerian, and gotu kola may increase CNS depression. Avoid St John's wort, yohimbe, kava kava, valerian, and gotu kola.

Preparation for Administration Per manufacturer, do not mix I.V. product with other medications.

Storage/Stability

Injection: Store at 20°C to 25°C (68°F to 77°F); excursions permitted to 15°C to 30°C (59°F to 86°F). Protect from light. Potency is retained for up to 3 months when kept at room temperature. Most stable at pH 4-8; hydrolysis occurs at pH <3.

Rectal gel: Store at 25°C (77°F); excursion permitted to 15°C to 30°C (59°F to 86°F).

Tablet: Store at 15°C to 30°C (59°F to 86°F).

Mechanism of Action Binds to stereospecific benzodiazepine receptors on the postsynaptic GABA neuron at several sites within the central nervous system, including the limbic system, reticular formation. Enhancement of the inhibitory effect of GABA on neuronal excitability results by increased neuronal membrane permeability to chloride ions. This shift in chloride ions results in hyperpolarization (a less excitable state) and stabilization.

Pharmacodynamics/Kinetics

Onset of action: I.V.: Almost immediate; Oral: Rapid

Duration: I.V.: 20-30 minutes; Oral: Variable (dose and frequency dependent)

Absorption: Oral: 85% to 100%, more reliable than I.M.

Distribution: V_d: Young healthy males: 0.8-1.0 L/kg

Protein binding: 98%

Metabolism: Hepatic

Half-life elimination: Parent drug: Adults: 20-50 hours; increased half-life in neonates, elderly, and those with severe hepatic disorders; Active major metabolite (desmethyldiazepam): 50-100 hours; may be prolonged in neonates

Time to peak: Oral: 15 minutes to 2 hours

Dosage Oral absorption is more reliable than I.M.

Children:

- Conscious sedation for procedures: Oral: 0.2-0.3 mg/kg (maximum: 10 mg) 45-60 minutes prior to procedure
- Muscle spasm associated with tetanus: I.V., I.M.:
  - Infants >30 days and Children <5 years: 1-2 mg/dose every 3-4 hours as needed
  - Children ≥5 years: 5-10 mg/dose every 3-4 hours as needed
- Sedation/muscle relaxant/anxiety:
  - Oral: 0.12-0.8 mg/kg/day in divided doses every 6-8 hours
  - I.M., I.V.: 0.04-0.3 mg/kg/dose every 2-4 hours to a maximum of 0.6 mg/kg within an 8-hour period if needed

Spasticity in cerebral palsy (unlabeled use): Oral: Dose should be individualized:
Children ≤5 years: <8.5 kg: 0.5-1 mg at bedtime; 8.5-15 kg: 1-2 mg at bedtime (Mathew, 2005)
Children 5-16 years: 1.25 mg 3 times daily to 5 mg 4 times daily (Engle, 1966)
Status epilepticus:
I.V.: Infants >30 days and Children: 0.1-0.3 mg/kg (maximum dose: 10 mg) given over ≤5 mg/minute; may repeat dose after 5-10 minutes (Hegenbarth, 2008)
Manufacturer's recommendations:
Infants >30 days and Children <5 years: 0.2-0.5 mg given slowly every 2-5 minutes (maximum total dose: 5 mg); repeat in 2-4 hours if needed
Children ≥5 years: 1 mg given slowly every 2-5 minutes (maximum total dose: 10 mg); repeat in 2-4 hours if needed
Rectal gel: 0.5 mg/kg, then 0.25 mg/kg in 10 minutes if needed (maximum dose: 20 mg) (Hegenbarth, 2008).
Anticonvulsant (acute treatment): Rectal gel:
Children <2 years: Safety and efficacy have not been studied
Children 2-5 years: 0.5 mg/kg (maximum dose: 20 mg)
Children 6-11 years: 0.3 mg/kg (maximum dose: 20 mg)
Children ≥12 years: 0.2 mg/kg (maximum dose: 20 mg)
Note: Dosage should be rounded upward to the next available dose, 2.5, 5, 7.5, 10, 12.5, 15, 17.5, and 20 mg/dose; dose may be repeated in 4-12 hours if needed; do not use for more than 5 episodes per month or more than one episode every 5 days
Adolescents: Conscious sedation for procedures:
Oral: 10 mg
I.V.: 5 mg, may repeat with 1/2 dose if needed
Adults:
Acute ethanol withdrawal: Oral: 10 mg 3-4 times during first 24 hours, then decrease to 5 mg 3-4 times/day as needed
Anticonvulsant (acute treatment): Rectal gel: 0.2 mg/kg
Note: Dosage should be rounded upward to the next available dose, 2.5, 5, 7.5, 10, 12.5, 15, 17.5, and 20 mg/dose; dose may be repeated in 4-12 hours if needed; do not use for more than 5 episodes per month or more than one episode every 5 days.
Anxiety (symptoms/disorders): Oral, I.M, I.V.: 2-10 mg 2-4 times/day if needed
Muscle spasm: I.V., I.M.: Initial: 5-10 mg; then 5-10 mg in 3-4 hours, if necessary. Larger doses may be required if associated with tetanus.
Sedation in the ICU patient: I.V.: Loading dose: 5-10 mg; Maintenance dose: 0.03-0.1 mg/kg every 30 minutes to 6 hours (Barr, 2013)
Skeletal muscle relaxant (adjunct therapy): Oral: 2-10 mg 3-4 times/day
Status epilepticus:
I.V.: 5-10 mg every 5-10 minutes given over ≤5 mg/minute; maximum dose: 30 mg
Rectal gel: Premonitory/Out-of-hospital treatment: 10 mg once; may repeat once if necessary (Kälviäinen, 2007)
Rapid tranquilization of agitated patient (administer every 30-60 minutes): Oral: 5-10 mg; average total dose for tranquilization: 20-60 mg
Elderly/debilitated patients:
Oral: 2-2.5 mg 1-2 times/day initially; increase gradually as needed and tolerated
Rectal gel: Due to the increased half-life in elderly and debilitated patients, consider reducing dose.

Dosing adjustment in renal impairment: No dose adjustment recommended; decrease dose if administered for prolonged periods.
I.V.: Risk of propylene glycol toxicity; monitor closely if using for prolonged periods or at high doses
Hemodialysis: Not dialyzable (0% to 5%); supplemental dose is not necessary

Dosing adjustment in hepatic impairment: Decrease maintenance dose by 50%; half-life significantly prolonged.

Administration Oral solution (Intensol™) should be diluted before use.
I.V.: Continuous infusion is not recommended because of precipitation in I.V. fluids and absorption of drug into infusion bags and tubing. In children, do not exceed 1-2 mg/minute IVP; adults 5 mg/minute.
Vesicant; ensure proper needle or catheter placement prior to and during infusion; avoid extravasation.
Extravasation management: If extravasation occurs, stop I.V. administration immediately and disconnect (leave cannula/needle in place); gently aspirate extravasated solution (do **NOT** flush the line); remove needle/cannula; elevate extremity. Apply dry cold compresses (Hurst, 2004).
Rectal gel: Prior to administration, confirm that prescribed dose is visible and correct, and that the green "ready" band is visible. Patient should be positioned on side (facing person responsible for monitoring), with top leg bent forward. Insert rectal tip (lubricated) into rectum and push in plunger gently over 3 seconds. Remove tip of rectal syringe after 3 additional seconds. Buttocks should be held together for 3 seconds after removal. Dispose of syringe appropriately.

Monitoring Parameters Respiratory, cardiovascular, and mental status; check for orthostasis

Critically-ill mechanically-ventilated patients: Monitor depth of sedation with either the Richmond Agitation-Sedation Scale (RASS) or Sedation-Agitation Scale (SAS) (Barr, 2013)

Reference Range Therapeutic: Diazepam: 0.2-1.5 mcg/mL (SI: 0.7-5.3 micromole/L); N-desmethyldiazepam (nordiazepam): 0.1-0.5 mcg/mL (SI: 0.35-1.8 micromole/L)

Test Interactions False-negative urinary glucose determinations when using Clinistix® or Diastix®

Additional Information Diazepam does not have any analgesic effects.
Diastat® AcuDial™: When dispensing, consult package information for directions on setting patient's dose; confirm green "ready" band is visible prior to dispensing product.

Dosage Forms Excipient information presented when available (limited, particularly for generics); consult specific product labeling.
Concentrate, Oral:
Diazepam Intensol: 5 mg/mL (30 mL) [contains alcohol, usp; unflavored flavor]
Device, Intramuscular:
Generic: 10 mg/2 mL (2 mL)
Gel, Rectal:
Diastat AcuDial: 10 mg (1 ea); 20 mg (1 ea) [contains alcohol, usp, benzoic acid, sodium benzoate]
Diastat Pediatric: 2.5 mg (1 ea) [contains alcohol, usp]
Generic: 2.5 mg (1 ea); 10 mg (1 ea); 20 mg (1 ea)
Solution, Injection:
Generic: 5 mg/mL (2 mL, 10 mL)
Solution, Oral:
Generic: 1 mg/mL (5 mL, 500 mL)
Tablet, Oral:
Valium: 2 mg, 5 mg, 10 mg [scored]
Generic: 2 mg, 5 mg, 10 mg

Controlled Substance C-IV

◆ **Diazepam Auto Injector (Can)** *see* Diazepam *on page 594*

◆ **Diazepam Injection USP (Can)** *see* Diazepam *on page 594*

◆ **Diazepam Intensol** *see* Diazepam *on page 594*

Diazoxide (dye az OKS ide)

Brand Names: U.S. Proglycem

Brand Names: Canada Proglycem®

Pharmacologic Category Antidote, Hypoglycemia; Vasodilator, Direct-Acting

Use Hypoglycemia related to islet cell adenoma, carcinoma, hyperplasia, or adenomatosis; nesidioblastosis; leucine sensitivity; extrapancreatic malignancy

Pregnancy Risk Factor C

Dosage Hyperinsulinemic hypoglycemia: Oral:

Neonates and Infants: Initial dose: 10 mg/kg/day in divided doses every 8 hours; dosing range: 8-15 mg/kg/day in divided doses every 8-12 hours. Discontinue if no effect after 2-3 weeks.

Children, Adolescents, and Adults: Initial dose: 3 mg/kg/day in divided doses every 8 hours; dosing range: 3-8 mg/kg/day in divided doses every 8-12 hours. **Note:** In certain instances, patients with refractory hypoglycemia may require higher doses. Discontinue if no effect after 2-3 weeks.

Dosage adjustment in renal impairment: Half-life may be prolonged with renal impairment; a reduced dose should be considered.

Dosage adjustment in hepatic impairment: No dosage adjustment provided in manufacturer's labeling.

Additional Information Complete prescribing information should be consulted for additional detail.

Dosage Forms Excipient information presented when available (limited, particularly for generics); consult specific product labeling.

Suspension, Oral:

Proglycem: 50 mg/mL (30 mL) [chocolate mint flavor]

Dosage Forms: Canada Excipient information presented when available (limited, particularly for generics); consult specific product labeling.

Capsule, oral:

Proglycem: 100 mg

◆ **Dibenzyline** *see* Phenoxybenzamine *on page 1632*

◆ **DIC** *see* Dacarbazine *on page 530*

◆ **Dicel® Chewable [OTC]** *see* Chlorpheniramine and Pseudoephedrine *on page 412*

◆ **Dicel® DM Chewables [OTC]** *see* Chlorpheniramine, Pseudoephedrine, and Dextromethorphan *on page 414*

◆ **Diclectin® (Can)** *see* Doxylamine and Pyridoxine *on page 673*

◆ **Diclegis®** *see* Doxylamine and Pyridoxine *on page 673*

Diclofenac (Systemic) (dye KLOE fen ak)

Brand Names: U.S. Cambia; Cataflam; Voltaren-XR; Zipsor; Zorvolex

Brand Names: Canada Apo-Diclo; Apo-Diclo Rapide; Apo-Diclo SR; Ava-Diclofenac; Ava-Diclofenac SR; Cambia; Cataflam; Diclofenac ECT; Diclofenac Sodium; Diclofenac Sodium SR; Diclofenac SR; Dom-Diclofenac; Dom-Diclofenac SR; NTP-Diclofenac; NTP-Diclofenac SR; Nu-Diclo; Nu-Diclo-SR; PMS-Diclofenac; PMS-Diclofenac SR; PMS-Diclofenac-K; PRO-Diclo-Rapide; Sandoz-Diclofenac; Sandoz-Diclofenac Rapide; Sandoz-Diclofenac SR; Teva-Diclofenac; Teva-Diclofenac K; Teva-Diclofenac SR; Voltaren; Voltaren Rapide; Voltaren SR

Index Terms Diclofenac Potassium; Diclofenac Sodium; Voltaren; Zorvolex

Pharmacologic Category Nonsteroidal Anti-inflammatory Drug (NSAID); Nonsteroidal Anti-inflammatory Drug (NSAID), Oral

Additional Appendix Information

Beers Criteria – Potentially Inappropriate Medications for Geriatrics *on page 2368*

Use

Capsule: Relief of mild-to-moderate acute pain

Immediate-release tablet: Relief of mild-to-moderate pain; primary dysmenorrhea; acute and chronic treatment of rheumatoid arthritis, osteoarthritis

Delayed-release tablet: Acute and chronic treatment of rheumatoid arthritis, osteoarthritis, ankylosing spondylitis

Extended-release tablet: Chronic treatment of osteoarthritis, rheumatoid arthritis

Oral solution: Treatment of acute migraine with or without aura

Suppository (CAN; not available in U.S.): Symptomatic treatment of rheumatoid arthritis and osteoarthritis (including degenerative joint disease of hip)

Unlabeled Use Juvenile idiopathic arthritis (JIA)

Pregnancy Risk Factor C (oral)/D (≥30 weeks gestation [oral])

Pregnancy Considerations Adverse events were not observed in the initial animal reproduction studies; therefore, manufacturers classify most dosage forms of diclofenac as pregnancy category C (oral: Category D ≥30 weeks gestation). Diclofenac crosses the placenta and can be detected in fetal tissue and amniotic fluid. NSAID exposure during the first trimester is not strongly associated with congenital malformations; however, cardiovascular anomalies and cleft palate have been observed following NSAID exposure in some studies. The use of a NSAID close to conception may be associated with an increased risk of miscarriage. Nonteratogenic effects have been observed following NSAID administration during the third trimester including: Myocardial degenerative changes, prenatal constriction of the ductus arteriosus, fetal tricuspid regurgitation, failure of the ductus arteriosus to close postnatally; renal dysfunction or failure, oligohydramnios; gastrointestinal bleeding or perforation, increased risk of necrotizing enterocolitis; intracranial bleeding (including intraventricular hemorrhage), platelet dysfunction with resultant bleeding; pulmonary hypertension. Because they may cause premature closure of the ductus arteriosus, use of NSAIDs late in pregnancy should be avoided (use after 31 or 32 weeks gestation is not recommended by some clinicians). Product labeling for Zipsor® specifically notes that use at ≥30 weeks gestation should be avoided and, therefore, classifies diclofenac as pregnancy category D at this time. Use in the third trimester is contraindicated in the Canadian labeling. The chronic use of NSAIDs in women of reproductive age may be associated with infertility that is reversible upon discontinuation of the medication. A registry is available for pregnant women exposed to autoimmune medications including diclofenac. For additional information contact the Organization of Teratology Information Specialists, OTIS Autoimmune Diseases Study, at 877-311-8972

Breast-Feeding Considerations Low concentrations of diclofenac can be found in breast milk. Breast-feeding is not recommended by the manufacturer. Use while breast-feeding is contraindicated in Canadian labeling.

Medication Guide Available Yes

Contraindications Hypersensitivity to diclofenac or any component of the formulation; hypersensitivity to bovine protein (capsule formulation only); patients who exhibit asthma, urticaria, or other allergic-type reactions after taking aspirin or other NSAIDs; perioperative pain in the setting of coronary artery bypass graft (CABG) surgery

Canadian labeling: Additional contraindications (not in U.S. labeling): Uncontrolled heart failure, active gastric/duodenal/peptic ulcer; active GI bleed or perforation; regional ulcer, gastritis, or ulcerative colitis; cerebrovascular bleeding or other bleeding disorders; inflammatory bowel disease; severe hepatic impairment; active hepatic disease; severe renal impairment (Cl_{cr} <30 mL/minute) or deteriorating renal disease; known hyperkalemia; patients <16 years of age; breast-feeding; pregnancy (third trimester); use of diclofenac suppository if recent history of bleeding or inflammatory lesions of rectum/anus

Warnings/Precautions [U.S. Boxed Warning]: NSAIDs are associated with an increased risk of adverse cardiovascular thrombotic events, including MI and stroke. Risk may be increased with duration of use or pre-existing cardiovascular risk factors or disease. Carefully evaluate individual cardiovascular risk profiles prior to prescribing. May cause new-onset hypertension or worsening of existing hypertension. Monitor blood pressure closely. Use caution with fluid retention. Avoid use in heart failure. Concurrent administration of ibuprofen, and potentially other nonselective NSAIDs, may interfere with aspirin's cardioprotective effect. **[U.S. Boxed Warning]: Use is contraindicated for treatment of perioperative pain in the setting of coronary artery bypass graft (CABG) surgery.** Risk of MI and stroke may be increased with use following CABG surgery.

NSAID use may compromise existing renal function; dose-dependent decreases in prostaglandin synthesis may result from NSAID use, reducing renal blood flow which may cause renal decompensation. NSAID use may increase the risk for hyperkalemia. Patients with impaired renal function, dehydration, heart failure, liver dysfunction, those taking diuretics and ACEI, and the elderly are at greater risk of renal toxicity and hyperkalemia. Rehydrate patient before starting therapy; monitor renal function closely. Not recommended for use in patients with advanced renal disease. Long-term NSAID use may result in renal papillary necrosis while persistent urinary symptoms (eg, dysuria, bladder pain), cystitis, or hematuria may occur anytime after initiating NSAID therapy. Discontinue therapy with symptom onset and evaluate for origin.

[U.S. Boxed Warning]: NSAIDs may increase risk of gastrointestinal irritation, inflammation, ulceration, bleeding, and perforation. These events may occur at any time during therapy and without warning. Use caution with a history of GI disease (bleeding or ulcers), concurrent therapy with aspirin, anticoagulants and/or corticosteroids, smoking, use of alcohol, the elderly or debilitated patients. When used concomitantly with ≤325 mg of aspirin, a substantial increase in the risk of gastrointestinal complications (eg, ulcer) occurs; concomitant gastroprotective therapy (eg, proton pump inhibitors) is recommended (Bhatt, 2008).

Use the lowest effective dose for the shortest duration of time, consistent with individual patient goals, to reduce risk of cardiovascular or GI adverse events. Alternate therapies should be considered for patients at high risk.

NSAIDs may cause photosensitivity or serious skin adverse events including exfoliative dermatitis, Stevens-Johnson syndrome (SJS), and toxic epidermal necrolysis (TEN); discontinue use at first sign of skin rash or hypersensitivity. Anaphylactoid reactions may occur, even without prior exposure; patients with "aspirin triad" (bronchial asthma, aspirin intolerance, rhinitis) may be at increased risk. Do not use in patients who experience bronchospasm, asthma, rhinitis, or urticaria with NSAID or aspirin therapy. Use caution in other forms of asthma. Platelet adhesion and aggregation may be decreased; may prolong bleeding time; patients with coagulation disorders or who are receiving anticoagulants should be monitored closely. Anemia may occur; patients on long-term NSAID therapy should be monitored for anemia. Rarely, NSAID use may cause severe blood dyscrasias (eg, agranulocytosis, aplastic anemia, thrombocytopenia).

Use with caution in patients with impaired hepatic function. Closely monitor patients with any abnormal LFT. Diclofenac can cause transaminase elevations; initiate monitoring 4-8 weeks into therapy. Rarely, severe hepatic reactions (eg, fulminant hepatitis, liver failure) have occurred; discontinue all formulations if signs or symptoms of liver disease develop, or if systemic manifestations occur. Use with caution in hepatic porphyria (may trigger attack).

NSAIDS may cause drowsiness, dizziness, blurred vision, and other neurologic effects which may impair physical or mental abilities; patients must be cautioned about performing tasks which require mental alertness (eg, operating machinery or driving). Discontinue use with blurred or diminished vision and perform ophthalmologic exam. Monitor vision with long-term therapy. May increase the risk of aseptic meningitis, especially in patients with systemic lupus erythematosus (SLE) and mixed connective tissue disorders. In the elderly, avoid chronic use (unless alternative agents ineffective and patient can receive concomitant gastroprotective agent); nonselective oral NSAID use is associated with an increased risk of GI bleeding and peptic ulcer disease in older adults in high risk category (eg, >75 years or age or receiving concomitant oral/parenteral corticosteroids, anticoagulants, or antiplatelet agents) (Beers Criteria).

Withhold for at least 4-6 half-lives prior to surgical or dental procedures. Safety and efficacy have not been established in children.

Capsule: Contains gelatin; use is contraindicated in patients with history of hypersensitivity to bovine protein.

Oral solution: Only indicated for the acute treatment of migraine; not indicated for migraine prophylaxis or cluster headache. Not bioequivalent to other forms of diclofenac (even same dose); do not interchange products. Contains phenylalanine.

Adverse Reactions

Oral:

1% to 10%:

- Cardiovascular: Edema
- Central nervous system: Dizziness, headache
- Dermatologic: Pruritus, rash
- Endocrine & metabolic: Fluid retention
- Gastrointestinal: Abdominal distension, abdominal pain, constipation, diarrhea, dyspepsia, flatulence, GI perforation, heartburn, nausea, peptic ulcer/GI bleed, vomiting
- Hematologic: Anemia, bleeding time increased
- Hepatic: Liver enzyme abnormalities (>3 x ULN; ≤4%)
- Otic: Tinnitus
- Renal: Renal function abnormal
- Miscellaneous: Diaphoresis increased

<1% (Limited to important or life-threatening): Agranulocytosis, alopecia, anaphylactoid reactions, anaphylaxis, angioedema, aplastic anemia, anxiety, appetite changes, arrhythmia, aseptic meningitis, asthma, azotemia, blurred vision, chest pain, CHF, colitis, coma, confusion, conjunctivitis, cystitis, depression, diplopia, disorientation, dreams abnormal, drowsiness, dyspnea, dysuria, ecchymosis, eosinophilia, eructation, erythema multiforme, esophageal lesions, esophagitis, exfoliative dermatitis, fever, fulminant hepatitis, gastritis, glossitis,hallucination, hearing impairment, hearing loss, hematemesis, hematuria, hemoglobin decreased, hemolytic anemia, hepatic failure, hepatic necrosis, hepatitis, hepatotoxicity, hyper-/hypotension, hyper-/hypoglycemia, infection, insomnia, interstitial nephritis, intestinal perforation, jaundice,

laryngeal edema, leukopenia, lymphadenopathy, malaise, melena, memory disturbance, meningitis, MI, nephrotic syndrome, nervousness, oliguria, palpitation, pancreatitis, pancytopenia, paresthesia, pharynx edema, photosensitivity, pneumonia, polyuria, proteinuria, psychotic reactions, purpura, rectal bleeding, renal failure, renal papillary necrosis, respiratory depression, seizure, sepsis, somnolence, Stevens-Johnson syndrome, stomatitis, stroke, swelling of lips and tongue, syncope, tachycardia, taste disorder, thrombocytopenia, toxic epidermal necrolysis, tremor, urticaria, vasculitis, vertigo, weight change, weakness, xerostomia

Rectal suppository (CAN; not available in U.S.):

Also refer to adverse reactions associated with oral formulations.

<1%, postmarketing, and/or case reports: Local: Bleeding, hemorrhoid exacerbation, proctitis, rectal irritation

Drug Interactions

Metabolism/Transport Effects Substrate of CYP1A2 (minor), CYP2B6 (minor), CYP2C19 (minor), CYP2C8 (minor), CYP2C9 (minor), CYP2D6 (minor), CYP3A4 (minor); **Note:** Assignment of Major/Minor substrate status based on clinically relevant drug interaction potential; **Inhibits** CYP1A2 (weak), CYP2C9 (weak), CYP2E1 (weak), CYP3A4 (weak), UGT1A6

Avoid Concomitant Use

Avoid concomitant use of Diclofenac (Systemic) with any of the following: Floctafenine; Ketorolac (Nasal); Ketorolac (Systemic); NSAID (COX-2 Inhibitor); Omacetaxine; Pimozide

Increased Effect/Toxicity

Diclofenac (Systemic) may increase the levels/effects of: 5-ASA Derivatives; Agents with Antiplatelet Properties; Aliskiren; Aminoglycosides; Anticoagulants; ARIPiprazole; Bisphosphonate Derivatives; Collagenase (Systemic); CycloSPORINE (Systemic); Dabigatran Etexilate; Deferasirox; Deferiprone; Desmopressin; Digoxin; Dofetilide; Eplerenone; Haloperidol; Ibritumomab; Lithium; Lomitapide; Methotrexate; Nonsteroidal Anti-Inflammatory Agents; NSAID (COX-2 Inhibitor); Omacetaxine; PEMEtrexed; Pimozide; Porfimer; Potassium-Sparing Diuretics; PRALAtrexate; Quinolone Antibiotics; Rivaroxaban; Salicylates; Tenofovir; Thrombolytic Agents; Tositumomab and Iodine I 131 Tositumomab; Vancomycin; Vitamin K Antagonists

The levels/effects of Diclofenac (Systemic) may be increased by: ACE Inhibitors; Angiotensin II Receptor Blockers; Antidepressants (Tricyclic, Tertiary Amine); Corticosteroids (Systemic); CycloSPORINE (Systemic); CYP2C9 Inhibitors (Strong); Dasatinib; Floctafenine; Glucosamine; Herbs (Anticoagulant/Antiplatelet Properties); Ibrutinib; Ketorolac (Nasal); Ketorolac (Systemic); Multivitamins/Fluoride (with ADE); Multivitamins/Minerals (with ADEK, Folate, Iron); Multivitamins/Minerals (with AE, No Iron); Nonsteroidal Anti-Inflammatory Agents; Omega-3 Fatty Acids; Pentosan Polysulfate Sodium; Pentoxifylline; Probenecid; Prostacyclin Analogues; Selective Serotonin Reuptake Inhibitors; Serotonin/Norepinephrine Reuptake Inhibitors; Sodium Phosphates; Tipranavir; Treprostinil; Vitamin E; Voriconazole

Decreased Effect

Diclofenac (Systemic) may decrease the levels/effects of: ACE Inhibitors; Agents with Antiplatelet Properties; Aliskiren; Angiotensin II Receptor Blockers; Beta-Blockers; Eplerenone; HydrALAZINE; Loop Diuretics; Potassium-Sparing Diuretics; Prostaglandins (Ophthalmic); Salicylates; Selective Serotonin Reuptake Inhibitors; Thiazide Diuretics

The levels/effects of Diclofenac (Systemic) may be decreased by: Bile Acid Sequestrants; CYP2C9 Inducers (Strong); Nonsteroidal Anti-Inflammatory Agents; Peginterferon Alfa-2b; Salicylates

Ethanol/Nutrition/Herb Interactions

Ethanol: Avoid ethanol (may enhance gastric mucosal irritation).

Herb/Nutraceutical: Avoid alfalfa, anise, bilberry, bladderwrack, bromelain, cat's claw, celery, chamomile, coleus, cordyceps, dong quai, evening primrose, fenugreek, feverfew, garlic, ginger, ginkgo biloba, grapeseed, green tea, ginseng (Siberian), guggul, horse chestnut, horseradish, licorice, prickly ash, red clover, reishi, SAMe (s-adenosylmethionine), sweet clover, turmeric, white willow (all have additional antiplatelet activity).

Preparation for Administration Oral solution: Empty contents of packet into 1-2 ounces (30-60 mL) of water (do not use other liquids), mix well and administer immediately.

Storage/Stability

Capsule, oral solution: Store at 25°C (77°F); excursions permitted to 15°C to 30°C (59°F to 86°F). Protect from moisture.

Suppository (CAN; not available in U.S.): Store at 15°C to 30°C (59°F to 86°F); protect from heat.

Tablet: Store below 30°C (86°F). Protect from moisture; store in tight container.

Mechanism of Action Reversibly inhibits cyclooxygenase-1 and 2 (COX-1 and 2) enzymes, which results in decreased formation of prostaglandin precursors; has antipyretic, analgesic, and anti-inflammatory properties

Other proposed mechanisms not fully elucidated (and possibly contributing to the anti-inflammatory effect to varying degrees), include inhibiting chemotaxis, altering lymphocyte activity, inhibiting neutrophil aggregation/activation, and decreasing proinflammatory cytokine levels.

Pharmacodynamics/Kinetics

Onset of action:

Cataflam® (potassium salt) is more rapid than the sodium salt because it dissolves in the stomach instead of the duodenum

Suppository: More rapid onset, but slower rate of absorption when compared to enteric coated tablet

Distribution: ~1.4 L/kg

Protein binding: >99%, primarily to albumin

Metabolism: Hepatic; undergoes first-pass metabolism; forms several metabolites (1 with weak activity)

Bioavailability: 55%

Half-life elimination: ~2 hours

Time to peak, serum:

Cambia™: ~0.25 hours

Cataflam®: ~1 hour

Voltaren® XR ~5 hours

Zipsor®: ~0.5 hour

Suppository: ≤1 hour; **Note:** Suppository: C_{max}: Approximately two-thirds of that observed with enteric coated tablet (equivalent 50 mg dose)

Tablet, delayed release (diclofenac sodium): ~2 hours

Excretion: Urine (~65%); feces (~35%)

Dosage Adults:

Oral:

Analgesia:

Immediate release tablet: Starting dose: 50 mg 3 times/day (maximum dose: 150 mg/day); may administer 100 mg loading dose, followed by 50 mg every 8 hours (maximum dose day 1: 200 mg/day; maximum dose day 2 and thereafter: 150 mg/day)

Canadian labeling: Maximum loading dose day 1: 200 mg/day; maximum dose day 2 and up to 7 days: 150 mg/day (50 mg every 6-8 hours)

Immediate release capsule: 25 mg 4 times/day

Primary dysmenorrhea: Immediate release tablet: Starting dose: 50 mg 3 times/day (maximum dose: 150 mg/day); may administer 100 mg loading dose, followed by 50 mg every 8 hours (maximum dose day 1: 200 mg/day; maximum dose day 2 and thereafter: 150 mg/day)

Canadian labeling: Maximum loading dose day 1: 200 mg/day; maximum dose day 2 and up to 7 days: 150 mg/day (50 mg every 6-8 hours)

Rheumatoid arthritis: Immediate release tablet: 150-200 mg/day in 3-4 divided doses; Delayed release tablet: 150-200 mg/day in 2-4 divided doses; Extended release tablet: 100 mg/day (may increase dose to 200 mg/day in 2 divided doses)

Canadian labeling: 150 mg/day in 3 divided doses (75-150 mg/day of slow release tablet)

Osteoarthritis: Immediate or delayed release tablet: 100-150 mg/day in 2-3 divided doses; Extended release tablet: 100 mg/day

Canadian labeling: 150 mg/day in 3 divided doses (75-150 mg/day of slow release tablet)

Ankylosing spondylitis: Delayed release tablet: 100-125 mg/day in 4-5 divided doses

Migraine: Oral solution: 50 mg (one packet) as a single dose at the time of migraine onset; safety and efficacy of a second dose have not been established

Rectal suppository (not available in U.S.):

Osteoarthritis: *Canadian labeling:* Insert 50 mg or 100 mg suppository rectally as single dose to substitute for final (third) oral daily dose; maximum combined dose (rectal and oral): 150 mg/day

Rheumatoid arthritis: *Canadian labeling:* Insert 50 mg or 100 mg suppository rectally as single dose to substitute for final (third) oral daily dose (maximum combined dose [rectal and oral]: 150 mg/day)

Dosage adjustment in renal impairment: Not recommended in patients with advanced renal disease or significant renal impairment

Dosage adjustment in hepatic impairment: May require dosage adjustment; use oral solution only if benefits outweigh risks

Elderly: No specific dosing recommendations; elderly may demonstrate adverse effects at lower doses than younger adults, and >60% may develop asymptomatic peptic ulceration with or without hemorrhage; monitor renal function

Dietary Considerations Oral formulations may be taken with food to decrease GI distress. Food may reduce effectiveness of oral solution. Some products may contain phenylalanine.

Diclofenac potassium = Cataflam®; potassium content: 5.8 mg (0.15 mEq) per 50 mg tablet

Administration

Oral: Do not crush delayed or extended release tablets. Administer with food or milk to avoid gastric distress. Take with full glass of water to enhance absorption.

Oral solution: Administer immediately after preparing; food may reduce effectiveness.

Rectal suppository: Remove entire plastic wrapping prior to inserting rectally.

Monitoring Parameters Monitor CBC, liver enzymes (periodically during chronic therapy starting 4-8 weeks after initiation), BUN/serum creatinine; monitor urine output; occult blood loss

Product Availability

Zorvolex: FDA approved October 2013; anticipated availability is first quarter of 2014. Zorvolex is indicated for the treatment of mild to moderate acute pain.

Zorvolex capsules contain diclofenac as submicron particles that are approximately 20 times smaller than their original size. The reduction in particle size provides an increased surface area, leading to faster dissolution. Refer to the prescribing information for additional information.

Dosage Forms Excipient information presented when available (limited, particularly for generics); consult specific product labeling. [DSC] = Discontinued product

Capsule, Oral:

Zorvolex: 18 mg, 35 mg [contains brilliant blue fcf (fd&c blue #1), fd&c blue #2 (indigotine)]

Capsule, Oral, as potassium:

Zipsor: 25 mg

Zipsor: 25 mg [DSC] [contains polysorbate 80]

Packet, Oral, as potassium:

Cambia: 50 mg (1 ea, 9 ea) [contains aspartame, saccharin sodium; flavored flavor]

Tablet, Oral, as potassium:

Cataflam: 50 mg

Generic: 50 mg

Tablet Delayed Release, Oral, as sodium:

Generic: 25 mg, 50 mg, 75 mg

Tablet Extended Release 24 Hour, Oral, as sodium:

Voltaren-XR: 100 mg

Generic: 100 mg

Dosage Forms: Canada Excipient information presented when available (limited, particularly for generics); consult specific product labeling.

Suppository:

Voltaren®: 50 mg, 100mg

Diclofenac (Ophthalmic) (dye KLOE fen ak)

Brand Names: Canada Voltaren Ophtha®

Index Terms Diclofenac Sodium

Pharmacologic Category Nonsteroidal Anti-inflammatory Drug (NSAID); Nonsteroidal Anti-inflammatory Drug (NSAID), Ophthalmic

Use Treatment of postoperative inflammation following cataract extraction; temporary relief of pain and photophobia in patients undergoing corneal refractive surgery

Pregnancy Risk Factor C

Dosage Ophthalmic: Adults:

Cataract surgery: Instill 1 drop into affected eye 4 times/day beginning 24 hours after cataract surgery and continuing for 2 weeks

Corneal refractive surgery: Instill 1-2 drops into affected eye within the hour prior to surgery, within 15 minutes following surgery, and then continue for 4 times/day, up to 3 days

Additional Information Complete prescribing information should be consulted for additional detail.

Dosage Forms Excipient information presented when available (limited, particularly for generics); consult specific product labeling.

Solution, Ophthalmic, as sodium:

Generic: 0.1% (2.5 mL, 5 mL)

Diclofenac and Misoprostol

(dye KLOE fen ak & mye soe PROST ole)

Brand Names: U.S. Arthrotec®

Brand Names: Canada Arthrotec®

Index Terms Misoprostol and Diclofenac

Pharmacologic Category Nonsteroidal Anti-inflammatory Drug (NSAID), Oral; Prostaglandin

Use Treatment of osteoarthritis and rheumatoid arthritis in patients at high risk for NSAID-induced gastric and duodenal ulceration

Pregnancy Risk Factor X

Medication Guide Available Yes

Dosage Oral:

Adults:

Osteoarthritis: Arthotec® 50: 1 tablet 3 times/day

Rheumatoid arthritis: Arthotec® 50: 1 tablet 3 or 4 times/day

Note: For both indications, may administer Arthrotec® 50 or Arthrotec® 75 one tablet twice daily if recommended dose is not tolerated; however, these options are less effective in preventing GI ulceration. May adjust dose using individual agents in combination with Arthrotec®. The maximum daily dose of misoprostal is 800 mcg and the maximum single dose of misoprostal is 200 mcg. The maximum daily dose of diclofenac is 150 mg/day (osteoarthritis) or 225 mg/day (rheumatoid arthritis).

Elderly: No specific dosage adjustment is recommended; may require reduced dosage due to lower body weight; monitor renal function

Dosage adjustment in renal impairment: Not recommended in patients with advanced renal disease. In renal insufficiency, diclofenac should be used with caution due to potential detrimental effects on renal function, and misoprostol dosage reduction may be required if adverse effects occur (misoprostol is renally eliminated).

Dosage adjustment in hepatic impairment: May require dosage adjustment.

Additional Information Complete prescribing information should be consulted for additional detail.

Dosage Forms Excipient information presented when available (limited, particularly for generics); consult specific product labeling.

Tablet, oral: Diclofenac sodium 50 mg and misoprostol 200 mcg; Diclofenac sodium 75 mg and misoprostol 200 mcg

Arthrotec® 50: Diclofenac sodium 50 mg and misoprostol 200 mcg

Arthrotec® 75: Diclofenac sodium 75 mg and misoprostol 200 mcg

- **Diclofenac ECT (Can)** *see* Diclofenac (Systemic) *on page 597*
- **Diclofenac Potassium** *see* Diclofenac (Systemic) *on page 597*
- **Diclofenac Sodium** *see* Diclofenac (Ophthalmic) *on page 600*
- **Diclofenac Sodium** *see* Diclofenac (Systemic) *on page 597*
- **Diclofenac Sodium SR (Can)** *see* Diclofenac (Systemic) *on page 597*
- **Diclofenac SR (Can)** *see* Diclofenac (Systemic) *on page 597*

Dicloxacillin (dye kloks a SIL in)

Index Terms Dicloxacillin Sodium

Pharmacologic Category Antibiotic, Penicillin

Use Treatment of systemic infections such as pneumonia, skin and soft tissue infections, and osteomyelitis caused by penicillinase-producing staphylococci

Pregnancy Risk Factor B

Dosage

Usual dosage range:

Newborns: Use not recommended

Children <40 kg: Oral: 12.5-100 mg/kg/day divided every 6 hours

Children >40 kg: Oral: 125-250 mg every 6 hours

Adults: Oral: 125-1000 mg every 6 hours

Indication-specific dosing:

Children: Oral:

Furunculosis: 25-50 mg/kg/day divided every 6 hours

Osteomyelitis: 50-100 mg/kg/day in divided doses every 6 hours

Adults: Oral:

Erysipelas, furunculosis, mastitis, otitis externa, septic bursitis, skin abscess: 500 mg every 6 hours

Impetigo: 250 mg every 6 hours

Prosthetic joint infection: Chronic suppression therapy: Staphylococci (oxacillin-susceptible) (unlabeled regimen): 500 mg every 6-8 hours (Osmon, 2013)

***Staphylococcus aureus*, methicillin susceptible infection if no I.V. access:** 500-1000 mg every 6-8 hours

Dosage adjustment in renal impairment: No specific adjustment provided in manufacturer's labeling; a reduction in total dosage should be considered in renal impairment.

Hemodialysis: Not dialyzable (0% to 5%); supplemental dosage not necessary

Peritoneal dialysis: Supplemental dosage not necessary

Continuous arteriovenous or venovenous hemofiltration: Supplemental dosage not necessary

Dosage adjustment in hepatic impairment: No dosage adjustment provided in manufacturer's labeling.

Additional Information Complete prescribing information should be consulted for additional detail.

Dosage Forms Excipient information presented when available (limited, particularly for generics); consult specific product labeling.

Capsule, Oral:

Generic: 250 mg, 500 mg

- **Dicloxacillin Sodium** *see* Dicloxacillin *on page 601*

Dicyclomine (dye SYE kloe meen)

Brand Names: U.S. Bentyl

Brand Names: Canada Bentylol; Dicyclomine Hydrochloride Injection; Formulex; Jamp-Dicyclomine; Protylol; Riva-Dicyclomine

Index Terms Dicyclomine Hydrochloride; Dicycloverine Hydrochloride

Pharmacologic Category Anticholinergic Agent

Additional Appendix Information

Beers Criteria – Potentially Inappropriate Medications for Geriatrics *on page 2368*

Use Treatment of functional bowel/irritable bowel syndrome

Pregnancy Risk Factor B

Dosage

Adults:

Oral: Initial: 20 mg 4 times daily for 7 days; after 1 week, may increase to 40 mg 4 times daily. If efficacy not achieved in 2 weeks or if adverse effects require a dose <80 mg/day, therapy should be discontinued. Safety data are not available for doses >80 mg daily for a duration that exceeds 2 weeks.

I.M. **(should not be used I.V.)**: 10-20 mg 4 times daily for 1-2 days; convert to oral therapy as soon as possible

Elderly: Refer to adult dosing. Use caution; lower dosages may be required.

Dosage adjustment in renal impairment: No dosage adjustment provided in the manufacturer's labeling (has not been studied); use with caution.

Dosage adjustment in hepatic impairment: No dosage adjustment provided in the manufacturer's labeling (has not been studied); use with caution.

Additional Information Complete prescribing information should be consulted for additional detail.

Dosage Forms Excipient information presented when available (limited, particularly for generics); consult specific product labeling.

Capsule, Oral, as hydrochloride:

Bentyl: 10 mg [contains brilliant blue fcf (fd&c blue #1), fd&c red #40]

Generic: 10 mg

Solution, Intramuscular, as hydrochloride:

Bentyl: 10 mg/mL (2 mL) [pyrogen free]

Solution, Oral, as hydrochloride:
Generic: 10 mg/5 mL (473 mL)
Tablet, Oral, as hydrochloride:
Bentyl: 20 mg
Generic: 20 mg

◆ **Dicyclomine Hydrochloride** *see* Dicyclomine *on page 601*

◆ **Dicyclomine Hydrochloride Injection (Can)** *see* Dicyclomine *on page 601*

◆ **Dicycloverine Hydrochloride** *see* Dicyclomine *on page 601*

◆ **Di-Dak-Sol [OTC]** *see* Sodium Hypochlorite Solution *on page 1918*

Didanosine (dye DAN oh seen)

Brand Names: U.S. Videx; Videx EC

Brand Names: Canada Videx®; Videx® EC

Index Terms ddI; Dideoxyinosine

Pharmacologic Category Antiretroviral, Reverse Transcriptase Inhibitor, Nucleoside (Anti-HIV)

Use Treatment of HIV infection; always to be used in combination with at least two other antiretroviral agents

Pregnancy Risk Factor B

Pregnancy Considerations Adverse events have not been observed in animal reproduction studies. Didanosine has been shown to cross the placenta. Based on data from the Antiretroviral Pregnancy Registry, an increased rate of birth defects has been observed following maternal use of didanosine during pregnancy; no pattern of defects has been observed and clinical relevance is uncertain. Pharmacokinetics are not significantly altered during pregnancy; dose adjustments are not needed. Cases of lactic acidosis/hepatic steatosis syndrome related to mitochondrial toxicity have been reported in pregnant women with prolonged use of nucleoside analogues. It is not known if pregnancy itself potentiates this known side effect; however, women may be at increased risk of lactic acidosis and liver damage. In addition, these adverse events are similar to other rare but life-threatening syndromes which occur during pregnancy (eg, HELLP syndrome). Hepatic enzymes and electrolytes should be monitored in women receiving nucleoside analogues and clinicians should watch for early signs of the syndrome. In addition, mitochondrial dysfunction may develop in infants following *in utero* exposure. Due to the reports of lactic acidosis, maternal, and neonatal mortality, didanosine and stavudine should **not** be used in combination during pregnancy. The DHHS Perinatal HIV Guidelines recommend didanosine to be used only in special circumstances during pregnancy.

Regardless of CD4 count or HIV RNA copy number, all HIV-infected pregnant women should receive a combination antepartum antiretroviral (ARV) drug regimen; this includes women who require therapy for their own health, as well as women who do not yet require therapy for their own health. ARV therapy should be started as soon as possible if required for the woman's health. Although earlier initiation may be more effective in reducing the perinatal transmission of HIV), also consider maternal conditions (eg, nausea and vomiting) and the potential risks of first trimester fetal exposure for specific agents. Plasma HIV RNA levels should be assessed at ~34-36 weeks gestation in order to help determine mode of delivery. If ARV therapy must be interrupted for <24 hours during the peripartum period, stop then restart all medications simultaneously in order to decrease the chance of developing resistance. Long-term follow-up is recommended for all infants exposed to ARV medications.

Healthcare providers are encouraged to enroll pregnant women exposed to antiretroviral medications in the Antiretroviral Pregnancy Registry (1-800-258-4263 or www.APRegistry.com). Healthcare providers caring for HIV-infected women and their infants may contact the National Perinatal HIV Hotline (888-448-8765) for clinical consultation (DHHS [perinatal], 2012).

Breast-Feeding Considerations Maternal or infant antiretroviral therapy does not completely eliminate the risk of postnatal HIV transmission. In addition, multiclass-resistant virus has been detected in breast-feeding infants despite maternal therapy. Therefore, in the United States, where formula is accessible, affordable, safe, and sustainable, and the risk of infant mortality due to diarrhea and respiratory infections is low, complete avoidance of breast-feeding by HIV-infected women is recommended to decrease potential transmission of HIV (DHHS [perinatal], 2012).

Medication Guide Available Yes

Contraindications Concurrent administration with allopurinol or ribavirin

Warnings/Precautions [U.S. Boxed Warning]: Pancreatitis (sometimes fatal) has been reported; incidence is dose related. Risk factors for developing pancreatitis may include a previous history of the condition, concurrent cytomegalovirus or *Mycobacterium avium-intracellulare* infection, renal impairment, advanced age, and concomitant use of stavudine, pentamidine, or hydroxyurea. Discontinue didanosine if clinical signs of pancreatitis occur. **[U.S. Boxed Warning]: Lactic acidosis, symptomatic hyperlactatemia, and severe hepatomegaly with steatosis (sometimes fatal) have occurred with antiretroviral nucleoside analogues, including didanosine.** Hepatotoxicity may occur even in the absence of marked transaminase elevations; suspend therapy in any patient developing clinical/laboratory findings which suggest hepatotoxicity. Hepatotoxicity and hepatic failure (including fatal cases) have been reported in HIV patients receiving combination drug therapy with didanosine and stavudine or hydroxyurea, or didanosine, stavudine, and hydroxyurea; avoid these combinations. Not currently recommended in combination with tenofovir due to failure and resistance. Noncirrhotic portal hypertension may develop within months to years of starting didanosine therapy. Signs may include elevated liver enzymes, esophageal varices, hematemesis, ascites, and splenomegaly. Noncirrhotic portal hypertension may lead to liver failure and/or death. Discontinue use in patients with evidence of this condition. Pregnant women may be at increased risk of lactic acidosis and liver damage. Use with caution in patients with hepatic impairment; safety and efficacy have not been established in patients with significant hepatic disease. Patients on combination antiretroviral therapy with hepatic impairment may be at increased risk of potentially severe and fatal hepatic toxicity; consider interruption or discontinuation of therapy if hepatic impairment worsens.

Peripheral neuropathy occurs in ~20% of patients receiving the drug. If symptomatic, discontinue therapy; after resolution of symptoms, reinitiation of therapy at a reduced dose may be tolerated. Permanently discontinue if neuropathy recurs. Retinal changes (including retinal depigmentation) and optic neuritis have been reported in adults and children using didanosine. Patients should undergo retinal examination every 6-12 months. Use caution in renal impairment; dose reduction recommended for Cl_{cr} <60 mL/minute. May cause redistribution of fat (eg, buffalo hump, peripheral wasting with increased abdominal girth, cushingoid appearance). Patients may develop immune reconstitution syndrome resulting in the occurrence of an inflammatory response to an indolent or residual opportunistic infection during initial HIV treatment or activation of autoimmune disorders (eg, Graves' disease, polymyositis, Guillain-Barré syndrome) later in therapy; further evaluation and treatment may be required. Didanosine delayed release capsules are indicated for once-daily use.

Adverse Reactions As reported in monotherapy studies; risk of toxicity may increase when combined with other agents.

>10%:
- Gastrointestinal: Diarrhea (19% to 28%), amylase increased (15% to 17%), abdominal pain (7% to 13%)
- Neuromuscular & skeletal: Peripheral neuropathy (17% to 20%)

1% to 10%:
- Dermatologic: Rash/pruritus (7% to 9%)
- Endocrine & metabolic: Uric acid increased (2% to 3%)
- Gastrointestinal: Pancreatitis (1% to 7% dose dependent); patients >65 years of age had a higher frequency of pancreatitis than younger patients patients (10% vs 5% in younger patients)
- Hepatic: AST increased (7% to 9%), ALT increased (6% to 9%), alkaline phosphatase increased (1% to 4%)

Postmarketing and/or case reports: Acute renal impairment, alopecia, anaphylactoid reaction, anemia, anorexia, arthralgia, chills/fever, diabetes mellitus, dry eyes, dyspepsia, flatulence, granulocytopenia, hepatic steatosis, hepatitis, hyper-/hypoglycemia, hyperlactatemia (symptomatic), hypersensitivity, immune reconstitution syndrome, lactic acidosis/hepatomegaly, leukopenia, lipodystrophy, liver failure, myalgia, myopathy, optic neuritis, pain, parotid gland enlargement, portal hypertension (noncirrhotic), retinal depigmentation, rhabdomyolysis, sialoadenitis, Stevens-Johnson syndrome, thrombocytopenia, weakness, xerostomia

Drug Interactions

Metabolism/Transport Effects None known.

Avoid Concomitant Use

Avoid concomitant use of Didanosine with any of the following: Alcohol (Ethyl); Allopurinol; Febuxostat; Hydroxyurea; Ribavirin; Tenofovir

Increased Effect/Toxicity

Didanosine may increase the levels/effects of: Hydroxyurea

The levels/effects of Didanosine may be increased by: Alcohol (Ethyl); Allopurinol; Febuxostat; Ganciclovir-Valganciclovir; Hydroxyurea; Ribavirin; Stavudine; Tenofovir

Decreased Effect

Didanosine may decrease the levels/effects of: Antifungal Agents (Azole Derivatives, Systemic); Atazanavir; Indinavir; Quinolone Antibiotics; Rilpivirine

The levels/effects of Didanosine may be decreased by: Atazanavir; Darunavir; Lopinavir; Methadone; Quinolone Antibiotics; Rilpivirine; Tenofovir; Tipranavir

Ethanol/Nutrition/Herb Interactions

Ethanol: Ethanol increases risk of pancreatitis. Management: Avoid ethanol.

Food: Food decreases AUC and C_{max}; serum levels may be decreased by 55%. Management: Administer on an empty stomach at least 30 minutes before or 2 hours after eating depending on dosage form.

Preparation for Administration Pediatric powder for oral solution: Prior to dispensing, add 100 mL or 200 mL purified water, USP to the 2 g or 4 g container, respectively, to achieve a 20 mg/mL solution. Immediately mix the resulting solution with an equal volume of Mylanta® Maximum Strength (or equivalent) to achieve a final concentration of 10 mg/mL.

Storage/Stability Delayed release capsules should be stored in tightly closed bottles at controlled room temperature of 25°C (77°F). Unreconstituted powder should be stored at 15°C to 30°C (59°F to 86°F); reconstituted pediatric solution is stable for 30 days if refrigerated.

Mechanism of Action Didanosine, a purine nucleoside (adenosine) analog and the deamination product of dideoxyadenosine (ddA), inhibits HIV replication *in vitro* in both T cells and monocytes. Didanosine is converted within the cell to the mono-, di-, and triphosphates of ddA. These ddA triphosphates act as substrate and inhibitor of HIV reverse transcriptase substrate and inhibitor of HIV reverse transcriptase thereby blocking viral DNA synthesis and suppressing HIV replication.

Pharmacodynamics/Kinetics

Absorption: Subject to degradation by acidic pH of stomach; some formulations are buffered to resist acidic pH; ≤55% reduction in peak plasma concentration is observed in presence of food. Delayed release capsules contain enteric-coated beadlets which dissolve in the small intestine.

Distribution: V_d: Children: 28 L/m²; Adults: 1.08 L/kg

Protein binding: <5%

Metabolism: Has not been evaluated in humans; studies conducted in dogs show extensive metabolism with allantoin, hypoxanthine, xanthine, and uric acid being the major metabolites found in urine

Bioavailability: Children: 25%; Adults: 42%

Half-life elimination:
- Children and Adolescents: 0.8 hour
- Adults: Normal renal function: 1.5 hours; active metabolite, ddATP, has an intracellular half-life >12 hours *in vitro*; Renal impairment: 2.5-5 hours

Time to peak: Delayed release capsules: 2 hours; Powder for suspension: 0.25-1.5 hours

Excretion: Urine (~55% as unchanged drug)
- Clearance: Total body: Averages 800 mL/minute

Dosage Oral: Treatment of HIV infection:

Pediatric powder for oral solution (Videx®): **Note:** Once-daily dosing of the oral solution is not FDA approved in children.
- Infants: 2 weeks to 8 months: 100 mg/m² twice daily is recommended by the manufacturer; 50 mg/m² may be considered in infants 2 weeks to <3 months (DHHS [pediatric], 2011)
- Infants and Children >8 months: 120 mg/m² twice daily, not to exceed adult dose, is recommended by the manufacturer. **Note:** DHHS guidelines suggest a range of 90-150 mg/m² twice daily
- Children 3-21 years (unlabeled dose): Treatment-naive: 240 mg/m²/dose once daily (maximum: 400 mg/dose) (DHHS [pediatric], 2011)
- Adolescents and Adults: Dosing based on patient weight:
  - <60 kg: 125 mg twice daily (preferred) or 250 mg once daily
  - ≥60 kg: 200 mg twice daily (preferred) or 400 mg once daily

Delayed release capsule (Videx® EC):
- Children ≥6 years and Adults:
  - 20 kg to <25 kg: 200 mg once daily
  - 25 kg to <60 kg: 250 mg once daily
  - ≥60 kg: 400 mg once daily
- Children 3-21 years (unlabeled dose): Treatment-naive: 240 mg/m²/dose once daily (maximum: 400 mg/dose) (DHHS [pediatric], 2011)

Elderly: Higher frequency of pancreatitis (10% versus 5% in younger patients); monitor renal function and dose accordingly

When taken with tenofovir: Adults:
- <60 kg and Cl_{cr} ≥60 mL/minute: 200 mg once daily
- ≥60 kg and Cl_{cr} ≥60 mL/minute: 250 mg once daily
- **Note:** Combined use of tenofovir with didanosine is no longer recommended (DHHS, 2013).

Dosage adjustment in renal impairment:
Children: No specific guidelines available; consider dosage reduction using adjustments for adults.
Adults: Dosing based on patient weight, creatinine clearance, and dosage form: See table.

Recommended Dose (mg) of Didanosine by Body Weight – Adults

Creatinine Clearance (mL/min)	≥60 kg		<60 kg	
	Powder for Oral Solution	Delayed Release Capsule	Powder for Oral Solution	Delayed Release Capsule
≥60	400 mg daily or 200 mg twice daily	400 mg daily	250 mg daily or 125 mg twice daily	250 mg daily
30-59	200 mg daily or 100 mg twice daily	200 mg daily	150 mg daily or 75 mg twice daily	125 mg daily
10-29	150 mg daily	125 mg daily	100 mg daily	125 mg daily
<10	100 mg daily	125 mg daily	75 mg daily	See **Note**

Note: Per manufacturer, not suitable for use in patients <60 kg with Cl_{cr} <10 mL/minute; use alternate formulation.

Patients requiring hemodialysis or CAPD: Dose per Cl_{cr} <10 mL/minute. Didanosine is not removed via CAPD and minimal amount of dose (≤7%) is removed by hemodialysis; no supplemental dosing necessary.

Dosing adjustment in hepatic impairment: No dosage adjustment needed

Dietary Considerations Take on an empty stomach; administer at least 30 minutes before or 2 hours after eating

Administration Pediatric powder for oral solution: Administer on an empty stomach at least 30 minutes before or 2 hours after eating. Shake well prior to use.
Videx® EC: Administer on an empty stomach at least 1 hour before or 2 hours after eating; swallow capsule whole.

Monitoring Parameters Serum potassium, uric acid, creatinine; hemoglobin, CBC with neutrophil and platelet count, CD4 cells; viral load; liver function tests, serum bilirubin, albumin, INR, amylase; weight gain; perform dilated retinal exam every 6 months, ultrasonography (if portal hypertension suspected)

Additional Information A high rate of early virologic nonresponse was observed when the combination of didanosine, lamivudine, and tenofovir or the triple NRTI combination of didanosine, tenofovir and emtricitabine were used as the initial regimen in treatment-naive patients. Use of either of these combinations is not recommended; patients currently on these regimens should be closely monitored for modification of therapy. Early virologic failure and increased toxicity was also observed with tenofovir and didanosine delayed release capsules, plus either efavirenz or nevirapine; use is not recommended.

Dosage Forms Excipient information presented when available (limited, particularly for generics); consult specific product labeling.
Capsule Delayed Release, Oral:
Videx EC: 125 mg, 200 mg, 250 mg, 400 mg
Generic: 125 mg, 200 mg, 250 mg, 400 mg
Solution Reconstituted, Oral:
Videx: 2 g (100 mL); 4 g (200 mL)

- **Dideoxyinosine** *see* Didanosine *on page 602*
- **Didronel [DSC]** *see* Etidronate *on page 798*
- **Dienogest and Estradiol** *see* Estradiol and Dienogest *on page 762*
- **Dietary Fiber Laxative [OTC]** *see* Psyllium *on page 1748*

Diethylpropion (dye eth il PROE pee on)

Index Terms Amfepramone; Diethylpropion Hydrochloride; Tenuate; Tenuate Dospan

Pharmacologic Category Anorexiant; Central Nervous System Stimulant; Sympathomimetic

Use Short-term (few weeks) adjunct in the management of exogenous obesity

Pharmacotherapy for weight loss is recommended only for obese patients with a body mass index ≥30 kg/m^2, or ≥27 kg/m^2 in the presence of other risk factors such as hypertension, diabetes, and/or dyslipidemia or a high waist circumference; therapy should be used in conjunction with a comprehensive weight management program.

Pregnancy Risk Factor B

Dosage Children >16 years and Adults: Oral:
Immediate release: 25 mg 3 times daily
Controlled release: 75 mg once daily at midmorning
Dosage adjustment in renal impairment: No dosage adjustment provided in manufacturer's labeling; use with caution.
Dosage adjustment in hepatic impairment: No dosage adjustment provided in manufacturer's labeling.

Additional Information Complete prescribing information should be consulted for additional detail.

Dosage Forms Excipient information presented when available (limited, particularly for generics); consult specific product labeling.
Tablet, Oral, as hydrochloride:
Generic: 25 mg
Tablet Extended Release 24 Hour, Oral, as hydrochloride:
Generic: 75 mg

Controlled Substance C-IV

- **Diethylpropion Hydrochloride** *see* Diethylpropion *on page 604*
- **Differin** *see* Adapalene *on page 48*
- **Differin® (Can)** *see* Adapalene *on page 48*
- **Differin® XP (Can)** *see* Adapalene *on page 48*
- **Dificid** *see* Fidaxomicin *on page 859*
- **Dificid™ (Can)** *see* Fidaxomicin *on page 859*
- **Difimicin** *see* Fidaxomicin *on page 859*

Diflorasone (dye FLOR a sone)

Brand Names: U.S. ApexiCon; ApexiCon E

Index Terms Diflorasone Diacetate

Pharmacologic Category Corticosteroid, Topical

Additional Appendix Information
Topical Corticosteroids *on page 2299*

Use Relieves inflammation and pruritic symptoms of corticosteroid-responsive dermatosis (high to very high potency topical corticosteroid)

Pregnancy Risk Factor C

Dosage Topical: Apply ointment sparingly 1-3 times/day; apply cream sparingly 2-4 times/day. Therapy should be discontinued when control is achieved; if no improvement is seen, reassessment of diagnosis may be necessary.

Additional Information Complete prescribing information should be consulted for additional detail.

Dosage Forms Excipient information presented when available (limited, particularly for generics); consult specific product labeling. [DSC] = Discontinued product
Cream, External, as diacetate:
ApexiCon E: 0.05% (30 g [DSC], 60 g)
ApexiCon E: 0.05% (30 g, 60 g) [contains cetyl alcohol, propylene glycol]
Generic: 0.05% (15 g, 30 g, 60 g)

Ointment, External, as diacetate:
ApexiCon: 0.05% (30 g, 60 g)
Generic: 0.05% (15 g, 30 g, 60 g)

◆ **Diflorasone Diacetate** *see* Diflorasone *on page* 604
◆ **Diflucan** *see* Fluconazole *on page* 868
◆ **Diflucan® (Can)** *see* Fluconazole *on page* 868

Diflunisal (dye FLOO ni sal)

Brand Names: Canada Apo-Diflunisal®; Novo-Diflunisal; Nu-Diflunisal

Index Terms Dolobid

Pharmacologic Category Nonsteroidal Anti-inflammatory Drug (NSAID), Oral

Additional Appendix Information

Beers Criteria – Potentially Inappropriate Medications for Geriatrics *on page* 2368

Use

Mild to moderate pain: For acute or long-term use for symptomatic treatment of mild to moderate pain

Osteoarthritis/Rheumatoid arthritis (RA): For acute or long-term use for symptomatic relief of osteoarthritis and RA

Pregnancy Risk Factor C

Medication Guide Available Yes

Dosage

Mild to moderate pain:

Adults: Oral: Initial: 1 g, followed by 500 mg every 12 hours; maintenance doses of 500 mg every 8 hours may be necessary in some patients; maximum daily dose: 1.5 g

Dosage adjustments: A lower dosage may be appropriate depending on pain severity, patient response, and weight: Initial: 500 mg, followed by 250 mg every 8-12 hours; maximum daily dose: 1.5 g

Elderly: Mild-to-moderate pain: Oral: Initial: 500 mg, followed by 250 mg every 8-12 hours; maximum daily dose: 1.5 g

Arthritis: Adults and Elderly: Oral: 500 mg to 1 g daily in 2 divided doses; maximum daily dose: 1.5 g

Dosage adjustment in renal impairment: No dosage adjustment provided in the manufacturer's labeling; however the following adjustments have been used by some clinicians (Aronoff, 2007):

Cl_{cr} <50 mL/minute: Administer 50% of normal dose
Hemodialysis: No supplement required
CAPD: No supplement required

Dosage adjustment in hepatic impairment: No dosage adjustment provided in manufacturer's labeling; use with caution.

Additional Information Complete prescribing information should be consulted for additional detail.

Dosage Forms Excipient information presented when available (limited, particularly for generics); consult specific product labeling.

Tablet, Oral:
Generic: 500 mg

◆ **Difluorodeoxycytidine Hydrochlorothiazide** *see* Gemcitabine *on page* 943

Difluprednate (dye floo PRED nate)

Brand Names: U.S. Durezol

Pharmacologic Category Corticosteroid, Ophthalmic

Use Treatment of inflammation and pain following ocular surgery; treatment of endogenous anterior uveitis

Pregnancy Risk Factor C

Dosage Ophthalmic: Children, Adolescents, and Adults:

Endogenous anterior uveitis: Instill 1 drop into conjunctival sac of the affected eye(s) 4 times daily for 14 days, then taper as clinically indicated

Inflammation associated with ocular surgery: Instill 1 drop in conjunctival sac of the affected eye(s) 4 times daily beginning 24 hours after surgery, continue for 2 weeks, then decrease to 2 times daily for 1 week, then taper based on response

Additional Information Complete prescribing information should be consulted for additional detail.

Dosage Forms Excipient information presented when available (limited, particularly for generics); consult specific product labeling.

Emulsion, Ophthalmic:
Durezol: 0.05% (5 mL) [contains edetate sodium (tetrasodium), polysorbate 80]

◆ **Digibind** *see* Digoxin Immune Fab *on page* 609
◆ **DigiFab** *see* Digoxin Immune Fab *on page* 609
◆ **DigiFab® (Can)** *see* Digoxin Immune Fab *on page* 609
◆ **Digitalis** *see* Digoxin *on page* 605
◆ **Digox** *see* Digoxin *on page* 605

Digoxin (di JOKS in)

Brand Names: U.S. Digox; Lanoxin; Lanoxin Pediatric

Brand Names: Canada Apo-Digoxin; Digoxin Injection CSD; Lanoxin; Pediatric Digoxin CSD; PMS-Digoxin; Toloxin

Index Terms Digitalis

Pharmacologic Category Antiarrhythmic Agent, Miscellaneous; Cardiac Glycoside

Additional Appendix Information

Beers Criteria – Potentially Inappropriate Medications for Geriatrics *on page* 2368

Use

Atrial fibrillation: For the control of ventricular response rate in adults with chronic atrial fibrillation.

Heart failure: For the treatment of mild-to-moderate (or stage C as recommended by the ACCF/AHA) heart failure (HF) in adults; to increase myocardial contractility in pediatric patients with heart failure

Note: In treatment of atrial fibrillation (AF), use is not considered first-line unless AF coexistent with heart failure or in sedentary patients (Anderson, 2013). In the treatment of heart failure, digoxin should be considered for use only in HF with reduced ejection fraction (HFrEF) when symptoms remain despite guideline-directed medical therapy or as initial therapy in patients with severe symptoms yet to respond to guideline-directed medical therapy (Yancy, 2013).

Unlabeled Use Fetal tachycardia with or without hydrops; to slow ventricular rate in supraventricular tachyarrhythmias such as supraventricular tachycardia (SVT) excluding atrioventricular reciprocating tachycardia (AVRT)

Pregnancy Risk Factor C

Pregnancy Considerations Animal reproduction studies have not been conducted. Digoxin crosses the placenta and serum concentrations are similar in the mother and fetus at delivery. Digoxin is recommended as first-line in the treatment of fetal tachycardia determined to be SVT. In pregnant women with atrial fibrillation or SVT, use of digoxin is recommended (Anderson, 2013; Blomström-Lundqvist, 2003).

Breast-Feeding Considerations Digoxin is excreted into breast milk and similar concentrations are found within mother's serum and milk. The manufacturer recommends that caution be used when administered to nursing women.

Contraindications Hypersensitivity to digoxin (rare) or other forms of digitalis, or any component of the formulation; ventricular fibrillation

Warnings/Precautions Watch for proarrhythmic effects (especially with digoxin toxicity). Withdrawal in clinically stable patients with HF may lead to recurrence of HF symptoms. During an episode of atrial fibrillation or flutter in patients with an accessory bypass tract (eg, Wolff-Parkinson-White syndrome), use has been associated with increased anterograde conduction down the accessory pathway leading to ventricular fibrillation; avoid use in such patients (Anderson, 2013; Neumar, 2010). Because digoxin slows sinoatrial and AV conduction, the drug commonly prolongs the PR interval. Digoxin may cause severe sinus bradycardia or sinoatrial block in patients with pre-existing sinus node disease. Avoid use in patients with second- or third-degree heart block (except in patients with a functioning artificial pacemaker) (Yancy, 2013); incomplete AV block (eg, Stokes-Adams attack) may progress to complete block with digoxin administration. HF patients with preserved left ventricular function including patients with restrictive cardiomyopathy, constrictive pericarditis, acute cor pulmonale, and amyloid heart disease may be susceptible to digoxin toxicity; avoid use unless used to control ventricular response with atrial fibrillation. Avoid use in patients with hypertrophic cardiomyopathy (HCM) and outflow tract obstruction unless used to control ventricular response with atrial fibrillation; outflow obstruction may worsen due to the positive inotropic effects of digoxin. Digoxin is potentially harmful in the treatment of dyspnea in patients with HCM in the absence of atrial fibrillation (Gersh, 2011). In a murine model of viral myocarditis, digoxin in high doses was shown to be detrimental (Matsumori, 1999). If used in humans, therefore, digoxin should be used with caution and only at low doses (Frishman, 2007). The manufacturer recommends avoiding the use of digoxin in patients with myocarditis.

Use with caution in patients with hyperthyroidism (increased digoxin clearance) and hypothyroidism (reduced digoxin clearance). Atrial arrhythmias associated with hypermetabolic (eg, hyperthyroidism) or hyperdynamic (hypoxia, arteriovenous shunt) states are very difficult to treat; treat underlying condition first. Use with caution in patients with an acute MI; may increase myocardial oxygen demand. During the immediate post-MI period, digoxin administered I.V. may be used to slow a rapid ventricular response and improve left ventricular (LV) function in the acute treatment of atrial fibrillation associated with severe LV function and heart failure (Anderson, 2013). Reduce dose with renal impairment and when amiodarone, propafenone, quinidine, or verapamil are added to a patient on digoxin; use with caution in patients taking strong inducers or inhibitors of P-glycoprotein (eg, cyclosporine). Avoid rapid I.V. administration of calcium in digitalized patients; may produce serious arrhythmias.

Atrial arrhythmias associated with hypermetabolic states are very difficult to treat; treat underlying condition first; if digoxin is used, ensure digoxin toxicity does not occur. Patients with beri beri heart disease may fail to adequately respond to digoxin therapy; treat underlying thiamine deficiency concomitantly. Correct electrolyte disturbances, especially hypokalemia or hypomagnesemia, prior to use and throughout therapy; toxicity may occur despite therapeutic digoxin concentrations. Hypercalcemia may increase the risk of digoxin toxicity; maintain normocalcemia. It is not necessary to routinely reduce or hold digoxin therapy prior to elective electrical cardioversion for atrial fibrillation; however, exclusion of digoxin toxicity (eg, clinical and ECG signs) is necessary prior to cardioversion. If signs of digoxin excess exist, withhold digoxin and delay cardioversion until toxicity subsides (Anderson, 2013). I.V. administration: Vesicant; ensure proper needle or catheter placement prior to and during administration; avoid extravasation. Use with caution in the elderly; decreases in renal clearance may result in toxic effects; in general, avoid doses >0.125 mg/day; in heart failure, higher doses may increase the risk of potential toxicity and have not been shown to provide additional benefit (Beers Criteria).

Adverse Reactions Incidence not always reported.

Cardiovascular: Accelerated junctional rhythm, asystole, atrial tachycardia with or without block, AV dissociation, first-, second- (Wenckebach), or third-degree heart block, facial edema, PR prolongation, PVCs (especially bigeminy or trigeminy), ST segment depression, ventricular tachycardia or ventricular fibrillation

Central nervous system: Dizziness (6%), mental disturbances (5%), headache (4%), apathy, anxiety, confusion, delirium, depression, fever, hallucinations

Dermatologic: Rash (erythematous, maculopapular [most common], papular, scarlatiniform, vesicular or bullous), pruritus, urticaria, angioneurotic edema

Gastrointestinal: Nausea (4%), vomiting (2%), diarrhea (4%), abdominal pain, anorexia

Neuromuscular & skeletal: Weakness

Ocular: Visual disturbances (blurred or yellow vision)

Respiratory: Laryngeal edema

<1% (Limited to important or life-threatening): Asymmetric chorea, gynecomastia, thrombocytopenia, palpitation, intestinal ischemia, hemorrhagic necrosis of the intestines, vaginal cornification, eosinophilia, sexual dysfunction, diaphoresis

Drug Interactions

Metabolism/Transport Effects **Substrate** of CYP3A4 (minor), P-glycoprotein; **Note:** Assignment of Major/Minor substrate status based on clinically relevant drug interaction potential

Avoid Concomitant Use There are no known interactions where it is recommended to avoid concomitant use.

Increased Effect/Toxicity

Digoxin may increase the levels/effects of: Adenosine; Carvedilol; Colchicine; Dronedarone; Midodrine

The levels/effects of Digoxin may be increased by: Aminoquinolines (Antimalarial); Amiodarone; Antithyroid Agents; AtorvaSTATin; Beta-Blockers; Boceprevir; Brimonidine (Topical); Calcium Channel Blockers (Nondihydropyridine); Calcium Polystyrene Sulfonate; Carvedilol; CloNIDine; Conivaptan; CycloSPORINE (Systemic); Dronedarone; Etravirine; Ezogabine; Flecainide; Glycopyrrolate; Itraconazole; Lenalidomide; Loop Diuretics; Macrolide Antibiotics; Mifepristone; Milnacipran; Mirabegron; Multivitamins/Fluoride (with ADE); Multivitamins/Minerals (with ADEK, Folate, Iron); Multivitamins/Minerals (with AE, No Iron); Nefazodone; Neuromuscular-Blocking Agents; NIFEdipine; Nonsteroidal Anti-Inflammatory Agents; Paricalcitol; P-glycoprotein/ABCB1 Inhibitors; Posaconazole; Potassium-Sparing Diuretics; Propafenone; Protease Inhibitors; QuiNIDine; QuiNINE; Ranolazine; Regorafenib; Reserpine; Simeprevir; SitaGLIPtin; Sodium Polystyrene Sulfonate; Spironolactone; Telaprevir; Telmisartan; Ticagrelor; Tolvaptan; Trimethoprim; Vitamin D Analogs

Decreased Effect

Digoxin may decrease the levels/effects of: Antineoplastic Agents (Anthracycline, Systemic)

The levels/effects of Digoxin may be decreased by: 5-ASA Derivatives; Acarbose; Aminoglycosides; Antineoplastic Agents; Antineoplastic Agents (Anthracycline, Systemic); Bile Acid Sequestrants; Kaolin; PenicillAMINE; P-glycoprotein/ABCB1 Inducers; Potassium-Sparing Diuretics; St Johns Wort; Sucralfate

Ethanol/Nutrition/Herb Interactions

Food: Digoxin peak serum concentrations may be decreased if taken with food. Meals containing increased fiber (bran) or foods high in pectin may decrease oral absorption of digoxin.

Herb/Nutraceutical: Avoid ephedra (risk of cardiac stimulation). Avoid natural licorice (causes sodium and water retention and increases potassium loss).

Preparation for Administration

I.M.: No dilution required.

I.V.: May be administered undiluted or diluted fourfold in D_5W, NS, or SWFI for direct injection. Less than fourfold dilution may lead to drug precipitation.

Storage/Stability Store at 25°C (77°F); excursions permitted to 15°C to 30°C (59°F to 86°F). Protect elixir, injection, and tablets from light.

Mechanism of Action

Heart failure: Inhibition of the sodium/potassium ATPase pump in myocardial cells results in a transient increase of intracellular sodium, which in turn promotes calcium influx via the sodium-calcium exchange pump leading to increased contractility.

Supraventricular arrhythmias: Direct suppression of the AV node conduction to increase effective refractory period and decrease conduction velocity positive inotropic effect, enhanced vagal tone, and decreased ventricular rate to fast atrial arrhythmias. Atrial fibrillation may decrease sensitivity and increase tolerance to higher serum digoxin concentrations.

Pharmacodynamics/Kinetics

Onset of action: Heart rate control: Oral: 1-2 hours; I.V.: 5-60 minutes

Peak effect: Heart rate control: Oral: 2-8 hours; I.V.: 1-6 hours; **Note:** In patients with atrial fibrillation, median time to ventricular rate control in one study was 6 hours (range: 3-15 hours) (Siu, 2009)

Duration: Adults: 3-4 days

Absorption: By passive nonsaturable diffusion in the upper small intestine; food may delay, but does not affect extent of absorption

Distribution:

Normal renal function: 6-7 L/kg

V_d: Extensive to peripheral tissues, with a distinct distribution phase which lasts 6-8 hours; concentrates in heart, liver, kidney, skeletal muscle, and intestines. Heart/serum concentration is 70:1. Pharmacologic effects are delayed and do not correlate well with serum concentrations during distribution phase.

Hyperthyroidism: Increased V_d

Hyperkalemia, hyponatremia: Decreased digoxin distribution to heart and muscle

Hypokalemia: Increased digoxin distribution to heart and muscles

Concomitant quinidine therapy: Decreased V_d

Chronic renal failure: 4-6 L/kg

Decreased sodium/potassium ATPase activity - decreased tissue binding

Neonates, full-term: 7.5-10 L/kg

Children: 16 L/kg

Adults: 7 L/kg, decreased with renal disease

Protein binding: ~25%; in uremic patients, digoxin is displaced from plasma protein binding sites

Metabolism: Via sequential sugar hydrolysis in the stomach or by reduction of lactone ring by intestinal bacteria (in ~10% of population, gut bacteria may metabolize up to 40% of digoxin dose); once absorbed, only ~16% is metabolized to 3-beta-digoxigenin, 3-keto-digoxigenin, and glucuronide and sulfate conjugates; metabolites may contribute to therapeutic and toxic effects of digoxin; metabolism is reduced with decompensated HF

Bioavailability: Oral (formulation dependent): Elixir: 70% to 85%; Tablet: 60% to 80%

Half-life elimination (age, renal and cardiac function dependent):

Neonates: Premature: 61-170 hours; Full-term: 35-45 hours

Infants: 18-25 hours

Children: 18-36 hours

Adults: 36-48 hours

Adults, anephric: 3.5-5 days

Half-life elimination: Parent drug: 38 hours; Metabolites: Digoxigenin: 4 hours; Monodigitoxoside: 3-12 hours

Time to peak, serum: Oral: 1-3 hours

Excretion: Urine (50% to 70% as unchanged drug)

Dosage

Children: When changing from oral (tablets or liquid) or I.M. to I.V. therapy, dosage should be reduced by 20% to 25%. Refer to the following: See table.

Dosage Recommendations for Digoxin[1]

Age	Total Digitalizing Dose[2,3] (mcg/kg)		Daily Maintenance Dose[3,4] (mcg/kg)	
	Oral	I.V. or I.M.[5]	Oral	I.V. or I.M.[5]
Preterm infant	20-30	15-25	5-7.5	4-6
Full-term infant	25-35	20-30	6-10	5-8
1 mo - 2 y	35-60	30-50	10-15	7.5-12
2-5 y	30-40	25-35	7.5-10	6-9
5-10 y	20-35	15-30	5-10	4-8
>10 y	10-15	8-12	2.5-5	2-3

[1]**Heart failure:** A lower serum digoxin concentration may be adequate to treat heart failure (compared to cardiac arrhythmias); consider doses at the lower end of the recommended range for treatment of heart failure; a digitalizing dose (loading dose) may not be necessary when treating heart failure (Ross, 2001).

[2]**Do not give full total digitalizing dose (TDD) at once.** Give one-half of the total digitalizing dose (TDD) in the initial dose, then give one-quarter of the TDD in each of two subsequent doses at 6- to 8-hour intervals. Obtain ECG 6 hours after each dose to assess potential toxicity.

[3]Based on lean body weight and normal renal function for age. Decrease dose in patients with decreased renal function; digitalizing dose often not recommended in infants and children.

[4]Divided every 12 hours in infants and children <10 years of age. Given once daily to children >10 years of age and adults.

[5]I.M. not preferred due to severe injection site pain. If I.M. route is necessary, administer as deep injection followed by massage of injection site.

Adults:

Heart failure: Daily maintenance dose (**Note:** Loading dose not recommended): Oral: 0.125-0.25 mg once daily; higher daily doses (eg, 0.375-0.5 mg/day) are rarely necessary. If patient is >70 years of age, has impaired renal function, or has a low lean body mass, low doses (eg, 0.125 mg daily or every other day) should be used initially (Yancy, 2013). **Note:** I.V. digoxin may be used to control ventricular response in patients with atrial fibrillation and heart failure who do not have an accessory pathway (Anderson, 2013). The addition of a beta-blocker to digoxin is usually more effective in controlling ventricular response, particularly during exercise (Yancy, 2013).

Supraventricular tachyarrhythmias (rate control):

Initial: Total digitalizing dose:

Oral: 0.75-1.5 mg

I.V., I.M.: 0.5-1 mg (**Note:** I.M. not preferred due to severe injection site pain.)

Give 1/2 (one-half) of the total digitalizing dose (TDD) as the initial dose, then give 1/4 (one-quarter) of the TDD in each of 2 subsequent doses at 6- to 8-hour intervals. Obtain ECG 6 hours after each dose to assess potential toxicity.

Daily maintenance dose:

Oral: 0.125-0.5 mg once daily

I.V., I.M.: 0.1-0.4 mg once daily (**Note:** I.M. not preferred due to severe injection site pain.)

Elderly: Dose is based on assessment of lean body mass and renal function. Elderly patients with low lean body mass may experience higher digoxin concentrations due to reduced volume of distribution (Cheng, 2010). Decrease dose in patients with decreased renal function.

Heart failure: If patient is >70 years, low doses (eg, 0.125 mg daily or every other day) should be used (Yancy, 2013).

Dosage adjustment in renal impairment: Adults: No dosage adjustment provided in manufacturer's labeling; however, the following adjustments have been recommended:

Loading dose:

ESRD: If loading dose necessary, reduce dose by 50% (Aronoff, 2007)

Acute renal failure: Based on expert opinion, if patient in acute renal failure requires ventricular rate control (eg, in atrial fibrillation), consider alternative therapy. If loading digoxin becomes necessary, patient volume of distribution may be increased and reduction in loading dose may not be necessary; however, maintenance dosing will require adjustment as long as renal failure persists.

Maintenance dose (Aronoff, 2007):

Cl_{cr} >50 mL/minute: No dosage adjustment necessary.

Cl_{cr} 10-50 mL/minute: Administer 25% to 75% of the normal daily dose or administer normal dose every 36 hours

Cl_{cr} <10 mL/minute: Administer 10% to 25% of the normal daily dose or administer normal dose every 48 hours

Continuous renal replacement therapy (CRRT): Administer 25% to 75% of the normal daily dose or administer normal dose every 36 hours; monitor serum concentrations.

Hemodialysis: Not dialyzable; no supplemental dose necessary.

Heart failure: Initial maintenance dose (Bauman, 2006; Koup, 1975; Jusko, 1974): **Note:** The following suggested dosing recommendations are intended to achieve a target digoxin concentration of 0.7 ng/mL. Renal function estimated using Cockcroft-Gault formula.

Cl_{cr} >120 mL/minute: 0.25 mg once daily

Cl_{cr} 80-120 mL/minute: 0.25 mg once daily, alternating with 0.125 mg once daily

Cl_{cr} 30-80 mL/minute: 0.125 mg once daily

Cl_{cr} <30 mL/minute: 0.125 mg every 48 hours

Note: A contemporary digoxin dosing nomogram using creatinine clearance and ideal body weight or height has been published for determining the initial maintenance dose in patients with heart failure to achieve a target digoxin concentration of 0.7 ng/mL (Bauman, 2006).

Dosage adjustment in hepatic impairment: No dosage adjustment provided in manufacturer's labeling.

Dietary Considerations Maintain adequate amounts of potassium in diet to decrease risk of hypokalemia (hypokalemia may increase risk of digoxin toxicity).

Administration

I.M.: I.V. route preferred. If I.M. injection necessary, administer by deep injection followed by massage at the injection site. Inject no more than 2 mL per injection site. May cause intense pain.

I.V.: May be administered undiluted or diluted. Inject slowly over ≥5 minutes.

Vesicant; ensure proper needle or catheter placement prior to and during administration; avoid extravasation.

Extravasation management: If extravasation occurs, stop I.V. administration immediately and disconnect (leave cannula/needle in place); gently aspirate extravasated solution (do **NOT** flush the line); remove needle/cannula; elevate extremity.

Monitoring Parameters

Heart rate and rhythm should be monitored along with periodic ECGs to assess desired effects and signs of toxicity; baseline and periodic serum creatinine. Periodically monitor serum potassium, magnesium, and calcium especially if on medications where these electrolyte disturbances can occur (eg, diuretics), or if patient has a history of hypokalemia or hypomagnesemia. Observe patients for noncardiac signs of toxicity, confusion, and depression.

When to draw serum digoxin concentrations: Digoxin serum concentrations are monitored because digoxin possesses a narrow therapeutic serum range; the therapeutic endpoint is difficult to quantify and digoxin toxicity may be life-threatening. Digoxin serum concentrations should be drawn **at least 6-8 hours after last dose, regardless of route of administration (optimally 12-24 hours after a dose). Note:** Serum digoxin concentrations may decrease in response to exercise due to increased skeletal muscle uptake; a period of rest (eg, ~2 hours) after exercise may be necessary prior to drawing serum digoxin concentrations.

Initiation of therapy:

If a loading dose is given: Digoxin serum concentration may be drawn within 12-24 hours after the initial loading dose administration. Concentrations drawn this early may confirm the relationship of digoxin plasma concentrations and response but are of little value in determining maintenance doses.

If a loading dose is not given: Digoxin serum concentration should be obtained after 3-5 days of therapy.

Maintenance therapy:

Trough concentrations should be followed just prior to the next dose or at a minimum of 6-8 hours after last dose.

Digoxin serum concentrations should be obtained within 5-7 days (approximate time to steady-state) after any dosage changes. Continue to obtain digoxin serum concentrations 7-14 days after any change in maintenance dose. **Note:** In patients with end-stage renal disease, it may take 15-20 days to reach steady-state.

Patients who are receiving electrolyte-depleting medications such as diuretics, serum potassium, magnesium, and calcium should be monitored closely.

Digoxin serum concentrations should be obtained whenever any of the following conditions occur:

Questionable patient compliance or to evaluate clinical deterioration following an initial good response

Changing renal function

Suspected digoxin toxicity

Initiation or discontinuation of therapy with drugs (eg, amiodarone, quinidine, verapamil) which potentially interact with digoxin.

Any disease changes (eg, thyroid disease)

Reference Range

Digoxin therapeutic serum concentrations:

Heart failure: 0.5-0.9 ng/mL (Yancy, 2013)

Adults: <0.5 ng/mL; probably indicates underdigitalization unless there are special circumstances

Toxic: >2 ng/mL

Digoxin-like immunoreactive substance (DLIS) may cross-react with digoxin immunoassay. DLIS has been found in patients with renal and liver disease, heart failure, neonates, and pregnant women (3rd trimester).

Test Interactions Spironolactone may interfere with digoxin radioimmunoassay.

Dosage Forms Excipient information presented when available (limited, particularly for generics); consult specific product labeling.

Solution, Injection:

Lanoxin: 0.25 mg/mL (2 mL) [contains alcohol, usp, propylene glycol]

Lanoxin Pediatric: 0.1 mg/mL (1 mL) [contains alcohol, usp, propylene glycol]

Generic: 0.25 mg/mL (1 mL, 2 mL)

Solution, Oral:

Generic: 0.05 mg/mL (60 mL)

Tablet, Oral:

Digox: 0.125 mg [scored; contains fd&c yellow #10 aluminum lake]

Digox: 0.25 mg [scored]

Lanoxin: 0.125 mg [scored; contains fd&c yellow #10 (quinoline yellow), fd&c yellow #6 (sunset yellow)]

Lanoxin: 0.25 mg [scored]

Generic: 0.125 mg, 0.25 mg

Dosage Forms: Canada Excipient information presented when available (limited, particularly for generics); consult specific product labeling.

Tablet, oral:

Apo-Digoxin®: 62.5 mcg, 125 mcg, 250 mcg

Digoxin Immune Fab (di JOKS in i MYUN fab)

Brand Names: U.S. DigiFab

Brand Names: Canada DigiFab®

Index Terms Antidigoxin Fab Fragments, Ovine; Digibind

Pharmacologic Category Antidote

Use Treatment of life-threatening or potentially life-threatening digoxin intoxication, including:

- acute digoxin ingestion (ie, >10 mg in adults; >0.1 mg/kg or >4 mg in children; ingestions resulting in serum concentrations >10 ng/mL)
- chronic ingestions leading to steady-state digoxin concentrations >6 ng/mL in adults or >4 ng/mL in children
- manifestations of digoxin toxicity due to overdose (eg, life-threatening ventricular arrhythmias, progressive bradycardia, second- or third-degree heart block not responsive to atropine, serum potassium >5.5 mEq/L in adults or >6 mEq/L in children)

Pregnancy Risk Factor C

Pregnancy Considerations Animal reproduction studies have not been conducted. Safety and efficacy in pregnant women have not been established. Use during pregnancy only if clearly needed. In general, medications used as antidotes should take into consideration the health and prognosis of the mother; antidotes should be administered to pregnant women if there is a clear indication for use and should not be withheld because of fears of teratogenicity (Bailey, 2003).

Breast-Feeding Considerations It is not known if digoxin immune fab is excreted into breast milk. The manufacturer recommends caution be used if administered to a nursing woman. Also consider the presence of digoxin in breast milk.

Contraindications There are no contraindications listed in the manufacturer's labeling.

Warnings/Precautions Digoxin immune Fab is derived from ovine (sheep) Fab immunoglobulin fragments; hypersensitivity reactions (eg, anaphylactic or anaphylactoid reactions, delayed allergic reactions) are possible. Patients with allergies to sheep proteins and patients with prior exposure to ovine antibodies or ovine Fab may be at a higher risk for hypersensitivity reactions. In patients who develop an anaphylactic reaction, discontinue the infusion and administer emergency care. Immediate treatment (eg, epinephrine 1:1000, corticosteroids, diphenhydramine) should be available. Processed with papain and may cause hypersensitivity reactions in patients allergic to papaya, other papaya extracts, papain, chymopapain, or the pineapple-enzyme bromelain. There may also be cross allergenicity with dust mite and latex allergens.

Total serum digoxin concentrations will rise precipitously following administration of digoxin immune Fab due to the presence of the Fab-digoxin complex; because digoxin bound to Fab fragments cannot result in toxicity, this rise has no clinical meaning. Therefore, avoid monitoring total serum digoxin concentrations until the Fab fragments have been eliminated completely. Patients experiencing acute digitalis toxicity may present with significant hyperkalemia due to shifting of potassium into the extracellular space. Upon treatment with digoxin immune Fab, potassium shifts back into the intracellular space and may result in hypokalemia. Monitor potassium closely, especially during the first few hours after administration; treat hypokalemia cautiously when clinically indicated.

In patients chronically maintained on digoxin for HF, administration of digoxin immune Fab may result in exacerbation of HF symptoms due to a reduction in digoxin serum concentration. If reinitiation is required, consider postponing until Fab fragments have been eliminated completely; elimination may take several days or longer, especially in patients with renal impairment. Use with caution in patients with renal failure (experience limited); the Fab-digoxin complex will be eliminated more slowly. Toxicity may recur; prolonged monitoring for recurrence of symptoms and evaluation of free (unbound) digoxin concentrations (if test available) may be warranted in this patient population.

Adverse Reactions Frequency not defined.

Cardiovascular: Heart failure exacerbation (due to withdrawal of digoxin), orthostatic hypotension, rapid ventricular response (patients with atrial fibrillation; due to withdrawal of digoxin)

Endocrine & metabolic: Hypokalemia

Local: Phlebitis

Miscellaneous: Allergic reactions, serum sickness

Drug Interactions

Metabolism/Transport Effects None known.

Avoid Concomitant Use There are no known interactions where it is recommended to avoid concomitant use.

Increased Effect/Toxicity There are no known significant interactions involving an increase in effect.

Decreased Effect There are no known significant interactions involving a decrease in effect.

Preparation for Administration Reconstitute to a final concentration of 10 mg/mL by adding 4 mL SWFI. Reconstituted solutions should be stored under refrigeration at 2°C to 8°C (36°F to 46°F) and used within 4 hours. For very small doses (eg, those required in infants and children), the reconstituted vial can be further diluted by adding an additional 36 mL NS to achieve a final concentration of 1 mg/mL.

Storage/Stability Store vials at 2°C to 8°C (36°F to 46°F); do not freeze.

Mechanism of Action Digoxin immune antigen-binding fragments (Fab) are specific antibodies for the treatment of digitalis intoxication in carefully selected patients; binds with molecules of digoxin or digitoxin and is then excreted by the kidneys and removed from the body

Pharmacodynamics/Kinetics

Onset of action: I.V.: Digitalis toxicity: Improvement may be seen in ≤30 minutes

Distribution: V_d: 0.3 L/kg

Half-life elimination: 15-20 hours; prolonged with renal impairment

Excretion: Urine; undetectable amounts within 5-7 days

Dosage Each vial of DigiFab™ 40 mg will bind ~0.5 mg of digoxin or digitoxin.

Note: Estimation of the dose is based on the body burden of digitalis. This may be calculated if the amount ingested is known or the post-distribution serum drug level is known (round the dose up to the nearest whole vial). If the amount ingested is unknown, general dosing guidelines should be used.

Acute ingestion of *unknown* amount: I.V.: Children and Adults: 20 vials is adequate to treat most life-threatening ingestions. May give as a single dose or give 10 vials, observe the response, and give a second dose of 10 vials if indicated.

Acute ingestion of *known* amount: I.V.:

Based on number of tablets or capsules ingested: Children and Adults:

Step 1: Calculate total body load (mg)

*Digoxin capsules **or** digitoxin:*

Total body load (mg) = Amount (mg) digoxin capsules **or** digitoxin ingested

Digoxin tablets:

Total body load (mg) = 0.8 x (amount [mg] digoxin tablets ingested)

Step 2: Calculate number of vials needed

Digoxin Immune Fab Dose (vials) = Total body load (mg) / (0.5)

Alternatively, the following table gives an estimation of the number of vials needed based on the number of **digoxin** tablets or capsules ingested.

Number of Digoxin Tablets or Capsules Ingested[1]	Dose of Digoxin Immune Fab (# of Vials)
25	10
50	20
75	30
100	40
150	60
200	80

[1]250 mcg tablets with 80% bioavailability or 200 mcg capsules with 100% bioavailability.

Based on steady-state serum digoxin concentration:

Infants and Children ≤20 kg: May require smaller doses; calculate the dose in milligrams (mg), consider dilution of the reconstituted vial with NS, and administer the dose via a tuberculin syringe

Digoxin Immune Fab Dose (mg) = [(serum digoxin concentration [ng/mL] x weight [kg]) / 100] x (digoxin immune Fab amount per vial [mg/vial])

Note: Digoxin immune Fab amount per vial: 40 mg/vial.

Alternatively, the following table gives an estimation of the amount of **DigiFab™** needed based on the steady-state serum digoxin concentration.

Infants and Small Children Dose Estimates of DigiFab™ (in mg) From Steady-State Serum Digoxin Concentration

Patient Weight (kg)	Serum Digoxin Concentration (ng/mL)						
	1	2	4	8	12	16	20
1	0.4 mg[1]	1 mg[1]	1.5 mg[1]	3 mg[1]	5 mg	6.5 mg	8 mg
3	1 mg[1]	2.5 mg[1]	5 mg	10 mg	14 mg	19 mg	24 mg
5	2 mg[1]	4 mg	8 mg	16 mg	24 mg	32 mg	40 mg
10	4 mg	8 mg	16 mg	32 mg	48 mg	64 mg	80 mg
20	8 mg	16 mg	32 mg	64 mg	96 mg	128 mg	160 mg

[1]Dilution of reconstituted vial to 1 mg/mL may be desirable.

Children >20 kg and Adults:

Digoxin Immune Fab Dose (vials) = [(serum digoxin concentration [ng/mL] x weight [kg]) / 100]

Alternatively, the following table gives an estimation of the number of vials needed based on the steady-state serum digoxin concentration.

Adult Dose Estimates of DigiFab™ (in # of Vials) From Steady-State Serum Digoxin Concentration

Patient Weight (kg)	Serum Digoxin Concentration (ng/mL)						
	1	2	4	8	12	16	20
40	0.5 vial	1 vial	2 vials	3 vials	5 vials	7 vials	8 vials
60	0.5 vial	1 vial	3 vials	5 vials	7 vials	10 vials	12 vials
70	1 vial	2 vials	3 vials	6 vials	9 vials	11 vials	14 vials
80	1 vial	2 vials	3 vials	7 vials	10 vials	13 vials	16 vials
100	1 vial	2 vials	4 vials	8 vials	12 vials	16 vials	20 vials

Based on steady-state digitoxin concentration: Children and Adults: If the calculated dose based on the **digitoxin** concentration is different than that for the digoxin concentration, use the higher dose.

Digoxin Immune Fab Dose (vials) = [serum **digitoxin** concentration (ng/mL) x weight (kg)] / 1000

Chronic toxicity (serum digoxin concentration unavailable): I.V.:

Infants and Children ≤20 kg: 1 vial is adequate to reverse most cases of toxicity

Children >20 kg and Adults: 6 vials is adequate to reverse most cases of toxicity

Dosage adjustment in renal impairment: No dosage adjustment necessary; however, use with caution since digoxin-digoxin immune Fab complex is renally eliminated. Patients should undergo prolonged monitoring for recurrence of toxicity.

Dosage adjustment in hepatic impairment: No dosage adjustment provided in manufacturer's labeling.

Administration I.V. infusion over at least 30 minutes is preferred. May also be given by bolus injection if cardiac arrest is imminent (infusion-related reaction may occur). Small doses (eg, those required in infants or small children) may be administered using a tuberculin syringe as undiluted digoxin immune Fab or diluted with NS to a concentration of 1 mg/mL digoxin immune Fab. Stopping the infusion and restarting at a slower rate may help if an infusion-related reaction occurs.

Monitoring Parameters Prior to the first dose of digoxin immune Fab evaluate serum potassium, serum digoxin concentration, and serum creatinine; closely monitor serum potassium (eg, hourly for 4-6 hours; at least daily thereafter), temperature, blood pressure, and electrocardiogram after administration. **Total serum digoxin concentrations will rise precipitously following administration of digoxin immune Fab due to the presence of the Fab-digoxin complex; because digoxin bound to Fab fragments cannot result in toxicity, this rise has no clinical meaning.** Therefore, avoid monitoring total serum digoxin concentrations until the Fab fragments have been eliminated completely; this may be several days to weeks in patients with renal impairment (Ujhelyi, 1995).

Patients with renal failure may experience a recurrence of toxicity; prolonged monitoring for recurrence of symptoms and evaluation of free (unbound) digoxin concentrations (if test available) may be warranted in this patient population.

Test Interactions Digoxin immune fab will interfere with digitalis immunoassay measurements, thereby resulting in clinically misleading total serum digoxin concentrations until all Fab fragments are eliminated from the body (may take several days to >1 week after administration).

Dosage Forms Excipient information presented when available (limited, particularly for generics); consult specific product labeling.

Solution Reconstituted, Intravenous [preservative free]:
DigiFab: 40 mg (1 ea)

◆ **Digoxin Injection CSD (Can)** *see* Digoxin *on page 605*
◆ **Dihematoporphyrin Ether** *see* Porfimer *on page 1679*
◆ **Dihydroartemisinin Hemisuccinate Sodium** *see* Artesunate *on page 171*

Dihydrocodeine, Aspirin, and Caffeine

(dye hye droe KOE deen, AS pir in, & KAF een)

Brand Names: U.S. Synalgos®-DC

Index Terms Aspirin, Dihydrocodeine, and Caffeine; Caffeine, Dihydrocodeine, and Aspirin; Dihydrocodeine Compound; Dihydrocodeine, Aspirin, and Caffeine

Pharmacologic Category Analgesic, Opioid

Use Management of mild-to-moderate pain

Dosage

Adults: Oral: 1-2 capsules every 4-6 hours as needed for pain

Elderly: Initial dosing should be cautious (low end of adult dosing range)

Dosage adjustment in renal impairment: No dosage adjustment provided in manufacturer's labeling.

Dosage adjustment in hepatic impairment: No dosage adjustment provided in manufacturer's labeling.

Additional Information Complete prescribing information should be consulted for additional detail.

Dosage Forms Excipient information presented when available (limited, particularly for generics); consult specific product labeling.

Capsule, oral:
Synalgos®-DC: Dihydrocodeine bitartrate 16 mg, aspirin 356.4 mg, and caffeine 30 mg
Generic: Dihydrocodeine bitartrate 16 mg, aspirin 356.4 mg, and caffeine 30 mg

Controlled Substance C-III

◆ **Dihydrocodeine, Aspirin, and Caffeine** *see* Dihydrocodeine, Aspirin, and Caffeine *on page 611*

Dihydrocodeine, Chlorpheniramine, and Phenylephrine

(dye hye droe KOE deen, klor fen IR a meen, & fen il EF rin)

Brand Names: U.S. Coldcough PD; Novahistine DH; Tusscough DHC™

Index Terms Chlorpheniramine Maleate, Dihydrocodeine Bitartrate, and Phenylephrine Hydrochloride; Phenylephrine, Chlorpheniramine, and Dihydrocodeine

Pharmacologic Category Alkylamine Derivative; Alpha-Adrenergic Agonist; Analgesic, Opioid; Antitussive; Decongestant; Histamine H_1 Antagonist; Histamine H_1 Antagonist, First Generation

Use Symptomatic relief of cough and congestion associated with the upper respiratory tract

Dosage Cough and congestion: Oral:

Children 2-6 years (Novahistine DH): 1.25-2.5 mL every 4-6 hours as needed (maximum: 10 mL/24 hours)

Children 6-12 years (Novahistine DH): 2.5-5 mL every 4-6 hours as needed (maximum: 20 mL/24 hours)

Children ≥12 years and Adults (Novahistine DH): 5-10 mL every 4-6 hours as needed (maximum: 40 mL/24 hours)

Additional Information Complete prescribing information should be consulted for additional detail.

Dosage Forms Excipient information presented when available (limited, particularly for generics); consult specific product labeling. [DSC] = Discontinued product

Liquid, oral:
Novahistine DH: Dihydrocodeine bitartrate 7.5 mg, chlorpheniramine maleate 2 mg and phenylephrine hydrochloride 5 mg per 5 mL (480 mL) [ethanol free, sugar free; contains propylene glycol; strawberry flavor; C-III]

Syrup, oral:
Coldcough PD: Dihydrocodeine bitartrate 3 mg, chlorpheniramine maleate 2 mg, and phenylephrine hydrochloride 7.5 mg per 5 mL (120 mL) [ethanol free, sugar free; grape flavor; C-V]
Tusscough DHC™: Dihydrocodeine bitartrate 3 mg, chlorpheniramine maleate 5 mg, and phenylephrine hydrochloride 20 mg per 5 mL (473 mL) [ethanol free, sugar free, dye free; contains benzoic acid, propylene glycol; grape flavor; C-III]

Controlled Substance C-III; C-V

◆ **Dihydrocodeine Compound** *see* Dihydrocodeine, Aspirin, and Caffeine *on page 611*

Dihydroergotamine (dye hye droe er GOT a meen)

Brand Names: U.S. D.H.E. 45; Migranal

Brand Names: Canada Migranal®

Index Terms DHE; Dihydroergotamine Mesylate

Pharmacologic Category Antimigraine Agent; Ergot Derivative

Use Treatment of migraine headache with or without aura; injection also indicated for treatment of cluster headaches

Unlabeled Use Adjunct for DVT prophylaxis for hip surgery, for orthostatic hypotension, xerostomia secondary to antidepressant use, and pelvic congestion with pain

Pregnancy Risk Factor X

Pregnancy Considerations Dihydroergotamine is oxytocic and should not be used during pregnancy.

Breast-Feeding Considerations Ergot derivatives inhibit prolactin and it is known that ergotamine is excreted in breast milk (vomiting, diarrhea, weak pulse, and unstable blood pressure have been reported in nursing infants). It is not known if dihydroergotamine would also cause these effects, however, it is likely that it is excreted in human breast milk. Do not use in nursing women.

Contraindications Hypersensitivity to dihydroergotamine or any component of the formulation; uncontrolled hypertension, ischemic heart disease, angina pectoris, history of MI, silent ischemia, or coronary artery vasospasm including Prinzmetal's angina; hemiplegic or basilar migraine; peripheral vascular disease; sepsis; severe hepatic or renal dysfunction; following vascular surgery; avoid use within 24 hours of sumatriptan, zolmitriptan, other serotonin agonists, or ergot-like agents; avoid during or within 2 weeks of discontinuing MAO inhibitors; concurrent use of peripheral and central vasoconstrictors; ergot alkaloids are contraindicated with potent inhibitors of CYP3A4 (includes protease inhibitors, azole antifungals, and some macrolide antibiotics); pregnancy, breast-feeding

Warnings/Precautions Hazardous agent - use appropriate precautions for handling and disposal (meets NIOSH, 2012 criteria). **[U.S. Boxed Warning]: Ergot alkaloids are contraindicated with potent inhibitors of CYP3A4 (includes protease inhibitors, azole antifungals, and some macrolide antibiotics); concomitant use associated with an increased risk of vasospasm leading to cerebral ischemia and/or ischemia of the extremities.** Do not give to patients with risk factors for CAD until a cardiovascular evaluation has been performed; if evaluation is satisfactory, the healthcare provider should administer the first dose and cardiovascular status should be periodically evaluated. May cause vasospastic reactions; persistent vasospasm may lead to gangrene or death in patients with compromised circulation. Discontinue if signs of vasoconstriction develop. Rare reports of increased blood pressure in patients without history of hypertension. Rare reports of adverse cardiac events (acute MI, life-threatening arrhythmias, death) have been reported following use of the injection. Cerebral hemorrhage, subarachnoid hemorrhage, and stroke have also occurred following use of the injection. Not for prolonged use. Pleural and peritoneal fibrosis have been reported with prolonged daily use. Cardiac valvular fibrosis has also been associated with ergot alkaloids. Use with caution in the elderly.

Migranal® Nasal Spray: Local irritation to nose and throat (usually transient and mild-moderate in severity) can occur; long-term consequences on nasal or respiratory mucosa have not been extensively evaluated.

Adverse Reactions

>10%: Nasal spray: Respiratory: Rhinitis (26%)

1% to 10%: Nasal spray:
- Central nervous system: Dizziness (4%), somnolence (3%)
- Endocrine & metabolic: Hot flashes (1%)
- Gastrointestinal: Nausea (10%), taste disturbance (8%), vomiting (4%), diarrhea (2%)
- Local: Application site reaction (6%)
- Neuromuscular & skeletal: Weakness (1%), stiffness (1%)
- Respiratory: Pharyngitis (3%)

<1% (Limited to important or life-threatening): Injection and nasal spray: Cerebral hemorrhage, coronary artery vasospasm, dyspnea, hypertension, MI, paresthesia, peripheral cyanosis, peripheral ischemia, stroke, subarachnoid hemorrhage, ventricular fibrillation, ventricular tachycardia. Pleural and retroperitoneal fibrosis have been reported following prolonged use of the injection; cardiac valvular fibrosis has been associated with ergot alkaloids.

Drug Interactions

Metabolism/Transport Effects **Substrate** of CYP3A4 (major); **Note:** Assignment of Major/Minor substrate status based on clinically relevant drug interaction potential; **Inhibits** CYP3A4 (weak)

Avoid Concomitant Use

Avoid concomitant use of Dihydroergotamine with any of the following: Alpha-/Beta-Agonists; Alpha1-Agonists; Boceprevir; Clarithromycin; Cobicistat; Conivaptan; Crizotinib; Efavirenz; Enzalutamide; Fusidic Acid (Systemic); Itraconazole; Ketoconazole (Systemic); Lorcaserin; Mifepristone; Nitroglycerin; Posaconazole; Protease Inhibitors; Serotonin 5-HT1D Receptor Agonists; Telaprevir; Voriconazole

Increased Effect/Toxicity

Dihydroergotamine may increase the levels/effects of: Alpha-/Beta-Agonists; Alpha1-Agonists; Antipsychotics; Dofetilide; Lomitapide; Metoclopramide; Serotonin 5-HT1D Receptor Agonists; Serotonin Modulators

The levels/effects of Dihydroergotamine may be increased by: Antipsychotics; Beta-Blockers; Boceprevir; Clarithromycin; Cobicistat; Conivaptan; Crizotinib; CYP3A4 Inhibitors (Moderate); CYP3A4 Inhibitors (Strong); Dasatinib; Efavirenz; Fusidic Acid (Systemic); Itraconazole; Ivacaftor; Ketoconazole (Systemic); Lorcaserin; Luliconazole; Macrolide Antibiotics; Mifepristone; Nitroglycerin; Posaconazole; Protease Inhibitors; Serotonin 5-HT1D Receptor Agonists; Simeprevir; Telaprevir; Voriconazole

Decreased Effect

Dihydroergotamine may decrease the levels/effects of: Nitroglycerin

The levels/effects of Dihydroergotamine may be decreased by: Enzalutamide

Storage/Stability

Injection: Store below 25°C (77°F); do not refrigerate or freeze; protect from heat. Protect from light.

Nasal spray: Prior to use, store below 25°C (77°F); do not refrigerate or freeze. Once spray applicator has been prepared, use within 8 hours; discard any unused solution.

Mechanism of Action Ergot alkaloid alpha-adrenergic blocker directly stimulates vascular smooth muscle to vasoconstrict peripheral and cerebral vessels; also has effects on serotonin receptors

Pharmacodynamics/Kinetics

Onset of action: I.M.: 15-30 minutes
Duration: I.M.: 3-4 hours
Distribution: V_d: ~800 L
Protein binding: 93%
Metabolism: Extensively hepatic
Half-life elimination: ~9-10 hours
Time to peak, serum: I.M.: 24 minutes; I.V.: 1-2 minutes; Intranasal: 30-60 minutes; SubQ 15-45 minutes
Excretion: Primarily feces; urine (6% to 7% as unchanged drug)

Dosage Adults:

I.M., SubQ: 1 mg at first sign of headache; repeat hourly to a maximum dose of 3 mg/day; maximum dose: 6 mg/week

I.V.: 1 mg at first sign of headache; repeat hourly up to a maximum dose of 2 mg/day; maximum dose: 6 mg/week

Raskin protocol (unlabeled dosing): Initial test dose: 0.5 mg (following premedication with metoclopramide); subsequent dosing is titrated (range: 0.2-1 mg) every 8 hours for 2-3 days and administered with or without metoclopramide based on response and tolerance (Raskin, 1986; Raskin, 1990). **Note:** Some clinicians use modified versions of this protocol, with additional adjunctive medications and/or alternate antiemetic agents.

Intranasal: 1 spray (0.5 mg) of nasal spray should be administered into each nostril; if needed, repeat after 15 minutes, up to a total of 4 sprays (2 mg). **Note:** Do not exceed 6 sprays (3 mg) in a 24-hour period and no more than 8 sprays (4 mg) in a week.

Elderly: Patients >65 years of age were not included in controlled clinical studies

Dosing adjustment in renal impairment: Contraindicated in severe renal impairment

Dosing adjustment in hepatic impairment: Dosage reductions are probably necessary but specific guidelines are not available; contraindicated in severe hepatic dysfunction

Administration

Intranasal: Prior to administration of nasal spray, the nasal spray applicator must be primed (pumped 4 times); in order to let the drug be absorbed through the skin in the nose, patients should not inhale deeply through the nose while spraying or immediately after spraying; for best results, treatment should be initiated at the first symptom or sign of an attack; however, nasal spray can be used at any stage of a migraine attack.

I.M., SubQ: May administer by intramuscular or subcutaneous injection.

I.V.: Administer slowly over 2-3 minutes (Raskin protocol)

Hazardous agent; use appropriate precautions for handling and disposal (meets NIOSH, 2012 criteria).

Reference Range Minimum concentration for vasoconstriction is reportedly 0.06 ng/mL

Dosage Forms Considerations

Migranal nasal solution contains caffeine 10 mg/mL

Dosage Forms Excipient information presented when available (limited, particularly for generics); consult specific product labeling.

Solution, Injection, as mesylate:

D.H.E. 45: 1 mg/mL (1 mL)

Generic: 1 mg/mL (1 mL)

Solution, Nasal, as mesylate:

Migranal: 4 mg/mL (1 mL)

Generic: 4 mg/mL (1 mL)

- ◆ **Dihydroergotamine Mesylate** *see* Dihydroergotamine *on page 611*
- ◆ **Dihydrohydroxycodeinone** *see* OxyCODONE *on page 1535*
- ◆ **Dihydromorphinone** *see* HYDROmorphone *on page 1013*
- ◆ **Dihydroqinghaosu Hemisuccinate Sodium** *see* Artesunate *on page 171*
- ◆ **Dihydroxyanthracenedione** *see* MitoXANtrone *on page 1386*
- ◆ **Dihydroxyanthracenedione Dihydrochloride** *see* MitoXANtrone *on page 1386*
- ◆ **1,25 Dihydroxycholecalciferol** *see* Calcitriol *on page 314*
- ◆ **Dihydroxydeoxynorvinkaleukoblastine** *see* Vinorelbine *on page 2196*
- ◆ **Diiodohydroxyquin** *see* Iodoquinol *on page 1109*
- ◆ **Dilacor XR** *see* Diltiazem *on page 613*
- ◆ **Dilantin** *see* Phenytoin *on page 1638*
- ◆ **Dilantin Infatabs** *see* Phenytoin *on page 1638*
- ◆ **Dilatrate-SR** *see* Isosorbide Dinitrate *on page 1126*
- ◆ **Dilaudid** *see* HYDROmorphone *on page 1013*
- ◆ **Dilaudid-HP** *see* HYDROmorphone *on page 1013*
- ◆ **Dilt-CD** *see* Diltiazem *on page 613*

Diltiazem (dil TYE a zem)

Brand Names: U.S. Cardizem; Cardizem CD; Cardizem LA; Cartia XT; Dilacor XR; Dilt-CD; Dilt-XR; Diltiazem HCl CD; Diltzac; Matzim LA; Taztia XT; Tiazac

Brand Names: Canada Apo-Diltiaz CD®; Apo-Diltiaz SR®; Apo-Diltiaz TZ®; Apo-Diltiaz®; Apo-Diltiaz® Injectable; Ava-Diltiazem; Cardizem® CD; CO Diltiazem CD; CO Diltiazem T; Diltiazem HCl ER®; Diltiazem Hydrochloride Injection; Diltiazem TZ; Diltiazem-CD; Nu-Diltiaz; Nu-Diltiaz-CD; PMS-Diltiazem CD; ratio-Diltiazem CD; Sandoz-Diltiazem CD; Sandoz-Diltiazem T; Teva-Diltiazem; Teva-Diltiazem CD; Teva-Diltiazem HCL ER Capsules; Tiazac®; Tiazac® XC

Index Terms Diltiazem Hydrochloride

Pharmacologic Category Antianginal Agent; Antiarrhythmic Agent, Class IV; Antihypertensive; Calcium Channel Blocker; Calcium Channel Blocker, Nondihydropyridine

Additional Appendix Information

Calcium Channel Blockers - Comparative Pharmacokinetics *on page 2296*

Dosing Considerations for the Critically-Ill Patient With Morbid Obesity *on page 2379*

Use

Oral: Primary hypertension; chronic stable angina or angina from coronary artery spasm

Injection: Control of rapid ventricular rate in patients with atrial fibrillation or atrial flutter; conversion of paroxysmal supraventricular tachycardia (PSVT)

Unlabeled Use ACLS guidelines: Injection: Stable narrow-complex tachycardia uncontrolled or unconverted by adenosine or vagal maneuvers or if SVT is recurrent

Hypertrophic cardiomyopathy; pediatric hypertension

Pregnancy Risk Factor C

Pregnancy Considerations Adverse events have been observed in animal reproduction studies. Untreated chronic maternal hypertension is associated with adverse events in the fetus, infant, and mother. If treatment for hypertension during pregnancy is needed, other agents are preferred (ACOG, 2012; Chobanian, 2003). The Canadian labeling contraindicates use in pregnant women or women of childbearing potential. Diltiazem may be used to control atrial fibrillation in pregnant women (Fuster, 2006). Women with hypertrophic cardiomyopathy who are controlled with diltiazem prior to pregnancy may continue therapy, but increased fetal monitoring is recommended (Gersh, 2011).

Breast-Feeding Considerations Diltiazem is excreted into breastmilk in concentrations similar to those in the maternal plasma (Okada, 1985). Breast-feeding is not recommended by the manufacturer. Breast-fed infants of mothers taking medications for hypertension should be monitored for adverse effects (Chobanian, 2003).

Contraindications

Oral: Hypersensitivity to diltiazem or any component of the formulation; sick sinus syndrome (except in patients with a functioning artificial pacemaker); second- or third-degree AV block (except in patients with a functioning artificial pacemaker); severe hypotension (systolic <90 mm Hg); acute MI and pulmonary congestion

Intravenous (I.V.): Hypersensitivity to diltiazem or any component of the formulation; sick sinus syndrome (except in patients with a functioning artificial pacemaker); second- or third-degree AV block (except in patients with a functioning artificial pacemaker); severe hypotension (systolic <90 mm Hg); cardiogenic shock; administration concomitantly or within a few hours of the administration of I.V. beta-blockers; atrial fibrillation or flutter associated with accessory bypass tract (eg, Wolff-Parkinson-White syndrome); ventricular tachycardia (with wide-complex tachycardia, must determine whether origin is supraventricular or ventricular)

Canadian labeling: Additional contraindications (not in U.S. labeling): I.V. and Oral: Pregnancy; use in women of childbearing potential

Warnings/Precautions Can cause first-, second-, and third-degree AV block or sinus bradycardia and risk increases with agents known to slow cardiac conduction. The most common side effect is peripheral edema; occurs within 2-3 weeks of starting therapy. Symptomatic hypotension with or without syncope can rarely occur; blood pressure must be lowered at a rate appropriate for the patient's clinical condition. Use caution when using diltiazem together with a beta-blocker; may result in conduction disturbances, hypotension, and worsened LV function. Simultaneous administration of I.V. diltiazem and an I.V. beta-blocker or administration within a few hours of each other may result in asystole and is contraindicated. Use with other agents known to either reduce SA node function and/or AV nodal conduction (eg, digoxin) or reduce sympathetic outflow (eg, clonidine) may increase the risk of serious bradycardia. Use caution in left ventricular dysfunction (may exacerbate condition). Avoid use of diltiazem in patients with heart failure and reduced ejection fraction (Hunt, 2009). Use with caution with hypertrophic obstructive cardiomyopathy; routine use is currently not recommended due to insufficient evidence (Maron, 2003). Use with caution in hepatic or renal dysfunction. Transient dermatologic reactions have been observed with use; if reaction persists, discontinue. May (rarely) progress to erythema multiforme or exfoliative dermatitis.

Adverse Reactions Note: Frequencies represent ranges for various dosage forms. Patients with impaired ventricular function and/or conduction abnormalities may have higher incidence of adverse reactions.

>10%:

Cardiovascular: Edema (2% to 15%)

Central nervous system: Headache (5% to 12%)

2% to 10%:

Cardiovascular: AV block (first degree 2% to 8%), edema (lower limb, 2% to 8%), pain (6%), bradycardia (2% to 6%), hypotension (<2% to 4%), vasodilation (2% to 3%), extrasystoles (2%), flushing (1% to 2%), palpitation (1% to 2%)

Central nervous system: Dizziness (3% to 10%), nervousness (2%)

Dermatologic: Rash (1% to 4%)

Endocrine & metabolic: Gout (1% to 2%)

Gastrointestinal: Dyspepsia (1% to 6%), constipation (<2% to 4%), vomiting (2%), diarrhea (1% to 2%)

Local: Injection site reactions: Burning, itching (4%)

Neuromuscular & skeletal: Weakness (1% to 4%), myalgia (2%)

Respiratory: Rhinitis (<2% to 10%), pharyngitis (2% to 6%), dyspnea (1% to 6%), bronchitis (1% to 4%), cough (≤3), sinus congestion (1% to 2%)

<2% (Limited to important or life-threatening): Alkaline phosphatase increased, allergic reaction, ALT increased, AST increased, amblyopia, amnesia, arrhythmia, AV block (second or third degree), bundle branch block, CHF, depression, dysgeusia, extrapyramidal symptoms, gingival hyperplasia, hemolytic anemia, petechiae, photosensitivity, Stevens-Johnson syndrome, syncope, tachycardia, thrombocytopenia, tremor, toxic epidermal necrolysis

Drug Interactions

Metabolism/Transport Effects Substrate of CYP2C9 (minor), CYP2D6 (minor), CYP3A4 (major), P-glycoprotein; **Note:** Assignment of Major/Minor substrate status based on clinically relevant drug interaction potential; **Inhibits** CYP2C9 (weak), CYP2D6 (weak), CYP3A4 (moderate)

Avoid Concomitant Use

Avoid concomitant use of Diltiazem with any of the following: Bosutinib; Conivaptan; Dantrolene; Fusidic Acid (Systemic); Ibrutinib; Ivabradine; Lomitapide; Pimozide; Simeprevir; Tolvaptan; Ulipristal

Increased Effect/Toxicity

Diltiazem may increase the levels/effects of: Alfentanil; Amifostine; Amiodarone; Antihypertensives; Aprepitant; ARIPiprazole; AtorvaSTATin; Atosiban; Avanafil; Benzodiazepines (metabolized by oxidation); Beta-Blockers; Bosentan; Bosutinib; Budesonide (Systemic, Oral Inhalation); BusPIRone; Calcium Channel Blockers (Dihydropyridine); CarBAMazepine; Cardiac Glycosides; Colchicine; Corticosteroids (Systemic); CycloSPORINE (Systemic); CYP3A4 Substrates; Dofetilide; Dronedarone; Eletriptan; Eplerenone; Everolimus; Fingolimod; Fosaprepitant; Fosphenytoin; Halofantrine; Hypotensive Agents; Ibrutinib; Imatinib; Ivabradine; Ivacaftor; Lithium; Lomitapide; Lovastatin; Lurasidone; Magnesium Salts; Midodrine; Neuromuscular-Blocking Agents (Nondepolarizing); Nitroprusside; Obinutuzumab; OxyCODONE; Phenytoin; Pimecrolimus; Pimozide; Propafenone; QuiNIDine; Ranolazine; Red Yeast Rice; RiTUXimab; Rivaroxaban; Salicylates; Salmeterol; Saxagliptin; Simeprevir; Simvastatin; Tacrolimus (Systemic); Tacrolimus (Topical); Tolvaptan; Ulipristal; Vilazodone; Zuclopenthixol

The levels/effects of Diltiazem may be increased by: Alpha1-Blockers; Anilidopiperidine Opioids; Antifungal Agents (Azole Derivatives, Systemic); Aprepitant; AtorvaSTATin; Brimonidine (Topical); Calcium Channel Blockers (Dihydropyridine); Cimetidine; CloNIDine; Conivaptan; CycloSPORINE (Systemic); CYP3A4 Inhibitors (Moderate); CYP3A4 Inhibitors (Strong); Dantrolene; Dasatinib; Diazoxide; Dronedarone; Fluconazole; Fosaprepitant; Fusidic Acid (Systemic); Grapefruit Juice; Herbs (Hypotensive Properties); Ivabradine; Ivacaftor; Lovastatin; Luliconazole; Macrolide Antibiotics; Magnesium Salts; MAO Inhibitors; Mifepristone; Pentoxifylline; P-glycoprotein/ABCB1 Inhibitors; Phosphodiesterase 5 Inhibitors; Prostacyclin Analogues; Protease Inhibitors; Regorafenib; Simeprevir; Simvastatin

Decreased Effect

Diltiazem may decrease the levels/effects of: Clopidogrel; Ifosfamide

The levels/effects of Diltiazem may be decreased by: Barbiturates; Bosentan; Calcium Salts; CarBAMazepine; Colestipol; CYP3A4 Inducers (Strong); Dabrafenib; Deferasirox; Herbs (CYP3A4 Inducers); Herbs (Hypertensive Properties); Methylphenidate; Mitotane; Nafcillin; Peginterferon Alfa-2b; P-glycoprotein/ABCB1 Inducers; Rifamycin Derivatives; Tocilizumab; Yohimbine

Ethanol/Nutrition/Herb Interactions

Ethanol: Ethanol may increase risk of hypotension or vasodilation. Management: Avoid ethanol.

Food: Diltiazem serum levels may be elevated if taken with food. Serum concentrations were not altered by grapefruit juice in small clinical trials.

Herb/Nutraceutical: St John's wort may decrease diltiazem levels. Some herbal medications may worsen hypertension (eg, licorice); others may increase the antihypertensive effect of diltiazem (eg, shepherd's purse). Management: Avoid St John's wort, bayberry, blue cohosh, cayenne, ephedra, ginger, ginseng (American), kola, licorice, and yohimbe. Avoid black cohosh, California poppy, coleus, golden seal, hawthorn, mistletoe, periwinkle, quinine, and shepherd's purse.

Storage/Stability

Capsule, tablet: Store at room temperature. Protect from light.

Solution for injection: Store in refrigerator at 2°C to 8°C (36°F to 46°F); do not freeze. May be stored at room temperature for up to 1 month. Following dilution to ≤1 mg/mL with $D_5{}^1/_2NS$, D_5W, or NS, solution is stable for 24 hours at room temperature or under refrigeration.

Mechanism of Action Nondihydropyridine calcium channel blocker which inhibits calcium ion from entering the "slow channels" or select voltage-sensitive areas of vascular smooth muscle and myocardium during depolarization, producing a relaxation of coronary vascular smooth muscle and coronary vasodilation; increases myocardial oxygen delivery in patients with vasospastic angina

Pharmacodynamics/Kinetics

Onset of action: Oral: Immediate release tablet: 30-60 minutes; I.V.: 3 minutes

Duration: I.V.: Bolus: 1-3 hours; Continuous infusion (after discontinuation): 0.5-10 hours
Absorption: Immediate release tablet: >90%; Extended release capsule: ~93%
Distribution: V_d: 3-13 L/kg
Protein binding: 70% to 80%
Metabolism: Hepatic (extensive first-pass effect); following single I.V. injection, plasma concentrations of N-monodesmethyldiltiazem and desacetyldiltiazem are typically undetectable; however, these metabolites accumulate to detectable concentrations following 24-hour constant rate infusion. N-monodesmethyldiltiazem appears to have 20% of the potency of diltiazem; desacetyldiltiazem is about 25% to 50% as potent as the parent compound.
Bioavailability: Oral: ~40% (undergoes extensive first-pass metabolism)
Half-life elimination: Immediate release tablet: 3-4.5 hours, may be prolonged with renal impairment; Extended release tablet: 6-9 hours; Extended release capsules: 5-10 hours; I.V.: single dose: ~3.4 hours; continuous infusion: 4-5 hours
Time to peak, serum: Immediate release tablet: 2-4 hours; Extended release tablet: 11-18 hours; Extended release capsule: 10-14 hours
Excretion: Urine (2% to 4% as unchanged drug; 6% to 7% as metabolites); feces

Dosage

Children (unlabeled use): Minimal information available; some centers use the following: Oral: Hypertension: Immediate release tablets: Initial: 1.5-2 mg/kg/day divided in 3 doses/day (maximum dose 6 mg/kg/day up to 360 mg/day) (Flynn, 2000)

Adults:
Oral:
Angina:
Capsule, extended release:
Dilacor XR®, Dilt-XR, Diltia XT®: Initial: 120 mg once daily; titrate over 7-14 days; usual dose range: 120-320 mg/day: maximum: 480 mg/day
Cardizem® CD, Cartia XT®, Dilt-CD: Initial: 120-180 mg once daily; titrate over 7-14 days; usual dose range: 120-320 mg/day; maximum: 480 mg/day
Tiazac®, Taztia XT®: Initial: 120-180 mg once daily; titrate over 7-14 days; usual dose range: 120-320 mg/day; maximum: 540 mg/day
Tablet, extended release (Cardizem® LA, Matzim® LA, Tiazac® XC [CAN; not available in U.S.]): 180 mg once daily; may increase at 7- to 14-day intervals; usual dose range: 120-320 mg/day; maximum: 360 mg/day
Tablet, immediate release (Cardizem®): Usual starting dose: 30 mg 4 times/day; titrate dose gradually at 1- to 2-day intervals; usual dose range: 120-320 mg/day
Hypertension:
Capsule, extended release (once-daily dosing):
Cardizem® CD, Cartia XT®, Dilt-CD: Initial: 180-240 mg once daily; dose adjustment may be made after 14 days; usual dose range (JNC 7): 180-420 mg/day; maximum: 480 mg/day
Dilacor® XR, Diltia XT®, Dilt-XR: Initial: 180-240 mg once daily; dose adjustment may be made after 14 days; usual dose range (JNC 7): 180-420 mg/day; maximum: 540 mg/day
Tiazac®, Taztia XT®: Initial: 120-240 mg once daily; dose adjustment may be made after 14 days; usual dose range (JNC 7): 180-420 mg/day; maximum: 540 mg/day
Capsule, extended release (twice-daily dosing): Initial: 60-120 mg twice daily; dose adjustment may be made after 14 days; usual range: 240-360 mg/day
Note: Diltiazem is available as a generic intended for either once- or twice-daily dosing, depending on the formulation; verify appropriate extended release capsule formulation is administered.
Tablet, extended release (Cardizem® LA, Matzim® LA, Tiazac® XC [CAN; not available in U.S.]): Initial: 180-240 mg once daily; dose adjustment may be made after 14 days; usual dose range (JNC 7): 120-540 mg/day
Note: Elderly: Consider lower initial doses (eg, 120 mg once daily using extended release capsule) and titrate to response (Aronow, 2011)
I.V.: *Atrial fibrillation, atrial flutter, PSVT:*
Initial bolus dose: 0.25 mg/kg actual body weight over 2 minutes (average adult dose: 20 mg); ACLS guideline recommends 15-20 mg
Repeat bolus dose (may be administered after 15 minutes if the response is inadequate): 0.35 mg/kg actual body weight over 2 minutes (average adult dose: 25 mg); ACLS guideline recommends 20-25 mg
Continuous infusion (infusions >24 hours or infusion rates >15 mg/hour are not recommended): Initial infusion rate of 10 mg/hour; rate may be increased in 5 mg/hour increments up to 15 mg/hour as needed; some patients may respond to an initial rate of 5 mg/hour.
If diltiazem injection is administered by continuous infusion for >24 hours, the possibility of decreased diltiazem clearance, prolonged elimination half-life, and increased diltiazem and/or diltiazem metabolite plasma concentrations should be considered.
Conversion from I.V. diltiazem to oral diltiazem:
Oral dose (mg/day) is approximately equal to [rate (mg/hour) x 3 + 3] x 10.
3 mg/hour = 120 mg/day
5 mg/hour = 180 mg/day
7 mg/hour = 240 mg/day
11 mg/hour = 360 mg/day

Dosing adjustment in renal impairment: Use with caution; no dosing adjustments recommended
Dialysis: Not removed by hemo- or peritoneal dialysis; supplemental dose is not necessary.
Dosing adjustment in hepatic impairment: Use with caution; no specific dosing recommendations available; extensively metabolized by the liver; half-life is increased in patients with cirrhosis

Usual Infusion Concentrations: Pediatric I.V. infusion: 1 mg/mL

Usual Infusion Concentrations: Adult I.V. infusion: 125 mg in 125 mL (total volume) (concentration: 1 mg/mL) of D_5W or NS

Administration

Oral:
Immediate release tablet (Cardizem®): Administer before meals and at bedtime.
Long acting dosage forms: Do not open, chew, or crush; swallow whole.
Cardizem® CD, Cardizem® LA, Cartia XT®, Dilt-CD, Matzim® LA: May be administered without regards to meals.
Dilacor XR®, Dilt-XR, Diltia XT®: Administer on an empty stomach.
Taztia XT™, Tiazac®: Capsules may be opened and sprinkled on a spoonful of applesauce. Applesauce should not be hot and should be swallowed without chewing, followed by drinking a glass of water.
Tiazac® XC [CAN; not available in U.S.]: Administer at bedtime
I.V.: Bolus doses given over 2 minutes with continuous ECG and blood pressure monitoring. Continuous infusion should be via infusion pump.

Monitoring Parameters Liver function tests, blood pressure, ECG, heart rate; consult individual institutional policies and procedures

Dosage Forms Excipient information presented when available (limited, particularly for generics); consult specific product labeling. [DSC] = Discontinued product

Capsule Extended Release 12 Hour, Oral, as hydrochloride:
- Generic: 60 mg, 90 mg, 120 mg

Capsule Extended Release 24 Hour, Oral, as hydrochloride:
- Cardizem CD: 120 mg, 180 mg, 240 mg, 300 mg, 360 mg [contains brilliant blue fcf (fd&c blue #1)]
- Cartia XT: 120 mg, 180 mg, 240 mg, 300 mg
- Dilacor XR: 240 mg
- Dilt-CD: 120 mg
- Dilt-CD: 180 mg, 240 mg [contains brilliant blue fcf (fd&c blue #1)]
- Dilt-CD: 300 mg
- Dilt-XR: 120 mg, 180 mg, 240 mg [contains brilliant blue fcf (fd&c blue #1), fd&c red #40, fd&c yellow #10 (quinoline yellow)]
- Diltiazem HCl CD: 360 mg [contains brilliant blue fcf (fd&c blue #1)]
- Diltzac: 120 mg [contains brilliant blue fcf (fd&c blue #1)]
- Diltzac: 180 mg
- Diltzac: 240 mg, 300 mg [contains brilliant blue fcf (fd&c blue #1)]
- Diltzac: 360 mg
- Taztia XT: 120 mg, 180 mg, 240 mg, 300 mg, 360 mg
- Tiazac: 120 mg, 180 mg, 240 mg, 300 mg, 360 mg, 420 mg
- Generic: 120 mg, 180 mg, 240 mg, 300 mg, 360 mg, 420 mg

Solution, Intravenous, as hydrochloride:
- Generic: 25 mg/5 mL (5 mL); 50 mg/10 mL (10 mL); 125 mg/25 mL (25 mL)

Solution, Intravenous, as hydrochloride [preservative free]:
- Generic: 25 mg/5 mL (5 mL); 50 mg/10 mL (10 mL); 125 mg/25 mL (25 mL)

Solution Reconstituted, Intravenous, as hydrochloride:
- Generic: 100 mg (1 ea)

Tablet, Oral, as hydrochloride:
- Cardizem: 30 mg
- Cardizem: 60 mg [scored]
- Cardizem: 60 mg [scored; contains fd&c blue #1 aluminum lake, fd&c yellow #10 aluminum lake, fd&c yellow #6 aluminum lake, methylparaben]
- Cardizem: 90 mg [DSC] [scored]
- Cardizem: 120 mg [scored; contains fd&c yellow #10 aluminum lake, fd&c yellow #6 aluminum lake, methylparaben]
- Generic: 30 mg, 60 mg, 90 mg, 120 mg

Tablet Extended Release 24 Hour, Oral, as hydrochloride:
- Cardizem LA: 120 mg, 180 mg, 240 mg, 300 mg, 360 mg, 420 mg
- Matzim LA: 180 mg, 240 mg, 300 mg, 360 mg, 420 mg

Dosage Forms: Canada Note: Also refer to Dosage Forms. Excipient information presented when available (limited, particularly for generics); consult specific product labeling.

Tablet, Extended Release, Oral, as hydrochloride:
- Tiazac XC: 120 mg, 180 mg, 240 mg, 300 mg, 360 mg

Extemporaneous Preparations A 12 mg/mL oral suspension may be made from tablets (regular, not extended release) and one of three different vehicles (cherry syrup, a 1:1 mixture of Ora-Sweet® and Ora-Plus®, or a 1:1 mixture of Ora-Sweet® SF and Ora-Plus®). Crush sixteen 90 mg tablets in a mortar and reduce to a fine powder. Add 10 mL of the chosen vehicle and mix to a uniform paste; mix while adding the vehicle in incremental proportions to **almost** 120 mL; transfer to a calibrated bottle, rinse mortar with vehicle, and add quantity of vehicle sufficient to make 120 mL. Label "shake well" and "protect from light". Stable for 60 days when stored in amber plastic prescription bottles in the dark at room temperature or refrigerated.

Allen LV and Erickson MA, "Stability of Baclofen, Captopril, Diltiazem Hydrochloride, Dipyridamole, and Flecainide Acetate in Extemporaneously Compounded Oral Liquids," *Am J Health Syst Pharm*, 1996, 53(18):2179-84.

- ◆ **Diltiazem-CD (Can)** *see* Diltiazem *on page 613*
- ◆ **Diltiazem HCl CD** *see* Diltiazem *on page 613*
- ◆ **Diltiazem HCl ER® (Can)** *see* Diltiazem *on page 613*
- ◆ **Diltiazem Hydrochloride** *see* Diltiazem *on page 613*
- ◆ **Diltiazem Hydrochloride Injection (Can)** *see* Diltiazem *on page 613*
- ◆ **Diltiazem TZ (Can)** *see* Diltiazem *on page 613*
- ◆ **Dilt-XR** *see* Diltiazem *on page 613*
- ◆ **Diltzac** *see* Diltiazem *on page 613*

DimenhyDRINATE (dye men HYE dri nate)

Brand Names: U.S. Dramamine [OTC]; Driminate [OTC]; Motion Sickness [OTC]

Brand Names: Canada Apo-Dimenhydrinate® [OTC]; Children's Motion Sickness Liquid [OTC]; Dimenhydrinate Injection; Dinate® [OTC]; Gravol IM; Gravol® [OTC]; Jamp-Dimenhydrinate [OTC]; Nauseatol [OTC]; Novo-Dimenate [OTC]; PMS-Dimenhydrinate [OTC]; Sandoz-Dimenhydrinate [OTC]; Travel Tabs [OTC]

Pharmacologic Category Ethanolamine Derivative; Histamine H_1 Antagonist; Histamine H_1 Antagonist, First Generation

Additional Appendix Information

Beers Criteria – Potentially Inappropriate Medications for Geriatrics *on page 2368*

Use Treatment and prevention of nausea, vertigo, and vomiting associated with motion sickness

Unlabeled Use Nausea and vomiting of pregnancy (NVP)

Pregnancy Risk Factor B

Dosage

Oral:
- Children:
  - 2-5 years: 12.5-25 mg every 6-8 hours, maximum: 75 mg/day
  - 6-12 years: 25-50 mg every 6-8 hours, maximum: 150 mg/day
- Adults: 50-100 mg every 4-6 hours, not to exceed 400 mg/day

I.M.:
- Children: 1.25 mg/kg **or** 37.5 mg/m^2 4 times/day; maximum: 300 mg/day
- Adults: 50 mg every 4 hours; maximum: 100 mg every 4 hours

I.V.: Adults: 50 mg every 4 hours; maximum: 100 mg every 4 hours

Additional Information Complete prescribing information should be consulted for additional detail.

Dosage Forms Excipient information presented when available (limited, particularly for generics); consult specific product labeling.

Solution, Injection:
- Generic: 50 mg/mL (1 mL)

Tablet, Oral:
- Dramamine: 50 mg
- Dramamine: 50 mg [scored]
- Driminate: 50 mg [scored]
- Motion Sickness: 50 mg
- Motion Sickness: 50 mg [scored]
- Generic: 50 mg

Tablet Chewable, Oral:
  Dramamine: 50 mg [contains aspartame, fd&c yellow #6 aluminum lake]
  Dramamine: 50 mg [scored; contains aspartame, fd&c yellow #6 aluminum lake]

◆ **Dimenhydrinate Injection (Can)** *see* DimenhyDRINATE *on page 616*

Dimercaprol (dye mer KAP role)

Brand Names: U.S. Bal in Oil

Index Terms 2,3-Dimercapto-1-Propanol; 2,3-Dimercapto-propan-1-Ol; 2,3-Dimercaptopropanol; BAL; British Anti-Lewisite; Dithioglycerol

Pharmacologic Category Antidote

Use Antidote to gold, arsenic (except arsine), or acute mercury poisoning (except nonalkyl mercury); adjunct to edetate CALCIUM disodium in acute lead poisoning

Pregnancy Risk Factor C

Pregnancy Considerations Animal reproduction studies have not been conducted. There are no adequate and well-controlled studies in pregnant women.

Lead poisoning: Lead is known to cross the placenta in amounts related to maternal plasma levels. Prenatal lead exposure may be associated with adverse events such as spontaneous abortion, preterm delivery, decreased birth weight, and impaired neurodevelopment. Some adverse outcomes may occur with maternal blood lead levels <10 mcg/dL. In addition, pregnant women exposed to lead may have an increased risk of gestational hypertension. Consider chelation therapy in pregnant women with confirmed blood lead levels ≥45 mcg/dL (pregnant women with blood lead levels ≥70 mcg/dL should be considered for chelation regardless of trimester); consultation with experts in lead poisoning and high-risk pregnancy is recommended. Encephalopathic pregnant women should be chelated regardless of trimester (CDC, 2010).

Breast-Feeding Considerations It is not known if dimercaprol is excreted in breast milk; however, it is not absorbed orally, which would limit the exposure to a nursing infant. When used for the treatment of lead poisoning, the amount of lead in breast milk may range from 0.6% to 3% of the maternal serum concentration. Women with confirmed blood lead levels ≥40 mcg/dL should not initiated breast-feeding; pumping and discarding breast milk is recommended until blood lead levels are <40 mcg/dL, at which point breast-feeding may resume (CDC, 2010). Calcium supplementation may reduce the amount of lead in breast milk.

Contraindications Hepatic insufficiency (unless due to arsenic poisoning)

Warnings/Precautions Potentially a nephrotoxic drug, use with caution in patients with oliguria; keep urine alkaline to protect the kidneys (prevents dimercaprol-metal complex breakdown). Discontinue or use with extreme caution if renal insufficiency develops during treatment. Hemodialysis may be used to remove dimercaprol-metal chelate in patients with renal dysfunction. Use with caution in patients with glucose 6-phosphate dehydrogenase deficiency; may increase the risk of hemolytic anemia. Administer all injections deep I.M. at different sites; **not** for I.V. administration. Fevers may occur in ~30% of children and may persistent for the duration of therapy. Product contains peanut oil; use caution in patients with peanut allergy; medication for the treatment of hypersensitivity reactions should be available for immediate use. When used in the treatment of lead poisoning, investigate, identify, and remove sources of lead exposure prior to treatment; do not permit patients to re-enter the contaminated environment until lead abatement has been completed. Primary care providers should consult experts in the chemotherapy of heavy metal toxicity before using chelation drug therapy. Dimercaprol is not indicated for the treatment of iron, cadmium, or selenium poisoning; use in these patients may result in toxic dimercaprol-metal complexes.

Adverse Reactions
Frequency not always defined.
Cardiovascular: Chest pain, hypertension (dose related), tachycardia (dose related)
Central nervous system: Anxiety, fever (children ~30%), headache, nervousness
Dermatologic: Abscess
Gastrointestinal: Abdominal pain, burning sensation (lips, mouth, throat), nausea, salivation, throat irritation/pain, vomiting
Genitourinary: Burning sensation (penis)
Hematologic: Leukopenia (polymorphonuclear)
Local: Injection site pain
Neuromuscular & skeletal: Paresthesias (hand), weakness
Ocular: Blepharospasm, conjunctivitis, lacrimation
Renal: Acute renal insufficiency
Respiratory: Rhinorrhea, throat constriction
Miscellaneous: Diaphoresis

Drug Interactions

Metabolism/Transport Effects None known.

Avoid Concomitant Use

Avoid concomitant use of Dimercaprol with any of the following: Iron Salts; Multivitamins/Minerals (with ADEK, Folate, Iron)

Increased Effect/Toxicity

Dimercaprol may increase the levels/effects of: Iron Salts; Multivitamins/Minerals (with ADEK, Folate, Iron)

Decreased Effect There are no known significant interactions involving a decrease in effect.

Storage/Stability Store at 20°C to 25°C (68°F to 77°F).

Mechanism of Action Sulfhydryl group combines with ions of various heavy metals to form relatively stable, nontoxic, soluble chelates which are excreted in urine

Pharmacodynamics/Kinetics
Absorption: I.M.: Rapid; Oral: Not absorbed
Distribution: To all tissues including the brain
Metabolism: Hepatic; rapid to inactive metabolites
Time to peak, serum: 0.5-1 hour
Excretion: Urine

Dosage Note: Premedication with a histamine H_1 antagonist (eg, diphenhydramine) is recommended.

Children and Adults: Deep I.M.:
  Arsenic or gold poisoning (acute, mild): 2.5 mg/kg every 6 hours for 2 days, then every 12 hours for 1 day, followed by once daily for 10 days
  Arsenic or gold poisoning (acute, severe): 3 mg/kg every 4 hours for 2 days, then every 6 hours for 1 day, followed every 12 hours for 10 days
  Mercury poisoning (acute): 5 mg/kg initially, followed by 2.5 mg/kg 1-2 times/day for 10 days
  Lead poisoning: **Note:** For the treatment of high blood lead levels in children, the CDC recommends chelation treatment when blood lead levels are >45 mcg/dL (CDC, 2002); however, dimercaprol is only recommended for use (in combination with edetate CALCIUM disodium) in children whose blood lead levels are >70 mcg/dL or in children with lead encephalopathy (AAP, 2005; Chandran, 2010). In adults, available guidelines recommend chelation therapy with blood lead levels >50 mcg/dL and significant symptoms; chelation therapy may also be indicated with blood lead levels ≥100 mcg/dL and/or symptoms (Kosnett, 2007).
    Blood lead levels ≥70 mcg/dL, symptomatic lead poisoning, or lead encephalopathy (in conjunction with edetate CALCIUM disodium): 4 mg/kg every 4 hours for 2-7 days; duration of therapy of at least 3 days is recommended by some experts (Chandran, 2010). **Note:** Begin treatment with edetate CALCIUM disodium with the second dimercaprol dose.

Dosage adjustment in renal impairment: No specific adjustment provided in manufacturer's labeling. Use with extreme caution or discontinue if acute renal insufficiency develops during therapy.

Dosage adjustment in hepatic impairment: Use is contraindicated in hepatic insufficiency (except in cases of postarsenical jaundice).

Administration Administer all injections by deep I.M. injection. Rotate injection sites. Keep urine alkaline to protect renal function. When used in the treatment of lead poisoning, administer in a separate site from edetate CALCIUM disodium.

Monitoring Parameters Renal function, urine pH, infusion-related reactions

For lead poisoning: Blood lead levels (baseline and 7-21 days after completing chelation therapy); hemoglobin or hematocrit, iron status, free erythrocyte protoporphyrin or zinc protoporphyrin; neurodevelopmental changes

For arsenic poisoning: Urine arsenic concentration

Test Interactions Iodine I^{131} thyroidal uptake values may be decreased

Dosage Forms Excipient information presented when available (limited, particularly for generics); consult specific product labeling.

Solution, Intramuscular:

Bal in Oil: 100 mg/mL (3 mL) [contains benzyl benzoate, peanut oil]

◆ **2,3-Dimercapto-1-Propanol** *see* Dimercaprol *on page 617*

◆ **2,3-Dimercaptopropan-1-Ol** *see* Dimercaprol *on page 617*

◆ **2,3-Dimercaptopropanol** *see* Dimercaprol *on page 617*

◆ **Dimetapp® Children's Long Acting Cough Plus Cold [OTC]** *see* Dextromethorphan and Chlorpheniramine *on page 591*

◆ **Dimetapp® Children's Nighttime Cold & Congestion [OTC]** *see* Diphenhydramine and Phenylephrine *on page 625*

Dimethyl Fumarate (dye meth il FYOO ma rate)

Brand Names: U.S. Tecfidera

Brand Names: Canada Tecfidera

Index Terms BG-12; Dimethylfumarate; DMF; FAG-201

Pharmacologic Category Fumaric Acid Derivative; Immunomodulator, Systemic

Use Treatment of relapsing forms of multiple sclerosis (MS)

Pregnancy Risk Factor C

Pregnancy Considerations Adverse events were observed in animal reproduction studies.

Women exposed to dimethyl fumarate during pregnancy are encouraged to enroll in the Pregnancy Registry by calling 800-456-2255.

Breast-Feeding Considerations It is not known if dimethyl fumarate is excreted into breast milk. The manufacturer recommends caution be used if administered to nursing women.

Contraindications There are no contraindications listed within the manufacturer's U.S. product labeling.

Canadian labeling: Hypersensitivity to dimethyl fumarate or any component of the formulation.

Warnings/Precautions Decreased lymphocyte counts may occur with use. Prior to initiation, a recent CBC (within 6 months) should be reviewed to identify patients with pre-existing low lymphocyte counts. Obtain CBC at least annually (or more frequently if indicated) during use. In trials, mean lymphocyte counts decreased ~30% over the first year of therapy (then stabilized), and lymphocyte counts increased (but did not return to baseline) 4 weeks following discontinuation. No difference in incidence of infection or series infections has been observed in treated patients when compared to placebo; consider temporarily discontinuing therapy in patients with serious infections. Canadian labeling recommends treatment not be initiated in patients with signs/symptoms of a serious infection. Has not been studied in patients with pre-existing low lymphocyte counts.

Use commonly causes GI events (eg, nausea, vomiting, diarrhea, abdominal pain, dyspepsia) and mild-to-moderate flushing (eg, warmth, redness, itching, burning sensation). GI events generally occur in the first month of use and decrease thereafter. To improve tolerability the Canadian labeling recommends administering with food or temporarily reducing the dosage. Flushing generally appears soon after initiation, and improves or resolves with subsequent dosing. Administration with food may decrease flushing incidence. The Canadian labeling suggests that a temporary dosage reduction or short-term (≤4 days) administration of aspirin (nonenteric coated) 30 minutes prior to dimethyl fumarate may also reduce the incidence and severity of flushing. Use of aspirin >4 days has not been studied; long-term use of aspirin is not recommended.

Transaminase elevations (usually <3 times ULN) were observed, generally occurring in the first 6 months of treatment. Use may cause rash, pruritus, or erythema. There are case reports of contact dermatitis resulting from dimethyl fumarate (DMF) exposure after use as a fungicide and desiccant in the shipping of furniture (Bruze, 2011; Giménez-Arnau, 2011; Ropper, 2012). In clinical trials, proteinuria was reported at a slightly higher incidence than that observed with placebo; significance of these findings is unknown. Canadian labeling does not recommend administration of live attenuated vaccines during therapy (has not been studied).

Adverse Reactions

>10%:

- Cardiovascular: Flushing (40%)
- Gastrointestinal: Abdominal pain (18%), diarrhea (14%), nausea (12%)
- Infection: Infection (60%; placebo: 58%)

1% to 10%:

- Dermatologic: Pruritus (8%), skin rash (8%), erythema (5%)
- Gastrointestinal: Vomiting (9%), dyspepsia (5%)
- Genitourinary: Proteinuria (6%)
- Hematologic: Lymphocytopenia (2% to 6%)
- Hepatic: Increased serum AST (4%)

<1% (Limited to important or life-threatening: Eosinophilia (transient)

Drug Interactions

Metabolism/Transport Effects None known.

Avoid Concomitant Use There are no known interactions where it is recommended to avoid concomitant use.

Increased Effect/Toxicity

Dimethyl Fumarate may increase the levels/effects of: Vaccines (Live)

Decreased Effect

Dimethyl Fumarate may decrease the levels/effects of: Vaccines (Live)

Storage/Stability Store at 15°C to 30°C (50°F to 86°F). Protect capsules from light and store in the original container. Once opened, discard after 90 days.

Mechanism of Action DMF and its active metabolite, monomethyl fumarate (MMF), have been shown to activate the nuclear factor (erythyroid-derived 2)-like 2 (Nrf2) pathway, which is involved in cellular response to oxidative stress. The mechanism by which dimethyl fumarate (DMF) exerts a therapeutic effect in MS is unknown, although it is believed to result from its anti-inflammatory and cytoprotective properties via activation of the Nrf2 pathway (Fox, 2012; Gold, 2012).

Pharmacodynamics/Kinetics

Distribution: V_d: MMF: 53-73 L

Protein binding: MMF: 27% to 45%

Metabolism: Undergoes rapid and extensive presystemic hydrolysis by esterases to its active metabolite, monomethyl fumarate (MMF); MMF is further metabolized via the tricarboxylic acid (TCA) cycle with no CYP involvement in metabolism. Major serum metabolites include: MMF, fumaric acid, citric acid, and glucose.

Half-life elimination: MMF: ~1 hour

Time to peak: 2-2.5 hours

Excretion: CO_2 via exhalation (~60%); urine (16%; trace amounts as unchanged MMF), feces (1%)

Dosage Multiple sclerosis (relapsing): Adults: Oral: Initial: 120 mg twice daily for 7 days; then increase to the maintenance dose: 240 mg twice daily

Dosing adjustment for toxicity:

U.S. labeling: Serious infection: Consider withholding treatment until infection resolves.

Canadian labeling:

Flushing or GI intolerance: Consider temporary dose reduction to 120 mg twice daily (resume recommended dose of 240 mg twice daily within 1 month)

Serious infection: Consider withholding treatment until infection resolves.

Dosing adjustment in renal impairment: No dosage adjustment necessary.

Dosing adjustment in hepatic impairment: No dosage adjustment necessary.

Dietary Considerations May take with or without food; taking with food may decrease the incidence of flushing.

Administration Swallow capsules whole (delayed release); do not crush, chew, open the capsule, or sprinkle contents on food. May administer orally with or without food however administering with food may decrease the incidence of flushing. Canadian labeling suggests that short-term (≤4 days) administration of aspirin (non-enteric coated) 30 minutes prior to dimethyl fumarate may reduce the incidence and severity of flushing. Missed doses may be taken if ≥4 hours lapse between the morning and evening doses.

Monitoring Parameters CBC (obtained within 6 months prior to use, then at least annually during therapy or as clinically necessary)

Canadian labeling recommends obtaining a CBC, hepatic transaminases, and a urinalysis within 6 months prior to use, after 6 months of therapy, then every 6-12 months during therapy and as clinically indicated.

Additional Information Dimethyl fumarate (DMF) has been implicated as the cause of an outbreak of contact dermatitis in Europe resulting from DMF's use as a fungicide and desiccant in the shipping of furniture (Bruze, 2011; Giménez-Arnau, 2011; Ropper, 2012); may be irritating to mucous membranes (do not crush, chew, or open capsule).

Dosage Forms Excipient information presented when available (limited, particularly for generics); consult specific product labeling.

Capsule Delayed Release, Oral:

Tecfidera: 120 mg, 240 mg [contains brilliant blue fcf (fd&c blue #1)]

Miscellaneous, Oral:

Tecfidera: Capsule, delayed release: 120 mg (14s) and Capsule, delayed release: 240 mg (46s) (60 ea) [contains brilliant blue fcf (fd&c blue #1)]

◆ **Dimethylfumarate** *see* Dimethyl Fumarate *on page 618*

◆ **Dimethyl Triazeno Imidazole Carboxamide** *see* Dacarbazine *on page 530*

◆ **Dinate® [OTC] (Can)** *see* DimenhyDRINATE *on page 616*

Dinoprostone (dye noe PROST one)

Brand Names: U.S. Cervidil; Prepidil; Prostin E2

Brand Names: Canada Cervidil®; Prepidil®; Prostin E_2®

Index Terms PGE_2; Prostaglandin E_2

Pharmacologic Category Abortifacient; Prostaglandin

Use

Endocervical gel (Prepidil®): Promote cervical ripening in patients at or near term in whom there is a medical or obstetrical indication for the induction of labor

Suppositories (Prostin E_2®): Terminate pregnancy from 12th through 20th week of gestation; evacuate uterus in cases of missed abortion or intrauterine fetal death up to 28 weeks of gestation; manage benign hydatidiform mole (nonmetastatic gestational trophoblastic disease)

Tablet (oral) (Prostin E_2®; Canadian availability): Elective induction of labor; when indications for induction of labor exist (eg, premature rupture of amniotic membranes, toxemia of pregnancy, Rh incompatibility, diabetes mellitus, hypertension, postmaturity, intrauterine death or fetal growth retardation)

Vaginal gel (Prostin E_2®; Canadian availability): Induction of labor in patients at or near term with singleton pregnancy, vertex presentation, and favorable induction features

Vaginal insert (Cervidil®): Initiation and/or continuation of cervical ripening in patients at or near term in whom there is a medical or obstetrical indication for the induction of labor

Pregnancy Risk Factor C

Pregnancy Considerations Skeletal anomalies and embryotoxicity have been observed in animal reproduction studies. Although these effects would not be expected in humans when administered after the period of organogenesis, a sustained increase in uterine tone may have increased risks of adverse events to the fetus.

Fetal distress without corresponding maternal uterine hyperstimulation was observed in 3% to 4% of infants exposed to Cervidil® *in utero.* No adverse effects on physical or psychomotor function were observed in a 3 year follow-up study of exposed infants. Abnormal fetal heart rates were observed in 17% of infants exposed to Prepidil® gel *in utero.* Deceleration, intrauterine fetal sepsis, fetal depression and fetal acidosis have also been reported with administration of the endocervical gel. Still births, abnormal fetal heart rate and fetal distress have been reported with administration of Prostin E_2® vaginal gel and oral tablets (Canadian availability).

When used for termination of pregnancy, dinoprostone is not considered feticidal, but is used to terminate pregnancy due to its ability to stimulate uterine contractions; do not use if fetus has reached the stage of viability.

Breast-Feeding Considerations Endogenous PGE_2 can be detected in breast milk. High levels have been associated with diarrhea in nursing infants.

Contraindications Generally, labor induction is contraindicated whenever spontaneous labor or vaginal delivery is contraindicated (ACOG 2009); manufacturer specific contraindications are listed by dosage form.

All dosage forms: Hypersensitivity to prostaglandins or any component of the formulation

Endocervical gel: Patients in whom oxytocic drugs are contraindicated; history of cesarean section or major uterine surgery; presence of cephalopelvic disproportion; fetal distress when delivery is not imminent; unexplained vaginal bleeding during this pregnancy; history of difficult labor and/or traumatic delivery; ≥6 previous term pregnancies with nonvertex presentation; hyperactive or hypertonic uterine patterns; obstetric emergencies when surgical intervention would be favorable; placenta previa; when vaginal delivery is not indicated (eg, vasa previa, active herpes genitalia)

Canadian labeling: Additional contraindications (not in U.S. labeling): History of epilepsy; fetal malpresentation; overdistention of the uterus (multiple pregnancies, polyhydramnios); ruptured amniotic membranes or suspected chorioamnionitis

Suppository: Acute pelvic inflammatory disease; active cardiac, pulmonary, renal, or hepatic disease

Tablet (oral) (Canadian availability; not available in the U.S.): Active cardiac, pulmonary, renal or hepatic disease; simultaneous use with other oxytocics; history of cesarean section or major uterine surgery; presence of cephalopelvic disproportion; history of difficult labor and/or traumatic delivery; ≥6 pregnancies; suspected or clinically evident pre-existing fetal distress; overdistention of the uterus (multiple pregnancy, polyhydramnios); pre-existing uterine hypertonus; situations where a responsible physician is unavailable; engagement of head not taken place; unexplained vaginal bleeding during this pregnancy; fetal malpresentation; gynecological, obstetrical or medical conditions that preclude vaginal delivery; pregnancy complicated by abnormal position of the placenta or umbilical cord; history of or existing pelvic inflammatory disease unless adequately treated

Vaginal gel (Canadian availability; not available in the U.S.): Active cardiac, pulmonary, renal or hepatic disease; simultaneous use with other oxytocics; history of cesarean section or major uterine surgery; presence of cephalopelvic disproportion; history of difficult labor and/or traumatic delivery; ≥6 term pregnancies; suspected or clinically evident pre-existing fetal distress; overdistention of the uterus (multiple pregnancy, polyhydramnios); pre-existing uterine hypertonus; situations where a responsible physician is unavailable; engagement of head not taken place; unexplained vaginal bleeding during this pregnancy; fetal malpresentation; gynecological, obstetrical or medical conditions that preclude vaginal delivery; pregnancy complicated by abnormal position of the placenta or umbilical cord; history of or existing pelvic inflammatory disease unless adequately treated; ruptured amniotic membranes or suspected chorioamnionitis

Vaginal insert: Patients in whom oxytocic drugs are contraindicated; history of cesarean section or major uterine surgery; presence of cephalopelvic disproportion; fetal distress when delivery is not imminent; unexplained vaginal bleeding during this pregnancy; patients already receiving I.V. oxytocic drugs; ≥6 previous term pregnancies

Canadian labeling: Additional contraindications (not in U.S. labeling): Placenta previa; history of difficult labor and/or traumatic delivery; overdistention of the uterus (multiple pregnancies, polyhydramnios); fetal malpresentation; history of uncontrolled epilepsy; history of or existing pelvic inflammatory disease unless adequately treated

Warnings/Precautions Hazardous agent - use appropriate precautions for handling and disposal (NIOSH, 2012).

[U.S. Boxed Warning]: Dinoprostone should be used only by medically-trained personnel in a hospital.

Postpartum DIC has been reported following dinoprostone for labor induction. Risk may be increased in women ≥30 years of age, gestation age >40 weeks, or women with pregnancy complications. Use caution in patients with hepatic or renal impairment. Intracervical placement of endocervical gel, vaginal gel or vaginal insert may lead to anaphylactoid syndrome of pregnancy (rare). Use with caution in patients with asthma or glaucoma. Use with caution in patients with cardiovascular or pulmonary disease and renal or hepatic impairment (manufacturer labeling for some dosage forms (eg, suppository, tablet, vaginal gel) contraindicate use in these patients. Use with caution in patients with epilepsy; Canadian labeling (depending on dosage form) either contraindicates use in patients with epilepsy or recommends avoiding use unless seizures are adequately controlled.

Endocervical gel: Use caution with ruptured membranes.

Vaginal gel: Canadian availability (not available in U.S.): Intended for intravaginal use only and is not for intracervical use; improper placement of gel may lead to uterine hyperstimulation or to anaphylactoid syndrome of pregnancy (rare). Avoid use in patients with uncontrolled epilepsy.

Vaginal insert: Use caution with ruptured membranes; nonvertex or nonsingleton pregnancy; previous uterine hypertony. Must be removed prior to administration of oxytocin, in case of hyperstimulation or if labor begins, fetal distress, maternal distress (eg, hypotension, nausea, tachycardia, vomiting), and prior to amniotomy.

Suppository: Transient pyrexia and decreased blood pressure may be observed with treatment. Use caution with history of hypotension or hypertension, anemia, jaundice, diabetes, compromised uteri, cervicitis, endocervical infections or acute vaginitis. Measures should be taken to ensure complete abortion. Commercially available suppositories should not be used for extemporaneous preparation of any other dosage form of drug. Do not use for cervical ripening or other indications in patients with term pregnancy.

Adverse Reactions

Endocervical gel:

1% to 10%:

- Central nervous system: Fever (1%)
- Gastrointestinal: GI upset (6%)
- Genitourinary: Abnormal uterine contractions (7%), warm feeling in vagina (2%)
- Neuromuscular & skeletal: Back pain (3%)

Postmarketing and/or case reports: Amnionitis, anaphylactoid syndrome of pregnancy (amniotic fluid embolism), postpartum DIC, premature rupture of membranes, uterine rupture (with intracervical administration)

Suppository:

Frequency not defined:

- Cardiovascular: Arrhythmia, chest pain, chest tightness, hypotension, syncope
- Central nervous system: Chills, dizziness, fever, headache, shivering, tension
- Dermatologic: Rash, skin discoloration
- Endocrine & metabolic: Breast tenderness, endometritis, hot flashes
- Gastrointestinal: Dehydration, diarrhea, nausea, vomiting
- Genitourinary: Uterine rupture, urinary retention, vaginal pain, vaginismus, vaginitis, vulvitis
- Neuromuscular & skeletal: Arthralgia, backache, joint inflammation/pain (new or exacerbated), leg cramps (nocturnal), muscle cramp/pain, myalgia, paresthesia, stiff neck, tremor, weakness
- Ocular: Blurred vision, eye pain
- Otic: Hearing impairment
- Respiratory: Cough, dyspnea, laryngitis, pharyngitis, wheezing
- Miscellaneous: Diaphoresis

Postmarketing and/or case reports: MI

Tablets (oral) (Canadian availability):

>10%: Gastrointestinal: Vomiting (with or without nausea/diarrhea): 21% to 50% (dose dependent)

1% to 10%: Genitourinary: Uterine hypertonus (3%)

<1%: Bronchospasm, chills, dizziness, dyspnea, fever, flushing, headache, hiccups, hyper-/hypotension, postpartum hemorrhage, rash, tachycardia

Frequency not defined:
Cardiovascular: Cardiac arrest
Central nervous system: Transient vasovagal symptoms
Genitourinary: Abnormal uterine contractions, placental abruption, rapid cervical dilation, uterine rupture
Neuromuscular & skeletal: Back pain
Respiratory: Asthma, pulmonary amniotic fluid embolism
Miscellaneous: Hypersensitivity reactions including anaphylaxis, anaphylactic shock, and nonimmunologic anaphylaxis (formerly known as anaphylactoid reaction)
Postmarketing and/or case reports: DIC

Vaginal gel (Canadian availability):
1% to 10%: Genitourinary: Uterine hypercontractility (3%), failed induction (2%)
Frequency not defined:
Cardiovascular: Cardiac arrest
Central nervous system: Fever
Gastrointestinal: Diarrhea, nausea, vomiting
Genitourinary: Abnormal uterine contractions, uterine rupture, warm feeling in vagina
Neuromuscular & skeletal: Back pain
Miscellaneous: Hypersensitivity reactions including anaphylaxis, anaphylactic shock, and nonimmunologic anaphylaxis (formerly known as anaphylactoid reaction)
Postmarketing and/or case reports: DIC

Vaginal insert:
1% to 10%: Genitourinary: Uterine hyperstimulation *without* fetal distress (2% to 5%), uterine hyperstimulation *with* fetal distress (3%)
<1% (Limited to important or life-threatening): Anaphylactoid syndrome of pregnancy (amniotic fluid embolism), postpartum DIC, hypersensitivity reactions, hypotension, uterine rupture

Drug Interactions

Metabolism/Transport Effects None known.

Avoid Concomitant Use

Avoid concomitant use of Dinoprostone with any of the following: Carbetocin

Increased Effect/Toxicity

Dinoprostone may increase the levels/effects of: Carbetocin; Oxytocin

Decreased Effect There are no known significant interactions involving a decrease in effect.

Storage/Stability

Endocervical gel should be stored under refrigeration at 2°C to 8°C (36°F to 46°F).
Suppositories must be kept frozen; store in freezer not above -20°C (-4°F).
Tablets (oral) (Canadian availability): Store under refrigeration at 2°C to 8°C (36°F to 46°F). Discard unused tablets 90 days after bottle is opened.
Vaginal gel (Canadian availability): Store under refrigeration at 2°C to 8°C (36°F to 46°F).
Vaginal insert should be stored in freezer between -20°C and -10°C (-4°F and 14°F).

Mechanism of Action Dinoprostone (prostaglandin E_2) is an endogenous hormone found in low concentrations in most tissues of the body. When administered as an abortifacient, it stimulates uterine contractions similar to those seen during natural labor. When administered for labor induction, it relaxes the smooth muscle of the cervix allowing dilation and passage of the fetus through the birth canal.

Pharmacodynamics/Kinetics

Onset of action (uterine contractions): Vaginal suppository: Within 10 minutes
Duration: Vaginal insert: 0.3 mg/hour over 12 hours; Vaginal suppository: Up to 2-3 hours
Absorption: Vaginal suppository: Slow
Metabolism: Metabolized in the lungs; forms metabolites which are further metabolized in the liver and kidney
Half-life elimination: 2.5-5 minutes
Time to peak, plasma: Endocervical gel: 30-45 minutes
Excretion: Primarily urine; feces (small amounts)

Dosage Females of reproductive age:

Abortifacient: Vaginal suppository: Insert 20 mg (1 suppository) high in vagina, repeat at 3- to 5-hour intervals until abortion occurs; continued administration for longer than 2 days is not advisable

Cervical ripening:

Endocervical gel: Using catheter supplied with gel, insert 0.5 mg into the cervical canal. May repeat every 6 hours if needed. Maximum cumulative dose: 1.5 mg/24 hours

Tablet (oral) (Canadian availability):

Induction: Initial: 0.5 mg and then repeat 0.5 mg dose 1 hour later; may give additional 0.5 mg dose on an hourly basis as needed for satisfactory uterine response. Maintain patient at the lowest effective dose. **Note:** Failure to induce regular contractions after 8 hours indicates failed induction and alternative management of patient should be considered. If patient vomits an intact tablet during therapy repeat dose. If patient vomits intact tablets following 2 successive doses, withhold therapy until next scheduled dose. If patient vomits a partial tablet or if no tablet is visible, continue at next regularly scheduled dose.

Parity ≥2 times or Bishop Score of ≥6: Administer 0.5 mg hourly throughout induction (discontinue hourly dose for excessive uterine activity)

Nulliparous or multiparous and resistant to induction (Bishop Score <6): If inadequate response after 2 hours of therapy may increase dose in 0.5 mg increments at hourly intervals up to a maximum single dose of 1.5 mg.

Maintenance of labor: 0.5 mg dose hourly; may occasionally withhold hourly dose to assess need for further dosing

Vaginal gel (Canadian labeling): Initial: Using prefilled syringe, insert 1 mg into the posterior fornix of the vaginal canal; may give 1 additional dose of 1-2 mg 6 hours later if needed.

Vaginal insert: Insert 10 mg transversely into the posterior fornix of the vagina (to be removed at the onset of active labor or after 12 hours)

Administration

Endocervical gel: Bring to room temperature just prior to use. Do not force the warming process (eg, water bath, microwave). Avoid contact with skin while handling; wash hands thoroughly with soap and water after administration. For cervical ripening, patient should be supine in the dorsal position. The appropriate catheter length should be based on degree of effacement; 20 mm for no effacement; 10 mm if 50% effaced. Patient should remain supine for 15-30 minutes following administration. The manufacturer recommends waiting 6-12 hours after dinoprostone gel administration before initiating oxytocin.

Tablet (oral) (Canadian availability): Administer with small amount of water. Use of oxytocin should be avoided until ≥1 hour after administration of the last oral tablet.

Vaginal gel: (Canadian availability): Using prefilled syringe, dose is placed in the posterior fornix of the vagina. Patient should remain in lateral or supine position for 30 minutes to prevent leakage. Syringe contains overfill. Syringe is for single use only. Use of oxytocin should be avoided for 12-24 hours after administration of vaginal gel.

Vaginal insert: One vaginal insert is placed transversely in the posterior fornix of the vagina immediately after removal from its foil package. Patients should remain in the recumbent position for 2 hours after insertion, but thereafter may be ambulatory. Do not use without retrieval system. Product does not need warmed prior to use. A water miscible lubricant may be used to facilitate insertion (avoid excessive use of lubricant).

Ensure complete removal of system at completion of therapy. The manufacturer recommends waiting ≥30 minutes after removing the dinoprostone vaginal insert before initiating oxytocin.

Vaginal suppository: Insert high into vagina after removal from its foil package. Bring to room temperature just prior to use. Patient should remain supine for 10 minutes following insertion.

Hazardous agent; use appropriate precautions for handling and disposal (NIOSH, 2012).

Monitoring Parameters

Gel, insert: Fetal heart rate, uterine activity, progression of cervical dilation and effacement

Suppository: Confirmation of fetal death

Dosage Forms Excipient information presented when available (limited, particularly for generics); consult specific product labeling.

Gel, Vaginal:
Prepidil: 0.5 mg/3 g (3 g)

Insert, Vaginal:
Cervidil: 10 mg (1 ea)

Suppository, Vaginal:
Prostin E2: 20 mg (5 ea)

Dosage Forms: Canada Excipient information presented when available (limited, particularly for generics); consult specific product labeling.

Gel, vaginal:
Prostin E_2®: 1 mg/3 g (3 g), 2 mg/3 g (3 g)

Tablet, oral:
Prostin E_2®: 0.5 mg [contains lactose]

◆ **Diocaine® (Can)** *see* Proparacaine *on page 1733*

◆ **Diocarpine (Can)** *see* Pilocarpine (Ophthalmic) *on page 1647*

◆ **Diochloram® (Can)** *see* Chloramphenicol *on page 405*

◆ **Diocto [OTC]** *see* Docusate *on page 644*

◆ **Dioctyl Calcium Sulfosuccinate** *see* Docusate *on page 644*

◆ **Dioctyl Sodium Sulfosuccinate** *see* Docusate *on page 644*

◆ **Diodex® (Can)** *see* Dexamethasone (Ophthalmic) *on page 583*

◆ **Diodoquin® (Can)** *see* Iodoquinol *on page 1109*

◆ **Diogent® (Can)** *see* Gentamicin (Ophthalmic) *on page 954*

◆ **Diomycin® (Can)** *see* Erythromycin (Ophthalmic) *on page 744*

◆ **Diopentolate® (Can)** *see* Cyclopentolate *on page 504*

◆ **Diopred® (Can)** *see* PrednisoLONE (Ophthalmic) *on page 1706*

◆ **Dioptic's Atropine Solution (Can)** *see* Atropine *on page 197*

◆ **Dioptimyd® (Can)** *see* Sulfacetamide and Prednisolone *on page 1957*

◆ **Dioptrol® (Can)** *see* Neomycin, Polymyxin B, and Dexamethasone *on page 1439*

◆ **Diosulf™ (Can)** *see* Sulfacetamide (Ophthalmic) *on page 1956*

◆ **Diotame [OTC]** *see* Bismuth *on page 260*

◆ **Diotrope® (Can)** *see* Tropicamide *on page 2132*

◆ **Diovan** *see* Valsartan *on page 2154*

◆ **Diovan HCT** *see* Valsartan and Hydrochlorothiazide *on page 2156*

◆ **Diovol® (Can)** *see* Aluminum Hydroxide and Magnesium Hydroxide *on page 90*

◆ **Diovol® Ex (Can)** *see* Aluminum Hydroxide and Magnesium Hydroxide *on page 90*

◆ **Diovol Plus® (Can)** *see* Aluminum Hydroxide, Magnesium Hydroxide, and Simethicone *on page 90*

◆ **Dipentum** *see* Olsalazine *on page 1500*

◆ **Dipentum® (Can)** *see* Olsalazine *on page 1500*

◆ **Diphen [OTC]** *see* DiphenhydrAMINE (Systemic) *on page 622*

◆ **Diphenhist [OTC]** *see* DiphenhydrAMINE (Systemic) *on page 622*

DiphenhydrAMINE (Systemic)

(dye fen HYE dra meen)

Brand Names: U.S. Aler-Dryl [OTC]; Allergy Relief Childrens [OTC]; Allergy Relief [OTC]; Altaryl [OTC]; Anti-Hist Allergy [OTC]; Anti-Hist [OTC]; Banophen [OTC]; Benadryl Allergy Childrens [OTC]; Benadryl Allergy [OTC]; Benadryl Dye-Free Allergy [OTC]; Benadryl [OTC]; Complete Allergy Medication [OTC]; Complete Allergy Relief [OTC]; Diphen [OTC]; Diphenhist [OTC]; Genahist [OTC]; Geri-Dryl [OTC]; Nighttime Sleep Aid [OTC]; Nytol Maximum Strength [OTC]; Nytol [OTC]; PediaCare Childrens Allergy [OTC]; Pharbedryl [OTC]; Q-Dryl [OTC]; Quenalin [OTC]; Scot-Tussin Allergy Relief [OTC]; Siladryl Allergy [OTC]; Silphen Cough [OTC]; Simply Allergy [OTC]; Simply Sleep [OTC]; Sleep Tabs [OTC]; Sominex Maximum Strength [OTC]; Sominex [OTC]; Tetra-Formula Nighttime Sleep [OTC]; Total Allergy Medicine [OTC]; Total Allergy [OTC]; Triaminic Cough/Runny Nose [OTC]; ZzzQuil [OTC]

Brand Names: Canada Allerdryl®; Allernix; Benadryl®; Nytol®; Nytol® Extra Strength; PMS-Diphenhydramine; Simply Sleep®; Sominex®

Index Terms Diphenhydramine Citrate; Diphenhydramine Hydrochloride; Diphenhydramine Tannate

Pharmacologic Category Ethanolamine Derivative; Histamine H_1 Antagonist; Histamine H_1 Antagonist, First Generation

Use Symptomatic relief of allergic symptoms caused by histamine release including nasal allergies and allergic dermatosis; adjunct to epinephrine in the treatment of anaphylaxis; nighttime sleep aid; prevention or treatment of motion sickness; antitussive; management of Parkinsonian syndrome including drug-induced extrapyramidal symptoms

Pregnancy Risk Factor B

Pregnancy Considerations Adverse events have not been observed in animal reproduction studies. Diphenhydramine crosses the placenta. Maternal diphenhydramine use has generally not resulted in an increased risk of birth defects; however, adverse events (withdrawal symptoms, respiratory depression) have been reported in newborns exposed to diphenhydramine *in utero*. Antihistamines are recommended for the treatment of rhinitis, urticaria, and pruritus with rash in pregnant women (although second generation antihistamines may be preferred). Antihistamines are not recommended for treatment of pruritus associated with intrahepatic cholestasis in pregnancy.

Breast-Feeding Considerations Diphenhydramine is excreted into breast milk; drowsiness has been reported in a breast-feeding infant. Premature infants and newborns have a higher risk of intolerance to antihistamines. Breast-feeding is contraindicated by the manufacturer. Antihistamines may decrease maternal serum prolactin concentrations when administered prior to the establishment of nursing.

Contraindications Hypersensitivity to diphenhydramine or any component of the formulation; acute asthma; neonates or premature infants; breast-feeding; use as a local anesthetic (injection)

Warnings/Precautions Causes sedation, caution must be used in performing tasks which require alertness (eg, operating machinery or driving). Sedative effects of CNS depressants or ethanol are potentiated. Antihistamines may cause excitation in young children. Use with caution in patients with angle-closure glaucoma, pyloroduodenal obstruction (including stenotic peptic ulcer), urinary tract obstruction (including bladder neck obstruction and symptomatic prostatic hyperplasia), asthma, hyperthyroidism, increased intraocular pressure, and cardiovascular disease (including hypertension and tachycardia). Some preparations contain soy protein; avoid use in patients with soy protein or peanut allergies. Some products may contain phenylalanine.

Oral products: In the elderly, avoid use of this potent anticholinergic agent due to increased risk of confusion, dry mouth, constipation, and other anticholinergic effects; clearance decreases in patients of advanced age; tolerance develops to hypnotic effects; when used for severe allergic reaction, use may be appropriate (Beers Criteria).

Self-medication (OTC use): Do not use with other products containing diphenhydramine, even ones used on the skin. Oral products are not for OTC use in children <6 years of age.

Adverse Reactions Frequency not defined.

Cardiovascular: Chest tightness, extrasystoles, hypotension, palpitation, tachycardia

Central nervous system: Chills, confusion, convulsion, disturbed coordination, dizziness, euphoria, excitation, fatigue, headache, insomnia, irritability, nervousness, paradoxical excitement, restlessness, sedation, sleepiness, vertigo

Endocrine & metabolic: Menstrual irregularities (early menses)

Gastrointestinal: Anorexia, constipation, diarrhea, dry mucous membranes, epigastric distress, nausea, throat tightness, vomiting, xerostomia

Genitourinary: Difficult urination, urinary frequency, urinary retention

Hematologic: Agranulocytosis, hemolytic anemia, thrombocytopenia

Neuromuscular & skeletal: Neuritis, paresthesia, tremor

Ocular: Blurred vision, diplopia

Otic: Labyrinthitis (acute), tinnitus

Respiratory: Nasal stuffiness, thickening of bronchial secretions, wheezing

Miscellaneous: Anaphylactic shock, diaphoresis

Drug Interactions

Metabolism/Transport Effects Inhibits CYP2D6 (moderate)

Avoid Concomitant Use

Avoid concomitant use of DiphenhydrAMINE (Systemic) with any of the following: Aclidinium; Azelastine (Nasal); Ipratropium (Oral Inhalation); Paraldehyde; Thioridazine; Tiotropium; Umeclidinium

Increased Effect/Toxicity

DiphenhydrAMINE (Systemic) may increase the levels/effects of: Alcohol (Ethyl); Analgesics (Opioid); Anticholinergics; ARIPiprazole; Azelastine (Nasal); Buprenorphine; CNS Depressants; CYP2D6 Substrates; Fesoterodine; Highest Risk QTc-Prolonging Agents; Hydrocodone; Methotrimeprazine; Metoprolol; Metyrosine; Mirtazapine; Moderate Risk QTc-Prolonging Agents; Nebivolol; Paraldehyde; Pramipexole; ROPINIRole; Rotigotine; Selective Serotonin Reuptake Inhibitors; Thioridazine; Tiotropium; Zolpidem

The levels/effects of DiphenhydrAMINE (Systemic) may be increased by: Aclidinium; Brimonidine (Topical); Doxylamine; Droperidol; HydrOXYzine; Ipratropium (Oral Inhalation); Magnesium Sulfate; Methotrimeprazine; Mifepristone; Perampanel; Pramlintide; Propafenone; Sodium Oxybate; Tapentadol; Umeclidinium

Decreased Effect

DiphenhydrAMINE (Systemic) may decrease the levels/effects of: Acetylcholinesterase Inhibitors (Central); Benzylpenicilloyl Polylysine; Betahistine; Codeine; Hyaluronidase; Tamoxifen; TraMADol

The levels/effects of DiphenhydrAMINE (Systemic) may be decreased by: Acetylcholinesterase Inhibitors (Central); Amphetamines

Ethanol/Nutrition/Herb Interactions

Ethanol: May increase CNS depression; monitor for increased effects with coadministration. Caution patients about effects.

Herb/Nutraceutical: Avoid valerian, St John's wort, kava kava, gotu kola (may increase CNS depression).

Storage/Stability Injection: Store at room temperature of 15°C to 30°C (59°F to 86°F); protect from freezing. Protect from light.

Mechanism of Action Competes with histamine for H_1-receptor sites on effector cells in the gastrointestinal tract, blood vessels, and respiratory tract; anticholinergic and sedative effects are also seen

Pharmacodynamics/Kinetics

Duration:

Histamine-induced wheal suppression: ≤10 hours (Simons, 1990)

Histamine-induced flare suppression: ≤12 hours (Simons, 1990)

Distribution: V_d: Children: 22 L/kg (range: 15-28 L/kg); Adults: 17 L/kg (range: 13-20 L/kg); Elderly: 14 L/kg (range: 7-20 L/kg) (Blyden, 1986; Simons, 1990)

Protein binding: 98.5% (Vozeh, 1988)

Metabolism: Extensively hepatic n-demethylation via CYP2D6; minor demethylation via CYP1A2, 2C9 and 2C19; smaller degrees in pulmonary and renal systems; significant first-pass effect (Akutsu, 2007)

Bioavailability: 42% to 62% (Paton, 1985)

Half-life elimination: Children: 5 hours (range: 4-7 hours); Adults: 9 hours (range: 7-12 hours); Elderly: 13.5 hours (range: 9-18 hours) (Blyden, 1986; Simons, 1990)

Time to peak, serum: ~2 hours (Blyden, 1986; Simons, 1990)

Excretion: Urine (as metabolites and unchanged drug) (Albert, 1975; Maurer, 1988)

Dosage Note: Dosages are expressed as the hydrochloride salt.

Children:

Allergic reactions or motion sickness: Oral, I.M., I.V.: 5 mg/kg/day or 150 mg/m²/day in divided doses every 6-8 hours, not to exceed 300 mg/day

Alternate dosing by age: Oral:

2 to <6 years: 6.25 mg every 4-6 hours; maximum: 37.5 mg/day

6 to <12 years: 12.5-25 mg every 4-6 hours; maximum: 150 mg/day

≥12 years: 25-50 mg every 4-6 hours; maximum: 300 mg/day

Night-time sleep aid: Oral: Children ≥12 years: 50 mg at bedtime

Antitussive: Oral:

2 to <6 years: 6.25 mg every 4 hours; maximum: 37.5 mg/day

6 to <12 years: 12.5 mg every 4 hours; maximum: 75 mg/day

≥12 years: 25 mg every 4 hours; maximum: 150 mg/day

Treatment of dystonic reactions: I.M., I.V.: 0.5-1 mg/kg/dose

Adults:

Allergic reactions or motion sickness: Oral: 25-50 mg every 6-8 hours

Antitussive: Oral: 25 mg every 4 hours; maximum: 150 mg/24 hours

Night-time sleep aid: Oral: 50 mg at bedtime

Allergic reactions or motion sickness: I.M., I.V.: 10-50 mg per dose; single doses up to 100 mg may be used if needed; not to exceed 400 mg/day

Dystonic reaction: I.M., I.V.: 50 mg in a single dose; may repeat in 20-30 minutes if necessary

Elderly: Initial: 25 mg 2-3 times/day increasing as needed

Dietary Considerations Some products may contain sodium and/or phenylalanine.

Administration When used to prevent motion sickness, first dose should be given 30 minutes prior to exposure. Injection solution is for I.V. or I.M. administration only; local necrosis may result with SubQ or intradermal use. For I.V. administration, inject at a rate ≤25 mg/minute.

Monitoring Parameters Relief of symptoms, mental alertness

Test Interactions May interfere with urine detection of methadone and PCP (false-positives); may cause false-positive serum TCA screen; may suppress the wheal and flare reactions to skin test antigens

Additional Information Diphenhydramine citrate 19 mg is equivalent to diphenhydramine hydrochloride 12.5 mg

Dosage Forms Excipient information presented when available (limited, particularly for generics); consult specific product labeling.

Capsule, Oral, as hydrochloride:

Allergy Relief: 25 mg [contains brilliant blue fcf (fd&c blue #1), butylparaben, edetate calcium disodium, fd&c blue #2 (indigotine), fd&c red #40, fd&c yellow #10 (quinoline yellow), methylparaben, polysorbate 80, propylparaben]

Anti-Hist: 25 mg

Banophen: 25 mg [contains brilliant blue fcf (fd&c blue #1), fd&c red #40, fd&c yellow #6 (sunset yellow), methylparaben, propylparaben]

Banophen: 50 mg [contains brilliant blue fcf (fd&c blue #1), fd&c red #40]

Benadryl: 25 mg

Benadryl Allergy: 25 mg [dye free]

Benadryl Dye-Free Allergy: 25 mg [dye free]

Diphenhist: 25 mg [contains brilliant blue fcf (fd&c blue #1), butylparaben, fd&c red #40, methylparaben, propylparaben]

Genahist: 25 mg

Geri-Dryl: 25 mg

Pharbedryl: 25 mg, 50 mg [contains brilliant blue fcf (fd&c blue #1), fd&c red #40]

Q-Dryl: 25 mg [contains brilliant blue fcf (fd&c blue #1), butylparaben, fd&c red #40, methylparaben, propylparaben]

ZzzQuil: 25 mg [contains brilliant blue fcf (fd&c blue #1), fd&c red #40]

Generic: 25 mg, 50 mg

Elixir, Oral, as hydrochloride:

Altaryl: 12.5 mg/5 mL (120 mL, 480 mL, 3840 mL) [contains alcohol, usp]

Generic: 12.5 mg/5 mL (5 mL, 10 mL)

Liquid, Oral, as hydrochloride:

Allergy Relief Childrens: 12.5 mg/5 mL (118 mL, 480 mL) [alcohol free; contains fd&c red #40, sodium benzoate]

Banophen: 12.5 mg/5 mL (118 mL) [alcohol free; cherry flavor]

Banophen: 12.5 mg/5 mL (473 mL) [alcohol free, sugar free; cherry flavor]

Benadryl Allergy Childrens: 12.5 mg/5 mL (118 mL, 236 mL) [alcohol free; contains fd&c red #40, sodium benzoate]

Benadryl Allergy Childrens: 12.5 mg/5 mL (5 mL, 236 mL) [alcohol free; contains fd&c red #40, sodium benzoate; cherry flavor]

Benadryl Allergy Childrens: 12.5 mg/5 mL (118 mL) [alcohol free, dye free, sugar free; contains saccharin sodium, sodium benzoate]

Diphenhist: 12.5 mg/5 mL (118 mL, 473 mL) [alcohol free; contains fd&c red #40, saccharin sodium, sodium benzoate; fruit flavor]

PediaCare Childrens Allergy: 12.5 mg/5 mL (118 mL) [alcohol free; contains fd&c red #40, sodium benzoate]

Q-Dryl: 12.5 mg/5 mL (118 mL, 237 mL, 473 mL) [alcohol free; contains fd&c red #40, saccharin sodium, sodium benzoate; cherry flavor]

Scot-Tussin Allergy Relief: 12.5 mg/5 mL (118.3 mL, 240 mL, 480 mL, 3780 mL) [alcohol free, dye free, saccharin free, sodium free, sorbitol free, sugar free]

Siladryl Allergy: 12.5 mg/5 mL (118 mL, 237 mL, 473 mL) [alcohol free, sugar free; contains fd&c red #40, methylparaben, propylene glycol, propylparaben, saccharin sodium; cherry flavor]

Total Allergy Medicine: 12.5 mg/5 mL (118 mL) [alcohol free]

ZzzQuil: 50 mg/30 mL (177 mL, 354 mL) [contains alcohol, usp, brilliant blue fcf (fd&c blue #1), fd&c red #40, propylene glycol, saccharin sodium, sodium benzoate; berry flavor]

Solution, Injection, as hydrochloride:

Generic: 50 mg/mL (1 mL, 10 mL)

Solution, Injection, as hydrochloride [preservative free]:

Generic: 50 mg/mL (1 mL)

Strip, Oral, as hydrochloride:

Triaminic Cough/Runny Nose: 12.5 mg (14 ea) [contains alcohol, usp, brilliant blue fcf (fd&c blue #1), fd&c red #40]

Triaminic Cough/Runny Nose: 12.5 mg (16 ea) [contains alcohol, usp, brilliant blue fcf (fd&c blue #1), fd&c red #40; grape flavor]

Syrup, Oral, as hydrochloride:

Altaryl: 12.5 mg/5 mL (120 mL, 480 mL, 3785 mL) [alcohol free; cherry flavor]

Quenalin: 12.5 mg/5 mL (120 mL) [fruit flavor]

Silphen Cough: 12.5 mg/5 mL (118 mL, 237 mL, 473 mL) [contains alcohol, usp, fd&c red #40, menthol, methylparaben, propylene glycol, propylparaben; strawberry flavor]

Tablet, Oral, as hydrochloride:

Aler-Dryl: 50 mg

Allergy Relief: 25 mg [contains polysorbate 80]

Anti-Hist Allergy: 25 mg

Banophen: 25 mg

Benadryl: 25 mg

Benadryl Allergy: 25 mg

Benadryl Allergy: 25 mg [contains edetate calcium disodium, fd&c red #40, methylparaben, polysorbate 80, propylparaben]

Complete Allergy Medication: 25 mg

Complete Allergy Relief: 25 mg

Diphen: 25 mg

Diphenhist: 25 mg

Geri-Dryl: 25 mg

Nighttime Sleep Aid: 25 mg [contains fd&c blue #1 aluminum lake, fd&c blue #2 aluminum lake, polysorbate 80]

Nighttime Sleep Aid: 50 mg [contains fd&c blue #1 aluminum lake]

Nytol: 25 mg

Nytol Maximum Strength: 50 mg

Simply Allergy: 25 mg

Simply Sleep: 25 mg [contains brilliant blue fcf (fd&c blue #1)]

Sleep Tabs: 25 mg [scored; contains fd&c blue #1 aluminum lake]

Sominex: 25 mg [contains fd&c blue #1 aluminum lake]
Sominex Maximum Strength: 50 mg [contains fd&c blue #1 aluminum lake, polysorbate 80]
Tetra-Formula Nighttime Sleep: 50 mg [contains fd&c blue #1 aluminum lake]
Total Allergy: 25 mg
Generic: 25 mg

Tablet Chewable, Oral, as hydrochloride:
Benadryl Allergy Childrens: 12.5 mg [contains aspartame, fd&c blue #1 aluminum lake; cherry flavor]
Benadryl Allergy Childrens: 12.5 mg [contains aspartame, fd&c blue #1 aluminum lake; grape flavor]

◆ **Diphenhydramine and Acetaminophen** *see* Acetaminophen and Diphenhydramine *on page 32*

◆ **Diphenhydramine and ASA** *see* Aspirin and Diphenhydramine *on page 182*

◆ **Diphenhydramine and Aspirin** *see* Aspirin and Diphenhydramine *on page 182*

Diphenhydramine and Phenylephrine

(dye fen HYE dra meen & fen il EF rin)

Brand Names: U.S. Aldex® CT; Benadryl-D® Allergy & Sinus [OTC]; Benadryl-D® Children's Allergy & Sinus [OTC]; Dimetapp® Children's Nighttime Cold & Congestion [OTC]; Triaminic® Children's Night Time Cold & Cough [OTC]

Index Terms Diphenhydramine Hydrochloride and Phenylephrine Hydrochloride; Diphenhydramine Tannate and Phenylephrine Tannate; Phenylephrine and Diphenhydramine; Phenylephrine Hydrochloride and Diphenhydramine Hydrochloride; Phenylephrine Tannate and Diphenhydramine Tannate

Pharmacologic Category Alpha-Adrenergic Agonist; Decongestant; Ethanolamine Derivative; Histamine H_1 Antagonist; Histamine H_1 Antagonist, First Generation

Use Temporary relief of symptoms of allergic rhinitis, sinusitis, and other upper respiratory conditions, including sinus/nasal congestion, sneezing, stuffy/runny nose, itchy/watery eyes, and cough

Dosage Oral:

Aldex® CT:
Children 6-11 years: One-half to 1 tablet every 6 hours
Children ≥12 years and Adults: 1-2 tablets every 6 hours

OTC labeling:
Children <6 years: Use not recommended
Children 6-11 years:
Benadryl-D® Children's Allergy & Sinus: 5 mL every 4 hours as needed (maximum: 6 doses/24 hours)
Dimetapp® Children's Nighttime Cold and Congestion, Triaminic® Children's Night Time Cold & Cough: 10 mL every 4 hours as needed (maximum: 6 doses/24 hours)
Children ≥12 years and Adults: **Note:** General dosing guidelines; refer to specific product labeling:
10-20 mL every 4 hours as needed (maximum: 6 doses/24 hours) **or** 1 tablet every 4 hours as needed (maximum: 6 doses/24 hours)

Additional Information Complete prescribing information should be consulted for additional detail.

Dosage Forms Excipient information presented when available (limited, particularly for generics); consult specific product labeling.

Liquid, oral:
Benadryl-D® Children's Allergy & Sinus: Diphenhydramine hydrochloride 12.5 mg and phenylephrine hydrochloride 5 mg per 5 mL (118 mL) [ethanol free, sugar free; contains sodium 10 mg/5 mL, sodium benzoate; grape flavor]

Syrup, oral:
Dimetapp® Children's Nighttime Cold and Congestion: Diphenhydramine hydrochloride 6.25 mg and phenylephrine hydrochloride 2.5 mg per 5 mL (120 mL) [ethanol free, sugar free; contains propylene glycol, sodium 4 mg/5 mL, sodium benzoate; grape flavor]
Triaminic® Children's Night Time Cold & Cough: Diphenhydramine hydrochloride 6.25 mg and phenylephrine hydrochloride 2.5 mg per 5 mL (118 mL) [contains ethanol, propylene glycol, sodium 6 mg/5 mL; grape flavor]

Tablet, oral:
Benadryl-D® Allergy & Sinus: Diphenhydramine hydrochloride 25 mg and phenylephrine hydrochloride 10 mg

Tablet, chewable, oral:
Aldex® CT: Diphenhydramine hydrochloride 12.5 mg and phenylephrine hydrochloride 5 mg [contains phenylalanine; strawberry flavor]

◆ **Diphenhydramine Citrate** *see* DiphenhydrAMINE (Systemic) *on page 622*

◆ **Diphenhydramine Citrate and Aspirin** *see* Aspirin and Diphenhydramine *on page 182*

◆ **Diphenhydramine Hydrochloride** *see* DiphenhydrAMINE (Systemic) *on page 622*

◆ **Diphenhydramine Hydrochloride and Phenylephrine Hydrochloride** *see* Diphenhydramine and Phenylephrine *on page 625*

◆ **Diphenhydramine Tannate** *see* DiphenhydrAMINE (Systemic) *on page 622*

◆ **Diphenhydramine Tannate and Phenylephrine Tannate** *see* Diphenhydramine and Phenylephrine *on page 625*

Diphenoxylate and Atropine

(dye fen OKS i late & A troe peen)

Brand Names: U.S. Lomotil®

Brand Names: Canada Lomotil®

Index Terms Atropine and Diphenoxylate

Pharmacologic Category Antidiarrheal

Use Treatment of diarrhea

Pregnancy Risk Factor C

Pregnancy Considerations Teratogenic effects were not noted in animal studies; decreased maternal weight, fertility and litter sizes were observed. There are no adequate and well-controlled studies in pregnant women.

Breast-Feeding Considerations Atropine is excreted in breast milk (refer to Atropine monograph); the manufacturer states that diphenoxylic acid may be excreted in breast milk.

Contraindications Hypersensitivity to diphenoxylate, atropine, or any component of the formulation; obstructive jaundice; diarrhea associated with pseudomembranous enterocolitis or enterotoxin-producing bacteria; not for use in children <2 years of age

Warnings/Precautions Use in conjunction with fluid and electrolyte therapy when appropriate. In case of severe dehydration or electrolyte imbalance, withhold diphenoxylate/atropine treatment until corrective therapy has been initiated. Inhibiting peristalsis may lead to fluid retention in the intestine aggravating dehydration and electrolyte imbalance. Reduction of intestinal motility may be deleterious in diarrhea resulting from *Shigella, Salmonella*, toxigenic strains of *E. coli*, and pseudomembranous enterocolitis associated with broad-spectrum antibiotics; use is not recommended.

Use with caution in children. Younger children may be predisposed to toxicity; signs of atropinism may occur even at recommended doses, especially in patients with Down syndrome. Overdose in children may result in severe respiratory depression, coma, and possibly permanent brain damage.

Use caution with acute ulcerative colitis, hepatic or renal dysfunction. If there is no response with 48 hours, this medication is unlikely to be effective and should be discontinued; if chronic diarrhea is not improved symptomatically within 10 days at maximum dosage, control is unlikely with further use. Physical and psychological dependence have been reported with higher than recommended dosing.

Adverse Reactions Frequency not defined.

Cardiovascular: Tachycardia

Central nervous system: Confusion, depression, dizziness, drowsiness, euphoria, flushing, headache, hyperthermia, lethargy, malaise, restlessness, sedation

Dermatologic: Angioneurotic edema, dry skin, pruritus, urticaria

Gastrointestinal: Abdominal discomfort, anorexia, gum swelling, nausea, pancreatitis, paralytic ileus, toxic megacolon, vomiting, xerostomia

Genitourinary: Urinary retention

Neuromuscular & skeletal: Numbness

Miscellaneous: Anaphylaxis

Drug Interactions

Metabolism/Transport Effects None known.

Avoid Concomitant Use

Avoid concomitant use of Diphenoxylate and Atropine with any of the following: Aclidinium; Azelastine (Nasal); Ipratropium (Oral Inhalation); Paraldehyde; Potassium Chloride; Tiotropium; Umeclidinium

Increased Effect/Toxicity

Diphenoxylate and Atropine may increase the levels/effects of: AbobotulinumtoxinA; Alcohol (Ethyl); Analgesics (Opioid); Anticholinergics; Azelastine (Nasal); Buprenorphine; Cannabinoids; CNS Depressants; Hydrocodone; Methotrimeprazine; Metyrosine; Mirabegron; Mirtazapine; OnabotulinumtoxinA; Paraldehyde; Potassium Chloride; Pramipexole; RimabotulinumtoxinB; ROPINIRole; Rotigotine; Selective Serotonin Reuptake Inhibitors; Thiazide Diuretics; Tiotropium; Topiramate; Zolpidem

The levels/effects of Diphenoxylate and Atropine may be increased by: Aclidinium; Brimonidine (Topical); Doxylamine; Droperidol; HydrOXYzine; Ipratropium (Oral Inhalation); Magnesium Sulfate; Methotrimeprazine; Perampanel; Pramlintide; Sodium Oxybate; Tapentadol; Umeclidinium

Decreased Effect

Diphenoxylate and Atropine may decrease the levels/effects of: Acetylcholinesterase Inhibitors (Central); Secretin

The levels/effects of Diphenoxylate and Atropine may be decreased by: Acetylcholinesterase Inhibitors (Central)

Ethanol/Nutrition/Herb Interactions Ethanol: May increase CNS depression; monitor for increased effects with coadministration. Caution patients about effects.

Mechanism of Action Diphenoxylate inhibits excessive GI motility and GI propulsion; commercial preparations contain a subtherapeutic amount of atropine to discourage abuse

Pharmacodynamics/Kinetics

Atropine: See Atropine monograph.

Diphenoxylate:

Onset of action: Antidiarrheal: 45-60 minutes

Duration: Antidiarrheal: 3-4 hours

Absorption: Well absorbed

Metabolism: Extensively hepatic via ester hydrolysis to diphenoxylic acid (active)

Half-life elimination: Diphenoxylate: 2.5 hours; Diphenoxylic acid: 12-14 hours

Time to peak, serum: 2 hours

Excretion: Primarily feces (49% as unchanged drug and metabolites); urine (~14%, <1% as unchanged drug)

Dosage Oral:

Children 2-12 years (use with caution in young children due to variable responses): Liquid: Diphenoxylate 0.3-0.4 mg/kg/day in 4 divided doses until control achieved (maximum: 10 mg/day), then reduce dose as needed; some patients may be controlled on doses as low as 25% of the initial daily dose

Adults: Diphenoxylate 5 mg 4 times/day until control achieved (maximum: 20 mg/day), then reduce dose as needed; some patients may be controlled on doses of 5 mg/day

Dosage adjustment in renal impairment: No adjustment provided in the manufacturer's labeling. Use with extreme caution in patients with advanced hepatorenal disease.

Dosage adjustment in hepatic impairment: No adjustment provided in the manufacturer's labeling. Use with extreme caution in patients with advanced hepatorenal disease or abnormal liver function tests.

Administration If there is no response within 48 hours of continuous therapy, this medication is unlikely to be effective and should be discontinued; if chronic diarrhea is not improved symptomatically within 10 days at maximum dosage, control is unlikely with further use. Use of the liquid preparation is recommended in children <13 years of age; use plastic dropper provided when measuring liquid.

Monitoring Parameters Watch for signs of atropinism (dryness of skin and mucous membranes, tachycardia, thirst, flushing); monitor number and consistency of stools; observe for signs of toxicity, fluid and electrolyte loss, hypotension, and respiratory depression

Dosage Forms Excipient information presented when available (limited, particularly for generics); consult specific product labeling. [DSC] = Discontinued product

Solution, oral: Diphenoxylate hydrochloride 2.5 mg and atropine sulfate 0.025 mg per 5 mL (5 mL, 10 mL, 60 mL)

Lomotil®: Diphenoxylate hydrochloride 2.5 mg and atropine sulfate 0.025 mg per 5 mL (60 mL) [contains alcohol 15%; cherry flavor] [DSC]

Tablet, oral: Diphenoxylate hydrochloride 2.5 mg and atropine sulfate 0.025 mg

Lomotil®: Diphenoxylate hydrochloride 2.5 mg and atropine sulfate 0.025 mg

Controlled Substance C-V

◆ **Diphenylhydantoin** *see* Phenytoin *on page* 1638

Diphtheria and Tetanus Toxoid

(dif THEER ee a & TET a nus TOKS oyds)

Brand Names: U.S. Tenivac

Brand Names: Canada Td Adsorbed

Index Terms DT; Td; Tetanus and Diphtheria Toxoid

Pharmacologic Category Vaccine, Inactivated (Bacterial)

Additional Appendix Information

Immunization Recommendations *on page* 2339

Use

Diphtheria and tetanus toxoids adsorbed for pediatric use (DT): Infants and children through 6 years of age: Active immunization against diphtheria and tetanus when pertussis vaccine is contraindicated

Tetanus and diphtheria toxoids adsorbed for adult use (Td) (Tenivac): Children ≥7 years of age and Adults: Active immunization against diphtheria and tetanus; tetanus prophylaxis in wound management

The Advisory Committee on Immunization Practices (ACIP) recommends routine vaccination for the following:
- Adults and children ≥7 years should receive a booster dose of Td every 10 years; may substitute a single Td booster dose with Tdap
- Children 7-10 years of age, adults, and the elderly (≥65 years) who are wounded in bombings or similar mass casualty events who have penetrating injuries or non-intact skin exposure and who cannot confirm receipt of a tetanus booster within the previous 5 years, may also receive a single dose of Td; children ≥11 years and adults may also receive Td if Tdap is unavailable

Pregnancy Risk Factor C

Pregnancy Considerations Reproduction studies have not been conducted. DT is not recommended for use in persons ≥7 years of age. Inactivated bacterial vaccines have not been shown to cause increased risks to the fetus (CDC, 60[2], 2011). The Advisory Committee on Immunization Practices (ACIP) recommends booster injections for previously vaccinated pregnant women who have not had Td vaccination within the past 10 years. Pregnant women who are not immunized or are only partially immunized should complete the primary series. Vaccination may be deferred until the postpartum period in women who are likely to have sufficient diphtheria and tetanus protection until delivery; Tdap may be substituted for Td after delivery to add extra protection against pertussis. Td should be administered during pregnancy to women who do not have sufficient tetanus immunity to protect against maternal and neonatal tetanus, and if booster protection for diphtheria is required (eg, travel to where diphtheria is endemic). Tetanus immune globulin and a tetanus toxoid containing vaccine are recommended by the ACIP as part of the standard wound management to prevent tetanus in pregnant women; the use of Td during pregnancy is recommended for wound management if ≥5 years have passed since the last Td vaccination.

Breast-Feeding Considerations Inactivated vaccines do not affect the safety of breast-feeding for the mother or the infant. Breast-feeding infants should be vaccinated according to the recommended schedules (CDC, 60[2], 2011).

Contraindications Hypersensitivity to diphtheria, tetanus toxoid, or any component of the formulation

Warnings/Precautions Do not confuse pediatric diphtheria and tetanus (DT) with adult tetanus and diphtheria (Td). Immediate treatment for anaphylactic/anaphylactoid reaction should be available during administration. Patients with a history of severe local reaction (Arthus-type) following a previous dose should not be given further routine or emergency doses of Td more frequently than every 10 years even if using for wound management with wounds that are not clean or minor; these patients generally have high serum antitoxin levels. Continue use with caution if Guillain-Barré syndrome occurs within 6 weeks of prior tetanus toxoid. Syncope has been reported with use of injectable vaccines and may be accompanied by transient visual disturbances, weakness, or tonic-clonic movements. Procedures should be in place to avoid injuries from falling and to restore cerebral perfusion if syncope occurs.

For I.M. administration; use caution with history of bleeding disorders or anticoagulant therapy. Defer administration during moderate or severe illness (with or without fever). Immune response may be decreased in immunocompromised patients; in general, household and close contacts of persons with altered immunocompetence may receive all age appropriate vaccines. Vaccination may not result in effective immunity in all patients. Response depends upon multiple factors (eg, type of vaccine, age of patient) and may be improved by administering the vaccine at the recommended dose, route, and interval. Vaccines may not be effective if administered during periods of altered immune competence (CDC, 2011). Safety and efficacy of DT have not been established in children <6 weeks of age; Td should be administered to children ≥7 years of age and adults. Some products may contain natural latex/natural rubber or thimerosal. In order to maximize vaccination rates, the ACIP recommends simultaneous administration of all age-appropriate vaccines (live or inactivated) for which a person is eligible at a single clinic visit, unless contraindications exist. The use of combination vaccines is generally preferred over separate injections, taking into consideration provider assessment, patient preference, and adverse events. When using combination vaccines, the minimum age for administration is the oldest minimum age for any individual component; the minimum interval between dosing is the greatest minimum interval between any individual component. Use of this vaccine for specific medical and/or other indications (eg, immunocompromising conditions, hepatic or kidney disease, diabetes) is also addressed in the ACIP Recommended Immunization Schedule (CDC, 2013a; CDC, 2013b).

Adverse Reactions All serious adverse reactions must be reported to the U.S. Department of Health and Human Services (DHHS) Vaccine Adverse Event Reporting System (VAERS) 1-800-822-7967 or online at https://vaers.hhs.gov/esub/index. In Canada, adverse reactions may be reported to local provincial/territorial health agencies or to the Vaccine Safety Section at Public Health Agency of Canada (1-866-844-0018).

Note: Percentages noted within 2 weeks following booster dose of Decavac® in persons ≥11 years of age:

>10%:
- Central nervous system: Headache (34% to 40%), tiredness (21% to 27%), chills (7% to 13%)
- Gastrointestinal: Nausea (8% to 12%), diarrhea (10% to 11%)
- Local: Injection site: Pain (63% to 71%), erythema (20% to 22%), swelling (17% to 18%)
- Neuromuscular & skeletal: Body ache/muscle weakness (19% to 30%), sore/swollen joints (7% to 12%)

1% to 10%:
- Central nervous system: Fever (1% to 3%)
- Dermatologic: Rash (2%)
- Endocrine & metabolic: Lymph node swelling (4% to 5%)
- Gastrointestinal: Vomiting (2% to 3%)

Postmarketing and/or case reports: Allergic reactions (angioedema, rash, urticaria), anaphylactic reactions, arthralgia, chills, dizziness, fatigue, injection site reactions (cellulitis, induration, nodules, warmth), lymphadenopathy, musculoskeletal stiffness, myalgia, pain, pain in extremities, paresthesia, peripheral edema, seizure, syncope, weakness

Drug Interactions

Metabolism/Transport Effects None known.

Avoid Concomitant Use There are no known interactions where it is recommended to avoid concomitant use.

Increased Effect/Toxicity There are no known significant interactions involving an increase in effect.

Decreased Effect

The levels/effects of Diphtheria and Tetanus Toxoids may be decreased by: Belimumab; Fingolimod; Immunosuppressants

Storage/Stability Store at 2°C to 8°C (35°F to 46°F). Do not freeze; discard if product has been frozen.

Dosage I.M.:

Children 6 weeks to <7 years (DT): Primary immunization: **Note:** For use when a pertussis-containing vaccine is contraindicated: 0.5 mL per dose, total of 5 doses administered as follows:

Three doses, usually given at 2-, 4-, and 6 months of age; may be given as early as 6 weeks of age and repeated every 4-8 weeks

Fourth dose: Given at ~15-18 months of age, but at least 6 months after third dose. The fourth dose may be given as early as 12 months of age, but at least 6 months must have elapsed between the third dose and the fourth dose.

Fifth dose: Given at 4-6 years of age, prior to starting school or kindergarten; if the fourth dose is given at ≥4 years of age, the fifth dose may be omitted

For children who start primary immunization series ≥4 months of age, refer to current ACIP "Catch-up Immunization Schedule"

Children ≥7 years and Adults (Td):

Primary immunization (Tenivac): Patients previously not immunized should receive 2 primary doses of 0.5 mL each, given at an interval of 8 weeks; third (reinforcing) dose of 0.5 mL 6-8 months later

Booster immunization: For routine booster in patients who have completed primary immunization series. The ACIP prefers Tdap for use in in some situations if no contraindications exist; refer to Diphtheria and Tetanus Toxoids, and Acellular Pertussis Vaccine monograph for additional information.

Children 11-12 years: A single dose when at least 5 years have elapsed since last dose of toxoid-containing vaccine. Subsequent routine doses are not recommended more often than every 10 years.

Adults: 0.5 mL every 10 years

Tetanus prophylaxis in wound management: Tetanus prophylaxis in patients with wounds should consider if the wound is clean or contaminated, the immunization status of the patient, proper use of tetanus toxoid and/or tetanus immune globulin (TIG), wound cleaning, and (if required) surgical debridement and the proper use of antibiotics. Patients with an uncertain or incomplete tetanus immunization status should have additional follow up to ensure a series is completed. Patients with a history of Arthus reaction following a previous dose of a tetanus toxoid-containing vaccine should not receive a tetanus toxoid-containing vaccine until >10 years after the most recent dose even if they have a wound that is neither clean nor minor. See table.

Tetanus Prophylaxis in Wound Management

History of Tetanus Immunization Doses	Clean, Minor Wounds		All Other Wounds[1]	
	Tetanus Toxoid[2]	TIG	Tetanus Toxoid[2]	TIG
Uncertain or <3 doses	Yes	No	Yes	Yes
3 or more doses	No[3]	No	No[4]	No

[1]Such as, but not limited to, wounds contaminated with dirt, feces, soil, and saliva; puncture wounds; wounds from crushing, tears, burns, and frostbite.

[2]Tetanus toxoid in this chart refers to a tetanus toxoid-containing vaccine. For children <7 years of age, DTaP (DT, if pertussis vaccine contraindicated) is preferred to tetanus toxoid alone. For children ≥7 years and adults, Td preferred to tetanus toxoid alone; Tdap may be preferred if the patient has not previously been vaccinated with Tdap.

[3]Yes, if ≥10 years since last dose.

[4]Yes, if ≥5 years since last dose.

Adapted from CDC "Yellow Book" (*Health Information for International Travel 2010*), "Routine Vaccine-Preventable Diseases, Tetanus" (available at http://www.cdc.gov/yellowbook) and *MMWR* 2006, 55 (RR-17).

Abbreviations: **DT** = Diphtheria and Tetanus Toxoids (formulation for age ≤6 years); **DTaP** = Diphtheria and Tetanus Toxoids, and Acellular Pertussis (formulation for age ≤6 years; Daptacel, Infanrix); **Td** = Diphtheria and Tetanus Toxoids (formulation for age ≥7 years; Tenivac); **TT**= Tetanus toxoid (adsorbed [formulation for age ≥7 years]); **Tdap** = Diphtheria and Tetanus Toxoids, and Acellular Pertussis (Adacel or Boostrix [formulations for age ≥7 years]); **TIG** = Tetanus Immune Globulin

Administration For I.M. administration; prior to use, shake suspension well

Td: Administer in the deltoid muscle; do not inject in the gluteal area

DT: Administer in the anterolateral aspect of the thigh or the deltoid muscle; do not inject in the gluteal area

For patients at risk of hemorrhage following intramuscular injection, the ACIP recommends "it should be administered intramuscularly if, in the opinion of the physician familiar with the patient's bleeding risk, the vaccine can be administered by this route with reasonable safety. If the patient receives antihemophilia or other similar therapy, intramuscular vaccination can be scheduled shortly after such therapy is administered. A fine needle (23 gauge or smaller) can be used for the vaccination and firm pressure applied to the site (without rubbing) for at least 2 minutes. The patient should be instructed concerning the risk of hematoma from the injection." Patients on anticoagulant therapy should be considered to have the same bleeding risks and treated as those with clotting factor disorders (CDC, 60[2], 2011).

Simultaneous administration of vaccines helps ensure the patients will be fully vaccinated by the appropriate age. Simultaneous administration of vaccines is defined as administering >1 vaccine on the same day at different anatomic sites. The use of licensed combination vaccines is generally preferred over separate injections of the equivalent components. Separate vaccines should not be combined in the same syringe unless indicated by product specific labeling. Separate needles and syringes should be used for each injection. The ACIP prefers each dose of a specific vaccine in a series come from the same manufacturer when possible. Adolescents and adults should be vaccinated while seated or lying down. In general, preterm infants should be vaccinated at the same chronological age as full-term infants (CDC, 60[2], 2011).

Antipyretics have not been shown to prevent febrile seizures. Antipyretics may be used to treat fever or discomfort following vaccination (CDC, 2011). One study reported that routine prophylactic administration of acetaminophen to prevent fever prior to vaccination decreased the immune response of some vaccines; the clinical significance of this reduction in immune response has not been established (Prymula, 2009).

Monitoring Parameters Monitor for syncope for 15 minutes following administration. If seizure-like activity associated with syncope occurs, maintain patient in supine or Trendelenburg position to reestablish adequate cerebral perfusion.

Additional Information Pediatric dosage form should only be used in patients ≤6 years of age. U.S. federal law requires that the name of medication, date of administration, the vaccine manufacturer, lot number of vaccine, and the administering person's name, title, and address be entered into the patient's permanent medical record.

DT contains higher proportions of diphtheria toxoid than Td.

Dosage Forms Excipient information presented when available (limited, particularly for generics); consult specific product labeling. [DSC] = Discontinued product

Injection, suspension [Td, adult; preservative free]: Diphtheria 2 Lf units and tetanus 2 Lf units per 0.5 mL (0.5 mL)

Tenivac: Diphtheria 2 Lf units and tetanus 5 Lf units per 0.5 mL (0.5 mL) [contains aluminum, may contain natural rubber/natural latex in prefilled syringe]

Injection, suspension [DT, pediatric; preservative free]: Diphtheria 6.7 Lf units and tetanus 5 Lf units per 0.5 mL (0.5 mL) [DSC]; Diphtheria 25 Lf units and tetanus 5 Lf units per 0.5 mL (0.5 mL) [contains aluminum]

Diphtheria and Tetanus Toxoids, Acellular Pertussis, and Poliovirus Vaccine

(dif THEER ee a & TET a nus TOKS oyds, ay CEL yoo lar per TUS sis & POE lee oh VYE rus vak SEEN)

Brand Names: U.S. Kinrix®

Brand Names: Canada Adacel®-Polio

Index Terms Diphtheria and Tetanus Toxoids and Acellular Pertussis Adsorbed, and Inactivated Poliovirus Vaccine Combined; Diphtheria, Tetanus Toxoids, Acellular Pertussis (DTaP); DTaP-IPV; Poliovirus, Inactivated (IPV)

Pharmacologic Category Vaccine, Inactivated (Bacterial); Vaccine, Inactivated (Viral)

Additional Appendix Information

Immunization Administration Recommendations *on page 2334*

Immunization Recommendations *on page 2339*

Use Kinrix®: Active immunization against diphtheria, tetanus, pertussis, and poliomyelitis, used as the fifth dose in the DTaP series and the 4th dose in the IPV series

The Advisory Committee on Immunization Practices (ACIP) recommends routine vaccination for use as the fifth dose in the DTaP series and the fourth dose in the IPV series in children who received DTaP (Infanrix®) and/or DTaP-Hepatitis B-IPV (Pediarix®) as the first 3 doses and DTaP (Infanrix®) as the fourth dose. Whenever feasible, the same manufacturer should be used to provide the pertussis component; however, vaccination should not be deferred if a specific brand is not known or is not available.

Adacel®-Polio (Canadian availability): Active booster immunization against diphtheria, tetanus, pertussis, and poliomyelitis; alternative to fifth dose of DTaP-IPV; May be used for wound management when a tetanus toxoid-containing vaccine is needed for wound management [refer to current National Advisory Committee on Immunization (NACI) guidelines]

Pregnancy Risk Factor C

Dosage I.M.:

Kinrix®: Children 4-6 years: Immunization: 0.5 mL; **Note:** For use as the fifth dose in the DTaP series and the fourth dose in the IPV series

Adacel®-Polio (Canadian availability): Children ≥4 years and Adults: Booster immunization: 0.5 mL; **Note:** May also be used as alternative to fifth dose of DTaP-IPV in children 4-6 years.

Dosage adjustment in renal impairment: No dosage adjustment provided in manufacturer's labeling.

Dosage adjustment in hepatic impairment: No dosage adjustment provided in manufacturer's labeling.

Additional Information Complete prescribing information should be consulted for additional detail.

Dosage Forms Excipient information presented when available (limited, particularly for generics); consult specific product labeling.

Injection, suspension [preservative free]:

Kinrix®: Diphtheria toxoid 25 Lf, tetanus toxoid 10 Lf, acellular pertussis antigens [inactivated pertussis toxin 25 mcg, filamentous hemagglutinin 25 mcg, pertactin 8 mcg], type 1 poliovirus 40 D-antigen units, type 2 poliovirus 8 D-antigen units, and type 3 poliovirus 32 D-antigen units per 0.5 mL (0.5 mL) [contains aluminum, neomycin sulfate, polymyxin B, polysorbate 80; may contain natural rubber/natural latex in prefilled syringe]

Dosage Forms: Canada Excipient information presented when available (limited, particularly for generics); consult specific product labeling.

Injection, suspension [preservative free]:

Adacel®-Polio: Diphtheria toxoid 2 Lf, tetanus toxoid 5 Lf, acellular pertussis antigens [inactivated pertussis toxoid 2.5 mcg, filamentous hemagglutinin 5 mcg, pertactin 3 mcg, types 2 and 3 fimbriae 5 mcg], type 1 poliovirus 40 D-antigen units, type 2 poliovirus 8 D-antigen units, and type 3 poliovirus 32 D-antigen units per 0.5 mL (0.5 mL) [contains aluminum, neomycin sulfate, polymyxin B, polysorbate 80]

Diphtheria and Tetanus Toxoids, Acellular Pertussis, Poliovirus and *Haemophilus* b Conjugate Vaccine

(dif THEER ee a & TET a nus TOKS oyds ay CEL yoo lar per TUS sis POE lee oh VYE rus & hem OF fi lus bee KON joo gate vak SEEN)

Brand Names: U.S. Pentacel®

Brand Names: Canada Pediacel®; Pentacel®

Index Terms *Haemophilus* B Conjugate (Hib); *Haemophilus* B Polysaccharide; Diphtheria Toxoid; Diphtheria, Tetanus Toxoids, Acellular Pertussis (DTaP); DTaP-IPV/Hib; Pertussis, Acellular (Adsorbed); Poliovirus, Inactivated (IPV); Tetanus Toxoid

Pharmacologic Category Vaccine, Inactivated (Bacterial); Vaccine, Inactivated (Viral)

Additional Appendix Information

Immunization Administration Recommendations *on page 2334*

Immunization Recommendations *on page 2339*

Use Active immunization against diphtheria, tetanus, pertussis, poliomyelitis, and invasive disease caused by *H. influenzae* type b in children 6 weeks through 4 years of age

Advisory Committee on Immunization Practices (ACIP) recommends that Pentacel® (DTaP-IPV/Hib) may be used to provide the recommended DTaP, IPV, and Hib immunization in children <5 years of age. Whenever feasible, the same manufacturer should be used to provide the pertussis component; however, vaccination should not be deferred if a specific brand is not known or is not available. The Hib component in Pentacel® contains a tetanus toxoid conjugate. A Hib vaccine containing the PRP-OMP conjugate (PedvaxHIB®) may provide a more rapid seroconversion following the first dose and may be preferable to use in certain populations (eg, American Indian or Alaska Native children).

Pregnancy Risk Factor C

Dosage I.M.: Children:

Primary immunization: Children 6 weeks to ≤4 years: 0.5 mL per dose administered at 2, 4, 6 and 15-18 months of age (total of 4 doses). The first dose may be administered as early as 6 weeks of age. Following completion of the 4-dose series, children should receive a dose of DTaP vaccine at 4-6 years of age (Daptacel® recommended due to same pertussis antigen used in both products).

Note: Per the ACIP, polio vaccine should not be administered more frequently than 4 weeks apart. Use of the minimum age and minimum intervals during the first 6 months of life should only be done when the vaccine recipient is at risk for imminent exposure to circulating poliovirus (shorter intervals and earlier start dates may lead to lower seroconversion. Pentacel® is not indicated for the polio booster dose given at 4-6 years of age; Kinrix® or IPV should be used.

Children previously vaccinated with ≥1 dose of Daptacel® or IPV vaccines: Pentacel® may be used to complete the first 4 doses of the DTaP or IPV series in children scheduled to receive the other components in the vaccine.

Children previously vaccinated with ≥1 dose of *Haemophilus* b conjugate vaccine: Pentacel® may be used to complete the series in children scheduled to receive the other components in the vaccine; however, if different brands of *Haemophilus* b conjugate vaccine are administered to complete the series, 3 primary immunizing doses are needed, followed by a booster dose.

Note: Completion of 3 doses of Pentacel® provides primary immunization against diphtheria, tetanus, *H. influenzae* type B, and poliomyelitis. Completion of the 4-dose series with Pentacel® provides primary immunization against pertussis. It also provides a booster vaccination against diphtheria, tetanus, *H. influenzae* type B, and poliomyelitis.

Dosage adjustment in renal impairment: No dosage adjustment provided in manufacturer's labeling.

Dosage adjustment in hepatic impairment: No dosage adjustment provided in manufacturer's labeling.

Additional Information Complete prescribing information should be consulted for additional detail.

Dosage Forms Excipient information presented when available (limited, particularly for generics); consult specific product labeling.

Injection, suspension:

Pentacel®: Diphtheria toxoid 15 Lf, tetanus toxoid 5 Lf, acellular pertussis antigens [pertussis toxin detoxified 20 mcg, filamentous hemagglutinin 20 mcg, pertactin 3 mcg, fimbriae (types 2 and 3) 5 mcg], type 1poliovirus 40 D-antigen units; type 2 poliovirus 8 D-antigen units; type 3 poliovirus 32 D-antigen units, and *Haemophilus* b capsular polysaccharide 10 mcg [bound to tetanus toxoid 24 mcg] per 0.5 mL (0.5 mL) [contains albumin, aluminum, neomycin, polymyxin B sulfate, and polysorbate 80; supplied in two vials, one containing DTaP-IPV liquid and one containing Hib powder]

◆ **Diphtheria and Tetanus Toxoids and Acellular Pertussis Adsorbed, and Inactivated Poliovirus Vaccine Combined** *see* Diphtheria and Tetanus Toxoids, Acellular Pertussis, and Poliovirus Vaccine *on page 629*

◆ **Diphtheria and Tetanus Toxoids and Acellular Pertussis Adsorbed, Hepatitis B (Recombinant) and Inactivated Poliovirus Vaccine Combined** *see* Diphtheria, Tetanus Toxoids, Acellular Pertussis, Hepatitis B (Recombinant), and Poliovirus (Inactivated) Vaccine *on page 634*

Diphtheria and Tetanus Toxoids, and Acellular Pertussis Vaccine

(dif THEER ee a & TET a nus TOKS oyds & ay CEL yoo lar per TUS sis vak SEEN)

Brand Names: U.S. Adacel®; Boostrix®; Daptacel®; Infanrix®

Brand Names: Canada Adacel®; Boostrix®

Index Terms DTaP; Tdap; Tetanus Toxoid, Reduced Diphtheria Toxoid, and Acellular Pertussis, Adsorbed; Tripedia

Pharmacologic Category Vaccine, Inactivated (Bacterial)

Additional Appendix Information

Immunization Administration Recommendations *on page 2334*

Immunization Recommendations *on page 2339*

Use

Daptacel®, Infanrix® (DTaP): Active immunization against diphtheria, tetanus, and pertussis from age 6 weeks through 6 years of age (prior to seventh birthday)

Adacel®, Boostrix® (Tdap): Active booster immunization against diphtheria, tetanus, and pertussis

The Advisory Committee on Immunization Practices (ACIP) recommends routine vaccination for the following:

Children 6 weeks to <7 years (DTaP):

- For primary immunization against diphtheria, tetanus and pertussis
- Pediatric patients who are wounded in bombings or similar mass casualty events and who have penetrating injuries or nonintact skin exposure, and have an uncertain vaccination history should receive a tetanus booster with DTaP (if no contraindications exist) (CDC, 57 [RR6], 2008)

Children 7-10 years (Tdap):

- Children not fully vaccinated against pertussis should receive a single dose of Tdap (if no contraindications exist) (CDC, 60[1], 2011)
- Children never vaccinated against diphtheria, tetanus, or pertussis, or whose vaccination status is not known should receive a series of three vaccinations containing tetanus and diphtheria toxoids and the first dose should be with Tdap (CDC, 60[1], 2011)

Adolescents 11-18 years (Tdap):

- A single dose of Tdap as a booster dose in adolescents who have completed the recommended childhood DTaP vaccination series (preferred age of administration is 11-12 years) (CDC, 60[1], 2011)

Adolescents ≥11 years and Adults (Tdap):

- Persons wounded in bombings or similar mass casualty events and who cannot confirm receipt of a tetanus booster within the previous 5 years and who have penetrating injuries or nonintact skin exposure should receive a single dose of Tdap (CDC, 57 [RR6] 2008; CDC, 61[25], 2012)

Adolescent and Adult females (Tdap): Pregnant females should receive a single dose with each pregnancy, preferably between 27-36 weeks gestation (CDC, 62 [7], 2013)

Adults ≥19 years (including adults ≥65 years) (Tdap): A single dose of Tdap should be given to all patients who have not previously received Tdap or for whom their vaccine status is unknown (CDC, 62[1], 2013). Following administration of Tdap, Td vaccine should be used for routine boosters. (CDC, 61[25], 2012). The following patients, who have not yet received Tdap or for whom vaccine status is not known, should receive a single dose of Tdap as soon as feasible:

- Close contacts of children <12 months of age; Tdap should ideally be administered at least 2 weeks prior to beginning close contact (CDC, 55[RR17], 2006; CDC, 60[41], 2011)
- Healthcare providers with direct patient contact (CDC, 55[RR17], 2006)

Note: Tdap is currently recommended for a single dose only (all age groups) (CDC, 60[1], 2011; CDC, 61[25], 2012), except pregnant females (CDC, 62 [7], 2013

Pregnancy Risk Factor B/C (manufacturer specific)

Pregnancy Considerations Animal reproduction studies have not been conducted with all products; when conducted, adverse effects to the fetus were not observed in developmental toxicity studies. Inactivated bacterial vaccines have not been shown to cause increased risks to the fetus (CDC, 60[2], 2011). Daptacel® and Infanrix® are not recommended for use in a pregnant woman or any patient

≥7 years of age. Using data collected from 2005-2010 VAERS, there were not any patterns of adverse maternal, fetal, or neonatal outcomes identified following maternal use of the Tdap vaccine (Zheteyeva, 2012). All pregnant females should receive a single dose of Tdap during each pregnancy, regardless of previous vaccination status, preferably between 27-36 weeks gestation. Alternately, administration of Tdap can be given immediately postpartum to all women who have not previously been vaccinated with Tdap in order to protect the mother and infant from pertussis (CDC, 62[7], 2013).

Pregnancy registries have been established for women who may become exposed to Boostrix® (888-452-9622) or Adacel® (800-822-2463) while pregnant.

Breast-Feeding Considerations It is not known if this vaccine is excreted into breast milk. The manufacturer recommends that caution be used if administered to a nursing woman. Breast-feeding is not a contraindication to vaccine administration. Women who have not previously had a dose of Tdap should receive a dose postpartum to help prevent pertussis in infants <12 months of age (CDC, 62[7], 2013). Inactivated vaccines do not affect the safety of breast-feeding for the mother or the infant. Breast-feeding infants should be vaccinated according to the recommended schedules (CDC, 60[2], 2011).

Contraindications Hypersensitivity to diphtheria, tetanus toxoids, pertussis, or any component of the formulation; history of any of the following effects from previous administration of pertussis-containing vaccine - progressive neurologic disorder, including infantile spasms, uncontrolled epilepsy or progressive epilepsy (postpone until condition stabilized); encephalopathy occurring within 7 days of administration and not attributable to another cause

Warnings/Precautions Defer administration during moderate or severe illness (with or without fever). Carefully consider use in patients with history of any of the following effects from previous administration of any pertussis-containing vaccine: Fever ≥105°F (40.5°C) within 48 hours of unknown cause; seizures with or without fever occurring within 3 days; persistent, inconsolable crying episodes lasting ≥3 hours and occurring within 48 hours; shock or collapse within 48 hours. Carefully consider use in patients with history of Guillain-Barré syndrome occurring within 6 weeks of a vaccine containing tetanus toxoid. Td or Tdap vaccines and emergency doses of Td vaccine should not be given more frequently than every 10 years in patients who have experienced a serious Arthus-type hypersensitivity reaction following a prior use of tetanus toxoid even if using for wound management with wounds that are not clean or minor; these patients generally have high serum antitoxin levels. Apnea has been reported following I.M. vaccine administration in premature infants; consider risk versus benefit in infants born prematurely. Syncope has been reported with use of injectable vaccines and may be accompanied by transient visual disturbances, weakness, or tonic-clonic movements. Procedures should be in place to avoid injuries from falling and to restore cerebral perfusion if syncope occurs.

Use caution in patients with coagulation disorders (including thrombocytopenia) where intramuscular injections should not be used. Patients who are immunocompromised may have reduced response; may be used in patients with HIV infection. In general, household and close contacts of persons with altered immunocompetence may receive all age appropriate vaccines. Vaccination may not result in effective immunity in all patients. Response depends upon multiple factors (eg, type of vaccine, age of patient) and may be improved by administering the vaccine at the recommended dose, route, and interval. Vaccines may not be effective if administered during periods of altered immune competence (CDC 60[2], 2011). Use caution in patients with history of seizure disorder, progressive neurologic disease, or conditions predisposing to seizures; ACIP and APP guidelines recommend deferring immunization until health status can be assessed and condition stabilized. Antipyretics may be considered at the time of and for 24 hours following vaccination to patients at high risk for seizures to reduce the possibility of postvaccination fever. Products may contain thimerosal or gelatin; packaging may contain natural latex rubber. Immediate treatment for anaphylactic/anaphylactoid reaction should be available during vaccine use. In order to maximize vaccination rates, the ACIP recommends simultaneous administration of all age-appropriate vaccines (live or inactivated) for which a person is eligible at a single clinic visit, unless contraindications exist. The use of combination vaccines is generally preferred over separate injections, taking into consideration provider assessment, patient preference, and adverse events. When using combination vaccines, the minimum age for administration is the oldest minimum age for any individual component; the minimum interval between dosing is the greatest minimum interval between any individual component. Use of this vaccine for specific medical and/or other indications (eg, immunocompromising conditions, hepatic or kidney disease, diabetes) is also addressed in the ACIP Recommended Immunization Schedule (CDC, 2013a; CDC, 2013b).

Adacel® is formulated with the same antigens found in Daptacel®, but with reduced quantities of tetanus and pertussis. Safety and efficacy have not been established in children <11 years of age.

Boostrix® is formulated with the same antigens found in Infanrix®, but in reduced quantities. Safety and efficacy have not been established in patients <10 years of age. Use of Adacel® or Boostrix® in the primary immunization series or to complete the primary series has not been evaluated.

Daptacel®, Infanrix®: Safety and efficacy in children <6 weeks of age or ≥7 years of age have not been established.

Adverse Reactions All serious adverse reactions must be reported to the U.S. Department of Health and Human Services (DHHS) Vaccine Adverse Event Reporting System (VAERS) 1-800-822-7967 or online at https://vaers.hhs.gov/esub/index. In Canada, adverse reactions may be reported to local provincial/territorial health agencies or to the Vaccine Safety Section at Public Health Agency of Canada (1-866-844-0018).

Daptacel®, Infanrix® (incidence of erythema, swelling, and fever increases with successive doses):

Frequency not defined:

Central nervous system: Drowsiness, fever, fussiness, irritability, lethargy

Gastrointestinal: Appetite decreased, vomiting

Local: Pain, redness, swelling, tenderness

Miscellaneous: Prolonged or persistent crying, refusal to play

Postmarketing and/or case reports: Allergic reaction, anaphylactic reactions, angioedema, apnea, bronchitis, cellulitis, cough, cyanosis, diarrhea, ear pain, encephalopathy, erythema, fatigue, headache, hypersensitivity, hypotonia, hypotonic-hyporesponsive episode, immune thrombocytopenia (ITP), infantile spasm, injection site reaction (abscess, cellulitis, induration, mass, nodule, rash), intussusception, limb swelling, lymphadenopathy, nausea, pruritus, rash, respiratory tract infection, seizure, screaming, somnolence, sudden infant death syndrome, thrombocytopenia, urticaria

Adacel®, Boostrix®: Note: Ranges presented, actual percent varies by product and age group

>10%:

Central nervous system: Fatigue, tiredness (24% to 37%; grade 3/severe: 1% to 4%), headache (12% to 44%; grade 3/severe: 1% to 4%), chills (8% to 15%; severe: <1%)

Gastrointestinal: Gastrointestinal symptoms, includes abdominal pain, diarrhea, nausea and/or vomiting (3% to 26%; grade 3/severe: ≤3%)

Local: Injection site pain (22% to 78%; grade 3/severe: ≤5%), arm circumference increased (28%; >40 mm: 0.5%), redness (11% to 25%; ≥50 mm: 2% to 4%), swelling (8% to 21%; ≥50 mm: ≤3%)

Neuromuscular & skeletal: Body aches/muscle weakness (22% to 30%; severe: 1%), soreness/swollen joints (9% to 11%; severe: <1%)

1% to 10%:

Central nervous system: Fever ≥38°C (≥100.4°F: 1% to 5%)

Dermatologic: Rash (2% to 3%)

Miscellaneous: Lymph node swelling (7%; severe: <1%)

Postmarketing and/or case reports: Anaphylactic reaction, arthralgia, back pain, diabetes mellitus, encephalitis, exanthema, facial palsy, GBS, Henoch-Schönlein purpura (IgA vasculitis), hypersensitivity reactions, hypoesthesia, injection site reaction (bruising, induration, inflammation, mass, nodule, pruritus, sterile abscess, warmth), limb swelling (extensive), lymphadenitis, lymphadenopathy, myalgia, myocarditis, myositis, nerve compression, paresthesia, pruritus, seizure, syncope, urticaria

Drug Interactions

Metabolism/Transport Effects None known.

Avoid Concomitant Use There are no known interactions where it is recommended to avoid concomitant use.

Increased Effect/Toxicity There are no known significant interactions involving an increase in effect.

Decreased Effect

The levels/effects of Diphtheria and Tetanus Toxoids, and Acellular Pertussis Vaccine may be decreased by: Belimumab; Fingolimod; Immunosuppressants

Storage/Stability Refrigerate at 2°C to 8°C (35°F to 46°F); do not freeze; discard if frozen. The following stability information has also been reported for Infanrix®: May be stored at room temperature for up to 72 hours (Cohen, 2007).

Mechanism of Action Promotes active immunity to diphtheria, tetanus, and pertussis by inducing production of specific antibodies.

Dosage Note: Tdap can be administered regardless of the interval between the last tetanus or diphtheria toxoid containing vaccine. Tdap is currently recommended for a single dose only (CDC, 60[1], 2011; CDC, 61[25], 2012), except pregnant females (CDC, 62 [7], 2013).

Immunization: I.M.:

Children 6 weeks to <7 years: Primary immunization: **Note:** Whenever possible, the same product should be used for all doses. Interruption of recommended schedule does not require starting the series over; a delay between doses should not interfere with final immunity.

Daptacel®, Infanrix®: 0.5 mL per dose, total of 5 doses administered as follows:

Three doses, usually given at 2-, 4-, and 6 months of age; may be given as early as 6 weeks of age and repeated every 4-8 weeks

Fourth dose: Given at ~15-20 months of age, but at least 6 months after third dose. The fourth dose may be given as early as 12 months of age, but at least 6 months must have elapsed between the third dose and the fourth dose.

Fifth dose: Given at 4-6 years of age, prior to starting school or kindergarten; if the fourth dose is given at ≥4 years of age, the fifth dose may be omitted

For children who start primary immunization series ≥4 months of age, refer to current ACIP "Catch-up Immunization Schedule".

Children 7-10 years: Not fully vaccinated against pertussis, or never vaccinated against diphtheria, tetanus, or pertussis, or whose vaccination status is not known: Administer a series of 3 vaccinations containing tetanus and diphtheria toxoids; the first dose should be with Tdap (CDC, 60[1], 2011).

Adolescents and Adults: Booster immunization: ACIP recommendations:

Adolescents 11-18 years: 0.5 mL per dose. Tdap should be given as a single booster dose at age 11 or 12 years in adolescents who have completed a childhood vaccination series, followed by booster doses of Td every 10 years. Adolescents who have not received Tdap at age 11 or 12 should receive a single dose of Tdap in place of a single Td booster dose (CDC, 55[3], 2006; CDC, 60 [1], 2011).

Adults ≥19 years: 0.5 mL per dose. A single dose of Tdap should be given to replace a single dose of the 10 year Td booster in patients who have not previously received Tdap or for whom vaccine status is not known. A single dose of Tdap is recommended for health care personnel who have not previously received Tdap and who have direct patient contact (CDC, 55[17], 2006). Tdap should be administered regardless of interval since last tetanus- or diphtheria-containing vaccine (CDC, 61 [25], 2012).

Adolescents and Adults: Booster immunization: Manufacturer's recommendations:

Children ≥10 years and Adults (Boostrix®): 0.5 mL as a single dose, administered 5 years after last dose of tetanus toxoid, diphtheria toxoid, and/or pertussis-containing vaccine

Children ≥11 years and Adults ≤64 years (Adacel®): 0.5 mL as a single dose, administered 5 years after last dose of tetanus toxoid, diphtheria toxoid and/or pertussis-containing vaccine

Elderly: Adults ≥65 years: Booster immunization:

ACIP recommendations: Refer to adult dosing. In adults ≥65 years Boostrix® should be used if feasible; however, ACIP has concluded that either Tdap vaccine (Boostrix® or Adacel®) may be used (CDC, 61 [25], 2012).

Manufacturer's recommendations: Boostrix®: 0.5 mL as a single dose, administered 5 years after last dose of tetanus toxoid, diphtheria toxoid, and/or pertussis-containing vaccine.

Wound management: I.M.: Children, Adolescents, Adults, and Elderly: Adacel® or Boostrix® may be used as an alternative to Td vaccine when a tetanus toxoid-containing vaccine is needed for wound management, and in whom the pertussis component is also indicated. Tetanus prophylaxis in patients with wounds should consider if the wound is clean or contaminated, the immunization status of the patient, proper use of tetanus toxoid and/or tetanus immune globulin (TIG), wound cleaning, and (if required) surgical debridement and the proper use of antibiotics.

Patients with an uncertain or incomplete tetanus immunization status should have additional follow up to ensure a series is completed. Patients with a history of Arthus reaction following a previous dose of a tetanus toxoid-containing vaccine should not receive a tetanus toxoid-containing vaccine until >10 years after the most recent dose even if they have a wound that is neither clean nor minor. See table.

Tetanus Prophylaxis in Wound Management

History of Tetanus Immunization Doses	Clean, Minor Wounds		All Other Wounds[1]	
	Tetanus Toxoid[2]	TIG	Tetanus Toxoid[2]	TIG
Uncertain or <3 doses	Yes	No	Yes	Yes
3 or more doses	No[3]	No	No[4]	No

[1]Such as, but not limited to, wounds contaminated with dirt, feces, soil, and saliva; puncture wounds; wounds from crushing, tears, burns, and frostbite.

[2]Tetanus toxoid in this chart refers to a tetanus toxoid-containing vaccine. For children <7 years of age, DTaP (DT, if pertussis vaccine contraindicated) is preferred to tetanus toxoid alone. For children ≥7 years and adults, Td preferred to tetanus toxoid alone; Tdap may be preferred if the patient has not previously been vaccinated with Tdap.

[3]Yes, if ≥10 years since last dose.

[4]Yes, if ≥5 years since last dose.

Adapted from CDC "Yellow Book" (*Health Information for International Travel 2010*), "Routine Vaccine-Preventable Diseases, Tetanus" (available at http://www.cdc.gov/yellowbook) and *MMWR* 2006, 55 (RR-17).

Abbreviations: **DT** = Diphtheria and Tetanus Toxoids (formulation for age ≤6 years); **DTaP** = Diphtheria and Tetanus Toxoids, and Acellular Pertussis (formulation for age ≤6 years; Daptacel®, Infanrix®); **Td** = Diphtheria and Tetanus Toxoids (formulation for age ≥7 years; Decavac®,Tenivac™); **TT**= Tetanus toxoid (adsorbed [formulation for age ≥7 years]); **Tdap** = Diphtheria and Tetanus Toxoids, and Acellular Pertussis (Adacel® or Boostrix® [formulations for age ≥7 years]); **TIG** = Tetanus Immune Globulin

Administration Shake suspension well.

Adacel®, Boostrix®: Administer only I.M. in deltoid muscle of upper arm.

Daptacel®, Infanrix®: Administer only I.M. in anterolateral aspect of thigh or deltoid muscle of upper arm.

If feasible, the same brand of DTaP should be used for all doses in the series (CDC, 60[2], 2011).

For patients at risk of hemorrhage following intramuscular injection, the ACIP recommends "it should be administered intramuscularly if, in the opinion of the physician familiar with the patient's bleeding risk, the vaccine can be administered by this route with reasonable safety. If the patient receives antihemophilia or other similar therapy, intramuscular vaccination can be scheduled shortly after such therapy is administered. A fine needle (23 gauge or smaller) can be used for the vaccination and firm pressure applied to the site (without rubbing) for at least 2 minutes. The patient should be instructed concerning the risk of hematoma from the injection." Patients on anticoagulant therapy should be considered to have the same bleeding risks and treated as those with clotting factor disorders (CDC, 60[2], 2011).

Simultaneous administration of vaccines helps ensure the patients will be fully vaccinated by the appropriate age. Simultaneous administration of vaccines is defined as administering >1 vaccine on the same day at different anatomic sites. The use of licensed combination vaccines is generally preferred over separate injections of the equivalent components. Separate vaccines should not be combined in the same syringe unless indicated by product specific labeling. Separate needles and syringes should be used for each injection. The ACIP prefers each dose of a specific vaccine in a series come from the same manufacturer when possible. Adolescents and adults should be vaccinated while seated or lying down. In general, preterm infants should be vaccinated at the same chronological age as full-term infants (CDC, 60[2], 2011).

Antipyretics have not been shown to prevent febrile seizures. Antipyretics may be used to treat fever or discomfort following vaccination (CDC, 2011). One study reported that routine prophylactic administration of acetaminophen to prevent fever prior to vaccination decreased the immune response of some vaccines; the clinical significance of this reduction in immune response has not been established (Prymula, 2009).

Monitoring Parameters Monitor for syncope for 15 minutes following administration. If seizure-like activity associated with syncope occurs, maintain patient in supine or Trendelenburg position to reestablish adequate cerebral perfusion.

Additional Information In patients who cannot be given pertussis vaccine, DT for pediatric use should be given to complete the series.

Adacel® is formulated with the same antigens found in Daptacel® but with reduced quantities of pertussis and tetanus. It is intended for use as a booster dose in children and adults, 11-64 years of age, and **not** for primary immunization.

Boostrix® is formulated with the same antigens found in Infanrix® but in reduced quantities. It is intended for use as a booster dose in children and adults, 10-64 years of age, and is **not** for primary immunization.

The ACIP considers Adacel® and Boostrix® to be interchangeable when administered to adolescents for childhood vaccination according to the Child and Adolescent Immunization Schedule.

The child's medical record should document that the small risk of postvaccination seizure and the benefits of the pertussis vaccination were discussed with the patient; parents or guardians should be questioned prior to administration of vaccine as to any adverse reactions from previous dose. Provide Vaccine Information Materials, as required by National Childhood Vaccine Injury Act of 1986, prior to immunization.

U.S. federal law requires that the name of medication, date of administration, the vaccine manufacturer, lot number of vaccine, and the administering person's name, title and address be entered into the patient's permanent medical record.

Dosage Forms Excipient information presented when available (limited, particularly for generics); consult specific product labeling.

Injection, suspension [Tdap, booster formulation]:

Adacel®: Diphtheria 2 Lf units, tetanus 5 Lf units, and acellular pertussis antigens [detoxified pertussis toxin 2.5 mcg, filamentous hemagglutinin 5 mcg, pertactin 3 mcg, fimbriae (types 2 and 3) 5 mcg] per 0.5 mL (0.5 mL) [contains aluminum; may contain natural rubber/natural latex in prefilled syringe]

Boostrix®: Diphtheria 2.5 Lf units, tetanus 5 Lf units, and acellular pertussis antigens [inactivated pertussis toxin 8 mcg, filamentous hemagglutinin 8 mcg, pertactin 2.5 mcg] per 0.5 mL (0.5 mL) [contains aluminum and polysorbate 80; may contain natural rubber/natural latex in prefilled syringe]

Injection, suspension [DTaP, active immunization formulation]:

Daptacel®: Diphtheria 15 Lf units, tetanus 5 Lf units, and acellular pertussis antigens [detoxified pertussis toxin 10 mcg, filamentous hemagglutinin 5 mcg, pertactin 3 mcg, fimbriae (types 2 and 3) 5 mcg] per 0.5 mL (0.5 mL) [preservative free; contains aluminum]

Infanrix®: Diphtheria 25 Lf units, tetanus 10 Lf units, and acellular pertussis antigens [inactivated pertussis toxin 25 mcg, filamentous hemagglutinin 25 mcg, pertactin 8 mcg] per 0.5 mL (0.5 mL) [preservative free; contains aluminum and polysorbate 80]

Infanrix®: Diphtheria 25 Lf units, tetanus 10 Lf units, and acellular pertussis antigens [inactivated pertussis toxin 25 mcg, filamentous hemagglutinin 25 mcg, pertactin 8 mcg] per 0.5 mL (0.5 mL) [preservative free; contains aluminum and polysorbate 80; prefilled syringes contain natural rubber/natural latex] [DSC]

◆ **Diphtheria, Tetanus Toxoids, Acellular Pertussis (DTaP)** *see* Diphtheria and Tetanus Toxoids, Acellular Pertussis, and Poliovirus Vaccine *on page 629*

◆ **Diphtheria, Tetanus Toxoids, Acellular Pertussis (DTaP)** *see* Diphtheria and Tetanus Toxoids, Acellular Pertussis, Poliovirus and *Haemophilus* b Conjugate Vaccine *on page 629*

Diphtheria, Tetanus Toxoids, Acellular Pertussis, Hepatitis B (Recombinant), and Poliovirus (Inactivated) Vaccine

(dif THEER ee a, TET a nus TOKS oyds, ay CEL yoo lar per TUS sis, hep a TYE tis bee ree KOM be nant, & POE lee oh VYE rus in ak ti VAY ted vak SEEN)

Brand Names: U.S. Pediarix®

Brand Names: Canada Pediarix®

Index Terms Diphtheria and Tetanus Toxoids and Acellular Pertussis Adsorbed, Hepatitis B (Recombinant) and Inactivated Poliovirus Vaccine Combined; Diphtheria, Tetanus Toxoids, Acellular Pertussis, Hepatitis B (Recombinant), and Poliovirus (Inactivated) Vaccine; Diphtheria, Tetanus Toxoids, Acellular Pertussis, Hepatitis B (Recombinant), and Poliovirus Vaccine; DTaP-HepB-IPV

Pharmacologic Category Vaccine, Inactivated (Bacterial); Vaccine, Inactivated (Viral)

Additional Appendix Information

Immunization Administration Recommendations *on page 2334*

Immunization Recommendations *on page 2339*

Use Combination vaccine for the active immunization against diphtheria, tetanus, pertussis, hepatitis B virus (all known subtypes), and poliomyelitis (caused by poliovirus types 1, 2, and 3)

The Advisory Committee on Immunization Practices (ACIP) recommends Pediarix® for the following:

- Primary vaccination for DTaP, Hep B, and IPV in children at 2, 4, and 6 months of age.
- To complete the primary vaccination series in children who have received DTaP (Infanrix®) and who are scheduled to receive the other components of the vaccine. Whenever feasible, the same manufacturer should be used to provide the pertussis component; however, vaccination should not be deferred if a specific brand is not known or is not available. HepB and IPV from different manufacturers are interchangeable.

Pregnancy Risk Factor C

Dosage I.M.: Children 6 weeks to <7 years:

Primary immunization: 0.5 mL/dose; administer as a 3-dose series at 2-, 4-, and 6 months of age in 6- to 8-week intervals (preferably 8-week intervals). Vaccination usually begins at 2 months, but may be started as early as 6 weeks of age.

Note: Pediarix® is approved for the first 3 doses of polio vaccine. Per the ACIP, polio vaccine is given at 2, 4 and 6 months of age and should not be administered more frequently than 4 weeks apart. Use of the minimum age and minimum intervals during the first 6 months of life should only be done when the vaccine recipient is at risk for imminent exposure to circulating poliovirus (shorter intervals and earlier start dates may lead to lower seroconversion).

Use in children previously vaccinated with one or more component, and who are also scheduled to receive all vaccine components:

Hepatitis B vaccine: Infants previously vaccinated with 1 or 2 doses of another hepatitis B vaccine may use Pediarix® to complete the 3-dose series. Not for use as birth dose of hepatitis B vaccine. Infants born to HB_sAg-positive women should begin dosing with DTaP-HepB-IPV by age 6-8 weeks after receiving the single antigen hepatitis B vaccine at birth.

Diphtheria and tetanus toxoids, and acellular pertussis vaccine (DTaP): Infants previously vaccinated with 1 or 2 doses of Infanrix® may use Pediarix® to complete the first 3 doses of the series; use of Pediarix® to complete DTaP vaccination started with products other than Infanrix® is not recommended.

Inactivated polio vaccine (IPV): Infants previously vaccinated with 1 or 2 doses of IPV may use Pediarix® to complete the first 3 doses of the series.

Dosage adjustment in renal impairment: No dosage adjustment provided in manufacturer's labeling.

Dosage adjustment in hepatic impairment: No dosage adjustment provided in manufacturer's labeling.

Additional Information Complete prescribing information should be consulted for additional detail.

Dosage Forms Excipient information presented when available (limited, particularly for generics); consult specific product labeling.

Injection, suspension [preservative free]:

Pediarix®: Diphtheria toxoid 25 Lf, tetanus toxoid 10 Lf, acellular pertussis antigens [inactivated pertussis toxin 25 mcg, filamentous hemagglutin 25 mcg, pertactin 8 mcg, HBsAg 10 mcg, type 1 poliovirus 40 D antigen units, type 2 poliovirus 8 D antigen units and type 3 poliovirus 32 D antigen units] per 0.5 mL (0.5 mL) [contains aluminum, neomycin sulfate (trace amounts), polymyxin B (trace amounts), polysorbate 80, and yeast protein ≤5%; may contain natural rubber/natural latex in prefilled syringe]

◆ **Diphtheria, Tetanus Toxoids, Acellular Pertussis, Hepatitis B (Recombinant), and Poliovirus (Inactivated) Vaccine** *see* Diphtheria, Tetanus Toxoids, Acellular Pertussis, Hepatitis B (Recombinant), and Poliovirus (Inactivated) Vaccine *on page 634*

◆ **Diphtheria, Tetanus Toxoids, Acellular Pertussis, Hepatitis B (Recombinant), and Poliovirus Vaccine** *see* Diphtheria, Tetanus Toxoids, Acellular Pertussis, Hepatitis B (Recombinant), and Poliovirus (Inactivated) Vaccine *on page 634*

◆ **Diphtheria Toxoid** *see* Diphtheria and Tetanus Toxoids, Acellular Pertussis, Poliovirus and *Haemophilus* b Conjugate Vaccine *on page 629*

◆ **Dipivalyl Epinephrine** *see* Dipivefrin *on page 634*

Dipivefrin (dye PI ve frin)

Brand Names: Canada Ophtho-Dipivefrin™; PMS-Dipivefrin; Propine®

Index Terms Dipivalyl Epinephrine; Dipivefrin Hydrochloride; DPE

Pharmacologic Category Alpha/Beta Agonist; Ophthalmic Agent, Antiglaucoma; Ophthalmic Agent, Vasoconstrictor

Use Reduces elevated intraocular pressure in chronic open-angle glaucoma; also used to treat ocular hypertension, low tension, and secondary glaucomas

Pregnancy Risk Factor B

Dosage Adults: Ophthalmic: Instill 1 drop every 12 hours into the eyes

Dosage adjustment in renal impairment: No dosage adjustment provided in manufacturer's labeling.

Dosage adjustment in hepatic impairment: No dosage adjustment provided in manufacturer's labeling.

Additional Information Complete prescribing information should be consulted for additional detail.

Dosage Forms Excipient information presented when available (limited, particularly for generics); consult specific product labeling. [DSC] = Discontinued product

Solution, ophthalmic, as hydrochloride [drops]:

Propine®: 0.1% (10 mL [DSC]) [contains benzalkonium chloride]

◆ **Dipivefrin Hydrochloride** *see* Dipivefrin *on page 634*

◆ **Diprivan** *see* Propofol *on page 1734*

◆ **Diprolene** *see* Betamethasone *on page 247*

◆ **Diprolene® (Can)** *see* Betamethasone *on page 247*

◆ **Diprolene AF** *see* Betamethasone *on page 247*

◆ **Diprolene® Glycol (Can)** *see* Betamethasone *on page 247*

◆ **Dipropylacetic Acid** *see* Valproic Acid and Derivatives *on page 2149*

◆ **Diprosone® (Can)** *see* Betamethasone *on page 247*

Dipyridamole (dye peer ID a mole)

Brand Names: U.S. Persantine

Brand Names: Canada Apo-Dipyridamole FC®; Dipyridamole For Injection; Persantine®

Pharmacologic Category Antiplatelet Agent; Vasodilator

Additional Appendix Information

Beers Criteria - Potentially Inappropriate Medications for Geriatrics *on page 2368*

Use

Oral: Used with warfarin to decrease thrombosis in patients after artificial heart valve replacement

I.V.: Diagnostic agent in CAD

Unlabeled Use Stroke prevention (in combination with aspirin); **Note:** For this indication, the use of aspirin/extended release dipyridamole is recommended (Guyatt, 2012).

Pregnancy Risk Factor B

Pregnancy Considerations Teratogenic effects were not observed in animal studies.

Breast-Feeding Considerations Excretion in breast milk is reported to be minimal.

Contraindications Hypersensitivity to dipyridamole or any component of the formulation

Warnings/Precautions Use with caution in patients with hypotension, unstable angina, and/or recent MI. Use with caution in hepatic impairment. Avoid use of oral dipyridamole in this age group due to risk of orthostatic hypotension and availability of more efficacious alternative agents (Beers Criteria). Use caution in patients on other antiplatelet agents or anticoagulation. Severe adverse reactions have occurred with I.V. administration (rarely); use the I.V. form with caution in patients with bronchospastic disease or unstable angina. Aminophylline should be available in case of urgency or emergency with I.V. use.

Adverse Reactions

Oral:

>10%: Dizziness (14%)

1% to 10%:

Central nervous system: Headache (2%)

Dermatologic: Rash (2%)

Gastrointestinal: Abdominal distress (6%)

Frequency not defined: Diarrhea, vomiting, flushing, pruritus, angina pectoris, liver dysfunction

Postmarketing and/or case reports: Alopecia, arthritis, cholelithiasis, dyspepsia, fatigue, hepatitis, hypersensitivity reaction, hypotension, larynx edema, malaise, myalgia, nausea, palpitation, paresthesia, tachycardia, thrombocytopenia

I.V.:

>10%:

Cardiovascular: Exacerbation of angina pectoris (20%)

Central nervous system: Dizziness (12%), headache (12%)

1% to 10%:

Cardiovascular: Hypotension (5%), hypertension (2%), blood pressure lability (2%), ECG abnormalities (ST-T changes, extrasystoles; 5% to 8%), pain (3%), tachycardia (3%)

Central nervous system: Flushing (3%), fatigue (1%)

Gastrointestinal: Nausea (5%)

Neuromuscular & skeletal: Paresthesia (1%)

Respiratory: Dyspnea (3%)

<1% (Limited to important or life-threatening): Abdominal pain, abnormal coordination, allergic reaction (pruritus, rash, urticaria), appetite increased, arrhythmia (ventricular tachycardia, bradycardia, AV block, SVT, atrial fibrillation, asystole), arthralgia, asthenia, back pain, breast pain, bronchospasm, cardiomyopathy, cough, depersonalization, diaphoresis, dry mouth, dysgeusia, dyspepsia, dysphagia, earache, ECG abnormalities (unspecified), edema, eructation, flatulence, hypertonia, hyperventilation, injection site reaction, intermittent claudication leg cramping, malaise, MI, myalgia, orthostatic hypotension, palpitation, perineal pain, pharyngitis, pleural pain, renal pain, rhinitis, rigor, syncope, tenesmus, thirst, tinnitus, tremor, vertigo, vision abnormalities, vomiting

Drug Interactions

Metabolism/Transport Effects Inhibits BCRP, P-glycoprotein

Avoid Concomitant Use

Avoid concomitant use of Dipyridamole with any of the following: Bosutinib; PAZOPanib; Pomalidomide; Riociguat; Silodosin; VinCRIStine (Liposomal)

Increased Effect/Toxicity

Dipyridamole may increase the levels/effects of: Adenosine; Afatinib; Agents with Antiplatelet Properties; Anticoagulants; Beta-Blockers; Bosutinib; Colchicine; Collagenase (Systemic); Dabigatran Etexilate; Everolimus; Hypotensive Agents; Ibritumomab; PAZOPanib; P-glycoprotein/ABCB1 Substrates; Pomalidomide; Prucalopride; Regadenoson; Riociguat; Rivaroxaban; Salicylates; Silodosin; Thrombolytic Agents; Topotecan; Tositumomab and Iodine I 131 Tositumomab; VinCRIStine (Liposomal)

The levels/effects of Dipyridamole may be increased by: Dasatinib; Glucosamine; Herbs (Anticoagulant/Antiplatelet Properties); Ibrutinib; Multivitamins/Fluoride (with ADE); Multivitamins/Minerals (with ADEK, Folate, Iron); Multivitamins/Minerals (with AE, No Iron); Nonsteroidal Anti-Inflammatory Agents; Omega-3 Fatty Acids; Pentosan Polysulfate Sodium; Pentoxifylline; Prostacyclin Analogues; Tipranavir; Vitamin E

Decreased Effect

Dipyridamole may decrease the levels/effects of: Acetylcholinesterase Inhibitors

The levels/effects of Dipyridamole may be decreased by: Nonsteroidal Anti-Inflammatory Agents

Ethanol/Nutrition/Herb Interactions

Food: Management: Administer with water 1 hour before meals.

Herb/Nutraceutical: Many herbal medications may have additional antiplatelet activity. Management: Avoid cat's claw, dong quai, evening primrose, feverfew, garlic, ginger, ginkgo, glucosamine, omega-3-acid ethyl esters (fish oil), red clover, horse chestnut, green tea, and ginseng.

Preparation for Administration Prior to administration, dilute solution for injection to a ≥1:2 ratio in NS, ½NS, or D_5W. Total volume should be ~20-50 mL.

Storage/Stability I.V.: Store between 15°C to 25°C (59°F to 77°F); do not freeze. Protect from light.

Mechanism of Action Inhibits the activity of adenosine deaminase and phosphodiesterase, which causes an accumulation of adenosine, adenine nucleotides, and cyclic AMP; these mediators then inhibit platelet aggregation and may cause vasodilation; may also stimulate release of prostacyclin or PGD_2; causes coronary vasodilation

Pharmacodynamics/Kinetics

Absorption: Readily, but variable

Distribution: Adults: V_d: 2-3 L/kg

Protein binding: 91% to 99%

Metabolism: Hepatic

Half-life elimination: Terminal: 10-12 hours

Time to peak, serum: 2-2.5 hours

Excretion: Feces (as glucuronide conjugates and unchanged drug)

Dosage

Oral: Children ≥12 years and Adults: Adjunctive therapy for prophylaxis of thromboembolism with cardiac valve replacement: 75-100 mg 4 times/day

I.V.: Adults: Evaluation of coronary artery disease: 0.14 mg/kg/minute for 4 minutes; maximum dose: 60 mg

Following dipyridamole infusion, inject thallium-201 within 5 minutes. **Note:** Aminophylline should be available for urgent/emergent use; dosing of 50-100 mg (range: 50-250 mg) I.V. push over 30-60 seconds.

Dosage adjustment in renal impairment: No dosage adjustment provided in manufacturer's labeling.

Dosage adjustment in hepatic impairment: No dosage adjustment provided in manufacturer's labeling.

Dietary Considerations Should be taken with water 1 hour before meals.

Administration

I.V.: Infuse diluted solution over 4 minutes.

Tablet: Administer with water 1 hour before meals.

Monitoring Parameters Blood pressure, heart rate, ECG (stress test)

Test Interactions Concurrent caffeine or theophylline use may demonstrate a false-negative result with dipyridamole-thallium myocardial imaging.

Dosage Forms Excipient information presented when available (limited, particularly for generics); consult specific product labeling.

Solution, Intravenous:

Generic: 5 mg/mL (2 mL, 10 mL)

Tablet, Oral:

Persantine: 25 mg, 50 mg, 75 mg [contains fd&c yellow #10 aluminum lake, methylparaben, propylparaben, sodium benzoate]

Generic: 25 mg, 50 mg, 75 mg

Extemporaneous Preparations A 10 mg/mL oral suspension may be made with tablets and one of three different vehicles (cherry syrup, a 1:1 mixture of Ora-Sweet® and Ora-Plus®, or a 1:1 mixture of Ora-Sweet® SF and Ora-Plus®). Crush twenty-four 50 mg tablets in a mortar and reduce to a fine powder. Add 20 mL of the chosen vehicle and mix to a uniform paste; mix while adding the vehicle in incremental proportions to **almost** 120 mL; transfer to a calibrated bottle, rinse mortar with vehicle, and add quantity of vehicle sufficient to make 120 mL. Label "shake well" and "protect from light". Stable for 60 days when stored in amber plastic prescription bottles in the dark at room temperature or refrigerated.

Allen LV and Erickson III MA, "Stability of Baclofen, Captopril, Diltiazem, Hydrochloride, Dipyridamole, and Flecainide Acetate in Extemporaneously Compounded Oral Liquids," *Am J Health Syst Pharm*, 1996, 53:2179-84.

- **Dipyridamole and Aspirin** *see* Aspirin and Dipyridamole *on page* 182
- **Dipyridamole For Injection (Can)** *see* Dipyridamole *on page* 635
- **Disalicylic Acid** *see* Salsalate *on page* 1873
- **DisCoVisc®** *see* Sodium Chondroitin Sulfate and Sodium Hyaluronate *on page* 1917
- **Disodium Cromoglycate** *see* Cromolyn (Nasal) *on page* 500
- **Disodium Cromoglycate** *see* Cromolyn (Ophthalmic) *on page* 501
- **Disodium Thiosulfate Pentahydrate** *see* Sodium Thiosulfate *on page* 1931
- ***d*-Isoephedrine Hydrochloride** *see* Pseudoephedrine *on page* 1746

Disopyramide (dye soe PEER a mide)

Brand Names: U.S. Norpace; Norpace CR

Brand Names: Canada Norpace®; Rythmodan®; Rythmodan®-LA

Index Terms Disopyramide Phosphate

Pharmacologic Category Antiarrhythmic Agent, Class Ia

Additional Appendix Information

Beers Criteria – Potentially Inappropriate Medications for Geriatrics *on page* 2368

Use Life-threatening ventricular arrhythmias (eg, sustained ventricular tachycardia)

Unlabeled Use Alternative agent for the prevention of recurrent symptomatic focal atrial tachycardia (in combination with an AV nodal blocking agent), atrial fibrillation (especially vagally-induced), or atrial flutter (in combination with an AV nodal-blocking agent); obstructive hypertrophic cardiomyopathy (HCM) in combination with ventricular rate-controlling agents (eg, beta blockers or verapamil) to control symptoms of angina or dyspnea who are unresponsive to rate-controlling agents alone; atrial fibrillation in patients with HCM in combination with rate-controlling agents

Pregnancy Risk Factor C

Dosage Oral:

Children: Arrhythmias: *Immediate release:*

<1 year: 10-30 mg/kg/24 hours in 4 divided doses

1-4 years: 10-20 mg/kg/24 hours in 4 divided doses

4-12 years: 10-15 mg/kg/24 hours in 4 divided doses

12-18 years: 6-15 mg/kg/24 hours in 4 divided doses

Adults:

Ventricular arrhythmias: **Note:** Since newer agents with less toxicity are available, the use of disopyramide for this indication has fallen out of favor. Controlled release formulation not to be used when rapid achievement of disopyramide plasma concentrations is desired. A maximum dose up to 400 mg every 6 hours (immediate release) may be required for patients with severe refractory ventricular tachycardia.

<50 kg:

Immediate release: An initial loading dose of 200 mg may be administered if rapid onset is required. Maintenance dose: 100 mg every 6 hours

Controlled release: Maintenance dose: 200 mg every 12 hours

≥50 kg:

Immediate release: An initial loading dose of 300 mg may be administered if rapid onset is required. Maintenance dose: 150 mg every 6 hours. If rapid control is necessary and no response seen within 6 hours of loading dose, may increase maintenance dose to 200 mg every 6 hours.

Controlled release: Maintenance dose: 300 mg every 12 hours

Hypertrophic cardiomyopathy (obstructive physiology) with or without atrial fibrillation (unlabeled use): Initial: *Controlled release:* 200-250 mg twice daily. If symptoms do not improve, increase by 100 mg/day at 2-week intervals to a maximum daily dose of 600 mg (Gersh, 2011; Sherrid, 2005).

Elderly: Dose with caution, starting at the lower end of dosing range

Dosing adjustment in renal impairment:

Manufacturer recommendations:

Immediate release:

Cl_{cr} >40 mL/minute: 100 mg every 6 hours
Cl_{cr} 30-40 mL/minute: 100 mg every 8 hours
Cl_{cr} 15-30 mL/minute: 100 mg every 12 hours
Cl_{cr} <15 mL/minute: 100 mg every 24 hours

Controlled release:

Cl_{cr} >40 mL/minute: 200 mg every 12 hours
Cl_{cr} ≤40 mL/minute: Not recommended for use

Alternative recommendations (Aronoff, 2007): *Immediate release:*

Cl_{cr} >50 mL/minute: 100-200 mg every 8 hours
Cl_{cr} 10-50 mL/minute: 100-200 mg every 12-24 hours
Cl_{cr} <10 mL/minute: 100-200 mg every 24-48 hours

Dialysis: Not dialyzable (0% to 5%) by hemo- or peritoneal methods; supplemental dose is not necessary.

Dosing interval in hepatic impairment: Manufacturer's recommendations:

Immediate release: 100 mg every 6 hours
Controlled release: 200 mg every 12 hours

Additional Information Complete prescribing information should be consulted for additional detail.

Dosage Forms Excipient information presented when available (limited, particularly for generics); consult specific product labeling.

Capsule, Oral:
Norpace: 100 mg, 150 mg
Generic: 100 mg, 150 mg

Capsule Extended Release 12 Hour, Oral:
Norpace CR: 100 mg, 150 mg

◆ **Disopyramide Phosphate** *see* Disopyramide *on page 636*

Disulfiram (dye SUL fi ram)

Brand Names: U.S. Antabuse

Pharmacologic Category Aldehyde Dehydrogenase Inhibitor

Use Management of chronic alcoholism

Dosage Adults: Oral: Do not administer until the patient has abstained from ethanol for at least 12 hours

Initial: 500 mg once daily for 1-2 weeks (maximum daily dose: 500 mg)

Average maintenance dose: 250 mg once daily (range: 125-500 mg; maximum daily dose: 500 mg); duration of therapy is to continue until the patient is fully recovered socially and a basis for permanent self-control has been established; maintenance therapy may be required for months or even years.

Dosage adjustment in renal impairment: No dosage adjustment provided in manufacturer's labeling. Use with extreme caution in chronic and acute nephritis.

Dosage adjustment in hepatic impairment: No dosage adjustment provided in manufacturer's labeling. Use with extreme caution in hepatic cirrhosis or insufficiency.

Additional Information Complete prescribing information should be consulted for additional detail.

Dosage Forms Excipient information presented when available (limited, particularly for generics); consult specific product labeling.

Tablet, Oral:
Antabuse: 250 mg
Antabuse: 500 mg [scored]
Generic: 250 mg, 500 mg

◆ **Dithioglycerol** *see* Dimercaprol *on page 617*
◆ **Dithranol** *see* Anthralin *on page 140*
◆ **Ditropan** *see* Oxybutynin *on page 1533*
◆ **Ditropan XL** *see* Oxybutynin *on page 1533*
◆ **Diuril** *see* Chlorothiazide *on page 411*
◆ **Divalproex Sodium** *see* Valproic Acid and Derivatives *on page 2149*
◆ **Divigel** *see* Estradiol (Systemic) *on page 754*
◆ **Dixarit® (Can)** *see* CloNIDine *on page 468*
◆ **5071-1DL(6)** *see* Megestrol *on page 1283*
◆ ***dl*-Alpha Tocopherol** *see* Vitamin E *on page 2202*
◆ **DLV** *see* Delavirdine *on page 565*
◆ ***D*-Mannitol** *see* Mannitol *on page 1266*
◆ **4-DMDR** *see* IDArubicin *on page 1039*
◆ **DMF** *see* Dimethyl Fumarate *on page 618*
◆ **DMSA** *see* Succimer *on page 1952*
◆ **D-Natural-5 [OTC]** *see* Vitamin A and Vitamin D (Systemic) *on page 2202*
◆ **Doans Extra Strength [OTC]** *see* Magnesium Salicylate *on page 1262*
◆ **Doans Pills [OTC]** *see* Magnesium Salicylate *on page 1262*

DOBUTamine (doe BYOO ta meen)

Brand Names: Canada Dobutamine Injection, USP; Dobutrex®

Index Terms Dobutamine Hydrochloride

Pharmacologic Category Adrenergic Agonist Agent

Additional Appendix Information

Vasoactive Agents, Intravenous *on page 2315*

Use Short-term management of patients with cardiac decompensation

Unlabeled Use Positive inotropic agent for use in myocardial dysfunction related to sepsis; stress echocardiography

Pregnancy Risk Factor B

Pregnancy Considerations Adverse events have not been observed in animal reproduction studies.

Breast-Feeding Considerations It is not known if dobutamine is excreted in breast milk. The manufacturer recommends that caution be exercised when administering dobutamine to nursing women.

Contraindications Hypersensitivity to dobutamine or sulfites (some contain sodium metabisulfate), or any component of the formulation; idiopathic hypertrophic subaortic stenosis (IHSS)

Warnings/Precautions May increase heart rate. Patients with atrial fibrillation may experience an increase in ventricular response. An increase in blood pressure is more common, but occasionally a patient may become hypotensive. May exacerbate ventricular ectopy. If needed, correct hypovolemia first to optimize hemodynamics. Ineffective therapeutically in the presence of mechanical obstruction such as severe aortic stenosis. Use caution post-MI (can increase myocardial oxygen demand). Use cautiously in the elderly starting at lower end of the dosage range. Use with extreme caution in patients taking MAO inhibitors. Dobutamine in combination with stress echo may be used diagnostically. Product may contain sodium sulfite.

Adverse Reactions Incidence of adverse events is not always reported.

Cardiovascular: Increased heart rate, increased blood pressure, increased ventricular ectopic activity, hypotension, premature ventricular beats (5%, dose related), anginal pain (1% to 3%), nonspecific chest pain (1% to 3%), palpitation (1% to 3%)

Central nervous system: Fever (1% to 3%), headache (1% to 3%), paresthesia

Endocrine & metabolic: Slight decrease in serum potassium

Gastrointestinal: Nausea (1% to 3%)

Hematologic: Thrombocytopenia (isolated cases)

Local: Phlebitis, local inflammatory changes and pain from infiltration, cutaneous necrosis (isolated cases)

Neuromuscular & skeletal: Mild leg cramps

Respiratory: Dyspnea (1% to 3%)

Drug Interactions

Metabolism/Transport Effects Substrate of COMT

Avoid Concomitant Use

Avoid concomitant use of DOBUTamine with any of the following: Iobenguane I 123

Increased Effect/Toxicity

DOBUTamine may increase the levels/effects of: Sympathomimetics

The levels/effects of DOBUTamine may be increased by: AtoMOXetine; Cannabinoids; COMT Inhibitors; Linezolid

Decreased Effect

DOBUTamine may decrease the levels/effects of: Iobenguane I 123

The levels/effects of DOBUTamine may be decreased by: Calcium Salts

Storage/Stability Store reconstituted solution under refrigeration for 48 hours or 6 hours at room temperature. Stability of parenteral admixture at room temperature (25°C) is 48 hours; at refrigeration (4°C) stability is 7 days. Remix solution every 24 hours. Pink discoloration of solution indicates slight oxidation but no significant loss of potency.

Mechanism of Action Stimulates $beta_1$-adrenergic receptors, causing increased contractility and heart rate, with little effect on $beta_2$- or alpha-receptors

Pharmacodynamics/Kinetics

Onset of action: I.V.: 1-10 minutes

Peak effect: 10-20 minutes

Metabolism: In tissues and hepatically to inactive metabolites

Half-life elimination: 2 minutes

Excretion: Urine (as metabolites)

Dosage Administration requires the use of an infusion pump; I.V. infusion: Children and Adults: 2.5-20 mcg/kg/minute; maximum: 40 mcg/kg/minute, titrate to desired response. **Note:** In patients with sepsis or septic shock, the recommended maximum dose is 20 mcg/kg/minute (Dellinger, 2013). See table.

Infusion Rates of Various Dilutions of Dobutamine

Desired Delivery Rate (mcg/kg/min)	Infusion Rate (mL/kg hour)	
	500 mcg/mL	1000 mcg/mL
2.5	0.3	0.15
5	0.6	0.3
7.5	0.9	0.45
10	1.2	0.6
12.5	1.5	0.75
15	1.8	0.9
20	2.4	1.2

Dosage adjustment in renal impairment: No dosage adjustment provided in manufacturer's labeling.

Dosage adjustment in hepatic impairment: No dosage adjustment provided in manufacturer's labeling.

Usual Infusion Concentrations: Pediatric Note: Premixed solutions available.

I.V. infusion: 1000 **mcg**/mL, 2000 **mcg**/mL, **or** 4000 **mcg**/mL

Usual Infusion Concentrations: Adult Note: Premixed solutions available.

I.V. infusion: 250 mg in 500 mL (concentration: 500 **mcg**/mL), 500 mg in 250 mL (concentration: 2000 **mcg**/mL), **or** 1000 mg in 250 mL (concentration: 4000 **mcg**/mL) of D_5W or NS

Administration Use infusion device to control rate of flow; administer into large vein. Do not administer through same I.V. line as heparin, hydrocortisone sodium succinate, cefazolin, or penicillin.

Monitoring Parameters Blood pressure, ECG, heart rate, CVP, RAP, MAP; serum glucose, renal function; urine output; if pulmonary artery catheter is in place, monitor CI, PCWP, and SVR

Consult individual institutional policies and procedures.

Additional Information Dobutamine lowers central venous pressure and wedge pressure but has little effect on pulmonary vascular resistance.

Dobutamine therapy should be avoided in patients with stable heart failure due to an increase in mortality. In patients with intractable heart failure, dobutamine may be used as a short-term infusion to provide symptomatic benefit. It is not known whether short-term dobutamine therapy in end-stage heart failure has any outcome benefit.

Dobutamine infusion during echocardiography is used as a cardiovascular stress. Wall motion abnormalities developing with increasing doses of dobutamine may help to identify ischemic and/or hibernating myocardium.

Dosage Forms Excipient information presented when available (limited, particularly for generics); consult specific product labeling.

Solution, Intravenous, as hydrochloride:

Generic: 1 mg/mL (250 mL); 2 mg/mL (250 mL); 4 mg/mL (250 mL); 250 mg/20 mL (20 mL); 500 mg/40 mL (40 mL)

Solution, Intravenous, as hydrochloride [preservative free]:

Generic: 250 mg/20 mL (20 mL)

◆ **Dobutamine Hydrochloride** *see* DOBUTamine *on page 637*

◆ **Dobutamine Injection, USP (Can)** *see* DOBUTamine *on page 637*

◆ **Dobutrex® (Can)** *see* DOBUTamine *on page 637*

◆ **Docefrez** *see* DOCEtaxel *on page 638*

DOCEtaxel (doe se TAKS el)

Brand Names: U.S. Docefrez; Taxotere

Brand Names: Canada Docetaxel for Injection; Taxotere

Index Terms RP-6976

Pharmacologic Category Antineoplastic Agent, Antimicrotubular; Antineoplastic Agent, Natural Source (Plant) Derivative; Antineoplastic Agent, Taxane Derivative

Use

U.S. labeling:

Docefrez: Treatment of breast cancer (locally-advanced/metastatic) after prior chemotherapy failure; treatment of locally-advanced or metastatic nonsmall cell lung cancer (NSCLC) after failure of prior platinum-based chemotherapy; treatment of hormone-refractory metastatic prostate cancer

Taxotere: Treatment of breast cancer (locally-advanced/metastatic) after prior chemotherapy failure, or adjuvant treatment of operable node-positive); locally-advanced or metastatic nonsmall cell lung cancer (NSCLC); hormone refractory, metastatic prostate cancer; advanced gastric adenocarcinoma; locally-advanced squamous cell head and neck cancer

Canadian labeling: Treatment of breast cancer (locally-advanced/metastatic or adjuvant treatment of operable node-positive); locally-advanced or metastatic nonsmall cell lung cancer (NSCLC); hormone refractory, metastatic prostate cancer; recurrent and/or metastatic squamous cell head and neck cancer; treatment of metastatic ovarian cancer following failure of first-line or subsequent chemotherapy

Unlabeled Use Treatment of bladder cancer (metastatic), ovarian cancer, cervical cancer (recurrent), esophageal cancer, small cell lung cancer (relapsed), soft tissue sarcoma, Ewing's sarcoma, osteosarcoma, and unknown-primary adenocarcinoma

Pregnancy Risk Factor D

Pregnancy Considerations Adverse events have been observed in animal reproduction studies. An *ex vivo* human placenta perfusion model illustrated that docetaxel crossed the placenta at term. Placental transfer was low and affected by the presence of albumin; higher albumin concentrations resulted in lower docetaxel placental transfer (Berveiller, 2012). Women of childbearing potential should avoid becoming pregnant. A pregnancy registry is available for all cancers diagnosed during pregnancy at Cooper Health (877-635-4499).

Breast-Feeding Considerations It is not known if docetaxel is excreted into breast milk. Due to the potential for serious adverse reactions in nursing the infant, the decision to discontinue docetaxel or to discontinue breast-feeding should take into account the importance of treatment to the mother.

Contraindications

Severe hypersensitivity to docetaxel or any component of the formulation; severe hypersensitivity to other medications containing polysorbate 80; neutrophil count <1500/mm^3

Canadian labeling: Additional contraindications (not in U.S. labeling): Severe hepatic impairment; pregnancy; breast-feeding

Warnings/Precautions Hazardous agent - use appropriate precautions for handling and disposal (NIOSH, 2012). **[U.S. Boxed Warning]: Avoid use in patients with bilirubin exceeding upper limit of normal (ULN) or AST and/or ALT >1.5 times ULN in conjunction with alkaline phosphatase >2.5 times ULN; patients with isolated transaminase elevations >1.5 times ULN also had a higher rate of neutropenic fever, although no increased incidence of toxic death.** Patients with abnormal liver function are also at increased risk of other treatment-related adverse events, including grade 4 neutropenia, infections, and severe thrombocytopenia, stomatitis, skin toxicity or toxic death; obtain liver function tests prior to each treatment cycle. Canadian labeling contraindicates use in severe hepatic impairment. Canadian labeling contraindicates use in severe hepatic impairment. **[U.S. Boxed Warnings]: Severe hypersensitivity reactions, characterized by generalized rash/erythema, hypotension, bronchospasms, or anaphylaxis may occur (may be fatal; has occurred in patients receiving corticosteroid premedication); minor reactions including flushing or localized skin reactions may also occur; do not administer to patients with a history of severe hypersensitivity to docetaxel or polysorbate 80 (component of formulation). Severe fluid retention, characterized by pleural effusion (requiring immediate drainage, ascites, peripheral edema (poorly tolerated), dyspnea at rest, cardiac tamponade, generalized edema, and weight gain, has been reported.** Fluid retention may begin as lower extremity peripheral edema and become generalized with a median weight gain of 2 kg. In patients with breast cancer, the median cumulative dose to onset of moderate or severe fluid retention was 819 mg/m^2; fluid retention resolves in a median of 16 weeks after discontinuation. Observe for hypersensitivity, especially with the first two infusions. Discontinue for severe reactions; do not rechallenge if severe. Patients should be premedicated with a corticosteroid (starting one day prior to administration) to prevent or reduce the severity of hypersensitivity reactions and fluid retention; severity is reduced with dexamethasone premedication starting one day prior to docetaxel administration.

[U.S. Boxed Warning]: Patients with abnormal liver function, those receiving higher doses, and patients with nonsmall cell lung cancer and a history of prior treatment with platinum derivatives who receive single-agent docetaxel at a dose of 100 mg/m^2 are at higher risk for treatment-related mortality.

Neutropenia is the dose-limiting toxicity. Patients with increased liver function tests experienced more episodes of neutropenia with a greater number of severe infections. **[U.S. Boxed Warning]: Patients with an absolute neutrophil count <1500/mm^3 should not receive docetaxel.** Platelets should recover to >100,000/mm^3 prior to treatment. Monitor blood counts and liver function tests frequently; dose reduction or therapy discontinuation may be necessary.

Cutaneous reactions including erythema (with edema) and desquamation have been reported; may require dose reduction. Cystoid macular edema (CME) has been reported; if vision impairment occurs, a prompt comprehensive ophthalmic exam is recommended. If CME is diagnosed, initiate appropriate CME management and discontinue docetaxel (consider non-taxane treatments). In a study of patients receiving docetaxel for the adjuvant treatment of breast cancer, a majority of patients experienced tearing, which occurred in patients with and without lacrimal duct obstruction at baseline; onset was generally after cycle 1, but subsided in most patients within 4 months after therapy completion (Chan, 2013). Dosage adjustment is recommended with severe neurosensory symptoms (paresthesia, dysesthesia, pain); persistent symptoms may require discontinuation; reversal of symptoms may be delayed after discontinuation. Treatment-related acute myeloid leukemia or myelodysplasia occurred in patients receiving docetaxel in combination with anthracyclines and/or cyclophosphamide. Fatigue and weakness (may be severe) have been reported; symptoms may last a few days up to several weeks; in patients with progressive disease, weakness may be associated with a decrease in performance status. Potentially significant drug-drug interactions may exist, requiring dose or frequency adjustment, additional monitoring, and/or selection of alternative therapy. Docetaxel is an irritant with vesicant-like properties; ensure proper needle or catheter placement prior to and during infusion; avoid extravasation.

Adverse Reactions Percentages reported for docetaxel monotherapy; frequency may vary depending on diagnosis, dose, liver function, prior treatment, and premedication. The incidence of adverse events was usually higher in patients with elevated liver function tests.

>10%:

Central nervous system: Central nervous system toxicity (20% to 58%; including neuropathy)

Dermatologic: Alopecia (56% to 76%), dermatological reaction (20% to 48%), nail disease (11% to 41%)

Endocrine & metabolic: Fluid retention (13% to 60%; dose dependent)

Gastrointestinal: Stomatitis (19% to 53%; severe 1% to 8%), diarrhea (23% to 43%; severe: 5% to 6%), nausea (34% to 42%), vomiting (22% to 23%)

Hematologic & oncologic: Neutropenia (84% to 99%; grade 4: 75% to 86%; nadir (median): 7 days, duration (severe neutropenia): 7 days; dose dependent), leukopenia (84% to 99%; grade 4: 32% to 44%), anemia (65% to 94%; dose dependent; grades 3/4: 8% to 9%), thrombocytopenia (8% to 14%; grade 4: 1%; dose dependent), febrile neutropenia (6% to 12%; dose dependent)

Hepatic: Increased serum transaminases (4% to 19%)

Hypersensitivity: Hypersensitivity (1% to 21%; with premedication 15%)

Infection: Increased susceptibility to infection (1% to 34%; dose dependent)

Neuromuscular & skeletal: Weakness (53% to 66%; severe 13% to 18%), myalgia (3% to 23%), neuromuscular reaction (16%)

Respiratory: Pulmonary events (41%)

Miscellaneous: Fever (31% to 35%)

1% to 10%:

Cardiovascular: Decreased left ventricular ejection fraction (prostate cancer: 10%; metastatic breast cancer: 8%), hypotension (3%)

Gastrointestinal: Taste perversion (6%)

Hepatic: Increased serum bilirubin (9%), increased serum alkaline phosphatase (4% to 7%)

Local: Infusion site reactions (4%, including hyperpigmentation, inflammation, redness, dryness, phlebitis, extravasation, swelling of the vein)

Neuromuscular and skeletal: Arthralgia (3% to 9%)

Ophthalmic: Epiphora (associated with canalicular stenosis [≤77% with weekly administration; ≤1% with every 3-week administration])

<1% (Limited to important or life-threatening): Acute myelocytic leukemia, acute respiratory distress, anaphylactic shock, ascites, atrial fibrillation, atrial flutter, atrioventricular block, bradycardia, bronchospasm, cardiac arrhythmia, cardiac failure, cardiac tamponade, chest pain, chest tightness, colitis, conjunctivitis, constipation, deep vein thrombosis, dehydration, disease of the lacrimal apparatus (duct obstruction), disseminated intravascular coagulation, drug fever, duodenal ulcer, dyspnea, ECG abnormality, erythema multiforme, esophagitis, gastrointestinal hemorrhage, gastrointestinal obstruction, gastrointestinal perforation, hearing loss, hemorrhagic diathesis, hepatitis, hypertension, intestinal obstruction, interstitial pulmonary disease, ischemic colitis, ischemic heart disease, loss of consciousness (transient), multi-organ failure, myelodysplastic syndrome, myocardial infarction, neutropenic enterocolitis, ototoxicity, palmar-plantar erythrodysesthesia, pericardial effusion, pleural effusion, pneumonia, pneumonitis, pruritus, pulmonary edema, pulmonary embolism, pulmonary fibrosis, radiation pneumonitis, radiation recall phenomenon, renal failure, renal insufficiency, respiratory failure, skin changes (scleroderma-like), seizure, sepsis, sinus tachycardia, Stevens-Johnson syndrome, subacute cutaneous lupus erythematosus, syncope, toxic epidermal necrolysis, tachycardia, thrombophlebitis, unstable angina pectoris, visual disturbance (transient)

Drug Interactions

Metabolism/Transport Effects Substrate of CYP3A4 (major), P-glycoprotein; **Note:** Assignment of Major/Minor substrate status based on clinically relevant drug interaction potential; **Inhibits** CYP3A4 (weak)

Avoid Concomitant Use

Avoid concomitant use of DOCEtaxel with any of the following: BCG; CloZAPine; Conivaptan; Fusidic Acid (Systemic); Natalizumab; Pimecrolimus; Pimozide; Tacrolimus (Topical); Tofacitinib; Vaccines (Live)

Increased Effect/Toxicity

DOCEtaxel may increase the levels/effects of: Antineoplastic Agents (Anthracycline, Systemic); ARIPiprazole; CloZAPine; Dofetilide; Leflunomide; Lomitapide; Natalizumab; Pimozide; Tofacitinib; Vaccines (Live)

The levels/effects of DOCEtaxel may be increased by: Antifungal Agents (Azole Derivatives, Systemic); Conivaptan; CYP3A4 Inhibitors (Moderate); CYP3A4 Inhibitors (Strong); Dasatinib; Denosumab; Dronedarone; Fusidic Acid (Systemic); Ivacaftor; Luliconazole; Mifepristone; P-glycoprotein/ABCB1 Inhibitors; Pimecrolimus; Platinum Derivatives; Roflumilast; Simeprevir; SORAfenib; Tacrolimus (Topical); Trastuzumab

Decreased Effect

DOCEtaxel may decrease the levels/effects of: BCG; Coccidioidin Skin Test; Sipuleucel-T; Vaccines (Inactivated); Vaccines (Live)

The levels/effects of DOCEtaxel may be decreased by: Bosentan; CYP3A4 Inducers (Strong); Dabrafenib; Deferasirox; Echinacea; Herbs (CYP3A4 Inducers); Mitotane; P-glycoprotein/ABCB1 Inducers; Tocilizumab

Ethanol/Nutrition/Herb Interactions

Ethanol: Avoid ethanol (due to GI irritation).

Herb/Nutraceutical: Avoid St John's wort (may decrease docetaxel levels).

Preparation for Administration Preparation instructions may vary by manufacturer, refer to specific prescribing information.

Note: Multiple concentrations: Docetaxel is available as a one-vial formulation at concentrations of 10 mg/mL (generic formulation) and 20 mg/mL (concentrate; Taxotere, and as a lyophilized powder (Docefrez) which is reconstituted (with provided diluent) to 20 mg/0.8 mL (20 mg vial) or 24 mg/mL (80 mg vial). Admixture errors have occurred due to the availability of various concentrations. Docetaxel was previously available as a two-vial formulation which included two vials (a concentrated docetaxel vial and a diluent vial), resulting in a reconstituted concentration of 10 mg/mL; the two-vial formulation has been discontinued by the Taxotere manufacturer (available generically).

Hazardous agent; use appropriate precautions for handling and disposal (NIOSH, 2012).

One-vial formulations: Further dilute for infusion in 250-500 mL of NS or D_5W in a non-DEHP container (eg, glass, polypropylene, polyolefin) to a final concentration of 0.3-0.74 mg/mL. Gently rotate and invert manually to mix thoroughly; avoid shaking or vigorous agitation.

Taxotere: Use **only** a 21 gauge needle to withdraw docetaxel from the vial (larger bore needles, such as 18 gauge or 19 gauge needles, may cause stopper coring and rubber precipitates). If intact vials were stored refrigerated, allow to stand at room temperature for 5 minutes prior to dilution. Inspect vials prior to dilution; solution is supersaturated and may crystalize over time; do not use if crystalized.

Lyophilized powder: Dilute with the provided diluent (contains ethanol in polysorbate 80); add 1 mL to each 20 mg vial (resulting concentration is 20 mg/0.8 mL) and 4 mL to each 80 mg vial (resulting concentration is 24 mg/mL). Shake well to dissolve completely. If air bubbles are present, allow to stand for a few minutes while air bubbles dissipate. Further dilute in 250 mL of NS or D_5W in a non-DEHP container (eg, glass, polypropylene, polyolefin) to a final concentration of 0.3-0.74 mg/mL (for doses >200 mg, use a larger volume of NS or D_5W, not to exceed a final concentration of 0.74 mg/mL). Mix thoroughly by manual agitation.

Two-vial formulation *(generic; concentrate plus diluent formulation):* Vials should be diluted with 13% (w/w) polyethylene glycol 400/water (provided with the drug) to a final concentration of 10 mg/mL. Do not shake. Further dilute for infusion in 250-500 mL of NS or D_5W in a non-DEHP container (eg, glass, polypropylene, polyolefin) to a final concentration of 0.3-0.74 mg/mL. Gently rotate to mix thoroughly. Do not use the two-vial formulation with the one-vial formulation for the same admixture product.

Storage/Stability

Storage and stability may vary by manufacturer, refer to specific prescribing information.

Docetaxel 10 mg/mL: Store intact vials between 2°C to 25°C (36°F to 77°F) (actual recommendations may vary by generic manufacturer; consult manufacturer's labeling). Protect from bright light. Freezing does not adversely affect the product. Multi-use vials (80 mg/8 mL and 160 mg/16 mL) are stable for up to 28 days after first entry when stored between 2°C to 8°C (36°F to 46°F) and protected from light. Solutions diluted for infusion should be used within 4 hours of preparation, including infusion time.

Docetaxel 20 mg/mL concentrate:

Taxotere: Store intact vials between 2°C to 25°C (36°F to 77°F). Protect from bright light. Freezing does not adversely affect the product. Solutions diluted for infusion in non-PVC containers should be used within 6 hours of preparation, including infusion time, when stored between 2°C to 25°C (36°F to 77°F) or within 48 hours when stored between 2°C to 8°C (36°F to 46°F).

Generic formulations: Store intact vials at 25°C (77°F); excursions permitted between 15°C to 30°C (59°F to 86°F). Protect from light. Solutions diluted for infusion should be used within 4 hours of preparation, including infusion time.

Docetaxel lyophilized powder (Docefrez): Store intact vials between 2°C to 8°C (36°F to 46°F). Protect from light. Allow vials (and provided diluent) to stand at room temperature for 5 minutes prior to reconstitution. After reconstitution, may be stored refrigerated or at room temperature for up to 8 hours. Solutions diluted for infusion should be used within 4 hours of preparation, including infusion time.

Two-vial formulation *(generic; concentrate plus diluent formulation):* Reconstituted solutions of the two-vial formulation are stable in the vial for 8 hours at room temperature or under refrigeration. Solutions diluted for infusion in polyolefin containers should be used within 4 hours of preparation, including infusion time.

Mechanism of Action Docetaxel promotes the assembly of microtubules from tubulin dimers, and inhibits the depolymerization of tubulin which stabilizes microtubules in the cell. This results in inhibition of DNA, RNA, and protein synthesis. Most activity occurs during the M phase of the cell cycle.

Pharmacodynamics/Kinetics Exhibits linear pharmacokinetics at the recommended dosage range

Distribution: Extensive extravascular distribution and/or tissue binding; V_{dss}: 113 L (mean steady state)

Protein binding: ~94% to 97%, primarily to alpha$_1$-acid glycoprotein, albumin, and lipoproteins

Metabolism: Hepatic; oxidation via CYP3A4 to metabolites

Half-life elimination: Terminal: ~11 hours

Excretion: Feces (~75%, <8% as unchanged drug); urine (~6%)

Dosage Note: Premedicate with corticosteroids for 3 days, beginning one day prior to docetaxel administration, to reduce the severity of hypersensitivity reactions and fluid retention. Details concerning dosing in combination regimens should also be consulted.

U.S. labeling:

Breast cancer: Adults: I.V.:

Locally-advanced or metastatic: 60-100 mg/m^2 every 3 weeks (as a single agent)

Operable, node-positive (adjuvant treatment): 75 mg/m^2 every 3 weeks for 6 courses (in combination with doxorubicin and cyclophosphamide)

Adjuvant treatment (unlabeled dosing): 75 mg/m^2 every 21 days (in combination with cyclophosphamide) for 4 cycles (Jones, 2006) **or** 75 mg/m^2 every 21 days (in combination with carboplatin and trastuzumab) for 6 cycles (Slamon, 2011)

Metastatic treatment (unlabeled dosing):

Every-3-week administration: 75 mg/m^2 (cycle 1; may increase to 100 mg/m2 in subsequent cycles) every 21 days for at least 6 cycles (in combination with trastuzumab and pertuzumab) (Baselga, 2012; Swain, 2013) **or** 100 mg/m^2 every 21 days (in combination with trastuzumab) for at least 6 cycles (Marty, 2005) **or** 75 mg/m^2 every 21 days (in combination with capecitabine) until disease progression or unacceptable toxicity (O'Shaughnessy, 2002) **or** 60 mg/m^2, 75 mg/m^2, or 100 mg/m^2 every 21 days for at least 6 cycles until disease progression, unacceptable toxicity, or discontinuation (Harvey, 2006)

Weekly administration: 40 mg/m^2/dose once a week (as a single agent) for 6 weeks followed by a 2-week rest, repeat until disease progression or unacceptable toxicity (Burstein, 2000) **or** 35 mg/m^2/dose once weekly for 3 weeks, followed by a 1-week rest, may increase to 40 mg/m^2 once weekly for 3 weeks followed by a 1-week rest with cycle 2 (Rivera, 2008) **or** 35 mg/m^2/dose once weekly (in combination with trastuzumab) for 3 weeks followed by a 1-week rest; repeat until disease progression or unacceptable toxicity (Esteva, 2002)

Nonsmall cell lung cancer: Adults: I.V.: 75 mg/m^2 every 3 weeks (as a single agent or in combination with cisplatin)

Prostate cancer: Adults: I.V.: 75 mg/m^2 every 3 weeks (in combination with prednisone)

Gastric adenocarcinoma: Adults: I.V.: 75 mg/m^2 every 3 weeks (in combination with cisplatin and fluorouracil)

Sequential chemotherapy and chemoradiation (unlabeled dosing): Induction: 75 mg/m^2 on days 1 and 22 (in combination with cisplatin) for 2 cycles, followed by chemoradiation: 20 mg/m^2 weekly for 5 weeks (in combination with cisplatin and radiation) (Ruhstaller, 2009)

Locally-advanced or metastatic disease (unlabeled dosing): 50 mg/m^2 on day 1 every 2 weeks (in combination with fluorouracil, leucovorin, and oxaliplatin) until disease progression or unacceptable toxicity up to a maximum of 8 cycles (Al-Batran, 2008)

Head and neck cancer: Adults: I.V.: 75 mg/m^2 every 3 weeks (in combination with cisplatin and fluorouracil) for 3 or 4 cycles, followed by radiation therapy

Canadian labeling:

Breast cancer: Adults: I.V.:

Locally-advanced or metastatic: 75 mg/m^2 (as combination therapy) **or** 100 mg/m^2 (as a single agent) every 3 weeks

Operable, node-positive (adjuvant treatment): 75 mg/m^2 every 3 weeks for 6 courses (in combination with doxorubicin and cyclophosphamide)

Nonsmall cell lung cancer (locally-advanced or metastatic), ovarian cancer (metastatic), head and neck cancer (recurrent and/or metastatic): Adults: I.V.: 75 mg/m^2 (as combination therapy) **or** 100 mg/m^2 (as a single agent) every 3 weeks

Prostate cancer (hormone-refractory, metastatic): Adults: I.V.: 75 mg/m^2 every 3 weeks (in combination with prednisone or prednisolone)

Unlabeled uses:

Bladder cancer, metastatic (unlabeled use): Adults: I.V.: 100 mg/m^2 every 3 weeks (as a single agent) (McCaffrey, 1997) **or** 35 mg/m^2 on days 1 and 8 of a 21-day cycle (in combination with gemcitabine and cisplatin) for at least 6 cycles or until disease progression or unacceptable toxicity (Pectasides, 2002)

Esophageal cancer (unlabeled use): Adults: I.V.:

Sequential chemotherapy and chemoradiation: Induction: 75 mg/m^2 on days 1 and 22 (in combination with cisplatin) for 2 cycles, followed by chemoradiation: 20 mg/m^2 weekly for 5 weeks (in combination with cisplatin and radiation) (Ruhstaller, 2009)

Definitive chemoradiation: 60 mg/m^2 on days 1 and 22 (in combination with cisplatin and radiation) for 1 cycle (Li, 2010)

Locally-advanced or metastatic disease: 75 mg/m^2 on day 1 every 3 weeks (in combination with cisplatin and fluorouracil) (Ajani, 2007; Van Cutsem, 2006) **or** 50 mg/m^2 on day 1 every 2 weeks (in combination with fluorouracil, leucovorin, and oxaliplatin) until disease progression or unacceptable toxicity up to a maximum of 8 cycles (Al-Batran, 2008) **or** 35 mg/m^2 weekly for 8 weeks (in combination with cisplatin, fluorouracil, and radiotherapy; neoadjuvant setting) (Pasini, 2013)

Ewing sarcoma, osteosarcoma (recurrent or progressive; unlabeled uses): Children ≥8 years, Adolescents, and Adults: I.V.: 100 mg/m^2 on day 8 of a 21-day cycle (in combination with gemcitabine) (Navid, 2008)

Ovarian cancer (unlabeled use in U.S.): Adults: I.V.: 60 mg/m^2 every 3 weeks (in combination with carboplatin) for up to 6 cycles (Markman, 2001) **or** 75 mg/m^2 every 3 weeks (in combination with carboplatin) for 6 to 9 cycles (Vasey, 2004) **or** 35 mg/m^2 (maximum dose: 70 mg) weekly for 3 weeks followed by a 1-week rest (in combination with carboplatin) (Kushner, 2007)

Small cell lung cancer, relapsed (unlabeled use): Adults: I.V.:100 mg/m^2 every 3 weeks (Smyth, 1994)

Soft tissue sarcoma (unlabeled use): Adults: I.V.: 100 mg/m^2 on day 8 of a 3-week treatment cycle (in combination with gemcitabine and filgrastim or pegfilgrastim) (Leu, 2004; Maki, 2007)

Unknown-primary, adenocarcinoma (unlabeled use): Adults: I.V.: 65 mg/m^2 every 3 weeks (in combination with carboplatin) (Greco, 2000) **or** 75 mg/m^2 on day 8 of a 3-week treatment cycle (in combination with gemcitabine) for up to 6 cycles (Pouessel, 2004) **or** 60 mg/m^2 on day 1 of a 3-week treatment cycle (in combination with cisplatin) (Mukai, 2010)

Dosing adjustment for concomitant CYP3A4 inhibitors: Avoid the concomitant use of strong CYP3A4 inhibitors with docetaxel. If concomitant use of a strong CYP3A4 inhibitor cannot be avoided, consider reducing the docetaxel dose by 50% (based on limited pharmacokinetic data).

Dosing adjustment for toxicity:

Note: Toxicity includes febrile neutropenia, neutrophils <500/mm^3 for >1 week, severe or cumulative cutaneous reactions; in nonsmall cell lung cancer, this may also include platelet nadir <25,000/mm^3 and other grade 3/4 nonhematologic toxicities.

Breast cancer (single agent): Patients dosed initially at 100 mg/m^2; reduce dose to 75 mg/m^2; **Note:** If the patient continues to experience these adverse reactions, the dosage should be reduced to 55 mg/m^2 or therapy should be discontinued; discontinue for peripheral neuropathy ≥ grade 3. Patients initiated at 60 mg/m^2 who do not develop toxicity may tolerate higher doses.

Breast cancer, adjuvant treatment (combination chemotherapy): TAC regimen should be administered when neutrophils are ≥1500/mm^3. Patients experiencing febrile neutropenia should receive G-CSF in all subsequent cycles. Patients with persistent febrile neutropenia (while on G-CSF), patients experiencing severe/cumulative cutaneous reactions, moderate neurosensory effects (signs/symptoms) or grade 3 or 4 stomatitis should receive a reduced dose (60 mg/m^2) of docetaxel. Discontinue therapy with persistent toxicities after dosage reduction.

Nonsmall cell lung cancer:

Monotherapy: Patients dosed initially at 75 mg/m^2 should have dose held until toxicity is resolved, then resume at 55 mg/m^2; discontinue for peripheral neuropathy ≥ grade 3.

Combination therapy (with cisplatin): Patients dosed initially at 75 mg/m^2 should have the docetaxel dosage reduced to 65 mg/m^2 in subsequent cycles; if further adjustment is required, dosage may be reduced to 50 mg/m^2

Prostate cancer: Reduce dose to 60 mg/m^2; discontinue therapy if toxicities persist at lower dose.

Gastric cancer, head and neck cancer: **Note:** Cisplatin may require dose reductions/therapy delays for peripheral neuropathy, ototoxicity, and/or nephrotoxicity. Patients experiencing febrile neutropenia, documented infection with neutropenia or neutropenia >7 days should receive G-CSF in all subsequent cycles. For neutropenic complications despite G-CSF use, further reduce dose to 60 mg/m^2. Dosing with neutropenic complications in subsequent cycles should be further reduced to 45 mg/m^2. Patients who experience grade 4 thrombocytopenia should receive a dose reduction from 75 mg/m^2 to 60 mg/m^2. Discontinue therapy for persistent toxicities.

Gastrointestinal toxicity for docetaxel in combination with cisplatin and fluorouracil for treatment of gastric cancer or head and neck cancer:

Diarrhea, grade 3:
- First episode: Reduce fluorouracil dose by 20%
- Second episode: Reduce docetaxel dose by 20%

Diarrhea, grade 4:
- First episode: Reduce fluorouracil and docetaxel doses by 20%
- Second episode: Discontinue treatment

Stomatitis, grade 3:
- First episode: Reduce fluorouracil dose by 20%
- Second episode: Discontinue fluorouracil for all subsequent cycles
- Third episode: Reduce docetaxel dose by 20%

Stomatitis, grade 4:
- First episode: Discontinue fluorouracil for all subsequent cycles
- Second episode: Reduce docetaxel dose by 20%

Canadian labeling: **Note:** Toxicity includes febrile neutropenia, neutrophils ≤500/mm^3 for >1 week, severe or cumulative cutaneous reactions, or severe neurosensory symptoms.

Patients initially dosed at 100 mg/m^2: Reduce dose to 75 mg/m^2; Patients initially dosed at 75 mg/m^2: Reduce dose to 60 mg/m^2. Discontinue therapy for persistent toxicities after dosage reduction.

Breast cancer, adjuvant treatment (combination chemotherapy): Patients experiencing febrile neutropenia should receive G-CSF in all subsequent cycles. Patients with persistent febrile neutropenia (while on G-CSF), patients experiencing severe/cumulative cutaneous reactions, severe neurosensory symptoms, or grade 3 or 4 stomatitis should receive a reduced dose (60 mg/m^2). Discontinue therapy with persistent toxicities after dosage reduction.

Concomitant use with capecitabine (treatment of metastatic breast cancer):

Grade 2 toxicities:

First episode: Interrupt therapy until resolution to < grade 2, then resume docetaxel and capecitabine at previous dose; consider prophylactic measures if appropriate and/or possible

Second episode of same toxicity: Interrupt therapy until resolution to < grade 2, then resume docetaxel at 55 mg/m^2; reduce capecitabine dose to 75% of original dose

Further episodes of same toxicity: Discontinue docetaxel; interrupt capecitabine until resolution to < grade 2, then resume at 50% of original dose (third episode) or discontinue therapy altogether (fourth episode)

Grade 3 toxicities:

First episode: Occurring at time treatment is due: Interrupt docetaxel until resolution to < grade 2 (maximum delay ≤2 weeks), then resume docetaxel at 55 mg/m^2; reduce capecitabine dose to 75% of original dose (consider prophylactic measure if appropriate); if no resolution to < grade 2 within 2 weeks, discontinue docetaxel but may resume capecitabine at 75% of original dose after resolution to < grade 2. Occurring between cycles and resolves to < grade 2 by time of next treatment: Administer docetaxel at 55 mg/m^2 and reduce capecitabine dose to 75% of original dose; consider prophylactic measures if appropriate and/or possible.

Further episodes of same toxicity: Discontinue docetaxel; interrupt capecitabine until resolution to < grade 2, then resume capecitabine at 50% of original dose (second episode) or discontinue therapy altogether (third episode)

Grade 4 toxicities: First episode: Discontinue docetaxel and capecitabine therapy or if deemed clinically necessary, capecitabine may be continued at 50% of original dose

Dosage adjustment in renal impairment: Renal excretion is minimal (~6%), therefore, the need for dosage adjustments for renal dysfunction is unlikely (Janus, 2010; Li, 2007). Not removed by hemodialysis, may be administered before or after hemodialysis (Janus, 2010).

Dosage adjustment in hepatic impairment:

U.S. labeling:

Total bilirubin greater than the ULN, or AST and/or ALT >1.5 times ULN concomitant with alkaline phosphatase >2.5 times ULN: Use is not recommended.

Hepatic impairment dosing adjustment specific for gastric or head and neck cancer:

AST/ALT >2.5 to ≤5 times ULN and alkaline phosphatase ≤2.5 times ULN: Administer 80% of dose

AST/ALT >1.5 to ≤5 times ULN and alkaline phosphatase >2.5 to ≤5 times ULN: Administer 80% of dose

AST/ALT >5 times ULN and /or alkaline phosphatase >5 times ULN: Discontinue docetaxel

Canadian labeling: **Note:** Dosing recommendations when used as a single agent; dosage adjustment when used as part of combination therapy not provided in manufacturer's labeling.

AST and/or ALT >1.5 times ULN and alkaline phosphatase >2.5 times ULN: Reduce dose from 100 mg/m^2 to 75 mg/m^2

Serum bilirubin >ULN and/or AST and ALT >3.5 times ULN associated with alkaline phosphatase >6 times ULN: Avoid use unless strictly indicated.

Severe hepatic impairment: Use is contraindicated.

The following adjustments have also been used (Floyd, 2006):

Transaminases 1.6-6 times ULN: Administer 75% of dose.

Transaminases >6 times ULN: Use clinical judgment.

Dosing in obesity: *ASCO Guidelines for appropriate chemotherapy dosing in obese adults with cancer:* Utilize patient's actual body weight (full weight) for calculation of body surface area- or weight-based dosing, particularly when the intent of therapy is curative; manage regimen-related toxicities in the same manner as for nonobese patients; if a dose reduction is utilized due to toxicity, consider resumption of full weight-based dosing with subsequent cycles, especially if cause of toxicity (eg, hepatic or renal impairment) is resolved (Griggs, 2012).

Administration Administer I.V. infusion over 1-hour through nonsorbing polyethylene lined (non-DEHP) tubing; in-line filter is not necessary (the use of a filter during administration is not recommended by the manufacturer). Infusion should be completed within 4 hours of final preparation. **Note:** Premedication with corticosteroids for 3 days, beginning the day before docetaxel administration, is recommended to reduce the incidence and severity of hypersensitivity reactions and fluid retention (see Additional Information).

Irritant with vesicant-like properties; avoid extravasation. Assure proper needle or catheter position prior to administration.

Extravasation management: If extravasation occurs, stop infusion immediately and disconnect (leave cannula/needle in place); gently aspirate extravasated solution (do **NOT** flush the line); remove needle/cannula; elevate extremity. Information conflicts regarding the use of warm or cold compresses (Perez Fidalgo, 2012; Polovich, 2009).

Hazardous agent; use appropriate precautions for handling and disposal (NIOSH, 2012).

Monitoring Parameters CBC with differential, liver function tests, bilirubin, alkaline phosphatase, renal function; monitor for hypersensitivity reactions, neurosensory symptoms, gastrointestinal toxicity (eg, diarrhea, stomatitis), cutaneous reactions, visual impairment, fluid retention, epiphora, and canalicular stenosis

Additional Information Premedication with oral corticosteroids is recommended to decrease the incidence and severity of fluid retention and severity of hypersensitivity reactions. The manufacturer recommends dexamethasone 16 mg/day (8 mg twice daily) orally for 3 days, starting the day before docetaxel administration; for prostate cancer, when prednisone is part of the antineoplastic regimen, dexamethasone 8 mg orally is administered at 12 hours, 3 hours, and 1 hour prior to docetaxel.

Dosage Forms Excipient information presented when available (limited, particularly for generics); consult specific product labeling.

Concentrate, Intravenous:

Taxotere: 20 mg/mL (1 mL); 80 mg/4 mL (4 mL) [contains alcohol, usp, polysorbate 80]

Generic: 20 mg/mL (1 mL); 80 mg/4 mL (4 mL); 160 mg/8 mL (8 mL); 20 mg/0.5 mL (0.5 mL); 80 mg/2 mL (2 mL)

Concentrate, Intravenous [preservative free]:

Generic: 20 mg/mL (1 mL); 80 mg/4 mL (4 mL); 140 mg/7 mL (7 mL)

Solution, Intravenous:

Generic: 20 mg/2 mL (2 mL); 80 mg/8 mL (8 mL); 160 mg/16 mL (16 mL)

Solution Reconstituted, Intravenous:

Docefrez: 20 mg (1 ea); 80 mg (1 ea) [contains alcohol, usp, polysorbate 80]

◆ Docetaxel for Injection (Can) *see* DOCEtaxel *on page 638*

◆ Docosahexaenoic Acid *see* Omega-3-Acid Ethyl Esters *on page 1504*

Docosanol (doe KOE san ole)

Brand Names: U.S. Abreva [OTC]

Index Terms *n*-Docosanol; Behenyl Alcohol

Pharmacologic Category Antiviral Agent, Topical

Use Treatment of herpes simplex of the face or lips

Dosage Children ≥12 years and Adults: Topical: Apply 5 times/day to affected area of face or lips. Start at first sign of cold sore or fever blister and continue until healed.

Additional Information Complete prescribing information should be consulted for additional detail.

Dosage Forms Excipient information presented when available (limited, particularly for generics); consult specific product labeling.

Cream, External:
Abreva: 10% (2 g) [contains benzyl alcohol]

◆ DocQLace [OTC] *see* Docusate *on page 644*

◆ Doc-Q-Lax [OTC] *see* Docusate and Senna *on page 645*

◆ Docu [OTC] *see* Docusate *on page 644*

◆ Docuprene [OTC] *see* Docusate *on page 644*

Docusate (DOK yoo sate)

Brand Names: U.S. Colace [OTC]; D.O.S. [OTC]; Diocto [OTC]; DocQLace [OTC]; Docu Soft [OTC]; Docu [OTC]; Docuprene [OTC]; Docusil [OTC]; DocuSol Mini [OTC]; DOK [OTC]; Dulcolax Stool Softener [OTC]; Enemeez Mini [OTC]; Kao-Tin [OTC]; KS Stool Softener [OTC]; Laxa Basic [OTC]; Pedia-Lax [OTC]; Promolaxin [OTC]; Silace [OTC]; Sof-Lax [OTC]; Stool Softener Laxative DC [OTC]; Stool Softener [OTC]; Sur-Q-Lax [OTC]; Vacuant Mini-Enema [OTC] [DSC]

Brand Names: Canada Apo-Docusate-Sodium®; Colace®; Colax-C®; Novo-Docusate Calcium; Novo-Docusate Sodium; PMS-Docusate Calcium; PMS-Docusate Sodium; Regulex®; Selax®; Soflax™

Index Terms Dioctyl Calcium Sulfosuccinate; Dioctyl Sodium Sulfosuccinate; Docusate Calcium; Docusate Potassium; Docusate Sodium; DOSS; DSS

Pharmacologic Category Stool Softener

Additional Appendix Information

Laxatives, Classification and Properties *on page 2304*

Use Stool softener in patients who should avoid straining during defecation and constipation associated with hard, dry stools; prophylaxis for straining (Valsalva) following myocardial infarction. A safe agent to be used in elderly; some evidence that doses <200 mg are ineffective; stool softeners are unnecessary if stool is well hydrated or "mushy" and soft; shown to be ineffective used long-term.

Unlabeled Use Ceruminolytic

Dosage Docusate salts are interchangeable; the amount of sodium or calcium per dosage unit is clinically insignificant

Infants and Children <3 years: Oral: 10-40 mg/day in 1-4 divided doses

Children: Oral:
3-6 years: 20-60 mg/day in 1-4 divided doses
6-12 years: 40-150 mg/day in 1-4 divided doses

Adolescents and Adults: Oral: 50-500 mg/day in 1-4 divided doses

Older Children and Adults: Rectal: Add 50-100 mg of docusate liquid to enema fluid (saline or water); administer as retention or flushing enema

Ceruminolytic (unlabeled use): Intra-aural: Administer 1 mL of docusate sodium in 2 mL syringes; if no clearance in 15 minutes, irrigate with 50-100 mL normal saline (this method is 80% effective)

Additional Information Complete prescribing information should be consulted for additional detail.

Dosage Forms Excipient information presented when available (limited, particularly for generics); consult specific product labeling. [DSC] = Discontinued product

Capsule, Oral, as calcium:
Kao-Tin: 240 mg [sodium free; contains fd&c red #40]
Stool Softener Laxative DC: 240 mg [contains fd&c red #40]
Sur-Q-Lax: 240 mg
Generic: 240 mg

Capsule, Oral, as sodium:
Colace: 50 mg, 100 mg
D.O.S.: 250 mg
DocQLace: 100 mg [contains fd&c red #40, fd&c yellow #6 (sunset yellow)]
Docu Soft: 100 mg
Docusil: 100 mg
DOK: 100 mg, 250 mg
Dulcolax Stool Softener: 100 mg [contains fd&c red #40, fd&c yellow #6 (sunset yellow)]
KS Stool Softener: 100 mg [stimulant free; contains brilliant blue fcf (fd&c blue #1), fd&c red #40, methylparaben, propylparaben, tartrazine (fd&c yellow #5)]
Laxa Basic: 100 mg, 250 mg
Sof-Lax: 100 mg
Stool Softener: 100 mg
Stool Softener: 100 mg, 250 mg [contains fd&c red #40, fd&c yellow #6 (sunset yellow)]
Stool Softener: 100 mg [stimulant free; contains brilliant blue fcf (fd&c blue #1), fd&c red #40, fd&c yellow #6 (sunset yellow)]
Generic: 100 mg, 250 mg

Enema, Rectal, as sodium:
DocuSol Mini: 283 mg (5 ea)
Enemeez Mini: 283 mg (5 mL)
Vacuant Mini-Enema: 283 mg (5 mL [DSC])

Liquid, Oral, as sodium:
Diocto: 50 mg/5 mL (473 mL) [contains fd&c red #40, methylparaben, polyethylene glycol, propylene glycol, propylparaben; vanilla flavor]
Diocto: 50 mg/5 mL (473 mL) [contains parabens, polyethylene glycol]
Docu: 50 mg/5 mL (10 mL, 473 mL) [contains methylparaben, polyethylene glycol, propylene glycol, propylparaben, sodium benzoate; vanilla flavor]
Pedia-Lax: 50 mg/15 mL (118 mL) [contains edetate disodium, methylparaben, polyethylene glycol, propylene glycol, propylparaben; fruit punch flavor]
Silace: 150 mg/15 mL (473 mL) [lemon-vanilla flavor]
Generic: 50 mg/5 mL (10 mL)

Syrup, Oral, as sodium:
Diocto: 60 mg/15 mL (473 mL) [contains fd&c red #40, menthol, methylparaben, polyethylene glycol, propylparaben, sodium benzoate; peppermint flavor]
Diocto: 60 mg/15 mL (473 mL [DSC]) [contains fd&c red #40, methylparaben, propylene glycol, propylparaben, sodium benzoate; peppermint flavor]
Diocto: 60 mg/15 mL (473 mL) [contains fd&c red #40, propylene glycol, saccharin sodium, sodium benzoate]
Silace: 60 mg/15 mL (473 mL) [contains alcohol, usp; peppermint flavor]

Tablet, Oral, as sodium:
Docuprene: 100 mg [contains sodium benzoate]
DOK: 100 mg [scored]
Promolaxin: 100 mg [scored; contains sodium benzoate]
Stool Softener: 100 mg [contains sodium benzoate]
Generic: 100 mg

Docusate and Senna (DOK yoo sate & SEN na)

Brand Names: U.S. Doc-Q-Lax [OTC]; Dok™ Plus [OTC]; Geri-Stool [OTC]; Peri-Colace® [OTC]; Senexon®-S [OTC]; Senna Plus [OTC]; SennaLax-S [OTC]; Senokot-S® [OTC]; SenoSol™-SS [OTC]

Index Terms Senna and Docusate; Senna-S

Pharmacologic Category Laxative, Stimulant; Stool Softener

Additional Appendix Information

Laxatives, Classification and Properties *on page 2304*

Use Short-term treatment of constipation

Unlabeled Use Evacuate the colon for bowel or rectal examinations; management/prevention of opioid-induced constipation

Dosage Oral: Constipation: OTC ranges:

Children:

2-6 years: Initial: 4.3 mg sennosides plus 25 mg docusate (1/2 tablet) once daily (maximum: 1 tablet twice daily)

6-12 years: Initial: 8.6 sennosides plus 50 mg docusate (1 tablet) once daily (maximum: 2 tablets twice daily)

Children ≥12 years and Adults: Initial: 2 tablets (17.2 mg sennosides plus 100 mg docusate) once daily (maximum: 4 tablets twice daily)

Elderly: Consider half the initial dose in older, debilitated patients

Additional Information Complete prescribing information should be consulted for additional detail.

Dosage Forms Excipient information presented when available (limited, particularly for generics); consult specific product labeling.

Tablet, oral: Docusate sodium 50 mg and sennosides 8.6 mg

Doc-Q-Lax: Docusate sodium 50 mg and sennosides 8.6 mg

Dok™ Plus: Docusate sodium 50 mg and sennosides 8.6 mg [contains sodium benzoate]

Geri-Stool: Docusate sodium 50 mg and sennosides 8.6 mg

Peri-Colace®: Docusate sodium 50 mg and sennosides 8.6 mg

Senexon®-S: Docusate sodium 50 mg and sennosides 8.6 mg [contains calcium 20 mg/tablet, sodium 6 mg/tablet]

SennaLax-S: Docusate sodium 50 mg and sennosides 8.6 mg [contains sodium benzoate]

Senna Plus: Docusate sodium 50 mg and sennosides 8.6 mg

Senokot-S®: Docusate sodium 50 mg and sennosides 8.6 mg [sugar free; contains sodium 4 mg/tablet]

SenoSol™-SS: Docusate sodium 50 mg and sennosides 8.6 mg [contains sodium 3 mg/tablet]

◆ **Docusate Calcium** *see* Docusate *on page 644*
◆ **Docusate Potassium** *see* Docusate *on page 644*
◆ **Docusate Sodium** *see* Docusate *on page 644*
◆ **Docusil [OTC]** *see* Docusate *on page 644*
◆ **Docu Soft [OTC]** *see* Docusate *on page 644*
◆ **DocuSol Mini [OTC]** *see* Docusate *on page 644*

Dofetilide (doe FET il ide)

Brand Names: U.S. Tikosyn

Brand Names: Canada Tikosyn®

Pharmacologic Category Antiarrhythmic Agent, Class III

Additional Appendix Information

Beers Criteria – Potentially Inappropriate Medications for Geriatrics *on page 2368*

Use Maintenance of normal sinus rhythm in patients with chronic atrial fibrillation/atrial flutter of longer than 1-week duration who have been converted to normal sinus rhythm; conversion of atrial fibrillation and atrial flutter to normal sinus rhythm

Unlabeled Use Alternative antiarrhythmic for the treatment of atrial fibrillation in patients with hypertrophic cardiomyopathy (HCM)

Pregnancy Risk Factor C

Pregnancy Considerations Adverse events have been observed in animal reproduction studies.

Breast-Feeding Considerations It is not known if dofetilide is excreted in breast milk. Breast-feeding is not recommended by the manufacturer.

Prescribing and Access Restrictions As a requirement of the REMS program, access to this medication is restricted. Tikosyn® is only available to prescribers and hospitals that have confirmed their participation in a designated Tikosyn® Education Program. The program provides comprehensive education about the importance of in-hospital treatment initiation and individualized dosing.

T.I.P.S. is the Tikosyn® In Pharmacy System designated to allow retail pharmacies to stock and dispense Tikosyn® once they have been enrolled. A participating pharmacy must confirm receipt of the T.I.P.S. program materials and educate its pharmacy staff about the procedures required to fill an outpatient prescription for Tikosyn®. The T.I.P.S. enrollment form is available at www.tikosyn.com. Tikosyn® is only available from a special mail order pharmacy, and enrolled retail pharmacies. Pharmacists must verify that the hospital/prescriber is a confirmed participant before Tikosyn® is provided. For participant verification, the pharmacist may call 1-800-788-7353 or use the web site located at www.tikosynlist.com. Further details and directions on the program are provided at www.tikosyn.com.

Dofetilide therapy must be initiated/adjusted in a hospital setting with proper monitoring under the guidance of experienced personnel.

Medication Guide Available Yes

Contraindications Hypersensitivity to dofetilide or any component of the formulation; patients with congenital or acquired long QT syndromes, do not use if baseline QT interval or QT_c is >440 msec (500 msec in patients with ventricular conduction abnormalities); severe renal impairment (Cl_{cr} <20 mL/minute [Cockcroft-Gault method]); concurrent use with verapamil, cimetidine, hydrochlorothiazide (alone or in combinations), trimethoprim (alone or in combination with sulfamethoxazole), itraconazole (according to itraconazole prescribing information) ketoconazole, prochlorperazine, dolutegravir, or megestrol

Warnings/Precautions **[U.S. Boxed Warning]: Must be initiated (or reinitiated) in a setting with continuous monitoring and staff familiar with the recognition and treatment of life-threatening arrhythmias. Patients must be monitored with continuous ECG for a minimum of 3 days,** or for a minimum of 12 hours after electrical or pharmacological cardioversion to normal sinus rhythm, whichever is greater. Patients should be readmitted for continuous monitoring if dosage is later increased.

Reserve for patients who are highly symptomatic with atrial fibrillation/atrial flutter; risk of torsade de pointes (TdP) significantly increases with doses >500 mcg twice daily; hold Class I or Class III antiarrhythmics for at least three half-lives prior to starting dofetilide; use in patients previously on amiodarone therapy only if serum amiodarone level is <0.3 mg/L or if amiodarone was discontinued ≥3 months ago; correct hypokalemia or hypomagnesemia before initiating dofetilide and maintain within normal limits ▶

during treatment. The risk of TdP may be higher in certain patient subgroups (eg, patients with heart failure). Most episodes of TdP occur within the first 3 days of therapy. Risk of hypokalemia and/or hypomagnesemia may be increased by potassium-depleting diuretics, increasing the risk of TdP. Concurrent use with other drugs known to prolong QT_c interval is not recommended.

In the treatment of atrial fibrillation in the elderly, avoid antiarrhythmics as first-line treatment. In older adults, data suggests rate control may provide more benefits than risks compared to rhythm control for most patients (Beers Criteria).

Patients with sick sinus syndrome or with second or third-degree heart block should not receive dofetilide unless a functional pacemaker is in place. Defibrillation threshold is reduced in patients with ventricular tachycardia or ventricular fibrillation undergoing implantation of a cardioverter-defibrillator device. Use with caution in renal impairment; **dose adjustment required for patients with Cl_{cr} ≤60 mL/minute.** Use with caution in patients with severe hepatic impairment; not studied.

Adverse Reactions

Supraventricular arrhythmia patients:

>10%: Central nervous system: Headache (11%)

2% to 10%:

- Central nervous system: Dizziness (8%), insomnia (4%)
- Cardiovascular: Ventricular tachycardia (2.6% to 3.7%), chest pain (10%), torsade de pointes (3.3% in HF patients and 0.9% in patients with a recent MI; up to 10.5% in patients receiving doses in excess of those recommended). Torsade de pointes occurs most frequently within the first 3 days of therapy.
- Dermatologic: Rash (3%)
- Gastrointestinal: Nausea (5%), diarrhea (3%), abdominal pain (3%)
- Neuromuscular & skeletal: Back pain (3%)
- Respiratory: Respiratory tract infection (7%), dyspnea (6%)
- Miscellaneous: Flu-like syndrome (4%)

<2%:

- Central nervous system: CVA, facial paralysis, flaccid paralysis, migraine, paralysis
- Cardiovascular: AV block (0.4% to 1.5%), bundle branch block (0.1% to 0.5%), heart block (0.1% to 0.5%), ventricular fibrillation (0% to 0.4%), bradycardia, cardiac arrest, edema, MI, sudden death, syncope
- Dermatologic: Angioedema
- Gastrointestinal: Liver damage
- Neuromuscular & skeletal: Paresthesia
- Respiratory: Cough

Drug Interactions

Metabolism/Transport Effects Substrate of CYP3A4 (minor); **Note:** Assignment of Major/Minor substrate status based on clinically relevant drug interaction potential

Avoid Concomitant Use

Avoid concomitant use of Dofetilide with any of the following: Antifungal Agents (Azole Derivatives, Systemic); Cimetidine; Dolutegravir; Fingolimod; Highest Risk QTc-Prolonging Agents; Ivabradine; Megestrol; Mifepristone; Moderate Risk QTc-Prolonging Agents; Prochlorperazine; Propafenone; Saquinavir; Thiazide Diuretics; Trimethoprim; Verapamil

Increased Effect/Toxicity

Dofetilide may increase the levels/effects of: Highest Risk QTc-Prolonging Agents; Lidocaine (Topical)

The levels/effects of Dofetilide may be increased by: AMILoride; Antifungal Agents (Azole Derivatives, Systemic); Cimetidine; CYP3A4 Inhibitors (Moderate); CYP3A4 Inhibitors (Strong); CYP3A4 Inhibitors (Weak); Dolutegravir; Fingolimod; Ivabradine; Lidocaine (Topical); Loop Diuretics; Megestrol; MetFORMIN; Mifepristone; Moderate Risk QTc-Prolonging Agents; Prochlorperazine; Propafenone; QTc-Prolonging Agents (Indeterminate Risk and Risk Modifying); Saquinavir; Thiazide Diuretics; Triamterene; Trimethoprim; Verapamil

Decreased Effect There are no known significant interactions involving a decrease in effect.

Ethanol/Nutrition/Herb Interactions Herb/Nutraceutical: St John's wort may decrease dofetilide levels. Avoid ephedra (may worsen arrhythmia).

Mechanism of Action Vaughan Williams Class III antiarrhythmic activity. Blockade of the cardiac ion channel carrying the rapid component of the delayed rectifier potassium current. Dofetilide has no effect on sodium channels, adrenergic alpha-receptors, or adrenergic beta-receptors. It increases the monophasic action potential duration due to delayed repolarization. The increase in the QT interval is a function of prolongation of both effective and functional refractory periods in the His-Purkinje system and the ventricles. Changes in cardiac conduction velocity and sinus node function have not been observed in patients with or without structural heart disease. PR and QRS width remain the same in patients with pre-existing heart block and or sick sinus syndrome.

Pharmacodynamics/Kinetics

Absorption: Well absorbed

Distribution: V_d: 3 L/kg

Protein binding: 60% to 70%

Metabolism: Hepatic via CYP3A4, but low affinity for it; metabolites formed by N-dealkylation and N-oxidation

Bioavailability: >90%

Half-life elimination: ~10 hours; prolonged with renal impairment

Time to peak, serum: Fasting: 2-3 hours

Excretion: Urine (80%; 80% as unchanged drug, 20% as inactive or minimally active metabolites); renal elimination consists of glomerular filtration and active tubular secretion via cationic transport system

Dosage Adults: Oral:

Note: QT or QT_c must be determined prior to first dose. If QT_c >440 msec (>500 msec in patients with ventricular conduction abnormalities), dofetilide is contraindicated.

Initial: 500 mcg twice daily. Initial dosage must be adjusted in patients with estimated Cl_{cr} <60 mL/minute (see dosage adjustment in renal impairment). Dofetilide may be initiated at lower doses than recommended based on physician discretion.

Modification of dosage in response to **initial** dose: QT_c interval should be measured 2-3 hours after the initial dose. If the QT_c is >15% of baseline, or if the QT_c is >500 msec (550 msec in patients with ventricular conduction abnormalities), dofetilide should be reduced. If the starting dose was 500 mcg twice daily, then reduce to 250 mcg twice daily. If the starting dose was 250 mcg twice daily, then reduce to 125 mcg twice daily. If the starting dose was 125 mcg twice daily, then reduce to 125 mcg once daily. If at any time after the second dose is given the QT_c is >500 msec (550 msec in patients with ventricular conduction abnormalities), dofetilide should be discontinued.

Dosage adjustment in renal impairment: Note: Using the Modification of Diet in Renal Disease (MDRD) equation and subsequent eGFR to determine dose may lead to overestimation of creatinine clearance and overdose of medication; use only the Cockcroft-Gault equation to estimate creatinine clearance (Denetclaw, 2011). Use actual body weight when using the Cockcroft-Gault equation to calculate creatinine clearance (weight range of patients enrolled in clinical trials: 40-134 kg).

Cl_{cr} >60 mL/minute: Administer 500 mcg twice daily.

Cl_{cr} 40-60 mL/minute: Administer 250 mcg twice daily.

Cl_{cr} 20-39 mL/minute: Administer 125 mcg twice daily.

Cl_{cr} <20 mL/minute: Contraindicated.

Dosage adjustment in hepatic impairment: No dosage adjustments required in Child-Pugh class A and B. Patients with severe hepatic impairment were not studied.

Elderly: No specific dosage adjustments are recommended based on age, however, careful assessment of renal function is particularly important in this population.

Monitoring Parameters ECG monitoring with attention to QT (if heart rate <60 beats per minute) or QT_c and occurrence of ventricular arrhythmias, baseline serum creatinine and changes in serum creatinine. Upon initiation (or reinitiation) continuous ECG monitoring recommended for a minimum of 3 days, or for at least 12 hours after electrical or pharmacological conversion to normal sinus rhythm, whichever is greater. Check serum potassium and magnesium levels at baseline and throughout therapy especially if on medications where these electrolyte disturbances can occur, or if patient has a history of hypokalemia or hypomagnesemia. QT or QT_c must be monitored at baseline prior to the first dose and 2-3 hours afterwards. If at baseline, QT_c >440 msec (>500 msec in patients with ventricular conduction abnormalities), dofetilide is contraindicated. If dofetilide initiated, QT_c interval must be determined 2-3 hours after each subsequent dose of dofetilide for in-hospital doses 2-5. Thereafter, QT or QT_c and creatinine clearance should be evaluated every 3 months. If at any time during therapy after the second dose the measured QT_c is >500 msec (550 msec in patients with ventricular conduction abnormalities), dofetilide should be discontinued.

Consult individual institutional policies and procedures.

Dosage Forms Excipient information presented when available (limited, particularly for generics); consult specific product labeling.

Capsule, Oral:

Tikosyn: 125 mcg, 250 mcg, 500 mcg

◆ **DOK [OTC]** *see* Docusate *on page 644*

◆ **Dok™ Plus [OTC]** *see* Docusate and Senna *on page 645*

Dolasetron (dol A se tron)

Brand Names: U.S. Anzemet

Brand Names: Canada Anzemet

Index Terms Dolasetron Mesylate; MDL 73,147EF

Pharmacologic Category Antiemetic; Selective 5-HT_3 Receptor Antagonist

Use

U.S. labeling:

Injection: Prevention and treatment of postoperative nausea and vomiting

Oral: Prevention of nausea and vomiting associated with emetogenic cancer chemotherapy (initial and repeat courses)

Canadian labeling: Oral: Prevention of nausea and vomiting associated with emetogenic cancer chemotherapy (initial and repeat courses)

Pregnancy Risk Factor B

Pregnancy Considerations Adverse events have not been observed in animal reproduction studies.

Breast-Feeding Considerations It is not known if dolasetron is excreted in breast milk. The manufacturer recommends that caution be exercised when administering dolasetron to nursing women.

Contraindications

U.S. labeling:

Injection: Hypersensitivity to dolasetron or any component of the formulation; intravenous administration is contraindicated when used for prevention of chemotherapy-associated nausea and vomiting

Tablet: Hypersensitivity to dolasetron or any component of the formulation

Canadian labeling: Hypersensitivity to dolasetron or any component of the formulation; use in children and adolescents <18 years of age; use for the prevention or treatment of postoperative nausea and vomiting; concomitant use with apomorphine

Warnings/Precautions Dolasetron is associated with a number of dose-dependent increases in ECG intervals (eg, PR, QRS duration, QT/QT_c, JT), usually occurring 1-2 hours after I.V. administration and usually lasting 6-8 hours; however, may last ≥24 hours and rarely lead to heart block or arrhythmia. Clinically relevant QT-interval prolongation may occur resulting in torsade de pointes, when used in conjunction with other agents that prolong the QT interval (eg, Class I and III antiarrhythmics). Avoid use in patients at greater risk for QT prolongation (eg, patients with congenital long QT syndrome, medications known to prolong QT interval, electrolyte abnormalities, and cumulative high-dose anthracycline therapy) and/or ventricular arrhythmia. Correct potassium or magnesium abnormalities prior to initiating therapy. I.V. formulations of 5-HT_3 antagonists have more association with ECG interval changes, compared to oral formulations. Reduction in heart rate may also occur with the 5-HT_3 antagonists. Use with caution in children and adolescents who have or may develop QT_c prolongation; rare cases of supraventricular and ventricular arrhythmias, cardiac arrest, and MI have been reported in this population. ECG monitoring is recommended in patients with renal impairment and in the elderly.

Use with caution in patients allergic to other 5-HT_3 receptor antagonists; cross-reactivity has been reported with other 5-HT_3 receptor antagonists. **For chemotherapy-associated nausea and vomiting, should be used on a scheduled basis, not on an "as needed" (PRN) basis,** since data support the use of this drug only in the prevention of nausea and vomiting (due to antineoplastic therapy) and not in the rescue of nausea and vomiting. Not intended for treatment of nausea and vomiting or for chronic continuous therapy. If the prophylaxis dolasetron dose for postoperative nausea and vomiting has failed, a repeat dose should not be administered as rescue or treatment for postoperative nausea and vomiting. Potentially significant drug-drug interactions may exist, requiring dose or frequency adjustment, additional monitoring, and/or selection of alternative therapy.

Adverse Reactions Adverse events may vary according to indication

>10%:

Central nervous system: Headache (7% to 24%)

Gastrointestinal: Diarrhea (2% to 12%)

1% to 10%:

Cardiovascular: Bradycardia (4% to 5%), hypertension (≤3%), tachycardia (2% to 3%)

Central nervous system: Dizziness (1% to 6%), fatigue (3% to 6%), fever (4%), pain (≤2%), chills/shivering (1% to 2%)

Gastrointestinal: Dyspepsia (≤3%), abdominal pain (≤3%)

Hepatic: Abnormal hepatic function (4%)

Renal: Oliguria (3%)

<1% (Limited to important or life-threatening): Abnormal vision, abnormal dreams, acute renal failure, alkaline phosphatase increased, ALT increased, anaphylactic reaction, anemia, anxiety, AST increased, ataxia, bronchospasm, cardiac arrest, chest pain, confusion, constipation, diaphoresis, dyspnea, dysuria, edema, epistaxis, facial edema, flushing, GGT increased, hematuria, hyperbilirubinemia, hypotension, ischemia (peripheral), local injection site reaction (pain/burning), MI, myocardial ischemia, orthostatic hypotension, palpitation, pancreatitis, paresthesia, peripheral edema, photophobia,

polyuria, prothrombin time increased, PTT increased, purpura/hematoma, rash, syncope, taste alteration, thrombocytopenia, thrombophlebitis/phlebitis, tinnitus, tremor, twitching, urticaria, vertigo

Note: Cardiac conduction abnormalities (including arrhythmia [sinus, supraventricular and ventricular], atrial flutter/fibrillation, AV block, bundle branch block, extrasystoles, poor R wave progression, prolonged PR, QRS, JT, and QT_c intervals, ST, T and U wave changes, torsade de pointes, ventricular tachycardia, wide complex tachycardia and ventricular fibrillation) have also been reported.

Drug Interactions

Metabolism/Transport Effects Substrate of CYP2C9 (minor), CYP3A4 (minor); **Note:** Assignment of Major/Minor substrate status based on clinically relevant drug interaction potential; **Inhibits** CYP2D6 (weak)

Avoid Concomitant Use

Avoid concomitant use of Dolasetron with any of the following: Apomorphine; Highest Risk QTc-Prolonging Agents; Ivabradine; Mifepristone

Increased Effect/Toxicity

Dolasetron may increase the levels/effects of: Apomorphine; ARIPiprazole; Highest Risk QTc-Prolonging Agents; Moderate Risk QTc-Prolonging Agents

The levels/effects of Dolasetron may be increased by: Ivabradine; Mifepristone; QTc-Prolonging Agents (Indeterminate Risk and Risk Modifying)

Decreased Effect

Dolasetron may decrease the levels/effects of: Tapentadol; TraMADol

Ethanol/Nutrition/Herb Interactions Food: Food does not affect the bioavailability of oral doses.

Preparation for Administration May be administered undiluted, or diluted in 50 mL of a compatible solution (ie, 0.9% NS, D_5W, $D_5{}^{1/2}NS$, D_5LR, LR, and 10% mannitol injection).

Storage/Stability

Injection: Store intact vials at 20°C to 25°C (68°F to 77°F); excursions are permitted to 15°C to 30°C (59°F to 86°F). Protect from light. Solutions diluted for infusion are stable under normal lighting conditions at room temperature for 24 hours or under refrigeration for 48 hours.

Tablets: Store at 20°C to 25°C (68°F to 77°F). Protect from light.

Mechanism of Action Selective serotonin receptor ($5\text{-}HT_3$) antagonist, blocking serotonin both peripherally (primary site of action) and centrally at the chemoreceptor trigger zone

Pharmacodynamics/Kinetics

Absorption: Oral: Rapid and complete

Distribution: Hydrodolasetron: 5.8 L/kg

Protein binding: Hydrodolasetron: 69% to 77% (50% bound to $alpha_1$-acid glycoprotein)

Metabolism: Hepatic; rapid reduction by carbonyl reductase to hydrodolasetron (active metabolite); further metabolized by CYP2D6, CYP3A, and flavin monooxygenase

Bioavailability: Oral: ~75% (not affected by food)

Half-life elimination: Dolasetron: ≤10 minutes; hydrodolasetron: Adults: 6-8 hours; Children: 4-6 hours; Severe renal impairment: 11 hours; Severe hepatic impairment: 11 hours

Time to peak, plasma: Hydrodolasetron: I.V.: 0.6 hours; Oral: ~1 hour

Excretion: Urine ~67% (53% to 61% of the total dose as active metabolite hydrodolasetron); feces ~33%

Dosage Note: Use of intravenous dolasetron is contraindicated in the prevention of chemotherapy-associated nausea and vomiting. In Canada, use of dolasetron is also contraindicated in children and adolescents <18 years of age and in the prevention and treatment of postoperative nausea and vomiting in adults.

U.S. labeling:

Prevention of chemotherapy-associated nausea and vomiting (including initial and repeat courses):

Children 2-16 years: Oral: 1.8 mg/kg within 1 hour before chemotherapy; maximum: 100 mg/dose

Adults: Oral: 100 mg within 1 hour before chemotherapy

Prevention of postoperative nausea and vomiting:

Children 2-16 years:

Oral: 1.2 mg/kg within 2 hours before surgery; maximum: 100 mg/dose

I.V.: 0.35 mg/kg ~15 minutes before cessation of anesthesia; maximum: 12.5 mg/dose

Adults: I.V.: 12.5 mg ~15 minutes before cessation of anesthesia (do not exceed the recommended dose)

Treatment of postoperative nausea and vomiting:

Children 2-16 years: I.V.: 0.35 mg/kg as soon as nausea or vomiting present; maximum: 12.5 mg/dose

Adults: I.V.: 12.5 mg as soon as nausea or vomiting present (do not exceed the recommended dose)

Canadian labeling: **Prevention of chemotherapy-associated nausea and vomiting (including initial and repeat courses):** Adults: Oral: 100 mg within 1 hour before chemotherapy

Dosing adjustment in renal impairment: No dosage adjustment necessary; however, ECG monitoring is recommended in patients with renal impairment.

Dosing adjustment in hepatic impairment: No dosage adjustment necessary

Administration

I.V. injection may be given either undiluted as an I.V. push over 30 seconds or diluted in 50 mL of compatible fluid and infused over 15 minutes. Flush line before and after dolasetron administration.

Oral: When unable to administer in tablet form, dolasetron injection may be diluted in apple or apple-grape juice and taken orally; this dilution is stable for 2 hours at room temperature (Anzemet prescribing information, 2013).

Monitoring Parameters ECG (in patients with cardiovascular disease, elderly, renally impaired, those at risk of developing hypokalemia and/or hypomagnesemia); potassium, magnesium

Additional Information Efficacy of dolasetron, for chemotherapy treatment, is enhanced with concomitant administration of dexamethasone 20 mg (increases complete response by 10% to 20%). Oral administration of the intravenous solution is equivalent to tablets.

Dosage Forms Excipient information presented when available (limited, particularly for generics); consult specific product labeling.

Solution, Intravenous, as mesylate:

Anzemet: 20 mg/mL (0.625 mL, 5 mL, 25 mL)

Tablet, Oral, as mesylate:

Anzemet: 50 mg, 100 mg

Extemporaneous Preparations Dolasetron injection may be diluted in apple or apple-grape juice and taken orally; this dilution is stable for 2 hours at room temperature (Anzemet prescribing information, 2013).

A 10 mg/mL oral suspension may be prepared with tablets and either a 1:1 mixture of Ora-Plus and Ora-Sweet SF or a 1:1 mixture of strawberry syrup and Ora-Plus. Crush twelve 50 mg tablets in a mortar and reduce to a fine powder. Slowly add chosen vehicle to **almost** 60 mL; transfer to a calibrated bottle, rinse mortar with vehicle, and add quantity of vehicle sufficient to make 60 mL. Label "shake well" and "refrigerate". Stable for 90 days refrigerated.

Anzemet® prescribing information, sanofi-aventis U.S. LLC, Bridgewater, NJ, 2013.

Johnson CE, Wagner DS, and Bussard WE, "Stability of Dolasetron in Two Oral Liquid Vehicles," *Am J Health Syst Pharm*, 2003, 60 (21):2242-4.

◆ **Dom-Terbinafine (Can)** *see* Terbinafine (Systemic) *on page 2017*

◆ **Dom-Ticlopidine (Can)** *see* Ticlopidine *on page 2059*

◆ **Dom-Timolol (Can)** *see* Timolol (Ophthalmic) *on page 2064*

◆ **Dom-Topiramate (Can)** *see* Topiramate *on page 2090*

◆ **Dom-Trazodone (Can)** *see* TraZODone *on page 2112*

◆ **Dom-Ursodiol C (Can)** *see* Ursodiol *on page 2142*

◆ **DOM-Valacyclovir (Can)** *see* ValACYclovir *on page 2145*

◆ **Dom-Valproic Acid (Can)** *see* Valproic Acid and Derivatives *on page 2149*

◆ **Dom-Valproic Acid E.C. (Can)** *see* Valproic Acid and Derivatives *on page 2149*

◆ **Dom-Venlafaxine XR (Can)** *see* Venlafaxine *on page 2178*

◆ **Dom-Verapamil SR (Can)** *see* Verapamil *on page 2182*

◆ **Dom-Zolmitriptan (Can)** *see* ZOLMitriptan *on page 2240*

Donepezil (doh NEP e zil)

Brand Names: U.S. Aricept; Aricept ODT

Brand Names: Canada Aricept®; Aricept® RDT

Index Terms E2020

Pharmacologic Category Acetylcholinesterase Inhibitor (Central)

Use Treatment of mild, moderate, or severe dementia of the Alzheimer's type

Unlabeled Use Behavioral syndromes in dementia; mild-to-moderate dementia associated with Parkinson's disease; Lewy body dementia

Pregnancy Risk Factor C

Pregnancy Considerations Adverse events have been observed in some animal reproduction studies.

Breast-Feeding Considerations It is not known if donepezil is excreted in breast milk. The manufacturer recommends that caution be used if administered to a nursing woman.

Contraindications Hypersensitivity to donepezil, piperidine derivatives, or any component of the formulation

Warnings/Precautions Cholinesterase inhibitors may have vagotonic effects which may cause bradycardia and/or heart block with or without a history of cardiac disease; syncopal episodes have been associated with donepezil. Alzheimer's treatment guidelines consider bradycardia to be a relative contraindication for use of centrally-active cholinesterase inhibitors. Use with caution with sick sinus syndrome or other supraventricular cardiac conduction abnormalities, COPD, or asthma. Use with caution in patients with a history of seizure disorder; cholinomimetics may potentially cause generalized seizures, although seizure activity may also result from Alzheimer's disease. Use with caution in patients at risk of ulcer disease (eg, previous history or NSAID use), or in patients with bladder outlet obstruction. May cause dose-related diarrhea, nausea, and/or vomiting, which usually resolves in 1-3 weeks. May cause anorexia and/or weight loss (dose-related). Patients weighing <55 kg may experience more nausea, vomiting, and weight loss than patients ≥55 kg. May exaggerate neuromuscular blockade effects of depolarizing neuromuscular-blocking agents (eg, succinylcholine). Potentially significant interactions may exist, requiring dose or frequency adjustment, additional monitoring, and/or selection of alternative therapy. Consult drug interactions database for more detailed information.

Adverse Reactions

>10%:

Central nervous system: Insomnia (2% to 14%)

Gastrointestinal: Nausea (3% to 19%; dose related), diarrhea (5% to 15%; dose related)

Miscellaneous: Accident (7% to 13%), infection (11%)

1% to 10%:

Cardiovascular: Hypertension (3%), chest pain (2%), hemorrhage (2%), syncope (2%), hypotension, atrial fibrillation, bradycardia, ECG abnormal, edema, heart failure, hot flashes, peripheral edema, vasodilation

Central nervous system: Headache (3% to 10%), pain (3% to 9%), fatigue (1% to 8%), dizziness (2% to 8%), abnormal dreams (3%), hostility (3%), nervousness (1% to 3%), hallucinations (3%), depression (2% to 3%), confusion (2%), emotional lability (2%), personality disorder (2%), fever (2%), somnolence (2%), abnormal crying, aggression, agitation, anxiety, aphasia, delusions, irritability, restlessness, seizure, vertigo

Dermatologic: Bruising (4% to 5%), eczema (3%), pruritus, rash, skin ulcer, urticaria

Endocrine & metabolic: Dehydration (1% to 2%), hyperlipemia (2%), libido increased

Gastrointestinal: Anorexia (2% to 8%), vomiting (3% to 9%; dose related), weight loss (3% to 5%; dose related), abdominal pain, bloating, constipation, dyspepsia, epigastric pain, fecal incontinence, gastroenteritis, GI bleeding, toothache

Genitourinary: Urinary frequency (2%), urinary incontinence (1% to 3%), cystitis, hematuria, glycosuria, nocturia, UTI

Hematologic: Contusion (≤2%), anemia

Hepatic: Alkaline phosphatase increased

Neuromuscular & skeletal: Muscle cramps (3% to 8%), back pain (3%), CPK increased (3%), arthritis (1% to 2%), ataxia, bone fracture, gait abnormal, lactate dehydrogenase increased, paresthesia, tremor, weakness (1% to 2%)

Ocular: Blurred vision, cataract, eye irritation

Respiratory: Bronchitis, cough increased, dyspnea, pharyngitis, pneumonia, sore throat

Miscellaneous: Diaphoresis, fungal infection, flu symptoms, wandering

<1% (Limited to important or life-threatening): Angina, cardiomegaly, cerebrovascular accident, cholecystitis, conjunctival hemorrhage, deep vein thrombosis, diabetes mellitus, diverticulitis, gastrointestinal ulcer, glaucoma, heart block, heart failure, hemolytic anemia, hepatitis, hyperglycemia, hypertonia, hypokalemia, hypokinesia, hyponatremia, hypoxia, intracranial hemorrhage, jaundice, LFTs increased, MI, neuroleptic malignant syndrome, pancreatitis, pleurisy, pulmonary collapse, pulmonary congestion, pyelonephritis, renal failure, retinal hemorrhage, SVT, thrombocythemia, thrombocytopenia, tongue edema, transient ischemic attack

Drug Interactions

Metabolism/Transport Effects Substrate of CYP2D6 (minor), CYP3A4 (minor); **Note:** Assignment of Major/Minor substrate status based on clinically relevant drug interaction potential

Avoid Concomitant Use There are no known interactions where it is recommended to avoid concomitant use.

Increased Effect/Toxicity

Donepezil may increase the levels/effects of: Antipsychotics; Beta-Blockers; Cholinergic Agonists; Succinylcholine

The levels/effects of Donepezil may be increased by: Corticosteroids (Systemic)

Decreased Effect

Donepezil may decrease the levels/effects of: Anticholinergics; Neuromuscular-Blocking Agents (Nondepolarizing)

The levels/effects of Donepezil may be decreased by: Anticholinergics; Dipyridamole; Peginterferon Alfa-2b

Ethanol/Nutrition/Herb Interactions

Ethanol: Avoid ethanol (may increase CNS adverse events).

Herb/Nutraceutical: St John's wort may decrease donepezil levels. Ginkgo biloba may increase adverse effects/ toxicity of acetylcholinesterase inhibitors.

Storage/Stability Store at 15°C to 30°C (59°F to 86°F).

Mechanism of Action Alzheimer's disease is characterized by cholinergic deficiency in the cortex and basal forebrain, which contributes to cognitive deficits. Donepezil reversibly and noncompetitively inhibits centrally-active acetylcholinesterase, the enzyme responsible for hydrolysis of acetylcholine. This appears to result in increased concentrations of acetylcholine available for synaptic transmission in the central nervous system.

Pharmacodynamics/Kinetics

Absorption: Well absorbed

Distribution: V_{dss}: 12-16 L/kg

Protein binding: 96%, primarily to albumin (75%) and α_1-acid glycoprotein (21%)

Metabolism: Extensively to four major metabolites (two are active) via CYP2D6 and 3A4; undergoes glucuronidation

Bioavailability: 100%

Half-life elimination: 70 hours; time to steady-state: 15 days

Time to peak, plasma: Tablet, 10 mg: 3 hours; Tablet, 23 mg: ~8 hours; **Note:** Peak plasma concentrations almost twofold higher for the 23 mg tablet compared to the 10 mg tablet

Excretion: Urine 57% (17% as unchanged drug); feces 15%

Dosage Oral:

Adults: Alzheimer's dementia:

Mild-to-moderate: Initial: 5 mg once daily; may increase to 10 mg once daily after 4-6 weeks; effective dosage range in clinical studies: 5-10 mg/day

Moderate-to-severe: Initial: 5 mg once daily; may increase to 10 mg once daily after 4-6 weeks; may increase further to 23 mg once daily after ≥3 months; effective dosage range in clinical studies: 10-23 mg/day

Elderly: Refer to adult dosing. **Note:** The Canadian labeling recommends a maximum dose of 5 mg once daily in elderly women of low body weight.

Dosage adjustment in renal impairment: No adjustment provided in manufacturer's labeling. Limited data suggest severe renal impairment does not adversely affect donepezil clearance.

Dosage adjustment in hepatic impairment: No adjustment provided in manufacturer's labeling.

Dietary Considerations May take with or without food.

Administration Administer at bedtime without regard to food.

Aricept® 5 mg or 10 mg tablet: Swallow whole with water.

Aricept® 23 mg tablet: Swallow whole with water; do **NOT** crush or chew due to an increased rate of absorption. The 23 mg strength is provided in a unique film-coated formulation different from the 5 mg or 10 mg tablet strengths, which results in an altered pharmacokinetic profile.

Aricept® ODT: Allow tablet to dissolve completely on tongue and follow with water.

Monitoring Parameters Behavior, mood, bowel function, cognitive function, general function (eg, activities of daily living)

Dosage Forms Excipient information presented when available (limited, particularly for generics); consult specific product labeling.

Tablet, Oral, as hydrochloride:

Aricept: 5 mg, 10 mg, 23 mg

Generic: 5 mg, 10 mg, 23 mg

Tablet Dispersible, Oral, as hydrochloride:

Aricept ODT: 5 mg, 10 mg

Generic: 5 mg, 10 mg

◆ **Donnatal®** *see* Hyoscyamine, Atropine, Scopolamine, and Phenobarbital *on page 1028*

◆ **Donnatal Extentabs®** *see* Hyoscyamine, Atropine, Scopolamine, and Phenobarbital *on page 1028*

DOPamine (DOE pa meen)

Index Terms Dopamine Hydrochloride; Intropin

Pharmacologic Category Adrenergic Agonist Agent

Additional Appendix Information

Adult ACLS Algorithms *on page 2363*

Vasoactive Agents, Intravenous *on page 2315*

Use Adjunct in the treatment of shock (eg, MI, open heart surgery, renal failure, cardiac decompensation) which persists after adequate fluid volume replacement

Unlabeled Use Symptomatic bradycardia or heart block unresponsive to atropine or pacing

Pregnancy Risk Factor C

Pregnancy Considerations Adverse events have been observed in some animal reproduction studies. It is not known if dopamine crosses the placenta.

Breast-Feeding Considerations It is not known if dopamine is excreted in breast milk. The manufacturer recommends that caution be exercised when administering dopamine to nursing women.

Contraindications Hypersensitivity to sulfites (commercial preparation contains sodium bisulfite); pheochromocytoma; ventricular fibrillation

Warnings/Precautions Use with caution in patients with cardiovascular disease or cardiac arrhythmias or patients with occlusive vascular disease. Correct hypovolemia and electrolytes when used in hemodynamic support. May cause increases in HR and arrhythmia. Use with caution in post-MI patients. Use has been associated with a higher incidence of adverse events (eg, tachyarrhythmias) in patients with shock compared to norepinephrine. Higher 28-day mortality was also seen in patients with septic shock; the use of norepinephrine in patients with shock may be preferred. The 2012 Surviving Sepsis Campaign (SSC) guidelines suggest dopamine use as an alternative to norepinephrine only in patients with low risk of tachyarrhythmias and absolute or relative bradycardia (Dellinger, 2013). Use with extreme caution in patients taking MAO inhibitors.

Vesicant; ensure proper needle or catheter placement prior to and during infusion. Avoid extravasation; infuse into a large vein if possible. Avoid infusion into leg veins. Watch I.V. site closely. **[U.S. Boxed Warning]: If extravasation occurs, infiltrate the area with diluted phentolamine (5-10 mg in 10-15 mL of saline) with a fine hypodermic needle. Phentolamine should be administered as soon as possible after extravasation is noted to prevent sloughing/necrosis.** Product may contain sodium metabisulfite.

Adverse Reactions Frequency not defined.

Most frequent:

Cardiovascular: Anginal pain, ectopic beats, hypotension, palpitation, tachycardia, vasoconstriction

Central nervous system: Headache

Gastrointestinal: Nausea and vomiting

Respiratory: Dyspnea

Infrequent:

Cardiovascular: Aberrant conduction, atrial fibrillation, bradycardia, gangrene (high dose), hypertension, ventricular arrhythmia, widened QRS complex

Central nervous system: Anxiety

Endocrine & metabolic: Piloerection, serum glucose increased (usually not above normal limits)

Local: Extravasation of dopamine can cause tissue necrosis and sloughing of surrounding tissues

Ocular: Dilated pupils, intraocular pressure increased

Renal: Azotemia, polyuria

Drug Interactions

Metabolism/Transport Effects **Substrate** of COMT

Avoid Concomitant Use

Avoid concomitant use of DOPamine with any of the following: Inhalational Anesthetics; Iobenguane I 123; Lurasidone

Increased Effect/Toxicity

DOPamine may increase the levels/effects of: Lurasidone; Sympathomimetics

The levels/effects of DOPamine may be increased by: AtoMOXetine; Cannabinoids; COMT Inhibitors; Hyaluronidase; Inhalational Anesthetics; Linezolid

Decreased Effect

DOPamine may decrease the levels/effects of: Iobenguane I 123

Storage/Stability Protect from light. Solutions that are darker than slightly yellow should not be used.

Mechanism of Action Stimulates both adrenergic and dopaminergic receptors, lower doses are mainly dopaminergic stimulating and produce renal and mesenteric vasodilation, higher doses also are both dopaminergic and beta$_1$-adrenergic stimulating and produce cardiac stimulation and renal vasodilation; large doses stimulate alpha-adrenergic receptors

Pharmacodynamics/Kinetics

Children: Dopamine has exhibited nonlinear kinetics in children; with dose changes, may not achieve steady-state for ~1 hour rather than 20 minutes

Onset of action: Adults: 5 minutes

Duration: Adults: <10 minutes

Metabolism: Renal, hepatic, plasma; 75% to inactive metabolites by monoamine oxidase and 25% to norepinephrine

Half-life elimination: 2 minutes

Excretion: Urine (as metabolites)

Clearance: Neonates: Varies and appears to be age related; clearance is more prolonged with combined hepatic and renal dysfunction

Dosage I.V. infusion (administration requires the use of an infusion pump):

Children: 1-20 mcg/kg/minute, maximum: 50 mcg/kg/minute continuous infusion, titrate to desired response.

Adults: 1-5 mcg/kg/minute up to 20 mcg/kg/minute, titrate to desired response (maximum: 50 mcg/kg/minute; however, doses >20 mcg/kg/minute may not have a beneficial effect on blood pressure and increase the risk of tachyarrhythmias). Infusion may be increased by 1-4 mcg/kg/minute at 10- to 30-minute intervals until optimal response is obtained.

If dosages >20-30 mcg/kg/minute are needed, a more direct-acting pressor may be more beneficial (ie, epinephrine, norepinephrine).

The hemodynamic effects of dopamine are dose dependent (however, this is relative and there is overlap of clinical effects between dosing ranges):

Low-dose: 1-3 mcg/kg/minute, increased renal blood flow and urine output

Intermediate-dose: 3-10 mcg/kg/minute, increased renal blood flow, heart rate, cardiac contractility, and cardiac output

High-dose: >10 mcg/kg/minute, alpha-adrenergic effects begin to predominate, vasoconstriction, increased blood pressure

Usual Infusion Concentrations: Pediatric Note: Premixed solutions available.

I.V. infusion: 1600 **mcg**/mL **or** 3200 **mcg**/mL

Usual Infusion Concentrations: Adult Note: Premixed solutions available.

I.V. infusion: 400 mg in 250 mL (concentration: 1600 **mcg**/mL) **or** 800 mg in 250 mL (concentration: 3200 **mcg**/mL) of D$_5$W or NS

Administration Administer as a continuous infusion with the use of an infusion pump. Administer into large vein to prevent the possibility of extravasation (central line administration); monitor continuously for free flow; use infusion device to control rate of flow; administration into an umbilical arterial catheter is not recommended; when discontinuing the infusion, gradually decrease the dose of dopamine (sudden discontinuation may cause hypotension). Vials (concentrated solution) must be diluted prior to use.

Vesicant; ensure proper needle or catheter placement prior to and during infusion; avoid extravasation.

Extravasation management: If extravasation occurs, stop infusion immediately and disconnect (leave cannula/needle in place); gently aspirate extravasated solution (do **NOT** flush the line); remove needle/cannula; elevate extremity. Initiate phentolamine (or alternative) antidote. Apply dry warm compresses (Hurst, 2004).

Phentolamine: Dilute 5-10 mg in 10-15 mL NS and administer into extravasation site as soon as possible after extravasation (Peberdy, 2010)

Alternatives to phentolamine:

Nitroglycerin topical 2% ointment (based on limited case reports in neonates/infants): Apply 4 mm/kg as a thin ribbon to the affected areas; may repeat after 8 hours if needed (Wong, 1992) **or** apply a 1-inch strip on the affected site (Denkler, 1989)

Terbutaline (based on limited case reports): Infiltrate extravasation area using a solution of terbutaline 1 mg diluted to 10 mL in NS (large extravasation site; administration volume varied from 3-10 mL) **or** 1 mg diluted in 1 mL NS (small/distal extravasation site; administration volume varied from 0.5-1 mL) (Stier, 1999)

Monitoring Parameters Blood pressure, ECG, heart rate, CVP, RAP, MAP; serum glucose, renal function; urine output; if pulmonary artery catheter is in place, monitor CI, PCWP, SVR, and PVR

Consult individual institutional policies and procedures.

Additional Information Dopamine is most frequently used for treatment of hypotension because of its peripheral vasoconstrictor action. In this regard, dopamine is often used together with dobutamine and minimizes hypotension secondary to dobutamine-induced vasodilation. Thus, pressure is maintained by increased cardiac output (from dobutamine) and vasoconstriction (by dopamine). It is critical neither dopamine nor dobutamine be used in patients in the absence of correcting any hypovolemia as a cause of hypotension.

Low-dose dopamine is often used in the intensive care setting for presumed beneficial effects on renal function. However, there is no clear evidence that low-dose dopamine confers any renal or other benefit. Indeed, dopamine may act on dopamine receptors in the carotid bodies causing chemoreflex suppression. In patients with heart failure, dopamine may inhibit breathing and cause pulmonary shunting. Both these mechanisms would act to decrease minute ventilation and oxygen saturation. This could potentially be deleterious in patients with respiratory compromise and patients being weaned from ventilators.

Dosage Forms Excipient information presented when available (limited, particularly for generics); consult specific product labeling.

Solution, Intravenous, as hydrochloride:

Generic: 0.8 mg/mL (250 mL, 500 mL); 1.6 mg/mL (250 mL, 500 mL); 3.2 mg/mL (250 mL); 40 mg/mL (5 mL, 10 mL); 80 mg/mL (5 mL); 160 mg/mL (5 mL)

◆ **Dopamine Hydrochloride** *see* DOPamine *on page 651*

◆ **Dopram** *see* Doxapram *on page 655*

◆ **Doral** *see* Quazepam *on page 1757*

◆ **Doribax** *see* Doripenem *on page 653*

Doripenem (dore i PEN em)

Brand Names: U.S. Doribax

Index Terms S-4661

Pharmacologic Category Antibiotic, Carbapenem

Use Treatment of complicated intra-abdominal infections and complicated urinary tract infections (including pyelonephritis) due to susceptible aerobic gram-positive, aerobic gram-negative (including *Pseudomonas aeruginosa*), and anaerobic bacteria

Unlabeled Use Treatment of intravascular catheter-related bloodstream infection due to extended-spectrum β-lactamase (ESBL)-producing *Escherichia coli* and *Klebsiella* spp; pneumonia (healthcare-associated [HAP], including ventilator-associated [VAP])

Pregnancy Risk Factor B

Pregnancy Considerations Adverse events have not been observed in animal reproduction studies. Information related to use during pregnancy has not been located.

Breast-Feeding Considerations It is not known if doripenem is excreted into breast milk. The manufacturer recommends that caution be exercised when administering doripenem to nursing women.

Contraindications Known serious hypersensitivity to doripenem or other carbapenems (eg, ertapenem, imipenem, meropenem) or any component of the formulation; anaphylactic reactions to beta-lactam antibiotics

Warnings/Precautions Serious hypersensitivity reactions, including anaphylaxis, and skin reactions have been reported in patients receiving beta-lactams. Use may result in fungal or bacterial superinfection, including *C. difficile*-associated diarrhea (CDAD) and pseudomembranous colitis; CDAD has been observed >2 months postantibiotic treatment. Not indicated for the treatment of pneumonia including ventilator-associated pneumonia; decreased efficacy and increased mortality observed in a phase 3 study using a higher dose and fixed 7-day administration (Kollef, 2012). Use with caution in patients with renal impairment; dosage adjustment required in patients with moderate-to-severe renal dysfunction. Carbapenems have been associated with CNS adverse effects, including confusional states and seizures (myoclonic); use caution with CNS disorders (eg, brain lesions, stroke, or history of seizures) and adjust dose in renal impairment to avoid drug accumulation, which may increase seizure risk. Patients receiving doses >500 mg every 8 hours may also be at increased risk of seizures. Potentially significant interactions may exist, requiring dose or frequency adjustment, additional monitoring, and/or selection of alternative therapy. Administer via intravenous infusion only. Per manufacturer's labeling, investigational experience of doripenem via inhalation resulted in pneumonitis.

Adverse Reactions

>10%:

Central nervous system: Headache (3% to 16%)

Gastrointestinal: Diarrhea (6% to 12%), nausea (4% to 12%)

1% to 10%:

Cardiovascular: Phlebitis (2% to 8%)

Dermatologic: Skin rash (2% to 7%; includes allergic/bullous dermatitis, erythema, macular/papular eruptions, urticaria, and erythema multiforme), pruritus (1% to 3%)

Gastrointestinal: Oral candidiasis (1% to 3%), pseudomembranous colitis (≤1%)

Hematologic & oncologic: Anemia (2% to 10%)

Hepatic: Increased serum transaminases (2% to 7%)

Renal: Renal insufficiency (≤1%)

Miscellaneous: Vaginal infection (1% to 2%)

<1% (Limited to important or life-threatening): Anaphylaxis, leukopenia, neutropenia, pneumonia, seizure, Stevens-Johnson syndrome, thrombocytopenia, toxic epidermal necrolysis

Drug Interactions

Metabolism/Transport Effects None known.

Avoid Concomitant Use

Avoid concomitant use of Doripenem with any of the following: BCG; Probenecid

Increased Effect/Toxicity

The levels/effects of Doripenem may be increased by: Probenecid

Decreased Effect

Doripenem may decrease the levels/effects of: BCG; Sodium Picosulfate; Typhoid Vaccine; Valproic Acid and Derivatives

Preparation for Administration Reconstitute 250 mg vial with 10 mL of SWFI or NS; further dilute for infusion with 50 mL or 100 mL of NS or D_5W. Shake gently until clear. Reconstitute 500 mg vial with 10 mL of SWFI or NS; further dilute for infusion with 100 mL of NS or D_5W. Shake gently until clear. Reconstituted vial may be stored for up to 1 hour prior to preparation of infusion solution. To prepare a 250 mg dose using a 500 mg vial, reconstitute the 500 mg vial with 10 mL of SWFI or NS and further dilute with 100 mL of compatible solution as above, but remove and discard 55 mL from the infusion bag to leave the remaining solution containing the 250 mg dose.

Storage/Stability Store dry powder vials at 15°C to 30°C (59°F to 86°F). Stability of solution when diluted in NS is 12 hours at room temperature or 72 hours under refrigeration; stability in D_5W is 4 hours at room temperature and 24 hours under refrigeration.

Mechanism of Action Inhibits bacterial cell wall synthesis by binding to several of the penicillin-binding proteins (PBP-2, PBP-3, PBP-4), which in turn inhibits the final transpeptidation step of peptidoglycan synthesis in bacterial cell walls, thus inhibiting cell wall biosynthesis; bacteria eventually lyse due to ongoing activity of cell wall autolytic enzymes (autolysins and murein hydrolases) while cell wall assembly is arrested.

Pharmacodynamics/Kinetics Note: As with other time-dependent antibiotics, doripenem shows bacteriostatic effects at T>MIC <40% and bactericidal effects at T>MIC>40%. Of note, prolonged infusion time (over 4 hours) was more effective in increasing T>MIC over 40% to up to 81%. Pharmacokinetics are linear (AUC directly proportional to dose) at doses administered over 1 hour.

Distribution: Penetrates well into body fluids and tissues, including peritoneal and retroperitoneal fluids, gallbladder, bile, and urine

V_d: 16.8 L

Protein binding: 8% to 9%

Metabolism: Non-CYP-mediated metabolism via hydrolysis by dehydropeptidase-I to doripenem-M1 (inactive metabolite)

Half-life elimination: ~1 hour

Excretion: Urine (71% as unchanged drug; 15% as doripenem-M1 metabolite); feces (<1%)

Dialyzable with reduction in systemic levels by 48% to 62%.

Dosage

Note: A switch to appropriate oral antimicrobial therapy may be considered after 3 days of parenteral therapy and demonstrated clinical improvement.

Usual dosage: Adults: I.V.: 500 mg every 8 hours

Indication-specific dosing: Adults: I.V.:

Intra-abdominal infection, complicated, severe: 500 mg every 8 hours for 5-14 days. **Note:** 2010 IDSA guidelines recommend treatment duration of 4-7 days (provided source controlled). Not recommended for mild-to-moderate, community-acquired intra-abdominal infections due to risk of toxicity and the development of resistant organisms (Solomkin, 2010).

Urinary tract infection (complicated) or pyelonephritis: 500 mg every 8 hours for 10-14 days

Intravenous catheter-related bloodstream infection (unlabeled use): 500 mg every 8 hours for 7-14 days (IDSA, 2009)

Pneumonia (healthcare-associated [HAP], including ventilator-associated [VAP]) (unlabeled use): 500 mg every 8 hours for 7-14 days (Chastre, 2008; Rea-Neto, 2008). **Note:** A VAP trial using a higher dose and fixed 7-day administration showed numerically lower cure rate (versus a comparator antibiotic) and increased mortality (Kollef, 2012).

Dosage adjustment in renal impairment:

Cl_{cr} >50 mL/minute: No adjustment necessary

Cl_{cr} 30-50 mL/minute: 250 mg every 8 hours

Cl_{cr} 11-29 mL/minute: 250 mg every 12 hours

Hemodialysis: Dialyzable (~52% of dose removed during 4-hour session in ESRD patients)

Intermittent HD: 250 mg every 24 hours; if treating infections caused by ***Pseudomonas aeruginosa***, administer 500 mg every 12 hours on day 1, followed by 500 mg every 24 hours (Tanoue, 2011)

CVVHDF: 250 mg every 12 hours (Hidaka, 2010).

Dosage adjustment in hepatic impairment: No dosage adjustment provided in manufacturer's labeling (has not been studied). However, doripenem undergoes minimal hepatic metabolism.

Administration Infuse intravenously over 1 hour. Use of 4-hour infusion has been studied in the treatment of VAP (unlabeled use) (Chastre, 2008).

Monitoring Parameters Monitor for signs of anaphylaxis during first dose; periodic renal assessment; consider hematologic monitoring during prolonged therapy

Additional Information One mechanism of resistance to doripenem is production of the Ambler's class B metallo-beta-lactamase, a potent carbapenemase produced by *Stenotrophomonas maltophilia*.

Dosage Forms Excipient information presented when available (limited, particularly for generics); consult specific product labeling.

Solution Reconstituted, Intravenous:

Doribax: 250 mg (1 ea); 500 mg (1 ea)

Dornase Alfa (DOOR nase AL fa)

Brand Names: U.S. Pulmozyme

Brand Names: Canada Pulmozyme®

Index Terms Recombinant Human Deoxyribonuclease; rhDNase

Pharmacologic Category Enzyme; Mucolytic Agent

Use Management of cystic fibrosis patients to reduce the frequency of respiratory infections that require parenteral antibiotics in patients with FVC ≥40% of predicted; in conjunction with standard therapies, to improve pulmonary function in patients with cystic fibrosis

Unlabeled Use Infected parapneumonic effusion (following alteplase administration)

Pregnancy Risk Factor B

Pregnancy Considerations Teratogenic effects were not observed in animal reproduction studies.

Breast-Feeding Considerations Measurable amounts would not be expected in breast milk following inhalation; however, it is not known if dornase alfa is excreted in human milk.

Contraindications Hypersensitivity to dornase alfa, Chinese hamster ovary cell products, or any component of the formulation

Warnings/Precautions Safety and efficacy have not been established for daily administration >12 months. In patients with pulmonary function <40% of normal, dornase alfa does not significantly reduce the risk of respiratory infections that require parenteral antibiotics. Safety studies included children ≥3 months, however experience is limited in children <5 years of age

Adverse Reactions Adverse events were similar in children using the PARI BABY™ nebulizer (facemask as opposed to mouthpiece) with the addition of cough (45% in children 3 months to <5 years; 30% in children 5 to ≤10 years).

>10%:

Cardiovascular: Chest pain (18% to 25%)

Central nervous system: Fever (32% in patients with FVC <40%)

Dermatologic: Rash (3% to 12%)

Respiratory: Pharyngitis (32% to 40%), rhinitis (30% in patients with FVC <40%); FVC decrease ≥10% of predicted (22% in patients with FVC <40%), dyspnea (17% in patients with FVC <40%)

Miscellaneous: Voice alteration (12% to 18%)

1% to 10%:

Gastrointestinal: Dyspepsia (≤3%)

Ocular: Conjunctivitis (1% to 5%)

Respiratory: Laryngitis (3% to 4%)

Miscellaneous: Dornase alfa serum antibodies (2% to 4%)

Postmarketing and/or case reports: Headache, urticaria

Drug Interactions

Metabolism/Transport Effects None known.

Avoid Concomitant Use There are no known interactions where it is recommended to avoid concomitant use.

Increased Effect/Toxicity There are no known significant interactions involving an increase in effect.

Decreased Effect There are no known significant interactions involving a decrease in effect.

Storage/Stability Must be stored in the refrigerator at 2°C to 8°C (36°F to 46°F) and protected from strong light. Do not expose to room temperature for ≥24 hours.

Mechanism of Action The hallmark of cystic fibrosis lung disease is the presence of abundant, purulent airway secretions composed primarily of highly polymerized DNA. The principal source of this DNA is the nuclei of degenerating neutrophils, which is present in large concentrations in infected lung secretions. The presence of this DNA produces a viscous mucous that may contribute to the decreased mucociliary transport and persistent infections that are commonly seen in this population. Dornase alfa is a deoxyribonuclease (DNA) enzyme produced by recombinant gene technology. Dornase selectively cleaves DNA, thus reducing mucous viscosity and as a result, airflow in the lung is improved and the risk of bacterial infection may be decreased.

Pharmacodynamics/Kinetics

Onset of action: Nebulization: Enzyme levels are measured in sputum in ~15 minutes

Duration: Rapidly declines

Dosage
Inhalation: Mucolytic (cystic fibrosis):
Infants and Children ≤5 years: Not approved for use; however, studies using this therapy in small numbers of children as young as 3 months of age have reported efficacy and similar side effects.
Children >5 years and Adults: 2.5 mg daily through selected nebulizers in conjunction with a Pulmo-Aide®, Pari-Proneb®, Mobilaire™, Porta-Neb®, or Pari Baby™ compressor system
Patients unable to inhale or exhale orally throughout the entire treatment period may use Pari-Baby™ nebulizer. Some patients may benefit from twice daily administration.
Intrapleural: Complicated parapneumonic effusion (unlabeled use): Adults: 5 mg (diluted in 30 mL sterile water) administered twice daily >2 hours after intrapleural alteplase administration (Rahman, 2011)
Dosage adjustment in renal impairment: No dosage adjustment provided in manufacturer's labeling.
Dosage adjustment in hepatic impairment: No dosage adjustment provided in manufacturer's labeling.
Administration
Nebulization: Prior to use, squeeze each ampul to check for leaks. Should not be diluted or mixed with any other drugs in the nebulizer, this may inactivate the drug
Parapneumonic effusion (unlabeled use): Intrapleural: **Note:** Each dose must be diluted in 30 mL of sterile water. Stability of dornase alfa diluted in sterile water has not been formally evaluated; use immediately after preparation. Instill dose into chest tube and clamp drain. After 1 hour dwell time, release clamp and connect chest tube to continuous suction (Rahman, 2011).
Dosage Forms Excipient information presented when available (limited, particularly for generics); consult specific product labeling.
Solution, Inhalation:
Pulmozyme: 1 mg/mL (2.5 mL)

◆ **Doryx** *see* Doxycycline *on page 668*

Dorzolamide (dor ZOLE a mide)

Brand Names: U.S. Trusopt
Brand Names: Canada Sandoz-Dorzolamide; Trusopt®
Index Terms Dorzolamide Hydrochloride
Pharmacologic Category Carbonic Anhydrase Inhibitor (Ophthalmic); Ophthalmic Agent, Antiglaucoma
Use Treatment of elevated intraocular pressure in patients with ocular hypertension or open-angle glaucoma
Pregnancy Risk Factor C
Dosage Children and Adults: Reduction of intraocular pressure: Instill 1 drop in the affected eye(s) 3 times/day
Dosage adjustment in renal impairment: Cl_{cr} <30 mL/minute: Use is not recommended (has not been studied).
Dosage adjustment in hepatic impairment: No dosage adjustment provided in manufacturer's labeling (has not been studied); use with caution.
Additional Information Complete prescribing information should be consulted for additional detail.
Dosage Forms Excipient information presented when available (limited, particularly for generics); consult specific product labeling.
Solution, Ophthalmic:
Trusopt: 2% (10 mL)
Generic: 2% (10 mL)
Dosage Forms: Canada Excipient information presented when available (limited, particularly for generics); consult specific product labeling.
Solution, ophthalmic [drops; preservative free]:
Trusopt®: 2% (0.2 mL)

Dorzolamide and Timolol
(dor ZOLE a mide & TYE moe lole)

Brand Names: U.S. Cosopt®; Cosopt® PF
Brand Names: Canada Apo-Dorzo-Timop; Cosopt®; Cosopt® Preservative Free; Sandoz-Dorzolamide/Timolol
Index Terms Cosopt® PF; Timolol and Dorzolamide
Pharmacologic Category Beta-Adrenergic Blocker, Nonselective; Carbonic Anhydrase Inhibitor (Ophthalmic); Ophthalmic Agent, Antiglaucoma
Use Treatment of elevated intraocular pressure in patients with ocular hypertension or open-angle glaucoma
Pregnancy Risk Factor C
Dosage Ophthalmic: Children ≥2 years and Adults: Instill 1 drop in affected eye(s) twice daily
Dosage adjustment in renal impairment: Cl_{cr} <30 mL/minute: Use is not recommended (has not been studied).
Dosage adjustment in hepatic impairment: No dosage adjustment provided in manufacturer's labeling (has not been studied): use with caution.
Additional Information Complete prescribing information should be consulted for additional detail.
Dosage Forms Excipient information presented when available (limited, particularly for generics); consult specific product labeling. [DSC] = Discontinued product
Solution, ophthalmic [drops]: Dorzolamide 2% and timolol 0.5% (10 mL)
Cosopt®: Dorzolamide 2% and timolol 0.5% (5 mL [DSC]; 10 mL) [contains benzalkonium chloride]
Solution, ophthalmic [drops, preservative free]:
Cosopt® PF: Dorzolamide 2% and timolol 0.5% (0.2 mL)

◆ **Dorzolamide Hydrochloride** *see* Dorzolamide *on page 655*
◆ **D.O.S. [OTC]** *see* Docusate *on page 644*
◆ **DOSS** *see* Docusate *on page 644*
◆ **Dostinex® (Can)** *see* Cabergoline *on page 309*
◆ **Double Tussin DM [OTC]** *see* Guaifenesin and Dextromethorphan *on page 976*
◆ **Dovobet® (Can)** *see* Calcipotriene and Betamethasone *on page 312*
◆ **Dovonex** *see* Calcipotriene *on page 311*
◆ **Dovonex® (Can)** *see* Calcipotriene *on page 311*

Doxapram (DOKS a pram)

Brand Names: U.S. Dopram
Index Terms Doxapram Hydrochloride
Pharmacologic Category Respiratory Stimulant
Use Respiratory stimulant for respiratory depression secondary to anesthesia, mild-to-moderate drug-induced respiratory and CNS depression; acute hypercapnia secondary to COPD

Note: In general, the use of doxapram as a respiratory stimulant in adults is limited; alternate therapies are preferred.

Pregnancy Risk Factor B
Dosage Note: Although manufacturer's dosing recommendations are presented for these FDA-approved indications, use of doxapram has largely been replaced by alternate preferred agents.
Respiratory depression following anesthesia: Children ≥12 years, Adolescents, and Adults: I.V.:
Intermittent injection: Initial: 0.5-1 mg/kg; may repeat at 5-minute intervals (only in patients who demonstrate initial response); maximum total dose: 2 mg/kg
I.V. infusion: Initial: 5 mg/minute until adequate response or adverse effects seen; decrease to 1-3 mg/minute; maximum total dose: 4 mg/kg

Drug-induced CNS depression: Children ≥12 years, Adolescents, and Adults:

Intermittent injection: Initial: Priming dose of 1-2 mg/kg, repeat after 5 minutes; may repeat at 1-2 hour intervals (until sustained consciousness); maximum: 3000 mg daily. May repeat in 24 hours if necessary.

I.V. infusion: Initial: Priming dose of 1-2 mg/kg, repeat after 5 minutes. If no response, wait 1-2 hours and repeat priming dose. If some stimulation is noted, initiate infusion at 1-3 mg/minute (depending on size of patient/depth of CNS depression); suspend infusion if patient begins to awaken. Infusion should not be continued for >2 hours. May reinstitute infusion as described above, including bolus, after rest interval of 30 minutes to 2 hours; maximum: 3000 mg daily.

Acute hypercapnia secondary to COPD: Children ≥12 years, Adolescents, and Adults: I.V. infusion: Initial: Initiate infusion at 1-2 mg/minute (depending on size of patient/depth of CNS depression); may increase to maximum rate of 3 mg/minute; infusion should not be continued for >2 hours. Monitor arterial blood gases prior to initiation of infusion and at 30-minute intervals during the infusion (to identify possible development of acidosis/ CO_2 retention). Additional infusions are not recommended (per manufacturer).

Dosage adjustment in renal impairment: No dosage adjustment provided in manufacturer's labeling (has not been studied); however, use caution in severe impairment due to the potential for altered pharmacokinetics.

Dosage adjustment in hepatic impairment: No dosage adjustment provided in manufacturer's labeling (has not been studied); however, use caution in severe impairment due to the potential for altered pharmacokinetics.

Additional Information Complete prescribing information should be consulted for additional detail.

Dosage Forms Excipient information presented when available (limited, particularly for generics); consult specific product labeling.

Solution, Intravenous, as hydrochloride:

Dopram: 20 mg/mL (20 mL) [contains benzyl alcohol]

Generic: 20 mg/mL (20 mL)

◆ **Doxapram Hydrochloride** *see* Doxapram *on page 655*

Doxazosin (doks AY zoe sin)

Brand Names: U.S. Cardura; Cardura XL

Brand Names: Canada Alti-Doxazosin; Apo-Doxazosin®; Cardura-1™; Cardura-2™; Cardura-4™; Gen-Doxazosin; Mylan-Doxazosin; Novo-Doxazosin

Index Terms Doxazosin Mesylate

Pharmacologic Category $Alpha_1$ Blocker; Antihypertensive

Additional Appendix Information

Beers Criteria - Potentially Inappropriate Medications for Geriatrics *on page 2368*

Use

Immediate release formulation: Treatment of hypertension as monotherapy or in conjunction with diuretics, ACE inhibitors, beta-blockers, or calcium antagonists; treatment of urinary outflow obstruction and/or obstructive and irritative symptoms associated with benign prostatic hyperplasia (BPH)

Extended release formulation: Treatment of urinary outflow obstruction and/or obstructive and irritative symptoms associated with BPH

Unlabeled Use Pediatric hypertension; facilitation of distal ureteral stone expulsion; erectile dysfunction in patients with concomitant BPH

Pregnancy Risk Factor C

Pregnancy Considerations Adverse events were observed in some animal reproduction studies. If treatment for hypertension during pregnancy is needed, other agents are preferred (Chobanian, 2003).

Breast-Feeding Considerations Doxazosin is excreted into breast milk. Information is available from a single case report following a maternal dose of doxazosin 4 mg every 24 hours for 2 doses. Milk samples were obtained at various intervals over 24 hours, beginning ~17 hours after the first dose. Maternal serum samples were obtained at nearly the same times, beginning ~1 hour later. The highest serum and milk concentrations of doxazosin were observed ~1 hour after the dose. Using the highest milk concentration (4.15 mcg/L), the estimated dose to the nursing infant was calculated to be <1% of the weight-adjusted maternal dose (Jensen, 2013). The manufacturer recommends that caution be used if administered to nursing women.

Contraindications Hypersensitivity to quinazolines (prazosin, terazosin), doxazosin, or any component of the formulation

Warnings/Precautions Can cause significant orthostatic hypotension and syncope, especially with first dose; anticipate a similar effect if therapy is interrupted for a few days, if dosage is rapidly increased, or if another antihypertensive drug (particularly vasodilators) or a PDE-5 inhibitor is introduced. Discontinue if symptoms of angina occur or worsen. Patients should be cautioned about performing hazardous tasks when starting new therapy or adjusting dosage upward. Priapism has been associated with use (rarely). Prostate cancer should be ruled out before starting for BPH. Use with caution in mild-to-moderate hepatic impairment; not recommended in severe dysfunction. Intraoperative floppy iris syndrome has been observed in cataract surgery patients who were on or were previously treated with $alpha_1$-blockers. Causality has not been established and there appears to be no benefit in discontinuing alpha-blocker therapy prior to surgery. In the elderly, avoid use as an antihypertensive due to high risk of orthostatic hypotension; alternative agents preferred due to a more favorable risk/benefit profile (Beers Criteria).

The extended release formulation consists of drug within a nondeformable matrix; following drug release/absorption, the matrix/shell is expelled in the stool. The use of nondeformable products in patients with known stricture/narrowing of the GI tract has been associated with symptoms of obstruction. Use caution in patients with increased GI retention (eg, chronic constipation) as doxazosin exposure may be increased. Extended release formulation is not indicated for use in women or for the treatment of hypertension.

Adverse Reactions Note: Type and frequency of adverse reactions reflect combined data from BPH and hypertension trials and immediate release and extended release products.

>10%: Central nervous system: Dizziness (5% to 19%), malaise (12%), fatigue (8% to 12%), headache (6% to 10%)

1% to 10%:

Cardiovascular: Edema (3% to 4%), hypotension (1% to 2%), orthostatic hypotension (dose related; 0.3% up to 2%), arrhythmia (1%), facial edema (1%), flushing (1%)

Central nervous system: Vertigo (2% to 4%), somnolence (1% to 5%), pain (2%), anxiety (1%), ataxia (1%), hypertonia (1%), insomnia (1%), movement disorder (1%)

Endocrine & metabolic: Sexual dysfunction (2%)

Gastrointestinal: Abdominal pain (2%), nausea (1% to 2%), dyspepsia (1%), xerostomia (1%)

Genitourinary: Polyuria (2%), impotence (1%), incontinence (1%), urinary tract infection (1%)

Neuromuscular & skeletal: Weakness (4% to 7%), arthritis (1%), muscle cramps (1%), muscle weakness (1%), myalgia (1%)
Ocular: Abnormal vision (2%)
Otic: Tinnitus (1%)
Respiratory: Respiratory tract infection (5%), rhinitis (3%), dyspnea (1% to 3%), epistaxis (1%)

<1% (Limited to important or life-threatening): Abnormal lacrimation, abnormal thinking, agitation, allergic reaction, alopecia, amnesia, angina, anorexia, appetite increased, arthralgia, back pain, blurred vision, bradycardia, breast pain, bronchospasm, cerebrovascular accident, chest pain, cholestasis, confusion, cough, depersonalization, diaphoresis increased, diarrhea, dry skin, dysuria, earache, eczema, emotional lability, fecal incontinence, fever, gastroenteritis, gout, gynecomastia, hematuria, hepatitis, hot flashes, hypoesthesia, hypokalemia, impaired concentration, impotence, infection, influenza-like syndrome, intraoperative floppy iris syndrome (cataract surgery), jaundice, leukopenia, liver function tests increased, libido decreased, lymphadenopathy, micturition abnormality, migraine, MI, neutropenia, nocturia, pallor, palpitation, paranoia, paresis, parosmia, peripheral ischemia, pharyngitis, photophobia, priapism, pruritus, purpura, renal calculus, rigors, sinusitis, skin rash, syncope, taste perversion, thirst, thrombocytopenia, tremor, twitching, urticaria, vomiting, weight gain/loss

Drug Interactions

Metabolism/Transport Effects **Substrate** of CYP2C19 (minor), CYP2D6 (minor), CYP3A4 (major); **Note:** Assignment of Major/Minor substrate status based on clinically relevant drug interaction potential

Avoid Concomitant Use

Avoid concomitant use of Doxazosin with any of the following: Alpha1-Blockers; Conivaptan; Fusidic Acid (Systemic)

Increased Effect/Toxicity

Doxazosin may increase the levels/effects of: Alpha1-Blockers; Amifostine; Antihypertensives; Calcium Channel Blockers; Hypotensive Agents; Obinutuzumab; RiTUXimab

The levels/effects of Doxazosin may be increased by: Beta-Blockers; Brimonidine (Topical); Conivaptan; CYP3A4 Inhibitors (Moderate); CYP3A4 Inhibitors (Strong); Dasatinib; Diazoxide; Fusidic Acid (Systemic); Herbs (Hypotensive Properties); Ivacaftor; Luliconazole; MAO Inhibitors; Mifepristone; Pentoxifylline; Phosphodiesterase 5 Inhibitors; Prostacyclin Analogues; Simeprevir

Decreased Effect

Doxazosin may decrease the levels/effects of: Alpha-/Beta-Agonists; Alpha1-Agonists

The levels/effects of Doxazosin may be decreased by: Bosentan; CYP3A4 Inducers (Strong); Dabrafenib; Deferasirox; Herbs (CYP3A4 Inducers); Herbs (Hypertensive Properties); Methylphenidate; Mitotane; Peginterferon Alfa-2b; Tocilizumab; Yohimbine

Ethanol/Nutrition/Herb Interactions Herb/Nutraceutical: Avoid dong quai if using for hypertension (has estrogenic activity). Avoid ephedra, yohimbe, ginseng (may worsen hypertension). Avoid saw palmetto when used for BPH (due to limited experience with this combination). Avoid garlic (may have increased antihypertensive effect).

Storage/Stability Store at 25°C (77°F); excursions permitted between 15°C to 30°C (59°F to 86°F).

Mechanism of Action

Hypertension: Competitively inhibits postsynaptic alpha$_1$-adrenergic receptors which results in vasodilation of veins and arterioles and a decrease in total peripheral resistance and blood pressure; ~50% as potent on a weight by weight basis as prazosin.

BPH: Competitively inhibits postsynaptic alpha$_1$-adrenergic receptors in prostatic stromal and bladder neck tissues. This reduces the sympathetic tone-induced urethral stricture causing BPH symptoms.

Pharmacodynamics/Kinetics Not significantly affected by increased age

Duration: >24 hours
Protein binding: ~98%
Metabolism: Extensively hepatic to active metabolites; primarily via CYP3A4; secondary pathways involve CYP2D6 and 2C19
Bioavailability: Immediate release: ~65%; Extended release relative to immediate release: 54% to 59%
Half-life elimination: Immediate release: ~22 hours; Extended release: 15-19 hours
Time to peak, serum: Immediate release: 2-3 hours; Extended release: 8-9 hours
Excretion: Feces (63%, primarily as metabolites); urine (9%, primarily as metabolites)

Dosage Oral:

Children and Adolescents 1-17 years (unlabeled use): Hypertension: Immediate release: Initial: 1 mg once daily; maximum: 4 mg daily (NHBPEP, 2004)

Adults:

Immediate release: 1 mg once daily in morning or evening; may be increased to 2 mg once daily. Thereafter titrate upwards, if needed, every 1-2 weeks, balancing therapeutic benefit with doxazosin-induced postural hypotension.

BPH: Goal: 4-8 mg daily; maximum dose: 8 mg daily
Hypertension: Maximum dose: 16 mg daily
Distal ureteral stone expulsion (unlabeled use): 4 mg once daily in evening (Gurbuz, 2011; Resorlu, 2011). **Note:** Patients with stones >10 mm were excluded from studies.
Reinitiation of therapy: If therapy is discontinued for several days, restart at 1 mg dose and titrate as before

Extended release: BPH: 4 mg once daily with breakfast; titrate based on response and tolerability every 3-4 weeks to maximum recommended dose of 8 mg daily

Reinitiation of therapy: If therapy is discontinued for several days, restart at 4 mg dose and titrate as before.
Conversion to extended release from immediate release: Omit final evening dose of immediate release prior to starting morning dosing with extended release product; initiate extended release product using 4 mg once daily

Elderly: Hypertension: Consider lower initial doses (eg, immediate release: 0.5 mg once daily) and titrate to response (Aronow, 2011)

Dosage adjustment in renal impairment: No dosage adjustment provided in the manufacturer's labeling (limited data suggest renal impairment does not significantly alter pharmacokinetic parameters).

Dosage adjustment in hepatic impairment: Use with caution in mild-to-moderate hepatic dysfunction. Do not use with severe impairment.

Dietary Considerations Cardura® XL: Take with morning meal.

Administration Cardura® XL: Tablets should be swallowed whole; do not crush, chew, or divide. Administer with morning meal.

Monitoring Parameters Blood pressure, standing and sitting/supine; syncope may occur usually within 90 minutes of the initial dose or dose increase

Additional Information First-dose hypotension occurs less frequently with doxazosin as compared to prazosin; this may be due to its slower onset of action.

Dosage Forms Excipient information presented when available (limited, particularly for generics); consult specific product labeling.

Tablet, Oral:

Cardura: 1 mg, 2 mg, 4 mg, 8 mg [scored]

Generic: 1 mg, 2 mg, 4 mg, 8 mg

Tablet Extended Release 24 Hour, Oral:

Cardura XL: 4 mg, 8 mg

Dosage Forms: Canada Note: Refer to Dosage Forms. Extended-release capsules are not available in Canada.

◆ Doxazosin Mesylate *see* Doxazosin *on page 656*

Doxepin (Systemic) (DOKS e pin)

Brand Names: U.S. Silenor

Brand Names: Canada Apo-Doxepin®; Doxepine; Novo-Doxepin; Silenor®; Sinequan®; Zonalon

Index Terms Doxepin Hydrochloride

Pharmacologic Category Antidepressant, Tricyclic (Tertiary Amine)

Additional Appendix Information

Antidepressant Agents *on page 2284*

Beers Criteria − Potentially Inappropriate Medications for Geriatrics *on page 2368*

Use Depression; treatment of insomnia (with difficulty of sleep maintenance)

Unlabeled Use Analgesic for certain chronic and neuropathic pain; anxiety

Pregnancy Risk Factor C

Pregnancy Considerations Adverse events were observed in animal reproduction studies. Tricyclic antidepressants may be associated with irritability, jitteriness, and convulsions (rare) in the neonate (Yonkers, 2009).

The ACOG recommends that therapy for depression during pregnancy be individualized; treatment should incorporate the clinical expertise of the mental health clinician, obstetrician, primary healthcare provider, and pediatrician (ACOG, 2008). According to the American Psychiatric Association (APA), the risks of medication treatment should be weighed against other treatment options and untreated depression. For women who discontinue antidepressant medications during pregnancy and who may be at high risk for postpartum depression, the medications can be restarted following delivery (APA, 2010). Treatment algorithms have been developed by the ACOG and the APA for the management of depression in women prior to conception and during pregnancy (Yonkers, 2009).

Breast-Feeding Considerations Doxepin and N-desmethyldoxepin are excreted into breast milk (Frey, 1999; Kemp, 1985). Drowsiness, vomiting, poor feeding, and muscle hypotonia were noted in a nursing infant following maternal use of doxepin. Symptoms began to resolve 24 hours after feedings with breast milk were discontinued (Frey, 1999). In addition, product labeling notes that drowsiness and apnea have been reported in a nursing infant following maternal use of doxepin for depression. The manufacturer recommends that caution be used if administered to a nursing woman.

Medication Guide Available Yes

Contraindications Hypersensitivity to doxepin, drugs from similar chemical class, or any component of the formulation; narrow-angle glaucoma; urinary retention; use of MAO inhibitors within 14 days

Warnings/Precautions [U.S. Boxed Warning]: Antidepressants increase the risk of suicidal thinking and behavior in children, adolescents, and young adults (18-24 years of age) with major depressive disorder (MDD) and other psychiatric disorders; consider risk prior to prescribing. Short-term studies did not show an increased risk in patients >24 years of age and showed a decreased risk in patients ≥65 years. Closely monitor for clinical worsening, suicidality, or unusual changes in behavior; the patient's family or caregiver should be instructed to closely observe the patient and communicate condition with healthcare provider. A medication guide should be dispensed with each prescription. **Doxepin is approved for treatment of depression in adolescents.**

The possibility of a suicide attempt is inherent in major depression and may persist until remission occurs. Monitor for worsening of depression or suicidality, especially during initiation of therapy (generally first 1-2 months) or with dose increases or decreases. Use caution in high-risk patients. Worsening depression and severe abrupt suicidality that are not part of the presenting symptoms may require discontinuation or modification of drug therapy. The patient's family or caregiver should be alerted to monitor patients for the emergence of suicidality and associated behaviors (such as agitation, irritability, hostility, impulsivity, and hypomania) and call healthcare provider.

Risk of suicidal behavior may be increased regardless of doxepin dose; antidepressant doses of doxepin are 10- to 100-fold higher than doses for insomnia.

May worsen psychosis in some patients or precipitate a shift to mania or hypomania in patients with bipolar disorder. Patients presenting with depressive symptoms should be screened for bipolar disorder. Monotherapy in patients with bipolar disorder should be avoided. **Doxepin is not FDA approved for the treatment of bipolar depression.**

Should only be used for insomnia after evaluation of potential causes of sleep disturbance. Failure of sleep disturbance to resolve after 7-10 days may indicate psychiatric or medical illness. An increased risk for hazardous sleep-related activities has been noted; discontinue use with any sleep-related episodes. The risks of sedative and anticholinergic effects are high relative to other antidepressant agents. Doxepin frequently causes sedation, which may result in impaired performance of tasks requiring alertness (eg, operating machinery or driving). Sedative effects may be additive with other CNS depressants and/or ethanol. Also use caution in patients with benign prostatic hyperplasia, xerostomia, visual problems, constipation, or history of bowel obstruction.

May cause orthostatic hypotension or conduction disturbances (risks are moderate relative to other antidepressants). Use with caution in patients with a history of cardiovascular disease (including previous MI, stroke, tachycardia, or conduction abnormalities). Use with caution in patients with respiratory compromise or sleep apnea; use is generally not recommended with severe sleep apnea.

Use caution in patients with a previous seizure disorder or condition predisposing to seizures such as brain damage, alcoholism, or concurrent therapy with other drugs which lower the seizure threshold. Bone fractures have been associated with antidepressant treatment. Consider the possibility of a fragility fracture if an antidepressant-treated patient presents with unexplained bone pain, point tenderness, swelling, or bruising (Rabenda, 2013; Rizzoli, 2012). Use with caution in hyperthyroid patients or those receiving thyroid supplementation. Use with caution in patients with hepatic or renal dysfunction.

In the elderly, avoid doses >6 mg/day in this age group due to its potent anticholinergic and sedative properties, and potential to cause orthostatic hypotension; safety of doses ≤6 mg/day is comparable to placebo. In addition, may also cause or exacerbate syndrome of inappropriate antidiuretic hormone secretion or hyponatremia; monitor sodium closely with initiation or dosage adjustments in older adults (Beers Criteria).

Abrupt discontinuation or interruption of antidepressant therapy has been associated with a discontinuation syndrome. Symptoms arising may vary with antidepressant however commonly include nausea, vomiting, diarrhea, headaches, light-headedness, dizziness, diminished appetite, sweating, chills, tremors, paresthesias, fatigue, somnolence, and sleep disturbances (eg, vivid dreams, insomnia). Greater risks for developing a discontinuation syndrome have been associated with antidepressants with shorter half-lives, longer durations of treatment, and abrupt discontinuation. For antidepressants of short or intermediate half-lives, symptoms may emerge within 2-5 days after treatment discontinuation and last 7-14 days (APA, 2010; Fava, 2006; Haddad, 2001; Shelton, 2001; Warner, 2006).

Adverse Reactions Actual frequency may be dependent on diagnosis.

Cardiovascular: Flushing, hypertension (<3%), hypotension, tachycardia

Central nervous system: Ataxia, chills, confusion, disorientation, dizziness, drowsiness, fatigue, hallucinations, headache, seizure, somnolence/sedation (6% to 9%)

Dermatologic: Alopecia, photosensitivity, pruritus, rash

Endocrine & metabolic: Blood sugar increased/decreased, breast enlargement, galactorrhea, gynecomastia, libido increased/decreased, SIADH

Gastrointestinal: Anorexia, aphthous stomatitis, constipation, diarrhea, gastroenteritis (≤2%), indigestion, nausea (2%), trouble with gums, unpleasant taste, vomiting, weight gain, xerostomia; lower esophageal sphincter tone decrease may cause GE reflux

Genitourinary: Testicular edema, urinary retention

Hematologic: Agranulocytosis, eosinophilia, leukopenia, purpura, thrombocytopenia, purpura

Hepatic: Jaundice

Neuromuscular & skeletal: Extrapyramidal symptoms, numbness, paresthesia, tardive dyskinesia, tremor, weakness

Ocular: Blurred vision

Otic: Tinnitus

Respiratory: Asthma exacerbation, nasopharyngitis/upper respiratory tract infection (≤4%)

Miscellaneous: Allergic reactions, diaphoresis (excessive)

<1% (Limited to important or life-threatening): Abdominal pain, anemia, arthralgia, atrioventricular block, back pain, blepharospasm, chest pain, complex sleep-related behavior (sleep-driving, cooking or eating food, making phone calls), diplopia, dyspepsia, gingival recession, hematochezia, hyperbilirubinemia, hypermagnesemia, hypersensitivity, hypoacusis, infection, lacrimation decreased, lip blister, motion sickness, myalgia, palpitations, peripheral edema, tympanic membrane perforation, ventricular extrasystoles

Drug Interactions

Metabolism/Transport Effects Substrate of CYP1A2 (minor), CYP2C19 (minor), CYP2D6 (major), CYP3A4 (minor); **Note:** Assignment of Major/Minor substrate status based on clinically relevant drug interaction potential

Avoid Concomitant Use

Avoid concomitant use of Doxepin (Systemic) with any of the following: Aclidinium; Iobenguane I 123; Ipratropium (Oral Inhalation); Linezolid; MAO Inhibitors; Methylene Blue; Moxonidine; Tiotropium; Umeclidinium

Increased Effect/Toxicity

Doxepin (Systemic) may increase the levels/effects of: Alpha-/Beta-Agonists (Direct-Acting); Alpha1-Agonists; Amphetamines; Analgesics (Opioid); Anticholinergics; Antipsychotics; Aspirin; Beta2-Agonists; Citalopram; Desmopressin; Escitalopram; Highest Risk QTc-Prolonging Agents; Methylene Blue; Metoclopramide; Moderate Risk QTc-Prolonging Agents; NSAID (COX-2 Inhibitor); NSAID (Nonselective); QuiNIDine; Serotonin Modulators; Sodium Phosphates; Sulfonylureas; Tiotropium; TraMADol; Vitamin K Antagonists; Yohimbine

The levels/effects of Doxepin (Systemic) may be increased by: Abiraterone Acetate; Aclidinium; Altretamine; Antipsychotics; BuPROPion; Cimetidine; Cinacalcet; Citalopram; Cobicistat; CYP2D6 Inhibitors (Moderate); CYP2D6 Inhibitors (Strong); Dexmethylphenidate; DULoxetine; Escitalopram; FLUoxetine; FluvoxaMINE; Ipratropium (Oral Inhalation); Linezolid; Lithium; MAO Inhibitors; Methylphenidate; Metoclopramide; Metyrosine; Mifepristone; PARoxetine; Pramlintide; Protease Inhibitors; QuiNIDine; Sertraline; Terbinafine (Systemic); Thyroid Products; TraMADol; Umeclidinium; Valproic Acid and Derivatives

Decreased Effect

Doxepin (Systemic) may decrease the levels/effects of: Acetylcholinesterase Inhibitors (Central); Alpha2-Agonists; Alpha2-Agonists (Ophthalmic); Iobenguane I 123; Moxonidine

The levels/effects of Doxepin (Systemic) may be decreased by: Acetylcholinesterase Inhibitors (Central); Barbiturates; CarBAMazepine; Peginterferon Alfa-2b; St Johns Wort

Ethanol/Nutrition/Herb Interactions

Ethanol: May increase CNS depression; monitor for increased effects with coadministration. Caution patients about effects.

Food: A high-fat meal increases the bioavailability of Silenor® and delays the peak plasma concentration by ~3 hours

Herb/Nutraceutical: Avoid valerian, St John's wort, SAMe, kava kava (may increase risk of serotonin syndrome and/or excessive sedation).

Storage/Stability Store at 20°C to 25°C (68°F to 77°F). Protect from light.

Mechanism of Action Increases the synaptic concentration of serotonin and norepinephrine in the central nervous system by inhibition of their reuptake by the presynaptic neuronal membrane; antagonizes the histamine (H_1) receptor for sleep maintenance

Pharmacodynamics/Kinetics

Onset of action: Peak effect: Antidepressant: Usually >2 weeks; Anxiolytic: may occur sooner

Protein binding: ~80%

Metabolism: Hepatic via CYP2C19 and 2D6; metabolites include N-desmethyldoxepin (active)

Half-life elimination: Adults: Doxepin: ~15 hours; N-desmethyldoxepin: 31 hours

Time to peak, serum: Hypnotic: 3.5 hours

Excretion: Urine (<3% as unchanged drug or N-desmethyldoxepin)

Dosage Oral:

Depression or anxiety (entire daily dose may be given at bedtime):

Adults: Initial: 25-150 mg/day at bedtime or in 2-3 divided doses; may gradually increase up to 300 mg/day; single dose should not exceed 150 mg; select patients may respond to 25-50 mg/day

Elderly: Initial: 10-25 mg at bedtime; increase by 10-25 mg every 3 days for inpatients and weekly for outpatients if tolerated. Rarely does the maximum dose required exceed 75 mg/day; a single bedtime dose is recommended.

Insomnia (Silenor®):

Adults: 3-6 mg once daily 30 minutes prior to bedtime; maximum dose: 6 mg/day

Elderly: 3 mg once daily; increase to 6 mg once daily if clinically needed

Discontinuation of therapy: Upon discontinuation of antidepressant therapy, gradually taper the dose to minimize the incidence of withdrawal symptoms and allow for the detection of re-emerging symptoms. Evidence supporting ideal taper rates is limited. APA and NICE guidelines suggest tapering therapy over at least several weeks with consideration to the half-life of the antidepressant; antidepressants with a shorter half-life may need to be tapered more conservatively. In addition for long-term treated patients, WFSBP guidelines recommend tapering over 4-6 months. If intolerable withdrawal symptoms occur following a dose reduction, consider resuming the previously prescribed dose and/or decrease dose at a more gradual rate (APA, 2010; Bauer, 2002; Haddad, 2001; NCCMH, 2010; Schatzberg, 2006; Shelton, 2001; Warner, 2006).

MAO inhibitor recommendations:

Switching to or from an MAO inhibitor intended to treat psychiatric disorders:

Allow 14 days to elapse between discontinuing an MAO inhibitor intended to treat psychiatric disorders and initiation of doxepin.

Allow 14 days to elapse between discontinuing doxepin and initiation of an MAO inhibitor intended to treat psychiatric disorders.

Use with other MAO inhibitors (such as linezolid or I.V. methylene blue):

Do not initiate doxepin in patients receiving linezolid or I.V. methylene blue; consider other interventions for psychiatric condition.

If urgent treatment with linezolid or I.V. methylene blue is required in a patient already receiving doxepin and potential benefits outweigh potential risks, discontinue doxepin promptly and administer linezolid or I.V. methylene blue. Monitor for serotonin syndrome for 2 weeks or until 24 hours after the last dose of linezolid or I.V. methylene blue, whichever comes first. May resume doxepin 24 hours after the last dose of linezolid or I.V. methylene blue.

Dosage adjustment in renal impairment: No dosage adjustment provided in manufacturer's labeling.

Dosage adjustment in hepatic impairment: Use a lower dose and adjust gradually

Silenor®: Initial: 3 mg once daily

Administration Oral: Do not mix oral concentrate with carbonated beverages (physically incompatible).

Silenor®: Administer within 30 minutes prior to bedtime; do not take within 3 hours of food

Monitoring Parameters Monitor blood pressure and pulse rate prior to and during initial therapy; monitor mental status, suicidal ideation (especially at the beginning of therapy or when doses are increased or decreased); weight; ECG in older adults

Insomnia: Re-evaluate diagnosis if insomnia does not remit within 7-10 days of treatment.

Reference Range Proposed therapeutic concentration (doxepin plus desmethyldoxepin): 110-250 ng/mL. Toxic concentration (doxepin plus desmethyldoxepin): >500 ng/mL. Utility of serum level monitoring is controversial.

Test Interactions Increased glucose

Dosage Forms Excipient information presented when available (limited, particularly for generics); consult specific product labeling.

Capsule, Oral:

Generic: 10 mg, 25 mg, 50 mg, 75 mg, 100 mg, 150 mg

Concentrate, Oral:

Generic: 10 mg/mL (118 mL, 120 mL)

Tablet, Oral:

Silenor: 3 mg [contains brilliant blue fcf (fd&c blue #1)]

Silenor: 6 mg [contains brilliant blue fcf (fd&c blue #1), fd&c yellow #10 (quinoline yellow)]

Doxepin (Topical) (DOKS e pin)

Brand Names: U.S. Prudoxin; Zonalon

Brand Names: Canada Zonalon®

Index Terms Doxepin Hydrochloride

Pharmacologic Category Topical Skin Product

Use Short-term (<8 days) management of moderate pruritus in adults with atopic dermatitis or lichen simplex chronicus

Unlabeled Use Cream: Treatment of burning mouth syndrome and neuropathic pain

Pregnancy Risk Factor B

Dosage

Oral: Topical: Burning mouth syndrome (unlabeled use): Cream: Apply 3-4 times daily

Topical: Pruritus: Adults and Elderly: Apply a thin film 4 times/day with at least 3- to 4-hour interval between applications; not recommended for use >8 days. **Note:** Low-dose (25-50 mg) oral administration has also been used to treat pruritus, but systemic effects are increased.

Additional Information Complete prescribing information should be consulted for additional detail.

Dosage Forms Excipient information presented when available (limited, particularly for generics); consult specific product labeling.

Cream, External, as hydrochloride:

Prudoxin: 5% (45 g)

Zonalon: 5% (30 g, 45 g)

◆ **Doxepine (Can)** *see* Doxepin (Systemic) *on page* 658

◆ **Doxepin Hydrochloride** *see* Doxepin (Systemic) *on page* 658

◆ **Doxepin Hydrochloride** *see* Doxepin (Topical) *on page* 660

Doxercalciferol (doks er kal si fe FEER ole)

Brand Names: U.S. Hectorol

Brand Names: Canada Hectorol®

Index Terms 1α-Hydroxyergocalciferol

Pharmacologic Category Vitamin D Analog

Use Treatment of secondary hyperparathyroidism in patients with chronic kidney disease

Pregnancy Risk Factor B

Dosage

Oral:

Dialysis patients: Dose should be titrated to lower iPTH to 150-300 pg/mL; dose is adjusted at 8-week intervals (maximum dose: 20 mcg 3 times/week)

Initial dose: iPTH >400 pg/mL: 10 mcg 3 times/week at dialysis

Dose titration:

iPTH level decreased by 50% and >300 pg/mL: Dose can be increased to 12.5 mcg 3 times/week for 8 more weeks; this titration process can continue at 8-week intervals; each increase should be by 2.5 mcg/dose

iPTH level 150-300 pg/mL: Maintain current dose

iPTH level <100 pg/mL: Suspend doxercalciferol for 1 week; resume at a reduced dose; decrease each dose (not weekly dose) by at least 2.5 mcg

Predialysis patients: Dose should be titrated to lower iPTH to 35-70 pg/mL with stage 3 disease or to 70-110 pg/mL with stage 4 disease: Dose may be adjusted at 2-week intervals (maximum dose: 3.5 mcg/day)

Initial dose: 1 mcg/day

Dose titration:

iPTH level >70 pg/mL with stage 3 disease or >110 pg/mL with stage 4 disease: Increase dose by 0.5 mcg every 2 weeks as necessary

iPTH level 35-70 pg/mL with stage 3 disease or 70-110 pg/mL with stage 4 disease: Maintain current dose

iPTH level is <35 pg/mL with stage 3 disease or <70 pg/mL with stage 4 disease: Suspend doxercalciferol for 1 week, then resume at a reduced dose (at least 0.5 mcg lower)

I.V.:

Dialysis patients: Dose should be titrated to lower iPTH to 150-300 pg/mL; dose is adjusted at 8-week intervals (maximum dose: 18 mcg/week)

Initial dose: iPTH level >400 pg/mL: 4 mcg 3 times/week after dialysis, administered as a bolus dose

Dose titration:

iPTH level decreased by <50% and >300 pg/mL: Dose can be increased by 1-2 mcg at 8-week intervals, as necessary

iPTH level decreased by >50% and >300 pg/mL: Maintain current dose

iPTH level 150-300 pg/mL: Maintain current dose

iPTH level <100 pg/mL: Suspend doxercalciferol for 1 week; resume at a reduced dose (at least 1 mcg lower)

Hypercalcemia, hyperphosphatemia, or serum calcium times phosphorus product >55 mg^2/dL^2: Decrease or suspend dose and/or adjust dose of phosphate binders; if dose is suspended, resume at a reduced dose (at least 1 mcg lower)

Dosage adjustment in renal impairment: No dosage adjustment necessary.

Dosage adjustment in hepatic impairment: No dosage adjustment provided in manufacturer's labeling. Use with caution and consider more frequent monitoring.

Additional Information Complete prescribing information should be consulted for additional detail.

Dosage Forms Excipient information presented when available (limited, particularly for generics); consult specific product labeling.

Capsule, Oral:

Hectorol: 0.5 mcg [contains alcohol, usp, fd&c red #40, fd&c yellow #10 (quinoline yellow)]

Hectorol: 1 mcg [contains fd&c yellow #6 (sunset yellow)]

Hectorol: 2.5 mcg [contains alcohol, usp, fd&c yellow #10 (quinoline yellow)]

Solution, Intravenous:

Hectorol: 2 mcg/mL (1 mL); 4 mcg/2 mL (2 mL) [contains alcohol, usp, disodium edta]

Hectorol: 4 mcg/2 mL (2 mL) [contains disodium edta]

◆ **Doxil** *see* DOXOrubicin (Liposomal) *on page 663*

DOXOrubicin (doks oh ROO bi sin)

Brand Names: U.S. Adriamycin

Brand Names: Canada Adriamycin; Doxorubicin Hydrochloride For Injection, USP; Doxorubicin Hydrochloride Injection

Index Terms ADR (error-prone abbreviation); Adria; Conventional Doxorubicin; Doxorubicin Hydrochloride; Hydroxydaunomycin Hydrochloride; Hydroxyldaunorubicin Hydrochloride

Pharmacologic Category Antineoplastic Agent, Anthracycline

Use Treatment of acute lymphocytic leukemia (ALL), acute myeloid leukemia (AML), Hodgkin's disease, malignant lymphoma, soft tissue and bone sarcomas, thyroid cancer, small cell lung cancer, breast cancer, gastric cancer, ovarian cancer, bladder cancer, neuroblastoma, and Wilms' tumor

Unlabeled Use Treatment of multiple myeloma, endometrial carcinoma, uterine sarcoma, head and neck cancer, liver cancer, kidney cancer

Pregnancy Risk Factor D

Pregnancy Considerations Teratogenicity and embryotoxicity were observed in animal studies. There are no adequate and well-controlled studies in pregnant women. Advise patients to avoid becoming pregnant (females) and to avoid causing pregnancy (males) during treatment. According to the National Comprehensive Cancer Network (NCCN) breast cancer guidelines, doxorubicin, if indicated, may be administered to pregnant women with breast cancer as part of a combination chemotherapy regimen, although chemotherapy should not be administered during the first trimester or after 35 weeks gestation.

Breast-Feeding Considerations Doxorubicin and its metabolites are found in breast milk. Due to the potential for serious adverse reactions in the nursing infant, breast-feeding should be discontinued during treatment.

Contraindications Hypersensitivity to doxorubicin, any component of the formulation, or to other anthracyclines or anthracenediones; recent MI, severe myocardial insufficiency, severe arrhythmia; previous therapy with high cumulative doses of doxorubicin, daunorubicin, idarubicin, or other anthracycline and anthracenediones; baseline neutrophil count <1500/mm^3; severe hepatic impairment

Warnings/Precautions Hazardous agent - use appropriate precautions for handling and disposal (NIOSH, 2012). **[U.S. Boxed Warning]: May cause cumulative, dose-related, myocardial toxicity (early or delayed).** Cardiotoxicity is dose-limiting. Total cumulative dose should take into account previous or concomitant treatment with cardiotoxic agents or irradiation of chest. The incidence of irreversible myocardial toxicity increases as the total cumulative (lifetime) dosages approach 450-500 mg/m^2. Although the risk increases with cumulative dose, irreversible cardiotoxicity may occur at any dose level. Patients with pre-existing heart disease, hypertension, concurrent administration of other antineoplastic agents, prior or concurrent chest irradiation, advanced age; and infants and children are at increased risk. Alternative administration schedules (weekly or continuous infusions) have are associated with less cardiotoxicity Baseline and periodic monitoring of ECG and LVEF (with either ECHO or MUGA scan) is recommended.

[U.S. Boxed Warnings]: For I.V. administration only. Potent vesicant; if extravasation occurs, severe local tissue damage leading to ulceration, necrosis, and pain may occur. Ensure proper needle or catheter placement prior to and during infusion. Avoid extravasation.

[U.S. Boxed Warning]: Dose-limiting severe myelosuppression (primarily leukopenia and neutropenia) may occur. Secondary acute myelogenous leukemia and myelodysplastic syndrome have been reported following treatment. May cause tumor lysis syndrome and hyperuricemia (in patients with rapidly growing tumors). **[U.S. Boxed Warning]: Reduce doses are recommended in patients with impaired hepatic function.**

Children are at increased risk for developing delayed cardiotoxicity; follow-up cardiac function monitoring is recommended. Doxorubicin may contribute to prepubertal growth failure in children; may also contribute to gonadal impairment (usually temporary). Radiation recall pneumonitis has been reported in children receiving concomitant dactinomycin and doxorubicin. **[U.S. Boxed Warning]: Should be administered under the supervision of an experienced cancer chemotherapy physician.** Use caution when selecting product for preparation and dispensing; indications, dosages and adverse event profiles differ between conventional doxorubicin hydrochloride solution and doxorubicin liposomal. Both formulations are the same concentration. As a result, serious errors have occurred.

Adverse Reactions Frequency not defined.

Cardiovascular:

Acute cardiotoxicity: Atrioventricular block, bradycardia, bundle branch block, ECG abnormalities, extrasystoles (atrial or ventricular), sinus tachycardia, ST-T wave changes, supraventricular tachycardia, tachyarrhythmia, ventricular tachycardia

Delayed cardiotoxicity: LVEF decreased, CHF (manifestations include ascites, cardiomegaly, dyspnea, edema, gallop rhythm, hepatomegaly, oliguria, pleural effusion, pulmonary edema, tachycardia); myocarditis, pericarditis

Central nervous system: Malaise

Dermatologic: Alopecia, itching, photosensitivity, radiation recall, rash; discoloration of saliva, sweat, or tears

Endocrine & metabolic: Amenorrhea, dehydration, infertility (may be temporary), hyperuricemia

Gastrointestinal: Abdominal pain, anorexia, colon necrosis, diarrhea, GI ulceration, mucositis, nausea, vomiting

Genitourinary: Discoloration of urine

Hematologic: Leukopenia/neutropenia (75%; nadir: 10-14 days; recovery: by day 21); thrombocytopenia and anemia

Local: Skin "flare" at injection site, urticaria

Neuromuscular & skeletal: Weakness

Postmarketing and/or case reports: Anaphylaxis, azoospermia, bilirubin increased, coma (when in combination with cisplatin or vincristine), conjunctivitis, fever, gonadal impairment (children), growth failure (prepubertal), hepatitis, hyperpigmentation (nail, skin & oral mucosa), infection, keratitis, lacrimation, myelodysplastic syndrome, neutropenic fever, neutropenic typhlitis, oligospermia, peripheral neurotoxicity (with intra-arterial doxorubicin), phlebosclerosis, radiation recall pneumonitis (children), secondary acute myelogenous leukemia, seizure (when in combination with cisplatin or vincristine), sepsis, shock, Stevens-Johnson syndrome, systemic hypersensitivity (including urticaria, pruritus, angioedema, dysphagia, and dyspnea), toxic epidermal necrolysis, transaminases increased, urticaria

Drug Interactions

Metabolism/Transport Effects **Substrate** of CYP2D6 (major), CYP3A4 (major), P-glycoprotein; **Note:** Assignment of Major/Minor substrate status based on clinically relevant drug interaction potential; **Inhibits** CYP2B6 (moderate), CYP2D6 (weak), CYP3A4 (weak); **Induces** P-glycoprotein

Avoid Concomitant Use

Avoid concomitant use of DOXOrubicin with any of the following: BCG; CloZAPine; Conivaptan; Dabigatran Etexilate; Fusidic Acid (Systemic); Natalizumab; Pimecrolimus; Pimozide; Pomalidomide; Sofosbuvir; Tacrolimus (Topical); Tofacitinib; Vaccines (Live); VinCRIStine (Liposomal)

Increased Effect/Toxicity

DOXOrubicin may increase the levels/effects of: ARIPiprazole; CloZAPine; CYP2B6 Substrates; Dofetilide; Leflunomide; Lomitapide; Natalizumab; Pimozide; Tofacitinib; Vaccines (Live); Vitamin K Antagonists; Zidovudine

The levels/effects of DOXOrubicin may be increased by: Abiraterone Acetate; Bevacizumab; Conivaptan; Cyclophosphamide; CycloSPORINE (Systemic); CYP2D6 Inhibitors (Moderate); CYP2D6 Inhibitors (Strong); CYP3A4 Inhibitors (Moderate); CYP3A4 Inhibitors (Strong); Darunavir; Dasatinib; Denosumab; Fusidic Acid (Systemic); Ivacaftor; Luliconazole; Mifepristone; P-glycoprotein/ABCB1 Inhibitors; Pimecrolimus; Roflumilast; Simeprevir; SORAfenib; Tacrolimus (Topical); Taxane Derivatives; Trastuzumab

Decreased Effect

DOXOrubicin may decrease the levels/effects of: Afatinib; BCG; Cardiac Glycosides; Coccidioidin Skin Test; Dabigatran Etexilate; Linagliptin; P-glycoprotein/ABCB1 Substrates; Pomalidomide; Sipuleucel-T; Sofosbuvir; Stavudine; Vaccines (Inactivated); Vaccines (Live); VinCRIStine (Liposomal); Vitamin K Antagonists; Zidovudine

The levels/effects of DOXOrubicin may be decreased by: Bosentan; Cardiac Glycosides; CYP3A4 Inducers (Strong); Dabrafenib; Deferasirox; Dexrazoxane; Echinacea; Herbs (CYP3A4 Inducers); Mitotane; Peginterferon Alfa-2b; P-glycoprotein/ABCB1 Inducers; Tocilizumab

Ethanol/Nutrition/Herb Interactions Herb/Nutraceutical: Avoid St John's wort (may decrease doxorubicin levels). Avoid black cohosh, dong quai in estrogen-dependent tumors.

Preparation for Administration Hazardous agent; use appropriate precautions for handling and disposal (NIOSH, 2012). Reconstitute lyophilized powder with NS to a final concentration of 2 mg/mL (may further dilute in 50-1000 mL D_5W or NS for infusion). Unstable in solutions with a pH <3 or >7.

Storage/Stability Store intact vials of solution under refrigeration at 2°C to 8°C. Protected from light. Store intact vials of lyophilized powder at room temperature (15°C to 30°C). Reconstituted vials are stable for 7 days at room temperature (25°C) and 15 days under refrigeration (5°C) when protected from light. Infusions are stable for 48 hours at room temperature (25°C) when protected from light. Solutions diluted in 50-1000 mL D_5W or NS are stable for 48 hours at room temperature (25°C) when protected from light.

Mechanism of Action Inhibition of DNA and RNA synthesis by intercalation between DNA base pairs by inhibition of topoisomerase II and by steric obstruction. Doxorubicin intercalates at points of local uncoiling of the double helix. Although the exact mechanism is unclear, it appears that direct binding to DNA (intercalation) and inhibition of DNA repair (topoisomerase II inhibition) result in blockade of DNA and RNA synthesis and fragmentation of DNA. Doxorubicin is also a powerful iron chelator; the iron-doxorubicin complex can bind DNA and cell membranes and produce free radicals that immediately cleave the DNA and cell membranes.

Pharmacodynamics/Kinetics

Absorption: Oral: Poor (<50%)

Distribution: V_d: 809-1214 L/m²; to many body tissues, particularly liver, spleen, kidney, lung, heart; does not distribute into the CNS; crosses placenta

Protein binding, plasma: 70% to 76%

Metabolism: Primarily hepatic to doxorubicinol (active), then to inactive aglycones, conjugated sulfates, and glucuronides

Half-life elimination:

- Distribution: 5-10 minutes
- Elimination: Doxorubicin: 1-3 hours; Metabolites: 3-3.5 hours
- Terminal: 17-48 hours
- Male: 54 hours; Female: 35 hours

Excretion: Feces (~40% to 50% as unchanged drug); urine (~5% to 12% as unchanged drug and metabolites)

- Clearance: Male: 113 L/hour; Female: 44 L/hour

Dosage I.V.: Refer to individual protocols. **Note:** Lower dosage should be considered for patients with inadequate marrow reserve (due to old age, prior treatment or neoplastic marrow infiltration)

Children:

- 35-75 mg/m²/dose every 21 days **or**
- 20-30 mg/m²/dose once weekly **or**
- 60-90 mg/m²/dose given as a continuous infusion over 96 hours every 3-4 weeks

Adults: Usual or typical dose: 60-75 mg/m²/dose every 21 days **or**

- 60 mg/m²/dose every 2 weeks (dose dense) **or**
- 40-60 mg/m²/dose every 3-4 weeks **or**
- 20-30 mg/m²/day for 2-3 days every 4 weeks **or**
- 20 mg/m²/dose once weekly

Dosing adjustment in toxicity: The following delays and/or dose reductions have been used:

Neutropenic fever/infection: Consider reducing to 75% of dose in subsequent cycles

ANC <1000/mm^3: Delay treatment until ANC recovers to ≥1000/mm^3
Platelets <100,000/mm^3: Delay treatment until platelets recover to ≥100,000/mm^3

Dosing adjustment in renal impairment:
Adjustments are not required.
Hemodialysis: Supplemental dose is not necessary.

Dosing adjustment in hepatic impairment:
The FDA-approved labeling recommends the following adjustments:
Serum bilirubin 1.2-3 mg/dL: Administer 50% of dose
Serum bilirubin 3.1-5 mg/dL: Administer 25% of dose
Severe hepatic impairment: Use is contraindicated
The following guidelines have been used by some clinicians: Floyd, 2006:
Transaminases 2-3 times ULN: Administer 75% of dose
Transaminases >3 times ULN or serum bilirubin 1.2-3 mg/dL: Administer 50% of dose
Serum bilirubin 3.1-5 mg/dL: Administer 25% of dose
Serum bilirubin >5 mg/dL: Do not administer

Dosing in obesity: *ASCO Guidelines for appropriate chemotherapy dosing in obese adults with cancer:* Utilize patient's actual body weight (full weight) for calculation of body surface area- or weight-based dosing, particularly when the intent of therapy is curative; manage regimen-related toxicities in the same manner as for nonobese patients; if a dose reduction is utilized due to toxicity, consider resumption of full weight-based dosing with subsequent cycles, especially if cause of toxicity (eg, hepatic or renal impairment) is resolved (Griggs, 2012).

Administration Administer I.V. push over at least 3-5 minutes or by continuous infusion (infusion via central venous line recommended). Flush with 5-10 mL of I.V. solution before and after drug administration. Incompatible with heparin. Monitor for local erythematous streaking along vein and/or facial flushing (may indicate rapid infusion rate). Do not administer I.M. or SubQ.

Vesicant; ensure proper needle or catheter placement prior to and during infusion; avoid extravasation.

Extravasation management: If extravasation occurs, stop infusion immediately and disconnect (leave cannula/needle in place); gently aspirate extravasated solution (do **NOT** flush the line); remove needle/cannula; elevate extremity. Initiate antidote (dexrazoxane or dimethyl sulfate [DMSO]). Apply dry cold compresses for 20 minutes 4 times daily for 1-2 days (Perez Fidalgo, 2012); withhold cooling beginning 15 minutes before dexrazoxane infusion; continue withholding cooling until 15 minutes after infusion is completed. Topical DMSO should not be administered in combination with dexrazoxane; may lessen dexrazoxane efficacy.

Dexrazoxane: Adults: 1000 mg/m^2 (maximum dose: 2000 mg) I.V. (administer in a large vein remote from site of extravasation) over 1-2 hours days 1 and 2, then 500 mg/m^2 (maximum dose: 1000 mg) I.V. over 1-2 hours day 3; begin within 6 hours of extravasation. Day 2 and day 3 doses should be administered at approximately the same time (± 3 hours) as the dose on day 1 (Mouridsen, 2007; Perez Fidalgo, 2012). **Note:** Reduce dexrazoxane dose by 50% in patients with moderate to severe renal impairment (Cl_{cr} <40 mL/minute).

DMSO: Children and Adults: Apply topically to a region covering twice the affected area every 8 hours for 7 days; begin within 10 minutes of extravasation; do not cover with a dressing (Perez Fidalgo, 2012).

Hazardous agent; use appropriate precautions for handling and disposal (NIOSH, 2012).

Monitoring Parameters CBC with differential and platelet count; liver function tests (bilirubin, ALT/AST, alkaline phosphatase); serum uric acid, calcium, potassium, phosphate and creatinine; cardiac function (baseline, periodic, and followup): ECG, left ventricular ejection fraction (echocardiography [ECHO] or multigated radionuclide angiography [MUGA])

Dosage Forms Excipient information presented when available (limited, particularly for generics); consult specific product labeling. [DSC] = Discontinued product
Solution, Intravenous, as hydrochloride:
Adriamycin: 2 mg/mL (5 mL, 10 mL, 25 mL, 100 mL)
Generic: 2 mg/mL (5 mL, 10 mL, 25 mL, 100 mL)
Solution, Intravenous, as hydrochloride [preservative free]:
Generic: 2 mg/mL (5 mL, 10 mL, 25 mL, 75 mL, 100 mL)
Solution Reconstituted, Intravenous, as hydrochloride:
Adriamycin: 10 mg (1 ea); 20 mg (1 ea); 50 mg (1 ea)
Generic: 10 mg (1 ea [DSC]); 50 mg (1 ea [DSC])
Solution Reconstituted, Intravenous, as hydrochloride [preservative free]:
Generic: 10 mg (1 ea); 50 mg (1 ea)

◆ **Doxorubicin Hydrochloride** *see* DOXOrubicin *on page 661*
◆ **DOXOrubicin Hydrochloride Encapsulated Liposomes (Myocet™)** *see* DOXOrubicin (Liposomal) *on page 663*
◆ **Doxorubicin Hydrochloride For Injection, USP (Can)** *see* DOXOrubicin *on page 661*
◆ **Doxorubicin Hydrochloride Injection (Can)** *see* DOXOrubicin *on page 661*
◆ **DOXOrubicin Hydrochloride (Liposomal)** *see* DOXOrubicin (Liposomal) *on page 663*
◆ **DOXOrubicin Hydrochloride Liposome** *see* DOXOrubicin (Liposomal) *on page 663*
◆ **DOXOrubicin Hydrochloride Liposomes (Myocet™)** *see* DOXOrubicin (Liposomal) *on page 663*

DOXOrubicin (Liposomal)

(doks oh ROO bi sin lye po SO mal)

Brand Names: U.S. Doxil; Lipodox; Lipodox 50
Brand Names: Canada Caelyx; Myocet
Index Terms DOXOrubicin Hydrochloride (Liposomal); DOXOrubicin Hydrochloride Encapsulated Liposomes (Myocet™); DOXOrubicin Hydrochloride Liposome; DOXOrubicin Hydrochloride Liposomes (Myocet™); Lipodox; Liposomal DOXOrubicin; Pegylated DOXOrubicin Liposomal; Pegylated Liposomal DOXOrubicin; Pegylated Liposomal DOXOrubicin Hydrochloride (Doxil®, Caelyx®)
Pharmacologic Category Antineoplastic Agent, Anthracycline
Use
U.S. labeling: Treatment of ovarian cancer (progressive or recurrent after platinum-based treatment); multiple myeloma (in combination with bortezomib in patients who are bortezomib naïve and after failure of at least 1 prior therapy); AIDS-related Kaposi's sarcoma (after failure of or intolerance to prior systemic therapy)
Canadian labeling: Treatment of metastatic breast cancer (as monotherapy [Caelyx®] or in combination with cyclophosphamide [Myocet™]); advanced ovarian cancer (after failure of first-line treatment [Caelyx®]); AIDS-related Kaposi's sarcoma (after failure of or intolerance to prior systemic therapy [Caelyx®])
Unlabeled Use Treatment of metastatic breast cancer, Hodgkin lymphoma (salvage treatment), cutaneous T-cell lymphomas (mycosis fungoides and Sézary syndrome), advanced soft tissue sarcomas; advanced or recurrent uterine sarcoma
Pregnancy Risk Factor D

Pregnancy Considerations Adverse events were observed in animal reproduction studies at doses less than the equivalent human dose (based on BSA). May cause fetal harm if administered during pregnancy. Women of childbearing potential should avoid becoming pregnant during treatment.

Breast-Feeding Considerations Due to the potential for serious adverse reactions in the nursing infant, breast-feeding should be discontinued during treatment.

Contraindications Hypersensitivity to doxorubicin liposomal, conventional doxorubicin, or any component of the formulation

Canadian labeling (Caelyx®): Additional contraindications (not in U.S. labeling): Breast-feeding

Warnings/Precautions Hazardous agent - use appropriate precautions for handling and disposal (NIOSH, 2012).

[U.S. Boxed Warning]: Doxorubicin may cause cumulative, dose-related myocardial toxicity may lead to congestive heart failure as the cumulative (lifetime) dose of pegylated doxorubicin liposomal approaches 550 mg/m². When calculating cumulative doses, also include prior dose of other anthracyclines and anthracenediones. Cardiotoxicity may occur at lower cumulative doses (400 mg/m²) in patients who have received prior mediastinal irradiation or are receiving concurrent cyclophosphamide treatment. For Myocet™ (Canadian availability), cardiotoxicity may occur as the cumulative (lifetime) dose approaches 750 mg/m². Anthracycline-induced cardiotoxicity may be delayed (after discontinuation of anthracycline treatment). Use only if potential benefits outweigh cardiovascular risk in patients with a history of cardiovascular disease. Monitor cardiac function with biopsy, echocardiography, or MUGA scan; evaluate left ventricular ejection fraction (LVEF) prior to treatment and periodically during treatment; if results indicate possible heart failure, carefully evaluate the potential effects of continued treatment.

[U.S. Boxed Warning]: Acute infusion reactions may occur, some may be serious/life-threatening (eg, allergic or anaphylactoid reactions). Reactions may include flushing, dyspnea, facial swelling, headache, chills, back pain, hypotension, and/or chest/throat tightness. Infusion reactions typically occur with the first dose and usually resolve with within several hours to a day after terminating the infusion; some have resolved with slowing the infusion rate. To minimize the risk of infusion reactions, infuse at an initial rate of 1 mg/minute. Medications for the treatment of reactions should be readily available in the event of severe reaction.

[U.S. Boxed Warning]: Use with caution in patients with hepatic impairment; dosage reduction is recommended. Use in patients with hepatic impairment has not been adequately studied; no dosing adjustment recommendations are available for multiple myeloma patients with hepatic impairment. **[U.S. Boxed Warning]: Severe myelosuppression may occur.** Monitor blood counts. Treatment delay, dosage modification, or discontinuation may be required. Leukopenia is usually transient, although persistent or severe neutropenia may result in superinfection or neutropenic fever; sepsis due to neutropenia has resulted in discontinuation (may rarely be fatal). Hemorrhage due to thrombocytopenia may occur. Hematologic toxicity may be more severe with combination chemotherapy. Palmar-plantar erythrodysesthesia (hand-foot syndrome) has been reported, more commonly in patients with ovarian cancer and multiple myeloma, and less commonly in patients with Kaposi's sarcoma. May occur early in treatment, but is usually seen after 2-3 treatment cycles. Dosage modification may be required; mild cases resolve within 1-2 weeks; in severe cases, treatment discontinuation may be required. Use of Caelyx® (Canadian availability) in splenectomized patients with AIDS-related Kaposi's sarcoma is not recommended (has not been studied). **[U.S. Boxed Warning]: Liposomal formulations of doxorubicin should NOT be substituted for conventional doxorubicin hydrochloride on a mg-per-mg basis.**

Cases of secondary oral cancers (primarily squamous cell carcinoma) have been reported with long-term (>1 year) doxorubicin liposomal exposure; these secondary oral malignancies have occurred during treatment and up to 6 years after treatment. The development of oral ulceration or discomfort should be monitored and further evaluated in patients with past or present use of doxorubicin liposomal. Tissue distribution of the liposomal doxorubicin compared to free doxorubicin may play a role in the development of oral secondary malignancies associated with long-term use.

Doxorubicin may potentiate the toxicity of cyclophosphamide (hemorrhagic cystitis) and mercaptopurine (hepatotoxicity). Radiation recall reaction has been reported with doxorubicin liposomal treatment after radiation therapy. Radiation-induced toxicity (to the myocardium, mucosa, skin, and liver) may be increased by doxorubicin.

Adverse Reactions

>10%:

- Cardiovascular: Peripheral edema (≤11%)
- Central nervous system: Fever (8% to 21%), headache (≤11%), pain (≤21%)
- Dermatologic: Palmar-plantar erythrodysesthesia/hand-foot syndrome (≤51% in ovarian cancer [grades 3/4: 24%]; 3% in Kaposi's sarcoma), rash (≤29% in ovarian cancer, ≤5% in Kaposi's sarcoma), alopecia (9% to 19%)
- Gastrointestinal: Nausea (17% to 46%), stomatitis (5% to 41%), vomiting (8% to 33%), constipation (≤30%), diarrhea (5% to 21%), anorexia (≤20%), mucositis (≤14%), dyspepsia (≤12%), intestinal obstruction (≤11%)
- Hematologic: Myelosuppression (onset: 7 days; nadir: 10-14 days; recovery: 21-28 days), thrombocytopenia (13% to 65%; grades 3/4: 1%), neutropenia (12% to 62%; grade 4: 4%), leukopenia (36%), anemia (6% to 74%; grade 4: <1%)
- Neuromuscular & skeletal: Weakness (7% to 40%), back pain (≤12%)
- Respiratory: Pharyngitis (≤16%), dyspnea (≤15%)
- Miscellaneous: Infection (≤12%)

1% to 10%:

- Cardiovascular: Cardiac arrest, chest pain, deep thrombophlebitis, edema, hypotension, pallor, tachycardia, vasodilation
- Central nervous system: Agitation, anxiety, chills, confusion, depression, dizziness, emotional lability, insomnia, somnolence, vertigo
- Dermatologic: Acne, bruising, dry skin (6%), exfoliative dermatitis, fungal dermatitis, furunculosis, maculopapular rash, pruritus, skin discoloration, vesiculobullous rash
- Endocrine & metabolic: Dehydration, hypercalcemia, hyperglycemia, hypokalemia, hyponatremia
- Gastrointestinal: Abdomen enlarged, anorexia, ascites, cachexia, dyspepsia, dysphagia, esophagitis, flatulence, gingivitis, glossitis, ileus, mouth ulceration, oral moniliasis, rectal bleeding, taste perversion, weight loss, xerostomia
- Genitourinary: Cystitis, dysuria, leukorrhea, pelvic pain, polyuria, urinary incontinence, urinary tract infection, urinary urgency, vaginal bleeding, vaginal moniliasis
- Hematologic: Hemolysis, prothrombin time increased
- Hepatic: ALT increased, alkaline phosphatase increased, hyperbilirubinemia

Local: Thrombophlebitis
Neuromuscular & skeletal: Arthralgia, hypertonia, myalgia, neuralgia, neuritis (peripheral), neuropathy, paresthesia (≤10%), pathological fracture
Ocular: Conjunctivitis, dry eyes, retinitis
Otic: Ear pain
Renal: Albuminuria, hematuria
Respiratory: Apnea, cough (≤10%), epistaxis, pleural effusion, pneumonia, rhinitis, sinusitis
Miscellaneous: Allergic reaction; infusion-related reactions (7%; includes bronchospasm, chest tightness, chills, dyspnea, facial edema, flushing, headache, herpes simplex/zoster, hypotension, pruritus); moniliasis, diaphoresis

<1% (Limited to important or life-threatening): Abscess, acute brain syndrome, abnormal vision, acute myeloid leukemia (secondary), alkaline phosphatase increased, anaphylactic or anaphylactoid reaction, asthma, balanitis, blindness, bronchitis, BUN increased, bundle branch block, cardiomegaly, cardiomyopathy, cellulitis, CHF, colitis, creatinine increased, cryptococcosis, diabetes mellitus, erythema multiforme, erythema nodosum, eosinophilia, fecal impaction, flu-like syndrome, gastritis, glucosuria, hemiplegia, hemorrhage, hepatic failure, hepatitis, hepatosplenomegaly, hyperkalemia, hypernatremia, hyperuricemia, hyperventilation, hypoglycemia, hypolipidemia, hypomagnesemia, hypophosphatemia, hypoproteinemia, hypothermia, injection site hemorrhage, injection site pain, jaundice, ketosis, lactic dehydrogenase increased, lymphadenopathy, lymphangitis, migraine, myositis, optic neuritis, oral cancers (squamous cell; long-term use), palpitation, pancreatitis, pericardial effusion, petechia, pneumonitis, pneumothorax, pulmonary embolism, radiation injury, reddish/orange discoloration of urine/body fluids, renal failure, sclerosing cholangitis, seizure, sepsis, skin necrosis, skin ulcer, syncope, Stevens-Johnson syndrome, tenesmus, thromboplastin decreased, thrombosis, tinnitus, toxic epidermal necrolysis, urticaria, visual field defect, ventricular arrhythmia

Drug Interactions

Metabolism/Transport Effects Substrate of CYP2D6 (major), CYP3A4 (major); **Note:** Assignment of Major/Minor substrate status based on clinically relevant drug interaction potential; **Inhibits** CYP2B6 (moderate)

Avoid Concomitant Use

Avoid concomitant use of DOXOrubicin (Liposomal) with any of the following: BCG; CloZAPine; Conivaptan; Fusidic Acid (Systemic); Natalizumab; Pimecrolimus; Tacrolimus (Topical); Tofacitinib; Vaccines (Live)

Increased Effect/Toxicity

DOXOrubicin (Liposomal) may increase the levels/effects of: CloZAPine; CYP2B6 Substrates; Leflunomide; Natalizumab; Tofacitinib; Vaccines (Live); Zidovudine

The levels/effects of DOXOrubicin (Liposomal) may be increased by: Abiraterone Acetate; Bevacizumab; Conivaptan; Cyclophosphamide; CYP2D6 Inhibitors (Moderate); CYP2D6 Inhibitors (Strong); CYP3A4 Inhibitors (Moderate); CYP3A4 Inhibitors (Strong); Darunavir; Dasatinib; Denosumab; Fusidic Acid (Systemic); Ivacaftor; Luliconazole; Mifepristone; Pimecrolimus; Roflumilast; Simeprevir; Tacrolimus (Topical); Taxane Derivatives; Trastuzumab

Decreased Effect

DOXOrubicin (Liposomal) may decrease the levels/effects of: BCG; Cardiac Glycosides; Coccidioidin Skin Test; Sipuleucel-T; Stavudine; Vaccines (Inactivated); Vaccines (Live); Zidovudine

The levels/effects of DOXOrubicin (Liposomal) may be decreased by: Bosentan; Cardiac Glycosides; CYP3A4 Inducers (Strong); Dabrafenib; Deferasirox; Echinacea; Herbs (CYP3A4 Inducers); Mitotane; Peginterferon Alfa-2b; Tocilizumab

Ethanol/Nutrition/Herb Interactions

Ethanol: Avoid ethanol (due to GI irritation).
Herb/Nutraceutical: St John's wort may decrease doxorubicin levels.

Preparation for Administration Hazardous agent; use appropriate precautions for handling and disposal (NIOSH, 2012).

Doxil®, Caelyx®: Doses ≤90 mg must be diluted in D_5W 250 mL prior to administration. Doses >90 mg should be diluted in D_5W 500 mL. Solution is not clear, but has a red, translucent appearance due to the liposomal dispersion. Dilute only in D_5W; do not use bacteriostatic agents; do not mix with other medications.
Myocet™: Refer to product labeling for detailed reconstitution and preparation information.

Storage/Stability Store intact vials refrigerated at 2°C to 8°C (36°F to 46°F); avoid freezing.

Doxil®, Caelyx®: Prolonged freezing may adversely affect liposomal drug products, however, short-term freezing (<1 month) does not appear to have a deleterious effect (Doxil®). Solutions diluted for infusion should be refrigerated at 2°C to 8°C (36°F to 46°F); administer within 24 hours. **Do not infuse with in-line filters.**
Myocet™: Refer to product labeling for detailed reconstitution and preparation information. Following reconstitution, may be stored up to 8 hours at room temperature or up to 72 hours refrigerated at 2°C to 8°C (36°F to 46°F); do not freeze.

Mechanism of Action Doxorubicin inhibits DNA and RNA synthesis by intercalating between DNA base pairs causing steric obstruction and inhibits topoisomerase-II at the point of DNA cleavage. Doxorubicin is also a powerful iron chelator. The iron-doxorubicin complex can bind DNA and cell membranes, producing free hydroxyl (OH) radicals that cleave DNA and cell membranes. Active throughout entire cell cycle. Doxorubicin liposomal is a pegylated formulation which protects the liposomes, and thereby increases blood circulation time.

Pharmacodynamics/Kinetics

Distribution: V_{dss}: 2.7-2.8 L/m^2
Protein binding, plasma: Unknown; nonliposomal (conventional) doxorubicin: 70%
Half-life elimination: Terminal: Distribution: 4.7-5.2 hours, Elimination: 44-55 hours
Metabolism: Hepatic and in plasma to doxorubicinol and the sulfate and glucuronide conjugates of 4-demethyl,7-deoxyaglycones
Excretion: Urine (5% as doxorubicin or doxorubicinol)

Dosage Details concerning dosing in combination regimens should also be consulted. **Liposomal formulations of doxorubicin should NOT be substituted for conventional doxorubicin hydrochloride on a mg-per-mg basis.**

U.S. labeling:

AIDS-related Kaposi's sarcoma: I.V.: 20 mg/m^2 once every 3 weeks; continue as long as responding and tolerating
Multiple myeloma: I.V.: 30 mg/m^2 on day 4 every 3 weeks (in combination with bortezomib) for up to 8 cycles until disease progression or unacceptable toxicity
Ovarian cancer, progressive or recurrent: I.V.: 50 mg/m^2 once every 4 weeks (minimum of 4 cycles is recommended)

Canadian labeling:
AIDS-related Kaposi's sarcoma (Caelyx®): I.V.: 20 mg/m^2 once every 2-3 weeks; continue as long as responding and tolerating
Breast cancer, metastatic: I.V.:
Caelyx®: 50 mg/m^2 once every 4 weeks until disease progression or unacceptable toxicity
Myocet™: 60-75 mg/m^2 once every 3 weeks (in combination with cyclophosphamide)
Ovarian cancer, advanced (Caelyx®): I.V.: 50 mg/m^2 once every 4 weeks until disease progression or unacceptable toxicity

Unlabeled uses/doses:
Breast cancer, metastatic (unlabeled use in U.S.): I.V.: 50 mg/m^2 every 4 weeks (Keller, 2004)
Cutaneous T-cell lymphomas (unlabeled use): I.V.: 20 mg/m^2 days 1 and 15 every 4 weeks for 6 cycles (Dummer, 2012) **or** 20 mg/m^2 every 4 weeks (Wollina, 2003)
Hodgkin lymphoma, salvage treatment (unlabeled use): I.V.: GVD regimen: 10 mg/m^2 (post-transplant patients) or 15 mg/m^2 (transplant-naive patients) days 1 and 8 every 3 weeks (in combination with gemcitabine and vinorelbine) for 2-6 cycles (Bartlett, 2007)
Multiple myeloma (unlabeled dosing): I.V.: 40 mg/m^2 on day 1 every 4 weeks (in combination with vincristine and dexamethasone) for at least 4 cycles (Rifkin, 2006)
Soft tissue sarcoma, advanced (unlabeled use): I.V.: 50 mg/m^2 every 4 weeks for 6 cycles (Judson, 2001)
Uterine sarcoma, advanced or recurrent (unlabeled use): I.V.: 50 mg/m^2 every 4 weeks until disease progression or unacceptable toxicity (Sutton, 2005)

Dosage adjustment in renal impairment: No dosage adjustment provided in manufacturer's labeling (has not been studied).
Dosage adjustment in hepatic impairment:
U.S. labeling:
Ovarian cancer and AIDS-related Kaposi's sarcoma:
Bilirubin 1.2-3 mg/dL: Administer 50% of normal dose
Bilirubin >3 mg/dL: Administer 25% of normal dose
Multiple myeloma: Dosage adjustment information is not available.
Canadian labeling:
AIDS-related Kaposi's sarcoma (Caelyx®):
Bilirubin 1.2-3 mg/dL: Administer 50% of normal dose
Bilirubin >3 mg/dL: Administer 25% of normal dose
Breast cancer:
Caelyx®:
Bilirubin 1.2-3 mg/dL: Initial dose: Administer 75% of normal dose; if tolerated and no change in bilirubin/hepatic enzymes, may increase to full dose with cycle 2
Bilirubin >3 mg/dL: Initial dose: Administer 50% of normal dose; if tolerated and no change in bilirubin/hepatic enzymes, may increase dose to 75% of normal dose for cycle 2; if cycle 2 dose tolerated, may increase to full dose for subsequent cycles.
Myocet™:
Bilirubin 1.2-3 mg/dL: Administer 50% of normal dose
Bilirubin >3 mg/dL: Administer 25% of normal dose
Ovarian cancer (Caelyx®):
Bilirubin 1.2-3 mg/dL: Initial dose: Administer 75% of normal dose; if tolerated and no change in bilirubin/hepatic enzymes, may increase to full dose with cycle 2
Bilirubin >3 mg/dL: Initial dose: Administer 50% of normal dose; if tolerated and no change in bilirubin/hepatic enzymes, may increase dose to 75% of normal dose for cycle 2; if cycle 2 dose tolerated, may increase to full dose for subsequent cycles.

Dosing in obesity: *ASCO Guidelines for appropriate chemotherapy dosing in obese adults with cancer:* Utilize patient's actual body weight (full weight) for calculation of body surface area- or weight-based dosing, particularly when the intent of therapy is curative; manage regimen-related toxicities in the same manner as for nonobese patients; if a dose reduction is utilized due to toxicity, consider resumption of full weight-based dosing with subsequent cycles, especially if cause of toxicity (eg, hepatic or renal impairment) is resolved (Griggs, 2012).

Dosing adjustment for toxicity:
U.S. labeling: **Note:** Once a dosage reduction is implemented, the dose should not be increased at a later time.

Recommended Dose Modification Guidelines

Toxicity Grade	Dose Adjustment
HAND FOOT SYNDROME (HFS)	
1 (Mild erythema, swelling, or desquamation not interfering with daily activities)	Redose unless patient has experienced previous Grade 3 or 4 HFS toxicity. If so, delay up to 2 weeks and decrease dose by 25%; return to original dosing interval.
2 (Erythema, desquamation, or swelling interfering with, but not precluding, normal physical activities; small blisters or ulcerations <2 cm in diameter)	Delay dosing up to 2 weeks or until resolved to Grade 0-1. If after 2 weeks there is no resolution, discontinue liposomal doxorubicin. Otherwise, if no prior Grade 3-4 HFS, continue treatment at previous dose and dosage interval. If a prior Grade 3-4 HFS has occurred, continue prior dosage interval, but decrease dose by 25%.
3 (Blistering, ulceration, or swelling interfering with walking or normal daily activities; cannot wear regular clothing)	Delay dosing up to 2 weeks or until resolved to Grade 0-1. Decrease dose by 25% and return to original dosing interval; if after 2 weeks there is no resolution, discontinue liposomal doxorubicin.
4 (Diffuse or local process causing infectious complications, or a bedridden state or hospitalization)	Delay dosing up to 2 weeks or until resolved to Grade 0-1. Decrease dose by 25% and return to original dosing interval. If after 2 weeks there is no resolution, discontinue liposomal doxorubicin.
STOMATITIS	
1 (Painless ulcers, erythema, or mild soreness)	Redose unless patient has experienced previous Grade 3 or 4 toxicity. If so, delay up to 2 weeks and decrease by 25%. Return to original dosing interval.
2 (Painful erythema, edema, or ulcers, but can eat)	Delay dosing up to 2 weeks or until resolved to Grade 0-1. If after 2 weeks there is no resolution, discontinue liposomal doxorubicin. Otherwise, if not prior Grade 3-4 stomatitis, continue treatment at previous dose and dosage interval. If prior Grade 3-4 toxicity, continue treatment with previous dosage interval, but decrease dose by 25%.
3 (Painful erythema, edema, or ulcers, and cannot eat)	Delay dosing up to 2 weeks or until resolved to Grade 0-1. Decrease dose by 25% and return to original dosing interval. If after 2 weeks there is no resolution, discontinue liposomal doxorubicin.
4 (Requires parenteral or enteral support)	Delay dosing up to 2 weeks or until resolved to Grade 0-1. Decrease dose by 25% and return to original dosing interval. If after 2 weeks there is no resolution, discontinue liposomal doxorubicin.

See table: "Hematologic Toxicity"

Hematologic Toxicity (see below for multiple myeloma)

Grade	ANC	Platelets	Modification
1	1500-1900	75,000-150,000	Resume treatment with no dose reduction.
2	1000-<1500	50,000-<75,000	Wait until ANC ≥1500 and platelets ≥75,000; redose with no dose reduction.
3	500-999	25,000-<50,000	Wait until ANC ≥1500 and platelets ≥75,000; redose with no dose reduction.
4	<500	<25,000	Wait until ANC ≥1500 and platelets ≥75,000; redose at 25% dose reduction or continue full dose with cytokine support.

Dosing Adjustment for Toxicity in Treatment with Bortezomib (for Multiple Myeloma) (see Bortezomib monograph for bortezomib dosage reduction with toxicity guidelines):

Fever ≥38°C and ANC <1000/mm³: If prior to doxorubicin liposomal treatment (day 4), do not administer; if after doxorubicin liposomal administered, reduce dose by 25% in next cycle.

ANC <500/mm³, platelets <25,000/mm³, hemoglobin <8 g/dL: If prior to doxorubicin liposomal treatment (day 4); do not administer; if after doxorubicin liposomal administered, reduce dose by 25% in next cycle if bortezomib dose reduction occurred for hematologic toxicity.

Grade 3 or 4 nonhematologic toxicity: Delay dose until resolved to grade <2; reduce dose by 25% for all subsequent doses.

Neuropathic pain or peripheral neuropathy: No dose reductions needed for doxorubicin liposomal, refer to Bortezomib monograph for bortezomib dosing adjustment.

Canadian labeling:

Caelyx®: Nonhematologic toxicity: Breast cancer, ovarian cancer:

Caelyx®: Recommended Dose Modification Guidelines

Toxicity Grade	Week After Prior Caelyx® Dose (Breast Cancer or Ovarian Cancer)	
	Weeks 4 and 5	Week 6
HAND FOOT SYNDROME (HFS)		
1 (Mild erythema, swelling, or desquamation not interfering with daily activities)	Redose unless patient has experienced previous Grade 3 or 4 HFS toxicity. If so, wait an additional week	Decrease dose by 25%; return to 4-week interval
2 (Erythema, desquamation, or swelling interfering with, but not precluding, normal physical activities; small blisters or ulcerations <2 cm in diameter)	Wait an additional week	Decrease dose by 25%; return to 4-week interval
3 (Blistering, ulceration, or swelling interfering with walking or normal daily activities; cannot wear regular clothing)	Wait an additional week	Discontinue therapy
4 (Diffuse or local process causing infectious complications, or a bedridden state or hospitalization)	Wait an additional week	Discontinue therapy
STOMATITIS		
1 (Painless ulcers, erythema, or mild soreness)	Redose unless patient has experienced previous Grade 3 or 4 stomatitis. If so, wait an additional week.	Decrease dose by 25%; return to 4-week interval or if warranted, discontinue therapy
2 (Painful erythema, edema, or ulcers, but can eat)	Wait an additional week	Decrease dose by 25%; return to 4-week interval or if warranted, discontinue therapy
3 (Painful erythema, edema, or ulcers, and cannot eat)	Wait an additional week	Discontinue therapy
4 (Requires parenteral or enteral support)	Wait an additional week	Discontinue therapy

Caelyx®: Hematologic toxicity: Breast cancer, ovarian cancer: Refer to U.S. dosage adjustment for hematologic toxicity section.

Caelyx®: Nonhematologic toxicity: AIDS-related Kaposi's sarcoma:

Caelyx®: Recommended Dose Modification Guidelines: Hand-Foot Syndrome (HFS) (AIDS-related Kaposi's Sarcoma)

Toxicity Grade	Weeks Since Last Caelyx® Dose (AIDS-related Kaposi's Sarcoma)	
	3 Weeks	4 Weeks
HAND-FOOT SYNDROME (HFS)		
1 (Mild erythema, swelling, or desquamation not interfering with daily activities)	Redose unless patient has experienced previous Grade 3 or 4 skin toxicity. If so, wait an additional week	Decrease dose by 25%; return to 3-week interval
2 (Erythema, desquamation, or swelling interfering with, but not precluding, normal physical activities; small blisters or ulcerations <2 cm in diameter)	Wait an additional week	Decrease dose by 50%; return to 3-week interval
3 (Blistering, ulceration, or swelling interfering with walking or normal daily activities; cannot wear regular clothing)	Wait an additional week	Discontinue therapy
4 (Diffuse or local process causing infectious complications, or a bedridden state or hospitalization)	Wait an additional week	Discontinue therapy

Caelyx®: Recommended Dose Modification Guidelines: Stomatitis (AIDS-related Kaposi's Sarcoma)

STOMATITIS Toxicity grade:	Caelyx® Dosage Adjustment (AIDS-related Kaposi's Sarcoma)
1 (Painless ulcers, erythema, or mild soreness)	No dosage adjustment
2 (Painful erythema, edema, or ulcers, but can eat)	Wait 1 week and if symptoms improve, redose at 100% dose
3 (Painful erythema, edema, or ulcers, and cannot eat)	Wait 1 week and if symptoms improve, redose with a 25% dose reduction
4 (Requires parenteral or enteral support)	Wait 1 week and if symptoms improve, redose with a 50% dose reduction

Caelyx®: Hematologic toxicity: AIDS-related Kaposi's sarcoma:

Caelyx®: Hematologic Toxicity (AIDS-related Kaposi's Sarcoma)

Grade	ANC	Platelets	Modification
1	1500-1900	75,000-150,000	None
2	1000-<1500	50,000-<75,000	None
3	500-999	25,000-<50,000	Wait until ANC ≥1000 and/or platelets ≥50,000; redose with a 25% dose reduction.
4	<500	<25,000	Wait until ANC ≥1000 and/or platelets ≥50,000; redose with a 50% dose reduction.

Myocet™: Hematologic or gastrointestinal toxicity: Dosage reduction: If initial dose was 75 mg/m^2, reduce dose to 60 mg/m^2; if initial dose was 60 mg/m^2, reduce dose to 50 mg/m^2. If toxicity persists with subsequent cycles, consider reducing dose further (from 60 mg/m^2 to 50 mg/m^2 or from 50 mg/m^2 to 40 mg/m^2).

Neutropenia: If grade 4 neutropenia (ANC <500/mm^3) without fever lasting ≥7 days or grade 4 neutropenia of any duration with concurrent fever (≥38.5°C) occurs, consider reducing dose with subsequent cycles. **Note:** Prior to dose reductions, prophylactic cytokine therapy may be considered.

Thrombocytopenia or anemia: If grade 4 thrombocytopenia or anemia occurs, hold therapy until recovery to ≤ grade 2. Reduce dose with subsequent cycles or consider discontinuing treatment.

Gastrointestinal toxicity or mucositis: Grade 3 mucositis persisting ≥3 days, or grade 4 mucositis of any duration, or grade 3 or 4 gastrointestinal toxicity not responsive to interventions and/or prophylaxis: Consider dose reduction with subsequent cycles.

Administration Do not administer as a bolus injection or I.M. or SubQ. Avoid extravasation (irritant); monitor infusion site; extravasation may occur without stinging or burning. Monitor for infusion reaction.

Doxil®, Caelyx®: Administer IVPB over 60 minutes; manufacturer recommends administering at initial rate of 1 mg/minute to minimize risk of infusion reactions until the absence of a reaction has been established, then increase the infusion rate for completion over 1 hour. Do **NOT** administer undiluted. Do **NOT** infuse with in-line filters. Incompatible with heparin flushes; flush with 5-10 mL of D_5W solution before and after drug administration (do not rapidly flush through the I.V. line). Monitor for local erythematous streaking along vein and/or facial flushing (may indicate rapid infusion rate).

Myocet™: Infuse over 1 hour.

Hazardous agent; use appropriate precautions for handling and disposal (NIOSH, 2012).

Monitoring Parameters CBC with differential and platelet count, liver function tests (ALT/AST, bilirubin, alkaline phosphatase); monitor for infusion reactions, hand-foot syndrome, stomatitis, and oral ulceration/discomfort suggestive of secondary oral malignancy

Cardiac function (left ventricular ejection fraction [LVEF]; baseline and periodic); echocardiography, or MUGA scan may be used. Endomyocardial biopsy is the most definitive test for anthracycline myocardial injury.

Dosage Forms Excipient information presented when available (limited, particularly for generics); consult specific product labeling.

Injectable, Intravenous:
- Generic: 2 mg/mL (10 mL, 25 mL)

Injectable, Intravenous, as hydrochloride:
- Doxil: 2 mg/mL (10 mL, 25 mL)
- Lipodox: 2 mg/mL (10 mL)
- Lipodox 50: 2 mg/mL (25 mL)

Dosage Forms: Canada

Excipient information presented when available (limited, particularly for generics); consult specific product labeling.

Injection, solution, as hydrochloride, pegylated:
- Caelyx®: 2 mg/mL (10 mL, 25 mL)

Injection, encapsulated liposomes:
- Myocet™: 3-vial kit (doxorubicin HCl for injection 50 mg/vial, liposomes for injection, and buffer for injection)

◆ **Doxy 100** *see* Doxycycline *on page* 668

◆ **Doxycin (Can)** *see* Doxycycline *on page* 668

Doxycycline (doks i SYE kleen)

Brand Names: U.S. Adoxa; Adoxa Pak 1/100; Adoxa Pak 1/150; Adoxa Pak 2/100; Alodox Convenience; Avidoxy; Doryx; Doxy 100; Monodox; Morgidox; NicAzelDoxy 30; NicAzelDoxy 60; Ocudox; Oracea; Oraxyl [DSC]; Vibramycin

Brand Names: Canada Apo-Doxy Tabs®; Apo-Doxy®; Apprilon™; Dom-Doxycycline; Doxycin; Doxytab; Novo-Doxylin; Periostat®; PHL-Doxycycline; PMS-Doxycycline; Vibra-Tabs®; Vibramycin®

Index Terms Doxycycline Calcium; Doxycycline Hyclate; Doxycycline Monohydrate

Pharmacologic Category Antibiotic, Tetracycline Derivative

Use Principally in the treatment of infections caused by susceptible *Rickettsia*, *Chlamydia*, *Chlamydophila*, and *Mycoplasma*; malaria prophylaxis (areas with chloroquine- or pyrimethamine-sulfadoxine resistant strains) for short-term travel (<4 months); treatment for syphilis, uncomplicated *Neisseria gonorrhoeae* (alternative agent), *Listeria*, *Actinomyces israelii*, and *Clostridium* infections in penicillin-allergic patients; used for community-acquired pneumonia and other common infections due to susceptible organisms; anthrax due to *Bacillus anthracis,* including inhalational anthrax (postexposure); treatment of infections caused by uncommon susceptible gram-negative and gram-positive organisms including *Borrelia recurrentis*, *Ureaplasma urealyticum*, *Haemophilus ducreyi*, *Yersinia pestis*, *Francisella tularensis*, *Vibrio cholerae*, *Campylobacter fetus*, *Brucella* spp, *Bartonella bacilliformis*, and *Klebsiella granulomatis,* Q fever, Lyme disease; intestinal amebiasis; severe acne

Oracea® (U.S. labeling), Apprilon™ (Canadian labeling): Treatment of inflammatory lesions associated with rosacea

Periostat® (Canadian labeling; not available in U.S.): Adjunctive periodontitis treatment to scaling and root planing to promote attachment level gain and reduce pocket depth

Unlabeled Use Sclerosing agent for pleural effusion (injection); vancomycin-resistant enterococci (VRE); alternate treatment for MRSA infections; treatment of periodontitis (refractory); localized juvenile periodontitis (LJP); treatment of acute bacterial rhinosinusitis (ABRS) (adults); oral phase treatment of prosthetic joint infection; chronic oral antimicrobial suppression of prosthetic joint infection; anorectal gonococcal infections

Pregnancy Risk Factor D

Pregnancy Considerations Tetracyclines cross the placenta and accumulate in developing teeth and long tubular bones. Therapeutic doses of doxycycline during pregnancy are unlikely to produce substantial teratogenic risk, but data are insufficient to say that there is no risk. In general, reports of exposure have been limited to short durations of therapy in the first trimester. Tetracyclines may discolor fetal teeth following maternal use during pregnancy; the specific teeth involved and the portion of the tooth affected depends on the timing and duration of exposure relative to tooth calcification. As a class, tetracyclines are generally considered second-line antibiotics in pregnant women and their use should be avoided. Tetracycline medications should be used during pregnancy only when other medications are contraindicated or ineffective (Mylonas, 2011).

Breast-Feeding Considerations Doxycycline is excreted in breast milk (Chung, 2002). According to the manufacturer, the decision to continue or discontinue breast-feeding during therapy should take into account the risk of exposure to the infant and the benefits of treatment to the mother. Although nursing is not specifically contraindicated, the effects of long-term exposure via breast milk are not known. Oral absorption of doxycycline is not markedly influenced by simultaneous ingestion of milk; therefore, oral absorption of doxycycline by the breast-feeding infant would not be expected to be diminished by the calcium in the maternal milk. Nondose-related effects could include modification of bowel flora.

Contraindications

U.S. labeling: Hypersensitivity to doxycycline, tetracycline or any component of the formulation

Canadian labeling: Hypersensitivity to doxycycline, tetracycline or any component of the formulation; myasthenia gravis

Periostat®, Apprilon™: Additional contraindications: Use in infants and children <8 years of age or during second or third trimester of pregnancy; breast-feeding

Warnings/Precautions Photosensitivity reaction may occur with this drug; avoid prolonged exposure to sunlight or tanning equipment. Antianabolic effects of tetracyclines can increase BUN (dose-related). Hypersensitivity syndromes have been reported, including drug rash with eosinophilia and systemic symptoms (DRESS), urticaria, angioneurotic edema, anaphylaxis, anaphylactoid purpura, serum sickness, pericarditis, and systemic lupus erythematosus exacerbation. Hepatotoxicity rarely occurs; if symptomatic, conduct LFT and discontinue drug. Intracranial hypertension (headache, blurred vision, diplopia, vision loss, and/or papilledema) has been associated with use. Women of childbearing age who are overweight or have a history of intracranial hypertension are at greater risk. Concomitant use of isotretinoin (known to cause pseudotumor cerebri) and doxycycline should be avoided. Intracranial hypertension typically resolves after discontinuation of treatment; however, permanent visual loss is possible. If visual symptoms develop during treatment, prompt ophthalmologic evaluation is warranted. Intracranial pressure can remain elevated for weeks after drug discontinuation; monitor patients until they stabilize. Prolonged use may result in fungal or bacterial superinfection, including *C. difficile*-associated diarrhea (CDAD) and pseudomembranous colitis; CDAD has been observed >2 months postantibiotic treatment. May cause tissue hyperpigmentation, tooth enamel hypoplasia, or permanent tooth discoloration; use of tetracyclines should be avoided during tooth development (last half or pregnancy, infancy, and children <8 years of age) unless other drugs are not likely to be effective or are contraindicated. However, recommended in treatment of anthrax exposure, tickborne rickettsial diseases, and Q fever. Do not use during pregnancy. In addition to affecting tooth development, tetracycline use has been associated with retardation of skeletal development and reduced bone growth. When used for malaria prophylaxis, does not completely suppress asexual blood stages of *Plasmodium* strains. Doxycycline does not suppress *Plasmodium falciparum*'s sexual blood stage gametocytes. Patients completing a regimen may still transmit the infection to mosquitoes outside endemic areas.

Oracea® (U.S. labeling) or Apprilon™ (Canadian labeling): Additional specific warnings: Should not be used for the treatment or prophylaxis of bacterial infections, since the lower dose of drug per capsule may be subefficacious and promote resistance. Syrup contains sodium metabisulfite. Effectiveness of products intended for use in periodontitis has not been established in patients with coexistent oral candidiasis; use with caution in patients with a history or predisposition to oral candidiasis.

Adverse Reactions Frequency not always defined.

Central nervous system: Headache (2%), bulging fontanel (infants), intracranial hypertension (adults), pericarditis

Dermatologic: Discoloration of thyroid gland (brown/black, no dysfunction reported), erythema multiforme, erythematous rash, exfoliative dermatitis, maculopapular rash, skin hyperpigmentation, skin photosensitivity, Stevens-Johnson syndrome, toxic epidermal necrolysis, urticaria

Endocrine & metabolic: Hypoglycemia

Gastrointestinal: Nausea (13%), vomiting (8%), diarrhea (3%), upper abdominal pain (2%), anorexia, *Clostridium difficile* associated diarrhea, dental discoloration (children), dysphagia, enterocolitis, esophageal ulcer, esophagitis, glossitis

Genitourinary: Vaginitis (bacterial, 3%), vulvovaginal disease (mycotic infection, 2%), inflammatory anogenital lesion

Hematologic & oncologic: Anaphylactoid purpura, eosinophilia, hemolytic anemia, neutropenia, thrombocytopenia

Hepatic: Hepatotoxicity (rare)

Hypersensitivity: Anaphylaxis, angioedema, serum sickness

Neuromuscular & skeletal: Exacerbation of systemic lupus erythematosus

Renal: Increased blood urea nitrogen (dose related)

Note: Additional adverse reactions not listed above that have been reported with Oracea or Periostat (Canadian availability; not available in the U.S.):

Periostat: Arthralgia (6%), dyspepsia (6%), dysmenorrhea (4%), pain (4%), bronchitis (3%)

Oracea: Nasopharyngitis (5%), hypertension (3%), sinusitis (3%), anxiety (2%), fungal infection (2%), increased blood pressure (2%), increased lactate dehydrogenase (2%), increased serum AST (2%), influenza (2%), pain (2%), abdominal pain (1% to 2%), back pain (1%), hyperglycemia (1%), sinus headache (1%), xerostomia (1%)

Drug Interactions

Metabolism/Transport Effects Inhibits CYP3A4 (weak)

Avoid Concomitant Use

Avoid concomitant use of Doxycycline with any of the following: BCG; Pimozide; Retinoic Acid Derivatives; Strontium Ranelate

Increased Effect/Toxicity

Doxycycline may increase the levels/effects of: ARIPiprazole; Dofetilide; Lomitapide; Mipomersen; Neuromuscular-Blocking Agents; Pimozide; Porfimer; Retinoic Acid Derivatives; Vitamin K Antagonists

Decreased Effect

Doxycycline may decrease the levels/effects of: BCG; Penicillins; Sodium Picosulfate; Typhoid Vaccine

The levels/effects of Doxycycline may be decreased by: Antacids; Barbiturates; Bile Acid Sequestrants; Bismuth; Bismuth Subsalicylate; Calcium Salts; CarBAMazepine; Fosphenytoin; Iron Salts; Lanthanum; Magnesium Salts; Multivitamins/Minerals (with ADEK, Folate, Iron); Multivitamins/Minerals (with AE, No Iron); Phenytoin; Quinapril; Rifampin; Strontium Ranelate; Sucralfate; Sucroferric Oxyhydroxide

Ethanol/Nutrition/Herb Interactions

Ethanol: Chronic ethanol ingestion may reduce the serum concentration of doxycycline.

Food: Doxycycline serum levels may be slightly decreased if taken with food or milk. Doryx® tablets can be administered without regard to meals. Administration with iron or calcium may decrease doxycycline absorption. May decrease absorption of calcium, iron, magnesium, zinc, and amino acids.

Herb/Nutraceutical: St John's wort may decrease doxycycline levels. Avoid dong quai, St John's wort (may also cause photosensitization).

Preparation for Administration I.V. infusion: Following reconstitution with sterile water for injection, dilute to a final concentration of 0.1-1 mg/mL using a compatible solution.

Storage/Stability

Syrup, oral suspension: All products are to be stored below 30°C (86°F) and dispensed in tight, light-resistant containers.

Capsule, tablet: Store at 20°C to 25°C (68°F to 77°F); excursions are permitted between 15°C and 30°C (59°F and 86°F). Dispense in a tight, light-resistant container.

I.V. infusion: Protect from light. Stability varies based on solution.

Mechanism of Action Inhibits protein synthesis by binding with the 30S and possibly the 50S ribosomal subunit(s) of susceptible bacteria; may also cause alterations in the cytoplasmic membrane

Periostat® capsules (Canadian availability; not available in the U.S.): Proposed mechanism: Has been shown to inhibit collagenase activity *in vitro*. Also has been noted to reduce elevated collagenase activity in the gingival crevicular fluid of patients with periodontal disease. Systemic levels do not reach inhibitory concentrations against bacteria.

Pharmacodynamics/Kinetics

Absorption: Oral: Almost complete

Distribution: Widely into body tissues and fluids including synovial, pleural, prostatic, seminal fluids, and bronchial secretions; saliva, aqueous humor, and CSF penetration is poor; Periostat® (Canadian availability; not available in the U.S.): ~53-134 L

Protein binding: 90%

Metabolism: Not hepatic; partially inactivated in GI tract by chelate formation

Bioavailability: Reduced at high pH; may be clinically significant in patients with gastrectomy, gastric bypass surgery or who are otherwise deemed achlorhydric

Half-life elimination: Single dose: 12-15 hours (usually increases to 22-24 hours with multiple doses); End-stage renal disease: 18-25 hours

Oracea® (U.S. labeling), Apprilon™ (Canadian labeling): Single dose: 21 hours

Periostat®: Single dose: 18 hours

Time to peak, serum: 1.5-4 hours

Excretion: Feces (30%); urine (23%)

Dosage

Usual dosage range:

Children >8 years (≤45 kg): Oral, I.V.: 2-5 mg/kg/day in 1-2 divided doses, not to exceed 200 mg/day

Children >8 years (>45 kg) and Adults: Oral, I.V.: 100-200 mg/day in 1-2 divided doses

Indication-specific dosing:

Children:

Anthrax: Doxycycline should be used in children if antibiotic susceptibility testing, exhaustion of drug supplies, or allergic reaction preclude use of penicillin or ciprofloxacin. For treatment, the consensus recommendation does not include a loading dose for doxycycline.

Inhalational (postexposure prophylaxis) (ACIP, 2010): Oral, I.V. (use oral route when possible):

≤8 years: 2.2 mg/kg every 12 hours for 60 days

>8 years and ≤45 kg: 2.2 mg/kg every 12 hours for 60 days

>8 years and >45 kg: 100 mg every 12 hours for 60 days

Cutaneous (treatment): Oral: See dosing for "Inhalational (postexposure prophylaxis)"

Note: In the presence of systemic involvement, extensive edema, and/or lesions on head/neck, doxycycline should initially be administered I.V.

Inhalational/gastrointestinal/oropharyngeal (treatment): I.V.: Refer to dosing for inhalational anthrax (postexposure prophylaxis); switch to oral therapy when clinically appropriate

Note: Initial treatment should include two or more agents predicted to be effective (CDC, 2001). Agents suggested for use in conjunction with doxycycline or ciprofloxacin include rifampin, vancomycin, imipenem, penicillin, ampicillin, chloramphenicol, clindamycin, and clarithromycin. May switch to oral antimicrobial therapy when clinically appropriate. Continue combined therapy for 60 days

Community-acquired pneumonia (CAP) (IDSA/PIDS, 2011): Oral: Children >7 years: **Note:** A beta-lactam antibiotic should be added if typical bacterial pneumonia cannot be ruled out.

Presumed atypical, mild atypical (*M. pneumoniae, C. pneumoniae, C. trachomatis*) infection or step-down therapy (alternative to azithromycin): 2-4 mg/kg/day in 2 divided doses (maximum: 200 mg/day)

Cellulitis (purulent) due to community-acquired MRSA (unlabeled use): Oral: Children >8 years and ≤45 kg: 2 mg/kg/dose every 12 hours for 5-10 days (Liu, 2011)

Localized juvenile periodontitis (LJP) (unlabeled use): Oral: 50-100 mg/day

Q fever: Oral:

Acute:

Children <8 years with high-risk criteria (eg, hospitalized or have severe illness, with pre-existing heart valvulopathy, immunocompromised, or with delayed Q fever diagnosis who have experienced illness for >14 days without resolution of symptoms): 2.2 mg/kg/dose (maximum: 100 mg per dose) twice daily for 14 days (CDC, 2013).

Children <8 years with mild or uncomplicated illness: 2.2 mg/kg/dose (maximum: 100 mg per dose) twice daily for 5 days. If patient remains febrile past 5 days of treatment, switch to sulfamethoxazole and trimethoprim (CDC, 2013). **Note:** Some clinicians may recommend initial treatment with sulfamethoxazole and trimethoprim for children <8 years with mild or uncomplicated illness (Hartzell, 2008; CDC, 2013).

Children ≥8 years and Adolescents: 2.2 mg/kg/dose (maximum: 100 mg per dose) twice daily for 14 days (CDC, 2013).

Chronic: ID consult recommended for treatment of chronic Q fever (CDC, 2013)

Tickborne rickettsial disease: Oral, I.V.: Children ≤8 years: 2.2 mg/kg (maximum dose: 100 mg) every 12 hours for 5-7 days; severe or complicated disease may require longer treatment; human granulocytotropic anaplasmosis (HGA) should be treated for 10-14 days. **Note:** The American Academy of Pediatrics Committee on Infectious Diseases identifies doxycycline as the drug of choice in children of any age.

Tularemia: I.V. (may transition to oral if clinically indicated) (Dennis, 2001):

Children <45 kg: 2.2 mg/kg every 12 hours for 14-21 days

Children ≥45 kg: 100 mg every 12 hours for 14-21 days

Children ≥8 years:

Lyme disease: Oral (Halperin, 2007; Wormser, 2006):

Prevention: 4 mg/kg (maximum: 200 mg) administered as a single dose; **Note:** Initiate within 72 hours of tick removal

Treatment (early Lyme disease without neurologic manifestations): 1-2 mg/kg twice daily for 10-21 days (maximum: 100 mg/dose)

Treatment (meningitis and other early neurologic manifestations): 4-8 mg/kg/day in 2 divided doses for 10-28 days (maximum: 200 mg/dose)

Malaria chemoprophylaxis: Oral:

Manufacturer's recommendation: 2 mg/kg/day (maximum: 100 mg daily). Start 1-2 days prior to travel to endemic area; continue daily during travel and for 4 weeks after leaving endemic area (CDC, 2012)

Alternative recommendation: 2.2 mg/kg/day (maximum: 100 mg daily). Start 1-2 days prior to travel to endemic area; continue daily during travel and for 4 weeks after leaving endemic area (CDC, 2012)

Malaria, severe, treatment (unlabeled use): Oral, I.V.:

<45 kg: 2.2 mg/kg (maximum dose: 100 mg) every 12 hours for 7 days with quinidine gluconate. **Note:** Quinidine gluconate duration is region specific; consult CDC for current recommendations (CDC, 2011).

≥45 kg: 100 mg every 12 hours for 7 days with quinidine gluconate. **Note:** Quinidine gluconate duration is region specific; consult CDC for current recommendations (CDC, 2011).

Malaria, uncomplicated, treatment (unlabeled use): Oral: 2.2 mg/kg (maximum dose: 100 mg) every 12 hours for 7 days with quinine sulfate. **Note:** Quinine sulfate duration is region specific; consult CDC for current recommendations (CDC, 2011).

Children >8 years (and >45 kg) and Adults:

Cellulitis (purulent) due to community-acquired MRSA (unlabeled use): Oral: 100 mg twice daily for 5-10 days (Liu, 2011)

Chlamydial infections, uncomplicated: Oral: *Manufacturer's recommendation:* 100 mg twice daily for 7 days; alternatively, for endocervical or urethral infections, may give 200 mg once daily for 7 days

Tickborne rickettsial disease: Oral, I.V.: 100 mg twice daily for 5-7 days; severe or complicated disease may require longer treatment; human granulocytotropic anaplasmosis (HGA) should be treated for 10-14 days. **Note:** The American Academy of Pediatrics Committee on Infectious Diseases identifies doxycycline as the drug of choice in children of any age.

Adults:

Acute bacterial rhinosinusitis (unlabeled use): Oral: 200 mg/day in 1-2 divided doses for 5-7 days (Chow, 2012)

Anthrax:

Inhalational (postexposure prophylaxis): Oral, I.V. (use oral route when possible): 100 mg every 12 hours for 60 days (ACIP, 2010)

Cutaneous (treatment): Oral: 100 mg every 12 hours for 60 days. **Note:** In the presence of systemic involvement, extensive edema, lesions on head/neck, refer to I.V. dosing for treatment of inhalational/gastrointestinal/oropharyngeal anthrax

Inhalational/gastrointestinal/oropharyngeal (treatment): I.V.: Initial: 100 mg every 12 hours; switch to oral therapy when clinically appropriate; some recommend initial loading dose of 200 mg, followed by 100 mg every 8-12 hours (Franz, 1997). **Note:** Initial treatment should include two or more agents predicted to be effective (CDC, 2001). Agents suggested for use in conjunction with doxycycline or ciprofloxacin include rifampin, vancomycin, imipenem, penicillin, ampicillin, chloramphenicol, clindamycin, and clarithromycin. May switch to oral antimicrobial therapy when clinically appropriate. Continue combined therapy for 60 days

Brucellosis: Oral: 100 mg twice daily for 6 weeks with rifampin or streptomycin

Community-acquired pneumonia, bronchitis: Oral, I.V.: 100 mg twice daily (Ailani, 1999; Mandell, 2007)

Epididymitis: Oral: 100 mg twice daily for 10 days (in combination with ceftriaxone) (CDC, 2010)

Gonococcal infection, uncomplicated: Oral: **Note:** Azithromycin is preferred over doxycycline as the second antimicrobial in combination with ceftriaxone in uncomplicated infections due to a high prevalence of tetracycline resistance in isolates (CDC, 2012).

Cervix, rectum (unlabeled use), urethra: 100 mg twice daily for 7 days in combination with ceftriaxone (preferred) or cefixime (only if ceftriaxone is not available and test-of-cure follow up in 7 days) (CDC, 2010; CDC, 2012).

Pharynx: 100 mg twice daily for 7 days in combination with ceftriaxone (CDC, 2012).

Alternatively, the manufacturer recommends a single-visit dose in nonanorectal infections in men: 300 mg initially, repeat dose in 1 hour (total dose: 600 mg)

Granuloma inguinale (donovanosis): Oral: 100 mg twice daily for at least 3 weeks (and until lesions have healed) (CDC, 2010)

Lyme disease: Oral (Halperin, 2007; Wormser, 2006):

Prevention: Initiate within 72 hours of tick removal: 200 mg administered as a single dose

Treatment (early Lyme disease without neurologic manifestations): 100 mg twice daily for 10-21 days

Treatment (meningitis or other early neurologic manifestations): 100-200 mg twice daily for 14 days (range: 10-28 days)

Lymphogranuloma venereum: Oral: 100 mg twice daily for 21 days (CDC, 2010)

Malaria chemoprophylaxis: Oral: 100 mg daily. Start 1-2 days prior to travel to endemic area; continue daily during travel and for 4 weeks after leaving endemic area

Malaria, severe, treatment (unlabeled use): Oral, I.V.: 100 mg every 12 hours for 7 days with quinidine gluconate. **Note:** Quinidine gluconate duration is region specific; consult CDC for current recommendations (CDC, 2011).

Malaria, uncomplicated, treatment (unlabeled use): Oral: 100 mg twice daily for 7 days with quinine sulfate. **Note:** Quinine sulfate duration is region specific; consult CDC for current recommendations (CDC, 2011).

Nongonococcal urethritis: Oral: 100 mg twice daily for 7 days (CDC, 2010)

Pelvic inflammatory disease:

Treatment, inpatient: Oral, I.V.: 100 mg twice daily (in combination with cefoxitin or cefotetan); may transition to oral doxycycline (add clindamycin or metronidazole if tubo-ovarian abscess present) to complete 14 days of treatment (CDC, 2010)

Treatment, outpatient: Oral: 100 mg twice daily for 14 days (with or without metronidazole); preceded by a single I.M. dose of cefoxitin (plus oral probenecid) or ceftriaxone (CDC, 2010)

Periodontitis: Oral (Periostat® [Canadian availability; not available in the U.S.]): 20 mg twice daily as an adjunct following scaling and root planing; may treat for up to 9 months

Periodontitis, refractory (unlabeled use): Oral: 100-200 mg daily (Jolkovsky, 2006)

Proctitis: Oral: 100 mg twice daily for 7 days (in combination with ceftriaxone) (CDC, 2010)

Prosthetic joint infection (unlabeled use): Oral:

Chronic oral antimicrobial suppression:

Propionibacterium spp (alternative to penicillin or amoxicillin): 100 mg twice daily (Osmon, 2013)

Staphylococci (oxacillin-resistant): 100 mg twice daily (Osmon, 2013)

Staphylococci (oxacillin-sensitive or –resistant) oral phase treatment (after completion of pathogen-specific I.V) following 1-stage exchange:

Total ankle, elbow, hip, or shoulder arthroplasty: 100 mg twice daily for 3 months; **Note:** Must be used in combination with rifampin (Osmon, 2013).

Total knee arthroplasty: 100 mg twice daily for 6 months; **Note:** Must be used in combination with rifampin (Osmon, 2013)

Q fever: Oral:

Acute: 100 mg every 12 hours for 14 days (CDC, 2013); **Note:** In patients who have valvular heart disease, consider increasing the duration of therapy to 1 year and adding hydroxychloroquine to the regimen to prevent endocarditis; consultation with an infectious disease expert is recommended (CDC, 2002; Fenollar, 2001).

Chronic (CDC, 2013):

Endocarditis or vascular infection: 100 mg every 12 hours in combination with hydroxychloroquine for ≥18 months

Noncardiac organ disease: 100 mg every 12 hours in combination with hydroxychloroquine (duration based on serologic response; ID consult recommended)

Postpartum with serologic evidence present >12 months after delivery: 100 mg every 12 hours in combination with hydroxychloroquine for 12 months

Rosacea Oral (Oracea® [U.S. labeling], Apprilon™ [Canadian labeling]): 40 mg once daily in the morning

Sclerosing agent for pleural effusion (unlabeled use): Intrapleural: 500 mg as a single dose in 100 mL NS (Porcel, 2006); may require a repeat dose (Kvale, 2007)

Syphilis:

Primary/secondary syphilis: Oral: 100 mg twice daily for 14 days (CDC, 2010)

Latent syphilis: Oral: 100 mg twice daily for 28 days (CDC, 2010)

Tularemia: I.V. (may transition to oral if clinically appropriate): Initial: 100 mg every 12 hours for 14-21 days (Dennis, 2001)

Vibrio cholerae: Oral: 300 mg as a single dose (WHO, 2004)

***Yersinia pestis* (plague):** Oral, I.V.: 200 mg initially then 100 mg twice daily **or** 200 mg once daily for 10 days (Daya, 2005; Inglesby, 2000)

Dosage adjustment in renal impairment: No dosage adjustment necessary in renal impairment.

Poorly dialyzed; no supplemental dose or dosage adjustment necessary, including patients on intermittent hemodialysis, peritoneal dialysis, or continuous renal replacement therapy (eg, CVVHD).

Dosage adjustment in hepatic impairment: No dosage adjustment provided in manufacturer's labeling.

Dietary Considerations

Tetracyclines (in general): Take with food if gastric irritation occurs. While administration with food may decrease GI absorption of doxycycline by up to 20%, administration on an empty stomach is not recommended due to GI intolerance. Of currently available tetracyclines, doxycycline has the least affinity for calcium.

Doryx® tablets: May be taken without regard to meals; nausea occurs more frequently when taken on an empty stomach.

Oracea® (U.S. labeling), Apprilon™ (Canadian labeling): Take on an empty stomach 1 hour before or 2 hours after meals.

Periostat® (Canadian availability; not available in the U.S.): Take at least 1 hour before morning and evening meals.

Some products may contain sodium.

Administration Oral administration is preferable unless patient has significant nausea and vomiting; I.V. and oral routes are bioequivalent.

Oral: May give with meals to decrease GI upset. Capsule and tablet: Administer with at least 8 ounces of water and have patient sit up for at least 30 minutes after taking to reduce the risk of esophageal irritation and ulceration.

Oracea® (U.S. labeling), Apprilon™ (Canadian labeling): Administer on an empty stomach 1 hour before or 2 hours after meals.

Doryx®: Administer without regard to meals; nausea occurs more frequently when taken on an empty stomach. May be administered by carefully breaking up the tablet and sprinkling tablet contents on a spoonful of cold applesauce. The delayed release pellets must not be crushed or damaged when breaking up tablet. Should be administered immediately after preparation and without chewing.

Periostat® (Canadian availability; not available in the U.S.): Administer 1 hour before breakfast and evening meal.

I.V.: Infuse I.V. doxycycline over 1-4 hours; avoid extravasation

Intrapleural (unlabeled route): Add to 100 mL NS and instill into chest tube (Porcel, 2006)

Monitoring Parameters Perform culture and sensitivity testing prior to initiating therapy. CBC, renal and liver function tests periodically with prolonged therapy. When used as part of alternative treatment for gonococcal infection, test of cure 7 days after dose (CDC, 2012).

Patients with no risk factors for chronic Q fever should undergo clinical and serological evaluation 6 months after diagnosis of acute Q fever to identify possible progression to chronic disease. Postpartum women treated during pregnancy for acute Q fever, others who are at high risk for progression to chronic disease or when used as part of treatment for chronic Q fever infection unrelated to endocarditis or vascular infection (eg, osteoarticular infections or chronic hepatitis), assess serologic response at 3, 6, 12, 18, and 24 months after diagnosis of acute Q fever (or after delivery in pregnant women) (CDC, 2013).

Test Interactions Injectable tetracycline formulations (if they contain large amounts of ascorbic acid) may result in a false-negative urine glucose using glucose oxidase tests (eg, Clinistix®, Diastix, Tes-Tape®); false elevations of urinary catecholamines with fluorescence

Additional Information Oracea® (U.S. labeling) or Apprilon™ (Canadian labeling) capsules are not bioequivalent to other doxycycline products.

Dosage Forms Considerations

NizAzel Doxy kits contain doxycycline tablets 100 mg, plus NicAzel FORTE dietary supplement tablets

Dosage Forms Excipient information presented when available (limited, particularly for generics); consult specific product labeling. [DSC] = Discontinued product

Capsule, Oral, as hyclate [strength expressed as base]:
- Morgidox: 100 mg [contains brilliant blue fcf (fd&c blue #1)]
- Oraxyl: 20 mg [DSC]
- Vibramycin: 100 mg [contains brilliant blue fcf (fd&c blue #1)]
- Generic: 50 mg, 100 mg

Capsule, Oral, as monohydrate [strength expressed as base]:
- Adoxa: 150 mg [contains fd&c red #40, fd&c yellow #6 (sunset yellow)]
- Monodox: 75 mg, 100 mg
- Generic: 50 mg, 75 mg, 100 mg, 150 mg

Capsule Delayed Release, Oral, as monohydrate [strength expressed as base]:
- Oracea: 40 mg

Capsule Delayed Release Particles, Oral, as hyclate [strength expressed as base]:
- Generic: 100 mg

Kit, Combination, as hyclate [strength expressed as base]:
- Alodox Convenience: 20 mg
- Morgidox: 1 x 100 MG, 2 x 100 MG [contains brilliant blue fcf (fd&c blue #1), cetyl alcohol, edetate disodium]
- Ocudox: 50 mg [contains brilliant blue fcf (fd&c blue #1)]

Kit, Oral, as monohydrate [strength expressed as base]:
- NicAzelDoxy 30: 100 mg [contains brilliant blue fcf (fd&c blue #1), fd&c yellow #10 aluminum lake, fd&c yellow #6 (sunset yellow), fd&c yellow #6 aluminum lake, tartrazine (fd&c yellow #5)]
- NicAzelDoxy 60: 100 mg [contains brilliant blue fcf (fd&c blue #1), fd&c yellow #10 aluminum lake, fd&c yellow #6 (sunset yellow), fd&c yellow #6 aluminum lake, tartrazine (fd&c yellow #5)]

Solution Reconstituted, Intravenous, as hyclate [strength expressed as base]:
- Generic: 100 mg (1 ea)

Solution Reconstituted, Intravenous, as hyclate [strength expressed as base, preservative free]:
- Doxy 100: 100 mg (1 ea)
- Generic: 100 mg (1 ea)

Suspension Reconstituted, Oral, as monohydrate [strength expressed as base]:
- Vibramycin: 25 mg/5 mL (60 mL) [contains brilliant blue fcf (fd&c blue #1), methylparaben, propylparaben; raspberry flavor]
- Generic: 25 mg/5 mL (60 mL)

Syrup, Oral, as calcium [strength expressed as base]:
- Vibramycin: 50 mg/5 mL (473 mL) [contains butylparaben, propylene glycol, propylparaben, sodium metabisulfite; raspberry-apple flavor]

Tablet, Oral, as hyclate [strength expressed as base]:
- Generic: 20 mg, 100 mg

Tablet, Oral, as monohydrate [strength expressed as base]:
- Adoxa: 50 mg
- Adoxa: 75 mg [contains fd&c yellow #10 aluminum lake, fd&c yellow #6 (sunset yellow)]
- Adoxa: 100 mg
- Adoxa Pak 1/100: 100 mg [contains fd&c yellow #10 aluminum lake, fd&c yellow #6 (sunset yellow)]
- Adoxa Pak 2/100: 100 mg [contains fd&c yellow #10 aluminum lake, fd&c yellow #6 (sunset yellow)]
- Adoxa Pak 1/150: 150 mg [scored; contains fd&c yellow #6 (sunset yellow)]
- Avidoxy: 100 mg [contains fd&c yellow #10 aluminum lake, fd&c yellow #6 aluminum lake]
- Generic: 50 mg, 75 mg, 100 mg, 150 mg

Tablet Delayed Release, Oral, as hyclate [strength expressed as base]:
- Doryx: 150 mg, 200 mg [scored]
- Generic: 75 mg, 100 mg, 150 mg

Dosage Forms: Canada Excipient information presented when available (limited, particularly for generics); consult specific product labeling.

Capsule, oral, as monohydrate [strength expressed as base]:
- Apprilon™: 40 mg [30 mg (immediate release) and 10 mg (delayed release)]

Capsule, oral, as hyclate [strength expressed as base]:
- Periostat®: 20 mg

Extemporaneous Preparations If a public health emergency is declared and liquid doxycycline is unavailable for the treatment of anthrax, emergency doses may be prepared for children or adults who cannot swallow tablets.

Add 20 mL of water to one 100 mg tablet. Allow tablet to soak in the water for 5 minutes to soften. Crush into a fine powder and stir until well mixed. Appropriate dose should be taken from this mixture. To increase palatability, mix with food or drink. If mixing with drink, add 15 mL of milk, chocolate milk, chocolate pudding, or apple juice to the appropriate dose of mixture. If using apple juice, also add 4 teaspoons of sugar. Doxycycline and water mixture may be stored at room temperature for up to 24 hours.

U.S. Food and Drug Administration, Center for Drug Evaluation and Research, "Public Health Emergency Home Preparation Instructions for Doxycycline." Available at http://www.fda.gov/Drugs/EmergencyPreparedness/BioterrorismandDrugPreparedness/ucm130996.htm

◆ **Doxycycline Calcium** *see* Doxycycline *on page 668*
◆ **Doxycycline Hyclate** *see* Doxycycline *on page 668*
◆ **Doxycycline Monohydrate** *see* Doxycycline *on page 668*

Doxylamine and Pyridoxine

(dox IL a meen & peer i DOX een)

Brand Names: U.S. Diclegis®

Brand Names: Canada Diclectin®

Index Terms Doxylamine Succinate and Pyridoxine Hydrochloride; Pyridoxine and Doxylamine

Pharmacologic Category Ethanolamine Derivative; Histamine H_1 Antagonist; Histamine H_1 Antagonist, First Generation; Vitamin, Water Soluble

Use Treatment of pregnancy-associated nausea and vomiting

Pregnancy Risk Factor A

Dosage Nausea and vomiting associated with pregnancy: Adults: Oral:

U.S. labeling: Day 1: Two delayed release tablets (a total of doxylamine 20 mg and pyridoxine 20 mg) at bedtime. If symptoms are controlled the next day, continue taking 2 tablets at bedtime. If symptoms persist into the afternoon of Day 2, take 2 tablets at bedtime, then 1 tablet in the morning of Day 3 and 2 tablets at bedtime. If ▶

symptoms are controlled on Day 4, continue with 1 tablet in the morning and 2 tablets at bedtime. If symptoms are **not** controlled on Day 4, increase dose to 1 tablet in the morning, 1 tablet midafternoon, and 2 tablets in the evening. Tablets should be taken as scheduled and not on an as needed basis. Maximum dose: Four tablets daily.

Canadian labeling: Take 2 delayed release tablets (a total of doxylamine 20 mg and pyridoxine 20 mg) at bedtime. One additional tablet may be taken in the morning or midafternoon; dose should be individualized to control symptoms. Tablets should not be taken on an as needed basis. Maximum dose: Four tablets daily. A gradual tapering of the dose is recommended to prevent a sudden onset of symptoms.

Dosage adjustment in renal impairment: No dosage adjustment provided in manufacturer's labeling (has not been studied).

Dosage adjustment in hepatic impairment: No dosage adjustment provided in manufacturer's labeling (has not been studied).

Additional Information Complete prescribing information should be consulted for additional detail.

Dosage Forms Excipient information presented when available (limited, particularly for generics); consult specific product labeling.

Tablet, delayed release:

Diclegis®: Doxylamine succinate 10 mg and pyridoxine hydrochloride 10 mg

Dosage Forms: Canada Excipient information presented when available (limited, particularly for generics); consult specific product labeling.

Tablet, delayed release:

Diclectin®: Doxylamine 10 mg and pyridoxine 10 mg

◆ **Doxylamine Succinate and Pyridoxine Hydrochloride** *see* Doxylamine and Pyridoxine *on page 673*

◆ **Doxytab (Can)** *see* Doxycycline *on page 668*

◆ **DPA** *see* Valproic Acid and Derivatives *on page 2149*

◆ **DPE** *see* Dipivefrin *on page 634*

◆ **D-Penicillamine** *see* PenicillAMINE *on page 1603*

◆ **DPH** *see* Phenytoin *on page 1638*

◆ **DPM [OTC]** *see* Urea *on page 2140*

◆ **Dramamine [OTC]** *see* DimenhyDRINATE *on page 616*

◆ **Dramamine Less Drowsy [OTC]** *see* Meclizine *on page 1277*

◆ **Dr Gs Clear Nail [OTC]** *see* Tolnaftate *on page 2087*

◆ **Driminate [OTC]** *see* DimenhyDRINATE *on page 616*

◆ **Drisdol** *see* Ergocalciferol *on page 733*

◆ **Drisdol® (Can)** *see* Ergocalciferol *on page 733*

◆ **Dristan® N.D. (Can)** *see* Acetaminophen and Pseudoephedrine *on page 33*

◆ **Dristan® N.D., Extra Strength (Can)** *see* Acetaminophen and Pseudoephedrine *on page 33*

◆ **Dritho-Creme HP** *see* Anthralin *on page 140*

◆ **Drixoral® ND (Can)** *see* Pseudoephedrine *on page 1746*

Dronabinol (droe NAB i nol)

Brand Names: U.S. Marinol

Brand Names: Canada Marinol®

Index Terms Delta-9 THC; Delta-9-tetrahydro-cannabinol; Tetrahydrocannabinol; THC

Pharmacologic Category Antiemetic; Appetite Stimulant

Use Chemotherapy-associated nausea and vomiting refractory to other antiemetic(s); AIDS-related anorexia

Unlabeled Use Cancer-related anorexia

Pregnancy Risk Factor C

Pregnancy Considerations Adverse events have been observed in animal reproduction studies.

Breast-Feeding Considerations Dronabinol is excreted in breast milk. Breast-feeding is not recommended by the manufacturer.

Contraindications Hypersensitivity to dronabinol, cannabinoids, sesame oil, or any component of the formulation, or marijuana; should be avoided in patients with a history of schizophrenia

Warnings/Precautions Use with caution in patients with hepatic disease or seizure disorders. Reduce dosage in patients with severe hepatic impairment. May cause additive CNS effects with sedatives, hypnotics or other psychoactive agents; patients must be cautioned about performing tasks which require mental alertness (eg, operating machinery or driving).

May have potential for abuse; drug is psychoactive substance in marijuana; use caution in patients with a history of substance abuse or potential. May cause withdrawal symptoms upon abrupt discontinuation. Use with caution in patients with mania, depression, or schizophrenia; careful psychiatric monitoring is recommended. Use caution in elderly; they are more sensitive to adverse effects.

Adverse Reactions Frequency not always specified.

>1%:

Cardiovascular: Palpitations, tachycardia, vasodilation/facial flushing

Central nervous system: Euphoria (8% to 24%, dose related), abnormal thinking (3% to 10%), dizziness (3% to 10%), paranoia (3% to 10%), somnolence (3% to 10%), amnesia, anxiety, ataxia, confusion, depersonalization, hallucination

Gastrointestinal: Abdominal pain (3% to 10%), nausea (3% to 10%), vomiting (3% to 10%)

Neuromuscular & skeletal: Weakness

<1% (Limited to important or life-threatening): Conjunctivitis, depression, diarrhea, fatigue, fecal incontinence, flushing, hypotension, myalgia, nightmares, seizure, speech difficulties, tinnitus, vision difficulties

Drug Interactions

Metabolism/Transport Effects **Substrate** of CYP2C9 (major), CYP3A4 (major); **Note:** Assignment of Major/Minor substrate status based on clinically relevant drug interaction potential

Avoid Concomitant Use

Avoid concomitant use of Dronabinol with any of the following: Azelastine (Nasal); Conivaptan; Fusidic Acid (Systemic); Paraldehyde

Increased Effect/Toxicity

Dronabinol may increase the levels/effects of: Alcohol (Ethyl); Analgesics (Opioid); Azelastine (Nasal); CNS Depressants; Methotrimeprazine; Metyrosine; Mirtazapine; Paraldehyde; Pramipexole; ROPINIRole; Rotigotine; Selective Serotonin Reuptake Inhibitors; Sympathomimetics; Zolpidem

The levels/effects of Dronabinol may be increased by: Anticholinergic Agents; Brimonidine (Topical); Cocaine; Conivaptan; CYP2C9 Inhibitors (Moderate); CYP2C9 Inhibitors (Strong); CYP3A4 Inhibitors (Moderate); CYP3A4 Inhibitors (Strong); Dasatinib; Doxylamine; Droperidol; Fusidic Acid (Systemic); HydrOXYzine; Ivacaftor; Luliconazole; Magnesium Sulfate; MAO Inhibitors; Methotrimeprazine; Mifepristone; Perampanel; Ritonavir; Simeprevir; Sodium Oxybate

Decreased Effect There are no known significant interactions involving a decrease in effect.

Ethanol/Nutrition/Herb Interactions

Ethanol: May increase CNS depression; monitor for increased effects with coadministration. Caution patients about effects.

Food: Administration with high-lipid meals may increase absorption.

Herb/Nutraceutical: St John's wort may decrease dronabinol levels.

Storage/Stability Store under refrigeration (or in a cool environment) between 8°C and 15°C (46°F and 59°F); protect from freezing.

Mechanism of Action Unknown, may inhibit endorphins in the brain's emetic center, suppress prostaglandin synthesis, and/or inhibit medullary activity through an unspecified cortical action. Some pharmacologic effects appear to involve sympathimometic activity; tachyphylaxis to some effect (eg, tachycardia) may occur, but appetite-stimulating effects do not appear to wane over time. Antiemetic activity may be due to effect on cannabinoid receptors (CB1) within the central nervous system.

Pharmacodynamics/Kinetics

Onset of action: Within 1 hour

Peak effect: 2-4 hours

Duration: 24 hours (appetite stimulation)

Absorption: Oral: 90% to 95%; 10% to 20% of dose gets into systemic circulation

Distribution: V_d: 10 L/kg; dronabinol is highly lipophilic and distributes to adipose tissue

Protein binding: 97% to 99%

Metabolism: Hepatic to at least 50 metabolites, some of which are active; 11-hydroxy-delta-9-tetrahydrocannabinol (11-OH-THC) is the major metabolite; extensive first-pass effect

Half-life elimination: Dronabinol: 25-36 hours (terminal); Dronabinol metabolites: 44-59 hours

Time to peak, serum: 0.5-4 hours

Excretion: Feces (50% as unconjugated metabolites, 5% as unchanged drug); urine (10% to 15% as acid metabolites and conjugates)

Dosage Refer to individual protocols. Oral:

Antiemetic: Children and Adults: 5 mg/m^2 1-3 hours before chemotherapy, then 5 mg/m^2/dose every 2-4 hours after chemotherapy for a total of 4-6 doses/day; increase doses in increments of 2.5 mg/m^2 to a maximum of 15 mg/m^2/dose.

Appetite stimulant: Adults: Initial: 2.5 mg twice daily (before lunch and dinner); titrate up to a maximum of 20 mg/day.

Dosage adjustment in renal impairment: No dosage adjustment provided in manufacturer's labeling.

Dosage adjustment in hepatic impairment: Usual dose should be reduced in patients with severe liver failure.

Dietary Considerations Capsules contain sesame oil.

Monitoring Parameters CNS effects, heart rate, blood pressure, behavioral profile

Reference Range Antinauseant effects: 5-10 ng/mL

Test Interactions Decreased FSH, LH, growth hormone, and testosterone

Dosage Forms Excipient information presented when available (limited, particularly for generics); consult specific product labeling.

Capsule, Oral:

Marinol: 2.5 mg, 5 mg, 10 mg [contains sesame oil]

Generic: 2.5 mg, 5 mg, 10 mg

Controlled Substance C-III

Dronedarone (droe NE da rone)

Brand Names: U.S. Multaq

Brand Names: Canada Multaq®

Index Terms Dronedarone Hydrochloride; SR33589

Pharmacologic Category Antiarrhythmic Agent, Class III

Additional Appendix Information

Beers Criteria – Potentially Inappropriate Medications for Geriatrics *on page 2368*

Use To reduce the risk of hospitalization for atrial fibrillation (AF) in patients in sinus rhythm with a history of paroxysmal or persistent AF

Unlabeled Use Alternative antiarrhythmic for the treatment of atrial fibrillation in patients with hypertrophic cardiomyopathy (HCM)

Pregnancy Risk Factor X

Medication Guide Available Yes

Dosage Oral: Adults: Atrial fibrillation/atrial flutter: 400 mg twice daily

Dosing adjustment in renal impairment: No dosage adjustment necessary.

Dosing adjustment in hepatic impairment:

Mild-to-moderate impairment: No dosage adjustment necessary

Severe impairment: Contraindicated

Additional Information Complete prescribing information should be consulted for additional detail.

Dosage Forms Excipient information presented when available (limited, particularly for generics); consult specific product labeling.

Tablet, Oral:

Multaq: 400 mg

◆ **Dronedarone Hydrochloride** *see* Dronedarone *on page 675*

Droperidol (droe PER i dole)

Brand Names: Canada Droperidol Injection, USP

Index Terms Dehydrobenzperidol

Pharmacologic Category Antiemetic; Antipsychotic Agent, Typical

Use Prevention and/or treatment of nausea and vomiting from surgical and diagnostic procedures

Pregnancy Risk Factor C

Pregnancy Considerations Adverse events were observed in some animal reproduction studies. Although use in pregnancy has been reported, due to cases of QT prolongation and torsade de pointes (some fatal), use of other agents in pregnant women is preferred (ACOG, 2004).

Breast-Feeding Considerations It is not known if droperidol is excreted in breast milk. The manufacturer recommends that caution be exercised when administering droperidol to nursing women.

Contraindications Hypersensitivity to droperidol or any component of the formulation; known or suspected QT prolongation, including congenital long QT syndrome (prolonged QT_c is defined as >440 msec in males or >450 msec in females)

Canadian labeling: Additional contraindications (not in U.S. labeling): Not for use in children ≤2 years of age

Warnings/Precautions May alter cardiac conduction. **[U.S. Boxed Warning]: Cases of QT prolongation and torsade de pointes, including some fatal cases, have been reported.** Use extreme caution in patients with bradycardia (<50 bpm), cardiac disease, concurrent MAO inhibitor therapy, Class I and Class III antiarrhythmics or other drugs known to prolong QT interval, and electrolyte disturbances (hypokalemia or hypomagnesemia), including concomitant drugs which may alter electrolytes (diuretics).

Use with caution in patients with seizures or severe liver disease. May be sedating, use with caution in disorders where CNS depression is a feature. Caution in patients with hemodynamic instability, predisposition to seizures, subcortical brain damage, pheochromocytoma or renal disease. Esophageal dysmotility and aspiration have been associated with antipsychotic use - use with caution in patients at risk of pneumonia (ie, Alzheimer's disease). Caution in breast cancer or other prolactin-dependent tumors (may elevate prolactin levels). May alter temperature regulation or mask toxicity of other drugs due to antiemetic effects. May cause orthostatic hypotension - use with caution in patients at risk of this effect or those who would tolerate transient hypotensive episodes (cerebrovascular disease, cardiovascular disease, or other medications which may predispose). Significant hypotension may occur.

May cause anticholinergic effects (confusion, agitation, constipation, xerostomia, blurred vision, urinary retention). Therefore, they should be used with caution in patients with decreased gastrointestinal motility, urinary retention, BPH, xerostomia, visual problems, or narrow-angle glaucoma (screening is recommended). Relative to other neuroleptics, droperidol has a low potency of cholinergic blockade.

May cause extrapyramidal symptoms (EPS), including pseudoparkinsonism, acute dystonic reactions, akathisia, and tardive dyskinesia. Risk of dystonia (and possibly other EPS) may be greater with increased doses, use of conventional antipsychotics, males, and younger patients. May be associated with neuroleptic malignant syndrome (NMS). May mask toxicity of other drugs or conditions (eg, intestinal obstruction, Reye's syndrome, brain tumor) due to antiemetic effects. Use with caution in the elderly; reduce initial dose.

Adverse Reactions Frequency not defined.

Cardiovascular: Cardiac arrest, hypertension, hypotension (especially orthostatic), QT_c prolongation (dose dependent), tachycardia, torsade de pointes, ventricular tachycardia

Central nervous system: Anxiety, chills, depression (postoperative, transient), dizziness, drowsiness (postoperative) increased, dysphoria, extrapyramidal symptoms (akathisia, dystonia, oculogyric crisis), hallucinations (postoperative), hyperactivity, neuroleptic malignant syndrome (NMS) (rare), restlessness

Respiratory: Bronchospasm, laryngospasm

Miscellaneous: Anaphylaxis, shivering

Drug Interactions

Metabolism/Transport Effects None known.

Avoid Concomitant Use

Avoid concomitant use of Droperidol with any of the following: Aclidinium; Amisulpride; Azelastine (Nasal); Highest Risk QTc-Prolonging Agents; Ipratropium (Oral Inhalation); Ivabradine; Metoclopramide; Mifepristone; Paraldehyde; Sulpiride; Tiotropium; Umeclidinium

Increased Effect/Toxicity

Droperidol may increase the levels/effects of: Alcohol (Ethyl); Amisulpride; Analgesics (Opioid); Anticholinergics; Azelastine (Nasal); Buprenorphine; CNS Depressants; Highest Risk QTc-Prolonging Agents; Hydrocodone; Methotrimeprazine; Methylphenidate; Metoclopramide; Moderate Risk QTc-Prolonging Agents; Paraldehyde; Serotonin Modulators; Sulpiride; Tiotropium; Zolpidem

The levels/effects of Droperidol may be increased by: Acetylcholinesterase Inhibitors (Central); Aclidinium; Brimonidine (Topical); Doxylamine; HydrOXYzine; Ipratropium (Oral Inhalation); Ivabradine; Lithium formulations; Magnesium Sulfate; MAO Inhibitors; Methotrimeprazine; Methylphenidate; Metyrosine; Mifepristone; Perampanel; Pramlintide; QTc-Prolonging Agents (Indeterminate Risk and Risk Modifying); Serotonin Modulators; Sodium Oxybate; Tetrabenazine; Umeclidinium

Decreased Effect

Droperidol may decrease the levels/effects of: Amphetamines; Anti-Parkinson's Agents (Dopamine Agonist); Quinagolide

The levels/effects of Droperidol may be decreased by: Anti-Parkinson's Agents (Dopamine Agonist); Lithium formulations

Preparation for Administration I.V. infusion: Dilute in 50-100 mL NS or D_5W.

Storage/Stability Store at 20°C to 25°C (68°F to 77°F); excursions permitted to 15°C to 30°C (59°F to 86°F). Protect from light. Solutions diluted in NS or D_5W are stable at room temperature for up to 7 days in PVC bags or glass bottles. Solutions diluted in LR are stable at room temperature for 24 hours in PVC bags and up to 7 days in glass bottles.

Mechanism of Action Droperidol is a butyrophenone antipsychotic; antiemetic effect is a result of blockade of dopamine stimulation of the chemoreceptor trigger zone. Other effects include alpha-adrenergic blockade, peripheral vascular dilation, and reduction of the pressor effect of epinephrine resulting in hypotension and decreased peripheral vascular resistance; may also reduce pulmonary artery pressure

Pharmacodynamics/Kinetics

Onset of action: 3-10 minutes
  Peak effect: ~30 minutes
Duration: 2-4 hours, may extend to 12 hours
Absorption: I.M.: Rapid
Distribution: Crosses blood-brain barrier and placenta
  V_d: Children: ~0.6 L/kg; Adults: ~1.5 L/kg
Protein binding: 85% to 90%
Metabolism: Hepatic, to *p*-fluorophenylacetic acid, benzimidazolone, *p*-hydroxypiperidine
Half-life elimination: ~2.3 hours
Excretion: Urine (75%, <1% as unchanged drug); feces (22%, 11% as unchanged drug)

Dosage Note: Titrate carefully to desired effect

I.M., I.V.:

Children 2-12 years: Prevention of postoperative nausea and vomiting (PONV):

Manufacturer labeling: Maximum dose: 0.1 mg/kg; additional doses may be repeated with caution to achieve desired effect

Consensus guideline recommendations: 0.01-0.015 mg/kg (maximum: 1.25 mg) I.V. administered at the end of surgery (Gan, 2007)

Adults: Prevention of PONV:

Manufacturer labeling: Maximum initial dose: 2.5 mg; additional doses of 1.25 mg may be administered with caution to achieve desired effect

Consensus guideline recommendations: 0.625-1.25 mg I.V. administered at the end of surgery (Gan, 2007)

Canadian labeling: I.V.: Prevention and treatment of PONV:

Children >2 years and Adolescents: 0.02-0.05 mg/kg (maximum dose: 1.25 mg) 30 minutes prior to anticipated end of surgery, and then every 6 hours as needed for breakthrough PONV

Adults: 0.625-1.25 mg 30 minutes prior to anticipated end of surgery, and then every 6 hours as needed for breakthrough PONV

Elderly: PONV: 0.625 mg 30 minutes prior to anticipated end of surgery and then every 6 hours as needed for breakthrough PONV; additional dosing should be administered with caution

Dosage adjustment in renal impairment:

U.S. labeling: Specific dosing recommendations are not provided; use with caution

Canadian labeling: I.V.: 0.625 mg; additional dosing should be administered with caution

Dosage adjustment in hepatic impairment:

U.S. labeling: Specific dosing recommendations are not provided; use with caution

Canadian labeling: I.V.: 0.625 mg; additional dosing should be administered with caution

Administration Administer I.M. or I.V.; according to the manufacturer, I.V. push administration should be slow. For I.V. infusion, further dilute.

Monitoring Parameters To identify QT prolongation, a 12-lead ECG prior to use is recommended; continued ECG monitoring for 2-3 hours following administration is recommended. Vital signs; serum magnesium and potassium; mental status, abnormal involuntary movement scale (AIMS); observe for dystonias, extrapyramidal side effects, and temperature changes

Dosage Forms Excipient information presented when available (limited, particularly for generics); consult specific product labeling.

Solution, Injection:

Generic: 2.5 mg/mL (2 mL)

DULoxetine (doo LOX e teen)

Brand Names: U.S. Cymbalta

Brand Names: Canada Cymbalta®

Index Terms (+)-(*S*)-*N*-Methyl-γ-(1-naphthyloxy)-2-thiophenepropylamine Hydrochloride; Duloxetine Hydrochloride; LY248686

Pharmacologic Category Antidepressant, Serotonin/Norepinephrine Reuptake Inhibitor

Additional Appendix Information

Antidepressant Agents *on page* 2284

Use Acute and maintenance treatment of major depressive disorder (MDD); treatment of generalized anxiety disorder (GAD); management of diabetic peripheral neuropathic pain (DPNP); management of fibromyalgia (FM); chronic musculoskeletal pain (eg, chronic low back pain, osteoarthritis)

Unlabeled Use Treatment of stress incontinence

Pregnancy Risk Factor C

Pregnancy Considerations Adverse events were observed in animal reproduction studies. Nonteratogenic effects in the newborn following SSRI/SNRI exposure late in the third trimester include respiratory distress, cyanosis, apnea, seizures, temperature instability, feeding difficulty, vomiting, hypoglycemia, hyper- or hypotonia, hyperreflexia, jitteriness, irritability, constant crying, and tremor. Symptoms may be due to the toxicity of the SNRIs/SSRIs or a discontinuation syndrome and may be consistent with serotonin syndrome associated with SSRI treatment. The long-term effects of *in utero* SNRI/SSRI exposure on infant development and behavior are not known.

The ACOG recommends that therapy with SSRIs or SNRIs during pregnancy be individualized; treatment of depression during pregnancy should incorporate the clinical expertise of the mental health clinician, obstetrician, primary healthcare provider, and pediatrician. According to the American Psychiatric Association (APA), the risks of medication treatment should be weighed against other treatment options and untreated depression. For women who discontinue antidepressant medications during pregnancy and who may be at high risk for postpartum depression, the medications can be restarted following delivery. Treatment algorithms have been developed by the ACOG and the APA for the management of depression in women prior to conception and during pregnancy.

Healthcare providers are encouraged to enroll women exposed to duloxetine during pregnancy in the Cymbalta® Pregnancy Registry (866-814-6975 or http://cymbaltapregnancyregistry.com).

Breast-Feeding Considerations Duloxetine is excreted in human milk and has been detected in the serum of a nursing infant. Breast-feeding is not recommended by the manufacturer. The long-term effects on neurobehavior have not been studied, thus one should prescribe duloxetine to a mother who is breast-feeding only when the benefits outweigh the potential risks.

Medication Guide Available Yes

Contraindications Concomitant use or within 14 days of discontinuing MAO inhibitor (intended to treat psychiatric disorders); concomitant use with linezolid or intravenous methylene blue; uncontrolled narrow-angle glaucoma

Note: Treatment with MAO inhibitors for psychiatric disorders should not be initiated until 5 days after the discontinuation of duloxetine. Although acceptable alternatives should be considered, there may be circumstances when it is necessary to initiate an MAO inhibitor (eg, linezolid or intravenous methylene blue) in a patient taking duloxetine; in this case, discontinue duloxetine prior to administering the MAO inhibitor.

Canadian labeling: Additional contraindications (not in U.S. labeling): Hypersensitivity to duloxetine or any component of the formulation; hepatic impairment; severe renal impairment (eg, Cl_{cr} <30 mL/minute) or end-stage renal disease (ESRD); concomitant use with thioridazine or with CYP1A2 inhibitors

Warnings/Precautions [U.S. Boxed Warning]: Antidepressants increase the risk of suicidal thinking and behavior in children, adolescents, and young adults (18-24 years of age) with major depressive disorder (MDD) and other psychiatric disorders; consider risk prior to prescribing. Short-term studies did not show an increased risk in patients >24 years of age and showed a decreased risk in patients ≥65 years. Closely monitor for clinical worsening, suicidality, or unusual changes in behavior; the patient's family or caregiver should be instructed to closely observe the patient and communicate condition with healthcare provider. A medication guide concerning the use of antidepressants in children and teenagers should be dispensed with each prescription. **Duloxetine is not FDA approved for use in children.**

The possibility of a suicide attempt is inherent in major depression and may persist until remission occurs. Patients treated with antidepressants should be observed for clinical worsening and suicidality, especially during the initial (generally first 1-2 months) few months of a course of drug therapy, or at times of dose changes, either increases or decreases. Use caution in high-risk patients. Worsening depression and severe abrupt suicidality that are not part of the presenting symptoms may require discontinuation or modification of drug therapy. The patient's family or caregiver should be alerted to monitor patients for the emergence of suicidality and associated behaviors (such as agitation, irritability, hostility, impulsivity, and hypomania) and call healthcare provider.

May worsen psychosis in some patients or precipitate a shift to mania or hypomania in patients with bipolar disorder. Patients presenting with depressive symptoms should be screened for bipolar disorder. Monotherapy in patients with bipolar disorder should be avoided. **Duloxetine is not FDA approved for the treatment of bipolar depression.**

May cause orthostatic hypotension/syncope at therapeutic doses especially within the first week of therapy and after dose increases. Monitor blood pressure with initiation of therapy, dose increases (especially in patients receiving >60 mg/day), or with concomitant use of vasodilators, CYP2D6 inhibitors/substrates, or CYP1A2 inhibitors. Use caution in patients with hypertension. May increase blood pressure. Rare cases of hypertensive crisis have been reported in patients with pre-existing hypertension; evaluate blood pressure prior to initiating therapy and periodically thereafter; consider dose reduction or gradual discontinuation of therapy in individuals with sustained hypertension during therapy.

Modest increases in serum glucose and hemoglobin A_{1c} (Hb A_{1c}) levels have been observed in some diabetic patients receiving duloxetine therapy for diabetic peripheral neuropathic pain (DPNP). Duloxetine may cause increased urinary resistance; advise patient to report symptoms of urinary hesitation/difficulty. Has a low potential to impair cognitive or motor performance. Use caution with a previous seizure disorder or condition predisposing to seizures such as brain damage or alcoholism. Avoid use in patients with substantial ethanol intake, evidence of chronic liver disease, or hepatic impairment (contraindicated in Canadian labeling). Rare cases of hepatic failure (including fatalities) have been reported with use. Hepatitis with abdominal pain, hepatomegaly, elevated transaminase levels >20 times the upper limit of normal (ULN) with and without jaundice have all been observed. Discontinue therapy with the presentation of jaundice or other signs of hepatic dysfunction and do not reinitiate therapy unless another source or cause is identified. Use caution in patients with impaired gastric motility (eg, some diabetics) may affect stability of the capsule's enteric coating.

Severe skin reactions (including Stevens-Johnson syndrome and erythema multiforme) have been reported; discontinue immediately if hypersensitivity reaction suspected. May cause hyponatremia/SIADH (elderly at increased risk); volume depletion (diuretics may increase risk). Use with caution in patients with controlled narrow angle glaucoma. May cause or exacerbate sexual dysfunction. Use caution with renal impairment (contraindicated in Canadian labeling for severe renal impairment or ESRD). Use caution with concomitant CNS depressants. May impair platelet aggregation; use caution with concomitant use of NSAIDs, ASA, or other drugs that affect coagulation; the risk of bleeding may be potentiated. Bone fractures have been associated with antidepressant treatment. Consider the possibility of a fragility fracture if an antidepressant-treated patient presents with unexplained bone pain, point tenderness, swelling, or bruising (Rabenda, 2013; Rizzoli, 2012).

Serotonin syndrome (SS) reactions have occurred with duloxetine when used alone and particularly when used in combination with other serotonergic agents (eg, triptans, tricyclic antidepressants, fentanyl, lithium, tramadol, tryptophan, buspirone, and St John's wort) and drugs that inhibit serotonin metabolism (eg, MAO inhibitors, specifically linezolid, methylene blue, and others used for psychiatric disorders). The diagnosis of SS can be made using the Hunter Serotonin Toxicity Criteria (Dunkley, 2003). Monitor patients closely for signs/symptoms of SS which may include mental status changes (eg, agitation, hallucinations, delirium), seizures, autonomic instability (eg, tachycardia, dizziness, diaphoresis), neuromuscular symptoms (eg, tremor, rigidity, myoclonus), or gastrointestinal symptoms (eg, nausea, vomiting, diarrhea). Discontinue treatment (and any concomitant serotonergic agents) immediately if signs/symptoms of SS arise. Concurrent use of serotonergic agents is not recommended; however, if clinically indicated, use with caution and advise patients of increased SS risk especially during initiation and dose increases.

Concurrent use with or within 14 days of MAO inhibitors is contraindicated. Allow 5 days to elapse after discontinuation of duloxetine before initiating an MAO inhibitor for psychiatric disorders. If already receiving duloxetine and urgent treatment with MAO inhibitors (eg, linezolid or I.V. methylene blue) is required, stop duloxetine and initiate linezolid or I.V. methylene blue if the potential benefits outweigh the risk of SS. Monitor for serotonin syndrome for 5 days or for 24 hours after the last dose of linezolid or methylene blue, whichever occurs first; may resume duloxetine 24 hours after the last dose of linezolid or methylene blue. The risks associated with methylene blue doses <1 mg/kg or when administered nonparenterally are unknown.

Use caution during concurrent therapy with drugs which lower the seizure threshold. May increase the risks associated with electroconvulsive therapy. Use caution in elderly patients; may cause or exacerbate syndrome of inappropriate antidiuretic hormone secretion or hyponatremia; monitor sodium closely with initiation or dosage adjustments in older adults (Beers Criteria). Formulation contains sucrose; patients with fructose intolerance, glucose-galactose malabsorption, or sucrase-isomaltase deficiency should avoid use.

Abrupt discontinuation or interruption of antidepressant therapy has been associated with a discontinuation syndrome. Symptoms arising may vary with antidepressant however commonly include nausea, vomiting, diarrhea, headaches, light-headedness, dizziness, diminished appetite, sweating, chills, tremors, paresthesias, fatigue, somnolence, and sleep disturbances (eg, vivid dreams, insomnia). Greater risks for developing a discontinuation syndrome have been associated with antidepressants with shorter half-lives, longer durations of treatment, and abrupt discontinuation. For antidepressants of short or intermediate half-lives, symptoms may emerge within 2-5 days after treatment discontinuation and last 7-14 days (APA, 2010; Fava, 2006; Haddad, 2001; Shelton, 2001; Warner, 2006).

Adverse Reactions

>10%:

Central nervous system: Headache (13% to 14%), somnolence (10% to 12%; dose related), fatigue (10% to 11%)

Gastrointestinal: Nausea (23% to 25%), xerostomia (11% to 15%; dose related)

1% to 10%:

Cardiovascular: Palpitation (1% to 2%)

Central nervous system: Dizziness (10%), insomnia (10%; dose related), agitation (3% to 5%), anxiety (3%), dreams abnormal (1% to 2%), yawning (1% to 2%), hypoesthesia (≥1%), lethargy (≥1%), vertigo (≥1%), chills (1%), sleep disorder (1%)

Dermatologic: Hyperhydrosis (6% to 7%)

Endocrine & metabolic: Libido decreased (2% to 4%), hot flushes (1% to 3%), orgasm abnormality (1% to 3%)

Gastrointestinal: Constipation (10%; dose related), diarrhea (9% to 10%), appetite decreased (7% to 9%; dose related), abdominal pain (4% to 6%), vomiting (3% to 5%), dyspepsia (2%), weight loss (2%), flatulence (≥1%), taste abnormal (≥1%), weight gain (≥1%)

Genitourinary: Erectile dysfunction (4% to 5%), ejaculation delayed (3%; dose related), ejaculatory dysfunction (2%)

Hepatic: ALT >3x ULN (1%)

Neuromuscular & skeletal: Muscle spasms (3%), tremor (2% to 3%; dose related), musculoskeletal pain (≥1%), paresthesia (≥1%), rigors (≥1%)

Ocular: Blurred vision (1% to 3%)

Respiratory: Nasopharyngitis (5%), cough (3%)

Miscellaneous: Influenza (3%)

<1% (Limited to important or life-threatening): Alkaline phosphatase increased, anaphylactic reaction, angioneurotic edema, apathy, bruxism, contact dermatitis, dehydration, dermatitis, diastolic blood pressure increased, diplopia, disorientation, dysarthria, dyskinesia, dysuria, eructation, erythema, erythema multiforme, EPS, gastritis, gastroenteritis, glaucoma, gynecological bleeding, hallucinations, Hb A_{1c} increased, hepatic failure, hepatitis, hepatomegaly, hyperbilirubinemia, hypercholesterolemia, hyperglycemia, hyperlipidemia, hypersensitivity, hypertensive crisis, hyponatremia, hypothyroidism, jaundice, malaise, mania, MI, micturition urgency, mood swings, muscle spasm, muscle tightness, muscle twitching, night sweats, nocturia, orthostatic hypotension, peripheral coldness, photosensitivity, polyuria, rash, restless leg syndrome, seizure, serotonin syndrome, SIADH, Stevens-Johnson syndrome, stomatitis, supraventricular arrhythmia, syncope, systolic blood pressure increased, tachycardia, thirst, throat tightness, transaminases increased, trismus, urinary retention, urticaria

Drug Interactions

Metabolism/Transport Effects Substrate of CYP1A2 (major), CYP2D6 (major); **Note:** Assignment of Major/Minor substrate status based on clinically relevant drug interaction potential; **Inhibits** CYP2D6 (moderate)

Avoid Concomitant Use

Avoid concomitant use of DULoxetine with any of the following: Iobenguane I 123; Linezolid; MAO Inhibitors; Methylene Blue; Thioridazine

Increased Effect/Toxicity

DULoxetine may increase the levels/effects of: Agents with Antiplatelet Properties; Alpha-/Beta-Agonists; Anticoagulants; Antipsychotics; ARIPiprazole; Aspirin; Collagenase (Systemic); CYP2D6 Substrates; Dabigatran Etexilate; Fesoterodine; FluvoxaMINE; Ibritumomab; Methylene Blue; Metoclopramide; Metoprolol; Nebivolol; NSAID (Nonselective); PARoxetine; Rivaroxaban; Salicylates; Serotonin Modulators; Thioridazine; Thrombolytic Agents; Tositumomab and Iodine I 131 Tositumomab; Tricyclic Antidepressants

The levels/effects of DULoxetine may be increased by: Abiraterone Acetate; Alcohol (Ethyl); Antipsychotics; ARIPiprazole; CYP1A2 Inhibitors (Moderate); CYP1A2 Inhibitors (Strong); CYP2D6 Inhibitors (Moderate); CYP2D6 Inhibitors (Strong); Darunavir; Dasatinib; Deferasirox; FluvoxaMINE; Glucosamine; Herbs (Anticoagulant/Antiplatelet Properties); Ibrutinib; Linezolid; MAO Inhibitors; Multivitamins/Fluoride (with ADE); Multivitamins/Minerals (with ADEK, Folate, Iron); Multivitamins/Minerals (with AE, No Iron); Nonsteroidal Anti-Inflammatory Agents; Omega-3 Fatty Acids; PARoxetine; Pentosan Polysulfate Sodium; Pentoxifylline; Propafenone; Prostacyclin Analogues; Tipranavir; Vemurafenib; Vitamin E

Decreased Effect

DULoxetine may decrease the levels/effects of: Alpha2-Agonists; Codeine; Iobenguane I 123; Ioflupane I 123; Tamoxifen

The levels/effects of DULoxetine may be decreased by: CYP1A2 Inducers (Strong); Cyproterone; Nonsteroidal Anti-Inflammatory Agents; Peginterferon Alfa-2b

Ethanol/Nutrition/Herb Interactions

Ethanol: Ethanol may increase hepatotoxic potential of duloxetine and increase CNS depression. Management: Avoid ethanol.

Herb/Nutraceutical: Some herbal medications may increase CNS depression. Management: Avoid valerian, St John's wort, SAMe, kava kava, and gotu kola.

Storage/Stability Store at 25°C (77°F); excursions permitted to 15°C to 30°C (59°F to 86°F)

Mechanism of Action Duloxetine is a potent inhibitor of neuronal serotonin and norepinephrine reuptake and a weak inhibitor of dopamine reuptake. Duloxetine has no significant activity for muscarinic cholinergic, H_1-histaminergic, or $alpha_2$-adrenergic receptors. Duloxetine does not possess MAO-inhibitory activity.

Pharmacodynamics/Kinetics

Absorption: Well absorbed, 2-hour delay in absorption after ingestion; food decreases extent of absorption ~10% (no effect on C_{max})

Distribution: 1640 L (range: 701-3800 L)

Protein binding: >90%; primarily to albumin and α_1-acid glycoprotein

Metabolism: Hepatic, via CYP1A2 and CYP2D6; forms multiple metabolites (inactive)

Half-life elimination: 12 hours (range: 8-17 hours)

Time to peak: 6 hours; 10 hours when ingested with food

Excretion: Urine (~70%; <1% of total dose as unchanged drug); feces (~20%)

Dosage Oral:

Adults:

Major depressive disorder: Initial: 40-60 mg/day; dose may be divided (ie, 20 or 30 mg twice daily) or given as a single daily dose of 60 mg; maintenance: 60 mg once daily; for doses >60 mg/day, titrate dose in increments of 30 mg/day over 1 week as tolerated to a maximum dose: 120 mg/day. **Note:** Doses >60 mg/day have not been demonstrated to be more effective.

Diabetic neuropathy: 60 mg once daily; lower initial doses may be considered in patients where tolerability is a concern and/or renal impairment is present. **Note:** Doses up to 120 mg/day administered in clinical trials offered no additional benefit and were less well tolerated than dose of 60 mg/day.

Fibromyalgia: 30 mg once daily for 1 week, then increase to 60 mg once daily as tolerated. **Note:** Doses up to 120 mg/day administered in clinical trials offered no additional benefit and were less well tolerated than dose of 60 mg/day.

Generalized anxiety disorder: Initial: 30-60 mg/day as a single daily dose; patients initiated at 30 mg/day should be titrated to 60 mg/day after 1 week; maximum dose: 120 mg/day. **Note:** Doses >60 mg/day have not been demonstrated to be more effective than 60 mg/day.

Chronic musculoskeletal pain: 30 mg once daily for 1 week, then increase to 60 mg once daily as tolerated

Stress incontinence (unlabeled use): 40 mg twice daily (Dmochowski, 2003)

Elderly:

Major depressive disorder: Manufacturer does not recommend specific dosage adjustment. Conservatively, may initiate at a dose of 20 mg 1-2 times/day; increase to 40-60 mg/day as a single daily dose or in divided doses **or** initiate therapy at 30 mg/day for 1 week then increase to 60 mg/day as tolerated.

Other indications: Refer to adult dosing

Discontinuation of therapy: Upon discontinuation of antidepressant therapy, gradually taper the dose to minimize the incidence of withdrawal symptoms and allow for the detection of re-emerging symptoms. Evidence supporting ideal taper rates is limited. APA and NICE guidelines suggest tapering therapy over at least several weeks with consideration to the half-life of the antidepressant; antidepressants with a shorter half-life may need to be tapered more conservatively. In addition for long-term treated patients, WFSBP guidelines recommend tapering over 4-6 months. If intolerable withdrawal symptoms occur following a dose reduction, consider resuming the previously prescribed dose and/or decrease dose at a more gradual rate (APA, 2010; Bauer, 2002; Haddad, 2001; NCCMH, 2010; Schatzberg, 2006; Shelton, 2001; Warner, 2006).

MAO inhibitor recommendations:

Switching to or from an MAO inhibitor intended to treat psychiatric disorders:

Allow 14 days to elapse between discontinuing an MAO inhibitor intended to treat psychiatric disorders and initiation of duloxetine.

Allow 5-14 days to elapse between discontinuing duloxetine and initiation of an MAO inhibitor intended to treat psychiatric disorders.

Use with other MAO inhibitors (such as linezolid or I.V. methylene blue):

Do not initiate duloxetine in patients receiving linezolid or I.V. methylene blue; consider other interventions for psychiatric condition.

If urgent treatment with linezolid or I.V. methylene blue is required in a patient already receiving duloxetine and potential benefits outweigh potential risks, discontinue duloxetine promptly and administer linezolid or I.V. methylene blue. Monitor for serotonin syndrome for 5 days or until 24 hours after the last dose of linezolid or I.V. methylene blue, whichever comes first. May resume duloxetine 24 hours after the last dose of linezolid or I.V. methylene blue.

Dosage adjustment in renal impairment: Not recommended for use in Cl_{cr} <30 mL/minute or ESRD (contraindicated in Canadian labeling); in mild-moderate impairment, lower initial doses may be considered with titration guided by response and tolerability

Dosage adjustment in hepatic impairment: Not recommended for use in hepatic impairment (contraindicated in Canadian labeling)

Dietary Considerations May be taken without regard to meals.

Administration Capsule should be swallowed whole; do not crush or chew. Although the manufacturer does not recommend opening the capsule to facilitate administration; the contents of capsule may be sprinkled on applesauce or in apple juice and swallowed (without chewing) immediately. Do not sprinkle contents on chocolate pudding (Wells, 2008). Administer without regard to meals.

Monitoring Parameters Blood pressure should be checked prior to initiating therapy and then regularly monitored, especially in patients with a high baseline blood pressure; mental status for depression, suicidal ideation (especially at the beginning of therapy or when doses are increased or decreased), anxiety, social functioning, mania, panic attacks; glucose levels and Hb A_{1c} levels in diabetic patients, creatinine, BUN, transaminases

For musculoskeletal pain: Pain relief

Dosage Forms Excipient information presented when available (limited, particularly for generics); consult specific product labeling.

Capsule Delayed Release Particles, Oral:

Cymbalta: 20 mg, 30 mg, 60 mg [contains fd&c blue #2 (indigotine)]

Generic: 20 mg, 30 mg, 60 mg

- ◆ Duloxetine Hydrochloride *see* DULoxetine *on page 677*
- ◆ Duodopa™ (Can) *see* Carbidopa and Levodopa *on page 340*
- ◆ Duodote™ *see* Atropine and Pralidoxime *on page 200*
- ◆ DuoNeb® *see* Ipratropium and Albuterol *on page 1113*
- ◆ DuP 753 *see* Losartan *on page 1247*
- ◆ Duraclon *see* CloNIDine *on page 468*
- ◆ Duragesic *see* FentaNYL *on page 842*
- ◆ Duragesic MAT (Can) *see* FentaNYL *on page 842*
- ◆ Duralith® (Can) *see* Lithium *on page 1229*
- ◆ Duramorph *see* Morphine (Systemic) *on page 1398*
- ◆ Durela (Can) *see* TraMADol *on page 2099*
- ◆ Durezol *see* Difluprednate *on page 605*
- ◆ Duricef *see* Cefadroxil *on page 361*
- ◆ Durolane (Can) *see* Hyaluronate and Derivatives *on page 1000*

Dutasteride (doo TAS teer ide)

Brand Names: U.S. Avodart

Brand Names: Canada Avodart®

Pharmacologic Category 5 Alpha-Reductase Inhibitor

Use Treatment of symptomatic benign prostatic hyperplasia (BPH) as monotherapy or combination therapy with tamsulosin

Unlabeled Use Treatment of male pattern baldness

Pregnancy Risk Factor X

Dosage Oral: Adults: Males: BPH: 0.5 mg once daily alone or in combination with tamsulosin

Dosage adjustment in renal impairment: No adjustment required

Dosage adjustment in hepatic impairment: Use caution; no specific adjustments recommended

Additional Information Complete prescribing information should be consulted for additional detail.

Dosage Forms Excipient information presented when available (limited, particularly for generics); consult specific product labeling.

Capsule, Oral:

Avodart: 0.5 mg

Dutasteride and Tamsulosin

(doo TAS teer ide & tam SOO loe sin)

Brand Names: U.S. Jalyn

Index Terms Tamsulosin and Dutasteride; Tamsulosin Hydrochloride and Dutasteride

Pharmacologic Category 5 Alpha-Reductase Inhibitor; Alpha$_1$ Blocker

Use Benign prostatic hyperplasia: Treatment of symptomatic benign prostatic hyperplasia (BPH) in men with an enlarged prostate

Pregnancy Risk Factor X

Dosage Benign prostatic hypertrophy (BPH): Adults: Males: Oral: One capsule (0.5 mg dutasteride/0.4 mg tamsulosin) once daily ~30 minutes after the same meal each day

Dosage adjustment in renal impairment:

Cl_{cr} 10-30 mL/minute/1.73 m^2: No dosage adjustment necessary.

Cl_{cr} <10 mL/minute/1.73 m^2: No dosage adjustment provided in the manufacturer's labeling (has not been studied).

Dosage adjustment in hepatic impairment: No dosage adjustment provided in the manufacturer's labeling.

Additional Information Complete prescribing information should be consulted for additional detail.

Dosage Forms Excipient information presented when available (limited, particularly for generics); consult specific product labeling.

Capsule, oral:

Jalyn™: Dutasteride 0.5 mg and tamsulosin hydrochloride 0.4 mg

- ◆ **Duvoid® (Can)** *see* Bethanechol *on page 250*
- ◆ **DW286** *see* Gemifloxacin *on page 948*
- ◆ **DX-88** *see* Ecallantide *on page 681*
- ◆ **Dyazide** *see* Hydrochlorothiazide and Triamterene *on page 1006*

Dyclonine (DYE kloe neen)

Brand Names: U.S. Sucrets® Children's [OTC]; Sucrets® Maximum Strength [OTC]; Sucrets® Regular Strength [OTC]

Index Terms Dyclonine Hydrochloride

Pharmacologic Category Local Anesthetic, Oral

Use Temporary relief of pain associated with oral mucosa

Dosage Oral: Children ≥2 years and Adults: Lozenge: One lozenge every 2 hours as needed (maximum: 10 lozenges/day)

Additional Information Complete prescribing information should be consulted for additional detail.

Dosage Forms Excipient information presented when available (limited, particularly for generics); consult specific product labeling. [DSC] = Discontinued product

Lozenge, oral, as hydrochloride:

Sucrets® Children's: 1.2 mg (18s) [cherry flavor]

Sucrets® Maximum Strength: 3 mg (18s) [black-cherry flavor]

Sucrets® Maximum Strength: 3 mg (18s) [wintergreen flavor]

Sucrets® Regular Strength: 2 mg (18s)

Sucrets® Regular Strength: 2 mg (18s [DSC]) [wild cherry flavor]

- ◆ **Dyclonine Hydrochloride** *see* Dyclonine *on page 681*
- ◆ **Dymista™** *see* Azelastine and Fluticasone *on page 211*
- ◆ **Dynacin [DSC]** *see* Minocycline *on page 1373*
- ◆ **Dyrenium** *see* Triamterene *on page 2124*
- ◆ **Dyspel [OTC]** *see* Ibuprofen *on page 1032*
- ◆ **Dysport** *see* AbobotulinumtoxinA *on page 26*
- ◆ **Dysport (Glabellar Lines)** *see* AbobotulinumtoxinA *on page 26*
- ◆ **7E3** *see* Abciximab *on page 22*
- ◆ **E-400 [OTC]** *see* Vitamin E *on page 2202*
- ◆ **E-400-Clear [OTC]** *see* Vitamin E *on page 2202*
- ◆ **E-400-Mixed [OTC]** *see* Vitamin E *on page 2202*
- ◆ **E2020** *see* Donepezil *on page 650*
- ◆ **E 2080** *see* Rufinamide *on page 1865*
- ◆ **E7389** *see* Eribulin *on page 734*
- ◆ **EACA** *see* Aminocaproic Acid *on page 100*
- ◆ **Ear Drops Earwax Aid [OTC]** *see* Carbamide Peroxide *on page 340*
- ◆ **Ear Wax Remover [OTC]** *see* Carbamide Peroxide *on page 340*
- ◆ **Earwax Treatment Drops [OTC]** *see* Carbamide Peroxide *on page 340*
- ◆ **Ebixa (Can)** *see* Memantine *on page 1289*

Ecallantide (e KAL lan tide)

Brand Names: U.S. Kalbitor

Index Terms DX-88

Pharmacologic Category Kallikrein Inhibitor

Use Treatment of acute attacks of hereditary angioedema (HAE)

Pregnancy Risk Factor C

Pregnancy Considerations Adverse effects were noted in animal reproduction studies. If treatment for HAE is needed during pregnancy, other agents are preferred (Caballero, 2012).

Breast-Feeding Considerations It is not known if ecallantide is excreted in breast milk. The manufacturer recommends that caution be exercised when administering ecallantide to nursing women.

Medication Guide Available Yes

Contraindications Hypersensitivity to ecallantide or any component of the formulation

Warnings/Precautions [U.S. Boxed Warning]: Serious hypersensitivity reactions, including anaphylaxis have been reported; administer only by healthcare provider in presence of appropriate medical support to manage anaphylaxis and hereditary angioedema. Do not administer to patients with known hypersensitivity to ecallantide. Reactions usually occur within 1 hour and may include chest discomfort, flushing, hypotension, nasal congestion, pharyngeal edema, pruritus, rash, rhinorrhea, sneezing, throat irritation, urticaria, and wheezing. Signs/symptoms of hypersensitivity reactions may be similar to those associated with hereditary angioedema attacks, therefore, consideration should be given to treatment methods; monitor patients closely.

Adverse Reactions

>10%:

Central nervous system: Headache (8% to 16%), fatigue (12%)

Gastrointestinal: Nausea (5% to 13%), diarrhea (4% to 11%)

1% to 10%:

Central nervous system: Fever (4% to 5%)

Dermatologic: Pruritus (5%), rash (3%), urticaria (2%)

Gastrointestinal: Vomiting (6%), upper abdominal pain (5%)

Local: Injection site reactions (3% to 7%; includes bruising, erythema, irritation, pain, pruritus, urticaria)

Respiratory: Upper respiratory infection (8%), nasopharyngitis (3% to 6%)

Miscellaneous: Antibody formation (5% to 7%), anaphylaxis (4%)

<1% (Limited to important or life-threatening) Hypersensitivity (chest discomfort, flushing, pharyngeal edema, rhinorrhea, sneezing, nasal congestion, wheezing, hypotension)

Drug Interactions

Metabolism/Transport Effects None known.

Avoid Concomitant Use There are no known interactions where it is recommended to avoid concomitant use.

Increased Effect/Toxicity There are no known significant interactions involving an increase in effect.

Decreased Effect There are no known significant interactions involving a decrease in effect.

Storage/Stability Store under refrigeration at 2°C to 8°C (36°F to 46°F). Protect from light. May be stored for up to 14 days at <30°C (<86°F). Do not use if solution is discolored or has particulate matter present.

Mechanism of Action Ecallantide is a recombinant protein which inhibits the conversion of high molecular weight kininogen to bradykinin by selectively and reversibly inhibiting plasma kallikrein. Unregulated bradykinin production is thought to contribute to the increased vascular permeability and angioedema observed in HAE.

Pharmacodynamics/Kinetics

Onset: 30 minutes to 4 hours

Distribution: 18.6-34.2 L

Half-life elimination: 1.5-2.5 hours

Time to peak: ~2-3 hours

Excretion: Primarily urine

Dosage SubQ: Children ≥16 years and adults: Treatment of HAE attacks: 30 mg (as three 10 mg [1 mL] injections); may repeat an additional 30 mg within 24 hours

Dosage adjustment in renal impairment: No dosage adjustment provided in manufacturer's labeling (has not been studied).

Dosage adjustment in hepatic impairment: No dosage adjustment provided in manufacturer's labeling (has not been studied).

Administration Administer as 3 (10 mg/mL each) injections subcutaneously into skin of abdomen, upper arm, or thigh (do not administer at site of attack). Recommended needle size is 27 gauge. Separate injections by 2 inches (5 cm). May inject all doses in same or different location; rotation of sites is not necessary. Monitor/observe for hypersensitivity.

Monitoring Parameters Monitor for hypersensitivity reaction

Dosage Forms Excipient information presented when available (limited, particularly for generics); consult specific product labeling.

Solution, Subcutaneous [preservative free]:

Kalbitor: 10 mg/mL (1 mL)

Echothiophate Iodide

(ek oh THYE oh fate EYE oh dide)

Brand Names: U.S. Phospholine Iodide

Index Terms Ecostigmine Iodide

Pharmacologic Category Acetylcholinesterase Inhibitor; Ophthalmic Agent, Antiglaucoma; Ophthalmic Agent, Miotic

Use Used as miotic in treatment of chronic, open-angle glaucoma; may be useful in specific cases of angle-closure glaucoma (postiridectomy or where surgery refused/contraindicated); postcataract surgery-related glaucoma; accommodative esotropia

Pregnancy Risk Factor C

Dosage Ophthalmic:

Children: Accommodative esotropia:

Diagnosis: Instill 1 drop (0.125%) once daily into both eyes at bedtime for 2-3 weeks

Treatment: Usual dose: Instill 1 drop of 0.06% once daily or 0.125% every other day (maximum: 0.125% daily). **Note:** Use lowest concentration and frequency which gives satisfactory response; if necessary, doses >0.125% daily may be used for short periods of time.

Adults: Open-angle or secondary glaucoma:

Initial: Instill 1 drop (0.03%) twice daily into eyes with 1 dose just prior to bedtime

Maintenance: Some patients have been treated with 1 dose daily or every other day

Conversion from other ophthalmic agents: If IOP control was unsatisfactory, patients may be expected to require higher doses of echothiophate (eg, ≥0.06%); however, patients should be initially started on the 0.03% strength for a short period to better tolerance.

Dosage adjustment in renal impairment: No dosage adjustment provided in manufacturer's labeling.

Dosage adjustment in hepatic impairment: No dosage adjustment provided in manufacturer's labeling.

Additional Information Complete prescribing information should be consulted for additional detail.

Dosage Forms Excipient information presented when available (limited, particularly for generics); consult specific product labeling.

Solution Reconstituted, Ophthalmic:

Phospholine Iodide: 0.125% (5 mL)

◆ **EC-Naprosyn** *see* Naproxen *on page* 1425

◆ ***E. coli* Asparaginase** *see* Asparaginase (*E. coli*) *on page* 174

Econazole (e KONE a zole)

Brand Names: U.S. Ecoza

Index Terms Econazole Nitrate; Ecoza

Pharmacologic Category Antifungal Agent, Topical

Use Topical treatment of tinea pedis (athlete's foot), tinea cruris (jock itch), tinea corporis (ringworm), tinea versicolor, and cutaneous candidiasis

Pregnancy Risk Factor C

Dosage Children and Adults: Topical:

Tinea pedis: Apply sufficient amount to cover affected areas once daily for 1 month

Tinea cruris, tinea corporis, tinea versicolor: Apply sufficient amount to cover affected areas once daily for 2 weeks

Cutaneous candidiasis: Apply sufficient quantity twice daily (morning and evening) for 2 weeks

Additional Information Complete prescribing information should be consulted for additional detail.

Product Availability Ecoza topical foam: FDA approved October 2013; anticipated availability currently unknown

Dosage Forms Excipient information presented when available (limited, particularly for generics); consult specific product labeling.

Cream, External, as nitrate:

Generic: 1% (15 g, 30 g, 85 g)

Foam, External:

Ecoza: 1% (70 g) [contains propylene glycol, trolamine (triethanolamine)]

- ◆ **Econazole Nitrate** *see* Econazole *on page 682*
- ◆ **Econopred** *see* PrednisoLONE (Ophthalmic) *on page 1706*
- ◆ **Ecostigmine Iodide** *see* Echothiophate Iodide *on page 682*
- ◆ **Ecotrin® [OTC]** *see* Aspirin *on page 177*
- ◆ **Ecotrin® Arthritis Strength [OTC]** *see* Aspirin *on page 177*
- ◆ **Ecotrin® Low Strength [OTC]** *see* Aspirin *on page 177*
- ◆ **Ecoza** *see* Econazole *on page 682*
- ◆ **Ectosone (Can)** *see* Betamethasone *on page 247*

Eculizumab (e kue LIZ oo mab)

Brand Names: U.S. Soliris

Brand Names: Canada Soliris®

Index Terms h5G1.1; Monoclonal Antibody 5G1.1; Monoclonal Antibody Anti-C5

Pharmacologic Category Monoclonal Antibody; Monoclonal Antibody, Complement Inhibitor

Use Treatment of paroxysmal nocturnal hemoglobinuria (PNH) to reduce hemolysis; treatment of atypical hemolytic uremic syndrome (aHUS) to inhibit complement-mediated thrombotic microangiopathy

Note: Not indicated for the treatment of hemolytic uremic syndrome related to Shiga toxin *E. coli* (STEC-HUS)

Pregnancy Risk Factor C

Pregnancy Considerations Animal studies have demonstrated fetal abnormalities. Eculizumab is a recombinant IgG molecule with IgG2 and IgG4 sequences; human IgG is known to cross the placenta, however IgG2 may have reduced placental transfer compared to other IgG subclasses. There are no adequate and well-controlled studies in pregnant women. Pregnant women with PNH and their fetuses have high rates of morbidity and mortality during pregnancy and the postpartum period. Limited information is available related to use during pregnancy. Use during pregnancy only if clearly needed.

Breast-Feeding Considerations It is not known if eculizumab is excreted in human milk. However, human IgG is excreted in breast milk, and therefore, eculizumab may also be excreted in milk. Although antibodies in human milk do not enter neonatal or infant circulation in substantial amounts, the risks to the infant from gastrointestinal or limited systemic exposure are unknown.

Prescribing and Access Restrictions Patients and providers must enroll with Soliris® OneSource™ (1-888-765-4747) program prior to treatment initiation.

Medication Guide Available Yes

Contraindications Unresolved serious *Neisseria meningitidis* infection; patients not currently vaccinated against *Neisseria meningitidis* (unless risks of treatment delay outweigh risk of meningococcal infection)

Warnings/Precautions [U.S. Boxed Warning]: Meningococcal *(Neisseria meningitides)* infections have occurred in patients receiving eculizumab; may be fatal or life-threatening if not detected and treated promptly. Monitor for early signs of meningococcal infection; evaluate and treat promptly if suspected. Follow current meningococcal immunization recommendations for patients with complement deficiencies. Vaccinate with meningococcal vaccine at least 2 weeks prior to initiation of treatment; revaccinate according to current guidelines. Polyvalent meningococcal vaccines are recommended. If urgent treatment is necessary in an unvaccinated patient, administer meningococcal vaccine as soon as possible. Although the risk/benefits of prophylactic meningococcal antibiotic therapy have not been determined, prophylactic antibiotics were administered in clinical studies until at least 2 weeks after vaccination. Meningococcal infections developed in some patients despite vaccination. Discontinue eculizumab during the treatment of serious meningococcal infections. In addition to meningitis, the risk of other infections, especially encapsulated bacteria (eg, *Streptococcus pneumoniae, H. influenzae*) is increased with eculizumab treatment (because eculizumab blocks terminal complement activation). Children should receive vaccination for prevention of *S. pneumoniae, H. influenzae* according to current ACIP guidelines. Use caution in patients with concurrent systemic infection. Patients should be up to date with all immunizations before initiating therapy. **[U.S. Boxed Warning]: Access is restricted through a REMS program. Prescribers must be enrolled in the program; enrollment information is available at 1-888-765-4747.** Counsel patients on the risk of meningococcal infection; ensure patients are vaccinated and provide educational materials.

Infusion reactions, including anaphylaxis or hypersensitivity, may occur; interrupt infusion for severe reaction. Continue monitoring for 1 hour after completion of infusion. Patients with PNH who discontinue treatment may be at increased risk for serious hemolysis; monitor closely for at least 8 weeks after treatment discontinuation. Consider RBC transfusion, exchange transfusion, anticoagulation, corticoids or reinitiation of eculizumab for serious hemolysis after discontinuation. When used for aHUS, monitor for at least 12 weeks after treatment discontinuation for signs/symptoms of thrombotic microangiopathy (TMA) complications (angina, dyspnea, mental status changes, seizure, serum creatinine elevation, serum LDH elevation, thrombocytopenia, or thrombosis). If TMA complications occur after stopping eculizumab, consider reinitiation of treatment, plasmapheresis, plasma exchange, fresh frozen plasma infusion, and/or appropriate organ-specific measures. In clinical trials, anticoagulant therapy was continued in patients who were receiving these agents (due to history of or risk for thromboembolism) prior to initiation of eculizumab. The effect of anticoagulant therapy withdrawal is unknown; treatment with eculizumab should not alter anticoagulation management

Adverse Reactions

>10%:

Cardiovascular: Hypertension (aHUS: 35%), tachycardia (aHUS: children 21%), peripheral edema (11%)

Central nervous system: Headache (30% to 44%; serious: 2%), insomnia (14%), fatigue (11% to 12%), fever (2% to 11%; children 47%), vertigo (11%)

Gastrointestinal: Diarrhea (32%), vomiting (21% to 22%), nausea (16% to 19%), abdominal pain (11%)

Genitourinary: Urinary tract infection (16%)

Hematologic: Anemia (24%; serious: 2%), leukopenia (16%)

Neuromuscular & skeletal: Back pain (19%), limb pain (7% to 11%)

Respiratory: Respiratory tract infection (7% to 35%), cough (12% to 26%), nasopharyngitis (23%), nasal congestion (aHUS: children 21%), pharyngolaryngeal pain (14%)

1% to 10%:

Gastrointestinal: Constipation (7%)

Neuromuscular & skeletal: Myalgia (7%)

Respiratory: Sinusitis (7%)

Miscellaneous: Herpes infections (7%), flu-like syndrome (5%), viral infection (serious: 2%), meningococcal infection (≤1%)

<1% (Limited to important or life-threatening): Abdominal distention, anxiety, arthralgia, cholangitis, dizziness, endometritis, hematoma (mild), infusion reaction, pyelonephritis, renal impairment, taste alteration

Drug Interactions

Metabolism/Transport Effects None known.

Avoid Concomitant Use

Avoid concomitant use of Eculizumab with any of the following: BCG; Natalizumab; Pimecrolimus; Tacrolimus (Topical); Tofacitinib; Vaccines (Live)

Increased Effect/Toxicity

Eculizumab may increase the levels/effects of: Leflunomide; Natalizumab; Tofacitinib; Vaccines (Live)

The levels/effects of Eculizumab may be increased by: Denosumab; Pimecrolimus; Roflumilast; Tacrolimus (Topical); Trastuzumab

Decreased Effect

Eculizumab may decrease the levels/effects of: BCG; Coccidioidin Skin Test; Sipuleucel-T; Vaccines (Inactivated); Vaccines (Live)

The levels/effects of Eculizumab may be decreased by: Echinacea

Preparation for Administration Add eculizumab to an infusion bag and dilute with an equal volume of D_5W, sodium chloride 0.9%, sodium chloride 0.45%, or Ringer's injection to a final concentration of 5 mg/mL (eg, 300 mg to a total volume of 60 mL, 600 mg in a total volume of 120 mL, 900 mg in a total volume of 180 mL, or 1200 mg to a total volume of 240 mL). Gently invert bag to mix thoroughly.

Storage/Stability Prior to dilution, store vials at 2°C to 8°C (36°F to 46°F); do not freeze. Protect from light; do not shake. Allow admixture to reach room temperature prior to administration (do not use a heat source or warming). Following dilution, store at room temperature or refrigerate; protect from light; use within 24 hours.

Mechanism of Action Terminal complement-mediated intravascular hemolysis is a key clinical feature of paroxysmal nocturnal hemoglobinuria (PNH); blocking the formation of membrane attack complex (MAC) results in stabilization of hemoglobin and a reduction in the need for RBC transfusions. Impairment of complement activity regulation leads to uncontrolled complement activation in atypical hemolytic uremic syndrome (aHUS). Eculizumab is a humanized monoclonal IgG antibody that binds to complement protein C5, preventing cleavage into C5a and C5b. Blocking the formation of C5b inhibits the subsequent formation of terminal complex C5b-9 or MAC.

Pharmacodynamics/Kinetics

Onset of action: PNH: Reduced hemolysis: ≤1 week

Distribution: PNH: 7.7 L; aHUS: 6.14 L

Half-life elimination: PNH: ~11 days (range: ~8-15 days); aHUS: ~12 days (during plasma exchange the half-life is reduced to 1.26 hours)

Dosage Note: Patients must receive meningococcal vaccine at least 2 weeks prior to treatment initiation; revaccinate according to current guidelines. Treatment should be administered at the recommended time interval although administration may be varied by ±2 days.

Atypical hemolytic uremic syndrome (aHUS): I.V.:

Children 5 kg to <10 kg: Induction: 300 mg weekly for 1 dose; Maintenance: 300 mg at week 2, then 300 mg every 3 weeks

Children 10 kg to <20 kg: Induction: 600 mg weekly for 1 dose; Maintenance: 300 mg at week 2, then 300 mg every 2 weeks

Children 20 kg to <30 kg: Induction: 600 mg weekly for 2 doses; Maintenance: 600 mg at week 3, then 600 mg every 2 weeks

Children 30 kg to <40 kg: Induction: 600 mg weekly for 2 doses; Maintenance: 900 mg at week 3, then 900 mg every 2 weeks

Children ≥40 kg and Adults: Induction: 900 mg weekly for 4 doses; Maintenance: 1200 mg at week 5, then 1200 mg every 2 weeks

Supplemental dosing for patients receiving plasmapheresis or plasma exchange:

If most recent dose was 300 mg, administer 300 mg within 60 minutes after each plasmapheresis or plasma exchange

If most recent dose was ≥600 mg, administer 600 mg within 60 minutes after each plasmapheresis or plasma exchange

Supplemental dosing for patients receiving fresh frozen plasma infusion: If most recent dose was ≥300 mg, administer 300 mg within 60 minutes prior to each 1 unit of fresh frozen plasma infusion

PNH: I.V.: Adults: 600 mg weekly for 4 doses, followed by 900 mg 1 week later, then 900 mg every 2 weeks

Dosage adjustment in renal impairment: No dosage adjustment is recommended in the manufacturer's labeling.

Dosage adjustment in hepatic impairment: Not studied in hepatic dysfunction

Administration I.V.: Allow to reach room temperature prior to administration. Infuse over 35 minutes. Decrease infusion rate or discontinue for infusion reactions; do not exceed a maximum 2-hour duration of infusion. Monitor for at least 1 hour following completion of infusion (for signs/symptoms of infusion reaction).

Monitoring Parameters Signs and symptoms of infusion reaction (during infusion and for 1 hour after infusion complete); CBC with differential, lactic dehydrogenase (LDH), serum creatinine, AST, urinalysis

Serum LDH levels greater than pretreatment level along with: >25% decrease in PNH clone size in ≤1 week, or hemoglobin level <5 g/dL, or a hemoglobin decrease of >4 g/dL in ≤1 week, or 50% increase in serum creatinine, or angina, mental status change, or thrombosis is indicative of serious hemolysis

After discontinuation:

aHUS: Signs/symptoms of thrombotic microangiopathy (TMA) complications (monitor for at least 12 weeks after treatment discontinuation), including angina, dyspnea, mental status changes, seizure, serum creatinine elevation, serum LDH elevation, thrombocytopenia, or thrombosis.

PNH: Signs and symptoms of intravascular hemolysis (monitor for at least 8 weeks after discontinuation), including serum LDH, hemoglobin, serum creatinine; signs of angina, mental status change, or thrombosis

Dosage Forms Excipient information presented when available (limited, particularly for generics); consult specific product labeling.

Solution, Intravenous [preservative free]:

Soliris: 10 mg/mL (30 mL)

◆ **Ed-A-Hist™ [OTC]** *see* Chlorpheniramine and Phenylephrine *on page 412*

- ◆ **Ed A-Hist DM [OTC]** *see* Chlorpheniramine, Phenylephrine, and Dextromethorphan *on page 413*
- ◆ **Edarbi** *see* Azilsartan *on page 212*
- ◆ **Edarbi™ (Can)** *see* Azilsartan *on page 212*
- ◆ **Edarbyclor** *see* Azilsartan and Chlorthalidone *on page 213*
- ◆ **Edarbyclor™ (Can)** *see* Azilsartan and Chlorthalidone *on page 213*
- ◆ **Ed ChlorPed D [OTC]** *see* Chlorpheniramine and Phenylephrine *on page 412*
- ◆ **Edecrin** *see* Ethacrynic Acid *on page 782*
- ◆ **Edecrin® (Can)** *see* Ethacrynic Acid *on page 782*

Edetate CALCIUM Disodium

(ED e tate KAL see um dye SOW dee um)

Index Terms CaEDTA; Calcium Disodium Edetate; Calcium Disodiumethylenediaminetetraacetic Acid; Edetate Disodium CALCIUM; EDTA (CALCIUM Disodium) (error-prone abbreviation)

Pharmacologic Category Chelating Agent

Use Treatment of symptomatic acute and chronic lead poisoning

Pregnancy Risk Factor B

Pregnancy Considerations Adverse events were observed in some animal reproduction studies; there are no well controlled studies of edetate CALCIUM disodium in pregnant women. Lead is known to cross the placenta in amounts related to maternal plasma levels. Prenatal lead exposure may be associated with adverse events such as spontaneous abortion, preterm delivery, decreased birth weight, and impaired neurodevelopment. Some adverse outcomes may occur with maternal blood lead levels <10 mcg/dL. In addition, pregnant women exposed to lead may have an increased risk of gestational hypertension. Consider chelation therapy in pregnant women with confirmed blood lead levels ≥45 mcg/dL (pregnant women with blood lead levels ≥70 mcg/dL should be considered for chelation regardless of trimester); consultation with experts in lead poisoning and high-risk pregnancy is recommended. Encephalopathic pregnant women should be chelated regardless of trimester (CDC, 2010).

Breast-Feeding Considerations If present in breast milk, oral absorption of edetate CALCIUM disodium is poor (<5%) which would limit exposure to a nursing infant. However, edetate CALCIUM disodium is not used orally because it may increase lead absorption from the GI tract. The amount of lead in breast milk may range from 0.6% to 3% of the maternal serum concentration. Women with confirmed blood lead levels ≥40 mcg/dL should not initiate breast-feeding; pumping and discarding breast milk is recommended until blood lead levels are <40 mcg/dL, at which point breast-feeding may resume (CDC, 2010). Calcium supplementation may reduce the amount of lead in breast milk.

Contraindications Active renal disease or anuria; hepatitis

Warnings/Precautions [U.S. Boxed Warning]: Use with extreme caution in patients with lead encephalopathy and cerebral edema. In these patients, I.V. infusion has been associated with lethal increase in intracranial pressure; I.M. injection is preferred.

Edetate CALCIUM disodium is potentially nephrotoxic. Renal tubular acidosis and fatal nephrosis may occur, especially with high doses; do not exceed the recommended daily dose. If anuria, increasing proteinuria, or hematuria occurs during therapy, discontinue use. Minimize nephrotoxicity by providing adequate hydration, establishment of good urine output, avoidance of excessive doses, and limit continuous administration to ≤5 days. Monitor for arrhythmias and ECG changes during I.V. therapy.

Exercise caution in the ordering, dispensing, and administration of this drug. Edetate CALCIUM disodium (CaEDTA) may be confused with edetate disodium (Na_2EDTA) (not commercially available in the U.S. or Canada). The CDC and FDA recommend that edetate disodium should never be used for chelation therapy (especially in children) (Mitka, 2008). Death has occurred following the use of edetate disodium for chelation therapy in pediatric patients with autism (Baxter, 2008). Fatal hypocalcemia may result if edetate disodium is used for the treatment of lead poisoning instead of edetate CALCIUM disodium (Baxter, 2008). Investigate, identify, and remove sources of lead exposure prior to treatment. Primary care providers should consult experts in chemotherapy of lead toxicity before using chelation drug therapy. Do not permit patients to re-enter the contaminated environment until lead abatement has been completed.

Adverse Reactions Frequency not defined.

Cardiovascular: Arrhythmia, ECG changes, hypotension

Central nervous system: Chills, fatigue, fever, headache, malaise

Dermatologic: Cheilosis, dermatitis, rash

Endocrine & metabolic: Hypercalcemia, hypokalemia

Gastrointestinal: Anorexia, GI upset, nausea, thirst (excessive), vomiting

Hematologic: Anemia, bone marrow suppression (transient)

Hepatic: Alkaline phosphatase decreased, liver function test increased (mild)

Local: Pain at injection site (I.M. injection), thrombophlebitis (I.V. infusion when concentration >5 mg/mL)

Neuromuscular & skeletal: Arthralgia, myalgia, numbness, paresthesia, tremor

Ocular: Lacrimation

Renal: Glucosuria, microscopic hematuria, nephrosis, nephrotoxicity, proteinuria, renal tubular necrosis, urinary frequency/urgency

Respiratory: Nasal congestion, sneezing

Miscellaneous: Iron, magnesium, and/or zinc deficiency (with chronic therapy)

Drug Interactions

Metabolism/Transport Effects None known.

Avoid Concomitant Use

Avoid concomitant use of Edetate CALCIUM Disodium with any of the following: CloZAPine

Increased Effect/Toxicity

Edetate CALCIUM Disodium may increase the levels/effects of: CloZAPine; Insulin

Decreased Effect There are no known significant interactions involving a decrease in effect.

Preparation for Administration For I.V. infusion, dilute total daily dose into 250-500 mL of 0.9% sodium chloride or D_5W. Concentrations >0.5% (5 mg/mL) should be avoided. Procaine or lidocaine may be added to solutions given by I.M. injection.

Storage/Stability Store at 25°C (77°F); excursion permitted to 15°C to 30°C (59°F to 86°F).

Mechanism of Action Calcium is displaced by divalent and trivalent heavy metals, forming a nonionizing soluble complex that is excreted in urine

Pharmacodynamics/Kinetics

Onset of action: Chelation of lead: I.V.: 1 hour

Absorption: I.M., SubQ: Well absorbed; Oral: <5%

Distribution: Into extracellular fluid; minimal CSF penetration (~5%)

Metabolism: Almost none of the drug is metabolized

Half-life elimination: 20-60 minutes

Excretion: Urine (as metal chelates or unchanged drug); decreased GFR decreases elimination

Dosage

I.M., I.V.:

Lead poisoning: **Note:** For the treatment of high blood lead levels in children, the CDC recommends chelation treatment when blood lead levels are >45 mcg/dL (CDC, 2002). The AAP recommends succimer as the drug used for initial management in asymptomatic children when blood lead levels are >45 mcg/dL and <70 mcg/dL. Edetate CALCIUM disodium can be used in children allergic to succimer (AAP, 2005; Chandran, 2010). Combination therapy with edetate CALCIUM disodium and dimercaprol is recommended for use in children whose blood lead levels are ≥70 mcg/dL or in children with lead encephalopathy (AAP, 2005; Chandran, 2010). In adults, available guidelines recommend chelation therapy with blood lead levels >50 mcg/dL and significant symptoms; chelation therapy may also be indicated with blood lead levels ≥100 mcg/dL and/or symptoms (Kosnett, 2007). Depending upon the blood lead level, additional courses may be necessary; at least 2-4 days should elapse before repeat treatment is initiated.

Blood lead levels <70 mcg/dL and asymptomatic:

Children: 1000 mg/m^2/day for 5 days or 50 mg/kg/day (maximum: 1000 mg/day) for 5 days (Chandran, 2010)

Adults: 1000 mg/m^2/day for 5 days

Blood lead levels ≥70 mcg/dL or symptomatic lead poisoning (in conjunction with dimercaprol): **Note:** Begin treatment with edetate CALCIUM disodium with the second dimercaprol dose:

Children: 1000 mg/m^2/day **or** 25-50 mg/kg/day (maximum: 1000 mg/day) for 5 days (Chandran, 2010; Howland, 2011)

Adults: 1000 mg/m^2/day **or** 25-50 mg/kg/day for 5 days; a maximum dose of 3000 mg has been suggested (Howland, 2011)

Lead encephalopathy (in conjunction with dimercaprol): **Note:** Begin treatment with edetate CALCIUM disodium with the second dimercaprol dose:

Children: 1500 mg/m^2/day **or** 50-75 mg/kg/day (maximum: 1000 mg/day) for 5 days (Chandran, 2010; Howland, 2011)

Adults: 1500 mg/m^2/day **or** 50-75 mg/kg/day for 5 days; a maximum dose of 3000 mg has been suggested (Howland, 2011)

Lead nephropathy: Adults: An alternative dosing regimen reflecting the reduction in renal clearance is based upon the serum creatinine; **Note:** Repeat regimen monthly until lead levels are reduced to an acceptable level:

S_{cr} 2-3 mg/dL: 500 mg/m^2 every 24 hours for 5 days

S_{cr} 3-4 mg/dL: 500 mg/m^2 every 48 hours for 3 doses

S_{cr} >4 mg/dL: 500 mg/m^2 once weekly

Dosage adjustment in renal impairment: Dose should be reduced with pre-existing mild renal disease. Limiting the daily dose to 1 g in children and 2 g in adults may decrease risk of nephrotoxicity, although larger doses may be needed in the treatment of lead encephalopathy (Howland, 2011).

Administration For I.M. or I.V. use; I.V. is generally preferred, however, the I.M. route is preferred when cerebral edema is present.

I.V. infusion: Administer the daily dose as a diluted solution over 8-12 hours or continuously over 24 hours (Howland, 2011)

For I.M. injection: Daily dose should be divided into 2-3 equal doses spaced 8-12 hours apart. Procaine hydrochloride or lidocaine may be added to the edetate CALCIUM disodium to minimize pain at injection site. Administer by deep I.M. injection. When used in conjunction with dimercaprol, inject into a separate site.

Monitoring Parameters Urinary output; urinalysis; renal function, hepatic function, serum electrolytes (baseline and daily [severe lead poisoning] or at days 2 and 5 [less severe lead poisoning]); ECG (with I.V. therapy); blood lead levels (baseline and 7-21 days after completing chelation therapy); hemoglobin or hematocrit; iron status; free erythrocyte protoporphyrin or zinc protoporphyrin; neurodevelopmental changes

Test Interactions If edetate CALCIUM disodium is given as a continuous I.V. infusion, stop the infusion for at least 1 hour before blood is drawn for lead concentration to avoid a falsely elevated value

Dosage Forms Excipient information presented when available (limited, particularly for generics); consult specific product labeling. [DSC] = Discontinued product

Solution, Injection:

Generic: 500 mg/2.5 mL (2.5 mL [DSC]); 1 g/5 mL (5 mL)

◆ **Edetate Disodium CALCIUM** *see* Edetate CALCIUM Disodium *on page* 685

◆ **Edex** *see* Alprostadil *on page* 83

◆ **Edluar** *see* Zolpidem *on page* 2242

Edrophonium (ed roe FOE nee um)

Brand Names: U.S. Enlon

Brand Names: Canada Enlon®; Tensilon®

Index Terms Edrophonium Chloride

Pharmacologic Category Acetylcholinesterase Inhibitor; Antidote; Diagnostic Agent

Use Diagnosis of myasthenia gravis; differentiation of cholinergic crises from myasthenia crises; reversal of nondepolarizing neuromuscular blockers

Pregnancy Considerations Animal reproduction studies have not been conducted.

Breast-Feeding Considerations It is not known if edrophonium is excreted in breast milk. According to the manufacturer, if administration is required, avoid breastfeeding the infant immediately after use due to the potential for adverse events in the nursing infant.

Contraindications Hypersensitivity to edrophonium, sulfites, or any component of the formulation; GI or GU obstruction

Warnings/Precautions Use with caution in patients with bronchial asthma and those receiving a cardiac glycoside; atropine sulfate should always be readily available as an antagonist. Overdosage can cause cholinergic crisis which may be fatal. I.V. atropine should be readily available for treatment of cholinergic reactions. Use with caution in patients with cardiac arrhythmias (eg, bradyarrhythmias). Avoid use in myasthenia gravis; may exacerbate muscular weakness. Products may contain sodium sulfite.

Adverse Reactions Frequency not defined.

Cardiovascular: Arrhythmias (especially bradycardia), AV block, carbon monoxide decreased, cardiac arrest, ECG changes (nonspecific), flushing, hypotension, nodal rhythm, syncope, tachycardia

Central nervous system: Convulsions, dizziness, drowsiness, dysarthria, dysphonia, headache, loss of consciousness

Dermatologic: Skin rash, thrombophlebitis (I.V.), urticaria

Gastrointestinal: Diarrhea, dysphagia, flatulence, hyperperistalsis, nausea, salivation, stomach cramps, vomiting

Genitourinary: Urinary urgency

Neuromuscular & skeletal: Arthralgias, fasciculations, muscle cramps, spasms, weakness

Ocular: Lacrimation, small pupils

Respiratory: Bronchiolar constriction, bronchospasm, dyspnea, bronchial secretions increased, laryngospasm, respiratory arrest, respiratory depression, respiratory muscle paralysis

Miscellaneous: Allergic reactions, anaphylaxis, diaphoresis increased

Drug Interactions

Metabolism/Transport Effects None known.

Avoid Concomitant Use There are no known interactions where it is recommended to avoid concomitant use.

Increased Effect/Toxicity

Edrophonium may increase the levels/effects of: Beta-Blockers; Cholinergic Agonists; Succinylcholine

The levels/effects of Edrophonium may be increased by: Corticosteroids (Systemic)

Decreased Effect

Edrophonium may decrease the levels/effects of: Neuromuscular-Blocking Agents (Nondepolarizing)

The levels/effects of Edrophonium may be decreased by: Dipyridamole

Mechanism of Action Inhibits destruction of acetylcholine by acetylcholinesterase. This facilitates transmission of impulses across myoneural junction and results in increased cholinergic responses such as miosis, increased tonus of intestinal and skeletal muscles, bronchial and ureteral constriction, bradycardia, and increased salivary and sweat gland secretions.

Pharmacodynamics/Kinetics

Onset of action: I.M.: 2-10 minutes; I.V.: 30-60 seconds

Duration: I.M.: 5-30 minutes: I.V.: 10 minutes

Distribution: V_d: Adults: 1.1 L/kg

Half-life elimination: Adults: 1.2-2.4 hours; Anephric patients: 2.4-4.4 hours

Excretion: Adults: Primarily urine (67%)

Dosage Usually administered I.V., however, if not possible, I.M. or SubQ may be used:

Infants:

I.M.: 0.5-1 mg

I.V.: Initial: 0.1 mg, followed by 0.4 mg if no response; total dose = 0.5 mg

Children:

Diagnosis: Initial: 0.04 mg/kg over 1 minute followed by 0.16 mg/kg if no response, to a maximum total dose of 5 mg for children <34 kg, or 10 mg for children >34 kg **or**

Alternative dosing (manufacturer's recommendation):

≤34 kg: 1 mg; if no response after 45 seconds, repeat dosage in 1 mg increments every 30-45 seconds, up to a total of 5 mg

>34 kg: 2 mg; if no response after 45 seconds, repeat dosage in 1 mg increments every 30-45 seconds, up to a total of 10 mg

I.M.:

<34 kg: 1 mg

>34 kg: 5 mg

Titration of oral anticholinesterase therapy: 0.04 mg/kg once given 1 hour after oral intake of the drug being used in treatment; if strength improves, an increase in neostigmine or pyridostigmine dose is indicated

Adults:

Diagnosis:

I.V.: 2 mg test dose administered over 15-30 seconds; 8 mg given 45 seconds later if no response is seen; test dose may be repeated after 30 minutes

I.M.: Initial: 10 mg; if no cholinergic reaction occurs, administer 2 mg 30 minutes later to rule out false-negative reaction

Titration of oral anticholinesterase therapy: 1-2 mg given 1 hour after oral dose of anticholinesterase; if strength improves, an increase in neostigmine or pyridostigmine dose is indicated

Reversal of nondepolarizing neuromuscular blocking agents (neostigmine with atropine usually preferred): I.V.: 10 mg over 30-45 seconds; may repeat every 5-10 minutes up to 40 mg

Termination of paroxysmal atrial tachycardia: I.V. rapid injection: 5-10 mg

Differentiation of cholinergic from myasthenic crisis: I.V.: 1 mg; may repeat after 1 minute. **Note:** Intubation and controlled ventilation may be required if patient has cholinergic crisis

Dosage adjustment in renal impairment: Dose may need to be reduced in patients with chronic renal failure

Dosage adjustment in hepatic impairment: No dosage adjustment provided in manufacturer's labeling.

Administration Edrophonium is administered by direct I.V. injection; see Dosage

Monitoring Parameters Pre- and postinjection strength (cranial musculature is most useful); heart rate, respiratory rate, blood pressure

Test Interactions Increased aminotransferase [ALT/AST] (S), amylase (S)

Additional Information Atropine should be administered along with edrophonium when reversing the effects of nondepolarizing agents to antagonize the cholinergic effects at the muscarinic receptors, especially bradycardia. It is important to recognize the difference in dose for diagnosis of myasthenia gravis versus reversal of muscle relaxant, a much larger dose is needed for desired effect of reversal of muscle paralysis.

Dosage Forms Excipient information presented when available (limited, particularly for generics); consult specific product labeling.

Solution, Injection, as chloride:

Enlon: 10 mg/mL (15 mL) [contains phenol]

Edrophonium and Atropine

(ed roe FOE nee um & A troe peen)

Brand Names: U.S. Enlon-Plus®

Index Terms Atropine Sulfate and Edrophonium Chloride; Edrophonium Chloride and Atropine Sulfate

Pharmacologic Category Acetylcholinesterase Inhibitor; Anticholinergic Agent; Antidote

Use Reversal of nondepolarizing neuromuscular blockers; adjunct treatment of respiratory depression caused by curare overdose

Pregnancy Risk Factor C

Dosage I.V.: Adults: Reversal of neuromuscular blockade: 0.05-0.1 mL/kg given over 45-60 seconds. The dose delivered is 0.5-1 mg/kg of edrophonium and 0.007-0.014 mg/kg of atropine. An edrophonium dose of 1 mg/kg should rarely be exceeded. **Note:** Monitor closely for bradyarrhythmias.

Dosage adjustment in renal impairment: Adjustment not required.

Dosage adjustment in hepatic impairment: Adjustment not required.

Additional Information Complete prescribing information should be consulted for additional detail.

Dosage Forms Excipient information presented when available (limited, particularly for generics); consult specific product labeling.

Injection, solution:

Enlon-Plus®: Edrophonium chloride 10 mg/mL and atropine sulfate 0.14 mg/mL (5 mL, 15 mL) [contains sodium sulfite; may contain natural rubber/natural latex in vial]

- **Edrophonium Chloride** *see* Edrophonium *on page* 686
- **Edrophonium Chloride and Atropine Sulfate** *see* Edrophonium and Atropine *on page* 687
- **Ed-Spaz** *see* Hyoscyamine *on page* 1026
- **EDTA (CALCIUM Disodium) (error-prone abbreviation)** *see* Edetate CALCIUM Disodium *on page* 685
- **Edurant** *see* Rilpivirine *on page* 1817
- **Edurant® (Can)** *see* Rilpivirine *on page* 1817

◆ EES (Can) *see* Erythromycin (Systemic) *on page 741*
◆ E.E.S. 400 *see* Erythromycin (Systemic) *on page 741*
◆ E.E.S. Granules *see* Erythromycin (Systemic) *on page 741*

Efavirenz (e FAV e renz)

Brand Names: U.S. Sustiva

Brand Names: Canada Mylan-Efavirenz; Sustiva; Teva-Efavirenz

Pharmacologic Category Antiretroviral, Reverse Transcriptase Inhibitor, Non-nucleoside (Anti-HIV)

Use Treatment of HIV-1 infections in combination with at least two other antiretroviral agents

Pregnancy Risk Factor D

Pregnancy Considerations Teratogenic effects have been observed in primates receiving efavirenz. Efavirenz crosses the placenta. Based on data from the Antiretroviral Pregnancy Registry, an increased risk of overall birth defects has not been observed following first trimester exposure to efavirenz; however, neural tube and other CNS defects have been reported. Due to the low number of first trimester exposures and the low incidence of neural tube defects in the general population, available data are insufficient to evaluate risk. Other antiretroviral agents should strongly be considered for use in women of childbearing potential who are planning to become pregnant or who are sexually active and not using effective contraception. Nonpregnant women of reproductive age should undergo pregnancy testing prior to initiation of efavirenz. Barrier contraception should be used in combination with other (hormonal) methods of contraception during therapy and for 12 weeks after efavirenz is discontinued. Neural tube defects would occur following exposure during the first 5-6 weeks of gestation (most pregnancies are not detected before 4-6 weeks gestation). For women who present in the first trimester already on an efavirenz-containing regimen and who have adequate viral suppression, efavirenz may be continued; changing regimens may lead to loss of viral control and increase the risk of perinatal transmission. Pharmacokinetic data from available studies do not suggest dose alterations are needed during pregnancy. Hypersensitivity reactions (including hepatic toxicity and rash) are more common in women on NNRTI therapy; it is not known if pregnancy increases this risk

Regardless of CD4 count or HIV RNA copy number, all HIV-infected pregnant women should receive a combination antepartum antiretroviral (ARV) drug regimen; this includes women who require therapy for their own health, as well as women who do not yet require therapy for their own health. ARV therapy should be started as soon as possible if required for the woman's health. Although earlier initiation may be more effective in reducing the perinatal transmission of HIV), also consider maternal conditions (eg, nausea and vomiting) and the potential risks of first trimester fetal exposure for specific agents. Plasma HIV RNA levels should be assessed at ~34-36 weeks gestation in order to help determine mode of delivery. If ARV therapy must be interrupted for <24 hours during the peripartum period, stop then restart all medications simultaneously in order to decrease the chance of developing resistance. Long-term follow-up is recommended for all infants exposed to ARV medications.

Healthcare providers are encouraged to enroll pregnant women exposed to antiretroviral medications in the Antiretroviral Pregnancy Registry (1-800-258-4263 or www.-APRegistry.com). Healthcare providers caring for HIV-infected women and their infants may contact the National Perinatal HIV Hotline (888-448-8765) for clinical consultation (DHHS [perinatal], 2012).

Breast-Feeding Considerations Efavirenz is excreted into breast milk. Although breast-feeding is not recommended, plasma concentrations of efavirenz in nursing infants have been reported as ~13% of maternal plasma concentrations.

Maternal or infant antiretroviral therapy does not completely eliminate the risk of postnatal HIV transmission. In addition, multiclass-resistant virus has been detected in breast-feeding infants despite maternal therapy. Therefore, in the United States, where formula is accessible, affordable, safe, and sustainable, and the risk of infant mortality due to diarrhea and respiratory infections is low, complete avoidance of breast-feeding by HIV-infected women is recommended to decrease potential transmission of HIV (DHHS [perinatal], 2012).

Prescribing and Access Restrictions Efavirenz oral solution is available only through an expanded access (compassionate use) program. Enrollment information may be obtained by calling 877-372-7097.

Contraindications Previous significant hypersensitivity (eg, Stevens-Johnson syndrome, erythema multiforme, toxic skin eruptions) to efavirenz or any component of the formulation; concurrent use of bepridil, cisapride, midazolam, pimozide, triazolam, St. John's wort, or ergot alkaloids (includes dihydroergotamine, ergotamine, ergonovine, methylergonovine)

Warnings/Precautions Do not use as single-agent therapy. Avoid pregnancy; women of childbearing potential should undergo pregnancy testing prior to initiation of therapy. Use caution with other agents metabolized by cytochrome P450 isoenzyme 3A4 (see Contraindications); concomitant use of other efavirenz-containing products should be avoided (unless needed for dosage adjustment with concomitant rifampin treatment). Use caution with history of mental illness/drug abuse (predisposition to psychological reactions); may cause CNS and psychiatric symptoms, which include impaired concentration, dizziness or drowsiness (avoid potentially hazardous tasks such as driving or operating machinery if these effects are noted); CNS effects may be potentiated when used with other sedative drugs or ethanol. Serious psychiatric side effects have been associated with efavirenz, including severe depression, suicide, paranoia, and mania; instruct patients to contact healthcare provider if serious psychiatric effects occur. May cause mild-to-moderate maculopapular rash; usually occurs within 2 weeks of starting therapy; discontinue if severe rash (involving blistering, desquamation, mucosal involvement, or fever) develops; contraindicated in patients with a history of a severe cutaneous reaction (eg, Stevens-Johnson syndrome). Children are more susceptible.

Caution in patients with known or suspected hepatitis B or C infection (monitoring of liver function is recommended) or Child-Pugh class A hepatic impairment; not recommended in Child-Pugh class B or C hepatic impairment. Persistent elevations of serum transaminases >5 times the upper limit of normal should prompt evaluation - benefit of continued therapy should be weighed against possible risk of hepatotoxicity. Increases in total cholesterol and triglycerides have been reported; screening should be done prior to therapy and periodically throughout treatment. May cause redistribution of fat (eg, buffalo hump, peripheral wasting with increased abdominal girth, cushingoid appearance). Patients may develop immune reconstitution syndrome resulting in the occurrence of an inflammatory response to an indolent or residual opportunistic infection during initial HIV treatment or activation of autoimmune disorders (eg, Graves' disease, polymyositis, Guillain-Barré syndrome) later in therapy; further evaluation and treatment may be required. Use with caution in patients with a history of seizure disorder; seizures have been associated with use. Efavirenz administered as monotherapy or added on to a failing regimen may result in rapid viral resistance to efavirenz. Consider cross-resistance when adding antiretroviral agents on to efavirenz therapy.

Adverse Reactions Unless otherwise noted, frequency of adverse events is as reported in adults receiving combination antiretroviral therapy.

>10%:

Central nervous system: Dizziness (2% to 28%; children 16%), fever (children 21%), depression (≤19%; severe: 1% to 2%), insomnia (≤16%), anxiety (2% to 13%), pain (1% to 13%; children 14%), headache (2% to 8%; children 11%)

Dermatologic: Rash (5% to 26%, grade 3/4: <1%; children ≤46%, grade 3/4: 2% to 4%)

Endocrine & metabolic: HDL increased (25% to 35%), total cholesterol increased (20% to 40%), triglycerides increased (≥751 mg/dL: 6% to 11%)

Gastrointestinal: Diarrhea (3% to 14%; children: ≤39%), nausea (2% to 10%; children 12%), vomiting (3% to 6%; children 12%)

Respiratory: Cough (children 16%)

1% to 10%:

Central nervous system: Impaired concentration (≤8%), somnolence (≤7%), fatigue (≤8%), abnormal dreams (1% to 6%), nervousness (2% to 7%), hallucinations (1%)

Dermatologic: Pruritus (≤9%)

Endocrine & metabolic: Hyperglycemia (>250 mg/dL: 2% to 5%)

Gastrointestinal: Dyspepsia (≤4%), abdominal pain (2% to 3%), anorexia (≤2%), amylase increased (grade 3/4: ≤6%)

Hematologic: Neutropenia (grade 3/4: 2% to 10%)

Hepatic: Incidence higher with hepatitis B and/or C coinfection: ALT increased (grades 3/4: 2% to 8%), AST increased (grades 3/4: 5% to 8%)

<1% (Limited to important or life-threatening): Allergic reaction, ataxia, body fat accumulation/redistribution, cerebellar coordination disturbances, delusions, dermatitis (photoallergic), erythema multiforme, gynecomastia, hepatic failure, hepatitis, immune reconstitution syndrome, malabsorption, mania, neuropathy, neurosis, palpitations, pancreatitis, paranoia, psychosis, seizures, Stevens-Johnson syndrome, suicide attempts, suicidal ideation, visual abnormalities

Drug Interactions

Metabolism/Transport Effects **Substrate** of CYP2B6 (major), CYP3A4 (major); **Note:** Assignment of Major/Minor substrate status based on clinically relevant drug interaction potential; **Inhibits** CYP2C19 (moderate), CYP2C9 (moderate), CYP3A4 (moderate); **Induces** CYP2B6 (weak/moderate), CYP3A4 (weak/moderate)

Avoid Concomitant Use

Avoid concomitant use of Efavirenz with any of the following: Atovaquone; Axitinib; Azelastine (Nasal); Bepridil [Off Market]; Boceprevir; Bosutinib; CarBAMazepine; Cisapride; Dihydroergotamine; Ergoloid Mesylates; Ergonovine; Ergotamine; Etravirine; Ibrutinib; Ivabradine; Lomitapide; Methylergonovine; Midazolam; Nevirapine; Paraldehyde; Pimozide; Posaconazole; Rilpivirine; Simeprevir; St Johns Wort; Tolvaptan; Triazolam; Ulipristal

Increased Effect/Toxicity

Efavirenz may increase the levels/effects of: Alcohol (Ethyl); ARIPiprazole; Avanafil; Azelastine (Nasal); Bepridil [Off Market]; Bosentan; Bosutinib; Budesonide (Systemic, Oral Inhalation); Carvedilol; Cisapride; Citalopram; CNS Depressants; Colchicine; CYP2C19 Substrates; CYP2C9 Substrates; CYP3A4 Substrates; Dihydroergotamine; Dofetilide; Eplerenone; Ergoloid Mesylates; Ergonovine; Ergotamine; Etravirine; FentaNYL; Fosphenytoin; Halofantrine; Hydrocodone; Ibrutinib; Imatinib; Ivabradine; Ivacaftor; Lomitapide; Lurasidone; Methotrimeprazine; Methylergonovine; Metyrosine; Midazolam; Mirtazapine; Nevirapine; OxyCODONE; Paraldehyde; Phenytoin; Pimecrolimus; Pimozide; Pramipexole; Propafenone; Ranolazine; Rilpivirine; Ritonavir; ROPINIRole; Rotigotine; Salmeterol; Saxagliptin; Selective Serotonin Reuptake Inhibitors; Simeprevir; Tolvaptan; Triazolam; Ulipristal; Vilazodone; Vitamin K Antagonists; Zolpidem; Zuclopenthixol

The levels/effects of Efavirenz may be increased by: Boceprevir; Brimonidine (Topical); CYP2B6 Inhibitors (Moderate); CYP2B6 Inhibitors (Strong); Darunavir; Doxylamine; Droperidol; HydrOXYzine; Magnesium Sulfate; Methotrimeprazine; Mifepristone; Nevirapine; Perampanel; Quazepam; Ritonavir; Saquinavir; Sodium Oxybate; Tapentadol; Voriconazole

Decreased Effect

Efavirenz may decrease the levels/effects of: Alcohol (Ethyl); ARIPiprazole; Atazanavir; AtorvaSTATin; Atovaquone; Axitinib; Boceprevir; Buprenorphine; BuPROPion; CarBAMazepine; Caspofungin; Clopidogrel; CycloSPORINE (Systemic); Darunavir; Dolutegravir; Etonogestrel; Etravirine; Everolimus; Fosamprenavir; Ibrutinib; Ifosfamide; Indinavir; Itraconazole; Lopinavir; Lovastatin; Methadone; Norgestimate; Posaconazole; Pravastatin; Proguanil; Raltegravir; Rifabutin; Rilpivirine; Saquinavir; Saxagliptin; Sertraline; Simeprevir; Simvastatin; Sirolimus; Tacrolimus (Systemic); Telaprevir; Vitamin K Antagonists; Voriconazole

The levels/effects of Efavirenz may be decreased by: Bosentan; CarBAMazepine; CYP3A4 Inducers (Strong); Dabrafenib; Deferasirox; Fosphenytoin; Mitotane; Nevirapine; Phenytoin; Rifabutin; Rifampin; St Johns Wort; Telaprevir; Tocilizumab

Ethanol/Nutrition/Herb Interactions

Ethanol: Ethanol may increase hepatotoxic potential of efavirenz and increase CNS depression. Management: Limit or avoid ethanol.

Food: High-fat meals increase the absorption of efavirenz. CNS effects are possible. Management: Avoid high-fat meals. Administer at or before bedtime on an empty stomach unless using capsule sprinkle method in patients unable to swallow capsules or tablets. If capsule sprinkle method is used, patient should not consume additional food for 2 hours after administration.

Herb/Nutraceutical: St John's wort may decrease efavirenz serum levels. Management: Avoid concurrent use.

Storage/Stability Store at 25°C (77°F); excursion permitted to 15°C to 30°C (59°F to 86°F).

Mechanism of Action As a non-nucleoside reverse transcriptase inhibitor, efavirenz has activity against HIV-1 by binding to reverse transcriptase. It consequently blocks the RNA-dependent and DNA-dependent DNA polymerase activities including HIV-1 replication. It does not require intracellular phosphorylation for antiviral activity.

Pharmacodynamics/Kinetics

Absorption: Increased by fatty meals

Distribution: CSF concentrations exceed free fraction in serum

Protein binding: >99%, primarily to albumin

Metabolism: Hepatic via CYP3A4 and 2B6 to inactive hydroxylated metabolites; may induce its own metabolism

Half-life elimination: Single dose: 52-76 hours; Multiple doses: 40-55 hours

Time to peak: 3-5 hours

Excretion: Feces (16% to 61% primarily as unchanged drug); urine (14% to 34% as metabolites)

Dosage Oral: HIV infection (as part of combination therapy):

Children ≥3 months and ≥3.5 kg: Dosage is based on body weight:

3.5 kg to <5 kg: 100 mg once daily
5 kg to <7.5 kg: 150 mg once daily
7.5 kg to <15 kg: 200 mg once daily
15 kg to <20 kg: 250 mg once daily
20 kg to <25 kg: 300 mg once daily
25 kg to <32.5 kg: 350 mg once daily
32.5 kg to <40 kg: 400 mg once daily
≥40 kg: 600 mg once daily; **Note:** Dosage adjustments may be necessary if patient receives certain concomitant medications. Refer to adult dosing.

Adults: 600 mg once daily; preferred regimen for therapy-naive patients with tenofovir and emtricitabine (DHHS, 2013)

Dosage adjustment for concomitant rifampin (only if patient weighs ≥50 kg): Increase efavirenz dose to 800 mg once daily

Dosage adjustment for concomitant voriconazole: Reduce efavirenz dose to 300 mg once daily and increase voriconazole to 400 mg every 12 hours

Dosing adjustment in renal impairment: No dosage adjustment provided in manufacturer's labeling (has not been studied); however, undergoes minimal renal excretion.

Dosing comments in hepatic impairment:

Mild impairment (Child-Pugh class A): No dosage adjustment necessary; use with caution.

Moderate-to-severe impairment (Child-Pugh class B or C): No dosage adjustment provided in manufacturer's labeling (has not been adequately studied); use not recommended.

Dietary Considerations Should be taken on an empty stomach unless using capsule sprinkle method in patients unable to swallow capsules or tablets. If capsule sprinkle method is used, do not consume additional food for 2 hours after administration.

Administration Administer on an empty stomach. Dosing at or before bedtime is recommended to limit central nervous system effects (DHHS, 2013). Tablets should not be broken.

Capsule contents may be sprinkled onto a small amount of soft food (eg, applesauce, grape jelly, yogurt) for pediatric or adult patients who cannot swallow capsules. Place 1-2 teaspoonfuls of food in a small container. Hold capsule horizontally over container and carefully twist in opposite directions to open, sprinkling contents over food. If more than 1 capsule is needed for a dose, add contents of all capsules needed to 1-2 teaspoonfuls of food; do not add more food. Use a small spoon to gently mix capsule contents with food and administer all of mixture to patient. To ensure entire capsule contents are administered, add another 2 teaspoonfuls of food to the container, mix to incorporate any drug residue, and administer.

Capsule contents may also be mixed with infant formula only for pediatric patients who cannot reliably consume solid foods. Combine entire contents of capsule(s) with 10 mL of reconstituted, room temperature infant formula in a 30 mL medicine cup, stir carefully, then draw up mixture in a 10 mL oral syringe for administration. If more than 1 capsule is needed for a dose, add contents of all capsules needed to 10 mL of formula; do not add more formula. To ensure entire capsule contents are administered, add another 10 mL of formula to the cup, stir to incorporate any drug residue, draw up in oral syringe and administer.

Administer within 30 minutes of mixing. Patient should not consume any additional food or administer additional formula for 2 hours after administration.

Monitoring Parameters Serum transaminases (discontinuation of treatment should be considered for persistent elevations >5 times the upper limit of normal); cholesterol and triglycerides (prior to therapy and periodically during); signs and symptoms of infection; psychiatric effects

Test Interactions False-positive tests for cannabinoids have been reported when the CEDIA DAU Multilevel THC assay is used. False-positive results with other assays for cannabinoids have not been observed. False-positive tests for benzodiazepines have been reported and are likely due to the 8-hydroxy-efavirenz major metabolite.

Additional Information Early virologic failure was observed with tenofovir and didanosine delayed release capsules, plus either efavirenz or nevirapine; use caution in treatment-naive patients with high baseline viral loads.

Dosage Forms Excipient information presented when available (limited, particularly for generics); consult specific product labeling.

Capsule, Oral:
Sustiva: 50 mg, 200 mg

Tablet, Oral:
Sustiva: 600 mg

Efavirenz, Emtricitabine, and Tenofovir

(e FAV e renz, em trye SYE ta been, & ten OF oh vir)

Brand Names: U.S. Atripla

Brand Names: Canada Atripla

Index Terms Emtricitabine, Efavirenz, and Tenofovir; FTC, TDF, and EFV; Tenofovir Disoproxil Fumarate, Efavirenz, and Emtricitabine

Pharmacologic Category Antiretroviral, Reverse Transcriptase Inhibitor, Non-nucleoside (Anti-HIV); Antiretroviral, Reverse Transcriptase Inhibitor, Nucleoside (Anti-HIV); Antiretroviral, Reverse Transcriptase Inhibitor, Nucleotide (Anti-HIV)

Use Treatment of HIV-1 infection

Pregnancy Risk Factor D

Dosage Note: Prior to initiation, patients should be tested for hepatitis B infection, and baseline estimated creatinine clearance, serum phosphorus, urine glucose, and urine protein should be assessed in all patients.

Oral: Children ≥12 years and ≥40 kg, Adolescents, and Adults: One tablet once daily. **Note:** Recommended as an initial regimen for antiretroviral-naive patients (DHHS, 2013).

Dosage adjustment in renal impairment: Moderate-to-severe renal impairment (Cl_{cr} <50 mL/minute): Use not recommended

Dosage adjustment in hepatic impairment:

Mild hepatic impairment (Child-Pugh class A): Use with caution

Moderate or severe hepatic impairment (Child-Pugh class B, C): Not recommended

Additional Information Complete prescribing information should be consulted for additional detail.

Dosage Forms Excipient information presented when available (limited, particularly for generics); consult specific product labeling.

Tablet:
Atripla®: Efavirenz 600 mg, emtricitabine 200 mg, and tenofovir disoproxil fumarate 300 mg

◆ **Effer-K®** *see* Potassium Bicarbonate and Potassium Citrate *on page* 1684
◆ **Effexor XR** *see* Venlafaxine *on page* 2178
◆ **Effient** *see* Prasugrel *on page* 1699
◆ **Effient® (Can)** *see* Prasugrel *on page* 1699

Eflornithine (ee FLOR ni theen)

Brand Names: U.S. Vaniqa
Brand Names: Canada Vaniqa®
Index Terms DFMO; Eflornithine Hydrochloride
Pharmacologic Category Antiprotozoal; Topical Skin Product
Use Reduce unwanted hair from face and adjacent areas under the chin
Unlabeled Use Injection: Treatment of meningoencephalitic stage of *Trypanosoma brucei gambiense* infection (sleeping sickness). **Note:** Eflornithine has specific activity against *T.b. gambiense* in early and late stages (not effective for *T.b. rhodesiense*).
Pregnancy Risk Factor C
Prescribing and Access Restrictions Injectable eflornithine is donated to World Health Organization (WHO) by the manufacturer. Further information may be found on WHO website at http://www.who.int/trypanosomiasis_african/diagnosis/en/index.html or by contacting the CDC Drug Service (404-639-3670).
Dosage
Children ≥12 years and Adults: Females: Topical: Unwanted facial hair: Apply thin layer of cream to affected areas of face and areas under the chin twice daily, at least 8 hours apart
Adults: I.V. infusion: Treatment of infections caused by *Trypanosoma brucei gambiense* infection (sleeping sickness) (unlabeled use): 100 mg/kg/dose given every 6 hours for 14 days (Kappagoda, 2011)
Dosing adjustment in renal impairment: Injection: Dose should be adjusted although no specific guidelines are available.
Additional Information Complete prescribing information should be consulted for additional detail.
Dosage Forms Excipient information presented when available (limited, particularly for generics); consult specific product labeling. [DSC] = Discontinued product
Cream, External, as hydrochloride:
Vaniqa: 13.9% (30 g [DSC], 45 g) [contains cetearyl alcohol, methylparaben, propylparaben]

- ◆ **Eflornithine Hydrochloride** *see* Eflornithine *on page 691*
- ◆ **Eformoterol and Budesonide** *see* Budesonide and Formoterol *on page 287*
- ◆ **Efudex** *see* Fluorouracil (Topical) *on page 885*
- ◆ **Efudex® (Can)** *see* Fluorouracil (Topical) *on page 885*
- ◆ **Egrifta** *see* Tesamorelin *on page 2025*
- ◆ **EHDP** *see* Etidronate *on page 798*
- ◆ **Eicosapentaenoic Acid** *see* Omega-3-Acid Ethyl Esters *on page 1504*
- ◆ **EL-970** *see* Dalfampridine *on page 534*
- ◆ **Elaprase** *see* Idursulfase *on page 1041*
- ◆ **Elavil** *see* Amitriptyline *on page 105*
- ◆ **Eldepryl** *see* Selegiline *on page 1884*
- ◆ **Eldopaque [OTC] [DSC]** *see* Hydroquinone *on page 1017*
- ◆ **Eldopaque® (Can)** *see* Hydroquinone *on page 1017*
- ◆ **Eldopaque Forte [DSC]** *see* Hydroquinone *on page 1017*
- ◆ **Eldoquin [OTC] [DSC]** *see* Hydroquinone *on page 1017*
- ◆ **Eldoquin® (Can)** *see* Hydroquinone *on page 1017*
- ◆ **Eldoquin Forte [DSC]** *see* Hydroquinone *on page 1017*
- ◆ **Electrolyte Lavage Solution** *see* Polyethylene Glycol-Electrolyte Solution *on page 1669*

Electrolyte Solution, Renal Replacement
(ee LEK trow lite soe LOO shun REE nil ree PLASE ment)

Brand Names: U.S. Normocarb HF® 25; Normocarb HF® 35; PrismaSol
Index Terms Continuous Renal Replacement Therapy; CRRT; Renal Replacement Solution
Pharmacologic Category Alkalinizing Agent; Electrolyte Supplement
Use Used as a replacement solution to replenish water, correct electrolytes, and adjust acid-base balance depleted by hemofiltration or hemodiafiltration (continuous renal replacement therapy [CRRT]); drug poisoning when CRRT is used to remove filterable substances
Dosage Note: If using PrismaSol™, ensure that compartment A and B are mixed.
Continuous renal replacement circuit: Children and Adults:
Pre- or post-filter: Volume of solution administered depends upon the patient's fluid balance, target fluid balance, body weight, and amount of fluid removed during hemofiltration process.
Post-filter replacement: Volume infused/hour should not be greater than 1/3 of blood flow rate (eg, blood flow rate 100 mL/minute [6000 mL/hour], post-filter replacement rate ≤2000 mL/hour)
Dosage adjustment in hepatic impairment: Ability to convert lactate to bicarbonate may be impaired; use solutions containing lactate cautiously.
Additional Information Complete prescribing information should be consulted for additional detail.
Dosage Forms Excipient information presented when available (limited, particularly for generics); consult specific product labeling.
Injection, solution [concentrate; preservative free]:
Normocarb HF® 25: Bicarbonate 25 mEq/L, chloride 116.5 mEq/L, magnesium 1.5 mEq/L, sodium 140 mEq/L (240 mL) [strength represents final solution after mixing; when diluted as directed, makes 3240 mL of infusate]
Normocarb HF® 35: Bicarbonate 35 mEq/L, chloride 106.5 mEq/L, magnesium 1.5 mEq/L, sodium 140 mEq/L (240 mL) [strength represents final solution after mixing; when diluted as directed, makes 3240 mL of infusate]
Injection, solution [preservative free]:
PrismaSol B22GK 2/0: Bicarbonate 22 mEq/L, chloride 118.5 mEq/L, dextrose 100 mg/dL, lactate 3 mEq/L, magnesium 1.5 mEq/L, potassium 2 mEq/L, sodium 140 mEq/L (5000 mL) [strength represents final solution after mixing]
PrismaSol BGK 2/0: Bicarbonate 32 mEq/L, chloride 108 mEq/L, dextrose 100 mg/dL, lactate 3 mEq/L, magnesium 1 mEq/L, potassium 2 mEq/L, sodium 140 mEq/L (5000 mL) [strength represents final solution after mixing]
PrismaSol BGK 2/3.5: Bicarbonate 32 mEq/L, calcium 3.5 mEq/L, chloride 111.5 mEq/L, dextrose 100 mg/dL, lactate 3 mEq/L, magnesium 1 mEq/L, potassium 2 mEq/L, sodium 140 mEq/L (5000 mL) [strength represents final solution after mixing]
PrismaSol BGK 4/0/1.2: Bicarbonate 32 mEq/L, chloride 110.2 mEq/L, dextrose 100 mg/dL, lactate 3 mEq/L, magnesium 1.2 mEq/L, potassium 4 mEq/L, sodium 140 mEq/L (5000 mL) [strength represents final solution after mixing]
PrismaSol BGK 4/2.5: Bicarbonate 32 mEq/L, calcium 2.5 mEq/L, chloride 113 mEq/L, dextrose 100 mg/dL, lactate 3 mEq/L, magnesium 1.5 mEq/L, potassium 4 mEq/L, sodium 140 mEq/L (5000 mL) [strength represents final solution after mixing]

PrismaSol BK 0/0/1.2: Bicarbonate 32 mEq/L, chloride 106.2 mEq/L, lactate 3 mEq/L, magnesium 1.2 mEq/L, sodium 140 mEq/L (5000 mL) [strength represents final solution after mixing]

◆ Elelyso *see* Taliglucerase Alfa *on page 1986*

◆ Elestrin *see* Estradiol (Systemic) *on page 754*

Eletriptan (el e TRIP tan)

Brand Names: U.S. Relpax

Brand Names: Canada Relpax®

Index Terms Eletriptan Hydrobromide

Pharmacologic Category Antimigraine Agent; Serotonin 5-$HT_{1B,\ 1D}$ Receptor Agonist

Additional Appendix Information

Antimigraine Drugs: 5-HT_1 Receptor Agonists *on page 2288*

Use Migraines: Acute treatment of migraine, with or without aura in adults

Pregnancy Risk Factor C

Pregnancy Considerations Adverse events were observed in animal reproduction studies. Information related to eletriptan use in pregnancy is limited (Källén, 2011; Nezvalová-Henriksen, 2010; Nezvalová-Henriksen, 2012). Until additional information is available, other agents are preferred for the initial treatment of migraine in pregnancy (Da Silva, 2012; MacGregor, 2012; Williams, 2012).

Breast-Feeding Considerations Eletriptan is excreted in breast milk. Eight women were given a single dose of eletriptan 80 mg. The amount of drug detected in breast milk over 24 hours was ~0.02% of the maternal dose and the milk-to-plasma ratio was variable. The presence of the active metabolite was not measured. The manufacturer recommends that caution be exercised when administering eletriptan to nursing women.

Contraindications

Ischemic coronary artery disease (eg, angina pectoris, history of myocardial infarction, documented silent ischemia); coronary artery vasospasm, including Prinzmetal's angina; Wolff-Parkinson-White syndrome or arrhythmias associated with other cardiac accessory conduction pathway disorders; history of stroke, transient ischemic attack, or history or current evidence of hemiplegic or basilar migraine; peripheral vascular disease; ischemic bowel disease; uncontrolled hypertension; recent use (within 24 hours) of treatment with another 5-HT_1 agonist, or an ergotamine-containing or ergot-type medication (eg, dihydroergotamine or methysergide); recent use (within at least 72 hours) of the following potent CYP3A4 inhibitors: ketoconazole, itraconazole, nefazodone, troleandomycin, clarithromycin, ritonavir, or nelfinavir; known hypersensitivity to eletriptan or any component of the formulation.

Canadian labeling: Additional contraindications (not in U.S. labeling): Cardiac arrhythmias (especially tachycardias), valvular heart disease, congenital heart disease, atherosclerotic disease; management of ophthalmoplegic migraine; Raynaud's syndrome; severe hepatic impairment.

Documentation of allergenic cross-reactivity for serotonin 5-HT_1 receptor agonists (triptans) in this class is limited. However, because of similarities in chemical structure and/or pharmacologic actions, the possibility of cross-sensitivity cannot be ruled out with certainty.

Warnings/Precautions Only indicated for treatment of acute migraine; not indicated for migraine prophylaxis, or for the treatment of cluster headache, hemiplegic or basilar migraine. If a patient does not respond to the first dose, the diagnosis of migraine should be reconsidered. Acute migraine agents (eg, triptans, opioids, ergotamine, or a combination of the agents) used for 10 or more days per month may lead to worsening of headaches (medication overuse headache); withdrawal treatment may be necessary in the setting of overuse. Do not give to patients with risk factors for CAD until a cardiovascular evaluation has been performed; if evaluation is satisfactory, the health care provider should administer the first dose (consider ECG monitoring) and cardiovascular status should be periodically evaluated. Cardiac events (coronary artery vasospasm, transient ischemia, MI, ventricular tachycardia/fibrillation, cardiac arrest, and death), cerebral/subarachnoid hemorrhage, stroke (some fatal), peripheral vascular ischemia, gastrointestinal vascular ischemia/infarction, and Raynaud's syndrome have been reported with 5-HT_1 agonist administration. Patients who experience sensations of chest pain/pressure/tightness or symptoms suggestive of angina following dosing should be evaluated for coronary artery disease or Prinzmetal's angina before receiving additional doses; if dosing is resumed and similar symptoms recur, monitor with ECG. Significant elevation in blood pressure, including hypertensive crisis with acute impairment of organ systems, has been reported on rare occasions in patients with and without a history of hypertension; monitor blood pressure.

Not recommended for use in patients with severe hepatic impairment; the Canadian labeling contraindicates use in patients with severe impairment. Symptoms of agitation, confusion, hallucinations, hyper-reflexia, myoclonus, shivering, and tachycardia (serotonin syndrome) may occur with concomitant proserotonergic drugs (ie, SSRIs/SNRIs or triptans) or agents which reduce eletriptan's metabolism. Concurrent use of serotonin precursors (eg, tryptophan) is not recommended. If concomitant administration with SSRIs is warranted, monitor closely, especially at initiation and with dose increases. Discontinue eletriptan if serotonin syndrome is suspected. Potentially significant drug-drug interactions may exist, requiring dose or frequency adjustment, additional monitoring, and/or selection of alternative therapy. Use is contraindicated within 72 hours of patients taking strong CYP3A4 inhibitors. Anaphylaxis, anaphylactoid, and hypersensitivity reactions (including angioedema) have occurred; may be life-threatening or fatal.

Adverse Reactions

1% to 10%:

Cardiovascular: Chest pain/tightness (1% to 4%; placebo 1%), palpitation

Central nervous system: Dizziness (3% to 7%; placebo 3%), somnolence (3% to 7%; placebo 4%), headache (3% to 4%; placebo 3%), chills, pain, vertigo

Gastrointestinal: Nausea (4% to 8%; placebo 5%), xerostomia (2% to 4%, placebo 2%), dysphagia (1% to 2%), abdominal pain/discomfort (1% to 2%; placebo 1%), dyspepsia (1% to 2%; placebo 1%)

Neuromuscular & skeletal: Weakness (4% to 10%), paresthesia (3% to 4%), back pain, hypertonia, hypoesthesia

Respiratory: Pharyngitis

Miscellaneous: Diaphoresis

<1% (Limited to important or life-threatening): Agitation, allergic reaction, angina, arrhythmia, ataxia, confusion, CPK increased, depersonalization, depression, dyspnea, edema, emotional lability, esophagitis, euphoria, hyperesthesia, hyperkinesia, hypertension, impotence, incoordination, insomnia, lacrimation disorder, liver function tests abnormal, myalgia, myasthenia, peripheral vascular disorder, photophobia, polyuria, pruritus, rash, seizure, shock, speech disorder, stupor, tachycardia, thrombophlebitis, tinnitus, tongue edema, tremor, urinary frequency, vasospasm, vision abnormal

Drug Interactions

Metabolism/Transport Effects **Substrate** of CYP3A4 (major); **Note:** Assignment of Major/Minor substrate status based on clinically relevant drug interaction potential

Avoid Concomitant Use

Avoid concomitant use of Eletriptan with any of the following: Conivaptan; Ergot Derivatives; Fusidic Acid (Systemic); Itraconazole; Ketoconazole (Systemic); Posaconazole; Voriconazole

Increased Effect/Toxicity

Eletriptan may increase the levels/effects of: Antipsychotics; Ergot Derivatives; Metoclopramide; Serotonin Modulators

The levels/effects of Eletriptan may be increased by: Antipsychotics; Calcium Channel Blockers (Nondihydropyridine); Conivaptan; CYP3A4 Inhibitors (Moderate); CYP3A4 Inhibitors (Strong); Dasatinib; Ergot Derivatives; Fluconazole; Fusidic Acid (Systemic); Itraconazole; Ivacaftor; Ketoconazole (Systemic); Luliconazole; Macrolide Antibiotics; Mifepristone; Posaconazole; Simeprevir; Voriconazole

Decreased Effect There are no known significant interactions involving a decrease in effect.

Ethanol/Nutrition/Herb Interactions Food: High-fat meal increases bioavailability.

Storage/Stability Store at 20°C to 25°C (68°F to77°F); excursions are permitted between 15°C and 30°C (59°F and 86°F).

Mechanism of Action Selective agonist for serotonin (5-HT_{1B}, 5-HT_{1D} and 5-HT_{1F} receptors) in cranial arteries; causes vasoconstriction and reduces sterile inflammation associated with antidromic neuronal transmission correlating with relief of migraine

Pharmacodynamics/Kinetics

Absorption: Well absorbed

Distribution: V_d: 138 L

Protein binding: ~85%

Metabolism: Hepatic via CYP3A4; forms one metabolite (active)

Bioavailability: ~50%, increased with high-fat meal

Half-life elimination: ~4 hours (Elderly: 4.4-5.7 hours); Metabolite: ~13 hours

Time to peak, plasma: 1.5-2 hours

Dosage Note: If the first dose is ineffective, diagnosis needs to be re-evaluated. Safety of treating >3 headaches/month has not been established.

U.S. labeling: Acute migraine: Adults: Oral: Initial: 20-40 mg as a single dose (maximum: 40 mg/dose); if the headache improves but returns, dose may be repeated after 2 hours have elapsed since first dose (maximum: 80 mg daily)

Canadian labeling: Acute migraine: Adults: Oral: Initial: 20-40 mg as a single dose (maximum: 40 mg/dose). If after an initial dose of 20 mg, the headache improves but returns a repeat 20 mg dose may be administered after 2 hours have elapsed since first dose. If an initial dose of 40 mg was administered, a repeat dose is not recommended (maximum: 40 mg daily).

Dosage adjustment in renal impairment: No dosing adjustment provided in manufacturer's labeling, however, dosage adjustment likely not needed based on pharmacokinetic analysis; monitor for increased blood pressure.

Dosage adjustment in hepatic impairment:

Mild-to-moderate impairment: No dosage adjustment necessary

Severe impairment:

U.S. labeling: Use is not recommended.

Canadian labeling: Use is contraindicated.

Administration Administer orally as soon as symptoms appear. May take with or without food.

Monitoring Parameters Headache severity; signs/symptoms suggestive of angina; blood pressure, heart rate, and/or ECG with first dose in patients with likelihood of unrecognized coronary disease, such as patients with significant hypertension, hypercholesterolemia, obese patients, patients with diabetes, smokers with other risk factors or strong family history of coronary artery disease; signs/symptoms of serotonin syndrome and hypersensitivity reactions

Dosage Forms Excipient information presented when available (limited, particularly for generics); consult specific product labeling.

Tablet, Oral:

Relpax: 20 mg, 40 mg

◆ **Eletriptan Hydrobromide** *see* Eletriptan *on page* 692

◆ **Elidel** *see* Pimecrolimus *on page* 1647

◆ **Elidel® (Can)** *see* Pimecrolimus *on page* 1647

◆ **Eligard** *see* Leuprolide *on page* 1189

◆ **Elimite** *see* Permethrin *on page* 1624

◆ **Eliphos** *see* Calcium Acetate *on page* 317

◆ **Eliquis** *see* Apixaban *on page* 152

◆ **Eliquis® (Can)** *see* Apixaban *on page* 152

◆ **Elitek** *see* Rasburicase *on page* 1788

◆ **Elixophyllin** *see* Theophylline *on page* 2042

◆ **ElixSure Congestion [OTC]** *see* Pseudoephedrine *on page* 1746

◆ **Ella** *see* Ulipristal *on page* 2138

◆ **Ellence** *see* Epirubicin *on page* 718

◆ **Ellence® (Can)** *see* Epirubicin *on page* 718

◆ **Elmiron** *see* Pentosan Polysulfate Sodium *on page* 1617

◆ **Elmiron® (Can)** *see* Pentosan Polysulfate Sodium *on page* 1617

◆ **Elocom (Can)** *see* Mometasone (Topical) *on page* 1395

◆ **Elocon** *see* Mometasone (Topical) *on page* 1395

◆ **Eloxatin** *see* Oxaliplatin *on page* 1524

◆ **Elspar** *see* Asparaginase (*E. coli*) *on page* 174

◆ **Eltor® (Can)** *see* Pseudoephedrine *on page* 1746

Eltrombopag (el TROM boe pag)

Brand Names: U.S. Promacta

Brand Names: Canada Revolade™

Index Terms Eltrombopag Olamine; Revolade®; SB-497115; SB-497115-GR

Pharmacologic Category Colony Stimulating Factor; Thrombopoietic Agent

Use Treatment of thrombocytopenia in patients with chronic immune thrombocytopenia (ITP) at risk for bleeding who have had insufficient response to corticosteroids, immune globulin, or splenectomy; treatment of thrombocytopenia in patients with chronic hepatitis C in order to allow and maintain interferon-based therapy

Pregnancy Risk Factor C

Pregnancy Considerations Adverse effects were observed in animal reproduction studies. Use during pregnancy only if the potential benefit to the mother outweighs the potential risk to the fetus. A Promacta® pregnancy registry has been established to monitor outcomes of women exposed to eltrombopag during pregnancy (1-888-825-5249).

Breast-Feeding Considerations It is not known if eltrombopag is excreted in breast milk. Due to the potential for serious adverse effects in the nursing infant, the decision to discontinue therapy or to discontinue breast-feeding should take into account the importance of treatment to the mother.

Medication Guide Available Yes

Contraindications There are no contraindications listed within the manufacturer's labeling.

Warnings/Precautions **[U.S. Boxed Warning]: May cause hepatotoxicity; obtain ALT, AST, and bilirubin prior to treatment initiation, every 2 weeks during adjustment phase, then monthly (after stable dose established); obtain fractionation for elevated bilirubin levels. Repeat abnormal liver function tests within 3-5 days; if confirmed abnormal, monitor weekly until resolves, stabilizes, or returns to baseline. Discontinue treatment for ALT levels ≥3 times the upper limit of normal (ULN) in patients with normal hepatic function, or ≥3 times baseline in those with pre-existing transaminase elevations and which are progressive, or persistent (≥4 weeks), or accompanied by increased direct bilirubin, or accompanied by clinical signs of liver injury or evidence of hepatic decompensation.** Reinitiation is not recommended; hepatotoxicity usually recurred with retreatment after therapy interruption; however, if the benefit of treatment outweighs the hepatotoxicity risk, initiate carefully, and monitor liver function tests weekly during the dose adjustment phase; permanently discontinue if hepatotoxicity recurs with rechallenge. Use with caution in patients with pre-existing hepatic impairment (clearance may be reduced); dosage reductions are recommended in patients with ITP who have hepatic dysfunction (no initial dose reductions are necessary in patients with chronic hepatitis C-related thrombocytopenia); monitor closely.

[U.S. Boxed Warning]: May increase risk of hepatic decompensation when used in combination with interferon and ribavirin in patients with chronic hepatitis C. In clinical trials, patients with low albumin (<3.5 g/dL) or a Model for End-Stage Liver Disease (MELD) score ≥10 at baseline had an increased risk of hepatic decompensation; closely monitor these patients during therapy. If antiviral therapy is discontinued for hepatic decompensation according to interferon/ribavirin recommendations, eltrombopag should also be discontinued. Indirect hyperbilirubinemia is commonly observed with eltrombopag when used in combination with peginterferon and ribavirin. In addition, ascites, encephalopathy, and thrombotic events were reported more frequently than placebo in chronic hepatitis C trials.

May increase the risk for bone marrow reticulin formation or progression; collagen fibrosis (not associated with cytopenias) was observed in clinical trials. In an extension study, myelofibrosis (≤ grade 1) was observed in a majority of bone marrow biopsies performed after 1 year of treatment. Monitor peripheral blood smear for cellular morphologic abnormalities; analyze CBC monthly; discontinue treatment with onset of new or worsening abnormalities (eg, teardrop and nucleated RBC, immature WBC) or cytopenias and consider bone marrow biopsy (with staining for fibrosis).

Thromboembolism may occur with excess increases in platelet levels. Use with caution in patients with known risk factors for thromboembolism (eg, Factor V Leiden, ATIII deficiency, antiphospholipid syndrome, chronic liver disease). Thrombotic events, primarily involving the portal venous system, were more commonly seen in eltrombopag-treated chronic hepatitis C patients with thrombocytopenia (when compared to placebo). In addition, portal venous thrombosis was reported in a study of non-ITP thrombocytopenic patients with chronic liver disease undergoing elective invasive procedures receiving eltrombopag 75 mg once daily for 14 days as a preparative regimen to reduce platelet transfusions (not an FDA-approved indication). Stimulation of cell surface thrombopoietin (TPO) receptors may increase the risk for hematologic malignancies.

Cataract formation or worsening was observed in clinical trials. Monitor regularly for signs and symptoms of cataracts; obtain ophthalmic exam at baseline and during therapy. Use with caution in patients at risk for cataracts (eg, advanced age, long-term glucocorticoid use). Allow at least 4 hours between dosing of eltrombopag and antacids, minerals (eg, iron, calcium, aluminum, magnesium, selenium, zinc), or foods high in calcium; may reduce eltrombopag levels. Patients of East-Asian ethnicity (eg, Chinese, Japanese, Korean, Taiwanese) may have greater drug exposure (compared to non-East Asians); therapy should be initiated with lower starting doses in ITP patients. Use with caution in renal impairment (any degree) and monitor closely; initial dosage adjustment is not necessary.

Do not use to normalize platelet counts. *ITP:* Indicated only when the degree of thrombocytopenia and clinical conditions increase the risk for bleeding in patients with chronic immune ITP; use the lowest dose necessary to achieve and maintain platelet count ≥50,000/mm^3. Discontinue if platelet count does not respond to a level to avoid clinically important bleeding after 4 weeks at the maximum recommended dose. *Chronic hepatitis C-associated thrombocytopenia:* Use only when thrombocytopenia prevents the initiation and maintenance of interferon-based therapy; discontinue if antiviral therapy is discontinued. Safety and efficacy have not been established when combined with direct acting antiviral medications approved for chronic hepatitis C genotype 1 infection therapy.

Adverse Reactions Adverse reactions and incidences reported are associated with ITP unless otherwise indicated.

>10%:

- Central nervous system: Fever (chronic hepatitis C 30%), fatigue (4%; chronic hepatitis C 28%), headache (10%; chronic hepatitis C 21%), insomnia (chronic hepatitis C 16%), chills (chronic hepatitis C 14%)
- Dermatologic: Pruritus (chronic hepatitis C 15%)
- Gastrointestinal: Diarrhea (9%; chronic hepatitis C 19%), nausea (4% to 9%; chronic hepatitis C 19%), appetite decreased (chronic hepatitis C 18%)
- Hematologic: Myelofibrosis (bone marrow biopsy: Grade ≤1: 93%; grade 2: 7%; grade 3: <3%) anemia (chronic hepatitis C 40%)
- Hepatic: Liver function tests abnormal (11%)
- Neuromuscular & skeletal: Weakness (chronic hepatitis C 16%), myalgia (5% to 12%)
- Respiratory: Cough (chronic hepatitis C 15%)
- Miscellaneous: Flu-like syndrome (3%; chronic hepatitis C 18%)

1% to 10%:

- Cardiovascular: Peripheral edema (chronic hepatitis C 10%), thrombosis (chronic hepatitis C 3%)
- Dermatologic: Alopecia (2%; chronic hepatitis C 10%), rash (3%)
- Gastrointestinal: Vomiting (6%), xerostomia (2%)
- Genitourinary: Urinary tract infection (5%)
- Hematologic: Rebound thrombocytopenia (8%)
- Hepatic: Ascites and encephalopathy (chronic hepatitis C 7%), hyperbilirubinemia (6% to 8%), ALT increased (5% to 6%), AST increased (4%), alkaline phosphatase increased (2%)
- Neuromuscular & skeletal: Back pain (3%), paresthesia (3%), musculoskeletal pain (2%)
- Ocular: Cataract (4% to 8%)

Respiratory: Upper respiratory infection (7%), oropharyngeal pain (4%), pharyngitis (4%)

<1% (Limited to important or life-threatening): Bone marrow fibrosis, bone marrow reticulin fiber deposits, hemorrhage (due to thrombocytopenia or rebound thrombocytopenia), non-Hodgkin's lymphoma, portal vein thrombosis, thrombotic/thromboembolic complications, visual acuity decreased

Drug Interactions

Metabolism/Transport Effects **Substrate** of CYP1A2 (minor), CYP2C8 (minor), UGT1A1, UGT1A3; **Note:** Assignment of Major/Minor substrate status based on clinically relevant drug interaction potential; **Inhibits** CYP2C8 (moderate), SLCO1B1, UGT1A1, UGT1A3, UGT1A4, UGT1A6, UGT1A9, UGT2B15, UGT2B7

Avoid Concomitant Use There are no known interactions where it is recommended to avoid concomitant use.

Increased Effect/Toxicity

Eltrombopag may increase the levels/effects of: CYP2C8 Substrates; Deferiprone; OATP1B1/SLCO1B1 Substrates; Rosuvastatin

Decreased Effect

The levels/effects of Eltrombopag may be decreased by: Aluminum Hydroxide; Calcium Salts; Iron Salts; Magnesium Salts; Multivitamins/Minerals (with ADEK, Folate, Iron); Multivitamins/Minerals (with AE, No Iron); Selenium; Sucralfate; Zinc Salts

Ethanol/Nutrition/Herb Interactions Food: Food, especially dairy products, may decrease the absorption of eltrombopag. Management: Take on an empty stomach at least 1 hour before or 2 hours after a meal. Separate intake from antacids, foods high in calcium, or minerals (eg, iron, calcium, aluminum, magnesium, selenium, zinc) by at least 4 hours.

Storage/Stability Store at room temperature between 20°C to 25°C (68°F to 77°F); excursions permitted to 15°C to 30°C (59°F to 86°F). If present, do not remove desiccant. Dispense in original bottle.

Mechanism of Action Thrombopoietin (TPO) nonpeptide agonist which increases platelet counts by binding to and activating the human TPO receptor. Activates intracellular signal transduction pathways to increase proliferation and differentiation of marrow progenitor cells. Does not induce platelet aggregation or activation.

Pharmacodynamics/Kinetics

Onset of action: Platelet count increase: Within 1-2 weeks
Peak platelet count increase: 14-16 days

Duration: Platelets return to baseline: 1-2 weeks after last dose

Protein binding: >99%

Metabolism: Extensive hepatic metabolism; via CYP 1A2, 2C8 oxidation and UGT 1A1, 1A3 glucuronidation

Bioavailability: ~52%

Half-life elimination: ~21-32 hours in healthy individuals; ~26-35 hours in patients with ITP

Time to peak, plasma: 2-6 hours

Excretion: Feces (~59%, 20% as unchanged drug, 21% glutathione-related conjugates); urine (31%, 20% glucuronide of the phenypyrazole moiety)

Dosage

Immune thrombocytopenia (ITP): Adults: Oral: **Note:** Use the lowest dose to achieve and maintain platelet count ≥50,000/mm^3 as needed to reduce the risk of bleeding. Discontinue if platelet count does not respond to a level that avoids clinically important bleeding after 4 weeks at the maximum daily dose of 75 mg.

Initial: 50 mg once daily (25 mg once daily for patients of East-Asian ethnicity [eg, Chinese, Japanese, Korean, Taiwanese]); dose should be titrated based on platelet response. Maximum dose: 75 mg once daily.

Dosage adjustment based on platelet response:

Platelet count <50,000/mm^3 (≥2 weeks after treatment initiation or a dose increase): Increase daily dose by 25 mg (if taking 12.5 mg once daily, increase dose to 25 mg once daily prior to increasing the dose amount by 25 mg daily); maximum: 75 mg once daily

Platelet count ≥200,000/mm^3 and ≤400,000/mm^3 (at any time): Reduce daily dose by 25 mg; reassess in 2 weeks

Platelet count >400,000/mm^3: Withhold dose; assess platelet count twice weekly; when platelet count <150,000/mm^3, resume with the daily dose reduced by 25 mg (if taking 25 mg once daily, resume with 12.5 mg once daily)

Platelet count >400,000/mm^3 after 2 weeks at the lowest dose: Discontinue treatment

Chronic hepatitis C-associated thrombocytopenia: Adults: Oral: **Note:** Use the lowest dose to achieve the target platelet count necessary to initiate antiviral therapy or to avoid dose reductions of peginterferon during antiviral therapy. Discontinue when antiviral therapy is stopped.

Initial: 25 mg once daily; dose should be titrated based on platelet response. Maximum dose: 100 mg once daily

Dosage adjustment based on platelet response:

Platelet count <50,000/mm^3 (after at least 2 weeks): Increase daily dose by 25 mg every 2 weeks; maximum dose: 100 mg once daily

Platelet count ≥200,000/mm^3 and ≤400,000/mm^3 (at any time): Reduce daily dose by 25 mg; reassess in 2 weeks

Platelet count >400,000/mm^3: Withhold dose; assess platelet count twice weekly; when platelet count <150,000/mm^3, resume with the daily dose reduced by 25 mg (if taking 25 mg once daily, resume with 12.5 mg once daily)

Platelet count >400,000/mm^3 after 2 weeks at the lowest dose: Discontinue treatment

Dosage adjustment in renal impairment: No dosage adjustment necessary.

Dosage adjustment in hepatic impairment:

Adjustment for hepatic impairment prior to initiating treatment:

ITP:

Mild, moderate, or severe impairment (Child-Pugh classes A, B, or C): Initial: 25 mg once daily

Patients of East-Asian ethnicity with hepatic impairment (Child-Pugh classes A, B, or C): Initial: 12.5 mg once daily

Chronic hepatitis C-associated thrombocytopenia: Initial: No dosage adjustment necessary.

Adjustment for hepatic impairment during treatment:

ITP: Hepatic impairment (Child-Pugh classes A, B, or C) after treatment initiation or after dose increases: Wait 3 weeks (instead of 2 weeks) prior to increasing dose for platelet count <50,000/mm^3

ITP and chronic hepatitis C-associated thrombocytopenia: ALT levels ≥3 times the upper limit of normal (ULN) in patients with normal hepatic function or ≥3 times baseline in those with pre-existing transaminase elevations **and** which are progressive, persistent (≥4 weeks), accompanied by increased direct bilirubin, or accompanied by clinical signs of liver injury or evidence of hepatic decompensation: Discontinue treatment. Treatment reinitiation is not recommended, but if determined to be clinically beneficial, may cautiously resume treatment; monitor ALT weekly during dosage titration; permanently discontinue if ALT elevations persist, worsen or recur.

Dietary Considerations Take on an empty stomach (1 hour before or 2 hours after a meal). Food, especially dairy products, may decrease the absorption of eltrombopag; allow at least 4 hours between dosing of eltrombopag and polyvalent cation intake (eg, dairy products, calcium-rich foods, multivitamins with minerals).

Administration Administer on an empty stomach, 1 hour before or 2 hours after a meal. Do not administer concurrently with antacids, foods high in calcium, or minerals (eg, iron, calcium, aluminum, magnesium, selenium, zinc); separate by at least 4 hours. Do not administer more than one dose within 24 hours.

Monitoring Parameters Liver function tests, including ALT, AST, and bilirubin (baseline, every 2 weeks during dosage titration, then monthly; evaluate abnormal liver function tests within 3-5 days; monitor weekly until abnormalities resolve, stabilize, or return to baseline or if retreating [not recommended] after therapy interruption for hepatotoxicity); bilirubin fractionation (for elevated bilirubin); CBC with differential and platelet count (weekly at initiation and during dosage titration, then monthly when stable; after cessation, monitor weekly for ≥4 weeks); peripheral blood smear (baseline and monthly when stable), bone marrow biopsy with staining for fibrosis (if peripheral blood smear reveals abnormality); ophthalmic exam (baseline and during treatment)

Reference Range Target platelet count (with treatment) of 50,000-200,000/mm^3; platelet life span: 8-11 days

Additional Information Restricted access to Promacta® was previously a REMS requirement via the Promacta® Cares™ program. Patients, prescribers, and pharmacies were required to be enrolled in this program. However, the FDA eliminated this REMS requirement in December 2011. There is currently no restricted access to obtaining Promacta®.

Dosage Forms Excipient information presented when available (limited, particularly for generics); consult specific product labeling.

Tablet, Oral:

Promacta: 12.5 mg

Promacta: 25 mg [contains fd&c yellow #6 aluminum lake]

Promacta: 50 mg [contains fd&c blue #2 aluminum lake]

Promacta: 75 mg

◆ **Eltrombopag Olamine** *see* Eltrombopag *on page 693*

◆ **Eltroxin® (Can)** *see* Levothyroxine *on page 1206*

Elvitegravir, Cobicistat, Emtricitabine, and Tenofovir

(el vi TEG ra vir, koe BIK i stat, em trye SYE ta been, & ten OF oh vir)

Brand Names: U.S. Stribild

Brand Names: Canada Stribild

Index Terms Cobicistat, Emtricitabine, Tenofovir, and Elvitegravir; Elvitegravir, Cobicistat, Emtricitabine, and Tenofovir Disoproxil Fumarate; Emtricitabine, Tenofovir, Elvitegravir, and Cobicistat; EVG/COBI/FTC/TDF; Quad Pill; Tenofovir, Elvitegravir, Cobicistat, and Emtricitabine

Pharmacologic Category Antiretroviral Agent, Integrase Inhibitor (Anti-HIV); Antiretroviral, Reverse Transcriptase Inhibitor, Nucleoside (Anti-HIV); Antiretroviral, Reverse Transcriptase Inhibitor, Nucleotide (Anti-HIV)

Use Treatment of human immunodeficiency virus type 1 (HIV-1) infection in antiretroviral treatment-naive adult patients

Pregnancy Risk Factor B

Pregnancy Considerations Adverse events were not observed in animal reproduction studies following administration of the individual agents contained in this combination product. Also see individual agents. Healthcare providers are encouraged to enroll pregnant women exposed to antiretroviral medications in the Antiretroviral Pregnancy Registry (1-800-258-4263 or www.APRegistry.com). Healthcare providers caring for HIV-infected women and their infants may contact the National Perinatal HIV Hotline (888-448-8765) for clinical consultation (DHHS [perinatal], 2012).

Breast-Feeding Considerations Maternal or infant antiretroviral therapy does not completely eliminate the risk of postnatal HIV transmission. In addition, multiclass-resistant virus has been detected in breast-feeding infants despite maternal therapy. Therefore, in the United States, where formula is accessible, affordable, safe, and sustainable, and the risk of infant mortality due to diarrhea and respiratory infections is low, complete avoidance of breast-feeding by HIV-infected women is recommended to decrease potential transmission of HIV (DHHS [perinatal], 2012).

Contraindications Concurrent use of alfuzosin, cisapride, ergot derivatives (eg, dihydroergotamine, ergotamine, methylergonovine); lovastatin, midazolam (oral), pimozide, rifampin, sildenafil (when used for pulmonary arterial hypertension), simvastatin, St John's wort, triazolam

Warnings/Precautions **[U.S. Boxed Warning]: Lactic acidosis and severe hepatomegaly with steatosis have been reported with nucleoside and nucleotide analogues (eg, tenofovir), including fatal cases.** Use with caution in patients with risk factors for liver disease (risk may be increased in obese patients or prolonged exposure) and suspend treatment in any patient who develops clinical or laboratory findings suggestive of lactic acidosis (transaminase elevation may/may not accompany hepatomegaly and steatosis). Use is not recommended in severe hepatic impairment (Child-Pugh Class C) and has not been studied in this population; no dosage adjustment is required in mild or moderate (Child-Pugh Class A or B) hepatic impairment.

Do not initiate therapy in patients with Cl_{cr} <70 mL/minute. Continued use is not recommended in patients with Cl_{cr} <50 mL/minute. May cause acute renal failure or Fanconi syndrome; use caution with other nephrotoxic agents (including high dose or multiple NSAID use or those which compete for active tubular secretion). Acute renal failure has occurred in HIV-infected patients with risk factors for renal impairment who were on a stable tenofovir regimen to which a high dose or multiple NSAID therapy was added. Consider alternatives to NSAIDS in patients taking tenofovir and at risk for renal impairment. Calculate creatinine clearance prior to initiation in all patients; monitor renal function during therapy (including recalculation of creatinine clearance, urine glucose, and protein and serum phosphorus) in patients at risk for renal impairment. Cobicistat component may cause modest declines in renal function without affecting glomerular filtration; closely monitor patients with >0.4 mg/dL increase of serum creatinine from baseline. In clinical trials, use has been associated with decreases in bone mineral density in HIV-1 infected adults and increases in bone metabolism markers. Serum parathyroid hormone and 1,25 vitamin D levels were also higher. Decreases in bone mineral density have also been observed in clinical trials of HIV-1 infected pediatric patients. Observations in chronic hepatitis B infected pediatric patients (aged 12-18 years) were similar. May cause osteomalacia with proximal renal tubulopathy. Bone pain, extremity pain, fractures, arthralgias, weakness and muscle pain have been reported. In patients at risk for renal dysfunction, persistent or worsening bone or muscle symptoms should be evaluated for hypophosphatemia and osteomalacia.

All patients with HIV should be tested for HBV prior to initiation of treatment. **[U.S. Boxed Warning]: Safety and efficacy during coinfection of HIV and HBV have not been established; acute, severe exacerbations of HBV**

have been reported following discontinuation of antiretroviral therapy. Not indicated for the treatment of chronic hepatitis B. In HBV-coinfected patients, monitor hepatic function closely for several months following discontinuation. May cause redistribution of fat (eg, buffalo hump, peripheral wasting with increased abdominal girth, cushingoid appearance). Patients may develop immune reconstitution syndrome resulting in the occurrence of an inflammatory response to an indolent or residual opportunistic infection during initial HIV treatment or activation of autoimmune disorders (eg, Graves' disease, polymyositis, Guillain-Barré syndrome) later in therapy; further evaluation and treatment may be required.

Adverse Reactions Percentages as reported for combination product.

>10%:

- Gastrointestinal: Nausea (16%), diarrhea (12%)
- Renal: Proteinuria (39%)

1% to 10%:

- Central nervous system: Abnormal dreams (9%), headache (7%), fatigue (5%), dizziness (3%), insomnia (3%), somnolence (1%)
- Dermatologic: Rash (3%)
- Endocrine & metabolic: Cholesterol increased (grades 3/4: ≤1%), triglycerides increased (grades 3/4: ≤1%)
- Gastrointestinal: Amylase increased (2%), flatulence (2%)
- Hepatic: AST increased (2%)
- Neuromuscular & skeletal: CPK increased (5%), fractures (1%)
- Renal: Creatinine increased (7%), hematuria (3%)

<1% (Limited to important or life-threatening): Fanconi syndrome, immune reconstitution syndrome, renal failure

Drug Interactions

Metabolism/Transport Effects Refer to individual components.

Avoid Concomitant Use

Avoid concomitant use of Elvitegravir, Cobicistat, Emtricitabine, and Tenofovir with any of the following: Adefovir; Ado-Trastuzumab Emtansine; Alfuzosin; Apixaban; Avanafil; Axitinib; Bosutinib; Cabozantinib; Cisapride; Conivaptan; Crizotinib; Dabigatran Etexilate; Didanosine; Dihydroergotamine; Dronedarone; Eplerenone; Ergotamine; Everolimus; Fluticasone (Oral Inhalation); Halofantrine; Ibrutinib; Imatinib; Ivabradine; LamiVUDine; Lapatinib; Lomitapide; Lovastatin; Lurasidone; Macitentan; Methylergonovine; Midazolam; Nilotinib; Nisoldipine; PAZOPanib; Pimozide; Pomalidomide; Ranolazine; Red Yeast Rice; Regorafenib; Rifabutin; Rifampin; Rifapentine; Rivaroxaban; Salmeterol; Sildenafil; Silodosin; Simeprevir; Simvastatin; St Johns Wort; Tamsulosin; Ticagrelor; Tolvaptan; Toremifene; Triazolam; Ulipristal; Vardenafil; Vemurafenib; VinCRIStine (Liposomal)

Increased Effect/Toxicity

Elvitegravir, Cobicistat, Emtricitabine, and Tenofovir may increase the levels/effects of: Adefovir; Ado-Trastuzumab Emtansine; Afatinib; Alfuzosin; Almotriptan; Alosetron; Aminoglycosides; Apixaban; ARIPiprazole; AtorvaSTATin; Avanafil; Axitinib; Bedaquiline; Bortezomib; Bosentan; Bosutinib; Brentuximab Vedotin; Brinzolamide; Budesonide (Nasal); Budesonide (Systemic, Oral Inhalation); Cabozantinib; Cisapride; Clarithromycin; ClonazePAM; Colchicine; Conivaptan; Contraceptives (Progestins); Corticosteroids (Orally Inhaled); Crizotinib; CYP3A4 Substrates; Dabigatran Etexilate; Darunavir; Didanosine; Dienogest; Dihydroergotamine; Dofetilide; Dronedarone; Dutasteride; Enzalutamide; Eplerenone; Ergotamine; Ethosuximide; Everolimus; FentaNYL; Fesoterodine; Fluticasone (Nasal); Fluticasone (Oral Inhalation); Ganciclovir-Valganciclovir; GuanFACINE; Halofantrine; Ibrutinib; Iloperidone; Imatinib; Itraconazole; Ivabradine; Ivacaftor; Ixabepilone; Ketoconazole (Systemic); Lacosamide; Lapatinib; Levomilnacipran; Lomitapide; Lovastatin; Lumefantrine; Lurasidone; Macitentan; Maraviroc; Methylergonovine; MethylPREDNISolone; Midazolam; Mifepristone; Nilotinib; Nisoldipine; Ospemifene; OxyCODONE; Paricalcitol; PAZOPanib; P-glycoprotein/ABCB1 Substrates; Pimecrolimus; Pimozide; Pomalidomide; PONATinib; Propafenone; Prucalopride; QUEtiapine; Ranolazine; Red Yeast Rice; Regorafenib; Repaglinide; Rilpivirine; Riociguat; Rivaroxaban; RomiDEPsin; Ruxolitinib; Salmeterol; Saxagliptin; Selective Serotonin Reuptake Inhibitors; Sildenafil; Silodosin; Simeprevir; Simvastatin; SORAfenib; Tadalafil; Tamsulosin; Telithromycin; Ticagrelor; Tofacitinib; Tolterodine; Tolvaptan; Topotecan; Toremifene; TraZODone; Triazolam; Tricyclic Antidepressants; Ulipristal; Vardenafil; Vemurafenib; Vilazodone; VinCRIStine (Liposomal); Voriconazole; Warfarin; Zuclopenthixol

The levels/effects of Elvitegravir, Cobicistat, Emtricitabine, and Tenofovir may be increased by: Acyclovir-Valacyclovir; Adefovir; Aminoglycosides; Atazanavir; Cidofovir; Clarithromycin; Darunavir; Diclofenac (Systemic); Ganciclovir-Valganciclovir; Itraconazole; Ketoconazole (Systemic); LamiVUDine; Lopinavir; Nonsteroidal Anti-Inflammatory Agents; Ribavirin; Simeprevir; Telaprevir; Telithromycin; Voriconazole

Decreased Effect

Elvitegravir, Cobicistat, Emtricitabine, and Tenofovir may decrease the levels/effects of: Afatinib; Atazanavir; Contraceptives (Estrogens); Dabigatran Etexilate; Didanosine; Ifosfamide; Linagliptin; P-glycoprotein/ABCB1 Substrates; Prasugrel; Simeprevir; Ticagrelor; Tipranavir; Warfarin

The levels/effects of Elvitegravir, Cobicistat, Emtricitabine, and Tenofovir may be decreased by: Adefovir; Antacids; CarBAMazepine; CYP3A4 Inducers (Strong); Dabrafenib; Deferasirox; Dexamethasone (Systemic); Fosphenytoin-Phenytoin; Mitotane; OXcarbazepine; PHENobarbital; Rifabutin; Rifampin; Rifapentine; St Johns Wort; Tipranavir; Tocilizumab

Storage/Stability Store tablets at 25°C (77°F); excursions permitted to 15°C to 30°C (59°F to 86°F). Keep container tightly closed. Dispense in original container.

Mechanism of Action Integrase strand transfer inhibitor, CYP3A enzyme inhibitor plus nucleoside and nucleotide reverse transcriptase inhibitor combination; the viral cDNA strand produced by reverse transcriptase is processed and inserted into the human genome by the enzyme HIV-1 integrase. Elvitegravir inhibits the catalytic activity of integrase, thus preventing integration of the proviral gene into human DNA. Cobicistat inhibits enzymes of the CYP3A subfamily and enhances systemic exposure to elvitegravir. Emtricitabine is a cytosine analogue and tenofovir disoproxil fumarate (TDF) is an analog of adenosine 5'-monophosphate. Emtricitabine and tenofovir interfere with HIV viral RNA dependent DNA polymerase activities resulting in inhibition of viral replication.

Pharmacodynamics/Kinetics

Absorption: AUC of elvitegravir and tenofovir increases with food; emtricitabine and cobicistat not affected

Protein binding: Elvitegravir (99%); cobicistat (98%); emtricitabine (<4%); tenofovir (<1%)

Metabolism:

- Elvitegravir: By CYP3A enzymes and also hepatic glucuronidation mediated by UGT1A1/3
- Cobicistat: By CYP3A enzymes and to a minor extent CYP2D6
- Emtricitabine and tenofovir: Not metabolized

Bioavailability: Not established

Half-life elimination: Elvitegravir ~13 hours; cobicistat ~4 hours; emtricitabine ~10 hours; tenofovir ~17 hours

Time to peak, plasma: ~3 hours (range: 2-4 hours)

Excretion: Elvitegravir: Feces (~95%), urine (~7%); cobicistat: Feces (~86%), urine (~8%); emtricitabine: Feces (14%), urine (86%); tenofovir: Urine (70% to 80%)

Dosage Note: Prior to initiation, patients should be tested for hepatitis B infection, and baseline estimated creatinine clearance, urine glucose, and urine protein should be assessed in all patients.

Oral: Adults: HIV-1: One tablet once daily. **Note:** Recommended as a preferred regimen for antiretroviral-naive patients with Cl_{cr} >70 mL/minute (DHHS [adult, INSTI], 2013).

Dosing adjustment in renal impairment:

Cl_{cr} ≥70 mL/minute: No dosage adjustments are recommended.

Cl_{cr} <70 mL/minute at initiation of therapy: Initial use is not recommended.

Cl_{cr} <50 mL/minute during therapy: Continued use is not recommended.

ESRD requiring dialysis: Use is not recommended.

Dosing adjustment in hepatic impairment:

Mild-to-moderate hepatic impairment (Child-Pugh class A or B): No dosage adjustments are recommended.

Severe hepatic impairment (Child-Pugh class C): Use is not recommended (has not been studied).

Dietary Considerations Take with a meal. Consider calcium and vitamin D supplementation in patients with history of bone fracture or osteopenia.

Administration Administer with food.

Monitoring Parameters CBC with differential, reticulocyte count, creatine kinase, CD4 count, HIV RNA plasma levels, serum phosphorus; serum creatinine, urine glucose and urine protein prior to initiation and as clinically indicated during therapy, hepatic function tests, bone density (patients with a history of bone fracture or have risk factors for bone loss); testing for HBV is recommended prior to the initiation of antiretroviral therapy; weight (children)

Patients with HIV and HBV coinfection should be monitored for several months following tenofovir discontinuation.

Dosage Forms Excipient information presented when available (limited, particularly for generics); consult specific product labeling.

Tablet, oral:

Stribild™: Elvitegravir 150 mg, cobicistat 150 mg, emtricitabine 200 mg, and tenofovir disoproxil fumarate 300 mg

- **Elvitegravir, Cobicistat, Emtricitabine, and Tenofovir Disoproxil Fumarate** *see* Elvitegravir, Cobicistat, Emtricitabine, and Tenofovir *on page* *696*
- **E-Max-1000 [OTC]** *see* Vitamin E *on page* *2202*
- **Emcyt** *see* Estramustine *on page* *763*
- **EMD 68843** *see* Vilazodone *on page* *2186*
- **Emend** *see* Aprepitant *on page* *158*
- **Emend** *see* Fosaprepitant *on page* *919*
- **Emend® (Can)** *see* Aprepitant *on page* *158*
- **Emend® IV (Can)** *see* Fosaprepitant *on page* *919*
- **EMLA®** *see* Lidocaine and Prilocaine *on page* *1213*
- **Emo-Cort® (Can)** *see* Hydrocortisone (Topical) *on page* *1011*
- **Emoquette** *see* Ethinyl Estradiol and Desogestrel *on page* *784*
- **Emsam** *see* Selegiline *on page* *1884*
- **Emtec** *see* Acetaminophen and Codeine *on page* *32*

Emtricitabine (em trye SYE ta been)

Brand Names: U.S. Emtriva

Brand Names: Canada Emtriva®

Index Terms BW524W91; Coviracil; FTC

Pharmacologic Category Antiretroviral, Reverse Transcriptase Inhibitor, Nucleoside (Anti-HIV)

Use Treatment of HIV infection in combination with at least two other antiretroviral agents

Pregnancy Risk Factor B

Pregnancy Considerations Adverse events were not observed in animal studies. Emtricitabine crosses the placenta; no increased risk of overall birth defects has been observed according to data collected by the antiretroviral pregnancy registry. Cases of lactic acidosis/hepatic steatosis syndrome related to mitochondrial toxicity have been reported in pregnant women with prolonged use of nucleoside analogues. It is not known if pregnancy itself potentiates this known side effect; however, women may be at increased risk of lactic acidosis and liver damage. In addition, these adverse events are similar to other rare but life-threatening syndromes which occur during pregnancy (eg, HELLP syndrome). Hepatic enzymes and electrolytes should be monitored in women receiving nucleoside analogues and clinicians should watch for early signs of the syndrome. In addition, mitochondrial dysfunction may develop in infants following *in utero* exposure. A pharmacokinetic study shows a slight decrease in emtricitabine serum levels during the third trimester; however, there is no clear need to adjust the dose. The DHHS Perinatal HIV Guidelines consider emtricitabine to be an alternative NRTI in dual nucleoside combination regimens. The DHHS Perinatal HIV Guidelines consider emtricitabine plus tenofovir a recommended dual NRTI/NtRTI backbone for HIV/HBV coinfected pregnant women.

Regardless of CD4 count or HIV RNA copy number, all HIV-infected pregnant women should receive a combination antepartum antiretroviral (ARV) drug regimen; this includes women who require therapy for their own health, as well as women who do not yet require therapy for their own health. ARV therapy should be started as soon as possible if required for the woman's health. Although earlier initiation may be more effective in reducing the perinatal transmission of HIV, also consider maternal conditions (eg, nausea and vomiting) and the potential risks of first trimester fetal exposure for specific agents. Plasma HIV RNA levels should be assessed at ~34-36 weeks gestation in order to help determine mode of delivery. If ARV therapy must be interrupted for <24 hours during the peripartum period, stop then restart all medications simultaneously in order to decrease the chance of developing resistance. Long-term follow-up is recommended for all infants exposed to ARV medications.

Healthcare providers are encouraged to enroll pregnant women exposed to antiretroviral medications in the Antiretroviral Pregnancy Registry (1-800-258-4263 or www.APRegistry.com). Healthcare providers caring for HIV-infected women and their infants may contact the National Perinatal HIV Hotline (888-448-8765) for clinical consultation (DHHS [perinatal], 2012).

Breast-Feeding Considerations Emtricitabine is excreted into breast milk. Maternal or infant antiretroviral therapy does not completely eliminate the risk of postnatal HIV transmission. In addition, multiclass-resistant virus has been detected in breast-feeding infants despite maternal therapy. Therefore, in the United States, where formula is accessible, affordable, safe, and sustainable, and the risk of infant mortality due to diarrhea and respiratory infections is low, complete avoidance of breast-feeding by HIV-infected women is recommended to decrease potential transmission of HIV (DHHS [perinatal], 2012).

Contraindications Hypersensitivity to emtricitabine or any component of the formulation

Warnings/Precautions [U.S. Boxed Warning]: Lactic acidosis, severe hepatomegaly with steatosis, and hepatic failure have occurred rarely with emtricitabine (similar to other nucleoside analogues). Some cases have been fatal; stop treatment if lactic acidosis or hepatotoxicity occur. Prior liver disease, obesity, extended duration of therapy, and female gender may represent risk factors for severe hepatic reactions. Testing for hepatitis B is recommended prior to the initiation of therapy; **[U.S. Boxed Warnings]: Hepatitis B may be exacerbated following discontinuation of emtricitabine; not indicated for treatment of chronic hepatitis B; safety and efficacy in HIV/HBV coinfected patients not established.** May be associated with fat redistribution (buffalo hump, increased abdominal girth, breast engorgement, facial atrophy, and dyslipidemia). Immune reconstitution syndrome may develop resulting in the occurrence of an inflammatory response to an indolent or residual opportunistic infection during initial HIV treatment or activation of autoimmune disorders (eg, Graves' disease, polymyositis, Guillain-Barré syndrome) later in therapy; further evaluation and treatment may be required. Use caution in patients with renal impairment (dosage adjustment required). Concomitant use of other emtricitabine-containing products should be avoided. Concomitant use of lamivudine or lamivudine-containing products should be avoided; cross-resistance may develop.

Adverse Reactions Clinical trials were conducted in patients receiving other antiretroviral agents, and it is not possible to correlate frequency of adverse events with emtricitabine alone. The range of frequencies of adverse events is generally comparable to comparator groups, with the exception of hyperpigmentation, which occurred more frequently in patients receiving emtricitabine. Unless otherwise noted, percentages are as reported in adults.

>10%:

Central nervous system: Dizziness (4% to 25%), headache (6% to 22%), fever (children 18%), insomnia (5% to 16%), abnormal dreams (2% to 11%)

Dermatologic: Hyperpigmentation (children 32%; adults 2% to 4%; primarily of palms and/or soles but may include tongue, arms, lip and nails; generally mild and nonprogressive without associated local reactions such as pruritus or rash); rash (17% to 30%; includes pruritus, maculopapular rash, vesiculobullous rash, pustular rash, and allergic reaction)

Gastrointestinal: Diarrhea (children 20%; adults 9% to 23%), vomiting (children 23%; adults 9%), nausea (13% to 18%), abdominal pain (8% to 14%), gastroenteritis (children 11%)

Neuromuscular & skeletal: Weakness (12% to 16%), CPK increased (grades 3/4: 11% to 12%)

Otic: Otitis media (children 23%)

Respiratory: Cough (children 28%; adults 14%), rhinitis (children 20%; adults 12% to 18%), pneumonia (children 15%)

Miscellaneous: Infection (children 44%)

1% to 10%:

Central nervous system: Depression (6% to 9%), neuropathy/neuritis (4%)

Endocrine & metabolic: Serum triglycerides increased (grades 3/4: 4% to 10%), disordered glucose homeostasis (grades 3/4: 2% to 3%), serum amylase increased (grades 3/4: children 9%; adults 2% to 5%), serum lipase increased (grades 3/4: ≤1%)

Gastrointestinal: Dyspepsia (4% to 8%), serum amylase increased (grades 3/4: 8%)

Genitourinary: Hematuria (grades 3/4: 3%)

Hematologic: Anemia (children: 7%), neutropenia (grades 3/4: children 2%; adults 5%)

Hepatic: Transaminases increased (grades 3/4: 2% to 6%), alkaline phosphatase increased (>550 units/L: 1%), bilirubin increased (grades 3/4: 1%)

Neuromuscular & skeletal: Creatinine kinase increased (grades 3/4: 9%), myalgia (4% to 6%), paresthesia (5% to 6%), arthralgia (3% to 5%)

Respiratory: Upper respiratory tract infection (8%), sinusitis (8%), pharyngitis (5%)

<1% (Limited to important or life-threatening): Immune reconstitution syndrome

Drug Interactions

Metabolism/Transport Effects None known.

Avoid Concomitant Use

Avoid concomitant use of Emtricitabine with any of the following: LamiVUDine

Increased Effect/Toxicity

The levels/effects of Emtricitabine may be increased by: Ganciclovir-Valganciclovir; LamiVUDine; Ribavirin

Decreased Effect There are no known significant interactions involving a decrease in effect.

Ethanol/Nutrition/Herb Interactions Food: Food decreases peak plasma concentrations, but does not alter the extent of absorption or overall systemic exposure.

Storage/Stability Store capsules at 15°C to 30°C (59°F to 86°F). Solution should be stored under refrigeration at 2°C to 8°C (36°F to 46°F). Once dispensed, may be stored at 15°C to 30°C (59°F to 86°F) if used within 3 months.

Mechanism of Action Nucleoside reverse transcriptase inhibitor; emtricitabine is a cytosine analogue which is phosphorylated intracellularly to emtricitabine 5'-triphosphate which interferes with HIV viral RNA dependent DNA polymerase resulting in inhibition of viral replication.

Pharmacodynamics/Kinetics

Absorption: Rapid, extensive

Protein binding: <4%

Metabolism: Limited, via oxidation and conjugation (not via CYP isoenzymes)

Bioavailability: Capsule: 93%; solution: 75%

Half-life elimination: Normal renal function: Adults: 10 hours; children: 5-18 hours

Time to peak, plasma: 1-2 hours

Excretion: Urine (86% primarily as unchanged drug, 13% as metabolites); feces (14%)

Dosage Oral:

Children:

0-3 months: Solution: 3 mg/kg/day

3 months to 17 years:

Capsule: Children >33 kg: 200 mg once daily

Solution: 6 mg/kg once daily; maximum: 240 mg/day

Note: Emtricitabine in combination with tenofovir is recommended as a component of first line regimens (with atazanavir/ritonavir, with darunavir/ritonavir, with efavirenz, or with raltegravir) in treatment-naive patients (DHHS, 2013).

Adults:

Capsule: 200 mg once daily

Solution: 240 mg once daily

Dosage adjustment in renal impairment: Adults (consider similar adjustments in children):

Cl_{cr} 30-49 mL/minute: Capsule: 200 mg every 48 hours; solution: 120 mg every 24 hours

Cl_{cr} 15-29 mL/minute: Capsule: 200 mg every 72 hours; solution: 80 mg every 24 hours

Cl_{cr} <15 mL/minute (including hemodialysis patients): Capsule: 200 mg every 96 hours; solution: 60 mg every 24 hours; administer after dialysis

Dosage adjustment in hepatic impairment: No adjustment required.

Dietary Considerations May be taken with or without food.

Administration May be administered with or without food.

Monitoring Parameters Viral load, CD4, liver function tests; hepatitis B testing is recommended prior to initiation of therapy

Dosage Forms Excipient information presented when available (limited, particularly for generics); consult specific product labeling.

Capsule, Oral:

Emtriva: 200 mg [contains fd&c blue #2 (indigotine)]

Solution, Oral:

Emtriva: 10 mg/mL (170 mL) [contains edetate disodium, fd&c yellow #6 (sunset yellow), methylparaben, propylene glycol, propylparaben; cotton candy flavor]

Emtricitabine and Tenofovir

(em trye SYE ta been & ten OF oh vir)

Brand Names: U.S. Truvada

Brand Names: Canada Truvada

Index Terms Tenofovir and Emtricitabine

Pharmacologic Category Antiretroviral, Reverse Transcriptase Inhibitor, Nucleoside (Anti-HIV); Antiretroviral, Reverse Transcriptase Inhibitor, Nucleotide (Anti-HIV)

Use

Treatment of HIV-1 infection in combination with other antiretroviral agents in adults and pediatric patients ≥12 years of age

Pre-exposure prophylaxis (PrEP) for prevention of HIV-1 infection in adults who are at high risk for acquiring HIV

High risk individuals include those with partners known to be HIV-1 infected or who engage in sexual activity within a high prevalence area or social network, and one or more of the following:

- Inconsistent or no condom use
- Diagnosis of sexually-transmitted infections
- Exchange of sex for commodities
- Use of illicit drugs or alcohol dependence
- Incarceration
- Partner of unknown HIV-1 status with any of the above risk factors

When prescribing PrEP healthcare providers **MUST**:

- Include PrEP as part of a comprehensive prevention strategy because PrEP alone is not always effective in preventing HIV-1 infection
- Counsel all uninfected patients to strictly adhere to the dosing schedule, because adherence was strongly correlated with effectiveness in clinical trials
- Confirm a negative HIV-1 test prior to starting PrEP; if a candidate has acute viral infection symptoms and unprotected exposure events <1 month prior, delay PrEP for at least 1 month and retest HIV-1 status or use an Food and Drug Administration (FDA) test approved for HIV-1 diagnosis, including acute or primary HIV-1 infection
- Retest for HIV-1 infection at least every 3 months while the patient receives PrEP

Unlabeled Use Treatment of hepatitis B in patients with antiviral-resistant HBV or coinfection with HIV; pre-exposure prophylaxis (PrEP) for prevention of HIV-1 infection in injecting drug users (IDU) who are at risk for parenteral acquisition of HIV but not at risk for sexual acquisition of HIV; postexposure prophylaxis (PEP) for occupational exposure to HIV

Pregnancy Risk Factor B

Medication Guide Available Yes

Dosage Note: Avoid concurrent use with adefovir or lamivudine-containing products or other emtricitabine- and/or tenofovir-containing products.

HIV-1 infection: Children ≥12 (and ≥35 kg), Adolescents (≥35 kg), and Adults: Oral: One tablet (emtricitabine 200 mg and tenofovir 300 mg) once daily. **Note:** Recommended as a component of preferred regimens (in combination with atazanavir/ritonavir or darunavir/ritonavir or efavirenz or raltegravir) in antiretroviral-naive patients (DHHS, 2013).

Preexposure prophylaxis (PrEP) for prevention of HIV infection in uninfected high-risk individuals: Adults: Oral: One tablet (emtricitabine 200 mg and tenofovir 300 mg) once daily

Hepatitis B treatment in patients with antiviral-resistant HBV or coinfection with HIV (unlabeled use): Adults: Oral: One tablet (emtricitabine 200 mg and tenofovir 300 mg) once daily (Lok, 2009)

Occupational HIV postexposure, prophylaxis (PEP) (unlabeled use): Adults: Oral: One tablet (emtricitabine 200 mg and tenofovir 300 mg) once daily for 4 weeks with concomitant raltegravir. Recommended as preferred therapy (Kuhar, 2013)

PrEP for prevention of HIV infection in injecting drug users (IDU) who are at risk for parenteral acquisition of HIV but not at risk for sexual acquisition of HIV (unlabeled use): Adults: Oral: One tablet (emtricitabine 200 mg and tenofovir 300 mg) once daily (CDC, 2013)

Dosage adjustment in renal impairment: Adults:

HIV-1 infection:

Cl_{cr} ≥50 mL/minute: No dosage adjustment necessary

Cl_{cr} 30-49 mL/minute: Increase interval to every 48 hours.

Cl_{cr} <30 mL/minute or hemodialysis: Not recommended.

PrEP:

Cl_{cr} ≥60 mL/minute: No dosage adjustment necessary

Cl_{cr} <60 mL/minute: Not recommended.

Dosage adjustment in hepatic impairment: No dosing adjustment necessary for tenofovir in moderate-to-severe hepatic compromise; no specific data available on emtricitabine in hepatic impairment, but given limited hepatic metabolism, dose adjustments are unlikely.

Additional Information Complete prescribing information should be consulted for additional detail.

Dosage Forms Excipient information presented when available (limited, particularly for generics); consult specific product labeling.

Tablet:

Truvada: Emtricitabine 200 mg and tenofovir disoproxil fumarate 300 mg

◆ **Emtricitabine, Efavirenz, and Tenofovir** *see* Efavirenz, Emtricitabine, and Tenofovir *on page 690*

Emtricitabine, Rilpivirine, and Tenofovir

(em trye SYE ta been, ril pi VIR een, & ten OF oh vir)

Brand Names: U.S. Complera

Brand Names: Canada Complera

Index Terms FTC/RPV/TDF; Rilpivirine, Emtricitabine, and Tenofovir; Tenofovir Disoproxil Fumarate, Rilpivirine, and Emtricitabine; Tenofovir, Emtricitabine, and Rilpivirine

Pharmacologic Category Antiretroviral, Reverse Transcriptase Inhibitor, Non-nucleoside (Anti-HIV); Antiretroviral, Reverse Transcriptase Inhibitor, Nucleoside (Anti-HIV); Antiretroviral, Reverse Transcriptase Inhibitor, Nucleotide (Anti-HIV)

Use

Treatment of human immunodeficiency virus type 1 (HIV-1) infection in antiretroviral treatment-naive patients with HIV-1 RNA ≤100,000 copies/mL at the start of therapy

Treatment (replacement of a current antiretroviral treatment regimen) in virologically-suppressed (HIV-1 RNA <50 copies/mL) patients who meet all of the following parameters:
- are on a stable antiretroviral regimen at start of therapy
- have no history of virologic failure
- prior to regimen replacement, have been suppressed for at least 6 months
- are currently on their first or second antiretroviral regimen
- have no history of resistance to emtricitabine, rilpivirine or tenofovir.

Pregnancy Risk Factor B

Dosage HIV: Adults: Oral: One tablet once daily

Dosage adjustment in renal impairment:

Cl_{cr} ≥50 mL/minute: No dosage adjustments necessary.

Cl_{cr} <50 mL/minute: Use is not recommended

ESRD requiring dialysis: Use is not recommended

Dosage adjustment in hepatic impairment:

Mild-to-moderate impairment (Child-Pugh class A or B): No dosage adjustments necessary.

Severe impairment (Child-Pugh class C): No dosage adjustment provided in manufacturer's labeling (has not been studied).

Additional Information Complete prescribing information should be consulted for additional detail.

Dosage Forms Excipient information presented when available (limited, particularly for generics); consult specific product labeling.

Tablet, oral:

Complera: Emtricitabine 200 mg, rilpivirine 25 mg, and tenofovir disoproxil fumarate 300 mg

◆ **Emtricitabine, Tenofovir, Elvitegravir, and Cobicistat** *see* Elvitegravir, Cobicistat, Emtricitabine, and Tenofovir *on page 696*

◆ **Emtriva** *see* Emtricitabine *on page 698*

◆ **Emtriva® (Can)** *see* Emtricitabine *on page 698*

◆ **ENA 713** *see* Rivastigmine *on page 1841*

◆ **Enablex** *see* Darifenacin *on page 546*

◆ **Enablex® (Can)** *see* Darifenacin *on page 546*

Enalapril (e NAL a pril)

Brand Names: U.S. Epaned; Vasotec

Brand Names: Canada Apo-Enalapril; Ava-Enalapril; CO Enalapril; Mylan-Enalapril; PMS-Enalapril; PRO-Enalapril; RAN-Enalapril; ratio-Enalapril; Riva-Enalapril; Sandoz-Enalapril; Sig-Enalapril; Taro-Enalapril; Teva-Enalapril; Vasotec

Index Terms Enalapril Maleate

Pharmacologic Category Angiotensin-Converting Enzyme (ACE) Inhibitor; Antihypertensive

Additional Appendix Information

Angiotensin Agents *on page 2280*

Use Treatment of hypertension; treatment of symptomatic heart failure; treatment of asymptomatic left ventricular dysfunction

Unlabeled Use To delay the progression of nephropathy and reduce risks of cardiovascular events in hypertensive patients with type 1 or 2 diabetes mellitus; hypertensive crisis, diabetic nephropathy, hypertension secondary to scleroderma renal crisis, diagnosis of aldosteronism, idiopathic edema, Bartter's syndrome, postmyocardial infarction for prevention of ventricular failure

Pregnancy Risk Factor D

Pregnancy Considerations **[U.S. Boxed Warning]: Drugs that act on the renin-angiotensin system can cause injury and death to the developing fetus. Discontinue as soon as possible once pregnancy is detected.** Enalaprilat, the active metabolite of enalapril, crosses the placenta; teratogenic effects may occur following maternal use during pregnancy. Drugs that act on the renin-angiotensin system are associated with oligohydramnios. Oligohydramnios, due to decreased fetal renal function, may lead to fetal lung hypoplasia and skeletal malformations. The use of these drugs in pregnancy is also associated with anuria, hypotension, renal failure, skull hypoplasia, and death in the fetus/neonate. Chronic maternal hypertension itself is also associated with adverse events in the fetus/infant. ACE inhibitors are not recommended during pregnancy to treat maternal hypertension or heart failure. Use of an ACE inhibitor should also be avoided in any woman of reproductive age. Women who are planning a pregnancy should be considered for other medication options if an ACE inhibitor is currently prescribed or the ACE inhibitor should be discontinued as soon as possible once pregnancy is detected. The exposed fetus should be monitored for fetal growth, amniotic fluid volume, and organ formation. Infants exposed to an ACE inhibitor *in utero* should be monitored for hyperkalemia, hypotension, and oliguria.

Breast-Feeding Considerations Enalapril and enalaprilat are excreted in breast milk. Breast-feeding is not recommended by the manufacturer.

Contraindications

Hypersensitivity to enalapril or enalaprilat; angioedema related to previous treatment with an ACE inhibitor; patients with idiopathic or hereditary angioedema; concomitant use with aliskiren in patients with diabetes mellitus

Canadian labeling: Additional contraindications (not in U.S. labeling): Concomitant use with aliskiren-containing drugs in patients with moderate-to-severe renal impairment (GFR <60 mL/minute/1.73m^2)

Warnings/Precautions Anaphylactic reactions may occur rarely with ACE inhibitors. At any time during treatment (especially following first dose) angioedema may occur rarely with ACE inhibitors; it may involve the head and neck (potentially compromising airway) or the intestine (presenting with abdominal pain). African-Americans may be at an increased risk. Prolonged frequent monitoring may be required especially if tongue, glottis, or larynx are involved as they are associated with airway obstruction. Patients with a history of airway surgery may have a higher risk of airway obstruction. Aggressive early and appropriate management is critical. Use in patients with idiopathic or hereditary angioedema or previous angioedema associated with ACE inhibitor therapy is contraindicated. Severe anaphylactoid reactions may be seen during hemodialysis (eg, CVVHD) with high-flux dialysis membranes (eg, AN69), and rarely, during low density lipoprotein apheresis with dextran sulfate cellulose. Rare cases of anaphylactoid reactions have been reported in patients undergoing sensitization treatment with hymenoptera (bee, wasp) venom while receiving ACE inhibitors.

Symptomatic hypotension with or without syncope can occur with ACE inhibitors (usually with the first several doses); effects are most often observed in volume depleted patients; correct volume depletion prior to initiation; close monitoring of patient is required especially with initial dosing and dosing increases; blood pressure must be lowered at a rate appropriate for the patient's clinical condition. Initiation of therapy in patients with ischemic heart disease or cerebrovascular disease warrants close observation due to the potential consequences posed by falling blood pressure (eg, MI, stroke). Use with caution in hypertrophic cardiomyopathy with outflow tract obstruction, severe aortic stenosis, or before, during, or immediately after major surgery. **[U.S. Boxed Warning]: Drugs that act on the renin-angiotensin system can cause injury and death to the developing fetus. Discontinue as soon as possible once pregnancy is detected.**

Hyperkalemia may occur with ACE inhibitors; risk factors include renal dysfunction, diabetes mellitus, concomitant use of potassium-sparing diuretics, potassium supplements, and/or potassium-containing salts. Use cautiously, if at all, with these agents and monitor potassium closely. Cough may occur with ACE inhibitors. Other causes of cough should be considered (eg, pulmonary congestion in patients with heart failure) and excluded prior to discontinuation.

May be associated with deterioration of renal function and/or increases in serum creatinine, particularly in patients with low renal blood flow (eg, renal artery stenosis, heart failure) whose glomerular filtration rate (GFR) is dependent on efferent arteriolar vasoconstriction by angiotensin II; deterioration may result in oliguria, acute renal failure, and progressive azotemia. Small increases in serum creatinine may occur following initiation; consider discontinuation only in patients with progressive and/or significant deterioration in renal function. Use with caution in patients with unstented unilateral/bilateral renal artery stenosis. When unstented bilateral renal artery stenosis is present, use is generally avoided due to the elevated risk of deterioration in renal function unless possible benefits outweigh risks. Potentially significant drug-drug interactions may exist, requiring dose or frequency adjustment, additional monitoring, and/or selection of alternative therapy.

Rare toxicities associated with ACE inhibitors include cholestatic jaundice (which may progress to fulminant hepatic necrosis), agranulocytosis, neutropenia or leukopenia with myeloid hypoplasia. Patients with collagen vascular diseases (especially with concomitant renal impairment) or renal impairment alone may be at increased risk for hematologic toxicity; periodically monitor CBC with differential in these patients.

Adverse Reactions Note: Frequency ranges include data from hypertension and heart failure trials. Higher rates of adverse reactions have generally been noted in patients with CHF. However, the frequency of adverse effects associated with placebo is also increased in this population.

1% to 10%:

Cardiovascular: Hypotension (1% to 7%), chest pain (2%), syncope (≤2%), orthostasis (2%), orthostatic hypotension (2%)

Central nervous system: Headache (2% to 5%), dizziness (4% to 8%), fatigue (2% to 3%)

Dermatologic: Rash (2%)

Gastrointestinal: Abnormal taste, abdominal pain, vomiting, nausea, diarrhea, anorexia, constipation

Neuromuscular & skeletal: Weakness

Renal: Serum creatinine increased (≤20%), worsening of renal function (in patients with bilateral renal artery stenosis or hypovolemia)

Respiratory (1% to 2%): Bronchitis, cough, dyspnea

<1% (Limited to important or life-threatening): Agranulocytosis, alopecia, anaphylactoid reaction, angina pectoris, angioedema, ataxia, atrial fibrillation, atrial tachycardia, bone marrow suppression, bradycardia, cardiac arrest, cerebral vascular accident, cholestatic jaundice, depression, eosinophilia, eosinophilic pneumonitis, erythema multiforme, erythrocyte sedimentation rate increased, exfoliative dermatitis, giant cell arteritis, gynecomastia, hallucinations, hemolysis with G6PD, Henoch-Schönlein purpura (IgA vasculitis), hepatitis, ileus, interstitial nephritis, lichen-form reaction, melena, MI, neutropenia, ototoxicity, pancreatitis, pemphigus, pemphigus foliaceus, peripheral neuropathy, photosensitivity, positive ANA, psychosis, pulmonary edema, pulmonary embolism, pulmonary infiltrates, Raynaud's phenomenon, sicca syndrome, Stevens-Johnson syndrome, systemic lupus erythematosus, thrombocytopenia, toxic epidermal necrolysis, toxic pustuloderma, vasculitis, visual hallucinations (Doane, 2013)

Drug Interactions

Metabolism/Transport Effects None known.

Avoid Concomitant Use There are no known interactions where it is recommended to avoid concomitant use.

Increased Effect/Toxicity

Enalapril may increase the levels/effects of: Allopurinol; Amifostine; Antihypertensives; AzaTHIOprine; CycloSPORINE (Systemic); Ferric Gluconate; Gold Sodium Thiomalate; Hypotensive Agents; Iron Dextran Complex; Lithium; Nonsteroidal Anti-Inflammatory Agents; Obinutuzumab; RiTUXimab; Sodium Phosphates

The levels/effects of Enalapril may be increased by: Alfuzosin; Aliskiren; Angiotensin II Receptor Blockers; Brimonidine (Topical); Canagliflozin; Diazoxide; DPP-IV Inhibitors; Eplerenone; Everolimus; Heparin; Heparin (Low Molecular Weight); Herbs (Hypotensive Properties); Loop Diuretics; MAO Inhibitors; Pentoxifylline; Phosphodiesterase 5 Inhibitors; Potassium Salts; Potassium-Sparing Diuretics; Prostacyclin Analogues; Sirolimus; Temsirolimus; Thiazide Diuretics; TiZANidine; Tolvaptan; Trimethoprim

Decreased Effect

The levels/effects of Enalapril may be decreased by: Antacids; Aprotinin; Herbs (Hypertensive Properties); Icatibant; Lanthanum; Methylphenidate; Nonsteroidal Anti-Inflammatory Agents; Salicylates; Yohimbine

Ethanol/Nutrition/Herb Interactions

Food: Potassium supplements and/or potassium-containing salts may cause or worsen hyperkalemia. Management: Consult prescriber before consuming a potassium-rich diet, potassium supplements, or salt substitutes.

Herb/Nutraceutical: Some herbal medications may worsen hypertension (eg, licorice); others may increase the antihypertensive effect of enalapril (eg, shepherd's purse). Management: Avoid bayberry, blue cohosh, cayenne, ephedra, ginger, ginseng (American), kola, licorice, and yohimbe. Avoid black cohosh, California poppy, coleus, golden seal, hawthorn, mistletoe, periwinkle, quinine, and shepherd's purse.

Preparation for Administration Epaned: Solution kit (for 150 mL, enalapril solution 1 mg/mL): Kit contains 1 bottle of enalapril powder and 1 bottle of Ora-Sweet SF dilution to be added to the enalapril powder prior to dispensing. Firmly tap the enalapril powder for oral solution bottle on a hard surface 5 times. Add approximately one-half (75 mL) of the Ora-Sweet SF diluent to the enalapril 150 mL oral solution bottle and shake well for 30 seconds. Add the remainder of the Ora-Sweet SF diluent and shake well for an additional 30 seconds. May be used for 60 days after reconstitution.

Storage/Stability

Solution kit: Store at 25°C (77°F); excursions are permitted between 15°C and 30°C (59°F and 86°F). Do not freeze. Protect from moisture. Once reconstituted, the solution should be refrigerated at 2°C to 8°C (36°F to 46°F) and can be stored for up to 60 days.

Tablet: Store below 30°C (86°F); avoid temperatures >50°C (122°F). Protect from moisture.

Mechanism of Action Competitive inhibitor of angiotensin-converting enzyme (ACE); prevents conversion of angiotensin I to angiotensin II, a potent vasoconstrictor; results in lower levels of angiotensin II which causes an increase in plasma renin activity and a reduction in aldosterone secretion

Pharmacodynamics/Kinetics

Onset of action: ~1 hour

Peak effect: 4-6 hours

Duration: 12-24 hours

Absorption: 55% to 75%

Protein binding: ~50% (Davies, 1984)

Metabolism: Prodrug, undergoes hepatic biotransformation to enalaprilat

Half-life elimination:

Enalapril: Adults: Healthy: 2 hours; Congestive heart failure: 3.4-5.8 hours

Enalaprilat: Infants 6 weeks to 8 months of age: 6-10 hours (Lloyd, 1989); Adults: ~35 hours (Till, 1984; Ulm, 1982)

Time to peak, serum: Oral: Enalapril: 0.5-1.5 hours; Enalaprilat (active metabolite): 3-4.5 hours

Excretion: Urine (61%; 18% of which was enalapril, 43% was enalaprilat); feces (33%; 6% of which was enalapril, 27% was enalaprilat) (Ulm, 1982)

Dosage Use lower listed initial dose in patients with hyponatremia, hypovolemia, severe congestive heart failure, decreased renal function, or in those receiving diuretics.

Oral:

Children ≥1 month and Adolescents: Hypertension: Initial: 0.08 mg/kg (up to 5 mg) once daily; adjust dosage based on patient response; doses >0.58 mg/kg (40 mg) have not been evaluated in pediatric patients

Infants and Children: Heart failure (unlabeled dosing): Initial: 0.1 mg/kg/day in 1-2 divided doses; increase as required over 2 weeks to maximum of 0.5 mg/kg/day. **Note:** Mean dose required for CHF improvement in 39 children (9 days to 17 years) was 0.36 mg/kg/day; select individuals have been treated with doses up to 0.94 mg/kg/day (Leversha, 1994).

Adults:

Asymptomatic left ventricular dysfunction: 2.5 mg twice daily, titrated as tolerated to 20 mg/day

Heart failure (with reduced ejection fraction): Initial: 2.5 mg once or twice daily (usual range: 5-40 mg daily in 2 divided doses); titrate slowly at 1- to 2-week intervals. Target dose: 10-20 mg twice daily (ACCF/AHA 2013 Heart Failure Guidelines)

Hypertension: 2.5-5 mg daily then increase as required, usually at 1- to 2-week intervals; usual dose range (JNC 7): 2.5-40 mg daily in 1-2 divided doses. **Note:** Initiate with 2.5 mg if patient is taking a diuretic which cannot be discontinued. May add a diuretic if blood pressure cannot be controlled with enalapril alone.

Conversion from I.V. **enalaprilat** to oral **enalapril** therapy: If not concurrently receiving diuretics, initiate enalapril 5 mg once daily; if concurrently receiving diuretics and responding to enalaprilat 0.625 mg I.V. every 6 hours, initiate with enalapril 2.5 mg once daily; subsequent titration as needed.

Dosing adjustment in renal impairment: Note: Use in infants and children ≤16 years of age with GFR <30 mL/minute/1.73 m^2 is not recommended (no dosing data exists).

Manufacturer's recommendations:

Cl_{cr} >30 mL/minute: No dosage adjustment necessary

Cl_{cr} ≤30 mL/minute: Administer 2.5 mg day; titrated upward until blood pressure is controlled.

Heart failure patients with sodium <130 mEq/L or serum creatinine >1.6 mg/dL: Initiate dosage with 2.5 mg daily, increasing to twice daily as needed. Increase further in increments of 2.5 mg/dose at >4-day intervals to a maximum daily dose of 40 mg.

Intermittent hemodialysis (IHD): Moderately dialyzable (20% to 50%): Initial: 2.5 mg on dialysis days; adjust dose on nondialysis days depending on blood pressure response.

Conversion from I.V. **enalaprilat** to oral **enalapril** therapy:

Cl_{cr} >30 mL/minute: May initiate enalapril 5 mg once daily.

Cl_{cr} ≤30 mL/minute: May initiate enalapril 2.5 mg once daily.

Alternate recommendations (Aronoff, 2007):

Cl_{cr} >50 mL/minute: No dosage adjustment necessary

Cl_{cr} 10-50 mL/minute: Administer 75% to 100% of usual dose

Cl_{cr} <10 mL/minute: Administer 50% of usual dose

Peritoneal dialysis: Supplemental dose is not necessary, although some removal of drug occurs.

Dosing adjustment in hepatic impairment: Hydrolysis of enalapril to enalaprilat may be delayed and/or impaired in patients with severe hepatic impairment, but the pharmacodynamic effects of the drug do not appear to be significantly altered; no dosage adjustment.

Dietary Considerations Limit salt substitutes or potassium-rich diet.

Monitoring Parameters Blood pressure; serum creatinine and potassium; if patient has collagen vascular disease and/or renal impairment, periodically monitor CBC with differential

Test Interactions Positive Coombs' [direct]; may cause false-positive results in urine acetone determinations using sodium nitroprusside reagent

Dosage Forms Excipient information presented when available (limited, particularly for generics); consult specific product labeling.

Solution Reconstituted, Oral, as maleate:

Epaned: 1 mg/mL (150 mL) [contains methylparaben, propylparaben, saccharin sodium; berry-citrus flavor]

Tablet, Oral, as maleate:

Vasotec: 2.5 mg, 5 mg, 10 mg, 20 mg [scored]

Generic: 2.5 mg, 5 mg, 10 mg, 20 mg

Dosage Forms: Canada Note: Refer to Dosage Forms. Oral solution for reconstitution is not available in Canada.

Extemporaneous Preparations Note: Commercial oral solution kit is available (1 mg/mL).

A 1 mg/mL oral suspension may be made with tablets, Bicitra [discontinued] or equivalent, and Ora-Sweet SF. Place ten 20 mg tablets in a 200 mL polyethylene terephthalate bottle; add 50 mL of Bicitra [discontinued] or equivalent and shake well for at least 2 minutes. Let stand for 1 hour then shake for 1 additional minute; add 150 mL of Ora-Sweet SF and shake well. Label "shake well" and "refrigerate". Stable for 30 days when stored in a polyethylene terephthalate bottle and refrigerated (Vasotec prescribing information, 2011).

A 1 mg/mL oral suspension may be made with tablets and one of three different vehicles (cherry syrup, a 1:1 mixture of Ora-Sweet and Ora-Plus, or a 1:1 mixture of Ora-Sweet SF and Ora-Plus). Crush six 20 mg tablets in a mortar and reduce to a fine powder. Add 15 mL of the chosen vehicle and mix to a uniform paste; mix while adding the vehicle in incremental proportions to **almost** 120 mL; transfer to a calibrated bottle, rinse mortar with vehicle, and add quantity of vehicle sufficient to make 120 mL. Label "shake well" and "protect from light". Stable for 60 days when stored in amber plastic prescription bottles in the dark at room temperature or refrigerated (Allen, 1998).

A 1 mg/mL oral suspension may be made with tablets and one of three different vehicles (deionized water, citrate buffer solution at pH 5.0, or a 1:1 mixture of Ora-Sweet and Ora-Plus). Crush twenty 10 mg tablets in a mortar and reduce to a fine powder. Add small portions of the chosen vehicle and mix to a uniform paste; mix while adding vehicle in incremental proportions to **almost** 200 mL; transfer to a graduated cylinder, rinse mortar with vehicle, and add quantity of vehicle sufficient to make 200 mL.

Label "shake well" and "protect from light". Preparations made in citrate buffer solution at pH 5.0 and the 1:1 mixture of Ora-Sweet and Ora-Plus are stable for 91 days when stored in plastic prescription bottles in the dark at room temperature or refrigerated. Preparation made in deionized water is stable for 91 days refrigerated or 56 days at room temperature when stored in plastic prescription bottles in the dark. **Note:** To prepare the isotonic citrate buffer solution (pH 5.0), see reference (Nahata, 1998).

A more dilute, 0.1 mg/mL oral suspension may be made with tablets and an isotonic buffer solution at pH 5.0. Grind one 20 mg tablet in a glass mortar and reduce to a fine powder; mix with isotonic citrate buffer (pH 5.0) and filter; add quantity of buffer solution sufficient to make 200 mL. Label "shake well", "protect from light", and "refrigerate". Stable for 90 days (Boulton, 1994).

Allen LV Jr and Erickson MA 3rd, "Stability of Alprazolam, Chloroquine Phosphate, Cisapride, Enalapril Maleate, and Hydralazine Hydrochloride in Extemporaneously Compounded Oral Liquids," *Am J Health Syst Pharm*, 1998, 55(18):1915-20.

Boulton DW, Woods DJ, Fawcett JP, et al, "The Stability of an Enalapril Maleate Oral Solution Prepared From Tablets," *Aust J Hosp Pharm*, 1994, 24(2):151-6.

Nahata MC, Morosco RS, and Hipple TF, "Stability of Enalapril Maleate in Three Extemporaneously Prepared Oral Liquids," *Am J Health Syst Pharm*, 1998, 55(11):1155-7.

Vasotec® prescribing information, Valeant Pharmaceuticals North America LLC, Bridgewater, NJ; 2011.

Enalapril and Hydrochlorothiazide

(e NAL a pril & hye droe klor oh THYE a zide)

Brand Names: U.S. Vaseretic

Brand Names: Canada Apo-Enalapril Maleate/Hctz; Novo-Enalapril/Hctz; Vaseretic

Index Terms Enalapril Maleate and Hydrochlorothiazide; Hydrochlorothiazide and Enalapril

Pharmacologic Category Angiotensin-Converting Enzyme (ACE) Inhibitor; Antihypertensive; Diuretic, Thiazide

Use Treatment of hypertension

Pregnancy Risk Factor D

Dosage Oral: Adults: Enalapril 5-10 mg and hydrochlorothiazide 12.5-25 mg once daily (maximum: 40 mg/day [enalapril]; 50 mg/day [hydrochlorothiazide])

Dosage adjustment in renal impairment:

Cl_{cr} >30 mL/minute: No dosage adjustment required.

Severe renal failure: Avoid; loop diuretics are recommended.

Dosage adjustment in hepatic impairment: No dosage adjustment provided in manufacturer's labeling; use with caution.

Additional Information Complete prescribing information should be consulted for additional detail.

Dosage Forms Excipient information presented when available (limited, particularly for generics); consult specific product labeling.

Tablet:

5/12.5: Enalapril maleate 5 mg and hydrochlorothiazide 12.5 mg

10/25: Enalapril maleate 10 mg and hydrochlorothiazide 25 mg

Vaseretic:

10/25: Enalapril maleate 10 mg and hydrochlorothiazide 25 mg

◆ Enalapril Maleate *see* Enalapril *on page* 701

◆ Enalapril Maleate and Hydrochlorothiazide *see* Enalapril and Hydrochlorothiazide *on page* 704

◆ Enbrel *see* Etanercept *on page* 780

◆ Enbrel SureClick *see* Etanercept *on page* 780

◆ Endocet *see* Oxycodone and Acetaminophen *on page* 1538

◆ Endodan® *see* Oxycodone and Aspirin *on page* 1539

◆ Endometrin *see* Progesterone *on page* 1725

◆ Enduron *see* Methyclothiazide *on page* 1332

◆ Enemeez Mini [OTC] *see* Docusate *on page* 644

◆ Enerjets [OTC] *see* Caffeine *on page* 309

Enfuvirtide (en FYOO vir tide)

Brand Names: U.S. Fuzeon

Brand Names: Canada Fuzeon®

Index Terms T-20

Pharmacologic Category Antiretroviral, Fusion Protein Inhibitor (Anti-HIV)

Use Treatment of HIV-1 infection in combination with other antiretroviral agents in treatment-experienced patients with evidence of HIV-1 replication despite ongoing antiretroviral therapy

Pregnancy Risk Factor B

Pregnancy Considerations Teratogenic effects were not observed in animal studies. Limited data suggest that enfuvirtide does not cross the placenta. The DHHS Perinatal HIV Guidelines note that data are insufficient to recommend use during pregnancy.

Regardless of CD4 count or HIV RNA copy number, all HIV-infected pregnant women should receive a combination antepartum antiretroviral (ARV) drug regimen; this includes women who require therapy for their own health, as well as women who do not yet require therapy for their own health. ARV therapy should be started as soon as possible if required for the woman's health. Although earlier initiation may be more effective in reducing the perinatal transmission of HIV, also consider maternal conditions (eg, nausea and vomiting) and the potential risks of first trimester fetal exposure for specific agents. Plasma HIV RNA levels should be assessed at ~34-36 weeks gestation in order to help determine mode of delivery. If ARV therapy must be interrupted for <24 hours during the peripartum period, stop then restart all medications simultaneously in order to decrease the chance of developing resistance. Long-term follow-up is recommended for all infants exposed to ARV medications.

Healthcare providers are encouraged to enroll pregnant women exposed to antiretroviral medications in the Antiretroviral Pregnancy Registry (1-800-258-4263 or www.APRegistry.com). Healthcare providers caring for HIV-infected women and their infants may contact the National Perinatal HIV Hotline (888-448-8765) for clinical consultation (DHHS [perinatal], 2012).

Breast-Feeding Considerations Maternal or infant antiretroviral therapy does not completely eliminate the risk of postnatal HIV transmission. In addition, multiclass-resistant virus has been detected in breast-feeding infants despite maternal therapy. Therefore, in the United States, where formula is accessible, affordable, safe, and sustainable, and the risk of infant mortality due to diarrhea and respiratory infections is low, complete avoidance of breast-feeding by HIV-infected women is recommended to decrease potential transmission of HIV (DHHS [perinatal], 2012).

Contraindications Hypersensitivity to enfuvirtide or any component of the formulation

Warnings/Precautions Use is not recommended in antiretroviral therapy-naive patients (DHHS, 2013). Monitor closely for signs/symptoms of pneumonia; associated with an increased incidence during clinical trials, particularly in patients with a low CD4 cell count, high initial viral load, I.V. drug use, smoking, or a history of lung disease. May cause hypersensitivity reactions (symptoms may include rash, fever, nausea, vomiting, hypotension, and elevated transaminases). In addition, local injection site reactions are common. Patients may develop immune reconstitution syndrome resulting in the occurrence of an inflammatory response to an indolent or residual opportunistic infection during initial HIV treatment or activation of autoimmune disorders (eg, Graves' disease, polymyositis, Guillain-Barré syndrome) later in therapy; further evaluation and treatment may be required. Administration using a needle-free device has been associated with nerve pain (including neuralgia and/or paresthesia lasting up to 6 months), bruising, and hematomas when administered at sites where large nerves are close to the skin; only administer medication in recommended sites and use caution in patients with coagulation disorders (eg, hemophilia) or receiving anticoagulants. Safety and efficacy have not been established in children <6 years of age.

Adverse Reactions

>10%:

Central nervous system: Fatigue (20%), insomnia (11%)

Gastrointestinal: Diarrhea (32%), nausea (23%)

Local: Injection site infection (children 11%), injection site reactions (98%; may include pain, erythema, induration, pruritus, ecchymosis, nodule or cyst formation)

1% to 10%:

Dermatologic: Folliculitis (2%)

Gastrointestinal: Weight loss (7%), abdominal pain (4%), appetite decreased (3%), pancreatitis (3%), anorexia (2%), xerostomia (2%)

Hematologic: Eosinophilia (2% to 9%)

Hepatic: Transaminases increased (4%, grade 4: 1%)

Local: Injection site infection (adults 2%)

Neuromuscular & skeletal: CPK increased (3% to 7%), limb pain (3%), myalgia (3%)

Ocular: Conjunctivitis (2%)

Respiratory: Sinusitis (6%), cough (4%), bacterial pneumonia (3%)

Miscellaneous: Infections (4% to 6%), herpes simplex (4%), flu-like syndrome (2%)

<1% (Limited to important or life-threatening): Abacavir hypersensitivity worsening, amylase increased, angina, anxiety, constipation, depression, GGT increased, glomerulonephritis, Guillain-Barré syndrome, hepatic steatosis, hyperglycemia; hypersensitivity reactions (symptoms may include rash, fever, nausea, vomiting, hypotension, and transaminase increases); insomnia, lipase increased, lymphadenopathy, neutropenia, peripheral neuropathy, pneumopathy, renal failure, renal insufficiency, respiratory distress, sepsis, sixth nerve palsy, suicide attempt, taste disturbances, thrombocytopenia, toxic hepatitis, triglycerides increased, tubular necrosis, weakness

Drug Interactions

Metabolism/Transport Effects None known.

Avoid Concomitant Use There are no known interactions where it is recommended to avoid concomitant use.

Increased Effect/Toxicity

Enfuvirtide may increase the levels/effects of: Protease Inhibitors

The levels/effects of Enfuvirtide may be increased by: Protease Inhibitors

Decreased Effect There are no known significant interactions involving a decrease in effect.

Preparation for Administration Reconstitute with 1.1 mL SWFI; tap vial for 10 seconds and roll gently to ensure contact with diluent; then allow to stand until solution is completed; may require up to 45 minutes to form solution (108 mg/1.2 mL).

Storage/Stability Store powder at 15°C to 30°C (59°F to 86°F). Reconstituted solutions should be refrigerated and must be used within 24 hours.

Mechanism of Action Binds to the first heptad-repeat (HR1) in the gp41 subunit of the viral envelope glycoprotein. Inhibits the fusion of HIV-1 virus with CD4 cells by blocking the conformational change in gp41 required for membrane fusion and entry into CD4 cells

Pharmacodynamics/Kinetics

Distribution: V_d: 5.5 L; CSF concentrations (2-18 hours after administration): nondetectable (<0.025 mcg/mL)

Protein binding: 92%

Metabolism: Proteolytic hydrolysis (CYP isoenzymes do not appear to contribute to metabolism)

Clearance: Adults: 24.8 mL/hour/kg

Bioavailability: 84% ± 16%

Half-life elimination: 3.8 hours

Time to peak: 4-8 hours

Dosage Note: Use is not recommended in antiretroviral therapy naïve patients (DHHS, 2013). SubQ:

Children 6-16 years: 2 mg/kg twice daily (maximum dose: 90 mg twice daily)

Adolescents ≥16 years and Adults: 90 mg twice daily

Dosage adjustment in renal impairment:

Cl_{cr} >35 mL/minute: Clearance not affected; no dosage adjustment required.

Cl_{cr} ≤35 mL/minute: Limited data showed decreased clearance; however, no dosage adjustment recommended.

End-stage renal disease (on dialysis): Limited data showed decreased clearance; however, no dosage adjustment recommended.

Dosage adjustment in hepatic impairment: No dosage adjustment required

Administration Inject subcutaneously into upper arm, abdomen, or anterior thigh. Do not inject into moles, the navel, over a blood vessel or skin abnormalities such as scar tissue, surgical scars, bruises, or tattoos. In addition, do not inject in or near sites where large nerves are close to the skin including the elbow, knee, groin, or buttocks. Rotate injection site, give injections at a site different from the preceding injection site; do not inject into any site where an injection site reaction is evident. Bioequivalence was found to be similar in a study comparing standard administration using a needle versus a needle-free device.

Additional Information If hypersensitivity reactions occur (symptoms may include rash, fever, nausea, vomiting, hypotension, and transaminase increases), enfuvirtide rechallenge is not recommended. If changing to an oral antiretroviral, raltegravir may be considered if not used previously.

Dosage Forms Excipient information presented when available (limited, particularly for generics); consult specific product labeling.

Solution Reconstituted, Subcutaneous:

Fuzeon: 90 mg (1 ea)

- **Engerix-B®** *see* Hepatitis B Vaccine (Recombinant) *on page 995*
- **Engerix-B® and Havrix®** *see* Hepatitis A and Hepatitis B Recombinant Vaccine *on page 990*
- **Enhanced-Potency Inactivated Poliovirus Vaccine** *see* Poliovirus Vaccine (Inactivated) *on page 1666*
- **Enjuvia** *see* Estrogens (Conjugated B/Synthetic) *on page 767*
- **Enlon** *see* Edrophonium *on page 686*
- **Enlon® (Can)** *see* Edrophonium *on page 686*
- **Enlon-Plus®** *see* Edrophonium and Atropine *on page 687*
- **EnovaRX-Ibuprofen** *see* Ibuprofen *on page 1032*

Enoxaparin (ee noks a PA rin)

Brand Names: U.S. Lovenox

Brand Names: Canada Enoxaparin Injection; Lovenox; Lovenox HP

Index Terms Enoxaparin Sodium

Pharmacologic Category Low Molecular Weight Heparin

Additional Appendix Information

Dosing Considerations for the Critically-Ill Patient With Morbid Obesity *on page 2379*

Use

Acute coronary syndromes: Unstable angina (UA), non-ST-elevation (NSTEMI), and ST-elevation myocardial infarction (STEMI)

DVT prophylaxis: Following hip or knee replacement surgery, abdominal surgery, or in medical patients with severely-restricted mobility during acute illness who are at risk for thromboembolic complications. **Note:** Patients at risk of thromboembolic complications who undergo abdominal surgery include those with one or more of the following risk factors: >40 years of age, obesity, general anesthesia lasting >30 minutes, malignancy, history of deep vein thrombosis or pulmonary embolism

DVT treatment (acute): Inpatient treatment (patients with or without pulmonary embolism) and outpatient treatment (patients without pulmonary embolism)

Unlabeled Use Prophylaxis and treatment of thromboembolism in children; anticoagulant bridge therapy during temporary interruption of vitamin K antagonist therapy in patients at high risk for thromboembolism; DVT prophylaxis following moderate-risk general surgery, major gynecologic surgery and following higher-risk general surgery for cancer; management of venous thromboembolism (VTE) during pregnancy; anticoagulant used during percutaneous coronary intervention (PCI)

Pregnancy Risk Factor B

Pregnancy Considerations Adverse events were not observed in animal reproduction studies. Low molecular weight heparin (LMWH) does not cross the placenta; increased risks of fetal bleeding or teratogenic effects have not been reported.

LMWH is recommended over unfractionated heparin for the treatment of acute venous thromboembolism (VTE) in pregnant women. LMWH is also recommended over unfractionated heparin for VTE prophylaxis in pregnant women with certain risk factors (eg, homozygous factor V Leiden, antiphospholipid antibody syndrome with ≥3 previous pregnancy losses). Prophylaxis is not routinely recommended for women undergoing assisted reproduction therapy; however, LMWH therapy is recommended for women who develop severe ovarian hyperstimulation syndrome. LMWH should be discontinued at least 24 hours prior to induction of labor or a planned cesarean delivery. For women undergoing cesarean section and who have additional risk factors for developing VTE, the prophylactic use of LMWH may be considered.

LMWH may also be used in women with mechanical heart valves (consult current ACCP guidelines for details). Women who require long-term anticoagulation with warfarin and who are considering pregnancy, LMWH substitution should be done prior to conception when possible. When choosing therapy, fetal outcomes (ie, pregnancy loss, malformations), maternal outcomes (ie, VTE, hemorrhage), burden of therapy, and maternal preference should be considered (Guyatt, 2012). Monitoring antifactor Xa levels is recommended.

Multiple-dose vials contain benzyl alcohol (avoid in pregnant women due to association with gasping syndrome in premature infants); use of preservative-free formulations is recommended.

Breast-Feeding Considerations Small amounts of LMWH have been detected in breast milk; however, because it has a low oral bioavailability, it is unlikely to cause adverse events in a nursing infant. Enoxaparin product labeling does not recommend use in nursing women; however, antithrombotic guidelines state that use of LMWH may be continued in breast-feeding women (Guyatt, 2012).

Contraindications

Hypersensitivity to enoxaparin, heparin, pork products, or any component of the formulation (including benzyl alcohol in multiple-dose vials); thrombocytopenia associated with a positive *in vitro* test for antiplatelet antibodies in the presence of enoxaparin; active major bleeding

Canadian labeling: Additional contraindications (not in U.S. labeling): Use of multiple-dose vials in newborns or premature neonates; history of confirmed or suspected immunologically-mediated heparin-induced thrombocytopenia; acute or subacute bacterial endocarditis; major blood clotting disorders; active gastric or duodenal ulcer; hemorrhagic cerebrovascular accident (except if there are systemic emboli); severe uncontrolled hypertension; diabetic or hemorrhagic retinopathy; other conditions or diseases involving an increased risk of hemorrhage; injuries to and operations on the brain, spinal cord, eyes, and ears; spinal/epidural anesthesia when repeated dosing of enoxaparin (1 mg/kg every 12 hours or 1.5 mg/kg daily) is required, due to increased risk of bleeding.

Note: Use of enoxaparin in patients with current heparin-induced thrombocytopenia (HIT) or HIT with thrombosis is **not** recommended and considered contraindicated due to high cross-reactivity to heparin-platelet factor-4 antibody (Guyatt [ACCP], 2012; Warkentin, 1999).

Warnings/Precautions [U.S. Boxed Warning]: Spinal or epidural hematomas, including subsequent long-term or permanent paralysis, may occur with recent or anticipated neuraxial anesthesia (epidural or spinal anesthesia) or spinal puncture in patients anticoagulated with LMWH or heparinoids. Consider risk versus benefit prior to spinal procedures; risk is increased by the use of concomitant agents which may alter hemostasis, the use of indwelling epidural catheters, a history of spinal deformity or spinal surgery, as well as a history of traumatic or repeated epidural or spinal punctures. Optimal timing between neuraxial procedures and enoxaparin administration is not known. Delay placement or removal of catheter for at least 12 hours after administration of low-dose enoxaparin (eg, 30-60 mg/day) and at least 24 hours after high-dose enoxaparin (eg, 0.75-1 mg/kg twice daily or 1.5 mg/kg once daily) and consider doubling these times in patients with creatinine clearance <30 mL/minute; risk of neuraxial hematoma may still exist since anti-factor Xa levels are still detectable at these time points. Patients receiving twice daily high-dose enoxaparin should have the second dose withheld to allow a longer time period prior to catheter placement or removal. Upon removal of catheter, consider withholding enoxaparin for at least 4 hours. **Patient should be observed closely for bleeding and signs and symptoms of neurological impairment if therapy is administered during or immediately following diagnostic lumbar puncture, epidural anesthesia, or spinal anesthesia. If neurological compromise is noted, urgent treatment is necessary.** If spinal hematoma is suspected, diagnose and treat immediately; spinal cord decompression may be considered although it may not prevent or reverse neurological sequelae.

Do not administer intramuscularly. Discontinue use 12-24 hours prior to CABG and dose with unfractionated heparin per institutional practice (Jneid, 2012). Not recommended for thromboprophylaxis in patients with prosthetic heart valves (especially pregnant women). Not to be used interchangeably (unit for unit) with heparin or any other low molecular weight heparins. Monitor patient closely for signs or symptoms of bleeding. Certain patients are at increased risk of bleeding. Risk factors include bacterial endocarditis; congenital or acquired bleeding disorders; active ulcerative or angiodysplastic GI diseases; severe uncontrolled hypertension; hemorrhagic stroke; use shortly after brain, spinal, or ophthalmic surgery; patients treated concomitantly with platelet inhibitors; recent GI bleeding or ulceration; renal dysfunction and hemorrhage; thrombocytopenia or platelet defects or history of heparin-induced thrombocytopenia; severe liver disease; hypertensive or diabetic retinopathy; or in patients undergoing invasive procedures. To minimize risk of bleeding following PCI, achieve hemostasis at the puncture site after PCI. If a closure device is used, sheath can be removed immediately. If manual compression is used, remove sheath 6 hours after the last I.V./SubQ dose of enoxaparin. Do not administer further doses until 6-8 hours after sheath removal; observe for signs of bleeding/hematoma formation. Cases of enoxaparin-induced thrombocytopenia and thrombosis (similar to heparin-induced thrombocytopenia [HIT]), some complicated by organ infarction, limb ischemia, or death, have been observed. Use with extreme caution or avoid in patients with history of HIT, especially if administered within 100 days of HIT episode (Warkentin, 2001); monitor platelet count closely. Use is contraindicated in patients with thrombocytopenia associated with a positive *in vitro* test for antiplatelet antibodies in the presence of enoxaparin. Discontinue therapy and consider alternative treatment if platelets are <100,000/mm^3 and/or thrombosis develops. Use caution in patients with congenital or drug-induced thrombocytopenia or platelet defects. Risk of bleeding may be increased in women <45 kg and in men <57 kg. Use caution in patients with renal failure; dosage adjustment needed if Cl_{cr} <30 mL/minute. Use with caution in the elderly (delayed elimination may occur); dosage alteration/adjustment may be required (eg, omission of I.V. bolus in acute STEMI in patients ≥75 years of age). Monitor for hyperkalemia; can cause hyperkalemia possibly by suppressing aldosterone production. Multiple-dose vials contain benzyl alcohol (use caution in pregnant women). In neonates, large amounts of benzyl alcohol (>100 mg/kg/day) have been associated with fatal toxicity (gasping syndrome). Use of multiple-dose vials is contraindicated in patients who have hypersensitivity to benzyl alcohol.

Safety and efficacy of prophylactic dosing of enoxaparin has not been established in patients who are obese (>30 kg/m^2) nor is there a consensus regarding dosage adjustments. The American College of Chest Physicians Practice Guidelines suggest consulting with a pharmacist regarding dosing in bariatric surgery patients and other obese patients who may require higher doses of LMWH (Gould, 2012).

Adverse Reactions As with all anticoagulants, bleeding is the major adverse effect of enoxaparin. Hemorrhage may occur at virtually any site. Risk is dependent on multiple variables. At the recommended doses, single injections of enoxaparin do not significantly influence platelet aggregation or affect global clotting time (ie, PT or aPTT).

1% to 10%:

Central nervous system: Confusion (2%), pain

Gastrointestinal: Nausea (3%), diarrhea (2%)

Hematologic & oncologic: Major hemorrhage (<1% to 4%; includes cases of intracranial, retroperitoneal, or intraocular hemorrhage; incidence varies with indication/population), thrombocytopenia (moderate 1%; severe 0.1%), anemia (<2%), bruise

Hepatic: Increased serum ALT (6%), increased serum AST (6%)

Local: Hematoma at injection site (9%), irritation at injection site, bruising at injection site, erythema at injection site, pain at injection site

Renal: Hematuria (≤2%)

Miscellaneous: Fever (5% to 8%)

<1% (limited to important or life-threatening): Alopecia, anaphylaxis, anaphylactoid reaction, eczematous rash (plaques), eosinophilia, epidural hematoma (spinal; after neuroaxial anesthesia or spinal puncture; risk may be increased with indwelling epidural catheter or concomitant use of other drugs affecting hemostasis), headache, hepatic injury (hepatocellular and cholestatic), hyperkalemia, hyperlipidemia (very rare), hypersensitivity angiitis, hypersensitivity reaction, hypertriglyceridemia, intracranial hemorrhage (up to 0.8%), osteoporosis (following long-term therapy), pruritic erythematous rash (patches), pruritus, purpura, retroperitoneal hemorrhage, severe anemia (hemorrhagic), shock, skin necrosis, thrombocythemia, thrombocytopenia, thrombosis (prosthetic value [in pregnant females] or associated with enoxaparin-induced thrombocytopenia; can cause limb ischemia or organ infarction), urticaria, vesicobullous rash

Drug Interactions

Metabolism/Transport Effects None known.

Avoid Concomitant Use

Avoid concomitant use of Enoxaparin with any of the following: Apixaban; Dabigatran Etexilate; Omacetaxine; Rivaroxaban

Increased Effect/Toxicity

Enoxaparin may increase the levels/effects of: ACE Inhibitors; Aliskiren; Angiotensin II Receptor Blockers; Anticoagulants; Canagliflozin; Collagenase (Systemic); Deferasirox; Eplerenone; Ibritumomab; Omacetaxine; Palifermin; Potassium Salts; Potassium-Sparing Diuretics; Rivaroxaban; Tositumomab and Iodine I 131 Tositumomab

The levels/effects of Enoxaparin may be increased by: 5-ASA Derivatives; Agents with Antiplatelet Properties; Apixaban; Dabigatran Etexilate; Dasatinib; Herbs (Anticoagulant/Antiplatelet Properties); Ibrutinib; Nonsteroidal Anti-Inflammatory Agents; Omega-3 Fatty Acids; Pentosan Polysulfate Sodium; Pentoxifylline; Prostacyclin Analogues; Salicylates; Sugammadex; Thrombolytic Agents; Tibolone; Tipranavir; Vitamin E

Decreased Effect

The levels/effects of Enoxaparin may be decreased by: Estrogen Derivatives; Progestins

Ethanol/Nutrition/Herb Interactions Herb/Nutraceutical: Avoid cat's claw, dong quai, evening primrose, feverfew, garlic, ginger, ginkgo, red clover, horse chestnut, green tea, ginseng (all have additional antiplatelet activity).

Storage/Stability Store at 25°C (77°F); excursions permitted to 15°C to 30°C (59°F to 86°F); do not freeze. Do not store multiple-dose vials for >28 days after first use.

Mechanism of Action Standard heparin consists of components with molecular weights ranging from 4000-30,000 daltons with a mean of 16,000 daltons. Heparin acts as an anticoagulant by enhancing the inhibition rate of clotting proteases by antithrombin III impairing normal hemostasis and inhibition of factor Xa. Low molecular weight heparins have a small effect on the activated partial thromboplastin time and strongly inhibit factor Xa. Enoxaparin is derived from porcine heparin that undergoes benzylation followed by alkaline depolymerization. The average molecular weight of enoxaparin is 4500 daltons which is distributed as (≤20%) 2000 daltons (≥68%) 2000-8000 daltons, and (≤15%) >8000 daltons. Enoxaparin has a higher ratio of antifactor Xa to antifactor IIa activity than unfractionated heparin.

Pharmacodynamics/Kinetics

Onset of action: Peak effect: SubQ: Antifactor Xa and antithrombin (antifactor IIa): 3-5 hours

Duration: 40 mg dose: Antifactor Xa activity: ~12 hours
Distribution: 4.3 L (based on antifactor Xa activity)
Protein binding: Does not bind to heparin binding proteins
Metabolism: Hepatic, to lower molecular weight fragments (little activity)
Half-life elimination, plasma: 2-4 times longer than standard heparin, independent of dose; based on anti-Xa activity: 4.5-7 hours
Excretion: Urine (40% of dose; 10% as active fragments)

Dosage Note: One mg of enoxaparin is equal to 100 units of anti-Xa activity (World Health Organization First International Low Molecular Weight Heparin Reference Standard).

Infants and Children (unlabeled use; Monagle, 2012):
SubQ:
Infants <2 months: Initial:
Prophylaxis: 0.75 mg/kg every 12 hours
Treatment: 1.5 mg/kg every 12 hours
Infants >2 months and Children ≤18 years: Initial:
Prophylaxis: 0.5 mg/kg every 12 hours
Treatment: 1 mg/kg every 12 hours
Maintenance: See **Dosage Titration** table:

Enoxaparin Pediatric Dosage Titration[1]

Anti-Xa Result	Dose Titration	Time to Repeat Anti-Xa Measurement
<0.35 units/mL	Increase dose by 25%	4 h after next dose
0.35-0.49 units/mL	Increase dose by 10%	4 h after next dose
0.5-1 unit/mL	Keep same dosage	Next day, then 1 wk later, then monthly (4 h after dose)
1.1-1.5 units/mL	Decrease dose by 20%	Before next dose
1.6-2 units/mL	Hold dose for 3 h and decrease dose by 30%	Before next dose, then 4 h after next dose
>2 units/mL	Hold all doses until anti-Xa is 0.5 units/mL, then decrease dose by 40%	Before next dose and every 12 h until anti-Xa <0.5 units/mL

[1]Nomogram to be used for treatment dosing.

Modified from Duplaga BA, et al, "Dosing and Monitoring of Low-Molecular-Weight Heparins in Special Populations," *Pharmacotherapy*, 2001, 21(2):218-34.

Adults: Note: Weight -based doses (eg, 1 mg/kg) are commonly rounded to the nearest 10 mg; also see institution-specific rounding protocols if available. Most available prefilled syringes are graduated in 10 mg increments.
SubQ:
DVT prophylaxis: SubQ:
Obesity: **Note:** In morbidly-obese patients (BMI ≥40 kg/m^2), increasing the prophylactic dose by 30% may be appropriate for some indications (Nutescu, 2009). For bariatric surgery, dose increases may be >30% based on clinical trial data.
Abdominal surgery: 40 mg once daily, with initial dose given 2 hours prior to surgery; continue until risk of DVT has diminished (usually 7-10 days).
Hip replacement surgery:
Twice-daily dosing: 30 mg every 12 hours, with initial dose within 12-24 hours after surgery, and every 12 hours for at least 10 days or until risk of DVT has diminished or the patient is adequately anticoagulated on warfarin. The American College of Chest Physicians recommends initiation ≥12 hours preoperatively **or** ≥12 hours postoperatively; extended duration of up to 35 days suggested (Guyatt, 2012).
Once-daily dosing: 40 mg once daily, with initial dose within 9-15 hours before surgery, and daily for at least 10 days (or up to 35 days postoperatively) or until risk of DVT has diminished or the patient is adequately anticoagulated on warfarin. The American College of Chest Physicians recommends initiation ≥12 hours preoperatively **or** ≥12 hours postoperatively; extended duration of up to 35 days suggested (Guyatt, 2012).
Knee replacement surgery: 30 mg every 12 hours, with initial dose within 12-24 hours after surgery, and every 12 hours for at least 10 days or until risk of DVT has diminished or the patient is adequately anticoagulated on warfarin. The American College of Chest Physicians recommends initiation ≥12 hours preoperatively **or** ≥12 hours postoperatively; extended duration of up to 35 days suggested (Guyatt, 2012).
Medical patients with severely-restricted mobility during acute illness: 40 mg once daily; continue until risk of DVT has diminished (usually 6-11 days).
Bariatric surgery (unlabeled use): Roux-en-Y gastric bypass: Appropriate dosing strategies have not been clearly defined (Borkgren-Okonek, 2008; Scholten, 2002):
BMI ≤50 kg/m^2: 40 mg every 12 hours
BMI >50 kg/m^2: 60 mg every 12 hours
Note: Bariatric surgery guidelines suggest initiation 30-120 minutes before surgery and postoperatively until patient is fully mobile (Mechanick, 2009). Alternatively, limiting administration to the postoperative period may reduce perioperative bleeding.
Prevention of recurrent venous thromboembolism in pregnancy (unlabeled use): 40 mg once daily. Therapy should continue for 6 weeks postpartum in high-risk women (Bates, 2012).
DVT treatment (acute): **Note:** Start warfarin on the first or second treatment day and continue enoxaparin until INR is ≥2 for at least 24 hours (usually 5-7 days) (Guyatt, 2012).
Inpatient treatment (with or without pulmonary embolism): 1 mg/kg/dose every 12 hours or 1.5 mg/kg once daily.
Outpatient treatment (without pulmonary embolism): 1 mg/kg/dose every 12 hours.
Obesity: Use actual body weight to calculate dose; dose capping not recommended; use of twice daily dosing preferred (Nutescu, 2009).
Pregnant women: 1 mg/kg/dose every 12 hours. Discontinue ≥24 hours prior to the induction of labor or cesarean section. Enoxaparin therapy may be substituted with heparin near term. Continue anticoagulation therapy for ≥6 weeks postpartum (minimum duration of therapy: 3 months). LMWH or heparin therapy is preferred over warfarin during pregnancy (Bates, 2012).
ST-elevation myocardial infarction (STEMI):
Patients <75 years of age: Initial: 30 mg I.V. single bolus plus 1 mg/kg (maximum 100 mg for the first 2 doses only) SubQ every 12 hours. The first SubQ dose should be administered with the I.V. bolus. Maintenance: After first 2 doses, administer 1 mg/kg SubQ every 12 hours.
Patients ≥75 years of age: Initial: SubQ: 0.75 mg/kg every 12 hours (**Note:** No I.V. bolus is administered in this population); a maximum dose of 75 mg is recommended for the first 2 doses. Maintenance: After first 2 doses, administer 0.75 mg/kg SubQ every 12 hours
Obesity: Use weight-based dosing; a maximum dose of 100 mg is recommended for the first 2 doses (Nutescu, 2009)

Additional notes on STEMI treatment: Therapy was continued for 8 days or until hospital discharge; optimal duration not defined. Unless contraindicated, all patients received aspirin (75-325 mg daily) in clinical trials. In patients with STEMI receiving thrombolytics, initiate enoxaparin dosing between 15 minutes before and 30 minutes after fibrinolytic therapy.

Unstable angina or non-ST-elevation myocardial infarction (NSTEMI): 1 mg/kg every 12 hours in conjunction with oral aspirin therapy (100-325 mg once daily); continue until clinical stabilization (a minimum of at least 2 days)

Obesity: Use actual body weight to calculate dose; dose capping not recommended (Nutescu, 2009)

I.V.: Percutaneous coronary intervention (PCI), adjunctive therapy (unlabeled dosing): In patients treated with multiple doses of enoxaparin undergoing PCI, if PCI occurs within 8 hours after the last SubQ enoxaparin dose, no additional dosing is needed. If PCI occurs 8-12 hours after the last SubQ enoxaparin dose or the patient received only 1 therapeutic SubQ dose (eg, 1 mg/kg), a single I.V. dose of 0.3 mg/kg should be administered. If PCI occurs >12 hours after the last SubQ dose, it is prudent to use an established anticoagulation regimen (eg, full-dose unfractionated heparin or bivalirudin) (Levine, 2011).

If patient has not received prior anticoagulant therapy: 0.5-0.75 mg/kg bolus dose (Levine, 2011)

Conversion from I.V. unfractionated heparin (UFH) infusion to SubQ enoxaparin (Nutescu, 2007): Calculate specific dose for enoxaparin based on indication, discontinue UFH and begin enoxaparin within 1 hour.

Conversion from SubQ enoxaparin to I.V. UFH infusion (Nutescu, 2007): Discontinue enoxaparin, calculate specific dose for I.V. UFH infusion based on indication, omit heparin bolus/loading dose:

Converting from SubQ enoxaparin dosed every 12 hours: Start I.V. UFH infusion 10-11 hours after last dose of enoxaparin

Converting from SubQ enoxaparin dosed every 24 hours: Start I.V. UFH infusion 22-23 hours after last dose of enoxaparin

Elderly: Refer to adult dosing. Increased incidence of bleeding with doses of 1.5 mg/kg/day or 1 mg/kg every 12 hours; injection-associated bleeding and serious adverse reactions are also increased in the elderly. Careful attention should be paid to elderly patients, particularly those <45 kg. **Note:** Dosage alteration/adjustment may be required.

Dosage adjustment in renal impairment: SubQ:

Cl_{cr} ≥30 mL/minute: No specific adjustment recommended (per manufacturer); monitor closely for bleeding

Cl_{cr} <30 mL/minute:

DVT prophylaxis in abdominal surgery, hip replacement, knee replacement, or in medical patients during acute illness: 30 mg once daily. **Note:** The Canadian labeling recommends 20-30 mg once daily (based on risk/benefit assessment) for prophylaxis in abdominal or colorectal surgery or in medical patients during acute illness.

DVT treatment (inpatient or outpatient treatment in conjunction with warfarin): 1 mg/kg once daily

STEMI:

<75 years: Initial: I.V.: 30 mg as a single dose with the first dose of the SubQ maintenance regimen administered at the same time as the I.V. bolus; Maintenance: SubQ: 1 mg/kg once daily

≥75 years of age: Omit I.V. bolus; Maintenance: SubQ: 1 mg/kg once daily

Unstable angina, NSTEMI: SubQ: 1 mg/kg once daily

Dialysis: Enoxaparin has not been FDA approved for use in dialysis patients. It's elimination is primarily via the renal route. Serious bleeding complications have been reported with use in patients who are dialysis dependent or have severe renal failure. LMWH administration at fixed doses without monitoring has greater unpredictable anticoagulant effects in patients with chronic kidney disease. If used, dosages should be reduced and anti-Xa levels frequently monitored, as accumulation may occur with repeated doses. Many clinicians would not use enoxaparin in this population especially without timely anti-Xa levels.

Hemodialysis: Supplemental dose is not necessary.

Peritoneal dialysis: Significant drug removal is unlikely based on physiochemical characteristics.

Dosage adjustment in hepatic impairment: No dosage adjustment provided in manufacturer's labeling (has not been studied); use with caution.

Administration Note: Enoxaparin is available in 100 mg/mL and 150 mg/mL concentrations.

SubQ: Administer by deep SubQ injection alternating between the left or right anterolateral and left or right posterolateral abdominal wall. Do not mix with other infusions or injections. In order to minimize bruising, do not rub injection site. To avoid loss of drug from the 30 mg and 40 mg prefilled syringes, do not expel the air bubble from the syringe prior to injection.

I.V.: STEMI and PCI only: The U.S. labeling recommends using the multiple-dose vial to prepare I.V. doses. The Canadian labeling recommends either the multiple-dose vial or a prefilled syringe. Do not mix or coadminister with other medications; may be administered with NS or D_5W. Flush I.V. access site with a sufficient amount of NS or D_5W prior to and following I.V. bolus administration. When used prior to percutaneous coronary intervention or as part of treatment for ST-elevation myocardial infarction (STEMI), a single dose may be administered I.V. except when the patient is ≥75 years of age and is experiencing STEMI then only administer by SubQ injection.

Monitoring Parameters Platelets, occult blood, anti-Xa levels, serum creatinine; monitoring of PT and/or aPTT is not necessary. Routine monitoring of anti-Xa levels is not required, but has been utilized in patients with obesity and/or renal insufficiency. Monitoring anti-Xa levels is recommended in pregnant women receiving therapeutic doses of enoxaparin or when receiving enoxaparin for the prevention of thromboembolism with mechanical heart valves (Guyatt, 2012). For patients >190 kg, if anti-Xa monitoring is available, adjusting dose based on anti-Xa levels is recommended; if anti-Xa monitoring is unavailable, reduce dose if bleeding occurs (Nutescu, 2009). Monitor obese patients closely for signs/symptoms of thromboembolism.

Reference Range The following therapeutic ranges for anti-Xa levels have been suggested, but have not been validated in a controlled trial. Anti-Xa level measured 4 hours postdose.

Treatment of venous thromboembolism: Anti-Xa concentration target (Garcia, 2012):

Once-daily dosing: >1 anti-Xa units/mL; the manufacturer recommends a range of 1-2 anti-Xa units/mL

Twice-daily dosing: 0.6-1 anti-Xa units/mL

Recurrent VTE prophylaxis in pregnant women: Peak anti-Xa concentrations: 0.2-0.6 units/mL (Bates, 2012)

Additional Information Neutralization of enoxaparin (in overdose) with protamine 1% solution: Manufacturer's recommendations:

Enoxaparin administered in ≤8 hours: Dose of protamine should equal the dose of enoxaparin administered. Therefore, 1 mg of protamine sulfate neutralizes 1 mg of enoxaparin

Enoxaparin administered in >8 hours or if it has been determined that a second dose is required (eg, if aPTT measured 2-4 hours after the first dose remains prolonged or if bleeding continues): 0.5 mg of protamine sulfate for every 1 mg of enoxaparin administered

Dosage Forms Excipient information presented when available (limited, particularly for generics); consult specific product labeling.

Solution, Injection, as sodium:
Lovenox: 300 mg/3 mL (3 mL) [contains benzyl alcohol]
Generic: 300 mg/3 mL (3 mL)

Solution, Subcutaneous, as sodium:
Lovenox: 30 mg/0.3 mL (0.3 mL); 40 mg/0.4 mL (0.4 mL); 60 mg/0.6 mL (0.6 mL); 80 mg/0.8 mL (0.8 mL); 100 mg/mL (1 mL); 120 mg/0.8 mL (0.8 mL); 150 mg/mL (1 mL)
Generic: 30 mg/0.3 mL (0.3 mL); 40 mg/0.4 mL (0.4 mL); 60 mg/0.6 mL (0.6 mL); 80 mg/0.8 mL (0.8 mL); 100 mg/mL (1 mL); 120 mg/0.8 mL (0.8 mL); 150 mg/mL (1 mL)

Solution, Subcutaneous, as sodium [preservative free]:
Lovenox: 30 mg/0.3 mL (0.3 mL); 40 mg/0.4 mL (0.4 mL); 60 mg/0.6 mL (0.6 mL); 80 mg/0.8 mL (0.8 mL); 100 mg/mL (1 mL); 120 mg/0.8 mL (0.8 mL); 150 mg/mL (1 mL)
Generic: 30 mg/0.3 mL (0.3 mL); 40 mg/0.4 mL (0.4 mL); 60 mg/0.6 mL (0.6 mL); 80 mg/0.8 mL (0.8 mL); 100 mg/mL (1 mL); 120 mg/0.8 mL (0.8 mL); 150 mg/mL (1 mL)

◆ Enoxaparin Injection (Can) *see* Enoxaparin *on page 705*
◆ Enoxaparin Sodium *see* Enoxaparin *on page 705*
◆ Enpresse *see* Ethinyl Estradiol and Levonorgestrel *on page 787*
◆ Enskyce *see* Ethinyl Estradiol and Desogestrel *on page 784*

Entacapone (en TA ka pone)

Brand Names: U.S. Comtan

Brand Names: Canada Comtan®; Sandoz-Entacapone; Teva-Entacapone

Pharmacologic Category Anti-Parkinson's Agent, COMT Inhibitor

Additional Appendix Information
Antiparkinsonian Agents *on page 2289*

Use Adjunct to levodopa/carbidopa therapy in patients with idiopathic Parkinson's disease who experience "wearing-off" symptoms at the end of a dosing interval

Pregnancy Risk Factor C

Pregnancy Considerations Adverse events were observed in some animal reproduction studies. The incidence of Parkinson's disease in pregnancy is relatively rare and information related to the use of entacapone in pregnant women is very limited (Kranick, 2010).

Breast-Feeding Considerations It is not known if entacapone is excreted in breast milk. The manufacturer recommends that caution be exercised when administering entacapone to nursing women.

Contraindications Hypersensitivity to entacapone or any of component of the formulation

Warnings/Precautions May cause orthostatic hypotension and syncope; Parkinson's disease patients appear to have an impaired capacity to respond to a postural challenge; use with caution in patients at risk of hypotension (such as those receiving antihypertensive drugs) or where transient hypotensive episodes would be poorly tolerated (cardiovascular disease or cerebrovascular disease). Parkinson's patients being treated with dopaminergic agonists ordinarily require careful monitoring for signs and symptoms of postural hypotension, especially during dose escalation, and should be informed of this risk. May cause hallucinations, which may improve with reduction in levodopa therapy. Use with caution in patients with pre-existing dyskinesias; exacerbation of pre-existing dyskinesia and severe rhabdomyolysis has been reported. Levodopa dosage reduction may be required, particularly in patients with levodopa dosages >600 mg daily or with moderate-to-severe dyskinesia prior to initiation. Entacapone, in conjunction with other drug therapy that alters brain biogenic amine concentrations (eg, MAO inhibitors, SSRIs), has been associated with a syndrome resembling neuroleptic malignant syndrome (hyperpyrexia and confusion - some fatal) on abrupt withdrawal or dosage reduction. Concomitant use of entacapone and nonselective MAO inhibitors should be avoided. Selegiline is a selective MAO type B inhibitor (when given orally at ≤10 mg/day) and can be taken with entacapone.

Dopaminergic agents have been associated with compulsive behaviors and/or loss of impulse control, which has manifested as pathological gambling, libido increases (hypersexuality), and/or binge eating. Causality has not been established, and controversy exists as to whether this phenomenon is related to the underlying disease, prior behaviors/addictions and/or drug therapy. Dose reduction or discontinuation of therapy has been reported to reverse these behaviors in some, but not all cases. Risk for melanoma development is increased in Parkinson's disease patients; drug causation or factors contributing to risk have not been established. Patients should be monitored closely and periodic skin examinations should be performed. Dopaminergic agents from the ergot class have also been associated with fibrotic complications, such as retroperitoneal fibrosis, pulmonary infiltrates or effusion and pleural thickening. It is unknown whether non-ergot, pro-dopaminergic agents like entacapone confer this risk. Use caution in patients with hepatic impairment or severe renal impairment. Do not withdraw therapy abruptly. Discoloration of urine, saliva, or sweat to dark colors (red, brown, black) may be observed during therapy. Use with caution in patients with lower gastrointestinal disease or an increased risk of dehydration; has been associated with delayed development of diarrhea (usual onset after 4-12 weeks). Diarrhea may be a sign of drug-induced colitis. Discontinue use with prolonged diarrhea.

Adverse Reactions

>10%:
Gastrointestinal: Nausea (14%)
Neuromuscular & skeletal: Dyskinesia (25%), placebo (15%)

1% to 10%:
Cardiovascular: Orthostatic hypotension (4.3%), syncope (1.2%)
Central nervous system: Dizziness (8%), fatigue (6%), hallucinations (4%), anxiety (2%), somnolence (2%), agitation (1%)
Dermatologic: Purpura (2%)
Gastrointestinal: Diarrhea (10%), abdominal pain (8%), constipation (6%), vomiting (4%), dry mouth (3%), dyspepsia (2%), flatulence (2%), gastritis (1%), taste perversion (1%)
Genitourinary: Brown-orange urine discoloration (10%)
Neuromuscular & skeletal: Hyperkinesia (10%), hypokinesia (9%), back pain (4%), weakness (2%)
Respiratory: Dyspnea (3%)
Miscellaneous: Diaphoresis increased (2%), bacterial infection (1%)

<1% (Limited to important or life-threatening): Hyperpyrexia and confusion (resembling neuroleptic malignant syndrome), pulmonary fibrosis, retroperitoneal fibrosis, rhabdomyolysis

Drug Interactions

Metabolism/Transport Effects Inhibits COMT, CYP1A2 (weak), CYP2A6 (weak), CYP2C19 (weak), CYP2C9 (weak), CYP2D6 (weak), CYP2E1 (weak), CYP3A4 (weak)

Avoid Concomitant Use

Avoid concomitant use of Entacapone with any of the following: Azelastine (Nasal); Paraldehyde; Pimozide

Increased Effect/Toxicity

Entacapone may increase the levels/effects of: Alcohol (Ethyl); ARIPiprazole; Azelastine (Nasal); Buprenorphine; CNS Depressants; COMT Substrates; Dofetilide; Hydrocodone; Lomitapide; MAO Inhibitors; Methotrimeprazine; Metyrosine; Mirtazapine; Paraldehyde; Pimozide; Pramipexole; ROPINIRole; Rotigotine; Selective Serotonin Reuptake Inhibitors; Zolpidem

The levels/effects of Entacapone may be increased by: Brimonidine (Topical); Doxylamine; Droperidol; HydrOXYzine; Magnesium Sulfate; Methotrimeprazine; Perampanel; Sodium Oxybate; Tapentadol

Decreased Effect There are no known significant interactions involving a decrease in effect.

Ethanol/Nutrition/Herb Interactions

Ethanol: May increase CNS depression; monitor for increased effects with coadministration. Caution patients about effects.

Food: Entacapone has been reported to chelate iron and decreasing serum iron levels were noted in clinical trials; however, clinically significant anemia has not been observed.

Mechanism of Action Entacapone is a reversible and selective inhibitor of catechol-O-methyltransferase (COMT). When entacapone is taken with levodopa, the pharmacokinetics are altered, resulting in more sustained levodopa serum levels compared to levodopa taken alone. The resulting levels of levodopa provide for increased concentrations available for absorption across the blood-brain barrier, thereby providing for increased CNS levels of dopamine, the active metabolite of levodopa.

Pharmacodynamics/Kinetics

Onset of action: Rapid

Peak effect: 1 hour

Absorption: Rapid

Distribution: I.V.: V_{dss}: 20 L

Protein binding: 98%, primarily to albumin

Metabolism: Isomerization to the *cis*-isomer, followed by direct glucuronidation of the parent and *cis*-isomer

Bioavailability: 35%

Half-life elimination: Β phase: 0.4-0.7 hours; Y phase: 2.4 hours

Time to peak, serum: 1 hour

Excretion: Feces (90%); urine (10%)

Dosage Oral: Adults: 200 mg with each dose of levodopa/carbidopa, up to a maximum of 8 times/day (maximum daily dose: 1600 mg/day). To optimize therapy, the dosage of levodopa may need reduced or the dosing interval may need extended. Patients taking levodopa ≥800 mg/day or who had moderate-to-severe dyskinesias prior to therapy required an average decrease of 25% in the daily levodopa dose.

Dosage adjustment in hepatic impairment: Treat with caution and monitor carefully; AUC and C_{max} can be possibly doubled

Dietary Considerations May be taken without regard to meals.

Administration Always administer in association with levodopa/carbidopa; can be combined with both the immediate and sustained release formulations of levodopa/carbidopa. May be administered without regard to meals. Should not be abruptly withdrawn from patient's therapy due to significant worsening of symptoms.

Monitoring Parameters Signs and symptoms of Parkinson's disease; liver function tests, blood pressure, patient's mental status; serum iron (if signs of anemia)

Dosage Forms Excipient information presented when available (limited, particularly for generics); consult specific product labeling.

Tablet, Oral:

Comtan: 200 mg

Generic: 200 mg

◆ **Entacapone, Carbidopa, and Levodopa** *see* Levodopa, Carbidopa, and Entacapone *on page 1197*

Entecavir (en TE ka veer)

Brand Names: U.S. Baraclude

Brand Names: Canada Baraclude®

Pharmacologic Category Antiviral Agent

Use Treatment of chronic hepatitis B virus (HBV) infection, with compensated or decompensated liver disease, in patients with evidence of active viral replication and either evidence of persistent transaminase elevations or histologically-active disease

Unlabeled Use HBV reinfection prophylaxis, post liver transplant; HIV/HBV coinfection

Pregnancy Risk Factor C

Pregnancy Considerations Teratogenic effects have been observed in animal studies. Information related to use in pregnancy is limited; use only if other options are inappropriate (DHHS [OI], 2013). Pregnant women taking entecavir should enroll in the pregnancy registry by calling 1-800-258-4263.

Breast-Feeding Considerations It is not known if entecavir is excreted in breast milk. Due to the potential for serious adverse reactions in the nursing infant, the manufacturer recommends a decision be made whether to discontinue nursing or to discontinue the drug, taking into account the importance of treatment to the mother.

Contraindications There are no contraindications listed in the manufacturer's U.S. labeling.

Canadian labeling: Hypersensitivity to entecavir or any component of the formulation

Warnings/Precautions Hazardous agent - use appropriate precautions for handling and disposal (NIOSH, 2012). **[U.S. Boxed Warning]: Lactic acidosis and severe hepatomegaly with steatosis (including fatal cases) have been reported. [U.S. Boxed Warning]: Severe, acute exacerbation of hepatitis B may occur upon discontinuation of antihepatitis B therapy, including entecavir. Monitor liver function for at least several months after stopping treatment; reinitiation of antihepatitis B therapy may be required.** Use caution in patients with renal impairment or in patients receiving concomitant therapy which may reduce renal function; dose adjustment recommended for Cl_{cr} <50 mL/minute. Cross-resistance may develop in patients failing previous therapy with lamivudine.

HIV: **[U.S. Boxed Warning]: May cause the development of HIV resistance in chronic hepatitis B patients with unrecognized or untreated HIV infection.** Determine HIV status prior to initiating treatment with entecavir. **Not recommended for HIV/HBV coinfected patients unless also receiving highly active antiretroviral therapy (HAART).** The manufacturer's labeling states that entecavir does not exhibit any clinically-relevant activity against human immunodeficiency virus (HIV type 1). However, a small number of case reports have indicated declines in virus levels during entecavir therapy. HIV resistance to a common HIV drug has been reported in an HIV/HBV-infected patient receiving entecavir as monotherapy for HBV.

Dose adjustment not required in patients with hepatic impairment. Limited data supporting treatment of chronic hepatitis B in patients with decompensated liver disease; observe for increased adverse reactions, including hepatorenal dysfunction.

Adverse Reactions

>10%:

Cardiovascular: Peripheral edema (16% with decompensated liver disease)

Central nervous system: Pyrexia (14% with decompensated liver disease)

Hepatic: Ascites (15% with decompensated liver disease), ALT increased (>5 x ULN: 11% to 12%; post-treatment flare [lamivudine refractory]: >10 x ULN and >2 x baseline: 12%)

1% to 10%:

Central nervous system: Headache (2% to 4%), fatigue (1% to 3%), dizziness

Endocrine & metabolic: Hyperglycemia (2% to 3%), blood bicarbonate decreased (2% with decompensated liver disease)

Gastrointestinal: Lipase increased (7%), amylase increased (2% to 3%), diarrhea (≤1%), dyspepsia (≤1%), nausea

Hepatic: Hepatic encephalopathy (10% with decompensated liver disease), bilirubin increased (2% to 3%), ALT increased (>10 x ULN and >2 x baseline: 2%; post-treatment flare [nucleoside-naive]: >10 x ULN and >2 x baseline: 2% to 8%)

Renal: Hematuria (9%), glycosuria (4%), creatinine increased (1% to 2%)

Respiratory: Upper respiratory tract infection (10% with decompensated liver disease)

<1% (Limited to important or life-threatening): Alopecia, anaphylactoid reaction, hepatomegaly, hypoalbuminemia, insomnia, lactic acidosis, macular edema (Muqit, 2011), rash, renal failure, somnolence, thrombocytopenia, vomiting

Drug Interactions

Metabolism/Transport Effects None known.

Avoid Concomitant Use There are no known interactions where it is recommended to avoid concomitant use.

Increased Effect/Toxicity

The levels/effects of Entecavir may be increased by: Ganciclovir-Valganciclovir; Ribavirin

Decreased Effect There are no known significant interactions involving a decrease in effect.

Ethanol/Nutrition/Herb Interactions Food: Food delays absorption and reduces AUC by 18% to 20%. Management: Administer on an empty stomach 2 hours before or after a meal.

Storage/Stability Store at controlled room temperature of 25°C (77°F); excursions permitted to 15°C to 30°C (59°F to 86°F). Protect oral solution from light.

Mechanism of Action Entecavir is intracellularly phosphorylated to guanosine triphosphate which competes with natural substrates to effectively inhibit hepatitis B viral polymerase; enzyme inhibition blocks reverse transcriptase activity thereby reducing viral DNA synthesis.

Pharmacodynamics/Kinetics

Absorption: Delayed with food; C_{max} decreased 44% to 46%, AUC decreased 18% to 20%

Distribution: Extensive (V_d in excess of body water)

Protein binding: ~13%

Metabolism: Minor hepatic glucuronide/sulfate conjugation

Half-life elimination: Terminal: ~5-6 days; accumulation: ~24 hours

Time to peak, plasma: 0.5-1.5 hours

Excretion: Urine (60% to 73% as unchanged drug)

Dosage

Hepatitis B virus (HBV) infection, treatment: Oral:

Adolescents ≥16 years and Adults:

Nucleoside treatment naive: 0.5 mg once daily

Lamivudine-refractory or -resistant viremia (or known lamivudine- or telbivudine-resistance mutations): 1 mg once daily

Adults: Decompensated liver disease: 1 mg once daily

HBV reinfection prophylaxis, post liver transplant (with or without HBIG) (unlabeled use): Adults: Oral: 0.5 mg once daily (Fung, 2011) or 1 mg once daily (Perrillo, 2012)

HIV/HBV coinfection (unlabeled use): Oral: Adults:

Nucleoside treatment naive: 0.5 mg once daily

Lamivudine refractory or resistant: 1 mg once daily

Note: Only recommended in patients who cannot take tenofovir; must be used in addition to a fully suppressive antiretroviral therapy regimen (DHHS, 2013).

Treatment duration (AASLD Practice Guidelines, 2009):

Hepatitis Be antigen (HBeAg) positive chronic hepatitis: Treat ≥1 year until HBeAg seroconversion and undetectable serum HBV DNA; continue therapy for ≥6 months after HBeAg seroconversion

HBeAg negative chronic hepatitis: Treat >1 year until hepatitis B surface antigen (HBsAg) clearance

Decompensated liver disease: Lifelong treatment is recommended

Note: Patients not achieving a primary response (<2 log decrease in serum HBV DNA) after at least 6 months of therapy should either receive additional treatment or be switched to an alternative therapy.

Dosage adjustment in renal impairment: Daily-dosage regimen preferred:

Cl_{cr} ≥50 mL/minute: No dosage adjustment necessary.

Cl_{cr} 30-49 mL/minute: Administer 50% of usual dose daily or administer the normal dose every 48 hours

Cl_{cr} 10-29 mL/minute: Administer 30% of usual dose daily or administer the normal dose every 72 hours

Cl_{cr} <10 mL/minute (including hemodialysis and CAPD): Administer 10% of usual dose daily or administer the normal dose every 7 days; administer after hemodialysis

Dosage adjustment in hepatic impairment: No dosage adjustment necessary.

Dietary Considerations Take on an empty stomach (2 hours before or after a meal).

Administration Administer on an empty stomach (2 hours before or after a meal). Do not dilute or mix oral solution with water or other beverages; use calibrated oral dosing syringe. Oral solution and tablet are bioequivalent on a mg-to-mg basis.

Hazardous agent; use appropriate precautions for handling and disposal (NIOSH, 2012).

Monitoring Parameters HIV status (prior to initiation of therapy); liver function tests, renal function; in HBV/HIV-coinfected patients, monitor HIV viral load and CD4 count; HBeAg, HBV DNA; in patients with lamivudine-refractory or -resistant viremia (or known lamivudine- or telbivudine-resistance mutations) entecavir resistance can develop rapidly. Monitor HBV DNA every 3 months (DHHS, 2013)

Dosage Forms Excipient information presented when available (limited, particularly for generics); consult specific product labeling.

Solution, Oral:

Baraclude: 0.05 mg/mL (210 mL) [contains methylparaben, propylparaben; orange flavor]

Tablet, Oral:

Baraclude: 0.5 mg, 1 mg

◆ **Entereg** *see* Alvimopan *on page 91*

◆ **Entex® LA (Can)** *see* Guaifenesin and Pseudoephedrine *on page 978*

◆ **Entocort® (Can)** *see* Budesonide (Systemic) *on page 282*

◆ **Entocort EC** *see* Budesonide (Systemic) *on page 282*

- **Entre-Cough** *see* Guaifenesin, Pseudoephedrine, and Dextromethorphan *on page 979*
- **Entrophen® (Can)** *see* Aspirin *on page 177*
- **Entsol [OTC]** *see* Sodium Chloride *on page 1914*
- **Entsol Nasal [OTC]** *see* Sodium Chloride *on page 1914*
- **Entsol Nasal Wash [OTC]** *see* Sodium Chloride *on page 1914*
- **Enulose** *see* Lactulose *on page 1161*

Enzalutamide (en za LOO ta mide)

Brand Names: U.S. Xtandi

Brand Names: Canada Xtandi

Index Terms MDV3100

Pharmacologic Category Antiandrogen; Antineoplastic Agent, Antiandrogen

Use Prostate cancer: Treatment of metastatic, castration-resistant prostate cancer in patients previously treated with docetaxel

Pregnancy Risk Factor X

Pregnancy Considerations Enzalutamide is an androgen receptor inhibitor. Although animal reproduction studies have not been conducted, it is expected to cause fetal harm based on its mechanism of action. Enzalutamide is not indicated for use in women and is specifically contraindicated for use in women who are or may become pregnant. Men using this medication should use a condom if having intercourse with a pregnant woman. A condom plus another effective method of birth control is recommended during therapy and for 3 months after treatment for men using this medication and who are having intercourse with a woman of reproductive potential.

Breast-Feeding Considerations Enzalutamide is not indicated for use in women.

Contraindications Women who are or may become pregnant

Canadian labeling: Additional contraindications (not in U.S. labeling): Hypersensitivity to enzalutamide or any component of the formulation; women who are lactating

Warnings/Precautions Hazardous agent - use appropriate precautions for handling and disposal (meets NIOSH, 2012 criteria). Seizures were observed in a clinical trial (onset: ~1-20 months after treatment initiation). Therapy was permanently discontinued and patients were not rechallenged; seizures resolved upon therapy cessation. Patients with predisposing factors for seizure were excluded from the trial; factors include seizure history, underlying brain injury with loss of consciousness, transient ischemic attack within the past 12 months, cerebral vascular accident, brain metastases, brain arteriovenous malformation, or the use of concomitant medications which may lower the seizure threshold. Enzalutamide should be used with caution in patients with a history of seizure disorders or other predisposing factors. Enzalutamide may cause hypospermatogenesis and may impair male fertility. Androgen-deprivation therapy may increase the risk of cardiovascular disease (Levine, 2010). An increase in systolic and diastolic blood pressures has been observed (Scher, 2012); may worsen pre-existing hypertension.

Potentially significant drug-drug interactions may exist, requiring dose or frequency adjustment, additional monitoring, and/or selection of alternative therapy. May contain sorbitol; Canadian product labeling recommends avoiding use in patients with fructose intolerance.

Adverse Reactions

>10%:

Cardiovascular: Peripheral edema (15%)
Central nervous system: Fatigue (51%), headache (12%)
Endocrine & metabolic: Hot flashes (20%)
Gastrointestinal: Diarrhea (22%)
Hematologic: Neutropenia (15%; grades 3/4: 1%)
Neuromuscular & skeletal: Back pain (26%), arthralgia (21%), musculoskeletal pain (15%)
Respiratory: Upper respiratory tract infection (11%)

1% to 10%:

Cardiovascular: Hypertension (6%)
Central nervous system: Dizziness (10%), insomnia (9%), anxiety (7%), hypoesthesia (4%), mental impairment (4%), hallucinations (2%)
Dermatologic: Dry skin (4%), pruritus (4%)
Genitourinary: Hematuria (7%), pollakiuria (5%)
Hepatic: Bilirubin increased (3%)
Neuromuscular & skeletal: Muscle weakness (10%), paresthesia (7%), falling (5%), fractures (4%), stiffness (3%)
Respiratory: Lower respiratory tract infection (9%), epistaxis (3%)
Miscellaneous: Infection (≤6%; including sepsis)

<1% (Limited to important or life-threatening): Seizures

Drug Interactions

Metabolism/Transport Effects Substrate of CYP2C8 (major), CYP3A4 (major); **Note:** Assignment of Major/Minor substrate status based on clinically relevant drug interaction potential; **Inhibits** P-glycoprotein; **Induces** CYP2C19 (weak/moderate), CYP2C9 (weak/moderate), CYP3A4 (strong)

Avoid Concomitant Use

Avoid concomitant use of Enzalutamide with any of the following: Abiraterone Acetate; Alfentanil; Apixaban; Artemether; Axitinib; Bedaquiline; Boceprevir; Bortezomib; Bosutinib; Cabozantinib; CloZAPine; Crizotinib; CycloSPORINE (Systemic); CYP2C8 Inducers (Strong); CYP2C8 Inhibitors (Strong); CYP3A4 Inducers (Strong); Dienogest; Dihydroergotamine; Dronedarone; Ergotamine; Everolimus; FentaNYL; Fosphenytoin-Phenytoin; Ibrutinib; Itraconazole; Ivacaftor; Lapatinib; Lumefantrine; Lurasidone; Macitentan; Mifepristone; NIFEdipine; Nilotinib; Nisoldipine; PAZOPanib; Perampanel; Pimozide; Pomalidomide; PONATinib; Praziquantel; QuiNIDine; Ranolazine; Regorafenib; Rivaroxaban; Roflumilast; RomiDEPsin; Simeprevir; Sirolimus; SORAfenib; St Johns Wort; Tacrolimus (Systemic); Telaprevir; Ticagrelor; Tofacitinib; Tolvaptan; Toremifene; Ulipristal; Vandetanib; Vemurafenib; VinCRIStine (Liposomal); Warfarin

Increased Effect/Toxicity

Enzalutamide may increase the levels/effects of: Clarithromycin; Ifosfamide

The levels/effects of Enzalutamide may be increased by: Clarithromycin; CYP2C8 Inhibitors (Moderate); CYP2C8 Inhibitors (Strong); CYP3A4 Inhibitors (Strong); Deferasirox

Decreased Effect

Enzalutamide may decrease the levels/effects of: Abiraterone Acetate; Alfentanil; Apixaban; ARIPiprazole; Artemether; Axitinib; Bedaquiline; Boceprevir; Bortezomib; Bosutinib; Brentuximab Vedotin; Cabozantinib; Clarithromycin; CloZAPine; Crizotinib; CycloSPORINE (Systemic); CYP3A4 Substrates; Dasatinib; Dienogest; Dihydroergotamine; Dronedarone; Ergotamine; Everolimus; Exemestane; FentaNYL; Fosphenytoin-Phenytoin; Gefitinib; GuanFACINE; Ibrutinib; Imatinib; Itraconazole; Ivacaftor; Ixabepilone; Lapatinib; Linagliptin; Lumefantrine; Lurasidone; Macitentan; Maraviroc; Mifepristone; NIFEdipine; Nilotinib; Nisoldipine; PAZOPanib; Perampanel; Pimozide; Pomalidomide; PONATinib; Praziquantel; QUEtiapine; QuiNIDine; Ranolazine; Regorafenib; Rivaroxaban; Roflumilast; RomiDEPsin; Saxagliptin; Simeprevir; Sirolimus; SORAfenib; SUNItinib; Tacrolimus (Systemic); Tadalafil; Telaprevir; Ticagrelor; Tofacitinib; Tolvaptan; Toremifene; Ulipristal; Vandetanib;

Vemurafenib; VinCRIStine (Liposomal); Vortioxetine; Warfarin; Zuclopenthixol

The levels/effects of Enzalutamide may be decreased by: Bosentan; CYP2C8 Inducers (Strong); CYP3A4 Inducers (Strong); Dabrafenib; Deferasirox; St Johns Wort; Tocilizumab

Storage/Stability Store at 20°C to 25°C (68°F to 77°F); excursions permitted to 15°C to 30°C (59°F to 86°F). Protect from moisture; keep bottle tightly closed.

Mechanism of Action Enzalutamide is a pure androgen receptor signaling inhibitor; unlike other antiandrogen therapies, it has no known agonistic properties. It inhibits androgen receptor nuclear translocation, DNA binding, and coactivator mobilization, leading to cellular apoptosis and decreased prostate tumor volume.

Pharmacodynamics/Kinetics

Absorption: Rapid

Distribution: 110 L

Protein binding: Parent drug: 97% to 98% to primarily albumin; active metabolite: 95% to plasma proteins

Metabolism: Primarily hepatic via CYP2C8 (responsible for formation of active metabolite N-desmethyl enzalutamide) and CYP3A4

Half-life elimination: 5.8 days (range: 2.8-10.2 days)

Time to peak: 1 hour (range: 0.5-3 hours)

Excretion: Urine (71%); feces (14%); primarily as inactive metabolite

Dosage Prostate cancer, metastatic, castration-resistant: Adults: Oral: 160 mg once daily

Dosage adjustment for concomitant strong CYP2C8 inhibitors: Avoid concomitant use if possible. If coadministration is necessary, reduce enzalutamide dose to 80 mg once daily. If the strong CYP2C8 inhibitor is discontinued, adjust the enzalutamide dose back up to the dose used prior to the initiation of the inhibitor.

Dosage adjustment for toxicity: If ≥grade 3 toxicity occurs, withhold treatment for 1 week or until symptom(s) improve to ≤grade 2, then resume at same dose, or reduce dose to 120 mg or 80 mg once daily, if necessary. *Seizures:* Discontinue treatment.

Dosage adjustment in renal impairment:

Pre-existing mild-to-moderate impairment (Cl_{cr} 30-89 mL/minute): No initial dosage adjustment necessary.

Pre-existing severe impairment (Cl_{cr} <30 mL/minute), including end-stage renal disease: No dosage adjustment provided in manufacturer's labeling (has not been studied).

Dosage adjustment in hepatic impairment:

Pre-existing mild-to-moderate impairment (Child-Pugh class A or B): No dosage adjustment necessary.

Pre-existing severe impairment (Child-Pugh class C): No dosage adjustment provided in manufacturer's U.S. labeling (has not been studied). Canadian labeling recommends to avoid use in severe impairment.

Dietary Considerations May be taken with or without food.

Administration May be administered with or without food; take at the same time each day. Swallow capsules whole; do not chew, dissolve, or open the capsules.

Hazardous agent; use appropriate precautions for handling and disposal (meets NIOSH, 2012 criteria).

Monitoring Parameters Monitor for signs/symptoms of seizure, loss of consciousness, dizziness, and hallucinations; CBC with differential and liver function tests (baseline and periodic); additional INR monitoring (if on warfarin); blood pressure (baseline and periodic)

Dosage Forms Excipient information presented when available (limited, particularly for generics); consult specific product labeling.

Capsule, Oral:

Xtandi: 40 mg

◆ **Epaned** *see* Enalapril *on page 701*

◆ **EPEG** *see* Etoposide *on page 802*

EPHEDrine (Systemic) (e FED rin)

Index Terms Ephedrine Sulfate

Pharmacologic Category Alpha/Beta Agonist

Additional Appendix Information

Contrast Media Reactions, Premedication for Prophylaxis *on page 2373*

Use Treatment of nasal congestion, anesthesia-induced hypotension

Unlabeled Use Postoperative nausea and vomiting (PONV) refractory to traditional antiemetics; idiopathic orthostatic hypotension

Pregnancy Risk Factor C

Dosage

Children: Hypotension: Slow I.V. push: 0.2-0.3 mg/kg/dose every 4-6 hours

Adults:

Hypotension induced by anesthesia: I.V.: 5-25 mg/dose slow I.V. push repeated after 5-10 minutes as needed, then every 3-4 hours (maximum: 150 mg/24 hours)

Idiopathic orthostatic hypotension (unlabeled use): Oral: 25-50 mg 3 times/day; maximum: 150 mg/day. **Note:** Not considered first-line for this indication.

PONV refractory to traditional antiemetics (unlabeled use): I.M.: 0.5 mg/kg at the end of surgery (Gan, 2007; Hagemann, 2000)

Additional Information Complete prescribing information should be consulted for additional detail.

Dosage Forms Excipient information presented when available (limited, particularly for generics); consult specific product labeling.

Capsule, Oral, as sulfate:

Generic: 25 mg

Solution, Injection, as sulfate:

Generic: 50 mg/mL (1 mL)

Solution, Injection, as sulfate [preservative free]:

Generic: 50 mg/mL (1 mL)

◆ **Ephedrine Sulfate** *see* EPHEDrine (Systemic) *on page 714*

◆ **E-Pherol [OTC]** *see* Vitamin E *on page 2202*

◆ **Epidoxorubicin** *see* Epirubicin *on page 718*

◆ **Epiduo®** *see* Adapalene and Benzoyl Peroxide *on page 48*

◆ **Epi E-Z Pen (Can)** *see* EPINEPHrine (Systemic, Oral Inhalation) *on page 714*

◆ **Epiflur™** *see* Fluoride *on page 880*

◆ **Epifoam®** *see* Pramoxine and Hydrocortisone *on page 1699*

EPINEPHrine (Systemic, Oral Inhalation)
(ep i NEF rin)

Brand Names: U.S. Adrenaclick; Adrenalin; Asthmanefrin Refill [OTC]; Asthmanefrin Starter Kit [OTC]; Auvi-Q; EpiPen 2-Pak; EpiPen Jr 2-Pak; Micronefrin [OTC]; S2 [OTC]

Brand Names: Canada Adrenalin; Epi E-Z Pen; EpiPen; EpiPen Jr; Twinject

Index Terms Adrenaline; Auvi-Q; Epinephrine Bitartrate; Epinephrine Hydrochloride; Racemic Epinephrine; Racepinephrine

Pharmacologic Category Alpha/Beta Agonist

Additional Appendix Information

Adult ACLS Algorithms *on page 2363*

Pediatric ALS (PALS) Algorithms *on page 2359*

Vasoactive Agents, Intravenous *on page 2315*

Use Treatment of bronchospasms, bronchial asthma, viral croup, anaphylactic reactions, cardiac arrest; added to local anesthetics to decrease systemic absorption of intraspinal and local anesthetics and increase duration of action; decrease superficial hemorrhage; induction and maintenance of mydriasis during intraocular surgery

Unlabeled Use ACLS guidelines: Ventricular fibrillation (VF) or pulseless ventricular tachycardia (VT) unresponsive to initial defibrillatory shocks; pulseless electrical activity; asystole; hypotension/shock unresponsive to volume resuscitation; symptomatic bradycardia unresponsive to atropine or pacing; inotropic support

Pregnancy Risk Factor C

Pregnancy Considerations Teratogenic effects have been observed in animal reproduction studies. Epinephrine crosses the placenta and may cause fetal anoxia. Use during pregnancy when the potential benefit to the mother outweighs the possible risk to the fetus.

Breast-Feeding Considerations It is not known if epinephrine is excreted in breast milk. The manufacturer recommends that caution be exercised when administering epinephrine to nursing women.

Contraindications There are no absolute contraindications to the use of injectable epinephrine (including Adrenaclick, Auvi-Q, EpiPen, EpiPen Jr, and Twinject) in a life-threatening situation.

Oral inhalation: Concurrent use or within 2 weeks of MAO inhibitors

Injectable solution: There are no contraindications listed in the manufacturer's labeling.

Warnings/Precautions Use with caution in elderly patients, patients with diabetes mellitus, cardiovascular diseases (eg, coronary artery disease, hypertension), thyroid disease, cerebrovascular disease, Parkinson's disease, or patients taking tricyclic antidepressants. Some products contain sulfites as preservatives; the presence of sulfites in some products should not deter administration during a serious allergic or other emergency situation even if the patient is sulfite-sensitive.

I.V. administration: Vesicant; ensure proper needle or catheter placement prior to and during infusion; avoid extravasation. Accidental injection into digits, hands, or feet may result in local reactions, including injection site pallor, coldness and hypoesthesia or injury, resulting in bruising, bleeding, discoloration, erythema or skeletal injury; patient should seek immediate medical attention if this occurs. Rapid I.V. administration may cause death from cerebrovascular hemorrhage or cardiac arrhythmias; however, rapid I.V. administration during pulseless arrest is necessary. Prior to intraocular use, must dilute 1:**1000** (1 mg/mL) solution to a concentration of 1:**100,000** to 1:**1,000,000** (10 **mcg**/mL to 1 **mcg**/mL) prior to intraocular use. When used undiluted, has been associated with corneal endothelial damage.

Oral inhalation: Use with caution in patients with prostate enlargement or urinary retention; may cause temporary worsening of symptoms.

Self medication (OTC use): Oral inhalation: Prior to self-medication, patients should contact healthcare provider. The product should only be used in persons with a diagnosis of asthma. If symptoms are not relieved in 20 minutes or become worse do not continue to use the product - seek immediate medical assistance. The product should not be used more frequently or at higher doses than recommended unless directed by a healthcare provider. This product should not be used in patients who have required hospitalization for asthma or if a patient is taking prescription medication for asthma. Do not use if you have taken a MAO inhibitor (certain drugs used for depression, Parkinson's disease, or other conditions) within 2 weeks.

Adverse Reactions Frequency not defined.

Cardiovascular: Angina, cardiac arrhythmia, chest pain, flushing, hypertension, pallor, palpitation, sudden death, tachycardia (parenteral), vasoconstriction, ventricular ectopy, ventricular fibrillation

Central nervous system: Anxiety (transient), apprehensiveness, cerebral hemorrhage, dizziness, headache, insomnia, lightheadedness, nervousness, restlessness

Gastrointestinal: Dry throat, loss of appetite, nausea, vomiting, xerostomia

Genitourinary: Acute urinary retention in patients with bladder outflow obstruction

Neuromuscular & skeletal: Tremor, weakness

Ocular: Allergic lid reaction, burning, corneal endothelial damage (intraocular use), eye pain, ocular irritation, precipitation of or exacerbation of narrow-angle glaucoma, transient stinging

Respiratory: Dyspnea, pulmonary edema

Miscellaneous: Diaphoresis

Drug Interactions

Metabolism/Transport Effects Substrate of COMT

Avoid Concomitant Use

Avoid concomitant use of EPINEPHrine (Systemic, Oral Inhalation) with any of the following: Ergot Derivatives; Iobenguane I 123; Lurasidone

Increased Effect/Toxicity

EPINEPHrine (Systemic, Oral Inhalation) may increase the levels/effects of: Lurasidone; Sympathomimetics

The levels/effects of EPINEPHrine (Systemic, Oral Inhalation) may be increased by: Antacids; AtoMOXetine; Beta-Blockers; Cannabinoids; Carbonic Anhydrase Inhibitors; COMT Inhibitors; Ergot Derivatives; Hyaluronidase; Inhalational Anesthetics; MAO Inhibitors; Serotonin/Norepinephrine Reuptake Inhibitors; Tricyclic Antidepressants

Decreased Effect

EPINEPHrine (Systemic, Oral Inhalation) may decrease the levels/effects of: Benzylpenicilloyl Polylysine; Iobenguane I 123

The levels/effects of EPINEPHrine (Systemic, Oral Inhalation) may be decreased by: Alpha1-Blockers; Promethazine; Spironolactone

Ethanol/Nutrition/Herb Interactions Herb/Nutraceutical: Avoid ephedra, yohimbe (may cause CNS stimulation).

Preparation for Administration

Endotracheal (unlabeled route): Dilute in NS or sterile water.

Intraocular: Dilute 1 mL of 1 mg/mL (1:**1000**) solution in 100 mL to 1000 mL of an ophthalmic irrigation fluid for a final concentration of 1:**100,000** to 1:**1,000,000** (10 **mcg**/mL to 1 **mcg**/mL); may use this solution as an irrigation as needed during the procedure. May also prepare a dilution of 1:**100,000** to 1:**400,000** (10 **mcg**/mL to 2.5 **mcg**/mL) for intracameral administration.

Oral inhalation: S2: If using jet nebulizer,must be diluted with 3-5 mL NS. If using handheld rubber bulb nebulizer, dilution is not required.

Storage/Stability Epinephrine is sensitive to light and air. Protection from light is recommended. Oxidation turns drug pink, then a brown color. **Solutions should not be used if they are discolored or contain a precipitate.**

Adrenaclick: Store between 20°C to 25°C (68°F to 77°F); excursions permitted to 15°C to 30°C (59°F to 86°F); do not freeze or refrigerate. Protect from light.

Adrenalin: Store between 20°C to 25°C (68°F to 77°F); do not freeze. Protect from light.

Auvi-Q: Store between 20°C to 25°C (68°F to 77°F); excursions permitted to 15°C to 30°C (59°F to 86°F); do not refrigerate. Protect from light by storing in outer case provided.

EpiPen and EpiPen Jr: Store at 25°C (77°F); excursions permitted to 15°C to 30°C (59°F to 86°F); do not freeze or refrigerate. Protect from light by storing in carrier tube provided.

Twinject: Store between 20°C to 25°C (68°F to 77°F); excursions permitted to 15°C to 30°C (59°F to 86°F); do not freeze or refrigerate. Protect from light.

Primatene Mist: Store between 20°C to 25°C (68°F to 77°F).

S2: Store between 2°C to 20°C (36°F to 68°F). Protect from light.

Stability of injection of parenteral admixture at room temperature (25°C) or refrigeration (4°C) is 24 hours.

Mechanism of Action Stimulates alpha-, beta$_1$-, and beta$_2$-adrenergic receptors resulting in relaxation of smooth muscle of the bronchial tree, cardiac stimulation (increasing myocardial oxygen consumption), and dilation of skeletal muscle vasculature; small doses can cause vasodilation via beta$_2$-vascular receptors; large doses may produce constriction of skeletal and vascular smooth muscle

Pharmacodynamics/Kinetics

Onset of action: Bronchodilation: SubQ: ~5-10 minutes; Inhalation: ~1 minute

Metabolism: Taken up into the adrenergic neuron and metabolized by monoamine oxidase and catechol-o-methyltransferase; circulating drug hepatically metabolized

Excretion: Urine (as inactive metabolites, metanephrine, and sulfate and hydroxy derivatives of mandelic acid, small amounts as unchanged drug)

Dosage

Infants and Children:

Asystole/pulseless arrest, pulseless VT/VF (after failed defibrillation attempts) (PALS, 2010):

I.V., I.O.: 0.01 mg/kg (0.1 mL/kg of **1:10,000** [0.1 mg/mL] solution) (maximum single dose: 1 mg) every 3-5 minutes until return of spontaneous circulation

Endotracheal: 0.1 mg/kg (0.1 mL/kg of **1:1000** [1 mg/mL] solution) (maximum single dose: 2.5 mg) every 3-5 minutes until I.V./I.O. access established or return of spontaneous circulation. Flush with 5 mL of NS immediately after administration. May cause false-negative reading with exhaled CO_2 detectors; use second method to confirm tube placement if CO_2 is not detected (Neumar, 2010).

Postresuscitation infusion to maintain cardiac output or stabilize: I.V., I.O.: 0.1-1 mcg/kg/minute; doses <0.3 mcg/kg/minute generally produce beta-adrenergic effects and higher doses (>0.3 mcg/kg/minute) generally produce alpha-adrenergic vasoconstriction; titrate dosage to desired effect

Bradycardia (symptomatic; unresponsive to atropine or pacing):

I.V., I.O.: 0.01 mg/kg (0.1 mL/kg of **1:10,000** [0.1 mg/mL] solution) (maximum single dose: 1 mg) every 3-5 minutes as needed

Endotracheal: 0.1 mg/kg or (0.1 mL/kg of **1:1000** [1 mg/mL] solution) (maximum single dose: 2.5 mg) every 3-5 minutes as needed until I.V./I.O. access established. Flush with 5 mL of NS immediately after administration. May cause false-negative reading with exhaled CO_2 detectors; use second method to confirm tube placement if CO_2 is not detected (Neumar, 2010).

Continuous infusion: I.V., I.O.: 0.1-1 mcg/kg/minute; doses <0.3 mcg/kg/minute generally produce beta-adrenergic effects and higher doses (>0.3 mcg/kg/minute) generally produce alpha-adrenergic vasoconstriction; titrate dosage to desired effect

Bronchodilator:

SubQ: 0.01 mg/kg (0.01 mL/kg of **1:1000** [1 mg/mL] solution) (maximum single dose: 0.5 mg) every 20 minutes for 3 doses

Nebulization: S2 (racepinephrine, OTC labeling):

Children <4 years: Jet nebulizer: Croup: 0.05 mL/kg (maximum dose: 0.5 mL); dilute in 3 mL of NS. Administer over ~15 minutes; do not administer more frequently than every 2 hours

Children ≥4 years: Refer to adult dosing.

Inhalation: Children ≥4 years: Primatene Mist: Refer to adult dosing.

Hypersensitivity reaction (eg, anaphylaxis): **Note:** SubQ administration results in slower absorption and is less reliable. I.M. administration in the anterolateral aspect of the middle third of the thigh is preferred in the setting of anaphylaxis (ACLS guidelines, 2010; Kemp, 2008).

I.M., SubQ: Larger I.M. or SubQ doses, use of I.V. route, or continuous I.V. infusion may be needed for severe anaphylactic reactions (Kemp, 2008; Lieberman, 2010). If clinician deems appropriate, the 5-minute interval between injections may be shortened to allow for more frequent administration (Lieberman, 2010).

Children <30 kg: 0.01 mg/kg (0.01 mL/kg of 1:**1000** [1 mg/mL] solution) (maximum single dose: 0.3 mg) every 5-10 minutes

Children ≥30 kg: 0.3-0.5 mg (0.3-0.5 mL of 1:**1000** [1 mg/mL] solution) every 5-10 minutes

Self-administration following severe allergic reactions (eg, insect stings, food): **Note:** World Health Organization (WHO) and Anaphylaxis Canada recommend the availability of 1 dose for every 10-20 minutes of travel time to a medical emergency facility. More than 2 sequential doses should only be administered under direct medical supervision.

Adrenaclick: I.M., SubQ:

Children 15-29 kg: 0.15 mg

Children ≥30 kg: 0.3 mg

Auvi-Q: I.M., SubQ:

Children 15-29 kg: 0.15 mg; if anaphylactic symptoms persist, dose may be repeated

Children ≥30 kg: 0.3 mg; if anaphylactic symptoms persist, dose may be repeated

EpiPen Jr: I.M., SubQ: Children 15-29 kg: 0.15 mg; if anaphylactic symptoms persist, dose may be repeated in 5-15 minutes using an additional EpiPen Jr

EpiPen: I.M., SubQ: Children ≥30 kg: 0.3 mg; if anaphylactic symptoms persist, dose may be repeated in 5-15 minutes using an additional EpiPen

Twinject: I.M. SubQ:

Children 15-29 kg: 0.15 mg; if anaphylactic symptoms persist, dose may be repeated in 5-15 minutes using the same device after partial disassembly

Children ≥30 kg: 0.3 mg; if anaphylactic symptoms persist, dose may be repeated in 5-15 minutes using the same device after partial disassembly

Alternate auto-injector dose: I.M. (Sicherer, 2007):

Children 10-25 kg: 0.15 mg

Children >25 kg: 0.3 mg

Hypotension/shock, fluid-resistant (unlabeled use): Continuous I.V. infusion: 0.1-1 mcg/kg/minute; doses up to 5 mcg/kg/minute may rarely be necessary (Hegenbarth, 2008)

Mydriasis during intraocular surgery, induction and maintenance: Intraocular: Must dilute 1:**1000** (1 mg/mL) solution to a concentration of 1:**100,000** to 1:**1,000,000** (10 **mcg**/mL to 1 **mcg**/mL) prior to intraocular use: May use as an irrigation solution as needed during the procedure or may administer intracamerally (ie, directly into the anterior chamber of the eye) with a bolus dose of 0.1 mL of a 1:**100,000** to 1:**400,000** (10 **mcg**/mL to 2.5 **mcg**/mL) dilution.

Adults:

Asystole/pulseless arrest, pulseless VT/VF (ACLS, 2010):

I.V., I.O.: 1 mg every 3-5 minutes until return of spontaneous circulation; if this approach fails, higher doses of epinephrine (up to 0.2 mg/kg) have been used for treatment of specific problems (eg, beta-blocker or calcium channel blocker overdose)

Endotracheal: 2-2.5 mg every 3-5 minutes until I.V./I.O. access established or return of spontaneous circulation; dilute in 5-10 mL NS or sterile water. **Note:** Absorption may be greater with sterile water (Naganobu, 2000). May cause false-negative reading with exhaled CO_2 detectors; use second method to confirm tube placement if CO_2 is not detected (Neumar, 2010).

Bradycardia (symptomatic; unresponsive to atropine or pacing): I.V. infusion: 2-10 mcg/minute **or** 0.1-0.5 mcg/kg/minute (7-35 mcg/minute in a 70 kg patient); titrate to desired effect (ACLS, 2010)

Bronchodilator:

SubQ: 0.3-0.5 mg (**1:1000** [1 mg/mL] solution) every 20 minutes for 3 doses

Nebulization: S2 (racepinephrine, OTC labeling):

Hand-bulb nebulizer: Add 0.5 mL (~10 drops) to nebulizer; 1-3 inhalations up to every 3 hours if needed

Jet nebulizer: Add 0.5 mL (~10 drops) to nebulizer and dilute with 3 mL of NS; administer over ~15 minutes every 3-4 hours as needed

Inhalation: Primatene Mist (OTC labeling): One inhalation, wait at least 1 minute; if not relieved, may use once more. Do not use again for at least 3 hours.

Hypersensitivity reaction (eg, anaphylaxis): **Note:** SubQ administration results in slower absorption and is less reliable. I.M. administration in the anterolateral aspect of the middle third of the thigh is preferred in the setting of anaphylaxis (ACLS guidelines, 2010; Kemp, 2008).

I.M., SubQ: 0.2-0.5 mg (**1:1000** [1 mg/mL] solution) every 5-15 minutes in the absence of clinical improvement (ACLS, 2010; Kemp, 2008; Lieberman, 2010). If clinician deems appropriate, the 5-minute interval between injections may be shortened to allow for more frequent administration (Lieberman, 2010).

I.V.: 0.1 mg (**1:10,000** [0.1 mg/mL] solution) over 5 minutes; may infuse at 1-4 mcg/minute to prevent the need to repeat injections frequently **or** may initiate with an infusion at 5-15 mcg/minute (with crystalloid administration) (ACLS, 2010; Brown, 2004). In general, I.V. administration should only be done in patients who are profoundly hypotensive or are in cardiopulmonary arrest refractory to volume resuscitation and several epinephrine injections (Lieberman, 2010).

Self-administration following severe allergic reactions (eg, insect stings, food): **Note:** The World Health Organization (WHO) and Anaphylaxis Canada recommend the availability of one dose for every 10-20 minutes of travel time to a medical emergency facility. More than 2 sequential doses should only be administered under direct medical supervision.

Adrenaclick: I.M., SubQ: 0.3 mg

Auvi-Q: I.M., SubQ: 0.3 mg; if anaphylactic symptoms persist, dose may be repeated

EpiPen: I.M., SubQ: 0.3 mg; if anaphylactic symptoms persist, dose may be repeated in 5-15 minutes using an additional EpiPen

Twinject: I.M., SubQ: 0.3 mg; if anaphylactic symptoms persist, dose may be repeated in 5-15 minutes using the same device after partial disassembly

Hypotension/shock, severe and fluid resistant (unlabeled use): I.V. infusion: Initial: 0.1-0.5 mcg/kg/minute (7-35 mcg/minute in a 70 kg patient); titrate to desired response (ACLS, 2010)

Mydriasis during intraocular surgery, induction and maintenance: Intraocular: Must dilute 1:**1000** (1 mg/mL) solution to a concentration of 1:**100,000** to 1:**1,000,000** (10 **mcg**/mL to 1 **mcg**/mL) prior to intraocular use: May use as an irrigation solution as needed during the procedure or may administer intracamerally (ie, directly into the anterior chamber of the eye) with a bolus dose of 0.1 mL of a 1:**100,000** to 1:**400,000** (10 **mcg**/mL to 2.5 **mcg**/mL) dilution.

Dosage adjustment in renal impairment: No dosage adjustment provided in manufacturer's labeling.

Dosage adjustment in hepatic impairment: No dosage adjustment provided in manufacturer's labeling.

Usual Infusion Concentrations: Pediatric I.V. infusion: 16 **mcg**/mL, 32 **mcg**/mL, or 64 **mcg**/mL

Usual Infusion Concentrations: Adult I.V. infusion: 1 mg in 250 mL (concentration: 4 **mcg**/mL) **or** 4 mg in 250 mL (concentration: 16 **mcg**/mL) of D_5W or NS

Administration Epinephrine solutions for injection can be administered I.M., I.O., endotracheally, I.V., or SubQ. **Note:** Adrenaclick, Auvi-Q, EpiPen and EpiPen Jr Auto-Injectors contain a single, fixed-dose of epinephrine and may only be administered I.M. (preferred) or SubQ. Twinject Auto-Injectors contain two doses; the first fixed-dose is available for auto-injection; the second dose is available for manual injection following partial disassembly of device.

I.V.: When administering as a continuous infusion, central line administration is preferred. I.V. infusions require an infusion pump.

Vesicant; ensure proper needle or catheter placement prior to and during infusion; avoid extravasation.

Extravasation management: If extravasation occurs, stop infusion immediately and disconnect (leave cannula/needle in place); gently aspirate extravasated solution (do **NOT** flush the line); remove needle/cannula; elevate extremity. Initiate phentolamine (or alternative antidote). Apply dry warm compresses (Hurst, 2004).

Phentolamine: Dilute 5-10 mg in 10-15 mL NS and administer into extravasation site as soon as possible after extravasation (Peberdy, 2010).

Alternatives to phentolamine (due to shortage):

Nitroglycerin topical 2% ointment (based on limited case reports in neonates/infants): Apply 4 mm/kg as a thin ribbon to the affected areas; may repeat after 8 hours if needed (Wong, 1992) **or** apply a 1-inch strip on the affected site (Denkler, 1989).

Terbutaline (based on limited case reports): Infiltrate extravasation area using a solution of terbutaline 1 mg diluted to 10 mL in NS (large extravasation site; administration volume varied from 3-10 mL) **or** 1 mg diluted in 1 mL NS (small/distal extravasation site; administration volume varied from 0.5-1 mL) (Stier, 1999).

Subcutaneous: SubQ administration results in slower absorption and is less reliable.

I.M.: I.M. administration in the anterolateral aspect of the middle third of the thigh is preferred in the setting of anaphylaxis (ACLS guidelines, 2010; Kemp, 2008). I.M. administration into the buttocks should be avoided. Adrenaclick, Auvi-Q, EpiPen, EpiPen Jr, and Twinject Auto-Injectors should only be injected into the anterolateral aspect of the thigh, through clothing if necessary.

Obesity: In overweight or obese children, because skin surface to muscle depth is greater in the upper half of the thigh, administration into the lower half of the thigh may be preferred. In very obese children, injection into the calf will provide an even greater chance of intramuscular administration (Arkwright, 2013).

Endotracheal (cardiac arrest): Dilute in NS or sterile water. Absorption may be greater with sterile water (Naganobu, 2000). Stop compressions, spray drug quickly down tube. Follow immediately with several quick insufflations and continue chest compressions. May cause false-negative reading with exhaled CO_2 detectors; use second method to confirm tube placement if CO_2 is not detected (Neumar, 2010).

Oral inhalation: S2: If using jet nebulizer: Administer diluted over ~15 minutes. If using handheld rubber bulb nebulizer, dilution is not required.

Monitoring Parameters Pulmonary function, heart rate, blood pressure, site of infusion for blanching, extravasation; cardiac monitor and blood pressure monitor required during continuous infusion. If using to treat hypotension, assess intravascular volume and support as needed.

Consult individual institutional policies and procedures.

Dosage Forms Excipient information presented when available (limited, particularly for generics); consult specific product labeling. [DSC] = Discontinued product

Device, Injection:
- Adrenaclick: 0.15 mg/0.15 mL (2 ea); 0.3 mg/0.3 mL (2 ea) [latex free; contains chlorobutanol (chlorobutol), sodium bisulfite]
- Auvi-Q: 0.15 mg/0.15 mL (2 ea); 0.3 mg/0.3 mL (2 ea) [contains sodium bisulfite]
- EpiPen 2-Pak: 0.3 mg/0.3 mL (2 ea) [latex free; contains sodium metabisulfite]
- EpiPen Jr 2-Pak: 0.15 mg/0.3 mL (2 ea) [contains sodium metabisulfite]
- Generic: 0.15 mg/0.15 mL (2 ea); 0.3 mg/0.3 mL (2 ea)

Nebulization Solution, Inhalation:
- Asthmanefrin Refill: 2.25% (1 ea) [contains edetate disodium]
- Asthmanefrin Starter Kit: 2.25% (1 ea) [contains edetate disodium]
- Micronefrin: 2.25% (15 mL, 30 mL)

Nebulization Solution, Inhalation [preservative free]:
- S2: 2.25% (1 ea) [sulfite free; contains edetate disodium]

Solution, Injection:
- Generic: 0.1 mg/mL (10 mL); 1 mg/mL (1 mL)

Solution, Injection, as hydrochloride:
- Adrenalin: 1 mg/mL (30 mL [DSC]) [contains chlorobutanol (chlorobutol), sodium bisulfite]
- Adrenalin: 1 mg/mL (1 mL [DSC]) [contains sodium bisulfite]
- Adrenalin: 1 mg/mL (1 mL) [contains sodium metabisulfite]
- Generic: 1 mg/mL (1 mL, 30 mL)

◆ Epinephrine and Lidocaine *see* Lidocaine and Epinephrine *on page 1213*

◆ Epinephrine Bitartrate *see* EPINEPHrine (Systemic, Oral Inhalation) *on page 714*

◆ Epinephrine Hydrochloride *see* EPINEPHrine (Systemic, Oral Inhalation) *on page 714*

◆ EpiPen (Can) *see* EPINEPHrine (Systemic, Oral Inhalation) *on page 714*

◆ EpiPen 2-Pak *see* EPINEPHrine (Systemic, Oral Inhalation) *on page 714*

◆ EpiPen Jr (Can) *see* EPINEPHrine (Systemic, Oral Inhalation) *on page 714*

◆ EpiPen Jr 2-Pak *see* EPINEPHrine (Systemic, Oral Inhalation) *on page 714*

◆ Epipodophyllotoxin *see* Etoposide *on page 802*

◆ Epipodophyllotoxin *see* Etoposide Phosphate *on page 805*

◆ EpiQuin Micro *see* Hydroquinone *on page 1017*

Epirubicin (ep i ROO bi sin)

Brand Names: U.S. Ellence

Brand Names: Canada Ellence®; Epirubicin for Injection; Epirubicin Hydrochloride Injection; Pharmorubicin®

Index Terms Epidoxorubicin; Epirubicin Hydrochloride; Pidorubicin; Pidorubicin Hydrochloride

Pharmacologic Category Antineoplastic Agent, Anthracycline

Use Adjuvant therapy component for primary breast cancer

Unlabeled Use Treatment of esophageal cancer, gastric cancer, soft tissue sarcoma, uterine sarcoma

Pregnancy Risk Factor D

Pregnancy Considerations Teratogenic effects and embryotoxicity were noted in animal studies. If a pregnant woman is treated with epirubicin, or if a woman becomes pregnant while receiving this drug, she should be informed of the potential hazard to the fetus. Limited information is available from retrospective studies of women who received epirubicin during the second or third (prior to week 35) trimester for the treatment of pregnancy-associated breast cancer; premature births and intrauterine growth retardation have been observed (Peccatori, 2009; Ring, 2005). Women of childbearing potential should be advised to use effective contraception and avoid becoming pregnant during treatment. Men undergoing treatment should use effective contraception. Epirubicin may cause irreversible amenorrhea in premenopausal women.

Breast-Feeding Considerations Excretion in human breast milk is unknown, however, other anthracyclines are excreted. According to the manufacturers, the decision to continue or discontinue breast-feeding during therapy should take into account the risk of exposure to the infant and the benefits of treatment to the mother.

Contraindications Hypersensitivity to epirubicin or any component of the formulation, other anthracyclines, or anthracenediones; previous anthracycline treatment up to maximum cumulative dose; cardiomyopathy and/or heart failure, severe arrhythmias, recent myocardial infarction

Warnings/Precautions Hazardous agent - use appropriate precautions for handling and disposal (NIOSH, 2012).

[U.S. Boxed Warning]: Myocardial toxicity, including heart failure (HF) may occur, particularly in patients who have received prior anthracyclines, prior or concomitant radiotherapy to the mediastinal/pericardial area, who have pre-existing cardiac disease (active or dormant), or with concomitant cardiotoxic medications. Cardiotoxicity may be concurrent or delayed (months to years after treatment). The risk of HF is ~0.9% at a cumulative dose of 550 mg/m^2, ~1.6% at a cumulative dose of 700 mg/m^2, and ~3.3% at a cumulative dose of 900 mg/m^2. Cardiotoxicity may also occur at lower cumulative doses or without risk factors. The risk of delayed cardiotoxicity increases more steeply with cumulative doses >900 mg/m^2 and this dose should be exceeded only with extreme caution. Acute toxicity, primarily sinus tachycardia and/or ECG abnormalities, including arrhythmia, and delayed toxicity, including decreased left ventricular ejection fraction (LVEF) and HF, have been described. Delayed toxicity usually develops late in the course of therapy or within 2-3 months after completion. Toxicity may be additive with other anthracyclines or anthracenediones, and may be increased in pediatric patients. Regular monitoring of LVEF and discontinuation at the first sign of impairment is recommended especially in patients with cardiac risk factors or impaired cardiac function. Discontinue treatment with signs of decreased LVEF. The half life of other cardiotoxic agents must be considered in sequential therapy; avoid epirubicin for up to 24 weeks after completing trastuzumab treatment.

[U.S. Boxed Warning]: May cause severe myelosuppression; neutropenia is the dose-limiting toxicity; severe thrombocytopenia or anemia may occur; obtain baseline and periodic blood counts. Patients should recover from myelosuppression due to prior chemotherapy treatment before beginning treatments. Thrombophlebitis and thromboembolic phenomena (including pulmonary embolism) have occurred.

[U.S. Boxed Warning]: Reduce dosage in patients with mild-to-moderate hepatic impairment (not recommended in severe hepatic impairment; predominantly hepatically eliminated) and in patients with serum creatinine >5 mg/dL (has not been studied in patients on dialysis); monitor hepatic and renal function at baseline and during treatment. May cause tumor lysis syndrome (TLS), although generally generally does not occur in patients with breast cancer; if TLS risk is suspected, consider monitoring serum uric acid, potassium, calcium, phosphate, and serum creatinine after initial administration; hydration and allopurinol prophylaxis may minimize potential TLS complications. Radiation recall (inflammatory) has been reported; epirubicin may have radiosensitizing activity. **[U.S. Boxed Warning]: Treatment with anthracyclines (including epirubicin) may increase the risk of secondary acute myelogenous leukemia (AML). AML is more common when given in combination with other antineoplastic agents, in patients who have received multiple courses of previous chemotherapy, or with escalated cumulative anthracycline doses (>720 mg/m^2 for epirubicin). In breast cancer patients, the risk for treatment-related AML or myelodysplastic syndrome (MDS) was estimated at 0.3% at 3 years, 0.5% at 5 years, and 0.6% at 8 years after treatment.** The latency period for secondary leukemias may be short (1-3 years).

[U.S. Boxed Warning]: For I.V. administration only, severe local tissue damage and necrosis will result if extravasation occurs (vesicant); not for I.M. or SubQ use. Injection in to a small vein or repeated administration in the same vein may result in venous sclerosis. Ensure proper needle or catheter placement prior to and during infusion. Avoid extravasation. Women ≥70 years of age should be closely monitored for toxicity. **[U.S. Boxed Warning]: Should be administered under the supervision of an experienced cancer chemotherapy physician.** Epirubicin is emetogenic; consider prophylactic antiemetics prior to administration. Patients should recover from acute toxicities (stomatitis, myelosuppression, infections) prior to initiating treatment. Assess baseline labs (blood counts, bilirubin, ALT, AST, serum creatinine) and cardiac function (with LVEF). Prophylactic antibiotics should be administered with the CDF-120 regimen. Patients should not be immunized with live viral vaccines during or shortly after treatment. Inactivated vaccines may be administered (response may be diminished).

Adverse Reactions Percentages reported as part of combination chemotherapy regimens.

>10%:

Central nervous system: Lethargy (1% to 46%)

Dermatologic: Alopecia (70% to 96%)

Endocrine & metabolic: Amenorrhea (69% to 72%), hot flashes (5% to 39%)

Gastrointestinal: Nausea/vomiting (83% to 92%; grades 3/4: 22% to 25%), mucositis (9% to 59%; grades 3/4: ≤9%), diarrhea (7% to 25%)

Hematologic: Leukopenia (50% to 80%; grades 3/4: 2% to 59%), neutropenia (54% to 80%; grades 3/4: 11% to 67%; nadir: 10-14 days; recovery: by day 21), anemia (13% to 72%; grades 3/4: ≤6%), thrombocytopenia (5% to 49%; grades 3/4: ≤5%)

Local: Injection site reactions (3% to 20%; grades 3/4: <1%)

Ocular: Conjunctivitis (1% to 15%)

Miscellaneous: Infection (15% to 22%; grades 3/4: ≤2%)

1% to 10%:

Cardiovascular: LVEF decreased (asymptomatic; delayed: 1% to 2%), HF (0.4% to 1.5%)

Central nervous system: Fever (1% to 5%)

Dermatologic: Rash (1% to 9%), skin changes (1% to 5%)

Gastrointestinal: Anorexia (2% to 3%)

Hematologic: Neutropenic fever (grades 3/4: ≤6%)

<1%, postmarketing, case reports, and/or frequency not defined: Acute lymphoid leukemia (ALL), acute myelogenous leukemia (AML), anaphylaxis, arrhythmia, arterial embolism, ascites, atrioventricular block, bradycardia, bundle-branch block, cardiomyopathy, chills, dehydration, dyspnea, ECG abnormalities, erythema, esophagitis, GI bleeding, GI burning sensation, GI erosions/ulcerations, GI pain, hepatomegaly, hyperpigmentation (oral mucosa, nails, skin), hypersensitivity, hyperuricemia, myelodysplastic syndrome, myocarditis, neutropenic typhlitis, phlebitis, photosensitivity, pneumonia, premature menopause, premature ventricular contractions, pulmonary edema, pulmonary embolism, radiation recall, sepsis, shock, sinus tachycardia, stomatitis, ST-T wave changes (nonspecific), tachyarrhythmias, thromboembolism, thrombophlebitis, toxic megacolon, transaminases increased, urine discoloration (red), urticaria, ventricular tachycardia

Drug Interactions

Metabolism/Transport Effects None known.

Avoid Concomitant Use

Avoid concomitant use of EPIrubicin with any of the following: BCG; Cimetidine; CloZAPine; Natalizumab; Pimecrolimus; Tacrolimus (Topical); Tofacitinib; Vaccines (Live)

Increased Effect/Toxicity

EPIrubicin may increase the levels/effects of: CloZAPine; Leflunomide; Natalizumab; Tofacitinib; Vaccines (Live)

The levels/effects of EPIrubicin may be increased by: Bevacizumab; Cimetidine; Cyclophosphamide; Denosumab; Pimecrolimus; Roflumilast; Tacrolimus (Topical); Taxane Derivatives; Trastuzumab

Decreased Effect

EPIrubicin may decrease the levels/effects of: BCG; Cardiac Glycosides; Coccidioidin Skin Test; Sipuleucel-T; Vaccines (Inactivated); Vaccines (Live)

The levels/effects of EPIrubicin may be decreased by: Cardiac Glycosides; Echinacea

Ethanol/Nutrition/Herb Interactions

Ethanol: Avoid ethanol (due to GI irritation).

Herb/Nutraceutical: Avoid black cohosh, dong quai in estrogen-dependent tumors.

Preparation for Administration Hazardous agent; use appropriate precautions for handling and disposal (NIOSH, 2012). Reconstitute lyophilized powder with SWFI (25 mL for the 50 mg vial or 100 mL for the 200 mg vial) to a final concentration of 2 mg/mL.

Storage/Stability Protect from light.

Solution: Store intact vials refrigerated at 2°C to 8°C (36°F to 46°F); do not freeze. Product may "gel" at refrigerated temperatures; will return to slightly viscous solution after 2-4 hours at room temperature (15°C to 30°C). Discard unused solution from single dose vials within 24 hours of entry.

Lyophilized powder: Store at room temperature of 25°C (77°F); excursions permitted to 15°C to 30°C (59°F to 86°F). Reconstituted solutions are stable for 24 hours when stored at 2°C to 8°C (36°F to 46°F) or at room temperature.

Mechanism of Action Epirubicin is an anthracycline antineoplastic agent; known to inhibit DNA and RNA synthesis by steric obstruction after intercalating between DNA base pairs; active throughout entire cell cycle. Intercalation triggers DNA cleavage by topoisomerase II, resulting in cytocidal activity. Also inhibits DNA helicase, and generates cytotoxic free radicals.

Pharmacodynamics/Kinetics

Distribution: V_{ss}: 21-27 L/kg

Protein binding: ~77% to albumin

Metabolism: Extensively via hepatic and extrahepatic (including RBCs) routes

Half-life elimination: Triphasic; Mean terminal: 33 hours

Excretion: Feces (34% to 35%); urine (20% to 27%)

Dosage Adults: I.V.: **Note:** Patients receiving 120 mg/m^2/cycle as part of combination therapy (CEF-120 regimen) should also receive prophylactic therapy with sulfamethoxazole/trimethoprim or a fluoroquinolone. Details concerning dosing in combination regimens should also be consulted. Lower starting doses may be necessary for heavily pretreated patients, patients with pre-existing myelosuppression, or with bone marrow involvement.

Breast cancer, adjuvant treatment: Usual dose: 100-120 mg/m^2 per 3- or 4-week treatment cycle as follows:

60 mg/m^2 on days 1 and 8 every 28 days for 6 cycles in combination with cyclophosphamide and fluorouracil (CEF-120 regimen; Levine, 2005) **or**

100 mg/m^2 on day 1 every 21 days for 6 cycles in combination with cyclophosphamide and fluorouracil (FEC-100 regimen; Bonneterre, 2005) **or**

Breast cancer (unlabeled regimens; as a part of combination chemotherapy):

60 mg/m^2 on day 1 every 21 days for 8 cycles (EC regimen; Piccart, 2001) **or**

75 mg/m^2 on day 1 every 21 days for 4 cycles (FEC regimen; Buzdar, 2005) **or**

75 mg/m^2 on day 1 every 21 days for 6 cycles (EP or EC regimen; Langley, 2005) **or**

90 mg/m^2 on day 1 every 21 days for 4 or 6 cycles (FEC regimen ± paclitaxel; Martin, 2008) **or**

50 mg/m^2 on days 1 and 8 every 21-28 days for 6-9 cycles (CEF regimen; Ackland, 2001)

Esophageal cancer (unlabeled use; as part of combination chemotherapy):

50 mg/m^2 on day 1 every 21 days for up to 8 cycles (ECF, ECX, EOF, and EOX regimens; Cunningham, 2008) **or**

50 mg/m^2 on day 1 every 21 days for 3 preoperative and 3 postoperative cycles (ECF regimen; Cunningham, 2006)

Gastric cancer (unlabeled use; as part of combination chemotherapy):

50 mg/m^2 on day 1 every 21 days for up to 8 cycles (ECF, ECX, EOF, and EOX regimens [Cunningham, 2008]; ECF regimen [Waters, 1999]) **or**

50 mg/m^2 on day 1 every 21 days for 3 preoperative and 3 postoperative cycles (ECF regimen; Cunningham, 2006)

Dosage modifications (breast cancer; labeled dosing):

Delay day 1 dose until platelets are ≥100,000/mm^3, ANC ≥1500/mm^3, and nonhematologic toxicities have recovered to ≤grade 1

Reduce day 1 dose in subsequent cycles to 75% of previous day 1 dose if patient experiences nadir platelet counts <50,000/mm^3, ANC <250/mm^3, neutropenic fever, or grade 3/4 nonhematologic toxicity during the previous cycle

For CEF-120 regimen, reduce day 8 dose to 75% of day 1 dose if platelet counts are 75,000-100,000/mm^3 and ANC is 1000-1499/mm^3; omit day 8 dose if platelets are <75,000/mm^3, ANC <1000/mm^3, or grade 3/4 nonhematologic toxicity

Elderly: Plasma clearance of epirubicin in elderly female patients was noted to be reduced by 35%. Although no initial dosage reduction is specifically recommended, particular care should be exercised in monitoring toxicity and adjusting subsequent dosage in elderly patients (particularly females >70 years of age).

Dosage adjustment in bone marrow dysfunction: Heavily-treated patients, patients with pre-existing bone marrow depression or neoplastic bone marrow infiltration: Lower starting doses (75-90 mg/m^2) should be considered.

Dosage adjustment in renal impairment: The manufacturer's labeling recommends lower doses (dose not specified) in patients with severe renal impairment (serum creatinine >5 mg/dL). Other sources (Aronoff, 2007) suggest no dosage adjustment is needed for Cl_{cr} <50 mL/minute.

Dosage adjustment in hepatic impairment: The manufacturer's labeling recommends the following adjustments (based on clinical trial information):

Bilirubin 1.2-3 mg/dL or AST 2-4 times the upper limit of normal: Administer 50% of recommended starting dose

Bilirubin >3 mg/dL or AST >4 times the upper limit of normal: Administer 25% of recommended starting dose

Severe hepatic impairment: Use is not recommended (has not been studied)

Dosing in obesity: *ASCO Guidelines for appropriate chemotherapy dosing in obese adults with cancer:* Utilize patient's actual body weight (full weight) for calculation of body surface area- or weight-based dosing, particularly when the intent of therapy is curative; manage regimen-related toxicities in the same manner as for nonobese patients; if a dose reduction is utilized due to toxicity, consider resumption of full weight-based dosing with subsequent cycles, especially if cause of toxicity (eg, hepatic or renal impairment) is resolved (Griggs, 2012).

Administration I.V.: Infuse over 15-20 minutes or slow I.V. push; if lower doses due to dose reduction are administered, may reduce infusion time proportionally. Do not infuse over <3 minutes. Infuse into a free-flowing I.V. solution. Avoid the use of veins over joints or in extremities with compromised venous or lymphatic drainage.

Vesicant; ensure proper needle or catheter placement prior to and during infusion; avoid extravasation.

Extravasation management: If extravasation occurs, stop infusion immediately and disconnect (leave cannula/needle in place); gently aspirate extravasated solution (do **NOT** flush the line); remove needle/cannula; elevate extremity. Initiate antidote (dexrazoxane or dimethyl sulfate [DMSO]). Apply dry cold compresses for 20 minutes 4 times daily for 1-2 days (Perez Fidalgo, 2012); withhold cooling beginning 15 minutes before dexrazoxane infusion; continue withholding cooling until 15 minutes after infusion is completed. Topical DMSO should not be administered in combination with dexrazoxane; may lessen dexrazoxane efficacy.

Dexrazoxane: Adults: 1000 mg/m² (maximum dose: 2000 mg) I.V. (administer in a large vein remote from site of extravasation) over 1-2 hours days 1 and 2, then 500 mg/m² (maximum dose: 1000 mg) I.V. over 1-2 hours day 3; begin within 6 hours of extravasation. Day 2 and day 3 doses should be administered at approximately the same time (± 3 hours) as the dose on day 1 (Mouridsen, 2007; Perez Fidalgo, 2012). **Note:** Reduce dexrazoxane dose by 50% in patients with moderate to severe renal impairment (Cl_{cr} <40 mL/minute).

DMSO: Children and Adults: Apply topically to a region covering twice the affected area every 8 hours for 7 days; begin within 10 minutes of extravasation; do not cover with a dressing (Perez Fidalgo, 2012).

Hazardous agent; use appropriate precautions for handling and disposal (NIOSH, 2012).

Monitoring Parameters Monitor injection site during infusion for possible extravasation or local reactions. Baseline and repeated measurements of CBC with differential, liver function tests, serum creatinine, ECG, and LVEF. The method used for assessment of LVEF (echocardiogram or MUGA) should be consistent during routine monitoring.

Dosage Forms Excipient information presented when available (limited, particularly for generics); consult specific product labeling.

Solution, Intravenous, as hydrochloride [preservative free]:
Ellence: 50 mg/25 mL (25 mL); 200 mg/100 mL (100 mL)
Generic: 50 mg/25 mL (25 mL); 200 mg/100 mL (100 mL)

Solution Reconstituted, Intravenous, as hydrochloride:
Generic: 50 mg (1 ea)

◆ **Epirubicin for Injection (Can)** *see* Epirubicin *on page 718*
◆ **Epirubicin Hydrochloride** *see* Epirubicin *on page 718*
◆ **Epirubicin Hydrochloride Injection (Can)** *see* Epirubicin *on page 718*
◆ **Epitol** *see* CarBAMazepine *on page 336*
◆ **Epival (Can)** *see* Valproic Acid and Derivatives *on page 2149*
◆ **Epivir** *see* LamiVUDine *on page 1162*
◆ **Epivir HBV** *see* LamiVUDine *on page 1162*

Eplerenone (e PLER en one)

Brand Names: U.S. Inspra

Brand Names: Canada Inspra™

Pharmacologic Category Antihypertensive; Diuretic, Potassium-Sparing; Selective Aldosterone Blocker

Use

U.S. labeling: Treatment of hypertension (may be used alone or in combination with other antihypertensive agents); treatment of heart failure (HF) (LVEF ≤40%) following acute MI

Canadian labeling: Treatment of NYHA class II chronic heart failure (HF) with left ventricular systolic dysfunction; treatment of HF following acute MI

Pregnancy Risk Factor B

Pregnancy Considerations Adverse events were observed in some animal reproduction studies. Information related to eplerenone use in pregnancy is limited (Cabassi, 2012; Morton, 2011).

Breast-Feeding Considerations It is not known if eplerenone is excreted in breast milk. Due to the potential for serious adverse reactions in the nursing infant, the manufacturer recommends a a decision be made whether to discontinue nursing or to discontinue the drug, taking into account the importance of treatment to the mother.

Contraindications

U.S. labeling: Serum potassium >5.5 mEq/L at initiation; Cl_{cr} ≤30 mL/minute; concomitant use of strong CYP3A4 inhibitors (see Drug Interactions for details)

The following additional contraindications apply to patients with hypertension: Type 2 diabetes mellitus (noninsulin dependent, NIDDM) with microalbuminuria; serum creatinine >2.0 mg/dL in males or >1.8 mg/dL in females; Cl_{cr} <50 mL/minute; concomitant use with potassium supplements or potassium-sparing diuretics

Canadian labeling: Hypersensitivity to eplerenone or any component of the formulation; serum potassium >5 mEq/L at initiation; severe hepatic impairment (Child-Pugh class C); severe renal impairment (eGFR <30 mL/minute/1.73 m²); clinically significant hyperkalemia; concomitant use with potassium supplements, potassium-sparing diuretics or strong CYP3A4 inhibitors

Warnings/Precautions Dosage adjustment needed for patients on moderate CYP3A4 inhibitors (U.S. labeling) or mild-to-moderate CYP3A4 inhibitors (Canadian labeling). Monitor closely for hyperkalemia; increases in serum potassium were dose related during clinical trials and rates of hyperkalemia also increased with declining renal function. Dose reduction or interruption of therapy may be necessary with development of hyperkalemia. Use is contraindicated in patients with potassium >5.5 mEq/L (U.S. labeling) or >5 mEq/L (Canadian labeling) at initiation of therapy. Safety and efficacy have not been established in patients with severe hepatic impairment (Canadian labeling contraindicates use in severe hepatic impairment). Use with caution in HF patients post-MI with diabetes (especially if patient has proteinuria); risk of hyperkalemia is increased. Risk of hyperkalemia is increased with declining renal function. Use with caution in patients with mild renal impairment; contraindicated with moderate-severe impairment (hypertension: Cl_{cr} <50 mL/minute; heart failure post-MI: Cl_{cr} ≤30 mL/minute). Canadian labeling contraindicates use in all patients with severe renal impairment.

Adverse Reactions

>10%: Endocrine & metabolic: Hyperkalemia ([HF post-MI: K >5.5 mEq/L: 16%; K ≥6 mEq/L: 6%] [HTN: K >5.5 mEq/L at doses ≤200 mg: ≤1%; dose of 400 mg: 9%]), hypertriglyceridemia (1% to 15%, dose related)

1% to 10%:

Central nervous system: Dizziness (3%), fatigue (2%)
Endocrine & metabolic: Hyponatremia (2%, dose related), breast pain (males <1% to 1%), gynecomastia (males <1% to 1%), hypercholesterolemia (<1% to 1%)
Gastrointestinal: Diarrhea (2%), abdominal pain (1%)
Genitourinary: Abnormal vaginal bleeding (<1% to 2%)
Renal: Creatinine increased (HF post-MI: 6%), albuminuria (1%)
Respiratory: Cough (2%)
Miscellaneous: Flu-like syndrome (2%)

<1%, postmarketing, and/or case reports: Angioneurotic edema, BUN increased, liver function tests increased, rash, uric acid increased

Drug Interactions

Metabolism/Transport Effects Substrate of CYP3A4 (major); **Note:** Assignment of Major/Minor substrate status based on clinically relevant drug interaction potential

Avoid Concomitant Use

Avoid concomitant use of Eplerenone with any of the following: CycloSPORINE (Systemic); CYP3A4 Inhibitors (Strong); Fusidic Acid (Systemic); Itraconazole; Ketoconazole (Systemic); Posaconazole; Tacrolimus (Systemic); Voriconazole

Increased Effect/Toxicity

Eplerenone may increase the levels/effects of: ACE Inhibitors; Amifostine; Angiotensin II Receptor Blockers; Antihypertensives; CycloSPORINE (Systemic); Hypotensive Agents; Lithium; Obinutuzumab; Potassium Salts; Potassium-Sparing Diuretics; RiTUXimab; Tacrolimus (Systemic)

The levels/effects of Eplerenone may be increased by: Alfuzosin; Brimonidine (Topical); Canagliflozin; CYP3A4 Inhibitors (Moderate); CYP3A4 Inhibitors (Strong); Dasatinib; Diazoxide; Fluconazole; Fusidic Acid (Systemic); Heparin; Heparin (Low Molecular Weight); Herbs (Hypotensive Properties); Itraconazole; Ivacaftor; Ketoconazole (Systemic); Luliconazole; MAO Inhibitors; Mifepristone; Nitrofurantoin; Nonsteroidal Anti-Inflammatory Agents; Pentoxifylline; Phosphodiesterase 5 Inhibitors; Posaconazole; Prostacyclin Analogues; Simeprevir; Trimethoprim; Voriconazole

Decreased Effect

The levels/effects of Eplerenone may be decreased by: Bosentan; CYP3A4 Inducers (Strong); Dabrafenib; Deferasirox; Herbs (CYP3A4 Inducers); Herbs (Hypertensive Properties); Methylphenidate; Mitotane; Nonsteroidal Anti-Inflammatory Agents; Tocilizumab; Yohimbine

Ethanol/Nutrition/Herb Interactions

Food: Grapefruit juice increases eplerenone AUC ~25%.

Herb/Nutraceutical: St John's wort may decrease levels of eplerenone. Avoid black cohosh, California poppy, coleus, golden seal, hawthorn, mistletoe, periwinkle, quinine, shepherd's purse (may have increased antihypertensive effect). Avoid bayberry, blue cohosh, cayenne, ephedra, ginger, ginseng (American), kola, licorice (may diminish the antihypertensive effect).

Storage/Stability Store at controlled room temperature of 25°C (77°F); excursions permitted to 15°C to 30°C (59°F to 86°F).

Mechanism of Action Aldosterone, a mineralocorticoid, increases blood pressure primarily by inducing sodium and water retention. Overexpression of aldosterone is thought to contribute to myocardial fibrosis (especially following myocardial infarction) and vascular fibrosis. Mineralocorticoid receptors are located in the kidney, heart, blood vessels, and brain. Eplerenone selectively blocks mineralocorticoid receptors reducing blood pressure in a dose-dependent manner and appears to prevent myocardial and vascular fibrosis.

Pharmacodynamics/Kinetics

Distribution: V_d: 43-90 L

Protein binding: ~50%; primarily to alpha$_1$-acid glycoproteins

Metabolism: Primarily hepatic via CYP3A4; metabolites inactive

Bioavailability: 69%

Half-life elimination: 4-6 hours

Time to peak, plasma: ~1.5 hours; may take up to 4 weeks for full antihypertensive effect

Excretion: Urine (~67%); feces (32%); <5% as unchanged drug in urine and feces

Dosage Oral: Adults:

U.S. labeling:

Hypertension: Initial: 50 mg once daily; may increase to 50 mg twice daily if response is not adequate; may take up to 4 weeks for full therapeutic response. Doses >100 mg/day are associated with increased risk of hyperkalemia and no greater therapeutic effect.

Concurrent use with **moderate** CYP3A4 inhibitors: Initial: 25 mg once daily

Heart failure (post-MI): Initial: 25 mg once daily; dosage goal: Titrate to 50 mg once daily within 4 weeks, as tolerated

Dosage adjustment per serum potassium concentrations for HF (post-MI):

<5 mEq/L:

Increase dose from 25 mg every other day to 25 mg daily **or**

Increase dose from 25 mg daily to 50 mg daily

5-5.4 mEq/L: No adjustment needed

5.5-5.9 mEq/L:

Decrease dose from 50 mg daily to 25 mg daily **or**

Decrease dose from 25 mg daily to 25 mg every other day **or**

Modify dose from 25 mg every other day to withhold medication

≥6 mEq/L: Withhold medication until potassium <5.5 mEq/L, then restart at 25 mg every other day

Canadian labeling: Chronic HF (NYHA class II) or HF (post-MI):

eGFR ≥50 mL/minute/1.73 m^2 and potassium ≤5 mEq/L: Initial: 25 mg once daily; may increase within 4 weeks as tolerated to a target dose of 50 mg once daily (maximum dose). **Note:** Treatment following MI should be initiated 3-14 days after MI.

Concurrent use with **mild-to-moderate** CYP3A4 inhibitors: Maximum dose: 25 mg once daily

eGFR 30-49 mL/minute/1.73 m^2 and potassium ≤5 mEq/L: Initial: 25 mg every other day; may increase within 4 weeks as tolerated to a target dose of 25 mg once daily (maximum dose). **Note:** Treatment following MI should be initiated 3-14 days after MI.

Concurrent use with **mild-to-moderate** CYP3A4 inhibitors: Avoid concurrent use (target dose <25 mg once daily has not been studied).

Dosage adjustment (after initiation) per serum potassium concentrations:

<5 mEq/L:

Current dose is 25 mg every other day: Increase to 25 mg daily

Current dose is 25 mg daily and eGFR ≥50 mL/minute/1.73 m^2 or **not taking** concurrent mild-to-moderate CYP3A4 inhibitor: Increase to 50 mg daily

Current dose is 25 mg daily and eGFR 30-49 mL/minute/1.73 m^2 or **if taking** concurrent mild-to-moderate CYP3A4 inhibitor: Do not increase dose.

5-5.4 mEq/L: No adjustment needed

5.5-5.9 mEq/L:

Current dose is 50 mg daily: Decrease to 25 mg daily

Current dose is 25 mg daily: Decrease to 25 mg every other day

Decrease dose is 25 mg every other day: Withhold further doses; reinitiate only if potassium <5 mEq/L

≥6 mEq/L: Withhold further doses until potassium <5 mEq/L, then may temporarily resume therapy at 25 mg every other day (dose efficacy has not been established); reassess potassium levels in 1 week and if within acceptable limits, increase dose to 25 mg once daily; reassess potassium levels again in 1 week to determine whether therapy should be continued or interrupted.

Dosage adjustment in renal impairment:

U.S. labeling:

Hypertension: Cl_{cr} <50 mL/minute or serum creatinine >2 mg/dL (males) or >1.8 mg/dL (females): Use is contraindicated; risk of hyperkalemia increases with declining renal function.

HF (post-MI):

Cl_{cr} 31-50 mL/minute or serum creatinine >2 mg/dL (males) or >1.8 mg/dL (females): No dosage adjustment provided in manufacturer's labeling; use with caution.

Cl_{cr} ≤30 mL/minute: Use is contraindicated.

Canadian labeling:

eGFR ≥50 mL/minute/1.73 m^2: No dosage adjustment necessary unless receiving concurrent mild-to-moderate CYP3A4 inhibitor, then maximum dose is 25 mg once daily.

eGFR 30-49 mL/minute/1.73 m^2: Initial: 25 mg every other day; titrate to 25 mg once daily (maximum dose) within 4 weeks, as tolerated. Avoid concurrent use with mild-to-moderate CYP3A4 inhibitors.

eGFR ≤30 mL/minute/1.73 m^2: Use is contraindicated.

Dosage adjustment in hepatic impairment:

U.S. labeling:

Mild-to-moderate impairment: No dosage adjustment necessary.

Severe impairment: No dosage adjustment provided in manufacturer's labeling (has not been studied).

Canadian labeling:

Mild-to-moderate impairment: No dosage adjustment necessary.

Severe impairment: Use is contraindicated.

Dietary Considerations May be taken with or without food. Do not use salt substitutes containing potassium.

Administration May be administered with or without food.

Monitoring Parameters Blood pressure; serum potassium (prior to therapy, within the first week, 1 month after start of treatment or dose adjustment, then periodically as clinically indicated); additionally, check serum potassium in 3-7 days after initiating concurrent therapy with moderate CYP3A4 inhibitor; serum creatinine

Dosage Forms Excipient information presented when available (limited, particularly for generics); consult specific product labeling.

Tablet, Oral:

Inspra: 25 mg, 50 mg

Generic: 25 mg, 50 mg

◆ **EPO** *see* Epoetin Alfa *on page* 723

Epoetin Alfa (e POE e tin AL fa)

Brand Names: U.S. Epogen; Procrit

Brand Names: Canada Eprex

Index Terms rHuEPO; rHuEPO-α; EPO; Erythropoiesis-Stimulating Agent (ESA); Erythropoietin

Pharmacologic Category Colony Stimulating Factor; Erythropoiesis-Stimulating Agent (ESA); Growth Factor; Recombinant Human Erythropoietin

Use Treatment of anemia due to concurrent myelosuppressive chemotherapy in patients with cancer (nonmyeloid malignancies) receiving chemotherapy (palliative intent) for a planned minimum of 2 additional months of chemotherapy; treatment of anemia due to chronic kidney disease (including patients on dialysis and not on dialysis) to decrease the need for RBC transfusion; treatment of anemia associated with HIV (zidovudine) therapy when endogenous erythropoietin levels ≤500 mUnits/mL; reduction of allogeneic RBC transfusion for elective, noncardiac, nonvascular surgery when perioperative hemoglobin is >10 to ≤13 g/dL and there is a high risk for blood loss

Note: Epoetin is **not** indicated for use under the following conditions:

- Cancer patients receiving hormonal therapy, therapeutic biologic products, or radiation therapy unless also receiving concurrent myelosuppressive chemotherapy
- Cancer patients receiving myelosuppressive chemotherapy when the expected outcome is curative
- Surgery patients who are willing to donate autologous blood
- Surgery patients undergoing cardiac or vascular surgery
- As a substitute for RBC transfusion in patients requiring immediate correction of anemia

Note: In clinical trials (and one meta-analysis), epoetin has not demonstrated improved quality of life, fatigue, or well-being.

Unlabeled Use Treatment of symptomatic anemia in myelodysplastic syndrome (MDS)

Pregnancy Risk Factor C

Pregnancy Considerations Adverse events were observed in animal reproduction studies. In vitro studies suggest that recombinant erythropoietin does not cross the human placenta (Reisenberger, 1997). Polyhydramnios and intrauterine growth retardation have been reported with use in women with chronic kidney disease (adverse effects also associated with maternal disease). Hypospadias and pectus excavatum have been reported with first trimester exposure (case report).

Recombinant erythropoietin alfa has been evaluated as adjunctive treatment for severe pregnancy associated iron deficiency anemia (Breymann, 2001; Krafft, 2009) and has been used in pregnant women with iron-deficiency anemia associated with chronic kidney disease (CKD) (Furaz-Czerpak 2012; Josephson, 2007).

Amenorrheic premenopausal women should be cautioned that menstruation may resume following treatment with recombinant erythropoietin (Furaz-Czerpak, 2012). Multi-dose formulations containing benzyl alcohol are contraindicated for use in pregnant women; if treatment during pregnancy is needed, single dose preparations should be used.

Women who become pregnant during treatment with epoetin are encouraged to enroll in Amgen's Pregnancy Surveillance Program (1-800-772-6436).

Breast-Feeding Considerations Endogenous erythropoietin is found in breast milk (Semba, 2002). It is not known if recombinant erythropoietin alfa is excreted into breast milk. The manufacturer recommends caution be used if the single dose vial preparation is administered to nursing women; use of the multiple dose vials containing benzyl alcohol is contraindicated in breast-feeding women. When administered enterally to neonates (mixed with human milk or infant formula), recombinant erythropoietin did not significantly increase serum EPO concentrations. If passage via breast milk does occur, risk to a nursing infant appears low (Juul, 2003).

Prescribing and Access Restrictions As a requirement of the REMS program, access to this medication is restricted. Healthcare providers and hospitals must be enrolled in the ESA APPRISE (Assisting Providers and Cancer Patients with Risk Information for the Safe use of ESAs) Oncology Program (866-284-8089; http://www.esa-apprise.com) to prescribe or dispense ESAs (ie, epoetin alfa, darbepoetin alfa) to patients with cancer.

Medication Guide Available Yes

Contraindications Hypersensitivity to epoetin or any component of the formulation; uncontrolled hypertension; pure red cell aplasia (due to epoetin or other epoetin protein drugs); multidose vials contain benzyl alcohol and are contraindicated in neonates, infants, pregnant women, and nursing women

Warnings/Precautions [U.S. Boxed Warning]: Erythropoiesis-stimulating agents (ESAs) increased the risk of serious cardiovascular events, thromboembolic events, stroke, mortality, and/or tumor progression in clinical studies when administered to target hemoglobin levels >11 g/dL (and provide no additional benefit); a rapid rise in hemoglobin (>1 g/dL over 2 weeks) may also contribute to these risks. **[U.S. Boxed Warning]: A shortened overall survival and/or increased risk of tumor progression or recurrence has been reported in studies with breast, cervical, head and neck, lymphoid, and nonsmall cell lung cancer patients.** It is of note that in these studies, patients received ESAs to a target hemoglobin of ≥12 g/dL; although risk has not been excluded when dosed to achieve a target hemoglobin of <12 g/dL. **[U.S. Boxed Warnings]: To decrease these risks, and risk of cardio- and thrombovascular events, use the lowest dose needed to avoid red blood cell transfusions. Use ESAs in cancer patients only for the treatment of anemia related to concurrent myelosuppressive chemotherapy; discontinue ESA following completion of the chemotherapy course. ESAs are not indicated for patients receiving myelosuppressive therapy when the anticipated outcome is curative.** A dosage modification is appropriate if hemoglobin levels rise >1 g/dL per 2-week time period during treatment (Rizzo, 2010). Use of ESAs has been associated with an increased risk of venous thromboembolism (VTE) without a reduction in transfusions in patients with cancer (Hershman, 2009). Improved anemia symptoms, quality of life, fatigue, or well-being have not been demonstrated in controlled clinical trials. **[U.S. Boxed Warning]: Because of the risks of decreased survival and increased risk of tumor growth or progression, all healthcare providers and hospitals are required to enroll and comply with the ESA APPRISE (Assisting Providers and Cancer Patients with Risk Information for the Safe use of ESAs) Oncology Program prior to prescribing or dispensing ESAs to cancer patients.** Prescribers and patients will have to provide written documentation of discussed risks prior to each epoetin course.

[U.S. Boxed Warning]: An increased risk of death, serious cardiovascular events, and stroke was reported in chronic kidney disease (CKD) patients administered ESAs to target hemoglobin levels ≥11 g/dL; use the lowest dose sufficient to reduce the need for RBC transfusions. An optimal target hemoglobin level, dose or dosing strategy to reduce these risks has not been identified in clinical trials. Hemoglobin rising >1 g/dL in a 2-week period may contribute to the risk (dosage reduction recommended). The American College of Physicians recommends against the use of ESAs in patients with mild to moderate anemia and heart failure or coronary heart disease (ACP [Qaseem, 2013]).

Chronic kidney disease patients who exhibit an inadequate hemoglobin response to ESA therapy may be at a higher risk for cardiovascular events and mortality compared to other patients. ESA therapy may reduce dialysis efficacy (due to increase in red blood cells and decrease in plasma volume); adjustments in dialysis parameters may be needed. Patients treated with epoetin may require increased heparinization during dialysis to prevent clotting of the extracorporeal circuit. **[U.S. Boxed Warning]: DVT prophylaxis is recommended in perisurgery patients due to the risk of DVT.** Increased mortality was also observed in patients undergoing coronary artery bypass surgery who received epoetin alfa; these deaths were associated with thrombotic events. Epoetin is **not** approved for reduction of red blood cell transfusion in patients undergoing cardiac or vascular surgery and is **not** indicated for surgical patients willing to donate autologous blood.

Use with caution in patients with hypertension (contraindicated in uncontrolled hypertension) or with a history of seizures; hypertensive encephalopathy and seizures have been reported. If hypertension is difficult to control, reduce or hold epoetin alfa. An excessive rate of rise of hemoglobin is associated with hypertension or exacerbation of hypertension; decrease the epoetin dose if the hemoglobin increase exceeds 1 g/dL in any 2-week period. Blood pressure should be controlled prior to start of therapy and monitored closely throughout treatment. The risk for seizures is increased with epoetin use in patients with CKD; monitor closely for neurologic symptoms during the first several months of therapy. Due to the delayed onset of erythropoiesis, epoetin alfa is **not** recommended for acute correction of severe anemia or as a substitute for emergency transfusion.

Prior to treatment, correct or exclude deficiencies of iron, vitamin B_{12}, and/or folate, as well as other factors which may impair erythropoiesis (inflammatory conditions, infections). Prior to and periodically during therapy, iron stores must be evaluated. Supplemental iron is recommended if serum ferritin <100 mcg/L or serum transferrin saturation <20%; most patients with chronic kidney disease will require iron supplementation. Poor response should prompt evaluation of these potential factors, as well as possible malignant processes and hematologic disease (thalassemia, refractory anemia, myelodysplastic disorder), occult blood loss, hemolysis, ostetis fibrosa cystic, and/or bone marrow fibrosis. Severe anemia and pure red cell aplasia (PRCA) with associated neutralizing antibodies to erythropoietin has been reported, predominantly in patients with CKD receiving SubQ epoetin (the I.V. route is preferred for hemodialysis patients). Cases have also been reported in patients with hepatitis C who were receiving ESAs, interferon, and ribavirin. Patients with a sudden loss of response to epoetin alfa (with severe anemia and a low reticulocyte count) should be evaluated for PRCA with associated neutralizing antibodies to erythropoietin; discontinue treatment (permanently) in patients with PRCA secondary to neutralizing antibodies to epoetin.

Potentially serious allergic reactions have been reported (rarely). Discontinue immediately (and permanently) in patients who experience serious allergic/anaphylactic reactions. Some products may contain albumin. Multidose vials contain benzyl alcohol; do not use in premature infants.

Adverse Reactions

>10%:

- Cardiovascular: Hypertension (3% to 28%)
- Central nervous system: Fever (10% to 42%), headache (5% to 18%)
- Dermatologic: Pruritus (12% to 21%), rash (2% to 19%)
- Gastrointestinal: Nausea (35% to 56%), vomiting (12% to 28%)
- Local: Injection site reaction (7% to 13%)
- Neuromuscular & skeletal: Arthralgia (10% to 16%)
- Respiratory: Cough (4% to 26%)

1% to 10%:

- Cardiovascular: Deep vein thrombosis, edema, thrombosis
- Central nervous system: Chills, depression, dizziness, insomnia
- Dermatologic: Urticaria
- Endocrine & metabolic: Hyperglycemia, hypokalemia
- Gastrointestinal: Dysphagia, stomatitis, weight loss
- Hematologic: Leukopenia
- Local: Clotted vascular access
- Neuromuscular & skeletal: Bone pain, muscle spasm, myalgia
- Respiratory: Pulmonary embolism, respiratory congestion, upper respiratory infection

<1% (Limited to important or life-threatening): Allergic reaction, anaphylactic reaction, angioedema, bronchospasm, erythema, hypersensitivity reactions, hypertensive encephalopathy, microvascular thrombosis, MI, neutralizing antibodies, porphyria, pure red cell aplasia (PRCA), renal vein thrombosis, retinal artery thrombosis, seizure, stroke, tachycardia, temporal vein thrombosis, thrombophlebitis, TIA, tumor progression

Drug Interactions

Metabolism/Transport Effects None known.

Avoid Concomitant Use There are no known interactions where it is recommended to avoid concomitant use.

Increased Effect/Toxicity There are no known significant interactions involving an increase in effect.

Decreased Effect There are no known significant interactions involving a decrease in effect.

Preparation for Administration Prior to SubQ administration, preservative free solutions may be mixed with bacteriostatic NS containing benzyl alcohol 0.9% in a 1:1 ratio.

Storage/Stability Vials should be stored at 2°C to 8°C (36°F to 46°F); **do not freeze or shake**. Protect from light.

Single-dose 1 mL vial contains no preservative: Use one dose per vial. Do not re-enter vial; discard unused portions.

Single-dose vials (except 40,000 units/mL vial) are stable for 2 weeks at room temperature (Cohen, 2007). Single-dose 40,000 units/mL vial is stable for 1 week at room temperature.

Multidose 1 mL or 2 mL vial contains preservative. Store at 2°C to 8°C after initial entry and between doses. Discard 21 days after initial entry.

Multidose vials (with preservative) are stable for 1 week at room temperature (Cohen, 2007).

Prefilled syringes containing the 20,000 units/mL formulation with preservative are stable for 6 weeks refrigerated (2°C to 8°C) (Naughton, 2003).

Dilutions of 1:10 and 1:20 (1 part epoetin:19 parts sodium chloride) are stable for 18 hours at room temperature (Ohls, 1996).

Prior to SubQ administration, preservative free solutions may be mixed with bacteriostatic NS containing benzyl alcohol 0.9% in a 1:1 ratio (Corbo, 1992).

Dilutions of 1:10 in $D_{10}W$ with human albumin 0.05% or 0.1% are stable for 24 hours.

Mechanism of Action Induces erythropoiesis by stimulating the division and differentiation of committed erythroid progenitor cells; induces the release of reticulocytes from the bone marrow into the bloodstream, where they mature to erythrocytes. There is a dose response relationship with this effect. This results in an increase in reticulocyte counts followed by a rise in hematocrit and hemoglobin levels.

Pharmacodynamics/Kinetics

Onset of action: Several days

Peak effect: Hemoglobin level: 2-6 weeks

Distribution: V_d: 9 L; rapid in the plasma compartment; concentrated in liver, kidneys, and bone marrow

Metabolism: Some degradation does occur

Bioavailability: SubQ: ~21% to 31%; intraperitoneal epoetin: 3% (Macdougall, 1989)

Half-life elimination: Cancer: SubQ: 16-67 hours; Chronic kidney disease: I.V.: 4-13 hours

Time to peak, serum: Chronic kidney disease: SubQ: 5-24 hours

Excretion: Feces (majority); urine (small amounts, 10% unchanged in normal volunteers)

Dosage

Anemia associated with chronic kidney disease: Individualize dosing and use the lowest dose necessary to reduce the need for RBC transfusions.

*Chronic kidney disease patients **ON dialysis*** (I.V. route is preferred for hemodialysis patients; initiate treatment when hemoglobin is <10 g/dL; reduce dose or interrupt treatment if hemoglobin approaches or exceeds 11 g/dL):

Children 1 month to 16 years: I.V., SubQ: Initial dose: 50 units/kg 3 times/week

Adults: I.V., SubQ: Initial dose: 50-100 units/kg 3 times/week

*Chronic kidney disease patients **NOT on dialysis*** (consider initiating treatment when hemoglobin is <10 g/dL; use only if rate of hemoglobin decline would likely result in RBC transfusion and desire is to reduce risk of alloimmunization or other RBC transfusion-related risks; reduce dose or interrupt treatment if hemoglobin exceeds 10 g/dL):

Adults: I.V., SubQ: Initial dose: 50-100 units/kg 3 times/week

Dosage adjustments for chronic kidney disease patients (either on dialysis or not on dialysis):

If hemoglobin does not increase by >1 g/dL after 4 weeks: Increase dose by 25%; do not increase the dose more frequently than once every 4 weeks

If hemoglobin increases >1 g/dL in any 2-week period: Reduce dose by ≥25%; dose reductions can occur more frequently than once every 4 weeks; avoid frequent dosage adjustments

Inadequate or lack of response over a 12-week escalation period: Further increases are unlikely to improve response and may increase risks; use the minimum effective dose that will maintain a Hgb level sufficient to avoid RBC transfusions and evaluate patient for other causes of anemia. Discontinue therapy if responsiveness does not improve.

Anemia due to chemotherapy in cancer patients: Initiate treatment only if hemoglobin <10 g/dL and anticipated duration of myelosuppressive chemotherapy is ≥2 months. Titrate dosage to use the minimum effective dose that will maintain a hemoglobin level sufficient to avoid red blood cell transfusions. Discontinue erythropoietin following completion of chemotherapy.

Children ≥5 years: I.V.: Initial dose: 600 units/kg once weekly until completion of chemotherapy.

Dosage adjustments:

If hemoglobin does not increase by >1 g/dL **and** remains <10 g/dL after initial 4 weeks: Increase to 900 units/kg (maximum dose: 60,000 units); discontinue after 8 weeks of treatment if RBC transfusions are still required or there is no hemoglobin response.

If hemoglobin exceeds a level needed to avoid red blood cell transfusion: Withhold dose; resume treatment with a 25% dose reduction when hemoglobin approaches a level where transfusions may be required.

If hemoglobin increases >1 g/dL in any 2-week period **or** hemoglobin reaches a level sufficient to avoid red blood cell transfusion: Reduce dose by 25%.

Adults: SubQ: Initial dose: 150 units/kg 3 times/week or 40,000 units once weekly until completion of chemotherapy

Dosage adjustments:

If hemoglobin does not increase by >1 g/dL **and** remains below 10 g/dL after initial 4 weeks: Increase to 300 units/kg 3 times/week or 60,000 units weekly; discontinue after 8 weeks of treatment if RBC transfusions are still required or there is no hemoglobin response

If hemoglobin exceeds a level needed to avoid red blood cell transfusion: Withhold dose; resume treatment with a 25% dose reduction when hemoglobin approaches a level where transfusions may be required.

If hemoglobin increases >1 g/dL in any 2-week period **or** hemoglobin reaches a level sufficient to avoid red blood cell transfusion: Reduce dose by 25%.

Anemia due to zidovudine in HIV-infected patients: Titrate dosage to use the minimum effective dose that will maintain a hemoglobin level sufficient to avoid red blood cell transfusions. Hemoglobin levels should not exceed 12 g/dL.

Children 8 months to 17 years (based on limited data): I.V., SubQ: Reported dosing range: 50-400 units/kg 2-3 times/week

Adults (with serum erythropoietin levels ≤500 mUnits/mL and zidovudine doses ≤4200 mg/week): I.V., SubQ: Initial: 100 units/kg 3 times/week; if hemoglobin does not increase after 8 weeks, increase dose by ~50-100 units/kg at 4-8 week intervals until hemoglobin reaches a level sufficient to avoid RBC transfusion; maximum dose: 300 units/kg. Withhold dose if hemoglobin exceeds 12 g/dL, may resume treatment with a 25% dose reduction once hemoglobin <11 g/dL. Discontinue if hemoglobin increase is not achieved with 300 units/kg for 8 weeks.

Surgery patients (perioperative hemoglobin should be >10 g/dL and ≤13 g/dL; DVT prophylactic anticoagulation is recommended): Adults: SubQ: Initial dose:

300 units/kg/day beginning 10 days before surgery, on the day of surgery, and for 4 days after surgery **or**

600 units/kg once weekly for 4 doses, given 21-, 14-, and 7 days before surgery, and on the day of surgery

Symptomatic anemia associated with MDS (unlabeled use): Adults: SubQ: 40,000-60,000 units 1-3 times/week (NCCN MDS guidelines v.2.2011)

Dosage adjustment in renal impairment: No dosage adjustment necessary.

Dosage adjustment in hepatic impairment: No dosage adjustment provided in manufacturer's labeling.

Administration

SubQ is the preferred route of administration **except** in patients with CKD on hemodialysis; 1:1 dilution with bacteriostatic NS (containing benzyl alcohol) acts as a local anesthetic to reduce pain at the injection site

Patients with CKD on hemodialysis: I.V. route preferred; it may be administered into the venous line at the end of the dialysis procedure

Monitoring Parameters Transferrin saturation and serum ferritin (prior to and during treatment); hemoglobin (weekly after initiation and following dose adjustments until stable and sufficient to minimize need for RBC transfusion, CKD patients should be also be monitored at least monthly following hemoglobin stability); blood pressure; seizures (CKD patients following initiation for first few months, includes new-onset or change in seizure frequency or premonitory symptoms)

Cancer patients: Examinations recommended by the ASCO/ASH guidelines (Rizzo, 2010) prior to treatment include: peripheral blood smear (in some situations a bone marrow exam may be necessary), assessment for iron, folate, or vitamin B_{12} deficiency, reticulocyte count, renal function status, and occult blood loss; during ESA treatment, assess baseline and periodic iron, total iron-binding capacity, and transferrin saturation or ferritin levels.

Reference Range Zidovudine-treated HIV patients: Available evidence indicates patients with endogenous serum erythropoietin levels >500 mU/mL are unlikely to respond

Additional Information Oncology Comment: The American Society of Clinical Oncology (ASCO) and American Society of Hematology (ASH) 2010 updates to the clinical practice guidelines for the use of erythropoiesis-stimulating agents (ESAs) in patients with cancer indicate that ESAs are most appropriate when used according to the parameters identified within the Food and Drug Administration (FDA) approved labeling for epoetin and darbepoetin (Rizzo, 2010). ESAs are an option for chemotherapy associated anemia when the hemoglobin has fallen to <10 g/dL to decrease the need for RBC transfusions. ESAs should only be used in conjunction with concurrent chemotherapy. Although the FDA label now limits ESA use to the palliative setting, the ASCO/ASH guidelines suggest using clinical judgment in weighing risks versus benefits as formal outcomes studies of ESA use defined by intent of chemotherapy treatment have not been conducted.

The ASCO/ASH guidelines continue to recommend following the FDA approved dosing (and dosing adjustment) guidelines as alternate dosing and schedules have not demonstrated consistent differences in effectiveness with regard to hemoglobin response. In patients who do not have a response within 6-8 weeks (hemoglobin rise <1-2 g/dL or no reduction in transfusions) ESA therapy should be discontinued.

Prior to the initiation of ESAs, other sources of anemia (in addition to chemotherapy or underlying hematologic malignancy) should be investigated. Examinations recommended prior to treatment include peripheral blood smear (in some situations a bone marrow exam may be necessary), assessment for iron, folate, or vitamin B_{12} deficiency, reticulocyte count, renal function status, and occult blood loss. During ESA treatment, assess baseline and periodic iron, total iron-binding capacity, and transferrin saturation or ferritin levels. Iron supplementation may be necessary

The guidelines note that patients with an increased risk of thromboembolism (generally includes previous history of thrombosis, surgery, and/or prolonged periods of immobilization) and patients receiving concomitant medications that may increase thromboembolic risk, should begin ESA therapy only after careful consideration. With the exception of low-risk myelodysplasia-associated anemia (which has evidence supporting the use of ESAs without concurrent chemotherapy), the guidelines do not support the use of ESAs in the absence of concurrent chemotherapy.

Dosage Forms Excipient information presented when available (limited, particularly for generics); consult specific product labeling.

Solution, Injection:

Epogen: 10,000 units/mL (2 mL); 20,000 units/mL (1 mL) [contains benzyl alcohol]

Procrit: 10,000 units/mL (2 mL); 20,000 units/mL (1 mL) [contains benzyl alcohol]

Solution, Injection [preservative free]:

Epogen: 2000 units/mL (1 mL); 3000 units/mL (1 mL); 4000 units/mL (1 mL); 10,000 units/mL (1 mL)

Procrit: 2000 units/mL (1 mL); 3000 units/mL (1 mL); 4000 units/mL (1 mL); 10,000 units/mL (1 mL); 40,000 units/mL (1 mL)

Dosage Forms: Canada Excipient information presented when available (limited, particularly for generics); consult specific product labeling.

Injection, solution [preservative free]:

Eprex: 1000 units/0.5 mL (0.5 mL), 2000 units/0.5 mL (0.5 mL), 3000 units/0.3 mL (0.3 mL), 4000 units/0.4 mL (0.4 mL), 5000 units/0.5 mL (0.5 mL), 6000 units/0.6 mL (0.6 mL), 8000 units/0.8 mL (0.8 mL), 10,000 units/mL (1 mL), 20,000 units/0.5 mL (0.5 mL), 30,000 units/0.75 mL (0.75 mL), 40,000 units/mL (1 mL) [contains polysorbate 80; prefilled syringe, free of human serum albumin]

◆ **Epogen** *see* Epoetin Alfa *on page 723*

Epoprostenol (e poe PROST en ole)

Brand Names: U.S. Flolan; Veletri

Brand Names: Canada Caripul; Flolan

Index Terms Epoprostenol Sodium; PGI_2; PGX; Prostacyclin

Pharmacologic Category Prostacyclin; Prostaglandin; Vasodilator

Use Treatment of pulmonary arterial hypertension (PAH) (WHO Group I) in patients with NYHA Class III or IV symptoms to improve exercise capacity

Unlabeled Use Acute vasodilator testing in pulmonary arterial hypertension (PAH)

Inhalation: Intraoperative treatment of pulmonary hypertension in patients undergoing cardiac surgery with cardiopulmonary bypass; post-cardiothoracic surgery pulmonary hypertension, right ventricular dysfunction, or refractory hypoxemia

Pregnancy Risk Factor B

Pregnancy Considerations Adverse events were not observed in animal reproduction studies. Women with PAH are encouraged to avoid pregnancy (McLaughlin, 2009).

Breast-Feeding Considerations It is not known if epoprostenol is excreted in breast milk. The manufacturer recommends that caution be exercised when administering epoprostenol to nursing women.

Prescribing and Access Restrictions Orders for epoprostenol are distributed by two sources in the United States. Information on orders or reimbursement assistance may be obtained from either Accredo Health, Inc (1-866-344-4874) or CVS Caremark (1-877-242-2738).

Contraindications Hypersensitivity to epoprostenol or to structurally-related compounds; chronic use in patients with heart failure due to severe left ventricular systolic dysfunction; patients who develop pulmonary edema during dose initiation

Warnings/Precautions Initiation or transition to epoprostenol requires specialized cardiopulmonary monitoring in a critical care setting where clinicians are experienced in advanced management of pulmonary arterial hypertension. Abrupt interruptions or large sudden reductions in dosage may result in rebound pulmonary hypertension; some patients with PAH have developed pulmonary edema during dosing adjustment and acute vasodilator testing (not an approved use), which may be associated with concomitant heart failure (LV systolic dysfunction with significantly elevated left heart filling pressures) or pulmonary veno-occlusive disease/pulmonary capillary hemangiomatosis. During chronic use, unless contraindicated, anticoagulants should be coadministered to reduce the risk of thromboembolism. Use cautiously in patients who have conditions that increase bleeding risk (inhibits platelet aggregation). Use with caution in patients receiving anticoagulants and antiplatelet agents. Chronic continuous I.V. infusion of epoprostenol via a chronic indwelling central venous catheter (CVC) has been associated with local infections and serious blood stream infections. Clinical studies of epoprostenol in pulmonary hypertension did not include sufficient numbers of patients ≥65 years of age to substantiate its safety and efficacy in the geriatric population. As a result, in general, dose selection for an elderly patient should be cautious usually starting at the low end of the dosing range.

Adverse Reactions

Note: Adverse events reported during dose initiation and escalation include flushing (58%), headache (49%), nausea/vomiting (32%), hypotension (16%), anxiety/nervousness/agitation (11%), chest pain (11%); dizziness, abdominal pain, bradycardia, musculoskeletal pain, dyspnea, back pain, diaphoresis, dyspepsia, hypoesthesia/paresthesia, and tachycardia are also reported. Although some adverse reactions may be related to the underlying disease state, abdominal pain, anxiety/nervousness/agitation, arthralgia, bleeding, bradycardia, diarrhea, diaphoresis, flu-like syndrome, flushing, headache, hypotension, jaw pain, nausea, pain, pulmonary edema, rash, tachycardia, thrombocytopenia, and vomiting are clearly contributed to epoprostenol. The following adverse events have been reported during chronic administration for idiopathic or heritable PAH:

>10%:

Cardiovascular: Tachycardia (35% to 43%), flushing (23% to 42%), hypotension (13%)

Central nervous system: Dizziness (83%), headache (46% to 83%), chills/fever/sepsis/flu-like syndrome (25%), anxiety/nervousness/tremor (21%)

Dermatologic: Skin ulcer (39%), eczema/rash/urticaria (25%)

Gastrointestinal: Nausea/vomiting (41% to 67%), anorexia (66%), diarrhea (37% to 50%)

Local: Injection site reactions: Infection (18%), pain (11%)

Neuromuscular & skeletal: Pain/neck pain/arthralgia (84%), jaw pain (54% to 75%), arthritis (52%), myalgia (44%), musculoskeletal pain (35%), hypoesthesia/hyperesthesia/paresthesia (5% to 12%)

<1%, postmarketing, and/or case reports: Anemia, fatigue, hepatic failure, hypersplenism, hyperthyroidism, pallor, pancytopenia, pulmonary embolism, splenomegaly, thrombocytopenia

Drug Interactions

Metabolism/Transport Effects None known.

Avoid Concomitant Use There are no known interactions where it is recommended to avoid concomitant use.

Increased Effect/Toxicity

Epoprostenol may increase the levels/effects of: Agents with Antiplatelet Properties; Anticoagulants; Antihypertensives

Decreased Effect There are no known significant interactions involving a decrease in effect.

Preparation for Administration

Preparation of Epoprostenol Infusion

To make solution with concentration:	Flolan Instructions	Veletri or Caripul Instructions
	Note: Flolan may only be prepared with sterile diluent provided.	**Note:** Veletri or Caripul may only be prepared with sterile water for injection (SWFI) or NS.
3000 ng/mL	Dissolve one 0.5 mg vial with 5 mL supplied diluent, withdraw 3 mL, and add to a sufficient volume of supplied diluent to make a total of 100 mL.	Dissolve one 0.5 mg vial with 5 mL of SWFI or NS, withdraw 3 mL, and add to a sufficient volume of the identical diluent to make a total of 100 mL.
5000 ng/mL	Dissolve one 0.5 mg vial with 5 mL supplied diluent, withdraw entire vial contents, and add to a sufficient volume of supplied diluent to make a total of 100 mL.	Dissolve one 0.5 mg vial with 5 mL of SWFI or NS, withdraw entire vial contents, and add to a sufficient volume of the identical diluent to make a total of 100 mL.
10,000 ng/mL	Dissolve two 0.5 mg vials each with 5 mL supplied diluent, withdraw entire vial contents, and add to a sufficient volume of supplied diluent to make a total of 100 mL.	Dissolve two 0.5 mg vials each with 5 mL of SWFI or NS, withdraw entire vial contents, and add to a sufficient volume of the identical diluent to make a total of 100 mL.
15,000 ng/mL	Dissolve one 1.5 mg vial with 5 mL supplied diluent, withdraw entire vial contents, and add to a sufficient volume of supplied diluent to make a total of 100 mL.	Dissolve one 1.5 mg vial with 5 mL of SWFI or NS, withdraw entire vial contents, and add to a sufficient volume of the identical diluent to make a total of 100 mL.
20,000 ng/mL	Dissolve two 0.5 mg vials each with 5 mL supplied diluent, withdraw entire vial contents, and add to a sufficient volume of supplied diluent to make a total of **50 mL** (DeWet, 2004).	
30,000 ng/mL		Dissolve two 1.5 mg vials each with 5 mL of SWFI or NS, withdraw entire vial contents, and add to a sufficient volume of the identical diluent to make a total of 100 mL.

Storage/Stability

Flolan: Prior to use, store vials at 15°C to 25°C (59°F to 77°F); do not freeze. Protect from light. Following reconstitution, solution must be stored under refrigeration at 2°C to 8°C (36°F to 46°F) if not used immediately; do not freeze. Protect from light. Total storage and infusion time must not exceed 48 hours for reconstituted solutions. Each reservoir of solution may be refrigerated for ≤40 hours and infused at room temperature over ≤8 hours; alternatively, each reservoir may be refrigerated for ≤24 hours and infused with the use of a cold pouch over ≤24 hours (gel packs must be changed every 12 hours).

Veletri: Prior to use, store vials at 20°C to 25°C (68°F to 77°F); do not freeze. Protect from light. Reconstituted vials must be further diluted prior to use.

Caripul (Canadian availability; not available in the U.S.): Prior to use, store vials at 15°C to 30°C (59°F to 86°F); do not freeze. Reconstituted vials must be further diluted prior to use.

Reconstituted solutions of Veletri or Caripul immediately diluted to a final concentration within a drug delivery reservoir may be administered immediately or stored at 2°C to 8°C (36°F to 46°F) for up to 8 days; do not freeze. Protect from light.

If administered immediately, the following maximum durations of administration at room temperature (25°C [77°F]) according to solution concentration are recommended:

U.S. labeling (Veletri):
3000 to <15,000 ng/mL: 48 hours
15,000 to <60,000 ng/mL: 48 hours
≥60,000 ng/mL: 72 hours

Canadian labeling (Caripul):
3000 to <15,000 ng/mL: 48 hours
≥15,000: 48 hours

If stored at 2°C to 8°C (36°F to 46°F) for up to 8 days, the following maximum durations of administration at room temperature (25°C [77°F]) according to solution concentration are recommended:
3000 to <15,000 ng/mL: 24 hours
15,000 to <60,000 ng/mL: 48 hours
≥60,000 ng/mL: 48 hours

Short excursions at 40°C (104°F) are permitted as follows:
Solution concentration <15,000 ng/mL: Up to 2 hours
Solution concentration 15,000 to <60,000 ng/mL: Up to 4 hours
Solution concentration ≥60,000 ng/mL: Up to 8 hours

The following maximum durations of administration at temperatures >25°C to 40°C (>77°F up to 104°F) administered either immediately or after up to 8 days storage at 2°C to 8°C (36°F to 46°F) according to solution concentration are recommended:

Use at temperature >25°C to 30°C (>77°F up to 86°F):
U.S. labeling (Veletri):
<60,000 ng/mL: 24 hours
≥60,000 ng/mL: 48 hours
Canadian labeling (Caripul): All concentrations: 24 hours

Use at temperature up to 40°C (104°F):
U.S. labeling (Veletri): ≥60,000 ng/mL: 24 hours (immediately administered after preparation)

Mechanism of Action Epoprostenol is also known as prostacyclin and PGI_2. It is a strong vasodilator of all vascular beds. In addition, it is a potent endogenous inhibitor of platelet aggregation. The reduction in platelet aggregation results from epoprostenol's activation of intracellular adenylate cyclase and the resultant increase in cyclic adenosine monophosphate concentrations within the platelets. Additionally, it is capable of decreasing thrombogenesis and platelet clumping in the lungs by inhibiting platelet aggregation.

Pharmacodynamics/Kinetics

Metabolism: Rapidly hydrolyzed; subject to some enzymatic degradation; forms two active metabolites (6-keto-prostaglandin $F_1\alpha$ and 6,15-diketo-13,14-dihydro-prostaglandin $F_1\alpha$) with minimal activity and 14 inactive metabolites

Half-life elimination: ~6 minutes

Excretion: Urine (84%); feces (4%)

Dosage

I.V.:

Pulmonary arterial hypertension (PAH): Children (unlabeled use), Adolescents (unlabeled use), and Adults: Initial: 2 ng/kg/minute; a lower initial dose may be used if patient is intolerant of starting dose. Increase dose in increments of 2 ng/kg/minute at intervals of ≥15 minutes until dose-limiting side effects (eg, flushing, jaw pain, headache, hypotension, nausea) are noted or response to epoprostenol plateaus. Usual optimal dose (monotherapy): 25-40 ng/kg/minute (McLaughlin, 2009); significant patient variability in optimal dose exists. Maximum dose with chronic therapy has not been defined; however, doses as high as 195 ng/kg/minute have been described in children (Rosenzweig, 1999).

Dose adjustment during chronic phase of treatment:

If PAH symptoms persist or recur following improvement, increase dose in 1-2 ng/kg/minute increments at intervals of ≥15 minutes. May also increase dose at intervals of 24-48 hours or longer (eg, every 1-2 weeks). **Note:** The need for increased doses should be expected with chronic use; incremental increases occur more frequently during the first few months after the drug is initiated.

In case of dose-limiting pharmacologic events (eg, hypotension, severe nausea, vomiting), decrease dose in 2 ng/kg/minute decrements at intervals of ≥15 minutes. Avoid abrupt withdrawal or sudden large dose reductions. **Note:** Adverse event may resolve without dosage adjustment.

Lung transplant: In patients receiving lung transplants, epoprostenol may be tapered after sequential lung transplantation once the allografts have been reperfused. If cardiopulmonary bypass utilized, epoprostenol may be tapered after pump perfusion has been initiated.

Acute vasodilator testing in patients with PAH (unlabeled use; McLaughlin, 2009): Adults: **Note:** Acute vasodilator testing should only be done in patients who might be considered candidates for calcium channel blocker therapy.

Initial: 2 ng/kg/minute; increase dose in increments of 2 ng/kg/minute every 10-15 minutes; dosing range during testing: 2-10 ng/kg/minute

Inhalation (unlabeled route): Adults:

Intraoperative pulmonary hypertension during cardiac surgery with cardiopulmonary bypass (CPB) (unlabeled use): **Note:** Institution-specific protocols vary.

Administration after induction of anesthesia before incision: 60 mcg (4 mL of 15,000 ng/mL concentration) via jet nebulizer; effect persists for ~25 minutes (Hache, 2003)

or

Intraoperative administration: Nebulization via ventilator circuit: Using a 15,000 ng/mL concentration and an oxygen flow of 8 L/minute, begin administration via jet nebulizer 5 minutes prior to weaning from CPB; discontinue at least 60 minutes after CPB weaned (Fattouch, 2006)

Post-cardiothoracic surgery pulmonary hypertension, right ventricular dysfunction, or refractory hypoxemia (unlabeled use) (DeWet, 2004): **Note:** May need to change ventilator filter every 2 hours due to glycine buffer diluent; may cause ventilator valve malfunction. Tidal volume delivered by ventilator may require adjustment.

Nebulization via ventilator circuit: Using a 20,000 ng/mL concentration, prime nebulizer chamber with 15 mL; administer remainder at a constant rate of 8 mL/hour; delivers ~38 ng/kg/minute (based on a 70 kg patient); set oxygen flow at 2-3 L/minute; wean as tolerated. **Note:** Although not achieved with this regimen, in general, doses >50 ng/kg/minute do not provide additional benefit and may increase the risk of hypotension.

or

Nebulization via facemask with Venturi attachment: Using a 20,000 ng/mL concentration, prime nebulizer chamber with 15 mL; set oxygen flow at 2-3 L/minute; 8 mL/hour will be nebulized; wean as tolerated.

Weaning procedure: Reduce dose by 50% every 2-4 hours (ie, 20,000 ng/mL to 10,000 ng/mL to 5000 ng/mL) until a concentration of 2500 ng/mL is reached; carefully discontinue once patient remains stable on this concentration for at least 4 hours.

Dosage adjustment in renal impairment: No dosage adjustment provided in manufacturer's labeling.

Dosage adjustment in hepatic impairment: No dosage adjustment provided in manufacturer's labeling.

Administration

I.V.: Use infusion sets with an in-line 0.22 micron filter for Veletri or Caripul infusions. Flolan labeling does not specifically recommend filtering; however, the use of an in-line 0.22 micron filter was used during clinical trials. The ambulatory infusion pump should be small and lightweight, be able to adjust infusion rates in 2 ng/kg/minute increments, have occlusion, end of infusion, and low battery alarms, have ± 6% accuracy of the programmed rate, and have positive continuous or pulsatile pressure with intervals ≤3 minutes between pulses. The reservoir should be made of polyvinyl chloride, polypropylene, or glass. Immediate access to back up pump, infusion sets and medication is essential to prevent treatment interruptions.

When administered on an ongoing basis, must be infused through a central venous catheter. Peripheral infusion may be used temporarily until central line is established. Infuse using an infusion pump. Avoid abrupt withdrawal (including interruptions in delivery) or sudden large reductions in dosing.

Inhalation (unlabeled route):

Intraoperative administration: Administer via jet nebulizer connected to the inspiratory limb of the ventilator near the endotracheal tube with a bypass oxygen flow of 8 L/minute to achieve administration of a high proportion of small particles (Fattouch, 2006; Hache, 2003).

Post-cardiothoracic surgery: May also be administered via jet nebulizer connected to the inspiratory limb of the ventilator near the endotracheal tube or via face mask with a Venturi attachment for aerosolization with a bypass oxygen flow of 2-3 L/minute (De Wet, 2004). **Note:** Glycine buffer diluent may cause ventilator valve malfunction; it has been recommended that filters be changed on the ventilator every 2 hours; may also use a ventilator heating coil (De Wet, 2004).

Monitoring Parameters Monitor for improvements in pulmonary function, decreased exertional dyspnea, fatigue, syncope and chest pain, pulmonary vascular resistance, pulmonary arterial pressure and quality of life. In addition, the pump device and catheters should be monitored frequently to avoid "system" related failure. Monitor arterial pressure; assess all vital functions. Hypoxia, flushing, and tachycardia may indicate overdose.

Dosage Forms Excipient information presented when available (limited, particularly for generics); consult specific product labeling.

Solution Reconstituted, Intravenous:
- Flolan: 0.5 mg (1 ea); 1.5 mg (1 ea)
- Veletri: 0.5 mg (1 ea); 1.5 mg (1 ea)
- Generic: 0.5 mg (1 ea); 1.5 mg (1 ea)

Dosage Forms: Canada Excipient information presented when available (limited, particularly for generics); consult specific product labeling.

Solution Reconstituted, Intravenous:
- Caripul: 0.5 mg (1 ea); 1.5 mg (1 ea)
- Flolan: 0.5 mg (1 ea); 1.5 mg (1 ea)

◆ **Epoprostenol Sodium** *see* Epoprostenol *on page 727*
◆ **Epothilone B Lactam** *see* Ixabepilone *on page 1139*
◆ **Eprex (Can)** *see* Epoetin Alfa *on page 723*

Eprosartan (ep roe SAR tan)

Brand Names: U.S. Teveten

Brand Names: Canada Teveten®

Pharmacologic Category Angiotensin II Receptor Blocker; Antihypertensive

Additional Appendix Information

Angiotensin Agents *on page 2280*

Use Treatment of hypertension; may be used alone or in combination with other antihypertensives

Pregnancy Risk Factor D

Pregnancy Considerations [U.S. Boxed Warning]: Drugs that act on the renin-angiotensin system can cause injury and death to the developing fetus. Discontinue as soon as possible once pregnancy is detected. The use of drugs which act on the renin-angiotensin system are associated with oligohydramnios. Oligohydramnios, due to decreased fetal renal function, may lead to fetal lung hypoplasia and skeletal malformations. Use is also associated with anuria, hypotension, renal failure, skull hypoplasia, and death in the fetus/neonate. The exposed fetus should be monitored for fetal growth, amniotic fluid volume, and organ formation. Infants exposed *in utero* should be monitored for hyperkalemia, hypotension, and oliguria.

Untreated chronic maternal hypertension is also associated with adverse events in the fetus, infant, and mother. If treatment for hypertension during pregnancy is needed, other agents are preferred (ACOG, 2012; Chobanian, 2003). In women of reproductive potential, angiotensin II receptor blockers should be discontinued prior to conception or as soon as pregnancy is confirmed (Chobanian, 2003).

Breast-Feeding Considerations It is not known if eprosartan is excreted into breast milk. Due to the potential for serious adverse reactions in the nursing infant, the manufacturer recommends a decision be made whether to discontinue nursing or to discontinue the drug, taking into account the importance of treatment to the mother. Breast-fed infants of mothers taking medications for hypertension should be monitored for adverse effects (Chobanian, 2003).

Contraindications Hypersensitivity to eprosartan or any component of the formulation; concomitant use with aliskiren in patients with diabetes mellitus

Warnings/Precautions [U.S. Boxed Warning]: Drugs that act on the renin-angiotensin system can cause injury and death to the developing fetus. Discontinue as soon as possible once pregnancy is detected. May cause hyperkalemia; avoid potassium supplementation unless specifically required by healthcare provider. Avoid use or use a smaller dose in patients who are volume depleted; correct depletion first. May be associated with deterioration of renal function and/or increases in serum creatinine, particularly in patients with low renal blood flow (eg, renal artery stenosis, heart failure) whose glomerular filtration rate (GFR) is dependent on efferent arteriolar vasoconstriction by angiotensin II. Use with caution in unstented unilateral/bilateral renal artery stenosis. When unstented bilateral renal artery stenosis is present, use is generally avoided due to the elevated risk of deterioration in renal function unless possible benefits outweigh risks. Use with caution in pre-existing renal insufficiency; significant aortic/mitral stenosis. Concomitant use of an angiotensin-converting enzyme (ACE) inhibitor or renin inhibitor (eg, aliskiren) is associated with an increased risk of hypotension, hyperkalemia, and renal dysfunction; concomitant use with aliskiren should be avoided in patients with GFR <60 mL/minute and is contraindicated in patients with diabetes mellitus (regardless of GFR).

Angioedema has been reported rarely with some angiotensin II receptor antagonists (ARBs) and may occur at any time during treatment (especially following first dose). It may involve the head and neck (potentially compromising airway) or the intestine (presenting with abdominal pain). Patients with idiopathic or hereditary angioedema or previous angioedema associated with ACE-inhibitor therapy may be at an increased risk. Prolonged frequent monitoring may be required, especially if tongue, glottis, or larynx are involved, as they are associated with airway obstruction. Patients with a history of airway surgery may have a higher risk of airway obstruction. Discontinue therapy immediately if angioedema occurs. Aggressive early management is critical. Intramuscular (I.M.) administration of epinephrine may be necessary. Do not readminister to patients who have had angioedema with ARBs.

Adverse Reactions

1% to 10%:

Central nervous system: Fatigue (2%), depression (1%)
Endocrine & metabolic: Hypertriglyceridemia (1%)
Gastrointestinal: Abdominal pain (2%)
Genitourinary: Urinary tract infection (1%)
Respiratory: Upper respiratory tract infection (8%), rhinitis (4%), pharyngitis (4%), cough (4%)
Miscellaneous: Viral infection (2%), injury (2%)

<1% (Limited to important or life-threatening): Abnormal ECG, angina, arthritis, asthma, ataxia, bradycardia, BUN increased, creatinine increased, eczema, edema, esophagitis, ethanol intolerance, gingivitis, gout, hypotension, influenza-like symptoms, leg cramps, leukopenia, maculopapular rash, migraine, neuritis, neutropenia, orthostasis, palpitation, paresthesia, peripheral ischemia, purpura, renal calculus, somnolence, tachycardia, tendonitis, thrombocytopenia, tinnitus, tremor, urinary incontinence, vertigo; rhabdomyolysis has been reported (rarely) with angiotensin-receptor antagonists.

Drug Interactions

Metabolism/Transport Effects Inhibits CYP2C9 (weak)

Avoid Concomitant Use There are no known interactions where it is recommended to avoid concomitant use.

Increased Effect/Toxicity

Eprosartan may increase the levels/effects of: ACE Inhibitors; Amifostine; Antihypertensives; CycloSPORINE (Systemic); Hypotensive Agents; Lithium; Nonsteroidal Anti-Inflammatory Agents; Obinutuzumab; Potassium-Sparing Diuretics; RiTUXimab; Sodium Phosphates

The levels/effects of Eprosartan may be increased by: Alfuzosin; Aliskiren; Brimonidine (Topical); Canagliflozin; Diazoxide; Eplerenone; Heparin; Heparin (Low Molecular Weight); Herbs (Hypotensive Properties); MAO Inhibitors; Pentoxifylline; Phosphodiesterase 5 Inhibitors; Potassium Salts; Prostacyclin Analogues; Tolvaptan; Trimethoprim

Decreased Effect

The levels/effects of Eprosartan may be decreased by: Herbs (Hypertensive Properties); Methylphenidate; Nonsteroidal Anti-Inflammatory Agents; Yohimbine

Ethanol/Nutrition/Herb Interactions Herb/Nutraceutical: Dong quai has estrogenic activity. Some herbal medications may worsen hypertension (eg, ephedra); garlic may have additional antihypertensive effects. Management: Avoid dong quai if using for hypertension. Avoid ephedra, yohimbe, ginseng, and garlic.

Mechanism of Action Angiotensin II is formed from angiotensin I in a reaction catalyzed by angiotensin-converting enzyme (ACE, kininase II). Angiotensin II is the principal pressor agent of the renin-angiotensin system, with effects that include vasoconstriction, stimulation of synthesis and release of aldosterone, cardiac stimulation, and renal reabsorption of sodium. Eprosartan blocks the vasoconstrictor and aldosterone-secreting effects of angiotensin II by selectively blocking the binding of angiotensin II to the AT1 receptor in many tissues, such as vascular smooth muscle and the adrenal gland. Its action is therefore independent of the pathways for angiotensin II synthesis. Blockade of the renin-angiotensin system with ACE inhibitors, which inhibit the biosynthesis of angiotensin II from angiotensin I, is widely used in the treatment of hypertension. ACE inhibitors also inhibit the degradation of bradykinin, a reaction also catalyzed by ACE. Because eprosartan does not inhibit ACE (kininase II), it does not affect the response to bradykinin. Whether this difference has clinical relevance is not yet known. Eprosartan does not bind to or block other hormone receptors or ion channels known to be important in cardiovascular regulation.

Pharmacodynamics/Kinetics

Protein binding: 98%
Metabolism: Minimally hepatic
Bioavailability: 300 mg dose: 13%
Half-life elimination: Terminal: 5-9 hours

Time to peak, serum: Fasting: 1-2 hours
Excretion: Feces (90%); urine (7%, mostly as unchanged drug)
Clearance: 7.9 L/hour

Dosage Adults: Oral: Dosage must be individualized; can administer once or twice daily with total daily doses of 400-800 mg. Usual starting dose is 600 mg once daily as monotherapy in patients who are euvolemic. Limited clinical experience with doses >800 mg.

Dosage adjustment in renal impairment: Moderate-to-severe impairment: No initial starting dosage adjustment is necessary; however, carefully monitor the patient. Maximum dose: 600 mg daily.

Hemodialysis: Poorly removed (Cl_{HD} <1 L/hour)

Dosage adjustment in hepatic impairment: No starting dosage adjustment is necessary; however, carefully monitor the patient

Elderly: No starting dosage adjustment is necessary; however, carefully monitor the patient

Monitoring Parameters Electrolytes, serum creatinine, BUN, urinalysis

Dosage Forms Excipient information presented when available (limited, particularly for generics); consult specific product labeling. [DSC] = Discontinued product

Tablet, Oral:
Teveten: 400 mg [DSC], 600 mg [contains polysorbate 80]
Generic: 600 mg

Eprosartan and Hydrochlorothiazide
(ep roe SAR tan & hye droe klor oh THYE a zide)

Brand Names: U.S. Teveten® HCT
Brand Names: Canada Teveten® Plus
Index Terms Eprosartan Mesylate and Hydrochlorothiazide; Hydrochlorothiazide and Eprosartan
Pharmacologic Category Angiotensin II Receptor Blocker; Antihypertensive; Diuretic, Thiazide
Use Treatment of hypertension (not indicated for initial treatment)
Pregnancy Risk Factor D
Dosage Oral: Adults: Dose is individualized (combination substituted for individual components)

Usual recommended dose: Eprosartan 600 mg/hydrochlorothiazide 12.5 mg once daily (maximum dose: Eprosartan 600 mg/hydrochlorothiazide 25 mg once daily)

Dosage adjustment in renal impairment: Moderate-to-severe impairment: Initial dose adjustments are not necessary per manufacturer; however carefully monitor patient. Do not exceed a maximum dose of eprosartan 600 mg daily. Hydrochlorothiazide is ineffective in patients with Cl_{cr} <30 mL/minute.

Dosage adjustment in hepatic impairment: Initial dose adjustments not recommended by manufacturer; carefully monitor patient.

Additional Information Complete prescribing information should be consulted for additional detail.

Dosage Forms Excipient information presented when available (limited, particularly for generics); consult specific product labeling.

Tablet:
600 mg/12.5 mg: Eprosartan 600 mg and hydrochlorothiazide 12.5 mg
600 mg/25 mg: Eprosartan 600 mg and hydrochlorothiazide 25 mg

- **Eprosartan Mesylate and Hydrochlorothiazide** *see* Eprosartan and Hydrochlorothiazide *on page 731*
- **Epsilon Aminocaproic Acid** *see* Aminocaproic Acid *on page 100*
- **Epsom Salt [OTC]** *see* Magnesium Sulfate *on page 1263*
- **Epsom Salts** *see* Magnesium Sulfate *on page 1263*
- **EPT** *see* Teniposide *on page 2012*
- **Eptacog Alfa (Activated)** *see* Factor VIIa (Recombinant) *on page 821*

Eptifibatide (ep TIF i ba tide)

Brand Names: U.S. Integrilin
Brand Names: Canada Integrilin®
Index Terms Intrifiban
Pharmacologic Category Antiplatelet Agent, Glycoprotein IIb/IIIa Inhibitor
Use Treatment of patients with acute coronary syndrome (unstable angina/non-ST-segment elevation myocardial infarction [UA/NSTEMI]), including patients who are to be managed medically and those undergoing percutaneous coronary intervention (PCI including angioplasty, intracoronary stenting)
Unlabeled Use To support PCI during ST-elevation myocardial infarction (administered at the time of primary PCI); elective PCI for stable ischemic heart disease (in combination with unfractionated heparin)
Pregnancy Risk Factor B
Pregnancy Considerations Teratogenic effects were not observed in animal studies.
Breast-Feeding Considerations It is not known if eptifibatide is excreted in breast milk. The manufacturer recommends that caution be exercised when administering eptifibatide to nursing women.
Contraindications Hypersensitivity to eptifibatide or any component of the product; active abnormal bleeding within the previous 30 days or a history of bleeding diathesis; history of stroke within 30 days or a history of hemorrhagic stroke; severe hypertension (systolic blood pressure >200 mm Hg or diastolic blood pressure >110 mm Hg) not adequately controlled on antihypertensive therapy; major surgery within the preceding 6 weeks; current or planned administration of another parenteral GP IIb/IIIa inhibitor; dependency on hemodialysis

Canadian labeling: Additional contraindications (not in U.S. labeling): PT >1.2 times control or INR ≥2.0; known history of intracranial disease (eg, neoplasm, arteriovenous malformation, aneurysm); severe renal impairment (Cl_{cr} <30 mL/minute); thrombocytopenia (<100,000 cells/mm^3); clinically significant liver disease

Warnings/Precautions Bleeding is the most common complication. Most major bleeding occurs at the arterial access site where the cardiac catheterization was done. When bleeding can not be controlled with pressure, discontinue infusion and heparin. Patients <70 kg may be at greater risk for major and minor bleeding. Discontinue ≥2-4 hours prior to coronary artery bypass graft surgery (Hillis, 2011). Use caution in patients with hemorrhagic retinopathy or with other drugs that affect hemostasis. Use with extreme caution in patients with platelet counts <100,000/mm^3 (contraindicated in the Canadian labeling). If platelet count decreases to <100,000/mm^3 during therapy, discontinue eptifibatide and heparin if administered concurrently.

Minimize invasive procedures, including arterial and venous punctures, I.M. injections, and nasogastric tube insertion. Prior to sheath removal, the aPTT or ACT should be checked (do not remove unless aPTT is <45 seconds or the ACT <150 seconds). Use caution in renal dysfunction (estimated Cl_{cr} <50 mL/minute, using Cockcroft-Gault equation); dosage adjustment required. Use is contraindicated in patients dependent upon hemodialysis.

Adverse Reactions Bleeding is the major drug-related adverse effect. Access site is often primary source of bleeding complications. Incidence of bleeding is also related to heparin intensity. Patients weighing <70 kg may have an increased risk of major bleeding.

>10%: Hematologic: Bleeding (major: 1% to 11%; minor: 3% to 14%; transfusion required: 2% to 13%)

1% to 10%:

Cardiovascular: Hypotension (up to 7%)

Hematologic: Thrombocytopenia (1% to 3%)

Local: Injection site reaction

<1% (Limited to important or life-threatening): Acute profound thrombocytopenia (including immune-mediated thrombocytopenia), fatal bleeding events, GI hemorrhage, pulmonary hemorrhage

Drug Interactions

Metabolism/Transport Effects None known.

Avoid Concomitant Use There are no known interactions where it is recommended to avoid concomitant use.

Increased Effect/Toxicity

Eptifibatide may increase the levels/effects of: Agents with Antiplatelet Properties; Anticoagulants; Collagenase (Systemic); Dabigatran Etexilate; Ibritumomab; Rivaroxaban; Salicylates; Thrombolytic Agents; Tositumomab and Iodine I 131 Tositumomab

The levels/effects of Eptifibatide may be increased by: Dasatinib; Glucosamine; Herbs (Anticoagulant/Antiplatelet Properties); Ibrutinib; Multivitamins/Fluoride (with ADE); Multivitamins/Minerals (with ADEK, Folate, Iron); Multivitamins/Minerals (with AE, No Iron); Nonsteroidal Anti-Inflammatory Agents; Omega-3 Fatty Acids; Pentosan Polysulfate Sodium; Pentoxifylline; Prostacyclin Analogues; Tipranavir; Vitamin E

Decreased Effect

The levels/effects of Eptifibatide may be decreased by: Nonsteroidal Anti-Inflammatory Agents

Ethanol/Nutrition/Herb Interactions Herb/Nutraceutical: Avoid alfalfa, anise, bilberry, bladderwrack, bromelain, cat's claw, celery, coleus, cordyceps, dong quai, evening primrose oil, fenugreek, feverfew, garlic, ginger, ginkgo biloba, ginseng (American), ginseng (Panax), ginseng (Siberian), grapeseed, green tea, guggul, horse chestnut seed, horseradish, licorice, prickly ash, red clover, reishi, same (s-adenosylmethionine), sweet clover, turmeric, and white willow (all have additional antiplatelet activity).

Storage/Stability Vials should be stored refrigerated at 2°C to 8°C (36°F to 46°F). Vials can be kept at room temperature for 2 months, after which they must be discarded. Protect from light until administration. Do not use beyond the expiration date. Discard any unused portion left in the vial.

Mechanism of Action Eptifibatide is a cyclic heptapeptide which blocks the platelet glycoprotein IIb/IIIa receptor, the binding site for fibrinogen, von Willebrand factor, and other ligands. Inhibition of binding at this final common receptor reversibly blocks platelet aggregation and prevents thrombosis.

Pharmacodynamics/Kinetics

Onset of action: Within 1 hour

Duration: Platelet function restored ~4 hours following discontinuation

Protein binding: ~25%

Half-life elimination: 2.5 hours

Excretion: Primarily urine (as eptifibatide and metabolites); significant renal impairment may alter disposition of this compound

Clearance: Total body: 55-58 mL/kg/hour; Renal: ~50% of total in healthy subjects

Dosage I.V.: Adults:

Acute coronary syndrome: Bolus of 180 mcg/kg (maximum: 22.6 mg) over 1-2 minutes, begun as soon as possible following diagnosis, followed by a continuous infusion of 2 mcg/kg/minute (maximum: 15 mg/hour) until hospital discharge or initiation of CABG surgery (discontinue ≥2-4 hours before surgery), up to 72 hours (if PCI performed during initial 72 hours, maintain continuous infusion at the time of PCI and continue until hospital discharge or for up to 18-24 hours, whichever comes first [total infusion time ≤96 hours]). Concurrent aspirin and heparin therapy (target aPTT 50-70 seconds) are recommended. **Note:** If UA/NSTEMI, administration ≥12 hours before angiography was shown not to be superior to provisional use at the time of PCI and has a higher incidence of bleeding (Giugliano, 2009).

Percutaneous coronary intervention (PCI) with or without stenting: Bolus of 180 mcg/kg (maximum: 22.6 mg) administered immediately before the initiation of PCI, followed by a continuous infusion of 2 mcg/kg/minute (maximum: 15 mg/hour). A second 180 mcg/kg bolus (maximum: 22.6 mg) should be administered 10 minutes after the first bolus. Infusion should be continued until hospital discharge or for up to 18-24 hours, whichever comes first; shorter infusion durations (ie, <2 hours) may be considered for nonemergent uncomplicated PCI in patients adequately pretreated with clopidogrel (Fung, 2007). Preprocedural aspirin and heparin therapy (ACT 200-250 seconds during PCI) are recommended. Heparin infusion after PCI is discouraged. In patients who undergo CABG surgery, discontinue infusion ≥2-4 hours prior to surgery.

Elderly: No dosing adjustment for the elderly appears to be necessary; adjust carefully to renal function.

Dosage adjustment in renal impairment: Dialysis is a contraindication to use.

Note: The Cockcroft-Gault equation using actual body weight should be used to estimate renal function.

Acute coronary syndrome: Cl_{cr} <50 mL/minute: 180 mcg/kg bolus (maximum: 22.6 mg) and 1 mcg/kg/minute infusion (maximum: 7.5 mg/hour)

Percutaneous coronary intervention (PCI) with or without stenting: Cl_{cr} <50 mL/minute: 180 mcg/kg bolus (maximum: 22.6 mg) administered immediately before the initiation of PCI and followed by a continuous infusion of 1 mcg/kg/minute (maximum: 7.5 mg/hour). Administer a second 180 mcg/kg (maximum: 22.6 mg) bolus 10 minutes after the first bolus.

Dosage adjustment in hepatic impairment: No dosage adjustment provided in manufacturer's labeling (has not been studied).

Administration Do not shake vial. Visually inspect for discoloration or particulate matter prior to administration. The bolus dose should be withdrawn from the 10 mL vial into a syringe and administered by I.V. push over 1-2 minutes. Begin continuous infusion immediately following bolus administration, administered directly from the 100 mL vial. The 100 mL vial should be spiked with a vented infusion set.

Monitoring Parameters Coagulation parameters, signs/symptoms of excessive bleeding. Laboratory tests at baseline and monitoring during therapy: hematocrit and hemoglobin, platelet count, serum creatinine, PT/aPTT (maintain aPTT between 50-70 seconds unless PCI is to be performed), and ACT with PCI (maintain ACT between 200-300 seconds during PCI).

Assess sheath insertion site and distal pulses of affected leg every 15 minutes for the first hour and then every 1 hour for the next 6 hours. Arterial access site care is important to prevent bleeding. Care should be taken when attempting vascular access that only the anterior wall of the femoral artery is punctured, avoiding a Seldinger (through and through) technique for obtaining sheath access. Femoral vein sheath placement should be avoided unless needed. While the vascular sheath is in place, patients should be maintained on complete bedrest with the head of the bed at a 30° angle and the affected limb restrained in a straight position.

Observe patient for mental status changes, hemorrhage, assess nose and mouth mucous membranes, puncture sites for oozing, ecchymosis and hematoma formation, and examine urine, stool and emesis for presence of occult or frank blood; gentle care should be provided when removing dressings.

Dosage Forms Excipient information presented when available (limited, particularly for generics); consult specific product labeling.

Solution, Intravenous:

Integrilin: 0.75 mg/mL (100 mL); 2 mg/mL (10 mL, 100 mL)

◆ **Epzicom®** *see* Abacavir and Lamivudine *on page* 20
◆ **Equanil** *see* Meprobamate *on page* 1300
◆ **Equetro** *see* CarBAMazepine *on page* 336
◆ **ER-086526** *see* Eribulin *on page* 734
◆ **Eraxis** *see* Anidulafungin *on page* 139
◆ **Erbitux** *see* Cetuximab *on page* 398
◆ **Erbitux® (Can)** *see* Cetuximab *on page* 398

Ergocalciferol (er goe kal SIF e role)

Brand Names: U.S. Calcidol [OTC]; Calciferol [OTC]; Drisdol; Drisdol [OTC]

Brand Names: Canada Drisdol®; Ostoforte®

Index Terms Activated Ergosterol; D2; Viosterol; Vitamin D2

Pharmacologic Category Vitamin D Analog

Use Treatment of refractory rickets, hypophosphatemia, hypoparathyroidism; dietary supplement

Unlabeled Use Prevention and treatment of vitamin D deficiency in patients with chronic kidney disease (CKD); osteoporosis prevention

Pregnancy Risk Factor C (manufacturer); A/C (dose exceeding RDA recommendation; per expert analysis)

Dosage Oral: **Note:** 1 mcg = 40 units

Dietary Reference Intake for Vitamin D:

0-12 months: Adequate intake: 400 units/day

1-18 years: RDA: 600 units/day

Adults:

19-70 years: RDA: 600 units/day

Female: Pregnancy/Lactating: RDA: 600 units/day

Elderly >70 years: RDA: 800 units/day

Adequate intake:

Breast-fed (fully or partially) Infants: 10 mcg/day (400 units/day) beginning in the first few days of life; continue supplementation until infant is weaned to ≥1 L/day or 1 quart/day of vitamin D-fortified formula or whole milk (after 12 months of age)

Nonbreast-fed Infants, Older Children ingesting <1000 mL of vitamin D-fortified formula or milk: 10 mcg/day (400 units/day)

Children with increased risk of vitamin D deficiency (chronic fat malabsorption, maintained on chronic antiseizure medications): Higher doses may be required; use laboratory testing (25 [OH]D, PTH, bone mineral status) to evaluate

Osteoporosis prevention (unlabeled use): Adults ≥50 years: 800-1000 units/day (NOF guidelines, 2013)

Vitamin D deficiency treatment (unlabeled dose): Adults: 50,000 units once per week for 8 weeks, followed by 50,000 units every 2-4 weeks thereafter for maintenance of adequate levels (Holick, 2007) **or** 50,000 units twice per week for 5 weeks (Stechschulte, 2009)

Vitamin D deficiency/insufficiency in patients with CKD stages 3-4 (K/DOQI guidelines): **Note:** Dose is based on 25-hydroxyvitamin D serum level (25[OH]D):

Children (treatment duration should be a total of 3 months):

Serum 25(OH)D <5 ng/mL:

8000 units/day for 4 weeks, then 4000 units/day for 2 months **or**

50,000 units/week for 4 weeks, then 50,000 units twice a month for 2 months

Serum 25(OH)D 5-15 ng/mL:

4000 int units/day **or**

50,000 int units every other week

Serum 25(OH)D 16-30 ng/mL:

2000 units/day **or**

50,000 units every 4 weeks

Adults (treatment duration should be a total of 6 months):

Serum 25(OH)D <5 ng/mL:

50,000 units/week for 12 weeks, then 50,000 units/month

Serum 25(OH)D 5-15 ng/mL:

50,000 units/week for 4 weeks, then 50,000 units/month

Serum 25(OH)D 16-30 ng/mL:

50,000 units/month

Hypoparathyroidism:

Children: 1.25-5 mg/day (50,000-200,000 units) and calcium supplements

Adults: 625 mcg to 5 mg/day (25,000-200,000 units) and calcium supplements

Nutritional rickets and osteomalacia:

Children and Adults (with normal absorption): 25-125 mcg/day (1000-5000 units)

Children with malabsorption: 250-625 mcg/day (10,000-25,000 units)

Adults with malabsorption: 250-7500 mcg (10,000-300,000 units)

Vitamin D-*dependent* rickets:

Children: 75-125 mcg/day (3000-5000 units); maximum: 1500 mcg/day

Adults: 250 mcg to 1.5 mg/day (10,000-60,000 units)

Vitamin D-*resistant* rickets: Children and Adults: 12,000-500,000 units/day

Familial hypophosphatemia:

Children: 40,000-80,000 units plus phosphate supplements; dose may be reduced once growth is complete

Adults: 10,000-60,000 units plus phosphate supplements

Dosage adjustment in renal impairment: No dosage adjustment necessary.

Dosage adjustment in hepatic impairment: No dosage adjustment provided in manufacturer's labeling.

Additional Information Complete prescribing information should be consulted for additional detail.

Dosage Forms Excipient information presented when available (limited, particularly for generics); consult specific product labeling.

Capsule, Oral:

Drisdol: 50,000 units [contains brilliant blue fcf (fd&c blue #1), soybean oil, tartrazine (fd&c yellow #5)]

Generic: 50,000 units

Solution, Oral:

Calcidol: 8000 units/mL (60 mL) [contains propylene glycol]

Calciferol: 8000 units/mL (60 mL)

Drisdol: 8000 units/mL (60 mL)

Generic: 8000 units/mL (60 mL)

Tablet, Oral:

Generic: 400 units, 2000 units

◆ **Ergomar** *see* Ergotamine *on page* 734

Ergotamine (er GOT a meen)

Brand Names: U.S. Ergomar

Index Terms Ergotamine Tartrate

Pharmacologic Category Antimigraine Agent; Ergot Derivative

Use Abort or prevent vascular headaches, such as migraine, migraine variants, or so-called "histaminic cephalalgia"

Pregnancy Risk Factor X

Dosage Migraine: Adults: Sublingual: 2 mg (1 tablet) under tongue at first sign of migraine, then 2 mg every 30 minutes if needed; maximum dose: 6 mg per 24 hours, 10 mg per week

Dosage adjustment in renal impairment: Use is contraindicated in patients with impaired renal function.

Dosage adjustment in hepatic impairment: Use is contraindicated in patients with impaired hepatic function.

Additional Information Complete prescribing information should be consulted for additional detail.

Dosage Forms Excipient information presented when available (limited, particularly for generics); consult specific product labeling.

Tablet Sublingual, Sublingual, as tartrate:

Ergomar: 2 mg [contains fd&c blue #1 aluminum lake, fd&c yellow #10 aluminum lake, saccharin sodium]

◆ Ergotamine Tartrate *see* Ergotamine *on page 734*

Eribulin (er i BUE lin)

Brand Names: U.S. Halaven

Brand Names: Canada Halaven™

Index Terms B1939; E7389; ER-086526; Eribulin Mesylate; Halichondrin B Analog

Pharmacologic Category Antineoplastic Agent, Antimicrotubular

Use Treatment of metastatic breast cancer in patients who have received at least 2 prior chemotherapy regimens

Pregnancy Risk Factor D

Pregnancy Considerations Teratogenicity and fetal loss were observed in animal studies. There are no adequate and well-controlled studies in pregnant women. Based on its mechanism of action, eribulin would be expected to cause fetal harm if administered during pregnancy.

Breast-Feeding Considerations Due to the potential for serious adverse reactions in the nursing infant, breast-feeding is not recommended.

Contraindications There are no contraindications listed within the manufacturer's labeling.

Canadian labeling (not in U.S. labeling): Hypersensitivity to eribulin mesylate, halichondrin B, or its chemical derivatives.

Warnings/Precautions Hazardous agent - use appropriate precautions for handling and disposal (meets NIOSH, 2012 criteria). Hematologic toxicity, including severe neutropenia, has occurred; may require treatment delay and dosage reduction. A higher incidence of grade 4 neutropenia and neutropenic fever occurred in patients with ALT or AST >3 x ULN or bilirubin >1.5 x ULN. Monitor complete blood counts prior to each dose; more frequently if severe cytopenias develop.

Peripheral neuropathy is a common toxicity; may be prolonged (>1 year in 5% of patients); may require treatment delay. Monitor for signs of motor or sensory neuropathy. Some patients may have pre-existing neuropathy due to prior chemotherapy; monitor closely for worsening.

QT prolongation was observed on day 8 (in an uncontrolled study); monitor ECG in patients with heart failure, bradyarrhythmia, and with concomitant medication known to prolong the QT interval; correct hypokalemia and hypomagnesemia prior to treatment; monitor electrolytes periodically during treatment. Avoid use in patients with congenital long QT syndrome.

Dosage reduction required in patients with mild-to-moderate (Child-Pugh class A or B) hepatic impairment; use has not been studied in patients with severe hepatic impairment; transaminase or bilirubin elevations are associated with a higher incidence of grade 4 neutropenia and neutropenic fever. Dosage reduction required in patients with renal impairment (Cl_{cr} 30-50 mL/minute); use has not been studied in patients with Cl_{cr} <30 mL/minute.

Adverse Reactions

>10%:

Central nervous system: Fatigue (54%), fever (21%), headache (19%)

Dermatologic: Alopecia (45%)

Gastrointestinal: Nausea (35%), stomatitis (5% to 18%), constipation (25%), weight loss (21%), anorexia (20%), diarrhea (18%), vomiting (18%)

Hematologic: Neutropenia (82%; grades 3: 28%; grade 4: 29%; nadir: 13 days; recovery: 8 days), anemia (58%; grades 3/4: 2%)

Hepatic: ALT increased (18%)

Neuromuscular & skeletal: Weakness (54%), peripheral neuropathy (35%; grades 3/4: ≤8%), arthralgia/myalgia (22%), back pain (16%), bone pain (12%), limb pain (11%)

Respiratory: Dyspnea (16%), cough (14%)

1% to 10%:

Cardiovascular: Peripheral edema

Central nervous system: Depression, dizziness, insomnia

Dermatologic: Rash

Endocrine & metabolic: Hypokalemia

Gastrointestinal: Mucosal inflammation (9%), abdominal pain, dyspepsia, taste alteration, xerostomia

Genitourinary: Urinary tract infection (10%)

Hematologic: Neutropenic fever (5%), thrombocytopenia (grades 3/4: 1%)

Neuromuscular & skeletal: Muscle spasm

Ocular: Lacrimation increased

Respiratory: Upper respiratory infection

<1% (Limited to important or life-threatening): Pharyngolaryngeal pain, sepsis

Drug Interactions

Metabolism/Transport Effects Substrate of CYP3A4 (minor); **Note:** Assignment of Major/Minor substrate status based on clinically relevant drug interaction potential; **Inhibits** CYP3A4 (weak)

Avoid Concomitant Use

Avoid concomitant use of EriBULin with any of the following: CloZAPine; Highest Risk QTc-Prolonging Agents; Ivabradine; Mifepristone

Increased Effect/Toxicity

EriBULin may increase the levels/effects of: ARIPiprazole; CloZAPine; Highest Risk QTc-Prolonging Agents; Lomitapide; Moderate Risk QTc-Prolonging Agents; Vitamin K Antagonists

The levels/effects of EriBULin may be increased by: Ivabradine; Mifepristone; QTc-Prolonging Agents (Indeterminate Risk and Risk Modifying)

Decreased Effect

EriBULin may decrease the levels/effects of: Cardiac Glycosides; Vitamin K Antagonists

Preparation for Administration Hazardous agent; use appropriate precautions for handling and disposal (meets NIOSH, 2012 criteria). No dilution required. May dilute in 100 mL normal saline.

Storage/Stability Store intact vials at 25°C (77°F); excursions permitted between 15°C and 30°C (59°F and 86°F); do not freeze. Store in original carton. Undiluted solutions in a syringe and solutions diluted in normal saline for infusion are stable for up to 4 hours at room temperature or up to 24 hours refrigerated.

Mechanism of Action Eribulin is a non-taxane microtubule inhibitor which is a halichondrin B analog. It inhibits the growth phase of the microtubule by inhibiting formation of mitotic spindles causing mitotic blockage and arresting the cell cycle at the G_2/M phase; suppresses microtubule polymerization yet does not affect depolymerization.

Pharmacodynamics/Kinetics

Distribution: V_d: 43-114 L/m²

Protein binding: 49% to 65%

Metabolism: Negligible

Half-life, elimination: ~40 hours

Excretion: Feces (82%; predominantly as unchanged drug); urine (9%, primarily as unchanged drug)

Dosage I.V.: Adults: Breast cancer, metastatic: 1.4 mg/m²/dose on days 1 and 8 of a 21-day treatment cycle

Dosing adjustment in toxicity:

ANC <1000/mm³ or platelets <75,000/mm³ or grade 3 or 4 nonhematologic toxicity on day 1 or 8: Withhold dose; may delay day 8 dose up to 1 week. If toxicity resolves to ≤grade 2 by day 15 administer a reduced dose and wait at least 2 weeks before beginning the next cycle. Omit dose if not resolved to ≤grade 2 by day 15. Do not re-escalate dose after reduction.

Permanently reduce dose from 1.4 mg/m² to 1.1 mg/m² for the following:

- ANC <500/mm³ for >7 days
- ANC <1000/mm³ with fever or infection
- Platelets <25,000/mm³
- Platelets <50,000/mm³ requiring transfusion
- Nonhematologic toxicity of grade 3 or 4
- Dose omission or delay due to toxicity on day 8 of prior cycle

Permanently reduce dose from 1.1 mg/m² to 0.7 mg/m² for occurrence of any of the above events; discontinue treatment if the above toxicities occur at the 0.7 mg/m² dose level.

Dosage adjustment in renal impairment:

Cl_{cr} >50 mL/minute: No adjustment required

Cl_{cr} 30-50 mL/minute: Reduce to 1.1 mg/m²/dose

Cl_{cr} <30 mL/minute: Use has not been studied

Dosage adjustment in hepatic impairment:

Mild hepatic impairment (Child-Pugh class A): Reduce to 1.1 mg/m²/dose

Moderate hepatic impairment (Child-Pugh class B): Reduce to 0.7 mg/m²/dose

Severe hepatic impairment (Child-Pugh class C): Use has not been studied

Dosing in obesity: *ASCO Guidelines for appropriate chemotherapy dosing in obese adults with cancer:* Utilize patient's actual body weight (full weight) for calculation of body surface area- or weight-based dosing, particularly when the intent of therapy is curative; manage regimen-related toxicities in the same manner as for nonobese patients; if a dose reduction is utilized due to toxicity, consider resumption of full weight-based dosing with subsequent cycles, especially if cause of toxicity (eg, hepatic or renal impairment) is resolved (Griggs, 2012).

Administration I.V.: Infuse over 2-5 minutes. May be administered undiluted or diluted.

Hazardous agent; use appropriate precautions for handling and disposal (meets NIOSH, 2012 criteria).

Monitoring Parameters CBC with differential prior to each dose; renal and liver function tests; serum electrolytes, including potassium and magnesium. Assess for peripheral neuropathy prior to each dose. Monitor ECG in patients with heart failure, bradyarrhythmia, and with concomitant medication known to prolong the QT interval, and electrolyte abnormalities (eg, hypokalemia, hypomagnesemia).

Dosage Forms Excipient information presented when available (limited, particularly for generics); consult specific product labeling.

Solution, Intravenous, as mesylate:

Halaven: 1 mg/2 mL (2 mL) [contains alcohol, usp]

◆ **Eribulin Mesylate** *see* Eribulin *on page 734*

◆ **Erivedge** *see* Vismodegib *on page 2199*

Erlotinib (er LOE tye nib)

Brand Names: U.S. Tarceva

Brand Names: Canada Tarceva®

Index Terms CP358774; Erlotinib Hydrochloride; OSI-774

Pharmacologic Category Antineoplastic Agent, Tyrosine Kinase Inhibitor; Epidermal Growth Factor Receptor (EGFR) Inhibitor

Use

Nonsmall cell lung cancer (NSCLC): First-line treatment of metastatic NSCLC in patients with known EGFR exon 19 deletions or exon 21 (L858R) substitution mutations; treatment (as monotherapy) of locally-advanced or metastatic NSCLC refractory to at least 1 prior chemotherapy regimen; maintenance treatment of locally-advanced or metastatic NCSLC which has not progressed after 4 cycles of first-line platinum-based chemotherapy

Note: Use in combination with platinum-based chemotherapy is not recommended. First-line treatment in patients with metastatic NSCLC with EGFR mutations other than exon 19 deletion or exon 21 (L858R) substitution has not been evaluated.

Pancreatic cancer (not an approved use in Canada): First-line treatment of locally-advanced, unresectable or metastatic pancreatic cancer (combination with gemcitabine)

Pregnancy Risk Factor D

Pregnancy Considerations Adverse events were observed in animal reproduction studies. Based on the mechanism of action, may cause fetal harm if administered in pregnancy. Females of reproductive potential should be advised to avoid pregnancy; adequate contraception is recommended during treatment and for at least 2 weeks after treatment has been completed.

Breast-Feeding Considerations It is not known if erlotinib is excreted in breast milk. Due to the potential for serious adverse reactions in the nursing infant, the decision to discontinue breast-feeding or discontinue erlotinib should take into account the benefits of treatment to the mother.

Contraindications There are no contraindications listed within the manufacturer's U.S. labeling.

Canadian labeling: Hypersensitivity to erlotinib or any component of the formulation

Warnings/Precautions Hazardous agent - use appropriate precautions for handling and disposal (meets NIOSH, 2012 criteria). Rare, sometimes fatal, interstitial lung disease (ILD) has occurred; symptoms include acute respiratory distress syndrome, interstitial pneumonia, obliterative bronchiolitis, pneumonitis (including radiation and hypersensitivity), pulmonary fibrosis, and pulmonary infiltrates. The onset of symptoms has been within 5 days to more than 9 months after treatment initiation (median: 39 days). Interrupt treatment for unexplained new or worsening pulmonary symptoms (dyspnea, cough, and fever); discontinue for confirmed ILD.

Liver enzyme elevations have been reported. Hepatic failure and hepatorenal syndrome have also been reported, particularly in patients with baseline hepatic impairment. Monitor liver function; patients with any hepatic impairment (total bilirubin >ULN; Child-Pugh class A, B, or C) should be closely monitored, including those with hepatic disease due to tumor burden; use with extreme caution in patients with total bilirubin >3 times ULN. Increased monitoring of liver function is required in patients with pre-existing hepatic impairment or biliary obstruction. Dosage reduction, interruption or discontinuation may be recommended for changes in hepatic function. Acute renal failure, renal insufficiency, and hepatorenal syndrome have been reported, either secondary to hepatic impairment at baseline or due to severe dehydration; use with caution in patients with or at risk for renal impairment. Monitor closely for dehydration; monitor renal function and electrolytes in patients at risk for dehydration. Gastrointestinal perforation has been reported with use; risk for perforation is increased with concurrent anti-angiogenic agents, corticosteroids, NSAIDs, and/or taxane based-therapy, and patients with history of peptic ulcers or diverticular disease; permanently discontinue in patients who develop perforation.

Bullous, blistering, or exfoliating skin conditions, some suggestive of Stevens-Johnson or toxic epidermal necrolysis (TEN) have been reported. An acne-like rash commonly appears on the face, back, and upper chest. Generalized or severe acneiform, erythematous or maculopapular rash may occur. Skin rash may correlate with treatment response and prolonged survival (Saif, 2008); management of skin rashes that are not serious should include alcohol-free lotions, topical antibiotics, or topical corticosteroids, or if necessary, oral antibiotics and systemic corticosteroids; avoid sunlight. Reduce dose or temporarily interrupt treatment for severe skin reactions; discontinue treatment for bullous, blistering or exfoliative skin toxicity. Corneal perforation and ulceration have been reported with use; abnormal eyelash growth, keratoconjunctivitis sicca, or keratitis have also been reported and are known risk factors for corneal ulceration/perforation. Interrupt or discontinue treatment in patients presenting with eye pain or other acute or worsening ocular symptoms.

MI, CVA, and microangiopathic hemolytic anemia with thrombocytopenia have been reported. Elevated INR and bleeding events (including fatal hemorrhage) have been reported; monitor for INR changes. Erlotinib levels may be lower in patients who smoke; advise patients to stop smoking. Smokers treated with 300 mg/day exhibited steady-state erlotinib levels comparable to former- and never-smokers receiving 150 mg/day (Hughes, 2009). Potentially significant drug-drug interactions may exist, requiring dose or frequency adjustment, additional monitoring, and/or selection of alternative therapy. Avoid concomitant use with proton pump inhibitors. If taken with an H_2-receptor antagonist (eg, ranitidine), administer erlotinib 10 hours after the H_2-receptor antagonist dose and at least 2 hours prior to the next H_2-receptor dose. If an antacid is necessary, separate dosing by several hours. In patients with NSCLC, EGFR mutations, specifically exon 19 deletions and exon 21 mutation (L858R), are associated with better response to erlotinib (Riely, 2006); erlotinib treatment is not recommended in patients with *K-ras* mutations; they are not likely to benefit from erlotinib treatment (Eberhard, 2005; Miller, 2008). Concurrent erlotinib plus platinum-based chemotherapy is not recommended for first line treatment of locally advanced or metastatic NSCLC due to a lack of clinical benefit. The cobas® EGFR mutation test has been approved to detect EGFR mutation for first-line NSCLC treatment. Product may contain lactose; avoid use in patients with Lapp lactase deficiency, glucose-galactose malabsorption, or glucose intolerance.

Adverse Reactions

Adverse reactions reported with monotherapy:

>10%:

- Cardiovascular: Chest pain (≤18%)
- Central nervous system: Fatigue (9% to 52%)
- Dermatologic: Skin rash (49% to 85%; grade 3: 5% to 13%; grade 4: <1%; median onset: 8 days), xeroderma (4% to 21%), paronychia (4% to 16%), alopecia (14% to 15%), pruritus (7% to 16%), acne vulgaris (6% to 12%)
- Gastrointestinal: Diarrhea (20% to 62%; grade 3: 2% to 6%; grade 4: <1%; median onset: 12 days), anorexia (9% to 52%), nausea (23% to 33%), decreased appetite (≤28%), vomiting (13% to 23%), stomatitis (11% to 17%), mucositis (≤18%), abdominal pain (3% to 11%), constipation (≤8%)
- Genitourinary: Urinary tract infection (≤4%)
- Hematologic & oncologic: Anemia (≤11%; grade 4: 1%)
- Infection: Increased susceptibility to infection (4% to 24%)
- Neuromuscular & skeletal: Weakness (≤53%), back pain (19%), arthralgia (≤13%), musculoskeletal pain (11%)
- Ophthalmic: Conjunctivitis (12% to 18%), keratoconjunctivitis sicca (12%)
- Respiratory: Cough (33% to 48%), dyspnea (41% to 45%; grades 3/4: 8% to 28%)
- Miscellaneous: Fever (≤11%)

1% to 10%:

- Cardiovascular: Peripheral edema (≤5%)
- Central nervous system: Pain (≤9%), headache (≤7%), anxiety (≤5%), dizziness (≤4%), insomnia (≤4%), neurotoxicity (≤4%), voice disorder (≤4%)
- Dermatologic: Folliculitis (≤8%), nail disease (≤7%), exfoliative dermatitis (5%), hypertrichosis (5%), skin fissure (5%), acneiform eruption (4% to 5%), erythema (≤5%), dermatitis (4%), erythematous rash (≤4%), palmar-plantar erythrodysesthesia (≤4%), bullous dermatitis
- Endocrine & metabolic: Weight loss (4% to 5%)
- Gastrointestinal: Dyspepsia (≤5%), xerostomia (≤3%), taste disorder (≤1%)
- Hematologic & oncologic: Lymphocytopenia (≤4%; grade 3: 1%), leukopenia (≤3%), thrombocytopenia (≤1%)
- Hepatic: Hyperbilirubinemia (7%; grade 3: ≤1%), increased serum ALT (grade 2: 2% to 4%; grade 3: 1% to 3%), increased gamma-glutamyl transferase (≤4%), hepatic failure (≤1%)
- Neuromuscular & skeletal: Ostealgia (≤4%), muscle spasm (≤4%), musculoskeletal chest pain (≤4%), paresthesia (≤4%)
- Otic: Tinnitus (≤1%)
- Renal: Renal failure (≤1%), increased serum creatinine (≤1%)
- Respiratory: Nasopharyngitis (≤7%), epistaxis (≤4%), pulmonary embolism (≤4%), respiratory tract infection (≤4%), pneumonitis (3%), pulmonary fibrosis (3%)

<1%: Interstitial pulmonary disease

Adverse reactions reported with combination (erlotinib plus gemcitabine) therapy:

>10%:

- Cardiovascular: Edema (37%), thrombosis (grades 3/4: 11%)
- Central nervous system: Fatigue (73% to 79%), depression (19%), dizziness (15%), headache (15%), anxiety (13%)
- Dermatologic: Skin rash (70%), alopecia (14%)
- Gastrointestinal: Nausea (60%), anorexia (52%), diarrhea (48%), abdominal pain (46%), vomiting (42%), weight loss (39%), stomatitis (22%), dyspepsia (17%), flatulence (13%)

Hepatic: Increased serum ALT (grade 2: 31%, grade 3: 13%, grade 4: <1%), increased serum AST (grade 2: 24%, grade 3: 10%, grade 4 <1%), hyperbilirubinemia (grade 2: 17%, grade 3: 10%, grade 4: <1%)
Infection: Increased susceptibility to infection (39%)
Neuromuscular & skeletal: Ostealgia (25%), myalgia (21%), neuropathy (13%), rigors (12%)
Respiratory: Dyspnea (24%), cough (16%)
Miscellaneous: Fever (36%)

1% to 10%:
Cardiovascular: Cardiac arrhythmia (<5%), syncope (<5%), deep vein thrombosis (4%), cerebrovascular accident (2%; including cerebral hemorrhage), myocardial infarction (2%)
Gastrointestinal: Intestinal obstruction (<5%), pancreatitis (<5%)
Hematologic: Hemolytic anemia (<5%; microangiopathic with thrombocytopenia: 1%)
Renal: Renal insufficiency (<5%), renal failure (1%)
Respiratory: Interstitial pulmonary disease (<3%)

<1%: Bullous dermatitis, exfoliative dermatitis, hepatic failure

Mono- or combination therapy: <1% (Limited to important or life-threatening): Acute peptic ulcer with hemorrhage, bronchiolitis, corneal perforation, corneal ulcer, episcleritis, gastritis, gastrointestinal hemorrhage, gastrointestinal perforation, hearing loss, hematemesis, hematochezia, hepatorenal syndrome, hepatotoxicity, hirsutism, hyperpigmentation, hypokalemia, increased eyelash thickness, increased growth in number of eyelashes, keratitis, melena, misdirected growth of eyelashes, myopathy (in combination with statin therapy), peptic ulcer, rhabdomyolysis (in combination with statin therapy), skin photosensitivity, skin rash (acneiform; sparing prior radiation field), Stevens-Johnson syndrome, toxic epidermal necrolysis, tympanic membrane perforation

Drug Interactions

Metabolism/Transport Effects **Substrate** of CYP1A2 (minor), CYP3A4 (major); **Note:** Assignment of Major/Minor substrate status based on clinically relevant drug interaction potential

Avoid Concomitant Use

Avoid concomitant use of Erlotinib with any of the following: Conivaptan; Fusidic Acid (Systemic); Proton Pump Inhibitors

Increased Effect/Toxicity

Erlotinib may increase the levels/effects of: Vitamin K Antagonists

The levels/effects of Erlotinib may be increased by: Ciprofloxacin (Systemic); Conivaptan; CYP3A4 Inhibitors (Moderate); CYP3A4 Inhibitors (Strong); Dasatinib; FluvoxaMINE; Fusidic Acid (Systemic); Ivacaftor; Luliconazole; Mifepristone; Simeprevir

Decreased Effect

Erlotinib may decrease the levels/effects of: Cardiac Glycosides; Vitamin K Antagonists

The levels/effects of Erlotinib may be decreased by: Antacids; Bosentan; CYP3A4 Inducers (Strong); Dabrafenib; Deferasirox; H2-Antagonists; Herbs (CYP3A4 Inducers); Mitotane; Proton Pump Inhibitors; Rifampin; Tocilizumab

Ethanol/Nutrition/Herb Interactions

Food: Erlotinib bioavailability is increased with food. Grapefruit or grapefruit juice may decrease metabolism and increase erlotinib plasma concentrations. Management: Take on an empty stomach at least 1 hour before or 2 hours after the ingestion of food. Avoid grapefruit and grapefruit juice. Maintain adequate nutrition and hydration, unless instructed to restrict fluid intake.

Herb/Nutraceutical: St John's wort may increase metabolism and decrease erlotinib concentrations. Management: Avoid St John's wort.

Storage/Stability Store at room temperature of 25°C (77°F); excursions permitted to 15°C and 30°C (59°F and 86°F).

Mechanism of Action Reversibly inhibits overall epidermal growth factor receptor (HER1/EGFR) - tyrosine kinase activity. Intracellular phosphorylation is inhibited which prevents further downstream signaling, resulting in cell death. Erlotinib has higher binding affinity for EGFR exon 19 deletion or exon 21 L858R mutations than for the wild type receptor.

Pharmacodynamics/Kinetics

Absorption: Oral: 60% on an empty stomach; almost 100% on a full stomach
Distribution: 94-232 L
Protein binding: 92% to 95% to albumin and α_1-acid glycoprotein
Metabolism: Hepatic, via CYP3A4 (major), CYP1A1 (minor), CYP1A2 (minor), and CYP1C (minor)
Bioavailability: Almost 100% when given with food; 60% without food
Half-life elimination: 24-36 hours
Time to peak, plasma: 1-7 hours
Excretion: Primarily as metabolites: Feces (83%; 1% as unchanged drug); urine (8%)

Dosage

Nonsmall cell lung cancer (NSCLC), metastatic, first-line therapy in patients with EGFR exon 19 deletions or exon 21 (L858R) substitution mutations: Adults: Oral: 150 mg once daily until disease progression or unacceptable toxicity (Rosell, 2012; Zhou, 2011).

NSCLC, refractory: Adults: Oral: 150 mg once daily until disease progression or unacceptable toxicity (Shepherd, 2005)

NSCLC, maintenance therapy: Adults: Oral: 150 mg once daily until disease progression or unacceptable toxicity (Capuzzo, 2010)

Pancreatic cancer: Adults: Oral: 100 mg once daily until disease progression or unacceptable toxicity (in combination with gemcitabine) (Moore, 2007)

Dosage adjustment for concomitant CYP3A4 inhibitors/inducers:

CYP3A4 inhibitors: Avoid concurrent use if possible; consider dose reductions for severe adverse reactions if erlotinib is administered concomitantly with strong CYP3A4 inhibitors (eg, azole antifungals, clarithromycin, erythromycin, nefazodone, protease inhibitors, telithromycin). Dose reduction (if required) should be done in decrements of 50 mg (after toxicity has resolved to baseline or ≤ grade 1).

Concomitant CYP3A4 and CYP1A2 inhibitor (eg, ciprofloxacin): Avoid concurrent use if possible; consider dose reductions in decrements of 50 mg if severe adverse reactions occur (after toxicity has resolved to baseline or ≤ grade 1).

CYP3A4 inducers: Alternatives to the enzyme-inducing agent should be utilized first. Concomitant administration with CYP3A4 inducers (eg, carbamazepine, phenobarbital, phenytoin, rifamycins, and St John's wort) may require increased erlotinib doses (increase as tolerated at 2-week intervals in 50 mg increments to a maximum of 450 mg); doses >150 mg daily should be considered with rifampin (the maximum erlotinib dose studied in combination with rifampin was 450 mg). Immediately reduce erlotinib dose to recommended starting dose when CYP3A4 inducer is discontinued.

Dosage adjustment for concomitant smoking: Increase dose at 2-week intervals in 50 mg increments to a maximum dose of 300 mg (with careful monitoring) in patients who continue to smoke; immediately reduce erlotinib dose to recommended starting dose upon smoking cessation.

Dosage adjustment for toxicity:

Dermatologic toxicity:

Bullous, blistering or exfoliative skin toxicity (severe): Discontinue treatment.

Severe rash (unresponsive to medical management): Withhold treatment; may reinitiate with a 50 mg dose reduction after toxicity has resolved to baseline or ≤ grade 1.

Gastrointestinal toxicity:

Diarrhea: Manage with loperamide; in severe diarrhea (unresponsive to loperamide) or dehydration due to diarrhea, withhold treatment; may reinitiate with a 50 mg dose reduction after toxicity has resolved to baseline or ≤ grade 1.

Gastrointestinal perforation: Discontinue treatment.

Ocular toxicities:

Acute or worsening ocular toxicities (eg, eye pain): Interrupt and consider discontinuing treatment. If therapy is resumed, reinitiate with a 50 mg dose reduction after toxicity has resolved to baseline or ≤ grade 1.

Corneal perforation or severe ulceration: Discontinue treatment.

Keratitis (grade 3 or 4 or grade 2 persisting >2 weeks): Withhold treatment; may reinitiate with a 50 mg dose reduction after toxicity has resolved to baseline or ≤ grade 1.

Pulmonary symptoms: Acute onset (or worsening) of pulmonary symptoms (eg, dyspnea, cough, fever): Interrupt treatment and evaluate for drug-induced interstitial lung disease; discontinue permanently with development of interstitial lung disease

Dosage adjustment in renal impairment:

Renal impairment at treatment initiation: No dosage adjustment provided in the manufacturer's labeling (has not been studied), although <9% of a single dose is excreted in the urine.

Renal toxicity during treatment: Withhold treatment for grades 3/4 renal toxicity (consider discontinuing) and for risk of renal failure due to dehydration; may resume after euvolemia re-established (at previous dose). If treatment withheld due to toxicity and therapy is resumed, reinitiate with a 50 mg dose reduction after toxicity has resolved to baseline or ≤ grade 1.

Dosage adjustment in hepatic impairment:

Hepatic impairment at treatment initiation:

U.S. labeling:

Total bilirubin > ULN or Child-Pugh classes A, B, and C: No dosage adjustment provided in manufacturer's labeling; use with caution and monitor closely during treatment.

Total bilirubin >3 times ULN: Use extreme caution.

Canadian labeling:

Moderate impairment: No dosage adjustment provided in manufacturer's labeling; however, a reduced dose should be considered.

Severe impairment (including total bilirubin >3 times ULN and/or transaminases >5 times ULN): Use is not recommended.

The following adjustments have also been studied: A reduced starting dose (75 mg once daily) has been recommended in patients with hepatic dysfunction (AST ≥3 times ULN or direct bilirubin 1-7 mg/dL), with individualized dosage escalation if tolerated (Miller, 2007); another study determined that pharmacokinetic and safety profiles were similar between patients with normal hepatic function and moderate hepatic impairment (O'Bryant, 2012).

Hepatotoxicity during treatment: U.S. labeling:

Patients with normal hepatic function at baseline: If total bilirubin >3 times ULN and/or transaminases >5 times ULN during use: Interrupt therapy (consider discontinuing); if treatment is resumed, reinitiate with a 50 mg dose reduction after bilirubin and transaminases return to baseline; discontinue treatment if there is no significant improvement or resolution within 3 weeks.

Patients with baseline hepatic impairment or biliary obstruction: If bilirubin doubles or transaminases triple over baseline during use: Interrupt therapy (consider discontinuing); if treatment is resumed, reinitiate with a 50 mg dose reduction after bilirubin and transaminases return to baseline; discontinue treatment if there is no significant improvement or resolution of hepatotoxicity within 3 weeks.

Dietary Considerations Take this medicine an empty stomach, 1 hour before or 2 hours after a meal. Avoid grapefruit juice.

Administration The manufacturer recommends administration on an empty stomach (at least 1 hour before or 2 hours after the ingestion of food). Avoid concomitant use with proton pump inhibitors. If taken with an H2-receptor antagonist (eg, ranitidine), administer erlotinib 10 hours after the H_2-receptor antagonist dose and at least 2 hours prior to the next H_2-receptor dose. If an antacid is necessary, separate dosing by several hours.

For patients unable to swallow whole, tablets may be dissolved in 100 mL water and administered orally or via feeding tube (silicone-based); to ensure full dose is received, rinse container with 40 mL water, administer residue and repeat rinse (data on file, Genentech; Siu, 2007; Soulieres, 2004).

Hazardous agent; use appropriate precautions for handling and disposal (meets NIOSH, 2012 criteria).

Monitoring Parameters Periodic liver function tests (transaminases, bilirubin, and alkaline phosphatase); monitor more frequently with worsening liver function; periodic renal function tests and serum electrolytes (in patients at risk for dehydration); hydration status; EGFR mutation status in patients with NSCLC adenocarcinoma (Keedy, 2011); the cobas® EGFR mutation test has been approved to detect EGFR mutation for first-line NSCLC treatment

Additional Information In patients with NSCLC, some factors which correlate positively with response to EGFR-tyrosine kinase inhibitor (TKI) therapy include patients who have never smoked, EGFR mutation, and patients of Asian origin. EGFR mutations, specifically exon 19 deletions and exon 21 mutation (L858R) correlate with response to tyrosine kinase inhibitors (Riely, 2006). *K-ras* mutations correlated with poorer outcome with EGFR-TKI therapy in patients with NSCLC (Cooley, 2008; Jackman, 2008; Masarelli, 2007; Shepherd, 2005).

Dosage Forms Excipient information presented when available (limited, particularly for generics); consult specific product labeling.

Tablet, Oral:

Tarceva: 25 mg [contains fd&c yellow #6 (sunset yellow)]

Tarceva: 100 mg, 150 mg

Extemporaneous Preparations Hazardous agent; use appropriate precautions for handling and disposal (meets NIOSH, 2012 criteria).

A suspension for oral or feeding tube (silicone-based) administration may be prepared by dissolving tablets needed for dose in 100 mL water. To ensure full dose is received, rinse container with 40 mL water, administer residue and repeat rinse. Administer immediately after preparation; stability of solution is unknown (Tarceva® data on file from Genentech).

Siu LL, Soulieres D, Chen EX, et al, "Phase I/II Trial of Erlotinib and Cisplatin in Patients With Recurrent or Metastatic Squamous Cell Carcinoma of the Head and Neck: A Princess Margaret Hospital Phase II Consortium and National Cancer Institute of Canada Clinical Trials Group Study," *J Clin Oncol*, 2007, 25(16):2178-83. [PubMed 17538162]

Soulieres D, Senzer NN, Vokes EE, et al, "Multicenter Phase II Study of Erlotinib, an Oral Epidermal Growth Factor Receptor Tyrosine Kinase Inhibitor, in Patients With Recurrent or Metastatic Squamous Cell Cancer of the Head and Neck," *J Clin Oncol*, 2004, 22(1):77-85. [PubMed 14701768]

◆ **Erlotinib Hydrochloride** *see* Erlotinib *on page 735*

◆ **E-R-O Ear Drops [OTC]** *see* Carbamide Peroxide *on page 340*

◆ **E-R-O Ear Wax Removal System [OTC]** *see* Carbamide Peroxide *on page 340*

◆ **Errin** *see* Norethindrone *on page 1472*

◆ **Ertaczo** *see* Sertaconazole *on page 1889*

Ertapenem (er ta PEN em)

Brand Names: U.S. INVanz

Brand Names: Canada Invanz

Index Terms Ertapenem Sodium; L-749,345; MK0826

Pharmacologic Category Antibiotic, Carbapenem

Use Moderate-to-severe infections:

Acute pelvic infections: For the treatment of acute pelvic infections, including postpartum endomyometritis, septic abortion, and postsurgical gynecologic infections caused by *Streptococcus agalactiae*, *Escherichia coli*, *Bacteroides fragilis*, *Porphyromonas asaccharolytica*, *Peptostreptococcus* spp, or *Prevotella bivia*.

Community-acquired pneumonia: For the treatment of community-acquired pneumonia (CAP) caused by *Streptococcus pneumoniae* (penicillin-susceptible isolates only), including cases with concurrent bacteremia; *Haemophilus influenzae* (beta-lactamase-negative isolates only); or *Moraxella catarrhalis*.

Complicated intra-abdominal infections: For the treatment of complicated intra-abdominal infections caused by *E. coli*, *Clostridium clostridioforme*, *Eubacterium lentum*, *Peptostreptococcus* spp, *B. fragilis*, *Bacteroides distasonis*, *Bacteroides ovatus*, *Bacteroides thetaiotaomicron*, or *Bacteroides uniformis*.

Complicated skin and skin structure infections: For the treatment of complicated skin and skin structure infections, including diabetic foot infections without osteomyelitis caused by *Staphylococcus aureus* (methicillin-susceptible isolates only), *S. agalactiae*, *Streptococcus pyogenes*, *E. coli*, *Klebsiella pneumoniae*, *Proteus mirabilis*, *B. fragilis*, *Peptostreptococcus* spp, *P. asaccharolytica*, or *P. bivia*. Ertapenem has not been studied in diabetic foot infections with concomitant osteomyelitis.

Complicated urinary tract infections: For the treatment of complicated urinary tract infections (UTIs), including pyelonephritis caused by *E. coli*, including cases with concurrent bacteremia or *K. pneumoniae*.

Prophylaxis of surgical-site infection in colorectal surgery: For the prophylaxis of surgical-site infection in adults following elective colorectal surgery.

Note: Methicillin-resistant *Staphylococcus aureus, Enterococcus* spp, penicillin-resistant strains of *Streptococcus pneumoniae*, *Acinetobacter*, and *Pseudomonas aeruginosa*, are **resistant** to ertapenem while most extended-spectrum beta-lactamase (ESBL)-producing bacteria remain sensitive to ertapenem.

Unlabeled Use Treatment of intravenous catheter-related bloodstream infection; treatment of prosthetic joint infection

Pregnancy Risk Factor B

Pregnancy Considerations Teratogenic effects were not observed in animal reproduction studies. Ertapenem is approved for the treatment of postpartum endomyometritis, septic abortion, and postsurgical infections. Information related to use during pregnancy has not been located.

Breast-Feeding Considerations Ertapenem is excreted in breast milk. The low concentrations in milk and low oral bioavailability suggest minimal exposure risk to the infant. The manufacturer recommends that caution be exercised when administering ertapenem to nursing women. Non-dose-related effects could include modification of bowel flora.

Contraindications Known hypersensitivity to any component of this product or to other drugs in the same class or in patients who have demonstrated anaphylactic reactions to beta-lactams; known hypersensitivity to local anesthetics of the amide type due to the use of lidocaine as a diluent (I.M. use only).

Warnings/Precautions Use caution with renal impairment. Dosage adjustment required in patients with moderate-to-severe renal dysfunction; elderly patients often require lower doses (based upon renal function). Use may result in fungal or bacterial superinfection, including *C. difficile*-associated diarrhea (CDAD) and pseudomembranous colitis; CDAD has been observed >2 months postantibiotic treatment. Carbapenems have been associated with CNS adverse effects, including confusional states and seizures (myoclonic); use caution with CNS disorders (eg, brain lesions and history of seizures) and adjust dose in renal impairment to avoid drug accumulation, which may increase seizure risk. Serious hypersensitivity reactions, including anaphylaxis, have been reported (some without a history of previous allergic reactions to beta-lactams). Doses for I.M. administration are mixed with lidocaine; consult Lidocaine (Systemic) information for associated Warnings/Precautions. May decrease divalproex sodium/valproic acid concentrations leading to breakthrough seizures; concomitant use not recommended. Safety and efficacy have not been established in children <3 months of age.

Adverse Reactions

>10%: Gastrointestinal: Diarrhea (2% to 12%)

1% to 10%:

Cardiovascular: Edema (3%), chest pain (1% to 2%), hypertension (1% to 2%), hypotension (1% to 2%), tachycardia (1% to 2%)

Central nervous system: Headache (4% to 7%); altered mental status (eg, agitation, confusion, disorientation, mental acuity decreased, somnolence, stupor) (3% to 5%); fever (2% to 5%), insomnia (3%), dizziness (2%), hypothermia (infants, children, and adolescents <2%), fatigue (1%), anxiety (1%)

Dermatologic: Diaper rash (infants and children 5%), rash (2% to 3%), pruritus (1% to 2%), erythema (1% to 2%), genital rash (infants, children, and adolescents <2%), skin lesions (infants, children, and adolescents <2%)

Endocrine & metabolic: Hypokalemia (2%), hyperglycemia (1% to 2%), hyperkalemia (≤1%)

Gastrointestinal: Vomiting (2% to 10%), nausea (6% to 9%), abdominal pain (4% to 5%), constipation (2% to 4%), acid regurgitation (1% to 2%), appetite decreased (infants, children, and adolescents <2%), dyspepsia (1%), oral candidiasis (≤1%)

Genitourinary: Urine WBCs increased (2% to 3%), urine RBCs increased (1% to 3%), vaginitis (1% to 3%)

Hematologic: Thrombocytosis (4% to 7%), hematocrit/hemoglobin decreased (3% to 5%), eosinophils increased (1% to 2%), leukopenia (1% to 2%), neutrophils decreased (1% to 2%), thrombocytopenia (1%), prothrombin time increased (≤1%)

Hepatic: Hepatic enzyme increased (7% to 9%), alkaline phosphatase increase (4% to 7%), albumin decreased (1% to 2%), bilirubin (total) increased (1% to 2%)

Local: Infused vein complications (5% to 7%), phlebitis/thrombophlebitis (2%), extravasation (1% to 2%)

Neuromuscular & skeletal: Arthralgia (infants, children, and adolescents <2%), weakness (1%), leg pain (≤1%)

Otic: Otitis media (infants, children, and adolescents <2%)

Renal: Serum creatinine increased (1%)

Respiratory: Cough (1% to 4%), dyspnea (1% to 3%), nasopharyngitis (infants, children, and adolescents <2%), rhinitis (infants, children, and adolescents <2%), rhinorrhea (infants, children, and adolescents <2%), upper respiratory tract infection (infants, children, and adolescents <2%), wheezing (infants, children, and adolescents <2%), pharyngitis (1%), rales/rhonchi (1%), respiratory distress (≤1%)

Miscellaneous: Herpes simplex (infants, children, and adolescents <2%)

<1% (Limited to important or life-threatening): Anaphylactoid reactions, anaphylaxis, arrhythmia, asthma, asystole, atrial fibrillation, bradycardia, bronchoconstriction, *C. difficile*-associated diarrhea, cardiac arrest, cholelithiasis, delirium, DRESS syndrome, gastrointestinal hemorrhage, gout, heart failure, heart murmur, hemoptysis, hypoxemia, ileus, jaundice, oliguria/anuria, pancreatitis, pleural effusion, renal insufficiency, seizure, septicemia, septic shock, subdural hemorrhage, ventricular tachycardia

Drug Interactions

Metabolism/Transport Effects None known.

Avoid Concomitant Use

Avoid concomitant use of Ertapenem with any of the following: BCG

Increased Effect/Toxicity

Ertapenem may increase the levels/effects of: Tacrolimus (Systemic)

The levels/effects of Ertapenem may be increased by: Probenecid

Decreased Effect

Ertapenem may decrease the levels/effects of: BCG; Sodium Picosulfate; Typhoid Vaccine; Valproic Acid and Derivatives

Preparation for Administration

I.M.: Reconstitute 1 g vial with 3.2 mL of 1% lidocaine HCl injection (without epinephrine). Shake well.

I.V.: Reconstitute 1 g vial with 10 mL of sterile water for injection, 0.9% sodium chloride injection, or bacteriostatic water for injection. Shake well. For adults, transfer dose to 50 mL of 0.9% sodium chloride injection; for children, dilute dose with NS to a final concentration ≤20 mg/mL.

Storage/Stability Prior to reconstitution, store vials at ≤25°C (77°F). The reconstituted I.M. solution should be used within 1 hour after preparation. The reconstituted I.V. solution may be stored at room temperature (25°C [77°F]) and used within 6 hours, or stored for 24 hours under refrigeration (5°C [41°F]) and used within 4 hours after removal from refrigeration. Do not freeze.

Mechanism of Action Inhibits bacterial cell wall synthesis by binding to one or more of the penicillin-binding proteins; which in turn inhibits the final transpeptidation step of peptidoglycan synthesis in bacterial cell walls, thus inhibiting cell wall biosynthesis. Bacteria eventually lyse due to ongoing activity of cell wall autolytic enzymes (autolysins and murein hydrolases) while cell wall assembly is arrested.

Pharmacodynamics/Kinetics

Absorption: I.M.: Almost complete

Distribution: V_{dss}:

Children 3 months to 12 years: ~0.2 L/kg

Children 13-17 years: ~0.16 L/kg

Adults: ~0.12 L/kg

Protein binding (concentration dependent, primarily to albumin): 85% at 300 mcg/mL, 95% at <100 mcg/mL

Metabolism: Non-CYP-mediated hydrolysis to inactive metabolite

Bioavailability: I.M.: ~90%

Half-life elimination:

Children 3 months to 12 years: ~2.5 hours

Children ≥13 years and Adults: ~4 hours

Time to peak: I.M.: ~2.3 hours

Excretion: Urine (~80% as unchanged drug and metabolite); feces (~10%)

Dosage Note: I.V. therapy may be administered for up to 14 days; I.M. therapy for up to 7 days

Usual dosage ranges:

Infants ≥3 months and Children: I.M., I.V.: 15 **mg**/kg twice daily (maximum: 1 g daily)

Adolescents and Adults: I.M., I.V.: 1 g once daily

Indication-specific dosing:

Infants ≥3 months and Children: I.M., I.V.:

Community-acquired pneumonia, complicated urinary tract infections (including pyelonephritis): 15 **mg**/kg twice daily (maximum: 1 g daily); duration of total antibiotic treatment: 10-14 days (**Note:** Duration includes possible switch to appropriate oral therapy after at least 3 days of parenteral treatment, once clinical improvement demonstrated.)

Intra-abdominal infection: 15 **mg**/kg twice daily (maximum: 1 g daily) for 5-14 days

Pelvic infections (acute): 15 **mg**/kg twice daily (maximum: 1 g daily) for 3-10 days

Skin and skin structure infections: 15 **mg**/kg twice daily (maximum: 1 g daily) for 7-14 days

Adolescents and Adults: I.M., I.V.:

Community-acquired pneumonia, complicated urinary tract infections (including pyelonephritis): 1 g once daily; duration of total antibiotic treatment: 10-14 days; duration includes possible switch to appropriate oral therapy after at least 3 days of parenteral treatment, once clinical improvement demonstrated. **Note:** The carbapenems, including ertapenem, are preferred agents for *Enterobacter* spp and *Burkholderia pseudomallei*, and are considered alternative agents for anaerobes in aspiration pneumonia (IDSA, 2007).

Intra-abdominal infection: 1 g once daily for 5-14 days; **Note:** 2010 IDSA guidelines recommend a treatment duration of 4-7 days (provided source controlled) for community-acquired, mild-to-moderate intra-abdominal infections (Solomkin, 2010)

Pelvic infections (acute): 1 g once daily for 3-10 days

Skin and skin structure infections (excluding diabetic foot infections with osteomyelitis): 1 g once daily for 7-14 days. **Notes:** For diabetic foot infections, recommended treatment duration is up to 4 weeks depending on severity of infection and response to therapy (Lipsky, 2012); guidelines recommend ertapenem as a preferred agent for animal bites. (IDSA, 2005).

Adults: I.V.:

Prophylaxis of surgical site following colorectal surgery: 1 g as a single dose given 1 hour preoperatively

Intravenous catheter-related bloodstream infection (unlabeled use): 1 g once daily (**Note:** Carbapenems, including ertapenem, are preferred agents for extended-spectrum β-lactamase [ESBL]-positive *Escherichia coli* and *Klebsiella, Enterobacter,* and *Serratia* [IDSA, 2009].)

Prosthetic joint infection, *Enterobacter* spp (unlabeled use): 1 g every 24 hours for 4-6 weeks (Osmon, 2013)

Dosage adjustment in renal impairment:

Children: No data available for pediatric patients with renal insufficiency.

Adults:

Cl_{cr} >30 mL/minute/1.73 m^2: No dosage adjustment necessary.

Cl_{cr} ≤30 mL/minute/1.73 m^2 and ESRD: 500 mg daily

Hemodialysis: Adults: When the daily dose is given within 6 hours prior to hemodialysis, a supplementary dose of 150 mg is required following hemodialysis. If ertapenem is given at least 6 hours prior to hemodialysis, no supplementary dose is needed.

CAPD: I.V.: 500 mg daily (Cardone, 2011)

Dosage adjustment in hepatic impairment: Adjustments cannot be recommended (lack of experience and research in this patient population).

Dietary Considerations Some products may contain sodium.

Administration

I.M.: Avoid injection into a blood vessel. Make sure patient does not have an allergy to lidocaine or another anesthetic of the amide type. Administer by deep I.M. injection into a large muscle mass (eg, gluteal muscle or lateral part of the thigh). Do not administer I.M. preparation or drug reconstituted for I.M. administration intravenously.

I.V.: Infuse over 30 minutes

Monitoring Parameters Periodic renal, hepatic, and hematopoietic assessment during prolonged therapy; neurological assessment

Dosage Forms Excipient information presented when available (limited, particularly for generics); consult specific product labeling.

Solution Reconstituted, Injection:

INVanz: 1 g (1 ea)

Solution Reconstituted, Intravenous:

INVanz: 1 g (1 ea)

- **Ertapenem Sodium** *see* Ertapenem *on page 739*
- **Erwinase® (Can)** *see* Asparaginase (*Erwinia*) *on page 176*
- **Erwinaze** *see* Asparaginase (*Erwinia*) *on page 176*
- ***Erwinia chrysanthemi*** *see* Asparaginase (*Erwinia*) *on page 176*
- **Ery** *see* Erythromycin (Topical) *on page 744*
- **Erybid (Can)** *see* Erythromycin (Systemic) *on page 741*
- **Eryc (Can)** *see* Erythromycin (Systemic) *on page 741*
- **Erygel** *see* Erythromycin (Topical) *on page 744*
- **EryPed 200** *see* Erythromycin (Systemic) *on page 741*
- **EryPed 400** *see* Erythromycin (Systemic) *on page 741*
- **Erysol® (Can)** *see* Erythromycin (Topical) *on page 744*
- **Ery-Tab** *see* Erythromycin (Systemic) *on page 741*
- **Erythrocin Lactobionate** *see* Erythromycin (Systemic) *on page 741*
- **Erythrocin Stearate** *see* Erythromycin (Systemic) *on page 741*

Erythromycin (Systemic) (er ith roe MYE sin)

Brand Names: U.S. E.E.S. 400; E.E.S. Granules; Ery-Tab; EryPed 200; EryPed 400; Erythrocin Lactobionate; Erythrocin Stearate; PCE

Brand Names: Canada Apo-Erythro Base; Apo-Erythro E-C; Apo-Erythro-ES; Apo-Erythro-S; EES; Erybid; Eryc; Novo-Rythro Estolate; Novo-Rythro Ethylsuccinate; Nu-Erythromycin-S; PCE

Index Terms Erythromycin Base; Erythromycin Ethylsuccinate; Erythromycin Lactobionate; Erythromycin Stearate

Pharmacologic Category Antibiotic, Macrolide

Use Treatment of susceptible bacterial infections including *S. pyogenes*, some *S. pneumoniae,* some *S. aureus*, *M. pneumoniae*, *Legionella pneumophila*, diphtheria, pertussis, *Chlamydia*, erythrasma, *N. gonorrhoeae*, *E. histolytica*, syphilis and nongonococcal urethritis, and *Campylobacter* gastroenteritis; used in conjunction with neomycin for decontaminating the bowel

Unlabeled Use Management of gastroparesis, chancroid; treatment of *Bartonella* spp infections

Pregnancy Risk Factor B

Pregnancy Considerations Adverse events were not observed in animal reproduction studies. Erythromycin crosses the placenta and low concentrations are found in the fetal serum. Most reports do not identify an increase in risk for congenital abnormalities due to prenatal exposure to erythromycin. Cardiovascular anomalies following exposure in early pregnancy have been reported in some observational studies. Most studies also do not support a link between prenatal exposure to erythromycin and pyloric stenosis in the neonate. In general, serum concentrations of erythromycin are lower in pregnant women. Erythromycin therapy in patients with preterm, premature rupture of membranes is associated with a range of health benefits to the neonate and no long-term adverse events to the child have been observed. However, maternal use of erythromycin in women with preterm labor, intact membranes, and no documented infection does not improve neonatal health and may have adverse effects in childhood (use is not recommended). In patients with acute infections during pregnancy, erythromycin may be given if an antibiotic is required and appropriate based on bacterial sensitivity. Erythromycin is the antibiotic of choice for preterm premature rupture of membranes (with membrane rupture prior to 34 weeks gestation), the treatment of granuloma inguinale and lymphogranuloma venereum in pregnancy, and the treatment of or long-term suppression of *Bartonella* infection in HIV-infected pregnant patients. Erythromycin may be appropriate as an alternative agent for the treatment of chlamydial infections in pregnant women (consult current guidelines).

Breast-Feeding Considerations Erythromycin is excreted in breast milk; therefore, the manufacturer recommends that caution be exercised when administering erythromycin to breast-feeding women.

Due to the low concentrations in human milk, minimal toxicity would be expected in the nursing infant. One case report and a cohort study raise the possibility for a connection with pyloric stenosis in neonates exposed to erythromycin via breast milk and an alternative antibiotic may be preferred for breast-feeding mothers of infants in this age group. Nondose-related effects could include modification of bowel flora.

Contraindications Hypersensitivity to erythromycin, any macrolide antibiotics, or any component of the formulation

Concomitant use with pimozide, cisapride, ergotamine or dihydroergotamine, terfenadine, astemizole, lovastatin, or simvastatin

Warnings/Precautions Use caution with hepatic impairment with or without jaundice has occurred, it may be accompanied by malaise, nausea, vomiting, abdominal colic, and fever; discontinue use if these occur. Use caution with other medication relying on CYP3A4 metabolism; high potential for drug interactions exists. Prolonged use may result in fungal or bacterial superinfection, including *C. difficile*-associated diarrhea (CDAD) and pseudomembranous colitis; CDAD has been observed >2 months postantibiotic treatment. Use in infants has been associated with infantile hypertrophic pyloric stenosis (IHPS). Macrolides have been associated with rare QT_c prolongation and ventricular arrhythmias, including torsade de pointes; avoid use in patients with prolonged QT interval, uncorrected hypokalemia or hypomagnesemia, clinically significant bradycardia, or concurrent use of Class IA (eg, quinidine, procainamide) or Class III (eg, amiodarone, dofetilide, sotalol) antiarrhythmic agents. Avoid concurrent use with strong CYP3A inhibitors; may increase the risk of sudden cardiac death (Ray, 2004). Use caution in elderly patients, as risk of adverse events may be increased. Use caution in myasthenia gravis patients; erythromycin may aggravate muscular weakness.

Adverse Reactions Frequency not defined. Incidence may vary with formulation.

Cardiovascular: QT_c prolongation, torsade de pointes, ventricular arrhythmia, ventricular tachycardia

Central nervous system: Seizure

Dermatologic: Erythema multiforme, pruritus, rash, Stevens-Johnson syndrome, toxic epidermal necrolysis

Gastrointestinal: Abdominal pain, anorexia, diarrhea, infantile hypertrophic pyloric stenosis, nausea, oral candidiasis, pancreatitis, pseudomembranous colitis, vomiting

Hepatic: Cholestatic jaundice (most common with estolate), hepatitis, liver function tests abnormal

Local: Phlebitis at the injection site, thrombophlebitis

Neuromuscular & skeletal: Weakness

Otic: Hearing loss

Miscellaneous: Allergic reactions, anaphylaxis, hypersensitivity reactions, interstitial nephritis, urticaria

Drug Interactions

Metabolism/Transport Effects Substrate of CYP2B6 (minor), CYP3A4 (major), P-glycoprotein; **Note:** Assignment of Major/Minor substrate status based on clinically relevant drug interaction potential; **Inhibits** CYP3A4 (moderate), P-glycoprotein

Avoid Concomitant Use

Avoid concomitant use of Erythromycin (Systemic) with any of the following: BCG; Bosutinib; Cisapride; Conivaptan; Disopyramide; Fusidic Acid (Systemic); Highest Risk QTc-Prolonging Agents; Ibrutinib; Ivabradine; Lincosamide Antibiotics; Lomitapide; Lovastatin; Mifepristone; Pimozide; Pomalidomide; QuiNIDine; QuiNINE; Silodosin; Simeprevir; Simvastatin; Terfenadine; Tolvaptan; Topotecan; Ulipristal

Increased Effect/Toxicity

Erythromycin (Systemic) may increase the levels/effects of: Afatinib; Alfentanil; ALPRAZolam; Antifungal Agents (Azole Derivatives, Systemic); Antineoplastic Agents (Vinca Alkaloids); ARIPiprazole; AtorvaSTATin; Avanafil; Bosentan; Bosutinib; Budesonide (Systemic, Oral Inhalation); BusPIRone; Calcium Channel Blockers; CarBAMazepine; Cardiac Glycosides; Cilostazol; Cisapride; CloZAPine; Colchicine; Corticosteroids (Systemic); CycloSPORINE (Systemic); CYP3A4 Substrates; Dabigatran Etexilate; Disopyramide; Eletriptan; Eplerenone; Ergot Derivatives; Estazolam; Everolimus; FentaNYL; Fexofenadine; Highest Risk QTc-Prolonging Agents; Ibrutinib; Imatinib; Ivacaftor; Lomitapide; Lovastatin; Lurasidone; Midazolam; Moderate Risk QTc-Prolonging Agents; OxyCODONE; P-glycoprotein/ABCB1 Substrates; Pimecrolimus; Pimozide; Pitavastatin; Pomalidomide; Pravastatin; QuiNIDine; QuiNINE; Repaglinide; Rifamycin Derivatives; Rilpivirine; Rivaroxaban; Salmeterol; Saxagliptin; Selective Serotonin Reuptake Inhibitors; Sildenafil; Silodosin; Simeprevir; Simvastatin; Sirolimus; Tacrolimus (Systemic); Tacrolimus (Topical); Telaprevir; Temsirolimus; Terfenadine; Theophylline Derivatives; Tolvaptan; Topotecan; Triazolam; Ulipristal; Vardenafil; Vitamin K Antagonists; Zopiclone

The levels/effects of Erythromycin (Systemic) may be increased by: Antifungal Agents (Azole Derivatives, Systemic); Conivaptan; CYP3A4 Inhibitors (Moderate); CYP3A4 Inhibitors (Strong); Dasatinib; Fusidic Acid (Systemic); Ivabradine; Ivacaftor; Luliconazole; Mifepristone; P-glycoprotein/ABCB1 Inhibitors; QTc-Prolonging Agents (Indeterminate Risk and Risk Modifying); Telaprevir

Decreased Effect

Erythromycin (Systemic) may decrease the levels/effects of: BCG; Clopidogrel; Ifosfamide; Sodium Picosulfate; Typhoid Vaccine; Zafirlukast

The levels/effects of Erythromycin (Systemic) may be decreased by: Bosentan; CYP3A4 Inducers (Strong); Dabrafenib; Deferasirox; Etravirine; Herbs (CYP3A4 Inducers); Lincosamide Antibiotics; Mitotane; P-glycoprotein/ABCB1 Inducers; Tocilizumab

Ethanol/Nutrition/Herb Interactions

Ethanol: Ethanol may decrease absorption of erythromycin or enhance effects of ethanol. Management: Avoid ethanol.

Food: Erythromycin serum levels may be altered if taken with food (formulation-dependent). GI upset, including diarrhea, is common. Management: May be taken with food to decrease GI upset, otherwise take around-the-clock with a full glass of water. Do not give with milk or acidic beverages (eg, soda, juice).

Herb/Nutraceutical: St John's wort may decrease erythromycin levels. Management: Avoid St John's wort.

Preparation for Administration Erythromycin lactobionate should be reconstituted with sterile water for injection without preservatives to avoid gel formation. I.V. form has the longest stability in NS and should be prepared in this base solution whenever possible. Do not use D_5W as a diluent unless sodium bicarbonate is added to solution. If I.V. must be prepared in D_5W, 0.5 mL of the 8.4% sodium bicarbonate solution should be added per each 100 mL of D_5W.

Standard diluent: 500 mg/250 mL D_5W/NS; 750 mg/250 mL D_5W/NS; 1 g/250 mL D_5W/NS.

Storage/Stability

Injection: Store unreconstituted vials at 15°C to 30°C (59°F to 86°F). Reconstituted solution is stable for 2 weeks when refrigerated or for 8 hours at room temperature. Erythromycin I.V. infusion solution is stable at pH 6-8; stability of lactobionate is pH dependent; I.V. form has longest stability in NS. Stability of parenteral admixture at room temperature (25°C) and at refrigeration temperature (4°C) is 24 hours.

Oral suspension:

Granules: Prior to mixing, store at <30°C (86°F). After mixing, store under refrigeration and use within 10 days.

Powder: Prior to mixing, store at <30°C (86°F). After mixing, store at ≤25°C (77°F) and use within 35 days.

Tablet and capsule formulations: Store at <30°C (86°F).

Mechanism of Action Inhibits RNA-dependent protein synthesis at the chain elongation step; binds to the 50S ribosomal subunit resulting in blockage of transpeptidation

Pharmacodynamics/Kinetics

Absorption: Oral: Variable but better with salt forms than with base form; 18% to 45%; ethylsuccinate may be better absorbed with food

Distribution:
Relative diffusion from blood into CSF: Minimal even with inflammation
CSF:blood level ratio: Normal meninges: 2% to 13%; Inflamed meninges: 7% to 25%
Protein binding: Base: 73% to 81%
Metabolism: Demethylation primarily via hepatic CYP3A4
Half-life elimination: Peak: 1.5-2 hours; End-stage renal disease: 5-6 hours
Time to peak, serum: Base: 4 hours; Ethylsuccinate: 0.5-2.5 hours; delayed with food due to differences in absorption
Excretion: Primarily feces; urine (2% to 15% as unchanged drug)

Dosage Note: Due to differences in absorption, 400 mg erythromycin ethylsuccinate produces the same serum levels as 250 mg erythromycin base or stearate.

Usual dosage range:
Infants and Children:
Oral:
Base: 30-50 mg/kg/day in 2-4 divided doses; maximum: 2 g daily
Ethylsuccinate: 30-50 mg/kg/day in 2-4 divided doses; maximum: 3.2 g daily
Stearate: 30-50 mg/kg/day in 2-4 divided doses; maximum: 2 g daily
I.V.: Lactobionate: 15-50 mg/kg/day divided every 6 hours, not to exceed 4 g daily
Adults:
Oral:
Base: 250-500 mg every 6-12 hours; maximum: 4 g daily
Ethylsuccinate: 400-800 mg every 6-12 hours; maximum: 4 g daily
I.V.: Lactobionate: 15-20 mg/kg/day divided every 6 hours or 500 mg to 1 g every 6 hours, or given as a continuous infusion over 24 hours; maximum: 4 g daily

Indication-specific dosing:
Infants and Children:
***Bartonella* spp infections (bacillary angiomatosis [BA], peliosis hepatis [PH]) (unlabeled use):** Oral: 40 mg/kg/day (ethylsuccinate) in 4 divided doses (maximum: 2 g daily) for 3 months (BA) or 4 months (PH) (Rolain, 2004)
Chlamydial infection *(C. trachomatis):* Children <45 kg: Oral: 50 mg/kg/day (base or ethylsuccinate) in 4 divided doses for 14 days (CDC, 2010)
Community-acquired pneumonia (CAP) (IDSA/PIDS, 2011): Infants >3 months and Children: **Note:** A beta-lactam antibiotic should be added if typical bacterial pneumonia cannot be ruled out.
Presumed atypical *(M. pneumoniae, C. pneumoniae, C. trachomatis)* infection, mild atypical infection or step-down therapy (alternative to azithromycin): Oral: 10 mg/kg/dose every 6 hours
Moderate-to-severe atypical infection (alternative to azithromycin): I.V.: 5 mg/kg/dose every 6 hours
Mild/moderate infection: Oral: 30-50 mg/kg/day in divided doses every 6-12 hours
Pertussis: Oral: 40-50 mg/kg/day in 4 divided doses for 14 days; maximum: 2 g daily (not preferred agent for infants <1 month due to IHPS)
Pharyngitis, tonsillitis (streptococcal): Oral: 20 mg (base)/kg/day or 40 mg (ethylsuccinate)/kg/day in 2 divided doses for 10 days. **Note:** No longer preferred therapy due to increased organism resistance.
Surgical (preoperative) prophylaxis (colorectal) (unlabeled use): Children ≥1 year: Oral: 20 mg (base)/kg (maximum dose: 1000 mg) at 1 PM, 2 PM, and 11 PM on the day before 8 AM surgery combined with mechanical cleansing of the large intestine, oral neomycin. Perioperative I.V. antibiotics are also given on the day of surgery (Bratzler, 2013).
Severe infection: I.V.: 15-50 mg/kg/day; maximum: 4 g daily
Adults:
***Bartonella* spp infections (bacillary angiomatosis [BA], peliosis hepatis [PH]) (unlabeled use):** Oral: 500 mg (base) 4 times daily for 3 months (BA) or 4 months (PH) (Koehler, 1992; Rolain, 2004; Stevens, 2005; Tappero, 1993)
Chancroid (unlabeled use): Oral: 500 mg (base) 3 times daily for 7 days; **Note:** Not a preferred agent; isolates with intermediate resistance have been documented (CDC, 2010)
Gastroparesis (unlabeled use):
I.V.: 3 mg/kg administered over 45 minutes every 8 hours (Camilleri, 2013)
Oral: Patients refractory/intolerant to other prokinetic agents (eg, metoclopramide, domperidone): 250-500 mg (base) 3 times daily before meals. Limit duration of therapy, tachyphylaxis may occur after 4 weeks (Camilleri, 2013).
Granuloma inguinale (donovanosis) (unlabeled use): Oral: 500 mg (base) 4 times daily for 21 days (CDC, 2010)
Legionnaires' disease: Oral: 1.6-4 g (ethylsuccinate) daily or 1-4 g (base) daily in divided doses for 21 days. **Note:** No longer preferred therapy and only used in nonhospitalized patients.
Lymphogranuloma venereum: Oral: 500 mg (base) 4 times daily for 21 days; **Note:** Preferred therapy for pregnant or lactating women (CDC, 2010)
Nongonococcal urethritis (including coinfection with *C. trachomatis*): Oral: 500 mg (base) 4 times daily for 7 days or 800 mg (ethylsuccinate) 4 times daily for 7 days. **Note:** May use 250 mg (base) or 400 mg (ethylsuccinate) 4 times daily for 14 days if gastrointestinal intolerance.
Pertussis: Oral: 500 mg (base) every 6 hours for 14 days
Surgical (preoperative) prophylaxis (colorectal) (unlabeled dose): Oral: 1 g erythromycin base per dose at 1 PM, 2 PM, and 11 PM on the day before 8 AM surgery combined with mechanical cleansing of the large intestine, oral neomycin. Perioperative I.V. antibiotics are also given on the day of surgery (Bratzler, 2013).

Dosage adjustment in renal impairment: Dialysis: Slightly dialyzable (5% to 20%); no supplemental dosage necessary in hemo- or peritoneal dialysis or in continuous arteriovenous or venovenous hemofiltration
Dosage adjustment in hepatic impairment: No dosage adjustment provided in manufacturer's labeling; use with caution.

Dietary Considerations Drug may cause GI upset; may take with food. Some products may contain sodium.

Administration
Oral: Do not crush enteric coated drug product. GI upset, including diarrhea, is common. May be administered with food to decrease GI upset. Do not give with milk or acidic beverages.
I.V.: Infuse 1 g over 20-60 minutes. I.V. infusion may be very irritating to the vein. If phlebitis/pain occurs with used dilution, consider diluting further (eg, 1:5) if fluid status of the patient will tolerate, or consider administering in larger available vein. The addition of lidocaine or bicarbonate does not decrease the irritation of erythromycin infusions.

Test Interactions False-positive urinary catecholamines, 17-hydroxycorticosteroids and 17-ketosteroids

Dosage Forms Excipient information presented when available (limited, particularly for generics); consult specific product labeling.

Capsule Delayed Release Particles, Oral, as base:
- Generic: 250 mg

Solution Reconstituted, Intravenous, as lactobionate:
- Erythrocin Lactobionate: 500 mg (1 ea); 1000 mg (1 ea)

Suspension Reconstituted, Oral, as ethylsuccinate:
- E.E.S. Granules: 200 mg/5 mL (100 mL, 200 mL) [cherry flavor]
- EryPed 200: 200 mg/5 mL (100 mL) [fruit flavor]
- EryPed 400: 400 mg/5 mL (100 mL) [banana flavor]

Tablet, Oral, as base:
- Generic: 250 mg, 500 mg

Tablet, Oral, as ethylsuccinate:
- E.E.S. 400: 400 mg [contains fd&c red #40, fd&c yellow #10 (quinoline yellow)]
- Generic: 400 mg

Tablet, Oral, as stearate:
- Erythrocin Stearate: 250 mg

Tablet Delayed Release, Oral, as base:
- Ery-Tab: 250 mg, 333 mg, 500 mg
- PCE: 333 mg
- PCE: 500 mg [dye free, no artificial color(s)]

Erythromycin (Ophthalmic) (er ith roe MYE sin)

Brand Names: U.S. Ilotycin; Romycin

Brand Names: Canada Diomycin®; PMS-Erythromycin

Index Terms Erythromycin Base

Pharmacologic Category Antibiotic, Macrolide; Antibiotic, Ophthalmic

Use Treatment of superficial eye infections involving the conjunctiva or cornea

Pregnancy Risk Factor B

Dosage Ophthalmic: Children and Adults: Usual dosage range: Instill 1/2" (1.25 cm) 2-6 times/day depending on the severity of the infection

Additional Information Complete prescribing information should be consulted for additional detail.

Dosage Forms Excipient information presented when available (limited, particularly for generics); consult specific product labeling.

Ointment, Ophthalmic:
- Ilotycin: 5 mg/g (1 g)
- Romycin: 5 mg/g (3.5 g)
- Generic: 5 mg/g (1 g, 3.5 g)

Dosage Forms: Canada Excipient information presented when available (limited, particularly for generics); consult specific product labeling.

Ointment, ophthalmic: 0.5% (1 g, 3.5 g)

Erythromycin (Topical) (er ith roe MYE sin)

Brand Names: U.S. Akne-Mycin; Ery; Erygel

Brand Names: Canada Erysol®

Pharmacologic Category Acne Products; Antibiotic, Macrolide; Antibiotic, Topical; Topical Skin Product; Topical Skin Product, Acne

Use Treatment of acne vulgaris

Pregnancy Risk Factor B

Dosage Acne: Topical:

Adolescents and Adults: Usual dosage range: Apply over the affected area twice daily (morning and evening) after the skin has been thoroughly washed and patted dry; drying and peeling may be controlled by reducing the frequency of application.

Erysol® (Canadian availability; not available in the U.S.): Children ≥12 years, Adolescents, and Adults: Apply thin film to affected area twice daily (morning and evening); may decrease to once daily if irritation develops at application site. Therapeutic response may take up to 6-8 weeks; discontinue use if no improvement after 6-8 weeks or if condition worsens. Maximum therapy duration: 3 months.

Dosage adjustment in renal impairment: No dosage adjustment necessary.

Dosage adjustment in hepatic impairment: No dosage adjustment necessary.

Additional Information Complete prescribing information should be consulted for additional detail.

Dosage Forms Excipient information presented when available (limited, particularly for generics); consult specific product labeling.

Gel, External:
- Erygel: 2% (30 g, 60 g)
- Generic: 2% (30 g, 60 g)

Ointment, External:
- Akne-Mycin: 2% (25 g) [contains cetostearyl alcohol]

Pad, External:
- Ery: 2% (60 ea) [contains propylene glycol]
- Generic: 2% (60 ea)

Solution, External:
- Generic: 2% (60 mL)

Dosage Forms: Canada Excipient information presented when available (limited, particularly for generics); consult specific product labeling.

Gel, topical:
- Erysol®: 2% (25 g) [contains ethanol, octinoxate and avobenzone]

Erythromycin and Benzoyl Peroxide
(er ith roe MYE sin & BEN zoe il per OKS ide)

Brand Names: U.S. Benzamycin®; Benzamycin® Pak

Brand Names: Canada Benzamycin®

Index Terms Benzoyl Peroxide and Erythromycin

Pharmacologic Category Acne Products; Topical Skin Product, Acne

Use Topical control of acne vulgaris

Pregnancy Risk Factor C

Dosage Adolescents ≥12 years and Adults: Apply twice daily, morning and evening

Additional Information Complete prescribing information should be consulted for additional detail.

Dosage Forms Excipient information presented when available (limited, particularly for generics); consult specific product labeling.

Gel, topical: Erythromycin 30 mg and benzoyl peroxide 50 mg per g (23 g, 47 g)
- Benzamycin®: Erythromycin 30 mg and benzoyl peroxide 50 mg per g (47 g) [contains alcohol 20%]
- Benzamycin® Pak: Erythromycin 30 mg and benzoyl peroxide 50 mg per 0.8 g packet (60s) [supplied with diluent containing alcohol]

Erythromycin and Sulfisoxazole
(er ith roe MYE sin & sul fi SOKS a zole)

Brand Names: U.S. E.S.P.®

Brand Names: Canada Pediazole®

Index Terms Sulfisoxazole and Erythromycin

Pharmacologic Category Antibiotic, Macrolide; Antibiotic, Macrolide Combination; Antibiotic, Sulfonamide Derivative

Use Treatment of otitis media caused by susceptible strains of *Haemophilus influenzae*

Pregnancy Risk Factor C

Dosage Oral: Otitis media: Infants ≥2 months and Children: Erythromycin 50 mg/kg/day and sulfisoxazole 150 mg/kg/day in divided doses every 6-8 hours for 10 days; maximum: Erythromycin 2 g/day or sulfisoxazole 6 g/day

Dosage adjustment in renal impairment: No dosage adjustment provided in the manufacturer's labeling.

Dosage adjustment in hepatic impairment: No dosage adjustment provided in manufacturer's labeling; use with caution.

Additional Information Complete prescribing information should be consulted for additional detail.

Dosage Forms Excipient information presented when available (limited, particularly for generics); consult specific product labeling.

Powder for oral suspension: Erythromycin ethylsuccinate 200 mg and sulfisoxazole acetyl 600 mg per 5 mL (100 mL, 150 mL, 200 mL)

E.S.P.®: Erythromycin ethylsuccinate 200 mg and sulfisoxazole acetyl 600 mg per 5 mL (100 mL, 150 mL, 200 mL) [cheri beri flavor]

◆ **Erythromycin Base** *see* Erythromycin (Ophthalmic) *on page 744*

◆ **Erythromycin Base** *see* Erythromycin (Systemic) *on page 741*

◆ **Erythromycin Ethylsuccinate** *see* Erythromycin (Systemic) *on page 741*

◆ **Erythromycin Lactobionate** *see* Erythromycin (Systemic) *on page 741*

◆ **Erythromycin Stearate** *see* Erythromycin (Systemic) *on page 741*

◆ **Erythropoiesis-Stimulating Agent (ESA)** *see* Darbepoetin Alfa *on page 543*

◆ **Erythropoiesis-Stimulating Agent (ESA)** *see* Epoetin Alfa *on page 723*

◆ **Erythropoiesis-Stimulating Agent (ESA)** *see* Peginesatide *on page 1589*

◆ **Erythropoiesis-Stimulating Protein** *see* Darbepoetin Alfa *on page 543*

◆ **Erythropoietin** *see* Epoetin Alfa *on page 723*

Escitalopram (es sye TAL oh pram)

Brand Names: U.S. Lexapro

Brand Names: Canada Cipralex®

Index Terms Escitalopram Oxalate; Lu-26-054; S-Citalopram

Pharmacologic Category Antidepressant, Selective Serotonin Reuptake Inhibitor

Additional Appendix Information

Antidepressant Agents *on page 2284*

Selective Serotonin Reuptake Inhibitors (SSRIs) Pharmacokinetics *on page 2314*

Use Treatment of major depressive disorder; generalized anxiety disorders (GAD)

Canadian labeling: Additional use (not in U.S. labeling): Treatment of obsessive-compulsive disorder (OCD)

Unlabeled Use Treatment of mild dementia-associated agitation in nonpsychotic patients; treatment of vasomotor symptoms associated with menopause

Pregnancy Risk Factor C

Pregnancy Considerations Adverse events have been observed in animal reproduction studies. Escitalopram crosses the placenta and is distributed into the amniotic fluid. An increased risk of teratogenic effects, including cardiovascular defects, may be associated with maternal use of escitalopram or other SSRIs; however, available information is conflicting. Nonteratogenic effects in the newborn following SSRI/SNRI exposure late in the third trimester include respiratory distress, cyanosis, apnea, seizures, temperature instability, feeding difficulty, vomiting, hypoglycemia, hypo- or hypertonia, hyper-reflexia, jitteriness, irritability, constant crying, and tremor. Symptoms may be due to the toxicity of the SSRIs/SNRIs or a discontinuation syndrome and may be consistent with serotonin syndrome associated with SSRI treatment. Persistent pulmonary hypertension of the newborn (PPHN) has also been reported with SSRI exposure. The long-term effects of *in utero* SSRI exposure on infant development and behavior are not known. Escitalopram is the S-enantiomer of the racemic derivative citalopram; also refer to the Citalopram monograph.

Due to pregnancy-induced physiologic changes, some pharmacokinetic parameters of escitalopram may be altered. The ACOG recommends that therapy with SSRIs or SNRIs during pregnancy be individualized; treatment of depression during pregnancy should incorporate the clinical expertise of the mental health clinician, obstetrician, primary healthcare provider, and pediatrician. According to the American Psychiatric Association (APA), the risks of medication treatment should be weighed against other treatment options and untreated depression. For women who discontinue antidepressant medications during pregnancy and who may be at high risk for postpartum depression, the medications can be restarted following delivery. Treatment algorithms have been developed by the ACOG and the APA for the management of depression in women prior to conception and during pregnancy.

Breast-Feeding Considerations Escitalopram and its metabolite are excreted into breast milk. Limited data is available concerning the effects escitalopram may have in the nursing infant and the long-term effects on development and behavior have not been studied. Adverse effects have been reported in nursing infants exposed to some SSRIs. According to the manufacturer, the decision to continue or discontinue breast-feeding during therapy should take into account the risk of exposure to the infant and the benefits of treatment to the mother. Maternal use of an SSRI during pregnancy may cause delayed milk secretion. Escitalopram is the S-enantiomer of the racemic derivative citalopram; also refer to the Citalopram monograph.

Medication Guide Available Yes

Contraindications Hypersensitivity to escitalopram, citalopram, or any component of the formulation; use of MAO inhibitors intended to treat psychiatric disorders (concurrently or within 14 days of discontinuing either escitalopram or the MAO inhibitor); initiation of escitalopram in a patient receiving linezolid or intravenous methylene blue

Canadian labeling: Additional contraindications (not in U.S. labeling): Known QT-interval prolongation or congenital long QT syndrome

Warnings/Precautions [U.S. Boxed Warning]: Antidepressants increase the risk of suicidal thinking and behavior in children, adolescents, and young adults (18-24 years of age) with major depressive disorder (MDD) and other psychiatric disorders; consider risk prior to prescribing. Short-term studies did not show an increased risk in patients >24 years of age and showed a decreased risk in patients ≥65 years. Closely monitor patients for clinical worsening, suicidality, or unusual changes in behavior, particularly during the initial 1-2 months of therapy or during periods of dosage adjustments (increases or decreases); the patient's family or caregiver should be instructed to closely observe the patient and communicate condition with healthcare provider. A medication guide concerning the use of antidepressants should be dispensed with each prescription. **Escitalopram is not FDA approved for use in children <12 years of age.**

The possibility of a suicide attempt is inherent in major depression and may persist until remission occurs. Use caution in high-risk patients. Worsening depression and severe abrupt suicidality that are not part of the presenting symptoms may require discontinuation or modification of drug therapy. The patient's family or caregiver should be alerted to monitor patients for the emergence of suicidality and associated behaviors (such as agitation, irritability, hostility, impulsivity, and hypomania) and call healthcare provider.

May worsen psychosis in some patients or precipitate a shift to mania or hypomania in patients with bipolar disorder. Patients presenting with depressive symptoms should be screened for bipolar disorder. Monotherapy in patients with bipolar disorder should be avoided. Escitalopram is not FDA approved for the treatment of bipolar depression.

Potentially life-threatening serotonin syndrome (SS) has occurred with serotonergic agents (eg, SSRIs, SNRIs), particularly when used in combination with other serotonergic agents (eg, triptans, TCAs, fentanyl, lithium, tramadol, buspirone, St John's wort, tryptophan) or agents that impair metabolism of serotonin (eg, MAO inhibitors intended to treat psychiatric disorders, other MAO inhibitors [ie, linezolid and intravenous methylene blue]). Discontinue treatment (and any concomitant serotonergic agent) immediately if signs/symptoms arise. May increase the risks associated with electroconvulsive therapy. Has a low potential to impair cognitive or motor performance; caution operating hazardous machinery or driving. Bone fractures have been associated with antidepressant treatment. Consider the possibility of a fragility fracture if an antidepressant-treated patient presents with unexplained bone pain, point tenderness, swelling, or bruising (Rabenda, 2013; Rizzoli, 2012).

Use with caution in patients with a recent history of MI or unstable heart disease. Use has been associated with dose-dependent QT-interval prolongation with doses of 10 mg and 30 mg/day in healthy subjects (mean change from baseline: 4.3 msec and 10.7 msec, respectively); prolongation of QT interval and ventricular arrhythmia (including torsade de pointes) have been reported, particularly in females with pre-existing QT prolongation or other risk factors (eg, hypokalemia, other cardiac disease).

Use caution with a previous seizure disorder or condition predisposing to seizures such as brain damage, alcoholism, or concurrent therapy with other drugs which lower the seizure threshold. May cause hyponatremia/SIADH (elderly at increased risk); volume depletion (diuretics may increase risk) may occur. Use caution in patients with metabolic disease. May cause or exacerbate sexual dysfunction. Use caution in elderly patients; may cause or exacerbate syndrome of inappropriate antidiuretic hormone secretion or hyponatremia; monitor sodium closely with initiation or dosage adjustments in older adults (Beers Criteria). Bioavailability and half-life are increased by 50% in the elderly. Use caution with severe renal impairment or liver impairment; concomitant CNS depressants. Use with caution in patients who are hemodynamically unstable. UPotentially significant interactions may exist, requiring dose or frequency adjustment, additional monitoring, and/or selection of alternative therapy. Consult drug interactions database for more detailed information.

Abrupt discontinuation or interruption of antidepressant therapy has been associated with a discontinuation syndrome. Symptoms arising may vary with antidepressant however commonly include nausea, vomiting, diarrhea, headaches, light-headedness, dizziness, diminished appetite, sweating, chills, tremors, paresthesias, fatigue, somnolence, and sleep disturbances (eg, vivid dreams, insomnia). Greater risks for developing a discontinuation syndrome have been associated with antidepressants with shorter half-lives, longer durations of treatment, and abrupt discontinuation. For antidepressants of short or intermediate half-lives, symptoms may emerge within 2-5 days after treatment discontinuation and last 7-14 days (APA, 2010; Fava, 2006; Haddad, 2001; Shelton, 2001; Warner, 2006).

Adverse Reactions

>10%:

Central nervous system: Headache (24%), somnolence (4% to 13%), insomnia (7% to 12%)

Gastrointestinal: Diarrhea (6% to 14%), nausea (15% to 18%)

Genitourinary: Ejaculation disorder (9% to 14%)

1% to 10%:

Central nervous system: Fatigue (2% to 8%), dizziness (4% to 7%), abnormal dreaming (3%), lethargy (3%), yawning (2%)

Endocrine & metabolic: Libido decreased (3% to 7%), anorgasmia (2% to 6%), menstrual disorder (2%)

Gastrointestinal: Xerostomia (4% to 9%), constipation (3% to 6%), indigestion (2% to 6%), appetite decreased (3%), vomiting (3%), abdominal pain (2%), flatulence (2%), toothache (2%)

Genitourinary: Impotence (2% to 3%), urinary tract infection (children ≥2%)

Neuromuscular & skeletal: Neck/shoulder pain (3%), back pain (children ≥2%), paresthesia (2%)

Respiratory: Rhinitis (5%), sinusitis (3%), nasal congestion (children ≥2%)

Miscellaneous: Diaphoresis (3% to 8%), flu-like syndrome (5%)

<1% (Limited to important or life-threatening): Abdominal cramps, acute renal failure, aggression, agitation, agranulocytosis, akathisia, allergic reaction, allergy, alopecia, amnesia, anaphylaxis, anemia, angioedema, anxiety, apathy, aplastic anemia, appetite increased, arthralgia, ataxia, atrial fibrillation, bilirubin increased, blurred vision, bradycardia, bronchitis, cardiac failure, cerebrovascular accident, chest pain, choreoathetosis, concentration impaired delirium, delusion, depersonalization, depression aggravated, dermatitis, diabetes mellitus, diplopia, DVT, dyskinesia, dysphagia, dyspnea, dystonia, dysuria, ecchymosis, edema, epistaxis, erythema multiforme, extrapyramidal symptoms, fever, flushing, gait abnormal, gastroenteritis, GERD, GI hemorrhage, glaucoma, hallucination, heartburn, hemolytic anemia, hepatic necrosis, hepatitis, hot flashes, hypercholesterolemia, hyper-/hypoglycemia, hypertensive crisis, hypertension, hypoesthesia, hypokalemia, hyponatremia, hypotension, INR increased, irritability, jaw stiffness, leukopenia, lightheadedness, limb pain, liver enzymes increased, liver failure, menorrhagia, menstrual cramps, migraine, muscle weakness, myalgia, mydriasis, myocardial infarction, myoclonus, nasal congestion, neuroleptic malignant syndrome, nightmares, nystagmus, orthostasis, palpitation, pancreatitis, panic reaction, paranoia, Parkinsonism, phlebitis, photosensitivity, priapism, prolactinemia, prothrombin decreased, psychosis, pulmonary embolism, QT prolonged, rash, rectal hemorrhage, rhabdomyolysis, seizures, serotonin syndrome, SIADH, sinus congestion, sinus headache, spontaneous abortion, Stevens-Johnson syndrome, suicidal tendency, suicide attempt, syncope, tachycardia, tardive dyskinesia, thrombocytopenia, thrombocytopenic purpura (idiopathic), thrombosis, tinnitus, torsade de pointes, toxic epidermal necrolysis, tremor, urinary frequency, urinary retention, urticaria, ventricular arrhythmia, ventricular tachycardia, vertigo, visual disturbance, withdrawal syndrome

Drug Interactions

Metabolism/Transport Effects Substrate of CYP2C19 (major), CYP3A4 (major); **Note:** Assignment of Major/ Minor substrate status based on clinically relevant drug interaction potential; **Inhibits** CYP2D6 (weak)

Avoid Concomitant Use

Avoid concomitant use of Escitalopram with any of the following: Conivaptan; Dosulepin; Fusidic Acid (Systemic); Highest Risk QTc-Prolonging Agents; Iobenguane I 123; Ivabradine; Linezolid; MAO Inhibitors; Methylene Blue; Mifepristone; Moderate Risk QTc-Prolonging Agents; Pimozide; Tryptophan

Increased Effect/Toxicity

Escitalopram may increase the levels/effects of: Agents with Antiplatelet Properties; Anticoagulants; Antidepressants (Serotonin Reuptake Inhibitor/Antagonist); Antipsychotics; Aspirin; BusPIRone; CarBAMazepine; CloZAPine; Collagenase (Systemic); Dabigatran Etexilate; Desmopressin; Dextromethorphan; Dosulepin; Highest Risk QTc-Prolonging Agents; Hypoglycemic Agents; Ibritumomab; Methadone; Methylene Blue; Metoclopramide; Mexiletine; NSAID (COX-2 Inhibitor); NSAID (Nonselective); Pimozide; RisperiDONE; Rivaroxaban; Salicylates; Serotonin Modulators; Thiazide Diuretics; Thrombolytic Agents; Tositumomab and Iodine I 131 Tositumomab; TraMADol; Tricyclic Antidepressants; Vitamin K Antagonists

The levels/effects of Escitalopram may be increased by: Alcohol (Ethyl); Analgesics (Opioid); Antipsychotics; BusPIRone; Cimetidine; CNS Depressants; Cobicistat; Conivaptan; CYP2C19 Inhibitors (Moderate); CYP2C19 Inhibitors (Strong); CYP3A4 Inhibitors (Moderate); CYP3A4 Inhibitors (Strong); Dasatinib; Fusidic Acid (Systemic); Glucosamine; Herbs (Anticoagulant/Antiplatelet Properties); Ibrutinib; Ivabradine; Ivacaftor; Linezolid; Lithium; Luliconazole; Macrolide Antibiotics; MAO Inhibitors; Metoclopramide; Metyrosine; Mifepristone; Moderate Risk QTc-Prolonging Agents; Multivitamins/Fluoride (with ADE); Multivitamins/Minerals (with ADEK, Folate, Iron); Multivitamins/Minerals (with AE, No Iron); Omega-3 Fatty Acids; Omeprazole; Pentosan Polysulfate Sodium; Pentoxifylline; Prostacyclin Analogues; QTc-Prolonging Agents (Indeterminate Risk and Risk Modifying); Tipranavir; TraMADol; Tricyclic Antidepressants; Tryptophan; Vitamin E

Decreased Effect

Escitalopram may decrease the levels/effects of: Iobenguane I 123; Ioflupane I 123; Simeprevir; Thyroid Products

The levels/effects of Escitalopram may be decreased by: Boceprevir; Bosentan; CarBAMazepine; CYP2C19 Inducers (Strong); CYP3A4 Inducers (Strong); Cyproheptadine; Dabrafenib; Deferasirox; Mitotane; NSAID (COX-2 Inhibitor); NSAID (Nonselective); Telaprevir; Tocilizumab

Ethanol/Nutrition/Herb Interactions

Ethanol: May increase CNS depression; monitor for increased effects with coadministration. Caution patients about effects.

Herb/Nutraceutical: Avoid valerian, St John's wort, tryptophan, SAMe, kava kava, and gotu kola (may increase CNS depression and/or increase risk of serotonin syndrome).

Storage/Stability Store at 25°C (77°F); excursions permitted to 15°C to 30°C (59°F to 86°F).

Mechanism of Action Escitalopram is the S-enantiomer of the racemic derivative citalopram, which selectively inhibits the reuptake of serotonin with little to no effect on norepinephrine or dopamine reuptake. It has no or very low affinity for 5-HT_{1-7}, alpha- and beta-adrenergic, D_{1-5}, H_{1-3}, M_{1-5}, and benzodiazepine receptors. Escitalopram does not bind to or has low affinity for Na^+, K^+, Cl^-, and Ca^{++} ion channels.

Pharmacodynamics/Kinetics

Onset of action: Depression: The onset of action is within a week; however, individual response varies greatly and full response may not be seen until 8-12 weeks after initiation of treatment.

Distribution: V_d: ~20 L/kg (Søgaard, 2005)

Protein binding: ~56% to plasma proteins

Metabolism: Hepatic via CYP2C19 and 3A4 to S-desmethylcitalopram (S-DCT); S-DCT is metabolized to S-didesmethylcitalopram (S-DDCT) via CYP2D6; *in vitro* data suggest metabolites do not contribute significantly to the antidepressant effects of escitalopram

Half-life elimination: ~27-32 hours (increased ~50% in the elderly and doubled in patients with hepatic impairment)

Time to peak: Escitalopram: ~5 hours

Excretion: Urine (8% as unchanged drug; S-DCT 10%)

Dosage Oral:

U.S. labeling:

Children ≥12 years: Major depressive disorder: Initial: 10 mg once daily; dose may be increased to a maximum of 20 mg once daily after at least 3 weeks

Adults: Major depressive disorder, generalized anxiety disorder: Initial: 10 mg once daily; dose may be increased to a maximum of 20 mg once daily after at least 1 week

Elderly: 10 mg once daily

Canadian labeling:

Adults: Major depressive disorder, generalized anxiety disorder (GAD), obsessive compulsive disorder (OCD): Initial: 10 mg once daily (may consider 5 mg once daily where sensitivity is a concern); dose may be increased as tolerated to a maximum of 20 mg once daily. Patients with GAD or OCD who require extended therapy should be maintained at the lowest effective dose and assessed periodically to determine the need for continued therapy. **Note:** Initiate treatment in poor CYP2C19 metabolizers at a dose of 5 mg once daily; may increase dose to a maximum of 10 mg once daily.

Elderly: Initial: 5 mg once daily; dose may be increased as tolerated to a maximum of 10 mg once daily

Unlabeled use: Adults: Vasomotor symptoms associated with menopause: Initial: 10 mg once daily, increase to 20 mg once daily after 4 weeks if symptoms not adequately controlled (Carpenter, 2012; Freeman, 2011).

Discontinuation of therapy: Upon discontinuation of antidepressant therapy, gradually taper the dose to minimize the incidence of withdrawal symptoms and allow for the detection of re-emerging symptoms. Evidence supporting ideal taper rates is limited. APA and NICE guidelines suggest tapering therapy over at least several weeks with consideration to the half-life of the antidepressant; antidepressants with a shorter half-life may need to be tapered more conservatively. In addition for long-term treated patients, WFSBP guidelines recommend tapering over 4-6 months. If intolerable withdrawal symptoms occur following a dose reduction, consider resuming the previously prescribed dose and/or decrease dose at a more gradual rate (APA, 2010; Bauer, 2002; Haddad, 2001; NCCMH, 2010; Schatzberg, 2006; Shelton, 2001; Warner, 2006).

MAO inhibitor recommendations: *U.S. labeling:*

Switching to or from an MAO inhibitor intended to treat psychiatric disorders:

Allow 14 days to elapse between discontinuing an MAO inhibitor intended to treat psychiatric disorders and initiation of escitalopram.

Allow 14 days to elapse between discontinuing escitalopram and initiation of an MAO inhibitor intended to treat psychiatric disorders.

Use with other MAO inhibitors (linezolid or I.V. methylene blue):

Do not initiate escitalopram in patients receiving linezolid or I.V. methylene blue; consider other interventions for psychiatric condition.

If urgent treatment with linezolid or I.V. methylene blue is required in a patient already receiving escitalopram and potential benefits outweigh potential risks, discontinue escitalopram promptly and administer linezolid or I.V. methylene blue. Monitor for serotonin syndrome for 2 weeks or until 24 hours after the last dose of linezolid or I.V. methylene blue, whichever comes first. May resume escitalopram 24 hours after the last dose of linezolid or I.V. methylene blue.

Dosage adjustment with concomitant medications: *Canadian labeling:* Escitalopram dose should not exceed 10 mg once daily in patients taking omeprazole or cimetidine.

Dosage adjustment in renal impairment:

Mild-to-moderate impairment: No dosage adjustment is necessary

Severe impairment: Cl_{cr} <20 mL/minute (U.S. labeling) or Cl_{cr} <30 mL/minute (Canadian labeling): Use with caution.

Dosage adjustment in hepatic impairment:

U.S. labeling: 10 mg once daily

Canadian labeling:

Mild or moderate impairment (Child-Pugh class A or B): Initial: 5 mg once daily; dose may be increased as tolerated to 10 mg once daily (maximum dose)

Severe Impairment (Child-Pugh class C): No dosage adjustment provided in manufacturer's labeling; has not been studied. Use with caution.

Dietary Considerations May be taken with or without food.

Administration Administer once daily (morning or evening), with or without food.

Monitoring Parameters Mental status for depression, suicidal ideation (especially at the beginning of therapy or when doses are increased or decreased), anxiety, social functioning, mania, panic attacks; akathisia; signs/symptoms of serotonin syndrome

Additional Information The tablet and oral solution dosage forms are bioequivalent. Clinically, escitalopram 20 mg is equipotent to citalopram 40 mg. Do not coadminister with citalopram.

Dosage Forms Excipient information presented when available (limited, particularly for generics); consult specific product labeling.

Solution, Oral:

Lexapro: 5 mg/5 mL (240 mL) [contains methylparaben, propylene glycol, propylparaben; peppermint flavor]

Generic: 5 mg/5 mL (240 mL)

Tablet, Oral:

Lexapro: 5 mg

Lexapro: 10 mg, 20 mg [scored]

Generic: 5 mg, 10 mg, 20 mg

Dosage Forms: Canada Excipient information presented when available (limited, particularly for generics); consult specific product labeling.

Tablet:

Cipralex®: 10 mg, 20 mg

◆ **Escitalopram Oxalate** *see* Escitalopram *on page 745*

◆ **Eserine Salicylate** *see* Physostigmine *on page 1643*

◆ **Esgic** *see* Butalbital, Acetaminophen, and Caffeine *on page 305*

◆ **Esgic-Plus** *see* Butalbital, Acetaminophen, and Caffeine *on page 305*

◆ **Eskalith** *see* Lithium *on page 1229*

Esmolol (ES moe lol)

Brand Names: U.S. Brevibloc; Brevibloc in NaCl

Brand Names: Canada Brevibloc®; Brevibloc® Premixed

Index Terms Esmolol Hydrochloride

Pharmacologic Category Antiarrhythmic Agent, Class II; Antihypertensive; Beta-Blocker, Beta-1 Selective

Additional Appendix Information

Beta-Blockers *on page 2294*

Dosing Considerations for the Critically-Ill Patient With Morbid Obesity *on page 2379*

Use Treatment of supraventricular tachycardia (SVT) and atrial fibrillation/flutter (control ventricular rate); treatment of intraoperative and postoperative tachycardia and/or hypertension; treatment of noncompensatory sinus tachycardia

Unlabeled Use

Children: SVT and postoperative hypertension

Adults: Arrhythmia/rate control during acute coronary syndrome (eg, acute myocardial infarction, unstable angina), aortic dissection, intubation, thyroid storm, pheochromocytoma, electroconvulsive therapy

Pregnancy Risk Factor C

Pregnancy Considerations Adverse events were observed in some animal reproduction studies. Esmolol has been shown to decrease fetal heart rate. Adverse fetal/neonatal events have also been observed with the chronic use of beta-blockers during pregnancy. Esmolol is a short-acting beta-blocker and not indicated for the chronic treatment of hypertension. Esmolol may be considered for the acute management of atrial fibrillation in pregnant women (Fuster, 2006). Esmolol has been evaluated for use during intubation as an agent to offset the exaggerated pressor response observed in pregnant women with hypertension undergoing surgery (Bansal, 2002).

Breast-Feeding Considerations It is not known if esmolol is excreted into breast milk. Due to the potential for serious adverse reactions in the nursing infant, the manufacturer recommends a decision be made whether to discontinue nursing or to discontinue the drug, taking into account the importance of treatment to the mother. The short half-life and the fact that it is not intended for chronic use should limit any potential exposure to the nursing infant.

Contraindications Hypersensitivity to esmolol or any component of the formulation; severe sinus bradycardia; heart block greater than first degree (except in patients with a functioning artificial ventricular pacemaker); sick sinus syndrome; cardiogenic shock; decompensated heart failure; I.V. administration of calcium channel blockers (eg, verapamil) in close proximity to esmolol (ie, while effects of other drug are still present); pulmonary hypertension

Canadian labeling: Additional contraindications (not in U.S. labeling): Patients requiring inotropic agents and/or vasopressors to maintain cardiac output and systolic blood pressure; hypotension; right ventricular failure secondary to pulmonary hypertension; untreated pheochromocytoma

Warnings/Precautions Can cause bradycardia including sinus pause, heart block, severe bradycardia, and cardiac arrest. Consider pre-existing conditions such as first degree AV block, sick sinus syndrome, or other conduction disorders before initiating; use is contraindicated in patients with sick sinus syndrome or second- or third-degree AV block (except in patients with a functioning artificial ventricular pacemaker). Bradycardia may be observed more frequently in elderly patients (>65 years of age); dosage reductions may be necessary. Hypotension is common; patients need close blood pressure monitoring. If an unacceptable drop in blood pressure occurs, reduction in dose or discontinuation may reverse hypotension (usually within 30 minutes). Avoid use in patients with hypovolemia; treat hypovolemia first, otherwise, use of esmolol may attenuate reflex tachycardia and further increase the risk of hypotension. Administer cautiously in compensated heart failure and monitor for a worsening of the condition; use is contraindicated in patients with decompensated heart failure.

Esmolol has been associated with elevations in serum potassium and development of hyperkalemia especially in patients with risk factors (eg, renal impairment); monitor serum potassium during therapy. Use with caution in patients with myasthenia gravis. Use caution in patients with renal dysfunction (active metabolite retained). Adequate alpha-blockade is required prior to use of any beta-blocker for patients with untreated pheochromocytoma; Canadian labeling contraindicates use in this patient population. Use beta-blockers cautiously in patients with bronchospastic disease; monitor pulmonary status closely. Use cautiously in patients with diabetes because it can mask prominent hypoglycemic symptoms. May mask signs of hyperthyroidism (eg, tachycardia); if hyperthyroidism is suspected, carefully manage and monitor; abrupt withdrawal may exacerbate symptoms of hyperthyroidism or precipitate thyroid storm. Use esmolol with caution in patients with hypertension associated with hypothermia; monitor vital signs closely and titrate esmolol slowly. Use caution with history of severe anaphylaxis to allergens; patients taking beta-blockers may become more sensitive to repeated challenges. Treatment of anaphylaxis (eg, epinephrine) in patients taking beta-blockers may be ineffective or promote undesirable effects. Can precipitate or aggravate symptoms of arterial insufficiency in patients with PVD and Raynaud's disease; use with caution and monitor for progression of arterial obstruction.

Use caution with concurrent use of digoxin, verapamil or diltiazem; bradycardia or heart block can occur (may be fatal). Use is contraindicated when I.V. calcium channel blockers have been administered in close proximity to esmolol (ie, while effects of other drug are still present). Beta-blocker therapy should not be withdrawn abruptly (particularly in patients with CAD), but gradually tapered to avoid acute tachycardia, hypertension, and/or ischemia. Vesicant; ensure proper needle or catheter placement prior to and during infusion; avoid extravasation. Extravasation can lead to skin necrosis and sloughing; avoid infusions into small veins or through a butterfly catheter.

Adverse Reactions

>10%: Cardiovascular: Blood pressure decreased (20% to 50%), asymptomatic hypotension (dose related: 25%), symptomatic hypotension (dose related: 12%)

1% to 10%:

- Cardiovascular: Peripheral ischemia (1%)
- Central nervous system: Dizziness (3%), somnolence (3%), confusion (2%), headache (2%), agitation (2%)
- Gastrointestinal: Nausea (7%), vomiting (1%)
- Local: Infusion site reaction (8%; including irritation, inflammation, and severe reactions associated with extravasation [eg, thrombophlebitis, necrosis, and blistering])

<1% (Limited to important or life-threatening): Abdominal discomfort, abnormal thinking, angioedema, anorexia, anxiety, bradycardia, bronchospasm, cardiac arrest, constipation, coronary arteriospasm, decompensated heart failure, depression, dyspepsia, flushing, heart block, hyperkalemia, lightheadedness, pallor, paresthesia, psoriasis, renal tubular acidosis, seizure, severe bradycardia/asystole (rare), syncope, urinary retention, urticaria, xerostomia

Drug Interactions

Metabolism/Transport Effects None known.

Avoid Concomitant Use

Avoid concomitant use of Esmolol with any of the following: Floctafenine; Methacholine

Increased Effect/Toxicity

Esmolol may increase the levels/effects of: Alpha-/Beta-Agonists (Direct-Acting); Alpha1-Blockers; Alpha2-Agonists; Amifostine; Antihypertensives; Antipsychotic Agents (Phenothiazines); Bupivacaine; Cardiac Glycosides; Cholinergic Agonists; Ergot Derivatives; Fingolimod; Hypotensive Agents; Insulin; Lidocaine (Systemic); Lidocaine (Topical); Mepivacaine; Methacholine; Midodrine; Obinutuzumab; RiTUXimab; Sulfonylureas

The levels/effects of Esmolol may be increased by: Acetylcholinesterase Inhibitors; Alpha2-Agonists; Aminoquinolines (Antimalarial); Amiodarone; Anilidopiperidine Opioids; Antipsychotic Agents (Phenothiazines); Brimonidine (Topical); Calcium Channel Blockers (Dihydropyridine); Calcium Channel Blockers (Nondihydropyridine); Diazoxide; Dipyridamole; Disopyramide; Dronedarone; Floctafenine; Herbs (Hypotensive Properties); MAO Inhibitors; Pentoxifylline; Phosphodiesterase 5 Inhibitors; Propafenone; Prostacyclin Analogues; Regorafenib; Reserpine

Decreased Effect

Esmolol may decrease the levels/effects of: Beta2-Agonists; Theophylline Derivatives

The levels/effects of Esmolol may be decreased by: Barbiturates; Herbs (Hypertensive Properties); Methylphenidate; Nonsteroidal Anti-Inflammatory Agents; Rifamycin Derivatives; Yohimbine

Storage/Stability Clear, colorless to light yellow solution which should be stored at 25°C (77°F); excursions permitted to 15°C to 30°C (59°F to 86°F); do not freeze. Protect from excessive heat.

Mechanism of Action Class II antiarrhythmic: Competitively blocks response to $beta_1$-adrenergic stimulation with little or no effect of $beta_2$-receptors except at high doses, no intrinsic sympathomimetic activity, no membrane stabilizing activity

Pharmacodynamics/Kinetics

- Onset of action: Beta-blockade: I.V.: 2-10 minutes (quickest when loading doses are administered)
- Duration of hemodynamic effects: 10-30 minutes; prolonged following higher cumulative doses, extended duration of use
- Distribution: V_d: Esmolol: ~3.4 L/kg; Acid metabolite: ~0.4 L/kg
- Protein binding: Esmolol: 55%; Acid metabolite: 10%
- Metabolism: In blood by red blood cell esterases; forms acid metabolite (negligible activity; produces no clinically important effects) and methanol (does not achieve concentrations associated with methanol toxicity)
- Half-life elimination: Adults: Esmolol: 9 minutes; Acid metabolite: 3.7 hours; elimination of metabolite decreases with end-stage renal disease
- Excretion: Urine (~73% to 88% as acid metabolite, <2% unchanged drug)

Dosage I.V.: Adults:

U.S. labeling:

Intraoperative and postoperative tachycardia and/or hypertension:

Immediate control: Initial bolus: 1 **mg**/kg over 30 seconds, followed by a 150 mcg/kg/minute infusion, if necessary. Adjust infusion rate as needed to maintain desired heart rate and/or blood pressure (up to 300 mcg/kg/minute)

Gradual control: Initial bolus: 0.5 **mg**/kg over 1 minute, followed by a 50 mcg/kg/minute infusion for 4 minutes. Infusion may be continued at 50 mcg/kg/minute or, if the response is inadequate, titrated upward in 50 mcg/kg/minute increments (increased no more frequently than every 4 minutes) to a maximum of 300 mcg/kg/minute; may administer an optional loading dose equal to the initial bolus (0.5 **mg**/kg over 1 minute) prior to each increase in infusion rate.

For control of tachycardia, doses >200 mcg/kg/minute provide minimal additional effect. *For control of postoperative hypertension,* as many as one-third of patients may require higher doses (250-300 mcg/kg/minute) to control blood pressure; the safety of doses >300 mcg/kg/minute has not been studied.

Supraventricular tachycardia (SVT) or noncompensatory sinus tachycardia: Loading dose (optional): 0.5 **mg**/kg over 1 minute; follow with a 50 mcg/kg/minute infusion for 4 minutes; response to this initial infusion rate may be a rough indication of the responsiveness of the ventricular rate.

Infusion may be continued at 50 mcg/kg/minute or, if the response is inadequate, titrated upward in 50 mcg/kg/minute increments (increased no more frequently than every 4 minutes) to a maximum of 200 mcg/kg/minute.

To achieve more rapid response, following the initial loading dose and 50 mcg/kg/minute infusion, rebolus with a second 0.5 **mg**/kg loading dose over 1 minute, and increase the maintenance infusion to 100 mcg/kg/minute for 4 minutes. If necessary, a third (and final) 0.5 **mg**/kg loading dose may be administered, prior to increasing to an infusion rate of 150 mcg/kg/minute. After 4 minutes of the 150 mcg/kg/minute infusion, the infusion rate may be increased to a maximum rate of 200 mcg/kg/minute (without a bolus dose).

Note: If a loading dose is not administered, a continuous infusion at a fixed dose reaches steady-state in ~30 minutes. In general, the usual effective dose is 50-200 mcg/kg/minute; doses as low as 25 mcg/kg/minute may be adequate. Maintenance infusions may be continued for up to 48 hours.

Acute coronary syndromes (when relative contraindications to beta-blockade exist; unlabeled use): 0.5 **mg**/kg over 1 minute; follow with a 50 mcg/kg/minute infusion; if tolerated and response inadequate, may titrate upward in 50 mcg/kg/minute increments every 5-15 minutes to a maximum of 300 mcg/kg/minute (Mitchell, 2002); an additional bolus (0.5 **mg**/kg over 1 minute) may be administered prior to each increase in infusion rate (Mooss, 1994)

Electroconvulsive therapy (unlabeled use): 1 **mg**/kg administered 1 minute prior to induction of anesthesia (Weinger, 1991)

Intubation (unlabeled use): 1-2 **mg**/kg given 1.5-3 minutes prior to intubation (Kindler, 1996)

Thyrotoxicosis or thyroid storm (unlabeled use): 50-100 mcg/kg/minute (Bahn, 2011)

Canadian labeling: **Note:** Not recommended for use >24 hours.

Perioperative tachycardia and/or hypertension:

Associated with intubation (unlabeled use): Bolus: 1.5 **mg**/kg (maximum dose: 100 **mg**) over 30 seconds given 1-2 minutes prior to intubation.

Intraoperative/postoperative tachycardia and/or hypertension: Initial bolus: 1.5 **mg**/kg (maximum dose: 100 **mg**) over 30 seconds, followed by 150 mcg/kg/minute infusion. Adjust infusion rate as needed to maintain desired heart rate or blood pressure (up to 300 mcg/kg/minute).

Atrial fibrillation/atrial flutter:

Loading dose: 0.5 **mg**/kg over 1 minute; follow with a 50 mcg/kg/minute infusion for 4 minutes; response to this initial infusion rate may be a rough indication of the responsiveness of the ventricular rate.

Infusion may be continued at 50 mcg/kg/minute or, if the response is inadequate, rebolus with a second 0.5 **mg**/kg loading dose over 1 minute, and increase the maintenance infusion to 100 mcg/kg/minute for 4 minutes. If necessary, repeat same procedure (ie, 0.5 **mg**/kg loading dose and increase maintenance infusion by 50 mcg/kg/minute for 4 minutes) until target heart rate or safety end point (eg, hypotension) begins to occur then omit subsequent loading dose and decrease dosing increment of maintenance infusion to ≤25 mcg/kg/minute or alternatively, the manufacturer labeling suggests that the titration interval may be extended from 5 minutes to 10 minutes. If safety endpoints are exceeded discontinue infusion and when appropriate, resume infusion at reduced dose.

Note: In general, the usual effective dose is 50-200 mcg/kg/minute; doses as low as 25 mcg/kg/minute may be adequate.

Guidelines for transfer to oral therapy (beta-blocker, calcium channel blocker):

Infusion should be reduced by 50% thirty minutes following the first dose of the alternative agent

Manufacturer suggests following the second dose of the alternative drug, patient's response should be monitored and if control is adequate for the first hour, esmolol may be discontinued.

Dosage adjustment in renal impairment: No dosage adjustment necessary. Dialysis: Not removed by hemo- or peritoneal dialysis; supplemental dose is not necessary.

Dosage adjustment in hepatic impairment: No dosage adjustment necessary

Usual Infusion Concentrations: Pediatric Note: Premixed solutions available.

I.V. infusion: 10,000 **mcg**/mL or 20,000 **mcg**/mL

Usual Infusion Concentrations: Adult Note: Premixed solutions available.

I.V. infusion: 2500 mg in 250 mL (concentration: 10,000 **mcg**/mL) **or** 2000 mg in 100 mL (concentration: 20,000 **mcg**/mL) of D_5W or NS

Administration I.V.: Loading doses (eg, 0.5 **mg**/kg) may be administered over 30 seconds to 1 minute depending on how urgent the need for effect. Infusion into small veins or through a butterfly catheter should be avoided (can cause thrombophlebitis). Medication port of premixed bags should be used to withdraw only the initial bolus, if necessary (not to be used for withdrawal of additional bolus doses).

Vesicant; ensure proper needle or catheter placement prior to and during infusion; avoid extravasation.

Extravasation management: If extravasation occurs, stop infusion immediately and disconnect (leave cannula/needle in place); gently aspirate extravasated solution (do **NOT** flush the line); remove needle/cannula; elevate extremity.

Monitoring Parameters Blood pressure, MAP, heart rate, continuous ECG, respiratory rate, I.V. site; serum potassium (especially with renal impairment); consult individual institutional policies and procedures

Dosage Forms Excipient information presented when available (limited, particularly for generics); consult specific product labeling.

Solution, Intravenous, as hydrochloride:
- Brevibloc: 10 mg/mL (10 mL)
- Brevibloc in NaCl: 2000 mg (100 mL); 2500 mg (250 mL)
- Generic: 10 mg/mL (10 mL)

Solution, Intravenous, as hydrochloride [preservative free]:
- Generic: 10 mg/mL (10 mL); 100 mg/10 mL (10 mL)

◆ **Esmolol Hydrochloride** *see* Esmolol *on page 748*

Esomeprazole (es oh ME pray zol)

Brand Names: U.S. NexIUM; NexIUM I.V.

Brand Names: Canada Apo-Esomeprazole; Mylan-Esomeprazole; Nexium

Index Terms Esomeprazole Magnesium; Esomeprazole Sodium; Esomeprazole Strontium

Pharmacologic Category Proton Pump Inhibitor; Substituted Benzimidazole

Use

Oral: Esomeprazole magnesium, esomeprazole strontium: Short-term (4-8 weeks) treatment of erosive esophagitis; maintaining symptom resolution and healing of erosive esophagitis; short-term (4-8 weeks) treatment of symptomatic gastroesophageal reflux disease (GERD); as part of a multidrug regimen for *Helicobacter pylori* eradication in patients with duodenal ulcer disease (active or history of within the past 5 years); prevention of gastric ulcers associated with continuous NSAID therapy in patients at risk (age ≥60 years and/or history of gastric ulcer); long-term treatment of pathological hypersecretory conditions including Zollinger-Ellison syndrome

Canadian labeling: Additional use (not in U.S. labeling): Oral: Treatment of nonerosive reflux disease (NERD); treatment of NSAID-induced gastric ulcers

I.V.: Esomeprazole sodium: Short-term (≤10 days) treatment of gastroesophageal reflux disease (GERD) when oral therapy is not possible or appropriate

Unlabeled Use I.V.: Esomeprazole sodium: Prevention of recurrent peptic ulcer bleeding postendoscopy

Pregnancy Risk Factor B/C (product specific)

Pregnancy Considerations Adverse events were observed in some animal reproduction studies. An increased risk of hypospadias was reported following maternal use of proton pump inhibitors (PPIs) during pregnancy (Anderka, 2012), but this was based on a small number of exposures and the same association was not found in another study (Erichsen, 2012). An increased risk of major birth defects following maternal use of PPIs during pregnancy was not observed in an additional study (Pasternak, 2010). Esomeprazole is the s-isomer of omeprazole; refer to the omeprazole monograph for additional information. When treating GERD in pregnancy, PPIs may be used when clinically indicated (Katz, 2013).

Breast-Feeding Considerations Limited data indicate esomeprazole and strontium are excreted in breast milk. Esomeprazole is the s-isomer of omeprazole and omeprazole is excreted in breast milk; refer to the omeprazole monograph for additional information. Due to the potential for serious adverse reactions in the nursing infant, the manufacturer recommends a decision be made whether to discontinue nursing or to discontinue the drug, taking into account the importance of treatment to the mother.

Medication Guide Available Yes

Contraindications Hypersensitivity to esomeprazole, other substituted benzimidazole proton pump inhibitors, or any component of the formulation

Warnings/Precautions Use of proton pump inhibitors (PPIs) may increase the risk of gastrointestinal infections (eg, *Salmonella, Campylobacter*). Relief of symptoms does not preclude the presence of a gastric malignancy. Atrophic gastritis (by biopsy) has been noted with long-term omeprazole therapy; this may also occur with esomeprazole. No reports of enterochromaffin-like (ECL) cell carcinoids, dysplasia, or neoplasia have occurred. Use of PPIs may increase risk of CDAD, especially in hospitalized patients; consider CDAD diagnosis in patients with persistent diarrhea that does not improve. Use the lowest dose and shortest duration of PPI therapy appropriate for the condition being treated. Safety and efficacy of I.V. therapy >10 days have not been established; transition from I.V. to oral therapy as soon possible. Bioavailability may be increased in Asian populations, the elderly, and patients with hepatic dysfunction. Decreased *H. pylori* eradication rates have been observed with short-term (≤7 days) combination therapy. The American College of Gastroenterology recommends 10-14 days of therapy (triple or quadruple) for eradication of *H. pylori* (Chey, 2007).

PPIs may diminish the therapeutic effect of clopidogrel, thought to be due to reduced formation of the active metabolite of clopidogrel. The manufacturer of clopidogrel recommends either avoidance of both omeprazole (even when scheduled 12 hours apart) and esomeprazole or use of a PPI with comparatively less effect on the active metabolite of clopidogrel (eg, pantoprazole). In contrast to these warnings, others have recommended the continued use of PPIs, regardless of the degree of inhibition, in patients with a history of GI bleeding or multiple risk factors for GI bleeding who are also receiving clopidogrel since no evidence has established clinically meaningful differences in outcome; however, a clinically-significant interaction cannot be excluded in those who are poor metabolizers of clopidogrel (Abraham, 2010; Levine, 2011). Additionally, potentially significant drug-drug interactions may exist, requiring dose or frequency adjustment, additional monitoring, and/or selection of alternative therapy.

Increased incidence of osteoporosis-related bone fractures of the hip, spine, or wrist may occur with PPI therapy. Patients on high-dose or long-term therapy should be monitored. Use the lowest effective dose for the shortest duration of time, use vitamin D and calcium supplementation, and follow appropriate guidelines to reduce risk of fractures in patients at risk.

Hypomagnesemia, reported rarely, usually with prolonged PPI use of >3 months (most cases >1 year of therapy); may be symptomatic or asymptomatic; severe cases may cause tetany, seizures, and cardiac arrhythmias. Consider obtaining serum magnesium concentrations prior to beginning long-term therapy, especially if taking concomitant digoxin, diuretics, or other drugs known to cause hypomagnesemia; and periodically thereafter. Hypomagnesemia may be corrected by magnesium supplementation, although discontinuation of esomeprazole may be necessary; magnesium levels typically return to normal within 1 week of stopping. Serum chromogranin A levels may be increased if assessed while patient on esomeprazole; may lead to diagnostic errors related to neuroendocrine tumors.

Severe liver dysfunction may require dosage reductions. Dosage adjustments are not necessary for any degree of renal impairment when using esomeprazole magnesium or esomeprazole sodium; however, since pharmacokinetics of the strontium may be reduced in mild to moderate renal impairment, esomeprazole strontium is not recommended for use in severe impairment (has not been studied). Esomeprazole strontium competes with calcium for intestinal absorption and is incorporated into bone; use of esomeprazole strontium in pediatric patients is not recommended.

Adverse Reactions Unless otherwise specified, percentages represent adverse reactions identified in clinical trials evaluating the oral formulation.

>10%: Central nervous system: Headache (I.V. 11%; oral 2% to 8%)

1% to 10%:

Central nervous system: Dizziness (I.V. 3%; oral <1%), somnolence (adults <1%; children 2%)

Dermatologic: Pruritus (I.V. 1%; oral <1%)

Gastrointestinal: Flatulence (I.V. 10%; oral ≤5%), diarrhea (I.V. 4%; oral 2% to <7%), abdominal pain (I.V. 6%; oral 1% to ≤6%), nausea (I.V. 6%; oral 2% to ≤6%), xerostomia (I.V. 4%; oral 3%), constipation (I.V. 3%; oral 2%)

Local: Injection site reaction (I.V. 2%)

<1% (Limited to important or life-threatening): Aggression, agranulocytosis, alopecia, anaphylaxis, anemia, angioedema, anorexia, arthritis exacerbation, asthma exacerbation, benign polyps/nodules, blurred vision, carcinoid tumor of stomach, cervical lymphadenopathy, chest pain, *Clostridium difficile*-associated diarrhea (CDAD), conjunctivitis, creatinine increased, cystitis, depression, dermatitis, dysmenorrhea, epistaxis, erythema multiforme, fibromyalgia syndrome, fracture, fungal infection, gastroenteritis, GI candidiasis, GI dysplasia, goiter, gynecomastia, hallucinations, hematuria, hepatic encephalopathy, hepatic failure, hepatitis, hernia, hyperhidrosis, hyperparathyroidism, hypersensitivity reactions, hypertension, hypertonia, hyperuricemia, hypoesthesia, hypokalemia, hypomagnesemia, hyponatremia, impotence, insomnia, interstitial nephritis, jaundice, leukocytosis, leukopenia, microscopic colitis, migraine, moniliasis, osteoporosis-related fracture, otitis media, pancreatitis, pancytopenia, parosmia, phlebitis, photosensitivity, pneumonia, polymyalgia rheumatica, proteinuria, pruritus ani, rash (erythematous and maculo-papular), rigors, serum gastrin increased, Stevens-Johnson syndrome, stomatitis, tachycardia, thrombocytopenia, thrombophlebitis, thyroid-stimulating hormone increased, tinnitus, toxic epidermal necrolysis, tremor, vaginitis, vertigo, visual field defect, vitamin B_{12} deficiency, weight changes

Drug Interactions

Metabolism/Transport Effects Substrate of CYP2C19 (major), CYP3A4 (minor); **Note:** Assignment of Major/Minor substrate status based on clinically relevant drug interaction potential; **Inhibits** CYP2C19 (moderate)

Avoid Concomitant Use

Avoid concomitant use of Esomeprazole with any of the following: Clopidogrel; Dasatinib; Delavirdine; Erlotinib; Nelfinavir; PONATinib; Rifampin; Rilpivirine; Risedronate; St Johns Wort

Increased Effect/Toxicity

Esomeprazole may increase the levels/effects of: Amphetamines; Benzodiazepines (metabolized by oxidation); Cilostazol; Citalopram; CYP2C19 Substrates; Dexmethylphenidate; Methotrexate; Methylphenidate; Raltegravir; Risedronate; Saquinavir; Tacrolimus (Systemic); Vitamin K Antagonists; Voriconazole

The levels/effects of Esomeprazole may be increased by: Fluconazole; Ketoconazole (Systemic); Voriconazole

Decreased Effect

Esomeprazole may decrease the levels/effects of: Atazanavir; Bisphosphonate Derivatives; Bosutinib; Cefditoren; Clopidogrel; Dabigatran Etexilate; Dabrafenib; Dasatinib; Delavirdine; Erlotinib; Gefitinib; Indinavir; Iron Salts; Itraconazole; Ketoconazole (Systemic); Mesalamine; Multivitamins/Minerals (with ADEK, Folate, Iron); Mycophenolate; Nelfinavir; Nilotinib; PONATinib; Posaconazole; Rilpivirine; Riociguat; Risedronate; Vismodegib

The levels/effects of Esomeprazole may be decreased by: CYP2C19 Inducers (Strong); Dabrafenib; Rifampin; St Johns Wort; Tipranavir

Ethanol/Nutrition/Herb Interactions

Food: Absorption is decreased by 43% to 53% when taken with food. Management: Take at least 1 hour before meals at the same time each day, best if before breakfast.

Herb/Nutraceutical: St John's wort may decrease the efficacy of esomeprazole. Management: Avoid St John's wort.

Preparation for Administration

Granules for oral administration: Empty the 2.5 mg or 5 mg packet into a container with 5 mL of water or empty the 10 mg, 20 mg, or 40 mg packet into a container with 15 mL of water and stir; leave 2-3 minutes to thicken.

Powder for injection:

For I.V. injection: Adults: Reconstitute powder with 5 mL NS.

For I.V. infusion:

Children: Initially reconstitute powder (20 mg or 40 mg) with 5 mL of NS, then further dilute to a final volume of 50 mL; withdraw the appropriate amount of the final solution to administer the intended dose.

Adults: Initially reconstitute powder with 5 mL of NS, LR, or D_5W, then further dilute to a final volume of 50 mL.

Storage/Stability

Capsules: Keep container tightly closed.

Esomeprazole magnesium: Store at 25°C (77°F); excursions permitted to 15°C to 30°C (59°F to 86°F).

Esomeprazole strontium: Store at 20°C to 25°C (68°F to 77°F); excursions permitted to 15°C to 30°C (59°F to 86°F).

Granules: Store at 25°C (77°F); excursions permitted to 15°C to 30°C (59°F to 86°F).

Powder for injection: Store at 25°C (77°F); excursions permitted to 15°C to 30°C (59°F to 86°F). Protect from light. Per the manufacturer, following reconstitution, solution for injection prepared in NS, and solution for infusion prepared in NS or LR should be used within 12 hours. Following reconstitution, solution for infusion prepared in D_5W should be used within 6 hours. Refrigeration is not required following reconstitution.

Additional stability data: Following reconstitution, solutions for infusion prepared in D_5W, NS, or LR in PVC bags are chemically and physically stable for 48 hours at room temperature (25°C) and for at least 120 hours under refrigeration (4°C) (Kupiec, 2008).

Mechanism of Action Proton pump inhibitor suppresses gastric acid secretion by inhibition of the H^+/K^+-ATPase in the gastric parietal cell. Esomeprazole is the S-isomer of omeprazole.

Pharmacodynamics/Kinetics

Distribution: V_{dss}: 16 L

Protein binding: 97%

Metabolism: Hepatic via CYP2C19 primarily and (to a lesser extent) via 3A4 to hydroxy, desmethyl, and sulfone metabolites (all inactive)

Bioavailability: Oral: 90% with repeat dosing

Half-life elimination: ~1-1.5 hours

Time to peak: Oral: 1.5-2 hours

Excretion: Urine (80%, primarily as inactive metabolites; <1% as active drug); feces (20%)

Dosage Note: All dosing is expressed in terms of esomeprazole base, regardless of the salt associated with the dosing information. Esomeprazole strontium 24.65 mg is equivalent to 20 mg of esomeprazole base; esomeprazole strontium 49.3 mg is equivalent to 40 mg of esomeprazole base. Esomeprazole strontium is not recommended for use in pediatrics.

Oral:

Children 1 month to <1 year: Erosive esophagitis (healing): Esomeprazole magnesium: **Note:** Safety and efficacy of doses >1.33 mg/kg/day and/or therapy beyond 6 weeks have not been established.

3-5 kg: 2.5 mg once daily for up to 6 weeks

>5-7.5 kg: 5 mg once daily for up to 6 weeks

>7.5 kg: 10 mg once daily for up to 6 weeks

Children 1-11 years: **Note:** Safety and efficacy of doses >1 mg/kg/day and/or therapy beyond 8 weeks have not been established.

Symptomatic GERD: Esomeprazole magnesium: 10 mg once daily for up to 8 weeks

Erosive esophagitis (healing): Esomeprazole magnesium:

<20 kg: 10 mg once daily for 8 weeks

≥20 kg: 10-20 mg once daily for 8 weeks

Nonerosive reflux disease (NERD) (Canadian labeling): Esomeprazole magnesium: 10 mg once daily for up to 8 weeks

Adolescents 12-17 years:

Erosive esophagitis (healing): Esomeprazole magnesium: 20-40 mg once daily for 4-8 weeks

Symptomatic GERD: Esomeprazole magnesium: 20 mg once daily for up to 4 weeks

NERD (Canadian labeling): Esomeprazole magnesium: 20 mg once daily for 2-4 weeks; lack of symptom control after 4 weeks warrants further evaluation

Adults:

Erosive esophagitis (healing): Esomeprazole magnesium, esomeprazole strontium: Initial: 20-40 mg once daily for 4-8 weeks; if incomplete healing, may continue for an additional 4-8 weeks; maintenance: 20 mg once daily (controlled studies did not extend beyond 6 months)

NERD (Canadian labeling): Esomeprazole magnesium: Initial: 20 mg once daily for 2-4 weeks; lack of symptom control after 4 weeks warrants further evaluation; maintenance (in patients with successful initial therapy): 20 mg once daily as needed

Symptomatic GERD: Esomeprazole magnesium, esomeprazole strontium: 20 mg once daily for 4 weeks; may continue an additional 4 weeks if symptoms persist

Helicobacter pylori eradication:

Manufacturer labeling: Esomeprazole magnesium, esomeprazole strontium: 40 mg once daily administered with amoxicillin 1000 mg *and* clarithromycin 500 mg twice daily for 10 days

American College of Gastroenterology guidelines (Chey, 2007):

Nonpenicillin allergy: 40 mg once daily administered with amoxicillin 1000 mg *and* clarithromycin 500 mg twice daily for 10-14 days

Penicillin allergy: 40 mg once daily administered with clarithromycin 500 mg *and* metronidazole 500 mg twice daily for 10-14 days **or** 40 mg once daily administered with bismuth subsalicylate 525 mg *and* metronidazole 250 mg *plus* tetracycline 500 mg 4 times daily for 10-14 days

Canadian labeling: Esomeprazole magnesium: 20 mg twice daily for 7 days; requires combination therapy

Prevention of NSAID-induced gastric ulcers:

U.S. labeling: Esomeprazole magnesium, esomeprazole strontium: 20-40 mg once daily for up to 6 months

Canadian labeling: Esomeprazole magnesium: 20 mg once daily for up to 6 months

Note: 40 mg daily did not show additional benefit over 20 mg daily in clinical trials.

Treatment of NSAID-induced gastric ulcers (Canadian labeling; unlabeled in U.S.): Esomeprazole magnesium: 20 mg once daily for 4-8 weeks (Goldstein, 2007)

Pathological hypersecretory conditions (Zollinger-Ellison syndrome): Esomeprazole magnesium, esomeprazole strontium: 40 mg twice daily; adjust regimen to individual patient needs; doses up to 240 mg daily have been administered

I.V.:

Treatment of GERD (short-term): **Note:** Indicated only in cases where oral therapy is inappropriate or not possible; safety/efficacy ≥10 days has not been established.

Children 1 month to <1 year: 0.5 mg/kg once daily

Children 1-17 years: <55 kg: 10 mg once daily; ≥55 kg: 20 mg once daily

Adults: 20 mg or 40 mg once daily

Prevention of recurrent peptic ulcer bleeding postendoscopy (unlabeled use; Sung, 2009): Adults: 80 mg over 30 minutes, followed by 8 mg/hour infusion for 72 hours, then 40 mg *orally* once daily for 27 additional days

Dosage adjustment in renal impairment:

Oral:

Esomeprazole magnesium: Mild to severe impairment: No dosage adjustment necessary.

Esomeprazole strontium:

Mild to moderate impairment: No dosage adjustment necessary.

Severe impairment: Use is not recommended (has not been studied).

I.V.: Mild-to-severe impairment: No dosage adjustment necessary.

Dosage adjustment in hepatic impairment: Oral, I.V.: Safety and efficacy not established in children with hepatic impairment.

Mild to moderate impairment (Child-Pugh class A or B): No dosage adjustment necessary

Severe impairment (Child-Pugh class C): Dose should not exceed 20 mg (esomeprazole base) daily.

Dietary Considerations Take at least 1 hour before meals; best if taken before breakfast.

Usual Infusion Concentrations: Pediatric I.V. infusion: 0.4 mg/mL **or** 0.8 mg/mL

Usual Infusion Concentrations: Adult I.V. infusion: 20 mg in 50 mL (concentration: 0.4 mg/mL) **or** 40 mg in 50 mL (concentration: 0.8 mg/mL) of D_5W, LR, or NS

Administration

Oral:

Capsule: Should be swallowed whole and taken at least 1 hour before eating (best if taken before breakfast). Capsule can be opened and contents mixed with 1 tablespoon of applesauce. Swallow immediately; mixture should not be chewed or warmed. For patients with difficulty swallowing, use of granules may be more appropriate.

Granules: Empty the 2.5 mg or 5 mg packet into a container with 5 mL of water or the 10 mg, 20 mg, or 40 mg packet into a container with 15 mL of water and stir; leave 2-3 minutes to thicken. Stir and drink within 30 minutes. If any medicine remains after drinking, add more water, stir and drink immediately.

Tablet (Canadian formulation, not available in U.S.): Swallow whole or may be dispersed in a half a glass of noncarbonated water. Stir until tablets disintegrate, leaving a liquid containing pellets. Drink contents within 30 minutes. Do not chew or crush pellets. After drinking, rinse glass with water and drink.

I.V.: Flush line prior to and after administration with NS, LR, or D_5W.

Children: Administer by intermittent infusion (10-30 minutes); the manufacturer recommends that children receive intravenous esomeprazole by intermittent infusion only.

Adults: May be administered by injection (≥3 minutes), intermittent infusion (10-30 minutes), or continuous infusion for up to 72 hours (Sung, 2009).

Nasogastric tube:

Capsule: Open capsule and place intact granules into a 60 mL catheter-tip syringe; mix with 50 mL of water. Replace plunger and shake vigorously for 15 seconds. Ensure that no granules remain in syringe tip. Do not administer if pellets dissolve or disintegrate. Use immediately after preparation. After administration, flush nasogastric tube with additional water.

Granules: Delayed release oral suspension granules can also be given by nasogastric or gastric tube. If using a 2.5 mg or 5 mg packet, first add 5 mL of water to a catheter-tipped syringe, then add granules from packet.

If using a 10 mg, 20 mg, or 40 mg packet, first add 15 mL of water to a catheter-tipped syringe, then add granules from packet. Shake the syringe, leave 2-3 minutes to thicken. Shake the syringe and administer through nasogastric or gastric tube (size 6 French or greater) within 30 minutes. Refill the syringe with equal amount (5 mL or 15 mL) of water, shake and flush nasogastric/gastric tube.

Tablet (Canadian formulation, not available in U.S.): Disperse tablets in 50 mL of noncarbonated water. Stir until tablets disintegrate leaving a liquid containing pellets. After administration, flush with additional 25-50 mL of water to clear the syringe and tube.

Monitoring Parameters Susceptibility testing recommended in patients who fail *H. pylori* eradication regimen. Monitor for rebleeding in patients with peptic ulcer bleed. For patients expected to be on prolonged therapy or who take PPIs with medications such as digoxin or drugs that may cause hypomagnesemia (eg, diuretics), consider monitoring magnesium levels prior to initiation of treatment and periodically thereafter.

Test Interactions Esomeprazole may falsely elevate serum chromogranin A (CgA) levels. The increased CgA level may cause false-positive results in the diagnosis of a neuroendocrine tumor. Temporarily stop esomeprazole if assessing CgA level; repeat level if initially elevated; use the same laboratory for all testing of CgA levels.

Dosage Forms Considerations
Esomeprazole strontium 24.65 mg is equivalent to 20 mg of esomeprazole base; esomeprazole strontium 49.3 mg is equivalent to 40 mg of esomeprazole base.

Dosage Forms Excipient information presented when available (limited, particularly for generics); consult specific product labeling.

Capsule Delayed Release, Oral, as magnesium [strength expressed as base]:
NexIUM: 20 mg, 40 mg [contains brilliant blue fcf (fd&c blue #1), fd&c red #40, fd&c yellow #10 (quinoline yellow)]

Capsule Delayed Release, Oral, as strontium:
Generic: 24.65 mg, 49.3 mg

Packet, Oral, as magnesium [strength expressed as base]:
NexIUM: 2.5 mg (30 ea); 5 mg (30 ea); 10 mg (30 ea); 20 mg (30 ea); 40 mg (30 ea)

Solution Reconstituted, Intravenous:
Generic: 20 mg (1 ea); 40 mg (1 ea)

Solution Reconstituted, Intravenous, as sodium [strength expressed as base]:
NexIUM I.V.: 20 mg (1 ea); 40 mg (1 ea)

Dosage Forms: Canada Excipient information presented when available (limited, particularly for generics); consult specific product labeling.

Note: Strength expressed as base

Granules, for oral suspension, delayed release, as magnesium:
Nexium®: 10 mg/packet (28s)

Tablet, extended release, as magnesium:
Nexium®: 20 mg, 40 mg

◆ **Esomeprazole Magnesium** *see* Esomeprazole *on page 750*

◆ **Esomeprazole Sodium** *see* Esomeprazole *on page 750*

◆ **Esomeprazole Strontium** *see* Esomeprazole *on page 750*

◆ **Esoterica Daytime [OTC]** *see* Hydroquinone *on page 1017*

◆ **Esoterica Facial [OTC]** *see* Hydroquinone *on page 1017*

◆ **Esoterica Fade Nighttime [OTC]** *see* Hydroquinone *on page 1017*

◆ **Esoterica Sensitive Skin [OTC]** *see* Hydroquinone *on page 1017*

◆ **E.S.P.®** *see* Erythromycin and Sulfisoxazole *on page 744*

◆ **Estalis (Can)** *see* Estradiol and Norethindrone *on page 763*

◆ **Estarylla** *see* Ethinyl Estradiol and Norgestimate *on page 795*

Estazolam (es TA zoe lam)

Index Terms ProSom

Pharmacologic Category Benzodiazepine

Additional Appendix Information
Beers Criteria – Potentially Inappropriate Medications for Geriatrics *on page 2368*
Benzodiazepine Comparison Table *on page 2292*

Use Short-term management of insomnia

Pregnancy Risk Factor X

Dosage Insomnia:
Adults: Oral: 1 mg at bedtime, some patients may require 2 mg
Elderly: Oral: Initial: 0.5-1 mg at bedtime; initiate at lower dose in debilitated or small elderly patients

Dosage adjustment in renal impairment: No dosage adjustment provided in manufacturer's labeling (has not been studied); use with caution.

Dosage adjustment in hepatic impairment: No dosage adjustment provided in manufacturer's labeling (has not been studied); use with caution.

Additional Information Complete prescribing information should be consulted for additional detail.

Dosage Forms Excipient information presented when available (limited, particularly for generics); consult specific product labeling.

Tablet, Oral:
Generic: 1 mg, 2 mg

Controlled Substance C-IV

◆ **Ester-C [OTC]** *see* Ascorbic Acid *on page 172*

◆ **Esterified Estrogens** *see* Estrogens (Esterified) *on page 775*

◆ **Estrace** *see* Estradiol (Systemic) *on page 754*

◆ **Estrace** *see* Estradiol (Topical) *on page 759*

◆ **Estrace® (Can)** *see* Estradiol (Topical) *on page 759*

◆ **Estraderm (Can)** *see* Estradiol (Systemic) *on page 754*

◆ **Estradiol** *see* Estradiol (Systemic) *on page 754*

◆ **17β-estradiol** *see* Estradiol (Topical) *on page 759*

Estradiol (Systemic) (es tra DYE ole)

Brand Names: U.S. Alora; Climara; Delestrogen; Depo-Estradiol; Divigel; Elestrin; Estrace; Estrasorb; Estrogel; Evamist; Femring; Menostar; Minivelle; Vivelle-Dot

Brand Names: Canada Climara; Depo-Estradiol; Estraderm; Estradot; EstroGel; Menostar; Oesclim; Sandoz-Estradiol Derm 100; Sandoz-Estradiol Derm 50; Sandoz-Estradiol Derm 75

Index Terms Estradiol; Estradiol Acetate; Estradiol Transdermal; Estradiol Valerate

Pharmacologic Category Estrogen Derivative

Additional Appendix Information
Beers Criteria – Potentially Inappropriate Medications for Geriatrics *on page 2368*

Use Treatment of moderate-to-severe vasomotor symptoms associated with menopause; treatment of moderate-to-severe vulvar and vaginal atrophy associated with menopause; hypoestrogenism (due to hypogonadism, castration, or primary ovarian failure); advanced prostatic cancer (palliation); metastatic breast cancer (palliation) in men and postmenopausal women; postmenopausal osteoporosis (prophylaxis)

Pregnancy Risk Factor X

Pregnancy Considerations In general, the use of estrogen and progestin as in combination hormonal contraceptives has not been associated with teratogenic effects when inadvertently taken early in pregnancy. These products are contraindicated for use during pregnancy.

Breast-Feeding Considerations Estrogens are excreted in breast milk and have been shown to decrease the quantity and quality of human milk. The manufacturer recommends that caution be used if administered to breast-feeding women. Monitor the growth of the infant closely.

Contraindications Angioedema or anaphylactic reaction to estradiol or any component of the formulation; undiagnosed abnormal vaginal bleeding; DVT or PE (current or history of); active or history of arterial thromboembolic disease (eg, stroke, MI); carcinoma of the breast (known, suspected or history of), except in appropriately selected patients being treated for metastatic disease; estrogen-dependent tumor; hepatic dysfunction or disease; known protein C, protein S, antithrombin deficiency or other known thrombophilic disorders; pregnancy

Warnings/Precautions Hazardous agent - use appropriate precautions for handling and disposal (NIOSH, 2012). **[U.S. Boxed Warning]: The use of unopposed estrogen in women with an intact uterus is associated with an increased risk of endometrial cancer. The addition of a progestin to estrogen therapy may decrease the risk of endometrial hyperplasia, a precursor to endometrial cancer.** The use of a progestin is not generally required when low doses of estrogen are used locally for vaginal atrophy (NAMS, 2012). **Adequate diagnostic measures, including endometrial sampling if indicated, should be performed to rule out malignancy in postmenopausal women with undiagnosed abnormal vaginal bleeding.** Estrogens may exacerbate endometriosis. Malignant transformation of residual endometrial implants has been reported posthysterectomy with unopposed estrogen therapy. Consider adding a progestin in women with residual endometriosis posthysterectomy. Postmenopausal estrogen therapy and combined estrogen/progesterone therapy may increase the risk of ovarian cancer; however, the absolute risk to an individual woman is small. Although results from various studies are not consistent, risk does not appear to be significantly associated with the duration, route, or dose of therapy. In one study, the risk decreased after 2 years following discontinuation of therapy (Mørch, 2009). Although the risk of ovarian cancer is rare, women who are at an increased risk (eg, family history) should be counseled about the association (NAMS, 2012). **[U.S. Boxed Warning]: Based on data from the Women's Health Initiative (WHI) studies, an increased risk of invasive breast cancer was observed in postmenopausal women using conjugated estrogens (CE) in combination with medroxyprogesterone acetate (MPA).** This risk may be associated with duration of use and declines once combined therapy is discontinued (Chlebowski, 2009). The risk of invasive breast cancer was decreased in postmenopausal women with a hysterectomy using CE only, regardless of weight. However, the risk was not significantly decreased in women at high risk for breast cancer (family history of breast cancer, personal history of benign breast disease) (Anderson, 2012). An increase in abnormal mammogram findings has also been reported with estrogen alone or in combination with progestin therapy. Estrogen use may lead to severe hypercalcemia in patients with breast cancer and bone metastases; discontinue estrogen if hypercalcemia occurs.

[U.S. Boxed Warning]: Estrogens with or without progestin should not be used to prevent coronary heart disease. Using data from the Women's Health Initiative (WHI) studies, an increased risk of deep vein thrombosis (DVT) and stroke has been reported with CE and an increased risk of DVT, stroke, pulmonary emboli (PE) and myocardial infarction (MI) has been reported with CE with MPA in postmenopausal women. Additional risk factors include diabetes mellitus, hypercholesterolemia, hypertension, SLE, obesity, tobacco use, and/or history of venous thromboembolism (VTE). Adverse cardiovascular events have also been reported in males taking estrogens for prostate cancer. Risk factors should be managed appropriately; discontinue use if adverse cardiovascular events occur or are suspected. Women with inherited thrombophilias (eg, protein C or S deficiency) may have increased risk of venous thromboembolism (DeSancho, 2010; van Vlijmen, 2011). Use is contraindicated in women with protein C, protein S, antithrombin deficiency or other known thrombophilic disorders.

[U.S. Boxed Warning]: Estrogens with or without progestin should not be used to prevent dementia. In the Women's Health Initiative Memory Study (WHIMS), an increased incidence of dementia was observed in women ≥65 years of age taking CE alone or in combination with MPA.

[U.S. Boxed Warning]: Estrogens with or without progestin should be used for the shortest duration possible at the lowest effective dose consistent with treatment goals. Before prescribing estrogen therapy to postmenopausal women, the risks and benefits must be weighed for each patient. Women should be informed of these risks and benefits, as well as possible effects of progestin when added to estrogen therapy. Patients should be reevaluated as clinically appropriate to determine if treatment is still necessary. Available data related to treatment risks are from Women's Health Initiative (WHI) studies, which evaluated oral CE 0.625 mg with or without MPA 2.5 mg relative to placebo in postmenopausal women. Other combinations and dosage forms of estrogens and progestins were not studied. **Outcomes reported from clinical trials using CE with or without MPA should be assumed to be similar for other doses and other dosage forms of estrogens and progestins until comparable data becomes available.**

Estrogen compounds are generally associated with lipid effects such as increased HDL-cholesterol and decreased LDL-cholesterol. Triglycerides may also be increased; use with caution in patients with familial defects of lipoprotein metabolism. Estrogens may increase thyroid-binding globulin (TBG) levels leading to increased circulating total thyroid hormone levels. Women on thyroid replacement therapy may require higher doses of thyroid hormone while receiving estrogens.

Estrogens may cause retinal vascular thrombosis; discontinue if migraine, loss of vision, proptosis, diplopia, or other visual disturbances occur; discontinue permanently if papilledema or retinal vascular lesions are observed on examination. Estrogens are poorly metabolized in patients with hepatic dysfunction. Use caution with a history of cholestatic jaundice associated with prior estrogen use or pregnancy. Discontinue if jaundice develops or if acute or chronic hepatic disturbances occur. Use is contraindicated with hepatic disease. Use caution in patients with asthma, epilepsy, hepatic hemangiomas, migraine, porphyria, or SLE; may exacerbate disease. May have adverse effects on glucose tolerance; use caution in women with diabetes. Use with caution in patients with diseases which may be exacerbated by fluid retention, including cardiac or renal dysfunction. Use of postmenopausal estrogen may be associated with an increased risk of gallbladder disease requiring surgery. Use with caution in patients with severe hypocalcemia. In the elderly, avoid oral and transdermal patch estrogen products (with or without progestins) due to potential of increased risk of breast and endometrial cancers, and lack of proven cardioprotection and cognitive protection (Beers Criteria). Prior to puberty, estrogens may cause premature closure of the epiphyses, premature breast development in girls or gynecomastia in boys. Vaginal bleeding and vaginal cornification may also be induced in girls. Whenever possible, estrogens should be discontinued at least 4-6 weeks prior to elective surgery associated with an increased risk of thromboembolism or during periods of prolonged immobilization. May exacerbate angioedema symptoms in women with hereditary angioedema. The use of estrogens and/or progestins may change the results of some laboratory tests (eg, coagulation factors, lipids, glucose tolerance, binding proteins). The dose, route, and the specific estrogen/progestin influences these changes. In addition, personal risk factors (eg, cardiovascular disease, smoking, diabetes, age) also contribute to adverse events; use of specific products may be contraindicated in women with certain risk factors.

Estradiol may be transferred to another person following skin-to-skin contact with the application site. **[U.S. Boxed Warning]: Breast budding and breast masses in prepubertal females and gynecomastia and breast masses in prepubertal males have been reported following unintentional contact with application sites of women using topical estradiol (Evamist). Patients should strictly adhere to instructions for use in order to prevent secondary exposure. In most cases, conditions resolved with removal of estradiol exposure.** If unexpected changes in sexual development occur in prepubertal children, the possibility of unintentional estradiol exposure should be evaluated by a healthcare provider. Discontinue if conditions for the safe use of the topical spray cannot be met.

Some products may contain chlorobutanol (a chloral derivative) as a preservative, which may be habit forming; some products may contain tartrazine.

Topical emulsion, gel, spray: Absorption of the topical emulsion (Estrasorb) and topical gel (Elestrin) is increased by application of sunscreen; do not apply sunscreen within close proximity of estradiol. When sunscreen is applied ~1 hour prior to the topical spray (Evamist), no change in absorption was observed (estradiol absorption was decreased when sunscreen is applied 1 hour after Evamist). Application of Divigel or EstroGel with sunscreen has not been evaluated.

Transdermal patch: May contain conducting metal (eg, aluminum); remove patch prior to MRI.

Vaginal ring: Use may not be appropriate in women with narrow vagina, vaginal stenosis, vaginal infections, cervical prolapse, rectoceles, cystoceles, or other conditions which may increase the risk of vaginal irritation, ulceration, or increase the risk of expulsion. Ring should be removed in case of ulceration, erosion, or adherence to vaginal wall; do not reinsert until healing is complete. Ensure proper vaginal placement of the ring to avoid inadvertent urinary bladder insertion.

Osteoporosis: For use only in women at significant risk of osteoporosis and for who other nonestrogen medications are not considered appropriate.

Vulvar and vaginal atrophy: When used solely for the treatment of vulvar and vaginal atrophy, topical vaginal products should be considered. Use caution applying topical products to severely atrophic vaginal mucosa. Use of a progestin is normally not required when low-dose estrogen is applied locally and only for this purpose (NAMS, 2007).

Adverse Reactions Frequency not defined. Some adverse reactions observed with estrogen and/or progestin combination therapy.

Cardiovascular: Chest pain, DVT, edema, hypertension, MI, stroke, syncope, TIA, vasodilation, venous thromboembolism

Central nervous system: Anxiety, dementia, dizziness, epilepsy exacerbation, headache, insomnia, irritability, mental depression, migraine, mood disturbances, nervousness

Dermatologic: Angioedema, chloasma, dermatitis, erythema multiforme, erythema nodosum, hemorrhagic eruption, hirsutism, loss of scalp hair, melasma, rash, pruritus, urticaria

Endocrine & metabolic: Breast cancer, breast enlargement, breast pain, breast tenderness, carbohydrate intolerance, fibrocystic breast changes, fluid retention, galactorrhea, hot flashes, hypocalcemia, libido changes, nipple discharge, nipple pain

Gastrointestinal: Abdominal cramps, abdominal pain, bloating, cholecystitis, cholelithiasis, constipation, diarrhea, dyspepsia, flatulence, gallbladder disease, gastritis, nausea, pancreatitis, vomiting, weight gain/loss

Genitourinary: Alterations in frequency and flow of bleeding patterns, breakthrough bleeding, cervical ectropion changes, cervical secretion changes, cystitis, dysmenorrhea, endometrial cancer, endometrial hyperplasia, genital eruption, menorrhagia, metrorrhagia, ovarian cancer, ovarian cyst, Pap smear suspicious, spotting, uterine leiomyomata size increased, leukorrhea, uterine cancer, uterine enlargement, uterine pain, urinary incontinence, urogenital pruritus, vaginal candidiasis, vaginal discharge, vaginal moniliasis, vaginitis

Hematologic: Aggravation of porphyria

Hepatic: Cholestatic jaundice, hepatic hemangioma enlargement

Local: Thrombophlebitis

Gel, spray: Application site reaction

Transdermal patches: Erythema, irritation

Neuromuscular & skeletal: Arthralgia, back pain, chorea, leg cramps, myalgia, muscle cramps, skeletal pain, weakness

Ocular: Blindness, contact lens intolerance, corneal curvature steepening, retinal vascular thrombosis

Respiratory: Asthma exacerbation, pulmonary thromboembolism

Miscellaneous: Anaphylactoid/anaphylactic reactions, hypersensitivity reactions

Postmarketing and/or case reports: Vaginal ring: Bowel obstruction, ring adherence to vaginal wall, toxic shock syndrome

Drug Interactions

Metabolism/Transport Effects Substrate of CYP1A2 (major), CYP2A6 (minor), CYP2B6 (minor), CYP2C19 (minor), CYP2C9 (minor), CYP2D6 (minor), CYP2E1 (minor), CYP3A4 (major), P-glycoprotein; **Note:** Assignment of Major/Minor substrate status based on clinically relevant drug interaction potential; **Inhibits** CYP1A2 (weak), CYP2C8 (weak); **Induces** CYP3A4 (weak/moderate)

Avoid Concomitant Use

Avoid concomitant use of Estradiol (Systemic) with any of the following: Anastrozole; Axitinib; Dehydroepiandrosterone; Ospemifene; Simeprevir

Increased Effect/Toxicity

Estradiol (Systemic) may increase the levels/effects of: Corticosteroids (Systemic); Ospemifene; ROPINIRole; Theophylline Derivatives; Tipranavir

The levels/effects of Estradiol (Systemic) may be increased by: Ascorbic Acid; Dehydroepiandrosterone; Herbs (Estrogenic Properties); NSAID (COX-2 Inhibitor); P-glycoprotein/ABCB1 Inhibitors

Decreased Effect

Estradiol (Systemic) may decrease the levels/effects of: Anastrozole; Anticoagulants; ARIPiprazole; Axitinib; Chenodiol; Hyaluronidase; Ibrutinib; Ospemifene; Saxagliptin; Simeprevir; Somatropin; Thyroid Products; Ursodiol

The levels/effects of Estradiol (Systemic) may be decreased by: Bosentan; CYP1A2 Inducers (Strong); CYP3A4 Inducers (Strong); Cyproterone; Dabrafenib; Deferasirox; Herbs (CYP3A4 Inducers); Mitotane; Peginterferon Alfa-2b; P-glycoprotein/ABCB1 Inducers; Tipranavir; Tocilizumab

Ethanol/Nutrition/Herb Interactions

Ethanol: Avoid ethanol (routine use increases estrogen level and risk of breast cancer). Ethanol may also increase the risk of osteoporosis.

Food: Folic acid absorption may be decreased

Herb/Nutraceutical: St John's wort may decrease levels. Herbs with estrogenic properties may enhance the adverse/toxic effect of estrogen derivatives; examples include alfalfa, black cohosh, bloodroot, hops, kudzu, licorice, red clover, saw palmetto, soybean, thyme, wild yam, yucca.

Storage/Stability Store all products at controlled room temperature. In addition:

Climara, Estraderm, Menostar: Do not store >30°C (>86°F); store in protective pouch.

Mechanism of Action Estrogens are responsible for the development and maintenance of the female reproductive system and secondary sexual characteristics. Estradiol is the principle intracellular human estrogen and is more potent than estrone and estriol at the receptor level; it is the primary estrogen secreted prior to menopause. Following menopause, estrone and estrone sulfate are more highly produced. Estrogens modulate the pituitary secretion of gonadotropins, luteinizing hormone, and follicle-stimulating hormone through a negative feedback system; estrogen replacement reduces elevated levels of these hormones in postmenopausal women.

Pharmacodynamics/Kinetics

Absorption: Well absorbed from the gastrointestinal tract, mucous membranes, and the skin. Average serum estradiol concentrations (C_{avg}) vary by product

Injection: Estradiol valerate and estradiol cypionate are absorbed over several weeks following I.M. injection

Topical:

- Alora: C_{avg}: 41-98 pg/mL
- Climara: C_{avg}: 22-106 pg/mL
- Divigel: C_{avg}: 9.8-30.5 pg/mL
- Elestrin: C_{avg}: 15.4-39.2 pg/mL; Exposure increased by 55% with application of sunscreen 10 minutes prior to dose
- Estraderm 0.1 mg/day: C_{avg}: 73 pg/mL
- Estrasorb: Mean serum concentration on day 22 of therapy: ~35-65 pg/mL; Exposure increased by 35% with application of sunscreen 10 minutes prior to dose
- Estrogel: C_{avg} on day 14 of therapy: 28.3 pg/mL
- Evamist: C_{avg}: 19.6-30.9 pg/mL
- Menostar: C_{avg}: 13.7 pg/mL
- Vivelle-Dot: C_{avg}: 34-104 pg/mL

Vaginal: Femring: Rapid during the first hour following application, then declines to a steady rate over 3 months; C_{avg}: 40.6-76 pg/mL

Distribution: Widely distributed; high concentrations in the sex hormone target organs

Protein binding: Bound to sex hormone-binding globulin and albumin

Metabolism: Hepatic; partial metabolism via CYP3A4 enzymes; estradiol is reversibly converted to estrone and estriol; oral estradiol also undergoes enterohepatic recirculation by conjugation in the liver, followed by excretion of sulfate and glucuronide conjugates into the bile, then hydrolysis in the intestine and estrogen reabsorption. Sulfate conjugates are the primary form found in postmenopausal women. With transdermal application, less estradiol is metabolized leading to higher circulating concentrations of estradiol and lower concentrations of estrone and conjugates.

Excretion: Primarily urine (as estradiol, estrone, estriol and their glucuronide and sulfate conjugates)

Dosage All dosage needs to be adjusted based upon the patient's response

Oral:

Prostate cancer, advanced (androgen-dependent) (Estrace): 1-2 mg 3 times/day

Breast cancer, metastatic (appropriately selected patients): Males and postmenopausal females (Estrace): 10 mg 3 times/day **or** (unlabeled dosing) postmenopausal women: 2 mg 3 times/day (Ellis, 2009)

Osteoporosis prophylaxis in postmenopausal females (Estrace): Lowest effective dose has not been determined; doses of 0.5 mg/day in a cyclic regimen for 23 days of a 28-week cycle were used in clinical studies

Female hypoestrogenism (due to hypogonadism, castration, or primary ovarian failure) (Estrace): 1-2 mg/day; titrate as necessary to control symptoms using minimal effective dose for maintenance therapy

Vasomotor symptoms associated with menopause (Estrace): 1-2 mg/day, adjusted as necessary to limit symptoms; administration should be cyclic (3 weeks on, 1 week off)

Vulvar and vaginal atrophy associated with menopause (Estrace): 1-2 mg/day, adjusted as necessary to limit symptoms; administration should be cyclic (3 weeks on, 1 week off)

I.M.:

Prostate cancer, advanced (androgen-dependent): Valerate (Delestrogen): 30 mg or more every 1-2 weeks

Vasomotor symptoms associated with menopause:

- Cypionate (Depo-Estradiol): 1-5 mg every 3-4 weeks
- Valerate (Delestrogen): 10-20 mg every 4 weeks

Female hypoestrogenism (due to hypogonadism): Cypionate (Depo-Estradiol): 1.5-2 mg monthly

Female hypoestrogenism (due to hypogonadism, castration, or primary ovarian failure): Valerate (Delestrogen): 10-20 mg every 4 weeks

Vulvar and vaginal atrophy associated with menopause: Valerate (Delestrogen): 10-20 mg every 4 weeks

Topical:

Emulsion: Vasomotor symptoms associated with menopause (Estrasorb): 3.48 g applied once daily in the morning

Gel:

Vasomotor symptoms associated with menopause:

- Divigel: 0.25 g/day; adjust dose based on patient response. Dosing range: 0.25-1 g/day
- Elestrin: 0.87 g/day applied at the same time each day; adjust dose based on patient response. Dosing range: 0.87-1.7 g/day.
- EstroGel: 1.25 g/day applied at the same time each day

Vulvar and vaginal atrophy associated with menopause (EstroGel): 1.25 g/day applied at the same time each day

Spray: Vasomotor symptoms associated with menopause (Evamist): Initial: One spray (1.53 mg) per day. Adjust dose based on patient response. Dosing range: 1-3 sprays per day.

Transdermal patch: **Note:** Indicated dose may be used continuously in patients without an intact uterus. Some product labeling states they may be given continuously or cyclically (3 weeks on, 1 week off) in patients with an intact uterus (**exception - Menostar, see specific dosing instructions**). When changing patients from oral to transdermal therapy, start transdermal patch 1 week after discontinuing oral hormone (may begin sooner if symptoms reappear within 1 week):

Once-weekly patch:

Vasomotor symptoms associated with menopause, vulvar and vaginal atrophy associated with menopause, female hypoestrogenism (due to hypogonadism, castration, or primary ovarian failure) (Climara): Apply 0.025 mg/day patch once weekly. Adjust dose as necessary to control symptoms.

Osteoporosis prophylaxis in postmenopausal women:

Climara: Apply patch once weekly; minimum effective dose 0.025 mg/day; adjust dosage based on response to therapy as indicated by biochemical markers and bone mineral density

Menostar: Apply patch once weekly (0.014 mg/day). In women with a uterus, also administer a progestin for 14 days every 6-12 months

Twice-weekly patch:

Vasomotor symptoms associated with menopause, vulvar/vaginal atrophy associated with menopause, female hypoestrogenism (due to hypogonadism, castration, or primary ovarian failure): Titrate to lowest dose possible to control symptoms, adjusting initial dose after the first month of therapy:

Alora, Estraderm: Apply 0.05 mg patch twice weekly

Vivelle-Dot: Apply 0.0375 mg patch twice weekly

Vasomotor symptoms associated with menopause: Titrate to lowest dose possible to control symptoms, adjusting initial dose after the first month of therapy:

Minivelle: Apply 0.0375 mg patch twice weekly

Prevention of osteoporosis in postmenopausal women:

Alora, Vivelle-Dot: Apply 0.025 mg patch twice weekly, increase dose as necessary

Estraderm: Apply 0.05 mg patch twice weekly

Vaginal ring: Vasomotor symptoms associated with menopause; vulvar and vaginal atrophy associated with menopause (Femring): Initial: 0.05 mg intravaginally; following insertion, ring should remain in place for 3 months; dose may be increased to 0.1 mg if needed

Dietary Considerations Ensure adequate calcium and vitamin D intake when used for the prevention of osteoporosis.

Administration The use of a progestin should be considered when administering estrogens to postmenopausal women with an intact uterus.

Injection formulation: Intramuscular use only. Estradiol valerate should be injected into the upper outer quadrant of the gluteal muscle; administer with a dry needle (solution may become cloudy with wet needle).

Emulsion (Estrasorb): Apply to clean, dry skin while in a sitting position. Contents of two pouches (total 3.48 g) are to be applied individually, once daily in the morning. Apply contents of first pouch to left thigh; massage into skin of left thigh and calf until thoroughly absorbed (~3 minutes). Apply excess from both hands to the buttocks. Apply contents of second pouch to the right thigh; massage into skin of right thigh and calf until thoroughly absorbed (~3 minutes). Apply excess from both hands to buttocks. Wash hands with soap and water. Allow skin to dry before covering legs with clothing. Do not apply to other areas of body. Do not apply to red or irritated skin.

Gel: Apply to clean, dry, unbroken skin at the same time each day. Allow to dry for 5 minutes prior to dressing. Gel is flammable; avoid fire or flame until dry. After application, wash hands with soap and water. Prior to the first use, pump must be primed. Do not apply gel to breast.

Divigel: Apply entire contents of packet to right or left upper thigh each day (alternate sites). Do not apply to face, breasts, vaginal area or irritated skin. Apply over an area ~5x7 inches. Do not wash application site for 1 hour. Allow gel to dry before dressing

Elestrin: Apply to upper arm and shoulder area using two fingers to spread gel. Apply after bath or shower; allow at least 2 hours between applying gel and going swimming. Wait at least 25 minutes before applying sunscreen to application area. Do not apply sunscreen to application area for ≥7 days (may increase absorption of gel).

EstroGel: Apply gel to the arm, from the wrist to the shoulder. Spread gel as thinly as possible over one arm.

Spray: Evamist: Prior to first use, prime pump by spraying 3 sprays with the cover on. To administer dose, hold container upright and vertical and rest the plastic cone flat against the skin while spraying. Spray to the inner surface of the forearm, starting near the elbow. If more than one spray is needed, apply to adjacent but not overlapping areas. Apply at the same time each day. Allow spray to dry for ~2 minutes; do not rub into skin; do not cover with clothing until dry. Do not wash application site for at least 60 minutes. Apply to clean, dry, unbroken skin. Do not apply to skin other than that of the forearm. Make sure that children do not come in contact with any skin area where the drug was applied. If contact with children is unavoidable, wear a garment with long sleeves that covers the site of application. If direct exposure should occur, wash the child in the area of exposure with soap and water as soon as possible. Solution contained in the spray is flammable; avoid fire, flame, or smoking until spray has dried. If needed, sunscreen should be applied ~1 hour prior to application of Evamist.

Transdermal patch: Do not apply transdermal system to breasts, but place on trunk of body (preferably abdomen). Rotate application sites allowing a 1-week interval between applications at a particular site. Do not apply to oily, damaged or irritated skin; avoid waistline or other areas where tight clothing may rub the patch off. Apply patch immediately after removing from protective pouch. In general, if patch falls off, the same patch may be reapplied or a new system may be used for the remainder of the dosing interval (not recommended with all products). When replacing patch, reapply to a new site. Swimming, bathing or showering are not expected to affect use of the patch. Note the following exceptions:

Estraderm: Do not apply to an area exposed to direct sunlight.

Climara, Menostar, Minivelle: Swimming, bathing, or wearing patch while in a sauna have not been studied; adhesion of patch may be decreased or delivery of estradiol may be affected. Showering is not expected to cause the Minivelle patch to fall off. Remove patch slowly after use to avoid skin irritation. If any adhesive remains on the skin after removal, first allow skin to dry for 15 minutes, then gently rub area with an oil-based cream or lotion. If patch falls off, a new patch should be applied for the remainder of the dosing interval.

Vaginal ring: Exact positioning is not critical for efficacy; however, patient should not feel anything once inserted. In case of discomfort, ring should be pushed further into vagina. If ring is expelled prior to 90 days, it may be rinsed off and reinserted. Ensure proper vaginal placement of the ring to avoid inadvertent urinary bladder insertion. If vaginal infection develops, Femring may remain in place during local treatment of a vaginal infection.

Hazardous agent; use appropriate precautions for handling and disposal (NIOSH, 2012).

Monitoring Parameters Routine physical examination that includes blood pressure and Papanicolaou smear, breast exam, mammogram. Monitor for signs of endometrial cancer in female patients with uterus. Adequate diagnostic measures, including endometrial sampling, if indicated, should be performed to rule out malignancy in all cases of undiagnosed abnormal vaginal bleeding. Monitor for loss of vision, sudden onset of proptosis, diplopia, migraine; signs and symptoms of thromboembolic disorders; glycemic control in patients with diabetes; lipid profiles in patients being treated for hyperlipidemias; thyroid function in patients on thyroid hormone replacement therapy.

Menostar: When used in a woman with a uterus, endometrial sampling is recommended at yearly intervals or when clinically indicated.

Menopausal symptoms, vulvar and vaginal atrophy: Assess need for therapy at 3- to 6-month intervals

Prevention of osteoporosis: Bone density measurement

Reference Range

Children 6 months to 10 years: <15 pg/mL (SI: <55 pmol/L)

Males: 10-50 pg/mL (SI: 37-184 pmol/L)

Females:

Premenopausal: 30-400 pg/mL (SI: 110-1468 pmol/L) (depending on phase of menstrual cycle)

Postmenopausal: 0-30 pg/mL (SI: 0-110 pmol/L)

Test Interactions Reduced response to metyrapone test.

Dosage Forms Excipient information presented when available (limited, particularly for generics); consult specific product labeling.

Emulsion, Transdermal, as hemihydrate:

Estrasorb: 4.35 mg/1.74 g (1.74 g) [contains polysorbate 80, soybean oil]

Gel, Transdermal:

Divigel: 0.25 mg/0.25 g (1 ea); 0.5 mg/0.5 g (1 ea); 1 mg/g (1 g) [contains alcohol, usp, trolamine (triethanolamine)]

Elestrin: 0.06% (26 g) [contains alcohol, usp, edetate disodium, propylene glycol, trolamine (triethanolamine)]

Estrogel: 0.06% (50 g) [contains alcohol, usp, trolamine (triethanolamine)]

Oil, Intramuscular, as cypionate:

Depo-Estradiol: 5 mg/mL (5 mL)

Oil, Intramuscular, as valerate:

Delestrogen: 10 mg/mL (5 mL) [contains chlorobutanol (chlorobutol), sesame oil]

Delestrogen: 20 mg/mL (5 mL); 40 mg/mL (5 mL) [contains benzyl alcohol]

Generic: 10 mg/mL (5 mL); 20 mg/mL (5 mL); 40 mg/mL (5 mL)

Patch Biweekly, Transdermal:

Alora: 0.025 mg/24 hr (1 ea, 8 ea); 0.05 mg/24 hr (1 ea, 8 ea); 0.075 mg/24 hr (1 ea, 8 ea); 0.1 mg/24 hr (1 ea, 8 ea)

Minivelle: 0.0375 mg/24 hr (8 ea); 0.05 mg/24 hr (8 ea); 0.075 mg/24 hr (8 ea); 0.1 mg/24 hr (8 ea)

Vivelle-Dot: 0.025 mg/24 hr (8 ea); 0.0375 mg/24 hr (1 ea, 8 ea); 0.05 mg/24 hr (1 ea, 8 ea); 0.075 mg/24 hr (1 ea, 8 ea); 0.1 mg/24 hr (1 ea, 8 ea)

Patch Weekly, Transdermal:

Climara: 0.025 mg/24 hr (4 ea); 0.0375 mg/24 hr (4 ea); 0.05 mg/24 hr (4 ea); 0.06 mg/24 hr (4 ea); 0.075 mg/24 hr (4 ea); 0.1 mg/24 hr (1 ea, 4 ea)

Menostar: 14 mcg/24 hr (4 ea)

Generic: 0.025 mg/24 hr (4 ea); 0.0375 mg/24 hr (4 ea); 0.05 mg/24 hr (4 ea); 0.06 mg/24 hr (4 ea); 0.075 mg/24 hr (4 ea); 0.1 mg/24 hr (4 ea)

Ring, Vaginal, as acetate:

Femring: 0.05 mg/24 hr (1 ea); 0.1 mg/24 hr (1 ea)

Solution, Transdermal:

Evamist: 1.53 mg/spray (8.1 mL) [contains alcohol, usp, octyl salicylate]

Tablet, Oral:

Estrace: 0.5 mg, 1 mg, 2 mg [scored]

Generic: 0.5 mg, 1 mg, 2 mg

Estradiol (Topical) (es tra DYE ole)

Brand Names: U.S. Estrace; Estring; Vagifem

Brand Names: Canada Estrace®; Estring®; Vagifem®; Vagifem® 10

Index Terms 17β-estradiol

Pharmacologic Category Estrogen Derivative

Additional Appendix Information

Beers Criteria – Potentially Inappropriate Medications for Geriatrics *on page 2368*

Use Treatment of moderate-to-severe vulvar and vaginal atrophy associated with menopause

Pregnancy Considerations In general, the use of estrogen and progestin as in combination hormonal contraceptives has not been associated with teratogenic effects when inadvertently taken early in pregnancy. These products are contraindicated for use during pregnancy.

Breast-Feeding Considerations Estrogen has been shown to decrease the quantity and quality of human milk; use only if clearly needed; monitor the growth of the infant closely.

Contraindications Angioedema or anaphylactic reaction to estradiol or any component of the formulation; undiagnosed abnormal vaginal bleeding; DVT or PE (current or history of); active or history of arterial thromboembolic disease (eg, stroke, MI); carcinoma of the breast (known, suspected or history of); estrogen-dependent tumor; hepatic dysfunction or disease; known protein C, protein S, antithrombin deficiency, or other known thrombophilic disorders; pregnancy

Warnings/Precautions Hazardous agent - use appropriate precautions for handling and disposal (NIOSH, 2012). **[U.S. Boxed Warning]: The use of unopposed estrogen in women with an intact uterus is associated with an increased risk of endometrial cancer. The addition of a progestin to estrogen therapy may decrease the risk of endometrial hyperplasia, a precursor to endometrial cancer. Adequate diagnostic measures, including endometrial sampling if indicated, should be performed to rule out malignancy in postmenopausal women with undiagnosed abnormal vaginal bleeding.** Estrogens may exacerbate endometriosis. Malignant transformation of residual endometrial implants has been reported posthysterectomy with unopposed estrogen therapy. Consider adding a progestin in women with residual endometriosis posthysterectomy. Postmenopausal estrogen therapy and combined estrogen/progesterone therapy may increase the risk of ovarian cancer; however, the absolute risk to an individual woman is small. Although results from various studies are not consistent, risk does not appear to be significantly associated with the duration, route, or dose of therapy. In one study, the risk decreased after 2 years following discontinuation of therapy (Mørch, 2009). Although the risk of ovarian cancer is rare, women who are at an increased risk (eg, family history) should be counseled about the association (NAMS, 2012).

[U.S. Boxed Warning]: Based on data from the Women's Health Initiative (WHI) studies, an increased risk of invasive breast cancer was observed in postmenopausal women using conjugated estrogens (CE) in combination with medroxyprogesterone acetate (MPA). This risk may be associated with duration of use and declines once combined therapy is discontinued (Chlebowski, 2009). The risk of invasive breast cancer was decreased in postmenopausal women with a hysterectomy using CE only, regardless of weight. However, the risk was not significantly decreased in women at high risk for breast cancer (family history of breast cancer, personal history of benign breast disease) (Anderson, 2012). An increase in abnormal mammogram findings has also been reported with estrogen alone or in combination with progestin therapy. Estrogen use may also lead to severe hypercalcemia in patients with breast cancer and bone metastases; discontinue estrogen if hypercalcemia occurs. Use is contraindicated in patients with known or suspected breast cancer.

[U.S. Boxed Warning]: Estrogens with or without progestin should not be used to prevent cardiovascular disease. Using data from the Women's Health Initiative (WHI) studies, an increased risk of deep vein thrombosis (DVT) and stroke has been reported with CE and an increased risk of DVT, stroke, pulmonary emboli (PE) and myocardial infarction (MI) has been reported with CE with MPA in postmenopausal women. Additional risk factors include diabetes mellitus, hypercholesterolemia, hypertension, SLE, obesity, tobacco use, and/or history of venous thromboembolism (VTE). Risk factors should be managed appropriately; discontinue use if adverse cardiovascular events occur or are suspected. Women with inherited thrombophilias (eg, protein C or S deficiency) may have increased risk of venous thromboembolism (DeSancho, 2010; van Vlijmen, 2011). Use is contraindicated in women with protein C, protein S, antithrombin deficiency, or other known thrombophilic disorders.

[U.S. Boxed Warning]: Estrogens with or without progestin should not be used to prevent dementia. In the Women's Health Initiative Memory Study (WHIMS), an increased incidence of dementia was observed in women ≥65 years of age taking CE alone or in combination with MPA.

[U.S. Boxed Warning]: Estrogens with or without progestin should be used for the shortest duration possible at the lowest effective dose consistent with treatment goals. Before prescribing estrogen therapy to postmenopausal women, the risks and benefits must be weighed for each patient. Women should be informed of these risks and benefits, as well as possible effects of progestin when added to estrogen therapy. Patients should be reevaluated as clinically appropriate to determine if treatment is still necessary. Available data related to treatment risks are from Women's Health Initiative (WHI) studies, which evaluated oral CE 0.625 mg with or without MPA 2.5 mg relative to placebo in postmenopausal women. Other combinations and dosage forms of estrogens and progestins were not studied. **Outcomes reported from clinical trials using CE with or without MPA should be assumed to be similar for other doses and other dosage forms of estrogens and progestins until comparable data becomes available.** Systemic absorption occurs following vaginal use; warnings, precautions, and adverse events observed with oral therapy should be considered.

Estrogen compounds are generally associated with lipid effects such as increased HDL-cholesterol and decreased LDL-cholesterol. Triglycerides may also be increased; discontinue if pancreatitis occurs. Estrogens may increase thyroid-binding globulin (TBG) levels leading to increased circulating total thyroid hormone levels. Women on thyroid replacement therapy may require higher doses of thyroid hormone while receiving estrogens.

In the elderly, low-dose intravaginal estrogen may be appropriate for use in the management of vaginal symptoms, lower urinary tract infections, and dyspareunia; in addition, evidence has shown that vaginal estrogens (particularly at estradiol doses of <25 mcg twice weekly) in the treatment of vaginal dryness is safe and effective in women with breast cancer (Beers Criteria).

Estrogens may cause retinal vascular thrombosis; discontinue if migraine, loss of vision, proptosis, diplopia, or other visual disturbances occur; discontinue permanently if papilledema or retinal vascular lesions are observed on examination. Estrogens are poorly metabolized in patients with hepatic dysfunction. Use caution with a history of cholestatic jaundice associated with prior estrogen use or pregnancy. Discontinue if jaundice develops or if acute or chronic hepatic disturbances occur. Use is contraindicated with hepatic disease. Exogenous estrogens may exacerbate angioedema symptoms in women with hereditary angioedema. Use caution in patients with asthma, epilepsy, hepatic hemangiomas, migraine, porphyria, or SLE; may exacerbate disease. May have adverse effects on glucose tolerance; use caution in women with diabetes. Use with caution in patients with diseases which may be exacerbated by fluid retention, including cardiac or renal dysfunction. Use of postmenopausal estrogen may be associated with an increased risk of gallbladder disease requiring surgery. Use caution in patients with hypoparathyroidism; estrogen-induced hypocalcemia may occur. Whenever possible, estrogens should be discontinued at least 4-6 weeks prior to elective surgery associated with an increased risk of thromboembolism or during periods of prolonged immobilization. The use of estrogens and/or progestins may change the results of some laboratory tests (eg, coagulation factors, lipids, glucose tolerance, binding proteins). The dose, route, and the specific estrogen/progestin influences these changes. In addition, personal risk factors (eg, cardiovascular disease, smoking, diabetes, age) also contribute to adverse events; use of specific products may be contraindicated in women with certain risk factors.

Vaginal ring: Use may not be appropriate in women with narrow vagina, vaginal stenosis, vaginal infections, cervical prolapse, rectoceles, cystoceles, or other conditions which may increase the risk of vaginal irritation, ulceration, or increase the risk of expulsion. Ring should be removed in case of ulceration, erosion, or adherence to vaginal wall; do not reinsert until healing is complete. Ensure proper vaginal placement of the ring to avoid inadvertent urinary bladder insertion.

Moderate-to-severe symptoms of vulvar and vaginal atrophy include vaginal dryness, dyspareunia, and atrophic vaginitis. Use caution applying topical products to severely atrophic vaginal mucosa. Local abrasion caused by the vaginal applicator has been reported in women with severely atrophic vaginal mucosa.

Adverse Reactions

>10%: Central nervous system: Headache (13%)

1% to 10%:

- Cardiovascular: Chest pain, edema, hypertension, leg edema, MI, stroke, syncope, venous thrombosis
- Central nervous system: Insomnia (4%), anxiety, migraine
- Dermatologic: Angioedema, chloasma, dermatitis, erythema multiforme, erythema nodosum, hemorrhagic eruption, hirsutism, loss of scalp hair, melasma, pruritus, rash, skin hypertrophy, urticaria
- Endocrine & metabolic: Hot flashes (2%), breast pain (1%), breast cancer, breast enlargement, breast tenderness, carbohydrate tolerance decreased, endometrial carcinoma, endometrial hyperplasia, fibrocystic breast changes, galactorrhea, hypocalcemia, libido changes, nipple discharge, ovarian cancer
- Gastrointestinal: Abdominal pain (4%), diarrhea (5%), nausea (3%), dyspepsia, flatulence, gastritis, hemorrhoids, toothache, weight changes

Genitourinary: Leukorrhea (7%), cervical ectropion changes, cervical secretion changes, cystitis, dysmenorrhea, dysuria, genital eruption, urinary incontinence, uterine leiomyomata change, vaginal bleeding pattern change (including abnormal flow, breakthrough bleeding, spotting)

Vaginal: Trauma from applicator insertion may occur in women with severely atrophic mucosa; burning, discomfort, hemorrhage, moniliasis, pain, pruritus, vaginitis, vulvovaginal infection

Hematologic: Porphyria aggravated

Local: Thrombophlebitis

Neuromuscular & skeletal: Back pain (6% to 7%), arthritis (4%), arthralgias (3%), skeletal pain (2%), leg cramps

Ocular: Contact lens intolerance, retinal vascular thrombosis

Otic: Otitis media

Respiratory: Respiratory tract infection: (5%), sinusitis (4%), pharyngitis (1%), asthma exacerbation, bronchitis, pulmonary embolism

Miscellaneous: Anaphylactoid/anaphylactic reactions, flu-like syndrome (3%), hypersensitivity

Postmarketing and/or case reports: Bowel obstruction (ring), ring adherence to vaginal wall (ring), toxic shock syndrome (ring)

Drug Interactions

Metabolism/Transport Effects Substrate of CYP1A2 (major), CYP2A6 (minor), CYP2B6 (minor), CYP2C19 (minor), CYP2C9 (minor), CYP2D6 (minor), CYP2E1 (minor), CYP3A4 (major), P-glycoprotein; **Note:** Assignment of Major/Minor substrate status based on clinically relevant drug interaction potential; **Inhibits** CYP1A2 (weak), CYP2C8 (weak); **Induces** CYP3A4 (weak/moderate)

Avoid Concomitant Use

Avoid concomitant use of Estradiol (Topical) with any of the following: Anastrozole; Axitinib; Dehydroepiandrosterone; Ospemifene; Simeprevir

Increased Effect/Toxicity

Estradiol (Topical) may increase the levels/effects of: Corticosteroids (Systemic); Ospemifene; ROPINIRole; Theophylline Derivatives; Tipranavir

The levels/effects of Estradiol (Topical) may be increased by: Ascorbic Acid; Dehydroepiandrosterone; Herbs (Estrogenic Properties); NSAID (COX-2 Inhibitor); P-glycoprotein/ABCB1 Inhibitors

Decreased Effect

Estradiol (Topical) may decrease the levels/effects of: Anastrozole; Anticoagulants; ARIPiprazole; Axitinib; Chenodiol; Hyaluronidase; Ibrutinib; Ospemifene; Saxagliptin; Simeprevir; Somatropin; Thyroid Products; Ursodiol

The levels/effects of Estradiol (Topical) may be decreased by: Bosentan; CYP1A2 Inducers (Strong); CYP3A4 Inducers (Strong); Cyproterone; Dabrafenib; Deferasirox; Herbs (CYP3A4 Inducers); Mitotane; Peginterferon Alfa-2b; P-glycoprotein/ABCB1 Inducers; Tipranavir; Tocilizumab

Storage/Stability

Vaginal cream (Estrace®): Store at room temperature; protect from temperatures in excess of 40°C (104°F).

Vaginal ring (Estring®): Store at 15°C to 30°C (59°F to 86°F).

Vaginal tablet (Vagifem®): Store at 25°C (77°F); do not refrigerate.

Mechanism of Action In studies for vulvar and vaginal atrophy in postmenopausal women, local estrogens have been shown to reduce vaginal pH levels and mature the vaginal and urethral mucosa after 12 weeks of therapy, thereby improving vaginal dryness and mucosal atrophy.

Pharmacodynamics/Kinetics

Absorption: Average serum estradiol concentrations (C_{avg}) vary by product

Vaginal: Vaginal absorption is typically low; any contribution to circulating estradiol concentrations via systemic absorption does not exceed normal postmenopausal ranges (Ulrich, 2010; Weisberg, 2005).

Estring®: Average steady state serum concentrations decrease from 11.2 pg/mL at 48 hours to 8 pg/mL at 12 weeks

Vagifem®: C_{avg}: 10.9 pg/mL on day 1, 5.5 pg/mL on day 83

Distribution: Widely distributed; high concentrations in the sex hormone target organs

Protein binding: Bound to sex hormone-binding globulin and albumin

Metabolism: Hepatic; partial metabolism via CYP3A4 enzymes; estradiol is reversibly converted to estrone and estriol. Sulfate conjugates are the primary form found in postmenopausal women.

Excretion: Primarily urine (as estradiol, estrone, estriol and their glucuronide and sulfate conjugates)

Dosage Adults: Topical: All dosage needs to be adjusted based upon the patient's response.

Vaginal cream: Vulvar and vaginal atrophy associated with menopause: (Estrace®): Insert 2-4 g/day intravaginally for 1-2 weeks, then gradually reduce to 1/2 the initial dose for 1-2 weeks, followed by a maintenance dose of 1 g 1-3 times/week

Vaginal ring (Estring®): Vulvar and vaginal atrophy associated with menopause: 2 mg intravaginally; following insertion, ring should remain in place for 90 days

Vaginal tablet (Vagifem®): Vulvar and vaginal atrophy associated with menopause: Initial: Insert 1 tablet (10 mcg) once daily for 2 weeks; Maintenance: Insert 1 tablet twice weekly

Administration

Vaginal ring: Exact positioning is not critical for efficacy; however, patient should not feel anything once inserted. In case of discomfort, ring should be pushed further into vagina. If ring is expelled prior to 90 days, it may be rinsed off and reinserted. Ensure proper vaginal placement of the ring to avoid inadvertent urinary bladder insertion. If vaginal infection develops, Estring® should be removed; reinsert only after infection has been appropriately treated.

Vaginal tablet: Insert tablet with supplied applicator at the same time each day. Once inserted, press plunger until fully depressed, then remove applicator and discard. If tablet comes out of applicator prior to insertion, do not replace; use a new tablet filled applicator instead.

Hazardous agent; use appropriate precautions for handling and disposal (NIOSH, 2012).

Monitoring Parameters Routine physical examination that includes blood pressure and Papanicolaou smear, breast exam, mammogram. Monitor for signs of endometrial cancer in female patients with uterus. Adequate diagnostic measures, including endometrial sampling, if indicated, should be performed to rule out malignancy in all cases of undiagnosed abnormal vaginal bleeding. Monitor for loss of vision, sudden onset of proptosis, diplopia, migraine; signs and symptoms of thromboembolic disorders; glycemic control in patients with diabetes; lipid profiles in patients being treated for hyperlipidemias; thyroid function in patients on thyroid hormone replacement therapy. Assess need for therapy at 3- to 6-month intervals.

Test Interactions Reduced response to metyrapone test.

Dosage Forms Excipient information presented when available (limited, particularly for generics); consult specific product labeling.

Cream, Vaginal:

Estrace: 0.1 mg/g (42.5 g)

Ring, Vaginal, as base:

Estring: 2 mg (1 ea)

Tablet, Vaginal, as base:

Vagifem: 10 mcg

◆ **Estradiol Acetate** *see* Estradiol (Systemic) *on page 754*

Estradiol and Dienogest

(es tra DYE ole & dye EN oh jest)

Brand Names: U.S. Natazia®

Index Terms Dienogest and Estradiol; Estradiol Valerate and Dienogest

Pharmacologic Category Contraceptive; Estrogen and Progestin Combination

Use Prevention of pregnancy; treatment of heavy menstrual bleeding

Unlabeled Use Pain associated with endometriosis; dysmenorrhea

Dosage Oral: Adults: Females: Contraception or treatment of heavy menstrual bleeding: Take 1 tablet daily in the order presented in the blister pack

Initial dosing: Start on day 1 of menstrual period (first day of bleeding). A nonhormonal contraceptive should be used for the first 9 days.

Switching from another combination oral contraceptive tablet: Take the first dark yellow tablet on the first day of withdrawal bleeding; do not continue taking tablets from previous contraceptive pack. If withdrawal bleeding does not occur, rule-out pregnancy before starting therapy. A non-hormonal contraceptive should be used for the first 9 days.

Switching from a vaginal ring or patch: Take the first dark yellow tablet on the day the ring or patch is removed. A nonhormonal contraceptive should be used for the first 9 days.

Switching from a progestin-only contraceptive: Take the first dark yellow tablet on the day the next progestin-only tablet would have been given, or the day the progestin implant or IUD is removed, or on the day the next injection would have been given. A nonhormonal contraceptive should be used for the first 9 days.

Missed doses: If ≤12 hours late, take tablet as soon as remembering and take the next tablet at the usual time. If >12 hours late, instructions vary by day of cycle and number of tablets missed:

If missed ONE dose:

Days 1-17: Take missed tablet immediately; take next tablet at usual time; use back-up (nonhormonal) contraception for the next 9 days; continue taking 1 tablet each day for the rest of the cycle

Days 18-24: Do not continue using current blister pack (throw away); take day 1 of new blister pack; use back-up (nonhormonal) contraception for the next 9 days; continue taking 1 tablet each day for the rest of the cycle

Days 25-28: Take missed tablet immediately; take next tablet at usual time; continue taking 1 tablet each day for the rest of the cycle; no backup method of contraception is needed.

If missed TWO doses in a row:

Days 1-17: Do not take missed tablets; start by taking the tablet for the day it was first noticed that the tablet was missed; use back-up (nonhormonal) contraception for the next 9 days; continue taking 1 tablet each day for the rest of the cycle. If tablets were missed on days 17 and 18, follow directions for missed tablets on days 17-25.

Days 17-25: Do not continue using current blister pack (throw away); take day 3 of new blister pack; use back-up (nonhormonal) contraception for the next 9 days; continue taking 1 tablet each day for the rest of the cycle. If tablets were missed on days 25 and 26, follow directions for missed tablets on days 25-28.

Days 25-28: Do not continue using current blister pack (throw away); start a new pack on the same day, or start a new pack the day it would normally be started; continue taking 1 tablet each day for the rest of the cycle; no backup method of contraception is needed.

Dosage adjustment in renal impairment: Safety and efficacy have not been evaluated; dose adjustment not expected to be required

Dosage adjustment in hepatic impairment: Use is contraindicated with hepatic disease. Discontinue if hepatic dysfunction occurs.

Additional Information Complete prescribing information should be consulted for additional detail.

Dosage Forms Excipient information presented when available (limited, particularly for generics); consult specific product labeling.

Tablet, oral [four-phasic formulation]:

Natazia®:

Days 1-2: Estradiol valerate 3 mg [2 dark yellow tablets]

Days 3-7: Estradiol valerate 2 mg and dienogest 2 mg [5 medium red tablets]

Days 8-24: Estradiol valerate 2 mg and dienogest 3 mg [17 light yellow tablets]

Days 25-26: Estradiol valerate 1 mg [2 dark red tablets]

Days 27-28: 2 white inactive tablets (28s)

Estradiol and Levonorgestrel

(es tra DYE ole & LEE voe nor jes trel)

Brand Names: U.S. ClimaraPro

Index Terms Levonorgestrel and Estradiol

Pharmacologic Category Estrogen and Progestin Combination

Use

Moderate to severe vasomotor symptoms: Treatment of moderate to severe vasomotor symptoms associated with menopause in women with an intact uterus

Osteoporosis prevention: Prevention of postmenopausal osteoporosis in women with an intact uterus

Limitations of use: Osteoporosis: For use only in women at significant risk of osteoporosis and for whom other nonestrogen medications are not considered appropriate

Dosage Note: Patients should be treated with the lowest effective dose and for the shortest duration, consistent with treatment goals.

Transdermal: Adult females with an intact uterus: Treatment of moderate to severe vasomotor symptoms associated with menopause or prevention of postmenopausal osteoporosis: Estradiol 0.045 mg/levonorgestrel 0.015 mg: Apply one patch weekly. When used for the treatment of vasomotor symptoms associated with menopause, evaluate to see if therapy is still needed/attempt to discontinue every 3-6 months.

Dosage adjustment in renal impairment: No dosage adjustment provided in manufacturer's labeling. Total estradiol serum concentrations may be excessive in women with end stage renal disease receiving hemodialysis.

Dosage adjustment in hepatic impairment: Use is contraindicated in women with known hepatic impairment or disease.

Additional Information Complete prescribing information should be consulted for additional detail.

Dosage Forms Excipient information presented when available (limited, particularly for generics); consult specific product labeling.

Patch, transdermal:

ClimaraPro: Estradiol 0.045 mg and levonorgestrel 0.015 mg per 24 hours (4s) [22 cm^2; contains estradiol 4.4 mg and levonorgestrel 1.39 mg]

Estradiol and Norethindrone

(es tra DYE ole & nor eth IN drone)

Brand Names: U.S. Activella; CombiPatch; Mimvey

Brand Names: Canada Estalis

Index Terms Norethindrone and Estradiol

Pharmacologic Category Estrogen and Progestin Combination

Use Women with an intact uterus:

Tablet: Treatment of moderate-to-severe vasomotor symptoms associated with menopause; treatment of moderate-to-severe symptoms of vulvar and vaginal atrophy associated with menopause; prophylaxis for postmenopausal osteoporosis

Transdermal patch: Treatment of moderate-to-severe vasomotor symptoms associated with menopause; treatment of moderate-to-severe symptoms of vulvar and vaginal atrophy associated with menopause; treatment of hypoestrogenism due to hypogonadism, castration, or primary ovarian failure

Dosage Note: Patients should be treated with the lowest effective dose and for the shortest duration, consistent with treatment goals. Adults: Females:

Oral:

Moderate-to-severe vasomotor symptoms of menopause, postmenopausal osteoporosis prophylaxis:

Activella: Estradiol 1 mg/norethindrone 0.5 mg or estradiol 0.5 mg/norethindrone 0.1 mg: One tablet daily

Mimvey: Estradiol 1 mg/ norethindrone 0.5 mg: One tablet daily

Vulvar and vaginal atrophy associated with menopause: Activella, Mimvey: Estradiol 1 mg/norethindrone 0.5 mg: One tablet daily

Transdermal patch:

CombiPatch: Hypoestrogenism, menopause (moderate-to-severe vasomotor symptoms; vulvar and vaginal atrophy):

Continuous combined regimen: Apply 1 patch twice weekly

Continuous sequential regimen: Apply estradiol-only patch for first 14 days of cycle, followed by one CombiPatch® applied twice weekly for the remaining 14 days of a 28-day cycle

Estalis [Canadian product]: Menopause (moderate-to-severe vasomotor symptoms; vulvar and vaginal atrophy): Continuous combined regimen: Apply a new patch twice weekly during a 28-day cycle

Dosage adjustment in renal impairment: No dosage adjustment provided in manufacturer's labeling (has not been studied); use with caution.

Dosage adjustment in hepatic impairment: No dosage adjustment provided in manufacturer's labeling (has not been studied). Use is contraindicated with hepatic dysfunction or disease.

Additional Information Complete prescribing information should be consulted for additional detail.

Dosage Forms Excipient information presented when available (limited, particularly for generics); consult specific product labeling.

Patch, transdermal:

CombiPatch:

0.05/0.14: Estradiol 0.05 mg and norethindrone acetate 0.14 mg per day (8s) [9 sq cm]

0.05/0.25: Estradiol 0.05 mg and norethindrone acetate 0.25 mg per day (8s) [16 sq cm]

Tablet, oral: 0.5/0.1: Estradiol 0.5 mg and norethindrone acetate 0.1 mg (28s); 1/0.5: Estradiol 1 mg and norethindrone acetate 0.5 mg (28s)

Activella: 0.5/0.1: Estradiol 0.5 mg and norethindrone acetate 0.1 mg (28s)

Activella: 1/0.5: Estradiol 1 mg and norethindrone acetate 0.5 mg (28s)

Mimvey: 1/0.5: Estradiol 1 mg and norethindrone acetate 0.5 mg (28s)

Dosage Forms: Canada Excipient information presented when available (limited, particularly for generics); consult specific product labeling.

Patch, transdermal:

Estalis:

140/50: Norethindrone acetate 140 mcg and estradiol 50 mcg per day (8s) [9 sq cm; total norethindrone acetate 2.7 mg, total estradiol 0.62 mg]

250/50 Norethindrone acetate 250 mcg and estradiol 50 mcg per day (8s) [16 sq cm; total norethindrone acetate 4.8 mg, total estradiol 0.51 mg]

◆ **Estradiol Transdermal** *see* Estradiol (Systemic) *on page 754*

◆ **Estradiol Valerate** *see* Estradiol (Systemic) *on page 754*

◆ **Estradiol Valerate and Dienogest** *see* Estradiol and Dienogest *on page 762*

◆ **Estradot (Can)** *see* Estradiol (Systemic) *on page 754*

◆ **Estragyn (Can)** *see* Estrogens (Esterified) *on page 775*

Estramustine (es tra MUS teen)

Brand Names: U.S. Emcyt

Brand Names: Canada Emcyt

Index Terms Estramustine Phosphate; Estramustine Phosphate Sodium

Pharmacologic Category Antineoplastic Agent, Alkylating Agent; Antineoplastic Agent, Hormone; Antineoplastic Agent, Hormone (Estrogen/Nitrogen Mustard)

Use Prostate cancer: Treatment (palliative) of progressive or metastatic prostate cancer

Pregnancy Considerations Estramustine is not indicated for use in women. Some men who were impotent on estrogen therapy have regained potency while taking estramustine; effective contraception should be used for male patients with partners of childbearing potential.

Breast-Feeding Considerations Estramustine is not indicated for use in women.

Contraindications Hypersensitivity to estramustine, estradiol, nitrogen mustard, or any component of the formulation; active thrombophlebitis or thromboembolic disorders (except where tumor mass is the cause of thromboembolic disorder and the benefit may outweigh the risk)

Canadian labeling: Additional contraindications (not in the U.S. labeling): Severe hepatic or cardiac disease

Warnings/Precautions Hazardous agent - use appropriate precautions for handling and disposal (NIOSH, 2012). Glucose tolerance may be decreased; use with caution in patients with diabetes. Hypertension (monitor blood pressure periodically), peripheral edema (new-onset or exacerbation), or congestive heart disease may occur; use with caution in patients where fluid accumulation may be poorly tolerated, including cardiovascular disease (HF or hypertension), migraine, seizure disorder or renal dysfunction. Estrogen treatment for prostate cancer is associated with an increased risk of thrombosis and MI; (including fatalities); use caution with history of thrombophlebitis, thrombosis, or thromboembolic disease or history of cerebrovascular or coronary artery disease. Liver enzyme and bilirubin abnormalities may occur; monitor during and for 2 months after treatment. Use with caution in patients with hepatic impairment (may be metabolized poorly) or with metabolic bone diseases. Allergic reactions and angioedema, including airway involvement, have been reported with use. Patients with prostate cancer and osteoblastic metastases are at risk for hypocalcemia; monitor calcium. Estrogenic effects may decrease testosterone levels; may cause gynecomastia and/or impotence. Potentially significant drug-drug/drug-food interactions may exist, requiring dose or frequency adjustment, additional monitoring, and/or selection of alternative therapy. Avoid vaccination with live vaccines during treatment (risk of infection may be increased due to immunosuppression). Although the response to vaccines may be diminished, inactivated vaccines may be administered during treatment. Estramustine is moderately emetogenic; antiemetics may be needed to prevent nausea and vomiting.

Adverse Reactions

>10%:
- Cardiovascular: Edema (20%)
- Endocrine & metabolic: Gynecomastia (75%), breast tenderness (71%), libido decreased
- Gastrointestinal: Nausea (16%), diarrhea (13%), gastrointestinal upset (12%)
- Hepatic: LDH increased (2% to 33%), AST increased (2% to 33%)
- Respiratory: Dyspnea (12%)

1% to 10%:
- Cardiovascular: CHF (3%), MI (3%), cerebrovascular accident (2%), chest pain (1%), flushing (1%)
- Central nervous system: Lethargy (4%), insomnia (3%), emotional lability (2%), anxiety (1%), headache (1%)
- Dermatologic: Bruising (3%), dry skin (2%), pruritus (2%), hair thinning (1%), rash (1%), skin peeling (1%)
- Gastrointestinal: Anorexia (4%), flatulence (2%), burning throat (1%), gastrointestinal bleeding (1%), thirst (1%), vomiting (1%)
- Hematologic: Leukopenia (4%), thrombocytopenia (1%)
- Hepatic: Bilirubin increased (1% to 2%)
- Local: Thrombophlebitis (3%)
- Neuromuscular & skeletal: Leg cramps (9%)
- Ocular: Tearing (1%)
- Respiratory: Pulmonary embolism (2%), upper respiratory discharge (1%), hoarseness (1%)

<1% (Limited to important or life-threatening): Allergic reactions, anemia, angina, angioedema, cerebrovascular ischemia, confusion, coronary ischemia, depression, glucose tolerance decreased, hyper-/hypocalcemia, hypertension, impotence, muscle weakness, venous thrombosis

Drug Interactions

Metabolism/Transport Effects None known.

Avoid Concomitant Use

Avoid concomitant use of Estramustine with any of the following: BCG; Natalizumab; Pimecrolimus; Tacrolimus (Topical); Tofacitinib; Vaccines (Live)

Increased Effect/Toxicity

Estramustine may increase the levels/effects of: Leflunomide; Natalizumab; Tofacitinib; Vaccines (Live)

The levels/effects of Estramustine may be increased by: Clodronate; Denosumab; Pimecrolimus; Roflumilast; Tacrolimus (Topical); Trastuzumab

Decreased Effect

Estramustine may decrease the levels/effects of: BCG; Coccidioidin Skin Test; Sipuleucel-T; Vaccines (Inactivated); Vaccines (Live)

The levels/effects of Estramustine may be decreased by: Calcium Salts; Echinacea

Ethanol/Nutrition/Herb Interactions Food: Estramustine serum levels may be decreased if taken with milk or other dairy products, calcium supplements, and vitamins containing calcium. Management: Take on an empty stomach at least 1 hour before or 2 hours after eating.

Storage/Stability Store refrigerated at 2°C to 8°C (36°F to 46°F).

Mechanism of Action Estradiol and nornitrogen mustard carbamate-linked combination which has antiandrogen effects (due to estradiol) and antimicrotubule effects (due to nornitrogen mustard); causes a marked decrease in plasma testosterone and an increase in estrogen levels.

Pharmacodynamics/Kinetics

Absorption: Incomplete (Bergenheim, 1998)

Metabolism: Initially dephosphorylated in the GI tract, then hepatically oxidated and hydrolyzed to estramustine, estromustine (oxidized isomer of estramustine), estrone, and estradiol.

Bioavailability: Oral: 44% to 75% (Bergenheim, 1998)

Half-life elimination: Estromustine: 13.6 hours (range: 9-23 hours); Estrone: 16.5 hours (Bergenheim, 1998)

Time to peak: 2-3 hours (Bergenheim, 1998)

Excretion: Feces (primarily); urine (trace amounts) (Bergenheim, 1998)

Dosage Prostate cancer, progressive or metastatic: Adults: Males: Oral: 14 mg/kg/day (range: 10-16 mg/kg/day) in 3 or 4 divided doses

Dosage adjustment in renal impairment: No dosage adjustment provided in manufacturer's labeling; use with caution.

Dosage adjustment in hepatic impairment: No dosage adjustment provided in manufacturer's labeling; use with caution (may be poorly metabolized).

Dosing in obesity: *ASCO Guidelines for appropriate chemotherapy dosing in obese adults with cancer:* Utilize patient's actual body weight (full weight) for calculation of body surface area- or weight-based dosing, particularly when the intent of therapy is curative; manage regimen-related toxicities in the same manner as for nonobese patients; if a dose reduction is utilized due to toxicity, consider resumption of full weight-based dosing with subsequent cycles, especially if cause of toxicity (eg, hepatic or renal impairment) is resolved (Griggs, 2012).

Dietary Considerations Should be taken at least 1 hour before or 2 hours after eating. Milk products and calcium-rich foods or supplements may impair the oral absorption of estramustine phosphate sodium.

Administration Administer on an empty stomach, at least 1 hour before or 2 hours after eating. Administer with water; do not administer with milk, milk-based products, or calcium products.

Hazardous agent; use appropriate precautions for handling and disposal (NIOSH, 2012).

Monitoring Parameters Serum calcium, liver function tests (during and for 2 months following treatment); blood pressure

Dosage Forms Excipient information presented when available (limited, particularly for generics); consult specific product labeling.

Capsule, Oral, as phosphate sodium:
  Emcyt: 140 mg

- ◆ **Estramustine Phosphate** *see* Estramustine *on page 763*
- ◆ **Estramustine Phosphate Sodium** *see* Estramustine *on page 763*
- ◆ **Estrasorb** *see* Estradiol (Systemic) *on page 754*
- ◆ **Estratab® (Can)** *see* Estrogens (Esterified) *on page 775*
- ◆ **Estring** *see* Estradiol (Topical) *on page 759*
- ◆ **Estring® (Can)** *see* Estradiol (Topical) *on page 759*

◆ **Estrogel** *see* Estradiol (Systemic) *on page 754*

◆ **EstroGel (Can)** *see* Estradiol (Systemic) *on page 754*

◆ **Estrogenic Substances, Conjugated** *see* Estrogens (Conjugated/Equine, Systemic) *on page 770*

◆ **Estrogenic Substances, Conjugated** *see* Estrogens (Conjugated/Equine, Topical) *on page 773*

Estrogens (Conjugated/Equine) and Bazedoxifene

(ES troe jenz, KON joo gate ed/EE kwine & ba ze DOX i feen)

Index Terms Bazedoxifene and Estrogens (Conjugated/Equine); Duavee; Estrogens (Conjugated/Equine) and Bazedoxifene Acetate

Pharmacologic Category Estrogen Derivative; Selective Estrogen Receptor Modulator (SERM); Tissue-Selective Estrogen Complex (TSEC)

Use

Postmenopausal osteoporosis prophylaxis: Prevention of postmenopausal osteoporosis in women with a uterus

Vasomotor symptoms: Treatment of moderate-to-severe vasomotor symptoms associated with menopause in women with a uterus

Pregnancy Risk Factor X

Dosage Menopause (moderate-to-severe vasomotor symptoms), prevention of postmenopausal osteoporosis: Adults: Females: Oral: One tablet daily

Dosage adjustment in renal impairment: No dosage adjustment provided in manufacturer's labeling (has not been studied). Use is not recommended.

Dosage adjustment in hepatic impairment: Use is contraindicated with hepatic dysfunction or disease.

Additional Information Complete prescribing information should be consulted for additional detail.

Product Availability Duavee: FDA approved October 2013; anticipated availability is first quarter of 2014. Consult prescribing information for additional information.

Dosage Forms

Tablet, oral:

Duavee: Conjugated estrogens 0.45 mg and bazedoxifene 20 mg

Estrogens (Conjugated A/Synthetic)

(ES troe jenz, KON joo gate ed, aye, sin THET ik)

Brand Names: U.S. Cenestin

Brand Names: Canada Cenestin

Pharmacologic Category Estrogen Derivative

Additional Appendix Information

Beers Criteria – Potentially Inappropriate Medications for Geriatrics *on page 2368*

Use Treatment of moderate-to-severe vasomotor symptoms of menopause; treatment of vulvar and vaginal atrophy

Pregnancy Considerations Use during pregnancy is contraindicated.

Breast-Feeding Considerations Estrogen has been shown to decrease the quantity and quality of human milk. Use only if clearly needed. Monitor the growth of the infant closely.

Contraindications Hypersensitivity to estrogens or any component of the formulation; undiagnosed abnormal vaginal bleeding; history of or current thrombophlebitis or venous thromboembolic disorders (including DVT, PE); active or recent (within 1 year) arterial thromboembolic disease (eg, stroke, MI); carcinoma of the breast; estrogen-dependent tumor; hepatic dysfunction or disease; pregnancy

Warnings/Precautions Hazardous agent - use appropriate precautions for handling and disposal (NIOSH, 2012).

Cardiovascular-related considerations: **[U.S. Boxed Warning]: Estrogens with or without progestin should not be used to prevent cardiovascular disease.** Using data from the Women's Health Initiative (WHI) studies, an increased risk of deep vein thrombosis (DVT) and stroke has been reported with conjugated estrogens [CE] and an increased risk of DVT, stroke, pulmonary emboli (PE) and myocardial infarction (MI) has been reported with CE with medroxyprogesterone acetate [MPA] in postmenopausal women. Additional risk factors include diabetes mellitus, hypercholesterolemia, hypertension, SLE, obesity, tobacco use, and/or history of venous thromboembolism (VTE). Adverse cardiovascular events have also been reported in males taking estrogens for prostate cancer. Risk factors should be managed appropriately; discontinue use if adverse cardiovascular events occur or are suspected. Estrogen compounds are generally associated with lipid effects such as increased HDL-cholesterol and decreased LDL-cholesterol. Triglycerides may also be increased; use with caution in patients with familial defects of lipoprotein metabolism. Whenever possible, estrogens should be discontinued at least 4-6 weeks prior to elective surgery associated with an increased risk of thromboembolism or during periods of prolonged immobilization. Women with inherited thrombophilias (eg, protein C or S deficiency) may have increased risk of venous thromboembolism (DeSancho, 2010; van Vlijmen, 2011).

Neurological considerations: **[U.S. Boxed Warning]: Estrogens with or without progestin should not be used to prevent dementia. In the Women's Health Initiative Memory Study (WHIMS), an increased incidence of dementia was observed in women ≥65 years of age taking CE alone or in combination with MPA.**

Cancer-related considerations: **[U.S. Boxed Warning]: Based on data from the Women's Health Initiative (WHI) studies, an increased risk of invasive breast cancer was observed in postmenopausal women using conjugated estrogens (CE) in combination with medroxyprogesterone acetate (MPA).** This risk may be associated with duration of use and declines once combined therapy is discontinued (Chlebowski, 2009). The risk of invasive breast cancer was decreased in postmenopausal women with a hysterectomy using CE only, regardless of weight. However, the risk was not significantly decreased in women at high risk for breast cancer (family history of breast cancer, personal history of benign breast disease) (Anderson, 2012). An increase in abnormal mammogram findings has also been reported with estrogen alone or in combination with progestin therapy. Estrogen use may also lead to severe hypercalcemia in patients with breast cancer and bone metastases; discontinue estrogen if hypercalcemia occurs. Use is contraindicated in patients with known or suspected breast cancer. **[U.S. Boxed Warning]: The use of unopposed estrogen in women with an intact uterus is associated with an increased risk of endometrial cancer. The addition of a progestin to estrogen therapy may decrease the risk of endometrial hyperplasia, a precursor to endometrial cancer. Adequate diagnostic measures, including endometrial sampling if indicated, should be performed to rule out malignancy in postmenopausal women with undiagnosed abnormal vaginal bleeding.** Estrogens may exacerbate endometriosis. Malignant transformation of residual endometrial implants has been reported posthysterectomy with unopposed estrogen therapy. Consider adding a progestin in women with residual endometriosis posthysterectomy. Postmenopausal estrogen therapy and combined estrogen/progesterone therapy may increase the risk of ovarian cancer; however, the absolute risk to an ▶

individual woman is small. Although results from various studies are not consistent, risk does not appear to be significantly associated with the duration, route, or dose of therapy. In one study, the risk decreased after 2 years following discontinuation of therapy (Mørch, 2009). Although the risk of ovarian cancer is rare, women who are at an increased risk (eg, family history) should be counseled about the association (NAMS, 2012).

Estrogens may cause retinal vascular thrombosis; discontinue if migraine, loss of vision, proptosis, diplopia, or other visual disturbances occur; discontinue permanently if papilledema or retinal vascular lesions are observed on examination. Use caution in patients with asthma, epilepsy, hepatic hemangiomas, hereditary angioedema, migraine, porphyria, or SLE; may exacerbate disease. May have adverse effects on glucose tolerance; use caution in women with diabetes. Use with caution in patients with diseases which may be exacerbated by fluid retention, including cardiac or renal dysfunction. Use of postmenopausal estrogen may be associated with an increased risk of gallbladder disease requiring surgery. Estrogens are poorly metabolized in patients with hepatic dysfunction. Use caution with a history of cholestatic jaundice associated with prior estrogen use or pregnancy. Discontinue if jaundice develops or if acute or chronic hepatic disturbances occur. Use is contraindicated with hepatic disease. Use with caution in patients with severe hypocalcemia. Estrogens may increase thyroid-binding globulin (TBG) levels leading to increased circulating total thyroid hormone levels. Women on thyroid replacement therapy may require higher doses of thyroid hormone while receiving estrogens.

Avoid use of oral estrogen (with or without progestins) in the elderly due to potential of increased risk of breast and endometrial cancers, and lack of proven cardioprotection and cognitive protection (Beers Criteria). Safety and efficacy have not been established in children. Prior to puberty, estrogens may cause premature closure of the epiphyses, premature breast development in girls or gynecomastia in boys. Vaginal bleeding and vaginal cornification may also be induced in girls. Whenever possible, estrogens should be discontinued at least 4-6 weeks prior to elective surgery associated with an increased risk of thromboembolism or during periods of prolonged immobilization. The use of estrogens and/or progestins may change the results of some laboratory tests (eg, coagulation factors, lipids, glucose tolerance, binding proteins). The dose, route, and the specific estrogen/progestin influences these changes. In addition, personal risk factors (eg, cardiovascular disease, smoking, diabetes, age) also contribute to adverse events; use of specific products may be contraindicated in women with certain risk factors.

[U.S. Boxed Warning]: Estrogens with or without progestin should be used for the shortest duration possible at the lowest effective dose consistent with treatment goals. Before prescribing estrogen therapy to postmenopausal women, the risks and benefits must be weighed for each patient. Women should be informed of these risks and benefits, as well as possible effects of progestin when added to estrogen therapy. Patients should be reevaluated as clinically appropriate to determine if treatment is still necessary. Available data related to treatment risks are from Women's Health Initiative (WHI) studies, which evaluated oral CE 0.625 mg with or without MPA 2.5 mg relative to placebo in postmenopausal women. Other combinations and dosage forms of estrogens and progestins were not studied. **Outcomes reported from clinical trials using CE with or without MPA should be assumed to be similar for other doses and other dosage forms of estrogens and progestins until comparable data becomes available.**

Vulvar and vaginal atrophy use: When used solely for the treatment of vulvar and vaginal atrophy, topical vaginal products should be considered.

Adverse Reactions

>10%:

- Central nervous system: Headache (11% to 68%), dizziness (11%), pain (11%)
- Endocrine & metabolic: Breast pain (29%), endometrial thickening (19%), metrorrhagia (14%)
- Gastrointestinal: Abdominal pain (9% to 28%), nausea (9% to 18%)
- Neuromuscular & skeletal: Paresthesia (8% to 33%), back pain (14%)
- Respiratory: Upper respiratory tract infection (13%)
- Miscellaneous: Infection (2% to 14%)

1% to 10%:

- Central nervous system: Anxiety (6%), fever (1%)
- Gastrointestinal: Dyspepsia (10%), vomiting (7%), constipation (6%), diarrhea (6%), weight gain (6%)
- Genitourinary: Vaginitis (8%)
- Neuromuscular & skeletal: Leg cramps (10%), hypertonia (6%)
- Respiratory: Rhinitis (6% to 8%), cough (6%)

In addition, the following have been reported with estrogen and/or progestin therapy:

- Cardiovascular: Edema, hypertension, MI, stroke, venous thromboembolism
- Central nervous system: Epilepsy exacerbation, irritability, mental depression, migraine, mood disturbances, nervousness
- Dermatologic: Angioedema, chloasma, erythema multiforme, erythema nodosum, hemorrhagic eruption, hirsutism, melasma, pruritus, rash, scalp hair loss, urticaria
- Endocrine & metabolic: Breast cancer, breast enlargement, breast tenderness, glucose tolerance impaired, HDL-cholesterol increased, hyper-/hypocalcemia, LDL-cholesterol decreased, libido changes, serum triglycerides/phospholipids increased, thyroid-binding globulin increased, total thyroid hormone (T_4) increased
- Gastrointestinal: Abdominal cramps, bloating, cholecystitis, cholelithiasis, gallbladder disease, pancreatitis, weight gain/loss
- Genitourinary: Alterations in frequency and flow of menses, cervical secretion changes, endometrial cancer, endometrial hyperplasia, uterine leiomyomata size increased, vaginal candidiasis
- Hematologic: Aggravation of porphyria, antithrombin III and antifactor Xa decreased, fibrinogen levels increased, platelet aggregability and platelet count increased; prothrombin and factors VII, VIII, IX, X increased
- Hepatic: Cholestatic jaundice, hepatic hemangiomas enlarged
- Neuromuscular & skeletal: Arthralgias, chorea, leg cramps
- Local: Thrombophlebitis
- Ocular: Contact lens intolerance, corneal curvature steepening, retinal vascular thrombosis
- Respiratory: Asthma exacerbation, pulmonary thromboembolism
- Miscellaneous: Anaphylactoid/anaphylactic reactions, carbohydrate intolerance

Drug Interactions

Metabolism/Transport Effects Substrate of CYP1A2 (major), CYP2A6 (minor), CYP2B6 (minor), CYP2C19 (minor), CYP2C9 (minor), CYP2D6 (minor), CYP2E1 (minor), CYP3A4 (major); **Note:** Assignment of Major/Minor substrate status based on clinically relevant drug interaction potential; **Inhibits** CYP1A2 (weak); **Induces** CYP3A4 (weak/moderate)

Avoid Concomitant Use

Avoid concomitant use of Estrogens (Conjugated A/Synthetic) with any of the following: Anastrozole; Axitinib; Dehydroepiandrosterone; Ospemifene; Simeprevir

Increased Effect/Toxicity

Estrogens (Conjugated A/Synthetic) may increase the levels/effects of: Corticosteroids (Systemic); Ospemifene; ROPINIRole; Theophylline Derivatives; Tipranavir

The levels/effects of Estrogens (Conjugated A/Synthetic) may be increased by: Ascorbic Acid; Dehydroepiandrosterone; Herbs (Estrogenic Properties); NSAID (COX-2 Inhibitor)

Decreased Effect

Estrogens (Conjugated A/Synthetic) may decrease the levels/effects of: Anastrozole; Anticoagulants; ARIPiprazole; Axitinib; Chenodiol; Hyaluronidase; Ibrutinib; Ospemifene; Saxagliptin; Simeprevir; Somatropin; Thyroid Products; Ursodiol

The levels/effects of Estrogens (Conjugated A/Synthetic) may be decreased by: Bosentan; CYP1A2 Inducers (Strong); CYP3A4 Inducers (Strong); Cyproterone; Dabrafenib; Deferasirox; Herbs (CYP3A4 Inducers); Mitotane; Peginterferon Alfa-2b; Tipranavir; Tocilizumab

Ethanol/Nutrition/Herb Interactions

Ethanol: Avoid ethanol (routine use increases estrogen plasma concentrations and risk of breast cancer).

Food: Grapefruit juice may increase estrogen plasma concentrations, leading to increased adverse effects.

Herb/Nutraceutical: St John's wort may decrease levels. Herbs with estrogenic properties may enhance the adverse/toxic effect of estrogen derivatives; examples include alfalfa, black cohosh, bloodroot, hops, kudzu, licorice, red clover, saw palmetto, soybean, thyme, wild yam, yucca.

Storage/Stability Store at room temperature of 25°C (77°F).

Mechanism of Action Conjugated A/synthetic estrogens contain a mixture of 9 synthetic estrogen substances, including sodium estrone sulfate, sodium equilin sulfate, sodium 17 alpha-dihydroequilin, sodium 17 alpha-estradiol and sodium 17 beta-dihydroequilin. Estrogens are responsible for the development and maintenance of the female reproductive system and secondary sexual characteristics. Estradiol is the principle intracellular human estrogen and is more potent than estrone and estriol at the receptor level; it is the primary estrogen secreted prior to menopause. Following menopause, estrone and estrone sulfate are more highly produced. Estrogens modulate the pituitary secretion of gonadotropins, luteinizing hormone, and follicle-stimulating hormone through a negative feedback system; estrogen replacement reduces elevated levels of these hormones in postmenopausal women.

Pharmacodynamics/Kinetics

Absorption: Well absorbed over a period of several hours

Protein-binding: Sex hormone-binding globulin (SHBG) and albumin

Metabolism: Hepatic via CYP3A4; estradiol is converted to estrone and estriol; also undergoes enterohepatic recirculation; estrone sulfate is the main metabolite in postmenopausal women

Excretion: Urine (primarily estriol, also as estradiol, estrone, and conjugates)

Dosage The lowest dose that will control symptoms should be used; medication should be discontinued as soon as possible. Oral:

Adults:

Moderate-to-severe vasomotor symptoms: 0.45 mg/day; may be titrated up to 1.25 mg/day. Attempts to discontinue medication should be made at 3- to 6-month intervals.

Vulvar and vaginal atrophy: 0.3 mg/day

Elderly: Refer to adult dosing. A higher incidence of stroke and invasive breast cancer were observed in women >75 years in a WHI substudy using conjugated equine estrogen.

Dosage adjustment in renal impairment: No dosage adjustment provided in manufacturer's labeling (has not been studied); use with caution.

Dosage adjustment in hepatic impairment: No dosage adjustment provided in manufacturer's labeling (has not been studied); use with caution.

Administration Hazardous agent; use appropriate precautions for handling and disposal (NIOSH, 2012).

Monitoring Parameters Yearly physical examination that includes blood pressure and Papanicolaou smear, breast exam, mammogram. Monitor for signs of endometrial cancer in female patients with uterus. Adequate diagnostic measures, including endometrial sampling, if indicated, should be performed to rule out malignancy in all cases of undiagnosed abnormal vaginal bleeding. Monitor for loss of vision, sudden onset of proptosis, diplopia, migraine; signs and symptoms of thromboembolic disorders; glycemic control in patients with diabetes; lipid profiles in patients being treated for hyperlipidemias; thyroid function in patients on thyroid hormone replacement therapy.

Menopausal symptoms: Assess need for therapy at 3- to 6-month intervals

Test Interactions Reduced response to metyrapone test observed with conjugated estrogens (equine).

Additional Information Not biologically equivalent to conjugated estrogens from equine source. Contains 9 unique estrogenic compounds (equine source contains at least 10 active estrogenic compounds).

Dosage Forms Excipient information presented when available (limited, particularly for generics); consult specific product labeling. [DSC] = Discontinued product

Tablet, Oral:

Cenestin: 0.3 mg [contains fd&c blue #2 aluminum lake, fd&c yellow #10 aluminum lake, polysorbate 80]

Cenestin: 0.45 mg [contains fd&c yellow #6 (sunset yellow), polysorbate 80]

Cenestin: 0.625 mg [contains fd&c red #40 aluminum lake, polysorbate 80]

Cenestin: 0.9 mg [contains polysorbate 80]

Cenestin: 1.25 mg [DSC] [contains fd&c blue #2 aluminum lake, polysorbate 80]

Estrogens (Conjugated B/Synthetic)

(ES troe jenz, KON joo gate ed, bee, sin THET ik)

Brand Names: U.S. Enjuvia

Pharmacologic Category Estrogen Derivative

Additional Appendix Information

Beers Criteria - Potentially Inappropriate Medications for Geriatrics *on page 2368*

Use Treatment of moderate-to-severe vasomotor symptoms of menopause; treatment of vulvar and vaginal atrophy associated with menopause; treatment of moderate-to-severe vaginal dryness and pain with intercourse associated with menopause

Pregnancy Considerations Use during pregnancy is contraindicated.

Breast-Feeding Considerations Estrogen has been shown to decrease the quantity and quality of human milk. Use only if clearly needed. Monitor the growth of the infant closely.

Contraindications Hypersensitivity to estrogens or any component of the formulation; undiagnosed abnormal vaginal bleeding; history of or current thrombophlebitis or venous thromboembolic disorders (including DVT, PE); active or recent (within 1 year) arterial thromboembolic disease (eg, stroke, MI); carcinoma of the breast;

estrogen-dependent tumor; hepatic dysfunction or disease; pregnancy

Warnings/Precautions Hazardous agent - use appropriate precautions for handling and disposal (NIOSH, 2012).

Cardiovascular-related considerations: **[U.S. Boxed Warning]: Estrogens with or without progestin should not be used to prevent cardiovascular disease.** Using data from the Women's Health Initiative (WHI) studies, an increased risk of deep vein thrombosis (DVT) and stroke has been reported with CE and an increased risk of DVT, stroke, pulmonary emboli (PE), and myocardial infarction (MI) has been reported with CE with MPA in postmenopausal women. Additional risk factors include diabetes mellitus, hypercholesterolemia, hypertension, SLE, obesity, tobacco use, and/or history of venous thromboembolism (VTE). Risk factors should be managed appropriately; discontinue use if adverse cardiovascular events occur or are suspected. Estrogen compounds are generally associated with lipid effects such as increased HDL-cholesterol and decreased LDL-cholesterol. Triglycerides may also be increased; use with caution in patients with familial defects of lipoprotein metabolism. Whenever possible, estrogens should be discontinued at least 4-6 weeks prior to elective surgery associated with an increased risk of thromboembolism or during periods of prolonged immobilization. Women with inherited thrombophilias (eg, protein C or S deficiency) may have increased risk of venous thromboembolism (DeSancho, 2010; van Vlijmen, 2011).

Neurological considerations: **[U.S. Boxed Warning]: Estrogens with or without progestin should not be used to prevent dementia.** In the Women's Health Initiative Memory Study (WHIMS), an increased incidence of dementia was observed in women ≥65 years of age taking CE alone or in combination with MPA.

Cancer-related considerations: **[U.S. Boxed Warning]: Based on data from the Women's Health Initiative (WHI) studies, an increased risk of invasive breast cancer was observed in postmenopausal women using conjugated estrogens (CE) in combination with medroxyprogesterone acetate (MPA).** This risk may be associated with duration of use and declines once combined therapy is discontinued (Chlebowski, 2009). The risk of invasive breast cancer was decreased in postmenopausal women with a hysterectomy using CE only, regardless of weight. However, the risk was not significantly decreased in women at high risk for breast cancer (family history of breast cancer, personal history of benign breast disease) (Anderson, 2012). An increase in abnormal mammogram findings has also been reported with estrogen alone or in combination with progestin therapy. Estrogen use may also lead to severe hypercalcemia in patients with breast cancer and bone metastases; discontinue estrogen if hypercalcemia occurs. Use is contraindicated in patients with known or suspected breast cancer. **[U.S. Boxed Warning]: The use of unopposed estrogen in women with an intact uterus is associated with an increased risk of endometrial cancer. The addition of a progestin to estrogen therapy may decrease the risk of endometrial hyperplasia, a precursor to endometrial cancer. Adequate diagnostic measures, including endometrial sampling if indicated, should be performed to rule out malignancy in postmenopausal women with undiagnosed abnormal vaginal bleeding.** Estrogens may exacerbate endometriosis. Malignant transformation of residual endometrial implants has been reported posthysterectomy with unopposed estrogen therapy. Consider adding a progestin in women with residual endometriosis posthysterectomy. Postmenopausal estrogen therapy and combined estrogen/progesterone therapy may increase the risk of ovarian cancer; however, the absolute risk to an individual woman is small. Although results from various studies are not consistent, risk does not appear to be significantly associated with the duration, route, or dose of therapy. In one study, the risk decreased after 2 years following discontinuation of therapy (Mørch, 2009). Although the risk of ovarian cancer is rare, women who are at an increased risk (eg, family history) should be counseled about the association (NAMS, 2012).

Estrogens may cause retinal vascular thrombosis; discontinue if migraine, loss of vision, proptosis, diplopia, or other visual disturbances occur; discontinue permanently if papilledema or retinal vascular lesions are observed on examination. Use caution in patients with asthma, epilepsy, hepatic hemangiomas, hereditary angioedema, migraine, porphyria, or SLE; may exacerbate disease. May have adverse effects on glucose tolerance; use caution in women with diabetes. Use with caution in patients with diseases which may be exacerbated by fluid retention, including cardiac or renal dysfunction. Use of postmenopausal estrogen may be associated with an increased risk of gallbladder disease requiring surgery. Estrogens are poorly metabolized in patients with hepatic dysfunction. Use caution with a history of cholestatic jaundice associated with prior estrogen use or pregnancy. Discontinue if jaundice develops or if acute or chronic hepatic disturbances occur. Use is contraindicated with hepatic disease. Use with caution in patients with severe hypocalcemia. Estrogens may increase thyroid-binding globulin (TBG) levels leading to increased circulating total thyroid hormone levels. Women on thyroid replacement therapy may require higher doses of thyroid hormone while receiving estrogens. Avoid use of oral estrogen (with or without progestins) in the elderly due to potential of increased risk of breast and endometrial cancers, and lack of proven cardioprotection and cognitive protection (Beers Criteria). Safety and efficacy have not been established in children. Prior to puberty, estrogens may cause premature closure of the epiphyses, premature breast development in girls or gynecomastia in boys. Vaginal bleeding and vaginal cornification may also be induced in girls. Whenever possible, estrogens should be discontinued at least 4-6 weeks prior to elective surgery associated with an increased risk of thromboembolism or during periods of prolonged immobilization. The use of estrogens and/or progestins may change the results of some laboratory tests (eg, coagulation factors, lipids, glucose tolerance, binding proteins). The dose, route, and the specific estrogen/progestin influences these changes. In addition, personal risk factors (eg, cardiovascular disease, smoking, diabetes, age) also contribute to adverse events; use of specific products may be contraindicated in women with certain risk factors.

[U.S. Boxed Warning]: Estrogens with or without progestin should be used for the shortest duration possible at the lowest effective dose consistent with treatment goals. Before prescribing estrogen therapy to postmenopausal women, the risks and benefits must be weighed for each patient. Women should be informed of these risks and benefits, as well as possible effects of progestin when added to estrogen therapy. Patients should be reevaluated as clinically appropriate to determine if treatment is still necessary. Available data related to treatment risks are from Women's Health Initiative (WHI) studies, which evaluated oral CE 0.625 mg with or without MPA 2.5 mg relative to placebo in postmenopausal women. Other combinations and dosage forms of estrogens and progestins were not studied. **Outcomes reported from clinical trials using CE with or without MPA should be assumed to be similar for other doses and other dosage forms of estrogens and progestins until comparable data becomes available.** When used solely for the treatment of vaginal dryness and pain with intercourse, or vulvar and vaginal atrophy, topical vaginal products should be considered.

Adverse Reactions

>10%:

Central nervous system: Headache (15% to 25%), pain (10% to 19%)

Endocrine & metabolic: Breast pain (up to 14%)

Gastrointestinal: Abdominal pain (4% to 15%), nausea (7% to 12%)

1% to 10%:

Central nervous system: Dizziness (1% to 7%)

Endocrine & metabolic: Dysmenorrhea (1% to 8%)

Gastrointestinal: Flatulence (4% to 7%)

Genitourinary: Vaginitis (2% to 7%)

Neuromuscular & skeletal: Paresthesia (up to 6%)

Respiratory: Bronchitis (up to 7%), rhinitis (4% to 7%), sinusitis (3% to 7%)

Miscellaneous: Flu-like syndrome (4% to 7%)

In addition, the following have been reported with estrogen and/or progestin therapy:

Cardiovascular: Edema, hypertension, MI, stroke, venous thromboembolism

Central nervous system: Epilepsy exacerbation, irritability, mental depression, migraine, mood disturbances, nervousness

Dermatologic: Angioedema, chloasma, erythema multiforme, erythema nodosum, hemorrhagic eruption, hirsutism, loss of scalp hair, melasma, pruritus, rash, urticaria

Endocrine & metabolic: Breast cancer, breast enlargement, breast tenderness, HDL-cholesterol increased, hyper-/hypocalcemia, impaired glucose tolerance, LDL-cholesterol decreased, libido (changes in), serum triglycerides/phospholipids increased, thyroid-binding globulin increased, total thyroid hormone (T_4) increased

Gastrointestinal: Abdominal cramps, bloating, cholecystitis, cholelithiasis, gallbladder disease, pancreatitis, weight gain/loss

Genitourinary: Alterations in frequency and flow of menses, changes in cervical secretions, endometrial cancer, endometrial hyperplasia, increased size of uterine leiomyomata, vaginal candidiasis

Hematologic: Aggravation of porphyria; antithrombin III and antifactor Xa decreased; fibrinogen levels increased; platelet aggregability and platelet count increased; prothrombin and factors VII, VIII, IX, X increased

Hepatic: Cholestatic jaundice, hepatic hemangiomas enlarged

Local: Thrombophlebitis

Neuromuscular & skeletal: Arthralgias, chorea, leg cramps

Ocular: Contact lens intolerance, corneal curvature steepening, retinal vascular thrombosis

Respiratory: Asthma exacerbation, pulmonary thromboembolism

Miscellaneous: Anaphylactoid/anaphylactic reactions, carbohydrate intolerance

Drug Interactions

Metabolism/Transport Effects Substrate of CYP3A4 (major); **Note:** Assignment of Major/Minor substrate status based on clinically relevant drug interaction potential

Avoid Concomitant Use

Avoid concomitant use of Estrogens (Conjugated B/Synthetic) with any of the following: Anastrozole; Dehydroepiandrosterone; Ospemifene

Increased Effect/Toxicity

Estrogens (Conjugated B/Synthetic) may increase the levels/effects of: Corticosteroids (Systemic); Ospemifene; ROPINIRole; Theophylline Derivatives; Tipranavir

The levels/effects of Estrogens (Conjugated B/Synthetic) may be increased by: Ascorbic Acid; Dehydroepiandrosterone; Herbs (Estrogenic Properties); NSAID (COX-2 Inhibitor)

Decreased Effect

Estrogens (Conjugated B/Synthetic) may decrease the levels/effects of: Anastrozole; Anticoagulants; Chenodiol; Hyaluronidase; Ospemifene; Somatropin; Thyroid Products; Ursodiol

The levels/effects of Estrogens (Conjugated B/Synthetic) may be decreased by: Bosentan; CYP3A4 Inducers (Strong); Dabrafenib; Deferasirox; Herbs (CYP3A4 Inducers); Mitotane; Tipranavir; Tocilizumab

Ethanol/Nutrition/Herb Interactions

Ethanol: Avoid ethanol (routine use increases estrogen plasma concentrations and risk of breast cancer).

Food: Grapefruit juice may increase estrogen plasma concentrations, leading to increased adverse effects.

Herb/Nutraceutical: St John's wort may decrease levels. Herbs with estrogenic properties may enhance the adverse/toxic effect of estrogen derivatives; examples include alfalfa, black cohosh, bloodroot, hops, kudzu, licorice, red clover, saw palmetto, soybean, thyme, wild yam, and yucca.

Storage/Stability Store at room temperature of 25°C (77°F).

Mechanism of Action Conjugated B/synthetic estrogens contain a mixture of 10 synthetic estrogen substances, including sodium estrone sulfate, sodium equilin sulfate, sodium 17-alpha-dihydroequilin, sodium 17-alpha-estradiol, and sodium 17-beta-dihydroequilin. Estrogens are responsible for the development and maintenance of the female reproductive system and secondary sexual characteristics. Estradiol is the principle intracellular human estrogen and is more potent than estrone and estriol at the receptor level; it is the primary estrogen secreted prior to menopause. Following menopause, estrone and estrone sulfate are more highly produced. Estrogens modulate the pituitary secretion of gonadotropins, luteinizing hormone, and follicle-stimulating hormone through a negative feedback system; estrogen replacement reduces elevated levels of these hormones in postmenopausal women.

Pharmacodynamics/Kinetics

Absorption: Well absorbed over a period of several hours

Protein-binding: Sex hormone-binding globulin (SHBG) and albumin

Metabolism: Hepatic via CYP3A4; estradiol is converted to estrone and estriol; also undergoes enterohepatic recirculation; estrone sulfate is the main metabolite in postmenopausal women

Half-life elimination: Conjugated estrone: 8-20 hours; conjugated equilin: 5-17 hours

Excretion: Urine (primarily estriol, also as estradiol, estrone, and conjugates)

Dosage The lowest dose that will control symptoms should be used; medication should be discontinued as soon as possible. Oral:

Adults:

Moderate-to-severe vasomotor symptoms associated with menopause: 0.3 mg/day; may be titrated up to 1.25 mg/day. Attempts to discontinue medication should be made at 3- to 6-month intervals.

Vaginal dryness/vulvar and vaginal atrophy associated with menopause: 0.3 mg/day. Attempts to discontinue medication should be made at 3- to 6-month intervals.

Elderly: A higher incidence of stroke and invasive breast cancer were observed in women >75 years in a WHI substudy using conjugated equine estrogen.

Administration Hazardous agent; use appropriate precautions for handling and disposal (NIOSH, 2012).

Monitoring Parameters Yearly physical examination that may include blood pressure and Papanicolaou smear, breast exam, mammogram. Monitor for signs of endometrial cancer in female patients with uterus. Adequate diagnostic measures, including endometrial sampling, if indicated, should be performed to rule out malignancy in all cases of undiagnosed abnormal vaginal bleeding. Monitor for loss of vision, sudden onset of proptosis, diplopia, migraine; signs and symptoms of thromboembolic disorders; glycemic control in patients with diabetes; lipid profiles in patients being treated for hyperlipidemias; thyroid function in patients on thyroid hormone replacement therapy.

Test Interactions Reduced response to metyrapone test observed with conjugated estrogens (equine).

Additional Information Not biologically equivalent to conjugated estrogens from equine source. Contains 10 unique estrogenic compounds (equine source contains at least 10 active estrogenic compounds).

Dosage Forms Excipient information presented when available (limited, particularly for generics); consult specific product labeling. [DSC] = Discontinued product

Tablet, Oral:

- Enjuvia: 0.3 mg, 0.45 mg, 0.625 mg [DSC] [contains edetate disodium, polysorbate 80]
- Enjuvia: 0.9 mg [contains edetate disodium, fd&c blue #1 aluminum lake, fd&c yellow #10 aluminum lake, fd&c yellow #6 aluminum lake, polysorbate 80]
- Enjuvia: 1.25 mg [contains edetate disodium, polysorbate 80]

Estrogens (Conjugated/Equine, Systemic) (ES troe jenz KON joo gate ed, EE kwine)

Brand Names: U.S. Premarin

Brand Names: Canada C.E.S.®; Congest; PMS-Conjugated Estrogens C.S.D.; Premarin®

Index Terms C.E.S.; CE; CEE; Conjugated Estrogen; Estrogenic Substances, Conjugated

Pharmacologic Category Estrogen Derivative

Additional Appendix Information

Beers Criteria – Potentially Inappropriate Medications for Geriatrics *on page 2368*

Use Treatment of moderate-to-severe vasomotor symptoms associated with menopause; treatment of vulvar and vaginal atrophy due to menopause; hypoestrogenism (due to hypogonadism, castration, or primary ovarian failure); prostatic cancer (palliation); breast cancer (palliation); postmenopausal osteoporosis (prophylaxis); abnormal uterine bleeding

Unlabeled Use Uremic bleeding

Pregnancy Considerations Estrogens are not indicated for use during pregnancy or immediately postpartum. In general, the use of estrogen and progestin as in combination hormonal contraceptives have not been associated with teratogenic effects when inadvertently taken early in pregnancy. These products are contraindicated for use during pregnancy.

Breast-Feeding Considerations Estrogen has been shown to decrease the quantity and quality of human milk. Use only if clearly needed. Monitor the growth of the infant closely.

Contraindications Angioedema or anaphylactic reaction to estrogens or any component of the formulation; undiagnosed abnormal vaginal bleeding; history of or current thrombophlebitis or venous thromboembolic disorders (including DVT, PE); active or history of arterial thromboembolic disease (eg, stroke, MI); carcinoma of the breast (except in appropriately selected patients being treated for metastatic disease); estrogen-dependent tumor; hepatic dysfunction or disease; known protein C, protein S, antithrombin deficiency or other known thrombophilic disorders; pregnancy

Canadian labeling: Additional contraindications (not in U.S. labeling): Endometrial hyperplasia; partial or complete vision loss due to ophthalmic vascular disease; migraine with aura

Warnings/Precautions

Hazardous agent - use appropriate precautions for handling and disposal (NIOSH, 2012). Anaphylaxis requiring emergency medical management has been reported within minutes to hours of taking conjugated estrogen (CE) tablets. Angioedema involving the face, feet, hands, larynx, and tongue has also been reported. Exogenous estrogens may exacerbate symptoms in women with hereditary angioedema.

[U.S. Boxed Warning]: Based on data from the Women's Health Initiative (WHI) studies, an increased risk of invasive breast cancer was observed in postmenopausal women using conjugated estrogens (CE) in combination with medroxyprogesterone acetate (MPA). This risk may be associated with duration of use and declines once combined therapy is discontinued (Chlebowski, 2009). The risk of invasive breast cancer was decreased in postmenopausal women with a hysterectomy using CE only, regardless of weight. However, the risk was not significantly decreased in women at high risk for breast cancer (family history of breast cancer, personal history of benign breast disease) (Anderson, 2012). An increase in abnormal mammogram findings has also been reported with estrogen alone or in combination with progestin therapy. Estrogen use may lead to severe hypercalcemia in patients with breast cancer and bone metastases; discontinue estrogen if hypercalcemia occurs. **[U.S. Boxed Warning]: The use of unopposed estrogen in women with an intact uterus is associated with an increased risk of endometrial cancer. The addition of a progestin to estrogen therapy may decrease the risk of endometrial hyperplasia, a precursor to endometrial cancer. Adequate diagnostic measures, including endometrial sampling if indicated, should be performed to rule out malignancy in postmenopausal women with undiagnosed abnormal vaginal bleeding.** Estrogens may exacerbate endometriosis. Malignant transformation of residual endometrial implants has been reported posthysterectomy with unopposed estrogen therapy. Consider adding a progestin in women with residual endometriosis posthysterectomy. Postmenopausal estrogen therapy and combined estrogen/progesterone therapy may increase the risk of ovarian cancer; however, the absolute risk to an individual woman is small. Although results from various studies are not consistent, risk does not appear to be significantly associated with the duration, route, or dose of therapy. In one study, the risk decreased after 2 years following discontinuation of therapy (Mørch, 2009). Although the risk of ovarian cancer is rare, women who are at an increased risk (eg, family history) should be counseled about the association (NAMS, 2012).

[U.S. Boxed Warning]: Estrogens with or without progestin should not be used to prevent cardiovascular disease. Using data from the Women's Health Initiative (WHI) studies, an increased risk of deep vein thrombosis (DVT) and stroke has been reported with CE and an increased risk of DVT, stroke, pulmonary emboli (PE) and myocardial infarction (MI) has been reported with CE with MPA in postmenopausal women. Additional risk factors include diabetes mellitus, hypercholesterolemia, hypertension, SLE, obesity, tobacco use, and/or history of venous thromboembolism (VTE). Adverse cardiovascular events have also been reported in males taking estrogens for prostate cancer. Risk factors should be managed appropriately; discontinue use if adverse cardiovascular events occur or are suspected. Women with inherited thrombophilias (eg, protein C or S deficiency) may have increased risk of venous thromboembolism (DeSancho,

2010; van Vlijmen, 2011). Use is contraindicated in women with protein C, protein S, antithrombin deficiency, or other known thrombophilic disorders.

[U.S. Boxed Warning]: Estrogens with or without progestin should not be used to prevent dementia. In the Women's Health Initiative Memory Study (WHIMS), an increased incidence of dementia was observed in women ≥65 years of age taking CE alone or in combination with MPA.

Estrogen compounds are generally associated with lipid effects such as increased HDL-cholesterol and decreased LDL-cholesterol. Triglycerides may also be increased; discontinue if pancreatitis occurs. Use with caution in patients with familial defects of lipoprotein metabolism. Estrogens may increase thyroid-binding globulin (TBG) levels leading to increased circulating total thyroid hormone levels. Women on thyroid replacement therapy may require higher doses of thyroid hormone while receiving estrogens. Use caution in patients with hypoparathyroidism; estrogen-induced hypocalcemia may occur. May have adverse effects on glucose tolerance; use caution in women with diabetes. Use caution in patients with asthma, epilepsy, hepatic hemangiomas, porphyria, or SLE; may exacerbate disease. Use with caution in patients with diseases which may be exacerbated by fluid retention, including cardiac or renal dysfunction. Use of postmenopausal estrogen may be associated with an increased risk of gallbladder disease requiring surgery. Use caution with migraine; may exacerbate disease. Canadian labeling contraindicates use in migraine with aura. Estrogens may cause retinal vascular thrombosis; discontinue if migraine, loss of vision, proptosis, diplopia, or other visual disturbances occur; discontinue permanently if papilledema or retinal vascular lesions are observed on examination.

Estrogens are poorly metabolized in patients with hepatic dysfunction. Use caution with a history of cholestatic jaundice associated with prior estrogen use or pregnancy. Discontinue if jaundice develops or if acute or chronic hepatic disturbances occur. Use is contraindicated with hepatic disease.

Whenever possible, estrogens should be discontinued at least 4-6 weeks prior to elective surgery associated with an increased risk of thromboembolism or during periods of prolonged immobilization. Avoid use of oral estrogen (with or without progestins) in the elderly due to potential of increased risk of breast and endometrial cancers, and lack of proven cardioprotection and cognitive protection (Beers Criteria). Prior to puberty, estrogens may cause premature closure of the epiphyses, premature breast development in girls or gynecomastia in boys. Vaginal bleeding and vaginal cornification may also be induced in girls. The use of estrogens and/or progestins may change the results of some laboratory tests (eg, coagulation factors, lipids, glucose tolerance, binding proteins). The dose, route, and the specific estrogen/progestin influences these changes. In addition, personal risk factors (eg, cardiovascular disease, smoking, diabetes, age) also contribute to adverse events; use of specific products may be contraindicated in women with certain risk factors.

[U.S. Boxed Warning]: Estrogens with or without progestin should be used for the shortest duration possible at the lowest effective dose consistent with treatment goals. Before prescribing estrogen therapy to postmenopausal women, the risks and benefits must be weighed for each patient. Women should be informed of these risks and benefits, as well as possible effects of progestin when added to estrogen therapy. Patients should be reevaluated as clinically appropriate to determine if treatment is still necessary. Available data related to treatment risks are from Women's Health Initiative (WHI) studies, which evaluated oral CE 0.625 mg with or without MPA 2.5 mg relative to placebo in postmenopausal women. Other combinations and dosage forms of estrogens and progestins were not studied. **Outcomes reported from clinical trials using CE with or without MPA should be assumed to be similar for other doses and other dosage forms of estrogens and progestins until comparable data becomes available.**

Vulvar and vaginal atrophy use: Moderate-to-severe symptoms of vulvar and vaginal atrophy include vaginal dryness, dyspareunia, and atrophic vaginitis. When used solely for the treatment of vulvar and vaginal atrophy, topical vaginal products should be considered (NAMS, 2007).

Osteoporosis use: For use only in women at significant risk of osteoporosis and for who other nonestrogen medications are not considered appropriate.

Adverse Reactions Note: Percentages reported in postmenopausal women following oral use.

>10%:

- Central nervous system: Headache (26% to 32%; placebo 28%), pain (17% to 20%; placebo 18%)
- Endocrine & metabolic: Breast pain (7% to 12%; placebo 9%)
- Gastrointestinal: Abdominal pain (15% to 17%), diarrhea (6% to 7%; placebo 6%)
- Genitourinary: Vaginal hemorrhage (2% to 14%)
- Neuromuscular & skeletal: Back pain (13% to 14%), arthralgia (7% to 14%; placebo 12%)
- Respiratory: Pharyngitis (10% to 12%; placebo 11%), sinusitis: (6% to 11%; placebo 7%)

1% to 10%:

- Central nervous system: Depression (5% to 8%), dizziness (4% to 6%), nervousness (2% to 5%)
- Dermatologic: Pruritus (4% to 5%)
- Gastrointestinal: Flatulence (6% to 7%)
- Genitourinary: Vaginitis (5% to 7%), leukorrhea (4% to 7%), vaginal moniliasis (5% to 6%)
- Neuromuscular & skeletal: Weakness (7% to 8%), leg cramps (3% to 7%)
- Respiratory: Cough increased (4% to 7%)

Additional adverse reactions reported with injection; frequency not defined: Local: injection site: Edema, pain, phlebitis

Postmarketing and/or case reports: Alopecia, anaphylaxis, angioedema, asthma exacerbation, benign meningioma (possible growth), bloating, breast cancer, breast discharge/enlargement/tenderness, cervical secretion changes, chloasma, cholestatic jaundice, contact lens intolerance, dementia, deep vein thrombosis (DVT), dysmenorrhea, edema, endometrial cancer, endometrial hyperplasia, epilepsy exacerbation, erythema multiforme, erythema nodosum, fibrocystic breast changes, galactorrhea, gallbladder disease, glucose intolerance, gynecomastia (males), hepatic hemangiomas (enlargement), hirsutism, hypersensitivity reactions, hypertension, irritability, ischemic colitis, libido changes, melasma, MI, migraine, mood disturbances, nausea, ovarian cancer, pancreatitis, pulmonary emboli (PE), pelvic pain, porphyria exacerbation, rash, retinal vascular thrombosis, stroke, superficial venous thrombosis, thrombophlebitis, triglyceride increase, urticaria, uterine bleeding (abnormal), uterine leiomyomata (increase in size), vaginal candidiasis, vomiting, weight changes

Drug Interactions

Metabolism/Transport Effects Substrate of CYP1A2 (major), CYP2A6 (minor), CYP2B6 (minor), CYP2C19 (minor), CYP2C9 (minor), CYP2D6 (minor), CYP2E1 (minor), CYP3A4 (major); **Note:** Assignment of Major/Minor substrate status based on clinically relevant drug interaction potential; **Inhibits** CYP1A2 (weak); **Induces** CYP3A4 (weak/moderate)

Avoid Concomitant Use

Avoid concomitant use of Estrogens (Conjugated/Equine, Systemic) with any of the following: Anastrozole; Axitinib; Dehydroepiandrosterone; Ospemifene; Simeprevir

Increased Effect/Toxicity

Estrogens (Conjugated/Equine, Systemic) may increase the levels/effects of: Corticosteroids (Systemic); Ospemifene; ROPINIRole; Theophylline Derivatives; Tipranavir

The levels/effects of Estrogens (Conjugated/Equine, Systemic) may be increased by: Ascorbic Acid; Dehydroepiandrosterone; Herbs (Estrogenic Properties); NSAID (COX-2 Inhibitor)

Decreased Effect

Estrogens (Conjugated/Equine, Systemic) may decrease the levels/effects of: Anastrozole; Anticoagulants; ARIPiprazole; Axitinib; Chenodiol; Hyaluronidase; Ibrutinib; Ospemifene; Saxagliptin; Simeprevir; Somatropin; Thyroid Products; Ursodiol

The levels/effects of Estrogens (Conjugated/Equine, Systemic) may be decreased by: Bosentan; CYP1A2 Inducers (Strong); CYP3A4 Inducers (Strong); Cyproterone; Dabrafenib; Deferasirox; Herbs (CYP3A4 Inducers); Mitotane; Peginterferon Alfa-2b; Tipranavir; Tocilizumab

Ethanol/Nutrition/Herb Interactions

Ethanol: Avoid ethanol (routine use increases estrogen plasma concentrations and risk of breast cancer). Ethanol may also increase the risk of osteoporosis.

Food: Folic acid absorption may be decreased.

Herb/Nutraceutical: St John's wort may decrease levels. Herbs with estrogenic properties may enhance the adverse/toxic effect of estrogen derivatives; examples include alfalfa, black cohosh, bloodroot, hops, kudzu, licorice, red clover, saw palmetto, soybean, thyme, wild yam, yucca.

Preparation for Administration Injection: Reconstitute with sterile water for injection; slowly inject diluent against side wall of the vial. Agitate gently; do not shake violently.

Hazardous agent; use appropriate precautions for handling and disposal (NIOSH, 2012).

Storage/Stability

Injection: Refrigerate at 2°C to 8°C (36°F to 46°F) prior to reconstitution. Use immediately following reconstitution.

Tablets: Store at room temperature 20°C to 25°C (68°F to 77°F).

Mechanism of Action Conjugated estrogens contain a mixture of estrone sulfate, equilin sulfate, 17 alpha-dihydroequilin, 17 alpha-estradiol and 17 beta-dihydroequilin. Estrogens are responsible for the development and maintenance of the female reproductive system and secondary sexual characteristics. Estradiol is the principle intracellular human estrogen and is more potent than estrone and estriol at the receptor level; it is the primary estrogen secreted prior to menopause. Following menopause, estrone and estrone sulfate are more highly produced. Estrogens modulate the pituitary secretion of gonadotropins, luteinizing hormone, and follicle-stimulating hormone through a negative feedback system; estrogen replacement reduces elevated levels of these hormones in postmenopausal women.

Pharmacodynamics/Kinetics

Absorption: Well absorbed

Protein binding: Binds to sex-hormone-binding globulin and albumin

Metabolism: Hepatic via CYP3A4; estradiol is converted to estrone and estriol; also undergoes enterohepatic recirculation (avoided with vaginal administration); estrone sulfate is the main metabolite in postmenopausal women

Half-life elimination: Total estrone: 27 hours

Time to peak, plasma: Total estrone: 7 hours

Excretion: Urine (primarily estriol, also as estradiol, estrone, and conjugates

Dosage Adults:

Males: Androgen-dependent prostate cancer palliation: Oral: 1.25-2.5 mg 3 times/day

Females:

Prevention of postmenopausal osteoporosis: Oral:

U.S. labeling: Initial: 0.3 mg/day cyclically* or daily, depending on medical assessment of patient. Dose may be adjusted based on bone mineral density and clinical response. The lowest effective dose should be used.

Canadian labeling: 0.625 mg once daily

Moderate-to-severe vasomotor symptoms associated with menopause: Oral: Initial: 0.3 mg/day, cyclically* or daily, depending on medical assessment of patient. Adjust dose based on patient's response. The lowest dose that will control symptoms should be used.

Vulvar and vaginal atrophy: Oral: Initial: 0.3 mg/day; the lowest dose that will control symptoms should be used. May be given cyclically* or daily, depending on medical assessment of patient. Adjust dose based on patient's response.

Abnormal uterine bleeding: Acute/heavy bleeding:

Oral (unlabeled route): 10-20 mg/day in 4 divided doses has been used in place of I.M./I.V. doses (ACOG, 2000)

I.M., I.V.: 25 mg, may repeat in 6-12 hours if needed (manufacturer's labeling) **or** 25 mg I.V. repeated every 4 hours for 24 hours (ACOG, 2000). Patients who do not respond to 1-2 doses should be re-evaluated (ACOG, 2000).

Note: Treatment should be followed by a low-dose oral contraceptive; medroxyprogesterone acetate along with or following estrogen therapy can also be given

Female hypogonadism: Oral: 0.3-0.625 mg/day given cyclically*; dose may be titrated in 6- to 12-month intervals; progestin treatment should be added to maintain bone mineral density once skeletal maturity is achieved.

Female castration, primary ovarian failure: Oral: 1.25 mg/day given cyclically*; adjust according to severity of symptoms and patient response. For maintenance, adjust to the lowest effective dose.

***Cyclic administration:** Either 3 weeks on, 1 week off **or** 25 days on, 5 days off

Males and Females:

Breast cancer palliation, metastatic disease in selected patients: Oral: 10 mg 3 times/day for at least 3 months

Uremic bleeding (unlabeled use): I.V.: 0.6 mg/kg/day for 5 days (Livio, 1986)

Elderly: Refer to adult dosing; a higher incidence of stroke and invasive breast cancer was observed in women >75 years in a WHI substudy.

Dosage adjustment in renal impairment: No dosage adjustment provided in manufacturer's labeling (has not been studied). Use with caution; may increase risk of fluid retention.

Dosage adjustment in hepatic impairment: Use is contraindicated with hepatic dysfunction or disease.

Dietary Considerations Ensure adequate calcium and vitamin D intake when used for the prevention of osteoporosis. Powder for reconstitution for injection (25 mg) contains lactose 200 mg.

Administration

Injection: May also be administered intramuscularly; when administered I.V., drug should be administered slowly to avoid the occurrence of a flushing reaction

Oral tablet: Administer at bedtime to minimize adverse effects. May be administered without regard to meals.

Abnormal uterine bleeding: High-dose therapy (eg, 10-20 mg/day) may cause nausea; consider concomitant use of an antiemetic

Hazardous agent; use appropriate precautions for handling and disposal (NIOSH, 2012).

Monitoring Parameters Routine physical examination that includes blood pressure and Papanicolaou smear, breast exam, mammogram. Monitor for signs of endometrial cancer in female patients with uterus. Adequate diagnostic measures, including endometrial sampling, if indicated, should be performed to rule out malignancy in all cases of undiagnosed abnormal vaginal bleeding. Monitor for loss of vision, sudden onset of proptosis, diplopia, migraine; signs and symptoms of thromboembolic disorders; glycemic control in patients with diabetes; lipid profiles in patients being treated for hyperlipidemias; thyroid function in patients on thyroid hormone replacement therapy.

Menopausal symptoms: Assess need for therapy at 3- to 6-month intervals

Prevention of osteoporosis: Bone density measurement

Uremic bleeding: Bleeding time

Reference Range

Children: <10 mcg/24 hours (SI: <35 µmol/day) (values at Mayo Medical Laboratories)

Adults:

Males: 15-40 mcg/24 hours (SI: 52-139 micromole/day)

Females:

Menstruating: 15-80 mcg/24 hours (SI: 52-277 micromole/day)

Postmenopausal: <20 mcg/24 hours (SI: <69 micromole/day)

Test Interactions Reduced response to metyrapone test.

Dosage Forms Excipient information presented when available (limited, particularly for generics); consult specific product labeling.

Solution Reconstituted, Injection:

Premarin: 25 mg (1 ea) [contains benzyl alcohol]

Tablet, Oral:

Premarin: 0.3 mg [contains fd&c blue #2 (indigotine), fd&c yellow #10 (quinoline yellow)]

Premarin: 0.45 mg [contains fd&c blue #2 (indigotine)]

Premarin: 0.625 mg [contains fd&c blue #2 (indigotine), fd&c red #40]

Premarin: 0.9 mg

Premarin: 1.25 mg [contains fd&c yellow #10 (quinoline yellow), fd&c yellow #6 (sunset yellow)]

Estrogens (Conjugated/Equine, Topical)

(ES troe jenz KON joo gate ed, EE kwine)

Brand Names: U.S. Premarin

Brand Names: Canada Premarin®

Index Terms C.E.S.; CE; CEE; Conjugated Estrogen; Estrogenic Substances, Conjugated

Pharmacologic Category Estrogen Derivative

Additional Appendix Information

Beers Criteria – Potentially Inappropriate Medications for Geriatrics *on page 2368*

Use Treatment of atrophic vaginitis and kraurosis vulvae; moderate-to-severe dyspareunia (pain during intercourse) due to vaginal/vulvar atrophy of menopause

Pregnancy Considerations Estrogens are not indicated for use during pregnancy or immediately postpartum. In general, the use of estrogen and progestin as in combination hormonal contraceptives have not been associated with teratogenic effects when inadvertently taken early in pregnancy. These products are contraindicated for use during pregnancy. Use of the vaginal cream may weaken latex found in condoms, diaphragms, or cervical caps.

Breast-Feeding Considerations Estrogen has been shown to decrease the quantity and quality of human milk. Use only if clearly needed. Monitor the growth of the infant closely.

Contraindications Undiagnosed abnormal vaginal bleeding; history of or current thrombophlebitis or venous thromboembolic disorders (including DVT, PE); active or history of arterial thromboembolic disease (eg, stroke, MI); carcinoma of the breast; estrogen-dependent tumor; hepatic dysfunction or disease; known protein C, protein S, antithrombin deficiency or other known thrombophilic disorders; pregnancy

Canadian labeling: Additional contraindications (not in U.S. labeling): Hypersensitivity to estrogens or any component of the formulation; endometrial hyperplasia; partial or complete vision loss due to ophthalmic vascular disease

Warnings/Precautions Hazardous agent - use appropriate precautions for handling and disposal (NIOSH, 2012).

[U.S. Boxed Warning]: Based on data from the Women's Health Initiative (WHI) studies, an increased risk of invasive breast cancer was observed in postmenopausal women using conjugated estrogens (CE) in combination with medroxyprogesterone acetate (MPA). This risk may be associated with duration of use and declines once combined therapy is discontinued (Chlebowski, 2009). The risk of invasive breast cancer was decreased in postmenopausal women with a hysterectomy using CE only, regardless of weight. However, the risk was not significantly decreased in women at high risk for breast cancer (family history of breast cancer, personal history of benign breast disease) (Anderson, 2012). An increase in abnormal mammogram findings has also been reported with estrogen alone or in combination with progestin therapy. Estrogen use may lead to severe hypercalcemia in patients with breast cancer and bone metastases; discontinue estrogen if hypercalcemia occurs. Use is contraindicated in patients with known or suspected breast cancer. **[U.S. Boxed Warning]: The use of unopposed estrogen in women with an intact uterus is associated with an increased risk of endometrial cancer. The addition of a progestin to estrogen therapy may decrease the risk of endometrial hyperplasia, a precursor to endometrial cancer. Adequate diagnostic measures, including endometrial sampling if indicated, should be performed to rule out malignancy in postmenopausal women with undiagnosed abnormal vaginal bleeding.** Estrogens may exacerbate endometriosis. Malignant transformation of residual endometrial implants has been reported posthysterectomy with unopposed estrogen therapy. Consider adding a progestin in women with residual endometriosis posthysterectomy. Postmenopausal estrogen therapy and combined estrogen/progesterone therapy may increase the risk of ovarian cancer; however, the absolute risk to an individual woman is small. Although results from various studies are not consistent, risk does not appear to be significantly associated with the duration, route, or dose of therapy. In one study, the risk decreased after 2 years following discontinuation of therapy (Mørch, 2009). Although the risk of ovarian cancer is rare, women who are at an increased risk (eg, family history) should be counseled about the association (NAMS, 2012).

[U.S. Boxed Warning]: Estrogens with or without progestin should not be used to prevent cardiovascular disease. Using data from the Women's Health Initiative (WHI) studies, an increased risk of deep vein thrombosis (DVT) and stroke has been reported with CE and an increased risk of DVT, stroke, pulmonary emboli (PE) and myocardial infarction (MI) has been reported with CE with MPA in postmenopausal women. Additional risk factors include diabetes mellitus, hypercholesterolemia, hypertension, SLE, obesity, tobacco use, and/or history of venous thromboembolism (VTE). Risk factors should be managed appropriately; discontinue use if adverse cardiovascular events occur or are suspected. Women with inherited thrombophilias (eg, protein C or S deficiency) may have increased risk of venous thromboembolism (DeSancho, 2010; van Vlijmen 2011). Use is contraindicated in women with protein C, protein S, antithrombin deficiency, or other known thrombophilic disorders.

[U.S. Boxed Warning]: Estrogens with or without progestin should not be used to prevent dementia. In the Women's Health Initiative Memory Study (WHIMS), an increased incidence of dementia was observed in women ≥65 years of age taking CE alone or in combination with MPA.

Estrogen compounds are generally associated with lipid effects such as increased HDL-cholesterol and decreased LDL-cholesterol. Triglycerides may also be increased; discontinue if pancreatitis occurs. Use with caution in patients with familial defects of lipoprotein metabolism. Estrogens may increase thyroid-binding globulin (TBG) levels leading to increased circulating total thyroid hormone levels. Women on thyroid replacement therapy may require higher doses of thyroid hormone while receiving estrogens. Use caution in patients with hypoparathyroidism; estrogen induced hypocalcemia may occur. May have adverse effects on glucose tolerance; use caution in women with diabetes. Use caution in patients with asthma, epilepsy, hepatic hemangiomas, migraine, porphyria or SLE; may exacerbate disease. Use with caution in patients with diseases which may be exacerbated by fluid retention, including cardiac or renal dysfunction. Use of postmenopausal estrogen may be associated with an increased risk of gallbladder disease requiring surgery. Estrogens may cause retinal vascular thrombosis; discontinue if migraine, loss of vision, proptosis, diplopia, or other visual disturbances occur; discontinue permanently if papilledema or retinal vascular lesions are observed on examination. Exogenous estrogens may exacerbate angioedema symptoms in women with hereditary angioedema. The use of estrogens and/or progestins may change the results of some laboratory tests (eg, coagulation factors, lipids, glucose tolerance, binding proteins). The dose, route, and the specific estrogen/progestin influences these changes. In addition, personal risk factors (eg, cardiovascular disease, smoking, diabetes, age) also contribute to adverse events; use of specific products may be contraindicated in women with certain risk factors.

Estrogens are poorly metabolized in patients with hepatic dysfunction. Use caution with a history of cholestatic jaundice associated with prior estrogen use or pregnancy. Discontinue if jaundice develops or if acute or chronic hepatic disturbances occur. Use is contraindicated with hepatic disease.

In the elderly, low-dose intravaginal estrogen may be appropriate for use in the management of vaginal symptoms, lower urinary tract infections, and dyspareunia; in addition, evidence has shown that vaginal estrogens (particularly at estradiol doses of <25 mcg twice weekly) in the treatment of vaginal dryness is safe and effective in women with breast cancer. (Beers Criteria).

Vulvar and vaginal atrophy use: When used solely for the treatment of vulvar and vaginal atrophy, topical vaginal products should be considered. Use caution applying topical products to severely atrophic vaginal mucosa.

Whenever possible, estrogens should be discontinued at least 4-6 weeks prior to elective surgery associated with an increased risk of thromboembolism or during periods of prolonged immobilization.

[U.S. Boxed Warning]: Estrogens with or without progestin should be used for the shortest duration possible at the lowest effective dose consistent with treatment goals. Before prescribing estrogen therapy to postmenopausal women, the risks and benefits must be weighed for each patient. Women should be informed of these risks and benefits, as well as possible effects of progestin when added to estrogen therapy. Patients should be reevaluated as clinically appropriate to determine if treatment is still necessary. Available data related to treatment risks are from Women's Health Initiative (WHI) studies, which evaluated oral CE 0.625 mg with or without MPA 2.5 mg relative to placebo in postmenopausal women. Other combinations and dosage forms of estrogens and progestins were not studied. **Outcomes reported from clinical trials using CE with or without MPA should be assumed to be similar for other doses and other dosage forms of estrogens and progestins until comparable data becomes available.**

Moderate-to-severe symptoms of vulvar and vaginal atrophy include vaginal dryness, dyspareunia, and atrophic vaginitis. When used solely for the treatment of vulvar and vaginal atrophy, topical vaginal products should be considered. Use caution applying topical products to severely atrophic vaginal mucosa. Use of a progestin is normally not required when low-dose estrogen is applied locally and only for this purpose (NAMS, 2007).

Use of the vaginal cream may weaken latex found in condoms, diaphragms or cervical caps. Systemic absorption occurs following vaginal use; warnings, precautions, and adverse events observed with oral therapy should be considered.

Adverse Reactions Due to systemic absorption, other adverse effects associated with systemic therapy may also occur. Frequency of adverse events reported with daily use:

1% to 10%:
- Cardiovascular: Vasodilatation (4%)
- Central nervous system: Pain (7%)
- Endocrine & metabolic: Breast pain (6%)
- Gastrointestinal: Abdominal pain (8%)
- Genitourinary: Vaginitis (6%)
- Neuromuscular & skeletal: Back pain (5%), weakness (6%)

<1% (Limited to important or life-threatening): Anaphylactic reactions, breast cancer, deep vein thrombosis (DVT), dementia, depression, endometrial cancer, gallbladder disease, gynecomastia (males), hypertension, leukorrhea, MI, pulmonary emboli (PE), retinal vascular thrombosis, stroke, uterine leiomyomata (increase in size)

Drug Interactions

Metabolism/Transport Effects **Substrate** of CYP1A2 (major), CYP2A6 (minor), CYP2B6 (minor), CYP2C19 (minor), CYP2C9 (minor), CYP2D6 (minor), CYP2E1 (minor), CYP3A4 (major); **Note:** Assignment of Major/Minor substrate status based on clinically relevant drug interaction potential; **Inhibits** CYP1A2 (weak); **Induces** CYP3A4 (weak/moderate)

Avoid Concomitant Use

Avoid concomitant use of Estrogens (Conjugated/Equine, Topical) with any of the following: Anastrozole; Axitinib; Dehydroepiandrosterone; Ospemifene; Simeprevir

Increased Effect/Toxicity

Estrogens (Conjugated/Equine, Topical) may increase the levels/effects of: Corticosteroids (Systemic); Ospemifene; ROPINIRole; Theophylline Derivatives; Tipranavir

The levels/effects of Estrogens (Conjugated/Equine, Topical) may be increased by: Ascorbic Acid; Dehydroepiandrosterone; Herbs (Estrogenic Properties); NSAID (COX-2 Inhibitor)

Decreased Effect

Estrogens (Conjugated/Equine, Topical) may decrease the levels/effects of: Anastrozole; Anticoagulants; ARIPiprazole; Axitinib; Chenodiol; Hyaluronidase; Ibrutinib; Ospemifene; Saxagliptin; Simeprevir; Somatropin; Thyroid Products; Ursodiol

The levels/effects of Estrogens (Conjugated/Equine, Topical) may be decreased by: Bosentan; CYP1A2 Inducers (Strong); CYP3A4 Inducers (Strong); Cyproterone; Dabrafenib; Deferasirox; Herbs (CYP3A4 Inducers); Mitotane; Peginterferon Alfa-2b; Tipranavir; Tocilizumab

Storage/Stability Vaginal cream: Store at room temperature of 20°C to 25°C (68°F to 77°F); excursions permitted to 15°C to 30°C (59°F to 86°F).

Mechanism of Action Conjugated estrogens contain a mixture of estrone sulfate, equilin sulfate, 17 alpha-dihydroequilin, 17 alpha-estradiol and 17 beta-dihydroequilin. Estrogens are responsible for the development and maintenance of the female reproductive system and secondary sexual characteristics. Estradiol is the principle intracellular human estrogen and is more potent than estrone and estriol at the receptor level; it is the primary estrogen secreted prior to menopause. Following menopause, estrone and estrone sulfate are more highly produced. Estrogens modulate the pituitary secretion of gonadotropins, luteinizing hormone, and follicle-stimulating hormone through a negative feedback system; estrogen replacement reduces elevated levels of these hormones in postmenopausal women.

Pharmacodynamics/Kinetics

Absorption: Systemic absorption occurs

Protein binding: Binds to sex-hormone-binding globulin and albumin

Metabolism: Hepatic via CYP3A4; estradiol is converted to estrone and estriol; also undergoes enterohepatic recirculation (avoided with vaginal administration); estrone sulfate is the main metabolite in postmenopausal women

Time to peak, plasma: Total estrone: 6 hours

Excretion: Urine (primarily estriol, also as estradiol, estrone, and conjugates

Dosage Adults: Females:

Atrophic vaginitis, kraurosis vulvae: Intravaginal: 0.5 g/day (range 0.5-2 g/day) administered cyclically (21 days on, 7 days off). Adjust dose based on patient response. **Note:** Canadian labeling recommends oral estrogen therapy (~1.25 mg/day for 10 days) prior to initiating topical estrogen in severe atrophic vaginitis.

Moderate-to-severe dyspareunia due to menopause: Intravaginal: 0.5 g twice weekly (eg, Monday and Thursday) **or** once daily cyclically (21 days on, 7 days off)

Dosage adjustment in renal impairment: No dosage adjustment provided in manufacturer's labeling (has not been studied). Use with caution; may increase risk of fluid retention.

Dosage adjustment in hepatic impairment: Use is contraindicated with hepatic dysfunction or disease.

Administration Administer at bedtime to minimize adverse effects. Applicator calibrated in 0.5 g increments up to 2 g. To clean applicator, remove plunger from barrel. Wash with mild soap and warm water; do not boil or use hot water.

Hazardous agent; use appropriate precautions for handling and disposal (NIOSH, 2012).

Monitoring Parameters Routine physical examination that includes blood pressure and Papanicolaou smear, breast exam, mammogram. Monitor for signs of endometrial cancer in female patients with uterus. Adequate diagnostic measures, including endometrial sampling, if indicated, should be performed to rule out malignancy in all cases of undiagnosed abnormal vaginal bleeding. Monitor for loss of vision, sudden onset of proptosis, diplopia, migraine; signs and symptoms of thromboembolic disorders; glycemic control in patients with diabetes; lipid profiles in patients being treated for hyperlipidemias; thyroid function in patients on thyroid hormone replacement therapy.

Test Interactions Reduced response to metyrapone test.

Dosage Forms Excipient information presented when available (limited, particularly for generics); consult specific product labeling.

Cream, Vaginal:

Premarin: 0.625 mg/g (30 g) [contains benzyl alcohol, cetyl alcohol, propylene glycol monostearate]

◆ **Estrogens (Conjugated/Equine) and Bazedoxifene Acetate** *see* Estrogens (Conjugated/Equine) and Bazedoxifene *on page 765*

Estrogens (Esterified) (ES troe jenz, es TER i fied)

Brand Names: U.S. Menest

Brand Names: Canada Estragyn; Estratab®; Menest®

Index Terms Esterified Estrogens

Pharmacologic Category Estrogen Derivative

Additional Appendix Information

Beers Criteria – Potentially Inappropriate Medications for Geriatrics *on page 2368*

Use Treatment of moderate-to-severe vasomotor symptoms associated with menopause; treatment of moderate-to-severe vulvar and vaginal atrophy associated with menopause; hypoestrogenism (due to hypogonadism, castration, or primary ovarian failure); advanced prostatic cancer (palliation), metastatic breast cancer (palliation) in men and postmenopausal women

Pregnancy Considerations In general, the use of estrogen and progestin as in combination hormonal contraceptives have not been associated with teratogenic effects when inadvertently taken early in pregnancy. This product is contraindicated for use during pregnancy.

Breast-Feeding Considerations Estrogen has been shown to decrease the quantity and quality of human milk; use only if clearly needed; monitor the growth of the infant closely.

Contraindications Hypersensitivity to estrogens or any component of the formulation; undiagnosed abnormal vaginal bleeding; DVT or PE (current or history of); active or recent (within 1 year) arterial thromboembolic disease (eg, stroke, MI); carcinoma of the breast (known, suspected or history of), except in appropriately selected patients being treated for metastatic disease; estrogen-dependent tumor; hepatic dysfunction or disease; pregnancy

Warnings/Precautions Hazardous agent - use appropriate precautions for handling and disposal (NIOSH, 2012).

[U.S. Boxed Warning]: Based on data from the Women's Health Initiative (WHI) studies, an increased risk of invasive breast cancer was observed in postmenopausal women using conjugated estrogens (CE) in combination with medroxyprogesterone acetate (MPA). This risk may be associated with duration of use and declines once combined therapy is discontinued (Chlebowski, 2009). The risk of invasive breast cancer was decreased in postmenopausal women with a hysterectomy using CE only, regardless of weight. However, the risk was not significantly decreased in women at high risk for breast cancer (family history of breast cancer, personal history of benign breast disease) (Anderson, 2012). An increase in abnormal mammogram findings has also been reported with estrogen alone or in combination with progestin therapy. Estrogen use may also lead to severe hypercalcemia in patients with breast cancer and bone metastases; discontinue estrogen if hypercalcemia occurs. **[U.S. Boxed Warning]: The use of unopposed estrogen in women with an intact uterus is associated with an**

increased risk of endometrial cancer. The addition of a progestin to estrogen therapy may decrease the risk of endometrial hyperplasia, a precursor to endometrial cancer. Adequate diagnostic measures, including endometrial sampling if indicated, should be performed to rule out malignancy in postmenopausal women with undiagnosed abnormal vaginal bleeding. Estrogens may exacerbate endometriosis. Malignant transformation of residual endometrial implants has been reported posthysterectomy with unopposed estrogen therapy. Consider adding a progestin in women with residual endometriosis posthysterectomy. Postmenopausal estrogen therapy and combined estrogen/progesterone therapy may increase the risk of ovarian cancer; however, the absolute risk to an individual woman is small. Although results from various studies are not consistent, risk does not appear to be significantly associated with the duration, route, or dose of therapy. In one study, the risk decreased after 2 years following discontinuation of therapy (Mørch, 2009). Although the risk of ovarian cancer is rare, women who are at an increased risk (eg, family history) should be counseled about the association (NAMS, 2012).

[U.S. Boxed Warning]: Estrogens with or without progestin should not be used to prevent cardiovascular disease. Using data from the Women's Health Initiative (WHI) studies, an increased risk of deep vein thrombosis (DVT) and stroke has been reported with CE and an increased risk of DVT, stroke, pulmonary emboli (PE) and myocardial infarction (MI) has been reported with CE with MPA in postmenopausal women. Additional risk factors include diabetes mellitus, hypercholesterolemia, hypertension, SLE, obesity, tobacco use, and/or history of venous thromboembolism (VTE). Adverse cardiovascular events have also been reported in males taking estrogens for prostate cancer. Risk factors should be managed appropriately; discontinue use if adverse cardiovascular events occur or are suspected. Women with inherited thrombophilias (eg, protein C or S deficiency) may have increased risk of venous thromboembolism (DeSancho, 2010; van Vlijmen, 2011).

[U.S. Boxed Warning]: Estrogens with or without progestin should not be used to prevent dementia. In the Women's Health Initiative Memory Study (WHIMS), an increased incidence of dementia was observed in women ≥65 years of age taking CE alone or in combination with MPA.

[U.S. Boxed Warning]: Estrogens with or without progestin should be used for the shortest duration possible at the lowest effective dose consistent with treatment goals. Before prescribing estrogen therapy to postmenopausal women, the risks and benefits must be weighed for each patient. Women should be informed of these risks and benefits, as well as possible effects of progestin when added to estrogen therapy. Patients should be reevaluated as clinically appropriate to determine if treatment is still necessary. Available data related to treatment risks are from Women's Health Initiative (WHI) studies, which evaluated oral CE 0.625 mg with or without MPA 2.5 mg relative to placebo in postmenopausal women. Other combinations and dosage forms of estrogens and progestins were not studied. **Outcomes reported from clinical trials using CE with or without MPA should be assumed to be similar for other doses and other dosage forms of estrogens and progestins until comparable data becomes available.**

Estrogen compounds are generally associated with lipid effects such as increased HDL-cholesterol and decreased LDL-cholesterol. Triglycerides may also be increased; use with caution in patients with familial defects of lipoprotein metabolism. Estrogens may increase thyroid-binding globulin (TBG) levels leading to increased circulating total thyroid hormone levels. Women on thyroid replacement therapy may require higher doses of thyroid hormone while receiving estrogens.

Estrogens may cause retinal vascular thrombosis; discontinue if migraine, loss of vision, proptosis, diplopia or other visual disturbances occur; discontinue permanently if papilledema or retinal vascular lesions are observed on examination. Estrogens are poorly metabolized in patients with hepatic dysfunction. Use caution with a history of cholestatic jaundice associated with prior estrogen use or pregnancy. Discontinue if jaundice develops or if acute or chronic hepatic disturbances occur. Use is contraindicated with hepatic disease. Use caution in patients with asthma, epilepsy, hepatic hemangiomas, migraine, porphyria, or SLE; may exacerbate disease. May have adverse effects on glucose tolerance; use caution in women with diabetes. Use with caution in patients with diseases which may be exacerbated by fluid retention, including cardiac or renal dysfunction. Use of postmenopausal estrogen may be associated with an increased risk of gallbladder disease requiring surgery. Use with caution in patients with severe hypocalcemia. Avoid use of oral estrogen (with or without progestins) in the elderly due to potential of increased risk of breast and endometrial cancers, and lack of proven cardioprotection and cognitive protection (Beers Criteria). Prior to puberty, estrogens may cause premature closure of the epiphyses, premature breast development in girls or gynecomastia in boys. Vaginal bleeding and vaginal cornification may also be induced in girls. Whenever possible, estrogens should be discontinued at least 4-6 weeks prior to elective surgery associated with an increased risk of thromboembolism or during periods of prolonged immobilization. The use of estrogens and/or progestins may change the results of some laboratory tests (eg, coagulation factors, lipids, glucose tolerance, binding proteins). The dose, route, and the specific estrogen/progestin influences these changes. In addition, personal risk factors (eg, cardiovascular disease, smoking, diabetes, age) also contribute to adverse events; use of specific products may be contraindicated in women with certain risk factors.

Adverse Reactions Frequency not defined.

Cardiovascular: Edema, hypertension, MI, stroke, venous thromboembolism

Central nervous system: Dementia exacerbation, dizziness, epilepsy exacerbation, headache, irritability, mental depression, migraine, mood disturbances, nervousness

Dermatologic: Angioedema, chloasma, erythema multiforme, erythema nodosum, hemorrhagic eruption, hirsutism, pruritus, loss of scalp hair, melasma, rash, urticaria

Endocrine & metabolic: Breast cancer, breast enlargement, breast tenderness, carbohydrate intolerance, fibrocystic breast changes, galactorrhea, hypocalcemia, libido (changes in), nipple discharge, premenstrual like syndrome

Gastrointestinal: Abdominal cramps, bloating, gallbladder disease, nausea, pancreatitis, vomiting, weight gain/loss

Genitourinary: Alterations in frequency and flow of menstrual patterns, breakthrough bleeding, changes in cervical secretions, cervical ectropion changes, cystitis-like syndrome, dysmenorrhea, endometrial hyperplasia, endometrial cancer, increased size of uterine leiomyomata, ovarian cancer, vaginal candidiasis, vaginitis

Hematologic: Aggravation of porphyria

Hepatic: Cholestatic jaundice, hemangioma enlargement

Local: Thrombophlebitis

Neuromuscular & skeletal: Arthralgia, chorea, leg cramps

Ocular: Contact lens intolerance, corneal curvature steepening, retinal vascular thrombosis

Respiratory: Asthma exacerbation, pulmonary embolism

Miscellaneous: Anaphylactoid/anaphylactic reactions

Drug Interactions

Metabolism/Transport Effects **Substrate** of CYP1A2 (major), CYP2B6 (minor), CYP2C9 (minor), CYP2E1 (minor), CYP3A4 (major); **Note:** Assignment of Major/Minor substrate status based on clinically relevant drug interaction potential

Avoid Concomitant Use

Avoid concomitant use of Estrogens (Esterified) with any of the following: Anastrozole; Dehydroepiandrosterone; Ospemifene

Increased Effect/Toxicity

Estrogens (Esterified) may increase the levels/effects of: Corticosteroids (Systemic); Ospemifene; ROPINIRole; Theophylline Derivatives; Tipranavir

The levels/effects of Estrogens (Esterified) may be increased by: Ascorbic Acid; Dehydroepiandrosterone; Herbs (Estrogenic Properties); NSAID (COX-2 Inhibitor)

Decreased Effect

Estrogens (Esterified) may decrease the levels/effects of: Anastrozole; Anticoagulants; Chenodiol; Hyaluronidase; Ospemifene; Somatropin; Thyroid Products; Ursodiol

The levels/effects of Estrogens (Esterified) may be decreased by: Bosentan; CYP1A2 Inducers (Strong); CYP3A4 Inducers (Strong); Cyproterone; Dabrafenib; Deferasirox; Herbs (CYP3A4 Inducers); Mitotane; Tipranavir; Tocilizumab

Ethanol/Nutrition/Herb Interactions

Ethanol: Avoid ethanol (routine use increases estrogen plasma concentrations and risk of breast cancer). Ethanol may also increase the risk of osteoporosis.

Food: Folic acid absorption may be decreased.

Herb/Nutraceutical: St John's wort may decrease levels. Herbs with estrogenic properties may enhance the adverse/toxic effect of estrogen derivatives; examples include alfalfa, black cohosh, bloodroot, hops, kudzu, licorice, red clover, saw palmetto, soybean, thyme, wild yam, yucca.

Mechanism of Action Esterified estrogens contain a mixture of estrogenic substances; the principle component is estrone. Preparations contain 75% to 85% sodium estrone sulfate and 6% to 15% sodium equilin sulfate such that the total is not <90%. Estrogens are responsible for the development and maintenance of the female reproductive system and secondary sexual characteristics. Estradiol is the principle intracellular human estrogen and is more potent than estrone and estriol at the receptor level; it is the primary estrogen secreted prior to menopause. In males and following menopause in females, estrone and estrone sulfate are more highly produced. Estrogens modulate the pituitary secretion of gonadotropins, luteinizing hormone, and follicle-stimulating hormone through a negative feedback system; estrogen replacement reduces elevated levels of these hormones.

Pharmacodynamics/Kinetics

Absorption: Readily

Distribution: Widely distributed; high concentrations in the sex hormone target organs

Protein binding: Bound to sex hormone-binding globulin and albumin

Metabolism: Hepatic; partial metabolism via CYP3A4 enzymes; estradiol is reversibly converted to estrone and estriol; oral estradiol also undergoes enterohepatic recirculation by conjugation in the liver, followed by excretion of sulfate and glucuronide conjugates into the bile, then hydrolysis in the intestine and estrogen reabsorption. Sulfate conjugates are the primary form found in postmenopausal women.

Excretion: Primarily urine (as estradiol, estrone, estriol, and their glucuronide and sulfate conjugates)

Dosage Oral: Adults:

Prostate cancer, advanced: 1.25-2.5 mg 3 times/day

Female hypoestrogenism due to hypogonadism: 2.5-7.5 mg/day in divided doses for 20 days followed by a 10-day rest period. Administer cyclically (3 weeks on and 1 week off). If bleeding does not occur by the end of the 10-day period, repeat the same dosing schedule; the number of courses is dependent upon the responsiveness of the endometrium. If bleeding occurs before the end of the 10-day period, begin an estrogen-progestin cyclic regimen of 2.5-7.5 mg/day in divided doses for 20 days; during the last 5 days of estrogen therapy, give an oral progestin. If bleeding occurs before regimen is concluded, discontinue therapy and resume on the fifth day of bleeding.

Female hypoestrogenism due to castration and primary ovarian failure: 1.25 mg/day, cyclically. Adjust dosage upward or downward, according to the severity of symptoms and patient response. For maintenance, adjust dosage to lowest level that will provide effective control.

Vasomotor symptoms associated with menopause: 1.25 mg/day administered cyclically (3 weeks on and 1 week off). If patient has not menstruated within the last 2 months or more, cyclic administration is started arbitrary. If the patient is menstruating, cyclical administration is started on day 5 of the bleeding. For short-term use only and should be discontinued as soon as possible. Re-evaluate at 3- to 6-month intervals for tapering or discontinuation of therapy.

Vulvar and vaginal atrophy associated with menopause: 0.3 to ≥1.25 mg/day, depending on the tissue response of the individual patient. Administer cyclically. For short-term use only and should be discontinued as soon as possible. Re-evaluate at 3- to 6-month intervals for tapering or discontinuation of therapy.

Breast cancer, metastatic (appropriately selected patients): Males and postmenopausal females: 10 mg 3 times/day for at least 3 months

Elderly: Refer to adult dosing.

Dosage adjustment in renal impairment: No dosage adjustment provided in manufacturer's labeling; use with caution.

Dosage adjustment in hepatic impairment: No dosage adjustment provided in manufacturer's labeling; use with caution.

Dietary Considerations Should be taken with food at same time each day.

Administration Administer with food at same time each day.

Hazardous agent; use appropriate precautions for handling and disposal (NIOSH, 2012).

Monitoring Parameters Routine physical examination that includes blood pressure and Papanicolaou smear, breast exam, mammogram. Monitor for signs of endometrial cancer in female patients with uterus. Adequate diagnostic measures, including endometrial sampling, if indicated, should be performed to rule out malignancy in all cases of undiagnosed abnormal vaginal bleeding. Monitor for loss of vision, sudden onset of proptosis, diplopia, migraine; signs and symptoms of thromboembolic disorders; glycemic control in patients with diabetes; lipid profiles in patients being treated for hyperlipidemias; thyroid function in patients on thyroid hormone replacement therapy.

Menopausal symptoms; vulvar and vaginal atrophy: Assess need for therapy at 3- to 6-month intervals

Test Interactions Reduced response to metyrapone test.

Dosage Forms Excipient information presented when available (limited, particularly for generics); consult specific product labeling.

Tablet, Oral:

Menest: 0.3 mg, 0.625 mg, 1.25 mg, 2.5 mg

Estropipate (ES troe pih pate)

Brand Names: U.S. Ortho-Est 0.625; Ortho-Est 1.25

Brand Names: Canada Ogen®

Index Terms Ortho Est; Piperazine Estrone Sulfate

Pharmacologic Category Estrogen Derivative

Use Treatment of moderate-to-severe vasomotor symptoms associated with menopause; treatment of vulvar and vaginal atrophy; hypoestrogenism (due to hypogonadism, castration, or primary ovarian failure); osteoporosis (prophylaxis)

Dosage Adults:

Oral:

Moderate-to-severe vasomotor symptoms associated with menopause: Usual dosage range: 0.75-6 mg estropipate daily; use the lowest dose and regimen that will control symptoms, and discontinue as soon as possible. Attempt to discontinue or taper medication at 3- to 6-month intervals. If a patient with vasomotor symptoms has not menstruated within the last ≥2 months, start the cyclic administration arbitrarily. If the patient has menstruated, start cyclic administration on day 5 of bleeding.

Female hypogonadism: 1.5-9 mg estropipate daily for the first 3 weeks, followed by a rest period of 8-10 days; use the lowest dose and regimen that will control symptoms. Repeat if bleeding does not occur by the end of the rest period. The duration of therapy necessary to product the withdrawal bleeding will vary according to the responsiveness of the endometrium. If satisfactory withdrawal bleeding does not occur, give an oral progestin in addition to estrogen during the third week of the cycle.

Female castration or primary ovarian failure: 1.5-9 mg estropipate daily for the first 3 weeks of a theoretical cycle, followed by a rest period of 8-10 days; use the lowest dose and regimen that will control symptoms

Osteoporosis prophylaxis: 0.75 mg estropipate daily for 25 days of a 31-day cycle

Atrophic vaginitis or kraurosis vulvae: 0.75-6 mg estropipate daily; administer cyclically. Use the lowest dose and regimen that will control symptoms; discontinue as soon as possible.

Elderly: Refer to adult dosing. A higher incidence of stroke and invasive breast cancer were observed in women >75 years in a WHI substudy using conjugated equine estrogen.

Dosage adjustment in renal impairment: No dosage adjustment provided in manufacturer's labeling; use with caution.

Dosage adjustment in hepatic impairment: No dosage adjustment provided in manufacturer's labeling; use with caution.

Additional Information Complete prescribing information should be consulted for additional detail.

Dosage Forms Excipient information presented when available (limited, particularly for generics); consult specific product labeling.

Tablet, Oral:

Ortho-Est 0.625: 0.75 mg [scored]

Ortho-Est 1.25: 1.5 mg [scored]

Generic: 0.75 mg, 1.5 mg, 3 mg

◆ Estrostep Fe *see* Ethinyl Estradiol and Norethindrone *on page 793*

Eszopiclone (es zoe PIK lone)

Brand Names: U.S. Lunesta

Pharmacologic Category Hypnotic, Miscellaneous

Additional Appendix Information

Beers Criteria – Potentially Inappropriate Medications for Geriatrics *on page 2368*

Use Treatment of insomnia (with difficulty of sleep onset and/or sleep maintenance)

Pregnancy Risk Factor C

Pregnancy Considerations Adverse effects were observed in animal reproduction studies. Eszopiclone is the S-isomer of the racemic derivative zopiclone.

Breast-Feeding Considerations It is not known if eszopiclone is excreted in breast milk. Eszopiclone is the S-isomer of the racemic derivative zopiclone. Zopiclone is excreted in human milk and is not recommended for use while breast-feeding.

Medication Guide Available Yes

Contraindications Hypersensitivity to eszopiclone or any component of the formulation.

Warnings/Precautions Symptomatic treatment of insomnia should be initiated only after careful evaluation of potential causes of sleep disturbance. Failure of sleep disturbance to resolve after 7-10 days may indicate psychiatric and/or medical illness. Administer only when the patient is able to stay in bed a full night (7-8 hours) before being active again. Tolerance did not develop over 6 months of use. May cause CNS depression impairing physical and mental capabilities; patients must be cautioned about performing tasks which require mental alertness (operating machinery or driving); dose adjustment may be necessary if taking concomitant CNS depressants. Potentially significant interactions may exist, requiring dose or frequency adjustment, additional monitoring, and/or selection of alternative therapy.

Use with caution in patients with depression; worsening of depression, including suicidal ideation has been reported with the use of hypnotics. Intentional overdose may be an issue with this population. The minimum dose that will effectively treat the individual patient should be used. Prescriptions should be written for the smallest quantity consistent with good patient care. Use caution in patients with a history of drug dependence. Hypnotics/sedatives have been associated with abnormal thinking and behavior changes including decreased inhibition, aggression, bizarre behavior, agitation, hallucinations, and depersonalization. These changes may occur unpredictably and may indicate previously unrecognized psychiatric disorders; evaluate appropriately. An increased risk for hazardous sleep-related activities such as sleep-driving, cooking and eating food, and making phone calls while asleep has also been noted; amnesia may also occur. The use of alcohol, other CNS depressants, and exceeding the recommended maximum dose may increase the risk of these activities. Discontinue treatment in patients who report any sleep-related episodes. Use caution in patients with respiratory compromise, COPD, sleep apnea, and hepatic dysfunction (dose adjustment recommended with severe impairment). Because of the rapid onset of action, administer immediately prior to bedtime or after the patient has gone to bed and is having difficulty falling asleep. Abrupt discontinuance may lead to withdrawal symptoms. Hypersensitivity reactions including anaphylaxis as well as angioedema have been reported, in some cases following initial dosing. Patients who develop severe reactions should not be rechallenged.

Use with caution in debilitated and elderly patients; dosage adjustment recommended. Closely monitor elderly or debilitated patients for impaired cognitive and/or motor performance, confusion, and potential for falling. Avoid chronic use (>90 days) in older adults; adverse events, including delirium, falls, fractures, have been observed with nonbenzodiazepine hypnotic use in the elderly similar to events observed with benzodiazepines. Data suggests improvements in sleep duration and latency are minimal (Beers Criteria).

Adverse Reactions

>10%:

Central nervous system: Headache (15% to 21%)

Gastrointestinal: Unpleasant taste (8% to 34%)

1% to 10%:

Cardiovascular: Cardiovascular: Chest pain (≥1%), peripheral edema (≥1%)

Central nervous system: Somnolence (8% to 10%), dizziness (5% to 7%), pain (4% to 5%), nervousness (up to 5%), depression (1% to 4%), confusion (up to 3%), hallucinations (1% to 3%), anxiety (1% to 3%), abnormal dreams (1% to 3%), migraine

Dermatologic: Rash (3% to 4%), pruritus (1% to 4%)

Endocrine & metabolic: Libido decreased (up to 3%), dysmenorrhea (up to 3%), gynecomastia (males up to 3%)

Gastrointestinal: Xerostomia (3% to 7%), dyspepsia (2% to 6%), nausea (4% to 5%), diarrhea (2% to 4%), vomiting (up to 3%)

Genitourinary: Urinary tract infection (up to 3%)

Neuromuscular & skeletal: Neuralgia (up to 3%)

Miscellaneous: Infection (5% to 10%), viral infection (3%), accidental injury (up to 3%)

<1% (Limited to important or life-threatening): Abnormal gait, abnormal thinking, agitation, alopecia, allergic reaction, amenorrhea, anaphylaxis, anemia, angioedema, anorexia, apathy, appetite increased, arthritis, asthma, ataxia, breast enlargement, breast neoplasm, breast pain, bronchitis, bursitis, cholelithiasis, colitis; complex sleep-related behavior (sleep-driving, cooking or eating food, making phone calls); conjunctivitis, contact dermatitis, cystitis, dehydration, diaphoresis, dry eyes, dyspnea, dysphagia, dysuria, eczema, emotional lability, epistaxis, erythema multiforme, euphoria, facial edema, fever, gastritis, gout, halitosis, heat stroke, hematuria, hepatitis, hepatomegaly, herpes zoster, hirsutism, hostility, hypercholesterolemia, hypertension, hypokalemia, incoordination, insomnia, kidney calculus, kidney pain, laryngitis, liver damage, lymphadenopathy, maculopapular rash, malaise, mastitis, melena, memory impairment, menorrhagia, metrorrhagia, myasthenia, mydriasis, myopathy, neck rigidity, neuritis, neuropathy, neurosis, nystagmus, oliguria, paresthesia, photophobia, photosensitivity, ptosis, pyelonephritis, rectal hemorrhage, reflexes decreased, skin discoloration, stomach ulcer, swelling, thirst, thrombophlebitis, tinnitus, tongue edema, tremor, twitching, ulcerative stomatitis, urethritis, urinary frequency, urinary incontinence, urticaria, uterine hemorrhage, vaginal hemorrhage, vaginitis, vestibular disorder, vertigo, vesiculobullous rash

Drug Interactions

Metabolism/Transport Effects **Substrate** of CYP2E1 (minor), CYP3A4 (major); **Note:** Assignment of Major/Minor substrate status based on clinically relevant drug interaction potential

Avoid Concomitant Use

Avoid concomitant use of Eszopiclone with any of the following: Azelastine (Nasal); Conivaptan; Fusidic Acid (Systemic); Paraldehyde; Sodium Oxybate

Increased Effect/Toxicity

Eszopiclone may increase the levels/effects of: Alcohol (Ethyl); Azelastine (Nasal); Buprenorphine; CNS Depressants; Hydrocodone; Methotrimeprazine; Metyrosine; Mirtazapine; Paraldehyde; Pramipexole; ROPINIRole; Rotigotine; Selective Serotonin Reuptake Inhibitors; Sodium Oxybate; Zolpidem

The levels/effects of Eszopiclone may be increased by: Brimonidine (Topical); Conivaptan; CYP3A4 Inhibitors (Moderate); CYP3A4 Inhibitors (Strong); Dasatinib; Doxylamine; Droperidol; Fusidic Acid (Systemic); HydrOXYzine; Ivacaftor; Luliconazole; Magnesium Sulfate; Methotrimeprazine; Mifepristone; Perampanel; Simeprevir; Tapentadol

Decreased Effect

The levels/effects of Eszopiclone may be decreased by: Bosentan; CYP3A4 Inducers (Strong); Dabrafenib; Deferasirox; Flumazenil; Herbs (CYP3A4 Inducers); Mitotane; Tocilizumab

Ethanol/Nutrition/Herb Interactions

Ethanol: Ethanol may increase CNS depression. Management: Avoid ethanol.

Food: Onset of action may be reduced if taken with or immediately after a heavy meal. Management: Take immediately prior to bedtime, not with or immediately after a heavy or high-fat meal.

Herb/Nutraceutical: Some herbal medications may increase CNS depression. Management: Avoid valerian, St John's wort, kava kava, and gotu kola.

Storage/Stability Store at 25°C (77°F); excursions permitted to 15°C to 30°C (59°F to 86°F).

Mechanism of Action May interact with GABA-receptor complexes at binding domains located close to or allosterically coupled to benzodiazepine receptors.

Pharmacodynamics/Kinetics

Absorption: Rapid; high-fat/heavy meal may delay absorption

Protein binding: 52% to 59%

Metabolism: Hepatic via oxidation and demethylation (CYP2E1, 3A4); (S)-N-desmethyl zopiclone metabolite has less activity than parent compound

Half-life elimination: ~6 hours; Elderly (≥65 years): ~9 hours

Time to peak, plasma: ~1 hour

Excretion: Urine (up to 75%, primarily as metabolites; <10% as parent drug)

Dosage Oral:

Adults: Insomnia: Initial: 2 mg immediately before bedtime (maximum dose: 3 mg daily)

Concurrent use with strong CYP3A4 inhibitor: Initial: 1 mg immediately before bedtime; if needed, dose may be increased to 2 mg daily

Elderly:

Difficulty **falling** asleep: Initial: 1 mg immediately before bedtime; maximum dose: 2 mg daily

Difficulty **staying** asleep: 2 mg immediately before bedtime

Dosage adjustment in renal impairment: No dosage adjustment necessary.

Dosage adjustment in hepatic impairment:

Mild-to-moderate impairment: No dosage adjustment necessary.

Severe impairment: Initial dose: 1 mg; use with caution; systemic exposure is doubled in severe impairment.

Dietary Considerations Avoid taking after a heavy meal; may delay onset.

Administration Because of the rapid onset of action, eszopiclone should be administered immediately prior to bedtime or after the patient has gone to bed and is having difficulty falling asleep. Do not take with, or immediately following, a high-fat meal.

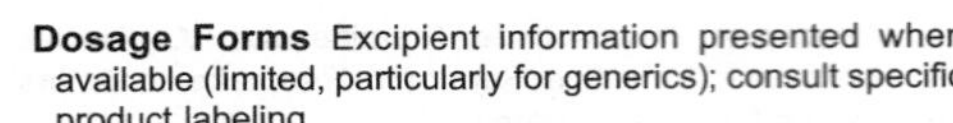

Dosage Forms Excipient information presented when available (limited, particularly for generics); consult specific product labeling.

Tablet, Oral:

Lunesta: 1 mg [contains fd&c blue #2 (indigotine)]

Lunesta: 2 mg

Lunesta: 3 mg [contains fd&c blue #2 (indigotine)]

Controlled Substance C-IV

Etanercept (et a NER sept)

Brand Names: U.S. Enbrel; Enbrel SureClick

Brand Names: Canada Enbrel

Pharmacologic Category Antirheumatic, Disease Modifying; Tumor Necrosis Factor (TNF) Blocking Agent

Use

Ankylosing spondylitis: For reducing signs and symptoms in patients with active ankylosing spondylitis.

Plaque psoriasis: For treatment of adults ≥18 years of age with chronic moderate to severe plaque psoriasis who are candidates for systemic therapy or phototherapy.

Polyarticular juvenile idiopathic arthritis: For reducing signs and symptoms of moderately to severely active polyarticular juvenile idiopathic arthritis in patients ≥2 years of age.

Psoriatic arthritis: For reducing signs and symptoms, inhibiting the progression of structural damage of active arthritis, and improving physical function in patients with psoriatic arthritis. Etanercept can be used in combination with methotrexate in patients who do not respond adequately to methotrexate alone.

Rheumatoid arthritis: For reducing signs and symptoms, inducing major clinical response, inhibiting the progression of structural damage, and improving physical function in patients with moderately to severely active rheumatoid arthritis (RA). Etanercept can be initiated in combination with methotrexate or used alone.

Unlabeled Use

Treatment of acute graft-versus-host disease (GVHD).

Pregnancy Risk Factor B

Pregnancy Considerations Adverse events were not observed in animal reproduction studies. Etanercept crosses the placenta. Following in utero exposure, concentrations in the newborn at delivery are 3-32% of the maternal serum concentration.

A pregnancy registry has been established to monitor outcomes of women exposed to etanercept during pregnancy (800-772-6436).

Breast-Feeding Considerations Etanercept is excreted into breast milk in low concentrations and is minimally absorbed by a nursing infant (limited data). The manufacturer recommends that caution be used if administered to a nursing woman, taking into account the importance of the drug to the mother and potential effects to the nursing infant. A lactation surveillance program has been established to monitor outcomes of breastfed infants exposed to etanercept (800-772-6436).

Medication Guide Available Yes

Contraindications Sepsis

Warnings/Precautions [U.S. Boxed Warning]: Patients receiving etanercept are at increased risk for serious infections which may result in hospitalization and/or fatality; infections usually developed in patients receiving concomitant immunosuppressive agents (eg, methotrexate or corticosteroids) and may present as disseminated (rather than local) disease. Active tuberculosis (or reactivation of latent tuberculosis), invasive fungal (including aspergillosis, blastomycosis, candidiasis, coccidioidomycosis, histoplasmosis, and pneumocystosis) and bacterial, viral or other opportunistic infections (including legionellosis and listeriosis) have been reported in patients receiving TNF-blocking agents, including etanercept. Monitor closely for signs/symptoms of infection. Discontinue for serious infection or sepsis. Consider risks versus benefits prior to use in patients with a history of chronic or recurrent infection. Consider empiric antifungal therapy in patients who are at risk for invasive fungal infection and develop severe systemic illness. Caution should be exercised when considering use in the elderly or in patients with conditions that predispose them to infections (eg, diabetes) or residence/travel from areas of endemic mycoses (blastomycosis, coccidioidomycosis, histoplasmosis), or with latent or localized infections. Do not initiate etanercept therapy with clinically important active infection. Patients who develop a new infection while undergoing treatment should be monitored closely. **[U.S. Boxed Warning]: Tuberculosis (disseminated or extrapulmonary) has been reported in patients receiving etanercept; both reactivation of latent infection and new infections have been reported.** Patients should be evaluated for tuberculosis risk factors and for latent tuberculosis infection with a tuberculin skin test prior to starting therapy. Treatment of latent tuberculosis should be initiated before etanercept therapy; consider antituberculosis treatment if adequate course of treatment cannot be confirmed in patients with a history of latent or active tuberculosis or with risk factors despite negative skin test. Some patients who tested negative prior to therapy have developed active infection; tests for latent tuberculosis infection may be falsely negative while on etanercept therapy. Monitor for signs and symptoms of tuberculosis in all patients. Rare reactivation of hepatitis B virus (HBV) has occurred in chronic virus carriers, usually in patients receiving concomitant immunosuppressants; evaluate for HBV prior to initiation in all patients. Monitor during and for several months following discontinuation of treatment in HBV carriers; interrupt therapy if reactivation occurs and treat appropriately with antiviral therapy; if resumption of therapy is deemed necessary, exercise caution and monitor patient closely. Patients should be brought up to date with all immunizations before initiating therapy. Live vaccines should not be given concurrently with etanercept; there is no data available concerning secondary transmission of live vaccines in patients receiving therapy. Patients with a significant exposure to varicella virus should temporarily discontinue etanercept. Treatment with varicella zoster immune globulin should be considered.

[U.S. Boxed Warning]: Lymphoma and other malignancies have been reported in children and adolescent patients receiving TNF-blocking agents, including etanercept. Half of the malignancies reported in children were lymphomas (Hodgkin and non-Hodgkin) while other cases varied and included malignancies not typically observed in this population. The impact of etanercept on the development and course of malignancy is not fully defined. Compared to the general population, an increased risk of lymphoma has been noted in clinical trials; however, rheumatoid arthritis alone has been previously associated with an increased rate of lymphoma. Lymphomas and other malignancies were also observed (at rates higher than expected for the general population) in adult patients receiving etanercept. Etanercept is not recommended for use in patients with Wegener's granulomatosis who are receiving immunosuppressive therapy due to higher incidence of noncutaneous solid malignancies. Hepatosplenic T-cell lymphoma (HSTCL), a rare T-cell lymphoma, has also been associated with TNF-blocking agents, primarily reported in adolescent and young adult males with Crohn's disease or ulcerative colitis. Melanoma, nonmelanoma skin cancer, and Merkel cell carcinoma have been reported in patients receiving TNF-blocking agents, including etanercept. Perform periodic skin examinations in all patients during therapy, particularly those at increased risk of skin cancer. Positive antinuclear antibody titers have been detected in patients (with negative baselines). Rare cases of autoimmune disorder, including lupus-like syndrome or autoimmune hepatitis, have been reported; monitor and discontinue if symptoms develop.

Allergic reactions may occur; if an anaphylactic reaction or other serious allergic reaction occurs, administration should be discontinued immediately and appropriate therapy initiated. Use with caution in patients with pre-existing or recent onset CNS demyelinating disorders; rare cases of new-onset or exacerbation of CNS demyelinating disorders have occurred; may present with mental status changes and some may be associated with permanent disability. Optic neuritis, transverse myelitis, multiple sclerosis, Guillain-Barré syndrome, other peripheral demyelinating neuropathies, and new-onset or exacerbation of seizures have been reported. Use with caution in patients with heart failure or decreased left ventricular function; worsening and new-onset heart failure has been reported, including in patients without known pre-existing cardiovascular disease. Use caution in patients with a history of significant hematologic abnormalities; has been associated with pancytopenia and aplastic anemia (rare). Patients must be advised to seek medical attention if they develop signs and symptoms suggestive of blood dyscrasias; discontinue if significant hematologic abnormalities are confirmed. Use with caution in patients with moderate to severe alcoholic hepatitis. Compared to placebo, the mortality rate in patients treated with etanercept was similar at one month but significantly higher after 6 months.

Due to a higher incidence of serious infections, concomitant use with anakinra is not recommended. Hypoglycemia has been reported in patients receiving concomitant therapy with etanercept and antidiabetic medications; dose reduction of antidiabetic medication may be necessary. Use with caution in patient with diabetes; monitor blood glucose as clinically necessary. Some dosage forms may contain dry natural rubber (latex). Some dosage forms may contain benzyl alcohol which has been associated with "gasping syndrome" in neonates.

Adverse Reactions

>10%:

- Central nervous system: Headache (17% to 19%)
- Dermatologic: Skin rash (3% to 13%)
- Gastrointestinal: Abdominal pain (5%; children 19%), diarrhea (3% to 16%), vomiting (3%; children 13%)
- Infection: Infection (50% to 81%; children 62%)
- Local: Injection site reaction (14% to 43%; bleeding, bruising, erythema, itching, pain, or swelling)
- Respiratory: Upper respiratory tract infection (38% to 65%), respiratory tract infection (21% to 54%), rhinitis (12%)
- Miscellaneous: Antibody development (positive antidouble-stranded DNA antibodies 15% by RIA, 3% by *Crithidia luciliae* assay), positive ANA titer (11%)

≥3% to 10%:

- Central nervous system: Dizziness (7%)
- Dermatologic: Pruritus (2% to 5%)
- Gastrointestinal: Nausea (children 9%), dyspepsia (4%)
- Neuromuscular & skeletal: Weakness (5%)
- Respiratory: Pharyngitis (7%), cough (6%), respiratory distress (5%), sinusitis (3%)
- Miscellaneous: Fever (2% to 3%)

<3% (Limited to important or life-threatening): Abscess, adenopathy, anemia, angioedema, anorexia, aplastic anemia, appendicitis, aseptic meningitis, aspergillosis, autoimmune hepatitis, blood coagulation disorder, bursitis, cardiac failure, cerebral ischemia, cerebrovascular accident, cholecystitis, cutaneous lupus erythematous, deep vein thrombosis, demyelinating disease of the central nervous system (suggestive of multiple sclerosis, transverse myelitis, or optic neuritis), depression, dermal ulcer, erythema multiforme, gastritis, gastroenteritis, gastrointestinal hemorrhage, glomerulopathy (membranous), herpes zoster, hydrocephalus (with normal pressure), hypersensitivity, hypersensitivity reaction, hypertension, hypotension, inflammatory bowel disease, interstitial pulmonary disease, intestinal perforation, ischemic heart disease, leukemia, leukopenia, lupus-like syndrome, lymphadenopathy, malignant lymphoma, malignant melanoma, malignant neoplasm, Merkel cell carcinoma, myocardial infarction, multiple sclerosis, nephrolithiasis, neutropenia, optic neuritis, oral mucosa ulcer, pancreatitis, pancytopenia, pneumonia due to *Pneumocystis carinii*, polymyositis, psoriasis (including new onset, palmoplantar, pustular, or exacerbation), pulmonary disease, pulmonary embolism, reactivation of HBV, sarcoidosis, scleritis, seizure, skin carcinoma, Stevens-Johnson syndrome, subcutaneous nodule, thrombocytopenia, thrombophlebitis, toxic epidermal necrolysis, tuberculosis, tuberculous arthritis, urinary tract infection, uveitis, varicella zoster infection, vasculitis (cutaneous and systemic), weight gain

Drug Interactions

Metabolism/Transport Effects None known.

Avoid Concomitant Use

Avoid concomitant use of Etanercept with any of the following: Abatacept; Anakinra; BCG; Belimumab; Canakinumab; Certolizumab Pegol; Cyclophosphamide; InFLIXimab; Natalizumab; Pimecrolimus; Rilonacept; Tacrolimus (Topical); Tocilizumab; Tofacitinib; Vaccines (Live)

Increased Effect/Toxicity

Etanercept may increase the levels/effects of: Abatacept; Anakinra; Belimumab; Canakinumab; Certolizumab Pegol; Cyclophosphamide; InFLIXimab; Leflunomide; Natalizumab; Rilonacept; Tofacitinib; Vaccines (Live)

The levels/effects of Etanercept may be increased by: Denosumab; Pimecrolimus; Roflumilast; Tacrolimus (Topical); Tocilizumab; Trastuzumab

Decreased Effect

Etanercept may decrease the levels/effects of: BCG; Coccidioidin Skin Test; Sipuleucel-T; Vaccines (Inactivated); Vaccines (Live)

The levels/effects of Etanercept may be decreased by: Echinacea

Ethanol/Nutrition/Herb Interactions Herb/Nutraceutical: Echinacea may decrease the therapeutic effects of etanercept (avoid concurrent use).

Preparation for Administration Reconstitute lyophilized powder aseptically with 1 mL sterile bacteriostatic water for injection, USP (supplied); swirl gently, do not shake. Do not filter reconstituted solution during preparation or administration.

Storage/Stability

Refrigerate at 2°C to 8°C (36°F to 46°F). Do not freeze. Do not store in extreme heat or cold. Store in the original carton to protect from light or physical damage until the time of use.

For convenience and a more comfortable injection, autoinjectors, prefilled syringes, or individual dose trays (containing multi-use vials and diluent syringes) may be stored at room temperature for a maximum single period of 14 days with protection from light and sources of heat, and humidity. Once an autoinjector, prefilled syringe or dose tray has been stored at room temperature, it should not be placed back into the refrigerator; discard after 14 days.

Once the multi-use vial has been reconstituted, use the reconstituted solution immediately or refrigerate at 2°C to 8°C (36°F to 46°F). Reconstituted solution must be used within 14 days; discard after 14 days.

Mechanism of Action Etanercept is a recombinant DNA-derived protein composed of tumor necrosis factor receptor (TNFR) linked to the Fc portion of human IgG1. Etanercept binds tumor necrosis factor (TNF) and blocks its interaction with cell surface receptors. TNF plays an important role in the inflammatory processes and the resulting joint pathology of rheumatoid arthritis (RA), polyarticular-course juvenile idiopathic arthritis (JIA), ankylosing spondylitis (AS), and plaque psoriasis.

Pharmacodynamics/Kinetics

Onset of action: ~2-3 weeks; RA: 1-2 weeks

Half-life elimination: RA: SubQ: 72-132 hours

Time to peak: RA: SubQ: 35-103 hours

Dosage SubQ:

Ankylosing spondylitis, psoriatic arthritis, rheumatoid arthritis: Adults: **Note:** Methotrexate, glucocorticoids, salicylates, NSAIDs, or analgesics may be continued during etanercept therapy: 50 mg once weekly **or** 25 mg given twice weekly (unlabeled dose; Bathon, 2000; Calin, 2004; Davis, 2003; Genovese, 2002; Mease, 2000; Mease, 2002)

Juvenile idiopathic arthritis: Children ≥2 years: **Note:** Glucocorticoids, NSAIDs, or analgesics may be continued during etanercept therapy: 0.8 mg/kg (maximum: 50 mg/dose) once weekly **or** 0.4 mg/kg (maximum: 25 mg/dose) twice weekly (unlabeled dose; Lovell, 2000; Lovell, 2006; Lovell, 2008)

Plaque psoriasis: Adults:

Initial: 50 mg twice weekly; maintain initial dose for 3 months (starting doses of 25 or 50 mg once weekly have also been used successfully)

Maintenance dose: 50 mg once weekly

Acute graft-versus-host disease (GVHD), treatment (unlabeled use): Children ≥1 year, Adolescents, and Adults: 0.4 mg/kg (maximum: 25 mg/dose) twice weekly for 8 weeks (in combination with methylprednisolone) (Levine, 2008)

Elderly: Refer to adult dosing. Although greater sensitivity of some elderly patients cannot be ruled out, no overall differences in safety or effectiveness were observed.

Dosage adjustment in renal impairment: No dosage adjustment provided in manufacturer's labeling (has not been studied).

Dosage adjustment in hepatic impairment: No dosage adjustment provided in manufacturer's labeling (has not been studied).

Administration Administer subcutaneously. Rotate injection sites; may inject into the thigh (preferred), abdomen (avoiding the 2-inch area around the navel), or upper arm. New injections should be given at least one inch from an old site and never into areas where the skin is tender, bruised, red, or hard or into any raised thick, red or scaly skin patches or lesions. For a more comfortable injection, autoinjectors, prefilled syringes, and dose trays may be allowed to reach room temperature by removing from the refrigerator 15-30 minutes prior to injection. **Note:** If the physician determines that it is appropriate, patients may self-inject after proper training in injection technique.

Monitoring Parameters Monitor improvement of symptoms and physical function assessments. Latent TB screening prior to initiating and during therapy; signs/symptoms of infection (prior to, during, and following therapy); CBC with differential; signs/symptoms/worsening of heart failure; HBV screening prior to initiating (all patients), HBV carriers (during and for several months following therapy); signs and symptoms of hypersensitivity reaction; symptoms of lupus-like syndrome; signs/symptoms of malignancy (eg, splenomegaly, hepatomegaly, abdominal pain, persistent fever, night sweats, weight loss).

Dosage Forms Excipient information presented when available (limited, particularly for generics); consult specific product labeling.

Kit, Subcutaneous [preservative free]:

Enbrel: 25 mg [contains benzyl alcohol, tromethamine]

Solution, Subcutaneous [preservative free]:

Enbrel: 25 mg/0.5 mL (0.51 mL); 50 mg/mL (0.98 mL)

Enbrel SureClick: 50 mg/mL (0.98 mL)

◆ Ethacrynate Sodium *see* Ethacrynic Acid *on page* 782

Ethacrynic Acid (eth a KRIN ik AS id)

Brand Names: U.S. Edecrin; Sodium Edecrin

Brand Names: Canada Edecrin®; Sodium Edecrin®

Index Terms Ethacrynate Sodium

Pharmacologic Category Diuretic, Loop

Use Management of edema associated with congestive heart failure; hepatic cirrhosis or renal disease; short-term management of ascites due to malignancy, idiopathic edema, and lymphedema

Pregnancy Risk Factor B

Dosage I.V. formulation should be diluted in D_5W or NS (1 mg/mL) and infused over several minutes.

Children: Oral: 1 mg/kg/dose once daily; increase at intervals of 2-3 days as needed, to a maximum of 3 mg/kg/day.

Adults:

Oral: 50-200 mg/day in 1-2 divided doses; may increase in increments of 25-50 mg at intervals of several days; doses up to 200 mg twice daily may be required with severe, refractory edema.

I.V.: 0.5-1 mg/kg/dose (maximum: 100 mg/dose); repeat doses not routinely recommended; however, if indicated, repeat doses every 8-12 hours.

Dosage adjustment in renal impairment: Cl_{cr} <10 mL/minute: Avoid use.

Dialysis: Not removed by hemo- or peritoneal dialysis; supplemental dose is not necessary.

Dosage adjustment in hepatic impairment: No dosage adjustment provided in manufacturer's labeling, use with caution.

Additional Information Complete prescribing information should be consulted for additional detail.

Dosage Forms Excipient information presented when available (limited, particularly for generics); consult specific product labeling.

Solution Reconstituted, Intravenous, as ethacrynate sodium:

Sodium Edecrin: 50 mg (1 ea)

Tablet, Oral:

Edecrin: 25 mg [scored]

Ethambutol (e THAM byoo tole)

Brand Names: U.S. Myambutol

Brand Names: Canada Etibi®

Index Terms Ethambutol Hydrochloride

Pharmacologic Category Antitubercular Agent

Use Treatment of pulmonary tuberculosis in conjunction with other antituberculosis agents

Unlabeled Use Other mycobacterial diseases in conjunction with other antimycobacterial agents

Pregnancy Risk Factor C

Pregnancy Considerations Teratogenic effects have been seen in animals. There are no adequate and well-controlled studies in pregnant women; there have been reports of ophthalmic abnormalities in infants born to women receiving ethambutol as a component of antituberculous therapy. Use only during pregnancy if benefits outweigh risks.

Breast-Feeding Considerations The manufacturer suggests use during breast-feeding only if benefits to the mother outweigh the possible risk to the infant. Some references suggest that exposure to the infant is low and does not produce toxicity, and breast-feeding should not be discouraged. Other references recommend if breast-feeding, monitor the infant for rash, malaise, nausea, or vomiting.

Contraindications Hypersensitivity to ethambutol or any component of the formulation; optic neuritis (risk vs benefit decision); use in young children, unconscious patients, or any other patient who may be unable to discern and report visual changes

Warnings/Precautions May cause optic neuritis (unilateral or bilateral), resulting in decreased visual acuity or other vision changes. Discontinue promptly in patients with changes in vision, color blindness, or visual defects (effects normally reversible, but reversal may require up to a year). Irreversible blindness has been reported. Monitor visual acuity prior to and during therapy. Evaluation of visual acuity changes may be more difficult in patients with cataracts, optic neuritis, diabetic retinopathy, and inflammatory conditions of the eye; consideration should be given to whether or not visual changes are related to disease progression or effects of therapy. Use only in children whose visual acuity can accurately be determined and monitored (not recommended for use in children <13 years of age unless the benefit outweighs the risk). Dosage modification is required in patients with renal insufficiency; monitor renal function prior to and during treatment. Hepatic toxicity has been reported, possibly due to concurrent therapy; monitor liver function prior to and during treatment.

Adverse Reactions Frequency not defined.

Cardiovascular: Myocarditis, pericarditis

Central nervous system: Confusion, disorientation, dizziness, fever, hallucinations, headache, malaise

Dermatologic: Dermatitis, erythema multiforme, exfoliative dermatitis, pruritus, rash

Endocrine & metabolic: Acute gout or hyperuricemia

Gastrointestinal: Abdominal pain, anorexia, GI upset, nausea, vomiting

Hematologic: Eosinophilia, leukopenia, lymphadenopathy, neutropenia, thrombocytopenia

Hepatic: Hepatitis, hepatotoxicity (possibly related to concurrent therapy), LFTs abnormal

Neuromuscular & skeletal: Arthralgia, peripheral neuritis

Ocular: Optic neuritis; symptoms may include decreased acuity, scotoma, color blindness, or visual defects (usually reversible with discontinuation, irreversible blindness has been described)

Renal: Nephritis

Respiratory: Infiltrates (with or without eosinophilia), pneumonitis

Miscellaneous: Anaphylaxis, anaphylactoid reaction; hypersensitivity syndrome (cutaneous reactions, eosinophilia, and organ-specific inflammation)

Drug Interactions

Metabolism/Transport Effects None known.

Avoid Concomitant Use There are no known interactions where it is recommended to avoid concomitant use.

Increased Effect/Toxicity There are no known significant interactions involving an increase in effect.

Decreased Effect

The levels/effects of Ethambutol may be decreased by: Aluminum Hydroxide

Storage/Stability Store at controlled room temperature of 20°C to 25°C (68°F to 77°F).

Mechanism of Action Inhibits arabinosyl transferase resulting in impaired mycobacterial cell wall synthesis

Pharmacodynamics/Kinetics

Absorption: ~80%

Distribution: Widely throughout body; concentrated in kidneys, lungs, saliva, and red blood cells

Relative diffusion from blood into CSF: Adequate with or without inflammation (exceeds usual MICs)

CSF:blood level ratio: Normal meninges: 0%; Inflamed meninges: 25%

Protein binding: 20% to 30%

Metabolism: Hepatic (20%) to inactive metabolite

Half-life elimination: 2.5-3.6 hours; End-stage renal disease: 7-15 hours

Time to peak, serum: 2-4 hours

Excretion: Urine (~50% as unchanged drug, 8% to 15% as metabolites); feces (~20% as unchanged drug)

Dosage

Usual dosage range: Oral:

Children: 15-20 mg/kg/day (maximum: 1 g/day) **or** 50 mg/kg/dose twice weekly (maximum: 2.5 g/dose)

Adults: 15-25 mg/kg daily (maximum dose: 1.5-2.5 g) **or** 25-30 mg/kg/dose 3 times/week (maximum: 2.4 g/dose) **or** 50 mg/kg/dose twice weekly (maximum: 4 g/dose)

Indication-specific dosing: Oral:

Infants and Children:

***Mycobacterium avium* (MAC), secondary prophylaxis or treatment: HIV-exposed/-infected:** 15-25 mg/kg/day once daily (maximum: 2.5 g/day) with clarithromycin (or azithromycin) with or without rifabutin (CDC, 2009)

Children:

Tuberculosis, active: Note: Used as part of a multidrug regimen; treatment regimens consist of an initial 2-month phase, followed by a continuation phase of 4 or 7 additional months; frequency of dosing may differ depending on phase of therapy.

HIV negative: Daily therapy: 15-20 mg/kg/day (maximum: 1 g/day); Twice weekly directly observed therapy (DOT): 50 mg/kg (maximum: 2.5 g/dose) (*MMWR*, 2003)

HIV-exposed/-infected: Daily therapy: 15-25 mg/kg/day (maximum: 2.5 g/day) (CDC, 2009)

Adolescents ≥13 years:

Tuberculosis, active: Refer to adult dosing.

Adults:

Disseminated *Mycobacterium avium* (MAC) treatment in patients with advanced HIV infection (unlabeled use; ATS/IDSA guidelines, 2007): 15 mg/kg ethambutol in combination with clarithromycin or azithromycin with/without rifabutin

Nontuberculous mycobacterium *(M. kansasii)* (unlabeled use; ATS/IDSA guidelines, 2007): 15 mg/kg/day ethambutol for duration to include 12 months of culture-negative sputum; typically used in combination with rifampin and isoniazid; **Note:** Previous recommendations stated to use 25 mg/kg/day for the initial 2 months of therapy; however, IDSA guidelines state this may be unnecessary given the success of rifampin-based regimens with ethambutol 15 mg/kg/day or omitted altogether.

Tuberculosis, active: Note: Used as part of a multidrug regimen; treatment regimens consist of an initial 2-month phase, followed by a continuation phase of 4 or 7 additional months; frequency of dosing may differ depending on phase of therapy.

FDA-approved labeling: Adolescents ≥13 years and Adults: Initial: 15 mg/kg once daily (maximum dose: 1.5 g); Retreatment (previous antituberculosis therapy): 25 mg/kg once daily (maximum dose: 2.5 g) for 60 days or until bacteriologic smears and cultures become negative, followed by 15 mg/kg daily.

Suggested doses by lean body weight (CDC, 2003)
Daily therapy: 15-25 mg/kg (maximum dose: 1.6 g)
40-55 kg: 800 mg
56-75 kg: 1200 mg
76-90 kg: 1600 mg
Twice weekly directly observed therapy (DOT): 50 mg/kg (maximum dose: 4 g)
40-55 kg: 2000 mg
56-75 kg: 2800 mg
76-90 kg: 4000 mg
Three times/week DOT: 25-30 mg/kg (maximum dose: 2.4 g)
40-55 kg: 1200 mg
56-75 kg: 2000 mg
76-90 kg: 2400 mg

Dosage adjustment in renal impairment:
MMWR, 2003: Cl_{cr} <30 mL/minute and hemodialysis: 15-25 mg/kg/dose 3 times weekly
Aronoff, 2007
Cl_{cr} 10-50 mL/minute: Administer every 24-36 hours
Cl_{cr} <10 mL/minute: Administer every 48 hours
Hemodialysis: Slightly dialyzable (5% to 20%); Administer dose postdialysis
Peritoneal dialysis: Dose for Cl_{cr} <10 mL/minute: Administer every 48 hours
Continuous arteriovenous or venovenous hemofiltration: Dose for Cl_{cr} 10-50 mL/minute: Administer every 24-36 hours
Dosage adjustment in hepatic impairment: No dosage adjustment provided in manufacturer's labeling; use with caution.

Dietary Considerations May be taken with food as absorption is not affected, may cause gastric irritation.

Monitoring Parameters Baseline and periodic (monthly) visual testing (each eye individually, as well as both eyes tested together) in patients receiving >15 mg/kg/day; baseline and periodic renal, hepatic, and hematopoietic tests

Dosage Forms Excipient information presented when available (limited, particularly for generics); consult specific product labeling.
Tablet, Oral, as hydrochloride:
Myambutol: 100 mg
Myambutol: 400 mg [scored]
Generic: 100 mg, 400 mg

◆ Ethambutol Hydrochloride *see* Ethambutol *on page 782*
◆ Ethamolin *see* Ethanolamine Oleate *on page 784*
◆ Ethanoic Acid *see* Acetic Acid *on page 35*

Ethanolamine Oleate (ETH a nol a meen OH lee ate)

Brand Names: U.S. Ethamolin
Index Terms Monoethanolamine
Pharmacologic Category Sclerosing Agent
Use Orphan drug: Sclerosing agent used for bleeding esophageal varices
Pregnancy Risk Factor C
Dosage Adults: 1.5-5 mL per varix, up to 20 mL total or 0.4 mL/kg for a 50 kg patient; doses should be decreased in patients with severe hepatic dysfunction and should receive less than recommended maximum dose
Dosage adjustment in renal impairment: No dosage adjustment provided in manufacturer's labeling.
Dosage adjustment in hepatic impairment: No dosage adjustment provided in manufacturer's labeling.
Additional Information Complete prescribing information should be consulted for additional detail.

Dosage Forms Excipient information presented when available (limited, particularly for generics); consult specific product labeling.
Solution, Intravenous:
Ethamolin: 5% (2 mL) [contains benzyl alcohol]

◆ Etherified Starch *see* Tetrastarch *on page 2036*

Ethinyl Estradiol and Desogestrel

(ETH in il es tra DYE ole & des oh JES trel)

Brand Names: U.S. Apri; Azurette; Caziant; Cyclessa; Desogen; Emoquette; Enskyce; Kariva; Mircette; Ortho-Cept; Pimtrea; Reclipsen; Velivet; Viorele
Brand Names: Canada Cyclessa; Linessa; Marvelon; Ortho-Cept
Index Terms Desogestrel and Ethinyl Estradiol; Ortho Cept
Pharmacologic Category Contraceptive; Estrogen and Progestin Combination
Use Contraception: For the prevention of pregnancy.
Unlabeled Use Treatment of heavy (excessive) menstrual bleeding (menorrhagia); dysmenorrhea; abnormal uterine bleeding
Pregnancy Risk Factor X
Dosage Oral: Adults: Females: Contraception:
Schedule 1 (Sunday starter): Dose begins on first Sunday after onset of menstruation; if the menstrual period starts on Sunday, take first tablet that very same day. **With a Sunday start, an additional method of contraception should be used until after the first 7 days of consecutive administration.**
For 21-tablet package: Dosage is 1 tablet daily for 21 consecutive days, followed by 7 days off of the medication; a new course begins on the 8th day after the last tablet is taken.
For 28-tablet package: Dosage is 1 tablet daily without interruption.
Schedule 2 (Day 1 starter): Dose starts on first day of menstrual cycle taking 1 tablet daily.
For 21-tablet package: Dosage is 1 tablet daily for 21 consecutive days, followed by 7 days off of the medication; a new course begins on the 8th day after the last tablet is taken.
For 28-tablet package: Dosage is 1 tablet daily without interruption.
If all doses have not been taken on schedule and one menstrual period is missed, the possibility of pregnancy should be considered. If two consecutive menstrual periods are missed, pregnancy test is required before new dosing cycle is started.
Missed doses **monophasic formulations** (refer to package insert for complete information):
One dose missed: Take as soon as remembered or take 2 tablets next day
Two consecutive doses missed in the first 2 weeks: Take 2 tablets as soon as remembered or 2 tablets next 2 days. **An additional method of contraception should be used for 7 days after missed dose.**
Two consecutive doses missed in week 3 or three consecutive doses missed at any time:
Schedule 1 (Sunday starter): Continue to take 1 tablet daily until Sunday, then discard the rest of the pack, and a new pack is started that same day. **An additional method of contraception should be used for 7 days after missed dose.**
Schedule 2 (Day 1 starter): Current pack should be discarded, and a new pack started that same day. **An additional method of contraception should be used for 7 days after missed dose.**
Missed doses **biphasic/triphasic formulations** (refer to package insert for complete information):
One dose missed: Take as soon as remembered.

Two consecutive doses missed in week 1 or week 2 of the pack: Take 2 tablets as soon as remembered and 2 tablets the next day. Resume taking 1 tablet daily until the pack is empty. **An additional method of contraception should be used for 7 days after a missed dose.**

Two consecutive doses missed in week 3 of the pack; **an additional method of contraception must be used for 7 days after a missed dose**:

Schedule 1 (Sunday starter): Take 1 tablet every day until Sunday. Discard the remaining pack and start a new pack of pills on the same day.

Schedule 2 (Day 1 starter): Discard the remaining pack and start a new pack the same day.

Three or more consecutive doses missed; **an additional method of contraception must be used for 7 days after a missed dose**:

Schedule 1 (Sunday starter): Take 1 tablet every day until Sunday; on Sunday, discard the pack and start a new pack.

Schedule 2 (Day 1 starter): Discard the remaining pack and begin new pack of tablets starting on the same day.

Dosage adjustment in renal impairment: No dosage adjustment provided in manufacturer's labeling; use with caution and monitor blood pressure closely. Consider other forms of contraception.

Dosage adjustment in hepatic impairment: Contraindicated in patients with hepatic impairment

Additional Information Complete prescribing information should be consulted for additional detail.

Dosage Forms Excipient information presented when available (limited, particularly for generics); consult specific product labeling. [DSC] = Discontinued product

Tablet, oral [low dose formulation]:

Azurette:

Day 1-21: Ethinyl estradiol 0.02 mg and desogestrel 0.15 mg [21 white tablets]

Day 22-23: 2 inactive green tablets

Day 24-28: Ethinyl estradiol 0.01 mg [5 blue tablets] (28s)

Kariva:

Day 1-21: Ethinyl estradiol 0.02 mg and desogestrel 0.15 mg [21 white tablets]

Day 22-23: 2 inactive light green tablets

Day 24-28: Ethinyl estradiol 0.01 mg [5 light blue tablets] (28s)

Mircette:

Day 1-21: Ethinyl estradiol 0.02 mg and desogestrel 0.15 mg [21 white tablets]

Day 22-23: 2 inactive green tablets

Day 24-28: Ethinyl estradiol 0.01 mg [5 yellow tablets] (28s)

Pimtrea:

Day 1-21: Ethinyl estradiol 0.02 mg and desogestrel 0.15 mg [21 dark blue tablets]

Day 22-23: 2 inactive white tablets

Day 24-28: Ethinyl estradiol 0.01 mg [5 green tablets] (28s)

Viorele:

Day 1-21: Ethinyl estradiol 0.02 mg and desogestrel 0.15 mg [21 white tablets]

Day 22-23: 2 inactive green tablets

Day 24-28: Ethinyl estradiol 0.01 mg [5 yellow tablets] (28s)

Tablet, oral [monophasic formulation]:

Apri 28: Ethinyl estradiol 0.03 mg and desogestrel 0.15 mg [21 rose tablets and 7 white inactive tablets] (28s)

Desogen, Reclipsen: Ethinyl estradiol 0.03 mg and desogestrel 0.15 mg [21 white tablets and 7 green inactive tablets] (28s)

Emoquette: Ethinyl estradiol 0.03 mg and desogestrel 0.15 mg [21 white tablets and 7 light green inactive tablets] (28s)

Enskyce: Ethinyl estradiol 0.03 mg and desogestrel 0.15 mg [21 light orange tablets and 7 green inactive tablets] (28s)

Ortho-Cept 28: Ethinyl estradiol 0.03 mg and desogestrel 0.15 mg [21 light orange tablets and 7 green inactive tablets] (28s)

Tablet, oral [triphasic formulation]:

Caziant:

Day 1-7: Ethinyl estradiol 0.025 mg and desogestrel 0.1 mg [7 white tablets]

Day 8-14: Ethinyl estradiol 0.025 mg and desogestrel 0.125 mg [7 light blue tablets]

Day 15-21: Ethinyl estradiol 0.025 mg and desogestrel 0.15 mg [7 blue tablets]

Day 22-28: 7 green inactive tablets (28s)

Cyclessa:

Day 1-7: Ethinyl estradiol 0.025 mg and desogestrel 0.1 mg [7 light yellow tablets]

Day 8-14: Ethinyl estradiol 0.025 mg and desogestrel 0.125 mg [7 orange tablets]

Day 15-21: Ethinyl estradiol 0.025 mg and desogestrel 0.15 mg [7 red tablets]

Day 22-28: 7 green inactive tablets (28s)

Velivet:

Day 1-7: Ethinyl estradiol 0.025 mg and desogestrel 0.1 mg [7 beige tablets]

Day 8-14: Ethinyl estradiol 0.025 mg and desogestrel 0.125 mg [7 orange tablets]

Day 15-21: Ethinyl estradiol 0.025 mg and desogestrel 0.15 mg [7 pink tablets]

Day 22-28: 7 white inactive tablets (28s)

Ethinyl Estradiol and Drospirenone

(ETH in il es tra DYE ole & droh SPYE re none)

Brand Names: U.S. Gianvi™; Loryna™; Ocella™; Syeda™; Vestura™; Yasmin®; Yaz®; Zarah®

Brand Names: Canada Yasmin®; Yaz®

Index Terms Drospirenone and Ethinyl Estradiol

Pharmacologic Category Contraceptive; Estrogen and Progestin Combination

Use Prevention of pregnancy; treatment of premenstrual dysphoric disorder (PMDD); treatment of acne

Unlabeled Use Treatment of hypermenorrhea (menorrhagia); pain associated with endometriosis; dysmenorrhea; dysfunctional uterine bleeding

Pregnancy Risk Factor X

Dosage Oral:

Children ≥14 years and Adults: Females: Acne (Yaz®): Refer to dosing for contraception

Adults: Females: Contraception (Yasmin®, Yaz®), PMDD (Yaz®): Dosage is 1 tablet daily for 28 consecutive days. Dosing may be started on the first day of menstrual period (Day 1 starter) or on the first Sunday after the onset of the menstrual period (Sunday starter). **An additional method of contraception should be used until after the first 7 days of consecutive administration.**

Day 1 starter: Dose starts on first day of menstrual cycle taking 1 tablet daily.

Sunday starter: Dose begins on first Sunday after onset of menstruation; if the menstrual period starts on Sunday, take first tablet that very same day.

Switching from a different contraceptive:

Oral contraceptive: Start on the same day that a new pack of the previous oral contraceptive would have been taken

Transdermal patch, vaginal ring, injection: Start on the day the next dose would have been due

IUD or implant: Start on the day of removal

Use after childbirth (in women who are not breast-feeding) or after second trimester abortion: Therapy may be started ≥4 weeks postpartum. Pregnancy should be ruled out prior to treatment if menstrual periods have not restarted and an additional method of contraception (nonhormonal) should be used until after the first 7 days of consecutive administration.

Missed doses:

If all doses have been taken on schedule and one menstrual period is missed, continue dosing cycle. If two consecutive menstrual periods are missed, pregnancy test is required before new dosing cycle is started.

If doses have been missed during the first 3 weeks and the menstrual period is missed, pregnancy should be ruled out prior to continuing treatment.

Missed doses (monophasic formulations) (refer to package insert for complete information):

One dose missed: Take as soon as remembered or take 2 tablets next day

Two consecutive doses missed in the first 2 weeks: Take 2 tablets as soon as remembered or 2 tablets next 2 days. **An additional method of contraception should be used for 7 days after missed dose.**

Two consecutive doses missed in week 3 or three consecutive doses missed at any time: **An additional method of contraception must be used for 7 days after a missed dose.**

Day 1 starter: Current pack should be discarded, and a new pack should be started that same day.

Sunday starter: Continue dose of 1 tablet daily until Sunday, then discard the rest of the pack, and a new pack should be started that same day.

Any number of doses missed in week 4: Continue taking one pill each day until pack is empty; no back-up method of contraception is needed

Dosage adjustment in renal impairment: Contraindicated in patients with renal dysfunction

Dosage adjustment in hepatic impairment: Contraindicated in patients with hepatic dysfunction

Additional Information Complete prescribing information should be consulted for additional detail.

Dosage Forms Excipient information presented when available (limited, particularly for generics); consult specific product labeling.

Tablet, oral: Ethinyl estradiol 0.03 mg and drospirenone 3 mg [21 active tablets and 7 inactive tablets] (28s)

Gianvi™: Ethinyl estradiol 0.02 mg and drospirenone 3 mg [24 light pink active tablets and 4 white inactive tablets] (28s)

Loryna™: Ethinyl estradiol 0.02 mg and drospirenone 3 mg [24 peach active tablets and 4 white inactive tablets] (28s)

Ocella™: Ethinyl estradiol 0.03 mg and drospirenone 3 mg [21 yellow active tablets and 7 white inactive tablets] (28s)

Syeda™: Ethinyl estradiol 0.03 mg and drospirenone 3 mg [21 yellow active tablets and 7 white inactive tablets] (28s)

Vestura™: Ethinyl estradiol 0.02 mg and drospirenone 3 mg [24 pink active tablets and 4 peach inactive tablets] (28s)

Yasmin®: Ethinyl estradiol 0.03 mg and drospirenone 3 mg [21 yellow active tablets and 7 white inactive tablets] (28s)

Yaz®: Ethinyl estradiol 0.02 mg and drospirenone 3 mg [24 light pink active tablets and 4 white inactive tablets] (28s)

Zarah®: Ethinyl estradiol 0.03 mg and drospirenone 3 mg [21 blue active tablets and 7 peach inactive tablets] (28s)

Ethinyl Estradiol and Ethynodiol Diacetate

(ETH in il es tra DYE ole & e thye noe DYE ole dye AS e tate)

Brand Names: U.S. Kelnor™; Zovia®

Brand Names: Canada Demulen® 30

Index Terms Ethynodiol Diacetate and Ethinyl Estradiol

Pharmacologic Category Contraceptive; Estrogen and Progestin Combination

Use Prevention of pregnancy

Unlabeled Use Treatment of hypermenorrhea (menorrhagia); pain associated with endometriosis; dysmenorrhea; dysfunctional uterine bleeding

Pregnancy Risk Factor X

Dosage Oral: Adults: Females: Contraception:

Schedule 1 (Sunday starter): Dose begins on first Sunday after onset of menstruation; if the menstrual period starts on Sunday, take first tablet that very same day. **With a Sunday start, an additional method of contraception should be used until after the first 7 days of consecutive administration.**

For 21-tablet package: 1 tablet/day for 21 consecutive days, followed by 7 days off of the medication; a new course begins on the 8th day after the last tablet is taken.

For 28-tablet package: 1 tablet/day without interruption.

Schedule 2 (Day 1 starter): Dose starts on first day of menstrual cycle taking 1 tablet daily.

For 21-tablet package: 1 tablet/day for 21 consecutive days, followed by 7 days off of the medication; a new course begins on the 8th day after the last tablet is taken.

For 28-tablet package: 1 tablet/day without interruption.

If all doses have been taken on schedule and one menstrual period is missed, continue dosing cycle. If two consecutive menstrual periods are missed, pregnancy test is required before new dosing cycle is started.

Missed doses **monophasic formulations** (refer to package insert for complete information):

One dose missed: Take as soon as remembered or take 2 tablets next day

Two consecutive doses missed in the first 2 weeks: Take 2 tablets as soon as remembered or 2 tablets next 2 days. **An additional method of contraception should be used for 7 days after missed dose.**

Two consecutive doses missed in week 3 or three consecutive doses missed at any time: **An additional method of contraception should be used for 7 days after missed dose:**

Schedule 1 (Sunday starter): Continue dose of 1 tablet daily until Sunday, then discard the rest of the pack, and a new pack should be started that same day.

Schedule 2 (Day 1 starter): Current package should be discarded, and a new pack should be started that same day.

Dosage adjustment in renal impairment: Specific guidelines not available; use with caution and monitor blood pressure closely. Consider other forms of contraception.

Dosage adjustment in hepatic impairment: Contraindicated in patients with hepatic impairment

Additional Information Complete prescribing information should be consulted for additional detail.

Dosage Forms Excipient information presented when available (limited, particularly for generics); consult specific product labeling.

Tablet, oral [monophasic formulation]:

Kelnor™ 1/35: Ethinyl estradiol 0.035 mg and ethynodiol diacetate 1 mg [21 light yellow tablets and 7 white inactive tablets] (28s)

Zovia® 1/35-28: Ethinyl estradiol 0.035 mg and ethynodiol diacetate 1 mg [21 light pink tablets and 7 white inactive tablets] (28s)

Zovia® 1/50-28: Ethinyl estradiol 0.05 mg and ethynodiol diacetate 1 mg [21 pink tablets and 7 white inactive tablets] (28s)

Ethinyl Estradiol and Etonogestrel

(ETH in il es tra DYE ole & et oh noe JES trel)

Brand Names: U.S. NuvaRing®

Brand Names: Canada NuvaRing®

Index Terms Etonogestrel and Ethinyl Estradiol

Pharmacologic Category Contraceptive; Estrogen and Progestin Combination

Use Contraception: For the prevention of pregnancy

Unlabeled Use Treatment of heavy (excessive) menstrual bleeding (menorrhagia); dysmenorrhea; abnormal uterine bleeding

Dosage Vaginal: Adults: Females: Contraception: One ring, inserted vaginally and left in place for 3 consecutive weeks, then removed for 1 week. A new ring is inserted 7 days after the last was removed (even if bleeding is not complete) and should be inserted at approximately the same time of day the ring was removed the previous week.

Initial treatment should begin as follows (pregnancy should always be ruled out first):

No hormonal contraceptive use in the past month: Insert ring on the first day of menstrual cycle ("Day 1"). May also insert on days 2-5 even if bleeding is not complete, however, **a spermicide or barrier method of contraception should be used for the following 7 days.***

Switching from combination oral contraceptive: Ring can be inserted on any day within 7 days after the last **active** tablet in the cycle was taken and no later than the first day a new cycle of tablets would begin. Additional forms of contraception are not needed.

Switching from progestin-only contraceptive: **A spermicide or barrier method of contraception should be used for the following 7 days with any of the following.***

If previously using a progestin-only mini-pill, insert the ring on any day of the month; insert the vaginal ring on the day after the last mini-pill; do not skip days between the last pill and insertion of the ring.

If previously using an implant, insert the ring on the same day of implant removal.

If previously using a progestin-containing IUD, insert the ring on day of IUD removal.

If previously using a progestin injection, insert the ring on the day the next injection would be given.

Following complete 1st trimester abortion or miscarriage: Insert ring within the first 5 days of abortion or miscarriage. If not inserted within 5 days, follow instructions for "No hormonal contraceptive use within the past month" and instruct patient to use a nonhormonal contraceptive in the interim.

Following delivery or 2nd trimester abortion or miscarriage: Insert ring no sooner than 4 weeks postpartum (in women who are not breast-feeding) or following 2nd trimester abortion or miscarriage. **A spermicide or barrier method of contraception should be used for the following 7 days.***

If the ring is accidentally removed from the vagina at any time during the 3-week period of use, it may be rinsed with cool or lukewarm water (not hot) and reinserted as soon as possible. If the ring is not reinserted within 3 hours, contraceptive effectiveness will be decreased. If the ring is accidently removed from the vagina for >3 hours during weeks 1 and 2, the ring should be reinserted as soon as the woman remembers and **a spermicide or barrier method of contraception should be used until the ring has been in place for 7 consecutive days.*** If the ring is accidently removed from the vagina for >3 hours during week 3, the ring should be discarded. A new ring may be inserted immediately, restarting a new 3-week cycle, OR a new ring may be inserted ≤7 days from the time the previous ring was removed or expelled (the second option should only be done if a vaginal ring was in continuous use for ≥7 days prior to the inadvertent expulsion/removal). With either option, a **spermicide or barrier method of contraception should be used until the ring has been in place for 7 consecutive days.*** Additional guidelines are available (CDC, 2013).

If the ring has been removed for longer than 1 week, pregnancy must be ruled out prior to restarting therapy. **A spermicide or barrier method of contraception should be used for the following 7 days.***

If the ring has been left in place for >3 weeks, a new ring should be inserted following a 1-week (ring-free) interval. Protection continues during week 4, however, if the ring is left in place >4 weeks, pregnancy must be ruled out prior to insertion and **a spermicide or barrier method of contraception should be used for the following 7 days.***

Disconnected ring: In the event the ring disconnects at the weld joint, discard and replace with a new ring.

***Note:** Diaphragms may interfere with proper ring placement, and therefore, are not recommended for use as an additional form of contraception.

Dosage adjustment in renal impairment: No dosage adjustment provided in manufacturer's labeling (has not been studied).

Dosage adjustment in hepatic impairment: No dosage adjustment provided in manufacturer's labeling (has not been studied). Use is contraindicated in patients with hepatic impairment.

Additional Information Complete prescribing information should be consulted for additional detail.

Dosage Forms Excipient information presented when available (limited, particularly for generics); consult specific product labeling.

Ring, vaginal:

NuvaRing®: Ethinyl estradiol 0.015 mg/day and etonogestrel 0.12 mg/day (3s) [3-week duration]

Ethinyl Estradiol and Levonorgestrel

(ETH in il es tra DYE ole & LEE voe nor jes trel)

Brand Names: U.S. Altavera; Amethia; Amethia Lo; Amethyst; Aubra; Aviane; camrese; Chateal; Daysee; Enpresse; Falmina; Introvale; Jolessa; Kurvelo; Lessina; Levonest; Levora; LoSeasonique; Lutera; Lybrel; Marlissa; Myzilra; Nordette 28 [DSC]; Orsythia; Portia; Quartette; Quasense; Seasonique; Sronyx; Trivora

Brand Names: Canada Alesse; Aviane; Min-Ovral; Seasonale; Triphasil; Triquilar

Index Terms Levonorgestrel and Ethinyl Estradiol

Pharmacologic Category Contraceptive; Estrogen and Progestin Combination

Use Prevention of pregnancy; postcoital contraception

Unlabeled Use Treatment of hypermenorrhea (menorrhagia); pain associated with endometriosis; dysmenorrhea; dysfunctional uterine bleeding

Pregnancy Risk Factor X

Pregnancy Considerations Pregnancy should be ruled out prior to treatment and discontinued if pregnancy occurs. In general, the use of combination hormonal contraceptives when inadvertently taken early in pregnancy have not been associated with teratogenic effects. Hormonal contraceptives may be less effective in obese patients. An increase in oral contraceptive failure was noted in women with a BMI >27.3 kg/m^2. Similar findings were noted in patients weighing ≥90 kg (198 lb) using the contraceptive patch.

Due to increased risk of venous thromboembolism (VTE) postpartum, combination hormonal contraceptives should not be started in any woman <21 days following delivery. Women without risk factors for VTE and who are not breast-feeding may start combination hormonal contraceptives during 21-42 days postpartum. After 42 days postpartum, restrictions for use are not related to postpartum status and should be based on other medical conditions (CDC, 2011). Some manufacturers recommend waiting ≥4 weeks postpartum before starting this combination.

Breast-Feeding Considerations Jaundice and breast enlargement in the nursing infant have been reported following the use of combination hormonal contraceptives. May decrease the quality and quantity of breast milk; alternative form of contraception is recommended (per manufacturer). The theoretical concerns about decreased milk production are greatest early in the postpartum period when milk production is being established. Postpartum risk status for VTE should be considered when initiating combination hormonal contraceptives after delivery. Combined hormonal contraceptives should not be started <21 days postpartum due to increased risk of VTE. Risk of VTE is still elevated in breast-feeding women until ~42 days postpartum and is greater in women with additional risk factors. After 42 days postpartum, restrictions for use are not related to postpartum VTE risk and should be based on other medical conditions (CDC, 2011). Some manufacturers recommend waiting ≥4 weeks postpartum before starting this combination.

Contraindications Breast cancer or other estrogen- or progestin-dependent neoplasms (current or a history of), hepatic tumors or disease, pregnancy, undiagnosed abnormal uterine bleeding

Use is also contraindicated in women at high risk of arterial or venous thrombotic diseases including: Cerebrovascular disease, coronary artery disease, diabetes mellitus with vascular disease, DVT or PE (current or history of), hypercoagulopathies (inherited or acquired), headaches with focal neurological symptoms, hypertension (uncontrolled), migraine headaches if >35 years of age, thrombogenic valvular or rhythm diseases of the heart (eg, subacute bacterial endocarditis with valvular disease or atrial fibrillation), women >35 years of age who smoke.

Canadian-labeling: Additional contraindication: Ocular lesions due to ophthalmic vascular disease including partial or complete loss of vision or defect in visual fields; severe dyslipoproteinemia; hereditary or acquired predisposition for venous or arterial thrombosis

Warnings/Precautions Hazardous agent - use appropriate precautions for handling and disposal (NIOSH, 2012). Combination hormonal contraceptives do not protect against HIV infection or other sexually-transmitted diseases. **[U.S. Boxed Warning]: The risk of cardiovascular side effects is increased in women who smoke cigarettes; risk increases with age (especially women >35 years of age) and the number of cigarettes smoked; women who use combination hormonal contraceptives should be strongly advised not to smoke. Use is contraindicated in patients >35 years of age who smoke.** Use with caution in patients with risk factors for coronary artery disease (eg, hypertension, hypercholesterolemia, morbid obesity, diabetes, or women who smoke); may lead to increased risk of myocardial infarction. May have a dose-related risk of vascular disease and hypertension; women with hypertension should be encouraged to use a nonhormonal form of contraception. Use is contraindicated with uncontrolled hypertension. May increase the risk of thromboembolism; discontinue use of combination hormonal contraceptives if an arterial or venous thrombotic event occurs. Women with inherited thrombophilias (eg, protein C or S deficiency) may have increased risk of venous thromboembolism (DeSancho, 2010; van Vlijmen, 2011). Use is contraindicated in women with hypercoagulopathies (inherited or acquired). Whenever possible, combination hormonal contraceptives should be discontinued at least 4 weeks prior to and for 2 weeks following elective surgery associated with an increased risk of thromboembolism or during periods of prolonged immobilization. Combination hormonal contraceptives may have a dose-related risk of gallbladder disease and may worsen existing gallbladder disease. Women with renal disease should be encouraged to use another form of contraception. May have adverse effects on glucose tolerance; use caution in women with diabetes.

Combination hormonal contraceptives may affect serum triglyceride and lipoprotein levels. Triglycerides may also be increased; use with caution in patients with familial defects of lipoprotein metabolism. The use of combination hormonal contraceptives has been associated with a slight increase in frequency of breast cancer; however, studies are not consistent. Use is contraindicated in women with (or history of) breast cancer. Use caution with conditions that may be aggravated by fluid retention, depression, or history of migraine. Evaluate new, recurrent, severe or persistent headaches. Use with migraine headaches with or without aura if >35 years of age is contraindicated. Not for use prior to menarche. Estrogens may cause retinal vascular thrombosis; discontinue if migraine, loss of vision, proptosis, diplopia or other visual disturbances occur; discontinue permanently if papilledema or retinal vascular lesions are observed on examination. Risk of chloasma may be increased with history of chloasma gravidarum. Women with history of chloasma should avoid exposure to sun or ultraviolet radiation during therapy. May induce or exacerbate symptoms of hereditary angioedema.

Presentation of irregular, unresolving vaginal bleeding warrants further evaluation including endometrial sampling, if indicated, to rule out malignancy; evaluate hypothalamic-pituitary-function in women with persistent (≥6 months) amenorrhea (especially associated with breast secretion) following discontinuation of therapy. Discontinue use with the onset of sudden enlargement, pain, or tenderness of fibroids (leiomyomata). Extremely rare adenomas and focal nodular hyperplasia resulting in fatal intra-abdominal hemorrhage have been reported in association with long-term oral contraceptive use. Presentation of an abdominal mass, acute abdominal pain, or intra-abdominal bleeding warrants further evaluation to rule out source. Combination hormonal contraceptives may be poorly metabolized in women with hepatic impairment. Discontinue if jaundice develops during therapy or if liver function becomes abnormal. Use is contraindicated with pre-existing hepatic tumors or disease. Risk of cholestasis may be increased with previous cholestatic jaundice of pregnancy or jaundice with prior oral contraceptive use. Estrogens may increase thyroid-binding globulin (TBG) levels leading to increased circulating total thyroid hormone levels. Women on thyroid replacement therapy may require higher doses of thyroid hormone while receiving estrogens. The use of estrogens and/or progestins may change the results of some laboratory tests (eg, coagulation factors, lipids, glucose tolerance, binding proteins). The dose, route, and the specific estrogen/progestin influences these changes. In addition, personal risk factors (eg, cardiovascular disease, smoking, diabetes, age) also contribute to adverse events; use of specific products may be contraindicated in women with certain risk factors. Some products may contain tartrazine, which may cause allergic reactions in certain individuals.

The minimum dosage combination of estrogen/progestin that will effectively treat the individual patient should be used. New patients should be started on products containing ≤0.035 mg of estrogen per tablet. Extended cycle regimen contraceptives provide more hormonal exposure per year than conventional monthly contraceptives.

Adverse Reactions The following reactions have been associated with oral contraceptive use:

Increased risk or evidence of association with use:

Cardiovascular: Arterial thromboembolism, cerebral hemorrhage, cerebral thrombosis, hypertension, mesenteric thrombosis, MI, venous thrombosis (with or without embolism)

Gastrointestinal: Gallbladder disease

Hepatic: Hepatic adenomas, liver tumors (benign)

Local: Thrombophlebitis

Ocular: Retinal thrombosis

Respiratory: Pulmonary embolism

Adverse reactions considered drug related:

Cardiovascular: Edema, varicose vein aggravation

Central nervous system: Depression, migraine, mood changes

Dermatologic: Chloasma, melasma, rash (allergic)

Endocrine & metabolic: Amenorrhea, breakthrough bleeding, breast changes (enlargement, pain, secretion, tenderness), carbohydrate tolerance decreased, fluid retention, infertility (temporary), lactation decreased (with use immediately postpartum), menstrual flow changes, spotting

Gastrointestinal: Abdominal bloating, abdominal cramps, abdominal pain, appetite changes, nausea, weight changes, vomiting

Genitourinary: Cervical ectropion, cervical secretion/erosion, endocervical hyperplasia, fibroid enlargement, vaginal candidiasis, vaginitis

Hematologic: Folate decreased, porphyria exacerbation

Hepatic: Cholestatic jaundice, focal nodular hyperplasia

Neuromuscular & skeletal: Chorea exacerbation

Ocular: Contact lens intolerance, corneal curvature changes (steepening)

Respiratory: Rhinitis

Miscellaneous: Anaphylactic/anaphylactoid reactions (including angioedema, circulatory collapse, respiratory collapse, urticaria), SLE exacerbation

Adverse reactions in which association is not confirmed or denied: Acne, auditory disturbances, Budd-Chiari syndrome, cataracts, cervical smear abnormal, colitis, cystitis-like syndrome, dizziness, dysmenorrhea, erythema multiforme, erythema nodosum, headache, hemolytic uremic syndrome, hemorrhagic eruption, hirsutism, libido changes, nervousness, optic neuritis (with or without partial or complete loss of vision), pancreatitis, premenstrual syndrome, renal function impaired, scalp hair loss

Drug Interactions

Metabolism/Transport Effects Refer to individual components.

Avoid Concomitant Use

Avoid concomitant use of Ethinyl Estradiol and Levonorgestrel with any of the following: Anastrozole; Dehydroepiandrosterone; Griseofulvin; Ospemifene; Pimozide; Pirfenidone; Tranexamic Acid; Ulipristal

Increased Effect/Toxicity

Ethinyl Estradiol and Levonorgestrel may increase the levels/effects of: Agomelatine; ARIPiprazole; Benzodiazepines (metabolized by oxidation); Corticosteroids (Systemic); CYP1A2 Substrates; Dofetilide; Lomitapide; Ospemifene; Pimozide; Pirfenidone; ROPINIRole; Selegiline; Theophylline Derivatives; Tipranavir; TiZANidine; Tranexamic Acid; Voriconazole

The levels/effects of Ethinyl Estradiol and Levonorgestrel may be increased by: Ascorbic Acid; Atazanavir; Boceprevir; Cobicistat; Dehydroepiandrosterone; Herbs (Estrogenic Properties); Herbs (Progestogenic Properties); Mifepristone; NSAID (COX-2 Inhibitor); Voriconazole

Decreased Effect

Ethinyl Estradiol and Levonorgestrel may decrease the levels/effects of: Anastrozole; Anticoagulants; Chenodiol; Hyaluronidase; LamoTRIgine; Ospemifene; Thyroid Products; Ursodiol; Vitamin K Antagonists

The levels/effects of Ethinyl Estradiol and Levonorgestrel may be decreased by: Acitretin; Aminoglutethimide; Aprepitant; Armodafinil; Artemether; Barbiturates; Bexarotene (Systemic); Bile Acid Sequestrants; Boceprevir; Bosentan; CarBAMazepine; CloBAZam; Cobicistat; Colesevelam; CYP3A4 Inducers (Strong); Dabrafenib; Deferasirox; Elvitegravir; Eslicarbazepine; Exenatide; Felbamate; Fosaprepitant; Fosphenytoin; Griseofulvin; LamoTRIgine; Mifepristone; Mitotane; Modafinil; Mycophenolate; Nafcillin; Nelfinavir; Nevirapine; OXcarbazepine; Perampanel; Phenytoin; Primidone; Protease Inhibitors; Prucalopride; Retinoic Acid Derivatives; Rifamycin Derivatives; Rufinamide; St Johns Wort; Sugammadex; Telaprevir; Tipranavir; Tocilizumab; Topiramate; Ulipristal

Ethanol/Nutrition/Herb Interactions

Food: CNS effects of caffeine may be enhanced if combination hormonal contraceptives are used concurrently with caffeine. Grapefruit juice increases ethinyl estradiol plasma concentrations and would be expected to increase progesterone serum levels as well; clinical implications are unclear.

Herb/Nutraceutical: St John's wort may decrease levels. Herbs with estrogenic properties may enhance the adverse/toxic effect of estrogen derivatives; examples include alfalfa, black cohosh, bloodroot, hops, kudzu, licorice, red clover, saw palmetto, soybean, thyme, wild yam, yucca. Herbs with progestogenic properties may enhance the adverse/toxic effect of progestins; examples include bloodroot, chasteberry, damiana, oregano, yucca. Impaired folate metabolism and reduced serum levels of cyanocobalamin have been reported with oral contraceptive use; increased dietary intake or supplementation may be necessary.

Storage/Stability Store at controlled room temperature of 20°C to 25°C (68°F to 77°F).

Mechanism of Action Combination hormonal contraceptives inhibit ovulation via a negative feedback mechanism on the hypothalamus, which alters the normal pattern of gonadotropin secretion of a follicle-stimulating hormone (FSH) and luteinizing hormone by the anterior pituitary. The follicular phase FSH and midcycle surge of gonadotropins are inhibited. In addition, combination hormonal contraceptives produce alterations in the genital tract, including changes in the cervical mucus, rendering it unfavorable for sperm penetration even if ovulation occurs. Changes in the endometrium may also occur, producing an unfavorable environment for nidation. Combination hormonal contraceptive drugs may alter the tubal transport of the ova through the fallopian tubes. Progestational agents may also alter sperm fertility.

Pharmacodynamics/Kinetics

Absorption: Rapid

Distribution: Ethinyl estradiol: 4.3 L/kg; Levonorgestrel: 1.8 L/kg

Protein binding:

Ethinyl estradiol: 95% to 97% to albumin

Levonorgestrel: 97% to 99% primarily to sex hormone binding globulin (SHBG), lesser amounts to albumin

Metabolism:

Ethinyl estradiol: Hepatic via CYP3A4; undergoes first-pass metabolism; forms metabolites

Levonorgestrel: Forms conjugated in unconjugated metabolites

Bioavailability: Ethinyl estradiol: 38% to 48%; Levonorgestrel: 100%

Half-life elimination: Ethinyl estradiol: 12-23 hours; Levonorgestrel: 22-49 hours

Excretion:

Ethinyl estradiol: Urine and feces

Levonorgestrel: Urine (40% to 68%, parent drug and metabolites); feces (16% to 48% as metabolites)

Dosage Oral: Adults: Females:

Contraception, 28-day cycle:

Schedule 1 (Sunday starter): Dose begins on first Sunday after onset of menstruation; if the menstrual period starts on Sunday, take first tablet that very same day. With a Sunday start, an additional method of contraception should be used until after the first 7 days of consecutive administration:

For 21-tablet package: 1 tablet/day for 21 consecutive days, followed by 7 days off of the medication; a new course begins on the 8th day after the last tablet is taken

For 28-tablet package: 1 tablet/day without interruption

Schedule 2 (Day 1 starter): Dose starts on first day of menstrual cycle taking 1 tablet/day:

For 21-tablet package: 1 tablet/day for 21 consecutive days, followed by 7 days off of the medication; a new course begins on the 8th day after the last tablet is taken

For 28-tablet package: 1 tablet/day without interruption

If all doses have been taken on schedule and one menstrual period is missed, continue dosing cycle. If two consecutive menstrual periods are missed, pregnancy test is required before new dosing cycle is started.

Missed doses **monophasic formulations** (refer to package insert for complete information):

One dose missed: Take as soon as remembered or take 2 tablets next day

Two consecutive doses missed in the first 2 weeks: Take 2 tablets as soon as remembered or 2 tablets next 2 days. An additional method of contraception should be used for 7 days after missed dose.

Two consecutive doses missed in week 3 or three consecutive doses missed at any time: An additional method of contraception must be used for 7 days after a missed dose:

Schedule 1 (Sunday starter): Continue dose of 1 tablet daily until Sunday, then discard the rest of the pack, and a new pack should be started that same day.

Schedule 2 (Day 1 starter): Current pack should be discarded, and a new pack should be started that same day.

Missed doses **biphasic/triphasic formulations** (refer to package insert for complete information):

One dose missed: Take as soon as remembered or take 2 tablets next day.

Two consecutive doses missed in week 1 or week 2 of the pack: Take 2 tablets as soon as remembered and 2 tablets the next day. Resume taking 1 tablet daily until the pack is empty. An additional method of contraception should be used for 7 days after a missed dose.

Two consecutive doses missed in week 3 of the pack: An additional method of contraception must be used for 7 days after a missed dose.

Schedule 1 (Sunday starter): Take 1 tablet every day until Sunday. Discard the remaining pack and start a new pack of pills on the same day.

Schedule 2 (Day 1 starter): Discard the remaining pack and start a new pack the same day.

Three or more consecutive doses missed: An additional method of contraception must be used for 7 days after a missed dose.

Schedule 1 (Sunday starter): Take 1 tablet every day until Sunday; on Sunday, discard the pack and start a new pack.

Schedule 2 (Day 1 starter): Discard the remaining pack and begin new pack of tablets starting on the same day.

Contraception, 91-day cycle (extended cycle regimen): Dose begins on first Sunday after onset of menstruation; if the menstrual period starts on Sunday, take first tablet that very same day. An additional method of contraception should be used until after the first 7 days of consecutive administration:

Introvale, Jolessa, Quasense, Seasonale [Canadian product]: One active tablet/day for 84 consecutive days, followed by 1 inactive tablet/day for 7 days; if all doses have been taken on schedule and one menstrual period is missed, pregnancy should be ruled out prior to continuing therapy.

Seasonique, LoSeasonique, Quartette: One active tablet/day for 84 consecutive days, followed by 1 low dose estrogen tablet/day for 7 days; if all doses have been taken on schedule and one menstrual period is missed, pregnancy should be ruled out prior to continuing therapy.

Missed doses:

One dose missed: Take as soon as remembered or take 2 tablets the next day

Two consecutive doses missed: Take 2 tablets as soon as remembered or 2 tablets the next 2 days. An additional nonhormonal method of contraception should be used for 7 consecutive days after the missed dose.

Three or more consecutive doses missed: Do not take the missed doses; continue taking 1 tablet/day until pack is complete. Bleeding may occur during the following week. An additional nonhormonal method of contraception should be used for 7 consecutive days after the missed dose.

Any number of pills during week 13: Throw away the missed pills and keep taking scheduled pills until the pack is finished. A back-up method of contraception is not needed

Contraception, continuous use (extended cycle regimen): Lybrel: Take one tablet daily, at the same time each day, without a tablet-free interval. Therapy should be initiated as follows:

No previous contraception: Begin on the first day of menstrual cycle. Back-up contraception is not needed.

Previously taking a 21-day or 28-day combination hormonal contraceptive: Begin on day 1 of the withdrawal bleed (at the latest, 7 days after the last active tablet). Back-up contraception is not needed.

Previously using a progestin-only pill: Begin the day after taking a progestin only pill. Back-up contraception is needed for the first 7 days of therapy.

Previously using contraceptive implant: Begin the day of implant removal. Back-up contraception is needed for the first 7 days of therapy.

Previously using contraceptive injection: Begin when the next injection is due. Back-up contraception is needed for the first 7 days of therapy.

Missed doses:

One dose missed: Take as soon as remembered then take the next tablet at the regular time (2 tablets in 1 day). An additional nonhormonal method of contraception should also be used for 7 consecutive days.

Two consecutive doses missed: If remembered the day of the second missed tablet, take 2 tablets as soon as remembered, then 1 tablet the next day. If remembered the day after the second tablet is missed, take 2 tablets the day remembered, then 2 tablets the next day. An additional nonhormonal method of contraception should also be used for 7 consecutive days.

Three or more consecutive doses missed: Take 1 tablet daily and contact healthcare provider; do not take the missed pills. An additional nonhormonal method of contraception should also be used for 7 consecutive days.

Dosage adjustment in renal impairment: Specific guidelines not available; use with caution and monitor blood pressure closely. Consider other forms of contraception.

Dosage adjustment in hepatic impairment: Contraindicated in patients with hepatic impairment

Dietary Considerations Should be taken at the same time each day.

Administration Administer at the same time each day.

Quartette: If severe diarrhea or vomiting occur within 3-4 hours after taking a light pink, pink, or purple tablet, it should be considered a missed dose; additional contraceptive measures are recommended.

Hazardous agent; use appropriate precautions for handling and disposal (NIOSH, 2012)

Monitoring Parameters Before starting therapy, a physical exam with reference to the breasts and pelvis are recommended, including a Papanicolaou smear. Exam may be deferred if appropriate; pregnancy should be ruled out prior to use. Monitor patient closely for loss of vision, sudden onset of proptosis, diplopia, migraine; blood pressure; signs and symptoms of thromboembolic disorders; signs or symptoms of depression; glycemic control in patients with diabetes; lipid profiles in patients being treated for hyperlipidemias. Adequate diagnostic measures, including endometrial sampling, if indicated, should be performed to rule out malignancy in all cases of undiagnosed abnormal vaginal bleeding.

Dosage Forms Excipient information presented when available (limited, particularly for generics); consult specific product labeling. [DSC] = Discontinued product

Tablet, oral [low-dose formulation]: Ethinyl estradiol 0.02 mg and levonorgestrel 0.1 mg [21 tablets and 7 inactive tablets] (28s)

Aubra: Ethinyl estradiol 0.02 mg and levonorgestrel 0.1 mg [21 light yellow tablets and 7 brown inactive tablets] (28s)

Aviane: Ethinyl estradiol 0.02 mg and levonorgestrel 0.1 mg [21 orange tablets and 7 light green inactive tablets] (28s)

Falmina: Ethinyl estradiol 0.02 mg and levonorgestrel 0.1 mg [21 orange tablets and 7 white inactive tablets] (28s) [contains soya lecithin, tartrazine]

Lessina: Ethinyl estradiol 0.02 mg and levonorgestrel 0.1 mg [21 pink tablets and 7 white inactive tablets] (28s)

Lutera, Sronyx: Ethinyl estradiol 0.02 mg and levonorgestrel 0.1 mg [21 white tablets and 7 peach inactive tablets] (28s)

Orsythia: Ethinyl estradiol 0.02 mg and levonorgestrel 0.1 mg [21 pink tablets and 7 light green inactive tablets] (28s)

Tablet, oral [monophasic formulation]: Ethinyl estradiol 0.03 mg and levonorgestrel 0.15 mg [21 tablets and 7 inactive tablets] (28s)

Altavera: Ethinyl estradiol 0.03 mg and levonorgestrel 0.15 mg [21 peach tablets and 7 white inactive tablets] (28s)

Chateal: Ethinyl estradiol 0.03 mg and levonorgestrel 0.15 mg [21 white tablets and 7 green inactive tablets] (28s)

Kurvelo: Ethinyl estradiol 0.03 mg and levonorgestrel 0.15 mg [21 light orange tablets and 7 pink inactive tablets] (28s)

Levora: Ethinyl estradiol 0.03 mg and levonorgestrel 0.15 mg [21 white tablets and 7 peach inactive tablets] (28s)

Marlissa: Ethinyl estradiol 0.03 mg and levonorgestrel 0.15 mg [21 light orange tablets and 7 pink inactive tablets] (28s)

Nordette 28: Ethinyl estradiol 0.03 mg and levonorgestrel 0.15 mg [21 light orange tablets and 7 pink inactive tablets] (28s) [DSC]

Portia 28: Ethinyl estradiol 0.03 mg and levonorgestrel 0.15 mg [21 pink tablets and 7 white inactive tablets] (28s)

Tablet, oral [extended cycle regimen]: Ethinyl estradiol 0.02 mg and levonorgestrel 0.1 mg [84 tablets] and ethinyl estradiol 0.01 mg [7 tablets] (91s); Ethinyl estradiol 0.03 mg and levonorgestrel 0.15 mg [84 tablets and 7 inactive tablets] (91s)

Amethia: Ethinyl estradiol 0.03 mg and levonorgestrel 0.15 mg [84 white tablets] and ethinyl estradiol 0.01 mg [7 light blue tablets] (91s)

Amethia Lo: Ethinyl estradiol 0.02 mg and levonorgestrel 0.1 mg [84 white tablets] and ethinyl estradiol 0.01 mg [7 blue tablets] (91s)

camrese: Ethinyl estradiol 0.03 mg and levonorgestrel 0.15 mg [84 light blue-green tablets] and ethinyl estradiol 0.01 mg [7 yellow tablets] (91s)

Daysee: Ethinyl estradiol 0.03 mg and levonorgestrel 0.15 mg [84 light blue tablets] and ethinyl estradiol 0.01 mg [7 mustard tablets] (91s)

Introvale: Ethinyl estradiol 0.03 mg and levonorgestrel 0.15 mg [84 peach tablets and 7 white inactive tablets] (91s)

Jolessa: Ethinyl estradiol 0.03 mg and levonorgestrel 0.15 mg [84 pink tablets and 7 white inactive tablets] (91s)

LoSeasonique: Ethinyl estradiol 0.02 mg and levonorgestrel 0.1 mg [84 orange tablets] and ethinyl estradiol 0.01 mg [7 yellow tablets] (91s)

Quartette:

Day 1-42: Ethinyl estradiol 0.02 mg and levonorgestrel 0.15 mg [42 light pink tablets]

Day 43-63: Ethinyl estradiol 0.025 mg and levonorgestrel 0.15 mg [21 pink tablets]

Day 64-84: Ethinyl estradiol 0.03 mg and levonorgestrel 0.15 mg [21 purple tablets]

Day 85-91: Ethinyl estradiol 0.01 mg [7 yellow tablets] (91s)

Quasense: Ethinyl estradiol 0.03 mg and levonorgestrel 0.15 mg [84 white tablets and 7 peach inactive tablets] (91s)

Seasonique: Ethinyl estradiol 0.03 mg and levonorgestrel 0.15 mg [84 light blue-green tablets] and ethinyl estradiol 0.01 mg [7 yellow tablets] (91s)

Tablet, oral [noncyclic regimen]:

Amethyst: Ethinyl estradiol 0.02 mg and levonorgestrel 0.09 mg [28 white tablets] (28s)

Lybrel: Ethinyl estradiol 0.02 mg and levonorgestrel 0.09 mg [28 yellow tablets] (28s)

Tablet, oral [triphasic formulation]:
Enpresse:
Day 1-6: Ethinyl estradiol 0.03 mg and levonorgestrel 0.05 mg [6 pink tablets]
Day 7-11: Ethinyl estradiol 0.04 mg and levonorgestrel 0.075 mg [5 white tablets]
Day 12-21: Ethinyl estradiol 0.03 mg and levonorgestrel 0.125 mg [10 orange tablets]
Day 22-28: 7 light green inactive tablets (28s)
Levonest:
Day 1-6: Ethinyl estradiol 0.03 mg and levonorgestrel 0.05 mg [6 yellow tablets]
Day 7-11: Ethinyl estradiol 0.04 mg and levonorgestrel 0.075 mg [5 green tablets]
Day 12-21: Ethinyl estradiol 0.03 mg and levonorgestrel 0.125 mg [10 light brown tablets]
Day 22-28: 7 white inactive tablets (28s)
Myzilra
Day 1-6: Ethinyl estradiol 0.03 mg and levonorgestrel 0.05 mg [6 beige tablets]
Day 7-11: Ethinyl estradiol 0.04 mg and levonorgestrel 0.075 mg [5 white tablets]
Day 12-21: Ethinyl estradiol 0.03 mg and levonorgestrel 0.125 mg [10 light yellow tablets]
Day 22-28: 7 light green inactive tablets (28s)
Trivora:
Day 1-6: Ethinyl estradiol 0.03 mg and levonorgestrel 0.05 mg [6 blue tablets]
Day 7-11: Ethinyl estradiol 0.04 mg and levonorgestrel 0.075 mg [5 white tablets]
Day 12-21: Ethinyl estradiol 0.03 mg and levonorgestrel 0.125 mg [10 pink tablets]
Day 22-28: 7 peach inactive tablets (28s)

◆ **Ethinyl Estradiol and NGM** *see* Ethinyl Estradiol and Norgestimate *on page 795*

Ethinyl Estradiol and Norelgestromin

(ETH in il es tra DYE ole & nor el JES troe min)

Brand Names: U.S. Ortho Evra®

Brand Names: Canada Evra®

Index Terms Norelgestromin and Ethinyl Estradiol; Ortho-Evra

Pharmacologic Category Contraceptive; Estrogen and Progestin Combination

Use Prevention of pregnancy

Pregnancy Risk Factor X

Dosage Topical: Adults: Females:

Contraception: Apply one patch each week for 3 weeks (21 total days); followed by one week that is patch-free. Each patch should be applied on the same day each week ("patch change day") and only one patch should be worn at a time. No more than 7 days should pass during the patch-free interval.

Schedule 1 (Sunday starter): Dose begins on first Sunday after onset of menstruation; if the menstrual period starts on Sunday, apply one patch that very same day. **With a Sunday start, an additional method of contraception (nonhormonal) must be used until after the first 7 days of consecutive administration.** Each patch change will then occur on Sunday.

Schedule 2 (Day 1 starter): Dose starts on first day of menstrual cycle, applying one patch during the first 24 hours of menstrual cycle. No back-up method of contraception is needed as long as the patch is applied on the first day of cycle. Each patch change will then occur on that same day of the week.

Additional dosing considerations:

No bleeding during patch-free week/missed menstrual period: If patch has been applied as directed, continue treatment on usual "patch change day". If used correctly, no bleeding during patch-free week does not necessarily indicate pregnancy. However, if no withdrawal bleeding occurs for 2 consecutive cycles, pregnancy should be ruled out. If patch has not been applied as directed, and one menstrual period is missed, pregnancy should be ruled out prior to continuing treatment.

If a patch becomes partially or completely detached for <24 hours: Try to reapply to same place, or replace with a new patch immediately. Do not reapply if patch is no longer sticky, if it is sticking to itself or another surface, or if it has material sticking to it.

If a patch becomes partially or completely detached for >24 hours (or time period is unknown): Apply a new patch and use this day of the week as the new "patch change day" from this point on. **An additional method of contraception (nonhormonal) must be used until after the first 7 days of consecutive administration.**

Switching from oral contraceptives or vaginal ring: Complete current cycle and apply the first patch on the day the next pill cycle would be started or ring would be inserted. If there is no menstrual bleeding within 7 days of taking the last active tablet, the patient can initiate the first patch application; however, pregnancy must be ruled out. If patch is applied later than 7 days after the last active pill or removal of the vaginal ring, **an additional method of contraception (nonhormonal) should be used until after the first 7 days of consecutive administration**

Use after childbirth: Therapy should not be started <4 weeks after childbirth. Pregnancy should be ruled out prior to treatment if menstrual periods have not restarted. **An additional method of contraception (nonhormonal) should be used until after the first 7 days of consecutive administration.**

Use after abortion or miscarriage: Therapy may be started immediately if abortion/miscarriage occurs within the first trimester. If therapy is not started within 5 days, follow instructions for first time use. An additional method of contraception (nonhormonal) should be used until after the first 7 days of consecutive administration. If abortion/miscarriage occurs during the second trimester, therapy should not be started for at least 4 weeks. Follow directions for use after childbirth.

Dosage adjustment in renal impairment: Specific guidelines not available; use with caution and monitor blood pressure closely. Consider other forms of contraception.

Dosage adjustment in hepatic impairment: Contraindicated in patients with hepatic impairment

Additional Information Complete prescribing information should be consulted for additional detail.

Dosage Forms Excipient information presented when available (limited, particularly for generics); consult specific product labeling.

Patch, transdermal:
Ortho Evra®: Ethinyl estradiol 0.75 mg and norelgestromin 6 mg [releases ethinyl estradiol 20 mcg and norelgestromin 150 mcg per day] (1s, 3s)

Dosage Forms: Canada Excipient information presented when available (limited, particularly for generics); consult specific product labeling.

Patch, transdermal:
Evra®: Ethinyl estradiol 0.6 mg and norelgestromin 6 mg [releases ethinyl estradiol 35 mcg and norelgestromin 200 mcg per day] (1s, 3s)

Ethinyl Estradiol and Norethindrone

(ETH in il es tra DYE ole & nor eth IN drone)

Brand Names: U.S. Alyacen 1/35; Alyacen 7/7/7; Aranelle; Balziva; Brevicon; Briellyn; Cyclafem 1/35; Cyclafem 7/7/7; Dasetta 1/35; Dasetta 7/7/7; Estrostep Fe; Femcon Fe; femhrt; Generess Fe; Gildess FE 1.5/30; Gildess FE 1/20; Jinteli; Junel 1.5/30; Junel 1/20; Junel Fe 1.5/30; Junel Fe 1/20; Larin Fe 1.5/30; Larin Fe 1/20; Leena; Lo Loestrin Fe; Lo Minastrin Fe; Loestrin 21 1.5/30; Loestrin 21 1/20; Loestrin 24 Fe; Loestrin Fe 1.5/30; Loestrin Fe 1/20; Lomedia 24 Fe; Microgestin 1.5/30; Microgestin 1/20; Microgestin Fe 1.5/30; Microgestin Fe 1/20; Minastrin 24 Fe; Modicon; Necon 0.5/35; Necon 1/35; Necon 10/11; Necon 7/7/7; Norinyl 1+35; Nortrel 0.5/35; Nortrel 1/35; Nortrel 7/7/7; Ortho-Novum 1/35; Ortho-Novum 7/7/7; Ovcon 35; Philith; Pirmella 1/35; Tilia Fe; Tri-Legest Fe; Tri-Norinyl; Wera; Wymzya Fe; Zenchent; Zenchent Fe

Brand Names: Canada Brevicon 0.5/35; Brevicon 1/35; FemHRT; Loestrin 1.5/30; Minestrin 1/20; Ortho 0.5/35; Ortho 1/35; Ortho 7/7/7; Select 1/35; Synphasic

Index Terms Norethindrone Acetate and Ethinyl Estradiol; Ortho Novum

Pharmacologic Category Contraceptive; Estrogen and Progestin Combination

Use

Acne vulgaris: For the treatment of moderate acne vulgaris in females at least 15 years of age.

Limitations of Use: When used for acne, use only in females ≥15 years of age who have achieved menarche, who also desire combination hormonal contraceptive therapy, are unresponsive to topical treatments, have no contraindications to combination hormonal contraceptive use, and plan to stay on therapy for ≥6 months.

Contraception: For the prevention of pregnancy.

Moderate to severe vasomotor symptoms: Treatment of moderate to severe vasomotor symptoms associated with menopause.

Osteoporosis prevention: For prevention of postmenopausal osteoporosis.

Limitations of use: For use only in women at significant risk of osteoporosis and for whom other nonestrogen medications are not considered appropriate.

Unlabeled Use Treatment of heavy (excessive) menstrual bleeding (menorrhagia); dysmenorrhea; abnormal uterine bleeding

Pregnancy Risk Factor X

Dosage Oral:

Adolescents ≥15 years and Adults: Females: Acne: Estrostep Fe: Refer to dosing for contraception

Adults: Females:

Moderate-to-severe vasomotor symptoms associated with menopause: Initial: femhrt 0.5/2.5: 1 tablet daily; patient should be re-evaluated at 3- to 6-month intervals to determine if treatment is still necessary; patient should be maintained at the lowest effective dose

Prevention of osteoporosis: Initial: femhrt 0.5/2.5: 1 tablet daily; patient should be maintained on the lowest effective dose

Contraception:

Schedule 1 (Sunday starter): Dose begins on first Sunday after onset of menstruation; if the menstrual period starts on Sunday, take first tablet that very same day. (This schedule is not preferred for all products [eg, Generess Fe, Lo Loestrin Fe, Lo Minastrin Fe]). With a Sunday start, an additional method of contraception should be used until after the first 7 days of consecutive administration (all products).

For 21-tablet package: Dosage is 1 tablet daily for 21 consecutive days, followed by 7 days off of the medication; a new course begins on the 8th day after the last tablet is taken.

For 28-tablet package: Dosage is 1 tablet daily without interruption.

Schedule 2 (Day 1 starter): Dose starts on first day of menstrual cycle taking 1 tablet daily.

For 21-tablet package: Dosage is 1 tablet daily for 21 consecutive days, followed by 7 days off of the medication; a new course begins on the 8th day after the last tablet is taken.

For 28-tablet package: Dosage is 1 tablet daily without interruption.

If all doses have not been taken on schedule and one menstrual period is missed, the possibility of pregnancy should be considered. If two consecutive menstrual periods are missed, pregnancy test is required before new dosing cycle is started.

Missed doses **monophasic formulations** (refer to package insert for complete information):

One dose missed: Take as soon as remembered. Take the next tablet at your regular time. You may take 2 tablets in 1 day.

Two consecutive doses missed in the first 2 weeks: Take 2 tablets as soon as remembered and 2 tablets the next day. An additional method of contraception should be used for 7 days after missed dose.

Two consecutive doses missed in week 3 (all products) or in week 4 (some products), or three consecutive doses missed at any time (all products): An additional method of contraception must be used for 7 days after a missed dose.

Schedule 1 (Sunday starter): Continue dose of 1 tablet daily until Sunday, then discard the rest of the pack, and a new pack should be started that same day.

Schedule 2 (Day 1 starter): Current pack should be discarded, and a new pack should be started that same day.

Missed doses **biphasic/triphasic formulations** (refer to package insert for complete information):

One dose missed: Take the next tablet at your regular time. You may take 2 tablets in 1 day.

Two consecutive doses missed in week 1 or week 2 of the pack: Take 2 tablets as soon as remembered and 2 tablets the next day. Resume taking 1 tablet daily until the pack is empty. An additional method of contraception should be used for 7 days after a missed dose.

Two consecutive doses missed in week 3 of the pack: An additional method of contraception must be used for 7 days after a missed dose.

Schedule 1 (Sunday Starter): Take 1 tablet every day until Sunday. Discard the remaining pack and start a new pack of pills on the same day.

Schedule 2 (Day 1 starter): Discard the remaining pack and start a new pack the same day.

Three or more consecutive doses missed: An additional method of contraception must be used for 7 days after a missed dose.

Schedule 1 (Sunday Starter): Take 1 tablet every day until Sunday; on Sunday, discard the pack and start a new pack.

Schedule 2 (Day 1 Starter): Discard the remaining pack and begin new pack of tablets starting on the same day.

Switching from a different contraceptive:

Oral contraceptive: Start on the same day that a new pack of the previous oral contraceptive would have been taken.

Transdermal patch, vaginal ring, injection: Start on the day the next dose would have been due.

IUD or implant: Start on the day of removal. A backup method of contraception may be required following IUD removal.

Use after childbirth (in women who are not breast-feeding) or after second trimester abortion: Therapy may be started ≥4 weeks postpartum. Pregnancy should be ruled out prior to treatment if menstrual periods have not restarted and an additional method of contraception (nonhormonal) should be used until after the first 7 days of consecutive administration.

Dosage adjustment in renal impairment: No dosage adjustment provided in manufacturer's labeling; use with caution and monitor blood pressure closely. Consider other forms of contraception.

Dosage adjustment in hepatic impairment: Contraindicated in patients with hepatic impairment.

Additional Information Complete prescribing information should be consulted for additional detail.

Dosage Forms Excipient information presented when available (limited, particularly for generics); consult specific product labeling. [DSC] = Discontinued product

Tablet, oral:

femhrt 0.5/2.5: Ethinyl estradiol 0.0025 mg and norethindrone acetate 0.5 mg [white tablets] (28s)

Jinteli: Ethinyl estradiol 0.005 mg and norethindrone acetate 1 mg [white tablets] (28s, 90s)

Tablet, oral [monophasic formulation]:

Alyacen 1/35: Ethinyl estradiol 0.035 mg and norethindrone 1 mg [21 peach tablets and 7 light green inactive tablets] (28s)

Balziva: Ethinyl estradiol 0.035 mg and norethindrone 0.4 mg [21 light peach tablets and 7 white inactive tablets] (28s)

Brevicon: Ethinyl estradiol 0.035 mg and norethindrone 0.5 mg [21 blue tablets and 7 orange inactive tablets] (28s)

Briellyn: Ethinyl estradiol 0.035 mg and norethindrone 0.4 mg [21 light peach tablets and 7 white-off-white inactive tablets] (28s)

Cyclafem 1/35: Ethinyl estradiol 0.035 mg and norethindrone 1 mg [21 pink tablets and 7 light green inactive tablets] (28s)

Dasetta 1/35: Ethinyl estradiol 0.035 mg and norethindrone 1 mg [21 orange tablets and 7 white inactive tablets] (28s) [contains soya lecithin, tartrazine]

Gildess FE 1/20: Ethinyl estradiol 0.02 mg and norethindrone acetate 1 mg [21 white tablets] and ferrous fumarate 75 mg [7 white-speckled brown tablets] (28s)

Gildess FE 1.5/30: Ethinyl estradiol 0.03 mg and norethindrone acetate 1.5 mg [21 light green tablets] and ferrous fumarate 75 mg [7 white-speckled brown tablets] (28s)

Junel 1/20: Ethinyl estradiol 0.02 mg and norethindrone acetate 1 mg [yellow tablets] (21s)

Junel 1.5/30: Ethinyl estradiol 0.03 mg and norethindrone acetate 1.5 mg [pink tablets] (21s)

Junel Fe 1/20: Ethinyl estradiol 0.02 mg and norethindrone acetate 1 mg [21 yellow tablets] and ferrous fumarate 75 mg [7 brown tablets] (28s)

Junel Fe 1.5/30: Ethinyl estradiol 0.03 mg and norethindrone acetate 1.5 mg [21 pink tablets] and ferrous fumarate 75 mg [7 brown tablets] (28s)

Larin Fe 1/20: Ethinyl estradiol 0.02 mg and norethindrone acetate 1 mg [21 pale yellow tablets] and ferrous fumarate 75 mg [7 brown tablets] (28s) [contains soya lecithin]

Larin Fe 1.5/30: Ethinyl estradiol 0.03 mg and norethindrone acetate 1.5 mg [21 green tablets] and ferrous fumarate 75 mg [7 brown tablets] (28s) [contains soya lecithin]

Loestrin 21 1/20: Ethinyl estradiol 0.02 mg and norethindrone acetate 1 mg [light yellow tablets] (21s)

Loestrin 21 1.5/30: Ethinyl estradiol 0.03 mg and norethindrone acetate 1.5 mg [pink tablets] (21s)

Loestrin 24 Fe: Ethinyl estradiol 0.02 mg and norethindrone acetate 1 mg [24 white tablets] and ferrous fumarate 75 mg [4 brown tablets] (28s)

Loestrin Fe 1/20: Ethinyl estradiol 0.02 mg and norethindrone acetate 1 mg [21 light yellow tablets] and ferrous fumarate 75 mg [7 brown tablets] (28s)

Loestrin Fe 1.5/30: Ethinyl estradiol 0.03 mg and norethindrone acetate 1.5 mg [21 pink tablets] and ferrous fumarate 75 mg [7 brown tablets] (28s)

Lomedia 24 Fe: Ethinyl estradiol 0.02 mg and norethindrone acetate 1 mg [24 white tablets] and ferrous fumarate 75 mg [4 brown tablets] (28s)

Microgestin 1/20: Ethinyl estradiol 0.02 mg and norethindrone acetate 1 mg [white tablets] (21s)

Microgestin 1.5/30: Ethinyl estradiol 0.03 mg and norethindrone acetate 1.5 mg [green tablets] (21s)

Microgestin Fe 1/20: Ethinyl estradiol 0.02 mg and norethindrone acetate 1 mg [21 white tablets] and ferrous fumarate 75 mg [7 brown tablets] (28s)

Microgestin Fe 1.5/30: Ethinyl estradiol 0.03 mg and norethindrone acetate 1.5 mg [21 green tablets] and ferrous fumarate 75 mg [7 brown tablets] (28s)

Modicon: Ethinyl estradiol 0.035 mg and norethindrone 0.5 mg [21 white tablets and 7 green inactive tablets] (28s)

Necon 0.5/35: Ethinyl estradiol 0.035 mg and norethindrone 0.5 mg [21 light yellow tablets and 7 white inactive tablets] (28s)

Necon 1/35: Ethinyl estradiol 0.035 mg and norethindrone 1 mg [21 dark yellow tablets and 7 white inactive tablets] (28s)

Norinyl 1+35: Ethinyl estradiol 0.035 mg and norethindrone 1 mg [21 yellow-green tablets and 7 orange inactive tablets] (28s)

Nortrel 0.5/35: Ethinyl estradiol 0.035 mg and norethindrone 0.5 mg [21 light yellow tablets and 7 white inactive tablets] (28s)

Nortrel 1/35:

Ethinyl estradiol 0.035 mg and norethindrone 1 mg [yellow tablets] (21s)

Ethinyl estradiol 0.035 mg and norethindrone 1 mg [21 yellow tablets and 7 white inactive tablets] (28s)

Ortho-Novum 1/35: Ethinyl estradiol 0.035 mg and norethindrone 1 mg [21 peach tablets and 7 green inactive tablets] (28s)

Ovcon 35: Ethinyl estradiol 0.035 mg and norethindrone 0.4 mg [21 light peach tablets and 7 green inactive tablets] (28s)

Philith: Ethinyl estradiol 0.035 mg and norethindrone 0.4 mg [21 tan tablets and 7 white inactive tablets] (28s)

Pirmella 1/35: Ethinyl estradiol 0.035 mg and norethindrone 1 mg [21 peach tablets and 7 green inactive tablets] (28s)

Wera: Ethinyl estradiol 0.035 mg and norethindrone 0.5 mg [21 light peach tablets and 7 white inactive tablets] (28s)

Zenchent: Ethinyl estradiol 0.035 mg and norethindrone 0.4 mg [21 orange tablets and 7 white inactive tablets] (28s)

Tablet, chewable, oral [monophasic formulation]: Ethinyl estradiol 0.035 mg and norethindrone 0.4 mg [21 tablets] and ferrous fumarate 75 mg [7 tablets] (28s)

Femcon Fe: Ethinyl estradiol 0.035 mg and norethindrone 0.4 mg [21 white tablets] and ferrous fumarate 75 mg [7 brown tablets] [spearmint flavor] (28s)

Generess Fe: Ethinyl estradiol 0.025 mg and norethindrone 0.8 mg [24 light green tablets] and ferrous fumarate 75 mg [4 brown tablets] (28s)

Minastrin 24 Fe: Ethinyl estradiol 0.02 mg and norethindrone 1 mg [24 white tablets] and ferrous fumarate 75 mg [4 brown tablets] [spearmint flavor] (28s)

Wymzya Fe: Ethinyl estradiol 0.035 mg and norethindrone 0.4 mg [21 white tablets] and ferrous fumarate 75 mg [7 brown tablets] (28s)

Zenchent Fe: Ethinyl estradiol 0.035 mg and norethindrone 0.4 mg [21 light yellow tablets] and ferrous fumarate 75 mg [7 brown tablets] [spearmint flavor] (28s)

Tablet, oral [biphasic formulation]:

Lo Loestrin Fe:

Day 1-24: Ethinyl estradiol 0.01 mg and norethindrone acetate 1 mg [24 blue tablets]

Day 25-26: Ethinyl estradiol 0.01 mg [2 white tablets]

Day 27-28: Ferrous fumarate 75 mg [2 brown tablets] (28s)

Lo Minastrin Fe:

Day 1-24: Ethinyl estradiol 0.01 mg and norethindrone acetate 1 mg [24 blue chewable tablets]

Day 25-26: Ethinyl estradiol 0.01 mg [2 white tablets]

Day 27-28: Ferrous fumarate 75 mg [2 brown tablets] (28s)

Necon 10/11:

Day 1-10: Ethinyl estradiol 0.035 mg and norethindrone 0.5 mg [10 light yellow tablets]

Day 11-21: Ethinyl estradiol 0.035 mg and norethindrone 1 mg [11 dark yellow tablets]

Day 22-28: 7 white inactive tablets (28s)

Tablet, oral [triphasic formulation]:

Alyacen 7/7/7:

Day 1-7: Ethinyl estradiol 0.035 mg and norethindrone 0.5 mg [7 white-off-white tablets]

Day 8-14: Ethinyl estradiol 0.035 mg and norethindrone 0.75 mg [7 light peach tablets]

Day 15-21: Ethinyl estradiol 0.035 mg and norethindrone 1 mg [7 peach tablets]

Day 22-28: 7 light green inactive tablets (28s)

Aranelle:

Day 1-7: Ethinyl estradiol 0.035 mg and norethindrone 0.5 mg [7 light yellow tablets]

Day 8-16: Ethinyl estradiol 0.035 mg and norethindrone 1 mg [9 white tablets]

Day 17-21: Ethinyl estradiol 0.035 mg and norethindrone 0.5 mg [5 light yellow tablets]

Day 22-28: 7 peach inactive tablets (28s)

Cyclafem 7/7/7:

Day 1-7: Ethinyl estradiol 0.035 mg and norethindrone 0.5 mg [7 white tablets]

Day 8-14: Ethinyl estradiol 0.035 mg and norethindrone 0.75 mg [7 light pink tablets]

Day 15-21: Ethinyl estradiol 0.035 mg and norethindrone 1 mg [7 pink tablets]

Day 22-28: 7 light green inactive tablets (28s)

Dasetta 7/7/7:

Day 1-7: Ethinyl estradiol 0.035 mg and norethindrone 0.5 mg [7 light peach tablets]

Day 8-14: Ethinyl estradiol 0.035 mg and norethindrone 0.75 mg [7 peach tablets]

Day 15-21: Ethinyl estradiol 0.035 mg and norethindrone 1 mg [7 orange tablets]

Day 22-28: 7 white inactive tablets (28s)

Estrostep Fe:

Day 1-5: Ethinyl estradiol 0.02 mg and norethindrone acetate 1 mg [5 white triangular tablets]

Day 6-12: Ethinyl estradiol 0.03 mg and norethindrone acetate 1 mg [7 white square tablets]

Day 13-21: Ethinyl estradiol 0.035 mg and norethindrone acetate 1 mg [9 white round tablets]

Day 22-28: Ferrous fumarate 75 mg [7 brown tablets] (28s)

Leena:

Day 1-7: Ethinyl estradiol 0.035 mg and norethindrone 0.5 mg [7 light blue tablets]

Day 8-16: Ethinyl estradiol 0.035 mg and norethindrone 1 mg [9 light yellow-green tablets]

Day 17-21: Ethinyl estradiol 0.035 mg and norethindrone 0.5 mg [5 light blue tablets]

Day 22-28: 7 orange inactive tablets (28s)

Necon 7/7/7, Ortho-Novum 7/7/7:

Day 1-7: Ethinyl estradiol 0.035 mg and norethindrone 0.5 mg [7 white tablets]

Day 8-14: Ethinyl estradiol 0.035 mg and norethindrone 0.75 mg [7 light peach tablets]

Day 15-21: Ethinyl estradiol 0.035 mg and norethindrone 1 mg [7 peach tablets]

Day 22-28: 7 green inactive tablets (28s)

Nortrel 7/7/7:

Day 1-7: Ethinyl estradiol 0.035 mg and norethindrone 0.5 mg [7 light yellow tablets]

Day 8-14: Ethinyl estradiol 0.035 mg and norethindrone 0.75 mg [7 blue tablets]

Day 15-21: Ethinyl estradiol 0.035 mg and norethindrone 1 mg [7 peach tablets]

Day 22-28: 7 white inactive tablets (28s)

Tilia Fe:

Day 1-5: Ethinyl estradiol 0.02 mg and norethindrone acetate 1 mg [5 white triangular tablets]

Day 6-12: Ethinyl estradiol 0.03 mg and norethindrone acetate 1 mg [7 white square tablets]

Day 13-21: Ethinyl estradiol 0.035 mg and norethindrone acetate 1 mg [9 white round tablets]

Day 22-28: Ferrous fumarate 75 mg [7 brown tablets] (28s)

Tri-Legest Fe:

Day 1-5: Ethinyl estradiol 0.02 mg and norethindrone acetate 1 mg [5 light pink tablets]

Day 6-12: Ethinyl estradiol 0.03 mg and norethindrone acetate 1 mg [7 light yellow tablets]

Day 13-21: Ethinyl estradiol 0.035 mg and norethindrone acetate 1 mg [9 light blue tablets]

Day 22-28: Ferrous fumarate 75 mg [7 brown tablets] (28s)

Tri-Norinyl:

Day 1-7: Ethinyl estradiol 0.035 mg and norethindrone 0.5 mg [7 blue tablets]

Day 8-16: Ethinyl estradiol 0.035 mg and norethindrone 1 mg [9 yellow-green tablets]

Day 17-21: Ethinyl estradiol 0.035 mg and norethindrone 0.5 mg [5 blue tablets]

Day 22-28: 7 orange inactive tablets (28s)

Ethinyl Estradiol and Norgestimate

(ETH in il es tra DYE ole & nor JES ti mate)

Brand Names: U.S. Estarylla; MonoNessa; Ortho Tri-Cyclen; Ortho Tri-Cyclen Lo; Ortho-Cyclen; Previfem; Sprintec; Tri-Estarylla; Tri-Previfem; Tri-Sprintec; TriNessa

Brand Names: Canada Cyclen; Tri-Cyclen; Tri-Cyclen Lo

Index Terms Ethinyl Estradiol and NGM; Norgestimate and Ethinyl Estradiol; Ortho Cyclen; Ortho Tri Cyclen

Pharmacologic Category Contraceptive; Estrogen and Progestin Combination

Use

Acne vulgaris: For the treatment of moderate acne vulgaris in females at least 15 years of age

Limitations of use: When used for acne, use only in females ≥15 years of age who achieved menarche, who also desire combination hormonal contraceptive therapy, are unresponsive to topical treatments, have no contraindications to combination hormonal contraceptive use, and plan to stay on therapy for ≥6 months

Contraception: For the prevention of pregnancy.

Unlabeled Use Treatment of heavy (excessive) menstrual bleeding (menorrhagia); dysmenorrhea; abnormal uterine bleeding

Pregnancy Risk Factor X

Dosage Oral:

Children ≥15 years and Adults: Females: Acne (Ortho Tri-Cyclen): Refer to dosing for contraception

Adults: Females:

Contraception:

Schedule 1 (Sunday starter): Dose begins on first Sunday after onset of menstruation; if the menstrual period starts on Sunday, take first tablet that very same day. **With a Sunday start, an additional method of contraception should be used until after the first 7 days of consecutive administration.**

For 21-tablet package: Dosage is 1 tablet daily for 21 consecutive days, followed by 7 days off of the medication; a new course begins on the 8th day after the last tablet is taken.

For 28-tablet package: Dosage is 1 tablet daily without interruption.

Schedule 2 (Day 1 starter): Dose starts on first day of menstrual cycle taking 1 tablet daily.

For 21-tablet package: Dosage is 1 tablet daily for 21 consecutive days, followed by 7 days off of the medication; a new course begins on the 8th day after the last tablet is taken.

For 28-tablet package: Dosage is 1 tablet daily without interruption.

If all doses have not been taken on schedule and one menstrual period is missed, the possibility of pregnancy should be considered. If two consecutive menstrual periods are missed, pregnancy test is required before new dosing cycle is started.

Missed doses **monophasic formulations** (refer to package insert for complete information):

One dose missed: Take as soon as remembered or take 2 tablets next day

Two consecutive doses missed in the first 2 weeks: Take 2 tablets as soon as remembered or 2 tablets next 2 days. **An additional method of contraception should be used for 7 days after missed dose.**

Two consecutive doses missed in week 3 or three consecutive doses missed at any time: **An additional method of contraception must be used for 7 days after a missed dose:**

Schedule 1 (Sunday starter): Continue dose of 1 tablet daily until Sunday, then discard the rest of the pack, and a new pack should be started that same day.

Schedule 2 (Day 1 starter): Current pack should be discarded, and a new pack should be started that same day.

Missed doses **biphasic/triphasic formulations** (refer to package insert for complete information):

One dose missed: Take as soon as remembered.

Two consecutive doses missed in week 1 or week 2 of the pack: Take 2 tablets as soon as remembered and 2 tablets the next day. Resume taking 1 tablet daily until the pack is empty. **An additional method of contraception must be used for 7 days after a missed dose.**

Two consecutive doses missed in week 3 of the pack. **An additional method of contraception must be used for 7 days after a missed dose.**

Schedule 1 (Sunday starter): Take 1 tablet every day until Sunday. Discard the remaining pack and start a new pack of pills on the same day.

Schedule 2 (Day 1 starter): Discard the remaining pack and start a new pack the same day.

Three or more consecutive doses missed. **An additional method of contraception must be used for 7 days after a missed dose.**

Schedule 1 (Sunday starter): Take 1 tablet every day until Sunday; on Sunday, discard the pack and start a new pack.

Schedule 2 (Day 1 starter): Discard the remaining pack and begin new pack of tablets starting on the same day.

Dosage adjustment in renal impairment: No dosage adjustment provided in manufacturer's labeling (has not been studied); use with caution and monitor blood pressure closely. Consider other forms of contraception.

Dosage adjustment in hepatic impairment: Contraindicated in patients with hepatic impairment.

Additional Information Complete prescribing information should be consulted for additional detail.

Dosage Forms Excipient information presented when available (limited, particularly for generics); consult specific product labeling.

Tablet, oral [monophasic formulation]:

Estarylla: Ethinyl estradiol 0.035 mg and norgestimate 0.25 mg [21 blue tablets and 7 green inactive tablets] (28s)

MonoNessa, Ortho-Cyclen: Ethinyl estradiol 0.035 mg and norgestimate 0.25 mg [21 blue tablets and 7 dark green inactive tablets] (28s)

Previfem: Ethinyl estradiol 0.035 mg and norgestimate 0.25 mg [21 blue tablets and 7 light green inactive tablets] (28s)

Sprintec: Ethinyl estradiol 0.035 mg and norgestimate 0.25 mg [21 blue tablets and 7 white inactive tablets] (28s)

Tablet, oral [triphasic formulation]:

Ortho Tri-Cyclen, TriNessa:

Day 1-7: Ethinyl estradiol 0.035 mg and norgestimate 0.18 mg [7 white tablets]

Day 8-14: Ethinyl estradiol 0.035 mg and norgestimate 0.215 mg [7 light blue tablets]

Day 15-21: Ethinyl estradiol 0.035 mg and norgestimate 0.25 mg [7 blue tablets]

Day 22-28: 7 dark green inactive tablets (28s)

Tri-Estarylla

Day 1-7: Ethinyl estradiol 0.035 mg and norgestimate 0.18 mg [7 white tablets]

Day 8-14: Ethinyl estradiol 0.035 mg and norgestimate 0.215 mg [7 light blue tablets]

Day 15-21: Ethinyl estradiol 0.035 mg and norgestimate 0.25 mg [7 blue tablets]

Day 22-28: 7 green inactive tablets (28s)

Tri-Previfem:

Day 1-7: Ethinyl estradiol 0.035 mg and norgestimate 0.18 mg [7 white tablets]

Day 8-14: Ethinyl estradiol 0.035 mg and norgestimate 0.215 mg [7 light blue tablets]

Day 15-21: Ethinyl estradiol 0.035 mg and norgestimate 0.25 mg [7 blue tablets]

Day 22-28: 7 light green inactive tablets (28s)

Tri-Sprintec:

Day 1-7: Ethinyl estradiol 0.035 mg and norgestimate 0.18 mg [7 gray tablets]

Day 8-14: Ethinyl estradiol 0.035 mg and norgestimate 0.215 mg [7 light blue tablets]

Day 15-21: Ethinyl estradiol 0.035 mg and norgestimate 0.25 mg [7 blue tablets]

Day 22-28: 7 white inactive tablets (28s)

Ortho Tri-Cyclen Lo:

Day 1-7: Ethinyl estradiol 0.025 mg and norgestimate 0.18 mg [7 white tablets]

Day 8-14: Ethinyl estradiol 0.025 mg and norgestimate 0.215 mg [7 light blue tablets]

Day 15-21: Ethinyl estradiol 0.025 mg and norgestimate 0.25 mg [7 dark blue tablets]

Day 22-28: 7 dark green inactive tablets (28s)

Ethinyl Estradiol and Norgestrel

(ETH in il es tra DYE ole & nor JES trel)

Brand Names: U.S. Cryselle 28; Low-Ogestrel; Ogestrel
Brand Names: Canada Lo-Femenal 21; Ovral®
Index Terms Lo Ovral; Morning After Pill; Norgestrel and Ethinyl Estradiol
Pharmacologic Category Contraceptive; Estrogen and Progestin Combination
Use Prevention of pregnancy; postcoital contraceptive or "morning after" pill
Unlabeled Use Treatment of hypermenorrhea (menorrhagia); pain associated with endometriosis; dysmenorrhea; dysfunctional uterine bleeding
Pregnancy Risk Factor X
Dosage Oral: Adults: Females:

Contraception:

Schedule 1 (Sunday starter): Dose begins on first Sunday after onset of menstruation; if the menstrual period starts on Sunday, take first tablet that very same day. **With a Sunday start, an additional method of contraception should be used until after the first 7 days of consecutive administration.**

For 21-tablet package: Dosage is 1 tablet daily for 21 consecutive days, followed by 7 days off of the medication; a new course begins on the 8th day after the last tablet is taken.

For 28-tablet package: Dosage is 1 tablet daily without interruption.

Schedule 2 (Day 1 starter): Dose starts on first day of menstrual cycle taking 1 tablet daily.

For 21-tablet package: Dosage is 1 tablet daily for 21 consecutive days, followed by 7 days off of the medication; a new course begins on the 8th day after the last tablet is taken.

For 28-tablet package: Dosage is 1 tablet daily without interruption.

If all doses have been taken on schedule and one menstrual period is missed, continue dosing cycle. If two consecutive menstrual periods are missed, pregnancy test is required before new dosing cycle is started.

Missed doses **monophasic formulations** (refer to package insert for complete information):

One dose missed: Take as soon as remembered or take 2 tablets next day

Two consecutive doses missed in the first 2 weeks: Take 2 tablets as soon as remembered or 2 tablets next 2 days. **An additional method of contraception should be used for 7 days after missed dose.**

Two consecutive doses missed in week 3 or three consecutive doses missed at any time:

Schedule 1 (Sunday starter): Continue to take 1 tablet daily until Sunday, then discard the rest of the pack, and a new pack is started that same day.

Schedule 2 (Day 1 starter): Current pack should be discarded, and a new pack started that same day. **An additional method of contraception should be used for 7 days after missed dose.**

Postcoital contraception:

Ethinyl estradiol 0.03 mg and norgestrel 0.3 mg formulation: 4 tablets within 72 hours of unprotected intercourse and 4 tablets 12 hours after first dose

Ethinyl estradiol 0.05 mg and norgestrel 0.5 mg formulation: 2 tablets within 72 hours of unprotected intercourse and 2 tablets 12 hours after first dose

Dosage adjustment in renal impairment: Specific guidelines not available; use with caution and monitor blood pressure closely. Consider other forms of contraception.
Dosage adjustment in hepatic impairment: Contraindicated in patients with hepatic impairment.

Additional Information Complete prescribing information should be consulted for additional detail.
Dosage Forms Excipient information presented when available (limited, particularly for generics); consult specific product labeling.

Tablet, oral [monophasic formulation]: Ethinyl estradiol 0.03 mg and norgestrel 0.3 mg [21 tablets and 7 inactive tablets] (28s)

Cryselle 28: Ethinyl estradiol 0.03 mg and norgestrel 0.3 mg [21 white tablets and 7 light green inactive tablets] (28s)

Low-Ogestrel: Ethinyl estradiol 0.03 mg and norgestrel 0.3 mg [21 white tablets and 7 peach inactive tablets] (28s)

Ogestrel: Ethinyl estradiol 0.05 mg and norgestrel 0.5 mg [21 white tablets and 7 peach inactive tablets] (28s)

Ethinyl Estradiol, Drospirenone, and Levomefolate

(ETH in il es tra DYE ole, droh SPYE re none, & lee voe me FOE late)

Brand Names: U.S. Beyaz; Safyral
Brand Names: Canada Yaz Plus
Index Terms Drospirenone, Ethinyl Estradiol, and Levomefolate Calcium; Ethinyl Estradiol, Drospirenone, and Levomefolate Calcium; Levomefolate Calcium, Drospirenone, and Ethinyl Estradiol; Levomefolate, Drospirenone, and Ethinyl Estradiol
Pharmacologic Category Contraceptive; Estrogen and Progestin Combination
Use Prevention of pregnancy; treatment of premenstrual dysphoric disorder (PMDD); treatment of acne; folate supplementation
Unlabeled Use Treatment of hypermenorrhea (menorrhagia); pain associated with endometriosis; dysmenorrhea; dysfunctional uterine bleeding
Dosage Oral:

Children ≥14 years and Adults: Females: Acne (Beyaz): Refer to dosing for contraception

Adults: Females: PMDD (Beyaz): Refer to dosing for contraception

Adults: Females: Contraception (Beyaz, Safyral): Dosage is 1 tablet daily

Beyaz: One pink tablet daily for 24 consecutive days, then one light orange tablet daily on days 25-28

Safyral: One orange tablet daily for 21 consecutive days, then one light orange tablet daily on days 22-28

Dose should be taken at the same time each day, either after the evening meal or at bedtime. Dosing may be started on the first day of menstrual period (Day 1 starter) or on the first Sunday after the onset of the menstrual period (Sunday starter).

Day 1 starter: Dose starts on first day of menstrual cycle taking 1 tablet daily. If first dose is taken later than the first day of the menstrual cycle, **an additional method of contraception should be used until after the first 7 days of consecutive administration.**

Sunday starter: Dose begins on first Sunday after onset of menstruation; if the menstrual period starts on Sunday, take first tablet that very same day. **With a Sunday start, an additional method of contraception should be used until after the first 7 days of consecutive administration.**

Switching from a different contraceptive:

Oral contraceptive: Start on the same day that a new pack of the previous oral contraceptive would have been taken

Transdermal patch, vaginal ring, injection: Start on the day the next dose would have been due

IUD or implant: Start on the day of removal

Use after childbirth (in women who are not breast-feeding) or after second trimester abortion: Therapy may be started ≥4 weeks postpartum. Pregnancy should be ruled out prior to treatment if menstrual periods have not restarted and an additional method of contraception (nonhormonal) should be used until after the first 7 days of consecutive administration.

Missed doses:

If all doses have been taken on schedule and one menstrual period is missed, continue dosing cycle. If two consecutive menstrual periods are missed, rule out pregnancy and discontinue if pregnancy is confirmed.

If doses have been missed during the first 3 weeks or if active tablets (pink tablets) were started later than as directed and the menstrual period is missed, pregnancy should be ruled out prior to continuing treatment.

Missed doses (monophasic formulations) (refer to package insert for complete information):

One dose missed: Take as soon as remembered or take 2 tablets next day

Two consecutive doses missed in the first 2 weeks: Take 2 tablets as soon as remembered or 2 tablets next 2 days. **An additional method of contraception should be used for 7 days after missed dose.**

Two consecutive doses missed in week 3 or three consecutive doses missed at any time: **An additional method of contraception must be used for 7 days after a missed dose.**

Day 1 starter: Current pack should be discarded, and a new pack should be started that same day.

Sunday starter: Continue dose of 1 tablet daily until Sunday, then discard the rest of the pack, and a new pack should be started that same day.

Any number of doses missed in week 4: Throw away the pills that were missed. Continue taking one pill each day until pack is empty; no back-up method of contraception is needed

Dosage adjustment in renal impairment: Contraindicated in patients with renal dysfunction

Dosage adjustment in hepatic impairment: Contraindicated in patients with hepatic disease. Exposure to drospirenone is ~3 times higher with moderate liver impairment; information not available for severe impairment.

Additional Information Complete prescribing information should be consulted for additional detail.

Dosage Forms Excipient information presented when available (limited, particularly for generics); consult specific product labeling.

Tablet, oral:

Beyaz: Ethinyl estradiol 0.02 mg, drospirenone 3 mg, and levomefolate calcium 0.451 mg [24 pink tablets] and levomefolate calcium 0.451 mg [4 light orange tablets] (28s)

Safyral: Ethinyl estradiol 0.03 mg, drospirenone 3 mg, and levomefolate calcium 0.451 mg [21 orange tablets] and levomefolate calcium 0.451 mg [7 light orange tablets] (28s)

- ◆ **Ethinyl Estradiol, Drospirenone, and Levomefolate Calcium** *see* Ethinyl Estradiol, Drospirenone, and Levomefolate *on page 797*
- ◆ **Ethiofos** *see* Amifostine *on page 96*

Ethosuximide (eth oh SUKS i mide)

Brand Names: U.S. Zarontin

Brand Names: Canada Zarontin®

Pharmacologic Category Anticonvulsant, Succinimide

Use Management of absence (petit mal) seizures

Medication Guide Available Yes

Dosage Oral:

Children 3-6 years: Initial: 250 mg/day; increase every 4-7 days; usual maintenance dose: 20 mg/kg/day; maximum dose: 1.5 g/day in divided doses

Children ≥6 years and Adults: Initial: 500 mg/day; increase by 250 mg as needed every 4-7 days, up to 1.5 g/day in divided doses; usual maintenance dose for most pediatric patients is 20 mg/kg/day.

Dosing comment in renal impairment: No dosage adjustment provided in manufacturer's labeling; use with caution.

Dosing comment in hepatic impairment: No dosage adjustment provided in manufacturer's labeling; use with caution.

Additional Information Complete prescribing information should be consulted for additional detail.

Dosage Forms Excipient information presented when available (limited, particularly for generics); consult specific product labeling.

Capsule, Oral:

Zarontin: 250 mg [contains fd&c yellow #10 (quinoline yellow)]

Generic: 250 mg

Solution, Oral:

Zarontin: 250 mg/5 mL (474 mL) [raspberry flavor]

Generic: 250 mg/5 mL (473 mL, 474 mL)

- ◆ **Ethoxynaphthamido Penicillin Sodium** *see* Nafcillin *on page 1417*
- ◆ **Ethyl Aminobenzoate** *see* Benzocaine *on page 240*
- ◆ **Ethyl Eicosapentaenoate** *see* Icosapent Ethyl *on page 1038*
- ◆ **Ethyl-Eicosapentaenoic Acid** *see* Icosapent Ethyl *on page 1038*
- ◆ **Ethyl-EPA** *see* Icosapent Ethyl *on page 1038*
- ◆ **Ethyl Esters of Omega-3 Fatty Acids** *see* Omega-3-Acid Ethyl Esters *on page 1504*
- ◆ **Ethyl Icosapentate** *see* Icosapent Ethyl *on page 1038*
- ◆ **Ethynodiol Diacetate and Ethinyl Estradiol** *see* Ethinyl Estradiol and Ethynodiol Diacetate *on page 786*
- ◆ **Ethyol** *see* Amifostine *on page 96*
- ◆ **Ethyol® (Can)** *see* Amifostine *on page 96*
- ◆ **Etibi® (Can)** *see* Ethambutol *on page 782*

Etidronate (e ti DROE nate)

Brand Names: U.S. Didronel [DSC]

Brand Names: Canada Co-Etidronate; Mylan-Etidronate

Index Terms EHDP; Etidronate Disodium; Sodium Etidronate

Pharmacologic Category Bisphosphonate Derivative

Use Symptomatic treatment of Paget's disease; prevention and treatment of heterotopic ossification due to spinal cord injury or after total hip replacement

Pregnancy Risk Factor C

Dosage Note: Patients should receive supplemental calcium and vitamin D if dietary intake is inadequate.

Paget's disease: Adults: Oral:

Initial: 5-10 mg/kg/day (not to exceed 6 months) or 11-20 mg/kg/day (not to exceed 3 months). The recommended initial dose is 5 mg/kg/day (not to exceed 6 months). Higher doses should be used only when lower doses are ineffective or there is a need to suppress rapid bone turnover (ie, potential for irreversible neurologic damage) or reduce elevated cardiac output. Doses >20 mg/kg/day are **not** recommended.

Retreatment: Initiate only after etidronate-free period ≥90 days. Monitor patients every 3-6 months. Retreatment regimens are the same as for initial treatment.

Heterotopic ossification: Adults: Oral:
Caused by spinal cord injury: 20 mg/kg/day for 2 weeks, then 10 mg/kg/day for 10 weeks; total treatment period: 12 weeks
Complicating total hip replacement: 20 mg/kg/day for 1 month preoperatively then 20 mg/kg/day for 3 months postoperatively; total treatment period is 4 months

Dosage adjustment in renal impairment: Manufacturer's labeling recommends decreasing the dose when GFR is reduced; however, no specific dosage adjustments are provided. Use with caution and monitor closely; etidronate is eliminated intact via the kidneys.

Dosage adjustment in hepatic impairment: No dosage adjustment provided in manufacturer's labeling.

Additional Information Complete prescribing information should be consulted for additional detail.

Dosage Forms Excipient information presented when available (limited, particularly for generics); consult specific product labeling. [DSC] = Discontinued product
Tablet, Oral, as disodium:
Didronel: 400 mg [DSC] [scored]
Generic: 200 mg, 400 mg

◆ Etidronate Disodium *see* Etidronate *on page 798*

Etodolac (ee toe DOE lak)

Brand Names: Canada Apo-Etodolac®; Utradol™

Index Terms Etodolic Acid; Lodine

Pharmacologic Category Nonsteroidal Anti-inflammatory Drug (NSAID), Oral

Additional Appendix Information
Beers Criteria – Potentially Inappropriate Medications for Geriatrics *on page 2368*

Use Acute and long-term use in the management of signs and symptoms of osteoarthritis; rheumatoid arthritis and juvenile idiopathic arthritis (JIA); management of acute pain

Pregnancy Risk Factor C

Pregnancy Considerations Adverse events were not observed in the initial animal reproduction studies; therefore, the manufacturer classifies etodolac as pregnancy category C. NSAID exposure during the first trimester is not strongly associated with congenital malformations; however, cardiovascular anomalies and cleft palate have been observed following NSAID exposure in some studies. The use of an NSAID close to conception may be associated with an increased risk of miscarriage. Nonteratogenic effects have been observed following NSAID administration during the third trimester including: Myocardial degenerative changes, prenatal constriction of the ductus arteriosus, fetal tricuspid regurgitation, failure of the ductus arteriosus to close postnatally; renal dysfunction or failure, oligohydramnios; gastrointestinal bleeding or perforation, increased risk of necrotizing enterocolitis; intracranial bleeding (including intraventricular hemorrhage), platelet dysfunction with resultant bleeding; pulmonary hypertension. Because they may cause premature closure of the ductus arteriosus, use of NSAIDs late in pregnancy should be avoided (use after 31 or 32 weeks gestation is not recommended by some clinicians). The chronic use of NSAIDs in women of reproductive age may be associated with infertility that is reversible upon discontinuation of the medication.

Breast-Feeding Considerations It is not known if etodolac is excreted into breast milk. Use of etodolac while breast-feeding is not recommended by the manufacturer.

Medication Guide Available Yes

Contraindications Hypersensitivity to etodolac, aspirin, other NSAIDs, or any component of the formulation; perioperative pain in the setting of coronary artery bypass graft (CABG) surgery

Warnings/Precautions [U.S. Boxed Warning]: NSAIDs are associated with an increased risk of adverse cardiovascular thrombotic events, including MI and stroke. Risk may be increased with duration of use or pre-existing cardiovascular risk factors or disease. Carefully evaluate individual cardiovascular risk profiles prior to prescribing. May cause new-onset hypertension or worsening of existing hypertension. Use caution with fluid retention. Avoid use in heart failure. Concurrent administration of ibuprofen, and potentially other nonselective NSAIDs, may interfere with aspirin's cardioprotective effect. **[U.S. Boxed Warning]: Use is contraindicated for treatment of perioperative pain in the setting of coronary artery bypass graft (CABG) surgery.** Risk of MI and stroke may be increased with use following CABG surgery.

[U.S. Boxed Warning]: NSAIDs may increase risk of gastrointestinal irritation, inflammation, ulceration, bleeding, and perforation. These events may occur at any time during therapy and without warning. Use caution with a history of GI disease (bleeding or ulcers), concurrent therapy with aspirin, anticoagulants and/or corticosteroids, smoking, use of alcohol, the elderly or debilitated patients. When used concomitantly with ≤325 mg of aspirin, a substantial increase in the risk of gastrointestinal complications (eg, ulcer) occurs; concomitant gastroprotective therapy (eg, proton pump inhibitors) is recommended (Bhatt, 2008).

Platelet adhesion and aggregation may be decreased; may prolong bleeding time; patients with coagulation disorders or who are receiving anticoagulants should be monitored closely. Anemia may occur; patients on long-term NSAID therapy should be monitored for anemia. Rarely, NSAID use may cause severe blood dyscrasias (eg, agranulocytosis, aplastic anemia, thrombocytopenia).

NSAID use may compromise existing renal function; dose-dependent decreases in prostaglandin synthesis may result from NSAID use, reducing renal blood flow which may cause renal decompensation. NSAID use may increase the risk for hyperkalemia. Patients with impaired renal function, dehydration, heart failure, liver dysfunction, those taking diuretics and ACE inhibitors, and the elderly are at greater risk for renal toxicity and hyperkalemia. Rehydrate patient before starting therapy; monitor renal function closely. Not recommended for use in patients with advanced renal disease. Long-term NSAID use may result in renal papillary necrosis.

Use the lowest effective dose for the shortest duration of time, consistent with individual patient goals, to reduce risk of cardiovascular or GI adverse events. Alternate therapies should be considered for patients at high risk.

NSAIDs may cause serious skin adverse events including exfoliative dermatitis, Stevens-Johnson syndrome (SJS), and toxic epidermal necrolysis (TEN); discontinue use at first sign of skin rash or hypersensitivity. Anaphylactoid reactions may occur, even without prior exposure; patients with "aspirin triad" (bronchial asthma, aspirin intolerance, rhinitis) may be at increased risk. Do not use in patients who experience bronchospasm, asthma, rhinitis, or urticaria with NSAID or aspirin therapy. Use caution in other forms of asthma.

Use with caution in patients with decreased hepatic function. Closely monitor patients with any abnormal LFT. Severe hepatic reactions (eg, fulminant hepatitis, liver failure) have occurred with NSAID use, rarely; discontinue if signs or symptoms of liver disease develop, or if systemic manifestations occur.

NSAIDS may cause drowsiness, dizziness, blurred vision and other neurologic effects which may impair physical or mental abilities; patients must be cautioned about performing tasks which require mental alertness (eg, operating machinery or driving). Discontinue use with blurred or diminished vision and perform ophthalmologic exam. Monitor vision with long-term therapy. In the elderly, avoid chronic use (unless alternative agents ineffective and patient can receive concomitant gastroprotective agent); nonselective oral NSAID use is associated with an increased risk of GI bleeding and peptic ulcer disease in older adults in high risk category (eg, >75 years or age or receiving concomitant oral/parenteral corticosteroids, anticoagulants, or antiplatelet agents) (Beers Criteria).

Withhold for at least 4-6 half-lives prior to surgical or dental procedures.

Use of extended release product consisting of a nondeformable matrix should be avoided in patients with stricture/narrowing of the GI tract; symptoms of obstruction have been associated with nondeformable products.

Adverse Reactions

1% to 10%:

Central nervous system: Dizziness (3% to 9%), chills/fever (1% to 3%), depression (1% to 3%), nervousness (1% to 3%)

Dermatologic: Rash (1% to 3%), pruritus (1% to 3%)

Gastrointestinal: Dyspepsia (10%), abdominal cramps (3% to 9%), diarrhea (3% to 9%), flatulence (3% to 9%), nausea (3% to 9%), vomiting (1% to 3%), constipation (1% to 3%), melena (1% to 3%), gastritis (1% to 3%)

Genitourinary: Dysuria (1% to 3%)

Neuromuscular & skeletal: Weakness (3% to 9%)

Ocular: Blurred vision (1% to 3%)

Otic: Tinnitus (1% to 3%)

Renal: Polyuria (1% to 3%)

<1% (Limited to important or life-threatening): Agranulocytosis, allergic reaction, allergic/necrotizing vasculitis, alopecia, anaphylactic/anaphylactoid reactions, anemia, angioedema, anorexia, arrhythmia, aseptic meningitis, asthma, bleeding time increased, CHF, confusion, conjunctivitis, CVA, cystitis, duodenitis, dyspnea, ecchymosis, edema, erythema multiforme, esophagitis (+/- stricture or cardiospasm), exfoliative dermatitis, GI ulceration, hallucination, headache, hearing decreased, hematemesis, hematuria, hepatic failure, hepatitis, hyperglycemia (in controlled patients with diabetes), hyperpigmentation, hypertension, infection, insomnia, interstitial nephritis, irregular uterine bleeding, jaundice, LFTs increased, leukopenia, MI, palpitation, pancreatitis, pancytopenia, paresthesia, peptic ulcer (+/- bleeding/perforation), peripheral neuropathy, photophobia, photosensitivity, pulmonary infiltration (eosinophilia), rectal bleeding, renal calculus, renal failure, renal insufficiency, shock, Stevens-Johnson syndrome, syncope, thrombocytopenia, toxic epidermal necrolysis, ulcerative stomatitis, urticaria, vesiculobullous rash, renal papillary necrosis, visual disturbances

Drug Interactions

Metabolism/Transport Effects None known.

Avoid Concomitant Use

Avoid concomitant use of Etodolac with any of the following: Floctafenine; Ketorolac (Nasal); Ketorolac (Systemic); NSAID (COX-2 Inhibitor); Omacetaxine

Increased Effect/Toxicity

Etodolac may increase the levels/effects of: 5-ASA Derivatives; Agents with Antiplatelet Properties; Aliskiren; Aminoglycosides; Anticoagulants; Bisphosphonate Derivatives; Collagenase (Systemic); CycloSPORINE (Systemic); Dabigatran Etexilate; Deferasirox; Desmopressin; Digoxin; Eplerenone; Haloperidol; Ibritumomab; Lithium; Methotrexate; Nonsteroidal Anti-Inflammatory Agents; NSAID (COX-2 Inhibitor); Omacetaxine; PEMEtrexed; Porfimer; Potassium-Sparing Diuretics; PRALAtrexate; Quinolone Antibiotics; Rivaroxaban; Salicylates; Tenofovir; Thrombolytic Agents; Tositumomab and Iodine I 131 Tositumomab; Vancomycin; Vitamin K Antagonists

The levels/effects of Etodolac may be increased by: ACE Inhibitors; Angiotensin II Receptor Blockers; Antidepressants (Tricyclic, Tertiary Amine); Corticosteroids (Systemic); CycloSPORINE (Systemic); Dasatinib; Floctafenine; Glucosamine; Herbs (Anticoagulant/Antiplatelet Properties); Ibrutinib; Ketorolac (Nasal); Ketorolac (Systemic); Multivitamins/Fluoride (with ADE); Multivitamins/Minerals (with ADEK, Folate, Iron); Multivitamins/Minerals (with AE, No Iron); Nonsteroidal Anti-Inflammatory Agents; Omega-3 Fatty Acids; Pentosan Polysulfate Sodium; Pentoxifylline; Probenecid; Prostacyclin Analogues; Selective Serotonin Reuptake Inhibitors; Serotonin/Norepinephrine Reuptake Inhibitors; Sodium Phosphates; Tipranavir; Treprostinil; Vitamin E

Decreased Effect

Etodolac may decrease the levels/effects of: ACE Inhibitors; Agents with Antiplatelet Properties; Aliskiren; Angiotensin II Receptor Blockers; Beta-Blockers; Eplerenone; HydrALAZINE; Loop Diuretics; Potassium-Sparing Diuretics; Prostaglandins (Ophthalmic); Salicylates; Selective Serotonin Reuptake Inhibitors; Thiazide Diuretics

The levels/effects of Etodolac may be decreased by: Bile Acid Sequestrants; Nonsteroidal Anti-Inflammatory Agents; Salicylates

Ethanol/Nutrition/Herb Interactions

Ethanol: Avoid ethanol (may enhance gastric mucosal irritation).

Food: Etodolac peak serum levels may be decreased if taken with food.

Herb/Nutraceutical: Avoid alfalfa, anise, bilberry, bladderwrack, bromelain, cat's claw, celery, chamomile, coleus, cordyceps, dong quai, evening primrose, fenugreek, feverfew, garlic, ginger, ginkgo biloba, ginseng (American, Panax, Siberian), grapeseed, green tea, guggul, horse chestnut seed, horseradish, licorice, prickly ash, red clover, reishi, SAMe (S-adenosylmethionine), sweet clover, turmeric, white willow (all have additional antiplatelet activity).

Storage/Stability Store at 20°C to 25°C (68°F to 77°F). Protect from moisture.

Mechanism of Action Reversibly inhibits cyclooxygenase-1 and 2 (COX-1 and 2) enzymes, which results in decreased formation of prostaglandin precursors; has antipyretic, analgesic, and anti-inflammatory properties

Other proposed mechanisms not fully elucidated (and possibly contributing to the anti-inflammatory effect to varying degrees), include inhibiting chemotaxis, altering lymphocyte activity, inhibiting neutrophil aggregation/activation, and decreasing proinflammatory cytokine levels.

Pharmacodynamics/Kinetics

Onset of action: Analgesic: 2-4 hours; Maximum anti-inflammatory effect: A few days

Absorption: ≥80%

Distribution: V_d:

Immediate release: Adults:0.4 L/kg

Extended release: Adults: 0.57 L/kg; Children (6-16 years): 0.08 L/kg

Protein binding: ≥99%, primarily albumin

Metabolism: Hepatic

Bioavailability: 100%

Half-life elimination: Terminal: Adults: 5-8 hours

Extended release: Children (6-16 years): 12 hours

Time to peak, serum:

Immediate release: Adults: 1-2 hours

Extended release: Extended release: 5-7 hours, increased 1.4-3.8 hours with food

Excretion: Urine 73% (1% unchanged); feces 16%

Dosage Note: For chronic conditions, response is usually observed within 2 weeks.

Children 6-16 years: Oral: Juvenile idiopathic arthritis (JIA):

Extended release formulation:

20-30 kg: 400 mg once daily

31-45 kg: 600 mg once daily

46-60 kg: 800 mg once daily

>60 kg: 1000 mg once daily

Adults: Oral:

Acute pain: Immediate release formulation: 200-400 mg every 6-8 hours, as needed, not to exceed total daily doses of 1000 mg

Rheumatoid arthritis, osteoarthritis:

Immediate release formulation: 400 mg 2 times/day **or** 300 mg 2-3 times/day **or** 500 mg 2 times/day (doses >1000 mg/day have not been evaluated)

Extended release formulation: 400-1000 mg once daily

Elderly: Refer to adult dosing; in patients ≥65 years, no dosage adjustment required based on pharmacokinetics. The elderly are more sensitive to antiprostaglandin effects and may need dosage adjustments.

Dosage adjustment in renal impairment:

Mild-to-moderate: No adjustment required

Severe: Use not recommended; use with caution

Hemodialysis: Not removed

Dosage adjustment in hepatic impairment: No adjustment required.

Dietary Considerations May be taken with food to decrease GI upset.

Administration May be administered with food to decrease GI upset.

Monitoring Parameters Monitor CBC and chemistry profile, liver enzymes; in patients with an increased risk for renal failure (CHF or decreased renal function, taking ACE inhibitors or diuretics, elderly), monitor urine output and BUN/serum creatinine

Test Interactions False-positive for urinary bilirubin and ketone

Dosage Forms Excipient information presented when available (limited, particularly for generics); consult specific product labeling.

Capsule, Oral:

Generic: 200 mg, 300 mg

Tablet, Oral:

Generic: 400 mg, 500 mg

Tablet Extended Release 24 Hour, Oral:

Generic: 400 mg, 500 mg, 600 mg

◆ **Etodolic Acid** *see* Etodolac *on page 799*

Etomidate (e TOM i date)

Brand Names: U.S. Amidate

Brand Names: Canada Amidate®

Pharmacologic Category General Anesthetic

Additional Appendix Information

Dosing Considerations for the Critically-Ill Patient With Morbid Obesity *on page 2379*

Use Induction and maintenance of general anesthesia

Unlabeled Use Sedation for diagnosis of seizure foci; procedural sedation

Pregnancy Risk Factor C

Pregnancy Considerations Adverse events have been observed in animal reproduction studies.

Breast-Feeding Considerations It is not known if etomidate is excreted in breast milk. The manufacturer recommends that caution be exercised when administering etomidate to nursing women.

Contraindications Hypersensitivity to etomidate or any component of the formulation

Warnings/Precautions Etomidate inhibits 11-B-hydroxylase, an enzyme important in adrenal steroid production. A single induction dose blocks the normal stress-induced increase in adrenal cortisol production for 4-8 hours, up to 24 hours in elderly and debilitated patients. Continuous infusion of etomidate for sedation in the ICU may increase mortality because patients may not be able to respond to stress. No increase in mortality has been identified with a single dose for induction of anesthesia. Consider exogenous corticosteroid replacement in patients undergoing severe stress. Safety and efficacy have not been established in children <10 years of age.

Adverse Reactions

>10%:

Gastrointestinal: Nausea, vomiting on emergence from anesthesia

Local: Pain at injection site (30% to 80%)

Neuromuscular & skeletal: Myoclonus (33%), transient skeletal movements, uncontrolled eye movements

1% to 10%: Hiccups

<1% (Limited to important or life-threatening): Apnea, arrhythmia, bradycardia, decreased cortisol synthesis, hypertension, hyperventilation, hypotension, hypoventilation, laryngospasm, tachycardia

Drug Interactions

Metabolism/Transport Effects None known.

Avoid Concomitant Use There are no known interactions where it is recommended to avoid concomitant use.

Increased Effect/Toxicity There are no known significant interactions involving an increase in effect.

Decreased Effect There are no known significant interactions involving a decrease in effect.

Storage/Stability Store at room temperature.

Mechanism of Action Ultrashort-acting nonbarbiturate hypnotic (benzylimidazole) used for the induction of anesthesia; chemically, it is a carboxylated imidazole which produces a rapid induction of anesthesia with minimal cardiovascular effects; produces EEG burst suppression at high doses

Pharmacodynamics/Kinetics

Onset of action: 30-60 seconds

Peak effect: 1 minute

Duration: 3-5 minutes; terminated by redistribution

Distribution: V_d: 2-4.5 L/kg

Protein binding: 76%

Metabolism: Hepatic and plasma esterases

Half-life elimination: Terminal: 2.6 hours

Dosage I.V.: Children >10 years and Adults:

Anesthesia: Initial: 0.2-0.6 mg/kg over 30-60 seconds for induction of anesthesia; maintenance: 5-20 mcg/kg/minute

Procedural sedation (unlabeled use): Initial: 0.1-0.2 mg/kg, followed by 0.05 mg/kg every 3-5 minutes as needed (Bahn, 2005; Miner, 2007; Vinson, 2002)

Dosage adjustment in renal impairment: No dosage adjustment provided in manufacturer's labeling.

Dosage adjustment in hepatic impairment: No dosage adjustment provided in manufacturer's labeling; use with caution.

Administration Administer I.V. push over 30-60 seconds. Solution is highly irritating; avoid administration into small vessels; in some cases, preadministration of lidocaine may be considered.

Monitoring Parameters Cardiac monitoring and blood pressure required

Additional Information Etomidate decreases cerebral metabolism and cerebral blood flow while maintaining perfusion pressure. Premedication with opioids or benzodiazepines can decrease myoclonus. Etomidate can enhance somatosensory evoked potential recordings.

Dosage Forms Excipient information presented when available (limited, particularly for generics); consult specific product labeling.

Solution, Intravenous:

Amidate: 2 mg/mL (10 mL, 20 mL) [contains propylene glycol]

Generic: 2 mg/mL (10 mL, 20 mL)

Solution, Intravenous [preservative free]:

Generic: 2 mg/mL (10 mL, 20 mL)

◆ **Etonogestrel and Ethinyl Estradiol** *see* Ethinyl Estradiol and Etonogestrel *on page 787*

◆ **ETOP** *see* Etoposide Phosphate *on page 805*

◆ **Etopophos** *see* Etoposide Phosphate *on page 805*

Etoposide (e toe POE side)

Brand Names: U.S. Toposar

Brand Names: Canada Etoposide Injection USP; Vepesid™

Index Terms EPEG; Epipodophyllotoxin; VePesid; VP-16; VP-16-213

Pharmacologic Category Antineoplastic Agent, Podophyllotoxin Derivative; Antineoplastic Agent, Topoisomerase II Inhibitor

Use Treatment of refractory testicular tumors (injectable formulation); treatment of small cell lung cancer (SCLC)

Canadian labeling: Treatment of small cell lung cancer (SCLC; first- and second-line); treatment of nonsmall cell lung cancer (NSCLC); treatment of non-Hodgkin lymphomas (first-line); treatment of testicular cancer (first-line [injectable formulation] and refractory)

Unlabeled Use Treatment of acute lymphocytic leukemia (ALL), refractory acute myeloid leukemia (AML), recurrent or metastatic breast cancer, central nervous system tumors, Ewing's sarcoma, gestational trophoblastic disease, Hodgkin lymphoma, merkel cell cancer, refractory multiple myeloma, neuroblastoma, neuroendocrine tumors (adrenal gland and carcinoid tumors), non-Hodgkin lymphomas, nonsmall cell lung cancer (NSCLC), osteosarcoma, ovarian cancer (refractory), prostate cancer, retinoblastoma, metastatic soft tissue sarcoma, thymic malignancies (locally advanced or metastatic), unknown-primary adenocarcinoma, Wilms' tumor; conditioning regimen for hematopoietic cell transplantation

Pregnancy Risk Factor D

Pregnancy Considerations Animal reproduction studies have demonstrated teratogenicity and fetal loss. There are no adequate and well-controlled studies in pregnant women. Women of childbearing potential should be advised to avoid pregnancy.

Breast-Feeding Considerations Due to the potential for serious adverse reactions in the nursing infant, the decision to discontinue etoposide or to discontinue breast-feeding during treatment should take into account the benefits of treatment to the mother.

Contraindications Hypersensitivity to etoposide or any component of the formulation

Canadian labeling: Additional contraindications (not in U.S. labeling): Severe leukopenia or thrombocytopenia; severe hepatic impairment; severe renal impairment

Warnings/Precautions Hazardous agent - use appropriate precautions for handling and disposal (NIOSH, 2012). **[U.S. Boxed Warning]: Severe dose-limiting and dose-related myelosuppression with resulting infection or bleeding may occur.** Treatment should be withheld for platelets <50,000/mm^3 or absolute neutrophil count (ANC) <500/mm^3. May cause anaphylactic-like reactions manifested by chills, fever, tachycardia, bronchospasm, dyspnea, and hypotension. In addition, facial/tongue swelling, coughing, chest tightness, cyanosis, laryngospasm, diaphoresis, hypertension, back pain, loss of consciousness, and flushing have also been reported less commonly. Incidence is primarily associated with intravenous administration (up to 2%) compared to oral administration (<1%). Infusion should be interrupted and medications for the treatment of anaphylaxis should be available for immediate use. High drug concentration and rate of infusion, as well as presence of polysorbate 80 and benzyl alcohol in the etoposide intravenous formulation have been suggested as contributing factors to the development of hypersensitivity reactions. Etoposide intravenous formulations may contain polysorbate 80 and/or benzyl alcohol, while etoposide phosphate (the water soluble prodrug of etoposide) intravenous formulation does not contain either vehicle. Case reports have suggested that etoposide phosphate has been used successfully in patients with previous hypersensitivity reactions to etoposide (Collier, 2008; Siderov, 2002). The use of concentrations higher than recommended were associated with higher rates of anaphylactic-like reactions in children.

Secondary acute leukemias have been reported with etoposide, either as monotherapy or in combination with other chemotherapy agents. Must be diluted; do not give I.V. push, infuse over at least 30-60 minutes; hypotension is associated with rapid infusion. If hypotension occurs, interrupt infusion and administer I.V. hydration and supportive care; decrease infusion upon reinitiation. Tissue irritation and inflammation have occurred following extravasation. Do not administer I.M. or SubQ. Dosage should be adjusted in patients with hepatic or renal impairment (Canadian labeling contraindicates use in severe hepatic and/or renal impairment). Use with caution in patients with low serum albumin; may increase risk for toxicities. Use with caution in elderly patients; may be more likely to develop severe myelosuppression and/or GI effects (eg, nausea/vomiting). **[U.S. Boxed Warning]: Should be administered under the supervision of an experienced cancer chemotherapy physician.** Injectable formulation contains polysorbate 80; do not use in premature infants. May contain benzyl alcohol; do not use in newborn infants. Injectable formulation also contains alcohol (~33% v/v); may contribute to adverse reactions, especially with higher etoposide doses.

Adverse Reactions Note: The following may occur with higher doses used in stem cell transplantation: Alopecia, ethanol intoxication, hepatitis, hypotension (infusion-related), metabolic acidosis, mucositis, nausea and vomiting (severe), secondary malignancy, skin lesions (resembling Stevens-Johnson syndrome).

>10%:

Dermatologic: Alopecia (8% to 66%)

Gastrointestinal: Nausea/vomiting (31% to 43%), anorexia (10% to 13%), diarrhea (1% to 13%)

Hematologic: Leukopenia (60% to 91%; grade 4: 3% to 17%; nadir: 7-14 days; recovery: by day 20), thrombocytopenia (22% to 41%; grades 3/4: 1% to 20%; nadir 9-16 days; recovery: by day 20), anemia (≤33%)

1% to 10%:

Cardiovascular: Hypotension (1% to 2%; due to rapid infusion)

Gastrointestinal: Stomatitis (1% to 6%), abdominal pain (up to 2%)

Hepatic: Hepatic toxicity (up to 3%)

Neuromuscular & skeletal: Peripheral neuropathy (1% to 2%)

Miscellaneous: Anaphylactic-like reaction (I.V. infusion 1% to 2%; oral capsules <1%; including chills, fever, tachycardia, bronchospasm, dyspnea)

<1% (Limited to important or life-threatening): Amenorrhea, blindness (transient/cortical), cyanosis, extravasation (induration/necrosis), facial swelling, hypersensitivity, hypersensitivity-associated apnea, interstitial pneumonitis, laryngospasm, maculopapular rash, metabolic

acidosis, MI, mucositis, myocardial ischemia, optic neuritis, perivasculitis, pruritus, pulmonary fibrosis, radiation-recall dermatitis, rash, reversible posterior leukoencephalopathy syndrome (RPLS), seizure, Stevens-Johnson syndrome, tongue swelling, toxic epidermal necrolysis, toxic megacolon, vasospasm

Drug Interactions

Metabolism/Transport Effects Substrate of CYP1A2 (minor), CYP2E1 (minor), CYP3A4 (major), P-glycoprotein; **Note:** Assignment of Major/Minor substrate status based on clinically relevant drug interaction potential; **Inhibits** CYP2C9 (weak), CYP3A4 (weak)

Avoid Concomitant Use

Avoid concomitant use of Etoposide with any of the following: BCG; CloZAPine; Conivaptan; Fusidic Acid (Systemic); Natalizumab; Pimecrolimus; Pimozide; Tacrolimus (Topical); Tofacitinib; Vaccines (Live)

Increased Effect/Toxicity

Etoposide may increase the levels/effects of: ARIPiprazole; CloZAPine; Dofetilide; Leflunomide; Lomitapide; Natalizumab; Pimozide; Tofacitinib; Vaccines (Live); Vitamin K Antagonists

The levels/effects of Etoposide may be increased by: Atovaquone; Conivaptan; CycloSPORINE (Systemic); CYP3A4 Inhibitors (Moderate); CYP3A4 Inhibitors (Strong); Dasatinib; Denosumab; Fusidic Acid (Systemic); Ivacaftor; Luliconazole; Mifepristone; P-glycoprotein/ABCB1 Inhibitors; Pimecrolimus; Roflumilast; Simeprevir; Tacrolimus (Topical); Trastuzumab

Decreased Effect

Etoposide may decrease the levels/effects of: BCG; Coccidioidin Skin Test; Sipuleucel-T; Vaccines (Inactivated); Vaccines (Live); Vitamin K Antagonists

The levels/effects of Etoposide may be decreased by: Barbiturates; Bosentan; CYP3A4 Inducers (Strong); Dabrafenib; Deferasirox; Fosphenytoin; Herbs (CYP3A4 Inducers); Mitotane; P-glycoprotein/ABCB1 Inducers; Phenytoin; Tocilizumab

Ethanol/Nutrition/Herb Interactions

Ethanol: Avoid ethanol (may increase GI irritation).

Herb/Nutraceutical: Avoid concurrent St John's wort; may decrease etoposide levels.

Preparation for Administration Hazardous agent; use appropriate precautions for handling and disposal (NIOSH, 2012). Etoposide should be diluted to a concentration of 0.2-0.4 mg/mL in D_5W or NS for administration. Diluted solutions have concentration-dependent stability: More concentrated solutions have shorter stability times. Precipitation may occur with concentrations >0.4 mg/mL.

Storage/Stability

Capsules: Store oral capsules under refrigeration at 2°C to 8°C (36°F to 46°F); do not freeze.

Injection: Store intact vials of injection at room temperature of 25°C (77°F); do not freeze. Protect from light. Diluted solutions for infusion, at room temperature, in D_5W or NS in polyvinyl chloride, are stable as follows, depending on the concentration:

0.2 mg/mL: 96 hours

0.4 mg/mL: 24 hours

Etoposide injection contains polysorbate 80 which may cause leaching of diethylhexyl phthalate (DEHP), a plasticizer contained in polyvinyl chloride (PVC) bags and tubing. Higher concentrations and longer storage time after preparation in PVC bags may increase DEHP leaching. Preparation in glass or polyolefin containers will minimize patient exposure to DEHP. When undiluted etoposide injection is stored in acrylic or ABS (acrylonitrile, butadiene and styrene) plastic containers, the containers may crack and leak.

Mechanism of Action Etoposide has been shown to delay transit of cells through the S phase and arrest cells in late S or early G_2 phase. The drug may inhibit mitochondrial transport at the NADH dehydrogenase level or inhibit uptake of nucleosides into HeLa cells. It is a topoisomerase II inhibitor and appears to cause DNA strand breaks. Etoposide does not inhibit microtubular assembly.

Pharmacodynamics/Kinetics

Absorption: Oral: Significant inter- and intrapatient variation

Distribution: Average V_d: 7-17 L/m^2; poor penetration across the blood-brain barrier; CSF concentrations <5% of plasma concentrations

Protein binding: 94% to 98%

Metabolism: Hepatic, via CYP3A4 and 3A5, to various metabolites; in addition, conversion of etoposide to the O-demethylated metabolites (catechol and quinine) via prostaglandin synthases or myeloperoxidase occurs, as well as glutathione and glucuronide conjugation via GSTT1/GSTP1 and UGT1A1 (Yang, 2009)

Bioavailability: Oral: ~50% (range: 25% to 75%)

Half-life elimination: Terminal: I.V.: 4-11 hours; Children: Normal renal/hepatic function: 6-8 hours

Excretion:

- Children: I.V.: Urine (~55% as unchanged drug) in 24 hours
- Adults: I.V.: Urine (56%; 45% as unchanged drug) within 120 hours; feces (44%) within 120 hours

Dosage Details concerning dosing in combination regimens should also be consulted:

Children (unlabeled uses): I.V.:

AML induction (combination chemotherapy; Woods, 1996):

- <3 years: 3.3 mg/kg/day continuous infusion for 4 days
- ≥3 years: 100 mg/m^2/day continuous infusion for 4 days

Central nervous system tumors (combination chemotherapy):

- <3 years: 6.5 mg/kg/dose days 3 and 4 of each 28-day "B" treatment cycle (Duffner, 1993)
- ≥3 years: 100 mg/m^2/day on days 1, 2, and 3 of a 3-week treatment cycle (Taylor, 2003)
- ≥6 years: 150 mg/m^2/day on days 3 and 4 of a 3-week treatment course (Kovnar, 1990)

Hematopoietic stem cell transplant conditioning regimen: 60 mg/kg/dose over 4 hours as a single dose 3 or 4 days prior to transplantation (Horning, 1994; Snyder, 1993)

Hodgkin lymphoma: 200 mg/m^2/day on days 1, 2, and 3 every 3 weeks (Kelly, 2002)

Neuroblastoma:

- Induction: 100 mg/m^2/day on days 1-5 of each cycle (Kaneko, 2002)
- Hematopoietic stem cell transplant conditioning regimen: 200 mg/m^2/day for 4 days beginning 8 or 9 days prior to transplantation (Kaneko, 2002)

Sarcoma, refractory: 100 mg/m^2/day on days 1-5 of cycle; repeat cycle every 21 days (Van Winkle, 2005)

Adults:

U.S. labeling:

Small cell lung cancer (combination chemotherapy):

- I.V.: 35 mg/m^2/day for 4 days, up to 50 mg/m^2/day for 5 days every 3-4 weeks
- Oral: Due to poor bioavailability, oral doses should be twice the I.V. dose (and rounded to the nearest 50 mg)

Testicular cancer (combination chemotherapy): I.V.: 50-100 mg/m^2/day for days 1-5 **or** 100 mg/m^2/day on days 1, 3, and 5 repeated every 3-4 weeks

Canadian labeling: Non-Hodgkin lymphoma (in combination with other agents), nonsmall cell lung cancer (alone or in combination), small cell lung cancer (first-line in combination; second-line alone or in combination), testicular cancer (in combination; oral therapy for refractory disease):

I.V.: 50-100 mg/m^2/day for 5 days

Oral: 100-200 mg/m^2/day for 5 days; administer daily doses >200 mg in 2 divided doses.

Adult unlabeled uses and/or dosing:

Hematopoietic stem cell transplant conditioning regimen, lymphoid malignancies: I.V.: 60 mg/kg over 4 hours as a single dose 3 or 4 days prior to transplantation (Horning, 1994; Snyder, 1993; Weaver, 1994)

Nonsmall cell lung cancer: I.V.: 100 mg/m^2 days 1, 2, and 3 every 3 weeks for 4 cycles or every 4 weeks for 3-4 cycles (in combination with cisplatin) (Arriagada, 2004) **or** 50 mg/m^2 days 1-5 and days 29-33 (in combination with cisplatin and radiation therapy) (Albain, 2009)

Ovarian cancer, refractory: Oral: 50 mg/m^2 once daily for 21 days every 4 weeks until disease progression or unacceptable toxicity (Rose, 1998)

Small cell lung cancer, limited stage (combination chemotherapy): I.V.: 120 mg/m^2/day on days 1, 2, and 3 every 3 weeks for 4 courses (Turrisi, 1999) **or** 100 mg/m^2/day on days 1, 2, and 3 for induction therapy, followed by consolidation chemotherapy (Saito, 2006) **or** 100 mg/m^2/day on days 1, 2, and 3 every 3 weeks up to a maximum of 6 cycles (Skarlos, 2001) **or** 100 mg/m^2/day I.V. on day 1, followed by 200 mg/m^2/day **orally** on days 2 through 4 every 3 weeks for a maximum of 5 courses (Sundstrom, 2002)

Small cell lung cancer, extensive stage (combination chemotherapy): 100 mg/m^2/day I.V. on days 1, 2, and 3 every 3 weeks for 4 cycles (Lara, 2009) **or** 100 mg/m^2/day I.V. on day 1, followed by 200 mg/m^2/day **orally** on days 2 through 4 every 3 weeks for a maximum of 5 courses (Sundstrom, 2002) **or** I.V.: 80 mg/m^2/day on days 1, 2, and 3 every 3 weeks up to 8 cycles (Ihede, 1994)

Testicular cancer (combination chemotherapy):

Nonseminoma: I.V.: 100 mg/m^2/day on days 1 through 5 every 21 days for 3-4 courses (Saxman, 1998)

Nonseminoma, metastatic (high-dose regimens): I.V.: 750 mg/m^2/day administered 5, 4, and 3 days before peripheral blood stem cell infusion, repeat for a second cycle after recovery of granulocyte and platelet counts (Einhorn, 2007) **or** 400 mg/m^2/day (beginning on cycle 3) on days 1, 2, and 3, with peripheral blood stem cell support, administered at 14- to 21-day intervals for 3 cycles (Kondagunta, 2007)

Thymoma, locally advanced or metastatic: I.V.: 120 mg/m^2 days 1, 2, and 3 every 3 weeks (in combination with cisplatin) for up to 8 cycles (Giaccone, 1996)

Unknown primary adenocarcinoma: Oral: 50 mg once daily on days 1, 3, 5, 7, and 9 alternating with 100 mg once daily on days 2, 4, 6, 8, and 10 every 3 weeks (in combination with paclitaxel and carboplatin) (Greco, 2000; Hainsworth, 2006)

Dosage adjustment for toxicity: Oral, I.V.:

Infusion (hypersensitivity) reactions: Interrupt infusion.

ANC <500/mm^3 or platelets <50,000/mm^3: Withhold treatment until recovery.

Severe adverse reactions (nonhematologic): Reduce dose or discontinue treatment.

WBC 2000-3000/mm^3 or platelets 75,000-100,000/mm^3: Canadian labeling (not in U.S. labeling): Reduce dose by 50%.

Dosing adjustment in renal impairment: Oral, I.V.:

U.S. labeling recommends the following adjustments:

Cl_{cr} >50 mL/minute: No adjustment required.

Cl_{cr} 15-50 mL/minute: Administer 75% of dose.

Cl_{cr} <15 mL minute: Data not available; consider further dose reductions.

The following adjustments have been recommended:

Aronoff, 2007:

Children:

Cl_{cr} 10-50 mL/minute/1.73 m^2: Administer 75% of dose.

Cl_{cr} <10 mL minute/1.73 m^2: Administer 50% of dose.

Hemodialysis: Administer 50% of dose.

Peritoneal dialysis: Administer 50% of dose.

Continuous renal replacement therapy (CRRT): Administer 75% of dose and reduce for hyperbilirubinemia.

Adults:

Cl_{cr} 10-50 mL/minute: Administer 75% of dose.

Cl_{cr} <10 mL minute: Administer 50% of dose.

Hemodialysis: Administer 50% of dose; supplemental posthemodialysis dose is not necessary.

Peritoneal dialysis: Administer 50% of dose; supplemental dose is not necessary.

Continuous renal replacement therapy (CRRT): Administer 75% of dose.

Janus, 2010: Hemodialysis: Reduce dose by 50%; not removed by hemodialysis so may be administered before or after dialysis.

Kintzel, 1995:

Cl_{cr} 46-60 mL/minute: Administer 85% of dose.

Cl_{cr} 31-45 mL/minute: Administer 80% of dose.

Cl_{cr} ≤30 mL/minute: Administer 75% of dose.

Dosing adjustment in hepatic impairment:

U.S. labeling: No dosage adjustment provided in manufacturer's labeling.

Canadian labeling:

Mild-to-moderate impairment: No dosage adjustment provided in manufacturer's labeling.

Severe impairment: Use is contraindicated.

The following adjustments have also been recommended:

Donelli, 1998: Liver dysfunction may reduce the metabolism and increase the toxicity of etoposide. Normal doses of I.V. etoposide should be given to patients with liver dysfunction (dose reductions may result in subtherapeutic concentrations); however, use caution with concomitant liver dysfunction (severe) and renal dysfunction as the decreased metabolic clearance cannot be compensated by increased renal clearance.

Floyd, 2006: Bilirubin 1.5-3 mg/dL or AST >3 times ULN: Administer 50% of dose

King, 2001; Koren, 1992: Bilirubin 1.5-3 mg/dL or AST >180 units/L: Administer 50% of dose

Dosing in obesity: *ASCO Guidelines for appropriate chemotherapy dosing in obese adults with cancer* (***Note:*** *Excludes HSCT dosing):* Utilize patient's actual body weight (full weight) for calculation of body surface area- or weight-based dosing, particularly when the intent of therapy is curative; manage regimen-related toxicities in the same manner as for nonobese patients; if a dose reduction is utilized due to toxicity, consider resumption of full weight-based dosing with subsequent cycles, especially if cause of toxicity (eg, hepatic or renal impairment) is resolved (Griggs, 2012).

Administration

Oral: Doses ≤200 mg/day as a single once daily dose; doses >200 mg should be given in 2-4 divided doses. If necessary, the injection may be used for oral administration (see Extemporaneous Preparations). Canadian labeling recommends administering capsule on an empty stomach.

I.V.: Administer standard doses over at least 30-60 minutes to minimize the risk of hypotension. Higher (unlabeled) doses used in transplantation may be infused over longer time periods depending on the protocol. Etoposide injection contains polysorbate 80 which may cause leaching of diethylhexyl phthalate (DEHP), a plasticizer contained in polyvinyl chloride (PVC) tubing. Administration through non-PVC (low sorbing) tubing will minimize patient exposure to DEHP. Tissue irritation and inflammation have occurred following extravasation.

Concentrations >0.4 mg/mL are very unstable and may precipitate within a few minutes. For large doses, where dilution to ≤0.4 mg/mL is not feasible, consideration should be given to slow infusion of the undiluted drug through a running normal saline, dextrose or saline/dextrose infusion; or use of etoposide phosphate. Etoposide solutions of 0.1-0.4 mg/mL may be filtered through a 0.22 micron filter without damage to the filter; etoposide solutions of 0.2 mg/mL may be filtered through a 0.22 micron filter without significant loss of drug.

Hazardous agent; use appropriate precautions for handling and disposal (NIOSH, 2012).

Monitoring Parameters CBC with differential; liver function (bilirubin, ALT, AST), albumin, renal function tests; vital signs (blood pressure)

Dosage Forms Excipient information presented when available (limited, particularly for generics); consult specific product labeling.

Capsule, Oral:
- Generic: 50 mg

Solution, Intravenous:
- Toposar: 20 mg/mL (5 mL); 500 mg/25 mL (25 mL); 1 g/50 mL (50 mL) [contains alcohol, usp, polyethylene glycol 300, polysorbate 80]
- Generic: 20 mg/mL (5 mL); 500 mg/25 mL (25 mL); 1 g/50 mL (50 mL)

Extemporaneous Preparations Hazardous agent: Use appropriate precautions for handling and disposal.

Etoposide 10 mg/mL oral solution: Dilute etoposide for injection 1:1 with normal saline to a concentration of 10 mg/mL. This solution is stable in plastic oral syringes for 22 days at room temperature. Prior to oral administration, further mix with fruit juice (orange, apple, or lemon; **NOT** grapefruit juice) to a concentration of <0.4 mg/mL; once mixed with fruit juice, use within 3 hours.

McLeod HL and Relling MV, "Stability of Etoposide Solution for Oral Use," *Am J Hosp Pharm*, 1992, 49(11):2784-5.

◆ **Etoposide Injection USP (Can)** *see* Etoposide *on page 802*

Etoposide Phosphate (e toe POE side FOS fate)

Brand Names: U.S. Etopophos

Index Terms Epipodophyllotoxin; ETOP

Pharmacologic Category Antineoplastic Agent, Podophyllotoxin Derivative; Antineoplastic Agent, Topoisomerase II Inhibitor

Use Treatment of refractory testicular tumors; treatment of small cell lung cancer

Pregnancy Risk Factor D

Pregnancy Considerations Animal studies have demonstrated teratogenicity and fetal loss. There are no adequate and well-controlled studies in pregnant women. Women of childbearing potential should be advised to avoid pregnancy.

Breast-Feeding Considerations Due to the potential for serious adverse reactions in the nursing infant, breast feeding is not recommended.

Contraindications Hypersensitivity to etoposide, etoposide phosphate, or any component of the formulation

Warnings/Precautions Hazardous agent - use appropriate precautions for handling and disposal (NIOSH, 2012). **[U.S. Boxed Warning]: Severe dose-limiting and dose-related myelosuppression with resulting infection or bleeding may occur.** Treatment should be withheld for platelets <50,000/mm^3 or absolute neutrophil count (ANC) <500/mm^3. May cause anaphylactic-like reactions manifested by chills, fever, tachycardia, bronchospasm, dyspnea, and hypotension. In addition, facial/tongue swelling, coughing, throat tightness, cyanosis, laryngospasm, diaphoresis, back pain, hypertension, flushing, apnea and loss of consciousness have also been reported less commonly. Anaphylactic-type reactions have occurred with the first infusion. Infusion should be interrupted and medications for the treatment of anaphylaxis should be available for immediate use. Underlying mechanisms behind the development of hypersensitivity reactions is unknown, but have been attributed to high drug concentration and rate of infusion. Another possible mechanism may be due to the differences between available etoposide intravenous formulations. Etoposide intravenous formulation contains polysorbate 80 and benzyl alcohol, while etoposide phosphate (the water soluble prodrug of etoposide) intravenous formulation does not contain either vehicle. Case reports have suggested that etoposide phosphate has been used successfully in patients with previous hypersensitivity reactions to etoposide (Collier, 2008; Siderov, 2002).

Secondary acute leukemias have been reported with etoposide, either as monotherapy or in combination with other chemotherapy agents. Dosage should be adjusted in patients with hepatic or renal impairment. Use with caution in patients with low serum albumin; may increase risk for toxicities. Doses of etoposide phosphate >175 mg/m^2 have not been evaluated. Use caution in elderly patients (may be more likely to develop severe myelosuppression and/or GI effects. Administer by slow I.V. infusion; hypotension has been reported with etoposide phosphate administration, generally associated with rapid I.V. infusion. Injection site reactions may occur; monitor infusion site closely. **[U.S. Boxed Warning]: Should be administered under the supervision of an experienced cancer chemotherapy physician.**

Adverse Reactions Note: Also see adverse reactions for **etoposide**; etoposide phosphate is converted to etoposide, adverse reactions experienced with etoposide would also be expected with etoposide phosphate.

>10%:
- Central nervous system: Chills/fever (24%)
- Dermatologic: Alopecia (33% to 44%)
- Gastrointestinal: Nausea/vomiting (37%), anorexia (16%), mucositis (11%)
- Hematologic: Leukopenia (91%; grade 4: 17%; nadir: day 15-22; recovery: usually by day 21), neutropenia (88%; grade 4: 37%; nadir: day 12-19; recovery: usually by day 21), anemia (72%; grades 3/4: 19%), thrombocytopenia (23%; grade 4: 9%; nadir: day 10-15; recovery: usually by day 21)
- Neuromuscular & skeletal: Weakness/malaise (39%)

1% to 10%:
- Cardiovascular: Hypotension (1% to 5%), hypertension (3%), facial flushing (2%)
- Central nervous system: Dizziness (5%)
- Dermatologic: Skin rash (3%)
- Gastrointestinal: Constipation (8%), abdominal pain (7%), diarrhea (6%), taste perversion (6%)

Local: Extravasation/phlebitis (5%; including swelling, pain, cellulitis, necrosis, and/or skin necrosis at site of infiltration)

Miscellaneous: Anaphylactic-type reactions (3%; including chills, diaphoresis, fever, rigor, tachycardia, bronchospasm, dyspnea, pruritus)

<1% (Limited to important or life-threatening): Acute leukemia (with/without preleukemia phase), anaphylactic-like reactions, blindness (transient, cortical), cyanosis, dysphagia, erythema, facial swelling, hepatic toxicity, hyperpigmentation, hypersensitivity-associated apnea, infection, interstitial pneumonitis, laryngospasm, maculopapular rash, neutropenic fever, optic neuritis, perivasculitis, pruritus, pulmonary fibrosis, radiation recall dermatitis, seizure, Stevens-Johnson syndrome, tongue swelling, toxic epidermal necrolysis, urticaria

Drug Interactions

Metabolism/Transport Effects **Substrate** of CYP1A2 (minor), CYP2E1 (minor), CYP3A4 (major), P-glycoprotein; **Note:** Assignment of Major/Minor substrate status based on clinically relevant drug interaction potential; **Inhibits** CYP2C9 (weak), CYP3A4 (weak)

Avoid Concomitant Use

Avoid concomitant use of Etoposide Phosphate with any of the following: BCG; CloZAPine; Conivaptan; Fusidic Acid (Systemic); Natalizumab; Pimecrolimus; Pimozide; Tacrolimus (Topical); Tofacitinib; Vaccines (Live)

Increased Effect/Toxicity

Etoposide Phosphate may increase the levels/effects of: ARIPiprazole; CloZAPine; Dofetilide; Leflunomide; Lomitapide; Natalizumab; Pimozide; Tofacitinib; Vaccines (Live)

The levels/effects of Etoposide Phosphate may be increased by: Conivaptan; CycloSPORINE (Systemic); CYP3A4 Inhibitors (Moderate); CYP3A4 Inhibitors (Strong); Dasatinib; Denosumab; Fusidic Acid (Systemic); Ivacaftor; Luliconazole; Mifepristone; P-glycoprotein/ABCB1 Inhibitors; Pimecrolimus; Roflumilast; Simeprevir; Tacrolimus (Topical); Trastuzumab

Decreased Effect

Etoposide Phosphate may decrease the levels/effects of: BCG; Coccidioidin Skin Test; Sipuleucel-T; Vaccines (Inactivated); Vaccines (Live)

The levels/effects of Etoposide Phosphate may be decreased by: Barbiturates; Bosentan; CYP3A4 Inducers (Strong); Dabrafenib; Deferasirox; Echinacea; Fosphenytoin; Herbs (CYP3A4 Inducers); Mitotane; P-glycoprotein/ABCB1 Inducers; Phenytoin; Tocilizumab

Ethanol/Nutrition/Herb Interactions

Ethanol: Avoid ethanol (may increase GI irritation).

Herb/Nutraceutical: Avoid St John's wort (may decrease etoposide levels).

Preparation for Administration Hazardous agent; use appropriate precautions for handling and disposal (NIOSH, 2012). Reconstitute vials with 5 mL or 10 mL SWFI, D_5W, NS, bacteriostatic SWFI, or bacteriostatic NS to a concentration of 20 mg/mL or 10 mg/mL etoposide equivalent. These solutions may be administered without further dilution or may be diluted in 50-500 mL of D_5W or NS to a concentration as low as 0.1 mg/mL.

Storage/Stability Store intact vials under refrigeration at 2°C to 8°C (36°F to 46°F). Protect from light. Reconstituted solution is stable refrigerated at 2°C to 8°C (36°F to 46°F) for 7 days. At room temperature of 20°C to 25°C (68°F to 77°F), reconstituted solutions are stable for 24 hours when reconstituted with SWFI, D_5W, or NS, or for 48 hours when reconstituted with bacteriostatic SWFI or bacteriostatic NS. Further diluted solutions for infusion are stable at room temperature 20°C to 25°C (68°F to 77°F) or under refrigeration 2°C to 8°C (36°F to 46°F) for up to 24 hours.

Mechanism of Action Etoposide phosphate is converted *in vivo* to the active moiety, etoposide, by dephosphorylation. Etoposide inhibits mitotic activity; inhibits cells from entering prophase; inhibits DNA synthesis. Initially thought to be mitotic inhibitors similar to podophyllotoxin, but actually have no effect on microtubule assembly. However, later shown to induce DNA strand breakage and inhibition of topoisomerase II (an enzyme which breaks and repairs DNA); etoposide acts in late S or early G2 phases.

Pharmacodynamics/Kinetics

Distribution: Average V_d: 7-17 L/m^2; poor penetration across blood-brain barrier; concentrations in CSF being <10% that of plasma

Protein binding: 97%

Metabolism:

Etoposide phosphate: Rapidly and completely converted to etoposide in plasma

Etoposide: Hepatic, via CYP3A4 and 3A5 to various metabolites; in addition, conversion of etoposide to the O-demethylated metabolites (catechol and quinine) via prostaglandin synthases or myeloperoxidase occurs, as well as glutathione and glucuronide conjugation via GSTT1/GSTP1 and UGT1A1 (Yang, 2009)

Half-life elimination: Terminal: 4-11 hours; Children: Normal renal/hepatic function: 6-8 hours

Excretion: Urine (56%; 45% as etoposide) within 120 hours; feces (44%) within 120 hours

Children: Urine (~55% as etoposide) in 24 hours

Dosage Adults: **Note:** Etoposide phosphate is a prodrug of etoposide; equivalent doses should be used when converting from etoposide to etoposide phosphate. Each 100 mg vial of etoposide phosphate is equivalent to 100 mg of etoposide.

Small cell lung cancer (in combination with other approved chemotherapeutic drugs): I.V.: Etoposide 35 mg/m^2/day for 4 days up to 50 mg/m^2/day for 5 days. Courses are repeated at 3- to 4-week intervals after adequate recovery from toxicity.

Testicular cancer (in combination with other approved chemotherapeutic agents): I.V.: Etoposide 50-100 mg/m^2/day on days 1-5 to 100 mg/m^2/day on days 1, 3, and 5. Courses are repeated at 3- to 4-week intervals after adequate recovery from toxicity.

Indication-specific unlabeled dosing: Refer to Etoposide monograph.

Dosage adjustment in renal impairment:

Manufacturer recommended guidelines:

Cl_{cr} >50 mL/minute: No adjustment required

Cl_{cr} 15-50 mL/minute: Administer 75% of dose

Cl_{cr} <15 mL minute: Data are not available; consider further dose reductions

Etoposide phosphate is rapidly and completely converted to etoposide in plasma, please refer to Etoposide monograph for additional renal dosing adjustments (for etoposide).

Dosage adjustment in hepatic impairment: The FDA-approved labeling does not contain dosing adjustment guidelines. Etoposide phosphate is rapidly and completely converted to etoposide in plasma; please refer to Etoposide monograph for etoposide hepatic dosing adjustments.

Dosing in obesity: *ASCO Guidelines for appropriate chemotherapy dosing in obese adults with cancer* (***Note:*** *Excludes HSCT dosing):* Utilize patient's actual body weight (full weight) for calculation of body surface area- or weight-based dosing, particularly when the intent of therapy is curative; manage regimen-related toxicities in the same manner as for nonobese patients; if a dose reduction is utilized due to toxicity, consider resumption of full weight-based dosing with subsequent cycles, especially if cause of toxicity (eg, hepatic or renal impairment) is resolved (Griggs, 2012).

Administration Infuse by slow I.V. infusion over 5-210 minutes; risk of hypotension may increase with rate of infusion. Do not administer as a bolus injection.

Hazardous agent; use appropriate precautions for handling and disposal (NIOSH, 2012).

Monitoring Parameters CBC with differential and platelets (prior to initial treatment and each cycle), vital signs (blood pressure), bilirubin, AST/ALT, renal function

Additional Information Each 100 mg vial of etoposide phosphate is equivalent to 100 mg of etoposide. Equivalent doses should be used when converting from etoposide to etoposide phosphate.

Dosage Forms Excipient information presented when available (limited, particularly for generics); consult specific product labeling.

Solution Reconstituted, Intravenous [strength expressed as base]:

Etopophos: 100 mg (1 ea)

◆ **ETR** *see* Etravirine *on page 807*

Etravirine (et ra VIR een)

Brand Names: U.S. Intelence

Brand Names: Canada Intelence®

Index Terms ETR; TMC125

Pharmacologic Category Antiretroviral, Reverse Transcriptase Inhibitor, Non-nucleoside (Anti-HIV)

Use Treatment of HIV-1 infection in combination with at least two additional antiretroviral agents in treatment-experienced patients exhibiting viral replication with documented non-nucleoside reverse transcriptase inhibitor (NNRTI) resistance

Pregnancy Risk Factor B

Dosage Oral:

Children 6 to <18 years:

≥16 kg to <20 kg: 100 mg twice daily

≥20 kg to <25 kg: 125 mg twice daily

≥25 kg to <30 kg: 150 mg twice daily

≥30 kg: 200 mg twice daily

Adults: 200 mg twice daily

Dosage adjustment in renal impairment: No dosage adjustment necessary

Due to extensive protein binding, significant removal by hemodialysis or peritoneal dialysis is unlikely.

Dosage adjustment in hepatic impairment:

Mild-to-moderate impairment (Child-Pugh class A or B): No dosage adjustment necessary.

Severe impairment (Child-Pugh class C): No dosage adjustment provided in manufacturer's labeling (has not been studied).

Additional Information Complete prescribing information should be consulted for additional detail.

Dosage Forms Excipient information presented when available (limited, particularly for generics); consult specific product labeling.

Tablet, Oral:

Intelence: 25 mg [scored]

Intelence: 100 mg, 200 mg

◆ **Euflex (Can)** *see* Flutamide *on page 892*

◆ **Euflexxa** *see* Hyaluronate and Derivatives *on page 1000*

◆ **Euglucon® (Can)** *see* GlyBURIDE *on page 963*

◆ **Eulexin** *see* Flutamide *on page 892*

◆ ***Euphorbia peplus*** **Derivative** *see* Ingenol Mebutate *on page 1085*

◆ **Eurax** *see* Crotamiton *on page 501*

◆ **Eurax Cream (Can)** *see* Crotamiton *on page 501*

◆ **Euro-Cyproheptadine (Can)** *see* Cyproheptadine *on page 515*

◆ **Euro-Lithium (Can)** *see* Lithium *on page 1229*

◆ **Eutectic Mixture of Lidocaine and Tetracaine** *see* Lidocaine and Tetracaine *on page 1215*

◆ **Euthyrox (Can)** *see* Levothyroxine *on page 1206*

◆ **Evac [OTC]** *see* Psyllium *on page 1748*

◆ **Evamist** *see* Estradiol (Systemic) *on page 754*

Everolimus (e ver OH li mus)

Brand Names: U.S. Afinitor; Afinitor Disperz; Zortress

Brand Names: Canada Afinitor

Index Terms RAD001

Pharmacologic Category Antineoplastic Agent, mTOR Kinase Inhibitor; Immunosuppressant Agent; mTOR Kinase Inhibitor

Use

Afinitor: Treatment of advanced hormone receptor-positive, HER2-negative breast cancer in postmenopausal women (in combination with exemestane and after letrozole or anastrozole failure); treatment of advanced renal cell cancer (RCC), after sunitinib or sorafenib failure; treatment of renal angiomyolipoma with tuberous sclerosis complex (TSC) not requiring immediate surgery; treatment of subependymal giant cell astrocytoma (SEGA) associated with TSC which requires intervention, but cannot be curatively resected; treatment of advanced, metastatic or unresectable pancreatic neuroendocrine tumors (PNET)

Afinitor Disperz: Treatment of subependymal giant cell astrocytoma (SEGA) associated with TSC which requires intervention, but cannot be curatively resected

Zortress: Prophylaxis of organ rejection in renal transplantation patients at low-moderate immunologic risk (in combination with basiliximab, cyclosporine, and corticosteroids); prophylaxis of organ rejection in liver transplantation (in combination with tacrolimus and corticosteroids)

Unlabeled Use Treatment of relapsed or refractory Waldenström's macroglobulinemia (WM); treatment of progressive advanced carcinoid tumors

Pregnancy Risk Factor D (Afinitor) / C (Zortress)

Pregnancy Considerations Embryotoxicity, fetotoxicity, malformations, and growth retardation were observed in animal reproduction studies with exposures lower than expected with human doses. Based on the mechanism of action, may cause fetal harm if administered during pregnancy. Women of childbearing potential should be advised to avoid pregnancy. Women of childbearing potential should use highly effective birth control during treatment, and continue for 8 weeks after everolimus discontinuation.

Breast-Feeding Considerations It is not known if everolimus is excreted in breast milk. Due to the potential for serious adverse reactions in the nursing infant, breast-feeding should be avoided.

Medication Guide Available Yes

Contraindications Hypersensitivity to everolimus, sirolimus, other rapamycin derivatives, or any component of the formulation.

Warnings/Precautions Hazardous agent - use appropriate precautions for handling and disposal (NIOSH, 2012). Noninfectious pneumonitis (sometimes fatal) has been observed with mTOR inhibitors including everolimus; symptoms include dyspnea, cough, hypoxia and/or pleural effusion; promptly evaluate worsening respiratory symptoms; may require treatment interruption followed by dose reduction (pneumonitis has developed even with reduced doses) and/or corticosteroid therapy; discontinue for grade 4 symptoms. Imaging may overestimate the incidence of clinical pneumonitis. **[U.S. Boxed Warning]: Everolimus has immunosuppressant properties which may result**

in infection; the risk of developing bacterial (including mycobacterial), viral, fungal and protozoal infections and for local, opportunistic (including polyomavirus infection), systemic infections, and/or sepsis is increased. Polyomavirus infection in transplant patients may be serious and/or fatal. Polyoma virus-associated nephropathy (due to BK virus), which may result in serious cases of deteriorating renal function and renal graft loss, has been observed with use. JC virus-associated progressive multiple leukoencephalopathy (PML) may also be associated with everolimus use in transplantation. Reduced immunosuppression (taking into account the risks of rejection) should be considered with evidence of polyoma virus infection or PML. Reactivation of hepatitis B has been observed in patients receiving everolimus. Resolve pre-existing invasive fungal infections prior to treatment initiation. Transplant recipient patients should receive prophylactic therapy for pneumocystis jiroveci pneumonia (PCP) and for cytomegalovirus (CMV). Monitor for signs and symptoms of infection during treatment. Discontinue if invasive systemic fungal infection is diagnosed (and manage with appropriate antifungal therapy).

[U.S. Boxed Warning]: Immunosuppressant use may result in the development of malignancy, including lymphoma and skin cancer. The risk is associated with treatment intensity and the duration of therapy. To minimize the risk for skin cancer, limit exposure to sunlight and ultraviolet light; wear protective clothing and use effective sunscreen.

[U.S. Boxed Warning]: Due to the increased risk for nephrotoxicity in renal transplantation, avoid standard doses of cyclosporine in combination with everolimus; reduced cyclosporine doses are recommended when everolimus is used in combination with cyclosporine. Therapeutic monitoring of cyclosporine and everolimus concentrations is recommended. Monitor for proteinuria; the risk of proteinuria is increased when everolimus is used in combination with cyclosporine, and with higher serum everolimus concentrations. Everolimus and cyclosporine combination therapy may increase the risk for thrombotic microangiopathy/thrombotic thrombocytopenic purpura/hemolytic uremic syndrome (TMA/TTP/HUS); monitor blood counts. Elevations in serum creatinine (generally mild), renal failure, and proteinuria have been also observed with everolimus use; monitor renal function (BUN, creatinine, and/or urinary protein). Risk of nephrotoxicity may be increased when administered with calcineurin inhibitors (eg, cyclosporine, tacrolimus); dosage adjustment of calcineurin inhibitor is necessary. An increased incidence of rash, infection and dose interruptions have been reported in patients with renal insufficiency (Cl_{cr} ≤60 mL/minute) who received mTOR inhibitors for the treatment of renal cell cancer (Gupta, 2011); pharmacokinetic studies have not been conducted; dosage adjustments are not required based on renal impairment. **[U.S. Boxed Warning]: An increased risk of renal arterial and venous thrombosis has been reported with use in renal transplantation, generally within the first 30 days after transplant; may result in graft loss.** MTOR inhibitors are associated with an increase in hepatic artery thrombosis, most cases have been reported within 30 days after transplant and usually proceeded to graft loss or death; do not use everolimus prior to 30 days post liver transplant.

Potentially significant drug-drug/drug-food interactions may exist, requiring dose or frequency adjustment, additional monitoring, and/or selection of alternative therapy. In transplant patients, avoid the use of certain HMG-CoA reductase inhibitors (eg, simvastatin, lovastatin); may increase the risk for rhabdomyolysis due to the potential interaction with cyclosporine (which may be given in combination with everolimus for transplantation).

Use is associated with mouth ulcers, mucositis and stomatitis; manage with topical therapy; avoid the use of alcohol-, peroxide-, iodine-, or thyme-based mouthwashes (due to the high potential for drug interactions, avoid the use of systemic antifungals unless fungal infection has been diagnosed). Everolimus is associated with the development of angioedema; concomitant use with other agents known to cause angioedema (eg, ACE inhibitors) may increase the risk. Everolimus use may delay wound healing and increase the occurrence of wound-related complications (eg, wound dehiscence, infection, incisional hernia, lymphocele, seroma); may require surgical intervention. Generalized edema, including peripheral edema and lymphedema, and local fluid accumulation (eg, pericardial effusion, pleural effusion, ascites) may also occur.

Everolimus exposure is increased in patients with hepatic impairment. For patients with breast cancer, PNET, RCC, or renal angiomyolipoma with mild and moderate hepatic impairment, reduced doses are recommended; in patients with severe hepatic impairment, use is recommended (at reduced doses) if the potential benefit outweighs risks. Reduced doses are recommended in transplant patients with hepatic impairment; pharmacokinetic information does not exist for renal transplant patients with severe impairment (Child-Pugh class B or C); monitor whole blood trough levels closely for patients with SEGA, reduced doses may be needed for mild and moderate hepatic impairment (based on therapeutic drug monitoring), and are recommended in severe hepatic impairment; monitor whole blood trough levels. The Canadian labeling recommends against the use of everolimus in patients <18 years of age with SEGA and hepatic impairment.

[U.S. Boxed Warning]: Increased mortality (usually associated with infections) within the first 3 months after transplant was noted in a study of patients with *de novo* heart transplant receiving immunosuppressive regimens containing everolimus (with or without induction therapy). Use in heart transplantation is not recommended. Use with caution in patients with hyperlipidemia; may increase serum lipids (cholesterol and triglycerides); higher serum concentrations are associated with an increased risk for hyperlipidemia; use has not been studied in patients with baseline cholesterol >350 mg/dL; antihyperlipidemic therapy may not normalize levels. Decreases in hemoglobin, neutrophils, platelets, and lymphocytes have been reported with use. Increases in serum glucose are common; may alter insulin and/or oral hypoglycemic therapy requirements in patients with diabetes; the risk for new onset diabetes is increased with everolimus use after transplantation; achieve optimal glucose levels prior to treatment. Patients should not be immunized with live viral vaccines during or shortly after treatment and should avoid close contact with recently vaccinated (live vaccine) individuals; consider the timing of routine immunizations prior to the start of therapy in pediatric patients treated for SEGA. Continue treatment with everolimus for renal cell cancer as long as clinical benefit is demonstrated or until occurrence of unacceptable toxicity. Safety and efficacy have not been established for the use of everolimus in the treatment of carcinoid tumors. Decreases in hemoglobin, neutrophils, platelets, and lymphocytes have been reported with use. Increases in serum glucose are common; may alter insulin and/or oral hypoglycemic therapy requirements in patients with diabetes; the risk for new onset diabetes is increased with everolimus use after transplantation. Patients should not be immunized with live viral vaccines during or shortly after treatment and should avoid close contact with recently vaccinated (live vaccine) individuals. In pediatric patients treated for SEGA, complete recommended series of live virus childhood vaccinations prior to treatment (if immediate everolimus treatment is not indicated); an accelerated vaccination schedule may be appropriate. Continue treatment with everolimus for renal cell cancer as long as clinical benefit is demonstrated or until occurrence of unacceptable toxicity.

Tablets (Afinitor®, Zortress®) and tablets for oral suspension (Afinitor® Disperz) are not interchangeable; Afinitor® Disperz is only indicated in conjunction with therapeutic monitoring for the treatment of SEGA. Do not combine formulations to achieve desired dose. Azoospermia and oligospermia have been observed in males. Avoid use in patients with hereditary galactose intolerance, Lapp lactase deficiency, or glucose-galactose malabsorption; may result in diarrhea and malabsorption. The safety and efficacy of everolimus in renal transplantation patients with high-immunologic risk or in solid organ transplant other than renal or liver have not been established. **[U.S. Boxed Warning]: In transplantation, everolimus should only be used by physicians experienced in immunosuppressive therapy and management of transplant patients. Adequate laboratory and supportive medical resources must be readily available.** For indications requiring whole blood trough concentrations to determine dosage adjustments, a consistent method should be used; concentration values from different assay methods may not be interchangeable.

Adverse Reactions

>10%:

Cardiovascular: Peripheral edema (4% to 45%), hypertension (4% to 30%; hypertensive crisis: 1%)

Central nervous system: Fatigue (7% to 45%), fever (13% to 32%), headache (18% to 30%), seizure (5% to 29%), behavioral changes (anxiety/aggression/behavioral disturbance; SEGA: 21%), insomnia (6% to 17%), dizziness (7% to 14%)

Dermatologic: Skin rash (18% to 59%), cellulitis (SEGA: 29%), acneiform eruption (3% to 25%), nail disease (including onychoclasis, 4% to 22%), acne vulgaris (3% to 22%), pruritus (13% to 21%), xeroderma (9% to 18%), contact dermatitis (14%), excoriation (14%)

Endocrine & metabolic: Hypercholesterolemia (17% to 85%), hyperglycemia (12% to 75%; grades 3/4: <1% to 17%), hypertriglyceridemia (≤73%), decreased serum bicarbonate (≤56%), hypophosphatemia (9% to 49%), hypocalcemia (17% to 37%), decreased serum albumin (≤33%), diabetes mellitus ([new onset] <10%; liver transplant: 32%), hypoglycemia (≤32%), hypokalemia (12% to 29%), hyperlipidemia (renal, liver transplant: 21% to 24%), hyperkalemia (renal transplant: 18%), amenorrhea (≤17%), hyponatremia (≤16%), lipid metabolism disorder (renal transplant: 15%), hypomagnesemia (renal transplant: 14%)

Gastrointestinal: Stomatitis (oncology uses: 44% to 86%; grade 3: 4% to 9%; grade 4: <1%; renal transplant: 8%), diarrhea (14% to 50%; grade 3: ≤5%; grade 4: <1%), constipation (10% to 38%), abdominal pain (3% to 36%), nausea (8% to 32%; grade 3: ≤2%; grade 4: <1%), decreased appetite (6% to 30%), anorexia (1% to 30%), vomiting (15% to 29%; grade 3: ≤2%; grade 4: <1%), weight loss (9% to 28%), dysgeusia (1% to 22%), gastroenteritis (1% to 18%), xerostomia (8% to 11%)

Genitourinary: Urinary tract infection (5% to 22%), hematuria (renal transplant: 12%), dysuria (renal transplant: 11%)

Hematologic & oncologic: Anemia (26% to 92%; grades 3/4: ≤15%; grade 4: <1%), prolonged partial thromboplastin time (SEGA: 72%), leukopenia (oncology uses: 26% to 58%; renal, liver transplant: 3% to 12%), lymphocytopenia (20% to 54%; grades 3/4: ≤18%), thrombocytopenia (oncology uses: 19% to 54%; grade 3: ≤3%; renal transplant: <10%), neutropenia (≤46%; grades 3/4: ≤9%)

Hepatic: Increased serum AST (23% to 89%; grade 3: ≤4%; grade 4: <1%), increased serum alkaline phosphatase (oncology uses: 32% to 74%; renal, liver transplant: <10%), increased serum ALT (18% to 51%; grade 3: ≤4%; grade 4: 1%)

Infection: Infection (13% to 62%; grade 3: 4% to 7%; grade 4: 1% to 3%)

Neuromuscular & skeletal: Weakness (13% to 33%), arthralgia (≤20%), back pain (11% to 15%), limb pain (8% to 14%)

Otic: Otitis (6% to 36%)

Renal: Increased serum creatinine (11% to 50%)

Respiratory: Upper respiratory tract infection (11% to 82%), sinusitis (3% to 39%), cough (7% to 30%), dyspnea (20% to 24%; grade 3: 2% to 6%; grade 4: ≤1%), epistaxis (≤22%), pneumonitis (including alveolitis, interstitial lung disease, lung infiltrate, pulmonary alveolar hemorrhage, pulmonary toxicity, 1% to 19%; grade 3: 3% to 4%; grade 4: <1%), nasal congestion (14%), rhinitis (14%), pharyngitis (4% to 11%)

Miscellaneous: Wound healing impairment (liver transplant: 11%; oncology uses: <1%)

1% to 10%:

Cardiovascular: Chest pain (5%), tachycardia (3%), cardiac failure (1%), angina pectoris, atrial fibrillation, chest discomfort, deep vein thrombosis, edema (generalized), hypotension, palpitations, syncope, venous thromboembolism

Central nervous system: Depression (5%), migraine (5%), paresthesia (5%), chills (4%), agitation, drowsiness, hallucination, hemiparesis, hypoesthesia, lethargy, malaise, neuralgia

Dermatologic: Eczema (10%), alopecia (≤10%), palmar-plantar erythrodysesthesia ([hand-foot syndrome] 5%), papule (5%), erythema (4%), pityriasis rosea (4%), skin lesion (4%), hirsutism, hyperhidrosis, hypertrichosis

Endocrine & metabolic: Hypermenorrhea (6% to 10%), menstrual disease (6% to 10%), dysmenorrhea (6%), irregular menses (6%), exacerbation of diabetes mellitus (2%), cushingoid appearance, cyanocobalamin deficiency, dehydration, gout, hypercalcemia, hyperparathyroidism, hyperphosphatemia, hyperuricemia, iron deficiency, ovarian cyst, scrotal edema

Gastrointestinal: Gastritis (7%), hemorrhoids (5%), dyspepsia (4%), dysphagia (4%), ageusia (1%), abdominal distention, epigastric distress, flatulence, gastroesophageal reflux disease, gingival hyperplasia, hematemesis, intestinal obstruction, oral herpes

Genitourinary: Vaginal hemorrhage (8%), bladder spasm, erectile dysfunction, pollakiuria, pyuria, urinary retention, urinary urgency

Hematologic & oncologic: Neoplasm (liver transplant: 4%), hemorrhage (3%), leukocytosis, lymphadenopathy, pancytopenia (renal, liver transplant)

Hepatic: Increased serum bilirubin (3% to 10%; grades 3/4: ≤1%), abnormal hepatic function tests (liver transplant: 7%), ascites (liver transplant: 4%), increased serum transaminases

Hypersensitivity: Hypersensitivity (including anaphylaxis, dyspnea, flushing, chest pain, angioedema, 3%)

Infection: BK virus infection, candidiasis, herpes infection, sepsis

Neuromuscular & skeletal: Muscle spasm (≤10%), tremor (8% to 9%), jaw pain (3%), joint swelling, musculoskeletal pain, myalgia, osteonecrosis, osteopenia, osteoporosis, spondylitis

Ophthalmic: Eyelid edema (4%), ocular hyperemia (4%), conjunctivitis (2%), blurred vision, cataract

Renal: Renal failure (3%), hydronephrosis, increased blood urea nitrogen, interstitial nephritis, polyuria, proteinuria, renal artery thrombosis, renal insufficiency

Respiratory: Pleural effusion (5% to 7%), nasopharyngitis (6%), pneumonia (6%), bronchitis (4%), pharyngolaryngeal pain (4%), rhinorrhea (3%), atelectasis, lower respiratory tract infection, oropharyngeal pain, pulmonary edema, pulmonary embolism, sinus congestion, wheezing

Miscellaneous: Night sweats, peritonitis, postoperative wound complication (including incisional hernia)

<1% (Limited to important or life-threatening): Aspergillosis, azoospermia, cardiac arrest, decreased plasma testosterone, fluid retention, hepatic artery thrombosis, hepatitis B reactivation, influenza, intrahepatic cholestasis, malignant lymphoma, oligospermia, pancreatitis, progressive multifocal leukoencephalopathy, pulmonary embolism, respiratory distress, skin neoplasm, synovitis (severe), thrombosis of vascular graft, thrombotic microangiopathy/thrombotic thrombocytopenic purpura/hemolytic uremic syndrome (TMA/TTP/HUS)

Drug Interactions

Metabolism/Transport Effects Substrate of CYP3A4 (major), P-glycoprotein; **Note:** Assignment of Major/Minor substrate status based on clinically relevant drug interaction potential

Avoid Concomitant Use

Avoid concomitant use of Everolimus with any of the following: BCG; CloZAPine; CYP3A4 Inducers (Strong); CYP3A4 Inhibitors (Strong); Fusidic Acid (Systemic); Grapefruit Juice; Natalizumab; Pimecrolimus; St Johns Wort; Tacrolimus (Topical); Tofacitinib; Vaccines (Live)

Increased Effect/Toxicity

Everolimus may increase the levels/effects of: ACE Inhibitors; CloZAPine; Leflunomide; Natalizumab; Tofacitinib; Vaccines (Live)

The levels/effects of Everolimus may be increased by: CycloSPORINE (Systemic); CYP3A4 Inhibitors (Moderate); CYP3A4 Inhibitors (Strong); Dasatinib; Denosumab; Fusidic Acid (Systemic); Grapefruit Juice; Ivacaftor; Luliconazole; Mifepristone; P-glycoprotein/ABCB1 Inhibitors; Pimecrolimus; Roflumilast; Simeprevir; Tacrolimus (Topical); Trastuzumab

Decreased Effect

Everolimus may decrease the levels/effects of: BCG; Coccidioidin Skin Test; Sipuleucel-T; Vaccines (Inactivated); Vaccines (Live)

The levels/effects of Everolimus may be decreased by: Bosentan; CYP3A4 Inducers (Strong); Dabrafenib; Deferasirox; Echinacea; Efavirenz; P-glycoprotein/ABCB1 Inducers; St Johns Wort; Tocilizumab

Ethanol/Nutrition/Herb Interactions

Food: Grapefruit juice may increase levels of everolimus. Absorption with food may be variable. Management: Avoid grapefruit juice. Take with or without food, but be consistent with regard to food.

Herb/Nutraceutical: St John's wort may decrease the levels of everolimus. Management: Avoid St John's wort.

Storage/Stability Tablets and tablets for suspension: Store at room temperature of 25°C (77°F); excursions permitted to 15°C to 30°C (59°F to 86°F). Protect from light; protect from moisture.

Mechanism of Action Everolimus is a macrolide immunosuppressant and an m-TOR inhibitor which has antiproliferative and antiangiogenic properties, and also reduces lipoma volume in patients with angiomyolipoma. Reduces protein synthesis and cell proliferation by binding to the FK binding protein-12 (FKBP-12), an intracellular protein, to form a complex that inhibits activation of mTOR (mammalian target of rapamycin) serine-threonine kinase activity. Also reduces angiogenesis by inhibiting vascular endothelial growth factor (VEGF) and hypoxia-inducible factor (HIF-1) expression. Angiomyolipomas may occur due to unregulated mTOR activity in TSC-associated renal angiomyolipoma (Budde, 2012); everolimus reduces lipoma volume (Bissler, 2012).

Pharmacodynamics/Kinetics

Absorption: Rapid, but moderate

Protein binding: ~74%

Metabolism: Extensively metabolized in the liver via CYP3A4; forms 6 weak metabolites

Bioavailability:

Tablets: ~30%; systemic exposure reduced by 22% with a high-fat meal and by 32% with a light-fat meal

Tablets for suspension: AUC equivalent to tablets although peak concentrations are 20% to 36% lower; steady state concentrations are similar

Half-life elimination: ~30 hours

Time to peak, plasma: 1-2 hours

Excretion: Feces (80%, based on solid organ transplant studies); Urine (~5%, based on solid organ transplant studies)

Dosage Note: Tablets (Afinitor, Zortress) and tablets for oral suspension (Afinitor Disperz) are not interchangeable; Afinitor Disperz is only indicated for the treatment of subependymal giant cell astrocytoma (SEGA), in conjunction with therapeutic monitoring. Do not combine formulations to achieve desired dose.

Breast cancer, advanced, hormone receptor-positive, HER2-negative: Adults: Oral: 10 mg once daily (in combination with exemestane), continue treatment until no longer clinically beneficial or until unacceptable toxicity

Liver transplantation, rejection prophylaxis (begin at least 30 days post-transplant): Adults: Oral: Initial: 1 mg twice daily; adjust maintenance dose if needed at a 4- to 5-day interval (from prior dose adjustment) based on serum concentrations, tolerability, and response; goal serum concentration is between 3 and 8 ng/mL (based on an LC/MS/MS assay method); administer in combination with tacrolimus (reduced dose required) and corticosteroids

Pancreatic neuroendocrine tumors (PNET), advanced: Adults: Oral: 10 mg once daily, continue treatment until no longer clinically beneficial or until unacceptable toxicity

Renal angiomyolipoma: Adults: Oral: 10 mg once daily, continue treatment until no longer clinically beneficial or until unacceptable toxicity

Renal cell cancer (RCC), advanced: Adults: Oral: 10 mg once daily, continue treatment until no longer clinically beneficial or until unacceptable toxicity

Renal transplantation, rejection prophylaxis: Adults: Oral: Initial: 0.75 mg twice daily; adjust maintenance dose if needed at a 4- to 5-day interval (from prior dose adjustment) based on serum concentrations, tolerability, and response; goal serum concentration is between 3 and 8 ng/mL (based on an LC/MS/MS assay method); administer in combination with basiliximab induction and concurrently with cyclosporine (dose adjustment required) and corticosteroids

Subependymal giant cell astrocytoma (SEGA; dosing based on body surface area [BSA]): Children ≥1 year (U.S. labeling) or ≥3 years (Canadian labeling) and Adults: Oral:

U.S. labeling: Initial dose: 4.5 mg/m^2 once daily; round to nearest tablet (tablet or tablet for oral suspension) size.

Canadian labeling: Initial dose:

0.5-1.2 m^2: 2.5 mg once daily

1.3-2.1 m^2: 5 mg once daily

≥2.2 m^2: 7.5 mg once daily

Assess whole blood trough concentrations ~2 weeks after everolimus initiation or with dosage modifications, initiation or changes to concurrent CYP3A4 inhibitor/inducer therapy, changes in hepatic impairment, and when changing dosage forms between Afinitor tablets and Afinitor Disperz; adjust maintenance dose if needed at 2-week intervals to achieve and maintain trough concentrations between 5 and 15 ng/mL; monitor trough concentrations routinely; once stable dose is attained and if BSA is stable throughout treatment, monitor trough concentrations every 6-12 months; monitor every 3-6 months if BSA is changing. Continue until disease progression or unacceptable toxicity.

If trough <5 ng/mL: Increase dose by 2.5 mg/day (tablets) or 2 mg/day (tablets for oral suspension)

If trough >15 ng/mL: Reduce dose by 2.5 mg/day (tablets) or 2 mg/day (tablets for oral suspension)

If dose reduction necessary in patients receiving the lowest strength available, administer every other day.

Carcinoid tumors, advanced (unlabeled use): Adults: Oral:10 mg once daily (in combination with octreotide LAR) until disease progression or toxicity (Pavel, 2011)

Waldenström's macroglobulinemia, relapsed or refractory (unlabeled use): Adults: Oral: 10 mg once daily until disease progression or toxicity (Ghobrial, 2010)

Dosage adjustment for toxicity:

Breast cancer (adjustments apply to everolimus), PNET, RCC, renal angiomyolipoma, SEGA: Reduce everolimus dose by ~50% if dosage adjustment is necessary:

Noninfectious pneumonitis:

Grade 1 (asymptomatic radiological changes suggestive of pneumonitis): No dosage adjustment necessary; monitor appropriately.

Grade 2 (symptomatic but not interfering with activities of daily living [ADL]): Consider interrupting treatment, rule out infection, and consider corticosteroids until symptoms improve to ≤grade 1; reinitiate at a lower dose. (Discontinue if recovery does not occur within 4 weeks.)

Grade 3 (symptomatic, interferes with ADL; oxygen indicated): Interrupt treatment until symptoms improve to ≤grade 1; rule out infection and consider corticosteroid treatment; may reinitiate at a lower dose. If grade 3 toxicity recurs, consider discontinuing.

Grade 4 (life-threatening; ventilatory support indicated): Discontinue treatment; rule out infection; consider corticosteroid treatment.

Stomatitis (avoid the use of products containing alcohol, hydrogen peroxide, iodine, or thyme derivatives):

Grade 1 (minimal symptoms, normal diet): No dosage adjustment necessary; manage with mouth wash (nonalcoholic or isotonic salt water) several times a day

Grade 2 (symptomatic but can eat and swallow modified diet): Interrupt treatment until symptoms improve to ≤grade 1; reinitiate at same dose; if stomatitis recurs at grade 2, interrupt treatment until symptoms improve to ≤grade 1 and then reinitiate at a lower dose. Also manage with topical (oral) analgesics (eg, benzocaine, butyl aminobenzoate, tetracaine, menthol, or phenol) ± topical (oral) corticosteroids (eg, triamcinolone).

Grade 3 (symptomatic and unable to orally aliment or hydrate adequately): Interrupt treatment until symptoms improve to ≤grade 1; then reinitiate at a lower dose. Also manage with topical (oral) analgesics (eg, benzocaine, butyl aminobenzoate, tetracaine, menthol, or phenol) ± topical (oral) corticosteroids (eg, triamcinolone).

Grade 4 (life-threatening symptoms): Discontinue treatment; initiate appropriate medical intervention.

Metabolic toxicity (eg, hyperglycemia, dyslipidemia):

Grade 1: No dosage adjustment necessary; initiate appropriate medical intervention and monitor.

Grade 2: No dosage adjustment necessary; manage with appropriate medical intervention and monitor.

Grade 3: Temporarily interrupt treatment; reinitiate at a lower dose; manage with appropriate medical intervention and monitor.

Grade 4: Discontinue treatment; manage with appropriate medical intervention.

Nonhematologic toxicities (excluding pneumonitis, stomatitis, or metabolic toxicity):

Grade 1: If toxicity is tolerable, no dosage adjustment necessary; initiate appropriate medical intervention and monitor.

Grade 2: If toxicity is tolerable, no dosage adjustment necessary; initiate appropriate medical intervention and monitor. If toxicity becomes intolerable, temporarily interrupt treatment until improvement to ≤grade 1 and reinitiate at the same dose; if toxicity recurs at grade 2, temporarily interrupt treatment until improvement to ≤grade 1 and then reinitiate at a lower dose.

Grade 3: Temporarily interrupt treatment until improvement to ≤grade 1; initiate appropriate medical intervention and monitor. May reinitiate at a lower dose; if toxicity recurs at grade 3, consider discontinuing.

Grade 4 (life-threatening symptoms): Discontinue treatment; initiate appropriate medical intervention.

Liver or renal transplantation:

Evidence of polyoma virus infection or PML: Consider reduced immunosuppression (taking into account the allograft risks associated with decreased immunosuppression)

Pneumonitis (grade 4 symptoms) or invasive systemic fungal infection: Discontinue

SEGA: *Other severe/intolerable adverse reactions:* Temporarily reduce dose (by ~50% from prior dose) and/or temporarily interrupt treatment; if dose reduction is required for patients receiving the lowest available strength, consider alternate day dosing.

Dosage adjustment for concomitant CYP3A4 inhibitors/inducers and/or P-gp inhibitors:

Breast cancer, PNET, RCC, renal angiomyolipoma:

CYP3A4 inducers: Strong inducers: Avoid concomitant administration with strong CYP3A4 inducers; if concomitant use cannot be avoided, consider adjusting everolimus dose upward in 5 mg increments up to 20 mg daily, with careful monitoring. If the strong CYP3A4 enzyme inducer is discontinued, reduce the everolimus to the recommended starting dose or to the dose used prior to initiation of the CYP3A4 inducer.

CYP3A4 or P-gp inhibitors:

Strong inhibitors: Avoid concomitant administration with strong CYP3A4 inhibitors.

Moderate CYP3A4 and/or P-gp inhibitors:

U.S. labeling: Reduce everolimus dose to 2.5 mg once daily; may consider increasing from 2.5 mg to 5 mg once daily based on patient tolerance. When the moderate inhibitor is discontinued, allow ~2-3 days to elapse prior to adjusting the everolimus upward to the recommended starting dose or to the dose used prior to initiation of the moderate inhibitor.

Canadian labeling: Reduce everolimus dose by 50%; further reductions may be necessary for adverse reactions. If dose reduction is required for patients receiving the lowest available strength, consider alternate day dosing.

Renal transplantation: Dosage adjustments may be necessary based on everolimus serum concentrations

SEGA:

CYP3A4 inducers: Strong inducers:

U.S. labeling: Avoid concomitant administration with strong CYP3A4 inducers; if concomitant use cannot be avoided, an initial starting everolimus dose of 9 mg/m^2 once daily is recommended, or, double the everolimus dose; individualize subsequent dose adjustments based on therapeutic drug monitoring. If the strong CYP3A4 enzyme inducer is discontinued, reduce the everolimus dose by ~50% or to the dose used prior to initiation of the CYP3A4 inducer; reassess trough concentration after ~2 weeks.

Canadian labeling: Avoid concomitant administration with strong CYP3A4 inducers; if concomitant use cannot be avoided and everolimus level <5 ng/mL, may increase daily dose by 2.5 mg every two weeks until target everolimus trough concentration is 5-10 ng/mL. Evaluate trough concentration and tolerability prior to each dosage adjustment. If the strong CYP3A4 enzyme inducer is discontinued, reduce everolimus to the dose used prior to initiation of the CYP3A4 inducer; reassess trough concentration after ~2 weeks.

CYP3A4 or P-gp inhibitors:

Strong inhibitors: Avoid concomitant administration with strong CYP3A4 inhibitors.

Moderate CYP3A4 and/or P-gp inhibitors: Initial everolimus dose:

U.S. labeling: 2.5 mg/m^2 once daily or reduce everolimus dose by ~50% (if dose reduction is required for patients receiving the lowest strength available, consider alternate day dosing)

Canadian labeling: Reduce everolimus dose by ~50% (if dose reduction is required for patients receiving the lowest strength available, consider alternate day dosing)

Assess trough concentrations after ~2 weeks; individualize dosing based on therapeutic drug monitoring. If the moderate inhibitor is discontinued, allow 2-3 days to elapse prior to adjusting the everolimus upward by ~50% or to the dose used prior to initiation of the moderate inhibitor; reassess trough concentrations after ~2 weeks.

Dosage adjustment in renal impairment: No dosage adjustment necessary.

Dosage adjustment in hepatic impairment:

Mild impairment (Child-Pugh class A):

Breast cancer, PNET, RCC, renal angiomyolipoma: Reduce dose to 7.5 mg once daily; if not tolerated, may further reduce to 5 mg once daily.

Liver or renal transplantation: Reduce initial dose by ~33%; individualize subsequent dosing based on therapeutic drug monitoring (target trough concentration: 3-8 ng/mL).

SEGA:

U.S. labeling: Adjustment to initial dose may not be necessary; subsequent dosing is based on therapeutic drug monitoring (monitor ~2 weeks after initiation, dosage modifications, or after any change in hepatic status; target trough concentration: 5-15 ng/mL).

Canadian labeling: Initial:

Patients ≥18 years of age: 75% of usual dose based on calculated BSA (rounded to the nearest strength)

Patients <18 years of age: Use is not recommended.

Moderate impairment (Child-Pugh class B):

Breast cancer, PNET, RCC, renal angiomyolipoma: Reduce dose to 5 mg once daily; if not tolerated, may further reduce to 2.5 mg once daily.

Liver or renal transplantation: Reduce initial dose by ~50%; individualize subsequent dosing based on therapeutic drug monitoring (target trough concentration: 3-8 ng/mL).

SEGA:

U.S. labeling: Adjustment to initial dose may not be necessary; subsequent dosing is based on therapeutic drug monitoring (monitor ~2 weeks after initiation, dosage modifications, or after any change in hepatic status; target trough concentration: 5-15 ng/mL).

Canadian labeling: Initial:

Patients ≥18 years of age: 50% of usual dose based on calculated BSA (rounded to the nearest strength)

Patients <18 years of age: Use is not recommended

Severe impairment (Child-Pugh class C):

Breast cancer, PNET, RCC, renal angiomyolipoma: If potential benefit outweighs risks, a maximum dose of 2.5 mg once daily may be used.

Liver or renal transplantation: Reduce initial dose by ~50%; individualize subsequent dosing based on therapeutic drug monitoring (target trough concentration: 3-8 ng/mL).

SEGA:

U.S. labeling: Reduce initial dose to 2.5 mg/m^2 once daily (or current dose by ~50%); subsequent dosing is based on therapeutic drug monitoring

Canadian labeling: Use is not recommended.

Dietary Considerations Avoid grapefruit juice. May be taken with or without food, although should be administered consistently with regard to food.

Administration May be taken with or without food; to reduce variability, take consistently with regard to food. Afinitor missed doses may be taken up to 6 hours after regularly scheduled time; if >6 hours, resume at next regularly scheduled time.

Tablets: Swallow whole with a glass of water. Do not break, chew, or crush (do not administer tablets that are crushed or broken). Avoid contact with or exposure to crushed or broken tablets.

Tablets for oral suspension: Administer as a suspension only. Administer immediately after preparation; discard if not administered within 60 minutes after preparation. Prepare suspension in water only. Do not break or crush tablets.

Preparation in an oral syringe: Place dose into 10 mL oral syringe (maximum: 10 mg/syringe; use an additional syringe for doses >10 mg). Draw ~5 mL of water and ~4 mL of air into oral syringe; allow to sit (tip up) in a container until tablets are in suspension (3 minutes). Gently invert syringe 5 times immediately prior to administration; administer contents, then add ~5 mL water and ~4 mL of air to same syringe, swirl to suspend remaining particles and administer entire contents.

Preparation in a small glass: Place dose into a small glass (≤100 mL) containing ~25 mL water (maximum 10 mg/glass; use and additional glass for doses >10 mg); allow to sit until tablets are in suspension (3 minutes). Stir gently with spoon immediately prior to administration; administer contents, then add ~25 mL water to same glass, swirl with same spoon to suspend remaining particles and administer entire contents.

Breast cancer, pancreatic neuroendocrine tumors, renal cell cancer, renal angiolipoma, SEGA: Administer at the same time each day.

Liver transplantation: Administer consistently ~12 hours apart; administer at the same time as tacrolimus.
Renal transplantation: Administer consistently ~12 hours apart; administer at the same time as cyclosporine.

Hazardous agent; use appropriate precautions for handling and disposal (NIOSH, 2012).

Monitoring Parameters CBC with differential (baseline and periodic), liver function; serum creatinine, urinary protein, and BUN (baseline and periodic); fasting serum glucose and lipid profile (baseline and periodic); monitor for signs and symptoms of infection, noninfectious pneumonitis, or malignancy

For liver or renal transplantation, monitor everolimus whole blood trough concentrations (based on an LC/MS/MS assay method), especially in patients with hepatic impairment, with concomitant CYP3A4 inhibitors and inducers, and when cyclosporine formulations or doses are changed; dosage adjustments should be made on trough concentrations obtained 4-5 days after a previous dosage adjustment; monitor cyclosporine concentrations; monitor for proteinuria

For SEGA, monitor everolimus whole blood trough concentrations ~2 weeks after treatment initiation, 2 weeks after dose modifications after initiation or dose modification of concomitant CYP3A4 and/or P-gp inducers or inhibitors, changes in hepatic function and when changing dosage forms between Afinitor tablets and Afinitor Disperz.

Reference Range Recommended range for everolimus whole blood trough concentrations:
Liver and renal transplantation: 3-8 ng/mL (based on an LCMSMS assay method)
Subependymal giant cell astrocytoma (SEGA): 5-15 ng/mL (high concentrations may be associated with larger reductions in SEGA volumes, responses have been observed at concentrations as low as 5 ng/mL)

Dosage Forms Excipient information presented when available (limited, particularly for generics); consult specific product labeling.
Tablet, Oral:
Afinitor: 2.5 mg, 5 mg, 7.5 mg, 10 mg
Zortress: 0.25 mg, 0.5 mg, 0.75 mg
Tablet Soluble, Oral:
Afinitor Disperz: 2 mg, 3 mg, 5 mg

Dosage Forms: Canada Excipient information presented when available (limited, particularly for generics); consult specific product labeling.
Tablet, Oral:
Afinitor: 2.5 mg, 5 mg, 10 mg

Extemporaneous Preparations
Hazardous agent: Use appropriate precautions for handling and disposal.

Tablets: An oral liquid may be prepared using tablets. Disperse tablet in ~30 mL (1 oz) of water; gently stir. Administer and rinse container with additional 30 mL (1 oz) water and administer to ensure entire dose is administered. Administer immediately after preparation.

Afinitor® prescribing information, East Hanover, NJ: Novartis Pharmaceuticals Corporation, July 2012.

Tablets for oral suspension: Administer as a suspension only. Administer immediately after preparation; discard if not administered within 60 minutes after preparation. Prepare suspension in water only. Do not break or crush tablets.

Preparation in an oral syringe: Place dose into 10 mL oral syringe (maximum 10 mg/syringe; use an additional syringe for doses >10 mg). Draw ~5 mL of water and ~4 mL of air into oral syringe; allow to sit (tip up) in a container until tablets are in suspension (3 minutes). Gently invert syringe 5 times immediately prior to administration; administer contents, then add ~5 mL water and ~4 mL of air to same syringe, swirl to suspend remaining particles and administer entire contents.

Preparation in a small glass: Place dose into a small glass (≤100 mL) containing ~25 mL water (maximum 10 mg/glass; use an additional glass for doses >10 mg); allow to sit until tablets are in suspension (3 minutes). Stir gently with spoon immediately prior to administration; administer contents, then add ~25 mL water to same glass, swirl with same spoon to suspend remaining particles and administer entire contents.

Administer immediately after preparation; discard if not administered within 60 minutes after preparation.

Afinitor® and Afinitor® Disperz prescribing information, East Hanover, NJ: Novartis Pharmaceuticals Corporation, August 2012

- ◆ **Everone® 200 (Can)** *see* Testosterone *on page 2026*
- ◆ **EVG/COBI/FTC/TDF** *see* Elvitegravir, Cobicistat, Emtricitabine, and Tenofovir *on page 696*
- ◆ **Evista** *see* Raloxifene *on page 1774*
- ◆ **Evista® (Can)** *see* Raloxifene *on page 1774*
- ◆ **Evoclin** *see* Clindamycin (Topical) *on page 454*
- ◆ **Evoxac** *see* Cevimeline *on page 400*
- ◆ **Evoxac® (Can)** *see* Cevimeline *on page 400*
- ◆ **Evra® (Can)** *see* Ethinyl Estradiol and Norelgestromin *on page 792*
- ◆ **Exactacain** *see* Benzocaine, Butamben, and Tetracaine *on page 242*
- ◆ **Exalgo** *see* HYDROmorphone *on page 1013*
- ◆ **Excedrin® Extra Strength [OTC]** *see* Acetaminophen, Aspirin, and Caffeine *on page 33*
- ◆ **Excedrin® Migraine [OTC]** *see* Acetaminophen, Aspirin, and Caffeine *on page 33*
- ◆ **Excedrin PM® [OTC]** *see* Acetaminophen and Diphenhydramine *on page 32*
- ◆ **Excedrin Tension Headache [OTC]** *see* Acetaminophen *on page 28*
- ◆ **ExeFen-DMX** *see* Guaifenesin, Pseudoephedrine, and Dextromethorphan *on page 979*
- ◆ **ExeFen-IR** *see* Guaifenesin and Pseudoephedrine *on page 978*
- ◆ **Exelderm** *see* Sulconazole *on page 1956*
- ◆ **Exelderm® (Can)** *see* Sulconazole *on page 1956*
- ◆ **Exelon** *see* Rivastigmine *on page 1841*

Exemestane (ex e MES tane)

Brand Names: U.S. Aromasin
Brand Names: Canada Aromasin®; CO Exemestane
Pharmacologic Category Antineoplastic Agent, Aromatase Inactivator
Use Treatment of advanced breast cancer in postmenopausal women whose disease has progressed following tamoxifen therapy; adjuvant treatment of postmenopausal estrogen receptor-positive early breast cancer following 2-3 years of tamoxifen (for a total of 5 years of adjuvant therapy)
Unlabeled Use Risk reduction for invasive breast cancer in postmenopausal women; treatment of endometrial cancer; treatment of uterine sarcoma
Pregnancy Risk Factor X
Pregnancy Considerations Adverse events were observed in animal reproduction studies. Exemestane is not indicated for use in premenopausal women and use during pregnancy is contraindicated. Based on the mechanism of action, exemestane is expected to cause fetal harm if administered to a pregnant woman.

Breast-Feeding Considerations Exemestane is indicated for use only in postmenopausal women. Due to the potential for serious adverse reactions in the nursing infant, the manufacturer recommends a decision be made whether to discontinue nursing or to discontinue the drug, taking into account the importance of treatment to the mother.

Contraindications Hypersensitivity to exemestane or any component of the formulation; use in women who are or may become pregnant; use in premenopausal women

Warnings/Precautions Hazardous agent - use appropriate precautions for handling and disposal (NIOSH, 2012). Due to decreased circulating estrogen levels, exemestane is associated with a reduction in bone mineral density; decreases (from baseline) in lumbar spine and femoral neck density have been observed. Due to high prevalence of vitamin D deficiency in women with breast cancer, assess 25-hydroxy vitamin D levels at baseline and supplement accordingly. Grade 3 or 4 lymphopenia has been observed with exemestane use, although most patients had pre-existing lower grade lymphopenia. Increases in bilirubin, alkaline phosphatase and serum creatinine have been observed. Not to be given with estrogen-containing agents. Dose adjustment recommended with concomitant CYP3A4 inducers.

Adverse Reactions

>10%:

Cardiovascular: Hypertension (5% to 15%)

Central nervous system: Fatigue (8% to 22%), insomnia (11% to 14%), pain (13%), headache (7% to 13%), depression (6% to 13%)

Dermatological: Hyperhidrosis (4% to 18%), alopecia (15%)

Endocrine & metabolic: Hot flashes (13% to 33%)

Gastrointestinal: Nausea (9% to 18%), abdominal pain (6% to 11%)

Hepatic: Alkaline phosphatase increased (14% to 15%)

Neuromuscular & skeletal: Arthralgia (15% to 29%)

1% to 10%:

Cardiovascular: Edema (6% to 7%); cardiac ischemic events (2%: MI, angina, myocardial ischemia); chest pain

Central nervous system: Dizziness (8% to 10%), anxiety (4% to 10%), fever (5%), confusion, hypoesthesia

Dermatologic: Dermatitis (8%), itching, rash

Endocrine & metabolic: Weight gain (8%)

Gastrointestinal: Diarrhea (4% to 10%), vomiting (7%), anorexia (6%), constipation (5%), appetite increased (3%), dyspepsia

Genitourinary: Urinary tract infection (2% to 5%)

Hepatic: Bilirubin increased (5% to 7%)

Neuromuscular & skeletal: Back pain (9%), limb pain (9%), myalgia (6%), osteoarthritis (6%), weakness (6%), osteoporosis (5%), pathological fracture (4%), paresthesia (3%), carpal tunnel syndrome (2%), cramps (2%)

Ocular: Visual disturbances (5%)

Renal: Creatinine increased (6%)

Respiratory: Dyspnea (10%), cough (6%), bronchitis, pharyngitis, rhinitis, sinusitis, upper respiratory infection

Miscellaneous: Flu-like syndrome (6%), lymphedema, infection

<1% (Limited to important or life-threatening): Cardiac failure, cholestatic hepatitis, endometrial hyperplasia, gastric ulcer, GGT increased, hepatitis, hypersensitivity, neuropathy, osteochondrosis, pruritus, thromboembolism, transaminases increased, trigger finger, urticaria, uterine polyps

A dose-dependent decrease in sex hormone-binding globulin has been observed with daily doses of ≥2.5 mg. Serum luteinizing hormone and follicle-stimulating hormone levels have increased with this medicine.

Drug Interactions

Metabolism/Transport Effects Substrate of CYP3A4 (major); **Note:** Assignment of Major/Minor substrate status based on clinically relevant drug interaction potential; **Induces** CYP3A4 (weak/moderate)

Avoid Concomitant Use

Avoid concomitant use of Exemestane with any of the following: Axitinib; Simeprevir

Increased Effect/Toxicity There are no known significant interactions involving an increase in effect.

Decreased Effect

Exemestane may decrease the levels/effects of: ARIPiprazole; Axitinib; Ibrutinib; Saxagliptin; Simeprevir

The levels/effects of Exemestane may be decreased by: Bosentan; CYP3A4 Inducers (Strong); Dabrafenib; Deferasirox; Herbs (CYP3A4 Inducers); Tocilizumab

Ethanol/Nutrition/Herb Interactions

Food: Plasma levels increased by 40% when exemestane was taken with a fatty meal.

Herb/Nutraceutical: St John's wort may decrease exemestane levels. Avoid black cohosh, dong quai in estrogen-dependent tumors.

Storage/Stability Store at 25°C (77°F); excursions permitted to 15°C to 30°C (59°F to 86°F).

Mechanism of Action Exemestane is an irreversible, steroidal aromatase inactivator. It is structurally related to androstenedione, and is converted to an intermediate that irreversibly blocks the active site of the aromatase enzyme, leading to inactivation ("suicide inhibition") and thus preventing conversion of androgens to estrogens in peripheral tissues. In postmenopausal breast cancers where growth is estrogen-dependent, this medicine will lower circulating estrogens.

Pharmacodynamics/Kinetics

Absorption: Rapid and moderate (~42%) following oral administration; absorption increases ~40% following high-fat meal

Distribution: Extensive into tissues

Protein binding: 90%, primarily to albumin and α_1-acid glycoprotein

Metabolism: Extensively hepatic; oxidation (CYP3A4) of methylene group, reduction of 17-keto group with formation of many secondary metabolites; metabolites are inactive

Half-life elimination: 24 hours

Time to peak: Women with breast cancer: 1.2 hours

Excretion: Urine (<1% as unchanged drug, 39% to 45% as metabolites); feces (36% to 48%)

Dosage Oral: Adults: Females: Postmenopausal:

Breast cancer, advanced: 25 mg once daily; continue until tumor progression

Breast cancer, early (adjuvant treatment): 25 mg once daily (following 2-3 years of tamoxifen therapy) for a total duration of 5 years of endocrine therapy (in the absence of recurrence or contralateral breast cancer)

Breast cancer, risk reduction (unlabeled use): 25 mg once daily for up to 5 years (Goss, 2011)

Dosage adjustment with CYP3A4 inducers: U.S. labeling: 50 mg once daily when used with potent inducers (eg, rifampin, phenytoin)

Dosing adjustment in renal impairment: No adjustment necessary (although the safety of chronic doses in patients with moderate-to-severe renal impairment has not been studied, dosage adjustment does not appear necessary).

Dosing adjustment in hepatic impairment: No adjustment necessary (although the safety of chronic doses in patients with moderate-to-severe hepatic impairment has not been studied, dosage adjustment does not appear necessary).

Dietary Considerations Take after a meal; patients on aromatase inhibitor therapy should receive vitamin D and calcium supplements.

Administration Administer after a meal.

Hazardous agent; use appropriate precautions for handling and disposal (NIOSH, 2012).

Monitoring Parameters 25-hydroxy vitamin D levels (at baseline); bone mineral density

Additional Information Oncology Comment: The American Society of Clinical Oncology (ASCO) guidelines for adjuvant endocrine therapy in postmenopausal women with HR-positive breast cancer (Burstein, 2010) recommend considering aromatase inhibitor (AI) therapy at some point in the treatment course (primary, sequentially, or extended). Optimal duration at this time is not known; however, treatment with an AI should not exceed 5 years in primary and extended therapies, and 2-3 years if followed by tamoxifen in sequential therapy (total of 5 years). If initial therapy with AI has been discontinued before the 5 years, consideration should be taken to receive tamoxifen for a total of 5 years. The optimal time to switch to an AI is also not known, but data supports switching after 2-3 years of tamoxifen (sequential) or after 5 years of tamoxifen (extended). If patient becomes intolerant or has poor adherence, consideration should be made to switch to another AI or initiate tamoxifen.

Dosage Forms Excipient information presented when available (limited, particularly for generics); consult specific product labeling.

Tablet, Oral:

Aromasin: 25 mg

Generic: 25 mg

Exenatide (ex EN a tide)

Brand Names: U.S. Bydureon; Byetta 10 MCG Pen; Byetta 5 MCG Pen

Brand Names: Canada Byetta®

Index Terms AC 2993; AC002993; Exendin-4; LY2148568

Pharmacologic Category Antidiabetic Agent, Glucagon-Like Peptide-1 (GLP-1) Receptor Agonist

Additional Appendix Information

Injectable Agents (Non-Insulin) for Type 2 Diabetes *on page 2302*

Use Treatment of type 2 diabetes mellitus (noninsulin dependent, NIDDM) to improve glycemic control

Pregnancy Risk Factor C

Pregnancy Considerations Adverse events were observed in some animal reproduction studies. Based on *in vitro* data, exenatide has a low potential to cross the placenta (Hiles, 2003). For women with diabetes, maternal hyperglycemia can be associated with adverse effects in the fetus, neonate, and mother. To prevent adverse events, prior to conception and throughout pregnancy, the maternal Hb A_{1c} should be kept close to normal but without causing significant hypoglycemia. The use of GLP-1 receptor agonists in pregnant women is not recommended; insulin is the drug of choice for the control of diabetes mellitus during pregnancy (ACOG, 2005; ADA, 2013; Kitzmiller, 2008; Metzger, 2007).

Breast-Feeding Considerations It is not known if exenatide is present in breast milk. According to the manufacturer, the decision to continue or discontinue breast-feeding during therapy should take into account the risk of exposure to the infant and the benefits of treatment to the mother; use caution if administering exenatide to nursing women.

Medication Guide Available Yes

Contraindications Hypersensitivity to exenatide or any component of the formulation

Bydureon™: Additional contraindications: History of or family history of medullary thyroid carcinoma (MTC); patients with multiple endocrine neoplasia syndrome type 2 (MEN2)

Byetta™: Canadian labeling: Additional contraindications (not in U.S. labeling): End-stage renal disease or severe renal impairment (Cl_{cr} <30 mL/minute) including dialysis patients; diabetic ketoacidosis, diabetic coma/precoma or type 1 diabetes mellitus

Warnings/Precautions Bydureon™: **[U.S. Boxed Warning] Dose- and duration- dependent thyroid C-cell tumors have developed in animal studies with exenatide extended release therapy; relevance in humans unknown.** Patients should be counseled on the risk and symptoms (eg, neck mass, dysphagia, dyspnea, persistent hoarseness) of thyroid tumors. Consultation with an endocrinologist is recommended in patients who develop elevated calcitonin concentrations or have thyroid nodules detected during imaging studies or physical exam. Use is contraindicated in patients with a personal or a family history of medullary thyroid cancer and in patients with multiple endocrine neoplasia syndrome type 2 (MEN2). All cases of MTC should be reported to the applicable state cancer registry.

Mechanism requires the presence of insulin, therefore use in type 1 diabetes (insulin dependent, IDDM) or diabetic ketoacidosis is not recommended (use is contraindicated in the Canadian labeling); it is not a substitute for insulin in insulin-requiring patients. Concurrent use with insulin therapy has not been evaluated and is not recommended. (Exception: Safety and efficacy of concurrent insulin glargine and immediate release exenatide has been demonstrated in a clinical trial.) May increase the risk of hypoglycemia in patients receiving concomitant insulin secretagogues (eg, sulfonylureas, meglitinides); dosage reduction of sulfonylureas may be required. Clinicians should note that the risk of hypoglycemia is not increased when exenatide is added to metformin monotherapy. Avoid concurrent use of extended release (weekly) and immediate release (daily) exenatide formulations. Bydureon™ is not recommended for first-line therapy in patients inadequately controlled on diet and exercise alone.

Exenatide is frequently associated with gastrointestinal adverse effects and is not recommended for use in patients with gastroparesis or severe gastrointestinal disease. Gastrointestinal effects may be dose-related and may decrease in frequency/severity with gradual titration and continued use. Due to its effects on gastric emptying, exenatide may reduce the rate and extent of absorption of orally-administered drugs; use with caution in patients receiving medications with a narrow therapeutic window or require rapid absorption from the GI tract. Administer medications 1 hour prior to the use of immediate release (daily) exenatide when optimal drug absorption and peak levels are important to the overall therapeutic effect (eg, antibiotics, oral contraceptives); effects of extended release (weekly) exenatide on drug absorption have not been evaluated; use caution. Cases of acute pancreatitis (including hemorrhagic and necrotizing with some fatalities) have been reported; monitor for unexplained severe abdominal pain and if pancreatitis suspected, discontinue use. Do not resume unless an alternative etiology of pancreatitis is confirmed. Consider alternative antidiabetic therapy in patients with a history of pancreatitis. Use may be associated with the development of anti-exenatide antibodies. Low titers are not associated with a loss of efficacy; however, high titers (observed in 6% to 12% of patients in clinical studies) may result in an attenuation of response. May be associated with weight loss (due to reduced intake) independent of the change in hemoglobin A_{1c}.

Not recommended in severe renal impairment (Cl_{cr} <30 mL/minute) or end-stage renal disease (ESRD) (use in these patients and in dialysis patients is contraindicated in the Canadian labeling). Patients with ESRD receiving dialysis may be more susceptible to GI effects (eg, nausea, vomiting) which may result in hypovolemia and further reductions in renal function. Use with caution in patients with renal transplantation or in patients with moderate renal impairment (Cl_{cr} 30-50 mL/minute). Cases of acute renal failure and chronic renal failure exacerbation, including severe cases requiring hemodialysis, have been reported, predominately in patients with nausea/vomiting/diarrhea or dehydration; renal dysfunction was usually reversible with appropriate corrective measures, including discontinuation of exenatide. Risk may be increased in patients receiving concomitant medications affecting renal function and/or hydration status.

According to the Centers for Disease Control and Prevention (CDC), pen-shaped injection devices should never be used for more than one person (even when the needle is changed) because of the risk of infection. The injection device should be clearly labeled with individual patient information to ensure that the correct pen is used (CDC, 2012).

Adverse Reactions

>10%:

Endocrine & metabolic: Hypoglycemia (monotherapy 2% to 5%; combination therapy with sulfonylurea 14% to 36%, with metformin ≤4%, with thiazolidinedione 11%)

Gastrointestinal: Nausea (monotherapy 8% to 11%; combination therapy 13% to 44%; dose-dependent), vomiting (monotherapy 4%; combination therapy 11% to 13%), diarrhea (monotherapy <2% to 11%; combination therapy 6% to 20%), constipation (monotherapy 9%; combination therapy 6% to 10%)

Local: Injection site nodule (Bydureon™ 6% to 77%), injection site reactions (2% to 18%; includes erythema, hematoma, pruritus)

Miscellaneous: Anti-exenatide antibodies (low titers 38% to 49%, high titers 6% to 12%)

1% to 10%:

Central nervous system: Central nervous system: Nervousness (9%), dizziness (monotherapy <2%; combination therapy 9%), headache (5% to 9%), fatigue (3% to 6%)

Dermatologic: Hyperhidrosis (3%)

Gastrointestinal: Viral gastroenteritis (6% to 9%), dyspepsia (monotherapy 3% to 7%; combination therapy 5% to 7%), GERD (3% to 7%), appetite decreased (1% to 5%)

Neuromuscular & skeletal: Weakness (4%)

Postmarketing and/or case reports (Limited to important or life-threatening): Alopecia, anaphylactic reaction, angioedema, hypersensitivity pneumonitis, influenza, pancreatitis (including hemorrhagic and necrotizing), rash, renal failure, renal impairment, upper respiratory tract infection

Drug Interactions

Metabolism/Transport Effects None known.

Avoid Concomitant Use There are no known interactions where it is recommended to avoid concomitant use.

Increased Effect/Toxicity

Exenatide may increase the levels/effects of: Sulfonylureas; Vitamin K Antagonists

The levels/effects of Exenatide may be increased by: Pegvisomant

Decreased Effect

Exenatide may decrease the levels/effects of: Contraceptives (Estrogens); Oral Contraceptive (Progestins)

The levels/effects of Exenatide may be decreased by: Corticosteroids (Orally Inhaled); Corticosteroids (Systemic); Luteinizing Hormone-Releasing Hormone Analogs; Somatropin; Thiazide Diuretics

Ethanol/Nutrition/Herb Interactions

Ethanol: Ethanol may cause hypoglycemia. Management: Consume ethanol with caution.

Food: Administer Byetta® within 60 minutes of meals, not after meals. May administer Bydureon™ without regard to meals or time of day.

Preparation for Administration Bydureon™: Reconstitute vial using provided diluent; use immediately.

Storage/Stability

Bydureon™: Store under refrigeration at 2°C to 8°C (36°F to 46°F); vials may be stored at ≤25°C (≤77°F) for up to 4 weeks. Do not freeze (discard if freezing occurs). Protect from light.

Byetta®: Prior to initial use, store under refrigeration at 2°C to 8°C (36°F to 46°F); after initial use, may store at ≤25°C (≤77°F). Do not freeze (discard if freezing occurs). Protect from light. Pen should be discarded 30 days after initial use.

Mechanism of Action Exenatide is an analog of the hormone incretin (glucagon-like peptide 1 or GLP-1) which increases glucose-dependent insulin secretion, decreases inappropriate glucagon secretion, increases B-cell growth/replication, slows gastric emptying, and decreases food intake. Exenatide administration results in decreases in hemoglobin A_{1c} by approximately 0.5% to 1% (immediate release) or 1.5% to 1.9% (extended release).

Pharmacodynamics/Kinetics

Distribution: V_d: 28.3 L

Metabolism: Minimal systemic metabolism; proteolytic degradation may occur following glomerular filtration

Half-life elimination:

Immediate release (daily) formulation: 2.4 hours

Extended release (weekly) formulation: ~2 weeks

Time to peak, plasma: SubQ:

Immediate release (daily) formulation: 2.1 hours

Extended release (weekly) formulation: Triphasic: Phase 1: 2-5 hours; Phase 2: ~2 weeks; Phase 3: ~7 weeks

Excretion: Urine (majority of dose)

Dosage SubQ: Adults:

Immediate release: Initial: 5 mcg twice daily within 60 minutes prior to a meal; after 1 month, may be increased to 10 mcg twice daily (based on response)

Extended release: 2 mg once weekly

Note: May administer a missed dose as soon as noticed if the next regularly scheduled dose is due in ≥3 days; resume normal schedule thereafter. To establish a new day of the week administration schedule, wait ≥3 days after last dose given, then administer next dose on new desired day of the week.

Conversion from immediate release to extended release: Initiate weekly administration of exenatide extended release the day after discontinuing exenatide immediate release. **Note:** May experience increased blood glucose levels for ~2 weeks after conversion. Pretreatment with immediate release exenatide is not required when initiating extended release exenatide.

Dosage adjustment in renal impairment:

Cl_{cr} ≥50 mL/minute: No dosage adjustment necessary

Cl_{cr} 30-50 mL/minute: No dosage adjustment provided in manufacturer's labeling; use caution.

Cl_{cr} <30 mL/minute:

U.S. labeling: Use is not recommended

Canadian labeling: Use is contraindicated.

Dosage adjustment in hepatic impairment: No dosage adjustment provided in manufacturer's labeling (has not been studied); however, hepatic dysfunction is not expected to affect exenatide pharmacokinetics.

Administration SubQ:

Immediate release: Use only if clear, colorless, and free of particulate matter. Administer via injection in the upper arm, thigh, or abdomen. Administer within 60 minutes prior to morning and evening meal (or prior to the 2 main meals of the day, approximately ≥6 hours apart). Set up each new pen before the first use by priming it. See pen user manual for further details. Dial the dose into the dose window before each administration.

Extended release: Administer via injection in the upper arm, thigh, or abdomen; rotate injection sites weekly. Administer immediately after reconstitution. May administer without regard to meals or time of day.

Monitoring Parameters Serum glucose, hemoglobin A_{1c}, and renal function

Reference Range Recommendations for glycemic control in nonpregnant adults with diabetes (ADA, 2013):

Hb A_{1c}: <7% (a more aggressive [<6.5%] or less aggressive [<8%] Hb A_{1c} goal may be targeted based on patient-specific characteristics)

Preprandial capillary plasma glucose: 70-130 mg/dL

Peak postprandial capillary blood glucose: <180 mg/dL

Additional Information A dosing strategy which employs progressive dose escalation of exenatide (initiating at 0.02 mcg/kg 3 times daily and increasing in increments of 0.02 mcg/kg every 3 days) has been described, limiting the frequency and severity of gastrointestinal adverse effects. The complexity of this regimen may limit its clinical application.

In animal models, exenatide has been a useful adjunctive therapy when added to immunotherapy protocols, resulting in recovery of beta cell function and sustained remission.

Dosage Forms Excipient information presented when available (limited, particularly for generics); consult specific product labeling.

Solution, Subcutaneous:

Byetta 10 MCG Pen: 10 mcg/0.04 mL (2.4 mL) [contains metacresol]

Byetta 5 MCG Pen: 5 mcg/0.02 mL (1.2 mL) [contains metacresol]

Suspension Reconstituted, Subcutaneous:

Bydureon: 2 mg (1 ea)

- **Exendin-4** *see* Exenatide *on page* 815
- **Exforge®** *see* Amlodipine and Valsartan *on page* 112
- **Exforge HCT®** *see* Amlodipine, Valsartan, and Hydrochlorothiazide *on page* 113
- **Exjade** *see* Deferasirox *on page* 558
- **Ex-Lax Ultra [OTC]** *see* Bisacodyl *on page* 259
- **Exparel™** *see* Bupivacaine (Liposomal) *on page* 290
- **Exparel** *see* Bupivacaine (Liposomal) *on page* 290
- **Extavia** *see* Interferon Beta-1b *on page* 1106
- **Extended Release Epidural Morphine** *see* Morphine (Liposomal) *on page* 1403
- **Extina** *see* Ketoconazole (Topical) *on page* 1149
- **Extraneal** *see* Icodextrin *on page* 1038
- **Extra Strength Allergy Relief [OTC] (Can)** *see* Cetirizine *on page* 396
- **Exuviance Lightening Complex [OTC]** *see* Hydroquinone *on page* 1017
- **EYE001** *see* Pegaptanib *on page* 1585
- **EyeFlur** *see* Fluorescein and Benoxinate *on page* 880
- **Eye-Sed [OTC]** *see* Zinc Sulfate *on page* 2230
- **Eylea** *see* Aflibercept (Ophthalmic) *on page* 56
- **EZ Char [OTC]** *see* Charcoal, Activated *on page* 401

Ezetimibe (ez ET i mibe)

Brand Names: U.S. Zetia

Brand Names: Canada Ezetrol

Pharmacologic Category Antilipemic Agent, 2-Azetidinone

Use Use in combination with dietary therapy for the treatment of primary hypercholesterolemia (as monotherapy or in combination with HMG-CoA reductase inhibitors); homozygous sitosterolemia; homozygous familial hypercholesterolemia (in combination with atorvastatin or simvastatin); mixed hyperlipidemia (in combination with fenofibrate)

Pregnancy Risk Factor C

Pregnancy Considerations Use is contraindicated in women who are or who may become pregnant.

Breast-Feeding Considerations It is not known if ezetimibe is excreted in breast milk. According to the manufacturer, the decision to continue or discontinue breastfeeding during therapy should take into account the risk of exposure to the infant and the benefits of treatment to the mother. Use is contraindicated in nursing women who require combination therapy with an HMG-CoA reductase inhibitor.

Contraindications Hypersensitivity to ezetimibe or any component of the formulation; concomitant use with an HMG-CoA reductase inhibitor in patients with active hepatic disease, unexplained persistent elevations in serum transaminases; pregnancy; breast-feeding

Warnings/Precautions Secondary causes of hyperlipidemia should be ruled out prior to therapy. Use caution with severe renal (Cl_{cr} <30 mL/minute); if using concurrent simvastatin in patients with moderate-to-severe renal impairment, the manufacturer of ezetimibe recommends that simvastatin doses exceeding 20 mg be used with caution and close monitoring for adverse events (eg, myopathy). Use caution with mild hepatic impairment (Child-Pugh class A); not recommended for use with moderate or severe hepatic impairment (Child-Pugh classes B and C). Concurrent use of ezetimibe and fibric acid derivatives may increase the risk of cholelithiasis.

Adverse Reactions

1% to 10%:

Central nervous system: Fatigue (2%)

Gastrointestinal: Diarrhea (4%)

Hepatic: Transaminases increased (with HMG-CoA reductase inhibitors) (≥3 x ULN, 1%)

Neuromuscular & skeletal: Arthralgia (3%), pain in extremity (3%)

Respiratory: Upper respiratory tract infection (4%), sinusitis (3%)

Miscellaneous: Influenza (2%)

Postmarketing and/or case reports: Abdominal pain, anaphylaxis, angioedema, autoimmune hepatitis (Stolk, 2006), cholecystitis, cholelithiasis, cholestatic hepatitis (Stolk, 2006), CPK increased, depression, dizziness, erythema multiforme, headache, hepatitis, hypersensitivity reactions, myalgia, myopathy, nausea, pancreatitis, paresthesia, rash, rhabdomyolysis, thrombocytopenia, urticaria

Drug Interactions

Metabolism/Transport Effects Substrate of SLCO1B1

Avoid Concomitant Use There are no known interactions where it is recommended to avoid concomitant use.

Increased Effect/Toxicity

Ezetimibe may increase the levels/effects of: CycloSPORINE (Systemic)

The levels/effects of Ezetimibe may be increased by: CycloSPORINE (Systemic); Eltrombopag; Fibric Acid Derivatives

Decreased Effect

The levels/effects of Ezetimibe may be decreased by: Bile Acid Sequestrants

Ethanol/Nutrition/Herb Interactions Food: Ezetimibe did not cause meaningful reductions in fat-soluble vitamin concentrations during a 2-week clinical trial. Effects of long-term therapy have not been evaluated.

Storage/Stability Store at controlled room temperature of 25°C (77°F). Protect from moisture.

Mechanism of Action Inhibits absorption of cholesterol at the brush border of the small intestine via the sterol transporter, Niemann-Pick C1-Like1 (NPC1L1). This leads to a decreased delivery of cholesterol to the liver, reduction of hepatic cholesterol stores and an increased clearance of cholesterol from the blood; decreases total C, LDL-cholesterol (LDL-C), ApoB, and triglycerides (TG) while increasing HDL-cholesterol (HDL-C).

Pharmacodynamics/Kinetics

Protein binding: >90% to plasma proteins

Metabolism: Undergoes glucuronide conjugation in the small intestine and liver; forms metabolite (active); may undergo enterohepatic recycling

Bioavailability: Variable

Half-life elimination: 22 hours (ezetimibe and metabolite)

Time to peak, plasma: 4-12 hours

Excretion: Feces (78%, 69% as ezetimibe); urine (11%, 9% as metabolite)

Dosage Oral:

Children ≥10 years and Adults: 10 mg/day

Elderly: Refer to adult dosing

Dosage adjustment in renal impairment: AUC increased with severe impairment (Cl_{cr} <30 mL/minute); no dosing adjustment necessary

Dosage adjustment in hepatic impairment: AUC increased with hepatic impairment

Mild impairment (Child-Pugh class A): No dosing adjustment necessary

Moderate-to-severe impairment (Child-Pugh class B or C): Use of ezetimibe not recommended

Dietary Considerations May be taken without regard to meals. Before initiation of therapy, patients should be placed on a standard cholesterol-lowering diet for 6 weeks and the diet should be continued during drug therapy.

Administration May be administered without regard to meals. May be taken at the same time as HMG-CoA reductase inhibitors. Administer ≥2 hours before or ≥4 hours after bile acid sequestrants.

Monitoring Parameters Total cholesterol profile prior to therapy, and when clinically indicated and/or periodically thereafter. When used in combination with fenofibrate, monitor LFTs and signs and symptoms of cholelithiasis.

2013 ACC/AHA Blood Cholesterol Guideline recommendations (Stone, 2013): Baseline LFTs (reasonable); when used in combination with statin therapy, monitor LFTs when clinically indicated; discontinue use of ezetimibe if ALT elevations >3 times upper limit of normal persist.

Additional Information When studied in combination with fenofibrate for mixed hyperlipidemia, the dose of fenofibrate was 160 mg daily.

Dosage Forms Excipient information presented when available (limited, particularly for generics); consult specific product labeling.

Tablet, Oral:

Zetia: 10 mg

Ezetimibe and Atorvastatin

(ez ET i mibe & a TORE va sta tin)

Brand Names: U.S. Liptruzet™

Index Terms Atorvastatin and Ezetimibe

Pharmacologic Category Antilipemic Agent, 2-Azetidinone; Antilipemic Agent, HMG-CoA Reductase Inhibitor

Use

Homozygous familial hypercholesterolemia: For the reduction of elevated total cholesterol (total-C) and low-density lipoprotein cholesterol (LDL-C) in patients with homozygous familial hypercholesterolemia, as an adjunct to other lipid-lowering treatments (eg, LDL apheresis), or if such treatments are unavailable.

Primary hyperlipidemia: For the reduction of elevated total-C, LDL-C, apolipoprotein B (apo B), triglycerides, and non–high-density lipoprotein cholesterol (non HDL-C), and to increase HDL-C in patients with primary (heterozygous familial and nonfamilial) hyperlipidemia or mixed hyperlipidemia

Pregnancy Risk Factor X

Dosage

Homozygous familial hypercholesterolemia: Adults: Oral: Ezetimibe 10 mg and atorvastatin 40-80 mg once daily

Hyperlipidemias: Adults: Oral: Initial: Ezetimibe 10 mg and atorvastatin 10-20 mg once daily; dosing range: Ezetimibe 10 mg and atorvastatin 10-80 mg once daily

Patients requiring >55% reduction in LDL-C: Initial: Ezetimibe 10 mg and atorvastatin 40 mg once daily

Dosage adjustment with concomitant medications:

Lopinavir plus ritonavir: Use lowest effective dose.

Clarithromycin, itraconazole, saquinavir plus ritonavir, darunavir plus ritonavir, fosamprenavir, or fosamprenavir plus ritonavir: Use lowest effective dose; atorvastatin dose should not exceed 20 mg once daily.

Nelfinavir or boceprevir: Use lowest effective dose; atorvastatin dose should not exceed 40 mg once daily.

Dosage adjustment in renal impairment: No dosage adjustment necessary.

Dosage adjustment in hepatic impairment: Contraindicated in active liver disease or in patients with unexplained persistent elevations of serum transaminases.

Additional Information Complete prescribing information should be consulted for additional detail.

Dosage Forms Excipient information presented when available (limited, particularly for generics); consult specific product labeling.

Tablet, oral:

Liptruzet™ 10/10: Ezetimibe 10 mg and atorvastatin 10 mg

Liptruzet™ 10/20: Ezetimibe 10 mg and atorvastatin 20 mg

Liptruzet™ 10/40: Ezetimibe 10 mg and atorvastatin 40 mg

Liptruzet™ 10/80: Ezetimibe 10 mg and atorvastatin 80 mg

Ezetimibe and Simvastatin

(ez ET i mibe & SIM va stat in)

Brand Names: U.S. Vytorin®

Index Terms Simvastatin and Ezetimibe

Pharmacologic Category Antilipemic Agent, 2-Azetidinone; Antilipemic Agent, HMG-CoA Reductase Inhibitor

Use

Homozygous familial hypercholesterolemia: As an adjunct to diet for the reduction of elevated total cholesterol (total-C) and low-density lipoprotein cholesterol (LDL-C) in patients with homozygous familial hypercholesterolemia, as an adjunct to other lipid-lowering treatments (eg, LDL apheresis), or if such treatments are unavailable

Primary hyperlipidemia: As an adjunct to diet for the reduction of elevated total-C, LDL-C, apolipoprotein B (apo B), triglycerides, and non-high-density lipoprotein cholesterol (HDL-C), and to increase HDL-C in patients with primary (heterozygous familial and nonfamilial) hyperlipidemia or mixed hyperlipidemia

Limitations of use: No incremental benefit of ezetimibe/simvastatin on cardiovascular morbidity and mortality over and above that demonstrated for simvastatin has been established. Ezetimibe/simvastatin has not been studied in Fredrickson type I, III, IV, and V dyslipidemias.

Pregnancy Risk Factor X

Dosage Oral: Adults:

Note: Dosing limitation: Simvastatin 80 mg is limited to patients that have been taking this dose for >12 consecutive months without evidence of myopathy and are not currently taking or beginning a simvastatin dose-limiting or contraindicated interacting medication. If patient is unable to achieve low-density lipoprotein-cholesterol (LDL-C) goal using the 40 mg dose of simvastatin, increasing to 80 mg dose is not recommended. Instead, switch patient to an alternative LDL-C-lowering treatment providing greater LDL-C reduction. After initiation or titration, monitor lipid response after ≥2 weeks and adjust dose as necessary.

Homozygous familial hypercholesterolemia: Ezetimibe 10 mg and simvastatin 40 mg once daily in the evening.

Hyperlipidemias: Initial: Ezetimibe 10 mg and simvastatin 10-20 mg once daily in the evening. Dosing range: Ezetimibe 10 mg and simvastatin 10-40 mg once daily

Patients who require less aggressive reduction in LDL-C: Initial: Ezetimibe 10 mg and simvastatin 10 mg once daily in the evening

Patients who require >55% reduction in LDL-C: Initial: Ezetimibe 10 mg and simvastatin 40 mg once daily in the evening

Dosage adjustment with concomitant medications: Note: Patients currently tolerating and requiring a dose of simvastatin 80 mg who require initiation of an interacting drug with a dose cap for simvastatin should be switched to an alternative statin with less potential for drug-drug interaction.

Amiodarone, amlodipine, or ranolazine: Simvastatin dose should **not** exceed 20 mg once daily

Diltiazem, dronedarone, or verapamil: Simvastatin dose should **not** exceed 10 mg once daily

Lomitapide: Reduce simvastatin dose by 50% when initiating lomitapide. Simvastatin dose should **not** exceed 20 mg once daily (or 40 mg once daily for those who previously tolerated simvastatin 80 mg daily for ≥1 year without evidence of muscle toxicity).

Dosage adjustment in Chinese patients on niacin doses ≥1 g/day: Use caution with simvastatin doses exceeding 20 mg/day; because of an increased risk of myopathy, do not administer simvastatin 80 mg

Dosage adjustment in renal impairment:

GFR ≥60 mL/minute/1.73 m^2: No dosage adjustment necessary.

GFR <60 mL/minute/1.73 m^2: Ezetimibe 10 mg and simvastatin 20 mg once daily in the evening (higher doses should be used with caution).

Dosage adjustment in hepatic impairment:

Mild impairment: No dosage adjustment necessary.

Moderate-to-severe impairment: Use not recommended.

Additional Information Complete prescribing information should be consulted for additional detail.

Dosage Forms Excipient information presented when available (limited, particularly for generics); consult specific product labeling.

Tablet:

Vytorin® 10/10: Ezetimibe 10 mg and simvastatin 10 mg
Vytorin® 10/20: Ezetimibe 10 mg and simvastatin 20 mg
Vytorin® 10/40: Ezetimibe 10 mg and simvastatin 40 mg
Vytorin® 10/80: Ezetimibe 10 mg and simvastatin 80 mg

◆ **Ezetrol (Can)** *see* Ezetimibe *on page 817*

◆ **EZFE 200 [OTC]** *see* Polysaccharide-Iron Complex *on page 1673*

◆ **EZG** *see* Ezogabine *on page 819*

Ezogabine (e ZOG a been)

Brand Names: U.S. Potiga

Index Terms D-23129; EZG; Retigabine; RTG

Pharmacologic Category Anticonvulsant, Neuronal Potassium Channel Opener

Use Adjuvant treatment of partial-onset seizures in patients ≥18 years of age who have responded inadequately to several alternative treatments and for whom the benefits outweigh the risk of retinal abnormalities and potential decline in visual acuity.

Pregnancy Risk Factor C

Pregnancy Considerations Adverse events were observed in animal reproduction studies. Patients exposed to ezogabine during pregnancy are encouraged to enroll themselves into the North American Antiepileptic Drug (NAAED) Pregnancy Registry by calling 1-888-233-2334. Additional information is available at www.-aedpregnancyregistry.org.

Breast-Feeding Considerations According to the manufacturer, due to the potential for serious adverse reactions in the nursing infant, the decision to continue or discontinue breast-feeding during therapy should take into account the risk of exposure to the infant and the benefits to the mother.

Medication Guide Available Yes

Contraindications There are no contraindications listed in the manufacturer's labeling.

Warnings/Precautions [U.S. Boxed Warning]: Retinal abnormalities that may progress to vision loss have been reported and were seen in about one-third of patients after approximately 4 years of treatment. These retinal abnormalities exhibited fundoscopic features similar to those of retinal pigment dystrophies. The rate of progression and reversibility of these retinal abnormalities is unknown. Limit use to patients who have responded inadequately to other treatments and in whom the benefits of therapy exceed the risk of vision loss. Visual monitoring (at least visual acuity and dilated fundus photography) by an ophthalmic professional is recommended at baseline and at 6-month intervals. Other visual tests may include fluorescein angiograms, ocular coherence tomography, perimetry, and electroretinograms. Discontinue use if there is no substantial benefit after adequate titration or if retinal pigmentary abnormalities or vision changes are detected. If no other treatment options are available and the benefits of treatment outweigh the potential risk of vision loss, then may cautiously continue treatment with ezogabine.

Skin discoloration has been reported; typically blue in color (but may also be grey-blue or brown) and is predominantly located on or around the lips, nail beds of the fingers or toes, face and legs; and discoloration of the palate, sclera, and conjunctiva may also occur. Skin discoloration developed in ~10% of patients, generally after ≥2 years of treatment and at higher doses (≥900 mg). If detected, consider other treatment options or discontinue use.

Urinary retention, including retention requiring catheterization, has been reported, generally within the first 6 months of treatment. All patients should be monitored for urologic symptoms; close monitoring is recommended in patients with other risk factors for urinary retention (eg, benign prostatic hyperplasia), patients unable to communicate clinical symptoms, or patients who use concomitant medications that may affect voiding (eg, anticholinergics). Dose-related neuropsychiatric disorders, including confusion, psychotic symptoms, and hallucinations, have been reported, generally within the first 8 weeks of treatment; some patients required hospitalization. Symptoms resolved in most patients within 7 days of discontinuation of ezogabine. The risk appears to be greatest with rapid titration at greater than the recommended doses. Dose-related dizziness and somnolence (generally mild-to-moderate) have been reported; effects generally occur during dose titration and appear to diminish with continued use. Patients must be cautioned about performing tasks which ▶

require mental alertness (eg, operating machinery or driving). QT prolongation has been observed; monitor ECG in patients with electrolyte abnormalities (eg, hypokalemia, hypomagnesemia), hypothyroidism, familial long QT syndrome, concomitant medications which may augment QT prolongation, or any underlying cardiac abnormality which may also potentiate risk (eg, heart failure, ventricular hypertrophy). Pooled analysis of trials involving various antiepileptics (regardless of indication) showed an increased risk of suicidal thoughts/behavior (incidence rate: 0.43% treated patients compared to 0.24% of patients receiving placebo); risk observed as early as 1 week after initiation and continued through duration of trials (most trials ≤24 weeks). Monitor all patients for notable changes in behavior that might indicate suicidal thoughts or depression; notify healthcare provider immediately if symptoms occur.

Dosage adjustment recommended in hepatic impairment; ezogabine exposure increases in moderate-to-severe impairment. Dosage adjustment recommended in renal impairment; ezogabine undergoes significant renal elimination. Use caution in elderly due to potential for urinary retention, particularly in older men with symptomatic BPH. Systemic exposure is increased in the elderly; dosage adjustment is recommended in patients ≥65 years of age.

Anticonvulsants should not be discontinued abruptly because of the possibility of increasing seizure frequency; therapy should be withdrawn gradually over a period of ≥3 weeks to minimize the potential of increased seizure frequency, unless safety concerns require a more rapid withdrawal.

Adverse Reactions

>10%: Central nervous system: Dizziness (dose related; 23%), drowsiness (dose related; 22%), fatigue (15%)

2% to 10%:

Central nervous system: Confusion (dose related; 9%), vertigo (8%), coordination impaired (dose related; 7%), lack of concentration (6%), memory impairment (dose related; 6%), abnormal gait (dose related; 4%), aphasia (dose related; 4%), dysarthria (4%), equilibrium disturbance (dose related; 4%), anxiety (3%), paresthesia (3%), amnesia (2%), disorientation (2%), dysphasia (2%), hallucination (2%)

Endocrine & metabolic: Weight gain (dose related; 3%)

Gastrointestinal: Nausea (7%), constipation (dose related; 3%), dysphagia (2%)

Genitourinary: Dysuria (dose related; 2%), hematuria (2%), urinary hesitancy (2%), urinary retention (2%), urine discoloration (dose related; 2%)

Infection: Influenza (3%)

Ophthalmic: Diplopia (7%), blurred vision (dose related; 5%)

Neuromuscular & skeletal: Tremor (dose related; 8%), weakness (5%)

<2% (Limited to important or life-threatening): Alopecia, brain disease, coma, euphoria, hydronephrosis, hyperhidrosis, hypokinesia, increased appetite, increased liver enzymes, leukopenia, muscle spasm, nephrolithiasis, neutropenia, nystagmus, peripheral edema, prolonged Q-T Interval on ECG (mean: 7.7 msec), psychotic symptoms, renal colic, skin rash, syncope, thrombocytopenia

Drug Interactions

Metabolism/Transport Effects None known.

Avoid Concomitant Use

Avoid concomitant use of Ezogabine with any of the following: Azelastine (Nasal); Highest Risk QTc-Prolonging Agents; Ivabradine; Mifepristone; Paraldehyde

Increased Effect/Toxicity

Ezogabine may increase the levels/effects of: Azelastine (Nasal); Buprenorphine; CNS Depressants; Digoxin; Highest Risk QTc-Prolonging Agents; Hydrocodone; Methotrimeprazine; Metyrosine; Mirtazapine; Moderate Risk QTc-Prolonging Agents; Paraldehyde; Pramipexole; ROPINIRole; Rotigotine; Selective Serotonin Reuptake Inhibitors; Zolpidem

The levels/effects of Ezogabine may be increased by: Alcohol (Ethyl); Brimonidine (Topical); Doxylamine; HydrOXYzine; Ivabradine; Magnesium Sulfate; Methotrimeprazine; Mifepristone; Perampanel; QTc-Prolonging Agents (Indeterminate Risk and Risk Modifying); Sodium Oxybate; Tapentadol

Decreased Effect

Ezogabine may decrease the levels/effects of: LamoTRIgine

The levels/effects of Ezogabine may be decreased by: CarBAMazepine; Ketorolac (Nasal); Ketorolac (Systemic); Mefloquine; Orlistat; Phenytoin

Storage/Stability Store at 25°C (77°F); excursions permitted to 15°C to 30°C (59°F to 86°F).

Mechanism of Action Ezogabine binds the KCNQ (Kv7.2-7.5) voltage-gated potassium channels, thereby stabilizing the channels in the open formation and enhancing the M-current. As a result, neuronal excitability is regulated and epileptiform activity is suppressed. In addition, ezogabine may also exert therapeutic effects through augmentation of GABA-mediated currents.

Pharmacodynamics/Kinetics

Absorption: Rapid

Distribution: V_{dss}: 2-3 L/kg

Protein binding: Ezogabine: 80%; N-acetyl active metabolite (NAMR): 45%

Metabolism: Glucuronidation via UGT1A4, UGT1A1, UGT1A3, and UGT1A9 and acetylation via NAT2 to an N-acetyl active metabolite (NAMR) and other inactive metabolites (eg, N-glucuronides, N-glucoside)

Bioavailability: Oral: ~60%

Half-life elimination: Ezogabine and NAMR: 7-11 hours; increased by ~30% in elderly patients

Time to peak, plasma: 0.5-2 hours; delayed by 0.75 hours when administered with high-fat food

Excretion: Urine (85%, 36% of total dose as unchanged drug, 18% of total dose as NAMR); feces (14%, 3% of total dose as unchanged drug)

Dosage Partial-onset seizures, adjunct: Oral:

Adults: Initial: 100 mg 3 times daily; may increase at weekly intervals in increments of ≤150 mg daily to a maintenance dose of 200-400 mg 3 times daily based on tolerability (maximum: 1200 mg daily). In clinical trials, no additional benefit and an increase in adverse effects was observed with doses >900 mg daily. **Note:** If there is no substantial benefit after adequate titration, then discontinue use and consider other treatment options.

Elderly: Initial: 50 mg 3 times daily; may increase at weekly intervals in increments of ≤150 mg daily to a maximum daily dose of 750 mg daily

Dosage adjustment in renal impairment:

Cl_{cr} ≥50 mL/minute: No dosage adjustment necessary.

Cl_{cr} <50 mL/minute: Initial: 50 mg 3 times daily; may increase at weekly intervals in increments of ≤150 mg daily to a maximum daily dose of 600 mg daily

ESRD requiring hemodialysis: Initial: 50 mg 3 times daily; may increase at weekly intervals in increments of ≤150 mg daily to a maximum daily dose of 600 mg daily

Dosage adjustment in hepatic impairment:

Mild impairment (Child-Pugh ≤7): No dosage adjustment necessary.

Moderate impairment (Child-Pugh 7-9): Initial: 50 mg 3 times daily; may increase at weekly intervals in increments of ≤150 mg daily to a maximum daily dose of 750 mg daily

Severe impairment (Child-Pugh >9): Initial: 50 mg 3 times daily; may increase at weekly intervals in increment of ≤150 mg daily to a maximum daily dose of 600 mg daily

Administration Oral: Swallow tablets whole. If therapy is discontinued, gradually reduce dose over ≥3 weeks unless safety concerns require abrupt withdrawal.

Monitoring Parameters Seizures; electrolytes, bilirubin, ALT, AST, serum creatinine, QT interval; urinary retention; observe patient for excessive sedation, confusion, psychotic symptoms, and hallucinations; suicidality (eg, suicidal thoughts, depression, behavioral changes); evaluate for signs/symptoms of ezogabine toxicity, including skin discoloration (blue, or grey-blue or brown in color) around the lips, nail beds of fingers or toes, face and legs.

Ophthalmic exams (at least visual acuity testing and dilated fundus photography) at baseline and 6-month intervals; fluorescein angiograms, ocular coherence tomography, perimetry, and electroretinograms may also be considered.

Test Interactions Falsely elevated: Bilirubin, serum; Bilirubin, urine

Dosage Forms Excipient information presented when available (limited, particularly for generics); consult specific product labeling.

Tablet, Oral:

Potiga: 50 mg [contains fd&c blue #2 (indigotine)]
Potiga: 200 mg
Potiga: 300 mg, 400 mg [contains fd&c blue #2 (indigotine)]

Controlled Substance C-V

- ◆ F_3T *see* Trifluridine *on page 2127*
- ◆ FA-8 [OTC] *see* Folic Acid *on page 907*
- ◆ FaBB *see* Folic Acid, Cyanocobalamin, and Pyridoxine *on page 908*
- ◆ Fabior *see* Tazarotene *on page 1994*
- ◆ Fabrazyme *see* Agalsidase Beta *on page 57*
- ◆ Fabrazyme® (Can) *see* Agalsidase Beta *on page 57*
- ◆ Factive *see* Gemifloxacin *on page 948*
- ◆ Factive® (Can) *see* Gemifloxacin *on page 948*

Factor VIIa (Recombinant)

(FAK ter SEV en aye ree KOM be nant)

Brand Names: U.S. NovoSeven RT

Brand Names: Canada Niastase®; Niastase® RT

Index Terms Coagulation Factor VIIa; Eptacog Alfa (Activated); rFVIIa

Pharmacologic Category Antihemophilic Agent

Use Treatment of bleeding episodes and prevention of bleeding in surgical interventions in patients with either hemophilia A or B with inhibitors to factor VIII or factor IX, acquired hemophilia, or congenital factor VII deficiency

Unlabeled Use Warfarin-related intracerebral hemorrhage; treatment of refractory bleeding after cardiac surgery in nonhemophiliac patients

Pregnancy Risk Factor C

Pregnancy Considerations Adverse events were observed in animal reproduction studies.

Breast-Feeding Considerations It is not known if factor VIIa (recombinant) is excreted in breast milk. Due to the potential for serious adverse reactions in the nursing infant, a decision should be made whether to discontinue nursing or to discontinue the drug, taking into account the importance of treatment to the mother.

Contraindications There are no contraindications listed within the FDA-approved labeling.

Warnings/Precautions [U.S. Boxed Warning]: Serious thrombotic events are associated with the use of factor VIIa outside labeled indications. Arterial and venous thrombotic and thromboembolic events, some fatal, following administration of factor VIIa have been reported during postmarketing surveillance. All patients receiving factor VIIa should be monitored for signs and symptoms of activation of the coagulation system or thrombosis; thrombotic events may be increased in patients with disseminated intravascular coagulation (DIC), advanced atherosclerotic disease, sepsis, crush injury, or concomitant treatment with prothrombin complex concentrates. Use with caution in patients with an increased risk of thromboembolic complications (eg, coronary heart disease, liver disease, DIC, postoperative immobilization, elderly patients, and neonates). Decreased dosage or discontinuation is warranted with confirmed intravascular coagulation or presence of clinical thrombosis. Use with caution in patients with known hypersensitivity to mouse, hamster, or bovine proteins, or factor VIIa, or any components of the product. Efficacy with prolonged infusions and data evaluating this agent's long-term adverse effects are limited.

Adverse Reactions

1% to 10%:

Cardiovascular: Hypertension (2%), bradycardia (1%), edema (1%), hypotension (1%)
Central nervous system: Fever (4%), headache (1%), pain (1%)
Dermatologic: Pruritus (1%), purpura (1%), rash (1%)
Gastrointestinal: Vomiting (1%)
Hematologic: Plasma fibrinogen decreased (2%), disseminated intravascular coagulation (1%), fibrinolysis increased (1%), prothrombin decreased (1%)
Local: Injection site reaction (1%)
Neuromuscular & skeletal: Arthrosis (1%)
Renal: Abnormal renal function (1%)
Respiratory: Pneumonia (1%)
Miscellaneous: Allergic reactions (1%)

<1% (Limited to important or life-threatening): Anaphylactic shock, angina, angioedema, antibody formation, arterial thrombosis, arterial thrombosis (limb), arthralgia, bowel infarction, cerebral artery occlusion, cerebral infarction and/or ischemia, consumptive coagulopathy, CVA, D-dimer elevation, deep vein thrombosis, fibrin degradation products increased, flushing, hepatic artery thrombosis, hypersensitivity, hypersensitivity reaction, injection site pain, intestinal infarction, I.V. site thrombosis, localized phlebitis, MI, myocardial ischemia, nausea, peripheral ischemia, portal vein thrombosis, pulmonary embolism, renal artery thrombosis, retinal artery embolism, retinal artery thrombosis, shock, thrombophlebitis, thrombosis, urticaria

Drug Interactions

Metabolism/Transport Effects None known.

Avoid Concomitant Use There are no known interactions where it is recommended to avoid concomitant use.

Increased Effect/Toxicity

The levels/effects of Factor VIIa (Recombinant) may be increased by: Factor XIII A-Subunit (Recombinant)

Decreased Effect There are no known significant interactions involving a decrease in effect.

Preparation for Administration Prior to reconstitution, bring vials to room temperature. Add recommended diluent along wall of vial; do not inject directly onto powder. Gently swirl until dissolved.

NovoSeven® RT: Reconstitute each vial to a final concentration of 1 mg/mL using the provided histidine diluent as follows:

1 mg vial: 1.1 mL histidine diluent
2 mg vial: 2.1 mL histidine diluent
5 mg vial: 5.2 mL histidine diluent
8 mg vial: 8.1 mL histidine diluent

Storage/Stability NovoSeven® RT: Prior to reconstitution, store under refrigeration or between 2°C to 25°C (36°F to 77°F); do not freeze. Protect from light. Reconstituted solutions may be stored at room temperature or under refrigeration, but must be infused within 3 hours of reconstitution. Do not freeze reconstituted solutions. Do not store reconstituted solutions in syringes.

Mechanism of Action Recombinant factor VIIa, a vitamin K-dependent glycoprotein, promotes hemostasis by activating the extrinsic pathway of the coagulation cascade. It replaces deficient activated coagulation factor VII, which complexes with tissue factor and may activate coagulation factor X to Xa and factor IX to IXa. When complexed with other factors, coagulation factor Xa converts prothrombin to thrombin, a key step in the formation of a fibrin-platelet hemostatic plug.

Pharmacodynamics/Kinetics

Distribution: V_d: 103 mL/kg (range: 78-139)

Half-life elimination: 2.3 hours (range: 1.7-2.7)

Excretion: Clearance: 33 mL/kg/hour (range: 27-49)

Dosage

Children and Adults: I.V. administration only:

Hemophilia A or B with inhibitors:

Bleeding episodes: 90 mcg/kg every 2 hours until hemostasis is achieved or until the treatment is judged ineffective. Doses between 35-120 mcg/kg have been used successfully in clinical trials. The dose, interval, and duration of therapy may be adjusted based upon the severity of bleeding and the degree of hemostasis achieved. For patients experiencing severe bleeds, dosing should be continued at 3- to 6-hour intervals after hemostasis has been achieved and the duration of dosing should be minimized.

Surgical interventions: 90 mcg/kg immediately before surgery; repeat at 2-hour intervals for the duration of surgery. Continue every 2 hours for 48 hours, then every 2-6 hours until healed for minor surgery; continue every 2 hours for 5 days, then every 4 hours until healed for major surgery.

Congenital factor VII deficiency: Bleeding episodes and surgical interventions: 15-30 mcg/kg every 4-6 hours until hemostasis is achieved. Doses as low as 10 mcg/kg have been effective.

Acquired hemophilia: 70-90 mcg/kg every 2-3 hours until hemostasis is achieved

Adults: I.V.:

Intracerebral hemorrhage (ICH) (warfarin-related) (unlabeled use; Freeman, 2004; Ilyas, 2008): 10-100 mcg/kg (see **"Note"** below) administered concurrently with I.V. vitamin K (to correct the nonfactor VII coagulation factors).

Note: Lower doses (10-20 mcg/kg) are generally preferred given the higher risk of thromboembolic complications with higher doses; response is highly variable; monitor INR frequently after administration since rebound increases in INR occur quickly given the short half-life of rFVIIa; duration of INR correction is dose dependent. Routine use as a sole agent is not recommended for warfarin-related ICH (Morgenstern, 2010).

Treatment of refractory bleeding after cardiac surgery in nonhemophiliac patients: Dosing not established; doses in the range of 35-70 mcg/kg have been recommended based on low-quality evidence (case series, observational studies) (Chapman, 2011; Ferraris, 2011; Karkouti, 2007); in patients with a left ventricular assist device, lower doses (ie, 10-20 mcg/kg) may be preferred to reduce thromboembolic events (Bruckner, 2009).

Dosage adjustment in renal impairment: No dosage adjustment provided in manufacturer's labeling.

Dosage adjustment in hepatic impairment: No dosage adjustment provided in manufacturer's labeling; use with caution.

Dietary Considerations Some products may contain sodium.

Administration I.V. administration only; bolus over 2-5 minutes. Administer within 3 hours after reconstitution.

Monitoring Parameters Monitor for evidence of hemostasis; although the prothrombin time/INR, aPTT, and factor VII clotting activity have no correlation with achieving hemostasis, these parameters may be useful as adjunct tests to evaluate efficacy and guide dose or interval adjustments

Additional Information The Hemophilia and Thrombosis Research Society (HTRS) Registry surveillance program is designed to collect data on the treatment of congenital and acquired bleeding disorders. All prescribers can obtain information regarding contribution of patient data to this program by calling 1-877-362-7355 or at www.novosevensurveillance.com.

Dosage Forms Excipient information presented when available (limited, particularly for generics); consult specific product labeling.

Solution Reconstituted, Intravenous [preservative free]:

NovoSeven RT: 1 mg (1 ea); 2 mg (1 ea); 5 mg (1 ea); 8 mg (1 ea) [contains polysorbate 80]

◆ **Factor Eight Inhibitor Bypassing Activity** *see* Anti-inhibitor Coagulant Complex (Human) *on page 147*

◆ **Factor VIII Concentrate** *see* Antihemophilic Factor/von Willebrand Factor Complex (Human) *on page 146*

◆ **Factor VIII (Human)** *see* Antihemophilic Factor (Human) *on page 143*

◆ **Factor VIII (Human)** *see* Antihemophilic Factor/von Willebrand Factor Complex (Human) *on page 146*

◆ **Factor VIII Inhibitor Bypassing Activity** *see* Anti-inhibitor Coagulant Complex (Human) *on page 147*

◆ **Factor VIII (Recombinant)** *see* Antihemophilic Factor (Recombinant) *on page 144*

Factor IX Complex (Human) [(Factors II, IX, X)] (FAK ter nyne KOM pleks HYU man FAKter too nyne ten)

Brand Names: U.S. Bebulin VH; Profilnine SD

Index Terms 3 Factor PCC; 3-Factor PCC; PCC (Caution: Confusion-prone synonym); Prothrombin Complex Concentrate (Caution: Confusion-prone synonym); Three-Factor PCC

Pharmacologic Category Antihemophilic Agent; Blood Product Derivative; Prothrombin Complex Concentrate (PCC)

Additional Appendix Information

Reversal of Oral Anticoagulants *on page 2308*

Use Prevention and control of bleeding in patients with factor IX deficiency (hemophilia B or Christmas disease)

Unlabeled Use Emergent correction of warfarin-induced coagulopathy (with clinically significant bleeding); **Note:** Products contain low or nontherapeutic levels of factor VII component; use of fresh frozen plasma (FFP) should be considered

Pregnancy Risk Factor C

Pregnancy Considerations Animal reproduction studies have not been conducted. Factor IX concentrations do not change significantly in pregnant women with coagulation disorders and women with factor IX deficiency may be at increased risk of postpartum hemorrhage. Pregnant women should have clotting factors monitored, particularly at 28 and 34 weeks gestation and prior to invasive procedures. Prophylaxis may be needed if factor IX concentrations are <50 units/mL at term and treatment should continue for 3-5 days postpartum depending on route of delivery. Because parvovirus infection may cause hydrops fetalis or fetal death, a recombinant product is preferred if prophylaxis or treatment is needed. The neonate may also be at an increased risk of bleeding following delivery and should be tested for the coagulation disorder (Chi, 2012; Kadir, 2009; Lee, 2006).

Contraindications There are no contraindications listed in the manufacturer's labeling.

Warnings/Precautions **Factor IX Complex (Human) [Factors II, IX, X] (Bebulin, Profilnine) contains low or nontherapeutic levels of factor VII component** and should not be confused with Prothrombin complex concentrate (Human) [(Factors II, VII, IX, X), Protein C, Protein S] (Kcentra, Octaplex) which contains therapeutic levels of factor VII. Factor IX Complex (Human) [Factors II, IX, X] (Bebulin, Profilnine) should not be used for the treatment of factor VII deficiency. When treating warfarin associated hemorrhage (unlabeled use), administration of additional fresh frozen plasma (FFP) or factor VIIa should be considered. Hypersensitivity and anaphylactic reactions have been reported with use. Delayed reactions (up to 20 days after infusion) in previously untreated patients may also occur. Due to potential for allergic reactions, the initial ~10-20 administrations should be performed under appropriate medical supervision. The development of factor IX antibodies (or inhibitors) has been reported with factor IX therapy (usually occurs within the first 10-20 exposure days); the risk of severe hypersensitivity reactions occurring may be greater in these patients. Patients experiencing allergic reactions should be evaluated for factor IX inhibitors. When clinical response is suboptimal or patient is to undergo surgical procedure, screen for inhibitors. Patients with severe gene defects (eg, gene deletion or inversion) are more likely to develop inhibitors (WFH, 2005).

Observe closely for signs or symptoms of intravascular coagulation or thrombosis. Use with caution when administering to patients with liver disease, postoperatively, neonates, or patients at risk of thromboembolic phenomena, disseminated intravascular coagulation or patients with signs of fibrinolysis due to the potential risk of thromboembolic complications. Use with caution in patients with liver dysfunction; may be at increased risk of developing thrombosis or DIC. Product of human plasma; may potentially contain infectious agents which could transmit disease. Screening of donors, as well as testing and/or inactivation or removal of certain viruses, reduces the risk. Infections thought to be transmitted by this product should be reported to the manufacturer. Some products may contain heparin. Use with caution in patients with a history of heparin-induced thrombocytopenia. Some product packaging may contain natural rubber latex.

Adverse Reactions Frequency not defined.

Cardiovascular: Flushing, thrombosis (sometimes fatal)

Central nervous system: Chills, fever, headache, lethargy, somnolence

Dermatologic: Rash, urticaria

Gastrointestinal: Nausea, vomiting

Hematologic: DIC

Neuromuscular & skeletal: Paresthesia

Respiratory: Dyspnea

Miscellaneous: Anaphylactic shock, clotting factor antibodies (development of), heparin-induced thrombocytopenia (with products containing heparin)

Drug Interactions

Metabolism/Transport Effects None known.

Avoid Concomitant Use

Avoid concomitant use of Factor IX Complex (Human) [(Factors II, IX, X)] with any of the following: Aminocaproic Acid

Increased Effect/Toxicity

The levels/effects of Factor IX Complex (Human) [(Factors II, IX, X)] may be increased by: Aminocaproic Acid

Decreased Effect There are no known significant interactions involving a decrease in effect.

Preparation for Administration Bring diluent and concentrate to room temperature; gently rotate or agitate to dissolve.

Storage/Stability

Bebulin® VH: Prior to use, store under refrigeration at 2°C to 8°C (36°F to 46°F); avoid freezing. Following reconstitution, do not refrigerate and use within 3 hours.

Profilnine® SD: Prior to use, store under refrigeration at 2°C to 8°C (36°F to 46°F); avoid freezing; may also stored at room temperature (not to exceed 30°C) for up to 3 months. Following reconstitution, do not refrigerate and use within 3 hours.

Mechanism of Action Replaces deficient clotting factor including factor X; hemophilia B, or Christmas disease, is an X-linked recessively inherited disorder of blood coagulation characterized by insufficient or abnormal synthesis of the clotting protein factor IX. Factor IX is a vitamin K-dependent coagulation factor which is synthesized in the liver. Factor IX is activated by factor XIa in the intrinsic coagulation pathway. Activated factor IX (IXa), in combination with factor VII:C, activates factor X to Xa, resulting ultimately in the conversion of prothrombin to thrombin and the formation of a fibrin clot. The infusion of exogenous factor IX to replace the deficiency present in hemophilia B temporarily restores hemostasis.

Pharmacodynamics/Kinetics Half-life elimination: IX component: ~24 hours

Dosage Note: Factor IX complex (Human) [Factors II, IX, X] (Bebulin, Profilnine) contains low or nontherapeutic levels of factor VII component and should not be confused with Prothrombin Complex Concentrate (Human) [(Factors II, VII, IX, X), Protein C, Protein S] (Kcentra, Octaplex)) which contains therapeutic levels of factor VII.

Children and Adults: Dosage is expressed in units of factor IX activity and must be individualized based on severity of factor IX deficiency, extent and location of bleeding, and clinical status of patient. When multiple doses are required, administer at 24-hour intervals unless otherwise specified. Administer I.V. only:

Formula for units required to raise blood level %:

Bebulin® VH: In general, factor IX 1 unit/kg will increase the plasma factor IX level by 0.8%

Number of Factor IX units required = body weight (kg) x desired factor IX increase (as %) x 1.2 units/kg

Profilnine® SD: In general, factor IX 1 unit/kg will increase the plasma factor IX level by 1%:

Number of factor IX units required = bodyweight (kg) x desired factor IX increase (as %) x 1 unit/kg

For example, to increase factor IX level to 25% of normal in a 70 kg patient: Number of factor IX units needed = 70 kg x 25 x 1 unit/kg = 1750 units

As a general rule, the level of factor IX required for treatment of different conditions is listed below:

Hemorrhage: I.V.:

Minor bleeding (early hemarthrosis, minor epistaxis, gingival bleeding, mild hematuria):

Bebulin® VH: Raise factor IX level to 20% of normal [typical initial dose: 25-35 units/kg]; generally a single dose is sufficient.

Profilnine® SD: Mild-to-moderate bleeding: Raise factor IX level to 20% to 30% of normal.

Moderate bleeding (severe joint bleeding, early hematoma, major open bleeding, minor trauma, minor hemoptysis, hematemesis, melena, major hematuria):

Bebulin® VH: Raise factor IX level to 40% of normal [typical initial dose: 40-55 units/kg]; average duration of treatment is 2 days or until adequate wound healing.

Profilnine® SD: Mild-to-moderate bleeding: raise factor IX level to 20% to 30% of normal.

Major bleeding (severe hematoma, major trauma, severe hemoptysis, hematemesis, melena):
Bebulin® VH: Raise factor IX level to ≥60% of normal [typical initial dose: 60-70 units/kg]; average duration of treatment is 2-3 days or until adequate wound healing. Do not raise >60% in patients who may be predisposed to thrombosis.
Profilnine® SD: Raise factor IX level to 30% to 50% of normal.

Surgical procedures: I.V.:
Dental surgery:
Bebulin® VH: Raise factor IX level to 40% to 60% of normal on day of surgery [typical dose: 50-60 units/kg]. One infusion, administered 1 hour prior to surgery, is generally sufficient for the extraction of one tooth; for the extraction of multiple teeth, replacement therapy may be required for up to 1 week (See dosing guidelines for *Minor Surgery*).
Profilnine® SD: Raise factor IX level to 50% of normal immediately prior to procedure.
Minor surgery:
Bebulin® VH: Raise factor IX level to 40% to 60% of normal on day of surgery [typical initial dose: 50-60 units/kg]. Decrease factor IX level from 40% of normal to 20% of normal during initial postoperative period (1-2 weeks or until adequate wound healing) [typical dose: 55 units/kg decreasing to 25 units/kg]. The preoperative dose should be given 1 hour prior to surgery. The average dosing interval may be every 12 hours initially, then every 24 hours later in the postoperative period.
Profilnine® SD: Raise factor IX level to 30% to 50% of normal for at least 1 week following surgery.
Major surgery:
Bebulin® VH: Raise factor IX level to ≥60% of normal on day of surgery [typical initial dose: 70-95 units/kg]; do not raise >60% in patients who may be predisposed to thrombosis. Decrease factor IX level from 60% of normal to 20% of normal during initial postoperative period (1-2 weeks) [typical dose: 70 units/kg decreasing to 35 units/kg]; further decrease to maintain a factor IX level of 20% of normal during late postoperative period (≥3 weeks) and continuing until adequate wound healing is achieved [typical dose: 35 units/kg decreasing to 25 units/kg]. The preoperative dose should be given 1 hour prior to surgery. The average dosing interval may be every 12 hours initially, then every 24 hours later in the postoperative period.
Profilnine® SD: Raise Factor IX level to 30% to 50% of normal for at least 1 week following surgery.

Hemorrhage: I.V.:
Long-term prophylactic treatment: Bebulin® VH: 20-30 units/kg once or twice a week may reduce frequency of spontaneous hemorrhage; dosing regimen should be individualized.

Warfarin associated hemorrhage (unlabeled use): I.V.:
Note: Products contain low or nontherapeutic levels of factor VII component; therefore, additional fresh frozen plasma (FFP) or factor VIIa may be considered (Masotti, 2011). When immediate INR reversal is required, concomitant use of 1-2 units of FFP should be considered to ensure acute INR reversal (Baker, 2004; Chong, 2010; Holland, 2009). Administer vitamin K (phytonadione) 5-10 mg by slow I.V. infusion (Guyatt, 2012); vitamin K may be repeated every 12 hours if INR is persistently elevated.
Adjusted-dose regimen, weight based (Chong, 2010):
Profilnine® SD:
INR <5: 30 units/kg
INR >5 (emergent): 50 units/kg
Note: If after administration, INR remains >1.2 consider repeating dose and administering more FFP until INR <1.2

The following 2 methods have also been suggested, but are not product specific:
Adjusted-dose regimen, weight based (Liumbruno, 2009):
INR <2.0: 20 units/kg
INR 2.0-4.0: 30 units/kg
INR >4.0: 50 units/kg
Note: If after administration, INR remains >1.5 consider repeating dose appropriate for INR.
May also determine dose based on presenting INR and estimated functional prothrombin complex (PC) expressed as percentage of normal plasma levels (see table; Masotti, 2011):
Units needed to be infused = (**target** % of functional PC to be reached – **current** estimated % of functional PC) x kg of body weight
Example:
Patient (weight: 70 kg) presents with INR of 4.5 which corresponds to an **estimated % functional PC** of 10% (see table). Target INR of 1.4 corresponds to an **estimated target % functional PC** of 40%.
Units needed to be infused = (40 - 10) x 70 kg = 2100 units

Conversion of the INR to Estimated Functional Prothrombin Complex (PC)

INR Value	Estimated Functional PC
≥5.0	5%
4-4.9	10%
2.6-3.2	15%
2.2-2.5	20%
1.9-2.1	25%
1.7-1.8	30%
1.4-1.6	40%
1.0-1.3	100%

Dosage adjustment in renal impairment: No dosage adjustment provided in manufacturer's labeling.
Dosage adjustment in hepatic impairment: No dosage adjustment provided in manufacturer's labeling; use with caution.

Administration I.V. administration only; should be infused **slowly**. Rate should not exceed 2 mL/minute for Bebulin® VH or 10 mL/minute for Profilnine® SD. Slowing the rate of infusion, changing the lot of medication, or administering antihistamines may relieve some adverse reactions

Monitoring Parameters Levels of factor IX; PT, PTT; INR (when used for warfarin reversal); signs and symptoms of hypersensitivity reactions, DIC, thrombosis

Reference Range Average normal factor IX levels are 50% to 150%; patients with severe hemophilia B will have factor IX levels <1%, often undetectable. Moderate forms of the disease have levels of 1% to 5% while some mild cases may have 5% to 49% of normal factor IX.

Additional Information Vaccination with hepatitis A and hepatitis B vaccines are recommended at diagnosis for patients with hemophilia.

Factor IX concentrate containing only factor IX is also available and preferable for hemophilia B (or Christmas disease). Prothrombin complex concentrates also contain factor II, factor VII, and factor X and are of intermediate purity. Heparin may be present in some products to decrease thrombotic effects.

Dosage Forms Excipient information presented when available (limited, particularly for generics); consult specific product labeling. [DSC] = Discontinued product

Injection, powder for reconstitution:

Bebulin® VH: Exact potency labeled on each vial [vapor heated; contains heparin and natural rubber/natural latex in packaging]

Profilnine® SD: ~500 units, ~1000 units, ~1500 units [exact potency labeled on each vial; solvent/detergent treated]

◆ **Factor IX Concentrate** *see* Factor IX (Human) *on page 825*

◆ **Factor IX Concentrate** *see* Factor IX (Recombinant) *on page 827*

Factor IX (Human) (FAK ter nyne HYU man)

Brand Names: U.S. AlphaNine SD; Mononine

Brand Names: Canada Immunine® VH

Index Terms Factor IX Concentrate

Pharmacologic Category Antihemophilic Agent; Blood Product Derivative

Use Prevention and control of bleeding in patients with hemophilia B (congenital factor IX deficiency or Christmas disease)

NOTE: Contains **nondetectable levels of factors II, VII, and X**. Therefore, **NOT INDICATED** for replacement therapy of any other clotting factor besides factor IX or for reversal of anticoagulation due to either vitamin K antagonists or other anticoagulants (eg, dabigatran), for hemophilia A patients with factor VIII inhibitors, or for patients in a hemorrhagic state caused by reduced production of liver-dependent coagulation factors (eg, hepatitis, cirrhosis).

Pregnancy Risk Factor C

Pregnancy Considerations Animal reproduction studies have not been conducted. Factor IX concentrations do not change significantly in pregnant women with coagulation disorders and women with factor IX deficiency may be at increased risk of postpartum hemorrhage. Pregnant women should have clotting factors monitored, particularly at 28 and 34 weeks gestation and prior to invasive procedures. Prophylaxis may be needed if factor IX concentrations are <50 units/mL at term and treatment should continue for 3-5 days postpartum depending on route of delivery. Because parvovirus infection may cause hydrops fetalis or fetal death, a recombinant product is preferred if prophylaxis or treatment is needed. The neonate may also be at an increased risk of bleeding following delivery and should be tested for the coagulation disorder (Chi, 2012; Kadir, 2009; Lee, 2006).

Contraindications

AlphaNine SD®: There are no contraindications listed in the manufacturer's labeling.

Mononine®: Hypersensitivity to mouse protein

Warnings/Precautions Hypersensitivity and anaphylactic reactions have been reported with use. Delayed reactions (up to 20 days after infusion) in previously untreated patients may also occur. Due to potential for allergic reactions, the initial ~10-20 administrations should be performed under appropriate medical supervision. Hypersensitivity reactions may be associated with factor IX inhibitor development; patients experiencing allergic reactions should be evaluated for factor IX inhibitors. The development of factor IX antibodies (or inhibitors) has been reported with factor IX therapy (usually occurs within the first 10-20 exposure days); the risk of severe hypersensitivity reactions occurring may be greater in these patients. When clinical response is suboptimal, the patient has reached a specified number of exposure days, or patient is to undergo surgical procedure, screen for inhibitors. Patients with severe hemophilia compared to those with mild or moderate hemophilia are more likely to develop inhibitors (WFH, 2012).

Observe closely for signs or symptoms of intravascular coagulation or thrombosis; risk is generally associated with the use of factor IX complex concentrates (containing therapeutic amounts of additional factors); however, potential risk exists with use of factor IX products (containing only factor IX). Use with caution when administering to patients with liver disease, postoperatively, neonates, or patients at risk of thromboembolic phenomena, disseminated intravascular coagulation or patients with signs of fibrinolysis due to the potential risk of thromboembolic complications.

Contains **nondetectable levels of factors II, VII, and X**. Therefore, **NOT INDICATED** for replacement therapy of any other clotting factor besides factor IX. In addition, factor IX concentrate is **NOT INDICATED** for reversal of anticoagulation due to either vitamin K antagonists or other anticoagulants (eg, dabigatran), hemophilia A patients with factor VIII inhibitors, or patients in a hemorrhagic state caused by reduced production of liver-dependent coagulation factors (eg, hepatitis, cirrhosis). Product of human plasma; despite purification methods (AlphaNine® SD - solvent detergent treated/virus filtered; Mononine® - virus filtered); products may potentially contain infectious agents which could transmit disease. Screening of donors, as well as testing and/or inactivation or removal of certain viruses, reduces the risk. Infections thought to be transmitted by this product should be reported to the manufacturer. Safety and efficacy have not been established with factor IX products in immune tolerance induction. Nephrotic syndrome has occurred following immune tolerance induction in patients with factor IX inhibitors and a history of allergic reactions to therapy.

Adverse Reactions Frequency not defined.

Cardiovascular: Cyanosis, flushing, hypotension, chest tightness, thrombosis

Central nervous system: Chills, dizziness, drowsiness, fever (including transient fever following rapid administration), headache, lethargy, lightheadedness, somnolence

Dermatologic: Angioedema, photosensitivity reaction, rash, urticaria

Gastrointestinal: Abnormal taste, diarrhea, nausea, vomiting

Hematologic: Disseminated intravascular coagulation (DIC)

Hepatic: Alkaline phosphatase increased, ALT increased, AST increased

Local: Injection site reactions: Cellulitis, discomfort, pain, phlebitis, stinging

Neuromuscular & skeletal: Neck tightness, paresthesia, rigors

Ocular: Visual disturbance

Respiratory: Allergic rhinitis, asthma, cough, dyspnea, hypoxia, laryngeal edema, lung disorder

Miscellaneous: Allergic reaction, anaphylaxis, burning sensation in jaw/skull, factor IX inhibitor development, hypersensitivity reaction

Postmarketing and/or case reports: HAV seroconversion, inadequate response/recovery, nephrotic syndrome (associated with immune tolerance induction), parvovirus B19 seroconversion, renal infarction, superior vena cava syndrome (neonates)

Drug Interactions

Metabolism/Transport Effects None known.

Avoid Concomitant Use

Avoid concomitant use of Factor IX (Human) with any of the following: Aminocaproic Acid

Increased Effect/Toxicity

The levels/effects of Factor IX (Human) may be increased by: Aminocaproic Acid

Decreased Effect There are no known significant interactions involving a decrease in effect.

Preparation for Administration Refer to instructions for individual products. Exact potency labeled on each vial. Diluent and factor IX should come to room temperature before combining.

Storage/Stability When stored at refrigerator temperature, 2°C to 8°C (36°F to 46°F), factor IX is stable for the period indicated by the expiration date on its label. Avoid freezing which may damage container for the diluent.

AlphaNine® SD: May also be stored at room temperature not to exceed 30°C (86°F) for up to 1 month. Reconstituted solution should be used within 3 hours of preparation.

Mononine®: May also be stored at room temperature not to exceed 25°C (77°F) for up to 1 month. Reconstituted solution should be at room temperature and used within 3 hours of preparation.

Mechanism of Action Replaces deficient clotting factor IX. Hemophilia B, or Christmas disease, is an X-linked inherited disorder of blood coagulation characterized by insufficient or abnormal synthesis of the clotting protein factor IX. Factor IX is a vitamin K-dependent coagulation factor which is synthesized in the liver. Factor IX is activated by factor XIa in the intrinsic coagulation pathway. Activated factor IX (IXa), in combination with factor VII:C activates factor X to Xa, resulting ultimately in the conversion of prothrombin to thrombin and the formation of a fibrin clot. The infusion of exogenous factor IX to replace the deficiency present in hemophilia B temporarily restores hemostasis.

Pharmacodynamics/Kinetics Half-life elimination: IX component: ~21-25 hours

Dosage NOTE: Contains **nondetectable levels of factors II, VII, and X**. Therefore, **NOT INDICATED** for replacement therapy of any other clotting factor besides factor IX or for reversal of anticoagulation due to either vitamin K antagonists or other anticoagulants (eg, dabigatran), for hemophilia A patients with factor VIII inhibitors, or for patients in a hemorrhagic state caused by reduced production of liver-dependent coagulation factors (eg, hepatitis, cirrhosis).

Control or prevention of bleeding in patients with factor IX deficiency (hemophilia B or Christmas disease): Infants, Children, Adolescents, and Adults: I.V.: *AlphaNine® SD, Mononine®:* Dosage is expressed in units of factor IX activity; dosing must be individualized based on severity of factor IX deficiency, extent and location of bleeding, and clinical status of patient. Refer to product information for specific manufacturer recommended dosing. Alternatively, the World Federation of Hemophilia (WFH) has recommended general dosing for factor IX products.

Formula to determine units required to obtain desired factor IX level: **Note:** If patient has severe hemophilia (ie, baseline factor IX level is or presumed to be <1%), then may just use "desired factor IX level" instead of "desired factor IX level increase".

Number of factor IX units required = patient weight (in kg) x desired factor IX level increase (as % or units/dL) x 1 unit/kg

For example, to attain an 80% level in a 70 kg patient who has a baseline level of 20%: Number of factor IX units needed = 70 kg x 60% x 1 unit/kg = 4200 units

World Federation of Hemophilia (WFH) Guidelines (2012): Note: The following recommendations may vary from those found within prescribing information or practitioner preference.

Prophylaxis: 15-30 units/kg twice weekly (WFH, 2012 [Utrecht protocol]) **or** 25-40 units/kg twice weekly (WFH, 2012 [Malmö protocol]) **or** 40-100 units/kg administered 2-3 times weekly (National Hemophilia Foundation, MASAC recommendation, 2007); optimum regimen has yet to be defined.

Treatment:

2012 World Federation of Hemophilia Treatment Recommendations (When No Significant Resource Constraint Exists):

Site of Hemorrhage/ Clinical Situation	Desired Factor IX Level to Maintain	Duration
Joint	40-60 units/dL	1-2 days, may be longer if response is inadequate
Superficial muscle/ no neurovascular compromise	40-60 units/dL	2-3 days, sometimes longer if response is inadequate
Iliopsoas and deep muscle with neurovascular injury, or substantial blood loss	*Initial:* 60-80 units/dL *Maintenance:* 30-60 units/dL	*Initial:* 1-2 days *Maintenance:* 3-5 days, sometimes longer as secondary prophylaxis during physiotherapy
CNS/head	*Initial:* 60-80 units/dL *Maintenance:* 30 units/dL	*Initial:* 1-7 days *Maintenance:* 8-21 days
Throat and neck	*Initial:* 60-80 units/dL *Maintenance:* 30 units/dL	*Initial:* 1-7 days *Maintenance:* 8-14 days
Gastrointestinal	*Initial:* 60-80 units/dL *Maintenance:* 30 units/dL	*Initial:* 7-14 days *Maintenance:* Not specified
Renal	40 units/dL	3-5 days
Deep laceration	40 units/dL	5-7 days
Surgery (major)	*Preop:* 60-80 units/dL	
	Postop: 40-60 units/dL 30-50 units/dL 20-40 units/dL	*Postop:* 1-3 days 4-6 days 7-14 days
Surgery (minor)	*Preop:* 50-80 units/dL	
	Postop: 30-80 units/dL	*Postop:* 1-5 days depending on procedure type

Note: Factor IX level may either be expressed as units/dL or as %. Dosing frequency most commonly corresponds to the half-life of factor IX but should be determined based on an assessment of factor IX levels before the next dose.

Continuous infusion (for patients who require prolonged periods of treatment [eg, intracranial hemorrhage or surgery] to avoid peaks and troughs associated with intermittent infusions) (Batorova, 2002; Poon, 2012; Rickard, 1995; WFH, 2012): Following initial bolus to achieve the desired factor IX level: Initiate 4-6 units/kg/hour; adjust dose based on frequent factor assays and calculation of factor IX clearance at steady-state using the following equations:

Factor IX clearance (mL/kg/hour) = (current infusion rate in units/kg/hour) divided by (plasma level in units/**mL**)

New infusion rate (units/kg/hour) = (factor IX clearance in mL/kg/hour) x (desired plasma level in units/**mL**)

Administration Solution should be infused at room temperature.

I.V. administration only: Should be infused **slowly over several minutes**: Rate of administration should be determined by the response and comfort of the patient.

AlphaNine® SD: Administer I.V. at a rate not exceeding 10 mL/minute

Mononine®: Administer I.V. at a rate of ~2 mL/minute. Administration rates of up to 225 **units**/minute have been regularly tolerated without incident (when reconstituted as directed to ~100 units/mL).

World Federation of Hemophilia (WFH) recommendations: Infuse at rate of 3 mL/minute for adults or 100 **units**/minute for young children; may also administer as a continuous infusion in select patients. With patients who have had allergic reactions during factor IX infusion, administration of hydrocortisone prior to infusion may be necessary (WFH, 2012).

Monitoring Parameters Factor IX levels (measure 15 minutes after infusion to verify calculated doses [WFH, 2012]), aPTT, BP, HR, signs of hypersensitivity reactions; screen for factor IX inhibitors if the patient experiences hypersensitivity reaction or when patient is to undergo surgery, if suboptimal response to treatment occurs, if patient is being intensively treated for >5 days within 4 weeks of the last infusion, or at the following intervals (WFH, 2012):

Children: Screen for inhibitors every 5 exposure days until 20 exposure days, every 10 exposure days between 21-50 exposure days, and at a minimum of twice a year until 150 exposure days is reached.

Adults (with >150 exposure days apart from a 6-12 monthly review): Screen for inhibitors when suboptimal response occurs.

Reference Range Average normal factor IX levels are 50% to 150%; patients with severe hemophilia B will have levels <1%, often undetectable. Moderate forms of the disease have levels of 1% to 5% while some mild cases may have 5% to 49% of normal factor IX.

Dosage Forms Excipient information presented when available (limited, particularly for generics); consult specific product labeling.

Solution Reconstituted, Intravenous [preservative free]:

AlphaNine SD: 500 units (1 ea); 1000 units (1 ea); 1500 units (1 ea) [contains polysorbate 80]

Mononine: 250 units (1 ea); 500 units (1 ea) [contains polysorbate 80]

Factor IX (Recombinant)

(FAK ter nyne ree KOM be nant)

Brand Names: U.S. BeneFIX; Rixubis

Brand Names: Canada BeneFix

Index Terms Factor IX Concentrate

Pharmacologic Category Antihemophilic Agent

Use Prevention and control of bleeding episodes in patients with hemophilia B (congenital factor IX deficiency or Christmas disease); perioperative management in patients with hemophilia B; routine prophylaxis in adults with hemophilia B to prevent or reduce the frequency of bleeding episodes (Rixubis)

NOTE: Contains **only factor IX**. Therefore, **NOT INDICATED** for replacement therapy of any other clotting factor besides factor IX or for reversal of anticoagulation due to either vitamin K antagonists or other anticoagulants (eg, dabigatran), for hemophilia A patients with factor VIII inhibitors, or for patients in a hemorrhagic state caused by reduced production of liver-dependent coagulation factors (eg, hepatitis, cirrhosis).

Pregnancy Risk Factor C

Pregnancy Considerations Animal reproduction studies have not been conducted. Factor IX concentrations do not change significantly in pregnant women with coagulation disorders and women with factor IX deficiency may be at increased risk of postpartum hemorrhage. Pregnant women should have clotting factors monitored, particularly at 28 and 34 weeks gestation and prior to invasive procedures. Prophylaxis may be needed if factor IX concentrations are <50 units/mL at term and treatment should continue for 3-5 days postpartum depending on route of delivery. Because parvovirus infection may cause hydrops fetalis or fetal death, a recombinant product is preferred if prophylaxis or treatment is needed. The neonate may also be at an increased risk of bleeding following delivery and should be tested for the coagulation disorder (Chi, 2012; Kadir, 2009; Lee, 2006).

Breast-Feeding Considerations It is not known if factor IX (recombinant) is excreted in breast milk. The manufacturer recommends that caution be exercised when administering factor IX (recombinant) to nursing women.

Contraindications Life-threatening, immediate hypersensitivity reactions (including anaphylaxis) to factor IX, hamster protein, or any component of the formulation; disseminated intravascular coagulation (Rixubis); signs of fibrinolysis (Rixubis)

Warnings/Precautions Contains **only factor IX**. Therefore, **NOT INDICATED** for replacement therapy of any other clotting factor besides factor IX or for reversal of anticoagulation due to either vitamin K antagonists or other anticoagulants (eg, dabigatran), for hemophilia A patients with factor VIII inhibitors, or for patients in a hemorrhagic state caused by reduced production of liver-dependent coagulation factors (eg, hepatitis, cirrhosis).

Hypersensitivity and anaphylactic reactions have been reported with use. Risk is highest during the early phases of initial exposure in previously untreated patients, especially those with high-risk gene mutations. Delayed reactions (up to 20 days after infusion) in previously untreated patients may also occur. Due to potential for allergic reactions, the initial ~10-20 administrations should be performed under appropriate medical supervision. Hypersensitivity reactions may be associated with factor IX inhibitor development; patients experiencing allergic reactions should be evaluated for factor IX inhibitors. If severe hypersensitivity reactions occur, consider the use of alternative hemostatic measures.

The development of factor IX antibodies (or inhibitors) has been reported with factor IX therapy (usually occurs within the first 10-20 exposure days); the risk of severe hypersensitivity reactions occurring may be greater in these patients. When clinical response is suboptimal, the patient has reached a specified number of exposure days, or patient is to undergo surgical procedure, screen for inhibitors. Patients with severe hemophilia compared to those with mild or moderate hemophilia are more likely to develop inhibitors (WFH, 2012).

Observe closely for signs or symptoms of intravascular coagulation or thrombosis; risk is generally associated with the use of factor IX complex concentrates (containing therapeutic amounts of additional factors); however, potential risk exists with use of factor IX products (containing only factor IX). Use with caution when administering to patients with liver disease, postoperatively, neonates, patients at risk of thromboembolic phenomena or disseminated intravascular coagulation, or patients with signs of fibrinolysis due to the potential risk of thromboembolic complications.

Safety and efficacy have not been established with factor IX products in immune tolerance induction. Nephrotic syndrome has occurred following immune tolerance induction in patients with factor IX inhibitors and a history of allergic reactions to therapy.

Adverse Reactions

>10%: Central nervous system: Headache (11%)

1% to 10%:

Cardiovascular: Flushing (3%), chest tightness (2%)

Central nervous system: Dizziness (8%), drowsiness (2%), chills (2%)

Dermatologic: Skin rash (2% to 6%), urticaria (3% to 5%)

Gastrointestinal: Nausea (6%), dysgeusia (1% to 5%), vomiting (2%)

Immunologic: Factor IX inhibitor development (2% to 3%), antibody development (furin: 1%)

Local: Injection site reaction (2% to 8%; including cellulitis, pain, phlebitis)

Neuromuscular & skeletal: Tremor (2%), limb pain (1%)

Ophthalmic: Blurred vision (2%)

Renal: Renal infarction (2%)

Respiratory: Dyspnea (3%), cough (2%), hypoxia (2%)

Miscellaneous: Fever (3%; including transient fever following rapid administration)

<1% (Limited to important or life-threatening): Anaphylaxis, angioedema, arterial thrombosis, deep vein thrombosis, hypersensitivity reaction, hypotension, nephrotic syndrome (associated with immune tolerance induction), peripheral thrombophlebitis, pulmonary embolism, superior vena cava syndrome (neonates), thrombosis

Drug Interactions

Metabolism/Transport Effects None known.

Avoid Concomitant Use

Avoid concomitant use of Factor IX (Recombinant) with any of the following: Aminocaproic Acid

Increased Effect/Toxicity

The levels/effects of Factor IX (Recombinant) may be increased by: Aminocaproic Acid

Decreased Effect There are no known significant interactions involving a decrease in effect.

Preparation for Administration Refer to instructions provided by the manufacturer. Diluent and factor IX should come to room temperature (if refrigerated) before combining.

Storage/Stability

BeneFIX:

Product labeled for room temperature storage: May either store at 2°C to 30°C (36°F to 86°F) or refrigerated at 2°C to 8°C (36°F to 46°F). Avoid freezing which may damage the diluent syringe. Reconstituted solution should be at room temperature and used within 3 hours of preparation.

Product labeled for refrigerated storage: Store at 2°C to 8°C (36°F to 46°F). May be stored at room temperature (not to exceed 30°C [86°F]) for up to 6 months; do not use after this 6-month period has elapsed even if the expiration date on the carton has not been exceeded. If date of removal from refrigeration is not recorded on the carton, the assigned expiration date (printed on the end flap of the carton) **must be reduced by 12 months**. Avoid freezing which may damage the diluent syringe. Reconstituted solution should be at room temperature and used within 3 hours of preparation.

Rixubis: Store at 2°C to 8°C (36°F to 46°F) for up to 18 months; do not freeze. After removal from refrigeration, may store at room temperature not to exceed 30°C (86°F) for up to 6 months within the 18-month time period; do not return to refrigerator. Following reconstitution, use within 3 hours and do not refrigerate.

Mechanism of Action Replaces deficient clotting factor IX. Hemophilia B, or Christmas disease, is an X-linked inherited disorder of blood coagulation characterized by insufficient or abnormal synthesis of the clotting protein factor IX. Factor IX is a vitamin K-dependent coagulation factor which is synthesized in the liver. Factor IX is activated by factor XIa in the intrinsic coagulation pathway. Activated factor IX (IXa) in combination with factor VII:C activates factor X to Xa, resulting ultimately in the conversion of prothrombin to thrombin and the formation of a fibrin clot. The infusion of exogenous factor IX to replace the deficiency present in hemophilia B temporarily restores hemostasis.

Pharmacodynamics/Kinetics

Distribution: V_{ss}: Rixubis: ~0.2 L/kg

Half-life elimination: Children: BeneFIX: 14: 14-28 hours; Adolescents ≥15 years and Adults: BeneFIX, Rixubis: 11-36 hours

Dosage NOTE: Contains **only factor IX**. Therefore, **NOT INDICATED** for replacement therapy of any other clotting factor besides factor IX or for reversal of anticoagulation due to either vitamin K antagonists or other anticoagulants (eg, dabigatran), for hemophilia A patients with factor VIII inhibitors, or for patients in a hemorrhagic state caused by reduced production of liver-dependent coagulation factors (eg, hepatitis, cirrhosis).

Control or prevention of bleeding in patients with factor IX deficiency (hemophilia B or Christmas disease): Dosage is expressed in units of factor IX activity; dosing must be individualized based on severity of factor IX deficiency, extent and location of bleeding, and clinical status of patient. Refer to product information for specific manufacturer recommended dosing. Alternatively, the World Federation of Hemophilia (WFH) has recommended general dosing for factor IX products.

Formula for units required to raise blood level %: **Note:** If patient has severe hemophilia (ie, baseline factor IX level is or presumed to be <1%), then may just use "desired factor IX level" instead of "desired factor IX level *increase*".

Infants, Children, and Adolescents <15 years: I.V.: Number of factor IX units required = patient weight (in kg) x desired factor IX level increase (as % or units/dL) x 1.4 (as units/kg per units/dL)

Adolescents ≥15 years and Adults: I.V.: Number of factor IX units required = patient weight (in kg) x desired factor IX level increase (as % or units/dL) x 1.3 (as units/kg per units/dL)

World Federation of Hemophilia (WFH) Guidelines (2012): Infants, Children, Adolescents, and Adults: **Note:** The following recommendations may vary from those found within prescribing information or practitioner preference.

Prophylaxis: 15-30 units/kg twice weekly (WFH, 2012 [Utrecht protocol]) **or** 25-40 units/kg twice weekly (WFH, 2012 [Malmö protocol]) **or** 40-100 units/kg administered 2-3 times weekly (National Hemophilia Foundation, MASAC recommendation, 2007); optimum regimen has yet to be defined.

Treatment:

2012 World Federation of Hemophilia Treatment Recommendations (When No Significant Resource Constraint Exists):

Site of Hemorrhage/ Clinical Situation	Desired Factor IX Level to Maintain	Duration
Joint	40-60 units/dL	1-2 days, may be longer if response is inadequate
Superficial muscle/ no neurovascular compromise	40-60 units/dL	2-3 days, sometimes longer if response is inadequate
Iliopsoas and deep muscle with neurovascular injury, or substantial blood loss	*Initial:* 60-80 units/dL *Maintenance:* 30-60 units/dL	*Initial:* 1-2 days *Maintenance:* 3-5 days, sometimes longer as secondary prophylaxis during physiotherapy
CNS/head	*Initial:* 60-80 units/dL *Maintenance:* 30 units/dL	*Initial:* 1-7 days *Maintenance:* 8-21 days
Throat and neck	*Initial:* 60-80 units/dL *Maintenance:* 30 units/dL	*Initial:* 1-7 days *Maintenance:* 8-14 days
Gastrointestinal	*Initial:* 60-80 units/dL *Maintenance:* 30 units/dL	*Initial:* 7-14 days *Maintenance:* Not specified
Renal	40 units/dL	3-5 days
Deep laceration	40 units/dL	5-7 days
Surgery (major)	*Preop:* 60-80 units/dL	
	Postop: 40-60 units/dL 30-50 units/dL 20-40 units/dL	*Postop:* 1-3 days 4-6 days 7-14 days
Surgery (minor)	*Preop:* 50-80 units/dL	
	Postop: 30-80 units/dL	*Postop:* 1-5 days depending on procedure type

Note: Factor IX level may either be expressed as units/dL or as %. Dosing frequency most commonly corresponds to the half-life of factor IX but should be determined based on an assessment of factor IX levels before the next dose.

Continuous infusion (For patients who require prolonged periods of treatment [eg, intracranial hemorrhage or surgery] to avoid peaks and troughs associated with intermittent infusions) (Batorova, 2002; Poon, 2012; Rickard, 1995; WFH, 2012): Following initial bolus to achieve the desired factor IX level: Initiate 4-6 units/kg/hour; adjust dose based on frequent factor assays and calculation of factor IX clearance at steady-state using the following equations:

Factor IX clearance (mL/kg/hour) = (current infusion rate in units/kg/hour)/(plasma level in units/**m**L)

New infusion rate (units/kg/hour) = (factor IX clearance in mL/kg/hour) x (desired plasma level in units/**m**L)

Routine prophylaxis to prevent bleeding episodes in patients with factor IX deficiency (hemophilia B or Christmas disease) (Rixubis): Adults: 40-60 units/kg twice weekly; may titrate dose depending upon age, bleeding pattern, and physical activity.

Administration Solution should be infused at room temperature. Safety and efficacy of continuous infusion administration have not been determined.

I.V. administration only:

BeneFIX: Should be infused **slowly over several minutes.** Rate of administration should be determined by the response and comfort of the patient.

Rixubis: Bolus infusion; maximum rate of administration is 10 mL/minute

Per the WFH, infuse at rate of 3 mL/minute for adults or 100 **units**/minute for young children; may also administer as a continuous infusion in select patients. With patients who have had allergic reactions during factor IX infusion, administration of hydrocortisone prior to infusion may be necessary (WFH, 2012).

Monitoring Parameters Factor IX levels (measure 15 minutes after infusion to verify calculated doses [WFH, 2012]), aPTT, BP, HR, signs of hypersensitivity reactions, DIC, and thrombosis; screen for factor IX inhibitors if the patient experiences hypersensitivity reaction or when patient is to undergo surgery, if suboptimal response to treatment occurs, if patient is being intensively treated for >5 days within 4 weeks of the last infusion, or at the following intervals (WFH, 2012):

Children: Screen for inhibitors every 5 exposure days until 20 exposure days, every 10 exposure days between 21-50 exposure days, and at a minimum of twice a year until 150 exposure days is reached.

Adults (with >150 exposure days apart from a 6-12 monthly review): Screen for inhibitors when suboptimal response occurs.

Reference Range Average normal factor IX levels are 50% to 150%; patients with severe hemophilia B will have levels <1%, often undetectable. Moderate forms of the disease have levels of 1% to 5% while some mild cases may have 5% to 49% of normal factor IX.

Dosage Forms Excipient information presented when available (limited, particularly for generics); consult specific product labeling.

Solution Reconstituted, Intravenous [preservative free]:

BeneFIX: 250 units (1 ea); 500 units (1 ea); 1000 units (1 ea); 2000 units (1 ea) [contains polysorbate 80]

Rixubis: 250 units (1 ea); 500 units (1 ea); 1000 units (1 ea); 2000 units (1 ea); 3000 units (1 ea) [contains polysorbate 80]

◆ **3 Factor PCC** *see* Factor IX Complex (Human) [(Factors II, IX, X)] *on page 822*

◆ **4 Factor PCC** *see* Prothrombin Complex Concentrate (Human) [(Factors II, VII, IX, X), Protein C, and Protein S] *on page 1743*

◆ **Factor 13** *see* Factor XIII Concentrate (Human) *on page 829*

Factor XIII Concentrate (Human)

(FAK ter THIR teen KON cen trate HYU man)

Brand Names: U.S. Corifact

Index Terms Activated Factor XIII; Corifact®; Factor 13; FXIII

Pharmacologic Category Antihemophilic Agent; Blood Product Derivative

Use Prophylaxis against bleeding episodes and management of perioperative surgical bleeding in patients with congenital factor XIII deficiency

Pregnancy Risk Factor C

Pregnancy Considerations Use in pregnant women only when benefit exceeds potential risk to the fetus. Thromboembolic events have been reported with use of factor XIII; pregnant women may be at increased risk due to hypercoagulable state.

Breast-Feeding Considerations It is not known if factor XIII concentrate (human) is excreted in breast milk. The manufacturer recommends that caution be exercised when administering factor XIII concentrate (human) to nursing women.

Contraindications History of anaphylaxis or severe systemic reactions to human plasma-derived products or hypersensitivity to any component of the formulation

Warnings/Precautions The development of factor XIII inhibitory antibodies has been reported. Factor XIII inhibitory antibodies should be measured when clinical response (breakthrough bleeding) and/or factor XIII trough levels are suboptimal after apparent adequate dosing. Hypersensitivity reactions have been reported with use; discontinue immediately if develops and initiate appropriate management. Thromboembolic events have been reported; pregnant women may be at increased risk due to hypercoagulable state. Use caution in patients with known risk factors for thrombosis. Product of human plasma; may potentially contain infectious agents which could transmit disease. Screening of donors, as well as testing and/or inactivation or removal of certain viruses, reduces the risk. Infections thought to be transmitted by this product should be reported to the manufacturer. Vaccination with hepatitis A and hepatitis B vaccines is recommended.

Adverse Reactions

>1%:

Central nervous system: Chills, fever, headache

Dermatologic: Bruising, erythema, pruritus, rash

Hematologic: Hematoma, thrombin-antithrombin levels increased

Hepatic: LDH increased

Neuromuscular & skeletal: Arthralgia, joint inflammation

Respiratory: Epistaxis

Miscellaneous: Hypersensitivity

<1% (Limited to important or life-threatening): Acute ischemia, anaphylaxis, factor XIII inhibitory antibodies, infection, thromboembolism

Drug Interactions

Metabolism/Transport Effects None known.

Avoid Concomitant Use There are no known interactions where it is recommended to avoid concomitant use.

Increased Effect/Toxicity There are no known significant interactions involving an increase in effect.

Decreased Effect There are no known significant interactions involving a decrease in effect.

Preparation for Administration Reconstitute with provided diluent (SWFI); gently swirl; do not shake. Product and diluent should be at room temperature prior to reconstitution. Reconstituted solution should be used within 4 hours; do not refrigerate or freeze.

Storage/Stability Store at 2°C to 8°C (36°F to 46°F); do not freeze. Protect from light. May be stored at room temperature (≤25°C [≤77°F]) for up to 6 months; do not return to refrigerator if stored at room temperature.

Mechanism of Action Factor XIII (FXIII) is an endogenous plasma glycoprotein found in platelets, monocytes and macrophages that is converted to activated factor XIII (FXIIIa) in the presence of calcium ions. Once activated, FXIIIa cross-links fibrin and cross-links plasmin inhibitor to protect and strengthen the hemostatic platelet plug.

Pharmacodynamics/Kinetics

Duration of effect: Plasma levels of FXIII: ~28 days; FXIII activity maintained at ≥5% in ≥97% of patients and ≥10% in ≥85% of patients

Distribution: V_d: 51.1 mL/kg

Metabolism: Factor XIII, a proenzyme, is converted to activated factor XIII

Half-life elimination: Children (<16): 5.7 days; Adults: 7.1 days

Time to peak: 1.7 hours postinfusion

Dosage Congenital factor XIII deficiency: Infants, Children, Adolescents, and Adults: I.V.:

Prophylaxis:

Initial: 40 units/kg

Maintenance: Dose adjustment should be based on factor XIII activity trough levels (target level of 5% to 20% using Berichrom® activity assay) and clinical response; repeat every 28 days

One trough level of <5%: Increase dosage by 5 units/kg

Trough level of 5% to 20%: No dosage change

Two trough levels of >20%: Decrease dosage by 5 units/kg

One trough level of >25%: Decrease dosage by 5 units/kg

Perioperative management of surgical bleeding: Individualize dosing based on factor XIII activity level, type of surgery, and clinical response; monitor factor XIII activity levels during and after surgery:

If time since last prophylactic dose ≤7 days: Additional dose may not be needed.

If time since last prophylactic dose 8-21 days: Additional partial or full dose may be necessary based on factor XIII activity level

If time since last prophylactic dose 21-28 days: Administer full prophylactic dose

Dosage adjustment in renal impairment: No dosage adjustment provided in the manufacturer's labeling.

Dosage adjustment in hepatic impairment: No dosage adjustment provided in the manufacturer's labeling.

Administration Administer by I.V. infusion at a rate not to exceed 4 mL/minute. Product should be brought to room temperature prior to infusing. Administer through a separate infusion line.

Monitoring Parameters Factor XIII trough levels in conjunction with clinical response to assess efficacy (ie, approximately every 28 days for prophylaxis, during and after surgery for perioperative management of surgical bleeding). Factor XIII inhibitory antibodies if inadequate clinical response and/or factor XIII trough levels are suboptimal. Signs/symptoms of hypersensitivity reactions, thrombotic events, and infection.

Dosage Forms Excipient information presented when available (limited, particularly for generics); consult specific product labeling.

Kit, Intravenous [preservative free]:

Corifact: 1000-1600 UNIT

◆ FAG-201 *see* Dimethyl Fumarate *on page 618*

◆ Falmina *see* Ethinyl Estradiol and Levonorgestrel *on page 787*

Famciclovir (fam SYE kloe veer)

Brand Names: U.S. Famvir

Brand Names: Canada Apo-Famciclovir®; Ava-Famciclovir; CO Famciclovir; Famvir®; PMS-Famciclovir; Sandoz-Famciclovir

Pharmacologic Category Antiviral Agent

Use Treatment of acute herpes zoster (shingles) in immunocompetent patients; treatment and suppression of recurrent episodes of genital herpes in immunocompetent patients; treatment of herpes labialis (cold sores) in immunocompetent patients; treatment of recurrent orolabial/ genital (mucocutaneous) herpes simplex in HIV-infected patients

Pregnancy Risk Factor B

Pregnancy Considerations Teratogenic effects were not observed in animal reproduction studies. Data in pregnant women is limited. A registry has been established for women exposed to famciclovir during pregnancy (888-669-6682).

Breast-Feeding Considerations There is no specific data describing the excretion of famciclovir in breast milk. Breast-feeding is not recommended by the manufacturer unless the potential benefits outweigh any possible risk. If herpes lesions are on breast, breast-feeding should be avoided in order to avoid transmission to infant.

Contraindications Hypersensitivity to famciclovir, penciclovir, or any component of the formulation

Warnings/Precautions Has not been established for use in immunocompromised patients (except HIV-infected patients with orolabial or genital herpes, patients with ophthalmic or disseminated zoster or with initial episode of genital herpes, and in Black and African American patients with recurrent episodes of genital herpes. Acute renal failure has been reported with use of inappropriate high doses in patients with underlying renal disease. Dosage adjustment is required in patients with renal insufficiency. Tablets contain lactose; do not use with galactose intolerance, severe lactase deficiency, or glucose-galactose malabsorption syndromes.

Adverse Reactions Note: Frequencies vary with dose and duration.

>10%:

Central nervous system: Headache (9% to 39%)

Gastrointestinal: Nausea (2% to 13%)

1% to 10%:

Central nervous system: Fatigue (1% to 5%), migraine (1% to 3%)

Dermatologic: Pruritus (≤4%), rash (≤3%)

Endocrine & metabolic: Dysmenorrhea (≤8%)

Gastrointestinal: Diarrhea (2% to 9%), abdominal pain (≤8%), vomiting (1% to 5%), flatulence (≤5%)

Hematologic: Neutropenia (3%)

Hepatic: Transaminases increased (2% to 3%), bilirubin increased (2%)

Neuromuscular & skeletal: Paresthesia (≤3%)

<1% (Limited to important or life-threatening): Anemia, angioedema (eyelid, face, periorbital, pharyngeal edema), cholestatic jaundice, confusion, delirium, disorientation, dizziness, erythema multiforme, hallucinations, leukocytoclastic vasculitis, palpitations, somnolence, Stevens-Johnson syndrome, thrombocytopenia, toxic epidermal necrolysis, urticaria

Drug Interactions

Metabolism/Transport Effects None known.

Avoid Concomitant Use

Avoid concomitant use of Famciclovir with any of the following: Zoster Vaccine

Increased Effect/Toxicity There are no known significant interactions involving an increase in effect.

Decreased Effect

Famciclovir may decrease the levels/effects of: Zoster Vaccine

Ethanol/Nutrition/Herb Interactions Food: Rate of absorption and/or conversion to penciclovir and peak concentration are reduced with food, but bioavailability is not affected.

Storage/Stability Store at 25°C (77°F); excursions permitted to 15°C to 30°C (59°F to 86°F).

Mechanism of Action Famciclovir undergoes rapid biotransformation to the active compound, penciclovir (prodrug), which is phosphorylated by viral thymidine kinase in HSV-1, HSV-2, and VZV-infected cells to a monophosphate form; this is then converted to penciclovir triphosphate and competes with deoxyguanosine triphosphate to inhibit HSV-2 polymerase, therefore, herpes viral DNA synthesis/replication is selectively inhibited.

Pharmacodynamics/Kinetics

Absorption: Food decreases maximum peak penciclovir concentration and delays time to penciclovir peak; AUC remains the same

Distribution: V_d: Penciclovir: 0.91-1.25 L/kg

Protein binding: Penciclovir: <20%

Metabolism: Famciclovir is rapidly deacetylated and oxidized to penciclovir (active prodrug); *in vitro* data demonstrate that metabolism does not occur via CYP isoenzymes

Bioavailability: Penciclovir: 69% to 85%

Half-life elimination: Penciclovir: 2-4 hours; Prolonged in renal impairment: Cl_{cr} 20-39 mL/minute: 5-8 hours, Cl_{cr} <20 mL/minute: 3-24 hours

Time to peak: Penciclovir: ~1 hour

Excretion: Urine (73% primarily as penciclovir); feces (27%)

Dosage Adults: Oral:

Immunocompetent patients:

Acute herpes zoster: 500 mg every 8 hours for 7 days (**Note:** Initiate therapy as soon as possible after diagnosis and within 72 hours of rash onset)

Genital herpes simplex virus (HSV) infection:

Initial episode: 250 mg 3 times/day for 7-10 days (CDC, 2010)

Recurrence: 1000 mg twice daily for 1 day (**Note:** Initiate therapy as soon as possible and within 6 hours of symptoms/lesions onset)

Alternatively, the following regimens are also recommended: 125 mg twice daily for 5 days or 500 mg as a single dose, followed by 250 mg twice daily for 2 days (CDC, 2010). **Note:** Canadian labeling recommends 125 mg twice daily for 5 days.

Suppressive therapy: 250 mg twice daily for up to 1 year; **Note:** Duration not established, but efficacy/safety have been demonstrated for 1 year (CDC, 2010)

Recurrent herpes labialis (cold sores): 1500 mg as a single dose; initiate therapy at first sign or symptom such as tingling, burning, or itching (initiated within 1 hour in clinical studies)

HIV patients (**Note:** Initiate therapy as soon as possible and within 48 hours of symptoms/lesions onset):

Recurrent orolabial/genital (mucocutaneous) HSV infection: 500 mg twice daily for 7 days or 5-10 days (CDC, 2010).

Prevention of HSV reactivation: 500 mg twice daily (CDC, 2010)

Dosing adjustment in renal impairment:

Herpes zoster:

Cl_{cr} ≥60 mL/minute: No dosage adjustment necessary

Cl_{cr} 40-59 mL/minute: Administer 500 mg every 12 hours

Cl_{cr} 20-39 mL/minute: Administer 500 mg every 24 hours

Cl_{cr} <20 mL/minute: Administer 250 mg every 24 hours

Hemodialysis: Administer 250 mg after each dialysis session.

Recurrent genital herpes: Treatment:

U.S. labeling (single-day regimen):

Cl_{cr} ≥60 mL/minute: No dosage adjustment necessary

Cl_{cr} 40-59 mL/minute: Administer 500 mg every 12 hours for 1 day

Cl_{cr} 20-39 mL/minute: Administer 500 mg as a single dose

Cl_{cr} <20 mL/minute: Administer 250 mg as a single dose

Hemodialysis: Administer 250 mg as a single dose after a dialysis session.

Canadian labeling:

Cl_{cr} >20 mL/minute/1.73 m^2: No dosage adjustment necessary

Cl_{cr} <20 mL/minute/1.73 m^2: Administer 125 mg every 24 hours

Hemodialysis: Administer 125 mg after each dialysis session.

Recurrent genital herpes: Suppression:

Cl_{cr} ≥40 mL/minute: No dosage adjustment necessary

Cl_{cr} 20-39 mL/minute: Administer 125 mg every 12 hours

Cl_{cr} <20 mL/minute: Administer 125 mg every 24 hours

Hemodialysis: Administer 125 mg after each dialysis session.

Recurrent herpes labialis: Treatment (single-dose regimen):

Cl_{cr} ≥60 mL/minute: No dosage adjustment necessary

Cl_{cr} 40-59 mL/minute: Administer 750 mg as a single dose

Cl_{cr} 20-39 mL/minute: Administer 500 mg as a single dose

Cl_{cr} <20 mL/minute: Administer 250 mg as a single dose

Hemodialysis: Administer 250 mg as a single dose after a dialysis session.

Recurrent orolabial/genital (mucocutaneous) herpes in HIV-infected patients:

Cl_{cr} ≥40 mL/minute: No dosage adjustment necessary

Cl_{cr} 20-39 mL/minute: Administer 500 mg every 24 hours

Cl_{cr} <20 mL/minute: Administer 250 mg every 24 hours

Hemodialysis: Administer 250 mg after each dialysis session.

Dosage adjustment in hepatic impairment:

Mild-to-moderate impairment: No dosage adjustment is necessary

Severe impairment: No dosage adjustment provided in manufacturer's labeling; has not been studied. However, a 44% decrease in the C_{max} of penciclovir (active metabolite) was noted in patients with mild-to-moderate impairment; impaired conversion of famciclovir to penciclovir may affect efficacy.

Dietary Considerations May be taken without regard to meals.

Administration May be administered without regard to meals.

Monitoring Parameters Periodic CBC during long-term therapy

Additional Information Most effective for herpes zoster if therapy is initiated within 48 hours of initial lesion. Resistance may occur by alteration of thymidine kinase, resulting in loss of or reduced penciclovir phosphorylation (cross-resistance occurs between acyclovir and famciclovir). When treatment for herpes labialis is initiated within 1 hour of symptom onset, healing time is reduced by ~2 days.

Dosage Forms Excipient information presented when available (limited, particularly for generics); consult specific product labeling.

Tablet, Oral:

Famvir: 125 mg, 250 mg, 500 mg

Generic: 125 mg, 250 mg, 500 mg

Famotidine (fa MOE ti deen)

Brand Names: U.S. Acid Reducer Maximum Strength [OTC]; Acid Reducer [OTC]; Heartburn Relief Max St [OTC]; Heartburn Relief [OTC]; Pepcid

Brand Names: Canada Acid Control; Apo-Famotidine®; Apo-Famotidine® Injectable; Famotidine Omega; Mylan-Famotidine; Novo-Famotidine; Nu-Famotidine; Pepcid®; Pepcid® AC; Pepcid® I.V.; Ulcidine

Pharmacologic Category Histamine H_2 Antagonist

Use Maintenance therapy and treatment of duodenal ulcer; treatment of gastroesophageal reflux disease (GERD), active benign gastric ulcer; pathological hypersecretory conditions

OTC labeling: Relief of heartburn, acid indigestion, and sour stomach

Unlabeled Use Part of a multidrug regimen for *H. pylori* eradication to reduce the risk of duodenal ulcer recurrence; stress ulcer prophylaxis in critically-ill patients; symptomatic relief in gastritis

Pregnancy Risk Factor B

Pregnancy Considerations Adverse events have not been observed in animal reproduction studies; therefore, famotidine is classified as pregnancy category B. Famotidine crosses the placenta. An increased risk of congenital malformations or adverse events in the newborn has generally not been observed following maternal use of famotidine during pregnancy. Histamine H_2 antagonists have been evaluated for the treatment of gastroesophageal reflux disease (GERD), as well as gastric and duodenal ulcers, during pregnancy. Although if needed, famotidine is not the agent of choice. Histamine H_2 antagonists may be used for aspiration prophylaxis prior to cesarean delivery.

Breast-Feeding Considerations Famotidine is excreted into breast milk with peak concentrations occurring ~6 hours after the maternal dose. According to the manufacturer, the decision to continue or discontinue breast-feeding during therapy should take into account the risk of exposure to the infant and the benefits of treatment to the mother.

Contraindications Hypersensitivity to famotidine, other H_2 antagonists, or any component of the formulation

Warnings/Precautions Modify dose in patients with moderate-to-severe renal impairment. Prolonged QT interval has been reported in patients with renal dysfunction. The FDA has received reports of torsade de pointes occurring with famotidine (Poluzzi, 2009). Relief of symptoms does not preclude the presence of a gastric malignancy. Reversible confusional states, usually clearing within 3-4 days after discontinuation, have been linked to use. Increased age (>50 years) and renal or hepatic impairment are thought to be associated. Multidose vials for injection contain benzyl alcohol.

OTC labeling: When used for self-medication, patients should be instructed not to use if they have difficulty swallowing, are vomiting blood, or have bloody or black stools. Not for use with other acid reducers.

Adverse Reactions

Note: Agitation and vomiting have been reported in up to 14% of pediatric patients <1 year of age.

1% to 10%:

Central nervous system: Headache (5%), dizziness (1%)

Gastrointestinal: Diarrhea (2%), constipation (1%), necrotizing enterocolitis (VLBW neonates; Guillet, 2006)

<1% (Limited to important or life-threatening): Abdominal discomfort, acne, agitation, agranulocytosis, allergic reaction, alopecia, anaphylaxis, angioedema, anorexia, anxiety, arrhythmia, arthralgia, AV block, bronchospasm, cholestatic jaundice, confusion, conjunctival injection, depression, dry skin, facial edema, fatigue, fever, flushing, hallucinations, hepatitis, injection site reactions, insomnia, interstitial pneumonia, leukopenia, libido decreased, liver function tests increased, muscle cramps, nausea, palpitation, pancytopenia, paresthesia, pruritus, QT-interval prolongation, rash, seizure, somnolence, Stevens-Johnson syndrome, taste disorder, tinnitus, thrombocytopenia, torsade de pointes, toxic epidermal necrolysis, urticaria, vomiting, weakness, xerostomia

Drug Interactions

Metabolism/Transport Effects None known.

Avoid Concomitant Use

Avoid concomitant use of Famotidine with any of the following: Dasatinib; Delavirdine; PONATinib; Risedronate

Increased Effect/Toxicity

Famotidine may increase the levels/effects of: Dexmethylphenidate; Highest Risk QTc-Prolonging Agents; Methylphenidate; Moderate Risk QTc-Prolonging Agents; Risedronate; Saquinavir; Varenicline

The levels/effects of Famotidine may be increased by: Mifepristone

Decreased Effect

Famotidine may decrease the levels/effects of: Atazanavir; Bosutinib; Cefditoren; Cefpodoxime; Cefuroxime; Dabrafenib; Dasatinib; Delavirdine; Erlotinib; Fosamprenavir; Gefitinib; Indinavir; Iron Salts; Itraconazole; Ketoconazole (Systemic); Mesalamine; Multivitamins/Minerals (with ADEK, Folate, Iron); Nelfinavir; Nilotinib; PONATinib; Posaconazole; Rilpivirine; Vismodegib

Ethanol/Nutrition/Herb Interactions

Ethanol: Avoid ethanol (may cause gastric mucosal irritation).

Food: Famotidine bioavailability may be increased if taken with food.

Preparation for Administration Solution for injection:

I.V. push: Dilute famotidine with NS (or another compatible solution) to a total of 5-10 mL (may also administer undiluted [Lipsy, 1995])

Infusion: Dilute with D_5W 100 mL or another compatible solution.

Storage/Stability

Oral:

Powder for oral suspension: Prior to mixing, dry powder should be stored at controlled room temperature of 25°C (77°F). Reconstituted oral suspension is stable for 30 days at room temperature; do not freeze.

Tablet: Store controlled room temperature. Protect from moisture.

I.V.:

Solution for injection: Prior to use, store at 2°C to 8°C (36°F to 46°F). If solution freezes, allow to solubilize at controlled room temperature. May be stored at room temperature for up to 3 months (data on file [Bedford Laboratories, 2011]).

I.V. push: Following preparation, solutions for I.V. push should be used immediately, or may be stored in refrigerator and used within 48 hours.

Infusion: Following preparation, the manufacturer states may be stored for up to 48 hours under refrigeration; however, solutions for infusion have been found to be physically and chemically stable for 7 days at room temperature.

Solution for injection, premixed bags: Store at controlled room temperature of 25°C (77°F); avoid excessive heat.

Mechanism of Action Competitive inhibition of histamine at H_2 receptors of the gastric parietal cells, which inhibits gastric acid secretion

Pharmacodynamics/Kinetics

Onset of action: Antisecretory effect: Oral: Within 1 hour; I.V.: Within 30 minutes

Peak effect: Antisecretory effect: Oral: Within 1-3 hours (dose-dependent)

Duration: Antisecretory effect: I.V., Oral: 10-12 hours

Absorption: Oral: Incompletely absorbed

Distribution: V_d:

Infants: 0-3 months: ~1.4-1.8 L/kg; >3-12 months: ~2.3 L/kg

Children: ~2 L/kg

Adults: ~1 L/kg

Protein binding: 15% to 20%

Metabolism: Minimal first-pass metabolism; forms one metabolite (S-oxide)

Bioavailability: Oral: 40% to 45%

Half-life elimination:

Infants: 0-3 months: ~8-10.5 hours; >3-12 months: ~4.5 hours

Children: 3.4 hours

Adults: 2.5-3.5 hours; prolonged with renal impairment; Oliguria: >20 hours

Time to peak, serum: Oral: ~1-3 hours

Excretion: Urine (25% to 30% [oral], 65% to 70% [I.V.] as unchanged drug)

Dosage

Children: Treatment duration and dose should be individualized

Peptic ulcer: 1-16 years:

Oral: 0.5 mg/kg/day at bedtime or divided twice daily (maximum dose: 40 mg/day); doses of up to 1 mg/kg/day have been used in clinical studies

I.V.: 0.25 mg/kg every 12 hours (maximum dose: 40 mg/day); doses of up to 0.5 mg/kg have been used in clinical studies

GERD: Oral:

<3 months: 0.5 mg/kg once daily

3-12 months: 0.5 mg/kg twice daily

1-16 years: 1 mg/kg/day divided twice daily (maximum dose: 40 mg twice daily); doses of up to 2 mg/kg/day have been used in clinical studies

Children ≥12 years and Adults: Heartburn, indigestion, sour stomach: OTC labeling: Oral: 10-20 mg every 12 hours; dose may be taken 15-60 minutes before eating foods known to cause heartburn

Adults:

Duodenal ulcer: Oral: Acute therapy: 40 mg/day at bedtime (or 20 mg twice daily) for 4-8 weeks; maintenance therapy: 20 mg/day at bedtime

Helicobacter pylori eradication (unlabeled use): Oral: 40 mg once daily; requires combination therapy with antibiotics

Gastric ulcer: Oral: Acute therapy: 40 mg/day at bedtime

GERD: Oral: 20 mg twice daily for 6 weeks

Hypersecretory conditions: Oral: Initial: 20 mg every 6 hours, may increase in increments up to 160 mg every 6 hours

Esophagitis and accompanying symptoms due to GERD: Oral: 20 mg or 40 mg twice daily for up to 12 weeks

Stress ulcer prophylaxis, ICU patients (unlabeled use): Oral, I.V., or nasogastric (NG) tube: 20 mg twice daily (ASHP, 1999; Baghaie, 1995); **Note:** Intended for patients with associated risk factors (eg, coagulopathy, mechanical ventilation for >48 hours, severe sepsis); discontinue use once risk factors have resolved. The Surviving Sepsis Campaign guidelines suggest the use of proton pump inhibitors rather than H_2 antagonist therapy (Dellinger, 2013).

Patients unable to take oral medication: I.V.: 20 mg every 12 hours

Dosage adjustment in renal impairment: Cl_{cr} <50 mL/minute: Manufacturer recommendation: Administer 50% of dose **or** increase the dosing interval to every 36-48 hours (to limit potential CNS adverse effects).

Dietary Considerations May be taken without regard to meals.

Administration

Oral: May administer with antacids.

Suspension: Shake vigorously before use. May be taken without regard to meals.

Tablet: May be taken without regard to meals.

I.V.:

I.V. push: Inject over at least 2 minutes.

Solution for infusion: Administer over 15-30 minutes.

Dosage Forms Excipient information presented when available (limited, particularly for generics); consult specific product labeling.

Solution, Intravenous:

Generic: 20 mg (50 mL); 10 mg/mL (2 mL, 4 mL, 20 mL, 50 mL)

Solution, Intravenous [preservative free]:

Generic: 10 mg/mL (2 mL)

Suspension Reconstituted, Oral:

Pepcid: 40 mg/5 mL (50 mL) [contains methylparaben sodium, propylparaben sodium, sodium benzoate; cherry banana mint flavor]

Generic: 40 mg/5 mL (50 mL)

Tablet, Oral:

Acid Reducer: 10 mg

Acid Reducer Maximum Strength: 20 mg

Heartburn Relief: 10 mg

Heartburn Relief Max St: 20 mg

Pepcid: 20 mg, 40 mg [scored]

Generic: 10 mg, 20 mg, 40 mg

Extemporaneous Preparations An 8 mg/mL oral suspension may be made with tablets. Crush seventy 40 mg tablets in a mortar and reduce to a fine powder. Add small portions of sterile water and mix to a uniform paste. Mix while adding a 1:1 mixture of Ora-Plus® and Ora-Sweet® in incremental proportions to **almost** 350 mL; transfer to a calibrated bottle, rinse mortar with vehicle, and add quantity of vehicle sufficient to make 350 mL. Label "shake well". Stable for 95 days at room temperature.

Dentinger PJ, Swenson CF, and Anaizi NH, "Stability of Famotidine in an Extemporaneously Compounded Oral Liquid," *Am J Health Syst Pharm*, 2000, 57(14):1340-2.

- Famotidine Omega (Can) *see* Famotidine *on page 832*
- Fampridine *see* Dalfampridine *on page 534*
- Fampridine-SR *see* Dalfampridine *on page 534*
- Fampyra™ (Can) *see* Dalfampridine *on page 534*
- Famvir *see* Famciclovir *on page 830*
- Famvir® (Can) *see* Famciclovir *on page 830*
- Fanapt *see* Iloperidone *on page 1045*
- Fanapt Titration Pack *see* Iloperidone *on page 1045*
- Fansidar® [DSC] *see* Sulfadoxine and Pyrimethamine *on page 1959*
- 2F-ara-AMP *see* Fludarabine *on page 872*
- Fareston *see* Toremifene *on page 2095*
- Fareston® (Can) *see* Toremifene *on page 2095*
- Faslodex *see* Fulvestrant *on page 930*
- Faslodex® (Can) *see* Fulvestrant *on page 930*
- Fasturtec® (Can) *see* Rasburicase *on page 1788*

Fat Emulsion (Plant Based)

(fat e MUL shun plant baste)

Brand Names: U.S. Intralipid; Liposyn II; Liposyn III

Brand Names: Canada Intralipid; Liposyn II

Index Terms Clinolipid; Intravenous Fat Emulsion

Pharmacologic Category Caloric Agent

Use Source of calories and essential fatty acids for patients requiring parenteral nutrition of extended duration; prevention and treatment of essential fatty acid deficiency (EFAD)

Unlabeled Use Treatment of local anesthetic-induced cardiac arrest unresponsive to conventional resuscitation

Pregnancy Risk Factor C

Dosage I.V.: **Note:** At the onset of therapy, the patient should be observed for any immediate allergic reactions (eg, dyspnea, cyanosis, and fever).

Caloric source: **Note:** Fat emulsion should not exceed 60% of the total daily calories.

Infants: Initial dose: 1-2 g/kg/day, increase by 0.5-1 g/kg/day to a maximum of 3 g/kg/day depending on needs/nutritional goals; daily dose may be infused over 24 hours if possible (ASPEN Guidelines, 2002; ASPEN Pediatric Nutrition Support Core Curriculum, 2010)

Children 1-10 years: Initial dose: 1-2 g/kg/day, increase by 0.5-1 g/kg/day to a maximum of 2-3 g/kg/day depending upon the needs/nutritional goals; daily dose may be infused over 24 hours if possible (ASPEN Guidelines, 2002; ASPEN Pediatric Nutrition Support Core Curriculum, 2010)

Adolescents and Adults: Initial dose: 1 g/kg/day (not to exceed 500 mL 20% fat emulsion on the first day of therapy), increase by 1 g/kg/day to a maximum of 2.5 g/kg/day (ASPEN Guidelines, 2002; ASPEN Pediatric Nutrition Support Core Curriculum, 2010)

Essential fatty acid deficiency (EFAD): Children and Adults: Administer 8% to 10% of total caloric intake as fat emulsion; infuse 2-3 times weekly. If EFAD occurs with stress, the dosage needed to correct EFAD may be increased.

Local anesthetic toxicity (unlabeled use): Adults: 20%: 1.5 **mL**/kg administered over 1 minute, followed immediately by an infusion of 0.25 **mL**/kg/minute. Continue chest compressions (lipid must circulate). Repeat the bolus 1-2 times as needed for persistent asystole, pulseless electrical activity, or re-emergence of hemodynamic instability. Increase the infusion rate to 0.5 **mL**/kg/minute if hemodynamic instability persists or recurs. Continue the infusion for at least 10 minutes after hemodynamic stability is restored; discontinue within 1 hour, if possible (ACMT, 2010; Neal, 2012).

Additional Information Complete prescribing information should be consulted for additional detail.

Product Availability Clinolipid: FDA approved October 2013; availability anticipated in the first quarter of 2014. Refer to the prescribing information for additional information.

Dosage Forms Considerations

Product oil components:

Soybean oil: Intralipid 20%, 30%; Liposyn III 10%, 20%, 30%

Soybean and safflower oil: Liposyn II 20% (10% each)

Dosage Forms Excipient information presented when available (limited, particularly for generics); consult specific product labeling.

Emulsion, Intravenous:

Intralipid: 20% (100 mL, 250 mL, 500 mL, 1000 mL); 30% (500 mL) [contains egg yolk phospholipids]

Liposyn II: 20% (200 mL, 250 mL) [contains egg phosphatides]

Liposyn III: 10% (200 mL, 250 mL, 500 mL) [contains egg phosphatides]

Liposyn III: 20% (200 mL, 250 mL, 500 mL) [contains egg yolk phospholipids]

Liposyn III: 30% (500 mL) [contains egg phosphatides]

- Father John's® Plus [OTC] *see* Chlorpheniramine, Phenylephrine, and Dextromethorphan *on page 413*
- FazaClo *see* CloZAPine *on page 477*
- 5-FC *see* Flucytosine *on page 871*
- FC1157a *see* Toremifene *on page 2095*
- FC1271a *see* Ospemifene *on page 1521*
- FE200486 *see* Degarelix *on page 564*

Febuxostat (feb UX oh stat)

Brand Names: U.S. Uloric

Brand Names: Canada Uloric®

Index Terms TEI-6720; TMX-67

Pharmacologic Category Antigout Agent; Xanthine Oxidase Inhibitor

Use Chronic management of hyperuricemia in patients with gout

Pregnancy Risk Factor C

Pregnancy Considerations Animal studies have demonstrated increased neonatal mortality and reduction in weight gain, but not teratogenic effects. There are no adequate and well-controlled studies in pregnant women. Use during pregnancy only if potential benefit to the mother outweighs potential risk to the fetus.

Breast-Feeding Considerations It is not known if febuxostat is excreted in breast milk.. The manufacturer recommends that caution be exercised when administering febuxostat to nursing women.

Contraindications Concurrent use with azathioprine or mercaptopurine

Canadian labeling: Additional contraindications (not in U.S. labeling): Hypersensitivity to febuxostat or any component of the formulation; concomitant administration with theophylline

Warnings/Precautions Administer concurrently with an NSAID or colchicine (up to 6 months) to prevent gout flare upon initiation of therapy. Do not use to treat asymptomatic or secondary hyperuricemia. Postmarketing cases of hepatic failure (both fatal and nonfatal) have been reported (causal relationship has not been established). Significant hepatic transaminase elevations (>3 x ULN), MI, stroke and cardiovascular deaths have been reported in controlled trials (causal relationship not established). Monitor patients for signs/symptoms of MI and stroke. Liver function tests should be evaluated at baseline, 2 and 4 months after initiation of therapy, and periodically thereafter; evaluate liver function tests in patients experiencing signs and symptoms of hepatic injury (eg, fatigue, anorexia, right upper quadrant pain, dark urine, jaundice). Interrupt therapy in patients who develop abnormal liver function tests (eg, ALT >3 x ULN); permanently discontinue use if no other explanation for the abnormalities is elucidated and in patients who develop ALT >3 x ULT **and** serum total bilirubin >2 x ULN. All other patients may be cautiously restarted on febuxostat. All other patients may be cautiously restarted on febuxostat. Use with caution in patients with severe renal impairment (Cl_{cr} <30 mL/minute); insufficient data.

Adverse Reactions

1% to 10%:

Dermatologic: Rash (1% to 2%)

Gastrointestinal: Nausea (1%)

Hepatic: Liver function abnormalities (5% to 7%)

Neuromuscular & skeletal: Arthralgia (1%)

<1% (Limited to important or life-threatening): Aggression, agitation, alkaline phosphatase increased, alopecia, amylase increased, anaphylactic reaction, anaphylaxis, anemia, angina, angioedema, anorexia, anxiety, aPTT prolonged, atrial fibrillation/flutter, bicarbonate decreased, blurred vision, bruising, BUN increased, cardiac murmur, cerebrovascular accident, cholecystitis, cholelithiasis, constipation, CPK increased, creatinine increased, deafness, dehydration, depression, dermatitis, dermographism, diabetes mellitus, dyspepsia, dyspnea, ECG abnormal, eczema, edema, EEG abnormal, epistaxis, erectile dysfunction, flushing, gait disturbance, gastritis, gastroesophageal reflux, gingival pain, Guillain-Barré syndrome, gynecomastia, hair color change, hair growth abnormal, hematemesis, hematochezia, hematocrit decreased, hematuria, hemiparesis, hepatic failure (fatal and nonfatal), hepatic steatosis, hepatitis, hepatomegaly, herpes zoster, hot flashes, hyperchlorhydria, hypercholesterolemia, hyperglycemia, hyperhidrosis, hyperkalemia, hyperlipidemia, hypernatremia, hypersensitivity, hyper/hypotension, hypertriglyceridemia, hypokalemia, immune thrombocytopenia (ITP), incontinence, influenza-like syndrome, jaundice, joint swelling, lacunar infarction, LDH increased, lethargy, leukocytosis, leukopenia, libido decreased, lymphocytopenia, MCV increased, MI, migraine, mouth ulceration, muscle spasm/twitching, myalgia, nephrolithiasis, neutropenia, pain, palpitation, pancreatitis, pancytopenia, panic attack, paresthesia, peptic ulcer, personality change, petechiae, pharyngeal edema, photosensitivity, pollakiuria, proteinuria, PSA increased, psychotic behavior, PT prolonged, renal failure, respiratory infection, rhabdomyolysis, sinus bradycardia, skin/pigmentation discoloration, splenomegaly, Stevens-Johnson syndrome, stroke, tachycardia, taste altered, thrombocytopenia, TIA, tinnitus, tremor, TSH increased, tubulointerstitial nephritis, urinary tract infection, urine output decreased/increased, urticaria, vertigo, vomiting, weakness, weight gain/loss

Drug Interactions

Metabolism/Transport Effects None known.

Avoid Concomitant Use

Avoid concomitant use of Febuxostat with any of the following: AzaTHIOprine; Didanosine; Mercaptopurine; Pegloticase

Increased Effect/Toxicity

Febuxostat may increase the levels/effects of: AzaTHIOprine; Didanosine; Mercaptopurine; Pegloticase; Theophylline Derivatives

Decreased Effect There are no known significant interactions involving a decrease in effect.

Storage/Stability Store at 25°C (77°F); excursions permitted to 15°C to 30°C (59°F to 86°F). Protect from light.

Mechanism of Action Selectively inhibits xanthine oxidase, the enzyme responsible for the conversion of hypoxanthine to xanthine to uric acid thereby decreasing uric acid. At therapeutic concentration does not inhibit other enzymes involved in purine and pyrimidine synthesis.

Pharmacodynamics/Kinetics

Absorption: ≥49%

Distribution: V_{ss}: ~50 L

Protein binding: ~99%, primarily to albumin

Metabolism: Extensive conjugation via uridine diphosphate glucuronosyltransferases (UGTs) 1A1, 1A3, 1A9, and 2B7 and oxidation via cytochrome P450 (CYP) 1A2, 2C8, and 2C9 as well as non-P450 enzymes. Oxidation leads to formation of active metabolites (67M-1, 67M-2, 67M-4)

Half-life elimination: ~5-8 hours

Time to peak, plasma: 1-1.5 hours

Excretion: Urine (~49% mostly as metabolites, 3% as unchanged drug); feces (~45% mostly as metabolites, 12% as unchanged drug)

Dosage Oral: Adults: **Note:** It is recommended to take an NSAID or colchicine with initiation of therapy and may continue for up to 6 months to help prevent gout flares. If a gout flare occurs, febuxostat does not need to be discontinued.

U.S. labeling: Initial: 40 mg once daily; may increase to 80 mg once daily in patients who do not achieve a serum uric acid level <6 mg/dL after 2 weeks

Canadian labeling: 80 mg once daily

Dosing adjustment in renal impairment:

Mild-to-moderate impairment (Cl_{cr} 30-89 mL/minute): No adjustment needed

Severe impairment (Cl_{cr} <30 mL/minute): Insufficient data; use caution (use not recommended in the Canadian labeling)

Dialysis: Not studied (use not recommended in the Canadian labeling)

Dosing adjustment in hepatic impairment:

Mild-to-moderate impairment (Child-Pugh class A or B): No adjustment needed

Severe impairment (Child-Pugh class C): Not studied; use caution (use not recommended in the Canadian labeling)

Dietary Considerations Take with or without meals or antacids.

Administration Administer with or without meals or antacids.

Monitoring Parameters Liver function tests at baseline, 2 and 4 months after initiation and then periodically, serum uric acid levels (as early as 2 weeks after initiation)

Reference Range Uric acid, serum: An increase occurs during childhood

Adults:

Males: 3.4-7 mg/dL or slightly more

Females: 2.4-6 mg/dL or slightly more

Target: <6 mg/dL

Values >7 mg/dL are sometimes arbitrarily regarded as hyperuricemia, but there is no sharp line between normals on the one hand, and the serum uric acid of those with clinical gout. Normal ranges cannot be adjusted for purine ingestion, but high purine diet increases uric acid. Uric acid may be increased with body size, exercise, and stress.

Dosage Forms Excipient information presented when available (limited, particularly for generics); consult specific product labeling.

Tablet, Oral:

Uloric: 40 mg, 80 mg

- ◆ Feiba NF *see* Anti-inhibitor Coagulant Complex (Human) *on page 147*
- ◆ FEIBA NF (Can) *see* Anti-inhibitor Coagulant Complex (Human) *on page 147*
- ◆ FEIBA VH *see* Anti-inhibitor Coagulant Complex (Human) *on page 147*
- ◆ Feiba VH Immuno *see* Anti-inhibitor Coagulant Complex (Human) *on page 147*

Felbamate (FEL ba mate)

Brand Names: U.S. Felbatol

Pharmacologic Category Anticonvulsant, Miscellaneous

Use Monotherapy or adjunctive therapy in the treatment of partial seizures (with and without generalization); adjunctive therapy in the treatment of partial and generalized seizures associated with Lennox-Gastaut syndrome; not indicated for use as first-line treatment

Pregnancy Risk Factor C

Prescribing and Access Restrictions A patient "informed consent" form should be completed and signed by the patient and physician. Copies are available from MEDA Pharmaceuticals by calling 800-526-3840.

Medication Guide Available Yes

Dosage Anticonvulsant:

Monotherapy: Children >14 years and Adults:

Initial: 1200 mg/day in divided doses 3 or 4 times/day; titrate previously untreated patients under close clinical supervision, increasing the dosage in 600 mg increments every 2 weeks to 2400 mg/day based on clinical response and thereafter to 3600 mg/day if clinically indicated

Conversion to monotherapy: Initiate at 1200 mg/day in divided doses 3 or 4 times/day, reduce the dosage of the concomitant anticonvulsant(s) by 33% at the initiation of felbamate therapy; at week 2, increase the felbamate dosage to 2400 mg/day while reducing the dosage of the other anticonvulsant(s) up to an additional 33% of their original dosage; at week 3, increase the felbamate dosage up to 3600 mg/day and continue to reduce the dosage of the other anticonvulsant(s) as clinically indicated

Adjunctive therapy: **Note:** Dose of concomitant carbamazepine, phenobarbital, phenytoin, or valproic acid should be decreased by 20% when initiating felbamate therapy. Further dosage reductions may be necessary as dose of felbamate is increased.

Children 2-14 years with Lennox-Gastaut syndrome: Initial: 15 mg/kg/day in divided doses 3 or 4 times/day; increase once per week by 15 mg/kg/day increments up to 45 mg/kg/day in divided doses 3 or 4 times/day.

Children >14 years and Adults: Initial: 1200 mg/day in divided doses 3 or 4 times/day; increase once per week by 1200 mg/day increments up to 3600 mg/day in divided doses 3 or 4 times/day.

Dosage adjustment in renal impairment: Use caution; reduce initial and maintenance doses by 50%.

Dosage adjustment in hepatic impairment: Use is contraindicated.

Additional Information Complete prescribing information should be consulted for additional detail.

Dosage Forms Excipient information presented when available (limited, particularly for generics); consult specific product labeling.

Suspension, Oral:

Felbatol: 600 mg/5 mL (237 mL, 946 mL)

Generic: 600 mg/5 mL (237 mL, 240 mL, 473 mL, 946 mL)

Tablet, Oral:

Felbatol: 400 mg, 600 mg [scored]

Generic: 400 mg, 600 mg

- ◆ Felbatol *see* Felbamate *on page 836*
- ◆ Feldene *see* Piroxicam *on page 1656*

Felodipine (fe LOE di peen)

Brand Names: Canada Plendil®; Renedil®; Sandoz-Felodipine

Index Terms Plendil

Pharmacologic Category Antihypertensive; Calcium Channel Blocker; Calcium Channel Blocker, Dihydropyridine

Additional Appendix Information

Calcium Channel Blockers – Comparative Pharmacokinetics *on page 2296*

Use Treatment of hypertension

Unlabeled Use Pediatric hypertension

Pregnancy Risk Factor C

Pregnancy Considerations Adverse events were observed in animal reproduction studies. Untreated chronic maternal hypertension is associated with adverse events in the fetus, infant, and mother. If treatment for hypertension during pregnancy is needed, other agents are preferred (ACOG, 2012; Chobanian, 2003).

Breast-Feeding Considerations It is not known if felodipine is excreted in breast milk. Due to the potential for serious adverse reactions in the nursing infant, the manufacturer recommends a decision be made whether to discontinue nursing or to discontinue the drug, taking into account the importance of treatment to the mother. Breast-fed infants of mothers taking medications for hypertension should be monitored for adverse effects (Chobanian, 2003).

Contraindications Hypersensitivity to felodipine, any component of the formulation, or other calcium channel blocker

Warnings/Precautions Increased angina and/or MI has occurred with initiation or dosage titration of dihydropyridine calcium channel blockers, reflex tachycardia may occur resulting in angina and/or MI in patients with obstructive coronary disease especially in the absence of concurrent beta-blockade. Use with extreme caution in patients with severe aortic stenosis. Use caution in patients with heart failure and/or hypertrophic cardiomyopathy with outflow tract obstruction. Elderly patients and patients with hepatic impairment should start off with a lower dose. Peripheral edema (dose dependent) is the most common side effect (occurs within 2-3 weeks of starting therapy). Symptomatic hypotension with or without syncope can rarely occur; blood pressure must be lowered at a rate appropriate for the patient's clinical condition. Dosage titration should occur after 14 days on a given dose.

Adverse Reactions

>10%: Central nervous system: Headache (11% to 15%)

2% to 10%: Cardiovascular: Peripheral edema (2% to 17%), tachycardia (0.4% to 2.5%), flushing (4% to 7%)

<1% (Limited to important or life-threatening): Angina, angioedema, anxiety, arrhythmia, CHF, CVA, libido decreased, depression, dizziness, gingival hyperplasia, dyspnea, dysuria, gynecomastia, hypotension, impotence, insomnia, irritability, leukocytoclastic vasculitis, MI, nervousness, paresthesia, somnolence, syncope, urticaria, vomiting

Drug Interactions

Metabolism/Transport Effects Substrate of CYP3A4 (major); **Note:** Assignment of Major/Minor substrate status based on clinically relevant drug interaction potential; **Inhibits** CYP2C8 (moderate), CYP2C9 (weak), CYP2D6 (weak), CYP3A4 (weak)

Avoid Concomitant Use

Avoid concomitant use of Felodipine with any of the following: Conivaptan; Fusidic Acid (Systemic); Itraconazole; Pimozide

Increased Effect/Toxicity

Felodipine may increase the levels/effects of: Amifostine; Antihypertensives; ARIPiprazole; Atosiban; Beta-Blockers; Calcium Channel Blockers (Nondihydropyridine); CYP2C8 Substrates; Dofetilide; Fosphenytoin; Hypotensive Agents; Lomitapide; Magnesium Salts; Neuromuscular-Blocking Agents (Nondepolarizing); Nitroprusside; Obinutuzumab; Phenytoin; Pimozide; RiTUXimab; Tacrolimus (Systemic)

The levels/effects of Felodipine may be increased by: Alpha1-Blockers; Antifungal Agents (Azole Derivatives, Systemic); Brimonidine (Topical); Calcium Channel Blockers (Nondihydropyridine); Cimetidine; Conivaptan; CycloSPORINE (Systemic); CYP3A4 Inhibitors (Moderate); CYP3A4 Inhibitors (Strong); Dasatinib; Diazoxide; Fluconazole; Fusidic Acid (Systemic); Grapefruit Juice; Herbs (Hypotensive Properties); Itraconazole; Ivacaftor; Luliconazole; Macrolide Antibiotics; Magnesium Salts; MAO Inhibitors; Mifepristone; Pentoxifylline; Phosphodiesterase 5 Inhibitors; Prostacyclin Analogues; Protease Inhibitors; Simeprevir

Decreased Effect

Felodipine may decrease the levels/effects of: Clopidogrel

The levels/effects of Felodipine may be decreased by: Barbiturates; Bosentan; Calcium Salts; CarBAMazepine; CYP3A4 Inducers (Strong); Dabrafenib; Deferasirox; Herbs (CYP3A4 Inducers); Herbs (Hypertensive Properties); Melatonin; Methylphenidate; Mitotane; Nafcillin; Rifamycin Derivatives; Tocilizumab; Yohimbine

Ethanol/Nutrition/Herb Interactions

Ethanol: Ethanol increases felodipine absorption. Management: Monitor for a greater hypotensive effect if ethanol is consumed.

Food: Compared to a fasted state, felodipine peak plasma concentrations are increased up to twofold when taken after a meal high in fat or carbohydrates. Grapefruit juice similarly increases felodipine C_{max} by twofold. Increased therapeutic and vasodilator side effects, including severe hypotension and myocardial ischemia, may occur. Management: May be taken with a small meal that is low in fat and carbohydrates; avoid grapefruit juice during therapy.

Herb/Nutraceutical: St John's wort may decrease felodipine levels. Dong quai has estrogenic activity. Some herbal medications may worsen hypertension (eg, ephedra); garlic may have additional antihypertensive effects. Management: Avoid dong quai if using for hypertension. Avoid ephedra, yohimbe, ginseng, and garlic.

Mechanism of Action Inhibits calcium ions from entering the "slow channels" or select voltage-sensitive areas of vascular smooth muscle and myocardium during depolarization, producing a relaxation of coronary vascular smooth muscle and coronary vasodilation; increases myocardial oxygen delivery in patients with vasospastic angina

Pharmacodynamics/Kinetics

Onset of action: Antihypertensive: 2-5 hours

Duration of antihypertensive effect: 24 hours

Absorption: 100%; Absolute: 20% due to first-pass effect

Protein binding: >99%

Metabolism: Hepatic; CYP3A4 substrate (major); extensive first-pass effect

Half-life elimination: Immediate release: 11-16 hours

Excretion: Urine (70% as metabolites); feces 10%

Dosage Oral: Hypertension:

Children (unlabeled use): Initial: 2.5 mg once daily; maximum: 10 mg/day

Adults: Oral: 2.5-10 mg once daily; usual initial dose: 5 mg; increase by 5 mg at 2-week intervals, as needed, to a maximum of 20 mg/day

Usual dose range (JNC 7) for hypertension: 2.5-20 mg once daily

Elderly: Consider lower initial doses (eg, 2.5 mg once daily) and titrate to response (Aronow, 2011)

Dosage adjustment in renal impairment: No dosage adjustment necessary.

Dosage adjustment in hepatic impairment: Initial: 2.5 mg/day; monitor blood pressure

Dietary Considerations May be taken with a small meal that is low in fat and carbohydrates.

Administration Swallow tablet whole; tablet should not be divided, crushed, or chewed. May be administered without food or with a small meal that is low in fat and carbohydrates.

Additional Information Felodipine maintains renal and mesenteric blood flow during hemorrhagic shock in animals.

Dosage Forms Excipient information presented when available (limited, particularly for generics); consult specific product labeling.

Tablet Extended Release 24 Hour, Oral:

Generic: 2.5 mg, 5 mg, 10 mg

◆ **Femara** *see* Letrozole *on page 1185*

◆ **Femcon Fe** *see* Ethinyl Estradiol and Norethindrone *on page 793*

◆ **femhrt** *see* Ethinyl Estradiol and Norethindrone *on page 793*

◆ **FemHRT (Can)** *see* Ethinyl Estradiol and Norethindrone *on page 793*

◆ **Fem-Prin® [OTC]** *see* Acetaminophen, Aspirin, and Caffeine *on page 33*

◆ **Femring** *see* Estradiol (Systemic) *on page 754*

◆ **Femstat® One (Can)** *see* Butoconazole *on page 306*

◆ **Fenesin DM IR [OTC]** *see* Guaifenesin and Dextromethorphan *on page 976*

◆ **Fenesin IR [OTC]** *see* GuaiFENesin *on page 974*

◆ **Fenesin PE IR** *see* Guaifenesin and Phenylephrine *on page 978*

Fenofibrate and Derivatives

(fen oh FYE brate & dah RIV ah tives)

Brand Names: U.S. Antara; Fenoglide; Fibricor; Lipofen; Lofibra; Tricor; Triglide; Trilipix

Brand Names: Canada Apo-Feno-Micro; Apo-Feno-Super; Apo-Fenofibrate; Ava-Fenofibrate Micro; Dom-Fenofibrate Micro; Feno-Micro-200; Fenofibrate Micro; Fenofibrate-S; Lipidil EZ; Lipidil Micro; Lipidil Supra;

Mylan-Fenofibrate Micro; Novo-Fenofibrate Micronized; PHL-Fenofibrate Micro; PMS-Fenofibrate Micro; PRO-Feno-Super; Q-Fenofibrate Micro; ratio-Fenofibrate MC; Riva-Fenofibrate Micro; Sandoz-Fenofibrate E; Sandoz-Fenofibrate S; Teva-Fenofibrate S

Index Terms ABT-335; Choline Fenofibrate; Fenofibric Acid; Procetofene; Proctofene

Pharmacologic Category Antilipemic Agent, Fibric Acid

Use

Hypercholesterolemia or mixed dyslipidemia: Adjunctive therapy to diet for the reduction of low-density lipoprotein cholesterol (LDL-C), total cholesterol (total-C), triglycerides, and apolipoprotein B (apo B), and to increase high-density lipoprotein cholesterol (HDL-C) in adults with primary hypercholesterolemia or mixed dyslipidemia (Fredrickson types IIa and IIb). Use lipid-altering agents in addition to a diet restricted in saturated fat and cholesterol when response to diet and nonpharmacological interventions alone has been inadequate.

Trilipix is also indicated as an adjunct to diet in combination with a statin to reduce triglycerides and increase HDL-C in patients with mixed dyslipidemia and coronary heart disease (CHD) or a CHD risk equivalent who are on optimal statin therapy.

Hypertriglyceridemia: Adjunctive therapy to diet for treatment of adult patients with severe hypertriglyceridemia (Fredrickson types IV and V hyperlipidemia).

Unlabeled Use Adjunctive therapy for the treatment of hyperuricemia in patients with gout

Pregnancy Risk Factor C

Pregnancy Considerations Maternal toxicity was observed in pregnant rats at doses approximately equivalent to the human dose; adverse events were not observed in reproduction studies done in rabbits. Reports of using fenofibrate during pregnancy are limited (Goldberg, 2012; Sunman, 2012; Whitten, 2011). Other agents are generally preferred if treatment for hypertriglyceridemia during pregnancy (Berglund, 2012) or treatment of lipid disorders in women of reproductive age (NCEP, 2001) is required. Use during pregnancy is specifically contraindicated in Canadian product labeling; some products recommend using effective birth control when treating women of reproductive age and discontinuing therapy several months prior to conception if planning a pregnancy.

Breast-Feeding Considerations It is not known if fenofibrate is excreted into breast milk. Use is contraindicated in nursing women. The manufacturer recommends a decision be made whether to discontinue nursing or to discontinue the drug, taking into account the importance of treatment to the mother.

Medication Guide Available Yes

Contraindications

Active liver disease, including primary biliary cirrhosis and unexplained, persistent liver function abnormality; severe renal dysfunction, including those receiving dialysis; pre-existing gallbladder disease; breast-feeding; hypersensitivity to fenofibrate or fenofibric acid.

Documentation of allergenic cross-reactivity for fibrates is limited. However, because of similarities in chemical structure and/or pharmacologic actions, the possibility of cross-sensitivity cannot be ruled out with certainty.

Canadian labeling: Additional contraindications (not in U.S. labeling): Pregnancy; known photoallergy or phototoxic reaction during treatment with fibrates or ketoprofen

Lipidil EZ, Lipidil Micro, Lipidil Supra: Additional contraindications: Allergy to soya lecithin or peanut or arachis oil; chronic or acute pancreatitis; patients <18 years of age; coadministration with HMG-CoA reductase inhibitors in patients with a predisposition for myopathy.

Warnings/Precautions Secondary causes of hyperlipidemia should be ruled out prior to therapy. Hepatic transaminases can become significantly elevated (dose-related); hepatocellular, chronic active, and cholestatic hepatitis have been reported. Regular monitoring of liver function tests is required; discontinue therapy in patients whose enzyme levels persist above 3 times the upper limit of normal. Use with caution in patients with mild-to-moderate renal impairment; dosage adjustment may be required. Contraindicated with severe renal impairment including those receiving dialysis. Contraindicated active liver disease, including primary biliary cirrhosis and unexplained persistent liver function abnormalities. Increases in serum creatinine (>2 mg/dL) have been observed with use; clinical significance unknown. Fenofibrate has been shown to increase creatinine production (unknown mechanism) resulting in an equal increase of creatinuria thereby demonstrating that the increase does not reflect a reduction in creatinine clearance (Hottelart, 2002). Monitor renal function in patients with renal impairment and consider monitoring patients with increased risk for developing renal impairment. May cause cholelithiasis.

Therapy should be discontinued in patients who develop markedly elevated CPK concentrations or if myopathy/myositis is suspected or diagnosed. No incremental benefit of combination therapy on cardiovascular morbidity and mortality over statin monotherapy has been established. In patients with type 2 diabetes mellitus, neither fenofibrate monotherapy nor the addition of fenofibrate to simvastatin compared to placebo has been shown to reduce cardiovascular disease morbidity and mortality in patients with type 2 diabetes. Potentially significant drug-drug interactions may exist, requiring dose or frequency adjustment, additional monitoring, and/or selection of alternative therapy. In combination with HMG-CoA reductase inhibitors, fenofibrate is generally regarded as safer than gemfibrozil due to limited pharmacokinetic interaction with statins. According to the 2013 ACC/AHA Blood Cholesterol Guidelines, fenofibrate may be considered in patients on low- or moderate-intensity statin therapy (ie, statin therapy intended to lower LDL-C by <30% or ~30% to 50%, respectively) only if the benefits from atherosclerotic cardiovascular disease (ASCVD) risk reduction or triglyceride lowering when triglycerides are >500 mg/dL, outweigh the potential risk for adverse effects (Stone, 2013). Therapy should be withdrawn if an adequate response is not obtained after 2-3 months of therapy at the maximal daily dose. In patients with severe hypertriglyceridemia, the occurrence of pancreatitis may represent a failure of efficacy, a direct effect of the drug, or obstruction of the common bile duct due to biliary tract stone or sludge formation. A paradoxical, severe, and reversible decrease in HDL-C (as low as 2 mg/dL) with a simultaneous decrease in apolipoprotein A1 has been reported within 2 weeks to years after initiation of fibrate therapy; clinical significance unknown. Monitor HDL-C within a few months of initiation of therapy and discontinue if HDL-C becomes severely depressed; do not restart therapy. The occurrence of pancreatitis may represent a failure of efficacy in patients with severely elevated triglycerides. May cause mild-to-moderate decreases in hemoglobin, hematocrit, and WBC upon initiation of therapy which usually stabilizes with long-term therapy. Agranulocytosis and thrombocytopenia have been reported (rare). Periodic monitoring of blood counts is recommended during the first year of therapy.

Rare hypersensitivity reactions may occur. Use has been associated with pulmonary embolism (PE) and deep vein thrombosis (DVT). Use with caution in patients with risk factors for VTE. Dose adjustment may be required for elderly patients.

Some products may contain soya lecithin or peanut or arachis oil; use is contraindicated in patients with a soya lecithin allergy or a peanut or arachis allergy for applicable formulations.

Adverse Reactions

>10%: Hepatic: Liver function tests increased (dose related; 3% to 13%; ALT/AST increased >3 x ULN: 5% to 13%)

1% to 10%:

Central nervous system: Headache (3%)

Dermatologic: Urticaria (1%)

Gastrointestinal: Abdominal pain (5%), constipation (2%), nausea (2%)

Neuromuscular & skeletal: Back pain (3%), CPK increased (3%)

Respiratory: Respiratory disorder (6%), rhinitis (2%)

<1% (Limited to important or life-threatening): Abnormal vision, acute renal failure, agranulocytosis, allergic reaction, alopecia, amblyopia, anemia, angina pectoris, anorexia, arrhythmia, arthralgia, arthritis, arthrosis, asthma, atrial fibrillation, bronchitis, bursitis, cataract, cholecystitis, cholelithiasis, cholestatic hepatitis, cirrhosis, colitis, conjunctivitis, contact dermatitis, cyst, cystitis, deep venous thrombosis, diabetes mellitus, diarrhea, duodenal ulcer, electrocardiogram abnormality, eosinophilia, esophagitis, extrasystoles, fatty liver deposits, gastritis, gastroenteritis, gout, gynecomastia, HDL-C decreased (paradoxical), hepatitis, hernia, herpes simplex, herpes zoster, homocysteine increased, hyper-/hypotension, hypersensitivity pneumonitis, hypersensitivity reaction, hypertonia, hyperuricemia, hypoglycemia, infection, leukopenia, lymphadenopathy, maculopapular rash, MI, migraine, myasthenia, myopathy, myositis, neuralgia, pancreatitis, peptic ulcer, photosensitivity reaction, pneumonia, pregnancy (unintended), prostate disorder, pulmonary embolus, rectal hemorrhage, refraction disorder, rhabdomyolysis, skin ulcer, Stevens-Johnson syndrome, tachycardia, tenosynovitis, thrombocytopenia, toxic epidermal necrolysis, urinary frequency, urolithiasis, vaginal moniliasis, vasodilatation, weight gain/loss

Drug Interactions

Metabolism/Transport Effects Inhibits CYP2A6 (weak), CYP2C8 (weak), CYP2C9 (weak)

Avoid Concomitant Use There are no known interactions where it is recommended to avoid concomitant use.

Increased Effect/Toxicity

Fenofibrate and Derivatives may increase the levels/effects of: Colchicine; Ezetimibe; HMG-CoA Reductase Inhibitors; Sulfonylureas; Vitamin K Antagonists; Warfarin

The levels/effects of Fenofibrate and Derivatives may be increased by: CycloSPORINE (Systemic); Raltegravir; Tacrolimus (Systemic)

Decreased Effect

Fenofibrate and Derivatives may decrease the levels/effects of: Chenodiol; CycloSPORINE (Systemic); Ursodiol

The levels/effects of Fenofibrate and Derivatives may be decreased by: Bile Acid Sequestrants

Ethanol/Nutrition/Herb Interactions

Food:

Antara (micronized): When administered under fasted conditions or with a low-fat meal, the extent of absorption and the time to peak did not change; however peak concentrations were increased in the presence of a low-fat meal. When administered with a high fat meal, a 26% increase in the AUC and 108% increase in the peak concentration were seen in comparison to the fasted state. Management: Administer with or without food.

Fenoglide: When administered with a high-fat meal, the peak concentration was increased by 44% as compared to fasting conditions. Management: Administer with meals.

Fibricor: When administered with a high-fat meal, the peak concentration was decreased by ~35% while AUC remained unchanged as compared to fasting conditions. Management: Administer with or without food.

Lipidil EZ [Canadian product]: Bioavailability was not significantly different when administered under fasting and nonfasting conditions. Management: Administer with or without food.

Lipidil Micro [Canadian product]: In comparison with non-micronized fenofibrate formulations, micronized fenofibrate is better absorbed when administered with a low-fat meal; absorption is less influenced by a higher fat content meal. Management: Administer with meals.

Lipidil Supra [Canadian product]: In general, fenofibrate absorption is low and variable when administered under fasting conditions; absorption is increased when administered with food. Management: Administer with meals.

Lipofen: When administered with a low-fat and high-fat meal, the extent of absorption is increased by ~25% and ~58%, respectively, as compared to fasting conditions. Management: Administer with meals.

Lofibra (micronized) capsules: Absorption is increased by ~35% under fed as compared to fasting conditions. Management: Administer with meals.

Lofibra tablets: Peak concentrations and AUC were not significantly different when a single dose was administered under fasting and nonfasting conditions. Management: Administer with or without food.

TriCor: Peak concentrations and AUC were not significantly different when a single dose was administered under fasting and nonfasting conditions. Management: Administer with or without food.

Triglide: When administered with food, the rate of absorption was increased ~55% as compared to fasting conditions; the AUC remained unchanged. Management: Administer with or without food.

Trilipix: Peak concentrations and AUC were not significantly different when a single dose was administered under fasting and nonfasting conditions. Management: Administer with or without food.

Storage/Stability Store at 25°C (77°F); excursions are permitted between 15°C and 30°C (59°F and 86°F). Protect Fibricor, Lipofen, Lofibra, TriCor, Triglide, and Trilipix from moisture. Protect Fibricor, Lofibra tablets, Lipofen, and Triglide from light.

Canadian products: Lipidil EZ, Lipidil Micro, Lipidil Supra: Store at 15°C to 25°C (59°F to 77°F). Protect Lipidil EZ, Lipidil Micro, and Lipidil Supra from moisture. Protect Lipidil EZ and Lipidil Supra from light.

Mechanism of Action Fenofibric acid, an agonist for the nuclear transcription factor peroxisome proliferator-activated receptor-alpha (PPAR-alpha), downregulates apoprotein C-III (an inhibitor of lipoprotein lipase) and upregulates the synthesis of apolipoprotein A-I, fatty acid transport protein, and lipoprotein lipase resulting in an increase in VLDL catabolism, fatty acid oxidation, and elimination of triglyceride-rich particles; as a result of a decrease in VLDL levels, total plasma triglycerides are reduced by 30% to 60%; modest increase in HDL occurs in some hypertriglyceridemic patients.

Pharmacodynamics/Kinetics

Absorption: Increased when taken with meals

Distribution: Widely to most tissues

Protein binding: ~99%

Metabolism: Fenofibrate is metabolized in the tissue and plasma via esterases to the active form, fenofibric acid; fenofibric acid then undergoes inactivation by glucuronidation hepatically or renally

Bioavailability: Fenofibric acid: ~81%
Half-life elimination: Fenofibric acid: Mean: 20 hours (range: 10-35 hours); half-life prolonged in patients with renal impairment
Time to peak: 2-8 hours
Excretion: Urine (60% as metabolites); feces (25%); hemodialysis has no effect on removal of fenofibric acid from plasma

Dosage Oral: **Note:** At least 2-3 months of therapy is required to determine efficacy.

Adults:

Hypertriglyceridemia: Initial:

Antara (micronized): 43-130 mg once daily; maximum dose: 130 mg once daily
Fenoglide: 40-120 mg once daily; maximum dose: 120 mg once daily
Fibricor: 35-105 mg once daily; maximum dose: 105 mg once daily
Lipidil EZ [Canadian product]: 145 mg once daily; maximum dose: 145 mg once daily
Lipidil Micro [Canadian product]: 200 mg once daily; maximum dose: 200 mg once daily
Lipidil Supra [Canadian product]: 160 mg once daily; maximum dose: 200 mg once daily
Lipofen: 50-150 mg once daily; maximum dose: 150 mg once daily
Lofibra (micronized): 67-200 mg once daily; maximum dose: 200 mg once daily
Lofibra (tablets): 54-160 mg once daily; maximum dose: 160 mg once daily
TriCor: 48-145 mg once daily; maximum dose: 145 mg once daily
Triglide: 50-160 mg once daily; maximum dose: 160 mg once daily
Trilipix: 45-135 mg once daily; maximum dose: 135 mg once daily

Hypercholesterolemia or mixed hyperlipidemia:

Antara (micronized): 130 mg once daily
Fenoglide: 120 mg once daily
Fibricor: 105 mg once daily
Lipidil EZ [Canadian product]: 145 mg once daily; maximum dose: 145 mg once daily
Lipidil Micro [Canadian product]: 200 mg once daily; maximum dose: 200 mg once daily
Lipidil Supra [Canadian product]: 160 mg once daily; maximum dose: 200 mg once daily
Lipofen: 150 mg once daily
Lofibra (micronized): 200 mg once daily
Lofibra (tablets): 160 mg once daily
TriCor: 145 mg once daily
Triglide: 160 mg once daily
Trilipix: 135 mg once daily; **Note:** Trilipix is approved for use with a statin in patients with mixed dyslipidemia; may be administered at the same time. Avoid coadministration with the maximum dose of a statin unless the benefits are expected to outweigh the risks

Elderly: Initial:

Antara (micronized): Adjust dosage based on renal function.
Fenoglide: Adjust dosage based on renal function.
Fibricor: Adjust dosage based on renal function.
Lipidil EZ [Canadian product]: 48 mg once daily
Lipidil Micro [Canadian product]: Adjust dosage based on creatinine clearance
Lipidil Supra [Canadian product]: Adjust dosage based on creatinine clearance
Lipofen: Adjust dosage based on renal function.
Lofibra (micronized): 67 mg once daily
Lofibra (tablets): 54 mg once daily
TriCor: Adjust dosage based on renal function.
Triglide: Adjust dosage based on renal function.
Trilipix: Adjust dosage based on renal function.

Dosage adjustment for toxicity:

Cholelithiasis: Discontinue if gallstones are found upon gallbladder studies.
CPK elevation, myopathy, and/or myositis: Discontinue therapy if the patient develops markedly elevated CPK concentrations or if myopathy/myositis is suspected or diagnosed.
HDL-C reductions: Permanently discontinue therapy if HDL-C becomes severely depressed; monitor HDL-C concentrations until returned to baseline.

Dosage adjustment in renal impairment: Monitor renal function and lipid panel before adjusting. **Note:** Use in severe renal impairment (including patients on dialysis) is contraindicated (see specific product labeling):

Antara (micronized):

Cl_{cr} >80 mL/minute or eGFR ≥60 mL/minute/1.73 m^2: No dosage adjustment necessary.
Cl_{cr} >30-80 mL/minute or eGFR 30-59 mL/minute/1.73 m^2: Initiate at 43 mg once daily
Cl_{cr} ≤30 mL/minute or eGFR <30 mL/minute/1.73 m^2: Use is contraindicated.
Dialysis: Use is contraindicated.

Fenoglide:

Cl_{cr} >80 mL/minute or eGFR ≥60 mL/minute/1.73 m^2: No dosage adjustment necessary.
Cl_{cr} >30-80 mL/minute or eGFR 30-59 mL/minute/1.73 m^2: Initiate at 40 mg once daily
Cl_{cr} ≤30 mL/minute or eGFR <30 mL/minute/1.73 m^2: Use is contraindicated.
Dialysis: Use is contraindicated.

Fibricor:

Cl_{cr} >80 mL/minute: No dosage adjustment necessary.
Cl_{cr} >30-80 mL/minute: Initiate at 35 mg once daily
Cl_{cr} ≤30 mL/minute: Use is contraindicated.
Dialysis: Use is contraindicated.

Lipidil EZ [Canadian product]: **Note:** Interrupt treatment in patients with an increase in creatinine concentrations >50% the upper limit of normal (ULN).

Cl_{cr} >50 mL/minute: No dosage adjustment necessary.
Cl_{cr} 20-50 mL/minute: Initiate at 48 mg once daily
Cl_{cr} <20 mL/minute: Use is contraindicated.
Dialysis: Use is contraindicated.

Lipidil Micro [Canadian product]: **Note:** Interrupt treatment in patients with an increase in creatinine concentrations >50% the upper limit of normal (ULN).

Cl_{cr} >85 mL/minute (women) or >95 mL/minute (men): No dosage adjustment necessary.
Cl_{cr} 20-85 mL/minute (women) or 20-95 mL/minute (men): Initiate therapy with Lipidil EZ formulation with a dose of 48 mg once daily.
Cl_{cr} <20 mL/minute: Use is contraindicated.
Dialysis: Use is contraindicated.

Lipidil Supra [Canadian product]: **Note:** Interrupt treatment in patients with an increase in creatinine concentrations >50% the upper limit of normal (ULN).

Cl_{cr} >100 mL/minute: No dosage adjustment necessary.
Cl_{cr} 20-100 mL/minute: Initiate at 100 mg once daily
Cl_{cr} <20 mL/minute: Use is contraindicated.
Dialysis: Use is contraindicated.

Lipofen:

eGFR ≥90 mL/minute/1.73 m^2: No dosage adjustment necessary.
eGFR 30-89 mL/minute/1.73 m^2: Initiate at 50 mg once daily
eGFR <30 mL/minute/1.73 m^2: Use is contraindicated.
Dialysis: Use is contraindicated.

Lofibra (micronized):

Cl_{cr} >80 mL/minute: No dosage adjustment necessary.
Cl_{cr} >30-80 mL/minute: Initiate at 67 mg once daily
Cl_{cr} ≤30 mL/minute: Use is contraindicated.
Dialysis: Use is contraindicated.

Lofibra (tablets):

eGFR ≥60 mL/minute/1.73 m^2: No dosage adjustment necessary.

eGFR 30-59 mL/minute/1.73 m^2: Initiate at 54 mg once daily

eGFR <30 mL/minute/1.73 m^2: Use is contraindicated.

Dialysis: Use is contraindicated.

TriCor:

eGFR ≥60 mL/minute/1.73 m^2: No dosage adjustment necessary.

eGFR 30-59 mL/minute/1.73 m^2: Initiate at 48 mg once daily

eGFR <30 mL/minute/1.73 m^2: Use is contraindicated.

Dialysis: Use is contraindicated.

Triglide:

Cl_{cr} >80 mL/minute or eGFR ≥60 mL/minute/1.73 m^2: No dosage adjustment necessary.

Cl_{cr} >30-80 mL/minute or eGFR 30-59 mL/minute/1.73 m^2: Initiate at 50 mg once daily

Cl_{cr} ≤30 mL/minute or eGFR <30 mL/minute/1.73 m^2: Use is contraindicated.

Dialysis: Use is contraindicated.

Trilipix:

eGFR ≥60 mL/minute/1.73 m^2: No dosage adjustment necessary.

eGFR 30-59 mL/minute/1.73 m^2: Initiate at 45 mg once daily

eGFR <30 mL/minute/1.73 m^2: Use is contraindicated.

Dialysis: Use is contraindicated.

Dosage adjustment in hepatic impairment: Use is contraindicated. Regular monitoring of liver function tests is required; discontinue therapy in patients whose enzyme levels persist above 3 times the upper limit of normal.

Dietary Considerations

Antara, Fibricor, Lipidil EZ [Canadian product], Lofibra tablets, TriCor, Triglide, Trilipix: May be taken with or without food.

Fenoglide, Lipidil Micro [Canadian product], Lipidil Supra [Canadian product], Lipofen, Lofibra (micronized capsules): Take with meals.

Administration

Antara, Fibricor, Lipidil EZ [Canadian product], Lofibra tablets, TriCor, Triglide, Trilipix: Administer with or without food. Swallow whole; do not open (capsules), crush, dissolve, or chew.

Lipidil Micro [Canadian product]; Lofibra (micronized) capsules: Administer with meals.

Fenoglide, Lipofen, Lipidil Supra [Canadian product]: Administer with meals. Swallow whole; do not open (capsules), crush, dissolve, or chew.

Monitoring Parameters Periodic blood counts during first year of therapy. Monitor lipid profile periodically. Monitor LFTs regularly and discontinue therapy if levels remain >3 times normal limits. Monitor renal function in patients with renal impairment or in those at increased risk for developing renal impairment.

2013 ACC/AHA Blood Cholesterol Guideline recommendations (Stone, 2013): Evaluate renal status at baseline, within 3 months after initiation, and every 6 months thereafter.

Dosage Forms Considerations

Micronized formulations: Antara, Lofibra capsules

Strength of choline fenofibrate products are expressed in terms of fenofibric acid.

Dosage Forms Excipient information presented when available (limited, particularly for generics); consult specific product labeling. [DSC] = Discontinued product

Capsule, Oral, as fenofibrate:

Antara: 30 mg, 43 mg [contains fd&c blue #2 (indigotine), fd&c yellow #10 (quinoline yellow)]

Antara: 90 mg [contains brilliant blue fcf (fd&c blue #1), fd&c yellow #10 (quinoline yellow), fd&c yellow #6 (sunset yellow)]

Antara: 130 mg [contains fd&c blue #2 (indigotine), fd&c yellow #10 (quinoline yellow)]

Lipofen: 50 mg [contains brilliant blue fcf (fd&c blue #1), fd&c blue #2 (indigotine), fd&c red #40, fd&c yellow #10 (quinoline yellow)]

Lipofen: 150 mg

Lofibra: 67 mg, 134 mg, 200 mg

Generic: 43 mg, 67 mg, 130 mg, 134 mg, 200 mg

Capsule Delayed Release, Oral, as choline fenofibrate:

Trilipix: 45 mg

Trilipix: 135 mg [contains fd&c blue #2 (indigotine)]

Generic: 45 mg, 135 mg

Tablet, Oral, as fenofibrate:

Fenoglide: 40 mg, 120 mg

Lofibra: 54 mg [contains fd&c yellow #10 aluminum lake]

Lofibra: 160 mg

Tricor: 48 mg [contains fd&c blue #2 aluminum lake, fd&c yellow #10 aluminum lake, fd&c yellow #6 aluminum lake, soybean lecithin]

Tricor: 145 mg [contains soybean lecithin]

Triglide: 50 mg [DSC], 160 mg

Generic: 48 mg, 54 mg, 145 mg, 160 mg

Tablet, Oral, as fenofibric acid:

Fibricor: 35 mg, 105 mg

Generic: 35 mg, 105 mg

◆ **Fenofibrate Micro (Can)** *see* Fenofibrate and Derivatives *on page 837*

◆ **Fenofibrate-S (Can)** *see* Fenofibrate and Derivatives *on page 837*

◆ **Fenofibric Acid** *see* Fenofibrate and Derivatives *on page 837*

◆ **Fenoglide** *see* Fenofibrate and Derivatives *on page 837*

Fenoldopam (fe NOL doe pam)

Brand Names: U.S. Corlopam

Index Terms Fenoldopam Mesylate

Pharmacologic Category Antihypertensive; Dopamine Agonist

Use Treatment of severe hypertension (up to 48 hours in adults), including in patients with renal compromise; short-term (up to 4 hours) blood pressure reduction in pediatric patients

Pregnancy Risk Factor B

Pregnancy Considerations Fetal harm was not observed in animal studies; however, safety and efficacy have not been established for use during pregnancy. Use during pregnancy only if clearly needed.

Breast-Feeding Considerations It is not known if fenoldopam is excreted in breast milk. The manufacturer recommends that caution be exercised when administering fenoldopam to nursing women.

Contraindications There are no contraindications listed within the manufacturer's approved labeling.

Warnings/Precautions Use with caution in patients with open-angle glaucoma or intraocular hypertension; fenoldopam causes a dose-dependent increase in intraocular pressure. Dose-related tachycardia can occur, especially at infusion rates >0.1 mcg/kg/minute. Use with extreme caution in patients with obstructive coronary disease or ongoing angina pectoris; can increase myocardial oxygen demand due to tachycardia leading to angina pectoris. Serum potassium concentrations <3 mEq/L were observed within 6 hours of fenoldopam initiation; monitor potassium concentrations appropriately. Use with caution in patients with increased intracranial pressure; use has not been studied in this population. For continuous infusion only (no bolus doses). Contains sulfites; may cause allergic reaction in susceptible individuals.

Adverse Reactions

≥5%:

Cardiovascular: Cutaneous flushing, hypotension

Central nervous system: Headache

Gastrointestinal: Nausea

<5%:

Cardiovascular: Angina, bradycardia, chest pain, extrasystoles, heart failure, MI, orthostatic hypotension, palpitation, ST-T abnormalities, T-wave inversion, tachycardia

Central nervous system: Anxiety, dizziness, fever, insomnia

Endocrine & metabolic: Hyperglycemia, hypokalemia, LDH increased

Gastrointestinal: Abdominal pain/fullness, constipation, diarrhea, vomiting

Genitourinary: Urinary tract infection

Hematologic: Bleeding, leukocytosis

Hepatic: Transaminases increased

Local: Injection site reactions

Neuromuscular & skeletal: Back pain, limb cramps

Ocular: Intraocular pressure increased

Renal: BUN increased, creatinine increased, oliguria

Respiratory: Dyspnea, nasal congestion

Miscellaneous: Diaphoresis

Drug Interactions

Metabolism/Transport Effects None known.

Avoid Concomitant Use There are no known interactions where it is recommended to avoid concomitant use.

Increased Effect/Toxicity There are no known significant interactions involving an increase in effect.

Decreased Effect There are no known significant interactions involving a decrease in effect.

Storage/Stability Store undiluted product at 2°C to 30°C (35°F to 86°F). Following dilution, store at room temperature and use solution within 24 hours.

Mechanism of Action A selective postsynaptic dopamine agonist (D_1-receptors) which exerts hypotensive effects by decreasing peripheral vasculature resistance with increased renal blood flow, diuresis, and natriuresis; 6 times as potent as dopamine in producing renal vasodilatation; has minimal adrenergic effects

Pharmacodynamics/Kinetics

Onset of action: I.V.: 10 minutes

Duration: I.V.: 1 hour

Distribution: V_d: 0.6 L/kg

Half-life elimination: I.V.: Children: 3-5 minutes; Adults: ~5 minutes

Metabolism: Hepatic via methylation, glucuronidation, and sulfation; the 8-sulfate metabolite may have some activity; extensive first-pass effect

Excretion: Urine (90%); feces (10%)

Dosage I.V.: Hypertension, severe:

Children: Initial: 0.2 mcg/kg/minute; may be increased to dosages of 0.3-0.5 mcg/kg/minute every 20-30 minutes (maximum dose: 0.8 mcg/kg/minute); limited to short-term (4 hours) use

Adults: Initial: 0.03-0.1 mcg/kg/minute (associated with less reflex tachycardia); may be increased in increments of 0.05-0.1 mcg/kg/minute every 15 minutes until target blood pressure is reached; the maximal infusion rate reported in clinical studies was 1.6 mcg/kg/minute

Dosing adjustment in renal impairment: No dosage adjustment required; the effects of hemodialysis on fenoldopam have not been evaluated.

Dosing adjustment in hepatic impairment: No dosage adjustment required.

Usual Infusion Concentrations: Pediatric I.V. infusion: 60 **mcg**/mL

Usual Infusion Concentrations: Adult I.V. infusion: 10 mg in 250 mL (concentration: 40 **mcg**/mL) of D_5W or NS

Administration For continuous I.V. infusion only.

Monitoring Parameters Blood pressure, heart rate, ECG; serum potassium concentrations (eg, every 6 hours)

Dosage Forms Excipient information presented when available (limited, particularly for generics); consult specific product labeling.

Solution, Intravenous:

Corlopam: 10 mg/mL (1 mL); 20 mg/2 mL (2 mL) [contains propylene glycol, sodium metabisulfite]

Generic: 10 mg/mL (1 mL); 20 mg/2 mL (2 mL)

◆ **Fenoldopam Mesylate** *see* Fenoldopam *on page* 841

◆ **Feno-Micro-200 (Can)** *see* Fenofibrate and Derivatives *on page* 837

Fenoprofen (fen oh PROE fen)

Brand Names: U.S. Nalfon

Brand Names: Canada Nalfon®

Index Terms Fenoprofen Calcium

Pharmacologic Category Nonsteroidal Anti-inflammatory Drug (NSAID), Oral

Additional Appendix Information

Beers Criteria – Potentially Inappropriate Medications for Geriatrics *on page* 2368

Use Symptomatic treatment of acute and chronic rheumatoid arthritis and osteoarthritis; relief of mild-to-moderate pain

Unlabeled Use Migraine prophylaxis

Pregnancy Risk Factor C

Medication Guide Available Yes

Dosage Adults: Oral:

Rheumatoid arthritis, osteoarthritis: 300-600 mg 3-4 times/day; maximum dose: 3.2 g/day

Mild-to-moderate pain: 200 mg every 4-6 hours as needed; maximum dose: 3.2 g/day

Dosage adjustment in renal impairment: Not recommended in patients with advanced renal disease

Dosage adjustment in hepatic impairment: No dosage adjustment provided in manufacturer's labeling.

Additional Information Complete prescribing information should be consulted for additional detail.

Dosage Forms Excipient information presented when available (limited, particularly for generics); consult specific product labeling.

Capsule, Oral:

Nalfon: 400 mg [contains brilliant blue fcf (fd&c blue #1), fd&c red #40]

Tablet, Oral:

Generic: 600 mg

◆ **Fenoprofen Calcium** *see* Fenoprofen *on page* 842

FentaNYL (FEN ta nil)

Brand Names: U.S. Abstral; Actiq; Duragesic; Fentora; Lazanda; Onsolis; Subsys

Brand Names: Canada Abstral; Actiq; Apo-Fentanyl Matrix; Duragesic; Duragesic MAT; Fentanyl Citrate Injection, USP; Novo-Fentanyl; Onsolis; PMS-Fentanyl MTX; RAN-Fentanyl Matrix Patch; RAN-Fentanyl Transdermal System; ratio-Fentanyl; Sandoz Fentanyl Patch; Teva-Fentanyl

Index Terms Fentanyl Citrate; Fentanyl Hydrochloride; Fentanyl Patch; OTFC (Oral Transmucosal Fentanyl Citrate)

Pharmacologic Category Analgesic, Opioid; Anilidopiperidine Opioid; General Anesthetic

Additional Appendix Information

Dosing Considerations for the Critically-Ill Patient With Morbid Obesity *on page 2379*

Opioid Conversion Table *on page 2306*

Patient Information for Disposal of Unused Medications *on page 2393*

Use

Injection: Relief of pain, preoperative medication, adjunct to general or regional anesthesia

Transdermal patch (eg, Duragesic): Management of persistent moderate-to-severe chronic pain in opioid-tolerant patients when around-the-clock analgesia is needed for an extended period of time

Transmucosal lozenge (eg, Actiq), buccal tablet (Fentora), buccal film (Onsolis), nasal spray (Lazanda), sublingual tablet (Abstral), sublingual spray (Subsys): Management of breakthrough cancer pain in opioid-tolerant patients who are already receiving and who are tolerant to around-the-clock opioid therapy for their underlying persistent cancer pain.

Note: "Opioid-tolerant" patients are defined as patients who are taking at least:

Oral morphine 60 mg/day, **or**

Transdermal fentanyl 25 mcg/hour, **or**

Oral oxycodone 30 mg/day, **or**

Oral hydromorphone 8 mg/day, **or**

Oral oxymorphone 25 mg/day, **or**

Equianalgesic dose of another opioid for at least 1 week

Pregnancy Risk Factor C

Pregnancy Considerations Adverse events were observed in some animal reproduction studies. Fentanyl crosses the placenta.

Fentanyl injection may be used for the management of pain during labor (ACOG, 2002). When used for pain relief during labor, opioids may temporarily affect the heart rate of the fetus (ACOG, 2002). Transient muscular rigidity has been observed in the neonate with fentanyl; symptoms of respiratory or neurological depression were not different than those observed in infants of untreated mothers.

If chronic opioid exposure occurs in pregnancy, adverse events in the newborn (including withdrawal) may occur; monitoring of the neonate is recommended. The minimum effective dose should be used if opioids are needed (Chou, 2009). Symptoms characteristic of neonatal abstinence syndrome have been observed following chronic fentanyl use in pregnant women. Neonatal abstinence syndrome following opioid exposure may present with autonomic (eg, fever, temperature instability), gastrointestinal (eg, diarrhea, vomiting, poor feeding/weight gain), or neurologic (eg, high pitched crying, increased muscle tone, irritability, seizure, tremor) symptoms (Dow, 2012; Hudak, 2012).

Transdermal patch, transmucosal lozenge, nasal spray (Lazanda), sublingual tablet, sublingual spray (Subsys), buccal tablet (Fentora), and buccal film (Onsolis) are not recommended for analgesia during labor and delivery.

Breast-Feeding Considerations Fentanyl is excreted in low concentrations into breast milk and breast-feeding is not recommended by the manufacturers.

Parenteral opioids used during labor have the potential to interfere with a newborn's natural reflex to nurse within the first few hours after birth. When needed, a short-acting opioid, such as fentanyl, is preferred for women who will be nursing (Montgomery, 2012)

Breast-feeding is considered acceptable following single doses to the mother; however, limited information is available when used long-term (Spigset, 2000). Nursing infants exposed to large doses of opioids should be monitored for apnea and sedation (Montgomery, 2012).

Note: Transdermal patch, transmucosal lozenge, sublingual tablet, sublingual spray (Subsys), buccal tablet (Fentora), and buccal film (Onsolis) are not recommended in nursing women due to potential for sedation and/or respiratory depression.

Prescribing and Access Restrictions As a requirement of the REMS program, access is restricted.

Transmucosal immediate-release fentanyl products (eg, sublingual tablets and spray, oral lozenges, buccal tablets and soluble film, nasal spray) are only available through the Transmucosal Immediate-Release Fentanyl (TIRF) REMS ACCESS program. Enrollment in the program is required for outpatients, prescribers for outpatient use, pharmacies (inpatient and outpatient), and distributors. Enrollment is not required for inpatient administration (eg, hospitals, hospices, long-term care facilities), inpatients, and prescribers who prescribe to inpatients. Further information is available at 1-866-822-1483 or at www.TIRFREMSaccess.com

Note: Effective December, 2011, individual REMs programs for TIRF products were combined into a single access program (TIRF REMS Access). Prescribers and pharmacies that were enrolled in at least one individual REMS program for these products will automatically be transitioned to the single access program.

Medication Guide Available Yes

Contraindications Hypersensitivity to fentanyl or any component of the formulation

Additional contraindications for transdermal patches (eg, Duragesic): Severe respiratory disease or depression including acute asthma (unless patient is mechanically ventilated); paralytic ileus; patients requiring short-term therapy, management of acute or intermittent pain, postoperative or mild pain, and in patients who are **not** opioid tolerant

Additional contraindications for transmucosal buccal tablets (Fentora), buccal films (Onsolis), lozenges (eg, Actiq), sublingual tablets (Abstral), sublingual spray (Subsys), nasal spray (Lazanda): Contraindicated in the management of acute or postoperative pain (including headache, migraine, or dental pain), and in patients who are **not** opioid tolerant. Abstral and Onsolis also are contraindicated for acute pain management in the emergency room.

Canadian labeling: Additional contraindication (not in U.S. labeling): Sublingual tablets (Abstral): Severe respiratory depression or severe obstructive lung disease

Warnings/Precautions An opioid-containing analgesic regimen should be tailored to each patient's needs and based upon the type of pain being treated (acute versus chronic), the route of administration, degree of tolerance for opioids (naive versus chronic user), age, weight, and medical condition. The optimal analgesic dose varies widely among patients. Doses should be titrated to pain relief/prevention. May cause CNS depression, which may impair physical or mental abilities; patients must be cautioned about performing tasks which require mental alertness (eg, operating machinery or driving). Fentanyl shares the toxic potentials of opioid agonists, and precautions of opioid agonist therapy should be observed; use with caution in patients with bradycardia or bradyarrhythmias; rapid I.V. infusion may result in skeletal muscle and chest wall rigidity leading to respiratory distress and/or apnea, bronchoconstriction, laryngospasm; inject slowly over 3-5 minutes. **[U.S. Boxed Warning]: Healthcare provider should be alert to problems of abuse, misuse, and diversion.** Tolerance or drug dependence may result from extended use. The elderly may be particularly susceptible to the CNS depressant and constipating effects of opioids. Use extreme caution in patients with COPD or other chronic respiratory conditions. Use caution with biliary tract impairment, pancreatitis, head injuries, morbid obesity, renal impairment, or hepatic dysfunction. **[U.S. Boxed Warning]: Use with strong or moderate CYP3A4 inhibitors may result in increased effects and potentially fatal respiratory depression.** Concurrent use of agonist/antagonist analgesics may precipitate withdrawal symptoms and/or reduced analgesic efficacy in patients following prolonged therapy with mu opioid agonists. Abrupt discontinuation following prolonged use may also lead to withdrawal symptoms. Potentially significant interactions may exist, requiring dose or frequency adjustment, additional monitoring, and/or selection of alternative therapy.

Pediatric patients: **[U.S. Boxed Warning]: Buccal film, buccal tablet, nasal spray, sublingual tablet, sublingual spray, transdermal patch, and lozenge preparations contain an amount of medication that can be fatal to children. Keep all used and unused products out of the reach of children at all times and discard products properly.** Patients and caregivers should be counseled on the dangers to children including the risk of exposure to partially-consumed products. After chronic maternal exposure to opioids, neonatal withdrawal syndrome may occur in the newborn; monitor neonate closely. Signs and symptoms include irritability, hyperactivity and abnormal sleep pattern, high pitched cry, tremor, vomiting, diarrhea and failure to gain weight. Onset, duration and severity depend on the drug used, duration of use, maternal dose, and rate of drug elimination by the newborn. Opioid withdrawal syndrome in the neonate, unlike in adults, may be life-threatening and should be treated according to protocols developed by neonatology experts.

[U.S. Boxed Warning] Abstral, Actiq, Duragesic, Fentora, Lazanda, Onsolis, Subsys: May cause potentially life-threatening hypoventilation, respiratory depression, and/or death; Abstral, Actiq, Duragesic, Fentora, Lazanda, Onsolis, or Subsys should only be prescribed for opioid-tolerant patients. Risk of respiratory depression increased in elderly patients, debilitated patients, and patients with conditions associated with hypoxia or hypercapnia; usually occurs after administration of initial dose in nontolerant patients or when given with other drugs that depress respiratory function.

Transmucosal (buccal film/tablet, sublingual spray/tablet, lozenge) and nasal spray: **[U.S. Boxed Warning]: Transmucosal and nasal fentanyl formulations are contraindicated in the management of acute or postoperative pain and in opioid nontolerant patients.** Should be used only for the care of opioid-tolerant cancer patients with breakthrough pain and is intended for use by specialists who are knowledgeable in treating cancer pain. **[U.S. Boxed Warning]: Substantial differences exist in the pharmacokinetic profile of fentanyl products. Do not convert patients on a mcg-per-mcg basis from one fentanyl product to another fentanyl product; the substitution of one fentanyl product for another fentanyl product may result in a fatal overdose. [U.S. Boxed Warning]: Available only through the TIRF REMS ACCESS program, a restricted distribution program with outpatients, prescribers who prescribe to outpatients, pharmacies (inpatient and outpatient), and distributor-required enrollment.** Avoid use of topical nasal decongestants (eg, oxymetazoline) during episodes of rhinitis when using fentanyl nasal spray; response to fentanyl may be delayed or reduced. Avoid use of sublingual spray in cancer patients with grade 2 or higher mucositis (fentanyl exposure increased); use with caution in patients with grade 1 mucositis, and closely monitor for respiratory and CNS depression.

Transdermal patch: **[U.S. Boxed Warning]: Transdermal patch is contraindicated in the management of short-term analgesia, or in the management of postoperative pain, and in patients who are opioid nontolerant. Should only be prescribed by healthcare professionals who are knowledgeable in the use of potent opioids in the management of chronic pain. Monitor closely for respiratory depression during use, particularly during first two applications after initiation of therapy or after dose increases. [U.S. Boxed Warning]: Avoid exposure of application site and surrounding area to direct external heat sources. Patients who experience fever or increase in core body temperature should be monitored closely.** Serum fentanyl concentrations may increase by approximately one-third for patients with a body temperature of 40°C (104°F) secondary to a temperature-dependent increase in fentanyl release from the patch and increased skin permeability. **[U.S. Boxed Warning]: Accidental exposure may lead to severe respiratory depression, including death, in children and adults; proper procedures for handling and disposal of patches should be followed.** Avoid unclothed/unwashed application site exposure, inadvertent person-to-person patch transfer (eg, while hugging), incidental exposure (eg, sharing same bed, sitting on patch), intentional exposure (eg, chewing), or accidental exposure by caregivers when applying/removing patch. Should be applied only to intact skin. Use of a patch that has been cut, damaged, or altered in any way may result in overdosage. Patients who experience adverse reactions should be monitored for at least 24 hours after removal of the patch. May contain conducting metal (eg, aluminum); remove patch prior to MRI.

Adverse Reactions

>10%:

Cardiovascular: Bradycardia, edema

Central nervous system: CNS depression, confusion, dizziness, drowsiness, fatigue, headache, sedation

Endocrine & metabolic: Dehydration

Gastrointestinal: Constipation, nausea, vomiting, xerostomia

Local: Application-site reaction erythema

Neuromuscular & skeletal: Chest wall rigidity (high dose I.V.), muscle rigidity, weakness

Ocular: Miosis

Respiratory: Dyspnea, respiratory depression

Miscellaneous: Diaphoresis

1% to 10%:

Cardiovascular: Cardiac arrhythmia, cardiorespiratory arrest, chest pain, DVT, flushing, hyper-/hypotension, orthostatic hypotension, pallor, palpitation, peripheral edema, sinus tachycardia, syncope, tachycardia, vasodilation

Central nervous system: Abnormal dreams, abnormal thinking, agitation, amnesia, anxiety, attention disturbance, chills, depression, disorientation, dysphoria, euphoria, fever, hallucinations, hypoesthesia, insomnia, irritability, lethargy, malaise, mental status change, migraine, nervousness, paranoid reaction, restlessness, somnolence, stupor, vertigo

Dermatologic: Alopecia, bruising, cellulitis, decubitus ulcer, erythema, hyperhidrosis, papules, pruritus, rash

Endocrine & metabolic: Breast pain, dehydration, hot flashes, hyper-/hypocalcemia, hyper-/hypoglycemia, hypoalbuminemia, hypokalemia, hypomagnesemia, hyponatremia

Gastrointestinal: Abdominal distension, abdominal pain, abnormal taste, anorexia, appetite decreased, biliary tract spasm, diarrhea, dyspepsia, dysphagia (buccal tablet/film/sublingual spray), flatulence, gastritis, gastroenteritis, gastroesophageal reflux, GI hemorrhage, gingival pain (buccal tablet), gingivitis (lozenge), glossitis (lozenge), hematemesis, ileus, intestinal obstruction (buccal film), periodontal abscess (lozenge/buccal tablet), proctalgia, stomatitis (lozenge/buccal tablet/sublingual tablet/sublingual spray), tongue disorder (sublingual tablet), ulceration (gingival, lip, mouth; transmucosal use/nasal spray), weight loss

Genitourinary: Dysuria, erectile dysfunction, urinary incontinence, urinary retention, urinary tract infection, vaginitis, vaginal hemorrhage

Hematologic: Anemia, leukopenia, neutropenia, thrombocytopenia

Hepatic: Alkaline phosphatase increased, ascites, AST increased, jaundice

Local: Application site pain, application site irritation

Neuromuscular & skeletal: Abnormal coordination, abnormal gait, arthralgia, back pain, limb pain, myalgia, neuropathy, paresthesia, rigors, tremor

Ocular: Blurred vision, diplopia, dry eye, swelling, ptosis, strabismus

Renal: Renal failure

Respiratory: Apnea, asthma, bronchitis, cough, dyspnea (exertional), epistaxis, hemoptysis, hypoventilation, hypoxia, laryngitis, nasal congestion (nasal spray), nasal discomfort (nasal spray), nasopharyngitis, pharyngolaryngeal pain, pharyngitis, pneumonia, postnasal drip (nasal spray), pulmonary embolism (nasal spray), rhinitis, rhinorrhea (nasal spray), sinusitis, upper respiratory infection, wheezing

Miscellaneous: Flu-like syndrome, hiccups, hypersensitivity, lymphadenopathy, night sweats, parosmia, speech disorder, withdrawal syndrome

<1% (Limited to important or life-threatening): Amblyopia, allergic reaction, anaphylaxis, angina, aphasia, bladder pain, bronchospasm, CNS excitation or delirium, depersonalization, dysesthesia, emotional lability, esophageal stenosis, exfoliative dermatitis, fecal impaction, gum line erosion (lozenge), gum hemorrhage (lozenge), hematuria, hostility, hyper-/hypotonia, laryngospasm, myasthenia, nocturia, oliguria, pancytopenia, paradoxical dizziness, physical and psychological dependence with prolonged use, pleural effusion, polyuria, pustules, speech disorder, stertorous breathing, seizure, tooth loss (lozenge), urinary tract spasm, urticaria, vertigo

Drug Interactions

Metabolism/Transport Effects Substrate of CYP3A4 (major); **Note:** Assignment of Major/Minor substrate status based on clinically relevant drug interaction potential; **Inhibits** CYP3A4 (weak)

Avoid Concomitant Use

Avoid concomitant use of FentaNYL with any of the following: Azelastine (Nasal); Crizotinib; Enzalutamide; Fusidic Acid (Systemic); MAO Inhibitors; Mifepristone; Paraldehyde; Pimozide

Increased Effect/Toxicity

FentaNYL may increase the levels/effects of: Alcohol (Ethyl); Alvimopan; ARIPiprazole; Azelastine (Nasal); Beta-Blockers; Calcium Channel Blockers (Nondihydropyridine); CNS Depressants; Desmopressin; Diuretics; Dofetilide; Hydrocodone; Lomitapide; MAO Inhibitors; Metyrosine; Mirtazapine; Paraldehyde; Pimozide; Pramipexole; ROPINIRole; Rotigotine; Selective Serotonin Reuptake Inhibitors; Zolpidem

The levels/effects of FentaNYL may be increased by: Amphetamines; Anticholinergics; Antipsychotic Agents (Phenothiazines); Brimonidine (Topical); Cannabinoids; Crizotinib; CYP3A4 Inhibitors (Moderate); CYP3A4 Inhibitors (Strong); Dasatinib; Doxylamine; Droperidol; Fusidic Acid (Systemic); HydrOXYzine; Ivacaftor; Luliconazole; Magnesium Sulfate; MAO Inhibitors; Mifepristone; Perampanel; Simeprevir; Sodium Oxybate; Succinylcholine; Tapentadol

Decreased Effect

FentaNYL may decrease the levels/effects of: Ioflupane I 123; Pegvisomant

The levels/effects of FentaNYL may be decreased by: Alpha-/Beta-Agonists (Indirect-Acting); Alpha1-Agonists; Ammonium Chloride; Enzalutamide; Mixed Agonist / Antagonist Opioids; Rifamycin Derivatives

Ethanol/Nutrition/Herb Interactions

Ethanol: Ethanol may increase CNS depression. Management: Monitor for increased effects with coadministration. Caution patients about effects.

Food: Fentanyl concentrations may be increased by grapefruit juice. Management: Avoid concurrent intake of large quantities (>1 quart/day) of grapefruit juice.

Herb/Nutraceutical: St John's wort may decrease fentanyl levels; gotu kola, valerian, and kava kava may increase CNS depression. Management: Avoid St John's wort, gotu kola, valerian, and kava kava.

Storage/Stability

Injection formulation: Store at controlled room temperature of 20°C to 25°C (68°F to 77°F). Protect from light.

Nasal spray: Do not store above 25°C (77°F); do not freeze. Protect from light. Bottle should be stored in the provided child-resistant container when not in use and kept out of the reach of children at all times.

Transdermal patch: Do not store above 25°C (77°F). Keep out of the reach of children.

Transmucosal (buccal film, buccal tablet, lozenge, sublingual spray, sublingual tablet): Store at controlled room temperature of 20°C to 25°C (68°F to 77°F). Protect from freezing and moisture. Keep out of the reach of children.

Mechanism of Action Binds with stereospecific receptors at many sites within the CNS, increases pain threshold, alters pain reception, inhibits ascending pain pathways

Pharmacodynamics/Kinetics

Onset of action: Analgesic: I.M.: 7-8 minutes; I.V.: Almost immediate (maximal analgesic and respiratory depressant effects may not be seen for several minutes); Transdermal (initial placement): 6 hours; Transmucosal: 5-15 minutes

Duration: I.M.: 1-2 hours; I.V.: 0.5-1 hour; Transdermal (removal of patch/no replacement): Related to blood level; some effects may last 72-96 hours due to extended half-life and absorption from the skin, fentanyl concentrations decrease by ~50% in 20-27 hours; Transmucosal: Related to blood level; respiratory depressant effect may last longer than analgesic effect

Absorption:

Transdermal: Initial application: Drug is released at a nearly constant rate from the transdermal matrix system into the skin, where it accumulates; this results in a depot of fentanyl in the outer layer of skin. Fentanyl is absorbed into systemic circulation from the depot. This results in a gradual increase in serum concentration over the first 12-24 hours, followed by fairly constant concentrations for the remainder of the dosing interval. Absorption is decreased in cachectic patients (compared to normal size patients). Exposure to external heat increases drug absorption from patch.

Transmucosal, buccal tablet and buccal film: Rapid, ~50% from the buccal mucosa; remaining 50% swallowed with saliva and slowly absorbed from GI tract.

Transmucosal, lozenge: Rapid, ~25% from the buccal mucosa; 75% swallowed with saliva and slowly absorbed from GI tract

Distribution: 4-6 L/kg; Highly lipophilic, redistributes into muscle and fat

Protein binding: 80% to 85%

Metabolism: Hepatic, primarily via CYP3A4

Bioavailability:

Buccal film: 71% (mucositis did not have a clinically significant effect on C_{max} and AUC; however, bioavailability is expected to decrease if film is inappropriately chewed and swallowed)

Buccal tablet: 65%

Lozenge: ~50%

Sublingual spray: 76%

Sublingual tablet: 54%

Half-life elimination:

I.V.: 2-4 hours; when administered as a continuous infusion, the half-life prolongs with infusion duration due to the large volume of distribution (Sessler, 2008)

Transdermal patch: 20-27 hours (apparent half-life is influenced by continued fentanyl absorption from skin)

Transmucosal products: 3-14 hours (dose dependent); Nasal spray: 15-25 hours (based on a multiple-dose pharmacokinetic study when doses are administered in the same nostril and separated by a 1-, 2-, or 4-hour time lapse)

Time to peak:

Buccal film: 0.75-4 hours (median: 1 hour)

Buccal tablet: 20-240 minutes (median: 47 minutes)

Lozenge: 20-480 minutes (median: 20-40 minutes)

Nasal spray: Median: 15-21 minutes

Sublingual spray: 10-120 minutes (median: 90 minutes)

Sublingual tablet: 15-240 minutes (median: 30-60 minutes)

Transdermal patch: 20-72 hours; steady state serum concentrations are reached after two sequential 72-hour applications

Excretion: Urine 75% (primarily as metabolites, <7% to 10% as unchanged drug); feces ~9%

Dosage Note: Ranges listed may not represent the maximum doses that may be required in all patients. Doses and dosage intervals should be titrated to pain relief/prevention. Monitor vital signs routinely. Single I.M. doses have duration of 1-2 hours, single I.V. doses last 0.5-1 hour.

Surgery:

Children ≥2 years and Adolescents: Adjunct to anesthesia (induction and maintenance): Slow I.V.: 2-3 mcg/**kg**/dose every 1-2 hours as needed

Adults:

Premedication: I.M.: 50-100 mcg administered 30-60 minutes prior to surgery **or** slow I.V.: 25-50 mcg given shortly before induction (Barash, 2009)

Adjunct to general anesthesia: Slow I.V.:

Low dose: 1-2 mcg/**kg** depending on the indication (Miller, 2010); additional maintenance doses are generally not needed

Moderate dose: Initial: 2-20 mcg/**kg**; Maintenance (bolus or infusion): 1-2 mcg/kg/**hour**. Discontinuing fentanyl infusion 30-60 minutes prior to the end of surgery will usually allow adequate ventilation upon emergence from anesthesia. For "fast-tracking" and early extubation following major surgery, total fentanyl doses are limited to 10-15 mcg/kg.

High dose: 20-50 mcg/**kg**; **Note:** High-dose fentanyl as an adjunct to general anesthesia is rarely used, but is still described in the manufacturer's labeling.

Adjunct to regional anesthesia: 50-100 mcg I.M. or slow I.V. over 1-2 minutes. **Note:** An I.V. should be in place with regional anesthesia so the I.M. route is rarely used but still maintained as an option in the manufacturer's labeling.

Postoperative recovery: I.M., slow I.V.: 50-100 mcg every 1-2 hours as needed.

Pain management:

Children <50 kg: Patient-controlled analgesia (PCA) (unlabeled use; American Pain Society, 2008): Opioid-naive: I.V.:

Usual concentration: 10-50 mcg/mL (varies by patient weight and institution)

Demand dose: 0.5-1 mcg/kg/dose

Lockout interval: 6-8 minutes

Usual basal rate: ≤0.5 mcg/kg/**hour**. **Note:** Due to safety concerns, continuous basal infusions are not recommended for initial programming and should rarely be used (Grass, 2005).

Adults: ***Severe pain:***

I.M., I.V.:

Intermittent dosing (unlabeled dose): Slow I.V.: 25-35 mcg (based on ~70 kg patient) **or** 0.35-0.5 mcg/kg every 30-60 minutes as needed (SCCM [Barr, 2013]). **Note:** After the first dose, if severe pain persists and adverse effects are minimal at the time of expected peak effect (eg, ~5 minutes after I.V. administration), may repeat dose (APS, 2008). In addition, since the duration of activity with I.V. administration is 30-60 minutes, more frequent administration may be necessary when administered by this route.

Patient-controlled analgesia (PCA) (unlabeled use; American Pain Society, 2008): Opioid-naive: I.V.:

Usual concentration: 10 mcg/mL

Demand dose: Usual: 20 mcg; range: 10-50 mcg

Lockout interval: 5-8 minutes

Usual basal rate: ≤50 mcg/hour. **Note:** Due to safety concerns, continuous basal infusions are not recommended for initial programming and should rarely be used; consider limiting infusion rate to 10 mcg/hour if used (Grass, 2005).

Critically-ill patients (unlabeled dose): Slow I.V.: 25-35 mcg (based on ~70 kg patient) **or** 0.35-0.5 mcg/kg every 30-60 minutes as needed (SCCM [Barr, 2013]). **Note:** More frequent dosing may be needed (eg, mechanically-ventilated patients).

Continuous infusion: 50-700 mcg/hour (based on ~70 kg patient) **or** 0.7-10 mcg/kg/**hour** (SCCM [Barr, 2013])

Alternative continuous infusion dosing: 1-2 mcg/kg bolus followed by an initial rate of 1-2 mcg/**kg**/hour (Peng, 1999) **or** 25-100 mcg bolus followed by an initial rate of 25-200 mcg/**hour** (Liu, 2003). **Note:** When pain is not controlled, may administer an additional small bolus dose (eg, 25-50 mcg) prior to increasing the infusion rate (Loper 1990; Peng, 1999; Salomaki, 1991).

Intrathecal (I.T.) (unlabeled use; American Pain Society, 2008): **Must be preservative-free.** Doses must be adjusted for age, injection site, and patient's medical condition and degree of opioid tolerance.

Single dose: 5-25 mcg; may provide adequate relief for up to 6 hours

Continuous infusion: Not recommended in acute pain management due to risk of excessive accumulation. For chronic cancer pain, infusion of very small doses may be practical (American Pain Society, 2008).

Epidural (unlabeled use; American Pain Society, 2008): **Must be preservative-free.** Doses must be adjusted for age, injection site, and patient's medical condition and degree of opioid tolerance

Single dose: 25-100 mcg; may provide adequate relief for up to 8 hours

Continuous infusion: 25-100 mcg/hour

Breakthrough cancer pain: For patients who are tolerant to and currently receiving opioid therapy for persistent cancer pain; dosing should be individually titrated to provide adequate analgesia with minimal side effects. Dose titration should be done if patient requires more than 1 dose/breakthrough pain episode for several consecutive episodes. Patients experiencing >4 breakthrough pain episodes per day should have the dose of their long-term opioid re-evaluated. **Patients must remain on around-the-clock opioids during use.**

Adolescents ≥16 years and Adults: Transmucosal: Lozenge (Actiq): **Note:** Do **not** convert patients from any other fentanyl product to Actiq on a mcg-per-mcg basis. Patients previously using another fentanyl product should be initiated at a dose of 200 mcg; individually titrate to provide adequate analgesia while minimizing adverse effects.

Initial dose: 200 mcg (consumed over 15 minutes) for all patients; if after 30 minutes from the start of the lozenge (ie, 15 minutes following the completion of the lozenge) the pain is unrelieved, a second 200 mcg dose may be given over 15 minutes. A maximum of 1 additional dose can be given per pain episode; **must wait at least 4 hours before treating another episode.** To limit the number of units in the home during titration, only prescribe an initial titration supply of six 200 mcg lozenges.

Dose titration: From the initial dose, closely follow patients and modify the dose until patient reaches a dose providing adequate analgesia using a single dosage unit per breakthrough cancer pain episode. If signs/symptoms of excessive opioid effects (eg, respiratory depression) occur, immediately remove the dosage unit from the patient's mouth, dispose of properly, and reduce subsequent doses. If adequate relief is not achieved 15 minutes after completion of the first dose (ie, 30 minutes after the start of the lozenge), only 1 additional lozenge of the same strength may be given for that episode; **must wait at least 4 hours before treating another episode.**

Maintenance dose: Once titrated to an effective dose, patients should generally use a single dosage unit per breakthrough pain episode. During any pain episode, if adequate relief is not achieved 15 minutes after completion of the first dose (ie, 30 minutes after the start of the lozenge), only 1 additional lozenge of the same strength may be given over 15 minutes for that episode; **must wait at least 4 hours before treating another episode.** Consumption should be limited to ≤4 units per day (once an effective breakthrough dose is found). If adequate analgesia is **not** provided after treating several episodes of breakthrough pain using the same dose, increase dose to next highest lozenge strength (initially dispense no more than 6 units of the new strength). Consider increasing the around-the-clock opioid therapy in patients experiencing >4 breakthrough pain episodes per day. If signs/symptoms of excessive opioid effects (eg, respiratory depression) occur, immediately remove the dosage unit from the patient's mouth, dispose of properly, and reduce subsequent doses.

Adults: Transmucosal:

Buccal film (Onsolis): **Note:** Do **not** convert patients from any other fentanyl product to Onsolis on a mcg-per-mcg basis. Patients previously using another fentanyl product should be initiated at a dose of 200 mcg; individually titrate to provide adequate analgesia while minimizing adverse effects.

Initial dose: 200 mcg for all patients; if after 30 minutes pain is unrelieved, the patient may use an alternative rescue medication as directed by their health care provider. Do **not** redose with Onsolis within an episode; buccal film should only be used once per breakthrough cancer pain episode. **Must wait at least 2 hours before treating another episode with buccal film.**

Dose titration: If titration required, increase dose in 200 mcg increments once per episode using multiples of the 200 mcg film (for doses up to 800 mcg); do not redose within a single episode of breakthrough pain and separate single doses by ≥2 hours. During titration, do not exceed 4 simultaneous applications of the 200 mcg films (800 mcg) (when using multiple films, do not place on top of each other; film may be placed on both sides of mouth); if >800 mcg required, treat next episode with one 1200 mcg film (maximum dose: 1200 mcg). Once maintenance dose is determined, all other unused films should be disposed of and that strength (using a single film) should be used. During any pain episode, if adequate relief is not achieved after 30 minutes following buccal film application, a rescue medication (as determined by health care provider) may be used.

Maintenance dose: Determined dose applied as a single film once per episode and separated by ≥2 hours (dose range: 200-1200 mcg); limit to 4 applications per day. Consider increasing the around-the-clock opioid therapy in patients experiencing >4 breakthrough pain episodes per day.

Buccal tablet (Fentora): **Note:** Do **not** convert patients from any other fentanyl product to Fentora on a mcg-per-mcg basis. Patients previously using another fentanyl product should be initiated at a dose of 100 mcg; individually titrate to provide adequate analgesia while minimizing adverse effects. For patients previously using the transmucosal lozenge (Actiq), the initial dose should be selected using the conversions listed; see *Conversion from lozenge (Actiq) to buccal tablet (Fentora)*.

Initial dose: 100 mcg for all patients unless patient already using Actiq; see *Conversion from lozenge (Actiq) to buccal tablet (Fentora)*; if after 30 minutes pain is unrelieved, may administer a second 100 mcg dose. **Must wait at least 4 hours before treating another episode with Fentora buccal tablet.**

Dose titration: If titration required, 100 mcg dose may be increased to 200 mcg using two 100 mcg tablets (one on each side of mouth) with the next breakthrough pain episode. If 200 mcg dose is not successful, patient can use four 100 mcg tablets (two on each side of mouth) with the next breakthrough pain episode. If titration requires >400 mcg per dose, titrate using 200 mcg tablets; do not use more than 4 tablets simultaneously. During any pain episode, if adequate relief is not achieved after 30 minutes following buccal tablet application, a second dose of same strength per breakthrough pain episode may be used. **Must wait at least 4 hours before treating another episode with Fentora buccal tablet.**

Maintenance dose: Following titration, the effective maintenance dose using 1 tablet of the appropriate strength should be administered once per episode; if after 30 minutes pain is unrelieved, may administer a second dose of the same strength; **must wait ≥4 hours before treating another episode.** Limit to 4 applications per day. Consider increasing the around-the-clock opioid therapy in patients experiencing >4 breakthrough pain episodes per day. Once an effective maintenance dose has been established, the buccal tablet may be administered sublingually (alternate route). To prevent confusion, patient should only have one strength available at a time. Once maintenance dose is determined, all other unused tablets should be disposed of and that strength (using a single tablet) should be used. Using more than four buccal tablets at a time has not been studied.

Conversion from lozenge (Actiq) to buccal tablet (Fentora):

Lozenge dose 200-400 mcg: Initial buccal tablet dose is 100 mcg; may titrate using multiples of 100 mcg

Lozenge dose 600-800 mcg: Initial buccal tablet dose is 200 mcg; may titrate using multiples of 200 mcg

Lozenge dose 1200-1600 mcg: Initial buccal tablet dose is 400 mcg (using two 200 mcg tablets); may titrate using multiples of 200 mcg

Nasal spray (Lazanda): **Note:** Do **not** convert patients from any other fentanyl product to Lazanda on a mcg-per-mcg basis. Patients previously using another fentanyl product should be initiated at a dose of 100 mcg; individually titrate to provide adequate analgesia while minimizing adverse effects.

Initial dose: 100 mcg (one 100 mcg spray in one nostril) for all patients; if after 30 minutes pain is unrelieved, an alternative rescue medication may be used as directed by their health care provider. **Must wait at least 2 hours before treating another episode with Lazanda nasal spray.** However, for the next pain episode, increase to a higher dose using the recommended dose titration steps.

Dose titration: If titration required, increase to a higher dose for the next pain episode using these titration steps **(Note: Must wait at least 2 hours before treating another episode with Lazanda nasal spray)**: If no relief with 100 mcg dose, increase to 200 mcg dose per episode (one 100 mcg spray in each nostril); if no relief with 200 mcg dose, increase to 400 mcg per episode (one 400 mcg spray in one nostril); if no relief with 400 mcg dose, increase to 800 mcg dose per episode (one 400 mcg spray in each nostril). **Note:** Single doses >800 mcg have not been evaluated. There are no data supporting the use of a combination of dose strengths.

Maintenance dose: Once maintenance dose for breakthrough pain episode has been determined, use that dose for subsequent episodes. For pain that is not relieved after 30 minutes of Lazanda administration or if a separate breakthrough pain episode occurs within the 2 hour window before the next Lazanda dose is permitted, a rescue medication may be used. Limit Lazanda use to ≤4 episodes of breakthrough pain per day. If patient is experiencing >4 breakthrough pain episodes per day, consider increasing the around-the-clock, long-acting opioid therapy; if long-acting opioid therapy dose is altered, re-evaluate and retitrate Lazanda dose as needed. If response to maintenance dose changes (increase in adverse reactions or alterations in pain relief), dose readjustment may be necessary.

Sublingual spray (Subsys): **Note:** Do **not** convert patients from any other fentanyl product to Subsys on a mcg-per-mcg basis. Patients previously using another fentanyl product should be initiated at a dose of 100 mcg; individually titrate to provide adequate analgesia while minimizing adverse effects. For patients previously using the transmucosal lozenge (Actiq), the initial dose should be selected using the conversions listed; see *Conversion from lozenge (Actiq) to sublingual spray (Subsys).*

Initial dose: 100 mcg for all patients unless patient already using Actiq; see *Conversion from lozenge (Actiq) to sublingual spray (Subsys).* If pain is unrelieved, 1 additional 100 mcg dose may be given 30 minutes after administration of the first dose. A maximum of 2 doses can be given per breakthrough pain episode. **Must wait at least 4 hours before treating another episode with sublingual spray.**

Dose titration: If titration required, titrate to a dose that provides adequate analgesia (with tolerable side effects) using the following titration steps: If no relief with 100 mcg dose, increase to 200 mcg dose (using one 200 mcg unit); if no relief with 200 mcg dose, increase to 400 mcg dose (using one 400 mcg unit); if no relief with 400 mcg dose, increase to 600 mcg dose (using one 600 mcg unit); if no relief with 600 mcg dose, increase to 800 mcg dose (using one 800 mcg unit); if no relief with 800 mcg dose, increase to 1200 mcg dose (using two 600 mcg units); if no relief with 1200 mcg dose, increase to 1600 mcg dose (using two 800 mcg units). During dose titration, if breakthrough pain unrelieved 30 minutes after Subsys administration, 1 additional dose using the same strength may be administered (maximum: 2 doses per breakthrough pain episode); **patient must wait 4 hours before treating another breakthrough pain episode with sublingual spray.**

Maintenance dose: Once maintenance dose for breakthrough pain episode has been determined, use that dose for subsequent episodes. If occasional episodes of unrelieved breakthrough pain occur following 30 minutes of Subsys administration, 1 additional dose using the same strength may be administered (maximum: 2 doses per breakthrough pain episode); **patient must wait 4 hours before treating another breakthrough pain episode with Subsys**. Once maintenance dose is determined, limit Subsys use to ≤4 episodes of breakthrough pain per day. If response to maintenance dose changes (increase in adverse reactions or alterations in pain relief), dose readjustment may be necessary. If patient is experiencing >4 breakthrough pain episodes per day, consider increasing the around-the-clock, long-acting opioid therapy.

Conversion from lozenge (Actiq) to sublingual spray (Subsys):

Lozenge dose 200-400 mcg: Initial sublingual spray dose is 100 mcg; may titrate using multiples of 100 mcg

Lozenge dose 600-800 mcg: Initial sublingual spray dose is 200 mcg; may titrate using multiples of 200 mcg

Lozenge dose 1200-1600 mcg: Initial sublingual spray dose is 400 mcg; may titrate using multiples of 400 mcg

Sublingual tablet (Abstral): **Note:** Do **not** convert patients from any other fentanyl product to Abstral on a mcg-per-mcg basis. Patients previously using another fentanyl product should be initiated at a dose of 100 mcg; individually titrate to provide adequate analgesia while minimizing adverse effects.

Initial dose:

U.S. labeling: 100 mcg for all patients; if pain is unrelieved, a second 100 mcg dose may be given 30 minutes after administration of the first dose. A maximum of 2 doses can be given per breakthrough pain episode. **Must wait at least 2 hours before treating another episode with sublingual tablet.**

Canadian labeling: 100 mcg for all patients; if pain is unrelieved 30 minutes after administration of Abstral, an alternative rescue medication (other than Abstral) may be given. Administer only 1 dose of

Abstral per breakthrough pain episode. **Must wait at least 2 hours before treating another episode with sublingual tablet.**

Dose titration: If titration required, increase in 100 mcg increments (up to 400 mcg) over consecutive breakthrough episodes. If titration requires >400 mcg per dose, increase in increments of 200 mcg, starting with 600 mcg dose and titrating up to 800 mcg. During titration, patients may use multiples of 100 mcg and/or 200 mcg tablets for any single dose; do not exceed 4 tablets at one time; safety and efficacy of doses >800 mcg have not been evaluated. During dose titration, if breakthrough pain unrelieved 30 minutes after sublingual tablet administration, 1 additional dose using the same strength may be administered (maximum: 2 doses per breakthrough pain episode); **patient must wait 2 hours before treating another breakthrough pain episode with sublingual tablet.**

Maintenance dose: Once maintenance dose for breakthrough pain episode has been determined, use only 1 tablet in the appropriate strength per episode; if pain is unrelieved with maintenance dose:

U.S. labeling: A second dose may be given after 30 minutes; maximum of 2 doses/episode of breakthrough pain; separate treatment of subsequent episodes by ≥2 hours; limit treatment to ≤4 breakthrough episodes per day.

Canadian labeling: Administer alternative rescue medication after 30 minutes; maximum of 1 Abstral dose/episode of breakthrough pain; separate treatment of subsequent episodes by ≥2 hours; limit treatment to ≤4 breakthrough episodes per day.

Consider increasing the around-the-clock long-acting opioid therapy in patients experiencing >4 breakthrough pain episodes per day; if long-acting opioid therapy dose altered, re-evaluate and retitrate Abstral dose as needed.

Elderly >65 years: Transmucosal lozenge (eg, Actiq): In clinical trials, patients who were >65 years of age were titrated to a mean dose that was 200 mcg less than that of younger patients.

Chronic pain management: Children ≥2 years and Adults (opioid-tolerant patients): Transdermal patch (Duragesic):

Initial: To convert patients from oral or parenteral opioids to transdermal patch, a 24-hour analgesic requirement should be calculated (based on prior opioid use). Using the tables, the appropriate initial dose can be determined. The initial fentanyl dosage may be approximated from the 24-hour morphine dosage equivalent and titrated to minimize adverse effects and provide analgesia. With the initial application, the absorption of transdermal fentanyl requires several hours to reach plateau; therefore transdermal fentanyl is inappropriate for management of acute pain. Change patch every 72 hours.

Conversion from continuous infusion of fentanyl: In patients who have adequate pain relief with a fentanyl infusion, fentanyl may be converted to transdermal dosing at a rate equivalent to the intravenous rate. A two-step taper of the infusion to be completed over 12 hours has been recommended (Kornick, 2001) after the patch is applied. The infusion is decreased to 50% of the original rate six hours after the application of the first patch, and subsequently discontinued twelve hours after application.

Titration: Short-acting agents may be required until analgesic efficacy is established and/or as supplements for "breakthrough" pain. The amount of supplemental doses should be closely monitored. Appropriate dosage increases may be based on daily supplemental dosage using the ratio of 45 mg/24 hours of oral morphine to a 12.5 mcg/hour increase in fentanyl dosage.

Frequency of adjustment: The dosage should not be titrated more frequently than every 3 days after the initial dose or every 6 days thereafter. Patients should wear a consistent fentanyl dosage through two applications (6 days) before dosage increase based on supplemental opioid dosages can be estimated. **Note:** Upon discontinuation, ~17 hours are required for a 50% decrease in fentanyl levels.

Frequency of application: The majority of patients may be controlled on every 72-hour administration; however, a small number of patients require every 48-hour administration.

Dose conversion guidelines for transdermal fentanyl (see tables below and on next page).

Note: U.S. and Canadian dose conversion guidelines differ. Consult appropriate table.

U.S. Labeling: Dose Conversion Guidelines: Recommended Initial Duragesic® Dose Based Upon Daily Oral Morphine Dose[1,2]

Oral 24-Hour Morphine (mg/day)	Duragesic® Dose[3] (mcg/h)
60-134	25
135-224	50
225-314	75
315-404	100
405-494	125
495-584	150
585-674	175
675-764	200
765-854	225
855-944	250
945-1034	275
1035-1124	300

[1]The table should NOT be used to convert from transdermal fentanyl (Duragesic®) to other opioid analgesics. Rather, following removal of the patch, titrate the dose of the new opioid until adequate analgesia is achieved.

[2]Recommendations are based on U.S. product labeling for Duragesic®.

[3]Pediatric patients initiating therapy on a 25 mcg/hour Duragesic® system should be opioid-tolerant and receiving at least 60 mg oral morphine equivalents per day.

U.S. Labeling: Dose Conversion Guidelines[1,2]

Current Analgesic	Daily Dosage (mg/day)			
Morphine (I.M./I.V.)	10-22	23-37	38-52	53-67
Oxycodone (oral)	30-67	67.5-112	112.5-157	157.5-202
Codeine (oral)	150-447	-	-	-
Hydromorphone (oral)	8-17	17.1-28	28.1-39	39.1-51
Hydromorphone (I.V.)	1.5-3.4	3.5-5.6	5.7-7.9	8-10
Meperidine (I.M.)	75-165	166-278	279-390	391-503
Methadone (oral)	20-44	45-74	75-104	105-134
Fentanyl transdermal recommended dose (mcg/h)	**25 mcg/h**	**50 mcg/h**	**75 mcg/h**	**100 mcg/h**

[1]The table should NOT be used to convert from transdermal fentanyl (Duragesic®) to other opioid analgesics. Rather, following removal of the patch, titrate the dose of the new opioid until adequate analgesia is achieved.

[2]Recommendations are based on U.S. product labeling for Duragesic®.

Transdermal patch (Duragesic MAT [Canada; not available in U.S.]): Adults:

Canadian Labeling: Dose Conversion Guidelines (Adults): Recommended Initial Duragesic® MAT Dose Based Upon Daily Oral Morphine Dose[1,2]

Oral 24-Hour Morphine (Current Dose in mg/day)	Duragesic® MAT Dose (Initial Dose in mcg/h)
45-59	12
60-134	25
135-179	37
180-224	50
225-269	62
270-314	75
315-359	87
360-404	100
405-494	125
495-584	150
585-674	175
675-764	200
765-854	225
855-944	250
945-1034	275
1035-1124	300

[1]The table should NOT be used to convert from transdermal fentanyl (Duragesic® MAT) to other opioid analgesics. Rather, following removal of the patch, titrate the dose of the new opioid until adequate analgesia is achieved.

[2]Recommendations are based on Canadian product labeling for Duragesic® MAT.

Note: The 12 mcg/hour dose included in this table is to be used for incremental dose adjustment and is generally not recommended for initial dosing, except for patients in whom lower starting doses are deemed clinically appropriate.

Canadian Labeling: Dose Conversion Guidelines (Adults)[1,2]

Current Analgesic	Daily Dosage (mg/day)						
Morphine[3] (I.M./I.V.)	20-44	45-60	61-75	76-90	n/a[4]	n/a[4]	n/a[4]
Oxycodone (oral)	30-66	67-90	91-112	113-134	135-157	158-179	180-202
Codeine (oral)	150-447	448-597	598-747	748-897	898-1047	1048-1197	1198-1347
Hydromorphone (oral)	8-16	17-22	23-28	29-33	34-39	40-45	46-51
Hydromorphone (I.V.)	4-8.4	8.5-11.4	11.5-14.4	14.5-16.5	16.6-19.5	19.6-22.5	22.6-25.5
Fentanyl transdermal recommended dose (mcg/h)	**25 mcg/h**	**37 mcg/h**	**50 mcg/h**	**62 mcg/h**	**75 mcg/h**	**87 mcg/h**	**100 mcg/h**

[1]The table should NOT be used to convert from transdermal fentanyl (Duragesic® MAT) to other opioid analgesics. Rather, following removal of the patch, titrate the dose of the new opioid until adequate analgesia is achieved.

[2]Recommendations are based on Canadian product labeling for Duragesic® MAT.

[3]Morphine dose conversion based upon I.M to oral dose ratio of 1:3.

[4]Insufficient data available to provide specific dosing recommendations. Use caution; adjust dose conservatively.

Dosage adjustment in renal impairment:

Injection: No dosage adjustment provided in manufacturer's labeling; use with caution.

Transdermal (patch): Degree of impairment (ie, Cl_{cr}) not defined in manufacturer's labeling.

Mild-to-moderate impairment: Initial: Reduce dose by 50%.

Severe impairment: Use not recommended.

Transmucosal (buccal film/tablet, sublingual spray/tablet, lozenge) and nasal spray: Although fentanyl pharmacokinetics may be altered in renal disease, fentanyl can be used successfully in the management of breakthrough cancer pain. Doses should be titrated to reach clinical effect with careful monitoring of patients with severe renal disease.

Dosage adjustment in hepatic impairment:

Injection: No dosage adjustment provided in manufacturer's labeling; use with caution.

Transdermal (patch):

Mild-to-moderate impairment: Initial: Reduce dose by 50%.

Severe impairment: Use not recommended.

Transmucosal (buccal film/tablet, sublingual spray/tablet, lozenge) and nasal spray: Although fentanyl pharmacokinetics may be altered in hepatic disease, fentanyl can be used successfully in the management of breakthrough cancer pain. Doses should be titrated to reach clinical effect with careful monitoring of patients with severe hepatic disease.

Dietary Considerations Transmucosal lozenge contains 2 g sugar per unit.

Usual Infusion Concentrations: Pediatric I.V. infusion: 10 **mcg**/mL

Usual Infusion Concentrations: Adult I.V. infusion: 10 **mcg**/mL

Administration

I.V.: Administer as slow I.V. infusion over 1-2 minutes. May also be administered as continuous infusion or PCA (unlabeled use) routes. Muscular rigidity may occur with rapid I.V. administration.

Transdermal patch (eg, Duragesic): Apply to nonirritated and nonirradiated skin, such as chest, back, flank, or upper arm. Do not shave skin; hair at application site should be clipped. Prior to application, clean site with clear water and allow to dry completely. Do not use damaged, cut or leaking patches; patch may be less effective. Skin exposure from fentanyl gel leaking from patch may lead to serious adverse effects; thoroughly wash affected skin surfaces with water (do not use soap). Firmly press in place and hold for 30 seconds. Change patch every 72 hours. Do **not** use soap, alcohol, or other solvents to remove transdermal gel if it accidentally touches skin; use copious amounts of water. Avoid exposing application site to external heat sources (eg, heating pad, electric blanket, heat lamp, hot tub). If there is difficulty with patch adhesion, the edges of the system may be taped in place with first-aid tape. If there is continued difficulty with adhesion, an adhesive film dressing (eg, Bioclusive, Tegaderm) may be applied over the system.

Lozenge: Foil overwrap should be removed just prior to administration. Place the unit in mouth between the cheek and gum and allow it to dissolve. Do not chew. Lozenge may be moved from one side of the mouth to the other. The unit should be consumed over a period of 15 minutes. Handle should be removed after the lozenge is consumed; early removal should be considered if the patient has achieved an adequate response and/or shows signs of respiratory depression.

Buccal film: Foil overwrap should be removed just prior to administration. Prior to placing film, wet inside of cheek using tongue or by rinsing with water. Place film inside mouth with the pink side of the unit against the inside of the moistened cheek. With finger, press the film against cheek and hold for 5 seconds. The film should stick to the inside of cheek after 5 seconds. The film should be left in place until it dissolves (usually within 15-30 minutes after application). Liquids may be consumed after 5 minutes of application. Food can be eaten after film dissolves. If using more than 1 film simultaneously (during titration period), apply films on either side of mouth (do not apply on top of each other). Do not chew or swallow film. Do not cut or tear the film. All patients must initiate therapy using the 200 mcg film.

Buccal tablet: Patient should not open blister until ready to administer. The blister backing should be peeled back to expose the tablet; tablet should not be pushed out through the blister. Immediately use tablet once removed from blister. Place entire tablet in the buccal cavity (above a rear molar, between the upper cheek and gum) or under the tongue (maintenance dosing only); should dissolve in about 14-25 minutes. If remnants remain after 30 minutes, they may be swallowed with water. Tablet should not be split, crushed, sucked, chewed, or swallowed whole. When possible, alternate sides of mouth with each dose.

Nasal spray: Prior to initial use, prime device by spraying 4 sprays into the provided pouch (the counting window will show a green bar when the bottle is ready for use). Insert nozzle a short distance into the nose (~1/2 inch or 1 cm) and point towards the bridge of the nose (while closing off the other nostril using 1 finger). Press on finger grips until a "click" sound is heard and the number in the counting window advances by one. The "click" sound and dose counter are the only reliable methods for ensuring a dose has been administered (spray is not always felt on the nasal mucosa). Patient should remain seated for at least 1 minute following administration. Do not blow nose for ≥30 minutes after administration. Wash hands before and after use. There are 8 full therapeutic sprays in each bottle; do not continue to use bottle after "8" sprays have been used. Dispose of bottle and contents if ≥5 days have passed since last use or if it has been ≥4 days since bottle was primed. Spray the remaining contents into the provided pouch, seal in the child-resistant container, and dispose of in the trash.

Sublingual spray: Open sealed blister unit with scissors immediately prior to administration. Contents of unit should be sprayed into mouth under the tongue.

Sublingual tablet: Remove from the blister unit immediately prior to administration. Place tablet directly under the tongue on the floor of the mouth and allow to completely dissolve; do not chew, suck, or swallow. Do not eat or drink anything until tablet is completely dissolved. In patients with a dry mouth, water may be used to moisten the buccal mucosa just before administration. All patients must initiate therapy using the 100 mcg tablet.

Monitoring Parameters Respiratory and cardiovascular status, blood pressure, heart rate; signs of misuse, abuse, or addiction

Transdermal patch: Monitor for 24 hours after application of first dose

Additional Information Fentanyl is 50-100 times as potent as morphine; morphine 10 mg I.M. is equivalent to fentanyl 0.1-0.2 mg I.M.; fentanyl has less hypotensive effects than morphine due to lack of histamine release. However, fentanyl may cause rigidity with high doses. If the patient has required high-dose analgesia or has used for a prolonged period (~7 days), taper dose to prevent withdrawal; monitor for signs and symptoms of withdrawal.

Transmucosal (nasal spray, Lazanda): Disposal of nasal spray: Before disposal, all unopened or partially used bottles must be completely emptied by spraying the contents into the provided pouch. After "8" therapeutic sprays has been reached on the counter, patients should continue to spray an additional four sprays into the pouch to ensure that any residual fentanyl has been expelled (an audible click will no longer be heard and the counter will not advance beyond "8"). The empty bottle and the sealed pouch must be put into the child-resistant container before placing in the trash. Wash hands with soap and water immediately after handling the pouch. If the pouch is lost, another one can be ordered by the patient or caregiver by calling 1-866-435-6775.

Transmucosal (oral lozenge, Actiq): Disposal of lozenge units: After consumption of a complete unit, the handle may be disposed of in a trash container that is out of the reach of children. For a partially-consumed unit, or a unit that still has any drug matrix remaining on the handle, the handle should be placed under hot running tap water until the drug matrix has dissolved. Special child-resistant containers are available to temporarily store partially consumed units that cannot be disposed of immediately.

Transmucosal (buccal film, Onsolis): Disposal of film: Remove foil overwrap from any unused, unneeded films and dispose by flushing in the toilet.

Transmucosal (sublingual spray, Subsys): Disposal of spray: Dispose of each unit dose immediately after use; place used unit into one of the provided small disposal bags. After sealing appropriately, discard in the trash. Also dispose of any unused unit as soon as no longer needed. Prior to disposal, empty all the medicine into the provided disposal bottle. The disposal bottle should then be placed into the large disposal bag (provided), seal appropriately, and discard in the trash.

Transmucosal (sublingual tablet, Abstral): Disposal of tablets: Remove any unused tablets from the blister cards and dispose by flushing in the toilet.

Transdermal patch (Duragesic): Upon removal of the patch, ~17 hours are required before serum concentrations fall to 50% of their original values. Opioid withdrawal symptoms are possible. Gradual downward titration (potentially by the sequential use of lower-dose patches) is recommended. Keep transdermal patch (both used and unused) out of the reach of children. Do **not** use soap, alcohol, or other solvents to remove transdermal gel if it accidentally touches skin as they may increase transdermal absorption, use copious amounts of water. Avoid exposure of direct external heat sources (eg, heating pads, electric blankets, heat lamps, saunas, hot tubs, heated water beds) to application site.

Dosage Forms Excipient information presented when available (limited, particularly for generics); consult specific product labeling.

Film, for buccal application, as citrate [strength expressed as base]:
  Onsolis: 200 mcg (30s); 400 mcg (30s); 600 mcg (30s); 800 mcg (30s); 1200 mcg (30s)

Injection, solution, as citrate [strength expressed as base, preservative free]: 0.05 mg/mL (2 mL, 5 mL, 10 mL, 20 mL, 50 mL)

Liquid, sublingual, as base [spray]:
  Subsys: 100 mcg (30s); 200 mcg (30s); 400 mcg (30s); 600 mcg (30s); 800 mcg (30s) [contains dehydrated ethanol 63.6%, propylene glycol]

Lozenge, oral, as citrate [strength expressed as base, transmucosal]: 200 mcg (30s); 400 mcg (30s); 600 mcg (30s); 800 mcg (30s); 1200 mcg (30s); 1600 mcg (30s)
  Actiq: 200 mcg (30s); 400 mcg (30s); 600 mcg (30s); 800 mcg (30s); 1200 mcg (30s); 1600 mcg (30s) [contains sugar 2 g/lozenge; berry flavor]

Patch, transdermal, as base: 12 [delivers 12.5 mcg/hr] (5s); 25 [delivers 25 mcg/hr] (5s); 50 [delivers 50 mcg/hr] (5s); 75 [delivers 75 mcg/hr] (5s); 100 [delivers 100 mcg/hr] (5s)
  Duragesic: 12 [delivers 12.5 mcg/hr] (5s) [contains ethanol 0.1 mL/10 cm^2; 5 cm^2]
  Duragesic: 25 [delivers 25 mcg/hr] (5s) [contains ethanol 0.1 mL/10 cm^2; 10 cm^2]
  Duragesic: 50 [delivers 50 mcg/hr] (5s) [contains ethanol 0.1 mL/10 cm^2; 20 cm^2]

Duragesic: 75 [delivers 75 mcg/hr] (5s) [contains ethanol 0.1 mL/10 cm^2; 30 cm^2]
Duragesic: 100 [delivers 100 mcg/hr] (5s) [contains ethanol 0.1 mL/10 cm^2; 40 cm^2]
Powder, for prescription compounding, as citrate: USP: 100% (1 g)
Solution, intranasal, as citrate [strength expressed as base, spray]:
Lazanda: 100 mcg/spray (5 mL); 400 mcg/spray (5 mL) [delivers 8 metered sprays]
Tablet, for buccal application, as citrate [strength expressed as base]:
Fentora: 100 mcg (28s); 200 mcg (28s); 400 mcg (28s); 600 mcg (28s); 800 mcg (28s)
Tablet, sublingual, as citrate [strength expressed as base]:
Abstral: 100 mcg (12s, 32s); 200 mcg (12s, 32s); 300 mcg (12s, 32s); 400 mcg (12s, 32s); 600 mcg (32s); 800 mcg (32s)

Dosage Forms: Canada Excipient information presented when available (limited, particularly for generics); consult specific product labeling.
Patch, transdermal, as base: 12 mcg/hr (5s); 25 mcg/hr (5s); 50 mcg/hr (5s); 75 mcg/hr (5s); 100 mcg/hr (5s)
Duragesic MAT: 12 mcg/hr (5s) [contains ethanol 0.1 mL/10 cm^2; 5 cm^2]
Duragesic MAT: 25 mcg/hr (5s) [contains ethanol 0.1 mL/10 cm^2; 10 cm^2]
Duragesic MAT: 50 mcg/hr (5s) [contains ethanol 0.1 mL/10 cm^2; 20 cm^2]
Duragesic MAT: 75 mcg/hr (5s) [contains ethanol 0.1 mL/10 cm^2; 30 cm^2]
Duragesic MAT: 100 mcg/hr (5s) [contains ethanol 0.1 mL/10 cm^2; 40 cm^2]

Controlled Substance C-II

- **Fentanyl Citrate** *see* FentaNYL *on page 842*
- **Fentanyl Citrate Injection, USP (Can)** *see* FentaNYL *on page 842*
- **Fentanyl Hydrochloride** *see* FentaNYL *on page 842*
- **Fentanyl Patch** *see* FentaNYL *on page 842*
- **Fentora** *see* FentaNYL *on page 842*
- **Feraheme** *see* Ferumoxytol *on page 855*
- **Feraheme® (Can)** *see* Ferumoxytol *on page 855*
- **Ferate [OTC]** *see* Ferrous Gluconate *on page 854*
- **Fergon [OTC]** *see* Ferrous Gluconate *on page 854*
- **Ferinject** *see* Ferric Carboxymaltose *on page 852*
- **Fer-In-Sol [OTC]** *see* Ferrous Sulfate *on page 854*
- **Fer-In-Sol® (Can)** *see* Ferrous Sulfate *on page 854*
- **Fer-Iron [OTC]** *see* Ferrous Sulfate *on page 854*
- **Ferodan™ (Can)** *see* Ferrous Sulfate *on page 854*
- **FeroSul [OTC]** *see* Ferrous Sulfate *on page 854*
- **Ferretts [OTC]** *see* Ferrous Fumarate *on page 854*
- **Ferrex 150 [OTC]** *see* Polysaccharide-Iron Complex *on page 1673*
- **Ferrex 150 Plus [OTC]** *see* Polysaccharide-Iron Complex *on page 1673*
- **Ferric (III) Hexacyanoferrate (II)** *see* Ferric Hexacyanoferrate *on page 853*

Ferric Carboxymaltose

(FER ik kar box ee MAWL tose)

Brand Names: U.S. Injectafer

Index Terms Ferinject; Iron Carboxymaltose; Iron Dextri-Maltose; VIT 45

Pharmacologic Category Iron Salt

Use Iron-deficiency anemia (IDA): Treatment of IDA in adults with intolerance to oral iron or unsatisfactory response to oral iron; treatment of IDA in adults with nondialysis-dependent chronic kidney disease (ND-CKD)

Pregnancy Risk Factor C

Pregnancy Considerations Adverse events were observed in some animal reproduction studies.

Breast-Feeding Considerations Ferric carboxymaltose is excreted into breast milk. Iron concentrations are higher than those following oral ferrous sulfate administration.

Contraindications Hypersensitivity to ferric carboxymaltose or any component of the formulation

Warnings/Precautions Serious hypersensitivity reactions, including anaphylactic-type reactions (some life-threatening and fatal) have been reported. Monitor during and for ≥30 minutes after administration and until clinically stable. Signs/symptoms of serious hypersensitivity reaction include shock, hypotension, loss of consciousness, and/or collapse. Equipment for resuscitation, medication, and trained personnel experienced in handling emergencies should be immediately available during infusion. Transient elevations in systolic blood pressure, (sometimes with facial flushing, dizziness, or nausea) were observed in studies; generally occurred immediately after dosing and resolved within 30 minutes. Monitor blood pressure following infusion. Lab assays may overestimate serum iron and transferrin bound irons for ~24 hours after infusion.

Adverse Reactions
>10%: Endocrine & metabolic: Decreased serum phosphate (27%; <2 mg/dL [0.65 mmol/L]; transient)
1% to 10%:
Cardiovascular: Increased blood pressure (6%; transient, systolic), flushing (4%), hypertension (4%), hypotension
Central nervous system: Dizziness (2%), headache (1%)
Dermatologic: Skin discoloration at injection site (1%)
Endocrine & metabolic: Hypophosphatemia (2%)
Gastrointestinal: Nausea (7%), vomiting (2%), constipation (1%), dysgeusia (1%)
Hepatic Increased serum ALT (1%)
<1% (Limited to important or life-threatening): Anaphylaxis, angioedema, hypersensitivity, syncope, tachycardia

Drug Interactions

Metabolism/Transport Effects None known.

Avoid Concomitant Use
Avoid concomitant use of Ferric Carboxymaltose with any of the following: Dimercaprol

Increased Effect/Toxicity
The levels/effects of Ferric Carboxymaltose may be increased by: Dimercaprol

Decreased Effect
Ferric Carboxymaltose may decrease the levels/effects of: Bisphosphonate Derivatives; Cefdinir; Deferiprone; Dolutegravir; Eltrombopag; Levodopa; Levothyroxine; Methyldopa; PenicillAMINE; Phosphate Supplements; Quinolone Antibiotics; Tetracycline Derivatives; Trientine

The levels/effects of Ferric Carboxymaltose may be decreased by: Antacids; H2-Antagonists; Pancrelipase; Proton Pump Inhibitors; Trientine

Preparation for Administration May administer undiluted (for I.V. push) or diluted (for infusion). When administering as an I.V. infusion, dilute up to 750 mg in a maximum of 250 mL of 0.9% sodium chloride injection to a concentration of 2-4 mg/mL; concentration should be ≥2 mg/mL. Discard unused portion of vial (single-use).

Storage/Stability Store intact vials at 20°C to 25°C (68°F to 77°F); excursions permitted between 15°C to 30°C (59°F to 86°F); do not freeze. Solutions diluted in 0.9% sodium chloride at concentrations of 2-4 mg/mL are stable for 72 hours at room temperature.

Mechanism of Action Ferric carboxymaltose is a colloidal iron (III) hydroxide in complex with carboxymaltose, a carbohydrate polymer that releases iron necessary to the function of hemoglobin, myoglobin, and specific enzyme systems; allows transport of oxygen via hemoglobin. Ferric carboxymaltose is a non-dextran formulation that allows for iron uptake (into reticuloendothelial system) without the release of free iron (Szczech, 2010).

Pharmacodynamics/Kinetics

Onset of action: Maximum iron levels (37-333 mcg/mL): 0.25-1.2 hours

Distribution: V_d: ~3 L

Half-life elimination: 7-12 hours

Excretion: Urine (negligible)

Dosage Note: Dose expressed as elemental iron.

Iron-deficiency anemia (IDA): Adults: I.V.:

<50 kg: 15 mg/kg on day 1; repeat dose after at least 7 days (maximum: 1500 mg per course). May repeat course if anemia reoccurs.

≥50 kg: 750 mg on day 1; repeat dose after at least 7 days (maximum: 1500 mg per course). May repeat course if anemia reoccurs.

Dosage adjustment in renal impairment: Chronic kidney disease (CKD), nondialysis dependent: No dosage adjustment necessary (indicated for use in nondialysis CKD)

Dosage adjustment in hepatic impairment: No dosage adjustment provided in manufacturer's labeling.

Administration

Administer as slow I.V. push (undiluted) at a rate of ~100 mg/minute or by I.V. infusion (diluted to ≥2 mg/mL) over at least 15 minutes.

Avoid extravasation (may cause persistent discoloration). Monitor; if extravasation occurs, discontinue administration at that site.

Monitoring Parameters Hemoglobin and hematocrit, serum ferritin, iron saturation; vital signs (including blood pressure); signs and symptoms of hypersensitivity (monitor for ≥30 minutes following the end of administration and until clinically stable); monitor infusion site for extravasation.

NKF KDOQI guidelines (2006) recommend monitoring iron status every 1-3 months, with more frequent monitoring after course of IV iron therapy.

Reference Range CKD patients should have sufficient iron to achieve and maintain hemoglobin of 11-12 g/dL; to achieve and maintain this target Hgb for patients with nondialysis dependent CKD, sufficient iron should be administered to maintain a transferrin saturation (TSAT) of 20%, and a serum ferritin level ≥100 ng/mL (NKF KDOQI, 2006)

Test Interactions Serum or transferrin bound iron levels may be falsely elevated if assessed within 24 hours of ferric carboxymaltose administration.

Dosage Forms Considerations

Each mL of Injectafer contains 50 mg of elemental iron

Dosage Forms Excipient information presented when available (limited, particularly for generics); consult specific product labeling.

Solution, Intravenous:

Injectafer: 750 mg/15 mL (15 mL)

Ferric Gluconate (FER ik GLOO koe nate)

Brand Names: U.S. Ferrlecit

Brand Names: Canada Ferrlecit

Index Terms Sodium Ferric Gluconate; Sodium Ferric Gluconate Complex

Pharmacologic Category Iron Salt

Use Iron deficiency anemia: Treatment of iron-deficiency anemia in patients undergoing hemodialysis in conjunction with erythropoietin therapy

Unlabeled Use Chemotherapy-associated anemia

Pregnancy Risk Factor B

Dosage

Iron-deficiency anemia, hemodialysis patients:

Children ≥6 years: I.V.: 1.5 mg/kg of elemental iron (maximum: 125 mg/dose) per dialysis session. Doses >1.5 mg/kg are associated with increased adverse events.

Adults: I.V.: 125 mg elemental iron per dialysis session. Most patients will require a cumulative dose of 1 g elemental iron over approximately 8 sequential dialysis treatments to achieve a favorable response.

Note: A test dose of 2 mL diluted in NS 50 mL administered over 60 minutes was previously recommended (not in current manufacturer labeling). Doses >125 mg are associated with increased adverse events.

Chemotherapy-associated anemia (unlabeled use): Adults: I.V. infusion: 125 mg once every week for 6 doses (Pedrazzoli, 2008) or for 8 doses (Henry, 2007).

Dosage adjustment in renal impairment: No dosage adjustment necessary. The ferric gluconate iron complex is not dialyzable.

Dosage adjustment in hepatic impairment: No dosage adjustment necessary.

Additional Information Complete prescribing information should be consulted for additional detail.

Dosage Forms Considerations

Strength of ferric gluconate injection is expressed as elemental iron.

Dosage Forms Excipient information presented when available (limited, particularly for generics); consult specific product labeling.

Solution, Intravenous:

Ferrlecit: 12.5 mg/mL (5 mL) [contains benzyl alcohol, sucrose]

Generic: 12.5 mg/mL (5 mL)

Ferric Hexacyanoferrate

(FER ik hex a SYE an oh fer ate)

Brand Names: U.S. Radiogardase®

Index Terms Ferric (III) Hexacyanoferrate (II); Insoluble Prussian Blue; Prussian Blue

Pharmacologic Category Antidote

Use Treatment of known or suspected internal contamination with radioactive cesium and/or radioactive or nonradioactive thallium

Pregnancy Risk Factor C

Dosage Oral: Internal contamination with radioactive cesium and/or radioactive or nonradioactive thallium:

Children 2-12 years: 1 g 3 times/day; treatment should begin as soon as possible following exposure, but is also effective if therapy is delayed

Children >12 years and Adults: 3 g 3 times/day; treatment should begin as soon as possible following exposure, but is also effective if therapy is delayed

Note: Cesium exposure: Once internal radioactivity is substantially decreased, dosage may be reduced to 1-2 g 3 times/day to improve gastrointestinal tolerance

Elderly: Refer to adult dosing

Dosage adjustment in renal impairment: Studies have not been conducted; however, ferric hexacyanoferrate is not renally eliminated.

Dosage adjustment in hepatic impairment: Studies have not been conducted; however, effectiveness may be decreased due to decreased bile excretion of cesium and thallium.

Additional Information Complete prescribing information should be consulted for additional detail.

Dosage Forms Excipient information presented when available (limited, particularly for generics); consult specific product labeling.

Capsule, oral:

Radiogardase®: 0.5 g

◆ **Ferrimin 150 [OTC]** *see* Ferrous Fumarate *on page* 854

◆ **Ferriprox®** *see* Deferiprone *on page* 561

◆ **Ferriprox** *see* Deferiprone *on page* 561

◆ **Ferrlecit** *see* Ferric Gluconate *on page* 853

◆ **Ferro-Bob [OTC]** *see* Ferrous Sulfate *on page* 854

◆ **Ferrocite [OTC]** *see* Ferrous Fumarate *on page* 854

Ferrous Fumarate (FER us FYOO ma rate)

Brand Names: U.S. Ferretts [OTC]; Ferrimin 150 [OTC]; Ferrocite [OTC]; Hemocyte [OTC]

Brand Names: Canada Palafer®

Index Terms Iron Fumarate

Pharmacologic Category Iron Salt

Use Prevention and treatment of iron-deficiency anemias

Dosage

Dietary Reference Intake: Dose is RDA presented as elemental iron unless otherwise noted:

0-6 months: 0.27 mg/day (adequate intake)
7-12 months: 11 mg/day
1-3 years: 7 mg/day
4-8 years: 10 mg/day
9-13 years: 8 mg/day
14-18 years: Males: 11 mg/day; Females: 15 mg/day; Pregnant females: 27 mg/day; Lactating females: 10 mg/day
19-50 years: Males: 8 mg/day; Females: 18 mg/day; Pregnant females: 27 mg/day; Lactating females: 9 mg/day
≥50 years: 8 mg/day

Doses expressed in terms of elemental iron; elemental iron content of ferrous fumarate is 33%. Oral:

Children:

Severe iron-deficiency anemia: 4-6 mg elemental iron/kg/day in 3 divided doses

Mild-to-moderate iron-deficiency anemia: 3 mg elemental iron/kg/day in 1-2 divided doses

Prophylaxis: 1-2 mg elemental iron/kg/day

Adults:

Iron deficiency: Usual range: 150-200 mg elemental iron/day in divided doses; 60-100 mg elemental iron twice daily, up to 60 mg elemental iron 4 times/day

Prophylaxis: 60-100 mg elemental iron/day

To avoid GI upset, start with a single daily dose and increase by 1 tablet/day each week or as tolerated until desired daily dose is achieved

Elderly: Lower doses (15-50 mg elemental iron/day) may have similar efficacy and less GI adverse events (eg, nausea,constipation) as compared to higher doses (eg, 150 mg elemental iron/day) (Rimon, 2005).

Additional Information Complete prescribing information should be consulted for additional detail.

Dosage Forms Excipient information presented when available (limited, particularly for generics); consult specific product labeling.

Tablet, Oral:

Ferretts: 325 mg [scored]
Ferrimin 150: 150 mg
Ferrocite: 324 mg [contains fd&c blue #1 aluminum lake, fd&c yellow #5 aluminum lake]
Hemocyte: 324 mg
Generic: 29 mg, 90 mg, 324 mg

Ferrous Gluconate (FER us GLOO koe nate)

Brand Names: U.S. Ferate [OTC]; Fergon [OTC]

Brand Names: Canada Apo-Ferrous Gluconate®; Novo-Ferrogluc

Index Terms Iron Gluconate

Pharmacologic Category Iron Salt

Use Prevention and treatment of iron-deficiency anemias

Dosage Oral:

Dietary Reference Intake: Dose is RDA presented as elemental iron unless otherwise noted:

0-6 months: 0.27 mg/day (adequate intake)
7-12 months: 11 mg/day
1-3 years: 7 mg/day
4-8 years: 10 mg/day
9-13 years: 8 mg/day
14-18 years: Males: 11 mg/day; Females: 15 mg/day; Pregnant females: 27 mg/day; Lactating females: 10 mg/day
19-50 years: Males: 8 mg/day; Females: 18 mg/day; Pregnant females: 27 mg/day; Lactating females: 9 mg/day
≥50 years: 8 mg/day

Dose expressed in terms of elemental iron:

Children:

Severe iron-deficiency anemia: 4-6 mg Fe/kg/day in 3 divided doses

Mild to moderate iron deficiency anemia: 3 mg Fe/kg/day in 1-2 divided doses

Prophylaxis: 1-2 mg Fe/kg/day

Adults:

Iron deficiency: 60 mg twice daily up to 60 mg 4 times/day

Prophylaxis: 60 mg/day

Elderly: Lower doses (15-50 mg elemental iron/day) may have similar efficacy and less GI adverse events (eg, nausea, constipation) as compared to higher doses (eg, 150 mg elemental iron/day) (Rimon, 2005).

Additional Information Complete prescribing information should be consulted for additional detail.

Dosage Forms Excipient information presented when available (limited, particularly for generics); consult specific product labeling.

Tablet, Oral:

Fergon: 240 (27 Fe) MG [contains tartrazine (fd&c yellow #5)]
Generic: 240 (27 Fe) MG, 324 (37.5 Fe) MG, 324 (38 Fe) MG, 325 (36 Fe) MG

Tablet, Oral [preservative free]:

Ferate: 256 (28 Fe) MG [gluten free, lactose free, milk free, no artificial color(s), no artificial flavor(s), sodium free, soy free, sugar free, wheat free, yeast free]

Ferrous Sulfate (FER us SUL fate)

Brand Names: U.S. BProtected Pedia Iron [OTC]; Fer-In-Sol [OTC]; Fer-Iron [OTC]; FeroSul [OTC]; Ferro-Bob [OTC]; FerrouSul [OTC]; Iron Supplement Childrens [OTC]; Slow Fe [OTC]; Slow Iron [OTC]; Slow Release Iron [OTC] [DSC]

Brand Names: Canada Apo-Ferrous Sulfate®; Fer-In-Sol®; Ferodan™

Index Terms $FeSO_4$; Iron Sulfate

Pharmacologic Category Iron Salt

Use Prevention and treatment of iron-deficiency anemias

Dosage Oral: **Note:** Multiple concentrations of ferrous sulfate oral liquid exist; close attention must be paid to the concentration when ordering and administering ferrous sulfate; incorrect selection or substitution of one ferrous sulfate liquid for another without proper dosage volume adjustment may result in serious over- or underdosing.

Dietary Reference Intake: Dose is RDA presented as elemental iron unless otherwise noted:
0-6 months: 0.27 mg/day (adequate intake)
7-12 months: 11 mg/day
1-3 years: 7 mg/day
4-8 years: 10 mg/day
9-13 years: 8 mg/day
14-18 years: Males: 11 mg/day; Females: 15 mg/day; Pregnant females: 27 mg/day; Lactating females: 10 mg/day
19-50 years: Males: 8 mg/day; Females: 18 mg/day; Pregnant females: 27 mg/day; Lactating females: 9 mg/day
≥50 years: 8 mg/day

Children **(dose expressed in terms of elemental iron)**:
Severe iron-deficiency anemia: 4-6 mg Fe/kg/day in 3 divided doses
Mild-to-moderate iron deficiency anemia: 3 mg Fe/kg/day in 1-2 divided doses
Prophylaxis: 1-2 mg Fe/kg/day up to a maximum of 15 mg/day
Adults **(dose expressed in terms of ferrous sulfate)**:
Iron deficiency: 300 mg twice daily up to 300 mg 4 times/day or 250 mg (extended release) 1-2 times/day
Prophylaxis: 300 mg/day
Elderly: Lower doses (15-50 mg elemental iron/day) may have similar efficacy and less GI adverse events (eg, nausea, constipation) as compared to higher doses (eg, 150 mg elemental iron/day) (Rimon, 2005).

Additional Information Complete prescribing information should be consulted for additional detail.

Dosage Forms Excipient information presented when available (limited, particularly for generics); consult specific product labeling. [DSC] = Discontinued product
Elixir, Oral:
FeroSul: 220 (44 Fe) MG/5ML (473 mL) [contains alcohol, usp, fd&c yellow #6 (sunset yellow), propylene glycol, saccharin sodium, sodium benzoate; lemon flavor]
Generic: 220 (44 Fe) MG/5ML (5 mL, 473 mL)
Liquid, Oral:
Generic: 220 (44 Fe) MG/5ML (473 mL)
Solution, Oral:
BProtected Pedia Iron: 75 (15 Fe) mg/mL (50 mL) [alcohol free, gluten free; contains sodium metabisulfite; citrus flavor]
Fer-In-Sol: 75 (15 Fe) mg/mL (50 mL) [contains alcohol, usp, sodium bisulfite]
Fer-Iron: 75 (15 Fe) mg/mL (50 mL) [contains sodium metabisulfite; lemon flavor]
Iron Supplement Childrens: 75 (15 Fe) mg/mL (50 mL) [alcohol free, dye free, gluten free, lactose free; contains sodium bisulfite]
Generic: 75 (15 Fe) mg/mL (50 mL)
Syrup, Oral:
Generic: 300 (60 Fe) MG/5ML (5 mL)
Tablet, Oral:
Ferro-Bob: 325 (65 Fe) MG
Generic: 325 (65 Fe) MG
Tablet, Oral [preservative free]:
FerrouSul: 325 (65 Fe) MG [sodium free, starch free]
Generic: 325 (65 Fe) MG
Tablet Delayed Release, Oral:
Generic: 324 (65 Fe) MG, 325 (65 Fe) MG
Tablet Extended Release, Oral:
Slow Fe: 160 (50 Fe) MG
Slow Fe: 142 (45 Fe) MG [contains fd&c blue #1 aluminum lake, fd&c red #40 aluminum lake, fd&c yellow #6 aluminum lake]
Slow Release Iron: 140 (45 Fe) MG [DSC] [contains brilliant blue fcf (fd&c blue #1), fd&c red #40 aluminum lake, fd&c yellow #6 aluminum lake]
Tablet Extended Release, Oral [preservative free]:
Slow Iron: 160 (50 Fe) MG [gluten free]
Generic: 140 (45 Fe) MG

◆ **FerrouSul [OTC]** *see* Ferrous Sulfate *on page 854*
◆ **Fertinorm® H.P. (Can)** *see* Urofollitropin *on page 2141*

Ferumoxytol (fer ue MOX i tol)

Brand Names: U.S. Feraheme
Brand Names: Canada Feraheme®
Pharmacologic Category Iron Salt
Use Treatment of iron-deficiency anemia in chronic kidney disease
Pregnancy Risk Factor C
Dosage Doses expressed in mg of **elemental** iron. **Note:** Test dose: Product labeling does not indicate need for a test dose.
I.V.: Adults: Iron-deficiency anemia in chronic kidney disease: 510 mg (17 mL) as a single dose, followed by a second 510 mg dose 3-8 days (U.S. labeling) or 2-8 days (Canadian labeling) after initial dose. Assess response at least 30 days following the second dose. U.S. manufacturer labeling states the recommended dose may be readministered in patients with persistent or recurrent iron-deficiency anemia.

Dosage adjustment in renal impairment: No dosage adjustment necessary.
Dosage adjustment in hepatic impairment: No dosage adjustment provided in manufacturer's labeling.

Additional Information Complete prescribing information should be consulted for additional detail.
Dosage Forms Considerations
Strength of ferumoxytol is expressed as elemental iron
Dosage Forms Excipient information presented when available (limited, particularly for generics); consult specific product labeling.
Solution, Intravenous [preservative free]:
Feraheme: 510 mg/17 mL (17 mL)

◆ **FerUS [OTC]** *see* Polysaccharide-Iron Complex *on page 1673*
◆ **FESO** *see* Fesoterodine *on page 855*
◆ **FeSO$_4$** *see* Ferrous Sulfate *on page 854*

Fesoterodine (fes oh TER oh deen)

Brand Names: U.S. Toviaz
Index Terms FESO; Fesoterodine Fumarate
Pharmacologic Category Anticholinergic Agent
Additional Appendix Information
Beers Criteria − Potentially Inappropriate Medications for Geriatrics *on page 2368*
Use Treatment of patients with an overactive bladder with symptoms of urinary frequency, urgency, or urge incontinence.

Pregnancy Risk Factor C
Pregnancy Considerations Teratogenic effects were observed in some animal reproduction studies.
Breast-Feeding Considerations It is not known if fesoterodine is excreted in breast milk. Breast-feeding is not recommended by the manufacturer.
Contraindications Hypersensitivity to fesoterodine or tolterodine (both are metabolized to 5-hydroxymethyl tolterodine) or any component of the formulation; urinary retention; gastric retention; uncontrolled narrow-angle glaucoma
Warnings/Precautions Cases of angioedema involving the face, lips, tongue, and/or larynx have been reported. Immediately discontinue if tongue, hypopharynx, or larynx are involved. May cause drowsiness and/or blurred vision,

which may impair physical or mental abilities; patients must be cautioned about performing tasks which require mental alertness (eg, operating machinery or driving). Consider dose reduction or discontinuation if CNS effects occur. Patients may experience decreased sweating; caution use in hot weather or during exercise. Use is not recommended in patients with severe hepatic impairment (Child-Pugh class C). Doses >4 mg are not recommended for patients with severe renal impairment (Cl_{cr} <30 mL/minute) or patients receiving concurrent therapy with strong CYP3A4 inhibitors (no dosing adjustments are recommended in patients receiving moderate CYP3A4 inhibitors). Use caution in patients with bladder flow obstruction, gastrointestinal obstructive disorders, myasthenia gravis, and treated narrow-angle glaucoma. This medication is associated with potent anticholinergic properties which may be inappropriate in older adults depending on comorbidities (eg, dementia, delirium) (Beers Criteria). In addition, risk of adverse effects may be increased in elderly patients.

Adverse Reactions

>10%: Gastrointestinal: Xerostomia (19% to 35%; dose related)

1% to 10%:

Central nervous system: Insomnia (1%)

Dermatological: Rash (1%)

Gastrointestinal: Constipation (4% to 6%), dyspepsia (2%), nausea (1% to 2%), abdominal pain (1%)

Genitourinary: Urinary tract infection (3% to 4%), dysuria (1% to 2%), urinary retention (1%)

Hepatic: ALT increased (1%), GGT increased (1%)

Neuromuscular & skeletal: Back pain (1% to 2%)

Ocular: Dry eyes (1% to 4%)

Respiratory: Upper respiratory tract infection (2% to 3%), cough (1% to 2%), dry throat (1% to 2%)

Miscellaneous: Peripheral edema (1%)

<1% (Limited to important or life-threatening): Angina, angioedema, diverticulitis, gastroenteritis, heat prostration, hypersensitivity reactions, irritable bowel syndrome, QT_c prolongation

Drug Interactions

Metabolism/Transport Effects **Substrate** of CYP2D6 (minor), CYP3A4 (major); **Note:** Assignment of Major/Minor substrate status based on clinically relevant drug interaction potential

Avoid Concomitant Use

Avoid concomitant use of Fesoterodine with any of the following: Aclidinium; Fusidic Acid (Systemic); Ipratropium (Oral Inhalation); Potassium Chloride; Tiotropium; Umeclidinium

Increased Effect/Toxicity

Fesoterodine may increase the levels/effects of: AbobotulinumtoxinA; Analgesics (Opioid); Anticholinergics; Cannabinoids; Mirabegron; OnabotulinumtoxinA; Potassium Chloride; RimabotulinumtoxinB; Thiazide Diuretics; Tiotropium; Topiramate

The levels/effects of Fesoterodine may be increased by: Aclidinium; CYP2D6 Inhibitors; CYP3A4 Inhibitors (Moderate); CYP3A4 Inhibitors (Strong); Dasatinib; Fusidic Acid (Systemic); Ipratropium (Oral Inhalation); Ivacaftor; Luliconazole; Mifepristone; Pramlintide; Simeprevir; Umeclidinium

Decreased Effect

Fesoterodine may decrease the levels/effects of: Acetylcholinesterase Inhibitors (Central); Secretin

The levels/effects of Fesoterodine may be decreased by: Acetylcholinesterase Inhibitors (Central); Bosentan; CYP3A4 Inducers (Strong); Dabrafenib; Deferasirox; Herbs (CYP3A4 Inducers); Mitotane; Peginterferon Alfa-2b; Tocilizumab

Ethanol/Nutrition/Herb Interactions Ethanol: Ethanol may potentiate adverse effects. Management: Avoid alcohol.

Storage/Stability Store at 20°C to 25°C (68°F to 77°F); excursions permitted between 15°C to 30°C (59°F to 86°F). Protect from moisture.

Mechanism of Action Fesoterodine acts as a prodrug and is converted to an active metabolite, 5-hydroxymethyl tolterodine (5-HMT); 5-HMT is responsible for fesoterodine's antimuscarinic activity and acts as a competitive antagonist of muscarinic receptors.

Urinary bladder contractions are mediated by muscarinic receptors; fesoterodine inhibits the receptors in the bladder preventing symptoms of urgency and frequency.

Pharmacodynamics/Kinetics

Absorption: Well absorbed

Distribution: I.V.: 5-HMT: V_d: 169 L

Protein binding: 5-HMT: ~50% (primarily to albumin and $alpha_1$-acid glycoprotein)

Metabolism: Fesoterodine is rapidly and extensively metabolized to its active metabolite (5-hydroxymethyl tolterodine; 5-HMT) by nonspecific esterases; 5-HMT is further metabolized via CYP2D6 and CYP3A4 to inactive metabolites.

Bioavailability: 5-HMT: 52%

Half-life elimination: ~7 hours

Time to peak, plasma: 5-HMT: ~5 hours; C_{max} higher in poor CYP2D6 metabolizers

Excretion: Urine (~70%; 16% as 5-HMT, ~53% as inactive metabolites); feces (7%)

Dosage Oral: Adults: Overactive bladder: 4 mg once daily; may be increased to 8 mg once daily based on individual response and tolerability

Dosing adjustment for concomitant strong CYP3A4 inhibitors (eg, ketoconazole, itraconazole, clarithromycin): 4 mg once daily; maximum dose: 4 mg once daily

Dosing adjustment in renal impairment:

Cl_{cr} ≥30 mL/minute: No dosage adjustment necessary

Cl_{cr} <30 mL/minute: 4 mg once daily; maximum dose: 4 mg once daily

Dosing adjustment in hepatic impairment:

Mild-to-moderate impairment (Child-Pugh class A or B): No dosage adjustment necessary

Severe impairment (Child-Pugh class C): Use is not recommended; has not been studied

Dietary Considerations May be taken with or without food.

Administration May be administered with or without food. Swallow whole; do not chew, crush, or divide.

Dosage Forms Excipient information presented when available (limited, particularly for generics); consult specific product labeling.

Tablet Extended Release 24 Hour, Oral, as fumarate:

Toviaz: 4 mg, 8 mg [contains fd&c blue #2 aluminum lake, soybean lecithin]

◆ Fesoterodine Fumarate *see* Fesoterodine *on page* 855

◆ Feverall [OTC] *see* Acetaminophen *on page* 28

◆ Fexmid *see* Cyclobenzaprine *on page* 502

Fexofenadine (feks oh FEN a deen)

Brand Names: U.S. Allegra Allergy Childrens [OTC]; Allegra Allergy [OTC]

Brand Names: Canada Allegra®

Index Terms Fexofenadine Hydrochloride

Pharmacologic Category Histamine H_1 Antagonist; Histamine H_1 Antagonist, Second Generation; Piperidine Derivative

Use Relief of symptoms associated with seasonal allergic rhinitis; treatment of chronic idiopathic urticaria

OTC labeling: Relief of symptoms associated with allergic rhinitis

Pregnancy Risk Factor C

Pregnancy Considerations Adverse events have been observed in animal reproduction studies; therefore, the manufacturer classifies fexofenadine as pregnancy category C. The use of antihistamines for the treatment of rhinitis during pregnancy is generally considered to be safe at recommended doses. Information related to the use of fexofenadine during pregnancy is limited; therefore, other agents are preferred.

Breast-Feeding Considerations It is not known if fexofenadine is excreted in breast milk. The manufacturer recommends that caution be exercised when administering fexofenadine to nursing women.

Contraindications Hypersensitivity to fexofenadine or any component of the formulation

Warnings/Precautions Use with caution in patients with renal impairment; dosage adjustment recommended. Safety and efficacy in children <6 months of age have not been established; orally disintegrating tablet not recommended for use in children <6 years of age. Orally disintegrating tablet contains phenylalanine.

Adverse Reactions

>10%:

Central nervous system: Headache (5% to 11%)

Gastrointestinal: Vomiting (children 6 months to 5 years: 4% to 12%)

1% to 10%:

Central nervous system: Fatigue (1% to 3%), somnolence (1% to 3%), dizziness (2%), fever (2%), pain (2%), drowsiness (1%)

Endocrine & metabolic: Dysmenorrhea (2%)

Gastrointestinal: Diarrhea (3% to 4%), nausea (2%), dyspepsia (1% to 2%)

Neuromuscular & skeletal: Myalgia (3%), back pain (2% to 3%), pain in extremities (2%)

Otic: Otitis media (2% to 4%)

Respiratory: Upper respiratory tract infection (3% to 4%), cough (2% to 4%), rhinorrhea (1% to 2%)

Miscellaneous: Viral infection (3%)

<1% (Limited to important or life-threatening): Hypersensitivity reactions (anaphylaxis, angioedema, chest tightness, dyspnea, flushing, pruritus, rash, urticaria); insomnia, nervousness, sleep disorders, paroniria

Drug Interactions

Metabolism/Transport Effects Substrate of CYP3A4 (minor), P-glycoprotein, SLCO1B1; **Note:** Assignment of Major/Minor substrate status based on clinically relevant drug interaction potential; **Inhibits** CYP2D6 (weak)

Avoid Concomitant Use

Avoid concomitant use of Fexofenadine with any of the following: Aclidinium; Azelastine (Nasal); Ipratropium (Oral Inhalation); Paraldehyde; Tiotropium; Umeclidinium

Increased Effect/Toxicity

Fexofenadine may increase the levels/effects of: Alcohol (Ethyl); Analgesics (Opioid); Anticholinergics; ARIPiprazole; Azelastine (Nasal); Buprenorphine; CNS Depressants; Hydrocodone; Methotrimeprazine; Metyrosine; Mirtazapine; Paraldehyde; Pramipexole; ROPINIRole; Rotigotine; Selective Serotonin Reuptake Inhibitors; Tiotropium; Zolpidem

The levels/effects of Fexofenadine may be increased by: Aclidinium; Brimonidine (Topical); Doxylamine; Droperidol; Eltrombopag; Erythromycin (Systemic); HydrOXYzine; Ipratropium (Oral Inhalation); Itraconazole; Ketoconazole (Systemic); Magnesium Sulfate; Methotrimeprazine; Perampanel; P-glycoprotein/ABCB1 Inhibitors; Pramlintide; Rifampin; Sodium Oxybate; Tapentadol; Umeclidinium; Verapamil

Decreased Effect

Fexofenadine may decrease the levels/effects of: Acetylcholinesterase Inhibitors (Central); Benzylpenicilloyl Polylysine; Betahistine; Hyaluronidase

The levels/effects of Fexofenadine may be decreased by: Acetylcholinesterase Inhibitors (Central); Amphetamines; Antacids; Grapefruit Juice; P-glycoprotein/ABCB1 Inducers; Rifampin

Ethanol/Nutrition/Herb Interactions

Ethanol: Ethanol may increase CNS depression. Management: Avoid ethanol.

Food: Fruit juice (apple, grapefruit, orange) may decrease bioavailability of fexofenadine by ~36%. Management: Administer with water only, avoid fruit juice.

Herb/Nutraceutical: St John's wort may decrease fexofenadine levels.

Storage/Stability Store at controlled room temperature of 20°C to 25°C (68°F to 77°F). Protect from excessive moisture.

Mechanism of Action Fexofenadine is an active metabolite of terfenadine and like terfenadine it competes with histamine for H_1-receptor sites on effector cells in the gastrointestinal tract, blood vessels and respiratory tract; it appears that fexofenadine does not cross the blood-brain barrier to any appreciable degree, resulting in a reduced potential for sedation

Pharmacodynamics/Kinetics

Onset of action: 60 minutes

Duration: Antihistaminic effect: ≥12 hours

Absorption: Rapid

Protein binding: 60% to 70%, primarily albumin and alpha$_1$-acid glycoprotein

Metabolism: Minimal (Hepatic ~5%)

Half-life elimination: 14.4 hours (31% to 72% longer in renal impairment)

Time to peak, serum: ODT: 2 hours (4 hours with high-fat meal); Tablet: ~2.6 hours; Suspension: ~1 hour

Excretion: Feces (~80%) and urine (~11%) as unchanged drug

Dosage Oral:

Chronic idiopathic urticaria: Children 6 months to <2 years: 15 mg twice daily

Chronic idiopathic urticaria, seasonal allergic rhinitis:

Children 2-11 years: 30 mg twice daily

Children ≥12 years and Adults: 60 mg twice daily **or** 180 mg once daily

Elderly: Starting dose: Use caution; adjust dose for renal impairment

Allergic rhinitis (OTC labeling):

Children 2-11 years: 30 mg twice daily

Children ≥12 years and Adults: 60 mg twice daily **or** 180 mg once daily

Dosage adjustment in renal impairment: Cl_{cr} <80 mL/minute:

Children 6 months to <2 years: Initial: 15 mg once daily

Children 2-11 years: Initial: 30 mg once daily

Children ≥12 years and Adults: Initial: 60 mg once daily

Hemodialysis: Not effectively removed by hemodialysis

Dosage adjustment in hepatic impairment: No dosage adjustment provided in manufacturer's labeling; however, need for adjustment not likely since undergoes minimal hepatic metabolism.

Dietary Considerations Some products may contain phenylalanine and/or sodium. Take suspension and tablets with water only; do not administer with fruit juices.

Administration

Suspension, tablet: Administer with water only; do not administer with fruit juices. Shake suspension well before use.

Orally disintegrating tablet: Take on an empty stomach. Do not remove from blister pack until administered. Using dry hands, place immediately on tongue. Tablet will dissolve within seconds, and may be swallowed with or without liquid (do not administer with fruit juices). Do not split or chew.

Monitoring Parameters Relief of symptoms

Test Interactions May suppress the wheal and flare reactions to skin test antigens.

Dosage Forms Excipient information presented when available (limited, particularly for generics); consult specific product labeling.

Suspension, Oral, as hydrochloride:

Allegra Allergy Childrens: 30 mg/5 mL (120 mL) [alcohol free, dye free; contains butylparaben, edetate disodium, propylene glycol, propylparaben; raspberry creme flavor]

Tablet, Oral, as hydrochloride:

Allegra Allergy: 60 mg, 180 mg

Allegra Allergy Childrens: 30 mg

Generic: 60 mg, 180 mg

Tablet Dispersible, Oral, as hydrochloride:

Allegra Allergy Childrens: 30 mg [contains aspartame; orange cream flavor]

Fexofenadine and Pseudoephedrine

(feks oh FEN a deen & soo doe e FED rin)

Brand Names: U.S. Allegra-D® 12 Hour; Allegra-D® 24 Hour

Brand Names: Canada Allegra-D®

Index Terms Pseudoephedrine and Fexofenadine

Pharmacologic Category Alpha/Beta Agonist; Decongestant; Histamine H_1 Antagonist; Histamine H_1 Antagonist, Second Generation; Piperidine Derivative

Use Relief of symptoms associated with seasonal allergic rhinitis in adults and children ≥12 years of age

Pregnancy Risk Factor C

Dosage Oral: Children ≥12 years and Adults:

Allegra-D® 12 Hour: One tablet twice daily

Allegra-D® 24 Hour: One tablet once daily

Dosage adjustment in renal impairment:

Allegra-D® 12 Hour: Cl_{cr} <80 mL/minute (based on fexofenadine component): One tablet once daily

Allegra-D® 24 Hour: Avoid use.

Dosage adjustment in hepatic impairment: No dosage adjustment provided in manufacturer's labeling; however, need for adjustment not likely since fexofenadine undergoes minimal hepatic metabolism; impact of hepatic impairment on pseudoephedrine pharmacokinetics are unknown.

Additional Information Complete prescribing information should be consulted for additional detail.

Dosage Forms Excipient information presented when available (limited, particularly for generics); consult specific product labeling.

Tablet, extended release: Fexofenadine hydrochloride 60 mg [immediate release] and pseudoephedrine hydrochloride 120 mg [extended release]; fexofenadine hydrochloride 180 mg [immediate release] and pseudoephedrine hydrochloride 240 mg [extended release]

Allegra-D® 12 Hour: Fexofenadine hydrochloride 60 mg [immediate release] and pseudoephedrine hydrochloride 120 mg [extended release]

Allegra-D® 24 Hour: Fexofenadine hydrochloride 180 mg [immediate release] and pseudoephedrine hydrochloride 240 mg [extended release]

◆ **Fexofenadine Hydrochloride** *see* Fexofenadine *on page 856*

◆ **Fiber Therapy [OTC]** *see* Psyllium *on page 1748*

◆ **Fibricor** *see* Fenofibrate and Derivatives *on page 837*

Fibrinogen Concentrate (Human)

(fi BRIN o gin KON suhn trate HYU man)

Brand Names: U.S. RiaSTAP®

Index Terms Coagulation Factor I

Pharmacologic Category Blood Product Derivative

Use Treatment of acute bleeding episodes in patients with congenital fibrinogen deficiency (afibrinogenemia and hypofibrinogenemia)

Pregnancy Risk Factor C

Pregnancy Considerations Animal reproduction studies have not been conducted. Increased pregnancy loss is associated with untreated congenital fibrinogen disorders.

Breast-Feeding Considerations The use of fibrinogen concentrate has not been studied in nursing women with congenital fibrinogen deficiency.

Contraindications Severe hypersensitivity reactions to fibrinogen concentrate or any component of the formulation

Warnings/Precautions Hypersensitivity reactions (eg, urticaria, hives, wheezing, hypotension, anaphylaxis) may occur. In the event of hypersensitivity reactions, treatment should be discontinued immediately. Thrombosis may occur in patients with congenital fibrinogen deficiency with or without fibrinogen replacement therapy. Consider potential risk of thrombosis with use. Product of human plasma; may potentially contain infectious agents which could transmit disease. Screening of donors, as well as testing and/or inactivation or removal of certain viruses, reduces the risk. Infections thought to be transmitted by this product should be reported to the manufacturer. Not for the treatment of dysfibrinogenemia.

Adverse Reactions

>1%: Central nervous system: Fever, headache

Postmarketing and/or case reports: Allergic reactions, anaphylaxis, arterial thrombosis, chills, DVT, dyspnea, MI, nausea, pulmonary embolism, rash, thromboembolism, vomiting

Drug Interactions

Metabolism/Transport Effects None known.

Avoid Concomitant Use There are no known interactions where it is recommended to avoid concomitant use.

Increased Effect/Toxicity

Fibrinogen Concentrate (Human) may increase the levels/effects of: Antifibrinolytic Agents

The levels/effects of Fibrinogen Concentrate (Human) may be increased by: Antifibrinolytic Agents

Decreased Effect There are no known significant interactions involving a decrease in effect.

Preparation for Administration Transfer sterile water for injection 50 mL into vial. Gently swirl until dissolved; do not shake.

Storage/Stability Store at 2°C to 25°C (36°F to 77°F) in original carton; do not freeze. Protect from light. Stable for 24 hours after reconstitution when stored at 20°C to 25°C (68°F to 77°F). Discard partially used vials.

Mechanism of Action Fibrinogen (coagulation factor I), a protein found in normal plasma, is required to clot blood. Fibrinogen concentrate made from pooled human plasma replaces this protein which is missing or reduced in patients with a congenital fibrinogen deficiency.

Pharmacodynamics/Kinetics

Distribution: V_d: 45-60 mL/kg (range 36-68 mL/kg)

Half-life elimination: 61-97 hours (range 56-117 hours); may be decreased in children <16 years of age

Dosage I.V.: Children and Adults: Congenital fibrinogen deficiency: **Note:** Adjust dose based on laboratory values and condition of patient. Maintain a target fibrinogen level of 100 mg/dL until hemostasis is achieved.

When baseline fibrinogen level is known:
Dose (mg/kg) = [Target level (mg/dL) - measured level (mg/dL)] **divided by** 1.7 (mg/dL per mg/kg body weight)
When baseline fibrinogen level is not known: 70 mg/kg

Dosage adjustment in renal impairment: No dosage adjustment provided in manufacturer's labeling.

Dosage adjustment in hepatic impairment: No dosage adjustment provided in manufacturer's labeling.

Administration For I.V. administration only; infuse at ≤5 mL/minute

Monitoring Parameters Signs and symptoms of hypersensitivity, thrombosis; fibrinogen level

Reference Range A target fibrinogen level of 100 mg/dL should be maintained until hemostasis occurs and wound healing is complete.
Normal fibrinogen levels: 200-450 mg/dL

Dosage Forms Excipient information presented when available (limited, particularly for generics); consult specific product labeling. [DSC] = Discontinued product
Injection, powder for reconstitution:
RiaSTAP®: 900-1300 mg [contains albumin (human); exact potency labeled on vial]

◆ **Fibristal (Can)** *see* Ulipristal *on page 2138*

Fidaxomicin (fye DAX oh mye sin)

Brand Names: U.S. Dificid

Brand Names: Canada Dificid™

Index Terms Difimicin; Lipiarrmycin; OPT-80; PAR-101; Tiacumicin B

Pharmacologic Category Antibiotic, Macrolide

Use Treatment of *Clostridium difficile*-associated diarrhea (CDAD)

Pregnancy Risk Factor B

Pregnancy Considerations Adverse events were not observed in animal reproduction studies. Due to the limited systemic absorption of fidaxomicin, exposure to the fetus is expected to be low.

Breast-Feeding Considerations It is not known if fidaxomicin is excreted in breast milk. The manufacturer recommends that caution be exercised when administering fidaxomicin to nursing women.

Contraindications Hypersensitivity to fidaxomicin

Warnings/Precautions Do not use for systemic infections; fidaxomicin systemic absorption is negligible. Hypersensitivity reactions (angioedema [mouth, face, throat], dyspnea, pruritus, and rash) to fidaxomicin have been reported. Patients with a history of macrolide allergy may be at increased risk. If a severe reaction occurs, discontinue drug and institute supportive care. Use only in patients with proven or strongly suspected *Clostridium difficile (C. difficile)* infections.

Adverse Reactions
>10%: Gastrointestinal: Nausea (11%)
2% to 10%:
Gastrointestinal: Gastrointestinal hemorrhage (4%), abdominal pain, vomiting
Hematologic: Anemia (2%), neutropenia (2%)
<2% (Limited to important or life-threatening): Abdominal distention, abdominal tenderness, angioedema, decreased platelet count, decreased serum bicarbonate, dyspepsia, dysphagia, dyspnea, fixed drug eruption, flatulence, hyperglycemia, hypersensitivity reaction, increased liver enzymes, increased serum alkaline phosphatase, intestinal obstruction, megacolon, metabolic acidosis, pruritus, skin rash

Drug Interactions

Metabolism/Transport Effects None known.

Avoid Concomitant Use There are no known interactions where it is recommended to avoid concomitant use.

Increased Effect/Toxicity
Fidaxomicin may increase the levels/effects of: Rilpivirine

Decreased Effect
Fidaxomicin may decrease the levels/effects of: Sodium Picosulfate

Storage/Stability Store at 20°C to 25°C (68°F to 77°F); excursions permitted to 15°C to 30°C (59°F to 86°F).

Mechanism of Action Inhibits RNA polymerase sigma subunit resulting in inhibition of protein synthesis and cell death in susceptible organisms including *C. difficile*; bactericidal

Pharmacodynamics/Kinetics
Absorption: Oral: Minimal systemic absorption
Distribution: Largely confined to the gastrointestinal tract; in single- and multiple-dose studies, fecal concentrations of fidaxomicin and its active metabolite (OP-1118) are very high while serum concentrations are minimally detectable to undetectable
Metabolism: Intestinal hydrolysis to less active metabolite (OP-1118)
Excretion: Feces (>92% as unchanged drug and metabolites); urine (<1% as metabolite)

Dosage Oral: Adults: Diarrhea due to *Clostridium difficile* (CDAD): 200 mg twice daily for 10 days

Dosing adjustment in renal impairment: No dosage adjustment necessary (minimal systemic absorption).

Dosing adjustment in hepatic impairment: No dosage adjustment provided in manufacturer's label (has not been studied); However, due to minimal systemic absorption no dosage adjustment predicted.

Administration May be administered with or without food.

Additional Information Fidaxomicin is bactericidal against gram-positive anaerobes (including *C. difficile* NAP1/B1/027 strain) and gram-positive aerobes. Fidaxomicin spectrum does **not** include gram-negative aerobes or gram-negative anaerobes (eg, *Bacteroides spp*). At the approved dose, concentrations in feces substantially exceed the 90% MIC of *C. difficile*. Postantibiotic effects against *C. difficile* in clinical studies range from 6-10 hours. Clinical studies excluded patients with a history of >1 recurrent *C. difficile*-associated diarrhea (CDAD) episode within 3 months.

Dosage Forms Excipient information presented when available (limited, particularly for generics); consult specific product labeling.
Tablet, Oral:
Dificid: 200 mg [contains soybean lecithin]

Filgrastim (fil GRA stim)

Brand Names: U.S. Granix; Neupogen

Brand Names: Canada Neupogen

Index Terms G-CSF; Granulocyte Colony Stimulating Factor; Tbo-Filgrastim; Tevagrastim

Pharmacologic Category Colony Stimulating Factor

Use

Myelosuppressive chemotherapy recipients with nonmyeloid malignancies:

Neupogen: To decrease the incidence of infection (neutropenic fever) in patients with nonmyeloid malignancies receiving myelosuppressive chemotherapy associated with a significant incidence of neutropenia with fever.

Granix: To decrease the duration of severe neutropenia in patients with nonmyeloid malignancies receiving myelosuppressive chemotherapy associated with a clinically significant incidence of neutropenic fever.

Acute myeloid leukemia (AML) patients following induction or consolidation chemotherapy (Neupogen): To reduce the time to neutrophil recovery and reduce the duration of fever following induction or consolidation chemotherapy in adults with AML.

Bone marrow transplantation (Neupogen): To reduce the duration of neutropenia and neutropenia-related events (eg, neutropenic fever) in patients with nonmyeloid malignancies receiving myeloablative chemotherapy followed by marrow transplantation.

Peripheral blood progenitor cell collection and therapy (Neupogen): Mobilization of hematopoietic progenitor cells into peripheral blood for apheresis collection (mobilization allows for collection of increased numbers of progenitor cells capable of engraftment, which may lead to more rapid engraftment).

Severe chronic neutropenia (Neupogen): Long-term administration to reduce the incidence and duration of neutropenic complications (eg, fever, infections, oropharyngeal ulcers) in symptomatic patients with congenital, cyclic, or idiopathic neutropenia.

Unlabeled Use Treatment of anemia in myelodysplastic syndrome (in combination with epoetin); mobilization of hematopoietic stem cells (HSC) for collection and subsequent autologous transplantation (in combination with plerixafor) in patients with non-Hodgkin's lymphoma (NHL) and multiple myeloma (MM); treatment of neutropenia in HIV-infected patients receiving zidovudine; hepatitis C treatment-associated neutropenia; treatment of radiation-induced myelosuppression of the bone marrow

Pregnancy Risk Factor C

Pregnancy Considerations Adverse events have been observed in animal reproduction studies. Filgrastim has been shown to cross the placenta in humans.

Women who become pregnant during Neupogen treatment are encouraged to enroll in the manufacturer's Pregnancy Surveillance Program (1-800-772-6436).

Breast-Feeding Considerations It is not known if filgrastim or tbo-filgrastim are is excreted in breast milk. The manufacturers recommend that caution be exercised when administering filgrastim or tbo-filgrastim to nursing women.

Women who are nursing during Neupogen treatment are encouraged to enroll in the manufacturer's Lactation Surveillance program (1-800-772-6436).

Contraindications

Neupogen: Hypersensitivity to filgrastim, *E. coli*-derived proteins, or any component of the formulation

Granix: There are no contraindications listed in the manufacturer's labeling

Warnings/Precautions Anaphylaxis, rash, urticaria, facial edema, wheezing, dyspnea, tachycardia, and/or hypotension have occurred with first or subsequent doses. Reactions tended to involve two or more body systems and occur more frequently with intravenous administration and generally within 30 minutes of administration. Symptoms recurred in >50% of patients when rechallenged. Management may include administration of antihistamines, steroids, bronchodilators, and/or epinephrine. Do not administer tbo-filgrastim to patients who experienced allergic reaction to filgrastim or pegfilgrastim. Permanently discontinue tbo-filgrastim in patients with serious allergic reactions. Rare cases of splenic rupture have been reported (may be fatal); in patients with left upper quadrant pain or shoulder tip pain, withhold treatment and evaluate for enlarged spleen or splenic rupture. Cutaneous vasculitis has been reported with filgrastim, generally occurring in patients with severe chronic neutropenia on chronic therapy; symptoms generally developed with increasing absolute neutrophil count (ANC) and subsided when the ANC decreased; dose reductions may improve symptoms to allow for continued therapy.

White blood cell counts of ≥100,000/mm^3 have been reported with filgrastim doses >5 mcg/kg/day. Monitor CBC twice weekly during therapy. Thrombocytopenia has also been reported with filgrastim; monitor platelet counts. Although the incidence of antibody development has not been determined, there is a potential for immunogenicity, which may result in cytopenias. Filgrastim should not be routinely used in the treatment of established neutropenic fever. Colony-stimulating factors may be considered in cancer patients with febrile neutropenia who are at high risk for infection-associated complications or who have prognostic factors indicative of a poor clinical outcome (eg, prolonged and severe neutropenia, age ≥65 years, pneumonia, sepsis syndrome, presence of invasive fungal infection) (Freifeld, 2011; Smith, 2006). Do not use filgrastim in the period 24 hours before to 24 hours after administration of cytotoxic chemotherapy because of the potential sensitivity of rapidly dividing myeloid cells to cytotoxic chemotherapy. Transient increase in neutrophil count is seen 1-2 days after filgrastim initiation; however, for sustained neutrophil response, continue until post-nadir ANC reaches 10,000/mm^3. Avoid simultaneous use of filgrastim with chemotherapy and radiation therapy. Safety and efficacy have not been established with patients receiving chemotherapy associated with delayed myelosuppression (eg, nitrosoureas, mitomycin). Avoid concurrent radiation therapy with filgrastim; safety and efficacy have not been established with patients receiving radiation therapy. May potentially act as a growth factor for any tumor type; caution should be exercised when using in any malignancy with myeloid characteristics. When used for stem cell mobilization, may release tumor cells from marrow which could be collected in leukapheresis product; potential effect of tumor cell reinfusion is unknown.

May precipitate severe sickle cell crises, sometimes resulting in fatalities, in patients with sickle cell disorders; carefully evaluate potential risks and benefits. Discontinue in patients undergoing sickle cell crisis. Cytogenic abnormalities and transformation to AML or myelodysplastic syndrome (MDS) have been reported in patients with severe chronic neutropenia (SCN), including patients receiving cytokine therapy; carefully consider the risks of continued filgrastim treatment if abnormal cytogenetics or myelodysplasia develop. Establish diagnosis prior to filgrastim initiation; use prior to appropriate diagnosis of SCN may impair or delay proper evaluation and treatment for neutropenia due to conditions other than SCN. Acute respiratory distress syndrome (ARDS) has been reported (possibly due to influx of neutrophils to sites of lung inflammation); patients must be instructed to report respiratory distress; monitor for fever, infiltrates, or respiratory distress; discontinue in patients with ARDS. Reports of alveolar hemorrhage, manifested as pulmonary infiltrates and hemoptysis, have occurred in healthy donors undergoing PBPC mobilization (unlabeled for use in healthy donors); hemoptysis resolved upon discontinuation. The packaging of some dosage forms may contain latex.

Adverse Reactions

>10%:

Central nervous system: Fever (12%)

Dermatologic: Petechiae (≤17%), rash (≤12%)

Endocrine & metabolic: LDH increased, uric acid increased

Gastrointestinal: Splenomegaly (severe chronic neutropenia: 30%; rare in other patients)

Hepatic: Alkaline phosphatase increased (21%)

Neuromuscular & skeletal: Bone/skeletal pain (22% to 33%; dose related), commonly in the lower back, posterior iliac crest, and sternum

Respiratory: Epistaxis (9% to 15%)

1% to 10%:

Cardiovascular: Hyper-/hypotension (4%), myocardial infarction/arrhythmias (3%)

Central nervous system: Headache (7%)

Gastrointestinal: Nausea (10%), vomiting (7%), peritonitis (≤2%)

Hematologic: Leukocytosis (2%)

Miscellaneous: Transfusion reaction (≤10%)

<1% (Limited to important or life-threatening): Acute respiratory distress syndrome (ARDS), allergic reactions, alopecia, alveolar hemorrhage, arthralgia, bone density decreased, capillary leak syndrome, cerebral hemorrhage, cutaneous vasculitis, dyspnea, edema (facial), erythema nodosum, hematuria, hemoptysis, hepatomegaly, hypersensitivity reaction, injection site reaction, osteoporosis, pericarditis, proteinuria, psoriasis exacerbation, pulmonary infiltrates, renal insufficiency, sickle cell crisis, splenic rupture, Sweet's syndrome (acute febrile dermatosis), tachycardia, thrombocytopenia (in PBPC mobilization), thrombophlebitis, transient supraventricular arrhythmia, urticaria, wheezing

Drug Interactions

Metabolism/Transport Effects None known.

Avoid Concomitant Use There are no known interactions where it is recommended to avoid concomitant use.

Increased Effect/Toxicity

Filgrastim may increase the levels/effects of: Bleomycin; Topotecan

Decreased Effect There are no known significant interactions involving a decrease in effect.

Preparation for Administration Visually inspect prior to use; discard if discolored or if particulates are present.

Neupogen: **Do not dilute with saline at any time; product may precipitate.** Filgrastim may be diluted with D_5W to a concentration of 5-15 mcg/mL for I.V. infusion administration (minimum concentration: 5 mcg/mL). Concentrations of 5-15 mcg/mL require addition of albumin (final albumin concentration of 2 mg/mL) to prevent adsorption to plastics. Dilution to <5 mcg/mL is not recommended. Do not shake. Discard unused portion of vial/prefilled syringe.

Granix: Remove needle shield and expel extra volume if needed (depending on dose). Prefilled syringe is single use; discard unused portion.

Storage/Stability

Neupogen: Store intact vials/prefilled syringes at 2°C to 8°C (36°F to 46°F). Do not shake. Protect from direct sunlight. Prior to injection, allow to reach room temperature for a maximum of 24 hours. Discard any vial or prefilled syringe left at room temperature for more than 24 hours.

Extended storage information may be available for undiluted filgrastim; contact product manufacturer to obtain current recommendations. Sterility has been assessed and maintained for up to 7 days when prepared under strict aseptic conditions (Jacobson, 1996; Singh, 1994). The manufacturer recommends using syringes within 24 hours due to the potential for bacterial contamination.

Granix: Store prefilled syringes at 2°C to 8°C (36°F to 46°F). Protect from light. Do not shake. May be removed from 2°C to 8°C (36°F to 46°F) storage for a single period of up to 5 days between 23°C to 27°C (73°F to 81°F). If not used within 5 days, the product may be returned to 2°C to 8°C (36°F to 46°F) up to the expiration date. Exposure to -1°C to -5°C (23°F to 30°F) for up to 72 hours and temperatures as low as -15°C to -25°C (5°F to -13°F) for up to 24 hours do not adversely affect stability. Discard unused product.

Mechanism of Action Filgrastim and tbo-filgrastim are granulocyte colony stimulating factors (G-CSF) produced by recombinant DNA technology. G-CSFs stimulate the production, maturation, and activation of neutrophils to increase both their migration and cytotoxicity.

Pharmacodynamics/Kinetics

Onset of action:

Filgrastim: ~24 hours; plateaus in 3-5 days

Tbo-filgrastim: Time to maximum ANC: 3-5 days

Duration:

Filgrastim: Neutrophil counts generally return to baseline within 4 days

Tbo-filgrastim: ANC returned to baseline by 21 days after completion of chemotherapy

Absorption: SubQ: 100%

Distribution: V_d: 150 mL/kg; no evidence of drug accumulation over a 11- to 20-day period

Metabolism: Systemically degraded

Bioavailability: Tbo-filgrastim: SubQ: 33%

Half-life elimination: Filgrastim: ~3.5 hours; Tbo-filgrastim: 3-4 hours

Time to peak, serum: SubQ: Filgrastim: 2-8 hours; Tbo-filgrastim: 4-6 hours

Dosage Note: May round the dose to the nearest vial size in adults for convenience and cost minimization (Ozer, 2000). Do not administer in the period 24 hours before to 24 hours after cytotoxic chemotherapy.

Myelosuppressive chemotherapy recipients with non-myeloid malignancies (Neupogen): Infants, Children, Adolescents, and Adults: SubQ, I.V.: 5 mcg/kg/day; doses may be increased by 5 mcg/kg (for each chemotherapy cycle) according to the duration and severity of the neutropenia; continue for up to 14 days until the ANC reaches 10,000/mm^3. Discontinue if the ANC surpasses 10,000/mm^3 after the expected chemotherapy-induced neutrophil nadir. In clinical studies, efficacy was observed at doses of 4-8 mcg/kg/day.

Myelosuppressive chemotherapy recipients with non-myeloid malignancies (Granix): Adults: SubQ: 5 mcg/kg/day; continue until anticipated nadir has passed and neutrophil count has recovered to normal range

Acute myeloid leukemia (AML) following induction or consolidation chemotherapy (Neupogen): Adults: SubQ, I.V.: 5 mcg/kg/day; doses may be increased by 5 mcg/kg (for each chemotherapy cycle) according to the duration and severity of the neutropenia; continue for up to 14 days until the ANC reaches 10,000/mm^3. Discontinue if the ANC surpasses 10,000/mm^3 after the expected chemotherapy-induced neutrophil nadir. In clinical studies, efficacy was observed at doses of 4-8 mcg/kg/day.

Bone marrow transplantation (Neupogen): Infants, Children, Adolescents, and Adults: SubQ, I.V.: 10 mcg/kg/day (administer ≥24 hours after chemotherapy and ≥24 hours after bone marrow infusion); adjust the dose according to the duration and severity of neutropenia; recommended steps based on neutrophil response:

When ANC >1000/mm^3 for 3 consecutive days: Reduce filgrastim dose to 5 mcg/kg/day

If ANC remains >1000/mm^3 for 3 more consecutive days: Discontinue filgrastim

If ANC decreases to <1000/mm^3: Resume at 5 mcg/kg/day

If ANC decreases to <1000/mm^3 during the 5 mcg/kg/day dose, increase filgrastim to 10 mcg/kg/day and follow the above steps

Peripheral blood progenitor cell collection and therapy (Neupogen): Infants, Children, Adolescents, and Adults: SubQ: 10 mcg/kg daily, usually for 6-7 days. Begin at least 4 days before the first apheresis and continue until the last apheresis; consider dose adjustment for WBC >100,000/mm^3

Severe chronic neutropenia (Neupogen): Infants ≥1 month, Children, Adolescents, and Adults: SubQ:

Congenital: Initial: 6 mcg/kg twice daily; adjust the dose based on ANC and clinical response; mean dose: 6 mcg/kg/day

Idiopathic: Initial: 5 mcg/kg/day; adjust the dose based on ANC and clinical response; mean dose: 1.2 mcg/kg/day

Cyclic: Initial: 5 mcg/kg/day; adjust the dose based on ANC and clinical response; mean dose: 2.1 mcg/kg/day

Anemia in myelodysplastic syndrome (unlabeled use; in combination with epoetin): Adults: SubQ: 300 mcg weekly in 2-3 divided doses (Malcovati, 2013) **or** 1 mcg/kg once daily (Greenberg, 2009) **or** 75 mcg, 150 mcg, or 300 mcg per dose 3 times weekly (Hellstrom-Lindberg, 2003)

Hematopoietic stem cell mobilization in autologous transplantation in patients with non-Hodgkin's lymphoma or multiple myeloma (in combination with plerixafor; unlabeled use): Adults: SubQ: 10 mcg/kg once daily; begin 4 days before initiation of plerixafor; continue G-CSF on each day prior to apheresis for up to 8 days (DiPersio, *JCO* 2009; DiPersio, *Blood* 2009)

Hepatitis C treatment-associated neutropenia (unlabeled use): Adults: SubQ: 150 mcg once weekly to 300 mcg 3 times weekly; titrate to maintain ANC between 750-10,000/mm^3 (Younossi, 2008)

Treatment of radiation-induced myelosuppression of the bone marrow (unlabeled use): Infants, Children, Adolescents, and Adults: SubQ: 5 mcg/kg/day; continue until ANC >1000/mm^3 (Smith, 2006; Waselenko, 2004).

Dosage adjustment in renal impairment:

Neupogen: No dosage adjustment provided in the manufacturer's labeling.

Granix:

Mild impairment: No dosage adjustment necessary.

Moderate to severe impairment: No dosage adjustment provided in the manufacturer's labeling (has not been studied).

Dosage adjustment in hepatic impairment: No dosage adjustment provided in the manufacturer's labeling.

Dietary Considerations Some products may contain sodium.

Administration

Do not administer earlier than 24 hours after or in the 24 hours prior to cytotoxic chemotherapy.

I.V. (Neupogen): May be administered I.V. as a short infusion over 15-30 minutes (chemotherapy-induced neutropenia) or by continuous infusion (chemotherapy-induced neutropenia) or as a 4- or 24-hour infusion (bone marrow transplantation).

SubQ: May be administered by SubQ, either as a bolus injection (chemotherapy-induced neutropenia, peripheral blood progenitor cell collection, severe chronic neutropenia) or as a continuous infusion (chemotherapy-induced neutropenia, bone marrow transplantation, and peripheral blood progenitor cell collection). Administer into the outer upper arm, abdomen (except within 2 inches of navel), front middle thigh, or the upper outer buttocks area.

Monitoring Parameters

Chemotherapy-induced neutropenia: CBC with differential and platelets prior to chemotherapy and twice weekly during growth factor treatment.

Bone marrow transplantation: CBC with differential and platelets at least 3 times a week.

Peripheral progenitor cell collection: Neutrophil counts after 4 days of filgrastim treatment.

Severe chronic neutropenia: CBC with differential and platelets twice weekly during the first month of therapy and for 2 weeks following dose adjustments; once clinically stable, monthly for 1 year and quarterly thereafter. Monitor bone marrow and karyotype prior to treatment; and monitor marrow and cytogenetics annually throughout treatment.

Reference Range No additional clinical benefit seen when filgrastim is used with ANC >10,000/mm^3

Test Interactions May interfere with bone imaging studies; increased hematopoietic activity of the bone marrow may appear as transient positive bone imaging changes

Dosage Forms Considerations

Prefilled syringes: Granix, Neupogen: 300 mcg/0.5 mL (0.5 mL); 480 mcg/0.8 mL (0.8 mL)

Vials: Neupogen: 300 mcg/mL (1 mL); 480 mcg/1.6 mL (1.6 mL)

Dosage Forms Excipient information presented when available (limited, particularly for generics); consult specific product labeling.

Solution, Injection:

Neupogen: 300 mcg/mL (1 mL); 480 mcg/1.6 mL (1.6 mL) [contains polysorbate 80]

Solution, Injection [preservative free]:

Neupogen: 300 mcg/0.5 mL (0.5 mL); 480 mcg/0.8 mL (0.8 mL) [contains polysorbate 80]

Solution Prefilled Syringe, Subcutaneous [preservative free]:

Granix: 300 mcg/0.5 mL (0.5 mL); 480 mcg/0.8 mL (0.8 mL) [contains polysorbate 80]

◆ Finacea *see* Azelaic Acid *on page 211*

◆ Finacea® (Can) *see* Azelaic Acid *on page 211*

Finasteride (fi NAS teer ide)

Brand Names: U.S. Propecia; Proscar

Brand Names: Canada Apo-Finasteride; CO Finasteride; JAMP-Finasteride; Mint-Finasteride; Mylan-Finasteride; PMS-Finasteride; Propecia®; Proscar®; ratio-Finasteride; Sandoz-Finasteride; Teva-Finasteride

Pharmacologic Category 5 Alpha-Reductase Inhibitor

Use

Propecia®: Treatment of male pattern hair loss in **men only**. Safety and efficacy were demonstrated in men between 18-41 years of age.

Proscar®: Treatment of symptomatic benign prostatic hyperplasia (BPH); can be used in combination with an alpha-blocker, doxazosin

Unlabeled Use Treatment of female hirsutism

Pregnancy Risk Factor X

Pregnancy Considerations Abnormalities of external male genitalia were reported in animal reproduction studies. Use is not indicated in women. Pregnant women are advised to avoid contact with crushed or broken tablets and the semen from a male partner exposed to finasteride.

Breast-Feeding Considerations It is not known if finasteride is excreted in breast milk. Use is contraindicated in women of childbearing potential.

Contraindications Hypersensitivity to finasteride or any component of the formulation; women of childbearing potential

Warnings/Precautions Hazardous agent - use appropriate precautions for handling and disposal (NIOSH, 2012). Other urological diseases (including prostate cancer) should be ruled out before initiating. For BPH, a minimum of 6 months of treatment may be necessary to determine whether an individual will respond to finasteride; for male pattern hair loss, daily use for 3 months or longer may be required before benefit is observed. Reduces prostate specific antigen (PSA) by ~50%; in patients treated for ≥6 months the PSA value should be doubled when comparing to normal ranges in untreated patients (for interpretation of serial PSAs, a new PSA baseline should be established ≥6 months after treatment initiation and PSA monitored periodically thereafter). Failure to demonstrate a meaningful PSA decrease (<50%) or a PSA increase while on this medication may be associated with an increased risk for prostate cancer (NCCN prostate cancer early detection guidelines, v.1.2011). Patients on a 5-alpha-reductase inhibitor (5-ARI) with any increase in PSA levels, even if within normal limits, should be evaluated; may indicate presence of prostate cancer. Use with caution in patients with hepatic dysfunction; finasteride is extensively metabolized in the liver. When compared to placebo, 5-ARIs have been shown to reduce the overall incidence of prostate cancer, although an increase in the incidence of high-grade prostate cancers has been observed; 5-ARIs are not approved in the U.S. or Canada for the prevention of prostate cancer. Carefully monitor patients with a large residual urinary volume or severely diminished urinary flow for obstructive uropathy; these patients may not be candidates for finasteride therapy. Rare reports of male breast cancer have been observed with finasteride use. Patients should promptly report any breast changes, including breast enlargement, lumps, tenderness, pain, or nipple discharge to their healthcare provider. Active ingredient of crushed or broken tablets can be absorbed through the skin; unbroken tablets are coated which prevents contact with the active ingredient during normal handling. Women should avoid contact with crushed or broken tablets and the semen from a male partner exposed to finasteride; finasteride may negatively impact fetal development.

Adverse Reactions Note: "Combination therapy" refers to finasteride and doxazosin.

>10%:

- Cardiovascular: Orthostatic hypotension (combination therapy 18%; monotherapy 9%)
- Central nervous system: Dizziness (combination therapy 23%; monotherapy 7%)
- Endocrine & metabolic: Decreased libido (combination therapy 12%; monotherapy 2% to 10%)
- Genitourinary: Impotence (combination therapy 23%; monotherapy 5% to 19%), ejaculatory disorder (combination therapy 14%; monotherapy <1% to 7%)
- Neuromuscular & skeletal: Weakness (combination therapy 17%; monotherapy 5%)

1% to 10%:

- Cardiovascular: Edema (combination therapy 3%; monotherapy 1%)
- Central nervous system: Drowsiness (combination therapy 3%; monotherapy 2%)
- Dermatologic: Skin rash (monotherapy 1%)
- Endocrine & metabolic: Gynecomastia (monotherapy 1% to 2%)
- Genitourinary: Decreased ejaculate volume (monotherapy 2% to 4%), breast tenderness (monotherapy ≤1%)
- Respiratory: Dyspnea (combination therapy 2%; monotherapy 1%), rhinitis (combination therapy 2%; monotherapy 1%)

<1% (Limited to important or life-threatening): Altered mental status, decreased testicular size, depression, disturbed sleep, hypersensitivity (pruritus, skin rash, urticaria, facial swelling, swelling of the lips), male infertility (temporary), malignant neoplasm of the male breast, prostate cancer - high grade, prostatitis, reduction in penile curvature, reduction in penile size, sexual disorder (may not be reversible with discontinuation), testicular pain

Drug Interactions

Metabolism/Transport Effects Substrate of CYP3A4 (minor); **Note:** Assignment of Major/Minor substrate status based on clinically relevant drug interaction potential

Avoid Concomitant Use There are no known interactions where it is recommended to avoid concomitant use.

Increased Effect/Toxicity There are no known significant interactions involving an increase in effect.

Decreased Effect There are no known significant interactions involving a decrease in effect.

Ethanol/Nutrition/Herb Interactions Herb/Nutraceutical: St John's wort may decrease finasteride levels. Avoid saw palmetto (concurrent use has not been adequately studied).

Storage/Stability

Propecia®: Store at 15°C to 30°C (59°F to 86°F). Protect from moisture.

Proscar®: Store below 30°C (86°F). Protect from light.

Mechanism of Action Finasteride is a competitive inhibitor of both tissue and hepatic 5-alpha reductase. This results in inhibition of the conversion of testosterone to dihydrotestosterone and markedly suppresses serum dihydrotestosterone levels

Pharmacodynamics/Kinetics

Onset of action: BPH: 6 months; Male pattern hair loss: ≥3 months of daily use

Duration:

- After a single oral dose as small as 0.5 mg: 65% depression of plasma dihydrotestosterone levels persists 5-7 days
- After 6 months of treatment with 5 mg/day: Circulating dihydrotestosterone levels are reduced to castrate levels without significant effects on circulating testosterone; levels return to normal within 14 days of discontinuation of treatment

Distribution: V_{dss}: 76 L

Protein binding: ~90%

Metabolism: Hepatic via CYP3A4; two active metabolites (<20% activity of finasteride)

Bioavailability: Mean: 65%

Half-life elimination, serum: 6 hours (range: 3-16 hours); Elderly: 8 hours (range: 6-15 hours)

Time to peak, serum: 1-2 hours

Excretion: Feces (57%) and urine (39%) as metabolites

Dosage Oral: Adults:

Males:

- Benign prostatic hyperplasia (Proscar®): 5 mg once daily as a single dose; clinical responses occur within 12 weeks to 6 months of initiation of therapy; long-term administration is recommended for maximal response
- Male pattern baldness (Propecia®): 1 mg daily

Female hirsutism (unlabeled use): 5 mg/day (Moghetti, 2000)

Dosing adjustment in renal impairment: No dosage adjustment is necessary

Dosing adjustment in hepatic impairment: Use with caution in patients with liver function abnormalities because finasteride is metabolized extensively in the liver

Dietary Considerations May be taken without regard to meals.

Administration May be administered without regard to meals. Women of childbearing age should not touch or handle broken tablets.

Hazardous agent; use appropriate precautions for handling and disposal (NIOSH, 2012).

Monitoring Parameters Objective and subjective signs of relief of benign prostatic hyperplasia, including improvement in urinary flow, reduction in symptoms of urgency, and relief of difficulty in micturition; for interpretation of serial PSAs, establish a new PSA baseline ≥6 months after treatment initiation and monitor PSA periodically thereafter. Finasteride does not interfere with free PSA levels.

Test Interactions PSA levels decrease in treated patients. After 6 months of therapy, PSA levels stabilize to a new baseline that is ~50% of pretreatment values. If following serial PSAs in a patient, re-establish a new baseline after ≥6 months of use.

Dosage Forms Excipient information presented when available (limited, particularly for generics); consult specific product labeling.

Tablet, Oral:

- Propecia: 1 mg
- Proscar: 5 mg [contains fd&c blue #2 aluminum lake]
- Generic: 1 mg, 5 mg

Fingolimod (fin GOL i mod)

Brand Names: U.S. Gilenya

Brand Names: Canada Gilenya®

Index Terms FTY720

Pharmacologic Category Sphingosine 1-Phosphate (S1P) Receptor Modulator

Use Treatment of relapsing forms of multiple sclerosis (MS) to reduce the frequency of clinical exacerbations and delay disability progression

Pregnancy Risk Factor C

Pregnancy Considerations Teratogenic and adverse effects have been observed in animal reproduction studies. Elimination of fingolimod takes approximately 2 months; to avoid potential fetal harm, women of childbearing potential should avoid pregnancy during and for 2 months after discontinuing treatment. Healthcare providers are encouraged to enroll pregnant women, or pregnant women may enroll themselves, in the Gilenya™ Pregnancy Registry (1-877-598-7237 or www.gilenyapregnancyregistry.com).

Breast-Feeding Considerations Due to the potential for serious adverse reactions in the nursing infant, breast-feeding is not recommended.

Medication Guide Available Yes

Contraindications Baseline QT_c interval ≥500 msec; concurrent use of a class Ia or III antiarrhythmic; Mobitz Type II second- or third-degree AV block or sick sinus syndrome (unless patient has functioning pacemaker); any of the following within 6 months prior to treatment initiation: MI, unstable angina, stroke, TIA, decompensated heart failure (requiring hospitalization) or NYHA class III/IV heart failure

Canadian labeling: Hypersensitivity to fingolimod or any component of the formulation; patients at increased risk for opportunistic infections (eg, immunosuppressed patients); severe active infections, active chronic bacterial, fungal or viral infections; known active malignancy (excluding basal cell carcinoma); severe hepatic impairment (Child-Pugh class C)

Warnings/Precautions Increased blood pressure may occur ~1 month after initiation of therapy; monitor blood pressure throughout treatment. Therapy may result in transient AV conduction delays; recurrence may be observed following discontinuation (>2 weeks) and subsequent resumption of therapy. Decreased heart rate may occur with initiation of therapy. **Initiation must occur in a setting with resources and personnel capable of appropriately managing symptomatic bradycardia.** Following the first dose, heart rate may decrease as soon as 1 hour postdose with the maximal decrease usually occurring ~6 hours postdose. Heart rate typically returns to baseline after 1 month of therapy. Due to the risk of bradycardia and AV conduction delays, ECG is required prior to initiation of therapy and after the initial observation period (6 hours) in all patients. Patients receiving concomitant antiarrhythmics including beta blockers and calcium channel blockers; patients with a prolonged QT interval at baseline (males: >450 msec; females: >470 msec), who develop QT prolongation during the first 6 hours of treatment initiation, or are at an increased risk of QT prolongation (eg, hypokalemia, hypomagnesemia, concomitant QT-prolonging drugs, congenital long-QT syndrome); or with other cardiac risk factors (eg, AV block, sick sinus syndrome, ischemic cardiac disease, heart failure, cerebrovascular disease, recurrent syncope, severe sleep apnea [untreated]), unless contraindicated, require continuous overnight ECG monitoring in a medical facility after the first dose.

May increase risk of infection due to dose-dependent reduction of lymphocytes; lymphocyte counts may be decreased for up to 2 months following discontinuation of therapy. Do not initiate treatment in patients with acute or chronic infections until the infection has resolved. Use with caution in patients receiving concomitant immunosuppressant, immune modulating, or antineoplastic medications.

Use with caution and closely monitor patients with severe hepatic impairment (contraindicated in the Canadian labeling). Macular edema may occur; use with caution in patients with a history of diabetes mellitus or uveitis. Ophthalmologic exams should be performed prior to therapy and 3-4 months after treatment initiation; more frequent examination is warranted in patients with diabetes or a history of uveitis. Reductions of FEV_1 and diffusion lung capacity for carbon monoxide (DLCO) are dose-dependent and may occur within the first month of therapy. FEV_1 changes may be reversible with drug discontinuation.

Consider varicella zoster virus (VZV) vaccination prior to initiation of treatment in VZV antibody negative patients; postpone fingolimod treatment for 1 month after varicella zoster vaccination.

Adverse Reactions

>10%:

- Central nervous system: Headache (25%)
- Gastrointestinal: Diarrhea (12%)
- Hepatic: ALT increased (14%), AST increased (14%)
- Neuromuscular & skeletal: Back pain (12%)
- Miscellaneous: Flu-like syndrome (13%)

1% to 10%:

- Cardiovascular: Hypertension (6%), bradycardia (4%)
- Central nervous system: Depression (8%), dizziness (7%), migraine (5%)
- Dermatologic: Alopecia (4%), eczema (3%), pruritus (3%)
- Endocrine & metabolic: Triglycerides increased (3%)
- Gastrointestinal: Gastroenteritis (5%), weight loss (5%)
- Hematologic: Lymphopenia (4%), leukopenia (3%)
- Hepatic: GGT increased (5%)
- Neuromuscular & skeletal: Paresthesia (5%), weakness (3%)
- Ocular: Blurred vision (4%), eye pain (3%)
- Respiratory: Cough (10%), bronchitis (8%), dyspnea (8%), sinusitis (7%)
- Miscellaneous: Herpes infection (9%), tinea infection (4%)

<1% (Limited to important or life-threatening): Asystole, AV block, death, lymphoma, macular edema (incidence increased in patients with uveitis or diabetes mellitus), QT prolongation, syncope

Drug Interactions

Metabolism/Transport Effects Substrate of CYP2D6 (minor), CYP2E1 (minor), CYP3A4 (minor); **Note:** Assignment of Major/Minor substrate status based on clinically relevant drug interaction potential

Avoid Concomitant Use

Avoid concomitant use of Fingolimod with any of the following: Antiarrhythmic Agents (Class Ia); Antiarrhythmic Agents (Class III); BCG; Highest Risk QTc-Prolonging Agents; Ivabradine; Mifepristone; Natalizumab; Pimecrolimus; Tacrolimus (Topical); Tofacitinib; Vaccines (Live)

Increased Effect/Toxicity

Fingolimod may increase the levels/effects of: Antiarrhythmic Agents (Class Ia); Antiarrhythmic Agents (Class III); Highest Risk QTc-Prolonging Agents; Leflunomide; Moderate Risk QTc-Prolonging Agents; Natalizumab; Tofacitinib; Vaccines (Live)

The levels/effects of Fingolimod may be increased by: Beta-Blockers; Denosumab; Diltiazem; Ivabradine; Ketoconazole (Systemic); Mifepristone; Pimecrolimus; QTc-Prolonging Agents (Indeterminate Risk and Risk Modifying); Roflumilast; Tacrolimus (Topical); Trastuzumab; Verapamil

Decreased Effect

Fingolimod may decrease the levels/effects of: BCG; Coccidioidin Skin Test; Sipuleucel-T; Vaccines (Inactivated); Vaccines (Live)

The levels/effects of Fingolimod may be decreased by: Echinacea; Peginterferon Alfa-2b

Storage/Stability Store at 25°C (77°F); excursions permitted to 15°C to 30°C (59°F to 86°F).

Mechanism of Action Fingolimod-phosphate, active metabolite of fingolimod, binds to sphingosine 1-phosphate receptors 1, 3, 4, and 5. The amount of lymphocytes available to the central nervous system are decreased which reduces central inflammation.

Pharmacodynamics/Kinetics

Distribution: V_d: 1200 ± 260 L: distributes into red blood cells (86%)

Protein binding: >99.7% (fingolimod and fingolimod-phosphate)

Metabolism: Hepatic via CYP4F2 to fingolimod-phosphate (active) and other metabolites (inactive); CYP2D6, 2E1, 3A4, and 4F12 also contribute to metabolism

Bioavailability: 93%

Half-life elimination: 6-9 days

Time to peak, plasma: 12-16 hours

Excretion: Urine (~81% as inactive metabolites); feces (fingolimod and fingolimod phosphate: <2.5% of dose)

Dosage Oral: Adults: Multiple sclerosis: 0.5 mg once daily; doses >0.5 mg/day associated with increased adverse events and no additional benefit

Dosage adjustment in renal impairment: No dosage adjustment necessary.

Dosage adjustment in hepatic impairment:

Mild-to-moderate impairment: No dosage adjustment necessary.

Severe impairment: No dosage adjustment provided in the manufacturer's labeling; use with caution and closely monitor; exposure is doubled in severe hepatic impairment. Use is contraindicated in the Canadian labeling.

Dietary Considerations May be taken with or without food.

Administration May be administered with or without food.

Monitoring Parameters CBC (baseline and periodically thereafter); ECG (baseline; repeat after initial dose observation period); heart rate, blood pressure and signs and symptoms of bradycardia (hourly for 6 hours following first dose; continued observation (until resolved) required if 6-hour postdose heart rate is either <45 bpm, is lowest post-baseline measurement, or new-onset second degree or higher AV block occurs on repeat ECG); continuous (until symptoms resolved) ECG monitoring if postdose symptomatic bradycardia occurs (overnight continuous ECG in a medical facility and repeat observation period for second dose if pharmacologic intervention for bradycardia necessary)

Initial monitoring procedures (ECG, heart rate, blood pressure) must be repeated for

- treatment interruption of ≥1 day during the first 2 weeks after treatment initiation, or
- treatment interruption of >7 days during weeks 3-4 after treatment initiation, or
- treatment interruption of >14 days after ≥1 month of treatment initiation

Ophthalmologic exam at baseline and 3-4 months after initiation of treatment (continue periodic examinations for duration of therapy in patients with diabetes or history of uveitis); baseline AST/ALT (obtained ≤6 months prior to treatment initiation) and bilirubin, repeat if clinically indicated; respiratory function (FEV_1, DLCO); VZV antibodies (patients with no history of chickenpox or previous VZV vaccination)

Dosage Forms Excipient information presented when available (limited, particularly for generics); consult specific product labeling.

Capsule, Oral:

Gilenya: 0.5 mg

- ◆ **Fioricet** *see* Butalbital, Acetaminophen, and Caffeine *on page 305*
- ◆ **Fiorinal®** *see* Butalbital, Aspirin, and Caffeine *on page 305*
- ◆ **Firazyr** *see* Icatibant *on page 1038*
- ◆ **Firmagon** *see* Degarelix *on page 564*
- ◆ **Firmagon® (Can)** *see* Degarelix *on page 564*
- ◆ **First-Hydrocortisone** *see* Hydrocortisone (Topical) *on page 1011*
- ◆ **First-Lansoprazole** *see* Lansoprazole *on page 1170*
- ◆ **First-Omeprazole** *see* Omeprazole *on page 1505*
- ◆ **First-Progesterone VGS 25** *see* Progesterone *on page 1725*
- ◆ **First-Progesterone VGS 50** *see* Progesterone *on page 1725*
- ◆ **First-Progesterone VGS 100** *see* Progesterone *on page 1725*
- ◆ **First-Progesterone VGS 200** *see* Progesterone *on page 1725*
- ◆ **First-Progesterone VGS 400** *see* Progesterone *on page 1725*
- ◆ **First-Testosterone** *see* Testosterone *on page 2026*
- ◆ **First-Testosterone MC** *see* Testosterone *on page 2026*
- ◆ **Fisalamine** *see* Mesalamine *on page 1305*
- ◆ **Fish Oil** *see* Omega-3-Acid Ethyl Esters *on page 1504*
- ◆ **FK228** *see* RomiDEPsin *on page 1848*
- ◆ **FK506** *see* Tacrolimus (Systemic) *on page 1976*
- ◆ **Flagyl** *see* MetroNIDAZOLE (Systemic) *on page 1351*
- ◆ **Flagyl ER** *see* MetroNIDAZOLE (Systemic) *on page 1351*
- ◆ **Flamazine® (Can)** *see* Silver Sulfadiazine *on page 1897*
- ◆ **Flanax Pain Relief [OTC]** *see* Naproxen *on page 1425*
- ◆ **Flarex** *see* Fluorometholone *on page 882*
- ◆ **Flarex® (Can)** *see* Fluorometholone *on page 882*

FlavoxATE (fla VOKS ate)

Brand Names: Canada Apo-Flavoxate®; Urispas®

Index Terms Flavoxate Hydrochloride; Urispas

Pharmacologic Category Antispasmodic Agent, Urinary

Additional Appendix Information

Beers Criteria – Potentially Inappropriate Medications for Geriatrics *on page 2368*

Use Antispasmodic to provide symptomatic relief of dysuria, nocturia, suprapubic pain, urgency, and incontinence in patients with cystitis, urethritis, urethrocystitis, urethrotrigonitis, and prostatitis

Pregnancy Risk Factor B

Dosage Children >12 years and Adults: Oral: 100-200 mg 3-4 times daily; reduce the dose when symptoms improve

Dosage adjustment in renal impairment: No dosage adjustment provided in manufacturer's labeling.

Dosage adjustment in hepatic impairment: No dosage adjustment provided in manufacturer's labeling.

Additional Information Complete prescribing information should be consulted for additional detail.

Dosage Forms Excipient information presented when available (limited, particularly for generics); consult specific product labeling.

Tablet, Oral, as hydrochloride:

Generic: 100 mg

◆ **Flavoxate Hydrochloride** *see* FlavoxATE *on page 865*

◆ **Flebogamma** *see* Immune Globulin *on page 1059*

◆ **Flebogamma DIF** *see* Immune Globulin *on page 1059*

Flecainide (fle KAY nide)

Brand Names: U.S. Tambocor [DSC]

Brand Names: Canada Apo-Flecainide®; Tambocor™

Index Terms Flecainide Acetate

Pharmacologic Category Antiarrhythmic Agent, Class Ic

Additional Appendix Information

Beers Criteria – Potentially Inappropriate Medications for Geriatrics *on page 2368*

Use Prevention and suppression of documented life-threatening ventricular arrhythmias (eg, sustained ventricular tachycardia); controlling symptomatic, disabling supraventricular tachycardias in patients without structural heart disease in whom other agents fail

Pregnancy Risk Factor C

Pregnancy Considerations Adverse events have been observed in some animal reproduction studies.

Breast-Feeding Considerations Flecainide is excreted in human breast milk at concentrations as high as 4 times corresponding plasma levels.

Contraindications Hypersensitivity to flecainide or any component of the formulation; pre-existing second- or third-degree AV block or with right bundle branch block when associated with a left hemiblock (bifascicular block) (except in patients with a functioning artificial pacemaker); cardiogenic shock; coronary artery disease (based on CAST study results); concurrent use of ritonavir or amprenavir

Warnings/Precautions [U.S. Boxed Warning]: In the Cardiac Arrhythmia Suppression Trial (CAST), recent (>6 days but <2 years ago) myocardial infarction patients with asymptomatic, non-life-threatening ventricular arrhythmias did not benefit and may have been harmed by attempts to suppress the arrhythmia with flecainide or encainide. An increased mortality or nonfatal cardiac arrest rate (7.7%) was seen in the active treatment group compared with patients in the placebo group (3%). The applicability of the CAST results to other populations is unknown. The risks of class 1C agents and the lack of improved survival make use in patients without life-threatening arrhythmias generally unacceptable. **[U.S. Boxed Warning]: Watch for proarrhythmic effects;** monitor and adjust dose to prevent QT_c prolongation. Not recommended for patients with chronic atrial fibrillation. In the treatment of atrial fibrillation in the elderly, avoid antiarrhythmics as first-line treatment. In older adults, data suggests rate control may provide more benefits than risks compared to rhythm control for most patients (Beers Criteria). **[U.S. Boxed Warning]: When treating atrial flutter, 1:1 atrioventricular conduction may occur; pre-emptive negative chronotropic therapy (eg, digoxin, beta-blockers) may lower the risk.** Pre-existing hypokalemia or hyperkalemia should be corrected before initiation (can alter drug's effect). A worsening or new arrhythmia may occur (proarrhythmic effect). Use caution in heart failure (may precipitate or exacerbate HF). Dose-related increases in PR, QRS, and QT intervals occur. Use with caution in sick sinus syndrome or with permanent pacemakers or temporary pacing wires (can increase endocardial pacing thresholds). Cautious use in significant hepatic impairment.

Adverse Reactions

>10%:

Central nervous system: Dizziness (19% to 30%)

Ocular: Visual disturbances (16%)

Respiratory: Dyspnea (~10%)

1% to 10%:

Cardiovascular: Palpitation (6%), chest pain (5%), edema (3.5%), tachycardia (1% to 3%), proarrhythmic (4% to 12%), sinus node dysfunction (1.2%), syncope

Central nervous system: Headache (4% to 10%), fatigue (8%), nervousness (5%) additional symptoms occurring at a frequency between 1% and 3%: fever, malaise, hypoesthesia, paresis, ataxia, vertigo, somnolence, tinnitus, anxiety, insomnia, depression

Dermatologic: Rash (1% to 3%)

Gastrointestinal: Nausea (9%), constipation (1%), abdominal pain (3%), anorexia (1% to 3%), diarrhea (0.7% to 3%)

Neuromuscular & skeletal: Tremor (5%), weakness (5%), paresthesia (1%)

Ocular: Diplopia (1% to 3%), blurred vision

<1% (Limited to important or life-threatening): Alopecia, alters pacing threshold, amnesia, angina, AV block, bradycardia, bronchospasm, CHF, corneal deposits, depersonalization, euphoria, exfoliative dermatitis, granulocytopenia, heart block, increased P-R, leukopenia, metallic taste, neuropathy, paradoxical increase in ventricular rate in atrial fibrillation/flutter, paresthesia, photophobia, pneumonitis, pruritus, QRS duration, swollen lips/tongue/mouth, tardive dyskinesia, thrombocytopenia, urinary retention, urticaria, ventricular arrhythmia

Drug Interactions

Metabolism/Transport Effects Substrate of CYP1A2 (minor), CYP2D6 (major); **Note:** Assignment of Major/Minor substrate status based on clinically relevant drug interaction potential; **Inhibits** CYP2D6 (weak)

Avoid Concomitant Use

Avoid concomitant use of Flecainide with any of the following: Fosamprenavir; Highest Risk QTc-Prolonging Agents; Ivabradine; Mifepristone; Ritonavir; Saquinavir; Tipranavir

Increased Effect/Toxicity

Flecainide may increase the levels/effects of: ARIPiprazole; Digoxin; Highest Risk QTc-Prolonging Agents; Moderate Risk QTc-Prolonging Agents

The levels/effects of Flecainide may be increased by: Abiraterone Acetate; Amiodarone; Boceprevir; Carbonic Anhydrase Inhibitors; CYP2D6 Inhibitors (Moderate); CYP2D6 Inhibitors (Strong); Darunavir; Fosamprenavir; Ivabradine; Mifepristone; Mirabegron; QTc-Prolonging Agents (Indeterminate Risk and Risk Modifying); Ritonavir; Saquinavir; Sodium Bicarbonate; Sodium Lactate; Telaprevir; Tipranavir; Tromethamine; Verapamil

Decreased Effect

The levels/effects of Flecainide may be decreased by: Etravirine; Peginterferon Alfa-2b; Sodium Bicarbonate

Ethanol/Nutrition/Herb Interactions Food: Clearance may be decreased in patients following strict vegetarian diets due to urinary pH ≥8. Dairy products (milk, infant formula, yogurt) may interfere with the absorption of flecainide in infants; there is one case report of a neonate (GA 34 weeks PNA >6 days) who required extremely large doses of oral flecainide when administered every 8 hours with feedings ("milk feeds"); changing the feedings from "milk feeds" to 5% glucose feeds alone resulted in a doubling of the flecainide serum concentration and toxicity.

Mechanism of Action Class Ic antiarrhythmic; slows conduction in cardiac tissue by altering transport of ions across cell membranes; causes slight prolongation of refractory periods; decreases the rate of rise of the action potential without affecting its duration; increases electrical stimulation threshold of ventricle, His-Purkinje system;

possesses local anesthetic and moderate negative inotropic effects

Pharmacodynamics/Kinetics

Absorption: Oral: Rapid

Distribution: Adults: V_d: 5-13.4 L/kg

Protein binding: $Alpha_1$ acid glycoprotein: 40% to 50%

Metabolism: Hepatic

Bioavailability: 85% to 90%

Half-life elimination: Infants: 11-12 hours; Children: 8 hours; Adults: 7-22 hours, increased with congestive heart failure or renal dysfunction; End-stage renal disease: 19-26 hours

Time to peak, serum: ~1.5-3 hours

Excretion: Urine (80% to 90%, 10% to 50% as unchanged drug and metabolites)

Dosage Oral:

Children:

Initial: 3 mg/kg/day or 50-100 mg/m²/day in 3 divided doses

Usual: 3-6 mg/kg/day or 100-150 mg/m²/day in 3 divided doses; up to 11 mg/kg/day or 200 mg/m²/day for uncontrolled patients with subtherapeutic levels

Adults:

Life-threatening ventricular arrhythmias:

Initial: 100 mg every 12 hours

Increase by 50-100 mg/day (given in 2 doses/day) every 4 days; maximum: 400 mg/day.

Use of higher initial doses and more rapid dosage adjustments have resulted in an increased incidence of proarrhythmic events and congestive heart failure, particularly during the first few days. Do not use a loading dose. Use very cautiously in patients with history of congestive heart failure or myocardial infarction.

Prevention of paroxysmal supraventricular arrhythmias in patients with disabling symptoms but no structural heart disease: Initial: 50 mg every 12 hours; increase by 50 mg twice daily at 4-day intervals; maximum: 300 mg/day

Paroxysmal atrial fibrillation: Outpatient: "Pill-in-the-pocket" dose (unlabeled dose): 200 mg (weight <70 kg), 300 mg (weight ≥70 kg). May not repeat in ≤24 hours. **Note:** An initial inpatient conversion trial should have been successful before sending patient home on this approach. Patient must be taking an AV nodal-blocking agent (eg, beta-blocker, nondihydropyridine calcium channel blocker) prior to initiation of antiarrhythmic.

Dosing adjustment in severe renal impairment: GFR ≤50 mL/minute: Decrease dose by 50%; dose increases should be made cautiously at intervals >4 days and serum levels monitored frequently.

Hemodialysis: No supplemental dose recommended.

Peritoneal dialysis: No supplemental dose recommended.

Dosing adjustment/comments in hepatic impairment: Monitoring of plasma levels is recommended because of significantly increased half-life.

When transferring from another antiarrhythmic agent, allow for 2-4 half-lives of the agent to pass before initiating flecainide therapy.

Administration Administer around-the-clock to promote less variation in peak and trough serum levels

Monitoring Parameters ECG, blood pressure, pulse, periodic serum concentrations, especially in patients with renal or hepatic impairment

Reference Range Therapeutic: 0.2-1 mcg/mL; pediatric patients may respond at the lower end of the recommended therapeutic range

Dosage Forms Excipient information presented when available (limited, particularly for generics); consult specific product labeling. [DSC] = Discontinued product

Tablet, Oral, as acetate:

Tambocor: 50 mg [DSC], 100 mg [DSC], 150 mg [DSC]

Generic: 50 mg, 100 mg, 150 mg

Extemporaneous Preparations A 20 mg/mL oral liquid suspension may be made from tablets and one of three different vehicles (cherry syrup, a 1:1 mixture of Ora-Sweet® and Ora-Plus®, or a 1:1 mixture of Ora-Sweet® SF and Ora-Plus®). Crush twenty-four 100 mg tablets in a mortar and reduce to a fine powder. Add 20 mL of the chosen vehicle and mix to a uniform paste; mix while adding the vehicle in incremental proportions to **almost** 120 mL; transfer to a calibrated bottle, rinse mortar with vehicle, and add quantity of vehicle sufficient to make 120 mL. Label "shake well" and "protect from light". Stable for 60 days when stored in amber plastic prescription bottles in the dark at room temperature or refrigerated.

Allen LV and Erickson III MA, "Stability of Baclofen, Captopril, Diltiazem, Hydrochloride, Dipyridamole, and Flecainide Acetate in Extemporaneously Compounded Oral Liquids," *Am J Health Syst Pharm*, 1996, 53:2179-84.

- **Flecainide Acetate** *see* Flecainide *on page 866*
- **Fleet Bisacodyl [OTC]** *see* Bisacodyl *on page 259*
- **Fleet Enema [OTC]** *see* Sodium Phosphates *on page 1923*
- **Fleet Enema (Can)** *see* Sodium Phosphates *on page 1923*
- **Fleet Enema Extra [OTC]** *see* Sodium Phosphates *on page 1923*
- **Fleet Laxative [OTC]** *see* Bisacodyl *on page 259*
- **Fleet Pedia-Lax Enema [OTC]** *see* Sodium Phosphates *on page 1923*
- **Flexbumin** *see* Albumin *on page 59*
- **Flexeril [DSC]** *see* Cyclobenzaprine *on page 502*
- **Flolan** *see* Epoprostenol *on page 727*
- **Flomax** *see* Tamsulosin *on page 1990*
- **Flomax® CR (Can)** *see* Tamsulosin *on page 1990*
- **Flonase** *see* Fluticasone (Nasal) *on page 896*
- **Flonase® (Can)** *see* Fluticasone (Nasal) *on page 896*
- **Flo-Pred** *see* PrednisoLONE (Systemic) *on page 1704*
- **Florical [OTC]** *see* Calcium Carbonate *on page 318*
- **Florinef** *see* Fludrocortisone *on page 875*
- **Florinef® (Can)** *see* Fludrocortisone *on page 875*
- **Flovent** *see* Fluticasone (Oral Inhalation) *on page 893*
- **Flovent Diskus** *see* Fluticasone (Oral Inhalation) *on page 893*
- **Flovent® Diskus® (Can)** *see* Fluticasone (Oral Inhalation) *on page 893*
- **Flovent HFA** *see* Fluticasone (Oral Inhalation) *on page 893*
- **Flovent® HFA (Can)** *see* Fluticasone (Oral Inhalation) *on page 893*
- **Floxin Otic Singles** *see* Ofloxacin (Otic) *on page 1492*
- **Fluad (Can)** *see* Influenza Virus Vaccine (Inactivated) *on page 1078*
- **Fluarix** *see* Influenza Virus Vaccine (Inactivated) *on page 1078*
- **Fluarix Quadrivalent** *see* Influenza Virus Vaccine (Inactivated) *on page 1078*
- **Flubenisolone** *see* Betamethasone *on page 247*
- **Flucaine** *see* Proparacaine and Fluorescein *on page 1734*

◆ **Flucelvax** *see* Influenza Virus Vaccine (Inactivated) *on page 1078*

◆ **Flucinom** *see* Flutamide *on page 892*

Fluconazole (floo KOE na zole)

Brand Names: U.S. Diflucan

Brand Names: Canada Apo-Fluconazole®; CanesOral®; CO Fluconazole; Diflucan®; Dom-Fluconazole; Fluconazole Injection; Fluconazole Omega; Monicure; Mylan-Fluconazole; Novo-Fluconazole; PHL-Fluconazole; PMS-Fluconazole; PRO-Fluconazole; Riva-Fluconazole; Taro-Fluconazole; ZYM-Fluconazole

Pharmacologic Category Antifungal Agent, Oral; Antifungal Agent, Parenteral

Additional Appendix Information

Antifungal Agents *on page 2286*

Dosing Considerations for the Critically-Ill Patient With Morbid Obesity *on page 2379*

Use Treatment of candidiasis (esophageal, oropharyngeal, peritoneal, urinary tract, vaginal); systemic candida infections (eg, candidemia, disseminated candidiasis, and pneumonia); cryptococcal meningitis; antifungal prophylaxis in allogeneic bone marrow transplant recipients

Unlabeled Use Cryptococcal pneumonia; candidal intertrigo

Pregnancy Risk Factor C (single dose for vaginal candidiasis)/D (all other indications)

Pregnancy Considerations Adverse events have been observed in some animal reproduction studies. When used in high doses, fluconazole is teratogenic in animal studies. Following exposure during the first trimester, case reports have noted similar malformations in humans when used in higher doses (400 mg/day) over extended periods of time (Aleck, 1997). Abnormalities reported include abnormal facies, abnormal calvarial development, arthrogryposis, brachycephaly, cleft palate, congenital heart disease, femoral bowing, thin ribs and long bones. Use of lower doses (150 mg as a single dose) does not suggest an increase risk to the fetus. Most azole antifungals, including fluconazole, are recommended to be avoided during pregnancy (Pappas, 2009).

Breast-Feeding Considerations Fluconazole is excreted in breast milk. The manufacturer recommends that caution be exercised when administering fluconazole to nursing women. Fluconazole is found in breast milk at concentrations similar to maternal plasma.

Contraindications Hypersensitivity to fluconazole or any component of the formulation (cross-reaction with other azole antifungal agents may occur, but has not been established; use caution); coadministration of terfenadine in patients receiving multiple doses of 400 mg or higher or with CYP3A4 substrates which may lead to QT_c prolongation (eg, astemizole, cisapride, pimozide, or quinidine)

Warnings/Precautions Serious (and sometimes fatal) hepatic toxicity (eg, hepatitis, cholestasis, fulminant hepatic failure) has been observed. Use with caution in patients with renal and hepatic dysfunction or previous hepatotoxicity from other azole derivatives. Patients who develop abnormal liver function tests during fluconazole therapy should be monitored closely and discontinued if symptoms consistent with liver disease develop. Rare exfoliative skin disorders have been observed; monitor closely if rash develops and discontinue if lesions progress. Cases of QT_c prolongation and torsade de pointes associated with fluconazole use have been reported (usually high dose or in combination with agents known to prolong the QT interval); use caution in patients with concomitant medications or conditions which are arrhythmogenic. Potentially significant drug-drug interactions may exist, requiring dose or frequency adjustment, additional monitoring, and/or selection of alternative therapy. May occasionally cause dizziness or seizures; use caution driving or operating machines. Powder for oral suspension contains sucrose; use caution with fructose intolerance, sucrose-isomaltase deficiency, or glucose-galactose malabsorption.

Adverse Reactions Frequency not always defined.

Cardiovascular: Angioedema (rare)

Central nervous system: Headache (2% to 13%), dizziness (1%)

Dermatologic: Rash (2%)

Gastrointestinal: Nausea (2% to 7%), abdominal pain (2% to 6%), vomiting (2% to 5%), diarrhea (2% to 3%), dysgeusia (1%), dyspepsia (1%)

Hepatic: Alkaline phosphatase increased, ALT increased, AST increased, hepatic failure (rare), hepatitis, jaundice

Miscellaneous: Anaphylactic reactions (rare)

Postmarketing and/or case reports: Agranulocytosis, alopecia, cholestasis, diaphoresis, drug eruption, exanthematous pustulosis, fatigue, fever, hypercholesterolemia, hypertriglyceridemia, hypokalemia, insomnia, leukopenia, malaise, myalgia, neutropenia, paresthesia, QT prolongation, seizure, somnolence, Stevens-Johnson syndrome, thrombocytopenia, torsade de pointes, toxic epidermal necrolysis, tremor, vertigo, weakness, xerostomia

Drug Interactions

Metabolism/Transport Effects Inhibits CYP1A2 (weak), CYP2C19 (strong), CYP2C9 (moderate), CYP3A4 (moderate)

Avoid Concomitant Use

Avoid concomitant use of Fluconazole with any of the following: Bosutinib; Cisapride; Citalopram; Conivaptan; Dofetilide; Highest Risk QTc-Prolonging Agents; Ibrutinib; Ivabradine; Lomitapide; Mifepristone; Ospemifene; Pimozide; QuiNIDine; Ranolazine; Simeprevir; Tolvaptan; Ulipristal; Voriconazole

Increased Effect/Toxicity

Fluconazole may increase the levels/effects of: Alfentanil; ARIPiprazole; AtorvaSTATin; Avanafil; Benzodiazepines (metabolized by oxidation); Bosentan; Bosutinib; Budesonide (Systemic, Oral Inhalation); BusPIRone; Busulfan; Calcium Channel Blockers; CarBAMazepine; Carvedilol; Cilostazol; Cisapride; Citalopram; Colchicine; Conivaptan; Corticosteroids (Systemic); CycloSPORINE (Systemic); CYP2C19 Substrates; CYP2C9 Substrates; CYP3A4 Substrates; DOCEtaxel; Dofetilide; Eletriptan; Eplerenone; Etravirine; Everolimus; FentaNYL; Fluvastatin; Fosphenytoin; Highest Risk QTc-Prolonging Agents; Ibrutinib; Imatinib; Irbesartan; Irinotecan; Ivacaftor; Lomitapide; Losartan; Lovastatin; Lurasidone; Macrolide Antibiotics; Methadone; Moderate Risk QTc-Prolonging Agents; Nevirapine; Ospemifene; OxyCODONE; Phenytoin; Pimecrolimus; Pimozide; Proton Pump Inhibitors; QuiNIDine; Ramelteon; Ranolazine; Red Yeast Rice; Rifamycin Derivatives; Salmeterol; Saxagliptin; Sildenafil; Simeprevir; Simvastatin; Sirolimus; Solifenacin; Sulfonylureas; SUNItinib; Tacrolimus (Systemic); Tacrolimus (Topical); Tadalafil; Temsirolimus; Tipranavir; Tofacitinib; Tolterodine; Tolvaptan; Ulipristal; Vardenafil; Vilazodone; Vitamin K Antagonists; Voriconazole; Zidovudine; Zolpidem

The levels/effects of Fluconazole may be increased by: Etravirine; Ivabradine; Macrolide Antibiotics; Mifepristone; QTc-Prolonging Agents (Indeterminate Risk and Risk Modifying)

Decreased Effect

Fluconazole may decrease the levels/effects of: Amphotericin B; Clopidogrel; Ifosfamide; Saccharomyces boulardii

The levels/effects of Fluconazole may be decreased by: Didanosine; Etravirine; Rifamycin Derivatives

Storage/Stability

Tablet: Store at <30°C (86°F).

Powder for oral suspension: Store dry powder at <30°C (86°F). Following reconstitution, store at 5°C to 30°C (41°F to 86°F). Discard unused portion after 2 weeks. Do not freeze.

Injection: Store injection in glass at 5°C to 30°C (41°F to 86°F). Store injection in plastic flexible containers at 5°C to 25°C (41°F to 77°F). Brief exposure of up to 40°C (104°F) does not adversely affect the product. Do not freeze. Do not unwrap unit until ready for use.

Mechanism of Action Interferes with fungal cytochrome P450 activity (lanosterol 14-α-demethylase), decreasing ergosterol synthesis (principal sterol in fungal cell membrane) and inhibiting cell membrane formation

Pharmacodynamics/Kinetics

Distribution: V_d: ~0.6 L/kg; widely throughout body with good penetration into CSF, eye, peritoneal fluid, sputum, skin, and urine

Relative diffusion blood into CSF: Adequate with or without inflammation (exceeds usual MICs)

CSF:blood level ratio: Normal meninges: 50% to 90%; Inflamed meninges: ~80%

Protein binding, plasma: 11% to 12%

Bioavailability: Oral: >90%

Half-life elimination: Normal renal function: ~30 hours (range: 20-50 hours); Elderly: ~46 hours

Time to peak, serum: Oral: 1-2 hours

Excretion: Urine (80% as unchanged drug)

Dosage The daily dose of fluconazole is the same for oral and I.V. administration

Usual dosage ranges: Oral, I.V:

Children: Loading dose: 6-12 mg/kg/dose; maintenance: 3-12 mg/kg/dose once daily; duration and dosage depend on location and severity of infection

Adults: 150 mg once **or** Loading dose: 200-800 mg; maintenance: 200-800 mg once daily; duration and dosage depend on location and severity of infection

Indication-specific dosing:

Children:

Candidiasis: Oral, I.V.:

Esophageal:

Manufacturer's recommendation: Loading dose: 6 mg/kg/dose; maintenance: 3-12 mg/kg/dose once daily for 21 days and for at least 2 weeks following resolution of symptoms (maximum: 600 mg/day)

HIV-exposed/-infected: Loading dose: 6 mg/kg/dose once on day 1; maintenance: 3-6 mg/kg/dose once daily for 4-21 days (maximum: 400 mg/day) (CDC, 2009)

Relapse suppression (HIV-exposed/-infected): 3-6 mg/kg/dose once daily (maximum: 200 mg/day) (CDC, 2009)

Invasive disease (alternative therapy): 5-6 mg/kg/dose every 12 hours for ≥28 days (maximum: 600 mg/day) (CDC, 2009)

Oropharyngeal:

Manufacturer's recommendation: Loading dose: 6 mg/kg/dose; maintenance: 3 mg/kg/dose once daily for ≥2 weeks (maximum: 600 mg/day)

HIV-exposed/-infected: 3-6 mg/kg/dose once daily for 7-14 days (maximum: 400 mg/day) (CDC, 2009)

Coccidiodomycosis: Oral, I.V.: *Meningeal infection, or in a stable patient with diffuse pulmonary or disseminated disease* (HIV-exposed/-infected):

Treatment: 5-6 mg/kg/dose twice daily (maximum daily dose: 800 mg/**day**) (CDC, 2009), followed by chronic suppressive therapy (see below)

Relapse suppression: 6 mg/kg/dose once daily (maximum daily dose: 400 mg/**day**) (CDC, 2009)

Cryptococcosis: Oral, I.V.:

Manufacturer's recommendation: Meningitis: 12 mg/kg/dose for 1 dose, then 6-12 mg/kg/day for 10-12 weeks following negative CSF culture

HIV-exposed/-infected:

CNS disease (alternative therapy in patients intolerant of amphotericin B): Induction: 12 mg/kg/dose for 1 dose, then 6-12 mg/kg/day (maximum: 800 mg/day) for ≥2 weeks (in combination with flucytosine) (CDC, 2009)

Consolidation: 10-12 mg/kg/day for 8 weeks (Perfect, 2010) **or** 12 mg/kg/dose for 1 dose, then 6-12 mg/kg/day (maximum: 800 mg/day) for 8 weeks (CDC, 2009)

Maintenance (suppression): 6 mg/kg/day (maximum: 200 mg/day) (CDC, 2009; Perfect, 2010)

Non-CNS disease, disseminated (including severe pulmonary disease) (alternative therapy; unlabeled use): Induction: 12 mg/kg/dose for 1 dose, then 6-12 mg/kg/day (maximum: 600 mg/day) (CDC, 2009)

Non-CNS disease, localized (including isolated pulmonary disease) (unlabeled use): 12 mg/kg/dose for 1 dose, then 6-12 mg/kg/day (maximum: 600 mg/day). **Note:** Duration depends upon infection site and severity (CDC, 2009). For patients with pulmonary disease (not delineated by severity), the IDSA recommends a duration of 6-12 months (Perfect, 2010).

Adults:

Blastomycosis (unlabeled use): Oral: *CNS disease:* Consolidation: 800 mg daily for ≥12 months and until resolution of CSF abnormalities (Chapman, 2008)

Candidiasis: Oral, I.V.:

Candidemia (neutropenic and non-neutropenic): Loading dose: 800 mg (12 mg/kg) on day 1, then 400 mg daily (6 mg/kg/day) for 14 days after first negative blood culture and resolution of signs/symptoms. **Note:** Not recommended for patients with recent azole exposure, critical illness, or if *C. krusei* or *C. glabrata* are suspected (Pappas, 2009).

Chronic, disseminated: 400 mg daily (6 mg/kg/day) until calcification or lesion resolution (Pappas, 2009)

CNS candidiasis (alternative therapy): 400-800 mg daily (6-12 mg/kg/day) until CSF/radiological abnormalities resolved. **Note:** Recommended as alternative therapy in patients intolerant of amphotericin B (Pappas, 2009).

Endocarditis, prosthetic valve (unlabeled use): 400-800 mg daily (6-12 mg/kg/day) for 6 weeks after valve replacement (as step-down in stable, culture-negative patients); long-term suppression in absence of valve replacement: 400-800 mg daily (Pappas, 2009)

Endophthalmitis (unlabeled use): 400-800 mg daily (6-12 mg/kg/day) for 4-6 weeks until examination indicates resolution (Pappas, 2009)

Esophageal:

Manufacturer's recommendation: Loading dose: 200 mg on day 1, then maintenance dose of 100-400 mg daily for 21 days and for at least 2 weeks following resolution of symptoms

Alternative dosing: 200-400 mg daily for 14-21 days; suppressive therapy of 100-200 mg 3 times weekly may be used for recurrent infections (Pappas, 2009)

Intertrigo (unlabeled use): 50 mg daily or 150 mg once weekly (Coldiron, 1991; Nozickova, 1998; Stengel, 1994)

Oropharyngeal:
Manufacturer's recommendation: Loading dose: 200 mg on day 1; maintenance dose 100 mg daily for ≥2 weeks. **Note:** Therapy with 100 mg daily is associated with resistance development (Rex, 1995).
Alternative dosing: 100-200 mg daily for 7-14 days for uncomplicated, moderate-to-severe disease; chronic therapy of 100 mg 3 times weekly is recommended in immunocompromised patients with history of oropharyngeal candidiasis (OPC) (Pappas, 2009)
Osteoarticular: 400 mg daily for 6-12 months (osteomyelitis) or 6 weeks (septic arthritis) (Pappas, 2009)
Pacemaker (or ICD, VAD) infection (unlabeled use): 400-800 mg daily (6-12 mg/kg/day) for 4- 6 weeks after device removal (as step-down in stable, culture-negative patients); long-term suppression when VAD cannot be removed: 400-800 mg daily (Pappas, 2009)
Pericarditis or myocarditis: 400-800 mg daily for several months (Pappas, 2009)
Peritonitis: 50-200 mg/day. **Note:** Some clinicians do not recommend using <200 mg daily (Chen, 2004).
Prophylaxis:
Bone marrow transplant: 400 mg once daily. Patients anticipated to have severe granulocytopenia should start therapy several days prior to the anticipated onset of neutropenia and continue for 7 days after the neutrophil count is >1000 mm^3.
High-risk ICU patients in units with high incidence of invasive candidiasis: 400 mg once daily (Pappas, 2009)
Neutropenic patients: 400 mg once daily for duration of neutropenia (Pappas, 2009)
Peritoneal dialysis associated infection (concurrently treated with antibiotics), prevention of secondary fungal infection: 200 mg every 48 hours (Restrepo, 2010)
Solid organ transplant: 200-400 mg once daily for at least 7-14 days (Pappas, 2009)
Thrombophlebitis, suppurative (unlabeled use): 400-800 mg daily (6-12 mg/kg/day) and as step-down in stable patients for ≥2 weeks (Pappas, 2009)
Urinary tract:
Cystitis:
Manufacturer's recommendation: UTI: 50-200 mg once daily
Asymptomatic, patient undergoing urologic procedure: 200-400 mg once daily several days before and after the procedure (Pappas, 2009)
Symptomatic: 200 mg once daily for 2 weeks (Pappas, 2009)
Fungus balls: 200-400 mg once daily (Pappas, 2009)
Pyelonephritis: 200-400 mg once daily for 2 weeks (Pappas, 2009)
Vaginal:
Uncomplicated: Manufacturer's recommendation: 150 mg as a single oral dose
Complicated: 150 mg every 72 hours for 3 doses (Pappas, 2009)
Recurrent: 150 mg once daily for 10-14 days, followed by 150 mg once weekly for 6 months (Pappas, 2009), **or** fluconazole (oral) 100 mg, 150 mg, or 200 mg every third day for a total of 3 doses (day 1, 4, and 7), then 100 mg, 150 mg, or 200 mg dose weekly for 6 months (CDC, 2010)

Coccidioidomycosis, treatment: Oral, I.V.:
HIV-infected (unlabeled use):
Meningitis: 400-800 mg once daily continued indefinitely (CDC, 2009)
Pneumonia, focal, mild or positive serology alone: 400 mg once daily continued indefinitely (CDC, 2009)
Pneumonia, diffuse or severe extrathoracic disseminated disease (after clinical improvement noted with amphotericin B): 400 mg once daily (CDC, 2009)
Non-HIV infected (unlabeled use):
Disseminated, extrapulmonary: 400 mg once daily (some experts use 2000 mg daily [Galgiani, 2005])
Meningitis: 400 mg once daily (some experts use initial doses of 800-1000 mg daily), lifelong duration (Galgiani, 2005)
Pneumonia, acute, uncomplicated: 200-400 mg daily for 3-6 months (Catanzaro, 1995; Galgiani, 2000)
Pneumonia, chronic progressive, fibrocavitary: 200-400 mg daily for 12 months (Catanzaro, 1995; Galgiani, 2000)
Pneumonia, diffuse: Consolidation after amphotericin B induction: 400 mg daily for 12 months (lifelong in chronically immunosuppressed) (Galgiani, 2005)

Coccidioidomycosis, prophylaxis: Oral:
HIV-infected, positive serology, CD4+ count <250 cells/microL (unlabeled use): 400 mg once daily (CDC, 2009)
Solid organ transplant (unlabeled use): **Note:** Prophylaxis regimens in this setting have not been established; the following regimen has been proposed for transplant recipients who maintain residence in a *Coccidioides* spp endemic area.
Previous history >12 months prior to transplant: 200 mg once daily for 6-12 months (Vikram, 2009; Vucicevic, 2011)
Previous history ≤12 months prior to transplant: 400 mg once daily, lifelong treatment (Vikram, 2009; Vucicevic, 2011)
Positive serology before or at transplant: 400 mg once daily, lifelong treatment; if serology is negative at 12 months, consider a dose reduction to 200 mg daily (Vikram, 2009; Vucicevic, 2011)
No history (at risk for *de novo* post-transplant disease): some clinicians treat with 200 mg daily for 6-12 months (Vucicevic, 2011)

Cryptococcosis: Oral, I.V.:
Meningitis: Manufacturer's recommendation: 400 mg for 1 dose, then 200-400 mg once daily for 10-12 weeks following negative CSF culture
HIV-infected:
Meningitis (in patients amphotericin B resistant or intolerant): Induction: 400-800 mg once daily for 4-6 weeks with concomitant flucytosine (CDC, 2009) **or** 800-1200 mg once daily with concomitant flucytosine for 6 weeks (Perfect, 2010)
Consolidation: 400 mg once daily for 8 weeks (CDC, 2009)
Maintenance (suppression): 200 mg once daily lifelong or until CD4+ count >200 (CDC, 2009)
Pulmonary (immunocompetent) (unlabeled use): 400 mg once daily for 6-12 months (Perfect, 2010)

Dosage adjustment in renal impairment:
Manufacturer's recommendation: **Note:** Renal function estimated using the Cockcroft-Gault formula
No adjustment for vaginal candidiasis single-dose therapy
For multiple dosing in adults, administer loading dose of 50-400 mg, then adjust daily doses as follows (dosage reduction in children should parallel adult recommendations): Cl_{cr} ≤50 mL/minute (no dialysis): Administer 50% of recommended dose daily

Intermittent hemodialysis (IHD): Dialyzable (50%): May administer 100% of daily dose (according to indication) after each dialysis session. Alternatively, doses of 200-400 mg every 48-72 hours **or** 100-200 mg every 24 hours have been recommended. **Note:** Dosing dependent on the assumption of 3 times/week, complete IHD sessions (Heintz, 2009).

Continuous renal replacement therapy (CRRT) (Heintz, 2009; Trotman, 2005): Drug clearance is highly dependent on the method of renal replacement, filter type, and flow rate. Appropriate dosing requires close monitoring of pharmacologic response, signs of adverse reactions due to drug accumulation, as well as drug concentrations in relation to target trough (if appropriate). The following are general recommendations only (based on dialysate flow/ultrafiltration rates of 1-2 L/hour and minimal residual renal function) and should not supersede clinical judgment:

CVVH: Loading dose of 400-800 mg followed by 200-400 mg every 24 hours

CVVHD/CVVHDF: Loading dose of 400-800 mg followed by 400-800 mg every 24 hours (CVVHD or CVVHDF) **or** 800 mg every 24 hours (CVVHDF)

Note: Higher maintenance doses of 400 mg every 24 hours (CVVH), 800 mg every 24 hours (CVVHD), and 500-600 mg every 12 hours (CVVHDF) may be considered when treating resistant organisms and/or when employing combined ultrafiltration and dialysis flow rates of ≥2 L/hour for CVVHD/CVVHDF (Heintz, 2009; Trotman, 2005).

Dosage adjustment in hepatic impairment: No dosage adjustment provided in manufacturer's labeling; use with caution.

Administration

I.V.: Do not use if cloudy or precipitated. Infuse over ~1-2 hours; do not exceed 200 mg/hour.

Oral: May be administered without regard to meals.

Monitoring Parameters Periodic liver function tests (AST, ALT, alkaline phosphatase) and renal function tests, potassium

Dosage Forms Excipient information presented when available (limited, particularly for generics); consult specific product labeling.

Solution, Intravenous:

Generic: 100 mg (50 mL); 200 mg (100 mL); 400 mg (200 mL)

Solution, Intravenous [preservative free]:

Generic: 200 mg (100 mL); 400 mg (200 mL)

Suspension Reconstituted, Oral:

Diflucan: 10 mg/mL (35 mL); 40 mg/mL (35 mL) [orange flavor]

Generic: 10 mg/mL (35 mL); 40 mg/mL (35 mL)

Tablet, Oral:

Diflucan: 50 mg, 100 mg, 150 mg, 200 mg

Generic: 50 mg, 100 mg, 150 mg, 200 mg

◆ **Fluconazole Injection (Can)** *see* Fluconazole *on page 868*

◆ **Fluconazole Omega (Can)** *see* Fluconazole *on page 868*

Flucytosine (floo SYE toe seen)

Brand Names: U.S. Ancobon

Index Terms 5-FC; 5-Fluorocytosine; 5-Flurocytosine

Pharmacologic Category Antifungal Agent, Oral

Additional Appendix Information

Antifungal Agents *on page 2286*

Dosing Considerations for the Critically-Ill Patient With Morbid Obesity *on page 2379*

Use Adjunctive treatment of systemic fungal infections (eg, septicemia, endocarditis, UTI, meningitis, or pulmonary) caused by susceptible strains of *Candida* or *Cryptococcus*

Pregnancy Risk Factor C

Pregnancy Considerations Adverse events have been observed in some animal reproduction studies. Flucytosine is metabolized to fluorouracil which may cause adverse events if administered during pregnancy; refer to the Fluorouracil (Systemic) monograph for additional information.

Breast-Feeding Considerations It is not known if flucytosine is excreted in breast milk. Due to the potential for serious adverse reactions in the nursing infant, a decision should be made whether to discontinue nursing or to discontinue the drug, taking into account the importance of treatment to the mother.

Contraindications Hypersensitivity to flucytosine or any component of the formulation

Warnings/Precautions [U.S. Boxed Warning]: Use with extreme caution in patients with renal dysfunction; dosage adjustment required. Avoid use as monotherapy; resistance rapidly develops. Use with caution in patients with bone marrow depression; patients with hematologic disease or who have been treated with radiation or drugs that suppress the bone marrow may be at greatest risk. Bone marrow toxicity may be irreversible. **[U.S. Boxed Warning]: Closely monitor hematologic, renal, and hepatic status.** Hepatotoxicity and bone marrow toxicity appear to be dose related; monitor levels closely and adjust dose accordingly.

Adverse Reactions Frequency not defined.

Cardiovascular: Cardiac arrest, myocardial toxicity, ventricular dysfunction, chest pain

Central nervous system: Ataxia, confusion, fatigue, hallucinations, headache, parkinsonism, psychosis, pyrexia, sedation, seizure, vertigo

Dermatologic: Rash, photosensitivity, pruritus, toxic epidermal necrolysis, urticaria

Endocrine & metabolic: Hypoglycemia, hypokalemia

Gastrointestinal: Abdominal pain, anorexia, diarrhea, duodenal ulcer, enterocolitis, hemorrhage, nausea, ulcerative colitis, vomiting, xerostomia

Hematologic: Agranulocytosis, anemia, aplastic anemia, bone marrow aplasia, eosinophilia, leukopenia, pancytopenia, thrombocytopenia

Hepatic: Acute hepatic injury, bilirubin increased, hepatic dysfunction, jaundice, liver enzymes increased

Neuromuscular & skeletal: Paresthesia, peripheral neuropathy, weakness

Otic: Hearing loss

Renal: Azotemia, BUN increased, crystalluria, renal failure, serum creatinine increased

Respiratory: Dyspnea, respiratory arrest

Miscellaneous: Allergic reaction

Drug Interactions

Metabolism/Transport Effects None known.

Avoid Concomitant Use

Avoid concomitant use of Flucytosine with any of the following: CloZAPine; Gimeracil

Increased Effect/Toxicity

Flucytosine may increase the levels/effects of: CloZAPine

The levels/effects of Flucytosine may be increased by: Amphotericin B; Gimeracil

Decreased Effect

Flucytosine may decrease the levels/effects of: Saccharomyces boulardii

The levels/effects of Flucytosine may be decreased by: Cytarabine (Conventional)

Ethanol/Nutrition/Herb Interactions Food: Food decreases the rate, but not the extent of absorption.

Storage/Stability Store at room temperature of 25°C (77°F); excursions permitted to 15°C to 30°C (59°F to 86°F).

Mechanism of Action Penetrates fungal cells and is converted to fluorouracil which competes with uracil interfering with fungal RNA and protein synthesis

Pharmacodynamics/Kinetics

Absorption: 78% to 89%

Distribution: Into CSF, aqueous humor, joints, peritoneal fluid; V_d: 0.6 L/kg

Protein binding: 3% to 4%

Metabolism: Minimally hepatic; deaminated both in yeasts and possibly via gut bacteria to 5-fluorouracil

Half-life elimination:

Normal renal function: 2-5 hours

Anuria: 85 hours (range: 30-250)

End stage renal disease: 75-200 hours

Time to peak, serum: ~1-2 hours

Excretion: Urine (>90% as unchanged drug)

Dosage

Usual dosage ranges: Children (unlabeled use) and Adults: Oral: 50-150 mg/kg/day in divided doses every 6 hours

Indication-specific dosing:

Children (unlabeled use) and Adults: Oral: **Meningoencephalitis, cryptococcal:** Induction: 25 mg/kg/dose (with amphotericin B) every 6 hours for at least 4 weeks, or if HIV-infected at least 2 weeks; if clinical improvement, may discontinue both amphotericin and flucytosine and follow with an extended course of fluconazole (Perfect, 2010)

Adults: Oral: **Endocarditis:** 100 mg/kg daily in 3 or 4 divided doses (with amphotericin B) for at least 4-6 weeks after valve replacement (Gould, 2012; Pappas, 2009)

Dosage adjustment in renal impairment: No dosage adjustment provided in manufacturer's labeling (**Note:** Manufacturer recommends dose reduction); however, the following adjustments have been recommended (Aronoff, 2007):

Adults (based upon dosing of 37.5 mg/kg every 6 hours):

Cl_{cr} >50 mL/minute: 37.5 mg/kg every 12 hours

Cl_{cr} 10-50 mL/minute: 37.5 mg/kg every 12-24 hours

Cl_{cr} <10 mL/minute: 37.5 mg/kg every 24-48 hours, but monitor drug concentrations frequently

Hemodialysis: Dialyzable (50% to 100%); administer dose posthemodialysis

Peritoneal dialysis: 0.5-1 g every 24 hours

Continuous renal replacement therapy: 37.5 mg/kg every 12-24 hours (monitor serum concentrations and adjust)

Children (based upon dosing of 100-150 mg/kg every 6 hours):

Cl_{cr} 30-50 mL/minute: 25-37.5 mg/kg every 8 hours

Cl_{cr} 10-29 mL/minute: 25-37.5 mg/kg every 12 hours

Cl_{cr} <10 mL/minute: 25-37.5 mg/kg every 24 hours

Hemodialysis: 25-37.5 mg/kg every 24 hours

Peritoneal dialysis: 25-37.5 mg/kg every 24 hours

Continuous renal replacement therapy: 25-37.5 mg/kg every 8 hours (monitor serum concentrations)

Dosage adjustment in hepatic impairment: No dosage adjustment provided in manufacturer's labeling; use with caution.

Administration Administer around-the-clock to promote less variation in peak and trough serum levels. To avoid nausea and vomiting, administer a few capsules at a time over 15 minutes until full dose is taken.

Monitoring Parameters

Pretreatment: Electrolytes (especially potassium), CBC with differential, BUN, renal function, blood culture

During treatment: CBC with differential, and LFTs (eg, alkaline phosphatase, AST/ALT) frequently, serum flucytosine concentration, renal function

Reference Range

Therapeutic: Trough: 25-50 mcg/mL; peak: 50-100 mcg/mL; peak levels should not exceed 100 mcg/mL to avoid bone marrow toxicity and hepatotoxicity

Trough: Draw just prior to dose administration

Peak: Draw 2 hours after an oral dose administration

Test Interactions Flucytosine causes markedly false elevations in serum creatinine values when the Ektachem® analyzer is used. The Jaffé reaction is recommended for determining serum creatinine.

Dosage Forms Excipient information presented when available (limited, particularly for generics); consult specific product labeling.

Capsule, Oral:

Ancobon: 250 mg, 500 mg

Generic: 250 mg, 500 mg

Extemporaneous Preparations A 10 mg/mL oral suspension may be made with capsules and distilled water. Empty the contents of ten 500 mg capsules in a mortar; add small portions of distilled water and mix to a uniform paste. Mix while adding distilled water in incremental proportions to **almost** 500 mL; transfer to a 500 mL volumetric flask, rinse mortar several times with distilled water, and add sufficient quantity of distilled water to make 500 mL. Store in glass or plastic prescription bottles and label "shake well". Stable for 70 days refrigerated and 14 days at room temperature.

Wintermeyer SM and Nahata MC, "Stability of Flucytosine in an Extemporaneously Compounded Oral Liquid," *Am J Health Syst Pharm*, 1996, 53(4):407-9.

◆ **Fludara** *see* Fludarabine *on page* 872

◆ **Fludara® (Can)** *see* Fludarabine *on page* 872

Fludarabine (floo DARE a been)

Brand Names: U.S. Fludara

Brand Names: Canada Fludara®

Index Terms 2F-ara-AMP; Fludarabine Phosphate

Pharmacologic Category Antineoplastic Agent, Antimetabolite (Purine Analog)

Use Treatment of progressive or refractory B-cell chronic lymphocytic leukemia (CLL)

Canadian labeling: Second-line treatment of chronic lymphocytic leukemia (CLL); second-line treatment of low-grade, refractory non-Hodgkin lymphoma (NHL)

Unlabeled Use Treatment of non-Hodgkin lymphomas (NHL); acute myeloid leukemia (AML), either refractory or in poor risk patients; relapsed acute lymphocytic leukemia (ALL) or AML in pediatric patients; Waldenström's macroglobulinemia (WM); reduced-intensity conditioning regimens prior to allogeneic hematopoietic stem cell transplantation (generally administered in combination with busulfan or cyclophosphamide and antithymocyte globulin or lymphocyte immune globulin, or in combination with melphalan and alemtuzumab)

Pregnancy Risk Factor D

Pregnancy Considerations Teratogenic effects were observed in animal studies. Based on the mechanism of action, fludarabine has the potential to cause fetal harm if administered during pregnancy. There are no adequate and well-controlled studies in pregnant women. Effective contraception is recommended during and for 6 months after treatment for women and men with female partners of reproductive potential.

Breast-Feeding Considerations Due to the potential for serious adverse reactions in the nursing infant, breast-feeding is not recommended.

Contraindications Hypersensitivity of fludarabine or any component of the formulation

Canadian labeling: Additional contraindications (not in U.S. labeling): Severe renal impairment (Cl_{cr} <30 mL/minute); decompensated hemolytic anemia; concurrent use with pentostatin

Warnings/Precautions Hazardous agent - use appropriate precautions for handling and disposal (NIOSH, 2012). Use with caution in patients with renal insufficiency (clearance of the primary metabolite 2-fluoro-ara-A is reduced); dosage reductions are recommended (monitor closely for excessive toxicity); use of the I.V. formulation is not recommended if Cl_{cr} <30 mL/minute. Canadian labeling contraindicates use of oral and I.V. formulations if Cl_{cr} <30 mL/minute. Use with caution in patients with pre-existing hematological disorders (particularly granulocytopenia) or pre-existing central nervous system disorder (epilepsy), spasticity, or peripheral neuropathy. **[U.S. Boxed Warning]: Higher than recommended doses are associated with severe neurologic toxicity (delayed blindness, coma, death); similar neurotoxicity (agitation, coma, confusion and seizure) has been reported with standard CLL doses.** Neurotoxicity symptoms due to high doses appear from 21-60 days following the last fludarabine dose, although neurotoxicity has been reported as early as 7 days and up to 225 days. Possible neurotoxic effects of chronic administration are unknown. Caution patients about performing tasks which require mental alertness (eg, operating machinery or driving).

[U.S. Boxed Warning]: Life-threatening (and sometimes fatal) autoimmune effects, including hemolytic anemia, autoimmune thrombocytopenia/thrombocytopenic purpura (ITP), Evans syndrome, and acquired hemophilia have occurred; monitor closely for hemolysis; discontinue fludarabine if hemolysis occurs; the hemolytic effects usually recur with fludarabine rechallenge. **[U.S. Boxed Warning]: Severe bone marrow suppression (anemia, thrombocytopenia, and neutropenia) may occur;** may be cumulative. Severe myelosuppression (trilineage bone marrow hypoplasia/aplasia) has been reported (rare) with a duration of significant cytopenias ranging from 2 months to 1 year. First-line combination therapy is associated with prolonged cytopenias, with anemia lasting up to 7 months, neutropenia up to 9 months, and thrombocytopenia up to 10 months; increased age is predictive for prolonged cytopenias (Gill, 2010).

Use with caution in patients with documented infection, fever, immunodeficiency, or with a history of opportunistic infection; prophylactic anti-infectives should be considered for patients with an increased risk for developing opportunistic infections. Progressive multifocal leukoencephalopathy (PML) due to JC virus (usually fatal) has been reported with use; usually in patients who had received prior and/or other concurrent chemotherapy; onset ranges from a few weeks to 1 year; evaluate any neurological change promptly. Avoid vaccination with live vaccines during and after fludarabine treatment. May cause tumor lysis syndrome; risk is increased in patients with large tumor burden prior to treatment. Patients receiving blood products should only receive irradiated blood products due to the potential for transfusion related GVHD. **[U.S. Boxed Warnings]: Do not use in combination with pentostatin; may lead to severe, even fatal pulmonary toxicity. Should be administered under the supervision of an experienced cancer chemotherapy physician.**

Adverse Reactions

>10%:

Cardiovascular: Edema (8% to 19%)

Central nervous system: Fever (60% to 69%), fatigue (10% to 38%), pain (20% to 22%), chills (11% to 19%)

Dermatologic: Rash (15%)

Gastrointestinal: Nausea/vomiting (31% to 36%), anorexia (7% to 34%), diarrhea (13% to 15%), gastrointestinal bleeding (3% to 13%)

Genitourinary: Urinary tract infection (2% to 15%)

Hematologic: Myelosuppression (nadir: 10-14 days; recovery: 5-7 weeks; dose-limiting toxicity), anemia (60%), neutropenia (grade 4: 59%; nadir: ~13 days), thrombocytopenia (55%; nadir: ~16 days)

Neuromuscular & skeletal: Weakness (9% to 65%), myalgia (4% to 16%), paresthesia (4% to 12%)

Ocular: Visual disturbance (3% to 15%)

Respiratory: Cough (10% to 44%), pneumonia (16% to 22%), dyspnea (9% to 22%), upper respiratory infection (2% to 16%)

Miscellaneous: Infection (33% to 44%), diaphoresis (1% to 13%)

1% to 10%:

Cardiovascular: Angina (≤6%), arrhythmia (≤3%), cerebrovascular accident (≤3%), heart failure (≤3%), MI (≤3%), supraventricular tachycardia (≤3%), deep vein thrombosis (1% to 3%), phlebitis (1% to 3%), aneurysm (≤1%), transient ischemic attack (≤1%)

Central nervous system: Malaise (6% to 8%), headache (≤3%), sleep disorder (1% to 3%), cerebellar syndrome (≤1%), depression (≤1%), mentation impaired (≤1%)

Dermatologic: Alopecia (≤3%), pruritus (1% to 3%), seborrhea (≤1%)

Endocrine & metabolic: Hyperglycemia (1% to 6%), dehydration (≤1%)

Gastrointestinal: Stomatitis (≤9%), esophagitis (≤3%), constipation (1% to 3%), mucositis (≤2%), dysphagia (≤1%)

Genitourinary: Dysuria (3% to 4%), hesitancy (≤3%)

Hematologic: Hemorrhage (≤1%)

Hepatic: Cholelithiasis (≤3%), liver function tests abnormal (1% to 3%), liver failure (≤1%)

Neuromuscular & skeletal: Osteoporosis (≤2%), arthralgia (≤1%)

Otic: Hearing loss (2% to 6%)

Renal: Hematuria (2% to 3%), renal failure (≤1%), renal function test abnormal (≤1%), proteinuria (≤1%)

Respiratory: Pharyngitis (≤9%), allergic pneumonitis (≤6%), hemoptysis (1% to 6%), sinusitis (≤5%), bronchitis (≤1%), epistaxis (≤1%), hypoxia (≤1%)

Miscellaneous: Anaphylaxis (≤1%), tumor lysis syndrome (≤1%)

<1% (Limited to important or life-threatening): Acute respiratory distress syndrome, blindness, bone marrow fibrosis, cerebral hemorrhage, coma, Epstein-Barr virus (EBV) associated lymphoproliferation, EBV reactivation, erythema multiforme, Evans syndrome, hemolytic anemia (autoimmune), hemophilia (acquired), hemorrhagic cystitis, herpes zoster reactivation, hyperkalemia, hyperphosphatemia, hyperuricemia, hypocalcemia, interstitial pulmonary infiltrate, metabolic acidosis, myelodysplastic syndrome/acute myeloid leukemia (usually associated with prior or concurrent treatment with other anticancer agents), opportunistic infection, optic neuritis, optic neuropathy, pancytopenia, pemphigus, pericardial effusion, peripheral neuropathy, pneumonitis, progressive multifocal leukoencephalopathy (PML), pulmonary fibrosis, pulmonary hemorrhage, respiratory distress, respiratory failure, Richter's syndrome, seizure, skin cancer (new onset or exacerbation), Stevens-Johnson syndrome, thrombocytopenia (autoimmune), thrombocytopenic purpura (autoimmune), toxic epidermal necrolysis, trilineage bone marrow aplasia, trilineage bone marrow hypoplasia, urate crystalluria, wrist drop

Also observed: Neurologic syndrome characterized by cortical blindness, coma, and paralysis [36% at doses >96 mg/m^2 for 5-7 days; <0.2% at doses <125 mg/m^2/cycle (onset of neurologic symptoms may be delayed for 3-4 weeks)]

Drug Interactions

Metabolism/Transport Effects None known.

Avoid Concomitant Use

Avoid concomitant use of Fludarabine with any of the following: BCG; CloZAPine; Natalizumab; Pentostatin; Pimecrolimus; Tacrolimus (Topical); Tofacitinib; Vaccines (Live)

Increased Effect/Toxicity

Fludarabine may increase the levels/effects of: CloZAPine; Leflunomide; Natalizumab; Pentostatin; Tofacitinib; Vaccines (Live)

The levels/effects of Fludarabine may be increased by: Denosumab; Pentostatin; Pimecrolimus; Roflumilast; Tacrolimus (Topical); Trastuzumab

Decreased Effect

Fludarabine may decrease the levels/effects of: BCG; Coccidioidin Skin Test; Sipuleucel-T; Vaccines (Inactivated); Vaccines (Live)

The levels/effects of Fludarabine may be decreased by: Echinacea; Imatinib

Ethanol/Nutrition/Herb Interactions Ethanol: Avoid ethanol (due to GI irritation).

Preparation for Administration Hazardous agent; use appropriate precautions for handling and disposal (NIOSH, 2012). Reconstitute vials with SWI, NS, or D_5W to a concentration of 10-25 mg/mL. Standard I.V. dilution: 100-125 mL D_5W or NS.

Storage/Stability

I.V.: Store intact vials under refrigeration at 2°C to 8°C (36°F to 46°F). Reconstituted vials are stable for 16 days at room temperature of 15°C to 30°C (59°F to 86°F) or refrigerated, although the manufacturer recommends use within 8 hours. Solutions diluted in saline or dextrose are stable for 48 hours at room temperature or under refrigeration.

Tablet: Store at 15°C to 30°C (59°F to 86°F); should be kept within packaging until use.

Mechanism of Action Fludarabine inhibits DNA synthesis by inhibition of DNA polymerase and ribonucleotide reductase; also inhibits DNA primase and DNA ligase I

Pharmacodynamics/Kinetics

Distribution: V_d: 38-96 L/m^2; widely with extensive tissue binding

Protein binding: 2-fluoro-ara-A: ~19% to 29%

Metabolism: I.V.: Fludarabine phosphate is rapidly dephosphorylated in the plasma to 2-fluoro-ara-A (active metabolite), which subsequently enters tumor cells and is phosphorylated by deoxycytidine kinase to the active triphosphate derivative (2-fluoro-ara-ATP)

Bioavailability: Oral: 2-fluoro-ara-A: 50% to 65%

Half-life elimination: 2-fluoro-ara-A: ~20 hours

Time to peak, plasma: Oral: 1-2 hours

Excretion: Urine (60%, 23% as 2-fluoro-ara-A) within 24 hours

Dosage Details concerning dosing in combination regimens should also be consulted.

I.V.:

Children (unlabeled use):

AML: 10.5 mg/m^2 bolus over 15 minutes followed by a continuous infusion of 30.5 mg/m^2/day for 48 hours (Lange, 2008)

ALL or AML, relapsed: 10.5 mg/m^2 bolus over 15 minutes followed by a continuous infusion of 30.5 mg/m^2/day for 48 hours (Avramis, 1998)

Stem cell transplant (allogeneic) conditioning regimen, reduced-intensity: 30 mg/m^2/dose for 6 doses beginning 7-10 days prior to transplant (in combination with busulfan and antithymocyte globulin) (Pulsipher, 2009)

Adults:

CLL: 25 mg/m^2/day for 5 days every 28 days

CLL combination regimens (unlabeled dosing):

CFAR: 20 mg/m^2/day for 3 days every 28 days for 6 cycles (in combination with cyclophosphamide, rituximab and alemtuzumab) (Wierda, 2008)

FC: 30 mg/m^2/day for 3 days every 28 days for 6 cycles (in combination with cyclophosphamide) (Eichhorst, 2006) **or** 20 mg/m^2/day for 5 days every 28 days for 6 cycles (in combination with cyclophosphamide) (Flinn, 2007)

FCR: 25 mg/m^2/day for 3 days every 28 days for 6 cycles (in combination with cyclophosphamide and rituximab) (Keating, 2005; Robak, 2010; Wierda, 2005)

FluCam: 30 mg/m^2/day for 3 days every 28 days for 4-6 cycles (in combination with alemtuzumab) (Elter, 2005)

FR: 25 mg/m^2/day for 5 days every 28 days for 6 cycles (in combination with rituximab) (Byrd, 2003)

OFAR: 30 mg/m^2/day for 2 days every 28 days for 6 cycles (in combination with oxaliplatin, cytarabine, and rituximab) (Tsimberidou, 2008)

AML, high-risk patients (unlabeled use): 30 mg/m^2/day for 5 days induction therapy, followed by post remission therapy of 30 mg/m^2/day for 4 days every other cycle (in combination with cytarabine with or without filgrastim) (Borthakur, 2008)

AML, refractory (unlabeled use): 30 mg/m^2/day for 5 days (in combination with cytarabine and filgrastim), may repeat once for partial remission (Montillo, 1998) **or** 30 mg/m^2/day for 5 days for 1 or 2 cycles (in combination with cytarabine, idarubicin, and filgrastim) (Virchis, 2004)

Non-Hodgkin lymphomas:

Canadian labeling: I.V.: 25 mg/m^2 for 5 days every 28 days; dosage adjustment may be necessary for hematologic or nonhematologic toxicity.

Follicular lymphoma (unlabeled use):

FCR: 25 mg/m^2/day for 3 days every 21 days for 4 cycles (in combination with cyclophosphamide and rituximab) (Sacchi, 2007)

FCMR: 25 mg/m^2/day for 3 days every 28 days for 4 cycles (in combination with cyclophosphamide, mitoxantrone, and rituximab) (Forstpointner, 2004; Forstpointner, 2006)

FND: 25 mg/m^2/day for 3 days every 28 days for up to 8 cycles (in combination with mitoxantrone and dexamethasone) (McLaughlin, 1996; Tsimberidou, 2002)

FNDR: 25 mg/m^2/day for 3 days every 28 days for up to 8 cycles (in combination with mitoxantrone, dexamethasone, and rituximab) (McLaughlin, 2000)

FR: 25 mg/m^2/day for 5 days every 28 days for 6 cycles (in combination with rituximab) (Czuczman, 2005)

Mantle cell lymphoma (unlabeled use):

FC: 20 mg/m^2/day for 4-5 days or 25 mg/m^2/day for 3-5 days (in combination with cyclophosphamide) (Cohen, 2001)

FCMR: 25 mg/m^2/day for 3 days every 28 days for 4 cycles (in combination with cyclophosphamide, mitoxantrone, and rituximab) (Forstpointner, 2004; Forstpointner, 2006)

Waldenstron's macroglobulinemia (unlabeled use): 25 mg/m^2/day for 5 days every 28 days (Foran, 1999) **or** 25 mg/m^2/day for 5 days every 28 days for 6 cycles (in combination with rituximab) (Treon, 2009)

Stem cell transplant (allogeneic) conditioning regimen, reduced-intensity, (unlabeled use): 30 mg/m^2/dose for 6 doses beginning 10 days prior to transplant **or** 30 mg/m^2/dose for 5 days beginning 6 days prior to transplant (in combination with busulfan with or without antithymocyte globulin) (Schetelig, 2003)

Stem cell transplant (allogeneic) nonmyeloablative conditioning regimen (unlabeled use): 30 mg/m²/dose for 3 doses beginning 5 days prior to transplant (in combination with cyclophosphamide and rituximab) (Khouri, 2008) **or** 30 mg/m²/dose for 3 doses beginning 4 days prior to transplant (in combination with total body irradiation) (Rezvani, 2008)

Oral (Canadian labeling; not available in U.S.): Adults: CLL: 40 mg/m² once daily for 5 days every 28 days

Dosage adjustment for toxicity:

Hematologic or nonhematologic toxicity (other than neurotoxicity): Consider treatment delay or dosage reduction

Hemolysis: Discontinue treatment

Neurotoxicity: Consider treatment delay or discontinuation

Dosage adjustment in renal impairment:

U.S. labeling: Adults: CLL: I.V.:

Cl_{cr} 50-79 mL/minute: Decrease dose to 20 mg/m²

Cl_{cr} 30-49 mL/minute: Decrease dose to 15 mg/m²

Cl_{cr} <30 mL/minute: Avoid use

Canadian labeling: CLL (Oral, I.V.), NHL (I.V.):

Cl_{cr} 30-70 mL/minute: Reduce dose by up to 50%

Cl_{cr} <30 mL/minute: Use is contraindicated

The following guidelines have been used by some clinicians: Aronoff, 2007: I.V.:

Children:

Cl_{cr} 30-50 mL/minute: Administer 80% of dose

Cl_{cr} <30 mL/minute: Not recommended

Hemodialysis: Administer 25% of dose

Continuous ambulatory peritoneal dialysis (CAPD): Not recommended

Continuous renal replacement therapy (CRRT): Administer 80% of dose

Adults:

Cl_{cr} 10-50 mL/minute: Administer 75% of dose

Cl_{cr} <10 mL/minute: Administer 50% of dose

Hemodialysis: Administer after dialysis

Continuous ambulatory peritoneal dialysis (CAPD): Administer 50% of dose

Continuous renal replacement therapy (CRRT): Administer 75% of dose

Dosage adjustment in hepatic impairment: No dosage adjustment provided in manufacturer's labeling.

Dosing in obesity: *ASCO Guidelines for appropriate chemotherapy dosing in obese adults with cancer* (**Note:** *Excludes HSCT dosing):* Utilize patient's actual body weight (full weight) for calculation of body surface area- or weight-based dosing, particularly when the intent of therapy is curative; manage regimen-related toxicities in the same manner as for nonobese patients; if a dose reduction is utilized due to toxicity, consider resumption of full weight-based dosing with subsequent cycles, especially if cause of toxicity (eg, hepatic or renal impairment) is resolved (Griggs, 2012).

Administration

Oral: Tablet may be administered with or without food; should be swallowed whole with water; do not chew, break, or crush.

I.V.: Usually administered as a 30-minute infusion; continuous infusions (unlabeled administration rate) are occasionally used

Hazardous agent; use appropriate precautions for handling and disposal (NIOSH, 2012).

Monitoring Parameters CBC with differential, platelet count, AST, ALT, serum creatinine, serum albumin, uric acid; monitor for signs of infection and neurotoxicity

Dosage Forms Excipient information presented when available (limited, particularly for generics); consult specific product labeling. [DSC] = Discontinued product

Solution, Intravenous, as phosphate:

Generic: 50 mg/2 mL (2 mL)

Solution, Intravenous, as phosphate [preservative free]:

Generic: 50 mg/2 mL (2 mL [DSC])

Solution Reconstituted, Intravenous, as phosphate:

Fludara: 50 mg (1 ea)

Generic: 50 mg (1 ea)

Solution Reconstituted, Intravenous, as phosphate [preservative free]:

Generic: 50 mg (1 ea)

Dosage Forms: Canada Excipient information presented when available (limited, particularly for generics); consult specific product labeling.

Tablet, as phosphate:

Fludara®: 10 mg

◆ **Fludarabine Phosphate** *see* Fludarabine *on page 872*

Fludrocortisone (floo droe KOR ti sone)

Brand Names: Canada Florinef®

Index Terms 9α-Fluorohydrocortisone Acetate; Florinef; Fludrocortisone Acetate; Fluohydrisone Acetate; Fluohydrocortisone Acetate

Pharmacologic Category Corticosteroid, Systemic

Additional Appendix Information

Corticosteroids Systemic Equivalencies *on page 2297*

Use Partial replacement therapy for primary and secondary adrenocortical insufficiency in Addison's disease; treatment of salt-losing adrenogenital syndrome (or congenital adrenal hyperplasia)

Unlabeled Use Treatment of idiopathic orthostatic hypotension in conjunction with increased sodium intake

Pregnancy Risk Factor C

Pregnancy Considerations Animal reproduction studies have not been conducted with fludrocortisone; adverse events have been observed with corticosteroids in animal reproduction studies. Some studies have shown an association between first trimester systemic corticosteroid use and oral clefts (Park-Wyllie, 2000; Pradat, 2003). Systemic corticosteroids may also influence fetal growth (decreased birth weight); however, information is conflicting (Lunghi, 2010). Hypoadrenalism may occur in newborns following maternal use of corticosteroids in pregnancy; monitor.

When systemic corticosteroids are needed in pregnancy, it is generally recommended to use the lowest effective dose for the shortest duration of time, avoiding high doses during the first trimester (Leachman, 2006; Lunghi, 2010). Fludrocortisone may be used to treat women during pregnancy who require therapy for congenital adrenal hyperplasia (Speiser, 2010).

Breast-Feeding Considerations Corticosteroids are excreted in human milk; information specific to fludrocortisone has not been located. The manufacturer recommends that caution be exercised when administering fludrocortisone to nursing women.

Contraindications Hypersensitivity to fludrocortisone, hypersensitivity to other corticosteroids, or any component of the formulation; systemic fungal infections

Warnings/Precautions May cause hypercorticism or suppression of hypothalamic-pituitary-adrenal (HPA) axis, particularly in younger children or in patients receiving high doses for prolonged periods. HPA axis suppression may lead to adrenal crisis. Withdrawal and discontinuation of a corticosteroid should be done slowly and carefully. Fludrocortisone is primarily a mineralocorticoid agonist, but may also inhibit the HPA axis. Prolonged use may increase risk of infection, mask acute infection, prolong or exacerbate viral infections, or limit response to vaccinations. Exposure to chickenpox should be avoided. Corticosteroids should not be used to treat ocular herpes simplex, cerebral malaria, or viral hepatitis. Close observation is required in patients with latent tuberculosis (TB) and/or TB reactivity. Restrict use in active TB (only in conjunction with antituberculosis treatment). Prolonged treatment with corticosteroids has been associated with the development of Kaposi's sarcoma (case reports); if noted, discontinuation of therapy should be considered. Acute myopathy has been reported with high-dose corticosteroids, usually in patients with neuromuscular transmission disorders; may involve ocular and/or respiratory muscles; monitor creatine kinase; recovery may be delayed.

Corticosteroid use may cause psychiatric disturbances, including depression, euphoria, insomnia, mood swings, and personality changes. Pre-existing psychiatric conditions may be exacerbated by corticosteroid use. Use with caution in patients with HF; use may be associated with fluid retention, edema, weight gain and hypertension. Use with caution in patients with sodium retention and potassium loss, diabetes mellitus, GI diseases (diverticulitis, peptic ulcer, ulcerative colitis), hepatic impairment, myasthenia gravis, post- myocardial infarction, osteoporosis, and/or renal impairment. Use with caution in patients with cataracts and/or glaucoma; increased intraocular pressure, open-angle glaucoma, and cataracts have occurred with prolonged use. Consider routine eye exams in chronic users. Use with caution in patients with a history of seizure disorder; seizures have been reported with adrenal crisis. Changes in thyroid status may necessitate dosage adjustments; metabolic clearance of corticosteroids increases in hyperthyroid patients and decreases in hypothyroid ones. Use with caution in the elderly. May affect growth velocity in pediatric patients. Withdraw therapy with gradual tapering of dose.

Adverse Reactions Frequency not defined.

Cardiovascular: Cardiac enlargement, CHF, edema, hypertension

Central nervous system: Delirium, depression, emotional instability, euphoria, hallucinations, headache, insomnia, intracranial pressure increased, malaise, mood swings, nervousness, personality changes, pseudotumor cerebri, psychiatric disorders, psychoses, seizure, vertigo

Dermatologic: Acne, bruising, erythema, hirsutism, hives, hyperpigmentation, maculopapular rash, petechiae, purpura, rash, skin test reaction impaired, striae, subcutaneous fat atrophy, thin fragile skin, urticaria, wound healing (impaired)

Endocrine & metabolic: Cushing's syndrome, diabetes mellitus, glucose intolerance, growth suppression, hyperglycemia, hypokalemia, hypokalemic alkalosis, menstrual irregularities, negative nitrogen balance, pituitary-adrenal axis suppression

Gastrointestinal: Abdominal distention, esophagitis ulceration, pancreatitis, peptic ulcer

Neuromuscular & skeletal: Fractures, necrosis (femoral and humeral heads), muscle mass loss, muscle weakness, myopathy, osteoporosis, vertebral compression fractures

Ocular: Cataracts, exophthalmos, glaucoma, increased intraocular pressure

Renal: Glycosuria

Miscellaneous: Anaphylaxis (generalized), diaphoresis

Drug Interactions

Metabolism/Transport Effects None known.

Avoid Concomitant Use

Avoid concomitant use of Fludrocortisone with any of the following: Aldesleukin; BCG; Mifepristone; Natalizumab; Pimecrolimus; Tacrolimus (Topical); Tofacitinib

Increased Effect/Toxicity

Fludrocortisone may increase the levels/effects of: Acetylcholinesterase Inhibitors; Amphotericin B; Deferasirox; Leflunomide; Loop Diuretics; Natalizumab; NSAID (COX-2 Inhibitor); NSAID (Nonselective); Thiazide Diuretics; Tofacitinib; Vaccines (Live); Warfarin

The levels/effects of Fludrocortisone may be increased by: Antifungal Agents (Azole Derivatives, Systemic); Aprepitant; Calcium Channel Blockers (Nondihydropyridine); Denosumab; Estrogen Derivatives; Fluconazole; Fosaprepitant; Indacaterol; Macrolide Antibiotics; Mifepristone; Neuromuscular-Blocking Agents (Nondepolarizing); Pimecrolimus; Quinolone Antibiotics; Roflumilast; Salicylates; Tacrolimus (Topical); Telaprevir; Trastuzumab

Decreased Effect

Fludrocortisone may decrease the levels/effects of: Aldesleukin; Antidiabetic Agents; BCG; Calcitriol; Coccidioidin Skin Test; Corticorelin; Hyaluronidase; Isoniazid; Salicylates; Sipuleucel-T; Telaprevir; Urea Cycle Disorder Agents; Vaccines (Inactivated)

The levels/effects of Fludrocortisone may be decreased by: Aminoglutethimide; Antacids; Barbiturates; Bile Acid Sequestrants; Echinacea; Mifepristone; Mitotane; Primidone; Rifamycin Derivatives

Storage/Stability Store at controlled room temperature at 20°C to 25°C (68°F 77°F); avoid excessive heat.

Mechanism of Action Very potent mineralocorticoid with high glucocorticoid activity; used primarily for its mineralocorticoid effects. Promotes increased reabsorption of sodium and loss of potassium from renal distal tubules.

Pharmacodynamics/Kinetics

Metabolism: Hepatic

Half-life elimination: Plasma: ~3.5 hours; Biological: 18-36 hours

Dosage Oral:

Infants, Children, and Adolescents: Congenital adrenal hyperplasia due to 21-hydroxylase deficiency (Endocrine Society guidelines): 0.05-0.2 mg daily in 1-2 divided doses in combination with sodium chloride supplementation (Speiser, 2010).

Adults:

Addison's disease: Initial: 0.1 mg daily; if transient hypertension develops, reduce dose to 0.05 mg daily; maintenance dosage range: 0.1 mg 3 times weekly to 0.2 mg daily. Preferred administration with cortisone (10-37.5 mg daily) or hydrocortisone (10-30 mg daily).

Salt-losing adrenogenital syndrome (or congenital adrenal hyperplasia): 0.1-0.2 mg daily

The Endocrine Society recommends a maintenance dose range of 0.05-0.2 mg once daily (in combination with hydrocortisone) for patients with congenital adrenal hyperplasia due to 21-hydroxylase deficiency (Speiser, 2010).

Orthostatic hypotension (unlabeled use; Kearney, 2009; Lahrmann, 2006; Lanier, 2011): Initial: 0.1 mg daily in conjunction with a high-salt diet and adequate fluid intake; may be increased in increments of 0.1 mg per week; maximum dose: 1 mg daily. **Note:** Doses exceeding 0.3 mg daily may not be beneficial and predispose patient to unwanted side effects (eg, hypertension, hypokalemia).

Dosage adjustment in renal impairment: No dosage adjustment provided in manufacturer's labeling; use with caution.

Dosage adjustment in hepatic impairment: No dosage adjustment provided in manufacturer's labeling.

Dietary Considerations Systemic use of mineralocorticoids/corticosteroids may require a diet with increased potassium, vitamins A, B_6, C, D, folate, calcium, zinc, and phosphorus, and decreased sodium. With fludrocortisone, a decrease in dietary sodium is often not required as the increased retention of sodium is usually the desired therapeutic effect.

Administration May be administered without regard to food.

Monitoring Parameters Monitor blood pressure and signs of edema when patient is on chronic therapy; very potent mineralocorticoid with high glucocorticoid activity; monitor serum electrolytes, plasma renin activity, blood pressure, and growth in children; monitor for evidence of infection; stop treatment if a significant increase in weight or blood pressure, edema, or cardiac enlargement occurs

Dosage Forms Excipient information presented when available (limited, particularly for generics); consult specific product labeling.

Tablet, Oral, as acetate:

Generic: 0.1 mg

◆ **Fludrocortisone Acetate** *see* Fludrocortisone *on page 875*

◆ **Flugerel** *see* Flutamide *on page 892*

◆ **Flulaval** *see* Influenza Virus Vaccine (Inactivated) *on page 1078*

◆ **Flulaval Quadrivalent** *see* Influenza Virus Vaccine (Inactivated) *on page 1078*

◆ **Flumadine** *see* Rimantadine *on page 1820*

◆ **Flumadine® (Can)** *see* Rimantadine *on page 1820*

Flumazenil (FLOO may ze nil)

Brand Names: Canada Anexate; Flumazenil Injection; Flumazenil Injection, USP; Romazicon

Pharmacologic Category Antidote

Use Benzodiazepine antagonist; reverses sedative effects of benzodiazepines used in conscious sedation and general anesthesia; treatment of benzodiazepine overdose

Pregnancy Risk Factor C

Pregnancy Considerations Teratogenic effects were not seen in animal reproduction studies. Embryocidal effects were seen at large doses. Use during labor and delivery is not recommended.In general, medications used as antidotes should take into consideration the health and prognosis of the mother; antidotes should be administered to pregnant women if there is a clear indication for use and should not be withheld because of fears of teratogenicity (Bailey, 2003).

Breast-Feeding Considerations It is not known if flumazenil is excreted in breast milk. The manufacturer recommends that caution be used if administering to breast-feeding women.

Contraindications Hypersensitivity to flumazenil, benzodiazepines, or any component of the formulation; patients given benzodiazepines for control of potentially life-threatening conditions (eg, control of intracranial pressure or status epilepticus); patients who are showing signs of serious cyclic-antidepressant overdosage

Warnings/Precautions [U.S. Boxed Warning]: Benzodiazepine reversal may result in seizures; seizures may occur more frequently in patients on benzodiazepines for long-term sedation or following tricyclic antidepressant overdose. Dose should be individualized and practitioners should be prepared to manage seizures. Seizures may also develop in patients with concurrent major sedative-hypnotic drug withdrawal, recent therapy with repeated doses of parenteral benzodiazepines, myoclonic jerking or seizure activity prior to flumazenil administration. Use with caution in patients relying on a benzodiazepine for seizure control. May cause CNS depression, which may impair physical or mental abilities; patients must be cautioned about performing tasks which require mental alertness (eg, operating machinery or driving) for 24 hours after discharge.

Flumazenil may not reliably reverse respiratory depression/hypoventilation. Flumazenil is not a substitute for evaluation of oxygenation; establishing an airway and assisting ventilation, as necessary, is always the initial step in overdose management. Resedation occurs more frequently in patients where a large single dose or cumulative dose of a benzodiazepine is administered along with a neuromuscular-blocking agent and multiple anesthetic agents. Flumazenil should be used with caution in the intensive care unit because of increased risk of unrecognized benzodiazepine dependence in such settings. Should not be used to diagnose benzodiazepine-induced sedation. Reverse neuromuscular blockade before considering use. Flumazenil does not antagonize the CNS effects of other GABA agonists (such as ethanol, barbiturates, or general anesthetics); nor does it reverse opioids. Flumazenil does not consistently reverse amnesia; patient may not recall verbal instructions after procedure.

Use with caution in patients with a history of panic disorder; may provoke panic attacks. Use caution in drug and ethanol-dependent patients; these patients may also be dependent on benzodiazepines. Not recommended for treatment of benzodiazepine dependence. Use with caution in patients with a head injury; may alter cerebral blood flow or precipitate convulsions in patients receiving benzodiazepines. Use caution in patients with mixed drug overdoses; toxic effects of other drugs taken may emerge once benzodiazepine effects are reversed. Use caution in hepatic dysfunction; repeated doses of the drug should be reduced in frequency or amount.

Adverse Reactions

>10%: Gastrointestinal: Vomiting (11%)

1% to 10%:

Cardiovascular: Palpitation (3% to 9%), flushing (1% to 3%), vasodilation (1% to 3%)

Central nervous system: Ataxia (10%), dizziness (10%), vertigo (10%), agitation (3% to 9%), anxiety (3% to 9%), insomnia (3% to 9%), nervousness (3% to 9%), abnormal crying (1% to 3%), depersonalization (1% to 3%), depression (1% to 3%), dysphoria (1% to 3%), emotional lability (1% to 3%), euphoria (1% to 3%), fatigue (1% to 3%), headache (1% to 3%), malaise (1% to 3%), paranoia (1% to 3%)

Endocrine & metabolic: Hot flashes (1% to 3%)

Gastrointestinal: Xerostomia (3% to 9%), nausea (1% to 3%)

Local: Pain at injection site (3% to 9%), injection site reaction (1% to 3%), rash (1% to 3%), skin abnormality (1% to 3%), thrombophlebitis (1% to 3%)

Neuromuscular & skeletal: Hypoesthesia (1% to 3%), paresthesia (1% to 3%), weakness (1% to 3%), tremor

Ocular: Blurred vision (3% to 9%), abnormal vision (1% to 3%), lacrimation (1% to 3%)

Respiratory: Dyspnea (3% to 9%), hyperventilation (3% to 9%)

Miscellaneous: Diaphoresis (1% to 3%)

<1% (Limited to important or life-threatening): Abnormal hearing, altered blood pressure increased/decreased, arrhythmia, bradycardia, chest pain, confusion, coldness sensation, delirium, difficulty concentrating, dysphonia, fear, generalized seizure, hiccups, hyperacusis, hypertension, junctional tachycardia, panic attacks, rigors, seizure, shivering, somnolence, stupor, tachycardia, thick tongue, tinnitus, transient hearing impairment, ventricular tachycardia, withdrawal syndrome

Drug Interactions

Metabolism/Transport Effects None known.

Avoid Concomitant Use There are no known interactions where it is recommended to avoid concomitant use.

Increased Effect/Toxicity There are no known significant interactions involving an increase in effect.

Decreased Effect

Flumazenil may decrease the levels/effects of: Hypnotics (Nonbenzodiazepine)

Storage/Stability Store at 20°C to 25°C (68°F to 77°F). For I.V. use only. Once drawn up in the syringe or mixed with solution use within 24 hours. Discard any unused solution after 24 hours.

Mechanism of Action Competitively inhibits the activity at the benzodiazepine receptor site on the GABA/benzodiazepine receptor complex. Flumazenil does not antagonize the CNS effect of drugs affecting GABA-ergic neurons by means other than the benzodiazepine receptor (ethanol, barbiturates, general anesthetics) and does not reverse the effects of opioids

Pharmacodynamics/Kinetics

Onset of action: 1-2 minutes; 80% response within 3 minutes

Peak effect: 6-10 minutes

Duration: Resedation occurs after ~1 hour (range: 19-50 minutes); duration related to dose given and benzodiazepine plasma concentrations; reversal effects of flumazenil may wear off before effects of benzodiazepine

Distribution: Initial V_d: 0.5 L/kg; V_{dss}: 0.9-1.1 L/kg

Protein binding: ~50% (~67% of which is bound to albumin)

Metabolism: Hepatic; dependent upon hepatic blood flow

Half-life elimination: Adults: Alpha: 4-11 minutes; Terminal: 40-80 minutes; Moderate hepatic dysfunction: 1.3 hours; Severe hepatic impairment: 2.4 hours

Excretion: Feces; urine (<1% as unchanged drug)

Dosage

I.V.:

Children ≥1 year: Reversal of conscious sedation:

Initial dose: 0.01 mg/kg over 15 seconds (maximum: 0.2 mg)

Repeat doses (maximum: 4 doses): If desired level of consciousness is not obtained, 0.01 mg/kg (maximum: 0.2 mg) repeated at 1-minute intervals

Maximum total cumulative dose: 1 mg or 0.05 mg/kg (whichever is lower)

Mean total dose: 0.65 mg (range: 0.08-1 mg)

Adults:

Reversal of conscious sedation and general anesthesia:

Initial dose: 0.2 mg over 15 seconds

Repeat doses (maximum: 4 doses): If desired level of consciousness is not obtained, 0.2 mg may be repeated at 1-minute intervals.

Maximum total cumulative dose: 1 mg (usual total dose: 0.6-1 mg). In the event of resedation: Repeat doses may be given at 20-minute intervals as needed at 0.2 mg per minute to a maximum of 1 mg total dose and 3 mg in 1 hour.

Suspected benzodiazepine overdose:

Initial dose: 0.2 mg over 30 seconds; if the desired level of consciousness is not obtained 30 seconds after the dose, 0.3 mg can be given over 30 seconds

Repeat doses: 0.5 mg over 30 seconds repeated at 1-minute intervals

Maximum total cumulative dose: 3 mg (usual total dose: 1-3 mg). Patients with a partial response at 3 mg may require (rare) additional titration up to a total dose of 5 mg (although doses >3 mg do not reliably produce additional effects). If a patient has not responded 5 minutes after cumulative dose of 5 mg, the major cause of sedation is not likely due to benzodiazepines. In the event of resedation, repeat doses may be given at 20-minute intervals if needed, at 0.5 mg per minute to a maximum of 1 mg total dose and 3 mg in 1 hour.

Elderly: No differences in safety or efficacy have been reported; however, increased sensitivity may occur in some elderly patients.

Dosing in renal impairment: No dosage adjustment provided in manufacturer's labeling; however, pharmacokinetics are not significantly affected by renal failure (Cl_{cr} <10 mL/minute) or hemodialysis.

Dosing in hepatic impairment: Initial reversal: No dosage adjustment necessary. Repeat doses: Reduce dose or frequency.

Dietary Considerations Avoid alcohol for the first 24 hours after administration or as long as the effects of benzodiazepines exist.

Administration I.V.: Administer in freely-running I.V. into large vein. Inject over 15 seconds for reversal of conscious sedation and general anesthesia and over 30 seconds for benzodiazepine overdose.

Monitoring Parameters Monitor for return of sedation, respiratory depression, and other residual effects of benzodiazepines for at least 2 hours and until the patient is stable and resedation is unlikely.

Dosage Forms Excipient information presented when available (limited, particularly for generics); consult specific product labeling.

Solution, Intravenous:

Generic: 0.5 mg/5 mL (5 mL); 1 mg/10 mL (10 mL)

◆ Flumazenil Injection (Can) *see* Flumazenil *on page 877*

◆ Flumazenil Injection, USP (Can) *see* Flumazenil *on page 877*

◆ FluMist *see* Influenza Virus Vaccine (Live/Attenuated) *on page 1082*

◆ FluMist® (Can) *see* Influenza Virus Vaccine (Live/Attenuated) *on page 1082*

◆ FluMist Quadrivalent *see* Influenza Virus Vaccine (Live/Attenuated) *on page 1082*

Flunisolide (Nasal) (floo NISS oh lide)

Brand Names: Canada Apo-Flunisolide®; Nasalide®; Rhinalar®

Pharmacologic Category Corticosteroid, Nasal

Use Seasonal or perennial rhinitis

Unlabeled Use Adjunct to antibiotics in empiric treatment of acute bacterial rhinosinusitis (ABRS) (Chow, 2012)

Pregnancy Risk Factor C

Dosage Intranasal: Rhinitis:

Children 6-14 years: 1 spray each nostril 3 times daily **or** 2 sprays in each nostril twice daily; not to exceed 4 sprays/day in each nostril

Children ≥15 years and Adults: 2 sprays each nostril twice daily (morning and evening); may increase to 2 sprays 3 times daily; maximum dose: 8 sprays/day in each nostril

Dosage adjustment in renal impairment: No dosage adjustment provided in manufacturer's labeling.

Dosage adjustment in hepatic impairment: No dosage adjustment provided in manufacturer's labeling.

Additional Information Complete prescribing information should be consulted for additional detail.

Dosage Forms Excipient information presented when available (limited, particularly for generics); consult specific product labeling. [DSC] = Discontinued product

Solution, Nasal:

Generic: 25 MCG/ACT (0.025%) (25 mL); 29 MCG/ACT (0.025%) (25 mL [DSC])

Fluocinolone (Topical) (floo oh SIN oh lone)

Brand Names: U.S. Capex; Derma-Smoothe/FS Body; Derma-Smoothe/FS Scalp; Fluocinolone Acetonide Body; Fluocinolone Acetonide Scalp; Synalar; Synalar (Cream); Synalar (Ointment); Synalar TS

Brand Names: Canada Capex®; Derma-Smoothe/FS®; Synalar®

Index Terms Fluocinolone Acetonide

Pharmacologic Category Corticosteroid, Topical

Additional Appendix Information
Topical Corticosteroids *on page 2299*
Use Relief of susceptible inflammatory dermatosis (low, medium corticosteroid); dermatitis or psoriasis of the scalp; atopic dermatitis in adults and children ≥3 months of age
Pregnancy Risk Factor C
Dosage Topical:
Atopic dermatitis (Derma-Smoothe/FS® body oil):
Children ≥3 months: Moisten skin; apply a thin film to affected area twice daily; do not use for longer than 4 weeks
Adults: Apply a thin film to affected area 3 times/day
Corticosteroid-responsive dermatoses: Children and Adults: Cream, ointment, solution: Apply a thin layer to affected area 2-4 times/day; may use occlusive dressings to manage psoriasis or recalcitrant conditions
Inflammatory and pruritic manifestations (dental use): Adults: Apply to oral lesion 4 times/day, after meals and at bedtime
Scalp psoriasis (Derma-Smoothe/FS® scalp oil): Adults: Massage thoroughly into wet or dampened hair/scalp; cover with shower cap. Leave on overnight (or for at least 4 hours). Remove by washing hair with shampoo and rinsing thoroughly.
Seborrheic dermatitis of the scalp (Capex®): Adults: Apply no more than 1 ounce to scalp once daily; work into lather and allow to remain on scalp for ~5 minutes. Remove from hair and scalp by rinsing thoroughly with water.
Additional Information Complete prescribing information should be consulted for additional detail.
Dosage Forms Excipient information presented when available (limited, particularly for generics); consult specific product labeling.
Cream, External, as acetonide:
Synalar: 0.025% (120 g) [contains cetyl alcohol, edetate disodium, methylparaben, propylene glycol, propylparaben]
Generic: 0.01% (15 g, 60 g); 0.025% (15 g, 60 g)
Kit, External, as acetonide:
Synalar (Cream): 0.025% [contains cetyl alcohol, edetate disodium, methylparaben, propylene glycol, propylparaben]
Synalar (Ointment): 0.025%
Synalar TS: 0.01% [contains propylene glycol]
Oil, External, as acetonide:
Derma-Smoothe/FS Body: 0.01% (118.28 mL) [contains isopropyl alcohol, peanut oil]
Derma-Smoothe/FS Scalp: 0.01% (118.28 mL) [contains isopropyl alcohol, peanut oil]
Fluocinolone Acetonide Body: 0.01% (118.28 mL) [contains isopropyl alcohol, peanut oil]
Fluocinolone Acetonide Scalp: 0.01% (118.28 mL) [contains isopropyl alcohol, peanut oil]
Ointment, External:
Synalar: 0.025% (120 g)
Ointment, External, as acetonide:
Generic: 0.025% (15 g, 60 g)
Shampoo, External, as acetonide:
Capex: 0.01% (120 mL)
Solution, External, as acetonide:
Synalar: 0.01% (60 mL, 90 mL) [contains propylene glycol]
Generic: 0.01% (60 mL)

◆ **Fluocinolone Acetonide** *see* Fluocinolone (Topical) *on page 878*

◆ **Fluocinolone Acetonide Body** *see* Fluocinolone (Topical) *on page 878*

◆ **Fluocinolone Acetonide Scalp** *see* Fluocinolone (Topical) *on page 878*

Fluocinolone, Hydroquinone, and Tretinoin

(floo oh SIN oh lone, HYE droe kwin one, & TRET i noyn)

Brand Names: U.S. Tri-Luma®
Index Terms Hydroquinone, Fluocinolone Acetonide, and Tretinoin; Tretinoin, Fluocinolone Acetonide, and Hydroquinone
Pharmacologic Category Corticosteroid, Topical; Depigmenting Agent; Retinoic Acid Derivative
Use Short-term treatment of moderate-to-severe melasma of the face
Pregnancy Risk Factor C
Dosage Topical: Adults: Melasma: Apply a thin film once daily to affected areas; not indicated for use beyond 8 weeks
Additional Information Complete prescribing information should be consulted for additional detail.
Dosage Forms Excipient information presented when available (limited, particularly for generics); consult specific product labeling.
Cream, topical:
Tri-Luma®: Fluocinolone acetonide 0.01%, hydroquinone 4%, and tretinoin 0.05% (30 g) [contains sodium metabisulfite]

Fluocinonide (floo oh SIN oh nide)

Brand Names: U.S. Vanos
Brand Names: Canada Lidemol®; Lidex®; Lyderm®; Tiamol®; Topactin; Topsyn®
Index Terms Lidex
Pharmacologic Category Corticosteroid, Topical
Additional Appendix Information
Topical Corticosteroids *on page 2299*
Use Anti-inflammatory, antipruritic; treatment of plaque-type psoriasis (up to 10% of body surface area) [high-potency topical corticosteroid]
Pregnancy Risk Factor C
Dosage
Children and Adults: Pruritus and inflammation: Topical (0.05% cream): Apply thin layer to affected area 2-4 times/day depending on the severity of the condition. Therapy should be discontinued when control is achieved; if no improvement is seen, reassessment of diagnosis may be necessary.
Children ≥12 years and Adults: Plaque-type psoriasis (Vanos™): Topical (0.1% cream): Apply a thin layer once or twice daily to affected areas (limited to <10% of body surface area). **Note:** Not recommended for use >2 consecutive weeks or >60 g/week total exposure. Discontinue when control is achieved.
Additional Information Complete prescribing information should be consulted for additional detail.
Dosage Forms Excipient information presented when available (limited, particularly for generics); consult specific product labeling.
Cream, External:
Vanos: 0.1% (30 g, 60 g, 120 g)
Generic: 0.05% (15 g, 30 g, 60 g, 120 g); 0.1% (30 g, 60 g, 120 g)
Gel, External:
Generic: 0.05% (15 g, 30 g, 60 g)
Ointment, External:
Generic: 0.05% (15 g, 30 g, 60 g)
Solution, External:
Generic: 0.05% (20 mL, 60 mL)

◆ **Fluohydrisone Acetate** *see* Fludrocortisone *on page 875*

- **Fluohydrocortisone Acetate** *see* Fludrocortisone *on page 875*
- **Fluor-I-Strips A.T.** *see* Fluorescein *on page 880*
- **Fluorabon™** *see* Fluoride *on page 880*
- **Fluor-A-Day®** *see* Fluoride *on page 880*
- **Fluor-A-Day (Can)** *see* Fluoride *on page 880*

Fluorescein (FLURE e seen)

Brand Names: U.S. AK-Fluor; Bio Glo; Fluor-I-Strips A.T.; Fluorescite; Fluorets; Ful-Glo

Brand Names: Canada Fluorescite®

Index Terms Fluorescein Sodium; Sodium Fluorescein; Soluble Fluorescein

Pharmacologic Category Diagnostic Agent

Use

Injection: Diagnostic aid in ophthalmic angiography and angioscopy

Ophthalmic: To stain the anterior segment of the eye for procedures (such as fitting contact lenses), disclosing corneal injury, and in applanation tonometry

Pregnancy Risk Factor C

Dosage

Diagnostic staining: Ophthalmic: Strips: Children and Adults: Moisten strip with sterile water, saline or ophthalmic fluid. Touch conjunctiva or fornix with tip of strip until adequately stained.

Ophthalmic angiography: Solution for injection: **Note:** Prior to use, an intradermal test dose of 0.05 mL may be used if an allergy is suspected. Evaluate 30-60 minutes following intradermal injection. A negative skin test does not exclude the potential for a reaction to occur.

I.V.:

Children: 3.5 mg/lb (7.7 mg/kg) as a single dose into antecubital vein; maximum 500 mg

Adults: 500 mg as a single dose into antecubital vein; a dose of 200 mg may be appropriate in cases when a highly sensitive imaging system (eg, scanning laser ophthalmoscope) is used.

Oral (unlabeled route): Adults: 1 g of injection solution has been administered orally; clarity of photographs, particularly during early arterial phase, is reportedly poorer than photographs obtained following I.V. administration (Hara, 1998)

Dosage adjustment in renal impairment: No dosage adjustment provided in manufacturer's labeling.

Dosage adjustment in hepatic impairment: No dosage adjustment provided in manufacturer's labeling.

Additional Information Complete prescribing information should be consulted for additional detail.

Dosage Forms Excipient information presented when available (limited, particularly for generics); consult specific product labeling.

Solution, Injection, as sodium:

AK-Fluor: 10% (5 mL); 25% (2 mL)

Fluorescite: 10% (5 mL)

Strip, Ophthalmic, as sodium:

Bio Glo: 1 mg (100 ea, 300 ea)

Fluor-I-Strips A.T.: 1 mg (300 ea)

Fluorets: 1 mg (100 ea)

Ful-Glo: 0.6 mg (300 ea); 1 mg (100 ea)

Fluorescein and Benoxinate
(FLURE e seen & ben OX i nate)

Brand Names: U.S. EyeFlur; Fluress®; Flurox™

Index Terms Benoxinate Hydrochloride and Fluorescein Sodium

Pharmacologic Category Anesthetic, Topical; Diagnostic Agent; Ophthalmic Agent

Use For use in ophthalmic procedures when a topical disclosing agent is needed along with an anesthetic

Pregnancy Risk Factor C

Dosage Ophthalmic: Adults:

Removal of foreign bodies, sutures, or tonometry: Instill 1 or 2 drops (single instillations) into each eye before operating

Deep ophthalmic anesthesia: Instill 2 drops into each eye every 90 seconds up to 3 doses

Dosage adjustment in renal impairment: No dosage adjustment provided in manufacturer's labeling.

Dosage adjustment in hepatic impairment: No dosage adjustment provided in manufacturer's labeling.

Additional Information Complete prescribing information should be consulted for additional detail.

Dosage Forms Excipient information presented when available (limited, particularly for generics); consult specific product labeling.

Solution, ophthalmic: Fluorescein sodium 0.25% and benoxinate hydrochloride 0.4% (5 mL)

EyeFlur, Fluress®, Flurox™: Fluorescein sodium 0.25% and benoxinate hydrochloride 0.4% (5 mL)

- **Fluorescein and Proparacaine** *see* Proparacaine and Fluorescein *on page 1734*
- **Fluorescein Sodium** *see* Fluorescein *on page 880*
- **Fluorescite** *see* Fluorescein *on page 880*
- **Fluorescite® (Can)** *see* Fluorescein *on page 880*
- **Fluorets** *see* Fluorescein *on page 880*

Fluoride (FLOR ide)

Brand Names: U.S. Act® Kids [OTC]; Act® Restoring™ [OTC]; Act® Total Care™ [OTC]; Act® [OTC]; CaviRinse™; Clinpro™ 5000; ControlRx™; ControlRx™ Multi; Denta 5000 Plus™; DentaGel™; Epiflur™; Fluor-A-Day®; Fluorabon™; Fluorinse®; Fluoritab; Flura-Drops®; Gel-Kam® Rinse; Gel-Kam® [OTC]; Just For Kids™ [OTC]; Lozi-Flur™; NeutraCare®; NeutraGard® Advanced; Omni Gel™ [OTC]; OrthoWash™; PerioMed™; Phos-Flur®; Phos-Flur® Rinse [OTC]; PreviDent®; PreviDent® 5000 Booster; PreviDent® 5000 Booster Plus; PreviDent® 5000 Dry Mouth; PreviDent® 5000 Plus®; PreviDent® 5000 Sensitive; StanGard® Perio; Stop®

Brand Names: Canada Fluor-A-Day

Index Terms Acidulated Phosphate Fluoride; Sodium Fluoride; Stannous Fluoride

Pharmacologic Category Nutritional Supplement

Use Prevention of dental caries

Pregnancy Risk Factor B

Dosage Oral:

The recommended daily dose of oral fluoride supplement (mg), based on fluoride ion content (ppm) in drinking water (2.2 mg of sodium fluoride is equivalent to 1 mg of fluoride ion): See table.

Fluoride Ion

Fluoride Content of Drinking Water	Daily Dose, Oral (mg)
<0.3 ppm	
Birth - 6 mo	None
6 mo - 3 y	0.25
3-6 y	0.5
6-16 y	1
0.3-0.6 ppm	
Birth - 6 mo	None
6 mo - 3 y	None
3-6 y	0.25
6-16 y	0.5

Adapted from Recommended Dosage Schedule of The American Dental Association, The American Academy of Pediatric Dentistry, and The American Academy of Pediatrics.

Cream: Children ≥6 years and Adults: Brush teeth with cream once daily regardless of fluoride content of drinking water

Dental rinse or gel:

Children 6-12 years: 5-10 mL rinse or apply to teeth and spit daily after brushing

Adults: 10 mL rinse or apply to teeth and spit daily after brushing

PreviDent® rinse: Children >6 years and Adults: Once weekly, rinse 10 mL vigorously around and between teeth for 1 minute, then spit; this should be done preferably at bedtime, after thoroughly brushing teeth; for maximum benefit, do not eat, drink, or rinse mouth for at least 30 minutes after treatment; do not swallow

Fluorinse®: Children >6 years and Adults: Once weekly, vigorously swish 5-10 mL in mouth for 1 minute, then spit

Lozenge (Lozi-Flur™): Adults: One lozenge daily regardless of fluoride content of drinking water

Additional Information Complete prescribing information should be consulted for additional detail.

Dosage Forms Excipient information presented when available (limited, particularly for generics); consult specific product labeling.

Cream, oral, as sodium [toothpaste]: 1.1% (51 g) [equivalent to fluoride 2.5 mg/dose]

Denta 5000 Plus™: 1.1% (51 g) [spearmint flavor; equivalent to fluoride 2.5 mg/dose]

PreviDent® 5000 Plus®: 1.1% (51 g) [contains sodium benzoate; fruitastic™ flavor; equivalent to fluoride 2.5 mg/dose]

PreviDent® 5000 Plus®: 1.1% (51 g) [contains sodium benzoate; spearmint flavor; equivalent to fluoride 2.5 mg/dose]

Gel, topical, as acidulated phosphate:

Phos-Flur®: 1.1% (51 g) [contains propylene glycol, sodium benzoate; mint flavor; equivalent to fluoride 0.5%]

Gel, oral, as sodium [toothpaste]:

PreviDent® 5000 Booster: 1.1% (100 mL, 106 mL) [contains sodium benzoate; fruitastic™ flavor; equivalent to fluoride 2.5 mg/dose]

PreviDent® 5000 Booster: 1.1% (100 mL, 106 mL) [contains sodium benzoate; spearmint flavor; equivalent to fluoride 2.5 mg/dose]

PreviDent® 5000 Booster Plus: 1.1% (100 mL) [contains sodium benzoate; fruitastic™ flavor; equivalent to fluoride 2.5 mg/dose]

PreviDent® 5000 Booster Plus: 1.1% (100 mL) [contains sodium benzoate; spearmint flavor; equivalent to fluoride 2.5 mg/dose]

PreviDent® 5000 Dry Mouth: 1.1% (100 mL) [mint flavor; equivalent to fluoride 2.5 mg/dose]

PreviDent® 5000 Sensitive: 1.1% (100 mL) [mild mint flavor; equivalent to fluoride 2.5 mg/dose]

Gel, topical, as sodium: 1.1% (56 g) [equivalent to fluoride 2 mg/dose]

DentaGel™: 1.1% (56 g) [fresh mint flavor; neutral pH; equivalent to fluoride 2 mg/dose]

NeutraCare®: 1.1% (60 g) [grape flavor; neutral pH]

NeutraCare®: 1.1% (60 g) [mint flavor; neutral pH]

NeutraGard® Advanced: 1.1% (60 g) [mint flavor; neutral pH]

NeutraGard® Advanced: 1.1% (60 g) [mixed berry flavor; neutral pH]

PreviDent®: 1.1% (56 g) [mint flavor; equivalent to fluoride 2 mg/dose]

PreviDent®: 1.1% (56 g) [very berry flavor; equivalent to fluoride 2 mg/dose]

Gel, topical, as stannous fluoride:

Gel-Kam®: 0.4% (129 g) [cinnamon flavor]

Gel-Kam®: 0.4% (129 g) [fruit & berry flavor]

Gel-Kam®: 0.4% (129 g) [mint flavor]

Just For Kids™: 0.4% (122 g) [bubblegum flavor]

Just For Kids™: 0.4% (122 g) [fruit-punch flavor]

Just For Kids™: 0.4% (122 g) [grapey grape flavor]

Omni Gel™: 0.4% (122 g) [cinnamon flavor]

Omni Gel™: 0.4% (122 g) [grape flavor]

Omni Gel™: 0.4% (122 g) [mint flavor]

Omni Gel™: 0.4% (122 g) [natural flavor]

Omni Gel™: 0.4% (122 g) [raspberry flavor]

Stop®: 0.4% (120 g) [bubblegum flavor]

Stop®: 0.4% (120 g) [mint flavor]

Liquid, oral, as base:

Fluoritab: 0.125 mg/drop [dye free]

Lozenge, oral, as sodium:

Lozi-Flur™: 2.21 mg (90s) [sugar free; cherry flavor; equivalent to fluoride 1 mg]

Paste, oral, as sodium [toothpaste]:

Clinpro™ 5000: 1.1% (113 g) [vanilla-mint flavor]

ControlRx™: 1.1% (57 g) [berry flavor]

ControlRx™: 1.1% (57 g) [vanilla-mint flavor]

ControlRx™ Multi: 1.1% (57 g) [vanilla-mint flavor]

Solution, oral, as fluoride [rinse]:

Act® Total Care™: 0.02% (1000 mL) [ethanol free; contains menthol, propylene glycol, sodium benzoate, tartrazine; fresh mint flavor; equivalent to fluoride 0.009%]

Solution, oral, as sodium [drops]: 1.1 mg/mL (50 mL) [equivalent to fluoride 0.5 mg/mL]

Fluor-A-Day®: 0.278 mg/drop (30 mL) [equivalent to fluoride 0.125 mg/drop]

Fluorabon™: 0.55 mg/0.6 mL (60 mL) [dye free, sugar free; equivalent to fluoride 0.25 mg/0.6 mL]

Flura-Drops®: 0.55 mg/drop (24 mL) [dye free, sugar free; equivalent to fluoride 0.25 mg/drop]

Solution, oral, as sodium [rinse]: 0.2% (473 mL)

Act®: 0.05% (532 mL) [contains benzyl alcohol, propylene glycol, sodium benzoate, tartrazine; cinnamon flavor; equivalent to fluoride 0.02%]

Act®: 0.05% (532 mL) [contains propylene glycol, sodium benzoate, tartrazine; mint flavor; equivalent to fluoride 0.02%]

Act® Kids: 0.05% (532 mL) [ethanol free; contains benzyl alcohol, propylene glycol, sodium benzoate; bubblegum flavor; equivalent to fluoride 0.02%]

Act® Kids: 0.05% (500 mL) [ethanol free; contains benzyl alcohol, propylene glycol, sodium benzoate; ocean berry flavor; equivalent to fluoride 0.02%]

Act® Restoring™: 0.02% (1000 mL) [contains ethanol 11%, propylene glycol, sodium benzoate; Cool Splash™ mint flavor; equivalent to fluoride 0.009%]

Act® Restoring™: 0.02% (1000 mL) [contains ethanol 11%, propylene glycol, sodium benzoate; Cool Splash™ spearmint flavor; equivalent to fluoride 0.009%]

Act® Restoring™: 0.05% (532 mL) [contains ethanol 11%, propylene glycol, sodium benzoate; Cool Splash™ mint flavor; equivalent to fluoride 0.02%]

Act® Restoring™: 0.05% (532 mL) [contains ethanol 11%, propylene glycol, sodium benzoate; Cool Splash™ spearmint flavor; equivalent to fluoride 0.02%]

Act® Restoring™: 0.05% (532 mL) [contains ethanol 11%, propylene glycol, sodium benzoate; Cool Splash™ vanilla-mint flavor; equivalent to fluoride 0.02%]

Act® Total Care™: 0.02% (1000 mL) [contains ethanol 11%, propylene glycol, sodium benzoate; icy clean mint flavor; equivalent to fluoride 0.009%]
Act® Total Care™: 0.05% (88 mL, 532 mL) [contains ethanol 11%, propylene glycol, sodium benzoate; icy clean mint flavor; equivalent to fluoride 0.02%]
Act® Total Care™: 0.05% (88 mL, 532 mL) [ethanol free; contains menthol, propylene glycol, sodium benzoate, tartrazine; fresh mint flavor; equivalent to fluoride 0.02%]
CaviRinse™: 0.2% (240 mL) [mint flavor]
Fluorinse®: 0.2% (480 mL) [ethanol free; cinnamon flavor]
Fluorinse®: 0.2% (480 mL) [ethanol free; mint flavor]
OrthoWash™: 0.044% (480 mL) [contains sodium benzoate; grape flavor]
OrthoWash™: 0.044% (480 mL) [contains sodium benzoate; strawberry flavor]
Phos-Flur® Rinse: 0.044% (473 mL) [ethanol free, sugar free; bubblegum flavor]
Phos-Flur® Rinse: 0.044% (473 mL) [ethanol free, sugar free; gushing grape flavor]
Phos-Flur® Rinse: 0.044% (500 mL) [sugar free; cool mint flavor]
PreviDent®: 0.2% (473 mL) [contains benzoic acid, ethanol 6%, sodium benzoate; cool mint flavor]

Solution, oral, as stannous fluoride [concentrated rinse]: 0.63% (300 mL) [equivalent to fluoride 7 mg/30 mL dose]
Gel-Kam® Rinse: 0.63% (300 mL) [mint flavor; equivalent to fluoride 7 mg/30 mL dose]
PerioMed™: 0.63% (284 mL) [ethanol free; cinnamon flavor; equivalent to fluoride 7 mg/30 mL dose]
PerioMed™: 0.63% (284 mL) [ethanol free; mint flavor; equivalent to fluoride 7 mg/30 mL dose]
PerioMed™: 0.63% (284 mL) [ethanol free; tropical fruit flavor; equivalent to fluoride 7 mg/30 mL dose]
StanGard® Perio: 0.63% (284 mL) [mint flavor]

Tablet, chewable, oral, as sodium: 0.55 mg [equivalent to fluoride 0.25 mg], 1.1 mg [equivalent to fluoride 0.5 mg], 2.2 mg [equivalent to fluoride 1 mg]
Epiflur™: 0.55 mg [sugar free; vanilla flavor; equivalent to fluoride 0.25 mg]
Epiflur™: 1.1 mg [sugar free; vanilla flavor; equivalent to fluoride 0.5 mg]
Epiflur™: 2.2 mg [sugar free; vanilla flavor; equivalent to fluoride 1 mg]
Fluor-A-Day®: 0.55 mg [raspberry flavor; equivalent to fluoride 0.25 mg]
Fluor-A-Day®: 1.1 mg [raspberry flavor; equivalent to fluoride 0.5 mg]
Fluor-A-Day®: 2.2 mg [raspberry flavor; equivalent to fluoride 1 mg]
Fluoritab: 2.2 mg [cherry flavor; equivalent to fluoride 1 mg]
Fluoritab: 1.1 mg [dye free; cherry flavor; equivalent to fluoride 0.5 mg]

◆ **Fluorinse®** *see* Fluoride *on page 880*
◆ **Fluoritab** *see* Fluoride *on page 880*
◆ **5-Fluorocytosine** *see* Flucytosine *on page 871*
◆ **9α-Fluorohydrocortisone Acetate** *see* Fludrocortisone *on page 875*

Fluorometholone (flure oh METH oh lone)

Brand Names: U.S. Flarex; FML; FML Forte; FML Liquifilm

Brand Names: Canada Flarex®; FML Forte®; FML®; PMS-Fluorometholone

Pharmacologic Category Corticosteroid, Ophthalmic

Use Treatment of steroid-responsive inflammatory conditions of the eye

Pregnancy Risk Factor C

Dosage Ophthalmic:

Children ≥2 years, Adolescents, and Adults: Re-evaluate therapy if improvement is not seen within 2 days; use care not to discontinue prematurely; in chronic conditions, gradually decrease dosing frequency prior to discontinuing treatment

Ointment (FML®): Apply small amount (~1/2 inch ribbon) to conjunctival sac 1-3 times daily; may increase application to every 4 hours during the initial 24-48 hours

Suspension (FML®, FML® Forte): Instill 1 drop into conjunctival sac 2-4 times daily; may instill 1 drop every 4 hours during initial 24-48 hours

Adults: Suspension (Flarex®): Instill 1-2 drops into conjunctival sac 4 times daily; may increase application to 2 drops every 2 hours during initial 24-48 hours

Dosage adjustment in renal impairment: No dosage adjustment provided in manufacturer's labeling.

Dosage adjustment in hepatic impairment: No dosage adjustment provided in manufacturer's labeling.

Additional Information Complete prescribing information should be consulted for additional detail.

Dosage Forms Excipient information presented when available (limited, particularly for generics); consult specific product labeling.

Ointment, Ophthalmic, as base:
FML: 0.1% (3.5 g) [contains phenylmercuric acetate]

Suspension, Ophthalmic, as acetate:
Flarex: 0.1% (5 mL)

Suspension, Ophthalmic, as base:
FML Forte: 0.25% (5 mL, 10 mL)
FML Liquifilm: 0.1% (5 mL, 10 mL)
Generic: 0.1% (5 mL, 10 mL, 15 mL)

◆ **Fluoroplex** *see* Fluorouracil (Topical) *on page 885*
◆ **Fluoroplex® (Can)** *see* Fluorouracil (Topical) *on page 885*
◆ **Fluoro Uracil** *see* Fluorouracil (Systemic) *on page 882*
◆ **5-Fluorouracil** *see* Fluorouracil (Systemic) *on page 882*
◆ **5-Fluorouracil** *see* Fluorouracil (Topical) *on page 885*

Fluorouracil (Systemic) (flure oh YOOR a sil)

Brand Names: U.S. Adrucil

Brand Names: Canada Fluorouracil Injection

Index Terms 5-Fluorouracil; 5-Fluracil; 5-FU; Fluoro Uracil; Flouracil; FU

Pharmacologic Category Antineoplastic Agent, Antimetabolite; Antineoplastic Agent, Antimetabolite (Pyrimidine Analog)

Use Treatment of breast cancer, colon cancer, rectal cancer, pancreatic cancer, and stomach (gastric) cancer

Unlabeled Use Treatment of anal cancer, bladder cancer, cervical cancer, esophageal cancer, head and neck cancer, hepatobiliary cancers, neuroendocrine tumors, penile cancer (metastatic), thymic cancers, and unknown primary cancer

Pregnancy Risk Factor D

Pregnancy Considerations Adverse effects (increased resorptions, embryolethality, and teratogenicity) have been observed in animal reproduction studies. Based on the mechanism of action, fluorouracil may cause fetal harm if administered during pregnancy (according to the manufacturer's labeling). The National Comprehensive Cancer Network (NCCN) breast cancer guidelines (v.3.2012) state that chemotherapy, if indicated, may be administered to pregnant women with breast cancer as part of a combination chemotherapy regimen (common regimens administered during pregnancy include doxorubicin, cyclophosphamide, and fluorouracil); chemotherapy should not be administered during the first trimester, after 35 weeks gestation, or within 3 weeks of planned delivery.

Breast-Feeding Considerations Based on the mechanism of action, the manufacturer's labeling recommends against breast-feeding if receiving fluorouracil.

Contraindications Hypersensitivity to fluorouracil or any component of the formulation; poor nutritional states; depressed bone marrow function; potentially serious infections

Warnings/Precautions Hazardous agent - use appropriate precautions for handling and disposal (NIOSH, 2012). Use with caution in patients with impaired kidney or liver function. Discontinue if intractable vomiting or diarrhea, precipitous falls in leukocyte or platelet counts, gastrointestinal ulcer or bleeding, stomatitis, or esophagopharyngitis, hemorrhage, or myocardial ischemia occurs. Use with caution in poor-risk patients who have had high-dose pelvic radiation or previous use of alkylating agents and in patients with widespread metastatic marrow involvement. Palmar-plantar erythrodysesthesia (hand-foot) syndrome has been associated with use (symptoms include a tingling sensation, which may progress to pain, and then to symmetrical swelling and erythema with tenderness; desquamation may occur; with treatment interruption, generally resolves over 5-7 days).

Administration to patients with a genetic deficiency of dihydropyrimidine dehydrogenase (DPD) has been associated with prolonged clearance and increased toxicity (diarrhea, neutropenia, and neurotoxicity) following administration; rechallenge has resulted in recurrent toxicity (despite dose reduction). **[U.S. Boxed Warning]: Should be administered under the supervision of an experienced cancer chemotherapy physician; the manufacturer's labeling recommends hospitalizing patients during the first treatment course due to the potential for severe toxicity.**

Adverse Reactions Toxicity depends on duration of treatment and/or rate of administration

Cardiovascular: Angina, arrhythmia, heart failure, MI, myocardial ischemia, vasospasm, ventricular ectopy

Central nervous system: Acute cerebellar syndrome, confusion, disorientation, euphoria, headache, nystagmus, stroke

Dermatologic: Alopecia, dermatitis, dry skin, fissuring, nail changes (nail loss), palmar-plantar erythrodysesthesia syndrome, pruritic maculopapular rash, photosensitivity, Stevens-Johnson syndrome, toxic epidermal necrolysis, vein pigmentation

Gastrointestinal: Anorexia, bleeding, diarrhea, esophagopharyngitis, mesenteric ischemia (acute), nausea, sloughing, stomatitis, ulceration, vomiting

Hematologic: Agranulocytosis, anemia, leukopenia (nadir: days 9-14; recovery by day 30), pancytopenia, thrombocytopenia

Local: Thrombophlebitis

Ocular: Lacrimation, lacrimal duct stenosis, photophobia, visual changes

Respiratory: Epistaxis

Miscellaneous: Anaphylaxis, generalized allergic reactions

Drug Interactions

Metabolism/Transport Effects **Inhibits** CYP2C9 (strong)

Avoid Concomitant Use

Avoid concomitant use of Fluorouracil (Systemic) with any of the following: BCG; CloZAPine; Gimeracil; Natalizumab; Pimecrolimus; Tacrolimus (Topical); Tofacitinib; Vaccines (Live)

Increased Effect/Toxicity

Fluorouracil (Systemic) may increase the levels/effects of: Bosentan; Carvedilol; CloZAPine; CYP2C9 Substrates; Diclofenac (Systemic); Fosphenytoin; Lacosamide; Leflunomide; Natalizumab; Ospemifene; Phenytoin; Tofacitinib; Vaccines (Live); Vitamin K Antagonists

The levels/effects of Fluorouracil (Systemic) may be increased by: Cimetidine; Denosumab; Gemcitabine; Gimeracil; Leucovorin Calcium-Levoleucovorin; MetroNIDAZOLE (Systemic); Pimecrolimus; Roflumilast; SORAfenib; Tacrolimus (Topical); Trastuzumab

Decreased Effect

Fluorouracil (Systemic) may decrease the levels/effects of: BCG; Coccidioidin Skin Test; Sipuleucel-T; Vaccines (Inactivated); Vaccines (Live); Vitamin K Antagonists

The levels/effects of Fluorouracil (Systemic) may be decreased by: Echinacea; SORAfenib

Ethanol/Nutrition/Herb Interactions

Ethanol: Avoid ethanol (due to GI irritation).

Herb/Nutraceutical: Avoid black cohosh, dong quai in estrogen-dependent tumors.

Preparation for Administration Hazardous agent; use appropriate precautions for handling and disposal (NIOSH, 2012). May dispense in a syringe or dilute in 50-1000 mL NS or D_5W for infusion.

Storage/Stability Store intact vials at room temperature. Do not refrigerate or freeze. Protect from light. Slight discoloration may occur during storage; does not usually denote decomposition. If exposed to cold, a precipitate may form; **gentle** heating to 60°C (140°F) will dissolve the precipitate without impairing the potency. According to the manufacturer, pharmacy bulk vials should be used within 4 hours of initial entry. Solutions for infusion should be used promptly. Fluorouracil 50 mg/mL in NS was stable in polypropylene infusion pump syringes for 7 days when stored at 30°C (86°F) (Stiles, 1996). Stability of fluorouracil 1 mg/mL or 10 mg/mL in NS or D_5W in PVC bags was demonstrated for up to 14 days at 4°C (39.2°F) and 21°C (69.8°F) (Martel, 1996). Stability of undiluted fluorouracil (50 mg/mL) in ethylene-vinyl acetate ambulatory pump reservoirs was demonstrated for 3 days at 4°C (39.2°F) (precipitate formed after 3 days) and for 14 days at 33°C (91.4°F) (Martel, 1996). Stability of undiluted fluorouracil (50 mg/mL) in PVC ambulatory pump reservoirs was demonstrated for 5 days at 4°C (39.2°F) (precipitate formed after 5 days) and for 14 days at 33°C (91.4°F) (Martel, 1996).

Mechanism of Action A pyrimidine analog antimetabolite that interferes with DNA and RNA synthesis; after activation, F-UMP (an active metabolite) is incorporated into RNA to replace uracil and inhibit cell growth; the active metabolite F-dUMP, inhibits thymidylate synthetase, depleting thymidine triphosphate (a necessary component of DNA synthesis).

Pharmacodynamics/Kinetics

Distribution: Penetrates extracellular fluid, CSF, and third space fluids (eg, pleural effusions and ascitic fluid), marrow, intestinal mucosa, liver and other tissues

Metabolism: Hepatic (90%); via a dehydrogenase enzyme; FU must be metabolized to be active metabolites, 5-fluoroxyuridine monophosphate (F-UMP) and 5-5-fluoro-2'-deoxyuridine-5'-O-monophosphate (F-dUMP)

Half-life elimination: 16 minutes (range: 8-20 minutes); two metabolites, F-dUMP and F-UMP, have prolonged half-lives depending on the type of tissue

Excretion: Primarily metabolized in the liver; excreted in lung (as expired CO_2) and urine (7% to 20% as unchanged drug within 6 hours; also as metabolites within 9-10 hours)

Dosage Details concerning dosing in combination regimens should be consulted: Adults:

Breast cancer (unlabeled dosing): I.V.:

CEF regimen: 500 mg/m^2 on days 1 and 8 every 28 days (in combination with cyclophosphamide and epirubicin) for 6 cycles (Levine, 1998)

CMF regimen: 600 mg/m^2 on days 1 and 8 every 28 days (in combination with cyclophosphamide and methotrexate) for 6 cycles (Goldhirsch, 1998; Levine, 1998)
FAC regimen: 500 mg/m^2 on days 1 and 8 every 21-28 days (in combination with cyclophosphamide and doxorubicin) for 6 cycles (Assikis, 2003)
Colorectal cancer (unlabeled dosing): I.V.:
FLOX regimen: 500 mg/m^2 bolus on days 1, 8, 15, 22, 29, and 36 (1 hour after leucovorin) every 8 weeks (in combination with leucovorin and oxaliplatin) for 3 cycles (Kuebler, 2007)
FOLFOX6 and mFOLFOX6 regimen: 400 mg/m^2 bolus on day 1, followed by 1200 mg/m^2/day continuous infusion for 2 days (over 46 hours) every 2 weeks (in combination with leucovorin and oxaliplatin) until disease progression or unacceptable toxicity (Cheeseman, 2002)
FOLFIRI regimens: 400 mg/m^2 bolus on day 1, followed by 1200 mg/m^2/day continuous infusion for 2 days (over 46 hours) every 2 weeks (in combination with leucovorin and irinotecan) until disease progression or unacceptable toxicity; after 2 cycles, may increase continuous infusion fluorouracil dose to 1500 mg/m^2/day (over 46 hours) (Andre, 1999)
Roswell Park regimen: 500 mg/m^2 (bolus) on days 1, 8, 15, 22, 29, and 36 (1 hour after leucovorin) every 8 weeks (in combination with leucovorin) for 4 cycles (Haller, 2005)
Gastric cancer (unlabeled dosing): I.V.:
CF regimen: 750-1000 mg/m^2/day continuous infusion days 1-4 and 29-32 of a 35-day treatment cycle (preoperative chemoradiation; in combination with cisplatin) (NCCN Gastric Cancer Guidelines v2.2012; Tepper, 2008)
ECF regimen (resectable disease): 200 mg/m^2/day continuous infusion days 1-21 every 3 weeks (in combination with epirubicin and cisplatin) for 6 cycles (3 cycles preoperatively and 3 cycles postoperatively) (Cunningham, 2006)
ECF or EOF regimen (advanced disease): 200 mg/m^2/day continuous infusion days 1-21 every 3 weeks (in combination with epirubicin and either cisplatin or oxaliplatin) for a planned duration of 24 weeks (Sumpter, 2005)
TCF or DCF regimen: 750 mg/m^2/day continuous infusion days 1-5 every 3 weeks or 1000 mg/m^2/day continuous infusion days 1-5 every 4 weeks (in combination with docetaxel and cisplatin) until disease progression or unacceptable toxicity (Ajani, 2007; NCCN Gastric Cancer Guidelines v2.2012; Van Cutsem, 2006)
ToGA regimen (HER2-positive): 800 mg/m^2/day continuous infusion days 1-5 every 3 weeks (in combination with cisplatin and trastuzumab) until disease progression or unacceptable toxicity (Bang, 2010)
Pancreatic cancer (unlabeled dosing): I.V.:
Chemoradiation therapy: 250 mg/m^2/day continuous infusion for 3 weeks prior to and then throughout radiation therapy (Regine, 2008)
Fluorouracil-Leucovorin: 425 mg/m^2/day (bolus) days 1-5 every 28 days (in combination with leucovorin) for 6 cycles (Neoptolemos, 2010)
FOLFIRINOX regimen: 400 mg/m^2 bolus on day 1, followed by 1200 mg/m^2/day continuous infusion for 2 days (over 46 hours) every 14 days (in combination with leucovorin, irinotecan, and oxaliplatin) until disease progression or unacceptable toxicity for a recommended 12 cycles (Conroy, 2011)
Anal carcinoma (unlabeled use): I.V.: 1000 mg/m^2/day continuous infusion days 1-4 and days 29-32 (in combination with mitomycin and radiation therapy) (Ajani, 2008)
Bladder cancer (unlabeled use): I.V.: 500 mg/m^2/day continuous infusion days 1-5 and days 16-20 (in combination with mitomycin and radiation therapy) (James, 2012)
Cervical cancer (unlabeled use): I.V.: 1000 mg/m^2/day continuous infusion days 1-4 (in combination with cisplatin and radiation therapy) every 3 weeks for 3 cycles (Eifel, 2004)
Esophageal cancer (unlabeled use): I.V.:
CF regimen: 750-1000 mg/m^2/day continuous infusion days 1-4 and 29-32 of a 35-day treatment cycle (preoperative chemoradiation; in combination with cisplatin) (NCCN Esophageal and Esophagogastric Junction Cancers Guidelines v2.2012; Tepper, 2008)
ECF regimen (resectable disease): 200 mg/m^2/day continuous infusion days 1-21 every 3 weeks (in combination with epirubicin and cisplatin) for 6 cycles (3 cycles preoperatively and 3 cycles postoperatively) (Cunningham, 2006)
ECF or EOF regimen (advanced disease): 200 mg/m^2/day continuous infusion days 1-21 every 3 weeks (in combination with epirubicin and either cisplatin or oxaliplatin) for a planned duration of 24 weeks (Sumpter, 2005)
TCF or DCF regimen: 750 mg/m^2/day continuous infusion days 1-5 every 3 weeks or 1000 mg/m^2/day continuous infusion days 1-5 every 4 weeks (in combination with docetaxel and cisplatin) until disease progression or unacceptable toxicity (Ajani, 2007; NCCN Esophageal and Esophagogastric Junction Cancers Guidelines v2.2012; Van Cutsem, 2006)
Head and neck cancer, squamous cell (unlabeled use): I.V.:
Platinum-Fluorouracil regimen: 1000 mg/m^2/day continuous infusion days 1-4 every 3 weeks (in combination with cisplatin) for at least 6 cycles (Gibson, 2005) **or** 600 mg/m^2/day continuous infusion days 1-4, 22-25, and 43-46 (in combination with carboplatin and radiation) (Bourhis, 2012; Denis, 2004)
TPF regimen: 1000 mg/m^2/day continuous infusion days 1-4 every 3 weeks (in combination with docetaxel and cisplatin) for 3 cycles, and followed by chemoradiotherapy (Posner, 2007) **or** 750 mg/m^2/day continuous infusion days 1-5 every 3 weeks (in combination with docetaxel and cisplatin) for up to 4 cycles (Vermorken, 2007)
Platinum, 5-FU, and cetuximab regimen: 1000 mg/m^2/day continuous infusion days 1-4 every 3 weeks (in combination with either cisplatin or carboplatin and cetuximab) for a total of up to 6 cycles (Vermorken, 2008)
Hepatobiliary cancer (unlabeled use): I.V.: 600 mg/m^2 (bolus) on days 1, 8, and 15 every 4 weeks (in combination with gemcitabine and leucovorin) (Alberts, 2005)

Dosage adjustment for toxicity: *According to the manufacturer, treatment should be discontinued for the following:* Stomatitis or esophagopharyngitis, leukopenia (WBC <3500/mm^3), rapidly falling white blood cell count, intractable vomiting, diarrhea, frequent bowel movements, watery stools, gastrointestinal ulcer or bleeding, thrombocytopenia (platelets <100,000/mm^3), hemorrhage

Dosage adjustment for renal impairment: No dosage adjustment provided in the manufacturer's labeling; however, extreme caution should be used in patients with renal impairment. The following adjustments have been recommended:
Cl_{cr} <50 mL/minute and continuous renal replacement therapy (CRRT): No dosage adjustment necessary (Aronoff, 2007).
Hemodialysis:
Administer standard dose following hemodialysis on dialysis days (Janus, 2010).

Administer 50% of standard dose following hemodialysis (Aronoff, 2007).

Dosage adjustment for hepatic impairment: No dosage adjustment provided in the manufacturer's labeling; however, extreme caution should be used in patients with hepatic impairment. The following adjustments have been recommended:

Floyd, 2006: Bilirubin >5 mg/dL: Avoid use.

Koren, 1992: Hepatic impairment (degree not specified): Administer <50% of dose, then increase if toxicity does not occur.

Dosing in obesity: *ASCO Guidelines for appropriate chemotherapy dosing in obese adults with cancer:* Utilize patient's actual body weight (full weight) for calculation of body surface area- or weight-based dosing, particularly when the intent of therapy is curative; manage regimen-related toxicities in the same manner as for nonobese patients; if a dose reduction is utilized due to toxicity, consider resumption of full weight-based dosing with subsequent cycles, especially if cause of toxicity (eg, hepatic or renal impairment) is resolved (Griggs, 2012).

Dietary Considerations Increase dietary intake of thiamine.

Administration I.V.: Administration rate varies by protocol; refer to specific reference for protocol. May be administered by I.V. push, I.V. bolus, or as a continuous infusion. Avoid extravasation (may be an irritant).

Hazardous agent; use appropriate precautions for handling and disposal (NIOSH, 2012).

Monitoring Parameters CBC with differential and platelet count, renal function tests, liver function tests, signs of palmar-plantar erythrodysesthesia syndrome, stomatitis, diarrhea, hemorrhage, or gastrointestinal ulcers or bleeding

Additional Information Oncology Comment: An investigational uridine prodrug, uridine triacetate (formerly called vistonuridine), has been studied in a limited number of cases of fluorouracil overdose. Of 17 patients receiving uridine triacetate beginning within 8-96 hours after fluorouracil overdose, all patients fully recovered (von Borstel, 2009). Updated data has described a total of 28 patients treated with uridine triacetate for fluorouracil overdose (including overdoses related to continuous infusions delivering fluorouracil at rates faster than prescribed), all of whom recovered fully (Bamat, 2010). Refer to Uridine Triacetate monograph.

Dosage Forms Excipient information presented when available (limited, particularly for generics); consult specific product labeling.

Solution, Intravenous:

Adrucil: 500 mg/10 mL (10 mL); 2.5 g/50 mL (50 mL); 5 g/100 mL (100 mL)

Generic: 500 mg/10 mL (10 mL); 1 g/20 mL (20 mL); 2.5 g/50 mL (50 mL); 5 g/100 mL (100 mL)

Fluorouracil (Topical) (flure oh YOOR a sil)

Brand Names: U.S. Carac; Efudex; Fluoroplex

Brand Names: Canada Efudex®; Fluoroplex®

Index Terms 5-Fluorouracil; 5-FU; FU

Pharmacologic Category Antineoplastic Agent, Antimetabolite; Antineoplastic Agent, Antimetabolite (Pyrimidine Analog); Topical Skin Product

Use Management of actinic or solar keratoses and superficial basal cell carcinomas

Pregnancy Risk Factor X

Dosage Topical: Refer to individual protocols: Adults:

Actinic keratoses:

Carac™: Apply thin film to lesions once daily for up to 4 weeks, as tolerated

Efudex®: Apply to lesions twice daily for 2-4 weeks; complete healing may not be evident for 1-2 months following treatment

Fluoroplex®: Apply to lesions twice daily for 2-6 weeks

Superficial basal cell carcinoma: Efudex® 5%: Apply to affected lesions twice daily for 3-6 weeks; treatment may be continued for up to 10-12 weeks

Additional Information Complete prescribing information should be consulted for additional detail.

Dosage Forms Excipient information presented when available (limited, particularly for generics); consult specific product labeling.

Cream, External:

Carac: 0.5% (30 g) [contains methylparaben, polysorbate 80, propylene glycol, propylparaben, trolamine (triethanolamine)]

Efudex: 5% (40 g)

Fluoroplex: 1% (30 g) [contains benzyl alcohol]

Generic: 5% (40 g)

Solution, External:

Generic: 2% (10 mL); 5% (10 mL)

◆ **Fluorouracil Injection (Can)** *see* Fluorouracil (Systemic) *on page 882*

◆ **Fluouracil** *see* Fluorouracil (Systemic) *on page 882*

FLUoxetine (floo OKS e teen)

Brand Names: U.S. PROzac; PROzac Weekly; Sarafem

Brand Names: Canada Apo-Fluoxetine; Ava-Fluoxetine; CO Fluoxetine; Dom-Fluoxetine; Fluoxetine Capsules BP; FXT 40; Gen-Fluoxetine; JAMP-Fluoxetine; Mint-Fluoxetine; Mylan-Fluoxetine; Novo-Fluoxetine; Nu-Fluoxetine; PHL-Fluoxetine; PMS-Fluoxetine; PRO-Fluoxetine; Prozac; Q-Fluoxetine; ratio-Fluoxetine; Riva-Fluoxetine; Sandoz-Fluoxetine; Teva-Fluoxetine; ZYM-Fluoxetine

Index Terms Fluoxetine Hydrochloride

Pharmacologic Category Antidepressant, Selective Serotonin Reuptake Inhibitor

Additional Appendix Information

Antidepressant Agents *on page 2284*

Selective Serotonin Reuptake Inhibitors (SSRIs) Pharmacokinetics *on page 2314*

Use Treatment of major depressive disorder (MDD); treatment of binge-eating and vomiting in patients with moderate-to-severe bulimia nervosa; obsessive-compulsive disorder (OCD); premenstrual dysphoric disorder (PMDD); panic disorder with or without agoraphobia; in combination with olanzapine for treatment-resistant or bipolar I depression

Unlabeled Use Selective mutism; treatment of mild dementia-associated agitation in nonpsychotic patients; post-traumatic stress disorder (PTSD); social anxiety disorder; fibromyalgia; Raynaud's phenomenon; treatment of paraphilia/hypersexuality

Pregnancy Risk Factor C

Pregnancy Considerations Adverse events have been observed in animal reproduction studies. Fluoxetine and its metabolite cross the human placenta. An increased risk of teratogenic effects, including cardiovascular defects, may be associated with maternal use of fluoxetine or other SSRIs; however, available information is conflicting. Nonteratogenic effects in the newborn following SSRI/SNRI exposure late in the third trimester include respiratory distress, cyanosis, apnea, seizures, temperature instability, feeding difficulty, vomiting, hypoglycemia, hypo- or hypertonia, hyper-reflexia, jitteriness, irritability, constant crying, and tremor. Symptoms may be due to the toxicity of the SSRIs/SNRIs or a discontinuation syndrome and may be consistent with serotonin syndrome associated with SSRI treatment. Persistent pulmonary hypertension of the newborn (PPHN) has also been reported with SSRI exposure. The long-term effects of *in utero* SSRI exposure on infant development and behavior are not known.

Due to pregnancy-induced physiologic changes, women who are pregnant may require dose adjustments of fluoxetine to achieve euthymia. The ACOG recommends that therapy with SSRIs or SNRIs during pregnancy be individualized; treatment of depression during pregnancy should incorporate the clinical expertise of the mental health clinician, obstetrician, primary healthcare provider, and pediatrician. According to the American Psychiatric Association (APA), the risks of medication treatment should be weighed against other treatment options and untreated depression. For women who discontinue antidepressant medications during pregnancy and who may be at high risk for postpartum depression, the medications can be restarted following delivery. Treatment algorithms have been developed by the ACOG and the APA for the management of depression in women prior to conception and during pregnancy.

Breast-Feeding Considerations Fluoxetine and its metabolite are excreted into breast milk and can be detected in the serum of breast-feeding infants. Concentrations in breast milk are variable. In comparison to other SSRIs, fluoxetine concentrations in breast milk are higher and adverse events have been observed in nursing infants. Maternal use of an SSRI during pregnancy may cause delayed milk secretion. Breast-feeding is not recommended by the manufacturer. Long-term effects on development and behavior have not been studied.

Medication Guide Available Yes

Contraindications Hypersensitivity to fluoxetine or any component of the formulation; use of MAO inhibitors intended to treat psychiatric disorders (concurrently, within 5 weeks of discontinuing fluoxetine, or within 2 weeks of discontinuing the MAO inhibitor); initiation of fluoxetine in a patient receiving linezolid or intravenous methylene blue; use with pimozide or thioridazine (**Note:** Thioridazine should not be initiated until 5 weeks after the discontinuation of fluoxetine)

Warnings/Precautions [U.S. Boxed Warning]: Antidepressants increase the risk of suicidal thinking and behavior in children, adolescents, and young adults (18-24 years of age) with major depressive disorder (MDD) and other psychiatric disorders; consider risk prior to prescribing. Short-term studies did not show an increased risk in patients >24 years of age and showed a decreased risk in patients ≥65 years. Closely monitor all patients for clinical worsening, suicidality, or unusual changes in behavior, particularly during the initial 1-2 months of therapy or during periods of dosage adjustments (increases or decreases); the patient's family or caregiver should be instructed to closely observe the patient and communicate condition with healthcare provider. A medication guide concerning the use of antidepressants should be dispensed with each prescription. **Fluoxetine is FDA approved for the treatment of OCD in children ≥7 years of age and MDD in children ≥8 years of age.**

The possibility of a suicide attempt is inherent in major depression and may persist until remission occurs. Use caution in high-risk patients. Worsening depression and severe abrupt suicidality that are not part of the presenting symptoms may require discontinuation or modification of drug therapy. Prescriptions should be written for the smallest quantity consistent with good patient care. The patient's family or caregiver should be alerted to monitor patients for the emergence of suicidality and associated behaviors (such as agitation, irritability, hostility, impulsivity, and hypomania) and call healthcare provider.

May worsen psychosis in some patients or precipitate a shift to mania or hypomania in patients with bipolar disorder. Patients presenting with depressive symptoms should be screened for bipolar disorder. Monotherapy in patients with bipolar disorder should be avoided. **Fluoxetine monotherapy is not FDA approved for the treatment of bipolar depression.** May cause insomnia, anxiety, nervousness, or anorexia. Use with caution in patients where weight loss is undesirable. May impair cognitive or motor performance; caution operating hazardous machinery or driving.

QT prolongation and ventricular arrhythmia including torsade de pointes has occurred. Use with caution in patients with risk factors for QT prolongation, under conditions that predispose to arrhythmias, or increased fluoxetine exposure. Consider discontinuation of fluoxetine if ventricular arrhythmia suspected and initiate cardiac evaluation. Avoid concurrent use with other medications that increase QT interval.

Potentially life-threatening serotonin syndrome (SS) has occurred with serotonergic agents (eg, SSRIs, SNRIs), particularly when used in combination with other serotonergic agents (eg, triptans, TCAs, fentanyl, lithium, tramadol, buspirone, St John's wort, tryptophan) or agents that impair metabolism of serotonin (eg, MAO inhibitors intended to treat psychiatric disorders, other MAO inhibitors [ie, linezolid and intravenous methylene blue]). Discontinue treatment (and any concomitant serotonergic agent) immediately if signs/symptoms arise. Fluoxetine use has been associated with occurrences of significant rash and allergic events, including vasculitis, lupus-like syndrome, laryngospasm, anaphylactoid reactions, and pulmonary inflammatory disease. Discontinue if underlying cause of rash cannot be identified.

Use caution in patients with a previous seizure disorder or condition predisposing to seizures such as brain damage, alcoholism, or concurrent therapy with other drugs which lower the seizure threshold. Use with caution in patients with hepatic or severe renal dysfunction and in elderly patients. Use caution in elderly patients; may cause or exacerbate syndrome of inappropriate antidiuretic hormone secretion or hyponatremia; monitor sodium closely with initiation or dosage adjustments in older adults (Beers Criteria). May also cause agitation, sleep disturbances, and excessive CNS stimulation. May cause hyponatremia/SIADH (elderly at increased risk); volume depletion (diuretics may increase risk). May increase the risks associated with electroconvulsive treatment. Use caution with history of MI or unstable heart disease; use in these patients is limited. May alter glycemic control in patients with diabetes. Due to the long half-life of fluoxetine and its metabolites, the effects and interactions noted may persist for prolonged periods following discontinuation. May cause or exacerbate sexual dysfunction. May cause mydriasis; use caution in patients at risk of acute narrow-angle glaucoma or with increased intraocular pressure. Bone fractures have been associated with antidepressant treatment. Consider the possibility of a fragility fracture if an antidepressant-treated patient presents with unexplained bone pain, point tenderness, swelling, or bruising (Rabenda, 2013; Rizzoli, 2012). Potentially significant drug-drug interactions may exist, requiring dose or frequency adjustment, additional monitoring, and/or selection of alternative therapy.

Abrupt discontinuation or interruption of antidepressant therapy has been associated with a discontinuation syndrome. Symptoms arising may vary with antidepressant however commonly include nausea, vomiting, diarrhea, headaches, light-headedness, dizziness, diminished appetite, sweating, chills, tremors, paresthesias, fatigue, somnolence, and sleep disturbances (eg, vivid dreams, insomnia). Greater risks for developing a discontinuation syndrome have been associated with antidepressants with shorter half-lives, longer durations of treatment, and abrupt discontinuation. For antidepressants of short or intermediate half-lives, symptoms may emerge within 2-5 days after treatment discontinuation and last 7-14 days (APA, 2010; Fava, 2006; Haddad, 2001; Shelton, 2001; Warner, 2006).

Adverse Reactions Percentages listed for adverse effects as reported in placebo-controlled trials and were generally similar in adults and children; actual frequency may be dependent upon diagnosis and in some cases the range presented may be lower than or equal to placebo for a particular disorder.

>10%:

Central nervous system: Insomnia (10% to 33%), headache (21%), somnolence (5% to 17%), anxiety (6% to 15%), nervousness (8% to 14%)

Endocrine & metabolic: Libido decreased (1% to 11%)

Gastrointestinal: Nausea (12% to 29%), diarrhea (8% to 18%), anorexia (4% to 17%), xerostomia (4% to 12%)

Neuromuscular & skeletal: Weakness (7% to 21%), tremor (3% to 13%)

Respiratory: Pharyngitis (3% to 11%), yawn (≤11%)

1% to 10%:

Cardiovascular: Vasodilation (1% to 5%), chest pain, hemorrhage, hypertension, palpitation

Central nervous system: Dizziness (9%), abnormal dreams (1% to 5%), abnormal thinking (2%), agitation, amnesia, chills, confusion, emotional lability, sleep disorder

Dermatologic: Rash (2% to 6%), pruritus (4%)

Endocrine & metabolic: Ejaculation abnormal (≤7%), impotence (≤7%), menorrhagia (≥2%)

Gastrointestinal: Dyspepsia (6% to 10%), constipation (5%), flatulence (3%), vomiting (3%), thirst (≥2%), weight loss (2%), appetite increased, taste perversion, weight gain

Genitourinary: Urinary frequency

Neuromuscular & skeletal: Hyperkinesia (≥2%)

Ocular: Vision abnormal (2%)

Otic: Ear pain, tinnitus

Respiratory: Sinusitis (1% to 6%)

Miscellaneous: Flu-like syndrome (3% to 10%), diaphoresis (2% to 8%), epistaxis (≥2%)

<1% (Limited to important or life-threatening): Acne, acute abdominal syndrome, akathisia, albuminuria, allergies, alopecia, amenorrhea, anaphylactoid reactions, anemia, angina, aphthous stomatitis, aplastic anemia, arrhythmia, arthritis, asthma, ataxia, atrial fibrillation, balance disorder, bone pain, bruising, bruxism, bursitis, cardiac arrest, cataract, cerebrovascular accident, CHF, cholelithiasis, cholestatic jaundice, colitis, dehydration, delusions, depersonalization, dyskinesia, dysphagia, dysuria, ecchymosis, edema, eosinophilic pneumonia, erythema multiforme, erythema nodosum, esophagitis, euphoria, exfoliative dermatitis, extrapyramidal symptoms (rare), gastritis, gastroenteritis, GI ulcer, glossitis, gout, gynecological bleeding, gynecomastia, hallucinations, hepatic failure/necrosis, hepatitis, hiccup, hostility, hypercholesteremia, hyperprolactinemia, hypertonia, hyperventilation, hypoglycemia, hypokalemia, hyponatremia (possibly in association with SIADH), hypotension, hypothyroidism, immune-related hemolytic anemia, kidney failure, laryngospasm, laryngeal edema, leg cramps, liver function test abnormalities, lupus-like syndrome, malaise, melena, migraine, misuse/abuse, MI, mydriasis, myoclonus, neuroleptic malignant syndrome (NMS), optic neuritis, orthostatic hypotension, pancreatitis, pancytopenia, paranoid reaction, petechia, photosensitivity reaction, priapism, pulmonary embolism, pulmonary fibrosis, pulmonary hypertension, purpuric rash, QT prolongation, serotonin syndrome, Stevens-Johnson syndrome, suicidal ideation, syncope, tachycardia, thrombocytopenia, thrombocytopenic purpura, toxic epidermal necrolysis, vasculitis, ventricular tachycardia (including torsade de pointes), violent behavior

Drug Interactions

Metabolism/Transport Effects **Substrate** of CYP1A2 (minor), CYP2B6 (minor), CYP2C19 (minor), CYP2C9 (major), CYP2D6 (major), CYP2E1 (minor), CYP3A4 (minor); **Note:** Assignment of Major/Minor substrate status based on clinically relevant drug interaction potential; **Inhibits** CYP1A2 (weak), CYP2B6 (weak), CYP2C19 (moderate), CYP2C9 (weak), CYP2D6 (strong)

Avoid Concomitant Use

Avoid concomitant use of FLUoxetine with any of the following: Dosulepin; Haloperidol; Highest Risk QTc-Prolonging Agents; Iobenguane I 123; Ivabradine; Linezolid; MAO Inhibitors; Methylene Blue; Mifepristone; Moderate Risk QTc-Prolonging Agents; Pimozide; Propafenone; Tamoxifen; Thioridazine; Tryptophan; Ziprasidone

Increased Effect/Toxicity

FLUoxetine may increase the levels/effects of: Agents with Antiplatelet Properties; Anticoagulants; Antidepressants (Serotonin Reuptake Inhibitor/Antagonist); Antipsychotics; ARIPiprazole; Aspirin; AtoMOXetine; Benzodiazepines (metabolized by oxidation); Beta-Blockers; BusPIRone; CarBAMazepine; CloZAPine; Collagenase (Systemic); CYP2C19 Substrates; CYP2D6 Substrates; Dabigatran Etexilate; Desmopressin; Dextromethorphan; Dosulepin; Fesoterodine; Fosphenytoin; Galantamine; Haloperidol; Highest Risk QTc-Prolonging Agents; Hypoglycemic Agents; Ibritumomab; Iloperidone; Methadone; Methylene Blue; Metoclopramide; Metoprolol; Mexiletine; Nebivolol; NIFEdipine; NiMODipine; NSAID (COX-2 Inhibitor); NSAID (Nonselective); Phenytoin; Pimozide; Propafenone; QuiNIDine; RisperiDONE; Rivaroxaban; Salicylates; Serotonin Modulators; Tetrabenazine; Thiazide Diuretics; Thioridazine; Thrombolytic Agents; Tositumomab and Iodine I 131 Tositumomab; TraMADol; Tricyclic Antidepressants; Vitamin K Antagonists; Vortioxetine; Ziprasidone

The levels/effects of FLUoxetine may be increased by: Abiraterone Acetate; Alcohol (Ethyl); Analgesics (Opioid); Antipsychotics; ARIPiprazole; BuPROPion; BusPIRone; Cimetidine; CNS Depressants; Cobicistat; CYP2C9 Inhibitors (Moderate); CYP2C9 Inhibitors (Strong); CYP2D6 Inhibitors (Moderate); CYP2D6 Inhibitors (Strong); Darunavir; Dasatinib; Fosphenytoin; Glucosamine; Herbs (Anticoagulant/Antiplatelet Properties); Ibrutinib; Ivabradine; Linezolid; Lithium; Macrolide Antibiotics; MAO Inhibitors; Metoclopramide; Metyrosine; Mifepristone; Moderate Risk QTc-Prolonging Agents; Multivitamins/Fluoride (with ADE); Multivitamins/Minerals (with ADEK, Folate, Iron); Multivitamins/Minerals (with AE, No Iron); Omega-3 Fatty Acids; Pentosan Polysulfate Sodium; Pentoxifylline; Propafenone; Prostacyclin Analogues; QTc-Prolonging Agents (Indeterminate Risk and Risk Modifying); Tipranavir; TraMADol; Tryptophan; Vitamin E; Ziprasidone

Decreased Effect

FLUoxetine may decrease the levels/effects of: Clopidogrel; Codeine; Iloperidone; Iobenguane I 123; Ioflupane I 123; Tamoxifen; Thyroid Products; TraMADol

The levels/effects of FLUoxetine may be decreased by: CarBAMazepine; CYP2C9 Inducers (Strong); Cyproheptadine; Dabrafenib; NSAID (COX-2 Inhibitor); NSAID (Nonselective); Peginterferon Alfa-2b

Ethanol/Nutrition/Herb Interactions

Ethanol: May increase CNS depression; monitor for increased effects with coadministration. Caution patients about effects.

Herb/Nutraceutical: Avoid valerian, St John's wort, tryptophan, kava kava, gotu kola (may increase CNS depression and/or risk of serotonin syndrome).

Storage/Stability All dosage forms should be stored at controlled room temperature. Protect from light.

Mechanism of Action Inhibits CNS neuron serotonin reuptake; minimal or no effect on reuptake of norepinephrine or dopamine; does not significantly bind to alpha-adrenergic, histamine, or cholinergic receptors

Pharmacodynamics/Kinetics

Onset of action: Depression: The onset of action is within a week; however, individual response varies greatly and full response may not be seen until 8-12 weeks after initiation of treatment.

Absorption: Well absorbed; delayed 1-2 hours with weekly formulation

Distribution: V_d: 12-43 L/kg

Protein binding: 95% to albumin and $alpha_1$ glycoprotein

Metabolism: Hepatic, via CYP2C19 and 2D6, to norfluoxetine (activity equal to fluoxetine)

Half-life elimination: Adults:

- Parent drug: 1-3 days (acute), 4-6 days (chronic), 7.6 days (cirrhosis)
- Metabolite (norfluoxetine): 9.3 days (range: 4-16 days), 12 days (cirrhosis)

Time to peak, serum: 6-8 hours

Excretion: Urine (10% as norfluoxetine, 2.5% to 5% as fluoxetine)

Note: Weekly formulation results in greater fluctuations between peak and trough concentrations of fluoxetine and norfluoxetine compared to once-daily dosing (24% daily/164% weekly; 17% daily/43% weekly, respectively). Trough concentrations are 76% lower for fluoxetine and 47% lower for norfluoxetine than the concentrations maintained by 20 mg once-daily dosing. Steady-state fluoxetine concentrations are ~50% lower following the once-weekly regimen compared to 20 mg once daily. Average steady-state concentrations of once-daily dosing were highest in children ages 6 to <13 (fluoxetine 171 ng/mL; norfluoxetine 195 ng/mL), followed by adolescents ages 13 to <18 (fluoxetine 86 ng/mL; norfluoxetine 113 ng/mL); concentrations were considered to be within the ranges reported in adults (fluoxetine 91-302 ng/mL; norfluoxetine 72-258 ng/mL).

Dosage Oral:

Children:

- Depression: 8-18 years: 10-20 mg/day; lower-weight children can be started at 10 mg/day, may increase to 20 mg/day after 1 week if needed
- Depression associated with bipolar I disorder (in combination with olanzapine): 10-17 years: Initial: 20 mg in the evening; adjust dose, if needed, as tolerated; safety of fluoxetine doses >50 mg in combination with doses >12 mg of olanzapine has not been studied in pediatrics. See **"Note"** below.
- Obsessive-compulsive disorder: 7-17 years: Initial: 10 mg/day; may increase after 2 weeks if inadequate clinical response to 20 mg/day; further increases may be considered after several weeks to recommended range of 20-30 mg/day (lower weight children) or 20-60 mg/day (adolescents and higher weight children)
- Selective mutism (unlabeled use): 5-18 years: Initial: 5-10 mg/day; titrate upwards as needed (usual maximum dose: 60 mg/day)

Adults: Depression, obessive-compulsive disorder: 20 mg/day in the morning; may increase after several weeks by 20 mg/day increments; maximum: 80 mg/day; doses >20 mg may be given once daily or divided twice daily. **Note:** Lower doses of 5-10 mg/day have been used for initial treatment.

Indication-specific dosing:

- Bulimia nervosa: 60 mg/day; may titrate dose to 60 mg over several days
- Depression: Initial: 20 mg/day; may increase after several weeks if inadequate response (maximum: 80 mg/day). Patients maintained on Prozac 20 mg/day may be changed to Prozac Weekly 90 mg/week, starting dose 7 days after the last 20 mg/day dose
- Depression associated with bipolar I disorder (in combination with olanzapine): Initial: 20 mg in the evening; adjust as tolerated to usual range of 20-50 mg/day. See **"Note"** below.
- Fibromyalgia (unlabeled use): Range: 20-80 mg/day (Arnold, 2002)
- Obsessive-compulsive disorder: Initial: 20 mg/day; may increase after several weeks if inadequate response; recommended range: 20-60 mg/day (maximum: 80 mg/day)
- Panic disorder: Initial: 10 mg/day; after 1 week, increase to 20 mg/day; may increase after several weeks; doses >60 mg/day have not been evaluated
- Post-traumatic stress disorder (PTSD) (unlabeled use): 20-40 mg/day
- Premenstrual dysphoric disorder (Sarafem): 20 mg/day continuously, **or** 20 mg/day starting 14 days prior to menstruation and through first full day of menses (repeat with each cycle)
- Raynaud's phenomena (unlabeled use): 20 mg/day (Coleiro, 2001)
- Social anxiety disorder (unlabeled use): Target dose: 40 mg/day; range 30-60 mg/day (Davidson, 2004)
- Treatment-resistant depression (in combination with olanzapine): Initial: 20 mg in the evening; adjust as tolerated to usual range of 20-50 mg/day. See **"Note."**

Note: When using individual components of fluoxetine with olanzapine rather than fixed-dose combination product (Symbyax), approximate dosage correspondence is as follows:

- Olanzapine 2.5 mg + fluoxetine 20 mg = Symbyax 3/25
- Olanzapine 5 mg + fluoxetine 20 mg = Symbyax 6/25
- Olanzapine 12.5 mg + fluoxetine 20 mg = Symbyax 12/25
- Olanzapine 5 mg + fluoxetine 50 mg = Symbyax 6/50
- Olanzapine 12.5 mg + fluoxetine 50 mg = Symbyax 12/50

Elderly: Depression: Some patients may require an initial dose of 10 mg/day with dosage increases of 10 and 20 mg every several weeks as tolerated; should not be taken at night unless patient experiences sedation

Discontinuation of therapy: Upon discontinuation of antidepressant therapy, gradually taper the dose to minimize the incidence of withdrawal symptoms and allow for the detection of re-emerging symptoms. Evidence supporting ideal taper rates is limited. APA and NICE guidelines suggest tapering therapy over at least several weeks with consideration to the half-life of the antidepressant; antidepressants with a shorter half-life may need to be tapered more conservatively. In addition for long-term treated patients, WFSBP guidelines recommend tapering over 4-6 months. If intolerable withdrawal symptoms occur following a dose reduction, consider resuming the previously prescribed dose and/or decrease dose at a more gradual rate (APA, 2010; Bauer, 2002; Haddad, 2001; NCCMH, 2010; Schatzberg, 2006; Shelton, 2001; Warner, 2006).

MAO inhibitor recommendations:

Switching to or from an MAO inhibitor intended to treat psychiatric disorders:

- Allow 14 days to elapse between discontinuing an MAO inhibitor intended to treat psychiatric disorders and initiation of fluoxetine.
- Allow 5 weeks to elapse between discontinuing fluoxetine and initiation of an MAO inhibitor intended to treat psychiatric disorders.

Use with other MAO inhibitors (linezolid or I.V. methylene blue):

Do not initiate fluoxetine in patients receiving linezolid or I.V. methylene blue; consider other interventions for psychiatric condition.

If urgent treatment with linezolid or I.V. methylene blue is required in a patient already receiving fluoxetine and potential benefits outweigh potential risks, discontinue fluoxetine promptly and administer linezolid or I.V. methylene blue. Monitor for serotonin syndrome for 5 weeks or until 24 hours after the last dose of linezolid or I.V. methylene blue, whichever comes first. May resume fluoxetine 24 hours after the last dose of linezolid or I.V. methylene blue.

Dosing adjustment in renal impairment:

Single dose studies: Pharmacokinetics of fluoxetine and norfluoxetine were similar among subjects with all levels of impaired renal function, including anephric patients on chronic hemodialysis

Chronic administration: Additional accumulation of fluoxetine or norfluoxetine may occur in patients with severely impaired renal function

Hemodialysis: Not removed by hemodialysis; use of lower dose or less frequent dosing is not usually necessary.

Dosing adjustment in hepatic impairment: Elimination half-life of fluoxetine is prolonged in patients with hepatic impairment; a lower or less frequent dose of fluoxetine should be used in these patients

Cirrhosis patients: Administer a lower dose or less frequent dosing interval

Compensated cirrhosis without ascites: Administer 50% of normal dose

Dietary Considerations May be taken without regard to meals.

Administration Administer without regard to meals.

Bipolar I disorder and treatment-resistant depression: Take once daily in the evening.

Major depressive disorder and obsessive compulsive disorder: Once daily doses should be taken in the morning, or twice daily (morning and noon).

Bulimia: Take once daily in the morning.

Monitoring Parameters Mental status for depression, suicidal ideation (especially at the beginning of therapy or when doses are increased or decreased), anxiety, social functioning, mania, panic attacks; signs/symptoms of serotonin syndrome; akathisia, sleep status; blood glucose (for diabetic patients), baseline liver function; ECG assessment and periodic monitoring in patients with risk factors for QT prolongation and ventricular arrhythmia

Reference Range Therapeutic levels have not been well established

Therapeutic: Fluoxetine: 100-800 ng/mL (SI: 289-2314 nmol/L); Norfluoxetine: 100-600 ng/mL (SI: 289-1735 nmol/L)

Toxic: Fluoxetine plus norfluoxetine: >2000 ng/mL

Additional Information ECG may reveal S-T segment depression. Not shown to be teratogenic in rodents; 15-60 mg/day, buspirone and cyproheptadine, may be useful in treatment of sexual dysfunction during treatment with a selective serotonin reuptake inhibitor.

Weekly capsules are a delayed release formulation containing enteric-coated pellets of fluoxetine hydrochloride, equivalent to 90 mg fluoxetine. Therapeutic equivalence of weekly formulation with daily formulation for delaying time to relapse has not been established.

Dosage Forms Excipient information presented when available (limited, particularly for generics); consult specific product labeling.

Capsule, Oral:

PROzac: 10 mg, 20 mg, 40 mg

Generic: 10 mg, 20 mg, 40 mg

Capsule Delayed Release, Oral:

PROzac Weekly: 90 mg

Generic: 90 mg

Solution, Oral:

Generic: 20 mg/5 mL (5 mL, 120 mL)

Tablet, Oral:

Sarafem: 10 mg, 20 mg [contains fd&c yellow #10 aluminum lake, fd&c yellow #6 aluminum lake]

Generic: 10 mg, 20 mg, 60 mg

Extemporaneous Preparations Note: Commercial oral solution is available (4 mg/mL)

A 1 mg/mL fluoxetine oral solution may be prepared using the commercially available preparation (4 mg/mL). In separate graduated cylinders, measure 5 mL of the commercially available fluoxetine preparation and 15 mL of Simple Syrup, NF. Mix thoroughly in incremental proportions. For a 2 mg/mL solution, mix equal proportions of both the commercially available fluoxetine preparation and Simple Syrup, NF. Label "refrigerate". Both concentrations are stable for up to 56 days.

Nahata MC, Pai VB, and Hipple TF, *Pediatric Drug Formulations*, 5th ed, Cincinnati, OH: Harvey Whitney Books Co, 2004.

◆ **Fluoxetine Capsules BP (Can)** *see* FLUoxetine *on page 885*

◆ **Fluoxetine Hydrochloride** *see* FLUoxetine *on page 885*

Fluoxymesterone (floo oks i MES te rone)

Brand Names: U.S. Androxy

Pharmacologic Category Androgen

Use Replacement therapy in the treatment of delayed male puberty; male hypogonadism (primary or hypogonadotropic); inoperable metastatic female breast cancer

Pregnancy Risk Factor X

Dosage Adults: Oral:

Male:

Hypogonadism: 5-20 mg daily

Delayed puberty: 2.5-20 mg daily for 4-6 months

Female: Inoperable breast carcinoma: 10-40 mg daily in divided doses for ≥3 months

Dosage adjustment in renal impairment: No dosage adjustment provided in manufacturer's labeling; use with caution.

Dosage adjustment in hepatic impairment: No dosage adjustment provided in manufacturer's labeling; use with caution.

Additional Information Complete prescribing information should be consulted for additional detail.

Dosage Forms Excipient information presented when available (limited, particularly for generics); consult specific product labeling.

Tablet, Oral:

Androxy: 10 mg [scored]

Controlled Substance C-III

FluPHENAZine (floo FEN a zeen)

Brand Names: Canada Apo-Fluphenazine Decanoate®; Apo-Fluphenazine®; Modecate®; Modecate® Concentrate; PMS-Fluphenazine Decanoate

Index Terms Fluphenazine Decanoate; Fluphenazine Hydrochloride

Pharmacologic Category Antipsychotic Agent, Typical, Phenothiazine

Additional Appendix Information

Antipsychotic Agents *on page 2290*

Beers Criteria – Potentially Inappropriate Medications for Geriatrics *on page 2368*

Use Management of manifestations of psychotic disorders and schizophrenia; depot formulation may offer improved outcome in individuals with psychosis who are nonadherent with oral antipsychotics

Unlabeled Use Psychosis/agitation related to Alzheimer's dementia

Pregnancy Considerations Jaundice or hyper-/hyporeflexia have been reported in newborn infants following maternal use of phenothiazines. Antipsychotic use during the third trimester of pregnancy has a risk for abnormal muscle movements (extrapyramidal symptoms [EPS]) and withdrawal symptoms in newborns following delivery. Symptoms in the newborn may include agitation, feeding disorder, hypertonia, hypotonia, respiratory distress, somnolence, and tremor; these effects may be self-limiting or require hospitalization.

Breast-Feeding Considerations Other phenothiazines are excreted in human milk; excretion of fluphenazine is not known.

Contraindications Hypersensitivity to fluphenazine or any component of the formulation (cross-reactivity between phenothiazines may occur); severe CNS depression; coma; subcortical brain damage; in patients receiving large doses of hypnotics; blood dyscrasias; hepatic disease

Warnings/Precautions [U.S. Boxed Warning]: Elderly patients with dementia-related psychosis treated with antipsychotics are at an increased risk of death compared to placebo. Most deaths appeared to be either cardiovascular (eg, heart failure, sudden death) or infectious (eg, pneumonia) in nature. Fluphenazine is not approved for the treatment of dementia-related psychosis. May be sedating; use with caution in disorders where CNS depression is a feature. Use with caution in Parkinson's disease. Caution in patients with hemodynamic instability; predisposition to seizures; or severe cardiac disease. Use caution in renal impairment; discontinue therapy if BUN abnormal. Use caution in hepatic impairment; use contraindicated in patients with liver damage. Esophageal dysmotility and aspiration have been associated with antipsychotic use; use with caution in patients at risk of pneumonia (ie, Alzheimer's disease). May alter temperature regulation or mask toxicity of other drugs due to antiemetic effects. May alter cardiac conduction; life-threatening arrhythmias have occurred with therapeutic doses of phenothiazines. Hypotension may occur, particularly with I.M. administration. May cause orthostatic hypotension; use with caution in patients at risk of this effect or those who would not tolerate transient hypotensive episodes (cerebrovascular disease, cardiovascular disease, or other medications which may predispose). Adverse effects of depot injections may be prolonged. Use associated with increased prolactin levels; clinical significance of hyperprolactinemia in patients with breast cancer or other prolactin-dependent tumors is unknown. May cause pigmentary retinopathy, and lenticular and corneal deposits, particularly with prolonged therapy.

Leukopenia, neutropenia, and agranulocytosis (sometimes fatal) have been reported in clinical trials and postmarketing reports with antipsychotic use; presence of risk factors (eg, pre-existing low WBC or history of drug-induced leuko-/neutropenia) should prompt periodic blood count assessment. Discontinue therapy at first signs of blood dyscrasias or if absolute neutrophil count <1000/mm^3.

Due to anticholinergic effects, use caution in patients with decreased gastrointestinal motility, urinary retention, BPH, xerostomia, visual problems, or narrow-angle glaucoma. Relative to other antipsychotics, fluphenazine has a low potency of cholinergic blockade.

May cause extrapyramidal symptoms, including pseudoparkinsonism, acute dystonic reactions, akathisia, and tardive dyskinesia (risk of these reactions is high relative to other antipsychotics). Risk of dystonia (and possibly other EPS) may be greater with increased doses, use of conventional antipsychotics, males, and younger patients. May also be associated with neuroleptic malignant syndrome (NMS).

Use in elderly patients with dementia is associated with an increased risk of mortality and cerebrovascular accidents; avoid antipsychotic use for behavioral problems associated with dementia unless alternative nonpharmacologic therapies have failed and patient may harm self or others. In addition, use may cause or exacerbate syndrome of inappropriate antidiuretic hormone secretion or hyponatremia; monitor sodium closely with initiation or dosage adjustments in older adults May also be inappropriate in older adults depending on comorbidities (eg, dementia, delirium) due to its potent anticholinergic effects (Beers Criteria). Increased risk for developing tardive dyskinesia, particularly elderly women.

Adverse Reactions Frequency not defined.

Cardiovascular: Tachycardia, fluctuations in blood pressure, hyper-/hypotension, arrhythmia, edema

Central nervous system: Parkinsonian symptoms, akathisia, dystonias, tardive dyskinesia, dizziness, hyperreflexia, headache, cerebral edema, drowsiness, lethargy, restlessness, excitement, bizarre dreams, EEG changes, depression, seizure, NMS, altered central temperature regulation

Dermatologic: Dermatitis, eczema, erythema, itching, photosensitivity, rash, seborrhea, skin pigmentation, urticaria

Endocrine & metabolic: Menstrual cycle changes, breast pain, amenorrhea, galactorrhea, gynecomastia, libido changes, prolactin increased, SIADH

Gastrointestinal: Weight gain, appetite loss, salivation, xerostomia, constipation, paralytic ileus, laryngeal edema

Genitourinary: Ejaculatory disturbances, impotence, polyuria, bladder paralysis, enuresis

Hematologic: Agranulocytosis, leukopenia, thrombocytopenia, nonthrombocytopenic purpura, eosinophilia, pancytopenia

Hepatic: Cholestatic jaundice, hepatotoxicity

Neuromuscular & skeletal: Trembling of fingers, SLE, facial hemispasm

Ocular: Pigmentary retinopathy, cornea and lens changes, blurred vision, glaucoma

Respiratory: Nasal congestion, asthma

Drug Interactions

Metabolism/Transport Effects Substrate of CYP2D6 (major); **Note:** Assignment of Major/Minor substrate status based on clinically relevant drug interaction potential; **Inhibits** CYP1A2 (weak), CYP2C9 (weak), CYP2D6 (weak), CYP2E1 (weak)

Avoid Concomitant Use

Avoid concomitant use of FluPHENAZine with any of the following: Aclidinium; Amisulpride; Azelastine (Nasal); Ipratropium (Oral Inhalation); Metoclopramide; Paraldehyde; Sulpiride; Tiotropium; Umeclidinium

Increased Effect/Toxicity

FluPHENAZine may increase the levels/effects of: Alcohol (Ethyl); Amisulpride; Analgesics (Opioid); Anticholinergics; Antidepressants (Serotonin Reuptake Inhibitor/Antagonist); ARIPiprazole; Azelastine (Nasal); Beta-Blockers; CNS Depressants; Methotrimeprazine; Methylphenidate; Paraldehyde; Porfimer; Serotonin Modulators; Sulpiride; Tiotropium; Zolpidem

The levels/effects of FluPHENAZine may be increased by: Abiraterone Acetate; Acetylcholinesterase Inhibitors (Central); Aclidinium; Antidepressants (Serotonin Reuptake Inhibitor/Antagonist); Antimalarial Agents; Beta-Blockers; Brimonidine (Topical); CYP2D6 Inhibitors (Moderate); CYP2D6 Inhibitors (Strong); Darunavir; Doxylamine; Droperidol; HydrOXYzine; Ipratropium (Oral Inhalation); Lithium formulations; Magnesium Sulfate;

Methotrimeprazine; Methylphenidate; Metoclopramide; Metyrosine; Perampanel; Pramlintide; Serotonin Modulators; Sodium Oxybate; Tetrabenazine; Umeclidinium

Decreased Effect

FluPHENAZine may decrease the levels/effects of: Amphetamines; Anti-Parkinson's Agents (Dopamine Agonist); Quinagolide

The levels/effects of FluPHENAZine may be decreased by: Antacids; Anti-Parkinson's Agents (Dopamine Agonist); Lithium formulations; Peginterferon Alfa-2b

Ethanol/Nutrition/Herb Interactions

Ethanol: May increase CNS depression; monitor for increased effects with coadministration. Caution patients about effects.

Herb/Nutraceutical: Avoid dong quai, St John's wort (may also cause photosensitization). Avoid kava kava, gotu kola, valerian, St John's wort (may increase CNS depression).

Preparation for Administration Oral liquid concentrate should be diluted into at least 60 mL (2 fl oz) of the following only: Water, saline, homogenized milk, carbonated orange beverages, pineapple, apricot, prune, orange, tomato, and grapefruit juices. Do not dilute in beverages containing caffeine, tannics (eg, tea), or pectinate (eg, apple juice).

Storage/Stability Store at room temperature; avoid freezing and excessive heat. Protect all dosage forms from light. Clear or slightly yellow solutions may be used. Should be dispensed in amber or opaque vials/bottles. Diluted oral solutions must be administered immediately after mixing. Do not prepare bulk dilutions or store bulk dilutions.

Mechanism of Action Fluphenazine is a piperazine phenothiazine antipsychotic which blocks postsynaptic mesolimbic dopaminergic D_1 and D_2 receptors in the brain; depresses the release of hypothalamic and hypophyseal hormones; believed to depress the reticular activating system, thus affecting basal metabolism, body temperature, wakefulness, vasomotor tone, and emesis

Pharmacodynamics/Kinetics

Onset of action: Decanoate: 24-72 hours;

Peak effect: Neuroleptic: Decanoate: 48-96 hours

Duration: Hydrochloride salt: 6-8 hours; Decanoate: ~4 weeks

Absorption: Oral: Erratic and variable

Half-life elimination (derivative dependent): Hydrochloride: ~14-16.4 hours; Decanoate: ~14 days

Time to peak, serum: Hydrochloride: Oral: 2 hours; Decanoate: 8-10 hours

Dosage

Adults: Psychoses:

Oral: Initial: 2.5-10 mg/day in divided doses at 6- to 8-hour intervals; Maintenance: 1-5 mg/day; **Note:** Some patients may require up to 40 mg/day for symptom control (long-term safety of higher doses not established)

PORT guidelines: Acute therapy: 6-20 mg/day for up to 6 weeks; Maintenance: 6-12 mg/day (Buchanan, 2009)

I.M. (hydrochloride): Initial: 1.25 mg as a single dose; depending on severity and duration, may need 2.5-10 mg/day in divided doses at 6- to 8-hour intervals (4 mg I.M. fluphenazine HCl is approximately equivalent to 10 mg oral fluphenazine HCl); use caution with doses >10 mg/day; once symptoms stabilized, transition to oral maintenance therapy

Long-acting maintenance injections (decanoate):

I.M., SubQ (decanoate): Initial: 12.5-25 mg every 2-4 weeks; response may last up to 6 weeks in some patients; titrate dose cautiously, if doses >50 mg are needed, increase in 12.5 mg increments (maximum dose: 100 mg)

Conversion from hydrochloride dosage forms to decanoate I.M.: 12.5 mg of decanoate every 2-4 weeks is approximately equivalent to 10 mg of oral hydrochloride/day; **Note:** Clinically, an every-2-week interval is frequently utilized

PORT guidelines: 6.25-25 mg every 2 weeks (Buchanan, 2009)

Elderly: Oral: Initial: 1-2.5 mg daily; titrated gradually based on patient response

Hemodialysis: Not dialyzable (0% to 5%)

Administration

I.M., SubQ: The hydrochloride or decanoate formulation may be administered intramuscularly. Watch for hypotension when administering I.M. Only the decanoate formulation may be administered subcutaneously. When administering fluphenazine decanoate, use a dry syringe and needle of ≥21 gauge to administer the fluphenazine decanoate; a wet needle/syringe may cause the solution to become cloudy.

Oral: Avoid contact of oral solution or injection with skin (contact dermatitis). Oral liquid concentrate should be diluted immediately prior to administration.

Monitoring Parameters CBC prior to and regularly during therapy; lipid profile, liver and kidney function, fasting blood glucose/Hgb A_{1c}; BMI; mental status, abnormal involuntary movement scale (AIMS), extrapyramidal symptoms (EPS). Monitor vital signs during administration.

Reference Range Therapeutic: 0.3-3 ng/mL (SI: 0.6-6.0 nmol/L); correlation of serum concentrations and efficacy is controversial; most often dosed to best response

Additional Information Less sedative and hypotensive effects than chlorpromazine.

Dosage Forms Excipient information presented when available (limited, particularly for generics); consult specific product labeling.

Concentrate, Oral, as hydrochloride:
Generic: 5 mg/mL (120 mL)

Elixir, Oral, as hydrochloride:
Generic: 2.5 mg/5 mL (60 mL, 473 mL)

Solution, Injection, as decanoate:
Generic: 25 mg/mL (5 mL)

Solution, Injection, as hydrochloride:
Generic: 2.5 mg/mL (10 mL)

Tablet, Oral, as hydrochloride:
Generic: 1 mg, 2.5 mg, 5 mg, 10 mg

◆ **Fluphenazine Decanoate** *see* FluPHENAZine *on page 889*

◆ **Fluphenazine Hydrochloride** *see* FluPHENAZine *on page 889*

◆ **5-Fluracil** *see* Fluorouracil (Systemic) *on page 882*

◆ **Flura-Drops®** *see* Fluoride *on page 880*

Flurandrenolide (flure an DREN oh lide)

Brand Names: U.S. Cordran; Cordran SP

Index Terms Flurandrenolone

Pharmacologic Category Corticosteroid, Topical

Additional Appendix Information

Topical Corticosteroids *on page 2299*

Use Dermatoses: Relief of inflammatory and pruritic manifestations of corticosteroid-responsive dermatoses

Pregnancy Risk Factor C

Dosage Topical: Therapy should be discontinued when control is achieved; if no improvement is seen within 2 weeks, reassessment of diagnosis may be necessary.

Children, Adolescents, and Adults:

Cream, lotion: Apply thin film to affected area 2-3 times per day

Tape: Apply 1-2 times per day

Additional Information Complete prescribing information should be consulted for additional detail.

Dosage Forms Excipient information presented when available (limited, particularly for generics); consult specific product labeling.

Cream, External:

Cordran SP: 0.05% (15 g, 30 g, 60 g, 120 g) [contains cetyl alcohol]

Lotion, External:

Cordran: 0.05% (15 mL, 60 mL, 120 mL) [contains benzyl alcohol, cetyl alcohol, menthol]

Tape, External:

Cordran: 4 mcg/cm^2 (1 ea)

◆ **Flurandrenolone** *see* Flurandrenolide *on page 891*

Flurazepam (flure AZ e pam)

Brand Names: Canada Apo-Flurazepam®; Dalmane®; Som Pam

Index Terms Flurazepam Hydrochloride

Pharmacologic Category Hypnotic, Benzodiazepine

Additional Appendix Information

Beers Criteria – Potentially Inappropriate Medications for Geriatrics *on page 2368*

Benzodiazepine Comparison Table *on page 2292*

Use Short-term treatment of insomnia

Medication Guide Available Yes

Dosage Oral: Insomnia:

Children:

<15 years: Dose not established

≥15 years: 15 mg at bedtime

Adults: 15-30 mg at bedtime

Elderly: 15 mg at bedtime; avoid use if possible

Dosage adjustment in renal impairment: No dosage adjustment provided in manufacturer's labeling; use with caution.

Dosage adjustment in hepatic impairment: No dosage adjustment provided in manufacturer's labeling; use with caution.

Additional Information Complete prescribing information should be consulted for additional detail.

Dosage Forms Excipient information presented when available (limited, particularly for generics); consult specific product labeling.

Capsule, Oral, as hydrochloride:

Generic: 15 mg, 30 mg

Controlled Substance C-IV

◆ **Flurazepam Hydrochloride** *see* Flurazepam *on page 892*

Flurbiprofen (Systemic) (flure BI proe fen)

Brand Names: Canada Alti-Flurbiprofen; Ansaid®; Apo-Flurbiprofen®; Froben-SR®; Froben®; Novo-Flurprofen; Nu-Flurprofen

Index Terms Flurbiprofen Sodium

Pharmacologic Category Nonsteroidal Anti-inflammatory Drug (NSAID), Oral

Use Treatment of rheumatoid arthritis and osteoarthritis

Unlabeled Use Management of postoperative pain

Pregnancy Risk Factor C

Medication Guide Available Yes

Dosage Oral:

Rheumatoid arthritis and osteoarthritis: 200-300 mg/day in 2, 3, or 4 divided doses; do not administer more than 100 mg for any single dose; maximum: 300 mg/day

Dental: Management of postoperative pain (unlabeled use): 100 mg every 12 hours

Dosage adjustment in renal impairment: Not recommended in patients with advanced renal disease.

Dosage adjustment in hepatic impairment: No dosage adjustment provided in manufacturer's labeling; patients with hepatic insufficiency may require reduced doses due to extensive hepatic metabolism.

Additional Information Complete prescribing information should be consulted for additional detail.

Dosage Forms Excipient information presented when available (limited, particularly for generics); consult specific product labeling.

Tablet, Oral:

Generic: 50 mg, 100 mg

Flurbiprofen (Ophthalmic) (flure BI proe fen)

Brand Names: U.S. Ocufen

Index Terms Flurbiprofen Sodium

Pharmacologic Category Nonsteroidal Anti-inflammatory Drug (NSAID), Ophthalmic

Use Inhibition of intraoperative miosis

Pregnancy Risk Factor C

Dosage Ophthalmic: Instill 1 drop every 30 minutes, beginning 2 hours prior to surgery for a total of 4 drops in each affected eye.

Dosage adjustment in renal impairment: No dosage adjustment provided in manufacturer's labeling.

Dosage adjustment in hepatic impairment: No dosage adjustment provided in manufacturer's labeling.

Additional Information Complete prescribing information should be consulted for additional detail.

Dosage Forms Excipient information presented when available (limited, particularly for generics); consult specific product labeling.

Solution, Ophthalmic, as sodium:

Ocufen: 0.03% (2.5 mL) [contains edetate disodium, thimerosal]

Generic: 0.03% (2.5 mL)

◆ **Flurbiprofen Sodium** *see* Flurbiprofen (Ophthalmic) *on page 892*

◆ **Flurbiprofen Sodium** *see* Flurbiprofen (Systemic) *on page 892*

◆ **Fluress®** *see* Fluorescein and Benoxinate *on page 880*

◆ **5-Flurocytosine** *see* Flucytosine *on page 871*

◆ **Flurox™** *see* Fluorescein and Benoxinate *on page 880*

Flutamide (FLOO ta mide)

Brand Names: Canada Apo-Flutamide; Euflex; PMS-Flutamide; Teva-Flutamide

Index Terms Eulexin; Flucinom; Flugerel; Niftolid; SCH 13521

Pharmacologic Category Antineoplastic Agent, Antiandrogen

Use Prostate cancer: Management of locally confined metastatic prostatic cancer (in combination with an LHRH agonist)

Pregnancy Risk Factor D

Dosage

Prostate cancer, metastatic: Adults (males): Oral: 250 mg 3 times daily (every 8 hours)

Dosage adjustment in renal impairment: No dosage adjustment necessary in patients with chronic renal insufficiency.

Dosage adjustment in hepatic impairment: No dosage adjustment provided in manufacturer's labeling; use is contraindicated in severe hepatic impairment.

Additional Information Complete prescribing information should be consulted for additional detail.

Dosage Forms Excipient information presented when available (limited, particularly for generics); consult specific product labeling.

Capsule, Oral:

Generic: 125 mg

Dosage Forms: Canada Excipient information presented when available (limited, particularly for generics); consult specific product labeling.

Tablet, Oral: 250 mg

Fluticasone (Oral Inhalation) (floo TIK a sone)

Brand Names: U.S. Flovent Diskus; Flovent HFA

Brand Names: Canada Flovent® Diskus®; Flovent® HFA

Index Terms Flovent; Fluticasone Propionate

Pharmacologic Category Corticosteroid, Inhalant (Oral)

Additional Appendix Information

Inhaled Corticosteroids *on page 2298*

Use Maintenance treatment of asthma as prophylactic therapy; also indicated for patients requiring oral corticosteroid therapy for asthma to assist in total discontinuation or reduction of total oral dose

Pregnancy Risk Factor C

Pregnancy Considerations Adverse events were observed in some animal reproduction studies. Hypoadrenalism may occur in infants born to mothers receiving corticosteroids during pregnancy. Based on available data, an overall increased risk of congenital malformations or a decrease in fetal growth has not been associated with maternal use of inhaled corticosteroids during pregnancy (Bakhireva, 2005; NAEPP, 2005; Namazy, 2004). Uncontrolled asthma is associated with adverse events in pregnancy (increased risk of perinatal mortality, pre-eclampsia, preterm birth, low birth weight infants). Inhaled corticosteroids are recommended for the treatment of asthma during pregnancy (most information available using budesonide) (ACOG, 2008; NAEPP, 2005).

Breast-Feeding Considerations Systemic corticosteroids are excreted in human milk. It is not known if sufficient quantities of fluticasone are absorbed following inhalation to produce detectable amounts in breast milk. The manufacturer recommends that caution be exercised when administering fluticasone to nursing women. The use of inhaled corticosteroids is not considered a contraindication to breast-feeding (NAEPP, 2005).

Contraindications Hypersensitivity to fluticasone or any component of the formulation; severe hypersensitivity to milk proteins or lactose (Flovent® Diskus®); primary treatment of status asthmaticus or other acute episodes of asthma requiring intensive measures

Canadian labeling: Additional contraindications (not in U.S. labeling): Moderate-to-severe bronchiectasis; untreated fungal, bacterial or tubercular infections of the respiratory tract

Warnings/Precautions May cause hypercorticism or suppression of hypothalamic-pituitary-adrenal (HPA) axis, particularly in younger children or in patients receiving high doses for prolonged periods. HPA axis suppression may lead to adrenal crisis. Withdrawal and discontinuation of a corticosteroid should be done slowly and carefully. Particular care is required when patients are transferred from systemic corticosteroids to inhaled products due to possible adrenal insufficiency or withdrawal from steroids, including an increase in allergic symptoms. Patients receiving ≥20 mg per day of prednisone (or equivalent) may be most susceptible. Fatalities have occurred due to adrenal insufficiency in asthmatic patients during and after transfer from systemic corticosteroids to aerosol steroids; aerosol steroids do **not** provide the systemic steroid needed to treat patients having trauma, surgery, or infections. Bronchospasm may occur with wheezing after inhalation; if this occurs, stop steroid and treat with a fast-acting bronchodilator. Supplemental steroids (oral or parenteral) may be needed during stress or severe asthma attacks. Corticosteroid use may cause psychiatric disturbances, including depression, euphoria, insomnia, mood swings, and personality changes. Pre-existing psychiatric conditions may be exacerbated by corticosteroid use. Prolonged use of corticosteroids may also increase the incidence of secondary infection, mask acute infection (including fungal infections), prolong or exacerbate viral infections, or limit response to vaccines. Avoid use in patients with ocular herpes or untreated viral, fungal, parasitic or bacterial systemic infections (Canadian labeling contraindicates use with untreated respiratory infections). Exposure to chickenpox should be avoided. Close observation is required in patients with latent tuberculosis and/or TB reactivity; restrict use in active TB (only in conjunction with antituberculosis treatment). Rare cases of vasculitis (Churg-Strauss syndrome) or other eosinophilic conditions can occur. Prolonged treatment with corticosteroids has been associated with the development of Kaposi's sarcoma (case reports); if noted, discontinuation of therapy should be considered.

Use with caution in patients with thyroid disease, hepatic impairment, renal impairment, cardiovascular disease, diabetes, glaucoma, cataracts, myasthenia gravis, patients at risk for osteoporosis, patients at risk for seizures, or GI diseases (diverticulitis, peptic ulcer, ulcerative colitis) due to perforation risk. Use caution following acute MI (corticosteroids have been associated with myocardial rupture). Because of the risk of adverse effects, systemic corticosteroids should be used cautiously in the elderly in the smallest possible effective dose for the shortest duration.

Orally-inhaled corticosteroids may cause a reduction in growth velocity in pediatric patients (~1 centimeter per year [range: 0.3-1.8 cm per year] and related to dose and duration of exposure). To minimize the systemic effects of orally-inhaled corticosteroids, each patient should be titrated to the lowest effective dose. Growth should be routinely monitored in pediatric patients.

Use with strong CYP3A4 inhibitors is not recommended (see Drug Interactions). Not to be used in status asthmaticus or for the relief of acute bronchospasm. Flovent® Diskus® contains lactose; very rare anaphylactic reactions have been reported in patients with severe milk protein allergy. There have been reports of systemic corticosteroid withdrawal symptoms (eg, joint/muscle pain, lassitude, depression) when withdrawing oral inhalation therapy. Local yeast infections (eg, oral pharyngeal candidiasis) may occur.

Adverse Reactions

>10%:

Central nervous system: Malaise/fatigue (16%), headache (2% to 14%)

Gastrointestinal: Oral candidiasis (≤31%)

Neuromuscular & skeletal: Arthralgia/articular rheumatism (17%), musculoskeletal pain (2% to 12%)

Respiratory: Sinusitis/sinus infection (≤33%), upper respiratory tract infection (≤31%), throat irritation (3% to 22%), nasal congestion/blockage (16%), rhinitis (≤13%)

1% to 10%:

Central nervous system: Pain (10%), fever (1% to 7%)

Dermatologic: Rash (8%), pruritus (6%)

Gastrointestinal: Nausea/vomiting (1% to 9%), gastrointestinal infection (including viral; 1% to 5%), gastrointestinal discomfort/pain (1% to 4%)

Neuromuscular & skeletal: Muscle injury (≤5%)

Respiratory: Hoarseness/dysphonia (2% to 9%), cough (1% to 9%), viral respiratory infection (1% to 9%), bronchitis (≤8%), upper respiratory tract inflammation (≤5%)

Miscellaneous: Viral infection (≤5%)

Postmarketing and/or case reports: Aggression, agitation, anaphylactic reaction (rare with both products; Diskus® - some patients with severe milk allergy), angioedema, anxiety, aphonia, asthma exacerbation, behavioral changes (eg, hyperactivity and irritability in children; rare), bone mineral density decreased, bronchospasm (immediate and delayed), cataracts, chest tightness, Churg-Strauss syndrome, contusion, Cushingoid features, cutaneous hypersensitivity, depression, dyspnea, ecchymoses, eosinophilia, facial edema, growth velocity reduction in children/adolescents, HPA axis suppression, hyperglycemia, hypersensitivity reactions (immediate and delayed), laryngitis, migraine, muscle rigidity/stiffness/tightness, oropharyngeal edema, osteoporosis, paradoxical bronchospasm, pneumonia, restlessness, throat soreness, tooth discoloration, urticaria, vasculitis, wheeze

Drug Interactions

Metabolism/Transport Effects Substrate of CYP3A4 (major); **Note:** Assignment of Major/Minor substrate status based on clinically relevant drug interaction potential

Avoid Concomitant Use

Avoid concomitant use of Fluticasone (Oral Inhalation) with any of the following: Aldesleukin; BCG; Cobicistat; Fusidic Acid (Systemic); Natalizumab; Pimecrolimus; Tacrolimus (Topical); Tofacitinib

Increased Effect/Toxicity

Fluticasone (Oral Inhalation) may increase the levels/effects of: Amphotericin B; Deferasirox; Leflunomide; Loop Diuretics; Natalizumab; Thiazide Diuretics; Tofacitinib

The levels/effects of Fluticasone (Oral Inhalation) may be increased by: Cobicistat; CYP3A4 Inhibitors (Moderate); CYP3A4 Inhibitors (Strong); Dasatinib; Denosumab; Fusidic Acid (Systemic); Ivacaftor; Luliconazole; Mifepristone; Pimecrolimus; Simeprevir; Tacrolimus (Topical); Telaprevir; Trastuzumab

Decreased Effect

Fluticasone (Oral Inhalation) may decrease the levels/effects of: Aldesleukin; Antidiabetic Agents; BCG; Coccidioidin Skin Test; Corticorelin; Hyaluronidase; Sipuleucel-T; Telaprevir; Vaccines (Inactivated)

The levels/effects of Fluticasone (Oral Inhalation) may be decreased by: Echinacea

Ethanol/Nutrition/Herb Interactions Herb/Nutraceutical: In theory, St John's wort may decrease serum levels of fluticasone by inducing CYP3A4 isoenzymes.

Storage/Stability

Flovent® HFA: Store at 15°C to 30°C (59°F to 86°F). Discard device when the dose counter reads "000". Store with mouthpiece down.

Flovent® Diskus®: Store at 20°C to 25°C (68°F to 77°F) in a dry place away from direct heat or sunlight. Discard after 6 weeks (50 mcg diskus) or after 2 months (100 mcg and 250 mcg diskus) from removal from protective foil pouch or when the dose counter reads "0" (whichever comes first); device is not reusable.

Mechanism of Action Fluticasone belongs to a group of corticosteroids which utilizes a fluorocarbothioate ester linkage at the 17 carbon position; extremely potent vasoconstrictive and anti-inflammatory activity. The effectiveness of inhaled fluticasone is due to its direct local effect.

Pharmacodynamics/Kinetics

Onset of action: Maximal benefit may take 1-2 weeks or longer

Absorption: Absorbed systemically (Flovent® Diskus®: ~8%) primarily via lungs, minimal GI absorption (<1%) due to presystemic metabolism

Distribution: 4.2 L/kg

Protein binding: 99%

Metabolism: Hepatic via CYP3A4 to 17β-carboxylic acid (negligible activity)

Half-life elimination: ~11-12 hours (Thorsson, 2001)

Excretion: Feces (as parent drug and metabolites); urine (<5% as metabolites)

Dosage Inhalation, oral: Asthma: **Note:** Titrate to lowest effective dose once asthma stability achieved.

Flovent® HFA:

U.S. labeling:

Children 4-11 years: Initial: 88 mcg twice daily; maximum: 88 mcg twice daily

Children ≥12 years and Adults: Dosing based on previous asthma therapy: **Note:** May increase dose after 2 weeks of therapy in patients who are not adequately controlled.

Bronchodilator alone: Initial: 88 mcg twice daily; maximum: 440 mcg twice daily

Inhaled corticosteroids: Initial: 88-220 mcg twice daily (initial dose >88 mcg twice daily may be considered in patients previously requiring higher doses of inhaled corticosteroids); maximum: 440 mcg twice daily

Oral corticosteroids (OCS): Initial: 440 mcg twice daily; maximum: 880 mcg twice daily

NIH Asthma Guidelines (NIH, 2007) (administer in divided doses twice daily):

"Low" dose:

0-4 years: 176 mcg/day

5-11 years: 88-176 mcg/day

≥12 years: 88-264 mcg/day

"Medium" dose:

0-4 years: >176-352 mcg/day

5-11 years: >176-352 mcg/day

≥12 years: >264-440 mcg/day

"High" dose:

0-4 years: >352 mcg/day

5-11 years: >352 mcg/day

≥12 years: >440 mcg/day

Canadian labeling:

Children 1-3 years: 100 mcg twice daily

Children 4-15 years: 100 mcg twice daily. **Note:** Canadian labeling recommends Flovent® HFA be administered as a minimum of 2 inhalations twice daily; therefore, patients requiring lower or higher dosages than 100 mcg twice daily should use Flovent® Diskus®.

Children ≥16 years and Adults: **Note:** May increase dose after ~1 week of therapy in patients who are not adequately controlled.

Mild asthma: 100-250 mcg twice daily

Moderate asthma: 250-500 mcg twice daily

Severe asthma: 500 mcg twice daily; may increase up to 1000 mcg twice daily in very severe patients (eg, patients using oral corticosteroids [OCS])

Flovent® Diskus®:

U.S. labeling:

Children 4-11 years: Initial: 50 mcg twice daily; may increase to maximum dose of 100 mcg twice daily in patients not adequately controlled after 2 weeks of therapy. Initial dose >50 mcg twice daily may be considered in patients with poorer asthma control or those previously requiring high ranges of inhaled corticosteroids

Children ≥12 years and Adults: **Note:** May increase dose after 2 weeks of therapy in patients who are not adequately controlled.

Dosing based on previous asthma therapy:
Bronchodilator alone: Initial: 100 mcg twice daily; maximum: 500 mcg twice daily
Inhaled corticosteroids: Initial: 100-250 mcg twice daily; maximum: 500 mcg twice daily; initial dose >100 mcg twice daily may be considered in patients with poorer asthma control or those previously requiring high ranges of inhaled corticosteroids
Oral corticosteroids (OCS): Initial: 500-1000 mcg twice daily; maximum: 1000 mcg twice daily

NIH Asthma Guidelines (NIH, 2007) (administer in divided doses twice daily):
"Low" dose:
5-11 years: 100-200 mcg/day
≥12 years: 100-300 mcg/day
"Medium" dose:
5-11 years: >200-400 mcg/day
≥12 years: >300-500 mcg/day
"High" dose:
5-11 years: >400 mcg/day
≥12 years: >500 mcg/day

Canadian labeling:
Children 4-16 years: Initial: 50-100 mcg twice daily; may increase up to 200 mcg twice daily after ~1 week of therapy in patients not adequately controlled
Children ≥16 years and Adults: **Note:** May increase dose after ~1 week of therapy in patients who are not adequately controlled.
Mild asthma: 100-250 mcg twice daily
Moderate asthma: 250-500 mcg twice daily
Severe asthma: 500 mcg twice daily; may increase up to 1000 mcg twice daily in very severe patients (eg, patients using oral corticosteroids [OCS])

Conversion from oral systemic corticosteroids to orally inhaled corticosteroids: When converting from oral corticosteroids (OCS) to orally inhaled corticosteroids, initiate oral inhalation therapy in patients whose asthma is previously stabilized on OCS. Gradual OCS dose reductions should begin ~7 days after starting inhaled therapy. U.S. labeling recommends reducing prednisone dose no more rapidly than 2.5-5 mg/day (or equivalent of other OCS) weekly in children ≥12 years but does not provide a recommendation for children <12 years. A similar approach to OCS dose reduction would however seem advisable. The Canadian labeling recommends decreasing the daily dose of prednisone by 1 mg (or equivalent of other OCS) no more rapidly than weekly (adults) or every 8 days (children) if closely monitored or every 10 days (adults) and 20 days (children) if not closely monitored. If adrenal insufficiency occurs, resume OCS therapy; initiate a more gradual withdrawal. When transitioning from systemic to inhaled corticosteroids, supplemental systemic corticosteroid therapy may be necessary during periods of stress or during severe asthma attacks.

Elderly: Refer to adult dosing.

Dosage adjustment in renal impairment: No dosage adjustment provided in manufacturer's labeling (has not been studied).

Dosage adjustment in hepatic impairment: No dosage adjustment provided in manufacturer's labeling (has not been studied); however, fluticasone is primarily cleared in the liver and plasma levels may be increased in patients with hepatic impairment. Use with caution; monitor.

Dietary Considerations Flovent® Diskus® contains lactose; very rare anaphylactic reactions have been reported in patients with severe milk protein allergy.

Administration

Aerosol inhalation: Flovent® HFA: Shake container thoroughly before using. Take 3-5 deep breaths. Use inhaler on inspiration. Allow 1 full minute between inhalations. Rinse mouth with water after use to reduce aftertaste and incidence of candidiasis; do not swallow. Inhaler must be primed before first use, when not used for 7 days, or if dropped. To prime the first time, release 4 sprays into air; shake well before each spray and spray away from face. If dropped or not used for 7 days, prime by releasing a single test spray. Patient should contact pharmacy for refill when the dose counter reads "020". Discard device when the dose counter reads "000". Do not use "float" test to determine contents.

Powder for oral inhalation: Flovent® Diskus®: Do not use with a spacer device. Do not exhale into Diskus®. Do not wash or take apart. Use in horizontal position. Mouth should be rinsed with water after use (do not swallow). Discard after 6 weeks (50 mcg diskus) or after 2 months (100 mcg and 250 mcg diskus) once removed from protective pouch or when the dose counter reads "0", whichever comes first (device is not reusable).

Monitoring Parameters Growth (adolescents and children); signs/symptoms of HPA axis suppression/adrenal insufficiency; possible eosinophilic conditions (including Churg-Strauss syndrome); FEV_1, peak flow, and/or other pulmonary function tests; asthma symptoms

Additional Information Effects of inhaled steroids on growth have been observed in the absence of laboratory evidence of HPA axis suppression, suggesting that growth velocity is a more sensitive indicator of systemic corticosteroid exposure in pediatric patients than some commonly used tests of HPA axis function. The long-term effects of this reduction in growth velocity associated with orally-inhaled corticosteroids, including the impact on final adult height, are unknown. The potential for "catch up" growth following discontinuation of treatment with inhaled corticosteroids has not been adequately studied.

In the United States, dosage for the metered dose inhaler (Flovent® HFA) is expressed as the amount of drug which leaves the actuater and is delivered to the patient. This differs from other countries, which express the dosage as the amount of drug which leaves the valve.

Dosage Forms Considerations

Flovent HFA 10.6 g and 12 g canisters contain 120 inhalations.

Dosage Forms Excipient information presented when available (limited, particularly for generics); consult specific product labeling.

Aerosol, Inhalation, as propionate:
Flovent HFA: 44 mcg/actuation (10.6 g); 110 mcg/actuation (12 g); 220 mcg/actuation (12 g)

Aerosol Powder Breath Activated, Inhalation, as propionate:
Flovent Diskus: 50 mcg/blister (60 ea); 100 mcg/blister (28 ea, 60 ea); 250 mcg/blister (28 ea, 60 ea) [contains lactose]

Dosage Forms: Canada Excipient information presented when available (limited, particularly for generics); consult specific product labeling.

Aerosol, for oral inhalation, as propionate:
Flovent® HFA: 50 mcg/inhalation (120 actuations); 125 mcg/inhalation (60 or 120 actuations); 250 mcg/inhalation (60 or 120 actuations)

Powder, for oral inhalation, as propionate:
Flovent® Diskus®: 50 mcg (60s) [contains lactose; prefilled blister pack]
Flovent® Diskus®: 100 mcg (60s) [contains lactose; prefilled blister pack]
Flovent® Diskus®: 250 mcg (60s) [contains lactose; prefilled blister pack]
Flovent® Diskus®: 500 mcg (60s) [contains lactose; prefilled blister pack]

Fluticasone (Nasal) (floo TIK a sone)

Brand Names: U.S. Flonase; Veramyst

Brand Names: Canada Apo-Fluticasone®; Avamys®; Flonase®; ratio-Fluticasone

Index Terms Fluticasone Furoate; Fluticasone Propionate

Pharmacologic Category Corticosteroid, Nasal

Additional Appendix Information

Inhaled Corticosteroids *on page 2298*

Use

Flonase®: Management of seasonal and perennial allergic rhinitis and nonallergic rhinitis

Veramyst®, Avamys® (Canadian availability; not available in the U.S.): Management of seasonal and perennial allergic rhinitis

Unlabeled Use Adjunct to antibiotics in empiric treatment of acute bacterial rhinosinusitis (ABRS) (Chow, 2012)

Pregnancy Risk Factor C

Dosage

Intranasal: Rhinitis:

Children:

Flonase® (fluticasone propionate): Children ≥4 years and Adolescents: Initial: 1 spray (50 mcg/spray) per nostril once daily (100 mcg/day); patients not adequately responding or patients with more severe symptoms may use 2 sprays per nostril once daily (200 mcg/day); once symptoms are controlled, dosage should be reduced to 1 spray per nostril once daily (100 mcg/day). Total daily dosage should not exceed 2 sprays in each nostril (200 mcg)/day. Dosing should be at regular intervals.

Veramyst® (fluticasone furoate):

Children 2-11 years: Initial: 1 spray (27.5 mcg/spray) per nostril once daily (55 mcg/day); patients not adequately responding may use 2 sprays per nostril once daily (110 mcg/day); once symptoms are controlled, dosage may be reduced to 55 mcg once daily. Total daily dosage should not exceed 2 sprays in each nostril (110 mcg)/day; once symptoms are controlled, dosage may be reduced to 1 spray per nostril once daily (55 mcg/day). Total daily dosage should not exceed 2 sprays in each nostril (110 mcg)/day.

Children ≥12 years and Adolescents: Initial: 2 sprays (27.5 mcg/spray) per nostril once daily (110 mcg/day). Once symptoms are controlled, dosage may be reduced to 1 spray per nostril once daily (55 mcg/day) for maintenance therapy.

Avamys® (fluticasone furoate) (Canadian availability; not available in the U.S.):

Children 2-11 years: Initial: 1 spray (27.5 mcg/spray) per nostril once daily (55 mcg/day); patients not adequately responding may use 2 sprays per nostril once daily (110 mcg/day); once symptoms are controlled, dosage should be reduced to 1 spray per nostril once daily (55 mcg/day). Total daily dosage should not exceed 2 sprays in each nostril (110 mcg)/day.

Children ≥12 years and Adolescents: Initial: 2 sprays (27.5 mcg/spray) per nostril once daily (110 mcg/day). Total daily dosage should not exceed 2 sprays in each nostril (110 mcg)/day.

Adults:

Flonase® (fluticasone propionate): Initial: 2 sprays (50 mcg/spray) per nostril once daily (200 mcg/day); alternatively, the same total daily dosage may be divided and given as 1 spray per nostril twice daily (200 mcg/day). After the first few days, dosage may be reduced to 1 spray per nostril once daily for maintenance therapy (100 mcg/day).

Veramyst® (fluticasone furoate): Initial: 2 sprays (27.5 mcg/spray) per nostril once daily (110 mcg/day); once symptoms are controlled, may reduce dosage to 1 spray per nostril once daily (55 mcg/day) for maintenance therapy.

Avamys® (fluticasone furoate) (Canadian availability; not available in the U.S.): 2 sprays (27.5 mcg/spray) in each nostril once daily (110 mcg/day). Total daily dosage should not exceed 2 sprays in each nostril (110 mcg)/day.

Additional Information Complete prescribing information should be consulted for additional detail.

Dosage Forms Considerations

Flonase 16 g bottles and Veramyst 10 g bottles contain 120 sprays each.

Dosage Forms Excipient information presented when available (limited, particularly for generics); consult specific product labeling.

Suspension, Nasal, as furoate:

Veramyst: 27.5 mcg/spray (10 g) [contains benzalkonium chloride]

Suspension, Nasal, as propionate:

Flonase: 50 mcg/actuation (16 g) [contains benzalkonium chloride, polysorbate 80]

Generic: 50 mcg/actuation (16 g); 50 mcg/actuation (16 g)

Dosage Forms: Canada Excipient information presented when available (limited, particularly for generics); consult specific product labeling.

Suspension, intranasal, as furoate [spray]:

Avamys®: 27.5 mcg/inhalation (4.5 g) [30 metered actuations; contains benzalkonium chloride]; (10 g) [120 metered actuations; contains benzalkonium chloride]

Fluticasone (Topical) (floo TIK a sone)

Brand Names: U.S. Cutivate

Brand Names: Canada Cutivate™

Index Terms Fluticasone Propionate

Pharmacologic Category Corticosteroid, Topical

Additional Appendix Information

Topical Corticosteroids *on page 2299*

Use Relief of inflammation and pruritus associated with corticosteroid-responsive dermatoses; atopic dermatitis

Pregnancy Risk Factor C

Dosage Topical:

Children:

Corticosteroid-responsive dermatoses: Children ≥3 months: Cream: Apply sparingly to affected area twice daily. If no improvement is seen within 2 weeks, reassessment of diagnosis may be necessary.

Atopic dermatitis

Children ≥3 months: Cream: Apply sparingly to affected area 1-2 times/day. If no improvement is seen within 2 weeks, reassessment of diagnosis may be necessary.

Children ≥1 year: Lotion: Apply sparingly to affected area once daily

Adults:

Corticosteroid-responsive dermatoses: Cream, lotion, ointment: Apply sparingly to affected area twice daily. If no improvement is seen within 2 weeks, reassessment of diagnosis may be necessary.

Atopic dermatitis: Cream, lotion: Apply sparingly to affected area once or twice daily. If no improvement is seen within 2 weeks, reassessment of diagnosis may be necessary.

Additional Information Complete prescribing information should be consulted for additional detail.

Dosage Forms Excipient information presented when available (limited, particularly for generics); consult specific product labeling.

Cream, External, as propionate:

Cutivate: 0.05% (30 g, 60 g) [contains cetyl alcohol, propylene glycol]

Generic: 0.05% (15 g, 30 g, 60 g)

Lotion, External, as propionate:

Cutivate: 0.05% (120 mL) [contains cetostearyl alcohol, methylparaben, propylene glycol, propylparaben]

Generic: 0.05% (60 mL, 120 mL)

Ointment, External, as propionate:

Cutivate: 0.005% (30 g, 60 g)

Generic: 0.005% (15 g, 30 g, 60 g)

Fluticasone and Salmeterol

(floo TIK a sone & sal ME te role)

Brand Names: U.S. Advair Diskus®; Advair® HFA

Brand Names: Canada Advair Diskus®; Advair®

Index Terms Fluticasone Propionate and Salmeterol Xinafoate; Salmeterol and Fluticasone

Pharmacologic Category $Beta_2$ Agonist; $Beta_2$-Adrenergic Agonist, Long-Acting; Corticosteroid, Inhalant (Oral)

Use Maintenance treatment of asthma; maintenance treatment of COPD

Pregnancy Risk Factor C

Pregnancy Considerations Adverse events were observed in animal reproduction studies using this combination. Refer to individual agents.

Breast-Feeding Considerations It is not known if fluticasone or salmeterol are excreted into breast milk. The manufacturer recommends that caution be used if administering this combination to breast-feeding women. Refer to individual agents.

Medication Guide Available Yes

Contraindications Hypersensitivity to fluticasone, salmeterol, or any component of the formulation; status asthmaticus; acute episodes of asthma or COPD; severe hypersensitivity to milk proteins (Advair Diskus®)

Warnings/Precautions See individual agents.

Adverse Reactions Percentages reported in patients with asthma; also see individual agents:

>10%:

Central nervous system: Headache (12% to 21%)

Respiratory: Upper respiratory tract infection (16% to 27%), pharyngitis (9% to 13%)

>3% to 10%:

Central nervous system: Dizziness (1% to 4%)

Endocrine & metabolic: Menstruation symptoms (3% to 5%)

Gastrointestinal: Nausea/vomiting (3% to 6%), diarrhea (2% to 4%), pain/discomfort (1% to 4%), oral candidiasis (1% to 4%), gastrointestinal infections (including viral, ≤4%)

Neuromuscular & skeletal: Musculoskeletal pain (2% to 7%), muscle pain (≤4%)

Respiratory: Throat irritation (7% to 9%), bronchitis (2% to 8%), upper respiratory tract inflammation (4% to 7%), lower respiratory tract infections/pneumonia (1% to 7%; COPD diagnosis and age >65 years increase risk), cough (3% to 6%), sinusitis (4% to 5%), hoarseness/dysphonia (1% to 5%), viral respiratory tract infection (3% to 5%)

1% to 3%:

Cardiovascular: Arrhythmia, chest symptoms, fluid retention, MI, palpitation, syncope, tachycardia

Central nervous system: Compressed nerve syndromes, hypnagogic effects, migraine, pain, sleep disorders, tremor

Dermatologic: Dermatitis, dermatosis, eczema, hives, skin flakiness, urticaria, viral skin infection

Endocrine & metabolic: Hypothyroidism

Gastrointestinal: Constipation, dental discomfort/pain, gastrointestinal infection, hemorrhoids, oral discomfort/pain, oral erythema/rash, oral ulcerations, unusual taste, weight gain

Genitourinary: Urinary tract infection

Hematologic: Contusions/hematomas

Hepatic: Abnormal liver function tests

Neuromuscular & skeletal: Arthralgia, articular rheumatism, bone/cartilage disorders, bone pain, cramps, fractures, muscle injuries (≤3%), muscle spasm, muscle stiffness, tightness/rigidity

Ocular: Conjunctivitis, edema, eye redness, keratitis, xerophthalmia

Respiratory: Blood in nasal mucosa, congestion, ear/nose/throat infection, epistaxis, laryngitis, lower respiratory hemorrhage, nasal irritation, rhinitis, rhinorrhea/postnasal drip, sneezing

Miscellaneous: Allergies/allergic reactions, bacterial infection, burns, candidiasis (≤3%), diaphoresis, sweat/sebum disorders, viral infection, wounds and lacerations

Postmarketing and/or case reports: Asthma exacerbation (serious and some fatal), abdominal pain, agitation, aggression, anaphylactic reaction (some in patients with severe milk allergy [Diskus®]), angioedema, aphonia, atrial fibrillation, bronchospasm, cataracts, chest congestion, chest tightness, choking, contact dermatitis, Cushing syndrome, Cushingoid features, depression, dysmenorrhea, dyspepsia, dyspnea, earache, ecchymoses, edema (facial, oropharyngeal), eosinophilic conditions, glaucoma, growth velocity reduction in children/adolescents, hyperactivity, hypercorticism, hyperglycemia, hypersensitivity reaction (immediate and delayed), hypertension, hypokalemia, hypothyroidism, influenza, intraocular pressure increased, irritability, laryngeal spasm/irritation, irregular menstruation, myositis, osteoporosis, pallor, paresthesia, paradoxical tracheitis, paranasal sinus pain, photodermatitis, PID, rash, restlessness, stridor, supraventricular tachycardia, syncope, vaginal candidiasis, vaginitis, vulvovaginitis, rare cases of vasculitis (Churg-Strauss syndrome), ventricular tachycardia, wheezing, xerostomia

Drug Interactions

Metabolism/Transport Effects Refer to individual components.

Avoid Concomitant Use

Avoid concomitant use of Fluticasone and Salmeterol with any of the following: Aldesleukin; BCG; Beta-Blockers (Nonselective); Cobicistat; CYP3A4 Inhibitors (Strong); Fusidic Acid (Systemic); Iobenguane I 123; Long-Acting Beta2-Agonists; Natalizumab; Pimecrolimus; Tacrolimus (Topical); Telaprevir; Tofacitinib

Increased Effect/Toxicity

Fluticasone and Salmeterol may increase the levels/effects of: Amphotericin B; Atosiban; Deferasirox; Highest Risk QTc-Prolonging Agents; Leflunomide; Long-Acting Beta2-Agonists; Loop Diuretics; Moderate Risk QTc-Prolonging Agents; Natalizumab; Sympathomimetics; Thiazide Diuretics; Tofacitinib

The levels/effects of Fluticasone and Salmeterol may be increased by: AtoMOXetine; Cannabinoids; Cobicistat; CYP3A4 Inhibitors (Moderate); CYP3A4 Inhibitors (Strong); Dasatinib; Denosumab; Fusidic Acid (Systemic); Ivacaftor; Luliconazole; MAO Inhibitors; Mifepristone; Pimecrolimus; Simeprevir; Tacrolimus (Topical); Telaprevir; Trastuzumab; Tricyclic Antidepressants

Decreased Effect

Fluticasone and Salmeterol may decrease the levels/effects of: Aldesleukin; Antidiabetic Agents; BCG; Coccidioidin Skin Test; Corticorelin; Hyaluronidase;

Iobenguane I 123; Sipuleucel-T; Telaprevir; Vaccines (Inactivated)

The levels/effects of Fluticasone and Salmeterol may be decreased by: Beta-Blockers (Beta1 Selective); Beta-Blockers (Nonselective); Betahistine; Echinacea

Storage/Stability

Advair Diskus®: Store at controlled room temperature of 20°C to 25°C (68°F to 77°F). Store in a dry place out of direct heat or sunlight. Diskus® device should be discarded 1 month after removal from foil pouch, or when dosing indicator reads "0" (whichever comes first); device is not reusable.

Advair® HFA: Store at controlled room temperature of 25°C (77°F). Store with mouthpiece down. Discard after 120 inhalations. Discard device when the dose counter reads "000". Device is not reusable.

Mechanism of Action Combination of fluticasone (corticosteroid) and salmeterol (long-acting beta$_2$-agonist) designed to improve pulmonary function and control over what is produced by either agent when used alone. Because fluticasone and salmeterol act locally in the lung, plasma levels do not predict therapeutic effect.

Fluticasone: The mechanism of action for all topical corticosteroids is believed to be a combination of three important properties: Anti-inflammatory activity, immunosuppressive properties, and antiproliferative actions. Fluticasone has extremely potent vasoconstrictive and anti-inflammatory activity.

Salmeterol: Relaxes bronchial smooth muscle by selective action on beta$_2$-receptors with little effect on heart rate

Pharmacodynamics/Kinetics See individual agents.

Dosage Oral inhalation: **Note:** Do not use to transfer patients from systemic corticosteroid therapy.

COPD: Adults:

Advair Diskus®: Fluticasone 250 mcg/salmeterol 50 mcg twice daily, 12 hours apart. **Note:** This is the maximum dose.

Advair Diskus® [Canadian labeling; not in approved U.S. labeling]: Fluticasone 250 mcg/salmeterol 50 mcg **or** fluticasone 500 mcg/salmeterol 50 mcg twice daily, 12 hours apart.

Maximum dose: Fluticasone 500 mcg/salmeterol 50 mcg per inhalation (2 inhalations/day)

Asthma:

Children 4-11 years: Advair Diskus®: Fluticasone 100 mcg/salmeterol 50 mcg twice daily, 12 hours apart. **Note:** This is the maximum dose.

Children ≥12 years and Adults:

Advair Diskus®: One inhalation twice daily, morning and evening, 12 hours apart

Maximum dose: Fluticasone 500 mcg/salmeterol 50 mcg per inhalation (2 inhalations/day)

Advair® HFA: Two inhalations twice daily, morning and evening, 12 hours apart

Maximum dose: Fluticasone 230 mcg/salmeterol 21 mcg per inhalation (4 inhalations/day)

Advair® 125 or Advair® 250 [Canadian labeling; not in approved U.S. labeling]: Two inhalations twice daily, morning and evening, 12 hours apart

Maximum dose: Fluticasone 250 mcg/salmeterol 25 mcg per inhalation (4 inhalations/day)

Note: Initial dose prescribed should be based upon previous dose of inhaled-steroid asthma therapy. Dose should be increased after 2 weeks if adequate response is not achieved. Patients should be titrated to lowest effective dose once stable. Each suggestion below specifies the product strength to use; remember to **use 1 inhalation for Diskus® and 2 inhalations for HFA.**

Patients not currently on inhaled corticosteroids:

Advair Diskus®: Fluticasone 100 mcg/salmeterol 50 mcg **or** fluticasone 250 mcg/salmeterol 50 mcg

Advair® HFA: Fluticasone 45 mcg/salmeterol 21 mcg **or** fluticasone 115 mcg/salmeterol 21 mcg

Patients currently using inhaled beclomethasone dipropionate:

≤160 mcg/day: Fluticasone 100 mcg/salmeterol 50 mcg **or** Advair® HFA: Fluticasone 45 mcg/salmeterol 21 mcg

320 mcg/day: Fluticasone 250 mcg/salmeterol 50 mcg **or** Advair® HFA: Fluticasone 115 mcg/salmeterol 21 mcg

640 mcg/day: Fluticasone 500 mcg/salmeterol 50 mcg **or** Advair® HFA: Fluticasone 230 mcg/salmeterol 21 mcg

Patients currently using inhaled budesonide:

≤400 mcg/day: Fluticasone 100 mcg/salmeterol 50 mcg **or** Advair® HFA: Fluticasone 45 mcg/salmeterol 21 mcg

800-1200 mcg/day: Fluticasone 250 mcg/salmeterol 50 mcg **or** Advair® HFA: Fluticasone 115 mcg/salmeterol 21 mcg

1600 mcg/day: Fluticasone 500 mcg/salmeterol 50 mcg **or** Advair® HFA: Fluticasone 230 mcg/salmeterol 21 mcg

Patients currently using inhaled flunisolide CFC aerosol:

≤1000 mcg/day: Fluticasone 100 mcg/salmeterol 50 mcg **or** Advair® HFA: Fluticasone 45 mcg/salmeterol 21 mcg

1250-2000 mcg/day: Fluticasone 250 mcg/salmeterol 50 mcg **or** Advair® HFA: Fluticasone 115 mcg/salmeterol 21 mcg

Patients currently using inhaled flunisolide HFA inhalation aerosol:

≤320 mcg/day: Fluticasone 100 mcg/salmeterol 50 mcg **or** Advair® HFA: Fluticasone 45 mcg/salmeterol 21 mcg

640 mcg/day: Fluticasone 250 mcg/salmeterol 50 mcg **or** Advair® HFA: Fluticasone 115 mcg/salmeterol 21 mcg

Patients currently using inhaled fluticasone HFA aerosol:

≤176 mcg/day: Fluticasone 100 mcg/salmeterol 50 mcg **or** Advair® HFA: Fluticasone 45 mcg/salmeterol 21 mcg

440 mcg/day: Fluticasone 250 mcg/salmeterol 50 mcg **or** Advair® HFA: Fluticasone 115 mcg/salmeterol 21 mcg

660-880 mcg/day: Fluticasone 500 mcg/salmeterol 50 mcg **or** Advair® HFA: Fluticasone 230 mcg/salmeterol 21 mcg

Patients currently using inhaled fluticasone propionate powder:

≤200 mcg/day: Fluticasone 100 mcg/salmeterol 50 mcg **or** Advair® HFA: Fluticasone 45 mcg/salmeterol 21 mcg

500 mcg/day: Fluticasone 250 mcg/salmeterol 50 mcg **or** Advair® HFA: Fluticasone 115 mcg/salmeterol 21 mcg

1000 mcg/day: Fluticasone 500 mcg/salmeterol 50 mcg **or** Advair® HFA: Fluticasone 230 mcg/salmeterol 21 mcg

Patients currently using inhaled mometasone furoate powder:

220 mcg/day: Fluticasone 100 mcg/salmeterol 50 mcg **or** Advair® HFA: Fluticasone 45 mcg/salmeterol 21 mcg

440 mcg/day: Fluticasone 250 mcg/salmeterol 50 mcg **or** Advair® HFA: Fluticasone 115 mcg/salmeterol 21 mcg

880 mcg/day: Fluticasone 500 mcg/salmeterol 50 mcg **or** Advair® HFA: Fluticasone 230 mcg/salmeterol 21 mcg

Patients currently using inhaled triamcinolone acetonide:
≤1000 mcg/day: Fluticasone 100 mcg/salmeterol 50 mcg **or** Advair® HFA: Fluticasone 45 mcg/salmeterol 21 mcg
1100-1600 mcg/day: Fluticasone 250 mcg/salmeterol 50 mcg **or** Advair® HFA: Fluticasone 115 mcg/salmeterol 21 mcg

Elderly: No differences in safety or effectiveness have been seen in studies of patients ≥65 years of age. However, increased sensitivity may be seen in the elderly. Use with caution in patients with concomitant cardiovascular disease.

Dosage adjustment in renal impairment: No dosage adjustment provided in manufacturer's labeling (has not been studied). However, fluticasone and salmeterol are predominately eliminated by hepatic metabolism.

Dosage adjustment in hepatic impairment: No dosage adjustment required; manufacturer suggests close monitoring of patients with hepatic impairment.

Dietary Considerations Advair Diskus® powder for oral inhalation contains lactose; very rare anaphylactic reactions have been reported in patients with severe milk protein allergy.

Administration

Advair Diskus®: After removing from box and foil pouch, write the "Pouch opened" and "Use by" dates on the label on top of the Diskus®. The "Use by" date is 1 month from date of opening the pouch. Every time the lever is pushed back, a dose is ready to be inhaled. Do not close or tilt the Diskus® after the lever is pushed back. Do not play with the lever or move the lever more than once. The dose indicator tells you how many doses are left. When the numbers 5 to 0 appear in red, only a few doses remain. Discard device 1 month after you remove it from the foil pouch or when the dose counter reads "0" (whichever comes first). Rinse mouth with water after use and spit to reduce risk of oral candidiasis.

Advair® HFA: Shake well for 5 seconds before each spray. Prime with 4 test sprays (into air and away from face) before using for the first time. If canister is dropped or not used for >4 weeks, prime with 2 sprays. Patient should contact pharmacy for refill when the dose counter reads "020". Discard device when the dose counter reads "000". Do not spray in eyes. Rinse mouth with water after use and spit to reduce risk of oral candidiasis.

Monitoring Parameters FEV_1, peak flow, and/or other pulmonary function tests; blood pressure, heart rate; CNS stimulation. Monitor for increased use of short-acting beta$_2$-agonist inhalers; may be marker of a deteriorating asthma condition. The growth of pediatric patients receiving inhaled corticosteroids should be monitored routinely (eg, via stadiometry).

Additional Information Effects of inhaled/intranasal steroids on growth have been observed in the absence of laboratory evidence of HPA axis suppression, suggesting that growth velocity is a more sensitive indicator of systemic corticosteroid exposure in pediatric patients than some commonly used tests of HPA axis function. The long-term effects of this reduction in growth velocity associated with orally-inhaled and intranasal corticosteroids, including the impact on final adult height, are unknown. The potential for "catch up" growth following discontinuation of treatment with inhaled corticosteroids has not been adequately studied.

Advair® HFA: Salmeterol (base) 21 mcg is equivalent to 30.45 mcg of salmeterol xinafoate.

Dosage Forms Excipient information presented when available (limited, particularly for generics); consult specific product labeling. [DSC] = Discontinued product

Aerosol, for oral inhalation:
Advair® HFA:
45/21: Fluticasone propionate 45 mcg and salmeterol 21 mcg per inhalation (8 g) [chlorofluorocarbon free; 60 metered actuations]
45/21: Fluticasone propionate 45 mcg and salmeterol 21 mcg per inhalation (12 g) [chlorofluorocarbon free; 120 metered actuations]
115/21: Fluticasone propionate 115 mcg and salmeterol 21 mcg per inhalation (8 g) [chlorofluorocarbon free; 60 metered actuations]
115/21: Fluticasone propionate 115 mcg and salmeterol 21 mcg per inhalation (12 g) [chlorofluorocarbon free; 120 metered actuations]
230/21: Fluticasone propionate 230 mcg and salmeterol 21 mcg per inhalation (8 g) [chlorofluorocarbon free; 60 metered actuations]
230/21: Fluticasone propionate 230 mcg and salmeterol 21 mcg per inhalation (12 g) [chlorofluorocarbon free; 120 metered actuations]

Powder, for oral inhalation:
Advair Diskus®:
100/50: Fluticasone propionate 100 mcg and salmeterol 50 mcg (14s, 28s [DSC], 60s) [contains lactose]
250/50: Fluticasone propionate 250 mcg and salmeterol 50 mcg (14s [DSC], 60s) [contains lactose]
500/50: Fluticasone propionate 500 mcg and salmeterol 50 mcg (14s [DSC], 60s) [contains lactose]

Dosage Forms: Canada Excipient information presented when available (limited, particularly for generics); consult specific product labeling.

Aerosol, for oral inhalation:
Advair®;
125/25: Fluticasone propionate 125 mcg and salmeterol 25 mcg per inhalation (12 g) [120 metered actuations]
250/25: Fluticasone propionate 250 mcg and salmeterol 25 mcg per inhalation (12 g) [120 metered actuations]

Fluticasone and Vilanterol

(floo TIK a sone & VYE lan ter ol)

Brand Names: U.S. Breo Ellipta

Index Terms Fluticasone Furoate and Vilanterol; Vilanterol and Fluticasone; Vilanterol and Fluticasone Furoate

Pharmacologic Category Beta$_2$ Agonist; Beta$_2$-Adrenergic Agonist, Long-Acting; Corticosteroid, Inhalant (Oral)

Use Maintenance treatment of airflow obstruction in patients with chronic obstructive pulmonary disease (COPD), including chronic bronchitis and/or emphysema; reduce exacerbations of COPD in patients with a history of exacerbations

Pregnancy Risk Factor C

Pregnancy Considerations Adverse events were not observed in animal reproduction studies. Hypoadrenalism may occur in infants born to mothers receiving corticosteroids during pregnancy (refer to the Fluticasone [Oral Inhalation] monograph for additional details). Beta-agonists have the potential to affect uterine contractility if administered during labor.

Breast-Feeding Considerations It is not known if sufficient quantities of fluticasone or vilanterol are absorbed following inhalation to produce detectable amounts in breast milk. The manufacturer recommends that caution be exercised when administering to nursing women.

Medication Guide Available Yes

Contraindications Hypersensitivity to fluticasone, vilanterol or any component of the formulation; severe hypersensitivity to milk proteins

Warnings/Precautions [U.S. Boxed Warning]: Long-acting beta$_2$-agonists (LABAs), such as vilanterol, increase the risk of asthma-related deaths. In a large, randomized, placebo-controlled U.S. clinical trial (SMART,

2006), salmeterol was associated with an increase in asthma-related deaths (when added to usual asthma therapy); risk is considered a class effect among all LABAs. Data are not available to determine if the addition of an inhaled corticosteroid lessens this increased risk of death associated with LABA use.

Do **not** use for acute bronchospasm or acute symptomatic COPD. Short-acting $beta_2$-agonist (eg, albuterol) should be used for acute symptoms and symptoms occurring between treatments. Do **not** initiate in patients with significantly worsening or acutely deteriorating COPD. Increased use and/or ineffectiveness of short-acting $beta_2$-agonists may indicate rapidly deteriorating disease and should prompt re-evaluation of the patient's condition. Patients must be instructed to seek medical attention in cases where acute symptoms are not relieved by short-acting beta-agonist (not vilanterol) or a previous level of response is diminished. Medical evaluation must not be delayed. Patients using inhaled, short acting $beta_2$-agonists should be instructed to discontinue routine use of these medications prior to beginning treatment with fluticasone/vilanterol; short acting agents should be reserved for symptomatic relief of acute symptoms. Data are not available to determine if LABA use increases the risk of death in patients with COPD.

Hypersensitivity reactions have been reported. Do not exceed recommended dose; serious adverse events, including fatalities, have been associated with excessive use of inhaled sympathomimetics. Rarely, paradoxical bronchospasm may occur with use of inhaled bronchodilating agents; this should be distinguished from inadequate response. Pneumonia and other lower respiratory tract infections have been reported in patients with COPD following the use of inhaled corticosteroids; monitor COPD patients closely since pneumonia symptoms may overlap symptoms of exacerbations.

Use caution in patients with cardiovascular disease (arrhythmia, hypertension or HF), seizure disorders, diabetes, ocular disease, osteoporosis, thyroid disease, or hypokalemia. Beta-agonists may cause elevation in blood pressure, heart rate, and result in CNS stimulation/excitation. $Beta_2$-agonists may increase risk of arrhythmia, increase serum glucose, or decrease serum potassium. Long-term use may affect bone mineral density in adults. Infections with *Candida albicans* in the mouth and throat (thrush) have been reported with use. Potentially significant drug-drug interactions may exist, requiring dose or frequency adjustment, additional monitoring, and/or selection of alternative therapy.

Fluticasone may cause hypercorticism and/or suppression of hypothalamic-pituitary-adrenal (HPA) axis. Caution is required when patients are transferred from systemic corticosteroids to products with lower systemic bioavailability (ie, inhalation). May lead to possible adrenal insufficiency or withdrawal symptoms, including an increase in allergic symptoms. Patients receiving prolonged therapy ≥20 mg per day of prednisone (or equivalent) may be most susceptible. Aerosol steroids do not provide the systemic steroid needed to treat patients having trauma, surgery, or infections.

Use increases susceptibility to infections (eg, chickenpox and measles, sometimes more serious or even fatal, in susceptible children or adults using corticosteroids). Avoid exposure in such patients who have not had these diseases or been properly immunized. How the dose, route, and duration of corticosteroid administration affect the risk of developing a disseminated infection is not known. The contribution of the underlying disease and/or prior corticosteroid treatment to the risk is also not known. Use with caution in patients with active or quiescent tuberculosis infections of the respiratory tract; systemic fungal, bacterial, viral, or parasitic infections; or ocular herpes simplex.

Adverse Reactions

1% to 10%:

Cardiovascular: Hypertension (≥3%), peripheral edema (≥3%)

Central nervous system: Headache (7%)

Gastrointestinal: Oropharyngeal candidiasis (5%), diarrhea (≥3%)

Infection: Influenza (≥3%)

Neuromuscular & skeletal: Arthralgia (≥3%), back pain (≥3%), bone fracture (2%)

Respiratory: Nasopharyngitis (9%), upper respiratory tract infection (7%), pneumonia (6%), bronchitis (≥3%), cough (≥3%), oropharyngeal pain (≥3%), pharyngitis (≥3%), sinusitis (≥3%)

Miscellaneous: Fever (≥3%)

<1% (Limited to important or life-threatening): Cataract, glaucoma

Drug Interactions

Metabolism/Transport Effects Refer to individual components.

Avoid Concomitant Use

Avoid concomitant use of Fluticasone and Vilanterol with any of the following: Aldesleukin; BCG; Beta-Blockers (Nonselective); Cobicistat; Fusidic Acid (Systemic); Iobenguane I 123; Long-Acting Beta2-Agonists; Natalizumab; Pimecrolimus; Tacrolimus (Topical); Tofacitinib

Increased Effect/Toxicity

Fluticasone and Vilanterol may increase the levels/effects of: Amphotericin B; Atosiban; Deferasirox; Highest Risk QTc-Prolonging Agents; Leflunomide; Long-Acting Beta2-Agonists; Loop Diuretics; Moderate Risk QTc-Prolonging Agents; Natalizumab; Sympathomimetics; Thiazide Diuretics; Tofacitinib

The levels/effects of Fluticasone and Vilanterol may be increased by: AtoMOXetine; Cannabinoids; Cobicistat; CYP3A4 Inhibitors (Moderate); CYP3A4 Inhibitors (Strong); Dasatinib; Denosumab; Fusidic Acid (Systemic); Ivacaftor; Luliconazole; MAO Inhibitors; Mifepristone; Pimecrolimus; Simeprevir; Tacrolimus (Topical); Telaprevir; Trastuzumab; Tricyclic Antidepressants

Decreased Effect

Fluticasone and Vilanterol may decrease the levels/effects of: Aldesleukin; Antidiabetic Agents; BCG; Coccidioidin Skin Test; Corticorelin; Hyaluronidase; Iobenguane I 123; Sipuleucel-T; Telaprevir; Vaccines (Inactivated)

The levels/effects of Fluticasone and Vilanterol may be decreased by: Beta-Blockers (Beta1 Selective); Beta-Blockers (Nonselective); Betahistine; Echinacea

Storage/Stability Store between 20°C and 25°C (68°F and 77°F); excursions permitted from 15° to 30°C (59° to 86°F). Store in a dry place away from heat and sunlight. Store inside the unopened foil tray prior to initial use. Discard 6 weeks after opening the foil tray or after the labeled number of inhalations have been used, whichever comes first.

Mechanism of Action

Fluticasone is a corticosteroid with anti-inflammatory activity, immunosuppressive properties, and antiproliferative actions.

Vilanterol, a long-acting $beta_2$-agonist, relaxes bronchial smooth muscle by selective action on $beta_2$-receptors with little effect on heart rate.

Pharmacodynamics/Kinetics

Absorption: Fluticasone and vilanterol: Systemic, primarily via lungs; minimal GI absorption due to presystemic metabolism

Distribution: Fluticasone: 661 L; Vilanterol: 165 L

Protein binding: Fluticasone: 99%; Vilanterol: 94%

Metabolism: Fluticasone and vilanterol: Hepatic via CYP3A4

Bioavailability: Fluticasone: 15%; Vilanterol: 27%

Half-life Elimination: Fluticasone: 24 hours; Vilanterol: 21 hours

Time to peak: Fluticasone: 0.5 to 1 hour; Vilanterol: 10 minutes

Excretion: Fluticasone: Primarily feces; Vilanterol: Urine (70%), feces (30%)

Dosage Chronic obstructive pulmonary disease (COPD): Adults: Oral inhalation: Fluticasone 100 mcg/vilanterol 25 mcg: One inhalation once daily; maximum: 1 inhalation once daily

Dosage adjustment in renal impairment: No dosage adjustment necessary.

Dosage adjustment in hepatic impairment:

Mild impairment: No dosage adjustment necessary.

Moderate-to-severe impairment: No dosage adjustment necessary. However, use with caution; systemic fluticasone exposure may be increased up to threefold.

Administration Oral inhalation: Administer at the same time each day. Discard device 6 weeks after it is removed from the foil tray or when the dose counter reads "0" (whichever comes first). Rinse mouth with water after use and spit.

Monitoring Parameters

FEV_1, peak flow, and/or other pulmonary function tests; bone mineral density (at baseline and periodically thereafter); blood pressure, heart rate; CNS stimulation; ocular changes (intraocular pressure, cataracts); signs/symptoms of oral or systemic infection, hypercorticism, or adrenal suppression

Dosage Forms Excipient information presented when available (limited, particularly for generics); consult specific product labeling.

Powder, for oral inhalation:

Breo Ellipta: Fluticasone furoate 100 mcg and vilanterol 25 mcg per actuation [contains lactose; blister pack]

- **Fluticasone Furoate** *see* Fluticasone (Nasal) *on page 896*
- **Fluticasone Furoate and Vilanterol** *see* Fluticasone and Vilanterol *on page 899*
- **Fluticasone Propionate** *see* Fluticasone (Nasal) *on page 896*
- **Fluticasone Propionate** *see* Fluticasone (Oral Inhalation) *on page 893*
- **Fluticasone Propionate** *see* Fluticasone (Topical) *on page 896*
- **Fluticasone Propionate and Azelastine Hydrochloride** *see* Azelastine and Fluticasone *on page 211*
- **Fluticasone Propionate and Salmeterol Xinafoate** *see* Fluticasone and Salmeterol *on page 897*

Fluvastatin (FLOO va sta tin)

Brand Names: U.S. Lescol; Lescol XL

Brand Names: Canada Lescol®; Lescol® XL; Teva-Fluvastatin

Pharmacologic Category Antilipemic Agent, HMG-CoA Reductase Inhibitor

Use To be used as a component of multiple risk factor intervention in patients at risk for atherosclerosis vascular disease due to hypercholesterolemia

Adjunct to dietary therapy to reduce elevated total cholesterol (total-C), LDL-C, triglyceride, and apolipoprotein B (apo-B) levels and to increase HDL-C in primary hypercholesterolemia and mixed dyslipidemia (Fredrickson types IIa and IIb); to slow the progression of coronary atherosclerosis in patients with coronary heart disease; reduce risk of coronary revascularization procedures in patients with coronary heart disease

Primary and secondary prevention of atherosclerotic cardiovascular disease (ASCVD) according to the American College of Cardiology/American Heart Association: To reduce the risk of ASCVD in patients with clinical ASCVD (eg, coronary heart disease, stroke/TIA, or peripheral arterial disease presumed to be of atherosclerotic origin) who are greater than 75 years of age or not a candidate for high-intensity statin therapy; in patients without clinical ASCVD if LDL-C is 190 mg/dL or greater and not a candidate for high-intensity statin therapy; in patients without clinical ASCVD who have type 1 or type 2 diabetes and are between 40 and 75 years of age; in patients with an estimated 10-year ASCVD risk 7.5% or greater and who are between 40 and 75 years of age (Stone, 2013).

Pregnancy Risk Factor X

Pregnancy Considerations Adverse events were not observed in animal reproduction studies. There are reports of congenital anomalies following maternal use of HMG-CoA reductase inhibitors in pregnancy; however, maternal disease, differences in specific agents used, and the low rates of exposure limit the interpretation of the available data (Godfrey, 2012; Lecarpentier, 2012). Cholesterol biosynthesis may be important in fetal development; serum cholesterol and triglycerides increase normally during pregnancy. The discontinuation of lipid lowering medications temporarily during pregnancy is not expected to have significant impact on the long term outcomes of primary hypercholesterolemia treatment.

Use of fluvastatin is contraindicated in pregnancy. HMG-CoA reductase inhibitors should be discontinued prior to pregnancy (ADA, 2013). If treatment of dyslipidemias is needed in pregnant women or in women of reproductive age, other agents are preferred (Berglund, 2012; Stone, 2013). The manufacturer recommends administration to women of childbearing potential only when conception is highly unlikely and patients have been informed of potential hazards.

Breast-Feeding Considerations It is not known if fluvastatin is excreted into breast milk. Due to the potential for serious adverse reactions in a nursing infant, use while breast-feeding is contraindicated by the manufacturer.

Contraindications Hypersensitivity to fluvastatin or any component of the formulation; active liver disease; unexplained persistent elevations of serum transaminases; pregnancy; breast-feeding

Warnings/Precautions Secondary causes of hyperlipidemia should be ruled out prior to therapy. Liver function must be monitored by periodic laboratory assessment. Rhabdomyolysis with acute renal failure has occurred with fluvastatin and other HMG-CoA reductase inhibitors. Risk may be increased with concurrent use of other drugs which may cause rhabdomyolysis (including colchicine, cyclosporine, erythromycin, fibric acid derivatives, or niacin at doses ≥1 g/day). Immune-mediated necrotizing myopathy (IMNM), an autoimmune-mediated myopathy, has been reported (rarely) with HMG-CoA reductase inhibitor therapy. IMNM presents as proximal muscle weakness with elevated CPK levels, which persists despite discontinuation of HMG-CoA reductase inhibitor therapy; additionally, muscle biopsy may show necrotizing myopathy with limited inflammation; immunosuppressive therapy (eg, corticosteroids, azathioprine) may be used for treatment. The manufacturer recommends temporary discontinuation for elective major surgery, acute medical or surgical conditions, or in any patient experiencing an acute or serious condition predisposing to renal failure (eg, sepsis, hypotension, trauma, uncontrolled seizures). However, based upon current evidence, HMG-CoA reductase inhibitor therapy should be continued in the perioperative period unless risk outweighs cardioprotective benefit. Use with caution in patients with advanced age; these patients are predisposed to myopathy. Use caution in patients with previous liver disease or heavy ethanol use.

If serious hepatotoxicity with clinical symptoms and/or hyperbilirubinemia or jaundice occurs during treatment, interrupt therapy. If an alternate etiology is not identified, do not restart fluvastatin. Liver enzyme tests should be obtained at baseline and as clinically indicated; routine periodic monitoring of liver enzymes is not necessary. Increases in Hb A_{1c} and fasting blood glucose have been reported with HMG-CoA reductase inhibitors; however, the benefits of statin therapy far outweigh the risk of dysglycemia. Use caution in patients with concurrent medications or conditions which reduce steroidogenesis.

Adverse Reactions As reported with fluvastatin capsules; in general, adverse reactions reported with fluvastatin extended release tablet were similar, but the incidence was less.

1% to 10%:

- Central nervous system: Headache (9%), fatigue (3%), insomnia (3%)
- Gastrointestinal: Dyspepsia (8%), diarrhea (5%), abdominal pain (5%), nausea (3%)
- Genitourinary: Urinary tract infection (2%)
- Neuromuscular & skeletal: Myalgia (5%)
- Respiratory: Sinusitis (3%), bronchitis (2%)

<1% (Limited to important or life-threatening) including additional class-related events (not necessarily reported with fluvastatin therapy): Alopecia, amnesia (reversible), anaphylaxis, angioedema, arthralgia, arthritis, blood glucose increased, cataracts, cholestatic jaundice, cirrhosis, cognitive impairment (reversible), confusion (reversible), CPK increased (>10x normal), depression, dermatomyositis, dyspnea, eosinophilia, erectile dysfunction, erythema multiforme, ESR increased, facial paresis, fatty liver, fever, fulminant hepatic necrosis, glycosylated hemoglobin (Hb A_{1c}) increased, gynecomastia, hemolytic anemia, hepatitis, hepatoma, hypersensitivity reaction, immune-mediated necrotizing myopathy (IMNM), impotence, interstitial lung disease, leukopenia, memory disturbance (reversible), memory impairment (reversible), muscle cramps, myopathy, nodules, ophthalmoplegia, pancreatitis, paresthesia, peripheral nerve palsy, peripheral neuropathy, photosensitivity, polymyalgia rheumatica, positive ANA, pruritus, psychic disturbance, purpura, rash, renal failure (secondary to rhabdomyolysis), rhabdomyolysis, skin discoloration, Stevens-Johnson syndrome, systemic lupus erythematosus-like syndrome, taste alteration, thrombocytopenia, thyroid dysfunction, toxic epidermal necrolysis, transaminases increased, tremor, urticaria, vasculitis, vertigo

Drug Interactions

Metabolism/Transport Effects Substrate of CYP2C9 (minor), CYP2D6 (minor), CYP3A4 (minor), SLCO1B1; **Note:** Assignment of Major/Minor substrate status based on clinically relevant drug interaction potential; **Inhibits** CYP1A2 (weak), CYP2C8 (weak), CYP2C9 (moderate), CYP2D6 (weak), CYP3A4 (weak)

Avoid Concomitant Use

Avoid concomitant use of Fluvastatin with any of the following: Fusidic Acid (Systemic); Gemfibrozil; Pimozide; Red Yeast Rice

Increased Effect/Toxicity

Fluvastatin may increase the levels/effects of: ARIPiprazole; Bosentan; Carvedilol; CYP2C9 Substrates; DAPTOmycin; Dofetilide; Lomitapide; PAZOPanib; Pimozide; Trabectedin; Vitamin K Antagonists

The levels/effects of Fluvastatin may be increased by: Amiodarone; Bezafibrate; Boceprevir; Colchicine; CycloSPORINE (Systemic); Cyproterone; Eltrombopag; Fenofibrate and Derivatives; Fluconazole; Fusidic Acid (Systemic); Gemfibrozil; Mifepristone; Niacin; Niacinamide; Raltegravir; Red Yeast Rice; Telaprevir

Decreased Effect

Fluvastatin may decrease the levels/effects of: Lanthanum

The levels/effects of Fluvastatin may be decreased by: Antacids; Cholestyramine Resin; Etravirine; Fosphenytoin; Peginterferon Alfa-2b; Phenytoin; Rifamycin Derivatives

Ethanol/Nutrition/Herb Interactions

Ethanol: Avoid excessive ethanol consumption (due to potential hepatic effects).

Food: Reduces rate but not the extent of absorption. Red yeast rice contains an estimated 2.4 mg lovastatin per 600 mg rice.

Storage/Stability Store at 15°C to 30°C (59°F to 86°F). Protect from light.

Mechanism of Action Acts by competitively inhibiting 3-hydroxyl-3-methylglutaryl-coenzyme A (HMG-CoA) reductase, the enzyme that catalyzes the reduction of HMG-CoA to mevalonate; this is an early rate-limiting step in cholesterol biosynthesis. HDL is increased while total, LDL, and VLDL cholesterols; apolipoprotein B; and plasma triglycerides are decreased.

Pharmacodynamics/Kinetics

Onset of action: Peak effect: Maximal LDL-C reductions achieved within 4 weeks

Distribution: V_d: 0.35 L/kg

Protein binding: >98%

Metabolism: To inactive and active metabolites (oxidative metabolism via CYP2C9 [75%], 2C8 [~5%], and 3A4 [~20%] isoenzymes); active forms do not circulate systemically; extensive (saturable) first-pass hepatic extraction

Bioavailability: Absolute: Capsule: 24%; Extended release tablet: 29%

Half-life elimination: Capsule: <3 hours; Extended release tablet: 9 hours

Time to peak: Capsule: 1 hour; Extended release tablet: 3 hours

Excretion: Feces (90%): urine (5%)

Dosage Oral:

Adolescents 10-16 years: Heterozygous familial hypercholesterolemia: Initial: 20 mg once daily; may increase every 6 weeks based on tolerability and response to a maximum recommended dose of 80 mg/day, given in 2 divided doses (immediate release capsule) or as a single daily dose (extended release tablet)

Note: Indicated only for adjunctive therapy when diet alone cannot reduce LDL-C below 190 mg/dL, or 160 mg/dL (with cardiovascular risk factors). Female patients must be 1 year postmenarche.

Concomitant use with cyclosporine or fluconazole: Refer to adult dosing.

Adults:

Patients requiring ≥25% decrease in LDL-C: 40 mg capsule once daily in the evening, 80 mg extended release tablet once daily (anytime), or 40 mg capsule twice daily

Patients requiring <25% decrease in LDL-C: Initial: 20 mg capsule once daily in the evening; may increase based on tolerability and response to a maximum recommended dose of 80 mg/day, given in 2 divided doses (immediate release capsule) or as a single daily dose (extended release tablet)

Concomitant use with cyclosporine or fluconazole: Immediate release: Do not exceed fluvastatin 20 mg twice daily

ACC/AHA Blood Cholesterol Guideline recommendations to reduce the risk of atherosclerotic cardiovascular disease (ASCVD) (Stone, 2013): Adults ≥21 years:

Primary prevention:

LDL-C ≥190 mg/dL: High-intensity therapy necessary; use alternate statin therapy (eg, atorvastatin, rosuvastatin)

Type 1 or 2 diabetes and age 40-75 years: Moderate intensity therapy:

Immediate release: 40 mg twice daily.

Extended release: 80 mg once daily.

Type 1 or 2 diabetes, age 40-75 years, and an estimated 10-year ASCVD risk ≥7.5%: High-intensity therapy necessary; use alternate statin therapy (eg, atorvastatin, rosuvastatin).

Age 40-75 years and an estimated 10-year ASCVD risk ≥7.5%: Moderate- to high-intensity therapy:

Immediate release: 40 mg twice daily or consider using high-intensity statin therapy (eg, atorvastatin, rosuvastatin).

Extended release: 80 mg once daily or consider using high-intensity statin therapy (eg, atorvastatin, rosuvastatin).

Secondary prevention:

Patient has clinical ASCVD (eg, coronary heart disease, stroke/TIA, or peripheral arterial disease presumed to be of atherosclerotic origin) **and**:

Age ≤75 years: High-intensity therapy necessary; use alternate statin therapy (eg, atorvastatin, rosuvastatin).

Age >75 years or not a candidate for high-intensity therapy: Moderate-intensity therapy:

Immediate release: 40 mg twice daily.

Extended release: 80 mg once daily.

Dosage adjustment for toxicity:

Severe muscle symptoms or fatigue: Promptly discontinue use; evaluate CPK, creatinine, and urinalysis for myoglobinuria (Stone, 2013).

Mild to moderate muscle symptoms: Discontinue use until symptoms can be evaluated; evaluate patient for conditions that may increase the risk for muscle symptoms (eg, hypothyroidism, reduced renal or hepatic function, rheumatologic disorders such as polymyalgia rheumatica, steroid myopathy, vitamin D deficiency, or primary muscle diseases). Upon resolution, resume the original or lower dose of fluvastatin. If muscle symptoms recur, discontinue fluvastatin use. After muscle symptom resolution, may then use a low dose of a different statin; gradually increase if tolerated. In the absence of continued statin use, if muscle symptoms or elevated CPK continues after 2 months, consider other causes of muscle symptoms. If determined to be due to another condition aside from statin use, may resume statin therapy at the original dose (Stone, 2013).

Dosage adjustment in renal impairment: Note: Less than 6% excreted renally

Mild-to-moderate renal impairment: No dosage adjustment necessary

Severe renal impairment: Use with caution (particularly at doses >40 mg/day; has not been studied)

Dosage adjustment in hepatic impairment: Manufacturer labeling does not provide specific dosing recommendations; however, systemic exposure may be increased in patients with liver disease (increased AUC and C_{max}); use is contraindicated in active liver disease or unexplained transaminase elevations.

Elderly: No dosage adjustment necessary based on age

Dietary Considerations Generally, patients should be placed on a standard cholesterol-lowering diet and other lifestyle modifications for 3-6 months prior to the initiation of drug therapy. The diet should be continued during drug therapy. However, for patients with advanced risk factors (eg, known coronary heart disease), drug therapy may be initiated concurrently with diet modification. May be taken without regard to meals. Red yeast rice contains an estimated 2.4 mg lovastatin per 600 mg rice.

Administration Patient should be placed on a standard cholesterol-lowering diet before and during treatment. Fluvastatin may be taken without regard to meals. Adjust dosage as needed in response to periodic lipid determinations during the first 4 weeks after a dosage change; lipid-lowering effects are additive when fluvastatin is combined with a bile-acid binding resin or niacin, however, it must be administered at least 2 hours following these drugs. Do not break, chew, or crush extended release tablets; do not open capsules.

Monitoring Parameters

2013 ACC/AHA Blood Cholesterol Guideline recommendations (Stone, 2013):

Lipid panel (total cholesterol, HDL, LDL, triglycerides): Baseline lipid panel; fasting lipid profile within 4-12 weeks after initiation or dose adjustment and every 3-12 months (as clinically indicated) thereafter. If 2 consecutive LDL levels are <40 mg/dL, consider decreasing the dose.

Hepatic transaminase levels: Baseline measurement of hepatic transaminase levels (ie, ALT); measure hepatic function if symptoms suggest hepatotoxicity (eg, unusual fatigue or weakness, loss of appetite, abdominal pain, dark-colored urine or yellowing of skin or sclera) during therapy.

CPK: CPK should not be routinely measured. Baseline CPK measurement is reasonable for some individuals (eg, family history of statin intolerance or muscle disease, clinical presentation, concomitant drug therapy that may increase risk of myopathy). May measure CPK in any patient with symptoms suggestive of myopathy (pain, tenderness, stiffness, cramping, weakness, or generalized fatigue).

Evaluate for new-onset diabetes mellitus during therapy; if diabetes develops, continue statin therapy and encourage adherence to a heart-healthy diet, physical activity, a healthy body weight, and tobacco cessation.

If patient develops a confusional state or memory impairment, may evaluate patient for nonstatin causes (eg, exposure to other drugs), systemic and neuropsychiatric causes, and the possibility of adverse effects associated with statin therapy.

Manufacturer recommendations: Liver enzyme tests at baseline and repeated when clinically indicated. Measure CPK when myopathy is being considered. Upon initiation or titration, lipid panel should be analyzed at 4 weeks.

Dosage Forms Excipient information presented when available (limited, particularly for generics); consult specific product labeling.

Capsule, Oral:

Lescol: 20 mg, 40 mg

Generic: 20 mg, 40 mg

Tablet Extended Release 24 Hour, Oral:

Lescol XL: 80 mg

◆ **Fluviral (Can)** *see* Influenza Virus Vaccine (Inactivated) *on page 1078*

◆ **Fluvirin** *see* Influenza Virus Vaccine (Inactivated) *on page 1078*

◆ **Fluvirin Preservative Free** *see* Influenza Virus Vaccine (Inactivated) *on page 1078*

FluvoxaMINE (floo VOKS a meen)

Brand Names: U.S. Luvox CR

Brand Names: Canada Apo-Fluvoxamine; Ava-Fluvoxamine; CO Fluvoxamine; Dom-Fluvoxamine; Luvox;

Novo-Fluvoxamine; PHL-Fluvoxamine; PMS-Fluvoxamine; ratio-Fluvoxamine; Riva-Fluvox; Sandoz-Fluvoxamine

Index Terms Luvox

Pharmacologic Category Antidepressant, Selective Serotonin Reuptake Inhibitor

Additional Appendix Information

Antidepressant Agents *on page 2284*

Selective Serotonin Reuptake Inhibitors (SSRIs) Pharmacokinetics *on page 2314*

Use Treatment of obsessive-compulsive disorder (OCD)

Unlabeled Use Treatment of major depression; panic disorder; anxiety disorders in children; treatment of mild dementia-associated agitation in nonpsychotic patients; post-traumatic stress disorder (PTSD); social anxiety disorder (SAD); patients; treatment of paraphilia/hypersexuality

Pregnancy Risk Factor C

Pregnancy Considerations Adverse events have been observed in animal reproduction studies. Fluvoxamine crosses the human placenta. An increased risk of teratogenic effects, including cardiovascular defects, may be associated with maternal use of fluvoxamine or other SSRIs; however, available information is conflicting. Nonteratogenic effects in the newborn following SSRI/SNRI exposure late in the third trimester include respiratory distress, cyanosis, apnea, seizures, temperature instability, feeding difficulty, vomiting, hypoglycemia, hypo- or hypertonia, hyper-reflexia, jitteriness, irritability, constant crying, and tremor. Symptoms may be due to the toxicity of the SSRIs/SNRIs or a discontinuation syndrome and may be consistent with serotonin syndrome associated with SSRI treatment. Persistent pulmonary hypertension of the newborn (PPHN) has also been reported with SSRI exposure. The long-term effects of *in utero* SSRI exposure on infant development and behavior are not known.

The ACOG recommends that therapy with SSRIs or SNRIs during pregnancy be individualized; treatment of depression during pregnancy should incorporate the clinical expertise of the mental health clinician, obstetrician, primary healthcare provider, and pediatrician. According to the American Psychiatric Association (APA), the risks of medication treatment should be weighed against other treatment options and untreated depression. For women who discontinue antidepressant medications during pregnancy and who may be at high risk for postpartum depression, the medications can be restarted following delivery. Treatment algorithms have been developed by the ACOG and the APA for the management of depression in women prior to conception and during pregnancy.

Breast-Feeding Considerations Fluvoxamine is excreted in breast milk. Based on case reports, the dose the infant receives is relatively small and adverse events have not been observed. Adverse events have been reported in nursing infants exposed to some SSRIs. According to the manufacturer, the decision to continue or discontinue breast-feeding during therapy should take into account the risk of exposure to the infant and the benefits of treatment to the mother.

The long-term effects on development and behavior have not been studied; therefore, fluvoxamine should be prescribed to a mother who is breast-feeding only when the benefits outweigh the potential risks. Maternal use of an SSRI during pregnancy may cause delayed milk secretion.

Medication Guide Available Yes

Contraindications Concurrent use with alosetron, pimozide, ramelteon, thioridazine, or tizanidine; use of MAO inhibitors intended to treat psychiatric disorders (concurrently or within 14 days of discontinuing either fluvoxamine or the MAO inhibitor); initiation of fluvoxamine in a patient receiving linezolid or intravenous methylene blue

Warnings/Precautions [U.S. Boxed Warning]: Antidepressants increase the risk of suicidal thinking and behavior in children, adolescents, and young adults (18-24 years of age) with major depressive disorder (MDD) and other psychiatric disorders; consider risk prior to prescribing. Short-term studies did not show an increased risk in patients >24 years of age and showed a decreased risk in patients ≥65 years. Closely monitor patients for clinical worsening, suicidality, or unusual changes in behavior, particularly during the initial 1-2 months of therapy or during periods of dosage adjustments (increases or decreases); the patient's family or caregiver should be instructed to closely observe the patient and communicate condition with healthcare provider. A medication guide concerning the use of antidepressants should be dispensed with each prescription. **Fluvoxamine is FDA approved for the treatment of OCD in children ≥8 years of age; extended release capsules are not FDA approved for use in children.**

The possibility of a suicide attempt is inherent in major depression and may persist until remission occurs. Use caution in high-risk patients. Worsening depression and severe abrupt suicidality that are not part of the presenting symptoms may require discontinuation or modification of drug therapy. The patient's family or caregiver should be alerted to monitor patients for the emergence of suicidality and associated behaviors (such as agitation, irritability, hostility, impulsivity, and hypomania) and call healthcare provider.

May worsen psychosis in some patients or precipitate a shift to mania or hypomania in patients with bipolar disorder. Patients presenting with depressive symptoms should be screened for bipolar disorder. Monotherapy in patients with bipolar disorder should be avoided. **Fluvoxamine is not FDA approved for the treatment of bipolar depression.**

Potentially life-threatening serotonin syndrome (SS) has occurred with serotonergic agents (eg, SSRIs, SNRIs), particularly when used in combination with other serotonergic agents (eg, triptans, TCAs, fentanyl, lithium, tramadol, buspirone, St John's wort, tryptophan) or agents that impair metabolism of serotonin (eg, MAO inhibitors intended to treat psychiatric disorders, other MAO inhibitors [ie, linezolid and intravenous methylene blue]). Discontinue treatment (and any concomitant serotonergic agent) immediately if signs/symptoms arise. Fluvoxamine has a low potential to impair cognitive or motor performance; caution operating hazardous machinery or driving. Use caution in patients with a previous seizure disorder or condition predisposing to seizures such as brain damage, alcoholism, or concurrent therapy with other drugs which lower the seizure threshold. Potentially significant drug-drug interactions may exist, requiring dose or frequency adjustment, additional monitoring, and/or selection of alternative therapy. Fluvoxamine levels may be lower in patients who smoke.

May increase the risks associated with electroconvulsive therapy. Bone fractures have been associated with antidepressant treatment. Consider the possibility of a fragility fracture if an antidepressant-treated patient presents with unexplained bone pain, point tenderness, swelling, or bruising (Rabenda, 2013; Rizzoli, 2012). Use with caution in patients with hepatic dysfunction and in elderly patients. May cause hyponatremia/SIADH (elderly at increased risk); volume depletion (diuretics may increase risk). Use with caution in patients at risk of bleeding or receiving concurrent anticoagulant therapy, although not consistently noted, fluvoxamine may cause impairment in platelet function. May cause or exacerbate sexual dysfunction. Use caution in elderly patients; monitor sodium closely with initiation or dosage adjustments in older adults (Beers Criteria).

Abrupt discontinuation or interruption of antidepressant therapy has been associated with a discontinuation syndrome. Symptoms arising may vary with antidepressant however commonly include nausea, vomiting, diarrhea, headaches, light-headedness, dizziness, diminished appetite, sweating, chills, tremors, paresthesias, fatigue, somnolence, and sleep disturbances (eg, vivid dreams, insomnia). Greater risks for developing a discontinuation syndrome have been associated with antidepressants with shorter half-lives, longer durations of treatment, and abrupt discontinuation. For antidepressants of short or intermediate half-lives, symptoms may emerge within 2-5 days after treatment discontinuation and last 7-14 days (APA, 2010; Fava, 2006; Haddad, 2001; Shelton, 2001; Warner, 2006).

Adverse Reactions Frequency varies by dosage form and indication. Adverse reactions reported as a composite of all indications.

>10%:

- Central nervous system: Headache (22% to 35%), insomnia (21% to 35%), somnolence (22% to 27%), dizziness (11% to 15%), nervousness (10% to 12%)
- Gastrointestinal: Nausea (34% to 40%), diarrhea (11% to 18%), xerostomia (10% to 14%), anorexia (6% to 14%)
- Genitourinary: Ejaculation abnormal (8% to 11%)
- Neuromuscular & skeletal: Weakness (14% to 26%)

1% to 10%:

- Cardiovascular: Chest pain (3%), palpitation (3%), vasodilation (2% to 3%), hypertension (1% to 2%), edema (≤1%), hypotension (≤1%), syncope (≤1%), tachycardia (≤1%)
- Central nervous system: Pain (10%), anxiety (5% to 8%), abnormal dreams (3%), abnormal thinking (3%), agitation (2% to 3%), apathy (≥1% to 3%), chills (2%), CNS stimulation (2%), depression (2%), neurosis (2%), amnesia, malaise, manic reaction, psychotic reaction
- Dermatologic: Bruising (4%), acne (2%)
- Endocrine & metabolic: Libido decreased (2% to 10%; incidence higher in males), anorgasmia (2% to 5%), sexual function abnormal (2% to 4%), menorrhagia (3%)
- Gastrointestinal: Dyspepsia (8% to 10%), constipation (4% to 10%), vomiting (4% to 6%), abdominal pain (5%), flatulence (4%), taste perversion (2% to 3%), toothache and dental caries (2% to 3%), dysphagia (2%), gingivitis (2%), weight loss (≤1% to 2%), weight gain
- Genitourinary: Polyuria (2% to 3%), impotence (2%), urinary tract infection (2%), urinary retention (1%)
- Hepatic: Liver function tests abnormal (≥1% to 2%)
- Neuromuscular & skeletal: Tremor (5% to 8%), myalgia (5%), paresthesia (3%), hypertonia (2%), twitching (2%), hyper-/hypokinesia, myoclonus
- Ocular: Amblyopia (2% to 3%)
- Respiratory: Upper respiratory infection (9%), pharyngitis (6%), yawn (2% to 5%), laryngitis (3%), bronchitis (2%), dyspnea (2%), epistaxis (2%), cough increased, sinusitis
- Miscellaneous: Diaphoresis (6% to 7%), flu-like syndrome (3%), viral infection (2%)

<1% (Limited to important or life-threatening): Acute renal failure, agranulocytosis, akinesia, allergic reaction, anaphylactic reaction, anemia, angina, angioedema, anuria, aplastic anemia, apnea, asthma, ataxia, AV block, bradycardia, bullous eruption, cardiomyopathy, cardiorespiratory arrest, cerebrovascular accident, cholecystitis, cholelithiasis, colitis, conduction delay, coronary artery disease, diplopia, dyskinesia, dystonia, extrapyramidal syndrome, embolus, GI bleeding, goiter, hallucinations, heart failure, hematemesis, hematuria, Henoch-Schönlein purpura (IgA vasculitis), hepatitis, hemoptysis, homicidal ideation, hypercholesterolemia, hyper-/hypoglycemia, hypokalemia, hyponatremia, hypothyroidism, ileus, interstitial lung disease, intestinal obstruction, jaundice, leukopenia, leukocytosis, loss of consciousness, lymphadenopathy, MI, myasthenia, myopathy, neuralgia, neuroleptic malignant syndrome, neuropathy, pancreatitis, paralysis, pericarditis, porphyria, purpura, QT prolongation, retinal detachment, rhabdomyolysis, serotonin syndrome, ST segment changes, seizure, Stevens-Johnson syndrome, suicidal tendencies, supraventricular extrasystoles, tardive dyskinesia, thrombocytopenia, toxic epidermal necrolysis, vasculitis, ventricular arrhythmia, ventricular tachycardia (including torsade de pointes), white blood cells decreased

Drug Interactions

Metabolism/Transport Effects Substrate of CYP1A2 (major), CYP2D6 (major); **Note:** Assignment of Major/Minor substrate status based on clinically relevant drug interaction potential; **Inhibits** CYP1A2 (strong), CYP2B6 (weak), CYP2C19 (strong), CYP2C9 (weak), CYP2D6 (weak), CYP3A4 (weak)

Avoid Concomitant Use

Avoid concomitant use of FluvoxaMINE with any of the following: Agomelatine; Alosetron; Dosulepin; Iobenguane I 123; Linezolid; MAO Inhibitors; Methylene Blue; Pimozide; Pirfenidone; Pomalidomide; Ramelteon; Thioridazine; TiZANidine; Tryptophan

Increased Effect/Toxicity

FluvoxaMINE may increase the levels/effects of: Agents with Antiplatelet Properties; Agomelatine; Alosetron; Anticoagulants; Antidepressants (Serotonin Reuptake Inhibitor/Antagonist); Antipsychotics; Asenapine; Aspirin; Bendamustine; Benzodiazepines (metabolized by oxidation); Bromazepam; BusPIRone; CarBAMazepine; Citalopram; CloZAPine; Collagenase (Systemic); CYP1A2 Substrates; CYP2C19 Substrates; Dabigatran Etexilate; Desmopressin; Dofetilide; Dosulepin; DULoxetine; Erlotinib; Fosphenytoin; Haloperidol; Hypoglycemic Agents; Ibritumomab; Lomitapide; Methadone; Methylene Blue; Metoclopramide; Mexiletine; NSAID (COX-2 Inhibitor); NSAID (Nonselective); OLANZapine; Phenytoin; Pimozide; Pirfenidone; Pomalidomide; Propafenone; Propranolol; QuiNIDine; Ramelteon; Rivaroxaban; Roflumilast; Ropivacaine; Salicylates; Serotonin Modulators; Theophylline Derivatives; Thiazide Diuretics; Thioridazine; Thrombolytic Agents; TiZANidine; Tositumomab and Iodine I 131 Tositumomab; TraMADol; Tricyclic Antidepressants; Vitamin K Antagonists; Zolpidem

The levels/effects of FluvoxaMINE may be increased by: Abiraterone Acetate; Alcohol (Ethyl); Analgesics (Opioid); Antipsychotics; BuPROPion; BusPIRone; Cimetidine; CNS Depressants; Cobicistat; CYP1A2 Inhibitors (Moderate); CYP1A2 Inhibitors (Strong); CYP2D6 Inhibitors (Moderate); CYP2D6 Inhibitors (Strong); Darunavir; Dasatinib; Deferasirox; DULoxetine; Glucosamine; Grapefruit Juice; Herbs (Anticoagulant/Antiplatelet Properties); Ibrutinib; Linezolid; Lithium; MAO Inhibitors; Metoclopramide; Metyrosine; Multivitamins/Fluoride (with ADE); Multivitamins/Minerals (with ADEK, Folate, Iron); Multivitamins/Minerals (with AE, No Iron); Omega-3 Fatty Acids; Pentosan Polysulfate Sodium; Pentoxifylline; Prostacyclin Analogues; Tipranavir; TraMADol; Tryptophan; Vemurafenib; Vitamin E

Decreased Effect

FluvoxaMINE may decrease the levels/effects of: Clopidogrel; Iobenguane I 123; Ioflupane I 123; Thyroid Products

The levels/effects of FluvoxaMINE may be decreased by: CarBAMazepine; CYP1A2 Inducers (Strong); Cyproheptadine; Cyproterone; NSAID (COX-2 Inhibitor); NSAID (Nonselective); Peginterferon Alfa-2b

Ethanol/Nutrition/Herb Interactions

Ethanol: May increase CNS depression; monitor for increased effects with coadministration. Caution patients about effects.

Herb/Nutraceutical: Avoid valerian, St John's wort, tryptophan, SAMe, kava kava (may increase risk of serotonin syndrome and/or excessive sedation). Avoid alfalfa, anise, bilberry, bladderwrack, bromelain, cat's claw, celery, chamomile, coleus, cordyceps, dong quai, evening primrose, fenugreek, feverfew, garlic, ginger, ginkgo biloba, ginseng (American), ginseng (Panax), ginseng (Siberian), grape seed, green tea, guggul, horse chestnuts, horseradish, licorice, prickly ash, red clover, reishi, SAMe (S-adenosylmethionine), sweet clover, turmeric, white willow (all have additional antiplatelet activity). Bioavailability of melatonin may be increased by fluvoxamine.

Storage/Stability Protect from high humidity and store at controlled room temperature 25°C (77°F).

Mechanism of Action Inhibits CNS neuron serotonin uptake; minimal or no effect on reuptake of norepinephrine or dopamine; does not significantly bind to alpha-adrenergic, histamine or cholinergic receptors

Pharmacodynamics/Kinetics

Onset of action: Depression: The onset of action is within a week; however, individual response varies greatly and full response may not be seen until 8-12 weeks after initiation of treatment.

Absorption: Steady-state plasma concentrations have been noted to be 2-3 times higher in children than those in adolescents; female children demonstrated a significantly higher AUC than males

Distribution: V_d: ~25 L/kg

Protein binding: ~80%, primarily to albumin

Metabolism: Extensively hepatic via oxidative demethylation and deamination

Bioavailability: Immediate release: 53%; not significantly affected by food

Half-life elimination: 15-16 hours; 17-26 hours in the elderly

Time to peak, plasma: 3-8 hours

Excretion: Urine (~85% as metabolites; ~2% as unchanged drug)

Dosage Oral:

Obsessive-compulsive disorder:

Children 8-17 years: Immediate release: Initial: 25 mg once daily at bedtime; may be increased in 25 mg increments at 4- to 7-day intervals, as tolerated, to maximum therapeutic benefit; usual dose range: 50-200 mg/day. **Note:** When total daily dose exceeds 50 mg, the dose should be given in 2 divided doses with larger portion administered at bedtime.

Maximum: Children: 8-11 years: 200 mg/day, adolescents: 300 mg/day; lower doses may be effective in female versus male patients

Adults:

Immediate release: Initial: 50 mg once daily at bedtime; may be increased in 50 mg increments at 4- to 7-day intervals, as tolerated; usual dose range: 100-300 mg/day; maximum dose: 300 mg/day. **Note:** When total daily dose exceeds 100 mg, the dose should be given in 2 divided doses with larger portion administered at bedtime.

Extended release: Initial: 100 mg once daily at bedtime; may be increased in 50 mg increments at intervals of at least 1 week; usual dosage range: 100-300 mg/day; maximum dose: 300 mg/day

Social anxiety disorder (unlabeled use): Adults: Extended release: Initial: 100 mg once daily at bedtime; may be increased in 50 mg increments at intervals of at least 1 week; usual dosage range: 100-300 mg/day; maximum dose: 300 mg/day (Davidson, 2004; Stein, 2003; Westenberg, 2004)

Post-traumatic stress disorder (PTSD) (unlabeled use): Adults: Immediate release: 75 mg twice daily (Spivak, 2006)

Elderly: Reduce dose, titrate slowly

Discontinuation of therapy: Upon discontinuation of antidepressant therapy, gradually taper the dose to minimize the incidence of withdrawal symptoms and allow for the detection of re-emerging symptoms. Evidence supporting ideal taper rates is limited. APA and NICE guidelines suggest tapering therapy over at least several weeks with consideration to the half-life of the antidepressant; antidepressants with a shorter half-life may need to be tapered more conservatively. In addition for long-term treated patients, WFSBP guidelines recommend tapering over 4-6 months. If intolerable withdrawal symptoms occur following a dose reduction, consider resuming the previously prescribed dose and/or decrease dose at a more gradual rate (APA, 2007; APA, 2010; Bauer, 2002; Haddad, 2001; NCCMH, 2010; Schatzberg, 2006; Shelton, 2001; Warner, 2006).

MAO inhibitor recommendations:

Switching to or from an MAO inhibitor intended to treat psychiatric disorders:

Allow 14 days to elapse between discontinuing an MAO inhibitor intended to treat psychiatric disorders and initiation of fluvoxamine.

Allow 14 days to elapse between discontinuing fluvoxamine and initiation of an MAO inhibitor intended to treat psychiatric disorders.

Use with other MAO inhibitors (linezolid or I.V. methylene blue):

Do not initiate fluvoxamine in patients receiving linezolid or I.V. methylene blue; consider other interventions for psychiatric condition.

If urgent treatment with linezolid or I.V. methylene blue is required in a patient already receiving fluvoxamine and potential benefits outweigh potential risks, discontinue fluvoxamine promptly and administer linezolid or I.V. methylene blue. Monitor for serotonin syndrome for 2 weeks or until 24 hours after the last dose of linezolid or I.V. methylene blue, whichever comes first. May resume fluvoxamine 24 hours after the last dose of linezolid or I.V. methylene blue.

Dosage adjustment in renal impairment: No dosage adjustment provided in manufacturer's labeling. Limited data suggest fluvoxamine does not accumulate in patients with renal impairment.

Dosage adjustment in hepatic impairment: No dosage adjustment provided in manufacturer's labeling. Limited data suggest fluvoxamine clearance is reduced in patients with hepatic impairment. Reduced initial dose and slow titration may be required.

Dietary Considerations May be taken with or without food.

Administration May be administered with or without food. Do not crush, open, or chew extended release capsules.

Monitoring Parameters Mental status for depression, suicide ideation (especially at the beginning of therapy or when doses are increased or decreased), anxiety, social functioning, mania, panic attacks; signs/symptoms of serotonin syndrome; akathisia; weight gain or loss, nutritional intake, sleep; liver function assessment prior to beginning drug therapy

Dosage Forms Excipient information presented when available (limited, particularly for generics); consult specific product labeling.

Capsule Extended Release 24 Hour, Oral, as maleate:
- Luvox CR: 100 mg, 150 mg [gluten free; contains fd&c blue #2 (indigotine)]
- Generic: 100 mg, 150 mg

Tablet, Oral, as maleate:
- Generic: 25 mg, 50 mg, 100 mg

- **Fluzone** *see* Influenza Virus Vaccine (Inactivated) *on page 1078*
- **Fluzone High-Dose** *see* Influenza Virus Vaccine (Inactivated) *on page 1078*
- **Fluzone Pediatric PF** *see* Influenza Virus Vaccine (Inactivated) *on page 1078*
- **Fluzone Preservative Free** *see* Influenza Virus Vaccine (Inactivated) *on page 1078*
- **Fluzone Quadrivalent** *see* Influenza Virus Vaccine (Inactivated) *on page 1078*
- **FML** *see* Fluorometholone *on page 882*
- **FML® (Can)** *see* Fluorometholone *on page 882*
- **FML Forte** *see* Fluorometholone *on page 882*
- **FML Forte® (Can)** *see* Fluorometholone *on page 882*
- **FML Liquifilm** *see* Fluorometholone *on page 882*
- **Focalin** *see* Dexmethylphenidate *on page 586*
- **Focalin XR** *see* Dexmethylphenidate *on page 586*
- **Foille [OTC]** *see* Benzocaine *on page 240*
- **Folacin** *see* Folic Acid *on page 907*
- **Folacin, Vitamin B_{12}, and Vitamin B_6** *see* Folic Acid, Cyanocobalamin, and Pyridoxine *on page 908*
- **Folastin [DSC]** *see* Folic Acid, Cyanocobalamin, and Pyridoxine *on page 908*
- **Folate** *see* Folic Acid *on page 907*
- **Folbee®** *see* Folic Acid, Cyanocobalamin, and Pyridoxine *on page 908*
- **Folbic™** *see* Folic Acid, Cyanocobalamin, and Pyridoxine *on page 908*
- **Folcaps™ [DSC]** *see* Folic Acid, Cyanocobalamin, and Pyridoxine *on page 908*
- **Folgard RX®** *see* Folic Acid, Cyanocobalamin, and Pyridoxine *on page 908*

Folic Acid (FOE lik AS id)

Brand Names: U.S. FA-8 [OTC]

Brand Names: Canada Apo-Folic®

Index Terms Folacin; Folate; Pteroylglutamic Acid

Pharmacologic Category Vitamin, Water Soluble

Use Treatment of megaloblastic and macrocytic anemias due to folate deficiency; dietary supplement to prevent neural tube defects

Unlabeled Use Adjunctive cofactor therapy in methanol toxicity (alternative to leucovorin calcium)

Pregnancy Risk Factor A

Pregnancy Considerations Water soluble vitamins cross the placenta. Folate requirements increase during pregnancy. Folate supplementation during the periconceptual period decreases the risk of neural tube defects. Folate supplementation (doses larger than the RDA) is recommended for women who may become pregnant (IOM, 1998).

Breast-Feeding Considerations Folate is found in breast milk; concentrations are not affected by dietary intake unless the mother has a severe deficiency (IOM, 1998).

Contraindications Hypersensitivity to folic acid or any component of the formulation

Warnings/Precautions Not appropriate for monotherapy with pernicious, aplastic, or normocytic anemias when anemia is present with vitamin B_{12} deficiency. Doses >0.1 mg/day may obscure pernicious anemia with continuing irreversible nerve damage progression. Resistance to treatment may occur with depressed hematopoiesis, alcoholism, and deficiencies of other vitamins. Injection contains benzyl alcohol (1.5%) as preservative (use care in administration to neonates).

Adverse Reactions Frequency not defined.
- Cardiovascular: Flushing (slight)
- Central nervous system: Malaise (general)
- Dermatologic: Erythema, pruritus, rash
- Respiratory: Bronchospasm
- Miscellaneous: Allergic reaction

Drug Interactions

Metabolism/Transport Effects None known.

Avoid Concomitant Use

Avoid concomitant use of Folic Acid with any of the following: Raltitrexed

Increased Effect/Toxicity There are no known significant interactions involving an increase in effect.

Decreased Effect

Folic Acid may decrease the levels/effects of: Fosphenytoin; PHENobarbital; Phenytoin; Primidone; Raltitrexed

The levels/effects of Folic Acid may be decreased by: Green Tea; SulfaSALAzine

Mechanism of Action Folic acid is necessary for formation of a number of coenzymes in many metabolic systems, particularly for purine and pyrimidine synthesis; required for nucleoprotein synthesis and maintenance in erythropoiesis; stimulates WBC and platelet production in folate deficiency anemia. Folic acid enhances the metabolism of formic acid, the toxic metabolite of methanol, to nontoxic metabolites (unlabeled use).

Pharmacodynamics/Kinetics
- Onset of action: Peak effect: Oral: 0.5-1 hour
- Absorption: Proximal part of small intestine
- Metabolism: Hepatic
- Excretion: Urine

Dosage

Oral, I.M., I.V., SubQ: Anemia:
- Infants: 0.1 mg/day
- Children <4 years: Up to 0.3 mg/day
- Children >4 years and Adults: 0.4 mg/day
- Pregnant and lactating women: 0.8 mg/day

Oral:

Adequate intake (AI) (IOM, 1998): Expressed as folate equivalents: Infants:
- 1-6 months: 65 mcg/day
- 7-12 months: 80 mcg/day

Recommended daily allowance (RDA) (IOM, 1998): Expressed as dietary folate equivalents:

Children:
- 1-3 years: 150 mcg/day
- 4-8 years: 200 mcg/day
- 9-13 years: 300 mcg/day

Children ≥14 years and Adults: 400 mcg/day
- Pregnancy: 600 mcg/day
- Lactation: 500 mcg/day

Elderly: Vitamin B_{12} deficiency must be ruled out before initiating folate therapy due to frequency of combined nutritional deficiencies: RDA requirements (1999): 400 mcg/day (0.4 mg) minimum

Prevention of neural tube defects:
- Females of childbearing potential: 400-800 mcg/day (USPSTF, 2009)
- Females at high risk or with family history of neural tube defects: 4 mg/day (ACOG, 2003)

Dietary Considerations As of January 1998, the FDA has required manufacturers of enriched flour, bread, corn meal, pasta, rice, and other grain products to add folic acid to their products. The intent is to help decrease the risk of neural tube defects by increasing folic acid intake. Other foods which contain folic acid include dark green leafy vegetables, citrus fruits and juices, and lentils.

Administration Oral preferred, but may also be administered by deep I.M., SubQ, or I.V. injection.

I.V. administration: May administer ≤5 mg dose undiluted over ≥1 minute **or** may dilute ≤5 mg in 50 mL of NS or D_5W and infuse over 30 minutes. May also be added to I.V. maintenance solutions and given as an infusion.

Reference Range Therapeutic: 0.005-0.015 mcg/mL

Test Interactions Falsely low serum concentrations may occur with the *Lactobacillus casei* assay method in patients on anti-infectives (eg, tetracycline)

Additional Information The RDA for folic acid is presented as dietary folate equivalents (DFE). DFE adjusts for the difference in bioavailability of folic acid from food as compared to dietary supplements.

Dosage Forms Excipient information presented when available (limited, particularly for generics); consult specific product labeling.

Capsule, Oral [preservative free]:
- FA-8: 0.8 mg [dye free, sugar free, yeast free]
- Generic: 5 mg, 20 mg

Solution, Injection, as sodium folate:
- Generic: 5 mg/mL (10 mL)

Tablet, Oral:
- Generic: 400 mcg, 800 mcg, 1 mg

Tablet, Oral [preservative free]:
- FA-8: 800 mcg [dye free]
- Generic: 400 mcg, 800 mcg

Extemporaneous Preparations A 1 mg/mL folic acid oral solution may be made with tablets. Heat 90 mL of purified water almost to boiling. Dissolve parabens (methylparaben 200 mg and propylparaben 20 mg) in the heated water; cool to room temperature. Crush one-hundred 1 mg tablets, then dissolve folic acid in the solution. Adjust pH to 8-8.5 with sodium hydroxide 10%; add sufficient quantity of purified water to make 100 mL; mix well. Stable for 30 days at room temperature (Allen, 2007).

A 0.05 mg/mL folic acid oral solution may be prepared using the injectable formulation (5 mg/mL). Mix 1 mL of injectable folic acid with 90 mL of purified water. Adjust pH to 8-8.5 with sodium hydroxide 10%; add sufficient quantity of purified water to make 100 mL; mix well. Stable for 30 days at room temperature (Nahata, 2004).

Allen LV Jr, "Folic Acid 1-mg/mL Oral Liquid," *Int J Pharm Compound*, 2007, 11(3):244.

Nahata MC, Pai VB, and Hipple TF, *Pediatric Drug Formulations*, 5th ed, Cincinnati, OH: Harvey Whitney Books Co, 2004.

Folic Acid, Cyanocobalamin, and Pyridoxine

(FOE lik AS id, sye an oh koe BAL a min, & peer i DOKS een)

Brand Names: U.S. FaBB; Folastin [DSC]; Folbee®; Folbic™; Folcaps™ [DSC]; Folgard RX®; Folplex 2.2; Foltabs™ 800 [OTC]; Foltx® [DSC]; Homocysteine Guard [OTC]; Lev-Tov [OTC]; Tri-B® [OTC]; Tricardio B; Virt-Vite Forte; Vita-Respa®

Index Terms Cyanocobalamin, Folic Acid, and Pyridoxine; Folacin, Vitamin B_{12}, and Vitamin B_6; Pyridoxine, Folic Acid, and Cyanocobalamin

Pharmacologic Category Vitamin

Use Nutritional supplement in end-stage renal failure, dialysis, hyperhomocysteinemia, homocystinuria, malabsorption syndromes, dietary deficiencies

Dosage Oral: Adults: One tablet daily

Additional Information Complete prescribing information should be consulted for additional detail.

Dosage Forms Excipient information presented when available (limited, particularly for generics); consult specific product labeling.

Tablet, oral: Folic acid 0.8 mg, cyanocobalamin 100 mcg, and pyridoxine hydrochloride 50 mg; Folic acid 0.8 mg, cyanocobalamin 1000 mcg, and pyridoxine hydrochloride 50 mg; Folic acid 2.2 mg, cyanocobalamin 500 mcg, and pyridoxine hydrochloride 25 mg
- FaBB: Folic acid 2.2 mg, cyanocobalamin 1000 mcg, and pyridoxine hydrochloride 25 mg
- Folastin: Folic acid 2.5 mg, cyanocobalamin 2000 mcg, and pyridoxine hydrochloride 25 mg [DSC]
- Folbee®: Folic acid 2.5 mg, cyanocobalamin 1000 mcg, and pyridoxine hydrochloride 25 mg [dye free, lactose free, and sugar free]
- Folbic™: Folic acid 2.5 mg, cyanocobalamin 2000 mcg, and pyridoxine hydrochloride 25 mg
- Folcaps™: Folic acid 2.2 mg, cyanocobalamin 500 mcg, and pyridoxine hydrochloride 25 mg [sugar free] [DSC]
- Folgard RX®: Folic acid 2.2 mg, cyanocobalamin 1000 mcg, and pyridoxine hydrochloride 25 mg
- Folplex 2.2: Folic acid 2.2 mg, cyanocobalamin 500 mcg, and pyridoxine hydrochloride 25 mg
- Foltabs™ 800: Folic acid 0.8 mg, cyanocobalamin 115 mcg, and pyridoxine hydrochloride 10 mg [gluten free]
- Foltx®: Folic acid 2.5 mg, cyanocobalamin 2000 mcg, and pyridoxine hydrochloride 25 mg [DSC]
- Homocysteine Guard: Folic acid 0.8 mg, cyanocobalamin 400 mcg, and pyridoxine hydrochloride 25 mg
- Lev-Tov: Folic acid 0.8 mg, cyanocobalamin 250 mcg, and pyridoxine hydrochloride 25 mg
- Tri-B®: Folic acid 0.8 mg, cyanocobalamin 400 mcg, and pyridoxine hydrochloride 25 mg
- Tricardio B: Folic acid 0.4 mg, cyanocobalamin 250 mcg, and pyridoxine hydrochloride 25 mg
- Virt-Vite Forte: Folic acid 2.5 mg, cyanocobalamin 2000 mcg, and pyridoxine hydrochloride 25 mg
- Vita-Respa®: Folic acid 2.2 mg, cyanocobalamin 1300 mcg, and pyridoxine hydrochloride 25 mg [dye free and sugar free]

◆ **Folinate Calcium** *see* Leucovorin Calcium *on page 1186*

◆ **Folinic Acid (error prone synonym)** *see* Leucovorin Calcium *on page 1186*

◆ **Follicle-Stimulating Hormone, Human** *see* Urofollitropin *on page 2141*

◆ **Follicle Stimulating Hormone, Recombinant** *see* Follitropin Alfa *on page 908*

◆ **Follicle Stimulating Hormone, Recombinant** *see* Follitropin Beta *on page 909*

◆ **Follistim AQ** *see* Follitropin Beta *on page 909*

Follitropin Alfa (foe li TRO pin AL fa)

Brand Names: U.S. Gonal-f; Gonal-f RFF; Gonal-f RFF Pen; Gonal-f RFF Rediject

Brand Names: Canada Gonal-f; Gonal-f Pen

Index Terms Follicle Stimulating Hormone, Recombinant; FSH; Gonal-f RFF Redi-ject; rFSH-alpha; rhFSH-alpha

Pharmacologic Category Gonadotropin; Ovulation Stimulator

Use

Gonal-f®: Induction of ovulation in anovulatory infertile patients in whom the cause of infertility is functional and not caused by primary ovarian failure; development of multiple follicles with Assisted Reproductive Technology (ART); induction of spermatogenesis in men with primary and secondary hypogonadotropic hypogonadism in whom the cause of infertility is not due to primary testicular failure.

Gonal-f® RFF: Induction of ovulation in oligo-anovulatory infertile patients in whom the cause of infertility is functional and not caused by primary ovarian failure; development of multiple follicles with ART

Pregnancy Risk Factor X

Dosage Adults: **Note:** Dose should be individualized. Use the lowest dose consistent with the expectation of good results. Over the course of treatment, doses may vary depending on individual patient response.

Gonal-f®, Gonal-f® RFF: Females:

Ovulation induction: SubQ: Initial: 75 units/day; incremental dose adjustments of up to 37.5 units may be considered after 14 days; further dose increases of the same magnitude can be made, if necessary, every 7 days (maximum dose: 300 units/day). If response to follitropin is appropriate, hCG is given 1 day following the last dose. Withhold hCG if serum estradiol is >2000 pg/mL, if the ovaries are abnormally enlarged, or if abdominal pain occurs. In general, therapy should not exceed 35 days.

ART: SubQ: Initiate therapy with follitropin alfa in the early follicular phase (cycle day 2 or day 3) at a dose of 150 units/day, until sufficient follicular development is attained. In most cases, therapy should not exceed 10 days. In patients ≥35 years whose endogenous gonadotropin levels are suppressed, initiate follitropin alfa at a dose of 225 units/day. Continue treatment until adequate follicular development is indicated as determined by ultrasound in combination with measurement of serum estradiol levels. Consider adjustments to dose after 5 days based on the patient's response; adjust subsequent dosage every 3-5 days by ≤75-150 units additionally at each adjustment. Doses >450 units/day are not recommended. Once adequate follicular development is evident, administer hCG to induce final follicular maturation in preparation for oocyte retrieval. Withhold hCG if the ovaries are abnormally enlarged.

Gonal-f®: Males: Spermatogenesis induction: SubQ: Therapy should begin with hCG pretreatment until serum testosterone is in normal range, then 150 units 3 times/week with hCG 3 times/week; continue with lowest dose needed to induce spermatogenesis (maximum dose: 300 units 3 times/week); may be given for up to 18 months

Dosage adjustment in renal impairment: No dosage adjustment provided in manufacturer's labeling (has not been studied).

Dosage adjustment in hepatic impairment: No dosage adjustment provided in manufacturer's labeling (has not been studied).

Additional Information Complete prescribing information should be consulted for additional detail.

Product Availability Gonal-f RFF Redi-ject: FDA approved October 2013; anticipated availability in December 2013. Refer to the prescribing information for additional information.

Dosage Forms Excipient information presented when available (limited, particularly for generics); consult specific product labeling.

Solution, Subcutaneous:

Gonal-f RFF Pen: 300 units/0.5 mL (0.5 mL); 450 units/0.75 mL (0.75 mL); 900 units/1.5 mL (1.5 mL) [contains metacresol]

Gonal-f RFF Rediject: 300 units/0.5 mL (0.5 mL); 450 units/0.75 mL (0.75 mL); 900 units/1.5 mL (1.5 mL) [contains metacresol]

Solution Reconstituted, Injection:

Gonal-f: 450 units (1 ea); 1050 units (1 ea)

Solution Reconstituted, Subcutaneous:

Gonal-f RFF: 75 units (1 ea)

Follitropin Beta (foe li TRO pin BAY ta)

Brand Names: U.S. Follistim AQ

Brand Names: Canada Puregon®

Index Terms Follicle Stimulating Hormone, Recombinant; FSH; rFSH-beta; rhFSH-beta

Pharmacologic Category Gonadotropin; Ovulation Stimulator

Use

Females: Induction of ovulation and pregnancy in anovulatory infertile patients in whom the cause of infertility is functional and not caused by primary ovarian failure; induction of pregnancy in normal ovulatory women undergoing Assisted Reproductive Technology (ART) (eg, *in vitro* fertilization [IVF], intracytoplasmic sperm injection [ICSI])

Males: Induction of spermatogenesis in men with primary and secondary hypogonadotropic hypogonadism in whom the cause of infertility is not due to primary testicular failure.

Pregnancy Risk Factor X

Dosage Adults: **Note:** Dose should be individualized. Use the lowest dose consistent with the expectation of good results. Over the course of treatment, doses may vary depending on individual patient response.

Females:

Ovulation induction:

Follistim® AQ: I.M., SubQ: Stepwise approach: Initiate therapy with 75 units/day for at least the first 7 days. Increase by 25 or 50 units at weekly intervals until follicular growth or serum estradiol levels indicate an adequate response. The maximum (individualized) daily dose that has been safely used for ovulation induction in patients during clinical trials is 300 units. If response to follitropin is appropriate, hCG is given 1 day following the last dose. Withhold hCG if the ovaries are abnormally enlarged, or if abdominal pain occurs.

Follistim® AQ Cartridge: SubQ: Stepwise approach: Initiate therapy with 50 units/day for at least the first 7 days. Increase by 25 or 50 units at weekly intervals until follicular growth or serum estradiol levels indicate an adequate response. The maximum (individualized) daily dose that has been safely used for ovulation induction in patients during clinical trials is 250 units. If response to follitropin is appropriate, hCG is given 1 day following the last dose. Withhold hCG if the ovaries are abnormally enlarged, or if abdominal pain occurs. See **"Note"** for dosage adjustment for this product.

ART:

Follistim® AQ: I.M., SubQ: Stepwise approach: A starting dose of 150-225 units is recommended for at least the first 4 days of treatment. The dose may be adjusted for the individual patient based upon their ovarian response. The maximum daily dose used in clinical studies is 600 units. When a sufficient number of follicles of adequate size are present, the final maturation of the follicles is induced by administering hCG. Oocyte retrieval is performed 34-36 hours later. Withhold hCG in cases where the ovaries are abnormally enlarged on the last day of follitropin beta therapy.

Follistim® AQ Cartridge: SubQ: Stepwise approach: A starting dose of 200 units is recommended for at least the first 7 days of treatment. The dose may be adjusted for the individual patient based upon their ovarian response. The maximum daily dose used in clinical studies is 500 units. When a sufficient number of follicles of adequate size are present, the final maturation of the follicles is induced by administering hCG. Oocyte retrieval is performed 34-36 hours later.

Withhold hCG in cases where the ovaries are abnormally enlarged on the last day of follitropin beta therapy. See **"Note"** for dosage adjustment for this product.

Males: Spermatogenesis induction (Follistim® AQ, Follistim® AQ Cartridge): **Note:** Pretreatment with hCG monotherapy is required prior to concomitant therapy with follitropin beta and hCG. Follitropin beta therapy may be initiated after normal serum testosterone levels have been reached. SubQ: 450 units/week (administered as 225 units twice weekly or 150 units 3 times/weekly). A lower dose of Follistim® AQ Cartridge may be considered. See **"Note"** for dosage adjustment for this product.

Note: Dose adjustment for Follistim® AQ Cartridge: When administered using the Follistim Pen®, the Follistim® AQ Cartridge delivers 18% more follitropin beta when compared to dissolved lyophilized follitropin beta administered by a conventional syringe. If the above starting doses were previously used when administering a recombinant lyophilized gonadotropin product via a conventional syringe, lower starting and maintenance doses should be considered when switching to Follistim® AQ Cartridge. The following dose conversion may be used:

Follistim® AQ Dosing Conversion[1]

Dose Administered Using Powder for Solution/Conventional Syringe	Follistim® AQ Dose Administered Using Follistim Pen®
75 units	50 units
150 units	125 units
225 units	175 units
300 units	250 units
375 units	300 units
450 units	375 units

[1]Values listed are rounded to the nearest 25 unit increment.

Dosage adjustment in renal impairment: No dosage adjustment provided in manufacturer's labeling (has not been studied).

Dosage adjustment in hepatic impairment: No dosage adjustment provided in manufacturer's labeling (has not been studied).

Additional Information Complete prescribing information should be consulted for additional detail.

Dosage Forms Excipient information presented when available (limited, particularly for generics); consult specific product labeling.

Solution, Injection:

Follistim AQ: 75 units/0.5 mL (0.5 mL); 150 units/0.5 mL (0.5 mL)

Solution, Subcutaneous:

Follistim AQ: 300 units/0.36 mL (0.42 mL); 600 units/0.72 mL (0.78 mL); 900 units/1.08 mL (1.17 mL) [contains benzyl alcohol]

◆ Folotyn *see* PRALAtrexate *on page 1692*

◆ Folplex 2.2 *see* Folic Acid, Cyanocobalamin, and Pyridoxine *on page 908*

◆ Foltabs™ 800 [OTC] *see* Folic Acid, Cyanocobalamin, and Pyridoxine *on page 908*

◆ Foltx® [DSC] *see* Folic Acid, Cyanocobalamin, and Pyridoxine *on page 908*

Fomepizole (foe ME pi zole)

Brand Names: U.S. Antizol

Brand Names: Canada Antizol

Index Terms 4-Methylpyrazole; 4-MP

Pharmacologic Category Antidote

Use Treatment of methanol or ethylene glycol poisoning alone or in combination with hemodialysis

Unlabeled Use Pediatric administration; treatment of propylene glycol toxicity

Pregnancy Risk Factor C

Pregnancy Considerations Animal reproduction studies have not been conducted. In general, medications used as antidotes should take into consideration the health and prognosis of the mother; antidotes should be administered to pregnant women if there is a clear indication for use and should not be withheld because of fears of teratogenicity (Bailey, 2003).

Breast-Feeding Considerations It is not known if fomepizole is excreted in breast milk. The manufacturer recommends that caution be exercised when administering fomepizole to nursing women.

Contraindications Hypersensitivity to fomepizole, other pyrazoles, or any component of the formulation

Warnings/Precautions Should not be given undiluted or by bolus injection. Fomepizole is metabolized in the liver and excreted in the urine; use caution with hepatic or renal impairment. Hemodialysis should be considered as an adjunct to fomepizole in patients with renal failure, significant acidosis (pH <7.25-7.3), worsening metabolic acidosis, or ethylene glycol or methanol concentrations ≥50 mg/dL. Pediatric administration is not FDA approved; however, safe and efficacious use in this patient population for ethylene glycol and methanol intoxication has been reported (Baum, 2000; Benitez, 2000; Boyer, 2001; Brown, 2001; De Brabander, 2005; Detaille, 2004; Fisher, 1998); consider consultation with a clinical toxicologist or poison control center.

Adverse Reactions

>10%:

Central nervous system: Headache (14%)

Gastrointestinal: Nausea (11%)

1% to 10% (≤3% unless otherwise noted):

Cardiovascular: Bradycardia, facial flush, hypotension, shock, tachycardia

Central nervous system: Dizziness (6%), drowsiness increased (6%), agitation, anxiety, fever, lightheadedness, seizure, vertigo

Dermatologic: Rash

Endocrine & metabolic: Liver function tests increased

Gastrointestinal: Bad/metallic taste (6%), abdominal pain, appetite decreased, diarrhea, heartburn, vomiting

Hematologic: Anemia, disseminated intravascular coagulation (DIC), eosinophilia, lymphangitis

Local: Application site reaction, injection site inflammation, pain during injection, phlebitis

Neuromuscular & skeletal: Backache

Ocular: Nystagmus, transient blurred vision, visual disturbances

Renal: Anuria

Respiratory: Abnormal smell, hiccups, pharyngitis

Miscellaneous: Multiorgan failure, speech disturbances

<1% (Limited to important or life-threatening): Mild allergic reactions (mild rash, eosinophilia)

Drug Interactions

Metabolism/Transport Effects None known.

Avoid Concomitant Use There are no known interactions where it is recommended to avoid concomitant use.

Increased Effect/Toxicity There are no known significant interactions involving an increase in effect.

Decreased Effect There are no known significant interactions involving a decrease in effect.

Ethanol/Nutrition/Herb Interactions Ethanol: Ethanol decreases the rate of fomepizole elimination by ~50%; conversely, fomepizole decreases the rate of elimination of ethanol by ~40%.

Preparation for Administration Prior to administration, dilute in at least 100 mL 0.9% sodium chloride or dextrose 5% water for injection. Diluted solution should be used within 24 hours and may be stored at room temperature or under refrigeration. Although, it is chemically and physically stable when diluted as recommended, sterile precautions should be observed because diluents generally do not contain preservatives.

Storage/Stability Store at controlled room temperature, 20°C to 25°C (68°F to 77°F); fomepizole solidifies at temperatures <25°C (77°F). If solution becomes solid in the vial, it be should be carefully warmed by running the vial under warm water or by holding in the hand. Solidification does not affect the efficacy, safety, or stability of the drug.

Mechanism of Action Fomepizole competitively inhibits alcohol dehydrogenase, an enzyme which catalyzes the metabolism of ethanol, ethylene glycol, and methanol to their toxic metabolites. Ethylene glycol is metabolized to glycoaldehyde, then oxidized to glycolate, glyoxylate, and oxalate. Glycolate and oxalate are responsible for metabolic acidosis and renal damage. Methanol is metabolized to formaldehyde, then oxidized to formic acid. Formic acid is responsible for metabolic acidosis and visual disturbances.

Pharmacodynamics/Kinetics

Onset of effect: Peak effect: Maximum: 1.5-2 hours

Absorption: Oral: Readily absorbed

Distribution: V_d: 0.6-1.02 L/kg; rapidly into total body water

Protein binding: Negligible

Metabolism: Hepatic to 4-carboxypyrazole (80% to 85% of dose), 4-hydroxymethylpyrazole, and their N-glucuronide conjugates; following multiple doses, induces its own metabolism via CYP oxidases after 30-40 hours

Half-life elimination: Has not been calculated; varies with dose

Excretion: Urine (1% to 3.5% as unchanged drug and metabolites)

Dosage Note: Fomepizole therapy should begin immediately upon suspicion of ethylene glycol or methanol ingestion.

Children (unlabeled use) and Adults: Ethylene glycol and methanol toxicity: I.V.: A loading dose of 15 mg/kg should be administered, followed by doses of 10 mg/kg every 12 hours for 4 doses, then 15 mg/kg every 12 hours thereafter until ethylene glycol or methanol concentrations have been reduced to <20 mg/dL and patient is asymptomatic with normal pH. **Note:** For severe toxicity requiring concomitant hemodialysis, see dosage adjustment in renal impairment.

Dosage adjustment in renal impairment: Note: Hemodialysis should be considered as an adjunct to fomepizole in patients with renal failure, significant or worsening metabolic acidosis, or ethylene glycol or methanol concentrations ≥50 mg/dL. The following dosing adjustments should be used for any patient receiving hemodialysis regardless of renal function.

Prior to the start of hemodialysis:

To determine if the patient requires a dose of fomepizole at the start of hemodialysis, determine when the last dose was administered.

If the last dose of fomepizole was given <6 hours ago, do not administer another dose upon beginning hemodialysis.

If the last dose of fomepizole was given ≥6 hours ago, administer next scheduled dose upon beginning hemodialysis.

During hemodialysis: During hemodialysis, administer fomepizole every 4 hours. Alternatively, a loading dose of 10-20 mg/kg followed by 1-1.5 mg/kg/hour continuous infusion during hemodialysis has been described in case reports (Jobard, 1996).

Upon completion of hemodialysis:

To determine if the patient requires a dose of fomepizole at the time of completion of hemodialysis, determine when the last dose was administered.

If the last dose of fomepizole was given <1 hour ago, do not administer a dose at the end of hemodialysis.

If the last dose of fomepizole was given >3 hours ago, administer the next scheduled dose at the end of hemodialysis.

Maintenance dose when off hemodialysis: Administer fomepizole every 12 hours (starting 12 hours from last dose administered).

Dosage adjustment in hepatic impairment: Fomepizole is metabolized in the liver; specific dosage adjustments have not been determined in patients with hepatic impairment

Administration The appropriate dose of fomepizole should be drawn from the vial with a syringe and injected into at least 100 mL of sterile 0.9% sodium chloride injection or dextrose 5% injection. All doses should be administered as a slow intravenous infusion (IVPB) over 30 minutes.

Monitoring Parameters Fomepizole plasma levels should be monitored; response to fomepizole; monitor plasma/urinary ethylene glycol or methanol levels, urinary oxalate (ethylene glycol), plasma/urinary osmolality, renal/hepatic function, serum electrolytes, arterial blood gases; anion and osmolar gaps, resolution of clinical signs and symptoms of ethylene glycol or methanol intoxication

Reference Range The manufacturer recommends concentrations 100-300 micromole/L (8.2-24.6 mg/L) to achieve enzyme inhibition of alcohol dehydrogenase; according to practice guidelines, serum fomepizole concentrations of ≥0.8 mg/L provide constant inhibition of alcohol dehydrogenase

Dosage Forms Excipient information presented when available (limited, particularly for generics); consult specific product labeling.

Solution, Intravenous [preservative free]:

Antizol: 1 g/mL (1.5 mL)

Generic: 1 g/mL (1.5 mL); 1.5 g/1.5 mL (1.5 mL)

Fondaparinux (fon da PARE i nuks)

Brand Names: U.S. Arixtra

Brand Names: Canada Arixtra®

Index Terms Fondaparinux Sodium

Pharmacologic Category Factor Xa Inhibitor

Use Prophylaxis of deep vein thrombosis (DVT) in patients undergoing surgery for hip replacement, knee replacement, hip fracture (including extended prophylaxis following hip fracture surgery), or abdominal surgery (in patients at risk for thromboembolic complications); treatment of acute pulmonary embolism (PE); treatment of acute DVT without PE

Canadian labeling: Additional uses (not approved in U.S.): Unstable angina or non-ST segment elevation myocardial infarction (UA/NSTEMI) for the prevention of death and subsequent MI; ST segment elevation MI (STEMI) for the prevention of death and myocardial reinfarction

Unlabeled Use Prophylaxis of DVT in patients with a history of heparin-induced thrombocytopenia (HIT); treatment of acute thrombosis (unrelated to HIT) in patients with a past history of HIT; acute symptomatic superficial vein thrombosis (≥5 cm in length) of the legs

Pregnancy Risk Factor B

Pregnancy Considerations Adverse events were not observed in animal reproduction studies. Based on case reports, small amounts of fondaparinux have been detected in the umbilical cord following multiple doses during pregnancy (Dempfle, 2004). Use of fondaparinux in pregnancy should be limited to those women who have severe allergic reactions to heparin, including heparin-induced thrombocytopenia, and who cannot receive danaparoid (Guyatt, 2012).

Breast-Feeding Considerations It is not known if fondaparinux is excreted into breast milk. The manufacturer recommends caution be used if administered to nursing women. The use of alternative anticoagulants is preferred (Guyatt, 2012).

Contraindications Serious hypersensitivity (eg, angioedema, anaphylactoid/anaphylactic reactions) to fondaparinux or any component of the formulation; severe renal impairment (Cl_{cr} <30 mL/minute); body weight <50 kg (prophylaxis); active major bleeding; bacterial endocarditis; thrombocytopenia associated with a positive *in vitro* test for antiplatelet antibody in the presence of fondaparinux

Warnings/Precautions **[U.S. Boxed Warning]: Spinal or epidural hematomas, including subsequent paralysis, may occur with recent or anticipated neuraxial anesthesia (epidural or spinal anesthesia) or spinal puncture in patients anticoagulated with LMWH, heparinoids, or fondaparinux.** Consider risk versus benefit prior to spinal procedures; risk is increased by the use of concomitant agents which may alter hemostasis, the use of indwelling epidural catheters for analgesia, a history of spinal deformity or spinal surgery, as well as a history of traumatic or repeated epidural or spinal punctures. Patient should be observed closely for bleeding and signs and symptoms of neurological impairment if therapy is administered during or immediately following diagnostic lumbar puncture, epidural anesthesia, or spinal anesthesia.

Discontinue use 24 hours prior to CABG and dose with unfractionated heparin per institutional practice (Jneid, 2012). Use caution in patients with moderate renal dysfunction (Cl_{cr} 30-50 mL/minute); contraindicated in patients with Cl_{cr} <30 mL/minute. Discontinue if severe dysfunction or labile function develops.

Use caution in congenital or acquired bleeding disorders; bacterial endocarditis; renal impairment; hepatic impairment; active ulcerative or angiodysplastic gastrointestinal disease; hemorrhagic stroke; shortly after brain, spinal, or ophthalmologic surgery; or in patients taking platelet inhibitors. Risk of major bleeding may be increased if initial dose is administered earlier than recommended (initiation recommended at 6-8 hours following surgery). Discontinue agents that may enhance the risk of hemorrhage if possible. Although considered an insensitive measure of fondaparinux activity, there have been postmarketing reports of bleeding associated with elevated aPTT. Has occurred with administration, including very rare reports of thrombocytopenia with thrombosis similar to heparin-induced thrombocytopenia (HIT); however, has been used in patients with current or history of HIT due to a lack of an immune-mediated effect on platelets (Guyatt [ACCP], 2012; Savi, 2005). Use is contraindicated in patients with thrombocytopenia associated with a positive *in vitro* test for antiplatelet antibodies in the presence of fondaparinux. Monitor patients closely and discontinue therapy if platelets fall to <100,000/mm^3 and/or thrombosis develops.

For subcutaneous administration; not for I.M. administration. Do not use interchangeably (unit for unit) with low molecular weight heparins, heparin, or heparinoids. Use caution in patients <50 kg who are being treated for DVT/PE; dosage reduction recommended. Contraindicated in patients <50 kg when used for prophylactic therapy. Use with caution in the elderly. The needle guard contains natural latex rubber.

The administration of fondaparinux as the sole anticoagulant is **not recommended** during PCI due to an increased risk for guiding-catheter thrombosis. Use of an anticoagulant with antithrombin activity (eg, unfractionated heparin) is recommended as adjunctive therapy to PCI even if prior treatment with fondaparinux (must take into account whether GP IIb/IIIa antagonists have been administered) (Levine, 2011). Do not administer with other agents that increase the risk of hemorrhage unless they are essential for the management of the underlying condition (eg, warfarin for treatment of VTE).

Adverse Reactions As with all anticoagulants, bleeding is the major adverse effect. Hemorrhage may occur at any site. Risk appears increased by a number of factors including renal dysfunction, age (>75 years), and weight (<50 kg).

>10%:

Central nervous system: Fever (4% to 14%)
Gastrointestinal: Nausea (3% to 11%)
Hematologic: Anemia (1% to 20%)

1% to 10%:

Cardiovascular: Edema (9%), hypotension (4%), hypertension (2%), chest pain (1%), thrombosis PCI catheter (without heparin 1%)
Central nervous system: Insomnia (4% to 5%), headache (2% to 5%), dizziness (4%), confusion (3%), pain (2%), anxiety (1%)
Dermatologic: Rash (8%), purpura (4%), bullous eruption (3%), bruising (1%)
Endocrine & metabolic: Hypokalemia (1% to 4%)
Gastrointestinal: Constipation (5% to 9%), vomiting (1% to 6%), diarrhea (2% to 3%), dyspepsia (2%), abdominal pain (1%)
Genitourinary: Urinary tract infection (2% to 4%), urinary retention (3%)
Hematologic: Minor bleeding (2% to 4%), moderate thrombocytopenia (50,000-100,000/mm^3: 3%), hematoma (3%), major bleeding (1% to 3%), prothrombin decreased (1%), risk of major bleeding increased as high as 5% in patients receiving initial dose <6 hours following surgery
Hepatic: ALT increased (≤3%), AST increased (≤2%)
Local: Injection site reaction (bleeding, rash, pruritus)
Neuromuscular & skeletal: Back pain (1%), leg pain (1%)
Respiratory: Cough (2%), pneumonia (2%), epistaxis (1%)
Miscellaneous: Wound drainage increased (5%)

<1% (Limited to important or life-threatening): aPTT increased (associated with bleeding), heparin-induced thrombocytopenia (1 case report), hepatic dysfunction, severe thrombocytopenia (<50,000/mm^3)

Drug Interactions

Metabolism/Transport Effects None known.

Avoid Concomitant Use

Avoid concomitant use of Fondaparinux with any of the following: Apixaban; Dabigatran Etexilate; Omacetaxine; Rivaroxaban

Increased Effect/Toxicity

Fondaparinux may increase the levels/effects of: Anticoagulants; Collagenase (Systemic); Deferasirox; Ibritumomab; Omacetaxine; Rivaroxaban; Tositumomab and Iodine I 131 Tositumomab

The levels/effects of Fondaparinux may be increased by: Agents with Antiplatelet Properties; Apixaban; Dabigatran Etexilate; Dasatinib; Herbs (Anticoagulant/Antiplatelet Properties); Ibrutinib; Nonsteroidal Anti-Inflammatory Agents; Omega-3 Fatty Acids; Pentosan Polysulfate Sodium; Prostacyclin Analogues; Salicylates; Sugammadex; Thrombolytic Agents; Tibolone; Tipranavir; Vitamin E

Decreased Effect

The levels/effects of Fondaparinux may be decreased by: Estrogen Derivatives; Progestins

Ethanol/Nutrition/Herb Interactions Herb/Nutraceutical: Avoid alfalfa, anise, bilberry, bladderwrack, bromelain, cat's claw, celery, coleus, cordyceps, dong quai, evening primrose oil, fenugreek, feverfew, garlic, ginger, ginkgo biloba, ginseng (American/Panax/Siberian), grapeseed, green tea, guggul, horse chestnut seed, horseradish, licorice, prickly ash, red clover, reishi, sweet clover, turmeric, white willow (all possess anticoagulant or antiplatelet activity and as such, may enhance the anticoagulant effects of fondaparinux).

Preparation for Administration Canadian labeling: For I.V. administration: May mix with 25 mL or 50 mL NS

Storage/Stability Store at 25°C (77°F); excursions permitted to 15°C to 30°C (59°F to 86°F).

Canadian labeling: For I.V. administration: Manufacturer recommends immediate use once diluted in NS, but is stable for up to 24 hours at 15°C to 30°C (59°F to 86°F).

Mechanism of Action Fondaparinux is a synthetic pentasaccharide that causes an antithrombin III-mediated selective inhibition of factor Xa. Neutralization of factor Xa interrupts the blood coagulation cascade and inhibits thrombin formation and thrombus development.

Pharmacodynamics/Kinetics

Absorption: SubQ: Rapid and complete

Distribution: V_d: 7-11 L; mainly in blood

Protein binding: ≥94% to antithrombin III

Bioavailability: SubQ: 100%

Half-life elimination: 17-21 hours; prolonged with renal impairment

Time to peak: SubQ: 2-3 hours

Excretion: Urine (~77%, unchanged drug)

Dosage SubQ: Adults:

DVT prophylaxis: Adults ≥50 kg: 2.5 mg once daily. **Note:** Prophylactic use contraindicated in patients <50 kg. Initiate dose after hemostasis has been established, 6-8 hours postoperatively.

DVT prophylaxis with history of HIT (unlabeled use): 2.5 mg once daily (Blackmer, 2009; Harenberg, 2004; Parody, 2003)

Usual duration: 5-9 days (up to 10 days following abdominal surgery or up to 11 days following hip replacement or knee replacement). The American College of Chest Physicians recommends a minimum of 10-14 days for patients undergoing total hip arthroplasty, total knee arthroplasty, or hip fracture surgery; extended duration of up to 35 days suggested (Guyatt, 2012).

Acute DVT/PE treatment: **Note:** Start warfarin on the first or second treatment day and continue fondaparinux until INR is ≥2 for at least 24 hours (usually 5-7 days) (Guyatt, 2012):

<50 kg: 5 mg once daily

50-100 kg: 7.5 mg once daily

>100 kg: 10 mg once daily

Usual duration: 5-9 days (has been administered up to 26 days)

Acute coronary syndrome (Canadian labeling; unlabeled use in U.S.):

UA/NSTEMI: SubQ: 2.5 mg once daily; initiate as soon as possible after presentation; treat for up to 8 days or until hospital discharge (Anderson, 2007; Yusuf 2006a)

STEMI: I.V.: 2.5 mg once; subsequent doses: SubQ: 2.5 mg once daily; treat for up to 8 days or until hospital discharge (Antman, 2007; Yusuf, 2006b)

Note: Discontinue fondaparinux 24 hours prior to coronary artery bypass graft (CABG) surgery; instead, administer unfractionated heparin per institutional practice (Anderson, 2007).

Acute symptomatic superficial vein thrombosis (≥5 cm in length) of the legs (unlabeled use): 2.5 mg once daily for 45 days (Decousus, 2010; Guyatt, 2012)

Acute thrombosis (unrelated to HIT) in patients with a past history of HIT (unlabeled use; Guyatt, 2012; Warkentin, 2011):

<50 kg: 5 mg once daily

50-100 kg: 7.5 mg once daily

>100 kg: 10 mg once daily

Dosage adjustment in renal impairment:

Cl_{cr} 30-50 mL/minute: Use caution; total clearance ~40% lower compared to patients with normal renal function. When used for thromboprophylaxis, the American College of Chest Physicians suggests a 50% reduction in dose or use of low-dose heparin instead of fondaparinux (Garcia, 2012).

Cl_{cr} <30 mL/minute: Use is contraindicated.

Dosage adjustment in hepatic impairment:

Mild-to-moderate impairment: Dosage adjustment not required; monitor for signs of bleeding.

Severe impairment: No dosage adjustment provided in manufacturer's labeling (has not been studied).

Administration Do **not** administer I.M.; intended for SubQ administration. Do not mix with other injections or infusions. Do not expel air bubble from syringe before injection. Administer according to recommended regimen; when used for DVT prophylaxis, early initiation (before 6 hours after orthopedic surgery) has been associated with increased bleeding. For STEMI patients (Canadian labeling; unlabeled use in U.S.) may administer initial dose as I.V. push or mix in 25-50 mL of NS (do not mix with other agents) and infuse over 2 minutes; flush tubing with NS after infusion to ensure complete administration for fondaparinux.

To convert from I.V. unfractionated heparin (UFH) infusion to SubQ fondaparinux (Nutescu, 2007): Calculate specific dose for fondaparinux based on indication, discontinue UFH, and begin fondaparinux within 1 hour

To convert from SubQ fondaparinux to I.V. UFH infusion (Nutescu, 2007): Discontinue fondaparinux; calculate specific dose for I.V. UFH infusion based on indication; omit heparin bolus/loading dose

For subQ fondaparinux dosed every 24 hours: Start I.V. UFH infusion 22-23 hours after last dose of fondaparinux

Monitoring Parameters Periodic monitoring of CBC, platelet count, serum creatinine, occult blood testing of stools recommended. Anti-Xa activity of fondaparinux can be measured by the assay if fondaparinux is used as the calibrator. PT and aPTT are insensitive measures of fondaparinux activity. If unexpected changes in coagulation parameters or major bleeding occur, discontinue fondaparinux (elevated aPTT associated with bleeding events have been reported in postmarketing data).

Reference Range Note: Routine monitoring is not recommended; the following fondaparinux-specific anti-Xa concentrations have been reported (Garcia, 2012):

Thromboprophylaxis dose: Anti-Xa activity at 3 hours post dose: ~0.39-0.5 mg/L

Therapeutic dosing (eg, 7.5 mg once daily): Anti-Xa activity at 3 hours post dose: 1.2-1.26 mg/L

Test Interactions International standards of heparin or LMWH are not the appropriate calibrators for antifactor Xa activity of fondaparinux.

Dosage Forms Excipient information presented when available (limited, particularly for generics); consult specific product labeling.

Solution, Subcutaneous, as sodium:

Generic: 2.5 mg/0.5 mL (0.5 mL); 5 mg/0.4 mL (0.4 mL); 7.5 mg/0.6 mL (0.6 mL); 10 mg/0.8 mL (0.8 mL)

Solution, Subcutaneous, as sodium [preservative free]:

Arixtra: 2.5 mg/0.5 mL (0.5 mL); 5 mg/0.4 mL (0.4 mL); 7.5 mg/0.6 mL (0.6 mL); 10 mg/0.8 mL (0.8 mL)

Generic: 2.5 mg/0.5 mL (0.5 mL); 5 mg/0.4 mL (0.4 mL); 7.5 mg/0.6 mL (0.6 mL); 10 mg/0.8 mL (0.8 mL)

◆ **Fondaparinux Sodium** *see* Fondaparinux *on page 911*
◆ **Foradil® (Can)** *see* Formoterol *on page 914*
◆ **Foradil Aerolizer** *see* Formoterol *on page 914*
◆ **Forfivo XL** *see* BuPROPion *on page 296*

Formoterol (for MOH te rol)

Brand Names: U.S. Foradil Aerolizer; Perforomist

Brand Names: Canada Foradil®; Oxeze® Turbuhaler®

Index Terms Formoterol Fumarate; Formoterol Fumarate Dihydrate

Pharmacologic Category $Beta_2$ Agonist; $Beta_2$-Adrenergic Agonist, Long-Acting

Use U.S. labeling: Treatment of asthma (only as concomitant therapy with an inhaled corticosteroid) in patients with reversible obstructive airway disease, including patients with symptoms of nocturnal asthma (Foradil® Aerolizer®); maintenance treatment of bronchoconstriction in patients with COPD (Foradil® Aerolizer®, Perforomist®); prevention of exercise-induced bronchospasm when administered on an as-needed basis (monotherapy may be indicated in patients without persistent asthma) (Foradil® Aerolizer®)

Canadian labeling: Treatment of asthma (only as concomitant therapy with an inhaled corticosteroid) in patients with reversible obstructive airway disease, including patients with symptoms of nocturnal asthma (Foradil®, Oxeze® Turbuhaler®); maintenance treatment of COPD (Foradil®); prevention of exercise-induced bronchospasm when administered on an as-needed basis (monotherapy may be indicated in patients without persistent asthma) (Oxeze® Turbuhaler®)

Pregnancy Risk Factor C

Pregnancy Considerations Adverse events were observed in some animal reproduction studies. Formoterol has the potential to affect uterine contractility if administered during labor.

Uncontrolled asthma is associated with adverse events on pregnancy (increased risk of perinatal mortality, preeclampsia, preterm birth, low birth weight infants). Although data related to its use in pregnancy is limited, formoterol may be used as an alternative agent when a long-acting beta agonist is needed to treat moderate persistent or severe persistent asthma in pregnant women (NAEPP, 2005).

Breast-Feeding Considerations
It is not known if formoterol is excreted into breast milk. The manufacturer recommends that caution be exercised when administering formoterol to nursing women. The use of $beta_2$-receptor agonists are not considered a contraindication to breast-feeding (NAEPP, 2005).

Medication Guide Available Yes

Contraindications Hypersensitivity to formoterol or any component of the formulation (Foradil® Aerolizer® only); treatment of status asthmaticus or other acute episodes of asthma or COPD (Foradil® Aerolizer® only); monotherapy in the treatment of asthma (ie, use without a concomitant long-term asthma control medication, such as an inhaled corticosteroid)

Canadian labeling: Additional contraindications (not in U.S. labeling): Presence of tachyarrhythmias

Warnings/Precautions [U.S. Boxed Warning]: Long-acting $beta_2$-agonists (LABAs) increase the risk of asthma-related deaths. Formoterol should only be used in asthma patients as adjuvant therapy in patients who are currently receiving but are not adequately controlled on a long-term asthma control medication (ie, an inhaled corticosteroid). Monotherapy with an LABA is contraindicated in the treatment of asthma. In a large, randomized, placebo-controlled U.S. clinical trial (SMART, 2006), salmeterol was associated with an increase in asthma-related deaths (when added to usual asthma therapy); risk is considered a class effect among all LABAs. Data are not available to determine if the addition of an inhaled corticosteroid lessens this increased risk of death associated with LABA use. Assess patients at regular intervals once asthma control is maintained on combination therapy to determine if step-down therapy is appropriate and the LABA can be discontinued (without loss of asthma control), and the patient can be maintained on an inhaled corticosteroid. LABAs are not appropriate in patients whose asthma is adequately controlled on low- or medium-dose inhaled corticosteroids. Do **not** use for acute bronchospasm. Short-acting $beta_2$-agonist (eg, albuterol) should be used for acute symptoms and symptoms occurring between treatments. Do **not** initiate in patients with significantly worsening or acutely deteriorating asthma; reports of severe (sometimes fatal) respiratory events have been reported when formoterol has been initiated in this situation. Corticosteroids should not be stopped or reduced when formoterol is initiated. Formoterol is not a substitute for inhaled or systemic corticosteroids and should not be used as monotherapy. During initiation, watch for signs of worsening asthma. **[U.S. Boxed Warning] (Foradil® Aerolizer®): LABAs may increase the risk of asthma-related hospitalization in pediatric and adolescent patients.** In general, a combination product containing a LABA and an inhaled corticosteroid is preferred in patients <18 years of age to ensure compliance.

Because LABAs may disguise poorly controlled persistent asthma, frequent or chronic use of LABAs for exercise-induced bronchospasm is discouraged by the NIH Asthma Guidelines (NIH, 2007). The safety and efficacy of Perforomist® in asthma patients have not been established and is not FDA approved for the treatment of asthma.

Do **not** use for acute episodes of COPD. Do **not** initiate in patients with significantly worsening or acutely deteriorating COPD. Data are not available to determine if LABA use increases the risk of death in patients with COPD. Increased use and/or ineffectiveness of short-acting $beta_2$-agonists may indicate rapidly deteriorating disease and should prompt re-evaluation of the patient's condition.

Immediate hypersensitivity reactions (urticaria, angioedema, rash, bronchospasm) have been reported. Do not exceed recommended dose or frequency; serious adverse events (including serious asthma exacerbations and fatalities) have been associated with excessive use of inhaled sympathomimetics. $Beta_2$-agonists may increase risk of arrhythmias, decrease serum potassium, prolong QT_c interval, or increase serum glucose. These effects may be exacerbated in hypoxemia. Use caution in patients with cardiovascular disease (arrhythmia, coronary insufficiency, hypertension, HF, or aneurysm), seizures, diabetes, hyperthyroidism, pheochromocytoma, or hypokalemia. Beta-agonists may cause elevation in blood pressure and heart rate, and result in CNS stimulation/excitation. Tolerance to the bronchodilator effect, measured by FEV_1, has been observed in studies.

Powder for oral inhalation contains lactose; very rare anaphylactic reactions have been reported in patients with severe milk protein allergy. The contents of the Foradil® Aerolizer® capsules are for inhalation only via the Aerolizer® device. There have been reports of incorrect administration (swallowing of the capsules).

Adverse Reactions
1% to 10%:
Cardiovascular: Chest pain (2% to 3%), palpitation
Central nervous system: Anxiety (2%), dizziness (2%), fever (2%), insomnia (2%), dysphonia (1%), headache
Dermatologic: Pruritus (2%), rash (1%)

Gastrointestinal: Diarrhea (5%), nausea (5%), xerostomia (1% to 3%), vomiting (2%), abdominal pain, dyspepsia, gastroenteritis

Neuromuscular & skeletal: Muscle cramps (2%), tremor

Respiratory: Infection (3% to 7%), asthma exacerbation (age 5-12 years: 5% to 6%; age >12 years: <4%), bronchitis (5%), pharyngitis (3% to 4%), sinusitis (3%), dyspnea (2%), tonsillitis (1%)

<1% (Limited to important or life-threatening): Acute asthma deterioration, anaphylactic reactions (severe hypotension/angioedema), agitation, angina, arrhythmia, atrial fibrillation, bronchospasm (paradoxical), cough, fatigue, hyperglycemia, hypertension, hypokalemia, glucose intolerance, malaise, metabolic acidosis, nervousness, QTc prolongation, tachycardia, ventricular extrasystoles

Drug Interactions

Metabolism/Transport Effects Substrate of CYP2C9 (minor); **Note:** Assignment of Major/Minor substrate status based on clinically relevant drug interaction potential

Avoid Concomitant Use

Avoid concomitant use of Formoterol with any of the following: Beta-Blockers (Nonselective); Highest Risk QTc-Prolonging Agents; Iobenguane I 123; Ivabradine; Long-Acting Beta2-Agonists; Mifepristone

Increased Effect/Toxicity

Formoterol may increase the levels/effects of: Atosiban; Highest Risk QTc-Prolonging Agents; Long-Acting Beta2-Agonists; Loop Diuretics; Moderate Risk QTc-Prolonging Agents; Sympathomimetics; Thiazide Diuretics

The levels/effects of Formoterol may be increased by: AtoMOXetine; Caffeine; Cannabinoids; Inhalational Anesthetics; Ivabradine; MAO Inhibitors; Mifepristone; QTc-Prolonging Agents (Indeterminate Risk and Risk Modifying); Theophylline Derivatives; Tricyclic Antidepressants

Decreased Effect

Formoterol may decrease the levels/effects of: Iobenguane I 123

The levels/effects of Formoterol may be decreased by: Beta-Blockers (Beta1 Selective); Beta-Blockers (Nonselective); Betahistine

Storage/Stability

Foradil® Aerolizer®: Prior to dispensing, store in refrigerator at 2°C to 8°C (36°F to 46°F). After dispensing, store at room temperature at 20°C to 25°C (68°F to 77°F). Protect from heat and moisture. Capsules should always be stored in the blister and only removed immediately before use.

Perforomist®: Prior to dispensing, store in refrigerator at 2°C to 8°C (36°F to 46°F). After dispensing, store at 2°C to 25°C (36°F to 77°F) for up to 3 months. Protect from heat. Unit-dose vials should always be stored in the foil pouch and only removed immediately before use.

Mechanism of Action Relaxes bronchial smooth muscle by selective action on $beta_2$ receptors with little effect on heart rate. Formoterol has a long-acting effect.

Pharmacodynamics/Kinetics

Onset of action: Powder for inhalation: Within 3 minutes

Peak effect: Powder for inhalation: 80% of peak effect within 15 minutes; Solution for nebulization: 2 hours

Duration: Improvement in FEV_1 observed for 12 hours in most patients

Absorption: Rapidly into plasma

Protein binding: 61% to 64% *in vitro* at higher concentrations than achieved with usual dosing

Metabolism: Hepatic via direct glucuronidation and O-demethylation; CYP2D6, CYP2C8/9, CYP2C19, CYP2A6 involved in O-demethylation

Half-life elimination: Powder: ~10-14 hours; Nebulized solution: ~7 hours

Time to peak: Maximum improvement in FEV_1 in 1-3 hours

Excretion:

Children 5-12 years: Urine (7% to 9% as direct glucuronide metabolites, 6% as unchanged drug)

Adults: Urine (15% to 18% as direct glucuronide metabolites, 2% to 10% as unchanged drug)

Dosage

Asthma treatment: **Note:** For asthma control, long-acting $beta_2$-agonists (LABAs) should be used in combination with inhaled corticosteroids and not as monotherapy.

U.S. labeling: Foradil® Aerolizer®: Inhalation: Children ≥5 years, Adolescents, and Adults: 12 mcg every 12 hours (maximum: 24 mcg daily)

Canadian labeling:

Foradil®:

Children 6-16 years: Inhalation: 12 mcg every 12 hours (maximum: 24 mcg daily)

Adolescents ≥17 years and Adults: Inhalation: 12 mcg every 12 hours; in severe cases, 24 mcg every 12 hours may be given (maximum: 48 mcg daily)

Oxeze® Turbuhaler®:

Children 6-16 years: Inhalation: 6 mcg or 12 mcg every 12 hours (maximum: 24 mcg daily)

Adolescents ≥17 years and Adults: Inhalation: 6 mcg or 12 mcg every 12 hours (maximum: 48 mcg daily)

Prevention of exercise-induced bronchospasm: **Note:** If already using for asthma maintenance, then should not use additional doses for exercise-induced bronchospasm. Because LABAs may disguise poorly controlled persistent asthma, frequent or chronic use of LABAs for exercise-induced bronchospasm is discouraged by the NIH Asthma Guidelines (NIH, 2007).

U.S. labeling: Foradil® Aerolizer®: Children ≥5 years, Adolescents, and Adults: Inhalation: 12 mcg at least 15 minutes before exercise on an occasional "as needed" basis; additional doses should not be used for another 12 hours

Canadian labeling: Oxeze® Turbuhaler®: Children ≥6 years, Adolescents, and Adults: Inhalation: 6 mcg or 12 mcg at least 15 minutes before exercise on an occasional "as needed" basis (maximum: Children and Adolescents: 24 mcg/24-hour period; Adults: 48 mcg/24-hour period)

COPD maintenance treatment: Adults: Inhalation:

U.S. labeling:

Foradil® Aerolizer®: 12 mcg every 12 hours (maximum: 24 mcg daily)

Perforomist®: 20 mcg twice daily (maximum dose: 40 mcg daily)

Canadian labeling: Foradil®: 12 mcg or 24 mcg twice daily (maximum dose: 48 mcg daily)

Dosage adjustment in renal impairment: No dosage adjustment provided in manufacturer's labeling (has not been studied).

Dosage adjustment in hepatic impairment: No dosage adjustment provided in manufacturer's labeling (has not been studied).

Administration

Foradil® Aerolizer®: Remove capsule from foil blister **immediately** before use. Place capsule in the capsule-chamber in the base of the Aerolizer® Inhaler. Capsules must not be swallowed whole; must only use the Aerolizer® Inhaler. Press both buttons **once only** and then release. Keep inhaler in a level, horizontal position. Exhale fully. Do not exhale into inhaler. Tilt head slightly back and inhale (rapidly, steadily, and deeply). Hold breath as long as possible. If any powder remains in capsule, exhale and inhale again. Repeat until capsule is empty. Throw away empty capsule; do not leave in inhaler. Do not use a spacer with the Aerolizer® Inhaler. Always keep capsules and inhaler dry.

Perforomist®: Remove unit-dose vial from foil pouch **immediately** before use. Solution does not require dilution prior to administration; do not mix other medications with formoterol solution. Place contents of unit-dose vial into the reservoir of a standard jet nebulizer connected to an air compressor; assemble nebulizer based on the manufacturer's instructions and turn nebulizer on; breathe deeply and evenly until all of the medication has been inhaled. Discard any unused medication immediately; do not ingest contents of vial. Clean nebulizer after use.

Oxeze® Turbuhaler® (Canadian availability): Hold inhaler upright. Turn colored grip as far as it will go in one direction and then turn back to original position; a clicking sound should be heard which means the inhaler is ready for use. Exhale fully. Do not exhale into mouthpiece of inhaler. Place mouthpiece to lips and inhale forcefully and deeply. Do not chew or bite on mouthpiece. Clean outside of mouthpiece once weekly with a dry tissue. Avoid getting inhaler wet. If the inhaler is accidently dropped or shaken, or if the patient exhales into the inhaler, the dose will be lost and a new dose should be loaded.

Monitoring Parameters FEV_1, peak flow, and/or other pulmonary function tests; blood pressure, heart rate; CNS stimulation; serum glucose, serum potassium

Dosage Forms Excipient information presented when available (limited, particularly for generics); consult specific product labeling.

Capsule, Inhalation, as fumarate:

Foradil Aerolizer: 12 mcg [contains milk protein]

Nebulization Solution, Inhalation, as fumarate dihydrate:

Perforomist: 20 mcg/2 mL (2 mL)

Dosage Forms: Canada Excipient information presented when available (limited, particularly for generics); consult specific product labeling.

Powder for oral inhalation, as fumarate:

Oxeze® Turbuhaler®: 6 mcg/inhalation [delivers 60 metered doses; contains lactose 600 mcg/dose]; 12 mcg/inhalation [delivers 60 metered doses; contains lactose 600 mcg/dose]

- ◆ **Formoterol and Budesonide** *see* Budesonide and Formoterol *on page 287*
- ◆ **Formoterol and Mometasone** *see* Mometasone and Formoterol *on page 1395*
- ◆ **Formoterol and Mometasone Furoate** *see* Mometasone and Formoterol *on page 1395*
- ◆ **Formoterol Fumarate** *see* Formoterol *on page 914*
- ◆ **Formoterol Fumarate Dihydrate** *see* Formoterol *on page 914*
- ◆ **Formoterol Fumarate Dihydrate and Budesonide** *see* Budesonide and Formoterol *on page 287*
- ◆ **Formoterol Fumarate Dihydrate and Mometasone** *see* Mometasone and Formoterol *on page 1395*
- ◆ **Formula E 400 [OTC]** *see* Vitamin E *on page 2202*
- ◆ **Formulex (Can)** *see* Dicyclomine *on page 601*
- ◆ **5-Formyl Tetrahydrofolate** *see* Leucovorin Calcium *on page 1186*
- ◆ **Fortamet** *see* MetFORMIN *on page 1310*
- ◆ **Fortaz** *see* CefTAZidime *on page 379*
- ◆ **Fortaz® (Can)** *see* CefTAZidime *on page 379*
- ◆ **Fortaz in D_5W** *see* CefTAZidime *on page 379*
- ◆ **Forteo** *see* Teriparatide *on page 2023*
- ◆ **Forteo® (Can)** *see* Teriparatide *on page 2023*
- ◆ **Fortesta** *see* Testosterone *on page 2026*
- ◆ **Fortical** *see* Calcitonin *on page 312*
- ◆ **Fosamax** *see* Alendronate *on page 69*
- ◆ **Fosamax® (Can)** *see* Alendronate *on page 69*
- ◆ **Fosamax Plus D®** *see* Alendronate and Cholecalciferol *on page 71*

Fosamprenavir (FOS am pren a veer)

Brand Names: U.S. Lexiva

Brand Names: Canada Telzir®

Index Terms Fosamprenavir Calcium; GW433908G

Pharmacologic Category Antiretroviral, Protease Inhibitor (Anti-HIV)

Use Treatment of HIV infections in combination with at least two other antiretroviral agents

Pregnancy Risk Factor C

Pregnancy Considerations Adverse events were observed in some animal reproduction studies. It is not known if fosamprenavir crosses the human placenta. A small increased risk of preterm birth has been associated with maternal use of protease inhibitor-based combination antiretroviral (ARV) therapy during pregnancy; however, the benefits of use generally outweigh this risk and protease inhibitors (PIs) should not be withheld if otherwise recommended. Hyperglycemia, new onset of diabetes mellitus, or diabetic ketoacidosis have been reported with PIs; it is not clear if pregnancy increases this risk. The DHHS Perinatal HIV Guidelines note there are insufficient data to recommend use during pregnancy; however, if used, they recommend that fosamprenavir be given with low-dose ritonavir boosting.

Regardless of CD4 count or HIV RNA copy number, all HIV-infected pregnant women should receive a combination antepartum ARV drug regimen; this includes women who require therapy for their own health, as well as women who do not yet require therapy for their own health. ARV therapy should be started as soon as possible if required for the woman's health. Although earlier initiation may be more effective in reducing the perinatal transmission of HIV, also consider maternal conditions (eg, nausea and vomiting) and the potential risks of first trimester fetal exposure for specific agents. Plasma HIV RNA levels should be assessed at ~34-36 weeks gestation in order to help determine mode of delivery. If ARV therapy must be interrupted for <24 hours during the peripartum period, stop then restart all medications simultaneously in order to decrease the chance of developing resistance. Long-term follow-up is recommended for all infants exposed to ARV medications.

Healthcare providers are encouraged to enroll pregnant women exposed to antiretroviral medications in the Antiretroviral Pregnancy Registry (1-800-258-4263 or www.APRegistry.com). Healthcare providers caring for HIV-infected women and their infants may contact the National Perinatal HIV Hotline (888-448-8765) for clinical consultation (DHHS [perinatal], 2012).

Breast-Feeding Considerations Maternal or infant antiretroviral therapy does not completely eliminate the risk of postnatal HIV transmission. In addition, multiclass-resistant virus has been detected in breast-feeding infants despite maternal therapy. Therefore, in the United States, where formula is accessible, affordable, safe, and sustainable, and the risk of infant mortality due to diarrhea and respiratory infections is low, complete avoidance of breast-feeding by HIV-infected women is recommended to decrease potential transmission of HIV (DHHS [perinatal], 2012).

Contraindications Clinically-significant hypersensitivity (eg, Stevens-Johnson syndrome) to fosamprenavir, amprenavir, or any component of the formulation; concurrent therapy with CYP3A4 substrates with a narrow therapeutic window; concomitant use with alfuzosin, cisapride, delavirdine, ergot derivatives, lovastatin, midazolam, pimozide, rifampin, simvastatin, St John's wort, and triazolam;

use of flecainide and propafenone with concomitant ritonavir therapy; sildenafil (when used for pulmonary artery hypertension [eg, Revatio®])

Warnings/Precautions Concomitant use of fosamprenavir with some drugs may require cautious use, may not be recommended, may require dosage adjustments, or may be contraindicated. Do not use with hormonal contraceptives. Do not coadminister colchicine in patient with renal or hepatic impairment.

Use with caution in patients with diabetes mellitus or sulfonamide allergy. Use caution with hepatic impairment (dosage adjustment required) or underlying hepatitis B or C. Redistribution of fat may occur (eg, buffalo hump, peripheral wasting, cushingoid appearance). Dosage adjustment is required for combination therapies (ritonavir and/or efavirenz); in addition, the risk of hyperlipidemia may be increased during concurrent therapy. Protease inhibitors have been associated with a variety of hypersensitivity events (some severe), including rash, anaphylaxis (rare), angioedema, bronchospasm, erythema multiforme, and/or Stevens-Johnson syndrome (rare). It is generally recommended to discontinue treatment if severe rash or moderate symptoms accompanied by other systemic symptoms occur. Acute hemolytic anemia has been reported in association with amprenavir use. Cases of nephrolithiasis have been reported in postmarketing surveillance; temporary or permanent discontinuation of therapy should be considered if symptoms develop. Spontaneous bleeding has been reported in patients with hemophilia A or B following treatment with protease inhibitors; use caution. Immune reconstitution syndrome may develop, resulting in the occurrence of an inflammatory response to an indolent or residual opportunistic infection during initial HIV treatment or activation of autoimmune disorders (eg, Graves' disease, polymyositis, Guillain-Barré syndrome) later in therapy; further evaluation and treatment may be required.

Adverse Reactions

>10%:

Dermatologic: Rash (≤19%; onset: ~11 days; duration: ~13 days)

Endocrine & metabolic: Hypertriglyceridemia (>750 mg/dL: ≤11%)

Gastrointestinal: Diarrhea (moderate-to-severe; 5% to 13%)

1% to 10%:

Central nervous system: Headache (moderate-to-severe; 2% to 4%), fatigue (moderate-to-severe; 2% to 4%)

Dermatologic: Pruritus (7% to 8%)

Endocrine & metabolic: Hyperglycemia (>251 mg/dL: ≤2%)

Gastrointestinal: Serum lipase increased (>2 times ULN: 5% to 8%), nausea (moderate-to-severe; 3% to 7%), vomiting (moderate-to-severe; 2% to 6%), abdominal pain (moderate-to-severe; ≤2%)

Hematologic: Neutropenia (<750 cells/mm^3: 3%)

Hepatic: Transaminases increased (>5 times ULN: 4% to 8%)

<1% (Limited to important or life-threatening): Angioedema, hypercholesterolemia, myocardial infarction, nephrolithiasis, oral paresthesia, QT prolongation (with amprenavir), Stevens-Johnson syndrome, stroke

Frequency not defined: Diabetes mellitus, fat redistribution, and immune reconstitution syndrome have been associated with protease inhibitor therapy. Spontaneous bleeding has been reported in patients with hemophilia A or B following treatment with protease inhibitors. Acute hemolytic anemia has been reported in association with amprenavir use.

Drug Interactions

Metabolism/Transport Effects **Substrate** of CYP2C9 (minor), CYP2D6 (minor), CYP3A4 (major), P-glycoprotein; **Note:** Assignment of Major/Minor substrate status based on clinically relevant drug interaction potential; **Inhibits** CYP2C19 (weak), CYP3A4 (strong)

Avoid Concomitant Use

Avoid concomitant use of Fosamprenavir with any of the following: Ado-Trastuzumab Emtansine; Alfuzosin; Amiodarone; Apixaban; Avanafil; Axitinib; Bosutinib; Cabozantinib; Cisapride; Conivaptan; Crizotinib; Delavirdine; Dronedarone; Eplerenone; Ergot Derivatives; Etravirine; Everolimus; Flecainide; Halofantrine; Ibrutinib; Imatinib; Ivabradine; Lapatinib; Lomitapide; Lovastatin; Lurasidone; Macitentan; Midazolam; Nilotinib; Nisoldipine; Pimozide; Pomalidomide; Propafenone; QuiNIDine; Ranolazine; Red Yeast Rice; Regorafenib; Rifampin; Rivaroxaban; Salmeterol; Silodosin; Simeprevir; Simvastatin; St Johns Wort; Tamsulosin; Telaprevir; Ticagrelor; Tolvaptan; Toremifene; Triazolam; Ulipristal; Vemurafenib; VinCRIStine (Liposomal)

Increased Effect/Toxicity

Fosamprenavir may increase the levels/effects of: Ado-Trastuzumab Emtansine; Alfuzosin; Almotriptan; Alosetron; ALPRAZolam; Amiodarone; Apixaban; ARIPiprazole; AtorvaSTATin; Avanafil; Axitinib; Bedaquiline; Bortezomib; Bosentan; Bosutinib; Brentuximab Vedotin; Brinzolamide; Budesonide (Nasal); Budesonide (Systemic, Oral Inhalation); Cabozantinib; Calcium Channel Blockers (Dihydropyridine); Calcium Channel Blockers (Nondihydropyridine); CarBAMazepine; Cisapride; Clarithromycin; Clorazepate; Colchicine; Conivaptan; Corticosteroids (Orally Inhaled); Crizotinib; CycloSPORINE (Systemic); CYP3A4 Substrates; Diazepam; Dienogest; Digoxin; Dofetilide; Dronedarone; Dutasteride; Enfuvirtide; Enzalutamide; Eplerenone; Ergot Derivatives; Everolimus; FentaNYL; Fesoterodine; Flecainide; Flurazepam; Fluticasone (Nasal); Fluticasone (Oral Inhalation); GuanFACINE; Halofantrine; Ibrutinib; Iloperidone; Imatinib; Itraconazole; Ivabradine; Ivacaftor; Ixabepilone; Ketoconazole (Systemic); Lacosamide; Lapatinib; Levomilnacipran; Lomitapide; Lovastatin; Lumefantrine; Lurasidone; Macitentan; Maraviroc; Meperidine; MethylPREDNISolone; Midazolam; Mifepristone; Nefazodone; Nilotinib; Nisoldipine; Ospemifene; OxyCODONE; Paricalcitol; PAZOPanib; Pimecrolimus; Pimozide; Pomalidomide; PONATinib; Propafenone; Protease Inhibitors; QUEtiapine; QuiNIDine; Ranolazine; Red Yeast Rice; Regorafenib; Repaglinide; Rifabutin; Rilpivirine; Riociguat; Rivaroxaban; RomiDEPsin; Rosuvastatin; Ruxolitinib; Salmeterol; Saxagliptin; Sildenafil; Silodosin; Simeprevir; Simvastatin; SORAfenib; Tacrolimus (Systemic); Tacrolimus (Topical); Tadalafil; Tamsulosin; Temsirolimus; Ticagrelor; Tofacitinib; Tolterodine; Tolvaptan; Toremifene; TraZODone; Triazolam; Tricyclic Antidepressants; Ulipristal; Vardenafil; Vemurafenib; Vilazodone; VinCRIStine (Liposomal); Voriconazole; Warfarin; Zuclopenthixol

The levels/effects of Fosamprenavir may be increased by: Clarithromycin; CycloSPORINE (Systemic); Delavirdine; Enfuvirtide; Etravirine; Fosphenytoin; Itraconazole; Ketoconazole (Systemic); P-glycoprotein/ABCB1 Inhibitors; Phenytoin; Posaconazole; Rifabutin; Simeprevir; Voriconazole

Decreased Effect

Fosamprenavir may decrease the levels/effects of: Abacavir; Boceprevir; Clarithromycin; Contraceptives (Estrogens); Delavirdine; Dolutegravir; Fosphenytoin; Ifosfamide; Lopinavir; Meperidine; Methadone; PARoxetine; Phenytoin; Posaconazole; Prasugrel; Raltegravir; Telaprevir; Ticagrelor; Valproic Acid and Derivatives; Zidovudine

The levels/effects of Fosamprenavir may be decreased by: Antacids; Boceprevir; Bosentan; CarBAMazepine; CYP3A4 Inducers (Strong); Dabrafenib; Deferasirox; Efavirenz; Garlic; H2-Antagonists; Methadone; Mitotane; Nevirapine; Peginterferon Alfa-2b; P-glycoprotein/ABCB1 Inducers; Raltegravir; Rifampin; St Johns Wort; Telaprevir; Tocilizumab

Ethanol/Nutrition/Herb Interactions

Food: Management:

Oral suspension: Administer without food to adults or with food to pediatric patients.

Tablet: Administer with food if taken with ritonavir. May be administered without regard to food if not taken with ritonavir.

Herb/Nutraceutical: Serum concentration may be decreased by St John's wort. Management: Avoid St John's wort; concurrent use is contraindicated.

Storage/Stability

Lexiva®: Store tablets at 25°C (77°F); excursions permitted to 15°C to 30°C (59°F to 86°F). Store oral suspension at 5°C to 30°C (41°F to 86°F). Do not freeze.

Telzir®: Store tablets 2°C to 30°C; do not freeze and discard 25 days after opening.

Mechanism of Action Fosamprenavir is rapidly and almost completely converted to amprenavir by cellular phosphatases *in vivo*. Amprenavir binds to the site of HIV-1 protease activity and inhibits cleavage of viral Gag-Pol polyprotein precursors into individual functional proteins required for infectious HIV. This results in the formation of immature, noninfectious viral particles.

Pharmacodynamics/Kinetics

Absorption: 63%

Protein-binding: ~90% (to alpha$_1$-acid glycoprotein); decreased in hepatic impairment

Metabolism: Fosamprenavir is rapidly and almost completely converted to amprenavir by cellular phosphatases in gut epithelium; amprenavir is hepatically metabolized via CYP isoenzymes (primarily CYP3A4)

Bioavailability: Not established; food does not have a significant effect on absorption of tablets. Administration of oral suspension with food reduced C_{max} by 46% and AUC by 28%.

Half-life elimination: ~7.7 hours (amprenavir)

Time to peak, plasma: 1.5-4 hours (median: 2.5 hours)

Excretion: Feces (75% as metabolites, <1% as unchanged drug); urine (14% as metabolites, ~1% as unchanged drug)

Dosage Oral: HIV infection:

Children:

U.S. labeling: Infants ≥4 weeks to Children <18 years: **Note:** Twice-daily dosing is recommended; once-daily dosing (without or without ritonavir) is **not** recommended in any pediatric patient.

Protease inhibitor (PI)-naive patients:

Ritonavir-boosted regimen: Infants ≥4 weeks: **Note:** Should not be administered to infants born <38 weeks gestation and who have not attained a postnatal age of 28 days.

<11 kg: Fosamprenavir 45 mg/kg/dose twice daily **plus** ritonavir 7 mg/kg/dose twice daily (maximum: fosamprenavir 700 mg/ritonavir 100 mg twice daily)

11 to <15 kg: Fosamprenavir 30 mg/kg/dose twice daily **plus** ritonavir 3 mg/kg/dose twice daily (maximum: fosamprenavir 700 mg/ritonavir 100 mg twice daily)

15 to <20 kg: Fosamprenavir 23 mg/kg/dose twice daily **plus** ritonavir 3 mg/kg/dose twice daily (maximum: fosamprenavir 700 mg/ritonavir 100 mg twice daily)

≥20 kg: Fosamprenavir 18 mg/kg/dose twice daily **plus** ritonavir 3 mg/kg/dose twice daily (maximum: fosamprenavir 700 mg/ritonavir 100 mg twice daily)

Note: When combined with ritonavir, the adult regimen of fosamprenavir 700 mg plus ritonavir 100 mg twice daily can be used in children who weigh ≥39 kg while ritonavir capsules may be used for children who weigh ≥33 kg.

Unboosted regimen:

Children <2 years: Fosamprenavir without ritonavir is not recommended

Children ≥2 years and <47 kg: Fosamprenavir 30 mg/kg/dose twice daily (not to exceed adult dosage of 1400 mg twice daily)

Children ≥2 years and ≥47 kg: The adult regimen of fosamprenavir 1400 mg twice daily may be used

Protease inhibitor (PI)-experienced patients:

Ritonavir-boosted regimen:

Infants <6 months: Not recommended in PI-experienced patients

Infants ≥6 months:

<11 kg: Fosamprenavir 45 mg/kg/dose twice daily **plus** ritonavir 7 mg/kg/dose twice daily (maximum: fosamprenavir 700 mg/ritonavir 100 mg twice daily)

11 to <15 kg: Fosamprenavir 30 mg/kg/dose twice daily **plus** ritonavir 3 mg/kg/dose twice daily (maximum: fosamprenavir 700 mg/ritonavir 100 mg twice daily)

15 to <20 kg: Fosamprenavir 23 mg/kg/dose twice daily **plus** ritonavir 3 mg/kg/dose twice daily (maximum: fosamprenavir 700 mg/ritonavir 100 mg twice daily)

≥20 kg: Fosamprenavir 18 mg/kg/dose twice daily **plus** ritonavir 3 mg/kg/dose twice daily (maximum: fosamprenavir 700 mg/ritonavir 100 mg twice daily)

Note: When combined with ritonavir, the adult regimen of fosamprenavir 700 mg plus ritonavir 100 mg twice daily can be used in children who weigh ≥39 while ritonavir capsules may be used for children who weigh ≥33 kg.

Unboosted regimen: **Note:** No information provided in manufacturer's labeling regarding unboosted fosamprenavir in PI-experienced pediatric patients except that fosamprenavir without ritonavir is not recommended in children <2 years of age and the adult unboosted regimen of 1400 mg twice daily may be used for pediatric patients who weigh ≥47 kg.

Canadian labeling: **Note:** Use of fosamprenavir without ritonavir (unboosted regimen) is not an approved use in the Canadian labeling.

PI-naive and PI-experienced patients: *Ritonavir boosted regimen:* Children ≥6 years: 18 mg/kg/dose **plus** ritonavir 3 mg/kg/dose twice daily; maximum dose: fosamprenavir 700 mg/ritonavir 100 mg twice daily; adult regimen of fosamprenavir 700 mg/ritonavir 100 mg twice daily can be used in children who weigh ≥39 kg while ritonavir tablets may be used for children who weigh ≥33 kg and can swallow tablets whole.

Adults:

Antiretroviral therapy-naive patients:

Unboosted regimen (per manufacturer's labeling): 1400 mg twice daily (without ritonavir); **Note:** This regimen is not recommended in adults due to inferior potency compared to other protease inhibitor based regimens and the potential for cross-resistance to darunavir (DHHS, 2013).

Ritonavir-boosted regimens:

Once-daily regimen: Fosamprenavir 1400 mg plus ritonavir 100-200 mg once daily

Twice-daily regimen: Fosamprenavir 700 mg plus ritonavir 100 mg twice daily

Protease inhibitor (PI)-experienced patients: Fosamprenavir 700 mg plus ritonavir 100 mg twice daily. **Note:** Once-daily administration is not recommended in protease inhibitor-experienced patients.

Dosage adjustments for concomitant therapy: Adults:
Combination therapy with efavirenz (ritonavir-boosted regimen):
Once-daily regimen (PI-naive patients only): Fosamprenavir 1400 mg plus ritonavir 300 mg plus efavirenz 600 mg once daily
Twice-daily regimen: Fosamprenavir 700 mg plus ritonavir 100 mg twice daily plus efavirenz 600 mg once daily
Combination therapy with maraviroc: Fosamprenavir 700 mg plus ritonavir 100 mg plus maraviroc 150 mg twice daily

Dosage adjustment in renal impairment: No dosage adjustment necessary.

Dosage adjustment in hepatic impairment: Adults (not established in pediatric patients):
Mild impairment (Child-Pugh score 5-6): Reduce dosage of fosamprenavir to 700 mg twice daily without concurrent ritonavir (therapy naive) **or** fosamprenavir 700 mg twice daily plus ritonavir 100 mg once daily (therapy naive or PI experienced)
Moderate impairment (Child-Pugh score 7-9): Reduce dosage of fosamprenavir to 700 mg twice daily without concurrent ritonavir (therapy naive) **or** fosamprenavir 450 mg twice daily plus ritonavir 100 mg once daily (therapy naive or PI experienced)
Severe impairment (Child-Pugh score 10-15): Reduce dosage of fosamprenavir to 350 mg twice daily without concurrent ritonavir (therapy naive) **or** fosamprenavir 300 mg twice daily plus ritonavir 100 mg once daily (therapy naive or PI experienced).

Dietary Considerations Tablets may be taken with or without food. Adults should take oral suspension **without** food; however, children should take oral suspension **with** food.

Administration
Oral suspension: Administer **without** food to adults; administer **with** food to pediatric patients. Readminister dose of suspension if emesis occurs within 30 minutes after dosing. Shake suspension vigorously prior to use.
Tablet: Administer with food if taken with ritonavir. May be administered without regard to food if not taken with ritonavir.

Monitoring Parameters Monitor viral load, CD4 count, glucose; triglycerides and cholesterol (prior to initiation and periodically during therapy)

Dosage Forms Excipient information presented when available (limited, particularly for generics); consult specific product labeling.
Suspension, Oral, as calcium:
Lexiva: 50 mg/mL (225 mL) [contains methylparaben, polysorbate 80, propylene glycol, propylparaben; grape bubblegum peppermint flavor]
Tablet, Oral, as calcium:
Lexiva: 700 mg

Dosage Forms: Canada Excipient information presented when available (limited, particularly for generics); consult specific product labeling.
Tablet, as calcium:
Telzir®: 700 mg
Suspension, oral, as calcium:
Telzir®: 50 mg/mL (225 mL)

◆ **Fosamprenavir Calcium** *see* Fosamprenavir *on page 916*

Fosaprepitant (fos a PRE pi tant)

Brand Names: U.S. Emend
Brand Names: Canada Emend® IV
Index Terms Aprepitant Injection; Fosaprepitant Dimeglumine; L-758,298; MK 0517

Pharmacologic Category Antiemetic; Substance P/Neurokinin 1 Receptor Antagonist

Use Prevention of acute and delayed nausea and vomiting associated with moderately- and highly-emetogenic chemotherapy (in combination with other antiemetics)

Pregnancy Risk Factor B

Pregnancy Considerations Teratogenic effects were not observed in animal reproduction studies for aprepitant. Use during pregnancy only if clearly needed. Efficacy of hormonal contraceptive may be reduced; alternative or additional methods of contraception should be used both during treatment with fosaprepitant or aprepitant and for at least 1 month following the last fosaprepitant/aprepitant dose.

Breast-Feeding Considerations It is not known if fosaprepitant is excreted in breast milk. Due to the potential for serious adverse reactions in the nursing infant, a decision should be made whether to discontinue nursing or to discontinue the drug, taking into account the importance of treatment to the mother.

Contraindications Hypersensitivity to fosaprepitant, aprepitant, polysorbate 80, or any component of the formulation; concurrent use with pimozide or cisapride
Canadian labeling: Additional contraindications (not in U.S. labeling): Concurrent use with astemizole or terfenadine

Warnings/Precautions Fosaprepitant is rapidly converted to aprepitant, which has a high potential for drug interactions. Potentially significant drug-drug interactions may exist, requiring dose or frequency adjustment, additional monitoring, and/or selection of alternative therapy. Immediate hypersensitivity has been reported (rarely) with fosaprepitant; stop infusion with hypersensitivity symptoms (dyspnea, erythema, flushing, or anaphylaxis); do not reinitiate. Contains polysorbate 80, which is associated with hypersensitivity reactions. Use caution with hepatic impairment; has not been studied in patients with severe hepatic impairment (Child-Pugh class C). Not studied for treatment of existing nausea and vomiting. Chronic continuous administration of fosaprepitant is not recommended.

Adverse Reactions Adverse reactions reported with aprepitant and fosaprepitant (as part of a combination chemotherapy regimen) occurring at a higher frequency than standard antiemetic therapy:
1% to 10%:
Central nervous system: Fatigue (1% to 3%), headache (2%)
Gastrointestinal: Anorexia (2%), constipation (2%), dyspepsia (2%), diarrhea (1%), eructation (1%)
Hepatic: ALT increased (1% to 3%), AST increased (1%)
Local: Injection site reactions (3%; includes erythema, induration, pain, pruritus, or thrombophlebitis)
Neuromuscular & skeletal: Weakness (3%)
Miscellaneous: Hiccups (5%)
<1% (Limited to important or life-threatening): Abdominal pain, alkaline phosphatase increased, anaphylactic reaction, anemia, angioedema, bradycardia, candidiasis, cardiovascular disorder, chest discomfort, chills, cognitive disorder, conjunctivitis, cough, disorientation, dizziness, duodenal ulcer (perforating), dyspnea, edema, erythema, flushing, gait disturbance, hematuria (microscopic), hyperglycemia, hyperhydrosis, hypersensitivity reaction, hypertension, hyponatremia, miosis, nausea, neutropenia, neutropenic colitis, neutropenic fever, palpitation, photosensitivity, pollakiuria, polyuria, pruritus, rash, sensory disturbance, somnolence, staphylococcal infection, Stevens-Johnson syndrome, stomatitis, subileus, tinnitus, toxic epidermal necrolysis, urticaria, visual acuity decreased, vomiting, wheezing

Drug Interactions

Metabolism/Transport Effects Substrate of CYP1A2 (minor), CYP2C19 (minor), CYP3A4 (major); **Note:** Assignment of Major/Minor substrate status based on clinically relevant drug interaction potential; **Inhibits** CYP2C19 (weak), CYP2C9 (weak), CYP3A4 (moderate); **Induces** CYP2C9 (weak/moderate), CYP3A4 (weak/moderate)

Avoid Concomitant Use

Avoid concomitant use of Fosaprepitant with any of the following: Astemizole; Axitinib; Bosutinib; Cisapride; Conivaptan; Fusidic Acid (Systemic); Ibrutinib; Ivabradine; Lomitapide; Pimozide; Simeprevir; Terfenadine; Tolvaptan; Ulipristal

Increased Effect/Toxicity

Fosaprepitant may increase the levels/effects of: ARIPiprazole; Astemizole; Avanafil; Benzodiazepines (metabolized by oxidation); Bosentan; Bosutinib; Budesonide (Systemic, Oral Inhalation); Cisapride; Colchicine; Corticosteroids (Systemic); CYP3A4 Substrates; Diltiazem; Dofetilide; Eplerenone; Everolimus; FentaNYL; Halofantrine; Ibrutinib; Imatinib; Ivabradine; Ivacaftor; Lomitapide; Lurasidone; OxyCODONE; Pimecrolimus; Pimozide; Propafenone; Ranolazine; Salmeterol; Saxagliptin; Simeprevir; Terfenadine; Tolvaptan; Ulipristal; Vilazodone; Zuclopenthixol

The levels/effects of Fosaprepitant may be increased by: Conivaptan; CYP3A4 Inhibitors (Moderate); CYP3A4 Inhibitors (Strong); Dasatinib; Diltiazem; Fusidic Acid (Systemic); Ivacaftor; Luliconazole; Mifepristone; Simeprevir

Decreased Effect

Fosaprepitant may decrease the levels/effects of: ARIPiprazole; Axitinib; Contraceptives (Estrogens); Contraceptives (Progestins); Ibrutinib; Ifosfamide; PARoxetine; Saxagliptin; Simeprevir; TOLBUTamide; Warfarin

The levels/effects of Fosaprepitant may be decreased by: Bosentan; CYP3A4 Inducers (Strong); Dabrafenib; Deferasirox; Herbs (CYP3A4 Inducers); Mitotane; PARoxetine; Rifampin; Tocilizumab

Ethanol/Nutrition/Herb Interactions

Food: Aprepitant serum concentration may be increased when taken with grapefruit juice; avoid concurrent use.

Herb/Nutraceutical: Avoid St John's wort (may decrease aprepitant levels).

Preparation for Administration Reconstitute vial with 5 mL of sodium chloride 0.9%, directing diluent down side of vial to avoid foaming; swirl gently. Add reconstituted contents of the 150 mg vial to 145 mL sodium chloride 0.9%, resulting in a final concentration of 1 mg/mL; gently invert bag to mix. Solutions may be diluted to a final volume of 250 mL (0.6 mg/mL) (data on file [Merck, 2013]).

Storage/Stability Store intact vials at 2°C to 8°C (36°F to 46°F). Solutions diluted to 1 mg/mL for infusion are stable for 24 hours at room temperature or at ≤25°C (≤77°F). Solutions diluted to a final volume of 250 mL (0.6 mg/mL) should be administered within 24 hours (data on file [Merck, 2013]).

Mechanism of Action Fosaprepitant is a prodrug of aprepitant, a substance P/neurokinin 1 (NK1) receptor antagonist. It is rapidly converted to aprepitant which prevents acute and delayed vomiting by inhibiting the substance P/neurokinin 1 (NK1) receptor; augments the antiemetic activity of the 5-HT_3 receptor antagonist and corticosteroid activity and inhibits chemotherapy-induced emesis.

Pharmacodynamics/Kinetics

Distribution: Fosaprepitant: ~5 L; Aprepitant: V_d: ~70 L; crosses the blood-brain barrier

Protein binding: Aprepitant: >95%

Metabolism:

Fosaprepitant: Hepatic and extrahepatic; rapidly (within 30 minutes after the end of infusion) converted to aprepitant (nearly complete conversion)

Aprepitant: Hepatic via CYP3A4 (major); CYP1A2 and CYP2C19 (minor); forms 7 weakly-active metabolites

Half-life elimination: Fosaprepitant: ~2 minutes; Aprepitant: ~9-13 hours

Time to peak, plasma: Fosaprepitant is converted to aprepitant within 30 minutes after the end of infusion

Excretion: Urine (57%); feces (45%)

Dosage Prevention of chemotherapy-induced nausea/vomiting: Adults: I.V.:

Single-dose regimen for highly-emetogenic chemotherapy: 150 mg ~30 minutes prior to chemotherapy on day 1 only (in combination with a 5-HT_3 antagonist on day 1 and dexamethasone on days 1 to 4)

Single-dose regimen for moderately-emetogenic chemotherapy: 150 mg ~30 minutes prior to chemotherapy on day 1 only (in combination with a 5-HT3 antagonist and dexamethasone on day 1, and either a 5-HT3 antagonist or dexamethasone on days 2 and 3) (NCCN Antiemesis guidelines v.1.2013)

Dosage adjustment in renal impairment:

Mild, moderate, or severe impairment: No dosage adjustment necessary.

Dialysis-dependent end-stage renal disease (ESRD): No dosage adjustment necessary.

Dosage adjustment in hepatic impairment:

Mild or moderate impairment (Child-Pugh class A or B): No dosage adjustment necessary.

Severe impairment (Child-Pugh class C): Has not been evaluated; use with caution.

Administration 150 mg: Infuse over 20-30 minutes ~30 minutes prior to chemotherapy

Dosage Forms Excipient information presented when available (limited, particularly for generics); consult specific product labeling.

Solution Reconstituted, Intravenous:

Emend: 150 mg (1 ea) [contains disodium edta, polysorbate 80]

- Fosaprepitant Dimeglumine *see* Fosaprepitant *on page 919*
- Fosavance (Can) *see* Alendronate and Cholecalciferol *on page 71*

Foscarnet (fos KAR net)

Brand Names: U.S. Foscavir

Brand Names: Canada Foscavir®

Index Terms PFA; Phosphonoformate; Phosphonoformic Acid

Pharmacologic Category Antiviral Agent

Use Treatment of acyclovir-resistant mucocutaneous herpes simplex virus (HSV) infections in immunocompromised persons (eg, with advanced AIDS); treatment of CMV retinitis in persons with HIV

Unlabeled Use Other CMV infections (eg, colitis, esophagitis, neurological disease); CMV prophylaxis for cancer patients receiving alemtuzumab therapy or allogeneic stem cell transplant

Pregnancy Risk Factor C

Pregnancy Considerations Associated with an increase in skeletal anomalies in animal studies at approximately the equivalent of 13% to 33% of the maximal daily human dose. There are no adequate and well controlled studies in pregnant women. A single case report of use during the third trimester with normal infant outcome was observed. Monitoring of amniotic fluid volumes by ultrasound is recommended weekly after 20 weeks of gestation to detect oligohydramnios.

Breast-Feeding Considerations The CDC recommends **not** to breast-feed if diagnosed with HIV to avoid postnatal transmission of the virus.

Contraindications Hypersensitivity to foscarnet or any component of the formulation

Warnings/Precautions [U.S. Boxed Warning]: Indicated only for immunocompromised patients with CMV retinitis and mucocutaneous acyclovir-resistant HSV infection. [U.S. Boxed Warning]: Renal impairment occurs to some degree in the majority of patients treated with foscarnet; renal impairment may occur at any time and is usually reversible within 1 week following dose adjustment or discontinuation of therapy, however, several patients have died with renal failure within 4 weeks of stopping foscarnet; therefore, renal function should be closely monitored. To reduce the risk of nephrotoxicity and the potential to administer a relative overdose, always calculate the creatine clearance even if serum creatinine is within the normal range. Adequate hydration may reduce the risk of nephrotoxicity; the manufacturer makes specific recommendations regarding this (see Administration).

Imbalance of serum electrolytes or minerals occurs in at least 15% of patients (hypocalcemia, low ionized calcium, hyper/hypophosphatemia, hypomagnesemia, or hypokalemia). Correct electrolytes before initiating therapy. Use caution when administering other medications that cause electrolyte imbalances. Patients who experience signs or symptoms of an electrolyte imbalance should be assessed immediately. **[U.S. Boxed Warning]: Seizures related to plasma electrolyte/mineral imbalance may occur;** incidence has been reported in up to 10% of HIV patients. Risk factors for seizures include impaired baseline renal function, low total serum calcium, and underlying CNS conditions. May cause anemia and granulocytopenia. May cause genital/vascular tissue irritation/ulceration; adequately hydrate and administer only into vein with adequate blood flow to minimize risk. Foscarnet is deposited in teeth and bone of young, growing animals; it has adversely affected tooth enamel development in rats.

Adverse Reactions

>10%:

Central nervous system: Fever (65%), headache (26%)

Endocrine & metabolic: Hypokalemia (16% to 48%), hypocalcemia (15% to 30%), hypomagnesemia (15% to 30%), hypophosphatemia (8% to 26%)

Gastrointestinal: Nausea (47%), diarrhea (30%), vomiting (26%)

Hematologic: Anemia (33%), granulocytopenia (17%)

Renal: Abnormal renal function/decreased creatinine clearance (12%; without adequate hydration 33%)

1% to 10%:

Cardiovascular: Chest pain (1% to 5%), edema (1% to 5%), facial edema (1% to 5%), flushing (1% to 5%), hyper-/hypotension (1% to 5%), palpitation (1% to 5%), ECG changes (1% to 5%)

Central nervous system: Seizures (8% to 10%), anxiety (≥5%), confusion (≥5%), depression (≥5%), dizziness (≥5%), fatigue (≥5%), hypoesthesia (≥5%), malaise (≥5%), pain (≥5%), aggressiveness (1% to 5%), agitation (1% to 5%), amnesia (1% to 5%), aphasia (1% to 5%), ataxia (1% to 5%), coordination abnormal (1% to 5%), dementia (1% to 5%), EEG abnormal (1% to 5%), hallucination (1% to 5%), insomnia (1% to 5%), meningitis (1% to 5%), nervousness (1% to 5%), somnolence (1% to 5%), stupor (1% to 5%)

Dermatologic: Rash (≥5%), erythematous rash (1% to 5%), maculopapular rash (1% to 5%), pruritus (1% to 5%), seborrhea (1% to 5%), skin discoloration (1% to 5%), skin ulceration (1% to 5%)

Endocrine & metabolic: Hyperphosphatemia (6%), acidosis (1% to 5%), hyponatremia (1% to 5%)

Gastrointestinal: Abdominal pain (≥5%), anorexia (≥5%), cachexia (1% to 5%), constipation (1% to 5%), dyspepsia (1% to 5%), dysphagia (1% to 5%), flatulence (1% to 5%), melena (1% to 5%), pancreatitis (1% to 5%), rectal hemorrhage (1% to 5%), taste perversion (1% to 5%), ulcerative stomatitis (1% to 5%), weight loss (1% to 5%), xerostomia (1% to 5%)

Genitourinary: Dysuria (1% to 5%), nocturia (1% to 5%), urinary retention (1% to 5%), urinary tract infection (1% to 5%)

Hematologic: Bone marrow suppression (10%), leukopenia (≥5%), lymphadenopathy (1% to 5%), thrombocytopenia (1% to 5%), thrombosis (1% to 5%)

Hepatic: Alkaline phosphatase increased (1% to 5%), ALT increased (1% to 5%), AST increased (1% to 5%), hepatic function abnormal (1% to 5%), LDH increased (1% to 5%)

Local: Abscess (1% to 5%), injection site pain/inflammation (1% to 5%)

Neuromuscular & skeletal: Paresthesia (≥5%), involuntary muscle contractions (≥5%), rigors (≥5%), neuropathy (peripheral; ≥5%), weakness (≥5%), arthralgia (1% to 5%), back pain (1% to 5%), leg cramps (1% to 5%), myalgia (1% to 5%), tremor (1% to 5%)

Ocular: Vision abnormalities (≥5%), conjunctivitis (1% to 5%), eye pain (1% to 5%)

Renal: Acute renal failure (1% to 5%), albuminuria (1% to 5%), BUN increased (1% to 5%), polyuria (1% to 5%)

Respiratory: Cough (≥5%), dyspnea (≥5%), bronchospasm (1% to 5%), hemoptysis (1% to 5%), pharyngitis (1% to 5%), pneumonia (1% to 5%), pneumothorax (1% to 5%), pulmonary infiltrates (1% to 5%), respiratory failure (1% to 5%), rhinitis (1% to 5%), sinusitis (1% to 5%), stridor (1% to 5%)

Miscellaneous: Diaphoresis (≥5%), sepsis (≥5%), flu-like syndrome (1% to 5%), infection (includes bacterial and fungal; 1% to 5%), malignancies (lymphoma/sarcoma 1% to 5%), thirst (1% to 5%)

<1% (Limited to important or life-threatening): Cardiac arrest, coma, diabetes insipidus (usually nephrogenic), erythema multiforme, hematuria, hypoproteinemia, myositis, neutropenia, pancytopenia, QT_c prolongation, renal calculus, rhabdomyolysis, Stevens-Johnson syndrome, syndrome of inappropriate antidiuretic hormone (SIADH), toxic epidermal necrolysis, ventricular arrhythmia

Drug Interactions

Metabolism/Transport Effects None known.

Avoid Concomitant Use There are no known interactions where it is recommended to avoid concomitant use.

Increased Effect/Toxicity

Foscarnet may increase the levels/effects of: Highest Risk QTc-Prolonging Agents; Moderate Risk QTc-Prolonging Agents

The levels/effects of Foscarnet may be increased by: Mifepristone; Pentamidine

Decreased Effect There are no known significant interactions involving a decrease in effect.

Preparation for Administration Foscarnet should be diluted in D_5W or NS. For peripheral line administration, foscarnet **must** be diluted to ≤12 mg/mL with D_5W or NS. For central line administration, foscarnet may be administered undiluted.

Storage/Stability Foscarnet injection is a clear, colorless solution. Store intact bottles at room temperature of 15°C to 30°C (59°F to 86°F) and protect from temperatures >40°C and from freezing. Diluted solution is stable for 24 hours at room temperature or under refrigeration.

Mechanism of Action Pyrophosphate analogue which acts as a noncompetitive inhibitor of many viral RNA and DNA polymerases as well as HIV reverse transcriptase. Similar to ganciclovir, foscarnet is a virostatic agent. Foscarnet does not require activation by thymidine kinase.

Pharmacodynamics/Kinetics

Distribution: V_d: ~0.5 L/kg; up to 28% of cumulative I.V. dose may be deposited in bone

Protein binding: 14% to 17%

Metabolism: Biotransformation does not occur

Half-life elimination: Elimination: ~3-4 hours; terminal: ~88 hours (due to bone deposition)

Excretion: Urine (≤28% as unchanged drug)

Dosage

CMV retinitis: I.V.:

Induction treatment: 60 mg/kg/dose every 8 hours **or** 90 mg/kg every 12 hours for 14-21 days

Maintenance therapy: 90-120 mg/kg/day as a single daily infusion

Herpes simplex infections (acyclovir-resistant): Induction: I.V.: 40 mg/kg/dose every 8-12 hours for 14-21 days

Therapy of CMV infection in cancer patients (unlabeled use): I.V.:

Prophylaxis: 60 mg/kg every 8-12 hours for 7 days, followed by 90-120 mg/kg daily until day 100 after HSCT

Pre-emptive treatment: 60 mg/kg every 12 hours for 14 days; if CMV still detectable, continue with 90 mg/kg daily for 5 days/week for 2 additional weeks

Treatment: 90 mg/kg every 12 hours for 2 weeks, followed by 120 mg/kg daily for ≥2 weeks

Dosage adjustment in renal impairment: Induction and maintenance dosing schedules based on creatinine clearance (mL/minute/kg): See tables.

Induction Dosing of Foscarnet in Patients With Abnormal Renal Function

Cl_{cr} (mL/min/kg)	HSV Equivalent to 40 mg/kg q12h	HSV Equivalent to 40 mg/kg q8h	CMV Equivalent to 60 mg/kg q8h	CMV Equivalent to 90 mg/kg q12h
<0.4	Not recommended	Not recommended	Not recommended	Not recommended
≥0.4-0.5	20 mg/kg every 24 hours	35 mg/kg every 24 hours	50 mg/kg every 24 hours	50 mg/kg every 24 hours
>0.5-0.6	25 mg/kg every 24 hours	40 mg/kg every 24 hours	60 mg/kg every 24 hours	60 mg/kg every 24 hours
>0.6-0.8	35 mg/kg every 24 hours	25 mg/kg every 12 hours	40 mg/kg every 12 hours	80 mg/kg every 24 hours
>0.8-1.0	20 mg/kg every 12 hours	35 mg/kg every 12 hours	50 mg/kg every 12 hours	50 mg/kg every 12 hours
>1.0-1.4	30 mg/kg every 12 hours	30 mg/kg every 8 hours	45 mg/kg every 8 hours	70 mg/kg every 12 hours
>1.4	40 mg/kg every 12 hours	40 mg/kg every 8 hours	60 mg/kg every 8 hours	90 mg/kg every 12 hours

Maintenance Dosing of Foscarnet in Patients With Abnormal Renal Function

Cl_{cr} (mL/min/kg)	CMV Equivalent to 90 mg/kg q24h	CMV Equivalent to 120 mg/kg q24h
<0.4	Not recommended	Not recommended
≥0.4-0.5	50 mg/kg every 48 hours	65 mg/kg every 48 hours
>0.5-0.6	60 mg/kg every 48 hours	80 mg/kg every 48 hours
>0.6-0.8	80 mg/kg every 48 hours	105 mg/kg every 48 hours
>0.8-1.0	50 mg/kg every 24 hours	65 mg/kg every 24 hours
>1.0-1.4	70 mg/kg every 24 hours	90 mg/kg every 24 hours
>1.4	90 mg/kg every 24 hours	120 mg/kg every 24 hours

Hemodialysis:

Foscarnet is highly removed by hemodialysis (up to ~38% in 2.5 hours HD with high-flux membrane)

Doses of 50 mg/kg/dose posthemodialysis have been found to produce similar serum concentrations as doses of 90 mg/kg twice daily in patients with normal renal function

Doses of 60-90 mg/kg/dose loading dose (posthemodialysis) followed by 45-60 mg/kg/dose posthemodialysis (3 times/week) with the monitoring of weekly plasma concentrations to maintain peak plasma concentrations in the range of 400-800 µMolar have been recommended by some clinicians

Continuous arteriovenous or venovenous hemodiafiltration effects: Dose as for Cl_{cr} 10-50 mL/minute

Dosage adjustment in hepatic impairment: No dosage adjustment provided in manufacturer's labeling.

Administration Foscarnet is administered by intravenous infusion, using an infusion pump, at a rate not exceeding 1 mg/kg/minute. Undiluted (24 mg/mL) solution can be administered without further dilution when using a central venous catheter for infusion. For peripheral vein administration, the solution **must** be diluted to a final concentration **not to exceed** 12 mg/mL. The manufacturer recommends 750-1000 mL of NS or D_5W be administered prior to first infusion to establish diuresis. With subsequent infusions of 90-120 mg/kg, this volume would be repeated. If the dose were 40-60 mg/kg, then the volume could be reduced to 500 mL. After the first dose, the hydration fluid should be administered concurrently with foscarnet.

Monitoring Parameters 24-hour creatinine clearance at baseline and periodically thereafter. During induction therapy: Obtain complete blood counts, and electrolytes (including serum creatinine, calcium, magnesium, potassium, and phosphorus) twice weekly and then one weekly during maintenance therapy. More frequent monitoring may be required in some patients. Check hydration status before and after infusion.

Additional Information CMV retinitis maintenance treatment may be discontinued if immune reconstitution occurs as a result of ART.

Dosage Forms Excipient information presented when available (limited, particularly for generics); consult specific product labeling.

Solution, Intravenous, as sodium:

Foscavir: 24 mg/mL (250 mL)

Generic: 24 mg/mL (500 mL)

◆ **Foscavir** *see* Foscarnet *on page* 920

◆ **Foscavir® (Can)** *see* Foscarnet *on page* 920

Fosfomycin (fos foe MYE sin)

Brand Names: U.S. Monurol

Brand Names: Canada Monurol®

Index Terms Fosfomycin Tromethamine

Pharmacologic Category Antibiotic, Miscellaneous

Use Single oral dose in the treatment of uncomplicated urinary tract infections in women due to susceptible strains of *E. coli* and *Enterococcus faecalis*

Unlabeled Use Multiple doses have been investigated for complicated urinary tract infections in men

Pregnancy Risk Factor B

Dosage Adults: Oral:

Females: Uncomplicated UTI: Single dose of 3 g in 3-4 oz (90-120 mL) of water

Males:

Complicated UTI (unlabeled): 3 g every 2-3 days for 3 doses

Prostatitis (unlabeled): 3 g every 3 days for a total of 21 days (Shrestha, 2000)

Dosage adjustment in renal impairment: No dosage adjustment provided in manufacturer's labeling.

Dosage adjustment in hepatic impairment: No dosage adjustment provided in manufacturer's labeling.

Additional Information Complete prescribing information should be consulted for additional detail.

Dosage Forms Excipient information presented when available (limited, particularly for generics); consult specific product labeling.

Packet, Oral:

Monurol: 3 g (3 ea) [orange flavor]

◆ Fosfomycin Tromethamine *see* Fosfomycin *on page 922*

Fosinopril (foe SIN oh pril)

Brand Names: Canada Apo-Fosinopril; Ava-Fosinopril; Jamp-Fosinopril; Mylan-Fosinopril; PMS-Fosinopril; RAN-Fosinopril; Riva-Fosinopril; Teva-Fosinopril

Index Terms Fosinopril Sodium; Monopril

Pharmacologic Category Angiotensin-Converting Enzyme (ACE) Inhibitor; Antihypertensive

Additional Appendix Information

Angiotensin Agents *on page 2280*

Use

Hypertension: Treatment of hypertension, either alone or in combination with other antihypertensive agents

Heart failure: Adjunctive treatment of heart failure (HF)

Pregnancy Risk Factor C (1st trimester); D (2nd and 3rd trimesters)

Pregnancy Considerations **[U.S. Boxed Warning]: Based on human data, ACE inhibitors can cause injury and death to the developing fetus when used in the second and third trimesters. ACE inhibitors should be discontinued as soon as possible once pregnancy is detected.** Teratogenic effects may occur following maternal use of an ACE inhibitor during pregnancy (ACOG, 2012). Drugs that act on the renin-angiotensin system are associated with oligohydramnios. Oligohydramnios, due to decreased fetal renal function, may lead to fetal lung hypoplasia and skeletal malformations. Their use in pregnancy is also associated with anuria, hypotension, renal failure, skull hypoplasia, and death in the fetus/neonate. Chronic maternal hypertension itself is also associated with adverse events in the fetus/infant. ACE inhibitors are not recommended during pregnancy to treat maternal hypertension or heart failure (ACOG, 2012; Chobanian, 2003; Yancy, 2013). Women who are planning a pregnancy should be considered for other medication options if an ACE inhibitor is currently prescribed or the ACE inhibitor should be discontinued as soon as possible once pregnancy is detected (ACOG, 2012; Chobanian, 2003). The exposed fetus should be monitored for fetal growth, amniotic fluid volume, and organ formation. Infants exposed to an ACE inhibitor *in utero*, especially during the second and third trimester, should be monitored for hyperkalemia, hypotension, and oliguria.

Breast-Feeding Considerations Fosinoprilat is excreted in breast milk. Breast-feeding is not recommended by the manufacturer.

Contraindications Hypersensitivity to fosinopril, any other ACE inhibitor, or any component of the formulation; angioedema related to previous treatment with an ACE inhibitor; concomitant use with aliskiren in patients with diabetes mellitus

Warnings/Precautions Anaphylactic reactions may occur rarely with ACE inhibitors. At any time during treatment (especially following first dose), angioedema may occur rarely with ACE inhibitors; it may involve the head and neck (potentially compromising airway) or the intestine (presenting with abdominal pain). African-Americans may be at an increased risk and patients with idiopathic or hereditary angioedema may be at an increased risk. Prolonged frequent monitoring may be required especially if tongue, glottis, or larynx are involved as they are associated with airway obstruction. Patients with a history of airway surgery may have a higher risk of airway obstruction. Aggressive early and appropriate management is critical. Use in patients with previous angioedema associated with ACE inhibitor therapy is contraindicated. Severe anaphylactoid reactions may be seen during hemodialysis (eg, CVVHD) with high-flux dialysis membranes (eg, AN69), and rarely, during low density lipoprotein apheresis with dextran sulfate cellulose. Rare cases of anaphylactoid reactions have been reported in patients undergoing sensitization treatment with hymenoptera (bee, wasp) venom while receiving ACE inhibitors.

Symptomatic hypotension with or without syncope can occur with ACE inhibitors (usually with the first several doses); effects are most often observed in volume-depleted patients; correct volume depletion prior to initiation; close monitoring of patient is required especially with initial dosing and dosing increases; blood pressure must be lowered at a rate appropriate for the patient's clinical condition. Initiation of therapy in patients with ischemic heart disease or cerebrovascular disease warrants close observation due to the potential consequences posed by falling blood pressure (eg, MI, stroke). Use with caution in hypertrophic cardiomyopathy with outflow tract obstruction, severe aortic stenosis, or before, during, or immediately after major surgery. **[U.S. Boxed Warning]: Based on human data, ACEIs can cause injury and death to the developing fetus when used in the second and third trimesters. ACEIs should be discontinued as soon as possible once pregnancy is detected.**

Hyperkalemia may occur with ACE inhibitors; risk factors include renal dysfunction, diabetes mellitus, concomitant use of potassium-sparing diuretics, potassium supplements, and/or potassium-containing salts. Use cautiously, if at all, with these agents and monitor potassium closely. Cough may occur with ACE inhibitors. Other causes of cough should be considered (eg, pulmonary congestion in patients with heart failure) and excluded prior to discontinuation. Use with caution in hepatic impairment; fosinopril undergoes hepatic and gut wall metabolism to its active form (fosinoprilat) and may accumulate in hepatic impairment. In patients with alcoholic or biliary cirrhosis, the rate of fosinoprilat formation was slowed, its total body clearance decreased and its AUC ~doubled.

May be associated with deterioration of renal function and/or increases in serum creatinine, particularly in patients with low renal blood flow (eg, renal artery stenosis, heart failure) whose glomerular filtration rate (GFR) is dependent on efferent arteriolar vasoconstriction by angiotensin II; deterioration may result in oliguria, acute renal failure, and progressive azotemia. Small increases in serum ▶

creatinine may occur following initiation; consider discontinuation only in patients with progressive and/or significant deterioration in renal function. Use with caution in patients with unstented unilateral/bilateral renal artery stenosis. When unstented bilateral renal artery stenosis is present, use is generally avoided due to the elevated risk of deterioration in renal function unless possible benefits outweigh risks. Potentially significant interactions may exist, requiring dose or frequency adjustment, additional monitoring, and/or selection of alternative therapy. Consult drug interactions database for more detailed information.

Rare toxicities associated with ACE inhibitors include cholestatic jaundice (which may progress to fulminant hepatic necrosis), agranulocytosis, neutropenia or leukopenia with myeloid hypoplasia. Patients with collagen vascular diseases (especially with concomitant renal impairment) or renal impairment alone may be at increased risk for hematologic toxicity; periodically monitor CBC with differential in these patients.

Adverse Reactions Note: Frequency ranges include data from hypertension and heart failure trials. Higher rates of adverse reactions have generally been noted in patients with CHF. However, the frequency of adverse effects associated with placebo is also increased in this population.

>10%: Central nervous system: Dizziness (1.6% to 11.9%)

1% to 10%:

- Cardiovascular: Orthostatic hypotension (1.4% to 1.9%), palpitation (1.4%)
- Central nervous system: Dizziness (1% to 2%; up to 12% in CHF patients), headache (3.2%), fatigue (1% to 2%)
- Endocrine & metabolic: Hyperkalemia (2.6%)
- Gastrointestinal: Diarrhea (2.2%), nausea/vomiting (1.2% to 2.2%)
- Hepatic: Transaminases increased
- Neuromuscular & skeletal: Musculoskeletal pain (<1% to 3.3%), noncardiac chest pain (<1% to 2.2%), weakness (1.4%)
- Renal: Serum creatinine increased, renal function worsening (in patients with bilateral renal artery stenosis or hypovolemia)
- Respiratory: Cough (2.2% to 9.7%)
- Miscellaneous: Upper respiratory infection (2.2%)

>1% but ≤ frequency in patients receiving placebo: Sexual dysfunction, fever, flu-like syndrome, dyspnea, rash, headache, insomnia

<1% (Limited to important or life-threatening): Anaphylactoid reaction, angina, angioedema, arthralgia, bronchospasm, cerebral infarction, cerebrovascular accident, gout, hepatitis, hepatomegaly, myalgia, MI, pancreatitis, paresthesia, photosensitivity, pleuritic chest pain, pruritus, rash, renal insufficiency, shock, sudden death, syncope, TIA, tinnitus, urticaria, vertigo. In a small number of patients, a symptom complex of cough, bronchospasm, and eosinophilia has been observed with fosinopril.

Other events reported with ACE inhibitors: Acute renal failure, agranulocytosis, anemia, aplastic anemia, bullous pemphigus, cardiac arrest, eosinophilic pneumonitis, exfoliative dermatitis, gynecomastia, hemolytic anemia, hepatic failure, jaundice, neutropenia, pancytopenia, Stevens-Johnson syndrome, symptomatic hyponatremia, thrombocytopenia. In addition, a syndrome which may include fever, myalgia, arthralgia, interstitial nephritis, vasculitis, rash, eosinophilia and positive ANA, and elevated ESR has been reported for other ACE inhibitors.

Drug Interactions

Metabolism/Transport Effects None known.

Avoid Concomitant Use There are no known interactions where it is recommended to avoid concomitant use.

Increased Effect/Toxicity

Fosinopril may increase the levels/effects of: Allopurinol; Amifostine; Antihypertensives; AzaTHIOprine; CycloSPORINE (Systemic); Ferric Gluconate; Gold Sodium Thiomalate; Hypotensive Agents; Iron Dextran Complex; Lithium; Nonsteroidal Anti-Inflammatory Agents; Obinutuzumab; RiTUXimab; Sodium Phosphates

The levels/effects of Fosinopril may be increased by: Alfuzosin; Aliskiren; Angiotensin II Receptor Blockers; Brimonidine (Topical); Canagliflozin; Diazoxide; DPP-IV Inhibitors; Eplerenone; Everolimus; Heparin; Heparin (Low Molecular Weight); Herbs (Hypotensive Properties); Loop Diuretics; MAO Inhibitors; Pentoxifylline; Phosphodiesterase 5 Inhibitors; Potassium Salts; Potassium-Sparing Diuretics; Prostacyclin Analogues; Sirolimus; Temsirolimus; Thiazide Diuretics; TiZANidine; Tolvaptan; Trimethoprim

Decreased Effect

The levels/effects of Fosinopril may be decreased by: Antacids; Aprotinin; Herbs (Hypertensive Properties); Icatibant; Lanthanum; Methylphenidate; Nonsteroidal Anti-Inflammatory Agents; Salicylates; Yohimbine

Ethanol/Nutrition/Herb Interactions

Food: Potassium supplements and/or potassium-containing salts may cause or worsen hyperkalemia. Management: Advise patient to consult prescriber before consuming a potassium-rich diet, potassium supplements, or salt substitutes.

Herb/Nutraceutical: Some herbal medications may worsen hypertension (eg, licorice); others may increase the antihypertensive effect of fosinopril (eg, shepherd's purse). Management: Avoid bayberry, blue cohosh, cayenne, ephedra, ginger, ginseng (American), kola, licorice, and yohimbe. Avoid black cohosh, california poppy, coleus, golden seal, hawthorn, mistletoe, periwinkle, quinine, and shepherd's purse.

Storage/Stability Store at 20°C to 25°C (68°F to 77°F). Protect from moisture.

Mechanism of Action Competitive inhibitor of angiotensin-converting enzyme (ACE); prevents conversion of angiotensin I to angiotensin II, a potent vasoconstrictor; results in lower levels of angiotensin II which causes an increase in plasma renin activity and a reduction in aldosterone secretion; a CNS mechanism may also be involved in hypotensive effect as angiotensin II increases adrenergic outflow from CNS; vasoactive kallikreins may be decreased in conversion to active hormones by ACE inhibitors, thus reducing blood pressure

Pharmacodynamics/Kinetics

Onset of action: 1 hour

Duration: 24 hours

Absorption: 36%

Protein binding: >99%

Metabolism: Prodrug, hydrolyzed to its active metabolite fosinoprilat by intestinal wall and hepatic esterases

Bioavailability: 36%

Half-life elimination, serum (fosinoprilat): 12 hours

Time to peak, serum: ~3 hours

Excretion: Urine and feces (as fosinoprilat and other metabolites in roughly equal proportions)

Dosage Oral:

Children ≥6 years and Adolescents >50 kg: Hypertension: Initial: 5-10 mg once daily (maximum: 40 mg once daily)

Adults:

Heart failure: Initial: 10 mg once daily (5 mg once daily if moderate-to-severe renal dysfunction is present or if aggressively diuresed); increase dose as needed and as tolerated over several weeks. Usual dosage range: 20-40 mg once daily (maximum dose: 40 mg once daily) If hypotension, orthostasis, or azotemia occur during titration, consider decreasing concomitant diuretic dose, if any.

Hypertension: Initial: 10 mg once daily; usual maintenance: 20-40 mg once daily (maximum: 80 mg once daily). May need to divide the dose into two if trough effect is inadequate. If patient is receiving a diuretic prior to initiation, consider discontinuation of the diuretic to reduce likelihood of hypotension, if possible 2-3 days before initiation of therapy. If blood pressure response is inadequate, resume diuretic therapy carefully.

Dosage adjustment in renal impairment:

Moderate-severe impairment: Initial dose reduction to 5 mg once daily recommended for heart failure patients. No other dose adjustments are required; hepatobiliary elimination partially compensates for diminished renal elimination.

Hemodialysis: Poorly dialyzed; supplemental dose not required (Gehr, 1993)

Peritoneal dialysis: Poorly dialyzed; supplemental dose not required (Gehr, 1991).

Dosage adjustment in hepatic impairment: No dosage adjustment provided in manufacturer's labeling.

Dietary Considerations Should not take a potassium salt supplement without the advice of healthcare provider.

Monitoring Parameters Blood pressure; BUN, serum creatinine and potassium; if patient has collagen vascular disease and/or renal impairment, periodically monitor CBC with differential

Test Interactions May cause false low serum digoxin levels with the Digi-Tab RIA kit for digoxin.

Dosage Forms Excipient information presented when available (limited, particularly for generics); consult specific product labeling.

Tablet, Oral, as sodium:

Generic: 10 mg, 20 mg, 40 mg

◆ **Fosinopril Sodium** *see* Fosinopril *on page 923*

Fosphenytoin (FOS fen i toyn)

Brand Names: U.S. Cerebyx

Brand Names: Canada Cerebyx®

Index Terms Cerebyx; Fosphenytoin Sodium

Pharmacologic Category Anticonvulsant, Hydantoin

Additional Appendix Information

Status Epilepticus *on page 2375*

Use Used for the control of generalized convulsive status epilepticus and prevention and treatment of seizures occurring during neurosurgery; indicated for short-term parenteral administration when other means of phenytoin administration are unavailable, inappropriate, or deemed less advantageous (the safety and effectiveness of fosphenytoin use for more than 5 days has not been systematically evaluated)

Pregnancy Risk Factor D

Pregnancy Considerations Fosphenytoin is the prodrug of phenytoin. Refer to Phenytoin on page 1638 for additional information.

Breast-Feeding Considerations Fosphenytoin is the prodrug of phenytoin. It is not known if fosphenytoin is excreted in breast milk prior to conversion to phenytoin. Refer to Phenytoin monograph for additional information.

Contraindications Hypersensitivity to phenytoin, other hydantoins, or any component of the formulation; patients with sinus bradycardia, sinoatrial block, second- and third-degree AV block, or Adams-Stokes syndrome; occurrence of rash during treatment (should not be resumed if rash is exfoliative, purpuric, or bullous); treatment of absence seizures; concurrent use of delavirdine (due to loss of virologic response and possible resistance to delavirdine or other non-nucleoside reverse transcriptase inhibitors [NNRTIs])

Warnings/Precautions [U.S. Boxed Warning]: Fosphenytoin administration should not exceed 150 mg phenytoin equivalents (PE)/minute in adult patients. Hypotension and severe cardiac arrhythmias (eg, heart block, ventricular tachycardia, ventricular fibrillation) may occur with rapid administration; adverse cardiac events have been reported at or below the recommended infusion rate. In the treatment of status epilepticus, the rate of administration is 150 mg PE/minute. In a nonemergent situation, administer more slowly or use oral phenytoin. Cardiac monitoring is necessary during and after administration of intravenous fosphenytoin; reduction in rate of administration or discontinuation of infusion may be necessary.

Doses of fosphenytoin are always expressed as their phenytoin sodium equivalent (PE). 1 mg PE is equivalent to 1 mg phenytoin sodium. Do not change the recommended doses when substituting fosphenytoin for phenytoin or vice versa as they are not equivalent on a mg to mg basis. Dosing errors have also occurred due to misinterpretation of vial concentrations resulting in two- or tenfold overdoses (some fatal); ensure correct volume of fosphenytoin is withdrawn from vial. Severe burning or itching, and/or paresthesias, mostly perineal, may occur upon administration, usually at the maximum administration rate and last from minutes to hours; occurrence and intensity may be lessened by slowing or temporarily stopping the infusion. Antiepileptic drugs should not be abruptly discontinued. Acute hepatotoxicity associated with a hypersensitivity syndrome characterized by fever, skin eruptions, and lymphadenopathy has been reported to occur within the first 2 months of treatment. Discontinue if skin rash or lymphadenopathy occurs. A spectrum of hematologic effects have been reported with use (eg, neutropenia, leukopenia, thrombocytopenia, pancytopenia, and anemias). Use with caution in patients with hypotension, severe myocardial insufficiency, diabetes mellitus, porphyria, hypoalbuminemia, hypothyroidism, fever, or hepatic dysfunction. Use with caution in patients with renal impairment; also consider the phosphate load of fosphenytoin (0.0037 mmol phosphate/mg PE fosphenytoin). Effects with other sedative drugs or ethanol may be potentiated. Severe reactions, including toxic epidermal necrolysis (TEN) and Stevens-Johnson syndromes, although rarely reported, have resulted in fatalities; drug should be discontinued if there are any signs of rash and patient should be evaluated for signs and symptoms of drug reaction with eosinophilia and systemic symptoms (DRESS). Patients of Asian descent with the variant *HLA-B*1502* may be at an increased risk of developing Stevens-Johnson syndrome and/or TEN.

The "purple glove syndrome" (ie, discoloration with edema and pain of distal limb) may occur following peripheral I.V. administration of fosphenytoin. This syndrome may or may not be associated with drug extravasation. Symptoms may resolve spontaneously; however, skin necrosis and limb ischemia may occur. In general, fosphenytoin has significantly less venous irritation and phlebitis compared with an equimolar dose of phenytoin (Jamerson, 1994). Sedation, confusional states, or cerebellar dysfunction (loss of motor coordination) may occur at higher total serum concentrations or at lower total serum concentrations when the free fraction of phenytoin is increased.

Adverse Reactions The more important adverse clinical events caused by the I.V. use of fosphenytoin or phenytoin are cardiovascular collapse and/or central nervous system depression. Hypotension can occur when either drug is administered rapidly by the I.V. route.

The adverse clinical events most commonly observed with the use of fosphenytoin in clinical trials were nystagmus, dizziness, pruritus, paresthesia, headache, somnolence, and ataxia. Paresthesia and pruritus were seen more often following fosphenytoin (versus phenytoin) administration and occurred more often with I.V. fosphenytoin than with I.M. administration. These events were dose and rate related (adult doses ≥15 mg/kg at a rate of 150 mg PE/minute) and occurred in up to 64% of patients. These sensations, generally described as itching, burning, or tingling are usually not at the infusion site. The location of the discomfort varied with the groin mentioned most frequently. The paresthesia and pruritus were transient events that occurred within several minutes of the start of infusion and generally resolved within 10 minutes after completion of infusion.

Transient pruritus, tinnitus, nystagmus, somnolence, and ataxia occurred 2-3 times more often at adult doses ≥15 mg/kg and rates ≥150 mg PE/minute.

Also refer to phenytoin monograph for additional adverse reactions.

I.V. and I.M. administration (as reported in clinical trials):

1% to 10%:

Cardiovascular: Facial edema, hypertension

Central nervous system: Chills, fever, intracranial hypertension, nervousness

Endocrine & metabolic: Hypokalemia

Neuromuscular & skeletal: Hyperreflexia, myasthenia

I.V. administration (maximum dose/rate):

>10%:

Central nervous system: Paresthesia (4% to 64%), nystagmus (44%), dizziness (31%), somnolence (20%), ataxia (11%)

Dermatologic: Pruritus (49% to 64%)

1% to 10%:

Cardiovascular: Hypotension (7%), vasodilation (6%), tachycardia (2%)

Central nervous system: Stupor (7%), extrapyramidal syndrome (4%), incoordination (4%), agitation (3%), tremor (3%), brain edema (2%), headache (2%), hypoesthesia (2%), vertigo (2%)

Gastrointestinal: Nausea (9%), tongue disorder (4%), xerostomia (4%), taste perversion (3%), vomiting (2%)

Neuromuscular & skeletal: Pelvic pain (4%), back pain (2%), dysarthria (2%), weakness (2%)

Ocular: Diplopia (3%), amblyopia (2%)

Otic: Tinnitus (9%), deafness (2%)

I.M. administration (substitute for oral phenytoin):

>10%: Central nervous system: Nystagmus (15%)

1% to 10%:

Central nervous system: Tremor (10%), headache (9%), ataxia (8%), incoordination (8%), somnolence (7%), dizziness (5%), paresthesia (4%), reflexes decreased (3%)

Dermatologic: Bruising (7%), pruritus (3%)

Gastrointestinal: Nausea (5%), vomiting (3%)

Neuromuscular & skeletal: Weakness (4%)

I.V. and I.M. administration: <1% (Limited to important or life-threatening): Acidosis, acute hepatic failure, acute hepatotoxicity, alkalosis, akathisia, amnesia, anemia, anorexia, aphasia, apnea, arthralgia, asthma, atrial flutter, Babinski sign positive, bundle branch block, cachexia, cardiac arrest, cardiomegaly, cerebral hemorrhage, cerebral infarct, CHF, circumoral paresthesia, CNS depression, cyanosis, dehydration, diabetes insipidus, dyskinesia, dysphagia, dyspnea, edema, emotional lability, encephalopathy, epistaxis, extrapyramidal symptoms, GI hemorrhage, hemiplegia, hemoptysis, hostility, hyperacusis, hyperesthesia, hyper-/hypokinesia, hyperkalemia, hyperventilation, hypochromic anemia, hypophosphatemia, hypotonia, hypoxia, ileus, injection site (edema, hemorrhage, inflammation), ketosis, leg cramps, leukocytosis, leukopenia, LFTs abnormal, malaise, migraine, myalgia, mydriasis, myopathy, neurosis, orthostatic hypotension, palpitation, paralysis, parosmia, petechia, photophobia, photosensitivity reaction, psychosis, pulmonary embolus, QT interval prolongation, rash (maculopapular or pustular), renal failure, sinus bradycardia, shock, subdural hematoma, syncope, Stevens-Johnson syndrome, tenesmus, thrombocytopenia, thrombophlebitis, tongue edema, toxic epidermal necrolysis, urticaria, ventricular extrasystoles, visual field defect

Drug Interactions

Metabolism/Transport Effects Substrate of CYP2C19 (major), CYP2C9 (major), CYP3A4 (minor); **Note:** Assignment of Major/Minor substrate status based on clinically relevant drug interaction potential; **Induces** CYP2B6 (strong), CYP2C19 (strong), CYP2C8 (strong), CYP2C9 (strong), CYP3A4 (strong), P-glycoprotein

Avoid Concomitant Use

Avoid concomitant use of Fosphenytoin with any of the following: Abiraterone Acetate; Apixaban; Artemether; Axitinib; Azelastine (Nasal); Bedaquiline; Boceprevir; Bortezomib; Bosutinib; Cabozantinib; CloZAPine; Crizotinib; Dabigatran Etexilate; Darunavir; Delavirdine; Dienogest; Dolutegravir; Dronedarone; Enzalutamide; Etravirine; Everolimus; Ibrutinib; Itraconazole; Ivacaftor; Lapatinib; Lumefantrine; Lurasidone; Macitentan; Mifepristone; NIFEdipine; Nilotinib; Nisoldipine; Paraldehyde; PAZOPanib; Pomalidomide; PONATinib; Praziquantel; Ranolazine; Regorafenib; Rilpivirine; Rivaroxaban; Roflumilast; RomiDEPsin; Simeprevir; Sofosbuvir; SORAfenib; Telaprevir; Ticagrelor; Tofacitinib; Tolvaptan; Toremifene; Ulipristal; Vandetanib; Vemurafenib; VinCRIStine (Liposomal)

Increased Effect/Toxicity

Fosphenytoin may increase the levels/effects of: Amiodarone; Azelastine (Nasal); Buprenorphine; Ciprofloxacin (Systemic); Clarithromycin; CNS Depressants; FLUoxetine; Fosamprenavir; Highest Risk QTc-Prolonging Agents; Hydrocodone; Ifosfamide; Lithium; Methotrimeprazine; Metyrosine; Mirtazapine; Moderate Risk QTc-Prolonging Agents; Neuromuscular-Blocking Agents (Nondepolarizing); Paraldehyde; PHENobarbital; Pramipexole; QuiNIDine; ROPINIRole; Rotigotine; Selective Serotonin Reuptake Inhibitors; Vitamin K Antagonists; Zolpidem

The levels/effects of Fosphenytoin may be increased by: Alcohol (Ethyl); Allopurinol; Amiodarone; Antifungal Agents (Azole Derivatives, Systemic); Benzodiazepines; Brimonidine (Topical); Calcium Channel Blockers; Capecitabine; CarBAMazepine; Carbonic Anhydrase Inhibitors; CeFAZolin; Chloramphenicol; Cimetidine; Clarithromycin; CYP2C19 Inhibitors (Moderate); CYP2C19 Inhibitors (Strong); CYP2C9 Inhibitors (Moderate); CYP2C9 Inhibitors (Strong); Delavirdine; Dexmethylphenidate; Disopyramide; Disulfiram; Doxylamine; Droperidol; Efavirenz; Eslicarbazepine; Ethosuximide; Felbamate; Floxuridine; Fluconazole; Fluorouracil (Systemic); Fluorouracil (Topical); FLUoxetine; FluvoxaMINE; Halothane; HydrOXYzine; Isoniazid; Luliconazole; Magnesium Sulfate; Methotrimeprazine; Methylphenidate; MetroNIDAZOLE (Systemic); Omeprazole; OXcarbazepine; Rufinamide; Sertraline; Sodium Oxybate; Tacrolimus (Systemic); Tapentadol; Tegafur; Telaprevir; Ticlopidine; Topiramate; TraZODone; Trimethoprim; Vitamin K Antagonists

Decreased Effect

Fosphenytoin may decrease the levels/effects of: Abiraterone Acetate; Acetaminophen; Afatinib; Amiodarone; Antifungal Agents (Azole Derivatives, Systemic); Apixaban; ARIPiprazole; Artemether; Axitinib; Bazedoxifene; Bedaquiline; Boceprevir; Bortezomib; Bosutinib; Brentuximab Vedotin; Busulfan; Cabozantinib; Canagliflozin; CarBAMazepine; Chloramphenicol; Clarithromycin; CloZAPine; Cobicistat; Contraceptives (Estrogens); Contraceptives (Progestins); Crizotinib; CycloSPORINE (Systemic); CYP2B6 Substrates; CYP2C19 Substrates; CYP2C8 Substrates; CYP2C9 Substrates; CYP3A4 Substrates; Dabigatran Etexilate; Darunavir; Dasatinib; Deferasirox; Delavirdine; Diclofenac (Systemic); Dienogest; Disopyramide; Dolutegravir; Doxycycline; Dronedarone; Efavirenz; Elvitegravir; Enzalutamide; Eslicarbazepine; Ethosuximide; Etoposide; Etoposide Phosphate; Etravirine; Everolimus; Exemestane; Felbamate; Flunarizine; Gefitinib; GuanFACINE; HMG-CoA Reductase Inhibitors; Ibrutinib; Imatinib; Irinotecan; Itraconazole; Ivacaftor; Ixabepilone; Lacosamide; LamoTRIgine; Lapatinib; Levodopa; Linagliptin; Loop Diuretics; Lopinavir; Lumefantrine; Lurasidone; Macitentan; Maraviroc; Mebendazole; Meperidine; Methadone; MethylPREDNISolone; MetroNIDAZOLE (Systemic); Metyrapone; Mexiletine; Mifepristone; Nelfinavir; Neuromuscular-Blocking Agents (Nondepolarizing); NIFEdipine; Nilotinib; Nisoldipine; Omeprazole; OXcarbazepine; PAZOPanib; Perampanel; P-glycoprotein/ABCB1 Substrates; Pomalidomide; PONATinib; Praziquantel; PrednisoLONE (Systemic); PredniSONE; Primidone; QUEtiapine; QuiNIDine; QuiNINE; Ranolazine; Regorafenib; Rilpivirine; Ritonavir; Rivaroxaban; Roflumilast; RomiDEPsin; Rufinamide; Saxagliptin; Sertraline; Simeprevir; Sirolimus; Sofosbuvir; SORAfenib; SUNItinib; Tacrolimus (Systemic); Tadalafil; Telaprevir; Temsirolimus; Teniposide; Theophylline Derivatives; Thyroid Products; Ticagrelor; Tipranavir; Tofacitinib; Tolvaptan; Topiramate; Topotecan; Toremifene; TraZODone; Treprostinil; Trimethoprim; Ulipristal; Valproic Acid and Derivatives; Vandetanib; Vemurafenib; VinCRIStine; VinCRIStine (Liposomal); Vortioxetine; Zonisamide; Zuclopenthixol

The levels/effects of Fosphenytoin may be decreased by: Alcohol (Ethyl); Antacids; CarBAMazepine; Ciprofloxacin (Systemic); CYP2C19 Inducers (Strong); CYP2C9 Inducers (Strong); Dabrafenib; Diazoxide; Enzalutamide; Folic Acid; Fosamprenavir; Ketorolac (Nasal); Ketorolac (Systemic); Leucovorin Calcium-Levoleucovorin; Levomefolate; Lopinavir; Mefloquine; Methotrexate; Methylfolate; Multivitamins/Minerals (with ADEK, Folate, Iron); Nelfinavir; Orlistat; Peginterferon Alfa-2b; PHENobarbital; Platinum Derivatives; Pyridoxine; Rifampin; Ritonavir; Theophylline Derivatives; Tipranavir; Valproic Acid and Derivatives; Vigabatrin; VinCRIStine

Ethanol/Nutrition/Herb Interactions Ethanol:

Acute use: Avoid or limit ethanol (inhibits metabolism of phenytoin). Ethanol may also increase CNS depression; monitor for increased effects with coadministration. Caution patients about effects.

Chronic use: Avoid or limit ethanol (stimulates metabolism of phenytoin).

Preparation for Administration Must be diluted to concentrations of 1.5-25 mg PE/mL, in normal saline or D_5W, for I.V. infusion.

Storage/Stability Refrigerate at 2°C to 8°C (36°F to 46°F). Do not store at room temperature for more than 48 hours. Do not use vials that develop particulate matter. Has been shown to be stable at 1, 8, and 20 mg PE/mL in normal saline or D_5W at 25°C (77°F) for 30 days in glass container and at 4°C to 20°C (39°F to 68°F) for 30 days in PVC bag (Fischer, 1997).

Mechanism of Action Diphosphate ester salt of phenytoin which acts as a water soluble prodrug of phenytoin; after administration, plasma esterases convert fosphenytoin to phosphate, formaldehyde, and phenytoin as the active moiety; phenytoin works by stabilizing neuronal membranes and decreasing seizure activity by increasing efflux or decreasing influx of sodium ions across cell membranes in the motor cortex during generation of nerve impulses

Pharmacodynamics/Kinetics Also refer to Phenytoin monograph for additional information.

Distribution: Fosphenytoin: V_d: 4.3-10.8 L

Protein binding: Fosphenytoin: 95% to 99% to albumin; can displace phenytoin and increase free fraction (up to 30% unbound) during the period required for conversion of fosphenytoin to phenytoin. **Note:** In patients with renal and/or hepatic impairment or hypoalbuminemia, the fraction of unbound phenytoin may be increased.

Metabolism: Fosphenytoin is rapidly converted via hydrolysis to phenytoin; phenytoin is metabolized in the liver and forms metabolites

Bioavailability: I.M.: Fosphenytoin: 100%

Half-life elimination:

- Fosphenytoin: Conversion half-life: 15 minutes
- Phenytoin: Variable (mean: 12-29 hours); kinetics of phenytoin are saturable

Time to peak: Conversion to phenytoin: Following I.V. administration (maximum rate of administration): 15 minutes; following I.M. administration, peak phenytoin levels are reached in 3 hours; therapeutic phenytoin concentrations may be achieved as early as 5-20 minutes following I.M. (gluteal) administration (Pryor, 2001)

Excretion: Phenytoin: Urine (as inactive metabolites)

Dosage The dose, concentration in solutions, and infusion rates for fosphenytoin are expressed as phenytoin sodium equivalents (PE); fosphenytoin should always be prescribed and dispensed in phenytoin sodium equivalents (PE)

Infants and Children (unlabeled use): I.V.: **Note:** A limited number of clinical studies have been conducted in pediatric patients; based on pharmacokinetic studies, experts recommend the following (Fischer, 2003): Use the pediatric I.V. phenytoin dosing guidelines to dose fosphenytoin using doses in **PE** equal to the phenytoin doses (ie, phenytoin 1 mg = fosphenytoin 1 mg **PE**). Further pediatric studies are needed.

Adults:

- Status epilepticus: I.V.: Loading dose: 15-20 mg PE/kg administered at 100-150 mg PE/minute
- Nonemergent loading and maintenance dosing: I.V. or I.M.:
  - Loading dose: 10-20 mg PE/kg (I.V. rate: Infuse more slowly [eg, over 30 minutes]; maximum rate: 150 mg PE/minute)
  - Initial daily maintenance dose: 4-6 mg PE/kg/day in divided doses

I.M. or I.V. substitution for oral phenytoin therapy: May be substituted for oral phenytoin sodium at the same total daily dose; however, Dilantin® capsules are ~90% bioavailable by the oral route; phenytoin, supplied as fosphenytoin, is 100% bioavailable by both the I.M. and I.V. routes; for this reason, plasma phenytoin concentrations may increase when I.M. or I.V. fosphenytoin is substituted for oral phenytoin sodium therapy; in clinical trials, I.M. fosphenytoin was administered as a single daily dose utilizing either 1 or 2 injection sites; some patients may require more frequent dosing

Dosage adjustment in renal impairment: No initial dosage adjustment necessary. Free (unbound) phenytoin concentrations should be monitored closely in patients with renal disease or in those with hypoalbuminemia; furthermore, fosphenytoin clearance to phenytoin may be increased without a similar increase in phenytoin clearance in these patients leading to increase frequency and severity of adverse events.

Dosage adjustment in hepatic impairment: No initial dosage adjustment necessary. Phenytoin clearance may be substantially reduced in cirrhosis and plasma level monitoring with dose adjustment advisable. Free (unbound) phenytoin concentrations should be monitored closely in patients with hepatic disease or in those with hypoalbuminemia; furthermore, fosphenytoin clearance to phenytoin may be increased without a similar increase in phenytoin clearance in these patients leading to increased frequency and severity of adverse events.

Dietary Considerations Provides phosphate 0.0037 mmol/mg PE fosphenytoin

Administration

I.M.: May be administered as a single daily dose using 1-4 injection sites (up to 20 mL per site well tolerated in adults) (Meek, 1999; Pryor, 2001).

I.V.: Rates of infusion:

Children: 1-3 mg PE/kg/minute (**maximum rate: 150 mg PE/minute**) (Pellock, 1996)

Adults: **Do not exceed 150 mg PE/minute.** Slower administration reduces incidence of cardiovascular events (eg, hypotension, arrhythmia) as well as severity of paresthesias and pruritus. For nonemergent situations, may administer loading dose more slowly (eg, over 30 minutes [~33 mg PE/minute for 1000 mg PE] **or** 50-100 mg PE/minute [Fischer, 2003]). Highly-sensitive patients (eg, elderly, patients with pre-existing cardiovascular conditions) should receive fosphenytoin more slowly (eg, 25-50 mg PE/minute) (Meek, 1999).

Monitoring Parameters Continuous blood pressure, ECG, and respiratory function monitoring with loading dose and for 10-20 minutes following infusion; vital signs, CBC, hepatic function tests, plasma phenytoin concentration monitoring (plasma concentrations should not be measured until conversion to phenytoin is complete, ~2 hours after an I.V. infusion or ~4 hours after an I.M. injection). **Note:** If available, free (unbound) phenytoin concentrations should be obtained in patients with renal impairment and/or hypoalbuminemia; if free phenytoin concentrations are unavailable, the adjusted total concentration may be determined based upon equations in adult patients. Trough concentrations are generally recommended for routine monitoring.

Consult individual institutional policies and procedures.

Reference Range

Therapeutic: 10-20 mcg/mL (SI: 40-79 micromole/L); toxicity is measured clinically, and some patients require levels outside the suggested therapeutic range

Toxic: >30 mcg/mL (SI: 120 micromole/L)

Lethal: >100 mcg/mL (SI: >400 micromole/L)

Manifestations of toxicity:

Nystagmus: 20 mcg/mL (SI: 79 micromole/L)

Ataxia: 30 mcg/mL (SI: 118.9 micromole/L)

Decreased mental status: 40 mcg/mL (SI: 159 micromole/L)

Coma: 50 mcg/mL (SI: 200 micromole/L)

Peak serum phenytoin level after a 375 mg I.M. fosphenytoin dose in healthy males: 5.7 mcg/mL

Peak serum fosphenytoin levels and phenytoin levels after a 1.2 g infusion (I.V.) in healthy subjects over 30 minutes were 129 mcg/mL and 17.2 mcg/mL, respectively

Test Interactions Falsely high plasma phenytoin concentrations (due to cross-reactivity with fosphenytoin) when measured by immunoanalytical techniques (eg, TD_X®, TD_XFL_X™, Emit® 2000) prior to complete conversion of fosphenytoin to phenytoin. Phenytoin may produce falsely low results for dexamethasone or metyrapone tests.

Additional Information 1.5 mg fosphenytoin is approximately equivalent to 1 mg phenytoin. Equimolar fosphenytoin dose is 375 mg (75 mg/mL solution) to phenytoin 250 mg (50 mg/mL). **However, doses of fosphenytoin are always expressed as their phenytoin sodium equivalent (PE). Thus, 1 mg PE is equivalent to 1 mg phenytoin sodium. Do not change the recommended doses when substituting fosphenytoin for phenytoin or vice versa as they are not equivalent on a mg to mg basis.**

Dosage Forms Excipient information presented when available (limited, particularly for generics); consult specific product labeling.

Solution, Injection, as sodium:

Cerebyx: 100 MG PE/2ML (2 mL); 500 MG PE/10ML (10 mL)

Generic: 100 MG PE/2ML (2 mL); 500 MG PE/10ML (10 mL)

- ◆ **Fosphenytoin Sodium** *see* Fosphenytoin *on page 925*
- ◆ **Fosrenol** *see* Lanthanum *on page 1173*
- ◆ **Fosrenol® (Can)** *see* Lanthanum *on page 1173*
- ◆ **Four-Factor PCC** *see* Prothrombin Complex Concentrate (Human) [(Factors II, VII, IX, X), Protein C, and Protein S] *on page 1743*
- ◆ **FR901228** *see* RomiDEPsin *on page 1848*
- ◆ **Fragmin** *see* Dalteparin *on page 534*
- ◆ **Fragmin® (Can)** *see* Dalteparin *on page 534*
- ◆ **Fresenius Propoven** *see* Propofol *on page 1734*
- ◆ **Frisium (Can)** *see* CloBAZam *on page 455*
- ◆ **Froben® (Can)** *see* Flurbiprofen (Systemic) *on page 892*
- ◆ **Froben-SR® (Can)** *see* Flurbiprofen (Systemic) *on page 892*
- ◆ **Frova** *see* Frovatriptan *on page 928*

Frovatriptan (froe va TRIP tan)

Brand Names: U.S. Frova

Brand Names: Canada Frova

Index Terms Frovatriptan Succinate

Pharmacologic Category Antimigraine Agent; Serotonin 5-$HT_{1B,\ 1D}$ Receptor Agonist

Additional Appendix Information

Antimigraine Drugs: 5-HT_1 Receptor Agonists *on page 2288*

Use Migraines: Acute treatment of migraine with or without aura in adults.

Unlabeled Use Short-term prevention of menstrually-associated migraines (MAMs)

Pregnancy Risk Factor C

Pregnancy Considerations Adverse events were observed in animal reproduction studies. Information related to the use of frovatriptan in pregnancy has not been located. Until additional information is available, other agents are preferred for the initial treatment of migraine in pregnancy (Da Silva, 2012; MacGregor, 2012; Williams, 2012).

Breast-Feeding Considerations It is not known if frovatriptan is excreted in breast milk. Due to the potential for serious adverse reactions in the nursing infant, the manufacturer recommends a decision be made whether to discontinue nursing or to discontinue the drug, taking into account the importance of treatment to the mother.

Contraindications

Ischemic coronary artery disease (eg, angina pectoris, history of MI, documented silent ischemia); coronary artery vasospasm, including Prinzmetal's angina; Wolff-Parkinson-White syndrome or arrhythmias associated with other cardiac accessory conduction pathway disorders; history of stroke, transient ischemic attack, or history of hemiplegic or basilar migraine; peripheral vascular disease; ischemic bowel disease; uncontrolled hypertension; recent use (within 24 hours) of another 5-HT_1 agonist, an ergotamine containing or ergot-type medication (eg, dihydroergotamine, methysergide); hypersensitivity to frovatriptan or any component of the formulation.

Canadian labeling: Additional contraindications (not in U.S. labeling): Cardiac arrhythmias, valvular heart disease (especially tachycardia), congenital heart disease, atherosclerotic disease; management of ophthalmoplegic migraine; severe hepatic impairment; Raynaud's syndrome

Documentation of allergenic cross-reactivity for triptans is limited. However, because of similarities in chemical structure and/or pharmacologic actions, the possibility of cross-sensitivity cannot be ruled out with certainty.

Warnings/Precautions Not intended for migraine prophylaxis, or treatment of cluster headaches, hemiplegic or basilar migraines. Rule out underlying neurologic disease in patients with atypical headache, migraine (with no prior history of migraine) or inadequate clinical response to initial dosing. Cardiac events (coronary artery vasospasm, transient ischemia, MI, ventricular tachycardia/fibrillation, cardiac arrest, and death), cerebral/subarachnoid hemorrhage, stroke (some fatal), peripheral vascular ischemia, gastrointestinal vascular ischemia and infarction, splenic infarction, and Raynaud's syndrome have been reported with 5-HT_1 agonist administration. Partial vision loss and blindness (transient and permanent) have been reported with use of 5-HT_1 agonists; a causal relationship between these events and 5-HT_1 agonist administration has not been clearly determined. Patients who experience sensations of chest pain/pressure/tightness or symptoms suggestive of angina following dosing should be evaluated for coronary artery disease or Prinzmetal's angina before receiving additional doses; if dosing is resumed and similar symptoms recur, monitor with ECG. Do not give to patients with risk factors for CAD until a cardiovascular evaluation has been performed; if evaluation is satisfactory, the healthcare provider should administer the first dose (consider ECG monitoring) and cardiovascular status should be periodically evaluated. Significant elevation in blood pressure, including hypertensive crisis with acute impairment of organ systems, has been reported on rare occasions in patients using other 5-HT_{1D} agonists with and without a history of hypertension; monitor blood pressure. Blood pressure was increased to a greater extent in elderly.

Use with caution in severe hepatic impairment (has not been studied) (Canadian labeling contraindicates use in severe impairment). Potentially significant drug-drug interactions may exist, requiring dose or frequency adjustment, additional monitoring, and/or selection of alternative therapy. Symptoms of agitation, confusion, hallucinations, hyper-reflexia, myoclonus, shivering, and tachycardia (serotonin syndrome) may occur with concomitant proserotonergic drugs (ie, SSRIs/SNRIs or triptans) or agents which reduce frovatriptan's metabolism. Concurrent use of serotonin precursors (eg, tryptophan) is not recommended. If concomitant administration with SSRIs is warranted, monitor closely, especially at initiation and with dose increases. Discontinue frovatriptan if serotonin syndrome is suspected. Anaphylaxis, anaphylactoid, and hypersensitivity reactions (including angioedema) have occurred; may be life-threatening or fatal.

Adverse Reactions

1% to 10%:

Cardiovascular: Flushing (4%), hot or cold flashes (3%), chest pain (2%), palpitations (1%)

Central nervous system: Dizziness (8%), fatigue (5%), headache (4%), paresthesia (4%), drowsiness (≥2%), anxiety (1%), dysesthesia (1%), hypoesthesia (1%), insomnia (1%), pain (1%)

Dermatologic: Diaphoresis (1%)

Gastrointestinal: Xerostomia (3%), nausea (≥2%), dyspepsia (2%), abdominal pain (1%), diarrhea (1%), vomiting (1%)

Neuromuscular & skeletal: Musculoskeletal pain (3%)

Ophthalmic: Visual disturbance (1%)

Otic: Tinnitus (1%)

Respiratory: Rhinitis (1%), sinusitis (1%)

<1% (Limited to important or life-threatening): Abnormal gait, abnormal lacrimation, abnormal reflexes, amnesia, anaphylactoid reactions, anaphylaxis, anorexia, ataxia, bradycardia, bullous rash, cheilitis, chest tightness, confusion, conjunctivitis, dehydration, depersonalization, depression, dysgeusia, ECG changes, emotional lability, epistaxis, esophageal spasm, euphoria, eye pain, gastroesophageal reflux disease, hyperacusis, hyperesthesia, hypersensitivity reaction (including angioedema), hypertonia, hyperventilation, hypocalcemia, hypoglycemia, hypotonia, involuntary muscle movements, jaw tightness, lack of concentration, laryngitis, myocardial infarction, nocturia, osteoarthritis, peptic ulcer, personality disorder, pharyngitis, polyuria, purpura, renal pain, rigors, salivary gland pain, seizure, sialorrhea, significant cardiovascular event, speech disturbance, stomatitis, syncope, tachycardia, tightness in chest and throat, tongue paralysis

Drug Interactions

Metabolism/Transport Effects **Substrate** of CYP1A2 (minor); **Note:** Assignment of Major/Minor substrate status based on clinically relevant drug interaction potential

Avoid Concomitant Use

Avoid concomitant use of Frovatriptan with any of the following: Ergot Derivatives

Increased Effect/Toxicity

Frovatriptan may increase the levels/effects of: Antipsychotics; Ergot Derivatives; Metoclopramide; Serotonin Modulators

The levels/effects of Frovatriptan may be increased by: Antipsychotics; Ergot Derivatives

Decreased Effect There are no known significant interactions involving a decrease in effect.

Ethanol/Nutrition/Herb Interactions Food: Food does not affect frovatriptan bioavailability.

Storage/Stability Store at 25°C (77°F); excursions are permitted between 15°C and 30°C (59°F and 86°F). Protect from moisture.

Mechanism of Action Selective agonist for serotonin (5-HT_{1B} and 5-HT_{1D} receptors) in cranial arteries; causes vasoconstriction and reduces sterile inflammation associated with antidromic neuronal transmission correlating with relief of migraine.

Pharmacodynamics/Kinetics

Distribution: Male: 4.2 L/kg; Female: 3 L/kg

Protein binding: ~15%

Metabolism: Primarily hepatic via CYP1A2

Bioavailability: Male: ~20%; Female: ~30%

Half-life elimination: ~26 hours

Time to peak: 2-4 hours

Excretion: Feces (62%); urine (32%)

Dosage Note: If the first dose is ineffective, diagnosis needs to be re-evaluated. The safety of treating >4 migraines/month has not been established.

Migraine: Adults: Oral:

U.S. labeling: Initial: 2.5 mg; if headache recurs, a second dose may be administered after 2 hours have elapsed since the first dose (maximum: 7.5 mg daily)

Canadian labeling: Initial: 2.5 mg; if headache recurs, a second dose may be administered after 4 hours have elapsed since the first dose (maximum: 5 mg daily)

Dosage adjustment in renal impairment: No dosage adjustment necessary

Dosage adjustment in hepatic impairment:

Mild-to-moderate impairment: No dosage adjustment necessary.

Severe impairment:

U.S. labeling: Use with caution (has not been studied).

Canadian labeling: Use is contraindicated.

Administration Administer orally with fluids as soon as symptoms appear.

Monitoring Parameters Headache severity, blood pressure, signs/symptoms suggestive of angina; perform a cardiovascular evaluation in triptan-naïve patients who have multiple cardiovascular risk factors (eg, increased age, diabetes, hypertension, smoking, obesity, strong family history of CAD), monitor ECG with first dose in patients with multiple cardiovascular risk factors who have a negative cardiovascular evaluation and consider periodic cardiovascular evaluation in such patients if they are intermittent long-term users; signs/symptoms of serotonin syndrome and hypersensitivity reactions.

Dosage Forms Excipient information presented when available (limited, particularly for generics); consult specific product labeling.

Tablet, Oral:

Frova: 2.5 mg

◆ **Frovatriptan Succinate** *see* Frovatriptan *on page* 928

◆ **Fruit C [OTC]** *see* Ascorbic Acid *on page* 172

◆ **Fruit C 500 [OTC]** *see* Ascorbic Acid *on page* 172

◆ **Fruity C [OTC]** *see* Ascorbic Acid *on page* 172

◆ **Frusemide** *see* Furosemide *on page* 931

◆ **FSH** *see* Follitropin Alfa *on page* 908

◆ **FSH** *see* Follitropin Beta *on page* 909

◆ **FSH** *see* Urofollitropin *on page* 2141

◆ **FTC** *see* Emtricitabine *on page* 698

◆ **FTC/RPV/TDF** *see* Emtricitabine, Rilpivirine, and Tenofovir *on page* 700

◆ **FTC, TDF, and EFV** *see* Efavirenz, Emtricitabine, and Tenofovir *on page* 690

◆ **FTY720** *see* Fingolimod *on page* 864

◆ **FU** *see* Fluorouracil (Systemic) *on page* 882

◆ **FU** *see* Fluorouracil (Topical) *on page* 885

◆ **5-FU** *see* Fluorouracil (Systemic) *on page* 882

◆ **5-FU** *see* Fluorouracil (Topical) *on page* 885

◆ **Ful-Glo** *see* Fluorescein *on page* 880

Fulvestrant (fool VES trant)

Brand Names: U.S. Faslodex

Brand Names: Canada Faslodex®

Index Terms ICI-182,780; ZD9238

Pharmacologic Category Antineoplastic Agent, Estrogen Receptor Antagonist

Use Treatment of hormone receptor positive metastatic breast cancer in postmenopausal women with disease progression following antiestrogen therapy

Pregnancy Risk Factor D

Pregnancy Considerations Fetal loss and abnormalities were observed in animal studies. Approved for use only in postmenopausal women. If used prior to confirmed menopause, women of reproductive potential should be advised not to become pregnant.

Breast-Feeding Considerations Approved for use only in postmenopausal women.

Contraindications Hypersensitivity to fulvestrant or any component of the formulation

Warnings/Precautions Hazardous agent - use appropriate precautions for handling and disposal (NIOSH, 2012). Use caution in hepatic impairment; dosage adjustment is recommended in patients with moderate hepatic impairment. Safety and efficacy have not been established in severe hepatic impairment. Use with caution in patients with a history of bleeding disorders (including thrombocytopenia) and/or patients on anticoagulant therapy; bleeding/hematoma may occur from I.M. administration.

Adverse Reactions Adverse reactions reported with 500 mg dose.

>10%:

Endocrine & metabolic: Hot flushes (7% to 13%)

Hepatic: Alkaline phosphatase increased (>15%; grades 3/4: 1% to 2%), transaminases increased (>15%; grades 3/4: 1% to 2%)

Local: Injection site pain (12% to 14%)

Neuromuscular & skeletal: Joint disorders (14% to 19%)

1% to 10%:

Cardiovascular: Ischemic disorder (1%)

Central nervous system: Fatigue (8%), headache (8%)

Gastrointestinal: Nausea (10%), anorexia (6%), vomiting (6%), constipation (5%), weight gain (≤1%)

Genitourinary: Urinary tract infection (2% to 4%)

Neuromuscular & skeletal: Bone pain (9%), arthralgia (8%), back pain (8%), extremity pain (7%), musculoskeletal pain (6%), weakness (6%)

Respiratory: Cough (5%), dyspnea (4%)

<1% (Limited to important or life-threatening; reported with 250 mg or 500 mg dose): Angioedema, hepatitis, hypersensitivity reactions, leukopenia, liver failure, osteoporosis, thrombosis, vaginal bleeding

Drug Interactions

Metabolism/Transport Effects Substrate of CYP3A4 (minor); **Note:** Assignment of Major/Minor substrate status based on clinically relevant drug interaction potential

Avoid Concomitant Use There are no known interactions where it is recommended to avoid concomitant use.

Increased Effect/Toxicity There are no known significant interactions involving an increase in effect.

Decreased Effect There are no known significant interactions involving a decrease in effect.

Storage/Stability Store in original carton under refrigeration at 2°C to 8°C (36°F to 46°F). Protect from light.

Mechanism of Action Estrogen receptor antagonist; competitively binds to estrogen receptors on tumors and other tissue targets, producing a nuclear complex that causes a dose-related down-regulation of estrogen receptors and inhibits tumor growth.

Pharmacodynamics/Kinetics

Duration: I.M.: Steady state concentrations reached within first month, when administered with additional dose given 2 weeks following the initial dose; plasma levels maintained for at least 1 month

Distribution: V_d: ~3-5 L/kg

Protein binding: 99%; to plasma proteins (VLDL, LDL and HDL lipoprotein fractions)

Metabolism: Hepatic via multiple biotransformation pathways (CYP3A4 substrate involved in oxidation pathway, although relative contribution to metabolism unknown); metabolites formed are either less active or have similar activity to parent compound

Half-life elimination: 250 mg: ~40 days
Excretion: Feces (~90%); urine (<1%)

Dosage I.M.: Adults (postmenopausal women): Breast cancer, metastatic: Initial: 500 mg on days 1, 15, and 29; Maintenance: 500 mg once monthly

Dosage adjustment in renal impairment: No dosage adjustment provided in manufacturer's labeling (has not been studied). However, renal elimination of fulvestrant is negligible.

Dosage adjustment in hepatic impairment:
Moderate impairment (Child-Pugh class B): Decrease initial and maintenance dose to 250 mg
Severe impairment (Child-Pugh class C): Use has not been evaluated.

Administration For I.M. administration only; do not administer I.V., SubQ, or intra-arterially. Administer 500 mg dose as two 5 mL injections (one in each buttocks) slowly over 1-2 minutes per injection.

Hazardous agent; use appropriate precautions for handling and disposal (NIOSH, 2012).

Dosage Forms Excipient information presented when available (limited, particularly for generics); consult specific product labeling.
Solution, Intramuscular:
Faslodex: 250 mg/5 mL (5 mL) [contains alcohol, usp, benzyl alcohol, benzyl benzoate, castor oil (ricine oil)]

◆ **Fulyzaq** *see* Crofelemer *on page 500*
◆ **Fungi-Guard [OTC]** *see* Tolnaftate *on page 2087*
◆ **Fungizone (Can)** *see* Amphotericin B (Conventional) *on page 123*
◆ **Fungoid-D [OTC]** *see* Tolnaftate *on page 2087*
◆ **Fungoid Tincture [OTC]** *see* Miconazole (Topical) *on page 1358*
◆ **Furadantin** *see* Nitrofurantoin *on page 1464*
◆ **Furazosin** *see* Prazosin *on page 1703*

Furosemide (fyoor OH se mide)

Brand Names: U.S. Lasix

Brand Names: Canada Apo-Furosemide®; AVA-Furosemide; Bio-Furosemide; Dom-Furosemide; Furosemide Injection Sandoz Standard; Furosemide Injection, USP; Furosemide Special; Furosemide Special Injection; Lasix®; Lasix® Special; Novo-Semide; NTP-Furosemide; Nu-Furosemide; PMS-Furosemide; Teva-Furosemide

Index Terms Frusemide

Pharmacologic Category Antihypertensive; Diuretic, Loop

Use Management of edema associated with heart failure and hepatic or renal disease; acute pulmonary edema; treatment of hypertension (alone or in combination with other antihypertensives)

Canadian labeling: Additional use: Furosemide Special Injection and Lasix® Special (products not available in the U.S.): Adjunctive treatment of oliguria in patients with severe renal impairment

Pregnancy Risk Factor C

Pregnancy Considerations Animal studies have demonstrated maternal death, fetal toxicity, and fetal loss. There are no adequate and well-controlled studies in pregnant women. Crosses the placenta. Increased fetal urine production, electrolyte disturbances reported. Generally, use of diuretics during pregnancy is avoided due to risk of decreased placental perfusion. Monitor fetal growth if used during pregnancy; may increase birth weight.

Breast-Feeding Considerations Crosses into breast milk; may suppress lactation

Contraindications Hypersensitivity to furosemide or any component of the formulation; anuria

Canadian labeling: Additional contraindications (not in U.S. labeling): Hypersensitivity to sulfonamide-derived drugs; complete renal shutdown; hepatic coma and precoma; uncorrected states of electrolyte depletion, hypovolemia, or hypotension; jaundiced newborn infants or infants with disease(s) capable of causing hyperbilirubinemia and possibly kernicterus; breast-feeding. **Note:** Manufacturer labeling for Lasix® Special and Furosemide Special Injection also includes: GFR <5 mL/minute or GFR >20 mL/minute; hepatic cirrhosis; renal failure accompanied by hepatic coma and precoma; renal failure due to poisoning with nephrotoxic or hepatotoxic substances.

Warnings/Precautions [U.S. Boxed Warning]: If given in excessive amounts, furosemide, similar to other loop diuretics, can lead to profound diuresis, resulting in fluid and electrolyte depletion; close medical supervision and dose evaluation are required. Watch for and correct electrolyte disturbances; adjust dose to avoid dehydration. When electrolyte depletion is present, therapy should not be initiated unless serum electrolytes, especially potassium, are normalized. In cirrhosis, avoid electrolyte and acid/base imbalances that might lead to hepatic encephalopathy; correct electrolyte and acid/base imbalances prior to initiation when hepatic coma is present. Coadministration of antihypertensives may increase the risk of hypotension.

Monitor fluid status and renal function in an attempt to prevent oliguria, azotemia, and reversible increases in BUN and creatinine; close medical supervision of aggressive diuresis is required. May increase risk of contrast-induced nephropathy. Rapid I.V. administration, renal impairment, excessive doses, hypoproteinemia, and concurrent use of other ototoxins is associated with ototoxicity. Asymptomatic hyperuricemia has been reported with use; rarely, gout may precipitate. Photosensitization may occur.

Use with caution in patients with prediabetes or diabetes mellitus; may see a change in glucose control. Use with caution in patients with systemic lupus erythematosus (SLE); may cause SLE exacerbation or activation. Use with caution in patients with prostatic hyperplasia/urinary stricture; may cause urinary retention. May lead to nephrocalcinosis or nephrolithiasis in premature infants or in children <4 years of age with chronic use. May prevent closure of patent ductus arteriosus in premature infants. Chemical similarities are present among sulfonamides, sulfonylureas, carbonic anhydrase inhibitors, thiazides, and loop diuretics (except ethacrynic acid). A risk of cross-reaction exists in patients with allergy to any of these compounds; avoid use when previous reaction has been severe. Discontinue if signs of hypersensitivity are noted.

Adverse Reactions Frequency not defined.
Cardiovascular: Acute hypotension, chronic aortitis, necrotizing angiitis, orthostatic hypotension, vasculitis
Central nervous system: Dizziness, fever, headache, hepatic encephalopathy, lightheadedness, restlessness, vertigo
Dermatologic: Bullous pemphigoid, cutaneous vasculitis, drug rash with eosinophilia and systemic symptoms (DRESS), erythema multiforme, exanthematous pustulosis (generalized), exfoliative dermatitis, photosensitivity, pruritus, purpura, rash, Stevens-Johnson syndrome, toxic epidermal necrolysis, urticaria
Endocrine & metabolic: Cholesterol and triglycerides increased, glucose tolerance test altered, gout, hyperglycemia, hyperuricemia, hypocalcemia, hypochloremia, hypokalemia, hypomagnesemia, hyponatremia, metabolic alkalosis
Gastrointestinal: Anorexia, constipation, cramping, diarrhea, nausea, oral and gastric irritation, pancreatitis, vomiting
Genitourinary: Urinary bladder spasm, urinary frequency

Hematological: Agranulocytosis (rare), anemia, aplastic anemia (rare), eosinophilia, hemolytic anemia, leukopenia, thrombocytopenia
Hepatic: Intrahepatic cholestatic jaundice, ischemic hepatitis, liver enzymes increased
Local: Injection site pain (following I.M. injection), thrombophlebitis
Neuromuscular & skeletal: Muscle spasm, paresthesia, weakness
Ocular: Blurred vision, xanthopsia
Otic: Hearing impairment (reversible or permanent with rapid I.V. or I.M. administration), tinnitus
Renal: Allergic interstitial nephritis, fall in glomerular filtration rate and renal blood flow (due to overdiuresis), glycosuria, transient rise in BUN
Miscellaneous: Anaphylaxis (rare), exacerbate or activate systemic lupus erythematosus

Drug Interactions

Metabolism/Transport Effects None known.

Avoid Concomitant Use

Avoid concomitant use of Furosemide with any of the following: Chloral Hydrate; Ethacrynic Acid

Increased Effect/Toxicity

Furosemide may increase the levels/effects of: ACE Inhibitors; Allopurinol; Amifostine; Aminoglycosides; Antihypertensives; Cardiac Glycosides; Chloral Hydrate; CISplatin; Dofetilide; Ethacrynic Acid; Hypotensive Agents; Ivabradine; Lithium; Methotrexate; Neuromuscular-Blocking Agents; Obinutuzumab; RisperiDONE; RiTUXimab; Salicylates; Sodium Phosphates; Topiramate

The levels/effects of Furosemide may be increased by: Alfuzosin; Analgesics (Opioid); Beta2-Agonists; Brimonidine (Topical); Corticosteroids (Orally Inhaled); Corticosteroids (Systemic); CycloSPORINE (Systemic); Diazoxide; Herbs (Hypotensive Properties); Licorice; MAO Inhibitors; Methotrexate; Pentoxifylline; Phosphodiesterase 5 Inhibitors; Probenecid; Prostacyclin Analogues

Decreased Effect

Furosemide may decrease the levels/effects of: Hypoglycemic Agents; Lithium; Neuromuscular-Blocking Agents

The levels/effects of Furosemide may be decreased by: Aliskiren; Bile Acid Sequestrants; Fosphenytoin; Herbs (Hypertensive Properties); Methotrexate; Methylphenidate; Nonsteroidal Anti-Inflammatory Agents; Phenytoin; Probenecid; Salicylates; Sucralfate; Yohimbine

Ethanol/Nutrition/Herb Interactions

Food: Furosemide serum levels may be decreased if taken with food.
Herb/Nutraceutical: Avoid bayberry, blue cohosh, cayenne, ephedra, ginger, ginseng (American), kola, licorice (may worsen hypertension). Avoid black cohosh, California poppy, coleus, golden seal, hawthorn, mistletoe, periwinkle, quinine, shepherd's purse (may increase antihypertensive effect). Licorice may also cause or worsen hypokalemia.

Preparation for Administration I.V. infusion solution mixed in NS or D_5W solution is stable for 24 hours at room temperature. May also be diluted for infusion to 1-2 mg/mL (maximum: 10 mg/mL).

Storage/Stability

Injection: Store at room temperature of 15°C to 30°C (59°F to 86°F). Protect from light. Exposure to light may cause discoloration; do not use furosemide solutions if they have a yellow color. Furosemide solutions are unstable in acidic media, but very stable in basic media. Refrigeration may result in precipitation or crystallization; however, resolubilization at room temperature or warming may be performed without affecting the drug's stability.
Tablet: Store at 25°C (77°F); excursions permitted to 15°C to 30°C (59°F to 89°F). Protect from light.

Mechanism of Action Inhibits reabsorption of sodium and chloride in the ascending loop of Henle and distal renal tubule, interfering with the chloride-binding cotransport system, thus causing increased excretion of water, sodium, chloride, magnesium, and calcium

Pharmacodynamics/Kinetics

Onset of action: Diuresis: Oral, S.L: 30-60 minutes; I.M.: 30 minutes; I.V.: ~5 minutes
Symptomatic improvement with acute pulmonary edema: Within 15-20 minutes; occurs prior to diuretic effect
Peak effect: Oral, S.L.: 1-2 hours
Duration: Oral, S.L.: 6-8 hours; I.V.: 2 hours
Protein binding: 91% to 99%; primarily to albumin
Metabolism: Minimally hepatic
Bioavailability: Oral tablet: 47% to 64%; Oral solution: 50%; S.L. administration of oral tablet: ~60%; results of a small comparative study (n=11) showed bioavailability of S.L. administration of tablet was ~12% higher than oral administration of tablet (Haegeli, 2007)
Half-life elimination: Normal renal function: 0.5-2 hours; End-stage renal disease: 9 hours
Excretion: Urine (Oral: 50%, I.V.: 80%) within 24 hours; feces (as unchanged drug); nonrenal clearance prolonged in renal impairment

Dosage

Infants and Children: Edema, heart failure:
Oral: Initial: 2 mg/kg/dose increased in increments of 1-2 mg/kg/dose with each succeeding dose at intervals of 6-8 hours until a satisfactory response is achieved; maximum dose: 6 mg/kg/dose
I.M., I.V.: Initial: 1 mg/kg/dose; if response not adequate, may increase dose in increments of 1 mg/kg/dose and administer not sooner than 2 hours after previous dose, until a satisfactory response is achieved; may administer maintenance dose at intervals of every 6-12 hours; maximum dose: 6 mg/kg/dose
Children 1-17 years: Hypertension, resistant (unlabeled; AAP, 2004): Oral: Initial: 0.5-2 mg/kg/dose once or twice daily; maximum dose: 6 mg/kg/dose
Adults:
Edema, heart failure:
Oral: Initial: 20-80 mg/dose; if response is not adequate, may repeat the same dose or increase dose in increments of 20-40 mg/dose at intervals of 6-8 hours; may be titrated up to 600 mg/day with severe edematous states; usual maintenance dose interval is once or twice daily. **Note:** Dosing frequency may be adjusted based on patient-specific diuretic needs.
I.M., I.V.: Initial: 20-40 mg/dose; if response is not adequate, may repeat the same dose or increase dose in increments of 20 mg/dose and administer 1-2 hours after previous dose (maximum dose: 200 mg/dose). Individually determined dose should then be given once or twice daily although some patients may initially require dosing as frequent as every 6 hours. **Note:** ACC/AHA 2009 guidelines for heart failure recommend a maximum single dose of 160-200 mg.
Continuous I.V. infusion (Howard, 2001; Hunt, 2009): Initial: I.V. bolus dose 20-40 mg over 1-2 minutes, followed by continuous I.V. infusion doses of 10-40 mg/hour. If urine output is <1 mL/kg/hour, double as necessary to a maximum of 80-160 mg/hour. The risk associated with higher infusion rates (80-160 mg/hour) must be weighed against alternative strategies. **Note:** ACC/AHA 2009 guidelines for heart failure recommend 40 mg I.V. load, then 10-40 mg/hour infusion.

Acute pulmonary edema: I.V.: 40 mg over 1-2 minutes. If response not adequate within 1 hour, may increase dose to 80 mg. **Note:** ACC/AHA 2009 guidelines for heart failure recommend a maximum single dose of 160-200 mg.

Hypertension, resistant (Chobanian, 2003; JNC 7): Oral: 20-80 mg/day in 2 divided doses

Refractory heart failure: Oral, I.V.: Doses up to 8 g/day have been used.

Elderly: Oral, I.M., I.V.: Initial: 20 mg/day; increase slowly to desired response.

Dosing adjustment/comments in renal impairment: Acute renal failure: High doses (up to 1-3 g/day - oral/I.V.) have been used to initiate desired response; avoid use in oliguric states.

Dialysis: Not removed by hemo- or peritoneal dialysis; supplemental dose is not necessary.

Dosing adjustment/comments in hepatic disease: Diminished natriuretic effect with increased sensitivity to hypokalemia and volume depletion in cirrhosis; monitor effects, particularly with high doses.

Dietary Considerations May cause potassium loss; potassium supplement or dietary changes may be required.

Usual Infusion Concentrations: Pediatric I.V. infusion: 1 mg/mL **or** 2 mg/mL **or** undiluted as 10 mg/mL

Usual Infusion Concentrations: Adult I.V. infusion: 1 mg/mL **or** 2 mg/mL **or** undiluted as 10 mg/mL

Administration

I.V.: I.V. injections should be given slowly. In adults, undiluted direct I.V. injections may be administered at a rate of 20-40 mg per minute; maximum rate of administration for short-term intermittent infusion is 4 mg/minute; exceeding this rate increases the risk of ototoxicity. In children, a maximum rate of 0.5 mg/kg/minute has been recommended.

Oral: Administer on an empty stomach (Bard, 2004). May be administered with food or milk if GI distress occurs; however, this may reduce diuretic efficacy.

Note: When I.V. or oral administration is not possible, the sublingual route may be used. Place 1 tablet under tongue for at least 5 minutes to allow for maximal absorption. Patients should be advised not to swallow during disintegration time (Haegeli, 2007).

Monitoring Parameters Monitor weight and I & O daily; blood pressure, orthostasis; serum electrolytes, renal function; monitor hearing with high doses or rapid I.V. administration

Dosage Forms Excipient information presented when available (limited, particularly for generics); consult specific product labeling.

Solution, Injection:
  Generic: 10 mg/mL (2 mL, 4 mL, 10 mL)

Solution, Injection [preservative free]:
  Generic: 10 mg/mL (10 mL)

Solution, Oral:
  Generic: 8 mg/mL (5 mL, 500 mL); 10 mg/mL (60 mL, 120 mL)

Tablet, Oral:
  Lasix: 20 mg
  Lasix: 40 mg, 80 mg [scored]
  Generic: 20 mg, 40 mg, 80 mg

Dosage Forms: Canada Excipient information presented when available (limited, particularly for generics); consult specific product labeling.

Injection, solution [preservative free]:
  Furosemide Special Injection: 10 mg/mL (25 mL)

Tablet, oral:
  Lasix® Special: 500 mg [scored]

◆ **Furosemide Injection Sandoz Standard (Can)** *see* Furosemide *on page* 931

◆ **Furosemide Injection, USP (Can)** *see* Furosemide *on page* 931

◆ **Furosemide Special (Can)** *see* Furosemide *on page* 931

◆ **Furosemide Special Injection (Can)** *see* Furosemide *on page* 931

◆ **Fusilev** *see* LEVOleucovorin *on page* 1201

◆ **Fuzeon** *see* Enfuvirtide *on page* 704

◆ **Fuzeon® (Can)** *see* Enfuvirtide *on page* 704

◆ **FVIII/vWF** *see* Antihemophilic Factor/von Willebrand Factor Complex (Human) *on page* 146

◆ **FXIII** *see* Factor XIII Concentrate (Human) *on page* 829

◆ **FXT 40 (Can)** *see* FLUoxetine *on page* 885

◆ **Fycompa** *see* Perampanel *on page* 1620

◆ **GA101** *see* Obinutuzumab *on page* 1482

◆ **GAA** *see* Alglucosidase Alfa *on page* 74

Gabapentin (GA ba pen tin)

Brand Names: U.S. Gralise; Gralise Starter; Neurontin

Brand Names: Canada Apo-Gabapentin; Auro-Gabapentin; CO Gabapentin; Dom-Gabapentin; Gabapentin Tablets USP; GD-Gabapentin; JAMP-Gabapentin; Mylan-Gabapentin; Neurontin; PHL-Gabapentin; PMS-Gabapentin; PRO-Gabapentin; RAN-Gabapentin; ratio-Gabapentin; Riva-Gabapentin; Teva-Gabapentin

Pharmacologic Category Anticonvulsant, Miscellaneous; GABA Analog

Use Adjunct for treatment of partial seizures with and without secondary generalized seizures in patients >12 years of age with epilepsy; adjunct for treatment of partial seizures in pediatric patients 3-12 years of age; management of postherpetic neuralgia (PHN) in adults

Unlabeled Use Neuropathic pain, diabetic peripheral neuropathy, fibromyalgia, postoperative pain (adjunct), restless legs syndrome (RLS), vasomotor symptoms

Pregnancy Risk Factor C

Pregnancy Considerations Adverse events have been observed in animal reproduction studies. Gabapentin crosses the placenta. In a small study (n=6), the umbilical/maternal plasma concentration ratio was ~1.74. Neonatal concentrations declined quickly after delivery and at 24 hours of life were ~27% of the cord blood concentrations at birth (gabapentin neonatal half-life ~14 hours) (Ohman, 2005). Outcome data following maternal use of gabapentin during pregnancy is limited (Holmes, 2012).

Patients exposed to gabapentin during pregnancy are encouraged to enroll in the North American Antiepileptic Drug (NAAED) Pregnancy Registry by calling 1-888-233-2334. Additional information is available at www.aedpregnancyregistry.org.

Breast-Feeding Considerations Gabapentin is excreted in human breast milk. Per the manufacturer, a nursed infant could be exposed to ~1 mg/kg/day of gabapentin; the effect on the child is not known. Use in breast-feeding women only if the benefits to the mother outweigh the potential risk to the infant.

In a small study of breast-feeding women (n=6), the estimated exposure of gabapentin to the nursing infants was ~1% to 4% of the weight-adjusted maternal dose (sampling occurred from 12-97 days after delivery and maternal doses ranged from 600-2100 mg daily). Gabapentin was detected in the serum of 2 nursing infants 2-3 weeks after delivery and in 1 infant after 3 months of breast-feeding. Serum concentrations were <12% of the maternal plasma concentrations and <5% of those measured in the umbilical cord. Adverse events were not reported in the breast-fed infants (Ohman, 2005).

Medication Guide Available Yes

Contraindications Hypersensitivity to gabapentin or any component of the formulation

Warnings/Precautions Antiepileptics are associated with an increased risk of suicidal behavior/thoughts with use (regardless of indication); patients should be monitored for signs/symptoms of depression, suicidal tendencies, and other unusual behavior changes during therapy and instructed to inform their healthcare provider immediately if symptoms occur. Avoid abrupt withdrawal, may precipitate seizures; Gralise™ should be withdrawn over ≥1 week. Use cautiously in patients with severe renal dysfunction; male rat studies demonstrated an association with pancreatic adenocarcinoma (clinical implication unknown). May cause CNS depression, which may impair physical or mental abilities. Patients must be cautioned about performing tasks which require mental alertness (eg, operating machinery or driving). Effects with other sedative drugs or ethanol may be potentiated. Pediatric patients (3-12 years of age) have shown increased incidence of CNS-related adverse effects, including emotional lability, hostility, thought disorder, and hyperkinesia. Gabapentin immediate release and extended release (Gralise™) products are not interchangeable with each other **or** with gabapentin enacarbil (Horizant™). The safety and efficacy of extended release gabapentin (Gralise™) has not been studied in patients with epilepsy. Potentially serious, sometimes fatal multiorgan hypersensitivity (also known as drug reaction with eosinophilia and systemic symptoms [DRESS]) has been reported with some antiepileptic drugs, including gabapentin; may affect lymphatic, hepatic, renal, cardiac, and/or hematologic systems; fever, rash, and eosinophilia may also be present. Discontinue immediately if suspected.

Adverse Reactions As reported for immediate release (IR) formulations in patients >12 years of age, unless otherwise noted in children (3-12 years) or with use of extended release (ER) formulation

>10%:

Central nervous system: Dizziness (IR: 17% to 28%; children 3%; ER: 11%), drowsiness (IR: 19% to 21%; children 8%; ER: 5%), ataxia (1% to 13%), fatigue (11%; children 3%)

Infection: Viral infection (children 11%)

1% to 10%:

Cardiovascular: Peripheral edema (IR: 2% to 8%; ER: 4%), vasodilatation (1%)

Central nervous system: Hostility (children 5% to 8%), tremor (7%), emotional lability (children 4% to 6%), hyperkinesia (children 3% to 5%), headache (ER: 4%; IR: 3%), abnormality in thinking (2% to 3%; children 2%), abnormal gait (2%), amnesia (2%), depression (2%), nervousness (2%), pain (ER: 1% to 2%), hyperesthesia (1%), lethargy (ER: 1%), twitching (1%), vertigo (ER: 1%)

Dermatologic: Pruritus (1%), skin rash (1%)

Endocrine & metabolic: Weight gain (IR: Adults and children 2% to 3%; ER: 2%), hyperglycemia (1%)

Gastrointestinal: Diarrhea (IR: 6%; ER: 3%), nausea and vomiting (3% to 4%; children 8%), xerostomia (IR: 2% to 5%; ER: 3%), constipation (IR: 1% to 4%; ER: 1%), abdominal pain (3%), dyspepsia (IR: 2%; ER: 1%), dry throat (2%), dental disease (2%), flatulence (2%), increased appetite (1%)

Genitourinary: Impotence (2%), urinary tract infection (ER: 2%)

Hematologic & oncologic: Decreased white blood cell count (1%), leukopenia (1%)

Infection: Infection (5%)

Neuromuscular & skeletal: Weakness (6%), back pain (IR: 2%; ER: 2%), dysarthria (2%), limb pain (ER: 2%), myalgia (2%), bone fracture (1%)

Ophthalmic: Nystagmus (8%), diplopia (1% to 6%), blurred vision (3% to 4%), conjunctivitis (1%)

Otic: Otitis media (1%)

Respiratory: Rhinitis (4%), bronchitis (children 3%), nasopharyngitis (ER: 3%), respiratory tract infection (children 3%), pharyngitis (1% to 3%), cough (2%)

Miscellaneous: Fever (children 10%)

Postmarketing and case reports (Limited to important or life-threatening): Acute renal failure, altered serum glucose, anemia, angina pectoris, angioedema, aphasia, aspiration pneumonia, blindness, blood coagulation disorder, bradycardia, brain disease, breast hypertrophy, cardiac arrhythmia (various), cardiac failure, cerebrovascular accident, CNS neoplasm, colitis, confusion, Cushingoid appearance, DRESS syndrome, drug abuse, drug dependence, erythema multiforme, facial paralysis, fecal incontinence, gastroenteritis, glaucoma, glycosuria, hearing loss, heart block, hematemesis, hematuria, hemiplegia, hemorrhage, hepatitis, hepatomegaly, herpes zoster, hyperlipidemia, hypertension, hyperthyroidism, hyperventilation, hyponatremia, hypotension, hypothyroidism, hypoventilation, increased creatine phosphokinase, increased liver enzymes, increased serum creatinine, jaundice, joint swelling, leukocytosis, lymphadenopathy, lymphocytosis, memory impairment, meningism, migraine, movement disorder, myocardial infarction, myoclonus (local), nephrolithiasis, nephrosis, nerve palsy, non-Hodgkin's lymphoma, ovarian failure, pancreatitis, peptic ulcer, pericardial effusion, pericardial rub, pericarditis, peripheral vascular disease, pneumonia, psychosis, pulmonary thromboembolism, purpura, retinopathy, rhabdomyolysis, seasonal allergy, skin necrosis, status epilepticus, Stevens-Johnson syndrome, subdural hematoma, suicidal ideation, suicidal tendencies, syncope, tachycardia, thrombocytopenia, thrombophlebitis, tumor growth, withdrawal syndrome

Drug Interactions

Metabolism/Transport Effects None known.

Avoid Concomitant Use

Avoid concomitant use of Gabapentin with any of the following: Azelastine (Nasal); Paraldehyde

Increased Effect/Toxicity

Gabapentin may increase the levels/effects of: Alcohol (Ethyl); Azelastine (Nasal); Buprenorphine; CNS Depressants; Hydrocodone; Methotrimeprazine; Metyrosine; Mirtazapine; Paraldehyde; Pramipexole; ROPINIRole; Rotigotine; Selective Serotonin Reuptake Inhibitors; Zolpidem

The levels/effects of Gabapentin may be increased by: Brimonidine (Topical); Doxylamine; Droperidol; HydrOXYzine; Methotrimeprazine; Perampanel; Sodium Oxybate; Tapentadol

Decreased Effect

The levels/effects of Gabapentin may be decreased by: Antacids; Ketorolac (Nasal); Ketorolac (Systemic); Magnesium Salts; Mefloquine; Orlistat

Ethanol/Nutrition/Herb Interactions

Ethanol: May increase CNS depression; monitor for increased effects with coadministration. Caution patients about effects.

Food: Tablet, solution (immediate release): No significant effect on rate or extent of absorption; tablet (extended release): Increases rate and extent of absorption.

Herb/Nutraceutical: Avoid evening primrose (seizure threshold decreased). Avoid valerian, St John's wort, kava kava, gotu kola (may increase CNS depression).

Storage/Stability

Capsules and tablets: Store at 25°C (77°F); excursions permitted to 15°C to 30°C (59°F to 86°F).

Oral solution: Store refrigerated at 2°C to 8°C (36°F to 46°F).

Mechanism of Action Gabapentin is structurally related to GABA. However, it does not bind to $GABA_A$ or $GABA_B$ receptors, and it does not appear to influence synthesis or uptake of GABA. High affinity gabapentin binding sites have been located throughout the brain; these sites correspond to the presence of voltage-gated calcium channels specifically possessing the alpha-2-delta-1 subunit. This channel appears to be located presynaptically, and may modulate the release of excitatory neurotransmitters which participate in epileptogenesis and nociception.

Pharmacodynamics/Kinetics

Absorption: Variable, from proximal small bowel by L-amino transport system

Distribution: V_d: 58 ± 6 L

Protein binding: <3%

Bioavailability: Inversely proportional to dose due to saturable absorption:

Immediate release:

900 mg/day: 60%

1200 mg/day: 47%

2400 mg/day: 34%

3600 mg/day: 33%

4800 mg/day: 27%

Extended release: Variable; increased with higher fat content meal

Half-life elimination: 5-7 hours; anuria 132 hours; during dialysis 3.8 hours

Time to peak: Immediate release: 2-4 hours; extended release: 8 hours

Excretion: Proportional to renal function; urine (as unchanged drug)

Dosage Oral:

Children: Immediate release: Anticonvulsant:

3-12 years: Initial: 10-15 mg/kg/day in 3 divided doses; titrate to effective dose over ~3 days; dosages of up to 50 mg/kg/day have been tolerated in clinical studies

3-4 years: Usual dose: 40 mg/kg/day in 3 divided doses

≥5-12 years: Usual dose: 25-35 mg/kg/day in 3 divided doses

See **"Note"** in adult dosing.

Children >12 years and Adults: Immediate release: Anticonvulsant: Initial: 300 mg 3 times/day; if necessary the dose may be increased up to 1800 mg/day; Maintenance: 900-1800 mg/day administered in 3 divided doses; doses of up to 2400 mg/day have been tolerated in long-term clinical studies; up to 3600 mg/day has been tolerated in short-term studies.

Note: If gabapentin is discontinued or if another anticonvulsant is added to therapy, it should be done slowly over a minimum of 1 week

Adults:

Immediate release:

Diabetic neuropathy (unlabeled use): 900-3600 mg/day (Bril, 2011)

Neuropathic pain (unlabeled use): 300-3600 mg/day (Attal, 2010; Dworkin, 2010)

Neuropathic pain, critically-ill patients (unlabeled use): Initial: 100 mg 3 times daily in combination with I.V. opioids; Maintenance: 300-1200 mg 3 times daily; maximum dose: 3600 mg daily (Barr, 2013)

Postherpetic neuralgia: Day 1: 300 mg, Day 2: 300 mg twice daily, Day 3: 300 mg 3 times/day; dose may be titrated as needed for pain relief (range: 1800-3600 mg/day in divided doses, daily doses >1800 mg do not generally show greater benefit)

Postoperative pain (adjunct) (unlabeled use): Usual dose: 300-1200 mg given the night before or 1-2 hours prior to surgery (Dauri, 2009)

Restless legs syndrome (RLS) (unlabeled use): Initial: 300 mg once daily 2 hours before bedtime. Doses ≥600 mg/day have been given in 2 divided doses (late afternoon and 2 hours before bedtime). Dose may be titrated every 2 weeks until symptom relief achieved (range: 300-1800 mg/day). Suggested maintenance dosing schedule: One-third of total daily dose given at 12 pm, remaining two-thirds total daily dose given at 8 pm. (Garcia-Borreguero, 2002; Happe, 2003; Saletu, 2010; Vignatelli, 2006)

Vasomotor symptoms associated with menopause (unlabeled use): Day 1: 300 mg at bedtime, Day 2: 300 mg twice daily, followed by 300 mg 3 times/day for 4 weeks and then tapered off (Butt, 2008)

Extended release (Gralise™): Postherpetic neuralgia: Day 1: 300 mg, Day 2: 600 mg, Days 3-6: 900 mg once daily, Days 7-10: 1200 mg once daily, Days 11-14: 1500 mg once daily, Days ≥15: 1800 mg once daily

Elderly: Studies in elderly patients have shown a decrease in clearance as age increases. This is most likely due to age-related decreases in renal function; dose reductions may be needed.

Dosing adjustment in renal impairment: Children ≥12 years and Adults: **Note:** Renal function may be estimated using the Cockcroft-Gault formula for dosage adjustment purposes.

Immediate release:

Cl_{cr} ≥60 mL/minute: 300-1200 mg 3 times/day

Cl_{cr} >30-59 mL/minute: 200-700 mg twice daily

Cl_{cr} >15-29 mL/minute: 200-700 mg once daily

Cl_{cr} 15 mL/minute: 100-300 mg once daily

Cl_{cr} <15 mL/minute: Reduce daily dose in proportion to creatinine clearance based on dose for creatinine clearance of 15 mL/minute (eg, reduce dose by one-half [range: 50-150 mg/day] for Cl_{cr} 7.5 mL/minute)

ESRD requiring hemodialysis: Dose for Cl_{cr} <15 mL/minute plus single supplemental dose of 125-350 mg (given after each 4 hours of hemodialysis)

Extended release: **Note:** Follow initial dose titration schedule if treatment-naive.

Cl_{cr} ≥60 mL/minute: 1800 mg once daily

Cl_{cr} >30-59 mL/minute: 600-1800 mg once daily; dependent on tolerability and clinical response

Cl_{cr} <30 mL/minute: Use is not recommended.

ESRD requiring hemodialysis: Use is not recommended.

Dosing adjustment in hepatic impairment: There are no dosage adjustments provided in the manufacturer's labeling; however, gabapentin is not hepatically metabolized.

Dietary Considerations Immediate release tablet and solution may be taken without regard to meals; extended release tablet should be taken with food.

Administration

Tablet, solution (immediate release): Administer first dose on first day at bedtime to avoid somnolence and dizziness. Dosage must be adjusted for renal function; when given 3 times daily, the maximum time between doses should not exceed 12 hours.

Tablet (extended release): Take with evening meal. Swallow whole; do not chew, crush, or split.

Monitoring Parameters Monitor serum levels of concomitant anticonvulsant therapy; suicidality (eg, suicidal thoughts, depression, behavioral changes)

Test Interactions False positives have been reported with the Ames N-Multistix SG® dipstick test for urine protein

Dosage Forms Excipient information presented when available (limited, particularly for generics); consult specific product labeling.

Capsule, Oral:

Neurontin: 100 mg, 300 mg, 400 mg

Generic: 100 mg, 300 mg, 400 mg

Miscellaneous, Oral:

Gralise Starter: 300 & 600 MG (78 ea) [contains soybean lecithin]

Solution, Oral:
Neurontin: 250 mg/5 mL (470 mL) [strawberry anise flavor]
Generic: 250 mg/5 mL (5 mL, 6 mL, 470 mL, 473 mL)
Tablet, Oral:
Gralise: 300 mg [contains soybean lecithin]
Gralise: 600 mg
Neurontin: 600 mg, 800 mg [scored]
Generic: 600 mg, 800 mg

Extemporaneous Preparations Note: Commercial oral solution is available (50 mg/mL)

A 100 mg/mL suspension may be made with tablets (immediate release) and either a 1:1 mixture of Ora-Sweet® (100 mL) and Ora-Plus® (100 mL) or 1:1 mixture of methylcellulose 1% (100 mL) and Simple Syrup N.F. (100 mL). Crush sixty-seven 300 mg tablets in a mortar and reduce to a fine powder. Add small portions of the chosen vehicle and mix to a uniform paste; mix while adding the vehicle in incremental proportions to **almost** 200 mL; transfer to a calibrated bottle, rinse mortar with vehicle, and add sufficient quantity of vehicle to make 200 mL. Label "shake well" and "refrigerate". Stable for 91 days refrigerated (preferred) or 56 days at room temperature.

Nahata MC, Pai VB, and Hipple TF, *Pediatric Drug Formulations*, 5th ed, Cincinnati, OH: Harvey Whitney Books Co, 2004.

Gabapentin Enacarbil (gab a PEN tin en a KAR bil)

Brand Names: U.S. Horizant

Index Terms GSK 1838262; Solzira; XP13512

Pharmacologic Category Anticonvulsant, Miscellaneous

Use Treatment of moderate-to-severe restless leg syndrome (RLS); management of postherpetic neuralgia (PHN)

Pregnancy Risk Factor C

Pregnancy Considerations Adverse events were observed in animal reproduction studies. Gabapentin enacarbil is the prodrug of gabapentin; bioavailability following gabapentin enacarbil is increased in comparison to gabapentin (Backonja, 2011). Refer to Gabapentin monograph for information related to gabapentin exposure during pregnancy.

Breast-Feeding Considerations It is not known if gabapentin enacarbil is excreted in human breast milk; however, other gabapentin products are excreted in human breast milk. Refer to Gabapentin monograph for additional information.

Medication Guide Available Yes

Contraindications There are no contraindications listed within the manufacturer's labeling.

Warnings/Precautions Potentially serious, sometimes fatal multiorgan hypersensitivity (also known as drug reaction with eosinophilia and systemic symptoms [DRESS]) has been reported with some antiepileptic drugs, including gabapentin. Monitor for signs and symptoms of possible disparate manifestations associated with lymphatic, hepatic, renal, cardiac, and/or hematologic systems; fever, rash, and eosinophilia may also be present. Discontinue immediately if suspected. Gabapentin and other antiepileptics are associated with an increased risk of suicidal behavior/thoughts with use (regardless of indication); gabapentin enacarbil is a prodrug of gabapentin and may also increase patient's risk. Patients should be monitored for signs/symptoms of depression, suicidal tendencies, and other unusual behavior changes during therapy and instructed to inform their healthcare provider immediately if symptoms occur. To avoid the potential for withdrawal seizure, dose reduction is recommended for patients with postherpetic neuralgia (PHN) receiving twice daily doses or patients with restless legs syndrome (RLS) receiving daily doses >600 mg (daily doses of ≤600 mg can be discontinued without tapering in patients with RLS). Rat studies demonstrated an association with pancreatic adenocarcinoma (clinical implication unknown). May cause CNS depression, which may impair physical or mental abilities. Patients must be cautioned about performing tasks which require mental alertness (eg, operating machinery or driving). Effects with other sedative drugs or ethanol may be potentiated. Use with caution in patients with renal impairment; dose adjustment is needed. Gabapentin enacarbil (Horizant®) and other gabapentin products are not interchangeable due to differences in formulation, indications, and pharmacokinetics.

Restless legs syndrome (RLS): Not recommended for use in patients who are required to sleep during the day and remain awake during the night.

Adverse Reactions Percentages reported are for restless leg syndrome (RLS) 600 mg daily and postherpetic neuralgia (PHN) 1200 mg daily.

>10%: Central nervous system: Sedation/somnolence (PHN 10%; RLS 20%), dizziness (13% to 17%), headache (10% to 12%)

1% to 10%:
Cardiovascular: Peripheral edema (PHN 6%; RLS <1%)
Central nervous system: Fatigue (6%), irritability (≤4%), insomnia (PHN 3%), balance disorder (<2%), depression (<2%), disorientation (<2%), lethargy (<2%), drunk feeling (<2%), vertigo (<2%)
Gastrointestinal: Nausea (6% to 8%), flatulence (≤3%), xerostomia (≤3%), weight gain (2% to 3%), appetite increased (≤2%)
Ocular: Blurred vision (≤2%)

<1%, postmarketing, and/or case reports (reported with gabapentin; limited to important or life-threatening): Creatine kinase increased, depression, feeling abnormal, libido decreased

Drug Interactions

Metabolism/Transport Effects None known.

Avoid Concomitant Use

Avoid concomitant use of Gabapentin Enacarbil with any of the following: Alcohol (Ethyl); Azelastine (Nasal); Paraldehyde

Increased Effect/Toxicity

Gabapentin Enacarbil may increase the levels/effects of: Azelastine (Nasal); Buprenorphine; CNS Depressants; Hydrocodone; Methotrimeprazine; Metyrosine; Mirtazapine; Paraldehyde; Pramipexole; ROPINIRole; Rotigotine; Selective Serotonin Reuptake Inhibitors; Zolpidem

The levels/effects of Gabapentin Enacarbil may be increased by: Alcohol (Ethyl); Brimonidine (Topical); Doxylamine; Droperidol; HydrOXYzine; Magnesium Sulfate; Methotrimeprazine; Perampanel; Sodium Oxybate; Tapentadol

Decreased Effect

The levels/effects of Gabapentin Enacarbil may be decreased by: Ketorolac (Nasal); Ketorolac (Systemic); Mefloquine; Orlistat

Ethanol/Nutrition/Herb Interactions

Ethanol: May increase CNS depression and cause rapid release of gabapentin enacarbil from the extended release tablet. Management: Avoid ethanol.

Herb/Nutraceutical: Avoid evening primrose (seizure threshold decreased). Avoid valerian, St John's wort, kava kava, gotu kola (may increase CNS depression).

Storage/Stability Store at 25°C (77°F); excursions permitted to 15°C to 30°C (59°F to 86°F). Protect from moisture. Do not remove from original container.

Mechanism of Action Gabapentin enacarbil is a prodrug of gabapentin. Gabapentin is structurally related to GABA. However, it does not bind to $GABA_A$ or $GABA_B$ receptors, and it does not appear to influence synthesis or uptake of GABA. High affinity gabapentin binding sites have been located throughout the brain; these sites correspond to the presence of voltage-gated calcium channels specifically possessing the alpha-2-delta-1 subunit. This channel appears to be located presynaptically, and may modulate the release of excitatory neurotransmitters. These effects on RLS are unknown.

Pharmacodynamics/Kinetics

Absorption: Mediated by active transport via proton-linked monocarboxylate transporter, MCT-1

Distribution: V_d: 76 L

Protein binding: <3%

Bioavailability: With food: ~75%; Fasting: 42% to 65%

Metabolism: Prodrug hydrolyzed primarily in the intestines to gabapentin (active metabolite)

Time to peak, plasma: With food: 7.3 hours; Fasting: 5 hours

Half-life elimination: 5-6 hours

Excretion: Urine (94%); feces (5%)

Dosage Oral: Adults:

Postherpetic neuralgia (PHN): Initial: 600 mg once daily in the morning for 3 days, then increase to 600 mg twice daily; increasing to >1200 mg daily provided no additional benefit and increased side effects

Restless legs syndrome (RLS): 600 mg once daily (at ~5:00 pm); increasing to 1200 mg daily provided no additional benefit and increased side effects

Dosage adjustment in renal impairment: Note: Estimation of renal function for the purpose of drug dosing should be done using the Cockcroft-Gault formula.

PHN:

Cl_{cr} 30-59 mL/minute: Initial: 300 mg every morning for 3 days, then increase to 300 mg twice daily. May increase to 600 mg twice daily as needed based on tolerability and efficacy. When discontinuing, reduce current dose to once daily in the morning for 1 week.

Cl_{cr} 15-29: Initial: 300 mg in the morning on day 1 and on day 3; then increase to 300 mg once daily. May increase to 300 mg twice daily if needed based on tolerability and efficacy. When discontinuing, if current dose is 300 mg twice daily, reduce to 300 mg once daily for 1 week. If current dose is 300 mg once daily, no taper is needed.

Cl_{cr} <15: 300 mg every other day in the morning; may increase dose to 300 mg once daily if needed based on tolerability and efficacy. When discontinuing, no taper is needed.

Cl_{cr} <15 and on hemodialysis: 300 mg following every dialysis. May increase to 600 mg following every dialysis if needed based on tolerability and efficacy. When discontinuing, no taper is needed.

RLS:

Cl_{cr} 30-59 mL/minute: Initial dose: 300 mg daily; increase to 600 mg daily as needed

Cl_{cr} 15-29: 300 mg daily

Cl_{cr} <15: 300 mg every other day

Cl_{cr} <15 and on hemodialysis: Use is not recommended.

Dosage adjustment in hepatic impairment: No dosage adjustment provided in manufacturer's labeling.

Dietary Considerations Take with food.

Administration Tablet should be swallowed whole; do not break, chew, cut, or crush. Administer with food.

Restless leg syndrome: Administer at ~5:00 pm daily.

Monitoring Parameters Suicidality (eg, suicidal thoughts, depression, behavioral changes)

Dosage Forms Excipient information presented when available (limited, particularly for generics); consult specific product labeling.

Tablet Extended Release 24 Hour, Oral:

Horizant: 300 mg, 600 mg

◆ **Gabapentin Tablets USP (Can)** *see* Gabapentin *on page 933*

◆ **Gabitril** *see* TiaGABine *on page 2053*

◆ **Gablofen** *see* Baclofen *on page 221*

Galantamine (ga LAN ta meen)

Brand Names: U.S. Razadyne; Razadyne ER

Brand Names: Canada Mylan-Galantamine ER; PAT-Galantamine ER; Reminyl®; Reminyl® ER

Index Terms Galantamine Hydrobromide

Pharmacologic Category Acetylcholinesterase Inhibitor (Central)

Use Treatment of mild-to-moderate dementia of Alzheimer's disease

Unlabeled Use Severe dementia associated with Alzheimer's disease; mild-to-moderate dementia associated with Parkinson's disease; Lewy body dementia

Pregnancy Risk Factor B

Pregnancy Considerations Adverse events have been observed in animal reproduction studies.

Breast-Feeding Considerations It is not known if galantamine is excreted in breast milk. Galantamine is not indicated in nursing mothers.

Contraindications Hypersensitivity to galantamine or any component of the formulation

Warnings/Precautions Use caution in patients with supraventricular conduction delays (without a functional pacemaker in place); Alzheimer's treatment guidelines consider bradycardia to be a relative contraindication for use of centrally-active cholinesterase inhibitors. Use caution in patients taking medicines that slow conduction through SA or AV node. Use caution in peptic ulcer disease (or in patients at risk); seizure disorder; asthma; COPD; mild-to-moderate liver dysfunction; moderate renal dysfunction. May cause bladder outflow obstruction. May exaggerate neuromuscular blockade effects of succinylcholine and like agents.

Adverse Reactions

>10%: Gastrointestinal: Nausea (13% to 24%), vomiting (6% to 13%), diarrhea (6% to 12%)

1% to 10%:

Cardiovascular: Bradycardia (2% to 3%), hypertension (≥2%), peripheral edema (≥2%), syncope (0.4% to 2.2%: dose related), chest pain (≥1% to 2%)

Central nervous system: Dizziness (9%), headache (8%), depression (7%), fatigue (5%), insomnia (5%), somnolence (4%), agitation (≥2%), anxiety (≥2%), confusion (≥2%), hallucination (≥2%), fever (≥1%), malaise (≥1%)

Dermatologic: Purpura (≥2%)

Gastrointestinal: Anorexia (7% to 9%), weight loss (5% to 7%), abdominal pain (5%), dyspepsia (5%), constipation (≥2%), flatulence (≥1%)

Genitourinary: Urinary tract infection (8%), hematuria (<1% to 3%), incontinence (≥1% to 2%)

Hematologic: Anemia (3%)

Neuromuscular & skeletal: Tremor (3%), back pain (≥2%), fall (≥2%), weakness (≥1% to 2%)

Respiratory: Rhinitis (4%), bronchitis (≥2%), cough (≥2%), upper respiratory tract infection (≥2%)

<1% (Limited to important or life-threatening): Aphasia, apraxia, ataxia, atrial fibrillation, AV block, bundle branch block, cystitis, dehydration, delirium, diverticulitis, dysphagia, epistaxis, esophageal perforation, gastrointestinal bleeding, heart failure, hepatitis, hyperglycemia, hyper-/hypokinesia, hypersensitivity reactions, hypertonia, hypokalemia, hypotension, libido increased, liver enzymes increased, MI, nightmares, nocturia, orthostatic hypotension, QT prolongation, rectal hemorrhage, renal calculi, renal failure (due to dehydration), seizure, stroke, suicide, supraventricular tachycardia, T-wave inversion, thrombocytopenia, TIA, urinary retention, ventricular tachycardia

Drug Interactions

Metabolism/Transport Effects **Substrate** of CYP2D6 (minor), CYP3A4 (minor); **Note:** Assignment of Major/Minor substrate status based on clinically relevant drug interaction potential

Avoid Concomitant Use There are no known interactions where it is recommended to avoid concomitant use.

Increased Effect/Toxicity

Galantamine may increase the levels/effects of: Antipsychotics; Beta-Blockers; Cholinergic Agonists; Highest Risk QTc-Prolonging Agents; Moderate Risk QTc-Prolonging Agents; Succinylcholine

The levels/effects of Galantamine may be increased by: Corticosteroids (Systemic); Mifepristone; Selective Serotonin Reuptake Inhibitors

Decreased Effect

Galantamine may decrease the levels/effects of: Anticholinergics; Neuromuscular-Blocking Agents (Nondepolarizing)

The levels/effects of Galantamine may be decreased by: Anticholinergics; Dipyridamole; Peginterferon Alfa-2b

Ethanol/Nutrition/Herb Interactions

Ethanol: Avoid ethanol (may increase CNS adverse events).

Herb/Nutraceutical: St John's wort may decrease galantamine serum levels; avoid concurrent use.

Storage/Stability Store at 25°C (77°F); excursions permitted to 15°C to 30°C (59°F to 86°F). Do not freeze oral solution.

Mechanism of Action Centrally-acting cholinesterase inhibitor (competitive and reversible). It elevates acetylcholine in cerebral cortex by slowing the degradation of acetylcholine. Modulates nicotinic acetylcholine receptor to increase acetylcholine from surviving presynaptic nerve terminals. May increase glutamate and serotonin levels.

Pharmacodynamics/Kinetics

Duration: 3 hours; maximum inhibition of erythrocyte acetylcholinesterase ~40% at 1 hour post 8 mg oral dose; levels return to baseline at 30 hours

Absorption: Rapid and complete

Distribution: 175 L; levels in the brain are 2-3 times higher than in plasma

Protein binding: 18%

Metabolism: Hepatic; linear, CYP2D6 and 3A4; metabolized to epigalanthaminone and galanthaminone both of which have acetylcholinesterase inhibitory activity 130 times less than galantamine

Bioavailability: ~90%

Half-life elimination: ~7 hours

Time to peak: Immediate release: 1 hour (2.5 hours with food); extended release: 4.5-5 hours

Excretion: Urine (20%)

Dosage Oral: Adults: **Note:** If therapy is interrupted for ≥3 days, restart at the lowest dose and increase to current dose.

Alzheimer's dementia (mild-to-moderate):

Immediate release tablet or solution: Initial: 4 mg twice a day for 4 weeks; if tolerated, increase to 8 mg twice daily for ≥4 weeks; if tolerated, increase to 12 mg twice daily. Range: 16-24 mg/day in 2 divided doses

Extended-release capsule: Initial: 8 mg once daily for 4 weeks; if tolerated, increase to 16 mg once daily for ≥4 weeks; if tolerated, increase to 24 mg once daily. Range: 16-24 mg once daily

Conversion from immediate release to extended release formulation: Patients may be switched from the immediate release formulation to the extended release formulation by taking the last immediate release dose in the evening and beginning the extended release dose the following morning; the same total daily dose should be used.

Conversion to galantamine from other cholinesterase inhibitors: Patients experiencing poor tolerability with donepezil or rivastigmine should wait until side effects subside or allow a 7-day washout period prior to beginning galantamine. Patients not experiencing side effects with donepezil or rivastigmine may begin galantamine therapy the day immediately following discontinuation of previous therapy (Morris, 2001).

Elderly: No dosage adjustment needed

Dosage adjustment in renal impairment:

Moderate renal impairment: Maximum dose: 16 mg/day.

Severe renal dysfunction (Cl_{cr} <9 mL/minute): Use is not recommended

Dosage adjustment in hepatic impairment:

Moderate liver dysfunction (Child-Pugh score 7-9): Maximum dose: 16 mg/day

Severe liver dysfunction (Child-Pugh score 10-15): Use is not recommended

Dietary Considerations Administration with food is preferred, but not required; should be taken with breakfast and dinner (tablet or solution) or with breakfast (capsule).

Administration Oral: Administer solution or tablet with breakfast and dinner; administer extended release capsule with breakfast. If therapy is interrupted for ≥3 days, restart at the lowest dose and increase to current dose. If using oral solution, mix dose with 3-4 ounces of any nonalcoholic beverage; mix well and drink immediately.

Monitoring Parameters Mental status

Dosage Forms Excipient information presented when available (limited, particularly for generics); consult specific product labeling.

Capsule Extended Release 24 Hour, Oral, as hydrobromide [strength expressed as base]:

Razadyne ER: 8 mg, 16 mg, 24 mg

Generic: 8 mg, 16 mg, 24 mg

Solution, Oral, as hydrobromide:

Razadyne: 4 mg/mL (100 mL) [contains methylparaben, propylparaben, saccharin sodium]

Generic: 4 mg/mL (100 mL)

Tablet, Oral, as hydrobromide [strength expressed as base]:

Razadyne: 4 mg, 8 mg

Razadyne: 12 mg [contains fd&c yellow #6 aluminum lake]

Generic: 4 mg, 8 mg, 12 mg

- ◆ **Galantamine Hydrobromide** *see* Galantamine *on page* 937
- ◆ **Galexos (Can)** *see* Simeprevir *on page* 1897
- ◆ **Galzin** *see* Zinc Acetate *on page* 2229
- ◆ **GamaSTAN S/D** *see* Immune Globulin *on page* 1059
- ◆ **Gamastan S/D (Can)** *see* Immune Globulin *on page* 1059
- ◆ **Gamma Benzene Hexachloride** *see* Lindane *on page* 1217
- ◆ **Gammagard** *see* Immune Globulin *on page* 1059
- ◆ **Gammagard Liquid (Can)** *see* Immune Globulin *on page* 1059
- ◆ **Gammagard S/D** *see* Immune Globulin *on page* 1059
- ◆ **Gammagard S/D Less IgA** *see* Immune Globulin *on page* 1059
- ◆ **Gamma Globulin** *see* Immune Globulin *on page* 1059
- ◆ **Gamma Hydroxybutyric Acid** *see* Sodium Oxybate *on page* 1922
- ◆ **Gammaked** *see* Immune Globulin *on page* 1059
- ◆ **Gammaphos** *see* Amifostine *on page* 96
- ◆ **Gammaplex** *see* Immune Globulin *on page* 1059
- ◆ **Gamunex (Can)** *see* Immune Globulin *on page* 1059

◆ **Gamunex-C** *see* Immune Globulin *on page 1059*

Ganciclovir (Systemic) (gan SYE kloe veer)

Brand Names: U.S. Cytovene

Brand Names: Canada Cytovene®

Index Terms DHPG Sodium; GCV Sodium; Nordeoxyguanosine

Pharmacologic Category Antiviral Agent

Use Treatment of CMV retinitis in immunocompromised individuals, including patients with acquired immunodeficiency syndrome; prophylaxis of CMV infection in transplant patients

Unlabeled Use CMV retinitis: May be given in combination with foscarnet in patients who relapse after monotherapy with either drug

Pregnancy Risk Factor C

Pregnancy Considerations [U.S. Boxed Warning]: Animal studies have demonstrated carcinogenic and teratogenic effects, and inhibition of spermatogenesis. Female patients should use effective contraception during therapy; male patients should use a barrier contraceptive during and for at least 90 days after therapy.

Breast-Feeding Considerations Due to the carcinogenic and teratogenic effects observed in animal studies, the possibility of adverse events in a nursing infant is considered likely. Therefore, nursing should be discontinued during therapy. In addition, the CDC recommends **not** to breast-feed if diagnosed with HIV to avoid postnatal transmission of the virus.

Contraindications Hypersensitivity to ganciclovir, acyclovir, or any component of the formulation

Warnings/Precautions Hazardous agent - use appropriate precautions for handling and disposal (NIOSH, 2012). **[U.S. Boxed Warning]: Granulocytopenia (neutropenia), anemia, and thrombocytopenia may occur.** Dosage adjustment or interruption of ganciclovir therapy may be necessary in patients with neutropenia and/or thrombocytopenia and patients with impaired renal function. **[U.S. Boxed Warning]: Animal studies have demonstrated carcinogenic and teratogenic effects, and inhibition of spermatogenesis;** contraceptive precautions for female and male patients need to be followed during and for at least 90 days after therapy with the drug; take care to administer only into veins with good blood flow. **[U.S. Boxed Warning]: Indicated only for treatment of CMV retinitis in the immunocompromised patient and CMV prevention in transplant patients at risk.**

Adverse Reactions

>10%:

Central nervous system: Fever (48%)

Gastrointestinal: Diarrhea (44%), anorexia (14%), vomiting (13%)

Hematologic: Thrombocytopenia (57%), leukopenia (41%), anemia (16% to 26%), neutropenia with ANC <500/mm^3 (12% to 14%)

Ocular: Retinal detachment (11%; relationship to ganciclovir not established)

Renal: Serum creatinine increased (2% to 14%)

Miscellaneous: Sepsis (15%), diaphoresis (12%)

1% to 10%:

Central nervous system: Chills (10%), neuropathy (9%)

Dermatologic: Pruritus (5%)

<1% (Limited to important or life-threatening): Allergic reaction (including anaphylaxis), alopecia, arrhythmia, bronchospasm, cardiac arrest, cataracts, cholestasis, coma, dyspnea, edema, encephalopathy, exfoliative dermatitis, extrapyramidal symptoms, hepatitis, hepatic failure, pancreatitis, pancytopenia, pulmonary fibrosis, psychosis, rhabdomyolysis, seizure, alopecia, urticaria, eosinophilia, hemorrhage, Stevens-Johnson syndrome, torsade de pointes, renal failure, SIADH, visual loss

Drug Interactions

Metabolism/Transport Effects None known.

Avoid Concomitant Use

Avoid concomitant use of Ganciclovir (Systemic) with any of the following: Imipenem

Increased Effect/Toxicity

Ganciclovir (Systemic) may increase the levels/effects of: Imipenem; Mycophenolate; Reverse Transcriptase Inhibitors (Nucleoside); Tenofovir

The levels/effects of Ganciclovir (Systemic) may be increased by: Mycophenolate; Probenecid; Tenofovir

Decreased Effect There are no known significant interactions involving a decrease in effect.

Preparation for Administration Hazardous agent; use appropriate precautions for handling and disposal (NIOSH, 2012). Reconstitute 500 mg vial with 10 mL unpreserved sterile water **not** bacteriostatic water because parabens may cause precipitation. Typically, dilute in 100 mL D_5W or NS to a concentration ≤10 mg/mL for infusion.

Storage/Stability Store intact vials at temperatures below 40°C (104°F). Reconstituted solution is stable for 12 hours at room temperature, however, conflicting data indicates that reconstituted solution is stable for 60 days under refrigeration (4°C). Stability of parenteral admixture at room temperature (25°C) and at refrigeration temperature (4°C) for 35 days has been reported. However, the manufacturer recommends use within 24 hours of preparation.

Mechanism of Action Ganciclovir is phosphorylated to a substrate which competitively inhibits the binding of deoxyguanosine triphosphate to DNA polymerase resulting in inhibition of viral DNA synthesis

Pharmacodynamics/Kinetics

Distribution: V_d: 15.26 L/1.73 m^2; widely to all tissues including CSF and ocular tissue

Protein binding: 1% to 2%

Half-life elimination: 1.7-5.8 hours; prolonged with renal impairment; End-stage renal disease: 5-28 hours

Excretion: Urine (80% to 99% as unchanged drug)

Dosage

CMV CNS infection in HIV-exposed/-infected patients (unlabeled use; CDC, 2009): Infants, Children, and Adults: I.V.: 5 mg/kg/dose every 12 hours plus foscarnet until symptoms improve followed by chronic suppression

CMV retinitis:

Children and Adults: I.V. (slow infusion):

Induction therapy: 5 mg/kg/dose every 12 hours for 14-21 days followed by maintenance therapy

Maintenance therapy: 5 mg/kg/day as a single daily dose for 7 days/week or 6 mg/kg/day for 5 days/week

Prevention (secondary) of CMV disease in HIV-exposed/-infected patients (unlabeled use; CDC, 2009): Infants, Children, and Adults: I.V.: 5 mg/kg/dose daily

Prevention (secondary) of CMV disease in transplant patients: Children and Adults: I.V. (slow infusion): 5 mg/kg/dose every 12 hours for 7-14 days; duration of maintenance therapy is dependent on clinical condition and degree of immunosuppression

Varicella zoster: Progressive outer retinal necrosis in HIV-exposed/-infected patients (unlabeled use; CDC, 2009): Infants, Children, and Adults: I.V.: 5 mg/kg/dose every 12 hours plus systemic foscarnet and intravitreal ganciclovir or intravitreal foscarnet

Elderly: Refer to adult dosing; in general, dose selection should be cautious, reflecting greater frequency of organ impairment

Dosage adjustment in renal impairment:

I.V. (Induction):

Cl_{cr} 50-69 mL/minute: Administer 2.5 mg/kg/dose every 12 hours

Cl_{cr} 25-49 mL/minute: Administer 2.5 mg/kg/dose every 24 hours

Cl_{cr} 10-24 mL/minute: Administer 1.25 mg/kg/dose every 24 hours
Cl_{cr} <10 mL/minute: Administer 1.25 mg/kg/dose 3 times/week following hemodialysis
I.V. (Maintenance):
Cl_{cr} 50-69 mL/minute: Administer 2.5 mg/kg/dose every 24 hours
Cl_{cr} 25-49 mL/minute: Administer 1.25 mg/kg/dose every 24 hours
Cl_{cr} 10-24 mL/minute: Administer 0.625 mg/kg/dose every 24 hours
Cl_{cr} <10 mL/minute: Administer 0.625 mg/kg/dose 3 times/week following hemodialysis

Intermittent hemodialysis (IHD) (administer after hemodialysis on dialysis days): Dialyzable (50%): CMV Infection: I.V.: Induction: 1.25 mg/kg every 48-72 hours; Maintenance: 0.625 mg/kg every 48-72 hours. **Note:** Dosing dependent on the assumption of 3 times/week, complete IHD sessions.

Peritoneal dialysis (PD): Dose as for Cl_{cr} <10 mL/minute.

Continuous renal replacement therapy (CRRT) (Heintz, 2009; Trotman, 2005): Drug clearance is highly dependent on the method of renal replacement, filter type, and flow rate. Appropriate dosing requires close monitoring of pharmacologic response, signs of adverse reactions due to drug accumulation, as well as drug concentrations in relation to target trough (if appropriate). The following are general recommendations only (based on dialysate flow/ultrafiltration rates of 1-2 L/hour and minimal residual renal function) and should not supersede clinical judgment: CMV Infection:
CVVH: I.V.: Induction: 2.5 mg/kg every 24 hours; Maintenance: 1.25 mg/kg every 24 hours
CVVHD/CVVHDF: I.V.: Induction: 2.5 mg/kg every 12 hours; Maintenance: 2.5 mg/kg every 24 hours

Dosage adjustment in hepatic impairment: No dosage adjustment provided in manufacturer's labeling.

Dietary Considerations Some products may contain sodium.

Administration Should not be administered by I.M., SubQ, or rapid IVP; administer by slow I.V. infusion over at least 1 hour. Too rapid infusion can cause increased toxicity and excessive plasma levels. Flush line well with NS before and after administration.

Hazardous agent; use appropriate precautions for handling and disposal (NIOSH, 2012).

Monitoring Parameters CBC with differential and platelet count, serum creatinine

Dosage Forms Excipient information presented when available (limited, particularly for generics); consult specific product labeling.
Solution Reconstituted, Intravenous:
Cytovene: 500 mg (1 ea)
Generic: 500 mg (1 ea)

Ganirelix (ga ni REL ix)

Brand Names: Canada Orgalutran®
Index Terms Antagon; Ganirelix Acetate
Pharmacologic Category Gonadotropin Releasing Hormone Antagonist
Use Inhibits premature luteinizing hormone (LH) surges in women undergoing controlled ovarian hyperstimulation
Pregnancy Risk Factor X
Dosage Adult: SubQ: 250 mcg/day during the mid-to-late phase after initiating follicle-stimulating hormone on day 2 or 3 of cycle. Treatment should be continued daily until the day of chorionic gonadotropin administration.

Dosage adjustment in renal impairment: No dosage adjustment provided in manufacturer's labeling (has not been studied).

Dosage adjustment in hepatic impairment: No dosage adjustment provided in manufacturer's labeling (has not been studied).

Additional Information Complete prescribing information should be consulted for additional detail.

Dosage Forms Excipient information presented when available (limited, particularly for generics); consult specific product labeling.
Solution, Subcutaneous, as acetate:
Generic: 250 mcg/0.5 mL (0.5 mL)

◆ Ganirelix Acetate *see* Ganirelix *on page 940*
◆ GAR-936 *see* Tigecycline *on page 2061*
◆ Garamycin *see* Gentamicin (Ophthalmic) *on page 954*
◆ Garamycin® (Can) *see* Gentamicin (Ophthalmic) *on page 954*
◆ Gardasil *see* Papillomavirus (Types 6, 11, 16, 18) Vaccine (Human, Recombinant) *on page 1567*

Gatifloxacin (gat i FLOKS a sin)

Brand Names: U.S. Zymaxid
Brand Names: Canada Zymar
Pharmacologic Category Antibiotic, Fluoroquinolone; Antibiotic, Ophthalmic
Use Treatment of bacterial conjunctivitis
Pregnancy Risk Factor C
Pregnancy Considerations Gatifloxacin has been shown to be fetotoxic in animal studies. Quinolone exposure during human pregnancy has been reported with other agents (refer to Ciprofloxacin (Systemic), Ofloxacin (Systemic), and Norfloxacin monographs). Following ophthalmic administration, serum concentrations of gatifloxacin are below the limits of quantification (<5 ng/mL). Systemic absorption would be required in order for gatifloxacin to cross the placenta.
Breast-Feeding Considerations Other quinolones are known to be excreted in breast milk. The manufacturer recommends using caution if gatifloxacin is administered while nursing.
Contraindications
Zymaxid: There are no contraindications listed in the manufacturer's labeling.
Zymar: Hypersensitivity to gatifloxacin, other quinolones, or any component of the formulation
Warnings/Precautions Severe hypersensitivity reactions, including anaphylaxis, have occurred with systemic quinolone therapy. Reactions may present as typical allergic symptoms after a single dose, or may manifest as severe idiosyncratic dermatologic, vascular, pulmonary, renal, hepatic, and/or hematologic events, usually after multiple doses. Prompt discontinuation of drug should occur if skin rash or other symptoms arise. Prolonged use may result in fungal or bacterial superinfection. For topical ophthalmic use only. Do not inject ophthalmic solution subconjunctivally or introduce directly into the anterior chamber of the eye. Contact lenses should not be worn during treatment of ophthalmic infections.
Adverse Reactions
1% to 10%:
Cardiovascular: Edema
Dermatologic: Contact dermatitis, erythema
Gastrointestinal: Taste disturbance
Ocular: Conjunctival irritation, discharge, dry eye, edema, irritation, keratitis, lacrimation increased, pain, papillary conjunctivitis, visual acuity decreased
Respiratory: Rhinorrhea
<1% (Limited to important or life-threatening): Angioedema, blepharitis (allergic), chemosis, conjunctival cyst, conjunctival hemorrhage, corneal deposits, corneal disorder, corneal ulcer, dermatitis, dizziness,

endophthalmitis, eye redness, iritis, keratoconjunctivitis, macular edema, nausea, paresthesia (oral), photophobia, pruritus, subepithelial opacities, tinnitus, tremor, urticaria, uveitis, vision blurred, throat sore

Drug Interactions

Metabolism/Transport Effects None known.

Avoid Concomitant Use There are no known interactions where it is recommended to avoid concomitant use.

Increased Effect/Toxicity There are no known significant interactions involving an increase in effect.

Decreased Effect There are no known significant interactions involving a decrease in effect.

Storage/Stability Store between 15°C to 25°C (59°F to 77°F); do not freeze.

Mechanism of Action Gatifloxacin is a DNA gyrase inhibitor, and also inhibits topoisomerase IV. DNA gyrase (topoisomerase II) is an essential bacterial enzyme that maintains the superhelical structure of DNA. DNA gyrase is required for DNA replication and transcription, DNA repair, recombination, and transposition; inhibition is bactericidal.

Pharmacodynamics/Kinetics Absorption: Ophthalmic: Not measurable (<5 ng/mL)

Dosage Ophthalmic: Children ≥1 year and Adults: Bacterial conjunctivitis:

Zymar:

Days 1 and 2: Instill 1 drop into affected eye(s) every 2 hours while awake (maximum: 8 times/day)

Days 3-7: Instill 1 drop into affected eye(s) 4 times/day while awake

Zymaxid:

Day 1: Instill 1 drop into affected eye(s) every 2 hours while awake (maximum: 8 times/day)

Days 2-7: Instill 1 drop into affected eye(s) 2-4 times/day while awake

Dosage adjustment in renal impairment: No dosage adjustment provided in manufacturer's labeling. However, dosage adjustment unlikely due to low systemic absorption.

Dosage adjustment in hepatic impairment: No dosage adjustment provided in manufacturer's labeling. However, dosage adjustment unlikely due to low systemic absorption.

Administration For topical ophthalmic use only; avoid touching tip of applicator to eye, fingers, or other surfaces.

Monitoring Parameters Signs of infection

Test Interactions Some quinolones may produce a false-positive urine screening result for opioids using commercially-available immunoassay kits. This has been demonstrated most consistently for levofloxacin and ofloxacin, but other quinolones have shown cross-reactivity in certain assay kits. Confirmation of positive opioid screens by more specific methods should be considered.

Dosage Forms Excipient information presented when available (limited, particularly for generics); consult specific product labeling.

Solution, Ophthalmic:

Zymaxid: 0.5% (2.5 mL) [contains benzalkonium chloride, edetate disodium]

Generic: 0.5% (2.5 mL)

Dosage Forms: Canada Excipient information presented when available (limited, particularly for generics); consult specific product labeling.

Solution, ophthalmic [drops]:

Zymar: 0.3% (1 mL, 2.5 mL, 5 mL) [contains benzalkonium chloride]

- ◆ Gattex *see* Teduglutide *on page 1995*
- ◆ GaviLAX [OTC] *see* Polyethylene Glycol 3350 *on page 1668*
- ◆ GaviLyte-C *see* Polyethylene Glycol-Electrolyte Solution *on page 1669*
- ◆ GaviLyte-G *see* Polyethylene Glycol-Electrolyte Solution *on page 1669*
- ◆ GaviLyte-N *see* Polyethylene Glycol-Electrolyte Solution *on page 1669*
- ◆ Gaviscon® Extra Strength [OTC] *see* Aluminum Hydroxide and Magnesium Carbonate *on page 89*
- ◆ Gaviscon® Liquid [OTC] *see* Aluminum Hydroxide and Magnesium Carbonate *on page 89*
- ◆ Gaviscon® Tablet [OTC] *see* Aluminum Hydroxide and Magnesium Trisilicate *on page 90*
- ◆ Gazyva *see* Obinutuzumab *on page 1482*
- ◆ G-CSF *see* Filgrastim *on page 859*
- ◆ G-CSF (PEG Conjugate) *see* Pegfilgrastim *on page 1588*
- ◆ GCV Sodium *see* Ganciclovir (Systemic) *on page 939*
- ◆ GD-Amlodipine (Can) *see* AmLODIPine *on page 109*
- ◆ GD-Atorvastatin (Can) *see* AtorvaSTATin *on page 190*
- ◆ GD-Azithromycin (Can) *see* Azithromycin (Systemic) *on page 214*
- ◆ GDC-0449 *see* Vismodegib *on page 2199*
- ◆ GD-Gabapentin (Can) *see* Gabapentin *on page 933*
- ◆ GD-Latanoprost (Can) *see* Latanoprost *on page 1178*
- ◆ GD-Mirtazapine (Can) *see* Mirtazapine *on page 1379*
- ◆ GD-Pregabalin (Can) *see* Pregabalin *on page 1710*
- ◆ GD-Sertraline (Can) *see* Sertraline *on page 1889*
- ◆ GD-Sildenafil (Can) *see* Sildenafil *on page 1894*
- ◆ GD-Terbinafine (Can) *see* Terbinafine (Systemic) *on page 2017*
- ◆ GD-Venlafaxine XR (Can) *see* Venlafaxine *on page 2178*

Gefitinib (ge FI tye nib)

Brand Names: U.S. Iressa®

Brand Names: Canada IRESSA®

Index Terms ZD1839

Pharmacologic Category Antineoplastic Agent, Tyrosine Kinase Inhibitor

Use Treatment of locally advanced or metastatic nonsmall cell lung cancer (NSCLC) after failure of platinum-based and docetaxel therapies. Treatment is limited to patients who are benefiting or have benefited from treatment with gefitinib.

Note: Due to the lack of improved survival data from clinical trials of gefitinib, and in response to positive survival data with another EGFR inhibitor, according to the U.S. labeling, physicians are advised to use treatment options other than gefitinib in patients with advanced nonsmall cell lung cancer following one or two prior chemotherapy regimens when they are refractory/intolerant to their most recent regimen.

Canada labeling: First-line treatment of locally advanced or metastatic NSCLC with activating mutations of EGFR-TK

Unlabeled Use First-line treatment of NSCLC with known EGFR mutation

Pregnancy Risk Factor D

Pregnancy Considerations Animal studies have demonstrated fetal harm; there are no well-controlled studies in pregnant women. The risk of fetal harm should be carefully weighed. Women of childbearing potential should be advised to avoid pregnancy.

Breast-Feeding Considerations Due to the potential for serious adverse reactions in the nursing infant, breast-feeding is not recommended.

Prescribing and Access Restrictions As of September 15, 2005, distribution of gefitinib (IRESSA®) is limited to patients enrolled in the IRESSA® Access Program. Under this program, access to gefitinib will be limited to the following groups:

Patients who are currently receiving and benefiting from gefitinib

Patients who have previously received and benefited from gefitinib

Previously-enrolled patients or new patients in non-Investigational New Drug (IND) clinical trials involving gefitinib if these protocols were approved by an IRB prior to June 17, 2005

New patients may also receive gefitinib if the manufacturer (AstraZeneca) decides to make it available under IND, and the patients meet the criteria for enrollment under the IND

Additional information on the IRESSA® Access Program, including enrollment forms, may be obtained by calling AstraZeneca at 1-800-601-8933.

Contraindications Hypersensitivity to gefitinib or any component of the formulation

Warnings/Precautions Hazardous agent - use appropriate precautions for handling and disposal (meets NIOSH, 2012 criteria). Rare, sometimes fatal, pulmonary toxicity, including interstitial lung disease (ILD) (eg, alveolitis, interstitial pneumonia, pneumonitis) has occurred. ILD has occurred in patients with prior radiation therapy, prior chemotherapy, and less commonly in treatment naïve patients. Therapy should be interrupted in patients with acute onset or worsening pulmonary symptoms (dyspnea, cough, fever); discontinue if interstitial pneumonitis is confirmed. An increase in mortality was observed in patients with concurrent idiopathic pulmonary fibrosis. Asymptomatic increases in transaminases have been reported; monitor liver function periodically and discontinue if elevations/changes are severe. Gefitinib exposure may be increased in patients with hepatic impairment. Interruption of therapy may be required in patients with poorly tolerated diarrhea or adverse skin reactions. Eye irritation should be promptly evaluated and therapy may be interrupted based on appropriate medical evaluation; may be reinitiated following resolution of symptoms or eye changes.

EGFR mutations, specifically exon 19 deletions and exon 21 mutation (L858R), are associated with better response to gefitinib in patients with NSCLC (Riely, 2006). There is a high potential for CYP3A4 mediated interactions with gefitinib. Concurrent use with CYP3A4 inducers may decrease gefitinib levels; consider increased gefitinib doses (to 500 mg) with close monitoring if concurrent use with inducers cannot be avoided. CYP3A4 inhibitors may increase gefitinib levels, use caution with concurrent administration.

Adverse Reactions

>10%:

Dermatologic: Rash (43% to 54%), acne (25% to 33%), dry skin (13% to 26%), paronychia (14%)

Gastrointestinal: Diarrhea (48% to 67%; grade 3: 1%), nausea (13% to 18%), vomiting (9% to 12%)

1% to 10%:

Cardiovascular: Peripheral edema (2%)

Dermatologic: Pruritus (8% to 9%)

Gastrointestinal: Anorexia (7% to 10%), weight loss (3% to 5%), mouth ulceration (1%)

Neuromuscular & skeletal: Weakness (4% to 6%)

Ocular: Amblyopia (2%), conjunctivitis (1%)

Respiratory: Dyspnea (2%), interstitial lung disease (1% to 2%; includes alveolitis, interstitial pneumonia, pneumonitis)

<1% (Limited to important or life-threatening): Aberrant eyelash growth, angioedema, CNS hemorrhage (pediatrics), corneal erosion/ulcer, corneal membrane sloughing, epistaxis, erythema multiforme, eye pain, fever, hematuria, hemorrhage, ocular hemorrhage, ocular ischemia, pancreatitis, toxic epidermal necrolysis, urticaria, vesiculobullous rash

Drug Interactions

Metabolism/Transport Effects Substrate of CYP2D6 (major), CYP3A4 (major); **Note:** Assignment of Major/Minor substrate status based on clinically relevant drug interaction potential; **Inhibits** BCRP, CYP2C19 (weak), CYP2D6 (weak)

Avoid Concomitant Use

Avoid concomitant use of Gefitinib with any of the following: Conivaptan; Fusidic Acid (Systemic); PAZOPanib

Increased Effect/Toxicity

Gefitinib may increase the levels/effects of: ARIPiprazole; PAZOPanib; Topotecan; Vinorelbine; Vitamin K Antagonists

The levels/effects of Gefitinib may be increased by: Abiraterone Acetate; Conivaptan; CYP2D6 Inhibitors (Moderate); CYP2D6 Inhibitors (Strong); CYP3A4 Inhibitors (Moderate); CYP3A4 Inhibitors (Strong); Darunavir; Dasatinib; Fusidic Acid (Systemic); Ivacaftor; Luliconazole; Mifepristone; Simeprevir

Decreased Effect

Gefitinib may decrease the levels/effects of: Cardiac Glycosides; Vitamin K Antagonists

The levels/effects of Gefitinib may be decreased by: Bosentan; CYP3A4 Inducers (Strong); Dabrafenib; Deferasirox; H2-Antagonists; Herbs (CYP3A4 Inducers); Peginterferon Alfa-2b; Proton Pump Inhibitors; Rifamycin Derivatives; Tocilizumab

Ethanol/Nutrition/Herb Interactions

Food: Grapefruit juice may increase serum gefitinib concentrations.

Herb/Nutraceutical: St John's wort may decrease serum gefitinib concentrations.

Storage/Stability Store tablets at controlled room temperature of 20°C to 25°C (68°F to 77°F). Protect from light and moisture.

Mechanism of Action Gefitinib is a tyrosine kinase inhibitor (TKI) which inhibits numerous tyrosine kinases associated with transmembrane cell surface receptors found on both normal and cancer cells, including the tyrosine kinase associated with the epidermal growth factor receptor, EGFR. Tyrosine kinase activity appears to be vitally important to cell proliferation and survival.

Pharmacodynamics/Kinetics

Absorption: Oral: Slow

Distribution: 1400 L

Protein binding: 90%, albumin and alpha$_1$-acid glycoprotein

Metabolism: Hepatic, primarily via CYP3A4; forms metabolites

Bioavailability: 60%

Half-life elimination: Oral: 41 hours

Time to peak, plasma: Oral: 3-7 hours

Excretion: Feces (86%); urine (<4%)

Dosage Oral: Adults:

Nonsmall cell lung cancer (NSCLC): 250 mg once daily

NSCLC, first-line therapy in patients with EGFR mutations (unlabeled use): 250 mg once daily (Maemondo, 2010; Mok, 2009; Sequist, 2008)

Dosage adjustment for concomitant CYP3A4 inducers (eg, phenytoin, rifampin): Consider increasing gefitinib dose to 500 mg once daily with close monitoring

Dosage adjustment for toxicity:

Worsening pulmonary symptoms (cough dyspnea, fever): Interrupt treatment and evaluate promptly; discontinue if interstitial lung disease is confirmed

Diarrhea (poorly tolerated or associated with dehydration) or skin toxicity: Interrupt treatment for up to 14 days; may reinitiate at 250 mg once daily

Ocular symptoms (eye pain): Evaluate and interrupt treatment based on symptoms; once symptoms or eye changes have resolved, may consider reinitiating at 250 mg once daily

Dosage adjustment in renal impairment: No adjustment necessary

Dosage adjustment in hepatic impairment:

Moderate-to-severe impairment due to metastases: No adjustment necessary

Hepatotoxicity during treatment (elevations in transaminases): Discontinue if severe

Dietary Considerations Food does not affect gefitinib absorption.

Administration May administer with or without food.

For patients unable to swallow tablets or for administration via NG tube: Tablets may be dispersed in noncarbonated drinking water. Drop whole tablet (do not crush) into 1/2 glass of water; stir until tablet is dispersed (~10 minutes). Drink immediately. Rinse glass with 1/2 glass of water and drink.

Hazardous agent; use appropriate precautions for handling and disposal (meets NIOSH, 2012 criteria).

Monitoring Parameters Periodic liver function tests (ALT, AST, bilirubin and alkaline phosphatase), INR or prothrombin time (with concurrently warfarin treatment), pulmonary symptoms

Additional Information Oncology Comment: Recent studies have demonstrated a subset of patients who are more likely to respond to treatment with gefitinib. This subset includes: patients of Asian origin, never-smokers, women, patients with bronchoalveolar adenocarcinoma, and patients with EGFR-mutated tumors. Deletion in exon 19 and mutation in exon 21 are the two most commonly found EGFR mutations; both mutations correlate with clinical response, resulting in increased response rates in patients with the mutation (Riely, 2006). Studies have compared gefitinib in treatment naïve patients to combination chemotherapy in the subsets of patients described above, resulting in a longer progression free survival in the gefitinib arm (Mok, 2009). Based on these data, the 2009 ASCO guidelines recommend the first-line use of gefitinib in stage IV with the known EGFR mutation (Azzoli, 2009). The NCCN guidelines recommend erlotinib as first-line therapy for EGFR mutation positive patients with stage IV NSCLC, and also states that gefitinib could be used in place of erlotinib in areas of the world where available. In patients with a kras mutation, however, EGFR-TKI therapy is not recommended.

Dosage Forms Excipient information presented when available (limited, particularly for generics); consult specific product labeling.

Tablet, oral:

Iressa®: 250 mg

Extemporaneous Preparations Hazardous agent: Use appropriate precautions for handling and disposal.

An oral suspension may be prepared by placing one tablet (whole, do not crush) in half a glass of noncarbonated drinking water. Stir until tablet is disintegrated (~10 minutes), then administer immediately. To ensure the full dose is administered, rinse with half a glass of water and administer residue.

Iressa® prescribing information, AstraZeneca Pharmaceuticals, Wilmington, DE, 2005.

◆ **Gel-Kam® [OTC]** *see* Fluoride *on page 880*

◆ **Gel-Kam® Rinse** *see* Fluoride *on page 880*

◆ **Gelnique** *see* Oxybutynin *on page 1533*

◆ **Gel-One** *see* Hyaluronate and Derivatives *on page 1000*

◆ **Gelucast®** *see* Zinc Gelatin *on page 2229*

◆ **Gelusil® [OTC]** *see* Aluminum Hydroxide, Magnesium Hydroxide, and Simethicone *on page 90*

◆ **Gelusil® (Can)** *see* Aluminum Hydroxide, Magnesium Hydroxide, and Simethicone *on page 90*

◆ **Gelusil® Extra Strength (Can)** *see* Aluminum Hydroxide and Magnesium Hydroxide *on page 90*

Gemcitabine (jem SITE a been)

Brand Names: U.S. Gemzar

Brand Names: Canada Gemcitabine For Injection; Gemcitabine For Injection, USP; Gemcitabine Hydrochloride For Injection; Gemcitabine Injection; Gemcitabine Sun For Injection; Gemzar

Index Terms dFdC; dFdCyd; Difluorodeoxycytidine Hydrochlorothiazide; Gemcitabine Hydrochloride; LY-188011

Pharmacologic Category Antineoplastic Agent, Antimetabolite; Antineoplastic Agent, Antimetabolite (Pyrimidine Analog)

Use

Breast cancer: First-line treatment of metastatic breast cancer (in combination with paclitaxel) after failure of adjuvant chemotherapy which contained an anthracycline (unless contraindicated)

Nonsmall cell lung cancer (NSCLC): First-line treatment of inoperable, locally-advanced (stage IIIA or IIIB) or metastatic (stage IV) NSCLC (in combination with cisplatin)

Ovarian cancer: Treatment of advanced ovarian cancer (in combination with carboplatin) that has relapsed at least 6 months following completion of platinum-based chemotherapy

Pancreatic cancer: First-line treatment of locally-advanced (nonresectable stage II or III) or metastatic (stage IV) pancreatic adenocarcinoma

Unlabeled Use Treatment of bladder cancer, cervical cancer (recurrent or persistent), Ewing's sarcoma (refractory), head and neck cancer (nasopharyngeal), hepatobiliary cancers (advanced), Hodgkin lymphoma (relapsed), non-Hodgkin lymphomas (refractory), malignant pleural mesothelioma, osteosarcoma (refractory), renal cell cancer (metastatic), small cell lung cancer (refractory or relapsed), soft tissue sarcoma (advanced), testicular cancer (refractory germ cell tumors), thymic malignancies, uterine sarcoma, and unknown-primary adenocarcinoma

Pregnancy Risk Factor D

Pregnancy Considerations Adverse events were observed in animal reproduction studies. May cause fetal harm if administered during pregnancy; adverse effects in reproduction are anticipated based on the mechanism of action.

Breast-Feeding Considerations It is not known if gemcitabine is excreted in breast milk. Due to the potential for serious adverse reactions in the nursing infant, the decision to discontinue gemcitabine or to discontinue breast-feeding should take into account the benefits of treatment to the mother.

Contraindications Hypersensitivity to gemcitabine or any component of the formulation

Warnings/Precautions Hazardous agent - use appropriate precautions for handling and disposal (NIOSH, 2012). Gemcitabine may suppress bone marrow function (neutropenia, thrombocytopenia, and anemia); myelosuppression is usually the dose-limiting toxicity; toxicity is increased when used in combination with other chemotherapy; monitor blood counts; dosage adjustments are frequently required.

Hemolytic uremic syndrome (HUS) has been reported; may lead to renal failure (including fatalities); monitor for evidence of anemia with microangiopathic hemolysis (elevation of bilirubin or LDH, reticulocytosis, severe thrombocytopenia, and/or renal failure) and monitor renal function at baseline and periodically during treatment. Permanently discontinue if HUS or severe renal impairment occurs; renal failure may not be reversible despite discontinuation. Serious hepatotoxicity (including liver failure and death) has been reported (when used alone or in combination with other hepatotoxic medications); use in patients with hepatic impairment (history of cirrhosis, hepatitis, or alcoholism) or in patients with hepatic metastases may lead to exacerbation of hepatic impairment. Monitor hepatic function at baseline and periodically during treatment; consider dose adjustments with elevated bilirubin; discontinue if severe liver injury develops. Capillary leak syndrome (CLS) with serious consequences has been reported, both with single-agent gemcitabine and with combination chemotherapy; discontinue if CLS develops.

Pulmonary toxicity, including adult respiratory distress syndrome, interstitial pneumonitis, pulmonary edema, and pulmonary fibrosis, has been observed; may lead to respiratory failure (some fatal) despite discontinuation. Onset for symptoms of pulmonary toxicity may be delayed up to 2 weeks beyond the last dose. Discontinue for unexplained dyspnea (with or without bronchospasm) or other evidence or pulmonary toxicity. Not indicated for use with concurrent radiation therapy; radiation toxicity, including tissue injury, severe mucositis, esophagitis, or pneumonitis, has been reported with concurrent and nonconcurrent administration; may have radiosensitizing activity when gemcitabine and radiation therapy are given ≤7 days apart; radiation recall may occur when gemcitabine and radiation therapy are given >7 days apart. Potentially significant drug-drug interactions may exist, requiring dose or frequency adjustment, additional monitoring, and/or selection of alternative therapy.

Prolongation of the infusion duration >60 minutes or more frequent than weekly dosing have been shown to alter the half-life and increase toxicity (hypotension, flu-like symptoms, myelosuppression, weakness); a fixed-dose rate (FDR) infusion rate of 10 mg/m^2/minute has been studied in order to optimize the pharmacokinetics (unlabeled); prolonged infusion times increase the intracellular accumulation of the active metabolite, gemcitabine triphosphate (Ko, 2006; Tempero, 2003); patients who receive gemcitabine FDR experience more grade 3/4 hematologic toxicity (Ko, 2006; Poplin, 2009).

Adverse Reactions Frequency of adverse reactions reported for single-agent use of gemcitabine only.

>10%:

Cardiovascular: Peripheral edema (20%), edema (13%)
Central nervous system: Drowsiness (11%)
Dermatologic: Skin rash (28% to 30%), alopecia (15% to 16%), pruritus (13%)
Gastrointestinal: Nausea/vomiting (69% to 71%), diarrhea (19% to 30%), stomatitis (10% to 11%)
Genitourinary: Proteinuria (32% to 45%), hematuria (23% to 35%), increased blood urea nitrogen (15% to 16%)
Hematologic & oncologic: Anemia (68% to 73%; grade 4: 1% to 3%), leukopenia (62% to 64%; grade 4: ≤1%), neutropenia (61% to 63%; grade 4: 6% to 7%), thrombocytopenia (24% to 36%; grade 4: 1%), hemorrhage (4% to 17%; grade 3: <1%; grade 4: <1%); bone marrow depression is the dose-limiting toxicity
Hepatic: Increased serum AST (67%; grade 3: 6%; grade 4: 2%), increased serum alkaline phosphatase (55%; grade 3: 7%; grade 4: 2%), increased serum ALT (68%; grade 3: 8%, grade 4: 2%), increased serum bilirubin (13%; grade 3: 2%, grade 4: <1%)
Infection: Localized infection (10% to 16%)
Respiratory: Dyspnea (10% to 23%; grade 3: 3%; grade 4: <1%)
Miscellaneous: Fever (16% to 41%), flu-like symptoms (19%)

1% to 10%:

Central nervous system: Paresthesia (10%; grade 3: <1%)
Local: Injection site reaction (4%)
Renal: Increased serum creatinine (6% to 8%)
Respiratory: Bronchospasm (<2%)

<1% (Limited to important or life-threatening; reported with single-agent use or with combination therapy): Adult respiratory distress syndrome (acute), anaphylactoid reaction, Budd-Chiari syndrome, bullous pemphigoid, capillary leak syndrome, cardiac arrhythmia, cardiac arrhythmia (supraventricular), cellulitis, cerebrovascular accident, congestive heart failure, desquamation, digital vasculitis, gangrene of skin or other tissue, hemolytic-uremic syndrome (HUS), hepatic necrosis, hepatotoxicity (rare), hypertension, hypotension, increased gamma-glutamyl transferase, interstitial pneumonitis, liver cirrhosis, myocardial infarction, neuropathy, petechiae, pulmonary edema, pulmonary fibrosis, radiation recall phenomenon, renal failure, respiratory failure, reversible posterior leukoencephalopathy syndrome (RPLS), sepsis, thrombotic thrombocytopenic purpura

Drug Interactions

Metabolism/Transport Effects None known.

Avoid Concomitant Use

Avoid concomitant use of Gemcitabine with any of the following: BCG; CloZAPine; Natalizumab; Pimecrolimus; Tacrolimus (Topical); Tofacitinib; Vaccines (Live)

Increased Effect/Toxicity

Gemcitabine may increase the levels/effects of: Bleomycin; CloZAPine; Fluorouracil (Systemic); Fluorouracil (Topical); Leflunomide; Natalizumab; Tofacitinib; Vaccines (Live); Vitamin K Antagonists

The levels/effects of Gemcitabine may be increased by: Denosumab; Pimecrolimus; Roflumilast; Tacrolimus (Topical); Trastuzumab

Decreased Effect

Gemcitabine may decrease the levels/effects of: BCG; Coccidioidin Skin Test; Sipuleucel-T; Vaccines (Inactivated); Vaccines (Live); Vitamin K Antagonists

The levels/effects of Gemcitabine may be decreased by: Echinacea

Preparation for Administration Hazardous agent; use appropriate precautions for handling and disposal (NIOSH, 2012). Reconstitute lyophilized powder with preservative free NS; add 5 mL to the 200 mg vial, add 25 mL to the 1000 mg vial, or add 50 mL to the 2000 mg vial, resulting in a reconstituted concentration of 38 mg/mL (solutions must be reconstituted to ≤40 mg/mL to completely dissolve).

Further dilute for infusion in NS 50-500 mL injection; to concentrations as low as 0.1 mg/mL.

Storage/Stability

Lyophilized powder: Store intact vials at room temperature of 20°C to 25°C (68°F to 77°F); excursions permitted to 15°C to 30°C (59°F to 86°F). Reconstituted vials are stable for 24 hours at room temperature. Do not refrigerate (may form crystals).

Solution for injection: Store intact vials refrigerated at 2°C to 8°C (36°F to 46°F); do not freeze.

Solutions diluted for infusion in NS are stable for 24 hours at room temperature. Do not refrigerate.

Mechanism of Action A pyrimidine antimetabolite that inhibits DNA synthesis by inhibition of DNA polymerase and ribonucleotide reductase, cell cycle-specific for the S-phase of the cycle (also blocks cellular progression at G1/S-phase). Gemcitabine is phosphorylated intracellularly by deoxycytidine kinase to gemcitabine monophosphate, which is further phosphorylated to active metabolites gemcitabine diphosphate and gemcitabine triphosphate. Gemcitabine diphosphate inhibits DNA synthesis by inhibiting ribonucleotide reductase; gemcitabine triphosphate incorporates into DNA and inhibits DNA polymerase.

Pharmacodynamics/Kinetics

Distribution: Infusions <70 minutes: 50 L/m^2; Long infusion times (70-285 minutes): 370 L/m^2

Protein binding: Negligible

Metabolism: Metabolized intracellularly by nucleoside kinases to the active diphosphate (dFdCDP) and triphosphate (dFdCTP) nucleoside metabolites

Half-life elimination:

Gemcitabine: Infusion time ≤70 minutes: 42-94 minutes; infusion time 3-4 hours: 4-10.5 hours (affected by age and gender)

Metabolite (gemcitabine triphosphate), terminal phase: 1.7-19.4 hours

Time to peak, plasma: 30 minutes after completion of infusion

Excretion: Urine (92% to 98%; primarily as inactive uracil metabolite); feces (<1%)

Dosage Details concerning dosing in combination regimens should also be consulted. **Note**: Prolongation of the infusion duration >60 minutes and administration more frequently than once weekly have been shown to increase toxicity.

Children (refer to specific references for ages of populations studied):

Germ cell tumor, refractory (unlabeled use): I.V.: 1000 mg/m^2 over 30 minutes days 1, 8, and 15 every 28 days (in combination with paclitaxel) for up to 6 cycles (Hinton, 2002)

Hodgkin lymphoma, relapsed (unlabeled use): I.V.: 1000 mg/m^2 over 100 minutes days 1 and 8; repeat cycle every 21 days (in combination with vinorelbine) (Cole; 2009) **or** 800 mg/m^2 days 1 and 4; repeat cycle every 21 days (in combination with ifosfamide, mesna, vinorelbine, and prednisolone) (Santoro, 2007)

Sarcomas (unlabeled use): I.V.:

Ewing's sarcoma, refractory: 675 mg/m^2 over 90 minutes days 1 and 8; repeat cycle every 21 days (in combination with docetaxel) (Navid, 2008)

Osteosarcoma, refractory: 675 mg/m^2 over 90 minutes days 1 and 8; repeat cycle every 21 days (in combination with docetaxel) (Navid, 2008) **or** 1000 mg/m^2 weekly for 7 weeks followed by 1 week rest; then weekly for 3 weeks out of every 4 weeks (Merimsky, 2000)

Adults:

Breast cancer, metastatic: I.V.: 1250 mg/m^2 over 30 minutes days 1 and 8; repeat cycle every 21 days (in combination with paclitaxel) **or** (unlabeled dosing; as a single agent) 800 mg/m^2 over 30 minutes days 1, 8, and 15 of a 28-day treatment cycle (Carmichael, 1995)

Nonsmall cell lung cancer, locally-advanced or metastatic: I.V.: 1000 mg/m^2 over 30 minutes days 1, 8, and 15; repeat cycle every 28 days (in combination with cisplatin) **or** 1250 mg/m^2 over 30 minutes days 1 and 8; repeat cycle every 21 days (in combination with cisplatin) **or** (unlabeled combination) 1000 mg/m^2 over 30 minutes days 1 and 8; repeat cycle every 21 days (in combination with carboplatin) for up to 4 cycles (Grønberg, 2009)

Ovarian cancer, advanced: I.V.: 1000 mg/m^2 over 30 minutes days 1 and 8; repeat cycle every 21 days (in combination with carboplatin) **or** (unlabeled dosing; as a single agent) 1000 mg/m^2 over 30-60 minutes days 1 and 8; repeat cycle every 21 days (Mutch, 2007)

Pancreatic cancer, locally advanced or metastatic: I.V.: Initial: 1000 mg/m^2 over 30 minutes once weekly for 7 weeks followed by 1 week rest; then once weekly for 3 weeks out of every 4 weeks **or** (unlabeled combinations) 1000 mg/m^2 over 30 minutes weekly for up to 7 weeks followed by 1 week rest; then weekly for 3 weeks out of every 4 weeks (in combination with erlotinib) (Moore, 2007) **or** 1000 mg/m^2 over 30 minutes days 1, 8, and 15 every 28 days (in combination with capecitabine) (Cunningham, 2009) **or** 1000 mg/m^2 over 30 minutes days 1 and 15 every 28 days (in combination with cisplatin) (Heinemann, 2006) **or** 1000 mg/m^2 infused at 10 mg/m^2/minute every 14 days (in combination with oxaliplatin) (Louvet, 2005) **or** 1000 mg/m^2 days 1, 8, and 15 every 28 days (in combination with paclitaxel [protein bound]) (Von Hoff, 2013)

Bladder cancer (unlabeled use):

Advanced or metastatic: I.V.: 1000 mg/m^2 over 30-60 minutes days 1, 8, and 15; repeat cycle every 28 days (in combination with cisplatin) (von der Maase, 2000)

Transitional cell carcinoma: Intravesicular instillation: 2000 mg (in 100 mL NS; retain for 1 hour) twice weekly for 3 weeks; repeat cycle every 4 weeks for at least 2 cycles (Dalbagni, 2006)

Cervical cancer, recurrent or persistent (unlabeled use): I.V.: 1000 mg/m^2 days 1 and 8; repeat cycle every 21 days (in combination with cisplatin) (Monk, 2009) **or** 1250 mg/m^2 over 30 minutes days 1 and 8; repeat cycle every 21 days (in combination with cisplatin) (Burnett, 2000) **or** 800 mg/m^2 over 30 minutes days 1, 8, and 15; repeat cycle every 28 days (as a single-agent) (Schilder, 2005) **or** 800 mg/m^2 days 1 and 8; repeat cycle every 28 days (in combination with cisplatin) (Brewer, 2006)

Head and neck cancer, nasopharyngeal (unlabeled use): I.V.: 1000 mg/m^2 over 30 minutes days 1, 8, and 15 every 28 days (Zhang, 2008) **or** 1000 mg/m^2 over 30 minutes days 1 and 8 every 21 days (in combination with vinorelbine) (Chen, 2012)

Hepatobiliary cancer, advanced (unlabeled use): I.V.: 1000 mg/m^2 over 30 minutes days 1 and 8; repeat cycle every 21 days (in combination with cisplatin) (Valle, 2010) **or** 1000 mg/m^2 over 30 minutes days 1 and 8; repeat cycle every 21 days (in combination with capecitabine) (Knox, 2005) **or** 1000 mg/m^2 infused at 10 mg/m^2/minute every 2 weeks (in combination with oxaliplatin) (Andre, 2004)

Hodgkin lymphoma, relapsed (unlabeled use): I.V.: 1000 mg/m^2 (800 mg/m^2 for post-transplant patients) over 30 minutes days 1 and 8; repeat cycle every 21 days (in combination with vinorelbine and doxorubicin liposomal) (Bartlett, 2007) **or** 800 mg/m^2 days 1 and 4; repeat cycle every 21 days (in combination with ifosfamide, mesna, vinorelbine, and prednisolone) (Santoro, 2007)

Malignant pleural mesothelioma (unlabeled use; in combination with cisplatin): I.V.: 1000 mg/m^2 over 30 minutes days 1, 8 and 15 every 28 days for up to 6 cycles (Nowak, 2002) **or** 1250 mg/m^2 over 30 minutes days 1 and 8 every 21 days for up to 6 cycles (van Haarst, 2002)

Non-Hodgkin lymphoma, refractory (unlabeled use): I.V.: 1000 mg/m^2 over 30 minutes days 1 and 8; repeat cycle every 21 days (in combination with cisplatin and dexamethasone) (Crump, 2004) **or** 1000 mg/m^2 every 15-21days (in combination with oxaliplatin and rituximab) (Lopez, 2008)

Sarcoma (unlabeled uses): I.V.:

Ewing's sarcoma, refractory: 675 mg/m^2 over 90 minutes days 1 and 8; repeat cycle every 21 days (in combination with docetaxel) (Navid, 2008)

Osteosarcoma, refractory: 675 mg/m^2 over 90 minutes days 1 and 8; repeat cycle every 21 days (in combination with docetaxel) (Navid, 2008) **or** 1000 mg/m^2 weekly for 7 weeks followed by 1 week rest; then weekly for 3 weeks out of every 4 weeks (Merimsky, 2000)

Soft tissue sarcoma, advanced: 800 mg/m^2 over 90 minutes days 1 and 8; repeat cycle every 21 days (in combination with vinorelbine) (Dileo, 2007) **or** 675 mg/m^2 over 90 minutes days 1 and 8; repeat cycle every 21 days (in combination with docetaxel) (Leu, 2004) **or** 900 mg/m^2 over 90 minutes days 1 and 8; repeat cycle every 21 days (in combination with docetaxel) (Maki, 2007)

Small cell lung cancer, refractory or relapsed (unlabeled use): I.V.: 1000-1250 mg/m^2 over 30 minutes days 1, 8, and 15 every 28 days (as a single agent) (Masters, 2003)

Testicular cancer, refractory germ cell (unlabeled use): I.V.: 1000-1250 mg/m^2 over 30 minutes days 1 and 8 every 21 days (in combination with oxaliplatin) (DeGiorgi, 2006; Kohllmannsberger, 2004; Pectasides, 2004) **or** 1000 mg/m^2 over 30 minutes days 1, 8, and 15 every 28 days for up to 6 cycles (in combination with paclitaxel) (Hinton, 2002) **or** 800 mg/m^2 over 30 minutes days 1 and 8 every 21 days (in combination with oxaliplatin and paclitaxel) (Bokemeyer, 2008)

Unknown-primary, adenocarcinoma (unlabeled use): I.V.: 1250 mg/m^2 days 1 and 8 every 21 days (in combination with cisplatin) (Culine, 2003) **or** 1000 mg/m^2 over 30 minutes days 1 and 8 every 21 days for up to 6 cycles (in combination with docetaxel) (Pouessel, 2004)

Uterine cancer (unlabeled use): I.V.: 900 mg/m^2 over 90 minutes days 1 and 8 every 21 days (in combination with docetaxel) (Hensley, 2008) **or** 1000 mg/m^2 over 30 minutes days 1, 8, and 15 every 28 days (Look, 2004)

Dosing adjustment for toxicity:

Nonhematologic toxicity (all indications):

Hold or decrease gemcitabine dose by 50% for the following: Severe (grade 3 or 4) nonhematologic toxicity until resolved (excludes nausea, vomiting, or alopecia [no dose modifications recommended])

Permanently discontinue gemcitabine for any of the following: Unexplained dyspnea (or other evidence of severe pulmonary toxicity), severe hepatotoxicity, hemolytic uremic syndrome (HUS), capillary leak syndrome (CLS)

Hematologic toxicity:

Breast cancer:

Day 1:

Absolute granulocyte count (AGC) ≥1500/mm^3 and platelet count ≥100,000/mm^3: Administer 100% of full dose

AGC <1500/mm^3 or platelet count <100,000/mm^3: Hold dose

Day 8:

AGC ≥1200/mm^3 and platelet count >75,000/mm^3: Administer 100% of full dose

AGC 1000-1199/mm^3 or platelet count 50,000-75,000/mm^3: Administer 75% of full dose

AGC 700-999/mm^3 and platelet count ≥50,000/mm^3: Administer 50% of full dose

AGC <700/mm^3 or platelet count <50,000/mm^3: Hold dose

Nonsmall cell lung cancer (cisplatin dosage may also require adjustment):

AGC ≥1000/mm^3 and platelet count ≥100,000/mm^3: Administer 100% of full dose

AGC 500-999/mm^3 or platelet count 50,000-99,999/mm^3: Administer 75% of full dose

AGC <500/mm^3 or platelet count <50,000/mm^3: Hold dose

Ovarian cancer:

Day 1:

AGC ≥1500/mm^3 and platelet count ≥100,000/mm^3: Administer 100% of full dose

AGC <1500/mm^3 or platelet count <100,000/mm^3: Delay treatment cycle

Day 8:

AGC ≥1500/mm^3 and platelet count ≥100,000/mm^3: Administer 100% of full dose

AGC 1000-1499/mm^3 or platelet count 75,000-99,999/mm^3: Administer 50% of full dose

AGC <1000/mm^3 or platelet count <75,000/mm^3: Hold dose

Hematologic toxicity in previous cycle (dosing adjustment for subsequent cycles):

Initial occurrence: AGC <500/mm^3 for >5 days, AGC <100/mm^3 for >3 days, febrile neutropenia, platelet count <25,000/mm^3, or cycle delay >1 week due to toxicity: Permanently reduce gemcitabine to 800 mg/m^2 on days 1 and 8.

Subsequent occurrence: AGC <500/mm^3 for >5 days, AGC <100/mm^3 for >3 days, neutropenic fever, platelet count <25,000/mm^3, or cycle delay >1 week due to toxicity: Permanently reduce gemcitabine to 800 mg/m^2 and administer on day 1 only.

Pancreatic cancer:

AGC ≥1000/mm^3 and platelet count ≥100,000/mm^3: Administer 100% of full dose

AGC 500-999/mm^3 or platelet count 50,000-99,999/mm^3: Administer 75% of full dose

AGC <500/mm^3 or platelet count <50,000/mm^3: Hold dose

Dosing adjustment in renal impairment: No dosage adjustment provided in manufacturer's labeling; use with caution in patients with pre-existing renal dysfunction. Discontinue if severe renal toxicity or hemolytic uremic syndrome (HUS) occur during gemcitabine treatment.

Mild-to-severe renal impairment: No dosage adjustment necessary (Janus, 2010; Li, 2007)

ESRD (on hemodialysis): Hemodialysis should begin 6-12 hours after gemcitabine infusion (Janus 2010; Li, 2007)

Dosing adjustment in hepatic impairment: No dosage adjustment provided in manufacturer's labeling; use with caution. Discontinue if severe hepatotoxicity occurs during gemcitabine treatment. The following adjustments have been reported:

Transaminases elevated (with normal bilirubin): No dosage adjustment necessary (Venook, 2000)

Serum bilirubin >1.6 mg/dL: Use initial dose of 800 mg/m^2; may escalate if tolerated (Ecklund, 2005; Floyd, 2006; Venook, 2000)

Dosing in obesity: *ASCO Guidelines for appropriate chemotherapy dosing in obese adults with cancer:* Utilize patient's actual body weight (full weight) for calculation of body surface area- or weight-based dosing, particularly when the intent of therapy is curative; manage regimen-related toxicities in the same manner as for nonobese patients; if a dose reduction is utilized due to toxicity, consider resumption of full weight-based dosing with subsequent cycles, especially if cause of toxicity (eg, hepatic or renal impairment) is resolved (Griggs, 2012).

Administration Infuse over 30 minutes; for unlabeled uses, infusion times may vary (refer to specific references). **Note:** Prolongation of the infusion time >60 minutes has been shown to increase toxicity. Gemcitabine has been administered at a fixed-dose rate (FDR) infusion rate of 10 mg/m^2/minute to optimize the pharmacokinetics (unlabeled); prolonged infusion times increase the intracellular accumulation of the active metabolite, gemcitabine triphosphate (Ko, 2006; Tempero, 2003). Patients who receive gemcitabine FDR experience more grade 3/4 hematologic toxicity (Ko, 2006; Poplin, 2009).

For intravesicular (bladder) instillation, gemcitabine was diluted in 50-100 mL normal saline; patients were instructed to retain in the bladder for 1 hour (Addeo, 2010; Dalbaghi, 2006)

Hazardous agent; use appropriate precautions for handling and disposal (NIOSH, 2012).

Monitoring Parameters CBC with differential and platelet count (prior to each dose); hepatic and renal function (prior to initiation of therapy and periodically, thereafter); monitor electrolytes, including potassium, magnesium, and calcium (when in combination therapy with cisplatin); monitor pulmonary function; signs/symptoms of capillary leak syndrome

Dosage Forms Excipient information presented when available (limited, particularly for generics); consult specific product labeling.

Solution, Intravenous:
- Generic: 200 mg/5.26 mL (5.26 mL); 1 g/26.3 mL (26.3 mL); 2 g/52.6 mL (52.6 mL)

Solution Reconstituted, Intravenous:
- Gemzar: 200 mg (1 ea); 1 g (1 ea)
- Generic: 200 mg (1 ea); 1 g (1 ea); 2 g (1 ea)

Solution Reconstituted, Intravenous [preservative free]:
- Generic: 200 mg (1 ea); 1 g (1 ea)

◆ **Gemcitabine For Injection (Can)** *see* Gemcitabine *on page 943*

◆ **Gemcitabine For Injection, USP (Can)** *see* Gemcitabine *on page 943*

◆ **Gemcitabine Hydrochloride** *see* Gemcitabine *on page 943*

◆ **Gemcitabine Hydrochloride For Injection (Can)** *see* Gemcitabine *on page 943*

◆ **Gemcitabine Injection (Can)** *see* Gemcitabine *on page 943*

◆ **Gemcitabine Sun For Injection (Can)** *see* Gemcitabine *on page 943*

Gemfibrozil (jem FI broe zil)

Brand Names: U.S. Lopid

Brand Names: Canada Apo-Gemfibrozil; Gen-Gemfibrozil; GMD-Gemfibrozil; Lopid; Mylan-Gemfibrozil; Novo-Gemfibrozil; Nu-Gemfibrozil; PMS-Gemfibrozil

Index Terms CI-719

Pharmacologic Category Antilipemic Agent, Fibric Acid

Use Treatment of hypertriglyceridemia in Fredrickson types IV and V hyperlipidemia for patients who are at greater risk for pancreatitis and who have not responded to dietary intervention; to reduce the risk of CHD development in Fredrickson type IIb patients without a history or symptoms of existing CHD who have not responded to dietary and other interventions (including pharmacologic treatment) and who have decreased HDL, increased LDL, and increased triglycerides

Pregnancy Risk Factor C

Pregnancy Considerations Adverse events were observed in animal reproduction studies. The Canadian product labeling specifically contraindicates use during pregnancy and recommends gemfibrozil be discontinued several months prior to conception.

Breast-Feeding Considerations It is not known if gemfibrozil is excreted in breast milk. Due to the potential for serious adverse reactions in the nursing infant, a decision should be made whether to discontinue nursing or to discontinue the drug, taking into account the importance of treatment to the mother. The Canadian product labeling specifically contraindicates use during breast-feeding.

Contraindications Hypersensitivity to gemfibrozil or any component of the formulation; hepatic or severe renal dysfunction; primary biliary cirrhosis; pre-existing gallbladder disease; concurrent use with repaglinide

Warnings/Precautions Secondary causes of hyperlipidemia should be ruled out prior to therapy. Possible increased risk of malignancy and cholelithiasis. Anemia, leukopenia, thrombocytopenia, and bone marrow hypoplasia have rarely been reported. Periodic monitoring recommended during the first year of therapy. Elevations in serum transaminases can be seen. Discontinue if lipid response not seen. Be careful in patient selection; this is not a first- or second-line choice. Other agents may be more suitable. Has been associated with rare myositis or rhabdomyolysis; patients should be monitored closely. Patients should be instructed to report unexplained muscle pain, tenderness, weakness, or brown urine. Potentially significant drug-drug interactions may exist, requiring dose or frequency adjustment, additional monitoring, and/or selection of alternative therapy. Use with caution in patients with mild-to-moderate renal impairment; contraindicated in patients with severe impairment. Renal function deterioration has been seen when used in patients with a serum creatinine >2 mg/dL.

Adverse Reactions

>10%: Gastrointestinal: Dyspepsia (20%)

1% to 10%:
- Cardiovascular: Atrial fibrillation (1%)
- Central nervous system: Fatigue (4%), vertigo (2%)
- Dermatologic: Eczema (2%), rash (2%)
- Gastrointestinal: Abdominal pain (10%), nausea/vomiting (3%)

<1% or case reports with probable causation (limited to important or life-threatening): Alkaline phosphatase increased, anemia, angioedema, arthralgia, bilirubin increased, blurred vision, bone marrow hypoplasia, cholelithiasis, cholecystitis, cholestatic jaundice, creatine phosphokinase increased, depression, dermatitis, dermatomyositis/polymyositis, dizziness, eosinophilia, exfoliative dermatitis, headache, hypoesthesia, hypokalemia, impotence, laryngeal edema, leukopenia, libido decreased, myalgia, myasthenia, myopathy, nephrotoxicity, painful extremities, paresthesia, peripheral neuritis, pruritus, Raynaud's phenomenon, rhabdomyolysis, somnolence, synovitis, taste perversion, transaminases increased, urticaria

Reports where causal relationship has not been established: Alopecia, anaphylaxis, cataracts, colitis, confusion, decreased fertility (male), drug-induced lupus-like syndrome, extrasystoles, hepatoma, intracranial hemorrhage, pancreatitis, peripheral vascular disease, photosensitivity, positive ANA, renal dysfunction, retinal edema, seizure, syncope, thrombocytopenia, vasculitis, weight loss

Drug Interactions

Metabolism/Transport Effects **Substrate** of CYP3A4 (minor); **Note:** Assignment of Major/Minor substrate status based on clinically relevant drug interaction potential; **Inhibits** CYP1A2 (moderate), CYP2C19 (strong), CYP2C8 (strong), CYP2C9 (strong)

Avoid Concomitant Use

Avoid concomitant use of Gemfibrozil with any of the following: AtorvaSTATin; Bexarotene (Systemic); Enzalutamide; Fluvastatin; Lovastatin; Pirfenidone; Pitavastatin; Pravastatin; Repaglinide; Rosuvastatin; Simvastatin

Increased Effect/Toxicity

Gemfibrozil may increase the levels/effects of: Agomelatine; Antidiabetic Agents (Thiazolidinedione); AtorvaSTATin; Bexarotene (Systemic); Bosentan; Carvedilol; Citalopram; Colchicine; CYP1A2 Substrates; CYP2C19 Substrates; CYP2C8 Substrates; CYP2C9 Substrates; Diclofenac (Systemic); Enzalutamide; Ezetimibe; Fluvastatin; Lacosamide; Lovastatin; Ospemifene; Pirfenidone;

Pitavastatin; Pravastatin; Repaglinide; Rosuvastatin; Simvastatin; Sulfonylureas; Treprostinil; Vitamin K Antagonists

The levels/effects of Gemfibrozil may be increased by: CycloSPORINE (Systemic); Raltegravir

Decreased Effect

Gemfibrozil may decrease the levels/effects of: Chenodiol; Clopidogrel; CycloSPORINE (Systemic); Imatinib; Ursodiol

The levels/effects of Gemfibrozil may be decreased by: Bile Acid Sequestrants

Ethanol/Nutrition/Herb Interactions

Ethanol: Avoid ethanol to decrease triglycerides.

Food: When given after meals, the AUC of gemfibrozil is decreased.

Storage/Stability Store at controlled room temperature of 20°C to 25°C (68°F to 77°F). Protect from light and moisture.

Mechanism of Action The exact mechanism of action of gemfibrozil is unknown, however, several theories exist regarding the VLDL effect; it can inhibit lipolysis and decrease subsequent hepatic fatty acid uptake as well as inhibit hepatic secretion of VLDL; together these actions decrease serum VLDL levels; increases HDL-cholesterol; the mechanism behind HDL elevation is currently unknown

Pharmacodynamics/Kinetics

Onset of action: May require several days

Absorption: Well absorbed

Protein binding: 99%

Metabolism: Hepatic via oxidation to two inactive metabolites; undergoes enterohepatic recycling

Half-life elimination: 1.5 hours

Time to peak, serum: 1-2 hours

Excretion: Urine (~70% primarily as conjugated drug); feces (6%)

Dosage Adults: Oral: 600 mg twice daily; administer 30 minutes before breakfast and dinner

Dosage adjustment in renal impairment:

Mild-to-moderate impairment: Use caution; deterioration of renal function has been reported in patients with baseline serum creatinine >2 mg/dL

Severe impairment: Use is contraindicated

Hemodialysis: Not removed by hemodialysis; supplemental dose is not necessary

Dosage adjustment in hepatic impairment: Use is contraindicated

Dietary Considerations Before initiation of therapy, patients should be placed on a standard cholesterol-lowering diet for 3-6 months and the diet should be continued during drug therapy. Should be taken 30 minutes prior to breakfast and dinner

Administration Administer 30 minutes prior to breakfast and dinner.

Monitoring Parameters Serum cholesterol, LFTs periodically, CBC periodically (first year)

Dosage Forms Excipient information presented when available (limited, particularly for generics); consult specific product labeling.

Tablet, Oral:

Lopid: 600 mg [scored]

Generic: 600 mg

Gemifloxacin (je mi FLOKS a sin)

Brand Names: U.S. Factive

Brand Names: Canada Factive®

Index Terms DW286; Gemifloxacin Mesylate; LA 20304a; SB-265805

Pharmacologic Category Antibiotic, Fluoroquinolone; Antibiotic, Respiratory Fluoroquinolone

Use Treatment of acute exacerbation of chronic bronchitis; treatment of community-acquired pneumonia (CAP), including pneumonia caused by multidrug-resistant strains of *S. pneumoniae* (MDRSP)

Unlabeled Use Acute sinusitis

Pregnancy Risk Factor C

Pregnancy Considerations Adverse events have been observed in some animal studies; therefore, the manufacturer classifies gemifloxacin as pregnancy category C. Quinolone exposure during human pregnancy has been reported with other agents (see Ciprofloxacin [Systemic], Ofloxacin [Systemic], and Norfloxacin monographs). To date, no specific teratogenic effect or increased pregnancy risk has been identified; however, because of concerns of cartilage damage in immature animals exposed to quinolones and the limited gemifloxacin specific data, gemifloxacin should only be used during pregnancy if a safer option is not available.

Breast-Feeding Considerations It is not known if gemifloxacin is excreted in breast milk. Breast-feeding is not recommended by the manufacturer. Nondose-related effects could include modification of bowel flora.

Medication Guide Available Yes

Contraindications Hypersensitivity to gemifloxacin, other fluoroquinolones, or any component of the formulation

Warnings/Precautions [U.S. Boxed Warning]: There have been reports of tendon inflammation and/or rupture with quinolone antibiotics; risk may be increased with concurrent corticosteroids, organ transplant recipients, and in patients >60 years of age. Rupture of the Achilles tendon sometimes requiring surgical repair has been reported most frequently; but other tendon sites (eg, rotator cuff, biceps) have also been reported. Strenuous physical activity, rheumatoid arthritis, and renal impairment may be an independent risk factor for tendonitis. Discontinue at first sign of tendon inflammation or pain. May occur even after discontinuation of therapy. Use with caution in patients with rheumatoid arthritis; may increase risk of tendon rupture. Fluoroquinolones may prolong QT_c interval; avoid use of gemifloxacin in patients with a history of QT_c prolongation, uncorrected hypokalemia, hypomagnesemia, or concurrent administration of other medications known to prolong the QT interval (including Class Ia and Class III antiarrhythmics, cisapride, erythromycin, antipsychotics, and tricyclic antidepressants). Use with caution in patients with significant bradycardia or acute myocardial ischemia. CNS effects may occur (tremor, restlessness, confusion, and very rarely hallucinations, increased intracranial pressure [including pseudotumor cerebri] or seizures). Use with caution in patients with known or suspected CNS disorder. Potential for seizures, although very rare, may be increased with concomitant NSAID therapy. Use with caution in individuals at risk of seizures. Use caution in renal dysfunction; dosage adjustment required for Cl_{cr} ≤40 mL/minute.

Fluoroquinolones have been associated with the development of serious, and sometimes fatal, hypoglycemia, most often in elderly diabetics, but also in patients without diabetes. This occurred most frequently with gatifloxacin (no longer available systemically) but may occur at a lower frequency with other quinolones.

Severe hypersensitivity reactions, including anaphylaxis, have occurred with quinolone therapy. Reactions may present as typical allergic symptoms after a single dose, or may manifest as severe idiosyncratic dermatologic, vascular, pulmonary, renal, hepatic, and/or hematologic events, usually after multiple doses. May cause maculopapular rash, usually 8-10 days after treatment initiation; risk factors may include age <40 years, female gender (including postmenopausal women on HRT), and treatment duration >7 days. Prompt discontinuation of drug should occur if skin rash or other symptoms arise. **[U.S. Boxed Warning]: Quinolones may exacerbate myasthenia gravis; avoid use (rare, potentially life-threatening weakness of respiratory muscles may occur).** Avoid excessive sunlight and take precautions to limit exposure (eg, loose fitting clothing, sunscreen); may cause moderate-to-severe phototoxicity reactions. Discontinue use if photosensitivity occurs. Prolonged use may result in fungal or bacterial superinfection, including *C. difficile*-associated diarrhea (CDAD) and pseudomembranous colitis; CDAD has been observed >2 months postantibiotic treatment. Peripheral neuropathy has been reported (rare); may occur soon after initiation of therapy and may be irreversible; discontinue if symptoms of sensory or sensorimotor neuropathy occur. Hemolytic reactions may (rarely) occur with quinolone use in patients with latent or actual G6PD deficiency.

Adverse Reactions

1% to 10%:

Central nervous system: Headache (4%), dizziness (2%)

Dermatologic: Rash (4%)

Gastrointestinal: Diarrhea (5%), nausea (4%), abdominal pain (2%), vomiting (2%)

Hematologic: Neutropenia/neutrophilia (1%), platelets increased (1%), thrombocythemia (1%)

Hepatic: Transaminases increased (1% to 4%), GGT increased (1%)

Neuromuscular & skeletal: CPK increased (1%)

<1% (Limited to important or life-threatening): Acute renal failure, alkaline phosphatase increased, anaphylactic reaction, anemia, anorexia, arthralgia, back pain, bilirubin increased, BUN increased, constipation, cramps (leg), dermatitis, dyspepsia, dyspnea, eczema, eosinophilia, erythema multiforme, facial edema, fatigue, flatulence, flushing, fungal infection, gastritis, gastroenteritis, genital moniliasis, granulocytopenia, hematocrit decreased/increased, hemoglobin decreased/increased, hemorrhage, hot flashes, hyperglycemia, hyper-/hypocalcemia, hyper-/hypokalemia, hyper-/hyponatremia, hypoalbuminemia, INR increased, insomnia, intracranial pressure increased, leukopenia, moniliasis, myalgia, myasthenia gravis exacerbation, nervousness, pain, pharyngitis, photosensitivity, pneumonia, pruritus, pseudomembranous colitis, pseudotumor cerebri, QT_c prolongation, retinal hemorrhage, serum creatinine increased, skin exfoliation, somnolence, supraventricular tachycardia, syncope, taste perversion, tendonitis, tendon rupture, thrombocytopenia, TIA, tremor, urticaria, vaginitis, vertigo, vision abnormal, weakness, xerostomia

Important adverse effects reported with other agents in this drug class include (not reported for gemifloxacin): Allergic reactions, CNS stimulation, hepatic necrosis/failure, hepatitis, hypersensitivity, jaundice, pancytopenia, peripheral neuropathy, pneumonitis (eosinophilic), seizure, sensorimotor-axonal neuropathy (paresthesia, hypoesthesias, dysesthesias, weakness), serum sickness, severe dermatologic reactions (toxic epidermal necrolysis, Stevens-Johnson syndrome), thrombotic thrombocytopenia purpura, torsade de pointes, vasculitis

Drug Interactions

Metabolism/Transport Effects None known.

Avoid Concomitant Use

Avoid concomitant use of Gemifloxacin with any of the following: BCG; Highest Risk QTc-Prolonging Agents; Ivabradine; Mifepristone; Strontium Ranelate

Increased Effect/Toxicity

Gemifloxacin may increase the levels/effects of: Corticosteroids (Systemic); Highest Risk QTc-Prolonging Agents; Moderate Risk QTc-Prolonging Agents; Porfimer; Sulfonylureas; Varenicline; Vitamin K Antagonists

The levels/effects of Gemifloxacin may be increased by: Insulin; Ivabradine; Mifepristone; Nonsteroidal Anti-Inflammatory Agents; Probenecid; QTc-Prolonging Agents (Indeterminate Risk and Risk Modifying)

Decreased Effect

Gemifloxacin may decrease the levels/effects of: BCG; Didanosine; Mycophenolate; Sodium Picosulfate; Sulfonylureas; Typhoid Vaccine

The levels/effects of Gemifloxacin may be decreased by: Antacids; Calcium Salts; Didanosine; Iron Salts; Magnesium Salts; Multivitamins/Minerals (with ADEK, Folate, Iron); Multivitamins/Minerals (with AE, No Iron); Quinapril; Sevelamer; Strontium Ranelate; Sucralfate; Zinc Salts

Ethanol/Nutrition/Herb Interactions Herb/Nutraceutical: Avoid dong quai, St John's wort (may also cause photosensitization).

Storage/Stability Store at 25°C (77°F). Protect from light.

Mechanism of Action Gemifloxacin is a DNA gyrase inhibitor and also inhibits topoisomerase IV. DNA gyrase (topoisomerase IV) is an essential bacterial enzyme that maintains the superhelical structure of DNA. DNA gyrase is required for DNA replication and transcription, DNA repair, recombination, and transposition; bactericidal

Pharmacodynamics/Kinetics

Absorption: Well absorbed from the GI tract

Distribution: V_{dss}: 4.2 L/kg

Protein binding: ~60% to 70%

Metabolism: Hepatic (minor); forms metabolites (CYP isoenzymes are not involved)

Bioavailability: ~71%

Half-life elimination: 7 hours (range 4-12 hours)

Time to peak, plasma: 0.5-2 hours

Excretion: Feces (61%); urine (36%)

Dosage

Usual dosage range:

Adults: Oral: 320 mg once daily

Indication-specific dosing:

Adults: Oral:

Acute exacerbations of chronic bronchitis: 320 mg once daily for 5 days

Community-acquired pneumonia (mild-to-moderate): 320 mg once daily for 5 or 7 days (decision to use 5- or 7-day regimen should be guided by initial sputum culture; 7 days are recommended for MDRSP, *Klebsiella*, or *M. catarrhalis* infection)

Sinusitis (unlabeled use): 320 mg once daily for 10 days

Elderly: Refer to adult dosing.

Dosage adjustment in renal impairment:

Cl_{cr} >40 mL/minute: No adjustment required

Cl_{cr} ≤40 mL/minute (or patients on hemodialysis/CAPD): 160 mg once daily (administer dose following hemodialysis)

Dosage adjustment in hepatic impairment: No adjustment required

Dietary Considerations May take tablets with or without food, milk, or calcium supplements. Gemifloxacin should be taken 3 hours before or 2 hours after supplements (including multivitamins) containing iron, zinc, or magnesium.

Administration May be administered with or without food, milk, or calcium supplements. Gemifloxacin should be taken 3 hours before or 2 hours after supplements (including multivitamins) containing iron, zinc, or magnesium.

Monitoring Parameters WBC, signs/symptoms of infection, renal function

Dosage Forms Excipient information presented when available (limited, particularly for generics); consult specific product labeling.

Tablet, Oral:

Factive: 320 mg [scored]

◆ **Gemifloxacin Mesylate** *see* Gemifloxacin *on page 948*

Gemtuzumab Ozogamicin

(gem TOO zoo mab oh zog a MY sin)

Index Terms CMA-676; Mylotarg

Pharmacologic Category Antineoplastic Agent, Monoclonal Antibody

Use Due to safety concerns, as well as lack of clinical benefit demonstrated in a post-approval clinical trial, gemtuzumab was withdrawn from the U.S. commercial market in 2010.

Unlabeled Use Treatment of relapsed or refractory CD33-positive acute myeloid leukemia (AML); salvage therapy for acute promyelocytic leukemia (APL)

Pregnancy Considerations Teratogenic effects have been observed in animal reproduction studies. May cause fetal harm when administered to a pregnant woman. Women of childbearing potential should avoid becoming pregnant while receiving treatment.

Breast-Feeding Considerations It is not known if gemtuzumab ozogamicin is excreted in breast milk. Because human IgG is secreted in breast milk and the potential for serious adverse reactions in the nursing infant exists, a decision should be made whether to discontinue nursing or to discontinue the drug, taking into account the importance of treatment to the mother.

Prescribing and Access Restrictions As of June 2010, gemtuzumab has been withdrawn from the U.S. market and is no longer commercially available to new patients; gemtuzumab is only available in the U.S. under an Investigational New Drug (IND) protocol.

In Canada, gemtuzumab is available through a special access program (access information is available from Health Canada).

Contraindications Hypersensitivity to gemtuzumab ozogamicin, calicheamicin derivatives, or any component of the formulation; patients with anti-CD33 antibody

Warnings/Precautions Hazardous agent - use appropriate precautions for handling and disposal (NIOSH, 2012).

Gemtuzumab has been associated with hepatotoxicity, including severe hepatic sinusoidal obstruction syndrome (SOS; formerly called veno-occlusive disease [VOD]). Symptoms of SOS include right upper quadrant pain, rapid weight gain, ascites, hepatomegaly, and bilirubin/transaminase elevations. Risk may be increased by combination chemotherapy, underlying hepatic disease, or hematopoietic stem cell transplant.

Severe hypersensitivity reactions (including anaphylaxis) and other infusion-related reactions may occur. Infusion-related events are common, generally reported to occur with the first dose after the end of the 2-hour intravenous infusion. These symptoms usually resolved after 2-4 hours with a supportive therapy of acetaminophen, diphenhydramine, and intravenous fluids. Other severe and potentially fatal infusion related pulmonary events (including dyspnea and hypoxia) have been reported infrequently. Symptomatic intrinsic lung disease or high peripheral blast counts may increase the risk of severe reactions. Fewer infusion-related events were observed after the second dose. Postinfusion reactions (may include fever, chills, hypotension, or dyspnea) may occur during the first 24 hours after administration. Consider discontinuation in patients who develop severe infusion-related reactions. In addition to infusion-related pulmonary events, gemtuzumab therapy is also associated with acute respiratory distress syndrome, pulmonary infiltrates, pleural effusion, noncardiogenic pulmonary edema, and pulmonary insufficiency.

Severe myelosuppression occurs in all patients at recommended dosages. Tumor lysis syndrome may occur as a consequence of leukemia treatment, adequate hydration and prophylactic allopurinol must be instituted prior to use. Other methods to lower WBC <30,000 cells/mm^3 may be considered (hydroxyurea or leukapheresis) to minimize the risk of tumor lysis syndrome, and/or severe infusion reactions. An increased number of deaths have been reported in patients receiving gemtuzumab in combination with chemotherapy, compared to those receiving chemotherapy alone.

Adverse Reactions Frequency not defined.

Cardiovascular: Cerebral hemorrhage, hyper-/hypotension, peripheral edema, tachycardia

Central nervous system: Anxiety, chills, depression, dizziness, fever, headache, insomnia, intracranial hemorrhage, pain

Dermatologic: Bruising, petechiae, pruritus, rash

Endocrine & metabolic: Hyperglycemia, hypocalcemia, hypokalemia, hypomagnesemia, hypophosphatemia

Gastrointestinal: Abdominal pain, anorexia, diarrhea, dyspepsia, gingival hemorrhage, melena, mucositis, nausea, stomatitis, vomiting

Genitourinary: Vaginal bleeding, vaginal hemorrhage

Hematologic: Anemia, disseminated intravascular coagulation (DIC), hemorrhage, leukopenia, lymphopenia, neutropenia (median recovery 40-51 days), neutropenic fever, thrombocytopenia (median recovery 36-51 days)

Hepatic: Alkaline phosphatase increased, ALT increased, ascites, AST increased, hyperbilirubinemia, LDH increased, prothrombin time increased, PTT increased, sinusoidal obstruction syndrome (SOS; veno-occlusive disease; higher frequency in patients with prior history of or subsequent hematopoietic stem cell transplant)

Local: Local reaction

Neuromuscular & skeletal: Arthralgia, back pain, myalgia, weakness

Renal: Creatinine increased, hematuria

Respiratory: Cough, dyspnea, epistaxis, hypoxia, pharyngitis, pneumonia, rhinitis

Miscellaneous: Cutaneous herpes simplex, infection, infusion reaction, sepsis

Infrequent and/or case reports (limited to important or life-threatening): Acute respiratory distress syndrome, anaphylaxis, bradycardia, Budd-Chiari syndrome, gastrointestinal hemorrhage, hepatic failure, hepatosplenomegaly, hypersensitivity reactions, jaundice, neutropenic sepsis, noncardiogenic pulmonary edema, portal vain thrombosis, pulmonary hemorrhage, renal impairment, renal failure (including renal failure secondary to tumor lysis syndrome)

Drug Interactions

Metabolism/Transport Effects None known.

Avoid Concomitant Use

Avoid concomitant use of Gemtuzumab Ozogamicin with any of the following: BCG; Belimumab; CloZAPine; Natalizumab; Pimecrolimus; Tacrolimus (Topical); Tofacitinib; Vaccines (Live)

Increased Effect/Toxicity

Gemtuzumab Ozogamicin may increase the levels/effects of: Belimumab; CloZAPine; Leflunomide; Natalizumab; Tofacitinib; Vaccines (Live)

The levels/effects of Gemtuzumab Ozogamicin may be increased by: Abciximab; Denosumab; Pimecrolimus; Roflumilast; Tacrolimus (Topical); Trastuzumab

Decreased Effect

Gemtuzumab Ozogamicin may decrease the levels/effects of: BCG; Coccidioidin Skin Test; Sipuleucel-T; Vaccines (Inactivated); Vaccines (Live)

The levels/effects of Gemtuzumab Ozogamicin may be decreased by: Echinacea

Preparation for Administration Hazardous agent; use appropriate precautions for handling and disposal (NIOSH, 2012). Protect from light during preparation (and administration). Prepare in biologic safety hood with shielded fluorescent light; (some institutions prepare in a darkened room with the lights in the biologic safety cabinet turned off). Allow to warm to room temperature prior to reconstitution. Reconstitute each 5 mg vial with sterile water for injection to a concentration of 1 mg/mL. Dilute in 100 mL of 0.9% sodium chloride injection.

Storage/Stability Light sensitive; protect from light (including direct and indirect sunlight, and unshielded fluorescent light). The infusion container should be placed in a UV protectant bag immediately after preparation. Store intact vials under refrigeration at 2°C to 8°C (36°F to 46°F). Reconstituted solutions may be stored for up to 2 hours at room temperature or under refrigeration. Following dilution for infusion, solutions are stable for up to 16 hours at room temperature. Administration requires 2 hours; therefore, the maximum elapsed time from initial reconstitution to completion of infusion should be 20 hours.

Mechanism of Action Antibody to CD33 antigen, which is expressed on leukemic blasts in 80% of AML patients. Binds to the CD33 antigen, resulting in internalization of the antibody-antigen complex. Following internalization, the calicheamicin derivative is released inside the myeloid cell. The calicheamicin derivative binds to DNA resulting in double strand breaks and cell death. Pluripotent stem cells and nonhematopoietic cells are not affected.

Pharmacodynamics/Kinetics

Distribution: V_{ss}: Adults: Initial dose: 21 L; Repeat dose: 10 L

Half-life elimination: Total calicheamicin: Initial: 41-45 hours, Repeat dose: 60-64 hours; Unconjugated: 100-143 hours (no change noted in repeat dosing)

Dosage I.V.: Adults: **Note:** Patients should receive diphenhydramine 50 mg orally and acetaminophen 650-1000 mg orally 1 hour prior to administration of each dose. Acetaminophen dosage should be repeated as needed every 4 hours for 2 additional doses. Pretreatment with methylprednisolone may ameliorate infusion-related symptoms.

AML (unlabeled/investigational use):

<60 years: 9 mg/m^2 infused over 2 hours. A full treatment course is a total of 2 doses administered with 14-28 days between doses (Larson, 2005).

≥60 years: 9 mg/m^2 infused over 2 hours. A full treatment course is a total of 2 doses administered with 14-28 days between doses (Larson, 2002; Larson, 2005).

APL (unlabeled/investigational use):

Single-agent therapy: 6 mg/m^2 infused over 2 hours on days 1 and 15; for patients testing PCR negative after 2 doses, a third dose was administered (LoCoco, 2004).

Combination therapy (high-risk patients; Ravandi, 2009):

Induction: 9 mg/m^2 as a single dose on day 1 (in combination with arsenic trioxide and tretinoin)

Post remission therapy (if arsenic trioxide or tretinoin discontinued due to toxicity): 9 mg/m^2 once every 4-5 weeks until 28 weeks after complete remission

Dosage adjustment for toxicity:

Dyspnea or significant hypotension: Interrupt infusion; monitor

Anaphylaxis, pulmonary edema, acute respiratory distress syndrome: Strongly consider discontinuing treatment

Dosage adjustment in renal impairment: No dosage adjustment provided in manufacturer's labeling (has not been studied).

Dosage adjustment in hepatic impairment: No dosage adjustment provided in manufacturer's labeling (has not been studied); use with caution.

Administration Do not administer as I.V. push or bolus. Administer via I.V. infusion, over at least 2 hours through a low protein-binding (0.2-1.2 micron) in-line filter. Protect from light during infusion. Premedicate with acetaminophen and diphenhydramine prior to each infusion.

Hazardous agent; use appropriate precautions for handling and disposal (NIOSH, 2012).

Monitoring Parameters Monitor vital signs during the infusion and for 4 hours following the infusion. Monitor for signs/symptoms of postinfusion reaction. Monitor electrolytes, liver function, CBC with differential and platelets frequently. Monitor for signs and symptoms of hepatic sinusoidal obstruction syndrome (SOS; veno-occlusive disease; weight gain, right upper quadrant abdominal pain, hepatomegaly, ascites).

Product Availability No longer commercially available in the U.S. market for new patients. Available in Canada through a special access program.

- **Gemzar** *see* Gemcitabine *on page 943*
- **Genahist [OTC]** *see* DiphenhydrAMINE (Systemic) *on page 622*
- **Genaphed [OTC]** *see* Pseudoephedrine *on page 1746*
- **Gen-Clozapine (Can)** *see* CloZAPine *on page 477*
- **Gen-Combo Sterinebs (Can)** *see* Ipratropium and Albuterol *on page 1113*
- **Gen-Doxazosin (Can)** *see* Doxazosin *on page 656*
- **Gene-Activated Human Acid-Beta-Glucosidase** *see* Velaglucerase Alfa *on page 2176*
- **Generess Fe** *see* Ethinyl Estradiol and Norethindrone *on page 793*
- **Generlac** *see* Lactulose *on page 1161*
- **Gen-Fluoxetine (Can)** *see* FLUoxetine *on page 885*
- **Gen-Gemfibrozil (Can)** *see* Gemfibrozil *on page 947*
- **Gengraf** *see* CycloSPORINE (Systemic) *on page 508*
- **Gen-Hydroxychloroquine (Can)** *see* Hydroxychloroquine *on page 1019*
- **Gen-Hydroxyurea (Can)** *see* Hydroxyurea *on page 1022*
- **Gen-Ipratropium (Can)** *see* Ipratropium (Systemic) *on page 1111*
- **Gen-Medroxy (Can)** *see* MedroxyPROGESTERone *on page 1278*
- **Gen-Nabumetone (Can)** *see* Nabumetone *on page 1413*
- **Gen-Nizatidine (Can)** *see* Nizatidine *on page 1470*
- **Genotropin** *see* Somatropin *on page 1934*
- **Genotropin MiniQuick** *see* Somatropin *on page 1934*
- **Genpril [OTC]** *see* Ibuprofen *on page 1032*
- **Gen-Selegiline (Can)** *see* Selegiline *on page 1884*
- **Gentak** *see* Gentamicin (Ophthalmic) *on page 954*
- **Gentak® (Can)** *see* Gentamicin (Ophthalmic) *on page 954*

Gentamicin (Systemic) (jen ta MYE sin)

Brand Names: Canada Gentamicin Injection, USP

Index Terms Gentamicin Sulfate

Pharmacologic Category Antibiotic, Aminoglycoside

Additional Appendix Information

Antibiotic Treatment of Adults With Infective Endocarditis *on page 2355*

Use Treatment of susceptible bacterial infections, normally gram-negative organisms, including *Pseudomonas*, *Proteus*, *Serratia*, and gram-positive *Staphylococcus*; treatment of bone infections, respiratory tract infections, skin and soft tissue infections, as well as abdominal and urinary tract infections, and septicemia; treatment of infective endocarditis

Unlabeled Use Surgical (preoperative) prophylaxis

Pregnancy Risk Factor D

Pregnancy Considerations Gentamicin crosses the placenta and produces detectable serum levels in the fetus. Renal toxicity has been described in two case reports following first trimester exposure. There are several reports of total irreversible bilateral congenital deafness in children whose mothers received streptomycin during pregnancy; therefore, the manufacturer classifies gentamicin as pregnancy category D. Although ototoxicity has not been reported following maternal use of gentamicin, a potential for harm exists. **[U.S. Boxed Warning]: Aminoglycosides may cause fetal harm if administered to a pregnant woman.**

Due to pregnancy induced physiologic changes, some pharmacokinetic parameters of gentamicin may be altered. Pregnant women have an average-to-larger volume of distribution which may result in lower serum peak levels than for the same dose in nonpregnant women. Serum half-life is also shorter.

Breast-Feeding Considerations Gentamicin is excreted into breast milk; however, it is not well absorbed when taken orally. This limited oral absorption may minimize exposure to the nursing infant. Nondose-related effects could include modification of bowel flora.

Contraindications Hypersensitivity to gentamicin or other aminoglycosides

Warnings/Precautions [U.S. Boxed Warning]: Aminoglycosides may cause neurotoxicity and/or nephrotoxicity; usual risk factors include pre-existing renal impairment, concomitant neuro-/nephrotoxic medications, advanced age and dehydration. Ototoxicity may be directly proportional to the amount of drug given and the duration of treatment; tinnitus or vertigo are indications of vestibular injury and impending hearing loss; renal damage is usually reversible. May cause neuromuscular blockade and respiratory paralysis; especially when given soon after anesthesia or muscle relaxants.

Not intended for long-term therapy due to toxic hazards associated with extended administration; use caution in pre-existing renal insufficiency, vestibular or cochlear impairment, myasthenia gravis, hypocalcemia, conditions which depress neuromuscular transmission. Dosage modification required in patients with impaired renal function. Prolonged use may result in fungal or bacterial superinfection, including *C. difficile*-associated diarrhea (CDAD) and pseudomembranous colitis; CDAD has been observed >2 months postantibiotic treatment.

Adverse Reactions Frequency not defined.

Cardiovascular: Edema, hyper/hypotension

Central nervous system: Ataxia, confusion, depression, dizziness, drowsiness, encephalopathy, fever, headache, lethargy, pseudomotor cerebri, seizures, vertigo

Dermatologic: Alopecia, erythema, itching, purpura, rash, urticaria

Endocrine & metabolic: Hypocalcemia, hypokalemia, hypomagnesemia, hyponatremia

Gastrointestinal: Anorexia, appetite decreased, *C. difficile*-associated diarrhea, enterocolitis, nausea, salivation increased, splenomegaly, stomatitis, vomiting, weight loss

Hematologic: Agranulocytosis, anemia, eosinophilia, granulocytopenia, leukopenia, reticulocytes increased/decreased, thrombocytopenia

Hepatic: Hepatomegaly, LFTs increased

Local: Injection site reactions, pain at injection site, phlebitis/thrombophlebitis

Neuromuscular & skeletal: Arthralgia, gait instability, muscle cramps, muscle twitching, muscle weakness, myasthenia gravis-like syndrome, numbness, paresthesia, peripheral neuropathy, tremor, weakness

Ocular: Visual disturbances

Otic: Hearing impairment, hearing loss (associated with persistently increased serum concentrations; early toxicity usually affects high-pitched sound), tinnitus

Renal: BUN increased, casts (hyaline, granular) in urine, creatinine clearance decreased, distal tubular dysfunction, Fanconi-like syndrome (high dose, prolonged course) (infants and adults), oliguria, renal failure (high trough serum concentrations), polyuria, proteinuria, serum creatinine increased, tubular necrosis, urine specific gravity decreased

Respiratory: Dyspnea, laryngeal edema, pulmonary fibrosis, respiratory depression

Miscellaneous: Allergic reaction, anaphylaxis, anaphylactoid reactions

Drug Interactions

Metabolism/Transport Effects None known.

Avoid Concomitant Use

Avoid concomitant use of Gentamicin (Systemic) with any of the following: Agalsidase Alfa; Agalsidase Beta; BCG; Gallium Nitrate

Increased Effect/Toxicity

Gentamicin (Systemic) may increase the levels/effects of: AbobotulinumtoxinA; Bisphosphonate Derivatives; CARBOplatin; Colistimethate; CycloSPORINE (Systemic); Gallium Nitrate; Neuromuscular-Blocking Agents; OnabotulinumtoxinA; RimabotulinumtoxinB; Tenofovir

The levels/effects of Gentamicin (Systemic) may be increased by: Amphotericin B; Capreomycin; Cephalosporins (2nd Generation); Cephalosporins (3rd Generation); Cephalosporins (4th Generation); CISplatin; Loop Diuretics; Nonsteroidal Anti-Inflammatory Agents; Tenofovir; Vancomycin

Decreased Effect

Gentamicin (Systemic) may decrease the levels/effects of: Agalsidase Alfa; Agalsidase Beta; BCG; Sodium Picosulfate; Typhoid Vaccine

The levels/effects of Gentamicin (Systemic) may be decreased by: Penicillins

Storage/Stability Gentamicin is a colorless to slightly yellow solution which should be stored between 2°C to 30°C, but refrigeration is not recommended. I.V. infusion solutions mixed in NS or D_5W solution are stable for 48 hours at room temperature and refrigeration (Goodwin, 1991). Premixed bag: Manufacturer expiration date; remove from overwrap stability: 30 days.

Mechanism of Action Interferes with bacterial protein synthesis by binding to 30S and 50S ribosomal subunits resulting in a defective bacterial cell membrane

Pharmacodynamics/Kinetics

Absorption:

Intramuscular: Rapid and complete

Oral: None

Distribution: Primarily into extracellular fluid (highly hydrophilic); high concentration in the renal cortex; minimal penetration to ocular tissues via I.V. route

V_d: Increased by edema, ascites, fluid overload; decreased with dehydration

Neonates: 0.4-0.6 L/kg

Children: 0.3-0.35 L/kg

Adults: 0.2-0.3 L/kg

Relative diffusion from blood into CSF: Minimal even with inflammation

CSF:blood level ratio: Normal meninges: Nil; Inflamed meninges: 10% to 30%

Protein binding: <30%

Half-life elimination:
Infants: <1 week: 3-11.5 hours; 1 week to 6 months: 3-3.5 hours
Adults: 1.5-3 hours; End-stage renal disease: 36-70 hours
Time to peak, serum: I.M.: 30-90 minutes; I.V.: 30 minutes after 30-minute infusion
Excretion: Urine (as unchanged drug)
Clearance: Directly related to renal function

Dosage Note: Dosage Individualization is **critical** because of the low therapeutic index.

In underweight and nonobese patients, use of total body weight (TBW) instead of ideal body weight for determining the initial mg/kg/dose is widely accepted (Nicolau, 1995). Ideal body weight (IBW) also may be used to determine doses for patients who are neither underweight nor obese (Gilbert, 2009).

Initial and periodic plasma drug levels (eg, peak and trough with conventional dosing, post dose level at a prespecified time with extended-interval dosing) should be determined, particularly in critically-ill patients with serious infections or in disease states known to significantly alter aminoglycoside pharmacokinetics (eg, cystic fibrosis, burns, or major surgery).

Usual dosage ranges:
Infants and Children <5 years: I.M., I.V.: 2.5 mg/kg/dose every 8 hours*
Children ≥5 years: I.M., I.V.: 2-2.5 mg/kg/dose every 8 hours*
***Note:** Higher individual doses and/or more frequent intervals (eg, every 6 hours) may be required in selected clinical situations (cystic fibrosis) or serum levels document the need.
Adults:
I.M., I.V.:
Conventional: 1-2.5 mg/kg/dose every 8-12 hours; to ensure adequate peak concentrations early in therapy, higher initial dosage may be considered in selected patients when extracellular water is increased (edema, septic shock, postsurgical, or trauma)
Once daily: 4-7 mg/kg/dose once daily; some clinicians recommend this approach for all patients with normal renal function; this dose is at least as efficacious with similar, if not less, toxicity than conventional dosing
Intrathecal: 4-8 mg/day

Indication-specific dosing:
Children ≥1 year: I.V.:
Surgical (preoperative) prophylaxis (unlabeled use): 2.5 mg/kg within 60 minutes prior to surgical incision with or without other antibiotics (procedure dependent). **Note:** Dose is based on actual body weight unless >20% above ideal body weight, then dosage requirement may best be estimated using a dosing weight of IBW + 0.4 (TBW - IBW) (Bratzler, 2013).
Children and Adults: I.M., I.V.:
Brucellosis: 240 mg (I.M.) daily or 5 mg/kg (I.V.) daily for 7 days; either regimen recommended in combination with doxycycline
Cholangitis: 4-6 mg/kg once daily with ampicillin
Diverticulitis (complicated): 1.5-2 mg/kg every 8 hours (with ampicillin and metronidazole)
Endocarditis: Treatment: 3 mg/kg/day in 1-3 divided doses
Meningitis: *Enterococcus* sp or *Pseudomonas aeruginosa*: Loading dose 2 mg/kg, then 1.7 mg/kg/dose every 8 hours (administered with another bacteriocidal drug)
Pelvic inflammatory disease: Loading dose: 2 mg/kg, then 1.5 mg/kg every 8 hours
Alternate therapy: 4.5 mg/kg once daily
Plague *(Yersinia pestis)*: Treatment: 5 mg/kg/day, followed by postexposure prophylaxis with doxycycline
Pneumonia, hospital- or ventilator-associated: 7 mg/kg/day (with antipseudomonal beta-lactam or carbapenem)
Synergy (for gram-positive infections): 3 mg/kg/day in 1-3 divided doses (with ampicillin)
Tularemia: 5 mg/kg/day divided every 8 hours for 1-2 weeks
Urinary tract infection: 1.5 mg/kg/dose every 8 hours
Adults: I.V.:
Surgical (preoperative) prophylaxis (unlabeled use): 5 mg/kg within 60 minutes prior to surgical incision with or without other antibiotics (procedure dependent). **Note:** Dose is based on actual body weight unless >20% above ideal body weight, then dosage requirement may best be estimated using a dosing weight of IBW + 0.4 (TBW - IBW) (Bratzler, 2013).

Dosing interval in renal impairment:
Conventional dosing:
Cl_{cr} ≥60 mL/minute: Administer every 8 hours
Cl_{cr} 40-60 mL/minute: Administer every 12 hours
Cl_{cr} 20-40 mL/minute: Administer every 24 hours
Cl_{cr} <20 mL/minute: Loading dose, then monitor levels
High-dose therapy: Interval may be extended (eg, every 48 hours) in patients with moderate renal impairment (Cl_{cr} 30-59 mL/minute) and/or adjusted based on serum level determinations.

Intermittent hemodialysis (IHD) (administer after hemodialysis on dialysis days) (Heintz, 2009): Dialyzable (~50%; variable; dependent on filter, duration, and type of IHD):
Loading dose of 2-3 mg/kg loading dose followed by:
Mild UTI or synergy: 1 mg/kg every 48-72 hours; consider redosing for pre-HD or post-HD concentrations <1 mg/L
Moderate-to-severe UTI: 1-1.5 mg/kg every 48-72 hours; consider redosing for pre-HD concentrations <1.5-2 mg/L or post-HD concentrations <1 mg/L
Systemic gram-negative rod infection: 1.5-2 mg/kg every 48-72 hours; consider redosing for pre-HD concentrations <3-5 mg/L or post-HD concentrations <2 mg/L
Note: Dosing dependent on the assumption of 3 times/week, complete IHD sessions.

Peritoneal dialysis (PD):
Administration via PD fluid:
Gram-positive infection (eg, synergy): 3-4 mg/L (3-4 mcg/mL) of PD fluid
Gram-negative infection: 4-8 mg/L (4-8 mcg/mL) of PD fluid
Administration via I.V., I.M. route during PD: Dose as for Cl_{cr} <10 mL/minute and follow levels

Continuous renal replacement therapy (CRRT) (Heintz, 2009; Trotman, 2005): Drug clearance is highly dependent on the method of renal replacement, filter type, and flow rate. Appropriate dosing requires close monitoring of pharmacologic response, signs of adverse reactions due to drug accumulation, as well as drug concentrations in relation to target trough (if appropriate). The following are general recommendations only (based on dialysate flow/ultrafiltration rates of 1-2 L/hour and minimal residual renal function) and should not supersede clinical judgment:
CVVH/CVVHD/CVVHDF: Loading dose of 2-3 mg/kg followed by:
Mild UTI or synergy: 1 mg/kg every 24-36 hours (redose when concentration <1 mg/L)
Moderate-to-severe UTI: 1-1.5 mg/kg every 24-36 hours (redose when concentration <1.5-2 mg/L)
Systemic gram-negative infection: 1.5-2.5 mg/kg every 24-48 hours (redose when concentration <3-5 mg/L)

Dosing adjustment/comments in hepatic disease: Monitor plasma concentrations

Dosing in obesity: In moderate obesity (TBW/IBW ≥1.25) or greater (eg, morbid obesity [TBW/IBW >2]), initial dosage requirement may be estimated using a dosing weight of IBW + 0.4 (TBW - IBW) (Traynor, 1995).

Dietary Considerations Calcium, magnesium, potassium: Renal wasting may cause hypocalcemia, hypomagnesemia, and/or hypokalemia.

Administration

I.M.: Administer by deep I.M. route if possible. Slower absorption and lower peak concentrations, probably due to poor circulation in the atrophic muscle, may occur following I.M. injection; in paralyzed patients, suggest I.V. route.

Some penicillins (eg, carbenicillin, ticarcillin, and piperacillin) have been shown to inactivate aminoglycosides *in vitro*. This has been observed to a greater extent with tobramycin and gentamicin, while amikacin has shown greater stability against inactivation. Concurrent use of these agents may pose a risk of reduced antibacterial efficacy *in vivo*, particularly in the setting of profound renal impairment. However, definitive clinical evidence is lacking. If combination penicillin/aminoglycoside therapy is desired in a patient with renal dysfunction, separation of doses (if feasible), and routine monitoring of aminoglycoside levels, CBC, and clinical response should be considered.

Monitoring Parameters Urinalysis, urine output, BUN, serum creatinine, plasma gentamicin levels (as appropriate to dosing method). Levels are typically obtained after the third dose in conventional dosing. Hearing should be tested before, during, and after treatment; particularly in those at risk for ototoxicity or who will be receiving prolonged therapy (>2 weeks)

Some penicillin derivatives may accelerate the degradation of aminoglycosides *in vitro*. This may be clinically-significant for certain penicillin (ticarcillin, piperacillin, carbenicillin) and aminoglycoside (gentamicin, tobramycin) combination therapy in patients with significant renal impairment. Close monitoring of aminoglycoside levels is warranted.

Reference Range

Timing of serum samples: Draw peak 30 minutes after 30-minute infusion has been completed or 1 hour after I.M. injection; draw trough immediately before next dose

Therapeutic levels:
- Peak:
  - Serious infections: 6-8 mcg/mL (12-17 micromole/L)
  - Life-threatening infections: 8-10 mcg/mL (17-21 micromole/L)
  - Urinary tract infections: 4-6 mcg/mL
  - Synergy against gram-positive organisms: 3-5 mcg/mL
- Trough:
  - Serious infections: 0.5-1 mcg/mL
  - Life-threatening infections: 1-2 mcg/mL
  - The American Thoracic Society (ATS) recommends trough levels of <1 mcg/mL for patients with hospital-acquired pneumonia.

Obtain drug levels after the third dose unless renal dysfunction/toxicity suspected

Test Interactions Some penicillin derivatives may accelerate the degradation of aminoglycosides *in vitro*, leading to a potential underestimation of aminoglycoside serum concentration.

Dosage Forms Excipient information presented when available (limited, particularly for generics); consult specific product labeling.

Solution, Injection:
Generic: 10 mg/mL (2 mL); 40 mg/mL (2 mL, 20 mL)

Solution, Injection [preservative free]:
Generic: 10 mg/mL (2 mL)

Solution, Intravenous:
Generic: 60 mg (50 mL); 70 mg (50 mL); 80 mg (50 mL, 100 mL); 90 mg (100 mL); 100 mg (50 mL, 100 mL); 120 mg (100 mL); 10 mg/mL (6 mL, 8 mL, 10 mL)

Gentamicin (Ophthalmic) (jen ta MYE sin)

Brand Names: U.S. Garamycin; Gentak

Brand Names: Canada Diogent®; Garamycin®; Gentak®; Gentocin; PMS-Gentamicin

Index Terms Gentamicin Sulfate

Pharmacologic Category Antibiotic, Aminoglycoside; Antibiotic, Ophthalmic

Use Treatment of ophthalmic infections caused by susceptible bacteria

Pregnancy Risk Factor C

Dosage Ophthalmic: Children and Adults:

Ointment: Instill 1/2" (1.25 cm) 2-3 times/day to every 3-4 hours

Solution: Instill 1-2 drops every 4 hours, up to 2 drops every hour for severe infections

Additional Information Complete prescribing information should be consulted for additional detail.

Dosage Forms Excipient information presented when available (limited, particularly for generics); consult specific product labeling.

Ointment, Ophthalmic:
Garamycin: 0.3% (3.5 g)
Gentak: 0.3% (3.5 g)
Generic: 0.3% (3.5 g)

Solution, Ophthalmic:
Garamycin: 0.3% (5 mL) [contains benzalkonium chloride]
Generic: 0.3% (5 mL, 15 mL)

◆ **Gentamicin and Prednisolone** *see* Prednisolone and Gentamicin *on page 1707*

◆ **Gentamicin Injection, USP (Can)** *see* Gentamicin (Systemic) *on page 951*

◆ **Gentamicin Sulfate** *see* Gentamicin (Ophthalmic) *on page 954*

◆ **Gentamicin Sulfate** *see* Gentamicin (Systemic) *on page 951*

Gentian Violet (JEN shun VYE oh let)

Index Terms Crystal Violet; Methylrosaniline Chloride

Pharmacologic Category Antibiotic, Topical; Antifungal Agent, Topical

Use Treatment of cutaneous or mucocutaneous infections caused by *Candida albicans* and other superficial skin infections; external treatment of minor abrasions or cuts

Dosage Children and Adults: Topical: Apply to affected area once or twice daily. Solutions diluted to 0.25% to 0.5% may be less irritating. Solutions diluted to 0.01% have been recommended for use in closed cavities.

Additional Information Complete prescribing information should be consulted for additional detail.

Dosage Forms Excipient information presented when available (limited, particularly for generics); consult specific product labeling.

Solution, External:
Generic: 1% (59 mL); 2% (59 mL)

◆ **Gen-Ticlopidine (Can)** *see* Ticlopidine *on page 2059*

◆ **Gen-Tizanidine (Can)** *see* TiZANidine *on page 2074*

◆ **Gentle Laxative [OTC]** *see* Bisacodyl *on page 259*

◆ **Gentocin (Can)** *see* Gentamicin (Ophthalmic) *on page 954*

◆ **Gen-Triazolam (Can)** *see* Triazolam *on page 2124*

- ◆ **Geodon** *see* Ziprasidone *on page 2230*
- ◆ **Geri-Dryl [OTC]** *see* DiphenhydrAMINE (Systemic) *on page 622*
- ◆ **Geri-Mox [OTC]** *see* Aluminum Hydroxide, Magnesium Hydroxide, and Simethicone *on page 90*
- ◆ **Geri-Mucil [OTC]** *see* Psyllium *on page 1748*
- ◆ **Geri-Stool [OTC]** *see* Docusate and Senna *on page 645*
- ◆ **Geri-Tussin [OTC]** *see* GuaiFENesin *on page 974*
- ◆ **GF196960** *see* Tadalafil *on page 1983*
- ◆ **GG** *see* GuaiFENesin *on page 974*
- ◆ **GHB** *see* Sodium Oxybate *on page 1922*
- ◆ **GI87084B** *see* Remifentanil *on page 1795*
- ◆ **Gianvi™** *see* Ethinyl Estradiol and Drospirenone *on page 785*
- ◆ **Giazo** *see* Balsalazide *on page 223*
- ◆ **Gildess FE 1.5/30** *see* Ethinyl Estradiol and Norethindrone *on page 793*
- ◆ **Gildess FE 1/20** *see* Ethinyl Estradiol and Norethindrone *on page 793*
- ◆ **Gilenya** *see* Fingolimod *on page 864*
- ◆ **Gilenya® (Can)** *see* Fingolimod *on page 864*
- ◆ **Gilotrif** *see* Afatinib *on page 54*
- ◆ **Glargine Insulin** *see* Insulin Glargine *on page 1089*

Glatiramer Acetate (gla TIR a mer AS e tate)

Brand Names: U.S. Copaxone

Brand Names: Canada Copaxone®

Index Terms Copolymer-1

Pharmacologic Category Biological, Miscellaneous

Use Management of relapsing-remitting type multiple sclerosis, including patients with a first clinical episode with MRI features consistent with multiple sclerosis

Pregnancy Risk Factor B

Pregnancy Considerations Adverse events were not observed in animal studies.

Breast-Feeding Considerations It is not known if glatiramer acetate is excreted in breast milk. The manufacturer recommends that caution be exercised when administering glatiramer acetate to nursing women.

Contraindications Hypersensitivity to glatiramer acetate, mannitol, or any component of the formulation

Warnings/Precautions For SubQ use only, **not for I.V. administration**. Glatiramer acetate is antigenic, and may interfere with recognition of foreign antigens affecting tumor surveillance and infection defense systems. Immediate postinjection systemic reactions occur in a substantial percentage of patients (~16% in studies); symptoms may begin within minutes of injection and are usually self-limiting. Most patients only have one reaction despite repeated administration. Chest pain (transient pain resolving in minutes) may occur as part of the postinjection systemic reaction, but can also occur alone. Lipoatrophy may occur at injection site; proper injection site rotation may prevent. Safety and efficacy has not been established in patients with renal impairment, in the elderly, or in patients <18 years of age.

Adverse Reactions

>10%:

Cardiovascular: Vasodilation (20%), chest pain (13%)

Central nervous system: Pain (20%), anxiety (13%)

Dermatologic: Rash (19%)

Gastrointestinal: Nausea (15%)

Local: Injection site reactions: Inflammation (49%), erythema (43%), pain (40%), pruritus (27%), mass (27%)

Neuromuscular & skeletal: Weakness (22%), back pain (12%)

Respiratory: Dyspnea (14%)

Miscellaneous: Infection (30%), flu-like syndrome (14%), diaphoresis (15%)

1% to 10%:

Cardiovascular: Edema (8%; includes peripheral and facial), palpitation (7%), tachycardia (5%), syncope (3%), hypertension (1%)

Central nervous system: Fever (6%), migraine (4%), chills (3%), nervousness (2%), speech disorder (2%), abnormal dreams (1%), emotional lability (1%), stupor (1%)

Dermatologic: Bruising (8%), pruritus (5%), erythema (4%), urticaria (3%), skin nodule (2%), eczema (1%), pustular rash (1%)

Endocrine & metabolic: Amenorrhea (1%), impotence (1%), menorrhagia (1%)

Gastrointestinal: Vomiting (7%), gastroenteritis (6%), weight gain (3%), dysphagia (2%), dental caries (1%)

Genitourinary: Urinary urgency (5%), vaginal moniliasis (4%)

Local: Injection site reactions: Hemorrhage (5%), hypersensitivity (4%), fibrosis (2%), lipoatrophy (2%), abscess (1%), edema (1%)

Neuromuscular & skeletal: Neck pain (8%), tremor (4%)

Ocular: Diplopia (3%), visual field defect (1%)

Respiratory: Rhinitis (7%), bronchitis (6%), cough (6%), laryngismus (5%), hyperventilation (1%)

Miscellaneous: Lymphadenopathy (7%), hypersensitivity (3%)

<1% (Limited to important or life-threatening): Allergic reaction, anaphylactoid reaction, anemia, angina, angioedema, aphasia, appetite increased, arrhythmia, arthritis, asthma, atrial fibrillation, blindness, bradycardia, carcinoma (breast, bladder, lung, ovarian), cardiomyopathy, cataract, cervical cancer, cholecystitis, cholelithiasis, cirrhosis, CNS neoplasm, colitis, corneal ulcer, Cushing's syndrome, dermatitis, dry eyes, dry skin, esophagitis, gastrointestinal carcinoma, gastrointestinal hemorrhage, gastrointestinal ulcer, glaucoma, gout, hallucination, heart failure, hepatitis, hepatomegaly, hypercholesterolemia, hypotension, injection site necrosis, leukemia, leukopenia, libido decreased, lupus erythematosus, lymphoma-like reaction, mania, meningitis, MI, mouth ulceration, neuralgia, optic neuritis, orthostatic hypotension, pancreatitis, pancytopenia, pericardial effusion, peripheral vascular disease, photophobia, pneumonia, priapism, pulmonary embolism, pyelonephritis, renal failure, seizures, sepsis, skin cancer, spasm, splenomegaly, stomatitis, stroke, thrombocytopenia, thrombophlebitis, thrombosis, urethritis

Drug Interactions

Metabolism/Transport Effects None known.

Avoid Concomitant Use

Avoid concomitant use of Glatiramer Acetate with any of the following: BCG; Natalizumab; Pimecrolimus; Tacrolimus (Topical); Tofacitinib; Vaccines (Live)

Increased Effect/Toxicity

Glatiramer Acetate may increase the levels/effects of: Leflunomide; Natalizumab; Tofacitinib; Vaccines (Live)

The levels/effects of Glatiramer Acetate may be increased by: Denosumab; Pimecrolimus; Roflumilast; Tacrolimus (Topical); Trastuzumab

Decreased Effect

Glatiramer Acetate may decrease the levels/effects of: BCG; Coccidioidin Skin Test; Sipuleucel-T; Vaccines (Inactivated); Vaccines (Live)

The levels/effects of Glatiramer Acetate may be decreased by: Echinacea

Storage/Stability Store in refrigerator at 2°C to 8°C (36°F to 46°F); excursions to room temperature for up to 1 month do not have a negative impact on potency. Avoid heat; protect from intense light.

Mechanism of Action Glatiramer is a mixture of random polymers of four amino acids; L-alanine, L-glutamic acid, L-lysine, and L-tyrosine, the resulting mixture is antigenically similar to myelin basic protein, which is an important component of the myelin sheath of nerves; glatiramer is thought to induce and activate T-lymphocyte suppressor cells specific for a myelin antigen, it is also proposed that glatiramer interferes with the antigen-presenting function of certain immune cells opposing pathogenic T-cell function

Pharmacodynamics/Kinetics

Distribution: Small amounts of intact and partial hydrolyzed drug enter lymphatic circulation

Metabolism: SubQ: Large percentage hydrolyzed locally

Dosage Adults: SubQ: 20 mg daily

Dosage adjustment in renal impairment: No dosage adjustment provided in manufacturer's labeling (has not been studied).

Dosage adjustment in hepatic impairment: No dosage adjustment provided in manufacturer's labeling.

Administration For SubQ administration in the arms, abdomen, hips, or thighs; rotate injection sites to prevent lipoatrophy. Bring to room temperature prior to use. Visually inspect the solution; discard if solution is cloudy or contains any particulate matter.

Dosage Forms Excipient information presented when available (limited, particularly for generics); consult specific product labeling.

Kit, Subcutaneous:

Copaxone: 20 mg/mL [contains mannitol]

- GlcCerase *see* Velaglucerase Alfa *on page* 2176
- Gleevec *see* Imatinib *on page* 1048
- Gliadel Wafer *see* Carmustine *on page* 352
- Gliadel Wafer® (Can) *see* Carmustine *on page* 352
- Glibenclamide *see* GlyBURIDE *on page* 963

Glimepiride (GLYE me pye ride)

Brand Names: U.S. Amaryl

Brand Names: Canada Amaryl; Apo-Glimepiride; Novo-Glimepiride; PMS-Glimepiride; ratio-Glimepiride; Sandoz-Glimepiride

Pharmacologic Category Antidiabetic Agent, Sulfonylurea

Additional Appendix Information

Oral Antidiabetic Agents Comparison Table *on page* 2312

Use Type 2 diabetes mellitus: As an adjunct to diet and exercise to improve glycemic control in adults with type 2 diabetes mellitus

Pregnancy Risk Factor C

Pregnancy Considerations Adverse events have been observed in some animal reproduction studies. Severe hypoglycemia lasting 4-10 days has been noted in infants born to mothers taking a sulfonylurea at the time of delivery. For women with diabetes, maternal hyperglycemia can be associated with adverse effects in the fetus, neonate, and mother. To prevent adverse events, prior to conception and throughout pregnancy, the maternal Hb A_{1c} should be kept close to normal but without causing significant hypoglycemia. The use of most oral antihyperglycemic agents in pregnant women is not recommended for routine management of GDM or type 2 diabetes mellitus in pregnant women; insulin is the drug of choice for the control of diabetes mellitus during pregnancy (ACOG, 2005; ADA, 2013; Kitzmiller, 2008; Metzger, 2007).

Breast-Feeding Considerations It is not known if glimepiride is excreted in breast milk. According to the manufacturer, due to the potential for hypoglycemia in the nursing infant, a decision should be made whether to discontinue nursing or to discontinue the drug, taking into account the importance of treatment to the mother.

Contraindications

Hypersensitivity to glimepiride, any component of the formulation, or sulfonamides; diabetic ketoacidosis (with or without coma)

Documentation of allergenic cross-reactivity for drugs in this class is limited. However, because of similarities in chemical structure and/or pharmacologic actions, the possibility of cross-sensitivity cannot be ruled out with certainty.

Canadian labeling: Additional contraindications (not in U.S. labeling): Pregnancy; breast-feeding; type 1 diabetes; severe renal or hepatic impairment

Warnings/Precautions All sulfonylurea drugs are capable of producing severe hypoglycemia. Hypoglycemia is more likely to occur when caloric intake is deficient, after severe or prolonged exercise, when ethanol is ingested, or when more than one glucose-lowering drug is used. It is also more likely in elderly patients, malnourished patients and in patients with impaired renal or hepatic function; use with caution. Reduce dosage in patients with renal impairment.

Loss of efficacy may be observed following prolonged use as a result of the progression of type 2 diabetes mellitus which results in continued beta cell destruction. In patients who were previously responding to sulfonylurea therapy, consider additional factors which may be contributing to decreased efficacy (eg, inappropriate dose, nonadherence to diet and exercise regimen). If no contributing factors can be identified, consider discontinuing use of the sulfonylurea due to secondary failure of treatment. Additional antidiabetic therapy (eg, insulin) will be required. It may be necessary to discontinue therapy and administer insulin if the patient is exposed to stress (fever, trauma, infection, surgery).

Chemical similarities are present among sulfonamides, sulfonylureas, carbonic anhydrase inhibitors, thiazides, and loop diuretics (except ethacrynic acid); a risk of cross-reaction exists in patients with allergy to any of these compounds. Use in patients with sulfonamide allergy is contraindicated. Patients with G6PD deficiency may be at an increased risk of sulfonylurea-induced hemolytic anemia; however, cases have also been described in patients without G6PD deficiency during postmarketing surveillance. Use with caution and consider a nonsulfonylurea alternative in patients with G6PD deficiency. Systemic exposure of glimepiride is increased in patients with CYP2C9*3 allele; dose reductions may be necessary (Niemi, 2002).

Product labeling states oral hypoglycemic drugs may be associated with an increased cardiovascular mortality as compared to treatment with diet alone or diet plus insulin. Data to support this association are limited, and several studies, including a large prospective trial (UKPDS) have not supported an association.

Adverse Reactions

>10%: Endocrine & metabolic: Hypoglycemia (4% to 20%)

1% to 10%:

Central nervous system: Dizziness (2%), headache

Gastrointestinal: Nausea (5%)

Hepatic: Increased serum ALT (2%)

Respiratory: Flu-like symptoms (5%)

Miscellaneous: Accidental injury (6%)

<1% (Limited to important or life-threatening): Abnormal hepatic function tests, accommodation disturbance (early treatment), agranulocytosis, anaphylaxis, angioedema, anorexia, aplastic anemia, cholestatic jaundice, disulfiram-like reaction, epigastric fullness, hemolytic anemia, hepatic failure, hepatic porphyria, hepatitis, hypersensitivity, hypersensitivity angiitis, hyponatremia,

hypotension, leukopenia, maculopapular rash, morbilliform rash, pancytopenia, porphyria cutanea tarda, shock, SIADH, skin photosensitivity, Stevens-Johnson syndrome, thrombocytopenia, weight gain

Drug Interactions

Metabolism/Transport Effects Substrate of CYP2C9 (major); **Note:** Assignment of Major/Minor substrate status based on clinically relevant drug interaction potential

Avoid Concomitant Use There are no known interactions where it is recommended to avoid concomitant use.

Increased Effect/Toxicity

Glimepiride may increase the levels/effects of: Alcohol (Ethyl); Carbocisteine; Hypoglycemic Agents; Porfimer; Vitamin K Antagonists

The levels/effects of Glimepiride may be increased by: Beta-Blockers; Chloramphenicol; Cimetidine; Cyclic Antidepressants; CYP2C9 Inhibitors (Moderate); CYP2C9 Inhibitors (Strong); Fibric Acid Derivatives; Fluconazole; GLP-1 Agonists; Herbs (Hypoglycemic Properties); MAO Inhibitors; Miconazole (Oral); Mifepristone; Pegvisomant; Probenecid; Quinolone Antibiotics; Ranitidine; Salicylates; Selective Serotonin Reuptake Inhibitors; Sulfonamide Derivatives; Vitamin K Antagonists; Voriconazole

Decreased Effect

The levels/effects of Glimepiride may be decreased by: Colesevelam; Corticosteroids (Orally Inhaled); Corticosteroids (Systemic); CYP2C9 Inducers (Strong); Dabrafenib; Loop Diuretics; Luteinizing Hormone-Releasing Hormone Analogs; Peginterferon Alfa-2b; Quinolone Antibiotics; Rifampin; Somatropin; Thiazide Diuretics

Ethanol/Nutrition/Herb Interactions

Ethanol: Caution with ethanol (may cause hypoglycemia).

Herb/Nutraceutical: Caution with chromium, garlic, gymnema (may cause hypoglycemia).

Storage/Stability Store at 25°C (77°F); excursions permitted between 20°C and 25°C (68°F and 77°F)

Mechanism of Action Stimulates insulin release from the pancreatic beta cells; reduces glucose output from the liver; insulin sensitivity is increased at peripheral target sites

Pharmacodynamics/Kinetics

Onset of action: Peak effect: Blood glucose reductions: 2-3 hours

Duration: 24 hours

Absorption: 100%; delayed when given with food

Distribution: V_d: 8.8 L

Protein binding: >99.5%

Metabolism: Hepatic oxidation via CYP2C9 to M1 metabolite (~33% activity of parent compound); further oxidative metabolism to inactive M2 metabolite

Half-life elimination: 5-9 hours

Time to peak, plasma: 2-3 hours

Excretion: Urine (60%, 80% to 90% as M1 and M2 metabolites); feces (40%, 70% as M1 and M2 metabolites)

Dosage Type 2 diabetes:

Adults: Oral: Initial: 1-2 mg once daily, administered with breakfast or the first main meal; based on response, may increase dose by 1-2 mg every 1-2 weeks up to maximum of 8 mg once daily. If inadequate response to maximal dose, combination therapy with other agents (eg, metformin, insulin) may be considered. Combination therapy is individualized based on glycemic response.

Conversion from therapy with long half-life agents: Observe patient carefully for 1-2 weeks when converting from a longer half-life agent (eg, chlorpropamide) to glimepiride due to overlapping hypoglycemic effects.

Elderly: Initial: 1 mg once daily; dose titration and maintenance dosing should be conservative to avoid hypoglycemia

Dosage adjustment in renal impairment:

U.S. labeling: Initial: 1 mg once daily; titrate carefully based on fasting blood glucose levels

Canadian labeling:

Mild-to-moderate impairment: Initial: 1 mg once daily; titrate carefully based on fasting blood glucose levels

Severe impairment: Use is contraindicated

Dosage adjustment in hepatic impairment:

U.S. labeling: No dosage adjustment provided in manufacturer's labeling (has not been studied).

Canadian labeling:

Mild-to-moderate impairment: No dosage adjustment provided in manufacturer's labeling (has not been studied).

Severe impairment: Use is contraindicated.

Dietary Considerations Take with breakfast or the first main meal of the day. Individualized medical nutrition therapy (MNT) based on ADA recommendations is an integral part of therapy.

Administration Administer once daily with breakfast or first main meal of the day. Patients that are NPO or require decreased caloric intake may need doses held to avoid hypoglycemia.

Monitoring Parameters Monitor for signs and symptoms of hypoglycemia (fatigue, excessive hunger, profuse sweating, numbness of extremities), fasting blood glucose, hemoglobin A_{1c}

Reference Range Recommendations for glycemic control in nonpregnant adults with diabetes (ADA, 2013):

Hb A_{1c}: <7% (a more aggressive [<6.5%] or less aggressive [<8%] Hb A_{1c} goal may be targeted based on patient-specific characteristics)

Preprandial capillary plasma glucose: 70-130 mg/dL

Peak postprandial capillary blood glucose: <180 mg/dL

Dosage Forms Excipient information presented when available (limited, particularly for generics); consult specific product labeling.

Tablet, Oral:

Amaryl: 1 mg [scored]

Amaryl: 2 mg, 4 mg [scored; contains fd&c blue #2 aluminum lake]

Generic: 1 mg, 2 mg, 4 mg

◆ **Glimepiride and Pioglitazone** *see* Pioglitazone and Glimepiride *on page 1652*

◆ **Glimepiride and Pioglitazone Hydrochloride** *see* Pioglitazone and Glimepiride *on page 1652*

◆ **Glimepiride and Rosiglitazone Maleate** *see* Rosiglitazone and Glimepiride *on page 1857*

GlipiZIDE (GLIP i zide)

Brand Names: U.S. GlipiZIDE XL; Glucotrol; Glucotrol XL

Index Terms Glydiazinamide

Pharmacologic Category Antidiabetic Agent, Sulfonylurea

Additional Appendix Information

Oral Antidiabetic Agents Comparison Table *on page 2312*

Use Management of type 2 diabetes mellitus (noninsulin dependent, NIDDM) as an adjunct to diet and exercise to lower blood glucose; may be used in combination with metformin or insulin in patients whose hyperglycemia cannot be controlled by diet and exercise in conjunction with a single oral hypoglycemic agent

Pregnancy Risk Factor C

Pregnancy Considerations Adverse events have been observed in some animal reproduction studies. Glipizide was found to cross the placenta in vitro (Elliott, 1994). Severe hypoglycemia lasting 4-10 days has been noted in infants born to mothers taking a sulfonylurea at the time of delivery.

For women with diabetes, maternal hyperglycemia can be associated with adverse effects in the fetus, neonate, and mother. To prevent adverse events, prior to conception and throughout pregnancy, the maternal Hb A_{1c} should be kept close to normal but without causing significant hypoglycemia. The use of most oral antihyperglycemic agents in pregnant women is not recommended for routine management of GDM or type 2 diabetes mellitus in pregnant women; insulin is the drug of choice for the control of diabetes mellitus during pregnancy (ACOG, 2005; ADA, 2013; Kitzmiller, 2008; Metzger, 2007). The manufacturer recommends if glipizide is used during pregnancy it should be discontinued at least 1 month before the expected delivery date.

Breast-Feeding Considerations Data from two mother-infant pairs note that glipizide was not detected in breast milk (Feig, 2005). Breast-feeding is encouraged for all women including those with diabetes; all types of insulin may be used while breast-feeding and some oral agents, including glipizide, may be acceptable for use as well (Metzger 2007). According to the manufacturer, due to the potential for hypoglycemia in the nursing infant, a decision should be made whether to discontinue nursing or to discontinue the drug, taking into account the importance of treatment to the mother.

Contraindications Hypersensitivity to glipizide or any component of the formulation; type 1 diabetes mellitus (insulin dependent, IDDM); diabetic ketoacidosis (with or without coma)

Warnings/Precautions All sulfonylurea drugs are capable of producing severe hypoglycemia. Hypoglycemia is more likely to occur when caloric intake is deficient, after severe or prolonged exercise, when ethanol is ingested, or when more than one glucose-lowering drug is used. It is also more likely in elderly patients, malnourished patients and in patients with impaired renal or hepatic function; use with caution. Autonomic neuropathy, advanced age, and concomitant use of beta-blockers or other sympatholytic agents may impair the patient's ability to recognize the signs and symptoms of hypoglycemia; use with caution.

Use with caution in patients with hepatic or renal impairment. It may be necessary to discontinue therapy and administer insulin if the patient is exposed to stress (fever, trauma, infection, surgery). Loss of efficacy may be observed following prolonged use as a result of the progression of type 2 diabetes mellitus which results in continued beta cell destruction. In patients who were previously responding to sulfonylurea therapy, consider additional factors which may be contributing to decreased efficacy (eg, inappropriate dose, nonadherence to diet and exercise regimen). If no contributing factors can be identified, consider discontinuing use of the sulfonylurea due to secondary failure of treatment. Additional antidiabetic therapy (eg, insulin) will be required.

Chemical similarities are present among sulfonamides, sulfonylureas, carbonic anhydrase inhibitors, thiazides, and loop diuretics (except ethacrynic acid). Use in patients with sulfonamide allergy is not specifically contraindicated in product labeling; however, a risk of cross-reaction exists in patients with allergy to any of these compounds; avoid use when previous reaction has been severe. Patients with G6PD deficiency may be at an increased risk of sulfonylurea-induced hemolytic anemia; however, cases have also been described in patients without G6PD deficiency during postmarketing surveillance. Use with caution and consider a nonsulfonylurea alternative in patients with G6PD deficiency.

Product labeling states oral hypoglycemic drugs may be associated with an increased cardiovascular mortality as compared to treatment with diet alone or diet plus insulin. Data to support this association are limited, and several studies, including a large prospective trial (UKPDS) have not supported an association. Avoid use of extended release tablets (Glucotrol XL®) in patients with known stricture/narrowing of the GI tract.

Adverse Reactions Frequency not always defined.

Cardiovascular: Syncope (<3%)

Central nervous system: Dizziness (2% to 7%), nervousness (4%), anxiety (<3%), depression (<3%), hypoesthesia (<3%), insomnia (<3%), pain (<3%), drowsiness (2%), headache (2%)

Dermatologic: Pruritus (1% to <3%), eczema (1%), erythema (1%), maculopapular eruptions (1%), morbilliform eruptions (1%), rash (1%), urticaria (1%)

Endocrine & metabolic: Hypoglycemia (<3%)

Gastrointestinal: Diarrhea (1% to 5%), flatulence (3%), constipation (1% to <3%), nausea (1% to <3%), dyspepsia (<3%), vomiting (<3%), abdominal pain (1%)

Hepatic: Alkaline phosphatase increased, AST increased, LDH increased

Neuromuscular & skeletal: Tremor (4%), arthralgia (<3%), leg cramps (<3%), myalgia (<3%), paresthesia (<3%)

Ocular: Blurred vision (<3%)

Renal: Blood urea nitrogen increased, creatinine increased

Respiratory: Rhinitis (<3%)

Miscellaneous: Diaphoresis (<3%)

<1% (Limited to important or life-threatening): Agranulocytosis, anorexia, aplastic anemia, arrhythmia, blood in stool, cholestatic jaundice, conjunctivitis, disulfiram-like reaction, edema, gait instability, hemolytic anemia, hypertension, hypertonia, hyponatremia, jaundice, leukopenia, liver injury, migraine, pancytopenia, photosensitivity, porphyria, retinal hemorrhage, SIADH, thrombocytopenia, vertigo

Drug Interactions

Metabolism/Transport Effects Substrate of CYP2C9 (major); **Note:** Assignment of Major/Minor substrate status based on clinically relevant drug interaction potential

Avoid Concomitant Use There are no known interactions where it is recommended to avoid concomitant use.

Increased Effect/Toxicity

GlipiZIDE may increase the levels/effects of: Alcohol (Ethyl); Carbocisteine; Hypoglycemic Agents; Porfimer; Vitamin K Antagonists

The levels/effects of GlipiZIDE may be increased by: Beta-Blockers; Chloramphenicol; Cimetidine; Clarithromycin; Cyclic Antidepressants; CYP2C9 Inhibitors (Moderate); CYP2C9 Inhibitors (Strong); Fibric Acid Derivatives; Fluconazole; GLP-1 Agonists; Herbs (Hypoglycemic Properties); MAO Inhibitors; Miconazole (Oral); Mifepristone; Pegvisomant; Posaconazole; Probenecid; Quinolone Antibiotics; Ranitidine; Salicylates; Selective Serotonin Reuptake Inhibitors; Sulfonamide Derivatives; Vitamin K Antagonists; Voriconazole

Decreased Effect

The levels/effects of GlipiZIDE may be decreased by: Colesevelam; Corticosteroids (Orally Inhaled); Corticosteroids (Systemic); CYP2C9 Inducers (Strong); Dabrafenib; Loop Diuretics; Luteinizing Hormone-Releasing Hormone Analogs; Peginterferon Alfa-2b; Quinolone Antibiotics; Rifampin; Somatropin; Thiazide Diuretics

Ethanol/Nutrition/Herb Interactions

Ethanol: Caution with ethanol (may cause hypoglycemia or rare disulfiram reaction).

Food: A delayed release of insulin may occur if glipizide is taken with food. Immediate release tablets should be administered 30 minutes before meals to avoid erratic absorption.

Herb/Nutraceutical: Herbs with hypoglycemic properties may enhance the hypoglycemic effect of glipizide. This includes alfalfa, aloe, bilberry, bitter melon, burdock, celery, damiana, fenugreek, garcinia, garlic, ginger, ginseng (American), gymnema, marshmallow, stinging nettle

Storage/Stability Store below 30°C (86°F)

Mechanism of Action Stimulates insulin release from the pancreatic beta cells; reduces glucose output from the liver; insulin sensitivity is increased at peripheral target sites

Pharmacodynamics/Kinetics

Duration: 12-24 hours

Absorption: Immediate release: Rapid and complete; delayed with food

Distribution: 10-11 L

Protein binding: 98% to 99%; primarily to albumin

Bioavailability: 90% to 100%

Metabolism: Hepatic via CYP2C9; forms metabolites (inactive)

Half-life elimination: 2-5 hours

Time to peak: 1-3 hours; extended release tablets: 6-12 hours

Excretion: Urine (<10% as unchanged drug; 80% as metabolites); feces (10%)

Dosage

Oral: Adults:

Immediate release tablet: Initial: 5 mg once daily; titrate in 2.5-5 mg increments no more frequently than every few days based on blood glucose response; if once-daily dose is ineffective, may divide the dose; doses >15 mg/day should be administered in divided doses. Maximum recommended once-daily dose: 15 mg; maximum recommended total daily dose: 40 mg (some clinicians recommend a maximum total daily dose of 20 mg [Defronzo, 1999]).

Extended release tablet (Glucotrol XL®): Initial: 5 mg once daily; usual dose: 5-10 mg once daily; maximum recommended dose: 20 mg/day; dosage adjustments based on blood glucose monitoring should be made no more frequently than every 7 days

When transferring from immediate release to extended release glipizide: May switch the total daily dose of immediate release to the nearest equivalent daily dose of the extended release tablet and administer once daily; alternatively, may initiate extended release at 5 mg once daily and titrate accordingly.

When transferring from insulin to glipizide immediate release or extended release tablet:

Current insulin requirement ≤20 units: Discontinue insulin and initiate glipizide at usual dose

Current insulin requirement >20 units: Decrease insulin by 50% and initiate glipizide at usual dose; gradually decrease insulin dose based on patient response

Conversion from therapy with long half-life agents: Observe patient carefully for 1-2 weeks when converting from a longer half-life agent (eg, chlorpropamide) to glipizide due to overlapping hypoglycemic effects.

Elderly:

Immediate release tablet: Initial: 2.5 mg once daily; consider titrating by 2.5-5 mg/day at 1- to 2-week intervals

Extended release tablet: Initial and maintenance dosing should be on the lower end of the recommended range.

Dosing adjustment in renal impairment: No dosage adjustment provided in manufacturer's labeling although caution is recommended.

The following guidelines have been used by some clinicians (Aronoff, 2007): GFR ≤50 mL/minute: Decrease dose by 50%

Dosing adjustment in hepatic impairment:

Immediate release tablet: Initial: 2.5 mg once daily

Extended release tablet: There are no dosage adjustments provided in manufacturer's labeling; however, drug undergoes hepatic metabolism and use of a lower initial and maintenance dose should be considered.

Dietary Considerations Take immediate release tablets 30 minutes before meals (preferably before breakfast if once-daily dosing); extended release tablets should be taken with breakfast. Individualized medical nutrition therapy (MNT) based on ADA recommendations is an integral part of therapy.

Administration Administer immediate release tablets 30 minutes before a meal (preferably before breakfast if once-daily dosing) to achieve greatest reduction in postprandial hyperglycemia. Extended release tablets should be given with breakfast. Patients that are NPO or require decreased caloric intake may need doses held to avoid hypoglycemia.

Monitoring Parameters Signs and symptoms of hypoglycemia (fatigue, excessive hunger, profuse sweating, numbness of extremities), blood glucose, hemoglobin A_{1c} every 3 months for unstable patients and twice yearly for stable patients

Reference Range Recommendations for glycemic control in nonpregnant adults with diabetes (ADA, 2013):

Hb A_{1c}: <7% (a more aggressive [<6.5%] or less aggressive [<8%] Hb A_{1c} goal may be targeted based on patient-specific characteristics)

Preprandial capillary plasma glucose: 70-130 mg/dL

Peak postprandial capillary blood glucose: <180 mg/dL

Dosage Forms Excipient information presented when available (limited, particularly for generics); consult specific product labeling.

Tablet, Oral:

Glucotrol: 5 mg, 10 mg [scored]

Generic: 5 mg, 10 mg

Tablet Extended Release 24 Hour, Oral:

GlipiZIDE XL: 2.5 mg, 5 mg, 10 mg

Glucotrol XL: 2.5 mg, 5 mg, 10 mg

Generic: 2.5 mg, 5 mg, 10 mg

◆ **GlipiZIDE XL** *see* GlipiZIDE *on page* 957

Glipizide and Metformin

(GLIP i zide & met FOR min)

Brand Names: U.S. Metaglip™

Index Terms Glipizide and Metformin Hydrochloride; Metformin and Glipizide

Pharmacologic Category Antidiabetic Agent, Biguanide; Antidiabetic Agent, Sulfonylurea

Use Indicated as an adjunct to diet and exercise to improve glycemic control in adults with type 2 diabetes mellitus (noninsulin dependent, NIDDM)

Pregnancy Risk Factor C

Dosage Oral: Type 2 diabetes:

Adults:

Patients inadequately controlled on diet and exercise alone: Initial dose: Glipizide 2.5 mg/metformin 250 mg once daily with a meal. In patients with fasting plasma glucose (FPG) 280-320 mg/dL, initiate therapy with glipizide 2.5 mg/metformin 500 mg twice daily.

Note: Increase dose by 1 tablet/day every 2 weeks (maximum daily dose: Glipizide 10 mg/metformin 2000 mg in divided doses)

Patients inadequately controlled on a sulfonylurea and/or metformin: Initial dose: Glipizide 2.5 mg/metformin 500 mg or glipizide 5 mg/metformin 500 mg twice daily with morning and evening meals; starting dose should not exceed current daily dose of glipizide (or sulfonylurea equivalent) and/or metformin.

Note: Increase dose in increments of no more than glipizide 5 mg/metformin 500 mg (maximum daily dose: Glipizide 20 mg/metformin 2000 mg)

Elderly: Conservative doses are recommended in the elderly due to potentially decreased renal function; **do not titrate to maximum dose**; should not be used in patients ≥80 years unless renal function is verified as normal

Dosage adjustment in renal impairment: Contraindicated in the presence of renal disease or renal dysfunction (serum creatinine ≥1.5 mg/dL [males], ≥1.4 mg/dL [females], or abnormal creatinine clearance)

Dosage adjustment in hepatic impairment: Avoid use in patients with impaired liver function

Additional Information Complete prescribing information should be consulted for additional detail.

Dosage Forms Excipient information presented when available (limited, particularly for generics); consult specific product labeling. [DSC] = Discontinued product

Tablet, oral: 2.5/250: Glipizide 2.5 mg and metformin hydrochloride 250 mg; 2.5/500: Glipizide 2.5 mg and metformin hydrochloride 500 mg; 5/500: Glipizide 5 mg and metformin hydrochloride 500 mg

Metaglip™ 2.5/250: Glipizide 2.5 mg and metformin hydrochloride 250 mg [DSC]

Metaglip™ 2.5/500: Glipizide 2.5 mg and metformin hydrochloride 500 mg

Metaglip™ 5/500: Glipizide 5 mg and metformin hydrochloride 500 mg

- ◆ Glipizide and Metformin Hydrochloride *see* Glipizide and Metformin *on page 959*
- ◆ Glivec *see* Imatinib *on page 1048*
- ◆ Gln *see* Glutamine *on page 962*
- ◆ GlucaGen *see* Glucagon *on page 960*
- ◆ GlucaGen® (Can) *see* Glucagon *on page 960*
- ◆ GlucaGen HypoKit *see* Glucagon *on page 960*
- ◆ GlucaGen® HypoKit® (Can) *see* Glucagon *on page 960*

Glucagon (GLOO ka gon)

Brand Names: U.S. GlucaGen; GlucaGen HypoKit; Glucagon Emergency

Brand Names: Canada GlucaGen®; GlucaGen® HypoKit®

Index Terms Glucagon Hydrochloride

Pharmacologic Category Antidote; Antidote, Hypoglycemia; Diagnostic Agent

Use Management of hypoglycemia; diagnostic aid in radiologic examinations to temporarily inhibit GI tract movement

Unlabeled Use Beta-blocker- or calcium channel blocker-induced myocardial depression (with or without hypotension) unresponsive to standard measures; suspected or documented hypoglycemia secondary to insulin or sulfonylurea overdose (as adjunct to dextrose)

Pregnancy Risk Factor B

Pregnancy Considerations Adverse events have not been observed in animal reproduction studies.

Breast-Feeding Considerations Glucagon is not absorbed from the GI tract and therefore, it is unlikely adverse effects would occur in a breast-feeding infant.

Contraindications Hypersensitivity to glucagon or any component of the formulation; insulinoma; pheochromocytoma

Warnings/Precautions Use of glucagon is contraindicated in insulinoma; exogenous glucagon may cause an initial rise in blood glucose followed by rebound hypoglycemia. Use of glucagon is contraindicated in pheochromocytoma; exogenous glucagon may cause the release of catecholamines, resulting in an increase in blood pressure. Use caution with prolonged fasting, starvation, adrenal insufficiency or chronic hypoglycemia; levels of glucose stores in liver may be decreased. Supplemental carbohydrates should be given to patients who respond to glucagon for severe hypoglycemia to prevent secondary hypoglycemia. Monitor blood glucose levels closely.

In patients with hypoglycemia secondary to insulin or sulfonylurea overdose, dextrose should be immediately administered; if I.V. access cannot be established or if dextrose is not available, glucagon may be considered as alternative acute treatment until dextrose can be administered.

May contain lactose; avoid administration in hereditary galactose intolerance, Lapp lactase deficiency, or glucose-galactose malabsorption.

Adverse Reactions Frequency not defined.

Cardiovascular: Hypotension (up to 2 hours after GI procedures), hypertension, tachycardia

Gastrointestinal: Nausea, vomiting (high incidence with rapid administration of high doses)

Miscellaneous: Hypersensitivity reactions, anaphylaxis

Drug Interactions

Metabolism/Transport Effects None known.

Avoid Concomitant Use There are no known interactions where it is recommended to avoid concomitant use.

Increased Effect/Toxicity

Glucagon may increase the levels/effects of: Vitamin K Antagonists

Decreased Effect There are no known significant interactions involving a decrease in effect.

Ethanol/Nutrition/Herb Interactions Glucagon depletes glycogen stores.

Preparation for Administration Reconstitute powder for injection by adding 1 mL of sterile diluent to a vial containing 1 unit of the drug, to provide solutions containing 1 mg of glucagon/mL. Gently roll vial to dissolve. Solution for infusion may be prepared by reconstitution with and further dilution in NS or D_5W (Love, 1998).

Storage/Stability Prior to reconstitution, store at controlled room temperature of 20°C to 25°C (69°F to 77°F); do not freeze. Use reconstituted solution immediately. May be kept at 5°C for up to 48 hours if necessary.

Mechanism of Action Stimulates adenylate cyclase to produce increased cyclic AMP, which promotes hepatic glycogenolysis and gluconeogenesis, causing a raise in blood glucose levels

Pharmacodynamics/Kinetics

Onset of action: Peak effect: Blood glucose levels: Parenteral:

I.V.: 5-20 minutes

I.M.: 30 minutes

SubQ: 30-45 minutes

Duration: Glucose elevation:

SubQ: 60-90 minutes

I.V.: 30 minutes

Metabolism: Primarily hepatic; some inactivation occurring renally and in plasma

Half-life elimination, plasma: 8-18 minutes

Dosage

Hypoglycemia: I.M., I.V., SubQ:

Children <20 kg: 0.5 mg or 20-30 mcg/kg/dose; repeated in 20 minutes as needed

Children ≥20 kg and Adults: 1 mg; may repeat in 20 minutes as needed

Note: I.V. dextrose should be administered as soon as it is available; if patient fails to respond to glucagon, I.V. dextrose must be given.

Beta-blocker- or calcium channel blocker-induced myocardial depression (with or without hypotension) unresponsive to standard measures (unlabeled use): I.V.:

Children: Initial bolus of 30-150 mcg/kg followed by an infusion of 70 mcg/kg/hour (maximum: 5 mg/hour) (Hegenbarth, 2008)

Adolescents: Initial: 5-10 mg over several minutes followed by infusion of 1-5 mg/hour (Hegenbarth, 2008)

Adults: 3-10 mg (or 0.05-0.15 mg/kg) bolus followed by an infusion of 3-5 mg/hour (or 0.05-0.1 mg/kg/hour); titrate infusion rate to achieve adequate hemodynamic response (ACLS, 2010)

Diagnostic aid: Adults:

I.M.: 1-2 mg 10 minutes prior to gastrointestinal procedure

I.V.: 0.25-2 mg 10 minutes prior to gastrointestinal procedure

Dosage adjustment in renal impairment: No dosage adjustment provided in manufacturer's labeling.

Dosage adjustment in hepatic impairment: No dosage adjustment provided in manufacturer's labeling.

Dietary Considerations Administer carbohydrates to patient as soon as possible after response to treatment.

Usual Infusion Concentrations: Adult I.V. infusion: 4 mg in 50 mL (concentration: 0.08 mg/mL) of D_5W

Administration I.V.: Bolus may be associated with nausea and vomiting.

Beta-blocker/calcium channel blocker toxicity: Administer bolus over 3-5 minutes; continuous infusions may be used. Ensure adequate supply available to continue therapy.

Monitoring Parameters Blood pressure, blood glucose, ECG, heart rate, mentation

Additional Information

1 unit = 1 mg

The American Diabetes Association (ADA) recommends that glucagon be prescribed for all patients at significant risk of severe hypoglycemia; caregivers or family members of these patients should be trained on how to administer glucagon (ADA, 2013).

Dosage Forms Excipient information presented when available (limited, particularly for generics); consult specific product labeling.

Kit, Injection:

Glucagon Emergency: 1 mg

Solution Reconstituted, Injection, as hydrochloride:

GlucaGen: 1 mg (1 ea)

GlucaGen HypoKit: 1 mg (1 ea)

◆ **Glucagon Emergency** *see* Glucagon *on page 960*

◆ **Glucagon Hydrochloride** *see* Glucagon *on page 960*

Glucarpidase (gloo KAR pid ase)

Brand Names: U.S. Voraxaze

Index Terms Carboxypeptidase-G2; CPDG2; CPG2; Voraxaze

Pharmacologic Category Antidote; Enzyme

Use Treatment of toxic plasma methotrexate concentrations (>1 micromole/L) in patients with delayed clearance due to renal impairment

Note: Due to the risk of subtherapeutic methotrexate exposure, glucarpidase is **NOT** indicated when methotrexate clearance is within expected range (plasma methotrexate concentration ≤2 standard deviations of mean methotrexate excretion curve specific for dose administered) **or** with normal renal function or mild renal impairment.

Unlabeled Use Rescue agent to reduce methotrexate toxicity in patients with accidental intrathecal methotrexate overdose

Pregnancy Risk Factor C

Pregnancy Considerations Animal reproduction studies have not been conducted. If administered to a pregnant woman, the risk to the fetus is unknown; use only if clearly needed. In general, medications used as antidotes should take into consideration the health and prognosis of the mother.

Breast-Feeding Considerations Caution should be used if administered to a breast-feeding woman.

Prescribing and Access Restrictions Voraxaze® is distributed through ASD Healthcare; procurement information is available (24 hours a day; 365 days a year) at 1-855-7-VORAXAZE (1-855-786-7292). Voraxaze® is also commercially available in the U.S. through certain pharmacy wholesalers on a drop-ship basis; orders will only be processed during business hours for overnight delivery. For additional information, refer to http://www.btgplc.com/products/specialty-pharmaceuticals/voraxaze.

Contraindications There are no contraindications listed in the manufacturer's labeling.

Warnings/Precautions Serious allergic reactions have been reported.

Leucovorin calcium administration should be continued after glucarpidase; the same dose as was given prior to glucarpidase should be continued for the first 48 hours after glucarpidase; after 48 hours, leucovorin doses should be based on methotrexate concentrations. A single methotrexate concentration should not determine when leucovorin should be discontinued; continue leucovorin until the methotrexate concentration remains below the threshold for leucovorin treatment for ≥3 days. Leucovorin calcium is a substrate for glucarpidase and may compete with methotrexate for binding sites; **do not administer leucovorin calcium within 2 hours before or after glucarpidase.** In addition to leucovorin, glucarpidase use should be accompanied with adequate hydration and urinary alkalinization. During the first 48 hours following glucarpidase administration, the only reliable method of measuring methotrexate concentrations is the chromatographic method. DAMPA, an inactive methotrexate metabolite with a half-life of 9 hours, may interfere with immunoassay and result in the overestimation of the methotrexate concentration (when collected within 48 hours of glucarpidase administration). Glucarpidase use for intrathecal methotrexate overdose (unlabeled route/use) should be used in conjunction with immediate lumbar drainage; concurrent dexamethasone (4 mg I.V. every 6 hours for 4 doses) may minimize methotrexate-induced chemical arachnoiditis; leucovorin calcium (100 mg I.V. every 6 hours for 4 doses) may prevent systemic methotrexate toxicity (Widemann, 2004).

Adverse Reactions

>10%: Immunologic: Antibody development (21%)

1% to 10%:

Cardiovascular: Flushing (2%), hypotension (1%)

Central nervous system: Headache (1%)

Gastrointestinal: Nausea/vomiting (2%)

Neuromuscular & skeletal: Paresthesia (2%)

<1%, postmarketing, and/or case reports: Blurred vision, diarrhea, hypersensitivity reaction, hypertension, localized warm feeling, skin rash, throat irritation, tremor

Drug Interactions

Metabolism/Transport Effects None known.

Avoid Concomitant Use There are no known interactions where it is recommended to avoid concomitant use.

Increased Effect/Toxicity There are no known significant interactions involving an increase in effect.

Decreased Effect

Glucarpidase may decrease the levels/effects of: Leucovorin Calcium-Levoleucovorin

Preparation for Administration

I.V.: Reconstitute each vial (1000 units/vial) with 1 mL normal saline. Mix gently by rolling or tilting vial; do not shake. Upon reconstitution, solution should be clear, colorless and free of particulate matter.

Intrathecal (unlabeled route/use): Reconstitute 2000 units with 12 mL preservative-free normal saline (Widemann, 2004)

Storage/Stability Store intact vials refrigerated at 2°C to 8°C (36°F to 46°F); do not freeze. Reconstituted solutions should be used immediately or may be stored for up to 4 hours under refrigeration.

Mechanism of Action Recombinant enzyme which rapidly hydrolyzes the carboxyl-terminal glutamate residue from extracellular methotrexate into inactive metabolites (DAMPA and glutamate), resulting in a rapid reduction of methotrexate concentrations independent of renal function

Pharmacodynamics/Kinetics

Onset of action: Methotrexate toxicity: Reduces methotrexate concentrations by ≥97% within 15 minutes of I.V. administration

Duration: Methotrexate toxicity: Maintains a >95% reduction of methotrexate concentrations for up to 8 days

Distribution: V_d: I.V.: 3.6 L; distribution restricted to plasma volume

Half-life elimination: I.V.: Normal renal function: 6-9 hours; impaired renal function (Cl_{cr} <30 mL/minute): 8-10 hours (Phillips, 2008)

Dosage Children and Adults:

I.V.: Methotrexate toxicity: 50 units/kg (Buchen, 2005; Widemann, 1997; Widemann, 2010)

Intrathecal: Intrathecal methotrexate overdose (unlabeled route/use): 2000 units as soon as possible after accidental overdose (Widemann, 2004)

Dosage adjustment in renal impairment: No dosage adjustment necessary

Dosage adjustment in hepatic impairment: No dosage adjustment provided in the manufacturer's labeling; has not been studied.

Administration

I.V.: Infuse over 5 minutes; flush I.V. line before and after glucarpidase administration

Intrathecal (for intrathecal methotrexate overdose; unlabeled route/use): Glucarpidase was administered within 3-9 hours of accidental intrathecal methotrexate overdose in conjunction with lumbar drainage or ventriculolumbar perfusion (Widemann, 2004). Administered over 5 minutes via lumbar route, ventriculostomy, Ommaya reservoir, or lumbar and ventriculostomy (O'Marcaigh, 1996; Widemann, 2004). In one case report, 1000 units was administered through the ventricular catheter over 5 minutes and another 1000 units was administered through the lumbar catheter (O'Marcaigh, 1996).

Monitoring Parameters

Serum methotrexate levels: Use chromatographic method if <48 hours from glucarpidase administration (DAMPA interferes with immunoassay results until >48 hours)

CBC with differential, bilirubin, ALT, AST, serum creatinine; evaluate for signs/symptoms of methotrexate toxicity

Test Interactions Methotrexate levels: During the first 48 hours following glucarpidase administration, the only reliable method of measuring methotrexate concentrations is the chromatographic method. DAMPA, an inactive methotrexate metabolite with a half-life of 9 hours, may interfere with immunoassay and result in the overestimation of the methotrexate concentration (when collected within 48 hours of glucarpidase administration).

Additional Information The utility of more than one glucarpidase dose in reducing plasma methotrexate levels was evaluated in a study of 100 patients with high-dose methotrexate-induced nephrotoxicity (Widemann, 2010). Glucarpidase 50 units/kg I.V. was administered either as a single dose (n=65), 2 doses given 24 hours apart (n=28), or 3 doses given at 4 hour intervals (n=7). Six of the 65 patients randomized to a single dose also received a second delayed glucarpidase dose (>24 hours later) due to persistent methotrexate concentrations ≥1 micromole/L in spite of a ≥90% decrease in the plasma methotrexate concentration after the initial dose. The use of scheduled second and third glucarpidase doses did not result in additional methotrexate concentration decreases; and only 2 of the 6 patients who received a second delayed glucarpidase dose (>24 hours later) experienced a ≥50% methotrexate concentration reduction.

Dosage Forms Excipient information presented when available (limited, particularly for generics); consult specific product labeling.

Solution Reconstituted, Intravenous [preservative free]:
Voraxaze: 1000 units (1 ea)

- ◆ Glucobay™ (Can) *see* Acarbose *on page 26*
- ◆ GlucoNorm® (Can) *see* Repaglinide *on page 1797*
- ◆ Glucophage *see* MetFORMIN *on page 1310*
- ◆ Glucophage® (Can) *see* MetFORMIN *on page 1310*
- ◆ Glucophage XR *see* MetFORMIN *on page 1310*
- ◆ Glucotrol *see* GlipiZIDE *on page 957*
- ◆ Glucotrol XL *see* GlipiZIDE *on page 957*
- ◆ Glucovance® *see* Glyburide and Metformin *on page 965*
- ◆ Glulisine Insulin *see* Insulin Glulisine *on page 1089*
- ◆ Glumetza *see* MetFORMIN *on page 1310*
- ◆ Glumetza® (Can) *see* MetFORMIN *on page 1310*

Glutamine (GLOO ta meen)

Brand Names: U.S. NutreStore; Sympt-X G.I. [OTC]; Sympt-X [OTC]

Index Terms Gln; L-Glutamine

Pharmacologic Category Amino Acid; Gastrointestinal Agent, Miscellaneous

Use

NutreStore™: Treatment of short bowel syndrome (SBS) when used in combination with specialized nutritional support and growth hormone therapy

OTC products: Medical food used to promote GI tract healing and nutritional supplementation with GI disorders, HIV/AIDS, cancer, and other critical illnesses

Pregnancy Risk Factor C

Dosage Oral: Adults:

Nutritional supplement (Enterex® Glutapak-10®, Resource® GlutaSolve®, Sympt-X, Sympt-X G.I.): Average dose: 10 g 3 times/day; dosing range: 5-30 g/day

Short bowel syndrome (NutreStore™): 30 g/day administered as 5 g 6 times/day (every 2-3 hours while awake) for up to 16 weeks; to be used in combination with growth hormone and nutritional support

Dosage adjustment in renal impairment: No dosage adjustment provided in manufacturer's labeling.

Dosage adjustment in hepatic impairment: No dosage adjustment provided in manufacturer's labeling; use with caution.

Additional Information Complete prescribing information should be consulted for additional detail.

Dosage Forms Excipient information presented when available (limited, particularly for generics); consult specific product labeling.

Capsule, Oral:
Generic: 500 mg

Packet, Oral:
NutreStore: 5 g (84 ea)
Sympt-X G.I.: 10 g (60 ea)

Powder, Oral:
Sympt-X: (480 g)

Tablet, Oral:
Generic: 500 mg

- ◆ Glybenclamide *see* GlyBURIDE *on page 963*
- ◆ Glybenzcyclamide *see* GlyBURIDE *on page 963*

GlyBURIDE (GLYE byoor ide)

Brand Names: U.S. Diabeta; Glynase

Brand Names: Canada Apo-Glyburide®; DiaBeta®; Dom-Glyburide; Euglucon®; Med-Glybe; Mylan-Glybe; Novo-Glyburide; Nu-Glyburide; PMS-Glyburide; PRO-Glyburide; ratio-Glyburide; Riva-Glyburide; Sandoz-Glyburide; Teva-Glyburide

Index Terms Diabeta; Glibenclamide; Glybenclamide; Glybenzcyclamide; Micronase

Pharmacologic Category Antidiabetic Agent, Sulfonylurea

Additional Appendix Information

Beers Criteria – Potentially Inappropriate Medications for Geriatrics *on page 2368*

Oral Antidiabetic Agents Comparison Table *on page 2312*

Use Adjunct to diet and exercise for the management of type 2 diabetes mellitus (noninsulin dependent, NIDDM)

Unlabeled Use Alternative to insulin in women for the treatment of gestational diabetes mellitus (GDM) (11-33 weeks gestation)

Pregnancy Risk Factor B/C (manufacturer dependent)

Pregnancy Considerations Outcomes of animal reproduction studies differ by manufacturer labeling. Glyburide crosses the placenta. Some pharmacokinetic properties of glyburide may change during pregnancy (Hebert, 2009).

Glyburide has been evaluated as an alternative for the treatment of GDM. The severity of GDM at diagnosis, the gestational age at diagnosis, and certain maternal characteristics may determine the appropriateness of this use. Most pregnancy outcome information is from studies evaluating glyburide in pregnant women with GDM when therapy was started after the period of organogenesis. Severe hypoglycemia lasting 4-10 days has been noted in infants born to mothers taking a sulfonylurea at the time of delivery. Additional adverse maternal and fetal events have been noted in some studies and may be influenced by maternal glycemic control and/or differences in study design (Bertini, 2005; Ekpebegh, 2007; Joy 2012; Langer, 2000; Langer 2005). Due to the potential for neonatal hypoglycemia, the manufacturer recommends that if glyburide is used during pregnancy, it should be discontinued at least 2 weeks before the expected delivery date

For women with diabetes, maternal hyperglycemia itself can be associated with adverse effects in the fetus, neonate, and mother. To prevent adverse events, prior to conception and throughout pregnancy, the maternal Hb A_{1c} should be kept close to normal but without causing significant hypoglycemia. Glyburide may be used as an adjunct to medical nutrition therapy in carefully selected patients for the treatment of GDM; maternal glucose and fetal markers should be monitored closely. Insulin is the drug of choice for the control of type 1 or type 2 diabetes mellitus during pregnancy (ACOG, 2005; ADA, 2013; Kitzmiller, 2008; Metzger, 2007).

Breast-Feeding Considerations Data from initial studies note that glyburide was not detected in breast milk (Feig, 2005). According to the manufacturer, due to the potential for hypoglycemia in the nursing infant, a decision should be made whether to discontinue nursing or to discontinue the drug, taking into account the importance of treatment to the mother. Current guidelines note that breast-feeding is encouraged for all women, including those with diabetes; all types of insulin may be used while breast-feeding and some oral agents, including glyburide, may be acceptable for use as well (Metzger, 2007).

Contraindications Hypersensitivity to glyburide or any component of the formulation; type 1 diabetes mellitus (insulin dependent, IDDM), diabetic ketoacidosis; concomitant use with bosentan

Warnings/Precautions All sulfonylurea drugs are capable of producing severe hypoglycemia. Hypoglycemia is more likely to occur when caloric intake is deficient, after severe or prolonged exercise, when ethanol is ingested, or when more than one glucose-lowering drug is used. It is also more likely in elderly patients, malnourished patients and in patients with impaired renal or hepatic function; use with caution.

It may be necessary to discontinue therapy and administer insulin if the patient is exposed to stress (fever, trauma, infection, surgery). Loss of efficacy may be observed following prolonged use as a result of the progression of type 2 diabetes mellitus which results in continued beta cell destruction. In patients who were previously responding to sulfonylurea therapy, consider additional factors which may be contributing to decreased efficacy (eg, inappropriate dose, nonadherence to diet and exercise regimen). If no contributing factors can be identified, consider discontinuing use of the sulfonylurea due to secondary failure of treatment. Additional antidiabetic therapy (eg, insulin) will be required.

Elderly: Avoid use in older adults due to increased risk of prolonged hypoglycemia (Beers Criteria). Rapid and prolonged hypoglycemia (>12 hours) despite hypertonic glucose injections have been reported; age and hepatic and renal impairment are independent risk factors for hypoglycemia; dosage titration should be made at weekly intervals.

Chemical similarities are present among sulfonamides, sulfonylureas, carbonic anhydrase inhibitors, thiazides, and loop diuretics (except ethacrynic acid). Use in patients with sulfonamide allergy is not specifically contraindicated in product labeling, however, a risk of cross-reaction exists in patients with allergy to any of these compounds; avoid use when previous reaction has been severe.

Product labeling states oral hypoglycemic drugs may be associated with an increased cardiovascular mortality as compared to treatment with diet alone or diet plus insulin. Data to support this association are limited, and several studies, including a large prospective trial (UKPDS) have not supported an association.

Patients with G6PD deficiency may be at an increased risk of sulfonylurea-induced hemolytic anemia; however, cases have also been described in patients without G6PD deficiency during postmarketing surveillance. Use with caution and consider a nonsulfonylurea alternative in patients with G6PD deficiency.

Micronized glyburide tablets are **not** bioequivalent to *conventional* glyburide tablets; retitration should occur if patients are being transferred to a different glyburide formulation (eg, micronized-to-conventional or vice versa) or from other hypoglycemic agents.

Adverse Reactions Frequency not defined.

Cardiovascular: Vasculitis

Central nervous system: Dizziness, headache

Dermatologic: Angioedema, erythema, maculopapular eruptions, morbilliform eruptions, photosensitivity reaction, pruritus, purpura, rash, urticaria

Endocrine & metabolic: Disulfiram-like reaction, hypoglycemia, hyponatremia (SIADH reported with other sulfonylureas)

Gastrointestinal: Anorexia, constipation, diarrhea, epigastric fullness, heartburn, nausea

Genitourinary: Nocturia

Hematologic: Agranulocytosis, aplastic anemia, hemolytic anemia, leukopenia, pancytopenia, porphyria cutanea tarda, thrombocytopenia

Hepatic: Cholestatic jaundice, hepatitis, liver failure, transaminase increased

Neuromuscular & skeletal: Arthralgia, myalgia, paresthesia

Ocular: Blurred vision
Renal: Diuretic effect (minor)
Miscellaneous: Allergic reaction

Drug Interactions

Metabolism/Transport Effects **Substrate** of CYP2C9 (major); **Note:** Assignment of Major/Minor substrate status based on clinically relevant drug interaction potential; **Inhibits** CYP2C8 (weak), CYP3A4 (weak)

Avoid Concomitant Use

Avoid concomitant use of GlyBURIDE with any of the following: Bosentan; Pimozide

Increased Effect/Toxicity

GlyBURIDE may increase the levels/effects of: Alcohol (Ethyl); ARIPiprazole; Bosentan; Carbocisteine; CycloSPORINE (Systemic); Dofetilide; Hypoglycemic Agents; Lomitapide; Pimozide; Porfimer; Vitamin K Antagonists

The levels/effects of GlyBURIDE may be increased by: Beta-Blockers; Chloramphenicol; Cimetidine; Clarithromycin; Cyclic Antidepressants; CYP2C9 Inhibitors (Moderate); CYP2C9 Inhibitors (Strong); Fibric Acid Derivatives; Fluconazole; GLP-1 Agonists; Herbs (Hypoglycemic Properties); MAO Inhibitors; Miconazole (Oral); Mifepristone; Pegvisomant; Probenecid; Quinolone Antibiotics; Ranitidine; Salicylates; Selective Serotonin Reuptake Inhibitors; Sulfonamide Derivatives; Vitamin K Antagonists; Voriconazole

Decreased Effect

GlyBURIDE may decrease the levels/effects of: Bosentan

The levels/effects of GlyBURIDE may be decreased by: Bosentan; Colesevelam; Corticosteroids (Orally Inhaled); Corticosteroids (Systemic); CycloSPORINE (Systemic); CYP2C9 Inducers (Strong); Dabrafenib; Loop Diuretics; Luteinizing Hormone-Releasing Hormone Analogs; Peginterferon Alfa-2b; Quinolone Antibiotics; Rifampin; Somatropin; Thiazide Diuretics

Ethanol/Nutrition/Herb Interactions

Ethanol: Caution with ethanol (may cause hypoglycemia).

Herb/Nutraceutical: Herbs with hypoglycemic properties may enhance the hypoglycemic effect of glyburide. This includes alfalfa, aloe, bilberry, bitter melon, burdock, celery, damiana, fenugreek, garcinia, garlic, ginger, ginseng (American), gymnema, marshmallow, stinging nettle

Mechanism of Action Stimulates insulin release from the pancreatic beta cells; reduces glucose output from the liver; insulin sensitivity is increased at peripheral target sites

Pharmacodynamics/Kinetics

Onset of action: Serum insulin levels begin to increase 15-60 minutes after a single dose
Duration: ≤24 hours
Absorption: Significant within 1 hour
Distribution: 9-10 L
Protein binding, plasma: >99% primarily to albumin
Metabolism: Hepatic; forms metabolites (weakly active)
Bioavailability: Variable among oral dosage forms
Half-life elimination: Diaβeta®: 10 hours; Glynase® PresTab®: ~4 hours; may be prolonged with renal or hepatic impairment
Time to peak, serum: Adults: 2-4 hours
Excretion: Feces (50%) and urine (50%) as metabolites

Dosage Oral: Micronized glyburide tablets are **not** bioequivalent to conventional glyburide tablets; retitration should occur if patients are being transferred to a different glyburide formulation (eg, micronized-to-conventional or vice versa) or from other hypoglycemic agents.

Diaβeta®: Adults:

Initial: 2.5-5 mg/day, administered with breakfast or the first main meal of the day. In patients who are more sensitive to hypoglycemic drugs, start at 1.25 mg/day. Increase in increments of no more than 2.5 mg/day at weekly intervals based on the patient's blood glucose response

Maintenance: 1.25-20 mg/day given as single or divided doses. Some patients (especially those receiving >10 mg/day) may have a more satisfactory response with twice-daily dosing. Maximum: 20 mg/day

Elderly: Initial: 1.25-2.5 mg/day, increase by 1.25-2.5 mg/day every 1-3 weeks

Micronized tablets (Glynase® PresTab®): Adults:

Initial: 1.5-3 mg/day, administered with breakfast or the first main meal of the day in patients who are more sensitive to hypoglycemic drugs, start at 0.75 mg/day. Increase in increments of no more than 1.5 mg/day in weekly intervals based on the patient's blood glucose response.

Maintenance: 0.75-12 mg/day given as a single dose or in divided doses. Some patients (especially those receiving >6 mg/day) may have a more satisfactory response with twice-daily dosing. Maximum: 12 mg/day

Management of noninsulin-dependent diabetes mellitus in patients previously maintained on insulin: Initial dosage dependent upon previous insulin dosage, see table.

Dose Conversion: Insulin to Glyburide

Previous Daily Insulin Dosage (units/day)	Initial Glyburide Dosage *Conventional Formulation* (mg/day)	Initial Glyburide Dosage *Micronized Formulation* (mg/day)	Insulin Dosage Change (after glyburide started)
<20	2.5-5	1.5-3	Discontinue
20-40	5	3	Discontinue
>40	5 (increase in increments of 1.25-2.5 mg every 2-10 days)	3 (increase in increments of 0.75-1.5 mg every 2-10 days)	Reduce insulin dosage by 50% (gradually taper off insulin as glyburide dosage increased)

Dosing adjustment/comments in renal impairment: Cl_{cr} <50 mL/minute: **Not recommended**

Dosing adjustment in hepatic impairment: Use conservative initial and maintenance doses and avoid use in severe disease

Dietary Considerations Should be taken with meals at the same time each day (twice-daily dosing may be beneficial if conventional glyburide doses are >10 mg or micronized glyburide doses are >6 mg). Individualized medical nutrition therapy (MNT) based on ADA recommendations is an integral part of therapy.

Administration Administer with meals at the same time each day (twice-daily dosing may be beneficial if conventional glyburide doses are >10 mg or micronized glyburide doses are >6 mg). Patients that are NPO or require decreased caloric intake may need doses held to avoid hypoglycemia.

Monitoring Parameters Signs and symptoms of hypoglycemia, fasting blood glucose, hemoglobin A_{1c}

Reference Range Recommendations for glycemic control in nonpregnant adults with diabetes (ADA, 2013):

Hb A_{1c}: <7% (a more aggressive [<6.5%] or less aggressive [<8%] Hb A_{1c} goal may be targeted based on patient-specific characteristics)
Preprandial capillary plasma glucose: 70-130 mg/dL
Peak postprandial capillary blood glucose: <180 mg/dL

Dosage Forms Excipient information presented when available (limited, particularly for generics); consult specific product labeling.

Tablet, Oral:
Diabeta: 1.25 mg, 2.5 mg, 5 mg [scored]
Glynase: 1.5 mg, 3 mg, 6 mg [scored]
Generic: 1.25 mg, 1.5 mg, 2.5 mg, 3 mg, 5 mg, 6 mg

Glyburide and Metformin

(GLYE byoor ide & met FOR min)

Brand Names: U.S. Glucovance®

Index Terms Glyburide and Metformin Hydrochloride; Metformin and Glyburide

Pharmacologic Category Antidiabetic Agent, Biguanide; Antidiabetic Agent, Sulfonylurea

Use Adjunct to diet and exercise for the management of type 2 diabetes mellitus (noninsulin dependent, NIDDM)

Pregnancy Risk Factor B

Dosage Note: Dose must be individualized. Dosages expressed as glyburide/metformin components.

Adults: Oral:

Initial therapy (no prior treatment with sulfonylurea or metformin): 1.25 mg/250 mg once daily with a meal; patients with Hb A_{1c} >9% or fasting plasma glucose (FPG) >200 mg/dL may start with 1.25 mg/250 mg twice daily with meals. **Note:** Doses of 5 mg/500 mg should not be used as initial therapy, due to risk of hypoglycemia.

Dosage may be increased in increments of 1.25 mg/250 mg, at intervals of not less than 2 weeks; maximum daily dose: 10 mg/2000 mg (limited experience with higher doses)

Previously treated with a sulfonylurea or metformin alone: Initial: 2.5 mg/500 mg or 5 mg/500 mg twice daily with meals; increase in increments no greater than 5 mg/500 mg; maximum daily dose: 20 mg/2000 mg

When switching patients previously on a sulfonylurea and metformin together, do not exceed the daily dose of glyburide (or glyburide equivalent) or metformin.

Note: May combine with a thiazolidinedione in patients with an inadequate response to glyburide/metformin therapy (risk of hypoglycemia may be increased). When adding thiazolidinedione, continue glyburide and metformin at current dose and initiate thiazolidinedione at recommended starting dose.

Elderly: Oral: Conservative doses are recommended in the elderly due to potentially decreased renal function; **do not titrate to maximum dose**; should not be used in patients ≥80 years of age unless renal function is verified as normal

Dosage adjustment in renal impairment: Use is contraindicated in patients with serum creatinine ≥1.5 mg/dL in males, or ≥1.4 mg/dL in females or abnormal creatinine clearance.

Dosage adjustment in hepatic impairment: No dosage adjustment provided in manufacturer's labeling (has not been studied).

Additional Information Complete prescribing information should be consulted for additional detail.

Dosage Forms Excipient information presented when available (limited, particularly for generics); consult specific product labeling. [DSC] = Discontinued product

Tablet, oral: 1.25 mg/250 mg: Glyburide 1.25 mg and metformin hydrochloride 250 mg; 2.5 mg/500 mg: Glyburide 2.5 mg and metformin hydrochloride 500 mg; 5 mg/500 mg: Glyburide 5 mg and metformin hydrochloride 500 mg

Glucovance®: 1.25 mg/250 mg: Glyburide 1.25 mg and metformin hydrochloride 250 mg [DSC]

Glucovance®: 2.5 mg/500 mg: Glyburide 2.5 mg and metformin hydrochloride 500 mg

Glucovance®: 5 mg/500 mg: Glyburide 5 mg and metformin hydrochloride 500 mg

◆ **Glyburide and Metformin Hydrochloride** *see* Glyburide and Metformin *on page 965*

◆ **Glycate** *see* Glycopyrrolate *on page 965*

◆ **Glycerol Guaiacolate** *see* GuaiFENesin *on page 974*

◆ **Glyceryl Trinitrate** *see* Nitroglycerin *on page 1466*

◆ **GlycoLax [OTC]** *see* Polyethylene Glycol 3350 *on page 1668*

◆ **Glycon (Can)** *see* MetFORMIN *on page 1310*

◆ **Glycophos** *see* Sodium Glycerophosphate Pentahydrate *on page 1918*

Glycopyrrolate

(glye koe PYE roe late)

Brand Names: U.S. Cuvposa; Glycate; Robinul; Robinul-Forte

Brand Names: Canada Glycopyrrolate Injection, USP; Seebri® Breezhaler®

Index Terms Glycopyrronium Bromide; NVA237

Pharmacologic Category Anticholinergic Agent

Use Inhibit salivation and excessive secretions of the respiratory tract preoperatively; control of upper airway secretions; intraoperatively to counteract drug-induced or vagal mediated bradyarrhythmias; adjunct in treatment of peptic ulcer (indication listed in product labeling but currently has no place in management of peptic ulcer disease)

Cuvposa™: Reduce chronic, severe drooling in those with neurologic conditions (eg, cerebral palsy) associated with drooling

Seebri® Breezhaler® (Canadian availability; not available in U.S.): Maintenance treatment of chronic obstructive pulmonary disease (COPD) including chronic bronchitis and emphysema

Unlabeled Use Adjunct with acetylcholinesterase inhibitors (eg, neostigmine, edrophonium, pyridostigmine) to antagonize cholinergic effects

Pregnancy Risk Factor B (injection) / C (oral solution)

Pregnancy Considerations Teratogenic effects were not observed in animal studies. Small amounts of glycopyrrolate cross the human placenta.

Breast-Feeding Considerations May suppress lactation

Contraindications Hypersensitivity to glycopyrrolate or any component of the formulation; medical conditions that preclude use of anticholinergic medication; severe ulcerative colitis, toxic megacolon complicating ulcerative colitis, paralytic ileus, obstructive disease of GI tract (eg, pyloric stenosis), intestinal atony in the elderly or debilitated patient; unstable cardiovascular status in acute hemorrhage; narrow-angle glaucoma; acute hemorrhage; tachycardia; obstructive uropathy; myasthenia gravis

Oral solution: Additional contraindication: Concomitant use of potassium chloride in a solid oral dosage form

Seebri® Breezhaler® (Canadian availability; not available in U.S.): Hypersensitivity to glycopyrronium bromide or any component of the formulation

Warnings/Precautions Diarrhea may be a sign of incomplete intestinal obstruction, treatment should be discontinued if this occurs. Use caution in elderly and in patients with autonomic neuropathy, narrow-angle glaucoma, renal disease, or ulcerative colitis; may precipitate/aggravate ileus or toxic megacolon, hyperthyroidism, CAD, CHF, arrhythmias, tachycardia, BPH, bladder neck obstruction, or hiatal hernia with reflux. Use of anticholinergics in gastric ulcer treatment may cause a delay in gastric emptying. Caution should be used in individuals demonstrating decreased pigmentation (skin and iris coloration, dark versus light) since there has been some evidence that these individuals have an enhanced sensitivity to the anticholinergic response. May cause drowsiness, eye sensitivity to light, or blurred vision; caution should be used when performing tasks which require mental alertness, such as driving. The risk of heat stroke with this medication may be increased during exercise or hot weather. Injection contains benzyl alcohol (associated with gasping syndrome in neonates). Seebri® Breezhaler® (Canadian availability; not available in U.S.) is not indicated for the initial (rescue) treatment of acute episodes of bronchospasm or with acutely deteriorating COPD; after initiation of therapy, patients should use short-acting bronchodilators only on an as needed basis for acute symptoms. Rarely, paradoxical bronchospasm may occur with use of inhaled bronchodilating agents; discontinue use of inhaler and consider other therapy if bronchospasm occurs. Patients using Seebri® Breezhaler® should avoid getting the powder into their eyes.

Adverse Reactions

>10% (as reported with Cuvposa™):

Cardiovascular: Flushing (30%)

Central nervous system: Headache (15%)

Gastrointestinal: Vomiting (40%), xerostomia (40%), constipation (35%)

Genitourinary: Urinary retention (15%)

Respiratory: Nasal congestion (30%), sinusitis (15%), upper respiratory tract infection (15%)

<10% (frequency not always defined):

Cardiovascular: Pallor (≤2%), arrhythmias, cardiac arrest, heart block, hyper-/hypotension, malignant hyperthermia, palpitation, QT_c-interval prolongation, tachycardia

Central nervous system: Aggressiveness (≤2%), agitation (≤2%), crying (abnormal; ≤2%), irritability (≤2%), mood changes (≤2%), pain(≤2%), restlessness(≤2%), confusion, dizziness, drowsiness, excitement, insomnia, nervousness, seizure

Dermatologic: Dry skin (≤2%), pruritus (≤2%), rash (≤2%), urticaria

Endocrine & metabolic: Dehydration (≤2%), lactation suppression

Gastrointestinal: Abdominal distention (≤2%), abdominal pain (≤2%), flatulence (≤2%), retching (≤2%), bloated feeling, intestinal obstruction, loss of taste, nausea, pseudo-obstruction

Genitourinary: Urinary tract infection (≤2%), impotence, urinary hesitancy

Local: Injection site reactions (edema, erythema, pain)

Neuromuscular & skeletal: Weakness

Ocular: Nystagmus (≤2%), blurred vision, cycloplegia, mydriasis, ocular tension increased, photophobia, sensitivity to light increased

Respiratory: Bronchial secretion (thickening; ≤2%), nasal dryness (≤2%), pneumonia (≤2%), respiratory depression

Miscellaneous: Anaphylactoid reactions, diaphoresis decreased, hypersensitivity reactions

As reported with Seebri® Breezhaler® (Canadian availability; not available in U.S.):

1% to 10%:

Central nervous system: Headache (elderly: 2%)

Gastrointestinal: Xerostomia (2% to 3%), gastroenteritis (1% to 3%), dyspepsia (1%), vomiting (1%)

Genitourinary: Urinary tract infection (elderly: 3%), dysuria (1%)

Neuromuscular & skeletal: Musculoskeletal pain (2%)

Respiratory: Nasopharyngitis (9%), rhinitis (2%)

<1% (Limited to important or life-threatening): Cough, cystitis, dental caries, diabetes mellitus, epistaxis, fatigue, hypoesthesia, palpitations, rash, throat irritation, urinary retention, weakness

Drug Interactions

Metabolism/Transport Effects None known.

Avoid Concomitant Use

Avoid concomitant use of Glycopyrrolate with any of the following: Aclidinium; Ipratropium (Oral Inhalation); Potassium Chloride; Tiotropium; Umeclidinium

Increased Effect/Toxicity

Glycopyrrolate may increase the levels/effects of: AbobotulinumtoxinA; Analgesics (Opioid); Anticholinergics; Atenolol; Cannabinoids; Digoxin; MetFORMIN; Mirabegron; OnabotulinumtoxinA; Potassium Chloride; RimabotulinumtoxinB; Thiazide Diuretics; Tiotropium; Topiramate

The levels/effects of Glycopyrrolate may be increased by: Aclidinium; Amantadine; Ipratropium (Oral Inhalation); MAO Inhibitors; Pramlintide; Umeclidinium

Decreased Effect

Glycopyrrolate may decrease the levels/effects of: Acetylcholinesterase Inhibitors (Central); Haloperidol; Levodopa; Secretin

The levels/effects of Glycopyrrolate may be decreased by: Acetylcholinesterase Inhibitors (Central)

Ethanol/Nutrition/Herb Interactions Food: Administration with a high-fat meal significantly reduced absorption; administer on an empty stomach.

Storage/Stability Store at 20°C to 25°C (68°F to 77°F).

Oral capsules for inhalation (Canadian availability; not available in U.S.): Store at 15°C to 25°C (59°F to 77°F) in blister. Capsules should be stored in the blister pack and only removed immediately before use. Once protective foil is peeled back and/or removed the capsule should be used immediately; if capsule is not used immediately, it should be discarded. Do not store capsules in Seebri® Breezhaler®. Protect from moisture.

Mechanism of Action Blocks the action of acetylcholine at parasympathetic sites in smooth muscle, secretory glands, and the CNS; indirectly reduces the rate of salivation by preventing the stimulation of acetylcholine receptors

In COPD, competitively and reversibly inhibits the action of acetylcholine at muscarinic receptor subtypes 1-3 (greater affinity for subtypes 1 and 3) in bronchial smooth muscle thereby causing bronchodilation

Pharmacodynamics/Kinetics

Note: Oral powder for inhalation is not available in the U.S.

Onset of action: Oral: 50 minutes; I.M.: 15-30 minutes; I.V.: ~1 minute

Peak effect: Oral: ~1 hour; I.M.: 30-45 minutes

Duration: Vagal effect: 2-3 hours; Inhibition of salivation: Up to 7 hours; Anticholinergic: Oral: 8-12 hours

Absorption: Oral tablet: Poor and erratic; Oral solution: 23% lower compared to tablet; Oral powder for inhalation: Rapid

Distribution: V_d: Children: 1.3-1.8 L/kg; Adults: 0.2-0.62 L/kg

Metabolism: Hepatic (minimal)

Bioavailability: Tablet: ~1% to 13%; Oral powder for inhalation: ~40%

Half-life elimination: Infants: 22-130 minutes; Children 19-99 minutes; Adults: ~60-75 minutes; Oral solution: Adults: 3 hours; Oral powder for inhalation: 13-22 hours (Sechaud, 2012)

Time to peak, plasma: Oral powder for inhalation: 5 minutes

Excretion: Urine (as unchanged drug, I.M.: 80%, I.V.: 85%); bile (as unchanged drug)

Dosage

Children:

Reduction of secretions (preanesthetic):

Oral (unlabeled): 40-100 mcg/kg/dose 3-4 times/day

I.M., I.V. (unlabeled): 4-10 mcg/kg/dose every 3-4 hours; maximum: 0.2 mg/dose or 0.8 mg/24 hours

Intraoperative: I.V.: 4 mcg/kg not to exceed 0.1 mg; repeat at 2- to 3-minute intervals as needed

Preoperative: I.M.:

<2 years: 4-9 mcg/kg 30-60 minutes before procedure

>2 years: 4 mcg/kg 30-60 minutes before procedure

Drooling, chronic: Children 3-16 years: Oral solution (Cuvposa™): Initial: 0.02 mg/kg 3 times/day; titrate in increments of 0.02 mg/kg every 5-7 days as tolerated, up to a maximum dose of 0.1 mg/kg 3 times/day, not to exceed 1.5-3 mg/dose

Children and Adults: Reverse neuromuscular blockade: I.V.: 0.2 mg for each 1 mg of neostigmine or 5 mg of pyridostigmine administered or 5-15 mcg/kg glycopyrrolate with 25-70 mcg/kg of neostigmine or 0.1-0.3 mg/kg of pyridostigmine (agents usually administered simultaneously, but glycopyrrolate may be administered first if bradycardia is present)

Adults:

COPD: Oral powder for inhalation: Seebri® Breezhaler® (Canadian availability; not available in the U.S.): 50 mcg (contents of one capsule) once daily

Reduction of secretions:

Intraoperative: I.V.: 0.1 mg repeated as needed at 2- to 3-minute intervals

Preoperative: I.M.: 4 mcg/kg 30-60 minutes before procedure

Dosage adjustment in renal impairment: No dosage adjustment provided in manufacturer's labeling. However, data suggest renal impairment reduces glycopyrrolate elimination; use with caution.

Dosage adjustment in hepatic impairment: No dosage adjustment provided in manufacturer's labeling (has not been studied).

Administration

I.V.: Administer I.V. at a rate of 0.2 mg over 1-2 minutes. May be administered I.M. or I.V. without dilution. May also be administered via the tubing of a running I.V. infusion of a compatible solution. May be administered I.V. in the same syringe with neostigmine or pyridostigmine.

Oral: Administer oral solution on an empty stomach, 1 hour before or 2 hours after meals

Oral inhalation (Canadian availability; not available in the U.S.): Administer once daily preferably at the same time each day using the Seebri® Breezhaler® only. Remove capsule from foil blister immediately before use. Do not swallow capsule. Avoid getting powder into eyes. Place capsule in the capsule-chamber in the base of the Seebri® Breezhaler®. A click is heard as it fully closes. Hold inhaler with mouthpiece in upright position and pierce capsule within chamber by simultaneously pressing piercing buttons on base of inhaler (click is heard as capsule is pierced). Release buttons. Exhale fully. Do not exhale into inhaler. Tilt head slightly back and place mouthpiece in mouth with piercing buttons on base of inhaler in horizontal position and not up and down. Do not press piercing buttons. Inhale (rapidly, steadily and deeply); the capsule vibration should be heard within the device. Hold breath for at least 5-10 seconds or as long as possible. Remove mouthpiece prior to exhalation. Patient should not breathe out through the mouthpiece. If any powder remains in capsule, exhale and inhale again. Repeat until capsule is empty. Throw away empty capsule; do not leave in inhaler. Always keep capsules and inhaler dry. **Note:** If a dose is missed, take as soon as possible on that day; do not take 2 doses on the same day.

Monitoring Parameters Heart rate; anticholinergic effects; bowel sounds; bowel movements; effects on drooling

Oral inhalation: FEV_1, peak flow (or other pulmonary function studies)

Dosage Forms Excipient information presented when available (limited, particularly for generics); consult specific product labeling.

Solution, Injection:

Robinul: 0.2 mg/mL (1 mL); 0.4 mg/2 mL (2 mL); 1 mg/5 mL (5 mL); 4 mg/20 mL (20 mL) [contains benzyl alcohol]

Generic: 0.2 mg/mL (1 mL); 0.4 mg/2 mL (2 mL); 1 mg/5 mL (5 mL); 4 mg/20 mL (20 mL)

Solution, Oral:

Cuvposa: 1 mg/5 mL (473 mL) [contains methylparaben, propylene glycol, propylparaben, saccharin sodium; cherry flavor]

Tablet, Oral:

Glycate: 1.5 mg [dye free]

Robinul: 1 mg [scored]

Robinul-Forte: 2 mg [scored]

Generic: 1 mg, 2 mg

Dosage Forms: Canada Excipient information presented when available (limited, particularly for generics); consult specific product labeling.

Powder, for oral inhalation:

Seebri® Breezhaler®: 50 mcg/capsule (30s) [contains lactose]

Extemporaneous Preparations A 0.5 mg/mL oral suspension may be made with 1 mg tablets and a 1:1 mixture of Ora-Plus® and either Ora-Sweet® or Ora-Sweet® SF. Crush thirty 1 mg tablets in a mortar and reduce to a fine powder. Prepare diluent by mixing 30 mL of Ora-Plus® with 30 mL of either Ora-Sweet® or Ora-Sweet® SF and stir vigorously. Add 30 mL of diluent (via geometric dilution) to powder until smooth suspension is obtained. Transfer suspension to 60 mL amber bottle. Rinse contents of mortar into bottle with sufficient quantity of remaining diluent to obtain 60 mL (final volume). Label "shake well". Stable at room temperature for 90 days. Due to bitter aftertaste, chocolate syrup may be administered prior to or mixed (1:1 v/v) with suspension immediately before administration (Cober, 2011).

A 0.5 mg/mL oral solution can be made from tablets. Crush fifty 1 mg tablets in a mortar and reduce to a fine powder. Add enough distilled water to make about 90 mL, mix well. Transfer to a bottle, rinse mortar with water, and add a quantity of water sufficient to make 100 mL. Label "shake well" and "protect from light". Stable at room temperature for 25 days (Gupta, 2001).

A 0.1 mg/mL oral solution may be made using glycopyrrolate 0.2 mg/mL injection without preservatives. Withdraw 50 mL from vials with a needle and syringe, add to 50 mL of a 1:1 mixture of Ora-Sweet® and Ora-Plus® in a bottle. Label "shake well", "protect from light," and "refrigerate". Stable refrigerated for 35 days (Landry, 2005).

Cober MP, Johnson CE, Sudekum D, et al, "Stability of Extemporaneously Prepared Glycopyrrolate Oral Suspensions," *Am J Health Syst Phar*,. 2011, 68(9):843-5.

Gupta VD, "Stability of an Oral Liquid Dosage Form of Glycopyrrolate Prepared from Tablets," *IJPC* 2001, 5(6):480-1.

Landry C, "Stability and Subjective Taste Acceptability of Four Glycopyrrolate Solutions for Oral Administration," *IJPC*, 2005, 9(5):396-98.

◆ **Glycopyrrolate Injection, USP (Can)** *see* Glycopyrrolate *on page 965*

◆ **Glycopyrronium Bromide** *see* Glycopyrrolate *on page 965*

◆ **Glydiazinamide** *see* GlipiZIDE *on page 957*

◆ **Glynase** *see* GlyBURIDE *on page 963*

◆ **Gly-Oxide [OTC]** *see* Carbamide Peroxide *on page 340*

◆ **Glyquin® XM (Can)** *see* Hydroquinone *on page 1017*

◆ **Glyset** *see* Miglitol *on page 1368*

◆ **GM-CSF** *see* Sargramostim *on page 1877*

◆ **GMD-Gemfibrozil (Can)** *see* Gemfibrozil *on page 947*

◆ GnRH Agonist *see* Histrelin *on page 998*

Golimumab (goe LIM ue mab)

Brand Names: U.S. Simponi; Simponi Aria

Brand Names: Canada Simponi; Simponi I.V.

Index Terms CNTO-148

Pharmacologic Category Antipsoriatic Agent; Antirheumatic, Disease Modifying; Monoclonal Antibody; Tumor Necrosis Factor (TNF) Blocking Agent

Use

Ankylosing spondylitis (Simponi): Treatment of active ankylosing spondylitis

Psoriatic arthritis (Simponi): Treatment of active psoriatic arthritis (either alone or in combination with methotrexate)

Rheumatoid arthritis (Simponi, Simponi Aria): Treatment of moderately-to-severely active rheumatoid arthritis (in combination with methotrexate)

Ulcerative colitis (Simponi): Treatment of moderately-to-severely active ulcerative colitis in patients with corticosteroid dependence or who are refractory or intolerant to oral aminosalicylates, oral corticosteroids, azathioprine, or 6-mercaptopurine (to induce and maintain clinical response, improve mucosal appearance during induction, induce clinical remission, and achieve and sustain remission in induction responders)

Pregnancy Risk Factor B

Pregnancy Considerations Adverse events were not observed in animal reproduction studies. Golimumab crosses the placenta. Based on data from other TNF-blockers, antibodies may be present in the newborn serum for up to 6 months and infants exposed to golimumab *in utero* may be at risk of increased infection. Administration of live vaccines to newborns is not recommended until 6 months after the last maternal dose. Canadian labeling recommends that women of childbearing potential use reliable contraception during and for at least 6 months after discontinuation of golimumab therapy.

Breast-Feeding Considerations It is not known whether golimumab is secreted in human milk. Because many immunoglobulins are secreted in milk and the potential for serious adverse reactions exists, a decision should be made whether to discontinue nursing or discontinue the drug, taking into account the importance of the drug to the mother.

Medication Guide Available Yes

Contraindications There are no contraindications listed in the manufacturer's U.S. labeling.

Canadian labeling: Hypersensitivity to golimumab, latex, or any other component of formulation or packaging; patients with severe infections (eg, sepsis, tuberculosis, opportunistic infections); moderate or severe heart failure (NYHA class III/IV)

Warnings/Precautions [U.S. Boxed Warning]: Patients receiving golimumab are at increased risk for serious infections which may result in hospitalization and/or fatality; infections usually developed in patients receiving concomitant immunosuppressive agents (eg, methotrexate or corticosteroids). Active tuberculosis (or reactivation of latent tuberculosis), invasive fungal (including aspergillosis, blastomycosis, candidiasis, coccidioidomycosis, histoplasmosis, and pneumocystosis) and bacterial, viral or other opportunistic infections (including legionellosis and listeriosis) have been reported in patients receiving TNF-blocking agents, including golimumab. May present as disseminated (rather than local) disease. Histoplasmosis testing (antigen or antibody) may be negative in some patients with active infection. Monitor closely for signs/symptoms of infection. Discontinue for serious infection or sepsis. Consider risks versus benefits prior to use in patients with a history of chronic or recurrent infection. Consider empiric antifungal therapy in patients who are at risk for invasive fungal infection and develop severe systemic illness. Discontinue in patients who develop a serious infection or an opportunistic infection. Caution should be exercised when considering use in the elderly, patients taking concomitant immunosuppressants, patients with a history of opportunistic infection, patients with comorbid conditions that predispose them to infections (eg, diabetes), or residence/travel from areas of endemic mycoses (blastomycosis, coccidioidomycosis, histoplasmosis). Do not initiate golimumab therapy in patients with with active infection, including localized infection which is clinically important. Patients who develop a new infection while undergoing treatment should be monitored closely.

[U.S. Boxed Warning]: Tuberculosis (disseminated or extrapulmonary) has been reported in patients receiving golimumab; both reactivation of latent infection and new infections have been reported. Patients should be evaluated for tuberculosis risk factors and latent tuberculosis infection (with a tuberculin skin test) prior to and during therapy. Treatment of latent tuberculosis should be initiated before use. Patients with initial negative tuberculin skin tests should receive continued monitoring for tuberculosis throughout treatment; active tuberculosis has developed in this population during treatment with TNF-blocking agents. Use with caution in patients who have resided in regions where tuberculosis is endemic. Consider antituberculosis therapy if an adequate course of treatment cannot be confirmed in patients with a history of latent or active tuberculosis or for patients with risk factors despite negative skin test.

Rare reactivation of hepatitis B virus (HBV) has occurred in chronic virus carriers (usually in patients receiving concomitant immunosuppressants); evaluate prior to initiation in all patients. Patients who test positive for HBV surface antigen should be referred for hepatitis B evaluation/treatment prior to golimumab initiation. Monitor during and for several months following discontinuation of treatment in HBV carriers; interrupt therapy if reactivation occurs and treat appropriately with antiviral therapy; if resumption of therapy is deemed necessary, exercise caution and monitor patient closely. Patients should be brought up to date with all immunizations before initiating therapy. Live vaccines should not be given concurrently. In clinical trials, humoral response to pneumococcal vaccine was not suppressed in psoriatic arthritis patients.

[U.S. Boxed Warning]: Lymphoma and other malignancies (some fatal) have been reported in children and adolescent patients receiving TNF-blocking agents. Half of the malignancies reported in children were lymphomas (Hodgkin's and non-Hodgkin's) while other cases varied and included malignancies not typically observed in this population. The onset of malignancy was after a median of 30 months (range: 1-84 months) after the initiation of the TNF-blocking agent. The impact of golimumab on the development and course of malignancy is not fully defined. Compared to the general population, an increased risk of lymphoma has been noted in clinical trials; however, rheumatoid arthritis alone has been previously associated with an increased rate of lymphoma. Lymphomas and other malignancies were also observed (at rates higher than expected for the general population) in adult patients receiving TNF-blocking agents. Hepatosplenic T-cell lymphoma (HSTCL), a rare T-cell lymphoma, has also been associated with TNF-blocking agents, primarily reported in adolescent and young adult males with Crohn's disease (or in some cases ulcerative colitis) treated with a TNF-blocking agent and concurrent or prior azathioprine or mercaptopurine. Melanoma and Merkel cell carcinoma have been reported in patients receiving TNF-blocking agents including golimumab. Perform periodic skin examinations in all patients during therapy, particularly those at increased risk for skin cancer. Consider risks versus benefits in patients with a known malignancy (other than a successfully treated nonmelanoma skin cancer) and if considering continuing treatment in a patient who develops a malignancy. Rare cases of pancytopenia and other significant cytopenias, including aplastic anemia, have been reported with TNF-blocking agents. Pancytopenia, leukopenia, neutropenia and thrombocytopenia have occurred with golimumab; use with caution in patients with underlying hematologic disorders. Consider discontinuing therapy with significant hematologic abnormalities. Treatment may result in the formation of autoimmune antibodies; cases of autoimmune disease have not been described.

Use with caution in patients with pre-existing or recent onset central or peripheral nervous system demyelinating disorders; rare cases of new-onset or exacerbation of demyelinating disorders (eg, multiple sclerosis, optic neuritis, Guillain-Barré syndrome, polyneuropathy) have been reported. Consider discontinuing use in patients who develop peripheral or central nervous system demyelinating disorders during treatment. Use with caution in patients with heart failure or decreased left ventricular function; monitor closely and discontinue with new-onset or worsening of symptoms. Canadian labeling contraindicates use in moderate or severe heart failure (NYHA class III/IV). Severe systemic hypersensitivity reactions (including anaphylaxis), have been reported (some have occurred with the first dose) following subcutaneous administration; discontinue immediately if signs develop and initiate appropriate treatment.

Avoid concomitant use with abatacept (increased incidence of serious infections) or anakinra (increased incidence of neutropenia and serious infection). Potentially significant drug-drug interactions may exist, requiring dose or frequency adjustment, additional monitoring, and/or selection of alternative therapy. Use caution when switching between biological disease-modifying antirheumatic drugs (DMARDs); overlapping of biological activity may increase the risk for infection. Use with caution in the elderly (general incidence of infection is higher). Packaging (prefilled syringe and needle cover) contains dry natural rubber (latex). Some dosage forms may contain dry natural rubber (latex) and/or polysorbate 80. The safety and efficacy of switching between the I.V. and SubQ formulations and routes have not been studied.

Adverse Reactions

>10%:

Respiratory: Upper respiratory tract infection (16%; includes laryngitis, nasopharyngitis, pharyngitis, and rhinitis)

Miscellaneous: Infection (28%)

1% to 10%:

Cardiovascular: Hypertension (3%)

Central nervous system: Dizziness (2%), fever (1%)

Gastrointestinal: Constipation (1%)

Hematologic & oncologic: Positive ANA titer (titer ≥1:160; 4%)

Hepatic: ALT increased (4%; ≥3 ULN: 2%), AST increased (3%)

Immunologic: Antibody development (3% to 7%)

Local: Injection site reactions (3% to 6%)

Neuromuscular & skeletal: Paresthesia (2%)

Respiratory: Bronchitis (2%), sinusitis (2%)

Miscellaneous: Viral infection (5%; includes herpes and influenza), antibody formation (4%), fungal infection (superficial; 2%)

<1% (Limited to important or life-threatening): Abscess, anaphylaxis, aspergillosis, atypical mycobacterial infection, bacterial arthritis, candidiasis, cellulitis, coccidioidomycosis, HBV reactivation, histoplasmosis, hypersensitivity reactions, infective bursitis, leukemia, leukopenia, listeriosis, lupus-like syndrome, lymphomas, malignancy (other than nonmelanoma skin cancer), malignant melanoma, Merkel cell carcinoma, multiple sclerosis, neutropenia, optic neuritis, pancytopenia, peripheral demyelinating polyneuropathy, pneumocystosis, pneumonia, psoriasis (including new onset, palmoplantar, pustular, or exacerbation), pyelonephritis, sarcoidosis, sepsis, septic shock, skin exfoliation, thrombocytopenia, tuberculosis (including reactivation of latent and new infection), vasculitis

Drug Interactions

Metabolism/Transport Effects None known.

Avoid Concomitant Use

Avoid concomitant use of Golimumab with any of the following: Abatacept; Anakinra; BCG; Belimumab; Canakinumab; Certolizumab Pegol; InFLIXimab; Natalizumab; Pimecrolimus; Rilonacept; Tacrolimus (Topical); Tocilizumab; Tofacitinib; Vaccines (Live)

Increased Effect/Toxicity

Golimumab may increase the levels/effects of: Abatacept; Anakinra; Belimumab; Canakinumab; Certolizumab Pegol; InFLIXimab; Leflunomide; Natalizumab; Rilonacept; Tofacitinib; Vaccines (Live)

The levels/effects of Golimumab may be increased by: Abciximab; Denosumab; Pimecrolimus; Roflumilast; Tacrolimus (Topical); Tocilizumab; Trastuzumab

Decreased Effect

Golimumab may decrease the levels/effects of: BCG; Coccidioidin Skin Test; Sipuleucel-T; Vaccines (Inactivated); Vaccines (Live)

The levels/effects of Golimumab may be decreased by: Echinacea

Preparation for Administration Intact solution should be colorless to light yellow.

SubQ: Bring to room temperature by allowing syringe/autoinjector to sit at room temperature outside the carton for 30 minutes prior to administration (do not warm in any other way). Do not use if discolored, cloudy, or if foreign particles are present.

I.V.: Do not use if solution in vial is discolored, or contains opaque or foreign particles. Dilute for infusion by slowly adding calculated dose/volume to sodium chloride 0.9% to a total volume of 100 mL. Gently mix. Visually inspect; do not use if particulate matter exists or if discolored.

Discard unused portion of vial/syringe/autoinjector.

Storage/Stability Store intact vials and syringes refrigerated at 2°C to 8°C (36°F to 46°F); do not freeze. Do not shake. Protect from light.

I.V.: Solutions diluted for infusion may be stored at room temperature for 4 hours.

Mechanism of Action Human monoclonal antibody that binds to human tumor necrosis factor alpha (TNFα), thereby interfering with endogenous TNFα activity. Biological activities of TNFα include the induction of proinflammatory cytokines (interleukin [IL]-6, IL-8, Granulocyte-colony stimulating factor, granulocyte-macrophage colony stimulating factor), expression of adhesion molecules (E-selectin, vascular cell adhesion molecule [VCAM]-1, intercellular adhesion molecule [ICAM]-1) necessary for leukocyte infiltration, activation of neutrophils and eosinophils.

Pharmacodynamics/Kinetics

Distribution: V_d: I.V: 151 ± 61 mL/kg (distributed primarily to circulatory system with limited extravascular distribution)

Bioavailability: SubQ: ~53%

Metabolism: Pathway unknown

Half-life elimination: ~2 weeks

Time to peak, serum: SubQ: 2-6 days

Dosage Note: Corticosteroids, *nonbiologic* disease-modifying antirheumatic drugs (DMARDs), and /or NSAIDs may be continued for the treatment of rheumatoid arthritis, psoriatic arthritis, or ankylosing spondylitis. Golimumab should not be used in combination with *biologic* DMARDs.

Ankylosing spondylitis: Adults: SubQ: 50 mg once a month (either alone or in combination with methotrexate or other nonbiologic DMARDs)

Psoriatic arthritis: Adults: SubQ: 50 mg once a month (either alone or in combination with methotrexate or other nonbiologic DMARDs)

Rheumatoid arthritis: Adults:

I.V.: 2 mg/kg at weeks 0, 4, and then every 8 weeks thereafter (in combination with methotrexate)

SubQ: 50 mg once a month (in combination with methotrexate)

Ulcerative colitis: Adults:

U.S. labeling: SubQ: Induction: 200 mg at week 0, then 100 mg at week 2, followed by maintenance therapy of 100 mg every 4 weeks

Canadian labeling: SubQ: Induction: 200 mg at week 0, then 100 mg at week 2, followed by maintenance therapy of 50 mg every 4 weeks (maintenance dose may be increased to 100 mg every 4 weeks if needed)

Dosage adjustment in renal impairment: No dosage adjustment provided in manufacturer's labeling (has not been studied).

Dosage adjustment in hepatic impairment: No dosage adjustment provided in manufacturer's labeling (has not been studied).

Administration

I.V.: Dilute prior to use. Infuse over 30 minutes, using an infusion set with an in-line low protein-binding 0.22 micron filter. Do not infuse in the same line with other medications.

Subcutaneous injection: Hold autoinjector firmly against skin and inject subcutaneously into thigh, lower abdomen (below navel), or upper arm. A loud click is heard when injection has begun. Continue to hold autoinjector against skin until second click is heard (may take 3-15 seconds). Following second click, lift autoinjector from injection site. Rotate injection sites and avoid injecting into tender, red, hard, or bruised skin. If multiple injections are required for a single dose, administer at different sites on body.

Monitoring Parameters CBC with differential; latent TB screening (prior to initiating and periodically during therapy); HBV screening (prior to initiating [all patients]; during and for several months following therapy [HBV carriers]); monitor improvement of symptoms and physical function assessments; signs/symptoms of infection (prior to, during, and following therapy); signs/symptoms/worsening of heart failure signs and symptoms of hypersensitivity reaction; symptoms of lupus-like syndrome; signs/symptoms of malignancy (eg, splenomegaly, hepatomegaly, abdominal pain, persistent fever, night sweats, weight loss) including periodic skin examination

Dosage Forms Excipient information presented when available (limited, particularly for generics); consult specific product labeling.

Solution, Intravenous [preservative free]:

Simponi Aria: 50 mg/4 mL (4 mL) [latex free; contains polysorbate 80]

Solution, Subcutaneous [preservative free]:

Simponi: 50 mg/0.5 mL (0.5 mL); 100 mg/mL (1 mL) [contains polysorbate 80]

- ◆ GoLYTELY *see* Polyethylene Glycol-Electrolyte Solution *on page 1669*
- ◆ Gonal-f *see* Follitropin Alfa *on page 908*
- ◆ Gonal-f Pen (Can) *see* Follitropin Alfa *on page 908*
- ◆ Gonal-f RFF *see* Follitropin Alfa *on page 908*
- ◆ Gonal-f RFF Pen *see* Follitropin Alfa *on page 908*
- ◆ Gonal-f RFF Redi-ject *see* Follitropin Alfa *on page 908*
- ◆ Gonal-f RFF Rediject *see* Follitropin Alfa *on page 908*
- ◆ GoodSense Mucus Relief [OTC] *see* GuaiFENesin *on page 974*
- ◆ Goody's® Extra Strength Headache Powder [OTC] *see* Acetaminophen, Aspirin, and Caffeine *on page 33*
- ◆ Goody's® Extra Strength Pain Relief [OTC] *see* Acetaminophen, Aspirin, and Caffeine *on page 33*
- ◆ Goody's PM® [OTC] *see* Acetaminophen and Diphenhydramine *on page 32*
- ◆ Gordon Boro-Packs [OTC] *see* Aluminum Sulfate and Calcium Acetate *on page 91*
- ◆ Gordons Urea *see* Urea *on page 2140*
- ◆ Gordons-Vite A [OTC] *see* Vitamin A *on page 2201*
- ◆ Gordons-Vite E [OTC] *see* Vitamin E *on page 2202*
- ◆ Gormel [OTC] *see* Urea *on page 2140*
- ◆ Gormel 10 [OTC] *see* Urea *on page 2140*

Goserelin (GOE se rel in)

Brand Names: U.S. Zoladex

Brand Names: Canada Zoladex®; Zoladex® LA

Index Terms Goserelin Acetate; ICI-118630; ZDX

Pharmacologic Category Antineoplastic Agent, Gonadotropin-Releasing Hormone Agonist; Gonadotropin Releasing Hormone Agonist

Use Treatment of locally confined prostate cancer; palliative treatment of advanced prostate cancer; palliative treatment of advanced breast cancer in pre- and perimenopausal women; treatment of endometriosis, including pain relief and reduction of endometriotic lesions; endometrial thinning agent as part of treatment for dysfunctional uterine bleeding

Pregnancy Risk Factor X (endometriosis, endometrial thinning); D (advanced breast cancer)

Pregnancy Considerations Goserelin has been found to be teratogenic and increases pregnancy loss in animal studies. Goserelin induces hormonal changes which increase the risk for fetal loss and use is contraindicated in pregnancy unless being used for palliative treatment of advanced breast cancer.

Breast cancer: If used for the palliative treatment of breast cancer during pregnancy, the potential for increased fetal loss should be discussed with the patient.

Endometriosis, endometrial thinning: Women of childbearing potential should not receive therapy until pregnancy has been excluded. Nonhormonal contraception is recommended for premenopausal women during therapy and for 12 weeks after therapy is discontinued. Although ovulation is usually inhibited and menstruation may stop, pregnancy prevention is not ensured during goserelin therapy. Changes in reproductive function may occur following chronic administration.

Breast-Feeding Considerations Goserelin is inactivated when used orally. Breast-feeding is not recommended by the manufacturer.

Contraindications Hypersensitivity to goserelin, GnRH, GnRH agonist analogues, or any component of the formulation; pregnancy (except if using for palliative treatment of advanced breast cancer)

Warnings/Precautions Hazardous agent - use appropriate precautions for handling and disposal (NIOSH, 2012). Allergic hypersensitivity reactions (including anaphylaxis) and antibody formation may occur; monitor. Androgen-deprivation therapy may increase the risk for cardiovascular disease (Levine, 2010). Transient increases in serum testosterone (in men with prostate cancer) and estrogen (in women with breast cancer) may result in a worsening of disease signs and symptoms (tumor flare) during the first few weeks of treatment. Urinary tract obstruction or spinal cord compression have been reported when used for prostate cancer; closely observe patients for weakness, paresthesias, and urinary tract obstruction in first few weeks of therapy. Decreased bone density has been reported in women and may be irreversible; use caution if other risk factors are present; evaluate and institute preventative treatment if necessary.

Women of childbearing potential should not receive therapy until pregnancy has been excluded. Nonhormonal contraception is recommended for premenopausal women during therapy and for 12 weeks after therapy is discontinued. Cervical resistance may be increased; use caution when dilating the cervix. The 3-month implant currently has no approved indications for use in women. Rare cases of pituitary apoplexy (frequently secondary to pituitary adenoma) have been observed with GnRH agonist administration (onset from 1 hour to usually <2 weeks); may present as sudden headache, vomiting, visual or mental status changes, and infrequently cardiovascular collapse; immediate medical attention required. Hyperglycemia has been reported in males and may manifest as diabetes or worsening of pre-existing diabetes. Decreased AUC may be observed when using the 3-month implant in obese patients. Monitor testosterone levels if desired clinical response is not observed. Safety and efficacy have not been established in pediatric patients.

Adverse Reactions Percentages reported with the 1-month implant:

>10%:

Cardiovascular: Vasodilatation (female 57%), peripheral edema (female 21%)

Central nervous system: Headache (female 32% to 75%; male 1% to 5%), emotional lability (female 60%), depression (female 54%; male 1% to 5%), pain (8% to 17%), dyspareunia (female 14%), insomnia (5% to 11%)

Dermatologic: Diaphoresis (female 16% to 45%; male 6%), acne vulgaris (female 42%; usually within 1 month after starting treatment), seborrhea (female 26%)

Endocrine & metabolic: Hot flash (female 57% to 96%; male 62%), decreased libido (female 48% to 61%), increased libido (female 12%)

Gastrointestinal: Abdominal pain (female 7% to 11%), nausea (5% to 11%)

Genitourinary: Vaginitis (75%), breast atrophy (female 33%), sexual disorder (male 21%), breast hypertrophy (female 18%), decrease in erectile frequency (18%), pelvic symptoms (female 9% to 18%), genitourinary signs and symptoms (lower; male 13%)

Hematologic & oncologic: Tumor flare (female 23%; male: Incidence not reported)

Infection: Infection (female 13%; male: Incidence not reported)

Neuromuscular & skeletal: Decreased bone mineral density (female 23%; ~4% decrease from baseline in 6 months; male: Incidence not reported), weakness (female 11%)

1% to 10%:

Cardiovascular: Cardiac arrhythmia, cardiac failure, cerebrovascular accident, chest pain, edema, hypertension, myocardial infarction, palpitations, peripheral vascular disease, tachycardia

Central nervous system: Abnormality in thinking, anxiety, chills, dizziness, drowsiness, lethargy, malaise, migraine, nervousness, paresthesia, voice disorder

Dermatologic: Alopecia, hair disease, pruritus, skin discoloration, skin rash, xeroderma

Endocrine & metabolic: Gout, hirsutism, hyperglycemia, weight gain, weight loss

Gastrointestinal: Anorexia, constipation, diarrhea, dyspepsia, flatulence, gastric ulcer, increased appetite, vomiting, xerostomia

Genitourinary: Breast swelling, breast tenderness, dysmenorrhea, mastalgia, urinary frequency, urinary tract infection, urinary tract obstruction, uterine hemorrhage, vaginal hemorrhage, vulvovaginitis

Hematologic & oncologic: Anemia, bruise, hemorrhage

Hypersensitivity: Hypersensitivity reaction

Local: Application site reaction

Neuromuscular & skeletal: Arthralgia, arthropathy, back pain, hypertonia, leg cramps, myalgia

Ophthalmic: Amblyopia, dry eye syndrome

Renal: Renal insufficiency

Respiratory: Bronchitis, chronic obstructive pulmonary disease, cough, epistaxis, flu-like symptoms, pharyngitis, rhinitis, sinusitis, upper respiratory tract infection

Miscellaneous: Fever

<1% (Limited to important or life-threatening): Anaphylaxis, bone fracture, convulsions, decreased glucose tolerance, decreased HDL cholesterol, deep vein thrombosis, diabetes mellitus, hypercalcemia, hypercholesterolemia, hyperlipidemia, hypotension, increased HDL cholesterol, increased LDL cholesterol, increased serum ALT, increased serum AST, increased serum triglycerides, osteoporosis, ovarian cyst, ovarian hyperstimulation syndrome, pituitary apoplexy, pituitary neoplasm (including adenoma), pulmonary embolism, psychotic reaction, transient ischemic attacks

Drug Interactions

Metabolism/Transport Effects None known.

Avoid Concomitant Use There are no known interactions where it is recommended to avoid concomitant use.

Increased Effect/Toxicity There are no known significant interactions involving an increase in effect.

Decreased Effect

Goserelin may decrease the levels/effects of: Antidiabetic Agents

Storage/Stability Zoladex® should be stored at room temperature not to exceed 25°C (77°F). Protect from light.

Mechanism of Action Goserelin (a gonadotropin-releasing hormone [GnRH] analog) causes an initial increase in luteinizing hormone (LH) and follicle stimulating hormone (FSH), chronic administration of goserelin results in a sustained suppression of pituitary gonadotropins. Serum testosterone falls to levels comparable to surgical castration. The exact mechanism of this effect is unknown, but may be related to changes in the control of LH or down-regulation of LH receptors.

Pharmacodynamics/Kinetics

Onset:

Females: Estradiol suppression reaches postmenopausal levels within 3 weeks and FSH and LH are suppressed to follicular phase levels within 4 weeks of initiation

Males: Testosterone suppression reaches castrate levels within 2-4 weeks after initiation

Duration:

Females: Estradiol, LH and FSH generally return to baseline levels within 12 weeks following the last monthly implant.

Males: Testosterone levels maintained at castrate levels throughout the duration of therapy.

Absorption: SubQ: Rapid and can be detected in serum in 30-60 minutes; 3.6 mg: released slowly in first 8 days, then rapid and continuous release for 28 days

Distribution: V_d: Male: 44.1 L; Female: 20.3 L

Protein binding: 27%

Time to peak, serum: SubQ: Male: 12-15 days, Female: 8-22 days

Half-life elimination: SubQ: Male: ~4 hours, Female: ~2 hours; Renal impairment: Male: 12 hours

Excretion: Urine (>90%; 20% as unchanged drug)

Dosage SubQ: Adults:

Prostate cancer, advanced:

28-day implant: 3.6 mg every 28 days

12-week implant: 10.8 mg every 12 weeks

Prostate cancer, locally confined (in combination with an antiandrogen and radiotherapy; begin 8 weeks prior to radiotherapy):

Combination 28-day/12-week implant: 3.6 mg implant, followed in 28 days by 10.8 mg implant

28-day implant (alternate dosing): 3.6 mg; repeated every 28 days for a total of 4 doses

Breast cancer, advanced: 3.6 mg every 28 days

Endometriosis: 3.6 mg every 28 days for 6 months

Endometrial thinning: 3.6 mg every 28 days for 1 or 2 doses

Dosing adjustment in renal impairment: No adjustment is necessary

Dosing adjustment in hepatic impairment: No adjustment is necessary

Administration SubQ: Administer implant by inserting needle at a 30-45 degree angle into the anterior abdominal wall below the navel line. Goserelin is an implant; therefore, do not attempt to eliminate air bubbles prior to injection (may displace implant). Do not attempt to aspirate prior to injection; if a large vessel is penetrated, blood will be visualized in the syringe chamber (if vessel is penetrated, withdraw needle and inject elsewhere with a new syringe). Do not penetrate into muscle or peritoneum. Implant may be detected by ultrasound if removal is required.

Hazardous agent; use appropriate precautions for handling and disposal (NIOSH, 2012).

Monitoring Parameters Bone mineral density, serum calcium, cholesterol/lipids

Prostate cancer: Weakness, paresthesias, and urinary tract obstruction in first few weeks of therapy; screen for diabetes

Test Interactions Interferes with pituitary gonadotropic and gonadal function tests during and for up to 12 weeks after discontinued

Additional Information If removal is necessary, implant may be located by ultrasound.

Dosage Forms Excipient information presented when available (limited, particularly for generics); consult specific product labeling.

Implant, Subcutaneous:

Zoladex: 3.6 mg (1 ea); 10.8 mg (1 ea)

◆ Goserelin Acetate *see* Goserelin *on page 970*

◆ GP 47680 *see* OXcarbazepine *on page 1530*

◆ GR38032R *see* Ondansetron *on page 1510*

◆ Gralise *see* Gabapentin *on page 933*

◆ Gralise Starter *see* Gabapentin *on page 933*

◆ Gramicidin, Neomycin, and Polymyxin B *see* Neomycin, Polymyxin B, and Gramicidin *on page 1440*

Granisetron (gra NI se tron)

Brand Names: U.S. Granisol; Sancuso

Brand Names: Canada Granisetron Hydrochloride Injection; Kytril®

Index Terms BRL 43694; Kytril

Pharmacologic Category Antiemetic; Selective 5-HT_3 Receptor Antagonist

Use Prophylaxis of nausea and vomiting associated with emetogenic chemotherapy and radiation therapy; prophylaxis and treatment of postoperative nausea and vomiting (PONV)

Unlabeled Use Breakthrough treatment of nausea and vomiting associated with chemotherapy

Pregnancy Risk Factor B

Pregnancy Considerations There are no adequate or well-controlled studies in pregnant women. Teratogenic effects were not observed in animal studies. Injection (1 mg/mL strength) contains benzyl alcohol which may cross the placenta. Use only if benefit exceeds the risk.

Breast-Feeding Considerations It is not known if granisetron is excreted in breast milk. The manufacturer recommends that caution be exercised when administering granisetron to nursing women.

Contraindications Hypersensitivity to granisetron or any component of the formulation

Warnings/Precautions Use with caution in patients with congenital long QT syndrome or other risk factors for QT prolongation (eg, medications known to prolong QT interval, electrolyte abnormalities, and cumulative high-dose anthracycline therapy). 5-HT_3 antagonists have been associated with a number of dose-dependent increases in ECG intervals (eg, PR, QRS duration, QT/QT_c, JT), usually occurring 1-2 hours after I.V. administration. In general, these changes are not clinically relevant, however, when used in conjunction with other agents that prolong these intervals, arrhythmia may occur. When used with agents that prolong the QT interval (eg, Class I and III antiarrhythmics), clinically relevant QT interval prolongation may occur resulting in torsade de pointes. I.V. formulations of 5-HT_3 antagonists have more association with ECG interval changes, compared to oral formulations.

For chemotherapy-related emesis, **granisetron should be used on a scheduled basis, not on an "as needed" (PRN) basis**, since data support the use of this drug in the prevention of nausea and vomiting and not in the rescue of nausea and vomiting. Granisetron should be used only in the first 24-48 hours of receiving chemotherapy or radiation. Data do not support any increased efficacy of granisetron in delayed nausea and vomiting.

Use with caution in patients allergic to other 5-HT_3 receptor antagonists; cross-reactivity has been reported. Routine prophylaxis for PONV is not recommended in patients where there is little expectation of nausea and vomiting postoperatively. In patients where nausea and vomiting must be avoided postoperatively, administer to all patients even when expected incidence of nausea and vomiting is low. Use caution following abdominal surgery or in chemotherapy-induced nausea and vomiting; may mask progressive ileus or gastric distention. Application site reactions, generally mild, have occurred with transdermal patch use; if skin reaction is severe or generalized, remove patch. Cover patch application site with clothing to protect from natural or artificial sunlight exposure while patch is applied and for 10 days following removal; granisetron may potentially be affected by natural or artificial sunlight. Do not apply patch to red, irritated, or damaged skin. Injection contains benzyl alcohol (1 mg/mL) and should not be used in neonates.

Adverse Reactions

>10%:

Central nervous system: Headache (3% to 21%; transdermal patch: 1%)

Gastrointestinal: Constipation (3% to 18%)

Neuromuscular & skeletal: Weakness (5% to 18%)

1% to 10%:

Cardiovascular: QT_c prolongation (1% to 3%), hypertension (1% to 2%)

Central nervous system: Pain (10%), fever (3% to 9%), dizziness (4% to 5%), insomnia (<2% to 5%), somnolence (1% to 4%), anxiety (2%), agitation (<2%), CNS stimulation (<2%)

Dermatologic: Rash (1%)

Gastrointestinal: Diarrhea (3% to 9%), abdominal pain (4% to 6%), dyspepsia (3% to 6%), taste perversion (2%)

Hepatic: Liver enzymes increased (5% to 6%)
Renal: Oliguria (2%)
Respiratory: Cough (2%)
Miscellaneous: Infection (3%)

<1% (Limited to important or life-threatening): Agitation, allergic reactions; anaphylaxis (including hypotension, dyspnea, urticaria); angina, application site reactions (transdermal patch), arrhythmias, atrial fibrillation, extrapyramidal syndrome, hot flashes, hypotension, hypersensitivity, syncope

Drug Interactions

Metabolism/Transport Effects Substrate of CYP3A4 (minor); **Note:** Assignment of Major/Minor substrate status based on clinically relevant drug interaction potential

Avoid Concomitant Use

Avoid concomitant use of Granisetron with any of the following: Apomorphine; Highest Risk QTc-Prolonging Agents; Ivabradine; Mifepristone

Increased Effect/Toxicity

Granisetron may increase the levels/effects of: Apomorphine; Highest Risk QTc-Prolonging Agents; Moderate Risk QTc-Prolonging Agents

The levels/effects of Granisetron may be increased by: Ivabradine; Mifepristone; QTc-Prolonging Agents (Indeterminate Risk and Risk Modifying)

Decreased Effect

Granisetron may decrease the levels/effects of: Tapentadol; TraMADol

Storage/Stability

I.V.: Store at 15°C to 30°C (59°F to 86°F). Protect from light. Do not freeze vials. Stable when mixed in NS or D_5W for 7 days under refrigeration and for 3 days at room temperature.

Oral: Store tablet or oral solution at 15°C to 30°C (59°F to 86°F). Protect from light.

Transdermal patch: Store at 20°C to 25°C (68°F to 77°F). Keep patch in original packaging until immediately prior to use.

Mechanism of Action Selective 5-HT_3-receptor antagonist, blocking serotonin, both peripherally on vagal nerve terminals and centrally in the chemoreceptor trigger zone

Pharmacodynamics/Kinetics

Duration: Oral, I.V.: Generally up to 24 hours
Absorption: Oral: Tablets and oral solution are bioequivalent; Transdermal patch: ~66% over 7 days
Distribution: V_d: 2-4 L/kg; widely throughout body
Protein binding: 65%
Metabolism: Hepatic via N-demethylation, oxidation, and conjugation; some metabolites may have 5-HT_3 antagonist activity
Half-life elimination: Oral: 6 hours; I.V.: 9 hours
Time to peak, plasma: Transdermal patch: Maximum systemic concentrations: ~48 hours after application (range: 24-168 hours)
Excretion: Urine (12% as unchanged drug, 48% to 49% as metabolites); feces (34% to 38% as metabolites)

Dosage

Oral: Adults:

Prophylaxis of chemotherapy-related emesis: 2 mg once daily up to 1 hour before chemotherapy or 1 mg twice daily; the first 1 mg dose should be given up to 1 hour before chemotherapy.

Prophylaxis of radiation therapy-associated emesis: 2 mg once daily given 1 hour before radiation therapy.

I.V.:

Children ≥2 years and Adults: Prophylaxis of chemotherapy-related emesis:

Within U.S.: 10 mcg/kg/dose (maximum: 1 mg/dose) given 30 minutes prior to chemotherapy; for some drugs (eg, carboplatin, cyclophosphamide) with a later onset of emetic action, 10 mcg/kg every 12 hours may be necessary

Outside U.S.: 40 mcg/kg/dose (or 3 mg/dose); maximum: 9 mg/24 hours

Breakthrough: Granisetron has not been shown to be effective in terminating nausea or vomiting once it occurs and should not be used for this purpose.

Adults: PONV:

Prevention: 1 mg given undiluted over 30 seconds; the manufacturer recommends administration before induction of anesthesia or immediately before reversal of anesthesia. **Note:** The Society for Ambulatory Anesthesia (SAMBA) Guidelines recommend a dosage range of 0.35-1.5 mg administered at the end of surgery (Gan, 2007). However, doses ≤1 mg are generally used since doses >1 mg are not more effective. Of note, 5 mcg/kg (~0.35 mg in a 70 kg adult) has been shown to be effective; doses >5 mcg/kg were not more effective (Mikawa, 1997).

Treatment: 1 mg given undiluted over 30 seconds

Transdermal patch: Adults: Prophylaxis of chemotherapy-related emesis: Apply 1 patch at least 24 hours prior to chemotherapy; do not apply ≥48 hours before chemotherapy. Remove patch a minimum of 24 hours after chemotherapy completion. Maximum duration: Patch may be worn up to 7 days, depending on chemotherapy regimen duration.

Dosing interval in renal impairment: No dosage adjustment required.

Dosing interval in hepatic impairment: Kinetic studies in patients with hepatic impairment showed that total clearance was approximately halved, however, standard doses were very well tolerated, and dose adjustments are not necessary.

Administration

Oral: Doses should be given up to 1 hour prior to initiation of chemotherapy/radiation

I.V.: Administer I.V. push over 30 seconds or as a 5- to 10-minute infusion

Prevention of PONV: Administer before induction of anesthesia or immediately before reversal of anesthesia.

Treatment of PONV: Administer undiluted over 30 seconds.

Transdermal (Sancuso®): Apply patch to clean, dry, intact skin on upper outer arm. Do not use on red, irritated, or damaged skin. Remove patch from pouch immediately before application. Do not cut patch.

Dosage Forms Excipient information presented when available (limited, particularly for generics); consult specific product labeling.

Patch, Transdermal:
Sancuso: 3.1 mg/24 hr (1 ea)
Solution, Intravenous:
Generic: 0.1 mg/mL (1 mL); 1 mg/mL (1 mL); 4 mg/4 mL (4 mL)
Solution, Intravenous [preservative free]:
Generic: 0.1 mg/mL (1 mL); 1 mg/mL (1 mL)
Solution, Oral:
Granisol: 2 mg/10 mL (30 mL) [contains fd&c yellow #6 (sunset yellow), sodium benzoate; orange flavor]
Tablet, Oral:
Generic: 1 mg

Extemporaneous Preparations Note: Commercial oral solution is available (0.2 mg/mL)

A 0.2 mg/mL oral suspension may be made with tablets. Crush twelve 1 mg tablets in a mortar and reduce to a fine powder. Add 30 mL distilled water, mix well, and transfer to a bottle. Rinse the mortar with 10 mL cherry syrup and add to bottle. Add sufficient quantity of cherry syrup to make a final volume of 60 mL. Label "shake well". Stable 14 days at room temperature or refrigerated (Quercia, 1997).

A 50 mcg/mL oral suspension may be made with tablets and one of three different vehicles (Ora-Sweet®, Ora-Plus®, or a mixture of methylcellulose 1% and Simple Syrup, N.F.). Crush one 1 mg tablet in a mortar and reduce to a fine powder. Add 20 mL of the chosen vehicle and mix to a uniform paste; transfer to a calibrated bottle. Label "shake well" and "refrigerate". Stable for 91 days refrigerated (Nahata, 1998).

Nahata MC, Morosco RS, and Hipple TF, "Stability of Granisetron Hydrochloride in Two Oral Suspensions," *Am J Health Syst Pharm*, 1998, 55(23):2511-3.

Quercia RA, Zhang J, Fan C, et al, "Stability of Granisetron Hydrochloride in an Extemporaneously Prepared Oral Liquid," *Am J Health Syst Pharm*, 1997, 54(12):1404-6.

- Granisetron Hydrochloride Injection (Can) *see* Granisetron *on page 972*
- Granisol *see* Granisetron *on page 972*
- Granix *see* Filgrastim *on page 859*
- Granulex® *see* Trypsin, Balsam Peru, and Castor Oil *on page 2133*
- Granulocyte Colony Stimulating Factor *see* Filgrastim *on page 859*
- Granulocyte Colony Stimulating Factor (PEG Conjugate) *see* Pegfilgrastim *on page 1588*
- Granulocyte-Macrophage Colony Stimulating Factor *see* Sargramostim *on page 1877*
- Gravol® [OTC] (Can) *see* DimenhyDRINATE *on page 616*
- Gravol IM (Can) *see* DimenhyDRINATE *on page 616*
- Grifulvin V *see* Griseofulvin *on page 974*

Griseofulvin (gri see oh FUL vin)

Brand Names: U.S. Grifulvin V; Gris-PEG

Index Terms Griseofulvin Microsize; Griseofulvin Ultramicrosize

Pharmacologic Category Antifungal Agent, Oral

Additional Appendix Information

Antifungal Agents *on page 2286*

Use Treatment of tinea infections of the skin, hair, and nails caused by susceptible species of *Microsporum, Epidermophyton,* or *Trichophyton*

Pregnancy Risk Factor X

Dosage Oral:

Children >2 years:

Microsize: 10-20 mg/kg/day in single or 2 divided doses (maximum: 1000 mg daily) (*Red Book*, 2012)

Tinea capitis: Higher dosages (20-25 mg/kg/day) have been recommended (Ali, 2007; Lipozenic, 2002; Sethi, 2006)

Ultramicrosize: 5-15 mg/kg/day in single dose or 2 divided doses (maximum: 750 mg daily) (*Red Book*, 2012)

Adults:

Microsize:

Tinea corporis, tinea cruris, tinea capitis: 500 mg daily in single or divided doses

Tinea pedis, tinea unguium: 1000 mg daily in single or divided doses

Ultramicrosize: 375 mg daily in single or divided doses; doses up to 750 mg daily in divided doses have been used for infections more difficult to eradicate such as tinea unguium and tinea pedis

Duration of therapy depends on the site of infection:

Children and Adults:

Tinea corporis: 2-4 weeks

Tinea cruris: 2-6 weeks (*Red Book*, 2012)

Tinea capitis:

Manufacturer's labeling: 4-6 weeks

Alternate recommendations: Children: 6-12 weeks; use up to 16 weeks may be required (AAP *Red Book®* recommends continuing treatment for 2 weeks after clinical resolution of symptoms) (Ali, 2007; Lipozenic, 2002; Sethi, 2006)

Tinea pedis: 4-8 weeks

Tinea unguium: 4-6 months or longer

Additional Information Complete prescribing information should be consulted for additional detail.

Dosage Forms Considerations

Microsized formulations: Suspensions, Grifulvin V tablets

Ultramicrosize formulation: Gris-PEG tablets

Dosage Forms Excipient information presented when available (limited, particularly for generics); consult specific product labeling.

Suspension, Oral:

Generic: 125 mg/5 mL (118 mL, 120 mL)

Tablet, Oral:

Grifulvin V: 500 mg [scored]

Gris-PEG: 125 mg, 250 mg [scored]

Generic: 125 mg, 250 mg, 500 mg

- Griseofulvin Microsize *see* Griseofulvin *on page 974*
- Griseofulvin Ultramicrosize *see* Griseofulvin *on page 974*
- Gris-PEG *see* Griseofulvin *on page 974*
- Growth Hormone, Human *see* Somatropin *on page 1934*
- GRx HiCort 25 *see* Hydrocortisone (Topical) *on page 1011*
- GSK-580299 *see* Papillomavirus (Types 16, 18) Vaccine (Human, Recombinant) *on page 1569*
- GSK1120212 *see* Trametinib *on page 2102*
- GSK 1838262 *see* Gabapentin Enacarbil *on page 936*
- GSK2118436 *see* Dabrafenib *on page 528*
- Guaiatussin AC *see* Guaifenesin and Codeine *on page 976*
- Guaicon DMS [OTC] *see* Guaifenesin and Dextromethorphan *on page 976*

GuaiFENesin (gwye FEN e sin)

Brand Names: U.S. Altarussin [OTC]; Bidex [OTC]; Buckleys Chest Congestion [OTC]; Cough Syrup [OTC]; Diabetic Siltussin DAS-Na [OTC]; Diabetic Tussin Mucus Relief [OTC]; Diabetic Tussin [OTC]; Fenesin IR [OTC]; Geri-Tussin [OTC]; GoodSense Mucus Relief [OTC]; Iophen-NR [OTC]; Liquibid [OTC]; Liquituss GG [OTC]; Mucinex Chest Congestion Child [OTC]; Mucinex For Kids [OTC]; Mucinex Maximum Strength [OTC]; Mucinex [OTC]; Mucosa [OTC]; Mucus Relief Childrens [OTC]; Mucus Relief [OTC]; Mucus-ER [OTC]; Organ-I NR [OTC]; Q-Tussin [OTC]; Refenesen 400 [OTC]; Refenesen [OTC]; Robafen [OTC]; Robitussin Chest Congestion [OTC]; Robitussin Mucus+Chest Congest [OTC]; Scot-Tussin Expectorant [OTC]; Siltussin DAS [OTC]; Siltussin SA [OTC]; Tussin [OTC]; Xpect [OTC]

Brand Names: Canada Balminil Expectorant; Benylin® E Extra Strength; Koffex Expectorant; Robitussin®

Index Terms Cheratussin; GG; Glycerol Guaiacolate

Pharmacologic Category Expectorant

Use Help loosen phlegm and thin bronchial secretions to make coughs more productive

Pregnancy Considerations Based on the limited available data, an increased risk of adverse birth outcomes has not been observed following maternal use of guaifenesin in pregnancy. Alcohol may be present in some liquid formulations of guaifenesin. If consumed in sufficient quantities during pregnancy, fetal alcohol syndrome may result.

Guaifenesin has been investigated as an agent to improve cervical mucus and improve fertility.

Breast-Feeding Considerations It is not known if guaifensin is excreted in breast milk. The manufacturer recommends that caution be exercised when administering guaifensin to nursing women.

Contraindications Hypersensitivity to guaifenesin or any component of the formulation

Warnings/Precautions When used for self medication (OTC) notify healthcare provider if symptoms do not improve within 7 days, or are accompanied by fever, rash, or persistent headache. Do not use for persistent or chronic cough (as with smoking, asthma, chronic bronchitis, emphysema) or if cough is accompanied by excessive phlegm unless directed to do so by healthcare provider. Not for OTC use in children <2 years of age. Some products may contain phenylalanine.

Adverse Reactions

Frequency not defined:

Central nervous system: Dizziness, drowsiness, headache

Dermatologic: Rash

Endocrine & metabolic: Uric acid levels decreased

Gastrointestinal: Nausea, stomach pain, vomiting

Postmarketing and/or case reports: Kidney stone formation (with consumption of large quantities)

Drug Interactions

Metabolism/Transport Effects None known.

Avoid Concomitant Use There are no known interactions where it is recommended to avoid concomitant use.

Increased Effect/Toxicity There are no known significant interactions involving an increase in effect.

Decreased Effect There are no known significant interactions involving a decrease in effect.

Mechanism of Action Thought to act as an expectorant by irritating the gastric mucosa and stimulating respiratory tract secretions, thereby increasing respiratory fluid volumes and decreasing mucous viscosity

Pharmacodynamics/Kinetics

Absorption: Well absorbed

Half-life elimination: ~1 hour

Excretion: Urine (as unchanged drug and metabolites)

Dosage Oral:

Children:

6 months to 2 years: 25-50 mg every 4 hours, not to exceed 300 mg/day

2-5 years: 50-100 mg every 4 hours, not to exceed 600 mg/day

6-11 years: 100-200 mg every 4 hours, not to exceed 1.2 g/day

Children >12 years and Adults: 200-400 mg every 4 hours to a maximum of 2.4 g/day

Extended release tablet: 600-1200 mg every 12 hours, not to exceed 2.4 g/day

Dietary Considerations Some products may contain phenylalanine and/or sodium.

Administration Do not crush, chew, or break extended release tablets. Administer with a full glass of water.

Test Interactions Possible color interference with determination of 5-HIAA and VMA; discontinue for 48 hours prior to test

Dosage Forms Excipient information presented when available (limited, particularly for generics); consult specific product labeling. [DSC] = Discontinued product

Liquid, Oral:

Buckleys Chest Congestion: 100 mg/5 mL (118 mL) [alcohol free, sugar free; contains butylparaben, menthol, propylene glycol, propylparaben]

Diabetic Siltussin DAS-Na: 100 mg/5 mL (118 mL) [alcohol free, color free, fructose free, sodium free, sorbitol free, sugar free; contains aspartame, benzoic acid, methylparaben, propylene glycol; strawberry flavor]

Diabetic Tussin: 100 mg/5 mL (118 mL) [alcohol free, dye free, fructose free, sodium free, sorbitol free, sugar free; contains aspartame, menthol, methylparaben]

Diabetic Tussin Mucus Relief: 200 mg/5 mL (118 mL) [alcohol free, dye free, fructose free, sodium free, sorbitol free, sugar free; contains aspartame, benzoic acid, menthol, polyethylene glycol, propylene glycol]

Iophen-NR: 100 mg/5 mL (473 mL) [contains propylene glycol, saccharin sodium, sodium benzoate; raspberry flavor]

Liquituss GG: 200 mg/5 mL (118 mL, 473 mL) [alcohol free, sugar free; contains methylparaben, propylene glycol, propylparaben, saccharin sodium]

Mucinex Chest Congestion Child: 100 mg/5 mL (118 mL) [alcohol free; contains brilliant blue fcf (fd&c blue #1), fd&c red #40, propylene glycol, saccharin sodium, sodium benzoate; grape flavor]

Mucus Relief Childrens: 100 mg/5 mL (118 mL) [alcohol free; contains brilliant blue fcf (fd&c blue #1), fd&c red #40, propylene glycol, saccharin sodium, sodium benzoate]

Robitussin Mucus+Chest Congest: 100 mg/5 mL (118 mL) [alcohol free; contains fd&c red #40, menthol, propylene glycol, saccharin sodium, sodium benzoate]

Scot-Tussin Expectorant: 100 mg/5 mL (30 mL, 118 mL, 240 mL, 480 mL, 3780 mL) [alcohol free, dye free, saccharin free, sodium free, sorbitol free, sugar free]

Siltussin DAS: 100 mg/5 mL (118 mL) [alcohol free, dye free, sugar free; strawberry flavor]

Packet, Oral:

Mucinex For Kids: 50 mg (12 ea) [contains aspartame; grape flavor]

Mucinex For Kids: 100 mg (12 ea) [contains aspartame; bubble-gum flavor]

Solution, Oral:

Generic: 100 mg/5 mL (5 mL, 10 mL, 15 mL); 200 mg/10 mL (10 mL); 300 mg/15 mL (15 mL)

Syrup, Oral:

Altarussin: 100 mg/5 mL (120 mL, 236 mL, 473 mL, 3840 mL)

Altarussin: 100 mg/5 mL (120 mL, 240 mL, 480 mL, 3840 mL) [contains alcohol, usp]

Cough Syrup: 100 mg/5 mL (118 mL, 473 mL) [alcohol free; contains fd&c red #40, menthol, propylene glycol, saccharin sodium, sodium benzoate; fruit flavor]

Geri-Tussin: 100 mg/5 mL (473 mL) [alcohol free, sugar free; contains fd&c red #40, menthol, saccharin sodium, sodium benzoate]

Q-Tussin: 100 mg/5 mL (118 mL, 240 mL, 473 mL) [alcohol free; contains fd&c red #40, saccharin sodium, sodium benzoate; cherry flavor]

Robafen: 100 mg/5 mL (118 mL, 240 mL [DSC], 473 mL) [contains alcohol, usp; cherry flavor]

Robitussin Chest Congestion: 100 mg/5 mL (118 mL, 237 mL) [alcohol free; contains fd&c red #40, saccharin sodium, sodium benzoate; flavored flavor]

Siltussin SA: 100 mg/5 mL (118 mL, 237 mL, 473 mL) [strawberry flavor]

Tussin: 100 mg/5 mL (118 mL, 237 mL) [alcohol free]

Generic: 100 mg/5 mL (480 mL)

Tablet, Oral:

Bidex: 400 mg [scored]

Bidex: 400 mg [scored; contains saccharin sodium]

Diabetic Tussin Mucus Relief: 400 mg [scored; dye free, sodium free, sugar free]

Fenesin IR: 400 mg

GoodSense Mucus Relief: 400 mg [scored]

Liquibid: 400 mg

Mucosa: 400 mg [scored]

Mucus Relief: 400 mg

Mucus Relief: 400 mg [scored; dye free]

Organ-I NR: 200 mg [scored]

Refenesen: 200 mg [scored; contains fd&c red #40 aluminum lake]
Refenesen 400: 400 mg [scored; dye free]
Xpect: 400 mg [scored; contains saccharin sodium]
Generic: 200 mg, 400 mg
Tablet Extended Release 12 Hour, Oral:
Mucinex: 600 mg [contains fd&c blue #1 aluminum lake]
Mucinex Maximum Strength: 1200 mg [contains fd&c blue #1 aluminum lake]
Mucus-ER: 600 mg [gluten free]
Generic: 600 mg

Guaifenesin and Codeine

(gwye FEN e sin & KOE deen)

Brand Names: U.S. Allfen CD; Allfen CDX; Codar® GF; Dex-Tuss; Guaiatussin AC; Iophen C-NR; M-Clear; M-Clear WC; Mar-Cof® CG; Robafen AC; Virtussin A/C

Index Terms Codeine and Guaifenesin; Robitussin AC

Pharmacologic Category Antitussive; Cough Preparation; Expectorant

Use Temporary control of cough due to minor throat and bronchial irritation

Dosage Oral:

Children 6-11 years:
Capsule: Guaifenesin 200 mg and codeine 9 mg: One capsule every 4 hours (maximum: 6 capsules/24 hours)
Liquid:
Guaifenesin 100 mg and codeine 6.33 mg per 5 mL: 7.5 mL every 4-6 hours (maximum: 45 mL/24 hours)
Guaifenesin 100-200 mg and codeine 8-10 mg per 5 mL: 5 mL every 4 hours (maximum: 30 mL/24 hours)
Guaifenesin 300 mg and codeine 10 mg per 5 mL: 2.5 mL every 4-6 hours (maximum: 20 mL/24 hours)
Tablet: Guaifenesin 400 mg and codeine 10-20 mg: One-half tablet every 4-6 hours (maximum: 3 tablets/24 hours)
Children ≥12 years and Adults:
Capsule: Guaifenesin 200 mg and codeine 9 mg: Two capsules every 4 hours (maximum: 12 capsules/24 hours)
Liquid:
Guaifenesin 100 mg and codeine 6.33 mg per 5 mL: 15 mL every 4-6 hours (maximum: 45 mL/24 hours)
Guaifenesin 100-200 mg and codeine 8-10 mg per 5 mL: 10 mL every 4 hours (maximum: 60 mL/24 hours)
Guaifenesin 300 mg and codeine 10 mg per 5 mL: 5 mL every 4-6 hours (maximum: 40 mL/24 hours)
Tablet: Guaifenesin 400 mg and codeine 10-20 mg: One tablet every 4-6 hours (maximum: 6 tablets/24 hours)

Additional Information Complete prescribing information should be consulted for additional detail.

Dosage Forms Excipient information presented when available (limited, particularly for generics); consult specific product labeling.

Capsule, oral:
M-Clear: Guaifenesin 200 mg and codeine phosphate 9 mg [contains tartrazine]
Liquid, oral:
Codar® GF: Guaifenesin 200 mg and codeine phosphate 8 mg per 5 mL (473 mL) [contains propylene glycol; cotton candy flavor]
Dex-Tuss: Guaifenesin 300 mg and codeine phosphate 10 mg per 5 mL (473 mL) [ethanol free, gluten free, sugar free; contains propylene glycol; grape flavor]
Iophen C-NR: Guaifenesin 100 mg and codeine phosphate 10 mg per 5 mL (473 mL) [contains propylene glycol, sodium benzoate; raspberry flavor]
M-Clear WC: Guaifenesin 100 mg and codeine phosphate 6.33 mg per 5 mL (473 mL) [contains propylene glycol; cotton candy flavor]
Solution, oral: Guaifenesin 100 mg and codeine phosphate 10 mg per 5 mL (5 mL, 10 mL, 118 mL, 473 mL)
Mar-Cof® CG: Guaifenesin 225 mg and codeine phosphate 7.5 mg per 5 mL (473 ml) [ethanol free, sugar free; contains propylene glycol, sodium benzoate, sodium 6 mg/5 mL]
Virtussin A/C: Guaifenesin 100 mg and codeine phosphate 10 mg per 5 mL (473 ml) [contains propylene glycol; cherry flavor]
Syrup, oral: Guaifenesin 100 mg and codeine phosphate 10 mg per 5 mL (473 mL)
Guaiatussin AC: Guaifenesin 100 mg and codeine phosphate 10 mg per 5 mL (5 mL, 10 mL, 118 mL, 473 mL) [sugar free; contains ethanol 3.5%, sodium 1 mg/5 mL, sodium benzoate; cherry flavor]
Robafen AC: Guaifenesin 100 mg and codeine phosphate 10 mg per 5 mL (120 mL, 480 mL) [contains ethanol 3.5%, sodium 4 mg/5 mL, sodium benzoate; cherry flavor]
Tablet, oral:
Allfen CD: Guaifenesin 400 mg and codeine phosphate 10 mg
Allfen CDX: Guaifenesin 400 mg and codeine phosphate 20 mg

Controlled Substance Capsule: C-V; Liquid products: C-V; Tablet: C-III

Guaifenesin and Dextromethorphan

(gwye FEN e sin & deks troe meth OR fan)

Brand Names: U.S. Cheracol D [OTC]; Cheracol Plus [OTC]; Coricidin HBP Chest Congestion and Cough [OTC]; Diabetic Siltussin-DM DAS-Na Maximum Strength [OTC]; Diabetic Siltussin-DM DAS-Na [OTC]; Diabetic Tussin DM Maximum Strength [OTC]; Diabetic Tussin DM [OTC]; Double Tussin DM [OTC]; Fenesin DM IR [OTC]; Guaicon DMS [OTC]; Iophen DM-NR [OTC]; Kolephrin GG/DM [OTC]; Mucinex DM Maximum Strength [OTC]; Mucinex DM [OTC]; Mucinex Kid's Cough Mini-Melts [OTC]; Mucinex Kid's Cough [OTC]; Q-Tussin DM [OTC]; Refenesen DM [OTC]; Robafen DM [OTC]; Robitussin Peak Cold Cough + Chest Congestion DM [OTC]; Robitussin Peak Cold Maximum Strength Cough + Chest Congestion DM [OTC]; Robitussin Peak Cold Sugar-Free Cough + Chest Congestion DM [OTC]; Safe Tussin DM [OTC]; Scot-Tussin Senior [OTC]; Silexin [OTC]; Siltussin DM DAS [OTC]; Siltussin DM [OTC]; Vicks 44E [OTC]; Vicks DayQuil Mucus Control DM [OTC]; Vicks Nature Fusion Cough & Chest Congestion [OTC]; Vicks Pediatric Formula 44E [OTC]; Zyncof [OTC]

Brand Names: Canada Balminil DM E; Benylin DM-E

Index Terms Dextromethorphan and Guaifenesin

Pharmacologic Category Antitussive; Cough Preparation; Expectorant

Use Temporary control of cough due to minor throat and bronchial irritation

Dosage Oral:

Children 2-6 years:
General dosing guidelines: Guaifenesin 50-100 mg and dextromethorphan 2.5-5 mg every 4 hours (maximum dose: Guaifenesin 600 mg and dextromethorphan 30 mg per day)
Product-specific labeling: Vicks Pediatric Formula 44E: 7.5 mL every 4 hours (maximum: 6 doses/24 hours)
Children: 6-12 years:
General dosing guidelines: Guaifenesin 100-200 mg and dextromethorphan 5-10 mg every 4 hours (maximum dose: Guaifenesin 1200 mg and dextromethorphan 60 mg per day)

Product-specific labeling:
Vicks 44E: 7.5 mL every 4 hours (maximum: 6 doses/24 hours)
Vicks Pediatric Formula 44E: 15 mL every 4 hours (maximum: 6 doses/24 hours)
Children ≥12 years and Adults:
General dosing guidelines: Guaifenesin 200-400 mg and dextromethorphan 10-20 mg every 4 hours (maximum dose: Guaifenesin 2400 mg and dextromethorphan 120 mg per day)
Product-specific labeling:
Mucinex DM: 1-2 tablets every 12 hours (maximum: 4 tablets/24 hours)
Vicks 44E: 15 mL every 4 hours (maximum: 6 doses/24 hours)
Vicks Pediatric Formula 44E: 30 mL every 4 hours (maximum: 6 doses/24 hours)

Additional Information Complete prescribing information should be consulted for additional detail.

Dosage Forms Excipient information presented when available (limited, particularly for generics); consult specific product labeling.

Caplet, oral:
Fenesin DM IR: Guaifenesin 400 mg and dextromethorphan hydrobromide 15 mg
Refenesen DM: Guaifenesin 400 mg and dextromethorphan hydrobromide 20 mg

Capsule, softgel, oral:
Coricidin HBP Chest Congestion and Cough: Guaifenesin 200 mg and dextromethorphan hydrobromide 10 mg

Granules, oral:
Mucinex Kid's Cough Mini-Melts: Guaifenesin 100 mg and dextromethorphan hydrobromide 5 mg per packet (12s) [contains magnesium 6 mg/pack, phenylalanine 2 mg/packet, sodium 3 mg/packet; orange crème flavor]

Liquid, oral: Guaifenesin 100 mg and dextromethorphan hydrobromide 10 mg per 5 mL (480 mL)
Diabetic Tussin DM: Guaifenesin 100 mg and dextromethorphan hydrobromide 10 mg per 5 mL (120 mL) [dye free, ethanol free, sugar free; contains phenylalanine 8.4 mg/5 mL]
Diabetic Tussin DM Maximum Strength: Guaifenesin 200 mg and dextromethorphan hydrobromide 10 mg per 5 mL (120 mL) [dye free, ethanol free, sugar free; contains phenylalanine 8.4 mg/5 mL]
Double Tussin DM: Guaifenesin 300 mg and dextromethorphan hydrobromide 20 mg per 5 mL (120 mL, 480 mL) [dye free, ethanol free, sugar free]
Iophen DM-NR: Guaifenesin 100 mg and dextromethorphan hydrobromide 10 mg per 5 mL (480 mL) [contains propylene glycol, sodium benzoate; raspberry flavor]
Kolephrin GG/DM: Guaifenesin 150 mg and dextromethorphan hydrobromide 10 mg per 5 mL (120 mL) [ethanol free; cherry flavor]
Mucinex Kid's Cough: Guaifenesin 100 mg and dextromethorphan hydrobromide 5 mg per 5 mL (120 mL) [contains propylene glycol, sodium 3 mg/5 mL; cherry flavor]
Safe Tussin DM: Guaifenesin 100 mg and dextromethorphan hydrobromide 15 mg per 5 mL (120 mL) [contains benzoic acid, phenylalanine 4.2 mg/5 mL, and propylene glycol; orange and mint flavors]
Scot-Tussin Senior: Guaifenesin 200 mg and dextromethorphan hydrobromide 15 mg per 5 mL (120 mL) [ethanol free, sodium free, sugar free]
Vicks 44E: Guaifenesin 200 mg and dextromethorphan hydrobromide 20 mg per 15 mL (120 mL, 235 mL) [contains ethanol, sodium 31 mg/15 mL, sodium benzoate]
Vicks DayQuil Mucus Control DM: Guaifenesin 200 mg and dextromethorphan hydrobromide 10 mg per 15 mL (295 mL) [contains propylene glycol, sodium 25 mg/15 mL, sodium benzoate; citrus blend flavor]
Vicks Nature Fusion Cough & Chest Congestion: Guaifenesin 200 mg and dextromethorphan hydrobromide 20 mg per 30 mL (236 mL) [dye free, ethanol free, gluten free; contains propylene glycol, sodium 36 mg/30 mL; honey flavor]
Vicks Pediatric Formula 44E: Guaifenesin 100 mg and dextromethorphan hydrobromide 10 mg per 15 mL (120 mL) [ethanol free; contains sodium 30 mg/15 mL, sodium benzoate; cherry flavor]

Syrup, oral: Guaifenesin 100 mg and dextromethorphan hydrobromide 10 mg per 5 mL (5 mL, 10 mL, 120 mL, 480 mL)
Cheracol D: Guaifenesin 100 mg and dextromethorphan hydrobromide 10 mg per 5 mL (120 mL, 180 mL) [contains benzoic acid, ethanol 4.75%]
Cheracol Plus: Guaifenesin 100 mg and dextromethorphan hydrobromide 10 mg per 5 mL (120 mL) [contains benzoic acid, ethanol 4.75%]
Diabetic Siltussin-DM DAS-Na: Guaifenesin 100 mg and dextromethorphan hydrobromide 10 mg per 5 mL (118 mL) [ethanol free, sugar free; contains benzoic acid, phenylalanine 3 mg/5 mL, propylene glycol; strawberry flavor]
Diabetic Siltussin-DM DAS-Na Maximum Strength: Guaifenesin 200 mg and dextromethorphan hydrobromide 10 mg per 5 mL (118 mL) [ethanol free, sugar free; contains benzoic acid, phenylalanine 3 mg/5 mL, propylene glycol; strawberry flavor]
Guaicon DMS: Guaifenesin 100 mg and dextromethorphan hydrobromide 10 mg per 5 mL (10 mL) [ethanol free, sugar free]
Q-Tussin DM: Guaifenesin 100 mg and dextromethorphan hydrobromide 10 mg per 5 mL (118 mL, 237 mL, 473 mL) [ethanol free, contains sodium benzoate; cherry flavor]
Robafen DM: Guaifenesin 100 mg and dextromethorphan hydrobromide 10 mg per 5 mL (120 mL, 240 mL, 480 mL) [cherry flavor]
Robitussin Peak Cold Cough + Chest Congestion DM: Guaifenesin 100 mg and dextromethorphan hydrobromide 10 mg per 5 mL (120 mL, 240 mL) [contains menthol, propylene glycol, sodium 7 mg/5 mL, sodium benzoate]
Robitussin Peak Cold Sugar-Free Cough + Chest Congestion DM: Guaifenesin 100 mg and dextromethorphan hydrobromide 10 mg per 5 mL (120 mL) [sugar free; contains propylene glycol, sodium 3 mg/5 mL, sodium benzoate]
Robitussin Peak Cold Maximum Strength Cough + Chest Congestion DM: Guaifenesin 200 mg and dextromethorphan hydrobromide 10 mg per 5 mL (120 mL, 240 mL) [contains menthol, propylene glycol, sodium 5 mg/5 mL, sodium benzoate]
Silexin: Guaifenesin 100 mg and dextromethorphan hydrobromide 10 mg per 5 mL (45 mL) [ethanol free, sugar free)]
Siltussin DM: Guaifenesin 100 mg and dextromethorphan hydrobromide 10 mg per 5 mL (120 mL, 240 mL, 480 mL) [strawberry flavor]
Siltussin DM DAS: Guaifenesin 100 mg and dextromethorphan hydrobromide 10 mg per 5 mL (120 mL) [dye free, ethanol free, sugar free; strawberry flavor]
Zyncof: Guaifenesin 400 mg and dextromethorphan hydrobromide 20 mg per 5 mL (120 mL, 480 mL) [dye free, ethanol free, sugar free; contains propylen glycol; grape flavor]

Tablet, oral: Guaifenesin 1000 mg and dextromethorphan hydrobromide 60 mg; guaifenesin 1200 mg and dextromethorphan hydrobromide 60 mg
Silexin: Guaifenesin 100 mg and dextromethorphan hydrobromide 10 mg
Tablet, extended release, oral:
Mucinex DM: Guaifenesin 600 mg and dextromethorphan hydrobromide 30 mg
Mucinex DM Maximum Strength: Guaifenesin 1200 mg and dextromethorphan hydrobromide 60 mg
Tablet, timed release, oral [scored]: Guaifenesin 1200 mg and dextromethorphan hydrobromide 60 mg

Guaifenesin and Phenylephrine

(gwye FEN e sin & fen il EF rin)

Brand Names: U.S. Ambi 10PEH/400GFN [OTC]; Fenesin PE IR; J-Max [OTC]; Liquibid® D-R [OTC]; Liquibid® PD-R [OTC]; Medent®-PEI [OTC]; Mucinex® Cold [OTC]; Mucus Relief Sinus [OTC]; Nu-COPD [OTC]; OneTab™ Congestion & Cold [OTC]; Refenesen™ PE [OTC]; Rescon GG [OTC]; Sudafed PE® Non-Drying Sinus [OTC]; Triaminic® Children's Chest & Nasal Congestion [OTC]

Index Terms Guaifenesin and Phenylephrine Tannate; Phenylephrine Hydrochloride and Guaifenesin

Pharmacologic Category Decongestant; Expectorant

Use Temporary relief of nasal congestion, sinusitis, rhinitis, and hay fever; temporary relief of cough associated with upper respiratory tract conditions, especially when associated with dry, nonproductive cough

Dosage Oral:
Children 2-5 years (Rescon GG): 2.5 mL every 4-6 hours; maximum: 10 mL/24 hours
Children 6-11 years (Rescon GG): 5 mL every 4-6 hours; maximum: 20 mL/24 hours
Children ≥12 years and Adults (Rescon GG): 10 mL every 4-6 hours; maximum: 40 mL/24 hours

Additional Information Complete prescribing information should be consulted for additional detail.

Dosage Forms Excipient information presented when available (limited, particularly for generics); consult specific product labeling. [DSC] = Discontinued product
Caplet, oral:
Fenesin PE IR: Guaifenesin 400 mg and phenylephrine hydrochloride 10 mg
OneTab™ Congestion & Cold: Guaifenesin 400 mg and phenylephrine hydrochloride 10 mg
Refenesen™ PE: Guaifenesin 400 mg and phenylephrine hydrochloride 10 mg
Sudafed PE® Non-Drying Sinus: Guaifenesin 200 mg and phenylephrine hydrochloride 5 mg
Liquid, oral:
Mucinex® Cold: Guaifenesin 100 mg and phenylephrine hydrochloride 2.5 mg per 5 mL (480 mL) [contains propylene glycol, sodium 3 mg/5 mL; mixed berry flavor]
Nu-COPD: Guaifenesin 200 mg and phenylephrine hydrochloride 10 mg per 5 mL (480 mL)
Rescon GG: Guaifenesin 100 mg and phenylephrine hydrochloride 5 mg per 5 mL (120 mL, 480 mL) [dye free, ethanol free; contains propylene glycol; wild cherry flavor]
Syrup, oral:
J-Max: Guaifenesin 200 mg and phenylephrine hydrochloride 5 mg per 5 mL (473 mL) [ethanol free, sugar free; contains propylene glycol; strawberry cream flavor]
Triaminic® Children's Chest & Nasal Congestion: Guaifenesin 50 mg and phenylephrine hydrochloride 2.5 mg per 5 mL (118 mL) [contains benzoic acid, propylene glycol, sodium 3 mg/5 mL; tropical flavor]
Tablet, oral:
Ambi 10PEH/400GFN: Guaifenesin 400 mg and phenylephrine hydrochloride 10 mg
Liquibid® D-R: Guaifenesin 400 mg and phenylephrine hydrochloride 10 mg
Liquibid® PD-R: Guaifenesin 200 mg and phenylephrine hydrochloride 5 mg
Medent®-PEI: Guaifenesin 400 mg and phenylephrine hydrochloride 10 mg
Mucus Relief Sinus: Guaifenesin 400 mg and phenylephrine hydrochloride 10 mg
Nu-COPD: Guaifenesin 400 mg and phenylephrine hydrochloride 10 mg

◆ Guaifenesin and Phenylephrine Tannate *see* Guaifenesin and Phenylephrine *on page 978*

Guaifenesin and Pseudoephedrine

(gwye FEN e sin & soo doe e FED rin)

Brand Names: U.S. Ambifed-G [OTC]; Congestac® [OTC]; ExeFen-IR; Maxifed [OTC]; Maxifed-G [OTC] [DSC]; Mucinex® D Maximum Strength [OTC]; Mucinex® D [OTC]; Refenesen Plus [OTC]

Brand Names: Canada Contac® Cold-Chest Congestion, Non Drowsy, Regular Strength; Entex® LA; Novahistex® Expectorant with Decongestant

Index Terms Pseudoephedrine and Guaifenesin

Pharmacologic Category Alpha/Beta Agonist; Expectorant

Use Temporary relief of nasal congestion and to help loosen phlegm and thin bronchial secretions in the treatment of cough

Dosage Oral:
Children 2-6 years (Maxifed-G®): One-third to 1/2 tablet every 12 hours (maximum: 1 tablet/12 hours)
Children 6-12 years:
Ambifed-G, Maxifed®: One-half caplet or tablet every 12 hours (maximum: 1 tablet/24 hours)
Congestac®: One-half caplet every 4-6 hours (maximum: 2 caplets/24 hours)
Maxifed-G®: One-half to 1 tablet every 12 hours (maximum: 2 tablets/24 hours)
Children >12 years and Adults:
Ambifed-G, Mucinex® D Maximum Strength: One tablet every 12 hours (maximum: 2 tablets/24 hours)
Congestac®: One caplet every 4-6 hours (maximum: 4 caplets in 24 hours)
Maxifed-G®, Mucinex® D: 1-2 tablets every 12 hours (maximum: 4 tablets/24 hours)
Maxifed®: One to 1 1/2 tablets every 12 hours (maximum: 3 tablets/24 hours)

Additional Information Complete prescribing information should be consulted for additional detail.

Dosage Forms Excipient information presented when available (limited, particularly for generics); consult specific product labeling.
Caplet, oral:
Congestac®, Refenesen Plus: Guaifenesin 400 mg and pseudoephedrine hydrochloride 60 mg
Tablet, oral:
Ambifed-G: Guaifenesin 400 mg and pseudoephedrine hydrochloride 20 mg
ExeFen-IR: Guaifenesin 400 mg and pseudoephedrine hydrochloride 30 mg
Maxifed: Guaifenesin 400 mg and pseudoephedrine hydrochloride 60 mg
Maxifed-G [DSC]: Guaifenesin 400 mg and pseudoephedrine hydrochloride 40 mg

Tablet, extended release, oral:

Mucinex® D: Guaifenesin 600 mg and pseudoephedrine hydrochloride 60 mg

Mucinex® D Maximum Strength: Guaifenesin 1200 mg and pseudoephedrine hydrochloride 120 mg

Guaifenesin, Pseudoephedrine, and Codeine (gwye FEN e sin, soo doe e FED rin, & KOE deen)

Brand Names: U.S. Cheratussin® DAC; Mytussin® DAC; Tricode® GF

Brand Names: Canada Benylin® 3.3 mg-D-E; Calmylin with Codeine

Index Terms Codeine, Guaifenesin, and Pseudoephedrine; Pseudoephedrine, Guaifenesin, and Codeine

Pharmacologic Category Antitussive/Decongestant/Expectorant

Use Temporarily relieves nasal congestion and controls cough associated with upper respiratory infections and related conditions (common cold, sinusitis, bronchitis, influenza)

Pregnancy Risk Factor C

Dosage Oral: **Note:** Products listed in dosage forms may contain differing amounts of active ingredients; however, the dosing volume and frequency are the same.

Children 6-12 years: 5 mL every 4 hours (maximum: 20 mL/24 hours)

Children >12 years and Adults: 10 mL every 4 hours (maximum: 40 mL/24 hours)

Additional Information Complete prescribing information should be consulted for additional detail.

Dosage Forms Excipient information presented when available (limited, particularly for generics); consult specific product labeling.

Syrup, oral: Guaifenesin 100 mg, pseudoephedrine hydrochloride 30 mg, and codeine phosphate 10 mg per 5 mL (473 mL)

Cheratussin® DAC: Guaifenesin 100 mg, pseudoephedrine 30 mg and codeine phosphate 10 mg per 5 mL (473 mL) [sugar free; contains ethanol 2.1% v/v, sodium benzoate; cherry flavor]

Mytussin® DAC: Guaifenesin 100 mg, pseudoephedrine hydrochloride 30 mg, and codeine phosphate 10 mg per 5 mL (118 mL, 473 mL) [sugar free; contains ethanol 1.7%; strawberry-raspberry flavor]

Tricode® GF: Guaifenesin 200 mg, pseudoephedrine hydrochloride 30 mg, and codeine phosphate 8 mg per 5 mL (473 mL) [ethanol free, dye free, gluten free, sugar free; contains propylene glycol; grape flavor]

Controlled Substance C-V

Guaifenesin, Pseudoephedrine, and Dextromethorphan
(gwye FEN e sin, soo doe e FED rin, & deks troe meth OR fan)

Brand Names: U.S. Ambifed DM; Ambifed-G DM; BP 8 Cough; Entre-Cough; ExeFen-DMX; Maxifed DM [DSC]; Maxifed DMX

Brand Names: Canada Balminil DM + Decongestant + Expectorant; Benylin® DM-D-E

Index Terms Dextromethorphan, Guaifenesin, and Pseudoephedrine; Pseudoephedrine, Dextromethorphan, and Guaifenesin

Pharmacologic Category Antitussive/Decongestant/Expectorant

Use Temporarily relieves nasal congestion and controls cough due to minor throat and bronchial irritation; helps loosen phlegm and thin bronchial secretions to make coughs more productive

Dosage Note: Also refer to specific product labeling.

Liquid (OTC labeling; Maxifed DM):

Children 6-11 years: 2.5 mL every 4-6 hours, not to exceed 15 mL/24 hours

Children ≥12 years and Adults: 5 mL every 4-6 hours, not to exceed 30 mL/24 hours

Tablet (OTC labeling; Ambifed-G DM, Maxifed DM):

Children 6-11 years: One-half tablet every 4-6 hours, not to exceed 3 tablets/24 hours

Children ≥12 years and Adults: One tablet every 4-6 hours, not to exceed 6 tablets/24 hours

Additional Information Complete prescribing information should be consulted for additional detail.

Dosage Forms Excipient information presented when available (limited, particularly for generics); consult specific product labeling.

Liquid, oral:

BP 8 Cough: Guaifenesin 175 mg, pseudoephedrine hydrochloride 30 mg, and dextromethorphan hydrobromide 15 mg per 5 mL (473 mL) [alcohol free, contains propylene glycol; grape flavor]

Maxifed DM: Guaifenesin 200 mg, pseudoephedrine hydrochloride 20 mg, and dextromethorphan hydrobromide 10 mg per 5 mL (473 mL) [sugar free, contains ethanol 0.1%, propylene glycol; orange cream flavor]

Suspension, oral:

Entre-Cough: Guaifenesin 175 mg, pseudoephedrine hydrochloride 30 mg, and dextromethorphan hydrobromide 15 mg per 5 mL (473 mL) [contains aspartame, sodium benzoate; cherry flavor]

Tablet, oral:

Ambifed DM: Guaifenesin 400 mg, pseudoephedrine hydrochloride 30 mg, and dextromethorphan hydrobromide 20 mg

Ambifed-G DM: Guaifenesin 400 mg, pseudoephedrine hydrochloride 20 mg, and dextromethorphan hydrobromide 20 mg

ExeFen-DMX: Guaifenesin 400 mg, pseudoephedrine hydrochloride 60 mg, and dextromethorphan hydrobromide 20 mg

Maxifed DM: Guaifenesin 400 mg, pseudoephedrine hydrochloride 40 mg, and dextromethorphan hydrobromide 20 mg [DSC]

Maxifed DMX: Guaifenesin 400 mg, pseudoephedrine hydrochloride 60 mg, and dextromethorphan hydrobromide 20 mg

GuanFACINE (GWAHN fa seen)

Brand Names: U.S. Intuniv; Tenex

Brand Names: Canada Intuniv XR

Index Terms Guanfacine Hydrochloride

Pharmacologic Category Alpha$_2$-Adrenergic Agonist; Antihypertensive

Additional Appendix Information

Beers Criteria - Potentially Inappropriate Medications for Geriatrics *on page 2368*

Use

Tablet, immediate release: Management of hypertension

Tablet, extended release: Treatment of attention-deficit/hyperactivity disorder (ADHD) as monotherapy or adjunctive therapy to stimulants

Unlabeled Use Tic disorder; Tourette's syndrome

Pregnancy Risk Factor B

Dosage Oral:

Extended release (Intuniv®): Children ≥6 years and Adolescents: ADHD, monotherapy or adjunct to stimulants: Initial: 1 mg once daily; may adjust by increments no larger than 1 mg/week as tolerated, based on clinical response; maximum dose: 4 mg/day.

Note: Clinical response is associated with doses of 0.05-0.08 mg/kg/day. Doses up to 0.12 mg/kg/day may provide additional benefit; however, doses >4 mg/day have not been evaluated.

Dosage adjustment for concomitant CYP3A4 inhibitors/inducers: Extended release:

Strong CYP3A4 inhibitors: If initiating guanfacine while taking a strong CYP3A4 inhibitor, do not exceed a maximum guanfacine dose of 2 mg/day. If continuing guanfacine and adding a strong CYP3A4 inhibitor, decrease guanfacine dose by 50%. If the strong CYP3A4 inhibitor is discontinued, double the guanfacine dose (maximum dose: 4 mg/day).

Strong CYP3A4 inducers: If initiating guanfacine while taking a strong CYP3A4 inducer, may titrate guanfacine up to 8 mg/day; consider faster titration (eg, 2 mg/week). If continuing guanfacine and adding a strong CYP3A4 inducer, consider increasing guanfacine gradually over 1-2 weeks to double the original dose. If the strong CYP3A4 inducer is discontinued, decrease guanfacine dose by 50% over 1-2 weeks (maximum dose: 4 mg/day).

Conversion from immediate release to extended release: Discontinue the immediate release formulation, and titrate according to extended release recommendations.

Missed doses of extended release: If ≥2 consecutive doses are missed, consider repeating dosage titration based on patient tolerability.

Discontinuation of extended release: Gradually discontinue by tapering dose in decrements of ≤1 mg every 3-7 days.

Immediate release:

Children ≥12 years and Adults: Hypertension: 1 mg usually at bedtime, may increase if needed at 3- to 4-week intervals; usual dose range (JNC 7): 0.5-2 mg once daily

Elderly: Hypertension: Consider lower initial doses and titrate to response (Aronow, 2011)

Dosage adjustment in renal impairment:

Extended release (Intuniv®): Children ≥6 years and Adolescents: No dosage adjustment provided in manufacturer's labeling (has not been studied); however, dosage adjustments may be necessary in patients with significant renal impairment.

Immediate release: Children ≥12 years and Adults: No dosage adjustment provided in manufacturer's labeling; however, the lower end of the dosing range is recommended in patients with renal impairment.

Hemodialysis: Immediate release or extended release: Dialysis clearance is low (~15% of total clearance).

Dosage adjustment in hepatic impairment:

Extended release (Intuniv®): Children ≥6 years and Adolescents: No dosage adjustment provided in manufacturer's labeling (has not been studied); however, dosage adjustments may be necessary in patients with significant hepatic impairment.

Immediate release: Children ≥12 years and Adults: No dosage adjustment provided in manufacturer's labeling; however, use with caution in chronic hepatic impairment.

Additional Information Complete prescribing information should be consulted for additional detail.

Dosage Forms Excipient information presented when available (limited, particularly for generics); consult specific product labeling.

Tablet, Oral:

Tenex: 1 mg [contains fd&c red #40 aluminum lake]

Tenex: 2 mg [contains fd&c yellow #10 aluminum lake]

Generic: 1 mg, 2 mg

Tablet Extended Release 24 Hour, Oral:

Intuniv: 1 mg, 2 mg, 3 mg, 4 mg

◆ Guanfacine Hydrochloride *see* GuanFACINE *on page 979*

◆ GW506U78 *see* Nelarabine *on page 1434*

◆ GW433908G *see* Fosamprenavir *on page 916*

◆ GW572016 *see* Lapatinib *on page 1174*

◆ GW786034 *see* PAZOPanib *on page 1581*

◆ Gynazole-1 *see* Butoconazole *on page 306*

◆ Gynazole-1® (Can) *see* Butoconazole *on page 306*

◆ Gyne-Lotrimin [OTC] *see* Clotrimazole (Topical) *on page 476*

◆ Gyne-Lotrimin 3 [OTC] *see* Clotrimazole (Topical) *on page 476*

◆ H1N1 Influenza Vaccine *see* Influenza Virus Vaccine (Inactivated) *on page 1078*

◆ H1N1 Influenza Vaccine *see* Influenza Virus Vaccine (Live/Attenuated) *on page 1082*

◆ h5G1.1 *see* Eculizumab *on page 683*

◆ H5N1 Influenza Vaccine *see* Influenza Virus Vaccine (H5N1) *on page 1076*

◆ Habitrol *see* Nicotine *on page 1453*

◆ Habitrol® (Can) *see* Nicotine *on page 1453*

Haemophilus b Conjugate and Hepatitis B Vaccine

(he MOF i lus bee KON joo gate & hep a TYE tis bee vak SEEN)

Brand Names: U.S. Comvax®

Index Terms *Haemophilus* b (meningococcal protein conjugate) Conjugate Vaccine; Hepatitis B Vaccine (Recombinant); Hib Conjugate Vaccine; Hib-HepB

Pharmacologic Category Vaccine, Inactivated (Bacterial); Vaccine, Inactivated (Viral)

Additional Appendix Information

Immunization Administration Recommendations *on page 2334*

Immunization Recommendations *on page 2339*

Use

Immunization against invasive disease caused by *H. influenzae* type b and against infection caused by all known subtypes of hepatitis B virus in infants 6 weeks to 15 months of age born of hepatitis B surface antigen (HB_sAg)-negative mothers

Infants born of HB_sAg-positive mothers or mothers of unknown HB_sAg status should receive hepatitis B vaccine (recombinant) at birth and should complete the hepatitis B vaccination series given according to a particular schedule (refer to current ACIP recommendations).

Pregnancy Risk Factor C

Dosage Infants: I.M.: 0.5 mL/dose; one dose at 2, 4, and 12-15 months of age (total of 3 doses)

If the recommended schedule cannot be followed, the interval between the first two doses should be at least 6 weeks and the interval between the second and third dose should be as close as possible to 8-11 months. Minimum age for first dose is 6 weeks.

Modified Schedule: Children who receive one dose of hepatitis B vaccine at or shortly after birth may receive Comvax® on a schedule of 2, 4, and 12-15 months of age

Dosage adjustment in renal impairment: No dosage adjustment provided in manufacturer's labeling.

Dosage adjustment in hepatic impairment: No dosage adjustment provided in manufacturer's labeling.

Additional Information Complete prescribing information should be consulted for additional detail.

Dosage Forms Excipient information presented when available (limited, particularly for generics); consult specific product labeling.

Injection, suspension [preservative free]:

Comvax®: *Haemophilus* b capsular polysaccharide 7.5 mcg (bound to *Neisseria meningitides* OMPC 125 mcg) and hepatitis B surface antigen 5 mcg per 0.5 mL (0.5 mL) [contains aluminum; contains natural rubber/natural latex in packaging]

◆ ***Haemophilus* B Conjugate (Hib)** *see* Diphtheria and Tetanus Toxoids, Acellular Pertussis, Poliovirus and *Haemophilus* b Conjugate Vaccine *on page 629*

Haemophilus b Conjugate Vaccine

(he MOF fi lus bee KON joo gate vak SEEN)

Brand Names: U.S. ActHIB®; Hiberix®; PedvaxHIB®

Brand Names: Canada ActHIB®; PedvaxHIB®

Index Terms *Haemophilus influenzae* Type b; Hib; PRP-OMP; PRP-T

Pharmacologic Category Vaccine, Inactivated (Bacterial)

Additional Appendix Information

Immunization Administration Recommendations *on page 2334*

Immunization Recommendations *on page 2339*

Use Routine immunization of children against invasive disease caused by *H. influenzae* type b

The Advisory Committee on Immunization Practices (ACIP) recommends routine vaccination of all children through age 59 months. Efficacy data are not available for use in older children and adults with chronic conditions associated with an increased risk of Hib disease. However, a single dose may also be considered for older children, adolescents, and adults who did not receive the childhood series and who have a chronic condition associated with an increased risk of Hib disease (eg, splenectomy, sickle cell disease, leukemia, HIV infection).

Pregnancy Risk Factor C

Pregnancy Considerations Animal reproduction studies have not been conducted.

Breast-Feeding Considerations Inactivated virus vaccines do not affect the safety of breast-feeding for the mother or the infant (CDC, 2011). Breast-feeding also appears to reduce the incidence of infant fever associated with routine childhood immunization (Piscane, 2010). Breast-feeding infants should be vaccinated according to the recommended schedules (CDC, 2011).

Contraindications Hypersensitivity to *Haemophilus* b polysaccharide vaccine or any component of the formulation

Warnings/Precautions Vaccination may not result in effective immunity in all patients. Response depends upon multiple factors (eg, type of vaccine, age of patient) and may be improved by administering the vaccine at the recommended dose, route, and interval. Vaccines may not be effective if administered during periods of altered immune competence (CDC, 2011). Infection may occur within the week of vaccination, prior to the onset of the vaccine. If used in persons with malignancies or those receiving immunosuppressive therapy or who are otherwise immunocompromised, the expected immune response may not be obtained; may be used in patients with HIV infection. In general, household and close contacts of persons with altered immunocompetence may receive all age appropriate vaccines. The decision to administer or delay vaccination because of current or recent febrile illness depends on the severity of symptoms and the etiology of the disease. Immunization should be delayed during the course of an acute febrile illness. Use caution in children with coagulation disorders (including thrombocytopenia) where intramuscular injections should not be used. Epinephrine 1:1000 should be readily available. Patients who develop symptoms suggestive of hypersensitivity after an injection should not receive further injections of the vaccine. Syncope has been reported with use of injectable vaccines and may be accompanied by transient visual disturbances, weakness, or tonic-clonic movements. Procedures should be in place to avoid injuries from falling and to restore cerebral perfusion if syncope occurs.

Children in whom DTP or DT vaccination is deferred: The carrier proteins used in PRP-T (ActHIB®, Hiberix®), but not PRP-OMP (PedvaxHIB®), are chemically and immunologically related to toxoids contained in DTP vaccine. Earlier or simultaneous vaccination with diphtheria or tetanus toxoids may be required to elicit an optimal anti-PRP antibody response. In contrast, the immunogenicity of PRP-OMP is not affected by vaccination with DTP. In infants in whom DTP or DT vaccination is deferred, PRP-OMP may be advantageous for *Haemophilus influenzae* type b vaccination. Immunization with Hiberix® is not a substitute for routine tetanus immunization.

Hiberix®: Use with caution in patients with history of Guillain-Barré syndrome (GBS); carefully consider risks and benefits to vaccination in patients known to have experienced GBS within 6 weeks following previous influenza vaccination.

In order to maximize vaccination rates, the ACIP recommends simultaneous administration of all age-appropriate vaccines (live or inactivated) for which a person is eligible at a single clinic visit, unless contraindications exist. The use of combination vaccines is generally preferred over separate injections, taking into consideration provider assessment, patient preference, and adverse events. When using combination vaccines, the minimum age for administration is the oldest minimum age for any individual component; the minimum interval between dosing is the greatest minimum interval between any individual component.

Packaging may contain latex. Some products may contain lactose.

Adverse Reactions All serious adverse reactions must be reported to the U.S. Department of Health and Human Services (DHHS) Vaccine Adverse Event Reporting System (VAERS) 1-800-822-7967 or online at https://vaers.hhs.gov/esub/index. In Canada, adverse reactions may be reported to local provincial/territorial health agencies or to the Vaccine Safety Section at Public Health Agency of Canada (1-866-844-0018).

Frequency not defined:

Central nervous system: Crying (unusual, high pitched, prolonged), fever, fussiness, irritability, pain, restlessness, sleepiness

Dermatologic: Rash

Gastrointestinal: Anorexia, diarrhea, vomiting

Local: Injection site: Erythema, induration, pain, soreness, swelling

Otic: Otitis media

Respiratory: Upper respiratory tract infection

Postmarketing and/or case reports: Allergic reactions, anaphylactoid reactions, angioedema, apnea, febrile seizure, Guillain-Barré syndrome, hypersensitivity, hyporesponsive episodes, hypotonia, injection site abscess (sterile), lethargy, lymphadenopathy, malaise, mass, pneumonia, seizure, swelling (extensive) of the injected limb, syncope, urticaria, vasovagal response

Drug Interactions

Metabolism/Transport Effects None known.

Avoid Concomitant Use There are no known interactions where it is recommended to avoid concomitant use.

Increased Effect/Toxicity There are no known significant interactions involving an increase in effect.

Decreased Effect

The levels/effects of Haemophilus b Conjugate Vaccine may be decreased by: Belimumab; Fingolimod; Immunosuppressants

Preparation for Administration Hiberix®: Dilute with provided saline diluent only. Transfer entire contents of prefilled syringe containing diluent into the vial; with needle still inserted, shake vigorously until it becomes a clear, colorless solution. Withdraw entire contents of vial (~0.5 mL) for administration.

Storage/Stability Store under refrigeration at 2°C to 8°C (36°F to 46°F); do not freeze.

ActHIB®: Use within 24 hours following reconstitution with saline.

Hiberix®: Prior to reconstitution, store powder under refrigeration at 2°C to 8°C (36°F to 46°F). Protect from light. Diluent may be stored under refrigeration or at room temperature; do not freeze, discard diluent if frozen. If not used immediately after reconstitution, may store under refrigeration for up to 24 hours. Shake well prior to use. Discard any unused portion.

Mechanism of Action Stimulates production of anticapsular antibodies and provides active immunity to *Haemophilus influenzae* type b

Pharmacodynamics/Kinetics Seroconversion following one dose of Hib vaccine for children 18 months or 24 months of age or older is 75% to 90%, respectively.

Onset of action: Serum antibody response: 1-2 weeks

Duration: Immunity: 1.5 years

Dosage I.M.:

Children: 0.5 mL as a single dose should be administered to previously unvaccinated children according to one of the following "brand-specific" schedules; number of doses in series is dependent upon age at first dose. ActHIB® and PedvaxHIB® are approved for a complete vaccine series; Hiberix® is approved only as a booster (final) dose in children who have received primary immunization.

ActHIB®: *Age at first dose:*

2 months of age: Immunization consists of 3 doses (0.5 mL/dose) administered at 2-, 4-, and 6 months of age (reconstitute with provided diluent). A booster dose is given at 15-18 months of age (may reconstitute with provided diluent).

7-11 months of age: Two doses (0.5 mL/dose) administered 8 weeks apart, with a booster dose at 15-18 months of age

12-14 months of age: One dose (0.5 mL) followed by a booster dose 2 months later

PedvaxHIB®: *Age at first dose:*

2-10 months of age: Two doses (0.5 mL/dose) administered 2 months apart; booster dose at 12-15 months of age

11-14 months of age: Two doses (0.5 mL/dose) administered 2 months apart

15-71 months of age: One 0.5 mL dose

Hiberix®: 15-59 months: One 0.5 mL booster dose (per manufacturer). The ACIP recommends booster dose administration at 12-15 months

Children ≥5 years of age, Adolescents, and Adults who have not received the childhood Hib series **and** are at increased risk for invasive Hib disease due to certain chronic conditions (eg, sickle cell disease, leukemia, HIV infection, or splenectomy) (ACIP recommendations): One dose (0.5 mL); may use any of the Hib conjugate vaccines

Dosage adjustment in renal impairment: No dosage adjustment provided in manufacturer's labeling.

Dosage adjustment in hepatic impairment: No dosage adjustment provided in manufacturer's labeling.

Administration For I.M. administration; do not inject I.V.

Hiberix®: Shake well prior to use. Administer into the anterolateral thigh or deltoid. If Hiberix® is inadvertently administered during the primary vaccination series, the dose can be counted as a valid PRP-T dose that does not need to be repeated if administered according to schedule. In this case, a total of 3 doses completes the primary series.

ActHIB®, PedvaxHIB®: Shake well prior to use. Administer into the anterolateral thigh or deltoid. Do not administer into buttocks due to potential risk of injury to sciatic nerve.

For patients at risk of hemorrhage following intramuscular injection, the ACIP recommends "it should be administered intramuscularly if, in the opinion of the physician familiar with the patient's bleeding risk, the vaccine can be administered by this route with reasonable safety. If the patient receives antihemophilia or other similar therapy, intramuscular vaccination can be scheduled shortly after such therapy is administered. A fine needle (23 gauge or smaller) can be used for the vaccination and firm pressure applied to the site (without rubbing) for at least 2 minutes. The patient should be instructed concerning the risk of hematoma from the injection." Patients on anticoagulant therapy should be considered to have the same bleeding risks and treated as those with clotting factor disorders (CDC, 2011).

Simultaneous administration of vaccines helps ensure the patients will be fully vaccinated by the appropriate age. Simultaneous administration of vaccines is defined as administering >1 vaccine on the same day at different anatomic sites. The use of licensed combination vaccines is generally preferred over separate injections of the equivalent components. Separate vaccines should not be combined in the same syringe unless indicated by product specific labeling. Separate needles and syringes should be used for each injection. The ACIP prefers each dose of a specific vaccine in a series come from the same manufacturer when possible. Adolescents and adults should be vaccinated while seated or lying down. In general, preterm infants should be vaccinated at the same chronological age as full-term infants (CDC, 2011).

Antipyretics have not been shown to prevent febrile seizures. Antipyretics may be used to treat fever or discomfort following vaccination (CDC, 2011). One study reported that routine prophylactic administration of acetaminophen to prevent fever prior to vaccination decreased the immune response of some vaccines; the clinical significance of this reduction in immune response has not been established (Prymula, 2009).

Monitoring Parameters Monitor for syncope for 15 minutes following administration. If seizure-like activity associated with syncope occurs, maintain patient in supine or Trendelenburg position to reestablish adequate cerebral perfusion.

Test Interactions May interfere with interpretation of urine antigen detection tests; antigenuria may occur up to 2 weeks following immunization

Additional Information U.S. federal law requires that the name of medication, date of administration, the vaccine manufacturer, lot number of vaccine, and the administering person's name, title, and address be entered into the patient's permanent medical record.

The conjugate vaccines currently available consist of *Haemophilus influenzae* type b (Hib) capsular polysaccharide (also referred to as PRP) linked to a carrier protein. PedvaxHIB® (PRP-OMP) is linked to the outer membrane protein complex from *Neisseria meningitidis*. ActHIB® and Hiberix® (PRP-T) use tetanus toxoid conjugate as the carrier protein.

Dosage Forms Excipient information presented when available (limited, particularly for generics); consult specific product labeling.

Injection, powder for reconstitution [preservative free]:

ActHIB®: *Haemophilus* b capsular polysaccharide 10 mcg [bound to tetanus toxoid 24 mcg] per 0.5 mL [contains sucrose; may be reconstituted with provided diluent (forms solution; contains natural rubber/natural latex in packaging)]

Hiberix®: *Haemophilus* b capsular polysaccharide 10 mcg [bound to tetanus toxoid 25 mcg] per 0.5 mL (0.5 mL) [contains lactose 12.6 mg]

Injection, suspension:

PedvaxHIB®: *Haemophilus* b capsular polysaccharide 7.5 mcg [bound to *Neisseria meningitidis* OMPC 125 mcg] per 0.5 mL (0.5 mL) [contains aluminum; natural rubber/natural latex in packaging]

◆ ***Haemophilus* b (meningococcal protein conjugate) Conjugate Vaccine** *see* *Haemophilus* b Conjugate and Hepatitis B Vaccine *on page 980*

◆ ***Haemophilus* B Polysaccharide** *see* Diphtheria and Tetanus Toxoids, Acellular Pertussis, Poliovirus and *Haemophilus* b Conjugate Vaccine *on page 629*

◆ ***Haemophilus influenzae* Type b** *see* *Haemophilus* b Conjugate Vaccine *on page 981*

◆ **Hair Regrowth Treatment Men [OTC]** *see* Minoxidil (Topical) *on page 1375*

◆ **Halaven** *see* Eribulin *on page 734*

◆ **Halaven™ (Can)** *see* Eribulin *on page 734*

Halcinonide (hal SIN oh nide)

Brand Names: U.S. Halog

Pharmacologic Category Corticosteroid, Topical

Additional Appendix Information

Topical Corticosteroids *on page 2299*

Use Relief of inflammatory and pruritic effects of corticosteroid-responsive dermatoses [high potency topical corticosteroid]

Pregnancy Risk Factor C

Dosage Children and Adults: Topical: Steroid-responsive dermatoses: Apply sparingly 2-3 times daily, occlusive dressing may be used for severe or resistant dermatoses; a thin film is effective; avoid excessive application. Therapy should be discontinued when control is achieved; if no improvement is seen, reassessment of diagnosis may be necessary.

Additional Information Complete prescribing information should be consulted for additional detail.

Dosage Forms Excipient information presented when available (limited, particularly for generics); consult specific product labeling.

Cream, External:

Halog: 0.1% (30 g, 60 g, 216 g) [contains cetyl alcohol, propylene glycol]

Ointment, External:

Halog: 0.1% (30 g, 60 g)

◆ **Halcion** *see* Triazolam *on page 2124*

◆ **Halcion® (Can)** *see* Triazolam *on page 2124*

◆ **Haldol** *see* Haloperidol *on page 983*

◆ **Haldol Decanoate** *see* Haloperidol *on page 983*

◆ **Haley's M-O** *see* Magnesium Hydroxide and Mineral Oil *on page 1261*

◆ **Halfprin® [OTC]** *see* Aspirin *on page 177*

◆ **Halichondrin B Analog** *see* Eribulin *on page 734*

Halobetasol (hal oh BAY ta sol)

Brand Names: U.S. Halonate; Ultravate

Brand Names: Canada Ultravate®

Index Terms Halobetasol Propionate

Pharmacologic Category Corticosteroid, Topical

Additional Appendix Information

Topical Corticosteroids *on page 2299*

Use Relief of inflammatory and pruritic manifestations of corticosteroid-response dermatoses [super high potency topical corticosteroid]

Pregnancy Risk Factor C

Dosage Topical: Children ≥12 years and Adults: Steroid-responsive dermatoses: Apply sparingly to skin once or twice daily, rub in gently and completely; treatment should not exceed 2 consecutive weeks and total dosage should not exceed 50 g/week. Therapy should be discontinued when control is achieved; if no improvement is seen, reassessment of diagnosis may be necessary.

Additional Information Complete prescribing information should be consulted for additional detail.

Dosage Forms Excipient information presented when available (limited, particularly for generics); consult specific product labeling.

Cream, External, as propionate:

Ultravate: 0.05% (50 g) [contains cetyl alcohol]

Generic: 0.05% (15 g, 50 g)

Kit, External, as propionate:

Halonate: 0.05 & 12% (Foam) [contains cetyl alcohol, propylene glycol, trolamine (triethanolamine)]

Ointment, External, as propionate:

Ultravate: 0.05% (50 g) [contains propylene glycol]

Generic: 0.05% (15 g, 50 g)

◆ **Halobetasol Propionate** *see* Halobetasol *on page 983*

◆ **Halog** *see* Halcinonide *on page 983*

◆ **Halonate** *see* Halobetasol *on page 983*

Haloperidol (ha loe PER i dole)

Brand Names: U.S. Haldol; Haldol Decanoate

Brand Names: Canada Apo-Haloperidol LA®; Apo-Haloperidol®; Haloperidol Injection, USP; Haloperidol Long Acting; Haloperidol-LA; Haloperidol-LA Omega; Novo-Peridol; PMS-Haloperidol; PMS-Haloperidol LA

Index Terms Haloperidol Decanoate; Haloperidol Lactate

Pharmacologic Category Antipsychotic Agent, Typical

Additional Appendix Information

Antipsychotic Agents *on page 2290*

Beers Criteria – Potentially Inappropriate Medications for Geriatrics *on page 2368*

Use Management of schizophrenia; control of tics and vocal utterances of Tourette's disorder in children and adults; severe behavioral problems in children

Unlabeled Use Treatment of nonschizophrenia psychosis; may be used for the emergency sedation of severely-agitated or delirious patients; treatment of ICU delirium; adjunctive treatment of ethanol dependence; postoperative nausea and vomiting (alternative therapy); psychosis/agitation related to Alzheimer's dementia

Pregnancy Risk Factor C

Pregnancy Considerations Adverse events were observed in animal reproduction studies. Haloperidol crosses the placenta in humans (Newport, 2007). Although haloperidol has not been found to be a major human teratogen, an association with limb malformations following first trimester exposure in humans cannot be ruled out (ACOG, 2008; Diav-Citrin, 2005). Antipsychotic use during the third trimester of pregnancy has a risk for abnormal muscle movements (extrapyramidal symptoms [EPS]) and withdrawal symptoms in newborns following delivery. Symptoms in the newborn may include agitation, feeding disorder, hypertonia, hypotonia, respiratory distress, somnolence, and tremor; these effects may be selflimiting or require hospitalization. If needed, the minimum effective maternal dose should be used in order to decrease the risk of EPS (ACOG, 2008).

Breast-Feeding Considerations Haloperidol is found in breast milk and has been detected in the plasma and urine of nursing infants (Whalley, 1981; Yoshida, 1999). Breast engorgement, gynecomastia, and lactation are known side effects with the use of haloperidol. Breast-feeding is not recommended by the manufacturer.

Contraindications Hypersensitivity to haloperidol or any component of the formulation; Parkinson's disease; severe CNS depression; coma

Warnings/Precautions [U.S. Boxed Warning]: Elderly patients with dementia-related psychosis treated with antipsychotics are at an increased risk of death compared to placebo. Most deaths appeared to be either cardiovascular (eg, heart failure, sudden death) or infectious (eg, pneumonia) in nature. Haloperidol is not approved for the treatment of dementia-related psychosis. Hypotension may occur, particularly with parenteral administration. Although the short-acting form (lactate) is used clinically, the I.V. use of the injection is not an FDA-approved route of administration; the decanoate form should never be administered intravenously.

May alter cardiac conduction and prolong QT interval; life-threatening arrhythmias have occurred with therapeutic doses of antipsychotics but risk may be increased with doses exceeding recommendations and/or intravenous administration (unlabeled route). Use caution or avoid use in patients with electrolyte abnormalities (eg, hypokalemia, hypomagnesemia), hypothyroidism, familial long QT syndrome, concomitant medications which may augment QT prolongation, or any underlying cardiac abnormality which may also potentiate risk. Monitor ECG closely for dose-related QT effects. Adverse effects of decanoate may be prolonged. Avoid in thyrotoxicosis.

Leukopenia, neutropenia, and agranulocytosis (sometimes fatal) have been reported in clinical trials and postmarketing reports with antipsychotic use; presence of risk factors (eg, pre-existing low WBC or history of drug-induced leuko-/neutropenia) should prompt periodic blood count assessment. Discontinue therapy at first signs of blood dyscrasias or if absolute neutrophil count <1000/mm^3.

May be sedating, use with caution in disorders where CNS depression is a feature. Effects may be potentiated when used with other sedative drugs or ethanol. Caution in patients with severe cardiovascular disease, predisposition to seizures, subcortical brain damage, or renal disease. Esophageal dysmotility and aspiration have been associated with antipsychotic use - use with caution in patients at risk of pneumonia (eg, Alzheimer's disease). Use associated with increased prolactin levels; clinical significance of hyperprolactinemia in patients with breast cancer or other prolactin-dependent tumors is unknown. May alter temperature regulation or mask toxicity of other drugs due to antiemetic effects. May cause orthostatic hypotension; use with caution in patients at risk of this effect or those who would tolerate transient hypotensive episodes (cerebrovascular disease, cardiovascular disease, or other medications which may predispose). Some tablets contain tartrazine. Antipsychotics have been associated with pigmentary retinopathy.

May cause anticholinergic effects (confusion, agitation, constipation, xerostomia, blurred vision, urinary retention). Therefore, they should be used with caution in patients with decreased gastrointestinal motility, urinary retention, BPH, xerostomia, visual problems, or narrow-angle glaucoma (screening is recommended). Relative to other neuroleptics, haloperidol has a low potency of cholinergic blockade.

May cause extrapyramidal symptoms (EPS), including pseudoparkinsonism, acute dystonic reactions, akathisia, and tardive dyskinesia. Risk of dystonia (and possibly other EPS) may be greater with increased doses, use of conventional antipsychotics, males, and younger patients. May be associated with neuroleptic malignant syndrome (NMS). Use in elderly patients with dementia is associated with an increased risk of mortality and cerebrovascular accidents; avoid antipsychotic use for behavioral problems associated with dementia unless alternative nonpharmacologic therapies have failed and patient may harm self or others. In addition, use may cause or exacerbate syndrome of inappropriate antidiuretic hormone secretion or hyponatremia; monitor sodium closely with initiation or dosage adjustments in older adults (Beers Criteria). Increased risk for developing tardive dyskinesia, particularly elderly women.

Adverse Reactions Frequency not defined.

Cardiovascular: Abnormal T waves with prolonged ventricular repolarization, arrhythmia, hyper-/hypotension, QT prolongation, sudden death, tachycardia, torsade de pointes

Central nervous system: Agitation, akathisia, altered central temperature regulation, anxiety, confusion, depression, drowsiness, dystonic reactions, euphoria, extrapyramidal reactions, headache, insomnia, lethargy, neuroleptic malignant syndrome (NMS), pseudoparkinsonian signs and symptoms, restlessness, seizure, tardive dyskinesia, tardive dystonia, vertigo

Dermatologic: Alopecia, contact dermatitis, hyperpigmentation, photosensitivity (rare), pruritus, rash

Endocrine & metabolic: Amenorrhea, breast engorgement, galactorrhea, gynecomastia, hyper-/hypoglycemia, hyponatremia, lactation, mastalgia, menstrual irregularities, sexual dysfunction

Gastrointestinal: Anorexia, constipation, diarrhea, dyspepsia, hypersalivation, nausea, vomiting, xerostomia

Genitourinary: Priapism, urinary retention

Hematologic: Agranulocytosis (rare), leukopenia, leukocytosis, neutropenia, anemia, lymphomonocytosis

Hepatic: Cholestatic jaundice, obstructive jaundice

Ocular: Blurred vision

Respiratory: Bronchospasm, laryngospasm

Miscellaneous: Diaphoresis, heat stroke

Drug Interactions

Metabolism/Transport Effects Substrate of CYP1A2 (minor), CYP2D6 (major), CYP3A4 (major); **Note:** Assignment of Major/Minor substrate status based on clinically relevant drug interaction potential; **Inhibits** CYP2D6 (moderate), CYP3A4 (moderate)

Avoid Concomitant Use

Avoid concomitant use of Haloperidol with any of the following: Aclidinium; Amisulpride; Azelastine (Nasal); Bosutinib; Conivaptan; FLUoxetine; Fusidic Acid (Systemic); Highest Risk QTc-Prolonging Agents; Ibrutinib; Ipratropium (Oral Inhalation); Ivabradine; Lomitapide; Metoclopramide; Mifepristone; Paraldehyde; QuiNIDine; Simeprevir; Sulpiride; Thioridazine; Tiotropium; Tolvaptan; Ulipristal; Umeclidinium

Increased Effect/Toxicity

Haloperidol may increase the levels/effects of: Alcohol (Ethyl); Amisulpride; Analgesics (Opioid); Anticholinergics; ARIPiprazole; Avanafil; Azelastine (Nasal); Bosentan; Bosutinib; Budesonide (Systemic, Oral Inhalation); Buprenorphine; ChlorproMAZINE; CNS Depressants; Colchicine; CYP2D6 Substrates; CYP3A4 Substrates; Eplerenone; Everolimus; FentaNYL; Fesoterodine; Highest Risk QTc-Prolonging Agents; Hydrocodone; Ibrutinib; Imatinib; Ivacaftor; Lomitapide; Lurasidone;

Methotrimeprazine; Methylphenidate; Metoprolol; Moderate Risk QTc-Prolonging Agents; Nebivolol; OxyCODONE; Paraldehyde; Pimecrolimus; QuiNIDine; Salmeterol; Saxagliptin; Serotonin Modulators; Simeprevir; Sulpiride; Thioridazine; Tiotropium; Tolvaptan; Ulipristal; Zolpidem

The levels/effects of Haloperidol may be increased by: Abiraterone Acetate; Acetylcholinesterase Inhibitors (Central); Aclidinium; ARIPiprazole; Brimonidine (Topical); ChlorproMAZINE; Conivaptan; CYP2D6 Inhibitors (Moderate); CYP2D6 Inhibitors (Strong); CYP3A4 Inhibitors (Moderate); CYP3A4 Inhibitors (Strong); Darunavir; Dasatinib; Doxylamine; FLUoxetine; FluvoxaMINE; Fusidic Acid (Systemic); HydrOXYzine; Ipratropium (Oral Inhalation); Ivabradine; Ivacaftor; Lithium formulations; Luliconazole; Magnesium Sulfate; Methotrimeprazine; Methylphenidate; Metoclopramide; Metyrosine; Mifepristone; Nonsteroidal Anti-Inflammatory Agents; Perampanel; Pramlintide; QTc-Prolonging Agents (Indeterminate Risk and Risk Modifying); QuiNIDine; Serotonin Modulators; Simeprevir; Sodium Oxybate; Tetrabenazine; Umeclidinium

Decreased Effect

Haloperidol may decrease the levels/effects of: Amphetamines; Anti-Parkinson's Agents (Dopamine Agonist); Codeine; Ifosfamide; Quinagolide; Tamoxifen; Urea Cycle Disorder Agents

The levels/effects of Haloperidol may be decreased by: Anti-Parkinson's Agents (Dopamine Agonist); ARIPiprazole; Bosentan; CarBAMazepine; CYP3A4 Inducers (Strong); Dabrafenib; Deferasirox; Glycopyrrolate; Lithium formulations; Mitotane; Peginterferon Alfa-2b; Tocilizumab

Ethanol/Nutrition/Herb Interactions

Ethanol: May increase CNS depression; monitor for increased effects with coadministration. Caution patients about effects.

Herb/Nutraceutical: Avoid valerian, St John's wort, kava kava, gotu kola (may increase CNS depression).

Preparation for Administration Haloperidol lactate may be administered IVPB or I.V. infusion in D_5W solutions. NS solutions should not be used due to reports of decreased stability and incompatibility.

Usual concentration range: 0.5-100 mg/50-100 mL D_5W.

Storage/Stability Protect oral dosage forms from light. Haloperidol lactate injection should be stored at controlled room temperature; do not freeze or expose to temperatures >40°C. Protect from light; exposure to light may cause discoloration and the development of a grayish-red precipitate over several weeks. Stability of standardized solutions is 38 days at room temperature (24°C).

Mechanism of Action Haloperidol is a butyrophenone antipsychotic which blocks postsynaptic mesolimbic dopaminergic D_1 and D_2 receptors in the brain; depresses the release of hypothalamic and hypophyseal hormones; believed to depress the reticular activating system thus affecting basal metabolism, body temperature, wakefulness, vasomotor tone, and emesis

Pharmacodynamics/Kinetics

Onset of action: Sedation: I.M., I.V.: 30-60 minutes

Duration: Decanoate: 2-4 weeks

Distribution: V_d: 8-18 L/kg

Protein binding: 90%

Metabolism: Hepatic: 50% to 60% glucuronidation (inactive); 23% CYP3A4-mediated reduction to inactive metabolites (some back-oxidation to haloperidol); and 20% to 30% CYP3A4-mediated N-dealkylation, including minor oxidation pathway to toxic pyridinium derivative (Kudo, 1999)

Bioavailability: Oral: 60% to 70%

Half-life elimination: 18 hours; Decanoate: 21 days

Time to peak, serum: Oral: 2-6 hours; I.M.: 20 minutes; Decanoate: 7 days

Excretion: Urine (30%, 1% as unchanged drug); feces (15%)

Dosage

Children: 3-12 years (15-40 kg): Oral:

Initial: 0.5 mg/day given in 2-3 divided doses; increase by 0.5 mg every 5-7 days; maximum: 0.15 mg/kg/day

Usual maintenance:

Nonpsychotic disorders, Tourette's disorder: 0.05-0.075 mg/kg/day in 2-3 divided doses

Psychotic disorders: 0.05-0.15 mg/kg/day in 2-3 divided doses

Children 6-12 years: Sedation/psychotic disorders: I.M. (as lactate): 1-3 mg/dose every 4-8 hours to a maximum of 0.15 mg/kg/day; convert to oral therapy as soon as able

Adults:

Psychosis:

Oral: 0.5-5 mg 2-3 times/day; usual maximum: 30 mg/day

I.M. (as lactate): 2-5 mg every 4-8 hours as needed

I.M. (as decanoate): Initial: 10-20 times the daily oral dose administered at 4-week intervals

Maintenance dose: 10-15 times initial oral dose; used to stabilize psychiatric symptoms

Delirium in the intensive care unit, treatment (unlabeled use, unlabeled route): **Note:** The optimal dose and regimen of haloperidol for the treatment of severe agitation and/or delirium has not been established. Currently, there are no studies evaluating the role of haloperidol on duration or severity of delirium. Haloperidol has been used for symptomatic treatment (severe agitation) of delirious patients. Current guidelines do not advocate use of haloperidol for the treatment or prevention of delirium due to insufficient evidence (Barr, 2013).

I.V.: Initial: 0.5-10 mg depending on degree of agitation; if inadequate response, may repeat bolus dose (with sequential doubling of initial bolus dose) every 15-30 minutes until calm achieved, then administer 25% of the last bolus dose every 6 hours; monitor ECG and QT_c interval. After the patient is controlled, haloperidol therapy should be tapered over several days. This strategy is based upon expert opinion; efficacy and safety have not been formally evaluated (Tesar, 1988).

Note: QT_c prolongation may occur with cumulative doses ≥35 mg per day and the risk of torsade de pointes is greater if ≥35 mg is received within <6 hours (Sharma, 1998). Continuous infusions have also been used with doses in the range of 0.5-2 mg/hour with an optional loading dose of 2.5 mg (Reade, 2009).

Delirium in the intensive care unit (patients at high risk of delirium), prevention (unlabeled use, unlabeled route): **Note:** The optimal dose and regimen of haloperidol for prevention of ICU delirium has not been established. Current guidelines do not advocate use of haloperidol for the treatment or prevention of delirium due to insufficient evidence (Barr, 2013). Haloperidol may decrease the incidence of delirium (Van den Boogaard, 2013; Wang, 2012).

I.V.: 0.5 mg followed by a continuous infusion of 0.1 mg/hour for 12 hours (Wang, 2012) **or** 0.5-1 mg every 8 hours (Van den Boogaard, 2013)

Rapid tranquilization of severely-agitated patient (unlabeled use): Administer every 30-60 minutes:

Oral: 5-10 mg

I.M. (as lactate): 5 mg

Average total dose (oral or I.M.) for tranquilization: 10-20 mg

Postoperative nausea and vomiting (PONV) (unlabeled use): I.M., I.V.: 0.5-2 mg (Gan, 2007)

Elderly: Nonpsychotic patient, dementia behavior (unlabeled use): Initial: Oral: 0.25-0.5 mg 1-2 times/day; increase dose at 4- to 7-day intervals by 0.25-0.5 mg/day; increase dosing intervals (twice daily, 3 times/day, etc) as necessary to control response or side effects

Dosage adjustment in renal impairment:
No dosage adjustment provided in manufacturer's labeling.
Hemodialysis/peritoneal dialysis: Supplemental dose is not necessary

Dosage adjustment in hepatic impairment: No dosage adjustment provided in manufacturer's labeling.

Administration
Injection oil (decanoate): The decanoate injectable formulation should be administered I.M. only, **do not administer decanoate I.V.**
Injection solution (lactate): The lactate injectable formulation may be administered I.V. (unlabeled route) or I.M.
Oral solution (lactate): Dilute the oral concentrate with water or juice before administration. Avoid skin contact with oral solution; may cause contact dermatitis.

Monitoring Parameters Vital signs; lipid profile, fasting blood glucose/Hgb A_{1c}; BMI; mental status, abnormal involuntary movement scale (AIMS), extrapyramidal symptoms (EPS); ECG (with off-label intravenous administration)

ICU delirium: Monitor either the Confusion Assessment Method for the ICU (CAM-ICU) or the Intensive Care Delirium Screening Checklist (ICDSC)

Reference Range
Therapeutic: 5-20 ng/mL (SI: 10-40 nmol/L) (psychotic disorders - less for Tourette's and mania)
Toxic: >42 ng/mL (SI: >84 nmol/L)

Dosage Forms Excipient information presented when available (limited, particularly for generics); consult specific product labeling.
Concentrate, Oral, as lactate [strength expressed as base]:
Generic: 2 mg/mL (5 mL, 15 mL, 120 mL)
Solution, Intramuscular, as decanoate [strength expressed as base]:
Haldol Decanoate: 50 mg/mL (1 mL); 100 mg/mL (1 mL) [contains benzyl alcohol, sesame oil]
Generic: 50 mg/mL (1 mL, 5 mL); 100 mg/mL (1 mL, 5 mL)
Solution, Injection, as lactate [strength expressed as base]:
Haldol: 5 mg/mL (1 mL)
Generic: 5 mg/mL (1 mL, 10 mL)
Solution, Injection, as lactate [strength expressed as base, preservative free]:
Generic: 5 mg/mL (1 mL)
Tablet, Oral:
Generic: 0.5 mg, 1 mg, 2 mg, 5 mg, 10 mg, 20 mg

◆ **Haloperidol Decanoate** *see* Haloperidol *on page 983*
◆ **Haloperidol Injection, USP (Can)** *see* Haloperidol *on page 983*
◆ **Haloperidol-LA (Can)** *see* Haloperidol *on page 983*
◆ **Haloperidol Lactate** *see* Haloperidol *on page 983*
◆ **Haloperidol-LA Omega (Can)** *see* Haloperidol *on page 983*
◆ **Haloperidol Long Acting (Can)** *see* Haloperidol *on page 983*
◆ **Harkoseride** *see* Lacosamide *on page 1159*
◆ **Havrix** *see* Hepatitis A Vaccine *on page 990*
◆ **HAVRIX (Can)** *see* Hepatitis A Vaccine *on page 990*
◆ **Havrix® and Engerix-B®** *see* Hepatitis A and Hepatitis B Recombinant Vaccine *on page 990*
◆ **HBIG** *see* Hepatitis B Immune Globulin (Human) *on page 993*
◆ **hBNP** *see* Nesiritide *on page 1443*
◆ **hCG** *see* Chorionic Gonadotropin (Human) *on page 419*
◆ **H-Chlor 12 [OTC]** *see* Sodium Hypochlorite Solution *on page 1918*
◆ **HCTZ (error-prone abbreviation)** *see* Hydrochlorothiazide *on page 1004*
◆ **HDCV** *see* Rabies Vaccine *on page 1772*
◆ **HealthyLax [OTC]** *see* Polyethylene Glycol 3350 *on page 1668*
◆ **Heartburn Relief [OTC]** *see* Famotidine *on page 832*
◆ **Heartburn Relief 24 Hour [OTC]** *see* Lansoprazole *on page 1170*
◆ **Heartburn Relief Max St [OTC]** *see* Famotidine *on page 832*
◆ **Heather** *see* Norethindrone *on page 1472*
◆ **Hecoria** *see* Tacrolimus (Systemic) *on page 1976*
◆ **Hectorol** *see* Doxercalciferol *on page 660*
◆ **Hectorol® (Can)** *see* Doxercalciferol *on page 660*
◆ **Hedgehog Antagonist GDC-0449** *see* Vismodegib *on page 2199*
◆ **Helixate FS** *see* Antihemophilic Factor (Recombinant) *on page 144*
◆ **Helixate® FS (Can)** *see* Antihemophilic Factor (Recombinant) *on page 144*
◆ **Hemabate** *see* Carboprost Tromethamine *on page 347*
◆ **Hemabate® (Can)** *see* Carboprost Tromethamine *on page 347*
◆ **Hematide** *see* Peginesatide *on page 1589*
◆ **Hemocyte [OTC]** *see* Ferrous Fumarate *on page 854*
◆ **Hemofil M** *see* Antihemophilic Factor (Human) *on page 143*
◆ **Hemorrhoidal HC** *see* Hydrocortisone (Topical) *on page 1011*
◆ **Hemril-30** *see* Hydrocortisone (Topical) *on page 1011*
◆ **HepA** *see* Hepatitis A Vaccine *on page 990*
◆ **HepaGam B** *see* Hepatitis B Immune Globulin (Human) *on page 993*
◆ **HepaGam B® (Can)** *see* Hepatitis B Immune Globulin (Human) *on page 993*
◆ **HepA-HepB** *see* Hepatitis A and Hepatitis B Recombinant Vaccine *on page 990*
◆ **Hepalean® (Can)** *see* Heparin *on page 986*
◆ **Hepalean® Leo (Can)** *see* Heparin *on page 986*
◆ **Hepalean®-LOK (Can)** *see* Heparin *on page 986*

Heparin (HEP a rin)

Brand Names: U.S. Hep Flush-10

Brand Names: Canada Hepalean®; Hepalean® Leo; Hepalean®-LOK

Index Terms Heparin Calcium; Heparin Lock Flush; Heparin Sodium

Pharmacologic Category Anticoagulant

Additional Appendix Information
Dosing Considerations for the Critically-Ill Patient With Morbid Obesity *on page 2379*
Reversal of Oral Anticoagulants *on page 2308*

Use Prophylaxis and treatment of thromboembolic disorders; as an anticoagulant for extracorporeal and dialysis procedures

Note: Heparin lock flush solution is intended only to maintain patency of I.V. devices and is **not** to be used for systemic anticoagulant therapy.

Unlabeled Use ST-elevation myocardial infarction (STEMI) as an adjunct to thrombolysis; unstable angina/non-STEMI (UA/NSTEMI); anticoagulant used during percutaneous coronary intervention (PCI)

Pregnancy Risk Factor C

Pregnancy Considerations Increased resorptions were observed in some animal reproduction studies. Heparin does not cross the placenta. Heparin may be used for the prevention and treatment of thromboembolism in pregnant women; however the use of low molecular weight heparin (LMWH) is preferred. Twice-daily heparin should be discontinued prior to induction of labor or a planned cesarean delivery. In pregnant women with mechanical heart valves, adjusted-dose LMWH or adjusted-dose heparin may be used throughout pregnancy or until week 13 of gestation when therapy can be changed to warfarin. LMWH or heparin should be resumed close to delivery. In women who are at a very high risk for thromboembolism (older generation prosthesis in mitral position or history of thromboembolism), warfarin can be used throughout pregnancy and replaced with LMWH or heparin near term; the use of low-dose aspirin is also recommended. When choosing therapy, fetal outcomes (ie, pregnancy loss, malformations), maternal outcomes (ie, VTE, hemorrhage), burden of therapy, and maternal preference should be considered (Guyatt, 2012).

Some products contain benzyl alcohol as a preservative; their use in pregnant women is contraindicated by some manufacturers; use of a preservative free formulation is recommended.

Breast-Feeding Considerations Heparin is not excreted into breast milk and can be used in breast-feeding women (Guyatt, 2012). Some products contain benzyl alcohol as a preservative; their use in breast-feeding women is contraindicated by some manufacturers due to the association of gasping syndrome in premature infants.

Contraindications Hypersensitivity to heparin or any component of the formulation (unless a life-threatening situation necessitates use and use of an alternative anticoagulant is not possible); severe thrombocytopenia; uncontrolled active bleeding except when due to disseminated intravascular coagulation (DIC); not for use when appropriate blood coagulation tests cannot be obtained at appropriate intervals (applies to full-dose heparin only)

Note: Some products contain benzyl alcohol as a preservative; their use in neonates, infants, or pregnant or nursing mothers is contraindicated by some manufacturers.

Warnings/Precautions Hypersensitivity reactions can occur. Only in life-threatening situations when use of an alternative anticoagulant is not possible should heparin be cautiously used in patients with a documented hypersensitivity reaction. Hemorrhage is the most common complication. Monitor for signs and symptoms of bleeding. Certain patients are at increased risk of bleeding. Risk factors for bleeding include bacterial endocarditis; congenital or acquired bleeding disorders; active ulcerative or angiodysplastic GI diseases; continuous GI tube drainage; severe uncontrolled hypertension; history of hemorrhagic stroke; or use shortly after brain, spinal, or ophthalmology surgery; patient treated concomitantly with platelet inhibitors; conditions associated with increased bleeding tendencies (hemophilia, vascular purpura); recent GI bleeding; thrombocytopenia or platelet defects; severe liver disease; hypertensive or diabetic retinopathy; renal failure; or in patients undergoing invasive procedures including spinal tap or spinal anesthesia. Many concentrations of heparin are available ranging from 1 unit/mL to 20,000 units/mL. Clinicians **must** carefully examine each prefilled syringe or vial prior to use ensuring that the correct concentration is chosen; fatal hemorrhages have occurred related to heparin overdose especially in pediatric patients. A higher incidence of bleeding has been reported in patients >60 years of age, particularly women. They are also more sensitive to the dose. Discontinue heparin if hemorrhage occurs; severe hemorrhage or overdosage may require protamine.

May cause thrombocytopenia; monitor platelet count closely. Patients who develop HIT may be at risk of developing a new thrombus (heparin-induced thrombocytopenia and thrombosis [HITT]). Discontinue therapy and consider alternatives if platelets are <100,000/mm^3 and/or thrombosis develops. HIT or HITT may be delayed and can occur up to several weeks after discontinuation of heparin. Use with extreme caution (for a limited duration) or avoid in patients with history of HIT, especially if administered within 100 days of HIT episode (Dager, 2007; Warkentin, 2001); monitor platelet count closely. Osteoporosis may occur with prolonged use (>6 months) due to a reduction in bone mineral density. Monitor for hyperkalemia; can cause hyperkalemia by suppressing aldosterone production. Patients >60 years of age may require lower doses of heparin.

[U.S. Boxed Warning]: Some products contain benzyl alcohol as a preservative; use of these products is contraindicated in neonates. In neonates, large amounts of benzyl alcohol (>100 mg/kg/day) have been associated with fatal toxicity (gasping syndrome). Use in neonates, infants, or pregnant or nursing mothers is contraindicated by some manufacturers; the use of preservative-free heparin is, therefore, recommended in these populations. Some preparations contain sulfite which may cause allergic reactions.

Heparin resistance may occur in patients with antithrombin deficiency, increased heparin clearance, elevations in heparin-binding proteins, elevations in factor VIII and/or fibrinogen; frequently encountered in patients with fever, thrombosis, thrombophlebitis, infections with thrombosing tendencies, MI, cancer, and in postsurgical patients; measurement of anticoagulant effects using antifactor Xa levels may be of benefit.

Adverse Reactions Note: Thrombocytopenia has been reported to occur at an incidence between 0% and 30%. It is often of no clinical significance. However, immunologically mediated heparin-induced thrombocytopenia (HIT) has been estimated to occur in 1% to 2% of patients, and is marked by a progressive fall in platelet counts and, in some cases, thromboembolic complications (skin necrosis, pulmonary embolism, gangrene of the extremities, stroke, or MI).

Frequency not defined.

Cardiovascular: Allergic vasospastic reaction (possibly related to thrombosis), chest pain, hemorrhagic shock, shock, thrombosis

Central nervous system: Chills, fever, headache

Dermatologic: Alopecia (delayed, transient), bruising (unexplained), cutaneous necrosis, dysesthesia pedis, erythematous plaques (case reports), eczema, urticaria, purpura

Endocrine & metabolic: Adrenal hemorrhage, hyperkalemia (suppression of aldosterone synthesis), ovarian hemorrhage, rebound hyperlipidemia on discontinuation

Gastrointestinal: Constipation, hematemesis, nausea, tarry stools, vomiting

Genitourinary: Frequent or persistent erection

Hematologic: Bleeding from gums, epistaxis, hemorrhage, ovarian hemorrhage, retroperitoneal hemorrhage, thrombocytopenia (see **"Note"**)

Hepatic: Liver enzymes increased

Local: Irritation, erythema, pain, hematoma, and ulceration have been rarely reported with deep SubQ injections; I.M. injection (not recommended) is associated with a high incidence of these effects

Neuromuscular & skeletal: Peripheral neuropathy, osteoporosis (chronic therapy effect)

Ocular: Conjunctivitis (allergic reaction), lacrimation

Renal: Hematuria

Respiratory: Asthma, bronchospasm (case reports), hemoptysis, pulmonary hemorrhage, rhinitis

Miscellaneous: Allergic reactions, anaphylactoid reactions, heparin resistance, hypersensitivity (including chills, fever, and urticaria)

Drug Interactions

Metabolism/Transport Effects None known.

Avoid Concomitant Use

Avoid concomitant use of Heparin with any of the following: Apixaban; Corticorelin; Dabigatran Etexilate; Omacetaxine; Palifermin; Rivaroxaban

Increased Effect/Toxicity

Heparin may increase the levels/effects of: ACE Inhibitors; Aliskiren; Angiotensin II Receptor Blockers; Anticoagulants; Canagliflozin; Collagenase (Systemic); Corticorelin; Deferasirox; Eplerenone; Ibritumomab; Omacetaxine; Palifermin; Potassium Salts; Potassium-Sparing Diuretics; Rivaroxaban; Tositumomab and Iodine I 131 Tositumomab

The levels/effects of Heparin may be increased by: 5-ASA Derivatives; Agents with Antiplatelet Properties; Apixaban; Aspirin; Dabigatran Etexilate; Dasatinib; Herbs (Anticoagulant/Antiplatelet Properties); Ibrutinib; Nonsteroidal Anti-Inflammatory Agents; Omega-3 Fatty Acids; Pentosan Polysulfate Sodium; Pentoxifylline; Prostacyclin Analogues; Salicylates; Sugammadex; Thrombolytic Agents; Tibolone; Tipranavir; Vitamin E

Decreased Effect

The levels/effects of Heparin may be decreased by: Estrogen Derivatives; Nitroglycerin; Progestins

Ethanol/Nutrition/Herb Interactions Herb/Nutraceutical: Avoid cat's claw, dong quai, evening primrose, feverfew, red clover, horse chestnut, garlic, green tea, ginseng, ginkgo (all have additional antiplatelet activity).

Storage/Stability Heparin solutions are colorless to slightly yellow. Minor color variations do not affect therapeutic efficacy. Heparin should be stored at controlled room temperature. Protect from freezing and temperatures >40°C.

Stability at room temperature and refrigeration:

Prepared bag: 24-72 hours (specific to solution, concentration, and/or study conditions)

Premixed bag: After seal is broken, 4 days.

Out of overwrap stability: 30 days.

Mechanism of Action Potentiates the action of antithrombin III and thereby inactivates thrombin (as well as activated coagulation factors IX, X, XI, XII, and plasmin) and prevents the conversion of fibrinogen to fibrin; heparin also stimulates release of lipoprotein lipase (lipoprotein lipase hydrolyzes triglycerides to glycerol and free fatty acids)

Pharmacodynamics/Kinetics

Onset of action: Anticoagulation: I.V.: Immediate; SubQ: ~20-30 minutes

Absorption: Oral, rectal: Erratic at best from these routes of administration; SubQ absorption is also erratic, but considered acceptable for prophylactic use

Metabolism: Hepatic; may be partially metabolized in the reticuloendothelial system

Half-life elimination:

Dose-dependent: I.V. bolus: 25 units/kg: 30 minutes; 100 units/kg: 60 minutes; 400 units/kg: 150 minutes (Hirsh, 2008)

Mean: 1.5 hours; Range: 1-2 hours; affected by obesity, renal function, malignancy, presence of pulmonary embolism, and infections

Note: At therapeutic doses, elimination occurs rapidly via nonrenal mechanisms. With very high doses, renal elimination may play more of a role; however, dosage adjustment remains unnecessary for patients with renal impairment (Hirsh, 2008).

Excretion: Urine (small amounts as unchanged drug)

Dosage Note: Many concentrations of heparin are available ranging from 1 unit/mL to 20,000 units/mL. Carefully examine each prefilled syringe or vial prior to use ensuring that the correct concentration is chosen. Heparin lock flush solution is intended only to maintain patency of I.V. devices and is not to be used for anticoagulant therapy.

Children >1 year:

Prophylaxis for cardiac catheterization (arterial approach): I.V.: Bolus: 100 units/kg (Freed, 1974; Monagle, 2012)

Systemic heparinization:

Intermittent I.V.: Initial: 50-100 units/kg, then 50-100 units/kg every 4 hours (**Note:** Continuous I.V. infusion is preferred)

I.V. infusion: Initial loading dose: 75 units/kg given over 10 minutes, then initial maintenance dose: 20 units/kg/hour; adjust dose to maintain aPTT of 60-85 seconds (assuming this reflects an antifactor Xa level of 0.35-0.7 units/mL); see table.

Pediatric Protocol For Systemic Heparin Adjustment

To be used after initial loading dose and maintenance I.V. infusion dose (see usual dosage listed above) to maintain aPTT of 60-85 seconds (assuming this reflects antifactor Xa level of 0.35-0.7 units/mL).

Obtain blood for aPTT 4 hours after heparin loading dose and 4 hours after every infusion rate change.

Obtain daily CBC and aPTT after aPTT is therapeutic.

aPTT (seconds)	Dosage Adjustment	Time to Repeat aPTT
<50	Give 50 units/kg bolus and increase infusion rate by 10%	4 h after rate change
50-59	Increase infusion rate by 10%	4 h after rate change
60-85	Keep rate the same	Next day
86-95	Decrease infusion rate by 10%	4 h after rate change
96-120	Hold infusion for 30 minutes and decrease infusion rate by 10%	4 h after rate change
>120	Hold infusion for 60 minutes and decrease infusion rate by 15%	4 h after rate change

Modified from Andrew M, et al, "Heparin Therapy in Pediatric Patients: A Prospective Cohort Study," *Pediatr Research*, 1994, 35(1):78-83.
Note: The aPTT range of 60-85 seconds corresponds to an anti-Xa level of 0.35-0.7 units/mL.

Adults:

Thromboprophylaxis (low-dose heparin): SubQ: 5000 units every 8-12 hours. **Note:** The American College of Chest Physicians recommends a minimum of 10-14 days for patients undergoing total hip arthroplasty, total knee arthroplasty, or hip fracture surgery (Guyatt, 2012).

Intermittent I.V.: Initial: 10,000 units, then 50-70 units/kg (5000-10,000 units) every 4-6 hours

Percutaneous coronary intervention (Levine, 2011):

No prior anticoagulant therapy:

If no GPIIb/IIIa inhibitor use planned: Initial bolus of 70-100 units/kg (target ACT 250-300 seconds for HemoTec®, 300-350 seconds for Hemochron®)

or

If planning GPIIb/IIIa inhibitor use: Initial bolus of 50-70 units/kg (target ACT 200-250 seconds regardless of device)

Prior anticoagulant therapy:

If no GPIIb/IIIa inhibitor use planned: Additional heparin as needed (eg, 2000-5000 units) (target ACT 250-300 seconds for HemoTec®, 300-350 seconds for Hemochron®)

or

If planning GPIIb/IIIa inhibitor use: Additional heparin as needed (eg, 2000-5000 units) (target ACT 200-250 seconds regardless of device)

I.V. infusion (weight-based dosing per institutional nomogram recommended):

Acute coronary syndromes:

STEMI: Adjunct to fibrinolysis (full-dose alteplase, reteplase, or tenecteplase) (Antman, 2008): Initial bolus of 60 units/kg (maximum: 4000 units), then 12 units/kg/hour (maximum: 1000 units/hour) as continuous infusion. Check aPTT every 4-6 hours; adjust to target of 1.5-2 times the upper limit of control (50-70 seconds). Duration of heparin therapy depends on concurrent therapy and the specific patient risks for systemic or venous thromboembolism.

Unstable angina (UA)/non-ST-elevation myocardial infarction (NSTEMI) (Anderson, 2007): Initial bolus of 60 units/kg (maximum: 4000 units), followed by an initial infusion of 12 units/kg/hour (maximum: 1000 units/hour). Check aPTT every 4-6 hours; adjust to target of 1.5-2 times the upper limit of control (50-70 seconds). Continue for 48 hours in low risk patients managed with a conservative strategy (ie, no diagnostic angiography or PCI) (Jneid, 2012).

Treatment of venous thromboembolism: **Note:** Start warfarin on the first or second treatment day and continue heparin until INR is ≥2 for at least 24 hours (usually 5-7 days) (Guyatt, 2012).

DVT/PE (unlabeled dosing): I.V.: 80 units/kg (or alternatively 5000 units) I.V. push followed by continuous infusion of 18 units/kg/hour (or alternatively 1000 units/hour) (Guyatt, 2012)

or

DVT/PE (unlabeled dosing): SubQ: *Unmonitored dosing regimen:* Initial: 333 units/kg then 250 units/kg every 12 hours (Guyatt, 2012; Kearon, 2006)

Line flushing: When using daily flushes of heparin to maintain patency of single and double lumen central catheters, 10 units/mL is commonly used for younger infants (eg, <10 kg) while 100 units/mL is used for older infants, children, and adults. Capped PVC catheters and peripheral heparin locks require flushing more frequently (eg, every 6-8 hours). Volume of heparin flush is usually similar to volume of catheter (or slightly greater). Additional flushes should be given when stagnant blood is observed in catheter, after catheter is used for drug or blood administration, and after blood withdrawal from catheter.

Addition of heparin (0.5-3 unit/mL) to peripheral and central parenteral nutrition has not been shown to decrease catheter-related thrombosis. The final concentration of heparin used for TPN solutions may need to be decreased to 0.5 units/mL in small infants receiving larger amounts of volume in order to avoid approaching therapeutic amounts. Arterial lines are heparinized with a final concentration of 1 unit/mL.

Dosing adjustments in the elderly: Patients >60 years of age may have higher serum levels and clinical response (longer aPTTs) as compared to younger patients receiving similar dosages; lower dosages may be required

Dosage adjustment in renal impairment: No dosage adjustment required; adjust therapeutic heparin according to aPTT or anti-Xa activity.

Dosage adjustment in hepatic impairment: No dosage adjustment required; adjust therapeutic heparin according to aPTT or anti-Xa activity.

Usual Infusion Concentrations: Pediatric Note: Premixed solutions available

I.V. infusion: 100 units/mL

Usual Infusion Concentrations: Adult Note: Premixed solutions available

I.V. infusion: 25,000 units in 250 mL (concentration: 100 units/mL) of D_5W, 1/2NS, or NS

Administration

SubQ: Inject in subcutaneous tissue only (not muscle tissue). Injection sites should be rotated (usually left and right portions of the abdomen, above iliac crest).

I.M.: Do not administer I.M. due to pain, irritation, and hematoma formation; central venous catheters must be flushed with heparin solution when newly inserted, daily (at the time of tubing change), after blood withdrawal or transfusion, and after an intermittent infusion through an injectable cap. A volume of at least 10 mL of blood should be removed and discarded from a heparinized line before blood samples are sent for coagulation testing.

Continuous I.V. infusion: Infuse via infusion pump. If preparing solution, mix thoroughly prior to administration.

Heparin lock: Inject via injection cap using positive pressure flushing technique. Heparin lock flush solution is intended only to maintain patency of I.V. devices and is **not** to be used for anticoagulant therapy.

Monitoring Parameters Hemoglobin, hematocrit, signs of bleeding; fecal occult blood test; aPTT (or antifactor Xa activity levels) or ACT depending upon indication

Platelet counts should be routinely monitored (eg, every 2-3 days on days 4-14 of heparin therapy) when the risk of HIT is >1% (eg, receiving therapeutic dose heparin, postoperative antithrombotic prophylaxis), if the patient has received heparin or low molecular weight heparin (eg, enoxaparin) within the past 100 days, if pre-exposure history is uncertain, or if anaphylactoid reaction to heparin occurs. When the risk of HIT is <1% (eg, medical/obstetrical patients receiving heparin flushes), routine platelet count monitoring is not recommended (Guyatt, 2012).

For intermittent I.V. injections, aPTT is measured 3.5-4 hours after I.V. injection.

Note: Continuous I.V. infusion is preferred over I.V. intermittent injections. For full-dose heparin (ie, nonlow-dose), the dose should be titrated according to aPTT results. For anticoagulation, an aPTT 1.5-2.5 times normal is usually desired. Because of variation among hospitals in the control aPTT values, nomograms should be established at each institution, designed to achieve aPTT values in the target range (eg, for a control aPTT of 30 seconds, the target range [1.5-2.5 times control] would be 45-75 seconds). Measurements should be made prior to heparin therapy, 6 hours (pediatric: 4 hours) after initiation, and 6 hours (pediatric: 4 hours) after any dosage change, and should be used to adjust the heparin infusion until the aPTT exhibits a therapeutic level. When two consecutive aPTT values are therapeutic, subsequent measurements may be made every 24 hours, and if necessary, dose adjustment carried out. In addition, a significant change in the patient's clinical condition (eg, recurrent ischemia, bleeding, hypotension) should prompt an immediate aPTT determination, followed by dose adjustment if necessary. In general, may increase or decrease infusion by 2-4 units/kg/hour dependent upon aPTT.

Heparin infusion dose adjustment: A number of dose-adjustment nomograms have been developed which target an aPTT range of 1.5-2.5 times control (Cruickshank, 1991; Flaker, 1994; Hull, 1992; Raschke, 1993). However, institution-specific and indication-specific nomograms should be consulted for dose adjustment. **Note:** aPTT values vary throughout the day with maximum values occurring during the night (Decousus, 1985).

Reference Range Venous thromboembolism: Heparin: 0.3-0.7 unit/mL (children: 0.35-0.7 unit/mL) anti-Xa activity (by chromogenic assay) or 0.2-0.4 unit/mL (by protamine titration); aPTT: 1.5-2.5 times control (usually reflects an aPTT of 60-85 seconds) (Garcia, 2012; Monagle, 2012)

When used with thrombolytic therapy in patients with acute MI, a lower therapeutic range corresponding to an aPTT of 1.5-2 times control (or approximately an aPTT of 50-70 seconds) is recommended (Antman, 2004).

Test Interactions Increased thyroxine (competitive protein binding methods); increased PT

Aprotinin significantly increases aPTT and celite Activated Clotting Time (ACT) which may not reflect the actual degree of anticoagulation by heparin. Kaolin-based ACTs are not affected by aprotinin to the same degree as celite ACTs. While institutional protocols may vary, a minimal celite ACT of 750 seconds or kaolin-ACT of 480 seconds is recommended in the presence of aprotinin. Consult the manufacturer's information on specific ACT test interpretation in the presence of aprotinin.

Dosage Forms Excipient information presented when available (limited, particularly for generics); consult specific product labeling.

Solution, Injection, as sodium:
- Generic: 1000 units (500 mL); 2000 units (1000 mL); 25,000 units (250 mL, 500 mL); 1000 units/mL (1 mL, 10 mL, 30 mL); 2500 units/mL (10 mL); 5000 units/mL (1 mL, 10 mL); 10,000 units/mL (1 mL, 4 mL, 5 mL); 20,000 units/mL (1 mL)

Solution, Injection, as sodium [preservative free]:
- Generic: 1000 units/mL (2 mL); 5000 units/0.5 mL (0.5 mL)

Solution, Intravenous, as sodium:
- Hep Flush-10: 10 units/mL (10 mL)
- Generic: 10,000 units (250 mL); 12,500 units (250 mL); 20,000 units (500 mL); 25,000 units (250 mL, 500 mL); 1 units/mL (1 mL, 2 mL, 2.5 mL, 3 mL, 5 mL, 10 mL); 2 units/mL (3 mL); 10 units/mL (1 mL, 2 mL, 2.5 mL, 3 mL, 5 mL, 10 mL, 30 mL); 100 units/mL (1 mL, 2 mL, 2.5 mL, 3 mL, 5 mL, 10 mL, 30 mL); 2000 units/mL (5 mL)

Solution, Intravenous, as sodium [preservative free]:
- Generic: 1 units/mL (3 mL); 10 units/mL (1 mL, 3 mL, 5 mL); 100 units/mL (1 mL, 3 mL, 5 mL)

◆ **Heparin Calcium** *see* Heparin *on page* 986
◆ **Heparin Lock Flush** *see* Heparin *on page* 986
◆ **Heparin Sodium** *see* Heparin *on page* 986

Hepatitis A and Hepatitis B Recombinant Vaccine

(hep a TYE tis aye & hep a TYE tis bee ree KOM be nant vak SEEN)

Brand Names: U.S. Twinrix®

Brand Names: Canada Twinrix®; Twinrix® Junior

Index Terms Engerix-B® and Havrix®; Havrix® and Engerix-B®; HepA-HepB; Hepatitis B and Hepatitis A Vaccine

Pharmacologic Category Vaccine, Inactivated (Viral)

Additional Appendix Information

Immunization Administration Recommendations *on page* 2334
Immunization Recommendations *on page* 2339

Use Active immunization against disease caused by hepatitis A virus and hepatitis B virus (all known subtypes) in populations desiring protection against or at high risk of exposure to these viruses.

Populations include travelers or people living in or relocating to areas of intermediate/high endemicity for **both** HAV and HBV and are at increased risk of HBV infection due to behavioral or occupational factors; patients with chronic liver disease; laboratory workers who handle live HAV and HBV; healthcare workers, police, and other personnel who render first-aid or medical assistance; workers who come in contact with sewage; employees of day care centers and correctional facilities; patients/staff of hemodialysis units; men who have sex with men; patients frequently receiving blood products; military personnel; users of injectable illicit drugs; close household contacts of patients with hepatitis A and hepatitis B infection; residents of drug and alcohol treatment centers

Pregnancy Risk Factor C

Dosage Primary immunization: I.M.:

U.S. labeling: Adults: Three doses (1 mL each) given on a 0-, 1-, and 6-month schedule

Alternative regimen: Accelerated regimen: Four doses (1 mL each) on day 0, 7, and 21-30, followed by a booster at 12 months

Canadian labeling:

Children ≥1 year and Adolescents (Twinrix Junior): Three doses (0.5 mL each) given on a 0-, 1-, and 6-month schedule

Alternative regimen: Children≥1 year and Adolescents ≤15 years (Twinrix): One dose (1 mL) given on elected date followed by second dose (1 mL) 6-12 months later

Adults (Twinrix): Three doses (1 mL each) given on a 0-, 1-, and 6-month schedule

Alternative regimen: Accelerated regimen: Four doses (1 mL each) on day 0, 7, and 21, followed by a booster at 12 months

Dosage adjustment in renal impairment: No dosage adjustment provided in manufacturer's labeling.

Dosage adjustment in hepatic impairment: No dosage adjustment provided in manufacturer's labeling.

Additional Information Complete prescribing information should be consulted for additional detail.

Dosage Forms Excipient information presented when available (limited, particularly for generics); consult specific product labeling.

Injection, suspension [preservative free]:
- Twinrix®: Hepatitis A virus antigen 720 ELISA units and hepatitis B surface antigen 20 mcg per mL (1 mL) [contains aluminum, yeast protein, and trace amounts of neomycin; may contain natural rubber/natural latex in prefilled syringe]

Dosage Forms: Canada Also refer to Dosage Forms. Excipient information presented when available (limited, particularly for generics); consult specific product labeling.

Injection, suspension [preservative free]:
- Twinrix® Junior: Hepatitis A virus antigen 360 ELISA units and hepatitis B surface antigen 10 mcg per 0.5 mL (0.5 mL) [contains aluminum and trace amounts of neomycin]

Hepatitis A Vaccine

(hep a TYE tis aye vak SEEN)

Brand Names: U.S. Havrix; VAQTA

Brand Names: Canada Avaxim; Avaxim-Pediatric; HAVRIX; VAQTA

Index Terms HepA

Pharmacologic Category Vaccine, Inactivated (Viral)

Additional Appendix Information

Immunization Administration Recommendations *on page 2334*

Immunization Recommendations *on page 2339*

Use Hepatitis A virus vaccination:

For active immunization of persons 12 months and older against disease caused by hepatitis A virus (HAV).

The Advisory Committee on Immunization Practices (ACIP) recommends routine vaccination (CDC, 2006) for:

- All children ≥12 months of age
- All unvaccinated adults requesting protection from HAV infection
- Unvaccinated persons with any of the following conditions: Men who have sex with men; injection and non-injection illicit drug users; persons who work with HAV-infected primates or with HAV in a research laboratory setting; persons with chronic liver disease; patients who receive clotting-factor concentrates; persons traveling to or work in countries with high or intermediate levels of endemic HAV infection
- Unvaccinated persons who anticipate close personal contact with international adoptee from a country of intermediate to high endemicity of HAV, during their first 60 days of arrival into the United States (eg, household contacts, babysitters) (CDC, 2009)

Pregnancy Risk Factor C

Pregnancy Considerations Animal reproduction studies have not been conducted. The safety of vaccination during pregnancy has not been determined, however, the theoretical risk to the infant is expected to be low. Inactivated vaccines have not been shown to cause increased risks to the fetus (CDC, 2011).

Breast-Feeding Considerations It is not known if this vaccine is excreted into breast milk. The manufacturer recommends that caution be used if administered to nursing women. Inactivated vaccines do not affect the safety of breast-feeding for the mother or the infant. Breast-feeding infants should be vaccinated according to the recommended schedules (CDC, 2011).

Contraindications Immediate and/or severe allergic or hypersensitivity reaction to hepatitis A containing vaccines or any component of the formulation, including neomycin.

Warnings/Precautions Use caution in patients on anticoagulants, with thrombocytopenia, or bleeding disorders (bleeding may occur following intramuscular injection) (CDC, 2011). Canadian product labeling suggests that subcutaneous administration may be considered in exceptional circumstances (eg, patients with thrombocytopenia or at risk for hemorrhage; however, this may convey a higher risk for local reactions (eg, injection site nodule). In healthy adults, seroconversion following an initial subcutaneous dose of VAQTA was slower than that historically observed following intramuscular administration (Linglöf, 2001).

Treatment for anaphylactic reactions should be immediately available. Postpone vaccination with acute infection or febrile illness. Use with caution in severely immunocompromised patients (eg, patients receiving chemo/radiation therapy or other immunosuppressive therapy (including high dose corticosteroids)); may have a reduced response to vaccination. In general, household and close contacts of persons with altered immunocompetence may receive all age appropriate vaccines (CDC, 2011). Vaccination may not result in effective immunity in all patients. Response depends upon multiple factors (eg, type of vaccine, age of patient) and is improved by administering the vaccine at the recommended dose, route, and interval. Vaccines may not be effective if administered during periods of altered immune competence (CDC, 2011). Due to the long incubation period for hepatitis A (15-50 days), unrecognized hepatitis A infection may be present; immunization may not prevent infection in these patients. Patients with chronic liver disease may have decreased antibody response.

Syncope has been reported with use of injectable vaccines and may be accompanied by transient visual disturbances, paresthesia, weakness, or tonic-clonic movements. Procedures should be in place to avoid injuries from falling and to restore cerebral perfusion if syncope occurs. Packaging may contain natural latex rubber; some products may contain neomycin. In order to maximize vaccination rates, the ACIP recommends simultaneous administration of all age-appropriate vaccines (live or inactivated) for which a person is eligible at a single clinic visit, unless contraindications exist. The use of combination vaccines is generally preferred over separate injections, taking into consideration provider assessment, patient preference, and adverse events (CDC, 2011). Use of this vaccine for specific medical and/or other indications (eg, immunocompromising conditions, hepatic or kidney disease, diabetes) is also addressed in the ACIP Recommended Immunization Schedule (CDC, 2013a; CDC, 2013b).

Adverse Reactions All serious adverse reactions must be reported to the U.S. Department of Health and Human Services (DHHS) Vaccine Adverse Event Reporting System (VAERS) at 1-800-822-7967 or online at https://vaers.hhs.gov/esub/index. In Canada, adverse reactions may be reported to local provincial/territorial health agencies or to the Vaccine Safety Section at Public Health Agency of Canada (1-866-844-0018).

Frequency dependent upon age, product used, and concomitant vaccine administration. In general, headache and injection site reactions were less common in younger children.

>10%:

Central nervous system: Drowsiness, headache, irritability

Gastrointestinal: Decreased appetite

Local: Erythema at injection site, injection site reaction (soreness, warmth), pain at injection site, swelling at injection site, tenderness at injection site

Neuromuscular & skeletal: Weakness

Miscellaneous: Fever (≥100.4°F [1-5 days postvaccination], >98.6°C [1-14 days postvaccination])

1% to 10%:

Central nervous system: Chills, fatigue, insomnia, malaise

Dermatologic: Skin rash

Endocrine & metabolic: Menstrual disease

Gastrointestinal: Abdominal pain, anorexia, constipation, diarrhea, gastroenteritis, nausea, vomiting

Local: Bruising at injection site, induration at injection site

Neuromuscular & skeletal: Arm pain, back pain, myalgia, stiffness

Ophthalmic: Conjunctivitis

Otic: Otitis media

Respiratory: Asthma, cough, nasal congestion, nasopharyngitis, pharyngitis, rhinitis, rhinorrhea, upper respiratory tract infection

Miscellaneous: Excessive crying, fever ≥102°F (1-5 days postvaccination)

<1% (Limited to important or life threatening): Anaphylaxis, angioedema, ataxia (cerebellar), bronchiolitis, bronchoconstriction, dehydration, dermatitis, encephalitis, erythema multiforme, Guillain-Barre syndrome, hematoma at injection site, hepatitis, hypersensitivity reaction, hypoesthesia, increased creatine kinase, increased serum transaminases (transient), injection site reaction (nodule), jaundice, lymphadenopathy, multiple sclerosis, myelitis, neuropathy, paresthesia, photophobia, pruritus, rash at injection site, seizure, serum sickness-like reaction, syncope, thrombocytopenia, vasculitis, wheezing

Drug Interactions

Metabolism/Transport Effects None known.

Avoid Concomitant Use There are no known interactions where it is recommended to avoid concomitant use.

Increased Effect/Toxicity There are no known significant interactions involving an increase in effect.

Decreased Effect

The levels/effects of Hepatitis A Vaccine may be decreased by: Belimumab; Fingolimod; Immunosuppressants

Storage/Stability

Store refrigerated between 2°C and 8°C (36°F and 46°F). Do not freeze; discard if the product has been frozen.

The following stability information has also been reported for Havrix: May be stored at room temperature for up to 72 hours (Cohen, 2007).

VAQTA: Canadian labeling suggests that the vaccine may be used if cumulative exposure to temperatures of 0°C to 2°C (32°F to 36°F) or 8°C to 25°C (46°F to 77°F) is ≤72 hours.

Mechanism of Action As an inactivated virus vaccine, hepatitis A vaccine induces active immunity against hepatitis A virus infection

Pharmacodynamics/Kinetics

Onset of action: Protective antibodies develop in 95% of adults after the first dose and in 100% of adults after the second dose of the vaccine; ≥97% of children and adolescents will be seropositive within 1 month of the first dose and 100% will develop protective antibodies after receiving two doses. The efficacy of preventing hepatitis A disease in children living in highly infected areas is 94-100% (CDC, 2012).

Duration: Protective antibodies induced by the vaccine may persist for ≥20 years (CDC, 2012).

Dosage I.M.: **Note:** When used for primary immunization, the vaccine should be given at least 2 weeks prior to expected HAV exposure. When used prior to an international adoption, the vaccination series should begin when adoption is being planned, but ideally ≥2 weeks prior to expected arrival of adoptee (CDC, 2009). When used for postexposure prophylaxis, the vaccine should be given as soon as possible (CDC, 2007).

Primary immunization: Advisory Committee on Immunization Practices (ACIP): Children ≥12 months: All children should receive primary immunization with a two-dose series. The series should be initiated at 12-23 months; the two doses should be separated by 6-18 months (CDC, 2006).

Manufacturer's labeling:

Avaxim [Canadian product]: Children ≥12 years, Adolescents, and Adults: 160 units (0.5 mL) with a booster dose of 160 units (0.5 mL) to be given 6-36 months following primary immunization

Avaxim-Pediatric [Canadian product]: Children ≥12 months and Adolescents ≤15 years: 80 units (0.5 mL) with a booster dose of 80 units (0.5 mL) to be given 6-12 months following primary immunization

Havrix:

Children ≥12 months and Adolescents: 720 ELISA units (0.5 mL) with a booster dose of 720 ELISA units to be given 6-12 months following primary immunization

Adults: 1440 ELISA units (1 mL) with a booster dose of 1440 ELISA units to be given 6-12 months following primary immunization

VAQTA:

Children ≥12 months and Adolescents: 25 units (0.5 mL) with a booster dose of 25 units (0.5 mL) to be given 6-18 months after primary immunization (6-12 months if initial dose was with Havrix).

Adults: 50 units (1 mL) with a booster dose of 50 units (1 mL) to be given 6-18 months after primary immunization (6-12 months if initial dose was with Havrix). **Note:** Canadian labeling recommends that adults with HIV receive a booster dose 6 months after primary immunization.

Dosage adjustment in renal impairment: No dosage adjustment provided in manufacturer's labeling.

Dosage adjustment in hepatic impairment: No specific recommendations provided in manufacturer's labeling. However, data suggest patients with chronic liver disease have a lower antibody response to HAVRIX than healthy subjects.

Administration For I.M. administration. The deltoid muscle is the preferred site for injection for older children and adults; administer to the anterolateral aspect of the thigh in infants and young children. Do not administer to the gluteal region; may decrease efficacy. Do not administer intravenously, intradermally, or subcutaneously. Shake well prior to use; discard if the suspension is discolored or does not appear homogenous after shaking, or if there are cracks in the vial or syringe. Do not dilute. When used for primary immunization, the vaccine should be given at least 2 weeks prior to expected HAV exposure. When used for postexposure prophylaxis, the vaccine should be given as soon as possible.

For patients at risk of hemorrhage following intramuscular injection, the ACIP recommends "it should be administered intramuscularly if, in the opinion of the physician familiar with the patient's bleeding risk, the vaccine can be administered by this route with reasonable safety. If the patient receives antihemophilia or other similar therapy, intramuscular vaccination can be scheduled shortly after such therapy is administered. A fine needle (23 gauge or smaller) can be used for the vaccination and firm pressure applied to the site (without rubbing) for at least 2 minutes. The patient should be instructed concerning the risk of hematoma from the injection." Patients on anticoagulant therapy should be considered to have the same bleeding risks and treated as those with clotting factor disorders (CDC, 2011). **Note:** Canadian product labeling suggests that subcutaneous administration may be considered in exceptional circumstances (eg, patients with thrombocytopenia or at risk for hemorrhage), although this may convey a higher risk for local reactions (eg, injection site nodule). In healthy adults, seroconversion following an initial subcutaneous dose of VAQTA was slower than that historically observed following intramuscular administration (Linglöf, 2001).

Simultaneous administration of vaccines helps ensure the patients will be fully vaccinated by the appropriate age. Simultaneous administration of vaccines is defined as administering >1 vaccine on the same day at different anatomic sites. The use of licensed combination vaccines is generally preferred over separate injections of the equivalent components. Separate vaccines should not be combined in the same syringe unless indicated by product specific labeling. Separate needles and syringes should be used for each injection. The ACIP prefers each dose of a specific vaccine in a series come from the same manufacturer when possible. Adolescents and adults should be vaccinated while seated or lying down. In general, preterm infants should be vaccinated at the same chronological age as full-term infants (CDC, 2011).

Antipyretics have not been shown to prevent febrile seizures. Antipyretics may be used to treat fever or discomfort following vaccination (CDC, 2011). One study reported that routine prophylactic administration of acetaminophen to prevent fever prior to vaccination decreased the immune response of some vaccines; the clinical significance of this reduction in immune response has not been established (Prymula, 2009).

Monitoring Parameters Liver function tests; monitor for syncope for 15 minutes following administration. If seizure-like activity associated with syncope occurs, maintain patient in supine or Trendelenburg position to reestablish adequate cerebral perfusion (CDC, 2011).

Additional Information The ACIP currently recommends that older adults, the immunocompromised, or persons with underlying medical conditions (including chronic liver disease) that are vaccinated <2 weeks from departure to an area with a high or intermediate risk of hepatitis A infection also receive immune globulin (CDC, 2007).

For postexposure prophylaxis, hepatitis A vaccine is preferred over immune globulin for people ages 12 months to 40 years who have recently been exposed to HAV and who have not previously received hepatitis A vaccine. Administer a single dose of hepatitis A vaccine as soon as possible. For people older than 40 years, immune globulin is preferred, although vaccine can be used if immune globulin is unavailable (CDC, 2007)

Although it is preferred to use the vaccines according to their approved labeling, Havrix and VAQTA are considered to be interchangeable (CDC, 2006).

U.S. federal law requires that the name of medication, date of administration, the vaccine manufacturer, lot number of vaccine, and the administering person's name, title, and address be entered into the patient's permanent medical record.

Dosage Forms Excipient information presented when available (limited, particularly for generics); consult specific product labeling. [DSC] = Discontinued product

Injection, suspension [adult, preservative free]:

- Havrix: Hepatitis A virus antigen 1440 ELISA units/mL (1 mL) [contains aluminum, neomycin (may have trace amounts); may contain natural rubber/natural latex in prefilled syringe]
- VAQTA: Hepatitis A virus antigen 50 units/mL (1 mL) [contains aluminum, natural rubber/natural latex in packaging]

Injection, suspension [pediatric, preservative free]:

- Havrix: Hepatitis A virus antigen 720 ELISA units/0.5 mL (0.5 mL) [contains aluminum, neomycin (may have trace amounts); may contain natural rubber/natural latex in prefilled syringe]

Injection, suspension [pediatric/adolescent, preservative free]:

- VAQTA: Hepatitis A virus antigen 25 units/0.5 mL (0.5 mL) [contains aluminum, natural rubber/natural latex in packaging]

Dosage Forms: Canada Also refer to Dosage Forms. Excipient information presented when available (limited, particularly for generics); consult specific product labeling.

Injection, suspension [pediatric/adolescent]:

- Avaxim-Pediatric: Hepatitis A virus antigen 80 units/0.5 mL [contains aluminum, polysorbate 80, neomycin (may have trace amounts)]

Injection, suspension [adolescent/adult]:

- Avaxim: Hepatitis A virus antigen 160 units/0.5 mL [contains aluminum, polysorbate 80, neomycin (may have trace amounts)]

◆ **Hepatitis B and Hepatitis A Vaccine** *see* Hepatitis A and Hepatitis B Recombinant Vaccine *on page 990*

Hepatitis B Immune Globulin (Human)

(hep a TYE tis bee i MYUN GLOB yoo lin YU man)

Brand Names: U.S. HepaGam B; HyperHEP B S/D; Nabi-HB

Brand Names: Canada HepaGam B®; HyperHEP B™ S/D

Index Terms HBIG

Pharmacologic Category Blood Product Derivative; Immune Globulin

Additional Appendix Information

Immunization Recommendations *on page 2339*

Use

Passive prophylactic immunity to hepatitis B following: Acute exposure to blood containing hepatitis B surface antigen (HB_sAg); perinatal exposure of infants born to HB_sAg-positive mothers; sexual exposure to HB_sAg-positive persons; household exposure to persons with acute HBV infection

Prevention of hepatitis B virus recurrence after liver transplantation in HB_sAg-positive transplant patients

Note: Hepatitis B immune globulin is not indicated for treatment of active hepatitis B infection and is ineffective in the treatment of chronic active hepatitis B infection.

Pregnancy Risk Factor C

Pregnancy Considerations Animal reproduction studies have not been conducted. Use of HBIG is not contraindicated in pregnant women and may be used for postexposure prophylaxis when indicated (CDC, 2001). In addition, use of HBIG has been evaluated to reduce maternal to fetal transmission of hepatis B virus during pregnancy (ACOG, 2007)

Breast-Feeding Considerations Infants born to HB_sAg-positive mothers may be breast fed (CDC, 2005). Use of HBIG is not contraindicated in breast-feeding women (CDC, 2001).

Contraindications

HepaGam B®: Anaphylactic or severe systemic reaction to human globulin preparations; postexposure prophylaxis in patients with severe thrombocytopenia or other coagulation disorders which would contraindicate I.M. injections (administer only if benefit outweighs the risk)

HyperHEP B™ S/D: No contraindications listed in manufacturer's labeling

Nabi-HB®: Anaphylactic or severe systemic reaction to human globulin preparations

Warnings/Precautions Hypersensitivity and anaphylactic reactions can occur; immediate treatment (including epinephrine 1:1000) should be available. Use with caution in patients with previous systemic hypersensitivity to human immunoglobulins. Use with caution in patients with thrombocytopenia or coagulation disorders; I.M. injections may be contraindicated. Use with caution in patients with IgA deficiency. When administered I.V., do not exceed recommended infusion rates; may increase risk of adverse events. Patients should be monitored for adverse events during and after the infusion. Thrombotic events have been reported with administration of intravenous immune globulin; use with caution in patients of advanced age, with a history of atherosclerosis or cardiovascular and/or thrombotic risk factors, patients with impaired cardiac output, coagulation disorders, prolonged immobilization, or patients with known/suspected hyperviscosity. Consider a baseline assessment of blood viscosity in patients at risk for hyperviscosity. Product of human plasma; may potentially contain infectious agents which could transmit disease. Screening of donors, as well as testing and/or inactivation or removal of certain viruses, reduces the risk. Infections thought to be transmitted by this product should be reported to the manufacturer. Some products may contain maltose, which may result in falsely-elevated blood glucose readings.

Adverse Reactions Reported with postexposure prophylaxis. Adverse events reported in liver transplant patients included tremor and hypotension, were associated with a single infusion during the first week of treatment, and did not recur with additional infusions.

Central nervous system: Dizziness, fainting, headache, lightheadedness, malaise
Dermatologic: Angioedema, bruising, urticaria
Gastrointestinal: Nausea, vomiting
Hematologic: WBC decreased
Hepatic: Alkaline phosphatase increased, AST increased
Local: Ache, erythema, pain, and/or tenderness at injection site
Neuromuscular & skeletal: Arthralgia, joint stiffness, myalgia
Renal: Creatinine increased
Respiratory: Cold symptoms
Miscellaneous: Anaphylaxis, flu-like syndrome

Drug Interactions

Metabolism/Transport Effects None known.

Avoid Concomitant Use There are no known interactions where it is recommended to avoid concomitant use.

Increased Effect/Toxicity There are no known significant interactions involving an increase in effect.

Decreased Effect

Hepatitis B Immune Globulin (Human) may decrease the levels/effects of: Vaccines (Live)

Preparation for Administration HepaGamB®: May dilute with NS prior to I.V. administration if preferred; do not dilute with D_5W.

Storage/Stability Refrigerate at 2°C to 8°C (36°F to 46°F); do not freeze. Do not shake vial; avoid foaming.
HepaGamB®: Use within 6 hours of entering vial.
HyperHEP B™ S/D: May be exposed to room temperature for a cumulative 7 days (Cohen, 2007).
Nabi-HB®: Use within 6 hours of entering vial.

Mechanism of Action Hepatitis B immune globulin (HBIG) is a nonpyrogenic sterile solution containing immunoglobulin G (IgG) specific to hepatitis B surface antigen (HB_sAg). HBIG differs from immune globulin in the amount of anti-HB_s. Immune globulin is prepared from plasma that is not preselected for anti-HB_s content. HBIG is prepared from plasma preselected for high titer anti-HB_s. In the U.S., HBIG has an anti-HB_s high titer >1:100,000 by IRA.

Pharmacodynamics/Kinetics
Duration: Postexposure prophylaxis: 3-6 months
Absorption: I.M.: Slow
Half-life: 17-25 days
Distribution: V_d: 7-15 L
Time to peak, serum: I.M.: 2-10 days

Dosage

I.M.:

Infants born to HB_sAg-positive mothers: 0.5 mL as soon after birth as possible (within 12 hours); active vaccination with hepatitis B vaccine may begin at the same time in a different site (if not contraindicated). If first dose of hepatitis B vaccine is delayed for as long as 3 months, dose may be repeated. If hepatitis B vaccine is refused, dose may be repeated at 3 and 6 months.

Infants born to mothers with unknown HB_sAg status at birth (CDC, 2005):

Birth weight <2 kg: 0.5 mL within 12 hours of birth (along with hepatitis B vaccine) if unable to determine maternal HB_sAg status within that time

Birth weight ≥2 kg: If the mother is determined to be HB_sAg positive, administer 0.5 mL as soon as possible, but within 7 days of birth

Infants <12 months: Household exposure prophylaxis: 0.5 mL (to be administered if mother or primary caregiver has acute HBV infection)

Children ≥12 months and Adults: Postexposure prophylaxis: 0.06 mL/kg as soon as possible after exposure (ie, within 24 hours of needlestick, ocular, or mucosal exposure or within 14 days of sexual exposure); repeat at 28-30 days after exposure in nonresponders to hepatitis B vaccine or in patients who refuse vaccination

Note: HBIG may be administered at the same time (but at a different site) or up to 1 month preceding hepatitis B vaccination without impairing the active immune response

I.V.: Adults: Prevention of hepatitis B virus recurrence after liver transplantation (HepaGam B™): 20,000 units/dose according to the following schedule:

Anhepatic phase (Initial dose): One dose given with the liver transplant

Week 1 postop: One dose daily for 7 days (days 1-7)

Weeks 2-12 postop: One dose every 2 weeks starting day 14

Month 4 onward: One dose monthly starting on month 4

Dose adjustment: Adjust dose to reach anti-HBs levels of 500 units/L within the first week after transplantation. In patients with surgical bleeding, abdominal fluid drainage >500 mL or those undergoing plasmapheresis, administer 10,000 units/dose every 6 hours until target anti-HBs levels are reached.

Dosage adjustment in renal impairment: No dosage adjustment provided in manufacturer's labeling.

Dosage adjustment in hepatic impairment: No dosage adjustment provided in manufacturer's labeling.

Administration

I.M.: Postexposure prophylaxis: I.M. injection only in anterolateral aspect of upper thigh and deltoid muscle of upper arm; to prevent injury from injection, care should be taken when giving to patients with thrombocytopenia or bleeding disorders

I.V.:

HepaGam B™: Liver transplant: Administer at 2 mL/minute. Decrease infusion to ≤1 mL/minute for patient discomfort or infusion-related adverse events. Actual volume of infusion is dependent upon potency labeled on each individual vial.

Nabi-HB®: Although not FDA-approved for this purpose, Nabi-HB® has been administered intravenously in hepatitis B-positive liver transplant patients (Dickson, 2006)

Monitoring Parameters Liver transplant: Serum HBsAg; infusion-related adverse events

Test Interactions

Glucose testing: HepaGam B™ contains maltose. Falsely-elevated blood glucose levels may occur when glucose monitoring devices and test strips utilizing the glucose dehydrogenase pyrroloquinolinequinone (GDH-PQQ) based methods are used.

Serological testing: Antibodies transferred following administration of immune globulins may provide misleading positive test results (eg, Coombs' test)

Additional Information Each vial contains anti-HB_s antibody equivalent to or exceeding the potency of anti-HB_s in a U.S. reference standard hepatitis B immune globulin (FDA). The U.S. reference standard has been tested against the WHO standard hepatitis B immune globulin with listed values between 207 units/mL and 220 units/mL (included in individual product information).

Dosage Forms Excipient information presented when available (limited, particularly for generics); consult specific product labeling.

Solution, Injection [preservative free]:
HepaGam B: (1 mL, 5 mL) [contains polysorbate 80]

Solution, Intramuscular:
HyperHEP B S/D: (0.5 mL, 1 mL, 5 mL)
Nabi-HB: (1 mL, 5 mL) [thimerosal free]

◆ **Hepatitis B Inactivated Virus Vaccine (recombinant DNA)** *see* Hepatitis B Vaccine (Recombinant) *on page* 995

Hepatitis B Vaccine (Recombinant)

(hep a TYE tis bee vak SEEN ree KOM be nant)

Brand Names: U.S. Engerix-B®; Recombivax HB®

Brand Names: Canada Engerix-B®; Recombivax HB®

Index Terms Hepatitis B Inactivated Virus Vaccine (recombinant DNA); HepB

Pharmacologic Category Vaccine, Inactivated (Viral)

Additional Appendix Information

Immunization Administration Recommendations *on page 2334*

Immunization Recommendations *on page 2339*

Use Immunization against infection caused by all known subtypes of hepatitis B virus (HBV)

The Advisory Committee on Immunization Practices (ACIP) recommends routine vaccination for the following (CDC, 2005; CDC, 2006; CDC, 2011):

- All infants at birth
- All infants and children (post-birth dose; refer to recommended vaccination schedule)
- All unvaccinated adults requesting protection from HBV infection
- All unvaccinated adults at risk for HBV infection such as those with:

Behavioral risks: Sexually-active persons with >1 partner in a 6-month period; persons seeking evaluation or treatment for a sexually-transmitted disease; men who have sex with men; injection drug users

Occupational risks: Healthcare and public safety workers with reasonably anticipated risk for exposure to blood or blood contaminated body fluids

Medical risks: Persons with end-stage renal disease (including predialysis, hemodialysis, peritoneal dialysis, and home dialysis); persons with HIV infection; persons with chronic liver disease. Adults (19 through 59 years of age) with diabetes mellitus type 1 or type 2 should be vaccinated as soon as possible following diagnosis. Adults ≥60 years with diabetes mellitus may also be vaccinated at the discretion of their treating clinician.

Other risks: Household contacts and sex partners of persons with chronic HBV infection; residents and staff of facilities for developmentally disabled persons; international travelers to regions with high or intermediate levels of endemic HBV infection

In addition, the ACIP recommends vaccination for any persons who are wounded in bombings or similar mass casualty events who have penetrating injuries or nonintact skin exposure, or who have contact with mucous membranes (exception - superficial contact with intact skin), and who cannot confirm receipt of a hepatitis B vaccination (CDC, 2008).

Pregnancy Risk Factor C

Pregnancy Considerations Animal reproduction studies have not been conducted. The ACIP recommends HB_sAg testing for all pregnant women. Based on limited data, there is no apparent risk to the fetus when the hepatitis B vaccine is administered during pregnancy. Pregnancy itself is not a contraindication to vaccination; vaccination should be considered if otherwise indicated (CDC, 2006).

Breast-Feeding Considerations Inactivated virus vaccines do not affect the safety of breast-feeding for the mother or the infant. Breast-feeding infants should be vaccinated according to the recommended schedules (CDC, 2011). Infants born to HB_sAg-positive mothers may be breast-fed (CDC, 2005).

Contraindications Hypersensitivity to yeast, hepatitis B vaccine, or any component of the formulation

Warnings/Precautions Immediate treatment for anaphylactic/anaphylactoid reaction should be available during vaccine use. Defer administration in patients with moderate or severe acute illness (with or without fever). Use caution with decreased cardiopulmonary function. Vaccination may not result in effective immunity in all patients. Response depends upon multiple factors (eg, type of vaccine, age of patient) and is improved by administering the vaccine at the recommended dose, route, and interval. Vaccines may not be effective if administered during periods of altered immune competence (CDC 60 [2], 2011). Due to the long incubation period for hepatitis, unrecognized hepatitis B infection may be present prior to vaccination; immunization may not prevent infection in these patients. Patients >65 years of age may have lower response rates. Use with caution in severely immunocompromised patients (eg, patients receiving chemo/radiation therapy or other immunosuppressive therapy [including high-dose corticosteroids]); may have a reduced response to vaccination. In general, household and close contacts of persons with altered immunocompetence may receive all age appropriate vaccines. Use caution in multiple sclerosis patients; rare exacerbations of symptoms have been observed. Apnea has been reported following I.M. vaccine administration in premature infants; consider risk versus benefit in infants born prematurely. Infants born to HB_sAg-negative mothers and weighing <2 kg at birth may have the initial dose deferred up to 30 days of chronological age or until hospital discharge. If the mothers HB_sAg status at delivery is unknown or positive, hepatitis B vaccine and hepatitis B immune globulin should be administered within 12 hours of life and the first dose of the vaccine should not be counted as part of the vaccine series.

Syncope has been reported with use of injectable vaccines and may be accompanied by transient visual disturbances, weakness, or tonic-clonic movements. Procedures should be in place to avoid injuries from falling and to restore cerebral perfusion if syncope occurs. Some dosage forms contain dry natural latex rubber. In order to maximize vaccination rates, the ACIP recommends simultaneous administration of all age-appropriate vaccines (live or inactivated) for which a person is eligible at a single clinic visit, unless contraindications exist. The use of combination vaccines is generally preferred over separate injections, taking into consideration provider assessment, patient preference, and adverse events. Use of this vaccine for specific medical and/or other indications (eg, immunocompromising conditions, hepatic or kidney disease, diabetes) is also addressed in the ACIP Recommended Immunization Schedule (CDC, 2013a; CDC, 2013b).

Adverse Reactions All serious adverse reactions must be reported to the U.S. Department of Health and Human Services (DHHS) Vaccine Adverse Event Reporting System (VAERS) at 1-800-822-7967 or online at https://vaers.hhs.gov/esub/index.

Frequency not defined. The most common adverse effects reported with both products included injection site reactions (>10%).

Cardiovascular: Flushing, hypotension

Central nervous system: Agitation, chills, dizziness, fatigue, fever (≥37.5°C/100°F), headache, insomnia, irritability, lightheadedness, malaise, somnolence, vertigo

Dermatologic: Angioedema, petechiae, pruritus, rash, urticaria

Gastrointestinal: Abdominal pain, appetite decreased, constipation, cramps, diarrhea, dyspepsia, nausea, vomiting

Genitourinary: Dysuria

Local: Injection site reactions: Ecchymosis, erythema, induration, pain, nodule formation, soreness, swelling, tenderness, warmth

Neuromuscular & skeletal: Achiness, arthralgia, back pain, myalgia, neck pain, neck stiffness, paresthesia, shoulder pain, tingling, weakness

Otic: Earache

Respiratory: Cough, pharyngitis, rhinitis, upper respiratory tract infection

Miscellaneous: Diaphoresis, lymphadenopathy, flu-like syndrome

Postmarketing and/or case reports: Allergic reactions, alopecia, anaphylaxis, apnea, Bell's palsy, bronchospasm, encephalitis, erythema nodosum, erythema multiforme, febrile seizure, Guillain-Barré syndrome, herpes zoster, hypoesthesia, keratitis, liver enzymes increased, lupus-like syndrome, migraine, multiple sclerosis, muscle weakness, neuropathy, optic neuritis, palpitation, paralysis, paresis, polyarteritis nodosa, purpura, seizure, serum-sickness like syndrome (may be delayed days to weeks), Stevens-Johnson syndrome, SLE, syncope, tachycardia, thrombocytopenia, tinnitus, transverse myelitis, uveitis, vasculitis, visual disturbances

Drug Interactions

Metabolism/Transport Effects None known.

Avoid Concomitant Use There are no known interactions where it is recommended to avoid concomitant use.

Increased Effect/Toxicity There are no known significant interactions involving an increase in effect.

Decreased Effect

The levels/effects of Hepatitis B Vaccine (Recombinant) may be decreased by: Belimumab; Fingolimod; Immunosuppressants

Storage/Stability Refrigerate at 2°C to 8°C (36°F to 46°F); do not freeze. The following stability information has also been reported for Engerix-B®: May be stored at room temperature for up to 72 hours (Cohen, 2007).

Mechanism of Action Recombinant hepatitis B vaccine is a noninfectious subunit viral vaccine, which confers active immunity via formation of antihepatitis B antibodies. The vaccine is derived from hepatitis B surface antigen (HB_sAg) produced through recombinant DNA techniques from yeast cells. The portion of the hepatitis B gene which codes for HB_sAg is cloned into yeast which is then cultured to produce hepatitis B vaccine.

Pharmacodynamics/Kinetics Duration: Following a 3-dose series in children, up to 50% of patients will have low or undetectable anti-HB antibody 5-15 years postvaccination. However, anamnestic increases in anti-HB have been shown up to 23 years later suggesting a lifelong immune memory response.

Dosage I.M.:

Primary immunization:

Infants: 0.5 mL/dose (pediatric/adolescent formulation) for 3 total doses administered at 0, 1, and 6 months. Alternate dosing regimens are also available for children who begin vaccination ≥1 year of age.

Note: Doses are presented using the pediatric/adolescent formulations. Pediatric/adolescent formulations of hepatitis B vaccine products differ by concentration (mcg/mL). However, when dosed in terms of volume (mL), the dose of Engerix-B® and Recombivax HB® are the same (both 0.5 mL).

Note: Combination vaccines (eg, vaccines containing HepB with DTaP, HIB) should not be used for the "birth" dose but may be used to complete the course beginning after the infant is ≥6 weeks of age (CDC, 2005). Please see combination vaccine monographs for dose and schedule details.

Infants (HB_sAg-**negative** mothers):

First dose: 0.5 mL at birth or before discharge (may be delayed in certain cases)

Second dose: 0.5 mL at 1-2 months of age

Third dose: 0.5 mL at 6-18 months of age, but no sooner than 24 weeks of age

Note: Premature neonates <2 kg may have the initial dose deferred up to 30 days of chronological age or at hospital discharge (CDC, 2005).

Infants (HB_sAg-**positive** mothers):

First dose: 0.5 mL within first 12 hours of life, even if premature and regardless of birth weight (hepatitis immune globulin should also be administered at the same time at a different site)

Second dose: 0.5 mL at 1-2 months of age

Third dose: 0.5 mL at 6 months of age but no sooner than 24 weeks of age

Note: Anti-HB_s and HB_sAg levels should be checked at 9-18 months of age (ie, next well-child visit after series completion). If HB_sAg negative and anti-HB_s levels <10 mIU/mL, reimmunize with 3 doses and reassess 1-2 months after the third dose.

Note: In premature neonates <2 kg, the birth dose should not be counted as part of the 3-dose vaccine series (CDC, 2005).

Infants (mother's HB_sAg status **unknown**):

First dose: 0.5 mL within 12 hours of birth even if premature and regardless of birth weight

Second dose: 0.5 mL at 1-2 months of age

Third dose: 0.5 mL at 6 months of age but no sooner than 24 weeks of age

Note: If mother is later determined to be HB_sAg-positive, the infant should receive hepatitis immune globulin as soon as possible (no later than age 1 week).

Note: In premature neonates <2 kg, the birth dose should not be counted as part of the 3-dose vaccine series (CDC, 2005).

Children: 0.5 mL/dose (pediatric/adolescent formulation) administered at 0, 1, and 6 months (for 3 total doses). Alternate dosing regimens are also available for children who begin vaccination ≥1 year of age.

Alternate dosing schedules (selection of schedule should optimize compliance with vaccination):

Children 1-10 years: 0.5 mL (pediatric/adolescent formulation) at the following intervals (two schedules presented):

0, 2, and 4 months (CDC, 2005)

0, 1, 2, and 12 months (Engerix-B®)

Children 5-10 years: 0.5 mL (pediatric/adolescent formulation) at 0, 12, and 24 months (Engerix-B®)

Children 11-15 years: 1 mL (adult formulation) at 0 and 4-6 months (Recombivax HB®)

Children 11-16 years: 0.5 mL (pediatric/adolescent formulation) at 0, 12, and 24 months (Engerix-B®)

Children 11-18 years: 0.5 mL (pediatric/adolescent formulation) at the following intervals (three schedules presented):

0, 1, and 4 months (CDC, 2005)

0, 2, and 4 months (CDC, 2005)

0, 12, and 24 months (CDC, 2005)

Children 11-18 years: 1 mL (adult formulation) at 0, 1, 2, and 12 months (Engerix-B®)

Adults: 1 mL/dose (adult formulation) for 3 total doses administered at 0, 1, and 6 months

Note: Adult formulations of hepatitis B vaccine products differ by concentration (mcg/mL) but when dosed in terms of volume (mL), the dose of Engerix-B® and Recombivax HB® are the same (both 1 mL).

Alternate dosing schedules (selection of schedule should optimize compliance with vaccination): All regimens use the adult formulation administered as one dose at the following intervals (three schedules presented):

0, 1, and 4 months (CDC, 2005)

0, 2, and 4 months (CDC, 2005)

0, 12, and 24 months (CDC, 2005)

Bombings or similar mass casualty events: In persons without a reliable history of vaccination against HepB and who have no known contraindications to the vaccine, vaccination should begin within 24 hours (but no later than 7 days) following the event (CDC, 2008).

Dosage adjustment for renal impairment: Adults on dialysis:

Engerix-B® 20 mcg/mL: Administer 2 mL per dose at 0, 1, 2, and 6 months

Recombivax HB® 40 mcg/mL: Administer 1 mL per dose at 0, 1, and 6 months

Note: Serologic testing is recommended 1-2 months after the final dose of the primary vaccine series and annually to determine the need for booster doses. Persons with anti-HB_s concentrations of <10 mIU/mL should be revaccinated with 3 doses of the vaccine (CDC, 2006).

Dosage adjustment in hepatic impairment: No dosage adjustment provided in manufacturer's labeling.

Administration Pediatric/adolescent formulations of hepatitis B vaccine products differ by concentration (mcg/mL). However, when dosed in terms of volume (mL), the dose of Engerix-B® and Recombivax HB® are the same (both 0.5 mL). Adult formulations of hepatitis B vaccine products also differ by concentration (mcg/mL), but when dosed in terms of volume (mL), the dose of Engerix-B® and Recombivax HB® are the same (both 1 mL). It is possible to interchange the vaccines for completion of a series or for booster doses; the antibody produced in response to each type of vaccine is comparable, however, the quantity of the vaccine will vary.

I.M. injection only; in adults, the deltoid muscle is the preferred site; the anterolateral thigh is the recommended site in infants and young children. Not for gluteal administration. Shake well prior to withdrawal and use.

For patients at risk of hemorrhage following intramuscular injection, hepatitis B vaccine may be administered subcutaneously although lower titers and/or increased incidence of local reactions may result. The ACIP recommends "it should be administered intramuscularly if, in the opinion of the physician familiar with the patient's bleeding risk, the vaccine can be administered by this route with reasonable safety. If the patient receives antihemophilia or other similar therapy, intramuscular vaccination can be scheduled shortly after such therapy is administered. A fine needle (23 gauge or smaller) can be used for the vaccination and firm pressure applied to the site (without rubbing) for at least 2 minutes. The patient should be instructed concerning the risk of hematoma from the injection." Patients on anticoagulant therapy should be considered to have the same bleeding risks and treated as those with clotting factor disorders (CDC, 2011).

Simultaneous administration of vaccines helps ensure the patients will be fully vaccinated by the appropriate age. Simultaneous administration of vaccines is defined as administering >1 vaccine on the same day at different anatomic sites. The use of licensed combination vaccines is generally preferred over separate injections of the equivalent components. Separate vaccines should not be combined in the same syringe unless indicated by product specific labeling. Separate needles and syringes should be used for each injection. The ACIP prefers each dose of a specific vaccine in a series come from the same manufacturer when possible. Adolescents and adults should be vaccinated while seated or lying down. In general, preterm infants should be vaccinated at the same chronological age as full-term infants (CDC, 2011).

Antipyretics have not been shown to prevent febrile seizures. Antipyretics may be used to treat fever or discomfort following vaccination (CDC, 2011). One study reported that routine prophylactic administration of acetaminophen to prevent fever prior to vaccination decreased the immune response of some vaccines; the clinical significance of this reduction in immune response has not been established (Prymula, 2009).

Vaccination at the time of HB_sAg testing: For persons in whom vaccination is recommended, the first dose of hepatitis B vaccine can be given after blood is drawn to test for HB_sAg.

Monitoring Parameters Monitor for syncope for 15 minutes following administration. If seizure-like activity associated with syncope occurs, maintain patient in supine or Trendelenburg position to reestablish adequate cerebral perfusion.

Additional Information U.S. federal law requires that the name of medication, date of administration, the vaccine manufacturer, lot number of vaccine, and the administering person's name, title, and address be entered into the patient's permanent medical record.

Dosage Forms Excipient information presented when available (limited, particularly for generics); consult specific product labeling. [DSC] = Discontinued product

Injection, suspension [adult, preservative free]:

Engerix-B®: Hepatitis B surface antigen 20 mcg/mL (1 mL) [contains aluminum, yeast protein, may contain natural rubber/natural latex in prefilled syringe]

Engerix-B®: Hepatitis B surface antigen 20 mcg/mL (1 mL) [contains aluminum, yeast protein; vial]

Recombivax HB®: Hepatitis B surface antigen 10 mcg/mL (1 mL) [contains aluminum, natural rubber/natural latex in packaging, yeast protein]

Injection, suspension [dialysis formulation, preservative free]:

Recombivax HB®: Hepatitis B surface antigen 40 mcg/mL (1 mL) [contains aluminum, natural rubber/natural latex in packaging, yeast protein]

Injection, suspension [pediatric/adolescent, preservative free]:

Engerix-B®: Hepatitis B surface antigen 10 mcg/0.5 mL (0.5 mL) [contains aluminum, yeast protein, may contain natural rubber/natural latex in prefilled syringe]

Recombivax HB®: Hepatitis B surface antigen 5 mcg/0.5 mL (0.5 mL) [contains aluminum, natural rubber/natural latex in packaging, yeast protein]

◆ **Hepatitis B Vaccine (Recombinant)** *see* Haemophilus b Conjugate and Hepatitis B Vaccine *on page* 980

◆ **HepB** *see* Hepatitis B Vaccine (Recombinant) *on page* 995

◆ **Hep Flush-10** *see* Heparin *on page* 986

◆ **Hepsera** *see* Adefovir *on page* 48

◆ **Hepsera™ (Can)** *see* Adefovir *on page* 48

◆ **Heptovir® (Can)** *see* LamiVUDine *on page* 1162

◆ **Herceptin** *see* Trastuzumab *on page* 2109

◆ **Herceptin® (Can)** *see* Trastuzumab *on page* 2109

◆ **Herpes Zoster Vaccine** *see* Zoster Vaccine *on page* 2247

◆ **HES** *see* Hetastarch *on page* 997

◆ **HES** *see* Tetrastarch *on page* 2036

◆ **HES 130/0.4** *see* Tetrastarch *on page* 2036

◆ **HES 450/0.7** *see* Hetastarch *on page* 997

◆ **Hespan** *see* Hetastarch *on page* 997

Hetastarch (HET a starch)

Brand Names: U.S. Hespan; Hextend

Brand Names: Canada Hextend

Index Terms HES; HES 450/0.7; Hydroxyethyl Starch

Pharmacologic Category Plasma Volume Expander, Colloid

Use Blood volume expander used in treatment of hypovolemia; adjunct in leukapheresis to improve harvesting and increase the yield of granulocytes by centrifugation (Hespan)

Unlabeled Use Priming fluid in pump oxygenators during cardiopulmonary bypass; plasma volume expansion during cardiopulmonary bypass

Pregnancy Risk Factor C

Dosage I.V. infusion: Adults:

Plasma volume expansion: 500-1000 mL (up to 1500 mL/day) or 20 mL/kg/day (up to 1500 mL/day). **Note:** With severe dehydration, administer crystalloid first. Daily dose and rate of infusion dependent on amount of blood lost, on maintenance or restoration of hemodynamics, and on amount of hemodilution. Titrate to individual colloid needs, hemodynamics, and hydration status. Do not use in the critically ill, those undergoing open heart surgery and cardiopulmonary bypass, or those with pre-existing renal dysfunction.

Leukapheresis (Hespan): 250-700 mL; **Note:** Citrate anticoagulant is added before use.

Dosage adjustment in renal impairment: Avoid use in patients with pre-existing renal dysfunction. Use is contraindicated in renal failure with oliguria or anuria (not related to hypovolemia). Discontinue use at the first sign of renal injury.

Dosage adjustment in hepatic impairment: No dosage adjustment provided in manufacturer's labeling; use with caution.

Additional Information Complete prescribing information should be consulted for additional detail.

Dosage Forms Excipient information presented when available (limited, particularly for generics); consult specific product labeling.

Solution, Intravenous:
- Hespan: 6% (500 mL)
- Hextend: 6% (500 mL)
- Generic: 6% (500 mL)

- ◆ **Hexachlorocyclohexane** *see* Lindane *on page 1217*
- ◆ **Hexamethylenetetramine** *see* Methenamine *on page 1319*
- ◆ **Hextend** *see* Hetastarch *on page 997*
- ◆ **hFSH** *see* Urofollitropin *on page 2141*
- ◆ **hGH** *see* Somatropin *on page 1934*
- ◆ **HHT** *see* Omacetaxine *on page 1501*
- ◆ **Hib** *see Haemophilus* b Conjugate Vaccine *on page 981*
- ◆ **Hib Conjugate Vaccine** *see Haemophilus* b Conjugate and Hepatitis B Vaccine *on page 980*
- ◆ **Hiberix®** *see Haemophilus* b Conjugate Vaccine *on page 981*
- ◆ **Hib-HepB** *see Haemophilus* b Conjugate and Hepatitis B Vaccine *on page 980*
- ◆ **Hibiclens [OTC]** *see* Chlorhexidine Gluconate *on page 408*
- ◆ **Hibidil® 1:2000 (Can)** *see* Chlorhexidine Gluconate *on page 408*
- ◆ **Hibistat [OTC]** *see* Chlorhexidine Gluconate *on page 408*
- ◆ **Hib-MenCY-TT** *see* Meningococcal Polysaccharide (Groups C and Y) and *Haemophilus* b Tetanus Toxoid Conjugate Vaccine *on page 1293*
- ◆ **High-Molecular-Weight Iron Dextran (DexFerrum)** *see* Iron Dextran Complex *on page 1119*
- ◆ **Hiprex** *see* Methenamine *on page 1319*
- ◆ **Hiprex® (Can)** *see* Methenamine *on page 1319*
- ◆ **Hirulog** *see* Bivalirudin *on page 262*
- ◆ **Histantil (Can)** *see* Promethazine *on page 1728*

Histrelin (his TREL in)

Brand Names: U.S. Supprelin LA; Vantas

Brand Names: Canada Vantas

Index Terms GnRH Agonist; Histrelin Acetate; LH-RH Agonist

Pharmacologic Category Gonadotropin Releasing Hormone Agonist

Use

Central precocious puberty (CPP): Treatment of CPP in children

Prostate cancer: Palliative treatment of advanced prostate cancer

Pregnancy Risk Factor X

Dosage

Central precocious puberty (CPP) (Supprelin LA): Children ≥2 years: SubQ: 50 mg implant surgically inserted every 12 months. Discontinue at the appropriate time for the onset of puberty.

Prostate cancer, advanced (Vantas): Adults: SubQ: 50 mg implant surgically inserted every 12 months

Elderly: Refer to adult dosing

Dosage adjustment in renal impairment:

Vantas: Cl_{cr} ≥15 mL/minute: No dosage adjustment necessary.

Supprelin LA: No dosage adjustment provided in manufacturer's labeling.

Dosage adjustment in hepatic impairment: No dosage adjustment is provided in manufacturers' labeling (has not been studied).

Additional Information Complete prescribing information should be consulted for additional detail.

Dosage Forms Excipient information presented when available (limited, particularly for generics); consult specific product labeling.

Kit, Subcutaneous:
- Supprelin LA: 50 mg
- Vantas: 50 mg

- ◆ **Histrelin Acetate** *see* Histrelin *on page 998*
- ◆ **Hizentra** *see* Immune Globulin *on page 1059*
- ◆ **Hizentra 20%** *see* Immune Globulin *on page 1059*
- ◆ **hMG** *see* Menotropins *on page 1295*
- ◆ **HMR1726** *see* Teriflunomide *on page 2021*
- ◆ **HMR 3647** *see* Telithromycin *on page 2000*
- ◆ **HN_2** *see* Mechlorethamine (Systemic) *on page 1274*
- ◆ **HOE 140** *see* Icatibant *on page 1038*
- ◆ **Homatropaire** *see* Homatropine *on page 998*

Homatropine (hoe MA troe peen)

Brand Names: U.S. Homatropaire; Isopto Homatropine

Index Terms Homatropine Hydrobromide

Pharmacologic Category Anticholinergic Agent, Ophthalmic; Ophthalmic Agent, Mydriatic

Additional Appendix Information

Beers Criteria – Potentially Inappropriate Medications for Geriatrics *on page 2368*

Use

Ciliary spasm: Relief of ciliary spasm.

Iritis/iridocyclitis: Treatment of iritis and iridocyclitis.

Mydriasis and cycloplegia for refraction: Producing cycloplegia and mydriasis for refraction; for pre- and postoperative states when cycloplegic and mydriasis is required.

Optical aid: Use as an optical aid in some cases of axial lens opacities.

Uveitis: Treatment of inflammatory conditions of the uveal tract.

Pregnancy Risk Factor C

Dosage

Children >3 months and Adults: Ophthalmic: **Note:** Children (>3 months of age) should only use the 2% strength solution; patients with heavily pigmented irides may require increased dose.

Ciliary spasm/iritis/iridocyclitis/uveitis: 2% or 5% solution: 1-2 drops 2-3 times daily, up to every 4 hours for severe uveitis (Alexander, 2004)

Refraction:

2% solution: 1-2 drops into eye(s); repeat every 10-15 minutes if necessary; maximum: 5 doses

5% solution: 1-2 drops into eye(s); repeat dose in 15 minutes.

Dosage adjustment in renal impairment: No dosage adjustment provided in manufacturer's labeling.

Dosage adjustment in hepatic impairment: No dosage adjustment provided in manufacturer's labeling.

Additional Information Complete prescribing information should be consulted for additional detail.

Dosage Forms Excipient information presented when available (limited, particularly for generics); consult specific product labeling.

Solution, Ophthalmic, as hydrobromide:

Homatropaire: 5% (5 mL)

Isopto Homatropine: 2% (5 mL); 5% (5 mL)

Generic: 5% (5 mL)

Hyaluronate and Derivatives

(hye al yoor ON ate & dah RIV ah tives)

Brand Names: U.S. Amvisc; Amvisc Plus; Bionect; Euflexxa; Gel-One; Hyalgan; Hylase Wound; Juvéderm Ultra; Juvéderm Ultra Plus; Juvéderm Ultra Plus XC; Juvéderm Ultra XC; Orthovisc; Perlane; Perlane-L; Provisc; Restylane; Restylane-L; Supartz; Synvisc; Synvisc-One

Brand Names: Canada Cystistat; Durolane; OrthoVisc; Suplasyn

Index Terms Hyaluronan; Hyaluronic Acid; Hylan G-F 20; Hylan Polymers; Sodium Hyaluronate

Pharmacologic Category Antirheumatic Miscellaneous; Ophthalmic Agent, Viscoelastic; Skin and Mucous Membrane Agent, Miscellaneous

Use

Intra-articular injection: Treatment of pain in osteoarthritis in knee in patients who have failed nonpharmacologic treatment and simple analgesics (Euflexxa, Gel-One, Hyalgan, OrthoVisc, Supartz, Synvisc, Synvisc-One) or nonsteroidal anti-inflammatory drugs (NSAIDS) (Gel-One)

Intradermal: Correction of moderate-to-severe facial wrinkles or folds (Juvederm [all formulations], Perlane, Perlane-L, Restylane, Restylane-L)

Ophthalmic: Surgical aid in cataract extraction (Amvisc, Amvisc Plus, Provisc); intraocular lens implantation (Amvisc, Amvisc Plus, Provisc); corneal transplant (Amvisc, Amvisc Plus); glaucoma filtration (Amvisc, Amvisc Plus); and retinal attachment surgery (Amvisc, Amvisc Plus)

Submucosal: Lip augmentation (Restylane, Restylane-L)

Topical cream, gel: Management of skin ulcers and wounds (Bionect, Hylase Wound)

Unlabeled Use Treatment of refractory interstitial cystitis

Pregnancy Considerations Adverse events were not observed in animal reproduction studies. Safety for use in pregnant women has not been established.

Breast-Feeding Considerations Safety for use in nursing women has not been established.

Contraindications Hypersensitivity to hyaluronate or any component of the formulation

Intradermal/Submucosal: Additional contraindications include history of anaphylaxis or presence of multiple severe allergies (Juvederm [all formulations], Perlane, Perlane-L, Restylane, Restylane-L); bleeding disorders (Perlane, Perlane-L, Restylane, Restylane-L); history of hypersensitivity to gram-positive bacterial proteins (Juvederm [all formulations], Perlane, Perlane-L, Restylane, Restylane-L) or lidocaine (Juvederm Ultra XC, Juvederm Ultra Plus XC); implantation/injection into sites other than the anatomical spaces recommended per labeling (Perlane, Perlane-L, Restylane, Restylane-L)

Intra-articular: Additional contraindications include knee joint infections or infections or skin diseases at the site of injection (Euflexxa, Gel-One, Hyalgan, OrthoVisc, Supartz, Synvisc, Synvisc-One); hypersensitivity to gram-positive bacterial proteins (Orthovisc)

Intraocular: There are no contraindications in the manufacturer's labeling (Amvisc, Amvisc Plus, Provisc).

Warnings/Precautions Not for I.V. injection. Do not inject into blood vessels; may cause occlusion, infarction, embolism, or other systemic adverse events.

Injection (gel): May be administered by intradermal (Juvederm [all formulations], Perlane, Restylane) or submucosal (Restylane) injection. Treatment may result in bruising/bleeding; use caution in patients receiving or recently exposed (≤3 weeks) to thrombolytics, anticoagulants, or platelet inhibitors. Do not inject into site of active inflammation or infection. Injection into a blood vessel may cause localized superficial necrosis or may cause occlusion and lead to embolism or infarction. Use of Juvederm in patients susceptible to keloid formation, hypertrophic scarring, or pigmentation disorders has not been studied; use cautiously. Following use of Perlane and Restylane, hyperpigmentation may occur at the injection site and may last for ≤6 weeks after treatment; keloid formation may also occur. Use caution in patients receiving immunosuppressive treatment. Use in patients with prior herpetic eruption may result in reactivation. Delayed inflammatory papules may result from injections, necessitating evaluation and treatment as soft tissue infection. Laser treatment or chemical peeling may cause acute inflammatory reaction at the injection site if performed following intradermal treatment. Patient must avoid exposure to ultraviolet rays (sun and UV lamp) or severe cold until swelling and redness is resolved. Treatment site reactions usually improve in <7 days (nasolabial folds) or <14 days (lips). Strenuous exercise and ethanol consumption should be avoided for 24 hours following use. Supplemental "touch up" treatments may be required. Use in lip augmentation has not been established for products other than Restylane. Use of larger than recommended volumes per injection result in an increase in adverse events; if larger amounts are needed, follow-up treatment sessions are recommended.

Injection (gel, solution): Intra-articular: Not for use in infected joints; do not use disinfectants containing quaternary ammonium salts for skin preparation (may cause precipitation of hyaluronate). Remove synovial fluid or effusion, if present, prior to injection. Do not inject extra-articularly or into synovium. Use with caution if venous or lymphatic stasis is present in the leg. Avoid strenuous activities for 48 hours after injection. Some products are produced from avian sources; use with caution in patients with hypersensitivity to avian proteins, feathers, or egg products. Use Gel-One with caution in patients allergic to cinnamon.

Ophthalmic: Do not overfill the anterior chamber. Postoperative increases in intraocular pressure have occurred following use of sodium hyaluronate; remove from the anterior chamber at the end of surgery and monitor intraocular pressure closely.

Topical: Bionect products (cream, gel): Do not use disinfectants containing quaternary ammonium salts for skin preparation (may cause precipitation of hyaluronate)

Packaging may contain natural latex rubber.

Adverse Reactions Frequencies and/or type of local reaction may vary by formulation and site of application/injection.

>10%:

Local: Injection site (intradermal): Erythema (75% to 93%), tenderness (61% to 92%), swelling (81% to 91%), pain (47% to 90%), firmness (86% to 89%), bruising (52% to 87%), lumps/bumps (56% to 83%), skin discoloration (33% to 78%), pruritus (25% to 36%)

Neuromuscular & skeletal: Arthralgia (intra-articular 25%)

1% to 10%:

Cardiovascular: Blood pressure increased (4%)

Central nervous system: Fatigue (1%)

Gastrointestinal: Nausea (≤2%)

Local: Injection site (intra-articular): Pain (3%)

Neuromuscular & skeletal: Back pain (intra-articular <1% to 7%), joint effusion (intra-articular 2% to 6%), tendonitis (intra-articular 2%), arthrosis (intra-articular 1%), limb pain (intra-articular 1%), parasthesia (intra-articular 1%)

Miscellaneous: Infection (intra-articular 1%)

<1% (Limited to important or life-threatening): Allergic reaction (intradermal), angioedema (intradermal), arthritis (intra-articular), dyspnea (intradermal), rash, effusion (intra-articular), facial swelling (intra-articular), gait disturbance(intra-articular), herpetic eruptions (intradermal), hives (intra-articular), infections/abscess/necrosis

(injection site; intradermal), peripheral edema (intra-articular), respiratory difficulty (intra-articular), thrombocytopenia (intra-articular; rare), urticarial (intradermal), vasovagal reaction (intradermal), visual abnormalities (intradermal)

Frequency not defined: Ocular (intraocular): Postoperative inflammatory reactions (iritis, hypopyon), corneal edema, corneal decompensation, postoperative increase in IOP (transient)

Drug Interactions

Metabolism/Transport Effects None known.

Avoid Concomitant Use There are no known interactions where it is recommended to avoid concomitant use.

Increased Effect/Toxicity There are no known significant interactions involving an increase in effect.

Decreased Effect There are no known significant interactions involving a decrease in effect.

Storage/Stability

Amvisc, Amvisc Plus: Store at 2°C to 8°C (36°F to 46°F); do not freeze.

Bionect products: Store at room temperature. Cream and gel may be stored up to 24 months.

Euflexxa: Store refrigerated or at room temperature, 2°C to 25°C (36°F to 77°F); do not freeze. Protect from light. If refrigerated, remove from refrigeration at least 20-30 minutes before use.

Gel-One: Store below 25°C (77°F); do not freeze.

Juvéderm (all formulations), Perlane, Perlane-L, Restylane, Restylane-L: Store at up to 25°C (77°F); do not freeze. Protect from light. Do not use if gel separates or becomes cloudy.

Hyalgan, Orthovisc: Store below 25°C (77°F); do not freeze. Protect from light.

Hylase Wound: Store at 15°C to 30°C (59°F to 86°F); do not freeze.

Provisc: Store refrigerated at 2°C to 8°C (36°F to 46°F); do not freeze. Prior to use, allow refrigerated product to reach room temperature (~20-40 minutes). Protect from light.

Supartz, Synvisc, Synvisc-One: Store at room temperature, below 30°C (86°C); do not freeze. Protect from light.

Mechanism of Action Sodium hyaluronate is a biological polysaccharide which is distributed widely in the extracellular matrix of connective tissue in man (vitreous and aqueous humor of the eye, synovial fluid, skin, and umbilical cord). Sodium hyaluronate and its derivatives form a viscoelastic solution in water (at physiological pH and ionic strength) which makes it suitable for aqueous and vitreous humor in ophthalmic surgery, and functions as a tissue and/or joint lubricant which plays an important role in modulating the interactions between adjacent tissues. Intradermal injection may decrease the depth of facial wrinkles. In the topical management of wounds and ulcers, sodium hyaluronate protects the skin against friction and abrasion.

Pharmacodynamics/Kinetics

Distribution: Intravitreous injection: Diffusion occurs slowly

Excretion: Ophthalmic: Via Canal of Schlemm

Dosage Adults:

Osteoarthritis of the knee: Intra-articular:

Euflexxa: Inject 20 mg (2 mL) once weekly for 3 weeks (total of 3 injections)

Gel-One: Inject 30 mg (3 mL) once

Hyalgan: Inject 20 mg (2 mL) once weekly for 5 weeks (total of 5 injections); some patients may benefit with a total of 3 injections

Orthovisc: Inject 30 mg (2 mL) once weekly for 3-4 weeks (total of 3-4 injections)

Supartz: Inject 25 mg (2.5 mL) once weekly for 5 weeks (total of 5 injections); some patients may benefit with a total of 3 injections

Synvisc: Inject 16 mg (2 mL) once weekly for 3 weeks (total of 3 injections)

Synvisc-One: Inject 48 mg (6 mL) once

Facial wrinkles/folds: Intradermal:

Note: Formulations differ in terms of recommended injection depth: Juvederm, Restylane, and Restylane-L are intended for mid to deep intradermal injection; Perlane and Perlane-L are intended for injection into the deep dermis to superficial subcutis

Juvéderm (all formulations): Inject as required for cosmetic result; typical treatment regimen requires 1.6 mL/treatment site typical volume for repeat treatment is 0.7 mL/treatment site; maximum: 20 mL/60 kg/year

Perlane, Perlane-L: Inject as required into deep dermis/superficial subcutis for cosmetic result; median total dose: 3 mL; maximum: 6 mL per treatment

Restylane, Restylane-L: Inject as required for cosmetic result; median total dose: 3 mL; maximum: 6 mL per treatment

Lip augmentation: Submucosal (Restylane, Restylane-L): Adults ≥21 years of age: Maximum 1.5 mL per lip (upper or lower) per treatment session

Surgical aid: Ophthalmic (Amvisc, Amvisc Plus, Provisc): Intraocular: Depends upon procedure (slowly introduce a sufficient quantity into eye)

Topical:

Bionect cream, gel: Apply a thin layer to clean and disinfected wound or ulcer 2-3 times daily

Hylase Wound gel: Apply liberally to ulcer cavity or wound and to surrounding areas once daily

Interstitial cystitis, refractory (unlabeled use): Intravesical (unlabeled route): 40 mg in 50 mL saline intravesically (retain in bladder for at least 30 minutes) once weekly for 4 weeks, then monthly for up to 1 year in patients showing an initial response (Morales, 1996)

Administration

Intra-articular: Inject directly into the knee joint; do not inject extra-articularly or into the synovial capsule or tissues. Do not use disinfectants containing quaternary ammonium salts for skin cleansing prior to injection. Remove synovial fluid or effusion, if present, prior to injection. If used for bilateral treatment, use a separate syringe for each knee. Refer to manufacturer's labeling for additional instructions on injection technique.

Intradermal/Submucosal: Do not inject into a blood vessel. Following injection, slowly massage area so that it conforms to the contour of the surrounding tissue. May apply ice pack to injection site for a short period immediately after administration if treatment area swollen. Refer to manufacturer's labeling for additional instructions on injection technique.

Juvéderm is intended for mid-to-deep intradermal injection.

Perlane and Perlane-L are intended for injection into the deep dermis to superficial subcutis.

Restylane and Restylane-L are intended for mid-to-deep intradermal injection (facial wrinkles) or submucosal injection (lip augmentation).

Ophthalmic: Allow to reach room temperature prior to use. Drug may become cloudy or form a slight precipitate after administration; clinical significance unknown, but cloudy or precipitated material should be removed by irrigation or aspiration

Topical:

Bionect products: Clean and disinfect wound prior to use (do not use quaternary ammonium salts due to potential for hyaluronic acid precipitation), and debride if necessary; apply a thin layer to wound or ulcer without extensive rubbing. After application, cover the area with a sterile gauze pad and if necessary, an elastic or compressive bandage.

Hylase Wound: Clean ulcer or wound with normal saline, remove excess moisture with dry gauze, then apply gel liberally to wound or ulcer and surrounding areas. After application, cover the area with a sterile nonstick gauze pad and adhesive tape/bandage.

Monitoring Parameters Intraocular pressure (ophthalmic formulations); signs and symptoms of excess local inflammation or infection (intradermal formulations)

Additional Information Perlane differs from Restylane in the size of its hyaluronate particles within the gel, allowing its use in deeper injections relative to other dermal fillers.

Dosage Forms Excipient information presented when available (limited, particularly for generics); consult specific product labeling.

Cream, topical [sodium hyaluronate]:
- Bionect: 0.2% (25 g)

Gel, topical [sodium hyaluronate]:
- Bionect: 0.2% (30 g, 60 g)
- Hylase Wound: 2.5% (75 g)

Injection, gel, intra-articular [cross-linked hyaluronate]:
- Gel-One: 10 mg/mL (3 mL) [derived from or manufactured using an avian source]

Injection, gel, intradermal [hyaluronic acid]:
- Juvéderm Ultra: 24 mg/mL (0.4 mL, 0.8 mL) [derived from or manufactured from bacterial source]
- Juvéderm Ultra Plus: 24 mg/mL (0.4 mL, 0.8 mL) [derived from or manufactured from bacterial source]
- Juvéderm Ultra Plus XC: Hyaluronic acid 24 mg/mL and lidocaine 0.3% (0.4 mL, 0.8 mL) [derived from or manufactured from bacterial source]
- Juvéderm Ultra XC: Hyaluronic acid 24 mg/mL and lidocaine 0.3% (0.4 mL, 0.8 mL) [derived from or manufactured from bacterial source]
- Perlane-L: Hyaluronic acid 20 mg/mL and lidocaine 0.3% (1 mL, 2 mL) [derived from or manufactured from bacterial source]
- Restylane-L: Hyaluronic acid 20 mg/mL and lidocaine 0.3% (0.5 mL, 1 mL, 2 mL) [derived from or manufactured from bacterial source]

Injection, gel, intradermal [sodium hyaluronate]:
- Perlane: 20 mg/mL (1 mL) [derived from or manufactured from bacterial source]
- Restylane: 20 mg/mL (0.4 mL, 1 mL, 2 mL) [derived from or manufactured from bacterial source]

Injection, solution, intra-articular [hylan polymers A and B]:
- Synvisc-One: 8 mg/mL (6 mL) [derived from or manufactured using an avian source]
- Synvisc: 8 mg/mL (2 mL) [derived from or manufactured using an avian source]

Injection, solution, intra-articular [sodium hyaluronate]:
- Euflexxa: 10 mg/mL (2 mL)
- Hyalgan: 10 mg/mL (2 mL) [derived from or manufactured using an avian source]
- Orthovisc: 15 mg/mL (2 mL) [derived from or manufactured from bacterial source]
- Supartz: 10 mg/mL (2.5 mL) [derived from or manufactured using an avian source]

Injection, solution, intraocular [sodium hyaluronate]:
- Amvisc: 12 mg/mL (0.5 mL, 0.8 mL)
- Amvisc Plus: 16 mg/mL (0.5 mL, 0.8 mL)
- Provisc: 10 mg/mL (0.4 mL, 0.55 mL, 0.85 mL) [contains natural rubber/natural latex in packaging]

◆ **Hyaluronic Acid** *see* Hyaluronate and Derivatives *on page 1000*

◆ **Hycamptamine** *see* Topotecan *on page 2093*

◆ **Hycamtin** *see* Topotecan *on page 2093*

◆ **hycet®** *see* Hydrocodone and Acetaminophen *on page 1006*

◆ **Hycodan** *see* Hydrocodone and Homatropine *on page 1008*

◆ **Hycort™ (Can)** *see* Hydrocortisone (Topical) *on page 1011*

◆ **Hydeltra T.B.A.® (Can)** *see* PrednisoLONE (Systemic) *on page 1704*

◆ **Hyderm (Can)** *see* Hydrocortisone (Topical) *on page 1011*

HydrALAZINE (hye DRAL a zeen)

Brand Names: Canada Apo-Hydralazine®; Apresoline®; Novo-Hylazin; Nu-Hydral

Index Terms Apresoline; Hydralazine Hydrochloride

Pharmacologic Category Antihypertensive; Vasodilator

Use Management of moderate-to-severe hypertension

Unlabeled Use Patients with heart failure with reduced ejection fraction (HFrEF) who do not tolerate an ACE inhibitor or an angiotensin receptor blocker (ARB) (in combination with isosorbide dinitrate); African-American (self-identified) patients with HFrEF NYHA Class III-IV remaining symptomatic despite optimal guideline directed medical therapy (in combination with isosorbide dinitrate); hypertensive emergency (with or without pre-eclampsia/eclampsia) in pregnancy; postoperative hypertension.

Pregnancy Risk Factor C

Pregnancy Considerations Adverse events were observed in some animal reproduction studies. Hydralazine crosses the placenta (Liedholm, 1982). Intravenous hydralazine is recommended for use in the management of acute onset severe hypertension in pregnancy and hypertension associated with pre-eclampsia (ACOG, 2011; ACOG, 2013). Untreated chronic maternal hypertension is associated with adverse events in the fetus, infant, and mother. If treatment for chronic hypertension in pregnancy is needed, other oral agents are preferred as initial therapy (ACOG, 2013).

Breast-Feeding Considerations Hydralazine is excreted into breast milk. In a case report, following a maternal dose of hydralazine 50 mg three times daily, exposure to the infant was calculated to be 0.013 mg per 75 mL breast milk (Liedholm, 1982). The manufacturer recommends that caution be used if administered to a nursing woman.

Contraindications Hypersensitivity to hydralazine or any component of the formulation; mitral valve rheumatic heart disease

Warnings/Precautions May cause peripheral neuritis or a drug-induced lupus-like syndrome (more likely on larger doses, longer duration). Discontinue hydralazine in patients who develop SLE-like syndrome or positive ANA. Use with caution in patients with severe renal disease or cerebral vascular accidents or with known or suspected coronary artery disease; monitor blood pressure closely with I.V. use. Slow acetylators, patients with decreased renal function, and patients receiving >200 mg/day (chronically) are at higher risk for SLE. Titrate dosage cautiously to patient's response. Hypotensive effect after I.V. administration may be delayed and unpredictable in some patients. Usually administered with diuretic and a beta-blocker to counteract side effects of sodium and water retention and reflex tachycardia.

Adjust dose in severe renal dysfunction. Use with caution in CAD (increase in tachycardia may increase myocardial oxygen demand). Use with caution in pulmonary hypertension (may cause hypotension). Patients may be poorly compliant because of frequent dosing. Hydralazine-induced fluid and sodium retention may require addition or increased dosage of a diuretic.

Adverse Reactions Frequency not defined.

Cardiovascular: Angina pectoris, flushing, orthostatic hypotension, palpitations, paradoxical hypertension, peripheral edema, tachycardia, vascular collapse

Central nervous system: Anxiety, chills, depression, disorientation, dizziness, fever, headache, increased intracranial pressure (I.V.; in patient with pre-existing increased intracranial pressure), psychotic reaction
Dermatologic: Pruritus, rash, urticaria
Gastrointestinal: Anorexia, constipation, diarrhea, nausea, paralytic ileus, vomiting
Genitourinary: Dysuria, impotence
Hematologic: Agranulocytosis, eosinophilia, erythrocyte count reduced, hemoglobin decreased, hemolytic anemia, leukopenia, thrombocytopenia (rare)
Neuromuscular & skeletal: Muscle cramps, peripheral neuritis, rheumatoid arthritis, tremor, weakness
Ocular: Conjunctivitis, lacrimation
Respiratory: Dyspnea, nasal congestion
Miscellaneous: Diaphoresis, drug-induced lupus-like syndrome (dose related; fever, arthralgia, splenomegaly, lymphadenopathy, asthenia, myalgia, malaise, pleuritic chest pain, edema, positive ANA, positive LE cells, maculopapular facial rash, positive direct Coombs' test, pericarditis, pericardial tamponade)

Drug Interactions

Metabolism/Transport Effects Inhibits CYP3A4 (weak)

Avoid Concomitant Use

Avoid concomitant use of HydrALAZINE with any of the following: Pimozide

Increased Effect/Toxicity

HydrALAZINE may increase the levels/effects of: Amifostine; Antihypertensives; ARIPiprazole; Dofetilide; Hypotensive Agents; Lomitapide; Obinutuzumab; Pimozide; RiTUXimab

The levels/effects of HydrALAZINE may be increased by: Alfuzosin; Brimonidine (Topical); Diazoxide; Herbs (Hypotensive Properties); MAO Inhibitors; Pentoxifylline; Phosphodiesterase 5 Inhibitors; Prostacyclin Analogues

Decreased Effect

The levels/effects of HydrALAZINE may be decreased by: Herbs (Hypertensive Properties); Methylphenidate; Nonsteroidal Anti-Inflammatory Agents; Yohimbine

Ethanol/Nutrition/Herb Interactions

Ethanol: Avoid ethanol (may increase CNS depression).
Food: Food enhances bioavailability of hydralazine.
Herb/Nutraceutical: Avoid dong quai if using for hypertension (has estrogenic activity). Avoid ephedra, yohimbe, ginseng (may worsen hypertension). Avoid garlic (may have increased antihypertensive effect).

Preparation for Administration Hydralazine should be diluted in NS for IVPB administration due to decreased stability in D_5W. Stability of IVPB solution in NS is 4 days at room temperature.

Storage/Stability Intact ampuls/vials of hydralazine should not be stored under refrigeration because of possible precipitation or crystallization.

Mechanism of Action Direct vasodilation of arterioles (with little effect on veins) with decreased systemic resistance

Pharmacodynamics/Kinetics

Onset of action: Oral: 20-30 minutes; I.V.: 5-20 minutes
Duration: Oral: Up to 8 hours; I.V.: 1-4 hours; **Note:** May vary depending on acetylator status of patient
Protein binding: 85% to 90%
Metabolism: Hepatically acetylated; extensive first-pass effect (oral)
Bioavailability: 30% to 50%; increased with food
Half-life elimination: Normal renal function: 2-8 hours; End-stage renal disease: 7-16 hours
Excretion: Urine (14% as unchanged drug)

Dosage

Children:
Oral: Initial: 0.75-1 mg/kg/day in 2-4 divided doses; increase over 3-4 weeks to maximum of 7.5 mg/kg/day in 2-4 divided doses; maximum daily dose: 200 mg/day
I.M., I.V.: 0.1-0.2 mg/kg/dose (not to exceed 20 mg) every 4-6 hours as needed, up to 1.7-3.5 mg/kg/day in 4-6 divided doses

Adults:
Oral:
Hypertension: Initial dose: 10 mg 4 times daily for the first 2-4 days; increase to 25 mg 4 times daily for the balance of the first week; further increase by 10-25 mg/dose gradually (every 2-5 days) to 50 mg 4 times daily (maximum: 300 mg daily in divided doses).
Heart failure (unlabeled use; ACCF/AHA [Yancy, 2013]): Initial dose: 25-50 mg 3 or 4 times daily; use in combination with isosorbide dinitrate; maximum dose: 300 mg daily in divided doses

I.M., I.V.:
Hypertensive emergency (unlabeled dose): **Note:** Use is generally not recommended due to unpredictable and prolonged antihypertensive effects (Marik, 2007): I.M., I.V.: 10-20 mg every 4-6 hours as needed (Rhoney, 2009)
Hypertensive emergency in pregnancy:
Without pre-eclampsia/eclampsia (unlabeled dose): I.V., I.M.: 5 mg followed by 5-10 mg I.V. administered every 20-40 minutes as needed to a maximum total dose of 30 mg (ACOG, 2013; Too, 2013). **Note:** May also initiate a continuous infusion of 0.5-10 mg/hour after the initial dose (ACOG, 2013).
With pre-eclampsia/eclampsia (unlabeled dose): I.V: 5-10 mg, repeat in 20 minutes with 10 mg as needed; if after an additional 20 minutes blood pressure still exceeds thresholds, consider switching to labetalol (ACOG, 2011).
Perioperative hypertension (unlabeled dose): I.V.: 3-20 mg every 20-60 minutes as needed (Varon, 2008). **Note:** The lower end of the dosage range is preferred in the immediate perioperative period and in patients with renal failure. The use of hydralazine in this setting especially in patients with ischemic heart disease, aortic dissection, or an intracranial process is best avoided due to unpredictable and prolonged antihypertensive effects (Lien, 2012; Varon, 2008).

Dosage interval in renal impairment:
Cl_{cr} 10-50 mL/minute: Administer every 8 hours.
Cl_{cr} <10 mL/minute: Administer every 8-16 hours in fast acetylators and every 12-24 hours in slow acetylators.
Hemodialysis: Supplemental dose is not necessary.
Peritoneal dialysis: Supplemental dose is not necessary.

Dosage adjustment in hepatic impairment: No dosage adjustment provided in manufacturer's labeling. However, hydralazine undergoes extensive hepatic metabolism.

Dietary Considerations Administer tablet with meals.

Administration Solution for injection: Administer as a slow I.V. push; maximum rate: 5 mg/minute

Monitoring Parameters Blood pressure (monitor closely with I.V. use), standing and sitting/supine, heart rate, ANA titer

Dosage Forms Excipient information presented when available (limited, particularly for generics); consult specific product labeling.
Solution, Injection, as hydrochloride:
Generic: 20 mg/mL (1 mL)
Tablet, Oral, as hydrochloride:
Generic: 10 mg, 25 mg, 50 mg, 100 mg

Extemporaneous Preparations A flavored suspension (1.25 mg/mL) may be made with tablets. Dissolve seventy-five 50 mg hydralazine hydrochloride tablets in 250 mL of distilled water with 2250 g of Lycasin® (75% w/w maltitol syrup vehicle). Add 3 g edetate disodium, then add 3 g sodium saccharin dissolved in 50 mL distilled water. Preserve solution with 30 mL of a solution containing methylparaben 10% (w/v) and propylparaben 2% (w/v) in propylene glycol. Flavor with 3 mL orange flavoring; add sufficient quantity of distilled water to make 3 L. Adjust to pH 3.7 with glacial acetic acid. Label "shake well" and "refrigerate". Stable for 5 days at room temperature and at least 2 weeks refrigerated (preferred).

Alexander KS, Pudipeddi M, and Parker GA, "Stability of Hydralazine Hydrochloride Syrup Compounded From Tablets," *Am J Hosp Pharm*, 1993, 50(4):683-6.

- **Hydralazine and Isosorbide Dinitrate** *see* Isosorbide Dinitrate and Hydralazine *on page 1127*
- **Hydralazine Hydrochloride** *see* HydrALAZINE *on page 1002*
- **Hydrated Chloral** *see* Chloral Hydrate *on page 403*
- **Hydrea** *see* Hydroxyurea *on page 1022*
- **Hydrea® (Can)** *see* Hydroxyurea *on page 1022*
- **Hydro 35** *see* Urea *on page 2140*
- **Hydro 40** *see* Urea *on page 2140*

Hydrochlorothiazide (hye droe klor oh THYE a zide)

Brand Names: U.S. Microzide

Brand Names: Canada Apo-Hydro; Bio-Hydrochlorothiazide; Dom-Hydrochlorothiazide; Novo-Hydrazide; Nu-Hydro; PMS-Hydrochlorothiazide

Index Terms HCTZ (error-prone abbreviation); Hydrodiuril

Pharmacologic Category Antihypertensive; Diuretic, Thiazide

Use Management of mild-to-moderate hypertension; treatment of edema due to heart failure, hepatic cirrhosis (see **"Note"**), various forms of renal dysfunction (eg, nephrotic syndrome, acute glomerulosclerosis, chronic renal failure) (see **"Note"**), corticosteroid and estrogen therapy

Note: The use of hydrochlorothiazide in the treatment of edema for hepatic cirrhosis has largely been replaced by spironolactone. The use of hydrochlorothiazide in the management of edema in patients with renal dysfunction has largely been replaced by the use of loop diuretics (eg, furosemide).

Unlabeled Use Treatment of lithium-induced diabetes insipidus

Pregnancy Risk Factor B

Pregnancy Considerations Adverse events were not observed in animal reproduction studies. Thiazide diuretics cross the placenta and are found in cord blood. Maternal use may cause may cause fetal or neonatal jaundice, thrombocytopenia, or other adverse events observed in adults. Use of thiazide diuretics to treat edema during normal pregnancies is not appropriate; use may be considered when edema is due to pathologic causes (as in the nonpregnant patient); monitor. Untreated chronic maternal hypertension is associated with adverse events in the fetus, infant, and mother (ACOG, 2012; Chobanian, 2003). Women who required thiazide diuretics for the treatment of hypertension prior to pregnancy may continue their use (ACOG, 2012).

Breast-Feeding Considerations Thiazide diuretics are found in breast milk. Following a single oral maternal dose of hydrochlorothiazide 50 mg, the mean breast milk concentration was 80 ng/mL (samples collected over 24 hours) and hydrochlorothiazide was not detected in the blood of the breast feeding infant (limit of detection 20 ng/mL) (Miller, 1982). Peak plasma concentrations reported in adults following hydrochlorothiazide 12.5-100 mg are 70-490 ng/mL. Due to the potential for serious adverse reactions in the nursing infant, the manufacturer recommends a decision be made whether to discontinue nursing or to discontinue the drug, taking into account the importance of treatment to the mother. Breast-fed infants of mothers taking medications for hypertension should be monitored for adverse effects (Chobanian, 2003). Diuretics have the potential to decrease milk volume and suppress lactation.

Contraindications Hypersensitivity to hydrochlorothiazide, any component of the formulation, or sulfonamide-derived drugs; anuria

Warnings/Precautions Hypersensitivity reactions may occur with hydrochlorothiazide. Risk is increased in patients with a history of allergy or bronchial asthma. Avoid in severe renal disease (ineffective as a diuretic). Electrolyte disturbances (hypokalemia, hypochloremic alkalosis, hypomagnesemia, hyponatremia) can occur. Development of electrolyte disturbances can be minimized when used in combination with other electrolyte sparing antihypertensives (eg, ACE inhibitors or angiotensin receptor blockers). (Sica, 2011) Use with caution in severe hepatic dysfunction; hepatic encephalopathy can be caused by electrolyte disturbances. Gout may be precipitated in certain patients with a history of gout, a familial predisposition to gout, or chronic renal failure. Thiazide diuretics reduce calcium excretion; pathologic changes in the parathyroid glands with hypercalcemia and hypophosphatemia have been observed with prolonged use. Should be discontinued prior to testing for parathyroid function. Use with caution in patients with prediabetes and diabetes; may alter glucose control. May cause SLE exacerbation or activation. Use with caution in patients with moderate or high cholesterol concentrations. Photosensitization may occur. Correct hypokalemia before initiating therapy. Thiazide diuretics may decrease renal calcium excretion; consider avoiding use in patients with hypercalcemia. May cause acute transient myopia and acute angle-closure glaucoma, typically occurring within hours to weeks following initiation; discontinue therapy immediately in patients with acute decreases in visual acuity or ocular pain. Risk factors may include a history of sulfonamide or penicillin allergy. Cumulative effects may develop, including azotemia, in patients with impaired renal function.

Chemical similarities are present among sulfonamides, sulfonylureas, carbonic anhydrase inhibitors, thiazides, and loop diuretics (except ethacrynic acid). Use in patients with sulfonamide allergy is specifically contraindicated in product labeling, however, a risk of cross-reaction exists in patients with allergy to any of these compounds; avoid use when previous reaction has been severe. Discontinue if signs of hypersensitivity are noted.

Adverse Reactions Frequency not defined; with capsule formulation, adverse events were observed at doses ≥25 mg in adults:

Cardiovascular: Hypotension, orthostatic hypotension

Central nervous system: Dizziness, fever, headache, vertigo

Dermatologic: Alopecia, erythema multiforme, exfoliative dermatitis, photosensitivity, purpura, rash, Stevens-Johnson syndrome, toxic epidermal necrolysis, urticaria

Endocrine & metabolic: Hyperglycemia, hypokalemia, hyperuricemia

Gastrointestinal: Anorexia, constipation, cramping, diarrhea, epigastric distress, gastric irritation, nausea, pancreatitis, sialadenitis, vomiting

Genitourinary: Glycosuria, impotence

Hematologic: Agranulocytosis, aplastic anemia, hemolytic anemia, leukopenia, thrombocytopenia

Hepatic: Jaundice

Neuromuscular & skeletal: Muscle spasm, paresthesia, restlessness, weakness
Ocular: Blurred vision (transient), xanthopsia
Renal: Interstitial nephritis, renal dysfunction, renal failure
Respiratory: Respiratory distress, pneumonitis, pulmonary edema
Miscellaneous: Anaphylactic reactions, necrotizing angiitis
<1% (Limited to important or life-threatening): Allergic myocarditis, eosinophilic pneumonitis, hepatic function impairment, hypercalcemia, lip cancer (Friedman, 2012)

Drug Interactions

Metabolism/Transport Effects None known.

Avoid Concomitant Use

Avoid concomitant use of Hydrochlorothiazide with any of the following: Dofetilide

Increased Effect/Toxicity

Hydrochlorothiazide may increase the levels/effects of: ACE Inhibitors; Allopurinol; Amifostine; Antihypertensives; Benazepril; Calcium Salts; CarBAMazepine; Diazoxide; Dofetilide; Hypotensive Agents; Ivabradine; Lithium; Multivitamins/Minerals (with ADEK, Folate, Iron); Multivitamins/Minerals (with AE, No Iron); Obinutuzumab; OXcarbazepine; Porfimer; RiTUXimab; Sodium Phosphates; Topiramate; Toremifene; Valsartan; Vitamin D Analogs

The levels/effects of Hydrochlorothiazide may be increased by: Alcohol (Ethyl); Alfuzosin; Analgesics (Opioid); Anticholinergic Agents; Barbiturates; Beta2-Agonists; Brimonidine (Topical); Corticosteroids (Orally Inhaled); Corticosteroids (Systemic); Herbs (Hypotensive Properties); Licorice; MAO Inhibitors; Multivitamins/Fluoride (with ADE); Pentoxifylline; Phosphodiesterase 5 Inhibitors; Prostacyclin Analogues; Selective Serotonin Reuptake Inhibitors; Valsartan

Decreased Effect

Hydrochlorothiazide may decrease the levels/effects of: Antidiabetic Agents

The levels/effects of Hydrochlorothiazide may be decreased by: Benazepril; Bile Acid Sequestrants; Herbs (Hypertensive Properties); Methylphenidate; Nonsteroidal Anti-Inflammatory Agents; Yohimbine

Ethanol/Nutrition/Herb Interactions

Food: Hydrochlorothiazide peak serum levels may be decreased if taken with food. This product may deplete potassium, sodium, and magnesium.
Herb/Nutraceutical: Avoid herbs with *hypertensive* properties (bayberry, blue cohosh, cayenne, ephedra, ginger, ginseng [American], kola, licorice); may diminish the antihypertensive effect of hydrochlorothiazide. Avoid herbs with *hypotensive* properties (black cohosh, California poppy, coleus, golden seal, hawthorn, mistletoe, periwinkle, quinine, shepherd's purse); may enhance the hypotensive effect of hydrochlorothiazide.

Storage/Stability Store at 20°C to 25°C (68°F to 77°F) (USP Controlled Room Temperature). Protect from light and moisture.

Mechanism of Action Inhibits sodium reabsorption in the distal tubules causing increased excretion of sodium and water as well as potassium and hydrogen ions

Pharmacodynamics/Kinetics

Onset of action: Diuresis: ~2 hours
Peak effect: 4-6 hours
Duration: 6-12 hours
Absorption: Well absorbed; when administered with food, time to maximum concentration increases from 1.6 to 2.9 hours. Absorption is reduced in patients with CHF.
Distribution: 3.6-7.8 L/kg (correlates with dose administered and concentration achieved)
Protein binding: ~40% to 68%
Metabolism: Not metabolized
Bioavailability: 65% to 75% (reduced by 10% when administered with food)
Half-life elimination: 6-15 hours
Time to peak: ~1-5 hours
Excretion: Urine (as unchanged drug)

Dosage Oral (effect of drug may be decreased when used every day):

Infants and Children (in pediatric patients, chlorothiazide may be preferred over hydrochlorothiazide as there are more dosage formulations [eg, suspension] available): Edema, hypertension:

Manufacturer's labeling: Usual dose:

<6 months: 1-3 mg/kg/day in 1-2 divided doses; maximum: 37.5 mg daily
>6 months to 2 years: 1-2 mg/kg/day in a single or 2 divided doses; maximum: 37.5 mg daily
>2-12 years: 1-2 mg/kg/day in a single or 2 divided doses; maximum: 100 mg daily

Alternate recommendations: Children and Adolescents: Initial: 1 mg/kg/day in a single dose once daily; maximum: 3 mg/kg/day not to exceed 50 mg daily (NHBPEP, 2005)

Adults:

Manufacturer recommendations:

Edema: 25-100 mg daily in 1-2 divided doses; may administer intermittently on alternate days or on 3-5 days each week.
Hypertension: Initial: 12.5-25 mg once daily administered alone or in combination with other antihypertensives; may increase up to 50 mg daily in 1-2 divided doses; minimal increase in response and more electrolyte disturbances are seen with doses >50 mg daily.

Alternate recommendations:

Mild fluid retention in heart failure: Initial: 25 mg once or twice daily; maximum dose: 200 mg daily (Yancy, 2013)
Hypertension in heart failure: Initial: 25 mg once or twice daily; maximum dose: 200 mg daily (Yancy, 2013)

Dosage adjustment in renal impairment: No dosage adjustment provided in manufacturer's labeling; however, the following adjustments have been recommended (Aronoff, 2007):

Cl_{cr} ≥10 mL/minute: No dosage adjustment necessary. Usually ineffective with Cl_{cr} <30 mL/minute unless in combination with a loop diuretic
Cl_{cr} <10 mL/minute: Use not recommended; use is contraindicated with anuria.

Dosage adjustment in hepatic impairment: No dosage adjustment provided in manufacturer's labeling. Use with caution and monitor for precipitation of hepatic coma.

Dietary Considerations May be taken with or without food.

Administration May be administered with or without food. Take early in day to avoid nocturia. Take the last dose of multiple doses no later than 6 PM unless instructed otherwise.

Monitoring Parameters Assess weight, I & O reports daily to determine fluid loss; blood pressure, serum electrolytes, BUN, creatinine

Test Interactions May interfere with parathyroid function tests and may decrease serum iodine (protein bound) without signs of thyroid disturbance.

Dosage Forms Excipient information presented when available (limited, particularly for generics); consult specific product labeling.

Capsule, Oral:
Microzide: 12.5 mg
Generic: 12.5 mg
Tablet, Oral:
Generic: 12.5 mg, 25 mg, 50 mg

◆ **Hydrochlorothiazide, Aliskiren, and Amlodipine** *see* Aliskiren, Amlodipine, and Hydrochlorothiazide *on page 76*

◆ **Hydrochlorothiazide, Amlodipine, and Aliskiren** *see* Aliskiren, Amlodipine, and Hydrochlorothiazide *on page 76*

◆ **Hydrochlorothiazide, Amlodipine, and Valsartan** *see* Amlodipine, Valsartan, and Hydrochlorothiazide *on page 113*

◆ **Hydrochlorothiazide and Aliskiren** *see* Aliskiren and Hydrochlorothiazide *on page 76*

◆ **Hydrochlorothiazide and Benazepril** *see* Benazepril and Hydrochlorothiazide *on page 236*

◆ **Hydrochlorothiazide and Bisoprolol** *see* Bisoprolol and Hydrochlorothiazide *on page 262*

◆ **Hydrochlorothiazide and Candesartan** *see* Candesartan and Hydrochlorothiazide *on page 329*

◆ **Hydrochlorothiazide and Captopril** *see* Captopril and Hydrochlorothiazide *on page 335*

◆ **Hydrochlorothiazide and Enalapril** *see* Enalapril and Hydrochlorothiazide *on page 704*

◆ **Hydrochlorothiazide and Eprosartan** *see* Eprosartan and Hydrochlorothiazide *on page 731*

◆ **Hydrochlorothiazide and Irbesartan** *see* Irbesartan and Hydrochlorothiazide *on page 1115*

◆ **Hydrochlorothiazide and Lisinopril** *see* Lisinopril and Hydrochlorothiazide *on page 1229*

◆ **Hydrochlorothiazide and Losartan** *see* Losartan and Hydrochlorothiazide *on page 1249*

◆ **Hydrochlorothiazide and Moexipril** *see* Moexipril and Hydrochlorothiazide *on page 1392*

◆ **Hydrochlorothiazide and Olmesartan Medoxomil** *see* Olmesartan and Hydrochlorothiazide *on page 1499*

◆ **Hydrochlorothiazide and Telmisartan** *see* Telmisartan and Hydrochlorothiazide *on page 2004*

Hydrochlorothiazide and Triamterene

(hye droe klor oh THYE a zide & trye AM ter een)

Brand Names: U.S. Dyazide; Maxzide; Maxzide-25

Brand Names: Canada Apo-Triazide; Pro-Triazide; Teva-Triamterene HCTZ

Index Terms Triamterene and Hydrochlorothiazide

Pharmacologic Category Antihypertensive; Diuretic, Potassium-Sparing; Diuretic, Thiazide

Use Treatment of hypertension or edema (not recommended for initial treatment) when hypokalemia has developed on hydrochlorothiazide alone or when the development of hypokalemia must be avoided

Pregnancy Risk Factor C

Dosage Oral: Adults:

Hydrochlorothiazide 25 mg and triamterene 37.5 mg: 1-2 tablets/capsules once daily

Hydrochlorothiazide 50 mg and triamterene 75 mg: 1/2-1 tablet daily

Dosage adjustment in renal impairment: Efficacy of hydrochlorothiazide is limited in patients with Cl_{cr} <30 mL/minute, contraindicated in patients with anuria, acute and chronic renal insufficiency, or significant renal impairment.

Dosage adjustment in hepatic impairment: No dosage adjustment provided in manufacturer's labeling; use with caution. Use with caution and monitor for precipitation of hepatic coma.

Additional Information Complete prescribing information should be consulted for additional detail.

Dosage Forms Excipient information presented when available (limited, particularly for generics); consult specific product labeling.

Capsule, oral: Hydrochlorothiazide 25 mg and triamterene 37.5 mg; hydrochlorothiazide 25 mg and triamterene 50 mg

Dyazide: Hydrochlorothiazide 25 mg and triamterene 37.5 mg

Tablet: Hydrochlorothiazide 25 mg and triamterene 37.5 mg; hydrochlorothiazide 50 mg and triamterene 75 mg

Maxzide: Hydrochlorothiazide 50 mg and triamterene 75 mg [scored]

Maxzide-25: Hydrochlorothiazide 25 mg and triamterene 37.5 mg [scored]

◆ **Hydrochlorothiazide and Valsartan** *see* Valsartan and Hydrochlorothiazide *on page 2156*

◆ **Hydrochlorothiazide, Olmesartan, and Amlodipine** *see* Olmesartan, Amlodipine, and Hydrochlorothiazide *on page 1498*

Hydrocodone and Acetaminophen

(hye droe KOE done & a seet a MIN oh fen)

Brand Names: U.S. hycet®; Lorcet® 10/650; Lorcet® Plus; Lortab®; Margesic® H; Maxidone®; Norco®; Stagesic™; Vicodin ES®; Vicodin HP®; Vicodin®; Xodol® 10/300; Xodol® 5/300; Xodol® 7.5/300; Zamicet™; Zolvit®; Zydone®

Index Terms Acetaminophen and Hydrocodone

Pharmacologic Category Analgesic Combination (Opioid)

Use Relief of moderate-to-severe pain

Pregnancy Risk Factor C

Dosage Oral (doses should be titrated to appropriate analgesic effect): Analgesic:

Children 2-13 years or <50 kg: Hydrocodone 0.1-0.2 mg/kg/dose every 4-6 hours; do not exceed 6 doses/day or the maximum recommended dose of acetaminophen

Children and Adults ≥50 kg: Average starting dose in opioid naive patients: Hydrocodone 5-10 mg 4 times/day; the dosage of acetaminophen should be limited to ≤4 g/day (and possibly less in patients with hepatic impairment or ethanol use).

Dosage ranges (based on specific product labeling): Hydrocodone 2.5-10 mg every 4-6 hours (maximum dose of hydrocodone may be limited by the acetaminophen content of specific product)

Elderly: Doses should be titrated to appropriate analgesic effect; 2.5-5 mg of the hydrocodone component every 4-6 hours. Do not exceed 4 g/day of acetaminophen.

Dosage adjustment in renal impairment: No dosage adjustment provided in manufacturer's labeling; use with caution.

Dosage adjustment in hepatic impairment: Use with caution. Limited, low-dose therapy usually well tolerated in hepatic disease/cirrhosis; however, cases of hepatotoxicity at daily acetaminophen dosages <4 g/day have been reported. Avoid chronic use in hepatic impairment.

Additional Information Complete prescribing information should be consulted for additional detail.

Dosage Forms Excipient information presented when available (limited, particularly for generics); consult specific product labeling.

Capsule, oral:

Margesic® H, Stagesic™: Hydrocodone bitartrate 5 mg and acetaminophen 500 mg

Elixir, oral:
Lortab®: Hydrocodone bitartrate 7.5 mg and acetaminophen 500 mg per 15 mL (480 mL) [contains ethanol 7%, propylene glycol; tropical fruit punch flavor] [DSC]
Lortab®: Hydrocodone bitartrate 10 mg and acetaminophen 300 mg per 15 mL (480 mL) [contains ethanol 7%, propylene glycol; tropical fruit punch flavor]
Solution, oral: Hydrocodone bitartrate 7.5 mg and acetaminophen 325 mg per 15 mL; hydrocodone bitartrate 7.5 mg and acetaminophen 500 mg per 15 mL (5 mL, 10 mL, 15 mL, 118 mL, 473 mL); hydrocodone bitartrate 10 mg and acetaminophen 325 mg per 15 mL (7.5 mL, 15 mL)
hycet®: Hydrocodone bitartrate 7.5 mg and acetaminophen 325 mg per 15 mL (473 mL) [contains ethanol 7%, propylene glycol; tropical fruit punch flavor]
Zamicet™: Hydrocodone bitartrate 10 mg and acetaminophen 325 mg per 15 mL (473 mL) [contains ethanol 6.7%, propylene glycol; fruit flavor]
Zolvit®: Hydrocodone bitartrate 10 mg and acetaminophen 300 mg per 15 mL (480 mL) [contains ethanol 7%, propylene glycol; tropical fruit punch flavor]
Tablet, oral:
Hydrocodone bitartrate 2.5 mg and acetaminophen 325 mg
Hydrocodone bitartrate 2.5 mg and acetaminophen 500 mg
Hydrocodone bitartrate 5 mg and acetaminophen 300 mg
Hydrocodone bitartrate 5 mg and acetaminophen 325 mg
Hydrocodone bitartrate 5 mg and acetaminophen 500 mg
Hydrocodone bitartrate 7.5 mg and acetaminophen 300 mg
Hydrocodone bitartrate 7.5 mg and acetaminophen 325 mg
Hydrocodone bitartrate 7.5 mg and acetaminophen 500 mg
Hydrocodone bitartrate 7.5 mg and acetaminophen 650 mg
Hydrocodone bitartrate 7.5 mg and acetaminophen 750 mg
Hydrocodone bitartrate 10 mg and acetaminophen 300 mg
Hydrocodone bitartrate 10 mg and acetaminophen 325 mg
Hydrocodone bitartrate 10 mg and acetaminophen 500 mg
Hydrocodone bitartrate 10 mg and acetaminophen 650 mg
Hydrocodone bitartrate 10 mg and acetaminophen 660 mg
Hydrocodone bitartrate 10 mg and acetaminophen 750 mg
Lorcet® 10/650: Hydrocodone bitartrate 10 mg and acetaminophen 650 mg
Lorcet® Plus: Hydrocodone bitartrate 7.5 mg and acetaminophen 650 mg
Lortab®:
5/500: Hydrocodone bitartrate 5 mg and acetaminophen 500 mg
7.5/500: Hydrocodone bitartrate 7.5 mg and acetaminophen 500 mg
10/500: Hydrocodone bitartrate 10 mg and acetaminophen 500 mg
Maxidone®: Hydrocodone bitartrate 10 mg and acetaminophen 750 mg
Norco®:
Hydrocodone bitartrate 5 mg and acetaminophen 325 mg
Hydrocodone bitartrate 7.5 mg and acetaminophen 325 mg
Hydrocodone bitartrate 10 mg and acetaminophen 325 mg
Vicodin®: Hydrocodone bitartrate 5 mg and acetaminophen 300 mg
Vicodin ES®: Hydrocodone bitartrate 7.5 mg and acetaminophen 300 mg
Vicodin HP®: Hydrocodone bitartrate 10 mg and acetaminophen 300 mg
Xodol®:
5/300: Hydrocodone bitartrate 5 mg and acetaminophen 300 mg
7.5/300: Hydrocodone bitartrate 7.5 mg and acetaminophen 300 mg
10/300: Hydrocodone bitartrate 10 mg and acetaminophen 300 mg
Zydone®:
Hydrocodone bitartrate 5 mg and acetaminophen 400 mg
Hydrocodone bitartrate 7.5 mg and acetaminophen 400 mg
Hydrocodone bitartrate 10 mg and acetaminophen 400 mg

Controlled Substance C-III

Hydrocodone and Chlorpheniramine

(hye droe KOE done & klor fen IR a meen)

Brand Names: U.S. TussiCaps; Tussionex Pennkinetic; Vituz

Index Terms Chlorpheniramine Maleate and Hydrocodone Bitartrate; Hydrocodone Polistirex and Chlorpheniramine Polistirex; Tussionex

Pharmacologic Category Alkylamine Derivative; Analgesic, Opioid; Antitussive; Histamine H_1 Antagonist; Histamine H_1 Antagonist, First Generation

Use Symptomatic relief of cough and upper respiratory symptoms associated with cold and allergy

Pregnancy Risk Factor C

Dosage Oral:
Children 6 to <12 years:
Capsules: Extended release: Hydrocodone 5 mg and chlorpheniramine 4 mg: One capsule every 12 hours (maximum: 2 capsules daily)
Suspension: Extended release: 2.5 mL every 12 hours; do not exceed 5 mL daily
Children ≥12 years, Adolescents, and Adults:
Capsules: Extended release: Hydrocodone 10 mg and chlorpheniramine 8 mg: One capsule every 12 hours (maximum: 2 capsules daily)
Suspension: Extended release: 5 mL every 12 hours; do not exceed 10 mL daily
Adults: Immediate release: Solution: 5 mL every 4-6 hours as needed; do not exceed 20 mL daily

Additional Information Complete prescribing information should be consulted for additional detail.

Dosage Forms Excipient information presented when available (limited, particularly for generics); consult specific product labeling.
Capsule, extended release, oral:
TussiCaps® 5/4: Hydrocodone polistirex [equivalent to hydrocodone bitartrate 5 mg] and chlorpheniramine polistirex [equivalent to chlorpheniramine maleate 4 mg]
TussiCaps® 10/8: Hydrocodone polistirex [equivalent to hydrocodone bitartrate 10 mg] and chlorpheniramine polistirex [equivalent to chlorpheniramine maleate 8 mg]
Solution, oral:
Vituz®: Hydrocodone bitartrate 5 mg and chlorpheniramine maleate 4 mg per 5 mL (480 mL) [contains propylene glycol; grape flavor]

Suspension, extended release, oral: Hydrocodone polistirex [equivalent to hydrocodone bitartrate 10 mg] and chlorpheniramine polistirex [equivalent to chlorpheniramine maleate 8 mg] per 5 mL (480 mL)

Tussionex® Pennkinetic®: Hydrocodone polistirex [equivalent to hydrocodone bitartrate 10 mg] and chlorpheniramine polistirex [equivalent to chlorpheniramine maleate 8 mg] per 5 mL (115 mL, 480 mL [DSC]) [contains propylene glycol]

Controlled Substance C-III

Hydrocodone and Homatropine

(hye droe KOE done & hoe MA troe peen)

Brand Names: U.S. Hydromet®; Tussigon®

Index Terms Homatropine and Hydrocodone; Hycodan; Hydrocodone Bitartrate and Homatropine Methylbromide

Pharmacologic Category Antitussive

Use Symptomatic relief of cough

Pregnancy Risk Factor C

Dosage Oral:

Children 6-11 years: 1/2 tablet or 2.5 mL every 4-6 hours as needed (maximum: 3 tablets or 15 mL/24 hours)

Children ≥12 years and Adults: 1 tablet or 5 mL every 4-6 hours as needed (maximum: 6 tablets/24 hours or 30 mL/24 hours)

Dosage adjustment in renal impairment: No dosage adjustment provided in manufacturer's labeling; use with caution.

Dosage adjustment in hepatic impairment: No dosage adjustment provided in manufacturer's labeling; use with caution.

Additional Information Complete prescribing information should be consulted for additional detail.

Dosage Forms Excipient information presented when available (limited, particularly for generics); consult specific product labeling. [DSC] = Discontinued product

Syrup:

Hydromet®: Hydrocodone bitartrate 5 mg and homatropine methylbromide 1.5 mg per 5 mL (480 mL) [cherry flavor]

Generic: Hydrocodone bitartrate 5 mg and homatropine methylbromide 1.5 mg per 5 mL (473 mL)

Tablet:

Tussigon®: Hydrocodone bitartrate 5 mg and homatropine methylbromide 1.5 mg

Generic: Hydrocodone bitartrate 5 mg and homatropine methylbromide 1.5 mg

Controlled Substance C-III

Hydrocodone and Ibuprofen

(hye droe KOE done & eye byoo PROE fen)

Brand Names: U.S. Ibudone; Reprexain; Vicoprofen

Brand Names: Canada Vicoprofen

Index Terms Hydrocodone Bitartrate and Ibuprofen; Ibuprofen and Hydrocodone

Pharmacologic Category Analgesic Combination (Opioid); Nonsteroidal Anti-inflammatory Drug (NSAID), Oral

Use Short-term (generally <10 days) management of moderate-to-severe acute pain; is not indicated for treatment of such conditions as osteoarthritis or rheumatoid arthritis

Pregnancy Risk Factor C

Medication Guide Available Yes

Dosage Oral:

Adults: 1 tablet every 4-6 hours as needed for pain; maximum: 5 tablets/day. **Note:** Short-term use is recommended (<10 days).

Elderly: Use with caution; consider reduced doses. Refer to dosing in individual monographs.

Additional Information Complete prescribing information should be consulted for additional detail.

Dosage Forms Excipient information presented when available (limited, particularly for generics); consult specific product labeling.

Tablet: Hydrocodone bitartrate 2.5 mg and ibuprofen 200 mg; Hydrocodone bitartrate 5 mg and ibuprofen 200 mg; Hydrocodone bitartrate 7.5 mg and ibuprofen 200 mg; Hydrocodone bitartrate 10 mg and ibuprofen 200 mg

Ibudone:

5/200: Hydrocodone bitartrate 5 mg and ibuprofen 200 mg

10/200: Hydrocodone bitartrate 10 mg and ibuprofen 200 mg

Reprexain:

2.5/200: Hydrocodone bitartrate 2.5 mg and ibuprofen 200 mg

5/200: Hydrocodone bitartrate 5 mg and ibuprofen 200 mg

10/200: Hydrocodone bitartrate 10 mg and ibuprofen 200 mg

Vicoprofen: 7.5/200: Hydrocodone bitartrate 7.5 mg and ibuprofen 200 mg

Controlled Substance C-III

◆ **Hydrocodone Bitartrate and Homatropine Methylbromide** *see* Hydrocodone and Homatropine *on page 1008*

◆ **Hydrocodone Bitartrate and Ibuprofen** *see* Hydrocodone and Ibuprofen *on page 1008*

◆ **Hydrocodone Polistirex and Chlorpheniramine Polistirex** *see* Hydrocodone and Chlorpheniramine *on page 1007*

Hydrocortisone (Systemic)

(hye droe KOR ti sone)

Brand Names: U.S. A-Hydrocort; Cortef; Solu-CORTEF

Brand Names: Canada Cortef®; Solu-Cortef®

Index Terms A-hydroCort; Compound F; Cortisol; Hydrocortisone Sodium Succinate

Pharmacologic Category Corticosteroid, Systemic

Additional Appendix Information

Contrast Media Reactions, Premedication for Prophylaxis *on page 2373*

Corticosteroids Systemic Equivalencies *on page 2297*

Use Management of adrenocortical insufficiency; anti-inflammatory or immunosuppressive

Unlabeled Use Management of septic shock when blood pressure is poorly responsive to fluid resuscitation and vasopressor therapy; treatment of thyroid storm

Pregnancy Risk Factor C

Pregnancy Considerations Adverse events have been observed with corticosteroids in animal reproduction studies. Some studies have shown an association between first trimester systemic corticosteroid use and oral clefts (Park-Wyllie, 2000; Pradat, 2003). Systemic corticosteroids may also influence fetal growth (decreased birth weight); however, information is conflicting (Lunghi, 2010). Hypoadrenalism may occur in newborns following maternal use of corticosteroids in pregnancy (monitor). When systemic corticosteroids are needed in pregnancy, it is generally recommended to use the lowest effective dose for the shortest duration of time, avoiding high doses during the first trimester (Leachman, 2006; Lunghi, 2010; Makol, 2011; Østensen, 2009).

Breast-Feeding Considerations Corticosteroids are excreted in breast milk. The manufacturer notes that when used systemically, maternal use of corticosteroids have the potential to cause adverse events in a nursing infant (eg, growth suppression, interfere with endogenous corticosteroid production). If there is concern about exposure to the infant, some guidelines recommend waiting 4 hours after the maternal dose of an oral systemic corticosteroid before breast-feeding in order to decrease potential exposure to the nursing infant (based on a study using prednisolone) (Bae, 2011; Leachman, 2006; Makol, 2011; Ost, 1985).

Contraindications Hypersensitivity to hydrocortisone or any component of the formulation; serious infections, except septic shock or tuberculous meningitis; viral, fungal, or tubercular skin lesions; I.M. administration contraindicated in idiopathic thrombocytopenia purpura; intrathecal administration of injection

Warnings/Precautions Use with caution in patients with thyroid disease, hepatic impairment, renal impairment, heart failure, hypertension, diabetes, glaucoma, cataracts, myasthenia gravis, patients at risk for osteoporosis, patients at risk for seizures, or GI diseases (diverticulitis, peptic ulcer, ulcerative colitis) due to perforation risk. Use caution following acute MI (corticosteroids have been associated with myocardial rupture). Because of the risk of adverse effects, systemic corticosteroids should be used cautiously in the elderly in the smallest possible effective dose for the shortest duration. May affect growth velocity; growth should be routinely monitored in pediatric patients. Withdraw therapy with gradual tapering of dose.

May cause hypercorticism or suppression of hypothalamic-pituitary-adrenal (HPA) axis, particularly in younger children or in patients receiving high doses for prolonged periods. HPA axis suppression may lead to adrenal crisis. Withdrawal and discontinuation of a corticosteroid should be done slowly and carefully. Particular care is required when patients are transferred from systemic corticosteroids to inhaled products due to possible adrenal insufficiency or withdrawal from steroids, including an increase in allergic symptoms. Patients receiving >20 mg per day of prednisone (or equivalent) may be most susceptible. Fatalities have occurred due to adrenal insufficiency in asthmatic patients during and after transfer from systemic corticosteroids to aerosol steroids; aerosol steroids do not provide the systemic steroid needed to treat patients having trauma, surgery, or infections.

Acute myopathy has been reported with high dose corticosteroids, usually in patients with neuromuscular transmission disorders; may involve ocular and/or respiratory muscles; monitor creatine kinase; recovery may be delayed. Corticosteroid use may cause psychiatric disturbances, including depression, euphoria, insomnia, mood swings, and personality changes. Pre-existing psychiatric conditions may be exacerbated by corticosteroid use. Prolonged use of corticosteroids may also increase the incidence of secondary infection, mask acute infection (including fungal infections), prolong or exacerbate viral infections, or limit response to vaccines. Exposure to chickenpox should be avoided; corticosteroids should not be used to treat ocular herpes simplex. Corticosteroids should not be used for cerebral malaria or viral hepatitis. Oral steroid treatment is not recommended for the treatment of acute optic neuritis. Close observation is required in patients with latent tuberculosis and/or TB reactivity; restrict use in active TB (only in conjunction with antituberculosis treatment). Prolonged treatment with corticosteroids has been associated with the development of Kaposi's sarcoma (case reports); if noted, discontinuation of therapy should be considered. High-dose corticosteroids should not be used to manage acute head injury. Some dosage forms contain benzyl alcohol which has been associated with "gasping syndrome" in neonates.

Adverse Reactions Frequency not defined.

Cardiovascular: Arrhythmias, bradycardia, cardiac arrest, cardiomegaly, circulatory collapse, congestive heart failure, edema, fat embolism, hypertension, hypertrophic cardiomyopathy (premature infants), myocardial rupture (post MI), syncope, tachycardia, thromboembolism, vasculitis

Central nervous system: Delirium, depression, emotional instability, euphoria, hallucinations, headache, insomnia, intracranial pressure increased, malaise, mood swings, nervousness, neuritis, neuropathy, personality changes, pseudotumor cerebri, psychic disorders, psychoses, seizure, vertigo

Dermatologic: Acne, allergic dermatitis, alopecia, bruising, burning/tingling, dry scaly skin, edema, erythema, hirsutism, hyper-/hypopigmentation, impaired wound healing, petechiae, rash, skin atrophy, skin test reaction impaired, sterile abscess, striae, urticaria

Endocrine & metabolic: Adrenal suppression, alkalosis, amenorrhea, carbohydrate intolerance increased, Cushing's syndrome, diabetes mellitus, glucose intolerance, growth suppression, hyperglycemia, hyperlipidemia, hypokalemia, hypokalemic alkalosis, menstrual irregularities, negative nitrogen balance, pituitary-adrenal axis suppression, potassium loss, protein catabolism, sodium and water retention, sperm motility increased/decreased, spermatogenesis increased/decreased

Gastrointestinal: Abdominal distention, appetite increased, bowel dysfunction (intrathecal administration), indigestion, nausea, pancreatitis, peptic ulcer, gastrointestinal perforation, ulcerative esophagitis, vomiting, weight gain

Genitourinary: Bladder dysfunction (intrathecal administration)

Hematologic: Leukocytosis (transient)

Hepatic: Hepatomegaly, transaminases increased

Local: Atrophy (at injection site), postinjection flare (intra-articular use), thrombophlebitis

Neuromuscular & skeletal: Arthralgia, necrosis (femoral and humoral heads), Charcot-like arthropathy, fractures, muscle mass loss, muscle weakness, myopathy, osteoporosis, tendon rupture, vertebral compression fractures

Ocular: Cataracts, exophthalmoses, glaucoma, intraocular pressure increased

Miscellaneous: Abnormal fat deposits, anaphylaxis, avascular necrosis, diaphoresis, hiccups, hypersensitivity reactions, infection, secondary malignancy

Drug Interactions

Metabolism/Transport Effects Substrate of CYP3A4 (minor), P-glycoprotein; **Note:** Assignment of Major/Minor substrate status based on clinically relevant drug interaction potential; **Induces** CYP3A4 (weak/moderate)

Avoid Concomitant Use

Avoid concomitant use of Hydrocortisone (Systemic) with any of the following: Aldesleukin; Axitinib; BCG; Mifepristone; Natalizumab; Pimecrolimus; Simeprevir; Tacrolimus (Topical); Tofacitinib

Increased Effect/Toxicity

Hydrocortisone (Systemic) may increase the levels/effects of: Acetylcholinesterase Inhibitors; Amphotericin B; Deferasirox; Leflunomide; Loop Diuretics; Natalizumab; NSAID (COX-2 Inhibitor); NSAID (Nonselective); Thiazide Diuretics; Tofacitinib; Vaccines (Live); Warfarin

The levels/effects of Hydrocortisone (Systemic) may be increased by: Antifungal Agents (Azole Derivatives, Systemic); Aprepitant; Calcium Channel Blockers (Nondihydropyridine); Denosumab; Estrogen Derivatives; Fluconazole; Fosaprepitant; Indacaterol; Macrolide Antibiotics; Mifepristone; Neuromuscular-Blocking Agents (Nondepolarizing); P-glycoprotein/ABCB1 Inhibitors; Pimecrolimus; Quinolone Antibiotics; Roflumilast; Salicylates; Tacrolimus (Topical); Telaprevir; Trastuzumab

Decreased Effect

Hydrocortisone (Systemic) may decrease the levels/effects of: Aldesleukin; Antidiabetic Agents; ARIPiprazole; Axitinib; BCG; Calcitriol; Coccidioidin Skin Test; Corticorelin; Hyaluronidase; Ibrutinib; Isoniazid; Salicylates; Simeprevir; Sipuleucel-T; Telaprevir; Urea Cycle Disorder Agents; Vaccines (Inactivated)

The levels/effects of Hydrocortisone (Systemic) may be decreased by: Aminoglutethimide; Antacids; Barbiturates; Bile Acid Sequestrants; Echinacea; Mifepristone; Mitotane; P-glycoprotein/ABCB1 Inducers; Primidone; Rifamycin Derivatives

Ethanol/Nutrition/Herb Interactions

Ethanol: Avoid ethanol (may enhance gastric mucosal irritation).

Food: Hydrocortisone interferes with calcium absorption.

Herb/Nutraceutical: St John's wort may decrease hydrocortisone levels. Avoid cat's claw, echinacea (have immunostimulant properties).

Preparation for Administration

Sodium succinate: I.V. bolus or I.M. administration: Reconstitute 100 mg vials with bacteriostatic water (not >2 mL). Act-O-Vial (self-contained powder for injection plus diluent) may be reconstituted by pressing the activator to force diluent into the powder compartment. Following gentle agitation, solution may be withdrawn via syringe through a needle inserted into the center of the stopper. May be administered (I.V. or I.M.) without further dilution.

Solutions for I.V. infusion: Reconstituted solutions may be added to an appropriate volume of compatible solution for infusion. Concentration should generally not exceed 1 mg/mL. However, in cases where administration of a small volume of fluid is desirable, 100-3000 mg may be added to 50 mL of D_5W or NS (stability limited to 4 hours).

Storage/Stability Store at controlled room temperature 20°C to 25°C (68°F to 77°F). Protect from light. Hydrocortisone sodium phosphate and hydrocortisone sodium succinate are clear, light yellow solutions which are heat labile.

Sodium succinate: After initial reconstitution, hydrocortisone sodium succinate solutions are stable for 3 days at room temperature or under refrigeration when protected from light. Stability of parenteral admixture (Solu-Cortef®) at room temperature (25°C) and at refrigeration temperature (4°C) is concentration-dependent:

Stability of concentration 1 mg/mL: 24 hours

Stability of concentration 2 mg/mL to 60 mg/mL: At least 4 hours

Mechanism of Action Decreases inflammation by suppression of migration of polymorphonuclear leukocytes and reversal of increased capillary permeability

Pharmacodynamics/Kinetics

Onset of action: Hydrocortisone sodium succinate (water soluble): Rapid

Absorption: Rapid

Metabolism: Hepatic

Half-life elimination: Biologic: 8-12 hours

Excretion: Urine (primarily as 17-hydroxysteroids and 17-ketosteroids)

Dosage Dose should be based on severity of disease and patient response

Adrenal insufficiency (acute): I.M., I.V.:

Infants and Young Children: 1-2 mg/kg/dose bolus, then 25-150 mg/day in divided doses every 6-8 hours

Older Children: 1-2 mg/kg bolus then 150-250 mg/day in divided doses every 6-8 hours

Adults: 100 mg I.V. bolus, then 300 mg/day in divided doses every 8 hours or as a continuous infusion for 48 hours; once patient is stable change to oral, 50 mg every 8 hours for 6 doses, then taper to 30-50 mg/day in divided doses

Adrenal insufficiency (chronic), physiologic replacement (unlabeled dosing): Adults: Oral: 15-25 mg/day in 2-3 divided doses. **Note:** Studies suggest administering one-half to two-thirds of the daily dose in the morning in order to mimic the physiological cortisol secretion pattern. If the twice-daily regimen is utilized, the second dose should be administered 6-8 hours following the first dose (Arlt, 2003).

Anti-inflammatory or immunosuppressive:

Infants and Children:

Oral: 2.5-10 mg/kg/day **or** 75-300 mg/m²/day every 6-8 hours

I.M., I.V.: 1-5 mg/kg/day **or** 30-150 mg/m²/day divided every 12-24 hours

Adolescents and Adults: Oral, I.M., I.V.: 15-240 mg every 12 hours

Congenital adrenal hyperplasia (unlabeled dosing): Oral: **Note:** Doses must be individualized by monitoring growth, bone age, and hormonal levels.

Children: 10-15 mg/m²/day in 3 divided doses; higher initial doses may be required to achieve initial target hormone serum concentrations in infancy (Speiser, 2010)

Adolescents and Adults: 15-25 mg/day in 2-3 divided doses (Speiser, 2010)

Physiologic replacement: Children: Oral: 8-10 mg/m²/day divided every 8 hours; up to 12 mg/m²/day in some patients (Ahmet, 2011; Gupta, 2008; Maguire, 2007)

Status asthmaticus: Children and Adults: I.V.: 1-2 mg/kg/dose every 6 hours for 24 hours, then maintenance of 0.5-1 mg/kg every 6 hours

Stress dosing (surgery) in patients known to be adrenally-suppressed or on chronic systemic steroids: I.V.: Adults:

Minor stress (ie, inguinal herniorrhaphy): 25 mg/day for 1 day

Moderate stress (ie, joint replacement, cholecystectomy): 50-75 mg/day (25 mg every 8-12 hours) for 1-2 days

Major stress (pancreatoduodenectomy, esophagogastrectomy, cardiac surgery): 100-150 mg/day (50 mg every 8-12 hours) for 2-3 days

Septic shock (unlabeled use): I.V.:

Children: Initial: 1-2 mg/kg/day (intermittent or as continuous infusion); may titrate up to 50 mg/kg/day for shock reversal (Brierley, 2009); alternative dosing suggests 50 mg/m²/day (Dellinger, 2013). **Note:** Use recommended only in fluid refractory, catecholamine-resistant shock, and suspected or proven absolute (classic) adrenal insufficiency.

Adults: 50 mg every 6 hours (Annane, 2002; COIITSS Study Investigators, 2010). Practice guidelines suggest administering 200 mg daily as a continuous infusion over 24 hours to prevent adverse effects (eg, hyperglycemia) (Dellinger, 2013; Weber-Carstens, 2007); however, the impact of continuous infusion on patient outcomes has not been formally evaluated. Taper slowly (over several days) when vasopressors are no longer required; do not stop abruptly. **Note:** Hydrocortisone should be used alone (ie, without fludrocortisone) (Dellinger, 2013).

Thyroid storm (unlabeled use): I.V.: 300 mg loading dose, followed by 100 mg every 8 hours (Bahn, 2011)

Dosage adjustment in renal impairment: No dosage adjustment provided in manufacturer's labeling; use with caution.

Dosage adjustment in hepatic impairment: No dosage adjustment provided in manufacturer's labeling.

Dietary Considerations Systemic use of corticosteroids may require a diet with increased potassium, vitamins A, B_6, C, D, folate, calcium, zinc, phosphorus, and decreased sodium. Some products may contain sodium.

Administration

Oral: Administer with food or milk to decrease GI upset.

Parenteral: Hydrocortisone sodium succinate may be administered by I.M. or I.V. routes. Dermal and/or subdermal skin depression may occur at the site of injection. Avoid injection into deltoid muscle (high incidence of subcutaneous atrophy).

I.V. bolus: Administer over 30 seconds or over 10 minutes for doses ≥500 mg

I.V. intermittent infusion: Administer over 20-30 minutes

Monitoring Parameters Serum glucose, electrolytes; blood pressure, weight, presence of infection; monitor IOP with therapy >6 weeks; bone mineral density, growth in children

Test Interactions Interferes with skin tests

Dosage Forms Excipient information presented when available (limited, particularly for generics); consult specific product labeling.

Solution Reconstituted, Injection, as sodium succinate [strength expressed as base]:

A-Hydrocort: 100 mg (1 ea)

Solu-CORTEF: 100 mg (1 ea)

Solution Reconstituted, Injection, as sodium succinate [strength expressed as base, preservative free]:

Solu-CORTEF: 100 mg (1 ea); 250 mg (1 ea); 500 mg (1 ea); 1000 mg (1 ea)

Tablet, Oral, as base:

Cortef: 5 mg, 10 mg, 20 mg [scored]

Generic: 5 mg, 10 mg, 20 mg

Extemporaneous Preparations A 2.5 mg/mL oral suspension may be made with either tablets or powder and a vehicle containing sodium carboxymethylcellulose (1 g), syrup BP (10 mL), hydroxybenzoate 0.1% preservatives (0.1 g), polysorbate 80 (0.5 mL), citric acid (0.6 g), and water. To make the vehicle, dissolve the hydroxybenzoate, citric acid, and syrup BP in hot water. Cool solution and add the carboxymethylcellulose; leave overnight. Crush twelve-and-one-half 20 mg hydrocortisone tablets (or use 250 mg of powder) in a mortar and reduce to a fine powder while adding polysorbate 80. Add small portions of vehicle and mix to a uniform paste; mix while adding the vehicle in incremental proportions to **almost** 100 mL; transfer to a calibrated bottle, rinse mortar with vehicle, and add sufficient quantity of vehicle to make 100 mL. Label "shake well" and "refrigerate". Stable for 90 days.

Fawcett JP, Boulton DW, Jiang R, et al, "Stability of Hydrocortisone Oral Suspensions Prepared From Tablets and Powder," *Ann Pharmacother*, 1995, 29(10):987-90.

Hydrocortisone (Topical) (hye droe KOR ti sone)

Brand Names: U.S. Ala Cort; Ala Scalp; Anti-Itch Maximum Strength [OTC]; Anucort-HC; Anusol-HC; Aquanil HC [OTC]; Beta HC [OTC]; Colocort; CortAlo; Cortenema; Corticool [OTC]; Cortifoam; Dermasorb HC; First-Hydrocortisone; GRx HiCort 25; Hemril-30; Hydro Skin Maximum Strength [OTC]; Hydrocortisone Max St [OTC]; Hydrocortisone Max St/12 Moist [OTC]; HydroSKIN [OTC]; Instacort 10 [OTC]; Instacort 5 [OTC]; Locoid; Locoid Lipocream; Med-Derm Hydrocortisone [OTC]; Medi-First Hydrocortisone [OTC]; NuCort; NuZon; Pandel; Pediaderm HC; Preparation H Hydrocortisone [OTC]; Procto-Pak; Proctocort; Proctocream HC [DSC]; Proctosol HC; Proctozone-HC; Recort Plus [OTC]; Rectacort-HC; Rederm [OTC]; Sarnol-HC [OTC]; Scalacort; Scalacort DK; Scalpicin Maximum Strength [OTC]; Texacort; TheraCort [OTC]; U-Cort; Westcort

Brand Names: Canada Aquacort®; Cortamed®; Cortenema®; Cortifoam™; Emo-Cort®; Hycort™; Hyderm; HydroVal®; Locoid®; Prevex® HC; Sarna® HC; Westcort®

Index Terms A-hydroCort; Compound F; Cortisol; Hemorrhoidal HC; Hydrocortisone Acetate; Hydrocortisone Butyrate; Hydrocortisone Probutate; Hydrocortisone Valerate; Nutracort

Pharmacologic Category Antihemorrhoidal Agent; Corticosteroid, Rectal; Corticosteroid, Topical

Use Relief of inflammation of corticosteroid-responsive dermatoses (low and medium potency topical corticosteroid); adjunctive treatment of ulcerative colitis; mild-to-moderate atopic dermatitis; inflamed hemorrhoids, postirradiation (factitial) proctitis, and other inflammatory conditions of anorectum and pruritus ani

Pregnancy Risk Factor C

Dosage

Topical:

Children 3 months to 18 years: Atopic dermatitis: Hydrocortisone butyrate (Locoid Lipocream®): Apply thin film to affected area twice daily

Children and Adults: Dermatosis: Apply thin film to affected area 2-4 times/day. Products labeled for OTC use (self-medication) should not be used in children <2 years of age.

Children ≥12 years and Adults: External anal and genital itching: (OTC labeling): Apply to clean dry skin up to 3-4 times/day

Adults: Dermatosis:

Hydrocortisone probutate (Pandel®): Apply thin film to affected area 1-2 times/day

Hydrocortisone valerate (Westcort®): Apply thin film to affected area 2-3 times/day

Rectal: Adults:

Hemorrhoids: Suppository: One suppository (30 mg) twice daily for 2 weeks. For severe cases of proctitis, 1 suppository 3 times/day or 2 suppositories twice daily may be needed. For factitial proctitis, duration of treatment may be up to 6-8 weeks.

Ulcerative colitis:

Foam: One applicatorful (80 mg) 1-2 times/day for 2-3 weeks, and then every other day thereafter; use lowest dose to maintain clinical response; taper dose to discontinue long-term therapy

Suspension: One enema (100 mg) every night for 21 days or until remission (clinical improvement may precede improvement of mucosal integrity); 2-3 months of therapy may be required; taper dose to discontinue long-term therapy

Additional Information Complete prescribing information should be consulted for additional detail.

Dosage Forms Excipient information presented when available (limited, particularly for generics); consult specific product labeling. [DSC] = Discontinued product

Cream, External, as acetate:

Hydrocortisone Max St: 1% (28.4 g)

U-Cort: 1% (28.35 g)

Cream, External, as acetate [strength expressed as base]:

Generic: 1% (30 g)

Cream, External, as base:

Ala Cort: 1% (28.4 g, 85.2 g) [contains cetyl alcohol, propylene glycol]

Anti-Itch Maximum Strength: 1% (28 g) [contains cetyl alcohol, methylparaben]

Anti-Itch Maximum Strength: 1% (28 g) [contains cetyl alcohol, methylparaben, propylene glycol, propylparaben]

Hydrocortisone Max St/12 Moist: 1% (28.4 g) [contains cetearyl alcohol, methylparaben, propylene glycol, propylparaben]

HydroSKIN: 1% (28 g) [contains benzyl alcohol]

Instacort 5: 0.5% (28.4 g)

Med-Derm Hydrocortisone: 0.5% (30 g); 1% (30 g)

Medi-First Hydrocortisone: 1% (1 ea) [contains trolamine (triethanolamine)]

Preparation H Hydrocortisone: 1% (26 g)

Recort Plus: 1% (30 g)

Generic: 0.5% (15 g, 28.35 g, 28.4 g, 30 g); 1% (1 g, 1.5 g, 15 g, 20 g, 28 g, 28.35 g, 28.4 g, 30 g, 120 g, 453.6 g, 454 g); 2.5% (20 g, 28 g, 28.35 g, 30 g, 453.6 g)
Cream, Rectal, as base:
Anusol-HC: 2.5% (30 g)
Procto-Pak: 1% (28.4 g)
Proctocort: 1% (28.35 g) [contains cetyl alcohol, propylene glycol]
Proctocream HC: 2.5% (30 g [DSC]) [contains benzyl alcohol]
Proctosol HC: 2.5% (28.35 g)
Proctozone-HC: 2.5% (30 g)
Cream, External, as butyrate:
Locoid: 0.1% (15 g [DSC], 45 g [DSC])
Locoid: 0.1% (15 g, 45 g) [contains butylparaben, propylparaben]
Locoid Lipocream: 0.1% (45 g, 60 g)
Generic: 0.1% (15 g, 45 g, 60 g)
Cream, External, as probutate:
Pandel: 0.1% (15 g, 45 g, 80 g) [contains butylparaben, methylparaben, propylene glycol]
Cream, External, as valerate:
Generic: 0.2% (15 g, 45 g, 60 g)
Enema, Rectal, as base:
Colocort: 100 mg/60 mL (60 mL)
Cortenema: 100 mg/60 mL (60 mL) [contains methylparaben, polysorbate 80]
Generic: 100 mg/60 mL (60 mL)
Foam, Rectal, as acetate:
Cortifoam: 90 mg (15 g) [contains cetyl alcohol, methylparaben, propylene glycol, propylparaben, trolamine (triethanolamine)]
Gel, External, as acetate:
CortAlo: 2% (43 g) [contains benzyl alcohol, menthol, trolamine (triethanolamine)]
NuZon: 2% (43 g) [contains menthol, trolamine (triethanolamine)]
Generic: 2% (43 g)
Gel, External, as base:
Corticool: 1% (42.53 g) [contains cremophor el, propylene glycol]
First-Hydrocortisone: 10% (60 g) [contains propylene glycol, simethicone]
Instacort 10: 1% (30 g)
Kit, External, as base:
Dermasorb HC: 2% [contains menthol, methylparaben, propylene glycol, propylparaben]
Pediaderm HC: 2% [contains benzalkonium chloride, cetyl alcohol, isopropyl alcohol, methylparaben, propylene glycol, propylparaben]
Scalacort DK: Hydrocortisone lotion 2% and Sal Acid 2% and sulfur 2% [contains benzalkonium chloride, isopropyl alcohol, methylparaben, propylene glycol, propylparaben, soybean lecithin]
Lotion, External, as acetate:
NuCort: 2% (60 g) [contains benzyl alcohol, cetyl alcohol, menthol, trolamine (triethanolamine)]
Lotion, External, as base:
Ala Scalp: 2% (29.6 mL) [contains benzalkonium chloride, isopropyl alcohol, propylene glycol]
Aquanil HC: 1% (120 mL)
Beta HC: 1% (60 mL)
Hydro Skin Maximum Strength: 1% (118 mL) [contains benzyl alcohol]
Rederm: 1% (120 mL)
Sarnol-HC: 1% (59 mL)
Scalacort: 2% (29.6 mL) [contains benzalkonium chloride, isopropyl alcohol, propylene glycol]
TheraCort: 1% (118 mL) [contains methylparaben, propylene glycol, propylparaben, trolamine (triethanolamine)]
Generic: 1% (114 g); 2.5% (59 mL, 118 mL)
Lotion, External, as butyrate:
Locoid: 0.1% (59 mL, 118 mL) [contains butylparaben, cetostearyl alcohol, propylparaben]
Ointment, External, as acetate [strength expressed as base]:
Generic: 1% (30 g)
Ointment, External, as base:
Generic: 0.5% (28.35 g, 30 g); 1% (25 g, 28 g, 28.35 g, 28.4 g, 30 g, 110 g, 430 g, 453.6 g); 2.5% (20 g, 28.35 g, 453.6 g, 454 g)
Ointment, External, as butyrate:
Locoid: 0.1% (15 g, 45 g)
Generic: 0.1% (15 g, 45 g)
Ointment, External, as valerate:
Westcort: 0.2% (15 g, 45 g, 60 g) [contains propylene glycol]
Generic: 0.2% (15 g, 45 g, 60 g)
Solution, External, as base:
Scalpicin Maximum Strength: 1% (44 mL) [contains disodium edta, menthol, propylene glycol]
Texacort: 2.5% (30 mL) [lipid free, paraben free; contains alcohol, usp]
Solution, External, as butyrate:
Locoid: 0.1% (60 mL) [contains isopropyl alcohol]
Generic: 0.1% (20 mL, 60 mL)
Suppository, Rectal, as acetate:
Anucort-HC: 25 mg (12 ea, 24 ea, 100 ea)
Anusol-HC: 25 mg (12 ea, 24 ea)
GRx HiCort 25: 25 mg (12 ea)
Hemril-30: 30 mg (12 ea, 24 ea)
Proctocort: 30 mg (12 ea)
Rectacort-HC: 25 mg (12 ea, 24 ea)
Generic: 25 mg (12 ea, 24 ea); 30 mg (12 ea)

- **Hydrocortisone Acetate** *see* Hydrocortisone (Topical) *on page 1011*
- **Hydrocortisone, Acetic Acid, and Propylene Glycol Diacetate** *see* Acetic Acid, Propylene Glycol Diacetate, and Hydrocortisone *on page 35*
- **Hydrocortisone and Benzoyl Peroxide** *see* Benzoyl Peroxide and Hydrocortisone *on page 243*
- **Hydrocortisone and Ciprofloxacin** *see* Ciprofloxacin and Hydrocortisone *on page 435*
- **Hydrocortisone and Iodoquinol** *see* Iodoquinol and Hydrocortisone *on page 1109*
- **Hydrocortisone and Pramoxine** *see* Pramoxine and Hydrocortisone *on page 1699*
- **Hydrocortisone and Urea** *see* Urea and Hydrocortisone *on page 2141*
- **Hydrocortisone, Bacitracin, Neomycin, and Polymyxin B** *see* Bacitracin, Neomycin, Polymyxin B, and Hydrocortisone *on page 221*
- **Hydrocortisone Butyrate** *see* Hydrocortisone (Topical) *on page 1011*
- **Hydrocortisone Max St [OTC]** *see* Hydrocortisone (Topical) *on page 1011*
- **Hydrocortisone Max St/12 Moist [OTC]** *see* Hydrocortisone (Topical) *on page 1011*
- **Hydrocortisone, Neomycin, and Polymyxin B** *see* Neomycin, Polymyxin B, and Hydrocortisone *on page 1440*
- **Hydrocortisone, Neomycin, Colistin, and Thonzonium** *see* Neomycin, Colistin, Hydrocortisone, and Thonzonium *on page 1439*
- **Hydrocortisone Probutate** *see* Hydrocortisone (Topical) *on page 1011*
- **Hydrocortisone Sodium Succinate** *see* Hydrocortisone (Systemic) *on page 1008*
- **Hydrocortisone Valerate** *see* Hydrocortisone (Topical) *on page 1011*

◆ **Hydrodiuril** *see* Hydrochlorothiazide *on page 1004*

◆ **Hydromet®** *see* Hydrocodone and Homatropine *on page 1008*

◆ **Hydromorph Contin (Can)** *see* HYDROmorphone *on page 1013*

HYDROmorphone (hye droe MOR fone)

Brand Names: U.S. Dilaudid; Dilaudid-HP; Exalgo

Brand Names: Canada Dilaudid; Dilaudid-HP; Hydromorph Contin; Hydromorphone HP; Hydromorphone HP 10; Hydromorphone HP 20; Hydromorphone HP 50; Hydromorphone HP Forte; Hydromorphone Hydrochloride Injection, USP; Jurnista; PMS-Hydromorphone; Teva-Hydromorphone

Index Terms Dihydromorphinone; Hydromorphone Hydrochloride

Pharmacologic Category Analgesic, Opioid

Additional Appendix Information

Opioid Conversion Table *on page 2306*

Patient Information for Disposal of Unused Medications *on page 2393*

Use Management of moderate-to-severe pain

Exalgo: Management of moderate-to-severe pain in opioid-tolerant patients (requiring around-the-clock analgesia for an extended period of time)

Pregnancy Risk Factor C

Pregnancy Considerations Adverse events were observed in some animal reproduction studies. Hydromorphone crosses the placenta. Some dosage forms are specifically contraindicated for use in obstetrical analgesia.

When used for pain relief during labor, opioids may temporarily affect the heart rate of the fetus (ACOG, 2002). Monitor the neonate for respiratory depression if hydromorphone is used during labor.

If chronic opioid exposure occurs in pregnancy, adverse events in the newborn (including withdrawal) may occur; monitoring of the neonate is recommended. The minimum effective dose should be used if opioids are needed (Chou, 2009). Neonatal abstinence syndrome following opioid exposure may present with autonomic (eg, fever, temperature instability), gastrointestinal (eg, diarrhea, vomiting, poor feeding/weight gain), or neurologic (eg, high pitched crying, increased muscle tone, irritability, seizure, tremor) symptoms (Dow, 2012; Hudak, 2012).

Breast-Feeding Considerations Low concentrations of hydromorphone can be found in breast milk. Withdrawal symptoms may be observed in breast-feeding infants when opioid analgesics are discontinued. Breast-feeding is not recommended by the manufacturer. Parenteral opioids used during labor have the potential to interfere with a newborn's natural reflex to nurse within the first few hours after birth. Nursing infants exposed to large doses of opioids should be monitored for apnea and sedation (Montgomery, 2012).

Prescribing and Access Restrictions Exalgo: As a requirement of the REMS program, healthcare providers who prescribe Exalgo need to receive training on the proper use and potential risks of Exalgo. For training, please refer to http://www.exalgorems.com. Prescribers will need retraining every 2 years or following any significant changes to the Exalgo REMS program.

Medication Guide Available Yes

Contraindications Hypersensitivity to hydromorphone, any component of the formulation; acute or severe asthma, severe respiratory depression (in absence of resuscitative equipment or ventilatory support)

Additional product-specific contraindications:

Dilaudid liquid and tablets: Obstetrical analgesia

Dilaudid injection, Dilaudid-HP injection: Opioid nontolerant patients (Dilaudid-HP injection only); patients with risk of developing GI obstruction, especially paralytic ileus

Exalgo: Opioid nontolerant patients, paralytic ileus (known or suspected), pre-existing GI surgery or diseases resulting in narrowing of GI tract, loops in the GI tract or GI obstruction

Suppository: Intracranial lesion associated with increased intracranial pressure; whenever ventilatory function is depressed (COPD, cor pulmonale, emphysema, kyphoscoliosis, status asthmaticus)

Warnings/Precautions [U.S. Boxed Warning]: May cause potentially life-threatening respiratory depression even with therapeutic use, especially with initiation or dose increases; instruct patients on proper administration of extended release tablets. The use of ethanol, other opioids, and other CNS depressants may increase the risk of adverse outcomes, including death. Critical respiratory depression may occur, even at therapeutic dosages, particularly in elderly, cachectic, or debilitated patients or in patients with pre-existing respiratory compromise (hypoxia and/or hypercapnia). Use caution in COPD or other obstructive pulmonary disease.

Use with caution in patients with hypersensitivity reactions to other phenanthrene derivative opioid agonists (codeine, hydrocodone, levorphanol, oxycodone, oxymorphone). Hydromorphone shares toxic potential of opioid agonists, including CNS depression and respiratory depression. Precautions associated with opioid agonist therapy should be observed. May cause CNS depression, which may impair physical or mental abilities; patients must be cautioned about performing tasks which require mental alertness (eg, operating machinery or driving). Myoclonus and seizures have been reported with high doses; use with caution in patients with a history of seizure disorder. Use with caution in patients with kyphoscoliosis, cardiovascular disease, morbid obesity, adrenocortical insufficiency, hypothyroidism, acute alcoholism, delirium tremens, toxic psychoses, prostatic hyperplasia and/or urinary stricture, or severe liver or renal failure. Avoid use in patients with CNS depression or coma as these patients are susceptible to intracranial effects of CO_2 retention. Use with caution in patients with biliary tract dysfunction. Hydromorphone may increase biliary tract pressure following spasm in sphincter of Oddi. Use caution in patients with inflammatory or obstructive bowel disorder, acute pancreatitis secondary to biliary tract disease, and patients undergoing biliary surgery. Use extreme caution in patients with head injury, intracranial lesions, or elevated intracranial pressure; exaggerated elevation of ICP may occur (in addition, hydromorphone may complicate neurologic evaluation due to pupillary dilation and CNS depressant effects). Use with caution in patients with depleted blood volume or drugs which may exaggerate hypotensive effects (including phenothiazines or general anesthetics). May obscure diagnosis or clinical course of patients with acute abdominal conditions. Severe and unpredictable potentiation by MAO inhibitors has been reported with opioid analgesics; use within 14 days of MAO inhibitors is not recommended.

[U.S. Boxed Warning]: Hydromorphone has a high potential for abuse; health care provider should be alert to problems of abuse, misuse, and diversion. Risk of opioid abuse is increased in patients with a history or family history of alcohol or drug abuse or mental illness. Tolerance or drug dependence may result from extended use; however, concerns for abuse should not prevent effective management of pain. In general, abrupt discontinuation of therapy in dependent patients should be avoided. After chronic maternal exposure to opioids, neonatal withdrawal syndrome may occur in the newborn; monitor neonate closely. Signs and symptoms include irritability, hyperactivity and abnormal sleep pattern, high pitched cry, tremor, vomiting, diarrhea and failure to gain weight. Onset, duration and severity depend on the drug used, duration of use, maternal dose, and rate of drug elimination by the newborn. Opioid withdrawal syndrome in the neonate, unlike in adults, may be life-threatening and should be treated according to protocols developed by neonatology experts.

An opioid-containing analgesic regimen should be tailored to each patient's needs and based upon the type of pain being treated (acute versus chronic), the route of administration, degree of tolerance for opioids (naive versus chronic user), age, weight, and medical condition. The optimal analgesic dose varies widely among patients. Doses should be titrated to pain relief/prevention. I.M. use may result in variable absorption and a lag time to peak effect.

Dosage form specific warnings:

[U.S. Boxed Warning]: Dilaudid-HP: Extreme caution should be taken to avoid confusing the highly-concentrated (Dilaudid-HP) injection with the less-concentrated (Dilaudid) injectable product. Dilaudid-HP should only be used in patients who are opioid-tolerant.

Controlled release: Capsules should only be used when continuous analgesia is required over an extended period of time. Controlled release products are not to be used on an "as needed" (PRN) basis.

Extended release tablets (Exalgo): **[U.S. Boxed Warning]: For use in opioid tolerant patients only; fatal respiratory depression may occur in patient who are not opioid tolerant. The highest risk of fatal respiratory depression is at initiation and with dose increases. Indicated for the management of moderate-to-severe pain when around the clock pain control is needed for an extended time period. Not for use as an as-needed analgesic or for the management of acute or postoperative pain. Tablets should be swallowed whole; do not crush, break, chew, dissolve or inject; doing so may lead to rapid release and absorption of a potentially fatal dose of hydromorphone. Accidental consumption may lead to fatal overdose, especially in children.** Exalgo tablets are nondeformable; do not administer to patients with pre-existing severe gastrointestinal narrowing (eg, esophageal motility, small bowel inflammatory disease, short gut syndrome, history of peritonitis, cystic fibrosis, chronic intestinal pseudo-obstruction, Meckel's diverticulum); obstruction may occur.

Some dosage forms contain trace amounts of sodium metabisulfite which may cause allergic reactions in susceptible individuals. Vial stoppers of single-dose injectable vials may contain latex.

Adverse Reactions
Frequency not defined.

Cardiovascular: Bradycardia, extrasystoles, flushing (facial), hypertension, hypotension, palpitations, peripheral edema, peripheral vasodilation, syncope, tachycardia

Central nervous system: Abnormal dreams, abnormal gait, abnormality in thinking, aggressive behavior, agitation, apprehension, ataxia, brain disease, burning sensation of skin (Exalgo), central nervous system depression, chills, cognitive dysfunction, confusion, decreased body temperature (Exalgo), depression, disruption of body temperature regulation (Exalgo), dizziness, drowsiness, drug dependence, dysarthria, dysphoria, equilibrium disturbance, euphoria, fatigue, hallucination, headache, hyperesthesia, hyperreflexia, hypoesthesia, hypothermia, increased intracranial pressure, insomnia, lack of concentration, lethargy, malaise, memory impairment, mood changes, myoclonus, nervousness, painful defecation, panic attack, paranoia, paresthesia, psychomotor agitation, restlessness, sedation, seizure, sleep disorder (Exalgo), suicidal ideation, uncontrolled crying, vertigo

Dermatologic: Diaphoresis, erythema (Exalgo), hyperhidrosis, pruritus, skin rash, urticaria

Endocrine & metabolic: Antidiuretic effect, decreased amylase, decreased libido, decreased plasma testosterone, dehydration, fluid retention, hyperuricemia, hypokalemia, weight loss

Gastrointestinal: Abdominal distention, anal fissure, anorexia, bezoar formation (Exalgo), biliary tract spasm, constipation, decreased appetite, decreased gastrointestinal motility (Exalgo), delayed gastric emptying, diarrhea, diverticulitis, diverticulosis, duodenitis, dysgeusia, dysphagia, eructation, flatulence, gastroenteritis, gastroesophageal reflux disease (aggravated; Exalgo), hematochezia, increased appetite, intestinal perforation (large intestine; Exalgo), nausea, paralytic ileus, stomach cramps, vomiting, xerostomia

Genitourinary: Bladder spasm, decreased urine output, difficulty in micturition, dysuria, erectile dysfunction, hypogonadism, sexual disorder, ureteral spasm, urinary frequency, urinary hesitancy, urinary retention

Hematologic & oncologic: Oxygen desaturation

Hepatic: Increased liver enzymes

Hypersensitivity: Histamine release

Local: Pain at injection site, post-injection flare

Neuromuscular & skeletal: Arthralgia, dyskinesia, laryngospasm, muscle rigidity, muscle spasm, myalgia, tremor, weakness

Ophthalmic: Blurred vision, diplopia, dry eye syndrome, miosis, nystagmus

Otic: Tinnitus

Respiratory: Apnea, bronchospasm, dyspnea, flu-like symptoms (Exalgo), hyperventilation, hypoxia, respiratory depression, respiratory distress, rhinorrhea

Postmarketing and/or case reports (Limited to important or life-threatening): Angioedema, hypersensitivity

Drug Interactions

Metabolism/Transport Effects
None known.

Avoid Concomitant Use

Avoid concomitant use of HYDROmorphone with any of the following: Azelastine (Nasal); MAO Inhibitors; Paraldehyde

Increased Effect/Toxicity

HYDROmorphone may increase the levels/effects of: Alcohol (Ethyl); Alvimopan; Azelastine (Nasal); CNS Depressants; Desmopressin; Diuretics; Hydrocodone; Metyrosine; Mirtazapine; Paraldehyde; Pramipexole; ROPINIRole; Rotigotine; Selective Serotonin Reuptake Inhibitors; Zolpidem

The levels/effects of HYDROmorphone may be increased by: Amphetamines; Anticholinergics; Antipsychotic Agents (Phenothiazines); Brimonidine (Topical); Cannabinoids; Doxylamine; Droperidol; HydrOXYzine; Magnesium Sulfate; MAO Inhibitors; Perampanel; Sodium Oxybate; Succinylcholine; Tapentadol

Decreased Effect

HYDROmorphone may decrease the levels/effects of: Pegvisomant

The levels/effects of HYDROmorphone may be decreased by: Ammonium Chloride; Mixed Agonist / Antagonist Opioids

Ethanol/Nutrition/Herb Interactions

Ethanol: Ethanol may increase CNS depression. Management: Monitor for increased effects with coadministration. Caution patients about effects.

Herb/Nutraceutical: Gotu kola, valerian, and kava kava may increase CNS depression. Management: Avoid gotu kola, valerian, and kava kava.

Storage/Stability

Injection: Store at 15°C to 30°C (59°F to 86°F). A slightly yellowish discoloration has not been associated with a loss of potency.

Oral dosage forms: Store at 15°C to 30°C (59°F to 86°F). Protect tablets from light.

Suppository: Store in refrigerator. Protect from light.

Mechanism of Action Binds to opioid receptors in the CNS, causing inhibition of ascending pain pathways, altering the perception of and response to pain; causes cough supression by direct central action in the medulla; produces generalized CNS depression

Pharmacodynamics/Kinetics

Onset of action: Analgesic:

Immediate release formulations:

Oral: 15-30 minutes; Peak effect: 30-60 minutes

I.V.: 5 minutes; Peak effect: 10-20 minutes

Extended release tablet: 6 hours; Peak effect: ~9 hours (Angst, 2001)

Duration:

Immediate release formulations: Oral, I.V.: 3-4 hours

Extended release tablet: ~13 hours (Angst, 2001)

Absorption: Extended release tablet: Delayed; I.M.: Variable and delayed

Distribution: V_d: 4 L/kg

Protein binding: ~8% to 19%

Metabolism: Hepatic via glucuronidation; to inactive metabolites

Bioavailability: 62%

Half-life elimination:

Immediate release formulations: 2-3 hours

Extended release tablets: Apparent half-life: ~11 hours (range: 8-15 hours)

Time to peak, plasma:

Immediate release tablet: ≤1 hour

Extended release tablet: 12-16 hours

Excretion: Urine (primarily as glucuronide conjugates)

Dosage

Acute pain (moderate-to-severe): Note: These are guidelines and do not represent the maximum doses that may be required in all patients. Doses should be titrated to provide adequate pain relief. When changing routes of administration, oral doses and parenteral doses are **NOT** equivalent; parenteral doses are up to 5 times more potent. Therefore, when administered parenterally, one-fifth of the oral dose will provide similar analgesia.

Children >50 kg and Adults:

Oral: Initial: Opioid-naive: 2-4 mg every 4-6 hours as needed; elderly/debilitated patients may require lower doses; patients with prior opioid exposure may require higher initial doses. **Note:** In adults with severe pain, the American Pain Society recommends an initial dose of 4-8 mg.

I.V.: Initial: Opioid-naive: 0.2-1 mg every 2-3 hours as needed; patients with prior opioid exposure may require higher initial doses

Critically ill patients (unlabeled dosing): 0.2-0.6 mg every 1-2 hours as needed **or** 0.5 mg every 3 hours as needed (Barr, 2013)

Continuous infusion: Usual dosage range: 0.5-3 mg/hour (Barr, 2013)

Patient-controlled analgesia (PCA) (unlabeled dosing) (American Pain Society, 2008): **Note:** Opioid-naive: Consider lower end of dosing range. A continuous (basal) infusion is not recommended in opioid-naive patients (ISMP, 2009):

Usual concentration: 0.2 mg/mL

Demand dose: Usual initial dose: 0.2 mg; range: 0.05-0.4 mg

Lockout interval: 5-10 minutes

Epidural PCA (unlabeled dosing) (de Leon-Casasola, 1996; Liu, 2010; Smith, 2009):

Usual concentration: 0.01 mg/mL

Bolus dose: 0.4-1 mg

Infusion rate: 0.03-0.3 mg/**hour**

Demand dose: 0.02-0.05 mg

Lockout interval: 10-15 minutes

I.M., SubQ: **Note:** I.M. use may result in variable absorption and lag time to peak effect; I.M. route not recommended for use (American Pain Society, 2008)

Initial: Opioid-naive: 0.8-1 mg every 3-4 hours as needed; patients with prior opioid exposure may require higher initial doses

Rectal: 3 mg every 6-8 hours as needed

Elderly: Acute pain, opioid-naive:

Oral: Use with caution; initiation at the low end of dosage range is recommended. For patients >70 years, The American Pain Society recommends consideration to lowering initial doses by 25% to 50% followed by upward or downward titration (APS, 2008).

I.V: Reduce initial dose to 0.2 mg

Chronic pain: Adults: Oral: **Note:** Patients taking opioids chronically may become tolerant and require doses higher than the usual dosage range to maintain the desired effect. Tolerance can be managed by appropriate dose titration. There is no optimal or maximal dose for hydromorphone in chronic pain. The appropriate dose is one that relieves pain throughout its dosing interval without causing unmanageable side effects.

Controlled release formulation (Hydromorph Contin, not available in U.S.): 3-30 mg every 12 hours. **Note:** A patient's hydromorphone requirement should be established using prompt release formulations; conversion to long acting products may be considered when chronic, continuous treatment is required. Higher dosages should be reserved for use only in opioid-tolerant patients.

Extended release formulation (Exalgo): Dosing range: 8-64 mg every 24 hours. For use in opioid-tolerant patients only; discontinue all other extended release opioids when starting therapy. Suggested recommendations for converting to Exalgo from other analgesics are presented, but when selecting the initial dose, other characteristics (eg, patient status, degree of opioid tolerance, concurrent medications, type of pain, risk factors for addiction or diversion, etc) should also be considered.

Individualization of dose: Pain relief and adverse events should be assessed frequently. Dose increases may occur not more often than every 3-4 days; consider titrating with increases of 25% to 50% of the current daily dose. If more than 2 doses of rescue medications are needed within 24 hours for 2 consecutive days, consider increasing the dose of Exalgo. Do not administer more frequently than every 24 hours.

Conversion from other oral hydromorphone formulations to Exalgo: Start with the equivalent total daily dose of immediate-release hydromorphone administered once daily. May titrate every 3-4 days until adequate pain relief with tolerable side effects have been achieved.

Conversion from other opioids to Exalgo: In general, start Exalgo at 50% of the calculated total daily dose every 24 hours (see Conversion Ratios to Exalgo table on next page). Titrate until adequate pain relief with tolerable side effects has been achieved. The following conversion ratios may be used to convert from **oral** opioid therapy to Exalgo.

Conversion ratios to Exalgo (see table): Select the opioid, sum the total daily dose, then multiply by the conversion ratio to calculate the *approximate* oral hydromorphone equivalent; start Exalgo at 50% of the calculated total daily dose every 24 hours. (**Note:** The conversion ratios and approximate equivalent doses in this conversion table are only to be used for the conversion from current opioid therapy to Exalgo).

Conversion Ratios to Exalgo[1]

Previous Opioid	Approximate Equivalent Oral Dose	Oral Conversion Ratio[2]
Hydromorphone	12 mg	1
Codeine	200 mg	0.06
Hydrocodone	30 mg	0.4
Methadone[3]	20 mg	0.6
Morphine	60 mg	0.2
Oxycodone	30 mg	0.4
Oxymorphone	20 mg	0.6

[1]*Approximate* equivalent doses for conversion from current opioid therapy to Exalgo®.

[2]Ratio for converting oral opioid dose to approximate hydromorphone equivalent dose.

[3]Monitor closely; ratio between methadone and other opioid agonists may vary widely as a function of previous drug exposure. Methadone has a long half-life and may accumulate in the plasma.

Conversion from transdermal fentanyl to Exalgo: Treatment with Exalgo can be started 18 hours after the removal of the transdermal fentanyl patch. For every fentanyl 25 mcg/hour transdermal dose, the equianalgesic dose of Exalgo is 12 mg every 24 hours. An appropriate starting dose is 50% of the calculated total daily dose given every 24 hours.

Discontinuing Exalgo: Taper by gradually decreasing the dose by 25% to 50% every 2-3 days to a dose of 8 mg every 24 hours before discontinuing therapy.

Dosing adjustment in renal impairment:

Oral (immediate release), injectable: Initiate with 25% to 50% of the usual starting dose depending on the degree of impairment. Monitor closely for respiratory and CNS depression.

Oral (extended release; Exalgo):

Moderate impairment (Cl_{cr} 30-60 mL/minute): Initiate with 50% of the usual starting dose for patients with normal renal function; monitor closely for respiratory and CNS depression.

Severe impairment (Cl_{cr} <30 mL/minute): Initiate with 25% of the usual starting dose for patients with normal renal function; monitor closely for respiratory and CNS depression. Consider use of an alternate analgesic with better dosing flexibility.

Dosing adjustment in hepatic impairment:

Oral (immediate release), injectable:

Moderate impairment: Initiate with 25% to 50% of the usual starting dose for patients with normal hepatic function.

Severe impairment: Has not been studied; initial dose should be more conservative as compared to those with moderate impairment; use with caution.

Oral (extended release; Exalgo):

Moderate impairment: Initiate with 25% of the usual starting dose for patients with normal hepatic function; monitor closely for respiratory and CNS depression.

Severe impairment: Use alternate analgesic.

Administration

Parenteral: **Note: Vial stopper may contain latex.** May be given SubQ or I.M.; I.M. route is not recommended (APS, 2008).

I.V.: For IVP, must be given slowly over 2-3 minutes (rapid IVP has been associated with an increase in side effects, especially respiratory depression and hypotension)

Oral: Hydromorphone is available in an 8 mg immediate release tablet and an 8 mg extended release tablet. Extreme caution should be taken to avoid confusing dosage forms.

Exalgo: Tablets should be swallowed whole; do not crush, break, chew, dissolve or inject. May be taken with or without food.

Hydromorph Contin: Capsule should be swallowed whole; do not crush or chew; contents may be sprinkled on soft food and swallowed

Monitoring Parameters Pain relief, respiratory and mental status, blood pressure

Test Interactions Some quinolones may produce a false-positive urine screening result for opioids using commercially-available immunoassay kits. This has been demonstrated most consistently for levofloxacin and ofloxacin, but other quinolones have shown cross-reactivity in certain assay kits. Confirmation of positive opioid screens by more specific methods should be considered.

Additional Information Equianalgesic doses: Morphine 10 mg I.M. = hydromorphone 1.5 mg I.M.

Exalgo is indicated for the management of moderate-to-severe pain in opioid-tolerant patients (requiring around-the-clock analgesia for an extended period of time). Patients are considered to be opioid tolerant if they have been taking oral morphine ≥60 mg/day, fentanyl transdermal ≥25 mcg/hour, oral oxycodone ≥30 mg/day, oral hydromorphone ≥8 mg/day, oral oxymorphone ≥25 mg/day, or an equianalgesic dose of another opioid for ≥1 week.

Dosage Forms Excipient information presented when available (limited, particularly for generics); consult specific product labeling.

Liquid, Oral, as hydrochloride:

Dilaudid: 1 mg/mL (473 mL) [contains methylparaben, propylparaben, sodium metabisulfite; sweet flavor]

Generic: 1 mg/mL (473 mL)

Solution, Injection, as hydrochloride:

Dilaudid: 1 mg/mL (1 mL); 2 mg/mL (1 mL); 4 mg/mL (1 mL)

Dilaudid-HP: 10 mg/mL (1 mL, 5 mL, 50 mL)

Generic: 1 mg/mL (0.5 mL, 1 mL); 2 mg/mL (1 mL, 20 mL); 4 mg/mL (1 mL); 10 mg/mL (1 mL); 50 mg/5 mL (5 mL); 500 mg/50 mL (50 mL)

Solution, Injection, as hydrochloride [preservative free]:

Generic: 10 mg/mL (1 mL); 50 mg/5 mL (5 mL); 500 mg/50 mL (50 mL)

Solution Reconstituted, Injection, as hydrochloride:

Dilaudid-HP: 250 mg (1 ea)

Suppository, Rectal, as hydrochloride:

Generic: 3 mg (6 ea)

Tablet, Oral, as hydrochloride:

Dilaudid: 2 mg, 4 mg [contains fd&c yellow #10 aluminum lake, sodium metabisulfite]

Dilaudid: 8 mg [scored; contains sodium metabisulfite]

Generic: 2 mg, 4 mg, 8 mg

Tablet ER 24 Hour Abuse-Deterrent, Oral, as hydrochloride:

Exalgo: 8 mg, 12 mg, 16 mg, 32 mg [contains sodium metabisulfite]

Dosage Forms: Canada Excipient information presented when available (limited, particularly for generics); consult specific product labeling.

Capsule, controlled release:

Hydromorph Contin: 3 mg, 6 mg, 12 mg, 18 mg, 24 mg, 30 mg

Controlled Substance C-II

- **Hydromorphone HP (Can)** *see* HYDROmorphone *on page 1013*
- **Hydromorphone HP 10 (Can)** *see* HYDROmorphone *on page 1013*
- **Hydromorphone HP 20 (Can)** *see* HYDROmorphone *on page 1013*
- **Hydromorphone HP 50 (Can)** *see* HYDROmorphone *on page 1013*
- **Hydromorphone HP Forte (Can)** *see* HYDROmorphone *on page 1013*
- **Hydromorphone Hydrochloride** *see* HYDROmorphone *on page 1013*
- **Hydromorphone Hydrochloride Injection, USP (Can)** *see* HYDROmorphone *on page 1013*
- **Hydroquinol** *see* Hydroquinone *on page 1017*

Hydroquinone (HYE droe kwin one)

Brand Names: U.S. Aclaro; Aclaro PD; Alphaquin HP; Eldopaque Forte [DSC]; Eldopaque [OTC] [DSC]; Eldoquin Forte [DSC]; Eldoquin [OTC] [DSC]; EpiQuin Micro; Esoterica Daytime [OTC]; Esoterica Facial [OTC]; Esoterica Fade Nighttime [OTC]; Esoterica Sensitive Skin [OTC]; Exuviance Lightening Complex [OTC]; Hydroquinone Time Release; Lustra; Lustra-AF; Lustra-Ultra; Melpaque HP; Melquin 3; Melquin HP; NAVA-SC; NeoCeuticals Post-Acne Fade [OTC]; NeoStrata HQ Skin Lightening [OTC]; Nuquin HP; Remergent HQ; Skin Bleaching; Skin Bleaching-Sunscreen; TL Hydroquinone

Brand Names: Canada Eldopaque®; Eldoquin®; Glyquin® XM; Lustra®; NeoStrata® HQ; Solaquin Forte®; Solaquin®; Ultraquin™

Index Terms Hydroquinol; Quinol

Pharmacologic Category Depigmenting Agent

Use Gradual bleaching of hyperpigmented skin conditions

Pregnancy Risk Factor C

Dosage Children >12 years and Adults: Topical: Apply thin layer and rub in twice daily

Additional Information Complete prescribing information should be consulted for additional detail.

Dosage Forms Excipient information presented when available (limited, particularly for generics); consult specific product labeling. [DSC] = Discontinued product

Cream, External:
- Alphaquin HP: 4% (28.4 g, 56.7 g)
- Eldopaque: 2% (28.35 g [DSC])
- Eldopaque Forte: 4% (28.35 g [DSC])
- Eldoquin: 2% (28.35 g [DSC])
- Eldoquin Forte: 4% (28.35 g [DSC]) [contains sodium metabisulfite]
- EpiQuin Micro: 4% (30 g) [contains benzyl alcohol, methylparaben, sodium metabisulfite, trolamine (triethanolamine), vitamin a, vitamin e]
- Esoterica Daytime: 2% (70 g) [contains disodium edta, methylparaben, propylene glycol, propylparaben, sodium bisulfite]
- Esoterica Daytime: 2% (70 g) [contains disodium edta, methylparaben, propylene glycol, propylparaben, sodium metabisulfite]
- Esoterica Facial: 2% (85 g)
- Esoterica Fade Nighttime: 2% (70 g) [contains disodium edta, methylparaben, propylene glycol, propylparaben, sodium metabisulfite]
- Esoterica Sensitive Skin: 1.5% (85 g)
- Hydroquinone Time Release: 4% (30 g) [contains benzyl alcohol, cetyl alcohol, edetate disodium, sodium metabisulfite, trolamine (triethanolamine)]
- Lustra: 4% (56.8 g) [contains sodium metabisulfite]
- Lustra-AF: 4% (56.8 g) [contains sodium metabisulfite, trolamine (triethanolamine)]
- Lustra-Ultra: 4% (28.4 g, 56.8 g) [contains methylparaben, octyl methoxycinnamate (octinoxate), propylparaben, sodium metabisulfite, vitamin a]
- Melpaque HP: 4% (28.4 g)
- Melquin HP: 4% (28.4 g)
- NAVA-SC: 4% (28.4 g) [contains propylene glycol, sodium metabisulfite]
- Nuquin HP: 4% (28.4 g, 56.7 g) [contains propylene glycol, sodium metabisulfite]
- Remergent HQ: 4% (30 mL) [contains sodium metabisulfite]
- Skin Bleaching: 4% (28.35 g)
- Skin Bleaching-Sunscreen: 4% (28.35 g) [contains cetostearyl alcohol, glycerin, isopropyl palmitate, propylene glycol, sodium lauryl sulfate, sodium metabisulfite, sorbic acid, water, purified]
- TL Hydroquinone: 4% (30 g) [contains benzyl alcohol, cetearyl alcohol, cetyl alcohol, edetate disodium, methylparaben, sodium metabisulfite, trolamine (triethanolamine)]
- Generic: 4% (28.35 g)

Emulsion, External:
- Aclaro: 4% (48.2 g) [contains benzyl alcohol, sodium metabisulfite]
- Aclaro PD: 4% (42.5 g)

Gel, External:
- Exuviance Lightening Complex: 2% (30 g) [contains denatured alcohol, propylene glycol, sodium bisulfite, sodium sulfite, tartrazine (fd&c yellow #5)]
- NeoCeuticals Post-Acne Fade: 2% (30 g) [contains denatured alcohol, propylene glycol, sodium bisulfite, sodium sulfite, tartrazine (fd&c yellow #5)]
- NeoStrata HQ Skin Lightening: 2% (30 g) [fragrance free, oil free; contains propylene glycol, sodium bisulfite, sodium sulfite]
- Nuquin HP: 4% (28.4 g)

Solution, External:
- Melquin 3: 3% (29.57 mL)

- **Hydroquinone, Fluocinolone Acetonide, and Tretinoin** *see* Fluocinolone, Hydroquinone, and Tretinoin *on page 879*
- **Hydroquinone Time Release** *see* Hydroquinone *on page 1017*
- **HydroSKIN [OTC]** *see* Hydrocortisone (Topical) *on page 1011*
- **Hydro Skin Maximum Strength [OTC]** *see* Hydrocortisone (Topical) *on page 1011*
- **HydroVal® (Can)** *see* Hydrocortisone (Topical) *on page 1011*

Hydroxocobalamin (hye droks oh koe BAL a min)

Brand Names: U.S. Cyanokit

Brand Names: Canada Cyanokit

Index Terms Vitamin B_{12a}

Pharmacologic Category Antidote; Vitamin, Water Soluble

Use

I.M. injection: Treatment of pernicious anemia; treatment of vitamin B_{12} deficiency due to dietary deficiencies or malabsorption diseases, inadequate secretion of intrinsic factor, competition for vitamin B_{12} by intestinal parasites/bacteria, or inadequate utilization of B_{12} (eg, during neoplastic treatment)

I.V. infusion (Cyanokit®): Treatment of cyanide poisoning (known or suspected)

Pregnancy Risk Factor C

Pregnancy Considerations Animal studies are insufficient to determine the effect, if any, on pregnancy or fetal development. There are no adequate and well-controlled studies in pregnant women. Data on the use of hydroxocobalamin in pregnancy for the treatment of cyanide poisoning and cobalamin defects are limited. In general, medications used as antidotes should take into consideration the health and prognosis of the mother; antidotes should be administered to pregnant women if there is a clear indication for use and should not be withheld because of fears of teratogenicity (Bailey, 2003).

Breast-Feeding Considerations It is not known if hydroxocobalamin is excreted in breast milk. Hydroxocobalamin may be administered in life-threatening situations; therefore, use in a breast-feeding woman is not contraindicated. Because of the unknown potential for adverse reactions in nursing infants, the patient should discontinue nursing.

Contraindications

I.M.: Hypersensitivity to hydroxocobalamin or any component of the formulation

I.V. (Cyanokit®): There are no contraindications listed in the manufacturer's labeling.

Warnings/Precautions

Solution for I.M. injection: Treatment of severe vitamin B_{12} megaloblastic anemia may result in thrombocytosis and severe hypokalemia, sometimes fatal, due to intracellular potassium shift upon anemia resolution. Use caution in folic acid deficient megaloblastic anemia; administration of vitamin B_{12} alone is not a substitute for folic acid and might mask true diagnosis. Vitamin B_{12} deficiency masks signs of polycythemia vera; vitamin B_{12} administration may unmask this condition. Neurologic manifestations of vitamin B_{12} deficiency will not be prevented with folic acid unless vitamin B_{12} is also given; spinal cord degeneration might also occur when folic acid is used as a substitute for vitamin B_{12} in anemia prevention. Blunted therapeutic response to vitamin B_{12} may occur in certain conditions (eg, infection, uremia, concurrent iron or folic acid deficiency) or in patients on medications with bone marrow suppressant properties (eg, chloramphenicol). Approved for use as I.M. injection only.

Cyanokit®: Use caution or consider alternatives in patients known to be allergic to, or who have experienced anaphylaxis,with hydroxocobalamin or cyanocobalamin. Increased blood pressure (≥180 mm Hg systolic or ≥110 mm Hg diastolic) may occur with infusion; elevations usually noted at the beginning of the infusion, peak toward the end of the infusion and return to baseline within 4 hours of the infusion. May offset hypotension induced by nitrite administration or cyanide. Collection of pretreatment blood cyanide concentrations does not preclude administration and should not delay administration in the emergency management of suspected or confirmed cyanide toxicity. Pretreatment cyanide concentrations may be useful as post infusion concentrations may be inaccurate. Treatment of cyanide poisoning should include external decontamination and supportive therapy. Fire victims may present with both cyanide and carbon monoxide poisoning. In this scenario, hydroxocobalamin is the agent of choice for cyanide intoxication. Hydroxocobalamin can discolor the skin and exudates, complicating the assessment of burn severity. Use caution with concurrent use of other cyanide antidotes; safety has not been established. Hydroxocobalamin may interfere with and/or trip alarms in patients who use hemodialysis machines that rely on colorimetric technology. Photosensitivity is a potential concern; avoid direct sunlight while skin remains discolored.

Adverse Reactions

I.M. injection: Frequency not defined:

Dermatologic: Exanthema (transient), itching

Gastrointestinal: Diarrhea (mild, transient)

Local: Injection site pain

Miscellaneous: Anaphylaxis, feeling of swelling of the entire body

I.V. infusion (Cyanokit®):

>10%:

Cardiovascular: Blood pressure increased (18% to 28%)

Central nervous system: Headache (6% to 33%)

Dermatologic: Erythema (94% to 100%; may last up to 2 weeks), rash (predominantly acneiform; 20% to 44%; can appear 7-28 days after administration and usually resolves within a few weeks)

Gastrointestinal: Nausea (6% to 11%)

Genitourinary: Chromaturia (100%; may last up to 5 weeks after administration)

Hematologic: Lymphocytes decreased (8% to 17%)

Local: Infusion site reaction (6% to 39%)

Frequency not defined:

Cardiovascular: Chest discomfort, hot flashes, peripheral edema

Central nervous system: Dizziness, memory impairment, restlessness

Dermatologic: Pruritus, urticaria

Gastrointestinal: Abdominal discomfort, diarrhea, dyspepsia, dysphagia, hematochezia, vomiting

Ocular: Irritation, redness, swelling

Respiratory: Dry throat, dyspnea, throat tightness

Miscellaneous: Allergic reaction (including anaphylaxis)

Postmarketing and/or case reports: Angioneurotic edema

Drug Interactions

Metabolism/Transport Effects None known.

Avoid Concomitant Use There are no known interactions where it is recommended to avoid concomitant use.

Increased Effect/Toxicity There are no known significant interactions involving an increase in effect.

Decreased Effect There are no known significant interactions involving a decrease in effect.

Preparation for Administration I.V. infusion (Cyanokit®): Reconstitute each 5 g vial with 200 mL of NS using provided sterile transfer spike. If NS is unavailable, may use LR or D_5W. Invert or rock each vial for 60 seconds prior to infusion; do not shake. Discard if solution is **not** dark red.

Storage/Stability

Solution for I.M. injection: Store at 20°C to 25°C (68°F to 77°F). Protect from light.

I.V. infusion (Cyanokit®): Prior to reconstitution, store at 25°C (77°F): excursions permitted to 15°C to 30°C (59°F to 86°F).

Temperature variation exposure allowed for transport of lyophilized form:

Usual transport: ≤15 days at 5°C to 40°C (41°F to 104°F)

Desert transport: ≤4 days at 5°C to 60°C (41°F to 140°F)

Freezing/defrosting cycles: ≤15 days at -20°C to 40°C (-4°F to 104°F)

Following reconstitution, store up to 6 hours at ≤40°C (104°F); do not freeze. Discard any remaining solution after 6 hours.

Mechanism of Action Hydroxocobalamin (vitamin B_{12a}) is a precursor to cyanocobalamin (vitamin B_{12}). Cyanocobalamin acts as a coenzyme for various metabolic functions, including fat and carbohydrate metabolism and protein synthesis, used in cell replication and hematopoiesis. In the presence of cyanide, each hydroxocobalamin molecule can bind one cyanide ion by displacing it for the hydroxo ligand linked to the trivalent cobalt ion, forming cyanocobalamin, which is then excreted in the urine.

Pharmacodynamics/Kinetics Following I.V. administration of Cyanokit®:

Protein binding: Significant; forms various cobalamin-(III) complexes

Half-life elimination: 26-31 hours

Excretion: Urine (50% to 60% within initial 72 hours)

Dosage

Cyanide poisoning: I.V.: **Note:** If cyanide poisoning is suspected, antidotal therapy must be given immediately.

Children (unlabeled use): Initial: 70 mg/kg (maximum: 5 **g**) as a single infusion; may repeat a second dose of 35 mg/kg depending on the severity of poisoning and clinical response (Shepherd, 2008).

Adults: Initial: 5 **g** as a single infusion; may repeat a second 5 **g** dose depending on the severity of poisoning and clinical response. Maximum cumulative dose: 10 **g**.

Vitamin B_{12} deficiency: I.M.:

Children: Initial: 100 mcg once daily for ≥2 weeks (total dose: 1-5 **mg**); maintenance: 30-50 mcg once per month

Adults: Initial: 30 mcg once daily for 5-10 days; maintenance: 100-200 mcg once per month

Note: Larger doses may be required in critically-ill patients or if patient has neurologic disease, an infectious disease, or hyperthyroidism.

Dosage adjustment in renal impairment: No dosage adjustments provided in manufacturer's labeling (has not been studied).

Dosage adjustment in hepatic impairment: No dosage adjustments provided in manufacturer's labeling (has not been studied).

Administration

I.M.: Administer 1000 mcg/mL solution I.M. only

I.V.: Cyanokit®: Administer initial dose by I.V. infusion over 15 minutes; if a second dose is needed, administer the second dose over 15 minutes to 2 hours; hydroxocobalamin is chemically incompatible with sodium thiosulfate and sodium nitrite and separate I.V. lines must be used if concomitant administration is desired **(the safety of coadministration is not established)**

Monitoring Parameters Vitamin B_{12}, hematocrit, hemoglobin, reticulocyte count, red blood cell counts, folate and iron levels should be obtained prior to treatment and periodically during treatment.

Cyanide poisoning: Blood pressure and heart rate during and after infusion, serum lactate levels, venous-arterial PO_2 gradient. Pretreatment cyanide levels may be useful as post infusion levels may be inaccurate.

Megaloblastic anemia: In addition to normal hematological parameters, serum potassium and platelet counts should be monitored during therapy, particularly in the first 48 hours of treatment.

Test Interactions The following values may be affected, *in vitro*, following hydroxocobalamin 5 g dose. Interference following hydroxocobalamin 10 g dose can be expected to last up to an additional 24 hours. **Note:** Extent and duration of interference dependent on analyzer used and patient variability.

Falsely elevated:

Basophils, hemoglobin, MCH, and MCHC [duration: 12-16 hours]

Albumin, alkaline phosphatase, cholesterol, creatinine, glucose, total protein, and triglycerides [duration: 24 hours]

Bilirubin [duration: up to 4 days]

Urinalysis: Glucose, protein, erythrocytes, leukocytes, ketones, bilirubin, urobilinogen, nitrite [duration: 2-8 days]

Falsely decreased: ALT and amylase [duration: 24 hours]

Unpredictable:

AST, CK, CKMB, LDH, phosphate, and uric acid [duration: 24 hours]

PT (quick or INR) and aPTT [duration: 24-48 hours]

Urine pH [duration: 2-8 days]

May also interfere with colorimetric tests and cause hemodialysis machines to shut down due to false detection of a blood leak from the blood-like appearance of the solution.

Dosage Forms Excipient information presented when available (limited, particularly for generics); consult specific product labeling.

Solution, Intramuscular:

Generic: 1000 mcg/mL (30 mL)

Solution Reconstituted, Intravenous:

Cyanokit: 5 g (1 ea)

◆ **4-Hydroxybutyrate** *see* Sodium Oxybate *on page 1922*

◆ **Hydroxycarbamide** *see* Hydroxyurea *on page 1022*

Hydroxychloroquine (hye droks ee KLOR oh kwin)

Brand Names: U.S. Plaquenil

Brand Names: Canada Apo-Hydroxyquine; Gen-Hydroxychloroquine; Mylan-Hydroxychloroquine; Plaquenil; PRO-Hydroxyquine

Index Terms Hydroxychloroquine Sulfate

Pharmacologic Category Aminoquinoline (Antimalarial)

Use Suppression and treatment of acute attacks of malaria; treatment of systemic lupus erythematosus (SLE) and rheumatoid arthritis

Unlabeled Use Porphyria cutanea tarda, polymorphous light eruptions, treatment of Q fever (*Coxiella burnetti*)

Pregnancy Considerations Hydroxychloroquine can be detected in the cord blood at delivery in concentrations similar to those in the maternal serum (Costedoat-Chalumeau, 2002). In animal reproduction studies with chloroquine, accumulation in fetal ocular tissues was observed and remained for several months following drug elimination from the rest of the body. Based on available human data, an increased risk of fetal ocular toxicity has not been observed following maternal use of hydroxychloroquine, but additional studies are needed to confirm (Osadchy, 2011).

Maternal lupus is associated with adverse maternal and fetal events; however, pregnancy outcomes may be improved if conception does not occur until the disease has been inactive for ≥6 months. Hydroxychloroquine is one of the medications recommended for the management of lupus and lupus nephritis in pregnant women. If pregnancy is detected during therapy, it should not be stopped (could precipitate a flare in maternal disease and exposure to the fetus will still continue for 6-8 weeks due to tissue binding) (Baer, 2011; Bertsias, 2012; Hahn, 2012; Levy, 2001). Maternal use of hydroxychloroquine may also decrease the incidence of cardiac malformations associated with neonatal lupus (Izmirly, 2012).

Malaria infection in pregnant women may be more severe than in nonpregnant women and has a high risk of maternal and perinatal morbidity and mortality. Therefore, pregnant women and women who are likely to become pregnant are advised to avoid travel to malaria-risk areas. Hydroxychloroquine is recommended as an alternative treatment of pregnant women for uncomplicated malaria in chloroquine-sensitive regions (refer to current guidelines) (CDC, 2011).

Women exposed to hydroxychloroquine for the treatment of rheumatoid arthritis or systemic lupus erythematosus during pregnancy may be enrolled in the Organization of Teratology Information Specialists (OTIS) Autoimmune Diseases Study pregnancy registry (877-311-8972).

Breast-Feeding Considerations Hydroxychloroquine is excreted into breast milk in low concentrations (Costedoat-Chalumeau, 2002; Ostensen, 1985). In a case report, hydroxychloroquine concentrations were ~100 ng/mL in the maternal serum and 3.2 ng/mL in breast milk 15-24 hours after an initial maternal dose of 200 mg twice daily;

the highest milk concentration was 10.6 ng/mL when measured 39-48 hours into the dosing regimen (Østensen, 1985)

Contraindications Hypersensitivity to hydroxychloroquine, 4-aminoquinoline derivatives, or any component of the formulation; retinal or visual field changes attributable to 4-aminoquinolines; long-term use in children

Warnings/Precautions May cause ophthalmic adverse effects (risk factors include daily doses >6.5 mg/kg lean body weight) or neuromyopathy; perform baseline and periodic (every 3 months) ophthalmologic examinations; test periodically for muscle weakness. Rare cardiomyopathy has been associated with long-term use of hydroxychloroquine. Aminoquinolines have been associated with rare hematologic reactions, including agranulocytosis, aplastic anemia, and thrombocytopenia; monitoring (CBC) is recommended in prolonged therapy. Use with caution in patients with hepatic disease, G6PD deficiency, psoriasis, and porphyria. Use caution in children due to increased sensitivity to adverse effects (long-term use in children is contraindicated). Not effective in the treatment of malaria caused by chloroquine resistant *P. falciparum.* **[U.S. Boxed Warning]: Should be prescribed by physicians familiar with its use.**

Adverse Reactions Frequency not defined.

Cardiovascular: Cardiomyopathy (rare, relationship to hydroxychloroquine unclear)

Central nervous system: Ataxia, dizziness, emotional changes, headache, irritability, lassitude, nervousness, nightmares, psychosis, seizure, vertigo

Dermatologic: Alopecia, angioedema, bleaching of hair, pigmentation changes (skin and mucosal; black-blue color), rash (acute generalized exanthematous pustulosis, erythema annulare centrifugum, exfoliative dermatitis, lichenoid, maculopapular, morbilliform, purpuric, Stevens-Johnson syndrome, urticarial), urticaria

Gastrointestinal: Abdominal cramping, anorexia, diarrhea, nausea, vomiting, weight loss

Hematologic: Agranulocytosis, aplastic anemia, hemolysis (in patients with glucose-6-phosphate deficiency), leukopenia, thrombocytopenia

Hepatic: Abnormal liver function/hepatic failure (isolated cases)

Neuromuscular & skeletal: Myopathy, palsy, or neuromyopathy leading to progressive weakness and atrophy of proximal muscle groups (may be associated with mild sensory changes, loss of deep tendon reflexes, and abnormal nerve conduction)

Ocular: Abnormal color vision, abnormal retinal pigmentation, atrophy, attenuation of retinal arterioles, corneal changes/deposits (visual disturbances, blurred vision, photophobia [reversible on discontinuation]), decreased visual acuity, disturbance in accommodation, keratopathy, macular edema, nystagmus, optic disc pallor/atrophy, pigmentary retinopathy, retinopathy (early changes reversible [may progress despite discontinuation if advanced]), scotoma

Otic: Deafness, tinnitus

Miscellaneous: Exacerbation of porphyria and nonlight sensitive psoriasis

Respiratory: Bronchospasm, respiratory failure (myopathy-related)

Drug Interactions

Metabolism/Transport Effects None known.

Avoid Concomitant Use

Avoid concomitant use of Hydroxychloroquine with any of the following: Artemether; BCG; Lumefantrine; Mefloquine; Natalizumab; Pimecrolimus; Tacrolimus (Topical); Tofacitinib

Increased Effect/Toxicity

Hydroxychloroquine may increase the levels/effects of: Antipsychotic Agents (Phenothiazines); Beta-Blockers; Cardiac Glycosides; Dapsone (Systemic); Dapsone (Topical); Leflunomide; Lumefantrine; Mefloquine; Natalizumab; Tofacitinib; Vaccines (Live)

The levels/effects of Hydroxychloroquine may be increased by: Artemether; Dapsone (Systemic); Denosumab; Mefloquine; Pimecrolimus; Roflumilast; Tacrolimus (Topical); Trastuzumab

Decreased Effect

Hydroxychloroquine may decrease the levels/effects of: Anthelmintics; BCG; Coccidioidin Skin Test; Sipuleucel-T; Vaccines (Inactivated)

The levels/effects of Hydroxychloroquine may be decreased by: Echinacea

Ethanol/Nutrition/Herb Interactions Ethanol: Avoid ethanol (due to GI irritation).

Mechanism of Action Interferes with digestive vacuole function within sensitive malarial parasites by increasing the pH and interfering with lysosomal degradation of hemoglobin; inhibits locomotion of neutrophils and chemotaxis of eosinophils; impairs complement-dependent antigen-antibody reactions

Pharmacodynamics/Kinetics

Onset of action: Rheumatic disease: May require 4-6 weeks to respond

Absorption: Rapid and complete

Protein binding: 55%

Metabolism: Hepatic; metabolites include desethylhydroxychloroquine and desethylchloroquine

Half-life elimination: 32-50 days

Time to peak: Rheumatic disease: Several months

Excretion: Urine (as metabolites and unchanged drug [up to 60%]); may be enhanced by urinary acidification

Dosage Note: Hydroxychloroquine sulfate 200 mg is equivalent to 155 mg hydroxychloroquine base and 250 mg chloroquine phosphate. All doses below expressed as hydroxychloroquine sulfate. Second-line alternative treatment for malaria (chloroquine is preferred).

Oral:

Children:

Malaria, chemoprophylaxis: 6.5 mg/kg once weekly (not to exceed 400 mg/dose); begin 2 weeks before exposure; continue for 4 weeks (per CDC guidelines) after leaving endemic area; if suppressive therapy is not begun prior to the exposure, double the initial dose and give in 2 doses, 6 hours apart and continue treatment for 8 weeks

Malaria, acute attack: 13 mg/kg initially (not to exceed 800 mg/dose), followed by 6.5 mg/kg (not to exceed 400 mg/dose) at 6, 24, and 48 hours

Adults:

Malaria, chemoprophylaxis: 400 mg weekly on same day each week; begin 2 weeks before exposure; continue for 4 weeks (per CDC guidelines) after leaving endemic area; if suppressive therapy is not begun prior to the exposure, double the initial dose and give in 2 doses, 6 hours apart and continue treatment for 8 weeks

Malaria, acute attack: 800 mg initially, followed by 400 mg at 6, 24, and 48 hours

Rheumatoid arthritis: Initial: 400-600 mg/day taken with food or milk; increase dose gradually until optimum response level is reached; usually after 4-12 weeks dose should be reduced by 1/2 to a maintenance dose of 200-400 mg/day

Lupus erythematosus: 400 mg every day or twice daily for several weeks-months depending on response; 200-400 mg/day for prolonged maintenance therapy

Q fever, chronic (unlabeled use; CDC, 2013): Oral:

Endocarditis or vascular infection: 200 mg every 8 hours in combination with doxycycline for ≥18 months

Noncardiac organ disease: 200 mg every 8 hours in combination with doxycycline (duration based on serologic response; ID consult recommended)

Postpartum with serologic evidence present >12 months after delivery: 200 mg every 8 hours in combination with doxycycline for 12 months

Dosage adjustment in renal impairment: Use with caution; dosage adjustment may be necessary in severe dysfunction (Bernstein, 1992); specific guidelines not available.

Dietary Considerations May be taken with food or milk.

Administration Administer with food or milk.

Monitoring Parameters CBC at baseline and periodically; liver function. Ophthalmologic exam at baseline and every 3 months during prolonged therapy (including visual acuity, slit-lamp, fundoscopic, and visual field exam); muscle strength (especially proximal, as a symptom of neuromyopathy) during long-term therapy

Dosage Forms Excipient information presented when available (limited, particularly for generics); consult specific product labeling.

Tablet, Oral, as sulfate:

Plaquenil: 200 mg

Generic: 200 mg

Extemporaneous Preparations A 25 mg/mL hydroxychloroquine sulfate oral suspension may be made with tablets. With a towel moistened with alcohol, remove the coating from fifteen 200 mg hydroxychloroquine sulfate tablets. Crush tablets in a mortar and reduce to a fine powder. Add 15 mL of Ora-Plus® and mix to a uniform paste; add an additional 45 mL of vehicle and mix until uniform. Mix while adding sterile water for irrigation in incremental proportions to **almost** 120 mL; transfer to a calibrated bottle, rinse mortar with sterile water, and add sufficient quantity of sterile water to make 120 mL. Label "shake well". A 30-day expiration date is recommended, although stability testing has not been performed.

Pesko LJ, "Compounding: Hydroxychloroquine," *Am Druggist*, 1993, 207(4):57.

◆ **Hydroxychloroquine Sulfate** *see* Hydroxychloroquine *on page 1019*

◆ **Hydroxydaunomycin Hydrochloride** *see* DOXOrubicin *on page 661*

◆ **Hydroxyethyl Starch** *see* Hetastarch *on page 997*

◆ **Hydroxyethyl Starch** *see* Tetrastarch *on page 2036*

◆ **Hydroxyldaunorubicin Hydrochloride** *see* DOXOrubicin *on page 661*

Hydroxyprogesterone Caproate

(hye droks ee proe JES te rone CAP ro ate)

Brand Names: U.S. Makena

Index Terms 17OHPC

Pharmacologic Category Progestin

Use To reduce the risk of preterm birth in women with singleton pregnancies who have a history of spontaneous preterm birth (delivery <37 weeks gestation) with previous singleton pregnancies

Pregnancy Risk Factor B

Pregnancy Considerations Teratogenic events were not observed in animal reproduction studies; embryolethality was observed in some species. Teratogenic effects were not observed in human studies following second or third trimester exposure; first trimester data not available.

Maternal serum concentrations of hydroxyprogesterone caproate are widely variable and may be decreased in women with increased BMI. Hydroxyprogesterone is metabolized by the placenta and reaches the fetal circulation. In one study, the cord:maternal concentration ratio averaged 0.2. Hydroxyprogesterone caproate was detected in cord blood when delivery occurred ≥44 days after the last injection (Cartitis, 2012; Hemauer, 2008).

Breast-Feeding Considerations Progestins have been detected in milk and have not been found to adversely affect breast-feeding, health, growth, or development of the infant. Use of hydroxyprogesterone caproate is not indicated following delivery.

Prescribing and Access Restrictions The Makena Care Connection™ is a comprehensive program for patients and healthcare providers which provides administrative support (including insurance benefit investigation and prescription fulfillment); financial and co-pay assistance for eligible patients; and treatment support (including educational information, home health care service and scheduled treatment reminders). The Makena Care Connection™ is available by calling 1-800-847-3418, Monday-Friday, 8 AM to 9 PM EST.

Contraindications Current or history of thrombosis or thromboembolic disorders; hepatic impairment, hepatic tumors or cholestatic jaundice of pregnancy; carcinoma of the breast (known or suspected) or other hormone sensitive cancers; undiagnosed vaginal bleeding unrelated to pregnancy; uncontrolled hypertension

Warnings/Precautions Hazardous agent - use appropriate precautions for handling and disposal (NIOSH, 2012). Not for use in women with multiple gestations or other risk factors for preterm birth. Clinical benefits related to improved neonatal mortality or morbidity following maternal use have not been demonstrated. Not intended to stop active preterm labor. May have adverse effects on glucose tolerance; use caution in women with diabetes. Use with caution in patients with depression; discontinue if depression occurs. Use with caution in patients with diseases which may be exacerbated by fluid retention, including asthma, epilepsy, migraine, diabetes, pre-eclampsia, cardiac or renal dysfunction. Specific studies have not been conducted in patients with hepatic impairment (use is contraindicated); elimination may be decreased. Monitor women who develop hypertension during therapy; consider risk versus benefit of continuation. Use is contraindicated with uncontrolled hypertension. Monitor women who develop jaundice during therapy; consider risk versus benefit of continuation. Use is contraindicated in women with cholestatic jaundice of pregnancy. Discontinue if arterial thrombosis, DVT, or thromboembolic events occur. Use is contraindicated with current or history of thrombosis or thromboembolic disorders. Limited numbers of pregnant women between 16 and 18 years of age were included in clinical trials. Contains castor oil. Discontinue if allergic reactions (eg, urticaria, pruritus, angioedema) occur.

Adverse Reactions

>10%:

Dermatologic: Urticaria (12%)

Genitourinary: Preterm labor (admission: 16%)

Local: Pain at injection site (35%), swelling at injection site (17%)

1% to 10%:

Cardiovascular: Preeclampsia (9%)

Dermatologic: Pruritus (8%)

Endocrine & metabolic: Gestational diabetes (6%)

Gastrointestinal: Nausea (6%), diarrhea (2%)

Genitourinary: Oligohydramnios (4%), stillborn infant (2%), spontaneous abortion (≤2%; <20 weeks gestation)

Local: Local pruritus (6%)

Miscellaneous: Nodule (5%)

<1% (Limited to important or life-threatening): Angioedema, cellulitis at injection site, cervical dilation, cervical shortening, decreased glucose tolerance, depression, fluid retention, headache, hypersensitivity reaction, hypertension, hot flash, jaundice, premature rupture of membranes, pulmonary embolism, skin rash, thromboembolic complications, urinary tract infection

Drug Interactions

Metabolism/Transport Effects **Substrate** of CYP3A4 (major); **Note:** Assignment of Major/Minor substrate status based on clinically relevant drug interaction potential; **Induces** CYP1A2 (weak/moderate), CYP2A6 (strong), CYP2B6 (weak/moderate)

Avoid Concomitant Use

Avoid concomitant use of Hydroxyprogesterone Caproate with any of the following: Conivaptan; Fusidic Acid (Systemic); Ulipristal

Increased Effect/Toxicity

The levels/effects of Hydroxyprogesterone Caproate may be increased by: Conivaptan; CYP3A4 Inhibitors (Moderate); CYP3A4 Inhibitors (Strong); Dasatinib; Fusidic Acid (Systemic); Herbs (Progestogenic Properties); Ivacaftor; Luliconazole; Mifepristone; Simeprevir

Decreased Effect

Hydroxyprogesterone Caproate may decrease the levels/effects of: Anticoagulants; CYP2A6 Substrates

The levels/effects of Hydroxyprogesterone Caproate may be decreased by: Aminoglutethimide; Bosentan; CYP3A4 Inducers (Strong); Dabrafenib; Deferasirox; Herbs (CYP3A4 Inducers); Mitotane; Tocilizumab; Ulipristal

Storage/Stability Store upright at controlled room temperature of 15°C to 30°C (59°F to 86°F); protect from light. Discard within 5 weeks of first use.

Pharmacodynamics/Kinetics

Distribution: Extensively bound to albumin and corticosteroid-binding globulins

Metabolism: Hepatic via CYP3A4 and 3A5; forms metabolites

Half-life elimination: Nonpregnant females: ~8 days; Pregnant females (singleton pregnancies): 16 days (range: 11-21 days) (Caritis, 2012)

Time to peak, serum: I.M.: Nonpregnant females: 3-7 days; Pregnant females (singleton pregnancies): 1-4 days (Caritis, 2012)

Excretion: Urine (~30%) and feces (~50%); primarily as metabolites

Dosage I.M.: Pregnant females ≥16 years: To reduce the risk of preterm birth: 250 mg once weekly (every 7 days). Treatment may begin between 16 weeks 0 days and 20 weeks 6 days of gestation. Continue weekly administration until 37 weeks gestation or until delivery, whichever comes first.

Dosage adjustment in renal impairment: No dosage adjustment provided in manufacturer's labeling (has not been studied).

Dosage adjustment in hepatic impairment: No dosage adjustment provided in manufacturer's labeling (has not been studied). However, hydroxyprogesterone caproate is extensively metabolized and hepatic impairment may reduce its elimination.

Administration For I.M. administration into the upper outer quadrant of the gluteus maximus. Withdraw dose using an 18 gauge needle; inject dose using a 21 gauge 1$^{1}/_{2}$ inch needle. Administer by slow injection (≥1 minute). Solution is viscous and oily; do not use if solution is cloudy or contains solid particles. Apply pressure to injection site to decrease bruising and swelling.

Hazardous agent; use appropriate precautions for handling and disposal (NIOSH, 2012).

Monitoring Parameters Signs and symptoms of thromboembolic disorders; signs or symptoms of depression; glucose in patients with diabetes; signs and symptoms of jaundice; or blood pressure

Dosage Forms Excipient information presented when available (limited, particularly for generics); consult specific product labeling.

Oil, Intramuscular:

Makena: 250 mg/mL (5 mL) [contains benzyl alcohol]

◆ 9-hydroxy-risperidone *see* Paliperidone *on page 1549*

Hydroxyurea (hye droks ee yoor EE a)

Brand Names: U.S. Droxia; Hydrea

Brand Names: Canada Apo-Hydroxyurea; Gen-Hydroxyurea; Hydrea®; Mylan-Hydroxyurea

Index Terms HU; Hydroxycarbamide; Hydurea

Pharmacologic Category Antineoplastic Agent, Antimetabolite

Use Treatment of melanoma, refractory chronic myelocytic leukemia (CML); recurrent, metastatic, or inoperable ovarian cancer; management (with concomitant radiation therapy) of squamous cell head and neck cancer (excluding lip cancer); management of sickle cell patients who have had at least three painful crises in the previous 12 months (to reduce frequency of these crises and the need for blood transfusions)

Unlabeled Use Treatment of essential thrombocythemia, polycythemia vera, hypereosinophilic syndrome; management of hyperleukocytosis due to acute myeloid leukemia (AML); treatment of AML in poor-risk patients; treatment of meningiomas

Pregnancy Risk Factor D

Pregnancy Considerations Animal reproduction studies have demonstrated teratogenicity and embryotoxicity at doses lower than the usual human dose (based on BSA). Hydroxyurea may cause fetal harm if administered during pregnancy. Women of childbearing potential should be advised to avoid becoming pregnant during treatment and should use effective contraception.

Breast-Feeding Considerations Hydroxyurea is excreted in breast milk. Due to the potential for serious adverse reactions in the nursing infant, the decision to discontinue hydroxyurea or to discontinue breast-feeding should take into account the importance of treatment to the mother.

Contraindications Hypersensitivity to hydroxyurea or any component of the formulation

Hydrea: Marked bone marrow suppression (WBC <2500/mm^3 or platelet count <100,000/mm^3) or severe anemia

Warnings/Precautions Hazardous agent - use appropriate precautions for handling and disposal (NIOSH, 2012); to decrease risk of exposure, wear gloves when handling and wash hands before and after contact. Leukopenia and neutropenia commonly occur (thrombocytopenia and anemia are less common); leukopenia/neutropenia occur first. Hematologic toxicity reversible (rapid) with treatment interruption. Correct severe anemia prior to initiating treatment. Hydrea® use is contraindicated in marked bone marrow suppression; should not be used in sickle cell anemia with severe bone marrow suppression (neutrophils <2000/mm^3, platelets <80,000/mm^3, hemoglobin <4.5 g/dL, or reticulocytes <80,000/mm^3 when hemoglobin <9 g/dL). Use with caution in patients with a history of prior chemotherapy or radiation therapy; myelosuppression is more common. Patients with a history of radiation therapy are also at risk for exacerbation of post irradiation erythema. Self-limiting megaloblastic erythropoiesis may be seen early in treatment (may resemble pernicious anemia, but is unrelated to vitamin B_{12} or folic acid deficiency). Plasma iron clearance may be delayed and iron utilization rate (by erythrocytes) may be reduced. Potentially significant drug-drug interactions may exist, requiring dose or frequency adjustment, additional monitoring, and/or selection of alternative therapy. When treated concurrently with hydroxyurea and antiretroviral agents (including didanosine and stavudine), HIV-infected patients are at higher risk for potentially fatal pancreatitis, hepatotoxicity, hepatic failure, and severe peripheral neuropathy; discontinue immediately if signs of these toxicities develop. Hyperuricemia may occur with antineoplastic treatment; adequate hydration and initiation or dosage adjustment of uricosuric agents (eg, allopurinol) may be necessary.

In patients with sickle cell anemia, use is not recommended if neutrophils <2000/mm^3, platelets <80,000/mm^3, hemoglobin <4.5 g/dL, or reticulocytes <80,000/mm^3 when hemoglobin <9 g/dL. May cause macrocytosis, which can mask folic acid deficiency; prophylactic fold acid supplementation is recommended. **[U.S. Boxed Warning]: Hydroxyurea is mutagenic and clastogenic; causes cellular transformation resulting in tumorigenicity; also considered genotoxic and may be carcinogenic. Treatment of myeloproliferative disorders (eg, polycythemia vera, thrombocythemia) with long-term hydroxyurea is associated with secondary leukemia;** it is unknown if this is drug-related or disease-related. Skin cancer has been reported with long-term hydroxyurea use. Cutaneous vasculitic toxicities (vasculitic ulceration and gangrene) have been reported with hydroxyurea treatment, most often in patients with a history of or receiving concurrent interferon therapy; discontinue hydroxyurea and consider alternate cytoreductive therapy if cutaneous vasculitic toxicity develops. Use caution with renal dysfunction; may require dose reductions. Elderly patients may be more sensitive to the effects of hydroxyurea; may require lower doses. **[U.S. Boxed Warning]: Should be administered under the supervision of a physician experienced in the treatment of sickle cell anemia** or in cancer chemotherapy.

Adverse Reactions Frequency not defined.

Cardiovascular: Edema

Central nervous system: Chills, disorientation, dizziness, drowsiness (dose-related), fever, hallucinations, headache, malaise, seizure

Dermatologic: Alopecia, cutaneous vasculitic toxicities, dermatomyositis-like skin changes, facial erythema, gangrene, hyperpigmentation, maculopapular rash, nail atrophy, nail discoloration, peripheral erythema, scaling, skin atrophy, skin cancer, skin ulcer, vasculitis ulcerations, violet papules

Endocrine & metabolic: Hyperuricemia

Gastrointestinal: Anorexia, constipation, diarrhea, gastrointestinal irritation and mucositis, (potentiated with radiation therapy), nausea, pancreatitis, stomatitis, vomiting

Genitourinary: Dysuria

Hematologic: Myelosuppression (anemia, leukopenia/neutropenia [common], thrombocytopenia; hematologic recovery: within 2 weeks); macrocytosis, megaloblastic erythropoiesis, secondary leukemias (long-term use)

Hepatic: Hepatic enzymes increased, hepatotoxicity

Neuromuscular & skeletal: Peripheral neuropathy, weakness

Renal: BUN increased, creatinine increased, renal tubular dysfunction

Respiratory: Acute diffuse pulmonary infiltrates (rare), dyspnea, pulmonary fibrosis (rare)

Drug Interactions

Metabolism/Transport Effects None known.

Avoid Concomitant Use

Avoid concomitant use of Hydroxyurea with any of the following: BCG; CloZAPine; Didanosine; Natalizumab; Pimecrolimus; Stavudine; Tacrolimus (Topical); Tofacitinib; Vaccines (Live)

Increased Effect/Toxicity

Hydroxyurea may increase the levels/effects of: CloZAPine; Didanosine; Leflunomide; Natalizumab; Stavudine; Tofacitinib; Vaccines (Live)

The levels/effects of Hydroxyurea may be increased by: Denosumab; Didanosine; Pimecrolimus; Roflumilast; Stavudine; Tacrolimus (Topical); Trastuzumab

Decreased Effect

Hydroxyurea may decrease the levels/effects of: BCG; Coccidioidin Skin Test; Sipuleucel-T; Vaccines (Inactivated); Vaccines (Live)

The levels/effects of Hydroxyurea may be decreased by: Echinacea

Storage/Stability Store at room temperature of 25°C (77°F); excursions permitted between 15°C and 30°C (59°F and 86°F).

Mechanism of Action Antimetabolite which selectively inhibits ribonucleoside diphosphate reductase, preventing the conversion of ribonucleotides to deoxyribonucleotides, halting the cell cycle at the G1/S phase and therefore has radiation sensitizing activity by maintaining cells in the G_1 phase and interfering with DNA repair. In sickle cell anemia, hydroxyurea increases red blood cell (RBC) hemoglobin F levels, RBC water content, deformability of sickled cells, and alters adhesion of RBCs to endothelium.

Pharmacodynamics/Kinetics

Onset: Sickle cell anemia: Fetal hemoglobin increase: 4-12 weeks

Absorption: Readily absorbed (≥80%)

Distribution: Distributes widely into tissues (including into the brain); estimated volume of distribution approximates total body water (Gwilt, 1998)

Metabolism: 60% via hepatic and GI tract

Protein binding: 75% to 80% bound to serum proteins (Gwilt, 1998)

Half-life elimination: 1.9-3.9 hours (Gwilt, 1998); Children: Sickle cell anemia: 1.7 hours (range: 0.7-3 hours) (Ware, 2011)

Time to peak: 1-4 hours

Excretion: Urine (sickle cell anemia: 40% of administered dose)

Dosage Oral: Doses should be based on ideal or actual body weight, whichever is less (per manufacturer):

Children ≥6 months: Sickle cell anemia (unlabeled use): Initial: 15-20 mg/kg once daily; may increase by 5 mg/kg/day every 2-6 months to a maximum dose of 30-35 mg/kg/day (Ferster, 2001; Hankins, 2005; Kinney, 1999; Thornburg, 2009; Wang, 2001; Wang, 2011; Zimmerman, 2004)

Adults:

Antineoplastic uses: Titrate dose to patient response; if WBC count falls to <2500/mm^3, or the platelet count to <100,000/mm^3, therapy should be stopped for at least 3 days and resumed when values rise toward normal

- Chronic myeloid leukemia (resistant): Continuous therapy: 20-30 mg/kg once daily
- Solid tumors (head and neck cancer, melanoma, ovarian cancer):
  - Intermittent therapy: 80 mg/kg as a single dose every third day
  - Continuous therapy: 20-30 mg/kg once daily
  - Concomitant therapy with irradiation (head and neck cancer): 80 mg/kg as a single dose every third day starting at least 7 days before initiation of irradiation

Sickle cell anemia: Initial: 15 mg/kg/day; if blood counts are in an acceptable range, may increase by 5 mg/kg every 12 weeks until the maximum tolerated dose of 35 mg/kg/day is achieved or the dose that does not produce toxic effects (do not increase dose if blood counts are between acceptable and toxic ranges). Monitor for toxicity every 2 weeks; if toxicity occurs, withhold treatment until the bone marrow recovers, then restart with a dose reduction of 2.5 mg/kg/day; if no toxicity occurs over the next 12 weeks, then the subsequent dose may be increased by 2.5 mg/kg/day every 12 weeks to a maximum tolerated dose (dose which does not produce hematologic toxicity for 24 consecutive weeks). If hematologic toxicity recurs a second time at a specific dose, do not retry that dose.

Acceptable hematologic ranges: Neutrophils ≥2500/mm³; platelets ≥95,000/mm³; hemoglobin >5.3 g/dL, and reticulocytes ≥95,000/mm³ if the hemoglobin concentration is <9 g/dL

Toxic hematologic ranges: Neutrophils <2000/mm³; platelets <80,000/mm³; hemoglobin <4.5 g/dL; and reticulocytes <80,000/mm³ if the hemoglobin concentration is <9 g/dL

Acute myeloid leukemia (AML), cytoreduction (unlabeled use): 50-100 mg/kg/day until WBC <100,000/mm³ (Grund, 1977) **or** 50-60 mg/kg/day until WBC <10,000-20,000/mm³ (Dohner, 2010)

Essential thrombocythemia, high-risk (unlabeled use): 500-1000 mg daily; adjust dose to maintain platelets <400,000/mm³ (Harrison, 2005)

Head and neck cancer (unlabeled dosing; with concurrent radiation therapy and fluorouracil): 1000 mg every 12 hours for 11 doses per cycle (Garden, 2004)

Hypereosinophilic syndrome (unlabeled use): 1000-3000 mg/day (Klion, 2006)

Meningioma (unlabeled use): 20 mg/kg once daily (Newton, 2000; Rosenthal, 2002)

Polycythemia vera, high-risk (unlabeled use): 15-20 mg/kg/day (Finazzi, 2007)

Elderly: May require lower doses.

Dosage adjustment for toxicity:

Cutaneous vasculitic ulcerations: Discontinue

Gastrointestinal toxicity (severe nausea, vomiting, anorexia): Temporarily interrupt treatment

Mucositis (severe): Temporarily interrupt treatment

Pancreatitis: Discontinue permanently

Hematologic toxicity:

Antineoplastic uses (CML, head and neck cancer, melanoma, ovarian cancer): WBC <2500/mm³ or platelets <100,000/mm³: Interrupt treatment (for at least 3 days), may resume when values rise toward normal

Sickle cell anemia: Neutrophils <2000/mm³, platelets <80,000/mm³, hemoglobin <4.5 g/dL, or reticulocytes <80,000/mm³ with hemoglobin <9 g/dL: Interrupt treatment; following recovery, may resume with a dose reduction of 2.5 mg/kg/day. If no toxicity occurs over the next 12 weeks, subsequent dose may be increased by 2.5 mg/kg/day every 12 weeks to a dose which does not produce hematologic toxicity for 24 consecutive weeks. If hematologic toxicity recurs a second time at a specific dose, do not retry that dose.

Dosage adjustment in renal impairment:

The manufacturer's labeling recommends the following adjustments:

Sickle cell anemia:

Cl_{cr} ≥60 mL/minute: No dosage adjustment (of initial dose) necessary.

Cl_{cr} <60 mL/minute: Reduce initial dose to 7.5 mg/kg/day (Yan, 2005); titrate to response/avoidance of toxicity (refer to usual dosing)

ESRD: Reduce initial dose to 7.5 mg/kg/dose (administer after dialysis on dialysis days); titrate to response/avoidance of toxicity

Other approved indications: Reduction in initial dose is recommended; however, no specific adjustments are available.

The following adjustments have also been reported:

Aronoff, 2007: Adults:

Cl_{cr} >50 mL/minute: No dosage adjustment necessary

Cl_{cr} 10-50 mL/minute: Administer 50% of dose

Cl_{cr} <10 mL/minute: Administer 20% of dose

Hemodialysis: Administer dose after dialysis on dialysis days

Continuous renal replacement therapy (CRRT): Administer 50% of dose

Kintzel, 1995:

Cl_{cr} 46-60 mL/minute: Administer 85% of dose

Cl_{cr} 31-45 mL/minute: Administer 80% of dose

Cl_{cr} <30 mL/minute: Administer 75% of dose

Dosing adjustment in hepatic impairment: No dosage adjustment provided in the manufacturer's labeling; closely monitor for bone marrow toxicity.

Dosing in obesity: *ASCO Guidelines for appropriate chemotherapy dosing in obese adults with cancer:* Utilize patient's actual body weight (full weight) for calculation of body surface area- or weight-based dosing, particularly when the intent of therapy is curative; manage regimen-related toxicities in the same manner as for nonobese patients; if a dose reduction is utilized due to toxicity, consider resumption of full weight-based dosing with subsequent cycles, especially if cause of toxicity (eg, hepatic or renal impairment) is resolved (Griggs, 2012). **Note:** The manufacturer recommends dosing based on ideal or actual body weight, whichever is less.

Dietary Considerations In sickle cell patients, supplemental administration of folic acid is recommended; hydroxyurea may mask development of folic acid deficiency.

Administration The manufacturer does not recommend opening the capsules.

Hazardous agent; use appropriate precautions for handling and disposal (NIOSH, 2012). Impervious gloves should be worn when handling; avoid exposure to crushed or open capsules.

Monitoring Parameters CBC with differential and platelets, renal function and liver function tests, serum uric acid; hemoglobin F levels (sickle cell disease); monitor for cutaneous toxicities

Sickle cell disease: Monitor for toxicity every 2 weeks. If toxicity occurs, stop treatment until the bone marrow recovers; restart at 2.5 mg/kg/day less than the dose at which toxicity occurs. If no toxicity occurs over the next 12 weeks, then the subsequent dose should be increased by 2.5 mg/kg/day. Reduced dosage of hydroxyurea alternating with erythropoietin may decrease myelotoxicity and increase levels of fetal hemoglobin in patients who have not been helped by hydroxyurea alone.

Acceptable range: Neutrophils ≥2500 cells/mm³, platelets ≥95,000/mm³, hemoglobin >5.3 g/dL, and reticulocytes ≥95,000/mm³ if the hemoglobin concentration is <9 g/dL

Toxic range: Neutrophils <2000 cells/mm³, platelets <80,000/mm³, hemoglobin <4.5 g/dL, and reticulocytes <80,000/mm³ if the hemoglobin concentration is <9 g/dL

Test Interactions False-negative triglyceride measurement by a glycerol oxidase method. An analytical interference between hydroxyurea and enzymes (lactate dehydrogenase, urease, and uricase) may result in false elevations of lactic acid, urea, and uric acid.

Dosage Forms Excipient information presented when available (limited, particularly for generics); consult specific product labeling.

Capsule, Oral:

Droxia: 200 mg, 300 mg, 400 mg

Hydrea: 500 mg

Generic: 500 mg

Extemporaneous Preparations Hazardous agent: Use appropriate precautions for handling and disposal.

A 40 mg/mL oral suspension may be prepared with capsules and either a 1:1 mixture of Ora-Sweet® and Ora-Plus® or a 1:1 mixture of methylcellulose 1% and simple syrup NF. Empty the contents of eight 500 mg capsules into a mortar. Add small portions of chosen vehicle and mix to a uniform paste; mix while incrementally adding the vehicle to **almost** 100 mL; transfer to a calibrated bottle, rinse mortar with vehicle, and add sufficient quantity of vehicle to make 100 mL. Label "shake well" and "refrigerate". Store in plastic prescription bottles. Stable for 14 days at room temperature or refrigerated (preferred) (Nahata, 2003).

A 100 mg/mL oral solution may be prepared with capsules. Mix the contents of twenty 500 mg capsules with enough room temperature sterile water (~50 mL) to initially result in a 200 mg/mL concentration. Stir vigorously using a magnetic stirrer for several hours, then filter to remove insoluble contents. Add 50 mL Syrpalta® (flavored syrup, HUMCO) to filtered solution, resulting in 100 mL of a 100 mg/mL hydroxyurea solution. Stable for 1 month at room temperature in amber plastic bottle (Heeney, 2004).

Heeney MM, Whorton MR, Howard TA, et al, "Chemical and Functional Analysis of Hydroxyurea Oral Solutions," *J Pediatr Hematol Oncol*, 2004, 26(3):179-84.

Nahata MC, Morosco RS, Boster EA, et al, "Stability of Hydroxyurea in Two Extemporaneously Prepared Oral Suspensions Stored at Two Temperatures," 2003, 38:P-161(E) [abstract from 2003 ASHP Midyear Clinical Meeting].

HydrOXYzine (hye DROKS i zeen)

Brand Names: U.S. Vistaril

Brand Names: Canada Apo-Hydroxyzine; Atarax; Hydroxyzine Hydrochloride Injection, USP; Novo-Hydroxyzin; Nu-Hydroxyzine; PMS-Hydroxyzine; Riva-Hydroxyzine

Index Terms Hydroxyzine Hydrochloride; Hydroxyzine Pamoate

Pharmacologic Category Antiemetic; Histamine H_1 Antagonist; Histamine H_1 Antagonist, First Generation; Piperazine Derivative

Additional Appendix Information

Beers Criteria – Potentially Inappropriate Medications for Geriatrics *on page 2368*

Use Treatment of anxiety/agitation (including adjunctive therapy in alcoholism); adjunct to pre- and postoperative analgesia and anesthesia; antipruritic; antiemetic

Pregnancy Considerations Adverse events were observed in animal reproduction studies. Hydroxyzine crosses the placenta. Maternal hydroxyzine use has generally not resulted in an increased risk of birth defects. Use of hydroxyzine early in pregnancy is contraindicated but hydroxyzine is approved for pre- and postpartum adjunctive therapy to reduce opioid dosage, treat anxiety, and control emesis. Antihistamines are recommended for the treatment pruritus with rash in pregnant women (although second generation antihistamines may be preferred). Antihistamines are not recommended for treatment of pruritus associated with intrahepatic cholestasis in pregnancy. Possible withdrawal symptoms have been observed in neonates following chronic maternal use of hydroxyzine during pregnancy.

Breast-Feeding Considerations It is not known if hydroxyzine is excreted in breast milk. Breast-feeding is not recommended by the manufacturer. Antihistamines may decrease maternal serum prolactin concentrations when administered prior to the establishment of nursing.

Contraindications Hypersensitivity to hydroxyzine or any component of the formulation; early pregnancy; SubQ, intra-arterial, or I.V. injection

Warnings/Precautions Causes sedation, caution must be used in performing tasks which require alertness (eg, operating machinery or driving). Sedative effects of CNS depressants or ethanol are potentiated. Use with caution with narrow-angle glaucoma, prostatic hyperplasia, bladder neck obstruction, asthma, or COPD. In the elderly, avoid use of this potent anticholinergic agent due to increased risk of confusion, dry mouth, constipation, and other anticholinergic effects; clearance decreases in patients of advanced age (Beers Criteria).

For I.M. use only. Subcutaneous, I.V., and intra-arterial routes of administration are contraindicated. Intravascular hemolysis, thrombosis, and digital gangrene have been reported with I.V. or intra-arterial administration (Baumgartner, 1979); subQ administration may result in significant tissue damage. If inadvertent I.V administration results in extravasation, stop infusion immediately and disconnect (leave cannula/needle in place); gently aspirate extravasated solution (do **NOT** flush the line); remove needle/cannula; elevate extremity.

Adverse Reactions Frequency not defined.

Central nervous system: Dizziness, drowsiness, fatigue, hallucination, headache, nervousness, seizure

Dermatologic: Pruritus, rash, urticaria

Gastrointestinal: Xerostomia

Neuromuscular & skeletal: Involuntary movements, paresthesia, tremor

Ocular: Blurred vision

Respiratory: Respiratory depression (at higher than recommended doses)

Miscellaneous: Allergic reaction

Drug Interactions

Metabolism/Transport Effects Inhibits CYP2D6 (weak)

Avoid Concomitant Use

Avoid concomitant use of HydrOXYzine with any of the following: Aclidinium; Azelastine (Nasal); Ipratropium (Oral Inhalation); Paraldehyde; Tiotropium; Umeclidinium

Increased Effect/Toxicity

HydrOXYzine may increase the levels/effects of: Alcohol (Ethyl); Analgesics (Opioid); Anticholinergics; ARIPiprazole; Azelastine (Nasal); Barbiturates; Buprenorphine; CNS Depressants; Hydrocodone; Meperidine; Methotrimeprazine; Metyrosine; Mirtazapine; Paraldehyde; Pramipexole; ROPINIRole; Rotigotine; Selective Serotonin Reuptake Inhibitors; Tiotropium; Zolpidem

The levels/effects of HydrOXYzine may be increased by: Aclidinium; Brimonidine (Topical); Doxylamine; Droperidol; Ipratropium (Oral Inhalation); Magnesium Sulfate; Methotrimeprazine; Perampanel; Pramlintide; Sodium Oxybate; Tapentadol; Umeclidinium

Decreased Effect

HydrOXYzine may decrease the levels/effects of: Acetylcholinesterase Inhibitors (Central); Benzylpenicilloyl Polylysine; Betahistine; Hyaluronidase

The levels/effects of HydrOXYzine may be decreased by: Acetylcholinesterase Inhibitors (Central); Amphetamines

Ethanol/Nutrition/Herb Interactions

Ethanol: May increase CNS depression; monitor for increased effects with coadministration. Caution patients about effects.

Herb/Nutraceutical: Avoid valerian, St John's wort, kava kava, gotu kola (may increase CNS depression).

Storage/Stability

Injection: Store at 20°C to 25°C (68°F to 77°F); excursions permitted to 15°C to 30°C (59°F to 86°F). Protect from light.

Tablets: Store at 20°C to 25°C (68°F to 77°F).

Mechanism of Action Competes with histamine for H_1-receptor sites on effector cells in the gastrointestinal tract, blood vessels, and respiratory tract. Possesses skeletal muscle relaxing, bronchodilator, antihistamine, antiemetic, and analgesic properties.

Pharmacodynamics/Kinetics

Onset of action: Oral: 15-30 minutes; Injection: Rapid

Duration: Decreased histamine-induced wheal and flare areas: 2 to ≥36 hours; Suppression of pruritus: 1-12 hours (Simons, 1984)

Absorption: Oral: Rapid

Distribution: Adults: V_d: ~16 L/kg (Simons, 1984); Elderly: ~23 L/kg (Simons K, 1989); Hepatic dysfunction: ~23 L/kg (Simons F, 1989)

Metabolism: Hepatic to multiple metabolites, including cetirizine (active) (Simons F, 1989)

Half-life elimination: Adults: ~20 hours (Simons, 1984); Elderly: ~29 hours (Simons K, 1989); Hepatic dysfunction: ~37 hours (Simons F, 1989)

Time to peak: Oral administration: Serum: ~2 hours; Peak suppression of antihistamine-induced wheal and flare: 4-12 hours (Simons, 1984)

Excretion: Urine

Dosage

Note: Adjust dose based on patient response.

Children:

- Preoperative sedation:
  - Oral: 0.6 mg/kg/dose
  - I.M.: 1.1 mg/kg/dose
- Pruritus, anxiety: Oral:
  - <6 years: 50 mg daily in divided doses
  - ≥6 years: 50-100 mg daily in divided doses
- Antiemetic: I.M.: 1.1 mg/kg/dose

Adults:

- Antiemetic: I.M.: 25-100 mg/dose
- Anxiety:
  - Oral: 50-100 mg 4 times/day
  - I.M.: Initial: 50-100 mg, then every 4-6 hours as needed
- Preoperative sedation:
  - Oral: 50-100 mg
  - I.M.: 25-100 mg
- Pruritus: Oral: 25 mg 3-4 times/day

Elderly: Initiate dosing using the lower end of the recommended dosage range due to an increased potential for anticholinergic side effects. Refer to adult dosing.

Dosing adjustment in renal impairment: No dosage adjustment provided in the manufacturer's labeling; however, the following guidelines have been used by some clinicians (Aronoff, 2007): Adults:

- GFR >50 mL/minute: No adjustment recommended.
- GFR ≤50 mL/minute: Administer 50% of normal dose.
- Continuous renal replacement therapy (CRRT), hemodialysis, peritoneal dialysis: Administer 50% of the normal dose.

Dosing interval in hepatic impairment: Change dosing interval to every 24 hours in patients with primary biliary cirrhosis (Simons F, 1989).

Administration

Injection: For I.M. use only. Do **NOT** administer I.V., SubQ, or intra-arterially. Administer I.M. deep in large muscle. In adults, the preferred site is the upper outer quadrant of the buttock or midlateral thigh. In children, the preferred site is the midlateral thigh. The upper outer quadrant of the gluteal region should be used only when necessary to minimize potential damage to the sciatic nerve.

Oral: Shake suspension vigorously prior to use.

Monitoring Parameters Relief of symptoms, mental status, blood pressure

Test Interactions May cause false-positive serum TCA screen.

Dosage Forms Excipient information presented when available (limited, particularly for generics); consult specific product labeling.

Capsule, Oral, as pamoate:
- Vistaril: 25 mg, 50 mg
- Generic: 25 mg, 50 mg, 100 mg

Solution, Intramuscular, as hydrochloride:
- Generic: 25 mg/mL (1 mL); 50 mg/mL (1 mL, 2 mL, 10 mL)

Solution, Oral, as hydrochloride:
- Generic: 10 mg/5 mL (473 mL)

Syrup, Oral, as hydrochloride:
- Generic: 10 mg/5 mL (118 mL, 473 mL)

Tablet, Oral, as hydrochloride:
- Generic: 10 mg, 25 mg, 50 mg

◆ **Hydroxyzine Hydrochloride** *see* HydrOXYzine *on page 1025*

◆ **Hydroxyzine Hydrochloride Injection, USP (Can)** *see* HydrOXYzine *on page 1025*

◆ **Hydroxyzine Pamoate** *see* HydrOXYzine *on page 1025*

◆ **Hydurea** *see* Hydroxyurea *on page 1022*

◆ **Hygroton** *see* Chlorthalidone *on page 417*

◆ **Hylan G-F 20** *see* Hyaluronate and Derivatives *on page 1000*

◆ **Hylan Polymers** *see* Hyaluronate and Derivatives *on page 1000*

◆ **Hylase Wound** *see* Hyaluronate and Derivatives *on page 1000*

◆ **HyoMax-SL** *see* Hyoscyamine *on page 1026*

◆ **Hyonatol** *see* Hyoscyamine, Atropine, Scopolamine, and Phenobarbital *on page 1028*

◆ **Hyophen™** *see* Methenamine, Phenyl Salicylate, Methylene Blue, Benzoic Acid, and Hyoscyamine *on page 1319*

◆ **Hyoscine Butylbromide** *see* Scopolamine (Systemic) *on page 1881*

Hyoscyamine (hye oh SYE a meen)

Brand Names: U.S. Anaspaz; Ed-Spaz; HyoMax-SL; Hyosyne; Levbid; Levsin; Levsin/SL; NuLev; Oscimin; Oscimin SR; Symax Duotab; Symax FasTabs; Symax-SL; Symax-SR

Brand Names: Canada Levsin

Index Terms *l*-Hyoscyamine Sulfate; Hyoscyamine Sulfate

Pharmacologic Category Anticholinergic Agent

Additional Appendix Information

Beers Criteria – Potentially Inappropriate Medications for Geriatrics *on page 2368*

Use

Anesthesia:

Preoperative antimuscarinic: Preoperative antimuscarinic to reduce salivary, tracheobronchial, and pharyngeal secretions; to reduce volume and acidity of gastric secretions; to block cardiac vagal inhibitory reflexes during induction of anesthesia and intubation

Reversal of neuromuscular blockade and associated muscarinic effects: Protects against peripheral muscarinic effects (such as bradycardia and excessive secretions produced by halogenated hydrocarbons and cholinergic agents [such as physostigmine, neostigmine, and pyridostigmine]) given to reverse actions of curariform agents

Antidote for anticholinesterase agent poisoning: Antidote for poisoning by anticholinesterase agents

Biliary and renal colic: Adjunctive therapy with morphine or other opioids for the symptomatic relief of biliary and renal colic

Diagnostic procedures: Reduces GI motility to facilitate diagnostic procedures such as endoscopy or hypotonic duodenography; may also improve radiologic visibility of the kidneys

GI disorders:

Aid in the control of acute episodes of gastric secretion, visceral spasm, hypermotility in spastic colitis, pylorospasm, and associated abdominal cramps; relieve symptoms in functional intestinal disorders (eg, mild dysenteries, diverticulitis) and infant colic (elixir and oral solution)

Adjunctive therapy for treatment in peptic ulcer; irritable bowel syndrome (irritable colon, spastic colon, acute enterocolitis, mucous colitis) and other functional GI disorders; neurogenic bowel disturbances (including splenic flexure syndrome and neurogenic colon)

Pancreatitis: Reduce pain and hypersecretion in pancreatitis

Parkinsonism: In parkinsonism, to reduce rigidity and tremors and to control associated sialorrhea and hyperhidrosis

Partial heart block: For use in certain cases of partial heart block associated with vagal activity

Rhinitis: "Drying agent" in the relief of symptoms of acute rhinitis

Urinary system disorder: To control hypermotility in spastic bladder and cystitis; adjunctive therapy in the treatment of neurogenic bladder

Pregnancy Risk Factor C

Dosage

Gastrointestinal disorders: Oral:

Children <2 years: Drops (Hyosyne [0.125 mg/**mL**]): Dose as listed, based on age and weight (kg); repeat dose every 4 hours or as needed:

3.4 kg: 4 **drops**; maximum: 24 **drops** daily
5 kg: 5 **drops**; maximum: 30 **drops** daily
7 kg: 6 **drops**; maximum: 36 **drops** daily
10 kg: 8 **drops**; maximum: 48 **drops** daily

Children 2 to <12 years:

Tablets (regular release [Levsin], dispersible [Anaspaz, ED-SPAZ, NuLev, Symax FasTab]): 0.0625 to 0.125 mg every 4 hours or as needed; maximum: 0.75 mg daily

Drops (Hyosyne [0.125 mg/**mL**]): 0.03125 mg (0.25 mL) to 0.125 mg (1 mL) every 4 hours or as needed; maximum: 0.75 mg (6 mL) daily

Elixir (Hyosyne [0.125 mg/**5 mL**]): Dose as listed, based on age and weight (kg); repeat dose every 4 hours or as needed:

10 kg: 0.03125 mg (1.25 mL); maximum: 0.75 mg (30 mL) daily
20 kg: 0.0625 mg (2.5 mL); maximum: 0.75 mg (30 mL) daily
40 kg: 0.09375 mg (3.75 mL); maximum: 0.75 mg (30 mL) daily
50 kg: 0.125 mg (5 mL); maximum: 0.75 mg (30 mL) daily

Children 6 to <12 years: Sublingual (HyoMax-SL): 0.0625 mg to 0.125 mg 3-4 times daily

Children ≥12 years, Adolescents, and Adults:

Tablet, dispersible:

Anaspaz, ED-SPAZ, NuLev, Symax FasTab: 0.125 to 0.25 mg every 4 hours or as needed; maximum: 1.5 mg daily

Oscimin: 0.125 to 0.25 mg 3-4 times daily

Tablet, extended release:

Levbid, Symax Duotab: 0.375 to 0.75 mg every 12 hours; maximum: 1.5 mg daily

Oscimin SR, Symax SR: 0.375 to 0.75 mg every 12 hours or 0.375 mg every 8 hours; maximum: 1.5 mg daily

Tablet, regular release:

Levsin: 0.125 to 0.25 mg every 4 hours or as needed; maximum: 1.5 mg daily

Oscimin: 0.125 to 0.25 mg 3-4 times daily

Tablet, sublingual (HyoMax-SL, Oscimin, Symax SL): 0.125 to 0.25 mg 3-4 times daily

Drops (Hyosyne [0.125 mg/**mL**]): 0.125 mg (1 mL) to 0.25 mg (2 mL) every 4 hours or as needed; maximum: 1.5 mg (12 mL) daily

Elixir (Hyosyne [0.125 mg/**5 mL**]): 0.125 mg (5 mL) to 0.25 mg (10 mL) every 4 hours or as needed; maximum: 1.5 mg (60 mL) daily

I.M., I.V., SubQ: 0.25 to 0.5 mg; may repeat as needed up to 4 times daily, at 4-hour intervals

Diagnostic procedures: Adults: I.V.: 0.25 to 0.5 mg given 5-10 minutes prior to procedure

Preanesthesia: Children >2 years, Adolescents, and Adults: I.M., I.V., SubQ: 5 **mcg**/kg given 30-60 minutes prior to induction of anesthesia or at the time preoperative opioids or sedatives are administered

Reduce drug-induced bradycardia during surgery: Adults: I.V.: 0.125 mg; repeat as needed

Reverse neuromuscular blockade: Adults: I.M., I.V., SubQ: 0.2 mg for every 1 mg neostigmine (or the physostigmine/pyridostigmine equivalent)

Dosage adjustment in renal impairment: No dosage adjustment provided in manufacturer's labeling, use with caution.

Dosage adjustment in hepatic impairment: No dosage adjustment provided in manufacturer's labeling.

Additional Information Complete prescribing information should be consulted for additional detail.

Dosage Forms Excipient information presented when available (limited, particularly for generics); consult specific product labeling.

Elixir, Oral, as sulfate:
Hyosyne: 0.125 mg/5 mL (473 mL) [contains alcohol, usp; lemon flavor]
Generic: 0.125 mg/5 mL (473 mL)

Solution, Injection, as sulfate:
Levsin: 0.5 mg/mL (1 mL) [contains benzyl alcohol]

Solution, Oral, as sulfate:
Hyosyne: 0.125 mg/mL (15 mL) [lemon flavor]
Generic: 0.125 mg/mL (15 mL)

Tablet, Oral, as sulfate:
Levsin: 0.125 mg
Oscimin: 0.125 mg [peppermint flavor]
Generic: 0.125 mg

Tablet Dispersible, Oral, as sulfate:
Anaspaz: 0.125 mg [scored]
Ed-Spaz: 0.125 mg [scored]
NuLev: 0.125 mg [peppermint flavor]
Oscimin: 0.125 mg [peppermint flavor]
Symax FasTabs: 0.125 mg [mint flavor]
Generic: 0.125 mg

Tablet Extended Release, Oral, as sulfate:
Symax Duotab: 0.375 mg [contains brilliant blue fcf (fd&c blue #1)]

Tablet Extended Release 12 Hour, Oral, as sulfate:
Levbid: 0.375 mg
Oscimin SR: 0.375 mg
Symax-SR: 0.375 mg [scored]
Generic: 0.375 mg

Tablet Sublingual, Sublingual, as sulfate:
HyoMax-SL: 0.125 mg
Levsin/SL: 0.125 mg
Oscimin: 0.125 mg [peppermint flavor]
Symax-SL: 0.125 mg [mint flavor]
Generic: 0.125 mg

Hyoscyamine, Atropine, Scopolamine, and Phenobarbital

(hye oh SYE a meen, A troe peen, skoe POL a meen, & fee noe BAR bi tal)

Brand Names: U.S. Donnatal Extentabs®; Donnatal®; Hyonatol

Index Terms Atropine, Hyoscyamine, Phenobarbital, and Scopolamine; Belladonna Alkaloids With Phenobarbital; Phenobarbital, Hyoscyamine, Atropine, and Scopolamine; Scopolamine, Hyoscyamine, Atropine, and Phenobarbital

Pharmacologic Category Anticholinergic Agent; Antispasmodic Agent, Gastrointestinal

Use Adjunct in treatment of irritable bowel syndrome, acute enterocolitis, duodenal ulcer

Pregnancy Risk Factor C

Dosage Oral:

Children ≥2 years: Elixir: To be given every 4-6 hours; initial dose based on weight:
- 9.1 kg: 1 mL every 4 hours **or** 1.5 mL every 6 hours
- 13.6 kg: 1.5 mL every 4 hours **or** 2 mL every 6 hours
- 22.7 kg: 2.5 mL every 4 hours **or** 3.75 mL every 6 hours
- 34 kg: 3.75 mL every 4 hours **or** 5 mL every 6 hours
- 45.4 kg: 5 mL every 4 hours **or** 7.5 mL every 6 hours

Adults:
- Immediate release: 1-2 tablets or 5-10 mL of elixir 3-4 times/day
- Extended release: One tablet every 12 hours; may increase to 1 tablet every 8 hours if needed

Additional Information Complete prescribing information should be consulted for additional detail.

Dosage Forms Excipient information presented when available (limited, particularly for generics); consult specific product labeling. [DSC] = Discontinued product

Elixir:
- Donnatal®: Hyoscyamine sulfate 0.1037 mg, atropine sulfate 0.0194 mg, scopolamine hydrobromide 0.0065 mg, and phenobarbital 16.2 mg per 5 mL (120 mL, 480 mL) [contains ethanol <23.8%; citrus flavor] [DSC]
- Donnatal®: Hyoscyamine sulfate 0.1037 mg, atropine sulfate 0.0194 mg, scopolamine hydrobromide 0.0065 mg, and phenobarbital 16.2 mg per 5 mL (120 mL, 480 mL) [contains ethanol <23.8%; grape flavor]

Tablet:
- Donnatal®: Hyoscyamine sulfate 0.1037 mg, atropine sulfate 0.0194 mg, scopolamine hydrobromide 0.0065 mg, and phenobarbital 16.2 mg
- Hyonatol: Hyoscyamine sulfate 0.1037 mg, atropine sulfate 0.0194 mg, scopolamine hydrobromide 0.0065 mg, and phenobarbital 16.2 mg

Tablet, extended release:
- Donnatal Extentabs®: Hyoscyamine sulfate 0.3111 mg, atropine sulfate 0.0582 mg, scopolamine hydrobromide 0.0195 mg, and phenobarbital 48.6 mg

◆ **Hyoscyamine, Methenamine, Benzoic Acid, Phenyl Salicylate, and Methylene Blue** *see* Methenamine, Phenyl Salicylate, Methylene Blue, Benzoic Acid, and Hyoscyamine *on page 1319*

◆ **Hyoscyamine, Methenamine, Methylene Blue, Phenyl Salicylate, and Sodium Biphosphate** *see* Methenamine, Sodium Biphosphate, Phenyl Salicylate, Methylene Blue, and Hyoscyamine *on page 1320*

◆ **Hyoscyamine, Methenamine, Sodium Biphosphate, Phenyl Salicylate, and Methylene Blue** *see* Methenamine, Sodium Biphosphate, Phenyl Salicylate, Methylene Blue, and Hyoscyamine *on page 1320*

◆ **Hyoscyamine Sulfate** *see* Hyoscyamine *on page 1026*

◆ **Hyosyne** *see* Hyoscyamine *on page 1026*

◆ **Hyperal** *see* Total Parenteral Nutrition *on page 2098*

◆ **Hyperalimentation** *see* Total Parenteral Nutrition *on page 2098*

◆ **HyperHEP B S/D** *see* Hepatitis B Immune Globulin (Human) *on page 993*

◆ **HyperHEP B™ S/D (Can)** *see* Hepatitis B Immune Globulin (Human) *on page 993*

◆ **HyperRAB S/D** *see* Rabies Immune Globulin (Human) *on page 1771*

◆ **HyperRAB® S/D (Can)** *see* Rabies Immune Globulin (Human) *on page 1771*

◆ **HyperRHO S/D** *see* Rh_o(D) Immune Globulin *on page 1801*

◆ **HyperSal** *see* Sodium Chloride *on page 1914*

◆ **HyperTET S/D** *see* Tetanus Immune Globulin (Human) *on page 2030*

◆ **HyperTET™ S/D (Can)** *see* Tetanus Immune Globulin (Human) *on page 2030*

◆ **Hypertonic Saline** *see* Sodium Chloride *on page 1914*

◆ **HySept [OTC]** *see* Sodium Hypochlorite Solution *on page 1918*

◆ **Hytrin** *see* Terazosin *on page 2015*

◆ **Hytrin® (Can)** *see* Terazosin *on page 2015*

◆ **Hyzaar®** *see* Losartan and Hydrochlorothiazide *on page 1249*

◆ **Hyzaar (Can)** *see* Losartan and Hydrochlorothiazide *on page 1249*

◆ **Hyzaar DS (Can)** *see* Losartan and Hydrochlorothiazide *on page 1249*

◆ **HZV** *see* Zoster Vaccine *on page 2247*

Ibandronate (eye BAN droh nate)

Brand Names: U.S. Boniva

Index Terms Ibandronate Sodium; Ibandronic Acid

Pharmacologic Category Bisphosphonate Derivative

Use Treatment and prevention of osteoporosis in postmenopausal females

Unlabeled Use Hypercalcemia of malignancy; reduce bone pain and skeletal complications from metastatic bone disease due to breast cancer

Pregnancy Risk Factor C

Pregnancy Considerations Adverse effects were observed in animal reproduction studies. It is not known if bisphosphonates cross the placenta, but fetal exposure is expected (Djokanovic, 2008; Stathopoulos, 2011). Bisphosphonates are incorporated into the bone matrix and gradually released over time. The amount available in the systemic circulation varies by dose and duration of therapy. Theoretically, there may be a risk of fetal harm when pregnancy follows the completion of therapy; however, available data have not shown that exposure to bisphosphonates during pregnancy significantly increases the risk of adverse fetal events (Djokanovic, 2008; Levy, 2009; Stathopoulos, 2011). Until additional data is available, most sources recommend discontinuing bisphosphonate therapy in women of reproductive potential as early as possible prior to a planned pregnancy; use in premenopausal women should be reserved for special circumstances when rapid bone loss is occurring (Bhalla, 2010; Pereira, 2012; Stathopoulos, 2011). Because hypocalcemia has been described following *in utero* bisphosphonate exposure, exposed infants should be monitored for hypocalcemia after birth (Djokanovic, 2008; Stathopoulos, 2011).

Breast-Feeding Considerations It is not known if ibandronate is excreted into breast milk. The manufacturer recommends caution be exercised when administering ibandronate to nursing women.

Medication Guide Available Yes

Contraindications Hypersensitivity to ibandronate or any component of the formulation; hypocalcemia; oral tablets are also contraindicated in patients unable to stand or sit upright for at least 60 minutes and in patients with abnormalities of the esophagus which delay esophageal emptying, such as stricture or achalasia

Warnings/Precautions Hypocalcemia must be corrected before therapy initiation. Ensure adequate calcium and vitamin D intake. Osteonecrosis of the jaw (ONJ) has been reported in patients receiving bisphosphonates. Risk factors include invasive dental procedures (eg, tooth extraction, dental implants, boney surgery); a diagnosis of cancer, with concomitant chemotherapy or corticosteroids; poor oral hygiene, ill-fitting dentures; and comorbid disorders (anemia, coagulopathy, infection, pre-existing dental disease); risk may increase with duration of bisphosphonate use. Most reported cases occurred after I.V. bisphosphonate therapy; however, cases have been reported following oral therapy. A dental exam and preventative dentistry should be performed prior to placing patients with risk factors on chronic bisphosphonate therapy. The manufacturer's labeling states that discontinuing bisphosphonates in patients requiring invasive dental procedures may reduce the risk of ONJ. However, other experts suggest that there is no evidence that discontinuing therapy reduces the risk of developing ONJ (Assael, 2009). The benefit/risk must be assessed by the treating physician and/or dentist/surgeon prior to any invasive dental procedure. Patients developing ONJ while on bisphosphonates should receive care by an oral surgeon.

Atypical femur fractures have been reported in patients receiving bisphosphonates for treatment/prevention of osteoporosis. The fractures include subtrochanteric femur (bone just below the hip joint) and diaphyseal femur (long segment of the thigh bone). Some patients experience prodromal pain weeks or months before the fracture occurs. It is unclear if bisphosphonate therapy is the cause for these fractures, although the majority of cases have been reported in patients taking bisphosphonates. Patients receiving long-term (>3-5 years) therapy may be at an increased risk. Discontinue bisphosphonate therapy in patients who develop a femoral shaft fracture.

Infrequently, severe (and occasionally debilitating) bone, joint, and/or muscle pain have been reported during bisphosphonate treatment. The onset of pain ranged from a single day to several months. Discontinue intravenous ibandronate therapy in patients who experience severe symptoms; symptoms usually resolve upon discontinuation. Some patients experienced recurrence when rechallenged with same drug or another bisphosphonate; avoid use in patients with a history of these symptoms in association with bisphosphonate therapy.

Oral bisphosphonates may cause dysphagia, esophagitis, esophageal or gastric ulcer; risk may increase in patients unable to comply with dosing instructions; discontinue use if new or worsening symptoms develop. Intravenous bisphosphonates may cause transient decreases in serum calcium and have also been associated with renal toxicity.

Use not recommended with severe renal impairment (Cl_{cr} <30 mL/minute). In the management of osteoporosis, re-evaluate the need for continued therapy periodically; the optimal duration of treatment has not yet been determined. Consider discontinuing after 3-5 years of use in patients at low-risk for fracture; following discontinuation, re-evaluate fracture risk periodically. Potentially significant drug-drug interactions may exist, requiring dose or frequency adjustment, additional monitoring, and/or selection of alternative therapy.

Adverse Reactions Percentages vary based on frequency of administration (daily vs monthly). Unless specified, percentages are reported with oral use.

>10%:

- Gastrointestinal: Dyspepsia (6% to 12%)
- Neuromuscular & skeletal: Back pain (4% to 14%)

1% to 10%:

- Cardiovascular: Hypertension (6% to 7%)
- Central nervous system: Headache (3% to 7%), dizziness (1% to 4%), insomnia (1% to 2%)
- Dermatologic: Rash (1% to 2%)
- Endocrine & metabolic: Hypercholesterolemia (5%)
- Gastrointestinal: Abdominal pain (5% to 8%), diarrhea (4% to 7%), nausea (5%), constipation (3% to 4%), vomiting (3%)
- Genitourinary: Urinary tract infection (2% to 6%)
- Hepatic: Alkaline phosphatase decreased (frequency not defined)
- Local: Injection site reaction (<2%)
- Neuromuscular & skeletal: Pain in extremity (1% to 8%), arthralgia (4% to 6%), myalgia (1% to 6%), joint disorder (4%), osteonecrosis of the jaw (4%), weakness (4%), osteoarthritis (localized; 1% to 3%), muscle cramp (2%)
- Respiratory: Bronchitis (3% to 10%), pneumonia (6%), pharyngitis/nasopharyngitis (3% to 4%), upper respiratory infection (2%)
- Miscellaneous: Acute phase reaction (I.V. 10%; oral 3% to 9%), infection (4%), flu-like syndrome (1% to 4%), allergic reaction (3%)

Postmarketing and/or case reports (Limited to important or life-threatening): Acute renal failure, anaphylactic shock, anaphylaxis, angioedema, bronchospasm, diaphyseal femur fracture, esophageal cancer, exacerbation of asthma, hypocalcemia; incapacitating bone, joint, or muscle pain; iritis, ocular inflammation, scleritis, subtrochanteric femur fracture, uveitis

Drug Interactions

Metabolism/Transport Effects None known.

Avoid Concomitant Use There are no known interactions where it is recommended to avoid concomitant use.

Increased Effect/Toxicity

Ibandronate may increase the levels/effects of: Deferasirox; Phosphate Supplements

The levels/effects of Ibandronate may be increased by: Aminoglycosides; Nonsteroidal Anti-Inflammatory Agents; Systemic Angiogenesis Inhibitors

Decreased Effect

The levels/effects of Ibandronate may be decreased by: Antacids; Calcium Salts; Iron Salts; Magnesium Salts; Multivitamins/Minerals (with ADEK, Folate, Iron); Multivitamins/Minerals (with AE, No Iron); Proton Pump Inhibitors; Sucroferric Oxyhydroxide

Ethanol/Nutrition/Herb Interactions

Ethanol: Ethanol may increase risk of osteoporosis. Management: Avoid ethanol.

Food: May reduce absorption; mean oral bioavailability is decreased up to 90% when given with food. Management: Take with a full glass (6-8 oz) of plain water, at least 60 minutes prior to any food, beverages, or medications. Mineral water with a high calcium content should be avoided. Wait at least 60 minutes after taking ibandronate before taking anything else.

Storage/Stability Store at controlled room temperature of 25°C (77°F); excursions permitted to 15°C to 30°C (59°F to 86°F).

Mechanism of Action A bisphosphonate which inhibits bone resorption via actions on osteoclasts or on osteoclast precursors; decreases the rate of bone resorption, leading to an indirect increase in bone mineral density.

Pharmacodynamics/Kinetics

Distribution: Terminal V_d: 90 L; 40% to 50% of circulating ibandronate binds to bone

Protein binding: 85.7% to 99.5%
Metabolism: Not metabolized
Bioavailability: Oral: Minimal; reduced ~90% following standard breakfast
Half-life elimination:
Oral: 150 mg dose: Terminal: 37-157 hours
I.V.: Terminal: ~5-25 hours
Time to peak, plasma: Oral: 0.5-2 hours
Excretion: Urine (50% to 60% of absorbed dose, excreted as unchanged drug); feces (unabsorbed drug)

Dosage

Postmenopausal osteoporosis (treatment): Adults: **Note:** Consider discontinuing after 3-5 years of use for osteoporosis in patients at low-risk for fracture. Patients should receive supplemental calcium and vitamin D if dietary intake is inadequate.
Oral: 150 mg once monthly
I.V.: 3 mg every 3 months
Postmenopausal osteoporosis (prevention): Adults: Oral: 150 mg once monthly. **Note:** Patients should receive supplemental calcium and vitamin D if dietary intake is inadequate.
Hypercalcemia of malignancy (unlabeled use): Adults: I.V.: 2-6 mg over 1-2 hours (Pecherstorfer, 2003; Ralston, 1997)
Metastatic bone disease due to breast cancer (unlabeled use): Adults: I.V.: 6 mg every 3-4 weeks (Diel, 2004)

Missed doses:
Oral: If once-monthly oral dose is missed, it should be given the next morning after remembered if the next month's scheduled dose is >7 days away. If the next month's scheduled dose is within 7 days, wait until the next month's scheduled dose. May then return to the original monthly schedule (original scheduled day of the month). Do not give >150 mg within 7 days.
I.V.: If an I.V. dose is missed, it should be administered as soon as it can be rescheduled. Thereafter, it should be given every 3 months from the date of the last injection.

Dosage adjustment in renal impairment:
Osteoporosis: Oral, I.V.:
Cl_{cr} ≥30 mL/minute: No dosage adjustment necessary.
Cl_{cr} <30 mL/minute: Use not recommended.
Oncologic uses (unlabeled): I.V.: Cl_{cr} <30 mL/minute: 2 mg every 3-4 weeks (von Moos, 2005)

Dosage adjustment in hepatic impairment: No dosage adjustment necessary (has not been studied); however, ibandronate does not undergo hepatic metabolism.

Dietary Considerations

Ensure adequate calcium and vitamin D intake; if dietary intake is inadequate, dietary supplementation is recommended. Women and men should consume:
Calcium: 1000 mg/day (men: 50-70 years) **or** 1200 mg/day (women ≥51 years and men ≥71 years) (IOM, 2011; NOF, 2013)
Vitamin D: 800-1000 IU/day (men and women ≥50 years) (NOF, 2013). Recommended Dietary Allowance (RDA): 600 IU/day (men and women ≤70 years) **or** 800 IU/day (men and women ≥71 years) (IOM, 2011).
Ibandronate tablet should be taken with a full glass (6-8 oz) of plain water, at least 60 minutes prior to any food, beverages, or medications. Mineral water with a high calcium content should be avoided.

Administration

Oral: Administer 60 minutes before the first food or drink of the day (other than water) and prior to taking any oral medications or supplements (eg, calcium, antacids, vitamins). Ibandronate should be taken in an upright position with a full glass (6-8 oz) of plain water and the patient should avoid lying down for 60 minutes to minimize the possibility of GI side effects. Mineral water with a high calcium content should be avoided. The tablet should be swallowed whole; do not chew or suck. Do not eat or drink anything (except water) for 60 minutes following administration of ibandronate.
I.V.: Administer as a 15-30 second bolus intravenously; avoid paravenous or intraarterial administration (may cause tissue damage). Do not mix with calcium-containing solutions or other drugs. For osteoporosis, do not administer more frequently than every 3 months. Infuse over 1 hour for metastatic bone disease due to breast cancer (Diel, 2004) and over 1-2 hours for hypercalcemia of malignancy (Pecherstorfer, 2003; Ralston, 1997).

Monitoring Parameters

Osteoporosis: Bone mineral density (BMD) should be re-evaluated every 2 years (or more frequently) after initiating therapy (NOF, 2013); annual measurements of height and weight, assessment of chronic back pain; serum calcium and 25(OH)D; may consider measuring biochemical markers of bone turnover

Serum creatinine prior to each I.V. dose

Reference Range

Calcium (total): Adults: 9.0-11.0 mg/dL (2.05-2.54 mmol/L), may slightly decrease with aging
Phosphorus: 2.5-4.5 mg/dL (0.81-1.45 mmol/L)
Vitamin D: There is no clear consensus on a reference range for total serum 25(OH)D concentrations or the validity of this level as it relates clinically to bone health. In addition, there is significant variability in the reporting of serum 25(OH)D levels as a result of different assay types in use; however, the following ranges have been suggested:
Adults (IOM, 2011): Sufficient levels in practically all persons: ≥20 ng/mL (50 nmol/L); concern for risk of toxicity: >50 ng/mL (125 nmol/L)
Osteoporosis patients (NOF, 2013): Recommended level to reach and maintain: ~30 ng/mL (75 nmol/L)

Test Interactions Bisphosphonates may interfere with diagnostic imaging agents such as technetium-99m-diphosphonate in bone scans.

Dosage Forms Excipient information presented when available (limited, particularly for generics); consult specific product labeling.
Solution, Intravenous:
Boniva: 3 mg/3 mL (3 mL)
Tablet, Oral:
Boniva: 150 mg
Generic: 150 mg

◆ **Ibandronate Sodium** *see* Ibandronate *on page* 1028
◆ **Ibandronic Acid** *see* Ibandronate *on page* 1028
◆ **Ibenzmethyzin** *see* Procarbazine *on page* 1720
◆ **Ibidomide Hydrochloride** *see* Labetalol *on page* 1156

Ibrutinib (eye BROO ti nib)

Brand Names: U.S. Imbruvica

Index Terms BTK inhibitor PCI-32765; CRA-032765; PCI-32765

Pharmacologic Category Antineoplastic Agent; Antineoplastic Agent, Bruton Tyrosine Kinase Inhibitor; Antineoplastic Agent, Tyrosine Kinase Inhibitor

Use Mantle cell lymphoma: Treatment of mantle cell lymphoma (MCL) in patients who have received at least 1 prior therapy

Pregnancy Risk Factor D

Pregnancy Considerations Adverse events were observed in animal reproduction studies. Women of reproductive potential should avoid pregnancy during therapy.

Breast-Feeding Considerations It is not known if ibrutinib is excreted into breast milk. Due to the potential for serious adverse reactions in the nursing infant, the manufacturer recommends a decision be made whether to discontinue nursing or to discontinue the drug, taking into account the importance of treatment to the mother.

Contraindications There are no contraindications listed within the manufacturer's labeling.

Warnings/Precautions Hazardous agent – use appropriate precautions for handling and disposal (meets NIOSH, 2012 criteria). Grade 3 and 4 neutropenia, thrombocytopenia, and anemia occurred commonly during clinical studies. Monitor blood counts monthly or as clinically necessary. Lymphocytosis (≥50% increase from baseline) may occur upon therapy initiation, generally within the first few weeks of therapy (median 1.1 weeks). The increase in lymphocytes is temporary, and resolves by a median of 8 weeks. Bleeding events (eg, bruising, petechiae) occurred during clinical trials; some events were grade 3 or higher (eg, subdural hematoma, gastrointestinal bleeding, and hematuria); monitor for bleeding. Evaluate the risk-benefit of using ibrutinib in patients receiving anticoagulant or antiplatelet medications. Consider interrupting therapy for 3-7 days prior to and after surgery, depending on the procedure type and risk of bleeding. Serious infections (some fatal) have been observed; monitor closely for fever and other signs/symptoms of infection. Evaluate promptly. Patients treated with ibrutinib have developed second primary malignancies during use, including skin cancers and other carcinomas. Evaluate for sign/symptoms of malignancy during treatment.

Atrial fibrillation, hypertension, infections (eg, pneumonia, cellulitis), and gastrointestinal toxicity (eg, diarrhea and dehydration) were observed more frequently in elderly patients. Use with caution in patients with pre-existing renal impairment; has not been studied in those with severe impairment or in patients on dialysis. Renal failure has been reported with use; some cases were fatal. Clinical trials report serum creatinine increases of up to 3 times ULN; monitor renal function periodically and maintain hydration. Increased uric acid levels have been observed, including grade 4 elevations. Use with caution in patients with any degree of hepatic impairment. Patients with AST or ALT levels ≥3 times ULN were excluded from clinical trials; ibrutinib is hepatically cleared, and exposure is expected to increase in patients with hepatic dysfunction. Monitor closely for toxicity. Potentially significant drug-drug/drug-food interactions may exist, requiring dose or frequency adjustment, additional monitoring, and/or selection of alternative therapy.

Adverse Reactions

>10%:

Cardiovascular: Peripheral edema (35%)

Central nervous system: Dizziness (14%), fatigue (41%), headache (13%)

Dermatologic: Skin rash (25%), skin infection (14%)

Endocrine & metabolic: Hyperuricemia (40%; >10 mg/dL: 13%), dehydration (12%)

Gastrointestinal: Diarrhea (51%), nausea (31%), constipation (25%), abdominal pain (24%), vomiting (23%), decreased appetite (21%), stomatitis (17%), dyspepsia (11%)

Genitourinary: Urinary tract infection (14%)

Hematologic & oncologic: Decreased platelet count (57%; grades 3/4:17%), hemorrhage (48%; grades 3/4: 5%, including subdural hematoma, gastrointestinal bleeding, hematuria), decreased hemoglobin (41%; grades 3/4: 9%), bruise (30%), neutropenia (47%; grades 3/4: 29%), petechia (11%)

Infection: Infection (grades 3/4: 25%)

Neuromuscular & skeletal: Musculoskeletal pain (37%), muscle spasm (14%), weakness (14%), arthralgia (11%)

Renal: Increased serum creatinine (<1.5 x ULN: 67%; 1.5-3 x ULN: 9%)

Respiratory: Upper respiratory tract infection (34%), dyspnea (27%), cough (19%), pneumonia (14%), sinusitis (13%), epistaxis (11%)

Miscellaneous: Fever (18%)

1% to 10%: Hematologic & oncologic: Malignant neoplasm of skin (4%), carcinoma (1%)

Frequency not defined: Renal failure

Drug Interactions

Metabolism/Transport Effects **Substrate** of CYP3A4 (major); **Note:** Assignment of Major/Minor substrate status based on clinically relevant drug interaction potential

Avoid Concomitant Use

Avoid concomitant use of Ibrutinib with any of the following: CYP3A4 Inducers (Strong); CYP3A4 Inhibitors (Moderate); CYP3A4 Inhibitors (Strong); Fusidic Acid (Systemic); Herbs (CYP3A4 Inducers)

Increased Effect/Toxicity

Ibrutinib may increase the levels/effects of: Agents with Antiplatelet Properties; Anticoagulants

The levels/effects of Ibrutinib may be increased by: CYP3A4 Inhibitors (Moderate); CYP3A4 Inhibitors (Strong); Dasatinib; Fusidic Acid (Systemic); Ivacaftor; Luliconazole; Mifepristone; Simeprevir

Decreased Effect

The levels/effects of Ibrutinib may be decreased by: Bosentan; CYP3A4 Inducers (Strong); CYP3A4 Inducers (Weakly to Moderately Effective); Dabrafenib; Deferasirox; Herbs (CYP3A4 Inducers); Tocilizumab

Ethanol/Nutrition/Herb Interactions Food: Grapefruit and Seville oranges moderately inhibit CYP3A and may increase ibrutinib exposure. Management: Avoid grapefruit and Seville oranges during therapy.

Storage/Stability Store at 20°C to 25°C (68°F to 77°F); excursions are permitted between 15°C and 30°C (59°F and 86°F). Keep in original container.

Mechanism of Action Ibrutinib is a potent and irreversible inhibitor of Bruton's tyrosine kinase (BTK), an integral component of the B-cell receptor (BCR) and cytokine receptor pathways. Constitutive activation of B-cell receptor signaling is important for survival of malignant B-cells; BTK inhibition results in decreased malignant B-cell proliferation and survival.

Pharmacodynamics/Kinetics

Distribution: ~10,000 L

Bioavailability: Administration with food increased exposure ~2-fold (compared to overnight fasting)

Protein binding: ~97%

Metabolism: Hepatic via CYP3A (major) and CYP2D6 (minor) to active metabolite PCI-45227

Half-life elimination: 4-6 hours

Time to peak: 1-2 hours

Excretion: Feces (80%; ~1% as unchanged drug); urine (<10%, as metabolites)

Dosage

Mantle cell lymphoma: Adults: Oral: 560 mg once daily (Wang, 2013)

Missed doses: Administer as soon as the missed dose is remembered; return to normal scheduling the following day. Do not take extra capsules to make up for the missed dose.

Dosage adjustment for concomitant therapy:

Moderate or strong CYP3A inhibitors: Avoid concurrent use with moderate or strong CYP3A inhibitors which are taken chronically; consider an alternative agent with less CYP3A inhibition. If short term use (≤7 days) of a strong inhibitor is necessary, consider withholding ibrutinib therapy until the strong CYP3A inhibitor is discontinued. If concomitant use of a moderate inhibitor is necessary, reduce ibrutinib dose to 140 mg once daily. Monitor closely for toxicity during concomitant use.

Strong CYP3A inducers: Avoid concurrent use with strong CYP3A inducers; consider alternative agents with less CYP3A induction.

Dosage adjustment for toxicity:

Hematologic toxicity: ≥ Grade 3 neutropenia with infection or fever, or grade 4 toxicity: Interrupt therapy; upon improvement to grade 1 toxicity or baseline, resume dosing at the starting dose. If toxicity recurs, reduce daily dose by 140 mg. If toxicity recurs after first dose reduction, reduce daily dose by an additional 140 mg. If toxicity persists following 2 dose reductions, discontinue therapy.

Nonhematologic toxicity: ≥ Grade 3 toxicity: Interrupt therapy; upon improvement to grade 1 toxicity or baseline, resume dosing at the starting dose. If toxicity recurs, reduce daily dose by 140 mg. If toxicity recurs after first dose reduction, reduce daily dose by an additional 140 mg. If toxicity persists following 2 dose reductions, discontinue therapy.

Recommend dose reductions for toxicity:

First occurrence: Restart at 560 mg once daily
Second occurrence: Restart at 420 mg once daily
Third occurrence: Restart at 280 mg once daily
Fourth occurrence: Discontinue

Dosage adjustment for renal impairment:

Mild to moderate impairment (Cl_{cr} ≥25 mL/minute): No dosage adjustment provided in manufacturer's labeling; however, renal excretion is minimal and drug exposure is not altered in patients with mild to moderate impairment.

Severe impairment (Cl_{cr} <25 mL/minute): No dosage adjustment provided in manufacturer's labeling (has not been studied).

End-stage renal disease (ESRD) requiring dialysis: No dosage adjustment provided in manufacturer's labeling (has not been studied).

Dosage adjustment for hepatic impairment: Mild, moderate, or severe impairment: No dosage adjustment provided in manufacturer's labeling. Ibrutinib is metabolized hepatically; significant increases in drug exposure are expected in patients with hepatic impairment. Patients with AST or ALT levels ≥3 times ULN were excluded from clinical trials.

Dietary Considerations Avoid grapefruit, grapefruit juice, and Seville oranges during therapy.

Administration Administer orally with water at approximately the same time every day. Swallow capsules whole; do not open, break, or chew the capsules. Hazardous agent; use appropriate precautions for handling and disposal (meets NIOSH, 2012 criteria).

Monitoring Parameters Monitor blood counts monthly or as clinically necessary; renal and hepatic function; sign/symptoms of bleeding, infections, and second primary malignancies.

Dosage Forms Excipient information presented when available (limited, particularly for generics); consult specific product labeling.

Capsule, Oral:

Imbruvica: 140 mg

◆ **IBU-200 [OTC]** *see* Ibuprofen *on page 1032*
◆ **Ibudone** *see* Hydrocodone and Ibuprofen *on page 1008*

Ibuprofen (eye byoo PROE fen)

Brand Names: U.S. Addaprin [OTC]; Advil Junior Strength [OTC]; Advil Migraine [OTC]; Advil [OTC]; Caldolor; Childrens Advil [OTC]; Childrens Ibuprofen [OTC]; Childrens Motrin Jr Strength [OTC]; Childrens Motrin [OTC]; Dyspel [OTC]; EnovaRX-Ibuprofen; Genpril [OTC]; I-Prin [OTC]; IBU-200 [OTC]; Ibuprofen Childrens [OTC]; Ibuprofen Comfort Pac; Ibuprofen Junior Strength [OTC]; Infants Advil [OTC]; Infants Ibuprofen [OTC]; KS Ibuprofen [OTC]; Motrin IB [OTC]; Motrin Infants Drops [OTC]; Motrin Junior Strength [OTC]; Motrin [OTC]; NeoProfen; Provil [OTC]

Brand Names: Canada Advil®; Advil® Children's; Apo-Ibuprofen®; Motrin® (Children's); Motrin® IB; Novo-Profen; Nu-Ibuprofen

Index Terms *p*-Isobutylhydratropic Acid; Ibuprofen Lysine

Pharmacologic Category Nonsteroidal Anti-inflammatory Drug (NSAID), Oral; Nonsteroidal Anti-inflammatory Drug (NSAID), Parenteral

Additional Appendix Information

Beers Criteria – Potentially Inappropriate Medications for Geriatrics *on page 2368*

Use

Oral: Inflammatory diseases and rheumatoid disorders including juvenile idiopathic arthritis (JIA), mild-to-moderate pain, fever, dysmenorrhea, osteoarthritis

Ibuprofen injection (Caldolor®): Management of mild-to-moderate pain; management moderate-to-severe pain when used concurrently with an opioid analgesic; reduction of fever

Ibuprofen lysine injection (NeoProfen®): To induce closure of a clinically-significant patent ductus arteriosus (PDA) in premature infants weighing between 500-1500 g and who are ≤32 weeks gestational age (GA) when usual treatments are ineffective

Unlabeled Use Ankylosing spondylitis, cystic fibrosis, gout, acute migraine headache, migraine prophylaxis, pericarditis

Pregnancy Risk Factor C/D ≥30 weeks gestation

Pregnancy Considerations Adverse events were not observed in the initial animal reproduction studies; therefore, the manufacturer classifies ibuprofen as pregnancy category C (category D: ≥30 weeks gestation). NSAID exposure during the first trimester is not strongly associated with congenital malformations; however, cardiovascular anomalies and cleft palate have been observed following NSAID exposure in some studies. The use of a NSAID close to conception may be associated with an increased risk of miscarriage. Nonteratogenic effects have been observed following NSAID administration during the third trimester including: Myocardial degenerative changes, prenatal constriction of the ductus arteriosus, fetal tricuspid regurgitation, failure of the ductus arteriosus to close postnatally; renal dysfunction or failure, oligohydramnios; gastrointestinal bleeding or perforation, increased risk of necrotizing enterocolitis; intracranial bleeding (including intraventricular hemorrhage), platelet dysfunction with resultant bleeding; pulmonary hypertension. Because they may cause premature closure of the ductus arteriosus, use of NSAIDs late in pregnancy should be avoided (use after 31 or 32 weeks gestation is not recommended by some clinicians). Product labeling for Caldolor® specifically notes that use at ≥30 weeks gestation should be avoided and therefore classifies ibuprofen as pregnancy category D at this time. The chronic use of NSAIDs in women of reproductive age may be associated with infertility that is reversible upon discontinuation of the medication. A registry is available for pregnant women exposed to autoimmune medications including ibuprofen. For additional information contact the Organization of Teratology Information Specialists, OTIS Autoimmune Diseases Study, at 877-311-8972.

Breast-Feeding Considerations Based on limited data, only very small amounts of ibuprofen are excreted into breast milk. Adverse events have not been reported in nursing infants. Because there is a potential for adverse events to occur in nursing infants, the manufacturer does not recommend the use of ibuprofen while breast-feeding.

Use with caution in nursing women with hypertensive disorders of pregnancy or pre-existing renal disease.

Medication Guide Available Yes

Contraindications Hypersensitivity to ibuprofen; history of asthma, urticaria, or allergic-type reaction to aspirin or other NSAIDs; aspirin triad (eg, bronchial asthma, aspirin intolerance, rhinitis); perioperative pain in the setting of coronary artery bypass graft (CABG) surgery

Ibuprofen lysine (NeoProfen®): Preterm infants with untreated proven or suspected infection; congenital heart disease where patency of the PDA is necessary for pulmonary or systemic blood flow; bleeding (especially with active intracranial hemorrhage or GI bleed); thrombocytopenia; coagulation defects; proven or suspected necrotizing enterocolitis (NEC); significant renal dysfunction

Warnings/Precautions [U.S. Boxed Warning]: NSAIDs are associated with an increased risk of adverse cardiovascular thrombotic events, including fatal MI and stroke. Risk may be increased with duration of use or pre-existing cardiovascular risk factors or disease. Carefully evaluate individual cardiovascular risk profiles prior to prescribing. May cause new-onset hypertension or worsening of existing hypertension. Response to ACE inhibitors, thiazides, or loop diuretics may be impaired with concurrent use of NSAIDs. Use caution with fluid retention. Avoid use in heart failure. Concurrent administration of ibuprofen, and potentially other nonselective NSAIDs, may interfere with aspirin's cardioprotective effect. **[U.S. Boxed Warning]: Use is contraindicated for treatment of perioperative pain in the setting of coronary artery bypass graft (CABG) surgery.** Risk of MI and stroke may be increased with use following CABG surgery.

May increase the risk of aseptic meningitis, especially in patients with systemic lupus erythematosus (SLE) and mixed connective tissue disorders. Platelet adhesion and aggregation may be decreased; may prolong bleeding time; patients with coagulation disorders or who are receiving anticoagulants should be monitored closely. Anemia may occur; patients on long-term NSAID therapy should be monitored for anemia. Rarely, NSAID use may cause severe blood dyscrasias (eg, agranulocytosis, aplastic anemia, thrombocytopenia).

NSAID use may compromise existing renal function; dose-dependent decreases in prostaglandin synthesis may result from NSAID use, reducing renal blood flow which may cause renal decompensation. NSAID use may increase the risk for hyperkalemia. Patients with impaired renal function, dehydration, heart failure, liver dysfunction, those taking diuretics, and ACE inhibitors, and the elderly are at greater risk of renal toxicity and hyperkalemia. Rehydrate patient before starting therapy; monitor renal function closely. Not recommended for use in patients with advanced renal disease. Long-term NSAID use may result in renal papillary necrosis.

NSAIDs may increase risk of gastrointestinal irritation, inflammation, ulceration, bleeding, and perforation. These events can be fatal and may occur at any time during therapy and without warning. Use caution with a history of GI disease (bleeding or ulcers), concurrent therapy with aspirin, anticoagulants and/or corticosteroids, smoking, use of ethanol, the elderly or debilitated patients. When used concomitantly with aspirin, a substantial increase in the risk of gastrointestinal complications (eg, ulcer) occurs; concomitant gastroprotective therapy (eg, proton pump inhibitors) is recommended (Bhatt, 2008).

Use the lowest effective dose for the shortest duration of time, consistent with individual patient goals, to reduce risk of cardiovascular or GI adverse events. Alternate therapies should be considered for patients at high risk.

NSAIDs may cause serious skin adverse events including exfoliative dermatitis, Stevens-Johnson Syndrome (SJS) and toxic epidermal necrolysis (TEN); discontinue use at first sign of skin rash or hypersensitivity. Anaphylactoid reactions may occur, even without prior exposure; patients with "aspirin triad" (bronchial asthma, aspirin intolerance, rhinitis) may be at increased risk. Do not use in patients who experience bronchospasm, asthma, rhinitis, or urticaria with NSAID or aspirin therapy. Use caution in other forms of asthma.

NSAIDS may cause drowsiness, dizziness, blurred vision and other neurologic effects which may impair physical or mental abilities; patients must be cautioned about performing tasks which require mental alertness (eg, operating machinery or driving). Monitor vision with long-term therapy. Blurred/diminished vision, scotomata, and changes in color vision have been reported. Discontinue use with altered vision and perform ophthalmologic exam.

Use with caution in patients with decreased hepatic function. Closely monitor patients with any abnormal LFT. Severe hepatic reactions (eg, fulminant hepatitis, liver failure) have occurred with NSAID use, rarely; discontinue if signs or symptoms of liver disease develop, or if systemic manifestations occur.

In the elderly, avoid chronic use (unless alternative agents ineffective and patient can receive concomitant gastroprotective agent); nonselective oral NSAID use is associated with an increased risk of GI bleeding and peptic ulcer disease in older adults in high risk category (eg, >75 years or age or receiving concomitant oral/parenteral corticosteroids, anticoagulants, or antiplatelet agents) (Beers Criteria).

Withhold for at least 4-6 half-lives prior to surgical or dental procedures. Some products may contain phenylalanine. Ibuprofen injection (Caldolor®) must be diluted prior to administration; hemolysis can occur if not diluted.

Ibuprofen lysine injection (NeoProfen®): Hold second or third doses if urinary output is <0.6 mL/kg/hour. May alter signs of infection. May inhibit platelet aggregation; monitor for signs of bleeding. May displace bilirubin; use caution when total bilirubin is elevated. Long-term evaluations of neurodevelopment, growth, or diseases associated with prematurity following treatment have not been conducted. A second course of treatment, alternative pharmacologic therapy or surgery may be needed if the ductus arteriosus fails to close or reopens following the initial course of therapy.

Self medication (OTC use): Prior to self-medication, patients should contact healthcare provider if they have had recurring stomach pain or upset, ulcers, bleeding problems, high blood pressure, heart or kidney disease, other serious medical problems, are currently taking a diuretic, aspirin, anticoagulant, or are ≥60 years of age. If patients are using for migraines, they should also contact healthcare provider if they have not had a migraine diagnosis by healthcare provider, a headache that is different from usual migraine, worst headache of life, fever and neck stiffness, headache from head injury or coughing, first headache at ≥50 years of age, daily headache, or migraine requiring bed rest. Recommended dosages should not be exceeded, due to an increased risk of GI bleeding. Stop use and consult a healthcare provider if symptoms get worse, newly appear, fever lasts for >3 days or pain lasts >3 days (children) and >10 days (adults). Do not give for >10 days unless instructed by healthcare provider. Consuming ≥3 alcoholic beverages/day or taking longer than recommended may increase the risk of GI bleeding.

Adverse Reactions

Oral:

1% to 10%:

Cardiovascular: Edema (1% to 3%)

Central nervous system: Dizziness (3% to 9%), headache (1% to 3%), nervousness (1% to 3%)

Dermatologic: Rash (3% to 9%), itching (1% to 3%)

Endocrine & metabolic: Fluid retention (1% to 3%)

Gastrointestinal: Epigastric pain (3% to 9%), heartburn (3% to 9%), nausea (3% to 9%), abdominal pain/cramps/distress (1% to 3%), appetite decreased (1% to 3%), constipation (1% to 3%), diarrhea (1% to 3%), dyspepsia (1% to 3%), flatulence (1% to 3%), vomiting (1% to 3%)

Otic: Tinnitus (3% to 9%)

<1% (Limited to important or life-threatening): Acute renal failure, agranulocytosis, anaphylaxis, aplastic anemia, azotemia, blurred vision, bone marrow suppression, confusion, creatinine clearance decreased, duodenal ulcer, edema, eosinophilia, epistaxis, erythema multiforme, gastric ulcer, GI bleed, GI hemorrhage, GI ulceration, hallucinations, hearing decreased, hematuria, hematocrit decreased, hemoglobin decreased, hemolytic anemia, hepatitis, hypertension, inhibition of platelet aggregation, jaundice, liver function tests abnormal, leukopenia, melena, neutropenia, pancreatitis, photosensitivity, Stevens-Johnson syndrome, thrombocytopenia, toxic amblyopia, toxic epidermal necrolysis, urticaria, vesiculobullous eruptions, vision changes

Injection: Ibuprofen (Caldolor®):

Cardiovascular: Edema, hypertension

Central nervous system: Dizziness, headache

Dermatologic: Pruritus

Endocrine & metabolic: Hypernatremia, hypokalemia

Gastrointestinal: Abdominal pain, dyspepsia, flatulence, nausea, vomiting

Genitourinary: Urinary retention

Hematologic: Anemia, hemorrhage, neutropenia

Renal: BUN increased

Respiratory: Cough

Injection: Ibuprofen lysine (NeoProfen®):

>10%:

Cardiovascular: Intraventricular hemorrhage (29%; grade 3/4: 15%)

Dermatologic: Skin irritation (16%)

Endocrine & metabolic: Hypocalcemia (12%), hypoglycemia (12%)

Gastrointestinal: GI disorders, non NEC (22%)

Hematologic: Anemia (32%)

Respiratory: Apnea (28%), respiratory infection (19%)

Miscellaneous: Sepsis (43%)

1% to 10%:

Cardiovascular: Edema (4%)

Endocrine & metabolic: Adrenal insufficiency (7%), hypernatremia (7%)

Genitourinary: Urinary tract infection (9%)

Renal: Urea increased (7%), renal impairment (6%), creatinine increased (3%), urine output decreased (3%; small decrease reported on days 2-6 with compensatory increase in output on day 9), renal failure (1%)

Respiratory: Respiratory failure (10%), atelectasis (4%)

Frequency not defined: Abdominal distension, cholestasis, feeding problems, gastritis, GI reflux, heart failure, hyperglycemia, hypotension, ileus, infection, inguinal hernia, injection site reaction, jaundice, neutropenia, seizure, tachycardia, thrombocytopenia

Postmarketing and/or case reports: GI perforation, necrotizing enterocolitis

Drug Interactions

Metabolism/Transport Effects Substrate of CYP2C19 (minor), CYP2C9 (minor); **Note:** Assignment of Major/Minor substrate status based on clinically relevant drug interaction potential; **Inhibits** CYP2C9 (weak)

Avoid Concomitant Use

Avoid concomitant use of Ibuprofen with any of the following: Floctafenine; Ketorolac (Nasal); Ketorolac (Systemic); NSAID (COX-2 Inhibitor); Omacetaxine

Increased Effect/Toxicity

Ibuprofen may increase the levels/effects of: 5-ASA Derivatives; Agents with Antiplatelet Properties; Aliskiren; Aminoglycosides; Anticoagulants; Bisphosphonate Derivatives; Collagenase (Systemic); CycloSPORINE (Systemic); Dabigatran Etexilate; Deferasirox; Desmopressin; Digoxin; Eplerenone; Haloperidol; Ibritumomab; Lithium; Methotrexate; Nonsteroidal Anti-Inflammatory Agents; NSAID (COX-2 Inhibitor); Omacetaxine; PEMEtrexed; Porfimer; Potassium-Sparing Diuretics; PRALAtrexate; Quinolone Antibiotics; Rivaroxaban; Salicylates; Tenofovir; Thrombolytic Agents; Tositumomab and Iodine I 131 Tositumomab; Vancomycin; Vitamin K Antagonists

The levels/effects of Ibuprofen may be increased by: ACE Inhibitors; Angiotensin II Receptor Blockers; Antidepressants (Tricyclic, Tertiary Amine); Corticosteroids (Systemic); CycloSPORINE (Systemic); Dasatinib; Floctafenine; Glucosamine; Herbs (Anticoagulant/Antiplatelet Properties); Ibrutinib; Ketorolac (Nasal); Ketorolac (Systemic); Multivitamins/Fluoride (with ADE); Multivitamins/Minerals (with ADEK, Folate, Iron); Multivitamins/Minerals (with AE, No Iron); Nonsteroidal Anti-Inflammatory Agents; Omega-3 Fatty Acids; Pentosan Polysulfate Sodium; Pentoxifylline; Probenecid; Prostacyclin Analogues; Selective Serotonin Reuptake Inhibitors; Serotonin/Norepinephrine Reuptake Inhibitors; Sodium Phosphates; Tipranavir; Treprostinil; Vitamin E; Voriconazole

Decreased Effect

Ibuprofen may decrease the levels/effects of: ACE Inhibitors; Agents with Antiplatelet Properties; Aliskiren; Angiotensin II Receptor Blockers; Beta-Blockers; Eplerenone; HydrALAZINE; Imatinib; Loop Diuretics; Potassium-Sparing Diuretics; Prostaglandins (Ophthalmic); Salicylates; Selective Serotonin Reuptake Inhibitors; Thiazide Diuretics

The levels/effects of Ibuprofen may be decreased by: Bile Acid Sequestrants; Nonsteroidal Anti-Inflammatory Agents; Salicylates

Ethanol/Nutrition/Herb Interactions

Ethanol: Avoid ethanol (may enhance gastric mucosal irritation).

Food: Ibuprofen peak serum levels may be decreased if taken with food.

Herb/Nutraceutical: Avoid alfalfa, anise, bilberry, bladderwrack, bromelain, cat's claw, celery, chamomile, coleus, cordyceps, dong quai, evening primrose, fenugreek, feverfew, garlic, ginger, ginkgo biloba, ginseng (American, Panax, Siberian), grapeseed, green tea, guggul, horse chestnut seed, horseradish, licorice, prickly ash, red clover, reishi, SAMe (S-adenosylmethionine), sweet clover, turmeric, white willow (all have additional antiplatelet activity).

Preparation for Administration

Ibuprofen injection (Caldolor®): Must be diluted prior to use. Dilute with D_5W, NS or LR to a final concentration ≤4 mg/mL.

Ibuprofen lysine injection (NeoProfen®): Dilute with dextrose or saline to an appropriate volume.

Storage/Stability

Ibuprofen injection (Caldolor®): Store intact vials at room temperature of 20°C to 25°C (68°F to 77°F). Must be diluted prior to use. Diluted solutions stable for 24 hours at room temperature.

Ibuprofen lysine injection (NeoProfen®): Store at room temperature of 20°C to 25°C (68°F to 77°F). Protect from light. Following dilution, administer within 30 minutes of preparation.

Mechanism of Action Reversibly inhibits cyclooxygenase-1 and 2 (COX-1 and 2) enzymes, which results in decreased formation of prostaglandin precursors; has antipyretic, analgesic, and anti-inflammatory properties

Other proposed mechanisms not fully elucidated (and possibly contributing to the anti-inflammatory effect to varying degrees), include inhibiting chemotaxis, altering lymphocyte activity, inhibiting neutrophil aggregation/activation, and decreasing proinflammatory cytokine levels.

Pharmacodynamics/Kinetics

Onset of action: Oral: Analgesic: 30-60 minutes; Anti-inflammatory: ≤7 days

Duration: Oral: 4-6 hours

Absorption: Oral: Rapid (85%)

Distribution: V_d: 6.35 L; premature infants with ductal closure (highly variable between studies):

Day 3: 145-349 mL/kg

Day 5: 72-222 mL/kg

Protein binding: 90% to 99%

Metabolism: Hepatic via oxidation

Half-life elimination:

Premature infants (highly variable between studies):

Day 3: 35-51 hours

Day 5: 20-33 hours

Children 3 months to 10 years: 1.6 ± 0.7 hours

Adults: 2-4 hours; End-stage renal disease: Unchanged

Time to peak: Oral: ~1-2 hours

Excretion: Urine (primarily as metabolites; 1% as unchanged drug); some feces

Dosage

I.V.:

Neonates: Ibuprofen lysine (NeoProfen®): Infants between 500-1500 g and ≤32 weeks GA: Patent ductus arteriosus: Initial dose: Ibuprofen 10 mg/kg, followed by two doses of 5 mg/kg at 24 and 48 hours. Dose should be based on birth weight.

Adults (Caldolor®): **Note**: Patients should be well hydrated prior to administration

Analgesic: 400-800 mg every 6 hours as needed (maximum: 3.2 g/day)

Antipyretic: Initial: 400 mg, then every 4-6 hours or 100-200 mg every 4 hours as needed (maximum: 3.2 g/day)

Oral:

Children:

Antipyretic: 6 months to 12 years: Temperature <102.5°F (39°C): 5 mg/kg/dose; temperature >102.5°F: 10 mg/kg/dose given every 6-8 hours (maximum daily dose: 40 mg/kg/day)

Juvenile idiopathic arthritis (JIA): 30-50 mg/kg/24 hours divided every 8 hours; start at lower end of dosing range and titrate upward (maximum: 2.4 g/day)

Analgesic: 4-10 mg/kg/dose every 6-8 hours

Cystic fibrosis (unlabeled use): Chronic (>4 years) twice daily dosing adjusted to maintain serum concentration of 50-100 mcg/mL has been associated with slowing of disease progression in younger patients with mild lung disease

OTC labeling (analgesic, antipyretic): **Note:** Treatment for >10 days is not recommended unless directed by healthcare provider.

Children 6 months to 11 years: See table; use of weight to select dose is preferred; doses may be repeated every 6-8 hours (maximum: 4 doses/day)

Children ≥12 years: 200 mg every 4-6 hours as needed (maximum: 1200 mg/24 hours)

Ibuprofen Dosing

Weight (lb)	Age	Dosage (mg)
12-17	6-11 mo	50
18-23	12-23 mo	75
24-35	2-3 y	100
36-47	4-5 y	150
48-59	6-8 y	200
60-71	9-10 y	250
72-95	11 y	300

Adults:

Inflammatory disease: 400-800 mg/dose 3-4 times/day (maximum dose: 3.2 g/day)

Analgesia/pain/fever/dysmenorrhea: 200-400 mg/dose every 4-6 hours (maximum daily dose: 1.2 g, unless directed by physician; under physician supervision daily doses ≤2.4 g may be used)

OTC labeling (analgesic, antipyretic): 200 mg every 4-6 hours as needed (maximum: 1200 mg/24 hours); treatment for >10 days is not recommended unless directed by healthcare provider.

Migraine: 400 mg at onset of symptoms (maximum: 400 mg/24 hours unless directed by healthcare provider)

Pericarditis (unlabeled use): 400-800 mg 3-4 times daily (maximum dose: 3.2 g daily) (Imazio, 2009); with pericarditis postmyocardial infarction, the ACCF/AHA prefers the use of aspirin (O'Gara, 2013).

Dosing adjustment/comments in renal impairment: If anuria or oliguria evident, hold dose until renal function returns to normal

Dosing adjustment/comments in severe hepatic impairment: Avoid use

Dietary Considerations Should be taken with food. Some products may contain phenylalanine and/or potassium.

Administration

Oral: Administer with food

I.V.:

Caldolor®: For I.V. administration only; infuse over at least 30 minutes

NeoProfen® (ibuprofen lysine): For I.V. administration only; administration via umbilical arterial line has not been evaluated. Infuse over 15 minutes through port closest to insertion site. Avoid extravasation. Do not administer simultaneously via same line with TPN. If needed, interrupt TPN for 15 minutes prior to and after ibuprofen administration, keeping line open with dextrose or saline.

Monitoring Parameters CBC, chemistry profile, occult blood loss and periodic liver function tests; monitor response (pain, range of motion, grip strength, mobility, ADL function), inflammation; observe for weight gain, edema; monitor renal function (urine output, serum BUN and creatinine); observe for bleeding, bruising; evaluate gastrointestinal effects (abdominal pain, bleeding, dyspepsia); mental confusion, disorientation; with long-term therapy, periodic ophthalmic exams; signs of infection (ibuprofen lysine)

Reference Range Plasma concentrations >200 mcg/mL may be associated with severe toxicity

PDA: Minimum effective concentration: 10-12 mg/L

Test Interactions May interfere with urine detection of PCP, cannabinoids, and barbiturates (false-positives)

Dosage Forms Excipient information presented when available (limited, particularly for generics); consult specific product labeling.

Capsule, Oral:
- Advil: 200 mg
- Advil Migraine: 200 mg
- KS Ibuprofen: 200 mg [contains fd&c blue #2 (indigotine)]
- Generic: 200 mg

Cream, External:
- EnovaRX-Ibuprofen: 10% (60 g) [contains cetearyl alcohol]

Kit, Combination:
- Ibuprofen Comfort Pac: 800 mg [contains methylparaben, trolamine (triethanolamine)]

Solution, Intravenous:
- Caldolor: 400 mg/4 mL (4 mL); 800 mg/8 mL (8 mL)

Solution, Intravenous, as lysine [preservative free]:
- NeoProfen: 10 mg/mL (2 mL)

Suspension, Oral:
- Childrens Advil: 100 mg/5 mL (120 mL) [fruit flavor]
- Childrens Advil: 100 mg/5 mL (120 mL) [alcohol free; grape flavor]
- Childrens Advil: 100 mg/5 mL (120 mL) [alcohol free; contains brilliant blue fcf (fd&c blue #1), edetate disodium, fd&c red #40, polysorbate 80, propylene glycol, sodium benzoate; grape flavor]
- Childrens Advil: 100 mg/5 mL (120 mL) [alcohol free; contains brilliant blue fcf (fd&c blue #1), propylene glycol, sodium benzoate; blue raspberry flavor]
- Childrens Advil: 100 mg/5 mL (30 mL, 120 mL) [alcohol free, dye free; contains edetate disodium, polysorbate 80, propylene glycol, sodium benzoate; white grape flavor]
- Childrens Advil: 50 mg/1.25 mL (15 mL) [dye free; contains propylene glycol, sodium benzoate; white grape flavor]
- Childrens Ibuprofen: 100 mg/5 mL (118 mL) [alcohol free; contains brilliant blue fcf (fd&c blue #1), fd&c red #40, polysorbate 80, sodium benzoate; grape flavor]
- Childrens Ibuprofen: 100 mg/5 mL (120 mL) [alcohol free; contains butylparaben, fd&c red #40, polysorbate 80, propylene glycol, sodium benzoate; bubble-gum flavor]
- Childrens Ibuprofen: 100 mg/5 mL (118 mL, 240 mL) [alcohol free; contains fd&c red #40, fd&c yellow #10 (quinoline yellow), polysorbate 80, sodium benzoate; berry flavor]
- Childrens Ibuprofen: 100 mg/5 mL (118 mL) [alcohol free; contains fd&c red #40, polysorbate 80, sodium benzoate]
- Childrens Ibuprofen: 40 mg/mL (15 mL) [alcohol free; berry flavor]
- Childrens Ibuprofen: 100 mg/5 mL (118 mL) [alcohol free, dye free; contains polysorbate 80, sodium benzoate]
- Childrens Motrin: 40 mg/mL (15 mL) [berry flavor]
- Childrens Motrin: 100 mg/5 mL (120 mL) [alcohol free]
- Childrens Motrin: 100 mg/5 mL (60 mL) [alcohol free; contains fd&c red #40, fd&c yellow #10 (quinoline yellow), polysorbate 80, sodium benzoate]
- Childrens Motrin: 100 mg/5 mL (120 mL) [alcohol free; contains fd&c red #40, fd&c yellow #10 (quinoline yellow), polysorbate 80, sodium benzoate; berry flavor]
- Childrens Motrin: 100 mg/5 mL (120 mL) [alcohol free; contains fd&c red #40, fd&c yellow #10 (quinoline yellow), sodium benzoate; berry flavor]
- Childrens Motrin: 100 mg/5 mL (120 mL) [alcohol free; contains fd&c red #40, polysorbate 80, sodium benzoate]
- Childrens Motrin: 100 mg/5 mL (120 mL) [alcohol free; contains fd&c red #40, sodium benzoate]
- Childrens Motrin: 100 mg/5 mL (120 mL) [alcohol free; contains fd&c red #40, sodium benzoate; bubble-gum flavor]
- Childrens Motrin: 100 mg/5 mL (120 mL) [alcohol free; contains fd&c red #40, sodium benzoate; tropical punch flavor]
- Childrens Motrin: 100 mg/5 mL (120 mL) [alcohol free, dye free; contains polysorbate 80, sodium benzoate]
- Childrens Motrin: 100 mg/5 mL (120 mL) [alcohol free, dye free; contains sodium benzoate; berry flavor]
- Ibuprofen Childrens: 100 mg/5 mL (120 mL) [alcohol free; contains butylparaben, fd&c red #40, fd&c yellow #6 (sunset yellow), polysorbate 80, propylene glycol, sodium benzoate; fruit flavor]
- Ibuprofen Childrens: 100 mg/5 mL (120 mL, 240 mL) [alcohol free; contains butylparaben, fd&c yellow #6 (sunset yellow), polysorbate 80, propylene glycol, sodium benzoate; berry flavor]
- Ibuprofen Childrens: 100 mg/5 mL (120 mL) [alcohol free, gluten free; contains brilliant blue fcf (fd&c blue #1), fd&c red #40, polysorbate 80, sodium benzoate; grape flavor]
- Infants Advil: 50 mg/1.25 mL (15 mL) [alcohol free, dye free; contains edetate disodium, polysorbate 80, propylene glycol, sodium benzoate; white grape flavor]
- Infants Ibuprofen: 50 mg/1.25 mL (15 mL) [alcohol free; contains butylparaben, fd&c red #40, polysorbate 80, propylene glycol, sodium benzoate; berry flavor]
- Infants Ibuprofen: 50 mg/1.25 mL (15 mL, 30 mL) [alcohol free, dye free; contains polysorbate 80, sodium benzoate; berry flavor]
- Motrin: 40 mg/mL (15 mL) [alcohol free, dye free; berry flavor]
- Motrin Infants Drops: 50 mg/1.25 mL (15 mL) [alcohol free; contains fd&c red #40, polysorbate 80, sodium benzoate; berry flavor]
- Motrin Infants Drops: 50 mg/1.25 mL (15 mL, 30 mL) [alcohol free, dye free; contains polysorbate 80, sodium benzoate]
- Generic: 100 mg/5 mL (5 mL, 118 mL, 120 mL, 473 mL)

Tablet, Oral:
- Addaprin: 200 mg
- Advil: 200 mg
- Advil Junior Strength: 100 mg
- Dyspel: 200 mg
- Genpril: 200 mg
- I-Prin: 200 mg
- IBU-200: 200 mg
- Motrin IB: 200 mg
- Motrin IB: 200 mg [contains fd&c yellow #6 (sunset yellow)]
- Motrin Junior Strength: 100 mg [scored]
- Provil: 200 mg
- Generic: 200 mg, 400 mg, 600 mg, 800 mg

Tablet Chewable, Oral:
- Advil Junior Strength: 100 mg [scored; contains aspartame, fd&c blue #2 aluminum lake; grape flavor]
- Childrens Motrin: 50 mg [scored; contains aspartame, fd&c yellow #6 (sunset yellow); orange flavor]
- Childrens Motrin Jr Strength: 100 mg [scored; contains aspartame, brilliant blue fcf (fd&c blue #1); grape flavor]
- Ibuprofen Junior Strength: 100 mg [contains aspartame, fd&c yellow #6 (sunset yellow), soybean oil, whey protein]
- Motrin Junior Strength: 100 mg [contains aspartame, brilliant blue fcf (fd&c blue #1)]
- Motrin Junior Strength: 100 mg [scored; contains aspartame, fd&c yellow #6 (sunset yellow); orange flavor]

◆ **Ibuprofen and Hydrocodone** *see* Hydrocodone and Ibuprofen *on page* 1008

◆ **Ibuprofen and Oxycodone** *see* Oxycodone and Ibuprofen *on page* 1539

◆ **Ibuprofen and Pseudoephedrine** *see* Pseudoephedrine and Ibuprofen *on page* 1748

◆ **Ibuprofen Childrens [OTC]** *see* Ibuprofen *on page* 1032

◆ **Ibuprofen Comfort Pac** *see* Ibuprofen *on page 1032*

◆ **Ibuprofen Junior Strength [OTC]** *see* Ibuprofen *on page 1032*

◆ **Ibuprofen Lysine** *see* Ibuprofen *on page 1032*

Ibutilide (i BYOO ti lide)

Brand Names: U.S. Corvert

Index Terms Ibutilide Fumarate

Pharmacologic Category Antiarrhythmic Agent, Class III

Additional Appendix Information

Beers Criteria – Potentially Inappropriate Medications for Geriatrics *on page 2368*

Use Acute termination of atrial fibrillation or flutter of recent onset; the effectiveness of ibutilide has not been determined in patients with arrhythmias >90 days in duration

Pregnancy Risk Factor C

Pregnancy Considerations Adverse events were observed in animal reproduction studies. Information related to the use of ibutilide in pregnancy is limited (Burkart, 2007; Kockova, 2007); other agents are generally preferred for initial treatment (Blomström-Lundqvist, 2003; Fuster, 2006).

Breast-Feeding Considerations It is not known if ibutilide is excreted in breast milk. The manufacturer does not recommend use in nursing women.

Contraindications Hypersensitivity to ibutilide or any component of the formulation; QT_c >440 msec

Warnings/Precautions [U.S. Boxed Warning]: Potentially fatal arrhythmias (eg, polymorphic ventricular tachycardia) can occur with ibutilide, usually in association with torsade de pointes (QT prolongation). Studies indicate a 1.7% incidence of arrhythmias in treated patients. The drug should be given in a setting of continuous ECG monitoring and by personnel trained in treating arrhythmias particularly polymorphic ventricular tachycardia. **[U.S. Boxed Warning]: Patients with chronic atrial fibrillation may not be the best candidates for ibutilide since they often revert after conversion and the risks of treatment may not be justified when compared to alternative management.** Dosing adjustments are not required in patients with renal or hepatic dysfunction. Safety and efficacy in children have not been established. In the treatment of atrial fibrillation in the elderly, avoid antiarrhythmics as first-line treatment. In older adults, data suggests rate control may provide more benefits than risks compared to rhythm control for most patients (Beers Criteria). Avoid concurrent use of any drug that can prolong QT interval. Correct hyperkalemia and hypomagnesemia before using. Monitor for heart block.

Adverse Reactions

1% to 10%:

Cardiovascular: Ventricular extrasystoles (5.1%), nonsustained monomorphic ventricular tachycardia (4.9%), nonsustained polymorphic ventricular tachycardia (2.7%), tachycardia/supraventricular tachycardia (2.7%), hypotension (2%), bundle branch block (1.9%), sustained polymorphic ventricular tachycardia (eg, torsade de pointes) (1.7%, often requiring cardioversion), AV block (1.5%), bradycardia (1.2%), QT segment prolongation, hypertension (1.2%), palpitation (1%)

Central nervous system: Headache (4%)

Gastrointestinal: Nausea (>1%)

<1% (Limited to important or life-threatening): CHF, erythematous bullous lesions, idioventricular rhythm, nodal arrhythmia, renal failure, supraventricular extrasystoles, sustained monomorphic ventricular tachycardia, syncope (0.3%, not > placebo)

Drug Interactions

Metabolism/Transport Effects None known.

Avoid Concomitant Use

Avoid concomitant use of Ibutilide with any of the following: Fingolimod; Highest Risk QTc-Prolonging Agents; Ivabradine; Mifepristone; Moderate Risk QTc-Prolonging Agents; Propafenone

Increased Effect/Toxicity

Ibutilide may increase the levels/effects of: Highest Risk QTc-Prolonging Agents; Lidocaine (Topical)

The levels/effects of Ibutilide may be increased by: Fingolimod; Ivabradine; Lidocaine (Topical); Mifepristone; Moderate Risk QTc-Prolonging Agents; Propafenone; QTc-Prolonging Agents (Indeterminate Risk and Risk Modifying)

Decreased Effect There are no known significant interactions involving a decrease in effect.

Preparation for Administration No dilution required. May dilute in 50 mL diluent (0.9% NS or D_5W).

Storage/Stability Admixtures are chemically and physically stable for 24 hours at room temperature and for 48 hours at refrigerated temperatures.

Mechanism of Action Exact mechanism of action is unknown; prolongs the action potential in cardiac tissue

Pharmacodynamics/Kinetics

Onset of action: ~90 minutes after start of infusion (1/2 of conversions to sinus rhythm occur during infusion)

Distribution: V_d: 11 L/kg

Protein binding: 40%

Metabolism: Extensively hepatic; oxidation

Half-life elimination: 2-12 hours (average: 6 hours)

Excretion: Urine (82%; 7% as unchanged drug and metabolites); feces (19%)

Dosage I.V.: Initial:

Adults:

<60 kg: 0.01 mg/kg over 10 minutes

≥60 kg: 1 mg over 10 minutes

Note: Discontinue infusion if arrhythmia terminates, if sustained or nonsustained ventricular tachycardia occurs, or if marked prolongation of QT/QT_c occurs. If the arrhythmia does not terminate within 10 minutes after the end of the initial infusion, a second infusion of equal strength may be infused over a 10-minute period.

Elderly: Refer to adult dosing. Dose selection should be cautious, usually starting at the lower end of the dosing range.

Dosage adjustment in renal impairment: No dosage adjustment necessary.

Dosage adjustment in hepatic impairment: No dosage adjustment necessary.

Administration Infuse undiluted or diluted over 10 minutes. Observe patient with continuous ECG monitoring for at least 4 hours (>4 hours in patients with abnormal hepatic function) following infusion or until QT_c has returned to baseline. Skilled personnel and proper equipment should be available during administration of ibutilide and subsequent monitoring of the patient.

Monitoring Parameters Electrolytes; observe patient with continuous ECG monitoring for at least 4 hours following infusion or until QT_c has returned to baseline; skilled personnel and proper equipment should be available during administration of ibutilide and subsequent monitoring of the patient

Consult individual institutional policies and procedures.

Dosage Forms Excipient information presented when available (limited, particularly for generics); consult specific product labeling.

Solution, Intravenous, as fumarate:

Corvert: 1 mg/10 mL (10 mL)

Generic: 1 mg/10 mL (10 mL)

◆ **Ibutilide Fumarate** *see* Ibutilide *on page 1037*

◆ IC51 *see* Japanese Encephalitis Virus Vaccine (Inactivated) *on page 1142*

Icatibant (eye KAT i bant)

Brand Names: U.S. Firazyr

Index Terms HOE 140; Icatibant Acetate

Pharmacologic Category Selective Bradykinin B2 Receptor Antagonist

Use Treatment of acute attacks of hereditary angioedema (HAE)

Pregnancy Risk Factor C

Pregnancy Considerations Adverse events were observed in animal reproduction studies with doses close to or less than the recommended human dose.

Breast-Feeding Considerations It is not known if icatibant is excreted in breast milk. The manufacturer recommends that caution be exercised when administering icatibant to nursing women.

Contraindications There are no contraindications listed in the manufacturer's labeling.

Warnings/Precautions Airway obstruction may occur during acute laryngeal attacks of HAE. Patients with laryngeal attacks should be instructed to seek medical attention immediately in addition to treatment with icatibant. Icatibant may potentially attenuate the antihypertensive effect of ACE inhibitors; patients taking ACE inhibitors were excluded from initial clinical trials.

Adverse Reactions

>10%: Local: Injection site reaction (97%)

1% to 10%:

Central nervous system: Pyrexia (4%), dizziness (3%)

Hepatic: Transaminase increased (4%)

<1% (Limited to important or life-threatening): Anti-icatibant antibody production (no association with efficacy observed), headache, nausea, rash

Drug Interactions

Metabolism/Transport Effects None known.

Avoid Concomitant Use There are no known interactions where it is recommended to avoid concomitant use.

Increased Effect/Toxicity There are no known significant interactions involving an increase in effect.

Decreased Effect

Icatibant may decrease the levels/effects of: ACE Inhibitors

Storage/Stability Store between 2°C to 25°C (36°F to 77°F); do not freeze. Store in original container until time of administration.

Mechanism of Action Icatibant is a selective competitive antagonist for the bradykinin B_2 receptor. Patients with HAE have an absence or dysfunction of C1-esterase-inhibitor which leads to the production of bradykinin. The presence of bradykinin may cause symptoms of localized swelling, inflammation, and pain. Icatibant inhibits bradykinin from binding at the B_2 receptor, thereby treating the symptoms associated with acute attack.

Pharmacodynamics/Kinetics

Onset: Median time to 50% decrease of symptoms: ~2 hours

Duration: Inhibits symptoms caused by bradykinin for ~6 hours

Distribution: V_{dss}: 20.3-37.7 L

Metabolism: Metabolized by proteolytic enzymes to metabolites (inactive)

Bioavailability: ~97%

Half-life elimination: 1-1.8 hours

Time to peak: 0.75 hours

Excretion: Urine (<10% unchanged)

Dosage SubQ: Adults: Hereditary angioedema (HAE): 30 mg/dose; may repeat one dose every 6 hours if response is inadequate or symptoms recur (maximum: 3 doses/24 hours)

Dosing adjustment in renal impairment: No dosage adjustments are recommended.

Dosing adjustment in hepatic impairment: No dosage adjustments are recommended.

Administration For SubQ injection only. Inject into the abdomen over ≥30 seconds, using the 25 gauge needle provided. Inject 2-4 inches below belly button and away from any scars; do not inject into an area that is bruised, swollen, or painful.

Monitoring Parameters Symptom relief; laryngeal symptoms or airway obstruction (immediate medical attention required in addition to icatibant therapy)

Dosage Forms Excipient information presented when available (limited, particularly for generics); consult specific product labeling.

Solution, Subcutaneous [preservative free]:

Firazyr: 30 mg/3 mL (3 mL)

◆ Icatibant Acetate *see* Icatibant *on page 1038*
◆ ICI-182,780 *see* Fulvestrant *on page 930*
◆ ICI-204,219 *see* Zafirlukast *on page 2219*
◆ ICI-46474 *see* Tamoxifen *on page 1987*
◆ ICI-118630 *see* Goserelin *on page 970*
◆ ICI-176334 *see* Bicalutamide *on page 258*
◆ ICI-D1033 *see* Anastrozole *on page 137*
◆ ICL670 *see* Deferasirox *on page 558*
◆ Iclusig *see* PONATinib *on page 1676*

Icodextrin (eye KOE dex trin)

Brand Names: U.S. Extraneal

Pharmacologic Category Adhesiolytic; Peritoneal Dialysate, Osmotic

Use

Adept®: Reduction of postsurgical adhesions in gynecologic laparoscopic procedures

Extraneal®: Daily exchange for the long dwell (8- to 16-hour) during continuous ambulatory peritoneal dialysis (CAPD) or automated peritoneal dialysis (APD) for the management of end-stage renal disease (ESRD); improvement of long-dwell ultrafiltration and clearance of creatinine and urea nitrogen (compared to 4.25% dextrose) in patients with high/average or greater transport characteristics as measured by peritoneal equilibration test (PET)

Pregnancy Risk Factor C

Medication Guide Available Yes

Dosage Intraperitoneal: Adults:

CAPD or APD (Extraneal®): Given as a single daily exchange in CAPD or APD; dwell time of 8-16 hours is suggested

Laparoscopic gynecologic surgery (Adept®): Irrigate with at least 100 mL every 30 minutes during surgery; aspirate remaining fluid after surgery is completed, then instill 1 L into the cavity

Additional Information Complete prescribing information should be consulted for additional detail.

Dosage Forms Excipient information presented when available (limited, particularly for generics); consult specific product labeling.

Solution, Intraperitoneal:

Extraneal: 7.5% (2000 mL, 2500 mL)

Icosapent Ethyl (eye KOE sa pent ETH il)

Brand Names: U.S. Vascepa

Index Terms AMR101; Ethyl Eicosapentaenoate; Ethyl Icosapentate; Ethyl-Eicosapentaenoic Acid; Ethyl-EPA

Pharmacologic Category Antilipemic Agent, Omega-3 Fatty Acids

Use Adjunct to dietary therapy in the treatment of hypertriglyceridemia (≥500 mg/dL)

Pregnancy Risk Factor C

Pregnancy Considerations Adverse events were observed in animal reproduction studies. Maternal dietary consumption of omega-3-fatty acids (containing eicosapentaenoic acid [EPA] and docosahexaenoic acid [DHA]) influences fetal concentrations (Coletta, 2010; Miles, 2011). Information specific to the therapeutic use of this product in pregnancy has not been located; however, the use of omega-3-fatty acids to manage elevated triglycerides in pregnancy has been described in case reports (Goldberg, 2012; Papadakis, 2011).

Breast-Feeding Considerations Maternal dietary consumption of omega-3-fatty acids (containing eicosapentaenoic acid [EPA] and docosahexaenoic acid [DHA]) influences milk concentrations (Coletta, 2010; Miles, 2011). Information specific to the therapeutic use of this product by nursing women has not been located.

Contraindications Hypersensitivity to icosapent ethyl or any component of the formulation

Warnings/Precautions Should be used as an adjunct to diet therapy and exercise and only in those with very high triglyceride levels (≥500 mg/dL). The effect, if any, of icosapent ethyl on the risk of pancreatitis or cardiovascular mortality and morbidity in patients with severe hypertriglyceridemia is not known. Treatment of primary metabolic disorders (eg, diabetes, thyroid disease) and/or evaluation of the patient's medication regimen for possible etiologic agents should be completed prior to a decision to initiate therapy. Secondary causes of hyperlipidemia should be ruled out prior to therapy. Medications known to worsen hypertriglyceridemia (eg, beta-blockers, thiazides, estrogens) should be discontinued or changed prior to initiation of triglyceride-lowering therapy if possible.

Use with caution in patients with known allergy or sensitivity to fish and/or shellfish. Studies have not been conducted in patients with hepatic impairment; however, ALT/AST levels should be monitored periodically during therapy in hepatically impaired patients. Prolongation of bleeding time not exceeding normal limits has been observed in some clinical studies of omega-3 fatty acids; clinically significant bleeding episodes did not occur. Use with caution in patients with coagulopathy or in those receiving therapeutic anticoagulation; monitor for changes in INR (with warfarin) or signs/symptoms of bleeding following initiation and dosage changes of icosapent ethyl and in patients receiving concomitant anticoagulant or antiplatelet therapy.

Adverse Reactions

1% to 10%: Neuromuscular & skeletal: Arthralgia (2%)

<1% (Limited to important or life-threatening): Oropharyngeal pain

Drug Interactions

Metabolism/Transport Effects None known.

Avoid Concomitant Use There are no known interactions where it is recommended to avoid concomitant use.

Increased Effect/Toxicity

Icosapent Ethyl may increase the levels/effects of: Agents with Antiplatelet Properties; Anticoagulants

Decreased Effect There are no known significant interactions involving a decrease in effect.

Ethanol/Nutrition/Herb Interactions Ethanol: Monitor ethanol use (alcohol use may increase triglycerides).

Storage/Stability Store at 20°C to 25°C (68°F to 77°F); excursions permitted to 15°C to 30°C (59°F to 86°F).

Mechanism of Action Icosapent ethyl, the ethyl ester of eicosapentaenoic acid (EPA), is an omega-3 fatty acid which aids in decreasing hepatic very low-density lipoprotein triglycerides (VLDL-TG) synthesis/secretion and increasing triglyceride clearance from VLDL particles. The mechanism has not been completely defined. Possible mechanisms include inhibition of acyl CoA: 1,2 diacylglycerol acyltransferase, increased hepatic beta-oxidation, a reduction in the hepatic synthesis of triglycerides, or an increase in plasma lipoprotein lipase activity.

Pharmacodynamics/Kinetics

Absorption: De-esterified to active metabolite (EPA) which is absorbed in the small intestine

Distribution: V_{dss}: EPA: ~88 L

Metabolism: Mainly hepatic via beta-oxidation; minor via CYP 450

Half-life Elimination: EPA: ~89 hours

Time to peak: EPA: ~5 hours

Excretion: Not renally excreted

Dosage Hypertriglyceridemia: Adults: Oral: 2 g twice daily

Dosage adjustment in renal impairment: No dosage adjustment provided in manufacturer's labeling (has not been studied); however, not renally eliminated.

Dosage adjustment in hepatic impairment: No dosage adjustment provided in manufacturer's labeling (has not been studied); periodic monitoring of ALT and AST is recommended in patients with hepatic impairment.

Dietary Considerations Take with food. Dietary modification is important in the control of severe hypertriglyceridemia. Maintain standard cholesterol-lowering diet during therapy.

Administration Administer with food. Swallow whole; do not chew, crush, or divide.

Monitoring Parameters Triglycerides and other lipids (LDL-C) should be monitored at baseline and periodically. In patients with hepatic impairment, monitor ALT and AST periodically during treatment.

Additional Information Icosapent ethyl contains ethyl esters of an omega-3 fatty acid, eicosapentaenoic acid (EPA), obtained from fish oil. It contains ≥96% EPA and does not contain docosahexaenoic acid (DHA). Historically, mixtures containing both EPA and DHA have increased LDL cholesterol in patients with severe hypertriglyceridemia. However, studies have suggested that icosapent ethyl has not caused significant increases in LDL cholesterol while significantly decreasing triglyceride levels (Bays, 2011; Miller, 2011).

Dosage Forms Excipient information presented when available (limited, particularly for generics); consult specific product labeling.

Capsule, Oral:

Vascepa: 1 g

◆ **ICRF-187** *see* Dexrazoxane *on page* 587

◆ **Icy Hot® [OTC]** *see* Methyl Salicylate and Menthol *on page* 1344

◆ **Idamycin® (Can)** *see* IDArubicin *on page* 1039

◆ **Idamycin PFS** *see* IDArubicin *on page* 1039

IDArubicin (eye da ROO bi sin)

Brand Names: U.S. Idamycin PFS

Brand Names: Canada Idamycin®

Index Terms 4-Demethoxydaunorubicin; 4-DMDR; Idarubicin Hydrochloride; IDR; IMI 30; SC 33428

Pharmacologic Category Antineoplastic Agent, Anthracycline; Antineoplastic Agent, Antibiotic

Use Treatment of acute myeloid leukemia (AML)

Unlabeled Use Acute lymphocytic leukemia (ALL)

Pregnancy Risk Factor D

Pregnancy Considerations Adverse events were observed in animal studies. Fetal fatality was noted in a case report following use in a pregnant woman during the second trimester. The manufacturer recommends that women of childbearing potential avoid pregnancy.

Breast-Feeding Considerations It is not known if idarubicin is excreted in breast milk. Breast-feeding is not recommended by the manufacturer.

Contraindications Hypersensitivity to idarubicin, other anthracyclines, or any component of the formulation; bilirubin >5 mg/dL

Warnings/Precautions Hazardous agent - use appropriate precautions for handling and disposal (NIOSH, 2012). **[U.S. Boxed Warning]: May cause myocardial toxicity; may lead to heart failure. Cardiotoxicity is more common in patients who have previously received anthracyclines or have pre-existing cardiac disease.** The risk of myocardial toxicity is also increased in patients with concomitant or prior mediastinal/pericardial irradiation, patients with anemia, bone marrow depression, infections, leukemic pericarditis or myocarditis. Acute arrhythmias (may be life-threatening) or other cardiomyopathies may also occur. Monitor cardiac function during treatment.

[U.S. Boxed Warning]: Vesicant; may cause severe local tissue damage and necrosis if extravasation occurs. For I.V. administration only. NOT for I.M. or SubQ administration. Administer through a rapidly flowing I.V. line. Ensure proper needle or catheter placement prior to and during infusion. Avoid extravasation.

[U.S. Boxed Warning]: May cause severe myelosuppression; use caution in patients with pre-existing myelosuppression from prior treatment or radiation. [U.S. Boxed Warning]: Dosage reductions are recommended in patients with renal or hepatic impairment. Rapid lysis of leukemic cells may lead to hyperuricemia. Systemic infections should be managed prior to initiation of treatment. **[U.S. Boxed Warning]: Should be administered under the supervision of an experienced cancer chemotherapy physician.**

Adverse Reactions

>10%:

Cardiovascular: CHF (dose related), transient ECG abnormalities (supraventricular tachycardia, S-T wave changes, atrial or ventricular extrasystoles); generally asymptomatic and self-limiting. The relative cardiotoxicity of idarubicin compared to doxorubicin is unclear. Some investigators report no increase in cardiac toxicity for adults at cumulative oral idarubicin doses up to 540 mg/m^2; other reports suggest a maximum cumulative intravenous dose of 150 mg/m^2.

Central nervous system: Headache

Dermatologic: Alopecia (25% to 30%), radiation recall, skin rash (11%), urticaria

Gastrointestinal: Nausea, vomiting (30% to 60%); diarrhea (9% to 22%); stomatitis (11%); GI hemorrhage (30%)

Emetic potential: Moderate (30% to 60%)

Genitourinary: Discoloration of urine (darker yellow)

Hematologic: Myelosuppression (nadir: 10-15 days; recovery: 21-28 days), primarily leukopenia; thrombocytopenia and anemia. Effects are generally less severe with oral dosing.

Hepatic: Bilirubin and transaminases increased (44%)

Local: Tissue necrosis upon extravasation, erythematous streaking

1% to 10%:

Central nervous system: Seizure

Neuromuscular & skeletal: Peripheral neuropathy

<1% (Limited to important or life-threatening): Cardiomyopathy, hyperuricemia, myocarditis, neutropenic typhlitis

Drug Interactions

Metabolism/Transport Effects Substrate of P-glycoprotein

Avoid Concomitant Use

Avoid concomitant use of IDArubicin with any of the following: BCG; CloZAPine; Natalizumab; Pimecrolimus; Tacrolimus (Topical); Tofacitinib; Vaccines (Live)

Increased Effect/Toxicity

IDArubicin may increase the levels/effects of: CloZAPine; Leflunomide; Natalizumab; Tofacitinib; Vaccines (Live)

The levels/effects of IDArubicin may be increased by: Bevacizumab; Cyclophosphamide; Denosumab; P-glycoprotein/ABCB1 Inhibitors; Pimecrolimus; Roflumilast; Tacrolimus (Topical); Taxane Derivatives; Trastuzumab

Decreased Effect

IDArubicin may decrease the levels/effects of: BCG; Cardiac Glycosides; Coccidioidin Skin Test; Sipuleucel-T; Vaccines (Inactivated); Vaccines (Live)

The levels/effects of IDArubicin may be decreased by: Cardiac Glycosides; Echinacea; P-glycoprotein/ABCB1 Inducers

Storage/Stability Store intact vials of solution under refrigeration at 2°C to 8°C (36°F to 46°F). Protect from light. Solutions diluted in D_5W or NS for infusion are stable for 4 weeks at room temperature, protected from light. Syringe and IVPB solutions are stable for 72 hours at room temperature and 7 days under refrigeration.

Mechanism of Action Similar to doxorubicin and daunorubicin; inhibition of DNA and RNA synthesis by intercalation between DNA base pairs

Pharmacodynamics/Kinetics

Absorption: Oral: Variable (4% to 77%; mean: ~30%)

Distribution: V_d: 64 L/kg (some reports indicate 2250 L); extensive tissue binding; CSF

Protein binding: 94% to 97%

Metabolism: Hepatic to idarubicinol (pharmacologically active)

Half-life elimination: Oral: 14-35 hours; I.V.: 12-27 hours

Time to peak, serum: 1-5 hours

Excretion:

Oral: Urine (~5% of dose; 0.5% to 0.7% as unchanged drug, 4% as idarubicinol); hepatic (8%)

I.V.: Urine (13% as idarubicinol, 3% as unchanged drug); hepatic (17%)

Dosage Refer to individual protocols. I.V.:

Children: AML (unlabeled use): 10-12 mg/m^2/day for 3 days every 3 weeks

Adults:

AML induction: 12 mg/m^2/day for 3 days

AML consolidation: 10-12 mg/m^2/day for 2 days

Dosing adjustment in renal impairment: The FDA-approved labeling does not contain specific dosing adjustment guidelines; however, it does reccomend that dosage reductions be made. Patients with S_{cr}: ≥2 mg/dL did not receive treatment in many clinical trials. The following guidelines have been used by some clinicians (Aronoff, 2007):

Children:

Cl_{cr} <50 mL/minute: Administer 75% of dose

Hemodialysis: Administer 75% of dose

Continuous ambulatory peritoneal dialysis (CAPD): Administer 75% of dose

Continuous renal replacement therapy (CRRT): Administer 75% of dose

Adults:

Cl_{cr} 10-50 mL/minute: Administer 75% of dose

Cl_{cr} <10 mL/minute: Administer 50% of dose

Hemodialysis/CAPD: Supplemental dose not needed

Dosing adjustment/comments in hepatic impairment:

Bilirubin 2.6-5 mg/dL: Administer 50% of dose

Bilirubin >5 mg/dL: Avoid use

Dosing in obesity: *ASCO Guidelines for appropriate chemotherapy dosing in obese adults with cancer:* Utilize patient's actual body weight (full weight) for calculation of body surface area- or weight-based dosing, particularly when the intent of therapy is curative; manage regimen-related toxicities in the same manner as for nonobese patients; if a dose reduction is utilized due to toxicity, consider resumption of full weight-based dosing with subsequent cycles, especially if cause of toxicity (eg, hepatic or renal impairment) is resolved (Griggs, 2012).

Administration For I.V. administration only. Do not administer I.M. or SubQ; administer as slow push over 3-5 minutes, preferably into the side of a freely-running saline or dextrose infusion **or** as intermittent infusion over 10-15 minutes into a free-flowing I.V. solution of NS or D_5W; also occasionally administered as a bladder lavage.

Vesicant; ensure proper needle or catheter placement prior to and during infusion; avoid extravasation.

Extravasation management: If extravasation occurs, stop infusion immediately and disconnect (leave cannula/needle in place); gently aspirate extravasated solution (do **NOT** flush the line); remove needle/cannula; elevate extremity. Initiate antidote (dexrazoxane or dimethyl sulfate [DMSO]). Apply dry cold compresses for 20 minutes 4 times daily for 1-2 days (Perez Fidalgo, 2012); withhold cooling beginning 15 minutes before dexrazoxane infusion; continue withholding cooling until 15 minutes after infusion is completed. Topical DMSO should not be administered in combination with dexrazoxane; may lessen dexrazoxane efficacy.

Dexrazoxane: Adults: 1000 mg/m^2 (maximum dose: 2000 mg) I.V. (administer in a large vein remote from site of extravasation) over 1-2 hours days 1 and 2, then 500 mg/m^2 (maximum dose: 1000 mg) I.V. over 1-2 hours day 3; begin within 6 hours of extravasation. Day 2 and day 3 doses should be administered at approximately the same time (± 3 hours) as the dose on day 1 (Mouridsen, 2007; Perez Fidalgo, 2012). **Note:** Reduce dexrazoxane dose by 50% in patients with moderate to severe renal impairment (Cl_{cr} <40 mL/minute).

DMSO: Children and Adults: Apply topically to a region covering twice the affected area every 8 hours for 7 days; begin within 10 minutes of extravasation; do not cover with a dressing (Perez Fidalgo, 2012).

Hazardous agent; use appropriate precautions for handling and disposal (NIOSH, 2012).

Monitoring Parameters CBC with differential, platelet count, cardiac function, serum electrolytes, creatinine, uric acid, ALT, AST, bilirubin, signs of extravasation

Dosage Forms Excipient information presented when available (limited, particularly for generics); consult specific product labeling.

Solution, Intravenous, as hydrochloride [preservative free]:
Idamycin PFS: 5 mg/5 mL (5 mL); 10 mg/10 mL (10 mL); 20 mg/20 mL (20 mL)
Generic: 5 mg/5 mL (5 mL); 10 mg/10 mL (10 mL); 20 mg/20 mL (20 mL)

◆ **Idarubicin Hydrochloride** *see* IDArubicin *on page 1039*
◆ **IDEC-C2B8** *see* RiTUXimab *on page 1833*
◆ **IDR** *see* IDArubicin *on page 1039*

Idursulfase (eye dur SUL fase)

Brand Names: U.S. Elaprase
Brand Names: Canada Elaprase
Pharmacologic Category Enzyme
Use Hunter syndrome: Replacement therapy in Hunter syndrome (mucopolysaccharidosis II; MPS II) for improvement of walking capacity
Pregnancy Risk Factor C
Dosage
Hunter syndrome (mucopolysaccharidosis II): Children ≥5 years, Adolescents, and Adults: I.V.: 0.5 mg/kg once weekly

Dosage adjustment in renal impairment: No dosage adjustment provided in manufacturer's labeling.
Dosage adjustment in hepatic impairment: No dosage adjustment provided in manufacturer's labeling.

Additional Information Complete prescribing information should be consulted for additional detail.

Dosage Forms Excipient information presented when available (limited, particularly for generics); consult specific product labeling.
Solution, Intravenous [preservative free]:
Elaprase: 6 mg/3 mL (3 mL)

◆ **IDV** *see* Indinavir *on page 1068*
◆ **iFerex 150 [OTC]** *see* Polysaccharide-Iron Complex *on page 1673*
◆ **Ifex** *see* Ifosfamide *on page 1041*

Ifosfamide (eye FOSS fa mide)

Brand Names: U.S. Ifex
Brand Names: Canada Ifex
Index Terms Isophosphamide; Z4942
Pharmacologic Category Antineoplastic Agent, Alkylating Agent; Antineoplastic Agent, Alkylating Agent (Nitrogen Mustard)
Use
U.S. labeling: Treatment (third-line) of germ cell testicular cancer (in combination with other chemotherapy drugs and with concurrent mesna)
Canadian labeling (not approved indications in the U.S.): Treatment of soft tissue sarcoma, pancreatic cancer (relapsed or refractory), cervical cancer (advanced or recurrent; as monotherapy or in combination with cisplatin and bleomycin)

Unlabeled Use Treatment of bladder cancer (metastatic), cervical cancer (recurrent or metastatic), head and neck cancers (recurrent or metastatic), ovarian cancer, small cell lung cancer (relapsed), Hodgkin lymphoma (relapsed or refractory), non-Hodgkin lymphomas, thymomas and thymic cancers (advanced), sarcomas (Ewing's sarcoma, osteosarcoma, and soft tissue sarcoma)

Pregnancy Risk Factor D

Pregnancy Considerations Embryotoxic and teratogenic effects have been observed in animal reproduction studies. Fetal growth retardation and neonatal anemia have been reported with exposure to ifosfamide-containing regimens during human pregnancy. Male and female fertility may be affected (dose and duration dependent). Ifosfamide interferes with oogenesis and spermatogenesis; amenorrhea, azoospermia, and sterility have been reported and may be irreversible. Avoid pregnancy during treatment; male patients should not father a child for at least 6 months after completion of therapy.

Breast-Feeding Considerations Breast-feeding should be avoided during ifosfamide treatment. According to the manufacturer, the decision to discontinue ifosfamide or discontinue breast-feeding should take into account the risk of exposure to the infant and the benefits of treatment to the mother.

Contraindications Hypersensitivity to ifosfamide or any component of the formulation; urinary outflow obstruction
Canadian labeling: Additional contraindications (not in U.S. labeling): Severe myelosuppression; severe renal or hepatic impairment; active infection (bacterial, fungal, viral); severe immunosuppression; urinary tract disease (eg, cystitis); advanced cerebral arteriosclerosis

Warnings/Precautions Hazardous agent: Use appropriate precautions for handling and disposal (NIOSH, 2012). **[U.S. Boxed Warning]: Hemorrhagic cystitis may occur; concomitant mesna reduces the risk of hemorrhagic cystitis.** Hydration (at least 2 L/day), dose fractionation, and/or mesna administration will reduce the incidence of hematuria and protect against hemorrhagic cystitis. Obtain urinalysis prior to each dose; if microscopic hematuria is detected, withhold until complete resolution. Exclude or correct urinary tract obstructions prior to treatment. Use with caution (if at all) in patients with active urinary tract infection. Hemorrhagic cystitis is dose-dependent and is increased with high single doses (compared with fractionated doses); past or concomitant bladder radiation or busulfan treatment may increase the risk for hemorrhagic cystitis. **[U.S. Boxed Warning]: May cause severe nephrotoxicity, resulting in renal failure.** Acute and chronic renal failure as well as renal parenchymal and tubular necrosis (including acute) have been reported; tubular damage may be delayed and may persist. Renal manifestations include decreased glomerular rate, increased creatinine, proteinuria, enzymuria, cylindruria, aminoaciduria, phosphaturia, and glycosuria. Syndrome of inappropriate antidiuretic hormone (SIADH), renal rickets, and Fanconi syndrome have been reported. Evaluate renal function prior to and during treatment; monitor urine for erythrocytes and signs of urotoxicity.

[U.S. Boxed Warning]: May cause CNS toxicity which may be severe, resulting in encephalopathy and death; monitor for CNS toxicity; discontinue for encephalopathy. Symptoms of CNS toxicity (somnolence, confusion, dizziness, disorientation, hallucinations, cranial nerve dysfunction, psychotic behavior, extrapyramidal symptoms, seizures, coma blurred vision, and/or incontinence) have been observed within a few hours to a few days after initial dose and generally resolve within 2-3 days of treatment discontinuation (although may persist longer); maintain supportive care until complete resolution. Risk factors may include hypoalbuminemia, renal dysfunction, and prior history of ifosfamide-induced encephalopathy. Concomitant centrally-acting medications may result in additive CNS effects. Peripheral neuropathy has been reported.

[U.S. Boxed Warning]: Severe bone marrow suppression may occur (dose-limiting toxicity); monitor blood counts before and after each cycle. Leukopenia, neutropenia, thrombocytopenia and anemia are associated with ifosfamide. Myelosuppression is dose dependent, increased with single high doses (compared to fractionated doses) and increased with decreased renal function. Severe myelosuppression may occur when administered in combination with other chemotherapy agents or radiation therapy. Use with caution in patients with compromised bone marrow reserve. Unless clinically necessary, avoid administering to patients with WBC <2000/mm^3 and platelets <50,000/mm^3. Antimicrobial prophylaxis may be necessary in some neutropenic patients; Administer antibiotics and/or antifungal agents for neutropenic fever. May cause significant suppression of the immune responses; may lead to serious infection, sepsis or septic shock; reported infections have included bacterial, viral, fungal, and parasitic; latent infections may be reactivated; use with caution with other immunosuppressants or in patients with infection.

Arrhythmias, ST-segment or T-wave changes, cardiomyopathy, pericardial effusion, pericarditis, and epicardial fibrosis have been observed; the risk for cardiotoxicity is dose-dependent; concomitant cardiotoxic agents (eg, anthracyclines), irradiation of the cardiac region, and renal impairment may also increase the risk; use with caution in patients with cardiac risk factors or pre-existing cardiac disease. Interstitial pneumonitis, pulmonary fibrosis, and pulmonary toxicity leading to respiratory failure have been reported; monitor for signs and symptoms of pulmonary toxicity.

Anaphylactic/anaphylactoid reactions have been associated with ifosfamide; cross sensitivity with similar agents may occur. Hepatic sinusoidal obstruction syndrome (SOS), formerly called veno-occlusive disease (VOD), has been reported with ifosfamide-containing regimens. Secondary malignancies may occur; the risk for myelodysplastic syndrome (which may progress to acute leukemia) is increased with treatment. May interfere with wound healing. Use with caution in patients with prior radiation therapy.

Adverse Reactions

>10%:

- Central nervous system: CNS toxicity or encephalopathy (12% to 15%)
- Dermatologic: Alopecia (83% to 90%; 100% with combination therapy)
- Endocrine & metabolic: Metabolic acidosis (31%)
- Gastrointestinal: Nausea/vomiting (47% to 58%)
- Hematologic: Leukopenia (50% to ≤100%; grade 4: ≤50%; nadir: 8-14 days), anemia (38%), thrombocytopenia (20%; grades 3/4: ≤8%)
- Renal: Hematuria (6% to 92%; reduced with mesna; grade 2 [gross hematuria]: 8% to 12%)

1% to 10%:

- Central nervous system: Fever (1%)
- Gastrointestinal: Anorexia (1%)
- Hematologic: Neutropenic fever (1%)
- Hepatic: Bilirubin increased (2% to 3%), liver dysfunction (2% to 3%), transaminases increased (2% to 3%)
- Local: Phlebitis (2% to 3%)
- Renal: Renal impairment (6%)
- Miscellaneous: Infection (8% to 10%)

<1% (Limited to important or life-threatening): Acute respiratory distress syndrome, acute tubular necrosis, agranulocytosis, alkaline phosphatase increased, allergic reaction, alveolitis (allergic), amenorrhea, aminoaciduria, amnesia, anaphylactic reaction, angina, angioedema, anuria, arrhythmia, arthralgia, asterixis, atrial ectopy, atrial fibrillation/flutter, azoospermia, bladder irritation, bleeding, blurred vision, bone marrow failure, bradycardia, bradyphrenia, bronchospasm, bundle branch block, BUN increased, capillary leak syndrome, cardiac arrest, cardiogenic shock, cardiomyopathy, cardiotoxicity, catatonia, cecitis, chest pain, cholestasis, coagulopathy, colitis, conjunctivitis, creatinine clearance decreased/increased, creatinine increased, cylindruria, cytolytic hepatitis, delirium, delusion, dermatitis, diarrhea, DIC, DVT, dysesthesia, dyspnea, dysuria, echolalia, edema, ejection fraction decreased, enterocolitis, enuresis, enzymuria, erythema, extrapyramidal disorder, facial swelling, Fanconi syndrome, fatigue, gait disturbance, GGT increased, GI hemorrhage, glycosuria, gonadotropin increased, granulocytopenia, growth retardation (children), hemolytic anemia, hemolytic uremic syndrome, hemorrhagic cystitis, hepatic failure, hepatic sinusoidal obstruction syndrome (SOS; formerly veno-occlusive disease [VOD]), hepatitis fulminant, hepatitis (viral), hepatorenal syndrome, herpes zoster, hyperglycemia, hyper-/hypotension, hypersensitivity reactions, hypocalcemia, hypokalemia, hyponatremia, hypophosphatemia, hypoxia, ileus, immunosuppression, infertility, infusion site reactions (erythema, inflammation, pain, pruritus, swelling, tenderness), interstitial lung disease, jaundice, LDH increased, leukoencephalopathy, lymphopenia, malaise, mania, mental status change, methemoglobinemia, MI, mucosal inflammation/ulceration, multiorgan failure, mutism, myocardial hemorrhage, myocarditis, nephrogenic diabetes insipidus, neuralgia, neutropenia, oligospermia, oliguria, osteomalacia (adults), ovarian failure, ovulation disorder, palmar-plantar erythrodysesthesia syndrome, pancreatitis, pancytopenia, panic attack, paranoia, paresthesia, pericardial effusion, pericarditis, peripheral neuropathy, petechiae, phosphaturia, pleural

effusion, *Pneumocystis jiroveci* pneumonia, pneumonia, pneumonitis, pollakiuria, polydipsia, polyneuropathy, polyuria, portal vein thrombosis, premature atrial contractions, premature menopause, progressive multifocal leukoencephalopathy, proteinuria, pruritus, pulmonary edema, pulmonary embolism, pulmonary fibrosis, pulmonary hypertension, QRS complex abnormal, radiation recall dermatitis, rash (including macular and papular), renal failure, renal parenchymal damage, renal tubular acidosis, respiratory failure, reversible posterior leukoencephalopathy syndrome (RPLS), rhabdomyolysis, rickets, salivation, secondary malignancy, seizure, sepsis, septic shock, SIADH, skin necrosis, spermatogenesis impaired, status epilepticus, sterility, Stevens-Johnson syndrome, stomatitis, ST segment abnormal, supraventricular extrasystoles, tachycardia, tinnitus, toxic epidermal necrolysis, tubulointerstitial nephritis, tumor lysis syndrome, T-wave inversion, uremia, urticaria, vasculitis, ventricular extrasystoles/fibrillation/tachycardia, ventricular failure, vertigo, visual impairment, wound healing impairment

Drug Interactions

Metabolism/Transport Effects **Substrate** of CYP2A6 (major), CYP2B6 (minor), CYP2C19 (major), CYP2C8 (minor), CYP2C9 (minor), CYP3A4 (minor); **Note:** Assignment of Major/Minor substrate status based on clinically relevant drug interaction potential; **Inhibits** CYP3A4 (weak); **Induces** CYP2C9 (weak/moderate)

Avoid Concomitant Use

Avoid concomitant use of Ifosfamide with any of the following: BCG; CloZAPine; Natalizumab; Pimecrolimus; Pimozide; Tacrolimus (Topical); Tofacitinib; Vaccines (Live)

Increased Effect/Toxicity

Ifosfamide may increase the levels/effects of: ARIPiprazole; CloZAPine; Dofetilide; Leflunomide; Lomitapide; Natalizumab; Pimozide; Tofacitinib; Vaccines (Live); Vitamin K Antagonists

The levels/effects of Ifosfamide may be increased by: Busulfan; CYP2A6 Inhibitors (Moderate); CYP2A6 Inhibitors (Strong); CYP2C19 Inhibitors (Moderate); CYP2C19 Inhibitors (Strong); CYP3A4 Inducers (Strong); Denosumab; Luliconazole; Pimecrolimus; Roflumilast; Tacrolimus (Topical); Trastuzumab

Decreased Effect

Ifosfamide may decrease the levels/effects of: BCG; Coccidioidin Skin Test; Sipuleucel-T; Vaccines (Inactivated); Vaccines (Live); Vitamin K Antagonists

The levels/effects of Ifosfamide may be decreased by: CYP2A6 Inducers (Strong); CYP2C19 Inducers (Strong); CYP3A4 Inhibitors (Moderate); CYP3A4 Inhibitors (Strong); Dabrafenib; Echinacea

Ethanol/Nutrition/Herb Interactions Herb/Nutraceutical: St John's wort may decrease ifosfamide levels.

Preparation for Administration Hazardous agent; use appropriate precautions for handling and disposal (NIOSH, 2012). Reconstitute powder with SWFI or bacteriostatic SWFI (1 g in 20 mL or 3 g in 60 mL) to a concentration of 50 mg/mL. Further dilution in 50-1000 mL D_5W, NS, or lactated Ringer's (to a final concentration of 0.6-20 mg/mL) is recommended for I.V. infusion (may also dilute in $D_{2.5}W$, 1/2NS, or D_5NS).

Storage/Stability Store intact vials of powder for injection at room temperature of 20°C to 25°C (68°F to 77°F); avoid temperatures >30°C (86°F). Store intact vials of solution under refrigeration at 2°C to 8°C (36°F to 46°F). Reconstituted solutions and solutions diluted for administration are stable for 24 hours refrigerated.

Mechanism of Action Causes cross-linking of strands of DNA by binding with nucleic acids and other intracellular structures; inhibits protein synthesis and DNA synthesis

Pharmacodynamics/Kinetics Pharmacokinetics are dose dependent

Distribution: V_d: Approximates total body water; penetrates CNS, but not in therapeutic levels

Protein binding: Negligible

Metabolism: Hepatic to active metabolites isofosforamide mustard, 4-hydroxy-ifosfamide, acrolein, and inactive dichloroethylated and carboxy metabolites; acrolein is the agent implicated in development of hemorrhagic cystitis

Half-life elimination (increased in the elderly):
- High dose (3800-5000 mg/m^2): ~15 hours
- Lower dose (1600-2400 mg/m^2): ~7 hours

Excretion:
- High dose (5000 mg/m^2): Urine (70% to 86%; 61% as unchanged drug)
- Lower dose (1600-2400 mg/m^2): Urine (12% to 18% as unchanged drug)

Dosage Also consult details concerning dosing in combination regimens. **Note:** To prevent bladder toxicity, ifosfamide should be given with the urinary protector mesna and hydration of at least 2 L of oral or I.V. fluid per day.

Children: I.V.:

Ewing sarcoma (unlabeled use):

VAC/IE regimen: IE: 1800 mg/m^2/day for 5 days (in combination with mesna and etoposide) alternate with VAC (vincristine, doxorubicin, and cyclophosphamide) every 3 weeks for a total of 17 courses (Grier, 2003)

ICE-CAV regimen: ICE: 1800 mg/m^2/day for 5 days every 3-4 weeks for 2 courses (in combination with carboplatin and etoposide [and mesna]), followed by CAV (cyclophosphamide, doxorubicin, and vincristine) (Milano, 2006)

VAIA regimen: 3000 mg/m^2/day on days 1, 2, 22, 23, 43, and 44 for 4 courses (in combination with vincristine, doxorubicin, dactinomycin, and mesna) (Paulussen, 2001) **or** 2000 mg/m^2/day for 3 days every 3 weeks for 14 courses (in combination with vincristine, doxorubicin, dactinomycin, and mesna) (Paulussen, 2008)

VIDE regimen: 3000 mg/m^2/day over 1-3 hours for 3 days every 3 weeks for 6 courses (in combination with vincristine, doxorubicin, etoposide, and mesna) (Juergens, 2006)

IE regimen: 1800 mg/m^2/day over 1 hour for 5 days every 3 weeks for 12 cycles (in combination with etoposide and mesna) (Miser, 1987)

ICE regimen: 1800 mg/m^2/day for 5 days every 3 weeks for up to 12 cycles (in combination with carboplatin and etoposide [and mesna]) (van Winkle, 2005)

Osteosarcoma (unlabeled use):

Ifosfamide/cisplatin/doxorubicin/HDMT regimen: 3000 mg/m^2/day continuous infusion for 5 days during weeks 4 and 10 (preop) and during weeks 16, 25, and 34 (postop) (in combination with cisplatin, doxorubicin, methotrexate [high-dose], and mesna) (Bacci, 2003)

Ifosfamide/cisplatin/epirubicin regimen: Children ≥15 years: 2000 mg/m^2/day over 4 hours for 3 days (days 2, 3, and 4) every 3 weeks for 3 cycles (preop) and every 4 weeks for 3 cycles (postop) (in combination with cisplatin, epirubicin, and mesna) (Basaran, 2007)

IE regimen: 3000 mg/m^2/day over 3 hours for 4 days every 3-4 weeks (in combination with etoposide and mesna) (Gentet, 1997)

ICE regimen: Children ≥1 year: 1800 mg/m^2/day for 5 days every 3 weeks for up to 12 cycles (in combination with carboplatin and etoposide [and mesna]) (van Winkle, 2005)

Ifosfamide/HDMT/etoposide regimen: 3000 mg/m^2/day over 3 hours for 4 days during weeks 4 and 9 (3 additional postop courses were administered in good responders) (in combination with methotrexate [high-dose], etoposide, and mesna) (Le Deley, 2007)

Adults: I.V.:

Testicular cancer:

U.S. manufacturer's labeling; as part of combination chemotherapy and with mesna: 1200 mg/m^2/day for 5 days every 3 weeks or after hematologic recovery

VIP regimen: 1200 mg/m^2/day for 5 days every 3 weeks for 4 cycles (in combination with etoposide, mesna, and cisplatin) (Nichols, 1998)

VeIP regimen: 1200 mg/m^2/day for 5 days every 3 weeks for 4 cycles (in combination with vinblastine, mesna, and cisplatin) (Loehrer, 1998)

Canadian labeling: I.V.: Soft tissue sarcoma, cervical cancer (advanced or recurrent), pancreatic cancer (relapsed or refractory): 2000-2400 mg/m^2/day for 5 consecutive days (with mesna), may repeat after 3-4 weeks (or longer depending on patient status) or if lower daily dosage or total dosage over a longer time period is indicated, administer every other day (eg, days 1, 3, 5, 7, 9) or over 10 consecutive days at reduced doses.

High **single-dose** infusions of up to 5000-8000 mg/m^2/24 hour with continuous mesna may also be feasible; may repeat after 3-4 weeks (or longer depending on patient's condition).

Adult unlabeled uses and/or dosing: I.V.:

Testicular cancer:

TIP regimen (unlabeled dosing): 1500 mg/m^2/day for 4 days (days 2-5) every 3 weeks for 4 cycles (in combination with paclitaxel, mesna, and cisplatin) (Kondagunta, 2005)

TICE regimen (unlabeled dosing): 2000 mg/m^2/day for 3 days (days 2-4) over 4 hours every 2 weeks for 2 cycles (in combination with paclitaxel and mesna; followed by carboplatin and etoposide) (Kondagunta, 2007)

Cervical cancer, recurrent or metastatic: 1500 mg/m^{2}day for 5 days every 3 weeks (with mesna) (Coleman, 1986; Sutton, 1993)

Hodgkin lymphoma, relapsed or refractory:

ICE regimen: 5000 mg/m^2 (over 24 hours) beginning on day 2 every 2 weeks for 2 cycles (in combination with mesna, carboplatin, and etoposide) (Moskowitz, 2001)

IGEV regimen: 2000 mg/m^2/day for 4 days every 3 weeks for 4 cycles (in combination with mesna, gemcitabine, vinorelbine, and prednisolone) (Santoro, 2007)

MINE-ESHAP regimen: 1500 mg/m^2/day for 3 days every 4 weeks for up to 2 cycles (MINE is combination with mesna, mitoxantrone, and etoposide; MINE alternates with ESHAP for up to 2 cycles of each) (Fernandez, 2010)

Non-Hodgkin lymphomas:

CODOX-M/IVAC regimen:

Adults ≤65 years: Cycles 2 and 4 (IVAC): 1500 mg/m^2/day for 5 days (IVAC is combination with cytarabine, mesna, and etoposide; IVAC alternates with CODOX-M) (Mead, 2008)

Adults >65 years: Cycles 2 and 4 (IVAC): 1000 mg/m^2/day for 5 days (IVAC is combination with cytarabine, mesna, and etoposide; IVAC alternates with CODOX-M) (Mead, 2008)

MINE-ESHAP regimen: 1330 mg/m^2/day for 3 days every 3 weeks for 6 cycles (MINE is combination with mesna, mitoxantrone, and etoposide; followed by ESHAP) (Rodriguez, 1995)

RICE regimen: 5000 mg/m^2 (over 24 hours) beginning on day 4 every 2 weeks for 3 cycles (in combination with mesna, carboplatin, etoposide, and rituximab) (Kewalramani, 2004)

Ewing sarcoma:

VAC/IE regimen: Adults ≤30 years: IE: 1800 mg/m^2/day for 5 days (in combination with mesna and etoposide) alternate with VAC (vincristine, doxorubicin, and cyclophosphamide) every 3 weeks for a total of 17 courses (Grier, 2003)

VAIA regimen: 3000 mg/m^{2}day on days 1, 2, 22, 23, 43, and 44 for 4 courses (in combination with vincristine, doxorubicin, dactinomycin, and mesna) (Paulussen, 2001) **or** Adults ≤35 years: 2000 mg/m^2/day for 3 days every 3 weeks for 14 courses (in combination with vincristine, doxorubicin, dactinomycin, and mesna) (Paulussen, 2008)

VIDE regimen: Adults ≤50 years: 3000 mg/m^2/day over 1-3 hours for 3 days every 3 weeks for 6 courses (in combination with vincristine, doxorubicin, etoposide, and mesna) (Juergens, 2006)

IE regimen: 1800 mg/m^2/day over 1 hour for 5 days every 3 weeks for 12 cycles (in combination with etoposide and mesna) (Miser, 1987)

ICE regimen: Adults ≤22 years: 1800 mg/m^2/day for 5 days every 3 weeks for up to 12 cycles (in combination with carboplatin and etoposide [and mesna]) (van Winkle, 2005)

Osteosarcoma:

Ifosfamide/cisplatin/doxorubicin/HDMT regimen: Adults <40 years: 3000 mg/m^2/day continuous infusion for 5 days during weeks 4 and 10 (preop) and during weeks 16, 25, and 34 (postop) (in combination with cisplatin, doxorubicin, methotrexate [high-dose], and mesna) (Bacci, 2003)

Ifosfamide/cisplatin/epirubicin regimen: 2000 mg/m^2/day over 4 hours for 3 days (days 2, 3, and 4) every 3 weeks for 3 cycles (preop) and every 4 weeks for 3 cycles (postop) (in combination with cisplatin, epirubicin, and mesna) (Basaran, 2007)

ICE regimen (adults ≤22 years): 1800 mg/m^2/day for 5 days every 3 weeks for up to 12 cycles (in combination with carboplatin and etoposide [and mesna]) (van Winkle, 2005)

Soft tissue sarcoma:

Single-agent ifosfamide: 3000 mg/m^2/day over 4 hours for 3 days every 3 weeks for at least 2 cycles or until disease progression (van Oosterom, 2002)

ICE regimen: 1500 mg/m^2/day for 4 days every 4 weeks for 4-6 cycles (in combination with carboplatin, etoposide, and regional hyperthermia) (Nickenig, 2009)

MAID regimen: 2000 mg/m^2/day continuous infusion for 3 days every 3 weeks (in combination with mesna, doxorubicin and dacarbazine) (Antman, 1993) **or** 2500 mg/m^2/day continuous infusion for 3 days every 3 weeks (in combination with mesna, doxorubicin, and dacarbazine); reduce ifosfamide to 1500mg/m^2/day if prior pelvic irradiation (Elias, 1989)

Ifosfamide/epirubicin: 1800 mg/m^2/day over 1 hour for 5 days every 3 weeks for 5 cycles (in combination with mesna and epirubicin) (Frustaci, 2001)

AIM regimens: 1500 mg/m^2/day over 2 hours for 4 days every 3 weeks for 4-6 cycles (in combination with mesna and doxorubicin) (Worden, 2005) **or** 2000-3000 mg/m^2/day over 3 hours for 3 days (in combination with mesna and doxorubicin) (Grobmyer, 2004)

Dosing adjustment in renal impairment:

U.S. labeling: Consider dosage reduction in patients with renal impairment; however, no dosage adjustment is provided in the manufacturer's labeling; ifosfamide (and metabolites) are excreted renally and may accumulate in patients with renal dysfunction. Ifosfamide and metabolites are dialyzable.

Canadian labeling:
Mild-moderate impairment: No dosage adjustment provided in the manufacturer's labeling.
Severe impairment: Use is contraindicated.
The following adjustments have also been recommended:
Aronoff, 2007:
Cl_{cr} ≥10 mL/minute: Children and Adults: No dosage adjustment necessary.
Cl_{cr} <10 mL/minute: Children and Adults: Administer 75% of dose.
Hemodialysis (supplement for dialysis):
Children: 1 g/m^2 followed by hemodialysis 6-8 hours later
Adults: No supplemental dose needed.
Kintzel, 1995:
Cl_{cr} 46-60 mL/minute: Administer 80% of dose.
Cl_{cr} 31-45 mL/minute: Administer 75% of dose.
Cl_{cr} <30 mL/minute: Administer 70% of dose.

Dosing adjustment in hepatic impairment: No dosage adjustment provided in the manufacturer's labeling; however, ifosfamide is extensively hepatically metabolized to both active and inactive metabolites; use with caution. The following adjustments have been recommended:
Floyd, 2006: Bilirubin >3 mg/dL: Administer 25% of dose.
Canadian labeling:
Mild-to-moderate impairment: No dosage adjustment provided in manufacturer labeling; use with caution.
Severe impairment: Use is contraindicated.

Dosing in obesity: *ASCO Guidelines for appropriate chemotherapy dosing in obese adults with cancer:* Utilize patient's actual body weight (full weight) for calculation of body surface area- or weight-based dosing, particularly when the intent of therapy is curative; manage regimen-related toxicities in the same manner as for nonobese patients; if a dose reduction is utilized due to toxicity, consider resumption of full weight-based dosing with subsequent cycles, especially if cause of toxicity (eg, hepatic or renal impairment) is resolved (Griggs, 2012).

Administration Administer I.V. over at least 30 minutes (infusion times may vary by protocol; refer to specific protocol for infusion duration)

Hazardous agent; use appropriate precautions for handling and disposal (NIOSH, 2012).

Monitoring Parameters CBC with differential (prior to each dose), urine output, urinalysis (prior to each dose), liver function, and renal function tests; signs and symptoms of neurotoxicity, pulmonary toxicity, and/or hemorrhagic cystitis

Dosage Forms Excipient information presented when available (limited, particularly for generics); consult specific product labeling.
Kit, Intravenous:
Generic: 1-1 GM
Solution, Intravenous:
Generic: 1 g/20 mL (20 mL); 3 g/60 mL (60 mL)
Solution, Intravenous [preservative free]:
Generic: 1 g/20 mL (20 mL); 3 g/60 mL (60 mL)
Solution Reconstituted, Intravenous:
Ifex: 1 g (1 ea); 3 g (1 ea)
Generic: 1 g (1 ea); 3 g (1 ea)

- ◆ **IG** *see* Immune Globulin *on page 1059*
- ◆ **IgG4-Kappa Monoclonal Antibody** *see* Natalizumab *on page 1431*
- ◆ **IGIM** *see* Immune Globulin *on page 1059*
- ◆ **IGIV** *see* Immune Globulin *on page 1059*
- ◆ **IGIVnex (Can)** *see* Immune Globulin *on page 1059*
- ◆ **IGSC** *see* Immune Globulin *on page 1059*
- ◆ **IIV** *see* Influenza Virus Vaccine (Inactivated) *on page 1078*
- ◆ **IIV3** *see* Influenza Virus Vaccine (Inactivated) *on page 1078*
- ◆ **IIV4** *see* Influenza Virus Vaccine (Inactivated) *on page 1078*
- ◆ **IL-1Ra** *see* Anakinra *on page 136*
- ◆ **IL-2** *see* Aldesleukin *on page 63*
- ◆ **IL-11** *see* Oprelvekin *on page 1514*
- ◆ **Ilaris** *see* Canakinumab *on page 326*
- ◆ **Ilevro** *see* Nepafenac *on page 1442*

Iloperidone (eye loe PER i done)

Brand Names: U.S. Fanapt; Fanapt Titration Pack

Pharmacologic Category Antipsychotic Agent, Atypical

Additional Appendix Information
Antipsychotic Agents *on page 2290*
Beers Criteria – Potentially Inappropriate Medications for Geriatrics *on page 2368*

Use Acute treatment of schizophrenia

Pregnancy Risk Factor C

Pregnancy Considerations Adverse events were observed in animal reproduction studies. Antipsychotic use during the third trimester of pregnancy has a risk for abnormal muscle movements (extrapyramidal symptoms [EPS]) and/or withdrawal symptoms in newborns following delivery. Symptoms in the newborn may include agitation, feeding disorder, hypertonia, hypotonia, respiratory distress, somnolence, and tremor; these effects may be self-limiting or require hospitalization. Iloperidone may cause hyperprolactinemia, which may decrease reproductive function in both males and females.

The ACOG recommends that therapy during pregnancy be individualized; treatment with psychiatric medications during pregnancy should incorporate the clinical expertise of the mental health clinician, obstetrician, primary healthcare provider, and pediatrician. Safety data related to atypical antipsychotics during pregnancy is limited and routine use is not recommended. However, if a woman is inadvertently exposed to an atypical antipsychotic while pregnant, continuing therapy may be preferable to switching to a typical antipsychotic that the fetus has not yet been exposed to; consider risk:benefit (ACOG, 2008).

Healthcare providers are encouraged to enroll women 18-45 years of age exposed to iloperidone during pregnancy in the Atypical Antipsychotics Pregnancy Registry (1-866-961-2388 or http://www.womensmentalhealth.org/pregnancyregistry).

Breast-Feeding Considerations It is not known if iloperidone is excreted into breast milk. Breast-feeding is not recommended by the manufacturer.

Contraindications Hypersensitivity to iloperidone or any component of the formulation

Warnings/Precautions [U.S. Boxed Warning]: Elderly patients with dementia-related psychosis treated with antipsychotics are at an increased risk of death compared to placebo. Most deaths appeared to be either cardiovascular (eg, heart failure, sudden death) or infectious (eg, pneumonia) in nature. In addition, an increased incidence of cerebrovascular effects (eg, transient ischemic attack, cerebrovascular accidents) has been reported in studies of placebo-controlled trials of antipsychotics in elderly patients with dementia-related psychosis. Iloperidone is not approved for the treatment of dementia-related psychosis.

May be sedating; use with caution in disorders where CNS depression is a feature. Caution in patients with predisposition to seizures. Use is not recommended in patients with hepatic impairment. Esophageal dysmotility and aspiration have been associated with antipsychotic use; use with caution in patients at risk of aspiration pneumonia (ie, Alzheimer's disease). Use is associated with increased prolactin levels; clinical significance of hyperprolactinemia in patients with breast cancer or other prolactin-dependent tumors is unknown. May alter temperature regulation. Leukopenia, neutropenia, and agranulocytosis (sometimes fatal) have been reported in clinical trials and postmarketing reports; presence of risk factors (eg, pre-existing low WBC or history of drug-induced leuko-/neutropenia) should prompt periodic blood count assessment and discontinuation at first signs of blood dyscrasias.

May alter cardiac conduction and prolong the QT_c interval; life-threatening arrhythmias have occurred with therapeutic doses of antipsychotics. Risks may be increased by conditions or concomitant medications which cause bradycardia, hypokalemia, and/or hypomagnesemia. Avoid use in combination with QT_c-prolonging drugs and in patients with congenital long QT syndrome, history of cardiac arrhythmia, recent MI, or uncompensated heart failure. Discontinue treatment in patients found to have persistent QT_c intervals >500 msec. Further cardiac evaluation is warranted in patients with symptoms of dizziness, palpitations, or syncope. May cause orthostatic hypotension; use with caution in patients at risk of this effect (eg, concurrent medication use which may predispose to hypotension/bradycardia or presence of hypovolemia) or in those who would not tolerate transient hypotensive episodes. Use with caution in patients with cardiovascular diseases (eg, heart failure, history of myocardial infarction or ischemia, cerebrovascular disease, conduction abnormalities).

May cause anticholinergic effects (confusion, agitation, constipation, xerostomia, blurred vision, urinary retention); therefore, use with caution in patients with decreased gastrointestinal motility, urinary retention, BPH, xerostomia, or visual problems (including narrow-angle glaucoma). May cause extrapyramidal symptoms (EPS), including pseudoparkinsonism, acute dystonic reactions, akathisia, and tardive dyskinesia. Risk of dystonia (and probably other EPS) may be greater with increased doses, use of conventional antipsychotics, males, and younger patients. Risk of neuroleptic malignant syndrome (NMS) may be increased in patients with Parkinson's disease or Lewy body dementia. May cause hyperglycemia; in some cases may be extreme and associated with ketoacidosis, hyperosmolar coma, or death. Use with caution in patients with diabetes or other disorders of glucose regulation; monitor for worsening of glucose control. Dyslipidemia has been reported with atypical antipsychotics; risk profile may differ between agents. In clinical trials, changes in triglyceride and total cholesterol levels observed with iloperidone were similar to those observed with placebo or were clinically insignificant. Small reductions in cholesterol and triglycerides have been observed in longer term iloperidone trials.

Significant weight gain has been observed with antipsychotic therapy; incidence varies with product. Monitor waist circumference and BMI. Rare cases of priapism have been reported.

Use in elderly patients with dementia is associated with an increased risk of mortality and cerebrovascular accidents; avoid antipsychotic use for behavioral problems associated with dementia unless alternative nonpharmacologic therapies have failed and patient may harm self or others. In addition, use may cause or exacerbate syndrome of inappropriate antidiuretic hormone secretion or hyponatremia; monitor sodium closely with initiation or dosage adjustments in older adults (Beers Criteria).

Dosage adjustments are recommended for iloperidone when given concomitantly with strong CYP2D6 or CYP3A4 inhibitors or in poor metabolizers of CYP2D6. The possibility of a suicide attempt is inherent in psychotic illness; use caution in high-risk patients during initiation of therapy. Prescriptions should be written for the smallest quantity consistent with good patient care. Continued use for >6 weeks has not been evaluated.

Adverse Reactions

>10%:

Cardiovascular: Tachycardia (3% to 12%; dose related)

Central nervous system: Dizziness (10% to 20%; dose related), somnolence (9% to 15%)

1% to 10%:

Cardiovascular: Orthostatic hypotension (3% to 5%), hypotension (<1% to 3%; dose related), palpitations (≥1%)

Central nervous system: Fatigue (4% to 6%), extrapyramidal symptoms (4% to 5%), tremor (3%), lethargy (1% to 3%), akathisia (2%), aggression (≥1%), delusion (≥1%), restlessness (≥1%)

Dermatologic: Rash (2% to 3%)

Gastrointestinal: Nausea (≤10%), xerostomia (8% to 10%), weight gain (1% to 9%; dose related), diarrhea (5% to 7%), abdominal discomfort (≤3%; dose related), weight loss (≥1%)

Genitourinary: Ejaculation failure (2%), erectile dysfunction (≥1%), urinary incontinence (≥1%)

Neuromuscular & skeletal: Arthralgia (3%), stiffness (1% to 3%; dose related), dyskinesia (<2%), muscle spasm (≥1%), myalgia (≥1%)

Ocular: Blurred vision (≤3%), conjunctivitis (≥1%)

Respiratory: Nasal congestion (5% to 8%), nasopharyngitis (≤4%), upper respiratory tract infection (2% to 3%), dyspnea (2%)

<1% (Limited to important or life-threatening): Acute renal failure, amenorrhea, amnesia, anemia, anorgasmia, aphthous stomatitis, appetite increased, arrhythmia, asthma, AV block (first degree), blepharitis, bradykinesia, breast pain, bulimia nervosa, cataract, catatonia, cholelithiasis, confusion, dehydration, delirium, difficulty walking, dry eye, duodenal ulcer, dystonia, dysuria, edema, enuresis, epistaxis, esophageal reflux, eyelid edema, eye swelling, fecal incontinence, fluid retention, gastric acid secretion increased, gastritis, gynecomastia, heart failure, hematocrit/hemoglobin decreased, hiatal hernia, hostility, hyperemia, hyperthermia, hypokalemia, hypothyroidism, impulse control disorder, lenticular opacities, leukopenia, libido decreased, major depression, mania, menorrhagia, menstrual irregularities, metrorrhagia, mood swings, mouth ulceration, nasal dryness, nephrolithiasis, neutrophils increased, nystagmus, obsessive compulsive disorder, panic attack, paraesthesia, paranoia, parkinsonism, pollakiuria, polydipsia psychogenic, postmenopausal hemorrhage, prostatitis, pruritus, psychomotor hyperactivity, QT_c interval prolongation, restless leg syndrome, retrograde ejaculation, rhinorrhea, salivation, sinus congestion, sleep apnea syndrome, stomatitis, testicular pain, thirst, tinnitus, torticollis, urinary retention, urticaria, vertigo

Drug Interactions

Metabolism/Transport Effects **Substrate** of CYP2D6 (major), CYP3A4 (minor); **Note:** Assignment of Major/Minor substrate status based on clinically relevant drug interaction potential; **Inhibits** CYP3A4 (moderate)

Avoid Concomitant Use

Avoid concomitant use of Iloperidone with any of the following: Amisulpride; Azelastine (Nasal); Bosutinib; Highest Risk QTc-Prolonging Agents; Ibrutinib; Ivabradine; Lomitapide; Metoclopramide; Mifepristone; Moderate Risk QTc-Prolonging Agents; Paraldehyde; Simeprevir; Sulpiride; Tolvaptan; Ulipristal

Increased Effect/Toxicity

Iloperidone may increase the levels/effects of: Alcohol (Ethyl); Amisulpride; ARIPiprazole; Avanafil; Azelastine (Nasal); Bosentan; Bosutinib; Budesonide (Systemic, Oral Inhalation); Buprenorphine; CNS Depressants; Colchicine; CYP3A4 Substrates; Eplerenone; Everolimus; FentaNYL; Highest Risk QTc-Prolonging Agents; Hydrocodone; Ibrutinib; Imatinib; Ivacaftor; Lomitapide; Lurasidone; Methylphenidate; OxyCODONE; Paraldehyde; Pimecrolimus; Salmeterol; Saxagliptin; Serotonin Modulators; Simeprevir; Sulpiride; Tolvaptan; Ulipristal; Zolpidem

The levels/effects of Iloperidone may be increased by: Abiraterone Acetate; Acetylcholinesterase Inhibitors (Central); Brimonidine (Topical); CYP2D6 Inhibitors (Moderate); CYP2D6 Inhibitors (Strong); CYP3A4 Inhibitors (Strong); Doxylamine; HydrOXYzine; Ivabradine; Lithium formulations; Magnesium Sulfate; MAO Inhibitors; Methylphenidate; Metoclopramide; Metyrosine; Mifepristone; Moderate Risk QTc-Prolonging Agents; Perampanel; QTc-Prolonging Agents (Indeterminate Risk and Risk Modifying); Serotonin Modulators; Sodium Oxybate; Tetrabenazine

Decreased Effect

Iloperidone may decrease the levels/effects of: Amphetamines; Anti-Parkinson's Agents (Dopamine Agonist); Ifosfamide; Quinagolide

The levels/effects of Iloperidone may be decreased by: CYP2D6 Inhibitors (Strong); Lithium formulations; Peginterferon Alfa-2b

Ethanol/Nutrition/Herb Interactions

Ethanol: May increase CNS depression; monitor for increased effects with coadministration. Caution patients about effects.

Herb/Nutraceutical: Avoid St John's wort (may decrease serum levels of iloperidone). Avoid kava kava, gotu kola, valerian, St John's wort (may increase CNS depression).

Storage/Stability Store at 25°C (77°F); excursions permitted to 15°C to 30°C (59°F to 86°F). Protect from light and moisture.

Mechanism of Action Iloperidone is a piperidinyl-benzisoxazole atypical antipsychotic with mixed D_2/5-HT_2 antagonist activity. It exhibits high affinity for 5-HT_{2A}, D_2, and D_3 receptors, low to moderate affinity for D_1, D_4, H_1, 5-HT_{1A}, 5-HT_6, 5-HT_7, and $NE_{\alpha1}$ receptors, and no affinity for muscarinic receptors. The addition of serotonin antagonism to dopamine antagonism (classic neuroleptic mechanism) is thought to improve negative symptoms of psychoses and reduce the incidence of extrapyramidal side effects. Iloperidone's low affinity for histamine H_1 receptors may decrease the risk for weight gain and somnolence while its affinity for $NE_{\alpha1/\alpha2C}$ may provide antidepressant and anxiolytic activity and improved cognitive function.

Pharmacodynamics/Kinetics

Absorption: Well absorbed

Distribution: V_d: 1340-2800 L

Protein binding: ~95% (iloperidone and active metabolites)

Metabolism: Hepatic via carbonyl reduction, hydroxylation (CYP2D6) and O-demethylation (CYP3A4); forms active metabolites (P88 and P95)

Bioavailability: Oral: Tablet (relative to solution): 96%

Half-life elimination:

Extensive metabolizers: Iloperidone: 18 hours; P88: 26 hours; P95: 23 hours

Poor metabolizers: Iloperidone: 33 hours; P88: 37 hours; P95: 31 hours

Time to peak, plasma: 2-4 hours

Excretion: Urine (58% extensive metabolizers, 45% poor metabolizers); feces (20% extensive metabolizers, 22% poor metabolizers)

Dosage Oral: Adults: Schizophrenia: Initial: 1 mg twice daily; titrate to the recommended dosage range with dosage adjustments not to exceed 2 mg twice daily (4 mg daily) every 24 hours; recommended dosage range: 6-12 mg twice daily (maximum: 24 mg daily)

Note: Titrate dose to effect (to avoid orthostatic hypotensive effects); treatment >6 weeks has not been evaluated; when reinitiating treatment after discontinuation (>3 days), the initial titration schedule should be followed.

Dosage adjustment in patients receiving strong CYP2D6 inhibitors (eg, paroxetine, fluoxetine, quinidine): Decrease iloperidone dose by 50%; when the CYP2D6 inhibitor is discontinued, return to previous dose.

Dosage adjustment in patients receiving strong CYP3A4 inhibitors (eg, ketoconazole, clarithromycin): Decrease iloperidone dose by 50%; when the CYP3A4 inhibitor is discontinued, return to previous dose.

Dosage adjustment in poor metabolizers of CYP2D6: Decrease iloperidone dose by 50%.

Dosage adjustment in renal impairment: No dosage adjustment provided in manufacturer's labeling; however, pharmacokinetics of iloperidone do not appear to be altered by renal impairment due to extensive hepatic metabolism.

Dosage adjustment in hepatic impairment: Use is not recommended in patients with hepatic impairment (has not been studied).

Dietary Considerations May be given with or without food.

Administration May be administered with or without food.

Monitoring Parameters Vital signs; fasting blood glucose/Hgb A_{1c} (prior to treatment and periodically during treatment); signs and symptoms of hyperglycemia; signs and symptoms of cardiac arrhythmia; CBC (frequently during first few months of therapy); serum potassium and magnesium levels (prior to treatment and periodically during treatment); orthostatic blood pressure changes; assess weight prior to and periodically during treatment;

Dosage Forms Excipient information presented when available (limited, particularly for generics); consult specific product labeling.

Tablet, Oral:

Fanapt: 1 mg, 2 mg, 4 mg, 6 mg, 8 mg, 10 mg, 12 mg

Fanapt Titration Pack: 1 & 2 & 4 & 6 MG

Iloprost (EYE loe prost)

Brand Names: U.S. Ventavis

Index Terms Iloprost Tromethamine; Prostacyclin PGI_2

Pharmacologic Category Prostacyclin; Prostaglandin; Vasodilator

Use Pulmonary arterial hypertension: Treatment of pulmonary arterial hypertension (World Health Organization [WHO] group I) in patients with New York Heart Association (NYHA) class III or IV symptoms to improve exercise tolerance, symptoms, and diminish clinical deterioration.

Unlabeled Use WHO group III and IV pulmonary arterial hypertension (PAH)

Pregnancy Risk Factor C

Dosage Inhalation: Adults: Pulmonary arterial hypertension (PAH): Initial: 2.5 mcg/dose; if tolerated, increase to 5 mcg/dose; administer 6-9 times daily (dosing at intervals ≥2 hours while awake according to individual need and tolerability); maintenance dose: 2.5-5 mcg/dose; maximum daily dose: 45 mcg (ie, 5 mcg/dose 9 times daily)

Dosage adjustment in renal impairment: Inhaled iloprost has not been studied in renal impairment; however, according to the manufacturer, no adjustment is required in patients with renal impairment who are not on dialysis (the effect of dialysis on iloprost is unknown).

Dosage adjustment in hepatic impairment: Child-Pugh class B or C: Consider increasing dosing interval (eg, every 3-4 hours) based on response at the end of the dose interval

Additional Information Complete prescribing information should be consulted for additional detail.

Dosage Forms Excipient information presented when available (limited, particularly for generics); consult specific product labeling.

Solution, Inhalation [preservative free]:

Ventavis: 10 mcg/mL (1 mL); 20 mcg/mL (1 mL) [contains alcohol, usp, tromethamine]

◆ Iloprost Tromethamine *see* Iloprost *on page 1047*

◆ Ilotycin *see* Erythromycin (Ophthalmic) *on page 744*

Imatinib (eye MAT eh nib)

Brand Names: U.S. Gleevec

Brand Names: Canada Apo-Imatinib; Gleevec; Teva-Imatinib

Index Terms CGP-57148B; Glivec; Imatinib Mesylate; STI-571

Pharmacologic Category Antineoplastic Agent, Tyrosine Kinase Inhibitor

Use Treatment of:

Gastrointestinal stromal tumors (GIST) kit-positive (CD117), including unresectable and/or metastatic malignant and adjuvant treatment following complete resection

Philadelphia chromosome-positive (Ph+) chronic myeloid leukemia (CML) in chronic phase (newly-diagnosed) in children and adults

Ph+ CML in blast crisis, accelerated phase, or chronic phase after failure of interferon therapy

Ph+ acute lymphoblastic leukemia (ALL) (relapsed or refractory)

Ph+ ALL (newly diagnosed; in combination with chemotherapy) in children

Aggressive systemic mastocytosis (ASM) without D816V c-Kit mutation (or c-Kit mutation status unknown)

Dermatofibrosarcoma protuberans (DFSP) (unresectable, recurrent and/or metastatic)

Hypereosinophilic syndrome (HES) and/or chronic eosinophilic leukemia (CEL)

Myelodysplastic/myeloproliferative disease (MDS/MPD) associated with platelet-derived growth factor receptor (PDGFR) gene rearrangements

Canadian labeling (not an approved indication in the U.S.): Ph+ ALL induction therapy (newly diagnosed; as a single agent)

Unlabeled Use Treatment of desmoid tumors or chordoma (soft tissue sarcomas); post-stem cell transplant (allogeneic) follow-up treatment for recurrence in CML; treatment of advanced or metastatic melanoma (C-KIT mutated tumors)

Pregnancy Risk Factor D

Pregnancy Considerations Animal reproduction studies have demonstrated teratogenic effects and fetal loss. Women of childbearing potential are advised not to become pregnant (female patients and female partners of male patients); highly effective contraception is recommended. Case reports of pregnancies while on therapy (both males and females) include reports of spontaneous abortion, minor abnormalities (hypospadias, pyloric stenosis, and small intestine rotation) at or shortly after birth, and other congenital abnormalities including skeletal malformations, hypoplastic lungs, exomphalos, kidney abnormalities, hydrocephalus, cerebellar hypoplasia, and cardiac defects.

Retrospective case reports of women with CML in complete hematologic response (CHR) with cytogenic response (partial or complete) who interrupted imatinib therapy due to pregnancy, demonstrated a loss of response in some patients while off treatment. At 18 months after treatment reinitiation following delivery, CHR was again achieved in all patients and cytogenic response was achieved in some patients. Cytogenetic response rates may not be at as high as compared to patients with 18 months of uninterrupted therapy (Ault, 2006; Pye, 2008).

Breast-Feeding Considerations Imatinib and its active metabolite are found in human breast milk; the milk/plasma ratio is 0.5 for imatinib and 0.9 for the active metabolite. Based on body weight, up to 10% of a therapeutic maternal dose could potentially be received by a breastfed infant, the decision to discontinue breast-feeding during therapy or to discontinue imatinib should take into account the benefits of treatment to the mother.

Contraindications There are no contraindications listed within the FDA-approved manufacturer's labeling.

Canadian labeling: Hypersensitivity to imatinib or any component of the formulation

Warnings/Precautions Hazardous agent - use appropriate precautions for handling and disposal (NIOSH, 2012). Often associated with fluid retention, weight gain, and edema (risk increases with higher doses and age >65 years); occasionally serious and may lead to significant complications, including pleural effusion, pericardial effusion, pulmonary edema, and ascites. Monitor regularly for rapid weight gain or other signs/symptoms of fluid retention. Use with caution in patients where fluid accumulation may be poorly tolerated, such as in cardiovascular disease (heart failure [HF] or hypertension) and pulmonary disease. Severe HF and left ventricular dysfunction (LVD) have been reported occasionally, usually in patients with comorbidities and/or risk factors; carefully monitor patients with pre-existing cardiac disease or risk factors for HF or history of renal failure. With initiation of imatinib treatment, cardiogenic shock and/or LVD have been reported in patients with hypereosinophilic syndrome and cardiac involvement (reversible with systemic steroids, circulatory support and temporary cessation of imatinib). Patients with high eosinophil levels and an abnormal echocardiogram or abnormal serum troponin level may benefit from prophylactic systemic steroids (for 1-2 weeks) with the initiation of imatinib.

Severe bullous dermatologic reactions (including erythema multiforme and Stevens-Johnson syndrome) have been reported; recurrence has been described with rechallenge. Case reports of successful resumption at a lower dose (with corticosteroids and/or antihistamine) have been described; however, some patients may experience recurrent reactions.

Hepatotoxicity may occur (may be severe); fatal hepatic failure and severe hepatic injury requiring liver transplantation have been reported with both short- and long-term use; monitor liver function prior to initiation and monthly or as needed thereafter; therapy interruption or dose reduction may be necessary. Transaminase and bilirubin elevations, and acute liver failure have been observed with imatinib in combination with chemotherapy. Use with caution in patients with pre-existing hepatic impairment; dosage adjustment recommended in patients with severe impairment. Use with caution in renal impairment; dosage adjustment recommended for moderate and severe impairment. Tumor lysis syndrome (TLS), including fatalities, has been reported in patients with ALL, CML eosinophilic leukemias, and GIST; risk for TLS is higher in patients with a high tumor burden or high proliferation rate; monitor closely; correct clinically significant dehydration and treat high uric acid levels prior to initiation of imatinib.

May cause GI irritation, severe hemorrhage (grades 3 and 4; including gastrointestinal hemorrhage and/or tumor hemorrhage; hemorrhage incidence is higher in patients with GIST [gastrointestinal tumors may have been hemorrhage source]), or hematologic toxicity (anemia, neutropenia, and thrombocytopenia; usually occurring within the first several months of treatment); monitor blood counts weekly for the first month, biweekly for the second month, and as clinically necessary thereafter; median duration of neutropenia is 2-3 weeks; median duration of thrombocytopenia is 3-4 weeks; in CML, cytopenias are more common in accelerated or blast phase than in chronic phase. Hypothyroidism has been reported in patients who were receiving thyroid hormone replacement therapy prior to the initiation of imatinib; monitor thyroid function; the average onset for imatinib-induced hypothyroidism is 2 weeks; consider doubling levothyroxine doses upon initiation of imatinib (Hamnvik, 2011). Potentially significant drug-drug interactions may exist, requiring dose or frequency adjustment, additional monitoring, and/or selection of alternative therapy. Imatinib exposure may be reduced in patients who have had gastric surgery (eg, bypass, major gastrectomy, or resection); monitor imatinib trough concentrations (Liu, 2011; Pavlovsky, 2009; Yoo, 2010). Growth retardation has been reported in children receiving imatinib for the treatment of CML; generally where treatment was initiated in prepubertal children; growth velocity was usually restored as pubertal age was reached (Shima, 2010); monitor growth closely. Reports of accidents have been received but it is unclear if imatinib has been the direct cause in any case; advise patients regarding side effects such as dizziness, blurred vision, or somnolence; use caution when driving/operating motor vehicles and heavy machinery.

Adverse Reactions Note: Adverse reactions listed as a composite of data across many trials, except where noted for a specific indication.

>10%:

Cardiovascular: Edema/fluid retention (11% to 86%; grades 3/4: 3% to 13%; includes aggravated edema, anasarca, ascites, pericardial effusion, peripheral edema, pulmonary edema, and superficial edema); facial edema (≤17%), chest pain (7% to 11%), hypotension (Ph+ ALL [pediatric] grades 3/4: 11%)

Central nervous system: Fatigue (29% to 75%), pain (≤47%), fever (6% to 41%), headache (8% to 37%), dizziness (5% to 19%), insomnia (10% to 15%), depression (≤15%), anxiety (8% to 12%), chills (≤11%)

Dermatologic: Rash (9% to 50%; grades 3/4: 1% to 9%), dermatitis (GIST ≤39%), pruritus (8% to 26%), alopecia (GIST 10% to 15%)

Endocrine & metabolic: LDH increased (GIST ≤60%), hypokalemia (6% to 13%; Ph+ ALL [pediatric] grades 3/4: 34%), hypoproteinemia (≤32%), albumin decreased (≤21%; grade 3: ≤4%)

Gastrointestinal: Nausea (42% to 73%; Ph+ ALL [pediatric] grades 3/4: 16%), diarrhea (25% to 59%; Ph+ ALL [pediatric] grades 3/4: 9%), vomiting (11% to 58%), abdominal pain (3% to 57%), anorexia (≤36%), weight gain (5% to 32%), dyspepsia (11% to 27%), flatulence (≤25%), abdominal distension (≤19%), stomatitis/mucositis (≤10% to 16%), constipation (9% to 16%), taste disturbance (≤13%)

Hematologic: Anemia (25% to 80%; grade 3: 1% to 42%; grade 4: ≤11%), leukopenia (GIST 5% to 47%; grades 3/4: 2%), hemorrhage (3% to 53%; grades 3/4: ≤19%), neutropenia (12% to 16%, grade 3: 7% to 27%; grade 4: 3% to 48%), thrombocytopenia (grade 3: 1% to 31%; grade 4: <1% to 33%)

Hepatic: Transaminases and/or bilirubin increased (Ph+ ALL [pediatric] grades 3/4: 57%), AST increased (≤38%; grade 3: 2% to 5%; grade 4: ≤3%), ALT increased (≤34%; grade 3: 2% to 7%; grade 4: <3%), alkaline phosphatase increased (≤17%; grade 3: ≤6%; grade 4: <1%), bilirubin increased (≤13%; grade 3: 1% to 4%; grade 4: ≤3%)

Neuromuscular & skeletal: Muscle cramps (16% to 62%), arthralgia (≤40%), musculoskeletal pain (children 21%; adults 38% to 49%), myalgia (9% to 32%), joint pain (11% to 31%), weakness (≤21%), rigors (10% to 12%), paresthesia (≤12%), bone pain (≤11%)

Ocular: Periorbital edema (29% to ≤74%), lacrimation increased (DFSP 25%; GIST ≤18%), blurred vision (≤11%)

Renal: Serum creatinine increased (≤44%; grade 3: ≤3%; DFSP: grade 4: 8%)

Respiratory: Nasopharyngitis (1% to 31%), cough (11% to 27%), dyspnea (≤21%), upper respiratory tract infection (3% to 21%), pharyngolaryngeal pain (≤18%), rhinitis (DFSP 17%), pharyngitis (CML 10% to 15%), pneumonia (CML 4% to 13%), sinusitis (4% to 11%)

Miscellaneous: Infection (Ph+ ALL [pediatric] grades 3/4: 53%; GIST ≤28%), night sweats (CML 13% to 17%), flu-like syndrome (1% to 14%), diaphoresis (GIST ≤13%)

1% to 10%:

Cardiovascular: Pleural effusion (Ph+ ALL [pediatric] grades 3/4: 7%), palpitation (≤5%), flushing

Central nervous system: CNS/cerebral hemorrhage (≤9%), depression (≤8%), hypoesthesia

Dermatologic: Photosensitivity reaction (4% to 7%), dry skin (≤7%), erythema

Endocrine & metabolic: Hyperglycemia (≤10%), hypocalcemia (GIST ≤6%)

Gastrointestinal: Appetite decreased (10%), weight loss (≤10%), gastrointestinal hemorrhage (2% to 8%), gastritis, gastroesophageal reflux, xerostomia

Hematologic: Lymphopenia (GIST ≤10%; grades 3/4: 1% to 2%), neutropenic fever, pancytopenia

Neuromuscular & skeletal: Back pain (GIST ≤7%), limb pain (GIST ≤7%), peripheral neuropathy, joint swelling

Ocular: Conjunctivitis (5% to 8%), conjunctival hemorrhage, dry eyes

Respiratory: Hypoxia (9%), pneumonitis (Ph+ ALL [pediatric] grades 3/4: 8%), epistaxis

<1% (Limited to important or life-threatening): Acute febrile neutropenic dermatosis (Sweet's syndrome), anaphylactic shock, angina, angioedema, aplastic anemia, arrhythmia, arthritis, ascites, atrial fibrillation, avascular necrosis, bullous eruption, cardiac arrest, cardiac tamponade, cardiogenic shock, cataract, cellulitis, cerebral edema, diverticulitis, embolism, eosinophilia, erythema multiforme, exanthematous pustulosis (acute generalized), exfoliative dermatitis, fungal infection, gastric ulcer, gastrointestinal obstruction, gastrointestinal perforation, glaucoma, gout, growth retardation (children), hearing loss, heart failure (severe), hematoma, hematemesis, hematuria, hemolytic anemia, hemorrhagic corpus luteum, hemorrhagic ovarian cyst, hepatic failure, hepatic necrosis, hepatitis, hepatotoxicity, herpes simplex, herpes zoster, hip osteonecrosis, hypercalcemia, hyperkalemia, hyperuricemia, hypertension, hypomagnesemia, hyponatremia, hypophosphatemia, hypothyroidism, ileus, inflammatory bowel disease, interstitial lung disease, interstitial pneumonitis, intracranial pressure increased, left ventricular dysfunction, leukocytoclastic vasculitis, lichen planus, lichenoid keratosis, lymphadenopathy,

macular edema, melena, memory impairment, menorrhagia, MI, migraine, myopathy, optic neuritis, ovarian cyst (hemorrhagic), palmar-plantar erythrodysesthesia syndrome, pancreatitis, papilledema, pericarditis, psoriasis, pulmonary fibrosis, pulmonary hemorrhage, pulmonary hypertension, Raynaud's phenomenon, renal failure, respiratory failure, respiratory tract (lower) infection, restless leg syndrome, retinal hemorrhage, rhabdomyolysis, sciatica, scleral hemorrhage, seizure, sepsis, skin pigment changes, Stevens-Johnson syndrome, subdural hematoma, syncope, tachycardia, thrombocythemia, thrombosis, toxic epidermal necrolysis, tumor hemorrhage (GIST), tumor lysis syndrome, tumor necrosis, urinary tract infection, vitreous hemorrhage

Drug Interactions

Metabolism/Transport Effects Substrate of CYP1A2 (minor), CYP2C19 (minor), CYP2C8 (minor), CYP2C9 (minor), CYP2D6 (minor), CYP3A4 (major), P-glycoprotein; **Note:** Assignment of Major/Minor substrate status based on clinically relevant drug interaction potential; **Inhibits** BCRP, CYP2C9 (weak), CYP2D6 (weak), CYP3A4 (moderate), P-glycoprotein

Avoid Concomitant Use

Avoid concomitant use of Imatinib with any of the following: BCG; Bosutinib; CloZAPine; CYP3A4 Inhibitors (Strong); Ibrutinib; Ivabradine; Lomitapide; Natalizumab; PAZOPanib; Pimecrolimus; Pimozide; Simeprevir; Tacrolimus (Topical); Tofacitinib; Tolvaptan; Ulipristal; Vaccines (Live)

Increased Effect/Toxicity

Imatinib may increase the levels/effects of: ARIPiprazole; Avanafil; Bosentan; Bosutinib; Budesonide (Systemic, Oral Inhalation); CloZAPine; Colchicine; CycloSPORINE (Systemic); CYP3A4 Substrates; Dofetilide; Eplerenone; Everolimus; FentaNYL; Halofantrine; Ibrutinib; Ivabradine; Ivacaftor; Leflunomide; Lomitapide; Lurasidone; Natalizumab; OxyCODONE; PAZOPanib; Pimozide; Propafenone; Ranolazine; Salmeterol; Saxagliptin; Simeprevir; Simvastatin; Tofacitinib; Tolvaptan; Topotecan; Ulipristal; Vaccines (Live); Vilazodone; Vitamin K Antagonists; Warfarin; Zuclopenthixol

The levels/effects of Imatinib may be increased by: Acetaminophen; CYP3A4 Inhibitors (Moderate); CYP3A4 Inhibitors (Strong); Denosumab; Lansoprazole; P-glycoprotein/ABCB1 Inhibitors; Pimecrolimus; Roflumilast; Tacrolimus (Topical); Trastuzumab

Decreased Effect

Imatinib may decrease the levels/effects of: BCG; Cardiac Glycosides; Coccidioidin Skin Test; Fludarabine; Ifosfamide; Sipuleucel-T; Vaccines (Inactivated); Vaccines (Live); Vitamin K Antagonists

The levels/effects of Imatinib may be decreased by: Bosentan; CYP3A4 Inducers (Strong); Dabrafenib; Deferasirox; Echinacea; Gemfibrozil; Ibuprofen; Peginterferon Alfa-2b; P-glycoprotein/ABCB1 Inducers; Rifamycin Derivatives; St Johns Wort; Tocilizumab

Ethanol/Nutrition/Herb Interactions

Ethanol: Management: Avoid ethanol.

Food: Food may reduce GI irritation. Grapefruit juice may increase imatinib plasma concentration. Management: Take with a meal and a large glass of water. Avoid grapefruit juice. Maintain adequate hydration, unless instructed to restrict fluid intake.

Herb/Nutraceutical: St John's wort may increase metabolism and decrease imatinib plasma concentration. Management: Avoid St John's wort.

Storage/Stability Store at 25°C (77°F); excursions permitted between 15°C to 30°C (59°F to 86°F). Protect from moisture.

Mechanism of Action Inhibits Bcr-Abl tyrosine kinase, the constitutive abnormal gene product of the Philadelphia chromosome in chronic myeloid leukemia (CML). Inhibition of this enzyme blocks proliferation and induces apoptosis in Bcr-Abl positive cell lines as well as in fresh leukemic cells in Philadelphia chromosome positive CML. Also inhibits tyrosine kinase for platelet-derived growth factor (PDGF), stem cell factor (SCF), c-Kit, and cellular events mediated by PDGF and SCF.

Pharmacodynamics/Kinetics

Absorption: Rapid

Protein binding: Parent drug and metabolite: ~95% to albumin and alpha$_1$-acid glycoprotein

Metabolism: Hepatic via CYP3A4 (minor metabolism via CYP1A2, CYP2D6, CYP2C9, CYP2C19); primary metabolite (active): N-demethylated piperazine derivative (CGP74588); severe hepatic impairment (bilirubin >3-10 times ULN) increases AUC by 45% to 55% for imatinib and its active metabolite, respectively

Bioavailability: 98%; may be decreased in patients who have had gastric surgery (eg, bypass, total or partial resection)

Half-life elimination: Adults: Parent drug: ~18 hours; N-desmethyl metabolite: ~40 hours; Children: Parent drug: ~15 hours

Time to peak: 2-4 hours

Excretion: Feces (68% primarily as metabolites, 20% as unchanged drug); urine (13% primarily as metabolites, 5% as unchanged drug)

Dosage Oral: **Note:** Treatment may be continued until disease progression or unacceptable toxicity. The optimal duration of therapy for chronic myeloid leukemia (CML) in complete remission is not yet determined. Discontinuing CML treatment is not recommended unless part of a clinical trial (Baccarani, 2009; NCCN CML guidelines v.3.2013).

Children ≥1 year and Adolescents:

- Ph+ ALL (newly diagnosed): 340 mg/m^2/day (in combination with chemotherapy); maximum: 600 mg daily
- Ph+ CML (chronic phase, newly diagnosed): 340 mg/m^2/day; maximum: 600 mg daily

Adults:

- Ph+ CML:
  - Chronic phase: 400 mg once daily; may be increased to 600 mg daily, if tolerated, for disease progression, lack of hematologic response after 3 months, lack of cytogenetic response after 6-12 months, or loss of previous hematologic or cytogenetic response; a range of up to 800 mg daily is included in the NCCN CML guidelines (v.3.2013)
    - *Canadian labeling:* 400 mg once daily; may be increased to 600-800 mg daily
  - Accelerated phase or blast crisis: 600 mg once daily; may be increased to 800 mg daily (400 mg twice daily), if tolerated, for disease progression, lack of hematologic response after 3 months, lack of cytogenetic response after 6-12 months, or loss of previous hematologic or cytogenetic response
- Ph+ ALL (relapsed or refractory): 600 mg once daily
- GIST (adjuvant treatment following complete resection): 400 mg once daily; recommended treatment duration: 3 years
- GIST (unresectable and/or metastatic malignant): 400 mg once daily; may be increased up to 800 mg daily (400 mg twice daily), if tolerated, for disease progression. **Note:** Significant improvement (progression-free survival, objective response rate) was demonstrated in patients with KIT exon 9 mutation with 800 mg (versus 400 mg), although overall survival (OS) was not impacted. The higher dose did not demonstrate a difference in time to progression or OS patients with Kit exon 11 mutation or wild-type status (Debiec-Rychter, 2006; Heinrich, 2009).

Canadian labeling: 400-600 mg daily (depending on disease stage/progression); may be increased to 600-800 mg daily

ASM with eosinophilia: Initiate at 100 mg once daily; titrate up to a maximum of 400 mg once daily (if tolerated) for insufficient response to lower dose

ASM without D816V c-Kit mutation or c-Kit mutation status unknown: 400 mg once daily

DFSP: 400 mg twice daily

HES/CEL: 400 mg once daily

HES/CEL with FIP1L1-PDGFRα fusion kinase: Initiate at 100 mg once daily; titrate up to a maximum of 400 mg once daily (if tolerated) if insufficient response to lower dose

MDS/MPD: 400 mg once daily

Ph+ ALL (induction, newly diagnosed): *Canadian labeling (not an approved use in the U.S.):* 600 mg once daily

Chordoma, progressive, advanced, or metastatic expressing PDGFRB and/or PDGFB (unlabeled use): 400 mg twice daily (Stacchiotti, 2012)

Desmoid tumors, unresectable and/or progressive (unlabeled use): 300 mg twice daily (BSA ≥1.5 m^2), 200 mg twice daily (BSA 1-1.49 m^2), 100 mg twice daily (BSA <1 m^2) (Chugh, 2010) **or** 400 mg once daily; may increase to 400 mg twice daily if progressive disease on 400 mg daily (Penel, 2011)

Melanoma, advanced or metastatic with C-KIT mutation (unlabeled use): 400 mg twice daily (Carvajal, 2011)

Stem cell transplant (SCT, unlabeled use) for CML (in patients who have not failed imatinib therapy prior to transplant):

Prophylactic use to prevent relapse post SCT: 400 mg daily starting after engraftment for 1 year post transplant (Carpenter, 2007) **or** 300 mg daily starting on day +35 post SCT (increased to 400 mg within 4 weeks) and continued until 12 months post transplant (Olavarria, 2007)

Relapse post SCT: Initial: 400 mg daily; if inferior response after 3 months, dose may be increased to 600-800 mg daily (Hess, 2005) **or** 400-600 mg daily (chronic phase) **or** 600 mg daily (blast or accelerated phase) (DeAngelo, 2004)

Dosage adjustment with concomitant strong CYP3A4 inducers: Avoid concomitant use of strong CYP3A4 inducers (eg, dexamethasone, carbamazepine, phenobarbital, phenytoin, rifabutin, rifampin); if concomitant use cannot be avoided, increase imatinib dose by at least 50% with careful monitoring.

Dosage adjustment for renal impairment:

U.S. labeling:

Mild impairment (Cl_{cr} 40-59 mL/minute): Maximum recommended dose: 600 mg

Moderate impairment (Cl_{cr} 20-39 mL/minute): Decrease recommended starting dose by 50%; dose may be increased as tolerated; maximum recommended dose: 400 mg

Severe impairment (Cl_{cr} <20 mL/minute): Use caution; a dose of 100 mg daily has been tolerated in a limited number of patients with severe impairment (Gibbons, 2008)

Canadian labeling:

Mild impairment (Cl_{cr} 40-59 mL/minute): Initial dose: 400 mg once daily (minimum effective dose); titrate to efficacy and tolerability

Moderate impairment (Cl_{cr} 20-39 mL/minute): Initial dose: 400 mg once daily (minimum effective dose); titrate to efficacy and tolerability; the use of 800 mg dose is not recommended

Severe impairment (Cl_{cr} <20 mL/minute): Use is not recommended

Dosage adjustment for hepatic impairment:

U.S. labeling:

Mild-to-moderate impairment: No dosage adjustment necessary

Severe impairment: Reduce dose by 25%

Canadian labeling:

Mild-to-moderate impairment: Initial dose: 400 mg once daily (minimum effective dose)

Severe impairment: Initial dose: 200 mg once daily; may increase up to 300 mg once daily in the absence of severe toxicity; decrease dose with unacceptable toxicity

Dosage adjustment for hepatotoxicity (during therapy): If elevations of bilirubin >3 times ULN or transaminases >5 times ULN occur, withhold treatment until bilirubin <1.5 times ULN and transaminases <2.5 times ULN. Resume treatment at a reduced dose as follows (**Note:** The decision to resume treatment should take into consideration the initial severity of hepatotoxicity):

Children ≥1 year and Adolescents: If current dose 340 mg/m^2/day, reduce dose to 260 mg/m^2/day

Adults:

If current dose 400 mg daily, reduce dose to 300 mg daily

If current dose 600 mg daily, reduce dose to 400 mg daily

If current dose 800 mg daily, reduce dose to 600 mg daily

Dosage adjustment for hematologic adverse reactions:

Chronic phase CML (initial dose 400 mg daily in adults or 340 mg/m^2/day in children); ASM, MDS/MPD, and HES/CEL (initial dose 400 mg daily); or GIST (initial dose 400 mg daily [U.S. labeling] or 400-600 mg daily [Canadian labeling]): If ANC <1 x 10^9/L and/or platelets <50 x 10^9/L: Withhold until ANC ≥1.5 x 10^9/L and platelets ≥75 x 10^9/L; resume treatment at original starting dose. For recurrent neutropenia and/or thrombocytopenia, withhold until recovery, and reinstitute treatment at a reduced dose as follows:

Children ≥1 year and Adolescents: If initial dose 340 mg/m^2/day, reduce dose to 260 mg/m^2/day

Adults:

If initial dose 400 mg daily, reduce dose to 300 mg daily

If initial dose 600 mg daily (Canadian labeling; not in U.S. labeling), reduce dose to 400 mg daily

CML (accelerated phase or blast crisis) and Ph+ ALL: Adults (initial dose 600 mg daily): If ANC <0.5 x 10^9/L and/or platelets <10 x 10^9/L, establish whether cytopenia is related to leukemia (bone marrow aspirate or biopsy). If unrelated to leukemia, reduce dose to 400 mg daily. If cytopenia persists for an additional 2 weeks, further reduce dose to 300 mg daily. If cytopenia persists for 4 weeks and is still unrelated to leukemia, withhold treatment until ANC ≥1 x 10^9/L and platelets ≥20 x 10^9/L, then resume treatment at 300 mg daily.

ASM associated with eosinophilia and HES/CEL with FIP1L1-PDGFRα fusion kinase: Adults (starting dose 100 mg daily): If ANC <1 x 10^9/L and/or platelets <50 x 10^9/L: Withhold until ANC ≥1.5 x 10^9/L and platelets ≥75 x 10^9/L; resume treatment at previous dose.

DFSP: Adults (initial dose 800 mg daily): If ANC <1 x 10^9/L and/or platelets <50 x 10^9/L, withhold until ANC ≥1.5 x 10^9/L and platelets ≥75 x 10^9/L; resume treatment at reduced dose of 600 mg daily. For recurrent neutropenia and/or thrombocytopenia, withhold until recovery, and reinstitute treatment with a further dose reduction to 400 mg daily.

Dosage adjustment for nonhematologic adverse reactions (eg, severe edema): Withhold treatment until toxicity resolves; may resume if appropriate (depending on initial severity of adverse event).

Dietary Considerations Should be taken with food and a large glass of water to decrease gastrointestinal irritation. Avoid grapefruit juice.

Administration Should be administered with a meal and a large glass of water; do not crush tablets. In adults, doses ≤600 mg may be given once daily; 800 mg dose should be administered as 400 mg twice daily. Dosing in children may be once or twice daily for CML and once daily for Ph+ ALL. Tablets may be dispersed in water or apple juice (using ~50 mL for 100 mg tablet, ~200 mL for 400 mg tablet); stir until dissolved and administer immediately. For daily dosing ≥800 mg, the 400 mg tablets should be used in order to reduce iron exposure.

Hazardous agent; use appropriate precautions for handling and disposal (NIOSH, 2012).

Monitoring Parameters CBC (weekly for first month, biweekly for second month, then periodically thereafter), liver function tests (at baseline and monthly or as clinically indicated; more frequently [at least weekly] in patients with moderate-to-severe hepatic impairment [Ramanathan, 2008]), renal function, serum electrolytes (including calcium, phosphorus, potassium and sodium levels); bone marrow cytogenetics (in CML; at 6-, 12-, and 18 months); fatigue, weight, and edema/fluid status; consider echocardiogram and serum troponin levels in patients with HES/CEL, and in patients with MDS/MPD or ASM with high eosinophil levels; in pediatric patients, also monitor serum glucose, albumin, and growth

Gastric surgery (eg, bypass, major gastrectomy, or resection) patients: Monitor imatinib trough concentrations (Liu, 2011; Pavlovsky, 2009, Yoo, 2010)

Thyroid function testing (Hamnvik, 2011):

Pre-existing levothyroxine therapy: Obtain baseline TSH levels, then monitor every 4 weeks until levels and levothyroxine dose are stable, then monitor every 2 months

Without pre-existing thyroid hormone replacement: TSH at baseline, then every 4 weeks for 4 months, then every 2-3 months

Monitor for signs/symptoms of CHF in patients with at risk for cardiac failure or patients with pre-existing cardiac disease. In Canada, a baseline evaluation of left ventricular ejection fraction is recommended prior to initiation of imatinib therapy in all patients with known underlying heart disease or in elderly patients. Monitor for signs/symptoms of gastrointestinal irritation or perforation and dermatologic toxicities.

Dosage Forms Excipient information presented when available (limited, particularly for generics); consult specific product labeling.

Tablet, Oral:

Gleevec: 100 mg, 400 mg [scored]

Extemporaneous Preparations Hazardous agent: Use appropriate precautions for handling and disposal.

An oral suspension may be prepared by placing tablets (whole, do not crush) in a glass of water or apple juice. Use ~50 mL for 100 mg tablet, or ~200 mL for 400 mg tablet. Stir until tablets are disintegrated, then administer immediately. To ensure the full dose is administered, rinse the glass and administer residue.

Gleevec® prescribing information, Novartis Pharmaceuticals Corporation, East Hanover, NJ, 2012.

◆ Imatinib Mesylate *see* Imatinib *on page* 1048
◆ Imbruvica *see* Ibrutinib *on page* 1030
◆ IMC-C225 *see* Cetuximab *on page* 398
◆ Imdur *see* Isosorbide Mononitrate *on page* 1128
◆ Imdur® (Can) *see* Isosorbide Mononitrate *on page* 1128
◆ Imferon *see* Iron Dextran Complex *on page* 1119
◆ IMI 30 *see* IDArubicin *on page* 1039
◆ IMid-1 *see* Lenalidomide *on page* 1180
◆ Imidazole Carboxamide *see* Dacarbazine *on page* 530
◆ Imidazole Carboxamide Dimethyltriazene *see* Dacarbazine *on page* 530

Imiglucerase (i mi GLOO ser ace)

Brand Names: U.S. Cerezyme
Brand Names: Canada Cerezyme
Pharmacologic Category Enzyme
Use

Gaucher disease:

U.S. labeling: Long-term enzyme replacement therapy for patients with type 1 Gaucher disease that results in at least one of the following: anemia, bone disease, hepatomegaly or splenomegaly, and thrombocytopenia

Canadian labeling: Long-term enzyme replacement therapy for patients with type 1 Gaucher disease or patients with type 3 Gaucher disease who display non-neurological manifestations (anemia, bone disease, hepatomegaly or splenomegaly, and thrombocytopenia) of the disease.

Pregnancy Risk Factor C

Dosage

Gaucher disease, type 1: Children ≥2 years, Adolescents, and Adults: I.V. (dose is individualized): Initial range: 2.5 units/kg 3 times weekly, up to 60 units/kg every 2 weeks. **Note:** Dosage adjustments are made based on assessment and therapeutic goals. Most benefits observed with doses of 30-60 units/kg every 2 weeks (Charrow, 2004).

Gaucher disease, type 3 (Canadian labeling; not in U.S. labeling): Children ≥2 years, Adolescents, and Adults: I.V. (dose is individualized): Initial range: 2.5 units/kg 3 times weekly, up to 60 units/kg every 2 weeks. Doses up to 120 units/kg every 2 weeks have been safely administered.

Dosage adjustment in renal impairment: No dosage adjustment provided in the manufacturer's labeling.

Dosage adjustment in hepatic impairment: No dosage adjustment provided in the manufacturer's labeling.

Additional Information Complete prescribing information should be consulted for additional detail.

Dosage Forms Excipient information presented when available (limited, particularly for generics); consult specific product labeling.

Solution Reconstituted, Intravenous:

Cerezyme: 200 units (1 ea); 400 units (1 ea)

◆ Imipemide *see* Imipenem and Cilastatin *on page* 1052

Imipenem and Cilastatin
(i mi PEN em & sye la STAT in)

Brand Names: U.S. Primaxin® I.V.
Brand Names: Canada Imipenem and Cilastatin for Injection; Primaxin® I.V. Infusion; RAN™-Imipenem-Cilastatin
Index Terms Imipemide; Primaxin® I.M. [DSC]
Pharmacologic Category Antibiotic, Carbapenem
Additional Appendix Information

Antibiotic Treatment of Adults With Infective Endocarditis *on page* 2355

Desensitization Protocols *on page* 2325

Use Treatment of lower respiratory tract, urinary tract, intra-abdominal, gynecologic, bone and joint, skin and skin structure, endocarditis (caused by *Staphylococcus aureus*) and polymicrobic infections as well as bacterial septicemia.

Antibacterial activity includes gram-positive bacteria (methicillin-sensitive *S. aureus* and *Streptococcus* spp), resistant gram-negative bacilli (including extended spectrum beta-lactamase-producing *Escherichia coli* and *Klebsiella* spp, *Enterobacter* spp, and *Pseudomonas aeruginosa*), and anaerobes.

Unlabeled Use Hepatic abscess; neutropenic fever; melioidosis

Pregnancy Risk Factor C

Pregnancy Considerations Teratogenic events have not been observed in animal reproduction studies. Due to pregnancy induced physiologic changes, some pharmacokinetic parameters of imipenem/cilastatin may be altered. Pregnant women have a larger volume of distribution resulting in lower serum peak levels than for the same dose in nonpregnant women. Clearance is also increased.

Breast-Feeding Considerations Imipenem is excreted in human milk. The low concentrations and low oral bioavailability suggest minimal exposure risk to the infant. The manufacturer recommends that caution be exercised when administering imipenem/cilastatin to nursing women. Nondose-related effects could include modification of bowel flora.

Contraindications Hypersensitivity to imipenem/cilastatin or any component of the formulation

Warnings/Precautions Dosage adjustment required in patients with impaired renal function; elderly patients often require lower doses (adjust to renal function). Prolonged use may result in fungal or bacterial superinfection, including *C. difficile*-associated diarrhea (CDAD) and pseudomembranous colitis; CDAD has been observed >2 months postantibiotic treatment. Carbapenems have been associated with CNS adverse effects, including confusional states and seizures (myoclonic); use caution with CNS disorders (eg, brain lesions and history of seizures) and adjust dose in renal impairment to avoid drug accumulation, which may increase seizure risk. Use with caution in patients with hypersensitivity to beta-lactams (including penicillins or cephalosporins); patients with impaired renal function are at increased risk of seizures if not properly dose adjusted. May decrease divalproex sodium/valproic acid concentrations leading to breakthrough seizures; concomitant use is not recommended. Not recommended in pediatric CNS infections due to seizure risk. Serious hypersensitivity reactions, including anaphylaxis, have been reported (some without a history of previous allergic reactions to beta-lactams).

Adverse Reactions

1% to 10%:

Cardiovascular: Tachycardia (infants 2%; adults <1%)

Central nervous system: Seizure (infants 6%; adults <1%)

Dermatologic: Rash (≤1%, children 2%)

Gastrointestinal: Nausea (1% to 2%), diarrhea (children 3% to 4%; adults 1% to 2%), vomiting (≤2%)

Genitourinary: Oliguria/anuria (infants 2%; adults <1%)

Local: Phlebitis/thrombophlebitis (3%)

<1% (Limited to important or life-threatening): Abdominal pain, abnormal urinalysis, acute renal failure, alkaline phosphatase increased, anaphylaxis, anemia, angioneurotic edema, asthenia, bilirubin increased, bone marrow depression, BUN/creatinine increased, candidiasis, confusion, cyanosis, dizziness, drug fever, dyspnea, encephalopathy, eosinophilia, erythema multiforme, fever, flushing, gastroenteritis, glossitis, hallucinations, hearing loss, hematocrit decreased, hemoglobin decreased, hemolytic anemia, hemorrhagic colitis, hepatitis (including fulminant onset), hepatic failure, hyperchloremia, hyperhidrosis, hyperkalemia, hypersensitivity, hyperventilation, hyponatremia, hypotension, jaundice, lactate dehydrogenase increased, leukocytosis, leukopenia, myoclonus, neutropenia (including agranulocytosis), palpitation, pancytopenia, paresthesia, pharyngeal pain, polyarthralgia, polyuria, positive Coombs' test, prothrombin time increased, pruritus vulvae, pseudomembranous colitis, psychic disturbances, rash, resistant *P. aeruginosa*, somnolence, Stevens-Johnson syndrome, thoracic spine pain, thrombocythemia, thrombocytopenia, tinnitus, tongue papillar hypertrophy, toxic epidermal necrolysis, transaminases increased, tremor, urticaria, vertigo

Drug Interactions

Metabolism/Transport Effects None known.

Avoid Concomitant Use

Avoid concomitant use of Imipenem and Cilastatin with any of the following: BCG; Ganciclovir-Valganciclovir

Increased Effect/Toxicity

Imipenem and Cilastatin may increase the levels/effects of: CycloSPORINE (Systemic)

The levels/effects of Imipenem and Cilastatin may be increased by: CycloSPORINE (Systemic); Ganciclovir-Valganciclovir; Probenecid

Decreased Effect

Imipenem and Cilastatin may decrease the levels/effects of: BCG; CycloSPORINE (Systemic); Sodium Picosulfate; Typhoid Vaccine; Valproic Acid and Derivatives

Preparation for Administration I.V.: Prior to use, dilute dose into 100-250 mL of an appropriate solution. Imipenem is inactivated at acidic or alkaline pH. Final concentration should not exceed 5 mg/mL.

Storage/Stability Imipenem/cilastatin powder for injection should be stored at <25°C (77°F).

I.V.: Reconstituted I.V. solutions are stable for 4 hours at room temperature and 24 hours when refrigerated. Do not freeze.

Mechanism of Action Inhibits bacterial cell wall synthesis by binding to one or more of the penicillin-binding proteins (PBPs); which in turn inhibits the final transpeptidation step of peptidoglycan synthesis in bacterial cell walls, thus inhibiting cell wall biosynthesis. Bacteria eventually lyse due to ongoing activity of cell wall autolytic enzymes (autolysins and murein hydrolases) while cell wall assembly is arrested. Cilastatin prevents renal metabolism of imipenem by competitive inhibition of dehydropeptidase along the brush border of the renal tubules.

Pharmacodynamics/Kinetics

Distribution: Rapidly and widely to most tissues and fluids including sputum, pleural fluid, peritoneal fluid, interstitial fluid, bile, aqueous humor, and bone; highest concentrations in pleural fluid, interstitial fluid, and peritoneal fluid; low concentrations in CSF

Protein binding: Imipenem: 20%; cilastatin: 40%

Metabolism: Imipenem is metabolized in the kidney by dehydropeptidase I; cilastatin prevents imipenem metabolism by this enzyme; cilastatin is partially metabolized renally

Half-life elimination: I.V.: Both drugs: 60 minutes; prolonged with renal impairment

Excretion: Both drugs: Urine (~70% as unchanged drug)

Dosage

Usual dosage ranges: Note: Dosage based on **imipenem** content:

Children >3 months: Non-CNS infections: I.V.: 15-25 mg/kg every 6 hours; maximum dosage: Susceptible infections: 2 g/day; moderately-susceptible organisms: 4 g/day

Adults: I.V.: Weight ≥70 kg: 250-1000 mg every 6-8 hours; maximum: 4 g/day. **Note:** For adults weighing <70 kg, refer to dosing adjustment in renal impairment

Indication-specific dosing: Note: Doses based on imipenem content.

Infants, Children, and Adolescents: I.V.:

Cystic fibrosis: Up to 100 mg/kg/day divided every 6 hours; maximum dose: 4 g daily has been used. **Note:** Efficacy in exacerbations may be limited due to rapid development of resistance (Zobell, 2013).

Children: I.V.:

Burkholderia pseudomallei (melioidosis) (unlabeled use): I.V.: Initial: 20 mg/kg every 8 hours for at least 10 days (White, 2003) **or** 25 mg/kg (up to 1 g) every 6 hours for at least 10 days (Currie, 2003); continue parenteral therapy until clinical improvement, then switch to oral therapy if tolerated and/or appropriate

Adults:

Burkholderia pseudomallei (melioidosis) (unlabeled use): Initial: 20 mg/kg every 8 hours for at least 10 days (White, 2003) **or** 25 mg/kg (up to 1 g) every 6 hours for at least 10 days (Currie, 2003); continue parenteral therapy until clinical improvement, then switch to oral therapy if tolerated and/or appropriate

Intra-abdominal infections: I.V.:

Mild infection: 250-500 mg every 6 hours

Severe infection: 500 mg every 6 hours **or** 1 g every 8 hours for 4-7 days (provided source controlled). **Note:** Not recommended for mild-to-moderate, community-acquired intra-abdominal infections due to risk of toxicity and the development of resistant organisms (Solomkin, 2010)

Liver abscess (unlabeled use): I.V.: 500 mg every 6 hours for 4-6 weeks (Ulug, 2010)

Mild infection: Note: Rarely a suitable option in mild infections; normally reserved for moderate-severe cases: I.V.:

Fully-susceptible organisms: 250 mg every 6 hours

Moderately-susceptible organisms: 500 mg every 6 hours

Moderate infection: I.V.:

Fully-susceptible organisms: 500 mg every 6-8 hours

Moderately-susceptible organisms: 500 mg every 6 hours or 1 g every 8 hours

Neutropenic fever (unlabeled use): I.V.: 500 mg every 6 hours (Paul, 2006)

***Pseudomonas* infections:** I.V.: 500 mg every 6 hours; **Note:** Higher doses may be required based on organism sensitivity.

Severe infection: I.V.:

Fully-susceptible organisms: 500 mg every 6 hours

Moderately-susceptible organisms: 1 g every 6-8 hours

Maximum daily dose should not exceed 50 mg/kg or 4 g/day, whichever is lower

Urinary tract infection: I.V.:

Uncomplicated: 250 mg every 6 hours

Complicated: 500 mg every 6 hours

Dosage adjustment in hepatic impairment: Hepatic dysfunction may further impair cilastatin clearance in patients receiving chronic renal replacement therapy; consider decreasing the dosing frequency.

Dosage adjustment in renal impairment: I.V.: **Note:**

Patients with a Cl_{cr} ≤5 mL/minute/1.73 m^2 should not receive imipenem/cilastatin unless hemodialysis is instituted within 48 hours.

Patients weighing <30 kg with impaired renal function should not receive imipenem/cilastatin.

Reduced I.V. dosage regimen based on creatinine clearance and/or body weight: See table.

Intermittent hemodialysis (IHD) (administer after hemodialysis on dialysis days): Use the dosing recommendation for patients with a Cl_{cr} 6-20 mL/minute; administer dose after dialysis session and every 12 hours thereafter **or** 250-500 mg every 12 hours (Heintz, 2009). **Note:** Dosing dependent on the assumption of 3 times/week, complete IHD sessions.

Peritoneal dialysis (unlabeled dosing): Dose as for Cl_{cr} 6-20 mL/minute (Somani, 1988)

Continuous renal replacement therapy (CRRT) (Heintz, 2009; Trotman, 2005): Drug clearance is highly dependent on the method of renal replacement, filter type, and flow rate. Appropriate dosing requires close monitoring of pharmacologic response, signs of adverse reactions due to drug accumulation, as well as drug concentrations in relation to target trough (if appropriate). The following are general recommendations only (based on dialysate flow/ultrafiltration rates of 1-2 L/hour and minimal residual renal function) and should not supersede clinical judgment:

CVVH: Loading dose of 1 g followed by either 250 mg every 6 hours **or** 500 mg every 8 hours

CVVHD: Loading dose of 1 g followed by either 250 mg every 6 hours **or** 500 mg every 6-8 hours

CVVHDF: Loading dose of 1 g followed by either 250 mg every 6 hours **or** 500 mg every 6 hours

Note: Data suggest that 500 mg every 8-12 hours may provide sufficient time above MIC to cover organisms with MIC values ≤2 mg/L; however, a higher dose of 500 mg every 6 hours is recommended for resistant organisms (particularly *Pseudomonas* spp) with MIC ≥4 mg/L or deep-seated infections (Fish, 2005).

Reduced I.V. dosage regimen based on creatinine clearance and/or body weight:

U.S. labeling: See table.

Imipenem and Cilastatin Dosage in Renal Impairment

Reduced I.V. Dosage Regimen Based on Creatinine Clearance (mL/minute/1.73 m^2) and/or Body Weight <70 kg					
	Body Weight (kg)				
	≥70	60	50	40	30
Total daily dose for normal renal function: 1 g/day					
Cl_{cr} ≥71	250 mg q6h	250 mg q8h	125 mg q6h	125 mg q6h	125 mg q8h
Cl_{cr} 41-70	250 mg q8h	125 mg q6h	125 mg q6h	125 mg q8h	125 mg q8h
Cl_{cr} 21-40	250 mg q12h	250 mg q12h	125 mg q8h	125 mg q12h	125 mg q12h
Cl_{cr} 6-20	250 mg q12h	125 mg q12h	125 mg q12h	125 mg q12h	125 mg q12h
Total daily dose for normal renal function: 1.5 g/day					
Cl_{cr} ≥71	500 mg q8h	250 mg q6h	250 mg q6h	250 mg q8h	125 mg q6h
Cl_{cr} 41-70	250 mg q6h	250 mg q8h	250 mg q8h	125 mg q6h	125 mg q8h
Cl_{cr} 21-40	250 mg q8h	250 mg q8h	250 mg q12h	125 mg q8h	125 mg q8h
Cl_{cr} 6-20	250 mg q12h	250 mg q12h	250 mg q12h	125 mg q12h	125 mg q12h
Total daily dose for normal renal function: 2 g/day					
Cl_{cr} ≥71	500 mg q6h	500 mg q8h	250 mg q6h	250 mg q6h	250 mg q8h
Cl_{cr} 41-70	500 mg q8h	250 mg q6h	250 mg q6h	250 mg q8h	125 mg q6h
Cl_{cr} 21-40	250 mg q6h	250 mg q8h	250 mg q8h	250 mg q12h	125 mg q8h
Cl_{cr} 6-20	250 mg q12h	250 mg q12h	250 mg q12h	250 mg q12h	125 mg q12h
Total daily dose for normal renal function: 3 g/day					
Cl_{cr} ≥71	1000 mg q8h	750 mg q8h	500 mg q6h	500 mg q8h	250 mg q6h
Cl_{cr} 41-70	500 mg q6h	500 mg q8h	500 mg q8h	250 mg q6h	250 mg q8h
Cl_{cr} 21-40	500 mg q8h	500 mg q8h	250 mg q6h	250 mg q8h	250 mg q8h
Cl_{cr} 6-20	500 mg q12h	500 mg q12h	250 mg q12h	250 mg q12h	250 mg q12h
Total daily dose for normal renal function: 4 g/day					
Cl_{cr} ≥71	1000 mg q6h	1000 mg q8h	750 mg q8h	500 mg q6h	500 mg q8h
Cl_{cr} 41-70	750 mg q8h	750 mg q8h	500 mg q6h	500 mg q8h	250 mg q6h
Cl_{cr} 21-40	500 mg q6h	500 mg q8h	500 mg q8h	250 mg q6h	250 mg q8h
Cl_{cr} 6-20	500 mg q12h	500 mg q12h	500 mg q12h	250 mg q12h	250 mg q12h

Canadian labeling: Reduced I.V. dosage regimen based on creatinine clearance (mL/minute/1.73 m^2) and body weight ≥70 kg (**Note:** The manufacturer labeling recommends further proportionate dose reductions for patients <70 kg, but does not provide specific dosing recommendations):

Mild renal impairment (Cl_{cr} 31-70 mL/minute/1.73 m^2):

Fully-susceptible organisms: Maximum dosage: 500 mg every 8 hours

Less susceptible organisms (primarily some *Pseudomonas* strains): Maximum dosage: 500 mg every 6 hours

Moderate renal impairment (Cl_{cr} 21-30 mL/minute/1.73 m^2):

Fully-susceptible organisms: Maximum dosage: 500 mg every 12 hours

Less susceptible organisms (primarily some *Pseudomonas* strains): Maximum dosage: 500 mg every 8 hours

Severe renal impairment (Cl_{cr} 0-20 mL/minute/1.73 m^2):

Fully-susceptible organisms: Maximum dosage: 250 mg every 12 hours

Less susceptible organisms (primarily some *Pseudomonas* strains): Maximum dosage: 500 mg every 12 hours

Note: Patients with Cl_{cr} 6-20 mL/minute/1.73 m^2 should receive 250 mg every 12 hours or 3.5 mg/kg (whichever is lower) every 12 hours for most pathogens; seizure risk may increase with higher dosing.

Dietary Considerations Some products may contain sodium.

Administration I.V.: Do not administer I.V. push. Infuse doses ≤500 mg over 20-30 minutes; infuse doses ≥750 mg over 40-60 minutes.

Monitoring Parameters Periodic renal, hepatic, and hematologic function tests; monitor for signs of anaphylaxis during first dose

Test Interactions Interferes with urinary glucose determination using Clinitest®; positive Coombs' [direct]

Dosage Forms Excipient information presented when available (limited, particularly for generics); consult specific product labeling.

Injection, powder for reconstitution: Imipenem 250 mg and cilastatin 250 mg; imipenem 500 mg and cilastatin 500 mg

Primaxin® I.V.: Imipenem 250 mg and cilastatin 250 mg [contains sodium 18.8 mg (0.8 mEq)]; imipenem 500 mg and cilastatin 500 mg [contains sodium 37.5 mg (1.6 mEq)]

◆ **Imipenem and Cilastatin for Injection (Can)** *see* Imipenem and Cilastatin *on page 1052*

Imipramine (im IP ra meen)

Brand Names: U.S. Tofranil; Tofranil-PM

Brand Names: Canada Apo-Imipramine®; Novo-Pramine; Tofranil®

Index Terms Imipramine Hydrochloride; Imipramine Pamoate

Pharmacologic Category Antidepressant, Tricyclic (Tertiary Amine)

Additional Appendix Information

Antidepressant Agents *on page 2284*

Beers Criteria – Potentially Inappropriate Medications for Geriatrics *on page 2368*

Use Treatment of depression; treatment of nocturnal enuresis in children

Unlabeled Use Analgesic for certain chronic and neuropathic pain (including diabetic neuropathy); panic disorder; attention-deficit/hyperactivity disorder (ADHD); post-traumatic stress disorder (PTSD)

Pregnancy Considerations Animal reproduction studies are inconclusive. Congenital abnormalities have been reported in humans; however, a causal relationship has not been established. Tricyclic antidepressants may be associated with irritability, jitteriness, and convulsions (rare) in the neonate (Yonkers, 2009). Due to pregnancy-induced physiologic changes, women who are pregnant may require dose adjustments late in pregnancy to achieve euthymia (Altshuler, 1996).

The ACOG recommends that therapy for depression during pregnancy be individualized; treatment should incorporate the clinical expertise of the mental health clinician, obstetrician, primary healthcare provider, and pediatrician (ACOG, 2008). According to the American Psychiatric Association (APA), the risks of medication treatment should be weighed against other treatment options and untreated depression. For women who discontinue antidepressant medications during pregnancy and who may be at high risk for postpartum depression, the medications can be restarted following delivery (APA, 2010). Treatment algorithms have been developed by the ACOG and the APA for the management of depression in women prior to conception and during pregnancy (Yonkers, 2009).

Breast-Feeding Considerations Imipramine and its active metabolite (desimpramine) are excreted into breast milk (Sovner, 1979). Concentrations of imipramine may be similar to those in the maternal plasma. Based on information from five mother/infant pairs, following maternal use of imipramine 75-200 mg/day, the estimated exposure to the breast-feeding infant would be 0.1% to 7.5% of the weight-adjusted maternal dose. Although adverse events were not reported, infants should be monitored for signs of adverse events (Fortinguerra, 2009). Imipramine can also be detected in the urine of nursing infants (Yoshida, 1997). Breast-feeding is not recommended by the manufacturer.

Medication Guide Available Yes

Contraindications Hypersensitivity to imipramine (cross-reactivity with other dibenzodiazepines may occur) or any component of the formulation; in a patient during acute recovery phase of MI; use of MAO inhibitors intended to treat psychiatric disorders (concurrently or within 14 days of discontinuing either imipramine or the MAO inhibitor); initiation of imipramine in a patient receiving linezolid or intravenous methylene blue

Warnings/Precautions [U.S. Boxed Warning]: Antidepressants increase the risk of suicidal thinking and behavior in children, adolescents, and young adults (18-24 years of age) with major depressive disorder (MDD) and other psychiatric disorders; consider risk prior to prescribing. Short-term studies did not show an increased risk in patients >24 years of age and showed a decreased risk in patients ≥65 years. Closely monitor for clinical worsening, suicidality, or unusual changes in behavior; the patient's family or caregiver should be instructed to closely observe the patient and communicate condition with healthcare provider. A medication guide should be dispensed with each prescription. **Imipramine is FDA approved for the treatment of nocturnal enuresis in children ≥6 years of age.**

The possibility of a suicide attempt is inherent in major depression and may persist until remission occurs. Monitor for worsening of depression or suicidality, especially during initiation of therapy (generally first 1-2 months) or with dose increases or decreases. Use caution in high-risk patients. Worsening depression and severe abrupt suicidality that are not part of the presenting symptoms may require discontinuation or modification of drug therapy. The patient's family or caregiver should be alerted to monitor patients for the emergence of suicidality and associated behaviors (such as agitation, irritability, hostility, impulsivity, and hypomania) and notify healthcare provider.

May worsen psychosis in some patients or precipitate a shift to mania or hypomania in patients with bipolar disorder. Patients presenting with depressive symptoms should be screened for bipolar disorder. Monotherapy in patients with bipolar disorder should be avoided. **Imipramine is not FDA approved for the treatment of bipolar depression.**

Potentially life-threatening serotonin syndrome (SS) has occurred with serotonergic agents (eg, SSRIs, SNRIs), particularly when used in combination with other serotonergic agents (eg, triptans, TCAs, fentanyl, lithium, tramadol, buspirone, St John's wort, tryptophan) or agents that impair metabolism of serotonin (eg, MAO inhibitors intended to treat psychiatric disorders, other MAO inhibitors such as linezolid and intravenous methylene blue). Discontinue treatment (and any concomitant serotonergic agent) immediately if signs/symptoms arise. TCAs may rarely cause bone marrow suppression; monitor for any signs of infection and obtain CBC if symptoms (eg, fever, sore throat) evident. The degree of sedation, anticholinergic effects, orthostasis, and conduction abnormalities are high relative to other antidepressants. Imipramine often causes drowsiness/sedation, resulting in impaired performance of tasks requiring alertness (eg, operating machinery or driving). Use with caution in patients with a history of cardiovascular disease (including previous MI, stroke, tachycardia, or conduction abnormalities). Use with caution in patients with urinary retention, benign prostatic hyperplasia, narrow-angle glaucoma, xerostomia, visual problems, constipation, or a history of bowel obstruction.

Consider discontinuing, when possible, prior to elective surgery. Therapy should not be abruptly discontinued in patients receiving high doses for prolonged periods. May lower seizure threshold - use caution in patients with a previous seizure disorder or condition predisposing to seizures such as brain damage, alcoholism, or concurrent therapy with other drugs which lower the seizure threshold. May increase the risks associated with electroconvulsive therapy. Bone fractures have been associated with antidepressant treatment. Consider the possibility of a fragility fracture if an antidepressant-treated patient presents with unexplained bone pain, point tenderness, swelling, or bruising (Rabenda, 2013; Rizzoli, 2012). Use with caution in hyperthyroid patients or those receiving thyroid supplementation. Use with caution in patients with diabetes mellitus; may alter glucose regulation. Use with caution in patients with hepatic or renal dysfunction and in elderly patients. Has been associated with photosensitization. Potentially significant interactions may exist, requiring dose or frequency adjustment, additional monitoring, and/or selection of alternative therapy. Consult drug interactions database for more detailed information.

Avoid use in the elderly due to its potent anticholinergic and sedative properties, and potential to cause orthostatic hypotension. In addition, may also cause or exacerbate syndrome of inappropriate antidiuretic hormone secretion or hyponatremia; monitor sodium closely with initiation or dosage adjustments in older adults (Beers Criteria).

Adverse Reactions Reported for tricyclic antidepressants in general. Frequency not defined.

Cardiovascular: Arrhythmia, CHF, ECG changes, heart block, hypertension, MI, orthostatic hypotension, palpitation, stroke, tachycardia

Central nervous system: Agitation, anxiety, confusion, delusions, disorientation, dizziness, drowsiness, fatigue, hallucination, headache, hypomania, insomnia, nightmares, psychosis, restlessness, seizure

Dermatologic: Alopecia, itching, petechiae, photosensitivity, purpura, rash, urticaria

Endocrine & metabolic: Breast enlargement, galactorrhea, gynecomastia, increase or decrease in blood sugar, increase or decrease in libido, SIADH

Gastrointestinal: Abdominal cramps, anorexia, black tongue, constipation, diarrhea, epigastric disorders, ileus, nausea, stomatitis, taste disturbance, vomiting, weight gain/loss, xerostomia

Genitourinary: Impotence, testicular swelling, urinary retention

Hematologic: Agranulocytosis, eosinophilia, thrombocytopenia

Hepatic: Cholestatic jaundice, transaminases increased

Neuromuscular & skeletal: Ataxia, extrapyramidal symptoms, incoordination, numbness, paresthesia, peripheral neuropathy, tingling, tremor, weakness

Ocular: Blurred vision, disturbances of accommodation, mydriasis

Otic: Tinnitus

Miscellaneous: Diaphoresis, falling, hypersensitivity (eg, drug fever, edema)

Drug Interactions

Metabolism/Transport Effects Substrate of CYP1A2 (minor), CYP2B6 (minor), CYP2C19 (major), CYP2D6 (major), CYP3A4 (minor); **Note:** Assignment of Major/Minor substrate status based on clinically relevant drug interaction potential; **Inhibits** CYP1A2 (weak), CYP2C19 (weak), CYP2D6 (moderate), CYP2E1 (weak)

Avoid Concomitant Use

Avoid concomitant use of Imipramine with any of the following: Aclidinium; Iobenguane I 123; Ipratropium (Oral Inhalation); Linezolid; MAO Inhibitors; Methylene Blue; Moxonidine; Thioridazine; Tiotropium; Umeclidinium

Increased Effect/Toxicity

Imipramine may increase the levels/effects of: Alpha-/Beta-Agonists (Direct-Acting); Alpha1-Agonists; Amphetamines; Analgesics (Opioid); Anticholinergics; Antipsychotics; Aspirin; Beta2-Agonists; Citalopram; CYP2D6 Substrates; Desmopressin; Escitalopram; Fesoterodine; Highest Risk QTc-Prolonging Agents; Methylene Blue; Metoclopramide; Metoprolol; Moderate Risk QTc-Prolonging Agents; Nebivolol; NSAID (COX-2 Inhibitor); NSAID (Nonselective); QuiNIDine; Serotonin Modulators; Sodium Phosphates; Sulfonylureas; Thioridazine; Tiotropium; TraMADol; Vitamin K Antagonists; Yohimbine

The levels/effects of Imipramine may be increased by: Abiraterone Acetate; Aclidinium; Altretamine; Antipsychotics; BuPROPion; Cimetidine; Cinacalcet; Citalopram; Cobicistat; CYP2C19 Inhibitors (Moderate); CYP2C19 Inhibitors (Strong); CYP2D6 Inhibitors (Moderate); CYP2D6 Inhibitors (Strong); Dexmethylphenidate; DULoxetine; Escitalopram; FLUoxetine; FluvoxaMINE; Ipratropium (Oral Inhalation); Linezolid; Lithium; Luliconazole; MAO Inhibitors; Methylphenidate; Metoclopramide; Metyrosine; Mifepristone; PARoxetine; Pramlintide; Propafenone; Protease Inhibitors; QuiNIDine; Sertraline; Terbinafine (Systemic); Thyroid Products; TraMADol; Umeclidinium; Valproic Acid and Derivatives

Decreased Effect

Imipramine may decrease the levels/effects of: Acetylcholinesterase Inhibitors (Central); Alpha2-Agonists; Alpha2-Agonists (Ophthalmic); Codeine; Iobenguane I 123; Moxonidine; Tamoxifen

The levels/effects of Imipramine may be decreased by: Acetylcholinesterase Inhibitors (Central); Barbiturates; CarBAMazepine; CYP2C19 Inducers (Strong); Dabrafenib; Peginterferon Alfa-2b; St Johns Wort

Ethanol/Nutrition/Herb Interactions

Ethanol: May increase CNS depression; monitor for increased effects with coadministration. Caution patients about effects.

Herb/Nutraceutical: St John's wort may decrease imipramine levels. Management: Avoid valerian, St John's wort, tryptophan, SAMe, kava kava (may increase risk of serotonin syndrome and/or excessive sedation).

Mechanism of Action Traditionally believed to increase the synaptic concentration of serotonin and/or norepinephrine in the central nervous system by inhibition of their reuptake by the presynaptic neuronal membrane. However, additional receptor effects have been found including desensitization of adenyl cyclase, down regulation of beta-adrenergic receptors, and down regulation of serotonin receptors.

Pharmacodynamics/Kinetics

Onset of action: Peak antidepressant effect: Usually after ≥2 weeks

Absorption: Well absorbed

Metabolism: Hepatic, primarily via CYP2D6 to desipramine (active) and other metabolites; significant first-pass effect

Half-life elimination: 6-18 hours

Excretion: Urine (as metabolites)

Dosage Oral:

Children:

Depression (unlabeled use): 1.5 mg/kg/day with dosage increments of 1 mg/kg every 3-4 days to a maximum dose of 5 mg/kg/day in 1-4 divided doses; monitor carefully especially with doses ≥3.5 mg/kg/day

Enuresis: ≥6 years: Initial: 25 mg at bedtime, if inadequate response still seen after 1 week of therapy, increase by 25 mg/day; dose should not exceed 2.5 mg/kg/day or 50 mg at bedtime if 6-12 years of age or 75 mg at bedtime if ≥12 years of age

Adjunct in the treatment of cancer pain (unlabeled use): Initial: 0.2-0.4 mg/kg at bedtime; dose may be increased by 50% every 2-3 days up to 1-3 mg/kg/dose at bedtime

Adolescents: Depression: Initial: 25-50 mg/day; increase gradually; maximum: 100 mg/day in single or divided doses

Adults:

Depression:

Outpatients: Initial: 75 mg/day; may increase gradually to 150 mg/day. May be given in divided doses or as a single bedtime dose; maximum: 200 mg/day

Inpatients: Initial: 100-150 mg/day; may increase gradually to 200 mg/day; if no response after 2 weeks, may further increase to 250-300 mg/day. May be given in divided doses or as a single bedtime dose; maximum: 300 mg/day.

Post-traumatic stress disorder (PTSD) (unlabeled use): 75-200 mg/day

Elderly: Depression: Initial: 25-50 mg at bedtime; may increase every 3 days for inpatients and weekly for outpatients if tolerated to a recommended maximum of 100 mg/day.

MAO inhibitor recommendations:

Switching to or from an MAO inhibitor intended to treat psychiatric disorders:

Allow 14 days to elapse between discontinuing an MAO inhibitor intended to treat psychiatric disorders and initiation of imipramine.

Allow 14 days to elapse between discontinuing imipramine and initiation of an MAO inhibitor intended to treat psychiatric disorders.

Use with other MAO inhibitors (linezolid or I.V. methylene blue):

Do not initiate imipramine in patients receiving linezolid or I.V. methylene blue; consider other interventions for psychiatric condition.

If urgent treatment with linezolid or I.V. methylene blue is required in a patient already receiving imipramine and potential benefits outweigh potential risks, discontinue imipramine promptly and administer linezolid or I.V. methylene blue. Monitor for serotonin syndrome for 2 weeks or until 24 hours after the last dose of linezolid or I.V. methylene blue, whichever comes first. May resume imipramine 24 hours after the last dose of linezolid or I.V. methylene blue.

Dosage adjustment in renal impairment: No dosage adjustment provided in manufacturer's labeling; use with caution.

Dosage adjustment in hepatic impairment: No dosage adjustment provided in manufacturer's labeling; use with caution.

Monitoring Parameters CBC, ECG in older adults, with high doses, and/or in patients with pre-existing cardiovascular disease; monitor blood pressure and pulse rate prior to and during initial therapy; evaluate mental status, suicide ideation (especially at the beginning of therapy or when doses are increased or decreased); signs/symptoms of serotonin syndrome; blood levels are useful for therapeutic monitoring

Reference Range Therapeutic: Imipramine and desipramine: 150-250 ng/mL (SI: 530-890 nmol/L); desipramine: 150-300 ng/mL (SI: 560-1125 nmol/L); Toxic: >500 ng/mL (SI: 446-893 nmol/L); utility of serum level monitoring controversial

Dosage Forms Excipient information presented when available (limited, particularly for generics); consult specific product labeling.

Capsule, Oral, as pamoate:

Tofranil-PM: 75 mg, 100 mg, 125 mg, 150 mg

Generic: 75 mg, 100 mg, 125 mg, 150 mg

Tablet, Oral, as hydrochloride:

Tofranil: 10 mg, 25 mg, 50 mg

Generic: 10 mg, 25 mg, 50 mg

◆ **Imipramine Hydrochloride** *see* Imipramine *on page 1055*

◆ **Imipramine Pamoate** *see* Imipramine *on page 1055*

Imiquimod (i mi KWI mod)

Brand Names: U.S. Aldara; Zyclara; Zyclara Pump

Brand Names: Canada Aldara®; Vyloma™; Zyclara®

Pharmacologic Category Skin and Mucous Membrane Agent; Topical Skin Product

Use

Aldara®: Treatment of external genital and perianal warts/condyloma acuminata; nonhyperkeratotic, nonhypertrophic actinic keratosis on face or scalp; superficial basal cell carcinoma (sBCC) with a maximum tumor diameter of 2 cm located on the trunk (excluding anogenital skin), neck, or extremities (excluding hands or feet)

Vyloma™ (Canadian availability; not available in the U.S.): Treatment of external genital and perianal warts/condyloma acuminata

Zyclara®:

U.S. labeling: Treatment of external genital and perianal warts/condyloma acuminata (3.75% formulation); treatment of clinically typical visible or palpable, actinic keratoses on face or scalp (2.5% or 3.75% formulation)

Canadian labeling: Treatment of clinically typical visible or palpable, actinic keratoses on face or scalp

Unlabeled Use Treatment of common warts

Pregnancy Risk Factor C

Dosage Topical: **Note:** Imiquimod treatment should not be prolonged beyond recommended period due to missed doses or rest periods.

U.S. labeling:

Actinic keratosis: Adults: **Note:** Prescribed course of therapy should be completed even if all lesions appear to be gone. Safety and efficacy of repeated use in a previously treated area has not been established.

Aldara®: Treatment should be limited to areas ≤25 cm^2; apply 2 times/week for 16 weeks to a treatment area on face or scalp (but not both concurrently); no more than 1 packet should be applied at each application and no more than 36 packets applied per 16 weeks; apply prior to bedtime and leave on skin for ~8 hours. Remove with mild soap and water.

Zyclara® 2.5%, 3.75%: Treatment consists of 2 cycles (14 days each) separated by 1 rest period (14 days) with no treatment. Apply up to 2 packets or 2 full actuations of pump once daily at bedtime to affected area on either face or balding scalp (but not both concurrently); leave on skin for ~8 hours. Remove with mild soap and water. Patient should not receive more than 56 packets or 2 x 7.5 g pumps or 1 x 15 g pump per 2 cycles of treatment.

External genital and/or perianal warts/condyloma acuminata: Children ≥12 years and Adults:

Aldara®: Apply a thin layer 3 times/week prior to bedtime and leave on skin for 6-10 hours. Remove with mild soap and water. Examples of 3 times/week application schedules are: Monday, Wednesday, Friday; or Tuesday, Thursday, Saturday. Continue treatment until there is total clearance of the warts or a maximum duration of therapy of 16 weeks.

Zyclara® 3.75%: Apply a thin layer using up to 1 packet or 1 full actuation of pump once daily prior to bedtime and leave on skin for ~8 hours. Remove with mild soap and water. Continue treatment until there is total clearance of the warts or a maximum duration of therapy of 8 weeks. Patient should not receive more than 56 packets or 2 x 7.5 g pumps or 1 x 15 g pump per course of treatment.

Superficial basal cell carcinoma: Adults: Aldara®: Apply once daily prior to bedtime, 5 days/week for 6 weeks. No more than 36 packets should be used during the 6-week treatment period. Tumor treatment area should not exceed 3 cm (maximum of 2 cm tumor diameter plus a 1 cm margin of skin around the tumor). The diameter of cream droplet applied should range from 4 mm to 7 mm for tumor areas of 0.5 cm to 2 cm, respectively. Leave on skin for ~8 hours. Remove with mild soap and water. Safety and efficacy of repeated use in a previously treated area have not been established.

Canadian labeling:

Actinic keratosis: Adults: **Note:** Prescribed course of therapy should be completed even if all lesions appear to be gone; safety and efficacy of repeated use in a previously treated area have not been established.

Aldara®: Treatment should be limited to areas ≤25 cm^2; apply 2 times/week for 16 weeks to a treatment area on face or scalp (but not both concurrently); no more than 1 packet should be applied at each application; apply prior to bedtime and leave on skin for ~8 hours. Remove with mild soap and water.

Zyclara®: Treatment should be limited to an area <200 cm^2 on the face or scalp and consists of 2 cycles (14 days each) separated by 1 rest period (14 days) with no treatment. Apply up to 2 packets or 2 full actuations of pump once daily at bedtime to affected area on either face or balding scalp (but not both concurrently). Leave on skin for ~8 hours. Remove with mild soap and water. Patient should not receive more than 56 packets or 2 x 7.5 g pumps or 1 x 15 g pump per 2 cycles of treatment.

External genital and/or perianal warts/condyloma acuminata: Adults:

Aldara®: Apply a thin layer 3 times/week prior to bedtime and leave on skin for 6-10 hours. Remove with mild soap and water. Examples of 3 times/week application schedules are: Monday, Wednesday, Friday; or Tuesday, Thursday, Saturday. Continue treatment until there is total clearance of the warts or a maximum duration of therapy of 16 weeks.

Vyloma™: Apply a thin layer once daily prior to bedtime and leave on skin for ~8 hours. Remove with mild soap and water. Continue treatment until there is total clearance of the warts or maximum duration of therapy of 8 weeks.

Superficial basal cell carcinoma: Adults: Aldara®: Apply once daily prior to bedtime, 5 days/week for 6 weeks. Tumor treatment area should not exceed 3 cm (maximum of 2 cm tumor diameter plus a 1 cm margin of skin around the tumor). The diameter of cream droplet applied should range from 4 mm to 7 mm for tumor areas of 0.5 cm to 2 cm, respectively. Leave on skin for ~8 hours. Remove with mild soap and water. Safety and efficacy of repeated use in a previously treated area have not been established.

Unlabeled uses: Common warts (5% cream): Apply once daily prior to bedtime for 5 days/week for up to 16 weeks (Hengge, 2000) or apply twice daily for up to 24 weeks (Grussendorf-Conen, 2002)

Dosing adjustment for toxicity:

Local skin reactions (eg, erythema, edema, scabbing, etc): Temporarily interrupt treatment for up to several days for severe or intolerable reactions; may consider resuming therapy once reaction subsides.

Systemic/flu-like reactions (eg, malaise, fever, rigors, etc): Consider temporary interruption of therapy.

Vulvar swelling: Interrupt or discontinue therapy for severe vulvar swelling.

Dosing adjustment in renal impairment: No dosage adjustment provided in manufacturer's labeling.

Dosing adjustment in hepatic impairment: No dosage adjustment provided in manufacturer's labeling.

Additional Information Complete prescribing information should be consulted for additional detail.

Dosage Forms Excipient information presented when available (limited, particularly for generics); consult specific product labeling.

Cream, External:

Aldara: 5% (12 ea) [contains benzyl alcohol, cetyl alcohol, methylparaben, propylparaben, sorbitan monostearate(sorbitan stearate)]

Zyclara: 3.75% (28 ea) [contains benzyl alcohol, cetyl alcohol, methylparaben, propylparaben]

Zyclara Pump: 2.5% (7.5 g); 3.75% (7.5 g) [contains benzyl alcohol, cetyl alcohol, methylparaben, propylparaben]

Generic: 5% (1 ea, 12 ea, 24 ea)

Dosage Forms: Canada Excipient information presented when available (limited, particularly for generics); consult specific product labeling.

Cream, topical:

Vyloma™: 3.75% (28s) [contains benzyl alcohol; 0.25 g/packet]

◆ **Imitrex** *see* SUMAtriptan *on page 1969*
◆ **Imitrex DF (Can)** *see* SUMAtriptan *on page 1969*
◆ **Imitrex Injection (Can)** *see* SUMAtriptan *on page 1969*
◆ **Imitrex Nasal Spray (Can)** *see* SUMAtriptan *on page 1969*
◆ **Imitrex STATdose Refill** *see* SUMAtriptan *on page 1969*
◆ **Imitrex STATdose System** *see* SUMAtriptan *on page 1969*
◆ **ImmuCyst® (Can)** *see* BCG *on page 226*

Immune Globulin (i MYUN GLOB yoo lin)

Brand Names: U.S. Bivigam; Carimune NF; Flebogamma; Flebogamma DIF; GamaSTAN S/D; Gammagard; Gammagard S/D; Gammagard S/D Less IgA; Gammaked; Gammaplex; Gamunex-C; Hizentra; Hizentra 20%; Octagam; Privigen

Brand Names: Canada Gamastan S/D; Gammagard Liquid; Gammagard S/D; Gamunex; Hizentra; IGIVnex; Octagam 10%; Privigen

Index Terms Gamma Globulin; IG; IGIM; IGIV; IGSC; Immune Globulin Subcutaneous (Human); Immune Serum Globulin; ISG; IV Immune Globulin; IVIG; Panglobulin; SCIG

Pharmacologic Category Blood Product Derivative; Immune Globulin

Additional Appendix Information

Immune Globulin Product Comparison *on page 2301*
Immunization Recommendations *on page 2339*

Use

Treatment of primary humoral immunodeficiency syndromes (congenital agammaglobulinemia, severe combined immunodeficiency syndromes [SCIDS], common variable immunodeficiency, X-linked immunodeficiency, Wiskott-Aldrich syndrome) (Bivigam, Carimune NF, Flebogamma DIF, Gammagard Liquid, Gammagard S/D, Gammaked, Gammaplex, Gamunex-C, Hizentra, Octagam, Privigen)

Treatment of acute and chronic immune thrombocytopenia (ITP) (Carimune NF, Gammagard S/D, Gammaked, Gammaplex [chronic only], Gamunex-C, Privigen [chronic only])

Treatment of chronic inflammatory demyelinating polyneuropathy (CIDP) (Gammaked, Gamunex-C)

Treatment of multifocal motor neuropathy (MMN) (Gammagard Liquid)

Prevention of coronary artery aneurysms associated with Kawasaki syndrome (in combination with aspirin) (Gammagard S/D)

Prevention of bacterial infection in patients with hypogammaglobulinemia and/or recurrent bacterial infections with B-cell chronic lymphocytic leukemia (CLL) (Gammagard S/D)

Prevention of serious infection in immunoglobulin deficiency (select agammaglobulinemias) (GamaSTAN S/D)

Provision of passive immunity in the following susceptible individuals (GamaSTAN S/D):

Hepatitis A: Pre-exposure prophylaxis; postexposure: within 14 days and/or prior to manifestation of disease

Measles: For use within 6 days of exposure in an unvaccinated person, who has not previously had measles

Rubella: Postexposure prophylaxis to reduce the risk of infection and fetal damage in exposed pregnant women who will not consider therapeutic abortion

Varicella: For immunosuppressed patients when varicella zoster immune globulin is not available

Unlabeled Use Acquired hypogammaglobulinemia secondary to malignancy; Guillain-Barré syndrome; hematopoietic stem cell transplantation (HSCT), to prevent bacterial infections among allogeneic recipients with severe hypogammaglobulinemia (IgG <400 mg/dL) at <100 days post transplant (CDC guidelines); HIV-associated thrombocytopenia; multiple sclerosis (relapsing, remitting when other therapies cannot be used); Lambert-Eaton myasthenic syndrome (LEMS); myasthenia gravis; refractory dermatomyositis/polymyositis

Pregnancy Risk Factor C

Pregnancy Considerations Animal reproduction studies have not been conducted. Immune globulins cross the placenta in increased amounts after 30 weeks gestation. Intravenous immune globulin has been recommended for use in fetal-neonatal alloimmune thrombocytopenia and pregnancy-associated ITP (Anderson, 2007). Intravenous immune globulin is recommended to prevent measles in nonimmune women exposed during pregnancy (CDC, 2013). May also be used in postexposure prophylaxis for rubella to reduce the risk of infection and fetal damage in exposed pregnant women who will not consider therapeutic abortion (per GamaSTAN S/D product labeling; use for postexposure rubella prophylaxis is not currently recommended [CDC, 2013]).

Breast-Feeding Considerations It is not known if immune globulin from these preparations is excreted in breast milk. The manufacturer recommends that caution be exercised when administering immune globulin to nursing women.

Contraindications Hypersensitivity to immune globulin or any component of the formulation; IgA deficiency (with antibodies against IgA and history of hypersensitivity); hyperprolinemia (Hizentra, Privigen); isolated IgA deficiency (GamaSTAN S/D); severe thrombocytopenia or coagulation disorders where I.M. injections are contraindicated (GamaSTAN S/D)

Warnings/Precautions [U.S. Boxed Warning]: I.V. administration only: Acute renal dysfunction (increased serum creatinine, oliguria, acute renal failure, osmotic nephrosis) can rarely occur and has been associated with fatalities; usually within 7 days of use (more likely with products stabilized with sucrose). Use with caution in the elderly, patients with renal disease, diabetes mellitus, volume depletion, sepsis, paraproteinemia, and nephrotoxic medications due to risk of renal dysfunction. In patients at risk of renal dysfunction, the rate of infusion and concentration of solution should be minimized. Discontinue if renal function deteriorates.

[U.S. Boxed Warning]: Thrombosis may occur with immune globulin products even in the absence of risk factors for thrombosis. For patients at risk of thrombosis (eg, advanced age, history of atherosclerosis, impaired cardiac output, prolonged immobilization, hypercoagulable conditions, history of venous or arterial thrombosis, use of estrogens, indwelling central vascular catheters, hyperviscosity, and cardiovascular risk factors), administer at the minimum dose and infusion rate practicable. Ensure adequate hydration before administration. Monitor for signs and symptoms of thrombosis and assess blood viscosity in patients at risk for hyperviscosity such as those with cryoglobulins, fasting chylomicronemia/severe hypertriglyceridemia, or monoclonal gammopathies.

High-dose regimens (1 g/kg for 1-2 days) are not recommended for individuals with fluid overload or where fluid volume may be of concern. Hypersensitivity and anaphylactic reactions can occur; a severe fall in blood pressure may rarely occur with anaphylactic reaction; immediate treatment (including epinephrine 1:1000) should be available. Product of human plasma; may potentially contain infectious agents which could transmit disease. Screening of donors, as well as testing and/or inactivation or removal of certain viruses, reduces the risk. Infections thought to be transmitted by this product should be reported to the manufacturer. Aseptic meningitis may occur with high doses (≥1-2 g/kg [product-dependent]) and/or rapid infusion; syndrome usually appears within several hours to 2 days following treatment; usually resolves within several days after product is discontinued; patients with a migraine history may be at higher risk for AMS. Increased risk of hypersensitivity, especially in patients with anti-IgA antibodies; use is contraindicated in patients with IgA deficiency (with antibodies against IgA and history of hypersensitivity) or isolated IgA deficiency (GamaSTAN S/D). Increased risk of hematoma formation when administered subcutaneously for the treatment of ITP.

Intravenous immune globulin has been associated with antiglobulin hemolysis (acute or delayed); monitor for signs of hemolytic anemia. Cases of hemolysis-related renal dysfunction/failure or disseminated intravascular coagulation (DIC) have been reported. Risk factors include high doses (≥2 g/kg) and non-O blood type. In chronic ITP, assess risk versus benefit of high-dose regimen in patients with increased risk of thrombosis, hemolysis, acute kidney injury, or volume overload.

Patients should be adequately hydrated prior to initiation of therapy. Hyperproteinemia, increased serum viscosity and hyponatremia may occur; distinguish hyponatremia from pseudohyponatremia to prevent volume depletion, a further increase in serum viscosity, and a higher risk of thrombotic events. Patients should be monitored for adverse events during and after the infusion. Stop administration with signs of infusion reaction (fever, chills, nausea, vomiting, and rarely shock). Risk may be increased with initial treatment, when switching brands of immune globulin, and with treatment interruptions of >8 weeks. Monitor for transfusion-related acute lung injury (TRALI); noncardiogenic pulmonary edema has been reported with immune globulin use. TRALI is characterized by severe respiratory distress, pulmonary edema, hypoxemia, and fever (in the presence of normal left ventricular function) and usually occurs within 1-6 hours after infusion. Response to live vaccinations may be impaired. Some clinicians may administer intravenous immune globulin products as a subcutaneous infusion based on patient tolerability and clinical judgment. SubQ infusion should begin 1 week after the last I.V. dose; dose should be individualized based on clinical response and serum IgG trough concentrations; consider premedicating with acetaminophen and diphenhydramine.

Some products may contain maltose, which may result in falsely-elevated blood glucose readings; maltose-containing products are contraindicated in patients with an allergy to corn. Some products may contain polysorbate 80, sodium, and/or sucrose. Some products may contain sorbitol; do not use in patients with fructose intolerance. Hizentra and Privigen contain the stabilizer L-proline and are contraindicated in patients with hyperprolinemia. Packaging of some products may contain natural latex/natural rubber; skin testing should not be performed with GamaSTAN S/D as local irritation can occur and be misinterpreted as a positive reaction.

Adverse Reactions Frequency not always defined.

Cardiovascular: Chest tightness (7%), hypertension (5% to 6%), angioedema, edema, flushing of the face, hypotension, palpitation, tachycardia

Central nervous system: Headache (16% to 48%), fever (6% to 16%), chills (3% to 6%), dizziness (1% to 6%), malaise (1%), anxiety, aseptic meningitis syndrome, drowsiness, fatigue, irritability, lethargy, lightheadedness, migraine, pain

Dermatologic: Bruising, contact dermatitis, eczema, erythema, hyperhidrosis, petechiae, pruritus, purpura, rash, urticaria

Endocrine & metabolic: Hyperglycemia (neuromuscular disease: 1%) dehydration

Gastrointestinal: Nausea (3% to 18%), anorexia (neuromuscular disease: 1%), abdominal cramps, abdominal pain, diarrhea, discomfort, dyspepsia, gastroenteritis, sore throat, toothache, vomiting

Hematologic: Anemia, autoimmune hemolytic anemia, hematocrit decreased, hematoma, hemolysis (mild), hemorrhage, thrombocytopenia

Hepatic: Bilirubin increased, LDH increased, liver function test increased

Local: Muscle stiffness at I.M. site; pain, swelling, redness or irritation at the infusion site

Neuromuscular & skeletal: Muscle spasm (MMN 7%), weakness (1%; MMN: 7%), arthralgia (1%), back or hip pain, leg cramps, muscle cramps, myalgia, neck pain, rigors

Ocular: Conjunctivitis

Otic: Ear pain

Renal: Acute renal failure, acute tubular necrosis, anuria, BUN increased, creatinine increased, oliguria, proximal tubular nephropathy, osmotic nephrosis

Respiratory: Oropharyngeal pain (7%), asthma aggravated, bronchitis, cough, dyspnea, epistaxis, nasal congestion, pharyngeal pain, pharyngitis, rhinitis, rhinorrhea, sinus headache, sinusitis, upper respiratory infection, wheezing

Miscellaneous: Anaphylaxis, diaphoresis, flu-like syndrome, hypersensitivity reactions, infusion reaction, thermal burn

<1% (Limited to important or life-threatening): Apnea, ARDS, autoimmune pure red cell aplasia (PRCA) exacerbation, bronchopneumonia, bullous dermatitis, cardiac arrest, coma, Coombs' test positive, cyanosis, epidermolysis, erythema multiforme, heart failure, hepatic dysfunction, hypoxemia, leukopenia, loss of consciousness, MI, pancytopenia, phlebitis, pulmonary edema, pulmonary embolism, seizures, Stevens-Johnson syndrome, stroke, thromboembolism, transfusion-related acute lung injury (TRALI), vascular collapse

Drug Interactions

Metabolism/Transport Effects None known.

Avoid Concomitant Use There are no known interactions where it is recommended to avoid concomitant use.

Increased Effect/Toxicity There are no known significant interactions involving an increase in effect.

Decreased Effect

Immune Globulin may decrease the levels/effects of: Vaccines (Live)

Preparation for Administration Dilution is dependent upon the manufacturer and brand. Gently swirl; do not shake; avoid foaming. Do not heat. Do not mix products from different manufacturers together. Discard unused portion of vials.

Bivigam: Dilution is not recommended.

Carimune NF: In a sterile laminar air flow environment, reconstitute with NS, D_5W, or SWFI. Complete dissolution may take up to 20 minutes. Begin infusion within 24 hours.

Flebogamma DIF: Dilution is not recommended.

Gammagard Liquid: May dilute in D_5W only.

Gammagard S/D: Reconstitute with SWFI.

Gammaked: May dilute in D_5W only.

Gamunex-C: May dilute in D_5W only.

Privigen: If necessary to further dilute, D_5W may be used.

Storage/Stability Stability is dependent upon the manufacturer and brand. Do not freeze (do not use if previously frozen). Do not shake. Do not heat (do not use if previously heated).

Bivigam: Store under refrigeration at 2°C to 8°C (36°F to 46°F). Dilution is not recommended.

Carimune NF: Prior to reconstitution, store at or below 30°C (86°F). Reconstitute with NS, D_5W, or SWFI. Following reconstitution in a sterile laminar air flow environment, store under refrigeration. Begin infusion within 24 hours.

Flebogamma DIF: Store at 2°C to 25°C (36°F to 77°F).

GamaSTAN S/D: Store under refrigeration at 2°C to 8°C (36°F to 46°F). The following stability information has also been reported for GamaSTAN S/D: May be exposed to room temperature for a cumulative 7 days (Cohen, 2007).

Gammagard Liquid: Prior to use, store at 2°C to 8°C (36°F to 46°F). May store at room temperature of 25°C (77°F) within the first 24 months of manufacturing. Storage time at room temperature varies with length of time previously refrigerated; refer to product labeling for details.

Gammagard S/D: Store at ≤25°C (≤77°F). May store diluted solution under refrigeration at 2°C to 8°C (36°F to 46°F) for up to 24 hours if originally prepared in a sterile laminar air flow environment.

Gammaked: Store at 2°C to 8°C (36°F to 46°F); may be stored at ≤25°C (≤77°F) for up to 6 months.

Gammaplex: Store at 2°C to 25°C (36°F to 77°F). Protect from light.

Gamunex-C: Store at 2°C to 8°C (36°F to 46°F); may be stored at ≤25°C (≤77°F) for up to 6 months.

Hizentra: Store at ≤25°C (≤77°F). Keep in original carton to protect from light.

Octagam: Store at 2°C to 25°C (36°F to 77°F).

Privigen: Store at ≤25°C (≤77°F). Protect from light.

Mechanism of Action Replacement therapy for primary and secondary immunodeficiencies, and IgG antibodies against bacteria, viral, parasitic and mycoplasma antigens; interference with F_c receptors on the cells of the reticuloendothelial system for autoimmune cytopenias and ITP; provides passive immunity by increasing the antibody titer and antigen-antibody reaction potential

Pharmacodynamics/Kinetics

Onset of action: I.V.: Provides immediate antibody levels

Duration: I.M., I.V.: Immune effect: 3-4 weeks (variable)

Distribution: V_d: 0.05-0.13 L/kg

Intravascular portion (primarily): Healthy subjects: 41% to 57%; Patients with congenital humoral immunodeficiencies: ~70%

Half-life elimination: I.M.: ~23 days; I.V.: IgG (variable among patients): Healthy subjects: 14-24 days; Patients with congenital humoral immunodeficiencies: 26-40 days; hypermetabolism associated with fever and infection have coincided with a shortened half-life

Time to peak:

Plasma: SubQ: Gammagard Liquid: 2.9 days; Hizentra: 2.9 days

Serum: I.M.: ~48 hours

Dosage Note: Some clinicians may administer IVIG formulations FDA approved only for intravenous administration as a subcutaneous infusion based on clinical judgment and patient tolerability.

Children and Adults:

B-cell chronic lymphocytic leukemia (CLL) (Gammagard S/D): I.V.: 400 mg/kg every 3-4 weeks

Chronic inflammatory demyelinating polyneuropathy (CIDP) (Gammaked, Gamunex-C): I.V.: Loading dose: 2000 mg/kg (given in divided doses over 2-4 consecutive days); Maintenance: 1000 mg/kg every 3 weeks. Alternatively, administer 500 mg/kg/day for 2 consecutive days every 3 weeks.

Hepatitis A (GamaSTAN S/D): I.M.:

Pre-exposure prophylaxis upon travel into endemic areas (hepatitis A vaccine preferred):

0.02 **mL**/kg for anticipated risk of exposure <3 months

0.06 **mL**/kg for anticipated risk of exposure ≥3 months; repeat every 4-6 months.

Postexposure prophylaxis: 0.02 **mL**/kg given within 14 days of exposure and/or prior to manifestation of disease; not needed if at least 1 dose of hepatitis A vaccine was given at ≥1 month before exposure

Immunoglobulin deficiency (GamaSTAN S/D): I.M.: 0.66 **mL**/kg (minimum dose should be 100 mg/kg) every 3-4 weeks. Administer a double dose at onset of therapy; some patients may require more frequent injections.

Immune thrombocytopenia (ITP):

Carimune NF: I.V.: Initial: 400 mg/kg/day for 2-5 days; Maintenance: 400 mg/kg as needed to maintain platelet count ≥30,000/mm^3 and/or to control significant bleeding; may increase dose if needed (range: 800-1000 mg/kg)

Gammagard S/D: I.V.: 1000 mg/kg; up to 3 additional doses may be given based on patient response and/or platelet count. **Note:** Additional doses should be given on alternate days.

Gammaked, Gamunex-C: I.V.: 1000 mg/kg/day for 2 consecutive days (second dose may be withheld if adequate platelet response in 24 hours) **or** 400 mg/kg once daily for 5 consecutive days

Privigen: I.V.: 1000 mg/kg/day for 2 consecutive days

Kawasaki syndrome: I.V.:

Gammagard S/D: 1000 mg/kg as a single dose **or** 400 mg/kg/day for 4 consecutive days. Begin within 7 days of onset of fever.

AHA guidelines (2004): 2000 mg/kg as a single dose within 10 days of disease onset

Note: Must be used in combination with aspirin: 80-100 mg/kg/day orally, divided every 6 hours for up to 14 days (until fever resolves for at least 48 hours); then decrease dose to 3-5 mg/kg/day once daily. In patients without coronary artery abnormalities, give lower dose for 6-8 weeks. In patients with coronary artery abnormalities, low-dose aspirin should be continued indefinitely.

Measles:

GamaSTAN S/D: I.M.:

Immunocompetent: 0.25 **mL**/kg given within 6 days of exposure

Immunocompromised children: 0.5 **mL**/kg (maximum dose: 15 **mL**) immediately following exposure

Postexposure prophylaxis, any nonimmune person (unlabeled): 0.5 **mL**/kg (maximum dose: 15 **mL**) within 6 days of exposure (CDC, 2013)

Gammaked, Gamunex-C, Octagam: I.V.:

Prophylaxis in patients with primary humoral immunodeficiency (**ONLY** if routine dose is <400 mg/kg): ≥400 mg/kg immediately before expected exposure

Treatment in patients with primary immunodeficiency: 400 mg/kg administered as soon as possible after exposure

Postexposure prophylaxis, any nonimmune person (unlabeled population): 400 mg/kg within 6 days of exposure (CDC, 2013)

Hizentra: SubQ infusion: Measles exposure in patients with primary humoral immunodeficiency: Weekly dose: ≥200 mg/kg for 2 consecutive weeks for patients at risk of measles exposure (eg, during an outbreak; travel to endemic area). Biweekly dose: ≥400 mg/kg single infusion. In patients who have been exposed to measles, administer the minimum dose as soon as possible following exposure.

ACIP recommendations: The Advisory Committee on Immunization Practices (ACIP) recommends postexposure prophylaxis with immune globulin (IG) to any nonimmune person exposed to measles. The following patient groups are at risk for severe measles complications and should receive IG therapy: Infants <12 months of age, pregnant women without evidence of immunity; severely compromised persons (eg, persons with severe primary immunodeficiency; some bone marrow transplant patients; some ALL patients; and some patients with AIDS or HIV infection [refer to guidelines for additional details]). IGIM is recommended for infants <12 months of age. IGIV is recommended for pregnant women and immunocompromised persons. Although prophylaxis may be given to any nonimmune person, priority should be given to those at greatest risk for measles complications and also to persons exposed in settings with intense, prolonged, close contact (eg, households, daycare centers, classrooms). Following IG administration, any nonimmune person should then receive the measles mumps and rubella (MMR) vaccine if the person is ≥12 months of age at the time of vaccine administration and the vaccine is not otherwise contraindicated. MMR should not be given until 6 months following IGIM or 8 months following IGIV administration. If a person is already receiving IGIV therapy, a dose of 400 mg/kg I.V. within 3 weeks prior to exposure (or 200 mg/kg SubQ for 2 consecutive weeks prior to exposure if previously on SubQ therapy) should be sufficient to prevent measles infection. IG therapy is not indicated for any person who already received one dose of a measles-containing vaccine at ≥12 months of age unless they are severely immunocompromised (CDC, 2013).

Primary humoral immunodeficiency disorders:

I.V. infusion dosing:

Bivigam: I.V.: 300-800 mg/kg every 3-4 weeks; dose adjusted based on monitored trough serum IgG concentrations and clinical response

Carimune NF: I.V.: 400-800 mg/kg every 3-4 weeks

Flebogamma DIF, Gammagard Liquid, Gammagard S/D, Gammaked, Gamunex-C, Octagam: I.V.: 300-600 mg/kg every 3-4 weeks; dose adjusted based on monitored trough serum IgG concentrations and clinical response

Privigen: I.V.: 200-800 mg/kg every 3-4 weeks; dose adjusted based on monitored trough serum IgG concentrations and clinical response

Switching to weekly subcutaneous infusion dosing:

Gammagard Liquid, Gammaked, Gamunex-C: SubQ infusion: Begin 1 week after last I.V. dose. Use the following equation to calculate initial dose:

Initial weekly dose (g) = [1.37 x IGIV dose (g)] divided by [I.V. dose interval (weeks)]

Note: For subsequent dose adjustments, refer to product labeling.

Hizentra: SubQ infusion: For weekly dosing, begin 1 week after last I.V. infusion. For biweekly dosing, begin 1 or 2 weeks after last I.V. infusion or 1 week after the last Hizentra weekly infusion. **Note:** Patient should have received an I.V. immune globulin routinely for at least 3 months before switching to SubQ. Use the following equation to calculate initial weekly dose:

Initial weekly dose (g) = [Previous IGIV dose (g)] divided by [I.V. dose interval (eg, 3 or 4 weeks)] then multiply by 1.53. To convert the dose (in g) to mL, multiply the calculated dose (in g) by 5.

Initial biweekly dose (g) = multiply the calculated weekly dose by 2.

Note: For subsequent dose adjustments, refer to product labeling.

Rubella (GamaSTAN S/D): I.M.: Prophylaxis during pregnancy: 0.55 **mL**/kg

Varicella (GamaSTAN S/D): I.M.: Prophylaxis: 0.6-1.2 **mL**/kg (varicella zoster immune globulin preferred) within 72 hours of exposure

Adults:

Immune thrombocytopenia (ITP) (Gammaplex): I.V.: 1000 mg/kg/day for 2 consecutive days

Multifocal motor neuropathy (MMN) (Gammagard liquid): I.V.: 500-2400 mg/kg/month based upon response

Primary humoral immunodeficiency disorders: *I.V. infusion dosing* (Gammaplex): I.V.: 300-800 mg/kg every 3-4 weeks; dose adjusted based on monitored trough serum IgG concentrations and clinical response

Unlabeled uses: I.V.:

Acquired hypogammaglobulinemia secondary to malignancy (unlabeled use): Adults: 400 mg/kg/dose every 3 weeks; reevaluate every 4-6 months (Anderson, 2007)

Guillain-Barré syndrome (unlabeled use): Children and Adults: Various regimens have been used, including:

400 mg/kg/day for 5 days (Hughes, 2003)

or

400 mg/kg/day for 6 days (Patwa, 2012)

or

2000 mg/kg in divided doses administered over 2-5 days (Feasby, 2007)

Hematopoietic stem cell transplantation with hypogammaglobulinemia (CDC guidelines, 2000; unlabeled use):

Children: 400 mg/kg per month; increase dose or frequency to maintain IgG levels >400 mg/dL

Adolescents and Adults: 500 mg/kg/week

HIV-associated thrombocytopenia (unlabeled use): Adults: 1000 mg/kg/day for 2 days (Anderson, 2007)

Lambert-Eaton myasthenic syndrome (LEMS) (unlabeled use): Adults: 1000 mg/kg/day for 2 days (Bain, 1996; Patwa, 2012)

Multiple sclerosis (relapsing-remitting, when other therapies cannot be used) (unlabeled use): Children and Adults: 1000 mg/kg per month, with or without an induction of 400 mg/kg/day for 5 days (Feasby, 2007)

Myasthenia gravis (severe exacerbation) (unlabeled use): Children and Adults: 2000 mg/kg per treatment course over 2-5 days (Feasby, 2007; Patwa, 2012)

Refractory dermatomyositis/polymyositis (unlabeled uses): Children and Adults: 2000 mg/kg per treatment course administered over 2-5 days (Feasby, 2007)

Dosage adjustment in renal impairment:

I.V.: Use with caution due to risk of immune globulin-induced renal dysfunction; the rate of infusion and concentration of solution should be minimized.

I.M., SubQ infusion: No dosage adjustment provided in the manufacturer's labeling; risk of immune globulin-induced renal dysfunction has not been identified with I.M. and SubQ infusion administration.

Dosage adjustment in hepatic impairment: I.M., I.V., SubQ infusion: No dosage adjustment provided in manufacturer's labeling.

Dosing in obesity: Some clinicians dose IVIG on ideal body weight or an adjusted ideal body weight in morbidly-obese patients (Siegel, 2010).

Dietary Considerations Some products may contain sodium.

Administration Note: If plasmapheresis employed for treatment of condition, administer immune globulin **after** completion of plasmapheresis session.

I.M.: Administer I.M. in the anterolateral aspects of the upper thigh or deltoid muscle of the upper arm. Avoid gluteal region due to risk of injury to sciatic nerve. Divide doses >10 mL and inject in multiple sites.

GamaSTAN S/D is for I.M. administration only.

I.V. infusion: Infuse over 2-24 hours; administer in separate infusion line from other medications; if using primary line, flush with NS or D_5W (product specific; consult product prescribing information) prior to administration. Decrease dose, rate and/or concentration of infusion in patients who may be at risk of renal failure. Decreasing the rate or stopping the infusion may help relieve some adverse effects (flushing, changes in pulse rate, changes in blood pressure). Epinephrine should be available during administration. For initial treatment or in the elderly, a lower concentration and/or a slower rate of infusion should be used. Initial rate of administration and titration is specific to each IVIG product. Refrigerated product should be warmed to room temperature prior to infusion. Some products require filtration; refer to individual product labeling. Antecubital veins should be used, especially with concentrations ≥10% to prevent injection site discomfort.

Bivigam 10%: Primary humoral immunodeficiency: Initial (first 10 minutes): 0.5 mg/kg/minute (0.3 **mL/kg/hour**); Maintenance: Increase every 20 minutes (if tolerated) by 0.8 mg/kg/minute (0.48 **mL/kg/hour)** up to 6 mg/kg/minute (3.6 **mL/kg/hour**)

Carimune NF: Refer to product labeling.

Flebogamma DIF 10%: Primary humoral immunodeficiency: Initial: 1 mg/kg/minute (0.6 **mL/kg/hour**); Maintenance: Increase slowly (if tolerated) up to 8 mg/kg/minute (4.8 **mL/kg/hour**)

Gammagard Liquid 10%:

Multifocal motor neuropathy (MMN): Initial: 0.8 mg/kg/minute (0.5 **mL/kg/hour**); Maintenance: Increase gradually (if tolerated) up to 9 mg/kg/minute (5.4 **mL/kg/hour**)

Primary humoral immunodeficiency: Initial (first 30 minutes): 0.8 mg/kg/minute (0.5 **mL/kg/hour**); Maintenance: Increase every 30 minutes (if tolerated) up to: 8 mg/kg/minute (5 **mL/kg/hour**)

Gammagard S/D: 5% solution: Initial: 0.5 **mL/kg/hour**; may increase (if tolerated) to a maximum rate of 4 **mL/kg/hour**. If 5% solution is tolerated at maximum rate, may administer 10% solution with an initial rate of 0.5 **mL/kg/hour**; may increase (if tolerated) to a maximum rate of 8 **mL/kg/hour**

Gammaked 10%:

CIDP: Initial (first 30 minutes): 2 mg/kg/minute (1.2 **mL/kg/hour**); Maintenance: Increase gradually (if tolerated) up to 8 mg/kg/minute (**4.8 mL/kg/hour**)

Primary humoral immunodeficiency or ITP: Initial (first 30 minutes): 1 mg/kg/minute (0.6 **mL/kg/hour**); Maintenance: Increase gradually (if tolerated) up to 8 mg/kg/minute (4.8 **mL/kg/hour**)

Gammaplex 5%: Primary humoral immunodeficiency or ITP: Initial (first 15 minutes): 0.5 mg/kg/minute (0.6 **mL/kg/hour**); Maintenance: Increase every 15 minutes (if tolerated) up to 4 mg/kg/minute (4.8 **mL/kg/hour**)

Gamunex-C 10%:

CIDP: Initial (first 30 minutes): 2 mg/kg/minute (1.2 **mL/kg/hour**); Maintenance: Increase gradually (if tolerated) up to 8 mg/kg/minute (4.8 **mL/kg/hour**)

Primary humoral immunodeficiency or ITP: Initial (first 30 minutes): 1 mg/kg/minute (0.6 **mL/kg/hour**); Maintenance: Increase gradually (if tolerated) up to 8 mg/kg/minute (4.8 **mL/kg/hour**)

Octagam 5%: Primary humoral immunodeficiency: Initial (first 30 minutes): 0.5 mg/kg/minute (0.6 **mL/kg/hour**); Maintenance: Double infusion rate (if tolerated) every 30 minutes up to a maximum rate of <3.33 mg/kg/minute (4.2 **mL/kg/hour**)

Privigen 10%

ITP: Initial: 0.5 mg/kg/minute (0.3 **mL/kg/hour**); Maintenance: Increase gradually (if tolerated) up to 4 mg/kg/minute (2.4 **mL/kg/hour**)

Primary humoral immunodeficiency: Initial: 0.5 mg/kg/minute (0.3 **mL/kg/hour**); Maintenance: Increase gradually (if tolerated) up to 8 mg/kg/minute (4.8 **mL/kg/hour**)

SubQ infusion: Initial dose should be administered in a healthcare setting capable of providing monitoring and treatment in the event of hypersensitivity. Using aseptic technique, follow the infusion device manufacturer's instructions for filling the reservoir and preparing the pump. Remove air from administration set and needle by priming. Appropriate injection sites include the abdomen, thigh, upper arm, lower back, and/or lateral hip; dose may be infused into multiple sites (spaced ≥2 inches apart) simultaneously. After the sites are clean and dry, insert subcutaneous needle and prime administration set. Attach sterile needle to administration set, gently pull back on the syringe to assure a blood vessel has not been inadvertently accessed (do not use needle and tubing if blood present). Repeat for each injection site; deliver the dose following instructions for the infusion device. Rotate the site(s) weekly. Treatment may be transitioned to the home/home care setting in the absence of adverse reactions.

Gammagard Liquid:

Injection sites: ≤8 simultaneous injection sites

Initial infusion rate:

<40 kg: 15 mL/hour per injection site (maximum volume: 20 mL per injection site)

≥40 kg: 20 mL/hour per injection site (maximum volume: 30 mL per injection site)

Maintenance infusion rate:

<40 kg: 15-20 mL/hour per injection site (maximum volume: 20 mL per injection site)

≥40 kg: 20-30 mL/hour per injection site (maximum volume: 30 mL per injection site)

Gammaked, Gamunex-C:

Injection sites: ≤8 simultaneous injection sites

Recommended infusion rate: 20 mL/hour per injection site

Hizentra:

Injection sites:

Weekly dosing: ≤4 simultaneous injection sites or ≤12 sites consecutively per infusion

Biweekly dosing: Increase the number of injection sites as needed.

Maximum infusion rate: First infusion: 15 mL/hour per injection site; subsequent infusions: 25 mL/hour per injection site

Maximum infusion volume: First 4 infusions: 15 mL per injection site; subsequent infusions: 20 mL per injection site (maximum: 25 mL per site as tolerated)

Monitoring Parameters Renal function, urine output, IgG concentrations, hemoglobin and hematocrit, platelets (in patients with ITP); infusion- or injection-related adverse reactions, anaphylaxis, signs and symptoms of hemolysis; blood viscosity (in patients at risk for hyperviscosity); presence of antineutrophil antibodies (if TRALI is suspected); volume status; neurologic symptoms (if AMS suspected); clinical response

For patients at high risk of hemolysis (dose ≥2 g/kg, given as a single dose or divided over several days, and non-O blood type): Hemoglobin or hematocrit prior to and 36 to 96 hours postinfusion.

SubQ infusion: Monitor IgG trough levels every 2-3 months before/after conversion from I.V.; subcutaneous infusions provide more constant IgG levels than usual I.V. immune globulin treatments.

Test Interactions Octagam contains maltose. Falsely-elevated blood glucose levels may occur when glucose monitoring devices and test strips utilizing the glucose dehydrogenase pyrroloquinolinequinone (GDH-PQQ) based methods are used. Glucose monitoring devices and test strips which utilize the glucose-specific method are recommended. Passively-transferred antibodies may yield false-positive serologic testing results; may yield false-positive direct and indirect Coombs' test. Skin testing should not be performed with GamaSTAN S/D as local chemical irritation can occur and be misinterpreted as a positive reaction.

Additional Information I.M.: When administering immune globulin for hepatitis A prophylaxis, use should be considered for the following close contacts of persons with confirmed hepatitis A: unvaccinated household and sexual contacts, persons who have shared illicit drugs, regular babysitters, staff and attendees of child care centers, food handlers within the same establishment (CDC, 2006).

For travelers, immune globulin is not an alternative to careful selection of foods and water; immune globulin can interfere with the antibody response to parenterally administered live virus vaccines. Frequent travelers should be tested for hepatitis A antibody, immune hemolytic anemia, and neutropenia (with ITP, I.V. route is usually used).

IgA content:

Bivigam: ≤200 mcg/mL
Carimune NF: 1000-2000 mcg/mL
Flebogamma 5% DIF: <50 mcg/mL
Flebogamma 10% DIF: <100 mcg/mL
Gammagard Liquid: 37 mcg/mL
Gammagard S/D 5% solution: <1 mcg/mL or <2.2 mcg/mL (product dependent) (see **"Note"**)
Gammaked: 46 mcg/mL
Gammaplex: <10 mcg/mL
Gamunex-C: 46 mcg/mL
Hizentra: ≤50 mcg/mL
Octagam: ≤200 mcg/mL
Privigen: ≤25 mcg/mL

Note: Manufacturer has discontinued Gammagard S/D 5% solution; however, the lower IgA product will remain available by special request for patients with known reaction to IgA or IgA deficiency with antibodies.

Dosage Forms Excipient information presented when available (limited, particularly for generics); consult specific product labeling.

Injectable, Intramuscular [preservative free]:
GamaSTAN S/D: 15% to 18% [150 to 180 mg/mL] (2 mL, 10 mL)
Solution, Injection:
Gamunex-C: 1 g/10 mL (10 mL); 2.5 g/25 mL (25 mL); 5 g/50 mL (50 mL); 10 g/100 mL (100 mL); 20 g/200 mL (200 mL) [latex free]
Solution, Injection [preservative free]:
Gammagard: 1 g/10 mL (10 mL); 2.5 g/25 mL (25 mL); 5 g/50 mL (50 mL); 10 g/100 mL (100 mL); 20 g/200 mL (200 mL); 30 g/300 mL (300 mL) [latex free]
Gammaked: 1 g/10 mL (10 mL); 2.5 g/25 mL (25 mL); 5 g/50 mL (50 mL); 10 g/100 mL (100 mL); 20 g/200 mL (200 mL) [latex free]
Solution, Intravenous:
Flebogamma: 0.5 g/10 mL (10 mL)
Flebogamma DIF: 0.5 g/10 mL (10 mL); 2.5 g/50 mL (50 mL); 5 g/100 mL (100 mL)
Flebogamma DIF: 5 g/50 mL (50 mL) [contains polyethylene glycol]
Flebogamma DIF: 10 g/200 mL (200 mL)
Flebogamma DIF: 10 g/100 mL (100 mL) [contains polyethylene glycol]
Flebogamma DIF: 20 g/400 mL (400 mL)
Flebogamma DIF: 20 g/200 mL (200 mL) [contains polyethylene glycol]
Octagam: 1 g/20 mL (20 mL); 2.5 g/50 mL (50 mL); 5 g/100 mL (100 mL); 10 g/200 mL (200 mL); 25 g/500 mL (500 mL)
Octagam: 1 g/20 mL (20 mL); 5 g/100 mL (100 mL); 10 g/200 mL (200 mL) [sucrose free]
Solution, Intravenous [preservative free]:
Bivigam: 5 g/50 mL (50 mL); 10 g/100 mL (100 mL) [sugar free; contains polysorbate 80]
Gammaplex: 2.5 g/50 mL (50 mL); 5 g/100 mL (100 mL); 10 g/200 mL (200 mL) [contains polysorbate 80]
Privigen: 5 g/50 mL (50 mL); 10 g/100 mL (100 mL); 20 g/200 mL (200 mL); 40 g/400 mL (400 mL)
Solution, Subcutaneous [preservative free]:
Hizentra 20%: 1 g/5 mL (5 mL); 2 g/10 mL (10 mL); 4 g/20 mL (20 mL); 10 g/50 mL (50 mL) [contains polysorbate 80]
Solution Reconstituted, Intravenous:
Carimune NF: 3 g (1 ea); 6 g (1 ea); 12 g (1 ea)
Gammagard S/D: 2.5 g (1 ea); 5 g (1 ea); 10 g (1 ea)
Solution Reconstituted, Intravenous [preservative free]:
Gammagard S/D Less IgA: 5 g (1 ea); 10 g (1 ea)

- ◆ **Immune Globulin Subcutaneous (Human)** *see* Immune Globulin *on page 1059*
- ◆ **Immune Serum Globulin** *see* Immune Globulin *on page 1059*
- ◆ **Immunine® VH (Can)** *see* Factor IX (Human) *on page 825*
- ◆ **Imodium® (Can)** *see* Loperamide *on page 1235*
- ◆ **Imodium A-D [OTC]** *see* Loperamide *on page 1235*
- ◆ **Imodium® Advanced Multi-Symptom (Can)** *see* Loperamide and Simethicone *on page 1237*
- ◆ **Imodium® Multi-Symptom Relief [OTC]** *see* Loperamide and Simethicone *on page 1237*
- ◆ **Imogam Rabies-HT** *see* Rabies Immune Globulin (Human) *on page 1771*
- ◆ **Imogam® Rabies Pasteurized (Can)** *see* Rabies Immune Globulin (Human) *on page 1771*
- ◆ **Imovax® Polio (Can)** *see* Poliovirus Vaccine (Inactivated) *on page 1666*
- ◆ **Imovax Rabies** *see* Rabies Vaccine *on page 1772*
- ◆ **Imuran** *see* AzaTHIOprine *on page 208*
- ◆ **Imuran® (Can)** *see* AzaTHIOprine *on page 208*
- ◆ **Inactivated Influenza Vaccine, Quadrivalent** *see* Influenza Virus Vaccine (Inactivated) *on page 1078*
- ◆ **Inactivated Influenza Vaccine, Trivalent** *see* Influenza Virus Vaccine (Inactivated) *on page 1078*
- ◆ **INCB424** *see* Ruxolitinib *on page 1867*
- ◆ **INCB 18424** *see* Ruxolitinib *on page 1867*
- ◆ **Incivek** *see* Telaprevir *on page 1996*
- ◆ **Incivek™ (Can)** *see* Telaprevir *on page 1996*

IncobotulinumtoxinA

(in kuh BOT yoo lin num TOKS in aye)

Brand Names: U.S. Xeomin
Brand Names: Canada Xeomin Cosmetic™; Xeomin®
Index Terms Botulinum Toxin Type A
Pharmacologic Category Neuromuscular Blocker Agent, Toxin; Ophthalmic Agent, Toxin
Use

U.S. labeling: Treatment of blepharospasm in patients previously treated with onabotulinumtoxinA (Botox®); treatment of cervical dystonia in botulinum toxin-naïve and previously treated patients; temporary improvement in the appearance of moderate-to-severe glabellar lines associated with corrugator and/or procerus muscle activity

Canadian labeling:
Xeomin®: Treatment of hypertonicity disorders of the seventh nerve (eg, blepharospasm, hemifacial spasm); treatment of poststroke spasticity of upper limb(s); treatment of cervical dystonia (spasmodic torticollis)
Xeomin Cosmetic™: Temporary improvement in the appearance of moderate-to-severe glabellar lines

Pregnancy Risk Factor C
Medication Guide Available Yes

Dosage I.M.: Adults:

Blepharospasm:

U.S. labeling: Initial: Total dose should be the same as previously administered onabotulinumtoxinA dose. If prior onabotulinumtoxinA dose is not known: 1.25-2.5 units/injection site (maximum initial dose: 35 units/eye or 70 units/both eyes). Number and location of injection sites based on disease severity and previous dose/ response to onabotulinumtoxinA (in clinical trials, a mean number of 6 injections per eye were administered). Cumulative dose should not exceed 35 units/ eye or 70 units/both eyes administered no more frequently than every 3 months.

Canadian labeling: Initial: 1.25-2.5 units/injection site (maximum initial dose: 25 units/eye). Dose may be increased up to twice the previous dose if the response from the initial dose lasted ≤2 months; maximum dose per site: 5 units. Cumulative dose should not exceed 35 units/eye or 70 units/both eyes administered no more frequently than every 3 months.

Cervical dystonia:

U.S. labeling: Initial total dose: 120 units (in clinical trials, similar efficacy was noted with initial total doses of 120 and 240 units and between treatment experienced and treatment naïve patients). Dose and number of injection sites should be individualized based on prior treatment, response, duration of effect, adverse events, number/ location of muscle(s) to be treated and disease severity. In clinical trials most patients received a total of 2-10 injections into treated muscles. Administer no more frequently than every 3 months

Canadian labeling: Usual total dose: 200 units (maximum: 300 units; maximum dose per injection site: 50 units); administer no more frequently than every 3 months

Reduction of glabellar lines: Inject 4 units into each of the 5 sites (2 injections in each corrugator muscle and 1 injection in the procerus muscle) for a total dose of 20 units per treatment session. Administer no more frequently than every 3 months.

Spasticity of upper limb (poststroke): Canadian labeling (not in U.S. labeling): Individualize dose based on patient size, extent, and location of muscle involvement, degree of spasticity, local muscle weakness, and response to prior treatment. In clinical trials, total doses up to 400 units were administered as separate injections typically divided among selected muscles; may repeat therapy at ≥3 months with appropriate dosage based upon the clinical condition of patient at time of retreatment.

Suggested guidelines for the treatment of stroke-related upper limb spasticity: Note: The lowest recommended starting dose should be used. Dosage and number of injection sites should be individualized. Multiple injections may minimize adverse effects. Dose listed is total dose administered to site:

Biceps: 80 units
Brachialis: 50 units
Brachioradialis: 60 units
Flexor carpi radialis: 50 units
Flexor carpi ulnaris: 40 units
Flexor digitorum profundus: 40 units
Flexor digitorum superficialis: 40 units
Adductor pollicis: 10 units
Flexor pollicis brevis: 10 units
Flexor pollicis longus: 20 units
Pronator quadratus 25 units
Pronator teres: 40 units

Elderly: Initiate therapy at lowest recommended dose and titrate upward cautiously.

Dosage adjustment in renal impairment: There are no dosage adjustments provided in manufacturer's labeling.

Dosage adjustment in hepatic impairment: There are no dosage adjustments provided in manufacturer's labeling.

Additional Information Complete prescribing information should be consulted for additional detail.

Dosage Forms Excipient information presented when available (limited, particularly for generics); consult specific product labeling.

Solution Reconstituted, Intramuscular [preservative free]:

Xeomin: 50 units (1 ea); 100 units (1 ea) [contains albumin human]

Dosage Forms: Canada Excipient information presented when available (limited, particularly for generics); consult specific product labeling.

Injection, powder for reconstitution:

Xeomin Cosmetic™: 100 units [contains albumin (human), sucrose 4.7 mg]

Indacaterol (in da KA ter ol)

Brand Names: U.S. Arcapta Neohaler

Brand Names: Canada Onbrez® Breezhaler®

Index Terms Indacaterol Maleate; QAB149

Pharmacologic Category $Beta_2$ Agonist; $Beta_2$-Adrenergic Agonist, Long-Acting

Use Long-term maintenance treatment of airflow obstruction in chronic obstructive pulmonary disease (COPD) including chronic bronchitis and/or emphysema

Pregnancy Risk Factor C

Pregnancy Considerations Adverse events were not observed in animal reproduction studies. Beta agonists may interfere with uterine contractility if administered during labor.

Breast-Feeding Considerations It is not known if indacaterol is excreted into breast milk. The manufacturer recommends that caution be exercised when administering indacaterol to nursing women. The use of $beta_2$-receptor agonists are not considered a contraindication to breast-feeding (NAEPP, 2005).

Medication Guide Available Yes

Contraindications Hypersensitivity to indacaterol or any component of the formulation; monotherapy in the treatment of asthma (ie, use without a concomitant long-term asthma control medication, such as an inhaled corticosteroid). **Note:** Indacaterol is not FDA approved for treatment of asthma.

Warnings/Precautions Asthma-related deaths: **[U.S. Boxed Warning]: Long-acting $beta_2$-agonists (LABAs) increase the risk of asthma-related deaths. Indacaterol is not indicated for treatment of asthma and should not be used.** In a large, randomized, placebo-controlled U.S. clinical trial (SMART, 2006), salmeterol was associated with an increase in asthma-related deaths (when added to usual asthma therapy); risk is considered a class effect among all LABAs. It is unknown if indacaterol increases asthma-related deaths. Do not use for acutely deteriorating COPD or as rescue therapy in acute episodes. Short-acting $beta_2$-agonists (eg, albuterol) should be used for acute symptoms and symptoms occurring between treatments. If deterioration develops, prompt evaluation of the COPD regimen is warranted. Do not increase the dose or frequency of indacaterol. Data are not available to determine if LABA use increases the risk of death in patients with COPD. Do not use more than once daily or at a higher dose than indicated; do not combine use with other long-acting $beta_2$-agonists. Deaths and significant cardiovascular effects have been reported with excessive sympathomimetic use. Rarely, paradoxical bronchospasm may occur with use of inhaled bronchodilators; this should be distinguished from inadequate response. Hypersensitivity reactions may occur; discontinue therapy if patient develops an allergic reaction.

Use caution in patients with cardiovascular disease (eg, arrhythmias, coronary insufficiency, hypertension), diabetes mellitus, hyperthyroidism, seizure disorders, or hypokalemia. Beta-agonists may cause elevation in blood pressure, heart rate, CNS stimulation/excitation, increased risk of arrhythmia, increase serum glucose, or decrease serum potassium.

Adverse Reactions

>10%: Respiratory: Cough (post inhalation 7% to 24%)

1% to 10%:

Central nervous system: Headache (5%)

Gastrointestinal: Nausea (2%)

Respiratory: Nasopharyngitis (5%), oropharyngeal pain (2%)

<1% (Limited to important or life-threatening): Dizziness, hypersensitivity reaction, palpitation, paradoxical bronchospasm, pruritus, rash, tachycardia

Drug Interactions

Metabolism/Transport Effects Substrate of CYP2D6 (minor), CYP3A4 (minor), P-glycoprotein, UGT1A1; **Note:** Assignment of Major/Minor substrate status based on clinically relevant drug interaction potential

Avoid Concomitant Use

Avoid concomitant use of Indacaterol with any of the following: Beta-Blockers (Nonselective); Highest Risk QTc-Prolonging Agents; Iobenguane I 123; Ivabradine; Long-Acting Beta2-Agonists; Mifepristone

Increased Effect/Toxicity

Indacaterol may increase the levels/effects of: Atosiban; Corticosteroids (Systemic); Highest Risk QTc-Prolonging Agents; Long-Acting Beta2-Agonists; Loop Diuretics; Moderate Risk QTc-Prolonging Agents; Sympathomimetics; Thiazide Diuretics

The levels/effects of Indacaterol may be increased by: AtoMOXetine; Caffeine; Cannabinoids; Ivabradine; MAO Inhibitors; Mifepristone; QTc-Prolonging Agents (Indeterminate Risk and Risk Modifying); Theophylline Derivatives; Tricyclic Antidepressants

Decreased Effect

Indacaterol may decrease the levels/effects of: Iobenguane I 123

The levels/effects of Indacaterol may be decreased by: Beta-Blockers (Beta1 Selective); Beta-Blockers (Nonselective); Betahistine; Peginterferon Alfa-2b

Storage/Stability Store capsules at controlled room temperature of 25°C (77°F); excursions permitted to 15°C to 30°C (59°F to 86°F). Protect from direct sunlight and moisture. Remove from blister pack immediately before use; discard capsule if not used immediately.

Mechanism of Action Relaxes bronchial smooth muscle by selective action on beta$_2$-receptors with little effect on heart rate; acts locally in the lung.

Pharmacodynamics/Kinetics

Onset of action: 5 minutes

Peak effect: 1-4 hours

Duration: 24 hours

Absorption: Systemic: Inhalation: 43% to 45% bioavailable

Protein binding: ~95%

Metabolism: Hepatic; hydroxylated via CYP3A4, CYP2D6, and CYP1A1

Half-life elimination: 40-56 hours

Time to peak, serum: ~15 minutes

Excretion: Feces (>90%; 54% as unchanged drug [after oral administration]); urine (<2% as unchanged drug)

Dosage Inhalation: Adults: COPD (maintenance): One inhalation (75 mcg/inhalation) once daily; maximum: 1 inhalation once daily. **Note:** A dose of 75-300 mcg once daily is recommended by the 2013 Updated GOLD Guidelines.

Dosage adjustment in renal impairment: No dosage adjustment necessary.

Dosage adjustment in hepatic impairment:

Mild-to-moderate impairment: No dosage adjustment necessary.

Severe impairment: No dosage adjustment provided in manufacturer's labeling.

Administration Inhalation: **For inhalation using Neohaler™ inhaler (U.S.) or Onbrez® Breezhaler® (Canada) only**. Do **not** swallow indacaterol capsules. Use the new inhaler included with each prescription. Do not remove capsules from blister until immediately before use. Use at the same time each day. Not to be used for the relief of acute attacks. Not for use with a spacer device. Do not wash mouthpiece; inhalation device should be kept dry. Discard any capsules that are exposed to air and not used immediately.

Monitoring Parameters FEV$_1$, FVC, and/or other pulmonary function tests; serum potassium, serum glucose; blood pressure, heart rate; CNS stimulation. Monitor for increased use of short-acting beta$_2$-agonist inhalers; may be marker of a deteriorating condition. Monitor for changes in risk factors (eg, environmental exposure, smoking status).

Additional Information In November 2009, the European Medicines Agency approved indacaterol (Onbrez® Breezhaler®) at a dose of 150-300 mcg/day. Indacaterol at a dose of 75-300 mcg/day, along with other long acting bronchodilators, is recommended by the 2013 Updated GOLD guidelines for maintenance treatment of moderate to very severe COPD. In reviewing the available data, the FDA concluded that the benefit of higher dosing (ie, >75 mcg/day) was not justified due to lack of additional benefit seen at the end of 2 weeks and a higher incidence of adverse reactions.

Dosage Forms Excipient information presented when available (limited, particularly for generics); consult specific product labeling.

Capsule, Inhalation:

Arcapta Neohaler: 75 mcg [contains lactose monohydrate, milk protein]

◆ **Indacaterol Maleate** *see* Indacaterol *on page 1065*

Indapamide (in DAP a mide)

Brand Names: Canada Apo-Indapamide®; Dom-Indapamide; Indapamide Hemihydrate; JAMP-Indapamide; Lozide®; Mylan-Indapamide; Novo-Indapamide; Nu-Indapamide; PHL-Indapamide; PMS-Indapamide; PRO-Indapamide; Riva-Indapamide

Pharmacologic Category Antihypertensive; Diuretic, Thiazide-Related

Use Management of mild-to-moderate hypertension; treatment of edema in heart failure

Unlabeled Use Nephrotic syndrome (Tanaka, 2005)

Pregnancy Risk Factor B

Pregnancy Considerations Adverse events were not observed in animal reproduction studies. Diuretics cross the placenta and are found in cord blood. Maternal use may cause may cause fetal or neonatal jaundice, thrombocytopenia, or other adverse events observed in adults. Use of diuretics during normal pregnancies is not appropriate; use may be considered when edema is due to pathologic causes (as in the nonpregnant patient); monitor.

Breast-Feeding Considerations It is not known if indapamide is excreted in breast milk. If therapy is needed, the manufacturer recommends that nursing be discontinued.

Contraindications Hypersensitivity to indapamide or any component of the formulation or sulfonamide-derived drugs; anuria

Canadian labeling: Additional contraindications (not in U.S. labeling): Severe renal failure (Cl_{cr} <30 mL/minute); hepatic encephalopathy; severe hepatic impairment; hypokalemia; concomitant use with nonantiarrhythmic agents causing torsade de pointes; breast-feeding

Warnings/Precautions Use with caution in severe renal disease; Canadian labeling contraindicates use in severe renal failure (Cl_{cr} <30 mL/minute). Electrolyte disturbances including severe hyponatremia (with hypokalemia, hypochloremic alkalosis, hypomagnesemia, or hypercalcemia) can occur; risk may be dose dependent. Correct hypokalemia before initiating therapy (Canadian labeling contraindicates use in hypokalemia). Use with caution in severe hepatic dysfunction; hepatic encephalopathy can be caused by electrolyte disturbances (Canadian labeling contraindicates use in severe hepatic impairment or hepatic encephalopathy). Gout may be precipitated in certain patients with a history of gout, a familial predisposition to gout, or chronic renal failure. Use caution in patients with prediabetes or diabetes; may alter glucose control. May cause SLE exacerbation or activation. Use with caution in patients with moderate or high cholesterol concentrations. Photosensitization may occur.

Chemical similarities are present among sulfonamides, sulfonylureas, carbonic anhydrase inhibitors, thiazides, and loop diuretics (except ethacrynic acid). Use in patients with sulfonamide allergy is specifically contraindicated in product labeling, however, a risk of cross-reaction exists in patients with allergy to any of these compounds; avoid use when previous reaction has been severe. Discontinue if signs of hypersensitivity are noted. Formulation may contain lactose; Canadian labeling recommends avoiding use in patients with hereditary conditions of galactose intolerance, glucose-galactose malabsorption, or lactase deficiency.

Adverse Reactions

≥5%:

- Central nervous system: Agitation, anxiety, dizziness, fatigue, headache, irritability, lethargy, malaise, nervousness (dose dependent), pain, tension, tiredness
- Endocrine & metabolic: Hypokalemia (<3.5 mEq/L: 20% to 72%, dose dependent)
- Neuromuscular & skeletal: Back pain, muscle cramps/spasm, paresthesia, weakness
- Respiratory: Rhinitis
- Miscellaneous: Infection

≥1% to <5%:

- Cardiovascular: Arrhythmia, chest pain, flushing, orthostatic hypotension, palpitation, peripheral edema, PVC, vasculitis
- Central nervous system: Depression, drowsiness, insomnia, lightheadedness, vertigo
- Dermatologic: Hives, pruritus, rash
- Endocrine & metabolic: Hyperglycemia, hyperuricemia, hypochloremia, hyponatremia, libido decreased
- Gastrointestinal: Abdominal pain, anorexia, constipation, cramping, diarrhea, dyspepsia, gastric irritation, nausea, vomiting, weight loss, xerostomia
- Genitourinary: Nocturia, polyuria
- Neuromuscular & skeletal: Hypertonia
- Ocular: Blurred vision, conjunctivitis
- Renal: BUN increased, creatinine increased, glycosuria
- Respiratory: Cough, pharyngitis, rhinorrhea, sinusitis
- Miscellaneous: Flu-like syndrome

<1% (Limited to important or life-threatening): Agranulocytosis, anaphylactic reaction, aplastic anemia, bullous eruptions, erythema multiforme, fever, hepatitis, hypercalcemia, jaundice (cholestatic jaundice), leukopenia, liver function test abnormality, pancreatitis, photosensitivity, pneumonitis, purpura, Stevens-Johnson syndrome, thrombocytopenia, torsade de pointes

Drug Interactions

Metabolism/Transport Effects None known.

Avoid Concomitant Use

Avoid concomitant use of Indapamide with any of the following: Dofetilide

Increased Effect/Toxicity

Indapamide may increase the levels/effects of: ACE Inhibitors; Allopurinol; Amifostine; Antihypertensives; Calcium Salts; CarBAMazepine; Diazoxide; Dofetilide; Highest Risk QTc-Prolonging Agents; Hypotensive Agents; Ivabradine; Lithium; Moderate Risk QTc-Prolonging Agents; Multivitamins/Minerals (with ADEK, Folate, Iron); Multivitamins/Minerals (with AE, No Iron); Obinutuzumab; OXcarbazepine; Porfimer; RiTUXimab; Sodium Phosphates; Topiramate; Toremifene; Vitamin D Analogs

The levels/effects of Indapamide may be increased by: Alcohol (Ethyl); Alfuzosin; Analgesics (Opioid); Anticholinergic Agents; Barbiturates; Beta2-Agonists; Brimonidine (Topical); Corticosteroids (Orally Inhaled); Corticosteroids (Systemic); Herbs (Hypotensive Properties); Licorice; MAO Inhibitors; Mifepristone; Multivitamins/Fluoride (with ADE); Pentoxifylline; Phosphodiesterase 5 Inhibitors; Prostacyclin Analogues; Selective Serotonin Reuptake Inhibitors

Decreased Effect

Indapamide may decrease the levels/effects of: Antidiabetic Agents

The levels/effects of Indapamide may be decreased by: Bile Acid Sequestrants; Herbs (Hypertensive Properties); Methylphenidate; Nonsteroidal Anti-Inflammatory Agents; Yohimbine

Ethanol/Nutrition/Herb Interactions Herb/Nutraceutical: Avoid herbs with *hypertensive* properties (bayberry, blue cohosh, cayenne, ephedra, ginger, ginseng [American], kola, licorice); may diminish the antihypertensive effect of indapamide. Avoid herbs with *hypotensive* properties (black cohosh, California poppy, coleus, golden seal, hawthorn, mistletoe, periwinkle, quinine, shepherd's purse); may enhance the hypotensive effect of indapamide.

Storage/Stability Store at 20°C to 25°C (68°F to 77°F).

Mechanism of Action Diuretic effect is localized at the proximal segment of the distal tubule of the nephron; it does not appear to have significant effect on glomerular filtration rate nor renal blood flow; like other diuretics, it enhances sodium, chloride, and water excretion by interfering with the transport of sodium ions across the renal tubular epithelium

Pharmacodynamics/Kinetics

- Absorption: Rapid and complete
- Distribution: V_d: 25 L (Grebow, 1982)
- Protein binding, plasma: 71% to 79%
- Metabolism: Extensively hepatic
- Bioavailability: 93% (Ernst, 2009)
- Half-life elimination: Biphasic: 14 and 25 hours
- Time to peak: 2 hours
- Excretion: Urine (~70%; 7% as unchanged drug within 48 hours); feces (23%)

Dosage Adults: Oral:

Edema: Initial: 2.5 mg/day; if inadequate response after 1 week, may increase dose to 5 mg/day. **Note:** There is little therapeutic benefit to increasing the dose >5 mg/day; there is, however, an increased risk of electrolyte disturbances

Hypertension: Initial: 1.25 mg/day; if inadequate response, may increase dose once every 4 weeks to 2.5 mg/day and then to 5 mg/day if needed. Consider adding another antihypertensive and decreasing the dose if response is not adequate. **Note:** Canadian labeling recommends a maximum dose of 2.5 mg/day.

Dosage adjustment in renal impairment: No dosage adjustment provided in manufacturer's labeling; use with caution.

Dosage adjustment in hepatic impairment: No dosage adjustment provided in manufacturer's labeling; use with caution.

Dietary Considerations May be taken without regard to meals (Caruso, 1983); however, administration with food or milk may to decrease GI adverse effects.

Administration May be administered without regard to meals (Caruso, 1983); however, administration with food or milk may decrease GI adverse effects. Administer early in day to avoid nocturia.

Monitoring Parameters Blood pressure (both standing and sitting/supine); serum electrolytes, hepatic function, renal function, uric acid; assess weight, I & O reports daily to determine fluid loss

Dosage Forms Excipient information presented when available (limited, particularly for generics); consult specific product labeling.

Tablet, Oral:

Generic: 1.25 mg, 2.5 mg

◆ Indapamide Hemihydrate (Can) *see* Indapamide *on page 1066*

◆ Inderal (Can) *see* Propranolol *on page 1737*

◆ Inderal LA *see* Propranolol *on page 1737*

Indinavir (in DIN a veer)

Brand Names: U.S. Crixivan

Brand Names: Canada Crixivan®

Index Terms IDV; Indinavir Sulfate

Pharmacologic Category Antiretroviral, Protease Inhibitor (Anti-HIV)

Use Treatment of HIV infection; should always be used as part of a multidrug regimen (at least three antiretroviral agents)

Pregnancy Risk Factor C

Pregnancy Considerations Adverse events were observed in some animal reproduction studies. Placental passage in humans is minimal. No increased risk of overall birth defects has been observed according to data collected by the antiretroviral pregnancy registry. A small increased risk of preterm birth has been associated with maternal use of protease inhibitor-based combination antiretroviral (ARV) therapy during pregnancy; however, the benefits of use generally outweigh this risk and protease inhibitors (PIs) should not be withheld if otherwise recommended. Hyperglycemia, new onset of diabetes mellitus, or diabetic ketoacidosis have been reported with PIs; it is not clear if pregnancy increases this risk. Hyperbilirubinemia may occur in neonates following *in utero* exposure to indinavir. Until optimal dosing during pregnancy has been established, the manufacturer does not recommend indinavir use in pregnant patients. The DHHS Perinatal HIV Guidelines consider indinavir an agent to be used in special circumstances when preferred and alternative agents cannot be used; however, if needed, indinavir must be used in combination with low-dose ritonavir during pregnancy (with ritonavir boosting, 82% of pregnant women reached target trough concentrations).

Regardless of CD4 count or HIV RNA copy number, all HIV-infected pregnant women should receive a combination antepartum ARV drug regimen; this includes women who require therapy for their own health, as well as women who do not yet require therapy for their own health. ARV therapy should be started as soon as possible if required for the woman's health. Although earlier initiation may be more effective in reducing the perinatal transmission of HIV, also consider maternal conditions (eg, nausea and vomiting) and the potential risks of first trimester fetal exposure for specific agents. Plasma HIV RNA levels should be assessed at ~34-36 weeks gestation in order to help determine mode of delivery. If ARV therapy must be interrupted for <24 hours during the peripartum period, stop then restart all medications simultaneously in order to decrease the chance of developing resistance. Long-term follow-up is recommended for all infants exposed to ARV medications.

Healthcare providers are encouraged to enroll pregnant women exposed to antiretroviral medications in the Antiretroviral Pregnancy Registry (1-800-258-4263 or www.APRegistry.com). Healthcare providers caring for HIV-infected women and their infants may contact the National Perinatal HIV Hotline (888-448-8765) for clinical consultation (DHHS [perinatal], 2012).

Breast-Feeding Considerations Maternal or infant antiretroviral therapy does not completely eliminate the risk of postnatal HIV transmission. In addition, multiclass-resistant virus has been detected in breast-feeding infants despite maternal therapy. Therefore, in the United States, where formula is accessible, affordable, safe, and sustainable, and the risk of infant mortality due to diarrhea and respiratory infections is low, complete avoidance of breast-feeding by HIV-infected women is recommended to decrease potential transmission of HIV (DHHS [perinatal], 2012).

Contraindications Hypersensitivity to indinavir or any component of the formulation; concurrent use of alfuzosin, alprazolam, amiodarone, cisapride, ergot alkaloids, lovastatin, midazolam (oral), pimozide, simvastatin, St John's wort, or triazolam; sildenafil (when used for pulmonary artery hypertension [eg, Revatio®])

Warnings/Precautions Because indinavir may cause nephrolithiasis/urolithiasis the drug should be discontinued if signs and symptoms occur. Adequate hydration is recommended. May cause tubulointerstitial nephritis (rare); severe asymptomatic leukocyturia may warrant evaluation. Indinavir has a high potential for drug interactions; concomitant use of indinavir with some drugs may require cautious use, may not be recommended, may require dosage adjustments, or may be contraindicated.

Patients with hepatic insufficiency due to cirrhosis should have dose reduction. Warn patients about fat redistribution that can occur. Indinavir has been associated with hemolytic anemia (discontinue if diagnosed), hepatitis, hyperbilirubinemia, and hyperglycemia (exacerbation or new-onset diabetes).

Patients may develop immune reconstitution syndrome resulting in the occurrence of an inflammatory response to an indolent or residual opportunistic infection during initial HIV treatment or activation of autoimmune disorders (eg, Graves' disease, polymyositis, Guillain-Barré syndrome) later in therapy; further evaluation and treatment may be required.

Use caution in patients with hemophilia; spontaneous bleeding has been reported.

Adverse Reactions

>10%:

Gastrointestinal: Abdominal pain (17%), nausea (12%)

Hepatic: Hyperbilirubinemia (14%; dose dependent)

Renal: Nephrolithiasis/urolithiasis, including flank pain with/without hematuria (29%, pediatric patients; 12% adult patients; dose dependent)

1% to 10%:

Central nervous system: Headache (5%), dizziness (3%), somnolence (2%), fever (2%), malaise (2%), fatigue (2%)

Dermatologic: Pruritus (4%), rash (1%)

Endocrine & metabolic: Hyperglycemia (1%)

Gastrointestinal: Vomiting (8%), diarrhea (3%), taste perversion (3%), acid reflux (3%), anorexia (3%), appetite increased (2%), dyspepsia (2%), serum amylase increased (2%)

Hematologic: Neutropenia (2%), anemia (1%), thrombocytopenia (1%)

Hepatic: Transaminases increased (4% to 5%), jaundice (2%)

Neuromuscular & skeletal: Back pain (8%), weakness (2%)

Renal: Dysuria (2%)

Respiratory: Cough (2%)

<1% (Limited to important or life-threatening): Abdominal distention, acute renal failure, alopecia, anaphylactoid reactions, angina, arthralgia, bleeding (spontaneous in patients with hemophilia A or B), cerebrovascular disorder, cholesterol increased, crystalluria, depression, dry skin, erythema multiforme, fat redistribution, hemolytic anemia, hepatic failure, hepatitis, hydronephrosis, hyperpigmentation, immune reconstitution syndrome, interstitial nephritis (with medullary calcification and cortical atrophy), leukocyturia (severe and asymptomatic), MI, new-onset diabetes, pancreatitis, paresthesia (oral), paronychia, pharyngitis, pyelonephritis, QT prolongation, renal insufficiency, renal failure, Stevens-Johnson syndrome, torsade de pointes, triglycerides increased, upper respiratory infection, urticaria, vasculitis

Drug Interactions

Metabolism/Transport Effects **Substrate** of CYP2D6 (minor), CYP3A4 (major), P-glycoprotein; **Note:** Assignment of Major/Minor substrate status based on clinically relevant drug interaction potential; **Inhibits** CYP2C19 (weak), CYP2C9 (weak), CYP2D6 (weak), CYP3A4 (strong)

Avoid Concomitant Use

Avoid concomitant use of Indinavir with any of the following: Ado-Trastuzumab Emtansine; Alfuzosin; ALPRAZolam; Amiodarone; Apixaban; Atazanavir; Avanafil; Axitinib; Bosutinib; Cabozantinib; Cisapride; Conivaptan; Crizotinib; Dronedarone; Eplerenone; Ergot Derivatives; Everolimus; Halofantrine; Ibrutinib; Imatinib; Ivabradine; Lapatinib; Lomitapide; Lovastatin; Lurasidone; Macitentan; Midazolam; Nilotinib; Nisoldipine; Pimozide; Pomalidomide; QuiNIDine; Ranolazine; Red Yeast Rice; Regorafenib; Rifampin; Rivaroxaban; Salmeterol; Silodosin; Simeprevir; Simvastatin; St Johns Wort; Tamsulosin; Ticagrelor; Tolvaptan; Toremifene; Triazolam; Ulipristal; Vemurafenib; VinCRIStine (Liposomal)

Increased Effect/Toxicity

Indinavir may increase the levels/effects of: Ado-Trastuzumab Emtansine; Alfuzosin; Almotriptan; Alosetron; ALPRAZolam; Amiodarone; Apixaban; ARIPiprazole; Atazanavir; AtorvaSTATin; Avanafil; Axitinib; Bedaquiline; Bortezomib; Bosentan; Bosutinib; Brentuximab Vedotin; Brinzolamide; Budesonide (Nasal); Budesonide (Systemic, Oral Inhalation); Cabozantinib; Calcium Channel Blockers (Dihydropyridine); Calcium Channel Blockers (Nondihydropyridine); CarBAMazepine; Cisapride; Clarithromycin; Colchicine; Conivaptan; Corticosteroids (Orally Inhaled); Crizotinib; CycloSPORINE (Systemic); CYP3A4 Substrates; Dienogest; Digoxin; Dofetilide; Dronedarone; Dutasteride; Enfuvirtide; Enzalutamide; Eplerenone; Ergot Derivatives; Everolimus; FentaNYL; Fesoterodine; Fluticasone (Nasal); Fluticasone (Oral Inhalation); GuanFACINE; Halofantrine; Ibrutinib; Iloperidone; Imatinib; Itraconazole; Ivabradine; Ivacaftor; Ixabepilone; Ketoconazole (Systemic); Lacosamide; Lapatinib; Levomilnacipran; Lomitapide; Lovastatin; Lumefantrine; Lurasidone; Macitentan; Maraviroc; Meperidine; MethylPREDNISolone; Midazolam; Mifepristone; Nefazodone; Nilotinib; Nisoldipine; Ospemifene; OxyCODONE; Paricalcitol; PAZOPanib; Pimecrolimus; Pimozide; Pomalidomide; PONATinib; Propafenone; Protease Inhibitors; QUEtiapine; QuiNIDine; Ranolazine; Red Yeast Rice; Regorafenib; Repaglinide; Rifabutin; Rilpivirine; Riociguat; Rivaroxaban; RomiDEPsin; Rosuvastatin; Ruxolitinib; Salmeterol; Saxagliptin; Sildenafil; Silodosin; Simeprevir; Simvastatin; SORAfenib; Tacrolimus (Systemic); Tacrolimus (Topical); Tadalafil; Tamsulosin; Temsirolimus; Ticagrelor; Tofacitinib; Tolterodine; Tolvaptan; Toremifene; TraZODone; Triazolam; Tricyclic Antidepressants; Ulipristal; Vardenafil; Vemurafenib; Vilazodone; VinCRIStine (Liposomal); Zuclopenthixol

The levels/effects of Indinavir may be increased by: Atazanavir; Clarithromycin; CycloSPORINE (Systemic); Delavirdine; Enfuvirtide; Etravirine; Itraconazole; Ketoconazole (Systemic); P-glycoprotein/ABCB1 Inhibitors; Simeprevir

Decreased Effect

Indinavir may decrease the levels/effects of: Abacavir; Boceprevir; Clarithromycin; Delavirdine; Etravirine; Ifosfamide; Meperidine; Prasugrel; Theophylline Derivatives; Ticagrelor; Valproic Acid and Derivatives; Zidovudine

The levels/effects of Indinavir may be decreased by: Antacids; Atovaquone; Boceprevir; Bosentan; CarBAMazepine; CYP3A4 Inducers (Strong); Dabrafenib; Deferasirox; Didanosine; Efavirenz; Garlic; H2-Antagonists; Mitotane; Nevirapine; Peginterferon Alfa-2b; P-glycoprotein/ABCB1 Inducers; Proton Pump Inhibitors; Rifabutin; Rifampin; St Johns Wort; Tocilizumab; Venlafaxine

Ethanol/Nutrition/Herb Interactions

Food: Indinavir bioavailability may be decreased if taken with food. Meals high in calories, fat, and protein result in a significant decrease in drug levels. Indinavir serum concentrations may be decreased by grapefruit juice. Management: Administer with water 1 hour before or 2 hours after a meal. May also be administered with other liquids (eg, skim milk, juice, coffee, tea) or a light meal (eg, toast, corn flakes). Administer around-the-clock to avoid significant fluctuation in serum levels. Drink at least 48 oz of water daily. May be taken with food when administered in combination with ritonavir.

Herb/Nutraceutical: Garlic may decrease the levels/effects of protease inhibitors. St John's wort appears to induce CYP3A enzymes and has lead to 57% reductions in indinavir AUCs and 81% reductions in trough serum concentrations, which may lead to treatment failures. Management: Avoid garlic and St John's wort while taking indinavir.

Storage/Stability Medication should be stored at 15°C to 30°C (59°F to 86°F), and used in the original container and the desiccant should remain in the bottle. Capsules are sensitive to moisture.

Mechanism of Action Binds to the site of HIV-1 protease activity and inhibits cleavage of viral Gag-Pol polyprotein precursors into individual functional proteins required for infectious HIV. This results in the formation of immature, noninfectious viral particles.

Pharmacodynamics/Kinetics

Absorption: Administration with a high fat, high calorie diet resulted in a reduction in AUC and in maximum serum concentration (77% and 84% respectively); lighter meal resulted in little or no change in these parameters.

Protein binding, plasma: 60%

Metabolism: Hepatic via CYP3A4; seven metabolites of indinavir identified

Bioavailability: Good

Half-life elimination: 1.8 ± 0.4 hour; hepatic insufficiency: 2.8 ± 0.5 hour

Time to peak: 0.8 ± 0.3 hour

Excretion: Feces (83%; 19% as unchanged drug); urine (19%; 9% as unchanged drug)

Dosage

Children 4-15 years (investigational): 500 mg/m^2 every 8 hours

Adults: Oral:
Unboosted regimen: 800 mg every 8 hours
Ritonavir-boosted regimen: Ritonavir 100-200 mg twice daily plus indinavir 800 mg twice daily

Dosage adjustments for indinavir when administered in combination therapy:
Delavirdine, itraconazole, or ketoconazole: Reduce indinavir dose to 600 mg every 8 hours
Efavirenz: Increase indinavir dose to 1000 mg every 8 hours
Lopinavir and ritonavir (Kaletra™): Indinavir 600 mg twice daily
Nelfinavir: Increase indinavir dose to 1200 mg twice daily
Nevirapine: Increase indinavir dose to 1000 mg every 8 hours
Rifabutin: Reduce rifabutin to 1/2 the standard dose plus increase indinavir to 1000 mg every 8 hours

Dosage adjustment in renal impairment: No dosage adjustment provided in manufacturer's labeling (has not been studied).

Dosage adjustment in hepatic impairment:
Mild-moderate impairment due to cirrhosis, monotherapy: 600 mg every 8 hours
Severe impairment: No dosage adjustment provided in the manufacturer's labeling (has not been studied).

Dietary Considerations Should be taken without food but with water 1 hour before or 2 hours after a meal. Administration with lighter meals (eg, dry toast, skim milk, corn flakes) resulted in little/no change in indinavir concentration. If taking with ritonavir, may take with food. Patient should drink at least 48 oz of water daily.

Administration Drink at least 48 oz of water daily. Administer with water, 1 hour before or 2 hours after a meal. May also be administered with other liquids (eg, skim milk, juice, coffee, tea) or a light meal (eg, toast, corn flakes). Administer around-the-clock to avoid significant fluctuation in serum levels. May be taken with food when administered in combination with ritonavir.

Monitoring Parameters Monitor viral load, CD4 count, triglycerides, cholesterol, glucose, liver function tests, CBC, urinalysis (severe leukocyturia should be monitored frequently).

Dosage Forms Excipient information presented when available (limited, particularly for generics); consult specific product labeling.
Capsule, Oral:
Crixivan: 200 mg, 400 mg

Extemporaneous Preparations A 10 mg/mL oral solution may be prepared using capsules. First, prepare a 100 mg/mL indinavir concentrate by adding the contents of fifteen 400 mg capsules and 60 mL purified water to a 100 mL amber glass bottle. Place bottle in an ultrasonic bath filled with water at 37°C for 60 minutes, stirring the solution every 10 minutes. Filter solution; wash bottle and filter with 6 mL purified water; cool solution to room temperature. Add 50 mL of 100 mg/mL indinavir concentrate to 360 mL viscous sweet base, 90 mL simple syrup, 1.8 g citric acid, 45 mg azorubine, 0.1M sodium hydroxide solution to pH 3, and 12 drops of lemon oil, to make a final volume of 500 mL. Mix to a uniform solution. Label "refrigerate". Stable for 2 weeks refrigerated.

Hugen PW, Burger DM, ter Hofstede HJ, et al, "Development of an Indinavir Oral Liquid for Children," *Am J Health Syst Pharm*, 2000, 57 (14):1332-9.

◆ **Indinavir Sulfate** *see* Indinavir *on page 1068*
◆ **Indocid® P.D.A. (Can)** *see* Indomethacin *on page 1070*
◆ **Indocin** *see* Indomethacin *on page 1070*
◆ **Indometacin** *see* Indomethacin *on page 1070*

Indomethacin (in doe METH a sin)

Brand Names: U.S. Indocin

Brand Names: Canada Apo-Indomethacin®; Indocid® P.D.A.; Novo-Methacin; Nu-Indo; Pro-Indo; ratio-Indomethacin; Sandoz-Indomethacin

Index Terms Indometacin; Indomethacin Sodium Trihydrate

Pharmacologic Category Nonsteroidal Anti-inflammatory Drug (NSAID), Oral; Nonsteroidal Anti-inflammatory Drug (NSAID), Parenteral

Additional Appendix Information
Beers Criteria – Potentially Inappropriate Medications for Geriatrics *on page 2368*

Use Acute gouty arthritis, acute bursitis/tendonitis, moderate-to-severe osteoarthritis, rheumatoid arthritis, ankylosing spondylitis; I.V. form used as alternative to surgery for closure of patent ductus arteriosus in neonates

Unlabeled Use Management of preterm labor; prevention of pancreatitis post-endoscopic retrograde cholangiopancreatography (ERCP)

Pregnancy Risk Factor C

Pregnancy Considerations Adverse events have been observed in animal reproduction studies; therefore, the manufacturer classifies indomethacin as pregnancy category C. Indomethacin crosses the placenta and can be detected in fetal plasma and amniotic fluid. Indomethacin exposure during the first trimester is not strongly associated with congenital malformations; however, cardiovascular anomalies and cleft palate have been observed following NSAID exposure in some studies. The use of an NSAID close to conception may be associated with an increased risk of miscarriage. Nonteratogenic effects have been observed following NSAID administration during the third trimester, including myocardial degenerative changes, prenatal constriction of the ductus arteriosus, failure of the ductus arteriosus to close postnatally, and fetal tricuspid regurgitation; renal dysfunction or failure, oligohydramnios; gastrointestinal bleeding or perforation, increased risk of necrotizing enterocolitis; intracranial bleeding (including intraventricular hemorrhage), platelet dysfunction with resultant bleeding; and pulmonary hypertension. The risk of fetal ductal constriction following maternal use of indomethacin is increased with gestational age and duration of therapy. Because they may cause premature closure of the ductus arteriosus, use of NSAIDs late in pregnancy should be avoided (use after 31 or 32 weeks gestation is not recommended by some clinicians). Indomethacin has been used in the management of preterm labor. Indomethacin should be used with caution in pregnant women with hypertension. The chronic use of NSAIDs in women of reproductive age may be associated with infertility that is reversible upon discontinuation of the medication.

Breast-Feeding Considerations Indomethacin is excreted into breast milk and low amounts have been measured in the plasma of nursing infants. Seizures in a nursing infant were observed in one case report, although adverse events have not been noted in other cases. Breast-feeding is not recommended by the manufacturer. (The therapeutic use of indomethacin is contraindicated in neonates with significant renal failure.) Hypertensive crisis and psychiatric side effects have been noted in case reports following use of indomethacin for analgesia in postpartum women. Use with caution in nursing women with hypertensive disorders of pregnancy or pre-existing renal disease.

Medication Guide Available Yes

Contraindications Hypersensitivity to indomethacin, aspirin, other NSAIDs, or any component of the formulation; perioperative pain in the setting of coronary artery bypass graft (CABG) surgery; patients with a history of proctitis or recent rectal bleeding (suppositories)

Neonates: Necrotizing enterocolitis; impaired renal function; active bleeding (including intracranial hemorrhage and gastrointestinal bleeding), thrombocytopenia, coagulation defects; untreated infection; congenital heart disease where patent ductus arteriosus is necessary

Warnings/Precautions [U.S. Boxed Warning]: NSAIDs are associated with an increased risk of adverse cardiovascular thrombotic events, including MI and stroke. Risk may be increased with duration of use or pre-existing cardiovascular risk factors or disease. May cause new-onset hypertension or worsening of existing hypertension. Use caution with fluid retention. Avoid use in heart failure. Concurrent administration of ibuprofen, and potentially other nonselective NSAIDs, may interfere with aspirin's cardioprotective effect. **[U.S. Boxed Warning]: Use is contraindicated for treatment of perioperative pain in the setting of coronary artery bypass graft (CABG) surgery.** Risk of MI and stroke may be increased with use following CABG surgery.

Platelet adhesion and aggregation may be decreased; may prolong bleeding time; patients with coagulation disorders or who are receiving anticoagulants should be monitored closely. Anemia may occur; patients on long-term NSAID therapy should be monitored for anemia. Rarely, NSAID use may cause severe blood dyscrasias (eg, agranulocytosis, aplastic anemia, thrombocytopenia).

NSAID use may compromise existing renal function; dose-dependent decreases in prostaglandin synthesis may result from NSAID use, reducing renal blood flow which may cause renal decompensation. NSAID use may increase the risk for hyperkalemia. Patients with impaired renal function, dehydration, heart failure, liver dysfunction, those taking diuretics, and ACE inhibitors are at greater risk of renal toxicity and hyperkalemia. Rehydrate patient before starting therapy; monitor renal function closely. Not recommended for use in patients with advanced renal disease. Long-term NSAID use may result in renal papillary necrosis.

[U.S. Boxed Warning]: NSAIDs may increase risk of gastrointestinal irritation, inflammation, ulceration, bleeding, and perforation. Use caution with a history of GI disease (bleeding or ulcers), concurrent therapy with aspirin, anticoagulants and/or corticosteroids, smoking, use of alcohol, the elderly or debilitated patients. When used concomitantly with ≤325 mg of aspirin, a substantial increase in the risk of gastrointestinal complications (eg, ulcer) occurs; concomitant gastroprotective therapy (eg, proton pump inhibitors) is recommended (Bhatt, 2008).

Use the lowest effective dose for the shortest duration of time, consistent with individual patient goals, to reduce risk of cardiovascular or GI adverse events. Alternate therapies should be considered for patients at high risk.

NSAIDS may cause drowsiness, dizziness, blurred vision and other neurologic effects which may impair physical or mental abilities; patients must be cautioned about performing tasks which require mental alertness (eg, operating machinery or driving). Discontinue use with blurred or diminished vision and perform ophthalmologic exam. Monitor vision with long-term therapy.

NSAIDs may cause serious skin adverse events including exfoliative dermatitis, Stevens-Johnson syndrome (SJS) and toxic epidermal necrolysis (TEN); discontinue use at first sign of skin rash or hypersensitivity. Anaphylactoid reactions may occur, even without prior exposure; patients with "aspirin triad" (bronchial asthma, aspirin intolerance, rhinitis) may be at increased risk. Do not use in patients who experience bronchospasm, asthma, rhinitis, or urticaria with NSAID or aspirin therapy. Use caution in other forms of asthma.

Use with caution in patients with decreased hepatic function. Closely monitor patients with any abnormal LFT. Severe hepatic reactions (eg, fulminant hepatitis, liver failure) have occurred with NSAID use, rarely; discontinue if signs or symptoms of liver disease develop, or if systemic manifestations occur. The elderly are at increased risk for adverse effects (especially peptic ulceration, CNS effects, renal toxicity) from NSAIDs even at low doses. Prolonged use may cause corneal deposits and retinal disturbances; discontinue if visual changes are observed. Use caution with depression, epilepsy, or Parkinson's disease.

Withhold for at least 4-6 half-lives prior to surgical or dental procedures.

Elderly: Nonselective oral NSAID use is associated with an increased risk of GI bleeding and peptic ulcer disease in older adults in high risk category (eg, >75 years or age or receiving concomitant oral/parenteral corticosteroids, anticoagulants, or antiplatelet agents). Risk of adverse events may be higher with indomethacin compared to other NSAIDs; avoid use in this age group (Beers Criteria).

Oral: Safety and efficacy have not been established in children <14 years of age. Hepatotoxicity has been reported in younger children treated for juvenile idiopathic arthritis (JIA). Closely monitor if use is needed in children ≥2 years of age.

Adverse Reactions

>10%: Central nervous system: Headache (12%)

1% to 10%:

Central nervous system: Dizziness (3% to 9%), depression (<3%), fatigue (<3%), malaise (<3%), somnolence (<3%), vertigo (<3%)

Gastrointestinal: Dyspepsia (3% to 9%), epigastric pain (3% to 9%), heartburn (3% to 9%), indigestion (3% to 9%), nausea (3% to 9%), abdominal pain/cramps/distress (<3%), constipation (<3%), diarrhea (<3%), rectal irritation (suppository), tenesmus (suppository), vomiting

Otic: Tinnitus (<3%)

<1% (Limited to important or life-threatening): Acute respiratory distress, agranulocytosis, allergic rhinitis, anaphylaxis, anemia, angiitis, angioedema, aplastic anemia, arrhythmia, aseptic meningitis, asthma, bone marrow suppression, bronchospasm, chest pain, cholestatic jaundice, coma, confusion, CHF, cystitis, depersonalization, depression, diplopia, disseminated intravascular coagulation (DIC), dysarthria, dyspnea, ecchymosis, edema, epistaxis, erythema multiforme, erythema nodosum, exfoliative dermatitis, fluid retention, flushing, hair loss, gastric perforation (rare), gastritis, GI bleeding, GI ulceration, glucosuria, gynecomastia, hearing decreased, hematuria, hemolytic anemia, hepatitis (including fatal cases), hot flashes, hyperglycemia, hyperkalemia, hypersensitivity reactions, hyper-/hypotension, interstitial nephritis, intestinal strictures, involuntary muscle movements, leukopenia, lightheadedness, necrotizing fasciitis, nephrotic syndrome, oliguria, paresthesia, parkinson's exacerbation, peptic ulcer, peripheral neuropathy, proctitis, psychosis, pulmonary edema, purpura, rectal bleeding, renal insufficiency, renal failure, retinal/macular disturbances, seizure exacerbation, shock, somnolence, Stevens-Johnson syndrome, stomatitis, syncope, thrombocytopenia, thrombocytopenic purpura, thrombophlebitis, toxic amblyopia, toxic epidermal necrolysis, ulcerative stomatitis

Drug Interactions

Metabolism/Transport Effects Substrate of CYP2C19 (minor), CYP2C9 (minor); **Note:** Assignment of Major/Minor substrate status based on clinically relevant drug interaction potential; **Inhibits** CYP2C19 (weak), CYP2C9 (weak)

Avoid Concomitant Use

Avoid concomitant use of Indomethacin with any of the following: Floctafenine; Ketorolac (Nasal); Ketorolac (Systemic); NSAID (COX-2 Inhibitor); Omacetaxine

Increased Effect/Toxicity

Indomethacin may increase the levels/effects of: 5-ASA Derivatives; Agents with Antiplatelet Properties; Aliskiren; Aminoglycosides; Anticoagulants; Bisphosphonate Derivatives; Collagenase (Systemic); CycloSPORINE (Systemic); Dabigatran Etexilate; Deferasirox; Desmopressin; Digoxin; Eplerenone; Haloperidol; Ibritumomab; Lithium; Methotrexate; Nonsteroidal Anti-Inflammatory Agents; NSAID (COX-2 Inhibitor); Omacetaxine; PEMEtrexed; Porfimer; Potassium-Sparing Diuretics; PRALAtrexate; Quinolone Antibiotics; Rivaroxaban; Salicylates; Tenofovir; Thrombolytic Agents; Tiludronate; Tositumomab and Iodine I 131 Tositumomab; Triamterene; Vancomycin; Vitamin K Antagonists

The levels/effects of Indomethacin may be increased by: ACE Inhibitors; Angiotensin II Receptor Blockers; Antidepressants (Tricyclic, Tertiary Amine); Corticosteroids (Systemic); CycloSPORINE (Systemic); Dasatinib; Floctafenine; Glucosamine; Herbs (Anticoagulant/Antiplatelet Properties); Ibrutinib; Ketorolac (Nasal); Ketorolac (Systemic); Multivitamins/Fluoride (with ADE); Multivitamins/Minerals (with ADEK, Folate, Iron); Multivitamins/Minerals (with AE, No Iron); Nonsteroidal Anti-Inflammatory Agents; Omega-3 Fatty Acids; Pentosan Polysulfate Sodium; Pentoxifylline; Probenecid; Prostacyclin Analogues; Selective Serotonin Reuptake Inhibitors; Serotonin/Norepinephrine Reuptake Inhibitors; Sodium Phosphates; Tipranavir; Treprostinil; Vitamin E

Decreased Effect

Indomethacin may decrease the levels/effects of: ACE Inhibitors; Agents with Antiplatelet Properties; Aliskiren; Angiotensin II Receptor Blockers; Beta-Blockers; Eplerenone; HydrALAZINE; Loop Diuretics; Potassium-Sparing Diuretics; Prostaglandins (Ophthalmic); Salicylates; Selective Serotonin Reuptake Inhibitors; Thiazide Diuretics

The levels/effects of Indomethacin may be decreased by: Bile Acid Sequestrants; Nonsteroidal Anti-Inflammatory Agents; Salicylates

Ethanol/Nutrition/Herb Interactions

Ethanol: Avoid ethanol (may enhance gastric mucosal irritation).

Food: Food may decrease the rate but not the extent of absorption. Indomethacin peak serum levels may be delayed if taken with food.

Herb/Nutraceutical: Avoid alfalfa, anise, bilberry, bladderwrack, bromelain, cat's claw, celery, chamomile, coleus, cordyceps, dong quai, evening primrose, fenugreek, feverfew, garlic, ginger, ginkgo biloba, ginseng (American, Panax, Siberian), grapeseed, green tea, guggul, horse chestnut seed, horseradish, licorice, prickly ash, red clover, reishi, SAMe (S-adenosylmethionine), sweet clover, turmeric, white willow (all have additional antiplatelet activity).

Preparation for Administration I.V.: Reconstitute with 1-2 mL preservative free NS or SWFI just prior to administration. Discard any unused portion. Do not use preservative-containing diluents for reconstitution.

Storage/Stability

Capsules: Store at controlled room temperature.

I.V.: Store below 30°C (86°F). Protect from light.

Suppositories: Store refrigerated at 2°C to 8°C (36°F to 46°F).

Suspension: Store at controlled room temperature.

Mechanism of Action Reversibly inhibits cyclooxygenase-1 and 2 (COX-1 and 2) enzymes, which results in decreased formation of prostaglandin precursors; has antipyretic, analgesic, and anti-inflammatory properties

Other proposed mechanisms not fully elucidated (and possibly contributing to the anti-inflammatory effect to varying degrees), include inhibiting chemotaxis, altering lymphocyte activity, inhibiting neutrophil aggregation/activation, and decreasing proinflammatory cytokine levels.

Pharmacodynamics/Kinetics

Onset of action: ~30 minutes

Duration: 4-6 hours

Absorption: Oral: Immediate release: Prompt and extensive; Extended release: 90% over 12 hours

Distribution: V_d: 0.34-1.57 L/kg; crosses blood-brain barrier

Protein binding: 99%

Metabolism: Hepatic; significant enterohepatic recirculation

Bioavailability: 100%

Half-life elimination: 4.5 hours; prolonged in neonates

Time to peak: Oral: Immediate release: 2 hours

Excretion: Urine (60%, primarily as glucuronide conjugates); feces (33%, primarily as metabolites)

Dosage

Patent ductus arteriosus:

Neonates: I.V.: Initial: 0.2 mg/kg, followed by 2 doses depending on postnatal age (PNA):

PNA **at time of first dose** <48 hours: 0.1 mg/kg at 12- to 24-hour intervals

PNA **at time of first dose** 2-7 days: 0.2 mg/kg at 12- to 24-hour intervals

PNA **at time of first dose** >7 days: 0.25 mg/kg at 12- to 24-hour intervals

In general, may use 12-hour dosing interval if urine output >1 mL/kg/hour after prior dose; use 24-hour dosing interval if urine output is <1 mL/kg/hour but >0.6 mL/kg/hour; doses should be withheld if patient has oliguria (urine output <0.6 mL/kg/hour) or anuria

Inflammatory/rheumatoid disorders: **Note:** Use lowest effective dose.

Children ≥2 years: Oral: 1-2 mg/kg/day in 2-4 divided doses; maximum dose: 4 mg/kg/day; not to exceed 150-200 mg/day

Children >14 years and Adults: Oral, rectal: 25-50 mg/dose 2-3 times/day; maximum dose: 200 mg/day; extended release capsule should be given on a 1-2 times/day schedule (maximum dose for extended release: 150 mg/day). In patients with arthritis and persistent night pain and/or morning stiffness may give the larger portion (up to 100 mg) of the total daily dose at bedtime.

Bursitis/tendonitis: Oral, rectal: Adults: Initial dose: 75-150 mg/day in 3-4 divided doses **or** 1-2 divided doses for extended release; usual treatment is 7-14 days

Acute gouty arthritis: Oral, rectal: Adults: 50 mg 3 times daily until pain is tolerable then reduce dose; usual treatment <3-5 days

Prevention of pancreatitis post-endoscopic retrograde cholangiopancreatography (ERCP) (unlabeled use): Rectal: Adults: 100 mg immediately after ERCP (Elmunzer, 2012)

Elderly: Refer to adult dosing. Use lowest recommended dose and frequency in elderly to initiate therapy for indications listed in adult dosing.

Dosage adjustment in renal impairment: No dosage adjustment provided in the manufacturer's labeling; not recommended in patients with advanced renal disease.

Dosage adjustment in hepatic impairment: No dosage adjustment provided in the manufacturer's labeling; use with caution.

Dietary Considerations May cause GI upset; take with food or milk to minimize

Administration

Oral: Administer with food, milk, or antacids to decrease GI adverse effects. Extended release capsules must be swallowed whole; do not crush.

I.V.: Administer over 20-30 minutes. Reconstitute I.V. formulation just prior to administration; discard any unused portion; avoid I.V. bolus administration or infusion via an umbilical catheter into vessels near the superior mesenteric artery as these may cause vasoconstriction and can compromise blood flow to the intestines. Do not administer intra-arterially.

Monitoring Parameters Monitor response (pain, range of motion, grip strength, mobility, ADL function), inflammation; observe for weight gain, edema; monitor renal function (serum creatinine, BUN); observe for bleeding, bruising; evaluate gastrointestinal effects (abdominal pain, bleeding, dyspepsia); mental confusion, disorientation, CBC, liver function tests (particularly with pediatric use); ophthalmologic exams with prolonged therapy

Test Interactions False-negative dexamethasone suppression test

Dosage Forms Excipient information presented when available (limited, particularly for generics); consult specific product labeling.

Capsule, Oral:
Generic: 25 mg, 50 mg

Capsule Extended Release, Oral:
Generic: 75 mg

Solution Reconstituted, Intravenous:
Indocin: 1 mg (1 ea)
Generic: 1 mg (1 ea)

Suppository, Rectal:
Indocin: 50 mg (30 ea)

Suspension, Oral:
Indocin: 25 mg/5 mL (237 mL) [contains alcohol, usp; pineapple-coconut-mint flavor]

◆ **Indomethacin Sodium Trihydrate** *see* Indomethacin *on page 1070*
◆ **INF-alpha 2** *see* Interferon Alfa-2b *on page 1099*
◆ **Infanrix®** *see* Diphtheria and Tetanus Toxoids, and Acellular Pertussis Vaccine *on page 630*
◆ **Infants Advil [OTC]** *see* Ibuprofen *on page 1032*
◆ **Infants Ibuprofen [OTC]** *see* Ibuprofen *on page 1032*
◆ **Infasurf** *see* Calfactant *on page 325*
◆ **Infed** *see* Iron Dextran Complex *on page 1119*
◆ **Infergen** *see* Interferon Alfacon-1 *on page 1103*

InFLIXimab (in FLIKS e mab)

Brand Names: U.S. Remicade

Brand Names: Canada Remicade®

Index Terms Avakine; Infliximab, Recombinant

Pharmacologic Category Antirheumatic, Disease Modifying; Gastrointestinal Agent, Miscellaneous; Immunosuppressant Agent; Monoclonal Antibody; Tumor Necrosis Factor (TNF) Blocking Agent

Use

Treatment of moderately- to severely-active rheumatoid arthritis (with methotrexate) (to reduce signs/symptoms of active arthritis and inhibit progression of structural damage and improve physical function)

Treatment of moderately- to severely-active Crohn's disease with inadequate response to conventional therapy (to reduce signs/symptoms and induce and maintain clinical remission) or to reduce the number of draining enterocutaneous and rectovaginal fistulas and maintain fistula closure

Treatment of psoriatic arthritis (to reduce signs/symptoms of active arthritis and inhibit progression of structural damage and improve physical function)

Treatment of chronic severe (extensive and/or disabling) plaque psoriasis as an alternative to other systemic therapy

Treatment of active ankylosing spondylitis (to reduce signs/symptoms)

Treatment of moderately- to severely-active ulcerative colitis with inadequate response to conventional therapy (to reduce signs/symptoms and induce and maintain clinical remission, mucosal healing and eliminate corticosteroid use)

Pregnancy Risk Factor B

Pregnancy Considerations Animal reproduction studies have not been conducted. Infliximab crosses the placenta and can be detected in the serum of infants for up to 6 months following *in utero* exposure. The safety of administering live or live-attenuated vaccines to exposed infants is not known. If a biologic agent such as infliximab is needed to treat inflammatory bowel disease during pregnancy, it is recommended to hold therapy after 30 weeks gestation (Habal, 2012).

Healthcare providers are also encouraged to enroll women exposed to infliximab during pregnancy in the MotherToBaby Autoimmune Diseases Study by contacting the Organization of Teratology Information Specialists (OTIS) (877-311-8972).

Breast-Feeding Considerations Small amounts of infliximab have been detected in breast milk. Information is available from three postpartum women who were administered infliximab 5 mg/kg 1-24 weeks after delivery. Infliximab was detected within 12 hours and the highest milk concentrations (0.09-0.105 mcg/mL) were seen 2-3 days after the dose. Corresponding maternal serum concentrations were 18-64 mcg/mL (Ben-Horin, 2011). Due to the potential for serious adverse reactions in the nursing infant, the manufacturer recommends a decision be made whether to discontinue nursing or to discontinue the drug, taking into account the importance of treatment to the mother.

Medication Guide Available Yes

Contraindications Hypersensitivity to infliximab, murine proteins or any component of the formulation; doses >5 mg/kg in patients with moderate or severe heart failure (NYHA Class III/IV)

Canadian labeling: Additional contraindications (not in U.S. labeling): Severe infections (eg, sepsis, abscesses, tuberculosis, and opportunistic infections)

Warnings/Precautions [U.S. Boxed Warning]: Patients receiving infliximab are at increased risk for serious infections which may result in hospitalization and/or fatality; infections usually developed in patients receiving concomitant immunosuppressive agents (eg, methotrexate or corticosteroids) and may present as disseminated (rather than local) disease. Active tuberculosis (or reactivation of latent tuberculosis), invasive fungal (including aspergillosis, blastomycosis, candidiasis, coccidioidomycosis, histoplasmosis, and pneumocystosis) and bacterial, viral or other opportunistic infections (including legionellosis and listeriosis) have been reported in patients receiving TNF-blocking agents, including infliximab. Monitor closely for signs/symptoms of infection. Discontinue for serious infection or sepsis. Consider risks versus benefits prior to use in patients with a history of chronic or recurrent infection. Consider empiric antifungal therapy in patients who are at risk for invasive fungal infection and develop severe systemic illness. Caution should be exercised when considering use the elderly or in patients with conditions that predispose them to infections (eg, diabetes) or residence/travel from areas of endemic mycoses (blastomycosis, coccidioidomycosis, histoplasmosis), or with latent or localized infections. Do not initiate infliximab therapy with an active infection, including clinically important localized infection. Patients who develop a new infection while undergoing treatment should be monitored closely. Serious infections and neutropenia have been reported when anakinra or abatacept have been used concurrently with other TNF-blocking agents; concurrent use of infliximab with anakinra or abatacept is not recommended. Concurrent use of infliximab and other biologic agents is not recommended due to possible increased risk of infection. Use caution when switching from one biologic disease-modifying antirheumatic drug (DMARD) to another; overlapping biological activities may further increase the risk of infection. Potentially significant drug interactions may exist, requiring dose or frequency adjustment, additional monitoring, and/or selection of alternative therapy.

[U.S. Boxed Warning]: Infliximab treatment has been associated with active tuberculosis (may be disseminated or extrapulmonary) or reactivation of latent infections; evaluate patients for tuberculosis risk factors and latent tuberculosis infection (with a tuberculin skin test) prior to and during therapy; treatment of latent tuberculosis should be initiated before use. Patients with initial negative tuberculin skin tests should receive continued monitoring for tuberculosis throughout treatment. Most cases of reactivation have been reported within the first 3-6 months of treatment. Caution should be exercised when considering the use of infliximab in patients who have been exposed to tuberculosis.

Patients should be brought up to date with all immunizations before initiating therapy. Live vaccines should not be given concurrently; there is no data available concerning secondary transmission of live vaccines in patients receiving therapy. Use caution when administering live vaccines to infants born to female patients who received infliximab therapy while pregnant; infliximab crosses the placenta and has been detected in infants' serum for up to 6 months. Rare reactivation of hepatitis B virus (HBV) has occurred in chronic virus carriers; use with caution; evaluate prior to initiation and during treatment.

[U.S. Boxed Warning]: Lymphoma and other malignancies have been reported in children and adolescent patients receiving TNF-blocking agents including infliximab. Half the cases are lymphomas (Hodgkin's and non-Hodgkin's). **[U.S. Boxed Warning]: Hepatosplenic T-cell lymphoma has been reported in patients with Crohn's disease or ulcerative colitis treated with infliximab and concurrent or prior azathioprine or mercaptopurine use, usually reported in adolescent and young adult males.** The impact of infliximab on the development and course of malignancies is not fully defined, but may be dose dependent. As compared to the general population, an increased risk of lymphoma has been noted in clinical trials; however, rheumatoid arthritis alone has been previously associated with an increased rate of lymphoma. Use caution in patients with a history of COPD, higher rates of malignancy were reported in COPD patients treated with infliximab. Psoriasis patients with a history of phototherapy had a higher incidence of nonmelanoma skin cancers. Melanoma and Merkel cell carcinoma have been reported in patients receiving TNF-blocking agents including infliximab. Perform periodic skin examinations in all patients during therapy, particularly those at increased risk for skin cancer.

Severe hepatic reactions (including hepatitis, jaundice, acute hepatic failure, and cholestasis) have been reported during treatment; discontinue with jaundice or marked increase in liver enzymes (≥5 times ULN). Use caution with heart failure; if a decision is made to use with heart failure, monitor closely and discontinue if exacerbated or new symptoms occur. Doses >5 mg/kg should not be administered in patients with moderate-to-severe heart failure (NYHA Class III/IV). Use caution with history of hematologic abnormalities; hematologic toxicities (eg, leukopenia, neutropenia, thrombocytopenia, pancytopenia) have been reported; discontinue if significant abnormalities occur. Autoimmune antibodies and a lupus-like syndrome have been reported. If antibodies to double-stranded DNA are confirmed in a patient with lupus-like symptoms, infliximab should be discontinued. Rare cases of optic neuritis and demyelinating disease (including multiple sclerosis, systemic vasculitis, and Guillain-Barré syndrome) have been reported; use with caution in patients with pre-existing or recent onset CNS demyelinating disorders, or seizures; discontinue if significant CNS adverse reactions develop.

Acute infusion reactions may occur. Hypersensitivity reaction may occur within 2 hours of infusion. Medication and equipment for management of hypersensitivity reaction should be available for immediate use. Interruptions and/or reinstitution at a slower rate may be required (consult protocols). Pretreatment may be considered, and may be warranted in all patients with prior infusion reactions. Serum sickness-like reactions have occurred; may be associated with a decreased response to treatment. The development of antibodies to infliximab may increase the risk of hypersensitivity and/or infusion reactions; concomitant use of immunosuppressants may lessen the development of anti-infliximab antibodies. The risk of infusion reactions may be increased with retreatment after an interruption or discontinuation of prior maintenance therapy. Retreatment in psoriasis patients should be resumed as a scheduled maintenance regimen without any induction doses; use of an induction regimen should be used cautiously for retreatment of all other patients.

Efficacy was not established in a study to evaluate infliximab use in juvenile idiopathic arthritis (JIA). Safety and efficacy for use in pediatric plaque psoriasis or pediatric ulcerative colitis have not been established. **Note:** For use in Crohn's disease: Safety and efficacy have not been established in children <6 years of age (U.S. labeling) and in children <9 years of age (Canadian labeling).

Adverse Reactions **Although profile is similar, frequency of adverse effects may vary with disease state. Except where noted, percentages reported in adults with rheumatoid arthritis:**

>10%:
- Central nervous system: Headache (18%)
- Gastrointestinal: Nausea (21%), diarrhea (12%), abdominal pain (12%, Crohn's 26%)
- Hepatic: ALT increased (risk increased with concomitant methotrexate)
- Respiratory: Upper respiratory tract infection (32%), sinusitis (14%), cough (12%), pharyngitis (12%)
- Miscellaneous: Development of antinuclear antibodies (~50%), infection (36%), infusion reactions (20%; severe <1%), development of antibodies to double-stranded DNA (20%), development of new abscess (Crohn's patients with fistulizing disease: 15%), anti-infliximab antibodies (variable; ~10% to 15% [range: 6% to 61%]; Mayer, 2006)

5% to 10%:
- Cardiovascular: Hypertension (7%)
- Central nervous system: Fatigue (9%), pain (8%), fever (7%)
- Dermatologic: Rash (1% to 10%), pruritus (7%)
- Gastrointestinal: Dyspepsia (10%)

Genitourinary: Urinary tract infection (8%)
Neuromuscular & skeletal: Arthralgia (1% to 8%), back pain (8%)
Respiratory: Bronchitis (10%), rhinitis (8%), dyspnea (6%)
Miscellaneous: Moniliasis (5%)
<5%: Abscess, adult respiratory distress syndrome, allergic reaction, anemia, arrhythmia, basal cell carcinoma, biliary pain, bradycardia, brain infarction, breast cancer, cardiac arrest, cellulitis, cholecystitis, cholelithiasis, circulatory failure, confusion, constipation, dehydration, delayed hypersensitivity (plaque psoriasis), diaphoresis increased, dizziness, edema, gastrointestinal hemorrhage, heart failure, hemolytic anemia, hepatitis, hypersensitivity reactions, hypotension, ileus, intervertebral disk herniation, intestinal obstruction, intestinal perforation, intestinal stenosis, leukopenia, lupus-like syndrome, lymphadenopathy, lymphoma, malignancies, meningitis, menstrual irregularity, MI, myalgia, neuritis, pancreatitis, pancytopenia, peripheral neuropathy, peritonitis, pleural effusion, pleurisy, proctalgia, pulmonary edema, pulmonary embolism, renal calculus, renal failure, respiratory insufficiency, sarcoidosis, seizure, sepsis, serum sickness, suicide attempt, syncope, tachycardia, tendon disorder, thrombocytopenia, thrombophlebitis (deep), ulceration

The following adverse events were reported in children with Crohn's disease and were found more frequently in children than adults:
>10%:
Hepatic: Liver enzymes increased (18%; ≥5 times ULN: 1%)
Hematologic: Anemia (11%)
Miscellaneous: Infections (56%; more common with every 8-week versus every 12-week infusions)
1% to 10%:
Central nervous system: Flushing (9%)
Gastrointestinal: Blood in stool (10%)
Hematologic: Leukopenia (9%), neutropenia (7%)
Neuromuscular & skeletal: Bone fracture (7%)
Respiratory: Respiratory tract allergic reaction (6%)
Miscellaneous: Viral infection (8%), bacterial infection (6%), antibodies to infliximab (3%)

Postmarketing and/or case reports (adults or children): Agranulocytosis, anaphylactic reactions, anaphylactic shock, angina, angioedema, autoimmune hepatitis, bronchospasm, central demyelinating disorders (eg, multiple sclerosis, optic neuritis); cholestasis, drug-induced lupus-like syndrome, erythema multiforme, heart failure (worsening), hepatic carcinoma, hepatitis B reactivation, hepatocellular damage, hepatosplenic T-cell lymphoma (HSTCL), Hodgkin's disease, idiopathic thrombocytopenia purpura, interstitial fibrosis, interstitial pneumonitis, jaundice, laryngeal/pharyngeal edema, latent tuberculosis reactivation, leiomyosarcoma, leukemias, liver failure, liver function tests increased, melanoma, Merkel cell carcinoma, neuropathy, numbness, opportunistic infection, pericardial effusion, peripheral demyelinating disorders (eg, Guillain-Barré syndrome, chronic inflammatory demyelinating polyneuropathy, multifocal motor neuropathy); pneumonia, psoriasis (including new onset, palmoplantar, pustular, or exacerbation), renal cell carcinoma, seizure, Stevens-Johnson syndrome, thrombotic thrombocytopenia purpura, taste abnormal, tingling, toxic epidermal necrolysis, transverse myelitis, tuberculosis, urticaria, vasculitis (systemic and cutaneous)

Drug Interactions

Metabolism/Transport Effects None known.

Avoid Concomitant Use

Avoid concomitant use of InFLIXimab with any of the following: Abatacept; Adalimumab; Anakinra; BCG; Belimumab; Canakinumab; Certolizumab Pegol; Etanercept; Golimumab; Natalizumab; Pimecrolimus; Rilonacept; Tacrolimus (Topical); Tocilizumab; Tofacitinib; Ustekinumab; Vaccines (Live)

Increased Effect/Toxicity

InFLIXimab may increase the levels/effects of: Abatacept; Anakinra; Belimumab; Canakinumab; Certolizumab Pegol; Leflunomide; Natalizumab; Rilonacept; Tofacitinib; Vaccines (Live)

The levels/effects of InFLIXimab may be increased by: Abciximab; Adalimumab; Denosumab; Etanercept; Golimumab; Pimecrolimus; Roflumilast; Tacrolimus (Topical); Tocilizumab; Trastuzumab; Ustekinumab

Decreased Effect

InFLIXimab may decrease the levels/effects of: BCG; Coccidioidin Skin Test; Sipuleucel-T; Vaccines (Inactivated); Vaccines (Live)

The levels/effects of InFLIXimab may be decreased by: Echinacea

Ethanol/Nutrition/Herb Interactions Herb/Nutraceutical: Avoid echinacea (may diminish the therapeutic effect of infliximab).

Preparation for Administration Reconstitute vials with 10 mL sterile water for injection. Swirl vial gently to dissolve powder; do not shake. Allow solution to stand for 5 minutes. Total dose of reconstituted product should be further diluted to 250 mL of 0.9% sodium chloride injection to a final concentration of 0.4-4 mg/mL. Infusion of dose should begin within 3 hours of preparation.

Storage/Stability Store vials at 2°C to 8°C (36°F to 46°F).

Mechanism of Action Infliximab is a chimeric monoclonal antibody that binds to human tumor necrosis factor alpha (TNFα), thereby interfering with endogenous TNFα activity. Elevated TNFα levels have been found in involved tissues/fluids of patients with rheumatoid arthritis, ankylosing spondylitis, psoriatic arthritis, plaque psoriasis, Crohn's disease and ulcerative colitis. Biological activities of TNFα include the induction of proinflammatory cytokines (interleukins), enhancement of leukocyte migration, activation of neutrophils and eosinophils, and the induction of acute phase reactants and tissue degrading enzymes. Animal models have shown TNFα expression causes polyarthritis, and infliximab can prevent disease as well as allow diseased joints to heal.

Pharmacodynamics/Kinetics
Onset of action: Crohn's disease: ~2 weeks
Distribution: V_d: 3-6 L
Half-life elimination: 7-12 days

Dosage I.V.: **Note:** Premedication with antihistamines (H_1-antagonist +/- H_2-antagonist), acetaminophen, and/or corticosteroids may be considered to prevent and/or manage infusion-related reactions:
Children and Adolescents: U.S. labeling ≥6 years, Canadian labeling ≥9 years: Crohn's disease: 5 mg/kg at 0, 2, and 6 weeks, followed by 5 mg/kg every 8 weeks thereafter; if no response by week 14, consider discontinuing therapy
Children ≥6 years and Adolescents: Ulcerative colitis: 5 mg/kg at 0, 2, and 6 weeks, followed by 5 mg/kg every 8 weeks thereafter
Adults:
Crohn's disease: 5 mg/kg at 0, 2, and 6 weeks, followed by 5 mg/kg every 8 weeks thereafter; dose may be increased to 10 mg/kg in patients who respond but then lose their response. If no response by week 14, consider discontinuing therapy.
Psoriatic arthritis (with or without methotrexate): 5 mg/kg at 0, 2, and 6 weeks, followed by 5 mg/kg every 8 weeks thereafter

Rheumatoid arthritis (in combination with methotrexate therapy): 3 mg/kg at 0, 2, and 6 weeks, followed by 3 mg/kg every 8 weeks thereafter; doses have ranged from 3-10 mg/kg repeated at 4- to 8-week intervals
Ankylosing spondylitis: 5 mg/kg at 0, 2, and 6 weeks, followed by 5 mg/kg every 6 weeks thereafter (Canadian labeling recommends every 6-8 weeks thereafter)
Plaque psoriasis: 5 mg/kg at 0, 2, and 6 weeks, followed by 5 mg/kg every 8 weeks thereafter
Ulcerative colitis: 5 mg/kg at 0, 2, and 6 weeks, followed by 5 mg/kg every 8 weeks thereafter

Dosage adjustment with heart failure (HF): Weigh risk versus benefits for individual patient:
Moderate-to-severe HF (NYHA Class III or IV): ≤5 mg/kg

Dosage adjustment in renal impairment: No dosage adjustment provided in manufacturer's labeling.

Dosage adjustment in hepatic impairment: No dosage adjustment provided in manufacturer's labeling.

Administration The infusion should begin within 3 hours of reconstitution and dilution. Infuse over at least 2 hours; do not infuse with other agents; use in-line low protein binding filter (≤1.2 micron). Temporarily discontinue or decrease infusion rate with infusion-related reactions. Antihistamines (H_1-antagonist +/- H_2-antagonist), acetaminophen and/or corticosteroids may be used to manage reactions. Infusion may be reinitiated at a lower rate upon resolution of mild-to-moderate symptoms.

Canadian labeling (not approved in U.S. labeling): Infusion of doses ≤6 mg/kg over not less than 1 hour may be considered in patients treated for rheumatoid arthritis who have initially tolerated 3 infusions each over 2 hours. Safety of shortened infusion has not been studied with doses >6 mg/kg.

Guidelines for the treatment and prophylaxis of infusion reactions: (**Note:** Limited to adult patients and dosages used in Crohn's; prospective data for other populations [pediatrics, other indications/dosing] are not available).

A protocol for the treatment of infusion reactions, as well as prophylactic therapy for repeat infusions, has been published (Mayer, 2006).

Treatment of infusion reactions: Medications for the treatment of hypersensitivity reactions should be available for immediate use. For mild reactions, the rate of infusion should be decreased to 10 mL/hour. Initiate a normal saline infusion (500-1000 mL/hour) and appropriate symptomatic treatment (eg, acetaminophen and diphenhydramine); monitor vital signs every 10 minutes until normal. After 20 minutes, the infusion may be increased at 15-minute intervals, as tolerated, to completion (initial increase to 20 mL/hour, then 40 mL/hour, then 80 mL/hour, etc [maximum of 125 mL/hour]). For moderate reactions, the infusion should be stopped or slowed. Initiate a normal saline infusion (500-1000 mL/hour) and appropriate symptomatic treatment. Monitor vital signs every 5 minutes until normal. After 20 minutes, the infusion may be reinstituted at 10 mL/hour; then increased at 15-minute intervals, as tolerated, to completion (initial increase 20 mL/hour, then 40 mL/hour, then 80 mL/hour, etc [maximum of 125 mL/hour]). For severe reactions, the infusion should be stopped with administration of appropriate symptomatic treatment (eg, hydrocortisone/methylprednisolone, diphenhydramine and epinephrine) and frequent monitoring of vitals (consult institutional policies, if available). Retreatment after a severe reaction should only be done if the benefits outweigh the risks and with appropriate prophylaxis. Delayed infusion reactions typically occur 1-7 days after an infusion. Treatment should consist of appropriate symptomatic treatment (eg, acetaminophen, antihistamine, methylprednisolone).

Prophylaxis of infusion reactions: Premedication with acetaminophen and diphenhydramine 90 minutes prior to infusion may be considered in all patients with prior infusion reactions, and in patients with severe reactions corticosteroid administration is recommended. Steroid dosing may be oral (prednisone 50 mg orally every 12 hours for 3 doses prior to infusion) or intravenous (a single dose of hydrocortisone 100 mg or methylprednisolone 20-40 mg administered 20 minutes prior to the infusion). On initiation of the infusion, begin with a test dose at 10 mL/hour for 15 minutes. Thereafter, the infusion may be increased at 15-minute intervals, as tolerated, to completion (initial increase 20 mL/hour, then 40 mL/hour, then 80 mL/hour, etc). A maximum rate of 125 mL/hour is recommended in patients who experienced prior mild-moderate reactions and 100 mL/hour is recommended in patients who experienced prior severe reactions. In patients with cutaneous flushing, aspirin may be considered (Becker, 2004). For delayed infusion reactions, premedicate with acetaminophen and diphenhydramine 90 minutes prior to infusion. On initiation of the infusion, begin with a test dose at 10 mL/hour for 15 minutes. Thereafter, the infusion may be increased to infuse over 3 hours. Postinfusion therapy with acetaminophen for 3 days and an antihistamine for 7 days is recommended.

Monitoring Parameters Monitor improvement of symptoms and physical function assessments. During infusion, if reaction is noted, monitor vital signs every 2-10 minutes, depending on reaction severity, until normal. Latent TB screening prior to initiating and during therapy; signs/symptoms of infection (prior to, during, and following therapy); CBC with differential; signs/symptoms/worsening of heart failure; HBV screening prior to initiating (all patients), HBV carriers (during and for several months following therapy); signs and symptoms of hypersensitivity reaction; symptoms of lupus-like syndrome; LFTs (discontinue if >5 times ULN); signs and symptoms of malignancy (eg, splenomegaly, hepatomegaly, abdominal pain, persistent fever, night sweats, weight loss).

Psoriasis patients with history of phototherapy should be monitored for nonmelanoma skin cancer.

Dosage Forms Excipient information presented when available (limited, particularly for generics); consult specific product labeling.
Solution Reconstituted, Intravenous [preservative free]:
Remicade: 100 mg (1 ea)

◆ **Infliximab, Recombinant** *see* InFLIXimab *on page 1073*

◆ **Influenza Vaccine** *see* Influenza Virus Vaccine (Inactivated) *on page 1078*

◆ **Influenza Vaccine** *see* Influenza Virus Vaccine (Live/Attenuated) *on page 1082*

Influenza Virus Vaccine (H5N1)

(in floo EN za VYE rus vak SEEN H5N1)

Index Terms Avian Influenza Virus Vaccine; Bird Flu Vaccine; H5N1 Influenza Vaccine; Influenza Virus Vaccine (Monovalent); Q-Pan H5N1 Influenza Vaccine

Pharmacologic Category Vaccine, Inactivated (Viral)

Additional Appendix Information

Immunization Administration Recommendations *on page 2334*

Immunization Recommendations *on page 2339*

Use Active immunization of adults at increased risk of exposure to the H5N1 viral subtype of influenza

Pregnancy Risk Factor C

Pregnancy Considerations Reproduction studies have not been conducted. Vaccine should be given only if clearly needed. Inactivated viral vaccines have not been shown to cause increased risks to the fetus (CDC, 2011).

Breast-Feeding Considerations Inactivated virus vaccines do not affect the safety of breast-feeding for the mother or the infant. Breast-feeding infants should be vaccinated according to the recommended schedules (CDC, 2011).

Prescribing and Access Restrictions Commercial distribution is not planned. The vaccine will be included as part of the U.S. Strategic National Stockpile. It will be distributed by public health officials if needed.

Contraindications Manufacturer states no contraindications

Warnings/Precautions Immediate treatment (including epinephrine 1:1000) for anaphylactoid and/or hypersensitivity reactions should be available during vaccine use. Use with caution in patients with a history of Guillain-Barré syndrome (GBS); these patients may have a greater likelihood of developing GBS. If recent occurrence of GBS (≤6 weeks), decision to administer vaccine should entail careful consideration of risk:benefit. Vaccination may not result in effective immunity in all patients. Response depends upon multiple factors (eg, type of vaccine, age of patient) and may be improved by administering the vaccine at the recommended dose, route, and interval. Vaccines may not be effective if administered during periods of altered immune competence (CDC, 2011). Use with caution in severely immunocompromised patients (eg, patients receiving chemo/radiation therapy or other immunosuppressive therapy [including high-dose corticosteroids]); may have a reduced response to vaccination. Syncope has been reported with use of injectable vaccines and may be accompanied by transient visual disturbances, weakness, or tonic-clonic movements. Procedures should be in place to avoid injuries from falling and to restore cerebral perfusion if syncope occurs. Safety and efficacy in children and patients >64 years of age have not been established. In general, household and close contacts of persons with altered immunocompetence may receive all age appropriate vaccines Manufactured with chicken egg protein. Contains thimerosal; hypersensitivity reactions may occur

Adverse Reactions All serious adverse reactions must be reported to the U.S. Department of Health and Human Services (DHHS) Vaccine Adverse Event Reporting System (VAERS) 1-800-822-7967 or online at https://vaers.hhs.gov/esub/index.

>10%:

- Central nervous system: Headache (3% to 35%), fatigue (34%), shivering (17%)
- Dermatologic: Diaphoresis (11%)
- Local: Pain at injection site (74% to 83%), tenderness at injection site (70%), erythema at injection site (9% to 20%), swelling at injection site (10% to 15%)
- Neuromuscular & skeletal: Myalgia (45%), arthralgia (25%)

1% to 10%:

- Gastrointestinal: Nausea (10%), diarrhea (6%)
- Local: Itching at injection site (2%), burning sensation at injection site (1%)
- Respiratory: Nasal congestion (1%)
- Miscellaneous: Fever (5%)

<1% (Limited to important or life-threatening): Celiac disease, cerebrovascular accident, convulsions, cranial nerve palsy (IV), Crohn's disease, erythema nodosum, facial paralysis, giant-cell arteritis, hepatitis, malignant neoplasm of thyroid, organ transplant rejection (corneal), polymyalgia rheumatica, psoriasis, pulmonary embolism, radiculopathy, rheumatoid arthritis, rheumatoid lung

Drug Interactions

Metabolism/Transport Effects None known.

Avoid Concomitant Use There are no known interactions where it is recommended to avoid concomitant use.

Increased Effect/Toxicity There are no known significant interactions involving an increase in effect.

Decreased Effect

The levels/effects of Influenza Virus Vaccine (H5N1) may be decreased by: Belimumab; Fingolimod; Immunosuppressants

Storage/Stability Store between 2°C to 8°C (36°F to 46°F). Potency is destroyed by freezing; do not use if product has been frozen. Protect from light.

Mechanism of Action A monovalent, split virus (inactivated) preparation of the H5N1 avian strain of influenza virus (A/Vietnam/1203/2004) which promotes active immunity to avian influenza.

Pharmacodynamics/Kinetics Onset of action: Fourfold increase in antibody titers occurred in up to 58% of patients 28 days after second dose.

Dosage I.M.: Adults 18-64 years: 1 mL, followed by second 1 mL dose given 28 days later (acceptable range: 21-35 days)

Dosage adjustment in renal impairment: No dosage adjustment provided in manufacturer's labeling.

Dosage adjustment in hepatic impairment: No dosage adjustment provided in manufacturer's labeling.

Administration For I.M. administration only. Inspect for particulate matter and discoloration prior to administration. Vaccinate in the deltoid muscle using a ≥1 inch needle length. Suspension should be shaken well prior to use. **Note:** For patients at risk of hemorrhage following intramuscular injection, the ACIP recommends "it should be administered intramuscularly if, in the opinion of the physician familiar with the patient's bleeding risk, the vaccine can be administered by this route with reasonable safety. If the patient receives antihemophilia or other similar therapy, intramuscular vaccination can be scheduled shortly after such therapy is administered. A fine needle (23 gauge or smaller) can be used for the vaccination and firm pressure applied to the site (without rubbing) for at least 2 minutes. The patient should be instructed concerning the risk of hematoma from the injection." Patients on anticoagulant therapy should be considered to have the same bleeding risks and treated as those with clotting factor disorders (CDC, 2011).

Simultaneous administration of vaccines helps ensure the patients will be fully vaccinated by the appropriate age. Simultaneous administration of vaccines is defined as administering >1 vaccine on the same day at different anatomic sites. Separate vaccines should not be combined in the same syringe unless indicated by product specific labeling. Separate needles and syringes should be used for each injection. The ACIP prefers each dose of a specific vaccine in a series come from the same manufacturer when possible. Adolescents and adults should be vaccinated while seated or lying down. In general, preterm infants should be vaccinated at the same chronological age as full-term infants (CDC, 2011).

Antipyretics have not been shown to prevent febrile seizures. Antipyretics may be used to treat fever or discomfort following vaccination (CDC, 2011). One study reported that routine prophylactic administration of acetaminophen to prevent fever prior to vaccination decreased the immune response of some vaccines; the clinical significance of this reduction in immune response has not been established (Prymula, 2009).

Monitoring Parameters Monitor for syncope for 15 minutes following administration. If seizure-like activity associated with syncope occurs, maintain patient in supine or Trendelenburg position to reestablish adequate cerebral perfusion.

Additional Information U.S. federal law requires that the name of medication, date of administration, the vaccine manufacturer, lot number of vaccine, and the administering person's name, title, and address be entered into the patient's permanent medical record.

The 2-dose regimen prompted antibody response consistent with a protective titer in up to 58% of patients (Treanor, 2006). However, there are no clinical data evaluating whether vaccination protects patients against development of infection. Therefore, protection against a pandemic avian flu strain cannot be assured. A study has shown that a third dose of the vaccine further increases the antibody response (Zangwill, 2008).

Healthcare workers involved in the care of patients with known or suspected H5N1 viral subtype influenza infection should be vaccinated with the most recent seasonal human influenza vaccine in order to reduce the risk of coinfection of human influenza A viruses.

Product Availability Influenza A (H5N1) Virus Monovalent Vaccine, Adjuvanted (also referred to as Q-Pan H5N1 influenza vaccine): FDA approved November 2013. Product will not be commercially available; distribution will be limited as part of the U.S. Strategic National Stockpile. Vaccine is indicated for the immunization of adults 18 and older for the prevention of disease caused by the influenza A virus H5N1 subtype contained in the vaccine.

Dosage Forms Excipient information presented when available (limited, particularly for generics); consult specific product labeling.

Injection, suspension [monovalent]: Hemagglutinin (H5N1strain) 90 mcg/mL (5 mL) [contains chicken, egg, and porcine protein, and thimerosal]

Influenza Virus Vaccine (Inactivated)

(in floo EN za VYE rus vak SEEN, in ak ti VAY ted)

Brand Names: U.S. Afluria; Afluria Preservative Free; Fluarix; Fluarix Quadrivalent; Flucelvax; Flulaval; Flulaval Quadrivalent; Fluvirin; Fluvirin Preservative Free; Fluzone; Fluzone High-Dose; Fluzone Pediatric PF; Fluzone Preservative Free; Fluzone Quadrivalent; Medical Provider EZ Flu PF; Physicians EZ Use Flu

Brand Names: Canada Agriflu; Fluad; Fluviral; Influvac; Intanza; Vaxigrip

Index Terms ccIIV3 [Flucelvax]; Cell Culture Inactivated Influenza Vaccine, Trivalent [Flucelvax]; H1N1 Influenza Vaccine; IIV; IIV3; IIV4; Inactivated Influenza Vaccine, Quadrivalent; Inactivated Influenza Vaccine, Trivalent; Influenza Vaccine; Influenza Virus Vaccine (Purified Surface Antigen); Influenza Virus Vaccine (Split-Virus); TIV (Trivalent Inactivated Influenza Vaccine)

Pharmacologic Category Vaccine, Inactivated (Viral)

Additional Appendix Information

Immunization Administration Recommendations *on page 2334*

Immunization Recommendations *on page 2339*

Use For active immunization against influenza disease caused by influenza virus subtypes A and type B contained in the vaccine

The Advisory Committee on Immunization Practices (ACIP) recommends routine annual vaccination with the seasonal influenza vaccine for all persons ≥6 months of age who do not otherwise have contraindications to the vaccine (CDC, 2013c).

The ACIP recommends use of any age and risk factor appropriate product and does not have a preferential recommendation for use of the trivalent inactivated influenza vaccine (IIV_3) or the quadrivalent inactivated influenza vaccine (IIV_4). In addition to the IIV products, other alternative products are available for certain patient populations: Healthy nonpregnant persons aged 2-49 years may receive vaccination with the live attenuated influenza vaccine (LAIV), and persons 18-49 years may receive vaccination with the recombinant influenza vaccine (RIV) (CDC, 2013c).

When vaccine supply is limited, target groups for vaccination (those at higher risk of complications from influenza infection and their close contacts) include the following:

- Children 6-59 months of age
- Persons ≥50 years of age
- Residents of nursing homes and other long-term care facilities
- Adults and children with chronic pulmonary disorders (including asthma) or cardiovascular systems disorders (except hypertension), renal, hepatic, neurologic, or metabolic disorders (including diabetes mellitus)
- Persons who have immunosuppression (including immunosuppression caused by medications or HIV)
- Children and adolescents (6 months to 18 years of age) who are receiving long-term aspirin therapy, and therefore, may be at risk for developing Reye's syndrome after influenza
- Women who are or will be pregnant during the influenza season
- Healthcare personnel
- Household contacts (including children) and caregivers of children <5 years (particularly children <6 months) and adults ≥50 years
- Household contacts (including children) and caregivers of persons with medical conditions which put them at high risk of complications from influenza infection
- American Indians/Alaska Natives
- Morbidly obese (BMI ≥40)

Pregnancy Risk Factor B/C (manufacturer specific)

Pregnancy Considerations Adverse events were not observed in animal reproduction studies. Inactivated influenza vaccine has not been shown to cause fetal harm when given to pregnant women, although information related to use in the first trimester is limited (CDC, 2013). Following maternal immunization with the inactivated influenza virus vaccine, vaccine specific antibodies are observed in the newborn (Englund, 1993; Steinhoff, 2010; Zaman, 2008; Zuccotti, 2010). Vaccination of pregnant women protects infants from influenza infection, including infants <6 months of age who are not able to be vaccinated (CDC, 2013).

Pregnant women are at an increased risk of complications from influenza infection (Rasmussen, 2008). Influenza vaccination with the inactivated influenza vaccine (IIV) is recommended for all women who are or will become pregnant during the influenza season and who do not otherwise have contraindications to the vaccine (CDC, 2013). Pregnant women should observe the same precautions as nonpregnant women to reduce the risk of exposure to influenza and other respiratory infections (CDC, 2010). When vaccine supply is limited, focus on delivering the vaccine should be given to women who are pregnant or will be pregnant during the flu season, as well as mothers of newborns and contacts or caregivers of children <5 years of age (CDC, 2013).

Healthcare providers are encouraged to refer women exposed to the influenza vaccine during pregnancy to the Vaccines and Medications in Pregnancy Surveillance System (VAMPSS) by contacting The Organization of Teratology Information Specialists (OTIS) at (877) 311-8972.

Women exposed to Flulaval, Flulaval Quadrivalent, Fluarix, or Fluarix Quadrivalent vaccine during pregnancy or their healthcare provider may also contact the GlaxoSmithKline registry at 888-452-9622.

Healthcare providers may enroll women exposed to Fluzone Intradermal or Fluzone Quadrivalent during pregnancy in the Sanofi Pasteur vaccination registry at 800-822-2463.

Breast-Feeding Considerations It is not known if inactivated influenza vaccine is excreted into breast milk. The manufacturers recommend that caution be used if administered to nursing women. Anti-influenza IgA antibodies can be detected in breast milk following maternal vaccination with the trivalent IIV vaccine (Schlaudecker, 2013). Inactivated vaccines do not affect the safety of breastfeeding for the mother or the infant (CDC, 2011). Postpartum women may be vaccinated with either IIV or LAIV (CDC, 2013). When vaccine supply is limited, focus on delivering the vaccine should be given to women who are pregnant or will be pregnant during the flu season, as well as mothers of newborns and contacts or caregivers of children <5 years of age (CDC, 2013). Breast-feeding infants should be vaccinated according to the recommended schedules (CDC, 2011).

Contraindications Severe allergic reaction (eg, anaphylaxis) to a previous influenza vaccination; hypersensitivity to any component of the formulation

Fluviral (not available in U.S.): Canadian labeling: Additional contraindications: Presence of acute respiratory infection, other active infections, or serious febrile illness

Warnings/Precautions Immediate treatment (including epinephrine 1:1000) for anaphylactoid and/or hypersensitivity reactions should be available during vaccine use. Oculorespiratory syndrome (ORS) is an acute, self-limiting reaction to IIV with one or more of the following symptoms appearing within 2-24 hours after the dose: Chest tightness, cough, difficulty breathing, facial swelling, red eyes, sore throat, or wheezing. Symptoms resolve within 48 hours of onset. The cause of ORS has not been established, but studies have suggested that it is not IgE-mediated. However, because ORS symptoms may be similar to those of an IgE-mediated hypersensitivity reaction, health care providers unsure of etiology of symptoms should seek advice from an allergist/immunologist when determining whether a patient may be revaccinated in subsequent seasons (CDC, 2013c).

Most products are manufactured with chicken egg protein (expressed as ovalbumin content when content is disclosed on prescribing information). The ovalbumin content may vary from season to season and lot to lot of vaccine. Allergy to eggs must be distinguished from allergy to the vaccine. Recommendations are available from the ACIP and NACI regarding influenza vaccination to persons who report egg allergies; however, ACIP states a prior severe allergic reaction to influenza vaccine, regardless of the component suspected, is a contraindication to vaccination. Patients with a history of egg allergy who have experienced only hives following egg exposure should receive influenza vaccine using IIV (egg- or cell-culture based) or RIV, if otherwise appropriate; however, the vaccine should only be administered by a health care provider familiar with the manifestations of egg allergy and patients be monitored for at least 30 minutes after vaccination (CDC, 2013c). Flucelvax (ccIIV$_3$) is an inactivated influenza vaccine manufactured using cell culture technology and provides an alternative to vaccines cultured with chicken egg protein but should not be considered egg free. It may be used in persons with a mild egg allergy if age appropriate and there are no other contraindications; appropriate precautions should be observed (CDC, 2013c). Some products are manufactured with gentamicin, kanamycin, neomycin, polymyxin or thimerosal; some packaging may contain natural latex rubber

May consider deferring administration in patients with moderate or severe acute illness (with or without fever); may administer to patients with mild acute illness (with or without fever) (CDC, 2011a). Postmarketing reports of increased incidence of fever and febrile seizures in children <5 years of age has been observed with the use of the 2010 Southern Hemisphere formulation of the Afluria vaccine. Febrile events have also been reported in children 5 to <9 years of age. Based on information from the CDC, an increased rate of febrile seizures has been reported in young children 6 months to 4 years who received vaccination with inactivated influenza vaccine (IIV) and the 13-valent pneumococcal conjugate vaccine (PCV13) simultaneously. However, due to the risks associated with delaying either vaccine, administering them at separate visits or deviating from the recommended vaccine schedule is not currently recommended. The ACIP does not recommend use of Afluria in children <9 years of age (CDC, 2013c). Syncope has been reported with use of injectable vaccines and may be accompanied by transient visual disturbances, weakness, or tonic-clonic movements. Procedures should be in place to avoid injuries from falling and to restore cerebral perfusion if syncope occurs (CDC, 2011a).

Use with caution in patients with history of Guillain-Barré syndrome (GBS); patients with history of GBS have a greater likelihood of developing GBS than those without. As a precaution, the ACIP recommends that patients with a history of GBS and who are at low risk for severe influenza complications, and patients known to have experienced GBS within 6 weeks following previous vaccination should generally not be vaccinated (consider influenza antiviral chemoprophylaxis in these patients). The benefits of vaccination may outweigh the potential risks in persons with a history of GBS who are also at high risk for complications of influenza (CDC, 2013c). Some Canadian product labeling recommends delaying therapy in patients with active neurologic disorders.

Use with caution in severely-immunocompromised patients (eg, patients receiving chemo/radiation therapy or other immunosuppressive therapy [including high-dose corticosteroid]); may have a reduced response to vaccination. Inactivated vaccine (IIV or RIV) is preferred over live virus vaccine for household members, healthcare workers and others coming in close contact with severely-immunosuppressed persons requiring care in a protected environment (CDC, 2011a; CDC, 2013c). Antigenic response may not be as great as expected in HIV-infected persons with CD4 cells <100/mm^3 and viral copies of HIV type 1 >30,000/mL, and a second dose does not improve immune response in these persons (CDC, 2013c). Antibody responses may be lower in older adults ≥65 years compared to younger adults (CDC, 2013c). Use of this vaccine for specific medical and/or other indications (eg, immunocompromising conditions, hepatic or kidney disease, diabetes) is also addressed in the ACIP Recommended Immunization Schedule (CDC, 2013a; CDC, 2013b).

Use with caution in patients with a history of bleeding disorders (including thrombocytopenia) and/or patients on anticoagulant therapy; bleeding/hematoma may occur from I.M. administration (CDC, 2011a). In order to maximize vaccination rates, the ACIP, as well as the Canadian National Advisory Committee on Immunization (NACI), recommends simultaneous administration of all age-appropriate vaccines (live or inactivated) for which a person is eligible at a single clinic visit, unless contraindications exist (CDC, 2011a; NACI, 2006). Vaccination may not result in effective immunity in all patients. Response depends upon multiple factors (eg, type of vaccine, age of patient) and may be improved by administering the vaccine at the recommended dose, route, and interval. Vaccines may not be effective if administered during periods of altered immune competence (CDC, 2011a). Influenza vaccines from previous seasons must not be used (CDC, 2013c).

Adverse Reactions All serious adverse reactions must be reported to the U.S. Department of Health and Human Services (DHHS) Vaccine Adverse Event Reporting System (VAERS) 1-800-822-7967 or online at https://vaers.hhs.gov/esub/index. In Canada, adverse reactions may be reported to local provincial/territorial health agencies or to the Vaccine Safety Section at Public Health Agency of Canada (1-866-844-0018).

Frequency not defined. Adverse reactions in adults ≥65 years of age may be greater using the high-dose vaccine, but are typically mild and transient.

Cardiovascular: Chest tightness, facial edema

Central nervous system: Chills, drowsiness, fatigue, fever, headache, irritability, malaise, migraine, shivering

Endocrine & metabolic: Dysmenorrhea

Gastrointestinal: Appetite decreased, diarrhea, nausea, sore throat, upper abdominal pain, vomiting

Local: Injection site reactions (including bruising, erythema, induration, inflammation, pain, soreness [≤64%; may last up to 2 days], pruritus, swelling, tenderness)

Neuromuscular & skeletal: Arthralgia, back pain, myalgia (may start within 6-12 hours and last 1-2 days; incidence generally equal to placebo in adults; occurs more frequently than placebo in children)

Ocular: Red eyes

Otic: Earache

Respiratory: Cough, nasal congestion, nasopharyngitis, pharyngolaryngeal pain, rhinitis, upper respiratory tract infection, wheezing

Miscellaneous: Diaphoresis

Postmarketing and/or case reports (limited to important or life-threatening): Allergic reactions, anaphylaxis, angioedema, convulsions, erythema multiforme, facial palsy (Bell's palsy), Guillain-Barré syndrome (GBS), Henoch-Schönlein purpura (IgA vasculitis), hypersensitivity reaction, limb paralysis, lymphadenopathy, myelitis (including encephalomyelitis and transverse myelitis), neuralgia, oculorespiratory syndrome (ORS; acute, self-limited reaction with ocular and respiratory symptoms), optic neuritis/neuropathy, paralysis, photophobia, serum sickness, Stevens-Johnson syndrome, syncope, tachycardia, thrombocytopenia, urticaria, vasculitis, vertigo

Drug Interactions

Metabolism/Transport Effects None known.

Avoid Concomitant Use There are no known interactions where it is recommended to avoid concomitant use.

Increased Effect/Toxicity There are no known significant interactions involving an increase in effect.

Decreased Effect

Influenza Virus Vaccine (Inactivated) may decrease the levels/effects of: Pneumococcal Conjugate Vaccine (13-Valent)

The levels/effects of Influenza Virus Vaccine (Inactivated) may be decreased by: Belimumab; Fingolimod; Immunosuppressants; Pneumococcal Conjugate Vaccine (13-Valent)

Storage/Stability Store all products between 2°C to 8°C (36°F to 46°F). Potency is destroyed by freezing; do not use if product has been frozen.

Agriflu, Fluad, Fluarix, Fluarix Quadrivalent, Flucelvax: Protect from light.

Afluria, FluLaval, Fluviral: Discard multiple dose vials 28 days after initial entry. Protect from light.

Fluvirin, Fluzone, Flulaval Quadrivalent: Between uses, the multiple dose vial should be stored at 2°C to 8°C (36°F to 46°F). Protect from light.

Vaxigrip: Between uses, the multiple dose vial should be stored at 2°C to 8°C (36°F to 46°F). Discard 7 days after initial entry. Protect from light.

Mechanism of Action Promotes immunity to seasonal influenza virus by inducing specific antibody production. Each year the formulation is standardized according to the U.S. Public Health Service. Preparations from previous seasons must not be used.

Pharmacodynamics/Kinetics

Onset of action: Most adults have antibody protection within 2 weeks of vaccination (CDC, 2013c)

Duration: ≥6-8 months when vaccine is antigenically similar to circulating virus; response may be diminished in persons ≥65 years and limited evidence suggests titers may decline significantly 6 months following vaccination in this population (CDC, 2013c)

Dosage It is important to note that influenza seasons vary in their timing and duration from year to year. In general, vaccination should begin soon after the vaccine becomes available (and, if possible, by October) and prior to onset of influenza activity in the community. However, vaccination should continue throughout the influenza season as long as vaccine is available. Unless noted, the ACIP does not have a preference for any given IIV formulation when used within their specified age indications.

Fluarix, Fluarix Quadrivalent, FluLaval, FluLaval Quadrivalent: I.M.:

Children 3-8 years: 0.5 mL/dose (1 or 2 doses per season; see **"Note"**)

Children ≥9 years years, Adolescents, and Adults: 0.5 mL/dose (1 dose per season)

Fluzone, Fluzone Quadrivalent: I.M.:

Children 6-35 months: 0.25 mL/dose (1 or 2 doses per season; see **"Note"**)

Children 3-8 years: 0.5 mL/dose (1 or 2 doses per season; see **"Note"**)

Children ≥9 years years, Adolescents, and Adults: 0.5 mL/dose (1 dose per season)

Fluzone High-Dose: I.M.: Adults ≥65 years: 0.5 mL/dose (1 dose per season)

Fluvirin: I.M.:

Children 4-8 years: 0.5 mL/dose (1 or 2 doses per season; see **"Note"**)

Children ≥9 years years, Adolescents, and Adults: 0.5 mL/dose (1 dose per season)

Afluria: I.M.: Although FDA-approved for use in children ≥5 years of age, the ACIP does not recommend use of Afluria in children <9 years due to an increased incidence of fever and febrile seizures noted during the 2010-2011 influenza season. However, if other age-appropriate vaccines are not available, children 5-8 years of age who are also considered at risk for influenza complications may be given Afluria. The benefits and risks of this vaccine should be discussed with parents or caregivers prior to administration (CDC, 2013c).

Children 5-8 years: 0.5 mL/dose (1 or 2 doses per season; see **"Note"**)

Children ≥9 years, Adolescents, and Adults: 0.5 mL/dose (1 dose per season)

Flucelvax: I.M.: Adults: 0.5 mL/dose (1 dose per season)

Fluzone Intradermal: Adults 18-64 years of age: 0.1 mL/dose (1 dose per season)

Canadian labeling (products not available in U.S.):

Agriflu, Fluviral, Vaxigrip: I.M.:

Children 6-35 months: Manufacturer labeling: 0.25 mL/dose; NACI recommendation: 0.5 mL/dose (NACI, 2011) (1 or 2 doses per season; see **Note**)

Children 3-8 years: 0.5 mL/dose (1 or 2 doses per season; see **"Note"**)

Children ≥9 years, Adolescents, and Adults: 0.5 mL/dose (1 dose per season)

Fluad: I.M.: Adults ≥65 years: 0.5 mL/dose (1 dose per season)

Influvac: I.M., SubQ: Adults: 0.5 mL/dose (1 per season).

Intanza 9 mcg/strain: Intradermal: Adults 18-59 years: 0.1 mL/dose (1 per season)

Intanza 15 mcg/strain: Intradermal: Adults ≥60 years: 0.1 mL/dose (1 per season)

Note: Children 6 months to <9 years who received a total of ≥2 doses of seasonal influenza vaccine since July 1, 2010, need only 1 dose of the 2013-2014 seasonal influenza vaccine. If a child did not receive a total of ≥2 doses of seasonal vaccine since July 1, 2010, if they have never received seasonal influenza vaccine (ie, this is their first season of vaccination), or if their vaccination status cannot be determined, they should receive 2 doses separated by ≥4 weeks, in order to achieve satisfactory antibody response. Additional dosing considerations are provided when vaccination history is available prior to the 2010-2011 season; see current guidelines for additional information (CDC, 2013c).

Dosage adjustment in renal impairment: No dosage adjustment provided in manufacturer's labeling.

Dosage adjustment in hepatic impairment: No dosage adjustment provided in manufacturer's labeling.

Administration

Fluzone Intradermal, Intanza (Canadian availability): For intradermal administration over the deltoid muscle only. Fluzone Intradermal should be shaken gently prior to use. Intanza should not be shaken prior to use. Hold system using the thumb and middle finger (do not place fingers on windows). Insert needle perpendicular to the skin; inject using index finger to push on plunger. Do not aspirate.

Afluria, Fluarix, Fluarix Quadrivalent, Flucelvax, FluLaval, FluLaval Quadrivalent, Fluvirin, Fluzone, Fluzone High-Dose, Fluzone Quadrivalent, Agriflu (Canadian availability), Fluad (Canadian availability), Fluviral (Canadian availability), Vaxigrip (Canadian availability): For I.M. administration only. Inspect for particulate matter and discoloration prior to administration. Adults and older children should be vaccinated in the deltoid muscle using a ≥1 inch needle length. Young children (≥6 months to <12 months of age) should be vaccinated in the anterolateral aspect of the thigh using a 1 inch needle length. Children ≥1 years with adequate deltoid muscle mass should be vaccinated using a 1 inch needle. A ⅝-inch needle may be adequate in younger children (refer to guidelines) (CDC, 2011a; CDC, 2013c). Do not inject into the gluteal region or areas where there may be a major nerve trunk. Suspensions should be shaken well prior to use. Some manufacturers recommend avoiding use if visible particles are present in the suspension after shaking. See manufacturer labeling for specific recommendations.

Influvac (Canadian availability): May be administered by I.M. or deep subcutaneous injection. Shake well prior to use.

Unless otherwise indicated in product labeling, jet injectors should **not** be used to administer inactivated influenza vaccines. Currently, there are no influenza vaccines licensed in the United States that can be given by a jet-injector device (2013c).

If a pediatric vaccine (0.25 mL) is inadvertently administered to an adult, an additional 0.25 mL should be administered to provide the full adult dose (0.5 mL). If the error is discovered after the patient has left, an adult dose should be given as soon as the patient can return. If an adult vaccine (0.5 mL) is inadvertently given to a child, no action needs to be taken (CDC, 2013c). *Agriflu (Canadian availability):* If 0.25 mL dose is to be given, discard half the contained syringe volume prior to administration.

Note: For patients at risk of hemorrhage following intramuscular injection, the ACIP recommends "it should be administered intramuscularly if, in the opinion of the physician familiar with the patient's bleeding risk, the vaccine can be administered by this route with reasonable safety. If the patient receives antihemophilia or other similar therapy, intramuscular vaccination can be scheduled shortly after such therapy is administered. A fine needle (23 gauge or smaller) can be used for the vaccination and firm pressure applied to the site (without rubbing) for at least 2 minutes. The patient should be instructed concerning the risk of hematoma from the injection." Patients on anticoagulant therapy should be considered to have the same bleeding risks and treated as those with clotting factor disorders (CDC, 2011a).

Simultaneous administration of vaccines helps ensure the patients will be fully vaccinated by the appropriate age. Simultaneous administration of vaccines is defined as administering >1 vaccine on the same day at different anatomic sites. Separate vaccines should not be combined in the same syringe unless indicated by product specific labeling. Separate needles and syringes should be used for each injection. However, in general, vaccination should not be deferred if the brand name or route of the previous dose is not available or not known (CDC, 2011a). Adolescents and adults should be vaccinated while seated or lying down. In general, preterm infants should be vaccinated at the same chronological age as full-term infants (CDC, 2011a).

Antipyretics have not been shown to prevent febrile seizures. Antipyretics may be used to treat fever or discomfort following vaccination (CDC, 2011b). One study reported that routine prophylactic administration of acetaminophen to prevent fever prior to vaccination decreased the immune response of some vaccines; the clinical significance of this reduction in immune response has not been established (Prymula, 2009).

Monitoring Parameters Monitor for syncope for 15 minutes following administration. If seizure-like activity associated with syncope occurs, maintain patient in supine or Trendelenburg position to reestablish adequate cerebral perfusion (CDC, 2011a). For those individuals who report a history of egg allergy but it is determined that the inactivated vaccine can be used, observe vaccine recipient for at least 30 minutes after receipt of vaccine (CDC, 2013c).

Additional Information Pharmacies will stock the formulations(s) standardized according to the USPHS requirements for the season. Influenza vaccines from previous seasons must not be used. U.S. federal law requires that the name of medication, date of administration, the vaccine manufacturer, lot number of vaccine, and the administering person's name, title, and address, and documentation of the vaccine information statement (VIS; date on VIS and date given to patient) be entered into the patient's permanent medical record.

It is important to note that influenza seasons vary in their timing and duration from year to year. In general, vaccination should begin soon after the vaccine becomes available and prior to onset of influenza activity in the community. However, vaccination should continue throughout the influenza season as long as vaccine is available.

Seasonal quadrivalent influenza vaccines contain two subtype A strains and two subtype B strains; trivalent influenza vaccines contain two subtype A strains and one subtype B strain.

When vaccine supply is not limited, either IIV or LAIV can be used in healthy, nonpregnant persons aged 2-49 years of age. RIV can be used in persons 18-49 years of age.

When vaccine supply is limited, administration should focus on the ACIP target groups. When IIV vaccine is in short supply, administering LAIV to eligible persons is encouraged to increase available IIV to those patients in whom LAIV cannot be used. During periods of inactivated influenza vaccine (IIV) shortage, the CDC and ACIP have recommended vaccination be prioritized based on the following three tiers. The grouping is based on influenza associated mortality and hospitalization rates. Those listed in group 1 should be vaccinated first, followed by persons in group 2, and then group 3. If the vaccine supply is extremely limited, group 1 has also been subdivided in three tiers, where those in group 1A should be vaccinated first, followed by 1B, then 1C.

Priority groups for vaccination with inactivated seasonal influenza vaccine during periods of vaccine shortage (CDC, 2005):

Tier 1A:
- Persons ≥65 years with comorbid conditions
- Residents of long-term-care facilities

Tier 1B:
- Persons 2-64 years with comorbid conditions
- Persons ≥65 years without comorbid conditions
- Children 6-23 months
- Pregnant women

Tier 1C:
- Healthcare personnel
- Household contacts and out-of-home caregivers of children <6 months

Tier 2:
- Household contacts of children and adults at increased risk of influenza-associated complications
- Healthy persons 50-64 years

Tier 3:
- Persons 2-49 years without high-risk conditions

Further information available at http://www.cdc.gov/mmwr/preview/mmwrhtml/mm5430a4.htm

Dosage Forms Excipient information presented when available (limited, particularly for generics); consult specific product labeling. [DSC] = Discontinued product

Device, Intradermal [preservative free]:
- Fluzone: 9 mcg/strain (0.1 mL [DSC]) [latex free; contains egg white (egg protein)]
- Fluzone: 9 mcg/strain (0.1 mL); 9 mcg/strain (0.1 mL) [contains egg white (egg protein)]

Injectable, Intramuscular:
- Flulaval: (5 mL) [contains egg white (egg protein), thimerosal]
- Fluvirin: (5 mL) [contains egg white (egg protein), neomycin, thimerosal]
- Fluzone: (5 mL) [contains egg white (egg protein), gelatin (pork), thimerosal]

Kit, Intramuscular:
- Physicians EZ Use Flu: [contains egg white (egg protein), neomycin, thimerosal]

Kit, Intramuscular [preservative free]:
- Medical Provider EZ Flu PF: [contains egg white (egg protein), neomycin]

Suspension, Intramuscular:
- Afluria: (5 mL) [contains egg white (egg protein), neomycin sulfate, thimerosal]
- Flulaval Quadrivalent: (5 mL) [contains egg white (egg protein), polysorbate 80, thimerosal]

Suspension, Intramuscular [preservative free]:
- Afluria Preservative Free: (0.5 mL) [contains egg white (egg protein), neomycin sulfate]
- Fluarix: (0.5 mL) [contains egg white (egg protein), polysorbate 80]
- Fluarix Quadrivalent: 0.5 mL (0.5 mL) [contains egg white (egg protein)]
- Flucelvax: (0.5 mL) [contains polysorbate 80]
- Fluvirin Preservative Free: (0.5 mL) [contains egg white (egg protein), neomycin]
- Fluzone High-Dose: (0.5 mL) [contains egg white (egg protein)]
- Fluzone Pediatric PF: (0.25 mL) [contains egg white (egg protein), gelatin (pork)]
- Fluzone Preservative Free: (0.5 mL) [contains egg white (egg protein), gelatin (pork)]
- Fluzone Quadrivalent: 0.25 mL (0.25 mL); 0.5 mL (0.5 mL) [contains egg white (egg protein)]

Dosage Forms: Canada Excipient information presented when available (limited, particularly for generics); consult specific product labeling.

Injection, suspension:
- Fluviral: Hemagglutinin 45 mcg/0.5 mL (5 mL) [contains chicken egg protein, thimerosal]
- Vaxigrip: Hemagglutinin 45 mcg/0.5 mL (5 mL) [contains chicken egg protein, neomycin (may have trace amounts), thimerosal]

Injection, suspension [preservative free]:
- Agriflu: Hemagglutinin 45 mcg/0.5 mL (0.5 mL) [contains chicken egg protein, neomycin (may have trace amounts), kanamycin (may have trace amounts), polysorbate 80]
- Fluad: Hemagglutinin 45 mcg/0.5 mL (0.5 mL) [contains chicken egg protein, neomycin (may have trace amounts), kanamycin (may have trace amounts), polysorbate 80]
- Influvac: Hemagglutinin 45 mcg/0.5 mL (0.5 mL) [contains chicken egg protein, gentamicin (may have trace amounts), polysorbate 80]
- Intanza: Hemagglutinin 27 mcg/0.1 mL (0.1 mL) [contains chicken egg protein, neomycin (may have trace amounts)]
- Intanza: Hemagglutinin 45 mcg/0.1 mL (0.1 mL) [contains chicken egg protein, neomycin (may have trace amounts)]
- Vaxigrip: Hemagglutinin 45 mcg/0.5 mL (0.25 mL, 0.5 mL) [contains chicken egg protein, neomycin (may have trace amounts)]

Influenza Virus Vaccine (Live/Attenuated)

(in floo EN za VYE rus vak SEEN live ah TEN yoo aye ted)

Brand Names: U.S. FluMist; FluMist Quadrivalent

Brand Names: Canada FluMist®

Index Terms H1N1 Influenza Vaccine; Influenza Vaccine; Influenza Virus Vaccine (Trivalent, Live); LAIV; $LAIV_4$; Live Attenuated Influenza Vaccine; Live Attenuated Influenza Vaccine (Quadrivalent)

Pharmacologic Category Vaccine, Live (Viral)

Additional Appendix Information

Immunization Administration Recommendations *on page 2334*

Immunization Recommendations *on page 2339*

Use For the active immunization against influenza disease caused by influenza virus subtypes A and type B contained in the vaccine.

The Advisory Committee on Immunization Practices (ACIP) recommends routine annual vaccination with seasonal influenza vaccine for all persons who do not otherwise have contraindications to the vaccine. ACIP recommends use of any age and risk factor appropriate product. Healthy, nonpregnant persons aged 2-49 years may receive vaccination with the seasonal live, attenuated influenza vaccine (LAIV) (nasal spray). In addition, other alternative products are available for certain patient populations: Persons ≥6 months of age may receive the trivalent inactivated influenza vaccine (IIV_3) or the quadrivalent inactivated influenza vaccine (IIV_4). Persons 18-49 years may also receive vaccination with the recombinant influenza vaccine (RIV) (CDC, 2013c).

Pregnancy Risk Factor B

Pregnancy Considerations Adverse events were not observed in animal reproduction studies. LAIV is not recommended for use during pregnancy. Influenza vaccination with the inactivated influenza vaccine (IIV) is recommended for all women who are or will become pregnant during the influenza season and who do not otherwise have contraindications to the vaccine (CDC, 2013c).

Healthy pregnant women do not need to avoid contact with persons vaccinated with LAIV (CDC, 2013). The nasal vaccine contains the same strains of influenza A and B found in the injection. Information specific to the use of LAIV in pregnancy has not been located. Refer to the Influenza Virus Vaccine (Inactivated) monograph for additional information.

Healthcare providers are encouraged to refer women exposed to the influenza vaccine during pregnancy to the Vaccines and Medications in Pregnancy Surveillance System (VAMPSS) by contacting The Organization of Teratology Information Specialists (OTIS) at (877) 311-8972.

Breast-Feeding Considerations It is not known if the vaccine is excreted into breast milk. LAIV should be used with caution in breast-feeding women (per manufacturer) due to the possibility of virus excretion into breast milk; however, LAIV may be administered to breast-feeding women unless contraindicated due to other reasons (per CDC). Postpartum women may be vaccinated with either IIV or LAIV. When vaccine supply is limited, focus on delivering the vaccine should be given to mothers of newborns and contacts or caregivers of children <5 years of age (CDC, 2013).

Contraindications Severe allergic reaction (eg, anaphylaxis) to previous influenza vaccination; hypersensitivity to any component of the formulation; children or adolescents 2-17 years of age receiving aspirin therapy

Warnings/Precautions Immediate treatment (including epinephrine 1:1000) for anaphylactoid and/or hypersensitivity reactions should be available during vaccine use. Manufactured with chicken egg protein. Allergy to eggs must be distinguished from allergy to the vaccine. Recommendations are available from the CDC regarding influenza vaccination to persons who report egg allergies; however, a prior severe allergic reaction to influenza vaccine, regardless of the component suspected, is a contraindication to vaccination. ACIP recommends use of IIV or RIV (if RIV is age appropriate) over LAIV when considering vaccination in persons reporting an egg allergy (due to lack of data of LAIV use in this setting) (CDC, 2013c). Also manufactured with arginine, gelatin, and gentamicin.

Use with caution in patients with history of Guillain-Barré syndrome (GBS); patients with history of GBS have a greater likelihood of developing GBS than those without. As a precaution, the ACIP recommends that patients with a history of GBS and who are at low risk for severe influenza complications, and patients known to have experienced GBS within 6 weeks following previous vaccination should generally not be vaccinated (consider influenza antiviral chemoprophylaxis in these patients). Based on limited data, the benefits of vaccinating persons with a history of GBS who are also at high risk for complications of influenza may outweigh the risks (CDC, 2013c).

Data on the use of the nasal spray in immunocompromised patients is limited. **Avoid contact with severely immunocompromised individuals for at least 7 days following vaccination (at least 14 days per Canadian labeling).** ACIP does not recommend the use of LAIV in immunosuppressed patients (CDC, 2013c). ACIP does not recommend the use of LAIV for persons who care for severely immunocompromised individuals who require a protective environment due to the theoretical risk of transmitting the live virus from the vaccine. Persons who care for the severely immunocompromised should receive either IIV or RIV. Persons who have received LAIV should avoid contact with severely immunocompromised individuals for at least 7 days following vaccination (at least 14 days per Canadian labeling) (CDC, 2013c).

Per the U.S. prescribing information, the nasal spray should not be used in patients with asthma or children <5 years of age with recurrent wheezing; risk of wheezing following vaccination is increased. Patients with severe asthma or active wheezing were not included in clinical trials. Children <24 months of age had increased wheezing and hospitalizations following administration in clinical trials; use of the nasal spray is not approved in this age group. ACIP does not recommend the use of LAIV in patients with chronic pulmonary disorders including asthma and children 2-4 years of age who have had asthma or wheezing episodes within the past year (CDC, 2013c).

May consider deferring administration in patients with moderate or severe acute illness (with or without fever); may administer to patients with mild acute illness (with or without fever) (CDC, 2011). ACIP does not recommend the use of LAIV in patients with chronic disorders of the cardiovascular system (except isolated hypertension), chronic metabolic diseases, hematologic disorders and hemoglobinopathies, hepatic disease, persons with HIV, neurologic or neuromuscular disorders, renal disease, or pregnant women (CDC, 2013c). Use of this vaccine for specific medical and/or other indications (eg, immunocompromising conditions, hepatic or kidney disease, diabetes) is also addressed in the ACIP Recommended Immunization Schedule (CDC, 2013a; CDC, 2013b).

Defer immunization if nasal congestion is present which may impede delivery of vaccine (CDC, 2013c). In order to maximize vaccination rates, the ACIP recommends simultaneous administration of all age-appropriate vaccines (live or inactivated) for which a person is eligible at a single clinic visit, unless contraindications exist (CDC, 2011).

Studies conducted in children using trivalent IIV and LAIV have shown significantly greater efficacy of LAIV in younger children. Information is not yet available for the quadrivalent LAIV vaccine (CDC, 2013c). The safety and efficacy of the nasal spray have not been established in adults ≥50 years of age (U.S. labeling) or ≥60 years of age (Canadian labeling). Vaccination may not result in effective immunity in all patients. Response depends upon multiple factors (eg, type of vaccine, age of patient) and may be improved by administering the vaccine at the recommended dose, route, and interval. Vaccines may not be effective if administered during periods of altered immune competence (CDC, 2011). Influenza vaccines from previous seasons must not be used (CDC, 2013c).

Adverse Reactions All serious adverse reactions must be reported to the U.S. Department of Health and Human Services (DHHS) Vaccine Adverse Event Reporting System (VAERS) 1-800-822-7967 or online at https://vaers.hhs.gov/esub/index. In Canada, adverse reactions may be reported to local provincial/territorial health agencies or to the Vaccine Safety Section at Public Health Agency of Canada (1-866-844-0018).

Frequency of events reported within 10 days.

>10%:

Central nervous system: Headache (children 3% to 9%; adults 40%), irritability (children 12% to 21%), lethargy (children 7% to 14%)

Gastrointestinal: Appetite decreased (children 13% to 21%), abdominal pain (children 2% to 12%)

Neuromuscular & skeletal: Tiredness/weakness (adults 26%), muscle aches (children 2% to 6%; adults 17%)

Respiratory: Cough (adults 14%), nasal congestion/runny nose (children 51% to 58%; adults 9% to 44%), sore throat (children 5% to 11%; adults 28%)

1% to 10%:

Central nervous system: Chills (children 2% to 4%, adults 9%), fever (100°F to 101°F: children 6% to 9%; >101°F: children 1% to 4%)

Otic: Otitis media (children 3%)

Respiratory: Sinusitis (adults 4%), sneezing (children 2%), wheezing (children 6-23 months 6%; children 24-59 months 2%)

Postmarketing and/or case reports: Anaphylactic reactions, asthma exacerbations, Bell's palsy, encephalitis (vaccine associated), epistaxis, Guillain-Barré syndrome, hypersensitivity reaction, meningitis (including eosinophilic meningitis), mitochondrial encephalomyopathy (Leigh syndrome) exacerbation, pericarditis

Drug Interactions

Metabolism/Transport Effects None known.

Avoid Concomitant Use

Avoid concomitant use of Influenza Virus Vaccine (Live/Attenuated) with any of the following: Belimumab; Fingolimod; Immunosuppressants; Salicylates

Increased Effect/Toxicity

Influenza Virus Vaccine (Live/Attenuated) may increase the levels/effects of: Salicylates

The levels/effects of Influenza Virus Vaccine (Live/Attenuated) may be increased by: AzaTHIOprine; Belimumab; Corticosteroids (Systemic); Dimethyl Fumarate; Fingolimod; Hydroxychloroquine; Immunosuppressants; Leflunomide; Mercaptopurine; Methotrexate

Decreased Effect

Influenza Virus Vaccine (Live/Attenuated) may decrease the levels/effects of: Tuberculin Tests

The levels/effects of Influenza Virus Vaccine (Live/Attenuated) may be decreased by: Antiviral Agents (Influenza A and B); Dimethyl Fumarate; Fingolimod; Immune Globulins; Immunosuppressants

Storage/Stability Store in refrigerator at 2°C to 8°C (36°F to 46°F). **Do not freeze.**

Mechanism of Action The vaccine contains live attenuated viruses which infect and replicate within the cells lining the nasopharynx. Promotes immunity to seasonal influenza virus by inducing specific antibody production. Each year the formulation is standardized according to the U.S. Public Health Service. Preparations from previous seasons must not be used.

Pharmacodynamics/Kinetics

Onset of action: Most adults have antibody protection within 2 weeks of vaccination (CDC, 2013c)

Duration: ≥6-8 months when vaccine is antigenically similar to circulating virus; response may be diminished in persons ≥65 years and limited evidence suggests titers may decline significantly 6 months following vaccination in this population (CDC, 2013c)

Distribution: Following nasal administration, vaccine is distributed in the nasal cavity (~90%), stomach (~3%), brain (~2%), and lung (0.4%)

Dosage It is important to note that influenza seasons vary in their timing and duration from year to year. In general, vaccination should begin soon after the vaccine becomes available (and, if possible, by October) and prior to onset of influenza activity in the community. However, vaccination should continue throughout the influenza season as long as vaccine is available (CDC, 2013c).

Intranasal (FluMist):

U.S. labeling:

Children 2-8 years: 0.2 mL/dose (1 or 2 doses per season; see **"Note"**)

Children ≥9 years, Adolescents, and Adults ≤49 years: 0.2 mL/dose (1 dose per season)

Elderly: Not indicated for use in patients ≥50 years

Canadian labeling:

Children 2-8 years: 0.2 mL/dose (1 or 2 doses per season; see **"Note"**)

Children ≥9 years, Adolescents, and Adults ≤59 years: 0.2 mL/dose (1 dose per season)

Elderly: Not indicated for use in patients ≥60 years

Note: Children 6 months to <9 years who received a total of ≥2 doses of seasonal influenza vaccine since July 1, 2010, need only 1 dose of the 2013-2014 seasonal influenza vaccine. If a child did not receive a total of ≥2 doses of seasonal vaccine since July 1, 2010, if they have never received seasonal influenza vaccine, (ie, this is their first season of vaccination), or if their vaccination status cannot be determined, they should receive 2 doses separated by ≥4 weeks, in order to achieve satisfactory antibody response. Additional dosing considerations are provided when vaccination history is available prior to the 2010-2011 season; see current guidelines for additional information (CDC, 2013c).

Dosage adjustment in renal impairment: No dosage adjustment provided in manufacturer's labeling.

Dosage adjustment in hepatic impairment: No dosage adjustment provided in manufacturer's labeling.

Administration LAIV: Intranasal: For intranasal administration only; do not inject. Half the dose (0.1 mL) is administered to each nostril; patient should be in upright position. A dose divider clip is provided to allow administration of 0.1 mL into each nostril. Place the tip of the sprayer inside the nostril and depress plunger as rapidly as possible to deliver the dose. Remove dose divider clip and repeat into opposite nostril. The patient does not need to inhale during administration (may breath normally). Severely immunocompromised persons should not administer the live vaccine. If recipient sneezes following administration, the dose should not be repeated. Defer immunization if nasal congestion is present which may impede delivery of vaccine (CDC, 2013c).

Simultaneous administration of vaccines helps ensure the patients will be fully vaccinated by the appropriate age. Simultaneous administration of vaccines is defined as administering >1 vaccine on the same day at different anatomic sites. The ACIP prefers each dose of a specific vaccine in a series come from the same manufacturer when possible. However, in general, vaccination should not be deferred if the brand name or route of the previous dose is not available or not known (CDC, 2011).

Antipyretics have not been shown to prevent febrile seizures. Antipyretics may be used to treat fever or discomfort following vaccination (CDC, 2011). One study reported that routine prophylactic administration of acetaminophen to prevent fever prior to vaccination decreased the immune response of some vaccines; the clinical significance of this reduction in immune response has not been established (Prymula, 2009). Aspirin-containing products should be avoided for 4 weeks following vaccination in children and adolescents ≤17 years of age.

Vaccine administration with oral influenza antiviral medications: Live influenza virus vaccine (LAIV) should not be given until 48 hours after the completion of influenza antiviral therapy (influenza A and B). Influenza antiviral therapy (influenza A and B) should not be administered for 2 weeks after receiving LAIV. If influenza antiviral therapy (influenza A and B) and LAIV are administered concomitantly, revaccination should be considered.

Test Interactions Administration of the intranasal influenza virus vaccine (live, LAIV) may cause a positive result on the rapid influenza diagnostic test for the 7 days after vaccine administration; for a person with influenza-like illness during this time, the positive test could be caused by either the live attenuated vaccine or wild-type influenza virus (Aly, 2004).

Additional Information Pharmacies will stock the formulations(s) standardized according to the USPHS requirements for the season. Influenza vaccines from previous seasons must not be used. U.S. federal law requires that the name of medication, date of administration, the vaccine manufacturer, lot number of vaccine, and the administering person's name, title, and address, and documentation of the vaccine information statement (VIS; date on VIS and date given to patient) be entered into the patient's permanent medical record.

It is important to note that influenza seasons vary in their timing and duration from year to year. In general, vaccination should begin soon after the vaccine becomes available and prior to onset of influenza activity in the community. However, vaccination should continue throughout the influenza season as long as vaccine is available.

Seasonal quadrivalent influenza vaccines contain two subtype A strains and two subtype B strains; trivalent influenza vaccines contain two subtype A strains and one subtype B strain.

When vaccine supply is not limited, either IIV or LAIV can be used in healthy, nonpregnant persons aged 2-49 years of age. RIV can be used in persons 18-49 years of age.

When vaccine supply is limited, administration should focus on the ACIP target groups. When IIV vaccine is in short supply, administering LAIV to eligible persons is encouraged to increase available IIV to those patients in whom LAIV cannot be used. During periods of inactivated influenza vaccine (IIV) shortage, the CDC and ACIP have recommended vaccination be prioritized based on the following three tiers. The grouping is based on influenza-associated mortality and hospitalization rates. Those listed in group 1 should be vaccinated first, followed by persons in group 2, and then group 3. If the vaccine supply is extremely limited, group 1 has also been subdivided in three tiers, where those in group 1A should be vaccinated first, followed by 1B, then 1C.

Priority groups for vaccination with inactivated seasonal influenza vaccine during periods of vaccine shortage (CDC, 2005):

Tier 1A:
- Persons ≥65 years with comorbid conditions
- Residents of long-term-care facilities

Tier 1B:
- Persons 2-64 years with comorbid conditions
- Persons ≥65 years without comorbid conditions
- Children 6-23 months
- Pregnant women

Tier 1C:
- Healthcare personnel
- Household contacts and out-of-home caregivers of children <6 months

Tier 2:
- Household contacts of children and adults at increased risk of influenza-associated complications
- Healthy persons 50-64 years

Tier 3:
- Persons 2-49 years without high-risk conditions

Further information available at http://www.cdc.gov/mmwr/preview/mmwrhtml/mm5430a4.htm

Dosage Forms Excipient information presented when available (limited, particularly for generics); consult specific product labeling.

Liquid, Nasal [preservative free]:
FluMist: (1 ea) [contains egg white (egg protein), gelatin (pork)]

Suspension, Nasal [preservative free]:
FluMist Quadrivalent: (1 ea) [latex free; contains egg white (egg protein), gelatin (pork)]

◆ **Influenza Virus Vaccine (Monovalent)** *see* Influenza Virus Vaccine (H5N1) *on page 1076*

◆ **Influenza Virus Vaccine (Purified Surface Antigen)** *see* Influenza Virus Vaccine (Inactivated) *on page 1078*

◆ **Influenza Virus Vaccine (Split-Virus)** *see* Influenza Virus Vaccine (Inactivated) *on page 1078*

◆ **Influenza Virus Vaccine (Trivalent, Live)** *see* Influenza Virus Vaccine (Live/Attenuated) *on page 1082*

◆ **Influvac (Can)** *see* Influenza Virus Vaccine (Inactivated) *on page 1078*

◆ **Infufer (Can)** *see* Iron Dextran Complex *on page 1119*

◆ **Infumorph 200** *see* Morphine (Systemic) *on page 1398*

◆ **Infumorph 500** *see* Morphine (Systemic) *on page 1398*

Ingenol Mebutate (IN je nol MEB u tate)

Brand Names: U.S. Picato

Index Terms *Euphorbia peplus* Derivative; PEP005

Pharmacologic Category Topical Skin Product

Use Topical treatment of actinic keratosis

Pregnancy Risk Factor C

Pregnancy Considerations Adverse events were observed in some animal reproduction studies following I.V. administration of ingenol mebutate. Absorption is limited in humans following topical application.

Breast-Feeding Considerations Excretion into breast milk is unknown; absorption is limited following topical application

Contraindications There are no contraindications listed in the manufacturer's labeling.

Warnings/Precautions Severe dermatologic reactions including erythema, crusting, swelling, vesiculation/pustulation, and erosion/ulceration can occur. Severe eye pain, eyelid edema, eyelid ptosis, and periorbital edema can occur after exposure; avoid contact with the periocular area (patients should wash hands immediately after applying and avoid transferring to the eye area).

Apply to intact and nonirritated skin only. Instruct patients to wash hands well after applying and to avoid contact with the periocular area during and after application. Avoid touching the treated area for 6 hours after application. If inadvertent exposure to other area(s) occurs, flush the area with water and seek medical care as soon as possible. Avoid inadvertent transfer to other individuals. Administration of ingenol mebutate gel is not recommended until the skin is healed from any previous drug or surgical treatment. For topical use only; not for oral, ophthalmic, or intravaginal use.

Adverse Reactions

>10%: Dermatologic: Erythema (92% to 94%), flaking/scaling (85% to 90%), crusting (74% to 80%), swelling (64% to 79%), vesiculation/pustulation (44% to 56%), erosion/ulceration (26% to 32%), application site pain (2% to 15%)

1% to 10%:
Central nervous system: Headache (2%)
Dermatologic: Application site pruritus (8%), application site irritation (4%), application site infection (3%)
Ocular: Periorbital edema (3%)
Respiratory: Nasopharyngitis (2%)
<1% (Limited to important or life-threatening): Eyelid edema, eye pain, conjunctivitis

Drug Interactions

Metabolism/Transport Effects None known.

Avoid Concomitant Use There are no known interactions where it is recommended to avoid concomitant use.

Increased Effect/Toxicity There are no known significant interactions involving an increase in effect.

Decreased Effect There are no known significant interactions involving a decrease in effect.

Storage/Stability Store in a refrigerator at 2°C to 8°C (36°F to 46°F); excursions are permitted to 0°C to 15°C (32°F to 59°F); do not freeze. Discard tubes after single use.

Mechanism of Action Ingenol mebutate appears to induce primary necrosis of actinic keratosis with a subsequent neutrophil-mediated inflammatory response with antibody-dependent cytotoxicity of residual disease cells; killing residual disease cells may prevent future relapse.

Pharmacodynamics/Kinetics Absorption: Absorption through the skin is minimal (with proper use); expected systemic exposure is <0.1 ng/mL.

Dosage Topical: Adults: Actinic keratoses:
Face and scalp: Apply 0.015% gel once daily to affected area for 3 consecutive days
Trunk/extremities: Apply 0.05% gel once daily to affected area for 2 consecutive days

Administration Apply to one contiguous affected area of skin using one unit-dose tube; one unit-dose tube will cover ~5 cm x 5 cm (~25 cm^2 or ~2 inch x 2 inch). Spread evenly then allow gel to dry for 15 minutes. Do not cover with bandages or occlusive dressings. Wash hands immediately after applying and avoid transferring gel to any other areas. Avoid washing or touching the treatment area for at least 6 hours, and following this period of time, patients may wash the area with a mild soap. Not for oral, ophthalmic, or intravaginal use.

Dosage Forms Excipient information presented when available (limited, particularly for generics); consult specific product labeling.
Gel, External:
Picato: 0.015% (3 ea); 0.05% (2 ea) [contains benzyl alcohol, isopropyl alcohol]

◆ INH *see* Isoniazid *on page* 1123
◆ Injectafer *see* Ferric Carboxymaltose *on page* 852
◆ Inlyta® *see* Axitinib *on page* 204
◆ Inlyta *see* Axitinib *on page* 204
◆ Innohep® (Can) *see* Tinzaparin *on page* 2066
◆ InnoPran XL *see* Propranolol *on page* 1737
◆ Insoluble Prussian Blue *see* Ferric Hexacyanoferrate *on page* 853
◆ Inspra *see* Eplerenone *on page* 721
◆ Inspra™ (Can) *see* Eplerenone *on page* 721
◆ Instacort 5 [OTC] *see* Hydrocortisone (Topical) *on page* 1011
◆ Instacort 10 [OTC] *see* Hydrocortisone (Topical) *on page* 1011

Insulin Aspart (IN soo lin AS part)

Brand Names: U.S. NovoLOG; NovoLOG FlexPen; NovoLOG PenFill

Brand Names: Canada NovoRapid®

Index Terms Aspart Insulin

Pharmacologic Category Insulin, Rapid-Acting

Additional Appendix Information
Insulin Products *on page* 2303

Use Treatment of type 1 diabetes mellitus (insulin dependent, IDDM) and type 2 diabetes mellitus (noninsulin dependent, NIDDM) to improve glycemic control

Unlabeled Use Diabetic ketoacidosis (DKA) (mild-to-moderate); gestational diabetes mellitus (GDM); hyperglycemia during critical illness; hyperosmolar hyperglycemic state (HHS) (mild-to-moderate)

Pregnancy Risk Factor B

Dosage Note: Insulin aspart is a rapid-acting insulin analog which is normally administered SubQ as a premeal component of the insulin regimen or as a continuous SubQ infusion and should be used with intermediate- or long-acting insulin. When compared to insulin regular, insulin aspart has a more rapid onset and shorter duration of activity. In carefully controlled clinical settings with close medical supervision and monitoring of blood glucose and potassium, insulin aspart may also be administered I.V. Insulin requirements vary dramatically between patients and dictate frequent monitoring and close medical supervision.

Diabetes mellitus: SubQ:

General insulin dosing:

Type 1: Children ≥2 years, Adolescents, and Adults: **Note:** Multiple daily doses or continuous subcutaneous infusions guided by blood glucose monitoring are the standard of diabetes care. Combinations of insulin formulations are commonly used. The daily doses presented below are expressed as the **total units/kg/day of all insulin formulations combined.**

Initial total insulin dose: 0.2-0.6 units/kg/day in divided doses. Conservative initial doses of 0.2-0.4 units/kg/day are often recommended to avoid the potential for hypoglycemia. A rapid-acting insulin may be the only insulin formulation used initially.

Usual maintenance range: 0.5-1 units/kg/day in divided doses. An estimate of anticipated needs may be based on body weight and/or activity factors as follows:
Nonobese: 0.4-0.6 units/kg/day
Obese: 0.8-1.2 units/kg/day
Pubescent Children and Adolescents: During puberty, requirements may substantially increase to >1 unit/kg/day and in some cases up to 2 units/kg/day (IDF-ISPAD, 2011).

Division of daily insulin requirement ("conventional therapy"): Generally, 50% to 75% of the total daily dose (TDD) is given as an intermediate- or long-acting form of insulin (in 1-2 daily injections). The remaining portion of the TDD is then divided and administered before or at mealtimes (depending on the formulation) as a rapid-acting (eg, insulin aspart) or short-acting form of insulin. Some patients may benefit from the use of CSII which delivers rapid-acting insulin (insulin aspart) as a continuous infusion throughout the day and as boluses at mealtimes via an external pump device.

Division of daily insulin requirement ("intensive therapy"): Basal insulin delivery with 1 or 2 doses of intermediate- or long-acting insulin formulations superimposed with doses of short- or rapid-acting insulin (eg, insulin aspart) formulations 3 or more times daily.

Adjustment of dose: Dosage must be titrated to achieve glucose control and avoid hypoglycemia. Adjust dose to maintain premeal and bedtime glucose in target range. Since combinations of agents are frequently used, dosage adjustment must address the individual component of the insulin regimen which most directly influences the blood glucose value in question, based on the known onset and duration of the insulin component. Treatment and monitoring regimens must be individualized.

Continuous SubQ insulin infusion (insulin pump): A combination of a "basal" continuous insulin infusion rate with preprogrammed, premeal bolus doses which are patient controlled. When converting from multiple daily SubQ doses of maintenance insulin, it is advisable to reduce the basal rate to less than the equivalent of the total daily units of the longer acting insulin (eg, NPH); divide the total number of units by 24 to get the basal rate in units/hour. Do not include the total units of regular insulin or other rapid-acting insulin formulations in this calculation. The same premeal regular insulin dosage may be used.

Type 2: Adults: Augmentation therapy (patients for which diet, exercise, weight reduction, and oral hypoglycemic agents have not been adequate): Initial dosage of 0.2 units/kg/day or 10 units/day of an intermediate-acting (eg, NPH) or long-acting insulin administered at bedtime has been recommended. As an alternative, regular insulin or rapid-acting insulin formulations administered before meals have also been used. Dosage must be carefully adjusted.

Diabetic ketoacidosis (DKA), mild-to-moderate (unlabeled use): Treatment should continue until reversal of acid-base derangement/ketonemia. Serum glucose is not a direct indicator of these abnormalities, and may decrease more rapidly than correction of the metabolic abnormalities. Also refer to institution-specific protocols where appropriate.

Children and Adolescents: SubQ (**Note:** Use of I.V. regular insulin is preferred; only use the SubQ route if I.V. infusion access is unavailable): 0.3 units/kg followed in 1 hour by 0.1 units/kg given every hour or 0.15-0.2 units/kg every 2 hours; continue until acidosis clears, then decrease to 0.05 units/kg given every hour until maintenance SubQ replacement dosing can be initiated (Kitabchi, 2004; Wolfsdorf, 2007).

Hyperglycemia, critically ill (unlabeled use): Adults: I.V. continuous infusion: Insulin therapy should be implemented when blood glucose ≥150 mg/dL with a goal to maintain blood glucose <150 mg/dL (with values absolutely <180 mg/dL) using a protocol that achieves a low rate of hypoglycemia (ie, ≤70 mg/dL). Before discontinuation, stable ICU patients should be transitioned to a protocol-driven basal/bolus insulin regimen, based on insulin infusion history and carbohydrate intake, to avoid loss of glycemic control. Subcutaneous insulin therapy may be considered for selected clinically stable ICU patients (Jacobi, 2012). **Note:** The Surviving Sepsis Campaign guidelines recommend initiating insulin dosing in patients with severe sepsis when 2 consecutive blood glucose concentrations are >180 mg/dL and to target an upper blood glucose ≤180 mg/dL (Dellinger, 2013).

Dosing adjustment in renal impairment: No dosage adjustment provided in manufacturer's labeling; insulin requirements may be reduced due to changes in insulin clearance or metabolism; monitor blood glucose closely.

Dosing adjustment in hepatic impairment: No dosage adjustment provided in manufacturer's labeling; insulin requirements may be reduced due to changes in insulin clearance or metabolism; monitor blood glucose closely.

Additional Information Complete prescribing information should be consulted for additional detail.

Dosage Forms Excipient information presented when available (limited, particularly for generics); consult specific product labeling.

Solution, Subcutaneous:

NovoLOG: 100 units/mL (10 mL) [contains metacresol, phenol]

NovoLOG FlexPen: 100 units/mL (3 mL) [contains metacresol, phenol]

NovoLOG PenFill: 100 units/mL (3 mL) [contains metacresol, phenol]

◆ **Insulin Aspart and Insulin Aspart Protamine** *see* Insulin Aspart Protamine and Insulin Aspart *on page 1087*

Insulin Aspart Protamine and Insulin Aspart (IN soo lin AS part PROE ta meen & IN soo lin AS part)

Brand Names: U.S. NovoLOG® Mix 70/30; NovoLOG® Mix 70/30 FlexPen®

Brand Names: Canada NovoMix® 30

Index Terms Insulin Aspart and Insulin Aspart Protamine; NovoLog 70/30

Pharmacologic Category Insulin, Combination

Additional Appendix Information

Insulin Products *on page 2303*

Use Treatment of type 1 diabetes mellitus (insulin dependent, IDDM) and type 2 diabetes mellitus (noninsulin dependent, NIDDM) to improve glycemic control

Pregnancy Risk Factor B

Dosage Note: Insulin aspart protamine is an intermediate-acting insulin and insulin aspart is a rapid-acting insulin administered by SubQ injection. Insulin aspart protamine and insulin aspart combination products are approximately equipotent to insulin NPH and insulin regular combination products with a similar duration of activity, but with a more rapid onset. With combination insulin products, the proportion of rapid-acting to long-acting insulin is fixed; basal vs prandial dose adjustments cannot be made. Fixed-ratio insulins (such as insulin aspart protamine and insulin aspart combination) are typically administered as 2 daily doses with each dose intended to cover two meals and a snack. Because of variability in the peak effect and individual patient variability in activities, meals, etc, it may be more difficult to achieve complete glycemic control using fixed combinations of insulins; frequent monitoring and close medical supervision may be necessary.

Diabetes mellitus: SubQ:

General insulin dosing:

Type 1: Children, Adolescents, and Adults: **Note:** Multiple daily doses are utilized and guided by blood glucose monitoring. Combinations of different insulin formulations are commonly used. The daily doses presented below are expressed as the **total units/kg/day of all insulin formulations combined.** Insulin aspart protamine and insulin aspart combination product is **not** intended for initial therapy; basal insulin requirements should be established **first** to direct dosing of combination insulin products.

Usual maintenance range: 0.5-1 units/kg/day in divided doses. An estimate of anticipated needs may be based on body weight and/or activity factors as follows:

Nonobese: 0.4-0.6 units/kg/day

Obese: 0.8-1.2 units/kg/day

Pubescent Children and Adolescents: During puberty, requirements may substantially increase to >1 unit/kg/day and in some cases up to 2 units/kg/day (IDF-ISPAD, 2011).

Division of daily insulin requirement ("conventional therapy"): Generally, 50% to 75% of the daily insulin dose is given as an intermediate- or long-acting form of insulin (in 1-2 daily injections). The remaining portion of the 24-hour insulin requirement is divided and administered as either regular insulin or a rapid-acting form of insulin at the same time before breakfast and dinner.

Adjustment of dose: Dosage must be titrated to achieve glucose control and avoid hypoglycemia. Adjust dose to maintain premeal and bedtime glucose in target range. Since combinations of agents are frequently used, dosage adjustment must address the individual component of the insulin regimen which most directly influences the blood glucose value in question, based on the known onset and duration of the insulin component. Treatment and monitoring regimens must be individualized.

Type 2: Adults: Augmentation therapy (patients for which diet, exercise, weight reduction, and oral hypoglycemic agents have not been adequate): **Note:** Insulin aspart protamine and insulin aspart combination product is **not** intended for initial therapy; basal insulin requirements should be established **first** to direct dosing of combination insulin products. Dosage must be carefully adjusted.

Dosing adjustment in renal impairment: No dosage adjustment provided in manufacturer's labeling; insulin requirements may be reduced due to changes in insulin clearance or metabolism; monitor blood glucose closely.

Dosing adjustment in hepatic impairment: No dosage adjustment provided in manufacturer's labeling; insulin requirements may be reduced due to changes in insulin clearance or metabolism; monitor blood glucose closely.

Additional Information Complete prescribing information should be consulted for additional detail.

Dosage Forms Excipient information presented when available (limited, particularly for generics); consult specific product labeling.

Injection, suspension:

NovoLOG® Mix 70/30: Insulin aspart protamine suspension 70% [intermediate acting] and insulin aspart solution 30% [rapid acting]: 100 units/mL (10 mL)

NovoLOG® Mix 70/30 FlexPen®: Insulin aspart protamine suspension 70% [intermediate acting] and insulin aspart solution 30% [rapid acting]: 100 units/mL (3 mL)

Insulin Detemir (IN soo lin DE te mir)

Brand Names: U.S. Levemir; Levemir FlexPen

Brand Names: Canada Levemir®

Index Terms Detemir Insulin

Pharmacologic Category Insulin, Intermediate- to Long-Acting

Additional Appendix Information

Insulin Products *on page 2303*

Use Treatment of type 1 diabetes mellitus (insulin dependent, IDDM) and type 2 diabetes mellitus (noninsulin dependent, NIDDM) to improve glycemic control

Pregnancy Risk Factor B

Dosage Note: Insulin detemir is an intermediate-acting insulin administered by SubQ injection. When compared to insulin NPH, insulin detemir has slower, more prolonged absorption; duration of activity is dose-dependent. Insulin detemir may be given once or twice daily when used as the basal insulin component of therapy. Changing the basal insulin component from another insulin to insulin detemir can be done on a unit-to-unit basis. Insulin requirements vary dramatically between patients and dictate frequent monitoring and close medical supervision.

Diabetes mellitus: SubQ:

General insulin dosing:

Type 1: Children, Adolescents, and Adults: **Note:** Multiple daily doses are utilized and guided by blood glucose monitoring. Combinations of insulin formulations are commonly used. The daily doses presented below are expressed as the **total units/kg/day of all insulin formulations combined.**

Usual maintenance range: 0.5-1 units/kg/day in divided doses. An estimate of anticipated needs may be based on body weight and/or activity factors as follows:

Nonobese: 0.4-0.6 units/kg/day

Obese: 0.8-1.2 units/kg/day

Pubescent Children and Adolescents: During puberty, requirements may substantially increase to >1 unit/kg/day and in some cases up to 2 units/kg/day (IDF-ISPAD, 2011).

Division of daily insulin requirement ("conventional therapy"): Generally, 50% to 75% of the total daily dose (TDD) is given as an intermediate-acting (eg, insulin detemir) or a long-acting form of insulin (in 1-2 daily injections). The remaining portion of the TDD is then divided and administered before or at mealtimes (depending on the formulation) as a rapid-acting or short-acting form of insulin.

Division of daily insulin requirement ("intensive therapy"): Basal insulin delivery with 1 or 2 doses of intermediate-acting (eg, insulin detemir) or long-acting insulin formulations superimposed with doses of short- or rapid-acting insulin formulations 3 or more times daily.

Adjustment of dose: Dosage must be titrated to achieve glucose control and avoid hypoglycemia. Adjust dose to maintain premeal and bedtime glucose in target range. Since combinations of agents are frequently used, dosage adjustment must address the individual component of the insulin regimen which most directly influences the blood glucose value in question, based on the known onset and duration of the insulin component. Treatment and monitoring regimens must be individualized.

Insulin detemir-specific dosing: Manufacturer recommendations:

Type 1: Children ≥2 years, Adolescents, and Adults: Initial dose: Approximately one-third of the total daily insulin requirement administered in 1-2 divided doses. A rapid- or short-acting insulin should be used to complete the balance (~2/3) of the total daily insulin requirement.

Conversion from insulin glargine or NPH insulin: May be substituted on an equivalent unit-per-unit basis; in one Type 2 diabetes clinical trial, higher doses of insulin detemir were required than insulin NPH.

Type 2: Adults: Initial:

Inadequately controlled on oral antidiabetic agents: 10 units (or 0.1-0.2 units/kg) once daily in the evening; may also administer total daily dose in 2 divided doses.

Inadequately controlled on GLP-1 receptor agonist: 10 units once daily in the evening.

Conversion from insulin glargine or NPH insulin: May be substituted on an equivalent unit-per-unit basis; in one Type 2 diabetes clinical trial, higher doses of insulin detemir were required than insulin NPH.

Dosing adjustment in renal impairment: No dosage adjustment provided in manufacturer's labeling; insulin requirements may be reduced due to changes in insulin clearance or metabolism; monitor blood glucose closely.

Dosing adjustment in hepatic impairment: No dosage adjustment provided in manufacturer's labeling; insulin requirements may be reduced due to changes in insulin clearance or metabolism; monitor blood glucose closely.

Additional Information Complete prescribing information should be consulted for additional detail.

Dosage Forms Excipient information presented when available (limited, particularly for generics); consult specific product labeling.

Solution, Subcutaneous:

Levemir: 100 units/mL (10 mL) [contains metacresol, phenol]

Levemir FlexPen: 100 units/mL (3 mL) [contains metacresol, phenol]

Insulin Glargine (IN soo lin GLAR jeen)

Brand Names: U.S. Lantus; Lantus SoloStar

Brand Names: Canada Lantus®; Lantus® OptiSet®

Index Terms Glargine Insulin

Pharmacologic Category Insulin, Long-Acting

Additional Appendix Information

Insulin Products *on page 2303*

Use Treatment of type 1 diabetes mellitus (insulin dependent, IDDM) and type 2 diabetes mellitus (noninsulin dependent, NIDDM) to improve glycemic control

Pregnancy Risk Factor C

Dosage Note: Insulin glargine is a long-acting insulin administered by SubQ injection. Insulin glargine is approximately equipotent to human insulin, but has a slower onset, no pronounced peak, and a longer duration of activity. Changing the basal insulin component from another insulin to insulin glargine can be done on a unit-to-unit basis. Insulin requirements vary dramatically between patients and dictates frequent monitoring and close medical supervision.

Diabetes mellitus: SubQ:

General insulin dosing:

Type 1: Children, Adolescents, and Adults: **Note:** Multiple daily doses are utilized and guided by blood glucose monitoring. Combinations of insulin formulations are commonly used. The daily doses presented below are expressed as the total units/kg/day of all insulin formulations used. Insulin glargine must be used in combination with a rapid- or short-acting insulin.

Usual maintenance range: 0.5-1 units/kg/day in divided doses. An estimate of anticipated needs may be based on body weight and/or activity factors as follows:

Nonobese: 0.4-0.6 units/kg/day

Obese: 0.8-1.2 units/kg/day

Pubescent Children and Adolescents: During puberty, requirements may substantially increase to >1 unit/kg/day and in some cases up to 2 units/kg/day (IDF-ISPAD, 2011).

Division of daily insulin requirement ("conventional therapy"): Generally, 50% to 75% of the total daily dose (TDD) is given as an intermediate-acting or a long-acting form of insulin (eg, insulin glargine) (in 1-2 daily injections). The remaining portion of the TDD is then divided and administered before or at mealtimes (depending on the formulation) as a rapid-acting or short-acting form of insulin.

Division of daily insulin requirement ("intensive therapy"): Basal insulin delivery with 1 or 2 doses of intermediate-acting or long-acting insulin formulations superimposed with doses of short- or rapid-acting insulin formulations 3 or more times daily.

Adjustment of dose: Dosage must be titrated to achieve glucose control and avoid hypoglycemia. Adjust dose to maintain premeal and bedtime glucose in target range. Since combinations of agents are frequently used, dosage adjustment must address the individual component of the insulin regimen which most directly influences the blood glucose value in question, based on the known onset and duration of the insulin component.

Insulin glargine-specific dosing: Manufacturer recommendations:

Type 1: Children ≥6 years, Adolescents, and Adults: Initial dose: Approximately one-third of the total daily insulin requirement administered once daily. A rapid-acting or short-acting insulin should also be used to complete the balance (~2/3) of the total daily insulin requirement.

Type 2: Adults: Initial basal insulin dose: 10 units (or 0.2 units/kg) once daily

Conversion to insulin glargine from other insulin therapies:

Converting from once-daily NPH insulin: May be substituted on an equivalent unit-per-unit basis

Converting from twice-daily NPH insulin: Initial dose: Use 80% of the total daily dose of NPH (eg, 20% reduction); administer once daily; adjust dosage according to patient response

Dosing adjustment in renal impairment: No dosage adjustment provided in manufacturer's labeling; insulin requirements may be reduced due to changes in insulin clearance or metabolism; monitor blood glucose closely.

Dosing adjustment in hepatic impairment: No dosage adjustment provided in manufacturer's labeling; insulin requirements may be reduced due to changes in insulin clearance or metabolism; monitor blood glucose closely.

Additional Information Complete prescribing information should be consulted for additional detail.

Dosage Forms Excipient information presented when available (limited, particularly for generics); consult specific product labeling.

Solution, Subcutaneous:

Lantus: 100 units/mL (10 mL) [contains metacresol]

Lantus SoloStar: 100 units/mL (3 mL)

Insulin Glulisine (IN soo lin gloo LIS een)

Brand Names: U.S. Apidra; Apidra SoloStar

Brand Names: Canada Apidra®

Index Terms Glulisine Insulin

Pharmacologic Category Insulin, Rapid-Acting

Additional Appendix Information

Insulin Products *on page 2303*

Use Treatment of type 1 diabetes mellitus (insulin dependent, IDDM) and type 2 diabetes mellitus (noninsulin dependent, NIDDM) to improve glycemic control

Unlabeled Use Hyperglycemia during critical illness

Pregnancy Risk Factor C

Dosage Note: Insulin glulisine is a rapid-acting insulin analog which is normally administered SubQ as a premeal component of the insulin regimen or as a continuous SubQ infusion and should be used with an intermediate- or long-acting insulin. When compared to insulin regular, insulin glulisine has a more rapid onset and shorter duration of activity. In carefully controlled clinical settings with close medical supervision and monitoring of blood glucose and potassium, insulin glulisine may be administered I.V. Insulin requirements vary dramatically between patients and dictate frequent monitoring and close medical supervision.

Diabetes mellitus: SubQ:

General insulin dosing:

Type 1: Children ≥4 years, Adolescents, and Adults: **Note:** Multiple daily doses or continuous subcutaneous infusions guided by blood glucose monitoring are the standard of diabetes care. Combinations of insulin formulations are commonly used. The daily doses presented below are expressed as the **total units/kg/day of all insulin formulations combined.**

Initial total insulin dose: 0.2-0.6 units/kg/day in divided doses. Conservative initial doses of 0.2-0.4 units/kg/day are often recommended to avoid the potential for hypoglycemia. A rapid-acting insulin may be the only insulin formulation used initially.

Usual maintenance range: 0.5-1 units/kg/day in divided doses. An estimate of anticipated needs may be based on body weight and/or activity factors as follows:

Nonobese: 0.4-0.6 units/kg/day

Obese: 0.8-1.2 units/kg/day

Pubescent Children and Adolescents: During puberty, requirements may substantially increase to >1 unit/kg/day and in some cases up to 2 units/kg/day (IDF-ISPAD, 2011).

Division of daily insulin requirement ("conventional therapy"): Generally, 50% to 75% of the total daily dose (TDD) is given as an intermediate- or long-acting form of insulin (in 1-2 daily injections). The remaining portion of the TDD is then divided and administered before or at mealtimes (depending on the formulation) as a rapid-acting insulin (eg, insulin glulisine) or short-acting form of insulin. Some patients may benefit from the use of CSII which delivers rapid-acting insulin (insulin aspart) as a continuous infusion throughout the day and as boluses at mealtimes via an external pump device.

Division of daily insulin requirement ("intensive therapy"): Basal insulin delivery with 1 or 2 doses of intermediate- or long-acting insulin formulations superimposed with doses of short- or rapid-acting insulin (eg, insulin glulisine) formulations 3 or more times daily.

Adjustment of dose: Dosage must be titrated to achieve glucose control and avoid hypoglycemia. Adjust dose to maintain premeal and bedtime glucose in target range. Since combinations of agents are frequently used, dosage adjustment must address the individual component of the insulin regimen which most directly influences the blood glucose value in question, based on the known onset and duration of the insulin component. Treatment and monitoring regimens must be individualized.

Continuous SubQ insulin infusion (insulin pump): A combination of a "basal" continuous insulin infusion rate with preprogrammed, premeal bolus doses which are patient controlled. When converting from multiple daily SubQ doses of maintenance insulin, it is advisable to reduce the basal rate to less than the equivalent of the total daily units of the longer-acting insulin (eg, NPH); divide the total number of units by 24 to get the basal rate in units/hour. Do not include the total units of regular insulin or other rapid-acting insulin formulations in this calculation. The same premeal regular insulin dosage may be used.

Type 2: Adults: Augmentation therapy (patients for which diet, exercise, weight reduction, and oral hypoglycemic agents have not been adequate): Initial dosage of 0.2 units/kg/day or 10 units/day of an intermediate-acting (eg, NPH) or long-acting insulin administered at bedtime has been recommended. As an alternative, regular insulin or rapid-acting insulin (eg, insulin glulisine) formulations administered before meals have also been used. Dosage must be carefully adjusted.

Hyperglycemia, critically ill (unlabeled use): Adults: I.V. continuous infusion: Insulin therapy should be implemented when blood glucose ≥150 mg/dL with a goal to maintain blood glucose <150 mg/dL (with values absolutely <180 mg/dL) using a protocol that achieves a low rate of hypoglycemia (ie, ≤70 mg/dL). Before discontinuation, stable ICU patients should be transitioned to a protocol-driven basal/bolus insulin regimen, based on insulin infusion history and carbohydrate intake, to avoid loss of glycemic control. Subcutaneous insulin therapy may be considered for selected clinically stable ICU patients (Jacobi, 2012). **Note:** The Surviving Sepsis Campaign guidelines recommend initiating insulin dosing in patients with severe sepsis when 2 consecutive blood glucose concentrations are >180 mg/dL and to target an upper blood glucose ≤180 mg/dL (Dellinger, 2013).

Dosing adjustment in renal impairment: No dosage adjustment provided in manufacturer's labeling; insulin requirements may be reduced due to changes in insulin clearance or metabolism; monitor blood glucose closely.

Dosing adjustment in hepatic impairment: No dosage adjustment provided in manufacturer's labeling; insulin requirements may be reduced due to changes in insulin clearance or metabolism; monitor blood glucose closely.

Additional Information Complete prescribing information should be consulted for additional detail.

Dosage Forms Excipient information presented when available (limited, particularly for generics); consult specific product labeling.

Solution, Injection:

Apidra: 100 units/mL (10 mL) [contains metacresol]

Solution, Subcutaneous:

Apidra SoloStar: 100 units/mL (3 mL) [contains metacresol]

Insulin Lispro (IN soo lin LYE sproe)

Brand Names: U.S. HumaLOG; HumaLOG KwikPen

Brand Names: Canada Humalog®

Index Terms Lispro Insulin

Pharmacologic Category Insulin, Rapid-Acting

Additional Appendix Information

Insulin Products *on page 2303*

Use Treatment of type 1 diabetes mellitus (insulin dependent, IDDM) and type 2 diabetes mellitus (noninsulin dependent, NIDDM) to improve glycemic control

Unlabeled Use Gestational diabetes mellitus (GDM); mild-to-moderate diabetic ketoacidosis (DKA); mild-to-moderate hyperosmolar hyperglycemic state (HHS)

Pregnancy Risk Factor B

Dosage Note: Insulin lispro is a rapid-acting insulin analog which is normally administered SubQ as a premeal component of the insulin regimen or as a continuous SubQ infusion and should be used with intermediate- or long-acting insulin. When compared to insulin regular, insulin lispro has a more rapid onset and shorter duration of activity. In carefully controlled clinical settings with close medical supervision and monitoring of blood glucose and potassium, insulin lispro may also be administered I.V. Insulin requirements vary dramatically between patients and dictate frequent monitoring and close medical supervision.

Diabetes mellitus: SubQ:

General insulin dosing:

Type 1: Children ≥3 years, Adolescents, and Adults: **Note:** Multiple daily doses or continuous subcutaneous infusions guided by blood glucose monitoring are the standard of diabetes care. Combinations of insulin formulations are commonly used. The daily doses presented below are expressed as the **total units/kg/day of all insulin formulations combined.**

Initial total insulin dose: 0.2-0.6 units/kg/day in divided doses. Conservative initial doses of 0.2-0.4 units/kg/day are often recommended to avoid the potential for hypoglycemia. A rapid-acting insulin may be the only insulin formulation used initially.

Usual maintenance range: 0.5-1 units/kg/day in divided doses. An estimate of anticipated needs may be based on body weight and/or activity factors as follows:

Nonobese: 0.4-0.6 units/kg/day

Obese: 0.8-1.2 units/kg/day

Pubescent Children and Adolescents: During puberty, requirements may substantially increase to >1 unit/kg/day and in some cases up to 2 units/kg/day (IDF-ISPAD, 2011).

Division of daily insulin requirement ("conventional therapy"): Generally, 50% to 75% of the total daily dose (TDD) is given as an intermediate- or long-acting form of insulin (in 1-2 daily injections). The remaining portion of the TDD is then divided and administered as either before or at mealtimes (depending on the formulation) as a rapid-acting insulin (eg, insulin lispro) or short-acting form of insulin. Some patients may benefit from the use of CSII which delivers rapid-acting insulin (insulin lispro) as a continuous infusion throughout the day and as boluses at mealtimes via an external pump device.

Division of daily insulin requirement ("intensive therapy"): Basal insulin delivery with 1 or 2 doses of intermediate- or long-acting insulin formulations superimposed with doses of short- or rapid-acting insulin (eg, insulin lispro) formulations 3 or more times daily.

Adjustment of dose: Dosage must be titrated to achieve glucose control and avoid hypoglycemia. Adjust dose to maintain premeal and bedtime glucose in target range. Since combinations of agents are frequently used, dosage adjustment must address the individual component of the insulin regimen which most directly influences the blood glucose value in question, based on the known onset and duration of the insulin component. Treatment and monitoring regimens must be individualized.

Continuous SubQ insulin infusion (insulin pump): A combination of a "basal" continuous insulin infusion rate with preprogrammed, premeal bolus doses which are patient controlled. When converting from multiple daily SubQ doses of maintenance insulin, it is advisable to reduce the basal rate to less than the equivalent of the total daily units of the longer-acting insulin (eg, NPH); divide the total number of units by 24 to get the basal rate in units/hour. Do not include the total units of regular insulin or other rapid-acting insulin formulations in this calculation. The same premeal regular insulin dosage may be used.

Type 2: Adults: Augmentation therapy (patients for which diet, exercise, weight reduction, and oral hypoglycemic agents have not been adequate): Initial dosage of 0.2 units/kg/day or 10 units/day of an intermediate- acting (eg, NPH) or long-acting insulin administered at bedtime has been recommended. As an alternative, regular insulin or rapid-acting insulin (eg, insulin lispro) formulations administered before meals have also been used. Dosage must be carefully adjusted.

Diabetic ketoacidosis (DKA), mild-to-moderate (unlabeled use): Treatment should continue until reversal of acid-base derangement/ketonemia. Serum glucose is not a direct indicator of these abnormalities, and may decrease more rapidly than correction of the metabolic abnormalities. Also refer to institution-specific protocols where appropriate.

Children and Adolescents: SubQ (**Note:** Use of I.V. regular insulin is preferred; only use the SubQ route if I.V. infusion access is unavailable): 0.3 units/kg followed in one hour by 0.1 units/kg given every hour or 0.15-0.2 units/kg every 2 hours; continue until acidosis clears, then decrease to 0.05 units/kg given every hour until maintenance SubQ replacement dosing can be initiated (Kitabchi, 2004; Wolfsdorf, 2007).

Dosing adjustment in renal impairment: Adults: Insulin requirements are reduced due to changes in insulin clearance or metabolism. No dosage adjustment provided in manufacturer's labeling; however, the following adjustments have been recommended (Aronoff, 2007):

Cl_{cr} >50 mL/minute: No adjustment necessary

Cl_{cr} 10-50 mL/minute: Administer at 75% of recommended dose

Cl_{cr} <10 mL/minute: Administer at 50% of recommended dose and monitor glucose closely

Hemodialysis: Because of a large molecular weight (6000 daltons), insulin is not significantly removed by either peritoneal or hemodialysis; supplemental dose is not necessary

Peritoneal dialysis: Supplemental dose is not necessary

Continuous renal replacement therapy: Administer at 75% of recommended dose

Dosing adjustment in hepatic impairment: No dosage adjustment provided in manufacturer's labeling; insulin requirements may be reduced due to changes in insulin clearance or metabolism; monitor blood glucose closely.

Additional Information Complete prescribing information should be consulted for additional detail.

Dosage Forms Excipient information presented when available (limited, particularly for generics); consult specific product labeling.

Solution, Subcutaneous:

HumaLOG: 100 units/mL (3 mL, 10 mL) [contains metacresol, phenol]

HumaLOG KwikPen: 100 units/mL (3 mL) [contains metacresol, phenol]

◆ **Insulin Lispro and Insulin Lispro Protamine** *see* Insulin Lispro Protamine and Insulin Lispro *on page 1091*

Insulin Lispro Protamine and Insulin Lispro

(IN soo lin LYE sproe PROE ta meen & IN soo lin LYE sproe)

Brand Names: U.S. HumaLOG® Mix 50/50™; HumaLOG® Mix 50/50™ KwikPen™; HumaLOG® Mix 75/25™; HumaLOG® Mix 75/25™ KwikPen™

Brand Names: Canada Humalog® Mix 25

Index Terms Insulin Lispro and Insulin Lispro Protamine

Pharmacologic Category Insulin, Combination

Additional Appendix Information

Insulin Products *on page 2303*

Use Treatment of type 1 diabetes mellitus (insulin dependent, IDDM) and type 2 diabetes mellitus (noninsulin dependent, NIDDM) to improve glycemic control

Pregnancy Risk Factor B

Dosage Note: Lispro protamine is an intermediate-acting insulin and lispro is a rapid-acting insulin administered by SubQ injection. Insulin lispro protamine and insulin lispro combination products are approximately equipotent to insulin NPH and insulin regular combination products with a similar duration of activity but a more rapid onset. With combination insulin products, the proportion of rapid-acting to long-acting insulin is fixed; basal vs prandial dose adjustments cannot be made. Fixed-ratio insulins (such as insulin lispro protamine and insulin lispro combination) are typically administered as 2 daily doses with each dose intended to cover two meals and a snack. Because of variability in the peak effect and individual patient variability in activities, meals, etc, it may be more difficult to achieve complete glycemic control using fixed combinations of insulins; frequent monitoring and close medical supervision may be necessary.

Diabetes mellitus: SubQ:

General insulin dosing:

Type 1: Adults: **Note:** Multiple daily doses are utilized and guided by blood glucose monitoring. Combinations of insulin formulations are commonly used. The daily doses presented below are expressed as the **total units/kg/day of all insulin formulations combined.** Insulin lispro protamine and insulin lispro combination product is **not** intended for initial therapy; basal insulin requirements should be established **first** to direct dosing of combination insulin products.

Usual maintenance range: 0.5-1 units/kg/day in divided doses. An estimate of anticipated needs may be based on body weight and/or activity factors as follows:

Nonobese: 0.4-0.6 units/kg/day

Obese: 0.8-1.2 units/kg/day

Pubescent Children and Adolescents: During puberty, requirements may substantially increase to >1 unit/kg/day and in some cases up to 2 units/kg/day (IDF-ISPAD, 2011).

Division of daily insulin requirement ("conventional therapy"): Generally, 50% to 75% of the daily insulin dose is given as an intermediate- or long-acting form of insulin (in 1-2 daily injections). The remaining portion of the 24-hour insulin requirement is divided and administered as either regular insulin or a rapid-acting form of insulin at the same time before breakfast and dinner.

Adjustment of dose: Dosage must be titrated to achieve glucose control and avoid hypoglycemia. Adjust dose to maintain premeal and bedtime glucose in target range. Since combinations of agents are frequently used, dosage adjustment must address the individual component of the insulin regimen which most directly influences the blood glucose value in question, based on the known onset and duration of the insulin component. Treatment and monitoring regimens must be individualized.

Type 2: Adults: Augmentation therapy (patients for which diet, exercise, weight reduction, and oral hypoglycemic agents have not been adequate): **Note:** Insulin lispro protamine and insulin lispro combination product is **not** intended for initial therapy; basal insulin requirements should be established **first** to direct dosing of combination insulin products. Dosage must be carefully adjusted.

Dosing adjustment in renal impairment: No dosage adjustment provided in manufacturer's labeling; insulin requirements may be reduced due to changes in insulin clearance or metabolism; monitor blood glucose closely.

Dosing adjustment in hepatic impairment: No dosage adjustment provided in manufacturer's labeling; insulin requirements may be reduced due to changes in insulin clearance or metabolism; monitor blood glucose closely.

Additional Information Complete prescribing information should be consulted for additional detail.

Dosage Forms Excipient information presented when available (limited, particularly for generics); consult specific product labeling.

Injection, suspension:

HumaLOG® Mix 50/50™: Insulin lispro protamine suspension 50% [intermediate acting] and insulin lispro solution 50% [rapid acting]: 100 units/mL (10 mL)

HumaLOG® Mix 50/50™ KwikPen™: Insulin lispro protamine suspension 50% [intermediate acting] and insulin lispro solution 50% [rapid acting]: 100 units/mL (3 mL)

HumaLOG® Mix 75/25™: Insulin lispro protamine suspension 75% [intermediate acting] and insulin lispro solution 25% [rapid acting]: 100 units/mL (10 mL)

HumaLOG® Mix 75/25™ KwikPen™: Insulin lispro protamine suspension 75% [intermediate acting] and insulin lispro solution 25% [rapid acting]: 100 units/mL (3 mL)

Insulin NPH (IN soo lin N P H)

Brand Names: U.S. HumuLIN N Pen [OTC]; HumuLIN N [OTC]; NovoLIN N ReliOn [OTC]; NovoLIN N [OTC]

Brand Names: Canada Humulin® N; Novolin® ge NPH

Index Terms Isophane Insulin; NPH Insulin

Pharmacologic Category Insulin, Intermediate-Acting

Additional Appendix Information

Insulin Products *on page 2303*

Use Treatment of type 1 diabetes mellitus (insulin dependent, IDDM) and type 2 diabetes mellitus (noninsulin dependent, NIDDM) to improve glycemic control

Unlabeled Use Gestational diabetes mellitus (GDM)

Dosage Note: Insulin NPH is an intermediate-acting insulin formulation which is usually administered subcutaneously once or twice daily. When compared to insulin regular, insulin NPH has a slower onset and longer duration of activity. Insulin requirements vary dramatically between patients and dictate frequent monitoring and close medical supervision.

Diabetes mellitus: SubQ:

General insulin dosing:

Type 1: Children, Adolescents, and Adults: **Note:** Multiple daily doses are utilized and guided by blood glucose monitoring. Combinations of insulin formulations are commonly used. The daily doses presented below are expressed as the **total units/kg/day of all insulin formulations combined.** Insulin NPH is **not** intended for initial therapy; basal insulin requirements should be established **first** to direct dosing.

Usual maintenance range: 0.5-1 units/kg/day in divided doses. An estimate of anticipated needs may be based on body weight and/or activity factors as follows:

Nonobese: 0.4-0.6 units/kg/day

Obese: 0.8-1.2 units/kg/day

Pubescent Children and Adolescents: During puberty, requirements may substantially increase to >1 unit/kg/day and in some cases up to 2 units/kg/day (IDF-ISPAD, 2011).

Division of daily insulin requirement ("conventional therapy"): Generally, 50% to 75% of the total daily dose (TDD) is given as an intermediate-acting (eg, NPH) or a long-acting form of insulin (in 1-2 daily injections). The remaining portion of the TDD is then divided and administered before or at mealtimes (depending on the formulation) as a rapid-acting or short-acting form of insulin.

Division of daily insulin requirement ("intensive therapy"): Basal insulin delivery with 1 or 2 doses of intermediate-acting (eg, NPH) or long-acting insulin formulations superimposed with doses of short- or rapid-acting insulin formulations 3 or more times daily.

Adjustment of dose: Dosage must be titrated to achieve glucose control and avoid hypoglycemia. Adjust dose to maintain premeal and bedtime glucose in target range. Since combinations of agents are frequently used, dosage adjustment must address the individual component of the insulin regimen which most directly influences the blood glucose value in question, based on the known onset and duration of the insulin component.

Type 2: Augmentation therapy (patients for which diet, exercise, weight reduction, and oral hypoglycemic agents have not been adequate): Adults: Initial dosage of 0.2 units/kg/day or 10 units/day of an intermediate-acting (eg, NPH) or long-acting insulin administered at bedtime has been recommended. As an alternative, regular insulin or rapid-acting insulin formulations administered before meals have also been used. Dosage must be carefully adjusted.

Dosing adjustment in renal impairment: No dosage adjustment provided in manufacturer's labeling; insulin requirements may be reduced due to changes in insulin clearance or metabolism; monitor blood glucose closely.

Dosing adjustment in hepatic impairment: No dosage adjustment provided in manufacturer's labeling; insulin requirements may be reduced due to changes in insulin clearance or metabolism; monitor blood glucose closely.

Additional Information Complete prescribing information should be consulted for additional detail.

Dosage Forms Excipient information presented when available (limited, particularly for generics); consult specific product labeling.

Suspension, Subcutaneous:

HumuLIN N: 100 units/mL (3 mL, 10 mL) [contains metacresol, phenol]

HumuLIN N Pen: 100 units/mL (3 mL) [contains metacresol, phenol]

NovoLIN N: 100 units/mL (10 mL) [contains metacresol, phenol]

NovoLIN N ReliOn: 100 units/mL (10 mL) [contains metacresol, phenol]

Dosage Forms: Canada Excipient information presented when available (limited, particularly for generics); consult specific product labeling.

Injection, suspension:

Novolin® ge NPH: 100 units/mL (3 mL) [NovolinSet® prefilled syringe or PenFill® prefilled cartridge]; 10 mL [vial]

Insulin NPH and Insulin Regular

(IN soo lin N P H & IN soo lin REG yoo ler)

Brand Names: U.S. HumuLIN® 70/30; NovoLIN® 70/30

Brand Names: Canada Humulin® 20/80; Humulin® 70/30; Novolin® ge 30/70; Novolin® ge 40/60; Novolin® ge 50/50

Index Terms Insulin Regular and Insulin NPH; Isophane Insulin and Regular Insulin; NPH Insulin and Regular Insulin

Pharmacologic Category Insulin, Combination

Additional Appendix Information

Insulin Products *on page 2303*

Use Treatment of type 1 diabetes mellitus (insulin dependent, IDDM) and type 2 diabetes mellitus (noninsulin dependent, NIDDM) to improve glycemic control

Unlabeled Use Gestational diabetes mellitus (GDM)

Dosage Note: Insulin NPH is an intermediate-acting insulin and regular insulin is a short-acting insulin administered by SubQ injection. When compared to insulin NPH, the combination product (insulin NPH and insulin regular) has a shorter onset of action and a similar duration of action. With combination insulin products, the proportion of short-acting to long-acting insulin is fixed; basal vs prandial dose adjustments cannot be made. Fixed-ratio insulins (such as insulin NPH and insulin regular combination) are typically administered as 2 daily doses with each dose intended to cover two meals and a snack. Because of variability in the peak effect and individual patient variability in activities, meals, etc, it may be more difficult to achieve complete glycemic control using fixed combinations of insulins; frequent monitoring and close medical supervision may be necessary.

Diabetes mellitus: SubQ:

General insulin dosing:

Type 1: Children, Adolescents, and Adults: **Note:** Multiple daily doses are utilized and guided by blood glucose monitoring. Combinations of different insulin formulations are commonly used. The daily doses presented below are expressed as the **total units/kg/day of all insulin formulations combined.** Insulin NPH and insulin regular combination product is **not** intended for initial therapy; basal insulin requirements should be established **first** to direct dosing of combination insulin products.

Usual maintenance range: 0.5-1 units/kg/day in divided doses. An estimate of anticipated needs may be based on body weight and/or activity factors as follows:

Nonobese: 0.4-0.6 units/kg/day

Obese: 0.8-1.2 units/kg/day

Pubescent Children and Adolescents: During puberty, requirements may substantially increase to >1 unit/kg/day and in some cases up to 2 units/kg/day (IDF-ISPAD, 2011).

Division of daily insulin requirement ("conventional therapy"): Generally, 50% to 75% of the total daily dose (TDD) is given as an intermediate-acting (eg, NPH) or a long-acting form of insulin (in 1-2 daily injections). The remaining portion of the TDD is then divided and administered before or at mealtimes (depending on the formulation) as a rapid-acting or short-acting form of insulin.

Adjustment of dose: Dosage must be titrated to achieve glucose control and avoid hypoglycemia. Adjust dose to maintain premeal and bedtime glucose in target range. Since combinations of agents are frequently used, dosage adjustment must address the individual component of the insulin regimen which most directly influences the blood glucose value in question, based on the known onset and duration of the insulin component.

Type 2: Augmentation therapy (patients for which diet, exercise, weight reduction, and oral hypoglycemic agents have not been adequate): Adults: **Note:** Insulin NPH and insulin regular combination product is **not** intended for initial therapy; basal insulin requirements should be established **first** to direct dosing of combination insulin products. Dosage must be carefully adjusted.

Dosing adjustment in renal impairment: No dosage adjustment provided in manufacturer's labeling; insulin requirements may be reduced due to changes in insulin clearance or metabolism; monitor blood glucose closely.

Dosing adjustment in hepatic impairment: No dosage adjustment provided in manufacturer's labeling; insulin requirements may be reduced due to changes in insulin clearance or metabolism; monitor blood glucose closely.

Additional Information Complete prescribing information should be consulted for additional detail.

Dosage Forms Excipient information presented when available (limited, particularly for generics); consult specific product labeling.

Injection, suspension:

HumuLIN® 70/30: Insulin NPH suspension 70% [intermediate acting] and insulin regular solution 30% [short acting]: 100 units/mL (3 mL) [prefilled pen, vial]

HumuLIN® 70/30: Insulin NPH suspension 70% [intermediate acting] and insulin regular solution 30% [short acting]: 100 units/mL (10 mL) [vial]

NovoLIN® 70/30: Insulin NPH suspension 70% [intermediate acting] and insulin regular solution 30% [short acting]: 100 units/mL (10 mL) [vial]

Dosage Forms: Canada Excipient information presented when available (limited, particularly for generics); consult specific product labeling.

Injection, suspension:

Humulin® 20/80: Insulin regular solution 20% [short acting] and insulin NPH suspension 80% [intermediate acting]: 100 units/mL (3 mL) [PenFill® prefilled cartridge]

Novolin® ge 30/70: Insulin regular solution 30% [short acting] and insulin NPH suspension 70% [intermediate acting]: 100 units/mL (3 mL) [prefilled syringe or PenFill® prefilled cartridge]; (10 mL) [vial]

Novolin® ge 40/60: Insulin regular solution 40% [short acting] and insulin NPH suspension 60% [intermediate acting]: 100 units/mL (3 mL) [PenFill® prefilled cartridge]

Novolin® ge 50/50: Insulin regular solution 50% [short acting] and insulin NPH suspension 50% [intermediate acting]: 100 units/mL (3 mL) [PenFill® prefilled cartridge]

Insulin Regular (IN soo lin REG yoo ler)

Brand Names: U.S. HumuLIN R U-500 (CONCENTRATED); HumuLIN R [OTC]; NovoLIN R ReliOn [OTC]; NovoLIN R [OTC]

Brand Names: Canada Humulin® R; Novolin® ge Toronto

Index Terms Regular Insulin

Pharmacologic Category Insulin, Short-Acting

Additional Appendix Information

Beers Criteria – Potentially Inappropriate Medications for Geriatrics *on page 2368*

Desensitization Protocols *on page 2325*

Insulin Products *on page 2303*

Use Treatment of type 1 diabetes mellitus (insulin dependent, IDDM) and type 2 diabetes mellitus (noninsulin dependent, NIDDM) to improve glycemic control

Unlabeled Use Adjunct of parenteral nutrition; diabetic ketoacidosis (DKA); gestational diabetes mellitus (GDM); hyperglycemia during critical illness; hyperkalemia; hyperosmolar hyperglycemic state (HHS)

Pregnancy Risk Factor B

Pregnancy Considerations Minimal amounts of endogenous insulin cross the placenta. Exogenous insulin bound to anti-insulin antibodies has been detected in cord blood. Maternal hyperglycemia can be associated with adverse effects in the fetus, including macrosomia, neonatal hyperglycemia, and hyperbilirubinemia; the risk of congenital malformations is increased when the Hb A_{1c} is >1% above the normal range. Insulin requirements tend to fall during the first trimester of pregnancy and increase in the later trimesters, peaking at 28-32 weeks of gestation. Following delivery, insulin requirements decrease rapidly. Diabetes can also be associated with adverse effects in the mother. Poorly treated diabetes may cause end-organ damage that may in turn negatively affect obstetric outcomes. Physiologic glucose levels should be maintained prior to and during pregnancy to decrease the risk of adverse events in the fetus and the mother. Insulin is the drug of choice for the control of diabetes mellitus during pregnancy.

Breast-Feeding Considerations Endogenous insulin can be found in breast milk. Plasma glucose concentrations in the mother affect glucose concentrations in breast milk. The gastrointestinal tract destroys insulin when administered orally; therefore, insulin is not expected to be absorbed intact by the breast-feeding infant. All types of insulin are safe for use while breast-feeding. Due to increased calorie expenditure, women with diabetes may require less insulin while nursing.

Contraindications Hypersensitivity to regular insulin or any component of the formulation; during episodes of hypoglycemia

Warnings/Precautions Hypoglycemia is the most common adverse effect of insulin. The timing of hypoglycemia differs among various insulin formulations. Hypoglycemia may result from increased work or exercise without eating; use of long-acting insulin preparations (eg, insulin detemir, insulin glargine) may delay recovery from hypoglycemia. Profound and prolonged episodes of hypoglycemia may result in convulsions, unconsciousness, temporary or permanent brain damage or even death. Insulin requirements may be altered during illness, emotional disturbances or other stressors. Insulin may produce hypokalemia which, if left untreated, may result in respiratory paralysis, ventricular arrhythmia and even death. Use with caution in patients at risk for hypokalemia (eg, I.V. insulin use). Use with caution in renal or hepatic impairment. In the elderly, avoid use of sliding scale insulin in this population due to increased risk of hypoglycemia without benefits in management of hyperglycemia regardless of care setting (Beers Criteria).

Human insulin differs from animal-source insulin. Any change of insulin should be made cautiously; changing manufacturers, type, and/or method of manufacture may result in the need for a change of dosage. U-500 regular insulin is a concentrated insulin formulation which contains 500 units of insulin per mL; for SubQ administration only using a U-100 insulin syringe or tuberculin syringe; **not for I.V. administration**. To avoid dosing errors when using a U-100 insulin syringe, the prescribed dose should be written in actual insulin units and as unit markings on the U-100 insulin syringe (eg, 50 units [10 units on a U-100 insulin syringe]). To avoid dosing errors when using a tuberculin syringe, the prescribed dose should be written in actual insulin units and as a volume (eg, 50 units [0.1 mL]). Mixing U-500 regular insulin with other insulin formulations is not recommended.

Regular insulin may be administered I.V. or I.M. in selected clinical situations; close monitoring of blood glucose and serum potassium, as well as medical supervision, is required.

The general objective of exogenous insulin therapy is to approximate the physiologic pattern of insulin secretion which is characterized by two distinct phases. Phase 1 insulin secretion suppresses hepatic glucose production and phase 2 insulin secretion occurs in response to carbohydrate ingestion; therefore, exogenous insulin therapy may consist of basal insulin (eg, intermediate- or long-acting insulin or via continuous subcutaneous insulin infusion [CSII]) and/or preprandial insulin (eg, short- or rapid-acting insulin) (see Related Information: Insulin Products). Patients with type 1 diabetes do not produce endogenous insulin; therefore, these patients require both basal and preprandial insulin administration. Patients with type 2 diabetes retain some beta-cell function in the early stages of their disease; however, as the disease progresses, phase 1 insulin secretion may become completely impaired and phase 2 insulin secretion becomes delayed and/or inadequate in response to meals. Therefore, patients with type 2 diabetes may be treated with oral antidiabetic agents, basal insulin, and/or preprandial insulin depending on the stage of disease and current glycemic control. Since treatment regimens often consist of multiple agents, dosage adjustments must address the specific phase of insulin release that is primarily contributing to the patient's impaired glycemic control. Diabetes self-management education (DSME) is essential to maximize the effectiveness of therapy. Treatment and monitoring regimens must be individualized.

Potentially significant drug-drug interactions may exist, requiring dose or frequency adjustment, additional monitoring, and/or selection of alternative therapy.

Adverse Reactions Primarily symptoms of hypoglycemia

Cardiovascular: Pallor, palpitation, tachycardia

Central nervous system: Fatigue, headache, hypothermia, loss of consciousness, mental confusion

Dermatologic: Redness, urticaria

Endocrine & metabolic: Hypoglycemia, hypokalemia

Gastrointestinal: Hunger, nausea, numbness of mouth

Local: Atrophy or hypertrophy of SubQ fat tissue; edema, itching, pain or warmth at injection site; stinging

Neuromuscular & skeletal: Muscle weakness, paresthesia, tremor

Ocular: Transient presbyopia or blurred vision

Miscellaneous: Anaphylaxis, diaphoresis, local and/or systemic hypersensitivity reactions

Drug Interactions

Metabolism/Transport Effects None known.

Avoid Concomitant Use There are no known interactions where it is recommended to avoid concomitant use.

Increased Effect/Toxicity

Insulin Regular may increase the levels/effects of: Antidiabetic Agents (Thiazolidinedione); Hypoglycemic Agents; Quinolone Antibiotics

The levels/effects of Insulin Regular may be increased by: Beta-Blockers; Edetate CALCIUM Disodium; Edetate Disodium; Herbs (Hypoglycemic Properties); MAO Inhibitors; Pegvisomant; Salicylates; Selective Serotonin Reuptake Inhibitors

Decreased Effect

The levels/effects of Insulin Regular may be decreased by: Corticosteroids (Orally Inhaled); Corticosteroids (Systemic); Loop Diuretics; Luteinizing Hormone-Releasing Hormone Analogs; Somatropin; Thiazide Diuretics

Ethanol/Nutrition/Herb Interactions

Ethanol: Use caution with ethanol; may increase risk of hypoglycemia.

Herb/Nutraceutical: Use caution with alfalfa, aloe, bilberry, bitter melon, burdock, celery, damiana, fenugreek, garcinia, garlic, ginger, ginseng (American), gymnema, marshmallow, stinging nettle; may increase risk of hypoglycemia.

Preparation for Administration

For SubQ administration:

Humulin® R: May be diluted with the universal diluent, Sterile Diluent for Humalog®, Humulin® N, Humulin® R, Humulin® 70/30, and Humulin® R U-500, to a concentration of 10 units/mL (U-10) or 50 units/mL (U-50).

Novolin® R: Insulin Diluting Medium for NovoLog® is **not** intended for use with Novolin® R or any insulin product other than insulin aspart.

For I.V. infusion:

Humulin® R: May be diluted in NS or D_5W to concentrations of 0.1-1 unit/mL.

Novolin® R: May be diluted in NS, D_5W, or $D_{10}W$ with 40 mEq/L potassium chloride at concentrations of 0.05-1 unit/mL.

Storage/Stability

Humulin® R, Humulin® R U-500: Store unopened vials in refrigerator between 2°C and 8°C (36°F to 46°F); do not freeze; keep away from heat and sunlight. Once punctured (in use), vials may be stored for up to 31 days in the refrigerator between 2°C and 8°C (36°F to 46°F) or at room temperature of ≤30°C (≤86°F).

Novolin® R: Store unopened vials in refrigerator between 2°C and 8°C (36°F to 46°F) until product expiration date or at room temperature ≤25°C (≤77°F) for up to 42 days; do not freeze; keep away from heat and sunlight. Once punctured (in use), store vials at room temperature ≤25°C (≤77°F) for up to 42 days (this includes any days stored at room temperature prior to opening vial); refrigeration of in-use vials is not recommended.

Canadian labeling (not in U.S. labeling): All products: Unopened vials, cartridges, and pens should be stored under refrigeration between 2°C and 8°C (36°F to 46°F) until the expiration date; do not freeze; keep away from heat and sunlight. Once punctured (in use), Humulin® vials, cartridges, and pens should be stored at room temperature <25°C (<77°F) for up to 4 weeks. Once punctured (in use), Novolin® ge vials, cartridges, and pens may be stored for up to 1 month at room temperature <25°C (<77°F) for vials or <30°C (<86°F) for pens/cartridges; do not refrigerate.

For SubQ administration:

Humulin® R: According to the manufacturer, diluted insulin should be stored at 30°C (86°F) and used within 14 days **or** at 5°C (41°F) and used within 28 days.

For I.V. infusion:

Humulin® R: Stable for 48 hours at room temperature or for 48 hours under refrigeration followed by 48 hours at room temperature.

Novolin® R: Stable for 24 hours at room temperature

Mechanism of Action Insulin acts via specific membrane-bound receptors on target tissues to regulate metabolism of carbohydrate, protein, and fats. Target organs for insulin include the liver, skeletal muscle, and adipose tissue.

Within the liver, insulin stimulates hepatic glycogen synthesis. Insulin promotes hepatic synthesis of fatty acids, which are released into the circulation as lipoproteins. Skeletal muscle effects of insulin include increased protein synthesis and increased glycogen synthesis. Within adipose tissue, insulin stimulates the processing of circulating lipoproteins to provide free fatty acids, facilitating triglyceride synthesis and storage by adipocytes; also directly inhibits the hydrolysis of triglycerides. In addition, insulin stimulates the cellular uptake of amino acids and increases cellular permeability to several ions, including potassium, magnesium, and phosphate. By activating sodium-potassium ATPases, insulin promotes the intracellular movement of potassium.

Normally secreted by the pancreas, insulin products are manufactured for pharmacologic use through recombinant DNA technology using either *E. coli* or *Saccharomyces cerevisiae*. Insulins are categorized based on the onset, peak, and duration of effect (eg, rapid-, short-, intermediate-, and long-acting insulin).

Pharmacodynamics/Kinetics Note: Rate of absorption, onset, and duration of activity may be affected by site of injection, exercise, presence of lipodystrophy, local blood supply, and/or temperature.

Onset of action: SubQ: 0.5 hours

Peak effect: SubQ: 2.5-5 hours

Duration: SubQ:

U-100: 4-12 hours (may increase with dose)

U-500: Up to 24 hours

Distribution: V_d: 0.26-0.36 L/kg

Bioavailability: SubQ: 55% to 77%

Half-life elimination: I.V.: ~0.5-1 hour (dose-dependent); SubQ: 1.5 hours

Time to peak, plasma: SubQ: 0.8-2 hours

Excretion: Urine

Dosage

Diabetes mellitus: SubQ: **Note:** Insulin requirements vary dramatically between patients and therapy requires dosage adjustments with careful medical supervision. Specific formulations may require distinct administration procedures; please see individual agents.

Type 1: Children and Adults: **Note:** Multiple daily injections (MDI) guided by blood glucose monitoring or the use of continuous subcutaneous insulin infusions (CSII) is the standard of care for patients with type 1 diabetes. Combinations of insulin formulations are commonly used.

Initial dose: 0.5-1.0 units/kg/day in divided doses. Conservative initial doses of 0.2-0.4 units/kg/day may be recommended to avoid the potential for hypoglycemia.

Division of daily insulin requirement: Generally, 50% to 75% of the total daily dose (TDD) is given as an intermediate- or long-acting form of insulin (in 1-2 daily injections). The remaining portion of the TDD is then divided and administered before or at mealtimes (depending on the formulation) as a rapid-acting or short-acting form of insulin.

Adjustment of dose: Dosage must be titrated to achieve glucose control and avoid hypoglycemia. Adjust dose to maintain preprandial plasma glucose between 70-130 mg/dL for most patients. Since treatment regimens often consist of multiple formulations, dosage adjustments must address the specific phase of insulin release that is primarily contributing to the patient's impaired glycemic control. Treatment and monitoring regimens must be individualized. Also see Additional Information.

Usual maintenance range: 0.5-1.2 units/kg/day in divided doses. Insulin requirements are patient-specific and may vary based on age, body weight, and/or activity factors:

Adolescents: May require as much as 1.5 units/kg/day during puberty (Silverstein, 2005)

Prepuberty: 0.7-1 unit/kg/day

Type 2: Children and Adults: The goal of therapy is to achieve an Hb A_{1c} <7% as quickly as possible using the safe titration of medications. According to a consensus statement by the ADA and European Association for the Study of Diabetes (EASD), basal insulin therapy (eg, intermediate- or long-acting insulin) should be considered in patients with type 2 diabetes who fail to achieve glycemic goals with lifestyle interventions and metformin ± a sulfonylurea. Pioglitazone or a GLP-1 agonist may also be considered prior to initiation of basal insulin therapy. In patients who continue to fail to achieve glycemic goals despite the addition of basal insulin, intensification of insulin therapy should be considered; this generally consists of multiple daily injections with a combination of insulin formulations (Nathan, 2009).

Intensification of therapy: Add a second injection of a short-, rapid-, or intermediate-acting insulin as needed based on blood glucose monitoring; the timing of administration and type of insulin added for intensification of therapy depends on the blood glucose level that is consistently out of the target range (eg, preprandial glucose levels before lunch or dinner, postprandial glucose levels, and/or bedtime glucose levels). Additional injections and subsequent dosage adjustments must address the specific phase of insulin release that is primarily contributing to the patient's impaired glycemic control. Intensification of therapy can usually begin with a second injection of ~4 units/day followed by adjustments of ~2 units/day every 3 days until the targeted blood glucose is within range (Nathan, 2009).

In the setting of glucose toxicity (loss of beta-cell sensitivity to glucose concentrations), insulin therapy may be used for short-term management to restore sensitivity of beta-cells; in these cases, the dose may need to be rapidly reduced/withdrawn when sensitivity is re-established.

Diabetic ketoacidosis (DKA) (unlabeled use): Only I.V. regular insulin should be used for severe DKA (Kitabchi, 2009). Treatment should continue until reversal of acid-base derangement/ketonemia. Serum glucose is not a direct indicator of these abnormalities, and may decrease more rapidly than correction of the metabolic abnormalities. Also, refer to institution-specific protocols where appropriate.

Children and Adults <20 years (Kitabchi, 2004):

I.V.:

Infusion: 0.1 units/kg/hour

Adjustment: If serum glucose does not fall by 50 mg/dL in the first hour, check hydration status; if acceptable, double insulin dose hourly until glucose levels fall at rate of 50-75 mg/dL per hour. Once serum glucose reaches 250 mg/dL, decrease dose to 0.05-0.1 units/kg/hour; dextrose-containing I.V. fluids should be administered to maintain serum glucose between 150-250 mg/dL until the acidosis clears. After resolution of DKA, supplement I.V. insulin with SubQ insulin as needed until the patient is able to eat and transition fully to a SubQ insulin regimen. An overlap of ~1-2 hours between discontinuation of I.V. insulin and administration of SubQ insulin is recommended to ensure adequate plasma insulin levels.

SubQ, I.M. (**Note:** Only use the SubQ and I.M route if I.V. infusion access is unavailable): 0.1-0.3 units/kg SubQ bolus, followed by 0.1 units/kg given every hour SubQ or I.M. or 0.15-0.2 units/kg every 2 hours SubQ; continue until acidosis clears, then decrease to 0.05 units/kg given every hour until SubQ replacement dosing can be initiated (Kitabchi, 2004; Wolfsdorf, 2007)

Adults ≥20 years (Kitabchi, 2009):

I.V.:

Bolus: 0.1 units/kg (optional)

Infusion: 0.1-0.14 units/kg/hour. **Note:** If no I.V. bolus was administered, patients should receive a continuous infusion of 0.14 units/kg/hour; lower doses may not achieve adequate insulin concentrations to suppress hepatic ketone body production.

Adjustment: If serum glucose does not fall by at least 10% in the first hour, give an I.V. bolus of 0.14 units/kg and continue previous regimen. In addition, if serum glucose does not fall by 50-70 mg/dL in the first hour, the insulin infusion dose should be increased hourly until a steady glucose decline is achieved Once serum glucose reaches 200 mg/dL, decrease infusion dose to 0.02-0.05 units/kg/hour or switch to SubQ rapid-acting insulin (eg, aspart, lispro) at 0.1 units/kg every 2 hours; dextrose-containing I.V. fluids should be administered to maintain serum glucose between 150-250 mg/dL until the acidosis clears. After resolution of DKA, supplement I.V. insulin with SubQ insulin as needed until the patient is able to eat and transition fully to a SubQ insulin regimen. An overlap of ~1-2 hours between discontinuation of I.V. insulin and administration of SubQ insulin is recommended to ensure adequate plasma insulin levels.

SubQ, I.M.: The following dosing regimen from the 2004 ADA position statement recommends regular insulin (Kitabchi, 2004):

Bolus: 0.4 units/kg; **Note:** Give half of the dose (0.2 units/kg) as an I.V. bolus and half of the dose (0.2 units/kg) as SubQ or I.M.

Intermittent: 0.1 units/kg given every hour SubQ or I.M.

Adjustment: If serum glucose does not fall by 50-70 mg/dL in the first hour, administer 10 units hourly by I.V. bolus until glucose levels fall at a rate of 50-70 mg/dL per hour. Once serum glucose reaches 250 mg/dL, decrease dose to 5-10 units SubQ every 2 hours; dextrose-containing I.V. fluids should be administered to maintain serum glucose between 150-250 mg/dL until the acidosis clears.

Gestational diabetes mellitus (unlabeled use): Insulin therapy should be considered when medical nutrition therapy has not achieved GDM glycemic goals (fasting plasma glucose: <95 mg/dL; 1-hour postprandial levels: <130-140 mg/dL; 2-hour postprandial levels: <120 mg/dL); dose and timing of administration should be based on frequent monitoring of plasma glucose levels (ACOG, 2001; ADA, 2004). Human insulin may be preferred (ADA, 2004); however, rapid-acting insulin analogues may also be considered (ACOG, 2001).

Hyperglycemia, critically ill (unlabeled use): Adults: I.V. continuous infusion: Insulin therapy should be implemented when blood glucose ≥150 mg/dL with a goal to maintain blood glucose <150 mg/dL (with values absolutely <180 mg/dL) using a protocol that achieves a low rate of hypoglycemia (ie, ≤70 mg/dL). Alternatively, other rapid acting insulin analogues (eg, insulin aspart or insulin glulisine) may also be used as a continuous infusion to maintain glycemic control (in place of regular insulin). Before discontinuation, stable ICU patients should be transitioned to a protocol-driven basal/bolus insulin regimen, based on insulin infusion history and carbohydrate intake, to avoid loss of glycemic control. Subcutaneous insulin therapy may be considered for selected clinically stable ICU patients (Jacobi, 2012). **Note:** The Surviving Sepsis Campaign guidelines recommend initiating insulin dosing in patients with severe sepsis when 2 consecutive blood glucose concentrations are >180 mg/dL and to target an upper blood glucose ≤180 mg/dL (Dellinger, 2013).

Hyperkalemia, moderate-to-severe (unlabeled use): I.V.:

Children: 0.1 units/kg regular insulin with dextrose 400 mg/kg infused over 15-30 minutes; ratio of ~1 unit of insulin to every 4 g of dextrose (Hegenbarth, 2008). **Note:** Dextrose monotherapy may be sufficient to correct hyperkalemia.

Adults: 10 units regular insulin mixed with 25 g dextrose (50 mL $D_{50}W$) given over 15-30 minutes (ACLS, 2010); alternatively, 50 mL $D_{50}W$ over 5 minutes followed by 10 units regular insulin I.V. push over seconds may be administered in the setting of imminent cardiac arrest. In patients with ongoing cardiac arrest (eg, PEA with presumed hyperkalemia), administration of $D_{50}W$ over <5 minutes is routine. Effects on potassium are temporary. As appropriate, consider methods of enhancing potassium removal/excretion.

Hyperosmolar hyperglycemic state (HHS) (unlabeled use): Only regular insulin should be used. Infusion should continue until reversal of mental status changes and hyperosmolality. Serum glucose is not a direct indicator of these abnormalities, and may decrease more rapidly than correction of the metabolic abnormalities. Also, refer to institution-specific protocols where appropriate.

Children and Adults <20 years (Kitabchi, 2004):

I.V.:

Infusion: 0.1 units/kg/hour

Adjustment: If serum glucose does not fall by 50 mg/dL in the first hour, check hydration status; if acceptable, double insulin dose hourly until glucose levels fall at rate of 50-75 mg/dL per hour. Once serum glucose reaches 300 mg/dL, decrease dose to 0.05-0.1 units/kg/hour; dextrose-containing I.V. fluids should be administered to maintain serum glucose between 250-300 mg/dL until hyperosmolality clears and mental status returns to normal. After resolution of HHS, supplement I.V. insulin with SubQ insulin as needed until the patient is able to eat and transition fully to a SubQ insulin regimen. An overlap of ~1-2 hours between discontinuation of I.V. insulin and administration of SubQ insulin is recommended to ensure adequate plasma insulin levels.

SubQ, I.M. (**Note:** Only use the SubQ and I.M route if I.V. infusion access is unavailable): 0.1-0.3 units/kg SubQ bolus, followed by 0.1 units/kg given every hour SubQ or I.M. or 0.15-0.2 units/kg every 2 hours SubQ; continue until resolution of hyperosmolality, then decrease to 0.05 units/kg given every hour until SubQ replacement dosing can be initiated (Kitabchi, 2004; Wolfsdorf, 2007)

Adults ≥20 years (Kitabchi, 2009):

I.V.:

Bolus: 0.1 units/kg bolus (optional)

Infusion: 0.1-0.14 units/kg/hour. **Note:** If no I.V. bolus was administered, patients should receive a continuous infusion of 0.14 units/kg/hour.

Adjustment: If serum glucose does not fall by at least 10% in the first hour, give an I.V. bolus of 0.14 units/kg and continue previous regimen. In addition, if serum glucose does not fall by 50-70 mg/dL in the first hour, the insulin infusion dose should be increased hourly until a steady glucose decline is achieved. Once serum glucose reaches 300 mg/dL, decrease dose to 0.02-0.05 units/kg/hour; dextrose-containing I.V. fluids should be administered to maintain serum glucose between 200-300 mg/dL until the patient is mentally alert. After resolution of HHS, supplement I.V. insulin with SubQ insulin as needed until the patient is able to eat and transition fully to a SubQ insulin regimen. An overlap of ~1-2 hours between discontinuation of I.V. insulin and administration of SubQ insulin is recommended to ensure adequate plasma insulin levels.

Dosing adjustment in renal impairment: Insulin requirements are reduced due to changes in insulin clearance or metabolism. Close monitoring of blood glucose and adjustment of therapy is required in renal impairment.

Cl_{cr} 10-50 mL/minute: Administer at 75% of normal dose and monitor glucose closely

Cl_{cr} <10 mL/minute: Administer at 25% to 50% of normal dose and monitor glucose closely

Hemodialysis: Because of a large molecular weight (6000 daltons), insulin is not significantly removed by hemodialysis; supplemental dose is not necessary

Peritoneal dialysis: Because of a large molecular weight (6000 daltons), insulin is not significantly removed by peritoneal dialysis; supplemental dose is not necessary

Continuous renal replacement therapy: Administer 75% of normal dose and monitor glucose closely; supplemental dose is not necessary

Dosing adjustment in hepatic impairment: Insulin requirements may be reduced. Close monitoring of blood glucose and adjustment of therapy is required in hepatic impairment.

Dietary Considerations Individualized medical nutrition therapy (MNT) based on ADA recommendations is an integral part of therapy.

Usual Infusion Concentrations: Pediatric I.V. infusion: 0.1 unit/mL, 0.5 unit/mL, **or** 1 unit/mL

Usual Infusion Concentrations: Adult I.V. infusion: 100 units in 100 mL (concentration: 1 unit/mL) of NS

Administration

SubQ administration: Do not use if solution is viscous or cloudy; use only if clear and colorless. Regular insulin should be administered within 30-60 minutes before a meal. Cold injections should be avoided. SubQ administration is usually made into the thighs, arms, buttocks, or abdomen; rotate injection sites. When mixing regular insulin with other preparations of insulin, regular insulin should be drawn into syringe first. Regular insulin is not recommended for use in external SubQ insulin infusion pump.

I.M. administration: Do not use if solution is viscous or cloudy; use only if clear and colorless. May be administered I.M. in selected clinical situations; close monitoring of blood glucose and serum potassium as well as medical supervision is required.

I.V. administration: Do not use if solution is viscous or cloudy; use only if clear and colorless. May be administered I.V. with close monitoring of blood glucose and serum potassium; appropriate medical supervision is required. If possible, avoid I.V. bolus administration in pediatric patients with DKA; may increase risk of cerebral edema. **Do not administer mixtures of insulin formulations intravenously.** I.V. administration of U-500 regular insulin is not recommended.

I.V. infusions: To minimize insulin adsorption to I.V. tubing: Flush the I.V. tubing with a priming infusion of 20 mL from the insulin infusion, whenever a new I.V. tubing set is added to the insulin infusion container. (Jacobi, 2012; Thompson, 2012).

Note: Also refer to institution-specific protocols where appropriate.

If insulin is required prior to the availability of the insulin drip, regular insulin should be administered by I.V. push injection.

Because of insulin adsorption to I.V. tubing or infusion bags, the actual amount of insulin being administered via I.V. infusion could be substantially less than the apparent amount. Therefore, adjustment of the I.V. infusion rate should be based on effect and not solely on the apparent insulin dose. The apparent dose may be used as a starting point for determining the subsequent SubQ dosing regimen (Moghissi, 2009); however, the transition to SubQ administration requires continuous medical supervision, frequent monitoring of blood glucose, and careful adjustment of therapy. In addition, SubQ insulin should be given 1-4 hours prior to the discontinuation of I.V. insulin to prevent hyperglycemia (Moghissi, 2009).

Monitoring Parameters

Critically-ill patients receiving insulin infusion: Blood glucose every 1-2 hours. **Note:** Every 4 hour blood glucose monitoring is not recommended unless a low hypoglycemia rate is demonstrated with the insulin protocol used. Arterial or venous whole blood sampling is recommended for patients in shock, on vasopressor therapy, or with severe edema, and when on a prolonged insulin infusion (Jacobi, 2012).

Diabetes mellitus: Plasma glucose, electrolytes, Hb A_{1c}

DKA/HHS: Serum electrolytes, glucose, BUN, creatinine, osmolality, venous pH (repeat arterial blood gases are generally unnecessary), anion gap, urine output, urinalysis, mental status

Hyperkalemia: Serum potassium and glucose must be closely monitored to avoid hypokalemia, rebound hyperkalemia, and hypoglycemia.

Reference Range

Therapeutic, serum insulin (fasting): 5-20 µIU/mL (SI: 35-145 pmol/L)

Glucose, fasting:

Newborns: 60-110 mg/dL

Adults: 60-110 mg/dL

Elderly: 100-180 mg/dL

Recommendations for glycemic control in nonpregnant adults with diabetes mellitus (ADA, 2013):

Hb A_{1c}: <7% (a more aggressive [<6.5%] or less aggressive [<8%] Hb A_{1c} goal may be targeted based on patient-specific characteristics)

Preprandial capillary plasma glucose: 70-130 mg/dL

Peak postprandial capillary plasma glucose: <180 mg/dL

Additional Information

Split-mixed or basal-bolus regimens: Combination regimens which optimize differences in the onset and duration of different insulin products are commonly used to approximate physiologic secretion. In split-mixed regimens, an intermediate-acting insulin (eg, NPH insulin) is administered once or twice daily and supplemented by short-acting (regular) or rapid-acting (lispro, aspart, or glulisine) insulin. Blood glucose measurements are completed several times daily. Dosages are adjusted emphasizing the individual component of the regimen which most directly influences the blood sugar in question (either the intermediate-acting component or the shorter-acting component). Fixed-ratio formulations (eg, 70/30 mix) may be used as twice daily injections in this scenario; however, the ability to titrate the dosage of an individual component is limited. An example of a "split-mixed" regimen would be 21 units of NPH plus 9 units of regular insulin in the morning and an evening meal dose consisting of 14 units of NPH plus 6 units of regular insulin.

Basal-bolus regimens are designed to more closely mimic physiologic secretion. These regimens employ a long-acting insulin (eg, glargine) to simulate basal insulin secretion. The basal component is frequently administered at bedtime or in the early morning. This is supplemented by multiple daily injections of rapid-acting products (lispro, aspart, or glulisine) immediately prior to a meal, which provides insulin at the time when nutrients are absorbed. An example of a basal-bolus regimen would be 30 units of glargine at bedtime and 12 units of lispro insulin prior to each meal.

Estimation of the effect per unit: A "Rule of 1500" has been frequently used as a means to estimate the change in blood sugar relative to each unit of insulin administered. In fact, the recommended values used in these calculations may vary from 1500-2200 (a value of 1500 is generally recommended for regular insulin while 1800 is recommended for "rapid-acting insulins"). The higher values lead to more conservative estimates of the effect per unit of insulin, and therefore lead to more cautious adjustments. The effect per unit of insulin is approximated by dividing the selected numerical value (eg, 1500-2200) by the number of units/day received by the patient. This may be used as a crude approximation of the patient's insulin sensitivity as adjustments to individual components of the regimen are made. Each additional unit of insulin added to the corresponding insulin dose may be expected to lower the blood glucose by this amount.

To illustrate, in the "basal-bolus" regimen example presented above, the rule of 1800 would indicate an expected change of 27 mg/dL per unit of lispro insulin (the total daily insulin dose is 66 units; using the formula: 1800/66 = 27). A patient may be instructed to add additional insulin if the preprandial glucose is >125 mg/dL. For a prelunch glucose of 195 mg/dL, this would mean the patient would administer the scheduled 12 units of lispro along with an additional "correctional" 3 units for a total of 15 units prior to the meal. If correctional doses are required on a consistent basis, an adjustment of the patients diet and/or scheduled insulin dose may be necessary.

Dosage Forms Excipient information presented when available (limited, particularly for generics); consult specific product labeling.

Solution, Injection:

HumuLIN R: 100 units/mL (3 mL, 10 mL) [contains metacresol, phenol]

NovoLIN R: 100 units/mL (10 mL) [contains metacresol]

NovoLIN R ReliOn: 100 units/mL (10 mL) [contains metacresol]

Solution, Subcutaneous:

HumuLIN R U-500 (CONCENTRATED): 500 units/mL (20 mL) [contains metacresol]

◆ **Insulin Regular and Insulin NPH** *see* Insulin NPH and Insulin Regular *on page 1093*

◆ **Intanza (Can)** *see* Influenza Virus Vaccine (Inactivated) *on page 1078*

◆ **Integrilin** *see* Eptifibatide *on page 731*

◆ **Integrilin® (Can)** *see* Eptifibatide *on page 731*

◆ **Intelence** *see* Etravirine *on page 807*

◆ **Intelence® (Can)** *see* Etravirine *on page 807*

◆ **α-2-interferon** *see* Interferon Alfa-2b *on page 1099*

◆ **Interferon Alfa-2a (PEG Conjugate)** *see* Peginterferon Alfa-2a *on page 1590*

◆ **Interferon Alfa-2b and Ribavirin Combination Pack** *see* Interferon Alfa-2b and Ribavirin *on page 1102*

◆ **Interferon Alfa-2b (PEG Conjugate)** *see* Peginterferon Alfa-2b *on page 1594*

Interferon Alfa-2b (in ter FEER on AL fa too bee)

Brand Names: U.S. Intron-A

Brand Names: Canada Intron® A

Index Terms INF-alpha 2; Interferon Alpha-2b; rLFN-α2; α-2-interferon

Pharmacologic Category Interferon

Use

Patients ≥1 year of age: Chronic hepatitis B

Patients ≥3 years of age: Chronic hepatitis C (in combination with ribavirin)

Patients ≥18 years of age: Condyloma acuminata, chronic hepatitis B, chronic hepatitis C, hairy cell leukemia, malignant melanoma (high-risk of recurrence), AIDS-related Kaposi's sarcoma, follicular non-Hodgkin lymphoma

Unlabeled Use Treatment of cutaneous ulcerations of Behçet's disease, neuroendocrine tumors (including carcinoid syndrome and islet cell tumor), cutaneous T-cell lymphoma, desmoid tumor, hepatitis D, chronic myelogenous leukemia (CML), non-Hodgkin lymphomas (other than follicular lymphoma, see approved use), multiple myeloma, renal cell carcinoma, West Nile virus

Pregnancy Risk Factor C / X in combination with ribavirin

Pregnancy Considerations Animal reproduction studies have demonstrated abortifacient effects. Disruption of the normal menstrual cycle was also observed in animal studies; therefore, the manufacturer recommends that reliable contraception is used in women of childbearing potential. Alfa interferon is endogenous to normal amniotic fluid. *In vitro* administration studies have reported that when administered to the mother, it does not cross the placenta. Case reports of use in pregnant women are limited. The Perinatal HIV Guidelines Working Group does not recommend that interferon-alfa be used during pregnancy. Interferon alfa-2b monotherapy should only be used in pregnancy when the potential benefit to the mother justifies the possible risk to the fetus. Combination therapy with ribavirin is contraindicated in pregnancy (refer to Ribavirin monograph); two forms of contraception should be used during combination therapy and patients should have monthly pregnancy tests. A pregnancy registry has been established for women inadvertently exposed to ribavirin while pregnant (800-593-2214).

Breast-Feeding Considerations Breast milk samples obtained from a lactating mother prior to and after administration of interferon alfa-2b showed that interferon alfa is present in breast milk and administration of the medication did not significantly affect endogenous levels. Breast-feeding is not linked to the spread of hepatitis C virus; however, if nipples are cracked or bleeding, breast-feeding is not recommended. Mothers coinfected with HIV are discouraged from breast-feeding to decrease potential transmission of HIV.

Medication Guide Available Yes

Contraindications Hypersensitivity to interferon alfa or any component of the formulation; decompensated liver disease; autoimmune hepatitis

Combination therapy with interferon alfa-2b and ribavirin is also contraindicated in pregnancy, males with pregnant partners; hemoglobinopathies (eg, thalassemia major, sickle-cell anemia); renal dysfunction (Cl_{cr} <50 mL/minute)

Warnings/Precautions [U.S. Boxed Warning]: May cause or aggravate fatal or life-threatening autoimmune disorders, neuropsychiatric symptoms (including depression and/or suicidal thoughts/behaviors), ischemic, and/or infectious disorders; monitor closely with clinical and lab evaluations (periodic); discontinue treatment for severe persistent or worsening symptoms; some cases may resolve with discontinuation.

Neuropsychiatric disorders: May cause neuropsychiatric events, including depression, psychosis, mania, suicidal behavior/ideation, homicidal ideation; may occur in patients with or without previous psychiatric symptoms. Careful neuropsychiatric monitoring is recommended during and for 6 months after treatment in patients who develop psychiatric disorders (including clinical depression). New or exacerbated neuropsychiatric or substance abuse disorders are best managed with early intervention. Use with caution in patients with a history of psychiatric disorders. Drug screening and periodic health evaluation (including monitoring of psychiatric symptoms) is recommended if initiating treatment in patients with coexisting psychiatric condition or substance abuse disorders. Suicidal ideation or attempts may occur more frequently in pediatric patients when compared to adults. Higher doses in elderly patients, or diseases other than hairy cell leukemia, may result in increased CNS toxicity.

Hepatic disease: May cause hepatotoxicity; monitor closely if abnormal liver function tests develop. A transient increase in ALT (≥2 times baseline) may occur in patients treated with interferon alfa-2b for chronic hepatitis B. Therapy generally may continue; monitor. Worsening and potentially fatal liver disease, including jaundice, hepatic encephalopathy, and hepatic failure have been reported in patients receiving interferon alfa for chronic hepatitis B and C with decompensated liver disease, autoimmune hepatitis, history of autoimmune disease, and immunosuppressed transplant recipients; avoid use in these patients. Chronic hepatitis B or C patients with a history of autoimmune disease or who are immunosuppressed transplant recipients should not receive interferon alfa-2b. Discontinue treatment (if appropriate) in any patient developing signs or symptoms of liver failure.

Bone marrow suppression: Causes bone marrow suppression, including potentially severe cytopenias, and very rarely, aplastic anemia. Discontinue treatment for severe neutropenia (ANC <500/mm^3) or thrombocytopenia (platelets <25,000/mm^3). Hemolytic anemia (hemoglobin <10 g/dL) was observed when combined with ribavirin; anemia occurred within 1-2 weeks of initiation of therapy.

Use caution in patients with pre-existing myelosuppression and in patients with concomitant medications which cause myelosuppression.

Autoimmune disorders: Avoid use in patients with history of autoimmune disorders; development of autoimmune disorders (thrombocytopenia, vasculitis, Raynaud's disease, rheumatoid arthritis, lupus erythematosus and rhabdomyolysis) has been associated with use. Monitor closely; consider discontinuing. Worsening of psoriasis and sarcoidosis (and the development of new sarcoidosis) have been reported; use caution.

Cardiovascular disease/coagulation disorders: Use caution and monitor closely in patients with cardiovascular disease (ischemic or thromboembolic), arrhythmias, hypertension, and in patients with a history of MI or prior therapy with cardiotoxic drugs. Patients with pre-existing cardiac disease and/or advanced cancer should have baseline and periodic ECGs. May cause hypotension (during administration or delayed), arrhythmia, tachycardia, cardiomyopathy (~2% in AIDS-related Kaposi's Sarcoma patients) and/or MI. Hemorrhagic cerebrovascular events have been observed with therapy. Use caution in patients with coagulation disorders.

Endocrine disorders: Thyroid disorders (possibly reversible) have been reported; use caution in patients with pre-existing thyroid disease. TSH levels should be within normal limits prior to initiating interferon. Discontinue interferon use in patients who cannot maintain normal ranges with thyroid medication. Diabetes mellitus has been reported; discontinue if cannot effectively manage with medication. Use with caution in patients with a history of diabetes mellitus, particularly if prone to DKA. Hypertriglyceridemia has been reported; discontinue if persistent and severe, and/or combined with symptoms of pancreatitis.

Pulmonary disease: Dyspnea, pulmonary infiltrates, pulmonary hypertension, interstitial pneumonitis, pneumonia, bronchiolitis obliterans, and sarcoidosis may be induced or aggravated by treatment, sometimes resulting in respiratory failure or fatality. Has been reported more in patients being treated for chronic hepatitis C, although has also occurred with use for oncology indications. Patients with fever, cough, dyspnea or other respiratory symptoms should be evaluated with a chest x-ray; monitor closely and consider discontinuing treatment with evidence of impaired pulmonary function. Use with caution in patients with a history of pulmonary disease.

Ophthalmic disorders: Decreased or loss of vision, macular edema, optic neuritis, retinal hemorrhages, cotton wool spots, papilledema, retinal detachment (serous), and retinal artery or vein thrombosis have occurred (or been aggravated) in patients receiving alpha interferons. Use caution in patients with pre-existing eye disorders; monitor closely; a complete eye exam should be done promptly in patients who develop ocular symptoms; discontinue with new or worsening ophthalmic disorders.

Commonly associated with fever and flu-like symptoms; rule out other causes/infection with persistent fever; use with caution in patients with debilitating conditions. Acute hypersensitivity reactions have been reported. Do not treat patients with visceral AIDS-related Kaposi's sarcoma associated with rapidly-progressing or life-threatening disease. Some formulations contain albumin, which may carry a remote risk of viral transmission. Due to differences in dosage, patients should not change brands of interferons without the concurrence of their healthcare provider. According to the Centers for Disease Control and Prevention (CDC), pen-shaped injection devices should never be used for more than one person (even when the needle is changed) because of the risk of infection. The injection device should be clearly labeled with individual patient information to ensure that the correct pen is used (CDC, 2012). Combination therapy with ribavirin is associated with birth defects and/or fetal mortality and hemolytic anemia. Do not use combination therapy with ribavirin in patients with renal dysfunction (Cl_{cr} <50 mL/minute).

Adverse Reactions Note: In a majority of patients, a flu-like syndrome (fever, chills, tachycardia, malaise, myalgia, headache), occurs within 1-2 hours of administration; may last up to 24 hours and may be dose limiting.

>10%:

- Cardiovascular: Chest pain (≤28%)
- Central nervous system: Fatigue (8% to 96%), fever (34% to 94%; more common in children), headache (21% to 62%), chills (≤54%), depression (3% to 40%; grades 3/4: 2%), somnolence (≤33%), dizziness (≤24%), irritability (≤22%), pain (≤18%), amnesia (≤14%), concentration impaired (≤14%), malaise (≤14%), confusion (≤12%), insomnia (≤12%)
- Dermatologic: Alopecia (≤38%), rash (≤25%), pruritus (≤11%)
- Endocrine & metabolic: Amenorrhea (≤12%)
- Gastrointestinal: Anorexia (1% to 69%), nausea, (17% to 66%), diarrhea (2% to 45%), xerostomia (≤28%), vomiting (children 27%; adults 7% to 10%), taste alteration (≤24%), abdominal pain (1% to 23%), constipation (≤14%), gingivitis (≤14%), weight loss (<1% to 13%)
- Hematologic: Neutropenia (≤92%; grade 4: 1% to 4%), leukopenia (≤68%), anemia (≤32%), thrombocytopenia (≤15%)
- Hepatic: AST increased (≤63%; grades 3/4: 14%), ALT increased (≤15%), pain (upper right quadrant: up to 15%); alkaline phosphatase increased (≤13%)
- Local: Injection site reaction (≤20%)
- Neuromuscular & skeletal: Myalgia (28% to 75%), weakness (≤63%), rigors (≤42%), paresthesia (1% to 21%), skeletal pain (≤21%), arthralgia (≤19%), back pain (≤19%)
- Renal: BUN increased (≤12%)
- Respiratory: Dyspnea (≤34%), cough (≤31%), pharyngitis (≤31%), sinusitis (≤21%)
- Miscellaneous: Flu-like syndrome (≤79%), diaphoresis (1% to 21%), moniliasis (≤17%)

5% to 10%:

- Cardiovascular: Edema (≤10%), hypertension (≤9%)
- Central nervous system: Hypoesthesia (≤10%), anxiety (≤9%), vertigo (≤8%), agitation (≤7%)
- Dermatologic: Dry skin (≤10%), dermatitis (≤8%), purpura (≤5%)
- Endocrine & metabolic: Libido decreased (≤5%)
- Gastrointestinal: Loose stools (≤10%), dyspepsia (≤8%)
- Genitourinary: Urinary tract infection (≤5%)
- Renal: Polyuria (≤10%), serum creatinine increased (≤6%)
- Respiratory: Bronchitis (≤10%), nasal congestion (≤10%), epistaxis (≤7%)
- Miscellaneous: Infection (≤7%), herpes virus infections (≤5%)

<5% (Limited to important or life-threatening): Acute hypersensitivity reaction, aggression, albuminuria, alcohol intolerance, allergic reactions, anaphylaxis, angina, angioedema, aphasia, aplastic anemia (rarely), arrhythmia, ascites, asthma, ataxia, atrial fibrillation, bell's palsy, bilirubinemia, blurred vision, bradycardia, bronchiolitis obliterans, bronchoconstriction, bronchospasm, cardiac failure, cardiomegaly, cardiomyopathy, cellulitis, colitis, coma, conjunctivitis, coronary artery disorder, cotton wool spots, cyanosis, cystitis, dehydration, diabetes mellitus, dysphasia, dysuria, eczema, ejection fraction decreased, epidermal necrolysis, erythema, erythema multiforme, erythematous rash, esophagitis, extrapyramidal disorder, extrasystoles, gastrointestinal hemorrhage, granulocytopenia, hallucination, hearing loss/impairment, heart valve

disorder, hematuria, hemolytic anemia, hemoptysis, hepatic encephalopathy, hepatic failure, hepatitis, hepatotoxicity, hot flashes, homicidal ideation, hyper-/hypothyroidism, hypercalcemia, hyperglycemia, hypertriglyceridemia, hypochromic anemia, hypopituitarism, hypotension, hypothermia, hypoventilation, impotence, incontinence, injection site necrosis, jaundice, lactate dehydrogenase increased, leukorrhea, liver function test abnormal, lupus erythematosus, lymphadenitis, lymphadenopathy, lymphocytosis, lymphopenia, maculopapular rash, macular edema, menorrhagia, MI, migraine, muscle atrophy, myositis, nephrotic syndrome, nervousness, neuralgia, neuropathy, neurosis, nystagmus, optic neuritis, palpitation, pancreatitis, pancytopenia, papilledema, paranoia, peripheral ischemia, peripheral neuropathy, photophobia, photosensitivity, pleural effusion, pneumonia, pneumonitis (interstitial), pneumothorax, proteinuria, psoriasis exacerbation, psychosis, pulmonary embolism, pulmonary fibrosis, pulmonary hypertension, pulmonary infiltrates, pure red cell aplasia, Raynaud's disease, renal failure, renal insufficiency, respiratory insufficiency, retinal artery thrombosis, retinal detachment (serous), retinal vein thrombosis, rhabdomyolysis, sarcoidosis exacerbation, sebaceous cyst, seizure, sepsis, sexual dysfunction, Stevens-Johnson syndrome, stomatitis, stroke, suicidal attempt/ideation, syncope, systemic lupus erythematosus, tachycardia, tendonitis, thrombocytopenia purpura (idiopathic and thrombotic), thrombosis, toxic epidermal necrolysis, upper respiratory tract infection, urticaria, uterine bleeding, vasculitis, Vogt-Koyanagi-Harada syndrome, wheezing

Drug Interactions

Metabolism/Transport Effects **Inhibits** CYP1A2 (weak)

Avoid Concomitant Use

Avoid concomitant use of Interferon Alfa-2b with any of the following: CloZAPine; Telbivudine

Increased Effect/Toxicity

Interferon Alfa-2b may increase the levels/effects of: Aldesleukin; CloZAPine; Methadone; Ribavirin; Telbivudine; Theophylline Derivatives; Zidovudine

Decreased Effect There are no known significant interactions involving a decrease in effect.

Preparation for Administration Powder for injection: The manufacturer recommends reconstituting vial with the diluent provided (SWFI). When reconstituted with SWFI 1 mL, the 10 million unit vial concentration is 10 million units/mL, the 18 million unit vial concentration is 18 million units/mL, and the 50 million unit vial concentration is 50 million units/mL. Swirl gently. To prepare solution for infusion, further dilute appropriate dose in NS 100 mL. Final concentration should be ≥10 million units/100 mL.

Storage/Stability Store powder and solution for injection (vials and pens) under refrigeration at 2°C to 8°C (36°F to 46°F); do not freeze.

Powder for injection: Following reconstitution, should be used immediately, but may be stored under refrigeration for up to 24 hours.

Prefilled pens: After first use, discard unused portion after 4 weeks.

Mechanism of Action Binds to a specific receptor on the cell wall to initiate intracellular activity; multiple effects can be detected including induction of gene transcription. Inhibits cellular growth, alters the state of cellular differentiation, interferes with oncogene expression, alters cell surface antigen expression, increases phagocytic activity of macrophages, and augments cytotoxicity of lymphocytes for target cells

Pharmacodynamics/Kinetics

Distribution: V_d: 31 L; but has been noted to be much greater (370-720 L) in leukemia patients receiving continuous infusion IFN; IFN does not penetrate the CSF

Metabolism: Primarily renal

Bioavailability: I.M.: 83%; SubQ: 90%

Half-life elimination: I.V.: ~2 hours; I.M., SubQ: ~2-3 hours

Time to peak, serum: I.M., SubQ: ~3-12 hours; I.V.: By the end of a 30-minute infusion

Dosage Details concerning dosing in combination regimens should also be consulted. Consider premedication with acetaminophen prior to administration to reduce the incidence of some adverse reactions. Not all dosage forms and strengths are appropriate for all indications; refer to product labeling for details.

Children 1-17 years: **Note:** The following dosing may also be used in **infants** in the setting of HIV-exposure/-infection (CDC, 2009).

Chronic hepatitis B (including HIV coinfection): SubQ: 3 million units/m^2 3 times weekly for 1 week, followed by 6 million units/m^2 3 times weekly (maximum: 10 million units per dose); total duration of therapy 16-24 weeks (treat for 24 weeks in HIV-exposure/-infection)

Chronic hepatitis C with HIV coinfection: I.M., SubQ: 3-5 million units/m^2 3 times weekly (maximum: 3 million units per dose) with ribavirin for 48 weeks, regardless of HCV genotype (CDC, 2009)

Adults:

Hairy cell leukemia: I.M., SubQ: 2 million units/m^2 3 times weekly for up to 6 months (may continue treatment with sustained treatment response); discontinue for disease progression or failure to respond after 6 months

Lymphoma (follicular): SubQ: 5 million units 3 times weekly for up to 18 months

Malignant melanoma: Induction: 20 million units/m^2 I.V. for 5 consecutive days per week for 4 weeks, followed by maintenance dosing of 10 million units/m^2 SubQ 3 times weekly for 48 weeks

AIDS-related Kaposi's sarcoma: I.M., SubQ: 30 million units/m^2 3 times weekly; continue until disease progression or until maximal response has been achieved after 16 weeks

Chronic hepatitis B: I.M., SubQ: 5 million units daily or 10 million units 3 times weekly for 16 weeks

Chronic hepatitis C: I.M., SubQ: 3 million units 3 times weekly. In patients with normalization of ALT at 16 weeks, continue treatment (if tolerated) for 18-24 months; consider discontinuation if normalization does not occur at 16 weeks. **Note:** May be used in combination therapy with ribavirin in previously untreated patients or in patients who relapse following alpha interferon therapy.

Condyloma acuminata: Intralesionally: 1 million units/lesion (maximum: 5 lesions per treatment) 3 times weekly (on alternate days) for 3 weeks; may administer a second course at 12-16 weeks

Dosage adjustment for toxicity:

Neuropsychiatric disorders (during treatment):

Clinical depression or other psychiatric problem: Monitor closely during and for 6 months after treatment.

Severe depression or other psychiatric disorder: Discontinue treatment.

Persistent or worsening psychiatric symptoms, suicidal ideation, aggression towards others: Discontinue treatment and follow with appropriate psychiatric intervention.

Hypersensitivity reaction (acute, serious), ophthalmic disorders (new or worsening), thyroid abnormality development (which cannot be normalized with medication), signs or symptoms of liver failure: Discontinue treatment.

Hematologic toxicity (also refer to indication specified adjustments below): ANC <500/mm^3 or platelets <25,000/mm^3: Discontinue treatment.

Liver function abnormality, pulmonary infiltrate development, evidence of pulmonary function impairment, or autoimmune disorder development, triglycerides >1000 mg/dL: Monitor closely and discontinue if appropriate.

Manufacturer-recommended adjustments, listed according to indication:

Lymphoma (follicular):

Neutrophils >1000/mm^3 to <1500/mm^3: Reduce dose by 50%; may re-escalate to starting dose when neutrophils return to >1500/mm^3

Severe toxicity (neutrophils <1000/mm^3 or platelets <50,000/mm^3): Temporarily withhold.

AST >5 times ULN or serum creatinine >2 mg/dL: Permanently discontinue.

Hairy cell leukemia:

Platelet count <50,000/mm^3: Do not administer intramuscularly (administer SubQ instead).

Severe toxicity: Reduce dose by 50% or temporarily withhold and resume with 50% dose reduction; permanently discontinue if persistent or recurrent severe toxicity is noted.

Chronic hepatitis B:

WBC <1500/mm^3, granulocytes <750/mm^3, or platelet count <50,000/mm^3, or other laboratory abnormality or severe adverse reaction: Reduce dose by 50%; may re-escalate to starting dose upon resolution of hematologic toxicity. Discontinue for persistent intolerance.

WBC <1000/mm^3, granulocytes <500/mm^3, or platelet count <25,000/mm^3: Permanently discontinue.

Chronic hepatitis C: Severe toxicity: Reduce dose by 50% or temporarily withhold until subsides; permanently discontinue for persistent toxicities after dosage reduction.

AIDS-related Kaposi sarcoma: Severe toxicity: Reduce dose by 50% or temporarily withhold; may resume at reduced dose with toxicity resolution; permanently discontinue for persistent/recurrent toxicities.

Malignant melanoma (induction and maintenance):

Severe toxicity, including neutrophils >250/mm^3 to <500/mm^3 or ALT/AST >5-10 times ULN: Temporarily withhold; resume with a 50% dose reduction when adverse reaction abates.

Neutrophils <250/mm^3, ALT/AST >10 times ULN, or severe/persistent adverse reactions: Permanently discontinue.

Dosage adjustment in renal impairment: Combination therapy with ribavirin (hepatitis C) should not be used in patients with reduced renal function (Cl_{cr} <50 mL/minute).

Dosage adjustment in hepatic impairment: No dosage adjustment provided in manufacturer's labeling.

Administration Administer dose in the evening (if possible) to enhance tolerability. Not all dosage forms are recommended for all administration routes; refer to manufacturer's labeling.

I.M.: Rotate injection sites. Some patients may be appropriate for self-administration with appropriate training. Allow to reach room temperature prior to injection. In hairy cell leukemia treatment, if platelets are <50,000/mm^3, do not administer intramuscularly (administer SubQ instead).

I.V.: Infuse over ~20 minutes

SubQ: Suggested for those who are at risk for bleeding or are thrombocytopenic. Rotate SubQ injection site. Patient should be well hydrated. Some patients may be appropriate for self-administration with appropriate training. Allow to reach room temperature prior to injection.

Intralesional: Inject at an angle nearly parallel to the plane of the skin, directing the needle to center of the base of the wart to infiltrate the lesion core and cause a small wheal. Only infiltrate the keratinized layer; avoid administration which is too deep or shallow. Allow to reach room temperature prior to injection.

Monitoring Parameters CBC with differential (baseline and periodic during treatment), liver function tests (baseline and periodic), electrolytes (baseline and periodic), serum creatinine (baseline), albumin, prothrombin time, triglycerides, thyroid-stimulating hormone (TSH) baseline and periodically during treatment (in patients with pre-existing thyroid disorders, repeat TSH at 3 months and 6 months); chest x-ray (baseline), weight; ophthalmic exam (baseline and periodic, or with new ocular symptoms); ECG (baseline and during treatment; in patients with pre-existing cardiac abnormalities or in advanced stages of cancer); neuropsychiatric changes during and for 6 months after therapy

Chronic hepatitis B: CBC with differential and platelets and liver function tests: Baseline, weeks 1, 2, 4, 8, 12, and 16, at the end of treatment, and then 3 and 6 months post treatment

Chronic hepatitis C:

CBC with differential and platelets: Baseline, weeks 1 and 2, then monthly

Liver function: Every 3 months

TSH: Baseline and periodically during treatment; in patients with pre-existing thyroid disorders also repeat at 3 months and 6 months

Malignant melanoma: CBC with differential and platelets and liver function tests: Weekly during induction phase, then monthly during maintenance

Oncology patients: Thyroid function monitoring (Hamnvik, 2011): TSH and anti-TPO antibodies at baseline; if TPO antibody positive, monitor TSH every 2 months; if TPO antibody negative, monitor TSH every 6 months

Dosage Forms Excipient information presented when available (limited, particularly for generics); consult specific product labeling.

Solution, Injection:

Intron-A: 6,000,000 units/mL (3.8 mL); 10,000,000 units/mL (3.2 mL)

Solution Reconstituted, Injection:

Intron-A: 10,000,000 units (1 ea) [contains benzyl alcohol]

Intron-A: 18,000,000 units (1 ea)

Intron-A: 50,000,000 units (1 ea) [contains benzyl alcohol]

Interferon Alfa-2b and Ribavirin

(in ter FEER on AL fa too bee & rye ba VYE rin)

Brand Names: U.S. Rebetron®

Index Terms Interferon Alfa-2b and Ribavirin Combination Pack; Ribavirin and Interferon Alfa-2b Combination Pack

Pharmacologic Category Antiviral Agent; Interferon

Use Combination therapy for the treatment of chronic hepatitis C in patients with compensated liver disease previously untreated with alpha interferon or who have relapsed after alpha interferon therapy

Pregnancy Risk Factor X

Dosage

Children ≥3 years: Chronic hepatitis C: **Note:** Treatment duration may vary. Consult current guidelines and literature. Combination therapy:

Intron® A: SubQ:

25-61 kg: 3 million int. units/m^2 3 times/week

>61 kg: Refer to adult dosing

Rebetol®: Oral: **Note:** Oral solution should be used in children 3-5 years of age, children ≤25 kg, or those unable to swallow capsules.

Capsule/solution: 15 mg/kg/day in 2 divided doses (morning and evening)

Capsule dosing recommendations:
26-36 kg: 400 mg/day (200 mg morning and evening)
37-49 kg: 600 mg/day (200 mg in the morning and two 200 mg capsules in the evening)
50-61 kg: 800 mg/day (two 200 mg capsules morning and evening)
>61 kg: Refer to adult dosing

Adults: Chronic hepatitis C: Recommended dosage of combination therapy:
Intron® A: SubQ: 3 million int. units 3 times/week **and**
Rebetol® capsule: Oral:
≤75 kg (165 lb): 1000 mg/day (two 200 mg capsules in the morning and three 200 mg capsules in the evening)
>75 kg: 1200 mg/day (three 200 mg capsules in the morning and three 200 mg capsules in the evening)
Note: Treatment duration may vary. Consult current guidelines and literature.

Dosing adjustment for toxicity: Note: Recommendations (per manufacturer labeling):
Anemia (RBC depression):
Patient **without** cardiac history:
Hemoglobin <10 g/dL:
Children: Decrease ribavirin dose by 1/2
Adults: Decrease ribavirin dose to 600 mg/day
Hemoglobin <8.5 g/dL: Permanently discontinue treatment
Patient **with** cardiac history:
Hemoglobin has ≥2 g/dL decrease during any 4-week period of treatment:
Children: Decrease ribavirin dose by 1/2 **and** decrease interferon alfa-2b to 1.5 million int. units 3 times/week
Adults: Decrease dose to ribavirin to 600 mg/day **and** decrease interferon-alfa 2b dose to 1.5 million int. units 3 times/week.
Hemoglobin <12 g/dL after 4 weeks of reduced dose: Permanently discontinue treatment
WBC, neutrophil, or platelet depression:
WBC <1500 cells/mm^3, neutrophils <750 cells/mm^3, or platelet count <50,000 cells/mm^3 (<80,000 cells/ mm^3 in children): Reduce interferon alfa-2b dose to 1.5 million int. units 3 times/week (50% reduction)
WBC <1000 cells/mm^3, neutrophils <500 cells/mm^3, or platelet count <25,000 cells/mm^3 (<50,000 cells/mm^3 in children): Permanently discontinue therapy

Dosage adjustment in renal impairment: Patients with Cl_{cr} <50 mL/minutes should not receive ribavirin.

Additional Information Complete prescribing information should be consulted for additional detail.

Dosage Forms Excipient information presented when available (limited, particularly for generics); consult specific product labeling.

Combination package:

For patients ≤75 kg [contains single-dose vials]:
Injection, solution: Interferon alfa-2b (Intron® A): 3 million units/0.5 mL (0.5 mL) [6 vials (3 million units/vial), 6 syringes, and alcohol swabs]
Capsule: Ribavirin (Rebetol®): 200 mg (70s)

For patients ≤75 kg [contains multidose vials]:
Injection, solution: Interferon alfa-2b (Intron® A): 3 million units/0.5 mL (3.8 mL) [1 multidose vial (18 million units/vial), 6 syringes, and alcohol swabs]
Capsule: Ribavirin (Rebetol®): 200 mg (70s)

For patients ≤75 kg [contains multidose pen]:
Injection, solution: Interferon alfa-2b (Intron® A): 3 million units/0.2 mL (1.5 mL) [1 multidose pen (18 million units/pen), 6 needles, and alcohol swabs]
Capsule: Ribavirin (Rebetol®): 200 mg (70s)

For patients >75 kg [contains single-dose vials]:
Injection, solution: Interferon alfa-2b (Intron® A): 3 million units/0.5 mL (0.5 mL) [6 vials (3 million units/vial), 6 syringes, and alcohol swabs]
Capsule: Ribavirin (Rebetol®): 200 mg (84s)

For patients >75 kg [contains multidose vials]:
Injection, solution: Interferon alfa-2b (Intron® A): 3 million units/0.5 mL (3.8 mL) [1 multidose vial (18 million units/vial), 6 syringes, and alcohol swabs]
Capsule: Ribavirin (Rebetol®): 200 mg (84s)

For patients >75 kg [contains multidose pen]:
Injection, solution: Interferon alfa-2b (Intron® A): 3 million units/0.2 mL (1.5 mL) [1 multidose pen (18 million units/pen), 6 needles, and alcohol swabs]
Capsule: Ribavirin (Rebetol®): 200 mg (84s)

For Rebetol® dose reduction [contains single-dose vials]:
Injection, solution: Interferon alfa-2b (Intron® A): 3 million units/0.5 mL (0.5 mL) [6 vials (3 million units/vial), 6 syringes, and alcohol swabs]
Capsule: Ribavirin (Rebetol®): 200 mg (42s)

For Rebetol® dose reduction [contains multidose vials]:
Injection, solution: Interferon alfa-2b (Intron® A): 3 million units/0.5 mL (3.8 mL) [1 multidose vial (18 million units/vial), 6 syringes, and alcohol swabs]
Capsule: Ribavirin (Rebetol®): 200 mg (42s)

For Rebetol® dose reduction [contains multidose pen]:
Injection, solution: Interferon alfa-2b (Intron® A): 3 million units/0.2 mL (1.5 mL) [1 multidose pen (18 million units/pen), 6 needles, and alcohol swabs]
Capsule: Ribavirin (Rebetol®): 200 mg (42s)

Interferon Alfacon-1 (in ter FEER on AL fa con one)

Brand Names: U.S. Infergen

Pharmacologic Category Interferon

Use Treatment of chronic hepatitis C virus (HCV) infection in patients ≥18 years of age with compensated liver disease and anti-HCV serum antibodies or HCV RNA; concurrent use with ribavirin in HCV-infected patients who have failed treatment with pegylated interferon/ribavirin (Bacon, 2009)

Pregnancy Risk Factor C

Medication Guide Available Yes

Dosage Adults ≥18 years: SubQ:
Chronic HCV infection: 9 mcg 3 times/week for 24 weeks; allow 48 hours between doses
Combination therapy with ribavirin: 15 mcg/day with ribavirin for up to 48 weeks
Patients who have previously tolerated interferon therapy but did not respond or relapsed: 15 mcg 3 times/week for up to 48 weeks
Dose reduction for toxicity: Dose should be held in patients who experience a severe adverse reaction, and treatment should be stopped or decreased if the reaction does not become tolerable.
Doses were reduced from 9 mcg to 7.5 mcg in the pivotal study.
For patients receiving 15 mcg/dose, doses were reduced in 3 mcg decrements. Efficacy is decreased with doses <7.5 mcg
Elderly: No information available.

Dosage adjustment in renal impairment: Cl_{cr} <50 mL/minute: Hepatitis C: Avoid combination therapy with ribavirin

Dosage adjustment in hepatic impairment: Use in decompensated hepatic disease (Child-Pugh class B or C) is contraindicated

Additional Information Complete prescribing information should be consulted for additional detail.

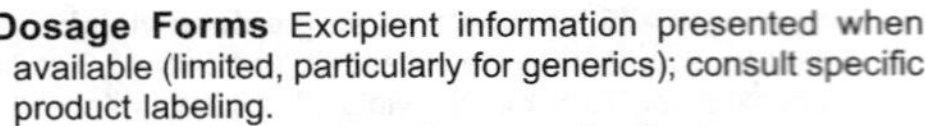

Dosage Forms Excipient information presented when available (limited, particularly for generics); consult specific product labeling.

Injectable, Subcutaneous [preservative free]:

Infergen: 9 mcg/0.3 mL (0.3 mL); 15 mcg/0.5 mL (0.5 mL)

Interferon Alfa-n3 (in ter FEER on AL fa en three)

Brand Names: U.S. Alferon N

Brand Names: Canada Alferon® N

Pharmacologic Category Interferon

Use Patients ≥18 years of age: Intralesional treatment of refractory or recurring genital or venereal warts (condylomata acuminata)

Pregnancy Risk Factor C

Medication Guide Available Yes

Dosage Adults: Inject 250,000 units (0.05 mL) in each wart twice weekly for a maximum of 8 weeks; therapy should not be repeated for at least 3 months after the initial 8-week course of therapy

Additional Information Complete prescribing information should be consulted for additional detail.

Dosage Forms Excipient information presented when available (limited, particularly for generics); consult specific product labeling.

Solution, Injection:

Alferon N: 5,000,000 units/mL (1 mL)

◆ Interferon Alpha-2b *see* Interferon Alfa-2b *on page 1099*

Interferon Beta-1a (in ter FEER on BAY ta won aye)

Brand Names: U.S. Avonex®; Avonex® Pen™; Rebif®; Rebif® Rebidose®; Rebif® Rebidose® Titration Pack; Rebif® Titration Pack

Brand Names: Canada Avonex®; Rebif®

Index Terms rIFN beta-1a

Pharmacologic Category Interferon

Use Treatment of relapsing forms of multiple sclerosis (MS)

Canadian labeling: Additional uses (not in U.S. labeling): Avonex®: To decrease the number and volume of active brain lesions, decrease overall disease burden, and delay onset of clinically definite MS in patients who have experienced a single demyelinating event.

Pregnancy Risk Factor C

Pregnancy Considerations Adverse events were observed in animal reproduction studies. Preliminary data from the Avonex® pregnancy registry (published in abstract) do not show an increased risk of adverse fetal events when exposure occurs during pregnancy (Richman, 2012; Tomczyk, 2013); however, other studies have reported conflicting results. Until additional information is available, consideration should be given to discontinuing treatment if a woman becomes pregnant, or 1 month prior to becoming pregnant in women with mild disease (Coyle, 2012; Houtchens, 2013; Lu, 2013).

Breast-Feeding Considerations Small amounts of interferon beta-1a are excreted in breast milk. Milk samples were obtained from six lactating women (6-23 months postpartum) receiving Avonex® 30 mcg I.M. once weekly; sampling occurred at intervals for 72 hours after the dose. The highest reported concentration was 179 pg/mL and the relative infant dose was calculated to be <1% of the maternal dose. Adverse events were not observed in the nursing infants (Hale, 2012). The manufacturer recommends that caution be exercised when administering interferon beta-1a to nursing women.

Medication Guide Available Yes

Contraindications Hypersensitivity to natural or recombinant interferons, human albumin (only for albumin-containing formulations), or any other component of the formulation

Canadian labeling: Additional contraindications (not in U.S. labeling): Rebif®: Pregnancy; decompensated liver disease

Warnings/Precautions Interferons have been associated with severe psychiatric adverse events (psychosis, mania, depression, suicidal behavior/ideation) in patients with and without previous psychiatric symptoms, avoid use in severe psychiatric disorders and use caution in patients with a history of depression; patients exhibiting depressive symptoms should be closely monitored and discontinuation of therapy should be considered.

Autoimmune disorders including idiopathic thrombocytopenia, hyper- and hypothyroidism and rarely autoimmune hepatitis have been reported. Allergic reactions, including anaphylaxis, have been reported; some reactions may occur after prolonged use. Rare cases of severe hepatic injury, including cases of hepatic failure requiring transplantation, have been reported in patients receiving interferon beta-1a; risk may be increased by ethanol use or concurrent therapy with hepatotoxic drugs. Some reports indicate symptoms began after 1-6 months of treatment. Transaminase elevations may be asymptomatic. Use with caution in patients with active or a history of liver disease, alcohol abuse, or increased serum ALT (>2.5 times ULN) at baseline. Obtain liver function tests at 1-, 3-, and 6 months post therapy initiation, or as clinically necessary. Treatment should be suspended immediately if jaundice or symptoms of hepatic dysfunction occur. Consider dose reductions or temporary discontinuation if ALT >5 times ULN. Hematologic effects, including pancytopenia (rare), leukopenia, and thrombocytopenia, have been reported. Use with caution in patients with bone marrow suppression; monitor blood counts at 1-, 3-, and 6 months post therapy initiation, or as clinically necessary. Associated with a high incidence of flu-like adverse effects; use of analgesics and/or antipyretics on treatment days may be helpful. Use caution in patients with pre-existing cardiovascular disease, including angina, HF, and/or arrhythmia. Rare cases of new-onset cardiomyopathy and/or HF have been reported. Use caution in patients with seizure disorders. Thyroid abnormalities may develop with use; may worsen pre-existing thyroid conditions. Monitor thyroid function tests every 6 months or as clinically necessary. Safety and efficacy in patients with chronic progressive MS have not been established. Albumin is a component of some formulations (contraindicated in albumin-sensitive patients); rare risk of CJD or viral transmission.

Adverse Reactions Note: Adverse reactions reported as a composite of both commercially-available products. Spectrum and incidence of reactions is generally similar between products, but consult individual product labels for specific incidence.

>10%:

Central nervous system: Headache (58% to 70%), fatigue (33% to 41%), fever (20% to 28%), pain (23%), chills (19%), depression (18% to 25%), dizziness (14%)

Gastrointestinal: Nausea (23%), abdominal pain (8% to 22%)

Genitourinary: Urinary tract infection (17%)

Hematologic: Leukopenia (28% to 36%)

Hepatic: ALT increased (20% to 27%), AST increased (10% to 17%)

Local: Injection site reaction (3% to 92%)

Neuromuscular & skeletal: Myalgia (25% to 29%), back pain (23% to 25%), weakness (24%), skeletal pain (10% to 15%), rigors (6% to 13%)

Ocular: Vision abnormal (7% to 13%)

Respiratory: Sinusitis (14%), upper respiratory tract infection (14%)

Miscellaneous: Flu-like syndrome (49% to 59%), neutralizing antibodies (significance not known; Avonex® 5%; Rebif® 24%), lymphadenopathy (11% to 12%)

1% to 10%:

Cardiovascular: Chest pain (5% to 6%), vasodilation (2%)

Central nervous system: Migraine (5%), somnolence (4% to 5%), malaise (4% to 5%), seizure (1% to 5%)

Dermatologic: Erythematous rash (5% to 7%), maculopapular rash (4% to 5%), alopecia (4%), urticaria

Endocrine & metabolic: Thyroid disorder (4% to 6%)

Gastrointestinal: Xerostomia (1% to 5%), toothache (3%)

Genitourinary: Micturition frequency (2% to 7%), urinary incontinence (2% to 4%)

Hematologic: Thrombocytopenia (2% to 8%), anemia (3% to 5%)

Hepatic: Bilirubinemia (2% to 3%)

Local: Injection site pain (8%), injection site bruising (6%), injection site necrosis (1% to 3%), injection site inflammation

Neuromuscular & skeletal: Arthralgia (9%), hypertonia (6% to 7%), coordination abnormal (4% to 5%)

Ocular: Eye disorder (4%), xerophthalmia (1% to 3%)

Respiratory: Bronchitis (8%)

Miscellaneous: Infection (7%)

<1% (Limited to important and life-threatening): Anaphylaxis, autoimmune hepatitis, cardiomyopathy, CHF, hepatic failure, hepatitis, hyper-/hypothyroidism, idiopathic thrombocytopenia, injection site abscess/cellulitis, menorrhagia, metrorrhagia, pancytopenia, psychiatric disorders (new or worsening; including suicidal ideation), vesicular rash

Drug Interactions

Metabolism/Transport Effects None known.

Avoid Concomitant Use There are no known interactions where it is recommended to avoid concomitant use.

Increased Effect/Toxicity

Interferon Beta-1a may increase the levels/effects of: Theophylline Derivatives; Zidovudine

Decreased Effect There are no known significant interactions involving a decrease in effect.

Preparation for Administration Avonex®: Reconstitute with 1.1 mL of diluent and swirl gently to dissolve. Do not shake. The reconstituted product contains no preservative and is for single-use only; discard unused portion.

Storage/Stability

Avonex®:

Prefilled syringe or pen: Store at 2°C to 8°C (36°F to 46°F); do not freeze. Protect from light. Allow to warm to room temperature prior to use (do not use external heat source). If refrigeration is not available, product may be stored at ≤25°C (77°F) for up to 7 days.

Vial: Store unreconstituted vial at 2°C to 8°C (36°F to 46°F). If refrigeration is not available, may be stored at 25°C (77°F) for up to 30 days; do not freeze. Protect from light. Following reconstitution, use immediately, but may be stored up to 6 hours at 2°C to 8°C (36°F to 46°F); do not freeze.

Rebif®, Rebif® Rebidose®: Store at 2°C to 8°C (36°F to 46°F); do not freeze. Protect from light. May also be stored ≤25°C (77°F) for up to 30 days if protected from heat and light.

Mechanism of Action Interferon beta differs from naturally occurring human protein by a single amino acid substitution and the lack of carbohydrate side chains; alters the expression and response to surface antigens and can enhance immune cell activities. Properties of interferon beta that modify biologic responses are mediated by cell surface receptor interactions; mechanism in the treatment of MS is unknown.

Pharmacodynamics/Kinetics

Onset of action: Avonex®: 12 hours (based on biological response markers)

Duration: Avonex®: 4 days (based on biological response markers)

Half-life elimination: Avonex®: 10 hours; Rebif®: 69 hours

Time to peak, serum: Avonex® (I.M.): ~15 hours (range: 6-36 hours); Rebif® (SubQ): 16 hours

Dosage

Multiple sclerosis (MS): Adults: **Note:** Analgesics and/or antipyretics may help decrease flu-like symptoms on treatment days:

I.M. (Avonex®):

U.S. labeling: 30 mcg once weekly; to decrease flu-like symptoms, may initiate once-weekly dosing with 7.5 mcg (week 1) then increase dose in increments of 7.5 mcg once weekly (weeks 2-4) up to recommended dose (30 mcg once weekly)

Canadian labeling: 30 mcg once weekly; may consider increasing to 60 mcg once weekly in progressive relapsing MS or secondary progressive MS with recurrent neurologic dysfunction

SubQ (Rebif®, Rebif® Rebidose®): Doses should be separated by at least 48 hours:

Target dose 44 mcg 3 times weekly:

Initial: 8.8 mcg (20% of final dose) 3 times weekly for 2 weeks

Titration: 22 mcg (50% of final dose) 3 times weekly for 2 weeks

Final dose: 44 mcg 3 times weekly

Target dose 22 mcg 3 times weekly:

Initial: 4.4 mcg (20% of final dose) 3 times weekly for 2 weeks

Titration: 11 mcg (50% of final dose) 3 times weekly for 2 weeks

Final dose: 22 mcg 3 times weekly

Single demyelinating event (Canadian labeling [Rebif®]; not in U.S. labeling): Adults: SubQ:

Target dose 44 mcg 3 times weekly: Note: Analgesics and/or antipyretics prior to and for 24 hours after dosing may help decrease flu-like symptoms:

Initial: 8.8 mcg (20% of final dose) 3 times weekly for 2 weeks

Titration: 22 mcg (50% of final dose) 3 times weekly for 2 weeks

Final dose: 44 mcg 3 times weekly

Dosage adjustment for toxicity:

Autoimmune disorder development: Consider discontinuing treatment.

Depression or other psychiatric symptoms: Consider discontinuing treatment.

Hepatotoxicity:

ALT >5 x ULN: Temporarily discontinue therapy or consider dose reduction until ALT normalizes, then may consider retitration of dose.

Symptomatic (eg, jaundice): Discontinue immediately.

Leukopenia: May require temporary discontinuation or dose reduction until resolution.

Dosage adjustment in renal impairment: No dosage adjustment provided in the manufacturer's labeling (has not been studied).

Dosage adjustment in hepatic impairment: Initial: No dosage adjustment provided in the manufacturer's labeling; use with caution in patients with a past or present history of active liver disease or ALT >2.5 x ULN.

Administration

Avonex®: Must be administered by I.M. injection; rotate injection site; do not inject into area where skin is irritated, red, bruised, scarred, or infected. Two hours after injection, examine site for redness, swelling, or tenderness. Discard any unused portion.

Rebif®, Rebif® Rebidose®: Administer SubQ at the same time of day on the same 3 days each week (ie, late afternoon/evening Mon, Wed, Fri; doses should be at least 48 hours apart); rotate injection site; do not inject into area where skin is sore, red, damaged, or infected. Discard any unused portion.

Monitoring Parameters Thyroid function tests, CBC with differential, transaminase levels, blood chemistries, symptoms of autoimmune disorders, signs/symptoms of psychiatric disorder (including depression and/or suicidal ideation), signs/symptoms of new onset/worsening cardiovascular disease

Avonex®: Frequency of monitoring for patients receiving Avonex® has not been specifically defined; in clinical trials, monitoring was at 6-month intervals. Canadian labeling recommends liver function testing monthly for first 6 months, then every 6 months thereafter or as clinically indicated.

Rebif®, Rebif® Rebidose®: CBC and liver function testing at 1-, 3-, and 6 months, then periodically thereafter. Thyroid function every 6 months (in patients with preexisting abnormalities and/or clinical indications). Canadian labeling recommends liver function testing monthly for first 6 months, then every 6 months thereafter or as clinically indicated.

Dosage Forms Excipient information presented when available (limited, particularly for generics); consult specific product labeling.

Injection, powder for reconstitution [preservative free]:

Avonex®: 33 mcg [contains albumin (human); provides 30 mcg/mL following reconstitution; derived from or manufactured using Chinese hamster ovary cells; supplied with diluent]

Injection, solution:

Avonex®: 30 mcg/0.5 mL (0.5 mL) [albumin free; derived from or manufactured using Chinese hamster ovary cells; prefilled syringe]

Avonex® Pen™: 30 mcg/0.5 mL (0.5 mL) [albumin free; derived from or manufactured using Chinese hamster ovary cells]

Injection, solution [preservative free]:

Rebif®: 22 mcg/0.5 mL (0.5 mL), 44 mcg/0.5 mL (0.5 mL) [contains albumin (human); derived from or manufactured using Chinese hamster ovary cells; prefilled syringe]

Rebif® Rebidose®: 22 mcg/0.5 mL (0.5 mL), 44 mcg/0.5 mL (0.5 mL) [contains albumin (human); derived from or manufactured using Chinese hamster ovary cells; autoinjector]

Injection, solution [preservative free, combination package]:

Rebif® Titration Pack: 8.8 mcg/0.2 mL (6s) and 22 mcg/0.5 mL (6s) [contains albumin (human); derived from or manufactured using Chinese hamster ovary cells; prefilled syringe]

Rebif® Rebidose® Titration Pack: 8.8 mcg/0.2 mL (6s) and 22 mcg/0.5 mL (6s) [contains albumin (human); derived from or manufactured using Chinese hamster ovary cells; autoinjector]

Interferon Beta-1b (in ter FEER on BAY ta won bee)

Brand Names: U.S. Betaseron; Extavia

Brand Names: Canada Betaseron; Extavia

Index Terms rIFN beta-1b

Pharmacologic Category Interferon

Use Treatment of relapsing forms of multiple sclerosis (MS); treatment of first clinical episode with MRI features consistent with MS

Canadian labeling: Additional use (not in U.S. labeling): Treatment of secondary-progressive MS

Pregnancy Risk Factor C

Pregnancy Considerations Adverse events have been observed in animal reproduction studies. Spontaneous abortions were reported in 4 women during a clinical trial. Women with multiple sclerosis are generally recommended to discontinue therapy prior to conception (Lu, 2012). The Canadian labeling contraindicates use in pregnant women.

Breast-Feeding Considerations It is not known if interferon beta-1b is excreted in breast milk. Due to the potential for serious adverse reactions in the nursing infant, the decision to continue or discontinue breastfeeding during therapy should take into account the risk of exposure to the infant and the benefits of treatment to the mother.

Medication Guide Available Yes

Contraindications Hypersensitivity to natural or recombinant interferon beta, albumin human or any other component of the formulation

Canadian labeling: Additional contraindication (not in U.S. labeling): Pregnancy; decompensated liver disease

Warnings/Precautions Allergic reactions (eg, bronchospasm, dyspnea, skin rash, tongue edema, urticaria), including anaphylaxis (rare), have been reported with use; discontinue use if anaphylaxis occurs. Associated with a high incidence of flu-like adverse effects; use of analgesics and/or antipyretics on treatment days may be helpful. Improvement in symptoms occurs over time. Hepatotoxicity has been reported with beta interferons, including rare reports of hepatitis (autoimmune) and hepatic failure requiring transplant; use with caution in patients with concurrent exposure to other hepatotoxic drugs. Monitor liver function tests as clinically necessary. Consider discontinuation if serum transaminase levels increase significantly or are associated with clinical symptoms (eg, jaundice). Interferons have been associated with severe psychiatric adverse events (psychosis, mania, depression, suicidal behavior/ideation) in patients with and without previous psychiatric symptoms; avoid use in severe psychiatric disorders and use caution in patients with a history of depression; patients exhibiting symptoms of depression should be closely monitored and discontinuation of therapy should be considered. Use with caution in patients with a history of seizure disorder.

Use with caution in patients with pre-existing cardiovascular disease. Rare cases of new-onset cardiomyopathy and/or HF have been reported. If HF worsens in the absence of another etiology, consider discontinuation of therapy. Use with caution in patients with hepatic impairment or in combination with alcohol. The Canadian labeling contraindicates use in patients with decompensated hepatic disease. Use with caution in patients with bone marrow suppression; may require increased monitoring. Leukopenia has also been observed; routine monitoring of complete blood counts with differentials is recommended. Dose reduction may be required. Thyroid abnormalities may develop with use; may worsen pre-existing thyroid conditions. Monitor thyroid function tests every 6 months or as clinically necessary.

Severe injection site reactions (necrosis) may occur, which may or may not heal with continued therapy. Reactions generally arise within the first 4 months of therapy, but have occurred ≥1 year after initiation. Incidence of reactions tend to improve over time. Patient and/or caregiver competency in injection technique should be confirmed and periodically re-evaluated. Do not inject into affected area until completely healed; if multiple lesions occur, discontinue use until they are fully healed. Contains albumin, which may carry a remote risk of transmitting viral diseases.

Adverse Reactions Note: Flu-like syndrome (including at least two of the following - headache, fever, chills, malaise, diaphoresis, and myalgia) are reported in the majority of patients (60%) and decrease over time (average duration ~1 week).

>10%:

Cardiovascular: Peripheral edema (12% to 15%), chest pain (9% to 11%)

Central nervous system: Headache (50% to 57%), pain (42% to 51%), hypertonia (40% to 50%), myasthenia (46%), chills (21% to 25%), dizziness (24%), insomnia (21% to 24%), ataxia (17% to 21%)

Dermatologic: Skin rash (21% to 24%), dermatological disease (10% to 12%)

Gastrointestinal: Nausea (27%), constipation (20%), diarrhea (19%), abdominal pain (16% to 19%), dyspepsia (14%)

Genitourinary: Urinary urgency (11% to 13%), uterine hemorrhage (9% to 11%)

Hematologic & oncologic: Lymphocytopenia (86% to 88%), leukopenia (13% to 18%), neutropenia (13% to 14%)

Immunologic: Antibody development (≤45%; neutralizing; significance not known)

Local: Injection site reaction (78% to 85%, including inflammation [53%], pain [18%], tissue necrosis [4% to 5%], hypersensitivity reaction [4%], swelling [2% to 3%], residual mass [2%])

Neuromuscular & skeletal: Weakness (53% to 61%), arthralgia (31%), myalgia (23% to 27%)

Respiratory: Flu-like symptoms (decreases over treatment course; 57% to 60%)

Miscellaneous: Fever (31% to 36%)

1% to 10%:

Cardiovascular: Vasodilatation (8%), hypertension (6% to 7%), peripheral vascular disease (6%), palpitations (4%), tachycardia (4%)

Central nervous system: Anxiety (10%), malaise (6% to 8%), nervousness (7%)

Dermatologic: Diaphoresis (8%), alopecia (4%)

Endocrine & metabolic: Hypermenorrhea (8%), dysmenorrhea (7%), weight gain (7%)

Genitourinary: Impotence (8% to 9%), cystitis (8%), urinary frequency (7%), pelvic pain (6%), prostatic disease (3%)

Hematologic & oncologic: Lymphadenopathy (6% to 8%)

Hepatic: Increased serum ALT (>5x baseline: 10% to 12%), increased serum AST (>5x baseline: 3% to 4%)

Hypersensitivity: Hypersensitivity (3%)

Neuromuscular & skeletal: Leg cramps (4%)

Respiratory: Dyspnea (6% to 7%)

<1% (Limited to important or life-threatening): Anaphylaxis, anorexia, apnea, ataxia, autoimmune hepatitis, capillary leak syndrome (in patients with pre-existing monoclonal gammopathy), cardiac arrest, cardiac arrhythmia, cardiac failure, cardiomegaly, cardiomyopathy, cerebral hemorrhage, coma, confusion, convulsion, deep vein thrombosis, delirium, depersonalization, depression, emotional lability, erythema nodosum, ethanol sensitization, exfoliative dermatitis, gastrointestinal hemorrhage, hallucinations, hematemesis, hepatic failure, hepatitis, hyperthyroidism, hyperuricemia, hypocalcemia, increased gamma-glutamyl transferase, increased serum triglycerides maculopapular rash, manic behavior, myocardial infarction, pancreatitis, pericardial effusion, pneumonia, pruritus, psychosis, pulmonary embolism, rash, sepsis, shock, skin discoloration, skin photosensitivity, suicidal ideation, syncope, SIADH, thrombocytopenia, thyroid dysfunction, urinary tract infection, urosepsis, vasculitis, vaginal hemorrhage, vesiculobullous dermatitis, weight loss

Drug Interactions

Metabolism/Transport Effects None known.

Avoid Concomitant Use There are no known interactions where it is recommended to avoid concomitant use.

Increased Effect/Toxicity

Interferon Beta-1b may increase the levels/effects of: Theophylline Derivatives; Zidovudine

Decreased Effect There are no known significant interactions involving a decrease in effect.

Preparation for Administration To reconstitute solution, inject 1.2 mL of diluent (provided); gently swirl to dissolve, do not shake. Reconstituted solution provides 0.25 mg/mL. Use product within 3 hours of reconstitution. Discard unused portion of vial. Foaming may occur if swirled or shaken too vigorously; allow vial to sit until foam settles.

Storage/Stability Store at room temperature of 25°C (77°F); excursions permitted to 15°C to 30°C (59°F to 86°F) for ≤3 months. If not used immediately following reconstitution, refrigerate solution at 2°C to 8°C (36°F to 46°F) and use within 3 hours; do not freeze or shake solution. Discard unused portion of vial.

Mechanism of Action Interferon beta-1b differs from naturally occurring human protein by a single amino acid substitution and the lack of carbohydrate side chains; mechanism in the treatment of MS is unknown; however, immunomodulatory effects attributed to interferon beta-1b include enhancement of suppressor T cell activity, reduction of proinflammatory cytokines, down-regulation of antigen presentation, and reduced trafficking of lymphocytes into the central nervous system. Improves MRI lesions, decreases relapse rate, and disease severity in patients with secondary progressive MS.

Pharmacodynamics/Kinetics Limited data due to small doses used

Half-life elimination: 8 minutes to 4.3 hours

Time to peak, serum: 1-8 hours

Dosage Note: Analgesics and/or antipyretics may help decrease flu-like symptoms on treatment days:

Multiple sclerosis (relapsing) or treatment of first clinical episode with MRI features consistent with MS: Adults: SubQ: Initial: 0.0625 mg (0.25 mL) every other day; gradually increase dose by 0.0625 mg every 2 weeks

Target dose: 0.25 mg (1 mL) every other day

Note: In clinical trials involving patients with a single clinical event suggestive of MS, dose was initiated at 0.0625 mg (2 million units [0.25 mL]) every other day and titrated weekly up to a target dose of 8 million units (1 mL) every other day (Kappos, 2006).

Multiple sclerosis (secondary-progressive) [Canadian labeling; not in U.S. labeling]: Adults: SubQ: Initial: 0.125 mg (4 million units [0.5 mL]) every other day for 2 weeks

Target dose: 0.25 mg (1 mL) every other day

Dosage adjustment in renal impairment: No dosage adjustment provided in manufacturer's labeling.

Dosage adjustment in hepatic impairment: No dosage adjustment provided in manufacturer's labeling. The Canadian labeling contraindicates use in decompensated liver disease.

Administration Withdraw dose of reconstituted solution from the vial into a sterile syringe fitted with a 27-gauge (Extavia) or 30-gauge (Betaseron) needle and inject the solution subcutaneously; sites for self-injection include outer surface of the arms, abdomen (**except** 2-inch area around the navel), hips, and thighs. Rotate SubQ injection site. Do not inject into area where skin is bruised, infected, or broken. Patient should be well hydrated. If a dose is missed, administer as soon as remembered; do not administer on 2 consecutive days. Time subsequent doses every 48 hours.

Monitoring Parameters Complete blood chemistries (including platelet count) and liver function tests are recommended at 1, 3, and 6 months following initiation of therapy and periodically thereafter. Thyroid function should be assessed every 6 months in patients with history of thyroid dysfunction or as clinically necessary. Monitor for flu-like symptoms, allergic or anaphylactic reactions, injection site reactions, and for sign/symptoms of depression.

Canadian labeling: Additional monitoring recommendations (not in U.S. labeling): Baseline pregnancy test, chest X-ray, and ECG

Additional Information American Academy of Neurology and MS Council guidelines suggest that, based upon published data, 6 million units of Avonex® (interferon beta-1a) (30 mcg) is equivalent to approximately 7-9 million units of Betaseron® (220-280 mcg).

Dosage Forms Excipient information presented when available (limited, particularly for generics); consult specific product labeling.

Kit, Subcutaneous:
  Betaseron: 0.3 mg [contains albumin human]

Kit, Subcutaneous [preservative free]:
  Extavia: 0.3 mg [contains albumin human]

Interferon Gamma-1b

(in ter FEER on GAM ah won bee)

Brand Names: U.S. Actimmune

Brand Names: Canada Actimmune®

Pharmacologic Category Interferon

Use Reduce frequency and severity of serious infections associated with chronic granulomatous disease; delay time to disease progression in patients with severe, malignant osteopetrosis

Pregnancy Risk Factor C

Pregnancy Considerations Teratogenic effects were not observed in animal studies. A dose-related abortifacient activity was reported in Rhesus monkeys. Safety and efficacy in pregnant women has not been established.

Breast-Feeding Considerations Potential for serious adverse reactions. Because its use has not been evaluated during lactation, breast-feeding is not recommended

Contraindications Hypersensitivity to interferon gamma, *E. coli* derived proteins, or any component of the formulation

Warnings/Precautions Hypersensitivity reactions have been reported (rarely). Transient cutaneous rashes may occur. Dose-related bone marrow toxicity has been reported; use caution in patients with myelosuppression. May cause hepatotoxicity and the incidence may be increased in children <1 year of age. Doses >10 times the weekly recommended dose (used in studies for unlabeled indications) have been associated with a different pattern/frequency of adverse effects. Flu-like symptoms which may exacerbate pre-existing cardiovascular disorders (including ischemia, HF, or arrhythmias) and the development of neurologic disorders have been noted at the higher doses. Caution should also be used in patients with seizure disorders or compromised CNS function.

Adverse Reactions Based on 50 mcg/m^2 dose administered 3 times weekly for chronic granulomatous disease

>10%:
  Central nervous system: Fever (52%), headache (33%), chills (14%), fatigue (14%)
  Dermatologic: Rash (17%)
  Gastrointestinal: Diarrhea (14%), vomiting (13%)
  Local: Injection site erythema or tenderness (14%)

1% to 10%:
  Central nervous system: Depression (3%)
  Gastrointestinal: Nausea (10%), abdominal pain (8%)
  Neuromuscular & skeletal: Myalgia (6%), arthralgia (2%), back pain (2%)

Postmarketing and/or case reports: Alkaline phosphatase elevated, atopic dermatitis, granulomatous colitis, hepatomegaly, hypersensitivity reactions, hypokalemia, neutropenia, Stevens-Johnson syndrome

Additional adverse reactions noted at doses >100 mcg/m^2 administered 3 times weekly: ALT increased, AST increased, autoantibodies increased, bronchospasm, chest discomfort, confusion, dermatomyositis exacerbation, disorientation, DVT, gait disturbance, GI bleeding, hallucinations, heart block, heart failure, hepatic insufficiency, hyperglycemia, hypertriglyceridemia, hyponatremia, hypotension, interstitial pneumonitis, lupus-like syndrome, MI, neutropenia, pancreatitis (may be fatal), Parkinsonian symptoms, PE, proteinuria, renal insufficiency (reversible), seizure, syncope, tachyarrhythmia, tachypnea, thrombocytopenia, TIA

Drug Interactions

Metabolism/Transport Effects **Inhibits** CYP1A2 (weak), CYP2E1 (weak)

Avoid Concomitant Use There are no known interactions where it is recommended to avoid concomitant use.

Increased Effect/Toxicity

Interferon Gamma-1b may increase the levels/effects of: Theophylline Derivatives; Zidovudine

Decreased Effect There are no known significant interactions involving a decrease in effect.

Storage/Stability Store in refrigerator at 2°C to 8°C (36°F to 46°F); do not freeze. Do not shake. Discard if left unrefrigerated for >12 hours.

Mechanism of Action Interferon gamma participates in immunoregulation by enhancing the oxidative metabolism of macrophages; it also enhances antibody dependent cellular cytotoxicity, activates natural killer cells and has a role in the expression of Fc receptors and histocompatibility antigens. The exact mechanism of action for the treatment of chronic granulomatous disease or osteopetrosis has not been defined.

Pharmacodynamics/Kinetics

Absorption: I.M., SubQ: >89%

Half-life elimination: I.V.: 38 minutes; I.M.: ~3 hours, SubQ: ~6 hours

Time to peak, plasma: I.M.: 4 hours (1.5 ng/mL); SubQ: 7 hours (0.6 ng/mL)

Dosage If severe reactions occur, reduce dose by 50% or therapy should be interrupted until adverse reaction abates.

Children: Severe, malignant osteopetrosis: SubQ:
  BSA ≤0.5 m^2: 1.5 mcg/kg/dose 3 times/week
  BSA >0.5 m^2: 50 mcg/m^2 (1 million units/m^2) 3 times/week

Children and Adults: Chronic granulomatous disease: SubQ:
  BSA ≤0.5 m^2: 1.5 mcg/kg/dose 3 times/week
  BSA >0.5 m^2: 50 mcg/m^2 (1 million units/m^2) 3 times/week

Note: Previously expressed as 1.5 million units/m^2; 50 mcg is equivalent to 1 million units/m^2.

Dosage adjustment in renal impairment: No dosage adjustment provided in manufacturer's labeling.

Dosage adjustment in hepatic impairment: No dosage adjustment provided in manufacturer's labeling.

Administration Administer by SubQ injection into the right and left deltoid or anterior thigh.

Monitoring Parameters CBC with differential, platelets, LFTs (monthly in children <1 year), electrolytes, BUN, creatinine, and urinalysis prior to therapy and at 3-month intervals

Dosage Forms Excipient information presented when available (limited, particularly for generics); consult specific product labeling.

Solution, Subcutaneous:

Actimmune: 2,000,000 units/0.5 mL (0.5 mL)

- **Interleukin-1 Receptor Antagonist** *see* Anakinra *on page 136*
- **Interleukin 2** *see* Aldesleukin *on page 63*
- **Interleukin-11** *see* Oprelvekin *on page 1514*
- **Intermezzo** *see* Zolpidem *on page 2242*
- **Intralipid** *see* Fat Emulsion (Plant Based) *on page 834*
- **Intrapleural Talc** *see* Talc (Sterile) *on page 1986*
- **Intravenous Fat Emulsion** *see* Fat Emulsion (Plant Based) *on page 834*
- **Intrifiban** *see* Eptifibatide *on page 731*
- **Intron-A** *see* Interferon Alfa-2b *on page 1099*
- **Intron® A (Can)** *see* Interferon Alfa-2b *on page 1099*
- **Intropin** *see* DOPamine *on page 651*
- **Introvale** *see* Ethinyl Estradiol and Levonorgestrel *on page 787*
- **Intuniv** *see* GuanFACINE *on page 979*
- **Intuniv XR (Can)** *see* GuanFACINE *on page 979*
- **INVanz** *see* Ertapenem *on page 739*
- **Invanz (Can)** *see* Ertapenem *on page 739*
- **Invega** *see* Paliperidone *on page 1549*
- **Invega Sustenna** *see* Paliperidone *on page 1549*
- **Invirase** *see* Saquinavir *on page 1875*
- **Invirase® (Can)** *see* Saquinavir *on page 1875*
- **Iodine and Potassium Iodide** *see* Potassium Iodide and Iodine *on page 1689*

Iodoquinol (eye oh doe KWIN ole)

Brand Names: U.S. Yodoxin

Brand Names: Canada Diodoquin®

Index Terms Diiodohydroxyquin

Pharmacologic Category Amebicide

Use Treatment of intestinal amebiasis due to trophozoite and cyst forms of *Entamoeba histolytica*

Unlabeled Use *Blastocystis hominis* infections, *Balantidium coli* infections, *Dientamoeba fragilis* infections

Dosage Oral:

Children: 30-40 mg/kg daily (maximum: 650 mg per dose) in 3 divided doses for 20 days; not to exceed 1.95 g daily

Adults: 650 mg 3 times daily after meals for 20 days; not to exceed 1.95 g daily

Additional Information Complete prescribing information should be consulted for additional detail.

Dosage Forms Excipient information presented when available (limited, particularly for generics); consult specific product labeling.

Tablet, Oral:

Yodoxin: 210 mg, 650 mg

Iodoquinol and Hydrocortisone

(eye oh doe KWIN ole & hye droe KOR ti sone)

Brand Names: U.S. Alcortin A; Dermazene; Vytone

Index Terms Hydrocortisone and Iodoquinol

Pharmacologic Category Antifungal Agent, Topical; Corticosteroid, Topical

Use Treatment of eczema (including impetiginized, nuchal, and nummular); acne urticata; anogenital pruritus, atopic and contact dermatitis, endogenous chronic infectious dermatitis; chronic eczematoid otitis externa; folliculitis, intertrigo; lichen simplex chronicus; moniliasis; dermatoses (mycotic or bacterial); neurodermatitis (localized or systemic); pyoderma, stasis dermatitis

Pregnancy Risk Factor C

Dosage Dermatoses: Children ≥12 years, Adolescents, and Adults: Topical: Apply 3-4 times daily to affected area(s)

Additional Information Complete prescribing information should be consulted for additional detail.

Dosage Forms Excipient information presented when available (limited, particularly for generics); consult specific product labeling.

Cream, topical: Iodoquinol 1% and hydrocortisone acetate 1% (30 g)

Dermazene: Iodoquinol 1% and hydrocortisone acetate 1% (30 g)

Vytone: Iodoquinol 1% and hydrocortisone 1.9% per 2 g packet (30s) [contains benzyl alcohol]

Gel, topical:

Alcortin A: Iodoquinol 1% and hydrocortisone 2% (2 g) [contains aloe, benzyl alcohol]

- **Iophen C-NR** *see* Guaifenesin and Codeine *on page 976*
- **Iophen DM-NR [OTC]** *see* Guaifenesin and Dextromethorphan *on page 976*
- **Iophen-NR [OTC]** *see* GuaiFENesin *on page 974*
- **Iopidine** *see* Apraclonidine *on page 158*
- **Iopidine® (Can)** *see* Apraclonidine *on page 158*

Ipilimumab (ip i LIM u mab)

Brand Names: U.S. Yervoy

Brand Names: Canada Yervoy®

Index Terms MDX-010; MDX-CTLA-4; MOAB-CTLA-4

Pharmacologic Category Antineoplastic Agent, Monoclonal Antibody; Monoclonal Antibody

Use Treatment of unresectable or metastatic melanoma

Pregnancy Risk Factor C

Pregnancy Considerations Adverse effects were observed in animal reproduction studies. Ipilimumab is an IgG1 immunoglobulin and human IgG1 is known to cross the placenta, therefore, ipilimumab may be expected to reach the fetus.

Breast-Feeding Considerations Due to the potential for serious adverse reactions in the nursing infant, the decision to discontinue ipilimumab or to discontinue breast-feeding should take into account the importance of treatment to the mother.

Medication Guide Available Yes

Contraindications There are no contraindications listed within the manufacturer's labeling.

Canadian labeling: Hypersensitivity to ipilimumab or any component of the formulation; active life-threatening auto-immune disease, or with organ transplantation graft where further immune activation is potentially imminently life-threatening

Warnings/Precautions **[U.S. Boxed Warning]: Severe and fatal immune-mediated adverse effects due to T-cell activation and proliferation may occur. While any organ system may be involved, common severe effects include dermatitis (including toxic epidermal necrolysis), endocrine disorder, enterocolitis, hepatitis, and neuropathy. Reactions generally occur during treatment, although some reactions have occurred weeks to months after treatment discontinuation. Discontinue treatment (permanently) and initiate high-dose corticosteroid treatment for severe immune mediated reactions. Evaluate liver function and thyroid function tests at baseline and prior to each dose. Assess for signs and symptoms of enterocolitis, dermatitis, neuropathy, and endocrine disorder at baseline and prior to each dose.** Initiate prednisone

1-2 mg/kg/day (or equivalent) for severe reactions. Uncommon immune-mediated adverse effects reported include hemolytic anemia, iritis, meningitis, nephritis, pericarditis, pneumonitis, and uveitis. Administer corticosteroid ophthalmic drops in patients who develop episcleritis, iritis, or uveitis; permanently discontinue ipilimumab if unresponsive to topical ophthalmic immunosuppressive treatments. For severe immune-mediated episcleritis or uveitis, initiate prednisone 1-2 mg/kg/day (or equivalent); taper over at least 1 month (Weber, 2012).

Immune-mediated enterocolitis was reported to occur at a median onset of 6-7 weeks. Monitor for signs and symptoms of enterocolitis (abdominal pain, blood in stool, diarrhea, or mucous in stool; with or without fever) and intestinal perforation (peritoneal signs, ileus). If enterocolitis develops, infectious causes should be ruled out; consider endoscopy for persistent or severe symptoms. Withhold ipilimumab treatment and administer antidiarrheals for moderate enterocolitis (diarrhea with ≤6 stools over baseline abdominal pain, mucous or blood in stool); if persists for >1 week, initiate prednisone at 0.5 mg/kg/day (or equivalent). If severe enterocolitis (diarrhea ≥7 stools above baseline, fever, ileus, peritoneal signs) develops, permanently discontinue ipilimumab and initiate prednisone 1-2 mg/kg/day (or equivalent); when resolved to ≤grade 1, taper corticosteroids slowly over ≥1 month (rapid tapering may worsen symptoms).

Severe, life-threatening or fatal hepatotoxicity and immune-mediated hepatitis have been observed. Monitor liver function tests (LFTs) and evaluate for signs of hepatotoxicity prior to each dose; if hepatotoxicity develops, infectious or malignant causes should be ruled out and liver function should be monitored more frequently until resolves. Withhold treatment for grade 2 hepatotoxicity (ALT or AST 2.5-5 times ULN or total bilirubin 1.5-3 times ULN). If severe hepatotoxicity develops (ALT or AST >5 times ULN or total bilirubin >3 times ULN), permanently discontinue ipilimumab and initiate prednisone 1-2 mg/kg/day (or equivalent). If transaminases do not decrease within 48 hours of steroid initiation, consider adding mycophenolate mofetil (Weber, 2012). May begin tapering corticosteroid (over 1 month) when LFTs show sustained improvement or return to baseline.

Severe, life-threatening, or fatal dermatitis has been reported. The median time to onset for dermatologic toxicity is 3 weeks (range: ≤17 weeks). Monitor for rash and pruritus; dermatitis should be considered immune-mediated unless identified otherwise. Mild-to-moderate dermatitis (localized rash and pruritus) should be treated symptomatically; topical or systemic corticosteroids should be administered if not resolved within 1 week. Withhold treatment for moderate to severe dermatologic symptoms. Permanently discontinue and initiate prednisone 1-2 mg/kg/day (or equivalent) for Stevens-Johnson syndrome, toxic epidermal necrolysis, or rash complicated by dermal ulceration (full thickness) or necrotic, bullous, or hemorrhagic manifestations; when dermatitis is controlled, taper corticosteroid over at least 1 month.

Severe or life-threatening endocrine disorders (hypopituitarism, adrenal insufficiency, hypogonadism and hypothyroidism) have been reported; may require hospitalization. Endocrine disorders of moderate severity (including hypothyroidism, adrenal insufficiency, hypopituitarism, and less commonly hyperthyroidism and Cushing's syndrome) which have required hormone replacement therapy or medical intervention have also been reported. The median onset for moderate-to-severe endocrine disorders was 11 weeks (range: ≤19 weeks); long-term hormone replacement therapy has been required in many cases. Monitor thyroid function tests and serum chemistries prior to each dose; also monitor for signs of hypophysitis, adrenal insufficiency and thyroid disorders (eg, abdominal pain, fatigue, headache, hypotension, mental status changes, unusual bowel habits); rule out other potential causes such as brain metastases. Endocrine disorders should be considered immune-mediated unless identified otherwise; consider endocrinology referral for further evaluation. If symptomatic, withhold ipilimumab treatment and initiate prednisone 1-2 mg/kg/day (or equivalent) and appropriate hormone replacement therapy.

Severe peripheral motor neuropathy and fatal Guillain-Barré syndrome have been reported (rare). Monitor for signs of motor or sensory neuropathy (unilateral or bilateral weakness, sensory changes or paresthesia). Withhold treatment in patients with neuropathy that does not interfere with daily activities (moderate neuropathy). Permanently discontinue for severe neuropathy (interferes with daily activities, including symptoms similar to Guillain-Barré syndrome). Consider initiating prednisone 1-2 mg/kg/day (or equivalent) for severe neuropathies.

Adverse Reactions

>10%:

- Central nervous system: Fatigue (41% to 42%; grades 3-5: 7%), headache (15%), fever (12%)
- Dermatologic: Pruritus (24% to 31%), rash (19% to 29%; grades 3-5: 2%), dermatitis (grade 2: 12%; grades 3-5: 2% to 3% [includes Stevens-Johnson syndrome, toxic epidermal necrolysis, dermal ulceration, necrotic, bullous or hemorrhagic dermatitis])
- Gastrointestinal: Nausea (35%), diarrhea (32% to 33%; grades 3-5: 5%), appetite decreased (27%), vomiting (24%), constipation (21%), abdominal pain (15%)
- Hematologic: Anemia (12%)
- Respiratory: Cough (16%), dyspnea (15%)

1% to 10%:

- Dermatologic: Urticaria (2%), vitiligo (2%)
- Endocrine & metabolic: Hypopituitarism (grade 2: 2%; grades 3-5: 4%), hypophysitis (2%), adrenal insufficiency (≤2%), hypothyroidism (≤2%)
- Gastrointestinal: Colitis (8%; grades 3-5: 5%), enterocolitis (grade 2: 5%; grades 3-5: 7%), intestinal perforation (1%)
- Hematologic: Eosinophilia (grades 3-5: 1%)
- Hepatic: Hepatotoxicity (grade 2: 3%; grades 3-5: 1% to 2%), ALT increased (2%)
- Renal: Nephritis (grades 3-5: 1%)
- Miscellaneous: Antibody formation (1%)

<1% (Limited to important or life-threatening): Acute respiratory distress syndrome, angiopathy, arthritis, AST increased, bilirubin increased, blepharitis, conjunctivitis, corticotrophin decreased, Cushing's syndrome, encephalitis, episcleritis, erythema multiforme, esophagitis, gastrointestinal ulcer, Guillain-Barré syndrome, hemolytic anemia, hepatic failure, hepatitis (immune-mediated), hyperthyroidism, hypogonadism, infusion reaction, iritis, leukocytoclastic vasculitis, meningitis, myasthenia gravis, myelofibrosis, myocarditis, myositis, neuropathy (sensory and motor), neurosensory hypoacusis, ocular myositis, pancreatitis, pericarditis, peritonitis, pneumonitis, polymyalgia rheumatica, polymyositis, psoriasis, renal failure, sarcoidosis, scleritis, sepsis, temporal arteritis, thyroiditis (autoimmune), thyrotropin increased, uveitis, vascular leak syndrome, vasculitis

Drug Interactions

Metabolism/Transport Effects None known.

Avoid Concomitant Use There are no known interactions where it is recommended to avoid concomitant use.

Increased Effect/Toxicity

Ipilimumab may increase the levels/effects of: Vemurafenib; Vitamin K Antagonists

Decreased Effect

Ipilimumab may decrease the levels/effects of: Cardiac Glycosides; Vitamin K Antagonists

Preparation for Administration Prior to preparation, allow vials to sit at room temperature for ~5 minutes. Inspect vial prior to use; solution may have a pale yellow color or may contain translucent or white amorphous ipilimumab particles; discard if cloudy or discolored. Withdraw appropriate ipilimumab volume and transfer to I.V. bag, dilute with NS or D_5W to a final concentration between 1-2 mg/mL. Mix by gently inverting, do not shake.

Storage/Stability Store intact vials refrigerated at 2°C to 8°C (36°F to 46°C); do not freeze. Protect from light. Prior to preparation, allow vials to sit at room temperature for ~5 minutes. Solutions diluted for infusion are stable for up to 24 hours refrigerated or at room temperature.

Mechanism of Action Ipilimumab is a recombinant human IgG1 immunoglobulin monoclonal antibody which binds to the cytotoxic T-lymphocyte associated antigen 4 (CTLA-4). CTLA-4 is a down-regulator of T-cell activation pathways. Blocking CTLA-4 allows for enhanced T-cell activation and proliferation. In melanoma, ipilimumab may indirectly mediate T-cell immune responses against tumors.

Pharmacodynamics/Kinetics

Distribution: V_{ss}: 7.21 L

Half-life elimination: Terminal: 15.4 days

Dosage I.V.: Adults: Melanoma, unresectable or metastatic: 3 mg/kg every 3 weeks for 4 doses

Dosage adjustment for toxicity:

Temporarily withhold scheduled dose for the following:

Moderate immune-mediated reactions

Symptomatic endocrine disorder

Grade 2 hepatotoxicity (AST or ALT >2.5 to ≤5 x ULN or bilirubin >1.5 to ≤3 x ULN)

Note: If receiving prednisone <7.5 mg daily (or equivalent), may resume with complete or partial resolution (to ≤grade 1) of symptoms. Resume ipilimumab treatment at 3 mg/kg every 3 weeks until all 4 planned doses have been administered or until 16 weeks from initial dose, whichever occurs first.

Permanently discontinue for the following:

Failure to complete treatment course within 16 weeks of initial dose

Persistent moderate adverse reactions or unable to reduce corticosteroid dose to prednisone 7.5 mg daily (or equivalent)

Severe or life-threatening adverse reactions including:

Central nervous system or neuromuscular toxicity: Severe motor or sensory neuropathy, Guillain-Barré syndrome, or myasthenia gravis

Dermatologic toxicities: Stevens-Johnson syndrome, toxic epidermal necrolysis, or rash complicated by full thickness dermal ulceration, or necrotic, bullous, or hemorrhagic manifestations

Gastrointestinal toxicities: Colitis with abdominal pain, fever, ileus, or peritoneal symptoms, increase in stool frequency (≥7 over baseline), stool incontinence, require I.V. hydration for >24 hours, or GI hemorrhage or perforation; grades 3/4 amylase or lipase increases (Weber, 2012)

Hepatotoxicities: ALT or AST >5 times ULN, or total bilirubin >3 times ULN

Ophthalmic toxicities: Immune-mediated ocular disease unresponsive to topical immunosuppressive treatment

Severe immune-mediated reactions involving any organ system (eg, myocarditis [noninfectious], nephritis, pancreatitis, pneumonitis)

Dosage adjustment in renal impairment: No dosage adjustment necessary.

Dosage adjustment in hepatic impairment:

Impairment at baseline:

Mild impairment (total bilirubin >1 to 1.5 x ULN **or** AST >ULN): No dosage adjustment necessary.

Moderate or severe impairment (total bilirubin >1.5 x ULN and any AST): No dosage adjustment provided in manufacturer's labeling (has not been studied).

Impairment during treatment:

AST or ALT >2.5 to ≤5 x ULN or bilirubin >1.5 to ≤3 x ULN: Temporarily withhold treatment.

ALT or AST >5 times ULN, or total bilirubin >3 times ULN: Permanently discontinue.

Administration I.V.: Infuse over 90 minutes through a low protein-binding in-line filter. Flush with NS or D_5W at the end of infusion

Monitoring Parameters Monitor liver function and evaluate for signs of hepatotoxicity prior to each dose; if hepatotoxicity develops, liver function should be monitored more frequently until resolves. If liver functions tests are >8 times ULN, monitor every other day until begin to fall, then weekly until normal (Weber, 2012). Monitor serum chemistries prior to each dose. Monitor for signs of hypophysitis, adrenal insufficiency and thyroid disorders (eg, abdominal pain, fatigue, headache, hypotension, mental status changes, unusual bowel habits). Monitor TSH, free T_4 and cortisol levels (morning) at baseline, prior to dose, and as clinically indicated. Monitor for signs and symptoms of enterocolitis (abdominal pain, blood or mucus in stool or diarrhea, and intestinal perforation (peritoneal signs, ileus). Monitor for rash and pruritus. Monitor for signs of motor or sensory neuropathy (unilateral or bilateral weakness, sensory changes or paresthesia). Monitor for ocular toxicity at baseline, then at 4-8 weeks with further evaluations as clinically indicated (Renouf, 2012).

Dosage Forms Excipient information presented when available (limited, particularly for generics); consult specific product labeling.

Solution, Intravenous [preservative free]:

Yervoy: 50 mg/10 mL (10 mL); 200 mg/40 mL (40 mL) [contains polysorbate 80]

◆ IPOL® *see* Poliovirus Vaccine (Inactivated) *on page 1666*

Ipratropium (Systemic) (i pra TROE pee um)

Brand Names: U.S. Atrovent HFA

Brand Names: Canada Atrovent HFA; Gen-Ipratropium; Mylan-Ipratropium Sterinebs; Novo-Ipramide; Nu-Ipratropium; PMS-Ipratropium; ratio-Ipratropium UDV; Teva-Ipratropium Sterinebs

Index Terms Ipratropium Bromide

Pharmacologic Category Anticholinergic Agent

Use Anticholinergic bronchodilator used in bronchospasm associated with COPD, bronchitis, and emphysema

Pregnancy Risk Factor B

Pregnancy Considerations Teratogenic effects were not observed in animal studies. Inhaled ipratropium is recommended for use as additional therapy for pregnant women with severe asthma exacerbations.

Breast-Feeding Considerations It is not known if ipratropium (oral inhalation) is excreted in breast milk. The manufacturer recommends that caution be exercised when administering ipratropium (oral inhalation) to nursing women.

Contraindications Hypersensitivity to ipratropium, atropine (and its derivatives), or any component of the formulation

Warnings/Precautions Immediate hypersensitivity reactions (urticaria, angioedema, rash, bronchospasm) have been reported. Rarely, paradoxical bronchospasm may occur with use of inhaled bronchodilating agents; this should be distinguished from inadequate response. Not indicated for the initial treatment of acute episodes of bronchospasm where rescue therapy is required for rapid response. Should only be used in acute exacerbations of asthma in conjunction with short-acting beta-adrenergic agonists for acute episodes. Use with caution in patients with myasthenia gravis, narrow-angle glaucoma, benign prostatic hyperplasia (BPH), or bladder neck obstruction

Adverse Reactions

>10%: Respiratory: Bronchitis (10% to 23%), COPD exacerbation (8% to 23%), sinusitis (1% to 11%)

1% to 10%:

Central nervous system: Headache (6% to 7%), dizziness (3%)

Gastrointestinal: Dyspepsia (1% to 5%), nausea (4%), xerostomia (2% to 4%), taste perversion (1%)

Genitourinary: Urinary tract infection (2% to 10%)

Neuromuscular & skeletal: Back pain (2% to 7%)

Respiratory: Dyspnea (7% to 8%), cough (>3%), rhinitis (>3%), upper respiratory infection (>3%)

Miscellaneous: Flu-like syndrome (4% to 8%)

<1% (Limited to important or life-threatening): Accommodation disorder, anaphylactic reaction, angioedema, bronchospasm, corneal edema, eye pain (acute), glaucoma, hypersensitivity reactions, hypotension, intraocular pressure increased, laryngospasm, palpitations, stomatitis, tachycardia, urinary retention

Drug Interactions

Metabolism/Transport Effects None known.

Avoid Concomitant Use

Avoid concomitant use of Ipratropium (Oral Inhalation) with any of the following: Aclidinium; Anticholinergics; Potassium Chloride; Tiotropium; Umeclidinium

Increased Effect/Toxicity

Ipratropium (Oral Inhalation) may increase the levels/effects of: AbobotulinumtoxinA; Analgesics (Opioid); Anticholinergics; Cannabinoids; Mirabegron; OnabotulinumtoxinA; Potassium Chloride; RimabotulinumtoxinB; Thiazide Diuretics; Tiotropium; Topiramate

The levels/effects of Ipratropium (Oral Inhalation) may be increased by: Aclidinium; Pramlintide; Umeclidinium

Decreased Effect

Ipratropium (Oral Inhalation) may decrease the levels/effects of: Acetylcholinesterase Inhibitors (Central); Secretin

The levels/effects of Ipratropium (Oral Inhalation) may be decreased by: Acetylcholinesterase Inhibitors (Central)

Storage/Stability

Aerosol: Store at controlled room temperature of 25°C (77°F). Do not store near heat or open flame.

Solution: Store at 15°C to 30°C (59°F to 86°F). Protect from light.

Mechanism of Action Blocks the action of acetylcholine at parasympathetic sites in bronchial smooth muscle causing bronchodilation; local application to nasal mucosa inhibits serous and seromucous gland secretions.

Pharmacodynamics/Kinetics

Onset of action: Bronchodilation: Within 15 minutes

Peak effect: 1-2 hours

Duration: 2-5 hours

Absorption: Negligible

Distribution: 15% of dose reaches lower airways

Protein Binding: ≤9%

Half-life elimination: 2 hours

Excretion: Urine

Dosage

Nebulization:

Children ≤12 years: Asthma exacerbation, acute (*NIH Asthma Guidelines, 2007*): 250-500 mcg every 20 minutes for 3 doses, then as needed. **Note:** Should be given in combination with a short-acting beta-adrenergic agonist.

Children >12 years and Adults:

Bronchodilator for COPD: 500 mcg (one unit-dose vial) 3-4 times/day with doses 6-8 hours apart

Asthma exacerbation, acute (*NIH Asthma Guidelines, 2007*): 500 mcg every 20 minutes for 3 doses, then as needed. **Note:** Should be given in combination with a short-acting beta-adrenergic agonist.

Oral inhalation: MDI:

Children ≤12 years: Asthma exacerbation, acute (*NIH Asthma Guidelines, 2007*): 4-8 inhalations every 20 minutes as needed for up to 3 hours. **Note:** Should be given in combination with a short-acting beta-adrenergic agonist.

Children >12 years and Adults:

Bronchodilator for COPD: 2 inhalations 4 times/day, up to 12 inhalations/24 hours

Asthma exacerbation, acute (*NIH Asthma Guidelines, 2007*): 8 inhalations every 20 minutes as needed for up to 3 hours. **Note:** Should be given in combination with a short-acting beta-adrenergic agonist.

Dosage adjustment in renal impairment: No dosage adjustment provided in manufacturer's labeling (has not been studied).

Dosage adjustment in hepatic impairment: No dosage adjustment provided in manufacturer's labeling (has not been studied).

Administration Avoid spraying into the eyes.

Atrovent® HFA: Prior to initial use, prime inhaler by releasing 2 test sprays into the air. If the inhaler has not been used for >3 days, reprime.

Dosage Forms Considerations

Atrovent HFA 12.9 g canister contains 200 inhalations.

Dosage Forms Excipient information presented when available (limited, particularly for generics); consult specific product labeling.

Aerosol Solution, Inhalation, as bromide:

Atrovent HFA: 17 mcg/actuation (12.9 g) [contains alcohol, usp]

Solution, Inhalation, as bromide:

Generic: 0.02% (2.5 mL)

Solution, Inhalation, as bromide [preservative free]:

Generic: 0.02% (2.5 mL)

Ipratropium (Nasal) (i pra TROE pee um)

Brand Names: U.S. Atrovent

Brand Names: Canada Alti-Ipratropium; Apo-Ipravent®; Atrovent®; Mylan-Ipratropium Solution

Index Terms Ipratropium Bromide

Pharmacologic Category Anticholinergic Agent

Use Symptomatic relief of rhinorrhea associated with the common cold and allergic and nonallergic rhinitis

Pregnancy Risk Factor B

Dosage Intranasal: Nasal spray:

Symptomatic relief of rhinorrhea associated with the common cold (safety and efficacy of use beyond 4 days in patients with the common cold have not been established):

Children 5-11 years: 0.06%: 2 sprays in each nostril 3 times/day

Children ≥12 years and Adults: 0.06%: 2 sprays in each nostril 3-4 times/day

Symptomatic relief of rhinorrhea associated with allergic/nonallergic rhinitis: Children ≥6 years and Adults: 0.03%: 2 sprays in each nostril 2-3 times/day

Symptomatic relief of rhinorrhea associated with seasonal allergic rhinitis (safety and efficacy of use beyond 3 weeks in patients with seasonal allergic rhinitis has not been established): Children ≥5 years and Adults: 0.06%: 2 sprays in each nostril 4 times/day

Dosage adjustment in renal impairment: No dosage adjustment provided in manufacturer's labeling (has not been studied); use with caution.

Dosage adjustment in hepatic impairment: No dosage adjustment provided in manufacturer's labeling (has not been studied); use with caution.

Additional Information Complete prescribing information should be consulted for additional detail.

Dosage Forms Considerations

Atrovent 0.03% (21 mcg/spray) nasal solution 30 mL bottles contain 345 sprays, and the 0.06% (42 mcg/spray) 15 mL bottles contain 165 sprays.

Dosage Forms Excipient information presented when available (limited, particularly for generics); consult specific product labeling.

Solution, Nasal, as bromide:

Atrovent: 0.03% (30 mL); 0.06% (15 mL)

Generic: 0.03% (30 mL); 0.06% (15 mL)

Ipratropium and Albuterol
(i pra TROE pee um & al BYOO ter ole)

Brand Names: U.S. Combivent® Respimat®; Combivent® [DSC]; DuoNeb®

Brand Names: Canada CO Ipra-Sal; Combivent UDV; Gen-Combo Sterinebs; ratio-Ipra Sal UDV; Teva-Combo Sterinebs

Index Terms Albuterol and Ipratropium; Salbutamol and Ipratropium

Pharmacologic Category Anticholinergic Agent; $Beta_2$-Adrenergic Agonist

Use Treatment of COPD in those patients who are currently on a regular bronchodilator who continue to have bronchospasms and require a second bronchodilator

Pregnancy Risk Factor C

Dosage COPD: Inhalation: Adults:

Aerosol for inhalation:

Combivent®: Two inhalations 4 times daily (maximum: 12 inhalations/24 hours)

Combivent® Respimat®: One inhalation 4 times daily (maximum: 6 inhalations/24 hours)

Solution for nebulization: Initial: 3 mL every 6 hours (maximum: 3 mL every 4 hours)

Dosage adjustment in renal impairment: No dosage adjustment provided in manufacturer's labeling (has not been studied); use with caution.

Dosage adjustment in hepatic impairment: No dosage adjustment provided in manufacturer's labeling (has not been studied); use with caution.

Additional Information Complete prescribing information should be consulted for additional detail.

Dosage Forms Excipient information presented when available (limited, particularly for generics); consult specific product labeling. [DSC] = Discontinued product

Aerosol, for oral inhalation:

Combivent®: Ipratropium bromide 18 mcg and albuterol (base) 90 mcg per inhalation (14.7 g) [contains chlorofluorocarbon, soya lecithin; 200 metered actuations] [DSC]

Solution, for nebulization: Ipratropium bromide 0.5 mg and albuterol (base) 2.5 mg per 3 mL (30s, 60s)

DuoNeb®: Ipratropium bromide 0.5 mg and albuterol (base) 2.5 mg per 3 mL (30s, 60s)

Solution, for oral inhalation [spray]:

Combivent® Respimat®: Ipratropium bromide 20 mcg and albuterol (base) 100 mcg per inhalation (4 g) [contains benzalkonium chloride; 120 metered actuations]

◆ **Ipratropium Bromide** *see* Ipratropium (Nasal) *on page 1112*

◆ **Ipratropium Bromide** *see* Ipratropium (Systemic) *on page 1111*

◆ **I-Prin [OTC]** *see* Ibuprofen *on page 1032*

◆ **Iprivask** *see* Desirudin *on page 574*

◆ **Iproveratril Hydrochloride** *see* Verapamil *on page 2182*

◆ **IPV** *see* Poliovirus Vaccine (Inactivated) *on page 1666*

Irbesartan (ir be SAR tan)

Brand Names: U.S. Avapro

Brand Names: Canada Apo-Irbesartan; Auro-Irbesartan; Ava-Irbesartan; Avapro; CO Irbesartan; Dom-Irbesartan; Mylan-Irbesartan; PMS-Irbesartan; ratio-Irbesartan; Sandoz-Irbesartan; Teva-Irbesartan

Pharmacologic Category Angiotensin II Receptor Blocker; Antihypertensive

Additional Appendix Information

Angiotensin Agents *on page 2280*

Use Treatment of hypertension alone or in combination with other antihypertensives; treatment of diabetic nephropathy in patients with type 2 diabetes mellitus (noninsulin dependent, NIDDM) and hypertension

Unlabeled Use To slow the rate of progression of aortic-root dilation in pediatric patients with Marfan's syndrome

Pregnancy Risk Factor D

Pregnancy Considerations [U.S. Boxed Warning]: Drugs that act on the renin-angiotensin system can cause injury and death to the developing fetus. Discontinue as soon as possible once pregnancy is detected. The use of drugs which act on the renin-angiotensin system are associated with oligohydramnios. Oligohydramnios, due to decreased fetal renal function, may lead to fetal lung hypoplasia and skeletal malformations. Use is also associated with anuria, hypotension, renal failure, skull hypoplasia, and death in the fetus/neonate. The exposed fetus should be monitored for fetal growth, amniotic fluid volume, and organ formation. Infants exposed *in utero* should be monitored for hyperkalemia, hypotension, and oliguria.

Untreated chronic maternal hypertension is also associated with adverse events in the fetus, infant, and mother. If treatment for hypertension during pregnancy is needed, other agents are preferred (ACOG, 2012; Chobanian, 2003). In women of reproductive potential, angiotensin II receptor blockers should be discontinued prior to conception or as soon as pregnancy is confirmed (Chobanian, 2003).

Breast-Feeding Considerations It is not known if irbesartan is excreted into breast milk. Due to the potential for serious adverse reactions in the nursing infant, the manufacturer recommends a decision be made whether to discontinue nursing or to discontinue the drug, taking into account the importance of treatment to the mother. Breast-fed infants of mothers taking medications for hypertension should be monitored for adverse effects (Chobanian, 2003).

Contraindications

Hypersensitivity to irbesartan or any component of the formulation; concomitant use with aliskiren in patients with diabetes mellitus

Canadian labeling: Additional contraindications (not in U.S. labeling): Hypersensitivity to irbesartan or any component of the formulation; concomitant use with aliskiren in patients with moderate to severe renal impairment (GFR <60 mL/minute/1.73 m^2)

Warnings/Precautions [U.S. Boxed Warning]: Drugs that act on the renin-angiotensin system can cause injury and death to the developing fetus. Discontinue as soon as possible once pregnancy is detected. May cause hyperkalemia; avoid potassium supplementation unless specifically required by healthcare provider. May be associated with deterioration of renal function and/or increases in serum creatinine, particularly in patients with low renal blood flow (eg, renal artery stenosis, heart failure) whose glomerular filtration rate (GFR) is dependent on efferent arteriolar vasoconstriction by angiotensin II. Avoid use or use a much smaller dose in patients who are intravascularly volume-depleted; use caution in patients with unstented unilateral or bilateral renal artery stenosis. When unstented bilateral renal artery stenosis is present, use is generally avoided due to the elevated risk of deterioration in renal function unless possible benefits outweigh risks. AUCs of irbesartan (not the active metabolite) are about 50% greater in patients with Cl_{cr} <30 mL/minute and are doubled in hemodialysis patients.

Potentially significant drug interactions may exist, requiring dose or frequency adjustment, additional monitoring, and/or selection of alternative therapy.

Angioedema has been reported rarely with some angiotensin II receptor antagonists (ARBs) and may occur at any time during treatment (especially following first dose). It may involve the head and neck (potentially compromising airway) or the intestine (presenting with abdominal pain). Patients with idiopathic or hereditary angioedema or previous angioedema associated with ACE-inhibitor therapy may be at an increased risk. Prolonged frequent monitoring may be required, especially if tongue, glottis, or larynx are involved, as they are associated with airway obstruction. Patients with a history of airway surgery may have a higher risk of airway obstruction. Discontinue therapy immediately if angioedema occurs. Aggressive early management is critical. Intramuscular (I.M.) administration of epinephrine may be necessary. Do not readminister to patients who have had angioedema with ARBs.

Adverse Reactions Unless otherwise indicated, percentage of incidence is reported for patients with hypertension.

>10%: Endocrine & metabolic: Hyperkalemia (19%, diabetic nephropathy; rarely seen in HTN)

1% to 10%:

Cardiovascular: Orthostatic hypotension (5%, diabetic nephropathy)

Central nervous system: Fatigue (4%), dizziness (10%, diabetic nephropathy)

Gastrointestinal: Diarrhea (3%), dyspepsia (2%)

Respiratory: Upper respiratory infection (9%), cough (2.8% versus 2.7% in placebo)

<1%, postmarketing, and/or case reports (Limited to important or life-threatening): Anemia (case report; Simonetti, 2007), angina, angioedema, arrhythmia, cardiopulmonary arrest, conjunctivitis, depression, dyspnea, ecchymosis, epistaxis, gout, heart failure, hepatitis, hypotension, jaundice, libido decreased, MI, orthostatic hypotension, paresthesia, renal failure, renal function impaired, sexual dysfunction, stroke, thrombocytopenia, transaminases increased, urticaria

Drug Interactions

Metabolism/Transport Effects Substrate of CYP2C9 (minor); **Note:** Assignment of Major/Minor substrate status based on clinically relevant drug interaction potential; **Inhibits** CYP2C8 (moderate), CYP2C9 (moderate), CYP2D6 (weak), CYP3A4 (weak)

Avoid Concomitant Use

Avoid concomitant use of Irbesartan with any of the following: Pimozide

Increased Effect/Toxicity

Irbesartan may increase the levels/effects of: ACE Inhibitors; Amifostine; Antihypertensives; ARIPiprazole; Bosentan; Carvedilol; CycloSPORINE (Systemic); CYP2C8 Substrates; CYP2C9 Substrates; Dofetilide; Hypotensive Agents; Lithium; Lomitapide; Nonsteroidal Anti-Inflammatory Agents; Obinutuzumab; Pimozide; Potassium-Sparing Diuretics; RiTUXimab; Sodium Phosphates

The levels/effects of Irbesartan may be increased by: Alfuzosin; Aliskiren; Brimonidine (Topical); Canagliflozin; Diazoxide; Eplerenone; Fluconazole; Heparin; Heparin (Low Molecular Weight); Herbs (Hypotensive Properties); MAO Inhibitors; Pentoxifylline; Phosphodiesterase 5 Inhibitors; Potassium Salts; Prostacyclin Analogues; Tolvaptan; Trimethoprim

Decreased Effect

The levels/effects of Irbesartan may be decreased by: Herbs (Hypertensive Properties); Methylphenidate; Nonsteroidal Anti-Inflammatory Agents; Rifamycin Derivatives; Yohimbine

Ethanol/Nutrition/Herb Interactions Herb/Nutraceutical: Dong quai has estrogenic activity. Some herbal medications may worsen hypertension (eg, ephedra); garlic may have additional antihypertensive effects. Management: Avoid dong quai if using for hypertension. Avoid ephedra, yohimbe, ginseng, and garlic.

Storage/Stability Store at room temperature of 15°C to 30°C (59°F to 86°F).

Mechanism of Action Irbesartan is an angiotensin receptor antagonist. Angiotensin II acts as a vasoconstrictor. In addition to causing direct vasoconstriction, angiotensin II also stimulates the release of aldosterone. Once aldosterone is released, sodium as well as water are reabsorbed. The end result is an elevation in blood pressure. Irbesartan binds to the AT1 angiotensin II receptor. This binding prevents angiotensin II from binding to the receptor thereby blocking the vasoconstriction and the aldosterone secreting effects of angiotensin II.

Pharmacodynamics/Kinetics

Onset of action: Peak effect: 1-2 hours

Duration: >24 hours

Distribution: V_d: 53-93 L

Protein binding, plasma: 90%

Metabolism: Hepatic, primarily CYP2C9

Bioavailability: 60% to 80%

Half-life elimination: Terminal: 11-15 hours

Time to peak, serum: 1.5-2 hours

Excretion: Feces (80%); urine (20%)

Dosage Oral:

Hypertension:

Children:

<6 years: Safety and efficacy have not been established.

≥6-12 years: Initial: 75 mg once daily; may be titrated to a maximum of 150 mg once daily

Children ≥13 years and Adults: 150 mg once daily; patients may be titrated to 300 mg once daily

Note: Starting dose in volume-depleted patients should be 75 mg

Aortic-root dilation with Marfan's syndrome (unlabeled use): Children 14 months to 16 years: Initial: 1.4 mg/kg/day; can be increased to a maximum of 2 mg/kg/day (not to exceed adult maximum of 300 mg/day)

Nephropathy in patients with type 2 diabetes and hypertension: Adults: Target dose: 300 mg once daily

Dosage adjustment in renal impairment: No dosage adjustment necessary with mild to severe impairment unless the patient is also volume depleted.

Dosage adjustment in hepatic impairment: No dosage adjustment necessary.

Dietary Considerations May be taken with or without food.

Monitoring Parameters Electrolytes, serum creatinine, BUN, urinalysis

Dosage Forms Excipient information presented when available (limited, particularly for generics); consult specific product labeling.

Tablet, Oral:

Avapro: 75 mg, 150 mg, 300 mg

Generic: 75 mg, 150 mg, 300 mg

Irbesartan and Hydrochlorothiazide

(ir be SAR tan & hye droe klor oh THYE a zide)

Brand Names: U.S. Avalide

Brand Names: Canada Apo-Irbesartan/HCTZ; AVA-Irbesartan/HCTZ; Avalide; CO Irbesartan HCT; Irbesartan-HCT; Irbesartan-HCTZ; Mint-Irbesartan/HCTZ; PMS-Irbesartan HCTZ; Ran-Irbesartan HCTZ; ratio-Irbesartan HCTZ; Sandoz-Irbesartan HCT; Teva-Irbesartan HCTZ

Index Terms Avapro® HCT; Hydrochlorothiazide and Irbesartan

Pharmacologic Category Angiotensin II Receptor Blocker; Antihypertensive; Diuretic, Thiazide

Use Combination therapy for the management of hypertension; may be used as initial therapy in patients likely to need multiple drugs to achieve blood pressure goals

Pregnancy Risk Factor D

Dosage Oral: Adults: **Note:** Maximum antihypertensive effects are attained within 2-4 weeks after initiation or a change in dose; however, if necessary, may carefully titrate dose as soon as after 1 week of treatment.

Add-on therapy: Dose must be individualized. A patient who is not controlled with either agent alone may be switched to the combination product. The lowest dosage available is irbesartan 150 mg/hydrochlorothiazide 12.5 mg.

Initial therapy: Irbesartan 150 mg/hydrochlorothiazide 12.5 mg once daily. If initial response is inadequate, may titrate dose after 1-2 weeks, to a maximum dose of irbesartan 300 mg/hydrochlorothiazide 25 mg once daily.

Dosing adjustment in renal impairment:

Mild-to-moderate impairment (Cl_{cr} >30 mL/minute): No dosage adjustment necessary; use with caution.

Severe impairment (Cl_{cr} ≤30 mL/minute): Use not recommended.

Dosage adjustment in hepatic impairment: No dosage adjustment necessary; use with caution.

Additional Information Complete prescribing information should be consulted for additional detail.

Dosage Forms Excipient information presented when available (limited, particularly for generics); consult specific product labeling. [DSC] = Discontinued product

Tablet, oral: 150/12.5: Irbesartan 150 mg and hydrochlorothiazide 12.5 mg; 300/12.5: Irbesartan 300 mg and hydrochlorothiazide 12.5 mg

Avalide 150/12.5: Irbesartan 150 mg and hydrochlorothiazide 12.5 mg

Avalide 300/12.5: Irbesartan 300 mg and hydrochlorothiazide 12.5 mg

Avalide 300/25: Irbesartan 300 mg and hydrochlorothiazide 25 mg [DSC]

◆ **Irbesartan-HCT (Can)** *see* Irbesartan and Hydrochlorothiazide *on page 1115*

◆ **Irbesartan-HCTZ (Can)** *see* Irbesartan and Hydrochlorothiazide *on page 1115*

◆ **Iressa®** *see* Gefitinib *on page 941*

◆ **IRESSA® (Can)** *see* Gefitinib *on page 941*

Irinotecan (eye rye no TEE kan)

Brand Names: U.S. Camptosar

Brand Names: Canada Camptosar®; Irinotecan Hydrochloride Trihydrate

Index Terms Camptothecin-11; CPT-11; Irinotecan HCl; Irinotecan Hydrochloride

Pharmacologic Category Antineoplastic Agent, Camptothecin; Antineoplastic Agent, Natural Source (Plant) Derivative; Antineoplastic Agent, Topoisomerase I Inhibitor

Use Treatment of metastatic carcinoma of the colon or rectum

Unlabeled Use Treatment of cervical cancer (recurrent or metastatic), central nervous system tumors (recurrent glioblastoma), esophageal cancer, Ewing's sarcoma (recurrent or progressive), gastric cancer (metastatic or locally advanced), nonsmall cell lung cancer (advanced), ovarian cancer (recurrent), pancreatic cancer (advanced), small cell lung cancer (extensive stage)

Pregnancy Risk Factor D

Pregnancy Considerations Teratogenic effects were noted in animal studies. There are no adequate and well-controlled studies in pregnant women. Women of child-bearing potential should avoid becoming pregnant while receiving treatment.

Breast-Feeding Considerations Due to the potential for serious adverse reactions in the nursing infant, breast-feeding is not recommended.

Contraindications Hypersensitivity to irinotecan or any component of the formulation

Warnings/Precautions Hazardous agent - use appropriate precautions for handling and disposal (NIOSH, 2012). Severe hypersensitivity reactions (including anaphylaxis) have occurred. For I.V. use only; monitor infusion site; may cause local tissue necrosis or thrombophlebitis if extravasation occurs (the manufacturer recommends flushing the site with sterile water and ice application).

[U.S. Boxed Warning]: Severe diarrhea may be dose-limiting and potentially fatal; early-onset and late-onset diarrhea may occur. Early diarrhea occurs during or within 24 hours of receiving irinotecan and is characterized by cholinergic symptoms (eg, increased salivation, rhinitis, miosis, diaphoresis, flushing, abdominal cramping, lacrimation); may be prevented or treated with atropine. Late diarrhea occurs more than 24 hours after treatment which may lead to dehydration, electrolyte imbalance, or sepsis; may be life-threatening and should be promptly treated with loperamide; dose reductions may be recommended for future doses within the current cycle. Antibiotics may be necessary if patient develops ileus, fever, or severe neutropenia. Patients with diarrhea should be carefully monitored and treated promptly; may require fluid and electrolyte therapy. Colitis, complicated by ulceration, bleeding, ileus, and infection has been reported; initiate antibiotics promptly in patients with ileus.

[U.S. Boxed Warning]: May cause severe myelosuppression. Deaths due to sepsis following severe neutropenia have been reported. Complications due to neutropenia should be promptly managed with antibiotics. Therapy should be temporarily discontinued if neutropenic fever occurs or if the absolute neutrophil count is <1000/mm^3. The dose of irinotecan should be reduced if there is a clinically significant decrease in the total WBC (<200/mm^3), neutrophil count (<1500/mm^3), hemoglobin (<8 g/dL), or platelet count (<100,000/mm^3). Routine administration of a colony-stimulating factor is generally not necessary, but may be considered for patients experiencing significant neutropenia. Fatal cases of interstitial pulmonary disease (IPD)-like events have been reported with single-agent and combination therapy. Promptly evaluate changes in baseline pulmonary symptoms or any new-onset pulmonary symptoms. Discontinue all chemotherapy if IPD is diagnosed.

Patients with even modest elevations in total serum bilirubin levels (1-2 mg/dL) have a significantly greater likelihood of experiencing first-course grade 3 or 4 neutropenia than those with bilirubin levels that were <1 mg/dL. Patients with abnormal glucuronidation of bilirubin, such as those with Gilbert's syndrome, may also be at greater risk of myelosuppression when receiving therapy with irinotecan. Use caution when treating patients with known hepatic dysfunction or hyperbilirubinemia exposure to the active metabolite (SN-38) is increased; toxicities may be increased. Dosage adjustments should be considered.

Patients homozygous for the UGT1A1*28 allele are at increased risk of neutropenia; initial one-level dose reduction should be considered for both single-agent and combination regimens. Heterozygous carriers of the UGT1A1*28 allele may also be at increased risk; however, most patients have tolerated normal starting doses. Avoid vaccination with live vaccines during treatment (risk of infection may be increased due to immunosuppression). Although the response to vaccines may be diminished, inactivated vaccines may be administered during treatment.

Renal impairment and acute renal failure have been reported, possibly due to dehydration secondary to diarrhea. Use with caution in patients with renal impairment; not recommended in patients on dialysis. Patients with bowel obstruction should not be treated with irinotecan until resolution of obstruction. Use caution in patients who previously received pelvic/abdominal radiation, elderly patients with comorbid conditions, or baseline performance status of 2; close monitoring and dosage adjustments are recommended. Contains sorbitol; do not use in patients with hereditary fructose intolerance. Thromboembolic events have been reported. **[U.S. Boxed Warning]: Should be administered under the supervision of an experienced cancer chemotherapy physician.** Except as part of a clinical trial, use in combination with fluorouracil and leucovorin "Mayo Clinic" regimen is not recommended. Increased toxicity has also been noted in patients with a baseline performance status of 2 in other combination regimens containing irinotecan, leucovorin, and fluorouracil. High potential for CYP-mediated drug interactions; enzyme inducers may decrease exposure to irinotecan and SN-38 (active metabolite); enzyme inhibitors may increase exposure; for use in patients with CNS tumors (unlabeled use), selection of antiseizure medications which are not enzyme inducers is preferred.

Adverse Reactions Frequency of adverse reactions reported for single-agent use of irinotecan only.

>10%:

Cardiovascular: Vasodilation (9% to 11%)

Central nervous system: Cholinergic toxicity (47% - includes rhinitis, increased salivation, miosis, lacrimation, diaphoresis, flushing and intestinal hyperperistalsis); fever (44% to 45%), pain (23% to 24%), dizziness (15% to 21%), insomnia (19%), headache (17%), chills (14%)

Dermatologic: Alopecia (46% to 72%), rash (13% to 14%)

Endocrine & metabolic: Dehydration (15%)

Gastrointestinal: Diarrhea, late (83% to 88%; grade 3/4: 14% to 31%), diarrhea, early (43% to 51%; grade 3/4: 7% to 22%), nausea (70% to 86%), abdominal pain (57% to 68%), vomiting (62% to 67%), cramps (57%), anorexia (44% to 55%), constipation (30% to 32%), mucositis (30%), weight loss (30%), flatulence (12%), stomatitis (12%)

Hematologic: Anemia (60% to 97%; grades 3/4: 5% to 7%), leukopenia (63% to 96%, grades 3/4: 14% to 28%), thrombocytopenia (96%, grades 3/4: 1% to 4%), neutropenia (30% to 96%; grades 3/4: 14% to 31%)

Hepatic: Bilirubin increased (84%), alkaline phosphatase increased (13%)

Neuromuscular & skeletal: Weakness (69% to 76%), back pain (14%)

Respiratory: Dyspnea (22%), cough (17% to 20%), rhinitis (16%)

Miscellaneous: Diaphoresis (16%), infection (14%)

1% to 10%:

Cardiovascular: Edema (10%), hypotension (6%), thromboembolic events (5%)

Central nervous system: Somnolence (9%), confusion (3%)

Gastrointestinal: Abdominal fullness (10%), dyspepsia (10%)

Hematologic: Neutropenic fever (grades 3/4: 2% to 6%), hemorrhage (grades 3/4: 1% to 5%), neutropenic infection (grades 3/4: 1% to 2%)

Hepatic: AST increased (10%), ascites and/or jaundice (grades 3/4: 9%)

Respiratory: Pneumonia (4%)

<1%, postmarketing, and/or case reports: ALT increased, amylase increased, anaphylactoid reaction, anaphylaxis, angina, arterial thrombosis, bleeding, bradycardia, cardiac arrest, cerebral infarct, cerebrovascular accident, circulatory failure, colitis, dysrhythmia, embolus, gastrointestinal bleeding, gastrointestinal obstruction, hepatomegaly, hyperglycemia, hypersensitivity, hyponatremia, ileus, interstitial pulmonary disease (IPD), intestinal perforation, ischemic colitis, lipase increased, lymphocytopenia, megacolon, MI, myocardial ischemia, neutropenic typhlitis, pancreatitis, paresthesia, peripheral vascular disorder, pulmonary embolus; pulmonary toxicity (dyspnea, fever, reticulonodular infiltrates on chest x-ray); renal failure (acute), renal impairment, thrombocytopenia (immune mediated), thrombophlebitis, thrombosis, typhlitis, ulcerative colitis

Note: In limited pediatric experience, dehydration (often associated with severe hypokalemia and hyponatremia) was among the most significant grade 3/4 adverse events, with a frequency up to 29%. In addition, grade 3/4 infection was reported in 24%.

Drug Interactions

Metabolism/Transport Effects Substrate of CYP2B6 (major), CYP3A4 (major), P-glycoprotein, SLCO1B1, UGT1A1; **Note:** Assignment of Major/Minor substrate status based on clinically relevant drug interaction potential

Avoid Concomitant Use

Avoid concomitant use of Irinotecan with any of the following: Atazanavir; BCG; CloZAPine; Conivaptan; Fusidic Acid (Systemic); Grapefruit Juice; Natalizumab; Pimecrolimus; St Johns Wort; Tacrolimus (Topical); Tofacitinib; Vaccines (Live)

Increased Effect/Toxicity

Irinotecan may increase the levels/effects of: CloZAPine; Leflunomide; Natalizumab; Tofacitinib; Vaccines (Live)

The levels/effects of Irinotecan may be increased by: Antifungal Agents (Azole Derivatives, Systemic); Atazanavir; Bevacizumab; Conivaptan; CYP2B6 Inhibitors (Moderate); CYP2B6 Inhibitors (Strong); CYP3A4 Inhibitors (Moderate); CYP3A4 Inhibitors (Strong); Dasatinib; Denosumab; Eltrombopag; Fusidic Acid (Systemic); Grapefruit Juice; Ivacaftor; Luliconazole; Mifepristone; P-glycoprotein/ABCB1 Inhibitors; Pimecrolimus; Quazepam; Regorafenib; Roflumilast; Simeprevir; SORAfenib; Tacrolimus (Topical); Trastuzumab

Decreased Effect

Irinotecan may decrease the levels/effects of: BCG; Coccidioidin Skin Test; Sipuleucel-T; Vaccines (Inactivated); Vaccines (Live)

The levels/effects of Irinotecan may be decreased by: Bosentan; CarBAMazepine; CYP3A4 Inducers (Strong); Dabrafenib; Deferasirox; Echinacea; Fosphenytoin; Mitotane; P-glycoprotein/ABCB1 Inducers; PHENobarbital; Phenytoin; St Johns Wort; Tocilizumab

Ethanol/Nutrition/Herb Interactions Herb/Nutraceutical: Avoid St John's wort (decreases the efficacy of irinotecan).

Preparation for Administration Hazardous agent; use appropriate precautions for handling and disposal (NIOSH, 2012). Dilute in 250-500 mL D_5W (preferred) or NS to a final concentration of 0.12-2.8 mg/mL. Due to the relatively acidic pH, irinotecan appears to be more stable in D_5W than NS.

Storage/Stability Store intact vials at room temperature. Protect from light. Solutions diluted in NS may precipitate if refrigerated. Solutions diluted in D_5W are stable for 24 hours at room temperature or 48 hours under refrigeration at 2°C to 8°C, although the manufacturer recommends use within 24 hours if refrigerated, within 6 hours at room temperature, and/or within 12 hours at room temperature (including infusion time) only if prepared under strict aseptic conditions (eg, laminar flow hood). Do not freeze.

Mechanism of Action Irinotecan and its active metabolite (SN-38) bind reversibly to topoisomerase I-DNA complex preventing religation of the cleaved DNA strand. This results in the accumulation of cleavable complexes and double-strand DNA breaks. As mammalian cells cannot efficiently repair these breaks, cell death consistent with S-phase cell cycle specificity occurs, leading to termination of cellular replication.

Pharmacodynamics/Kinetics

Distribution: V_d: 33-150 L/m^2

Protein binding, plasma: Predominantly albumin; Irinotecan: 30% to 68%, SN-38 (active metabolite): ~95%

Metabolism: Primarily hepatic to SN-38 (active metabolite) by carboxylesterase enzymes; SN-38 undergoes conjugation by UDP-glucuronosyl transferase 1A1 (UGT1A1) to form a glucuronide metabolite. Conversion of irinotecan to SN-38 is decreased and glucuronidation of SN-38 is increased patients who smoke cigarettes, resulting in lower levels of the metabolite and overall decreased systemic exposure. SN-38 is increased by UGT1A1*28 polymorphism (10% of North Americans are homozygous for UGT1A1*28 allele). The lactones of both irinotecan and SN-38 undergo hydrolysis to inactive hydroxy acid forms.

Half-life elimination: Irinotecan: 6-12 hours; SN-38: ~10-20 hours

Time to peak: SN-38: Following 90-minute infusion: ~1 hour

Excretion: Urine: Irinotecan (11% to 20%), metabolites (SN-38 <1%, SN-38 glucuronide, 3%)

Dosage I.V.: **Note:** A reduction in the starting dose by one dose level should be considered for prior pelvic/abdominal radiotherapy, performance status of 2, or known homozygosity for UGT1A1*28 allele. Consider premedication of atropine 0.25-1 mg I.V. or SubQ in patients with cholinergic symptoms (eg, increased salivation, rhinitis, miosis, diaphoresis, abdominal cramping) or early onset diarrhea. Details concerning dosage in combination regimens should also be consulted.

Children and Adults: **Ewing's sarcoma, recurrent or progressive (unlabeled use):** 20 mg/m^2/dose days 1-5 and days 8-12 every 3 weeks (in combination with temozolomide) (Casey, 2009)

Adults:

Colorectal cancer, metastatic (single-agent therapy):

Weekly regimen: 125 mg/m^2 over 90 minutes on days 1, 8, 15, and 22 of a 6-week treatment cycle (may adjust upward to 150 mg/m^2 if tolerated)

Adjusted dose level -1: 100 mg/m^2

Adjusted dose level -2: 75 mg/m^2

Further adjust to 50 mg/m^2 (in decrements of 25-50 mg/m^2) if needed

Once-every-3-week regimen: 350 mg/m^2 over 90 minutes, once every 3 weeks

Adjusted dose level -1: 300 mg/m^2

Adjusted dose level -2: 250 mg/m^2

Further adjust to 200 mg/m^2 (in decrements of 25-50 mg/m^2) if needed

Colorectal cancer, metastatic (in combination with fluorouracil and leucovorin): Six-week (42-day) cycle:

Regimen 1: 125 mg/m^2 over 90 minutes on days 1, 8, 15, and 22; to be given in combination with bolus leucovorin and fluorouracil (leucovorin administered immediately following irinotecan; fluorouracil immediately following leucovorin)

Adjusted dose level -1: 100 mg/m^2

Adjusted dose level -2: 75 mg/m^2

Further adjust if needed in decrements of ~20%

Regimen 2: 180 mg/m^2 over 90 minutes on days 1, 15, and 29; to be given in combination with infusional leucovorin and bolus/infusion fluorouracil (leucovorin administered immediately following irinotecan; fluorouracil immediately following leucovorin)

Adjusted dose level -1: 150 mg/m^2

Adjusted dose level -2: 120 mg/m^2

Further adjust if needed in decrements of ~20%

Colorectal cancer, metastatic (unlabeled dosing): FOLFOXIRI regimen: 165 mg/m^2 over 1 hour once every 2 weeks (Falcone, 2007)

Cervical cancer, recurrent or metastatic (unlabeled use): 125 mg/m^2 over 90 minutes once weekly for 4 consecutive weeks followed by a 2-week rest during each 6 week treatment cycle (Verschraegen, 1997)

CNS tumor, recurrent glioblastoma (unlabeled use): 125 mg/m^2 over 90 minutes once every 2 weeks (in combination with bevacizumab). **NOTE:** in patients taking concurrent antiepileptic enzyme-inducing medications irinotecan dose was increased to 340 mg/m^2 (Friedman, 2009; Vredenburgh, 2007).

Esophageal cancer, metastatic or locally advanced (unlabeled use): 65 mg/m^2/dose over 90 minutes days 1, 8, 15, and 22 of a 6-week treatment cycle (in combination with cisplatin) (Ajani, 2002; Ilson, 1999) **or** 80 mg/m^2/dose weekly for 6 weeks of a 7-week treatment cycle (in combination with leucovorin and fluorouracil) (Dank, 2008) **or** 250 mg/m^2/dose every 3 weeks (in combination with capecitabine) (Leary, 2009; Moehler, 2010)

Gastric cancer, metastatic or locally advanced (unlabeled use): 65 mg/m^2/dose over 90 minutes days 1, 8, 15, and 22 of a 6-week treatment cycle (in combination with cisplatin) (Ajani, 2002) **or** 180 mg/m^2/dose over 90 minutes every 2 weeks (in combination with leucovorin and fluorouracil) (Bouche, 2004) **or** 80 mg/m^2/dose weekly for 6 weeks of a 7-week treatment cycle (in combination with leucovorin and fluorouracil) (Dank, 2008) **or** 250 mg/m^2/dose every 3 weeks (in combination with capecitabine) (Moehler, 2010)

Nonsmall cell lung cancer, advanced (unlabeled use): 60 mg/m^2 days 1, 8, and 15 every 4 weeks (in combination with cisplatin) (Ohe, 2007)

Pancreatic cancer, advanced (unlabeled use): FOLFIRINOX regimen: 180 mg/m^2/dose over 90 minutes every 2 weeks (Conroy, 2005; Conroy, 2010)

Small cell lung cancer, extensive stage (unlabeled use): 60 mg/m^2 days 1, 8, and 15 every 4 weeks (in combination with cisplatin) (Noda, 2002) **or** 65 mg/m^2 days 1 and 8 every 3 weeks (in combination with cisplatin) (Hanna, 2006) **or** 175 mg/m^2 day 1 every 3 weeks (in combination with carboplatin) (Hermes, 2008) **or** 50 mg/m^2 days 1, 8 and 15 every 4 weeks (in combination with carboplatin) (Schmittel, 2006)

Elderly:

Weekly dosing schedule: No dosing adjustment is recommended

Every 3-week dosing colorectal cancer schedule: Recommended initial dose is 300 mg/m^2/dose for patients ≥70 years

Dosing adjustment in renal impairment:

Renal impairment: No dosage adjustment provided in manufacturer's labeling (has not been studied); use with caution.

Dialysis: Use in patients with dialysis is not recommended by the manufacturer; however, literature suggests reducing weekly dose from 125 mg/m^2 to 50 mg/m^2 and administer after hemodialysis or on nondialysis days (Janus, 2010).

Dosing adjustment in hepatic impairment:

Manufacturer's recommendations:

Liver metastases with normal hepatic function: No dosage adjustment necessary.

Bilirubin >ULN to ≤2 mg/dL: Consider reducing initial dose by one dose level

Bilirubin >2 mg/dL: Use is not recommended

Alternate recommendations: The following adjustments have been used by some clinicians:

Bilirubin 1.5-3 mg/dL: Administer 75% of dose (Floyd, 2006)

Bilirubin 1.51 to 3 times ULN: Reduce dose from 350 mg/m^2 every 3 weeks to 200 mg/m^2 every 3 weeks (Raymond, 2002)

Dosing in obesity: *ASCO Guidelines for appropriate chemotherapy dosing in obese adults with cancer:* Utilize patient's actual body weight (full weight) for calculation of body surface area- or weight-based dosing, particularly when the intent of therapy is curative; manage regimen-related toxicities in the same manner as for nonobese patients; if a dose reduction is utilized due to toxicity, consider resumption of full weight-based dosing with subsequent cycles, especially if cause of toxicity (eg, hepatic or renal impairment) is resolved (Griggs, 2012).

Dosage adjustment for toxicities: It is recommended that new courses begin only after the granulocyte count recovers to ≥1500/mm^3, the platelet counts recovers to ≥100,000/mm^3, and treatment-related diarrhea has fully resolved. Depending on the patient's ability to tolerate therapy, doses should be adjusted in increments of 25-50 mg/m^2. Treatment should be delayed 1-2 weeks to allow for recovery from treatment-related toxicities. If the patient has not recovered after a 2-week delay, consider discontinuing irinotecan. See tables.

Colorectal Cancer: Single-Agent Schedule: Recommended Dosage Modifications[1]

Toxicity NCI Grade[2] (Value)	During a Cycle of Therapy	At Start of Subsequent Cycles of Therapy (After Adequate Recovery), Compared to Starting Dose in Previous Cycle[1]	
	Weekly	Weekly	Once Every 3 Weeks
No toxicity	Maintain dose level	↑ 25 mg/m^2 up to a maximum dose of 150 mg/m^2	Maintain dose level
Neutropenia			
1 (1500-1999/mm^3)	Maintain dose level	Maintain dose level	Maintain dose level
2 (1000-1499/mm^3)	↓ 25 mg/m^2	Maintain dose level	Maintain dose level
3 (500-999/mm^3)	Omit dose until resolved to ≤ grade 2, then ↓ 25 mg/m^2	↓ 25 mg/m^2	↓ 50 mg/m^2
4 (<500/mm^3)	Omit dose until resolved to ≤ grade 2, then ↓ 50 mg/m^2	↓ 50 mg/m^2	↓ 50 mg/m^2
Neutropenic Fever (grade 4 neutropenia and ≥ grade 2 fever)	Omit dose until resolved, then ↓ 50 mg/m^2	↓ 50 mg/m^2	↓ 50 mg/m^2
Other Hematologic Toxicities	Dose modifications for leukopenia, thrombocytopenia, and anemia during a course of therapy and at the start of subsequent courses of therapy are also based on NCI toxicity criteria and are the same as recommended for neutropenia above.		
Diarrhea			
1 (2-3 stools/day > pretreatment)	Maintain dose level	Maintain dose level	Maintain dose level
2 (4-6 stools/day > pretreatment)	↓ 25 mg/m^2	Maintain dose level	Maintain dose level
3 (7-9 stools/day > pretreatment)	Omit dose until resolved to ≤ grade 2, then ↓ 25 mg/m^2	↓ 25 mg/m^2	↓ 50 mg/m^2
4 (≥10 stools/day > pretreatment)	Omit dose until resolved to ≤ grade 2, then ↓ 50 mg/m^2	↓ 50 mg/m^2	↓ 50 mg/m^2
Other Nonhematologic Toxicities[3]			
1	Maintain dose level	Maintain dose level	Maintain dose level
2	↓ 25 mg/m^2	↓ 25 mg/m^2	↓ 50 mg/m^2
3	Omit dose until resolved to ≤ grade 2, then ↓ 25 mg/m^2	↓ 25 mg/m^2	↓ 50 mg/m^2
4	Omit dose until resolved to ≤ grade 2, then ↓ 50 mg/m^2	↓ 50 mg/m^2	↓ 50 mg/m^2

[1]All dose modifications should be based on the worst preceding toxicity.

[2]National Cancer Institute Common Toxicity Criteria (version 1.0).

[3]Excludes alopecia, anorexia, asthenia.

Colorectal Cancer: Combination Schedules: Recommended Dosage Modifications[1]

Toxicity NCI[2] Grade (Value)	During a Cycle of Therapy	At the Start of Subsequent Cycles of Therapy (After Adequate Recovery), Compared to the Starting Dose in the Previous Cycle[1]
No toxicity	Maintain dose level	Maintain dose level
Neutropenia		
1 (1500-1999/mm^3)	Maintain dose level	Maintain dose level
2 (1000-1499/mm^3)	↓ 1 dose level	Maintain dose level
3 (500-999/mm^3)	Omit dose until resolved to ≤ grade 2, then ↓ 1 dose level	↓ 1 dose level
4 (<500/mm^3)	Omit dose until resolved to ≤ grade 2, then ↓ 2 dose levels	↓ 2 dose levels
Neutropenic Fever (grade 4 neutropenia and ≥ grade 2 fever)	Omit dose until resolved, then ↓ 2 dose levels	
Other Hematologic Toxicities	Dose modifications for leukopenia or thrombocytopenia during a course of therapy and at the start of subsequent courses of therapy are also based on NCI toxicity criteria and are the same as recommended for neutropenia above.	
Diarrhea		
1 (2-3 stools/day > pretreatment)	Delay dose until resolved to baseline, then give same dose	Maintain dose level
2 (4-6 stools/day > pretreatment)	Omit dose until resolved to baseline, then ↓ 1 dose level	Maintain dose level
3 (7-9 stools/day > pretreatment)	Omit dose until resolved to baseline, then ↓ by 1 dose level	↓ 1 dose level
4 (≥10 stools/day > pretreatment)	Omit dose until resolved to baseline, then ↓ 2 dose levels	↓ 2 dose levels
Other Nonhematologic Toxicities[3]		
1	Maintain dose level	Maintain dose level
2	Omit dose until resolved to ≤ grade 1, then ↓ 1 dose level	Maintain dose level
3	Omit dose until resolved to ≤ grade 2, then ↓ 1 dose level	↓ 1 dose level
4	Omit dose until resolved to ≤ grade 2, then ↓ 2 dose levels	↓ 2 dose levels
Mucositis and/or stomatitis	Decrease only 5-FU, not irinotecan	Decrease only 5-FU, not irinotecan

[1]All dose modifications should be based on the worst preceding toxicity.

[2]National Cancer Institute Common Toxicity Criteria (version 1.0).

[3]Excludes alopecia, anorexia, asthenia.

Dietary Considerations Contains sorbitol; do not use in patients with hereditary fructose intolerance.

Administration Administer by I.V. infusion, usually over 90 minutes. Premedication with dexamethasone and a 5-HT$_3$ blocker is recommended 30 minutes prior to administration; prochlorperazine may be considered for subsequent use (if needed). Consider atropine 0.25-1 mg I.V. or SubQ as premedication for or treatment of cholinergic symptoms (eg, increased salivation, rhinitis, miosis, diaphoresis, abdominal cramping) or early onset diarrhea.

The recommended regimen to manage late diarrhea is loperamide 4 mg orally at onset of late diarrhea, followed by 2 mg every 2 hours (or 4 mg every 4 hours at night) until 12 hours have passed without a bowel movement. If diarrhea recurs, then repeat administration. Loperamide should not be used for more than 48 consecutive hours.

Hazardous agent; use appropriate precautions for handling and disposal (NIOSH, 2012).

Monitoring Parameters CBC with differential, platelet count, and hemoglobin with each dose; bilirubin, electrolytes (with severe diarrhea); bowel movements and hydration status; monitor infusion site for signs of inflammation and avoid extravasation

A test is available for genotyping of UGT1A1; however, guidelines for use are not established and not recommended in patients who have experienced toxicity as a dose reduction is already recommended (NCCN Colon Cancer Guidelines v.1.2011)

Additional Information Patients who are homozygous for the UGT1A1*28 allele are at increased risk for neutropenia; a decreased dose is recommended. Clinical research of patients who are heterozygous for UGT1A1*28 have been variable for increased neutropenic risk and such patients have tolerated normal starting doses. An FDA-approved test (Invader® Molecular Assay) is available for clinical determination of UGT phenotype.

Dosage Forms Excipient information presented when available (limited, particularly for generics); consult specific product labeling.

Solution, Intravenous, as hydrochloride:

Camptosar: 40 mg/2 mL (2 mL); 100 mg/5 mL (5 mL); 300 mg/15 mL (15 mL)

Generic: 40 mg/2 mL (2 mL); 100 mg/5 mL (5 mL); 500 mg/25 mL (25 mL)

Solution, Intravenous, as hydrochloride [preservative free]:

Generic: 40 mg/2 mL (2 mL); 100 mg/5 mL (5 mL)

◆ **Irinotecan HCl** *see* Irinotecan *on page 1115*

◆ **Irinotecan Hydrochloride** *see* Irinotecan *on page 1115*

◆ **Irinotecan Hydrochloride Trihydrate (Can)** *see* Irinotecan *on page 1115*

◆ **Iron Carboxymaltose** *see* Ferric Carboxymaltose *on page 852*

◆ **Iron Dextran** *see* Iron Dextran Complex *on page 1119*

Iron Dextran Complex

(EYE ern DEKS tran KOM pleks)

Brand Names: U.S. Dexferrum; Infed

Brand Names: Canada Dexiron; Infufer

Index Terms High-Molecular-Weight Iron Dextran (DexFerrum); Imferon; Iron Dextran; Low-Molecular-Weight Iron Dextran (INFeD)

Pharmacologic Category Iron Salt

Use Iron deficiency: Treatment of iron deficiency in patients in whom oral administration is unsatisfactory or infeasible

Pregnancy Risk Factor C

Pregnancy Considerations Adverse events have been observed in animal reproduction studies. It is not known if iron dextran (as iron dextran) crosses the placenta. It is recommended that pregnant women meet the dietary requirements of iron with diet and/or supplements in order to prevent adverse events associated with iron deficiency anemia in pregnancy. Treatment of iron deficiency anemia in pregnant women is the same as in nonpregnant women and in most cases, oral iron preparations may be used. Except in severe cases of maternal anemia, the fetus achieves normal iron stores regardless of maternal concentrations.

Breast-Feeding Considerations Trace amounts of iron dextran (as iron dextran) are found in human milk. Iron is normally found in breast milk. Breast milk or iron fortified formulas generally provide enough iron to meet the recommended dietary requirements of infants. The amount of iron in breast milk is generally not influenced by maternal iron status.

Contraindications Hypersensitivity to iron dextran or any component of the formulation; any anemia not associated with iron deficiency

Warnings/Precautions [U.S. Boxed Warning]: Deaths associated with parenteral administration following anaphylactic-type reactions have been reported (use only where resuscitation equipment and personnel are available). A test dose should be administered to all patients prior to the first therapeutic dose. Fatal reactions have occurred even in patients who tolerated the test dose. Monitor patients for signs/symptoms of anaphylactic reactions during any iron dextran administration; fatalities have occurred with the test dose. A history of drug allergy (including multiple drug allergies) and/or the concomitant use of an ACE inhibitor may increase the risk of anaphylactic-type reactions. Adverse events (including life-threatening) associated with iron dextran usually occur with the high-molecular-weight formulation (Dexferrum), compared to low-molecular-weight (INFeD) (Chertow, 2006). Delayed (1-2 days) infusion reaction (including arthralgia, back pain, chills, dizziness, and fever) may occur with large doses (eg, total dose infusion) of I.V. iron dextran; usually subsides within 3-4 days. Delayed reaction may also occur (less commonly) with I.M. administration; subsiding within 3-7 days. Use with caution in patients with a history of significant allergies, asthma, serious hepatic impairment, pre-existing cardiac disease (may exacerbate cardiovascular complications), and rheumatoid arthritis (may exacerbate joint pain and swelling). Avoid use during acute kidney infection.

In patients with chronic kidney disease (CKD) requiring iron supplementation, the I.V. route is preferred for hemodialysis patients; either oral iron or I.V. iron may be used for nondialysis and peritoneal dialysis CKD patients. In patients with cancer-related anemia (either due to cancer or chemotherapy-induced) requiring iron supplementation, the I.V. route is superior to oral therapy; I.M. administration is not recommended for parenteral iron supplementation.

[U.S. Boxed Warning]: Use only in patients where the iron deficient state is not amenable to oral iron therapy. Discontinue oral iron prior to initiating parenteral iron therapy. Exogenous hemosiderosis may result from excess iron stores; patients with refractory anemias and/or hemoglobinopathies may be prone to iron overload with unwarranted iron supplementation. Anemia in the elderly is often caused by "anemia of chronic disease" or associated with inflammation rather than blood loss. Iron stores are usually normal or increased, with a serum ferritin >50 ng/mL and a decreased total iron binding capacity. I.V. administration of iron dextran is often preferred over I.M. in the elderly secondary to a decreased muscle mass and the need for daily injections. Intramuscular injections of iron-carbohydrate complexes may have a risk of delayed injection site tumor development. Iron dextran products differ in chemical characteristics. The high-molecular-weight formulation (Dexferrum) and the low-molecular-weight formulation (INFeD) are not clinically interchangeable. Not recommended in children <4 months of age. Intramuscular iron dextran use in neonates may be associated with an increased incidence of gram-negative sepsis.

Adverse Reactions Frequency not defined. **Note:** Adverse event risk is reported to be higher with the high-molecular-weight iron dextran formulation.

Cardiovascular: Arrhythmia, bradycardia, cardiac arrest, chest pain, chest tightness, cyanosis, flushing, hyper-/hypotension, shock, syncope, tachycardia

Central nervous system: Chills, disorientation, dizziness, fever, headache, malaise, seizure, unconsciousness, unresponsiveness

Dermatologic: Pruritus, purpura, rash, urticaria

Gastrointestinal: Abdominal pain, diarrhea, nausea, taste alteration, vomiting

Genitourinary: Discoloration of urine

Hematologic: Leukocytosis, lymphadenopathy

Local: Injection site reactions (cellulitis, inflammation, pain, phlebitis, soreness, swelling), muscle atrophy/fibrosis (with I.M. injection), skin/tissue staining (at the site of I.M. injection), sterile abscess

Neuromuscular & skeletal: Arthralgia, arthritis/arthritis exacerbation, back pain, myalgia, paresthesia, weakness

Respiratory: Bronchospasm, dyspnea, respiratory arrest, wheezing

Renal: Hematuria

Miscellaneous: Anaphylactic reactions (sudden respiratory difficulty, cardiovascular collapse), diaphoresis

Postmarketing and/or case reports: Angioedema, tumor formation (at former injection site)

Drug Interactions

Metabolism/Transport Effects None known.

Avoid Concomitant Use

Avoid concomitant use of Iron Dextran Complex with any of the following: Dimercaprol

Increased Effect/Toxicity

The levels/effects of Iron Dextran Complex may be increased by: ACE Inhibitors; Dimercaprol

Decreased Effect There are no known significant interactions involving a decrease in effect.

Preparation for Administration Solutions for infusion should be diluted in 250-1000 mL NS.

Storage/Stability Store at controlled room temperature.

Mechanism of Action The released iron, from the plasma, eventually replenishes the depleted iron stores in the bone marrow where it is incorporated into hemoglobin

Pharmacodynamics/Kinetics

Onset of action: I.V.: Serum ferritin peak: 7-9 days after dose

Absorption:

I.M.: 50% to 90% is promptly absorbed, balance is slowly absorbed over month

I.V.: Uptake of iron by the reticuloendothelial system appears to be constant at about 10-20 mg/hour

Excretion: Urine and feces via reticuloendothelial system

Dosage I.M. (INFeD; Z-track method should be used for I.M. injection), I.V. (Dexferrum, INFeD):

A 0.5 mL test dose (0.25 mL in infants) should be given prior to starting iron dextran therapy; total dose should be divided into a daily schedule for I.M., total dose may be given as a single continuous infusion. Individual doses of ≤2 mL may be administered daily until calculated total dose is received.

Iron-deficiency anemia:

Children 5-15 kg: Should not normally be given in the first 4 months of life:

Dose (mL) = 0.0442 (desired hemoglobin - observed hemoglobin) x W + (0.26 x W)

Desired hemoglobin: Usually 12 g/dL

W = Total body weight in kg

Children >15 kg and Adults:

Dose (mL) = 0.0442 (desired hemoglobin - observed hemoglobin) x LBW + (0.26 x LBW)

Desired hemoglobin: Usually 14.8 g/dL

LBW = Lean body weight in kg

Iron replacement therapy for blood loss: Replacement iron (mg) = blood loss (mL) x hematocrit

Maximum daily dosage: Manufacturer's labeling: **Note:** Replacement of larger estimated iron deficits may be achieved by serial administration of smaller incremental dosages. Daily dosages should be limited to:

Children:

<5 kg: 25 mg iron (0.5 mL)

5-10 kg: 50 mg iron (1 mL)

Children ≥10 kg and Adults: 100 mg iron (2 mL)

Cancer-/chemotherapy-associated anemia: Adults: I.V.: **Note:** Use the iron-deficiency anemia equation for determining a calculated dose, when applicable.

Weekly administration (unlabeled dosing; INFed):

Weeks 1-3: Test dose of 25 mg (over 1-2 minutes), followed by 75 mg (bolus) once weekly

Weeks 4 and after: 100 mg over 5 minutes once weekly until the calculated dose is reached (Auerbach, 2004)

or

Week 1: Test dose of 25 mg (slow I.V. push), followed 1 hour later by 75 mg over 5 minutes

Weeks 2-10: 100 mg over 5 minutes once weekly for a total cumulative dose of 1000 mg (NCCN anemia guidelines v.2.2014)

Total dose infusion (unlabeled dosing; INFeD):

Test dose of 25 mg (over 1-2 minutes), followed 1 hour later by the balance of the calculated total dose mixed in 500 mL NS and infused at 175 mL/hour (Auerbach, 2004)

or

Test dose of 25 mg (slow I.V. push) followed 1 hour later by the balance of the total dose as a single infusion over several hours; if calculated dose exceeds 1000 mg, administer remaining dose in excess of 1000 mg after 4 weeks if inadequate hemoglobin response (NCCN anemia guidelines v.2.2014)

Dosage adjustment in renal impairment: No dosage adjustment provided in manufacturer's labeling.

Dosage adjustment in hepatic impairment: No dosage adjustment provided in manufacturer's labeling.

Administration Note: A test dose should be given on the first day of therapy; patient should be observed for 1 hour for hypersensitivity reaction, then the remainder of the day's dose (dose minus test dose) should be given. Resuscitation equipment, medication, and trained personnel should be available. An uneventful test dose does not ensure an anaphylactic-type reaction will not occur during administration of the therapeutic dose.

I.M. (INFeD): Use Z-track technique (displacement of the skin laterally prior to injection); injection should be deep into the upper outer quadrant of buttock; alternate buttocks with subsequent injections. Administer test dose at same recommended site using the same technique.

I.V.: Test dose should be given gradually over at least 30 seconds (INFeD) or 5 minutes (Dexferrum), or over 1-2 minutes (INFeD) for cancer-/chemotherapy-associated anemia (Auerbach, 2004). Subsequent dose(s) may be administered by I.V. bolus undiluted at a rate not to exceed 50 mg/minute (maximum 100 mg). For total dose infusion in patients with cancer-/chemotherapy-associated anemia (unlabeled dose): 1 hour after the test dose, administer the balance of the dose diluted in 500 mL NS and infuse at 175 mL/hour (Auerbach, 2004) or administer over several hours (NCCN Anemia guidelines v.2.2104). Avoid dilutions with dextrose (increased incidence of local pain and phlebitis).

Monitoring Parameters Hemoglobin, hematocrit, reticulocyte count, serum ferritin, serum iron, TIBC; monitor for anaphylaxis/hypersensitivity reaction (during test dose and therapeutic dose)

Reference Range

Hemoglobin: Adults:

Males: 13.5-16.5 g/dL

Females: 12.0-15.0 g/dL

Serum iron: 40-160 mcg/dL

Total iron binding capacity: 230-430 mcg/dL

Transferrin: 204-360 mg/dL

Percent transferrin saturation: 20% to 50%

Test Interactions May cause falsely elevated values of serum bilirubin and falsely decreased values of serum calcium. Residual iron dextran may remain in reticuloendothelial cells; may affect accuracy of examination of bone marrow iron stores. Bone scans with 99m Tc-labeled bone seeking agents may show reduced bony uptake, marked renal activity, and excess blood pooling and soft tissue accumulation following I.V. iron dextran infusion or with high serum ferritin levels. Following I.M. iron dextran, bone scans with 99m Tc-diphosphonate may show dense activity in the buttocks.

Dosage Forms Considerations

Strength of iron dextran complex is expressed as elemental iron.

Dosage Forms Excipient information presented when available (limited, particularly for generics); consult specific product labeling.

Solution, Injection:

Dexferrum: 50 mg/mL (1 mL, 2 mL)

Infed: 50 mg/mL (2 mL)

◆ **Iron Dextri-Maltose** *see* Ferric Carboxymaltose *on page 852*

◆ **Iron Fumarate** *see* Ferrous Fumarate *on page 854*

◆ **Iron Gluconate** *see* Ferrous Gluconate *on page 854*

◆ **Iron-Polysaccharide Complex** *see* Polysaccharide-Iron Complex *on page 1673*

Iron Sucrose (EYE ern SOO krose)

Brand Names: U.S. Venofer

Brand Names: Canada Venofer

Pharmacologic Category Iron Salt

Use Iron deficiency anemia: Treatment of iron-deficiency anemia in chronic kidney disease (CKD)

Unlabeled Use Chemotherapy-associated anemia

Pregnancy Risk Factor B

Pregnancy Considerations Teratogenic effects were not observed in animal studies. There are no adequate and well-controlled studies in pregnant women. Based on limited data, iron sucrose may be effective for the treatment of iron-deficiency anemia in pregnancy. It is recommended that pregnant women meet the dietary requirements of iron with diet and/or supplements in order to prevent adverse events associated with iron deficiency anemia in pregnancy. Treatment of iron deficiency anemia in pregnant women is the same as in nonpregnant women and in most cases, oral iron preparations may be used. Except in severe cases of maternal anemia, the fetus achieves normal iron stores regardless of maternal concentrations.

Breast-Feeding Considerations Iron is normally found in breast milk. Breast milk or iron fortified formulas generally provide enough iron to meet the recommended dietary requirements of infants. The amount of iron in breast milk is generally not influenced by maternal iron status.

Contraindications Known hypersensitivity to iron sucrose or any component of the formulation

Warnings/Precautions Hypersensitivity reactions, including rare postmarketing anaphylactic and anaphylactoid reactions (some fatal), have been reported; monitor patients during and for ≥30 minutes postadministration; discontinue immediately for signs/symptoms of a hypersensitivity reaction (shock, hypotension, loss of consciousness). Equipment for resuscitation and trained personnel experienced in handling medical emergencies should always be immediately available. Significant hypotension has been reported frequently in hemodialysis-dependent patients. Hypotension has also been reported in peritoneal dialysis and nondialysis patients. Hypotension may be related to total dose or rate of administration (avoid rapid I.V. injection), follow recommended guidelines. Withhold iron in the presence of tissue iron overload; periodic monitoring of hemoglobin, hematocrit, serum ferritin, and transferrin saturation is recommended.

Adverse Reactions Events and incidences are associated with use in adults unless otherwise specified.

>10%:

Cardiovascular: Hypotension (2% to 3%; children 2%; 39% in hemodialysis patients; may be related to total dose or rate of administration)

Central nervous system: Headache (3% to 13%; children 6%)

Gastrointestinal: Nausea (5% to 15%; children 3%)

Neuromuscular & skeletal: Muscle cramps (1% to 3%; 29% in hemodialysis patients)

Respiratory: Nasopharyngitis (2% to 16%), pharyngitis (2% to 16%), sinusitis (2% to 16%), upper respiratory infection (2% to 16%; children 4%)

1% to 10%:

Cardiovascular: Hypertension (7% to 8%; children 2%), peripheral edema (3% to 7%), chest pain (1% to 6%), arteriovenous fistula thrombosis (children 2%), heart failure (>1%)

Central nervous system: Dizziness (1% to 7%; children 4%), fever (1% to 3%; children 4%)

Dermatologic: Pruritus (2% to 4%)

Endocrine & metabolic: Hypoglycemia (≤4%), fluid overload (1% to 3%), gout (≤3%), hyperglycemia (≤3%)

Gastrointestinal: Vomiting (5% to 9%; children 4%), diarrhea (5% to 8%), taste perversion (≤8%), peritonitis (children 4%), abdominal pain (1% to 4%)

Local: Injection site reaction (≤6%)

Neuromuscular & skeletal: Extremity pain (3% to 6%), arthralgia (1% to 4%), myalgia (≤4%), weakness (1% to 3%), back pain (1% to 2%)

Ocular: Conjunctivitis (≤3%)

Otic: Ear pain (≤2%)

Respiratory: Dyspnea (1% to 6%), cough (1% to 3%; children 4%), nasal congestion (≤1%)

Miscellaneous: Graft complication (≤10%), sepsis (>1%)

<1% (Limited to important or life-threatening): Anaphylactic shock, anaphylactoid reactions, angioedema, bradycardia, cardiovascular collapse, hypersensitivity (including wheezing), loss of consciousness, necrotizing enterocolitis (reported in premature infants, no causal relationship established), seizure, shock, urine discoloration

Drug Interactions

Metabolism/Transport Effects None known.

Avoid Concomitant Use

Avoid concomitant use of Iron Sucrose with any of the following: Dimercaprol

Increased Effect/Toxicity

The levels/effects of Iron Sucrose may be increased by: Dimercaprol

Decreased Effect There are no known significant interactions involving a decrease in effect.

Preparation for Administration

Children: May administer undiluted or diluted in 25 mL of NS. Do not dilute to concentrations <1 mg/mL.

Adults: Doses ≤200 mg may be administered undiluted or diluted in a maximum of 100 mL NS. Doses >200 mg should be diluted in a maximum of 250 mL NS. Do not dilute to concentrations <1 mg/mL.

Storage/Stability Store intact vials at controlled room temperature of 20°C to 25°C (68°F to 77°F); excursions permitted to 15°C to 30°C (59°F to 86°F); do not freeze. Iron sucrose is stable for 7 days at room temperature or under refrigeration when undiluted in a plastic syringe or following dilution in normal saline in a plastic syringe (2-10 mg/mL) or I.V. bag (1-2 mg/mL).

Mechanism of Action Iron sucrose is dissociated by the reticuloendothelial system into iron and sucrose. The released iron increases serum iron concentrations and is incorporated into hemoglobin.

Pharmacodynamics/Kinetics

Distribution: V_{dss}: Healthy adults: 7.9 L

Metabolism: Dissociated into iron and sucrose by the reticuloendothelial system

Half-life elimination: Healthy adults: 6 hours; Nondialysis-dependent adolescents: 8 hours

Excretion: Healthy adults: Urine (5%) within 24 hours

Dosage Doses expressed in mg of **elemental** iron. **Note:** Test dose: Product labeling does not indicate need for a test dose in product-naive patients.

Children ≥2 years and Adolescents: Iron-deficiency anemia in chronic kidney disease (CKD): I.V.: **Note:** Not indicated for iron replacement treatment in children and adolescents.

Hemodialysis-dependent patient: Maintenance therapy: 0.5 mg/kg/dose (maximum: 100 mg) every 2 weeks for 6 doses; may repeat if clinically indicated.

Nondialysis-dependent patient: Maintenance therapy: 0.5 mg/kg/dose (maximum: 100 mg) every 4 weeks for 3 doses; may repeat if clinically indicated

Peritoneal dialysis-dependent patient: Maintenance therapy: 0.5 mg/kg/dose (maximum: 100 mg) every 4 weeks for 3 doses; may repeat if clinically indicated

Adults:

Iron-deficiency anemia in CKD: I.V.:

Hemodialysis-dependent patient: 100 mg administered during consecutive dialysis sessions to a cumulative total dose of 1000 mg (10 doses); may repeat treatment if clinically indicated.

Peritoneal dialysis-dependent patient: Two infusions of 300 mg administered 14 days apart, followed by a single 400 mg infusion 14 days later (total cumulative dose of 1000 mg in 3 divided doses); may repeat treatment if clinically indicated.

Nondialysis-dependent patient: 200 mg administered on 5 different occasions within a 14-day period (total cumulative dose: 1000 mg in 14-day period); may repeat treatment if clinically indicated. **Note:** Dosage has also been administered as 2 infusions of 500 mg on day 1 and day 14 (limited experience).

Chemotherapy-associated anemia (unlabeled use): I.V.: 200 mg once every 3 weeks for 5 doses (Bastit, 2008) **or** 100 mg once weekly during weeks 0 to 6, followed by 100 mg every other week from weeks 8 to 14 (Hedenus, 2007)

Elderly: Refer to adult dosing.

Dosage adjustment in renal impairment: No dosage adjustment provided in manufacturer's labeling.

Dosage adjustment in hepatic impairment: No dosage adjustment provided in manufacturer's labeling.

Administration Administer intravenously as a slow I.V. injection (**not** for rapid I.V. injection) or as an I.V. infusion. Can be administered through dialysis line.

Children and Adolescents:

Slow I.V. injection: Administer undiluted over 5 minutes

Infusion: Infuse diluted solution over 5-60 minutes

Adults:

Slow I.V. injection: May administer doses ≤200 mg undiluted by slow I.V. injection over 2-5 minutes. When administering to hemodialysis-dependent patients, give iron sucrose early during the dialysis session.

Infusion: Infuse diluted doses ≤200 mg over at least 15 minutes; infuse diluted 300 mg dose over 1.5 hours; infuse diluted 400 mg dose over 2.5 hours; infuse diluted 500 mg dose over 3.5-4 hours (limited experience). When administering to hemodialysis-dependent patients, give iron sucrose early during the dialysis session.

Monitoring Parameters

CKD patients: Hematocrit, hemoglobin, serum ferritin, serum iron, transferrin, percent transferrin saturation, TIBC (takes ~4 weeks of treatment to see increased serum iron and ferritin, and decreased TIBC); iron status should be assessed ≥48 hours after last dose (due to rapid increase in values following administration); signs/ symptoms of hypersensitivity reactions (during and ≥30 minutes following infusion); hypotension (following infusion)

Chemotherapy-associated anemia (unlabeled use): Iron, total iron-binding capacity, transferrin saturation, or ferritin levels at baseline and periodically (Rizzo, 2011)

Reference Range

Hemoglobin: Adults:

Males: 13.5-16.5 g/dL

Females: 12.0-15.0 g/dL

Serum iron: 40-160 mcg/dL

Total iron binding capacity: 230-430 mcg/dL

Transferrin: 204-360 mg/dL

Percent transferrin saturation: 20% to 50%

Dosage Forms Considerations

Strength of iron sucrose is expressed as elemental iron.

Dosage Forms Excipient information presented when available (limited, particularly for generics); consult specific product labeling.

Solution, Intravenous [preservative free]:

Venofer: 20 mg/mL (2.5 mL, 5 mL, 10 mL)

- ◆ **Iron Sulfate** *see* Ferrous Sulfate *on page 854*
- ◆ **Iron Supplement Childrens [OTC]** *see* Ferrous Sulfate *on page 854*
- ◆ **ISD** *see* Isosorbide Dinitrate *on page 1126*
- ◆ **ISDN** *see* Isosorbide Dinitrate *on page 1126*
- ◆ **Isentress** *see* Raltegravir *on page 1776*
- ◆ **ISG** *see* Immune Globulin *on page 1059*
- ◆ **ISIS 301012** *see* Mipomersen *on page 1376*
- ◆ **ISMN** *see* Isosorbide Mononitrate *on page 1128*
- ◆ **Isoamyl Nitrite** *see* Amyl Nitrite *on page 135*
- ◆ **Isobamate** *see* Carisoprodol *on page 351*
- ◆ **IsoDitrate ER** *see* Isosorbide Dinitrate *on page 1126*

Isoniazid (eye soe NYE a zid)

Brand Names: Canada Isotamine®; PMS-Isoniazid

Index Terms INH; Isonicotinic Acid Hydrazide

Pharmacologic Category Antitubercular Agent

Additional Appendix Information

Tyramine Content of Foods *on page 2394*

Use Treatment of susceptible tuberculosis infections; treatment of latent tuberculosis infection (LTBI)

Pregnancy Risk Factor C

Pregnancy Considerations Isoniazid was found to be embryocidal in animal studies; teratogenic effects were not noted. Isoniazid crosses the human placenta. Due to the risk of tuberculosis to the fetus, treatment is recommended when the probability of maternal disease is moderate to high. The CDC recommends isoniazid as part of the initial treatment regimen (CDC, 2003). Pyridoxine supplementation is recommended (25 mg/day).

Breast-Feeding Considerations Small amounts of isoniazid are excreted in breast milk. However, women with tuberculosis should not be discouraged from breast-feeding. Pyridoxine supplementation is recommended for the mother and infant.

Contraindications Hypersensitivity to isoniazid or any component of the formulation; acute liver disease; previous history of hepatic damage during isoniazid therapy; previous severe adverse reaction (drug fever, chills, arthritis) to isoniazid

Warnings/Precautions Use with caution in patients with severe renal impairment and liver disease. **[U.S. Boxed Warning]: Severe and sometimes fatal hepatitis may occur; usually occurs within the first 3 months of treatment, although may develop even after many months of treatment.** The risk of developing hepatitis is age-related, although isoniazid-induced hepatotoxicity has been reported in children; daily ethanol consumption may also increase the risk. Patients must report any prodromal symptoms of hepatitis, such as fatigue, weakness, malaise, anorexia, nausea, abdominal pain, jaundice, or vomiting. Patients should be instructed to immediately discontinue therapy if any of these symptoms occur, even if a clinical evaluation has yet to be conducted. Treatment with isoniazid for latent tuberculosis infection should be deferred in patients with acute hepatic diseases. Periodic ophthalmic examinations are recommended even when usual symptoms do not occur. Pyridoxine (10-50 mg/day) is recommended in individuals at risk for development of peripheral neuropathies (eg, HIV infection, nutritional deficiency, diabetes, pregnancy). Children with low milk and low meat intake should receive concomitant pyridoxine therapy. Multidrug regimens should be utilized for the treatment of active tuberculosis to prevent the emergence of drug resistance.

Adverse Reactions Frequency not defined.

Cardiovascular: Hypertension, palpitation, tachycardia, vasculitis

Central nervous system: Depression, dizziness, encephalopathy, fever, lethargy, memory impairment, psychosis, seizure, slurred speech, toxic encephalopathy

Dermatologic: Flushing, rash (morbilliform, maculopapular, pruritic, or exfoliative)

Endocrine & metabolic: Gynecomastia, hyperglycemia, metabolic acidosis, pellagra, pyridoxine deficiency

Gastrointestinal: Anorexia, epigastric distress, nausea, stomach pain, vomiting

Hematologic: Agranulocytosis, anemia (sideroblastic, hemolytic, or aplastic), eosinophilia, thrombocytopenia

Hepatic: LFTs mildly increased (10% to 20%), hyperbilirubinemia, bilirubinuria, jaundice, hepatic dysfunction, hepatitis (may involve progressive liver damage; risk increases with age; 2.3% in patients >50 years)

Neuromuscular & skeletal: Arthralgia, hyper-reflexia, paresthesia, peripheral neuropathy (dose-related incidence, 10% to 20% incidence with 10 mg/kg/day), weakness

Ocular: Blurred vision, loss of vision, optic neuritis and atrophy

Miscellaneous: Lupus-like syndrome, lymphadenopathy, rheumatic syndrome

Drug Interactions

Metabolism/Transport Effects Substrate of CYP2E1 (major); **Note:** Assignment of Major/Minor substrate status based on clinically relevant drug interaction potential; **Inhibits** CYP1A2 (weak), CYP2A6 (moderate), CYP2C19 (moderate), CYP2C9 (weak), CYP2D6 (moderate), CYP2E1 (moderate), CYP3A4 (weak); **Induces** CYP2E1 (weak/moderate)

Avoid Concomitant Use

Avoid concomitant use of Isoniazid with any of the following: Pimozide; Tegafur; Thioridazine

Increased Effect/Toxicity

Isoniazid may increase the levels/effects of: Acetaminophen; ARIPiprazole; Benzodiazepines (metabolized by oxidation); CarBAMazepine; Chlorzoxazone; Citalopram; CycloSERINE; CYP2A6 Substrates; CYP2C19 Substrates; CYP2D6 Substrates; CYP2E1 Substrates; Dofetilide; Fesoterodine; Fosphenytoin; Lomitapide; Metoprolol; Nebivolol; Phenytoin; Pimozide; Theophylline Derivatives; Thioridazine

The levels/effects of Isoniazid may be increased by: Disulfiram; Ethionamide; Propafenone; Rifamycin Derivatives

Decreased Effect

Isoniazid may decrease the levels/effects of: Clopidogrel; Codeine; Itraconazole; Ketoconazole (Systemic); Tamoxifen; Tegafur; TraMADol

The levels/effects of Isoniazid may be decreased by: Antacids; Corticosteroids (Systemic); Cyproterone

Ethanol/Nutrition/Herb Interactions

Ethanol: Ethanol increases the risk of hepatitis. Management: Avoid ethanol.

Food: Bioavailability is decreased if taken with food. Isoniazid may also decrease folic acid absorption and alters pyridoxine metabolism. Management: Take on an empty stomach 1 hour before or 2 hours after a meal, increase dietary intake of folate, niacin, and magnesium.

Tyramine-containing food: Isoniazid has weak monoamine oxidase inhibiting activity and may potentially inhibit tyramine metabolism. Several case reports of mild reactions (flushing, palpitations, headache, mild increase in blood pressure, diaphoresis) after ingestion of certain types of cheese or red wine, have been reported (Self, 1999; Toutoungi, 1985). Management: Manufacturer's labeling recommends avoiding tyramine-containing foods (eg, aged or matured cheese, air-dried or cured meats including sausages and salamis; fava or broad bean pods, tap/draft beers, Marmite concentrate, sauerkraut, soy sauce, and other soybean condiments). However, the clinical relevance of the tyramine reaction for the vast majority of patients receiving isoniazid has been questioned due to isoniazid's weak MAO inhibition and the relatively few published case reports of the interaction. Although not fully investigated, it has been proposed that the reaction has a genetic component and may only be significant in poor or intermediate acetylators since isoniazid is primarily inactivated by acetylation (DiMartini, 1995; Toutoungi, 1985).

Histamine-containing food: Isoniazid may also inhibit diamine oxidase resulting in headache, sweating, palpitations, flushing, hypotension to histamine-containing foods (eg, skipjack, tuna, other tropical fish). Management: Manufacturer's labeling recommends avoiding histamine-containing foods.

Storage/Stability

Tablet: Store at 20°C to 25°C (68°F to 77°F). Protect from light.

Oral solution: Store at 15°C to 30°C (59°F to 86°F). Protect from light.

Mechanism of Action Unknown, but may include the inhibition of mycolic acid synthesis resulting in disruption of the bacterial cell wall

Pharmacodynamics/Kinetics

Absorption: Rapid and complete; rate can be slowed with food

Distribution: All body tissues and fluids including CSF; crosses placenta; enters breast milk

Protein binding: 10% to 15%

Metabolism: Hepatic with decay rate determined genetically by acetylation phenotype

Half-life elimination: Fast acetylators: 30-100 minutes; Slow acetylators: 2-5 hours; may be prolonged with hepatic or severe renal impairment

Time to peak, serum: 1-2 hours

Excretion: Urine (75% to 95%); feces; saliva

Dosage

Usual dosage ranges: Oral, I.M.:

Infants and Children: 10-15 mg/kg/day once daily (maximum: 300 mg/day) or 20-40 mg/kg given 2-3 times per week (maximum: 900 mg/dose)

Adults: 5 mg/kg/day (usual: 300 mg/day) as a single daily dose or 15 mg/kg (maximum: 900 mg/dose) given 2-3 times per week

Indication-specific dosing: Oral, I.M.: Recommendations often change due to resistant strains and newly-developed information; consult *MMWR* for current CDC recommendations. Intramuscular injection is available for patients who are unable to either take or absorb oral therapy.

Infants and Children:

Tuberculosis, active:

Daily therapy: CDC recommendations: 10-15 mg/kg/day once daily (maximum: 300 mg/day) (*MMWR*, 2003)

Directly observed therapy (DOT): CDC recommendations: 20-30 mg/kg (maximum: 900 mg/dose) twice weekly (*MMWR*, 2003); Manufacturer's labeling: 20-40 mg/kg (maximum: 900 mg/dose) twice weekly or 3 times/week

Tuberculosis, latent infection (LTBI):

Daily therapy: CDC recommendations: 10-20 mg/kg/day once daily (maximum: 300 mg/dose) (*MMWR*, 2000); Manufacturer's labeling: 10 mg/kg/day once daily (maximum: 300 mg/dose)

Directly observed therapy (DOT): CDC recommendations: 20-40 mg/kg (maximum: 900 mg/dose) twice weekly for 9 months (*MMWR*, 2000); Manufacturer's labeling: 20-30 mg/kg twice weekly (maximum: 900 mg/dose)

Adults: **Note:** Concomitant administration of 10-50 mg/day pyridoxine is recommended in malnourished patients or those prone to neuropathy (eg, alcoholics, patients with diabetes).

Nontuberculous mycobacterium *(M. kansasii)* (unlabeled use): 5 mg/kg/day (maximum: 300 mg/day) for duration to include 12 months of culture-negative sputum; typically used in combination with ethambutol and rifampin

Tuberculosis, active:

Daily therapy: CDC recommendations: 5 mg/kg/day once daily (usual dose: 300 mg/day) (*MMWR*, 2003)

Directly observed therapy (DOT): CDC recommendations: 15 mg/kg (maximum: 900 mg/dose) twice weekly or 3 times/week; **Note:** CDC guidelines state that once-weekly therapy (15 mg/kg/dose) may be considered, but only after the first 2 months of initial therapy in HIV-negative patients, and only in combination with rifapentine (*MMWR*, 2003).

Note: Treatment may be defined by the number of doses administered (eg, "six-month" therapy involves 182 doses of INH and rifampin, and 56 doses of pyrazinamide). Six months is the shortest interval of time over which these doses may be administered, assuming no interruption of therapy.

Tuberculosis, latent infection (LTBI): CDC recommendations: 5 mg/kg (maximum: 300 mg/dose) once daily or 15 mg/kg (maximum: 900 mg/dose) twice weekly by directly observed therapy (DOT) 6-9 months in patients who do not have HIV infection (9 months is optimal, 6 months may be considered to reduce costs of therapy) and 9 months in patients who have HIV infection. Extend to 12 months of therapy if interruptions in treatment occur (*MMWR*, 2000).

Dosing adjustment in renal impairment: No adjustment necessary

Hemodialysis: Dialyzable (50% to 100%); administer dose post dialysis

Dosing adjustment in hepatic impairment: No adjustment required, however, use with caution; may accumulate and additional liver damage may occur in patients with pre-existing liver disease. For ALT or AST >3 times the ULN: discontinue or temporarily withhold treatment.

Treatment with isoniazid for latent tuberculosis infection should be deferred in patients with acute hepatic diseases.

Dietary Considerations Should be taken 1 hour before or 2 hours after meals on an empty stomach; increase dietary intake of folate, niacin, magnesium.

Administration Should be administered 1 hour before or 2 hours after meals on an empty stomach.

Monitoring Parameters Baseline and periodic (more frequently in patients with higher risk for hepatitis) liver function tests (ALT and AST); sputum cultures monthly (until 2 consecutive negative cultures reported); monitoring for prodromal signs of hepatitis

LTBI therapy: American Thoracic Society/Centers for Disease Control (ATS/CDC) recommendations: Monthly clinical evaluation, including brief physical exam for adverse events. Baseline serum AST or ALT and bilirubin should be considered for patients at higher risk for adverse events (eg, history of liver disease, chronic ethanol use, HIV-infected patients, women who are pregnant or postpartum ≤3 months, older adults with concomitant medications or diseases). Routine, periodic monitoring is recommended for any patient with an abnormal baseline or at increased risk for hepatotoxicity.

Test Interactions False-positive urinary glucose with Clinitest®

Additional Information The AAP recommends that pyridoxine supplementation (1-2 mg/kg/day) should be administered to malnourished patients, children or adolescents on meat or milk-deficient diets, breast-feeding infants, and those predisposed to neuritis to prevent peripheral neuropathy; administration of isoniazid syrup has been associated with diarrhea

Dosage Forms Excipient information presented when available (limited, particularly for generics); consult specific product labeling.

Solution, Injection:
  Generic: 100 mg/mL (10 mL)
Syrup, Oral:
  Generic: 50 mg/5 mL (473 mL)
Tablet, Oral:
  Generic: 100 mg, 300 mg

Extemporaneous Preparations **Note:** Commercial oral solution is available (50 mg/mL)

A 10 mg/mL oral suspension may be made with tablets, purified water, and sorbitol. Crush ten 100 mg tablets in a mortar and reduce to a fine powder. Add 10 mL of purified water and mix to a uniform paste. Mix while adding sorbitol in incremental proportions to **almost** 100 mL; transfer to a graduated cylinder, rinse mortar with sorbitol, and add quantity of sorbitol sufficient to make 100 mL (do not use sugar-based solutions). Label "shake well" and "refrigerate". Stable for 21 days refrigerated.

Nahata MC, Pai VB, and Hipple TF, *Pediatric Drug Formulations*, 5th ed, Cincinnati, OH: Harvey Whitney Books Co, 2004.

◆ **Isonicotinic Acid Hydrazide** *see* Isoniazid *on page 1123*

◆ **Isonipecaine Hydrochloride** *see* Meperidine *on page 1297*

◆ **Isophane Insulin** *see* Insulin NPH *on page 1092*

◆ **Isophane Insulin and Regular Insulin** *see* Insulin NPH and Insulin Regular *on page 1093*

◆ **Isophosphamide** *see* Ifosfamide *on page 1041*

Isoproterenol (eye soe proe TER e nole)

Brand Names: U.S. Isuprel

Index Terms Isoproterenol Hydrochloride

Pharmacologic Category Beta$_1$- & Beta$_2$-Adrenergic Agonist Agent

Use Manufacturer's labeled indications (see **"Note"**): Mild or transient episodes of heart block that do not require electric shock or pacemaker therapy; serious episodes of heart block and Adams-Stokes attacks (except when caused by ventricular tachycardia or fibrillation); cardiac arrest until electric shock or pacemaker therapy is available; bronchospasm during anesthesia; adjunct to fluid and electrolyte replacement therapy and other drugs and procedures in the treatment of hypovolemic or septic shock and low cardiac output states (eg, decompensated heart failure, cardiogenic shock)

Note: The use of isoproterenol in advanced cardiac life support (ACLS) has largely been supplanted by the use of other adrenergic agents (eg, epinephrine and dopamine). The use of isoproterenol for bronchospasm during anesthesia and cardiogenic, hypovolemic, or septic shock is no longer recommended. See *Unlabeled Use* for more appropriate, yet unlabeled, uses.

Unlabeled Use Pharmacologic overdrive pacing for refractory torsade de pointes; pharmacologic provocation during tilt table testing for syncope; temporary control of bradycardia in denervated heart transplant patients unresponsive to atropine; ventricular arrhythmias due to AV nodal block; beta-blocker overdose; electrical storm associated with Brugada syndrome

Pregnancy Risk Factor C

Pregnancy Considerations Animal reproduction studies have not been conducted by the manufacturer. Use of isoproterenol may interfere with uterine contractions at term (Mahon, 1967).

Breast-Feeding Considerations It is not known if isoproterenol is excreted in breast milk. The manufacturer recommends that caution be exercised when administering isoproterenol to nursing women.

Contraindications Angina, pre-existing ventricular arrhythmias, tachyarrhythmias; cardiac glycoside intoxication

Warnings/Precautions Use with extreme caution; not currently a treatment of choice; use with caution in elderly patients, patients with diabetes, cardiovascular disease, or hyperthyroidism; excessive or prolonged use may result in decreased effectiveness. Contains sulfites; may cause allergic reaction in susceptible individuals.

Adverse Reactions Frequency not defined.

Cardiovascular: Angina, flushing, hyper-/hypotension, pallor, palpitation, paradoxical bradycardia (with tilt table testing), premature ventricular beats, Stokes-Adams attacks, tachyarrhythmia, ventricular arrhythmia
Central nervous system: Dizziness, headache, nervousness, restlessness, Stokes-Adams seizure
Endocrine & metabolic: Hypokalemia, serum glucose increased
Gastrointestinal: Nausea, vomiting
Neuromuscular & skeletal: Tremor, weakness
Ocular: Blurred vision
Respiratory: Dyspnea, pulmonary edema
Miscellaneous: Diaphoresis

Drug Interactions

Metabolism/Transport Effects Substrate of COMT

Avoid Concomitant Use

Avoid concomitant use of Isoproterenol with any of the following: Inhalational Anesthetics

Increased Effect/Toxicity

The levels/effects of Isoproterenol may be increased by: COMT Inhibitors; Inhalational Anesthetics

Decreased Effect

Isoproterenol may decrease the levels/effects of: Theophylline Derivatives

Ethanol/Nutrition/Herb Interactions Herb/Nutraceutical: Avoid ephedra, yohimbe (may cause CNS stimulation).

Storage/Stability Store undiluted solution at 20°C to 25°C (68°F to 77°F). Solution should not be used if a color or precipitate is present. Exposure to air, light, or increased temperature may cause a pink to brownish pink color to develop. Stability of parenteral admixture at room temperature (25°C) or at refrigeration (4°C) is 24 hours.

Mechanism of Action Stimulates $beta_1$- and $beta_2$-receptors resulting in relaxation of bronchial, GI, and uterine smooth muscle, increased heart rate and contractility, vasodilation of peripheral vasculature

Pharmacodynamics/Kinetics

Onset of action: I.V.: Immediate

Duration: I.V.: 10-15 minutes

Metabolism: Via conjugation in many tissues including hepatic and pulmonary

Half-life elimination: 2.5-5 minutes

Excretion: Urine (primarily as sulfate conjugates)

Dosage I.V.: **Note:** Patients may exhibit dose-dependent vasodilation due to unopposed $beta_2$-agonism elicited by isoproterenol.

Bradyarrhythmias, AV nodal block, or refractory torsade de pointes:

Children: Continuous infusion: Usual range: 0.05-2 mcg/**kg**/minute; titrate to patient response

Adults: Continuous infusion: Usual range: 2-10 mcg/minute; titrate to patient response

Brugada syndrome with electrical storm (unlabeled use): Adults: I.V. bolus: Initial: 1-2 mcg, followed by a continuous infusion of 0.15-0.3 mcg/minute for 1 day; may repeat sequence if ventricular tachycardia/fibrillation recurs (Watanabe, 2006; Zipes, 2006).

Tilt table testing for syncope (Benditt, 1996; Brignole, 2004): Adults: Continuous infusion: Initial: 1 mcg/minute; increase as necessary based on response; maximum dose: 5 mcg/minute. **Note:** Timing of initiation and dose adjustment during test may be institution-specific.

Dosage adjustment in renal impairment: No dosage adjustment provided in manufacturer's labeling.

Dosage adjustment in hepatic impairment: No dosage adjustment provided in manufacturer's labeling.

Usual Infusion Concentrations: Pediatric I.V. infusion: 20 **mcg**/mL

Usual Infusion Concentrations: Adult I.V. infusion: 1 mg in 100 mL (10 **mcg**/mL), 1 mg in 500 mL (2 **mcg**/mL), **or** 4 mg in 250 mL (16 **mcg**/mL) of D_5W or NS

Administration I.V. infusion administration requires the use of an infusion pump.

Monitoring Parameters ECG, heart rate, respiratory rate, arterial blood gas, arterial blood pressure, CVP; serum glucose, serum potassium, serum magnesium

Dosage Forms Excipient information presented when available (limited, particularly for generics); consult specific product labeling. [DSC] = Discontinued product

Solution, Injection, as hydrochloride:

Isuprel: 0.2 mg/mL (1 mL, 5 mL) [contains disodium edta]

Isuprel: 0.2 mg/mL (1 mL [DSC], 5 mL [DSC]) [contains sodium metabisulfite]

- ◆ **Isoproterenol Hydrochloride** *see* Isoproterenol *on page 1125*
- ◆ **Isoptin SR** *see* Verapamil *on page 2182*
- ◆ **Isoptin® SR (Can)** *see* Verapamil *on page 2182*
- ◆ **Isopto Atropine** *see* Atropine *on page 197*
- ◆ **Isopto® Atropine (Can)** *see* Atropine *on page 197*
- ◆ **Isopto Carbachol** *see* Carbachol *on page 335*
- ◆ **Isopto® Carbachol (Can)** *see* Carbachol *on page 335*
- ◆ **Isopto Carpine** *see* Pilocarpine (Ophthalmic) *on page 1647*
- ◆ **Isopto® Carpine (Can)** *see* Pilocarpine (Ophthalmic) *on page 1647*
- ◆ **Isopto Homatropine** *see* Homatropine *on page 998*
- ◆ **Isordil Titradose** *see* Isosorbide Dinitrate *on page 1126*
- ◆ **Isosorbide (Can)** *see* Isosorbide Dinitrate *on page 1126*

Isosorbide Dinitrate (eye soe SOR bide dye NYE trate)

Brand Names: U.S. Dilatrate-SR; IsoDitrate ER; Isordil Titradose

Brand Names: Canada ISDN; Isosorbide; Novo-Sorbide; PMS-Isosorbide

Index Terms ISD; ISDN

Pharmacologic Category Antianginal Agent; Vasodilator

Additional Appendix Information

Nitrates *on page 2305*

Use Prevention and treatment of angina pectoris

Note: Due to slower onset of action, not the drug of choice to abort an acute anginal episode.

Unlabeled Use Patients with heart failure (HF) who do not tolerate an ACE inhibitor or an angiotensin receptor blocker (ARB); African-American (self-identified) patients with HF remaining symptomatic despite optimal standard therapy; esophageal spastic disorders

Pregnancy Risk Factor C

Pregnancy Considerations Adverse events were observed in some animal reproduction studies. Nitric oxide donors, such as isosorbide, have been evaluated for pre-eclampsia and cervical ripening; isosorbide dinitrate use in these conditions is not currently recommended (Kalidindi, 2012; Ramirez, 2011).

Breast-Feeding Considerations It is not known if isosorbide dinitrate is excreted in breast milk. The manufacturer recommends that caution be exercised when administering isosorbide dinitrate to nursing women.

Contraindications Hypersensitivity to isosorbide dinitrate or any component of the formulation; hypersensitivity to organic nitrates; concurrent use with phosphodiesterase-5 (PDE-5) inhibitors (sildenafil, tadalafil, or vardenafil)

Warnings/Precautions Severe hypotension can occur; paradoxical bradycardia and increased angina pectoris can accompany hypotension. Postural hypotension can also occur; ethanol may potentiate this effect. Use with caution in volume depletion and moderate hypotension, and use with extreme caution with inferior wall MI and suspected right ventricular infarctions. Avoid use in patients with hypertrophic cardiomyopathy (HCM) with outflow tract obstruction; nitrates may reduce preload, exacerbating obstruction and cause hypotension or syncope and/or worsening of heart failure (Gersh, 2011).

Use of isosorbide dinitrate sublingual tablets to treat acute angina attacks is recommended only in patients unresponsive to sublingual nitroglycerin; however, current clinical practice guidelines do not recommend use during an acute anginal episode. Avoid use of extended release formulations in acute MI or acute HF; cannot easily reverse effects if adverse events develop. Nitrates may precipitate or aggravate increased intracranial pressure and subsequently may worsen clinical outcomes in patients with neurologic injury (eg, intracranial hemorrhage, traumatic brain injury). Appropriate dosing intervals are needed to minimize tolerance development. Tolerance can only be overcome by short periods of nitrate absence from the body. Dose escalation does not overcome this effect. When used for HF in combination with hydralazine, tolerance is less of a concern (Gogia, 1995).

Avoid concurrent use with PDE-5 inhibitors (eg, sildenafil, tadalafil, vardenafil). When nitrate administration becomes medically necessary, may administer nitrates only if 24 hours have elapsed after use of sildenafil or vardenafil (48 hours after tadalafil use) (Trujillo, 2007).

Adverse Reactions Frequency not defined.

Cardiovascular: Crescendo angina (uncommon), hypotension, orthostatic hypotension, rebound hypertension (uncommon), syncope (uncommon)

Central nervous system: Headache (most common), lightheadedness (related to blood pressure changes)

Hematologic: Methemoglobinemia (rare, overdose)

Drug Interactions

Metabolism/Transport Effects Substrate of CYP3A4 (major); **Note:** Assignment of Major/Minor substrate status based on clinically relevant drug interaction potential

Avoid Concomitant Use

Avoid concomitant use of Isosorbide Dinitrate with any of the following: Conivaptan; Fusidic Acid (Systemic); Phosphodiesterase 5 Inhibitors; Riociguat

Increased Effect/Toxicity

Isosorbide Dinitrate may increase the levels/effects of: Hypotensive Agents; Prilocaine; Riociguat; Rosiglitazone; Sodium Nitrite

The levels/effects of Isosorbide Dinitrate may be increased by: Conivaptan; CYP3A4 Inhibitors (Moderate); CYP3A4 Inhibitors (Strong); Dasatinib; Fusidic Acid (Systemic); Ivacaftor; Luliconazole; Mifepristone; Nitric Oxide; Phosphodiesterase 5 Inhibitors; Simeprevir

Decreased Effect

The levels/effects of Isosorbide Dinitrate may be decreased by: Bosentan; CYP3A4 Inducers (Strong); Dabrafenib; Deferasirox; Herbs (CYP3A4 Inducers); Mitotane; Tocilizumab

Ethanol/Nutrition/Herb Interactions

Ethanol: Caution with ethanol (may increase risk of hypotension).

Herb/Nutraceutical: Avoid black cohosh, California poppy, coleus, golden seal, hawthorn, mistletoe, periwinkle, quinine, shepherd's purse (may cause hypotension).

Mechanism of Action Stimulation of intracellular cyclic-GMP results in vascular smooth muscle relaxation of both arterial and venous vasculature with more prominent effects on the veins. Primarily reduces cardiac oxygen demand by decreasing preload (left ventricular end-diastolic pressure); may modestly reduce afterload. Additionally, coronary artery dilation improves collateral flow to ischemic regions.

Pharmacodynamics/Kinetics

Onset of action: Sublingual tablet: ~3 minutes; Oral tablet and capsule (includes extended-release formulations): ~1 hour

Duration: Sublingual tablet: 1-2 hours; Oral tablet and capsule (includes extended-release formulations): Up to 8 hours

Distribution: V_d: 2-4 L/kg

Metabolism: Extensively hepatic to conjugated metabolites, including isosorbide 5-mononitrate (active) and 2-mononitrate (active)

Bioavailability: Sublingual tablet: 40% to 50%; Oral immediate release formulations: Highly variable (10% to 90%); increases with chronic therapy

Half-life elimination: Parent drug: ~1 hour; Metabolites (5-mononitrate: 5 hours; 2-mononitrate: 2 hours)

Excretion: Urine and feces

Dosage Note: Due to slower onset of action, not the drug of choice to abort an acute anginal episode. Tolerance to nitrate effects develops with chronic exposure: Dose escalation does not overcome this effect. Tolerance can only be overcome by short periods of nitrate absence from the body. Nitrate-free intervals of ≥14 hours (immediate release products) or >18 hours (sustained release products) may help minimize tolerance.

Adults (elderly should be given lowest recommended daily doses initially and titrate upward):

Angina:

Oral:

Immediate release: Initial: 5-20 mg 2-3 times/day; Maintenance: 10-40 mg 2-3 times/day **or** 5-80 mg 2-3 times/day (Anderson, 2011)

Sustained release: 40-160 mg/day has been used in clinical trials (a nitrate free interval of at least 18 hours is recommended; however, a clinically efficacious dosage interval has not been clearly established) **or** 40 mg 1-2 times/day (Anderson, 2011)

Sublingual:

Prophylactic use: 2.5-5 mg administered 15 minutes prior to activities which may provoke an anginal episode

Treatment of acute anginal episode (use only if patient has failed sublingual nitroglycerin): 2.5-5 mg every 5-10 minutes for maximum of 3 doses in 15-30 minutes

Heart failure (unlabeled use; Cohn, 1991; HFSA, 2010; Hunt, 2009): Oral:

Immediate release (**Note:** Use in combination with hydralazine):

Initial dose: 20 mg 3-4 times per day

Target dose: 160 mg/day in 4 divided doses

Esophageal spastic disorders (unlabeled use; Goyal, 1998): Oral (immediate release), sublingual: 10-30 mg before meals

Dosage adjustment in renal impairment: No dosage adjustment provided in manufacturer's labeling.

Hemodialysis: Supplemental dose is not necessary

Peritoneal dialysis: Supplemental dose is not necessary

Dosage adjustment in hepatic impairment: No dosage adjustment provided in manufacturer's labeling.

Administration May consider administration of first dose in physician office; observe for maximal cardiovascular dynamic effects and adverse effects (orthostatic hypotension, headache). Do not administer around the clock; allow nitrate-free interval ≥14 hours (immediate release products) and >18 hours (sustained release products). Do not crush sublingual tablets or extended release formulations.

Immediate release products: When prescribed twice daily, consider administering at 8 AM and 1 PM. For 3 times/day dosing, consider 8 AM, 1 PM, and 6 PM.

Sustained release products: Consider once daily in morning or twice-daily dosing at 8 AM and between 1-2 PM.

Monitoring Parameters Blood pressure, heart rate

Dosage Forms Excipient information presented when available (limited, particularly for generics); consult specific product labeling. [DSC] = Discontinued product

Capsule Extended Release, Oral:

Dilatrate-SR: 40 mg [contains fd&c yellow #10 (quinoline yellow)]

Tablet, Oral:

Isordil Titradose: 5 mg [scored; contains fd&c red #40]

Isordil Titradose: 40 mg [scored; contains brilliant blue fcf (fd&c blue #1), fd&c yellow #10 (quinoline yellow), fd&c yellow #6 (sunset yellow)]

Generic: 5 mg, 10 mg, 20 mg, 30 mg

Tablet Extended Release, Oral:

IsoDitrate ER: 40 mg

Generic: 40 mg

Tablet Sublingual, Sublingual:

Generic: 2.5 mg [DSC]

Isosorbide Dinitrate and Hydralazine

(eye soe SOR bide dye NYE trate & hye DRAL a zeen)

Brand Names: U.S. BiDil®

Index Terms Hydralazine and Isosorbide Dinitrate

Pharmacologic Category Antihypertensive; Vasodilator

Use Treatment of heart failure, adjunct to standard therapy, in self-identified African-Americans

Pregnancy Risk Factor C

Dosage Oral: Adults: Initial: 1 tablet 3 times/day; may titrate to a maximum dose of 2 tablets 3 times/day

Dosage adjustment for toxicity: If patient experiences intolerable side effects, dose may be reduced to as little as one-half tablet 3 times/day; dose should be titrated upward as soon as tolerated.

Dosage adjustment in renal impairment: No dosage adjustment provided in manufacturer's labeling (has not been studied).

Dosage adjustment in hepatic impairment: No dosage adjustment provided in manufacturer's labeling (has not been studied).

Additional Information Complete prescribing information should be consulted for additional detail.

Dosage Forms

Tablet, oral:

BiDil®: Isosorbide dinitrate 20 mg and hydralazine hydrochloride 37.5 mg

Isosorbide Mononitrate

(eye soe SOR bide mon oh NYE trate)

Brand Names: U.S. Imdur

Brand Names: Canada Apo-ISMN®; Imdur®; PMS-ISMN; PRO-ISMN

Index Terms ISMN

Pharmacologic Category Antianginal Agent; Vasodilator

Additional Appendix Information

Nitrates *on page 2305*

Use Prevention of angina pectoris

Pregnancy Risk Factor B/C (manufacturer dependent)

Pregnancy Considerations Adverse events were observed in some animal reproduction studies. Nitric oxide donors, such as isosorbide, have been evaluated for pre-eclampsia and cervical ripening; isosorbide mononitrate use in these conditions is not currently recommended (Kalidindi, 2012; Ramirez, 2011).

Breast-Feeding Considerations It is not known if isosorbide mononitrate is excreted in breast milk. The manufacturer recommends that caution be exercised when administering isosorbide mononitrate to nursing women.

Contraindications Hypersensitivity to isosorbide mononitrate or any component of the formulation; hypersensitivity to organic nitrates; concurrent use with phosphodiesterase-5 (PDE-5) inhibitors (sildenafil, tadalafil, or vardenafil)

Warnings/Precautions Avoid use in hypertrophic cardiomyopathy with outflow tract obstruction; nitrates may reduce preload, exacerbating obstruction and cause hypotension or syncope and/or worsening of heart failure (Gersh, 2011). Use with caution in volume depletion, moderate hypotension, and extreme caution with inferior wall MI and suspected right ventricular infarctions. Nitrates may precipitate or aggravate increased intracranial pressure and subsequently may worsen clinical outcomes in patients with neurologic injury (eg, intracranial hemorrhage, traumatic brain injury). Postural hypotension, transient episodes of weakness, dizziness, or syncope may occur even with small doses; ethanol accentuates these effects; tolerance and cross-tolerance to nitrate antianginal and hemodynamic effects may occur during prolonged isosorbide mononitrate therapy; (minimized by using the smallest effective dose, by alternating coronary vasodilators or offering drug-free intervals of as little as 12 hours). Excessive doses may result in severe headache, blurred vision, or xerostomia; increased anginal symptoms may be a result of dosage increases. Avoid concurrent use with PDE-5 inhibitors (eg, sildenafil, tadalafil, vardenafil). When nitrate administration becomes medically necessary, may administer nitrates only if 24 hours have elapsed after use of sildenafil or vardenafil (48 hours after tadalafil use) (O'Connor, 2010).

Adverse Reactions

>10%: Central nervous system: Headache (13% to 35%)

1% to 10%:

Cardiovascular: Angina (≤2%), flushing (≤2%)

Central nervous system: Dizziness (≤4%), fatigue (≤4%), pain (≤4%), emotional lability (≤2%)

Dermatologic: Pruritus (≤2%), rash (≤2%)

Gastrointestinal: Nausea (≤3%), abdominal pain (≤2%), diarrhea (≤2%)

Respiratory: Upper respiratory infection (≤4%), cough increased (≤2%)

Miscellaneous: Allergic reaction (≤2%)

<1% (Limited to important or life-threatening): Apoplexy, arrhythmia, bradycardia, dyspnea, edema, hyper-/hypotension, methemoglobinemia (rare, overdose), MI, orthostatic hypotension, pallor, palpitation, paresthesia, tachycardia

Drug Interactions

Metabolism/Transport Effects Substrate of CYP3A4 (major); **Note:** Assignment of Major/Minor substrate status based on clinically relevant drug interaction potential

Avoid Concomitant Use

Avoid concomitant use of Isosorbide Mononitrate with any of the following: Conivaptan; Fusidic Acid (Systemic); Phosphodiesterase 5 Inhibitors; Riociguat

Increased Effect/Toxicity

Isosorbide Mononitrate may increase the levels/effects of: Hypotensive Agents; Prilocaine; Riociguat; Rosiglitazone; Sodium Nitrite

The levels/effects of Isosorbide Mononitrate may be increased by: Conivaptan; CYP3A4 Inhibitors (Moderate); CYP3A4 Inhibitors (Strong); Dasatinib; Fusidic Acid (Systemic); Ivacaftor; Luliconazole; Mifepristone; Nitric Oxide; Phosphodiesterase 5 Inhibitors; Simeprevir

Decreased Effect

The levels/effects of Isosorbide Mononitrate may be decreased by: Bosentan; CYP3A4 Inducers (Strong); Dabrafenib; Deferasirox; Herbs (CYP3A4 Inducers); Mitotane; Tocilizumab

Ethanol/Nutrition/Herb Interactions Ethanol: Caution with ethanol (may increase risk of hypotension).

Storage/Stability Tablets should be stored in a tight container at room temperature of 15°C to 30°C (59°F to 86°F).

Mechanism of Action Nitroglycerin and other nitrates form free radical nitric oxide. In smooth muscle, nitric oxide activates guanylate cyclase which increases guanosine 3'5' monophosphate (cGMP) leading to dephosphorylation of myosin light chains and smooth muscle relaxation. Produces a vasodilator effect on the peripheral veins and arteries with more prominent effects on the veins. Primarily reduces cardiac oxygen demand by decreasing preload (left ventricular end-diastolic pressure); may modestly reduce afterload; dilates coronary arteries and improves collateral flow to ischemic regions.

Pharmacodynamics/Kinetics

Onset of action: 30-60 minutes

Duration: Immediate release: ≥6 hours (Thadani, 1987); Extended release: ≥12-24 hours (Anderson, 2007)

Absorption: Nearly complete and low intersubject variability in its pharmacokinetic parameters and plasma concentrations

Distribution: V_d: ~0.6 L/kg

Protein binding: <5%

Metabolism: Hepatic

Bioavailability: ~100%

Half-life elimination: Mononitrate: ~5-6 hours

Excretion: Predominantly urine (2% as unchanged drug); feces (1% of dose)

Dosage Oral:
Adults:
Regular release tablet: Initial: 5-20 mg twice daily with the 2 doses given 7 hours apart (eg, 8 AM and 3 PM) to decrease tolerance development; patients initiating therapy with 5 mg twice daily (eg, small stature) should be titrated up to 10 mg twice daily in first 2-3 days.
Extended release tablet: Initial: 30-60 mg given once daily in the morning; titrate upward as needed, giving at least 3 days between increases; maximum daily single dose: 240 mg
Elderly: Start with lowest recommended adult dose.

Dosing adjustment in renal impairment: Dose adjustment not necessary
Hemodialysis: Dose supplementation is not necessary.
Peritoneal dialysis: Dose supplementation is not necessary.
Dosing adjustment in hepatic impairment: Dose adjustment not necessary

Note: Tolerance to nitrate effects develops with chronic exposure. Dose escalation does not overcome this effect. Tolerance can only be overcome by short periods of nitrate absence from the body. Short periods of nitrate withdrawal may help minimize tolerance. Recommended twice daily dosage regimens incorporate this interval. Administer sustained release tablet once daily in the morning.

Administration Do not administer around-the-clock. Immediate release tablet should be scheduled twice daily with doses 7 hours apart (8 AM and 3 PM); extended release tablet may be administered once daily in the morning upon rising with a half-glassful of fluid and should not be chewed or crushed.

Monitoring Parameters Monitor for orthostasis, increased hypotension

Dosage Forms Excipient information presented when available (limited, particularly for generics); consult specific product labeling.
Tablet, Oral:
Generic: 10 mg, 20 mg
Tablet Extended Release 24 Hour, Oral:
Imdur: 30 mg, 60 mg [scored]
Imdur: 120 mg
Generic: 30 mg, 60 mg, 120 mg

◆ Isotamine® (Can) *see* Isoniazid *on page 1123*

ISOtretinoin (eye soe TRET i noyn)

Brand Names: U.S. Absorica; Amnesteem; Claravis; Myorisan; Zenatane

Brand Names: Canada Accutane®; Clarus™

Index Terms 13-*cis*-Retinoic Acid; 13-*cis*-Vitamin A Acid; 13-CRA; *Cis*-Retinoic Acid; Accutane; Isotretinoinum

Pharmacologic Category Acne Products; Antineoplastic Agent, Miscellaneous; Retinoic Acid Derivative

Use Treatment of severe recalcitrant nodular acne unresponsive to conventional therapy

Unlabeled Use Management of moderate degrees of treatment-resistant acne, management of acne that produces physical or psychological scarring; treatment of cutaneous T-cell lymphomas (mycosis fungoides and Sézary syndrome); prevention of squamous cell skin cancers (in high-risk patients); treatment of high-risk neuroblastoma in children

Pregnancy Risk Factor X

Pregnancy Considerations Isotretinoin and its metabolites can be detected in fetal tissue following maternal use during pregnancy (Benifla, 1995; Kraft, 1989). **[U.S. Boxed Warnings]: Use of isotretinoin is contraindicated in females who are or may become pregnant. Birth defects (facial, eye, ear, skull, central nervous system, cardiovascular, thymus and parathyroid gland abnormalities) have been noted following isotretinoin exposure during pregnancy and the risk for severe birth defects is high, with any dose or even with short treatment duration. Low IQ scores have also been reported. The risk for spontaneous abortion and premature births is increased. Because of the high likelihood of teratogenic effects, all patients (male and female), prescribers, wholesalers, and dispensing pharmacists must register and be active in the iPLEDGE™ risk evaluation and mitigation strategy (REMS) program; do not prescribe isotretinoin for women who are or who are likely to become pregnant while using the drug. If pregnancy occurs during therapy, isotretinoin should be discontinued immediately and the patient referred to an obstetrician-gynecologist specializing in reproductive toxicity.** This medication is contraindicated in females of childbearing potential unless they are able to comply with the guidelines of the iPLEDGE™ pregnancy prevention program. Females of childbearing potential must have two negative pregnancy tests with a sensitivity of at least 25 mIU/mL prior to beginning therapy and testing should continue monthly during therapy. Females of childbearing potential should not become pregnant during therapy or for 1 month following discontinuation of isotretinoin. Upon discontinuation of treatment, females of childbearing potential should have a pregnancy test after their last dose and again one month after their last dose. Two forms of contraception should be continued during this time. Any pregnancies should be reported to the iPLEDGE™ program (www.-ipledgeprogram.com or 866-495-0654) and the FDA through MedWatch (800-FDA-1088).

Breast-Feeding Considerations It is not known if isotretinoin is excreted in breast milk. A case report describes a green discharge from the breast of a nonlactating woman which was determined to be iatrogenic galactorrhea due to isotretinoin (Larsen, 1985). Due to the potential for serious adverse reactions in the nursing infant, the manufacturer recommends a decision be made whether to discontinue nursing or to discontinue the drug, taking into account the importance of treatment to the mother.

Prescribing and Access Restrictions As a requirement of the REMS program, access to this medication is restricted. All patients (male and female), prescribers, wholesalers, and dispensing pharmacists must register and be active in the iPLEDGE™ risk management program, designed to eliminate fetal exposures to isotretinoin. This program covers all isotretinoin products (brand and generic). The iPLEDGE™ program requires that all patients meet qualification criteria and monthly program requirements (eg, pregnancy testing). Healthcare providers can only prescribe a maximum 30-day supply at each monthly visit and must counsel patients on the iPLEDGE™ program requirements and confirm counseling via the iPLEDGE™ automated system. Registration, activation, and additional information are provided at www.-ipledgeprogram.com or by calling 866-495-0654.

Medication Guide Available Yes

Contraindications Hypersensitivity to isotretinoin or any component of the formulation; sensitivity to parabens, vitamin A, or other retinoids; pregnant women or those who may become pregnant

Warnings/Precautions Hazardous agent - use appropriate precautions for handling and disposal (meets NIOSH, 2012 criteria). This medication should only be prescribed by prescribers competent in treating severe recalcitrant nodular acne and experienced with the use of systemic retinoids. Anaphylaxis and other types of allergic reactions, including cutaneous reactions and allergic vasculitis, have been reported. **[U.S. Boxed Warnings]: Birth defects (facial, eye, ear, skull, central nervous system,**

cardiovascular, thymus and parathyroid gland abnormalities) have been noted following isotretinoin exposure during pregnancy and the risk for severe birth defects is high, with any dose or even with short treatment duration. Low IQ scores have also been reported. The risk for spontaneous abortion and premature births is increased. Because of the high likelihood of teratogenic effects, all patients (male and female), prescribers, wholesalers, and dispensing pharmacists must register and be active in the iPLEDGE™ risk evaluation and mitigation strategy (REMS) program; do not prescribe isotretinoin for women who are or who are likely to become pregnant while using the drug. If pregnancy occurs during therapy, isotretinoin should be discontinued immediately and the patient referred to an obstetrician-gynecologist specializing in reproductive toxicity (see Additional Information for details). Women of childbearing potential must be capable of complying with effective contraceptive measures. Patients must select and commit to two forms of contraception. Therapy is begun after two negative pregnancy tests; effective contraception must be used for at least 1 month before beginning therapy, during therapy, and for 1 month after discontinuation of therapy. Prescriptions should be written for no more than a 30-day supply, and pregnancy testing and counseling should be repeated monthly.

May cause depression, psychosis, aggressive or violent behavior, and changes in mood; use with extreme caution in patients with psychiatric disorders. Rarely, suicidal thoughts and actions have been reported during isotretinoin usage. All patients should be observed closely for symptoms of depression or suicidal thoughts. Discontinuation of treatment alone may not be sufficient, further evaluation may be necessary. Cases of pseudotumor cerebri (benign intracranial hypertension) have been reported, some with concomitant use of tetracycline (avoid using together). Patients with papilledema, headache, nausea, vomiting, and visual disturbances should be referred to a neurologist and treatment with isotretinoin discontinued. Hearing impairment, which can continue after therapy is discontinued, may occur. Clinical hepatitis, elevated liver enzymes, inflammatory bowel disease, skeletal hyperostosis, premature epiphyseal closure, vision impairment, corneal opacities, decreased tolerance to contact lenses (due to dry eyes), and decreased night vision have also been reported with the use of isotretinoin. Rare postmarketing cases of severe skin reactions (eg, Stevens-Johnson syndrome, erythema multiforme) have been reported with use.

Use with caution in patients with diabetes mellitus; impaired glucose control has been reported. Use caution in patients with hypertriglyceridemia; acute pancreatitis and fatal hemorrhagic pancreatitis (rare) have been reported. Bone mineral density may decrease; use caution in patients with a genetic predisposition to bone disorders (ie, osteoporosis, osteomalacia) and with disease states or concomitant medications that can induce bone disorders. Patients may be at risk when participating in activities with repetitive impact (such as sports). Patients should be instructed not to donate blood during therapy and for 1 month following discontinuation of therapy due to risk of donated blood being given to a pregnant female. Safety of long-term use is not established and is not recommended.

Absorica™: Absorption is ~83% greater than Accutane® when administered under fasting conditions; they are bioequivalent when taken with a high-fat meal. Absorica™ is **not** interchangeable with other generic isotretinoin products. Isotretinoin and tretinoin (which is also known as all-*trans* retinoic acid, or ATRA) may be confused, while both products may be used in cancer treatment, they are **not** interchangeable; verify product prior to dispensing and administration to prevent medication errors.

Adverse Reactions Frequency not always defined.

Cardiovascular: Chest pain, edema, flushing, palpitation, stroke, syncope, tachycardia, vascular thrombotic disease

Central nervous system: Aggressive behavior, depression, dizziness, drowsiness, emotional instability, fatigue, headache, insomnia, lethargy, malaise, nervousness, paresthesia, pseudotumor cerebri, psychosis, seizure, stroke, suicidal ideation, suicide attempts, suicide, violent behavior

Dermatologic: Abnormal wound healing acne fulminans, alopecia, bruising, cheilitis, cutaneous allergic reactions, dry nose, dry skin, eczema, eruptive xanthomas, facial erythema, fragility of skin, hair abnormalities, hirsutism, hyperpigmentation, hypopigmentation, increased sunburn susceptibility, nail dystrophy, paronychia, peeling of palms, peeling of soles, photoallergic reactions, photosensitizing reactions, pruritus, purpura, rash

Endocrine & metabolic: Triglycerides increased (25%), abnormal menses, blood glucose increased, cholesterol increased, HDL decreased, hyperuricemia

Gastrointestinal: Bleeding and inflammation of the gums, colitis, esophagitis, esophageal ulceration, inflammatory bowel disease, nausea, nonspecific gastrointestinal symptoms, pancreatitis, weight loss, xerostomia

Genitourinary: Nonspecific urogenital findings

Hematologic: Agranulocytosis (rare), anemia, neutropenia, pyogenic granuloma, thrombocytopenia

Hepatic: Alkaline phosphatase increased, ALT increased, AST increased, GGTP increased, hepatitis, LDH increased

Neuromuscular & skeletal: Back pain (29% in pediatric patients), arthralgia, arthritis, bone abnormalities, bone mineral density decreased, calcification of tendons and ligaments, CPK increased, myalgia, premature epiphyseal closure, skeletal hyperostosis, tendonitis, weakness

Ocular: Conjunctivitis (4%), blepharitis (1%), chalazion (1%), hordeolum (1%), cataracts, color vision disorder, corneal opacities, eyelid inflammation, keratitis, night vision decreased, optic neuritis, photophobia, visual disturbances

Otic: Hearing impairment, tinnitus

Renal: Glomerulonephritis, hematuria, proteinuria, pyuria, vasculitis

Respiratory: Bronchospasms, epistaxis, respiratory infection, voice alteration, Wegener's granulomatosis

Miscellaneous: Allergic reactions, anaphylactic reactions, disseminated herpes simplex, diaphoresis, infection, lymphadenopathy

<1% (Limited to important or life-threatening): Abnormal meibomian gland secretion, erythema multiforme, meibomian gland atrophy, myopia, pseudotumor cerebri, Stevens-Johnson syndrome, toxic epidermal necrolysis, visual acuity decreased

Drug Interactions

Metabolism/Transport Effects None known.

Avoid Concomitant Use

Avoid concomitant use of ISOtretinoin with any of the following: Multivitamins/Fluoride (with ADE); Multivitamins/Minerals (with ADEK, Folate, Iron); Multivitamins/Minerals (with AE, No Iron); Tetracycline Derivatives; Vitamin A

Increased Effect/Toxicity

ISOtretinoin may increase the levels/effects of: Mipomersen; Porfimer; Vitamin A

The levels/effects of ISOtretinoin may be increased by: Alcohol (Ethyl); Multivitamins/Fluoride (with ADE); Multivitamins/Minerals (with ADEK, Folate, Iron); Multivitamins/Minerals (with AE, No Iron); Tetracycline Derivatives

Decreased Effect

ISOtretinoin may decrease the levels/effects of: Contraceptives (Estrogens); Contraceptives (Progestins)

Ethanol/Nutrition/Herb Interactions

Ethanol: Avoid or limit ethanol (may increase triglyceride levels if taken in excess).

Food: Isotretinoin bioavailability increased if taken with food or milk.

Herb/Nutraceutical: Avoid dong quai, St John's wort (may also cause photosensitization and may decrease the effectiveness of oral contraceptives). Additional vitamin A supplements may lead to vitamin A toxicity (dry skin, irritation, arthralgias, myalgias, abdominal pain, hepatic changes); avoid use.

Storage/Stability Store at room temperature of 59°F to 86°F (15°C to 30°C). Protect from light.

Mechanism of Action Reduces sebaceous gland size and reduces sebum production in acne treatment; in neuroblastoma, decreases cell proliferation and induces differentiation

Pharmacodynamics/Kinetics

Absorption: Enhanced with a high-fat meal; Absorica™ absorption is ~83% greater than Accutane® when administered under fasting conditions; they are bioequivalent when taken with a high-fat meal.

Protein binding: 99% to 100%; primarily albumin

Metabolism: Hepatic via CYP2B6, 2C8, 2C9, 2D6, 3A4; forms metabolites; major metabolite: 4-oxo-isotretinoin (active)

Half-life elimination: Terminal: Parent drug: 21 hours; Metabolite: 21-24 hours

Time to peak, serum: 3-5 hours

Excretion: Urine and feces (equal amounts)

Dosage Oral:

Children 1-17 years: Neuroblastoma, high-risk (unlabeled use): 160 mg/m²/day (in 2 divided doses) days 1 through 14 every 28 days for 6 cycles, beginning after continuation chemotherapy or transplantation (Matthay, 1999)

Children 12-17 years and Adults:

Acne, severe recalcitrant nodular: 0.5-1 mg/kg/day in 2 divided doses for 15-20 weeks; may discontinue earlier if the total cyst count decreases by 70%. Adults with very severe disease/scarring or primarily involves the trunk may require dosage adjustment up to 2 mg/kg/day. A second course of therapy may be initiated after a period of ≥2 months off therapy. A dose of ≤0.5 mg/kg/day may be used to minimize initial flaring (Strauss, 2007).

Acne, moderate (unlabeled use): 20 mg/day (~0.3-0.4 mg/kg/day) for 6 months (Amichai, 2006)

Dosing adjustment in renal impairment: No dosage adjustment provided in the manufacturer's labeling.

Dosing adjustment in hepatic impairment:

Hepatic impairment prior to treatment: No dosage adjustment provided in the manufacturer's labeling.

Hepatotoxicity during treatment: Liver enzymes may normalize with dosage reduction or with continued treatment; discontinue if normalization does not readily occur or if hepatitis is suspected.

Dietary Considerations Should be taken with food, except Absorbica™ which may be taken without regard to meals. Limit intake of vitamin A; avoid use of other vitamin A products. Some formulations may contain soybean oil.

Administration Administer orally with a meal (except Absorica™ which may be taken without regard to meals). According to the manufacturers' labeling, capsules should be swallowed whole with a full glass of liquid. For patients unable to swallow capsule whole, an oral liquid may be prepared; may irritate esophagus if contents are removed from the capsule.

Hazardous agent; use appropriate precautions for handling and disposal (meets NIOSH, 2012 criteria).

Monitoring Parameters CBC with differential and platelet count, baseline sedimentation rate, glucose, CPK; signs of depression, mood alteration, psychosis, aggression, severe skin reactions

Pregnancy test (for all female patients of childbearing potential): Two negative tests with a sensitivity of at least 25 mIU/mL prior to beginning therapy (the second performed at least 19 days after the first test and performed during the first 5 days of the menstrual period immediately preceding the start of therapy); monthly tests to rule out pregnancy prior to refilling prescription.

Lipids: Prior to treatment and at weekly or biweekly intervals until response to treatment is established. Test should not be performed <36 hours after consumption of ethanol.

Liver function tests: Prior to treatment and at weekly or biweekly intervals until response to treatment is established.

Additional Information All patients (male and female), must be registered in the iPLEDGE™ risk management program. Females of childbearing potential must receive oral and written information reviewing the hazards of therapy and the effects that isotretinoin can have on a fetus. Therapy should not begin without two negative pregnancy tests at least 19 days apart. Two forms of contraception (a primary and secondary form as described in the iPLEDGE™ program materials) must be used simultaneously beginning 1 month prior to treatment, during treatment, and for 1 month after therapy is discontinued; limitations to their use must be explained. Microdosed progesterone products that do not contain an estrogen ("mini-pills") are not an acceptable form of contraception during isotretinoin treatment. Prescriptions should be written for no more than a 30-day supply, and pregnancy testing and counseling should be repeated monthly. During therapy, pregnancy tests must be conducted by a CLIA-certified laboratory. Prescriptions must be filled and picked up from the pharmacy within 7 days of specimen collection for pregnancy test for women of childbearing potential. Prescriptions for males and females of nonchildbearing potential must be filled and picked up within 30 days of prescribing.

Any cases of accidental pregnancy should be reported to the iPLEDGE™ program or FDA MedWatch. All patients (male and female) must read and sign the informed consent material provided in the pregnancy prevention program.

Dosage Forms Excipient information presented when available (limited, particularly for generics); consult specific product labeling.

Capsule, Oral:

Absorica: 10 mg, 20 mg, 30 mg, 40 mg [contains soybean oil]

Amnesteem: 10 mg, 20 mg, 40 mg [contains soybean oil]

Claravis: 10 mg [contains fd&c yellow #6 (sunset yellow), soybean oil]

Claravis: 20 mg [contains soybean oil]

Claravis: 30 mg

Claravis: 40 mg [contains fd&c yellow #6 (sunset yellow), soybean oil]

Myorisan: 10 mg, 20 mg [contains soybean oil]

Myorisan: 40 mg [contains fd&c yellow #6 (sunset yellow), soybean oil]

Zenatane: 10 mg [contains brilliant blue fcf (fd&c blue #1), edetate disodium, fd&c yellow #10 (quinoline yellow), methylparaben, propylparaben, soybean oil]

Zenatane: 20 mg [contains edetate disodium, methylparaben, propylparaben, soybean oil]

Zenatane: 40 mg [contains brilliant blue fcf (fd&c blue #1), edetate disodium, fd&c blue #2 (indigotine), fd&c yellow #10 (quinoline yellow), methylparaben, propylparaben, soybean oil]

Extemporaneous Preparations Hazardous agent: Use appropriate precautions for handling and disposal of teratogenic capsule contents.

For patients unable to swallow the capsules whole, an oral liquid may be prepared with softgel capsules (not recommended by the manufacturers) by one of the following methods:

Place capsules (softgel formulations only) in small container and add warm (~37°C [97°F]) water or milk to cover capsule(s); wait 2-3 minutes until capsule is softened and then drink the milk or water with the softened capsule, or swallow softened capsule.

Puncture capsule (softgel formulations only) with needle or cut with scissors; squeeze capsule contents into 5-10 mL of milk or tube feed formula; draw mixture up into oral syringe and administer via feeding tube; flush feeding tube with ≥30 mL additional milk or tube feeding formula.

Puncture capsule (softgel formulations only) with needle or cut with scissors and draw contents into oral syringe; add 1-5 mL of medium chain triglyceride, soybean, or safflower oil to the oral syringe; mix gently and administer via feeding tube; flush feeding tube with ≥30 mL milk or tube feeding formula.

Lam MS, "Extemporaneous Compounding of Oral Liquid Dosage Formulations and Alternative Drug Delivery Methods for Anticancer Drugs," *Pharmacotherapy*, 2011, 31(2):164-92.

◆ Isotretinoinum *see* ISOtretinoin *on page 1129*

Isradipine (iz RA di peen)

Pharmacologic Category Antihypertensive; Calcium Channel Blocker; Calcium Channel Blocker, Dihydropyridine

Additional Appendix Information

Calcium Channel Blockers - Comparative Pharmacokinetics *on page 2296*

Use Management of hypertension (may be used alone or concurrently with thiazide-type diuretics).

Unlabeled Use Pediatric hypertension

Pregnancy Risk Factor C

Dosage Hypertension: Oral:

Children (unlabeled use): Initial: 0.15-0.2 mg/kg/day in 3-4 divided doses; maximum 0.8 mg/kg/day, up to 20 mg daily (NHBPEP, 2004).

Adults: 2.5 mg twice daily; antihypertensive response occurs in 2-3 hours; maximal response in 2-4 weeks; increase dose at 2- to 4-week intervals at 2.5-5 mg increments; usual dose range (JNC 7): 2.5-10 mg daily in 2 divided doses. **Note:** Most patients show no improvement with doses >10 mg daily except adverse reaction rate increases; therefore, maximal dose in older adults should be 10 mg daily.

Elderly: Refer to adult dosing.

Dosage adjustment in renal impairment: No dosage adjustment provided in manufacturer's labeling; however, bioavailability is increased with mild renal impairment and decreased with severe renal impairment. Other sources recommend that no initial dosage adjustment is required (Aronoff, 2007). Isradipine is not removed by hemodialysis; therefore, supplemental doses after hemodialysis are not necessary (Schonholzer, 1992).

Dosage adjustment in hepatic impairment: No dosage adjustment provided in manufacturer's labeling; however, peak serum concentrations are increased by 32% and bioavailability is increased by 52%.

Additional Information Complete prescribing information should be consulted for additional detail.

Dosage Forms Excipient information presented when available (limited, particularly for generics); consult specific product labeling.

Capsule, Oral:

Generic: 2.5 mg, 5 mg

◆ Istalol *see* Timolol (Ophthalmic) *on page 2064*

◆ Istodax *see* RomiDEPsin *on page 1848*

◆ Isuprel *see* Isoproterenol *on page 1125*

Itraconazole (i tra KOE na zole)

Brand Names: U.S. Onmel; Sporanox; Sporanox Pulsepak

Brand Names: Canada Sporanox

Pharmacologic Category Antifungal Agent, Oral

Additional Appendix Information

Antifungal Agents *on page 2286*

Use

Oral capsules: Treatment of susceptible fungal infections in immunocompromised and immunocompetent patients including blastomycosis and histoplasmosis; indicated for aspergillosis (in patients intolerant/refractory to amphotericin B), and onychomycosis of the toenail and fingernail (in nonimmunocompromised patients)

Oral solution: Treatment of oral and esophageal candidiasis

Oral tablets: Treatment of onychomycosis of the toenail (in nonimmunocompromised patients)

Canadian labeling: Oral capsules: Additional indications (not in U.S. labeling): Treatment of oral and esophageal candidiasis; treatment of cutaneous and lymphatic sporotrichosis, chromomycosis, or paracoccidioidomycosis in immunocompetent and immunosuppressed patients; treatment of onychomycosis in immunosuppressed patients; treatment of dermatomycoses due to tinea pedis, tinea cruris, tinea corporis and of pityriasis versicolor in immunocompetent and immunocompromised patients in whom oral therapy is appropriate

Pregnancy Risk Factor C

Pregnancy Considerations Dose related adverse events were observed in animal reproduction studies. Use is contraindicated for the treatment of onychomycosis during pregnancy. If used for the treatment of onychomycosis in women of reproductive potential, effective contraception should be used during treatment and for 2 months following treatment. Therapy should begin on the second or third day following menses. Congenital abnormalities have been reported during postmarketing surveillance, but a causal relationship has not been established.

Breast-Feeding Considerations Itraconazole is excreted in breast milk. According to the manufacturer, the decision to continue or discontinue breast-feeding during therapy should take into account the risk of exposure to the infant and the benefits of treatment to the mother.

Contraindications Hypersensitivity to itraconazole (use caution in patients with a history of hypersensitivity to other azoles), any component of the formulation; concurrent administration with cisapride, dofetilide, ergot derivatives, felodipine, levomethadyl, lovastatin, methadone, midazolam (oral), nisoldipine, pimozide, quinidine, simvastatin, or triazolam; treatment of onychomycosis (or other non-life-threatening indications) in patients with evidence of ventricular dysfunction, heart failure (HF) or a history of HF; treatment of onychomycosis in patients who are pregnant or intend on becoming pregnant

Canadian labeling: Oral capsule: Additional contraindications (not in U.S. labeling): Concurrent administration with eletriptan; treatment of dermatomycosis (tinea pedis, tinea cruris, tinea corporis) and of pityriasis versicolor in patients who are pregnant or intend on becoming pregnant

Warnings/Precautions [U.S. Boxed Warning]: Negative inotropic effects have been observed following intravenous administration. Discontinue or reassess use if signs or symptoms of HF (heart failure) occur during treatment. [U.S. Boxed Warning]: Use is contraindicated for treatment of onychomycosis in patients with ventricular dysfunction or a history of HF. Cases of HF, peripheral edema, and pulmonary edema have occurred in patients treated for onychomycosis. HF has been reported, particularly in patients receiving a total daily oral dose of 400 mg. Use with caution in patients with risk factors for HF (COPD, renal failure, edematous disorders, ischemic or valvular disease). Discontinue if signs or symptoms of HF or neuropathy occur during treatment. Due to potential toxicity, the manufacturer recommends confirmation of diagnosis testing of nail specimens prior to treatment of onychomycosis.

[U.S. Boxed Warning]: Serious cardiovascular adverse events including, QT prolongation, ventricular tachycardia, torsade de pointes, cardiac arrest and/or sudden death have been observed due to itraconazole-induced increased serum concentrations of the following: cisapride, dofetilide, ergot alkaloids (dihydroergotamine, ergonovine, ergotamine, methylergonovine), felodipine, levomethadyl, lovastatin, methadone, midazolam (oral), nisoldipine, pimozide, quinidine, simvastatin, or triazolam; concurrent use contraindicated. Other potentially significant interactions may exist, requiring dose or frequency adjustment, additional monitoring, and/or selection of alternative therapy.

Use with caution in patients with renal impairment. Rare cases of serious hepatotoxicity (including liver failure and death) have been reported (including some cases occurring within the first week of therapy); hepatotoxicity was reported in some patients without pre-existing liver disease or risk factors. Use with caution in patients with pre-existing hepatic impairment; monitor liver function closely. Not recommended for use in patients with active liver disease, elevated liver enzymes, or prior hepatotoxic reactions to other drugs unless the expected benefit exceeds the risk of hepatotoxicity. Discontinue treatment if signs or symptoms of hepatotoxicity develop. Transient or permanent hearing loss has been reported. Quinidine (a contraindicated drug) was used concurrently in several of these cases. Hearing loss usually resolves after discontinuation, but may persist in some patients.

Large differences in itraconazole pharmacokinetic parameters have been observed in cystic fibrosis patients receiving the solution; if a patient with cystic fibrosis does not respond to therapy, alternate therapies should be considered. Due to differences in bioavailability, oral capsules and oral solution cannot be used interchangeably. Only the oral solution has proven efficacy for oral and esophageal candidiasis. Initiation of treatment with oral solution is not recommended in patients at immediate risk for systemic candidiasis (eg, patients with severe neutropenia).

Adverse Reactions

>10%: Gastrointestinal: Nausea (3% to 11%), diarrhea (3% to 11%)

1% to 10%:

Cardiovascular: Edema (4%), hypertension (3%), chest pain (3%)

Central nervous system: Headache (4% to 10%), fever (2% to 7%), dizziness (2% to 4%), anxiety (3%), depression (2% to 3%), fatigue (2% to 3%), pain (2% to 3%), malaise (1% to 3%), dreams abnormal (2%)

Dermatologic: Rash (3% to 9%), pruritus (≤5%)

Endocrine & metabolic: Hypertriglyceridemia (≤3%), hypokalemia (2%)

Gastrointestinal: Vomiting (5% to 7%), abdominal pain (2% to 6%), dyspepsia (≤4%), flatulence (≤4%), gingivitis (3%), stomatitis (ulcerative) (≤3%), constipation (2% to 3%), appetite increased (2%), gastritis (2%), gastroenteritis (2%)

Hepatic: LFTs abnormal (≤4%)

Neuromuscular & skeletal: Bursitis (3%), myalgia (≤3%), tremor (2%), weakness (≤2%)

Renal: Cystitis (3%), urinary tract infection (3%)

Respiratory: Rhinitis (5% to 9%), upper respiratory tract infection (8%), sinusitis (2% to 7%), cough (4%), dyspnea (2%), pharyngitis (≤2%), pneumonia (2%), sputum increased (2%)

Miscellaneous: Diaphoresis increased (3%), herpes zoster (2%)

<2% (Limited to important or life-threatening): Adrenal insufficiency, albuminuria, allergic reactions, alopecia, anaphylactoid reactions, anaphylaxis, angioedema, anorexia, arrhythmia, arthralgia, blurred vision, dehydration, diplopia, dysgeusia, dysphagia, erythema multiforme, exanthematous pustulosis, exfoliative dermatitis, gynecomastia, hearing loss, heart failure, hematuria, hepatic failure, hepatitis, hepatotoxicity, hot flashes, hypoesthesia, impotence, insomnia, leukocytoclastic dermatitis, leukopenia, libido decreased, menstrual disorders, neutropenia, pancreatitis, paresthesia, peripheral edema, photosensitivity, pollakiuria, pulmonary edema, rigors, serum sickness, somnolence, Stevens-Johnson syndrome, thrombocytopenia, taste perversion, tinnitus, toxic epidermal necrolysis, urinary incontinence, urticaria, vasculitis

Drug Interactions

Metabolism/Transport Effects Substrate of CYP3A4 (major); **Note:** Assignment of Major/Minor substrate status based on clinically relevant drug interaction potential; **Inhibits** CYP3A4 (strong), P-glycoprotein

Avoid Concomitant Use

Avoid concomitant use of Itraconazole with any of the following: Ado-Trastuzumab Emtansine; Alfuzosin; Aliskiren; ALPRAZolam; Apixaban; Avanafil; Axitinib; Bosutinib; Cabozantinib; Cisapride; Conivaptan; Crizotinib; CYP3A4 Inducers (Strong); Dihydroergotamine; Dofetilide; Dronedarone; Eletriptan; Eplerenone; Ergoloid Mesylates; Ergonovine; Ergotamine; Estazolam; Everolimus; Felodipine; Halofantrine; Ibrutinib; Imatinib; Ivabradine; Lapatinib; Lomitapide; Lovastatin; Lurasidone; Macitentan; Methadone; Methylergonovine; Midazolam; Nevirapine; Nilotinib; Nisoldipine; Pimozide; Pomalidomide; QuiNIDine; Ranolazine; Red Yeast Rice; Regorafenib; Rivaroxaban; Salmeterol; Silodosin; Simeprevir; Simvastatin; Tamsulosin; Ticagrelor; Tolvaptan; Topotecan; Toremifene; Triazolam; Ulipristal; Vemurafenib; VinCRIStine (Liposomal)

Increased Effect/Toxicity

Itraconazole may increase the levels/effects of: Ado-Trastuzumab Emtansine; Afatinib; Alfentanil; Alfuzosin; Aliskiren; Almotriptan; Alosetron; ALPRAZolam; Apixaban; ARIPiprazole; AtorvaSTATin; Avanafil; Axitinib; Bedaquiline; Benzodiazepines (metabolized by oxidation); Boceprevir; Bortezomib; Bosentan; Bosutinib; Brentuximab Vedotin; Brinzolamide; Budesonide (Nasal); Budesonide (Systemic, Oral Inhalation); BusPIRone; Busulfan; Cabozantinib; Calcium Channel Blockers; Cardiac Glycosides; Cilostazol; Cisapride; Cobicistat; Colchicine; Conivaptan; Corticosteroids (Orally Inhaled); Corticosteroids (Systemic); Crizotinib; CycloSPORINE

(Systemic); CYP3A4 Substrates; Dabigatran Etexilate; Darunavir; Dienogest; Dihydroergotamine; DOCEtaxel; Dofetilide; Dronedarone; Dutasteride; Eletriptan; Elvitegravir; Enzalutamide; Eplerenone; Ergoloid Mesylates; Ergonovine; Ergotamine; Estazolam; Etravirine; Everolimus; Felodipine; FentaNYL; Fesoterodine; Fexofenadine; Fluticasone (Nasal); Fluticasone (Oral Inhalation); Fosamprenavir; Fosphenytoin; GuanFACINE; Halofantrine; Highest Risk QTc-Prolonging Agents; Ibrutinib; Iloperidone; Imatinib; Indinavir; Irinotecan; Ivabradine; Ivacaftor; Ixabepilone; Lacosamide; Lapatinib; Levomilnacipran; Lomitapide; Losartan; Lovastatin; Lumefantrine; Lurasidone; Macitentan; Macrolide Antibiotics; Maraviroc; Methadone; Methylergonovine; MethylPREDNISolone; Midazolam; Mifepristone; Moderate Risk QTc-Prolonging Agents; Nilotinib; Nisoldipine; Ospemifene; OxyCODONE; Paliperidone; Paricalcitol; PAZOPanib; P-glycoprotein/ABCB1 Substrates; Phenytoin; Pimecrolimus; Pimozide; Pomalidomide; PONATinib; Pravastatin; Propafenone; Prucalopride; QUEtiapine; QuiNIDine; Ranolazine; Red Yeast Rice; Regorafenib; Repaglinide; Rifamycin Derivatives; Rilpivirine; Riociguat; Rivaroxaban; RomiDEPsin; Rosuvastatin; Ruxolitinib; Salmeterol; Saquinavir; Saxagliptin; Sildenafil; Silodosin; Simeprevir; Simvastatin; Sirolimus; Solifenacin; SORAfenib; SUNItinib; Tacrolimus (Systemic); Tacrolimus (Topical); Tadalafil; Tamsulosin; Telaprevir; Temsirolimus; Ticagrelor; Tofacitinib; Tolterodine; Tolvaptan; Topotecan; Toremifene; Triazolam; Ulipristal; Vardenafil; Vemurafenib; Vilazodone; VinBLAStine; VinCRIStine; VinCRIStine (Liposomal); Vinorelbine; Vitamin K Antagonists; Zolpidem; Zuclopenthixol

The levels/effects of Itraconazole may be increased by: Boceprevir; Cobicistat; Darunavir; Etravirine; Fosamprenavir; Grapefruit Juice; Indinavir; Lopinavir; Macrolide Antibiotics; Ritonavir; Saquinavir; Telaprevir; Tipranavir

Decreased Effect

Itraconazole may decrease the levels/effects of: Amphotericin B; Ifosfamide; Prasugrel; Saccharomyces boulardii; Ticagrelor

The levels/effects of Itraconazole may be decreased by: Antacids; CYP3A4 Inducers (Strong); Dabrafenib; Deferasirox; Didanosine; Efavirenz; Etravirine; Fosphenytoin; Grapefruit Juice; H2-Antagonists; Herbs (CYP3A4 Inducers); Isoniazid; Nevirapine; Phenytoin; Proton Pump Inhibitors; Rifamycin Derivatives; Sucralfate; Tocilizumab

Ethanol/Nutrition/Herb Interactions

Food:

Capsules: Absorption enhanced by food and possibly by gastric acidity. Cola drinks have been shown to increase the absorption of the capsules in patients with achlorhydria or those taking H_2-receptor antagonists or other gastric acid suppressors. Grapefruit/grapefruit juice may increase serum levels. Management: Take capsules immediately after meals. Avoid grapefruit juice.

Solution: Food decreases the bioavailability and increases the time to peak concentration. Management: Take solution on an empty stomach 1 hour before or 2 hours after meals.

Herb/Nutraceutical: St John's wort may decrease itraconazole levels.

Storage/Stability

Capsule: Store at room temperature of 15°C to 25°C (59°F to 77°F). Protect from light and moisture.

Oral solution: Store at ≤25°C (77°F); do not freeze.

Tablet: Store at room temperature 15°C to 25°C (59°F to 77°F); excursions are permitted between 15°C and 30°C (59°F and 86°F). Protect from light and moisture.

Mechanism of Action Interferes with cytochrome P450 activity, decreasing ergosterol synthesis (principal sterol in fungal cell membrane) and inhibiting cell membrane formation

Pharmacodynamics/Kinetics

Absorption: Requires gastric acidity; capsule better absorbed with food, solution better absorbed on empty stomach

Distribution: V_d (average): 796 ± 185 L or 10 L/kg; highly lipophilic and tissue concentrations are higher than plasma concentrations. The highest concentrations: adipose, omentum, endometrium, cervical and vaginal mucus, and skin/nails. Aqueous fluids (eg, CSF and urine) contain negligible amounts.

Protein binding, plasma: 99.8%; metabolite hydroxy-itraconazole: 99.5%

Metabolism: Extensively hepatic via CYP3A4 into >30 metabolites including hydroxy-itraconazole (major metabolite); appears to have *in vitro* antifungal activity. Main metabolic pathway is oxidation; may undergo saturation metabolism with multiple dosing.

Bioavailability: Variable, ~55% (oral solution) in 1 small study; **Note:** Oral solution has a higher degree of bioavailability (149% ± 68%) relative to oral capsules; should not be interchanged

Half-life elimination: Oral: Single dose: ~21 hours, steady state: 64 hours; Cirrhosis (single dose): 37 hours (range: 20-54 hours)

Time to peak, plasma: Capsules: 3-5 hours; Oral solution: 2-3 hours

Excretion: Urine (<0.03% active drug, 40% as inactive metabolites); feces (~3% to 18%)

Dosage

Children: Oral: Manufacturer labeling states that a small number of patients 3-16 years of age have been treated with 100 mg daily for systemic fungal infections with no serious adverse effects reported. A dose of 5 mg/kg once daily was used in a pharmacokinetic study using the oral solution in patients 6 months to 12 years; duration of study was 2 weeks.

Indication-specific dosing:

Infants and Children (HIV-exposed/-positive; unlabeled use): **Note:** Doses >200 mg daily should be administered in 2 divided doses.

Candidiasis:

Oropharyngeal: Oral solution: 2.5 mg/kg/dose twice daily (maximum: 200 mg daily [400 mg daily if fluconazole-refractory]) for 7-14 days (CDC, 2009a)

Esophageal: Oral solution: 5 mg/kg/day once daily or divided twice daily for 4-21 days (CDC, 2009a)

Coccidioidomycosis:

Treatment: Oral: 5-10 mg/kg/dose twice daily for 3 days, followed by 2-5 mg/kg/dose orally twice daily (maximum: 400 mg daily) (CDC, 2009a)

Relapse prevention: Oral: 2-5 mg/kg/dose twice daily (maximum: 400 mg daily) (CDC, 2009a)

Cryptococcus:

Treatment, consolidation therapy: Oral solution (preferred): Initial: 2.5-5 mg/kg/dose 3 times daily (maximum daily dose: 600 mg daily) for 3 days (9 doses) followed by 5-10 mg/kg/day divided once or twice daily (maximum daily dose: 400 mg daily) for a minimum of 8 weeks (CDC, 2009a)

Relapse prevention: Oral solution: 5 mg/kg/dose once daily (maximum: 200 mg daily) (CDC, 2009a)

Histoplasmosis:

Treatment of mild disseminated disease: Oral solution: 2-5 mg/kg/dose 3 times daily for 3 days (9 doses), followed by twice daily for 12 months (maximum: 200 mg per dose) (CDC, 2009a)

Consolidation treatment for moderate-severe to severe disseminated disease, including CNS infection (following appropriate induction therapy): Oral solution: 2-5 mg/kg/dose 3 times daily for 3 days, followed by 2-5 mg/kg/dose (maximum: 200 mg per dose) twice daily for 12 months for non-CNS-disseminated disease or for ≥12 months for CNS infection as determined by clinical response (CDC, 2009a)

Relapse prevention: Oral solution: 5 mg/kg/dose twice daily (maximum: 400 mg daily) (CDC, 2009a)

Adults: **Note:** Doses >200 mg daily should be administered in 2 divided doses.

Aspergillosis: Oral capsule: 200-400 mg daily. **Note:** For life-threatening infections, administer a loading dose of 200 mg 3 times daily (total: 600 mg daily) for the first 3 days of therapy. Continue treatment for at least 3 months and until clinical and laboratory evidence suggest that infection has resolved.

Aspergillosis, invasive (salvage therapy): Duration of therapy should be a minimum of 6-12 weeks or throughout period of immunosuppression: Oral capsule: 200-400 mg daily; **Note:** 2008 IDSA guidelines recommend 600 mg daily for 3 days, followed by 400 mg daily (Walsh, 2008)

Appropriate use: Itraconazole should **NOT** be used for voriconazole-refractory aspergillosis since the same antifungal and/or resistance mechanism(s) may be shared by both agents. Itraconazole oral solution and capsule formulations are not bioequivalent or interchangeable. Due to variable bioavailability of oral preparations, therapeutic drug monitoring is advisable (Walsh, 2008).

Aspergillosis, allergic (ABPA, sinusitis): Oral: 200 mg daily; may be used in conjunction with corticosteroids (Andes, 2000; Walsh, 2008)

Blastomycosis: Oral capsule: Initial: 200 mg once daily; if no clinical improvement or evidence of progressive infection, may increase dose in increments of 100 mg up to maximum of 400 mg daily. **Note:** For life-threatening infections, administer a loading dose of 200 mg 3 times daily (total 600 mg daily) for the first 3 days of therapy. Continue treatment for at least 3 months and until clinical and laboratory evidence suggest that infection has resolved.

Alternative dosing: 200 mg 3 times daily for 3 days, then 200 mg twice daily for 6-12 months; in moderately-severe to severe infection, therapy should be initiated with ~2 weeks of amphotericin B (Chapman, 2008).

Candidiasis:

Esophageal:

Oral solution: 100-200 mg once daily for a minimum of 3 weeks; continue dosing for 2 weeks after resolution of symptoms

Oral capsule: Canadian labeling (not in U.S. labeling): 100 mg once daily for 4 weeks; increase dose to 200 mg once daily in patients with AIDS and neutropenic patients

Oropharyngeal:

Oral solution: 200 mg once daily for 1-2 weeks; in patients unresponsive or refractory to fluconazole: 100 mg twice daily (clinical response expected in 2-4 weeks)

Oral capsule: Canadian labeling (not in U.S. labeling): 100 mg once daily for 2 weeks; increase dose to 200 mg once daily in patients with AIDS and neutropenic patients

Chromomycosis: Canadian labeling (not in U.S. labeling): Oral capsule: 200 mg once daily for 6 months (when due to *Fonsecaea pedrosoi*) or 100 mg once daily for 3 months (when due to *Cladosporium carrioni*)

Coccidioidomycosis (nonprogressive, nondisseminated disease): Oral: 200 mg twice daily or 3 times daily (Galgiani, 2005)

Histoplasmosis: Manufacturer labeling: Oral capsule: Initial: 200 mg once daily; if no clinical improvement or evidence of progressive infection, may increase dose in increments of 100 mg up to maximum of 400 mg daily. **Note:** For life-threatening infections, administer a loading dose of 200 mg 3 times daily (total: 600 mg daily) for the first 3 days of therapy. Continue treatment for at least 3 months and until clinical and laboratory evidence suggest that infection has resolved.

Alternative dosing: 200 mg 3 times daily for 3 days, then 200 mg twice daily (or once daily in mild-moderate disease) for 6-12 weeks in mild-moderate disease or ≥12 months in progressive disseminated or chronic cavitary pulmonary histoplasmosis; in moderately-severe to severe infection, therapy should be initiated with ~2 weeks of a lipid formation of amphotericin B (Wheat, 2007).

Long-term suppression therapy: 200 mg daily (CDC, 2009b)

Meningitis: Oral:

Coccidioides: 400-600 mg daily (Galgiani, 2005)

Coccidioides, HIV-positive (unlabeled use): 200 mg 3 times daily for 3 days, then 200 mg twice daily; maintenance: 200 mg twice daily life-long (CDC, 2009b)

Appropriate use: Fluconazole is preferred for meningeal infections (CDC, 2009b; Galgiani, 2005)

Onychomycosis (fingernail involvement only): Oral capsule: 200 mg twice daily for 1 week; repeat 1-week course after 3-week off-time

Onychomycosis (toenails due to *Trichophyton rubrum* or *T. mentagrophytes*): Oral tablet: 200 mg once daily for 12 consecutive weeks.

Onychomycosis (toenails with or without fingernail involvement): Oral capsule: 200 mg once daily for 12 consecutive weeks

Canadian labeling (not in U.S. labeling): "Pulse-dosing": 200 mg twice daily for 1 week; repeat 1-week course twice with 3-week off-time between each course

Paracoccidioidomycosis: Canadian labeling (not in U.S. labeling): Oral capsule: 100 mg once daily for 6 months

Penicilliosis, HIV-positive (unlabeled use): Oral capsule: 400 mg daily for 8 weeks (mild disease) or 10 weeks (severe infections). In severely-ill patients, initiate therapy with 2 weeks of amphotericin B. Maintenance: 200 mg daily (CDC, 2009b)

Pityriasis versicolor: Canadian labeling (not in U.S. labeling): Oral capsule: 200 mg once daily for 7 days

Pneumonia: Oral:

Coccidioides: Mild-to-moderate: 200 mg twice daily (Galgiani, 2005)

Coccidioides, HIV-positive (focal pneumonia): 200 mg 3 times daily for 3 days, then 200 mg twice daily (CDC, 2009b)

Sporotrichosis: Oral:

Lymphocutaneous: 200 mg daily for 3-6 months (Kauffman, 2007)

Canadian labeling (not in U.S. labeling): 100 mg once daily for 3 months

Osteoarticular and pulmonary: 200 mg twice daily for ≥1 years (may use amphotericin B initially for stabilization) (Kauffman, 2007)

Tinea corporis or tinea cruris: Canadian labeling (not in U.S. labeling): Oral capsule: 100 mg once daily for 14 consecutive days or 200 mg once daily for 7 consecutive days. **Note:** Equivalency between regimens not established.

Tinea pedis: Canadian labeling (not in U.S. labeling): Oral capsule: 100 mg once daily for 28 consecutive days or 200 mg twice daily for 7 consecutive days. **Note:** Equivalency between regimens not established. Patients with chronic resistant infection may benefit from lower dose and extended treatment time (100 mg once daily for 28 days).

Dosage adjustment in renal impairment: The manufacturer's labeling states to use with caution in patients with renal impairment. Limited data suggests that no dosage adjustments are required in renal impairment; wide variations observed in plasma concentrations versus time profiles in patients with uremia, or receiving hemodialysis or continuous ambulatory peritoneal dialysis (Boelaert, 1988).

Dosage adjustment in hepatic impairment: No dosage adjustment provided in manufacturer's labeling; however, use caution and monitor closely for signs/symptoms of toxicity.

Dietary Considerations

Capsule, tablet: Take with food.

Solution: Take without food, if possible.

Administration Doses >200 mg/day are given in 2 divided doses; do not administer with antacids. Capsule and oral solution formulations are not bioequivalent and thus are not interchangeable. Capsule and tablet absorption is best if taken with food, therefore, it is best to administer itraconazole after meals at the same time each day; solution should be taken on an empty stomach. When treating oropharyngeal and esophageal candidiasis, solution should be swished vigorously in mouth (10 mL at a time), then swallowed.

Monitoring Parameters Liver function in patients with pre-existing hepatic dysfunction, and in all patients being treated for longer than 1 month; serum concentrations particularly for oral therapy (due to erratic bioavailability with capsule formulation); renal function

Reference Range Serum concentrations may be performed to assure therapeutic levels. Itraconazole plus the metabolite hydroxyitraconazole concentrations should be >1 mcg/mL (not to exceed 10 mcg/mL).

Timing of serum samples: Obtain level after ~2 weeks of therapy, level may be drawn anytime during the dosing interval.

Dosage Forms Excipient information presented when available (limited, particularly for generics); consult specific product labeling.

Capsule, Oral:

Sporanox: 100 mg [contains brilliant blue fcf (fd&c blue #1), d&c red #22 (eosine), fd&c blue #2 (indigotine)]

Sporanox Pulsepak: 100 mg [contains brilliant blue fcf (fd&c blue #1), d&c red #22 (eosine), fd&c blue #2 (indigotine)]

Generic: 100 mg

Solution, Oral:

Sporanox: 10 mg/mL (150 mL)

Tablet, Oral:

Onmel: 200 mg

Extemporaneous Preparations Note: Commercial oral solution is available (10 mg/mL)

A 20 mg/mL oral suspension may be made with capsules. Empty the contents of forty 100 mg capsules and add 15 mL of Alcohol, USP. Let stand for 5 minutes. Crush the beads in a mortar and reduce to a fine powder. Mix while adding a 1:1 mixture of Ora-Sweet and Ora-Plus in incremental proportions to **almost** 200 mL; transfer to a calibrated bottle, rinse mortar with vehicle, and add quantity of vehicle sufficient to make 200 mL. Label "shake well" and "refrigerate". Stable for 56 days refrigerated.

Nahata MC, Pai VB, and Hipple TF, *Pediatric Drug Formulations*, 5th ed, Cincinnati, OH: Harvey Whitney Books Co, 2004.

Ivacaftor (eye va KAF tor)

Brand Names: U.S. Kalydeco

Brand Names: Canada Kalydeco™

Index Terms VX-770

Pharmacologic Category Cystic Fibrosis Transmembrane Conductance Regulator Potentiator

Use Treatment of cystic fibrosis (CF) in patients who have a G551D mutation in the cystic fibrosis transmembrane conductance regulator (CFTR) gene

Note: Not effective in patients with CF who are homozygous for the F508del mutation in the CTFR gene

Pregnancy Risk Factor B

Pregnancy Considerations Adverse events were not observed in animal reproduction studies.

Breast-Feeding Considerations Although human data is not available, excretion of ivacaftor into breast milk is expected.

Contraindications There are no contraindications listed in the manufacturer's U.S. labeling.

Canadian labeling: Hypersensitivity to ivacaftor or any component of the formulation

Warnings/Precautions May increase hepatic transaminases; temporarily discontinue treatment if ALT or AST >5 times ULN. Use with caution in patients with moderate or severe hepatic impairment. Ivacaftor has a high potential for interactions with moderate or strong CYP3A4 inhibitors (eg, erythromycin, ketoconazole), strong CYP3A4 inducers (eg, rifampin, St John's wort), or CYP3A4/P-gp substrates (eg, digoxin, cyclosporine). Avoid use in patients homozygous for the CFTR gene F508del mutation (not effective). Cataracts have been observed in animal studies using juvenile rats exposed to ivacaftor (at doses approximately one-tenth the MRHD); cataracts have not been observed in studies involving older animals. It is unknown if this potential concern seen in animals studies is relevant to humans.

Adverse Reactions

>10%:

Central nervous system: Headache (4% to 24%)

Dermatologic: Rash (10% to 13%)

Gastrointestinal: Abdominal pain (16%), diarrhea (13%), nausea (10% to 12%)

Respiratory: Oropharyngeal pain (22%), upper respiratory tract infection (16% to 22%), nasal congestion (16% to 20%), nasopharyngitis (15%)

1% to 10%:

Central nervous system: Dizziness (5% to 9%)

Dermatologic: Acne (4% to 7%)

Endocrine & metabolic: Hyperglycemia (4% to 7%)

Hepatic: Transaminases increased (4% to 7%; >5 x ULN: 3%)

Neuromuscular & skeletal: Arthralgia (4% to 7%), musculoskeletal chest pain (4% to 7%), myalgia (4% to 7%)

Respiratory: Pharyngeal erythema (4% to 7%), pleuritic chest pain (4% to 7%), rhinitis (4% to 7%), sinus congestion (4% to 7%), wheezing (4% to 7%)

Miscellaneous: Bacteria in sputum (4% to 7%)

<1% (Limited to important or life-threatening): Hypoglycemia

Drug Interactions

Metabolism/Transport Effects Substrate of CYP3A4 (major); **Note:** Assignment of Major/Minor substrate status based on clinically relevant drug interaction potential; **Inhibits** CYP2C8 (weak), CYP2C9 (weak), CYP3A4 (weak), P-glycoprotein

Avoid Concomitant Use

Avoid concomitant use of Ivacaftor with any of the following: Bosutinib; CYP3A4 Inducers (Strong); Fusidic Acid (Systemic); Grapefruit Juice; PAZOPanib; Pimozide; Pomalidomide; Silodosin; St Johns Wort; Topotecan; VinCRIStine (Liposomal)

Increased Effect/Toxicity

Ivacaftor may increase the levels/effects of: Afatinib; ARIPiprazole; Bosutinib; Colchicine; CYP3A4 Substrates; Dabigatran Etexilate; Dofetilide; Everolimus; Lomitapide; PAZOPanib; P-glycoprotein/ABCB1 Substrates; Pimozide; Pomalidomide; Prucalopride; Rivaroxaban; Silodosin; Topotecan; VinCRIStine (Liposomal)

The levels/effects of Ivacaftor may be increased by: CYP3A4 Inhibitors (Moderate); CYP3A4 Inhibitors (Strong); Dasatinib; Fusidic Acid (Systemic); Grapefruit Juice; Luliconazole; Mifepristone; Simeprevir

Decreased Effect

The levels/effects of Ivacaftor may be decreased by: Bosentan; CYP3A4 Inducers (Strong); Dabrafenib; Deferasirox; St Johns Wort; Tocilizumab

Ethanol/Nutrition/Herb Interactions

Food: Ivacaftor serum concentrations may be increased when taken with grapefruit or Seville oranges. Management: Avoid concurrent use.

Herb/Nutraceutical: St John's wort may decrease ivacaftor serum concentrations. Management: Avoid concurrent use.

Storage/Stability Store at 20°C to 25°C (68°F to 77°F); excursions permitted to 15°C to 30°C (59°F to 86°F).

Mechanism of Action Potentiates epithelial cell chloride ion transport of defective (G551D mutant) cell-surface CFTR protein thereby improving the regulation of salt and water absorption and secretion in various tissues (eg, lung, gastrointestinal tract).

Pharmacodynamics/Kinetics

Onset of action: FEV_1 increased, sweat chloride decreased within ~2 weeks

Absorption: Variable; increased (by two- to fourfold) with fatty foods

Distribution: V_d: 353 L

Protein binding: ~99%; primarily to $alpha_1$ acid glycoprotein, albumin

Metabolism: Hepatic; extensive via CYP3A4; forms 2 major metabolites (M1 [active; 1/6 potency] and M6 [inactive])

Half-life elimination: ~12 hours

Time to peak: ~4 hours

Excretion: Feces (88%, 65% of administered dose as metabolites); urine (minimal, as unchanged drug)

Dosage Oral: Children ≥6 years and Adults: 150 mg every 12 hours

Dosage adjustment for ivacaftor with concomitant medications:

CYP3A4 strong inhibitors (eg, ketoconazole, itraconazole, posaconazole, voriconazole, clarithromycin, telithromycin): 150 mg twice **weekly**

CYP3A4 moderate inhibitors (eg, erythromycin, fluconazole): 150 mg once daily

Dosage adjustment for toxicity: ALT or AST >5 times ULN: Hold ivacaftor; may resume if elevated transaminases resolved and after assessing benefits vs risks of continued treatment

Dosage adjustment in renal impairment:

Cl_{cr} >30 mL/minute: No dosage adjustment necessary.

Cl_{cr} ≤30 mL/minute: No dosage adjustment provided in manufacturer's labeling (not studied); use with caution.

Dosage adjustment in hepatic impairment:

Mild impairment (Child-Pugh class A): No dosage adjustment necessary.

Moderate impairment (Child-Pugh class B): 150 mg once daily.

Severe impairment (Child-Pugh class C): Has not been studied; use with caution.

U.S. labeling: Initial: 150 mg once daily or less frequently.

Canadian labeling: Initial: 150 mg once every other day; adjust for tolerance and/or response.

Dietary Considerations Take with high-fat-containing foods (eg, butter, cheese pizza, eggs, peanut butter). Avoid grapefruit or Seville oranges.

Administration Oral: Administer with high-fat-containing foods (eg, butter, cheese pizza, eggs, peanut butter).

Monitoring Parameters CF mutation test (prior to therapy initiation if G551D mutation status unknown); ALT/AST at baseline, every 3 months for 1 year, then annually thereafter or as clinically indicated; FEV_1

Additional Information G551D mutation is present in approximately 4% to 5% of patients with CF. When used in addition to standard therapy (eg, dornase alfa, inhaled tobramycin), ivacaftor may provide further improvements in FEV_1, a reduction in pulmonary exacerbations, and a beneficial weight gain in CF patients. Long-term benefits on disease progression have not been established.

Dosage Forms Excipient information presented when available (limited, particularly for generics); consult specific product labeling.

Tablet, Oral:

Kalydeco: 150 mg [contains fd&c blue #2 (indigotine)]

Ivermectin (Systemic) (eye ver MEK tin)

Brand Names: U.S. Stromectol

Pharmacologic Category Anthelmintic

Use Treatment of the following infections: Strongyloidiasis of the intestinal tract due to the nematode parasite *Strongyloides stercoralis*. Onchocerciasis due to the immature form of the nematode parasite *Onchocerca volvulus*

Unlabeled Use Treatment of other parasitic infections, including *Ancylostoma braziliense, Ascaris lumbricoides, Sarcoptes scabiei* (in immunocompromised patients), *Gnathostoma spinigerum, Mansonella ozzardi, Mansonella streptocerca, Pediculus humanus capitis, Pediculus humanus corporis, Phthirus pubis, Trichuris trichiura, Wucheria bancrofti*; treatment of demodicosis due to hair follicle mites *Demodex folliculorum* and *Demodex brevis*

Pregnancy Risk Factor C

Pregnancy Considerations Teratogenic effects have been observed in animal reproduction studies; therefore, the manufacturer classifies ivermectin as pregnancy category C. Ivermectin is not recommended for use in pregnancy. Although studies during pregnancy are limited, several mass treatment programs have not identified an increased risk of adverse fetal, neonatal, or maternal outcomes following ivermectin use in the first and second trimesters.

Breast-Feeding Considerations Ivermectin is measurable in low concentrations in breast milk and is less than maternal plasma concentrations. Peak concentrations of ivermectin in breast milk may occur 4-12 hours after the oral dose. In one study, the calculated infant daily dose was 2.75 mcg/kg in a 1-month-old infant and would not be expected to cause adverse effects in the infant. The manufacturer and the CDC do not have safety data in children <15 kg and the CDC does not recommend the use of ivermectin in lactating women.

Contraindications Hypersensitivity to ivermectin or any component of the formulation

Warnings/Precautions Data have shown that antihelmintic drugs like ivermectin may cause cutaneous and/or systemic reactions (Mazzoti reaction) of varying severity including ophthalmological reactions in patients with onchocerciasis. These reactions are probably due to allergic and inflammatory responses to the death of microfilariae. Patients with hyper-reactive onchodermatitis may be more likely than others to experience severe adverse reactions, especially edema and aggravation of the onchodermatitis. Repeated treatment may be required in immunocompromised patients (eg, HIV); control of extraintestinal strongyloidiasis may necessitate suppressive (once monthly) therapy. Pretreatment assessment for *Loa loa* infection is recommended in any patient with significant exposure to endemic areas (West and Central Africa); serious and/or fatal encephalopathy has been reported (rarely) during treatment in patients with loiasis. Ivermectin has no activity against adult *Onchocerca volvulus* parasites.

Adverse Reactions

>10%: Miscellaneous: Mazzotti-type reaction (with onchocerciasis): Pruritus (28%), fever (23%), skin involvement (23%; including edema/urticarial rash), lymph node tenderness (1% to 14%), lymph node enlargement (3% to 13%), arthralgia/synovitis (9%)

1% to 10%:

Cardiovascular: Tachycardia (4%), peripheral edema (3%), facial edema (1%), orthostatic hypotension (1%)

Central nervous system: Dizziness (3%)

Dermatologic: Pruritus (3%)

Gastrointestinal: Diarrhea (2%), nausea (2%)

Hematologic: Eosinophilia (3%), leukocytes decreased (3%), hemoglobin increased (1%)

Hepatic: ALT increased (2%), AST increased (2%)

<1% (Limited to important or life-threatening): Abdominal distention, abdominal pain, anemia, anorexia, anterior uveitis, asthma exacerbation, back pain, bilirubin increased, chest discomfort, chorioretinitis, choroiditis, coma, confusion, conjunctival hemorrhage (associated with onchocerciasis), conjunctivitis, constipation, dyspnea, encephalopathy (rare; associated with loiasis), eyelid edema, eye sensation abnormal, fatigue, fecal incontinence, headache, hepatitis, hypotension, INR increased (with concomitant warfarin), keratitis, lethargy, leukopenia, mental status changes, myalgia, neck pain, rash, red eye, seizure, somnolence, standing/walking difficulty, Stevens-Johnson syndrome, stupor, toxic epidermal necrolysis, tremor, urinary incontinence, urticaria, vertigo, vision loss (transient), vomiting, weakness

Drug Interactions

Metabolism/Transport Effects Substrate of CYP3A4 (minor), P-glycoprotein; **Note:** Assignment of Major/Minor substrate status based on clinically relevant drug interaction potential

Avoid Concomitant Use

Avoid concomitant use of Ivermectin (Systemic) with any of the following: BCG

Increased Effect/Toxicity

Ivermectin (Systemic) may increase the levels/effects of: Vitamin K Antagonists

The levels/effects of Ivermectin (Systemic) may be increased by: Azithromycin (Systemic); P-glycoprotein/ABCB1 Inhibitors

Decreased Effect

Ivermectin (Systemic) may decrease the levels/effects of: BCG; Sodium Picosulfate; Typhoid Vaccine

The levels/effects of Ivermectin (Systemic) may be decreased by: P-glycoprotein/ABCB1 Inducers

Ethanol/Nutrition/Herb Interactions Food: Bioavailability is increased 2.5-fold when administered following a high-fat meal.

Storage/Stability Store at <30°C (86°F).

Mechanism of Action Ivermectin is a semisynthetic anthelminthic agent; it binds selectively and with strong affinity to glutamate-gated chloride ion channels which occur in invertebrate nerve and muscle cells. This leads to increased permeability of cell membranes to chloride ions then hyperpolarization of the nerve or muscle cell, and death of the parasite.

Pharmacodynamics/Kinetics

Onset of action:

Peak effect in treatment of onchocerciasis: 3-6 months

Peak effect in treatment of strongyloides: 3 months

Absorption: Well absorbed

Distribution: V_d: 3-3.5 L/kg (healthy males); does not cross blood-brain barrier

Protein binding: ~93%

Metabolism: Hepatic via CYP3A4 (major), CYP2D6 (minor), and CYP2E1 (minor)

Bioavailability: Increased with high-fat meal

Half-life elimination: ~18 hours

Time to peak, serum: ~4 hours

Excretion: Feces; urine (<1%)

Dosage

Onchocerciasis: Children ≥15 kg and Adults: Oral: 150 mcg/kg as a single dose; retreatment may be required every 3-12 months until asymptomatic

Strongyloidiasis: Children ≥15 kg and Adults: Oral:

Manufacturer recommendations: 200 mcg/kg as a single dose; perform follow-up stool examinations.

Alternative dosing: 200 mcg/kg/day for 2 days (CDC, 2012)

Ascariasis due to *Ascaris lumbricoides* (unlabeled use): Children ≥15 kg and Adults: Oral: 200 mcg/kg as a single dose (Marti, 1996; Naquira, 1989)

Cutaneous larva migrans (CLM) due to *Ancylostoma braziliense* (unlabeled use): Children ≥15 kg and Adults: Oral: 200 mcg/kg as a single dose (Vanhaecke, 2013)

Demodicosis due to *Demodex folliculorum* and *Demodex brevis* (unlabeled use): Children ≥15 kg and Adults: Oral: 200 mcg/kg as a single dose, followed by topical permethrin (Eismann, 2010)

Filariasis due to *Mansonella ozzardi* (unlabeled use): Adults: Oral: 6 mg as a single dose (Gonzales, 1999)

Filariasis due to *Mansonella streptocerca* (unlabeled use): Children ≥15 kg and Adults: Oral: 150 mcg/kg as a single dose (Fischer, 1997)

Filariasis due to *Wucheria bancrofti* (unlabeled use): Children ≥15 kg and Adults: Oral: 200-400 mcg/kg as a single dose in combination with albendazole (Addiss, 1997; Ismail, 2001)

Gnathostomiasis due to *Gnathostoma spinigerum* (unlabeled use): Children ≥15 kg and Adults: Oral: 200 mcg/kg as a single dose (Nontasut, 2000; Kraivichian, 2004)

Lice due to *Pediculus humanus capitis, Pediculus humanus corporis, Phthirus pubis* (unlabeled use): Children ≥15 kg and Adults: Oral: 200 mcg/kg/dose; generally requires >1 dose; number of doses and dosage intervals have not been established

Pediculus humanus capitis: Children ≥15 kg and Adults: Oral: 400 mcg/kg/dose every 7 days for 2 doses (Chosidow, 2010)

Pediculus humanus corporis: Children ≥15 kg and Adults: Oral: 200 mcg/kg/dose every 7 days for 3 doses (Foucault, 2006)

Phthirus pubis: Children ≥15 kg and Adults: Oral: 250 mcg/kg/dose every 7 days for 2 doses (Burkhart, 2004)

Scabies due to *Sarcoptes scabiei* in immunocompromised patients (unlabeled use): Children ≥15 kg and Adults: Oral: 200 mcg/kg as a single dose; may repeat dose in 14 days (Meinking, 1995). **Note:** Preferred drug for immunocompromised patients with crusted scabies.

Trichuriasis due to *Trichuris trichiura* (unlabeled use): Children ≥15 kg and Adults: Oral: 200 mcg/kg as a single dose on day 1; may repeat dose on day 4 (Naquira, 1989)

Dosage adjustment in renal impairment: No dosage adjustment provided in manufacturer's labeling.

Dosage adjustment in hepatic impairment: No dosage adjustment provided in manufacturer's labeling.

Dietary Considerations Take on an empty stomach with water.

Administration Administer on an empty stomach with water.

Monitoring Parameters Skin and eye microfilarial counts, periodic ophthalmologic exams; follow up stool examinations

Dosage Forms Excipient information presented when available (limited, particularly for generics); consult specific product labeling.

Tablet, Oral:

Stromectol: 3 mg

Ivermectin (Topical) (eye ver MEK tin)

Brand Names: U.S. Sklice

Pharmacologic Category Antiparasitic Agent, Topical; Pediculocide

Use Topical treatment of head lice (*Pediculus capitis*) infestation

Pregnancy Risk Factor C

Pregnancy Considerations Teratogenic effects have been observed in animal reproduction studies following oral administration. Refer to the Ivermectin (Systemic) monograph for additional information. Systemic absorption is less following topical application than with oral administration.

Breast-Feeding Considerations Following oral administration, ivermectin is measurable in low concentrations in breast milk. Refer to Ivermectin (Systemic) monograph for additional information. Systemic absorption is less following topical application than with oral administration.

Contraindications There are no contraindications listed in the manufacturer's labeling.

Warnings/Precautions For topical use on scalp and scalp hair only; avoid contact with eyes. Wash hands after application.

Adverse Reactions <1% (Limited to important or life-threatening): Burning sensation on skin, conjunctivitis, dandruff, dry skin, eye irritation, ocular hyperemia

Drug Interactions

Metabolism/Transport Effects None known.

Avoid Concomitant Use There are no known interactions where it is recommended to avoid concomitant use.

Increased Effect/Toxicity There are no known significant interactions involving an increase in effect.

Decreased Effect There are no known significant interactions involving a decrease in effect.

Storage/Stability Store at 20°C to 25°C (68°F to 77°F); excursions permitted between 15°C to 30°C (59°F to 86°F); do not freeze.

Mechanism of Action Ivermectin is a semisynthetic anthelminthic agent; it binds selectively and with strong affinity to glutamate-gated chloride ion channels which occur in invertebrate nerve and muscle cells. This leads to increased permeability of cell membranes to chloride ions then hyperpolarization of the nerve or muscle cell, and death of the parasite.

Dosage Topical: Children ≥6 months and Adults: Head Lice: Apply sufficient amount (up to 1 tube) to completely cover dry scalp and hair; for single-dose use only

Administration Topical lotion. For external use only. Apply to dry scalp and hair closest to scalp first, then apply outward towards ends of hair; completely covering scalp and hair. Leave on for 10 minutes (start timing treatment after the scalp and hair have been completely covered). The hair should then be rinsed thoroughly with warm water. Avoid contact with the eyes. Nit combing is not required, although a fine-tooth comb may be used to remove treated lice and nits. Lotion is for one-time use; discard any unused portion.

Ivermectin should be a portion of a whole lice removal program, which should include washing or dry cleaning all clothing, hats, bedding, and towels recently worn or used by the patient and washing combs, brushes, and hair accessories in hot soapy water.

Monitoring Parameters Monitor scalp for live lice.

Dosage Forms Excipient information presented when available (limited, particularly for generics); consult specific product labeling.

Lotion, External:

Sklice: 0.5% (117 g) [contains methylparaben, propylparaben]

- **IVIG** *see* Immune Globulin *on page 1059*
- **IV Immune Globulin** *see* Immune Globulin *on page 1059*
- **Ivy Block [OTC]** *see* Bentoquatam *on page 240*
- **Ivy-Rid [OTC]** *see* Benzocaine *on page 240*

Ixabepilone (ix ab EP i lone)

Brand Names: U.S. Ixempra Kit

Index Terms Azaepothilone B; BMS-247550; Epothilone B Lactam

Pharmacologic Category Antineoplastic Agent, Antimicrotubular; Antineoplastic Agent, Epothilone B Analog

Use Treatment of metastatic or locally-advanced breast cancer (refractory or resistant)

Unlabeled Use Treatment (second-line) of endometrial cancer

Pregnancy Risk Factor D

Pregnancy Considerations In animal studies, ixabepilone caused maternal toxicity and embryo/fetal toxicity at doses ~1/10 the human dose. There are no adequate and well-controlled studies in pregnant women. Women of childbearing potential should be advised to use effective contraception during treatment.

Breast-Feeding Considerations Due to the potential for serious adverse reactions in the nursing infant, breast-feeding is not recommended.

Contraindications History of severe hypersensitivity to polyoxyethylated castor oil or its derivatives (eg, Cremophor® EL); neutrophil count <1500/mm^3 or platelet count <100,000/mm^3; combination therapy with ixabepilone and capecitabine in patients with AST or ALT >2.5 times ULN or bilirubin >1 times ULN

Warnings/Precautions Hazardous agent - use appropriate precautions for handling and disposal (NIOSH, 2012). **[U.S. Boxed Warning]: Due to increased risk of toxicity and neutropenia-related mortality, combination therapy with capecitabine is contraindicated in patients with AST or ALT >2.5 times ULN or bilirubin >1 times ULN.** Use (as monotherapy) is not recommended if AST or ALT >10 times ULN or bilirubin >3 times ULN; use caution in patients with AST or ALT >5 times ULN. Toxicities and serious adverse reactions are increased (in mono- and combination therapy) with hepatic dysfunction; dosage reductions are necessary. Diluent contains Cremophor® EL, which is associated with hypersensitivity reactions; use is contraindicated in patients with a history of severe hypersensitivity to Cremophor® EL or its derivatives. Medications for the treatment of reaction should be available for immediate use; reactions may also be managed with a reduction of infusion rate. Premedicate with an H_1- and H_2-antagonist 1 hour prior to infusion; patients who experience hypersensitivity (eg, bronchospasm, dyspnea, flushing, rash) should also be premedicated with a corticosteroid for all subsequent cycles if treatment is continued.

Dose-dependent myelosuppression, particularly neutropenia, may occur with mono- or combination therapy. Neutropenic fever and infection have been reported with use. The risk for neutropenia is increased with hepatic dysfunction, especially when used in combination with capecitabine. Severe neutropenia and/or thrombocytopenia may require dosage adjustment and/or treatment delay. Peripheral (sensory and motor) neuropathy occurs commonly; may require dose reductions, treatment delays or discontinuation. Usually occurs during the first 3 cycles. Use with caution in patients with pre-existing neuropathy. Patients with diabetes may have an increased risk for severe peripheral neuropathy. Use with caution in patients with a history of cardiovascular disease; the incidence of MI, ventricular dysfunction, and supraventricular arrhythmias is higher when ixabepilone is used in combination with capecitabine (as compared to capecitabine alone). Consider discontinuing ixabepilone in patients who develop cardiac ischemia or impaired cardiac function.

Avoid concurrent use with strong CYP3A4 inhibitors (eg, itraconazole, ketoconazole, voriconazole, clarithromycin, telithromycin, nefazodone, amprenavir, atazanavir, delavirdine, indinavir, nelfinavir, ritonavir, saquinavir); dosage reductions are recommended if concurrent use cannot be avoided; allow ~1 week to elapse prior to adjusting ixabepilone dose upward after a strong CYP3A4 inhibitor is discontinued. Avoid strong CYP3A4 inducers (eg, dexamethasone, phenytoin, carbamazepine, rifampin, phenobarbital); may decrease the ixabepilone level; alternative agents should be considered; dosage increases of ixabepilone (with careful monitoring) may be recommended if concomitant administration with CYP3A4 inducers cannot be avoided. Due to the ethanol content in the diluent, may cause cognitive impairment; patients must be cautioned about performing tasks which require mental alertness (eg, operating machinery or driving). Toxicities or serious adverse events with combination therapy may be increased in the elderly.

Adverse Reactions

Percentages reported with monotherapy:

>10%:

Central nervous system: Headache (11%)

Dermatologic: Alopecia (48%)

Gastrointestinal: Nausea (42%), vomiting (29%), mucositis/stomatitis (29%), diarrhea (22%), anorexia (19%), constipation (16%), abdominal pain (13%)

Hematologic: Leukopenia (grade 3: 36%; grade 4: 13%), neutropenia (grade 3: 31%; grade 4: 23%)

Neuromuscular & skeletal: Peripheral neuropathy (63%; grades 3/4: 14%; grade 3/4 median onset: cycle 4), sensory neuropathy (62%; grades 3/4: 14%), weakness (56%), myalgia/arthralgia (49%), musculoskeletal pain (20%)

1% to 10%:

Cardiovascular: Edema (9%), chest pain (5%)

Central nervous system: Fever (8%), pain (8%), dizziness (7%), insomnia (5%)

Dermatologic: Nail disorder (9%), rash (9%), palmar-plantar erythrodysesthesia/hand-and-foot syndrome (8%), pruritus (6%), skin exfoliation (2%), hyperpigmentation (2%)

Endocrine & metabolic: Hot flush (6%), dehydration (2%)

Gastrointestinal: Gastroesophageal reflux disease (6%), taste perversion (6%), weight loss (6%)

Hematologic: Anemia (grade 3: 6%; grade 4: 2%), neutropenic fever (3%; grade 3: 3%), thrombocytopenia (grade 3: 5%; grade 4: 2%)

Neuromuscular & skeletal: Motor neuropathy (10%; grade 3: 1%)

Ocular: Lacrimation increased (4%)

Respiratory: Dyspnea (9%), upper respiratory tract infection (6%), cough (2%)

Miscellaneous: Hypersensitivity (5%; grade 3: 1%), infection (5%)

Mono- and combination therapy: <1% (Limited to important or life-threatening): Alkaline phosphatase increased, angina, atrial flutter, autonomic neuropathy, cardiomyopathy, cerebral hemorrhage, coagulopathy, colitis, dysphagia, dysphonia, embolism, enterocolitis, erythema multiforme, gastrointestinal hemorrhage, gastroparesis, GGT increased, hemorrhage, hepatic failure (acute), hypokalemia, hyponatremia, hypotension, hypovolemia, hypovolemic shock, hypoxia, ileus, interstitial pneumonia, jaundice, left ventricular dysfunction, metabolic acidosis, MI, nephrolithiasis, neutropenic infection, orthostatic hypotension, pneumonia, pneumonitis, pulmonary edema (acute), radiation recall, renal failure, respiratory failure, sepsis, septic shock, supraventricular arrhythmia, syncope, thrombosis, transaminases increased, trismus, urinary tract infection, vasculitis

Drug Interactions

Metabolism/Transport Effects Substrate of CYP3A4 (major); **Note:** Assignment of Major/Minor substrate status based on clinically relevant drug interaction potential

Avoid Concomitant Use

Avoid concomitant use of Ixabepilone with any of the following: CloZAPine; Fusidic Acid (Systemic); St Johns Wort

Increased Effect/Toxicity

Ixabepilone may increase the levels/effects of: CloZAPine

The levels/effects of Ixabepilone may be increased by: CYP3A4 Inhibitors (Moderate); CYP3A4 Inhibitors (Strong); Dasatinib; Fusidic Acid (Systemic); Ivacaftor; Luliconazole; Mifepristone; Simeprevir

Decreased Effect

The levels/effects of Ixabepilone may be decreased by: Bosentan; CYP3A4 Inducers (Strong); Dabrafenib; Deferasirox; St Johns Wort; Tocilizumab

Ethanol/Nutrition/Herb Interactions

Food: Grapefruit juice may increase plasma concentrations of ixabepilone. Management: Avoid grapefruit juice.

Herb/Nutraceutical: St John's wort may decrease ixabepilone levels. Management: Avoid St John's wort.

Preparation for Administration Hazardous agent; use appropriate precautions for handling and disposal (NIOSH, 2012). Allow to reach room temperature for ~30 minutes prior to reconstitution. Diluent vial may contain a white precipitate which should dissolve upon reaching room temperature. **Reconstitute only with the provided diluent.** Dilute the 15 mg vial with 8 mL and the 45 mg vial with 23.5 mL (using provided diluent) to a concentration of 2 mg/mL (contains overfill). Gently swirl and invert vial until dissolved completely. Prior to administration, further dilute using a non-DEHP container (eg, glass, polypropylene or polyolefin), to a final concentration of 0.2-0.6 mg/mL in ~250 mL lactated Ringer's, adjusted sodium chloride 0.9% (pH adjusted prior to ixabepilone addition with 2 mEq sodium bicarbonate per 250-500 mL sodium chloride) or PLASMA-LYTE A Injection pH 7.4®. Mix thoroughly.

Storage/Stability Store intact vials under refrigeration at 2°C to 8°C (36°F to 46°F); protect from light. Reconstituted solution (in the vial) is stable for 1 hour at room temperature; infusion solution diluted in appropriate solution for infusion is stable for 6 hours at room temperature if a pH range of 6-9 is maintained.

Mechanism of Action Epothilone B analog; binds to the beta-tubulin subunit of the microtubule, stabilizing microtubular promoting tubulin polymerization and stabilizing microtubular function, thus arresting the cell cycle (at the G2/M phase) and inducing apoptosis. Activity in taxane-resistant cells has been demonstrated.

Pharmacodynamics/Kinetics

Distribution: >1000 L

Protein binding: 67% to 77%

Metabolism: Extensively hepatic, via CYP3A4; >30 metabolites (inactive) formed

Half-life elimination: ~52 hours

Time to peak, plasma: At the end of infusion (3 hours)

Excretion: Feces (65%; 2% of the total dose as unchanged drug); urine (21%; 6% of the total dose as unchanged drug)

Dosage Details concerning dosing in combination regimens should also be consulted. **Note:** Premedicate with an H_1-antagonist (eg, oral diphenhydramine 50 mg) and H_2-antagonist (eg, oral ranitidine 150-300 mg) ~1 hour prior to infusion. Patients with a history of hypersensitivity should also be premedicated with corticosteroids (orally 1 hour before or I.V. 30 minutes before infusion). For dose calculation, body surface area (BSA) is capped at a maximum of 2.2 m^2.

I.V.: Adults:

Breast cancer (metastatic or locally advanced): 40 mg/m^2/dose over 3 hours every 3 weeks (maximum dose: 88 mg) either as monotherapy or in combination with capecitabine

Endometrial cancer (unlabeled use): 40 mg/m^2/dose over 3 hours every 3 weeks (Dizon, 2009)

Dosage adjustment with concomitant strong CYP3A4 inhibitors/inducers:

CYP3A4 inhibitors: Avoid concomitant administration with strong CYP3A4 inhibitors; if concomitant administration with a strong CYP3A4 inhibitor cannot be avoided, consider a dose reduction to 20 mg/m^2. When a strong CYP3A4 inhibitor is discontinued, allow ~1 week to elapse prior to adjusting ixabepilone dose upward to the indicated dose.

CYP3A4 inducers: Avoid concomitant administration with strong CYP3A4 inducers; if concomitant administration with a strong CYP3A4 inducer cannot be avoided and after maintenance on the strong CYP3A4 inducer is established, consider adjusting the ixabepilone dose gradually up to 60 mg/m^2 (as a 4-hour infusion), with careful monitoring. If the strong CYP3A4 enzyme inducer is discontinued, reduce ixabepilone dose to the dose used prior to initiation of the CYP3A4 inducer.

Ixabepilone dosage adjustments for toxicity for monotherapy or combination therapy:

Hematologic:

Neutrophils <500/mm^3 for ≥7 days: Reduce dose by 20%

Neutropenic fever: Reduce dose by 20%

Platelets <25,000/mm^3 (or <50,000/mm^3 with bleeding): Reduce dose by 20%

Nonhematologic:

Neuropathy:

Grade 2 (moderate) for ≥7 days: Reduce dose by 20%

Grade 3 (severe) for <7 days: Reduce dose by 20%

Grade 3 (severe or disabling) for ≥7 days: Discontinue treatment

Grade 3 toxicity (severe; other than neuropathy): Reduce dose by 20%

Grade 3 arthralgia/myalgia or fatigue (transient): Continue at current dose

Grade 3 hand-foot syndrome: Continue at current dose

Grade 4 toxicity (disabling): Discontinue treatment

Note: Adjust dosage at the start of a cycle are based on toxicities (hematologic and nonhematologic) from the previous cycle; delay new cycles until neutrophils have recovered to ≥1500/mm^3, platelets have recovered to ≥100,000/mm^3 and nonhematologic toxicities have resolved or improved to at least grade 1. If toxicities persist despite initial dose reduction, reduce dose an additional 20%.

Capecitabine dosage adjustments for toxicity in combination therapy with ixabepilone:

Hematologic:

Neutrophils <500/mm^3 for ≥7 days or neutropenic fever: Hold for concurrent diarrhea or stomatitis until neutrophils recover to >1000/mm^3, then continue at same dose

Platelets <25,000/mm^3 (or <50,000/mm^3 with bleeding): Hold for concurrent diarrhea or stomatitis until platelets recover to >50,000/mm^3, then continue at same dose

Nonhematologic: Refer to Capecitabine monograph.

Dosage adjustment in renal impairment: Pharmacokinetics (monotherapy) are not affected in patients with mild-to-moderate renal insufficiency (Cl_{cr} >30 mL/minute); monotherapy has not been studied in patients with serum creatinine >1.5 times ULN. Combination therapy with capecitabine has not been studied in patients with Cl_{cr} <50 mL/minute.

Dosage adjustment in hepatic impairment:

Ixabepilone monotherapy (initial cycle; adjust doses for subsequent cycles based on toxicity):

AST and ALT ≤2.5 times ULN and bilirubin ≤1 times ULN: No adjustment necessary

AST and ALT >2.5 to ≤10 times ULN and bilirubin >1 to ≤1.5 times ULN: Reduce dose to 32 mg/m^2

AST and ALT ≤10 times ULN and bilirubin >1.5 to ≤3 times ULN: Reduce dose to 20-30 mg/m^2 (initiate treatment at 20 mg/m^2, may escalate up to a maximum of 30 mg/m^2 in subsequent cycles if tolerated)

AST or ALT >10 times ULN or bilirubin >3 times ULN: Use is not recommended

Combination therapy of ixabepilone with capecitabine:

AST and ALT ≤2.5 times ULN and bilirubin ≤1 times ULN: No adjustment necessary

AST or ALT >2.5 times ULN or bilirubin >1 times ULN: Use is contraindicated

Dosing in obesity: *ASCO Guidelines for appropriate chemotherapy dosing in obese adults with cancer:* In general, utilize patient's actual body weight (full weight) for calculation of body surface area- or weight-based dosing, particularly when the intent of therapy is curative; manage regimen-related toxicities in the same manner as for nonobese patients; if a dose reduction is utilized due to toxicity, consider resumption of full weight-based dosing with subsequent cycles, especially if cause of toxicity (eg, hepatic or renal impairment) is resolved (Griggs, 2012). **Note:** According to the manufacturer, patients with a body surface area (BSA) >2.2 m^2 should be dosed based upon a maximum BSA of 2.2 m^2

Dietary Considerations Avoid grapefruit juice (may increase plasma concentrations of ixabepilone).

Administration I.V.: Infuse over 3 hours. Use non-DEHP administration set (eg, polyethylene); filter with a 0.2-1.2 micron inline filter. Administration should be completed within 6 hours of preparation. If the dose is increased (above 40 mg/m^2) due to concomitant CYP3A4 inducer use, infuse over 4 hours.

Hazardous agent; use appropriate precautions for handling and disposal (NIOSH, 2012).

Monitoring Parameters CBC with differential; hepatic function (ALT, AST, bilirubin); monitor for hypersensitivity, neuropathy

Dosage Forms Excipient information presented when available (limited, particularly for generics); consult specific product labeling.

Solution Reconstituted, Intravenous:

Ixempra Kit: 15 mg (1 ea); 45 mg (1 ea) [contains alcohol, usp, cremophor el]

- ◆ **Ixempra Kit** *see* Ixabepilone *on page 1139*
- ◆ **Ixiaro** *see* Japanese Encephalitis Virus Vaccine (Inactivated) *on page 1142*
- ◆ **Jakafi** *see* Ruxolitinib *on page 1867*
- ◆ **Jakavi™ (Can)** *see* Ruxolitinib *on page 1867*
- ◆ **Jalyn** *see* Dutasteride and Tamsulosin *on page 681*
- ◆ **JAMP-ACET-Tramadol (Can)** *see* Acetaminophen and Tramadol *on page 33*
- ◆ **JAMP-Alendronate (Can)** *see* Alendronate *on page 69*
- ◆ **JAMP-Amlodipine (Can)** *see* AmLODIPine *on page 109*
- ◆ **JAMP-Anastrozole (Can)** *see* Anastrozole *on page 137*
- ◆ **JAMP-Atenolol (Can)** *see* Atenolol *on page 186*
- ◆ **JAMP-Bicalutamide (Can)** *see* Bicalutamide *on page 258*
- ◆ **JAMP-Candesartan (Can)** *see* Candesartan *on page 327*
- ◆ **JAMP-Carvedilol (Can)** *see* Carvedilol *on page 355*
- ◆ **JAMP-Ciprofloxacin (Can)** *see* Ciprofloxacin (Systemic) *on page 430*
- ◆ **JAMP-Citalopram (Can)** *see* Citalopram *on page 440*
- ◆ **Jamp-Colchicine (Can)** *see* Colchicine *on page 485*
- ◆ **JAMP-Cyclobenzaprine (Can)** *see* Cyclobenzaprine *on page 502*
- ◆ **Jamp-Dicyclomine (Can)** *see* Dicyclomine *on page 601*
- ◆ **Jamp-Dimenhydrinate [OTC] (Can)** *see* DimenhyDRINATE *on page 616*
- ◆ **JAMP-Finasteride (Can)** *see* Finasteride *on page 862*
- ◆ **JAMP-Fluoxetine (Can)** *see* FLUoxetine *on page 885*
- ◆ **Jamp-Fosinopril (Can)** *see* Fosinopril *on page 923*
- ◆ **JAMP-Gabapentin (Can)** *see* Gabapentin *on page 933*
- ◆ **JAMP-Indapamide (Can)** *see* Indapamide *on page 1066*
- ◆ **JAMP-Letrozole (Can)** *see* Letrozole *on page 1185*
- ◆ **JAMP-Levetiracetam (Can)** *see* LevETIRAcetam *on page 1194*
- ◆ **JAMP-Lisinopril (Can)** *see* Lisinopril *on page 1226*
- ◆ **JAMP-Losartan (Can)** *see* Losartan *on page 1247*
- ◆ **JAMP-Metformin (Can)** *see* MetFORMIN *on page 1310*
- ◆ **JAMP-Metformin Blackberry (Can)** *see* MetFORMIN *on page 1310*
- ◆ **JAMP-Metoprolol-L (Can)** *see* Metoprolol *on page 1348*
- ◆ **Jamp-Mirtazapine (Can)** *see* Mirtazapine *on page 1379*
- ◆ **Jamp-Montelukast (Can)** *see* Montelukast *on page 1396*
- ◆ **JAMP-Mycophenolate (Can)** *see* Mycophenolate *on page 1407*
- ◆ **JAMP-Ondansetron (Can)** *see* Ondansetron *on page 1510*
- ◆ **JAMP-Paroxetine (Can)** *see* PARoxetine *on page 1575*
- ◆ **JAMP-Pioglitazone (Can)** *see* Pioglitazone *on page 1649*
- ◆ **JAMP-Pravastatin (Can)** *see* Pravastatin *on page 1700*
- ◆ **JAMP-Quetiapine (Can)** *see* QUEtiapine *on page 1757*
- ◆ **JAMP-Ramipril (Can)** *see* Ramipril *on page 1778*
- ◆ **JAMP-Risperidone (Can)** *see* RisperiDONE *on page 1826*
- ◆ **JAMP-Rizatriptan (Can)** *see* Rizatriptan *on page 1844*
- ◆ **JAMP-Ropinirole (Can)** *see* ROPINIRole *on page 1851*
- ◆ **Jamp-Rosuvastatin (Can)** *see* Rosuvastatin *on page 1858*
- ◆ **JAMP-Sertraline (Can)** *see* Sertraline *on page 1889*
- ◆ **JAMP-Simvastatin (Can)** *see* Simvastatin *on page 1899*
- ◆ **JAMP-Tamsulosin (Can)** *see* Tamsulosin *on page 1990*
- ◆ **JAMP-Terbinafine (Can)** *see* Terbinafine (Systemic) *on page 2017*
- ◆ **Jantoven** *see* Warfarin *on page 2211*
- ◆ **Janumet** *see* Sitagliptin and Metformin *on page 1907*
- ◆ **Janumet XR** *see* Sitagliptin and Metformin *on page 1907*
- ◆ **Januvia** *see* SitaGLIPtin *on page 1906*
- ◆ **Januvia® (Can)** *see* SitaGLIPtin *on page 1906*

Japanese Encephalitis Virus Vaccine (Inactivated)

(jap a NEESE en sef a LYE tis VYE rus vak SEEN, in ak ti VAY ted)

Brand Names: U.S. Ixiaro

Brand Names: Canada Ixiaro

Index Terms IC51; JE-VC (Ixiaro)

Pharmacologic Category Vaccine, Inactivated (Viral)

Additional Appendix Information

Immunization Administration Recommendations *on page 2334*

Immunization Recommendations *on page 2339*

Use Japanese encephalitis vaccination: For active immunization against Japanese encephalitis (JE) for persons 2 months of age and older

The Advisory Committee on Immunization Practices (ACIP) recommends vaccination for (CDC, 2010; CDC, 2013):

- Persons spending ≥1 month in endemic areas during transmission season
- Research laboratory workers who may be exposed to the Japanese encephalitis virus

Vaccination should also be considered for the following:

- Travelers to areas with an ongoing outbreak
- Travelers spending <30 days in endemic areas during the transmission season and planning to go outside of urban areas and have an increased risk of exposure. For example, high-risk activities include extensive outdoor activity in rural areas especially at night; extensive outdoor activities such as camping, hiking, etc; staying in accommodations without air conditioning, screens or bed nets.
- Travelers to endemic areas who are unsure of specific destination, activities, or duration of travel

Japanese encephalitis vaccine is not recommended for short-term travelers whose visit will be restricted to urban areas or periods outside of the well-defined JE virus transmission season.

Pregnancy Risk Factor B

Pregnancy Considerations Adverse events were not observed in animal reproduction studies. Risks of vaccine administration should be carefully considered and in general, pregnant women should only be vaccinated if they are at high risk for exposure. Infection from Japanese encephalitis during the first or second trimesters of pregnancy may increase risk of miscarriage. Intrauterine transmission of the Japanese encephalitis virus has been reported (CDC, 2010). To report inadvertent use of Ixiaro® during pregnancy, contact Novartis Vaccines (877-683-4732).

Breast-Feeding Considerations It is not known if the vaccine is excreted into breast milk; however, the ACIP does not consider breast-feeding to be a contraindication to (CDC, 2010). The manufacturer recommends that caution be used if administered to nursing women.

Contraindications

U.S. labeling: Severe allergic reaction to a previous dose of the vaccine, any other Japanese encephalitis virus vaccine, or any component of the vaccine, including protamine sulfate

Canadian labeling: Hypersensitivity to a previous dose of the vaccine or to any component of the formulation; acute severe febrile conditions

Warnings/Precautions Because of the potential for severe adverse reactions, Japanese encephalitis vaccine is not recommended for all persons traveling to or residing in Asia. Use is not recommended for short-term travelers (<30 days) who will not be outside of an urban area or when the visit is outside of a well-defined Japanese encephalitis virus transmission season. Risk of exposure to the Japanese encephalitis virus may vary from year to year for a particular area. Immediate treatment for anaphylactic/anaphylactoid reaction should be available during vaccine use (CDC, 2010).

Use of vaccine should also include other means to reduce the risk of mosquito exposure (bed nets, insect repellents, protective clothing, avoidance of travel in endemic areas, and avoidance of outdoor activity during twilight and evening periods) (CDC, 2010).

May contain protamine sulfate which may cause hypersensitivity reactions in certain individuals. Immunization should be completed ≥7 days prior to potential exposure.

In general, the decision to administer or delay vaccination because of current or recent febrile illness depends on the severity of symptoms and the etiology of the disease. Immunocompromised patients may have a reduced response to vaccines; information not available specific to this vaccine. In general, household and close contacts of persons with altered immunocompetence may receive all age appropriate vaccines. Vaccination may not result in effective immunity in all patients. Response depends upon multiple factors (eg, type of vaccine, age of patient) and may be improved by administering the vaccine at the recommended dose, route, and interval. Vaccines may not be effective if administered during periods of altered immune competence (CDC 60[2], 2011). In order to maximize vaccination rates, the ACIP recommends simultaneous administration of all age-appropriate vaccines (live or inactivated) for which a person is eligible at a single clinic visit, unless contraindications exist (CDC 60[2], 2011). Canadian labeling recommends avoiding I.M. administration in patients with bleeding disorders (eg, thrombocytopenia, hemophilia) and suggests that SubQ administration may be considered in these patients. Clinical efficacy data regarding this route is lacking and the U.S. labeling does not recommend SubQ administration.

Adverse Reactions Report allergic or unusual adverse reactions to the Vaccine Adverse Event Reporting System (VAERS) 1-800-822-7967 or online at https://vaers.hhs.gov/esub/index. In Canada, adverse reactions may be reported to local provincial/territorial health agencies or to the Vaccine Safety Section at Public Health Agency of Canada (1-866-844-0018).

Percentage of adverse reactions reported over days 0-56 in adults and 0-7 in pediatric patients. In general, incidence decreased with subsequent dosing.

>10%:

Central nervous system: Headache (adults 28%; infants, children, and adolescents 2% to 5%), irritability (infants and children <3 years 8% to 15%; children ≥3 years and adolescents ≤2%), fatigue (adults 11%; infants, children, and adolescents 2% to 3%)

Gastrointestinal: Diarrhea (infants and children <3 years 7% to 12%; children ≥3 years, adolescents, and adults <1% to 2%)

Local: Tenderness at injection site (adults 36%; children ≥3 years and adolescents 4% to 10%; infants and children <3 years 3%), pain at injection site (adults 33%; children ≥3 years and adolescents 6% to 15%; infants and children <3 years 4%), erythema at injection site (infants and children <3 years 6% to 18%; adults 10%; children ≥3 years and adolescents ≤3%)

Neuromuscular & skeletal: Myalgia (adults 16%; infants, children, and adolescents 2% to 3%)

Respiratory: Flu-like symptoms (adults 12%; infants, children, and adolescents 1% to 8%)

Miscellaneous: Fever (infants and children <3 years 20% to 24%; children ≥3 years and adolescents 4% to 11%; adults 3%)

1% to 10%:

Dermatologic: Skin rash (infants and children <3 years 4% to 8%; children ≥3 years, adolescents, and adults ≤1%)

Gastrointestinal: Nausea (adults 7%, infants, children, and adolescents ≤2%), vomiting (infants and children <3 years 4% to 8%; children ≥3 years, adolescents, and adults 1% to 2%), decreased appetite (infants, children, and adolescents 1% to 6%)

Infection: Influenza (adults ≥1%)

Local: Induration at injection site (adults 8%; infants, children, and adolescents ≤1%), swelling at injection site (≤2% to 4%), itching at injection site (adults 4%; infants, children, and adolescents ≤1%)

Neuromuscular & skeletal: Back pain (adults 1%)

Respiratory: Nasopharyngitis (adults 5%), pharyngolaryngeal pain (adults 2%), upper respiratory tract infection (adults 2%), sinusitis (adults ≥1%), cough (adults 1%), rhinitis (adults 1%)

Miscellaneous: Febrile seizures (children <3 years 1%)

<1%, postmarketing, and/or case reports (Limited to important or life-threatening): Appendicitis, cerebral infarction, chest pain, dermatomyositis, disseminated intravascular coagulation, encephalitis, epilepsy, herpes zoster, iritis, labyrinthitis, limb abscess, limb pain, musculoskeletal injury, neuritis, oropharyngeal spasm, ovarian torsion, paresthesia, rectal hemorrhage, rupture of ovarian cyst, seizure, syncope

Drug Interactions

Metabolism/Transport Effects None known.

Avoid Concomitant Use There are no known interactions where it is recommended to avoid concomitant use.

Increased Effect/Toxicity There are no known significant interactions involving an increase in effect.

Decreased Effect

The levels/effects of Japanese Encephalitis Virus Vaccine (Inactivated) may be decreased by: Belimumab; Fingolimod; Immunosuppressants

Storage/Stability Store in original packaging under refrigeration at 2°C to 8°C (35°F to 46°F); do not freeze. Protect from light.

Mechanism of Action This vaccine induces antibodies to neutralize the Japanese encephalitis virus. Antibody response is measured using a 50% plaque-reduction neutralization antibody test ($PRNT_{50}$); a threshold of ≥1:10 is considered protective immunity.

Pharmacodynamics/Kinetics

Onset: Protective immunity was observed in ~21% of adults 10 days after the first vaccine dose and in 96% to 100% of children and adults 28 days after the second vaccine dose.

Duration: Protective immunity was observed in ~80% to 85% of adults 12-36 months after the initiation of the two-dose series.

Dosage U.S. recommended primary immunization schedule:

Children 2 months to <3 years: I.M.: 0.25 mL/dose; a total of 2 doses given on days 0 and 28. Series should be completed at least 1 week prior to potential exposure.

Children ≥3 years, Adolescents, and Adults: I.M.: 0.5 mL/dose; a total of 2 doses given on days 0 and 28. Series should be completed at least 1 week prior to potential exposure.

Booster dose: Adults ≥17 years: Booster dose may be given prior to potential re-exposure if the primary series was completed >1 year previously. The safety of booster doses in children and adolescents <17 years has not been established.

Note: If the second dose is missed, limited data from one clinical trial in adults demonstrate a 99% seroconversion rate when the second dose was administered 11 months after the initial dose.

Elderly: Refer to adult dosing.

Dosage adjustment in renal impairment: No dosage adjustment provided in manufacturer's labeling.

Dosage adjustment in hepatic impairment: No dosage adjustment provided in manufacturer's labeling.

Administration For I.M. injection. Do not inject I.V., SubQ, or intradermally. Shake well prior to use to form a homogeneous suspension. Do not use if discolored or if particulate matter remains.

When administering to children 2-11 months of age, the preferred site for administration is the anterolateral aspect of the thigh; for children 1 to <3 years of age, the anterolateral aspect of the thigh or deltoid muscle may be used (if mass is adequate); the deltoid muscle is the preferred site in children ≥3 years, adolescents, and adults.

Ixiaro is available only in a prefilled syringe containing 0.5 mL. In order to administer a 0.25 mL dose in children 2 months to <3 years, first shake the syringe to form a homogenous suspension. Attach a sterile needle to the prefilled syringe and while holding the syringe upright, discard 0.25 mL of the suspension. Attach a new sterile needle prior to administration.

Canadian labeling recommends avoiding I.M. administration in patients with bleeding disorders (eg, thrombocytopenia, hemophilia) and suggests that SubQ administration may be considered in these patients. Clinical efficacy data regarding this route is lacking and the U.S. labeling does not recommend SubQ administration. For patients at risk of hemorrhage following intramuscular injection, the ACIP recommends "it should be administered intramuscularly if, in the opinion of the physician familiar with the patient's bleeding risk, the vaccine can be administered by this route with reasonable safety. If the patient receives antihemophilia or other similar therapy, intramuscular vaccination can be scheduled shortly after such therapy is administered. A fine needle (23 gauge or smaller) can be used for the vaccination and firm pressure applied to the site (without rubbing) for at least 2 minutes. The patient should be instructed concerning the risk of hematoma from the injection." Patients on anticoagulant therapy should be considered to have the same bleeding risks and treated as those with clotting factor disorders (CDC 60[2], 2011).

Simultaneous administration of vaccines helps ensure the patients will be fully vaccinated by the appropriate age. Simultaneous administration of vaccines is defined as administering >1 vaccine on the same day at different anatomic sites. Separate vaccines should not be combined in the same syringe unless indicated by product specific labeling. Separate needles and syringes should be used for each injection. The ACIP prefers each dose of a specific vaccine in a series come from the same manufacturer when possible. Adolescents and adults should be vaccinated while seated or lying down. In general, preterm infants should be vaccinated at the same chronological age as full-term infants (CDC 60[2], 2011).

Antipyretics have not been shown to prevent febrile seizures. Antipyretics may be used to treat fever or discomfort following vaccination (CDC 60[2], 2011). One study reported that routine prophylactic administration of acetaminophen to prevent fever prior to vaccination decreased the immune response of some vaccines; the clinical significance of this reduction in immune response has not been established (Prymula, 2009).

Monitoring Parameters Observe patients for 30 minutes after vaccination for anaphylactic/hypersensitivity reactions and syncope

Additional Information U.S. federal law requires that the name of medication, date of administration, the vaccine manufacturer, lot number of vaccine, and the administering person's name, title, and address be entered into the patient's permanent medical record.

Ixiaro is a purified Japanese encephalitis vaccine made from the SA14-14-2 strain grown in Vero cells (JE-VC). It was developed due to neurologic side effects observed with Je-Vax, a vaccine derived from mice-brain cells (JE-MB) that contains additives which may contribute to the adverse effects (Je-Vax is no longer available in the U.S. as of May 2011). In studies comparing the two vaccines, seroconversion rates were similar following two doses of Ixiaro as opposed to three doses of Je-Vax. Safety profile of Ixiaro was found to be similar to placebo.

Adults who previously received Je-Vax vaccine and require further immunization against Japanese encephalitis should be administered a 2-dose primary series of Ixiaro (CDC, 60 [20], 2011).

Dosage Forms Excipient information presented when available (limited, particularly for generics); consult specific product labeling.

Suspension, Intramuscular:

Ixiaro: (0.5 mL) [latex free; contains albumin bovine, protamine sulfate, sodium metabisulfite]

- ◆ **Jencycla** *see* Norethindrone *on page 1472*
- ◆ **Jentadueto** *see* Linagliptin and Metformin *on page 1217*
- ◆ **Jetrea** *see* Ocriplasmin *on page 1484*
- ◆ **JE-VC (Ixiaro)** *see* Japanese Encephalitis Virus Vaccine (Inactivated) *on page 1142*
- ◆ **Jevtana** *see* Cabazitaxel *on page 307*
- ◆ **Jinteli** *see* Ethinyl Estradiol and Norethindrone *on page 793*
- ◆ **J-Max [OTC]** *see* Guaifenesin and Phenylephrine *on page 978*
- ◆ **Jock Itch Spray [OTC]** *see* Tolnaftate *on page 2087*
- ◆ **Jolessa** *see* Ethinyl Estradiol and Levonorgestrel *on page 787*
- ◆ **Jolivette** *see* Norethindrone *on page 1472*
- ◆ **J-Tan PD [OTC]** *see* Brompheniramine *on page 282*
- ◆ **Junel 1.5/30** *see* Ethinyl Estradiol and Norethindrone *on page 793*
- ◆ **Junel 1/20** *see* Ethinyl Estradiol and Norethindrone *on page 793*

Kanamycin (kan a MYE sin)

Index Terms Kanamycin Sulfate

Pharmacologic Category Antibiotic, Aminoglycoside

Use Treatment of serious infections caused by susceptible strains of *E. coli*, *Proteus* species, *Enterobacter aerogenes*, *Klebsiella pneumoniae*, *Serratia marcescens*, and *Acinetobacter* species; second-line treatment of *Mycobacterium tuberculosis*

Pregnancy Risk Factor D

Dosage Note: Dosing should be based on ideal body weight

Children: Infections: I.M., I.V.: 15 mg/kg/day in divided doses every 8-12 hours

Adults:

Infections: I.M., I.V.: 5-7.5 mg/kg/dose in divided doses every 8-12 hours (<15 mg/kg/day)

Intraperitoneal: After contamination in surgery: 500 mg

Irrigating solution: 0.25%; maximum 1.5 g/day (via all administration routes)

Aerosol: 250 mg 2-4 times/day

Dosage adjustment in renal impairment: Adults: I.V.: The following adjustments have been recommended (Aronoff, 2007). **Note:** Renally adjusted dose recommendations are based on a dose of 7.5 mg/kg every 12 hours.

Cl_{cr} >50 mL/minute: Administer every 12-24 hours

Cl_{cr} 10-50 mL/minute: Administer every 24-72 hours; monitor levels.

Cl_{cr} <10 mL/minute: Administer every 48-72 hours; monitor levels.

Intermittent hemodialysis (IHD): One-half the dose administered after hemodialysis on dialysis days.

Peritoneal dialysis (PD): Administration via PD fluid: 15-20 mg/L/day of PD fluid

Continuous renal replacement therapy (CRRT): Administer every 24-72 hours; monitor levels. **Note:** Drug clearance is highly dependent on the method of renal replacement, filter type, and flow rate. Appropriate dosing requires close monitoring of pharmacologic response, signs of adverse reactions due to drug accumulation, as well as drug concentrations in relation to target trough (if appropriate).

Dosage adjustment in hepatic impairment: No dosage adjustment provided in manufacturer's labeling.

Additional Information Complete prescribing information should be consulted for additional detail.

Dosage Forms Excipient information presented when available (limited, particularly for generics); consult specific product labeling. [DSC] = Discontinued product

Solution, Injection, as sulfate:

Generic: 333 mg/mL (3 mL [DSC])

Ketamine (KEET a meen)

Brand Names: U.S. Ketalar

Brand Names: Canada Ketalar®; Ketamine Hydrochloride Injection, USP

Index Terms Ketamine Hydrochloride

Pharmacologic Category General Anesthetic

Additional Appendix Information

Dosing Considerations for the Critically-Ill Patient With Morbid Obesity *on page 2379*

Use Induction and maintenance of general anesthesia

Unlabeled Use Analgesia, sedation

Pregnancy Considerations Adverse events have not been observed in animal reproduction studies. Ketamine crosses the placenta and can be detected in fetal tissue. Ketamine produces dose dependent increases in uterine contractions; effects may vary by trimester. The plasma clearance of ketamine is reduced during pregnancy. Dose related neonatal depression and decreased APGAR scores have been reported with large doses administered at delivery (Ghoneim, 1977; Little, 1972; White, 1982).

Breast-Feeding Considerations It is not known if ketamine is excreted in breast milk.

Contraindications Hypersensitivity to ketamine or any component of the formulation; conditions in which an increase in blood pressure would be hazardous

Warnings/Precautions Use with caution in patients with coronary artery disease, catecholamine depletion, hypertension, and tachycardia. Cardiac function should be continuously monitored in patients with increased blood pressure or cardiac decompensation. Postanesthetic emergence reactions which can manifest as vivid dreams, hallucinations, and/or frank delirium occur; these reactions are less common in patients <15 years of age and >65 years and when given intramuscularly. Emergence reactions, confusion, or irrational behavior may occur up to 24 hours postoperatively and may be reduced by pretreatment with a benzodiazepine and the use of ketamine at the lower end of the dosing range. Rapid I.V. administration or overdose may cause respiratory depression, apnea, and enhanced pressor response. Resuscitative equipment should be available during use. Use with caution in patients with CSF pressure elevation, the chronic alcoholic or acutely alcohol-intoxicated. May cause dependence (withdrawal symptoms on discontinuation) and tolerance with prolonged use. May cause CNS depression, which may impair physical or mental abilities; patients must be cautioned about performing tasks which require mental alertness (eg, operating machinery or driving). When used for outpatient surgery, the patient be accompanied by a responsible adult. Should be administered under the supervision of a physician experienced in administering general anesthetics.

Adverse Reactions Frequency not always defined.

Cardiovascular: Arrhythmia, bradycardia/tachycardia, hyper-/hypotension

Central nervous system: Intracranial pressure increased

Dermatologic: Erythema (transient), morbilliform rash (transient)

Gastrointestinal: Anorexia, nausea, salivation increased, vomiting

Local: Pain at the injection site, exanthema at the injection site

Neuromuscular & skeletal: Skeletal muscle tone enhanced (tonic-clonic movements)

Ocular: Diplopia, intraocular pressure increased, nystagmus

Respiratory: Airway obstruction, apnea, bronchial secretions increased, respiratory depression, laryngospasm

Miscellaneous: Anaphylaxis, dependence with prolonged use, emergence reactions (~12%; includes confusion, delirium, dreamlike state, excitement, hallucinations, irrational behavior, vivid imagery)

Drug Interactions

Metabolism/Transport Effects Substrate of CYP2B6 (major), CYP2C9 (major), CYP3A4 (major); **Note:** Assignment of Major/Minor substrate status based on clinically relevant drug interaction potential

Avoid Concomitant Use

Avoid concomitant use of Ketamine with any of the following: Conivaptan; Fusidic Acid (Systemic)

Increased Effect/Toxicity

The levels/effects of Ketamine may be increased by: Conivaptan; CYP2B6 Inhibitors (Moderate); CYP2B6 Inhibitors (Strong); CYP2C9 Inhibitors (Moderate); CYP2C9 Inhibitors (Strong); CYP3A4 Inhibitors (Moderate); CYP3A4 Inhibitors (Strong); Dasatinib; Fusidic Acid (Systemic); Ivacaftor; Luliconazole; Mifepristone; Quazepam; Simeprevir

Decreased Effect

The levels/effects of Ketamine may be decreased by: CYP2C9 Inducers (Strong); Dabrafenib; Peginterferon Alfa-2b

Preparation for Administration The 50 mg/mL and 100 mg/mL vials may be further diluted in D_5W or NS to prepare a maintenance infusion with a final concentration of 1 mg/mL (or 2 mg/mL in patients with fluid restrictions). The 10 mg/mL vials are not recommended to be further diluted. Do not mix with barbiturates or diazepam (precipitation may occur). **Note:** The 100 mg/mL concentration should not be administered I.V. unless properly diluted with an equal volume of SWFI, NS, or D_5W.

Storage/Stability Store at 20°C to 25°C (68°F to 77°F). Protect from light.

Mechanism of Action Produces a cataleptic-like state in which the patient is dissociated from the surrounding environment by direct action on the cortex and limbic system. Ketamine is a noncompetitive NMDA receptor antagonist that blocks glutamate. Low (subanesthetic) doses produce analgesia, and modulate central sensitization, hyperalgesia and opioid tolerance. Reduces polysynaptic spinal reflexes.

Pharmacodynamics/Kinetics

Onset of action:

I.V.: Anesthetic effect: 30 seconds

I.M.: Anesthetic effect: 3-4 minutes

Duration: Anesthetic effect: I.V.: 5-10 minutes; I.M.: 12-25 minutes

Distribution: V_d: 3 L/kg

Metabolism: Hepatic via hydroxylation and N-demethylation; the metabolite norketamine is 33% as potent as parent compound; greater conversion to norketamine occurs after oral administration as compared to parenteral administration

Bioavailability: Oral: 16%; Intranasal: 50%

Half-life elimination: Alpha: 10-15 minutes; Beta: 2.5 hours

Excretion: Primarily urine

Dosage May be used in combination with anticholinergic agents to decrease hypersalivation.

Children: Note: Titrate dose for desired effect.

Sedation (unlabeled use): Oral (unlabeled route): 5-8 mg/kg for 1 dose (mixed in 0.2-0.3 mL/kg of cola or other beverage) given 30 minutes before the procedure (Sacchetti, 1994; Rosenberg, 1991)

Sedation/analgesia (unlabeled use):

I.M.: 2-5 mg/kg/dose (Green, 2011; Krause, 2000; McGlone, 2004; White, 1982)

I.V.: 0.5-1 mg/kg/dose (Sacchetti, 1994; Tobias, 1990)

Continuous I.V. infusion: 5-20 mcg/kg/minute (Tobias, 1990; White, 1982)

Children ≥16 years and Adults: Note: Titrate dose for desired effect.

Sedation/analgesia (unlabeled use):

I.M.: 2-4 mg/kg (White, 1982)

I.V.: 0.2-0.75 mg/kg (White, 1982)

Continuous I.V. infusion: 2-7 mcg/kg/minute (Hocking, 2003; Remérand, 2009; Zakine, 2008)

Critically-ill patients: Loading dose: 0.1-0.5 mg/kg; followed by 0.83-6.7 mcg/kg/minute (equivalent to 0.05-0.4 mg/kg/**hour**) (Barr, 2013)

Induction of anesthesia (unlabeled dosing):

I.M.: 4-10 mg/kg (Green, 1990; Miller, 2010; White, 1982)

I.V.: 0.5-2 mg/kg (Miller, 2010; White, 1982)

Maintenance of anesthesia: May administer supplemental doses of one-half to the full induction dose or a continuous infusion of 0.1-0.5 mg/minute (per manufacturer). **Note:** To maintain an adequate concentration of ketamine for maintenance of anesthesia, 1-2 mg/minute has been recommended (White, 1982); doses in the range of 15-90 mcg/kg/minute (~1-6 mg/minute in a 70-kg patient) have also been suggested (Miller, 2010). Concurrent use of nitrous oxide reduces ketamine requirements.

Dosage adjustment in renal impairment: No dosage adjustment provided in manufacturer's labeling.

Dosage adjustment in hepatic impairment: No dosage adjustment provided in manufacturer's labeling.

Administration

Oral: Mix the appropriate dose (using the 100 mg/mL injectable solution) in cola or other beverage; administer immediately after preparation.

Parenteral: I.V.: Administer bolus doses over 1 minute; more rapid administration may result in respiratory depression and enhanced pressor response.

Monitoring Parameters Heart rate, blood pressure, respiratory rate, transcutaneous O_2 saturation, emergence reactions; cardiac function should be continuously monitored in patients with increased blood pressure or cardiac decompensation

Test Interactions May interfere with urine detection of PCP (false-positive).

Additional Information May produce emergence psychosis including auditory and visual hallucinations, restlessness, disorientation, vivid dreams, and irrational behavior in ~12% of patients; pretreatment with a benzodiazepine reduces incidence of psychosis by >50%. Spontaneous involuntary movements, nystagmus, hypertonus, and vocalizations are also common.

The analgesia outlasts the general anesthetic component. Bronchodilation is beneficial in asthmatic or COPD patients. Laryngeal reflexes may remain intact or may be obtunded. The direct myocardial depressant action of ketamine can be seen in stressed, catecholamine-deficient patients. Ketamine increases cerebral metabolism and cerebral blood flow while producing a noncompetitive block of the glutaminergic postsynaptic NMDA receptor. It lowers seizure threshold and stimulates salivary secretions (atropine/scopolamine treatment is recommended).

Dosage Forms Excipient information presented when available (limited, particularly for generics); consult specific product labeling.

Solution, Injection:

Ketalar: 10 mg/mL (20 mL); 50 mg/mL (10 mL); 100 mg/mL (5 mL)

Generic: 10 mg/mL (20 mL); 50 mg/mL (10 mL); 100 mg/mL (5 mL, 10 mL)

Controlled Substance C-III

◆ **Ketamine Hydrochloride** *see* Ketamine *on page 1146*

◆ **Ketamine Hydrochloride Injection, USP (Can)** *see* Ketamine *on page 1146*

◆ **Ketek** *see* Telithromycin *on page 2000*

◆ **Ketek® (Can)** *see* Telithromycin *on page 2000*

Ketoconazole (Systemic) (kee toe KOE na zole)

Brand Names: Canada Apo-Ketoconazole; Novo-Ketoconazole

Index Terms Nizoral

Pharmacologic Category Antifungal Agent, Oral

Use Fungal infections:

U.S. labeling: Systemic fungal infections: Treatment of susceptible fungal infections, including blastomycosis, histoplasmosis, paracoccidioidomycosis, coccidioidomycosis, and chromomycosis in patients who have failed or who are intolerant to other antifungal therapies

Canadian labeling: Treatment of serious or life-threatening systemic fungal infections (eg, systemic candidiasis, chronic mucocutaneous candidiasis, coccidioidomycosis, paracoccidioidomycosis, histoplasmosis, and chromomycosis) where alternate therapy is inappropriate or ineffective; may be considered for severe dermatophytoses unresponsive to other therapy

Unlabeled Use Treatment of advanced prostate cancer

Pregnancy Risk Factor C

Pregnancy Considerations Adverse effects were noted in animal reproduction studies.

Breast-Feeding Considerations In a case report, ketoconazole in concentrations of ≤0.22 mcg/mL were detected in the breast milk of a woman 1 month postpartum. She had been taking oral ketoconazole 200 mg/day for 5 days at the time of sampling. The maximum milk concentration occurred 3.25 hours after the dose and concentrations were undetectable 24 hours after the dose. Based on the highest milk concentration, the estimated dose to the nursing infant was 1.4% of the maternal dose. Breast-feeding is not recommended by the manufacturer.

Medication Guide Available Yes

Contraindications

Hypersensitivity to ketoconazole or any component of the formulation; acute or chronic liver disease; coadministration with alprazolam, cisapride, dofetilide, eplerenone, ergot derivatives, HMG-CoA reductase inhibitors (eg, lovastatin, simvastatin), midazolam, nisoldipine, pimozide, quinidine, triazolam

Canadian labeling: Additional contraindications (not in U.S. labeling): Women of childbearing potential unless effective forms of contraception are used; coadministration with astemizole or terfenadine

Warnings/Precautions [U.S. Boxed Warning]: Use only when other effective antifungal therapy is unavailable or not tolerated and the benefits of ketoconazole treatment are considered to outweigh the risks. Ketoconazole has poor penetration into cerebral-spinal fluid and should not be used to treat fungal meningitis.

[U.S. Boxed Warning]: Ketoconazole has been associated with hepatotoxicity, including fatal cases and cases requiring liver transplantation; some patients had no apparent risk factors for hepatic disease. Patients should be advised of the hepatotoxicity risks and monitored closely. Toxicity was observed after a median duration of therapy of ~4 weeks but has also been noted after as little as 3 days; may occur when patients receive high doses for short durations or low doses for long durations. Most cases have been observed in the treatment of onychomycosis. Use with caution in patients with pre-existing hepatic impairment, those on prolonged therapy and/or taking other hepatotoxic drugs concurrently. Hepatic dysfunction is typically (but not always) reversible upon discontinuation. Obtain liver function tests at baseline and frequently throughout therapy; serum ALT should be monitored weekly throughout therapy. Discontinue therapy for elevated hepatic enzymes that persist or worsen or if accompanied by signs/symptoms (eg, jaundice, nausea/vomiting, dark urine) of hepatic injury.

High doses of ketoconazole may depress adrenocortical function; returns to baseline upon discontinuation of therapy. Recommended maximum dosing should not be exceeded. Monitor adrenal function as clinically necessary, particularly in patients with adrenal insufficiency and in patients under prolonged stress (eg, intensive care, major surgery). In European clinical trials of men with metastatic prostate cancer, fatalities were reported in a small number of study participants within 14 days of initiating high-dose ketoconazole (1200 mg daily); a causal effect has not been established. In animal studies, increased long bone fragility with cases of fracture has been observed with high-dose ketoconazole. Careful dose selection may be advisable for patients susceptible to bone fragility (eg, postmenopausal women, elderly). Cases of hypersensitivity reactions (including rare cases of anaphylaxis) have been reported; some reactions occurred after the initial dose.

[U.S. Boxed Warning]: Concomitant use with cisapride, dofetilide, pimozide, and quinidine is contraindicated due to the possible occurrence of life-threatening ventricular arrhythmias such as torsade de pointes. Concomitant use with HMG-CoA reductase inhibitors (eg, lovastatin, simvastatin) or with midazolam, triazolam, and alprazolam is contraindicated. Absorption is reduced in patients with achlorhydria; administer with acidic liquids (eg, soda pop). Avoid concomitant use of drugs that decrease gastric acidity (eg, proton pump inhibitors, antacids, H_2-blockers). Other potentially significant interactions may exist, requiring dose or frequency adjustment, additional monitoring, and/or selection of alternative therapy.

Adverse Reactions Frequency not always defined.

Cardiovascular: Orthostatic hypotension, peripheral edema

Central nervous system: Fatigue, insomnia, malaise, nervousness, paresthesia

Dermatologic: Pruritus (2%), alopecia, dermatitis, erythema, erythema multiforme, skin rash, urticaria, xeroderma

Endocrine & metabolic: Hot flash, hyperlipidemia, menstrual disease

Gastrointestinal: Nausea (3%), vomiting (3%), abdominal pain (1%), anorexia, constipation, dysgeusia, dyspepsia, flatulence, increased appetite, tongue discoloration, upper abdominal pain, xerostomia

Hematologic & oncologic: Decreased platelet count

Hepatic: Jaundice

Hypersensitivity: Anaphylactoid reaction

Neuromuscular & skeletal: Myalgia, weakness

Respiratory: Epistaxis

Miscellaneous: Alcohol intolerance

<1% (Limited to important or life-threatening): Acute generalized exanthematous pustulosis, adrenocortical insufficiency (≥400 mg/day), anaphylactic shock, anaphylaxis, angioedema, azoospermia, bulging fontanel (infants), cholestatic hepatitis, cirrhosis, decreased plasma testosterone (impaired at 800 mg/day), depression, erectile dysfunction (doses >200-400 mg/day), gynecomastia, hemolytic anemia, hepatic failure, hepatic necrosis, hepatitis, hepatotoxicity, hypertriglyceridemia, hypersensitivity reaction, impotence, increased intracranial pressure (reversible), leukopenia, myopathy, papilledema, photophobia, prolonged Q-T interval on ECG, skin photosensitivity, suicidal tendencies, thrombocytopenia

Drug Interactions

Metabolism/Transport Effects Substrate of CYP3A4 (major); **Note:** Assignment of Major/Minor substrate status based on clinically relevant drug interaction potential; **Inhibits** CYP1A2 (weak), CYP2A6 (moderate), CYP2B6 (weak), CYP2C19 (moderate), CYP2C8 (weak), CYP2C9 (moderate), CYP2D6 (moderate), CYP3A4 (strong), P-glycoprotein

Avoid Concomitant Use

Avoid concomitant use of Ketoconazole (Systemic) with any of the following: Ado-Trastuzumab Emtansine; Alfuzosin; ALPRAZolam; Apixaban; Astemizole; Avanafil; Axitinib; Bosutinib; Cabozantinib; Cisapride; Conivaptan; Crizotinib; Dihydroergotamine; Dofetilide; Domperidone; Dronedarone; Eletriptan; Eplerenone; Ergoloid Mesylates; Ergonovine; Ergotamine; Estazolam; Everolimus; Halofantrine; Ibrutinib; Imatinib; Ivabradine; Lapatinib; Lomitapide; Lovastatin; Lurasidone; Macitentan; Methylergonovine; Midazolam; Nevirapine; Nilotinib; Nisoldipine; Pimozide; Pomalidomide; QuiNIDine; Ranolazine; Red Yeast Rice; Regorafenib; Rivaroxaban; Salmeterol; Silodosin; Simeprevir; Simvastatin; Tamsulosin; Tegafur; Terfenadine; Thioridazine; Ticagrelor; Tipranavir; Tolvaptan; Topotecan; Toremifene; Triazolam; Ulipristal; Vemurafenib; VinCRIStine (Liposomal)

Increased Effect/Toxicity

Ketoconazole (Systemic) may increase the levels/effects of: Ado-Trastuzumab Emtansine; Afatinib; Alfentanil; Alfuzosin; Aliskiren; Almotriptan; Alosetron; ALPRAZolam; Apixaban; ARIPiprazole; Astemizole; AtorvaSTATin; Avanafil; Axitinib; Bedaquiline; Benzodiazepines (metabolized by oxidation); Boceprevir; Bortezomib; Bosentan; Bosutinib; Brentuximab Vedotin; Brinzolamide; Budesonide (Nasal); Budesonide (Systemic, Oral Inhalation); BusPIRone; Busulfan; Cabozantinib; Calcium Channel Blockers; Carvedilol; Cilostazol; Cisapride; Citalopram; Cobicistat; Colchicine; Conivaptan; Corticosteroids (Orally Inhaled); Corticosteroids (Systemic); Crizotinib; CycloSPORINE (Systemic); CYP2A6 Substrates; CYP2C19 Substrates; CYP2C9 Substrates; CYP2D6 Substrates; CYP3A4 Substrates; Dabigatran Etexilate; Darunavir; Dienogest; Dihydroergotamine; DOCEtaxel; Dofetilide; Domperidone; Dronedarone; Dutasteride; Eletriptan; Elvitegravir; Enzalutamide; Eplerenone; Ergoloid Mesylates; Ergonovine; Ergotamine; Estazolam; Etravirine; Everolimus; FentaNYL; Fesoterodine; Fexofenadine; Fingolimod; Fluticasone (Nasal); Fluticasone (Oral Inhalation); Fosamprenavir; Fosphenytoin; GuanFACINE; Halofantrine; Highest Risk QTc-Prolonging Agents; Ibrutinib; Iloperidone; Imatinib; Indinavir; Irinotecan; Ivabradine; Ivacaftor; Ixabepilone; Lacosamide; Lapatinib; Levomilnacipran; Lomitapide; Lopinavir; Losartan; Lovastatin; Lumefantrine; Lurasidone; Macitentan; Macrolide Antibiotics; Maraviroc; Methadone; Methylergonovine; MethylPREDNISolone; Metoprolol; Midazolam; Mifepristone; Mirabegron; Moderate Risk QTc-Prolonging Agents; Nebivolol; Nilotinib; Nisoldipine; Ospemifene; OxyCODONE; Paricalcitol; PAZOPanib; P-glycoprotein/ABCB1 Substrates; Phenytoin; Pimecrolimus; Pimozide; Pomalidomide; PONATinib; Praziquantel; Propafenone; Proton Pump Inhibitors; Prucalopride; QUEtiapine; QuiNIDine; Ramelteon; Ranolazine; Red Yeast Rice; Regorafenib; Repaglinide; Rifamycin Derivatives; Rilpivirine; Riociguat; Rivaroxaban; RomiDEPsin; Ruxolitinib; Salmeterol; Saquinavir; Saxagliptin; Sildenafil; Silodosin; Simeprevir; Simvastatin; Sirolimus; Solifenacin; SORAfenib; SUNItinib; Tacrolimus (Systemic); Tacrolimus (Topical); Tadalafil; Tamsulosin; Telaprevir; Temsirolimus; Terfenadine; Thioridazine; Ticagrelor; Tofacitinib; Tolterodine; Tolvaptan; Topotecan; Toremifene; Triazolam; Ulipristal; Vardenafil; Vemurafenib; Vilazodone; VinCRIStine (Liposomal); Vitamin K Antagonists; Zolpidem; Zuclopenthixol

The levels/effects of Ketoconazole (Systemic) may be increased by: AtorvaSTATin; Boceprevir; Cobicistat; Darunavir; Domperidone; Etravirine; Fosamprenavir; Indinavir; Lopinavir; Macrolide Antibiotics; Ritonavir; Saquinavir; Telaprevir; Tipranavir

Decreased Effect

Ketoconazole (Systemic) may decrease the levels/effects of: Amphotericin B; Clopidogrel; Codeine; Ifosfamide; Prasugrel; Saccharomyces boulardii; Tamoxifen; Tegafur; Ticagrelor; TraMADol

The levels/effects of Ketoconazole (Systemic) may be decreased by: Antacids; CYP3A4 Inducers (Strong); Dabrafenib; Deferasirox; Didanosine; Etravirine; Fosphenytoin; H2-Antagonists; Herbs (CYP3A4 Inducers); Isoniazid; Mitotane; Nevirapine; Phenytoin; Proton Pump Inhibitors; Rifamycin Derivatives; Rilpivirine; Sucralfate; Tocilizumab

Ethanol/Nutrition/Herb Interactions

Food: Ketoconazole peak serum levels may be prolonged if taken with food.

Herb/Nutraceutical: St John's wort may decrease ketoconazole levels.

Storage/Stability Store at 15°C to 25°C (59°F to 77°F). Protect from light and moisture.

Mechanism of Action Alters the permeability of the cell wall by blocking fungal cytochrome P450; inhibits biosynthesis of triglycerides and phospholipids by fungi; inhibits several fungal enzymes that results in a build-up of toxic concentrations of hydrogen peroxide; for management of prostate cancer, ketoconazole inhibits androgen synthesis

Pharmacodynamics/Kinetics

Distribution: Well into inflamed joint fluid, saliva, bile, urine, sebum, cerumen, feces, tendons, skin and soft tissue, and testes; crosses blood-brain barrier poorly; only negligible amounts reach CSF

Protein binding: ~99% (mainly albumin)

Metabolism: Partially hepatic via CYP3A4 to inactive metabolites

Bioavailability: Decreases as gastric pH increases

Half-life elimination: Biphasic: Initial: 2 hours; Terminal: 8 hours

Time to peak, serum: 1-2 hours

Excretion: Feces (57%); urine (13%)

Dosage

Fungal infections: Oral:

Children ≥2 years: 3.3-6.6 mg/kg once daily

Adults: 200-400 mg once daily

Therapy duration: Continue therapy until active fungal infection has resolved (based on clinical and laboratory parameters); some infections may require at least 6 months of therapy.

Prostate cancer, advanced (unlabeled use): Adults: Oral: 400 mg 3 times daily (in combination with oral hydrocortisone) until disease progression (Ryan, 2007; Small, 2004)

Dosage adjustment in renal impairment: No dosage adjustment provided in manufacturer's labeling. Some clinicians suggest that no dosage adjustment is necessary in mild-to-severe impairment (Aronoff, 2007).

Hemodialysis: Not dialyzable

Dosage adjustment in hepatic impairment: No dosage adjustment provided in manufacturer's labeling; use with caution due to risks of hepatotoxicity.

Hepatotoxicity during treatment:

U.S. labeling: If ALT >ULN or 30% above baseline (or if patient is symptomatic), interrupt therapy and obtain full hepatic function panel. Upon normalization of liver function, may consider resuming therapy if benefit outweighs risk (hepatotoxicity has been reported on rechallenge).

Canadian labeling: Discontinue therapy for liver function tests >3 times ULN or if abnormalities persist, worsen, or are associated with hepatotoxicity symptoms.

Dietary Considerations May be taken with food or milk to decrease GI adverse effects.

Administration Administer oral tablets 2 hours prior to antacids to prevent decreased absorption due to the high pH of gastric contents. Patients with achlorhydria should administer with acidic liquid (eg, soda pop).

Monitoring Parameters Hepatic function tests (baseline and frequently during therapy); Canadian labeling recommends monitoring hepatic function at baseline, at weeks 2 and 4, and monthly thereafter; calcium and phosphorous (periodically with long-term use); adrenal function as clinically necessary

Dosage Forms Excipient information presented when available (limited, particularly for generics); consult specific product labeling.

Tablet, Oral:

Generic: 200 mg

Extemporaneous Preparations A 20 mg/mL oral suspension may be made with tablets and one of three different vehicles (a 1:1 mixture of Ora-Sweet® and Ora-Plus®, a 1:1 mixture of Ora-Sweet® SF and Ora-Plus®, or a 1:4 mixture of cherry syrup and Simple Syrup, NF). Crush twelve 200 mg tablets in a mortar and reduce to a fine powder. Add 20 mL of chosen vehicle and mix to a uniform paste; mix while adding the vehicle in incremental proportions to **almost** 120 mL; transfer to a calibrated bottle, rinse mortar with vehicle, and add quantity of vehicle sufficient to make 120 mL. Label "shake well" and "refrigerate". Stable for 60 days.

Nahata MC, Pai VB, and Hipple TF, *Pediatric Drug Formulations*, 5th ed, Cincinnati, OH: Harvey Whitney Books Co, 2004.

Ketoconazole (Topical) (kee toe KOE na zole)

Brand Names: U.S. Extina; Ketodan; Nizoral; Nizoral A-D [OTC]; Xolegel

Brand Names: Canada Ketoderm®; Xolegel®

Pharmacologic Category Antifungal Agent, Topical

Additional Appendix Information

Antifungal Agents *on page 2286*

Use

Cream: Treatment of tinea corporis, tinea cruris, tinea versicolor, cutaneous candidiasis, seborrheic dermatitis

Foam, gel: Treatment of seborrheic dermatitis

Shampoo: Treatment of dandruff, seborrheic dermatitis, tinea versicolor

Unlabeled Use Cream: Treatment of susceptible fungal infections in the oral cavity including candidiasis, oral thrush, and chronic mucocutaneous candidiasis

Pregnancy Risk Factor C

Dosage

Shampoo:

Seborrheic dermatitis (ketoconazole 1%): Children ≥12 years and Adults: Apply twice weekly for up to 8 weeks with at least 3 days between each shampoo

Tinea versicolor (ketoconazole 2%): Adults: Apply to damp skin, lather, leave on 5 minutes, and rinse (one application should be sufficient)

Topical:

Tinea infections: Adults: Cream: Rub gently into the affected area once daily. Duration of treatment: Tinea corporis, cruris: 2 weeks; tinea pedis: 6 weeks

Seborrheic dermatitis: Children ≥12 years and Adults:

Cream: Rub gently into the affected area twice daily for 4 weeks or until clinical response is noted

Foam: Apply to affected area twice daily for 4 weeks

Gel: Rub gently into the affected area once daily for 2 weeks

Susceptible fungal infections in the oral cavity (candidiasis, oral thrush, and chronic mucocutaneous candidiasis) (unlabeled use): Adults: Cream: Apply locally as directed with a thin coat to inner surface of denture and affected areas after meals

Additional Information Complete prescribing information should be consulted for additional detail.

Dosage Forms Excipient information presented when available (limited, particularly for generics); consult specific product labeling. [DSC] = Discontinued product

Cream, External:
Generic: 2% (15 g, 30 g, 60 g)

Foam, External:
Extina: 2% (50 g, 100 g) [contains alcohol, usp, cetyl alcohol, propylene glycol]
Ketodan: 2% (100 g) [contains alcohol, usp, cetyl alcohol, propylene glycol]
Generic: 2% (50 g [DSC], 100 g [DSC])

Gel, External:
Xolegel: 2% (45 g) [contains alcohol, usp, fd&c yellow #10 (quinoline yellow), fd&c yellow #6 (sunset yellow), propylene glycol]

Kit, External:
Ketodan: 2% [contains cetyl alcohol, edetate disodium, propylene glycol]

Shampoo, External:
Nizoral: 2% (120 mL) [contains fd&c red #40]
Nizoral A-D: 1% (125 mL, 200 mL)
Generic: 2% (120 mL)

◆ Ketodan *see* Ketoconazole (Topical) *on page 1149*

◆ Ketoderm® (Can) *see* Ketoconazole (Topical) *on page 1149*

Ketoprofen (kee toe PROE fen)

Brand Names: Canada Apo-Keto SR®; Apo-Keto-E®; Apo-Keto®; Ketoprofen SR; Ketoprofen-E; Nu-Ketoprofen; Nu-Ketoprofen-E; PMS-Ketoprofen; PMS-Ketoprofen-E

Pharmacologic Category Nonsteroidal Anti-inflammatory Drug (NSAID), Oral

Additional Appendix Information

Beers Criteria – Potentially Inappropriate Medications for Geriatrics *on page 2368*

Use Acute and long-term treatment of rheumatoid arthritis and osteoarthritis; primary dysmenorrhea; mild-to-moderate pain

Unlabeled Use Migraine prophylaxis

Pregnancy Risk Factor C

Pregnancy Considerations Adverse events were not observed in the initial animal reproduction studies; therefore, the manufacturer classifies ketoprofen as pregnancy category C. Ketoprofen crosses the placenta. NSAID exposure during the first trimester is not strongly associated with congenital malformations; however, cardiovascular anomalies and cleft palate have been observed following NSAID exposure in some studies. The use of an NSAID close to conception may be associated with an increased risk of miscarriage. Nonteratogenic effects have been observed following NSAID administration during the third trimester including myocardial degenerative changes, prenatal constriction of the ductus arteriosus, fetal tricuspid regurgitation, failure of the ductus arteriosus to close postnatally; renal dysfunction or failure, oligohydramnios; gastrointestinal bleeding or perforation, increased risk of necrotizing enterocolitis; intracranial bleeding (including intraventricular hemorrhage), platelet dysfunction with resultant bleeding; pulmonary hypertension. Because they may cause premature closure of the ductus arteriosus, use of NSAIDs late in pregnancy should be avoided (use after 31or 32 weeks gestation is not recommended by some clinicians). The chronic use of NSAIDs in women of reproductive age may be associated with infertility that is reversible upon discontinuation of the medication.

Breast-Feeding Considerations Small amounts of ketoprofen are found in breast milk. Breast-feeding is not recommended by the manufacturer.

Medication Guide Available Yes

Contraindications Hypersensitivity to ketoprofen, aspirin, other NSAIDs, or any component of the formulation; perioperative pain in the setting of coronary artery bypass graft (CABG) surgery

Warnings/Precautions [U.S. Boxed Warning]: NSAIDs are associated with an increased risk of adverse cardiovascular thrombotic events, including MI and stroke Risk may be increased with duration of use or pre-existing cardiovascular risk factors or disease. Carefully evaluate individual cardiovascular risk profiles prior to prescribing. May cause new-onset hypertension or worsening of existing hypertension. Use caution with fluid retention. Avoid use in heart failure. Concurrent administration of ibuprofen, and potentially other nonselective NSAIDs, may interfere with aspirin's cardioprotective effect. **[U.S. Boxed Warning]: Use is contraindicated for treatment of perioperative pain in the setting of coronary artery bypass graft (CABG) surgery.** Risk of MI and stroke may be increased with use following CABG surgery.

NSAID use may compromise existing renal function; dose-dependent decreases in prostaglandin synthesis may result from NSAID use, reducing renal blood flow which may cause renal decompensation. NSAID use may increase the risk for hyperkalemia. Patients with impaired renal function, dehydration, heart failure, liver dysfunction, those taking diuretics, and ACE inhibitors, and the elderly are at greater risk of renal toxicity and hyperkalemia. Rehydrate patient before starting therapy; monitor renal function closely. Not recommended for use in patients with advanced renal disease. Long-term NSAID use may result in renal papillary necrosis.

[U.S. Boxed Warning]: NSAIDs may increase risk of gastrointestinal irritation, inflammation, ulceration, bleeding, and perforation. These events may occur at any time during therapy and without warning. Use caution with a history of GI disease (bleeding or ulcers), concurrent therapy with aspirin, anticoagulants and/or corticosteroids, smoking, use of alcohol, the elderly or debilitated patients. When used concomitantly with ≤325 mg of aspirin, a substantial increase in the risk of gastrointestinal complications (eg, ulcer) occurs; concomitant gastroprotective therapy (eg, proton pump inhibitors) is recommended (Bhatt, 2008). Platelet adhesion and aggregation may be decreased; may prolong bleeding time; patients with coagulation disorders or who are receiving anticoagulants should be monitored closely. Anemia may occur; patients on long-term NSAID therapy should be monitored for anemia. Rarely, NSAID use may cause severe blood dyscrasias (eg, agranulocytosis, aplastic anemia, thrombocytopenia).

In the elderly, avoid chronic use (unless alternative agents ineffective and patient can receive concomitant gastroprotective agent); nonselective oral NSAID use is associated with an increased risk of GI bleeding and peptic ulcer disease in older adults in high risk category (eg, >75 years or age or receiving concomitant oral/parenteral corticosteroids, anticoagulants, or antiplatelet agents) (Beers Criteria).

Use the lowest effective dose for the shortest duration of time, consistent with individual patient goals, to reduce risk of cardiovascular or GI adverse events. Alternate therapies should be considered for patients at high risk.

NSAIDS may cause drowsiness, dizziness, blurred vision and other neurologic effects which may impair physical or mental abilities; patients must be cautioned about performing tasks which require mental alertness (eg, operating machinery or driving). Discontinue use with blurred or diminished vision and perform ophthalmologic exam. Monitor vision with long-term therapy.

NSAIDs may cause serious skin adverse events including exfoliative dermatitis, Stevens-Johnson syndrome (SJS), and toxic epidermal necrolysis (TEN); discontinue use at first sign of skin rash or hypersensitivity. Anaphylactoid reactions may occur, even without prior exposure; patients with "aspirin triad" (bronchial asthma, aspirin intolerance, rhinitis) may be at increased risk. Do not use in patients who experience bronchospasm, asthma, rhinitis, or urticaria with NSAID or aspirin therapy. Use caution in other forms of asthma.

Use with caution in patients with decreased hepatic function. Closely monitor patients with any abnormal LFT. Severe hepatic reactions (eg, fulminant hepatitis, liver failure) have occurred with NSAID use, rarely; discontinue if signs or symptoms of liver disease develop, or if systemic manifestations occur. The elderly are at increased risk for adverse effects (especially peptic ulceration, CNS effects, renal toxicity) from NSAIDs, even at low doses.

Withhold for at least 4-6 half-lives prior to surgical or dental procedures. Safety and efficacy have not been established in pediatric patients.

Adverse Reactions

>10%:

Gastrointestinal: Dyspepsia (11%)

Hepatic: Liver function test abnormal (≤15%)

1% to 10%:

Cardiovascular: Peripheral edema (2%)

Central nervous system: Headache (3% to 9%), depression, dizziness (>1%), dreams, insomnia, malaise, nervousness, somnolence

Dermatologic: Rash (>1%)

Gastrointestinal: Abdominal pain (3% to 9%), constipation (3% to 9%), diarrhea (3% to 9%), flatulence (3% to 9%), nausea (3% to 9%), gastrointestinal bleeding (>2%), peptic ulcer (>2%), anorexia (>1%), stomatitis (>1%), vomiting (>1%)

Genitourinary: Urinary tract irritation (>1%)

Ocular: Visual disturbances (>1%)

Otic: Tinnitus (>1%)

Renal: Renal dysfunction (3% to 9%)

<1% (Limited to important or life-threatening): Agranulocytosis, allergic reaction, allergic rhinitis, alopecia, anaphylaxis, anemia, angioedema, arrhythmia, aseptic meningitis, blurred vision, bone marrow suppression, bronchospasm, buccal necrosis, bullous rash, chills, cholestatic hepatitis, confusion, CHF, conjunctivitis, cystitis, diabetes mellitus (aggravated), drowsiness, dysphoria, dyspnea, eczema, edema, epistaxis, erythema multiforme, exfoliative dermatitis, facial edema, fecal occult blood, fluid retention, gastritis, gastrointestinal perforation, GI ulceration, gynecomastia, hallucinations, hearing decreased, hematemesis, hematuria, hemolytic anemia, hemoptysis, hepatic dysfunction, hepatitis, hot flashes, hypertension, hyponatremia, impotence, infection, interstitial nephritis, intestinal ulceration, jaundice, laryngeal edema, leukopenia, libido disturbance, melena, microvesicular steatosis, migraine, myocardial infarction, nephrotic syndrome, onycholysis, palpitation, pancreatitis, peptic ulcer, peripheral neuropathy, peripheral vascular disease, photosensitivity, polydipsia, polyuria, pruritus, purpura, purpuric rash, renal failure, renal papillary necrosis, retinal hemorrhage, septicemia, shock, Stevens-Johnson syndrome, tachycardia, thrombocytopenia, toxic amblyopia, toxic epidermal necrolysis, tubulopathy, ulcerative colitis, urticaria, vasodilation, xerostomia

Drug Interactions

Metabolism/Transport Effects Inhibits CYP2C9 (weak)

Avoid Concomitant Use

Avoid concomitant use of Ketoprofen with any of the following: Floctafenine; Ketorolac (Nasal); Ketorolac (Systemic); NSAID (COX-2 Inhibitor); Omacetaxine

Increased Effect/Toxicity

Ketoprofen may increase the levels/effects of: 5-ASA Derivatives; Agents with Antiplatelet Properties; Aliskiren; Aminoglycosides; Anticoagulants; Bisphosphonate Derivatives; Collagenase (Systemic); CycloSPORINE (Systemic); Dabigatran Etexilate; Deferasirox; Desmopressin; Digoxin; Eplerenone; Haloperidol; Ibritumomab; Lithium; Methotrexate; Nonsteroidal Anti-Inflammatory Agents; NSAID (COX-2 Inhibitor); Omacetaxine; PEMEtrexed; Porfimer; Potassium-Sparing Diuretics; PRALAtrexate; Quinolone Antibiotics; Rivaroxaban; Salicylates; Tenofovir; Thrombolytic Agents; Tositumomab and Iodine I 131 Tositumomab; Vancomycin; Vitamin K Antagonists

The levels/effects of Ketoprofen may be increased by: ACE Inhibitors; Angiotensin II Receptor Blockers; Antidepressants (Tricyclic, Tertiary Amine); Corticosteroids (Systemic); CycloSPORINE (Systemic); Dasatinib; Floctafenine; Glucosamine; Herbs (Anticoagulant/Antiplatelet Properties); Ibrutinib; Ketorolac (Nasal); Ketorolac (Systemic); Multivitamins/Fluoride (with ADE); Multivitamins/Minerals (with ADEK, Folate, Iron); Multivitamins/Minerals (with AE, No Iron); Nonsteroidal Anti-Inflammatory Agents; Omega-3 Fatty Acids; Pentosan Polysulfate Sodium; Pentoxifylline; Probenecid; Prostacyclin Analogues; Selective Serotonin Reuptake Inhibitors; Serotonin/Norepinephrine Reuptake Inhibitors; Sodium Phosphates; Tipranavir; Treprostinil; Vitamin E

Decreased Effect

Ketoprofen may decrease the levels/effects of: ACE Inhibitors; Agents with Antiplatelet Properties; Aliskiren; Angiotensin II Receptor Blockers; Beta-Blockers; Eplerenone; HydrALAZINE; Loop Diuretics; Potassium-Sparing Diuretics; Prostaglandins (Ophthalmic); Salicylates; Selective Serotonin Reuptake Inhibitors; Thiazide Diuretics

The levels/effects of Ketoprofen may be decreased by: Bile Acid Sequestrants; Nonsteroidal Anti-Inflammatory Agents; Salicylates

Ethanol/Nutrition/Herb Interactions

Ethanol: Avoid ethanol (due to GI irritation).

Food: Food slows rate of absorption resulting in delayed and reduced peak serum concentrations; total bioavailability is not affected by food.

Herb/Nutraceutical: Avoid alfalfa, anise, bilberry, bladderwrack, bromelain, cat's claw, celery, chamomile, coleus, cordyceps, dong quai, evening primrose, fenugreek, feverfew, garlic, ginger, ginkgo biloba, ginseng (American, Panax, Siberian), grapeseed, green tea, guggul, horse chestnut seed, horseradish, licorice, prickly ash, red clover, reishi, SAMe (S-adenosylmethionine), sweet clover, turmeric, and white willow (all have additional antiplatelet activity).

Storage/Stability Store at room temperature of 25°C (77°F). Protect from light; avoid excessive heat and humidity.

Mechanism of Action Reversibly inhibits cyclooxygenase-1 and 2 (COX-1 and 2) enzymes, which results in decreased formation of prostaglandin precursors; has antipyretic, analgesic, and anti-inflammatory properties

Other proposed mechanisms not fully elucidated (and possibly contributing to the anti-inflammatory effect to varying degrees), include inhibiting chemotaxis, altering lymphocyte activity, inhibiting neutrophil aggregation/activation, and decreasing proinflammatory cytokine levels.

Pharmacodynamics/Kinetics

Onset of action: Regular release: <30 minutes

Duration: Regular release: Up to 6 hours

Absorption: Almost complete

Distribution: 0.1 L/kg

Protein binding: >99%, primarily to albumin; Hepatic impairment: Unbound fraction is approximately doubled

Metabolism: Hepatic via glucuronidation; metabolite (inactive) can be converted back to parent compound; may have enterohepatic recirculation

Bioavailability: ~90%

Half-life elimination:

Regular release: 2-4 hours; Renal impairment: Mild: 3 hours; moderate-to-severe: 5-9 hours

Extended release: ~3-7.5 hours

Time to peak, serum:

Regular release: 0.5-2 hours

Extended release: 6-7 hours

Excretion: Urine (~80%, primarily as glucuronide conjugates)

Dosage Note: The extended release formulation is not recommended for the treatment of acute pain. Oral:

Adults:

Rheumatoid arthritis, osteoarthritis (lower doses may be used in small patients or in the elderly, or debilitated):

Regular release: 50 mg 4 times/day **or** 75 mg 3 times/day; up to a maximum of 300 mg/day

Extended release: 200 mg once daily

Dysmenorrhea, mild-to-moderate pain: Regular release: 25-50 mg every 6-8 hours up to a maximum of 300 mg/day

Elderly: Initial dose should be decreased in patients >75 years; use caution when dosage changes are made

Dosage adjustment in renal impairment: In general, NSAIDs are not recommended for use in patients with advanced renal disease, but the manufacturer of ketoprofen does provide some guidelines for adjustment in renal dysfunction:

Mild impairment: Maximum dose: 150 mg/day

Severe impairment: Cl_{cr} <25 mL/minute: Maximum dose: 100 mg/day

Dosage adjustment in hepatic impairment and serum albumin <3.5 g/dL: Maximum dose: 100 mg/day

Dietary Considerations In order to minimize gastrointestinal effects, ketoprofen can be prescribed to be taken with food or milk.

Administration May take with food to reduce GI upset. Do not crush or break extended release capsules.

Monitoring Parameters CBC, chemistry profile, occult blood loss, periodic liver function; renal function (urine output, serum BUN, creatinine)

Dosage Forms Excipient information presented when available (limited, particularly for generics); consult specific product labeling.

Capsule, Oral:

Generic: 50 mg, 75 mg

Capsule Extended Release 24 Hour, Oral:

Generic: 200 mg

◆ Ketoprofen-E (Can) *see* Ketoprofen *on page 1150*

◆ Ketoprofen SR (Can) *see* Ketoprofen *on page 1150*

Ketorolac (Systemic) (KEE toe role ak)

Brand Names: Canada Apo-Ketorolac Injectable®; Apo-Ketorolac®; Ketorolac Tromethamine Injection, USP; Novo-Ketorolac; Toradol®; Toradol® IM

Index Terms Ketorolac Tromethamine; Toradol

Pharmacologic Category Nonsteroidal Anti-inflammatory Drug (NSAID), Oral; Nonsteroidal Anti-inflammatory Drug (NSAID), Parenteral

Additional Appendix Information

Beers Criteria – Potentially Inappropriate Medications for Geriatrics *on page 2368*

Use Short-term (≤5 days) management of moderate-to-severe acute pain requiring analgesia at the opioid level

Pregnancy Risk Factor C

Pregnancy Considerations Adverse events were observed in some animal reproduction studies. Ketorolac crosses the placenta (Walker, 1988). NSAID exposure during the first trimester is not strongly associated with congenital malformations; however, cardiovascular anomalies and cleft palate have been observed following NSAID exposure in some studies (Ericson, 2001). The use of an NSAID close to conception may be associated with an increased risk of miscarriage (Li, 2003; Nielsen, 2001). Nonteratogenic effects have been observed following NSAID administration during the third trimester, including myocardial degenerative changes, prenatal constriction of the ductus arteriosus, fetal tricuspid regurgitation, failure of the ductus arteriosus to close postnatally; renal dysfunction or failure, oligohydramnios; gastrointestinal bleeding or perforation, increased risk of necrotizing enterocolitis; intracranial bleeding (including intraventricular hemorrhage), platelet dysfunction with resultant bleeding; pulmonary hypertension (Van den Veyver, 1993). Because they may cause premature closure of the ductus arteriosus, use of NSAIDs late in pregnancy should be avoided (use after 31 or 32 weeks gestation is not recommended by some clinicians) (Moise, 1993). **[U.S. Boxed Warning]: Ketorolac is contraindicated during labor and delivery (may inhibit uterine contractions and adversely affect fetal circulation).** The chronic use of NSAIDs in women of reproductive age may be associated with infertility that is reversible upon discontinuation of the medication.

Breast-Feeding Considerations Low concentrations of ketorolac are found in breast milk (milk concentrations were <1% of the weight-adjusted maternal dose in one study [Wischnik, 1989]). The manufacturer recommends that caution be used if administered to nursing women.

Medication Guide Available Yes

Contraindications Hypersensitivity to ketorolac, aspirin, other NSAIDs, or any component of the formulation; active or history of peptic ulcer disease; recent or history of GI bleeding or perforation; patients with advanced renal disease or risk of renal failure (due to volume depletion); prophylaxis before major surgery; suspected or confirmed cerebrovascular bleeding; hemorrhagic diathesis, incomplete hemostasis, or high risk of bleeding; concurrent use with ASA, other NSAIDs, probenecid or pentoxifylline; epidural or intrathecal administration; perioperative pain in the setting of coronary artery bypass graft (CABG) surgery; labor and delivery

Warnings/Precautions [U.S. Boxed Warning]: Inhibits platelet function; contraindicated in patients with cerebrovascular bleeding (suspected or confirmed), hemorrhagic diathesis, incomplete hemostasis and patients at high risk for bleeding. Effects on platelet adhesion and aggregation may prolong bleeding time. Anemia may occur; patients on long-term NSAID therapy should be monitored for anemia. Rarely, NSAID use has been associated with potentially severe blood dyscrasias (eg, agranulocytosis, thrombocytopenia, aplastic anemia).

[U.S. Boxed Warning]: NSAIDs are associated with an increased risk of adverse cardiovascular thrombotic events, including MI and stroke. Risk may be increased with duration of use or pre-existing cardiovascular risk factors or disease. Carefully evaluate individual cardiovascular risk profiles prior to prescribing. May cause new-onset hypertension or worsening of existing hypertension. Use caution with fluid retention. Avoid use in heart failure. Concurrent use of aspirin has not been shown to consistently reduce thromboembolic events. **[U.S. Boxed Warning]: Use is contraindicated as prophylactic analgesic before any major surgery and is contraindicated for treatment of perioperative pain in the setting of coronary artery bypass graft (CABG) surgery.** Risk of MI and stroke may be increased with use following CABG surgery. Wound bleeding and postoperative hematomas have been associated with ketorolac use in the perioperative setting.

[U.S. Boxed Warning]: Ketorolac is contraindicated in patients with advanced renal impairment and in patients at risk for renal failure due to volume depletion. NSAID use may compromise existing renal function; dose-dependent decreases in prostaglandin synthesis may result from NSAID use, reducing renal blood flow which may cause renal decompensation. NSAID use may increase the risk for hyperkalemia. Patients with impaired renal function, dehydration, heart failure, liver dysfunction, those taking diuretics and ACE inhibitors, and the elderly are at greater risk of renal toxicity. Use with caution in patients with impaired renal function or history of kidney disease; dosage adjustment is required in patients with moderate elevation in serum creatinine. Monitor renal function closely. Acute renal failure, interstitial nephritis, and nephrotic syndrome have been reported with ketorolac use; papillary necrosis and renal injury have been reported with the use of NSAIDs. Use of NSAIDs can compromise existing renal function. Rehydrate patient before starting therapy.

[U.S. Boxed Warning]: NSAIDs may increase risk of gastrointestinal irritation, inflammation, ulceration, bleeding, and perforation. These events may occur at any time during therapy and without warning. Use is contraindicated in patients with active/history of peptic ulcer disease and recent/history of GI bleeding or perforation. Use caution with a history of inflammatory bowel disease, concurrent therapy with anticoagulants, and/or corticosteroids, smoking, use of alcohol, the elderly, or debilitated patients.

[U.S. Boxed Warning]: Ketorolac injection is contraindicated in patients with prior hypersensitivity reaction to aspirin or NSAIDs. NSAIDs may cause serious skin adverse events including exfoliative dermatitis, Stevens-Johnson syndrome (SJS), and toxic epidermal necrolysis (TEN); discontinue use at first sign of skin rash or hypersensitivity. Hypersensitivity or anaphylactoid reactions may occur, even without prior exposure; patients with "aspirin triad" (bronchial asthma, aspirin intolerance, rhinitis) may be at increased risk. Do not use in patients who experience bronchospasm, asthma, rhinitis, or urticaria with NSAID or aspirin therapy. Use caution in other forms of asthma.

Use with caution in patients with hepatic impairment or a history of liver disease. Closely monitor patients with any abnormal LFT. Rarely, severe hepatic reactions (eg, fulminant hepatitis, hepatic necrosis, liver failure) have occurred with NSAID use; discontinue if signs or symptoms of liver disease develop, or if systemic manifestations occur.

[U.S. Boxed Warning]: Dosage adjustment is required for patients ≥65 years of age. Avoid use in older adults; use is associated with an increased risk of GI bleeding and peptic ulcer disease in older adults in high risk category (eg, >75 years or age or receiving concomitant oral/parenteral corticosteroids, anticoagulants, or antiplatelet agents) (Beers Criteria). **[U.S. Boxed Warning]: Dosage adjustment is required for patients weighing <50 kg (<110 pounds). [U.S. Boxed Warning]: Ketorolac is contraindicated during labor and delivery (may inhibit uterine contractions and adversely affect fetal circulation). [U.S. Boxed Warning]: Concurrent use of ketorolac with aspirin or other NSAIDs is contraindicated due to the increased risk of adverse reactions.**

[U.S. Boxed Warning]: Contraindicated for epidural or intrathecal administration (formulation contains alcohol). [U.S. Boxed Warning]: Systemic ketorolac is indicated for short term (≤5 days) use in adults for treatment of moderately severe acute pain requiring opioid-level analgesia. Low doses of opioids may be needed for breakthrough pain. **[U.S. Boxed Warning]: Oral therapy is only indicated for use as continuation treatment, following parenteral ketorolac and is not indicated for minor or chronic painful conditions. Do not exceed maximum daily recommended doses; does not improve efficacy but may increase the risk of serious adverse effects.** The combined therapy duration (oral and parenteral) should not exceed 5 days. Use the lowest effective dose for the shortest duration of time, consistent with individual patient goals, to reduce risk of cardiovascular or GI adverse events. Alternate therapies should be considered for patients at high risk. **[U.S. Boxed Warning]: Ketorolac is not indicated for use in children.**

Potentially significant drug-drug interactions may exist, requiring dose or frequency adjustment, additional monitoring, and/or selection of alternative therapy.

NSAIDS may cause drowsiness, dizziness, blurred vision and other neurologic effects which may impair physical or mental abilities; patients must be cautioned about performing tasks which require mental alertness (eg, operating machinery or driving). Discontinue use with blurred or diminished vision and perform ophthalmologic exam.

Adverse Reactions Frequencies noted for parenteral administration:

>10%:

Central nervous system: Headache (17%)

Gastrointestinal: Gastrointestinal pain (13%), dyspepsia (12%), nausea (12%)

>1% to 10%:

Cardiovascular: Edema (4%), hypertension

Central nervous system: Dizziness (7%), drowsiness (6%)

Dermatologic: Diaphoresis, pruritus, skin rash

Gastrointestinal: Diarrhea (7%), constipation, flatulence, gastrointestinal fullness, gastrointestinal hemorrhage, gastrointestinal perforation, gastrointestinal ulcer, heartburn, stomatitis, vomiting

Hematologic & oncologic: Anemia, prolonged bleeding time, purpura

Hepatic: Increased liver enzymes

Local: Pain at injection site (2%)

Otic: Tinnitus

Renal: Renal function abnormality

<1% (Limited to important or life-threatening): Abnormality in thinking, acute pancreatitis, acute renal failure, agranulocytosis, alopecia, anaphylactoid reaction, anaphylaxis, angioedema, aplastic anemia, aseptic meningitis, asthma, azotemia, bradycardia, bronchospasm, bruise, cardiac arrhythmia, cholestatic jaundice, coma, confusion, congestive heart failure, conjunctivitis, cough,

cystitis, depression, dysuria, eosinophilia, epistaxis, eructation, erythema multiforme, euphoria, exacerbation of urinary frequency, exfoliative dermatitis, extrapyramidal reaction, flank pain, gastritis, glossitis, hallucination, hearing loss, hematemesis, hematuria, hemolytic anemia, hemolytic-uremic syndrome, hepatic failure, hepatitis, hyperglycemia, hyperkalemia, hyperkinesis, hypersensitivity reaction, hyponatremia, hypotension, increased susceptibility to infection, increased thirst, infertility, inflammatory bowel disease, insomnia, interstitial nephritis, jaundice, lack of concentration, laryngeal edema, leukopenia, lymphadenopathy, maculopapular rash, melena, myocardial infarction, nephritis, oliguria, palpitations, pancytopenia, paresthesia, pneumonia, polyuria, proteinuria, psychosis, pulmonary edema, rectal hemorrhage, renal failure, respiratory depression, rhinitis, seizure, sepsis, skin photosensitivity, Stevens-Johnson syndrome, stomatitis (ulcerative), stupor, syncope, tachycardia, thrombocytopenia, tongue edema, toxic epidermal necrolysis, urinary retention, urticaria, vasculitis, weight gain, wound hemorrhage (postoperative)

Drug Interactions

Metabolism/Transport Effects None known.

Avoid Concomitant Use

Avoid concomitant use of Ketorolac (Systemic) with any of the following: Aspirin; Floctafenine; Ketorolac (Nasal); Nonsteroidal Anti-Inflammatory Agents; NSAID (COX-2 Inhibitor); Omacetaxine; Pentoxifylline; Probenecid

Increased Effect/Toxicity

Ketorolac (Systemic) may increase the levels/effects of: 5-ASA Derivatives; Agents with Antiplatelet Properties; Aliskiren; Aminoglycosides; Anticoagulants; Aspirin; Bisphosphonate Derivatives; Collagenase (Systemic); CycloSPORINE (Systemic); Dabigatran Etexilate; Deferasirox; Desmopressin; Digoxin; Eplerenone; Haloperidol; Ibritumomab; Lithium; Methotrexate; Neuromuscular-Blocking Agents (Nondepolarizing); Nonsteroidal Anti-Inflammatory Agents; NSAID (COX-2 Inhibitor); Omacetaxine; PEMEtrexed; Pentoxifylline; Porfimer; Potassium-Sparing Diuretics; PRALAtrexate; Quinolone Antibiotics; Rivaroxaban; Salicylates; Tenofovir; Thrombolytic Agents; Tositumomab and Iodine I 131 Tositumomab; Vancomycin; Vitamin K Antagonists

The levels/effects of Ketorolac (Systemic) may be increased by: ACE Inhibitors; Angiotensin II Receptor Blockers; Antidepressants (Tricyclic, Tertiary Amine); Corticosteroids (Systemic); CycloSPORINE (Systemic); Dasatinib; Floctafenine; Glucosamine; Herbs (Anticoagulant/Antiplatelet Properties); Ibrutinib; Ketorolac (Nasal); Multivitamins/Fluoride (with ADE); Multivitamins/Minerals (with ADEK, Folate, Iron); Multivitamins/Minerals (with AE, No Iron); Omega-3 Fatty Acids; Pentosan Polysulfate Sodium; Probenecid; Prostacyclin Analogues; Selective Serotonin Reuptake Inhibitors; Serotonin/Norepinephrine Reuptake Inhibitors; Sodium Phosphates; Tipranavir; Treprostinil; Vitamin E

Decreased Effect

Ketorolac (Systemic) may decrease the levels/effects of: ACE Inhibitors; Agents with Antiplatelet Properties; Aliskiren; Angiotensin II Receptor Blockers; Anticonvulsants; Aspirin; Beta-Blockers; Eplerenone; HydrALAZINE; Loop Diuretics; Potassium-Sparing Diuretics; Prostaglandins (Ophthalmic); Salicylates; Selective Serotonin Reuptake Inhibitors; Thiazide Diuretics

The levels/effects of Ketorolac (Systemic) may be decreased by: Bile Acid Sequestrants; Salicylates

Ethanol/Nutrition/Herb Interactions

Ethanol: Avoid ethanol (may enhance gastric mucosal irritation).

Food: Oral: High-fat meals may delay time to peak (by ~1 hour) and decrease peak concentrations.

Herb/Nutraceutical: Avoid alfalfa, anise, bilberry, bladderwrack, bromelain, cat's claw, celery, chamomile, coleus, cordyceps, dong quai, evening primrose, fenugreek, feverfew, garlic, ginger, ginkgo biloba, ginseng (American, Panax, Siberian), grapeseed, green tea, guggul, horse chestnut seed, horseradish, licorice, prickly ash, red clover, reishi, SAMe (S-adenosylmethionine), sweet clover, turmeric, and white willow (all have additional antiplatelet activity).

Storage/Stability

Injection: Store at room temperature of 15°C to 30°C (59°F to 86°F). Protect from light. Injection is clear and has a slight yellow color. Precipitation may occur at relatively low pH values.

Tablet: Store at room temperature of 15°C to 30°C (59°F to 86°F).

Mechanism of Action Reversibly inhibits cyclooxygenase-1 and 2 (COX-1 and 2) enzymes, which results in decreased formation of prostaglandin precursors; has antipyretic, analgesic, and anti-inflammatory properties

Other proposed mechanisms not fully elucidated (and possibly contributing to the anti-inflammatory effect to varying degrees), include inhibiting chemotaxis, altering lymphocyte activity, inhibiting neutrophil aggregation/activation, and decreasing proinflammatory cytokine levels.

Pharmacodynamics/Kinetics

Onset of action: Analgesic: I.M., I.V.: ~30 minutes

Peak effect: Analgesic: ≤2-3 hours

Duration: Analgesic: 4-6 hours

Absorption: Oral: Well absorbed (100%)

Distribution: ~13 L; poor penetration into CSF

Protein binding: 99%

Metabolism: Hepatic

Half-life elimination: 2-6 hours; prolonged 30% to 50% in elderly; up to 19 hours in renal impairment

Time to peak, serum: I.M.: 30-60 minutes

Excretion: Urine (92%, ~60% as unchanged drug); feces ~6%

Dosage Pain management (acute; moderately severe): **Note:** The maximum combined duration of treatment (for parenteral and oral) is 5 days; do not increase dose or frequency; supplement with low-dose opioids if needed for breakthrough pain.

Adolescents ≥17 years and Adults ≥50 kg:

I.M.: 60 mg as a single dose or 30 mg every 6 hours (maximum daily dose: 120 mg)

I.V.: 30 mg as a single dose or 30 mg every 6 hours (maximum daily dose: 120 mg)

Oral: 20 mg, followed by 10 mg every 4-6 hours as needed; do not exceed 40 mg daily; oral dosing is intended to be a continuation of I.M. or I.V. therapy only

Adults, critically-ill (unlabeled dose): I.M., I.V.: 30 mg once, followed by 15-30 mg every 6 hours for up to 5 days (maximum daily dose: 120 mg) (Barr, 2013)

Elderly ≥65 years: **Note:** May have an increased incidence of GI bleeding, ulceration, and perforation. The maximum combined duration of treatment (for parenteral and oral) is 5 days.

I.M.: 30 mg as a single dose or 15 mg every 6 hours (maximum daily dose: 60 mg)

I.V.: 15 mg as a single dose or 15 mg every 6 hours (maximum daily dose: 60 mg)

Oral: 10 mg, followed by 10 mg every 4-6 hours as needed; do not exceed 40 mg daily; oral dosing is intended to be a continuation of I.M. or I.V. therapy only

Dosage adjustments for low body weight (<50 kg): Refer to elderly dosing.

Dosage adjustment in renal impairment: Use is contraindicated in patients with advanced renal impairment or patients at risk for renal failure due to volume depletion.

Mild-to-moderate impairment:

I.M.: 30 mg as a single dose or 15 mg every 6 hours (maximum daily dose: 60 mg)

I.V.: 15 mg as a single dose or 15 mg every 6 hours (maximum daily dose: 60 mg)

Oral: 10 mg, followed by 10 mg every 4-6 hours as needed; do not exceed 40 mg daily; oral dosing is intended to be a continuation of I.M. or I.V. therapy only

Note: The maximum combined duration of treatment (for parenteral and oral) is 5 days.

Advanced impairment or patients at risk for renal failure due to volume depletion: Use is contraindicated.

Dosage adjustment in hepatic impairment: No dosage adjustment provided in manufacturer's labeling. Use with caution, may cause elevation of liver enzymes; discontinue if clinical signs and symptoms of liver disease develop.

Dietary Considerations Administer tablet with food or milk to decrease gastrointestinal distress.

Administration

Oral: May take with food to reduce GI upset.

I.M.: Administer slowly and deeply into the muscle.

I.V.: Administer I.V. bolus over a minimum of 15 seconds.

Monitoring Parameters Monitor response (pain, range of motion, grip strength, mobility, ADL function), inflammation; observe for weight gain, edema; monitor renal function (serum creatinine, BUN, urine output); CBC and platelets, liver function tests; chemistry profile; blood pressure; observe for bleeding, bruising; evaluate gastrointestinal effects (abdominal pain, bleeding, dyspepsia); mental confusion, disorientation

Reference Range Serum concentration: Therapeutic: 0.3-5 mcg/mL; Toxic: >5 mcg/mL

Additional Information Ketorolac 30 mg I.M. provides analgesia comparable to morphine ≤12 mg or meperidine ≤100 mg (Buckley, 1990).

Dosage Forms Excipient information presented when available (limited, particularly for generics); consult specific product labeling.

Solution, Injection, as tromethamine:

Generic: 15 mg/mL (1 mL); 30 mg/mL (1 mL); 60 mg/2 mL (2 mL); 300 mg/10 mL (10 mL)

Solution, Intramuscular, as tromethamine:

Generic: 30 mg/mL (1 mL); 60 mg/2 mL (2 mL)

Tablet, Oral, as tromethamine:

Generic: 10 mg

Ketorolac (Nasal) (KEE toe role ak)

Brand Names: U.S. Sprix

Index Terms Ketorolac Tromethamine

Pharmacologic Category Nonsteroidal Anti-inflammatory Drug (NSAID), Nasal

Use Short-term (≤5 days) management of moderate-to-moderately-severe acute pain requiring analgesia at the opioid level

Pregnancy Risk Factor C/D ≥30 weeks gestation

Medication Guide Available Yes

Dosage Intranasal: **Note:** The maximum combined duration of treatment (for nasal spray or other ketorolac formulations) is 5 days.

Adults<65 years and ≥50 kg: One spray (15.75 mg) in each nostril (total dose: 31.5 mg) every 6-8 hours; maximum dose: 4 doses (126 mg)/day

Dosage adjustments in adults with low body weight (<50 kg): One spray (15.75 mg) in 1 nostril (total dose: 15.75 mg) every 6-8 hours; maximum dose: 4 doses (63 mg)/day

Elderly (≥65 years): Intranasal: One spray (15.75 mg) in 1 nostril (total dose: 15.75 mg) every 6-8 hours; maximum dose: 4 doses (63 mg)/day

Dosage adjustment in renal impairment:

Renal insufficiency: Intranasal: One spray (15.75 mg) in 1 nostril (total dose: 15.75 mg) every 6-8 hours; maximum dose: 4 doses (63 mg)/day

Advanced renal impairment (or at risk for renal failure due to volume depletion): Use is contraindicated

Dosage adjustment in hepatic impairment: Use with caution with hepatic impairment or history of hepatic disease; use may cause elevation of liver enzymes; discontinue if clinical signs and symptoms of liver disease develop.

Additional Information Complete prescribing information should be consulted for additional detail.

Dosage Forms Excipient information presented when available (limited, particularly for generics); consult specific product labeling.

Solution, Nasal, as tromethamine [preservative free]:

Sprix: 15.75 mg/spray (1 ea) [contains edetate disodium]

Ketorolac (Ophthalmic) (KEE toe role ak)

Brand Names: U.S. Acular; Acular LS; Acuvail

Brand Names: Canada Acular LS®; Acular®; Apo-Ketorolac® Ophthalmic; ratio-Ketorolac

Index Terms Ketorolac Tromethamine

Pharmacologic Category Nonsteroidal Anti-inflammatory Drug (NSAID), Ophthalmic

Use Temporary relief of ocular itching due to seasonal allergic conjunctivitis; postoperative pain and/or inflammation following cataract extraction; reduction of ocular pain, burning, and stinging following corneal refractive surgery

Pregnancy Risk Factor C

Dosage Ophthalmic:

Children ≥2 years, Adolescents, and Adults: Acular®:

Allergic conjunctivitis (relief of ocular itching): Instill 1 drop to affected eye(s) 4 times daily

Inflammation following cataract extraction: Instill 1 drop to affected eye(s) 4 times daily beginning 24 hours after surgery; continue for 2 weeks

Children ≥3 years, Adolescents, and Adults: Acular LS®: Pain, burning/stinging following corneal refractive surgery: Instill 1 drop to affected eye(s) 4 times daily as needed for up to 4 days after surgery

Adults: Acuvail®: Pain and inflammation associated with cataract surgery: Instill 1 drop to affected eye(s) 2 times daily 24 hours before surgery and on the day of surgery; continue for 2 weeks

Dosage adjustment in renal impairment: No dosage adjustment provided in manufacturer's labeling.

Dosage adjustment in hepatic impairment: No dosage adjustment provided in manufacturer's labeling.

Additional Information Complete prescribing information should be consulted for additional detail.

Dosage Forms Excipient information presented when available (limited, particularly for generics); consult specific product labeling.

Solution, Ophthalmic, as tromethamine:

Acular: 0.5% (5 mL) [contains benzalkonium chloride, edetate disodium]

Acular LS: 0.4% (5 mL) [contains benzalkonium chloride, edetate disodium]

Generic: 0.4% (5 mL); 0.5% (3 mL, 5 mL, 10 mL)

Solution, Ophthalmic, as tromethamine [preservative free]:

Acuvail: 0.45% (30 ea)

◆ **Ketorolac Tromethamine** *see* Ketorolac (Nasal) *on page 1155*

◆ **Ketorolac Tromethamine** *see* Ketorolac (Ophthalmic) *on page 1155*

◆ **Ketorolac Tromethamine** *see* Ketorolac (Systemic) *on page 1152*

- **Ketorolac Tromethamine Injection, USP (Can)** *see* Ketorolac (Systemic) *on page 1152*

Ketotifen (Ophthalmic) (kee toe TYE fen)

Brand Names: U.S. Alaway Childrens Allergy [OTC]; Alaway [OTC]; Claritin Eye [OTC]; Refresh Eye Itch Relief [OTC] [DSC]; Zaditor [OTC]; ZyrTEC Itchy Eye [OTC]

Brand Names: Canada Zaditor®

Index Terms Ketotifen Fumarate

Pharmacologic Category Histamine H_1 Antagonist; Histamine H_1 Antagonist, Second Generation; Mast Cell Stabilizer; Piperidine Derivative

Use Temporary relief of eye itching due to allergic conjunctivitis

Pregnancy Risk Factor C

Dosage Ophthalmic: Allergic conjunctivitis: Children ≥3 years and Adults: Instill 1 drop into the affected eye(s) twice daily, every 8-12 hours

Additional Information Complete prescribing information should be consulted for additional detail.

Dosage Forms Excipient information presented when available (limited, particularly for generics); consult specific product labeling. [DSC] = Discontinued product

Solution, Ophthalmic:

- Alaway: 0.025% (10 mL) [contains benzalkonium chloride]
- Alaway Childrens Allergy: 0.025% (5 mL) [contains benzalkonium chloride]
- Claritin Eye: 0.025% (5 mL) [contains benzalkonium chloride]
- Refresh Eye Itch Relief: 0.025% (5 mL [DSC]) [contains benzalkonium chloride]
- Zaditor: 0.025% (5 mL) [contains benzalkonium chloride]
- ZyrTEC Itchy Eye: 0.025% (5 mL) [contains benzalkonium chloride]
- Generic: 0.025% (5 mL)

Dosage Forms: Canada Excipient information presented when available (limited, particularly for generics); consult specific product labeling.

Solution, ophthalmic [drops]:

- Zaditor®: 0.025% (5 mL) [contains benzalkonium chloride]

Solution, ophthalmic [drops], preservative free:

- Zaditor®: 0.025% (0.4 mL) (30s)

- **Ketotifen Fumarate** *see* Ketotifen (Ophthalmic) *on page 1156*
- **Khedezla** *see* Desvenlafaxine *on page 579*
- **Khloditan** *see* Mitotane *on page 1385*
- **KI** *see* Potassium Iodide *on page 1687*
- **Kidkare Children's Cough/Cold [OTC]** *see* Chlorpheniramine, Pseudoephedrine, and Dextromethorphan *on page 414*
- **Kidrolase (Can)** *see* Asparaginase (*E. coli*) *on page 174*
- **Kineret** *see* Anakinra *on page 136*
- **Kineret® (Can)** *see* Anakinra *on page 136*
- **Kinrix®** *see* Diphtheria and Tetanus Toxoids, Acellular Pertussis, and Poliovirus Vaccine *on page 629*
- **Kionex** *see* Sodium Polystyrene Sulfonate *on page 1927*
- **Kivexa™ (Can)** *see* Abacavir and Lamivudine *on page 20*
- **Klaron** *see* Sulfacetamide (Topical) *on page 1957*
- **Klean-Prep (Can)** *see* Polyethylene Glycol-Electrolyte Solution *on page 1669*
- **KlonoPIN** *see* ClonazePAM *on page 465*
- **K-Lor** *see* Potassium Chloride *on page 1684*
- **Klor-Con** *see* Potassium Chloride *on page 1684*
- **Klor-Con 10** *see* Potassium Chloride *on page 1684*
- **Klor-Con®/EF** *see* Potassium Bicarbonate and Potassium Citrate *on page 1684*
- **Klor-Con M10** *see* Potassium Chloride *on page 1684*
- **Klor-Con M15** *see* Potassium Chloride *on page 1684*
- **Klor-Con M20** *see* Potassium Chloride *on page 1684*
- **K-Lyte/Cl** *see* Potassium Bicarbonate and Potassium Chloride *on page 1684*
- **KMD 3213** *see* Silodosin *on page 1896*
- **Koffex DM-D (Can)** *see* Pseudoephedrine and Dextromethorphan *on page 1748*
- **Koffex Expectorant (Can)** *see* GuaiFENesin *on page 974*
- **Kogenate FS** *see* Antihemophilic Factor (Recombinant) *on page 144*
- **Kogenate® FS (Can)** *see* Antihemophilic Factor (Recombinant) *on page 144*
- **Kogenate FS Bio-Set** *see* Antihemophilic Factor (Recombinant) *on page 144*
- **Kolephrin GG/DM [OTC]** *see* Guaifenesin and Dextromethorphan *on page 976*
- **Kombiglyze™ XR** *see* Saxagliptin and Metformin *on page 1881*
- **Komboglyze™ (Can)** *see* Saxagliptin and Metformin *on page 1881*
- **Konakion (Can)** *see* Phytonadione *on page 1644*
- **Konsyl [OTC]** *see* Psyllium *on page 1748*
- **Konsyl-D [OTC]** *see* Psyllium *on page 1748*
- **Korlym** *see* Mifepristone *on page 1364*
- **Koāte®-DVI** *see* Antihemophilic Factor (Human) *on page 143*
- **K-Phos** *see* Potassium Acid Phosphate *on page 1683*
- **K-Phos® Neutral** *see* Potassium Phosphate and Sodium Phosphate *on page 1691*
- **K-Phos® No. 2** *see* Potassium Phosphate and Sodium Phosphate *on page 1691*
- **Kristalose** *see* Lactulose *on page 1161*
- **Krystexxa** *see* Pegloticase *on page 1599*
- **KS Ibuprofen [OTC]** *see* Ibuprofen *on page 1032*
- **KS Stool Softener [OTC]** *see* Docusate *on page 644*
- **K-Tabs** *see* Potassium Chloride *on page 1684*
- **Kurvelo** *see* Ethinyl Estradiol and Levonorgestrel *on page 787*
- **Kuvan** *see* Sapropterin *on page 1875*
- **K-Vescent** *see* Potassium Chloride *on page 1684*
- **Kwell** *see* Lindane *on page 1217*
- **Kwellada-P™ (Can)** *see* Permethrin *on page 1624*
- **Kynamro** *see* Mipomersen *on page 1376*
- **Kyprolis** *see* Carfilzomib *on page 348*
- **Kytril** *see* Granisetron *on page 972*
- **Kytril® (Can)** *see* Granisetron *on page 972*
- **L-749,345** *see* Ertapenem *on page 739*
- **L-758,298** *see* Fosaprepitant *on page 919*
- **L 754030** *see* Aprepitant *on page 158*
- **LA 20304a** *see* Gemifloxacin *on page 948*

Labetalol (la BET a lole)

Brand Names: U.S. Trandate

Brand Names: Canada Apo-Labetalol®; Labetalol Hydrochloride Injection, USP; Normodyne®; Trandate®

Index Terms Ibidomide Hydrochloride; Labetalol Hydrochloride

Pharmacologic Category Antihypertensive; Beta-Blocker With Alpha-Blocking Activity

Additional Appendix Information

Beta-Blockers *on page 2294*

Dosing Considerations for the Critically-Ill Patient With Morbid Obesity *on page 2379*

Use Treatment of mild-to-severe hypertension; I.V. for severe hypertension (eg, hypertensive emergencies)

Unlabeled Use Pediatric hypertension; management of pre-eclampsia; severe hypertension in pregnancy; hypertension during acute ischemic stroke

Pregnancy Risk Factor C

Pregnancy Considerations Because adverse events were observed in some animal reproduction studies, labetalol is classified as pregnancy category C. Labetalol crosses the placenta and can be detected in cord blood and infant serum after delivery. It has been shown to decrease maternal blood pressure without significantly effecting placental blood flow. In a cohort study, an increased risk of cardiovascular defects was observed following maternal use of beta-blockers during pregnancy. Intrauterine growth restriction (IUGR), small placentas, as well as fetal/neonatal bradycardia, hypoglycemia, and/or respiratory depression have been observed following *in utero* exposure to beta-blockers as a class. Adequate facilities for monitoring infants at birth should be available. Untreated chronic maternal hypertension and pre-eclampsia are also associated with adverse events in the fetus, infant, and mother. The pharmacokinetics of labetalol are not significantly changed during the third trimester of pregnancy. Labetalol is considered an appropriate agent for the treatment of hypertension in pregnancy; intravenous labetalol is also used for the management of pre-eclampsia.

Breast-Feeding Considerations Low amounts of labetalol are found in breast milk and can be detected in the serum of nursing infants. The manufacturer recommends that caution be exercised when administering labetalol to nursing women.

Contraindications Hypersensitivity to labetalol or any component of the formulation; severe bradycardia; heart block greater than first degree (except in patients with a functioning artificial pacemaker); cardiogenic shock; bronchial asthma; uncompensated cardiac failure; conditions associated with severe and prolonged hypotension

Warnings/Precautions Consider pre-existing conditions such as sick sinus syndrome before initiating. Symptomatic hypotension with or without syncope may occur with labetalol; close monitoring of patient is required especially with initial dosing and dosing increases; blood pressure must be lowered at a rate appropriate for the patient's clinical condition. Initiation with a low dose and gradual up-titration may help to decrease the occurrence of hypotension or syncope. Patients should be advised to avoid driving or other hazardous tasks during initiation of therapy due to the risk of syncope. Orthostatic hypotension may occur with I.V. administration; patient should remain supine during and for up to 3 hours after I.V. administration. Use with caution in impaired hepatic function; bioavailability is increased due to decreased first-pass metabolism. Severe hepatic injury including some fatalities have also been rarely reported with use: periodically monitor LFTs with prolonged use. Use with caution in patients with diabetes mellitus; may potentiate hypoglycemia and/or mask signs and symptoms. Bradycardia may be observed more frequently in elderly patients (>65 years of age); dosage reductions may be necessary. May also reduce release of insulin in response to hyperglycemia; dosage of antidiabetic agents may need to be adjusted. May mask signs of hyperthyroidism (eg, tachycardia); if hyperthyroidism is suspected, carefully manage and monitor; abrupt withdrawal may exacerbate symptoms of hyperthyroidism or precipitate thyroid storm. Elimination of labetalol is reduced in elderly patients; lower maintenance doses may be required.

Use only with extreme caution in compensated heart failure and monitor for a worsening of the condition. Beta-blocker therapy should not be withdrawn abruptly (particularly in patients with CAD), but gradually tapered to avoid acute tachycardia, hypertension, and/or ischemia. Chronic beta-blocker therapy should not be routinely withdrawn prior to major surgery. Use caution with concurrent use of digoxin, verapamil, or diltiazem; bradycardia or heart block can occur. Use with caution in patients receiving inhaled anesthetic agents known to depress myocardial contractility. Patients with bronchospastic disease should not receive beta-blockers; if used at all, should be used cautiously with close monitoring. Use with caution in patients with myasthenia gravis or psychiatric disease (may cause or exacerbate CNS depression). Can precipitate or aggravate symptoms of arterial insufficiency in patients with PVD and Raynaud's disease; use with caution and monitor for progression of arterial obstruction. If possible, obtain diagnostic tests for pheochromocytoma prior to use. May induce or exacerbate psoriasis. Labetalol has been shown to be effective in lowering blood pressure and relieving symptoms in patients with pheochromocytoma. However, some patients have experienced paradoxical hypertensive responses; use with caution in patients with pheochromocytoma. Additional alpha-blockade may be required during use of labetalol. Use caution with history of severe anaphylaxis to allergens; patients taking beta-blockers may become more sensitive to repeated challenges. Treatment of anaphylaxis (eg, epinephrine) in patients taking beta-blockers may be ineffective or promote undesirable effects.

Intraoperative floppy iris syndrome has been observed in cataract surgery patients who were on or were previously treated with alpha$_1$-blockers; causality has not been established and there appears to be no benefit in discontinuing alpha-blocker therapy prior to surgery. Instruct patients to inform ophthalmologist of labetalol use when considering eye surgery.

Adverse Reactions

>10%:

- Cardiovascular: Orthostatic hypotension (I.V. use; ≤58%)
- Central nervous system: Dizziness (1% to 20%), fatigue (1% to 11%)
- Gastrointestinal: Nausea (≤19%)

1% to 10%:

- Cardiovascular: Hypotension (1% to 5%), edema (≤2%), flushing (1%), ventricular arrhythmia (I.V. use; 1%)
- Central nervous system: Somnolence (3%), headache (2%), vertigo (1% to 2%)
- Dermatologic: Scalp tingling (≤7%), pruritus (1%), rash (1%)
- Gastrointestinal: Dyspepsia (≤4%), vomiting (≤3%), taste disturbance (1%)
- Genitourinary: Ejaculatory failure (≤5%), impotence (1% to 4%)
- Hepatic: Transaminases increased (4%)
- Neuromuscular & skeletal: Paresthesia (≤5%), weakness (1%)
- Ocular: Vision abnormal (1%)
- Renal: BUN increased (≤8%)
- Respiratory: Nasal congestion (1% to 6%), dyspnea (2%)
- Miscellaneous: Diaphoresis (≤4%)

<1% (Limited to important or life-threatening): Alopecia (reversible), anaphylactoid reaction, ANA positive, angioedema, bradycardia, bronchospasm, cholestatic jaundice, CHF, diabetes insipidus, heart block, hepatic necrosis, hepatitis, hypersensitivity, Peyronie's disease,

psoriaform rash, Raynaud's syndrome, syncope, systemic lupus erythematosus, toxic myopathy, urinary retention, urticaria

Other adverse reactions noted with beta-adrenergic blocking agents include mental depression, catatonia, disorientation, short-term memory loss, emotional lability, clouded sensorium, intensification of pre-existing AV block, laryngospasm, respiratory distress, agranulocytosis, thrombocytopenic purpura, nonthrombocytopenic purpura, mesenteric artery thrombosis, and ischemic colitis.

Drug Interactions

Metabolism/Transport Effects None known.

Avoid Concomitant Use

Avoid concomitant use of Labetalol with any of the following: Beta2-Agonists; Floctafenine; Methacholine

Increased Effect/Toxicity

Labetalol may increase the levels/effects of: Alpha-/Beta-Agonists (Direct-Acting); Alpha1-Blockers; Alpha2-Agonists; Amifostine; Antihypertensives; Antipsychotic Agents (Phenothiazines); Bupivacaine; Cardiac Glycosides; Cholinergic Agonists; Ergot Derivatives; Fingolimod; Hypotensive Agents; Insulin; Lidocaine (Systemic); Lidocaine (Topical); Mepivacaine; Methacholine; Midodrine; Obinutuzumab; RiTUXimab; Sulfonylureas

The levels/effects of Labetalol may be increased by: Acetylcholinesterase Inhibitors; Alpha2-Agonists; Aminoquinolines (Antimalarial); Amiodarone; Anilidopiperidine Opioids; Antipsychotic Agents (Phenothiazines); Brimonidine (Topical); Calcium Channel Blockers (Dihydropyridine); Calcium Channel Blockers (Nondihydropyridine); Diazoxide; Dipyridamole; Disopyramide; Dronedarone; Floctafenine; Herbs (Hypotensive Properties); MAO Inhibitors; Pentoxifylline; Phosphodiesterase 5 Inhibitors; Propafenone; Prostacyclin Analogues; Regorafenib; Reserpine

Decreased Effect

Labetalol may decrease the levels/effects of: Beta2-Agonists; Theophylline Derivatives

The levels/effects of Labetalol may be decreased by: Barbiturates; Herbs (Hypertensive Properties); Methylphenidate; Nonsteroidal Anti-Inflammatory Agents; Rifamycin Derivatives; Yohimbine

Ethanol/Nutrition/Herb Interactions

Food: Labetalol serum concentrations may be increased if taken with food.

Herb/Nutraceutical: Avoid dong quai if using for hypertension (has estrogenic activity). Avoid ephedra, yohimbe, ginseng (may worsen hypertension). Avoid natural licorice (causes sodium and water retention and increases potassium loss). Avoid garlic (may have increased antihypertensive effect).

Storage/Stability

Tablets: Store at room temperature (refer to manufacturer's labeling for detailed storage requirements). Protect from light and excessive moisture.

Injectable: Store at room temperature (refer to manufacturer's labeling for detailed storage requirements); do not freeze. Protect from light. The solution is clear to slightly yellow.

Parenteral admixture: Stability of parenteral admixture at room temperature (25°C) and refrigeration temperature (4°C): 3 days.

Mechanism of Action Blocks alpha-, beta$_1$-, and beta$_2$-adrenergic receptor sites; elevated renins are reduced. The ratios of alpha- to beta-blockade differ depending on the route of administration: 1:3 (oral) and 1:7 (I.V.).

Pharmacodynamics/Kinetics

Onset of action: Oral: 20 minutes to 2 hours; I.V.: 2-5 minutes

Peak effect: Oral: 1-4 hours; I.V.: 5-15 minutes

Duration: Blood pressure response:

Oral: 8-12 hours (dose dependent)

I.V.: 2-18 hours (dose dependent; based on single and multiple sequential doses of 0.25-0.5 mg/kg with cumulative dosing up to 3.25 mg/kg)

Absorption: Complete

Distribution: V_d: Adults: 3-16 L/kg; mean: <9.4 L/kg; moderately lipid soluble, therefore, can enter CNS

Protein binding: 50%

Metabolism: Hepatic, primarily via glucuronide conjugation; extensive first-pass effect

Bioavailability: Oral: 25%; increased with liver disease, elderly, and concurrent cimetidine

Half-life elimination: Oral: 6-8 hours; I.V.: ~5.5 hours

Time to peak, plasma: Oral: 1-2 hours

Excretion: Urine (55% to 60% as glucuronide conjugates, <5% as unchanged drug)

Clearance: Possibly decreased in neonates/infants

Dosage

Children: Due to limited documentation of its use, labetalol should be initiated cautiously in pediatric patients with careful dosage adjustment and blood pressure monitoring.

Oral: Hypertension (unlabeled use): Initial: 1-3 mg/kg/day, in 2 divided doses; maximum: 10-12 mg/kg/day, up to 1200 mg/day

I.V., intermittent bolus doses of 0.3-1 mg/kg/dose have been reported.

For treatment of pediatric hypertensive emergencies, initial continuous infusions of 0.4-1 mg/kg/hour with a maximum of 3 mg/kg/hour have been used. Administration requires the use of an infusion pump.

Adults:

Hypertension: Oral: Initial: 100 mg twice daily, may increase as needed every 2-3 days by 100 mg twice daily (titration increments not to exceed 200 mg twice daily) until desired response is obtained; usual dose: 100-400 mg twice daily (JNC 7); may require up to 2.4 g/day.

Acute hypertension (hypertensive emergency/urgency):

I.V. bolus: Per the manufacturer: Initial: 20 mg I.V. push over 2 minutes; may administer 40-80 mg at 10-minute intervals, up to 300 mg total cumulative dose; as appropriate, follow with oral antihypertensive regimen

I.V. infusion (acute loading): Per the manufacturer: Initial: 2 mg/minute; titrate to response up to 300 mg total cumulative dose (eg, discontinue after 2.5 hours of 2 mg/minute); usual total dose required: 50-200 mg; as appropriate, follow with oral antihypertensive regimen

Note: Although loading infusions are well described in the product labeling, the labeling is silent in specific clinical situations, such as in the patient who has an initial response to labetalol infusions but cannot be converted to an oral route for subsequent dosing. There is limited documentation of prolonged continuous infusions (ie, >300 mg/day). In rare clinical situations, higher continuous infusion doses up to 6 mg/minute have been used in the critical care setting (eg, aortic dissection) and up to 8 mg/minute (eg, hypertension with ongoing acute ischemic stroke). At these doses, it may be best to consider an alternative agent if the labetalol infusion is not meeting the goals of therapy. At the other extreme, continuous infusions at relatively low doses (0.03-0.1 mg/minute) have been used in some settings (following loading infusion in patients who are unable to be converted to oral regimens or in some cases as a continuation of outpatient oral regimens). These prolonged infusions should not be confused with loading infusions. Because of wide variation in the use of infusions, an awareness of institutional policies and practices is extremely important. Careful clarification of orders and specific infusion rates/units is required to avoid confusion. Due to the prolonged duration of action, careful monitoring should be extended for the duration of the infusion and for several hours after the infusion. Excessive administration may result in prolonged hypotension and/or bradycardia.

Arterial hypertension in acute ischemic stroke (unlabeled use [Jauch, 2013]): I.V.:

Patient otherwise eligible for reperfusion treatment (eg, alteplase) except blood pressure (BP) >185/110 mm Hg: 10-20 mg over 1-2 minutes; may repeat once. If BP does not decline and remains >185/110 mm Hg, alteplase should not be administered.

Management of BP during and after reperfusion treatment (eg, alteplase) to maintain BP ≤180/105 mm Hg: If systolic BP >180-230 mm Hg or diastolic >105-120 mm Hg, then administer 10 mg over 1-2 minutes followed by an infusion of 2-8 mg/minute. If hypertension is refractory or diastolic BP >140 mm Hg, consider other I.V. antihypertensives (eg, nitroprusside).

I.V. to oral conversion: Upon discontinuation of I.V. infusion, may initiate oral dose of 200 mg followed in 6-12 hours with an additional dose of 200-400 mg. Thereafter, dose patients with 400-2400 mg/day in divided doses depending on blood pressure response.

Elderly: Refer to adult dosing.

Hypertension: Oral:

Manufacturer's recommendations: Initial: 100 mg twice daily; may titrate in increments of 100 mg twice daily; usual maintenance: 100-200 mg twice daily

ACCF/AHA Expert Consensus recommendations: Consider lower initial doses and titrating to response (Aronow, 2011)

Dosage adjustment in renal impairment: No dosage adjustment provided in manufacturer's labeling. Not removed by hemo- or peritoneal dialysis; supplemental dose is not necessary.

Dosage adjustment in hepatic impairment: No dosage adjustment provided in manufacturer's labeling. However, dosage reduction may be necessary in hepatic impairment due to decreased metabolism and increased oral bioavailability, use with caution.

Usual Infusion Concentrations: Pediatric I.V. infusion: 1 mg/mL

Usual Infusion Concentrations: Adult I.V. infusion: 500 mg in 250 mL (concentration: 2 mg/mL) of D_5W

Administration Bolus dose may be administered I.V. push at a rate of 10 mg/minute; may follow with continuous I.V. infusion

Monitoring Parameters Blood pressure, standing and sitting/supine, pulse, cardiac monitor and blood pressure monitor required for I.V. administration; consult individual institutional policies and procedures

Test Interactions False-positive urine catecholamines, vanillylmandelic acid (VMA) if measured by fluorometric or photometric methods; use HPLC or specific catecholamine radioenzymatic technique; false-positive amphetamine if measured by thin-layer chromatography or radioenzymatic assay (gas chromatographic-mass spectrometer technique should be used)

Dosage Forms Excipient information presented when available (limited, particularly for generics); consult specific product labeling.

Solution, Intravenous, as hydrochloride:

Generic: 5 mg/mL (4 mL, 20 mL, 40 mL)

Tablet, Oral, as hydrochloride:

Trandate: 100 mg, 200 mg, 300 mg [scored]

Generic: 100 mg, 200 mg, 300 mg

Extemporaneous Preparations A 40 mg/mL labetalol hydrochloride oral suspension may be made with tablets and one of three different vehicles (cherry syrup, a 1:1 mixture of Ora-Sweet® and Ora-Plus®, or a 1:1 mixture of Ora-Sweet® SF and Ora-Plus®). Crush sixteen 300 mg tablets in a mortar and reduce to a fine powder. Add 20 mL of the chosen vehicle and mix to a uniform paste; mix while adding the vehicle in incremental proportions to **almost** 120 mL; transfer to a calibrated bottle, rinse mortar with vehicle, and add quantity of vehicle sufficient to make 120 mL. Label "shake well" and "protect from light". Stable for 60 days when stored in amber plastic prescription bottles in the dark at room temperature or refrigerated (Allen, 1996).

Extemporaneously prepared solutions of labetalol hydrochloride (approximate concentrations 7-10 mg/mL) prepared in distilled water, simple syrup, apple juice, grape juice, and orange juice were stable for 4 weeks when stored in amber glass or plastic prescription bottles at room temperature or refrigerated (Nahata, 1991).

Allen LV Jr and Erickson MA 3rd, "Stability of Labetalol Hydrochloride, Metoprolol Tartrate, Verapamil Hydrochloride, and Spironolactone with Hydrochlorothiazide in Extemporaneously Compounded Oral Liquids," *Am J Health Syst Pharm*, 1996, 53(19):2304-9.

Nahata MC, "Stability of Labetalol Hydrochloride in Distilled Water, Simple Syrup, and Three Fruit Juices," *DICP*, 1991, 25(5):465-9.

◆ **Labetalol Hydrochloride** *see* Labetalol *on page* 1156

◆ **Labetalol Hydrochloride Injection, USP (Can)** *see* Labetalol *on page* 1156

Lacosamide (la KOE sa mide)

Brand Names: U.S. Vimpat

Brand Names: Canada Vimpat®

Index Terms ADD 234037; Harkoseride; LCM; SPM 927

Pharmacologic Category Anticonvulsant, Miscellaneous

Use Adjunctive therapy in the treatment of partial-onset seizures

Pregnancy Risk Factor C

Pregnancy Considerations Adverse events were observed in animal reproduction studies. Available information related to use in pregnancy is limited; if inadvertent exposure occurs during pregnancy, close monitoring of the mother and fetus/newborn is recommended (Hoeltzenbein, 2011). Two registries are available for women exposed to lacosamide during pregnancy:

Pregnant women may contact the North American Antiepileptic Drug (AED) Pregnancy Registry (888-233-2334 or http://www.aedpregnancyregistry.org)

The healthcare provider or patient may contact the UCB AED Pregnancy Registry (888-537-7734)

Breast-Feeding Considerations It is unknown if lacosamide is excreted in human milk. The manufacturer recommends a decision be made whether to discontinue nursing or to discontinue the drug, taking into account the importance of treatment to the mother.

Medication Guide Available Yes

Contraindications

U.S. labeling: There are no contraindications listed in manufacturer's labeling.

Canadian labeling: Hypersensitivity to lacosamide or any component of the formulation; second- or third-degree atrioventricular (AV) block (current or history of).

Warnings/Precautions Antiepileptics are associated with an increased risk of suicidal behavior/thoughts with use (regardless of indication); patients should be monitored for signs/symptoms of depression, suicidal tendencies, and other unusual behavior changes during therapy and instructed to inform their healthcare provider immediately if symptoms occur. CNS effects may occur; patients should be cautioned about performing tasks which require ▶

alertness (eg, operating machinery or driving). Lacosamide may prolong PR interval; second degree and complete AV block has also been reported. Use caution in patients with conduction problems (eg, first/second degree atrioventricular block and sick sinus syndrome without pacemaker), sodium channelopathies (eg, Brugada Syndrome), myocardial ischemia, heart failure, structural heart disease, or if concurrent use with other drugs that prolong the PR interval; ECG is recommended prior to initiating therapy and when at steady state. Instruct patients to contact their healthcare provider if signs or symptoms of conduction problems occur (eg, low or irregular pulse, feeling of lightheadedness and fainting). During investigational trials, atrial fibrillation/flutter, or syncope occurred slightly more often in patients with diabetic neuropathy and/or cardiovascular disease. Use caution with renal or hepatic impairment and if these patients are taking strong inhibitors of CYP3A4 and CYP2C9; dosage adjustment may be necessary. Multiorgan hypersensitivity reactions can occur (rare); monitor patient and discontinue therapy if necessary. Withdraw therapy gradually (≥1 week) to minimize the potential of increased seizure frequency. Blurred vision and diplopia may occur during therapy. If visual disturbances persist, further assessment, including dose reduction and discontinuation should be considered. Monitor patients with known vision-related issues or ocular conditions. Effects with ethanol may be potentiated. Some products may contain phenylalanine.

Adverse Reactions The majority of adverse events are dose-dependent.

>10%:

Central nervous system: Dizziness (16% to 53%), fatigue (7% to 15%), ataxia (4% to 15%), headache (11% to 14%)

Gastrointestinal: Nausea (7% to 17%), vomiting (6% to 16%)

Neuromuscular & skeletal: Tremor (4% to 12%)

Ophthalmic: Diplopia (6% to 16%), blurred vision (2% to 16%)

1% to 10%:

Cardiovascular: Syncope (adults 1%; dose-related: >400 mg/day)

Central nervous system: Drowsiness (5% to 8%), memory impairment (1% to 6%), vertigo (3% to 5%), abnormal gait (<1% to 4%), depression (2%)

Dermatologic: Pruritus (2% to 3%)

Gastrointestinal: Diarrhea (3% to 5%)

Hepatic: Increased serum ALT (1%)

Local: Pain at injection site (3%), local irritation (1%)

Neuromuscular & skeletal: Weakness (2% to 4%)

Ophthalmic: Nystagmus (2% to 10%)

Miscellaneous: Ecchymosis (2% to 4%), laceration (2% to 3%)

<1% (Limited to important or life-threatening): Agranulocytosis, anemia, atrial fibrillation, atrial flutter, atrioventricular block, bradycardia, cerebellar syndrome, cognitive dysfunction, DRESS syndrome, euphoria, falling, hallucination, hepatitis, nephritis, neutropenia

Drug Interactions

Metabolism/Transport Effects Substrate of CYP2C19 (minor); **Note:** Assignment of Major/Minor substrate status based on clinically relevant drug interaction potential; **Inhibits** CYP2C19 (weak)

Avoid Concomitant Use There are no known interactions where it is recommended to avoid concomitant use.

Increased Effect/Toxicity

The levels/effects of Lacosamide may be increased by: CYP2C9 Inhibitors (Strong); CYP3A4 Inhibitors (Strong); Delavirdine; NiCARdipine

Decreased Effect

The levels/effects of Lacosamide may be decreased by: CarBAMazepine; Fosphenytoin; PHENobarbital; Phenytoin

Ethanol/Nutrition/Herb Interactions Ethanol: Avoid ethanol (may increase CNS depression).

Preparation for Administration Injection: May be mixed with compatible diluents (NS, LR, D_5W) in glass or PVC.

Storage/Stability

Injection: Store at 20°C to 25°C (68°F to 77°F); excursions permitted between 15°C to 30°C (59°F to 86°F). Do not freeze. Stable when mixed with compatible diluents (NS, LR, D_5W) for at least 24 hours in glass or PVC at room temperature of 15°C to 30°C (59°F to 86°F). Discard any unused portion.

Oral solution, tablets: Store at 20°C to 25°C (68°F to 77°F); excursions permitted between 15°C to 30°C (59°F to 86°F). Do not freeze oral solution. Discard any unused portion of oral solution after 7 weeks.

Mechanism of Action *In vitro* studies have shown that lacosamide stabilizes hyperexcitable neuronal membranes and inhibits repetitive neuronal firing by enhancing the slow inactivation of sodium channels (with no effects on fast inactivation of sodium channels).

Pharmacodynamics/Kinetics

Absorption: Oral: Completely

Distribution: V_d: ~0.6 L/kg

Protein binding: <15%

Metabolism: Hepatic via CYP3A4, CYP2C9, and CYP2C19; forms metabolite, O-desmethyl-lacosamide (inactive)

Bioavailability: ~100%

Half-life elimination: ~13 hours

Time to peak, plasma: Oral: 1-4 hours

Excretion: Urine (95%; 40% as unchanged drug, 30% as inactive metabolite, 20% as uncharacterized metabolite); feces (<0.5%)

Dosage Oral, I.V.: Adolescents ≥17 years and Adults: Partial onset seizure:

Initial: 50 mg twice daily; may be increased at weekly intervals by 100 mg daily

Maintenance dose: 200-400 mg daily

Note: When switching from oral to I.V. formulations, the total daily dose and frequency should be the same; I.V. therapy should only be used temporarily.

Dosing adjustment in renal impairment: Use caution when titrating dose.

Mild-to-moderate renal impairment: No dose adjustment necessary. However, in patients with renal impairment taking concomitant strong CYP3A4 and/or CYP2C9 inhibitors, dosage reduction may be necessary.

Severe renal impairment (Cl_{cr} ≤30 mL/minute): Maximum dose: 300 mg daily. Further dosage reduction/limitation may be necessary with concomitant use of strong CYP3A4 and/or CYP2C9 inhibitors.

Hemodialysis: Removed by hemodialysis; after 4-hour HD treatment, a supplemental dose of up to 50% should be considered.

Dosing adjustment in hepatic impairment: Use caution when titrating dose.

Mild-to-moderate hepatic impairment: Maximum dose: 300 mg daily. Further dosage reduction/limitation may be necessary in patients taking concomitant strong CYP3A4 and/or CYP2C9 inhibitors.

Severe hepatic impairment: Use is not recommended.

Dietary Considerations Some products may contain phenylalanine.

Administration

Injection: Administer over 30-60 minutes. Twice daily I.V. infusions have been used for up to 5 days. Can be administered without further dilution or may be mixed with compatible diluents (NS, LR, D_5W).

Oral solution, tablets: May be administered with or without food. Oral solution should be administered with a calibrated measuring device (not a household teaspoon or tablespoon).

Monitoring Parameters Patients with conduction problems or severe cardiac disease should have ECG tracing prior to start of therapy and when at steady-state; suicidality (eg, suicidal thoughts, depression, behavioral changes)

Dosage Forms Excipient information presented when available (limited, particularly for generics); consult specific product labeling.

Solution, Intravenous:

Vimpat: 200 mg/20 mL (20 mL)

Solution, Oral:

Vimpat: 10 mg/mL (200 mL, 465 mL) [contains aspartame, methylparaben, polyethylene glycol, propylene glycol; strawberry flavor]

Tablet, Oral:

Vimpat: 50 mg [contains fd&c blue #2 aluminum lake]

Vimpat: 100 mg, 150 mg

Vimpat: 200 mg [contains fd&c blue #2 aluminum lake]

Controlled Substance C-V

◆ LaCrosse Complete [OTC] *see* Sodium Phosphates *on page 1923*

◆ Lactoflavin *see* Riboflavin *on page 1809*

Lactulose (LAK tyoo lose)

Brand Names: U.S. Constulose; Enulose; Generlac; Kristalose

Brand Names: Canada Acilac; Apo-Lactulose®; Laxilose; PMS-Lactulose

Pharmacologic Category Ammonium Detoxicant; Laxative, Osmotic

Additional Appendix Information

Laxatives, Classification and Properties *on page 2304*

Use Prevention and treatment of portal-systemic encephalopathy (including hepatic precoma and coma); treatment of constipation

Pregnancy Risk Factor B

Pregnancy Considerations Adverse events have not been observed in animal reproduction studies. Lactulose is poorly absorbed following oral administration. Use of dietary fiber or bulk-forming laxatives along with increased fluid intake is generally considered first line therapy for treating constipation in pregnant women. Short-term use of lactulose is also considered to be safe/low risk when therapy is needed; however, side effects may limit its use (Cullen, 2007; Mahadevan, 2006; Prather, 2004; Wald, 2003).

Breast-Feeding Considerations It is not known if lactulose is excreted into breast milk; however, lactulose is poorly absorbed following oral administration. The manufacturer recommends that caution be used if administered to a nursing woman.

Contraindications Use in patients requiring a low galactose diet

Warnings/Precautions Use with caution in patients with diabetes mellitus; solution contains galactose and lactose. Monitor periodically for electrolyte imbalance when lactulose is used >6 months or in patients predisposed to electrolyte abnormalities (eg, elderly). Hepatic disease may predispose patients to electrolyte imbalance. Infants receiving lactulose may develop hyponatremia and dehydration. Patients receiving lactulose and an oral anti-infective agent should be monitored for possible inadequate response to lactulose. During proctoscopy or colonoscopy procedures involving electrocautery, a theoretical risk of reaction between H_2 gas accumulation and electrical spark may exist; thorough bowel cleansing with a nonfermentable solution is recommended.

Adverse Reactions Frequency not defined.

Endocrine & metabolic: Dehydration, hypernatremia, hypokalemia

Gastrointestinal: Abdominal discomfort, abdominal distention, belching, cramping, diarrhea (excessive dose), flatulence, nausea, vomiting

Drug Interactions

Metabolism/Transport Effects None known.

Avoid Concomitant Use There are no known interactions where it is recommended to avoid concomitant use.

Increased Effect/Toxicity There are no known significant interactions involving an increase in effect.

Decreased Effect There are no known significant interactions involving a decrease in effect.

Storage/Stability Store at room temperature; do not freeze. Protect from light. Discard solution if cloudy or very dark. Prolonged exposure to cold temperatures will cause thickening which will return to normal upon warming to room temperature.

Mechanism of Action The bacterial degradation of lactulose resulting in an acidic pH inhibits the diffusion of NH_3 into the blood by causing the conversion of NH_3 to NH_4^+; also enhances the diffusion of NH_3 from the blood into the gut where conversion to NH_4^+ occurs; produces an osmotic effect in the colon with resultant distention promoting peristalsis; reduces blood ammonia concentration to reduce the degree of portal systemic encephalopathy

Pharmacodynamics/Kinetics

Onset:

Constipation: Up to 24-48 hours to produce a normal bowel movement

Encephalopathy: At least 24-48 hours

Absorption: Not appreciable

Metabolism: Via colonic flora to lactic acid and acetic acid; requires colonic flora for drug activation

Excretion: Primarily feces; urine (≤3%)

Dosage

Constipation: Oral:

Children (unlabeled use): 0.7-2 g/kg/day (1-3 mL/kg/day) in divided doses, maximum: 40 g/day (60 mL/day) (NASPGHAN, 2006)

Adults: 10-20 g (15-30 mL) daily; may increase to 40 g (60 mL) daily if necessary

Prevention of portal systemic encephalopathy (PSE): Oral:

Infants: 1.7-6.7 g/day (2.5-10 mL/day) in divided doses; adjust dosage to produce 2-3 stools/day

Children: 26.7-60 g/day (40-90 mL/day) in divided doses; adjust dosage to produce 2-3 stools/day

Adults: 20-30 g (30-45 mL) 3-4 times/day; adjust dose every 1-2 days to produce 2-3 soft stools/day

Treatment of acute PSE: Adults:

Oral: 20-30 g (30-45 mL) every 1 hour to induce rapid laxation; reduce to 20-30 g (30-45 mL) 3-4 times/day after laxation is achieved titrate to produce 2-3 soft stools/day

Rectal administration (retention enema): 200 g (300 mL) diluted with 700 mL of water or NS via rectal balloon catheter; retain for 30-60 minutes; may repeat every 4-6 hours; transition to oral treatment prior to discontinuing rectal administration

Dosage adjustment in renal impairment: No dosage adjustment provided in manufacturer's labeling.

Dosage adjustment in hepatic impairment: No dosage adjustment provided in manufacturer's labeling.

Dietary Considerations Contraindicated in patients on galactose-restricted diet; may be mixed with fruit juice, milk, water, or citrus-flavored carbonated beverages.

Administration

Oral solution: May mix with fruit juice, water or milk.

Crystals for oral solution: Dissolve contents of packet in 120 mL water.

Rectal: Mix with water or normal saline; administer as retention enema using a rectal balloon catheter; retain for 30-60 minutes. Transition to oral lactulose when appropriate (able to take oral medication and no longer a risk for aspiration) prior to discontinuing rectal administration

Monitoring Parameters Blood pressure, standing/supine; serum electrolytes, serum ammonia; bowel movement patterns, fluid status

Dosage Forms Excipient information presented when available (limited, particularly for generics); consult specific product labeling.

Packet, Oral:

Kristalose: 10 g (30 ea); 20 g (30 ea)

Solution, Oral:

Constulose: 10 g/15 mL (237 mL, 946 mL) [unflavored flavor]

Enulose: 10 g/15 mL (473 mL) [unflavored flavor]

Generlac: 10 g/15 mL (473 mL, 1892 mL) [unflavored flavor]

Generic: 10 g/15 mL (15 mL, 30 mL, 236 mL, 237 mL, 473 mL, 500 mL, 946 mL, 1892 mL); 20 g/30 mL (30 mL)

- Ladakamycin *see* AzaCITIDine *on page 206*
- LAIV *see* Influenza Virus Vaccine (Live/Attenuated) *on page 1082*
- $LAIV_4$ *see* Influenza Virus Vaccine (Live/Attenuated) *on page 1082*
- L-AmB *see* Amphotericin B (Liposomal) *on page 128*
- LaMICtal *see* LamoTRIgine *on page 1165*
- Lamictal® (Can) *see* LamoTRIgine *on page 1165*
- LaMICtal ODT *see* LamoTRIgine *on page 1165*
- LaMICtal Starter *see* LamoTRIgine *on page 1165*
- LaMICtal XR *see* LamoTRIgine *on page 1165*
- LamISIL *see* Terbinafine (Systemic) *on page 2017*
- Lamisil (Can) *see* Terbinafine (Systemic) *on page 2017*
- Lamisil® (Can) *see* Terbinafine (Topical) *on page 2018*
- LamISIL Advanced [OTC] *see* Terbinafine (Topical) *on page 2018*
- LamISIL AF Defense [OTC] *see* Tolnaftate *on page 2087*
- LamISIL AT [OTC] *see* Terbinafine (Topical) *on page 2018*
- LamISIL AT Jock Itch [OTC] *see* Terbinafine (Topical) *on page 2018*
- LamISIL AT Spray [OTC] *see* Terbinafine (Topical) *on page 2018*

LamiVUDine (la MI vyoo deen)

Brand Names: U.S. Epivir; Epivir HBV

Brand Names: Canada 3TC®; Apo-Lamivudine®; Apo-Lamivudine® HBV; Heptovir®

Index Terms 3TC

Pharmacologic Category Antiretroviral, Reverse Transcriptase Inhibitor, Nucleoside (Anti-HIV)

Use

Epivir®: Treatment of HIV infection when antiretroviral therapy is warranted; should always be used as part of a multidrug regimen (at least three antiretroviral agents)

Epivir-HBV®: Treatment of chronic hepatitis B associated with evidence of hepatitis B viral replication and active liver inflammation. Resistance develops rapidly in hepatitis B; consider use only if other anti-HBV antiviral agents with more favorable resistance patterns cannot be used.

Unlabeled Use Postexposure prophylaxis for HIV exposure as part of a multidrug regimen

Pregnancy Risk Factor C

Pregnancy Considerations Adverse events were observed in some animal reproduction studies. Lamivudine crosses the human placenta. No increased risk of overall birth defects has been observed following first trimester exposure according to data collected by the antiretroviral pregnancy registry. The pharmacokinetics of lamivudine during pregnancy are not significantly altered and dosage adjustment is not required. Cases of lactic acidosis/hepatic steatosis syndrome related to mitochondrial toxicity have been reported in pregnant women with prolonged use of nucleoside analogues. It is not known if pregnancy itself potentiates this known side effect; however, women may be at increased risk of lactic acidosis and liver damage. In addition, these adverse events are similar to other rare but life-threatening syndromes which occur during pregnancy (eg, HELLP syndrome). Hepatic enzymes and electrolytes should be monitored in women receiving nucleoside analogues and clinicians should watch for early signs of the syndrome. In addition, mitochondrial dysfunction may develop in infants following in utero exposure The DHHS Perinatal HIV Guidelines recommend lamivudine for use during pregnancy; the combination of lamivudine with zidovudine is the recommended dual combination NRTI in pregnancy. The DHHS Perinatal HIV Guidelines consider lamivudine plus tenofovir a recommended dual NRTI/NtRTI backbone for HIV/HBV coinfected pregnant women. Use caution with hepatitis B coinfection; hepatitis B flare may occur if lamivudine is discontinued postpartum.

Regardless of CD4 count or HIV RNA copy number, all HIV-infected pregnant women should receive a combination antepartum antiretroviral (ARV) drug regimen; this includes women who require therapy for their own health, as well as women who do not yet require therapy for their own health. ARV therapy should be started as soon as possible if required for the woman's health. Although earlier initiation may be more effective in reducing the perinatal transmission of HIV), also consider maternal conditions (eg, nausea and vomiting) and the potential risks of first trimester fetal exposure for specific agents. Plasma HIV RNA levels should be assessed at ~34-36 weeks gestation in order to help determine mode of delivery. If ARV therapy must be interrupted for <24 hours during the peripartum period, stop then restart all medications simultaneously in order to decrease the chance of developing resistance. Long-term follow-up is recommended for all infants exposed to ARV medications.

Healthcare providers are encouraged to enroll pregnant women exposed to antiretroviral medications in the Antiretroviral Pregnancy Registry (1-800-258-4263 or www.APRegistry.com). Healthcare providers caring for HIV-infected women and their infants may contact the National Perinatal HIV Hotline (888-448-8765) for clinical consultation (DHHS [perinatal], 2012).

Breast-Feeding Considerations Lamivudine is excreted into breast milk and can be detected in the serum of nursing infants.

Maternal or infant antiretroviral therapy does not completely eliminate the risk of postnatal HIV transmission. In addition, multiclass-resistant virus has been detected in breast-feeding infants despite maternal therapy. Therefore, in the United States, where formula is accessible, affordable, safe, and sustainable, and the risk of infant mortality due to diarrhea and respiratory infections is low, complete avoidance of breast-feeding by HIV-infected women is recommended to decrease potential transmission of HIV (DHHS [perinatal], 2012).

Contraindications Hypersensitivity to lamivudine or any component of the formulation

Warnings/Precautions Use caution with renal impairment; dosage reduction recommended. Use with extreme caution in children with history of pancreatitis or risk factors for development of pancreatitis. Pancreatitis has been reported, particularly in HIV-infected children with a history of nucleoside use. Do not use as monotherapy in treatment of HIV. Lamivudine combined with emtricitabine is not recommended as a dual-NRTI combination due to similar resistance patterns and negligible additive antiviral activity; lamivudine and tenofovir combination is preferred as the NRTIs in a fully suppressive antiretroviral regimen (DHHS, 2013). Treatment of HBV in patients with unrecognized/ untreated HIV may lead to rapid HIV resistance. In addition, treatment of HIV in patients with unrecognized/ untreated HBV may lead to rapid HBV resistance. Use with caution in combination with interferon alfa with or without ribavirin in HIV/HBV coinfected patients; monitor closely for hepatic decompensation, anemia, or neutropenia; dose reduction or discontinuation of interferon and/or ribavirin may be required if toxicity evident. In HIV/HBV coinfection, lamivudine and tenofovir are a preferred NRTI backbone in a fully suppressive antiretroviral regimen to provide activity against both HIV and HBV (DHHS, 2013). **[U.S. Boxed Warning]: Do not use Epivir-HBV® tablets or Epivir-HBV® oral solution for the treatment of HIV.**

[U.S. Boxed Warning]: Lactic acidosis and severe hepatomegaly with steatosis have been reported, including fatal cases. Use caution in hepatic impairment. Pregnancy, obesity, and/or prolonged therapy may increase the risk of lactic acidosis and liver damage.

Immune reconstitution syndrome may develop resulting in the occurrence of an inflammatory response to an indolent or residual opportunistic infection during initial HIV treatment or activation of autoimmune disorders (eg, Graves' disease, polymyositis, Guillain-Barré syndrome) later in therapy. May be associated with fat redistribution. Concomitant use of other lamivudine-containing products should be avoided.

[U.S. Boxed Warning]: Monitor patients closely for several months following discontinuation of therapy for chronic hepatitis B; clinical exacerbations may occur.

Not recommended as first-line therapy of chronic HBV due to high rate of resistance. Consider use only if other anti-HBV antiviral regimens with more favorable resistance patterns cannot be used. May be appropriate for short-term treatment of acute HBV (Lok, 2009). Potential compliance problems, frequency of administration, and adverse effects should be discussed with patients before initiating therapy to help prevent the emergence of resistance.

Adverse Reactions Incidence data include patients on combination therapy with other antiretroviral agents.

>10%:

Central nervous system: Headache (21% to 35%), fatigue (24% to 27%), insomnia (11%)

Gastrointestinal: Nausea (15% to 33%), diarrhea (14% to 18%), pancreatitis (range: 0.3% to 18%; higher percentage in pediatric patients), abdominal pain (9% to 16%), vomiting (13% to 15%)

Hematologic: Neutropenia (7% to 15%)

Hepatic: Transaminases increased (2% to 11%)

Neuromuscular & skeletal: Myalgia (8% to 14%), neuropathy (12%), musculoskeletal pain (12%)

Respiratory: Nasal signs and symptoms (20%), cough (18%), sore throat (13%)

Miscellaneous: Infections (25%; includes ear, nose, and throat)

1% to 10%:

Central nervous system: Dizziness (10%), depression (9%), fever (7% to 10%), chills (7% to 10%)

Dermatologic: Rash (5% to 9%)

Gastrointestinal: Anorexia (10%), lipase increased (10%), abdominal cramps (6%), dyspepsia (5%), amylase increased (<1% to 4%), heartburn

Hematologic: Thrombocytopenia (1% to 4%), hemoglobinemia (2% to 3%)

Neuromuscular & skeletal: Creatine phosphokinase increased (9%), arthralgia (5% to 7%)

<1% (Limited to important or life-threatening): Alopecia, anaphylaxis, anemia, body fat redistribution, hepatitis B exacerbation, hepatomegaly, hyperbilirubinemia, hyperglycemia, immune reconstitution syndrome, lactic acidosis, lymphadenopathy, muscle weakness, paresthesia, peripheral neuropathy, pruritus, red cell aplasia, rhabdomyolysis, splenomegaly, steatosis, stomatitis, urticaria, weakness, wheezing

Drug Interactions

Metabolism/Transport Effects None known.

Avoid Concomitant Use

Avoid concomitant use of LamiVUDine with any of the following: Emtricitabine

Increased Effect/Toxicity

LamiVUDine may increase the levels/effects of: Emtricitabine

The levels/effects of LamiVUDine may be increased by: Ganciclovir-Valganciclovir; Ribavirin; Trimethoprim

Decreased Effect There are no known significant interactions involving a decrease in effect.

Ethanol/Nutrition/Herb Interactions Food: Food decreases the rate of absorption and C_{max}; however, there is no change in the systemic AUC. Therefore, may be taken with or without food.

Storage/Stability

Oral solution:

Epivir®: Store at 25°C (77°F) tightly closed.

Epivir-HBV®: Store at 20°C to 25°C (68°F to 77°F) tightly closed.

Tablet: Store at 25°C (77°F); excursions permitted to 15°C to 30°C (59°F to 86°F).

Mechanism of Action Lamivudine is a cytosine analog. After lamivudine is triphosphorylated, the principle mode of action is inhibition of HIV reverse transcription via viral DNA chain termination; inhibits RNA- and DNA-dependent DNA polymerase activities of reverse transcriptase. The monophosphate form of lamivudine is incorporated into the viral DNA by hepatitis B virus polymerase, resulting in DNA chain termination.

Pharmacodynamics/Kinetics

Absorption: Rapid

Distribution: V_d: 1.3 L/kg

Protein binding, plasma: <36%

Metabolism: 4.2% to trans-sulfoxide metabolite

Bioavailability: Absolute; Cp_{max} decreased with food although AUC not significantly affected

Children: 66%

Adults: 86% to 87%

Half-life elimination: Children: 2 hours; Adults: 5-7 hours

Time to peak, plasma: Fed: 3.2 hours; Fasted: 0.9 hours

Excretion: Primarily urine (as unchanged drug)

Dosage Oral: **Note:** Use with at least two other antiretroviral agents when treating HIV.

HIV:

Infants 1-3 months (DHHS [pediatric], 2010): 4 mg/kg/dose twice daily

Infants and Children 3 months to 16 years: 4 mg/kg/dose twice daily (maximum: 150 mg/dose twice daily)

Alternate weight-based dosing using scored 150 mg tablets (DHHS [pediatric], 2010):

14-21 kg: 75 mg/dose twice daily (150 mg/day)

22-29 kg: 75 mg in the morning, 150 mg in the evening (225 mg/day)
≥30 kg: 150 mg/dose twice daily (300 mg/day)
Adults: 150 mg twice daily or 300 mg once daily
<50 kg (DHHS [pediatric], 2010): 4 mg/kg/dose twice daily (maximum: 150 mg/dose twice daily)

Treatment of hepatitis B (Epivir-HBV®): Note: Not a preferred agent in chronic HBV treatment due to high rates of resistance; consider alternative agents:
Children 2-17 years: 3 mg/kg/dose once daily (maximum: 100 mg/day)
Adults: 100 mg/day
Treatment duration (AASLD practice guidelines):
Hepatitis Be antigen (HBeAg) positive chronic hepatitis: Treat ≥1 year until HBeAg seroconversion and undetectable serum HBV DNA; continue therapy for ≥6 months after HBeAg seroconversion
HBeAg negative chronic hepatitis: Treat >1 year until hepatitis B surface antigen (HBsAg) clearance
Note: Patients not achieving <2 log decrease in serum HBV DNA after at least 6 months of therapy should either receive additional treatment or be switched to an alternative therapy (Lok, 2009).

Treatment of hepatitis B/HIV coinfection (in patients with both infections requiring treatment): Note: The formulation and dosage of Epivir-HBV® are not appropriate for patients infected with both HBV and HIV. Tenofovir and lamivudine are a preferred NRTI backbone in a fully suppressive antiretroviral regimen for the treatment of HIV/HBV coinfection (DHHS, 2013).
Infants and Children: 4 mg/kg/dose (maximum: 150 mg/dose) twice daily, in combination with other antiretrovirals in an antiretroviral (ARV) regimen (CDC, 2009).
Adolescents and Adults: 150 mg/dose twice daily or 300 mg/dose once daily, in combination with other antiretrovirals in an ARV regimen (DHHS, 2013)

Postexposure prophylaxis for HIV exposure (unlabeled use [CDC, 2005]): Adolescents ≥16 years and Adults: 150 mg/dose twice daily or 300 mg/dose once daily, in combination with zidovudine, tenofovir, stavudine, or didanosine, with or without a protease inhibitor depending on risk

Dosage adjustment in renal impairment: HIV:
Patients ≤16 years: Insufficient data; however, dose reduction should be considered.
Patients >16 years:
Cl_{cr} 30-49 mL/minute: Administer 150 mg once daily
Cl_{cr} 15-29 mL/minute: Administer 150 mg first dose, then 100 mg once daily
Cl_{cr} 5-14 mL/minute: Administer 150 mg first dose, then 50 mg once daily
Cl_{cr} <5 mL/minute: Administer 50 mg first dose, then 25 mg once daily

Dosage adjustment in renal impairment: Hepatitis B:
Adults:
Cl_{cr} 30-49: Administer 100 mg first dose then 50 mg once daily
Cl_{cr} 15-29: Administer 100 mg first dose then 25 mg once daily
Cl_{cr} 5-14: Administer 35 mg first dose then 15 mg once daily
Cl_{cr} <5: Administer 35 mg first dose then 10 mg once daily
Dialysis: Negligible amounts are removed by 4-hour hemodialysis or peritoneal dialysis. Supplemental dosing not needed; however, dosing after dialysis is recommended (DHHS, 2013).

Dosage adjustment in hepatic impairment: No dosage adjustment necessary. However, has not been studied in the setting of decompensated liver disease.

Dietary Considerations May be taken without regard to meals. Some products may contain sucrose.

Administration May be administered without regard to meals. Adjust dosage in renal failure.

Monitoring Parameters Amylase, bilirubin, liver enzymes (every 3 months during therapy), hematologic parameters, HIV viral load, and CD4 count; signs/symptoms of pancreatitis, HBV DNA (every 3-6 months during therapy), HBeAg and anti-HBe (after 1 year of therapy and every 3-6 months thereafter); signs/symptoms of HBV relapse/exacerbation (every 1-3 months for 6 months after discontinuation and every 3-6 months thereafter)

Dosage Forms Excipient information presented when available (limited, particularly for generics); consult specific product labeling.
Solution, Oral:
Epivir: 10 mg/mL (240 mL) [contains methylparaben, propylene glycol, propylparaben; strawberry-banana flavor]
Epivir HBV: 5 mg/mL (240 mL) [contains methylparaben, propylene glycol, propylparaben; strawberry-banana flavor]
Tablet, Oral:
Epivir: 150 mg, 300 mg
Epivir HBV: 100 mg
Generic: 100 mg, 150 mg, 300 mg

- **Lamivudine, Abacavir, and Zidovudine** *see* Abacavir, Lamivudine, and Zidovudine *on page 20*
- **Lamivudine and Abacavir** *see* Abacavir and Lamivudine *on page 20*

Lamivudine and Zidovudine

(la MI vyoo deen & zye DOE vyoo deen)

Brand Names: U.S. Combivir®

Brand Names: Canada Combivir®; Teva-Lamivudine/Zidovudine

Index Terms AZT + 3TC (error-prone abbreviation); Zidovudine and Lamivudine

Pharmacologic Category Antiretroviral, Reverse Transcriptase Inhibitor, Nucleoside (Anti-HIV)

Use Treatment of HIV infection when therapy is warranted based on clinical and/or immunological evidence of disease progression

Pregnancy Risk Factor C

Dosage Adolescents ≥30 kg and Adults: Oral: One tablet twice daily
Note: Because this is a fixed-dose combination product, avoid use in patients requiring dosage reduction including children <30 kg, renally-impaired patients with a creatinine clearance <50 mL/minute, hepatic impairment, or those patients experiencing dose-limiting adverse effects.
Dosage adjustment in renal impairment: Cl_{cr} <50 mL/min: Fixed-dose combination lamivudine/zidovudine is not recommended; use individual components for patients requiring dose adjustments.
Dosage adjustment in hepatic impairment: Fixed-dose combination lamivudine/zidovudine is not recommended; use individual components for patients requiring dose adjustments.

Additional Information Complete prescribing information should be consulted for additional detail.

Dosage Forms Excipient information presented when available (limited, particularly for generics); consult specific product labeling.
Tablet, oral: Lamivudine 150 mg and zidovudine 300 mg
Combivir®: Lamivudine 150 mg and zidovudine 300 mg [scored]

LamoTRIgine (la MOE tri jeen)

Brand Names: U.S. LaMICtal; LaMICtal ODT; LaMICtal Starter; LaMICtal XR

Brand Names: Canada Apo-Lamotrigine®; Auro-Lamotrigine; Lamictal®; Mylan-Lamotrigine; PMS-Lamotrigine; ratio-Lamotrigine; Teva-Lamotrigine

Index Terms BW-430C; LTG

Pharmacologic Category Anticonvulsant, Miscellaneous

Use

U.S. labeling:

Immediate release: Adjunctive therapy in the treatment of generalized seizures of Lennox-Gastaut syndrome, primary generalized tonic-clonic seizures, and partial seizures; conversion to monotherapy in patients with partial seizures who are receiving treatment with a single antiepileptic drug (AED) (specifically carbamazepine, phenytoin, phenobarbital, primidone, or valproic acid); maintenance treatment of bipolar I disorder

Extended release: Adjunctive therapy for primary generalized tonic-clonic seizures and partial seizures (with or without secondary generalization); conversion to monotherapy in patients with partial seizures who are receiving treatment with a single antiepileptic drug AED

Canadian labeling: Immediate release: Adjunctive therapy for epilepsy uncontrolled by conventional therapy; monotherapy of epilepsy following withdrawal of concurrent antiepileptic agents; adjunctive therapy for Lennox-Gastaut syndrome

Pregnancy Risk Factor C

Pregnancy Considerations Although teratogenic effects were not observed in animal reproduction studies, lamotrigine has been found to decrease folate concentrations in animals. Lamotrigine crosses the human placenta and can be measured in the plasma of exposed newborns (Harden and Pennell, 2009; Ohman, 2000). An overall increase in major congenital malformations has not been observed in available studies; however, an increased risk for cleft lip or cleft palate has not been ruled out (Cunnington, 2011; Hernández-Díaz, 2012; Holmes, 2012). An increased risk of malformations following maternal lamotrigine use may be associated with larger doses (Cunnington, 2007; Tomson, 2011). Polytherapy may increase the risk of congenital malformations; monotherapy with the lowest effective dose is recommended (Harden and Meader, 2009).

Due to pregnancy-induced physiologic changes, women who are pregnant may require dose adjustments of lamotrigine in order to maintain clinical response; monitoring during pregnancy should be considered (Harden and Pennell, 2009). For women with epilepsy who are planning a pregnancy in advance, baseline serum concentrations should be measured once or twice prior to pregnancy during a period when seizure control is optimal. Monitoring can then be continued up to once a month during pregnancy and every second day during the first week postpartum (Patsalos, 2008). In women taking lamotrigine who are trying to avoid pregnancy, potentially significant interactions may exist with hormone-containing contraceptives; consult drug interactions database for more detailed information.

Pregnancy registries are available for women who have been exposed to lamotrigine. Patients may enroll themselves in the North American Antiepileptic Drug (NAAED) Pregnancy Registry by calling (888) 233-2334. Additional information is available at www.aedpregnancyregistry.org.

Breast-Feeding Considerations Lamotrigine is found in breast milk and may be as high as 50% of the maternal serum concentration. Adverse events observed in breast-feeding infants include apnea, drowsiness, and poor sucking. The manufacturer recommends that caution be used if administered to a breast-feeding woman and to monitor the nursing infant.

Medication Guide Available Yes

Contraindications Hypersensitivity to lamotrigine or any component of the formulation

Warnings/Precautions [U.S. Boxed Warning]: Severe and potentially life-threatening skin rashes requiring hospitalization have been reported; incidence of serious rash is higher in pediatric patients than adults; risk may be increased by coadministration with valproic acid, higher than recommended starting doses, and exceeding recommended dose titration. The majority of cases occur in the first 8 weeks; however, isolated cases may occur after prolonged treatment or in patients without these risk factors. Discontinue at first sign of rash and do not reinitiate therapy unless rash is clearly not drug related. Rare cases of Stevens-Johnson syndrome, toxic epidermal necrolysis, and angioedema have been reported.

Antiepileptics are associated with an increased risk of suicidal behavior/thoughts with use (regardless of indication); patients should be monitored for signs/symptoms of depression, suicidal tendencies, and other unusual behavior changes during therapy and instructed to inform their healthcare provider immediately if symptoms occur.

A spectrum of hematologic effects have been reported with use (eg, neutropenia, leukopenia, thrombocytopenia, pancytopenia, anemias, and rarely, aplastic anemia and pure red cell aplasia); patients with a previous history of adverse hematologic reaction to any drug may be at increased risk. Early detection of hematologic change is important; advise patients of early signs and symptoms including fever, sore throat, mouth ulcers, infections, easy bruising, petechial or purpuric hemorrhage. May be associated with hypersensitivity syndrome (eg, anticonvulsant hypersensitivity syndrome). Multiorgan hypersensitivity reactions (drug reaction with eosinophilia and systemic symptoms [DRESS]) have been reported. Symptoms may include fever, rash, and/or lymphadenopathy; monitor for signs and symptoms of possible disparate manifestations associated with lymphatic, hepatic, renal, and/or hematologic organ systems. Evaluate patient with fever and lymphadenopathy, even if rash is not present; discontinuation and conversion to alternate therapy may be required. Increased risk of developing aseptic meningitis has been reported; symptoms (eg, headache, nuchal rigidity, fever, nausea/vomiting, rash, photophobia) have generally occurred within 1-45 days following therapy initiation. Use caution in patients with renal or hepatic impairment. Avoid abrupt cessation, taper over at least 2 weeks if possible.

May cause CNS depression, which may impair physical or mental abilities. Patients must be cautioned about performing tasks which require mental alertness (eg, operating machinery or driving). Effects with other sedative drugs or ethanol may be potentiated. Binds to melanin and may accumulate in the eye and other melanin-rich tissues; the clinical significance of this is not known. Safety and efficacy have not been established for use as initial monotherapy, conversion to monotherapy from antiepileptic drugs (AED) other than carbamazepine, phenytoin, phenobarbital, primidone or valproic acid or conversion to monotherapy from two or more AEDs. Patients treated for bipolar disorder should be monitored closely for clinical worsening or suicidality; prescriptions should be written for the smallest quantity consistent with good patient care. Hormonal contraceptives may cause a decrease in lamotrigine levels; dose adjustment of the lamotrigine maintenance dose may be required when initiating or discontinuing estrogen-containing oral contraceptives. Valproic acid may cause an increase in lamotrigine levels requiring dose adjustment. There is a potential for medication errors with similar-sounding medications and among different lamotrigine formulations; medication errors have occurred.

Adverse Reactions Percentages reported in adults on monotherapy for epilepsy or bipolar disorder.

>10%: Gastrointestinal: Nausea (7% to 14%)

1% to 10%:

Cardiovascular: Chest pain (5%), peripheral edema (2% to 5%), edema (1% to 5%)

Central nervous system: Insomnia (5% to 10%), somnolence (9%), fatigue (8%), coordination impaired (7%), dizziness (7%), anxiety (5%), pain (5%), ataxia (2% to 5%), irritability (2% to 5%), suicidal ideation (2% to 5%), agitation (1% to 5%), amnesia (1% to 5%), depression (1% to 5%), dream abnormality (1% to 5%), emotional lability (1% to 5%), fever (1% to 5%), hypoesthesia (1% to 5%), migraine (1% to 5%), thought abnormality (1% to 5%), confusion (1%)

Dermatologic: Rash (nonserious: 7%), dermatitis (2% to 5%), dry skin (2% to 5%)

Endocrine & metabolic: Dysmenorrhea (5%), libido increased (2% to 5%)

Gastrointestinal: Vomiting (5% to 9%), dyspepsia (7%), abdominal pain (6%), xerostomia (2% to 6%), constipation (5%), weight loss (5%), anorexia (2% to 5%), peptic ulcer (2% to 5%), rectal hemorrhage (2% to 5%), flatulence (1% to 5%), weight gain (1% to 5%)

Genitourinary: Urinary frequency (1% to 5%)

Neuromuscular & skeletal: Back pain (8%), weakness (2% to 5%), arthralgia (1% to 5%), myalgia (1% to 5%), neck pain (1% to 5%), paresthesia (1%)

Ocular: Nystagmus (2% to 5%), vision abnormal (2% to 5%), amblyopia (1%)

Respiratory: Rhinitis (7%), cough (5%), pharyngitis (5%), bronchitis (2% to 5%), dyspnea (2% to 5%), epistaxis (2% to 5%), sinusitis (1% to 5%)

Miscellaneous: Infection (5%), diaphoresis (2% to 5%), reflexes increased/decreased (2% to 5%), dyspraxia (1% to 5%)

<1%: Any indication (limited to important or life-threatening): Accommodation abnormality, agranulocytosis, alcohol intolerance, allergic reaction, alopecia, anemia, angina, angioedema, aphasia, aplastic anemia, apnea, appetite increased, arthritis, aseptic meningitis, atrial fibrillation, bruising, cerebellar syndrome, cerebral sinus thrombosis, cerebrovascular accident, chills, choreoathetosis, CNS depression/stimulation, conjunctivitis, deafness, deep thrombophlebitis, delirium, delusions, dermatitis (exfoliative, fungal), disseminated intravascular coagulation, dysphagia, dysphoria, dystonia, ECG abnormality, ejaculation abnormal, eructation, erythema multiforme, esophagitis, euphoria, extrapyramidal syndrome, flushing, gastritis, gingivitis, goiter, hallucinations, hematuria, hemiplegia, hemolytic anemia, hemorrhage, hepatitis, hiccup, hirsutism, hot flashes, hyperalgesia, hyperglycemia, hypersensitivity reactions, hypertension, hyperventilation, hypokinesia, hypothyroidism, hypotonia, impotence, kidney failure (acute), leg cramps, leukopenia, liver function tests abnormal, lupus-like reaction, lymphadenopathy, maculopapular rash, menorrhagia, MI, mouth ulceration, movement disorder, multiorgan failure, muscle spasm, myasthenia, neuralgia, neurosis, neutropenia, orthostatic hypotension, palpitation, pancreatitis, pancytopenia, paralysis, parkinsonian exacerbation, peripheral neuritis, photophobia, polyuria, progressive immunosuppression, pruritus, pure red cell aplasia, rhabdomyolysis, salivation increased, skin discoloration, status epilepticus, Stevens-Johnson syndrome, sudden unexplained death in epilepsy (SUDEP), suicidal behavior, suicide, syncope, tachycardia, taste loss/perversion, thrombocytopenia, tic, tinnitus, tongue edema, toxic epidermal necrolysis, twitching, urinary incontinence, urticaria, vasculitis, vasodilation, withdrawal seizures

Also observed: Rash requiring hospitalization: Children <16 years 0.8% (epilepsy adjunctive therapy), 1.2% (with concurrent valproic acid use); Adults 0.3% (epilepsy adjunctive therapy), 0.13% (epilepsy monotherapy), 1% (with concurrent valproic acid use), 0.8% (bipolar disorder, monotherapy)

Drug Interactions

Metabolism/Transport Effects None known.

Avoid Concomitant Use

Avoid concomitant use of LamoTRIgine with any of the following: Azelastine (Nasal); Paraldehyde

Increased Effect/Toxicity

LamoTRIgine may increase the levels/effects of: Alcohol (Ethyl); Azelastine (Nasal); Buprenorphine; CarBAMazepine; CNS Depressants; Desmopressin; Hydrocodone; MetFORMIN; Methotrimeprazine; Metyrosine; Mirtazapine; OLANZapine; Paraldehyde; Pramipexole; Procainamide; ROPINIRole; Rotigotine; Selective Serotonin Reuptake Inhibitors; Zolpidem

The levels/effects of LamoTRIgine may be increased by: Brimonidine (Topical); Doxylamine; Droperidol; HydrOXYzine; Magnesium Sulfate; Methotrimeprazine; Perampanel; Sodium Oxybate; Tapentadol; Valproic Acid and Derivatives

Decreased Effect

LamoTRIgine may decrease the levels/effects of: Contraceptives (Progestins)

The levels/effects of LamoTRIgine may be decreased by: Barbiturates; CarBAMazepine; Contraceptives (Estrogens); Ezogabine; Fosphenytoin; Ketorolac (Nasal); Ketorolac (Systemic); Mefloquine; Orlistat; Phenytoin; Primidone; Rifampin; Ritonavir

Ethanol/Nutrition/Herb Interactions

Ethanol: May increase CNS depression; monitor for increased effects with coadministration. Caution patients about effects.

Food: Has no effect on absorption.

Herb/Nutraceutical: Avoid evening primrose (seizure threshold decreased).

Storage/Stability Store at 25°C (77°F); excursions permitted to 15°C to 30°C (59°F to 86°F). Protect from light.

Mechanism of Action A triazine derivative which inhibits release of glutamate (an excitatory amino acid) and inhibits voltage-sensitive sodium channels, which stabilizes neuronal membranes. Lamotrigine has weak inhibitory effect on the 5-HT_3 receptor; *in vitro* inhibits dihydrofolate reductase.

Pharmacodynamics/Kinetics

Absorption: Immediate release: Rapid and complete

Distribution: V_d: 0.9-1.3 L/kg

Protein binding: ~55%

Metabolism: Hepatic and renal; metabolized primarily by glucuronic acid conjugation to inactive metabolites

Bioavailability: Immediate release: 98%; **Note:** AUCs were similar for immediate release and extended release preparations in patients receiving nonenzyme-inducing AEDs. In subjects receiving concomitant enzyme-inducing AEDs, bioavailability of extended release product was ~21% lower than immediate release product; in some of these subjects, a decrease in AUC of up to 70% was observed when switching from immediate release to extended release tablets.

Half-life elimination: Immediate release: Adults: 25-33 hours, Elderly: 25-43 hours; Extended release: Similar to immediate release

Concomitant valproic acid therapy: 48-70 hours

Concomitant phenytoin, phenobarbital, primidone, or carbamazepine therapy: 13-14 hours

Chronic renal failure: 43 hours

Hemodialysis: 13 hours during dialysis; 57 hours between dialysis (~20% of a dose is eliminated in a 4-hour dialysis session)

Hepatic impairment:

Mild: 26-66 hours

Moderate: 28-116 hours

Severe without ascites: 56-78 hours

Severe with ascites: 52-148 hours

Time to peak, plasma: Immediate release: 1-1.5 hours; Extended release: 4-11 hours (dependent on adjunct therapy)

Excretion: Urine (94%, ~90% as glucuronide conjugates and ~10% unchanged); feces (2%)

Dosage Oral: **Note:** Extended release formulation not FDA approved for children ≤12 years of age.

U.S. labeling:

Children 2-12 years: Lennox-Gastaut syndrome (adjunctive), partial seizures (adjunctive), or primary generalized tonic-clonic seizures (adjunctive): **Note:** Whole tablets should be used for dosing, round calculated dose down to the nearest whole tablet. Alternatively, a suspension may be prepared using immediate release tablets (see also Extemporaneous Preparations). Children <30 kg will likely require maintenance doses to be increased by as much as 50% based on clinical response regardless of regimen below:

Immediate release formulation:

Regimens **not containing** carbamazepine, phenytoin, phenobarbital, primidone, or valproic acid: Initial: Weeks 1 and 2: 0.3 mg/kg/day in 1-2 divided doses; Weeks 3 and 4: 0.6 mg/kg/day in 2 divided doses; Week 5 and beyond: Increase by 0.6 mg/kg/day every 1-2 weeks; Usual maintenance: 4.5-7.5 mg/kg/day (maximum: 300 mg daily) in 2 divided doses

Regimens **containing** valproic acid: Initial: Weeks 1 and 2: 0.15 mg/kg/day in 1-2 divided doses (if calculated dose is equal to or rounds down to 1 mg daily, give 2 mg every other day instead); Weeks 3 and 4: 0.3 mg/kg/day in 1-2 divided doses; Week 5 and beyond: Increase by 0.3 mg/kg/day every 1-2 weeks; Usual maintenance: 1-5 mg/kg/day (maximum: 200 mg daily) in 1 or 2 divided doses or 1-3 mg/kg/day (maximum: 200 mg daily) (valproic acid alone)

Regimens **containing** carbamazepine, phenytoin, phenobarbital, or primidone and without valproic acid: Initial: Weeks 1 and 2: 0.6 mg/kg/day in 2 divided doses; Weeks 3 and 4: 1.2 mg/kg/day in 2 divided doses; Week 5 and beyond: Increase by 1.2 mg/kg/day every 1-2 weeks; Usual maintenance: 5-15 mg/kg/day (maximum: 400 mg daily) in 2 divided doses

Adolescents >12 years:

Lennox-Gastaut syndrome (adjunctive): *Immediate release formulation:* Refer to adult dosing.

Partial seizures (adjunctive) or primary generalized tonic-clonic seizures (adjunctive): *Immediate release or extended release formulation*: Refer to adult dosing.

Conversion from adjunctive therapy with a single AED (eg, carbamazepine, phenytoin, phenobarbital, primidone, or valproic acid) for partial seizures to monotherapy with lamotrigine:

Immediate release formulation: Adolescents ≥16 years: Refer to adult dosing.

Extended release formulation: Adolescents ≥13 years: Refer to adult dosing.

Adults:

Lennox-Gastaut syndrome (adjunctive): *Immediate release formulation:*

Regimens **not containing** carbamazepine, phenytoin, phenobarbital, primidone, or valproic acid: Initial: Weeks 1 and 2: 25 mg once daily; Weeks 3 and 4: 50 mg once daily; Week 5 and beyond: Increase by 50 mg daily every 1-2 weeks; Usual maintenance: 225-375 mg daily in 2 divided doses

Regimens **containing** valproic acid: Initial: Weeks 1 and 2: 25 mg every other day; Weeks 3 and 4: 25 mg once daily; Week 5 and beyond: Increase by 25-50 mg daily every 1-2 weeks; Usual maintenance: 100-200 mg daily (valproic acid alone) or 100-400 mg daily (valproic acid and other drugs that induce glucuronidation) in 1 or 2 divided doses

Regimens **containing** carbamazepine, phenytoin, phenobarbital, or primidone and without valproic acid: Initial: Weeks 1 and 2: 50 mg once daily; Weeks 3 and 4: 100 mg daily in 2 divided doses; Week 5 and beyond: Increase by 100 mg daily every 1-2 weeks; Usual maintenance: 300-500 mg daily in 2 divided doses; maximum daily dose: 700 mg

Partial seizures (adjunctive) and primary generalized tonic-clonic seizures (adjunctive):

Immediate release formulation:

Regimens **not containing** carbamazepine, phenytoin, phenobarbital, primidone, or valproic acid: Initial: Weeks 1 and 2: 25 mg once daily; Weeks 3 and 4: 50 mg once daily; Week 5 and beyond: Increase by 50 mg daily every 1-2 weeks; Usual maintenance: 225-375 mg daily in 2 divided doses

Regimens **containing** valproic acid: Initial: Weeks 1 and 2: 25 mg every other day; Weeks 3 and 4: 25 mg once daily; Week 5 and beyond: Increase by 25-50 mg daily every 1-2 weeks; Usual maintenance: 100-200 mg daily (valproic acid alone) or 100-400 mg daily (valproic acid and other drugs that induce glucuronidation) in 1 or 2 divided doses

Regimens **containing** carbamazepine, phenytoin, phenobarbital, or primidone and without valproic acid: Initial: Weeks 1 and 2: 50 mg once daily; Weeks 3 and 4: 100 mg daily in 2 divided doses; Week 5 and beyond: Increase by 100 mg daily every 1-2 weeks; Usual maintenance: 300-500 mg daily in 2 divided doses; maximum daily dose: 700 mg

Extended release formulation:

Regimens **not containing** carbamazepine, phenytoin, phenobarbital, primidone, or valproic acid: Initial: Weeks 1 and 2: 25 mg once daily; Weeks 3 and 4: 50 mg once daily; Week 5: 100 mg once daily; Week 6: 150 mg once daily; Week 7: 200 mg once daily; Week 8 and beyond: Dose increases should not exceed 100 mg daily at weekly intervals; Usual maintenance: 300-400 mg once daily

Regimens **containing** valproic acid: Initial: Weeks 1 and 2: 25 mg every other day; Weeks 3 and 4: 25 mg once daily; Week 5: 50 mg once daily; Week 6: 100 mg once daily; Week 7: 150 mg once daily; Week 8 and beyond: Dose increases should not exceed 100 mg daily at weekly intervals; Usual maintenance: 200-250 mg once daily

Regimens **containing** carbamazepine, phenytoin, phenobarbital, or primidone and without valproic acid: Initial: Weeks 1 and 2: 50 mg once daily; Weeks 3 and 4: 100 mg once daily; Week 5: 200 mg once daily; Week 6: 300 mg once daily; Week 7: 400 mg once daily; Week 8 and beyond: Dose increases should not exceed 100 mg daily at weekly intervals; Usual maintenance: 400-600 mg once daily

Conversion strategy from adjunctive therapy with valproic acid to monotherapy with lamotrigine:

Immediate release formulation:

- Initiate and titrate as per escalation recommendations for adjunctive therapy to a lamotrigine dose of 200 mg daily.
- Then taper valproic acid dose in decrements of not >500 mg/day/week to a valproic acid dosage of 500 mg daily; this dosage should be maintained for 1 week. The lamotrigine dosage should then be increased to 300 mg daily while valproic acid is simultaneously decreased to 250 mg daily; this dosage should be maintained for 1 week.
- Valproic acid may then be discontinued, while the lamotrigine dose is increased by 100 mg daily at weekly intervals to achieve a lamotrigine maintenance dose of 500 mg daily in 2 divided doses.

Extended release formulation:

- Initiate and titrate as per escalation recommendations for adjunctive therapy to a lamotrigine dose of 150 mg daily.
- Then taper valproic acid dose in decrements of not >500 mg/day/week to a valproic acid dose of 500 mg daily; this dosage should be maintained for 1 week. The lamotrigine dosage should then be increased to 200 mg daily while valproic acid is simultaneously decreased to 250 mg daily; this dosage should be maintained for 1 week.
- Valproic acid may then be discontinued, while the lamotrigine dose is increased to achieve a maintenance dosage range of 250-300 mg once daily.

Conversion strategy from adjunctive therapy with carbamazepine, phenytoin, phenobarbital, or primidone to monotherapy with lamotrigine: *Immediate release formulation and extended release formulation:*

- Initiate and titrate as per escalation recommendations for adjunctive therapy to a lamotrigine dose of 500 mg daily.
- Concomitant enzyme-inducing AED should then be withdrawn by 20% decrements each week over a 4-week period.
- Following withdrawal of the enzyme-inducing AED (eg, ~2 weeks later for extended release; 1 week later for immediate release), the dosage of lamotrigine may be tapered in decrements of not >100 mg daily at 1-week intervals to achieve a maintenance dosage range of 250-300 mg once daily (extended release) or 200 mg daily (immediate release) as clinically indicated.

Conversion strategy from adjunctive therapy with AED other than carbamazepine, phenytoin, phenobarbital, primidone or valproic acid to monotherapy with lamotrigine:

Immediate release formulation: No specific guidelines available

Extended release formulation: Initiate and titrate as per escalation recommendations for adjunctive therapy to a lamotrigine dose of 250-300 mg daily. Concomitant AED should then be withdrawn by 20% decrements each week over a 4-week period.

Conversion from immediate release to extended release (Lamictal® XR™): Initial dose of the extended release tablet should match the total daily dose of the immediate-release formulation. Adjust dose as needed within the recommended dosing guidelines.

Bipolar disorder: *Immediate release formulation:*

Regimens **not containing** carbamazepine, phenytoin, phenobarbital, primidone, or valproic acid: Initial: Weeks 1 and 2: 25 mg once daily; Weeks 3 and 4: 50 mg once daily; Week 5: 100 mg once daily; Week 6 and maintenance: 200 mg once daily

Regimens **containing** valproic acid: Initial: Weeks 1 and 2: 25 mg every other day; Weeks 3 and 4: 25 mg once daily; Week 5: 50 mg once daily; Week 6 and maintenance: 100 mg once daily

Regimens **containing** carbamazepine, phenytoin, phenobarbital, or primidone and without valproic acid: Initial: Weeks 1 and 2: 50 mg once daily; Weeks 3 and 4: 100 mg daily in divided doses; Week 5: 200 mg daily in divided doses; Week 6: 300 mg daily in divided doses; Maintenance: Up to 400 mg daily in divided doses

Adjustment following discontinuation of psychotropic medication:

Discontinuing valproic acid with current dose of lamotrigine 100 mg daily: 150 mg daily for week 1, then increase to 200 mg daily beginning week 2

Discontinuing carbamazepine, phenytoin, phenobarbital, primidone, or rifampin with current dose of lamotrigine 400 mg daily: 400 mg daily for week 1, then decrease to 300 mg daily for week 2, then decrease to 200 mg daily beginning week 3

Canadian labeling:

Children ≤12 years (and ≥9 kg): Lennox-Gastaut syndrome (adjunctive therapy): **Note:** Whole tablets should be used for dosing, round calculated dose down to the nearest whole tablet. Alternatively, a suspension may be prepared using immediate release tablets (see also Extemporaneous Preparations). Several weeks to months may be required to achieve individualized maintenance dose. Use is not recommended in children <9 kg.

Regimens **containing** valproic acid regardless of any other concomitant medication: Initial: Weeks 1 and 2: 0.15 mg/kg once daily (if calculated dose is equal to or rounds down to 1 mg daily give 2 mg every other day instead); Weeks 3 and 4: 0.3 mg/kg once daily; Week 5 and beyond: Increase dose by 0.3 mg/kg every 1-2 weeks (usual maintenance dose: 1-5 mg/kg daily in 1 or 2 divided doses) up to a maximum dose of 200 mg daily. **Note:** Alternatively, refer to manufacturer's labeling for recommended weight-based rounding regimen.

Regimens **containing** carbamazepine, phenytoin, phenobarbital, primidone, or other drugs that induce glucuronidation and without valproic acid: Initial: Weeks 1 and 2: 0.3 mg/kg twice daily; Weeks 3 and 4: 0.6 mg/kg twice daily; Week 5 and beyond: Increase dose by 1.2 mg/kg every 1-2 weeks (usual maintenance dose: 2.5-7.5 mg/kg twice daily) up to a maximum dose of 400 mg daily. **Note:** When necessary, round doses down to closest 5 mg interval (eg, calculated dose >5 mg and <10 mg would be rounded to 5 mg; calculated dose >10 mg and <15 mg would be rounded to 10 mg). For week 5 and beyond, dose increases made every 1-2 weeks should not exceed previous daily dose administered in week 4 (eg, if week 4 dose was 20 mg daily than dose increase in week 5 or beyond should not exceed 20 mg daily). Manufacturer labeling suggests that insufficient data exists to support weight based dosing in patients >59 kg.

Adolescents >12 years: Lennox-Gastaut syndrome (adjunctive therapy): Refer to adult dosing.

Adolescents ≥16 years: Uncontrolled epilepsy (adjunctive therapy); conversion from adjunctive therapy with concomitant AEDs for epilepsy to monotherapy with lamotrigine: Refer to adult dosing

Adults: Uncontrolled epilepsy (adjunctive) or Lennox-Gastaut syndrome (adjunctive): **Note:** AED that induce lamotrigine glucuronidation include carbamazepine, phenytoin, phenobarbital, and primidone. Antiepileptic agents that do not induce or inhibit lamotrigine glucuronidation include oxcarbazepine, felbamate, levetiracetam, gabapentin, topiramate, zonisamide, pregabalin. Valproic acid inhibits lamotrigine glucuronidation.

Regimens **containing** inducers of lamotrigine glucuronidation and valproic acid or regimens not containing agents that induce or inhibit lamotrigine glucuronidation: Initial: Weeks 1 and 2: 25 mg once daily; Weeks 3 and 4: 25 mg twice daily; Week 5 and beyond: Increase dose by 25-50 mg every 1-2 weeks until maintenance dose established (usual maintenance dose: 100-200 mg daily in 2 divided doses)

Regimens **containing** inducers of lamotrigine glucuronidation and without valproic acid: Initial: Weeks 1 and 2: 50 mg once daily; Weeks 3 and 4: 50 mg twice daily; Week 5 and beyond: Increase dose by 100 mg every 1-2 weeks until maintenance dose established (usual maintenance dose: 300-500 mg daily in 2 divided doses)

Conversion from adjunctive therapy with concomitant AEDs for epilepsy to lamotrigine monotherapy: Decrease dose of concomitant antiepileptic agent by ~20% of original dose every week for 5 weeks (slower taper may be considered if clinically indicated). Lamotrigine dosage adjustments during this period should be determined by changes in lamotrigine pharmacokinetics due to withdrawal of the concomitant AED, and by the clinical response of patient.

Additional considerations:

Discontinuing therapy: Decrease dose by ~50% per week, over at least 2 weeks unless safety concerns require a more rapid withdrawal. Discontinuing carbamazepine, phenytoin, phenobarbital, primidone, or rifampin should prolong the half-life of lamotrigine; discontinuing valproic acid should shorten the half-life of lamotrigine

Restarting therapy after discontinuation: If lamotrigine has been withheld for >5 half-lives, consider restarting according to initial dosing recommendations. **Note:** Concomitant medications may affect the half-life of lamotrigine; consider pharmacokinetic interactions when restarting therapy.

Dosage adjustment with estrogen-containing hormonal contraceptives: Follow initial lamotrigine dosing guidelines, maintenance dose should be adjusted as follows, based on concomitant medications:

Patients taking concomitant carbamazepine, phenytoin, phenobarbital, primidone or rifampin: No dosing adjustment required

Patients **not** taking concomitant carbamazepine, phenytoin, phenobarbital, primidone or rifampin: Lamotrigine maintenance dose may need increased by twofold over target dose. If already taking a stable dose of lamotrigine and starting contraceptive, maintenance dose may need increased by twofold. Dose increases should start when contraceptive is started and titrated to clinical response increasing no more rapidly than 50-100 mg daily every week. Gradual increases of lamotrigine plasma levels may occur during the inactive "pill-free" week and will be greater when dose increases are made the week before. If increased adverse events consistently occur during "pill-free" week, overall maintenance dose adjustments may be required. When discontinuing estrogen-containing hormonal contraceptive, dose of lamotrigine may need decreased by as much as 50%; do not decrease by more than 25% of total daily dose over a 2-week period unless clinical response or plasma levels indicate otherwise. Dose adjustments during "pill-free" week are not recommended.

Dosage adjustment in renal impairment: Decreased maintenance dosage may be effective in patients with significant renal impairment; has not been adequately studied; use with caution

Dosage adjustment in hepatic impairment:

U.S. labeling:

Mild impairment: No adjustment required

Moderate-to-severe impairment without ascites: Decrease initial, escalation, and maintenance doses by ~25%; adjust according to clinical response and tolerance.

Moderate-to-severe impairment with ascites: Decrease initial, escalation, and maintenance doses by ~50%; adjust according to clinical response and tolerance.

Canadian labeling:

Mild and moderate impairment (Child-Pugh classes A and B): Reduce initial, escalation, and maintenance dosing by ~50%; adjust according to clinical response and tolerance.

Severe impairment (Child-Pugh class C): Reduce initial, escalation, and maintenance dosing by ~75%; adjust according to clinical response and tolerance.

Administration Doses should be rounded down to the nearest whole tablet.

Lamictal® chewable/dispersible tablets: May be chewed, dispersed in water or diluted fruit juice, or swallowed whole. To disperse tablets, add to a small amount of liquid (just enough to cover tablet); let sit ~1 minute until dispersed; swirl solution and consume immediately. Do not administer partial amounts of liquid. If tablets are chewed, a small amount of water or diluted fruit juice should be used to aid in swallowing.

Lamictal® ODT™: Place tablets on tongue and move around in the mouth. Tablets will dissolve rapidly and can be swallowed with or without food or water.

Lamictal® XR™: Administer without regard to meals. Swallow whole; do not chew, crush, or cut.

Monitoring Parameters Serum levels of concurrent anticonvulsants, LFTs, renal function, hypersensitivity reactions (especially rash); seizure, frequency and duration; suicidality (eg, suicidal thoughts, depression, behavioral changes); signs/symptoms of aseptic meningitis

Reference Range A therapeutic serum concentration range has not been established for lamotrigine. Dosing should be based on therapeutic response. Lamotrigine plasma concentrations of 0.25-29.1 mcg/mL have been reported in the literature.

Dosage Forms Excipient information presented when available (limited, particularly for generics); consult specific product labeling.

Kit, Oral:

LaMICtal ODT: 25 (21)-50 (7) MG, 50 (42)-100(14) MG, 25 & 50 & 100 MG

LaMICtal Starter: 25 (35) MG

LaMICtal Starter: 25 (42)-100 (7) MG, 25 (84)-100(14) MG [contains fd&c yellow #6 aluminum lake]

LaMICtal XR: 50 & 100 & 200 MG [contains fd&c blue #2 aluminum lake, polysorbate 80]

LaMICtal XR: 25 (21)-50 (7) MG, 25 & 50 & 100 MG [contains polysorbate 80]

Tablet, Oral:

LaMICtal: 25 mg, 100 mg, 150 mg, 200 mg [scored]

Generic: 25 mg, 100 mg, 150 mg, 200 mg

Tablet Chewable, Oral:

LaMICtal: 2 mg [contains saccharin sodium]

LaMICtal: 5 mg [scored; berry flavor]

LaMICtal: 25 mg [berry flavor]

Generic: 5 mg, 25 mg

Tablet Dispersible, Oral:

LaMICtal ODT: 25 mg, 50 mg, 100 mg, 200 mg

Tablet Extended Release 24 Hour, Oral:
LaMICtal XR: 25 mg, 50 mg, 100 mg [contains polysorbate 80]
LaMICtal XR: 200 mg [contains fd&c blue #2 aluminum lake, polysorbate 80]
LaMICtal XR: 250 mg [contains fd&c blue #2 aluminum lake]
LaMICtal XR: 300 mg [contains polysorbate 80]
Generic: 25 mg, 50 mg, 100 mg, 200 mg, 250 mg, 300 mg

Extemporaneous Preparations A 1 mg/mL oral suspension may be made with tablets and one of two different vehicles (a 1:1 mixture of Ora-Sweet® and Ora-Plus® or a 1:1 mixture of Ora-Sweet® SF and Ora-Plus®). Crush one 100 mg tablet in a mortar and reduce to a fine powder. Add small portions of the chosen vehicle and mix to a uniform paste; mix while adding the vehicle in incremental proportions to **almost** 100 mL; transfer to a graduated cylinder, rinse mortar with vehicle, and add quantity of vehicle sufficient to make 100 mL. Label "shake well" and "protect from light". Stable for 91 days when stored in amber plastic prescription bottles in the dark at room temperature or refrigerated.

Nahata M, Morosco R, Hipple T. "Stability of Lamotrigine in Two Extemporaneously Prepared Oral Suspensions at 4 and 25 Degrees C," *Am J Health Syst Pharm*, 1999, 56(3):240-2.

◆ Lanaphilic/Urea [OTC] *see* Urea *on page 2140*
◆ Lanoxin *see* Digoxin *on page 605*
◆ Lanoxin Pediatric *see* Digoxin *on page 605*

Lanreotide (lan REE oh tide)

Brand Names: U.S. Somatuline Depot
Brand Names: Canada Somatuline® Autogel®
Index Terms Lanreotide Acetate
Pharmacologic Category Somatostatin Analog
Use Long-term treatment of acromegaly in patients who are not candidates for or are unresponsive to surgery and/or radiotherapy
Pregnancy Risk Factor C
Dosage Acromegaly: Adults (per U.S. labeling) **or** Children ≥16 years and Adults (per Canadian labeling): SubQ: 90 mg once every 4 weeks for 3 months; after initial 90 days of therapy, adjust dose based on clinical response of patient, growth hormone (GH) levels, and/or insulin-like growth factor 1 (IGF-1) levels as follows:
GH ≤1 ng/mL, IGF-1 normal, symptoms stable: 60 mg once every 4 weeks; once stabilized on 60 mg every 4 weeks, may consider regimen of 120 mg every 6-8 weeks (extended-interval dosing)
GH >1-2.5 ng/mL, IGF-1 normal, symptoms stable: 90 mg once every 4 weeks; once stabilized on 90 mg every 4 weeks, may consider regimen of 120 mg every 6-8 weeks (extended-interval dosing)
GH >2.5 ng/mL, IGF-1 elevated and/or uncontrolled symptoms: 120 mg once every 4 weeks

Dosing adjustment in renal impairment:
U.S. labeling: Moderate-to-severe impairment: Recommended starting dose: 60 mg; use of an extended-interval dose of 120 mg every 6-8 weeks should be done with caution
Canadian labeling: Moderate-to-severe impairment: Recommended starting dose: 60 mg every 4 weeks for 3 months then adjust dose based on clinical response of patient, growth hormone (GH) levels, and/or insulin-like growth factor 1 (IGF-1) levels as described in adult dosing; however, extended-interval dosing is **not** recommended.

Dosing adjustment in hepatic impairment:
U.S. labeling: Moderate-to-severe impairment: Recommended starting dose: 60 mg; use of an extended-interval dose of 120 mg every 6-8 weeks should be done with caution
Canadian labeling: Moderate-to-severe impairment: Recommended starting dose: 60 mg every 4 weeks for 3 months then adjust dose based on clinical response of patient, growth hormone (GH) levels, and/or insulin-like growth factor 1 (IGF-1) levels as described in adult dosing; however, extended-interval dosing is **not** recommended.

Additional Information Complete prescribing information should be consulted for additional detail.
Dosage Forms Excipient information presented when available (limited, particularly for generics); consult specific product labeling.
Solution, Subcutaneous:
Somatuline Depot: 120 mg/0.5 mL (0.5 mL); 60 mg/0.2 mL (0.2 mL); 90 mg/0.3 mL (0.3 mL)
Dosage Forms: Canada Excipient information presented when available (limited, particularly for generics); consult specific product labeling.
Injection, solution:
Somatuline® Autogel®: 60 mg/~0.3 mL (~0.3 mL); 90 mg/~0.4 mL (~0.4 mL); 120 mg/~0.5 mL (~0.5 mL) [packaging contains natural rubber/natural latex]

◆ Lanreotide Acetate *see* Lanreotide *on page 1170*

Lansoprazole (lan SOE pra zole)

Brand Names: U.S. First-Lansoprazole; Heartburn Relief 24 Hour [OTC]; Prevacid; Prevacid 24HR [OTC]; Prevacid SoluTab
Brand Names: Canada Apo-Lansoprazole®; Mylan-Lansoprazole; Prevacid®; Prevacid® FasTab; Teva-Lansoprazole
Pharmacologic Category Proton Pump Inhibitor; Substituted Benzimidazole
Use Short-term (4 weeks) treatment of active duodenal ulcers; maintenance treatment of healed duodenal ulcers; as part of a multidrug regimen for *H. pylori* eradication to reduce the risk of duodenal ulcer recurrence; short-term (up to 8 weeks) treatment of active benign gastric ulcer; treatment of NSAID-associated gastric ulcer; to reduce the risk of NSAID-associated gastric ulcer in patients with a history of gastric ulcer who require an NSAID; short-term treatment of symptomatic GERD; short-term (up to 8 weeks) treatment for all grades of erosive esophagitis; to maintain healing of erosive esophagitis; long-term treatment of pathological hypersecretory conditions, including Zollinger-Ellison syndrome

OTC labeling: Relief of frequent heartburn (≥2 days/week)
Unlabeled Use Stress ulcer prophylaxis in the critically-ill
Pregnancy Risk Factor B
Pregnancy Considerations Adverse events were not observed in animal reproduction studies. An increased risk of hypospadias was reported following maternal use of proton pump inhibitors (PPIs) during pregnancy (Anderka, 2012), but this was based on a small number of exposures and the same association was not found in another study (Erichsen, 2012). Most available studies have not shown an increased risk of major birth defects following maternal use of PPIs during pregnancy (Diav-Citrin, 2005; Matok, 2012; Pasternak, 2010). When treating GERD in pregnancy, PPIs may be used when clinically indicated (Katz, 2013).

Breast-Feeding Considerations It is not known if lansoprazole is excreted into breast milk. Due to the potential for serious adverse reactions in the nursing infant, the manufacturer recommends a decision be made whether to discontinue nursing or to discontinue the drug, taking into account the importance of treatment to the mother.

Medication Guide Available Yes

Contraindications Hypersensitivity to lansoprazole or any component of the formulation

Warnings/Precautions Use of proton pump inhibitors (PPIs) may increase the risk of gastrointestinal infections (eg, *Salmonella, Campylobacter*). Relief of symptoms does not preclude the presence of a gastric malignancy. Atrophic gastritis (by biopsy) has been noted with long-term omeprazole therapy; this may also occur with lansoprazole. No reports of enterochromaffin-like (ECL) cell carcinoids, dysplasia, or neoplasia have occurred. Use of proton pump inhibitors (PPIs) may increase risk of CDAD, especially in hospitalized patients; consider CDAD diagnosis in patients with persistent diarrhea that does not improve. Use the lowest dose and shortest duration of PPI therapy appropriate for the condition being treated. Severe liver dysfunction may require dosage reductions. Decreased *H. pylori* eradication rates have been observed with short-term (≤7 days) combination therapy. The American College of Gastroenterology recommends 10-14 days of therapy (triple or quadruple) for eradication of *H. pylori* (Chey, 2007).

PPIs may diminish the therapeutic effect of clopidogrel thought to be due to reduced formation of the active metabolite of clopidogrel. The manufacturer of clopidogrel recommends either avoidance of both omeprazole (even when scheduled 12 hours apart) and esomeprazole or use of a PPI with comparatively less effect on the active metabolite of clopidogrel (eg, pantoprazole). Although lansoprazole exhibits the most potent CYP2C19 inhibition *in vitro* (Li, 2004; Ogilvie, 2011), an *in vivo* study of extensive CYP2C19 metabolizers showed less reduction of the active metabolite of clopidogrel by lansoprazole/dexlansoprazole compared to esomeprazole/omeprazole (Frelinger, 2012). The manufacturer of lansoprazole states that no dosage adjustment is necessary for clopidogrel when used concurrently. In contrast to these warnings, others have recommended the continued use of PPIs, regardless of the degree of inhibition, in patients with a history of GI bleeding or multiple risk factors for GI bleeding who are also receiving clopidogrel since no evidence has established clinically meaningful differences in outcome; however, a clinically-significant interaction cannot be excluded in those who are poor metabolizers of clopidogrel (Abraham, 2010; Levine, 2011). Additionally, concomitant use of lansoprazole with some drugs may require cautious use, may not be recommended, or may require dosage adjustments.

Increased incidence of osteoporosis-related bone fractures of the hip, spine, or wrist may occur with PPI therapy. Patients on high-dose or long-term therapy should be monitored. Use the lowest effective dose for the shortest duration of time, use vitamin D and calcium supplementation, and follow appropriate guidelines to reduce risk of fractures in patients at risk. Lansoprazole has been shown to be ineffective for the treatment of symptomatic GERD in children 1 month to <1 year.

Hypomagnesemia, reported rarely, usually with prolonged PPI use of >3 months (most cases >1 year of therapy); may be symptomatic or asymptomatic; severe cases may cause tetany, seizures, and cardiac arrhythmias. Consider obtaining serum magnesium concentrations prior to beginning long-term therapy, especially if taking concomitant digoxin, diuretics, or other drugs known to cause hypomagnesemia; and periodically thereafter. Hypomagnesemia may be corrected by magnesium supplementation, although discontinuation of lansoprazole may be necessary; magnesium levels typically return to normal within 1 week of stopping.

When used for self-medication, patients should be instructed not to use if they have difficulty swallowing, are vomiting blood, or have bloody or black stools. Prior to use, patients should contact healthcare provider if they have liver disease, heartburn for >3 months, heartburn with dizziness, lightheadedness, or sweating, MI symptoms, frequent chest pain, frequent wheezing (especially with heartburn), unexplained weight loss, nausea/vomiting, stomach pain, or are taking antifungals, atazanavir, digoxin, tacrolimus, theophylline, or warfarin. Patients should stop use and consult a healthcare provider if heartburn continues or worsens, or if they need to take for >14 days or more often than every 4 months. Patients should be informed that it may take 1-4 days for full effect to be seen; should not be used for immediate relief.

Adverse Reactions

1% to 10%:

Central nervous system: Headache (children 1-11 years 3%, 12-17 years 7%), dizziness (children 12-17 years 3%; adults <1%)

Gastrointestinal: Diarrhea (1% to 5%; 60 mg/day: 7%), abdominal pain (children 12-17 years 5%; adults 2%), constipation (children 1-11 years 5%; adults 1%), nausea (children 12-17 years 3%; adults 1%)

<1% (Limited to important or life-threatening): Abdomen enlarged, abnormal dreams, abnormal menses, abnormal stools, abnormal vision, agitation, agranulocytosis, albuminuria, allergic reaction, alkaline phosphatase increased, ALT increased, alopecia, amblyopia, amnesia, anaphylactoid reaction, anemia, angina, anorexia, anxiety, aplastic anemia, appetite increased, arrhythmia, AST increased, arthralgia, arthritis, asthma, avitaminosis, bezoar, bilirubinemia, blepharitis, blurred vision, bradycardia, breast enlargement, breast pain, breast tenderness, bronchitis, candidiasis, carcinoma, cardiospasm, cataract, cerebrovascular accident, cerebral infarction, chest pain, chills, cholelithiasis, cholesterol increased/decreased, *Clostridium difficile*-associated diarrhea (CDAD), colitis, confusion, conjunctivitis, cough increased, creatinine increased, deafness, dehydration, dementia, depersonalization, depression, diabetes mellitus, diaphoresis, diplopia, dry eyes, dry skin, dyspepsia, dysphagia, dyspnea, dysmenorrhea, dysuria, edema, electrolyte imbalance, emotional lability, enteritis, eosinophilia, epistaxis, eructation, erythema multiforme, esophageal stenosis, esophageal ulcer, esophagitis, fecal discoloration, fever, fixed eruption, flatulence, flu-like syndrome, fracture, fundic gland polyps, gastric nodules, gastrin levels increased, gastritis, gastroenteritis, gastrointestinal anomaly, gastrointestinal hemorrhage, GGTP increased/decreased, glaucoma, glucocorticoid levels increased, glossitis, glycosuria, goiter, gout, gum hemorrhage, gynecomastia, halitosis, hallucinations, hematemesis, hematuria, hemiplegia, hemolysis, hemolytic anemia, hemoptysis, hepatotoxicity, hostility aggravated, hyper-/hypoglycemia, hyperkinesia, hyperlipemia, hypertonia, hypoesthesia, hyper-/hypotension, hypomagnesemia, hypothyroidism, impotence, infection, insomnia, interstitial nephritis, kidney calculus, laryngeal neoplasia, LDH increased, leg cramps, leukopenia, leukorrhea, libido decreased/increased, liver function test abnormal, lung fibrosis, lymphadenopathy, maculopapular rash, malaise, melena, menorrhagia, migraine, moniliasis (oral), mouth ulceration, musculoskeletal pain, myalgia, myasthenia, myositis, MI, nervousness, neurosis, neutropenia, pain, palpitation, pancreatitis, pancytopenia, paresthesia, parosmia, pelvic pain, peripheral edema, pharyngitis, photophobia, platelet abnormalities,

pneumonia, polyuria, pruritus, ptosis, rash, rectal hemorrhage, retinal degeneration, rhinitis, salivation increased, seizure, shock, sinusitis, skin carcinoma, sleep disorder, somnolence, speech disorder, Stevens-Johnson syndrome, stomatitis, stridor, syncope, synovitis, tachycardia, taste loss, taste perversion, tenesmus, thirst, thrombocytopenia, thrombotic thrombocytopenic purpura, tinnitus, tremor, tongue disorder, toxic epidermal necrolysis, ulcerative colitis, ulcerative stomatitis, upper respiratory inflammation, upper respiratory infection, urethral pain, urinary frequency/urgency, urination impaired, urinary retention, urinary tract infection, urticaria, vaginitis, vasodilation, vertigo, visual field defect, vomiting, weakness, WBC abnormal, weight gain/loss, xerostomia

Drug Interactions

Metabolism/Transport Effects Substrate of CYP2C19 (major), CYP2C9 (minor), CYP3A4 (major); **Note:** Assignment of Major/Minor substrate status based on clinically relevant drug interaction potential; **Inhibits** CYP2C19 (weak), CYP2C9 (weak), CYP2D6 (weak), CYP3A4 (weak); **Induces** CYP1A2 (weak/moderate)

Avoid Concomitant Use

Avoid concomitant use of Lansoprazole with any of the following: Dasatinib; Delavirdine; Erlotinib; Nelfinavir; Pimozide; PONATinib; Rilpivirine; Risedronate

Increased Effect/Toxicity

Lansoprazole may increase the levels/effects of: Amphetamines; ARIPiprazole; Dexmethylphenidate; Dofetilide; Imatinib; Lomitapide; Methotrexate; Methylphenidate; Pimozide; Raltegravir; Risedronate; Saquinavir; Tacrolimus (Systemic); Vitamin K Antagonists; Voriconazole

The levels/effects of Lansoprazole may be increased by: Fluconazole; Ketoconazole (Systemic); Voriconazole

Decreased Effect

Lansoprazole may decrease the levels/effects of: Atazanavir; Bisphosphonate Derivatives; Bosutinib; Cefditoren; Clopidogrel; Dabigatran Etexilate; Dabrafenib; Dasatinib; Delavirdine; Erlotinib; Gefitinib; Indinavir; Iron Salts; Itraconazole; Ketoconazole (Systemic); Mesalamine; Multivitamins/Minerals (with ADEK, Folate, Iron); Mycophenolate; Nelfinavir; Nilotinib; PONATinib; Posaconazole; Rilpivirine; Riociguat; Risedronate; Vismodegib

The levels/effects of Lansoprazole may be decreased by: Bosentan; CYP2C19 Inducers (Strong); CYP3A4 Inducers (Strong); Dabrafenib; Deferasirox; Herbs (CYP3A4 Inducers); Mitotane; Tipranavir; Tocilizumab

Ethanol/Nutrition/Herb Interactions

Ethanol: Avoid ethanol (may cause gastric mucosal irritation).

Food: Lansoprazole serum concentrations may be decreased if taken with food.

Herb/Nutraceutical: Avoid St John's wort (may decrease the levels/effect of lansoprazole).

Storage/Stability Store at 25°C (77°F); excursions permitted to 15°C to 30°C (59°F to 86°F).

Mechanism of Action Decreases acid secretion in gastric parietal cells through inhibition of (H+, K+)-ATPase enzyme system, blocking the final step in gastric acid production.

Pharmacodynamics/Kinetics

Onset of action: Gastric acid suppression: Oral: 1-3 hours

Duration: Gastric acid suppression: Oral: >1 day

Absorption: Rapid

Distribution: V_d: 14-18 L

Protein binding: 97%

Metabolism: Hepatic via CYP2C19 and 3A4, and in parietal cells to two active metabolites that are not present in systemic circulation

Bioavailability: ≥80%; decreased 50% to 70% if given 30 minutes after food

Half-life elimination: 1.5 ± 1 hours; Elderly: 2-3 hours; Hepatic impairment: 3-7 hours

Time to peak, plasma: 1.7 hours

Excretion: Feces (67%); urine (33%)

Dosage

Children 1-11 years: GERD, erosive esophagitis: Oral:

≤30 kg: 15 mg once daily for up to 12 weeks

>30 kg: 30 mg once daily for up to 12 weeks

Note: Doses were increased in some pediatric patients if still symptomatic after 2 or more weeks of treatment (maximum dose: 30 mg twice daily)

Children 12-17 years: Oral:

Nonerosive GERD: 15 mg once daily for up to 8 weeks

Erosive esophagitis: 30 mg once daily for up to 8 weeks

Adults: Oral:

Duodenal ulcer: Short-term treatment: 15 mg once daily for 4 weeks; maintenance therapy: 15 mg once daily

Gastric ulcer: Short-term treatment: 30 mg once daily for up to 8 weeks

NSAID-associated gastric ulcer (healing): 30 mg once daily for 8 weeks; controlled studies did not extend past 8 weeks of therapy

NSAID-associated gastric ulcer (to reduce risk): 15 mg once daily for up to 12 weeks; controlled studies did not extend past 12 weeks of therapy

Symptomatic GERD: Short-term treatment: 15 mg once daily for up to 8 weeks

Erosive esophagitis: Short-term treatment: 30 mg once daily for up to 8 weeks; continued treatment for an additional 8 weeks may be considered for recurrence or for patients who do not heal after the first 8 weeks of therapy; maintenance therapy: 15 mg once daily

Hypersecretory conditions: Initial: 60 mg once daily; adjust dose based upon patient response and to reduce acid secretion to <10 mEq/hour (5 mEq/hour in patients with prior gastric surgery); doses of 90 mg twice daily have been used; administer doses >120 mg/day in divided doses

Helicobacter pylori eradication:

Manufacturer labeling: 30 mg 3 times daily administered with amoxicillin 1000 mg 3 times daily for 14 days **or** 30 mg twice daily administered with amoxicillin 1000 mg *and* clarithromycin 500 mg twice daily for 10-14 days

American College of Gastroenterology guidelines (Chey, 2007):

Nonpenicillin allergy: 30 mg twice daily administered with amoxicillin 1000 mg *and* clarithromycin 500 mg twice daily for 10-14 days

Penicillin allergy: 30 mg twice daily administered with clarithromycin 500 mg *and* metronidazole 500 mg twice daily for 10-14 days **or** 30 mg once or twice daily administered with bismuth subsalicylate 525 mg *and* metronidazole 250 mg *plus* tetracycline 500 mg 4 times daily for 10-14 days

Heartburn: OTC labeling: 15 mg once daily for 14 days; may repeat 14 days of therapy every 4 months. Do not take for >14 days or more often than every 4 months, unless instructed by healthcare provider.

Stress ulcer prophylaxis, ICU patients (unlabeled use): 30 mg once daily (Brophy, 2010; Olsen, 2008). **Note:** Intended for patients with associated risk factors (eg, coagulopathy, mechanical ventilation for ≥48 hours, severe sepsis); discontinue use once risk factors have resolved (Dellinger, 2013).

Dosage adjustment in renal impairment: No dosage adjustment necessary.

Dosage adjustment in hepatic impairment: Bioavailability increased in hepatic impairment. Consider dose reduction in severe impairment.

Dietary Considerations Should be taken before eating; best if taken before breakfast. Some products may contain phenylalanine.

Administration

Oral: Administer before food; best if taken before breakfast. The intact granules should not be chewed or crushed; however, several options are available for those patients unable to swallow capsules:

Capsules may be opened and the intact granules sprinkled on 1 tablespoon of applesauce, Ensure® pudding, cottage cheese, yogurt, or strained pears. The granules should then be swallowed immediately.

Capsules may be opened and emptied into ~60 mL orange juice, apple juice, or tomato juice; mix and swallow immediately. Rinse the glass with additional juice and swallow to assure complete delivery of the dose.

Orally-disintegrating tablets: Should not be swallowed whole, broken, cut, or chewed. Place tablet on tongue; allow to dissolve (with or without water) until particles can be swallowed. Orally-disintegrating tablets may also be administered via an oral syringe: Place the 15 mg tablet in an oral syringe and draw up ~4 mL water, or place the 30 mg tablet in an oral syringe and draw up ~10 mL water. After tablet has dispersed, administer within 15 minutes. Refill the syringe with water (2 mL for the 15 mg tablet; 5 mL for the 30 mg tablet), shake gently, then administer any remaining contents.

Nasogastric tube administration:

Capsule: Capsule can be opened, the granules mixed (not crushed) with 40 mL of apple juice and then administered through the NG tube into the stomach, then flush tube with additional apple juice. Do not mix with other liquids. Thirty milligrams has also been suspended in 10 mL of 8.4% sodium bicarbonate solution (or apple juice) and administered via NG tube (Brophy, 2010).

Orally-disintegrating tablet: Nasogastric tube ≥8 French: Place a 15 mg tablet in a syringe and draw up ~4 mL water, or place the 30 mg tablet in a syringe and draw up ~10 mL water. After tablet has dispersed, administer within 15 minutes. Refill the syringe with ~5 mL water, shake gently, and then flush the nasogastric tube.

Monitoring Parameters Patients with Zollinger-Ellison syndrome should be monitored for gastric acid output, which should be maintained at ≤10 mEq/hour during the last hour before the next lansoprazole dose; lab monitoring should include CBC, liver function, renal function, and serum gastrin levels

Dosage Forms Excipient information presented when available (limited, particularly for generics); consult specific product labeling.

Capsule Delayed Release, Oral:

Heartburn Relief 24 Hour: 15 mg [sodium free; contains brilliant blue fcf (fd&c blue #1), fd&c red #40, fd&c yellow #10 (quinoline yellow)]

Prevacid: 15 mg, 30 mg [contains brilliant blue fcf (fd&c blue #1), fd&c red #40]

Prevacid 24HR: 15 mg [sodium free; contains brilliant blue fcf (fd&c blue #1), fd&c red #40]

Generic: 15 mg, 30 mg

Suspension, Oral:

First-Lansoprazole: 3 mg/mL (90 mL, 150 mL, 300 mL) [contains benzyl alcohol, fd&c red #40, saccharin sodium; strawberry flavor]

Tablet Dispersible, Oral:

Prevacid SoluTab: 15 mg, 30 mg [contains aspartame]

Extemporaneous Preparations A 3 mg/mL oral solution (Simplified Lansoprazole Solution [SLS]) may be made with capsules and sodium bicarbonate. Empty the contents of ten lansoprazole 30 mg capsules into a beaker. Add 100 mL sodium bicarbonate 8.4% and gently stir until dissolved (about 15 minutes). Transfer solution to an amber-colored syringe or bottle. A prior study showed that SLS was stable for 8 hours at room temperature or for 14 days refrigerated (DiGiancinto, 2000). However, a more recent study, demonstrated SLS to be stable for 48 hours at room temperature in oral syringes and for only 7 days when refrigerated (Morrison, 2013).

Note: A more palatable lansoprazole (3 mg/mL) suspension is commercially available as a compounding kit (First-Lansoprazole).

DiGiancinto JL, Olsen KM, Bergman KL, et al, "Stability of Suspension Formulations of Lansoprazole and Omeprazole Stored in Amber-Colored Plastic Oral Syringes," *Ann Pharmacother*, 2000, 34(5):600-5

Morrison JT, Lugo RA, Thigpen JC, et al, "Stability of Extemporaneously Prepared Lansoprazole Suspension at Two Temperatures," *J Pediatr Pharmacol Ther*, 2013, 18(2):122-7.

Sharma V, "Comparison of 24-hour Intragastric pH Using Four Liquid Formulations of Lansoprazole and Omeprazole," *Am J Health Syst Pharm*, 1999, 56(Suppl 4):18-21.

Sharma VK, Vasudeva R, and Howden CW, "Simplified Lansoprazole Suspension - Liquid Formulations of Lansoprazole - Effectively Suppresses Intragastric Acidity When Administered Through a Gastrostomy," *Am J Gastroenterol*, 1999, 94(7):1813-7.

Lansoprazole, Amoxicillin, and Clarithromycin

(lan SOE pra zole, a moks i SIL in, & kla RITH roe mye sin)

Brand Names: U.S. Prevpac®

Brand Names: Canada Hp-PAC®

Index Terms Amoxicillin, Clarithromycin, and Lansoprazole; Clarithromycin, Lansoprazole, and Amoxicillin; Lansoprazole, Amoxicillin, and Clarithromycin

Pharmacologic Category Antibiotic, Macrolide Combination; Antibiotic, Penicillin; Gastrointestinal Agent, Miscellaneous; Proton Pump Inhibitor; Substituted Benzimidazole

Use Eradication of *H. pylori* to reduce the risk of recurrent duodenal ulcer

Pregnancy Risk Factor C

Dosage Oral: Adults: Lansoprazole 30 mg, amoxicillin 1 g, and clarithromycin 500 mg taken together twice daily for 10 or 14 days

Dosage adjustment in renal impairment: Cl_{cr} <30 mL/minute: Use is not recommended.

Dosage adjustment in hepatic impairment: Bioavailability of lansoprazole increased in hepatic impairment. Consider dose reduction in severe hepatic impairment

Additional Information Complete prescribing information should be consulted for additional detail.

Dosage Forms Excipient information presented when available (limited, particularly for generics); consult specific product labeling.

Combination package [each administration card contains]:

Prevpac®:

Capsule: Amoxicillin 500 mg (4 capsules/day)

Capsule, delayed release (Prevacid®): Lansoprazole 30 mg (2 capsules/day)

Tablet (Biaxin®): Clarithromycin 500 mg (2 tablets/day)

Generic:

Capsule: Amoxicillin 500 mg (4 capsules/day)

Capsule, delayed release: Lansoprazole 30 mg (2 capsules/day)

Tablet: Clarithromycin 500 mg (2 tablets/day)

◆ **Lansoprazole, Amoxicillin, and Clarithromycin** *see* Lansoprazole, Amoxicillin, and Clarithromycin *on page 1173*

Lanthanum (LAN tha num)

Brand Names: U.S. Fosrenol

Brand Names: Canada Fosrenol®

Index Terms Lanthanum Carbonate

Pharmacologic Category Phosphate Binder

Use Reduction of serum phosphate in patients with stage 5 chronic kidney disease (end-stage renal disease [ESRD]; kidney failure: GFR <15 mL/minute/1.73 m^2 or dialysis)

Pregnancy Risk Factor C

Medication Guide Available Yes

Dosage Oral: Adults: Reduction of serum phosphorous: Initial: 1500 mg/day divided and taken with meals; typical increases of 750 mg/day every 2-3 weeks are suggested as needed to reduce the serum phosphate level <6 mg/dL; usual dosage range: 1500-3000 mg; doses of up to 4500 mg have been evaluated

Dosage adjustment in renal impairment: No dosage adjustment necessary.

Dosage adjustment in hepatic impairment: No dosage adjustment provided in manufacturer's labeling.

Additional Information Complete prescribing information should be consulted for additional detail.

Dosage Forms Excipient information presented when available (limited, particularly for generics); consult specific product labeling.

Tablet Chewable, Oral:

Fosrenol: 500 mg, 750 mg, 1000 mg

- Lanthanum Carbonate *see* Lanthanum *on page 1173*
- Lantus *see* Insulin Glargine *on page 1089*
- Lantus® (Can) *see* Insulin Glargine *on page 1089*
- Lantus® OptiSet® (Can) *see* Insulin Glargine *on page 1089*
- Lantus SoloStar *see* Insulin Glargine *on page 1089*
- Lanvis® (Can) *see* Thioguanine *on page 2045*

Lapatinib (la PA ti nib)

Brand Names: U.S. Tykerb

Brand Names: Canada Tykerb®

Index Terms GW572016; Lapatinib Ditosylate

Pharmacologic Category Antineoplastic Agent, Anti-HER2; Antineoplastic Agent, Tyrosine Kinase Inhibitor; Epidermal Growth Factor Receptor (EGFR) Inhibitor

Use

Breast cancer: Treatment of human epidermal growth receptor type 2 (HER2) overexpressing advanced or metastatic breast cancer (in combination with capecitabine) in patients who have received prior therapy (with an anthracycline, a taxane, and trastuzumab); HER2 overexpressing hormone receptor–positive metastatic breast cancer in postmenopausal women where hormone therapy is indicated (in combination with letrozole)

Limitations of use: Patients should have disease progression on trastuzumab prior to initiation of treatment with lapatinib in combination with capecitabine.

Unlabeled Use Treatment (in combination with trastuzumab) of HER2 overexpressing metastatic breast cancer which had progressed on prior trastuzumab containing therapy; treatment of HER2 overexpressing metastatic breast cancer with brain metastases

Pregnancy Risk Factor D

Pregnancy Considerations Adverse events were demonstrated in animal reproduction studies. Lapatinib may cause fetal harm if administered during pregnancy. Women of childbearing potential should be advised to avoid pregnancy during treatment.

Breast-Feeding Considerations It is not known if lapatinib is excreted in breast milk. Due to the potential for serious adverse reactions in the nursing infant, the decision to discontinue lapatinib or discontinue breast-feeding during treatment should take in account the benefits of treatment to the mother.

Prescribing and Access Restrictions Lapatinib is available through specialty pharmacies only. Information is available at www.gskcta.com or 1-866-265-6491.

Contraindications Hypersensitivity to lapatinib or any component of the formulation

Warnings/Precautions Hazardous agent - use appropriate precautions for handling and disposal (meets NIOSH, 2012 criteria). Decreases in left ventricular ejection fraction (LVEF) have been reported (usually within the first 3 months of treatment); baseline and periodic LVEF evaluations are recommended; interrupt treatment with decreased LVEF ≥grade 2 or LVEF <LLN; may reinitiate with a reduced dose after a minimum of 2 weeks if the LVEF recovers and the patient is asymptomatic. QT_c prolongation has been observed; use caution in patients with a history of QT_c prolongation or with medications known to prolong the QT interval; a baseline and periodic 12-lead ECG should be considered; correct electrolyte (potassium, calcium and magnesium) abnormalities prior to and during treatment. Use with caution in conditions which may impair left ventricular function and in patients with a history of or predisposed to (prior treatment with anthracyclines, chest wall irradiation) left ventricular dysfunction. Interstitial lung disease (ILD) and pneumonitis have been reported (with lapatinib monotherapy and with combination chemotherapy); monitor for pulmonary symptoms which may indicate ILD or pneumonitis; discontinue treatment for grade 3 (or higher) pulmonary symptoms indicative of ILD or pneumonitis (eg, dyspnea, dry cough).

[U.S. Boxed Warning]: Hepatotoxicity (ALT or AST >3 times ULN and total bilirubin >2 times ULN) has been reported with lapatinib; may be severe and/or fatal. Onset of hepatotoxicity may occur within days to several months after treatment initiation. Monitor (at baseline and every 4-6 weeks during treatment, and as clinically indicated); discontinue with severe changes in liver function; do not reinitiate. Use caution in patients with hepatic dysfunction; dose reductions should be considered in patients with pre-existing severe (Child-Pugh class C) hepatic impairment. Potentially significant drug-drug interactions may exist, requiring dose or frequency adjustment, additional monitoring, and/or selection of alternative therapy. Patients who carry the HLA alleles DQA1*02:01 and DRB1*07:01 may experience a greater incidence of severe liver injury than patients who are noncarriers. These alleles are present in ~15% to 25% of Caucasian, Asian, African, and Hispanic patient populations and 1% in Japanese populations. May cause diarrhea (onset is generally within 6 days and duration is 4-5 days); may be severe and/or fatal; instruct patients to immediately report any bowel pattern changes. After first unformed stool, administer antidiarrheal agents; severe diarrhea may require hydration, electrolytes, antibiotics (if duration >24 hours, fever, or grade 3/4 neutropenia), and/or treatment interruption, dose reduction, or discontinuation.

Adverse Reactions Percentages reported for combination therapy.

>10%:

Central nervous system: Fatigue (10% to 20%), headache (≤14%)

Dermatologic: Palmar-plantar erythrodysesthesia (hand-and-foot syndrome) (with capecitabine: 53%; grade 3: 12%), rash (28% to 44%), dry skin (10% to 13%), alopecia (≤13%), pruritus (≤12%), nail disorder (≤11%)

Gastrointestinal: Diarrhea (64% to 65%; grade 3: 9% to 13%; grade 4: ≤1%), nausea (31% to 44%), vomiting (17% to 26%), abdominal pain (≤15%), mucosal inflammation (≤15%), stomatitis (≤14%), anorexia (≤11%), dyspepsia (≤11%)

Hematologic: Anemia (with capecitabine: 56%; grade 3: <1%), neutropenia (with capecitabine: 22%; grade 3: 3%; grade 4: <1%), thrombocytopenia (with capecitabine: 18%; grade 3: <1%)

Hepatic: AST increased (49% to 53%; grade 3: 2% to 6%; grade 4: <1%), ALT increased (37% to 46%; grade 3: 2% to 5%; grade 4<1%) total bilirubin increased (22% to 45%; grade 3: ≤4%; grade 4: <1%)

Neuromuscular & skeletal: Limb pain (≤12%), weakness (≤12%), back pain (≤11%)

Respiratory: Dyspnea (≤12%), epistaxis (≤11%)

1% to 10%:

Cardiovascular: LVEF decreased (grades 1/2: 2% to 4%; grades 3/4: <1%)

Central nervous system: Insomnia (≤10%)

<1% (Limited to important or life-threatening): Anaphylaxis, hepatotoxicity, hypersensitivity, interstitial lung disease, paronychia, pneumonitis, Prinzmetal's angina, QTc prolongation

Drug Interactions

Metabolism/Transport Effects **Substrate** of CYP3A4 (major), P-glycoprotein; **Note:** Assignment of Major/Minor substrate status based on clinically relevant drug interaction potential; **Inhibits** BCRP, CYP2C8 (moderate), CYP3A4 (weak), P-glycoprotein

Avoid Concomitant Use

Avoid concomitant use of Lapatinib with any of the following: Bosutinib; CYP3A4 Inducers (Strong); CYP3A4 Inhibitors (Strong); Fusidic Acid (Systemic); Grapefruit Juice; Highest Risk QTc-Prolonging Agents; Ivabradine; Mifepristone; PAZOPanib; Pomalidomide; Silodosin; St Johns Wort; VinCRIStine (Liposomal)

Increased Effect/Toxicity

Lapatinib may increase the levels/effects of: Afatinib; ARIPiprazole; Bosutinib; Colchicine; CYP2C8 Substrates; Dabigatran Etexilate; Everolimus; Highest Risk QTc-Prolonging Agents; Lomitapide; Moderate Risk QTc-Prolonging Agents; PAZOPanib; P-glycoprotein/ABCB1 Substrates; Pomalidomide; Prucalopride; Rivaroxaban; Silodosin; Topotecan; VinCRIStine (Liposomal); Vitamin K Antagonists

The levels/effects of Lapatinib may be increased by: CYP3A4 Inhibitors (Moderate); CYP3A4 Inhibitors (Strong); Dasatinib; Fusidic Acid (Systemic); Grapefruit Juice; Ivabradine; Ivacaftor; Luliconazole; Mifepristone; P-glycoprotein/ABCB1 Inhibitors; QTc-Prolonging Agents (Indeterminate Risk and Risk Modifying); Simeprevir

Decreased Effect

Lapatinib may decrease the levels/effects of: Cardiac Glycosides; Vitamin K Antagonists

The levels/effects of Lapatinib may be decreased by: Bosentan; CYP3A4 Inducers (Strong); Dabrafenib; Deferasirox; P-glycoprotein/ABCB1 Inducers; St Johns Wort; Tocilizumab

Ethanol/Nutrition/Herb Interactions

Food: Systemic exposure of lapatinib is increased when administered with food (AUC three- to fourfold higher). Grapefruit juice may increase the levels/effects of lapatinib. Management: Administer once daily on an empty stomach, 1 hour before or 1 hour after a meal at the same time each day. Avoid grapefruit juice. Maintain adequate hydration, unless instructed to restrict fluid intake.

Herb/Nutraceutical: St John's wort may increase metabolism and decrease lapatinib concentrations. Management: Avoid St John's wort.

Storage/Stability Store at room temperature of 25°C (77°F); excursions permitted between 15°C and 30°C (59°F and 86°F).

Mechanism of Action Tyrosine kinase (dual kinase) inhibitor; inhibits EGFR (ErbB1) and HER2 (ErbB2) by reversibly binding to tyrosine kinase, blocking phosphorylation and activation of downstream second messengers (Erk1/2 and Akt), regulating cellular proliferation and survival in ErbB- and ErbB2-expressing tumors. Combination therapy with lapatinib and endocrine therapy may overcome endocrine resistance occurring in HER2+ and hormone receptor positive disease.

Pharmacodynamics/Kinetics

Absorption: Incomplete and variable

Protein binding: >99% to albumin and alpha$_1$-acid glycoprotein

Metabolism: Hepatic; extensive via CYP3A4 and 3A5, and to a lesser extent via CYP2C19 and 2C8 to oxidized metabolites

Half-life elimination: ~24 hours

Time to peak, plasma: ~4 hours (Burris, 2009)

Excretion: Feces (27% as unchanged drug; range 3% to 67%); urine (<2%)

Dosage Details concerning dosing in combination regimens should also be consulted. **Note:** Patients should have disease progression on trastuzumab prior to initiation of treatment with lapatinib in combination with capecitabine.

Breast cancer, metastatic, HER2+ (with prior anthracycline, taxane and trastuzumab therapy): Adults: Oral: 1250 mg once daily (in combination with capecitabine) until disease progression or unacceptable toxicity (Geyer, 2006)

Breast cancer, metastatic, HER2+, hormonal therapy indicated: Adults: Oral: 1500 mg once daily (in combination with letrozole) until disease progression (Johnston, 2009)

Breast cancer, metastatic, HER2+ with brain metastases, first-line therapy (unlabeled use): Adults: Oral: 1250 mg once daily (in combination with capecitabine) until disease progression or unacceptable toxicity (Bachelot, 2013)

Breast cancer, metastatic, HER2+, with progression on prior trastuzumab therapy (unlabeled use): Adults: Oral: 1000 mg once daily (in combination with trastuzumab) (Blackwell, 2010; Blackwell, 2012)

Missed doses: If a dose is missed, resume with the next scheduled daily dose; do not double the dose the next day.

Dosage adjustment for concomitant CYP3A4 inhibitors/inducers:

CYP3A4 inhibitors: Avoid the use of concomitant strong CYP3A4 inhibitors. If concomitant use cannot be avoided, consider reducing lapatinib to 500 mg once daily with careful monitoring. When a strong CYP3A4 inhibitor is discontinued, allow ~1 week to elapse prior to adjusting the lapatinib dose upward.

CYP3A4 inducers: Avoid the use of concomitant strong CYP3A4 inducers.

U.S. labeling: If concomitant use cannot be avoided, consider gradually titrating lapatinib from 1250 mg once daily up to 4500 mg daily (in combination with capecitabine) **or** from 1500 mg once daily up to 5500 mg daily (in combination with letrozole), based on tolerability and with careful monitoring. If the strong CYP3A4 enzyme inducer is discontinued, reduce the lapatinib dose to the indicated dose.

Canadian labeling: If concomitant use cannot be avoided, titrate lapatinib dose gradually upward based on tolerability. If the strong CYP3A4 enzyme inducer is discontinued, reduce the lapatinib dose over 2 weeks.

Dosage adjustment for toxicity:

Cardiac toxicity: Discontinue treatment for at least 2 weeks for LVEF < LLN or decreased LVEF ≥ grade 2 (U.S. labeling) or decreased LVEF ≥ grade 3 (Canadian labeling); may be restarted at 1000 mg once daily (in combination with capecitabine) **or** 1250 mg once daily (in combination with letrozole) if LVEF recovers to normal and patient is asymptomatic.

Diarrhea:

Grade 3 diarrhea or grade 1 or 2 diarrhea with complicating features (moderate-to-severe abdominal cramping, grade 2 or higher nausea/vomiting, decreased performance status, fever, sepsis, neutropenia, frank bleeding, or dehydration):

U.S. labeling: Interrupt treatment; may restart at a reduced dose (from 1500 mg once daily to 1250 mg once daily or from 1250 mg once daily to 1000 mg once daily) when diarrhea resolves to ≤ grade 1.

Canadian labeling: Interrupt treatment; may restart at a reduced dose (from 1500 mg once daily to 1250 mg once daily or from 1250 mg once daily to 1000 mg once daily or from 1000 mg once daily to 750 mg once daily) when diarrhea resolves to ≤ grade 1.

Grade 4 diarrhea: Permanently discontinue.

Pulmonary toxicity: Discontinue treatment with pulmonary symptoms indicative of interstitial lung disease or pneumonitis which are ≥ grade 3

Other toxicities: Withhold for any toxicity (other than cardiac) ≥ grade 2 until toxicity resolves to ≤ grade 1 and reinitiate at the standard dose of 1250 mg or 1500 mg once daily; for persistent toxicity, reduce dosage to 1000 mg once daily (in combination with capecitabine) **or** 1250 mg once daily (in combination with letrozole)

Dosage adjustment in renal impairment: No dosage adjustment provided in the manufacturer's labeling (has not been studied); however, due to the minimal renal elimination (<2%), dosage adjustments may not be necessary.

Dosage adjustment in hepatic impairment:

Severe pre-existing impairment (Child-Pugh class C):

In combination with capecitabine: Reduce dose from 1250 mg once daily to 750 mg once daily

In combination with letrozole: Reduce dose from 1500 mg once daily to 1000 mg once daily

Severe hepatotoxicity during treatment: Discontinue permanently (do not rechallenge).

Dietary Considerations Take on an empty stomach, 1 hour before or 1 hour after a meal. (**Note:** For combination with capecitabine treatment, capecitabine should be taken with food, or within 30 minutes after a meal.) Avoid grapefruit juice.

Administration Administer once daily, on an empty stomach, 1 hour before or 1 hour after a meal. Take full dose at the same time each day; dividing doses throughout the day is not recommended.

Hazardous agent; use appropriate precautions for handling and disposal (meets NIOSH, 2012 criteria).

Monitoring Parameters LVEF (baseline and periodic), CBC with differential, liver function tests, including transaminases, bilirubin, and alkaline phosphatase (baseline and every 4-6 weeks during treatment); electrolytes including calcium, potassium, magnesium; monitor for fluid retention; ECG monitoring if at risk for QT_c prolongation; symptoms of ILD or pneumonitis; monitor for diarrhea

Dosage Forms Excipient information presented when available (limited, particularly for generics); consult specific product labeling.

Tablet, Oral:

Tykerb: 250 mg [contains fd&c yellow #6 (sunset yellow), fd&c yellow #6 aluminum lake]

◆ **Lapatinib Ditosylate** *see* Lapatinib *on page 1174*

◆ **L-Arginine** *see* Arginine *on page 163*

◆ **L-Arginine Hydrochloride** *see* Arginine *on page 163*

◆ **Larin Fe 1.5/30** *see* Ethinyl Estradiol and Norethindrone *on page 793*

◆ **Larin Fe 1/20** *see* Ethinyl Estradiol and Norethindrone *on page 793*

Laronidase (lair OH ni days)

Brand Names: U.S. Aldurazyme

Brand Names: Canada Aldurazyme®

Index Terms Recombinant α-L-Iduronidase (Glycosaminoglycan α-L-Iduronohydrolase)

Pharmacologic Category Enzyme

Use Treatment of Hurler and Hurler-Scheie forms of mucopolysaccharidosis I (MPS I); treatment of Scheie form of MPS I in patients with moderate-to-severe symptoms

Pregnancy Risk Factor B

Pregnancy Considerations Teratogenic effects were not observed in animal reproduction studies. Patients are encouraged to enroll in the MPS I registry (800-745-4447 or www.MPSIregistry.com).

Breast-Feeding Considerations It is not known if laronidase is excreted in breast milk. The manufacturer recommends that caution be exercised when administering laronidase to nursing women.

Contraindications

There are no contraindications listed within the manufacturer's U.S. labeling.

Canadian labeling: Severe hypersensitivity to laronidase or any component of the formulation

Warnings/Precautions [U.S. Boxed Warning]: Anaphylactic reactions have been observed during infusion, immediate treatment for hypersensitivity reactions should be available during administration. Additional monitoring may be required in patients with compromised respiratory function or acute respiratory disease; may be at increased risk for acute exacerbation of respiratory symptoms due to infusion reaction. Reactions, which may include airway obstruction, bradycardia, bronchospasm, hypotension, hypoxia, respiratory distress/failure, stridor, tachypnea, and urticaria, may be severe and tend to occur during or within 3 hours after administration. Immediately discontinue infusion if severe reactions occur; medical support should be available during administration. Risks and benefits should be carefully considered prior to readministration following a severe hypersensitivity reaction. Patients who initially experience severe reactions may require prolonged monitoring. In the case of anaphylaxis, caution should be used if epinephrine is being considered; many patients with MPS I have pre-existing heart disease.

Infusion reactions may occur; use caution and consider delaying treatment in patients with acute febrile/respiratory illness; may result in increased risk for infusion-related reactions. Pretreatment with antipyretics and antihistamines is recommended. Decrease infusion rate, temporarily discontinue infusion, and/or administer additional antipyretics and antihistamines to manage infusion reactions.

Use with caution in patients at risk for fluid overload or in conditions where fluid restriction is indicated (eg, acute underlying respiratory illness, compromised cardiac and/or respiratory function); conditions may be exacerbated during infusion. Extended observation may be necessary for some patients. Use with caution in patients with sleep apnea; evaluate patients prior to initiation of therapy. Apnea treatment options should be readily available (eg, CPAP or supplemental oxygen) during infusion or with use of sedating antihistamines.

Use has not been studied in patients with mild symptoms of the Scheie form of MPS I. Not indicated for the CNS manifestations of the disorder. A patient registry has been established and all patients are encouraged to participate. Registry information may be obtained at www.-MPSIregistry.com or by calling 800-745-4447.

Adverse Reactions Note: Unless otherwise noted, frequency of adverse reactions is reported for patients ≥6 years of age.

>10%:

Cardiovascular: Flushing (11% to 23%), poor venous access (14%)

Central nervous system: Fever 11% (infants and children 6 months to 5 years: 30%), chills (infants and children 6 months to 5 years: 20%)

Dermatologic: Rash (13% to 36%; infants and children 6 months to 5 years: ≥5%)

Immunologic: Antibody development (93% to 97%; children 6 months to 5 years: 100%)

Local: Injection site reaction (18%)

Neuromuscular & skeletal: Hyper-reflexia (14%), paresthesia (14%)

Otic: Otitis media (infants and children 6 months to 5 years: 20%)

Respiratory: Upper respiratory tract infection (32%)

Miscellaneous: Infusion reactions (32% to 49%; may be severe; infants and children 6 months to 5 years: 35%)

1% to 10%:

Cardiovascular: Hypertension (infants and children 6 months to 5 years: 10%), tachycardia (infants and children 6 months to 5 years: 10%), chest pain (9%), edema (9%), facial edema (9%), hypotension (9%), pallor (infants and children 6 months to 5 years: ≥5%)

Central nervous system: Headache (9%)

Dermatologic: Pruritus (4%), urticaria (4%), hyperhidrosis

Gastrointestinal: Abdominal pain/discomfort (9%), diarrhea (7%), vomiting (4%)

Hematologic: Thrombocytopenia (9%)

Hepatic: Bilirubinemia (9%)

Local: Abscess (9%), injection site pain (9%)

Neuromuscular & skeletal: Tremor (infants and children 6 months to 5 years: ≥5%), arthralgia (4%), back pain, musculoskeletal pain

Ocular: Corneal opacity (9%)

Respiratory: Oxygen saturation decreased (infants and children 6 months to 5 years: 10%), crepitations (infants and children 6 months to 5 years: ≥5%), respiratory distress (infants and children 6 months to 5 years: ≥5%), wheezing (infants and children 6 months to 5 years: ≥5%), bronchospasm, cough, dyspnea

Miscellaneous: Feeling warm/cold (7%), allergic reaction (severe/serious 1%)

<1% (Limited to important or life-threatening): Anaphylaxis, angioedema, cardiac failure, cardiorespiratory arrest, cyanosis, erythema, extravasation, pneumonia, respiratory failure

Drug Interactions

Metabolism/Transport Effects None known.

Avoid Concomitant Use There are no known interactions where it is recommended to avoid concomitant use.

Increased Effect/Toxicity There are no known significant interactions involving an increase in effect.

Decreased Effect There are no known significant interactions involving a decrease in effect.

Preparation for Administration Allow vials to come to room temperature prior to admixture. Prepare the infusion using a low protein-binding container (there is no compatability information of diluted laronidase in glass containers). Total volume of infusion is determined by body weight. For patients weighing ≤20 kg (or weighing up to 30 kg and with cardiac or respiratory compromise), dilute the required dose in 100 mL NS; for patients weighing >20 kg, dilute required dose in 250 mL NS. Determine the number of vials to dilute by calculating the required dose and rounding up to the nearest whole vial. Remove and discard a volume of NS from the infusion bag equal to the volume of the calculated dose of laronidase. Slowly withdraw from vial(s) and slowly add laronidase to the NS; avoid excessive agitation, do not use filter needle. Gently rotate infusion bag to mix (do not shake).

Storage/Stability Store vials under refrigeration at 2°C to 8°C (36°F to 46°F); do not freeze. Protect from light. Do not shake. Following dilution, solution for infusion should be used immediately; however, if not used immediately, refrigerate. Infusion of solution should be completed within 36 hours of preparation.

Mechanism of Action Laronidase is a recombinant (replacement) form of α-L-iduronidase derived from Chinese hamster cells. α-L-iduronidase is an enzyme needed to break down endogenous glycosaminoglycans (GAGs) within lysosomes. A deficiency of α-L-iduronidase leads to an accumulation of GAGs, causing cellular, tissue, and organ dysfunction as seen in MPS I. Improved pulmonary function and walking capacity have been demonstrated with the administration of laronidase to patients with Hurler, Hurler-Scheie, or Scheie (with moderate-to-severe symptoms) forms of MPS.

Pharmacodynamics/Kinetics

Distribution:

Infants and Children 6 months to 5 years: V_d: 0.12-0.56 L/kg

Children ≥6 years and Adults: V_d: 0.24-0.6 L/kg

Half-life elimination:

Infants and Children 6 months to 5 years: 0.3-1.9 hours

Children ≥6 years and Adults: 1.5-3.6 hours

Excretion:

Infants and Children 6 months to 5 years: Clearance: 2.2-7.7 mL/minute/kg

Children ≥6 years and Adults: Clearance: 1.7-2.7 mL/minute/kg; during the first 12 weeks of therapy the clearance of laronidase increases proportionally to the amount of antibodies a given patient develops against the enzyme. However, with long-term use (≥26 weeks) antibody titers have no effect on laronidase clearance.

Dosage Note: Premedicate with antipyretic and/or antihistamines 1 hour prior to start of infusion.

I.V.: Children ≥6 months and Adults: 0.58 mg/kg once weekly; dose should be rounded up to the nearest whole vial

Dosage adjustment in renal impairment: No dosage adjustment provided in manufacturer's labeling.

Dosage adjustment in hepatic impairment: No dosage adjustment provided in manufacturer's labeling.

Administration Administer using an infusion set with low protein-binding and 0.2 micrometer in-line filter. Antipyretics and/or antihistamines should be administered 60 minutes prior to infusion. Volume and infusion rate are based on body weight; deliver infusion over ~3-4 hours. Vital signs should be monitored every 15 minutes, if stable; rate may be increased as follows:

≤20 kg: Total infusion volume: 100 mL

2 mL/hour for 15 minutes

4 mL/hour for 15 minutes

8 mL/hour for 15 minutes

16 mL/hour for 15 minutes

32 mL/hour for remainder of infusion (~3 hours)

>20 kg: Total infusion volume: 250 mL

5 mL/hour for 15 minutes

10 mL/hour for 15 minutes

20 mL/hour for 15 minutes

40 mL/hour for 15 minutes

80 mL/hour for remainder of infusion (~3 hours)

Note: A total infusion volume of 100 mL NS and slower infusion rate may be considered for patients with cardiac or respiratory compromise who weigh up to 30 kg. In case of infusion-related reaction in any patient, decrease the rate of infusion, temporarily discontinue the infusion, and/or administer additional antipyretics/antihistamines.

Monitoring Parameters Vital signs; injection site reactions, infusion reactions

Dosage Forms Excipient information presented when available (limited, particularly for generics); consult specific product labeling.

Solution, Intravenous:

Aldurazyme: 2.9 mg/5 mL (5 mL) [contains mouse protein (murine) (hamster), polysorbate 80]

- **Lasix** *see* Furosemide *on page* 931
- **Lasix® (Can)** *see* Furosemide *on page* 931
- **Lasix® Special (Can)** *see* Furosemide *on page* 931
- **L-ASP** *see* Asparaginase (*E. coli*) *on page* 174
- **L-asparaginase (*E. coli*)** *see* Asparaginase (*E. coli*) *on page* 174
- **L-asparaginase (*Erwinia*)** *see* Asparaginase (*Erwinia*) *on page* 176
- **L-asparaginase with Polyethylene Glycol** *see* Pegaspargase *on page* 1586
- **Lassar's Zinc Paste** *see* Zinc Oxide *on page* 2230

Latanoprost (la TA noe prost)

Brand Names: U.S. Xalatan

Brand Names: Canada Apo-Latanoprost®; CO Latanoprost; GD-Latanoprost; Xalatan®

Pharmacologic Category Ophthalmic Agent, Antiglaucoma; Prostaglandin, Ophthalmic

Use Reduction of elevated intraocular pressure in patients with open-angle glaucoma or ocular hypertension

Pregnancy Risk Factor C

Dosage Adults: Ophthalmic: 1 drop (1.5 mcg) in the affected eye(s) once daily in the evening; do not exceed the once daily dosage because it has been shown that more frequent administration may decrease the IOP lowering effect

Note: A medication delivery device (Xal-Ease™) is available for use with Xalatan®.

Dosage adjustment in renal impairment: No dosage adjustment provided in manufacturer's labeling. However, dosage adjustment unlikely due to low systemic absorption.

Dosage adjustment in hepatic impairment: No dosage adjustment provided in manufacturer's labeling. However, dosage adjustment unlikely due to low systemic absorption.

Additional Information Complete prescribing information should be consulted for additional detail.

Dosage Forms Excipient information presented when available (limited, particularly for generics); consult specific product labeling.

Solution, Ophthalmic:

Xalatan: 0.005% (2.5 mL) [contains benzalkonium chloride]

Generic: 0.005% (2.5 mL)

- **Latisse** *see* Bimatoprost *on page* 259
- **Latisse® (Can)** *see* Bimatoprost *on page* 259
- **Latrix XM** *see* Urea *on page* 2140
- **Latuda** *see* Lurasidone *on page* 1255
- **Laxa Basic [OTC]** *see* Docusate *on page* 644
- **Laxative [OTC]** *see* Bisacodyl *on page* 259
- **Laxilose (Can)** *see* Lactulose *on page* 1161
- **Laxmar Natural Vegetable Laxat [OTC]** *see* Psyllium *on page* 1748
- **Lazanda** *see* FentaNYL *on page* 842
- ***l*-Bunolol Hydrochloride** *see* Levobunolol *on page* 1196
- **LC-4 Lidocaine [OTC]** *see* Lidocaine (Topical) *on page* 1212
- **LC-5 Lidocaine [OTC]** *see* Lidocaine (Topical) *on page* 1212
- **LCM** *see* Lacosamide *on page* 1159
- **L-Deprenyl** *see* Selegiline *on page* 1884
- **LDP-341** *see* Bortezomib *on page* 270
- **LEA29Y** *see* Belatacept *on page* 231
- **Lederle Leucovorin (Can)** *see* Leucovorin Calcium *on page* 1186
- **Leena** *see* Ethinyl Estradiol and Norethindrone *on page* 793

Leflunomide (le FLOO noh mide)

Brand Names: U.S. Arava

Brand Names: Canada Apo-Leflunomide®; Arava®; Mylan-Leflunomide; Novo-Leflunomide; PHL-Leflunomide; PMS-Leflunomide; Sandoz-Leflunomide

Pharmacologic Category Antirheumatic, Disease Modifying

Use Treatment of active rheumatoid arthritis; indicated to reduce signs and symptoms, and to inhibit structural damage and improve physical function

Unlabeled Use Treatment of cytomegalovirus (CMV) disease in transplant recipients resistant to standard antivirals; prevention of acute and chronic rejection in recipients of solid organ transplants

Pregnancy Risk Factor X

Pregnancy Considerations Has been associated with teratogenic and embryolethal effects in animal models at low doses. Leflunomide is contraindicated in pregnant women or women of childbearing potential who are not using reliable contraception. Pregnancy must be excluded prior to initiating treatment. **[U.S. Boxed Warning]: Women of childbearing potential should not receive therapy until pregnancy has been excluded,** they have been counseled concerning fetal risk, and reliable contraceptive measures have been confirmed. Following treatment, pregnancy should be avoided until undetectable serum concentrations (<0.02 mg/L) are verified. This may be accomplished by the use of an enhanced drug elimination procedure using cholestyramine. Serum concentrations <0.02 mg/L should be verified by two separate tests performed at least 14 days apart. If serum concentrations are >0.02 mg/L, additional cholestyramine treatment should be considered. Pregnant women exposed to leflunomide should be registered with the pregnancy registry (877-311-8972). It is not known if males taking leflunomide may contribute to fetal toxicity. Males taking leflunomide who wish to father a child should consider discontinuing therapy and using the cholestyramine procedure to eliminate the medication.

Breast-Feeding Considerations It is not known whether leflunomide is secreted in human milk. Because the potential for serious adverse reactions exists in the nursing infant, a decision should be made whether to discontinue nursing or discontinue the drug, taking into account the importance of the drug to the mother.

Contraindications Hypersensitivity to leflunomide or any component of the formulation; pregnancy

Warnings/Precautions Hazardous agent - use appropriate precautions for handling and disposal (NIOSH, 2012). **[U.S. Boxed Warning]: Use has been associated with rare reports of hepatotoxicity, hepatic failure, and**

death. Treatment should not be initiated in patients with pre-existing acute or chronic liver disease or ALT >2 x ULN. Use caution in patients with concurrent exposure to potentially hepatotoxic drugs. Monitor ALT levels during therapy; discontinue if ALT >3 x ULN occurs and, if hepatotoxicity is likely leflunomide-induced, start drug elimination procedures (eg, cholestyramine, activated charcoal).

Use has been associated (rarely) with interstitial lung disease; discontinue in patients who develop new onset or worsening of pulmonary symptoms. Drug elimination procedures should be considered (eg, cholestyramine, activated charcoal) if interstitial lung disease occurs; fatal outcomes have been reported. May increase susceptibility to infection, including opportunistic pathogens. Severe infections, sepsis, and fatalities have been reported. Not recommended in patients with severe immunodeficiency, bone marrow dysplasia, or severe, uncontrolled infections. Caution should be exercised when considering the use in patients with a history of new/recurrent infections, with conditions that predispose them to infections, or with chronic, latent, or localized infections. Patients who develop a new infection while undergoing treatment should be monitored closely; consider discontinuation of therapy and drug elimination procedures if infection is serious.

Use may affect defenses against malignancies; impact on the development and course of malignancies is not fully defined. As compared to the general population, an increased risk of lymphoma has been noted in clinical trials; however, rheumatoid arthritis has been previously associated with an increased rate of lymphoma. Use with caution in patients with a prior history of significant hematologic abnormalities; avoid use with bone marrow dysplasia. Use has been associated with rare pancytopenia, agranulocytosis, and thrombocytopenia, generally when given concurrently or recently with methotrexate or other immunosuppressive agents. Monitoring of hematologic function is required; discontinue if evidence of bone marrow suppression and begin drug elimination procedures (eg, cholestyramine or activated charcoal). Rare cases of dermatologic reactions (including Stevens-Johnson syndrome and toxic epidermal necrolysis) have been reported; discontinue if evidence of severe dermatologic reaction occurs, and begin drug elimination procedures (eg, cholestyramine or activated charcoal). Cases of peripheral neuropathy have been reported; use with caution in patients >60 years of age, receiving concomitant neurotoxic medications, or patients with diabetes; discontinue if evidence of peripheral neuropathy occurs and begin drug elimination procedures (eg, cholestyramine, activated charcoal).

Safety has not been established in patients with latent tuberculosis infection. Patients should be screened for tuberculosis and if necessary, treated prior to initiating therapy. Use with caution in patients with renal impairment. **[U.S. Boxed Warning]: Women of childbearing potential should not receive therapy until pregnancy has been excluded,** they have been counseled concerning fetal risk and reliable contraceptive measures have been confirmed. Women of childbearing potential should also undergo drug elimination procedures (eg, cholestyramine, activated charcoal) following discontinuation of therapy. Patients should be brought up to date with all immunizations before initiating therapy. Live vaccines should not be given concurrently; there is no data available concerning secondary transmission of live vaccines in patients receiving therapy. Due to variations in clearance, it may take up to 2 years to reach low levels of leflunomide metabolite serum concentrations. A drug elimination procedure using cholestyramine or activated charcoal is recommended when a more rapid elimination is needed.

Adverse Reactions

>10%:

- Gastrointestinal: Diarrhea (17%)
- Respiratory: Respiratory tract infection (4% to 15%)

1% to 10%:

- Cardiovascular: Hypertension (10%), chest pain (2%), edema (peripheral), palpitation, tachycardia, varicose vein, vasculitis, vasodilation
- Central nervous system: Headache (7%), dizziness (4%), pain (2%), anxiety, depression, fever, insomnia, malaise, migraine, sleep disorder, vertigo
- Dermatologic: Alopecia (10%), rash (10%), pruritus (4%), dry skin (2%), eczema (2%), acne, bruising, dermatitis, hair discoloration, hematoma, nail disorder, skin disorder/discoloration, skin ulcer, subcutaneous nodule
- Endocrine & metabolic: Hypokalemia (1%), diabetes mellitus, hyperglycemia, hyperlipidemia, hyperthyroidism, menstrual disorder
- Gastrointestinal: Nausea (9%), abdominal pain (5% to 6%), dyspepsia (5%), weight loss (4%), anorexia (3%), gastroenteritis (3%), mouth ulceration (3%), vomiting (3%), candidiasis (oral), colitis, constipation, esophagitis, flatulence, gastritis, gingivitis, melena, salivary gland enlarged, stomatitis, taste disturbance, xerostomia
- Genitourinary: Urinary tract infection (5%), albuminuria, cystitis, dysuria, prostate disorder, urinary frequency, vaginal candidiasis
- Hematologic: Anemia
- Hepatic: Abnormal LFTs (5%), cholelithiasis
- Local: Abscess
- Neuromuscular & skeletal: Back pain (5%), joint disorder (4%), tenosynovitis (3%), weakness (3%), paresthesia (2%), synovitis (2%), arthralgia (1%), leg cramps (1%), arthrosis, bone necrosis, bone pain, bursitis, CPK increased, myalgia, neck pain, neuralgia, neuritis, pelvic pain, tendon rupture
- Ocular: Blurred vision, cataract, conjunctivitis, eye disorder
- Renal: Hematuria
- Respiratory: Bronchitis (7%), cough (3%), pharyngitis (3%), pneumonia (2%), rhinitis (2%), sinusitis (2%), asthma, dyspnea, epistaxis
- Miscellaneous: Accidental injury (5%), allergic reactions (2%), flu-like syndrome (2%), cyst, diaphoresis, hernia, herpes infection

<1% (Limited to important or life-threatening): Agranulocytosis, anaphylaxis, angioedema, cholestasis, cutaneous lupus erythematosus, cutaneous necrotizing vasculitis, eosinophilia, erythema multiforme, hepatitis, hepatotoxicity (rare, including hepatic necrosis and hepatic failure, some fatalities reported), interstitial lung disease, jaundice, leukopenia, neutropenia, opportunistic infection, pancreatitis, pancytopenia, peripheral neuropathy, pneumonitis (interstitial), psoriasis exacerbation, pulmonary fibrosis, pustular psoriasis, sepsis, Stevens-Johnson syndrome, thrombocytopenia, toxic epidermal necrolysis, urticaria

Drug Interactions

Metabolism/Transport Effects Inhibits CYP2C9 (moderate)

Avoid Concomitant Use

Avoid concomitant use of Leflunomide with any of the following: BCG; Natalizumab; Pimecrolimus; Tacrolimus (Topical); Teriflunomide; Tofacitinib

Increased Effect/Toxicity

Leflunomide may increase the levels/effects of: Bosentan; Carvedilol; CYP2C9 Substrates; Natalizumab; Teriflunomide; Tofacitinib; TOLBUTamide; Vaccines (Live); Vitamin K Antagonists

The levels/effects of Leflunomide may be increased by: Denosumab; Immunosuppressants; Methotrexate; Pimecrolimus; Rifampin; Roflumilast; Tacrolimus (Topical); TOLBUTamide; Trastuzumab

Decreased Effect

Leflunomide may decrease the levels/effects of: BCG; Coccidioidin Skin Test; Sipuleucel-T; Vaccines (Inactivated)

The levels/effects of Leflunomide may be decreased by: Bile Acid Sequestrants; Charcoal, Activated; Echinacea

Ethanol/Nutrition/Herb Interactions

Food: No interactions with food have been noted. Management: Maintain adequate hydration, unless instructed to restrict fluid intake.

Herb/Nutraceutical: Echinacea may diminish the therapeutic effect of leflunomide.

Storage/Stability Store at 25°C (77°F); excursions permitted to 15°C to 30°C (59°F to 86°F). Protect from light.

Mechanism of Action Leflunomide is an immunodulatory agent that inhibits pyrimidine synthesis, resulting in antiproliferative and anti-inflammatory effects. Leflunomide is a prodrug; the active metabolite is responsible for activity. For CMV, may interfere with virion assembly.

Pharmacodynamics/Kinetics

Distribution: V_d: M1: 0.13 L/kg

Protein binding: M1: >99% to albumin

Metabolism: Hepatic to an active metabolite M1 (also known as A77 1726 or teriflunomide), which accounts for nearly all pharmacologic activity; further metabolism to multiple inactive metabolites; undergoes enterohepatic recirculation

Bioavailability: 80% (relative to oral solution)

Half-life elimination: M1: Mean: 14-15 days; enterohepatic recycling appears to contribute to the long half-life of this agent, since activated charcoal and cholestyramine substantially reduce plasma half-life

Time to peak: M1: 6-12 hours

Excretion: Feces (48%); urine (43%)

Dosage Oral:

Adults:

Rheumatoid arthritis: Loading dose: 100 mg/day for 3 days, followed by 20 mg/day; **Note:** The loading dose may be omitted in patients at increased risk of hepatic or hematologic toxicity (eg, recent concomitant methotrexate). Dosage may be decreased to 10 mg/day in patients who have difficulty tolerating the 20 mg dose. Due to the long half-life of the active metabolite, serum concentrations may require a prolonged period to decline after dosage reduction.

CMV disease, resistant to standard antivirals (unlabeled use): Some authors recommend 100-200 mg/day for 5-7 days, followed by 40-60 mg/day (Avery, 2004; Avery, 2010). Others have utilized the standard rheumatoid arthritis dosing (John, 2004). Adjust dose based on serum concentrations of metabolite and adverse events (Avery, 2008; Avery, 2010; Williams, 2002).

Elderly: Although hepatic function may decline with age, no specific dosage adjustment is recommended. Patients should be monitored closely for adverse effects which may require dosage adjustment.

Dosing adjustment in renal impairment: No specific dosage adjustment is recommended. There is no clinical experience in the use of leflunomide in patients with renal impairment. The free fraction of M1 is doubled in dialysis patients. Patients should be monitored closely for adverse effects requiring dosage adjustment.

Dosing adjustment in hepatic impairment: Not recommended for use in patients with pre-existing liver disease or in patients with significant hepatic impairment (ALT >2 times ULN). Patients should have LFTs monitored closely. Discontinue leflunomide if ALT >3 times ULN.

Dosing adjustment in hepatic toxicity: ALT elevations >3 times ULN: Discontinue leflunomide and initiate cholestyramine to enhance elimination

Drug elimination procedure: To achieve nondetectable serum concentrations (<0.02 mg/L) of the active metabolite (M1) of leflunomide administer the following:

Cholestyramine: 8 g administered 3 times/day for 11 days. The 11 days do not need to be consecutive unless plasma concentrations need to be lowered rapidly. Verify serum concentrations by 2 separate tests ≥14 days apart. If plasma concentrations are still high, additional cholestyramine treatment may be considered. In healthy volunteers, cholestyramine 8 g administered 3 times/day for 24 hours decreased M1 concentrations by 40% in 24 hours and 49% to 65% in 48 hours.

Activated charcoal: 50 g every 6 hours for 24 hours was shown to decrease plasma concentrations of M1 by 37% in 24 hours and 48% in 48 hours.

Dietary Considerations May be taken without regard to meals.

Administration Administer without regard to meals.

Hazardous agent; use appropriate precautions for handling and disposal (NIOSH, 2012).

Monitoring Parameters A complete blood count (WBC, platelet count, hemoglobin or hematocrit), serum phosphate, as well as serum transaminase determinations should be monitored at baseline and monthly during the initial 6 months of treatment; if stable, monitoring frequency may be decreased to every 6-8 weeks thereafter (continue monthly when used in combination with other immunosuppressive agents). ALT should be monitored at least monthly for the first 6 months of treatment, then every 6-8 weeks thereafter (discontinue if ALT >3 x ULN, treat with cholestyramine, and monitor liver function at least weekly until normal). In addition, monitor for signs/symptoms of severe infection, abnormalities in hepatic function tests, symptoms of hepatotoxicity, and blood pressure. If coadministered with methotrexate, monthly transaminases (ALT, AST) and serum albumin levels are recommended. Screen for tuberculosis and pregnancy prior to therapy.

When used for CMV disease, monitor serum trough concentrations of active metabolite (also see Reference Range).

Reference Range CMV disease:

Timing of serum samples: Initial: Obtain 24 hours after last dose of loading regimen and periodically thereafter

Therapeutic concentration: Active metabolite (A77 1726, M1, or teriflunomide): Trough: 50-80 mcg/mL (Avery, 2010) or up to 100 mcg/mL (Williams, 2002)

Dosage Forms Excipient information presented when available (limited, particularly for generics); consult specific product labeling.

Tablet, Oral:

Arava: 10 mg, 20 mg

Generic: 10 mg, 20 mg

◆ Legatrin PM® [OTC] *see* Acetaminophen and Diphenhydramine *on page 32*

◆ Lemtrada *see* Alemtuzumab *on page 66*

Lenalidomide (le na LID oh mide)

Brand Names: U.S. Revlimid

Brand Names: Canada Revlimid®

Index Terms CC-5013; IMid-1

Pharmacologic Category Angiogenesis Inhibitor; Antineoplastic Agent; Immunomodulator, Systemic

Use

Mantle cell lymphoma (MCL): Treatment of patients with MCL which has relapsed or progressed after two prior therapies (one of which included bortezomib)

Multiple myeloma: Treatment of multiple myeloma (in combination with dexamethasone) in patients who have received at least one prior therapy

Myelodysplastic syndromes (MDS): Treatment of low- or intermediate-1-risk MDS in patients with deletion 5q (del 5q) cytogenetic abnormality (with or without other cytogenetic abnormalities) with transfusion-dependent anemia

Unlabeled Use Treatment of non-Hodgkin lymphoma (diffuse large B-cell lymphoma); relapsed or refractory chronic lymphocytic leukemia (CLL), systemic light chain amyloidosis; lower-risk myelodysplastic syndrome (MDS) in transfusion-dependent patients without deletion 5q (del 5q); maintenance treatment for multiple myeloma (after response to primary treatment or following autologous stem cell transplant)

Pregnancy Risk Factor X

Pregnancy Considerations [U.S. Boxed Warning]: Lenalidomide is an analogue of thalidomide (a human teratogen) and could potentially cause birth defects in humans; do not use during pregnancy (contraindication); avoid pregnancy while taking lenalidomide. Obtain 2 negative pregnancy tests prior to initiation of treatment; 2 forms of contraception (or abstain from heterosexual intercourse) must be used at least 4 weeks prior to, during, and for 4 weeks after lenalidomide treatment (and during treatment interruptions). Distribution is restricted; physicians, pharmacies, and patients must be registered with the Revlimid REMS™ program. Animal reproduction studies with lenalidomide in nonhuman primates have demonstrated malformations similar to those observed in humans with thalidomide.

Women of childbearing potential should be treated only if they are able to comply with the conditions of the Revlimid REMS™ program. Women of reproductive potential must avoid pregnancy 4 weeks prior to therapy, during therapy, during therapy interruptions, and for ≥4 weeks after therapy is discontinued. Two forms of effective contraception or total abstinence from heterosexual intercourse must be used by females who are not infertile or who have not had a hysterectomy. A negative pregnancy test (sensitivity of at least 50 mIU/mL) 10-14 days prior to therapy, within 24 hours prior to beginning therapy, weekly during the first 4 weeks, and every 4 weeks (every 2 weeks for women with irregular menstrual cycles) thereafter is required for women of childbearing potential. Lenalidomide must be immediately discontinued for a missed period, abnormal pregnancy test or abnormal menstrual bleeding; refer patient to a reproductive toxicity specialist if pregnancy occurs during treatment.

Lenalidomide is also present in the semen of males. Males (including those vasectomized) should use a latex or synthetic condom during any sexual contact with women of childbearing age during treatment, during treatment interruptions, and for 4 weeks after discontinuation. Male patients should not donate sperm during, and for 4 weeks after treatment, and during therapy interruptions.

The parent or legal guardian for patients between 12 and 18 years of age must agree to ensure compliance with the required guidelines. Any suspected fetal exposure should be reported to the FDA via the MedWatch program (1-800-FDA-1088) and to Celgene Corporation (1-888-423-5436).

Breast-Feeding Considerations It is not known if lenalidomide is excreted in breast milk. Due to the potential for serious adverse reactions in the infant, a decision should be made to discontinue nursing or discontinue treatment. Use in breast-feeding women is contraindicated in the Canadian labeling.

Prescribing and Access Restrictions As a requirement of the REMS program, access to this medication is restricted. Lenalidomide is approved for marketing in the U.S. only under a Food and Drug Administration (FDA) approved, restricted distribution program called Revlimid REMS™ (www.celgeneriskmanagment.com or 1-888-423-5436). Prescriptions must be filled within 7 days (for females of reproductive potential) or within 30 days (for all other patients) after authorization number obtained. Subsequent prescriptions may be filled only if fewer than 7 days of therapy remain on the previous prescription. A new prescription is required for further dispensing (a telephone prescription may not be accepted). Pregnancy testing is required for females of childbearing potential. In Canada, distribution is restricted through RevAid® (www.RevAid.ca or 1-888-738-2431).

Medication Guide Available Yes

Contraindications Hypersensitivity (eg, angioedema, Stevens-Johnson syndrome, toxic epidermal necrolysis) to lenalidomide or any component of the formulation; pregnancy

Canadian labeling: Additional contraindications (not in U.S. labeling): Platelet count <50,000/mm^3 (in MDS patients); hypersensitivity to thalidomide; women capable of becoming pregnant; breast-feeding women

Warnings/Precautions Hazardous agent - use appropriate precautions for handling and disposal (NIOSH, 2012). **[U.S. Boxed Warning]: Hematologic toxicity (neutropenia and thrombocytopenia) occurs in a majority of patients (grade 3/4: 80% in patients with del 5q myelodysplastic syndrome) and may require dose reductions and/or delays; the use of blood product support and/or growth factors may be needed. CBC should be monitored weekly for the first 8 weeks and at least monthly thereafter in patients being treated for del 5q myelodysplastic syndromes.** In patients being treated for multiple myeloma, monitor CBC every 2 weeks for 12 weeks and monthly thereafter. In patients receiving lenalidomide for mantle cell lymphoma (MCL), monitor CBC weekly for the first cycle, every 2 weeks during cycles 2-4, and monthly thereafter. **[U.S. Boxed Warning]: Lenalidomide has been associated with a significant increase in risk for thrombosis and embolism in multiple myeloma patients treated with lenalidomide and dexamethasone combination therapy. Deep vein thrombosis (DVT) and pulmonary embolism (PE) have occurred; monitor for signs and symptoms of thromboembolism (shortness of breath, chest pain, or arm or leg swelling) and seek prompt medical attention with development of these symptoms.** The NCCN multiple myeloma guidelines (v1.2013) recommend anticoagulant prophylaxis when used in combination with dexamethasone. Anticoagulant prophylaxis should be individualized and selected based on the venous thromboembolism risk of the combination treatment regimen, using the safest and easiest to administer (Palumbo, 2008).

Second primary malignancies (SPMs), including hematologic (AML and lymphoma) and solid tumor malignancies, and skin cancers, have been reported with lenalidomide when used for the treatment of MDS and multiple myeloma; the incidence may be higher when lenalidomide is used in combination with an alkylating agent.

Angioedema, Stevens-Johnson syndrome (SJS), and toxic epidermal necrolysis (TEN) have been reported; may be fatal. Consider interrupting or discontinuing treatment with grade 2 or 3 skin rash; discontinue and do not reinitiate treatment with grade 4 rash, exfoliative or bullous rash, or for suspected SJS or TEN. Patients with a history of grade 4 rash with thalidomide should not receive lenalidomide. Discontinue treatment with angioedema. Use caution in renal impairment; may experience an increased rate of toxicities (due to reduced clearance and increased half-life); initial dosage adjustments are recommended for moderate-to-severe and dialysis-dependent renal impairment. Tumor lysis syndrome (with fatalities) has been reported with lenalidomide; patients with a high tumor burden may be at risk for tumor lysis syndrome; monitor closely; institute appropriate management for hyperuricemia. Tumor flare reaction has been observed in studies of lenalidomide for the treatment of chronic lymphocytic leukemia (CLL) and lymphoma; clinical presentation includes low grade fever, pain, rash, and tender lymph node swelling. In patients with MCL, tumor flare may mimic disease progression; monitor closely. In clinical trials, the majority of tumor flare events occurred in the first cycle of therapy. Treatment with corticosteroids, nonsteroidal anti-inflammatory drugs (NSAIDs), and/or analgesics may be considered; therapy interruption may be necessary as well. Hepatic failure, including fatalities, has occurred in patients treated with combination lenalidomide and dexamethasone therapy; may have hepatocellular, cholestatic, or mixed characteristics. Risk factors may include pre-existing viral liver disease, elevated liver enzymes at baseline, and concomitant medications. Monitor closely; interrupt therapy in patients with abnormal hepatic function tests. May consider resuming treatment at a lower dose upon return to baseline. Certain adverse reactions (DVT, pulmonary embolism, atrial fibrillation, renal failure) are more likely in elderly patients.

[U.S. Boxed Warning]: Lenalidomide is an analogue of thalidomide (a human teratogen) and could potentially cause birth defects in humans; do not use during pregnancy (contraindication); avoid pregnancy while taking lenalidomide. Obtain 2 negative pregnancy testes prior to initiation of treatment; 2 forms of contraception (or abstain from heterosexual intercourse) must be used at least 4 weeks prior to, during and for 4 weeks after lenalidomide treatment (and during treatment interruptions). Distribution is restricted; physicians, pharmacies, and patients must be registered with the Revlimid REMS™ program. Males taking lenalidomide (even those vasectomized) must use a latex or synthetic condom during any sexual contact with women of childbearing potential and for up to 28 days following discontinuation of therapy. Males taking lenalidomide must not donate sperm. Patients should be advised not to donate blood during therapy and for 1 month following completion of therapy. May cause dizziness or fatigue; caution patients about performing tasks which require mental alertness (eg, operating machinery or driving). Potentially significant drug-drug interactions may exist, requiring dose or frequency adjustment, additional monitoring, and/or selection of alternative therapy. Formulation contains lactose; avoid use in patients with Lapp lactase deficiency, glucose-galactose malabsorption, or glucose intolerance. Lenalidomide should only be prescribed to patients (male and female) who can understand and comply with the conditions of the Revlimid REMS™ program. If used in patients between 12-18 years of age, the parent or legal guardian must agree to ensure compliance with the Revlimid REMS™ program.

Adverse Reactions

>10%:

Cardiovascular: Peripheral edema (8% to 26%)

Central nervous system: Fatigue (31% to 44%), dizziness (20% to 23%), headache (20%)

Dermatologic: Pruritus (8% to 42%), skin rash (21% to 36%), xeroderma (9% to 14%)

Endocrine & metabolic: Weight loss (13% to 20%), hypokalemia (11% to 14%)

Gastrointestinal: Diarrhea (31% to 49%), constipation (16% to 41%), nausea (24% to 30%), anorexia (10% to 16%), dysgeusia (6% to 15%), decreased appetite (7% to 14%), vomiting (10% to 12%), abdominal pain (8% to 12%)

Genitourinary: Urinary tract infection (4% to 11%)

Hematologic & oncologic: Thrombocytopenia (22% to 62%; grades 3/4: 12% to 50%; MDS: Onset: 28 days [range: 8-290 days]; recovery: 22 days [range: 5-224 days]), neutropenia (42% to 59%; grades 3/4: 33% to 53%; MDS: Onset: 42 days [range: 14-411 days]; recovery: 17 days [range: 2-170 days]), anemia (12% to 31%; grades 3/4: 6% to 11%), leukopenia (8% to 15%; grades 3/4: 5% to 7%)

Neuromuscular & skeletal: Muscle cramps (18% to 33%), back pain (13% to 26%), arthralgia (8% to 22%), tremor (21%), weakness (14% to 15%), ostealgia (1% to 14%), muscle spasm (13%), limb pain (5% to 12%)

Ophthalmic: Blurred vision (17%)

Respiratory: Cough (20% to 28%), upper respiratory tract infection (13% to 25%), dyspnea (7% to 24%), nasopharyngitis (18% to 23%), pharyngitis (14% to 16%), epistaxis (15%), pneumonia (9% to 14%), bronchitis (6% to 11%)

Miscellaneous: Fever (21% to 28%)

1% to 10%:

Cardiovascular: Edema (10%), deep vein thrombosis (4% to 9%; grades 3/4: ≤8%), hypertension (6% to 8%), chest pain (5% to 8%), hypotension (7%), palpitations (5%), pulmonary embolism (2% to 4%), atrial fibrillation (3%; grades 3/4: ≤4%), syncope (grades 3/4: 1% to 3%), cerebrovascular accident (2%), tachycardia (grades 3/4: 2%), angina pectoris (≥1%), bradycardia (≥1%), cerebral ischemia (≥1%), myocardial infarction (≥1%), cardiac failure (1%)

Central nervous system: Insomnia (10%), hypoesthesia (7% to 10%), lethargy (7%), local pain (7%), peripheral neuropathy (5% to 7%), rigors (6%), depression (5%), emotional lability (≥1%), glossalgia (≥1%), hallucination (≥1%), malaise (≥1%)

Dermatologic: Diaphoresis (7% to 10%), night sweats (8%), ecchymoses (5%), erythema (5%), cellulitis (2% to 5%), hyperpigmentation (≥1%)

Endocrine & metabolic: Hypothyroidism (7%), hypomagnesemia (6% to 7%), dehydration (7%), hypophosphatemia (grades 3/4: 3%), hyponatremia (2%), hirsutism (≥1%), loss of libido (≥1%)

Gastrointestinal: Hypocalcemia (3% to 9%), xerostomia (7%), loose stools (6%), gastrointestinal hemorrhage (≥1%)

Genitourinary: Dysuria (7%), erectile dysfunction (≥1%)

Hematologic & oncologic: Tumor flare (10%), lymphocytopenia (5% to 7%; grades 3/4: 3% to 4%), febrile neutropenia (2% to 6%; grades 3/4: 2% to 6%), squamous cell carcinoma of skin (3%; grades 3/4: 3%), granulocytopenia (grades 3/4: 2%), pancytopenia (≥1%; grades 3/4: 2%), autoimmune hemolytic anemia (≥1%)

Hepatic: Increased serum ALT (8%), abnormal hepatic function tests (≥1%)

Infection: Sepsis (grades 3/4: 3%), bacteremia (1%)

Neuromuscular & skeletal: Myalgia (9%)

Ophthalmic: Cataract (grades 3/4: 1% to 2%), blindness (≥1%), ocular hypertension (≥1%)

Renal: Renal failure (4%)

Respiratory: Sinusitis (7% to 8%), pleural effusion (7%; grades 3/4: 1%), rhinitis (7%), hypoxia (2%; grades 3/4: 1%), hoarseness (≥1%), pneumonitis (grades 3/4: 1%), pulmonary hypertension (grades 3/4: 1%), respiratory distress (1%; grades 3/4: 1% to 2%)

Miscellaneous: Physical health deterioration (2%), multi-organ failure (grades 3/4: 1%)

<1% (Limited to important or life-threatening): Abnormal gait, acute leukemia, adrenocortical insufficiency, angioedema, aphasia, arthritis, atrial flutter, azotemia, bacterial infection, biliary obstruction, bone fracture, bone marrow depression, calcium pyrophosphate deposition disease, cardiogenic shock, cardiorespiratory arrest, cerebral edema, cholecystitis, chronic obstructive pulmonary disease, circulatory shock, clostridial infection, colonic polyps, decreased hemoglobin, delirium, desquamation, diabetes mellitus, diabetic ketoacidosis, diverticulitis, drug overdose, dysphagia, encephalitis, erythema multiforme, falling, Fanconi's syndrome, fungal infection, gastritis, gastroenteritis, gastroesophageal reflux disease, gout, Graves' disease, hematuria, hemolysis, hemolytic anemia, hemorrhage, hemorrhagic diathesis, hepatic failure, hepatitis, hyperbilirubinemia, hypernatremia, hypersensitivity reaction, hypoglycemia, impaired consciousness, increased cardiac enzymes (troponin I), increased serum creatinine, influenza, inguinal hernia, interstitial pulmonary disease, intestinal obstruction, intestinal perforation, intracranial hemorrhage, irritable bowel syndrome, ischemia, ischemic colitis, Klebsiella infection, leukoencephalopathy, localized infection, lung carcinoma, malignant lymphoma, melena, migraine, myelocytic leukemia, myopathy, neck pain, nephrolithiasis, neutropenic infection, nodule, orthostatic hypotension, otic infection, pancreatitis, pelvic pain, peripheral ischemia, perirectal abscess, prostate carcinoma, pseudomembranous colitis, pseudomonas infection, pulmonary edema, pulmonary infiltrates, rectal hemorrhage, renal cyst, renal tubular necrosis, respiratory failure, second primary malignant neoplasms (AML, lymphomas, solid tumors), septic shock, spinal cord compression, splenic infarction, staphylococcal infection, Stevens-Johnson syndrome, stomatitis, subarachnoid hemorrhage, supraventricular cardiac, Sweet's Syndrome, tachyarrhythmia, thrombophlebitis, toxic epidermal necrolysis, transfusion reaction, transient ischemic attacks, tumor lysis syndrome, urinary retention, urosepsis, urticaria, ventricular dysfunction, viral infection

Drug Interactions

Metabolism/Transport Effects **Substrate** of P-glycoprotein

Avoid Concomitant Use

Avoid concomitant use of Lenalidomide with any of the following: Abatacept; Anakinra; BCG; Canakinumab; Certolizumab Pegol; CloZAPine; Natalizumab; Pimecrolimus; Rilonacept; Tacrolimus (Topical); Tocilizumab; Tofacitinib; Vaccines (Live)

Increased Effect/Toxicity

Lenalidomide may increase the levels/effects of: Abatacept; Anakinra; Bisphosphonate Derivatives; Canakinumab; Certolizumab Pegol; CloZAPine; Digoxin; Leflunomide; Natalizumab; Rilonacept; Tofacitinib; Vaccines (Live)

The levels/effects of Lenalidomide may be increased by: Denosumab; Dexamethasone (Systemic); Pimecrolimus; Roflumilast; Tacrolimus (Topical); Tocilizumab; Trastuzumab

Decreased Effect

Lenalidomide may decrease the levels/effects of: BCG; Coccidioidin Skin Test; Sipuleucel-T; Vaccines (Inactivated); Vaccines (Live)

The levels/effects of Lenalidomide may be decreased by: Echinacea

Ethanol/Nutrition/Herb Interactions Herb/Nutraceutical: Avoid echinacea (has immunostimulant properties; consider therapy modifications).

Storage/Stability Store at 20°C to 25°C (68°F to 77°F); excursions permitted to 15°C and 30°C (59°F and 86°F).

Mechanism of Action Immunomodulatory, antiangiogenic, and antineoplastic characteristics via multiple mechanisms. Selectively inhibits secretion of proinflammatory cytokines (potent inhibitor of tumor necrosis factor-alpha secretion); enhances cell-mediated immunity by stimulating proliferation of anti-CD3 stimulated T cells (resulting in increased IL-2 and interferon gamma secretion); inhibits trophic signals to angiogenic factors in cells. Inhibits the growth of myeloma cells by inducing cell cycle arrest and cell death.

Pharmacodynamics/Kinetics

Absorption: Rapid

Protein binding: ~30%

Half-life elimination: 3-5 hours; Moderate-to-severe renal impairment: Increased threefold; Hemodialysis patients: Increased ~4.5-fold

Time, to peak, plasma: MDS or myeloma patients: 0.5-6 hours

Excretion: Urine (~82%; as unchanged drug)

Hemodialysis effect: ~40% of a dose is removed in a single dialysis session

Dosage

Mantle cell lymphoma (MCL): Adults: Oral: 25 mg once daily for 21 days of a 28-day treatment cycle; continue until disease progression or unacceptable toxicity

Multiple myeloma: Adults: Oral: 25 mg once daily for 21 days of a 28-day treatment cycle (in combination with dexamethasone)

Myelodysplastic syndrome (MDS) with deletion 5q: Adults: Oral: 10 mg once daily

Chronic lymphocytic leukemia (CLL), relapsed/refractory (unlabeled use): Adults: Oral: 10 mg once daily beginning on day 9 of cycle 1; administer continuously in combination with cyclic rituximab (Badoux, 2013)

Diffuse large B-cell lymphoma, relapsed/refractory (unlabeled use): Adults: Oral: 25 mg once daily for 21 days of a 28-day treatment cycle for up to 1 year (Wiernik, 2008)

Multiple myeloma, induction (unlabeled use): Adults: Oral: 25 mg once daily for 14 days of a 21-day cycle (in combination with bortezomib and dexamethasone) for 8 cycles (Kumar, 2012; Richardson, 2010)

Multiple myeloma, maintenance (following autologous stem cell transplant; unlabeled use): Adults: Oral: 10 mg once daily for 3 months, then increased to 15 mg daily if tolerated; continue until relapse (Attal, 2012; McCarthy, 2012) **or** 10 mg once daily for 21 days of a 28-day treatment cycle until relapse (Palumbo, 2010)

Myelodysplastic syndrome (MDS), lower risk, without deletion 5q (unlabeled use): Adults: Oral: 10 mg once daily (Raza, 2008)

Systemic light chain amyloidosis (unlabeled use): Adults: Oral: 15 mg once daily for 21 days of a 28-day cycle (in combination with dexamethasone) (Nair, 2012; Sanchorawala, 2007)

Elderly: Refer to adult dosing; due to the potential for decreased renal function in the elderly, select dose carefully and closely monitor renal function

Dosage adjustment in renal impairment:

Recommended initial dose adjustment in the FDA-approved labeling; further individualize based on tolerance:

MCL:

Cl_{cr} >60 mL/minute: No adjustment required

Cl_{cr} 30-60 mL/minute: 10 mg once daily

Cl_{cr} <30 mL/minute (nondialysis dependent): 15 mg every 48 hours

ESRD: Cl_{cr} <30 mL/minute and dialysis dependent: 5 mg once daily (administer after dialysis on dialysis days)

MDS:

Cl_{cr} >60 mL/minute: No adjustment required

Cl_{cr} 30-60 mL/minute: 5 mg once daily

Cl_{cr} <30 mL/minute (nondialysis dependent): 2.5 mg once daily

ESRD: Cl_{cr} <30 mL/minute and dialysis dependent: 2.5 mg once daily (administer after dialysis on dialysis days)

Multiple myeloma:

Cl_{cr} >60 mL/minute: No adjustment required

Cl_{cr} 30-60 mL/minute: 10 mg once daily (may increase to 15 mg once daily after 2 cycles if nonresponsive but tolerating treatment; Chen, 2007)

Cl_{cr} <30 mL/minute (nondialysis dependent): 15 mg every 48 hours

ESRD: Cl_{cr} <30 mL/minute and dialysis dependent: 5 mg once daily (administer after dialysis on dialysis days)

Recommended adjustment in Canadian labeling:

MDS:

Cl_{cr} ≥60 mL/minute: No adjustment required

Cl_{cr} 30-59 mL/minute: 5 mg once daily

Cl_{cr} <30 mL/minute (nondialysis dependent): 5 mg every 48 hours

ESRD: Cl_{cr} <30 mL/minute and dialysis dependent: 5 mg 3 times weekly (administer after each dialysis)

Multiple myeloma:

Cl_{cr} ≥60 mL/minute: No adjustment required

Cl_{cr} 30-59 mL/minute: 10 mg once daily; (may increase to 15 mg once daily after 2 cycles if nonresponsive but tolerating treatment; Chen, 2007)

Cl_{cr} <30 mL/minute (nondialysis dependent): 15 mg every 48 hours

ESRD: Cl_{cr} <30 mL/minute and dialysis dependent: 5 mg once daily (administer after dialysis on dialysis days)

Dosage adjustment in hepatic impairment: No dosage adjustment provided in manufacturer's labeling (has not been studied). However, lenalidomide undergoes minimal hepatic metabolism.

Dosage adjustment for NONHEMATOLOGIC toxicities:

Dermatologic toxicities:

Skin rash, grade 2 or 3: Consider interrupting or discontinuing treatment

Angioedema, grade 4 rash, exfoliative or bullous rash, or suspected Stevens-Johnson syndrome or toxic epidermal necrolysis: Discontinue treatment; do not rechallenge

Tumor flare reaction:

Grade 1 or 2: Continue therapy at physician's discretion; may consider symptom management with corticosteroids, nonsteroidal anti-inflammatory drugs (NSAIDs) and/or analgesic therapy.

Grade 3 or 4: Interrupt therapy until resolved to ≤ grade 1; consider symptom management with corticosteroids, nonsteroidal anti-inflammatory drugs (NSAIDs) and/or analgesic therapy.

Other toxicities: For additional treatment-related grade 3/4 toxicities, hold treatment and restart at next lower dose level when toxicity has resolved to ≤ grade 2.

Dosage adjustment for HEMATOLOGIC toxicities:

Adjustment for thrombocytopenia in MCL:

Platelets <50,000/mm^3: Hold treatment, check CBC weekly

When platelets return to ≥50,000/mm^3: Resume treatment at 5 mg below previous dose; do not dose below 5 mg daily

Adjustment for neutropenia in MCL:

ANC <1000/mm^3 for at least 7 days or associated with fever: Hold treatment, check CBC weekly

ANC <500/mm^3: Hold treatment, check CBC weekly

When ANC returns to ≥1000/mm^3: Resume treatment at 5 mg below previous dose; do not dose below 5 mg daily

Adjustment for thrombocytopenia in MDS:

Thrombocytopenia developing within 4 weeks of beginning treatment at 10 mg daily:

Baseline platelets ≥100,000/mm^3:

If platelets <50,000/mm^3: Hold treatment

When platelets return to ≥50,000/mm^3: Resume treatment at 5 mg daily

Baseline platelets <100,000/mm^3:

If platelets fall to 50% of baseline: Hold treatment

If baseline ≥60,000/mm^3 and platelet level returns to ≥50,000/mm^3: Resume at 5 mg daily

If baseline <60,000/mm^3 and platelet level returns to ≥30,000/mm^3: Resume at 5 mg daily

Thrombocytopenia developing after 4 weeks of beginning treatment at 10 mg daily:

Platelets <30,000/mm^3 **or** <50,000/mm^3 with platelet transfusions: Hold treatment

When platelets return to ≥30,000/mm^3 (without hemostatic failure): Resume at 5 mg daily

Thrombocytopenia developing with treatment at 5 mg daily:

Platelets <30,000/mm^3 **or** <50,000/mm^3 with platelet transfusions: Hold treatment

When platelets return to ≥30,000/mm^3 (without hemostatic failure):

U.S. labeling: Resume at 2.5 mg once daily

Canadian labeling: Resume at 5 mg every other day

Adjustment for neutropenia in MDS:

Neutropenia developing within 4 weeks of beginning treatment at 10 mg daily:

For baseline absolute neutrophil count (ANC) ≥1000/mm^3:

ANC <750/mm^3: Hold treatment

When ANC returns to ≥1000/mm^3: Resume at 5 mg daily

For baseline absolute neutrophil count (ANC) <1000/mm^3:

ANC <500/mm^3: Hold treatment

When ANC returns to ≥500/mm^3: Resume at 5 mg daily

Neutropenia developing after 4 weeks of beginning treatment at 10 mg daily:

ANC <500/mm^3 for ≥7 days or associated with fever: Hold treatment

When ANC returns to ≥500/mm^3: Resume at 5 mg daily

Neutropenia developing with treatment at 5 mg daily:

ANC <500/mm^3 for ≥7 days or associated with fever: Hold treatment

When ANC returns to ≥500/mm^3:

U.S. labeling: Resume at 2.5 mg once daily

Canadian labeling: Resume at 5 mg every other day

Adjustment for thrombocytopenia in multiple myeloma:

Platelets <30,000/mm^3: Hold treatment, check CBC weekly

When platelets return to ≥30,000/mm^3: Resume at 15 mg daily

Additional occurrence of platelets <30,000/mm^3: Hold treatment

When platelets return to ≥30,000/mm^3: Resume treatment at 5 mg below previous dose; do not dose below 5 mg daily

Adjustment for neutropenia in multiple myeloma:

ANC <1000/mm^3: Hold treatment, add G-CSF, check CBC weekly

When ANC returns to ≥1000/mm^3 (with neutropenia as only toxicity): Resume at 25 mg daily

When ANC returns to ≥1000/mm^3 (with additional toxicities): Resume at 15 mg daily

Additional occurrence of ANC <1000/mm^3: Hold treatment

When ANC returns to ≥1000/mm^3: Resume treatment at 5 mg below previous dose; do not dose below 5 mg daily.

Administration Administer at about the same time each day with water; administer with or without food. Swallow capsule whole; do not break, open, or chew.

Missed doses: May administer a missed dose if within 12 hours of usual dosing time. If greater than 12 hours, patient should skip dose for that day and resume usual dosing the following day. Patient should **not** take 2 doses to make up for a missed dose.

Hazardous agent; use appropriate precautions for handling and disposal (NIOSH, 2012).

Monitoring Parameters CBC with differential (MCL - weekly for the first cycle, every 2 weeks during cycles 2-4; MDS - weekly for first 8 weeks; multiple myeloma - every 2 weeks for the first 3 months), then monthly thereafter; serum creatinine, liver function tests, thyroid function tests (TSH at baseline then every 2-3 months during lenalidomide treatment [Hamnvik, 2011]); ECG when clinically indicated; monitor for signs and symptoms of thromboembolism, tumor lysis syndrome, or tumor flare reaction

Women of childbearing potential: Pregnancy test 10-14 days **and** 24 hours prior to initiating therapy, weekly during the first 4 weeks of treatment, then every 2-4 weeks through 4 weeks after therapy discontinued

Dosage Forms Excipient information presented when available (limited, particularly for generics); consult specific product labeling.

Capsule, Oral:

Revlimid: 2.5 mg [contains fd&c blue #2 (indigotine)]

Revlimid: 5 mg

Revlimid: 10 mg, 15 mg, 20 mg [contains fd&c blue #2 (indigotine)]

Revlimid: 25 mg

- **Lepargylic Acid** *see* Azelaic Acid *on page 211*
- **Lescol** *see* Fluvastatin *on page 901*
- **Lescol® (Can)** *see* Fluvastatin *on page 901*
- **Lescol XL** *see* Fluvastatin *on page 901*
- **Lescol® XL (Can)** *see* Fluvastatin *on page 901*
- **Lessina** *see* Ethinyl Estradiol and Levonorgestrel *on page 787*
- **Letairis** *see* Ambrisentan *on page 94*

Letrozole (LET roe zole)

Brand Names: U.S. Femara

Brand Names: Canada Apo-Letrozole; Auro-Letrozole; Bio-Letrozole; Femara; JAMP-Letrozole; Letrozole Tablets, USP; Mar-Letrozole; MED-Letrozole; Myl-Letrozole; PMS-Letrozole; RAN-Letrozole; Sandoz-Letrozole; Teva-Letrozole; Zinda-Letrozole

Index Terms CGS-20267

Pharmacologic Category Antineoplastic Agent, Aromatase Inhibitor

Use For use in postmenopausal women in the adjuvant treatment of hormone receptor positive early breast cancer, extended adjuvant treatment of early breast cancer after 5 years of tamoxifen, advanced breast cancer with disease progression following antiestrogen therapy, hormone receptor positive or hormone receptor unknown, locally-advanced, or first-line (or second-line) treatment of advanced or metastatic breast cancer

Unlabeled Use Treatment of ovarian (epithelial) cancer, endometrial cancer

Pregnancy Risk Factor X

Pregnancy Considerations Adverse events were observed in animal reproduction studies. Letrozole is FDA indicated for postmenopausal women only (no clinical benefit for breast cancer has been demonstrated in premenopausal women). Use in women who are or who may become pregnant is contraindicated. Women who are perimenopausal or recently postmenopausal should use adequate contraception until postmenopausal status is fully established.

Breast-Feeding Considerations It is not known if letrozole is excreted in breast milk. Due to the potential for serious adverse reactions in the nursing infant, a decision should be made whether to discontinue nursing or to discontinue the drug, taking into account the importance of treatment to the mother.

Contraindications Use in women who are or may become pregnant

Canadian labeling: Additional contraindications (not in U.S. labeling): Hypersensitivity to letrozole, other aromatase inhibitors, or any component of the formulation; use in patients <18 years of age; breast-feeding

Warnings/Precautions Hazardous agent - use appropriate precautions for handling and disposal (NIOSH, 2012). Use caution with hepatic impairment; dose adjustment recommended in patients with cirrhosis or severe hepatic dysfunction. May cause dizziness, fatigue, and somnolence; patients should be cautioned before performing tasks which require mental alertness (eg, operating machinery or driving). May increase total serum cholesterol; in patients treated with adjuvant therapy and cholesterol levels within normal limits, an increase of >1.5 x ULN in total cholesterol has been demonstrated in 8.2% of letrozole-treated patients (25% requiring lipid-lowering medications) vs 3.2% of tamoxifen-treated patients (16% requiring medications); monitor cholesterol panel; may require antihyperlipidemics. May cause decreases in bone mineral density (BMD); a decrease in hip BMD by 3.8% from baseline in letrozole-treated patients vs 2% in placebo at 2 years has been demonstrated; however, there was no statistical difference in changes to the lumbar spine BMD scores; monitor BMD.

Adverse Reactions

>10%:

Cardiovascular: Edema (7% to 18%)

Central nervous system: Headache (4% to 20%), dizziness (3% to 14%), fatigue (8% to 13%)

Endocrine & metabolic: Hypercholesterolemia (3% to 52%), hot flashes (6% to 50%)

Gastrointestinal: Nausea (9% to 17%), weight gain (2% to 13%), constipation (2% to 11%)

Neuromuscular & skeletal: Weakness (4% to 34%), arthralgia (8% to 25%), arthritis (7% to 25%), bone pain (5% to 22%), back pain (5% to 18%), bone mineral density decreased/osteoporosis (5% to 15%), bone fracture (10% to 14%)

Respiratory: Dyspnea (6% to 18%), cough (6% to 13%)

Miscellaneous: Diaphoresis (≤24%), night sweats (15%)

1% to 10%:

Cardiovascular: Chest pain (6% to 8%), hypertension (5% to 8%), chest wall pain (6%), peripheral edema (5%); cerebrovascular accident including hemorrhagic stroke, thrombotic stroke (2% to 3%); thromboembolic event including venous thrombosis, thrombophlebitis, portal vein thrombosis, pulmonary embolism (2% to 3%); MI (1% to 2%), angina (1% to 2%), transient ischemic attack

Central nervous system: Insomnia (6% to 7%), pain (5%), anxiety (<5%), depression (<5%), vertigo (<5%), somnolence (3%)
Dermatologic: Rash (5%), alopecia (3% to 5%), pruritus (1%)
Endocrine & metabolic: Breast pain (2% to 7%), hypercalcemia (<5%)
Gastrointestinal: Diarrhea (5% to 8%), vomiting (3% to 7%), weight loss (6% to 7%), abdominal pain (6%), anorexia (1% to 5%), dyspepsia (3%)
Genitourinary: Urinary tract infection (6%), vaginal bleeding (5%), vaginal dryness (5%), vaginal hemorrhage (5%), vaginal irritation (5%)
Neuromuscular & skeletal: Limb pain (4% to 10%), myalgia (7% to 9%)
Ocular: Cataract (2%)
Renal: Renal disorder (5%)
Respiratory: Pleural effusion (<5%)
Miscellaneous: Infection (7%), influenza (6%), viral infection (6%), secondary malignancy (2% to 4%)

<1%, postmarketing, and/or case reports (Limited to important or life-threatening): Anaphylactic reaction, angioedema, arterial thrombosis, cardiac failure, carpal tunnel syndrome, endometrial cancer, endometrial hyperplasia, endometrial proliferation, erythema multiforme, hepatitis, leukopenia, memory impairment, stomatitis, tachycardia, thrombocytopenia, toxic epidermal necrolysis, trigger finger

Drug Interactions

Metabolism/Transport Effects Substrate of CYP2A6 (minor), CYP3A4 (minor); **Note:** Assignment of Major/Minor substrate status based on clinically relevant drug interaction potential; **Inhibits** CYP2A6 (strong), CYP2C19 (weak)

Avoid Concomitant Use

Avoid concomitant use of Letrozole with any of the following: Tegafur

Increased Effect/Toxicity

Letrozole may increase the levels/effects of: CYP2A6 Substrates; Methadone; Vitamin K Antagonists

Decreased Effect

Letrozole may decrease the levels/effects of: Cardiac Glycosides; Tegafur; Vitamin K Antagonists

The levels/effects of Letrozole may be decreased by: Tamoxifen

Storage/Stability Store at room temperature of 25°C (77°F); excursions permitted to 15°C to 30°C (59°F to 86°F).

Mechanism of Action Nonsteroidal competitive inhibitor of the aromatase enzyme system which binds to the heme group of aromatase, a cytochrome P450 enzyme which catalyzes conversion of androgens to estrogens (specifically, androstenedione to estrone and testosterone to estradiol). This leads to inhibition of the enzyme and a significant reduction in plasma estrogen (estrone, estradiol and estrone sulfate) levels. Does not affect synthesis of adrenal or thyroid hormones, aldosterone, or androgens.

Pharmacodynamics/Kinetics

Absorption: Rapid and well absorbed; not affected by food
Distribution: V_d: ~1.9 L/kg
Protein binding, plasma: Weak
Metabolism: Hepatic via CYP3A4 and 2A6 to an inactive carbinol metabolite
Half-life elimination: Terminal: ~2 days
Time to steady state, plasma: 2-6 weeks
Excretion: Urine (90%; 6% as unchanged drug, 75% as glucuronide carbinol metabolite, 9% as unidentified metabolites)

Dosage Oral: Adults: Females: Postmenopausal:
Breast cancer, advanced (first- or second-line treatment): 2.5 mg once daily; continue until tumor progression
Breast cancer, early (adjuvant treatment): 2.5 mg once daily; optimal duration unknown, duration in clinical trial is 5 years; discontinue at relapse
Breast cancer, early (extended adjuvant treatment): 2.5 mg once daily; optimal duration unknown, duration in clinical trials is 5 years (after 5 years of tamoxifen); discontinue at relapse
Ovarian (epithelial) cancer (unlabeled use): 2.5 mg once daily; continue until disease progression (Ramirez, 2008)
Elderly: No dosage adjustments required

Dosage adjustment in renal impairment: No dosage adjustment is required in patients with renal impairment if Cl_{cr} ≥10 mL/minute

Dosage adjustment in hepatic impairment:
Mild-to-moderate impairment (Child-Pugh class A or B): No adjustment recommended
Severe impairment (Child-Pugh class C) and cirrhosis: 2.5 mg every other day

Dietary Considerations May be taken without regard to meals. Calcium and vitamin D supplementation are recommended.

Administration Administer with or without food.

Hazardous agent; use appropriate precautions for handling and disposal (NIOSH, 2012).

Monitoring Parameters Monitor periodically during therapy: Complete blood counts, thyroid function tests; serum electrolytes, cholesterol, transaminases, and creatinine; blood pressure; bone density

Additional Information Oncology Comment: The American Society of Clinical Oncology (ASCO) guidelines for adjuvant endocrine therapy in postmenopausal women with HR-positive breast cancer (Burstein, 2010) recommend considering aromatase inhibitor (AI) therapy at some point in the treatment course (primary, sequentially, or extended). Optimal duration at this time is not known; however, treatment with an AI should not exceed 5 years in primary and extended therapies, and 2-3 years if followed by tamoxifen in sequential therapy (total of 5 years). If initial therapy with AI has been discontinued before the 5 years, consideration should be taken to receive tamoxifen for a total of 5 years. The optimal time to switch to an AI is also not known, but data supports switching after 2-3 years of tamoxifen (sequential) or after 5 years of tamoxifen (extended). If patient becomes intolerant or has poor adherence, consideration should be made to switch to another AI or initiate tamoxifen.

Dosage Forms Excipient information presented when available (limited, particularly for generics); consult specific product labeling.
Tablet, Oral:
Femara: 2.5 mg
Generic: 2.5 mg

◆ **Letrozole Tablets, USP (Can)** *see* Letrozole *on page 1185*

◆ **Leucovorin** *see* Leucovorin Calcium *on page 1186*

Leucovorin Calcium (loo koe VOR in KAL see um)

Brand Names: Canada Lederle Leucovorin

Index Terms 5-Formyl Tetrahydrofolate; Calcium Folinate; Calcium Leucovorin; Citrovorum Factor; Folinate Calcium; Folinic Acid (error prone synonym); Leucovorin

Pharmacologic Category Antidote; Chemotherapy Modulating Agent; Rescue Agent (Chemotherapy); Vitamin, Water Soluble

Use Antidote for folic acid antagonists (methotrexate, trimethoprim, pyrimethamine) and rescue therapy following high-dose methotrexate; in combination with fluorouracil in the treatment of colon cancer; treatment of megaloblastic anemias when folate is deficient as in infancy, sprue, pregnancy, and nutritional deficiency when oral folate therapy is not possible

Unlabeled Use Adjunctive cofactor therapy in methanol toxicity; prevention of pyrimethamine hematologic toxicity in HIV-positive patients

Pregnancy Risk Factor C

Pregnancy Considerations Animal reproduction studies have not been conducted. Leucovorin is a biologically active form of folic acid. Adequate amounts of folic acid are recommended during pregnancy. Refer to Folic Acid monograph.

Breast-Feeding Considerations Leucovorin is a biologically active form of folic acid. Adequate amounts of folic acid are recommended in breast-feeding women. Refer to Folic Acid monograph.

Contraindications Pernicious anemia or vitamin B_{12}-deficient megaloblastic anemias

Warnings/Precautions When used for the treatment of accidental weak folic acid antagonist overdose, administer as soon as possible. When used for the treatment of a methotrexate overdose, administer as soon as possible. Do not wait for the results of a methotrexate level before initiating therapy. It is important to adjust the leucovorin dose once a methotrexate level is known. When used for methotrexate rescue therapy, methotrexate serum concentrations should be monitored to determine dose and duration of leucovorin therapy. The dose may need to be increased or administration prolonged in situations where methotrexate excretion may be delayed (eg, ascites, pleural effusion, renal insufficiency, inadequate hydration); **never administer leucovorin intrathecally.** Combination of leucovorin and sulfamethoxazole-trimethoprim for the acute treatment of PCP in patients with HIV infection has been reported to cause increased rates of treatment failure. Leucovorin may increase the toxicity of 5-fluorouracil; dose of 5-fluorouracil may need decreased.

Powder for injection: When doses >10 mg/m^2 are required, reconstitute using sterile water for injection, not a solution containing benzyl alcohol.

Injection: Due to calcium content, do not administer I.V. solutions at a rate >160 mg/minute. Not intended for intrathecal use.

Adverse Reactions Frequency not defined. Toxicities (especially gastrointestinal toxicity) of fluorouracil is higher when used in combination with leucovorin.

Dermatologic: Rash, pruritus, erythema, urticaria
Hematologic: Thrombocytosis
Respiratory: Wheezing
Miscellaneous: Allergic reactions, anaphylactoid reactions

Drug Interactions

Metabolism/Transport Effects None known.

Avoid Concomitant Use

Avoid concomitant use of Leucovorin Calcium with any of the following: Raltitrexed; Trimethoprim

Increased Effect/Toxicity

Leucovorin Calcium may increase the levels/effects of: Capecitabine; Fluorouracil (Systemic); Fluorouracil (Topical); Tegafur

Decreased Effect

Leucovorin Calcium may decrease the levels/effects of: Fosphenytoin; PHENobarbital; Phenytoin; Primidone; Raltitrexed; Trimethoprim

The levels/effects of Leucovorin Calcium may be decreased by: Glucarpidase

Preparation for Administration Powder for injection: Reconstitute with SWFI or BWFI; dilute in 100-1000 mL NS, D_5W for infusion. When doses >10 mg/m^2 are required, reconstitute using sterile water for injection, not a solution containing benzyl alcohol.

Storage/Stability

Powder for injection: Store at room temperature of 25°C (77°F). Protect from light. Solutions reconstituted with bacteriostatic water for injection U.S.P., must be used within 7 days. Solutions reconstituted with SWFI must be used immediately. Parenteral admixture is stable for 24 hours stored at room temperature (25°C) and for 4 days when stored under refrigeration (4°C).

Solution for injection: Prior to dilution, store vials under refrigeration at 2°C to 8°C (36°F to 46°F). Protect from light.

Tablet: Store at room temperature of 15°C to 30°C (59°F to 86°F).

Mechanism of Action A reduced form of folic acid, leucovorin supplies the necessary cofactor blocked by methotrexate. Leucovorin actively competes with methotrexate for transport sites, displaces methotrexate from intracellular binding sites, and restores active folate stores required for DNA/RNA synthesis. Stabilizes the binding of 5-dUMP and thymidylate synthetase, enhancing the activity of fluorouracil. When administered with pyrimethamine for the treatment of opportunistic infections, leucovorin reduces the risk for hematologic toxicity.

Methanol toxicity treatment: Formic acid (methanol's toxic metabolite) is normally metabolized to carbon dioxide and water by 10-formyltetrahydrofolate dehydrogenase after being bound to tetrahydrofolate. Administering a source of tetrahydrofolate may aid the body in eliminating formic acid.

Pharmacodynamics/Kinetics

Absorption: Oral, I.M.: Well absorbed
Metabolism: Intestinal mucosa and hepatically to 5-methyltetrahydrofolate (5MTHF; active)
Bioavailability: Saturable at oral doses >25 mg; 25 mg (97%), 50 mg (75%), 100 mg (37%)
Half-life elimination: ~4-8 hours
Time to peak: Oral: ~2 hours; I.V.: Total folates: 10 minutes; 5MTHF: ~1 hour
Excretion: Urine (primarily); feces

Dosage

Treatment of weak folic acid antagonist overdosage (eg, trimethoprim, pyrimethamine): Children and Adults: Oral: 5-15 mg/day

Folate-deficient megaloblastic anemia: Children and Adults: I.M.: ≤1 mg/day

High-dose methotrexate-rescue dose: Children and Adults: Initial: Oral, I.M., I.V.: 15 mg (~10 mg/m^2); start 24 hours after beginning methotrexate infusion; continue every 6 hours for 10 doses, until methotrexate level is <0.05 micromole/L. Adjust dose as follows:

Normal methotrexate elimination: Oral, I.M., I.V.: 15 mg every 6 hours

Delayed early methotrexate elimination: I.V.: 150 mg every 3 hours until methotrexate level is <1 micromole/L, then 15 mg every 3 hours until methotrexate level is <0.05 micromole/L

Methotrexate overdose: Children and Adults: **Note:** The amount of leucovorin administered should equal the amount of methotrexate inadvertently administered.

I.V.: 1 mg per mg of methotrexate inadvertently administered; 100-1000 mg/m^2 every 3-6 hours has been used; administer until methotrexate levels decrease to goal level or longer if methotrexate levels are unavailable or if patient has renal dysfunction or third-space storage (ascites, pleural effusion)

A nomogram for leucovorin rescue in cancer patients receiving high-dose methotrexate based upon a 48-hour methotrexate level may be helpful (Widemann, 2006). Methotrexate level:
≥80 micromole/L: 1000 mg/m^2 every 6 hours
≥8 to <80 micromole/L: 100 mg/m^2 every 3 hours
≥2 to <8 micromole/L: 10 mg/m^2 every 3 hours
≥0.1 to <2 micromole/L: 10 mg/m^2 every 6 hours
Use of I.T. leucovorin is not advised (Jardine, 1996; Smith, 2008).

Cofactor therapy in methanol toxicity (unlabeled use): Children and Adults: I.V.: 1 mg/kg (maximum dose: 50 mg) over 30-60 minutes every 4-6 hours. Therapy should continue until methanol and formic acid have been completely eliminated (Barceloux, 2002)

Colorectal cancer (also refer to Combination Regimens): Adults:
I.V.: 200 mg/m^2 over at least 3 minutes (used in combination with fluorouracil 370 mg/m^2)
or
I.V.: 20 mg/m^2 (used in combination with fluorouracil 425 mg/m^2)

Pemetrexed toxicity (unlabeled dose): Adults: I.V.: 100 mg/m^2 once, followed by 50 mg/m^2 every 6 hours for 8 days (used in clinical trial for CTC grade 4 leukopenia ≥3 days; CTC grade 4 neutropenia ≥3 days; immediately for CTC grade 4 thrombocytopenia, bleeding associated with grade 3 thrombocytopenia, or grade 3 or 4 mucositis)

Prevention of pyrimethamine hematologic toxicity in HIV-positive patients (unlabeled uses; CDC, 2009):
Infants and Children >1 month of age: **Note:** Leucovorin should continue for 1 week after pyrimethamine is discontinued.
Toxoplasmosis (*Toxoplasma gondii*):
Primary prophylaxis: Oral: 5 mg once every 3 days (in combination with pyrimethamine [with either dapsone or atovaquone])
Secondary prophylaxis: Oral: 5 mg once every 3 days (in combination with pyrimethamine [with either sulfadiazine, atovaquone, or clindamycin])
Treatment (congenital): Oral or I.M.: 10 mg with every pyrimethamine dose (in combination with either sulfadiazine or clindamycin); treatment duration: 12 months
Treatment (acquired): Acute induction: Oral: 10-25 mg once daily (in combination with pyrimethamine [with either sulfadiazine, clindamycin, or atovaquone]) for ≥6 weeks
Chronic maintenance (secondary prophylaxis): 10-25 mg once daily (in combination with pyrimethamine [with either sulfadiazine or clindamycin]) **or** 10 mg once daily (in combination with pyrimethamine [with atovaquone])

Adults: Oral:
Isosporiasis (*Isospora belli*):
Treatment: 10-25 mg once daily (in combination with pyrimethamine)
Chronic maintenance (secondary prophylaxis): 5-10 mg once daily (in combination with pyrimethamine)
Pneumocystis jirovecii pneumonia (PCP): Prophylaxis (primary and secondary): 25 mg once weekly (in combination with pyrimethamine [with dapsone]) **or** 10 mg once daily (in combination with pyrimethamine [with atovaquone])
Toxoplasmosis (*Toxoplasma gondii*):
Primary prophylaxis: 25 mg once weekly (in combination with pyrimethamine [with dapsone]) **or** 10 mg once daily (in combination with pyrimethamine [with atovaquone])
Treatment: 10-25 mg once daily (in combination with pyrimethamine [with either sulfadiazine, clindamycin, atovaquone, or azithromycin]). **Note:** May increase leucovorin to 50-100 mg/day in divided doses in cases of pyrimethamine toxicity (rash, nausea, bone marrow suppression).
Chronic maintenance (secondary prophylaxis): 10-25 mg once daily (in combination with pyrimethamine [with either sulfadiazine or clindamycin]) **or** 10 mg once daily (in combination with pyrimethamine [with atovaquone])

Dosage adjustment in renal impairment: No dosage adjustment provided in manufacturer's labeling.

Dosage adjustment in hepatic impairment: No dosage adjustment provided in manufacturer's labeling.

Dietary Considerations Solutions for injection contain calcium 0.004 mEq per leucovorin 1 mg

Administration Due to calcium content, do not administer I.V. solutions at a rate >160 mg/minute; not intended for intrathecal use.
Refer to individual protocols. Should be administered I.M., I.V. push, or I.V. infusion (15 minutes to 2 hours). Leucovorin should not be administered concurrently with methotrexate. It is commonly initiated 24 hours after the start of methotrexate. Toxicity to normal tissues may be irreversible if leucovorin is not initiated by ~40 hours after the start of methotrexate.
As a rescue after folate antagonists: Administer by I.V. bolus, I.M., or orally.
Do not administer orally in the presence of nausea or vomiting. Doses >25 mg should be administered parenterally.
In combination with fluorouracil: Fluorouracil activity, the fluorouracil is usually given after, or at the midpoint, of the leucovorin infusion. Leucovorin is usually administered by I.V. bolus injection or short (10-120 minutes) I.V. infusion. Other administration schedules have been used; refer to individual protocols.

Monitoring Parameters
High-dose methotrexate therapy: Plasma methotrexate concentration; leucovorin is continued until the plasma methotrexate level <0.05 micromole/L. With 4- to 6-hour high-dose methotrexate infusions, plasma drug values in excess of 50 and 1 micromole/L at 24 and 48 hours after starting the infusion, respectively, are often predictive of delayed methotrexate clearance.
Fluorouracil therapy: CBC with differential and platelets, liver function tests, electrolytes

Dosage Forms Excipient information presented when available (limited, particularly for generics); consult specific product labeling. [DSC] = Discontinued product
Solution, Injection [strength expressed as base]:
Generic: 100 mg/10 mL (10 mL [DSC]); 300 mg/30 mL (30 mL)
Solution, Intravenous [strength expressed as base]:
Generic: 10 mg/mL (50 mL)
Solution Reconstituted, Injection [strength expressed as base]:
Generic: 50 mg (1 ea); 100 mg (1 ea); 200 mg (1 ea); 350 mg (1 ea); 500 mg (1 ea)
Solution Reconstituted, Injection [strength expressed as base, preservative free]:
Generic: 50 mg (1 ea); 100 mg (1 ea); 200 mg (1 ea); 350 mg (1 ea)
Tablet, Oral [strength expressed as base]:
Generic: 5 mg, 10 mg, 15 mg, 25 mg

Extemporaneous Preparations A 5 mg/mL oral suspension may be prepared with tablets, Cologel®, and a 2:1 mixture of simple syrup and wild cherry syrup. Crush twenty-four 25 mg tablets in a glass mortar and reduce to a fine powder; transfer powder to amber bottle. Add 30 mL Cologel® and shake mixture thoroughly. Add a quantity of syrup mixture sufficient to make 120 mL. Label "shake well" and "refrigerate". Stable for 28 days refrigerated.

Lam MS, "Extemporaneous Compounding of Oral Liquid Dosage Formulations and Alternative Drug Delivery Methods for Anticancer Drugs," *Pharmacotherapy*, 2011, 31(2):164-92.

◆ **Leukeran** *see* Chlorambucil *on page 403*

◆ **Leukeran® (Can)** *see* Chlorambucil *on page 403*
◆ **Leukine** *see* Sargramostim *on page 1877*

Leuprolide (loo PROE lide)

Brand Names: U.S. Eligard; Lupron Depot; Lupron Depot-Ped

Brand Names: Canada Eligard; Lupron; Lupron Depot

Index Terms Abbott-43818; Leuprolide Acetate; Leuprorelin Acetate; TAP-144

Pharmacologic Category Antineoplastic Agent, Gonadotropin-Releasing Hormone Agonist; Gonadotropin Releasing Hormone Agonist

Use Palliative treatment of advanced prostate cancer; management of endometriosis; treatment of anemia caused by uterine leiomyomata (fibroids); central precocious puberty

Unlabeled Use Treatment of breast cancer; infertility; treatment of paraphilia/hypersexuality

Pregnancy Risk Factor X

Pregnancy Considerations Adverse events were observed in animal reproduction studies. Pregnancy must be excluded prior to the start of treatment. Although leuprolide usually inhibits ovulation and stops menstruation, contraception is not ensured and a nonhormonal contraceptive should be used. Use is contraindicated in pregnant women.

Breast-Feeding Considerations It is not known if leuprolide is excreted into breast milk; use is contraindicated in nursing women.

Contraindications Hypersensitivity to leuprolide, GnRH, GnRH-agonist analogs, or any component of the formulation; undiagnosed abnormal vaginal bleeding; pregnancy; breast-feeding

Lupron Depot 22.5 mg, 30 mg, and 45 mg are also not indicated for use in women

Warnings/Precautions Hazardous agent - use appropriate precautions for handling and disposal (NIOSH, 2012). Transient increases in testosterone serum levels (~50% above baseline) occur at the start of treatment. Androgen-deprivation therapy (ADT) may increase the risk for cardiovascular disease (Levine, 2010); sudden cardiac death and stroke have been reported in men receiving GnRH agonists; long-term ADT may prolong the QT interval; consider the benefits of ADT versus the risk for QT prolongation in patients with a history of QT_c prolongation, with medications known to prolong the QT interval, or with pre-existing cardiac disease. Tumor flare, bone pain, neuropathy, urinary tract obstruction, and spinal cord compression have been reported when used for prostate cancer; closely observe patients for weakness, paresthesias, hematuria, and urinary tract obstruction in first few weeks of therapy. Observe patients with metastatic vertebral lesions or urinary obstruction closely. Exacerbation of endometriosis or uterine leiomyomata may occur initially. Decreased bone density has been reported when used for ≥6 months; use caution in patients with additional risk factors for bone loss (eg, chronic alcohol use, corticosteroid therapy). In patients with prostate cancer, androgen deprivation therapy may increase the risk for cardiovascular disease, diabetes, insulin resistance, obesity, alterations in lipids, and fractures; monitor as clinically necessary. Use caution in patients with a history of psychiatric illness; alteration in mood, memory impairment, and depression have been associated with use. Rare cases of pituitary apoplexy (frequently secondary to pituitary adenoma) have been observed with GnRH agonist administration (onset from 1 hour to usually <2 weeks); may present as sudden headache, vomiting, visual or mental status changes, and infrequently cardiovascular collapse; immediate medical attention required. Convulsions have been observed in postmarketing reports; patients affected included both those with and without a history of cerebrovascular disorders, central nervous system anomalies or tumors, epilepsy, seizures, and those on concomitant medications which may lower the seizure threshold. If seizures occur, manage accordingly. Females treated for precocious puberty may experience menses or spotting during the first 2 months of treatment; notify healthcare provider if bleeding continues after the second month.

Some dosage forms may contain benzyl alcohol which has been associated with "gasping syndrome" in neonates; patients with benzyl alcohol allergy may demonstrate a hypersensitivity reaction (usually local) in the form of erythema and induration at the injection site. Vehicle used in depot injectable formulations (polylactide-co-glycolide microspheres) has rarely been associated with retinal artery occlusion in patients with abnormal arteriovenous anastomosis. Due to different release properties, combinations of dosage forms or fractions of dosage forms should not be interchanged.

Adverse Reactions

Children (percentages based on 1-month and 3-month pediatric formulations combined):

>10%: Local: Pain at injection site (≤20%)

2% to 10%:

Cardiovascular: Vasodilatation (2%)

Central nervous system: Emotional lability (5%), mood changes (5%), headache (3% to 5%), pain (3%)

Dermatologic: Acne vulgaris (3%), skin rash (3% including erythema multiforme), seborrhea (3%)

Endocrine & metabolic: Weight gain (≤7%)

Genitourinary: Vaginal hemorrhage (3%), vaginal discharge (3%), vaginitis (3%)

Local: Injection site reaction (≤9%)

<2% (Limited to important or life-threatening): Abnormal gait, alopecia, arthralgia, asthma, body odor, bradycardia, cervix disease, decreased visual acuity, depression, dysmenorrhea, dysphagia, epistaxis, excessive crying, feminization, gingivitis, goiter, growth suppression, gynecomastia, hirsutism, hyperhidrosis, hyperkinesia, hypersensitivity reaction, hypertension, infection, leukoderma, myopathy, obesity, peripheral edema, personality disorder, precocious puberty, purpura, skin striae, syncope, urinary incontinence

Adults: Note: For prostate cancer treatment, an initial rise in serum testosterone concentrations may cause "tumor flare" or worsening of symptoms, including bone pain, neuropathy, hematuria, or ureteral or bladder outlet obstruction during the first 2 weeks. Similarly, an initial increase in estradiol levels, with a temporary worsening of symptoms, may occur in women treated with leuprolide.

Delayed release formulations:

>10%:

Cardiovascular: Edema (≤14%)

Central nervous system: Headache (≤65%), pain (<2% to 33%), depression (≤31%), insomnia (≤31%), fatigue (≤17%), dizziness (≤16%)

Dermatologic: Allergic skin reaction (≤12%)

Endocrine & metabolic: Hot flash (25% to 98%), weight changes (≤13%), hyperlipidemia (≤12%), libido decreased (≤11%)

Gastrointestinal: Nausea and vomiting (≤25%), change in bowel habits (≤14%)

Genitourinary: Vaginitis (11% to 28%), testicular atrophy (≤20%), genitourinary complaint (13% to 15%)

Local: Burning sensation at injection site burning (transient: ≤35%)

Neuromuscular & skeletal: Weakness (≤18%), arthropathy (≤12%)

Respiratory: Flu-like symptoms (≤12%)

1% to 10% (limited to important or life-threatening):

Cardiovascular: Angina pectoris (<5%), atrial fibrillation (<5%), bradycardia (<5%), cardiac arrhythmia (<5%), cardiac failure (<5%), deep thrombophlebitis (<5%), hyper-/hypotension (<5%), palpitations (<5%), syncope (<5%), tachycardia (<5%)

Central nervous system: Nervousness (≤8%), paresthesia (≤8%), anxiety (≤6%), confusion (<5%), delusions (<5%), dementia (<5%), neuropathy (<5%), paralysis (<5%), seizure (<5%), ostealgia (<2%)

Dermatologic: Acne vulgaris (≤10%), alopecia (≤5%), diaphoresis (≤5%), cellulitis (<5%), pruritus (≤3%), skin rash (≤2%)

Endocrine & metabolic: Dehydration (≤8%), gynecomastia (≤7%), decreased prostatic acid phosphatase (≥5%), decreased serum bicarbonate (≥5%), hypercholesterolemia (≥5%), hyperglycemia (≥5%), hyperphosphatemia (≥5%), hyperuricemia (≥5%), hypoalbuminemia (≥5%), hypocholesterolemia (≥5%), hypoproteinemia (≥5%), increased prostatic acid phosphatase (≥5%), menstrual disorder (≤2%), hirsutism (<2%)

Gastrointestinal: Anorexia (<5%), dysphagia (<5%), gastrointestinal hemorrhage (<5%), intestinal obstruction (<5%), gastric ulcer (<5%), constipation (≤3%), gastroenteritis (≤3%), diarrhea (≤2%)

Genitourinary: Mastalgia (≤6%), impotence (≤5%), balanitis (<5%), urinary incontinence (<5%), lactation (<5%), penile disease (<5%), testicular disease (<5%), urinary tract infection (<5%), nocturia (≤4%), testicular pain (≤4%), dysuria (≤2%), bladder spasm (<2%), erectile dysfunction (<2%), hematuria (<2%), urinary retention (<2%), urinary urgency (<2%)

Hematologic & oncologic: Eosinophilia (≥5%), leukopenia (≥5%), change in platelet count (increased; ≥5%), bruise (≤5%), lymphadenopathy (<5%), anemia

Hepatic: Abnormal hepatic function tests (≥5%), prolonged partial thromboplastin time (≥5%), prolonged prothrombin time (≥5%), hepatomegaly (<5%)

Hypersensitivity: Hypersensitivity reaction (<5%)

Infection: Infection (5%)

Local: Pain at injection site (2% to 5%), erythema at injection site (1% to 3%)

Neuromuscular & skeletal: Myalgia (≤8%), pathological fracture (<5%), arthralgia (≤1%)

Renal: Increased blood urea nitrogen (≥5%), increased serum creatinine (≥5%), decreased urine specific gravity (≥5%), increased urine specific gravity (≥5%), polyuria (2% to 4%)

Respiratory: Emphysema (<5%), epistaxis (<5%), hemoptysis (<5%), pleural effusion (<5%), pulmonary edema (<5%), dyspnea (≤2%), cough (≤1%)

Miscellaneous: Fever (<5%)

Immediate release formulation:

>10%:

Cardiovascular: ECG changes (19%), peripheral edema (12%)

Central nervous system: Pain (13%)

Endocrine & metabolic: Hot flash (55%)

1% to 10% (limited to important or life-threatening):

Cardiovascular: Hypertension (8%), heart murmur (3%), thrombophlebitis (2%), cardiac failure (1%), angina pectoris, cardiac arrhythmia, myocardial infarction, pulmonary embolism, syncope

Central nervous system: Headache (7%), insomnia (7%), dizziness (5%), ostealgia (5%), anxiety, depression, fatigue, fever, nervousness, peripheral neuropathy

Dermatologic: Dermatitis (5%), alopecia, hyperpigmentation, pruritus, skin lesion

Endocrine & metabolic: Decreased libido, diabetes mellitus, goiter, gynecomastia, hypercalcemia, hypoglycemia

Gastrointestinal: Constipation (7%), anorexia (6%), nausea and vomiting (5%), diarrhea, dysphagia, gastrointestinal hemorrhage, peptic ulcer, rectal polyps

Genitourinary: Decreased testicular size (7%), hematuria (6%), urinary frequency (6%), impotence (4%), urinary tract infection (3%), bladder spasm, dysuria, incontinence, mastalgia, testicular pain, urinary tract obstruction

Hematologic & oncologic: Anemia (5%), bruise

Infection: Infection

Local: Injection site reaction

Neuromuscular & skeletal: Weakness (10%)

Ophthalmic: Blurred vision

Renal: Increased blood urea nitrogen, increased serum creatinine

Respiratory: Dyspnea (2%), cough, pneumonia, pulmonary fibrosis

Miscellaneous: Fever, inflammation

Children and Adults: *Any formulations:* Postmarketing and/or case reports (Limited to important or life-threatening): Abscess at injection site, anaphylaxis, anaphylactoid reaction, asthma, bone fracture (spine), cerebrovascular accident, convulsions, coronary artery disease, decreased white blood cell count, diabetes mellitus, fibromyalgia syndrome (arthralgia/myalgia, headaches, GI distress), hemoptysis, hepatic injury, hepatic insufficiency, hepatotoxicity, hyperuricemia, hypokalemia, hypoproteinemia, induration at injection site, interstitial pulmonary disease, leukocytosis, myocardial infarction, osteopenia, paralysis, penile swelling, peripheral neuropathy; pituitary apoplexy (cardiovascular collapse, mental status altered, ophthalmoplegia, sudden headache, visual changes, vomiting); prolonged QT interval on ECG, prostate pain, pulmonary embolism, pulmonary infiltrates, retroperitoneal fibrosis (pelvic), seizure, skin photosensitivity, suicidal ideation (rare), tenosynovitis (symptoms), thrombocytopenia, transient ischemic attacks

Drug Interactions

Metabolism/Transport Effects None known.

Avoid Concomitant Use There are no known interactions where it is recommended to avoid concomitant use.

Increased Effect/Toxicity There are no known significant interactions involving an increase in effect.

Decreased Effect

Leuprolide may decrease the levels/effects of: Antidiabetic Agents

Preparation for Administration

Hazardous agent; use appropriate precautions for handling and disposal (NIOSH, 2012).

Eligard: Packaged in two syringes; one contains the Atrigel polymer system and the second contains leuprolide acetate powder; follow package instructions for mixing

Lupron Depot, Lupron Depot-Ped: Reconstitute only with diluent provided

Storage/Stability

Eligard: Store at 2°C to 8°C (36°F to 46°C). Allow to reach room temperature prior to using; once mixed, must be administered within 30 minutes.

Lupron Depot, Lupron Depot-Ped: Store at room temperature of 25°C (77°F); excursions permitted to 15°C to 30°C (59°F to 86°F). Upon reconstitution, the suspension does not contain a preservative and should be used immediately; discard if not used within 2 hours.

Leuprolide acetate 5 mg/mL solution: Store at 20°C to 25°C (68°F to 77°F); excursions permitted to 15°C to 30°C (59°F to 86°F). Protect from light and store vial in carton until use. Do not freeze.

Mechanism of Action Leuprolide, is an agonist of luteinizing hormone-releasing hormone (LHRH). Acting as a potent inhibitor of gonadotropin secretion; continuous administration results in suppression of ovarian and testicular steroidogenesis due to decreased levels of LH and FSH with subsequent decrease in testosterone (male) and estrogen (female) levels. In males, testosterone levels are reduced to below castrate levels. Leuprolide may also have a direct inhibitory effect on the testes, and act by a different mechanism not directly related to reduction in serum testosterone.

Pharmacodynamics/Kinetics

Onset of action: Following transient increase, testosterone suppression occurs in ~2-4 weeks of continued therapy

Distribution: Males: V_d: 27 L

Protein binding: 43% to 49%

Metabolism: Major metabolite, pentapeptide (M-1)

Bioavailability: SubQ: 94%

Excretion: Urine (<5% as parent and major metabolite)

Dosage

Children: Precocious puberty (consider discontinuing by age 11 for females and by age 12 for males):

I.M.:

Lupron Depot-Ped (monthly):

≤25 kg: 7.5 mg every month

>25-37.5 kg: 11.25 mg every month

>37.5 kg: 15 mg every month

Titrate dose upward in increments of 3.75 mg every 4 weeks if down-regulation is not achieved.

Lupron Depot-Ped (3 month): 11.25 mg or 30 mg every 12 weeks

SubQ (leuprolide acetate 5 mg/mL solution): Initial: 50 mcg/kg/day; titrate dose upward by 10 mcg/kg/day if down-regulation is not achieved. **Note:** Higher mg/kg doses may be required in younger children.

Adults:

Prostate cancer, advanced:

I.M.:

Lupron Depot 7.5 mg (monthly): 7.5 mg every month **or**

Lupron Depot 22.5 mg (3 month): 22.5 mg every 12 weeks **or**

Lupron Depot 30 mg (4 month): 30 mg every 16 weeks **or**

Lupron Depot 45 mg (6 month): 45 mg every 24 weeks

SubQ:

Eligard: 7.5 mg monthly **or** 22.5 mg every 3 months **or** 30 mg every 4 months **or** 45 mg every 6 months

Leuprolide acetate 5 mg/mL solution: 1 mg daily

Endometriosis: I.M.: Initial therapy may be with leuprolide alone or in combination with norethindrone; if retreatment for an additional 6 months is necessary, concomitant norethindrone should be used. Retreatment is not recommended for longer than one additional 6-month course.

Lupron Depot: 3.75 mg every month for up to 6 months **or**

Lupron Depot-3 month: 11.25 mg every 3 months for up to 2 doses (6 months total duration of treatment)

Uterine leiomyomata (fibroids): I.M. (in combination with iron):

Lupron Depot: 3.75 mg every month for up to 3 months **or**

Lupron Depot-3 month: 11.25 mg as a single injection

Breast cancer, premenopausal ovarian ablation (unlabeled use): I.M.:

Lupron Depot: 3.75 mg every 28 days for up to 24 months (Boccardo, 1999) **or**

Lupron Depot-3 month: 11.25 mg every 3 months for up to 24 months (Boccardo, 1999; Schmid, 2007)

Adults: Males: Treatment of paraphilia/hypersexuality (unlabeled use; Guay, 2009; Reilly, 2000):

Note: May cause an initial increase in androgen concentrations which may be treated with an antiandrogen (eg, flutamide, cyproterone) for 1-2 months (Guay, 2009). Avoid use in patients with osteoporosis or active pituitary pathology.

SubQ: Test dose: 1 mg (observe for hypersensitivity)

Depot I.M.: 3.75-7.5 mg monthly

Dosage adjustment in renal impairment: No dosage adjustment provided in manufacturer's labeling (has not been studied).

Dosage adjustment in hepatic impairment: No dosage adjustment provided in manufacturer's labeling (has not been studied).

Administration

I.M.: Lupron Depot, Lupron Depot-Ped: Administer as a single injection. Vary injection site periodically

SubQ:

Eligard: Vary injection site; choose site with adequate subcutaneous tissue (eg, upper or mid-abdomen, upper buttocks); avoid areas that may be compressed or rubbed (eg, belt or waistband)

Leuprolide acetate 5 mg/mL solution: Vary injection site; if an alternate syringe from the syringe provided is required, insulin syringes should be used

Hazardous agent; use appropriate precautions for handling and disposal (NIOSH, 2012).

Monitoring Parameters Bone mineral density

Precocious puberty: GnRH testing (blood LH and FSH levels), measurement of height and bone age every 6-12 months, testosterone in males and estradiol in females (I.M. [monthly] and SubQ formulations: 1-2 months after initiation of therapy or with dosage change; I.M. [3 month] formulation: 2-3 months after initiation of therapy, month 6, and as clinically indicated thereafter); Tanner staging

Prostatic cancer: LH and FSH levels, serum testosterone (~4 weeks after initiation of therapy), PSA; weakness, paresthesias, and urinary tract obstruction in first few weeks of therapy. Screen for diabetes (blood glucose and Hb A_{1c}) and cardiovascular risk prior to initiating and periodically during treatment.

Treatment of paraphilia/hypersexuality (unlabeled use; Reilly, 2000): CBC (baseline, monthly for 4 months then every 6 months); serum testosterone (baseline, monthly for 4 months then every 6 months); serum LH (baseline and every 6 months), FSH (baseline), serum BUN and creatinine (baseline and every 6 months); bone density (baseline and yearly); ECG (baseline)

Test Interactions Interferes with pituitary gonadotropic and gonadal function tests during and up to 3 months after monthly administration of leuprolide therapy.

Additional Information

Eligard Atrigel: A nongelatin-based, biodegradable, polymer matrix

Oncology Comment: Guidelines from the American Society of Clinical Oncology (ASCO) for hormonal management of advanced prostate cancer which is androgen-sensitive (Loblaw, 2007) recommend either orchiectomy or luteinizing hormone-releasing hormone (LHRH) agonists as initial treatment for androgen deprivation.

Dosage Forms Excipient information presented when available (limited, particularly for generics); consult specific product labeling.

Kit, Injection, as acetate:

Generic: 1 mg/0.2 mL

Kit, Intramuscular, as acetate:

Lupron Depot: 7.5 mg, 45 mg [latex free; contains polysorbate 80]

Kit, Intramuscular, as acetate [preservative free]:
Lupron Depot: 3.75 mg, 11.25 mg, 22.5 mg, 30 mg [latex free; contains polysorbate 80]
Lupron Depot-Ped: 7.5 mg, 11.25 mg, 15 mg, 30 mg (Ped), 11.25 MG (Ped) [latex free; contains polysorbate 80]
Kit, Subcutaneous, as acetate:
Eligard: 7.5 mg, 22.5 mg, 30 mg, 45 mg

◆ **Leuprolide Acetate** *see* Leuprolide *on page 1189*

◆ **Leuprolide Acetate and Norethindrone Acetate** *see* Leuprolide and Norethindrone *on page 1192*

Leuprolide and Norethindrone

(loo PROE lide & nor eth IN drone)

Index Terms Leuprolide Acetate and Norethindrone Acetate; Lupaneta Pack; Norethindrone and Leuprolide

Pharmacologic Category Gonadotropin Releasing Hormone Agonist; Progestin

Use Endometriosis: Management of initial and recurrent painful symptoms of endometriosis

Pregnancy Risk Factor X

Dosage Endometriosis: Adults: Females: **Note:** Treatment consists of an oral norethindrone tablet used in conjunction with an I.M. leuprolide injection. The initial therapy should be limited to 6 months duration; a single retreatment of not more than 6 additional months may be administered if symptoms recur. Maximum total duration of therapy is 12 months.

1 month:
Injection: I.M.: Leuprolide 3.75 mg as a single dose administered by healthcare provider once every month for up to 6 doses (maximum initial therapy: 6 months; maximum cumulative therapy: 12 months)
Tablet: Oral: Norethindrone 5 mg once daily for up to 6 months (maximum initial therapy: 6 months; maximum cumulative therapy: 12 months)

3 month:
Injection: I.M.: Leuprolide 11.25 mg as a single dose administered by healthcare provider once every 3 months for up to 2 doses (maximum initial therapy: 6 months; maximum cumulative therapy: 12 months)
Tablet: Oral: Norethindrone 5 mg once daily for up to 6 months (maximum initial therapy: 6 months; maximum cumulative therapy: 12 months)

Dosage adjustment in renal Impairment: No dosage adjustment provided in manufacturer's labeling (has not been studied).

Dosage adjustment in hepatic Impairment: No dosage adjustment provided in manufacturer's labeling (has not been studied). Use is contraindicated with hepatic tumors or disease.

Additional Information Complete prescribing information should be consulted for additional detail.

Product Availability Lupaneta Pack: FDA approved December 2012: anticipated availability is fourth quarter of 2013. Refer to prescribing information for additional information.

◆ **Leuprorelin Acetate** *see* Leuprolide *on page 1189*

◆ **Leurocristine Sulfate** *see* VinCRIStine *on page 2191*

◆ **Leustatin** *see* Cladribine *on page 444*

Levalbuterol

(leve al BYOO ter ole)

Brand Names: U.S. Xopenex; Xopenex Concentrate; Xopenex HFA

Brand Names: Canada Xopenex®

Index Terms Levalbuterol Hydrochloride; Levalbuterol Tartrate; Levosalbutamol; R-albuterol

Pharmacologic Category $Beta_2$ Agonist

Use Treatment or prevention of bronchospasm in children and adults with reversible obstructive airway disease

Pregnancy Risk Factor C

Pregnancy Considerations Teratogenic effects were not observed in animal reproduction studies; however, racemic albuterol was teratogenic in some species. Beta-agonists may interfere with uterine contractility if administered during labor.

Uncontrolled asthma is associated with adverse events on pregnancy (increased risk of perinatal mortality, pre-eclampsia, preterm birth, low birth weight infants). Other $beta_2$-receptor agonists are currently preferred for the treatment of asthma during pregnancy (NAEPP, 2005).

Breast-Feeding Considerations It is not known whether levalbuterol is excreted in human milk. Although breast-feeding is not recommended by the manufacturer, the use of $beta_2$-receptor agonists are not considered a contra-indication to breast-feeding (NAEPP, 2005).

Contraindications Hypersensitivity to levalbuterol, albuterol, or any component of the formulation

Warnings/Precautions Optimize anti-inflammatory treatment before initiating maintenance treatment with levalbuterol. Do not use as a component of chronic therapy without an anti-inflammatory agent. Only the mildest form of asthma (Step 1 and/or exercise-induced) would not require concurrent use based upon asthma guidelines. Patient must be instructed to seek medical attention in cases where acute symptoms are not relieved or a previous level of response is diminished. The need to increase frequency of use may indicate deterioration of asthma, and treatment must not be delayed. A spacer device or valved holding chamber is recommended when using a metered-dose inhaler.

Use caution in patients with cardiovascular disease (arrhythmia or hypertension or HF), convulsive disorders, diabetes, glaucoma, hyperthyroidism, or hypokalemia. Beta-agonists may cause elevation in blood pressure, heart rate, and result in CNS stimulation/excitation. $Beta_2$-agonists may increase risk of arrhythmia, increase serum glucose, or decrease serum potassium.

Immediate hypersensitivity reactions (urticaria, angioedema, rash, bronchospasm) have been reported. Do not exceed recommended dose; serious adverse events including fatalities, have been associated with excessive use of inhaled sympathomimetics. Rarely, paradoxical bronchospasm may occur with use of inhaled bronchodilating agents; this should be distinguished from inadequate response. Use with caution during labor and delivery. Safety and efficacy have not been established in patients <4 years of age.

Adverse Reactions

>10%:
Endocrine & metabolic: Serum glucose increased, serum potassium decreased
Neuromuscular & skeletal: Tremor (≤7%)
Respiratory: Rhinitis (3% to 11%)
Miscellaneous: Viral infection (7% to 12%)

>2% to 10%:
Central nervous system: Headache (8% to 12%), nervousness (3% to 10%), dizziness (1% to 3%), anxiety (≤3%), migraine (≤3%), weakness (3%)
Cardiovascular: Tachycardia (~3%)
Dermatologic: Rash (≤8%)
Gastrointestinal: Diarrhea (2% to 6%), dyspepsia (1% to 3%)
Neuromuscular & skeletal: Leg cramps (≤3%)
Respiratory: Asthma (9%), pharyngitis (3% to 10%), cough (1% to 4%), sinusitis (1% to 4%), nasal edema (1% to 3%)

Miscellaneous: Flu-like syndrome (1% to 4%), accidental injury (≤3%)

<2% (Limited to important or life-threatening): Abnormal ECG, acne, anaphylaxis, angina, angioedema, arrhythmia, atrial fibrillation, chest pain, chills, constipation, conjunctivitis, cough, diaphoresis, dysmenorrhea, dyspnea, epistaxis, extrasystole, gastroenteritis, hematuria, hyper-/hypotension, hypoesthesia (hand), hypokalemia, insomnia, itching eyes, lymphadenopathy, metabolic acidosis, myalgia, nausea, oropharyngeal dryness, paresthesia, supraventricular arrhythmia, syncope, vaginal moniliasis, vertigo, vomiting, wheezing, xerostomia

Note: Immediate hypersensitivity reactions have occurred (including angioedema, oropharyngeal edema, urticaria, and anaphylaxis).

Drug Interactions

Metabolism/Transport Effects None known.

Avoid Concomitant Use

Avoid concomitant use of Levalbuterol with any of the following: Beta-Blockers (Nonselective); Iobenguane I 123

Increased Effect/Toxicity

Levalbuterol may increase the levels/effects of: Atosiban; Loop Diuretics; Sympathomimetics; Thiazide Diuretics

The levels/effects of Levalbuterol may be increased by: AtoMOXetine; Cannabinoids; MAO Inhibitors; Tricyclic Antidepressants

Decreased Effect

Levalbuterol may decrease the levels/effects of: Iobenguane I 123

The levels/effects of Levalbuterol may be decreased by: Beta-Blockers (Beta1 Selective); Beta-Blockers (Nonselective); Betahistine

Preparation for Administration Concentrated solution should be diluted with 2.5 mL NS prior to use.

Storage/Stability

Aerosol: Store at room temperature of 20°C to 25°C (68°F to 77°F); protect from freezing and direct sunlight. Store with mouthpiece down. Discard after 200 actuations.

Solution for nebulization: Store in protective foil pouch at room temperature of 20°C to 25°C (68°F to 77°F). Protect from light and excessive heat. Vials should be used within 2 weeks after opening protective pouch. Use within 1 week and protect from light if removed from pouch. Vials of concentrated solution should be used immediately after removing from protective pouch.

Mechanism of Action Relaxes bronchial smooth muscle by action on beta$_2$-receptors with little effect on heart rate

Pharmacodynamics/Kinetics

Onset of action (as measured by a 15% increase in FEV_1):
- Aerosol: 5.5-10.2 minutes
  - Peak effect: ~77 minutes
- Nebulization: 10-17 minutes
  - Peak effect: 1.5 hours

Duration (as measured by a 15% increase in FEV_1):
- Aerosol: 3-4 hours (up to 6 hours in some patients)
- Nebulization: 5-6 hours (up to 8 hours in some patients)

Absorption: A portion of inhaled dose is absorbed to systemic circulation

Half-life elimination: 3.3-4 hours

Time to peak, serum:
- Aerosol: Children: 0.8 hours, Adults: 0.5 hours
- Nebulization: Children: 0.3-0.6 hours, Adults: 0.2 hours

Dosage

Metered-dose inhaler (45 mcg/puff):

Children 5-11 years:

Bronchospasm, quick relief: 1-2 puffs every 4-6 hours as needed

Exacerbation of asthma (acute, severe) *(NIH Guidelines, 2007)*: 4-8 puffs every 20 minutes for 3 doses, then every 1-4 hours as needed

Children ≥12 years and Adults:

Bronchospasm, quick relief: 1-2 puffs every 4-6 hours

Exacerbation of asthma (acute, severe) *(NIH Guidelines, 2007)*: 4-8 puffs every 20 minutes for up to 4 hours, then every 1-4 hours as needed

Solution for nebulization:

Children: ≤4 years:

Bronchospasm, quick relief *(NIH Guidelines, 2007)*: 0.31-1.25 mg every 4-6 hours as needed

Exacerbation of asthma (acute, severe) *(NIH Guidelines, 2007)*: 0.075 mg/kg (minimum: 1.25 mg) every 20 minutes for 3 doses, then 0.075-0.15 mg/kg (maximum: 5 mg) every 1-4 hours as needed

Children 5-11 years:

Bronchospasm, quick relief: 0.31-0.63 mg every 8 hours as needed

Exacerbation of asthma (acute severe) *(NIH Guidelines, 2007)*: 0.075 mg/kg (minimum: 1.25 mg) every 20 minutes for 3 doses, then 0.075-0.15 mg/kg (maximum: 5 mg) every 1-4 hours as needed

Children ≥12 years and Adults:

Bronchospasm, quick relief: 0.63-1.25 mg every 8 hours as needed

Exacerbation of asthma (acute, severe) *(NIH Guidelines, 2007)*: 1.25-2.5 mg every 20 minutes for 3 doses, then 1.25-5 mg every 1-4 hours as needed

Elderly: Only a small number of patients have been studied. Although greater sensitivity of some elderly patients cannot be ruled out, no overall differences in safety or effectiveness were observed. An initial dose of 0.63 mg should be used in all patients >65 years of age.

Dosage adjustment in renal impairment: No dosage adjustment provided in manufacturer's labeling. Use with caution.

Dosage adjustment in hepatic impairment: No dosage adjustment provided in manufacturer's labeling (has not been studied).

Administration Inhalation:

Metered-dose inhaler: Shake well before use; prime with 4 test sprays prior to first use or if inhaler has not been used for more than 3 days. Clean actuator (mouthpiece) weekly. A spacer device or valved holding chamber is recommended when using a metered-dose inhaler.

Solution for nebulization: Safety and efficacy were established when administered with the following nebulizers: PARI LC Jet™, PARI LC Plus™, as well as the following compressors: PARI Master®, Dura-Neb® 2000, and Dura-Neb® 3000. Concentrated solution should be diluted prior to use. Blow-by administration is not recommended, use a mask device if patient unable to hold mouthpiece in mouth for administration.

Monitoring Parameters Asthma symptoms; FEV_1, peak flow, and/or other pulmonary function tests; heart rate, blood pressure, CNS stimulation; arterial blood gases (if condition warrants); serum potassium, serum glucose (in selected patients)

Dosage Forms Considerations

Xopenex HFA 15 g canisters contain 200 inhalations.

Dosage Forms Excipient information presented when available (limited, particularly for generics); consult specific product labeling.

Aerosol, Inhalation, as tartrate [strength expressed as base]:

Xopenex HFA: 45 mcg/actuation (15 g)

Nebulization Solution, Inhalation, as hydrochloride [strength expressed as base]:

Xopenex: 0.63 mg/3 mL (3 mL); 1.25 mg/3 mL (3 mL)

Generic: 0.63 mg/3 mL (3 mL)

Nebulization Solution, Inhalation, as hydrochloride [strength expressed as base, preservative free]:
Xopenex: 0.31 mg/3 mL (3 mL)
Xopenex Concentrate: 1.25 mg/0.5 mL (30 ea)
Generic: 0.31 mg/3 mL (3 mL); 0.63 mg/3 mL (3 mL); 1.25 mg/3 mL (3 mL); 1.25 mg/0.5 mL (1 ea, 30 ea)

- **Levalbuterol Hydrochloride** *see* Levalbuterol *on page 1192*
- **Levalbuterol Tartrate** *see* Levalbuterol *on page 1192*
- **Levaquin** *see* Levofloxacin (Systemic) *on page 1198*
- **Levaquin® (Can)** *see* Levofloxacin (Systemic) *on page 1198*
- **Levarterenol Bitartrate** *see* Norepinephrine *on page 1471*
- **Levate® (Can)** *see* Amitriptyline *on page 105*
- **Levbid** *see* Hyoscyamine *on page 1026*
- **Levemir** *see* Insulin Detemir *on page 1088*
- **Levemir® (Can)** *see* Insulin Detemir *on page 1088*
- **Levemir FlexPen** *see* Insulin Detemir *on page 1088*

LevETIRAcetam (lee va tye RA se tam)

Brand Names: U.S. Keppra; Keppra XR

Brand Names: Canada Apo-Levetiracetam; Auro-Levetiracetam; Ava-Levetiracetam; CO Levetiracetam; Dom-Levetiracetam; JAMP-Levetiracetam; Keppra; PHL-Levetiracetam; PMS-Levetiracetam; PRO-Levetiracetam; RAN-Levetiracetam

Pharmacologic Category Anticonvulsant, Miscellaneous

Additional Appendix Information

Status Epilepticus *on page 2375*

Use Adjunctive therapy in the treatment of partial onset, myoclonic, and/or primary generalized tonic-clonic seizures

Pregnancy Risk Factor C

Pregnancy Considerations Developmental toxicities were observed in animal reproduction studies. Levetiracetam crosses the placenta and can be detected in the neonate at birth. Concentrations in the umbical cord at delivery are similar to those in the maternal plasma. Serum concentrations of levetiracetam may decrease as pregnancy progresses; monitor carefully throughout pregnancy and postpartum (Tomson, 2007).

Two registries are available for women exposed to levetiracetam during pregnancy: Pregnant women may enroll themselves into the North American Antiepileptic Drug (AED) Pregnancy Registry (888-233-2334 or http://www.-mgh.harvard.edu/aed/). The patient or healthcare provider may contact the UCB AED Pregnancy Registry (888-537-7734).

The North American AED registry has published data collected from pregnant women taking levetiracetam monotherapy from 1997-2011 (n=450). Eleven major malformations were diagnosed within 12 weeks of birth. The relative risk of major malformations was not increased in comparison to women with epilepsy not taking AEDs (n=442; RR 2.2, 95% CI 0.8-6.4) or in comparison to women using lamotrigine monotherapy (n=1562; RR 1.2, 95% CI 0.6-2.5) (Hernández-Díaz, 2012).

Breast-Feeding Considerations Levetiracetam can be detected in breast milk. Using data from 11 women collected 4-23 days after delivery, the estimated exposure of levetiracetam to the breast-feeding infant would be ~2 mg/kg/day (relative infant dose 7.9% of the weight-adjusted maternal dose). Adverse events were not reported in the nursing infants (Tomson, 2007). Breast-feeding is not recommended by the manufacturer.

Medication Guide Available Yes

Contraindications There are no contraindications listed in the U.S. manufacturer's labeling.

Canadian labeling: Hypersensitivity to levetiracetam or any component of the formulation

Warnings/Precautions Antiepileptics are associated with an increased risk of suicidal behavior/thoughts with use (regardless of indication); patients should be monitored for signs/symptoms of depression, suicidal tendencies, and other unusual behavior changes during therapy and instructed to inform their healthcare provider immediately if symptoms occur.

Severe dermatologic reactions (toxic epidermal necrolysis and Stevens-Johnson syndrome) have been reported; onset usually within ~2 weeks of treatment initiation but may be delayed (>4 months); discontinue for any signs of a hypersensitivity reaction or unspecified rash.

Psychotic symptoms (psychosis, hallucinations) and behavioral symptoms (including aggression, anger, anxiety, depersonalization, depression, personality disorder) may occur; incidence may be increased in children. Dose reduction or discontinuation may be required. Levetiracetam should be withdrawn gradually, when possible, to minimize the potential of increased seizure frequency. Use caution with renal impairment; dosage adjustment may be necessary. Impaired coordination, weakness, dizziness, and somnolence may occur, most commonly during the first month of therapy; use caution when driving or operating heavy machinery. Although rare, decreases in red blood cell counts, hemoglobin, hematocrit, white blood cell counts and neutrophils have been observed. Safety and efficacy of I.V. and extended release tablet formulations have not been established in children <16 years of age. Isolated elevations in diastolic blood pressure measurements have been reported in children <4 years of age; however, no observable differences were noted in mean diastolic measurements of children receiving levetiracetam vs placebo. Similar effects have not been observed in older children and adults.

Adverse Reactions

>10%:

Cardiovascular: Increased blood pressure (diastolic; infants and children <4 years: 17%)

Central nervous system: Behavioral problems (including aggression, anger, apathy, depersonalization, hyperkinesias, neurosis: adults 5% to 13%; children 5% to 38%), drowsiness (2% to 23%), headache (14% to 19%), psychotic symptoms (infants and children <4 years: 17%; children 4-16 years: 2%; adults 1%), hostility (2% to 12%), irritability (2% to12%), fatigue (10% to 11%)

Gastrointestinal: Vomiting (children and adolescents 4-16 years: 15%), anorexia (3% to 13%)

Infection: Infection (2% to 13%)

Neuromuscular & skeletal: Weakness (9% to 15%)

Respiratory: Nasopharyngitis (7% to 15%), pharyngitis (6% to 14%), rhinitis (2% to 13%), cough (2% to 11%)

1% to 10%:

Cardiovascular: Facial edema (2%)

Central nervous system: Aggressive behavior (children and adolescents 4-16 years: 10%), nervousness (2% to 10%), dizziness (5% to 9%), personality disorder (8%), pain (6% to 7%), agitation (4% to 6%), emotional lability (2% to 6%), lethargy (children and adolescents 4-16 years: 6%), insomnia (children and adolescents 4-16 years: 5%), depression (2% to 5%), vertigo (3% to 5%), ataxia (3%), falling (children and adolescents 4-16 years: 3%), amnesia (2%), anxiety (2% to 3%), confusion (2%), paranoia (children and adolescents 4-16 years: 2%), paresthesia (2%), sedation (children 2%)

Dermatologic: Bruise (3% to 4%), pruritus (2%), skin discoloration (2%), skin rash (2%)

Endocrine & metabolic: Dehydration (2%)

Gastrointestinal: Upper abdominal pain (children and adolescents 4-16 years: 9%), decreased appetite (children and adolescents 4-16 years: 8%), diarrhea (6% to 8%), nausea (5%), gastroenteritis (2% to 4%), constipation (children and adolescents 4-16 years: 3%)

Genitourinary: Urine abnormality (2%)

Hematologic & oncologic: Eosinophilia (children and adolescents 4-16 years: 8%), decreased white blood cell count (3%)

Infection: Influenza (3% to 8%), viral infection (2%)

Neuromuscular & skeletal: Neck pain (2% to 8%), arthralgia (children and adolescents 4-16 years: 2%), hyperreflexia (2%), sprain (children and adolescents 4-16 years: 2%)

Ophthalmic: Conjunctivitis (2% to 3%), diplopia (2%), amblyopia (2%)

Otic: Otalgia (2%)

Renal: Albuminuria (4%)

Respiratory: Nasal congestion (children and adolescents 4-16 years: 9%), flu-like symptoms (3% to 8%), pharyngolaryngeal pain (children and adolescents 4-16 years: 7%), asthma (2%), sinusitis (2%)

Miscellaneous: Accidental injury (children and adolescents 4-16 years: 2% to 4%)

<1% (Limited to important or life-threatening): Abnormal hepatic function tests, alopecia, anemia, catatonia, choreoathetosis, decreased hematocrit, decreased hemoglobin, decreased red blood cells, dyskinesia, eczema, equilibrium disturbance, erythema multiforme, hepatic failure, hepatitis, leukopenia, neutropenia, pancreatitis, pancytopenia (with bone marrow suppression), psychotic symptoms, Stevens-Johnson syndrome, suicidal ideation, suicidal tendencies, thrombocytopenia, toxic epidermal necrolysis, weight loss

Drug Interactions

Metabolism/Transport Effects None known.

Avoid Concomitant Use

Avoid concomitant use of LevETIRAcetam with any of the following: Azelastine (Nasal); Paraldehyde

Increased Effect/Toxicity

LevETIRAcetam may increase the levels/effects of: Alcohol (Ethyl); Azelastine (Nasal); Buprenorphine; CNS Depressants; Hydrocodone; Methotrimeprazine; Metyrosine; Mirtazapine; Paraldehyde; Pramipexole; ROPINIRole; Rotigotine; Selective Serotonin Reuptake Inhibitors; Zolpidem

The levels/effects of LevETIRAcetam may be increased by: Brimonidine (Topical); Doxylamine; Droperidol; HydrOXYzine; Magnesium Sulfate; Methotrimeprazine; Perampanel; Sodium Oxybate; Tapentadol

Decreased Effect

The levels/effects of LevETIRAcetam may be decreased by: Ketorolac (Nasal); Ketorolac (Systemic); Mefloquine; Orlistat

Ethanol/Nutrition/Herb Interactions

Ethanol: May increase CNS depression; monitor for increased effects with coadministration. Caution patients about effects.

Food: Food may delay, but does not affect the extent of absorption.

Preparation for Administration Vials for injection: Must dilute dose in 100 mL of NS, LR, or D_5W.

Storage/Stability

Oral solution, tablets: Store at 25°C (77°F); excursions permitted to 15°C to 30°C (59°F to 86°F).

Premixed solution for infusion: Store at 20°C to 25°C (68°F to 77°F).

Vials for injection: Store at 25°C (77°F); excursions permitted to 15°C to 30°C (59°F to 86°F). Admixed solution is stable for 24 hours in PVC bags kept at room temperature.

Mechanism of Action The precise mechanism by which levetiracetam exerts its antiepileptic effect is unknown. However, several studies have suggested the mechanism may involve one or more of the following central pharmacologic effects: inhibition of voltage-dependent N-type calcium channels; facilitation of GABA-ergic inhibitory transmission through displacement of negative modulators; reduction of delayed rectifier potassium current; and/or binding to synaptic proteins which modulate neurotransmitter release.

Pharmacodynamics/Kinetics

Absorption: Oral: Rapid and almost complete

Distribution: V_d: Similar to total body water

Protein binding: <10%

Metabolism: Not extensive; primarily by enzymatic hydrolysis; forms metabolites (inactive)

Bioavailability: 100%

Half-life elimination: ~6-8 hours; extended release tablet: ~7 hours; half-life increased in renal dysfunction

Time to peak, plasma: Oral: Immediate release: ~1 hour; Extended release: ~4 hours

Excretion: Urine (66% as unchanged drug)

Dosage

Oral: **Note:** Use oral solution in children ≤20 kg; oral solution or immediate release tablets may be used in children >20 kg.

Children 1 to <6 months: Partial onset seizures: Immediate release: Initial: 7 mg/kg/dose twice daily; may increase every 2 weeks by 7 mg/kg/dose to a maximum of 21 mg/kg/dose twice daily

Children 6 months to <4 years: Partial onset seizures: Immediate release: Initial: 10 mg/kg/dose twice daily; may increase every 2 weeks by 10 mg/kg/dose to a maximum of 25 mg/kg/dose twice daily

Children 4 to <16 years: Partial onset seizures: Immediate release: Initial: 10 mg/kg/dose twice daily; may increase every 2 weeks by 10 mg/kg/dose to a maximum of 30 mg/kg/dose twice daily (maximum daily dose: 3000 mg/day)

Children 6 to <16 years: Tonic-clonic seizures: Immediate release: Initial: 10 mg/kg/dose twice daily; may increase every 2 weeks by 10 mg/kg/dose to the recommended dose of 30 mg/kg twice daily. Efficacy of doses other than 60 mg/kg/day has not been established.

Children ≥12 years and Adults: Myoclonic seizures: Immediate release: Initial: 500 mg twice daily; may increase every 2 weeks by 500 mg/dose to the recommended dose of 1500 mg twice daily. Efficacy of doses other than 3000 mg/day has not been established.

Children ≥16 years and Adults:

Partial onset seizure:

Immediate release: Initial: 500 mg twice daily; may increase every 2 weeks by 500 mg/dose to a maximum of 1500 mg twice daily. Doses >3000 mg/day have been used in trials; however, there is no evidence of increased benefit.

Extended release: Initial: 1000 mg once daily; may increase every 2 weeks by 1000 mg/day to a maximum of 3000 mg once daily.

Tonic-clonic seizures: Immediate release: Initial: 500 mg twice daily; may increase every 2 weeks by 500 mg/dose to the recommended dose of 1500 mg twice daily. Efficacy of doses other than 3000 mg/day has not been established.

Adults: Loading dose (unlabeled): Immediate release: Initial doses of 1500-2000 mg have been well-tolerated (Betts, 2000; Koubeissi, 2008), although the necessity of a loading dose has not been established.

I.V.:

Children ≥16 years and Adults: **Note:** When switching from oral to I.V. formulations, the total daily dose should be the same.

Myoclonic seizures: Initial: 500 mg twice daily; may increase every 2 weeks by 500 mg/dose to the recommended dose of 1500 mg twice daily. Efficacy of doses other than 3000 mg /day has not been established.

Partial onset seizure: Initial: 500 mg twice daily; may increase every 2 weeks by 500 mg/dose to a maximum of 1500 mg twice daily. Doses >3000 mg/day have been used in trials; however, there is no evidence of increased benefit.

Tonic-clonic seizures: Initial: 500 mg twice daily; may increase every 2 weeks by 500 mg/dose to the recommended dose of 1500 mg twice daily. Efficacy of doses other than 3000 mg/day has not been established.

Adults: Refractory status epilepticus (unlabeled use): 1000-3000 mg administered over 15 minutes (Meierkord, 2010); 2500 mg has been safely administered over 5 minutes in one report (Uges, 2009). **Note:** Levetiracetam has not been well studied in comparison to other agents routinely used in this setting.

Dosing adjustment in renal impairment: Adults:

Immediate release and I.V. formulations:

Cl_{cr} >80 mL/minute/1.73 m^2: 500-1500 mg every 12 hours

Cl_{cr} 50-80 mL/minute/1.73 m^2: 500-1000 mg every 12 hours

Cl_{cr} 30-50 mL/minute/1.73 m^2: 250-750 mg every 12 hours

Cl_{cr} <30 mL/minute/1.73 m^2: 250-500 mg every 12 hours

End-stage renal disease (ESRD) requiring hemodialysis: 500-1000 mg every 24 hours; supplemental dose of 250-500 mg is recommended posthemodialysis

Peritoneal dialysis (PD): 500-1000 mg every 24 hours (Aronoff, 2007)

Continuous renal replacement therapy (CRRT): 250-750 mg every 12 hours (Arnoff, 2007)

Extended release tablets:

Cl_{cr} >80 mL/minute/1.73 m^2: 1000-3000 mg every 24 hours

Cl_{cr} 50-80 mL/minute/1.73 m^2: 1000-2000 mg every 24 hours

Cl_{cr} 30-50 mL/minute/1.73 m^2: 500-1500 mg every 24 hours

Cl_{cr} <30 mL/minute/1.73 m^2: 500-1000 mg every 24 hours

End-stage renal disease (ESRD) requiring hemodialysis: Use of immediate release formulation is recommended

Dosing adjustment in hepatic impairment:

U.S. labeling: No dosage adjustment necessary

Canadian labeling:

Mild-to-moderate impairment: No dosage adjustment necessary

Severe impairment: Reduce maintenance dose by 50% in patients who **also** have Cl_{cr} <60 mL/minute/1.73 m^2

Dietary Considerations May be taken without regard to meals.

Administration

I.V.: Infuse over 15 minutes

Oral: May be administered without regard to meals.

Oral solution: Should be administered with a calibrated measuring device (not a household teaspoon or tablespoon)

Tablet (immediate release and extended release): Only administer as whole tablet; do not crush, break or chew.

Monitoring Parameters Suicidality (eg, suicidal thoughts, depression, behavioral changes)

Dosage Forms Excipient information presented when available (limited, particularly for generics); consult specific product labeling.

Solution, Intravenous:

Keppra: 500 mg/5 mL (5 mL)

Generic: 500 mg/100 mL (100 mL); 1000 mg/100 mL (100 mL); 1500 mg/100 mL (100 mL); 500 mg/5 mL (5 mL)

Solution, Intravenous [preservative free]:

Generic: 500 mg/5 mL (5 mL)

Solution, Oral:

Keppra: 100 mg/mL (473 mL) [gluten free, lactose free; contains acesulfame potassium, methylparaben, propylparaben; grape flavor]

Generic: 100 mg/mL (5 mL, 473 mL, 500 mL)

Tablet, Oral:

Keppra: 250 mg [scored; contains fd&c blue #2 (indigotine)]

Keppra: 500 mg [scored]

Keppra: 750 mg [scored; contains fd&c yellow #6 (sunset yellow)]

Keppra: 1000 mg [scored]

Generic: 250 mg, 500 mg, 750 mg, 1000 mg

Tablet Extended Release 24 Hour, Oral:

Keppra XR: 500 mg, 750 mg

Generic: 500 mg, 750 mg

◆ Levitra *see* Vardenafil *on page 2164*

Levobunolol (lee voe BYOO noe lole)

Brand Names: U.S. Betagan

Brand Names: Canada Apo-Levobunolol®; Betagan®; Novo-Levobunolol; PMS-Levobunolol; Ratio-Levobunolol; Sandoz-Levobunolol

Index Terms *l*-Bunolol Hydrochloride; Levobunolol Hydrochloride

Pharmacologic Category Beta-Adrenergic Blocker, Nonselective; Ophthalmic Agent, Antiglaucoma

Use To lower intraocular pressure in chronic open-angle glaucoma or ocular hypertension

Pregnancy Risk Factor C

Dosage Glaucoma (open-angle, chronic), intraocular hypertension: Adults: Ophthalmic:

0.25% solution: Instill 1-2 drops into affected eye(s) twice daily

0.5% solution: Instill 1-2 drops into affected eye(s) once daily; may increase to 1 drop twice daily in patients with severe or uncontrolled glaucoma; Maximum dose: Doses >1 drop twice daily (0.5%) are generally not more effective.

Dosage adjustment in renal impairment: No dosage adjustment provided in manufacturer's labeling.

Dosage adjustment in hepatic impairment: No dosage adjustment provided in manufacturer's labeling.

Additional Information Complete prescribing information should be consulted for additional detail.

Dosage Forms Excipient information presented when available (limited, particularly for generics); consult specific product labeling.

Solution, Ophthalmic, as hydrochloride:

Betagan: 0.5% (5 mL, 10 mL, 15 mL)

Generic: 0.25% (5 mL, 10 mL); 0.5% (5 mL, 10 mL, 15 mL)

◆ Levobunolol Hydrochloride *see* Levobunolol *on page 1196*

◆ Levocarb CR (Can) *see* Carbidopa and Levodopa *on page 340*

Levocetirizine (LEE vo se TI ra zeen)

Brand Names: U.S. Xyzal

Index Terms Levocetirizine Dihydrochloride

Pharmacologic Category Histamine H_1 Antagonist; Histamine H_1 Antagonist, Second Generation; Piperazine Derivative

Use Relief of symptoms of perennial and seasonal allergic rhinitis; treatment of skin manifestations (uncomplicated) of chronic idiopathic urticaria

Pregnancy Risk Factor B

Dosage Oral:

Perennial allergic rhinitis, chronic urticaria:

Children 6 months to 5 years: 1.25 mg once daily (in the evening); maximum: 1.25 mg

Children 6-11 years: 2.5 mg once daily (in the evening); maximum: 2.5 mg/day

Children ≥12 years and Adults: 5 mg once daily (in the evening); some patients may experience relief of symptoms with 2.5 mg once daily

Seasonal allergic rhinitis:

Children 2-5 years: 1.25 mg once daily (in the evening); maximum: 1.25 mg

Children 6-11 years: 2.5 mg once daily (in the evening); maximum: 2.5 mg/day

Children ≥12 years and Adults: 5 mg once daily (in the evening); some patients may experience relief of symptoms with 2.5 mg once daily

Elderly: Refer to adult dosing; dosing should begin at the lower end of the dosing range

Dosage adjustments in renal impairment:

Children 6 months to 11 years with renal impairment: Contraindicated

Children ≥12 and Adults:

Cl_{cr} 50-80 mL/minute: 2.5 mg once daily

Cl_{cr} 30-50 mL/minute: 2.5 mg once every other day

Cl_{cr} 10-30 mL/minute: 2.5 mg twice weekly (every 3 or 4 days)

Cl_{cr} <10 mL/minute, hemodialysis patients: Contraindicated

Dosage adjustments in hepatic impairment: No adjustment required.

Additional Information Complete prescribing information should be consulted for additional detail.

Dosage Forms Excipient information presented when available (limited, particularly for generics); consult specific product labeling.

Solution, Oral, as dihydrochloride:

Xyzal: 2.5 mg/5 mL (148 mL) [contains methylparaben, propylparaben, saccharin]

Generic: 2.5 mg/5 mL (148 mL)

Tablet, Oral, as dihydrochloride:

Xyzal: 5 mg [scored]

Generic: 5 mg

◆ Levocetirizine Dihydrochloride *see* Levocetirizine *on page 1197*

◆ Levodopa and Carbidopa *see* Carbidopa and Levodopa *on page 340*

Levodopa, Carbidopa, and Entacapone

(lee voe DOE pa, kar bi DOE pa, & en TA ka pone)

Brand Names: U.S. Stalevo®

Brand Names: Canada Stalevo®

Index Terms Carbidopa, Entacapone, and Levodopa; Carbidopa, Levodopa, and Entacapone; Entacapone, Carbidopa, and Levodopa

Pharmacologic Category Anti-Parkinson's Agent, COMT Inhibitor; Anti-Parkinson's Agent, Decarboxylase Inhibitor; Anti-Parkinson's Agent, Dopamine Precursor

Additional Appendix Information

Antiparkinsonian Agents *on page 2289*

Use Treatment of idiopathic Parkinson's disease

Pregnancy Risk Factor C

Dosage Oral: Adults: Parkinson's disease:

Note: All strengths of Stalevo® contain a carbidopa/levodopa ratio of 1:4 plus entacapone 200 mg.

Dose should be individualized based on therapeutic response; doses may be adjusted by changing strength or adjusting interval. Fractionated doses are not recommended and only 1 tablet should be given at each dosing interval; maximum daily dose: 8 tablets of Stalevo® 50, 75, 100, 125, or 150, **or** 6 tablets of Stalevo® 200.

Patients previously treated with carbidopa/levodopa immediate release tablets (ratio of 1:4):

With current entacapone therapy: May switch directly to corresponding strength of combination tablet. No data available on transferring patients from controlled release preparations or products with a 1:10 ratio of carbidopa/levodopa.

Without entacapone therapy:

If current levodopa dose is >600 mg/day: Levodopa dose reduction may be required when adding entacapone to therapy; therefore, titrate dose using individual products first (carbidopa/levodopa immediate release with a ratio of 1:4 plus entacapone 200 mg); then transfer to combination product once stabilized.

If current levodopa dose is <600 mg without dyskinesias: May transfer to corresponding dose of combination product; monitor, dose reduction of levodopa may be required.

Patients previously treated with benserazide/levodopa immediate release tablets (Canadian labeling, not in U.S. labeling): With current entacapone therapy: Prior to switching to combination product (carbidopa/levodopa/entacapone), withhold treatment for 1 night, then initiate (carbidopa/levodopa/entacapone) therapy the following morning at a dose that provides either an equivalent amount or ~5% to 10% more levodopa.

Dosage adjustment in renal impairment: No dosage adjustment provided in manufacturer's labeling (has not been studied); use caution with severe renal impairment.

Dosage adjustment in hepatic impairment: No dosage adjustment provided in manufacturer's labeling (has not been studied); use with caution in biliary obstruction or hepatic disease.

Additional Information Complete prescribing information should be consulted for additional detail.

Dosage Forms Excipient information presented when available (limited, particularly for generics); consult specific product labeling.

Tablet:

Stalevo® 50: Levodopa 50 mg, carbidopa 12.5 mg, and entacapone 200 mg

Stalevo® 75: Levodopa 75 mg, carbidopa 18.75 mg, and entacapone 200 mg

Stalevo® 100: Levodopa 100 mg, carbidopa 25 mg, and entacapone 200 mg

Stalevo® 125: Levodopa 125 mg, carbidopa 31.25 mg, and entacapone 200 mg

Stalevo® 150: Levodopa 150 mg, carbidopa 37.5 mg, and entacapone 200 mg

Stalevo® 200: Levodopa 200 mg, carbidopa 50 mg, and entacapone 200 mg

Generic: Levodopa 50 mg, carbidopa 12.5 mg, and entacapone 200 mg; Levodopa 75 mg, carbidopa 18.75 mg, and entacapone 200 mg; Levodopa 100 mg, carbidopa 25 mg, and entacapone 200 mg; Levodopa 125 mg, carbidopa 31.25 mg, and entacapone 200 mg; Levodopa 150 mg, carbidopa 37.5 mg, and entacapone 200 mg; Levodopa 200 mg, carbidopa 50 mg, and entacapone 200 mg

◆ Levo-Dromoran *see* Levorphanol *on page 1205*

Levofloxacin (Systemic) (lee voe FLOKS a sin)

Brand Names: U.S. Levaquin

Brand Names: Canada APO-Levofloxacin; AVA-Levofloxacin; CO Levofloxacin; Levaquin®; Mylan-Levofloxacin; Novo-Levofloxacin; PMS-Levofloxacin; Sandoz-Levofloxacin

Pharmacologic Category Antibiotic, Fluoroquinolone; Antibiotic, Respiratory Fluoroquinolone

Additional Appendix Information

Antibiotic Treatment of Adults With Infective Endocarditis *on page 2355*

Use Treatment of community-acquired pneumonia, including multidrug resistant strains of *S. pneumoniae* (MDRSP); nosocomial pneumonia; chronic bronchitis (acute bacterial exacerbation); acute bacterial rhinosinusitis (ABRS); prostatitis (chronic bacterial), urinary tract infection (uncomplicated or complicated); acute pyelonephritis; skin or skin structure infections (uncomplicated or complicated); reduce incidence or disease progression of inhalational anthrax (postexposure); prophylaxis and treatment of plague (pneumonic and septicemic) due to *Y. pestis*

Unlabeled Use Diverticulitis, enterocolitis (*Shigella* spp), epididymitis (nongonococcal), urethritis (nongonococcal), complicated intra-abdominal infections (in combination with metronidazole), Legionnaires' disease, peritonitis, PID (alternative therapy); traveler's diarrhea; oral phase treatment of prosthetic joint infection

Note: As of April 2007, the CDC no longer recommends the use of fluoroquinolones for the treatment of gonococcal disease due to increased prevalence of fluoroquinolone-resistant *Neisseria gonorrhoeae*.

Pregnancy Risk Factor C

Pregnancy Considerations Adverse events have been observed in some animal studies; therefore, the manufacturer classifies levofloxacin as pregnancy category C. Levofloxacin crosses the placenta. Quinolone exposure during human pregnancy has been reported with other agents (see Ciprofloxacin [Systemic], Ofloxacin [Systemic], and Norfloxacin monographs). To date, no specific teratogenic effect or increased pregnancy risk has been identified; however, because of concerns of cartilage damage in immature animals exposed to quinolones and the limited levofloxacin specific data, levofloxacin should only be used during pregnancy if a safer option is not available.

Breast-Feeding Considerations Based on data from a case report, small amounts of levofloxacin are excreted in breast milk. Breast-feeding is not recommended by the manufacturer. Levofloxacin is the L-isomer of ofloxacin. Ofloxacin has also been shown to have minimal concentrations in human milk. Nondose-related effects could include modification of bowel flora.

Medication Guide Available Yes

Contraindications Hypersensitivity to levofloxacin, any component of the formulation, or other quinolones

Canadian labeling: Additional contraindications (not in U.S. labeling): History of tendonitis or tendon rupture associated with use of any quinolone antimicrobial agent

Warnings/Precautions **[U.S. Boxed Warning]: There have been reports of tendon inflammation and/or rupture with quinolone antibiotics; risk may be increased with concurrent corticosteroids, organ transplant recipients, and in patients >60 years of age.** Rupture of the Achilles tendon sometimes requiring surgical repair has been reported most frequently; but other tendon sites (eg, rotator cuff, biceps) have also been reported. Strenuous physical activity, rheumatoid arthritis, and renal impairment may be an independent risk factor for tendonitis. Discontinue at first sign of tendon inflammation or pain. May occur even after discontinuation of therapy. Use with caution in patients with rheumatoid arthritis; may increase risk of tendon rupture. Safety of use in pediatric patients for >14 days of therapy has not been studied; increased incidence of musculoskeletal disorders (eg, arthralgia, tendon rupture) has been observed in children. CNS effects may occur (toxic psychoses, tremor, restlessness, anxiety, lightheadedness, paranoia, depression, nightmares, confusion, and very rarely hallucinations increased intracranial pressure (including pseudotumor cerebri, seizures, or toxic psychosis). Potential for seizures, although very rare, may be increased with concomitant NSAID therapy. Use with caution in individuals at risk of seizures, with known or suspected CNS disorders or renal dysfunction. Avoid excessive sunlight and take precautions to limit exposure (eg, loose fitting clothing, sunscreen); may cause moderate-to-severe phototoxicity reactions. Discontinue use if photosensitivity occurs.

Rare cases of torsade de pointes have been reported in patients receiving levofloxacin. Use caution in patients with known prolongation of QT interval, bradycardia, hypokalemia, hypomagnesemia, or in those receiving concurrent therapy with Class Ia or Class III antiarrhythmics.

Severe hypersensitivity reactions, including anaphylaxis, have occurred with quinolone therapy. Reactions may present as typical allergic symptoms after a single dose, or may manifest as severe idiosyncratic dermatologic, vascular, pulmonary, renal, hepatic, and/or hematologic events, usually after multiple doses. Prompt discontinuation of drug should occur if skin rash or other symptoms arise. Prolonged use may result in fungal or bacterial superinfection, including *C. difficile*-associated diarrhea (CDAD) and pseudomembranous colitis; CDAD has been observed >2 months postantibiotic treatment. Peripheral neuropathy has been reported (rare); may occur soon after initiation of therapy and may be irreversible; discontinue if symptoms of sensory or sensorimotor neuropathy occur. **[U.S. Boxed Warning]: Quinolones may exacerbate myasthenia gravis; avoid use (rare, potentially life-threatening weakness of respiratory muscles may occur).** Unrelated to hypersensitivity, severe hepatotoxicity (including acute hepatitis and fatalities) has been reported. Elderly patients may be at greater risk. Discontinue therapy immediately if signs and symptoms of hepatitis occur. Hemolytic reactions may (rarely) occur with quinolone use in patients with latent or actual G6PD deficiency.

Fluoroquinolones have been associated with the development of serious, and sometimes fatal, hypoglycemia, most often in elderly diabetics, but also in patients without diabetes. This occurred most frequently with gatifloxacin (no longer available systemically) but may occur at a lower frequency with other quinolones.

Adverse Reactions

1% to 10%:

Cardiovascular: Chest pain (1%), edema (1%)

Central nervous system: Headache (6%), insomnia (4%), dizziness (3%)

Dermatologic: Rash (2%), pruritus (1%)

Gastrointestinal: Nausea (7%), diarrhea (5%), constipation (3%), abdominal pain (2%), dyspepsia (2%), vomiting (2%)

Genitourinary: Vaginitis (1%)

Local: Injection site reaction (1%)

Respiratory: Dyspnea (1%)

Miscellaneous: Moniliasis (1%)

<1% (Limited to important or life-threatening): Abnormal taste, acute renal failure, agitation, agranulocytosis, alkaline phosphatase increased, altered sense of smell, allergic reaction (including anaphylaxis, angioedema, rash, pneumonitis, and serum sickness); anaphylactoid

reaction, anemia (including aplastic and hemolytic) anorexia, anxiety, arrhythmia (including ventricular tachycardia/fibrillation and torsade de pointes), arthralgia, bronchospasm, cardiac arrest, *C. difficile*-associated diarrhea (CDAD), confusion, depression, dysphonia, EEG abnormalities, encephalopathy (rare), eosinophilia, epistaxis, erythema multiforme, esophagitis, fever, gait abnormal, gastritis (including gastroenteritis), glossitis, granulocytopenia, hallucination, hepatic failure (some fatal), hepatic function abnormal, hepatitis, hyper-/hypoglycemia, hyperkalemia, hyperkinesias, hyper-/hypotension, hypertonia, hypoacusis, INR increased, intestinal obstruction, intracranial pressure increased, involuntary muscle contractions, jaundice, leukocytosis, leukopenia, leukorrhea, loss of taste perception, lymphadenopathy, multiple organ failure, muscle injury, myalgia, myasthenia gravis exacerbation, nephritis (interstitial), palpitation, pancreatitis, pancytopenia, paralysis, paranoia, paresthesia, peripheral neuropathy, phlebitis,photosensitivity/phototoxicity, pneumonitis, prothrombin time increased, pseudotumor cerebri, psychosis, QT_c prolongation, renal function abnormal, rhabdomyolysis, seizure, skeletal pain, skin disorder, sleep disorders (including abnormal dreams and nightmares) somnolence, Stevens-Johnson syndrome, stomatitis, suicide attempt/ideation, syncope, tachycardia, tendonitis, tendon rupture, tinnitus, toxic epidermal necrolysis, transaminases increased, thrombocytopenia, tremor, urticaria, vasculitis (leukocytoclastic), vasodilatation, vertigo, visual disturbances

Drug Interactions

Metabolism/Transport Effects None known.

Avoid Concomitant Use

Avoid concomitant use of Levofloxacin (Systemic) with any of the following: BCG; Highest Risk QTc-Prolonging Agents; Ivabradine; Mifepristone; Strontium Ranelate

Increased Effect/Toxicity

Levofloxacin (Systemic) may increase the levels/effects of: Corticosteroids (Systemic); Highest Risk QTc-Prolonging Agents; Moderate Risk QTc-Prolonging Agents; Porfimer; Sulfonylureas; Tacrolimus (Systemic); Varenicline; Vitamin K Antagonists

The levels/effects of Levofloxacin (Systemic) may be increased by: Insulin; Ivabradine; Mifepristone; Nonsteroidal Anti-Inflammatory Agents; Probenecid; QTc-Prolonging Agents (Indeterminate Risk and Risk Modifying)

Decreased Effect

Levofloxacin (Systemic) may decrease the levels/effects of: BCG; Didanosine; Mycophenolate; Sodium Picosulfate; Sulfonylureas; Typhoid Vaccine

The levels/effects of Levofloxacin (Systemic) may be decreased by: Antacids; Calcium Salts; Didanosine; Iron Salts; Lanthanum; Magnesium Salts; Multivitamins/Minerals (with ADEK, Folate, Iron); Multivitamins/Minerals (with AE, No Iron); Quinapril; Sevelamer; Strontium Ranelate; Sucralfate; Zinc Salts

Preparation for Administration Solution for injection: Single-use vials must be further diluted in compatible solution to a final concentration of 5 mg/mL prior to infusion.

Storage/Stability

Solution for injection:

Vial: Store at room temperature. Protect from light. Diluted solution (5 mg/mL) is stable for 72 hours when stored at room temperature; stable for 14 days when stored under refrigeration. When frozen, stable for 6 months; do not refreeze. Do not thaw in microwave or by bath immersion.

Premixed: Store at ≤25°C (77°F); do not freeze. Brief exposure to 40°C (104°F) does not affect product. Protect from light.

Tablet, oral solution: Store at 25°C (77°F); excursions permitted to 15°C to 30°C (59°F to 86°F).

Mechanism of Action As the S(-) enantiomer of the fluoroquinolone, ofloxacin, levofloxacin, inhibits DNA-gyrase in susceptible organisms thereby inhibits relaxation of supercoiled DNA and promotes breakage of DNA strands. DNA gyrase (topoisomerase II), is an essential bacterial enzyme that maintains the superhelical structure of DNA and is required for DNA replication and transcription, DNA repair, recombination, and transposition.

Pharmacodynamics/Kinetics

Absorption: Rapid and complete

Distribution: V_d: 74-112 L; CSF concentrations ~15% of serum levels; high concentrations are achieved in prostate, lung, and gynecological tissues, sinus, saliva

Protein binding: ~24% to 38%; primarily to albumin

Metabolism: Minimally hepatic

Bioavailability: ~99%

Half-life elimination: ~6-8 hours

Time to peak, serum: Oral: 1-2 hours

Excretion: Urine (~87% as unchanged drug, <5% as metabolites); feces (<4%)

Dosage Note: Sequential therapy (intravenous to oral) may be instituted based on prescriber's discretion.

Usual dosage range: Adults: Oral, I.V.: 250-500 mg every 24 hours; severe or complicated infections: 750 mg every 24 hours

Indication-specific dosing:

Infants ≥6 months and Children ≤4 years:

Community-acquired pneumonia (CAP) (IDSA/PIDS, 2011): Note: May consider addition of vancomycin or clindamycin to empiric therapy if community-acquired MRSA suspected; alternative to ceftriaxone or cefotaxime in patients not fully immunized for *H. influenzae* type b and *S. pneumoniae*, or significant local resistance to penicillin in invasive pneumococcal strains.

S. pneumoniae (MICs to penicillin ≤2.0 mcg/mL), mild infection or step-down therapy (alternative to amoxicillin): Oral: 8-10 mg/kg/dose every 12 hours (maximum: 750 mg daily)

S. pneumoniae (MICs to penicillin ≥4.0 mcg/mL):

Moderate-to-severe infection (alternative to ceftriaxone): I.V.: 8-10 mg/kg/dose every 12 hours (maximum: 750 mg daily)

Mild infection, step-down therapy (preferred): Oral: 8-10 mg/kg/dose every 12 hours (maximum: 750 mg daily)

H. influenzae, moderate-to-severe infection (alternative to ampicillin, ceftriaxone, or cefotaxime): I.V.: 8-10 mg/kg/dose every 12 hours (maximum: 750 mg daily)

Atypical pathogens, moderate-to-severe infection (alternative to azithromycin) or empiric treatment (alternative to azithromycin +/- beta-lactam; should be limited to macrolide allergic/intolerant patients): Oral, I.V.: 8-10 mg/kg/dose every 12 hours (maximum: 750 mg daily)

Infants ≥6 months, Children, and Adults: Oral, I.V.:

Anthrax (inhalational, postexposure):

≤50 kg: 8 mg/kg every 12 hours for 60 days (do not exceed 250 mg/dose), beginning as soon as possible after exposure

>50 kg and Adults: 500 mg every 24 hours for 60 days, beginning as soon as possible after exposure

Plague (prophylaxis and treatment):

≤50 kg: 8 mg/kg every 12 hours for 10-14 days (do not exceed 250 mg/dose), beginning as soon as possible after exposure

>50 kg and Adults: 500 mg every 24 hours for 10-14 days, beginning as soon as possible after exposure. **Note:** Dose of 750 mg once daily may be considered if clinically warranted.

Children:

Acute bacterial rhinosinusitis (unlabeled use): Oral, I.V.: 10-20 mg/kg/day divided every 12-24 hours for 10-14 days (maximum: 500 mg daily). **Note:** Recommended in patients with a type I penicillin allergy, after failure of initial therapy or in patients at risk for antibiotic resistance (eg, daycare attendance, age <2 years, recent hospitalization, antibiotic use within the past month) (Chow, 2012).

Children 5-16 years:

Community-acquired pneumonia (CAP) (IDSA/PIDS, 2011): Note: May consider addition of vancomycin or clindamycin to empiric therapy if community-acquired MRSA suspected; alternative to ceftriaxone or cefotaxime in patients not fully immunized for *H. influenzae* type b and *S. pneumoniae*, or significant local resistance to penicillin in invasive pneumococcal strains.

S. pneumoniae (MICs to penicillin ≤2.0 mcg/mL), mild infection or step-down therapy (alternative to amoxicillin): Oral: 8-10 mg/kg/dose once daily (maximum: 750 mg daily)

S. pneumoniae (MICs to penicillin ≥4.0 mcg/mL):

Moderate-to-severe infection (alternative to ceftriaxone): I.V.: 8-10 mg/kg/dose once daily (maximum: 750 mg daily)

Mild infection, step-down therapy (preferred): Oral: 8-10 mg/kg/dose once daily (maximum: 750 mg daily)

H. influenzae, moderate-to-severe infection (alternative to ampicillin, ceftriaxone, or cefotaxime): I.V.: 8-10 mg/kg/dose once daily (maximum: 750 mg daily)

Atypical pathogens:

Moderate-to-severe infection (alternative to azithromycin): I.V.: 8-10 mg/kg/dose once daily (maximum: 750 mg daily)

Mild infection, step-down therapy (alternative to azithromycin in adolescents with skeletal maturity): Oral: 500 mg once daily

Adults: Oral, I.V.:

Acute bacterial rhinosinusitis:

Manufacturer's recommendations: 750 mg every 24 hours for 5 days or 500 mg every 24 hours for 10-14 days

Alternate recommendations: 500 mg every 24 hours for 5-7 days (Chow, 2012)

***Chlamydia trachomatis* sexually-transmitted infections (unlabeled use) (CDC, 2010):** Oral: 500 mg every 24 hours for 7 days

Chronic bronchitis (acute bacterial exacerbation): Oral: 500 mg every 24 hours for 7 days; Canadian labeling (not in U.S. labeling) also includes a dosage regimen of 750 mg every 24 hours for 5 days

Diverticulitis, peritonitis (unlabeled use) (Solomkin, [IDSA] 2010): 750 mg every 24 hours for 7-10 days; use adjunctive metronidazole therapy

Epididymitis, nongonococcal (unlabeled use) (CDC, 2010): Oral: 500 mg once daily for 10 days

Gonococcal infection (unlabeled use) (CDC, 2010): As of April 2007, the CDC no longer recommends the use of fluoroquinolones for the treatment of uncomplicated or more serious gonococcal disease, unless no other options exist and susceptibility can be confirmed via culture.

Intra-abdominal infection, complicated, community-acquired (in combination with metronidazole) (unlabeled use) (Solomkin, [IDSA] 2010): I.V.: 750 mg once daily for 4-7 days (provided source controlled). **Note:** Avoid using in settings where *E. coli* susceptibility to fluoroquinolones is <90%.

Pelvic inflammatory disease (unlabeled use) (CDC, 2010): Oral: 500 mg once daily for 14 days with or without concomitant metronidazole; **Note:** The CDC recommends use as an alternative therapy only if standard parenteral cephalosporin therapy is not feasible and community prevalence of quinolone-resistant gonococcal organisms is low. Culture sensitivity must be confirmed.

Pneumonia:

Community-acquired (CAP): 500 mg every 24 hours for 7-14 days or 750 mg every 24 hours for 5 days (efficacy of 5-day regimen for MDRSP not established)

Healthcare-associated (HAP): 750 mg every 24 hours for 7-14 days

Prostatitis (chronic bacterial): Oral: 500 mg every 24 hours for 28 days

Skin and skin structure infections:

Uncomplicated: 500 mg every 24 hours for 7-10 days

Complicated: 750 mg every 24 hours for 7-14 days

Traveler's diarrhea (unlabeled use): Oral: 500 mg for one dose (Sanders, 2007)

Tuberculosis, drug-resistant tuberculosis, or intolerance to first-line agents (unlabeled use): Oral: 500-1000 mg every 24 hours (CDC, 2003)

Urethritis, nongonococcal (unlabeled use) (CDC, 2010): Oral: 500 mg every 24 hours for 7 days

Urinary tract infections:

Uncomplicated: 250 mg once daily for 3 days

Complicated, including pyelonephritis: 250 mg once daily for 10 days **or** 750 mg once daily for 5 days

Dosage adjustment in renal impairment: I.V., Oral:

Normal renal function dosing of 750 mg daily:

Cl_{cr} 20-49 mL/minute: Administer 750 mg every 48 hours

Cl_{cr} 10-19 mL/minute: Administer 750 mg initial dose, followed by 500 mg every 48 hours

Hemodialysis/chronic ambulatory peritoneal dialysis (CAPD): Administer 750 mg initial dose, followed by 500 mg every 48 hours; supplemental doses are not required following either hemodialysis or CAPD.

Normal renal function dosing of 500 mg daily:

Cl_{cr} 20-49 mL/minute: Administer 500 mg initial dose, followed by 250 mg every 24 hours

Cl_{cr} 10-19 mL/minute: Administer 500 mg initial dose, followed by 250 mg every 48 hours

Hemodialysis/chronic ambulatory peritoneal dialysis (CAPD): Administer 500 mg initial dose, followed by 250 mg every 48 hours; supplemental doses are not required following either hemodialysis or CAPD.

Normal renal function dosing of 250 mg daily:

Cl_{cr} 20-49 mL/minute: No dosage adjustment required

Cl_{cr} 10-19 mL/minute: Administer 250 mg every 48 hours (except in uncomplicated UTI, where no dosage adjustment is required)

Hemodialysis/chronic ambulatory peritoneal dialysis (CAPD): No information available

Continuous renal replacement therapy (CRRT) (Heintz, 2009; Trotman, 2005): Drug clearance is highly dependent on the method of renal replacement, filter type, and flow rate. Appropriate dosing requires close monitoring of pharmacologic response, signs of adverse reactions due to drug accumulation, as well as drug concentrations in relation to target trough (if appropriate). The following are general recommendations only (based on dialysate flow/ultrafiltration rates of 1-2 L/hour and minimal residual renal function) and should not supersede clinical judgment:

CVVH: Loading dose of 500-750 mg followed by 250 mg every 24 hours

CVVHD: Loading dose of 500-750 mg followed by 250-500 mg every 24 hours

CVVHDF: Loading dose of 500-750 mg followed by 250-750 mg every 24 hours

Dosage adjustment in hepatic impairment: I.V., Oral: No dosage adjustment provided in manufacturer's labeling (has not been studied). However, dosage adjustment unlikely due to limited hepatic metabolism.

Dietary Considerations Tablets may be taken without regard to meals. Oral solution should be administered on an empty stomach (1 hour before or 2 hours after a meal). Take 2 hours before or 2 hours after multiple vitamins, antacids, or other products containing magnesium, aluminum, iron, or zinc.

Administration

Oral: Tablets may be administered without regard to meals. Oral solution should be administered 1 hour before or 2 hours after meals. Maintain adequate hydration of patient to prevent crystalluria.

I.V.: Infuse 250-500 mg I.V. solution over 60 minutes; infuse 750 mg I.V. solution over 90 minutes. Too rapid of infusion can lead to hypotension. Avoid administration through an intravenous line with a solution containing multivalent cations (eg, magnesium, calcium). Maintain adequate hydration of patient to prevent crystalluria or cylindruria.

Monitoring Parameters Evaluation of organ system functions (renal, hepatic, and hematopoietic) is recommended periodically during therapy; the possibility of crystalluria should be assessed; WBC and signs of infection

Test Interactions Some quinolones may produce a false-positive urine screening result for opioids using commercially-available immunoassay kits. This has been demonstrated most consistently for levofloxacin and ofloxacin, but other quinolones have shown cross-reactivity in certain assay kits. Confirmation of positive opioid screens by more specific methods should be considered.

Dosage Forms Excipient information presented when available (limited, particularly for generics); consult specific product labeling.

Solution, Intravenous [preservative free]:

Levaquin: 250 mg/50 mL (50 mL); 500 mg/100 mL (100 mL); 750 mg/150 mL (150 mL)

Generic: 250 mg/50 mL (50 mL); 500 mg/100 mL (100 mL); 750 mg/150 mL (150 mL); 25 mg/mL (20 mL, 30 mL)

Solution, Oral:

Levaquin: 25 mg/mL (480 mL) [contains propylene glycol]

Generic: 25 mg/mL (10 mL, 20 mL, 100 mL, 200 mL, 480 mL)

Tablet, Oral:

Levaquin: 250 mg, 500 mg, 750 mg

Generic: 250 mg, 500 mg, 750 mg

Extemporaneous Preparations Note: Commercial oral solution is available (25 mg/mL)

A 50 mg/mL oral suspension may be made with tablets and a 1:1 mixture of Ora-Plus® and strawberry syrup NF. Crush six 500 mg levofloxacin tablets in a mortar and reduce to a fine powder. Add small portions of the vehicle and mix to a uniform paste; mix while adding the vehicle in incremental proportions to **almost** 60 mL; transfer to a graduated cylinder, rinse mortar with vehicle, and add quantity of vehicle sufficient to make 60 mL. Label "shake well". Stable for 57 days when stored in amber plastic prescription bottles at room temperature or refrigerated.

VandenBussche HL, Johnson CE, and Fontana EM, et al, "Stability of Levofloxacin in an Extemporaneously Compounded Oral Liquid," *Am J Health Syst Pharm*, 1999, 56(22):2316-8.

Levofloxacin (Ophthalmic) (lee voe FLOKS a sin)

Pharmacologic Category Antibiotic, Fluoroquinolone; Antibiotic, Ophthalmic

Use Treatment of bacterial conjunctivitis caused by susceptible organisms (Quixin® 0.5% ophthalmic solution); treatment of corneal ulcer caused by susceptible organisms (Iquix® 1.5% ophthalmic solution)

Pregnancy Risk Factor C

Dosage

Ophthalmic:

Usual dosage range:

Children ≥1 year: 1-2 drops every 2-6 hours

Adults: 1-2 drops every 2-6 hours

Indication-specific dosing:

Children ≥1 year and Adults:

Conjunctivitis (0.5% ophthalmic solution):

Treatment day 1 and day 2: Instill 1-2 drops into affected eye(s) every 2 hours while awake, up to 8 times/day

Treatment day 3 through day 7: Instill 1-2 drops into affected eye(s) every 4 hours while awake, up to 4 times/day

Children ≥6 years and Adults:

Corneal ulceration (1.5% ophthalmic solution):

Treatment day 1 through day 3: Instill 1-2 drops into affected eye(s) every 30 minutes to 2 hours while awake and 4-6 hours after retiring

Treatment day 4 through completion: Instill 1-2 drops into affected eye(s) every 1-4 hours while awake

Dosage adjustment in renal impairment: No dosage adjustment provided in manufacturer's labeling. However, dosage adjustment unlikely due to low systemic absorption.

Dosage adjustment in hepatic impairment: No dosage adjustment provided in manufacturer's labeling. However, dosage adjustment unlikely due to low systemic absorption.

Additional Information Complete prescribing information should be consulted for additional detail.

Dosage Forms Excipient information presented when available (limited, particularly for generics); consult specific product labeling.

Solution, Ophthalmic:

Generic: 0.5% (5 mL)

◆ Levo-folinic Acid *see* LEVOleucovorin *on page 1201*

LEVOleucovorin (lee voe loo koe VOR in)

Brand Names: U.S. Fusilev

Index Terms 6S-leucovorin; Calcium Levoleucovorin; L-leucovorin; Levo-folinic Acid; Levo-leucovorin; Levoleucovorin Calcium Pentahydrate; S-leucovorin

Pharmacologic Category Antidote; Chemotherapy Modulating Agent; Rescue Agent (Chemotherapy)

Use Treatment of advanced, metastatic colorectal cancer (palliative) in combination with fluorouracil; rescue agent after high-dose methotrexate therapy in osteosarcoma; antidote for impaired methotrexate elimination and for inadvertent overdosage of folic acid antagonists

Pregnancy Risk Factor C

Dosage Note: Levoleucovorin, when substituted in place of leucovorin calcium (the racemic form), is dosed at **one-half** the usual dose of leucovorin calcium:

Colorectal cancer: Adults I.V.: The following regimens have been used (in combination with fluorouracil; fluorouracil doses may need to be adjusted for toxicity; no adjustment required for the levoleucovorin dose):

100 mg/m^2/day over at least 3 minutes (followed by fluorouracil 370 mg/m^2/day) for 5 days every 4 weeks ▶

for 2 cycles, then every 4-5 weeks depending on recovery from toxicities, **or**

10 mg /m²/day (followed by fluorouracil 425 mg/m²/day) for 5 days every 4 weeks for 2 cycles, then every 4-5 weeks depending on recovery from toxicities, **or**

Alternative dosing: Levoleucovorin, when substituted in place of leucovorin calcium within a chemotherapy regimen, is dosed at **one-half** the usual dose of leucovorin calcium (Goldberg, 1997; NCCN colon cancer guidelines v.2.2013)

High-dose methotrexate rescue: Children and Adults: I.V.: Usual dose: 7.5 mg (~5 mg/m²) every 6 hours for 10 doses, beginning 24 hours after the start of the methotrexate infusion (based on a methotrexate dose of 12 g/m² I.V. over 4 hours). Levoleucovorin (and hydration and urinary alkalinization) should be continued and/or adjusted until the methotrexate level is <0.05 micromolar (5 x 10^{-8} M) as follows:

Normal methotrexate elimination (serum methotrexate levels ~10 micromolar at 24 hours post administration, 1 micromolar at 48 hours and <0.2 micromolar at 72 hours post infusion): 7.5 mg I.V. every 6 hours for 10 doses

Delayed late methotrexate elimination (serum methotrexate levels >0.2 micromolar at 72 hours and >0.05 micromolar at 96 hours post methotrexate infusion): Continue 7.5 mg I.V. every 6 hours until methotrexate level is <0.05 micromolar

Delayed early methotrexate elimination and/or evidence of acute renal injury (serum methotrexate level ≥50 micromolar at 24 hours, ≥5 micromolar at 48 hours or a doubling or more of the serum creatinine level at 24 hours post methotrexate infusion): 75 mg I.V. every 3 hours until methotrexate level is <1 micromolar, followed by 7.5 mg I.V. every 3 hours until methotrexate level is <0.05 micromolar

Significant clinical toxicity in the presence of less severe abnormalities in methotrexate elimination or renal function (as described above): Extend levoleucovorin treatment for an additional 24 hours (total of 14 doses) in subsequent treatment cycles.

Delayed methotrexate elimination due to third space fluid accumulation, renal insufficiency, or inadequate hydration: May require higher levoleucovorin doses or prolonged administration.

Methotrexate overdose (inadvertent): Children and Adults: I.V.: 7.5 mg (~5 mg/m²) every 6 hours; continue until the methotrexate level is <0.01 micromolar (10^{-8} M). Initiate treatment as soon as possible after methotrexate overdose. Increase the levoleucovorin dose to 50 mg/m² I.V. every 3 hours if the 24 hour serum creatinine has increased 50% over baseline, or if the 24-hour methotrexate level is >5 micromolar (5 x 10^{-6} M), or if the 48-hour methotrexate level is >0.9 micromolar (9 x 10^{-7} M); continue levoleucovorin until the methotrexate level is <0.01 micromolar (10^{-8} M). Hydration (aggressive) and urinary alkalinization (with sodium bicarbonate) should also be maintained.

Dosage adjustment in renal impairment: No dosage adjustment provided in manufacturer's labeling.

Dosage adjustment in hepatic impairment: No dosage adjustment provided in manufacturer's labeling.

Additional Information Complete prescribing information should be consulted for additional detail.

Dosage Forms Excipient information presented when available (limited, particularly for generics); consult specific product labeling.

Solution Reconstituted, Intravenous:

Fusilev: 50 mg (1 ea)

◆ **Levo-leucovorin** *see* LEVOleucovorin *on page 1201*

◆ **Levoleucovorin Calcium Pentahydrate** *see* LEVOleucovorin *on page 1201*

◆ **Levomefolate Calcium, Drospirenone, and Ethinyl Estradiol** *see* Ethinyl Estradiol, Drospirenone, and Levomefolate *on page 797*

◆ **Levomefolate, Drospirenone, and Ethinyl Estradiol** *see* Ethinyl Estradiol, Drospirenone, and Levomefolate *on page 797*

◆ **Levonest** *see* Ethinyl Estradiol and Levonorgestrel *on page 787*

Levonorgestrel (LEE voe nor jes trel)

Brand Names: U.S. Mirena; My Way; Next Choice One Dose; Next Choice [DSC]; Plan B; Plan B One-Step; Plan B One-Step [OTC]; Skyla

Brand Names: Canada Mirena; Next Choice; NorLevo; Plan B

Index Terms LNg 20; Plan B

Pharmacologic Category Contraceptive; Progestin

Use

Intrauterine device (IUD): Prevention of pregnancy; treatment of heavy menstrual bleeding in women who also choose to use an IUD for contraception

Oral: Emergency contraception following unprotected intercourse or possible contraceptive failure

Pregnancy Considerations Use during pregnancy is contraindicated. When pregnancies have continued following levonorgestrel exposure, congenital anomalies have been infrequent. Significant adverse effects on infant growth and development have not been observed (limited data). In doses larger than those used for oral contraception, progestins have been reported to increase the risk of masculinization of female genitalia.

Intrauterine device: Pregnancy should be ruled out prior to insertion. Women who become pregnant with an IUD in place risk septic abortion (septic shock and death may occur). Removal of the device is recommended, however, removal or manipulation of IUD may result in pregnancy loss. In addition, miscarriage, premature labor, and premature delivery may occur if pregnancy is continued with IUD in place. Following pregnancy, insertion of the device should not take place until 6 weeks postpartum or until involution of the uterus is complete. Consider waiting until 12 weeks postpartum if involution is substantially delayed. The device may be inserted immediately following a first trimester abortion. Following removal of the device, ~80% of women who wished to conceive became pregnant within 12 months.

Oral tablet: A rapid return of fertility is expected following use for emergency contraception; routine contraceptive measures should be initiated or continued following use to ensure ongoing prevention of pregnancy. Barrier contraception is recommended immediately following emergency contraception. Short-term contraception (eg, oral hormonal contraceptive pills, patches, rings) may be started with barrier contraception or after the next menstrual period. Long term contraception (eg, IUD, depot medroxyprogesterone, progestin implant) should be started after the next menstrual period (ACOG, 2010).

Breast-Feeding Considerations Following maternal use of the oral tablets or intrauterine device, levonorgestrel is found in breast milk and can be detected in the serum of nursing infants (Shikary, 1987). In general, no adverse effects on the growth or development if the infant have been observed. Isolated cases of decreased milk production have been reported. Risk of perforation with IUD is increased in lactating women. Following pregnancy, insertion of the device should not take place until 6 weeks postpartum or until involution of the uterus is complete.

Consider waiting until 12 weeks postpartum if involution is substantially delayed. Women who are breast-feeding may use levonorgestrel for emergency contraception (ACOG, 2010).

Contraindications Hypersensitivity to levonorgestrel or any component of the formulation; pregnancy

Additional product-specific contraindications:

Intrauterine device: Congenital or acquired uterine anomaly including fibroids that distort the uterine cavity, acute pelvic inflammatory disease, history of pelvic inflammatory disease (unless there has been a subsequent intrauterine pregnancy), postpartum endometritis or infected abortion within past 3 months, known or suspected uterine or cervical neoplasia, unresolved/abnormal Pap smear, untreated acute cervicitis or vaginitis or other lower genital tract infections until infection is controlled, conditions which increase susceptibility to pelvic infections, unremoved IUD, undiagnosed abnormal genital bleeding, active hepatic disease or hepatic tumors, current or history of known or suspected carcinoma of the breast or other progestin-sensitive cancer

Canadian labeling: Additional contraindications (not in U.S. labeling): Bacterial endocarditis, known immunodeficiency, hematologic malignancy, recent trophoblastic disease while human chorionic gonadotropin (hCG) hormone levels are elevated

Oral: It is not known if the same contraindications associated with long-term progestin-only contraceptives apply to the levonorgestrel emergency contraception dose regimens. A history of ectopic pregnancy is not a contraindication to use in emergency contraception. Canadian labeling contraindicates use in patients with undiagnosed vaginal bleeding.

Warnings/Precautions Hazardous agent - use appropriate precautions for handling and disposal (NIOSH, 2012). These products do not protect against HIV infection or other sexually transmitted diseases (CDC, 2013). Menstrual bleeding patterns may be altered with use of the intrauterine device; the possibility of pregnancy should be considered if menstruation does not occur within 6 weeks of the previous menstrual period. If bleeding irregularities continue with prolonged use, appropriate diagnostic measures should be taken to rule out endometrial pathology. An increase in menstrual bleeding may indicate a partial or complete expulsion of the IUD. If expulsion occurs, device may be replaced within 7 days of a menstrual period once pregnancy is ruled out. When using the oral tablet, spotting may occur following use; the possibility of pregnancy should be considered if menstruation is delayed for >7 days of the expected menstrual period.

Patients taking progestin-only contraceptives and presenting with lower abdominal pain should be evaluated for delayed follicular atresia (ovarian cysts) and ectopic pregnancy. Use caution in patients with previous ectopic pregnancy. Women with history of ectopic pregnancy were excluded from clinical trials; women with previous ectopic pregnancy, tubal surgery, or pelvic infection may be at increased risk for ectopic pregnancy. The possibility of ectopic pregnancy should be considered in patients with abdominal pain or vaginal bleeding in women with prior amenorrhea. May have adverse effects on glucose tolerance; use caution in women with diabetes. Use of the IUD is contraindicated with active hepatic disease or hepatic tumors. Use with caution in patients with depression; may be more susceptible to recurrence of depressive episodes; consider removal of IUD for serious recurrence. Depression is not a contraindication to use of the intrauterine device (CDC, 2010). Not indicated for use in postmenopausal women.

The use of combination hormonal contraceptives has been associated with a slight increase in the frequency of breast cancer, however, studies are not consistent. Data is insufficient to determine if progestin only contraceptives also increase this risk. Use of the intrauterine device is contraindicated in patients who have or who have had breast cancer or other progestin-sensitive cancers. The risk of cardiovascular side effects increases in women using estrogen containing combined hormonal contraceptives and who smoke cigarettes, especially those who are >35 years of age. This risk relative to progestin-only contraceptives has not been established. Women who take contraceptives should be advised not to smoke. Smoking is not a contraindication to use of the intrauterine device (CDC, 2010). The use of estrogens and/or progestins may change the results of some laboratory tests (eg, coagulation factors, lipids, glucose tolerance, binding proteins). The dose, route, and the specific estrogen/progestin influences these changes. In addition, personal risk factors (eg, cardiovascular disease, smoking, diabetes, age) also contribute to adverse events; use of specific products may be contraindicated in women with certain risk factors.

Additional formulation-specific warnings:

Intrauterine device: Bradycardia or syncope may occur during insertion or removal of the intrauterine device. An increased incidence of group A streptococcal sepsis, pelvic inflammatory disease (may be asymptomatic), and actinomycosis have been reported with use. Using aseptic technique during insertion is essential to minimizing the risk of serious infections. The highest risk of pelvic inflammatory disease is within 20 days of insertion; risk is increased with multiple sexual partners. May perforate uterus or cervix; risk of perforation is increased in lactating women, women with a fixed retroverted uteri, and during the postpartum period. Pregnancy may result if perforation occurs; delayed detection of perforation may result in migration of IUD outside of uterine cavity. Partial penetration or embedment in the myometrium may decrease effectiveness and lead to difficult removal. Use caution in patients with coagulopathy or receiving anticoagulants. Use caution in patients with congenital heart disease or other heart conditions which may increase the risk of infective endocarditis during insertion of the device (prophylactic antibiotics may be required at time of insertion and removal). Insertion should be done by a trained healthcare provider. Removal of the device may be necessary for the following reasons: Bleeding which causes anemia; coagulopathy or use of anticoagulants; marked increase in blood pressure; severe arterial disease (eg, stroke, MI); if the patient or her partner acquire a sexually transmitted disease; pelvic infection, endometritis, symptomatic genital actinomycosis; migraine, focal migraine with asymmetrical visual loss or other symptoms indicating transient cerebral ischemia; exceptionally severe headache; intractable pelvic pain, pain during intercourse; endometrial or cervical cancer; uterine or cervical perforation; jaundice; pregnancy. Embedded devices should also be removed. Use is contraindicated in patients with vaginitis or cervicitis. Postpone insertion until after treatment for infection is complete and cause of the cervicitis is proven not to be due to gonorrhea or chlamydia. Not effective for emergency contraception.

Skyla: Only under specific conditions may this device be scanned safely by MRI. Image quality may also be impaired if area of interest is relatively close to the device

Oral tablet: Not intended to be used for routine contraception and will not terminate an existing pregnancy. Barrier contraception is recommended immediately following emergency contraception and throughout the same menstrual cycle; efficacy of hormonal contraception may be decreased.

Adverse Reactions Frequency not always defined.

Intrauterine device:

>10%:

Central nervous system: Headache (12%)

Dermatologic: Acne (15%)

Endocrine & metabolic: Ovarian cysts (13%), enlarged follicles (12%), amenorrhea (<1% to 12%, increases with duration of treatment)

Gastrointestinal: Abdominal pain (12%)

Genitourinary: Uterine/vaginal bleeding alterations (52%), intermenstrual bleeding/spotting (23%), vulvovaginitis (20%)

Miscellaneous: Ectopic pregnancy (≤50%)

1% to 10%:

Cardiovascular: Edema

Central nervous system: Depression (4%), migraine (2%), nervousness

Dermatologic: Alopecia (1%), eczema, hirsutism, pruritus, rash, urticaria

Endocrine & metabolic: Dysmenorrhea (9%), menorrhagia (6%), breast pain/tenderness (3% to 9%), libido decreased

Gastrointestinal: Nausea (6%), abdominal distension, weight gain

Genitourinary: Pelvic pain (6%), leukorrhea (5%), vaginal discharge (4%), pelvic infection (1%), cervicitis, dyspareunia, vaginitis

Hematologic: Anemia

Neuromuscular & skeletal: Back pain

Miscellaneous: IUD expulsion (3%)

<1% (Limited to important or life-threatening): Angioedema, cervical wall perforation, device breakage, failed insertion, hypersensitivity reactions, jaundice, sepsis, uterine bleeding, uterine wall perforation

Oral tablets:

>10%:

Central nervous system: Fatigue (13% to 17%), headache (10% to 17%), dizziness (10% to 11%)

Endocrine & metabolic: Heavier menstrual bleeding (14% to 31%), lighter menstrual bleeding (12%), breast tenderness (8% to 11%)

Gastrointestinal: Nausea (14% to 23%), abdominal pain (13% to 18%)

1% to 10%:

Endocrine & metabolic: Menses delayed (5%)

Gastrointestinal: Vomiting (6%), diarrhea (5%)

Postmarketing and/or case reports: Dysmenorrhea, menstruation irregularities, oligomenorrhea, pelvic pain

Drug Interactions

Metabolism/Transport Effects **Substrate** of CYP3A4 (major); **Note:** Assignment of Major/Minor substrate status based on clinically relevant drug interaction potential

Avoid Concomitant Use

Avoid concomitant use of Levonorgestrel with any of the following: Griseofulvin; Tranexamic Acid; Ulipristal

Increased Effect/Toxicity

Levonorgestrel may increase the levels/effects of: Benzodiazepines (metabolized by oxidation); Selegiline; Tranexamic Acid; Voriconazole

The levels/effects of Levonorgestrel may be increased by: Atazanavir; Boceprevir; Cobicistat; Herbs (Progestogenic Properties); Mifepristone; Voriconazole

Decreased Effect

Levonorgestrel may decrease the levels/effects of: Anticoagulants; Vitamin K Antagonists

The levels/effects of Levonorgestrel may be decreased by: Acitretin; Aminoglutethimide; Aprepitant; Artemether; Barbiturates; Bexarotene (Systemic); Bile Acid Sequestrants; Bosentan; CarBAMazepine; CloBAZam; CYP3A4 Inducers (Strong); Dabrafenib; Deferasirox; Eslicarbazepine; Exenatide; Felbamate; Fosaprepitant; Fosphenytoin; Griseofulvin; LamoTRIgine; Mifepristone; Mitotane; Mycophenolate; Nelfinavir; Nevirapine; OXcarbazepine; Perampanel; Phenytoin; Primidone; Prucalopride; Retinoic Acid Derivatives; Rifamycin Derivatives; St Johns Wort; Sugammadex; Telaprevir; Tocilizumab; Topiramate; Ulipristal

Ethanol/Nutrition/Herb Interactions Herb/Nutraceutical: St John's wort (an enzyme inducer) may decrease serum levels of levonorgestrel.

Storage/Stability

Intrauterine device: Store at 25°C (77°F); excursions permitted between 15°C to 30°C (59°F to 86°F).

Oral tablet: Store at 20°C to 25°C (68°F to 77°F).

Mechanism of Action Pregnancy may be prevented through several mechanisms: Thickening of cervical mucus, which inhibits sperm passage through the uterus and sperm survival; inhibition of ovulation, from a negative feedback mechanism on the hypothalamus, leading to reduced secretion of follicle stimulating hormone (FSH) and luteinizing hormone (LH); and inhibition of implantation. Levonorgestrel is not effective once the implantation process has begun.

Pharmacodynamics/Kinetics

Duration: Intrauterine device: Mirena®: Up to 5 years; Skyla™: Up to 3 years

Absorption: Oral: Rapid and complete

Distribution: V_d: ~1.8 L/kg

Protein binding: Highly bound to albumin (~50%) and sex hormone-binding globulin (~47%) (Fotherby, 1995)

Metabolism: Hepatic via CYP3A4; forms inactive metabolites

Half-life elimination: Oral: ~24 hours

Time to peak: Oral: ~2 hours

Excretion: Urine (45%); feces (32%)

Dosage Adults: Females:

Long-term prevention of pregnancy: Intrauterine device (Skyla): To be inserted into uterine cavity; should be inserted within 7 days of onset of menstruation or immediately after first trimester abortion; releases levonorgestrel ~6 mcg per day over 3 years. May be removed and replaced with a new unit at anytime during menstrual cycle; do not leave any one system in place for >3 years.

Long-term prevention of pregnancy, treatment of heavy menstrual bleeding: Intrauterine device (Mirena): To be inserted into uterine cavity; should be inserted within 7 days of onset of menstruation or immediately after first trimester abortion; initially releases levonorgestrel 20 mcg per day, then rate subsequently decreases; mean release rate over 5 years is levonorgestrel ~14 mcg per day. May be removed and replaced with a new unit at anytime during menstrual cycle; do not leave any one system in place for >5 years.

Back up contraception: If the intrauterine device is inserted within the first 7 days of the onset of menstruation, back-up contraception is not needed. However, the device may be inserted at any time once it is determined that the woman is not pregnant. If insertion occurs >7 days after menstrual bleeding started, an additional form of contraception must be used for 7 days unless the woman abstains from sexual intercourse (CDC, 2013).

Continuation of therapy or switching to different contraceptive (Skyla, Mirena): At the time of device removal, a new device may be inserted immediately if continuation of therapy is desired. If the patient wishes to change to a different method of birth control, remove the device during the first 7 days of menstrual cycle and begin the new therapy. If the device is not removed during menstruation (or if the patient has irregular menstrual cycles) and wants to start a different method of birth control, consider starting the new method 7 days prior to device removal.

Emergency contraception: Oral: May be used at any time during menstrual cycle:

Two-dose regimen: One 0.75 mg tablet as soon as possible within 72 hours of unprotected sexual intercourse; a second 0.75 mg tablet should be taken 12 hours after the first dose

Single-dose regimen: One 1.5 mg tablet as soon as possible within 72 hours of unprotected sexual intercourse

Elderly: Not indicated for use in postmenopausal women

Dosage adjustment in renal impairment: No dosage adjustment provided in manufacturer's labeling (has not been studied).

Dosage adjustment in hepatic impairment: No dosage adjustment provided in manufacturer's labeling (has not been studied); use of the intrauterine device is contraindicated with active hepatic disease or hepatic tumor.

Administration

Intrauterine device: Insert into the uterine cavity to the recommended depth with the provided insertion device; should not be forced into the uterus. Transvaginal ultrasound may be used to check proper placement. Remove if not positioned properly and insert a new IUD; do not reinsert removed IUD. Exclude perforation if exceptional pain or bleeding occurs after insertion.

Oral: Consider repeating the dose if vomiting occurs within 2 hours. If severe vomiting occurs, may consider administering the oral tablets vaginally (ACOG, 2010).

Hazardous agent; use appropriate precautions for handling and disposal (NIOSH, 2012).

Monitoring Parameters

IUD: Prior to insertion: Assessment of pregnancy status; cervical examination; weight (optional; BMI at baseline may be helpful to monitor changes during therapy); STD screen (unless already screened according to CDC STD Treatment guidelines) (CDC, 2013). Re-examine following insertion (4-12 weeks Mirena; 4-6 weeks Skyla) and then yearly or more frequently if necessary. Threads should be visible; if length of thread has changed device may have become displaced, broken, perforated the uterus, or expelled. Transvaginal ultrasound may be used to check placement. Monitor for prolonged menstrual bleeding, amenorrhea, irregularity of menses, Pap smear, blood pressure, serum glucose in patients with diabetes, LDL levels in patients with hyperlipidemias; re-examine following first menses postinsertion of IUD. Patients presenting with lower abdominal pain should be evaluated for follicular atresia and ectopic pregnancy. Signs of infection following IUD insertion, especially in patients at increased risk (eg, patients on chronic corticosteroids, patients with type 1 diabetes mellitus).

Oral tablet: Evaluate for pregnancy, spontaneous abortion or ectopic pregnancy if menses is delayed for ≥1 week following emergency contraception, or if lower abdominal pain or persistent irregular bleeding develops.

Reference Range Intrauterine device:

Mirena®: Plasma concentrations range from 150-200 pg/mL

Skyla™: Plasma concentrations range from a peak of 192 pg/mL (2 days following insertion) to 61 pg/mL (after 3 years)

Additional Information

Intrauterine device (IUD):

Mirena: The cumulative 5-year pregnancy rate is ~0.7 pregnancies/100 users. Over 70% of women in the trials had previously used IUDs. The reported pregnancy rate after 12 months was ≤0.2 pregnancies/100 users. Approximately 80% of women who wish to conceive have become pregnant within 12 months of device removal. The recommended patient profile for this product: A woman who has at least one child, is in a stable and mutually-monogamous relationship, no history of pelvic inflammatory disease, and no history of ectopic pregnancy or predisposition to ectopic pregnancy. Keep a copy of the consent form and record lot number of device.

Skyla: The cumulative 3-year pregnancy rate is ~0.9 pregnancies/100 users. Approximately 77% of women who wish to conceive have become pregnant within 12 months of device removal.

Oral tablet: Treatment for emergency contraception should begin as soon as possible; however, treatment is still moderately effective if used within 5 days and should be made available to women up to 5 days after unprotected or inadequately protected intercourse. May be used in women with contraindications to conventional oral contraceptive agents (eg, cardiovascular disease, migraines, liver disease). When used as directed for emergency contraception, the expected pregnancy rate is decreased from 8% to 1%. Approximately 87% of women have their next menstrual period at approximately the expected time. A rapid return to fertility following use is expected. When using the two-dose emergency contraceptive regimen, the second dose is equally effective if taken 12-24 hours after the first (ACOG, 2010).

Dosage Forms Excipient information presented when available (limited, particularly for generics); consult specific product labeling. [DSC] = Discontinued product

Intrauterine Device, Intrauterine:

Mirena: 20 mcg/24 hr

Skyla: 13.5 mg

Tablet, Oral:

My Way: 1.5 mg

Next Choice: 0.75 mg [DSC] [contains fd&c yellow #6 (sunset yellow)]

Next Choice One Dose: 1.5 mg [contains fd&c yellow #6 (sunset yellow)]

Plan B: 0.75 mg

Plan B One-Step: 1.5 mg

Generic: 0.75 mg, 1.5 mg

◆ **Levonorgestrel and Estradiol** *see* Estradiol and Levonorgestrel *on page 762*

◆ **Levonorgestrel and Ethinyl Estradiol** *see* Ethinyl Estradiol and Levonorgestrel *on page 787*

◆ **Levophed** *see* Norepinephrine *on page 1471*

◆ **Levophed® (Can)** *see* Norepinephrine *on page 1471*

◆ **Levora** *see* Ethinyl Estradiol and Levonorgestrel *on page 787*

Levorphanol (lee VOR fa nole)

Index Terms Levo-Dromoran; Levorphan Tartrate; Levorphanol Tartrate

Pharmacologic Category Analgesic, Opioid

Additional Appendix Information

Opioid Conversion Table *on page 2306*

Use Relief of moderate-to-severe pain; preoperative sedation/analgesia; management of chronic pain (eg, cancer) requiring opioid therapy

Pregnancy Risk Factor C

Dosage Adults: **Note:** These are guidelines and do not represent the maximum doses that may be required in all patients. Doses should be titrated to pain relief/prevention.

Acute pain (moderate-to-severe): Oral: Initial: Opioid-naive: 2 mg every 6-8 hours as needed; patients with prior opioid exposure may require higher initial doses; usual dosage range: 2-4 mg every 6-8 hours as needed

Note: The American Pain Society recommends an initial dose of 4 mg for severe pain in adults (APS, 6th ed)

Chronic pain: Patients taking opioids chronically may become tolerant and require doses higher than the usual dosage range to maintain the desired effect. Tolerance can be managed by appropriate dose titration. **There is no optimal or maximal dose for levorphanol in chronic pain. The appropriate dose is one that relieves pain throughout its dosing interval without causing unmanageable side effects.**

Dosing adjustment in renal impairment: Use with caution; initial dose should be reduced in severe renal impairment

Dosing adjustment in hepatic impairment: Use with caution; initial dose should be reduced in severe hepatic impairment

Additional Information Complete prescribing information should be consulted for additional detail.

Dosage Forms Excipient information presented when available (limited, particularly for generics); consult specific product labeling.

Tablet, Oral, as tartrate:

Generic: 2 mg

Controlled Substance C-II

◆ Levorphanol Tartrate *see* Levorphanol *on page 1205*

◆ Levorphan Tartrate *see* Levorphanol *on page 1205*

◆ Levosalbutamol *see* Levalbuterol *on page 1192*

◆ Levothroid [DSC] *see* Levothyroxine *on page 1206*

Levothyroxine (lee voe thye ROKS een)

Brand Names: U.S. Levothroid [DSC]; Levoxyl [DSC]; Synthroid; Tirosint; Unithroid; Unithroid Direct

Brand Names: Canada Eltroxin®; Euthyrox; Levothyroxine Sodium; Levothyroxine Sodium for Injection; Synthroid®

Index Terms *L*-Thyroxine Sodium; Levothyroxine Sodium; T_4

Pharmacologic Category Thyroid Product

Use Replacement or supplemental therapy in hypothyroidism; pituitary TSH suppression

Unlabeled Use Management of hemodynamically unstable potential organ donors increasing the quantity of organs available for transplantation

Pregnancy Risk Factor A

Pregnancy Considerations Endogenous thyroid hormones minimally cross the placenta; the fetal thyroid becomes active around the end of the first trimester. Levothyroxine has not been shown to increase the risk of congenital abnormalities.

Uncontrolled maternal hypothyroidism may result in adverse neonatal outcomes (eg, premature birth, low birth weight, and respiratory distress) and adverse maternal outcomes (eg, spontaneous abortion, pre-eclampsia, stillbirth, and premature delivery). To prevent adverse events, normal maternal thyroid function should be maintained prior to conception and throughout pregnancy. Levothyroxine is considered the treatment of choice for the control of hypothyroidism during pregnancy. Due to alterations of endogenous maternal thyroid hormones, the levothyroxine dose may need to be increased during pregnancy and the dose usually needs to be decreased after delivery.

Breast-Feeding Considerations Endogenous thyroid hormones are minimally found in breast milk. The amount of endogenous thyroxine found in breast milk does not influence infant plasma thyroid values. Levothyroxine was not found to cause adverse events to the infant or mother during breast-feeding. Adequate thyroid hormone concentrations are required to maintain normal lactation. Appropriate levothyroxine doses should be continued during breast-feeding.

Contraindications Hypersensitivity to levothyroxine sodium or any component of the formulation; acute MI; thyrotoxicosis of any etiology; uncorrected adrenal insufficiency

Capsule: Additional contraindication: Inability to swallow capsules

Warnings/Precautions [U.S. Boxed Warning]: Thyroid supplements are ineffective and potentially toxic when used for the treatment of obesity or for weight reduction, especially in euthyroid patients. High doses may produce serious or even life-threatening toxic effects particularly when used with some anorectic drugs (eg, sympathomimetic amines). Routine use of T_4 for TSH suppression is not recommended in patients with benign thyroid nodules. In patients deemed appropriate candidates, treatment should never be fully suppressive (TSH <0.1 mIU/L). Use with caution and reduce dosage in patients with angina pectoris or other cardiovascular disease; decrease initial dose. Use cautiously in the elderly since they may be more likely to have compromised cardiovascular functions. Patients with adrenal insufficiency, myxedema, diabetes mellitus and insipidus may have symptoms exaggerated or aggravated. Chronic hypothyroidism predisposes patients to coronary artery disease. Long-term therapy can decrease bone mineral density. Levoxyl® may rapidly swell and disintegrate causing choking or gagging (should be administered with a full glass of water); use caution in patients with dysphagia or other swallowing disorders.

Adverse Reactions Frequency not defined.

Cardiovascular: Angina pectoris, cardiac arrest, cardiac arrhythmia, congestive heart failure, flushing, hypertension, increased pulse, myocardial infarction, palpitations, tachycardia

Central nervous system: Anxiety, choking sensation (Levoxyl), emotional lability, fatigue, headache, heat intolerance, hyperactivity, insomnia, irritability, myasthenia, nervousness, pseudotumor cerebri (children), seizure (rare)

Dermatologic: Alopecia, diaphoresis

Endocrine & metabolic: Menstrual disease, weight loss

Gastrointestinal: Abdominal cramps, diarrhea, dysphagia (Levoxyl), gag reflex (Levoxyl), increased appetite, vomiting

Genitourinary: Infertility

Hepatic: Increased liver enzymes

Hypersensitivity: Hypersensitivity (to inactive ingredients; symptoms include urticaria, pruritus, rash, flushing, angioedema, GI symptoms, fever, arthralgia, serum sickness, wheezing)

Neuromuscular & skeletal: Decreased bone mineral density, slipped capital femoral epiphysis (children), tremor

Respiratory: Dyspnea

Miscellaneous: Fever

Drug Interactions

Metabolism/Transport Effects None known.

Avoid Concomitant Use

Avoid concomitant use of Levothyroxine with any of the following: Sodium Iodide I131; Sucroferric Oxyhydroxide

Increased Effect/Toxicity

Levothyroxine may increase the levels/effects of: Tricyclic Antidepressants; Vitamin K Antagonists

The levels/effects of Levothyroxine may be increased by: Piracetam

Decreased Effect

Levothyroxine may decrease the levels/effects of: Sodium Iodide I131; Theophylline Derivatives

The levels/effects of Levothyroxine may be decreased by: Aluminum Hydroxide; Bile Acid Sequestrants; Calcium Polystyrene Sulfonate; Calcium Salts; CarBAMazepine; Estrogen Derivatives; Fosphenytoin; Iron Salts; Lanthanum; Multivitamins/Minerals (with ADEK, Folate,

Iron); Orlistat; Phenytoin; Raloxifene; Rifampin; Selective Serotonin Reuptake Inhibitors; Sevelamer; Sodium Polystyrene Sulfonate; Sucralfate; Sucroferric Oxyhydroxide

Ethanol/Nutrition/Herb Interactions Food: Taking levothyroxine with enteral nutrition may cause reduced bioavailability and may lower serum thyroxine levels leading to signs or symptoms of hypothyroidism. Soybean flour (infant formula), cottonseed meal, walnuts, and dietary fiber may decrease absorption of levothyroxine from the GI tract. Management: Take in the morning on an empty stomach at least 30 minutes before food. Consider an increase in dose if taken with enteral tube feed.

Preparation for Administration Dilute vial for injection with 5 mL normal saline. Reconstituted concentrations for the 100 mcg, 200 mcg and 500 mcg vials are 20 mcg/mL, 40 mcg/mL, and 100 mcg/mL, respectively. Shake well and use immediately after reconstitution (manufacturer recommendation); discard any unused portions.

Storage/Stability Store capsules, tablets, and injection at room temperature; excursions permitted to 15°C to 30°C (59°F to 86°F). Protect from light and moisture.

Additional stability data:

Stability in polypropylene syringes (100 mcg/mL in NS) at 5°C ± 1°C is 7 days (Gupta, 2000).

Stability in latex-free, PVC minibags protected from light and stored at 15°C to 30°C (59°F to 86°F) was 12 hours for a 2 mcg/mL concentration or 18 hours for a 0.4 mcg/mL concentration in NS. May be exposed to light; however, stability time is significantly reduced, especially for the 2 mcg/mL concentration (Strong, 2010).

Mechanism of Action Levothyroxine (T_4) is a synthetic form of thyroxine, an endogenous hormone secreted by the thyroid gland. T_4 is converted to its active metabolite, L-triiodothyronine (T_3). Thyroid hormones (T_4 and T_3) then bind to thyroid receptor proteins in the cell nucleus and exert metabolic effects through control of DNA transcription and protein synthesis; involved in normal metabolism, growth, and development; promotes gluconeogenesis, increases utilization and mobilization of glycogen stores, and stimulates protein synthesis, increases basal metabolic rate

Pharmacodynamics/Kinetics

Onset of action: Therapeutic: Oral: 3-5 days; I.V. 6-8 hours

Peak effect: I.V.: 24 hours

Absorption: Oral: Erratic (40% to 80% [per manufacturer]); may be decreased by age and specific foods and drugs

Protein binding: >99% bound to plasma proteins including thyroxine-binding globulin, thyroxine-binding prealbumin, and albumin

Metabolism: Hepatic to triiodothyronine (T_3; active); ~80% thyroxine (T_4) deiodinated in kidney and periphery; glucuronidation/conjugation also occurs; undergoes enterohepatic recirculation

Bioavailability: Oral tablets: 64% (nonfasting state) to 79% to 81% (fasting state)

Time to peak, serum: 2-4 hours

Half-life elimination: Euthyroid: 6-7 days; Hypothyroid: 9-10 days; Hyperthyroid: 3-4 days

Excretion: Urine (major route of elimination; decreases with age); feces (~20%)

Dosage Doses should be adjusted based on clinical response and laboratory parameters.

Oral:

Infants and Children: Hypothyroidism: Daily dosage based on body weight and age as listed below:

1-3 months: 10-15 mcg/kg/day; if the infant is at risk for development of cardiac failure, use a lower starting dose of 25 mcg/day; if the initial serum T_4 is very low (<5 mcg/dL) begin treatment at a higher dosage of 50 mcg/day

3-6 months: 8-10 mcg/kg/day **or** 25-50 mcg/day

6-12 months: 6-8 mcg/kg/day **or** 50-75 mcg/day

1-5 years: 5-6 mcg/kg/day **or** 75-100 mcg/day

6-12 years: 4-5 mcg/kg/day **or** 100-125 mcg/day

>12 years: 2-3 mcg/kg/day **or** ≥150 mcg/day

Growth and puberty complete: 1.7 mcg/kg/day; refer to Adult dosing.

Dosing modifications:

Hyperactivity in older children may be minimized by starting at 1/4 of the recommended dose and increasing each week by that amount until the full dose is achieved (4 weeks).

Children with severe or chronic hypothyroidism should be started at 25 mcg/day; adjust dose by 25 mcg every 2-4 weeks.

Adults (including children in whom growth and puberty are complete, healthy adults <50 years of age, and older adults who have been recently treated for hyperthyroidism or who have been hypothyroid for only a few months):

Hypothyroidism: ~1.7 mcg/kg/day; usual doses are ≤200 mcg/day (range: 100-125 mcg/day [70 kg adult]); doses ≥300 mcg/day are rare (consider poor compliance, malabsorption, and/or drug interactions). Titrate dose every 6 weeks.

Patients >50 years or patients with cardiac disease: Refer to Elderly dosing.

Severe hypothyroidism: Initial: 12.5-25 mcg/day; adjust dose by 25 mcg/day every 2-4 weeks as appropriate

Myxedema: Oral agents are not recommended for myxedema: Refer to I.V. dosing.

Subclinical hypothyroidism (if treated): 1 mcg/kg/day

TSH suppression:

Well-differentiated thyroid cancer: Highly individualized; Doses >2 mcg/kg/day may be needed to suppress TSH to <0.1 mIU/L in intermediate- to high-risk tumors. Low-risk tumors may be maintained at or slightly below the lower limit of normal (0.1-0.5 mIU/L) (Cooper, 2009).

Benign nodules and nontoxic multinodular goiter: Routine use of T_4 for TSH suppression is not recommended in patients with benign thyroid nodules. In patients deemed appropriate candidates, treatment should never be fully suppressive (TSH <0.1 mIU/L) (Cooper, 2009; Gharib, 2010). Avoid use if TSH is already suppressed.

Elderly: Hypothyroidism (elderly patients may require <1 mcg/kg/day):

>50 years without cardiac disease **or** <50 years with cardiac disease: Initial: 25-50 mcg/day; adjust dose by 12.5-25 mcg increments at 6- to 8-week intervals as needed

>50 years with cardiac disease: Initial: 12.5-25 mcg/day; adjust dose by 12.5-25 mcg increments at 4- to 6-week intervals (many clinicians prefer to adjust at 6- to 8-week intervals)

Note: Patients with combined hypothyroidism and cardiac disease should be monitored carefully for changes in stability.

I.M., I.V.: Children, Adults, Elderly: Hypothyroidism: 50% of the oral dose; alternatively, some clinicians administer up to 80% of the oral dose. **Note:** Bioavailability of the oral formulation is highly variable, but absorption has been measured to be ~80%, when the oral tablet formulation was administered in the recommended fasting state (Dickerson, 2010; Fish, 1987).

I.V.:

Adults: Myxedema coma or stupor: 200-500 mcg, then 100-300 mcg the next day if necessary; smaller doses should be considered in patients with cardiovascular disease

Elderly: Myxedema coma: Refer to adult dosing; lower doses may be needed

Dosage adjustment in renal impairment: No dosage adjustment provided in manufacturer's labeling.

Dosage adjustment in hepatic impairment: No dosage adjustment provided in manufacturer's labeling.

Dietary Considerations Should be taken on an empty stomach, at least 30 minutes before food.

Administration

Oral: Administer in the morning on an empty stomach, at least 30 minutes before food.

Capsule: Must be swallowed whole; do not cut, crush, or attempt to dissolve capsules in water to prepare a suspension.

Tablet: May be crushed and suspended in 5-10 mL of water; suspension should be used immediately. Levoxyl® should be administered with a full glass of water to prevent gagging (due to tablet swelling).

Nasogastric tube: Bioavailability of levothyroxine is reduced if administered with enteral tube feeds. Since holding feedings for at least 1 hour before and after levothyroxine administration may not completely resolve the interaction, an increase in dose (eg, additional 25 mcg) may be necessary (Dickerson, 2010).

Parenteral: Administer doses ≤100 mcg I.V. over 1 minute.

Monitoring Parameters Thyroid function test (serum thyroxine, thyrotropin concentrations), resin triiodothyronine uptake (rT_3U), free thyroxine index (FTI), T_4, TSH, heart rate, blood pressure, clinical signs of hypo- and hyperthyroidism; TSH is the most reliable guide for evaluating adequacy of thyroid replacement dosage. TSH may be elevated during the first few months of thyroid replacement despite patients being clinically euthyroid. In cases where T_4 remains low and TSH is within normal limits, an evaluation of "free" (unbound) T_4 is needed to evaluate further increase in dosage

Infants: Monitor closely for cardiac overload, arrhythmias, and aspiration from avid suckling

Infants/children: Monitor closely for under/overtreatment. Undertreatment may decrease intellectual development and linear growth, and lead to poor school performance due to impaired concentration and slowed mentation. Overtreatment may adversely affect brain maturation, accelerate bone age (leading to premature closure of the epiphyses and reduced adult height); craniosynostosis has been reported in infants. Treated children may experience a period of catch-up growth. Monitor TSH and total or free T_4 at 2 and 4 weeks after starting treatment; every 1-2 months for first year of life; every 2-3 months during years 1-3; every 3-12 months until growth completed. Perform routine clinical examinations at regular intervals (to assess mental and physical growth and development).

Adults: Monitor TSH every 6-8 weeks until normalized; 8-12 weeks after dosage changes; every 6-12 months throughout therapy

Reference Range Pediatrics: Cord T_4 and values in the first few weeks are much higher, falling over the first months and years. ≥10 years: ~5.8-11 mcg/dL (SI: 75-142 nmol/L). Borderline low: ≤4.5-5.7 mcg/dL (SI: 58-73 nmol/L); low: ≤4.4 mcg/dL (SI: 57 nmol/L); results <2.5 mcg/dL (SI: <32 nmol/L) are strong evidence for hypothyroidism.

Approximate adult normal range: 4-12 mcg/dL (SI: 51-154 nmol/L). Borderline high: 11.1-13 mcg/dL (SI: 143-167 nmol/L); high: ≥13.1 mcg/dL (SI: 169 nmol/L). Normal range is increased in women on birth control pills (5.5-12 mcg/dL); normal range in pregnancy: ~5.5-16 mcg/dL (SI: ~71-206 nmol/L). TSH: 0.4-10 (for those ≥80 years) mIU/L; T_4: 4-12 mcg/dL (SI: 51-154 nmol/L); T_3 (RIA) (total T_3): 80-230 ng/dL (SI: 1.2-3.5 nmol/L); T_4 free (free T_4): 0.7-1.8 ng/dL (SI: 9-23 pmol/L).

Test Interactions Many drugs may have effects on thyroid function tests (see Additional Information). Pregnancy, infectious hepatitis, and acute intermittent porphyria may increase TBG concentrations; nephrosis, severe hypoproteinemia, severe liver disease, and acromegaly may decrease TBG concentrations.

Additional Information Equivalent doses: The following statement on relative potency of thyroid products is included in a joint statement by American Thyroid Association (ATA), American Association of Clinical Endocrinologists (AACE) and The Endocrine Society (TES): For purposes of conversion, levothyroxine sodium (T_4) 100 mcg is usually considered equivalent to desiccated thyroid 60 mg, thyroglobulin 60 mg, or liothyronine sodium (T_3) 25 mcg. However, these are rough guidelines only and do not obviate the careful re-evaluation of a patient when switching thyroid hormone preparations, including a change from one brand of levothyroxine to another. Joint position statement is available at http://www.thyroid.org/thyroxine-products-joint-position-statement/.

Note: Several medications have effects on thyroid production or conversion. The impact in thyroid replacement has not been specifically evaluated, but patient response should be monitored:

Methimazole: Decreases thyroid hormone secretion, while propylthiouracil decrease thyroid hormone secretion and decreases conversion of T_4 to T_3.

Beta-adrenergic antagonists: Decrease conversion of T_4 to T_3 (dose related, propranolol ≥160 mg/day); patients may be clinically euthyroid.

Iodide, iodine-containing radiographic contrast agents may decrease thyroid hormone secretion; may also increase thyroid hormone secretion, especially in patients with Graves' disease.

Other agents reported to impact on thyroid production/conversion include aminoglutethimide, amiodarone, chloral hydrate, diazepam, ethionamide, interferon-alpha, interleukin-2, lithium, lovastatin (case report), glucocorticoids (dose-related), mercaptopurine, sulfonamides, thiazide diuretics, and tolbutamide.

In addition, a number of medications have been noted to cause transient depression in TSH secretion, which may complicate interpretation of monitoring tests for levothyroxine, including corticosteroids, octreotide, and dopamine. Metoclopramide may increase TSH secretion

Dosage Forms Excipient information presented when available (limited, particularly for generics); consult specific product labeling. [DSC] = Discontinued product

Capsule, Oral, as sodium:

Tirosint: 13 mcg, 25 mcg, 50 mcg, 75 mcg, 88 mcg, 100 mcg, 112 mcg, 125 mcg, 137 mcg, 150 mcg

Solution Reconstituted, Intravenous, as sodium [preservative free]:

Generic: 100 mcg (1 ea); 200 mcg (1 ea); 500 mcg (1 ea)

Tablet, Oral, as sodium:

Levothroid: 25 mcg [DSC] [scored; contains fd&c yellow #6 aluminum lake]

Levothroid: 50 mcg [DSC] [scored]

Levothroid: 75 mcg [DSC] [scored; contains fd&c blue #2 aluminum lake, fd&c red #40 aluminum lake]

Levothroid: 88 mcg [DSC] [scored; contains fd&c blue #1 aluminum lake, fd&c yellow #10 aluminum lake, fd&c yellow #6 aluminum lake]

Levothroid: 100 mcg [DSC] [scored; contains fd&c yellow #10 aluminum lake, fd&c yellow #6 aluminum lake]

Levothroid: 112 mcg [DSC] [scored]

Levothroid: 125 mcg [DSC] [scored; contains fd&c blue #1 aluminum lake, fd&c red #40 aluminum lake, fd&c yellow #6 aluminum lake]

Levothroid: 137 mcg [DSC] [scored; contains fd&c blue #1 aluminum lake]

Levothroid: 150 mcg [DSC] [scored; contains fd&c blue #2 aluminum lake]
Levothroid: 175 mcg [DSC] [scored; contains fd&c blue #1 aluminum lake]
Levothroid: 200 mcg [DSC] [scored; contains fd&c red #40 aluminum lake]
Levothroid: 300 mcg [DSC] [scored; contains fd&c blue #1 aluminum lake, fd&c yellow #10 (quinoline yellow), fd&c yellow #6 aluminum lake]
Levoxyl: 25 mcg [DSC] [scored; contains fd&c yellow #6 aluminum lake]
Levoxyl: 50 mcg [DSC] [scored]
Levoxyl: 75 mcg [DSC] [scored; contains fd&c blue #1 aluminum lake]
Levoxyl: 88 mcg [DSC] [scored; contains fd&c blue #1 aluminum lake, fd&c yellow #10 aluminum lake, fd&c yellow #6 aluminum lake]
Levoxyl: 100 mcg [DSC] [scored; contains fd&c yellow #10 aluminum lake, fd&c yellow #6 aluminum lake]
Levoxyl: 112 mcg [DSC] [scored; contains fd&c red #40 aluminum lake, fd&c yellow #6 aluminum lake]
Levoxyl: 125 mcg [DSC] [scored; contains fd&c red #40 aluminum lake, fd&c yellow #10 aluminum lake]
Levoxyl: 137 mcg [DSC], 150 mcg [DSC] [scored; contains fd&c blue #1 aluminum lake]
Levoxyl: 175 mcg [DSC] [scored; contains fd&c blue #1 aluminum lake, fd&c yellow #10 aluminum lake]
Levoxyl: 200 mcg [DSC] [scored; contains fd&c yellow #10 aluminum lake]
Synthroid: 25 mcg [scored; contains fd&c yellow #6 aluminum lake]
Synthroid: 50 mcg [scored]
Synthroid: 75 mcg [scored; contains fd&c blue #2 aluminum lake, fd&c red #40 aluminum lake]
Synthroid: 88 mcg [scored; contains fd&c blue #1 aluminum lake, fd&c yellow #10 aluminum lake, fd&c yellow #6 aluminum lake]
Synthroid: 100 mcg [scored; contains fd&c yellow #10 aluminum lake, fd&c yellow #6 aluminum lake]
Synthroid: 112 mcg [scored]
Synthroid: 125 mcg [scored; contains fd&c blue #1 aluminum lake, fd&c red #40 aluminum lake, fd&c yellow #6 aluminum lake]
Synthroid: 137 mcg [scored; contains fd&c blue #1 aluminum lake]
Synthroid: 150 mcg [scored; contains fd&c blue #2 aluminum lake]
Synthroid: 175 mcg [scored; contains fd&c blue #1 aluminum lake]
Synthroid: 200 mcg [scored; contains fd&c red #40 aluminum lake]
Synthroid: 300 mcg [scored; contains fd&c blue #1 aluminum lake, fd&c yellow #10 aluminum lake, fd&c yellow #6 aluminum lake]
Unithroid: 25 mcg [scored; contains fd&c yellow #6 aluminum lake]
Unithroid: 50 mcg, 75 mcg, 88 mcg [scored]
Unithroid: 100 mcg [scored; contains fd&c yellow #10 aluminum lake, fd&c yellow #6 aluminum lake]
Unithroid: 112 mcg [scored]
Unithroid: 125 mcg [scored; contains fd&c blue #1 aluminum lake, fd&c red #40 aluminum lake, fd&c yellow #6 aluminum lake]
Unithroid: 137 mcg [scored; contains fd&c blue #1 aluminum lake]
Unithroid: 150 mcg [scored; contains fd&c blue #2 aluminum lake]
Unithroid: 175 mcg, 200 mcg [scored]
Unithroid: 300 mcg [scored; contains fd&c blue #1 aluminum lake, fd&c yellow #10 aluminum lake, fd&c yellow #6 aluminum lake]
Unithroid Direct: 25 mcg [scored; contains fd&c yellow #6 aluminum lake]
Unithroid Direct: 50 mcg [scored]
Unithroid Direct: 75 mcg, 88 mcg [scored; contains fd&c blue #1 aluminum lake, fd&c blue #2 aluminum lake, fd&c red #40 aluminum lake, fd&c yellow #10 aluminum lake, fd&c yellow #6 aluminum lake]
Unithroid Direct: 100 mcg [scored; contains fd&c yellow #10 aluminum lake, fd&c yellow #6 aluminum lake]
Unithroid Direct: 112 mcg [scored]
Unithroid Direct: 125 mcg [scored; contains fd&c blue #1 aluminum lake, fd&c red #40 aluminum lake, fd&c yellow #6 aluminum lake]
Unithroid Direct: 150 mcg [scored; contains fd&c blue #2 aluminum lake]
Unithroid Direct: 175 mcg [scored; contains fd&c blue #1 aluminum lake]
Unithroid Direct: 200 mcg [scored; contains fd&c red #40 aluminum lake]
Unithroid Direct: 300 mcg [scored; contains fd&c blue #1 aluminum lake, fd&c yellow #10 aluminum lake, fd&c yellow #6 aluminum lake]
Generic: 25 mcg, 50 mcg, 75 mcg, 88 mcg, 100 mcg, 112 mcg, 125 mcg, 137 mcg, 150 mcg, 175 mcg, 200 mcg, 300 mcg

Extemporaneous Preparations A 25 mcg/mL oral suspension may be made with tablets and 40 mL glycerol. Crush twenty-five 0.1 mg levothyroxine tablets in a mortar and reduce to a fine powder. Add small portions of glycerol and mix to a uniform suspension. Transfer to a calibrated 100 mL amber bottle; rinse the mortar with about 10 mL of glycerol and pour into the bottle; repeat until all 40 mL of glycerol is used. Add quantity of water sufficient to make 100 mL. Label "shake well" and "refrigerate". Stable for 8 days refrigerated.

Boulton DW, Fawcett JP, and Woods DJ, "Stability of an Extemporaneously Compounded Levothyroxine Sodium Oral Liquid," *Am J Health Syst Pharm*, 1996, 53(10):1157-61.

◆ **Levothyroxine and Liothyronine** *see* Liotrix *on page 1222*

◆ **Levothyroxine and Liothyronine** *see* Thyroid, Desiccated *on page 2052*

◆ **Levothyroxine Sodium** *see* Levothyroxine *on page 1206*

◆ **Levothyroxine Sodium for Injection (Can)** *see* Levothyroxine *on page 1206*

◆ **Levoxyl [DSC]** *see* Levothyroxine *on page 1206*

◆ **Levsin** *see* Hyoscyamine *on page 1026*

◆ **Levsin/SL** *see* Hyoscyamine *on page 1026*

◆ **Lev-Tov [OTC]** *see* Folic Acid, Cyanocobalamin, and Pyridoxine *on page 908*

◆ **Levulan Kerastick** *see* Aminolevulinic Acid *on page 100*

◆ **Levulan® Kerastick® (Can)** *see* Aminolevulinic Acid *on page 100*

◆ **Lexapro** *see* Escitalopram *on page 745*

◆ **Lexiva** *see* Fosamprenavir *on page 916*

◆ **L-Glutamine** *see* Glutamine *on page 962*

◆ **LH-RH Agonist** *see* Histrelin *on page 998*

◆ ***l*-Hyoscyamine Sulfate** *see* Hyoscyamine *on page 1026*

◆ **Lialda** *see* Mesalamine *on page 1305*

◆ **Librax®** *see* Clidinium and Chlordiazepoxide *on page 451*

◆ **Librium** *see* ChlordiazePOXIDE *on page 406*

◆ **Licide® [OTC]** *see* Pyrethrins and Piperonyl Butoxide *on page 1752*

◆ **Lidemol® (Can)** *see* Fluocinonide *on page 879*

◆ **Lidex** *see* Fluocinonide *on page 879*

◆ **Lidex® (Can)** *see* Fluocinonide *on page 879*

Lidocaine (Systemic) (LYE doe kane)

Brand Names: U.S. Xylocaine; Xylocaine (Cardiac); Xylocaine-MPF

Brand Names: Canada Xylocard®

Index Terms Lidocaine Hydrochloride; Lignocaine Hydrochloride

Pharmacologic Category Antiarrhythmic Agent, Class Ib; Local Anesthetic

Additional Appendix Information

Dosing Considerations for the Critically-Ill Patient With Morbid Obesity *on page 2379*

Use Local and regional anesthesia by infiltration, nerve block, epidural, or spinal techniques; acute treatment of ventricular arrhythmias from myocardial infarction or cardiac manipulation (eg, cardiac surgery)

Note: The routine prophylactic use of lidocaine to prevent arrhythmia associated with fibrinolytic administration or to suppress isolated ventricular premature beats, couplets, runs of accelerated idioventricular rhythm, and nonsustained VT is not recommended (Antman, 2004).

Unlabeled Use

ACLS guidelines: Hemodynamically stable monomorphic ventricular tachycardia (VT) (preserved ventricular function); polymorphic VT (preserved ventricular function); drug-induced monomorphic VT; when amiodarone is not available, pulseless VT or ventricular fibrillation (VF) (unresponsive to defibrillation, CPR, and vasopressor administration)

PALS guidelines: When amiodarone is not available, pulseless VT or VF (unresponsive to defibrillation, CPR, and epinephrine administration); consider in patients with cocaine overdose to prevent arrhythmias secondary to MI

I.V. infusion for chronic pain syndrome

Pregnancy Risk Factor B

Pregnancy Considerations Adverse events were not observed in animal reproduction studies. Lidocaine and its metabolites cross the placenta and can be detected in the fetal circulation following injection (Cavalli, 2004; Mitani, 1987). Adverse reactions in the fetus/neonate may affect the CNS, heart, or peripheral vascular tone. Fetal heart monitoring is recommended. Lidocaine injection is approved for obstetric analgesia. Lidocaine administered by local infiltration is used to provide analgesia prior to episiotomy and during repair of obstetric lacerations (ACOG, 2002). Administration by the perineal route may result in greater absorption than administration by the epidural route (Cavalli, 2004). Cumulative exposure from all routes of administration should be considered. When used as an antiarrhythmic, ACLS guidelines recommend using the same dose that would be used in a nonpregnant woman (Vanden Hoek, 2010).

Breast-Feeding Considerations Lidocaine is excreted into breast milk. The manufacturer recommends that caution be used when administered to a nursing woman. When administered by injection for dental or obstetric analgesia, small amounts are detected in breast milk; oral bioavailability to the nursing infant is expected to be low and the amount of lidocaine available to the nursing infant would not be expected to cause adverse events (Lebedevs, 1993; Ortega, 1999). Cumulative exposure from all routes of administration should be considered.

Contraindications Hypersensitivity to lidocaine or any component of the formulation; hypersensitivity to another local anesthetic of the amide type; Adam-Stokes syndrome; Wolff-Parkinson-White syndrome; severe degrees of SA, AV, or intraventricular heart block (except in patients with a functioning artificial pacemaker); premixed injection may contain corn-derived dextrose and its use is contraindicated in patients with allergy to corn or corn-related products

Warnings/Precautions Use caution in patients with severe hepatic dysfunction or pseudocholinesterase deficiency; may have increased risk of lidocaine toxicity.

Intravenous: Constant ECG monitoring is necessary during I.V. administration. Use cautiously in hepatic impairment, HF, marked hypoxia, severe respiratory depression, hypovolemia, history of malignant hyperthermia, or shock. Increased ventricular rate may be seen when administered to a patient with atrial fibrillation. Correct electrolyte disturbances, especially hypokalemia or hypomagnesemia, prior to use and throughout therapy. Use is contraindicated in patients with Wolff-Parkinson-White syndrome and severe degrees of SA, AV, or intraventricular heart block (except in patients with a functioning artificial pacemaker). Correct any underlying causes of ventricular arrhythmias. Monitor closely for signs and symptoms of CNS toxicity. The elderly may be prone to increased CNS and cardiovascular side effects. Reduce dose in hepatic dysfunction and CHF.

Injectable anesthetic: Follow appropriate administration techniques so as not to administer any intravascularly. Continuous intra-articular infusion of local anesthetics after arthroscopic or other surgical procedures is **not** an approved use; chondrolysis (primarily in the shoulder joint) has occurred following infusion, with some cases requiring arthroplasty or shoulder replacement. Solutions containing antimicrobial preservatives should not be used for epidural or spinal anesthesia. Some solutions contain a bisulfite; avoid in patients who are allergic to bisulfite. Resuscitative equipment, medicine and oxygen should be available in case of emergency. Use products containing epinephrine cautiously in patients with significant vascular disease, compromised blood flow, or during or following general anesthesia (increased risk of arrhythmias). Adjust the dose for the elderly, pediatric, acutely ill, and debilitated patients.

Adverse Reactions Effects vary with route of administration. Many effects are dose related.

Frequency not defined.

Cardiovascular: Arrhythmia, bradycardia, arterial spasms, cardiovascular collapse, defibrillator threshold increased, edema, flushing, heart block, hypotension, sinus node supression, vascular insufficiency (periarticular injections)

Central nervous system: Agitation, anxiety, apprehension, coma, confusion, disorientation, dizziness, drowsiness, euphoria, hallucinations, headache, hyperesthesia, hypoesthesia, lethargy, lightheadedness, nervousness, psychosis, seizure, slurred speech, somnolence, unconsciousness

Gastrointestinal: Metallic taste, nausea, vomiting

Local: Thrombophlebitis

Neuromuscular & skeletal: Paresthesia, transient radicular pain (subarachnoid administration; up to 1.9%), tremor, twitching, weakness

Otic: Tinnitus

Respiratory: Bronchospasm, dyspnea, respiratory depression or arrest

Miscellaneous: Allergic reactions, anaphylactic reaction, anaphylactoid reaction, sensitivity to temperature extremes

Following spinal anesthesia: Positional headache (3%), shivering (2%), double vision (<1%), cauda equina syndrome, hypotension, nausea, peripheral nerve symptoms, respiratory inadequacy

Postmarketing and/or case reports: Asystole, disorientation, methemoglobinemia, skin reaction

Drug Interactions

Metabolism/Transport Effects **Substrate** of CYP1A2 (major), CYP2A6 (minor), CYP2B6 (minor), CYP2C9 (minor), CYP3A4 (major); **Note:** Assignment of Major/Minor substrate status based on clinically relevant drug interaction potential; **Inhibits** CYP1A2 (weak)

Avoid Concomitant Use

Avoid concomitant use of Lidocaine (Systemic) with any of the following: Conivaptan; Fusidic Acid (Systemic); Saquinavir

Increased Effect/Toxicity

Lidocaine (Systemic) may increase the levels/effects of: Prilocaine; Sodium Nitrite

The levels/effects of Lidocaine (Systemic) may be increased by: Abiraterone Acetate; Amiodarone; Beta-Blockers; Conivaptan; CYP1A2 Inhibitors (Moderate); CYP1A2 Inhibitors (Strong); CYP3A4 Inhibitors (Moderate); CYP3A4 Inhibitors (Strong); Dasatinib; Deferasirox; Disopyramide; Fusidic Acid (Systemic); Hyaluronidase; Ivacaftor; Luliconazole; Mifepristone; Nitric Oxide; Saquinavir; Simeprevir; Telaprevir; Vemurafenib

Decreased Effect

Lidocaine (Systemic) may decrease the levels/effects of: Technetium Tc 99m Tilmanocept

The levels/effects of Lidocaine (Systemic) may be decreased by: Bosentan; CYP1A2 Inducers (Strong); CYP3A4 Inducers (Strong); Cyproterone; Dabrafenib; Deferasirox; Etravirine; Herbs (CYP3A4 Inducers); Mitotane; Tocilizumab

Ethanol/Nutrition/Herb Interactions Herb/Nutraceutical: St John's wort may decrease lidocaine levels; avoid concurrent use.

Preparation for Administration Local infiltration: Buffered lidocaine for injectable local anesthetic may be prepared: Add 2 mL of sodium bicarbonate 8.4% to 18 mL of lidocaine 1% (Christoph, 1988).

Storage/Stability Injection: Stable at room temperature. Stability of parenteral admixture at room temperature (25°C) is the expiration date on premixed bag; out of overwrap stability is 30 days.

Mechanism of Action Class Ib antiarrhythmic; suppresses automaticity of conduction tissue, by increasing electrical stimulation threshold of ventricle, His-Purkinje system, and spontaneous depolarization of the ventricles during diastole by a direct action on the tissues; blocks both the initiation and conduction of nerve impulses by decreasing the neuronal membrane's permeability to sodium ions, which results in inhibition of depolarization with resultant blockade of conduction

Pharmacodynamics/Kinetics

Onset of action: Single bolus dose: 45-90 seconds

Duration: 10-20 minutes

Distribution: V_d: 1.1-2.1 L/kg; alterable by many patient factors; decreased in CHF and liver disease; crosses blood-brain barrier

Protein binding: 60% to 80% to alpha$_1$ acid glycoprotein

Metabolism: 90% hepatic; active metabolites monoethylglycinexylidide (MEGX) and glycinexylidide (GX) can accumulate and may cause CNS toxicity

Half-life elimination: Biphasic: Prolonged with congestive heart failure, liver disease, shock, severe renal disease; Initial: 7-30 minutes; Terminal: Infants, premature: 3.2 hours, Adults: 1.5-2 hours

Excretion: Urine (<10% as unchanged drug, ~90% as metabolites)

Dosage

Antiarrhythmic:

Children:

I.V., intraosseous (I.O.): **Note:** For use in VF or pulseless VT if amiodarone is not available; give after defibrillation attempts, CPR, and epinephrine:

Loading dose: 1 mg/kg (maximum: 100 mg); follow with continuous infusion; may administer second bolus of 0.5-1 mg/kg if delay between bolus and start of infusion is >15 minutes (PALS, 2000; PALS, 2010)

Continuous infusion: 20-50 mcg/kg/minute (PALS, 2010). Per the manufacturer, do not exceed 20 mcg/kg/minute in patients with shock, hepatic disease, cardiac arrest, or CHF.

Endotracheal: 2-3 mg/kg; flush with 5 mL of NS and follow with 5 assisted manual ventilations (PALS, 2010)

Adults (ACLS, 2010):

VF or pulseless VT (after defibrillation attempts, CPR, and vasopressor administration) if amiodarone is not available: I.V., intraosseous (I.O.): Initial: 1-1.5 mg/kg. If refractory VF or pulseless VT, repeat with 0.5-0.75 mg/kg bolus every 5-10 minutes (maximum cumulative dose: 3 mg/kg). Follow with continuous infusion (1-4 mg/minute) after return of perfusion. Reappearance of arrhythmia during constant infusion: 0.5 mg/kg bolus and reassessment of infusion (Zipes, 2000).

Endotracheal (loading dose only): 2-3.75 mg/kg (2-2.5 times the recommended I.V. dose); dilute in 5-10 mL NS or sterile water. **Note:** Absorption is greater with sterile water and results in less impairment of PaO_2.

Hemodynamically stable monomorphic VT: I.V.: 1-1.5 mg/kg; repeat with 0.5-0.75 mg/kg every 5-10 minutes as necessary (maximum cumulative dose: 3 mg/kg). Follow with continuous infusion of 1-4 mg/minute (or 14-57 mcg/kg/minute).

Note: Reduce maintenance infusion in patients with CHF, shock, or hepatic disease; initiate infusion at 10 mcg/kg/minute (maximum dose: 1.5 mg/minute or 20 mcg/kg/minute).

Anesthetic, local injectable: Children and Adults: Varies with procedure, degree of anesthesia needed, vascularity of tissue, duration of anesthesia required, and physical condition of patient; maximum: 4.5 mg/kg/dose not to exceed 300 mg; do not repeat within 2 hours.

Dosage adjustment in renal impairment: No dosage adjustment provided in manufacturer's labeling. However, accumulation of metabolites may be increased in renal dysfunction. Not dialyzable (0% to 5%) by hemo- or peritoneal dialysis; supplemental dose is not necessary.

Dosage adjustment in hepatic impairment: Use with caution; reduce maintenance infusion. Initial: 0.75 mg/minute or 10 mcg/kg/minute; maximum dose: 1.5 mg/minute or 20 mcg/kg/minute. Monitor lidocaine concentrations closely and adjust infusion rate as necessary; consider alternative therapy.

Dietary Considerations Premixed injection may contain corn-derived dextrose and its use is contraindicated in patients with allergy to corn-related products.

Usual Infusion Concentrations: Pediatric Note: Premixed solutions available

I.V. infusion: 8000 **mcg**/mL

Usual Infusion Concentrations: Adult Note: Premixed solutions available

I.V. infusion: 1000 mg in 250 mL (concentration: 4 mg/mL) **or** 2000 mg in 250 mL (concentration: 8 mg/mL) of D_5W

Administration

I.V.: Local thrombophlebitis may occur in patients receiving prolonged I.V. infusions.

Endotracheal (unlabeled administration route): Dilute in NS or sterile water. Absorption is greater with sterile water and results in less impairment of PaO_2 (Hahnel, 1990). Stop compressions, spray drug quickly down tube. Flush with 5 mL of NS and follow immediately with several quick insufflations and continue chest compressions.

Intraosseous (I.O.; unlabeled administration route): Intraosseous administration is a safe and effective alternative to venous access in children with cardiac arrest; the onset for most medications is similar to that of I.V. administration (PALS, 2010). In adults, I.O. administration is a reasonable alternative when quick I.V. access is not feasible (ACLS, 2010).

Monitoring Parameters Liver function tests, lidocaine concentrations, ECG; consult individual institutional policies and procedures

Reference Range

Therapeutic: 1.5-5.0 mcg/mL (SI: 6-21 micromole/L)

Potentially toxic: >6 mcg/mL (SI: >26 micromole/L)

Toxic: >9 mcg/mL (SI: >38 micromole/L)

Dosage Forms Excipient information presented when available (limited, particularly for generics); consult specific product labeling.

Solution, Injection, as hydrochloride:

Xylocaine: 0.5% (50 mL); 1% (20 mL, 50 mL); 2% (10 mL, 20 mL, 50 mL) [contains methylparaben]

Xylocaine-MPF: 0.5% (50 mL); 1% (2 mL, 5 mL, 10 mL, 30 mL); 1.5% (10 mL, 20 mL); 2% (2 mL, 5 mL, 10 mL); 4% (5 mL) [methylparaben free]

Generic: 0.5% (50 mL); 1% (2 mL, 5 mL, 10 mL, 20 mL, 30 mL, 50 mL); 1.5% (20 mL); 2% (2 mL, 5 mL, 20 mL, 50 mL)

Solution, Injection, as hydrochloride [preservative free]:

Generic: 0.5% (50 mL); 1% (2 mL, 5 mL, 30 mL); 1.5% (20 mL); 2% (2 mL, 5 mL, 10 mL); 4% (5 mL)

Solution, Intravenous, as hydrochloride:

Xylocaine (Cardiac): 20 mg/mL (5 mL)

Generic: 10 mg/mL (5 mL); 20 mg/mL (5 mL); 0.4% [4 mg/mL] (250 mL, 500 mL); 0.8% [8 mg/mL] (250 mL); 2% (5 mL); 5% [50 mg/mL] (2 mL)

Solution, Intravenous, as hydrochloride [preservative free]:

Generic: 10 mg/mL (5 mL); 20 mg/mL (5 mL)

Lidocaine (Topical) (LYE doe kane)

Brand Names: U.S. AneCream [OTC]; AneCream5 [OTC]; LC-4 Lidocaine [OTC]; LC-5 Lidocaine [OTC]; Lidoderm; LidoRx; LMX 4 Plus [OTC]; LMX 4 [OTC]; LMX 5 [OTC]; LTA 360 Kit; Predator [OTC]; RectiCare [OTC]; Tecnu First Aid [OTC]; Topicaine 5 [OTC]; Topicaine [OTC]; Xylocaine

Brand Names: Canada Betacaine®; Lidodan™; Lidoderm®; Maxilene®; Xylocaine®

Index Terms Lidocaine Hydrochloride; Lidocaine Patch; Lignocaine Hydrochloride; Viscous Lidocaine; Xylocaine Viscous

Pharmacologic Category Analgesic, Topical; Local Anesthetic

Use

Rectal: Temporary relief of pain and itching due to anorectal disorders

Topical: Local anesthetic for oral mucous membrane; use in laser/cosmetic surgeries; minor burns, cuts, and abrasions of the skin

Oral topical solution (viscous): Topical anesthesia of irritated oral mucous membranes and pharyngeal tissue

Patch (Lidoderm®): Relief of allodynia (painful hypersensitivity) and chronic pain in postherpetic neuralgia

Patch (LidoPatch™): Temporary relief of localized pain

Pregnancy Risk Factor B

Dosage Anesthesia, topical:

Cream:

LidaMantle®: Skin irritation: Children and Adults: Apply a thin film to affected area 2-3 times/day as needed

L-M-X® 4: Skin irritation: Children ≥2 years and Adults: Apply up to 3-4 times daily to intact skin

L-M-X® 5: Relief of anorectal pain and itching: Children ≥12 years and Adults: Apply to affected area up to 6 times/day

Gel, ointment: Adults: Apply to affected area ≤4 times/day as needed (maximum dose: 4.5 mg/kg, not to exceed 300 mg)

Topical solution: Adults: Apply 1-5 mL (40-200 mg) to affected area

Jelly:

Children: Dose varies with age and weight (maximum dose: 4.5 mg/kg)

Adults (maximum dose: 30 mL [600 mg] in any 12-hour period):

Anesthesia of male urethra: 5-30 mL (100-600 mg)

Anesthesia of female urethra: 3-5 mL (60-100 mg)

Oral topical solution (viscous):

Infants and Children <3 years: 1.25 mL applied to area with a cotton-tipped applicator no more frequently than every 3 hours (maximum: 4 doses per 12-hour period)

Children ≥3 years: Should not exceed 4.5 mg/kg/dose (or 300 mg/dose); swished in the mouth and spit out no more frequently than every 3 hours (maximum: 4 doses per 12-hour period)

Adults:

Anesthesia of the mouth: 15 mL swished in the mouth and spit out no more frequently than every 3 hours (maximum: 8 doses per 24-hour period)

Anesthesia of the pharynx: 15 mL gargled no more frequently than every 3 hours (maximum: 8 doses per 24-hour period); may be swallowed

Patch: Adults:

Lidoderm®: Postherpetic neuralgia: Apply patch to most painful area. Up to 3 patches may be applied in a single application. Patch(es) may remain in place for up to 12 hours in any 24-hour period.

LidoPatch™: Pain (localized): Apply patch to painful area. Patch may remain in place for up to 12 hours in any 24-hour period. No more than 1 patch should be used in a 24-hour period.

Additional Information Complete prescribing information should be consulted for additional detail.

Dosage Forms Excipient information presented when available (limited, particularly for generics); consult specific product labeling.

Cream, External:

AneCream: 4% (5 g, 15 g, 30 g) [contains benzyl alcohol, polysorbate 80, propylene glycol, trolamine (triethanolamine)]

AneCream5: 5% (15 g, 30 g) [contains benzyl alcohol, polysorbate 80, propylene glycol, trolamine (triethanolamine)]

LC-4 Lidocaine: 4% (45 g) [contains cetyl alcohol]

LC-5 Lidocaine: 5% (45 g) [contains cetyl alcohol]

LMX 4: 4% (5 g, 15 g, 30 g) [contains benzyl alcohol]

LMX 5: 5% (15 g, 30 g) [contains benzyl alcohol]

RectiCare: 5% (30 g) [contains benzyl alcohol, polysorbate 80, propylene glycol, trolamine (triethanolamine)]

Cream, External, as hydrochloride:

Predator: 4% (63 g) [contains propylene glycol, trolamine (triethanolamine)]

Generic: 3% (28.3 g, 28.35 g, 85 g)

Gel, External:

Tecnu First Aid: 0.2-2.5% (56.7 g) [contains disodium edta]

Topicaine: 4% (10 g, 30 g, 113 g) [contains benzyl alcohol, disodium edta]

Topicaine 5: 5% (10 g, 30 g, 113 g) [contains benzyl alcohol, disodium edta]
Gel, External, as hydrochloride:
LidoRx: 3% (10 mL, 30 mL) [contains isopropyl alcohol, trolamine (triethanolamine)]
Generic: 2% (5 mL, 20 mL, 30 mL)
Gel, External, as hydrochloride [preservative free]:
Generic: 2% (5 mL, 10 mL)
Kit, External:
AneCream: 4% [contains benzyl alcohol, polysorbate 80, propylene glycol, trolamine (triethanolamine)]
LMX 4 Plus: 4% [contains benzyl alcohol]
Lotion, External, as hydrochloride:
Generic: 3% (177 mL)
Ointment, External:
Generic: 5% (30 g, 50 g)
Ointment, External, as hydrochloride:
Generic: 5% (35.44 g, 50 g)
Patch, External:
Lidoderm: 5% (30 ea) [contains disodium edta, methylparaben, propylene glycol, propylparaben]
Generic: 5% (1 ea, 30 ea)
Solution, External, as hydrochloride:
Xylocaine: 4% (50 mL) [contains methylparaben]
Generic: 4% (50 mL)
Solution, Mouth/Throat, as hydrochloride:
Generic: 2% (15 mL, 100 mL)
Solution, Mouth/Throat, as hydrochloride [preservative free]:
LTA 360 Kit: 4% (4 mL)
Generic: 4% (4 mL)

Lidocaine and Epinephrine

(LYE doe kane & ep i NEF rin)

Brand Names: U.S. Lignospan® Forte; Lignospan® Standard; Xylocaine® MPF With Epinephrine; Xylocaine® With Epinephrine

Brand Names: Canada Xylocaine® With Epinephrine

Index Terms Epinephrine and Lidocaine

Pharmacologic Category Local Anesthetic

Use Local infiltration anesthesia; AVS for nerve block

Pregnancy Risk Factor B

Dosage Dosage varies with the anesthetic procedure, degree of anesthesia needed, vascularity of tissue, duration of anesthesia required, and physical condition of patient.

Dental anesthesia, infiltration, or conduction block:

Children <12 years: 20-30 mg (1-1.5 mL) of lidocaine hydrochloride as a 2% solution with epinephrine 1:100,000; maximum: 4.5 mg of lidocaine hydrochloride/kg of body weight or 100-150 mg as a single dose

Children ≥12 years and Adults: Do not exceed 7 mg/kg body weight up to a maximum range of 300 mg (usual dental practice) to 500 mg (approved product labeling) of lidocaine hydrochloride and 3 mcg (0.003 mg) of epinephrine/kg of body weight or 0.2 mg epinephrine per dental appointment. The effective anesthetic dose varies with procedure, intensity of anesthesia needed, duration of anesthesia required, and physical condition of the patient. Always use the lowest effective dose along with careful aspiration.

Note: For most routine dental procedures, lidocaine hydrochloride 2% with epinephrine 1:100,000 is preferred. When a more pronounced hemostasis is required, a 1:50,000 epinephrine concentration should be used.

Dosage adjustment in renal impairment: No dosage adjustment provided in manufacturer's labeling. However, accumulation of metabolites may be increased in renal dysfunction.

Dosage adjustment in hepatic impairment: No dosage adjustment provided in manufacturer's labeling; use with caution.

Additional Information Complete prescribing information should be consulted for additional detail.

Dosage Forms Excipient information presented when available (limited, particularly for generics); consult specific product labeling. [DSC] = Discontinued product

Injection, solution:
0.5% / 1:200,000: Lidocaine hydrochloride 0.5% [5 mg/mL] and epinephrine 1:200,000 (50 mL)
1% / 1:100,000: Lidocaine hydrochloride 1% [10 mg/mL] and epinephrine 1:100,000 (20 mL, 30 mL, 50 mL)
2% / 1:100,000: Lidocaine hydrochloride 2% [20 mg/mL] and epinephrine 1:100,000 (30 mL, 50 mL)
Xylocaine® with Epinephrine:
0.5% / 1:200,000: Lidocaine hydrochloride 0.5% [5 mg/mL] and epinephrine 1:200,000 (50 mL) [contains methylparaben]
1% / 1:100,000: Lidocaine hydrochloride 1% [10 mg/mL] and epinephrine 1:100,000 (10 mL, 20 mL, 50 mL) [contains methylparaben]
2% / 1:100,000: Lidocaine hydrochloride 2% [20 mg/mL] and epinephrine 1:100,000 (10 mL, 20 mL, 50 mL) [contains methylparaben]

Injection, solution [preservative free]:
1.5% / 1:200,000: Lidocaine hydrochloride 1.5% [15 mg/mL] and epinephrine 1:200,000 (5 mL, 30 mL)
2% / 1:200,000: Lidocaine hydrochloride 2% [20 mg/mL] and epinephrine 1:200,000 (20 mL)
Xylocaine®-MPF with Epinephrine:
1% / 1:200,000: Lidocaine hydrochloride 1% [10 mg/mL] and epinephrine 1:200,000 (5 mL, 10 mL, 30 mL) [contains sodium metabisulfite]
1.5% / 1:200,000: Lidocaine hydrochloride 1.5% [15 mg/mL] and epinephrine 1:200,000 (5 mL, 10 mL, 30 mL) [contains sodium metabisulfite]
2% / 1:200,000: Lidocaine hydrochloride 2% [20 mg/mL] and epinephrine 1:200,000 (5 mL, 10 mL, 20 mL) [contains sodium metabisulfite]

Injection, solution [for dental use]:
2% / 1:50,000: Lidocaine hydrochloride 2% [20 mg/mL] and epinephrine 1:50,000 (1.7 mL, 1.8 mL)
2% / 1:100,000: Lidocaine hydrochloride 2% [20 mg/mL] and epinephrine 1:100,000 (1.7 mL, 1.8 mL)
Lignospan® Forte: 2% / 1:50,000: Lidocaine hydrochloride 2% [20 mg/mL] and epinephrine 1:50,000 (1.7 mL) [contains edetate disodium, potassium metabisulfite]
Lignospan® Standard: 2% / 1:100,000: Lidocaine hydrochloride 2% [20 mg/mL] and epinephrine 1:100,000 (1.7 mL) [contains edetate disodium, potassium metabisulfite]
Xylocaine® Dental with Epinephrine:
2% / 1:50,000: Lidocaine hydrochloride 2% [20 mg/mL] and epinephrine 1:50,000 (1.7 mL; 1.8 mL [DSC]) [contains sodium metabisulfite]
2% / 1:100,000: Lidocaine hydrochloride 2% [20 mg/mL] and epinephrine 1:100,000 (1.7 mL; 1.8 mL [DSC]) [contains sodium metabisulfite]

Lidocaine and Prilocaine

(LYE doe kane & PRIL oh kane)

Brand Names: U.S. EMLA®; Oraqix®

Brand Names: Canada EMLA®; Oraqix®

Index Terms Prilocaine and Lidocaine

Pharmacologic Category Local Anesthetic

Use

U.S. labeling:

Cream: Topical anesthetic for use on normal intact skin to provide local analgesia for minor procedures such as I.V. cannulation or venipuncture; has also been used for painful procedures such as lumbar puncture and skin graft harvesting; for superficial minor surgery of genital mucous membranes and as an adjunct for local infiltration anesthesia in genital mucous membranes.

Periodontal gel: Topical anesthetic for use in periodontal pockets during scaling or root planing procedures

Canadian labeling:

Cream: Topical anesthetic to provide local analgesia for the following: minor procedures on intact skin such as I.V. cannulation or venipuncture, superficial procedures such as skin grafting and electrolysis, laser treatment for superficial skin surgery (eg, warts, moles, skin nodules, scar tissue); superficial minor surgery of genital mucous membranes and as an adjunct for local infiltration anesthesia in genital mucous membranes; mechanical cleansing/debridement of leg ulcers; vaccination with measles-mumps-rubella (MMR), diphtheria-pertussis-tetanus-poliovirus (DPTP), *Haemophilus influenzae* b, and hepatitis B.

Patch: Topical anesthetic of intact skin for I.V. cannulation or venipuncture; vaccination with measles-mumps-rubella (MMR), diphtheria-pertussis-tetanus-poliovirus (DPTP), *Haemophilus influenzae* b, and hepatitis B.

Periodontal gel: Topical anesthetic for use in periodontal pockets during scaling or root planing procedures

Pregnancy Risk Factor B

Dosage Although the incidence of systemic adverse effects is very low, caution should be exercised, particularly when applying over large areas and leaving on for >2 hours

Infants and Children (intact skin): **Note:** If a patient >3 months of age does not meet the minimum weight requirement, the maximum total dose should be restricted to the corresponding maximum based on patient weight.

Cream: Should **not** be used in neonates with a gestation age <37 weeks nor in infants <12 months of age who are receiving treatment with methemoglobin-inducing agents

Dosing is based on child's age and weight:

Age 0-3 months or <5 kg: Apply a maximum of 1 g over no more than 10 cm^2 of skin; leave on for no longer than 1 hour

Age 3 months to 12 months and >5 kg: Apply no more than a maximum 2 g total over no more than 20 cm^2 of skin; leave on for no longer than 4 hours

Age 1-6 years and >10 kg: Apply no more than a maximum of 10 g total over no more than 100 cm^2 of skin; leave on for no longer than 4 hours. U.S. labeling recommends leaving on for no longer than 4 hours. Canadian labeling recommends leaving on for no longer than 5 hours.

Age 7-12 years and >20 kg: Apply no more than a maximum 20 g total over no more than 200 cm^2 of skin; leave on for no longer than 4 hours. U.S. labeling recommends leaving on for no longer than 4 hours. Canadian labeling recommends leaving on for no longer than 5 hours.

Transdermal patch: Canadian availability (not available in U.S.): **Note:** Should not be used in neonates with a gestation age <37 weeks nor in infants <12 months of age who are receiving treatment with methemoglobin-inducing agents

Dosing is based on child's age and weight: Apply patch(es) to skin area(s) <10 cm^2:

Age 0-3 months or <5 kg: Apply 1 patch and leave on for ~1 hour (do not exceed 1-hour application time); do not apply more than 1 patch at same time; safety of repeated dosing not established

Age 3 months to 12 months and >5 kg: Apply 1-2 patches for ~1 hour (maximum application time: 4 hours); do not apply more than 2 patches at the same time

Age 1-6 years and >10 kg: Apply 1 or more patches for minimum of 1 hour (maximum application time: 5 hours); maximum dose: 10 patches

Age 7-12 years and >20 kg: Apply 1 or more patches for a minimum of 1 hour (maximum application time: 5 hours); maximum dose: 20 patches

Adults (intact skin):

Cream: **Note:** Apply a thick layer to intact skin and cover with an occlusive dressing. Dermal analgesia can be expected to increase for up to 3 hours under occlusive dressing and persist for 1-2 hours after removal of the cream.

U.S. labeling:

Minor dermal procedures (eg, I.V. cannulation or venipuncture): Apply 2.5 g of cream (1/2 of the 5 g tube) over 20-25 cm^2 of skin surface area) for at least 1 hour

Major dermal procedures (eg, more painful dermatological procedures involving a larger skin area such as split thickness skin graft harvesting): Apply 2 g of cream per 10 cm^2 of skin and allow to remain in contact with the skin for at least 2 hours.

Adult male genital skin (eg, pretreatment prior to local anesthetic infiltration): Apply a thick layer of cream (1 g per 10 cm^2) to the skin surface for 15 minutes. Local anesthetic infiltration should be performed immediately after removal of cream.

Adult female genital mucous membranes: Minor procedures (eg, removal of condylomata acuminata, pretreatment for local anesthetic infiltration): Apply a thick layer of cream (5-10 g) for 5-10 minutes. The local anesthetic infiltration or procedure should be performed immediately after removal of cream.

Canadian labeling:

Minor dermal procedures (eg, I.V. cannulation, venipuncture, surgical or laser treatment): Apply 2 g (~1/2 of the 5 g tube) over ~13.5 cm^2 for at least 1 hour but no longer than 5 hours

Major dermal procedures (eg, split-skin grafting): 1.5-2 g per 10 cm^2 (maximum: 60 g per 400 cm^2) for at least 2 hours but no longer than 5 hours

Genital mucosa (eg, surgical procedures ≤10 minutes such as localized wart removal, and prior to local anesthetic infiltration): Apply 2 g (~1/2 of 5 g tube) per lesion (maximum: 10 g) for 5-10 minutes. Initiate procedure immediately after removing cream.

Leg ulcers (eg, mechanical cleansing/surgical debridement): Apply ~1-2 g per 10 cm^2 (maximum: 10 g) for at least 30 minutes and up to 60 minutes for necrotic tissue that is more difficult to penetrate. Initiate procedure immediately after removing cream.

Periodontal gel (Oraqix®): Apply on gingival margin around selected teeth using the blunt-tipped applicator included in package. Wait 30 seconds, then fill the periodontal pockets using the blunt-tipped applicator until gel becomes visible at the gingival margin. Wait another 30 seconds before starting treatment. May reapply; maximum recommended dose: One treatment session: 5 cartridges (8.5 g)

Transdermal patch: Canadian availability (not available in U.S.): Apply 1 or more patches to intact skin surface area <10 cm^2 for at least 1 hour (maximum application time: 5 hours)

Elderly: Smaller areas of treatment may be necessary depending on status of patient (eg, debilitated, impaired hepatic function). Refer to adult dosing.

Dosage adjustment in renal impairment: No dosage adjustment provided in manufacturer labeling. Lidocaine and prilocaine primarily undergo hepatic metabolism and their pharmacokinetics are not expected to be changed significantly in renal impairment.

Dosage adjustment in hepatic impairment: Smaller areas of treatment are recommended for patients with severe hepatic impairment.

Additional Information Complete prescribing information should be consulted for additional detail.

Dosage Forms Excipient information presented when available (limited, particularly for generics); consult specific product labeling.

Cream, topical: Lidocaine 2.5% and prilocaine 2.5% (5 g, 30 g)

EMLA®: Lidocaine 2.5% and prilocaine 2.5% (5 g, 30 g)

Gel, periodontal:

Oraqix®: Lidocaine 2.5% and prilocaine 2.5% (1.7 g)

Dosage Forms: Canada Excipient information presented when available (limited, particularly for generics); consult specific product labeling.

Patch, transdermal:

EMLA® Patch: Lidocaine 2.5% and prilocaine 2.5% per patch (2s, 20s) [active contact surface area of each 1 g patch: 10 cm^2; surface area of entire patch: 40 cm^2]

Lidocaine and Tetracaine

(LYE doe kane & TET ra kane)

Brand Names: U.S. Synera®

Index Terms Eutectic Mixture of Lidocaine and Tetracaine; Tetracaine and Lidocaine

Pharmacologic Category Analgesic, Topical; Local Anesthetic

Use Topical anesthetic for use on normal intact skin for minor procedures (eg, I.V. cannulation or venipuncture) and superficial dermatologic procedures

Pregnancy Risk Factor B

Dosage Transdermal patch: Children ≥3 years and Adults:

Venipuncture or intravenous cannulation: Prior to procedure, apply to intact skin for 20-30 minutes; **Note:** Adults can use another patch at a new location to facilitate venous access after a failed attempt; remove previous patch.

Superficial dermatological procedures: Prior to procedure, apply to intact skin for 30 minutes

Dosage adjustment in hepatic impairment: Use caution in patients with severe hepatic dysfunction.

Additional Information Complete prescribing information should be consulted for additional detail.

Dosage Forms Excipient information presented when available (limited, particularly for generics); consult specific product labeling.

Patch, transdermal:

Synera®: Lidocaine 70 mg and tetracaine 70 mg (10s) [contains heating component, metal; each patch is ~50 cm^2]

- **Lidocaine Hydrochloride** *see* Lidocaine (Systemic) *on page 1210*
- **Lidocaine Hydrochloride** *see* Lidocaine (Topical) *on page 1212*
- **Lidocaine Patch** *see* Lidocaine (Topical) *on page 1212*
- **Lidodan™ (Can)** *see* Lidocaine (Topical) *on page 1212*
- **Lidoderm** *see* Lidocaine (Topical) *on page 1212*
- **Lidoderm® (Can)** *see* Lidocaine (Topical) *on page 1212*
- **LidoRx** *see* Lidocaine (Topical) *on page 1212*
- **LID-Pack® (Can)** *see* Bacitracin and Polymyxin B *on page 220*
- **Lignocaine Hydrochloride** *see* Lidocaine (Systemic) *on page 1210*
- **Lignocaine Hydrochloride** *see* Lidocaine (Topical) *on page 1212*
- **Lignospan® Forte** *see* Lidocaine and Epinephrine *on page 1213*
- **Lignospan® Standard** *see* Lidocaine and Epinephrine *on page 1213*
- **Limbitrol** *see* Amitriptyline and Chlordiazepoxide *on page 107*

Linaclotide (lin AK loe tide)

Brand Names: U.S. Linzess

Index Terms Linaclotide Acetate

Pharmacologic Category Gastrointestinal Agent, Miscellaneous

Use Treatment of chronic idiopathic constipation (CIC); treatment of irritable bowel syndrome with constipation (IBS-C) in adults

Pregnancy Risk Factor C

Pregnancy Considerations Adverse events were observed in some animal reproduction studies. Linaclotide and its metabolite are not measurable in plasma when used at recommended doses.

Breast-Feeding Considerations It is not known if linaclotide is excreted in breast milk; linaclotide and its metabolite are not measurable in plasma when used at recommended doses. The manufacturer recommends to use caution if administered to breast-feeding women.

Medication Guide Available Yes

Contraindications Use in pediatric patients ≤6 years of age; known or suspected mechanical gastrointestinal obstruction

Warnings/Precautions [U.S. Boxed Warning]: Use is contraindicated in pediatric patients ≤6 years of age. Use in pediatric patients 6-17 years of age should be avoided. Deaths were observed in young juvenile animals during nonclinical studies; deaths were not observed in older juvenile animals. There are not sufficient safety and efficacy data to support use in pediatric patients. May cause severe diarrhea; consider dose suspension if necessary. Patients should be instructed to discontinue use and contact their healthcare provider if severe diarrhea occurs. Administration with a high-fat meal may worsen diarrhea.

Adverse Reactions Adverse reactions reported with use in IBS-C and CIC.

>10%: Gastrointestinal: Diarrhea (16% to 20%; severe diarrhea: 2%)

1% to 10%:

Central nervous system: Headache (4%), fatigue (<2%)

Endocrine & metabolic: Dehydration (≤1%)

Gastrointestinal: Abdominal pain (7%), flatulence (4% to 6%), abdominal distension (2% to 3%), viral gastroenteritis (≤3%), dyspepsia (<2%), fecal incontinence (<2%), gastroesophageal reflux disease (<2%), vomiting (<2%)

Respiratory: Upper respiratory tract infection (5%), sinusitis (3%)

<1% (Limited to important or life-threatening): Hematochezia, hypersensitivity reaction, rectal hemorrhage

Drug Interactions

Metabolism/Transport Effects None known.

Avoid Concomitant Use There are no known interactions where it is recommended to avoid concomitant use.

Increased Effect/Toxicity There are no known significant interactions involving an increase in effect.

Decreased Effect There are no known significant interactions involving a decrease in effect.

Storage/Stability Store at 25°C (77°F) in tightly closed, original container with included desiccant packet; excursions permitted between 15°C and 30°C (59°F and 86°F). Do not repackage; protect from moisture.

Mechanism of Action Linaclotide and its active metabolite bind and agonize guanylate cyclase-C on the luminal surface of intestinal epithelium. Intracellular and extracellular cyclic guanosine monophosphate (cGMP) concentrations are subsequently increased resulting in chloride and bicarbonate secretion into the intestinal lumen. Intestinal fluid increases and transit time is decreased. Extracellular cGMP may decrease visceral pain by reducing pain-sensing nerve activity.

Pharmacodynamics/Kinetics

Absorption: Minimal systemic availability; plasma concentrations are not measurable when used at recommended doses.

Distribution: Minimal tissue distribution is expected given immeasurable plasma concentrations when used at recommended doses.

Metabolism: Metabolized within GI tract to active metabolite; parent drug and metabolite undergo proteolytic degradation within the intestinal lumen to smaller peptides and amino acids

Excretion: Primarily feces (3% to 5% as the active metabolite)

Dosage

Adults: Oral:

Chronic idiopathic constipation (CIC): 145 mcg once daily

Irritable bowel syndrome with constipation (IBS-C): 290 mcg once daily

Elderly: Not adequately studied in the elderly. Refer to adult dosing.

Dosage adjustment in renal impairment: No dosage adjustment necessary.

Dosage adjustment in hepatic impairment: No dosage adjustment necessary.

Dietary Considerations Take at least 30 minutes before breakfast on an empty stomach. Loose stools and greater stool frequency may occur after administration with a high-fat breakfast.

Administration Oral: Administer at least 30 minutes before breakfast on an empty stomach; loose stools and greater stool frequency may occur after administration with a high-fat breakfast. Swallow capsule whole; do not break or chew capsules.

Monitoring Parameters

IBS-C: Abdominal pain, spontaneous bowel movement quality and frequency

CIC: Frequency of straining during bowel movements; spontaneous bowel movement quality and frequency

Dosage Forms Excipient information presented when available (limited, particularly for generics); consult specific product labeling.

Capsule, Oral:

Linzess: 145 mcg, 290 mcg

◆ Linaclotide Acetate *see* Linaclotide *on page* 1215

Linagliptin (lin a GLIP tin)

Brand Names: U.S. Tradjenta

Brand Names: Canada Trajenta

Index Terms BI-1356; Trajenta

Pharmacologic Category Antidiabetic Agent, Dipeptidyl Peptidase IV (DPP-IV) Inhibitor

Additional Appendix Information

Oral Antidiabetic Agents Comparison Table *on page* 2312

Use Management of type 2 diabetes mellitus (noninsulin dependent, NIDDM) as an adjunct to diet and exercise as monotherapy or in combination with other antidiabetic agents

Pregnancy Risk Factor B

Pregnancy Considerations Adverse events were not observed in animal reproduction studies, except with doses that were also maternally toxic. For women with diabetes, maternal hyperglycemia can be associated with adverse effects in the fetus, neonate, and mother. To prevent adverse events, prior to conception and throughout pregnancy, the maternal Hb A_{1c} should be kept close to normal but without causing significant hypoglycemia. The use of dipeptidyl peptidase IV (DPP-IV) inhibitors in pregnant women is not currently recommended; insulin is the drug of choice for the control of diabetes mellitus during pregnancy (ACOG, 2005; ADA, 2013; Kitzmiller, 2008; Metzger, 2007).

Breast-Feeding Considerations It is not known if linagliptin is excreted in breast milk. The manufacturer recommends that caution be used if administered to breast-feeding women.

Medication Guide Available Yes

Contraindications Hypersensitivity to linagliptin or any component of the formulation

Canadian labeling: Additional contraindications: Use in type 1 diabetes mellitus or diabetic ketoacidosis

Warnings/Precautions Avoid use in type 1 diabetes mellitus (insulin dependent, IDDM) and diabetic ketoacidosis (DKA) due to lack of efficacy in these populations. Diabetes self-management education (DSME) is essential to maximize the effectiveness of therapy. Cases of acute pancreatitis, including fatalities, have been reported with use. Monitor for signs/symptoms of pancreatitis; discontinue use immediately if pancreatitis is suspected and initiate appropriate management. Use with caution in patients with a history of pancreatitis as it is not known if this population is at greater risk. Clinical trials included only a limited number of patients with heart failure (HF). No specific recommendations regarding this population are provided in the approved U.S. labeling (Canadian labeling recommends against use in this population). Potentially significant drug-drug interactions may exist, requiring dose or frequency adjustment, additional monitoring, and/or selection of alternative therapy.

Adverse Reactions

>10%: Endocrine & metabolic: Hypoglycemia (combined with metformin and/or sulfonylurea [15% to 23%]; monotherapy [<1% to 7%]; metformin [<1%], pioglitazone [<1%])

1% to 10%:

Central nervous system: Headache (6%)

Endocrine & metabolic: Hyperuricemia (3%), lipids increased (3%), triglycerides increased (2% to 3%), weight gain (2%)

Gastrointestinal: Constipation (2%)

Genitourinary: Urinary tract infection (3%)

Neuromuscular & skeletal: Arthralgia (6%), back pain (6%)

Respiratory: Nasopharyngitis (6% to 7%), cough (2%)

<1% (Limited to important or life-threatening): Angioedema, hypersensitivity, pancreatitis

Drug Interactions

Metabolism/Transport Effects Substrate of CYP3A4 (major), P-glycoprotein; **Note:** Assignment of Major/Minor substrate status based on clinically relevant drug interaction potential

Avoid Concomitant Use There are no known interactions where it is recommended to avoid concomitant use.

Increased Effect/Toxicity

Linagliptin may increase the levels/effects of: ACE Inhibitors; Hypoglycemic Agents

The levels/effects of Linagliptin may be increased by: Herbs (Hypoglycemic Properties); MAO Inhibitors; Pegvisomant; P-glycoprotein/ABCB1 Inhibitors; Ritonavir; Salicylates; Selective Serotonin Reuptake Inhibitors

Decreased Effect
The levels/effects of Linagliptin may be decreased by: Bosentan; Corticosteroids (Orally Inhaled); Corticosteroids (Systemic); CYP3A4 Inducers (Strong); Dabrafenib; Deferasirox; Herbs (CYP3A4 Inducers); Loop Diuretics; Luteinizing Hormone-Releasing Hormone Analogs; P-glycoprotein/ABCB1 Inducers; Somatropin; Thiazide Diuretics; Tocilizumab

Ethanol/Nutrition/Herb Interactions
Ethanol: Caution with ethanol (may cause hypoglycemia).
Herb/Nutraceutical: Herbs with hypoglycemic properties may enhance the hypoglycemic effect of linagliptin. This includes alfalfa, aloe, bilberry, bitter melon, burdock, celery, damiana, fenugreek, garcinia, garlic, ginger, ginseng (American), gymnema, marshmallow, stinging nettle.

Storage/Stability Store at 25°C (77°F); excursions permitted between 15°C to 30°C (59°F to 86°F).

Mechanism of Action Linagliptin inhibits dipeptidyl peptidase IV (DPP-IV) enzyme resulting in prolonged active incretin levels. Incretin hormones (eg, glucagon-like peptide-1 [GLP-1] and glucose-dependent insulinotropic polypeptide [GIP]) regulate glucose homeostasis by increasing insulin synthesis and release from pancreatic beta cells and decreasing glucagon secretion from pancreatic alpha cells. Decreased glucagon secretion results in decreased hepatic glucose production. Under normal physiologic circumstances, incretin hormones are released by the intestine throughout the day and levels are increased in response to a meal; incretin hormones are rapidly inactivated by the DPP-IV enzyme.

Pharmacodynamics/Kinetics
Absorption: Rapid
Distribution: Extensive
Protein binding: 70% to 80%; concentration dependent
Metabolism: Not extensively metabolized
Bioavailability: 30%
Half-life elimination: Effective (therapeutic): ~12 hours; Terminal (DPP-IV saturable binding): >100 hours
Time to peak: 1.5 hours
Excretion: 80% feces unchanged; 5% urine unchanged

Dosage Oral: Adults: Type 2 diabetes: 5 mg once daily
Concomitant use with insulin and/or insulin secretagogues (eg, sulfonylureas): Reduced dose of insulin and/or insulin secretagogues may be needed.

Dosage adjustment in renal impairment: No dosage adjustment necessary.
Dosage adjustment in hepatic impairment: No dosage adjustment necessary. **Note:** Canadian labeling does not recommend use in severe hepatic impairment.

Dietary Considerations May be taken without regard to food. Individualized medical nutrition therapy (MNT) based on ADA recommendations is an integral part of therapy.

Administration May be administered with or without food.

Monitoring Parameters Hb A_{1c}, serum glucose

Reference Range Recommendations for glycemic control in nonpregnant adults with diabetes (ADA, 2013):
Hb A_{1c}: <7% (a more aggressive [<6.5%] or less aggressive [<8%] Hb A_{1c} goal may be targeted based on patient-specific characteristics)
Preprandial capillary plasma glucose: 70-130 mg/dL
Peak postprandial capillary blood glucose: <180 mg/dL

Dosage Forms Excipient information presented when available (limited, particularly for generics); consult specific product labeling.
Tablet, Oral:
Tradjenta: 5 mg

Linagliptin and Metformin
(lin a GLIP tin & met FOR min)

Brand Names: U.S. Jentadueto

Brand Names: Canada Jentadueto

Index Terms Linagliptin and Metformin Hydrochloride; Metformin and Linagliptin; Metformin Hydrochloride and Linagliptin

Pharmacologic Category Antidiabetic Agent, Biguanide; Antidiabetic Agent, Dipeptidyl Peptidase IV (DPP-IV) Inhibitor

Use Management of type 2 diabetes mellitus (noninsulin dependent, NIDDM) as an adjunct to diet and exercise in patients when treatment with both linagliptin and metformin is appropriate

Pregnancy Risk Factor B

Medication Guide Available Yes

Dosage Oral: Type 2 diabetes mellitus:
Adults: Initial doses should be based on current dose of linagliptin and metformin.
Patients inadequately controlled on metformin (with or without sulfonylurea): Initial dose: Linagliptin 5 mg daily plus current daily dose of metformin given in 2 equally divided doses; maximum: linagliptin 5 mg/metformin 2000 mg daily.
Patients inadequately controlled on linagliptin alone: Initial dose: Metformin 1000 mg daily plus linagliptin 5 mg daily given in 2 equally divided doses.
Concomitant use with insulin and/or insulin secretagogues (eg, sulfonylureas): Reduced dose of insulin and/or insulin secretagogues may be needed.
Dosing adjustment: Metformin component may be gradually increased up to the maximum dose. Maximum dose: Linagliptin 5 mg/metformin 2000 mg daily.
Elderly: The initial and maintenance dosing should be conservative, due to the potential for decreased renal function (monitor). Do not use in patients ≥80 years of age unless normal renal function has been established.

Dosage adjustment in renal impairment: Use is contraindicated in patients with renal disease or renal dysfunction (serum creatinine ≥1.5 mg/dL [≥136 micromole/L] in males or ≥1.4 mg/dL [≥124 micromole/L] in females or abnormal clearance [<60 mL/minute]).
Dosage adjustment in hepatic impairment: Avoid metformin; liver disease is a risk factor for the development of lactic acidosis during metformin therapy.

Additional Information Complete prescribing information should be consulted for additional detail.

Dosage Forms Excipient information presented when available (limited, particularly for generics); consult specific product labeling.
Tablet, oral:
Jentadueto 2.5/500: Linagliptin 2.5 mg and metformin hydrochloride 500 mg
Jentadueto 2.5/850: Linagliptin 2.5 mg and metformin hydrochloride 850 mg
Jentadueto 2.5/1000: Linagliptin 2.5 mg and metformin hydrochloride 1000 mg

◆ **Linagliptin and Metformin Hydrochloride** *see* Linagliptin and Metformin *on page 1217*

Lindane (LIN dane)

Index Terms Benzene Hexachloride; Gamma Benzene Hexachloride; Hexachlorocyclohexane; Kwell

Pharmacologic Category Antiparasitic Agent, Topical; Pediculocide; Scabicidal Agent

Use
Lotion: Treatment of *Sarcoptes scabiei* (scabies)
Shampoo: Treatment of *Pediculus capitis* (head lice) and *Phthirus pubis* (crab lice)
Note: Not recommended for first line-treatment; use should be reserved for patients who are intolerant to or have failed first-line agents.

Pregnancy Risk Factor C

Pregnancy Considerations Adverse events have been observed in animal reproduction studies. Animal studies suggest possible neurologic abnormalities due to the increased susceptibility of drug and the immature central nervous system of the fetus. Lindane is lipophilic and may accumulate in the placenta. Use in pregnant women is contraindicated in some guidelines (CDC, 2010).

Breast-Feeding Considerations Lindane is excreted in breast milk. Nursing mothers should interrupt breast-feeding, express and discard milk for at least 24 hours following use. In addition, skin-to-skin contact between the infant and affected area should be avoided. Use in nursing women is contraindicated in some guidelines (CDC, 2010).

Medication Guide Available Yes

Contraindications Hypersensitivity to lindane or any component of the formulation; premature infants; uncontrolled seizure disorders; crusted (Norwegian) scabies or other skin conditions (eg, atopic dermatitis, psoriasis) which may increase systemic absorption

Warnings/Precautions Hazardous agent - use appropriate precautions for handling and disposal (EPA, U-listed). **[U.S. Boxed Warning]: Not a drug of first choice; use only in patients who have failed or cannot tolerate first-line agents. Instruct patients on proper use, including the amount to apply, how long to leave on, and to avoid retreatment. Itching may occur as a result of killing lice and does not necessarily indicate treatment failure or need for retreatment.** Because of the potential for systemic absorption and CNS side effects, lindane should be used with caution; consider permethrin or crotamiton agent first. Oil-based hair dressing may increase toxic potential. For external use only; avoid contact with face, eyes, mucous membranes, and urethral meatus. For treatment only; not to be used to prevent infestation. Should be used as a part of an overall lice management program.

[U.S. Boxed Warning]: May be associated with severe neurologic toxicities. Seizures and death have been reported with use (may occur with prolonged, repeated, or single use). Use is contraindicated in patients with uncontrolled seizure disorders and in premature infants. Use with caution in infants, small children, the elderly, patients with other skin conditions, patients weighing <50 kg, or patients with a history of seizures, head trauma, or HIV infection; use caution with conditions which may increase risk of seizures or medications which decrease seizure threshold.

[U.S. Boxed Warning]: Use is contraindicated in premature infants; the skin of premature infants may be more permeable and their liver enzymes may not be fully developed when compared to full-term infants. Use with caution in patients with hepatic impairment. A lindane medication use guide must be given to all patients along with instructions for proper use.

Adverse Reactions Frequency not defined.

Central nervous system: Ataxia, dizziness, localized burning, neurotoxicity (risk greater in patients <110 lbs [50 kg]), restlessness, seizure, stinging sensation

Dermatologic: Contact dermatitis, eczematous rash

Hematologic & oncologic: Aplastic anemia (CDC, 2010)

Limited to important or life-threatening: Alopecia, dermatitis, headache, pain, paresthesia, pruritus, urticaria

Drug Interactions

Metabolism/Transport Effects None known.

Avoid Concomitant Use There are no known interactions where it is recommended to avoid concomitant use.

Increased Effect/Toxicity There are no known significant interactions involving an increase in effect.

Decreased Effect There are no known significant interactions involving a decrease in effect.

Storage/Stability Store at 20°C to 25°C (68°F to 77°F).

Mechanism of Action Directly absorbed by parasites and ova through the exoskeleton; stimulates the nervous system resulting in seizures and death of parasitic arthropods

Pharmacodynamics/Kinetics

Absorption: ~10% systemically

Metabolism: Hepatic

Half-life elimination: Children: ~18 hours

Time to peak, serum: Children: 6 hours

Dosage Infants, Children, Adolescents, and Adults: Topical:

Scabies: Apply a thin layer of lotion and massage it on skin from the neck to the toes; after 8-12 hours, bathe and remove the drug; most patients will require 30 mL; larger adults may require up to 60 mL. Do not retreat. Do not leave on for more than 12 hours.

Head lice, crab lice: Apply shampoo to dry hair and massage into hair for 4 minutes; add small quantities of water to hair until lather forms, then rinse hair thoroughly and comb with a fine tooth comb to remove nits. Amount of shampoo needed is based on length and density of hair; most patients will require 30 mL (maximum: 60 mL). Do not retreat.

Administration Shake well prior to use. For topical use only; never administer orally. Caregivers should apply with gloves (avoid natural latex, may be permeable to lindane). Rinse off with warm (not hot) water.

Lotion: Apply to dry, cool skin; do not apply to face or eyes. Wait at least 1 hour after bathing or showering (wet or warm skin increases absorption). Skin should be clean and free of any other lotions, creams, or oil prior to lindane application. Do not use on open wounds or sores. Do not use occlusive dressings.

Shampoo: Apply to clean, dry hair. Wait at least 1 hour after washing hair before applying lindane shampoo. Hair should be washed with a shampoo not containing a conditioner; hair and skin of head and neck should be free of any lotions, oils, or creams prior to lindane application. Do not cover with shower cap or towel.

Hazardous agent; use appropriate precautions for handling and disposal (EPA, U-listed).

Additional Information Lindane shampoo should be used with a lice management program including visual inspection of live lice, manual removal of nits using a fine tooth comb, evaluation and treatment of recent contacts, and washing recently worn clothing, underwear, sheets, pillowcases and towels in very hot water or dry-cleaned.

Dosage Forms Excipient information presented when available (limited, particularly for generics); consult specific product labeling.

Lotion, External:

Generic: 1% (60 mL)

Shampoo, External:

Generic: 1% (60 mL)

◆ Linessa (Can) *see* Ethinyl Estradiol and Desogestrel *on page 784*

Linezolid (li NE zoh lid)

Brand Names: U.S. Zyvox

Brand Names: Canada Zyvoxam

Pharmacologic Category Antibiotic, Oxazolidinone

Additional Appendix Information

Antibiotic Treatment of Adults With Infective Endocarditis *on page 2355*

Dosing Considerations for the Critically-Ill Patient With Morbid Obesity *on page 2379*

Tyramine Content of Foods *on page 2394*

Use Treatment of vancomycin-resistant *Enterococcus faecium* (VRE) infections, nosocomial pneumonia caused by *Staphylococcus aureus* (including MRSA) or *Streptococcus pneumoniae* (including multidrug-resistant strains

[MDRSP]), complicated and uncomplicated skin and skin structure infections (including diabetic foot infections without concomitant osteomyelitis), and community-acquired pneumonia caused by susceptible gram-positive organisms

Unlabeled Use Treatment of prosthetic joint infection

Pregnancy Risk Factor C

Pregnancy Considerations Adverse effects were observed in some animal reproduction studies at doses that were also maternally toxic. Information related to linezolid use during pregnancy is limited.

Breast-Feeding Considerations Linezolid is excreted into breast milk. The manufacturer advises caution if administering linezolid to a breast-feeding woman. Non-dose-related effects could include modification of bowel flora.

Contraindications Hypersensitivity to linezolid or any other component of the formulation; concurrent use or within 2 weeks of MAO inhibitors

Warnings/Precautions Myelosuppression has been reported and may be dependent on duration of therapy (generally >2 weeks of treatment); use with caution in patients with pre-existing myelosuppression, in patients receiving other drugs which may cause bone marrow suppression, or in chronic infection (previous or concurrent antibiotic therapy). Weekly CBC monitoring is recommended. Consider discontinuation in patients developing myelosuppression (or in whom myelosuppression worsens during treatment).

Lactic acidosis has been reported with use. Linezolid exhibits mild MAO inhibitor properties and has the potential to have the same interactions as other MAO inhibitors; use with caution and monitor closely in patients with uncontrolled hypertension, pheochromocytoma, carcinoid syndrome, or untreated hyperthyroidism; do not use in the absence of close monitoring. Hypoglycemic episodes have been reported; use with caution and closely monitor glucose in diabetic patients. Dose reductions/discontinuation of concurrent hypoglycemic agents or discontinuation of linezolid may be required. Symptoms of agitation, confusion, hallucinations, hyper-reflexia, myoclonus, shivering, and tachycardia may occur with concomitant proserotonergic drugs (eg, SSRIs/SNRIs, tricyclic antidepressants, triptans, meperidine, bupropion) or agents which reduce linezolid's metabolism; these medications should not be used concurrently unless patient is closely monitored for signs/symptoms of serotonin syndrome or neuroleptic malignant syndrome-like reactions. Patients maintained on proserotonergic drugs requiring urgent treatment with linezolid may receive linezolid if the other proserotonergic drug is discontinued promptly and the benefits of linezolid outweigh risks; monitor for 2 weeks (5 weeks for fluoxetine) after discontinuation of maintenance drug or 24 hours after last linezolid dose, whichever comes first. Unnecessary use may lead to the development of resistance to linezolid; consider alternatives before initiating outpatient treatment.

Peripheral and optic neuropathy (with vision loss) has been reported in adults and children and may occur primarily with extended courses of therapy >28 days; any symptoms of visual change or impairment warrant immediate ophthalmic evaluation and possible discontinuation of therapy. Seizures have been reported; use with caution in patients with a history of seizures. Prolonged use may result in fungal or bacterial superinfection, including *C. difficile*-associated diarrhea (CDAD) and pseudomembranous colitis; CDAD has been observed >2 months post-antibiotic treatment.

Due to inconsistent concentrations in the CSF, empiric use in pediatric patients with CNS infections is not recommended by the manufacturer; however, there are multiple case reports describing successful treatment of documented VRE and *Staphylococcus aureus* CNS and shunt infections in the literature. Linezolid should not be used in the empiric treatment of catheter-related bloodstream infection (CRBSI), but may be appropriate for targeted therapy (Mermel, 2009). Oral suspension contains phenylalanine.

Adverse Reactions Percentages as reported in adults; frequency similar in pediatric patients unless otherwise noted.

>10%:

- Central nervous system: Headache (<1% to 11%)
- Gastrointestinal: Diarrhea (3% to 11%)
- Hematologic & oncologic: Decreased hemoglobin (1% to 16%), thrombocytopenia (<1% to 13%), leukopenia (children 1% to 12%; adults <1% to 2%)

1% to 10%:

- Central nervous system: Insomnia (3%), dizziness (≤2%), vertigo (children 1%)
- Dermatologic: Skin rash (2%)
- Endocrine & metabolic: Increased amylase (<1% to 2%), increased lactate dehydrogenase (<1% to 2%)
- Gastrointestinal: Nausea (1% to 10%), increased serum lipase (3% to 4%), vomiting (1% to 4%), constipation (2%), dysgeusia (1% to 2%), loose stools (children 1% to 2%), abdominal pain (≤2%), oral candidiasis (≤1%), tongue discoloration (≤1%), pancreatitis
- Genitourinary: Vulvovaginal candidiasis (1% to 2%)
- Hematologic & oncologic: Neutropenia (children 1% to 6%; adults ≤1%), anemia (≤1%), eosinophilia (children ≤1%)
- Hepatic: Increased serum ALT (≤10%), increased serum bilirubin (children ≤6%; adults ≤1%), increased serum AST (adults 2% to 5%), increased serum alkaline phosphatase (<1% to 4%), abnormal hepatic function tests (≤1%)
- Infection: Fungal infection (≤1% to 2%)
- Renal: Increased blood urea nitrogen (≤2%), increased serum creatinine (<1% to 2%)
- Miscellaneous: Fever (2%)

<1% (Limited to important or life-threatening): Anaphylaxis, angioedema, bullous skin disease, *Clostridium difficile* associated diarrhea, convulsions, dental discoloration, dyspepsia, hypertension, hypoglycemia, lactic acidosis, optic neuropathy, pancytopenia, peripheral neuropathy, pruritis, rhabdomyolysis, seizures, serotonin syndrome (with concurrent use of other serotonergic agents), Stevens-Johnson syndrome, vision loss

Drug Interactions

Metabolism/Transport Effects **Inhibits** Monoamine Oxidase

Avoid Concomitant Use

Avoid concomitant use of Linezolid with any of the following: Anilidopiperidine Opioids; Apraclonidine; AtoMOXetine; Bezafibrate; Buprenorphine; BuPROPion; BusPIRone; CarBAMazepine; CloZAPine; Cyclobenzaprine; Dexmethylphenidate; Dextromethorphan; Diethylpropion; Hydrocodone; HYDROmorphone; Isometheptene; Levonordefrin; MAO Inhibitors; Maprotiline; Meperidine; Methyldopa; Methylene Blue; Methylphenidate; Mirtazapine; Morphine (Liposomal); Morphine (Systemic); Nefazodone; Oxymorphone; Pizotifen; Selective Serotonin Reuptake Inhibitors; Serotonin 5-HT1D Receptor Agonists; Serotonin/Norepinephrine Reuptake Inhibitors; Tapentadol; Tetrabenazine; Tetrahydrozoline (Nasal); TraZODone; Tricyclic Antidepressants; Tryptophan

Increased Effect/Toxicity

Linezolid may increase the levels/effects of: Antihypertensives; Antipsychotics; Apraclonidine; AtoMOXetine; Beta2-Agonists; Betahistine; Bezafibrate; Brimonidine (Ophthalmic); Brimonidine (Topical); BuPROPion; CloZAPine; Dexmethylphenidate; Dextromethorphan; Diethylpropion; Domperidone; Doxapram; Doxylamine;

EPINEPHrine (Nasal); Epinephrine (Racemic); EPINEPHrine (Systemic, Oral Inhalation); Hydrocodone; HYDROmorphone; Hypoglycemic Agents; Isometheptene; Levonordefrin; Lithium; Meperidine; Methadone; Methyldopa; Methylene Blue; Methylphenidate; Metoclopramide; Mirtazapine; Morphine (Liposomal); Morphine (Systemic); Nefazodone; Norepinephrine; Orthostatic Hypotension Producing Agents; OxyCODONE; Pizotifen; Reserpine; Selective Serotonin Reuptake Inhibitors; Serotonin 5-HT1D Receptor Agonists; Serotonin Modulators; Serotonin/Norepinephrine Reuptake Inhibitors; Sympathomimetics; Tetrahydrozoline (Nasal); TraZODone; Tricyclic Antidepressants

The levels/effects of Linezolid may be increased by: Altretamine; Anilidopiperidine Opioids; Antipsychotics; Buprenorphine; BusPIRone; CarBAMazepine; COMT Inhibitors; Cyclobenzaprine; Levodopa; MAO Inhibitors; Maprotiline; Oxymorphone; Tapentadol; Tetrabenazine; TraMADol; Tryptophan

Decreased Effect

Linezolid may decrease the levels/effects of: Domperidone

The levels/effects of Linezolid may be decreased by: Domperidone

Ethanol/Nutrition/Herb Interactions

Ethanol: May cause additional CNS depressant effects and provide potential source of additional tyramine content. Management: Avoid ethanol.

Food: Concurrent ingestion of foods rich in tyramine may cause sudden and severe high blood pressure (hypertensive crisis). Food's freshness is also an important concern; improperly stored or spoiled food can create an environment where tyramine concentrations may increase. Management: Avoid tyramine-containing foods with MAOIs.

Herb/Nutraceutical: Ingestion of large quantities of supplements containing caffeine, tyrosine, tryptophan, or phenylalanine. May increase the risk of severe side effects (eg, hypertensive reactions, serotonin syndrome). Management: Avoid supplements containing caffeine, tyrosine, tryptophan, or phenylalanine.

Preparation for Administration Oral suspension: Reconstitute with 123 mL of distilled water (in 2 portions); shake vigorously. Concentration is 100 mg/5 mL. Prior to administration mix gently by inverting bottle; do not shake.

Storage/Stability

Infusion: Store at 25°C (77°F); excursions permitted to 15°C to 30°C (59°F to 86°F). Protect from light. Keep infusion bags in overwrap until ready for use. Protect infusion bags from freezing.

Oral suspension: Following reconstitution, store at 25°C (77°F); excursions permitted to 15°C to 30°C (59°F to 86°F). Use reconstituted suspension within 21 days. Protect from light.

Tablet: Store at 25°C (77°F); excursions permitted to 15°C to 30°C (59°F to 86°F). Protect from light; protect from moisture.

Mechanism of Action Inhibits bacterial protein synthesis by binding to bacterial 23S ribosomal RNA of the 50S subunit. This prevents the formation of a functional 70S initiation complex that is essential for the bacterial translation process. Linezolid is bacteriostatic against enterococci and staphylococci and bactericidal against most strains of streptococci.

Pharmacodynamics/Kinetics

Absorption: Rapid and extensive

Distribution: V_{dss}: Adults: 40-50 L

Protein binding: Adults: 31%

Metabolism: Hepatic via oxidation of the morpholine ring, resulting in two inactive metabolites (aminoethoxyacetic acid, hydroxyethyl glycine); minimally metabolized, may be mediated by cytochrome P450

Bioavailability: Oral: ~100%

Half-life elimination: Children ≥1 week (full-term) to 11 years: 1.5-3 hours; Adults: 4-5 hours

Time to peak: Adults: Oral: 1-2 hours

Excretion: Urine (~30% of total dose as parent drug, ~50% of total dose as metabolites); feces (~9% of total dose as metabolites)

Nonrenal clearance: Adults: ~65%

Dosage

Usual dosage: Oral, I.V.:

Children ≤11 years: 10 mg/kg (maximum: 600 mg/dose) every 8 hours

Children ≥12 years and Adults: 600 mg every 12 hours

Indication-specific dosing:

Pneumonia:

Community-acquired pneumonia (CAP):

Manufacturer's recommendation (includes concurrent bacteremia): Oral, I.V.:

Infants (excluding preterm neonates <1 week) and Children ≤11 years: 10 mg/kg/dose every 8 hours for 10-14 days

Children ≥12 years and Adults: 600 mg every 12 hours for 10-14 days. **Note**: May consider 7-day treatment course (versus manufacturer recommended 10-14 days) in patients with healthcare-, hospital-, and ventilator-associated pneumonia who have demonstrated good clinical response (ATS/IDSA, 2005).

Alternate recommendations:

Infants >3 months and Children ≤11 years (IDSA/PIDS, 2011):

S. pneumoniae (MICs to penicillin ≤2.0 mcg/mL), mild infection or step-down therapy (alternative to amoxicillin): Oral: 10 mg/kg/dose every 8 hours

S. pneumoniae (MICs to penicillin ≥4.0 mcg/mL):

Severe infection (alternative to ceftriaxone): I.V.: 10 mg/kg/dose every 8 hours

Mild infection, step-down therapy (preferred): Oral: 10 mg/kg/dose every 8 hours

S. aureus (methicillin-resistant/clindamycin-susceptible):

Severe infection (alternative to vancomycin or clindamycin): I.V.: 10 mg/kg/dose every 8 hours

Mild infection, step-down therapy (alternative to clindamycin): Oral: 10 mg/kg/dose every 8 hours

S. aureus (methicillin- and clindamycin-resistant):

Severe infection (alternative to vancomycin): I.V.: 10 mg/kg/dose every 8 hours

Mild infection, step-down therapy (preferred): Oral: 10 mg/kg/dose every 8 hours

Children ≤11 years (Liu, 2011): Oral, I.V.: *S. aureus* (methicillin-resistant): 10 mg/kg/dose every 8 hours for 7-21 days (maximum: 600 mg/dose)

Children ≥12 years (IDSA/PIDS, 2011):

S. pneumoniae (MICs to penicillin ≤2.0 mcg/mL), mild infection or step-down therapy (alternative to amoxicillin): Oral: 10 mg/kg/dose every 12 hours

S. pneumoniae (MICs to penicillin ≥4.0 mcg/mL)

Severe infection (alternative to ceftriaxone): I.V.: 10 mg/kg/dose every 12 hours

Mild infection, step-down therapy (preferred): Oral: 10 mg/kg/dose every 12 hours

S. aureus (methicillin-resistant/clindamycin-susceptible):

Severe infection (alternative to vancomycin/clindamycin): I.V.: 10 mg/kg/dose every 12 hours

Mild infection, step-down therapy (alternative to clindamycin): Oral: 10 mg/kg/dose every 12 hours

S. aureus (methicillin- and clindamycin-resistant):
Severe infection (alternative to vancomycin): I.V.: 10 mg/kg/dose every 12 hours
Mild infection, step-down therapy (preferred): Oral: 10 mg/kg/dose every 12 hours
Children ≥12 years and Adults: (Liu, 2011): Oral, I.V.: *S. aureus* (methicillin-resistant): 600 mg every 12 hours for 7-21 days
Healthcare-associated (HA) pneumonia: Oral, I.V.:
Manufacturer's recommendation:
Infants (excluding preterm neonates <1 week) and Children ≤11 years: 10 mg/kg every 8 hours for 10-14 days
Children ≥12 years and Adults: 600 mg every 12 hours for 10-14 days.
Note: May consider 7-day treatment course (versus manufacturer recommended 10-14 days) in patients with healthcare-, hospital-, and ventilator-associated pneumonia who have demonstrated good clinical response (ATS/IDSA, 2005).
Alternate recommendations (Liu, 2011): *S. aureus* (methicillin-resistant):
Children ≤11 years: 10 mg/kg/dose every 8 hours for 7-21 days (maximum: 600 mg/dose)
Children ≥12 years and Adults: 600 mg every 12 hours for 7-21 days

Skin and skin structure infections, complicated: Oral, I.V.:
Infants (excluding preterm neonates <1 week) and Children ≤11 years: 10 mg/kg every 8 hours for 10-14 days
Children ≥12 years and Adults: 600 mg every 12 hours for 10-14 days. **Note:** For diabetic foot infections, initial treatment duration is up to 4 weeks depending on severity of infection and response to therapy (Lipsky, 2012).

Skin and skin structure infections, uncomplicated: Oral:
Infants (excluding preterm neonates <1 week) and Children <5 years: 10 mg/kg every 8 hours for 10-14 days
Children 5-11 years: 10 mg/kg every 12 hours for 10-14 days
Children ≥12-18 years: 600 mg every 12 hours for 10-14 days
Adults: 400 mg every 12 hours for 10-14 days; **Note:** 400 mg dose is recommended in the product labeling; however, 600 mg dose is commonly employed clinically; consider 5- to 10-day treatment course as opposed to the manufacturer recommended 10-14 days (Liu, 2011; Stevens, 2005). For diabetic foot infections, may extend treatment duration up to 4 weeks if slow to resolve (Lipsky, 2012).

VRE infections including concurrent bacteremia: Oral, I.V.:
Infants (excluding preterm neonates <1 week) and Children ≤11 years: 10 mg/kg every 8 hours for 14-28 days
Children ≥12 years and Adults: 600 mg every 12 hours for 14-28 days

Brain abscess, subdural empyema, spinal epidural abscess (*S. aureus* [methicillin-resistant]) (unlabeled use; Liu, 2011): Oral, I.V.:
Children ≤11 years: 10 mg/kg every 8 hours for 4-6 weeks (maximum: 600 mg/dose)
Children ≥12 years and Adults: 600 mg every 12 hours for 4-6 weeks

Meningitis (*S. aureus* [methicillin-resistant]) (unlabeled use; Liu, 2011): Oral, I.V.: Children ≥12 years and Adults: 600 mg every 12 hours for 2 weeks

Osteomyelitis (*S. aureus* [methicillin-resistant]) (unlabeled use; Liu, 2011): Oral, I.V.:
Infants (excluding preterm neonates <1 week) and Children ≤11 years: 10 mg/kg every 8 hours for a minimum of 4-6 weeks (maximum: 600 mg/dose)
Children ≥12 years and Adults: 600 mg every 12 hours for a minimum of 8 weeks (some experts combine with rifampin)

Prosthetic joint infection (unlabeled use): Oral, I.V.:
Enterococcus spp (penicillin-susceptible or -resistant) (alternative treatment): 600 mg every 12 hours for 4-6 weeks (consider adding an aminoglycoside) followed by an oral antibiotic suppressive regimen (Osmon, 2013)
Staphylococci (oxacillin-sensitive or -resistant) (alternative treatment): 600 mg every 12 hours for 2-6 weeks used in combination with rifampin followed by oral antibiotic treatment and suppressive regimens (Osmon, 2013)

Septic arthritis (*S. aureus* [methicillin-resistant]) (unlabeled use; Liu, 2011): Oral, I.V.:
Infants (excluding preterm neonates <1 week) and Children ≤11 years: 10 mg/kg every 8 hours for 3-4 weeks (maximum: 600 mg/dose)
Children ≥12 years and Adults: 600 mg every 12 hours for 3-4 weeks

Septic thrombosis of cavernous or dural venous sinus (*S. aureus* [methicillin-resistant]) (unlabeled use; Liu, 2011): Oral, I.V.:
Children ≤11 years: 10 mg/kg every 8 hours for 4-6 weeks (maximum: 600 mg/dose)
Children ≥12 years and Adults: 600 mg every 12 hours for 4-6 weeks

Elderly: No dosage adjustment required

Dosage adjustment in renal impairment: No adjustment is recommended. The two primary metabolites may accumulate in patients with renal impairment but the clinical significance is unknown. Weigh the risk of accumulation of metabolites versus the benefit of therapy. Monitor for hematopoietic (eg, anemia, leukopenia, thrombocytopenia) and neuropathic (eg, peripheral neuropathy) adverse events when administering for extended periods.

Intermittent hemodialysis (administer after hemodialysis on dialysis days): Dialyzable (~30% removed during 3-hour dialysis session): If administration time is not immediately after dialysis session, may consider administration of a supplemental dose especially early in the treatment course to maintain levels above the MIC (Brier, 2003). Others have recommended no supplemental dose or dosage adjustment for patients on intermittent hemodialysis, peritoneal dialysis, or continuous renal replacement therapy (eg, CVVHD) (Heintz, 2009; Trotman, 2005)

Dosage adjustment in hepatic impairment:
Mild-to-moderate hepatic impairment (Child-Pugh class A or B): No dosage adjustment required
Severe hepatic impairment (Child-Pugh class C): Use has not been adequately evaluated

Dietary Considerations Take without regard to meals. Some products may contain sodium and/or phenylalanine. Avoid consuming large amounts of tyramine-containing foods/beverages. Some examples include aged or matured cheese, air-dried or cured meats (including sausages and salamis), fava or broad bean pods, tap/draft beers, Marmite concentrate, sauerkraut, soy sauce, and other soybean condiments.

Administration
I.V.: Administer intravenous infusion over 30-120 minutes. Do not mix or infuse with other medications. When the same intravenous line is used for sequential infusion of other medications, flush line with D_5W, NS, or LR before and after infusing linezolid. The yellow color of the injection may intensify over time without affecting potency.
Oral suspension: Invert gently to mix prior to administration, do not shake. Administer without regard to meals.

Monitoring Parameters Weekly CBC, particularly in patients at increased risk of bleeding, with pre-existing myelosuppression, on concomitant medications that cause bone marrow suppression, in those who require >2 weeks of therapy, or in those with chronic infection who have received previous or concomitant antibiotic therapy; visual function with extended therapy (≥3 months) or in patients with new onset visual symptoms, regardless of therapy length

Dosage Forms Excipient information presented when available (limited, particularly for generics); consult specific product labeling.

Solution, Intravenous:
Zyvox: 2 mg/mL (100 mL, 300 mL)
Suspension Reconstituted, Oral:
Zyvox: 100 mg/5 mL (150 mL) [orange flavor]
Tablet, Oral:
Zyvox: 600 mg

- **Linzess** *see* Linaclotide *on page 1215*
- **Lioresal** *see* Baclofen *on page 221*
- **Lioresal® (Can)** *see* Baclofen *on page 221*
- **Lioresal® D.S. (Can)** *see* Baclofen *on page 221*
- **Lioresal® Intrathecal (Can)** *see* Baclofen *on page 221*

Liothyronine (lye oh THYE roe neen)

Brand Names: U.S. Cytomel; Triostat
Brand Names: Canada Cytomel®
Index Terms Liothyronine Sodium; Sodium *L*-Triiodothyronine; T_3 Sodium (error-prone abbreviation)
Pharmacologic Category Thyroid Product
Use

Oral: Replacement or supplemental therapy in hypothyroidism; management of nontoxic goiter; a diagnostic aid
I.V.: Treatment of myxedema coma/precoma

Unlabeled Use Management of hemodynamically unstable potential organ donors increasing the quantity of organs available for transplantation
Pregnancy Risk Factor A
Dosage Doses should be adjusted based on clinical response and laboratory parameters.

Children: Congenital hypothyroidism: Oral: 5 mcg/day increase by 5 mcg every 3-4 days until the desired response is achieved. Usual maintenance dose: 20 mcg/day for infants, 50 mcg/day for children 1-3 years of age, and adult dose for children >3 years.

Adults:

Hypothyroidism: Oral: 25 mcg/day increase by increments of 12.5-25 mcg/day every 1-2 weeks to a maximum of 100 mcg/day; usual maintenance dose: 25-75 mcg/day.

Patients with cardiovascular disease: Refer to Elderly dosing.

T_3 suppression test: Oral: 75-100 mcg/day for 7 days; use lowest dose for elderly

Myxedema: Oral: Initial: 5 mcg/day; increase in increments of 5-10 mcg/day every 1-2 weeks. When 25 mcg/day is reached, dosage may be increased at intervals of 5-25 mcg/day every 1-2 weeks. Usual maintenance dose: 50-100 mcg/day.

Myxedema coma: I.V.: 25-50 mcg

Patients with known or suspected cardiovascular disease: 10-20 mcg

Note: Normally, at least 4 hours should be allowed between doses to adequately assess therapeutic response and no more than 12 hours should elapse between doses to avoid fluctuations in hormone levels. Oral therapy should be resumed as soon as the clinical situation has been stabilized and the patient is able to take oral medication. If levothyroxine rather than liothyronine sodium is used in initiating oral therapy, the physician should bear in mind that there is a delay of several days in the onset of levothyroxine activity and that I.V. therapy should be discontinued gradually.

Simple (nontoxic) goiter: Oral: Initial: 5 mcg/day; increase by 5-10 mcg every 1-2 weeks; after 25 mcg/day is reached, may increase dose by 12.5-25 mcg. Usual maintenance dose: 75 mcg/day

Elderly: Oral: 5 mcg/day; increase by 5 mcg/day every 2 weeks

Dosage adjustment in renal impairment: No dosage adjustment provided in manufacturer's labeling.

Dosage adjustment in hepatic impairment: No dosage adjustment provided in manufacturer's labeling.

Additional Information Complete prescribing information should be consulted for additional detail.

Dosage Forms Excipient information presented when available (limited, particularly for generics); consult specific product labeling.

Solution, Intravenous:
Triostat: 10 mcg/mL (1 mL) [contains alcohol, usp]
Generic: 10 mcg/mL (1 mL)
Tablet, Oral:
Cytomel: 5 mcg
Cytomel: 25 mcg, 50 mcg [scored]
Generic: 5 mcg, 25 mcg, 50 mcg

- **Liothyronine and Levothyroxine** *see* Liotrix *on page 1222*
- **Liothyronine Sodium** *see* Liothyronine *on page 1222*

Liotrix (LYE oh triks)

Brand Names: U.S. Thyrolar®
Brand Names: Canada Thyrolar®
Index Terms Levothyroxine and Liothyronine; Liothyronine and Levothyroxine; T_3/T_4 Liotrix
Pharmacologic Category Thyroid Product
Use

Replacement or supplemental therapy in hypothyroidism (uniform mixture of T_4:T_3 in 4:1 ratio by weight)

Thyroid-stimulating hormone (TSH) suppressant therapy used in the management of thyroid cancer (levothyroxine is generally recommended for this indication); prevention or treatment of euthyroid goiters (eg, thyroid nodules, subacute or chronic lymphocytic thyroiditis [Hashimoto's], multinodular goiters)

Diagnostic agent in suppression tests to diagnose suspected mild hyperthyroidism or to demonstrate thyroid gland autonomy

Pregnancy Risk Factor A
Dosage Oral:

Congenital hypothyroidism:

Children: **Note:** In newly diagnosed infants, begin therapy with full dose.

0-6 months: Levothyroxine 12.5-25 mcg/Liothyronine 3.1-6.25 mcg once daily

6-12 months: Levothyroxine 25-37.5 mcg/Liothyronine 6.25-9.35 mcg once daily

1-5 years: Levothyroxine 37.5-50 mcg/Liothyronine 9.35-12.5 mcg once daily

6-12 years: Levothyroxine 50-75 mcg/Liothyronine 12.5-18.75 mcg once daily

>12 years: Levothyroxine 75 mcg/Liothyronine 18.75 mcg once daily

Also see individual agents.

Hypothyroidism:

Adults: Initial: Levothyroxine 25 mcg/Liothyronine 6.25 mcg once daily; may increase by levothyroxine 12.5 mcg/Liothyronine 3.1 mcg every 2-3 weeks. A lower initial dose (levothyroxine 12.5 mcg/Liothyronine 3.1 mcg) is recommended in patients with long-standing myxedema, especially if cardiovascular impairment coexists. If angina occurs, reduce dose (usual maintenance dose: levothyroxine 50-100 mcg/Liothyronine 12.5-25 mcg)

Elderly: Initial: Levothyroxine 12.5-25 mcg/Liothyronine 3.1-6.25 mcg once daily; may increase by levothyroxine 12.5 mcg/Liothyronine 3.1 mcg every 2-3 weeks

Additional Information Complete prescribing information should be consulted for additional detail.

Dosage Forms Excipient information presented when available (limited, particularly for generics); consult specific product labeling.

Tablet, oral:

Thyrolar®: 1/4 [levothyroxine sodium 12.5 mcg and liothyronine sodium 3.1 mcg]

Thyrolar®: 1/2 [levothyroxine sodium 25 mcg and liothyronine sodium 6.25 mcg]

Thyrolar®: 1 [levothyroxine sodium 50 mcg and liothyronine sodium 12.5 mcg]

Thyrolar®: 2 [levothyroxine sodium 100 mcg and liothyronine sodium 25 mcg]

Thyrolar®: 3 [levothyroxine sodium 150 mcg and liothyronine sodium 37.5 mcg]

◆ **Lipancreatin** *see* Pancrelipase *on page 1558*
◆ **Lipase, Protease, and Amylase** *see* Pancrelipase *on page 1558*
◆ **Lipiarrmycin** *see* Fidaxomicin *on page 859*
◆ **Lipidil EZ (Can)** *see* Fenofibrate and Derivatives *on page 837*
◆ **Lipidil Micro (Can)** *see* Fenofibrate and Derivatives *on page 837*
◆ **Lipidil Supra (Can)** *see* Fenofibrate and Derivatives *on page 837*
◆ **Lipitor** *see* AtorvaSTATin *on page 190*
◆ **Lipodox** *see* DOXOrubicin (Liposomal) *on page 663*
◆ **Lipodox 50** *see* DOXOrubicin (Liposomal) *on page 663*
◆ **Lipofen** *see* Fenofibrate and Derivatives *on page 837*
◆ **Liposomal Bupivacaine** *see* Bupivacaine (Liposomal) *on page 290*
◆ **Liposomal Cytarabine** *see* Cytarabine (Liposomal) *on page 522*
◆ **Liposomal DAUNOrubicin** *see* DAUNOrubicin (Liposomal) *on page 555*
◆ **Liposomal DOXOrubicin** *see* DOXOrubicin (Liposomal) *on page 663*
◆ **Liposomal Vincristine** *see* VinCRIStine (Liposomal) *on page 2194*
◆ **Liposome Vincristine** *see* VinCRIStine (Liposomal) *on page 2194*
◆ **Liposyn II** *see* Fat Emulsion (Plant Based) *on page 834*
◆ **Liposyn III** *see* Fat Emulsion (Plant Based) *on page 834*
◆ **Liptruzet™** *see* Ezetimibe and Atorvastatin *on page 818*
◆ **Liqua-Cal [OTC]** *see* Calcium and Vitamin D *on page 318*
◆ **Liquibid [OTC]** *see* GuaiFENesin *on page 974*
◆ **Liquibid® D-R [OTC]** *see* Guaifenesin and Phenylephrine *on page 978*
◆ **Liquibid® PD-R [OTC]** *see* Guaifenesin and Phenylephrine *on page 978*
◆ **Liquid Antidote** *see* Charcoal, Activated *on page 401*
◆ **Liquituss GG [OTC]** *see* GuaiFENesin *on page 974*

Liraglutide (lir a GLOO tide)

Brand Names: U.S. Victoza

Brand Names: Canada Victoza

Index Terms NN2211

Pharmacologic Category Antidiabetic Agent, Glucagon-Like Peptide-1 (GLP-1) Receptor Agonist

Additional Appendix Information

Injectable Agents (Non-Insulin) for Type 2 Diabetes *on page 2302*

Use Treatment of type 2 diabetes mellitus (noninsulin dependent, NIDDM) to improve glycemic control as an adjunct to diet and exercise

Pregnancy Risk Factor C

Pregnancy Considerations Adverse events were observed in animal reproduction studies. For women with diabetes, maternal hyperglycemia can be associated with adverse effects in the fetus, neonate, and mother. To prevent adverse events, prior to conception and throughout pregnancy, the maternal Hb A_{1c} should be kept close to normal but without causing significant hypoglycemia. The use of GLP-1 receptor agonists in pregnant women is not recommended; insulin is the drug of choice for the control of diabetes mellitus during pregnancy (ACOG, 2005; ADA, 2013; Kitzmiller, 2008; Metzger, 2007).

Breast-Feeding Considerations It is not known if liraglutide is excreted into breast milk. Because tumors were observed in animal studies, the manufacturer recommends that a decision be made whether to discontinue nursing or to discontinue the drug, taking into account the importance of treatment to the mother.

Medication Guide Available Yes

Contraindications Hypersensitivity to liraglutide or any component of the formulation; history of or family history of medullary thyroid carcinoma (MTC); patients with multiple endocrine neoplasia syndrome type 2 (MEN2)

Canadian labeling: Additional contraindications (not in U.S. labeling): Pregnancy; breast-feeding

Warnings/Precautions [U.S. Boxed Warning] Dose- and duration- dependent thyroid C-cell tumors have developed in animal studies with liraglutide therapy; relevance in humans unknown. Due to the finding in animal studies, patients were monitored with serum calcitonin or thyroid ultrasound during clinical trials; however, it is unknown if this is beneficial in decreasing the risk of thyroid tumors. Patients should be counseled on the risk and symptoms (eg, neck mass, dysphagia, dyspnea, persistent hoarseness) of thyroid tumors. Use is contraindicated in patients with or a family history of medullary thyroid cancer and in patients with multiple endocrine neoplasia syndrome type 2 (MEN2). During clinical studies, a few cases of thyroid C-cell hyperplasia were reported. Consultation with an endocrinologist is recommended in patients who develop elevated calcitonin concentrations.

Serious hypersensitivity reactions, including anaphylactic reactions and angioedema, have been reported with use; discontinue therapy in the event of a hypersensitivity reaction. Use with caution in patients with a history of angioedema to other GLP-1 receptor agonists (angioedema has been reported with other GLP-1 receptor agonists); potential for cross-sensitivity is unknown. Cases of acute and chronic pancreatitis (including one case of fatal necrotizing pancreatitis) have been reported although conclusive evidence to liraglutide therapy has not been established; monitor for signs and symptoms of pancreatitis (eg, persistent severe abdominal pain which may radiate to the back and which may or may not be accompanied by vomiting. If pancreatitis is suspected, discontinue use. Do not resume unless an alternative etiology of pancreatitis is confirmed. Use with caution in patients with a history of pancreatitis or consider antidiabetic therapies other than liraglutide. Use with caution in patients with cholelithiasis and/or alcohol abuse. Most common reactions are gastrointestinal related; these symptoms may be dose-related and may decrease in frequency/severity with gradual titration and continued use. Slows gastric emptying; has not been studied in patients with pre-existing gastroparesis. Use may be associated with weight loss (likely due to reduced intake) independent of the change in hemoglobin A_{1c}. Use with caution in patients with hepatic impairment. Use with caution in renal impairment, particularly during initiation of therapy and dose escalation; cases of acute renal failure and chronic renal failure exacerbation have been reported; some cases have been reported in patients with no known pre-existing renal disease.

Concomitant use of an insulin secretagogue (eg, sulfonylurea, meglitinide) or insulin may increase the risk of hypoglycemia; dosage reduction of secretagogues or insulin may be required. Concurrent use with prandial insulin therapy has not been evaluated. Due to its effects on gastric emptying, liraglutide may reduce the rate and extent of absorption of orally-administered drugs; use with caution in patients receiving medications with a narrow therapeutic window or require rapid absorption from the GI tract. Not recommended for first-line therapy; use as adjunct to diet and exercise. Do not use in patients with type 1 diabetes mellitus or for the treatment of diabetic ketoacidosis; not a substitute for insulin. Diabetes self-management education (DSME) is essential to maximize the effectiveness of therapy. According to the Centers for Disease Control and Prevention (CDC), pen-shaped injection devices should never be used for more than one person (even when the needle is changed) because of the risk of infection. The injection device should be clearly labeled with individual patient information to ensure that the correct pen is used (CDC, 2012).

Adverse Reactions Incidence reported in monotherapy trials unless otherwise specified.

>10%: Gastrointestinal: Nausea (28%), diarrhea (17%), vomiting (11%)

1% to 10%:

Central nervous system: Headache (9%)

Gastrointestinal: Constipation (10%), dyspepsia (combination trials: 9%)

Hepatic: Hyperbilirubinemia (monotherapy and combination trials: 4%)

Immunologic: Antibody development: Antiliraglutide antibodies (low titers [concentrations not requiring dilution of serum]; monotherapy and combination trials: 9%), cross-reacting antiliraglutide antibodies to native GLP-1 (monotherapy: 7%; combination trials: 5%)

Local: Injection site reactions (monotherapy and combination trials: 2% [includes rash, erythema])

<1% (Limited to important or life-threatening): Acute renal failure, anaphylaxis, angioedema, carcinoma (papillary thyroid), chronic renal failure (exacerbation), hypersensitivity reaction, hypoglycemia (most reports in patients receiving combination therapy), increased susceptibility to infection, malignant neoplasm, pancreatitis (including acute, chronic, hemorrhagic, and necrotizing), thyroid disease (C-cell hyperplasia), upper respiratory tract infection

Drug Interactions

Metabolism/Transport Effects None known.

Avoid Concomitant Use There are no known interactions where it is recommended to avoid concomitant use.

Increased Effect/Toxicity

Liraglutide may increase the levels/effects of: Sulfonylureas

The levels/effects of Liraglutide may be increased by: Pegvisomant

Decreased Effect

The levels/effects of Liraglutide may be decreased by: Corticosteroids (Orally Inhaled); Corticosteroids (Systemic); Luteinizing Hormone-Releasing Hormone Analogs; Somatropin; Thiazide Diuretics

Ethanol/Nutrition/Herb Interactions Ethanol: Ethanol may cause hypoglycemia. Management: Avoid ethanol.

Storage/Stability Prior to initial use, store under refrigeration at 2°C to 8°C (36°F to 46°F); after initial use, may be stored in refrigerator or at room temperature of 15°C to 30°C (59°F to 86°F). Do not freeze (discard if freezing occurs). Protect from heat and light. Pen should be discarded 30 days after initial use.

Mechanism of Action Liraglutide is a long acting analog of human glucagon-like peptide-1 (GLP-1) (an incretin hormone) which increases glucose-dependent insulin secretion, decreases inappropriate glucagon secretion, increases B-cell growth/replication, slows gastric emptying, and decreases food intake. Liraglutide administration results in decreases in hemoglobin A_{1c} by approximately 1%.

Pharmacodynamics/Kinetics

Distribution: V_d: SubQ: ~13 L; I.V.: 0.07 L/kg

Protein binding: >98%

Metabolism: Endogenously metabolized by dipeptidyl peptidase IV (DPP-IV) and endogenous endopeptidases (Croom, 2009); metabolism occurs slower than that seen with native GLP-1

Bioavailability: SubQ: ~55%

Half-life, elimination: ~13 hours

Time to peak, plasma: 8-12 hours

Excretion: Urine (6%, as metabolites); feces (5%, as metabolites)

Dosage Note: Initial dose is intended to reduce GI symptoms; does not provide effective glycemic control.

SubQ: Adults: Initial: 0.6 mg once daily for 1 week; then increase to 1.2 mg once daily; may increase further to 1.8 mg once daily if optimal glycemic response not achieved with 1.2 mg/day

Missed doses: In the event of a missed dose, the once daily regimen can be resumed with the next scheduled dose (an extra dose or an increase in the next dose should **not** be attempted); if >3 days have passed since the last liraglutide dose, reinitiate therapy at 0.6 mg/day to avoid GI symptoms and titrate according to prescriber discretion.

Dosage adjustment in renal impairment:

U.S. labeling: Mild-to-severe impairment: No dosage adjustment provided in manufacturer's labeling; however, use with caution, due to limited experience and reports of acute renal failure and exacerbation of chronic renal failure.

Canadian labeling:

Mild impairment: No dosage adjustment necessary.

Moderate-to-severe impairment: Use is not recommended.

Dosage adjustment in hepatic impairment:

U.S. labeling: Mild-to-severe impairment: No dosage adjustment provided in manufacturer's labeling; use with caution, due to limited experience.

Canadian labeling: Mild-to-severe impairment: Use is not recommended.

Dietary Considerations Individualized medical nutrition therapy (MNT) based on ADA recommendations is an integral part of therapy.

Administration SubQ: Use only if clear, colorless, and free of particulate matter. Administer via injection in the upper arm, thigh, or abdomen. Administer without regard to meals or time of day. Change needle with each administration. Do not share pens between patients even if needle is changed. If using concomitantly with insulin, administer as separate injections (do **not** mix); may inject in the same body region as insulin, but not adjacent to one another.

Monitoring Parameters Plasma glucose, Hb A_{1c}; renal function; signs/symptoms of pancreatitis

Reference Range Recommendations for glycemic control in nonpregnant adults with diabetes (ADA, 2013):

Hb A_{1c}: <7% (a more aggressive [<6.5%] or less aggressive [<8%] Hb A_{1c} goal may be targeted based on patient-specific characteristics)

Preprandial capillary plasma glucose: 70-130 mg/dL

Peak postprandial capillary blood glucose: <180 mg/dL

Dosage Forms Excipient information presented when available (limited, particularly for generics); consult specific product labeling.

Solution, Subcutaneous:

Victoza: 18 mg/3 mL (3 mL) [contains phenol, propylene glycol]

Lisdexamfetamine (lis dex am FET a meen)

Brand Names: U.S. Vyvanse

Brand Names: Canada Vyvanse

Index Terms Lisdexamfetamine Dimesylate; Lisdexamphetamine; NRP104

Pharmacologic Category Central Nervous System Stimulant

Use Treatment of attention-deficit/hyperactivity disorder (ADHD)

Pregnancy Risk Factor C

Pregnancy Considerations Adverse effects have not been observed in animal reproduction studies. Lisdexamfetamine is converted to dextroamphetamine. The majority of human data is based on illicit amphetamine/methamphetamine exposure and not from therapeutic maternal use (Golub, 2005). Use of amphetamines during pregnancy may lead to an increased risk of premature birth and low birth weight; newborns may experience symptoms of withdrawal. Behavioral problems may also occur later in childhood (LaGasse, 2012).

Breast-Feeding Considerations The majority of human data is based on illicit amphetamine/methamphetamine exposure and not from therapeutic maternal use (Golub, 2005). Amphetamines are excreted into breast milk and use may decrease milk production. Increased irritability, agitation, and crying have been reported in nursing infants (ACOG, 2011). According to the manufacturer, the decision to continue or discontinue breast-feeding during therapy should take into account the risk of exposure to the infant and the benefits of treatment to the mother.

Medication Guide Available Yes

Contraindications

Hypersensitivity to amphetamine products or any component of the formulation; use during or within 14 days following MAO inhibitor therapy

Canadian labeling: Additional contraindications (not in U.S. labeling): Known hypersensitivity or idiosyncrasy to sympathomimetic amines; advanced arteriosclerosis; symptomatic cardiovascular disease; moderate-to-severe hypertension; hyperthyroidism; glaucoma; agitated states; history of drug abuse

Warnings/Precautions Sudden death, stroke, and myocardial infarction have been reported in adults receiving the recommended doses of CNS stimulants. In children and adolescents with pre-existing structural cardiac abnormalities or other serious heart problems, sudden death has been reported while receiving the recommended doses of CNS stimulants for ADHD. These products should be avoided in the patients with known serious structural cardiac abnormalities, cardiomyopathy, serious heart rhythm abnormalities, coronary artery disease (adults), or other serious cardiac problems that could increase the risk of sudden death that these conditions alone carry. Patients should be carefully evaluated for these cardiac disorders prior to initiation of therapy. Patients who develop chest pain, syncope, or arrhythmias during therapy should be evaluated promptly. CNS stimulants may increase heart rate (approximate mean increase: 3-6 bpm) and blood pressure (approximate mean increase: 2-4 mm Hg); monitor for adverse events related to tachycardia or hypertension. Stimulants are associated with peripheral vasculopathy, including Raynaud's phenomenon; signs/symptoms are usually mild and intermittent, and generally improve with dose reduction or discontinuation. Digital ulceration and/or soft tissue breakdown have been observed rarely; monitor for digital changes during therapy and seek further evaluation (eg, rheumatology) if necessary.

Use with caution in patients with psychiatric or seizure disorders. May exacerbate symptoms of behavior and thought disorder in psychotic patients. Stimulants may unmask tics in individuals with coexisting Tourette's syndrome. **[U.S. Boxed Warning]: CNS stimulants (including lisdexamfetamine) have a high potential for abuse and dependence; assess for abuse potential prior to use and monitor for signs of abuse and dependence during therapy.** Use with caution in patients with history of ethanol or drug abuse (Canadian labeling contraindicates use if history of drug abuse). Prescriptions should be written for the smallest quantity consistent with good patient care to minimize possibility of overdose. Abrupt discontinuation following high doses or for prolonged periods may result in symptoms for withdrawal (eg, depression, extreme fatigue). Recommended to be used as part of a comprehensive treatment program for attention deficit disorders. When used for extended periods, therapy should be periodically re-evaluated to determine if continued treatment is necessary; if possible, interrupt therapy to assess if behavioral symptoms recur.

Use with caution in the elderly due to CNS stimulant adverse effects. Appetite suppression may occur; monitor weight during therapy, particularly in children. Use of stimulants has been associated with slowing of growth rate; monitor growth rate during treatment. Treatment interruption may be necessary in patients who are not growing or gaining weight as expected. Potentially significant drug-drug interactions may exist, requiring dose or frequency adjustment, additional monitoring, and/or selection of alternative therapy.

Adverse Reactions

>10%:

Central nervous system: Insomnia (13% to 27%)

Gastrointestinal: Decreased appetite (children and adolescents 34% to 39%; adults 27%), xerostomia (adults 26%; children and adolescents 4% to 5%), abdominal pain (children 12%)

1% to 10%:

Cardiovascular: Increased blood pressure (adults 3%), increased heart rate (adults 2%)

Central nervous system: Irritability (children 10%), anxiety (adults 6%), dizziness (children 5%), akathisia (adults 4%), agitation (adults 3%), emotional lability (children 3%), restlessness (adults 3%), drowsiness (children 2%), tics (children 2%)

Dermatologic: Hyperhidrosis (adults 3%), skin rash (children 3%)

Endocrine & metabolic: Weight loss (children and adolescents 9%; adults 3%)

Gastrointestinal: Vomiting (children 9%), diarrhea (adults 7%), nausea (6% to 7%), anorexia (adults 5%)

Genitourinary: Erectile dysfunction (adults 3%), decreased libido (adults <2%)

Neuromuscular & skeletal: Tremor (adults 2%)

Respiratory: Dyspnea (adults 2%)
Miscellaneous: Fever (children 2%)
<1%, postmarketing, and/or case reports (Limited to important or life-threatening): Accommodation disturbance, anaphylaxis, angioedema, cardiomyopathy, depression, diplopia, excoriation, hallucination, hepatitis (eosinophilic), hostility, hypersensitivity, hypertension, mania, mydriasis, overstimulation, peripheral vascular insufficiency, psychotic reaction, Raynaud's phenomenon, seizure, Stevens-Johnson syndrome, tachycardia, Tourette's syndrome

Drug Interactions

Metabolism/Transport Effects None known.

Avoid Concomitant Use

Avoid concomitant use of Lisdexamfetamine with any of the following: Iobenguane I 123; MAO Inhibitors

Increased Effect/Toxicity

Lisdexamfetamine may increase the levels/effects of: Analgesics (Opioid); Sympathomimetics

The levels/effects of Lisdexamfetamine may be increased by: Alkalinizing Agents; Antacids; AtoMOXetine; Cannabinoids; Carbonic Anhydrase Inhibitors; MAO Inhibitors; Proton Pump Inhibitors; Tricyclic Antidepressants

Decreased Effect

Lisdexamfetamine may decrease the levels/effects of: Antihistamines; Ethosuximide; Iobenguane I 123; Ioflupane I 123; PHENobarbital; Phenytoin

The levels/effects of Lisdexamfetamine may be decreased by: Ammonium Chloride; Antipsychotics; Ascorbic Acid; Gastrointestinal Acidifying Agents; Lithium; Methenamine; Multivitamins/Fluoride (with ADE); Multivitamins/Minerals (with ADEK, Folate, Iron); Multivitamins/Minerals (with AE, No Iron); Urinary Acidifying Agents

Ethanol/Nutrition/Herb Interactions

Ethanol: Ethanol may increase CNS depression. Caffeine use may worsen problems with sleeping, headache, irritability, dizziness, nausea, vomiting, abdominal pain, and decreased appetite. Management: Avoid ethanol and caffeine.

Food: High-fat meal prolongs T_{max} by ~1 hour.

Storage/Stability Store at controlled room temperature of 25°C (77°F) excursions permitted to 15°C to 30°C (59°F to 86°F). Protect from light.

Mechanism of Action Lisdexamfetamine dimesylate is a prodrug that is converted to the active component dextroamphetamine (a noncatecholamine, sympathomimetic amine). Amphetamines are noncatecholamine, sympathomimetic amines that cause release of catecholamines (primarily dopamine and norepinephrine) from their storage sites in the presynaptic nerve terminals. A less significant mechanism may include their ability to block the reuptake of catecholamines by competitive inhibition.

Pharmacodynamics/Kinetics

Absorption: Rapid

Distribution: Dextroamphetamine: V_d: Adults: 3.5-4.6 L/kg; distributes into CNS; mean CSF concentrations are 80% of plasma

Metabolism: Metabolized in the blood by hydrolytic activity of red blood cells to dextroamphetamine and l-lysine; does not undergo CYP mediated metabolism

Half-life elimination: Lisdexamfetamine: <1 hour; Dextroamphetamine: 10-13 hours

Time to peak, serum: T_{max}: Lisdexamfetamine: ~1 hour; Dextroamphetamine: ~3.5 hours

Excretion: Urine (96%, 42% as amphetamine-related compounds, 2% as lisdexamfetamine, 25% hippuric acid); feces (minimal)

Dosage Note: Individualize dosage based on patient need and response to therapy. Administer at the lowest effective dose.

Attention-deficit/hyperactivity disorder (ADHD): Children ≥6 years, Adolescents, and Adults: Oral:

U.S. labeling: Initial: 30 mg once daily in the morning; may increase in increments of 10 mg or 20 mg daily at weekly intervals until optimal response is obtained; maximum: 70 mg daily

Canadian labeling: Initial: 20-30 mg once daily in the morning; per clinical discretion, dose may be increased at weekly intervals up to a maximum dose of 60 mg daily. **Note:** For patients requiring dose titration, the Canadian ADHD Resource Alliance (CADDRA) 2011 practice guidelines recommend weekly increases of 10 mg daily up to a maximum of 60 mg daily for children or 70 mg daily for adolescent and adult patients.

Administration Administer in the morning without regard to meals; swallow capsule whole, do not chew; capsule may be opened and the entire contents dissolved in glass of water; stir until dispersed completely and consume the resulting solution immediately; do not store solution.

Monitoring Parameters Cardiac evaluation should be completed on any patient who develops chest pain, unexplained syncope, and any symptom of cardiac disease during treatment with stimulants; growth (height and weight) in children; CNS activity in all patients; signs of peripheral vasculopathy (eg, digital changes); signs of misuse, abuse, or addiction

When used for the treatment of ADHD, thoroughly evaluate for cardiovascular risk. Monitor heart rate, blood pressure, and consider obtaining ECG prior to initiation (Vetter, 2008).

Test Interactions Amphetamines may elevate plasma corticosteroid levels; may interfere with urinary steroid determinations.

Dosage Forms Excipient information presented when available (limited, particularly for generics); consult specific product labeling.

Capsule, Oral, as dimesylate:

Vyvanse: 20 mg, 30 mg, 40 mg, 50 mg, 60 mg, 70 mg [contains brilliant blue fcf (fd&c blue #1), fd&c red #40, fd&c yellow #10 (quinoline yellow)]

Dosage Forms: Canada Refer to Dosage Forms. **Note:** Vyvanse 70 mg capsule is not available in Canada.

Controlled Substance C-II

◆ **Lisdexamfetamine Dimesylate** *see* Lisdexamfetamine *on page 1225*

◆ **Lisdexamphetamine** *see* Lisdexamfetamine *on page 1225*

Lisinopril (lyse IN oh pril)

Brand Names: U.S. Prinivil; Zestril

Brand Names: Canada Apo-Lisinopril; Auro-Lisinopril; CO Lisinopril; Dom-Lisinopril; JAMP-Lisinopril; Mylan-Lisinopril; PMS-Lisinopril; Prinivil; PRO-Lisinopril; RAN-Lisinopril; ratio-Lisinopril P; ratio-Lisinopril Z; Riva-Lisinopril; Sandoz-Lisinopril; Teva-Lisinopril (Type P); Teva-Lisinopril (Type Z); Zestril

Pharmacologic Category Angiotensin-Converting Enzyme (ACE) Inhibitor; Antihypertensive

Additional Appendix Information

Angiotensin Agents *on page 2280*

Use Treatment of hypertension, either alone or in combination with other antihypertensive agents; adjunctive therapy in treatment of heart failure (afterload reduction); treatment of acute myocardial infarction within 24 hours in hemodynamically-stable patients to improve survival; treatment of left ventricular dysfunction after myocardial infarction

Pregnancy Risk Factor D

Pregnancy Considerations [U.S. Boxed Warning]: Drugs that act on the renin-angiotensin system can cause injury and death to the developing fetus. Discontinue as soon as possible once pregnancy is detected. Lisinopril crosses the placenta; teratogenic effects may occur following maternal use during pregnancy. Drugs that act on the renin-angiotensin system are associated with oligohydramnios. Oligohydramnios, due to decreased fetal renal function, may lead to fetal lung hypoplasia and skeletal malformations. Their use in pregnancy is also associated with anuria, hypotension, renal failure, skull hypoplasia, and death in the fetus/neonate. Chronic maternal hypertension itself is also associated with adverse events in the fetus/infant. ACE inhibitors are not recommended during pregnancy to treat maternal hypertension or heart failure. Use of an ACE inhibitor should also be avoided in any woman of reproductive age. Women who are planning a pregnancy should be considered for other medication options if an ACE inhibitor is currently prescribed or the ACE inhibitor should be discontinued as soon as possible once pregnancy is detected. The exposed fetus should be monitored for fetal growth, amniotic fluid volume, and organ formation. Infants exposed to an ACE inhibitor *in utero* should be monitored for hyperkalemia, hypotension, and oliguria.

Breast-Feeding Considerations It is not known if lisinopril is excreted in breast milk. Breast-feeding is not recommended by the manufacturer.

Contraindications

Hypersensitivity to lisinopril or any component of the formulation; angioedema related to previous treatment with an ACE inhibitor; patients with idiopathic or hereditary angioedema; concomitant use with aliskiren in patients with diabetes mellitus

Canadian labeling: Additional contraindications (not in U.S. labeling): Concomitant use with aliskiren-containing drugs in patients with moderate-to-severe renal impairment (GFR <60 mL/minute/1.73 m^2)

Warnings/Precautions Anaphylactic reactions may occur rarely with ACE inhibitors. At any time during treatment (especially following first dose), angioedema may occur rarely with ACE inhibitors; it may involve the head and neck (potentially compromising airway) or the intestine (presenting with abdominal pain). African-Americans may be at an increased risk. Prolonged frequent monitoring may be required especially if tongue, glottis, or larynx are involved as they are associated with airway obstruction. Patients with a history of airway surgery may have a higher risk of airway obstruction. Aggressive early and appropriate management is critical. Use in patients with idiopathic or hereditary angioedema or previous angioedema associated with ACE inhibitor therapy is contraindicated. Severe anaphylactoid reactions may be seen during hemodialysis (eg, CVVHD) with high-flux dialysis membranes (eg, AN69), and rarely, during low density lipoprotein apheresis with dextran sulfate cellulose. Rare cases of anaphylactoid reactions have been reported in patients undergoing sensitization treatment with hymenoptera (bee, wasp) venom while receiving ACE inhibitors.

Symptomatic hypotension with or without syncope can occur with ACE inhibitors (usually with the first several doses); effects are most often observed in volume depleted patients; correct volume depletion prior to initiation; close monitoring of patient is required especially with initial dosing and dosing increases; blood pressure must be lowered at a rate appropriate for the patient's clinical condition. Initiation of therapy in patients with ischemic heart disease or cerebrovascular disease warrants close observation due to the potential consequences posed by falling blood pressure (eg, MI, stroke). Use with caution in hypertrophic cardiomyopathy with outflow tract obstruction, severe aortic stenosis, or before, during, or immediately after major surgery. **[U.S. Boxed Warning]: Drugs that act on the renin-angiotensin system can cause injury and death to the developing fetus. Discontinue as soon as possible once pregnancy is detected.**

Hyperkalemia may occur with ACE inhibitors; risk factors include renal dysfunction, diabetes mellitus, concomitant use of potassium-sparing diuretics, potassium supplements, and/or potassium-containing salts. Use cautiously, if at all, with these agents and monitor potassium closely. Cough may occur with ACE inhibitors. Other causes of cough should be considered (eg, pulmonary congestion in patients with heart failure) and excluded prior to discontinuation.

May be associated with deterioration of renal function and/or increases in serum creatinine, particularly in patients with low renal blood flow (eg, renal artery stenosis, heart failure) whose glomerular filtration rate (GFR) is dependent on efferent arteriolar vasoconstriction by angiotensin II; deterioration may result in oliguria, acute renal failure, and progressive azotemia. Small increases in serum creatinine may occur following initiation; consider discontinuation only in patients with progressive and/or significant deterioration in renal function. Use with caution in patients with unstented unilateral/bilateral renal artery stenosis. When unstented bilateral renal artery stenosis is present, use is generally avoided due to the elevated risk of deterioration in renal function unless possible benefits outweigh risks. Potentially significant drug-drug interactions may exist, requiring dose or frequency adjustment, additional monitoring, and/or selection of alternative therapy.

Rare toxicities associated with ACE inhibitors include cholestatic jaundice (which may progress to fulminant hepatic necrosis), agranulocytosis, neutropenia, or leukopenia with myeloid hypoplasia. Patients with collagen vascular diseases (especially with concomitant renal impairment) or renal impairment alone may be at increased risk for hematologic toxicity; periodically monitor CBC with differential in these patients. Safety and efficacy have not been established in children <6 years of age or children with a Cl_{cr} ≤30 mL/minute.

Adverse Reactions Note: Frequency ranges include data from hypertension and heart failure trials. Higher rates of adverse reactions have generally been noted in patients with heart failure. However, the frequency of adverse effects associated with placebo is also increased in this population.

1% to 10%:

- Cardiovascular: Orthostatic effects (1%), hypotension (1% to 4%)
- Central nervous system: Headache (4% to 6%), dizziness (5% to 12%), fatigue (3%)
- Dermatologic: Rash (1% to 2%)
- Endocrine & metabolic: Hyperkalemia (2% to 5%)
- Gastrointestinal: Diarrhea (3% to 4%), nausea (2%), vomiting (1%), abdominal pain (2%)
- Genitourinary: Impotence (1%)
- Hematologic: Decreased hemoglobin (small)
- Neuromuscular & skeletal: Chest pain (3%), weakness (1%)
- Renal: BUN increased (2%); deterioration in renal function (in patients with bilateral renal artery stenosis or hypovolemia); serum creatinine increased (often transient)
- Respiratory: Cough (4% to 9%), upper respiratory infection (1% to 2%)

<1% (Limited to important or life-threatening): Acute renal failure, alopecia, anaphylactoid reactions, angioedema, anuria, arrhythmia, arthralgia, arthritis, asthma, ataxia, atrial fibrillation, atrial tachycardia, azotemia, bone

marrow suppression, bradycardia, cardiac arrest, cutaneous pseudolymphoma, diabetes mellitus, eosinophilia, eosinophilic pneumonitis, erythrocyte sedimentation rate increased, gout, hemolytic anemia, hemoptysis, hepatic necrosis, hepatitis, herpes zoster, hypersomnia, hyponatremia, interstitial nephritis, intestinal angioedema, leukopenia, lung neoplasms (malignant), memory impairment, MI, mood changes, neutropenia, oliguria, orthostatic hypotension, pancreatitis, pemphigus, peripheral neuropathy, photosensitivity, pleural effusion, pneumonia, positive ANA, psoriasis, pulmonary embolism, pulmonary infarction, SIADH, skin infections, Stevens-Johnson syndrome, stroke, syncope, systemic lupus erythematosus, thrombocytopenia, TIA, toxic epidermal necrolysis, urinary tract infection, vasculitis, ventricular tachycardia, viral infection, vision loss, visual hallucinations (Doane, 2013)

Drug Interactions

Metabolism/Transport Effects None known.

Avoid Concomitant Use There are no known interactions where it is recommended to avoid concomitant use.

Increased Effect/Toxicity

Lisinopril may increase the levels/effects of: Allopurinol; Amifostine; Antihypertensives; AzaTHIOprine; CycloSPORINE (Systemic); Ferric Gluconate; Gold Sodium Thiomalate; Hypotensive Agents; Iron Dextran Complex; Lithium; Nonsteroidal Anti-Inflammatory Agents; Obinutuzumab; RiTUXimab; Sodium Phosphates

The levels/effects of Lisinopril may be increased by: Alfuzosin; Aliskiren; Angiotensin II Receptor Blockers; Brimonidine (Topical); Canagliflozin; Diazoxide; DPP-IV Inhibitors; Eplerenone; Everolimus; Heparin; Heparin (Low Molecular Weight); Herbs (Hypotensive Properties); Loop Diuretics; MAO Inhibitors; Pentoxifylline; Phosphodiesterase 5 Inhibitors; Potassium Salts; Potassium-Sparing Diuretics; Prostacyclin Analogues; Sirolimus; Temsirolimus; Thiazide Diuretics; TiZANidine; Tolvaptan; Trimethoprim

Decreased Effect

The levels/effects of Lisinopril may be decreased by: Antacids; Aprotinin; Herbs (Hypertensive Properties); Icatibant; Lanthanum; Methylphenidate; Nonsteroidal Anti-Inflammatory Agents; Salicylates; Yohimbine

Ethanol/Nutrition/Herb Interactions

Food: Potassium supplements and/or potassium-containing salts may cause or worsen hyperkalemia. Management: Consult prescriber before consuming a potassium-rich diet, potassium supplements, or salt substitutes.

Herb/Nutraceutical: Some herbal medications may worsen hypertension (eg, licorice); others may increase the antihypertensive effect of lisinopril (eg, shepherd's purse). Management: Avoid bayberry, blue cohosh, cayenne, ephedra, ginger, ginseng (American), kola, licorice, and yohimbe. Avoid black cohosh, California poppy, coleus, golden seal, hawthorn, mistletoe, periwinkle, quinine, and shepherd's purse.

Mechanism of Action Competitive inhibitor of angiotensin-converting enzyme (ACE); prevents conversion of angiotensin I to angiotensin II, a potent vasoconstrictor; results in lower levels of angiotensin II which causes an increase in plasma renin activity and a reduction in aldosterone secretion; a CNS mechanism may also be involved in hypotensive effect as angiotensin II increases adrenergic outflow from CNS; vasoactive kallikreins may be decreased in conversion to active hormones by ACE inhibitors, thus reducing blood pressure

Pharmacodynamics/Kinetics

Onset of action: 1 hour
 Peak effect: Hypotensive: Oral: ~6 hours
Duration: 24 hours
Absorption: Well absorbed; unaffected by food
Protein binding: 25%
Metabolism: Not metabolized
Bioavailability: Decreased with NYHA Class II-IV heart failure
Half-life elimination: 11-12 hours
Time to peak: ~7 hours
Excretion: Primarily urine (as unchanged drug)

Dosage Oral:

Heart failure: Adults: Initial: 2.5-5 mg once daily; then increase by no more than 10 mg increments at intervals no less than 2 weeks to a maximum daily dose of 40 mg. Usual maintenance: 5-40 mg/day as a single dose. Target dose: 20-40 mg once daily (ACC/AHA 2009 Heart Failure Guidelines)

Note: If patient has hyponatremia (serum sodium <130 mEq/L) or renal impairment (Cl_{cr} <30 mL/minute or creatinine >3 mg/dL), then initial dose should be 2.5 mg/day

Hypertension:

Children ≥6 years: Initial: 0.07 mg/kg once daily (up to 5 mg); increase dose at 1- to 2-week intervals; doses >0.61 mg/kg or >40 mg have not been evaluated.

Adults: Usual dosage range (JNC 7): 10-40 mg/day

Not maintained on diuretic: Initial: 10 mg/day

Maintained on diuretic: Initial: 5 mg/day

Note: Antihypertensive effect may diminish toward the end of the dosing interval especially with doses of 10 mg/day. An increased dose may aid in extending the duration of antihypertensive effect. Doses up to 80 mg/day have been used, but do not appear to give greater effect.

Patients taking diuretics should have them discontinued 2-3 days prior to initiating lisinopril if possible. Restart diuretic after blood pressure is stable if needed. If diuretic cannot be discontinued prior to therapy, begin with 5 mg with close supervision until stable blood pressure. In patients with hyponatremia (<130 mEq/L), start dose at 2.5 mg/day

Elderly: Consider lower initial doses (eg, 2.5-5 mg/day) and titrate to response (Aronow, 2011)

Acute myocardial infarction (within 24 hours in hemodynamically stable patients): Adults: 5 mg immediately, then 5 mg at 24 hours, 10 mg at 48 hours, and 10 mg every day thereafter for 6 weeks. Patients should continue to receive standard treatments such as thrombolytics, aspirin, and beta-blockers.

Dosage adjustment in renal impairment:

Heart failure: Adults: Cl_{cr} <30 mL/minute or creatinine >3 mg/dL: Initial: 2.5 mg/day

Hypertension:

Adults: Initial doses should be modified and upward titration should be cautious, based on response (maximum: 40 mg/day)

Cl_{cr} >30 mL/minute: Initial: 10 mg/day

Cl_{cr} 10-30 mL/minute: Initial: 5 mg/day

Hemodialysis: Initial: 2.5 mg/day; dialyzable (50%)

Children: Use in not recommended in pediatric patients with GFR <30 mL/minute/1.73 m^2

Dosage adjustment in hepatic impairment: No dosage adjustment provided in manufacturer's labeling.

Dietary Considerations Use potassium-containing salt substitutes cautiously in patients with diabetes, patients with renal dysfunction, or those maintained on potassium supplements or potassium-sparing diuretics.

Administration Watch for hypotensive effects within 1-3 hours of first dose or new higher dose.

Monitoring Parameters BUN, serum creatinine, renal function, WBC, and potassium; if patient has collagen vascular disease and/or renal impairment, periodically monitor CBC with differential

Test Interactions May cause false-positive results in urine acetone determinations using sodium nitroprusside reagent

Dosage Forms Excipient information presented when available (limited, particularly for generics); consult specific product labeling.

Tablet, Oral:

Prinivil: 5 mg, 10 mg, 20 mg [scored]

Zestril: 2.5 mg

Zestril: 5 mg [scored]

Zestril: 10 mg, 20 mg, 30 mg, 40 mg

Generic: 2.5 mg, 5 mg, 10 mg, 20 mg, 30 mg, 40 mg

Extemporaneous Preparations A 1 mg/mL lisinopril oral suspension may be made with tablets and a 1:1 mixture of Ora-Plus® and Ora-Sweet®. Crush ten 10 mg tablets in a mortar and reduce to a fine powder. Add small portions of the vehicle and mix to a uniform paste; mix while adding the vehicle in incremental proportions to **almost** 100 mL; transfer to a graduated cylinder; rinse mortar with vehicle, and add quantity of vehicle sufficient to make 100 mL. Store in amber plastic prescription bottles; label "shake well". Stable for 13 weeks at room temperature or refrigerated (Nahata, 2004).

A 1 mg/mL lisinopril oral suspension also be made with tablets, methylcellulose 1% with parabens, and simple syrup NF. Crush ten 10 mg tablets in a mortar and reduce to a fine powder. Add 7.7 mL of methylcellulose gel and mix to a uniform paste; mix while adding the simple syrup in incremental proportions to **almost** 100 mL; transfer to a graduated cylinder; rinse mortar with vehicle, and add quantity of vehicle sufficient to make 100 mL. Store in amber plastic prescription bottles; label "shake well". Stable for 13 weeks refrigerated or 8 weeks at room temperature (Nahata, 2004).

A 2 mg/mL lisinopril syrup may be made with powder (Sigma Chemical Company, St. Louis, MO) and simple syrup. Dissolve 1 g of lisinopril powder in 30 mL of distilled water. Mix while adding simple syrup in incremental proportions in a quantity sufficient to make 500 mL. Label "shake well" and "refrigerate". Stable for 30 days when stored in amber plastic prescription bottles at room temperature or refrigerated. **Note:** Although no visual evidence of microbial growth was observed, the authors recommend refrigeration to inhibit microbial growth (Webster, 1997).

Nahata MC and Morosco RS, "Stability of Lisinopril in Two Liquid Dosage Forms," *Ann Pharmacother*, 2004, 38(3):396-9.

Prinivil® prescribing information, Merck & Co, Inc, Whitehouse Station, NJ, 2008.

Thompson KC, Zhao Z, Mazakas JM, et al, "Characterization of an Extemporaneous Liquid Formulation of Lisinopril," *Am J Health Syst Pharm*, 2003, 60(1):69-74.

Webster AA, English BA, and Rose DJ, "The Stability of Lisinopril as an Extemporaneous Syrup," *Intr J Pharmaceut Compound*, 1997, 1:352-3.

Zestril® prescribing information, AstraZeneca Pharmaceuticals, Wilmington, DE, 2007.

Lisinopril and Hydrochlorothiazide

(lyse IN oh pril & hye droe klor oh THYE a zide)

Brand Names: U.S. Prinzide; Zestoretic

Brand Names: Canada Apo-Lisinopril/Hctz; Ava-Lisinopril/Hctz; Mylan-Lisinopril/Hctz; Prinzide; Sandoz-Lisinopril/Hctz; Teva-Lisinopril/Hctz (Type P); Teva-Lisinopril/Hctz (Type Z); Zestoretic

Index Terms Hydrochlorothiazide and Lisinopril

Pharmacologic Category Angiotensin-Converting Enzyme (ACE) Inhibitor; Antihypertensive; Diuretic, Thiazide

Use Treatment of hypertension

Pregnancy Risk Factor D

Dosage Adults: Oral: Dosage is individualized; see each component for appropriate dosing suggestions; doses >80 mg/day lisinopril or >50 mg/day hydrochlorothiazide are not recommended.

Dosage adjustment in renal impairment: Dosage adjustments should be made with caution. Usual regimens of therapy need not be adjusted as long as patient's Cl_{cr} >30 mL/minute. In patients with more severe renal impairment, loop diuretics are preferred.

Dosage adjustment in hepatic impairment: No dosage adjustment provided in manufacturer's labeling; use with caution.

Additional Information Complete prescribing information should be consulted for additional detail.

Dosage Forms Excipient information presented when available (limited, particularly for generics); consult specific product labeling.

Tablet, oral: 10/12.5: Lisinopril 10 mg and hydrochlorothiazide 12.5 mg; 20/12.5: Lisinopril 20 mg and hydrochlorothiazide 12.5 mg; 20/25: Lisinopril 20 mg and hydrochlorothiazide 25 mg

Prinzide®:

10/12.5: Lisinopril 10 mg and hydrochlorothiazide 12.5 mg

Zestoretic®:

10/12.5: Lisinopril 10 mg and hydrochlorothiazide 12.5 mg

20/12.5: Lisinopril 20 mg and hydrochlorothiazide 12.5 mg

20/25: Lisinopril 20 mg and hydrochlorothiazide 25 mg

◆ **Lispro Insulin** *see* Insulin Lispro *on page 1090*

◆ **Lithane™ (Can)** *see* Lithium *on page 1229*

Lithium (LITH ee um)

Brand Names: U.S. Lithobid

Brand Names: Canada Apo-Lithium® Carbonate; Apo-Lithium® Carbonate SR; Carbolith™; Duralith®; Euro-Lithium; Lithane™; Lithmax; PHL-Lithium Carbonate; PMS-Lithium Carbonate; PMS-Lithium Citrate

Index Terms Eskalith; Lithium Carbonate; Lithium Citrate

Pharmacologic Category Antimanic Agent

Use Management of bipolar disorders; treatment of mania in individuals with bipolar disorder (maintenance treatment prevents or diminishes intensity of subsequent episodes)

Unlabeled Use Potential augmenting agent for antidepressants; aggression, post-traumatic stress disorder, conduct disorder in children

Pregnancy Risk Factor D

Pregnancy Considerations Adverse events have been observed in animal reproduction studies. Lithium crosses the placenta in concentrations similar to those in the maternal plasma (Newport, 2005). Cardiac malformations in the infant, including Ebstein's anomaly, are associated with use of lithium during the first trimester of pregnancy. Other adverse events including polyhydramnios, fetal/neonatal cardiac arrhythmias, hypoglycemia, diabetes insipidus, changes in thyroid function, premature delivery, floppy infant syndrome, or neonatal lithium toxicity are associated with lithium exposure when used later in pregnancy (ACOG, 2008). The incidence of adverse events may be associated with higher maternal doses (Newport, 2005).

Due to pregnancy-induced physiologic changes, women who are pregnant may require dose adjustments of lithium to achieve euthymia and avoid toxicity (ACOG, 2008; Grandjean, 2009; Yonkers, 2011).

For planned pregnancies, use of lithium during the first trimester should be avoided if possible (Grandjean, 2009). If lithium is needed during pregnancy, the minimum effective dose should be used, maternal serum concentrations should be monitored, and consideration should be given to start therapy after the period of organogenesis; lithium should be suspended 24-48 hours prior to delivery or at ▶

the onset of labor when delivery is spontaneous, then restarted when the patient is medically stable after delivery (ACOG, 2008; Grandjean, 2009; Newport, 2005). Fetal echocardiography should be considered if first trimester exposure occurs (ACOG, 2008).

Breast-Feeding Considerations Lithium is excreted into breast milk and serum concentrations of nursing infants may be 10% to 50% of the maternal serum concentration (Grandjean, 2009). Hypotonia, hypothermia, cyanosis, electrocardiogram changes, and lethargy have been reported in nursing infants (ACOG, 2008). It is generally recommended that breast-feeding be avoided during maternal use of lithium; however, treatment may be continued in appropriately selected patients (Grandjean, 2009; Sharma, 2009; Viguera, 2007). The hydration status of the nursing infant and maternal serum concentrations of lithium should be monitored (ACOG, 2008). In addition, monitor the infant for lethargy, growth, and feeding problems; obtain infant serum concentrations only if clinical concerns arise (Bogen, 2012; Yonkers, 2011). Long-term effects on development and behavior have not been studied (ACOG, 2008; Grandjean, 2009).

Contraindications Hypersensitivity to lithium or any component of the formulation; avoid use in patients with severe cardiovascular or renal disease, or with severe debilitation, dehydration, or sodium depletion

Warnings/Precautions [U.S. Boxed Warning]: Lithium toxicity is closely related to serum levels and can occur at therapeutic doses; serum lithium determinations are required to monitor therapy. Use with caution in patients with thyroid disease, mild-moderate renal impairment, or mild-moderate cardiovascular disease. Use caution in patients receiving medications which alter sodium excretion (eg, diuretics, ACE inhibitors, NSAIDs), or in patients with significant fluid loss (protracted sweating, diarrhea, or prolonged fever); temporary reduction or cessation of therapy may be warranted. Some elderly patients may be extremely sensitive to the effects of lithium, see Dosage and Reference Range. Chronic therapy results in diminished renal concentrating ability (nephrogenic DI); this is usually reversible when lithium is discontinued. Changes in renal function should be monitored, and re-evaluation of treatment may be necessary. Use caution in patients at risk of suicide (suicidal thoughts or behavior).

Use with caution in patients receiving neuroleptic medications - a syndrome resembling NMS has been associated with concurrent therapy. Lithium may impair the patient's alertness, affecting the ability to operate machinery or driving a vehicle. Neuromuscular-blocking agents should be administered with caution; the response may be prolonged.

Higher serum concentrations may be required and tolerated during an acute manic phase; however, the tolerance decreases when symptoms subside. Normal fluid and salt intake must be maintained during therapy.

Adverse Reactions Frequency not defined.

Cardiovascular: Cardiac arrhythmia, hypotension, sinus node dysfunction, flattened or inverted T waves (reversible), edema, bradycardia, syncope

Central nervous system: Blackout spells, coma, confusion, dizziness, dystonia, fatigue, headache, lethargy, pseudotumor cerebri, psychomotor retardation, restlessness, sedation, seizure, slowed intellectual functioning, slurred speech, stupor, tics, vertigo

Dermatologic: Dry or thinning of hair, folliculitis, alopecia, exacerbation of psoriasis, rash

Endocrine & metabolic: Euthyroid goiter and/or hypothyroidism, hyperthyroidism, hyperglycemia, diabetes insipidus

Gastrointestinal: Polydipsia, anorexia, nausea, vomiting, diarrhea, xerostomia, metallic taste, weight gain, salivary gland swelling, excessive salivation

Genitourinary: Incontinence, polyuria, glycosuria, oliguria, albuminuria

Hematologic: Leukocytosis

Neuromuscular & skeletal: Tremor, muscle hyperirritability, ataxia, choreoathetoid movements, hyperactive deep tendon reflexes, myasthenia gravis (rare)

Ocular: Nystagmus, blurred vision, transient scotoma

Miscellaneous: Coldness and painful discoloration of fingers and toes

Postmarketing and/or case reports: Drug-induced Brugada syndrome

Drug Interactions

Metabolism/Transport Effects None known.

Avoid Concomitant Use There are no known interactions where it is recommended to avoid concomitant use.

Increased Effect/Toxicity

Lithium may increase the levels/effects of: Antipsychotics; Highest Risk QTc-Prolonging Agents; Metoclopramide; Moderate Risk QTc-Prolonging Agents; Neuromuscular-Blocking Agents; Selective Serotonin Reuptake Inhibitors; Serotonin Modulators; Tricyclic Antidepressants

The levels/effects of Lithium may be increased by: ACE Inhibitors; Angiotensin II Receptor Blockers; Antipsychotics; Calcium Channel Blockers (Nondihydropyridine); CarBAMazepine; Desmopressin; Eplerenone; Fosphenytoin; Loop Diuretics; MAO Inhibitors; Methyldopa; Mifepristone; Nonsteroidal Anti-Inflammatory Agents; Phenytoin; Potassium Iodide; Thiazide Diuretics; Topiramate

Decreased Effect

Lithium may decrease the levels/effects of: Amphetamines; Antipsychotics; Desmopressin

The levels/effects of Lithium may be decreased by: Calcitonin; Calcium Polystyrene Sulfonate; Carbonic Anhydrase Inhibitors; Loop Diuretics; Sodium Bicarbonate; Sodium Chloride; Sodium Polystyrene Sulfonate; Theophylline Derivatives

Ethanol/Nutrition/Herb Interactions Food: Limit caffeine.

Mechanism of Action Alters cation transport across cell membrane in nerve and muscle cells and influences reuptake of serotonin and/or norepinephrine; second messenger systems involving the phosphatidylinositol cycle are inhibited; postsynaptic D2 receptor supersensitivity is inhibited

Pharmacodynamics/Kinetics

Absorption: Rapid and complete

Distribution: V_d: Initial: 0.3-0.4 L/kg; V_{dss}: 0.7-1 L/kg

CSF, liver concentrations: 1/3 to 1/2 of serum concentration

Erythrocyte concentration: ~1/2 of serum concentration

Heart, lung, kidney, muscle concentrations: Equivalent to serum concentration

Saliva concentration: 2-3 times serum concentration

Thyroid, bone, brain tissue concentrations: Increase 50% over serum concentrations

Protein binding: Not protein bound

Metabolism: Not metabolized

Bioavailability: Not affected by food; Capsule, immediate release tablet: 95% to 100%; Extended release tablet: 60% to 90%; Syrup: 100%

Half-life elimination: 18-24 hours; can increase to more than 36 hours in elderly or with renal impairment

Time to peak, serum: Immediate release: ~0.5-2 hours; extended release: 4-12 hours; syrup: 15-60 minutes

Excretion: Urine (90% to 98% as unchanged drug); sweat (4% to 5%); feces (1%)

Clearance: 80% of filtered lithium is reabsorbed in the proximal convoluted tubules; therefore, clearance approximates 20% of GFR or 20-40 mL/minute

Dosage Oral: **Note:** Monitor serum concentrations and clinical response (efficacy and toxicity) to determine proper dose. Each 5 mL of lithium citrate oral solution contains 8 mEq of lithium ion, equivalent to the amount of lithium in 300 mg of lithium carbonate immediate release capsules/ tablets.

Children 6-12 years:

Bipolar disorder (unlabeled use): 15-60 mg/kg/day in 3-4 divided doses; dose not to exceed usual adult dosage

Conduct disorder (unlabeled use): 15-30 mg/kg/day in 3-4 divided doses; dose not to exceed usual adult dosage

Adults: Bipolar disorder: 900-2400 mg/day in 3-4 divided doses or 900-1800 mg/day (extended release) in 2 divided doses

Elderly: Bipolar disorder: Initial dose: 300 mg once or twice daily; increase weekly in increments of 300 mg/day, monitoring levels; rarely need >900-1200 mg/day

Dosage adjustment in renal impairment:

Cl_{cr} 10-50 mL/minute: Administer 50% to 75% of normal dose

Cl_{cr} <10 mL/minute: Administer 25% to 50% of normal dose

Hemodialysis: Dialyzable (50% to 100%); 4-7 times more efficient than peritoneal dialysis

Dosage adjustment in hepatic impairment: No dosage adjustment provided in manufacturer's labeling.

Dietary Considerations May be taken with meals to avoid GI upset; maintain adequate fluid intake.

Administration Administer with meals to decrease GI upset. Extended release tablets must be swallowed whole; do not crush or chew.

Monitoring Parameters Serum lithium every 4-5 days during initial therapy; draw lithium serum concentrations 8-12 hours postdose; renal, thyroid, and cardiovascular function; fluid status; serum electrolytes; CBC with differential, urinalysis; monitor for signs of toxicity; beta-hCG pregnancy test for all females not known to be sterile

Reference Range Levels should be obtained twice weekly until both patient's clinical status and levels are stable then levels may be obtained every 1-3 months

Timing of serum samples: Draw trough just before next dose (8-12 hours after previous dose)

Therapeutic levels:

Acute mania: 0.6-1.2 mEq/L (SI: 0.6-1.2 mmol/L)

Protection against future episodes in most patients with bipolar disorder: 0.8-1 mEq/L (SI: 0.8-1.0 mmol/L); a higher rate of relapse is described in subjects who are maintained at <0.4 mEq/L (SI: 0.4 mmol/L)

Elderly patients can usually be maintained at lower end of therapeutic range (0.6-0.8 mEq/L)

Toxic concentration: >1.5 mEq/L (SI: >1.5 mmol/L)

Adverse effect levels:

GI complaints/tremor: 1.5-2 mEq/L

Confusion/somnolence: 2-2.5 mEq/L

Seizures/death: >2.5 mEq/L

Dosage Forms Excipient information presented when available (limited, particularly for generics); consult specific product labeling.

Capsule, Oral, as carbonate:

Generic: 150 mg, 300 mg, 600 mg

Solution, Oral, as citrate:

Generic: 8 mEq/5 mL (5 mL, 500 mL)

Tablet, Oral, as carbonate:

Generic: 300 mg

Tablet Extended Release, Oral, as carbonate:

Lithobid: 300 mg [contains fd&c blue #2 aluminum lake, fd&c red #40 aluminum lake, fd&c yellow #6 aluminum lake]

Generic: 300 mg, 450 mg

◆ **Lithium Carbonate** *see* Lithium *on page 1229*
◆ **Lithium Citrate** *see* Lithium *on page 1229*
◆ **Lithmax (Can)** *see* Lithium *on page 1229*
◆ **Lithobid** *see* Lithium *on page 1229*
◆ **Little Colds Decongestant [OTC]** *see* Phenylephrine (Systemic) *on page 1636*
◆ **Little Fevers [OTC]** *see* Acetaminophen *on page 28*
◆ **Little Noses Decongestant [OTC]** *see* Sodium Chloride *on page 1914*
◆ **Livalo** *see* Pitavastatin *on page 1657*
◆ **Live Attenuated Influenza Vaccine** *see* Influenza Virus Vaccine (Live/Attenuated) *on page 1082*
◆ **Live Attenuated Influenza Vaccine (Quadrivalent)** *see* Influenza Virus Vaccine (Live/Attenuated) *on page 1082*
◆ **Live Smallpox Vaccine** *see* Smallpox Vaccine *on page 1909*
◆ **L-leucovorin** *see* LEVOleucovorin *on page 1201*
◆ **LM3100** *see* Plerixafor *on page 1657*
◆ **10% LMD** *see* Dextran *on page 587*
◆ **LMD in D_5W** *see* Dextran *on page 587*
◆ **LMD in NaCl** *see* Dextran *on page 587*
◆ **L-methylfolate, Methylcobalamin, and N-acetylcysteine** *see* Methylfolate, Methylcobalamin, and Acetylcysteine *on page 1335*
◆ **LMX 4 [OTC]** *see* Lidocaine (Topical) *on page 1212*
◆ **LMX 4 Plus [OTC]** *see* Lidocaine (Topical) *on page 1212*
◆ **LMX 5 [OTC]** *see* Lidocaine (Topical) *on page 1212*
◆ **LNg 20** *see* Levonorgestrel *on page 1202*
◆ **Locoid** *see* Hydrocortisone (Topical) *on page 1011*
◆ **Locoid® (Can)** *see* Hydrocortisone (Topical) *on page 1011*
◆ **Locoid Lipocream** *see* Hydrocortisone (Topical) *on page 1011*
◆ **Lodalis (Can)** *see* Colesevelam *on page 487*
◆ **Lodine** *see* Etodolac *on page 799*
◆ **Lodosyn** *see* Carbidopa *on page 340*

Lodoxamide (loe DOKS a mide)

Brand Names: U.S. Alomide

Brand Names: Canada Alomide®

Index Terms Lodoxamide Tromethamine

Pharmacologic Category Mast Cell Stabilizer

Use Treatment of vernal keratoconjunctivitis, vernal conjunctivitis, and vernal keratitis

Pregnancy Risk Factor B

Dosage Ophthalmic: Children >2 years and Adults: Instill 1-2 drops in eye(s) 4 times/day for up to 3 months

Dosage adjustment in renal impairment: No dosage adjustment provided in manufacturer's labeling. However, dosage adjustment unlikely due to low systemic absorption.

Dosage adjustment in hepatic impairment: No dosage adjustment provided in manufacturer's labeling. However, dosage adjustment unlikely due to low systemic absorption.

Additional Information Complete prescribing information should be consulted for additional detail.

Dosage Forms Excipient information presented when available (limited, particularly for generics); consult specific product labeling.

Solution, Ophthalmic:

Alomide: 0.1% (10 mL)

- **Lodoxamide Tromethamine** *see* Lodoxamide *on page 1231*
- **Loestrin 1.5/30 (Can)** *see* Ethinyl Estradiol and Norethindrone *on page 793*
- **Loestrin 21 1.5/30** *see* Ethinyl Estradiol and Norethindrone *on page 793*
- **Loestrin 21 1/20** *see* Ethinyl Estradiol and Norethindrone *on page 793*
- **Loestrin 24 Fe** *see* Ethinyl Estradiol and Norethindrone *on page 793*
- **Loestrin Fe 1.5/30** *see* Ethinyl Estradiol and Norethindrone *on page 793*
- **Loestrin Fe 1/20** *see* Ethinyl Estradiol and Norethindrone *on page 793*
- **Lo-Femenal 21 (Can)** *see* Ethinyl Estradiol and Norgestrel *on page 797*
- **Lofibra** *see* Fenofibrate and Derivatives *on page 837*
- **LoHist-D [OTC]** *see* Chlorpheniramine and Pseudoephedrine *on page 412*
- **L-OHP** *see* Oxaliplatin *on page 1524*
- **LoKara** *see* Desonide *on page 578*
- **Lo Loestrin Fe** *see* Ethinyl Estradiol and Norethindrone *on page 793*
- **Lomedia 24 Fe** *see* Ethinyl Estradiol and Norethindrone *on page 793*
- **Lo Minastrin Fe** *see* Ethinyl Estradiol and Norethindrone *on page 793*

Lomitapide (loe MI ta pide)

Brand Names: U.S. Juxtapid

Index Terms AEGR-733; BMS 201038; Lomitapide Mesylate

Pharmacologic Category Antilipemic Agent, Microsomal Triglyceride Transfer Protein (MTP) Inhibitor

Use Adjunct to dietary therapy and other lipid-lowering treatments, including LDL apheresis where available, to reduce low-density lipoprotein cholesterol (LDL-C), total cholesterol, apolipoprotein B, and non-high-density lipoprotein cholesterol (non-HDL-C) in patients with homozygous familial hypercholesterolemia (HoFH)

Pregnancy Risk Factor X

Pregnancy Considerations Teratogenic effects have been observed in animal reproduction studies using doses lower than equivalent human doses. Use is contraindicated in pregnant women. Discontinue immediately if pregnancy occurs during treatment. Women of reproductive potential should have a negative pregnancy test prior to therapy and effective contraception must be used during treatment. Dose adjustment may be required for women using oral contraceptives.

Breast-Feeding Considerations It is not known if lomitapide is excreted into breast milk. Due to the potential for serious adverse reactions in the nursing infant, a decision should be made whether to discontinue nursing or to discontinue the drug, taking into account the importance of treatment to the mother.

Prescribing and Access Restrictions As a requirement of the REMS program, access to this medication is restricted. Prescribers must enroll in the Juxtapid™ REMS program and complete the Prescriber Training Module and complete, sign, and submit the Prescriber Enrollment Form to the Juxtapid™ REMS program. Pharmacies must educate all pharmacy staff involved in the dispensing of Juxtapid™ on the REMS program requirements, put processes in place to verify (prior to dispensing Juxtapid™) that the prescriber is certified and the Prescription Authorization Form is received with each new prescription. Pharmacies must also agree to be audited to ensure that all processes and procedures in place are being followed in accordance with the program and be able to provide prescription data to the REMS program. Additional information is available at www.JUXTAPIDREMSProgram.com or at 1-855-898-2743.

Medication Guide Available Yes

Contraindications Pregnancy; concomitant use with moderate or strong CYP3A4 inhibitors; moderate or severe (Child-Pugh class B or C) hepatic impairment; active liver disease including unexplained persistent elevations of serum transaminases

Warnings/Precautions **[U.S. Boxed Warning]: May cause transaminase elevations; elevations in ALT or AST ≥3 times upper limit of normal occurred during clinical trials (no clinically meaningful concomitant bilirubin, INR, or alkaline phosphatase elevation was observed). Lomitapide also increases hepatic fat, with or without concomitant transaminase elevations. Hepatic steatosis associated with lomitapide (reversible upon discontinuation) may be a risk factor for progressive liver disease including steatohepatitis and cirrhosis. Monitor hepatic function (ALT, AST, alkaline phosphatase and total bilirubin) prior to treatment; monitor ALT and AST regularly as recommended during treatment; dosage adjustment or discontinuation may be necessary; transaminases typically reduce within 1-4 weeks after discontinuation.** Alcohol ingestion may increase the risk of hepatic steatosis; alcohol consumption should be limited to ≤1 drink/day. Use caution when administered concomitantly with other hepatotoxic medications (eg, acetaminophen (>4 g/day for ≥3 days/week), amiodarone, isotretinoin, methotrexate, tetracyclines, and tamoxifen); may require more frequent monitoring of liver function tests. Concomitant administration with other LDL-lowering agents that also have the potential to increase hepatic fat is not recommended (has not been studied). Use with caution in patients with mild (Child-Pugh class A) hepatic impairment due to increased drug exposure; a reduced maximum dose is recommended. Use is contraindicated in patients with moderate to severe (Child-Pugh class B or C) impairment or active liver disease including unexplained persistent elevations of serum transaminases. Monitor liver function as recommended. Use with caution in patients with mild-to-severe renal impairment including end-stage renal disease (ESRD) not receiving dialysis (has not been evaluated); drug exposure may significantly increase. Use with caution in patients with ESRD receiving dialysis; a reduced maximum dose of 40 mg daily is recommended.

Significant gastrointestinal events (eg, diarrhea, nausea, dyspepsia, vomiting) occurred during treatment with lomitapide; absorption of other oral medications may be affected; adherence to a low-fat diet (<20% of energy from fat) and gradual titration of dosage will reduce the risk of gastrointestinal adverse events. Lomitapide may reduce the absorption of fat-soluble nutrients (eg, vitamin E, linoleic acid, alpha-linolenic acid, eicosapentaenoic acid, and docosahexaenoic acid); supplementation is recommended; patients with chronic bowel or pancreatic diseases predisposed to malabsorption are at increased risk for deficiency.

Potentially significant drug-drug interactions may exist, requiring dose or frequency adjustment, additional monitoring, and/or selection of alternative therapy. Contains lactose; avoid use in patients with hereditary galactose intolerance, Lapp lactase deficiency, or glucose-galactose malabsorption; may result in diarrhea and malabsorption. **[U.S. Boxed Warning]: Due to the risk for hepatotoxicity, access is restricted through a REMS program (Juxtapid™ REMS program).** Only certified healthcare providers and pharmacies may prescribe and dispense lomitapide.

Adverse Reactions

>10%:

Cardiovascular: Chest pain (24%)

Central nervous system: Fatigue (17%)

Gastrointestinal: Diarrhea (79%; severe: 14%), nausea (65%), dyspepsia (38%), vomiting (34%; severe: 10%), abdominal pain (34%; severe: 7%), weight loss (24%), abdominal discomfort (21%; severe: 7%), abdominal distension (21%; severe: 7%), constipation (21%), flatulence (21%), gastroenteritis (14%)

Hepatic: Hepatic steatosis (increase in hepatic fat >5%: 78%; >20% fat increase: 13%), ALT increased (17%; severe: 10%), ALT and/or AST ≥3 times upper limit of normal (34%)

Neuromuscular & skeletal: Back pain (14%)

Respiratory: Nasopharyngitis (17%), pharyngolaryngeal pain (14%)

Miscellaneous: Influenza (21%)

1% to 10%:

Cardiovascular: Angina pectoris (10%), palpitation (10%)

Central nervous system: Dizziness (10%), fever (10%), headache (10%)

Gastrointestinal: Defecation urgency (10%), gastroesophageal reflux disease (10%), rectal tenesmus (10%)

Hepatic: Hepatotoxicity (severe: 10%)

Respiratory: Nasal congestion (10%)

Drug Interactions

Metabolism/Transport Effects Substrate of CYP1A2 (minor), CYP2B6 (minor), CYP2C19 (minor), CYP2C8 (minor), CYP3A4 (major); **Note:** Assignment of Major/Minor substrate status based on clinically relevant drug interaction potential; **Inhibits** CYP3A4 (moderate), P-glycoprotein

Avoid Concomitant Use

Avoid concomitant use of Lomitapide with any of the following: Bosutinib; CYP3A4 Inhibitors (Moderate); CYP3A4 Inhibitors (Strong); Fusidic Acid (Systemic); Ibrutinib; Ivabradine; Lovastatin; PAZOPanib; Pimozide; Pomalidomide; Silodosin; Simeprevir; Tolvaptan; Topotecan; Ulipristal; VinCRIStine (Liposomal)

Increased Effect/Toxicity

Lomitapide may increase the levels/effects of: Afatinib; ARIPiprazole; Avanafil; Bosentan; Bosutinib; Budesonide (Systemic, Oral Inhalation); Colchicine; CYP3A4 Substrates; Dabigatran Etexilate; Dofetilide; Eplerenone; Everolimus; FentaNYL; Halofantrine; Ibrutinib; Imatinib; Ivabradine; Ivacaftor; Lovastatin; Lurasidone; OxyCODONE; PAZOPanib; P-glycoprotein/ABCB1 Substrates; Pimecrolimus; Pimozide; Pomalidomide; Propafenone; Prucalopride; Ranolazine; Rivaroxaban; Salmeterol; Saxagliptin; Silodosin; Simeprevir; Simvastatin; Tolvaptan; Topotecan; Ulipristal; Vilazodone; VinCRIStine (Liposomal); Warfarin; Zuclopenthixol

The levels/effects of Lomitapide may be increased by: Alcohol (Ethyl); CYP3A4 Inhibitors (Moderate); CYP3A4 Inhibitors (Strong); CYP3A4 Inhibitors (Weak); Dasatinib; Fusidic Acid (Systemic); Ivacaftor; Luliconazole; Mifepristone; Simeprevir

Decreased Effect

Lomitapide may decrease the levels/effects of: Ifosfamide

The levels/effects of Lomitapide may be decreased by: Bile Acid Sequestrants; Bosentan; CYP3A4 Inducers (Strong); Dabrafenib; Deferasirox; Herbs (CYP3A4 Inducers); Mitotane; Tocilizumab

Ethanol/Nutrition/Herb Interactions

Ethanol: May increase the risk for hepatic steatosis. Management: Limit alcohol consumption to 1 drink per day.

Food:

Grapefruit juice may increase lomitapide plasma concentration. Management: Avoid grapefruit juice.

High-fat diet: Diets containing ≥20% of total calories from fat may increase the risk of gastrointestinal adverse reactions (eg, abdominal pain/discomfort, constipation, diarrhea, flatulence, and nausea/vomiting).

Herb/Nutraceutical: Absorption of fat-soluble nutrients may be reduced. Management: Take recommended daily supplements of vitamin E, alpha-linolenic acid (ALA), linoleic acid, eicosapentaenoic acid (EPA), and docosahexaenoic acid (DHA).

Storage/Stability Store at 20°C to 25°C (68°F to 77°F); excursions permitted between 15°C to 30°C (59°F to 86°F). Brief exposure up to 40°C (104°F) may be tolerated provided the mean temperature does not exceed 25°C (77°F); minimize this type of exposure. Protect from moisture.

Mechanism of Action Lomitapide directly binds to and inhibits microsomal triglyceride transfer protein (MTP) which is located in the lumen of the endoplasmic reticulum. MTP inhibition prevents the assembly of apo-B containing lipoproteins in enterocytes and hepatocytes resulting in reduced production of chylomicrons and VLDL and subsequently reduces plasma LDL-C concentrations.

Pharmacodynamics/Kinetics

Distribution: Mean V_d: 985-1292 L

Protein binding: 99.8% to plasma proteins

Metabolism: Primarily hepatic (extensive) through CYP3A4 to M1 and M3 (major [inactive *in vitro*] metabolites); CYP1A2, CYP2B6, CYP2C8, and CYP2C19 are also involved in metabolism to a minor degree.

Bioavailability: ~7%

Half-life elimination: 39.7 hours

Time to peak: ~6 hours

Excretion: Urine (53% to 60%; major component: M1 metabolite); feces (33% to 35%; major component: parent drug)

Dosage Homozygous familial hypercholesterolemia (HoFH):

Note: Transaminases should be measured prior to initiation and any dose increase. Maintenance dose should be individualized, taking into account patient characteristics such as goal of therapy and response to treatment. To reduce development of fat-soluble nutrient deficiency, administer daily supplements containing vitamin E 400 units, linoleic acid ≥200 mg, alpha-linolenic acid (ALA) ≥210 mg, eicosapentaenoic acid (EPA) ≥110 mg, and docosahexaenoic acid (DHA) ≥80 mg. Initiate and maintain a low-fat diet supplying <20% of energy from fat.

Adults: Oral: Initial: 5 mg once daily; after 2 weeks of therapy, may increase dose to 10 mg once daily, as tolerated; *then at 4-week intervals,* the dose may be increased to 20 mg once daily, *then* to 40 mg once daily, *and finally* to a maximum dose of 60 mg once daily.

Dosage adjustment for lomitapide with ***weak*** *CYP3A inhibitors (eg, amiodarone, amlodipine, atorvastatin, cyclosporine, fluoxetine, oral contraceptives):* Maximum dose: 30 mg once daily

Dosage adjustment for toxicity: *Hepatotoxicity:* **Note:** If patient experiences clinical symptoms of liver injury (eg, nausea, vomiting, abdominal pain, fever, jaundice, lethargy, flu-like symptoms) with transaminase elevation, increases in bilirubin ≥2 times ULN, or active liver disease, discontinue use and investigate for probable cause.

AST or ALT ≥3 to <5 times ULN: Confirm measurement (within 1 week); once confirmed, reduce dose and obtain additional liver function tests (LFTs) (eg, alkaline phosphatase, total bilirubin, and INR); repeat tests weekly and withhold subsequent doses if signs of abnormal liver function (eg, increased bilirubin or INR), if transaminases rise to >5 times ULN, or if they do not fall to <3 times ULN within ~4 weeks; investigate for probable cause. If resuming after transaminase resolution to <3 times ULN, consider reducing dose and monitor LFTs more frequently.

AST or ALT ≥5 times ULN: Withhold doses, obtain additional LFTs (eg, alkaline phosphatase, total bilirubin, and INR); investigate for probable cause. If resuming after transaminase resolution to <3 times ULN, reduce dose and monitor LFTs more frequently.

Dosage adjustment for renal impairment:

Mild-to-severe impairment (not receiving dialysis): No dosage adjustment provided in manufacturer's labeling (has not been studied); however, it is possible that patients with renal impairment not receiving dialysis may experience increases in lomitapide exposure exceeding 50%.

End stage renal disease (ESRD; receiving dialysis): Maximum dose: 40 mg once daily

Dosage adjustment for hepatic impairment:

Mild impairment (Child-Pugh class A): Maximum dose: 40 mg once daily

Moderate-to-severe impairment (Child-Pugh class B or C), active liver disease (including unexplained persistent transaminase elevations): Use is contraindicated.

Administration Oral: Administer with a glass of water and without food; administer at least 2 hours after the evening meal since administration with food may increase risk of gastrointestinal adverse effects. Swallow capsules whole (do not open, crush, dissolve, or chew).

Monitoring Parameters Baseline: ALT, AST, alkaline phosphatase, total bilirubin; pregnancy test in females of reproductive potential; measure transaminases prior to any increase in dose or monthly (whichever occurs first) during the first year, and then at least every 3 months and prior to dosage increases (also see dosage adjustment for toxicity in Dosage)

Dosage Forms Excipient information presented when available (limited, particularly for generics); consult specific product labeling.

Capsule, Oral:

Juxtapid: 5 mg, 10 mg, 20 mg

◆ Lomitapide Mesylate *see* Lomitapide *on page 1232*

◆ Lomotil® *see* Diphenoxylate and Atropine *on page 625*

Lomustine (loe MUS teen)

Brand Names: U.S. CeeNU

Brand Names: Canada CeeNU

Index Terms CCNU; Lomustinum

Pharmacologic Category Antineoplastic Agent; Antineoplastic Agent, Alkylating Agent; Antineoplastic Agent, Alkylating Agent (Nitrosourea)

Use Treatment of primary and metastatic brain tumors (after surgery and/or radiation therapy); treatment of relapsed or refractory Hodgkin's disease (as part of a combination chemotherapy regimen)

Unlabeled Use Treatment of gastric cancer, metastatic melanoma

Pregnancy Risk Factor D

Pregnancy Considerations Teratogenic effects and embryotoxicity have been observed in animal studies. There are no adequate and well-controlled studies in pregnant women. May cause fetal harm when administered to a pregnant woman. Women of childbearing potential should be advised to avoid pregnancy and should be advised of the potential harm to the fetus.

Breast-Feeding Considerations Due to the potential for serious adverse reactions in the nursing infant, breast-feeding is not recommended.

Contraindications Hypersensitivity to lomustine or any component of the formulation

Warnings/Precautions Hazardous agent - use appropriate precautions for handling and disposal (NIOSH, 2012). **[U.S. Boxed Warnings]: Cumulative and delayed bone marrow suppression, particularly thrombocytopenia and leukopenia, commonly occur; may lead to bleeding and overwhelming infections in an already compromised patient.** Do not administer courses more frequently than every 6 weeks due to delayed myelotoxicity. Use with caution in patients with depressed platelet, leukocyte, or erythrocyte counts. Because bone marrow toxicity is cumulative, dose adjustments should be based on nadir counts from prior dose.

May cause delayed pulmonary toxicity (infiltrates and/or fibrosis); usually related to cumulative doses >1100 mg/m^2; may be delayed (has been reported up to 17 years after childhood administration in combination with radiation therapy); patients with baseline below 70% of predicted forced vital capacity or carbon monoxide diffusing capacity are in increased risk. Long-term use may be associated with the development of secondary malignancies. Reversible hepatotoxicity (transaminase, alkaline phosphatase and bilirubin elevations) has been reported; use with caution in patients with hepatic impairment. Kidney damage has been observed and azotemia, decreased kidney size and renal failure have been reported with long-term use; use with caution in patients with renal impairment; may require dosage adjustment. **[U.S. Boxed Warning]: Should be administered under the supervision of an experienced cancer chemotherapy physician.** Lomustine should only be administered as a single dose once every 6 weeks; serious errors have occurred when lomustine was inadvertently administered daily.

Adverse Reactions

>10%:

Gastrointestinal: Nausea and vomiting, (onset: 3-6 hours after oral administration; duration: <24 hours)

Hematologic: Myelosuppression (dose-limiting, delayed, cumulative); leukopenia (65%; nadir: 5-6 weeks; recovery 6-8 weeks); thrombocytopenia (nadir: 4 weeks; recovery 5-6 weeks)

Frequency not defined: Acute leukemia, alkaline phosphatase increased, alopecia, anemia, ataxia, azotemia (progressive), bilirubin increased, blindness, bone marrow dysplasia, disorientation, dysarthria, hepatotoxicity, kidney size decreased, lethargy, optic atrophy, pulmonary fibrosis, pulmonary infiltrates, renal damage, renal failure, stomatitis, transaminases increased, visual disturbances

Drug Interactions

Metabolism/Transport Effects Substrate of CYP2D6 (minor); **Note:** Assignment of Major/Minor substrate status based on clinically relevant drug interaction potential; **Inhibits** CYP2D6 (weak), CYP3A4 (weak)

Avoid Concomitant Use

Avoid concomitant use of Lomustine with any of the following: BCG; CloZAPine; Natalizumab; Pimecrolimus; Pimozide; Tacrolimus (Topical); Tofacitinib; Vaccines (Live)

Increased Effect/Toxicity

Lomustine may increase the levels/effects of: ARIPiprazole; CloZAPine; Dofetilide; Leflunomide; Lomitapide; Natalizumab; Pimozide; Tofacitinib; Vaccines (Live)

The levels/effects of Lomustine may be increased by: Denosumab; Pimecrolimus; Roflumilast; Tacrolimus (Topical); Trastuzumab

Decreased Effect

Lomustine may decrease the levels/effects of: BCG; Coccidioidin Skin Test; Sipuleucel-T; Vaccines (Inactivated); Vaccines (Live)

The levels/effects of Lomustine may be decreased by: Echinacea; Peginterferon Alfa-2b

Ethanol/Nutrition/Herb Interactions Ethanol: Avoid ethanol (due to GI irritation).

Storage/Stability Store at room temperature of 25°C (77°F); excursions permitted to 15°C to 30°C (59°F to 86°F).

Mechanism of Action Inhibits DNA and RNA synthesis via carbamylation of DNA polymerase, alkylation of DNA, and alteration of RNA, proteins, and enzymes

Pharmacodynamics/Kinetics

Duration: Marrow recovery: ~5-8 weeks

Absorption: Complete

Distribution: Crosses blood-brain barrier to a greater degree than BCNU; CNS concentrations are ≥50% of plasma concentrations

Metabolism: Rapidly hepatic via hydroxylation producing at least two active metabolites; enterohepatically recycled

Half-life elimination: Parent drug: 16-24 hours; Active metabolite: 16-48 hours

Time to peak, serum: Active metabolite: ~3 hours

Excretion: Urine (~50%, as metabolites); feces (<5%); expired air (<10%)

Dosage Note: Repeat courses should only be administered after adequate recovery of leukocytes to >4000/mm^3 and platelets to >100,000/mm^3. Details concerning dosage in combination regimens should also be consulted. Oral: Children and Adults: Brain tumors, Hodgkin's lymphoma: 130 mg/m^2 as a single dose once every 6 weeks (dosage reductions may be recommended for combination chemotherapy regimens)

Compromised marrow function: Reduce dose to 100 mg/m^2 as a single dose once every 6 weeks

Dosing adjustment (based on nadir) for subsequent cycles:

Leukocytes >3000/mm^3, platelets >75,000/mm^3: No adjustment required

Leukocytes 2000-2999/mm^3, platelets 25,000-74,999/mm^3: Administer 70% of prior dose

Leukocytes <2000/mm^3, platelets <25,000/mm^3: Administer 50% of prior dose

Dosage adjustment in renal impairment: No dosage adjustment provided in manufacturer's labeling. The following adjustments have been recommended:

Aronoff, 2007: Adults:

Cl_{cr} 10-50 mL/minute: Administer 75% of dose

Cl_{cr} <10 mL/minute: Administer 25% to 50% of dose

Hemodialysis: Supplemental dose is not necessary

Continuous ambulatory peritoneal dialysis (CAPD): Administer 25% to 50% of dose

Kintzel, 1995:

Cl_{cr} 46-60 mL/minute: Administer 75% of normal dose

Cl_{cr} 31-45 mL/minute: Administer 70% of normal dose

Cl_{cr} ≤30 mL/minute: Avoid use

Dosage adjustment in hepatic impairment: No dosage adjustment provided in manufacturer's labeling. However, lomustine is hepatically metabolized and caution should be used in patients with hepatic dysfunction.

Dosing in obesity: *ASCO Guidelines for appropriate chemotherapy dosing in obese adults with cancer:* Utilize patient's actual body weight (full weight) for calculation of body surface area- or weight-based dosing, particularly when the intent of therapy is curative; manage regimen-related toxicities in the same manner as for nonobese patients; if a dose reduction is utilized due to toxicity, consider resumption of full weight-based dosing with subsequent cycles, especially if cause of toxicity (eg, hepatic or renal impairment) is resolved (Griggs, 2012).

Dietary Considerations Should be taken with fluids on an empty stomach; no food or drink for 2 hours after administration to decrease nausea.

Administration Oral: Administer with fluids on an empty stomach; no food or drink for 2 hours after administration. Administering on an empty stomach will reduce the incidence of nausea and vomiting. Standard antiemetics may be administered if needed. Varying strengths of capsules may be required to obtain necessary dose.

Do not break capsules; use appropriate precautions (eg, gloves) when handling; avoid exposure to broken capsules.

Hazardous agent; use appropriate precautions for handling and disposal (NIOSH, 2012).

Monitoring Parameters CBC with differential and platelet count (for at least 6 weeks after dose), hepatic and renal function tests (periodic), pulmonary function tests (baseline and periodic)

Dosage Forms Excipient information presented when available (limited, particularly for generics); consult specific product labeling.

Capsule, Oral:

CeeNU: 10 mg, 40 mg, 100 mg

Generic: 10 mg, 40 mg, 100 mg

◆ **Lomustinum** *see* Lomustine *on page* 1234

◆ **Longastatin** *see* Octreotide *on page* 1485

◆ **Loniten® (Can)** *see* Minoxidil (Systemic) *on page* 1375

◆ **Lo Ovral** *see* Ethinyl Estradiol and Norgestrel *on page* 797

◆ **Loperacap (Can)** *see* Loperamide *on page* 1235

Loperamide (loe PER a mide)

Brand Names: U.S. Anti-Diarrheal [OTC]; Diamode [OTC]; Imodium A-D [OTC]; Loperamide A-D [OTC]

Brand Names: Canada Apo-Loperamide®; Diarr-Eze; Dom-Loperamide; Imodium®; Loperacap; Novo-Loperamide; PMS-Loperamine; Rhoxal-loperamide; Rho®-Loperamine; Riva-Loperamide; Sandoz-Loperamide

Index Terms Loperamide Hydrochloride

Pharmacologic Category Antidiarrheal

Use Control and symptomatic relief of chronic diarrhea associated with inflammatory bowel disease and of acute nonspecific diarrhea; to reduce volume of ileostomy discharge

OTC labeling: Control of symptoms of diarrhea, including Traveler's diarrhea

Unlabeled Use Cancer treatment-induced diarrhea (eg, irinotecan induced); chronic diarrhea caused by bowel resection

Pregnancy Risk Factor C

Pregnancy Considerations Teratogenic effects were not observed in animal reproduction studies. Information related to loperamide use in pregnancy is limited and data is conflicting (Einarson, 2000; Källén, 2008). For acute diarrhea in pregnant women, some clinicians recommend oral rehydration and dietary changes; loperamide in small amounts may be used only if symptoms are disabling (Wald, 2003).

Breast-Feeding Considerations Small amounts of loperamide are excreted in human breast milk (information is based on studies using loperamide oxide, the prodrug of loperamide [Nikodem, 1992]). The manufacturer does not recommend use in nursing women.

Contraindications Hypersensitivity to loperamide or any component of the formulation; abdominal pain without diarrhea; children <2 years of age

Avoid use as primary therapy in patients with acute dysentery (bloody stools and high fever), acute ulcerative colitis, bacterial enterocolitis (caused by *Salmonella*, *Shigella*, and *Campylobacter*), pseudomembranous colitis associated with broad-spectrum antibiotic use

Warnings/Precautions Loperamide is a symptom-directed treatment; if an underlying diagnosis is made, other disease-specific treatment may be indicated. Rare cases of anaphylaxis and anaphylactic shock have been reported. Use is contraindicated if diarrhea is accompanied by high fever or blood in stool. Use caution in young children as response may be variable because of dehydration; contraindicated in children <2 years of age. Concurrent fluid and electrolyte replacement is often necessary in all age groups depending upon severity of diarrhea. Should not be used when inhibition of peristalsis is undesirable or dangerous. Discontinue promptly if constipation, abdominal pain, abdominal distension, blood in stool, or ileus develop. Do not use when peristalsis inhibition should be avoided due to potential for ileus, megacolon, and/or toxic megacolon. Stop therapy in AIDS patients at the first sign of abdominal distention; cases of toxic megacolon have occurred in AIDS patients with infectious colitis (due to viral or bacterial pathogens). Use caution in patients with hepatic impairment due to reduced first-pass metabolism; monitor for signs of CNS toxicity. May cause drowsiness or dizziness, which may impair physical or mental abilities; patients must be cautioned about performing tasks which require mental alertness (eg, operating machinery or driving). Discontinue use and consult healthcare provider if diarrhea lasts longer than 2 days, symptoms worsen, or abdominal swelling or bulging develops.

Adverse Reactions 1% to 10%:

Central nervous system: Dizziness (1%)

Gastrointestinal: Constipation (2% to 5%), abdominal cramping (≤3%), nausea (≤3%)

Postmarketing and/or case reports: Abdominal distention, abdominal pain, allergic reactions, anaphylactic shock, anaphylactoid reactions, angioedema, bullous eruption (rare), drowsiness, dyspepsia, erythema multiforme (rare), fatigue, flatulence, hypersensitivity, paralytic ileus, megacolon, pruritus, rash, Stevens-Johnson syndrome (rare), toxic epidermal necrolysis (rare), toxic megacolon, urinary retention, urticaria, vomiting, xerostomia

Drug Interactions

Metabolism/Transport Effects **Substrate** of P-glycoprotein

Avoid Concomitant Use There are no known interactions where it is recommended to avoid concomitant use.

Increased Effect/Toxicity

The levels/effects of Loperamide may be increased by: P-glycoprotein/ABCB1 Inhibitors

Decreased Effect

The levels/effects of Loperamide may be decreased by: P-glycoprotein/ABCB1 Inducers

Storage/Stability Store at 20°C to 25°C (68°F to 77°F).

Mechanism of Action Acts directly on circular and longitudinal intestinal muscles, through the opioid receptor, to inhibit peristalsis and prolong transit time; reduces fecal volume, increases viscosity, and diminishes fluid and electrolyte loss; demonstrates antisecretory activity. Loperamide increases tone on the anal sphincter

Pharmacodynamics/Kinetics

Absorption: Poor

Distribution: Poor penetration into brain

Metabolism: Hepatic via oxidative N-demethylation

Half-life elimination: 9-14 hours

Time to peak, plasma: Liquid: 2.5 hours; Capsule: 5 hours

Dosage Oral:

Children:

Acute diarrhea: Initial doses (in first 24 hours):

2-5 years (13-20 kg): 1 mg 3 times/day

6-8 years (20-30 kg): 2 mg twice daily

8-12 years (>30 kg): 2 mg 3 times/day

Maintenance: After initial dosing, 0.1 mg/kg doses after each loose stool, daily dose should not exceed the recommended dose for the initial 24 hours

Traveler's diarrhea:

6-8 years: 2 mg after first loose stool, followed by 1 mg after each subsequent stool (maximum dose: 4 mg/day)

9-11 years: 2 mg after first loose stool, followed by 1 mg after each subsequent stool (maximum dose: 6 mg/day)

≥12 years: Refer to adult dosing.

Adults:

Acute diarrhea: Initial: 4 mg, followed by 2 mg after each loose stool, up to 16 mg/day

Chronic diarrhea: Initial: Follow acute diarrhea; maintenance dose should be slowly titrated downward to minimum required to control symptoms (typically, 4-8 mg/day as a single dose or in divided doses)

Traveler's diarrhea: Initial: 4 mg after first loose stool, followed by 2 mg after each subsequent stool (maximum dose: 8 mg/day)

Cancer treatment-induced diarrhea (unlabeled use): 4 mg followed by 2 mg every 4 hours or after each unformed stool; Maximum 16 mg/day (Benson, 2004) **or** 4 mg followed by 2 mg every 2 hours (4 mg every 4 hours at night) until 12 hours have passed without a loose bowel movement (Sharma, 2005)

Irinotecan-induced delayed diarrhea (unlabeled use): 4 mg after first loose or frequent bowel movement, then 2 mg every 2 hours (4 mg every 4 hours at night) until 12 hours have passed without a bowel movement (Rothenberg, 1996)

Dosage adjustment in renal impairment: No dosage adjustment necessary.

Dosage adjustment in hepatic impairment: No dosage adjustment provided in manufacturer's labeling; use with caution.

Dietary Considerations Some products may contain sodium.

Dosage Forms Excipient information presented when available (limited, particularly for generics); consult specific product labeling.

Capsule, Oral, as hydrochloride:

Generic: 2 mg

Liquid, Oral, as hydrochloride:

Imodium A-D: 1 mg/7.5 mL (120 mL, 240 mL) [contains brilliant blue fcf (fd&c blue #1), fd&c yellow #10 (quinoline yellow), propylene glycol, sodium benzoate]

Imodium A-D: 1 mg/7.5 mL (30 mL, 120 mL, 240 mL, 360 mL) [contains brilliant blue fcf (fd&c blue #1), fd&c yellow #10 (quinoline yellow), propylene glycol, sodium benzoate; mint flavor]

Generic: 1 mg/5 mL (5 mL, 10 mL, 118 mL)

Suspension, Oral, as hydrochloride:

Generic: 1 mg/7.5 mL (120 mL)

Tablet, Oral, as hydrochloride:

Anti-Diarrheal: 2 mg

Anti-Diarrheal: 2 mg [scored]

Anti-Diarrheal: 2 mg [contains brilliant blue fcf (fd&c blue #1), fd&c yellow #10 (quinoline yellow)]

Anti-Diarrheal: 2 mg [scored; contains brilliant blue fcf (fd&c blue #1), fd&c yellow #10 (quinoline yellow)]

Anti-Diarrheal: 2 mg [contains fd&c blue #1 aluminum lake, fd&c yellow #10 (quinoline yellow)]

Diamode: 2 mg [scored]

Imodium A-D: 2 mg [scored; contains brilliant blue fcf (fd&c blue #1), fd&c yellow #10 (quinoline yellow)]
Imodium A-D: 2 mg [scored; contains fd&c blue #1 aluminum lake, fd&c yellow #10 aluminum lake]
Loperamide A-D: 2 mg
Tablet Chewable, Oral, as hydrochloride:
Imodium A-D: 2 mg [contains fd&c blue #1 aluminum lake, fd&c yellow #10 aluminum lake; cool mint flavor]

◆ **Loperamide A-D [OTC]** *see* Loperamide *on page 1235*

Loperamide and Simethicone

(loe PER a mide & sye METH i kone)

Brand Names: U.S. Imodium® Multi-Symptom Relief [OTC]

Brand Names: Canada Imodium® Advanced Multi-Symptom

Index Terms Simethicone and Loperamide Hydrochloride

Pharmacologic Category Antidiarrheal; Antiflatulent

Use Control of symptoms of diarrhea and gas (bloating, pressure, and cramps)

Dosage Oral: Acute diarrhea (weight-based dosing is preferred):

Children:

6-8 years (48-59 lbs): 1 caplet or tablet after first loose stool, followed by 1/2 caplet/tablet with each subsequent loose stool (maximum: 2 caplets or tablets/24 hours)

9-11 years (60-95 lbs): 1 caplet or tablet after first loose stool, followed by 1/2 caplet or tablet with each subsequent loose stool (maximum: 3 caplets or tablets/24 hours)

Children >12 years and Adults: One caplet or tablet after first loose stool, followed by 1 caplet or tablet with each subsequent loose stool (maximum: 4 caplets or tablets/ 24 hours)

Additional Information Complete prescribing information should be consulted for additional detail.

Dosage Forms Excipient information presented when available (limited, particularly for generics); consult specific product labeling.

Caplet:

Imodium® Multi-Symptom Relief: Loperamide hydrochloride 2 mg and simethicone 125 mg [contains calcium 65 mg/caplet, sodium 4 mg/caplet]

Tablet, chewable:

Imodium® Multi-Symptom Relief: Loperamide hydrochloride 2 mg and simethicone 125 mg [contains calcium 50 mg/tablet; mint flavor]

◆ **Loperamide Hydrochloride** *see* Loperamide *on page 1235*

◆ **Lopid** *see* Gemfibrozil *on page 947*

Lopinavir and Ritonavir

(loe PIN a veer & rit ON uh veer)

Brand Names: U.S. Kaletra®

Brand Names: Canada Kaletra®

Index Terms Ritonavir and Lopinavir

Pharmacologic Category Antiretroviral, Protease Inhibitor (Anti-HIV)

Use Treatment of HIV infection in combination with other antiretroviral agents

Pregnancy Risk Factor C

Pregnancy Considerations Adverse events were not seen in animal reproduction studies, except at doses which were also maternally toxic. Lopinavir/ritonavir crosses the placenta; however, based on information collected by the Antiretroviral Pregnancy Registry, an increased risk of teratogenic effects has not been observed in humans. The DHHS Perinatal HIV Guidelines consider lopinavir/ritonavir to be the preferred protease inhibitor for use in antiretroviral-naive pregnant women. Due to a decrease in bioavailability, a dose increase is suggested during the second and third trimesters of pregnancy, especially in PI-experienced women. Monitor virologic response (and lopinavir serum concentrations if available) if the standard dose is used. Once-daily dosing is not recommended during pregnancy. A small increased risk of preterm birth has been associated with maternal use of protease inhibitor-based combination antiretroviral (ARV) therapy during pregnancy; however, the benefits of use generally outweigh this risk and protease inhibitors (PIs) should not be withheld if otherwise recommended. Hyperglycemia, new onset of diabetes mellitus, or diabetic ketoacidosis have been reported with PIs; it is not clear if pregnancy increases this risk.

Regardless of CD4 count or HIV RNA copy number, all HIV-infected pregnant women should receive a combination antepartum ARV drug regimen; this includes women who require therapy for their own health, as well as women who do not yet require therapy for their own health. ARV therapy should be started as soon as possible if required for the woman's health. Although earlier initiation may be more effective in reducing the perinatal transmission of HIV, also consider maternal conditions (eg, nausea and vomiting) and the potential risks of first trimester fetal exposure for specific agents. Plasma HIV RNA levels should be assessed at ~34-36 weeks gestation in order to help determine mode of delivery. If ARV therapy must be interrupted for <24 hours during the peripartum period, stop then restart all medications simultaneously in order to decrease the chance of developing resistance. Long-term follow-up is recommended for all infants exposed to ARV medications.

Healthcare providers are encouraged to enroll pregnant women exposed to antiretroviral medications in the Antiretroviral Pregnancy Registry (1-800-258-4263 or www.-APRegistry.com). Healthcare providers caring for HIV-infected women and their infants may contact the National Perinatal HIV Hotline (888-448-8765) for clinical consultation (DHHS [perinatal], 2012).

Breast-Feeding Considerations It is not known if lopinavir or ritonavir is excreted in breast milk. Maternal or infant antiretroviral therapy does not completely eliminate the risk of postnatal HIV transmission. In addition, multiclass-resistant virus has been detected in breast-feeding infants despite maternal therapy. Therefore, in the United States, where formula is accessible, affordable, safe, and sustainable, and the risk of infant mortality due to diarrhea and respiratory infections is low, complete avoidance of breast-feeding by HIV-infected women is recommended to decrease potential transmission of HIV (DHHS [perinatal], 2012).

Medication Guide Available Yes

Contraindications Hypersensitivity (eg, toxic epidermal necrolysis, Stevens-Johnson syndrome, erythema multiforme, urticaria, angioedema) to any of the ingredients, including ritonavir; coadministration with drugs that are highly dependent on CYP3A for clearance and for which elevated plasma concentrations are associated with serious and/or life-threatening reactions; coadministration with the potent CYP3A inducers (where significantly decreased lopinavir levels may be associated with a potential for loss of virologic response and resistance and cross-resistance to develop): Alfuzosin, cisapride, ergot derivatives (eg, dihydroergotamine, ergotamine, methylergonovine), lovastatin, oral midazolam, pimozide, rifampin, sildenafil (when used to treat pulmonary arterial hypertension), simvastatin, St John's wort, and triazolam.

Warnings/Precautions Potentially significant interactions may exist, requiring dose or frequency adjustment, additional monitoring, and/or selection of alternative therapy. Cases of pancreatitis, some fatal, have been associated with lopinavir/ritonavir; use caution in patients with a history of pancreatitis or advanced HIV-1 disease (may be at increased risk). Patients with signs or symptoms of pancreatitis should be evaluated and therapy suspended as clinically appropriate. May alter cardiac conduction and prolong the QT_c and/or PR interval; second and third degree AV block and torsade de pointes have been observed. Possible higher risk of myocardial infarction associated with the cumulative use of lopinavir/ritonavir. Use with caution in patients with underlying structural heart disease, pre-existing conduction system abnormalities, ischemic heart disease or cardiomyopathies. Avoid use in combination with QT_c- or PR-interval prolonging drugs or in patients with hypokalemia or congenital long QT syndrome.

Changes in glucose tolerance, hyperglycemia, exacerbation of diabetes, DKA, and new-onset diabetes mellitus have been reported in patients receiving protease inhibitors. May cause hepatitis or exacerbate pre-existing hepatic dysfunction; use with caution in patients with hepatitis B or C and in hepatic disease; patients with hepatitis or elevations in transaminases prior to the start of therapy may be at increased risk for further increases in transaminases or hepatic dysfunction (rare fatalities reported postmarketing). Consider more frequent liver function test monitoring during therapy initiation in patients with preexisting hepatic dysfunction. Large increases in total cholesterol and triglycerides have been reported; screening should be done prior to therapy and periodically throughout treatment. Increased bleeding may be seen in patients with hemophilia A or B who are taking protease inhibitors. Redistribution or accumulation of body fat has been observed in patients using antiretroviral therapy. Patients may develop immune reconstitution syndrome resulting in the occurrence of an inflammatory response to an indolent or residual opportunistic infection during initial HIV treatment or activation of autoimmune disorders (eg, Graves' disease, polymyositis, Guillain-Barré syndrome) later in therapy; further evaluation and treatment may be required.

The oral solution is highly concentrated and contains large amounts of alcohol. Healthcare providers should pay special attention to accurate calculation, measurement, and administration of dose. Overdose in a child may lead to lethal ethanol or propylene glycol toxicity. Once-daily dosing is not recommended in patients with ≥3 lopinavir-resistance-associated substitutions; those receiving efavirenz, nevirapine, or nelfinavir, carbamazepine, phenobarbital, phenytoin, or in children <18 years of age. Safety, efficacy, and pharmacokinetic profiles of lopinavir and ritonavir have not been established for neonates <14 days of age. Neonates <14 days of age, particularly preterm neonates, are at risk for developing propylene glycol toxicity with use of the lopinavir/ritonavir oral solution. Oral solution contains ethanol and propylene glycol; ethanol competitively inhibits propylene glycol metabolism. Postmarketing reports in preterm neonates following use of the oral solution include cardiotoxicity (complete AV block, bradycardia, cardiomyopathy), lactic acidosis, CNS depression, respiratory complications, acute renal failure, and death. The oral solution should not be used in the immediate postnatal period, including full term neonates age <14 days or preterm neonates until 14 days after their due date, unless the infant is closely monitored and benefits clearly outweigh risk.

Adverse Reactions Data presented for short- and long-term combination antiretroviral therapy in both protease inhibitor experienced and naïve patients.

>10%:

Dermatologic: Rash (children 12%; adults ≤5%)

Endocrine & metabolic: Hypercholesterolemia (3% to 39%), triglycerides increased (3% to 36%)

Gastrointestinal: Diarrhea (7% to 28%; greater with once-daily dosing), abnormal taste/taste perversion (children 22%; adults <2%), vomiting (children 21%; adults 2% to 6%), nausea (5% to 16%), abdominal pain (1% to 11%)

Hepatic: GGT increased (10% to 29%), ALT increased (grade 3/4: 1% to 11%)

>2% to 10%:

Cardiovascular: Vasodilation (≤3%)

Central nervous system: Headache (2% to 6%), insomnia (≤3%)

Endocrine & metabolic: Hyperglycemia (≤5%), hyperuricemia (≤5%), sodium decreased or increased (children 3%),

Gastrointestinal: Amylase increased (3% to 8%), dyspepsia (≤6%), lipase increased (3% to 5%), flatulence (1% to 4%), weight loss (≤3%)

Hematologic: Platelets decreased (grade 3/4: 4% children), neutropenia (grade 3/4: 1% to 5%)

Hepatic: AST increased (grade 3/4: 2% to 10%), bilirubin increased (children 3%; adults 1%)

Neuromuscular & skeletal: Weakness (≤9%)

≤2% (Limited to important or life-threatening): Abdominal distension, abnormal dreams, abnormal ejaculation, abnormal thinking, abnormal vision, acne, agitation, allergic reaction, alopecia, amnesia, anemia, anorexia, anxiety, apathy, appetite increased/decreased, arthralgia, asthma, ataxia, atrial fibrillation, atrioventricular block, AV block (second and third degree), avitaminosis, back pain, bacterial infection, benign neoplasm, body fat redistribution, bone necrosis, bradyarrhythmia, breast enlargement, bronchitis, cellulitis, cerebral infarction, chest pain, chills, cholangitis, cholecystitis, confusion, constipation, cough, creatinine clearance decreased, Cushing's syndrome, cyst, deep vein thrombosis, dehydration, depression, diabetes mellitus, dizziness, dry skin, dyskinesia, dysphagia, dyspnea, eczema, edema, emotional lability, encephalopathy, enteritis, enterocolitis, eructation, erythema multiforme, esophagitis, exfoliative dermatitis, extrapyramidal symptoms, facial edema, facial paralysis, fatigue, fatty deposits, fecal incontinence, fever, flu-like syndrome, folliculitis, furunculosis, gastritis, gastroenteritis, GERD, glucose intolerance, gynecomastia, hemorrhagic colitis, hemorrhoids, hepatic dysfunction, hepatitis, hepatomegaly, hyperacusis, hyperhidrosis, hypertension, hypertonia, hypertrophy, hypogonadism (males), hypothyroidism, immune reconstitution syndrome, impotence, inorganic phosphorus decreased, jaundice, lactic acidosis, leukopenia, libido decreased, liver tenderness, lung edema, lymphadenopathy, maculopapular rash, malaise, MI, migraine, mouth ulceration, myalgia, neoplasm, nephritis, nervousness, neuropathy, obesity, orthostatic hypotension, otitis media, palpitation, pancreatitis, paresthesia, periodontitis, peripheral edema, peripheral neuropathy, pharyngitis, propylene glycol toxicity (preterm neonates [includes cardiomyopathy, lactic acidosis, acute renal failure, respiratory complications]), PR prolongation, pruritus, QT prolongation, rhinitis, seborrhea, seizure, sialadenitis, sinusitis, skin discoloration, skin ulcer, somnolence, splenomegaly, Stevens-Johnson syndrome, stomatitis, striae, thrombophlebitis, tinnitus, torsade de pointes, tremor, vasculitis, vertigo, viral infection, weight gain, xerostomia

Drug Interactions

Metabolism/Transport Effects Refer to individual components.

Avoid Concomitant Use

Avoid concomitant use of Lopinavir and Ritonavir with any of the following: Ado-Trastuzumab Emtansine; Alfuzosin; Amiodarone; Apixaban; Atovaquone; Avanafil;

Axitinib; Bosutinib; Cabozantinib; Cisapride; Conivaptan; Crizotinib; Darunavir; Disulfiram; Dronedarone; Eplerenone; Ergot Derivatives; Etravirine; Everolimus; Flecainide; Fluticasone (Nasal); Fusidic Acid (Systemic); Halofantrine; Highest Risk QTc-Prolonging Agents; Ibrutinib; Imatinib; Ivabradine; Lapatinib; Lomitapide; Lovastatin; Lurasidone; Macitentan; Methadone; Midazolam; Mifepristone; Moderate Risk QTc-Prolonging Agents; Nilotinib; Nisoldipine; Pimozide; Pomalidomide; Propafenone; QuiNIDine; QuiNINE; Ranolazine; Red Yeast Rice; Regorafenib; Rifampin; Rivaroxaban; Salmeterol; Silodosin; Simeprevir; Simvastatin; St Johns Wort; Tamoxifen; Tamsulosin; Telaprevir; Thioridazine; Ticagrelor; Tolvaptan; Topotecan; Toremifene; Triazolam; Ulipristal; Vemurafenib; VinCRIStine (Liposomal); Voriconazole

Increased Effect/Toxicity

Lopinavir and Ritonavir may increase the levels/effects of: Ado-Trastuzumab Emtansine; Afatinib; Alfuzosin; Almotriptan; Alosetron; ALPRAZolam; Amiodarone; Apixaban; ARIPiprazole; AtoMOXetine; AtorvaSTATin; Avanafil; Axitinib; Bedaquiline; Bortezomib; Bosentan; Bosutinib; Brentuximab Vedotin; Brinzolamide; Budesonide (Nasal); Budesonide (Systemic, Oral Inhalation); Cabozantinib; Calcium Channel Blockers (Dihydropyridine); Calcium Channel Blockers (Nondihydropyridine); CarBAMazepine; Cisapride; Clarithromycin; Clorazepate; Colchicine; Conivaptan; Corticosteroids (Orally Inhaled); Crizotinib; CycloSPORINE (Systemic); CYP2C8 Substrates; CYP2D6 Substrates; CYP3A4 Substrates; Dabigatran Etexilate; Diazepam; Dienogest; Digoxin; Dofetilide; Dronabinol; Dronedarone; Dutasteride; Efavirenz; Enfuvirtide; Enzalutamide; Eplerenone; Ergot Derivatives; Estazolam; Everolimus; FentaNYL; Fesoterodine; Flecainide; Flurazepam; Fluticasone (Nasal); Fluticasone (Oral Inhalation); Fusidic Acid (Systemic); GuanFACINE; Halofantrine; Highest Risk QTc-Prolonging Agents; Ibrutinib; Iloperidone; Imatinib; Itraconazole; Ivabradine; Ivacaftor; Ixabepilone; Ketoconazole (Systemic); Lacosamide; Lapatinib; Levomilnacipran; Linagliptin; Lomitapide; Lovastatin; Lumefantrine; Lurasidone; Macitentan; Maraviroc; Meperidine; MethylPREDNISolone; Metoprolol; Midazolam; Mifepristone; Nebivolol; Nefazodone; Nelfinavir; Nilotinib; Nisoldipine; Ospemifene; OxyCODONE; Paricalcitol; PAZOPanib; P-glycoprotein/ABCB1 Substrates; Pimecrolimus; Pimozide; Pioglitazone; Pomalidomide; PONATinib; PrednisoLONE (Systemic); PredniSONE; Propafenone; Protease Inhibitors; Prucalopride; QUEtiapine; QuiNIDine; QuiNINE; Ranolazine; Red Yeast Rice; Regorafenib; Repaglinide; Rifabutin; Rilpivirine; Riociguat; Rivaroxaban; RomiDEPsin; Rosuvastatin; Ruxolitinib; Salmeterol; Saxagliptin; Sildenafil; Silodosin; Simeprevir; Simvastatin; SORAfenib; Tacrolimus (Systemic); Tacrolimus (Topical); Tadalafil; Tamsulosin; Telaprevir; Temsirolimus; Tenofovir; Tetrabenazine; Thioridazine; Ticagrelor; Tofacitinib; Tolterodine; Tolvaptan; Topotecan; Toremifene; TraZODone; Treprostinil; Triamcinolone (Systemic); Triazolam; Tricyclic Antidepressants; Ulipristal; Vardenafil; Vemurafenib; Vilazodone; VinBLAStine; VinCRIStine; VinCRIStine (Liposomal); Vortioxetine; Zuclopenthixol

The levels/effects of Lopinavir and Ritonavir may be increased by: ARIPiprazole; Clarithromycin; CycloSPORINE (Systemic); Delavirdine; Disulfiram; Efavirenz; Enfuvirtide; Etravirine; Fusidic Acid (Systemic); Ivabradine; Ketoconazole (Systemic); Methadone; MetroNIDAZOLE (Topical); Mifepristone; Moderate Risk QTc-Prolonging Agents; P-glycoprotein/ABCB1 Inhibitors; Posaconazole; QTc-Prolonging Agents (Indeterminate Risk and Risk Modifying); QuiNINE; Rifabutin; Rifampin; Simeprevir

Decreased Effect

Lopinavir and Ritonavir may decrease the levels/effects of: Abacavir; Atovaquone; Boceprevir; BuPROPion; Canagliflozin; Clarithromycin; Codeine; Contraceptives (Estrogens); CYP2C19 Substrates; Darunavir; Deferasirox; Delavirdine; Didanosine; Etravirine; Fosphenytoin; Ifosfamide; Iloperidone; LamoTRIgine; Meperidine; Methadone; Phenytoin; Prasugrel; Proguanil; QuiNINE; Tamoxifen; Telaprevir; Theophylline Derivatives; Ticagrelor; TraMADol; Valproic Acid and Derivatives; Voriconazole; Warfarin; Zidovudine

The levels/effects of Lopinavir and Ritonavir may be decreased by: Antacids; Boceprevir; Bosentan; CarBAMazepine; CYP3A4 Inducers (Strong); Dabrafenib; Efavirenz; Fosamprenavir; Fosphenytoin; Garlic; Mitotane; Nelfinavir; Nevirapine; Peginterferon Alfa-2b; P-glycoprotein/ABCB1 Inducers; PHENobarbital; Phenytoin; Rifampin; St Johns Wort; Tocilizumab

Ethanol/Nutrition/Herb Interactions

Food: Moderate- to high-fat meals increase the C_{max} and AUC of lopinavir/ritonavir oral solution; no significant changes observed with oral tablets. Management: Take oral solution with food; take tablet with or without food.

Herb/Nutraceutical: St John's wort may decrease levels of protease inhibitors and lead to possible resistance. Garlic may decrease the serum concentration of protease inhibitors. Management: Concurrent use of St John's wort is contraindicated. Avoid garlic.

Storage/Stability

Oral solution: Store at 2°C to 8°C (36°F to 46°F). Avoid exposure to excessive heat. If stored at room temperature (25°C or 77°F), use within 2 months.

Tablet: Store at USP controlled room temperature of 20°C to 25°C (68°F to 77°F). Exposure to high humidity outside of the original container for >2 weeks is not recommended.

Mechanism of Action A coformulation of lopinavir and ritonavir. The lopinavir component binds to the site of HIV-1 protease activity and inhibits the cleavage of viral Gag-Pol polyprotein precursors into individual functional proteins required for infectious HIV. This results in the formation of immature, noninfectious viral particles. The ritonavir component inhibits the CYP3A metabolism of lopinavir, allowing increased plasma levels of lopinavir.

Pharmacodynamics/Kinetics

Ritonavir: See Ritonavir monograph.

Lopinavir:

Protein binding: 98% to 99%; decreased with mild-to-moderate hepatic dysfunction

Metabolism: Hepatic via CYP3A4; 13 metabolites identified

Half-life elimination: 5-6 hours

Time to peak, plasma: ~4 hours

Excretion: Feces (83%, 20% as unchanged drug); urine (10%; <3% as unchanged drug)

Dosage Oral:

Children: Dosage based on weight or body surface area (BSA), **presented based on lopinavir component** (maximum dose: Lopinavir 400 mg/ritonavir 100 mg).

14 days to 6 months: 16 mg/kg or 300 mg/m² twice daily; **Note:** Should not be administered to neonates age <14 days (defined as postmenstrual age of 42 weeks [first day of mother's last menstrual period to birth plus postnatal age]) and a postnatal age of at least 14 days

6 months to 18 years: **Note:** FDA-approved dose is approximately equivalent to lopinavir 230 mg/m² per dose.

<15 kg: 12 mg/kg twice daily

15-40 kg: 10 mg/kg twice daily

>40 kg: Lopinavir 400 mg/ritonavir 100 mg twice daily

Adults:

Twice-daily dosing:

Therapy-naive or therapy-experienced: Lopinavir 400 mg/ritonavir 100 mg twice daily.

Therapy-naive or therapy-experienced patients receiving efavirenz, fosamprenavir, nelfinavir, nevirapine: Lopinavir 500 mg/ritonavir 125 mg tablets twice daily **or** lopinavir 533 mg/ritonavir 133 mg solution twice daily

Once-daily dosing: Therapy-naive or experienced patients with <3 lopinavir resistance-associated substitutions: Lopinavir 800 mg/ritonavir 200 mg once daily

Elderly: Initial studies did not include enough elderly patients to determine effects based on age. Use with caution due to possible decreased hepatic, renal, and cardiac function.

Dosage adjustment for combination therapy with efavirenz, fosamprenavir, nelfinavir, or nevirapine:

Twice-daily dosing:

Children 14 days to 6 months: Combination therapy with these agents is not recommended due to lack of data.

Children 6 months to 18 years: Solution or tablet (**based on mg of lopinavir component**): FDA-approved dose is approximately equivalent to lopinavir 300 mg/m^2 per dose:

<15 kg: 13 mg/kg twice daily (**Note:** Tablets are not recommended)

15-45 kg: 11 mg/kg twice daily

>45 kg: Refer to adult dosing

Children >45 kg and Adults: Therapy-naive and therapy-experienced patients:

Solution: Lopinavir 533 mg/ritonavir 133 mg (6.5 mL) twice daily

Tablet: Lopinavir 500 mg/ritonavir 125 mg twice daily

Once-daily dosing:

Children: Not recommended

Adults: Not recommended in those receiving efavirenz, fosamprenavir, nevirapine, nelfinavir, carbamazepine, phenobarbital, phenytoin.

Dosage adjustment in renal impairment: Has not been studied in patients with renal impairment; however, a decrease in clearance is not expected

Hemodialysis: Do not use once-daily dosing in hemodialysis patients (DHHS, 2013)

Dosage adjustment in hepatic impairment: Use caution in hepatic impairment (metabolized primarily by the liver)

Mild-to-moderate impairment: Lopinavir AUC may be increased ~30%

Severe impairment: No data available

Dietary Considerations Solution must be taken with food. Tablet may be taken with or without food

Administration

Solution: Must be administered with food; if using didanosine, take didanosine 1 hour before or 2 hours after lopinavir/ritonavir. Administer using calibrated dosing syringe.

Tablet: May be taken with or without food. Swallow whole, do not break, crush, or chew. May be taken with didanosine when taken without food. Tablets are not recommended in patients <15 kg.

Monitoring Parameters Triglycerides, cholesterol, LFTs, electrolytes, basic HIV monitoring, viral load and CD4 count, glucose

Dosage Forms Excipient information presented when available (limited, particularly for generics); consult specific product labeling.

Solution, oral:

Kaletra®: Lopinavir 80 mg and ritonavir 20 mg per 1 mL (160 mL) [contains ethanol 42.4%, menthol, propylene glycol; cotton candy flavor]]

Tablet:

Kaletra®:

Lopinavir 100 mg and ritonavir 25 mg

Lopinavir 200 mg and ritonavir 50 mg

◆ Lopresor® (Can) *see* Metoprolol *on page 1348*

◆ Lopresor SR® (Can) *see* Metoprolol *on page 1348*

◆ Lopressor *see* Metoprolol *on page 1348*

◆ Loprox *see* Ciclopirox *on page 423*

◆ Loradamed [OTC] *see* Loratadine *on page 1240*

Loratadine (lor AT a deen)

Brand Names: U.S. Alavert [OTC]; Allergy Relief For Kids [OTC]; Allergy Relief [OTC]; Allergy [OTC]; Childrens Loratadine [OTC]; Claritin Reditabs [OTC]; Claritin [OTC]; Loradamed [OTC]; Loratadine Childrens [OTC]; Loratadine Hives Relief [OTC]; Triaminic Allerchews [OTC]

Brand Names: Canada Apo-Loratadine®; Claritin®; Claritin® Kids

Index Terms Tavist ND

Pharmacologic Category Histamine H_1 Antagonist; Histamine H_1 Antagonist, Second Generation; Piperidine Derivative

Additional Appendix Information

Beers Criteria – Potentially Inappropriate Medications for Geriatrics *on page 2368*

Use Relief of nasal and non-nasal symptoms of seasonal allergic rhinitis; treatment of chronic idiopathic urticaria

Pregnancy Considerations Maternal use of loratadine has not been associated with an increased risk of major malformations. The use of antihistamines for the treatment of rhinitis during pregnancy is generally considered to be safe at recommended doses. Although safety data is limited, loratadine may be the preferred second generation antihistamine for the treatment of rhinitis or urticaria during pregnancy.

Breast-Feeding Considerations Small amounts of loratadine and its active metabolite, desloratadine, are excreted into breast milk.

Contraindications Hypersensitivity to loratadine or any component of the formulation

Warnings/Precautions Use with caution in patients with liver or renal impairment; dosage adjustment recommended. Some products may contain phenylalanine. May be inappropriate in older adults depending on comorbidities (eg, dementia, delirium) due to its potent anticholinergic effects (Beers Criteria).

Adverse Reactions

Central nervous system: Headache (12% adults), somnolence (8% adults), nervousness (4% ages 6-12 years), fatigue (4% adults; 3% ages 6-12 years, 2% to 3% ages 2-5 years), malaise (2% ages 6-12 years)

Dermatologic: Rash (2% to 3% ages 2-5 years)

Gastrointestinal: Xerostomia (3% adults), stomatitis (2% to 3% ages 2-5 years), abdominal pain (2% ages 6-12 years)

Neuromuscular & skeletal: Hyperkinesia (3% ages 6-12 years)

Ocular: Conjunctivitis (2% ages 6-12 years)

Respiratory: Wheezing (4% ages 6-12 years), epistaxis (2% to 3% ages 2-5 years), pharyngitis (2% to 3% ages 2-5 years), dysphonia (2% ages 6-12 years), upper respiratory infection (2% ages 6-12 years)

Miscellaneous: Flu-like syndrome (2% to 3% ages 2-5 years), viral infection (2% to 3% ages 2-5 years)

<2% (Limited to important or life-threatening): Abnormal hepatic function, agitation, alopecia, altered lacrimation, altered micturition, altered salivation, altered taste, amnesia, anaphylaxis, angioneurotic edema, anorexia, arthralgia, back pain, blepharospasm, blurred vision, breast

enlargement, breast pain, bronchospasm, chest pain, confusion, depression, dizziness, dysmenorrhea, dyspnea, erythema multiforme, hemoptysis, hepatic necrosis, hepatitis, hypotension, impaired concentration, impotence, insomnia, irritability, jaundice, menorrhagia, migraine, nausea, palpitation, paresthesia, paroniria, peripheral edema, photosensitivity, pruritus, purpura, rigors, seizure, supraventricular tachyarrhythmia, syncope, tachycardia, tremor, urinary discoloration, urticaria, thrombocytopenia, vaginitis, vertigo, vomiting, weight gain

Drug Interactions

Metabolism/Transport Effects **Substrate** of CYP2D6 (minor), CYP3A4 (minor), P-glycoprotein; **Note:** Assignment of Major/Minor substrate status based on clinically relevant drug interaction potential; **Inhibits** CYP2C19 (weak), CYP2C8 (weak), CYP2D6 (weak)

Avoid Concomitant Use

Avoid concomitant use of Loratadine with any of the following: Aclidinium; Azelastine (Nasal); Ipratropium (Oral Inhalation); Paraldehyde; Tiotropium; Umeclidinium

Increased Effect/Toxicity

Loratadine may increase the levels/effects of: Alcohol (Ethyl); Analgesics (Opioid); Anticholinergics; ARIPiprazole; Azelastine (Nasal); Buprenorphine; CNS Depressants; Hydrocodone; Methotrimeprazine; Metyrosine; Mirtazapine; Paraldehyde; Pramipexole; ROPINIRole; Rotigotine; Selective Serotonin Reuptake Inhibitors; Tiotropium; Zolpidem

The levels/effects of Loratadine may be increased by: Aclidinium; Amiodarone; Brimonidine (Topical); Doxylamine; Droperidol; HydrOXYzine; Ipratropium (Oral Inhalation); Magnesium Sulfate; Methotrimeprazine; Perampanel; P-glycoprotein/ABCB1 Inhibitors; Pramlintide; Sodium Oxybate; Tapentadol; Umeclidinium

Decreased Effect

Loratadine may decrease the levels/effects of: Acetylcholinesterase Inhibitors (Central); Benzylpenicilloyl Polylysine; Betahistine; Hyaluronidase

The levels/effects of Loratadine may be decreased by: Acetylcholinesterase Inhibitors (Central); Amphetamines; Peginterferon Alfa-2b; P-glycoprotein/ABCB1 Inducers

Ethanol/Nutrition/Herb Interactions

Ethanol: May increase CNS depression; monitor for increased effects with coadministration. Caution patients about effects.

Food: Increases bioavailability and delays peak.

Herb/Nutraceutical: St John's wort may decrease loratadine levels.

Storage/Stability Store at 2°C to 25°C (36°F to 77°F).

Rapidly-disintegrating tablets: Use within 6 months of opening foil pouch, and immediately after opening individual tablet blister. Store in a dry place.

Mechanism of Action Long-acting tricyclic antihistamine with selective peripheral histamine H_1-receptor antagonistic properties

Pharmacodynamics/Kinetics

Onset of action: 1-3 hours

Peak effect: 8-12 hours

Duration: >24 hours

Absorption: Rapid

Metabolism: Extensively hepatic via CYP2D6 and 3A4 to active metabolite

Half-life elimination: 12-15 hours

Excretion: Urine (40%) and feces (40%) as metabolites

Dosage Oral: Seasonal allergic rhinitis, chronic idiopathic urticaria:

Children 2-5 years: 5 mg once daily

Children ≥6 years and Adults: 10 mg once daily

Elderly: Peak plasma levels are increased; elimination half-life is slightly increased; specific dosing adjustments are not available

Dosage adjustment in renal impairment: Cl_{cr} ≤30 mL/minute:

Children 2-5 years: 5 mg every other day

Children ≥6 years and Adults: 10 mg every other day

Dosage adjustment in hepatic impairment: Elimination half-life increases with severity of disease

Children 2-5 years: 5 mg every other day

Children ≥6 years and Adults: 10 mg every other day

Dietary Considerations May be taken without regard to meals. Some products may contain phenylalanine and/or sodium.

Administration May be administered without regard to meals.

Test Interactions May suppress the wheal and flare reactions to skin test antigens

Dosage Forms Excipient information presented when available (limited, particularly for generics); consult specific product labeling.

Capsule, Oral:

Claritin: 10 mg [contains brilliant blue fcf (fd&c blue #1), polysorbate 80]

Solution, Oral:

Childrens Loratadine: 5 mg/5 mL (120 mL) [alcohol free, dye free, sugar free; contains propylene glycol, sodium benzoate; grape flavor]

Loratadine Childrens: 5 mg/5 mL (120 mL) [alcohol free, dye free, sugar free; contains propylene glycol, sodium benzoate; fruit flavor]

Loratadine Hives Relief: 5 mg/5 mL (120 mL) [alcohol free, dye free, sugar free; contains propylene glycol, sodium benzoate; grape flavor]

Syrup, Oral:

Allergy Relief: 5 mg/5 mL (236 mL) [alcohol free; contains propylene glycol, sodium benzoate]

Allergy Relief For Kids: 5 mg/5 mL (120 mL) [contains propylene glycol, sodium benzoate; fruit flavor]

Childrens Loratadine: 5 mg/5 mL (120 mL) [fruit flavor]

Childrens Loratadine: 5 mg/5 mL (120 mL) [alcohol free, dye free; contains propylene glycol, sodium benzoate, sodium metabisulfite; grape flavor]

Claritin: 5 mg/5 mL (60 mL, 120 mL) [alcohol free, color free, dye free, sugar free; contains edetate disodium, propylene glycol, sodium benzoate; grape flavor]

Loratadine Childrens: 5 mg/5 mL (120 mL) [sugar free; contains polyethylene glycol, propylene glycol, sodium benzoate, sodium metabisulfite; grape flavor]

Tablet, Oral:

Alavert: 10 mg

Allergy: 10 mg

Allergy Relief: 10 mg

Claritin: 10 mg

Loradamed: 10 mg

Generic: 10 mg

Tablet Chewable, Oral:

Claritin: 5 mg [contains aspartame, fd&c blue #2 aluminum lake; grape flavor]

Tablet Dispersible, Oral:

Alavert: 10 mg [contains aspartame]

Alavert: 10 mg [contains aspartame; bubble-gum flavor]

Alavert: 10 mg [contains aspartame; citrus flavor]

Allergy: 10 mg [contains aspartame]

Allergy Relief: 10 mg [contains aspartame]

Allergy Relief: 10 mg [contains aspartame; fruit flavor]

Claritin Reditabs: 5 mg, 10 mg

Triaminic Allerchews: 10 mg

◆ **Loratadine-D 12 Hour [OTC]** *see* Loratadine and Pseudoephedrine *on page 1242*

Loratadine and Pseudoephedrine

(lor AT a deen & soo doe e FED rin)

Brand Names: U.S. Alavert™ Allergy and Sinus [OTC]; Claritin-D® 12 Hour Allergy & Congestion [OTC]; Claritin-D® 24 Hour Allergy & Congestion [OTC]; Loratadine-D 12 Hour [OTC]

Brand Names: Canada Chlor-Tripolon ND®; Claritin® Extra; Claritin® Liberator

Index Terms Pseudoephedrine and Loratadine

Pharmacologic Category Alpha/Beta Agonist; Decongestant; Histamine H_1 Antagonist; Histamine H_1 Antagonist, Second Generation; Piperidine Derivative

Use Temporary relief of symptoms of seasonal allergic rhinitis, other upper respiratory allergies, or the common cold

Dosage Children ≥12 years and Adults: Oral:

Claritin-D® 12-Hour: 1 tablet every 12 hours

Alavert™ Allergy and Sinus, Claritin-D® 24-Hour: 1 tablet daily

Dosage adjustment in renal impairment: Cl_{cr} ≤30 mL/minute:

Claritin-D® 12-Hour: 1 tablet daily

Claritin-D® 24-Hour: 1 tablet every other day

Dosage adjustment in hepatic impairment: Should be avoided

Additional Information Complete prescribing information should be consulted for additional detail.

Dosage Forms Excipient information presented when available (limited, particularly for generics); consult specific product labeling.

Tablet, extended release: Loratadine 10 mg and pseudoephedrine sulfate 240 mg

Alavert™ Allergy and Sinus: Loratadine 5 mg and pseudoephedrine sulfate 120 mg

Claritin-D® 12 Hour Allergy & Congestion: Loratadine 5 mg and pseudoephedrine sulfate 120 mg [contains calcium 30 mg/tablet]

Claritin-D® 24 Hour Allergy & Congestion: Loratadine 10 mg and pseudoephedrine sulfate 240 mg [contains calcium 25 mg/tablet]

Loratadine-D 12 Hour: Loratadine 5 mg and pseudoephedrine sulfate 120 mg

◆ **Loratadine Childrens [OTC]** *see* Loratadine *on page 1240*

◆ **Loratadine Hives Relief [OTC]** *see* Loratadine *on page 1240*

LORazepam (lor A ze pam)

Brand Names: U.S. Ativan; LORazepam Intensol

Brand Names: Canada Apo-Lorazepam; Ativan; Dom-Lorazepam; Lorazepam Injection, USP; Novo-Lorazem; Nu-Loraz; PHL-Lorazepam; PMS-Lorazepam; PRO-Lorazepam

Pharmacologic Category Benzodiazepine

Additional Appendix Information

Beers Criteria − Potentially Inappropriate Medications for Geriatrics *on page 2368*

Benzodiazepine Comparison Table *on page 2292*

Status Epilepticus *on page 2375*

Use

Anxiety (oral): Management of anxiety disorders, short-term (≤4 months) relief of anxiety symptoms, or anxiety associated with depressive symptoms, or anxiety/stress-associated insomnia

Anesthesia premedication (parenteral): Anesthesia premedication to relieve anxiety or to produce amnesia (diminish recall) or sedation

Status epilepticus (parenteral): Treatment of status epilepticus

Unlabeled Use Agitation in ICU patient (I.V.); alcohol withdrawal delirium; alcohol withdrawal syndrome; chemotherapy-associated nausea and vomiting (either as an adjunct to standard antiemetics or for breakthrough nausea/vomiting); partial complex seizures (refractory); psychogenic catatonia; rapid tranquilization of the agitated patient; status epilepticus (in pediatrics)

Pregnancy Risk Factor D

Pregnancy Considerations Teratogenic effects have been observed in some animal reproduction studies. Lorazepam and its metabolite cross the human placenta. Teratogenic effects in humans have been observed with some benzodiazepines (including lorazepam); however, additional studies are needed. The incidence of premature birth and low birth weights may be increased following maternal use of benzodiazepines; hypoglycemia and respiratory problems in the neonate may occur following exposure late in pregnancy. Neonatal withdrawal symptoms may occur within days to weeks after birth and "floppy infant syndrome" (which also includes withdrawal symptoms) have been reported with some benzodiazepines (including lorazepam). Elimination of lorazepam in the newborn infant is slow; following *in utero* exposure, term infants may excrete lorazepam for up to 8 days (Bergman, 1992; Iqbal, 2002; Wikner, 2007).

Breast-Feeding Considerations Lorazepam can be detected in breast milk. Drowsiness, lethargy, or weight loss in nursing infants have been observed in case reports following maternal use of some benzodiazepines (Iqbal, 2002). Breast-feeding is not recommended by the manufacturer.

Contraindications Hypersensitivity to lorazepam, any component of the formulation, or other benzodiazepines (cross-sensitivity with other benzodiazepines may exist); acute narrow-angle glaucoma; sleep apnea (parenteral); intra-arterial injection of parenteral formulation; severe respiratory insufficiency (except during mechanical ventilation)

Warnings/Precautions Use with caution in elderly or debilitated patients, patients with hepatic disease (including alcoholics) or renal impairment. In older adults, benzodiazepines increase the risk of impaired cognition, delirium, falls, fractures, and motor vehicle accidents. Due to increased sensitivity in this age group, avoid use for treatment of insomnia, agitation, or delirium. (Beers Criteria). Use with caution in patients with respiratory disease (COPD or sleep apnea) or limited pulmonary reserve, or impaired gag reflex. Initial doses in elderly or debilitated patients should be at the lower end of the dosing range. May worsen hepatic encephalopathy.

Causes CNS depression (dose-related) resulting in sedation, dizziness, confusion, or ataxia which may impair physical and mental capabilities. Patients must be cautioned about performing tasks which require mental alertness (eg, operating machinery or driving). Potentially significant drug-drug interactions may exist, requiring dose or frequency adjustment, additional monitoring, and/or selection of alternative therapy. Use with caution in patients receiving other CNS depressants or psychoactive agents. Effects with other sedative drugs or ethanol may be potentiated. Benzodiazepines have been associated with falls and traumatic injury and should be used with extreme caution in patients who are at risk of these events.

Lorazepam may cause anterograde amnesia. Paradoxical reactions, including hyperactive or aggressive behavior have been reported with benzodiazepines, particularly in adolescent/pediatric or psychiatric patients. Does not have analgesic, antidepressant, or antipsychotic properties.

Pre-existing depression may worsen or emerge during therapy. Not recommended for use in primary depressive or psychotic disorders. Should not be used in patients at risk for suicide without adequate antidepressant treatment. Risk of dependence increases in patients with a history of alcohol or drug abuse and those with significant personality disorders; use with caution in these patients. Tolerance, psychological and physical dependence may also occur with higher dosages and prolonged use. The risk of dependence is decreased with short-term treatment (2-4 weeks); evaluate the need for continued treatment prior to extending therapy duration. Benzodiazepines have been associated with dependence and acute withdrawal symptoms on discontinuation or reduction in dose. Acute withdrawal, including seizures, may be precipitated after administration of flumazenil to patients receiving long-term benzodiazepine therapy.

As a hypnotic agent, should be used only after evaluation of potential causes of sleep disturbance. Failure of sleep disturbance to resolve after 7-10 days may indicate psychiatric or medical illness. A worsening of insomnia or the emergence of new abnormalities of thought or behavior may represent unrecognized psychiatric or medical illness and requires immediate and careful evaluation.

Status epilepticus should not be treated with injectable benzodiazepines alone; requires close observation and management and possibly ventilatory support. When used as a component of preanesthesia, monitor for heavy sedation and airway obstruction; equipment necessary to maintain airway and ventilatory support should be available. Parenteral formulation of lorazepam contains polyethylene glycol which has resulted in toxicity during high-dose and/or longer-term infusions. Parenteral formulation also contains propylene glycol (PG); may be associated with dose-related toxicity and can occur ≥48 hours after initiation of lorazepam. Limited data suggest increased risk of PG accumulation at doses of ≥6 mg/hour for 48 hours or more (Nelson, 2008). Monitor for signs of toxicity which may include acute renal failure, lactic acidosis, and/or osmol gap. May consider using enteral delivery of lorazepam tablets to decrease the risk of PG toxicity (Lugo, 1999). Parenteral formulation also contains benzyl alcohol; avoid in neonates.

Adverse Reactions Frequency not always defined.

Cardiovascular: Hypotension (≤2%)

Central nervous system: Sedation (≤16%), dizziness (≤7%), drowsiness (2% to 4%), unsteadiness (3%), headache (1%), coma (≤1%), stupor (≤1%), aggressive behavior, agitation, akathisia, amnesia, anxiety, central nervous system stimulation, disinhibition, disorientation, dysarthria, euphoria, excitement, extrapyramidal reaction, fatigue, hostility, hypothermia, irritability, mania, memory impairment, outbursts of anger, psychosis, seizures, sleep apnea (exacerbation), sleep disturbances, slurred speech, suicidal behavior, suicidal ideation, vertigo

Dermatologic: Alopecia, skin rash

Gastrointestinal: Changes in appetite, constipation

Endocrine & metabolic: Change in libido, hyponatremia, SIADH

Genitourinary: Impotence, orgasm disturbance

Hematologic & oncologic: Agranulocytosis, pancytopenia, thrombocytopenia

Hepatic: Increased serum alkaline phosphatase, increased serum bilirubin, increased serum transaminases, jaundice

Hypersensitivity: Anaphylaxis, anaphylactoid reaction, hypersensitivity reaction

Local: Pain at injection site (I.M.: 1% to 17%; I.V.: ≤2%), erythema at injection site (≤2%)

Neuromuscular & skeletal: Weakness (≤4%)

Ophthalmic: Visual disturbances (including diplopia and blurred vision)

Respiratory: Respiratory failure (1% to 2%), apnea (1%), hypoventilation (≤1%), exacerbation of obstructive pulmonary disease, nasal congestion, respiratory depression, worsening of sleep apnea

<1% (Limited to important or life-threatening): Abnormal gait, abnormal hepatic function tests, abnormality in thinking, acidosis, cardiac arrhythmia, ataxia, blood coagulation disorder, bradycardia, cardiac arrest, cardiac failure, cerebral edema, confusion, convulsions, cystitis, decreased mental acuity, delirium, depression, drug dependence (with prolonged use), drug toxicity (polyethylene glycol or propylene glycol poisoning [prolonged I.V. infusion]), excessive crying, gastrointestinal hemorrhage, hallucinations, hearing loss, heart block, hematologic abnormality, hepatotoxicity, hypertension, hyperventilation, hyporeflexia, infection, injection site reaction, myoclonus, neuroleptic malignant syndrome, paralysis, pericardial effusion, pheochromocytoma (aggravation), pneumothorax, pulmonary edema, pulmonary hemorrhage, pulmonary hypertension, seizure, tachycardia, urinary incontinence, ventricular arrhythmia, withdrawal syndrome

Drug Interactions

Metabolism/Transport Effects None known.

Avoid Concomitant Use

Avoid concomitant use of LORazepam with any of the following: Azelastine (Nasal); OLANZapine; Paraldehyde; Sodium Oxybate

Increased Effect/Toxicity

LORazepam may increase the levels/effects of: Alcohol (Ethyl); Azelastine (Nasal); Buprenorphine; CloZAPine; CNS Depressants; Fosphenytoin; Hydrocodone; Methotrimeprazine; Metyrosine; Mirtazapine; Paraldehyde; Phenytoin; Pramipexole; ROPINIRole; Rotigotine; Selective Serotonin Reuptake Inhibitors; Sodium Oxybate; Zolpidem

The levels/effects of LORazepam may be increased by: Brimonidine (Topical); Doxylamine; Droperidol; HydrOXYzine; Loxapine; Magnesium Sulfate; Methotrimeprazine; OLANZapine; Perampanel; Probenecid; Tapentadol; Valproic Acid and Derivatives

Decreased Effect

The levels/effects of LORazepam may be decreased by: Theophylline Derivatives; Yohimbine

Ethanol/Nutrition/Herb Interactions

Ethanol: May increase CNS depression; monitor for increased effects with coadministration. Caution patients about effects.

Herb/Nutraceutical: Avoid valerian, St John's wort, kava kava, gotu kola (may increase CNS depression).

Preparation for Administration

I.V. injection: Dilute I.V. dose prior to use with an equal volume of compatible diluent (D_5W, NS, SWFI).

Infusion: Use 2 mg/mL injectable vial to prepare; there may be decreased stability when using 4 mg/mL vial. Dilute to ≤1 mg/mL and mix in glass bottle. Precipitation may occur. Can also be administered undiluted via infusion.

I.M.: Administer undiluted.

Storage/Stability

Parenteral: Intact vials should be refrigerated (room temperature storage information may be available; contact product manufacturer to obtain current recommendations). Protect from light. Do not use discolored or precipitate-containing solutions. Parenteral admixture is stable at room temperature (25°C) for 24 hours.

Oral concentrate: Store at colder room temperature or refrigerate at 2°C to 8°C (36°F to 46°F). Discard open bottle after 90 days.

Tablet: Store at room temperature. Protect from light.

Mechanism of Action Binds to stereospecific benzodiazepine receptors on the postsynaptic GABA neuron at several sites within the central nervous system, including the limbic system, reticular formation. Enhancement of the inhibitory effect of GABA on neuronal excitability results by increased neuronal membrane permeability to chloride ions. This shift in chloride ions results in hyperpolarization (a less excitable state) and stabilization.

Pharmacodynamics/Kinetics

Onset of action:

Hypnosis: I.M.: 20-30 minutes

Sedation: I.V.: Within 2-3 minutes (Greenblatt, 1983)

Anticonvulsant: I.V.: Within 10 minutes; Oral: 30-60 minutes

Duration: Up to 8 hours

Absorption: I.M.: Rapid and complete absorption; Oral: Readily absorbed

Distribution: V_d: Neonates: 0.78 L/kg; Children and Adolescents: 1.9 L/kg; Adults: 1.3 L/kg

Protein binding: ~85% to 93%; free fraction may be significantly higher in elderly

Metabolism: Hepatic; rapidly conjugated to inactive compounds

Bioavailability: Oral: 90%

Half-life elimination: Neonates: ~42 hours; Children 2-12 years: ~18 hours; Adolescents: ~28 hours; Adults: Oral: ~14 hours; End-stage renal disease (ESRD): ~18 hours

Time to peak: I.M.: ≤3 hours; Oral: ~2 hours

Excretion: Urine (~88%; predominantly as inactive metabolites); feces (~7%)

Dosage

Anxiety disorder:

Adults: Oral: 1-10 mg daily in 2-3 divided doses; usual dose: 2-6 mg daily in divided doses

Elderly: Oral: Initial: 1-2 mg daily in divided doses; Beers Criteria: Avoid maintenance doses >3 mg daily

Insomnia due to anxiety or stress: Adults: Oral: 2-4 mg at bedtime

Premedication for anesthesia: Adults:

I.M.: 0.05 mg/kg administered 2 hours before surgery (maximum dose: 4 mg)

I.V.: 0.044 mg/kg administered 15-20 minutes before surgery (usual dose: 2 mg; maximum dose: 4 mg)

Status epilepticus:

Infants, Children, and Adolescents (unlabeled use):

I.V.: 0.1 mg/kg (maximum dose: 4 mg) slow I.V. (maximum rate: 2 mg/minute); may repeat in 5-10 minutes (Brophy, 2012)

or

I.V., I.M.: 0.05-0.1 mg/kg; repeat doses every 10-15 minutes for clinical effect (American Academy of Pediatrics, 1998)

Adults: I.V.: 4 mg slow I.V. (maximum rate: 2 mg/minute); may repeat in 5-10 minutes (Brophy, 2012). May be given I.M., but I.V. preferred.

Agitation in the ICU patient (unlabeled use): Adults: I.V.: Loading dose: 0.02-0.04 mg/kg (maximum single dose: 2 mg); Maintenance: 0.02-0.06 mg/kg every 2-6 hours as needed **or** 0.01-0.1 mg/kg/hour; maximum dose: ≤10 mg/hour (Barr, 2013)

Alcohol withdrawal delirium (unlabeled use) (Mayo-Smith, 2004): Adults:

I.V.: 1-4 mg every 5-15 minutes until calm, then every hour as needed to maintain light somnolence

I.M.: 1-4 mg every 30-60 minutes until calm, then every hour as needed to maintain light somnolence

Alcohol withdrawal syndrome (unlabeled use) (Mayo-Smith, 1997): Adults:

Oral, I.M., I.V. (fixed-dose regimen): 2 mg every 6 hours for 4 doses, then 1 mg every 6 hours for 8 additional doses

Oral, I.M., I.V. (symptom-triggered regimen): 2-4 mg every 1 hour as needed; dose determined by a validated severity assessment scale

Chemotherapy-associated nausea and vomiting (unlabeled use):

Breakthrough nausea/vomiting: Children ≥2 years and Adolescents: I.V.: 0.025-0.05 mg/kg/dose (maximum dose: 2 mg) every 6 hours as needed (Dupuis, 2003)

Breakthrough nausea/vomiting or as adjunct to standard antiemetics: Adults: Oral, I.V., Sublingual (unlabeled route): 0.5-2 mg every 4-6 hours as needed (NCCN Antiemesis guidelines v.1.2013)

Partial complex seizures, refractory (unlabeled use): Adults: Oral: 1 mg twice daily; increase biweekly in increments of 1 mg twice daily until seizures stop or side effects occur (Walker, 1984)

Psychogenic catatonia (unlabeled use): Adults:

I.M., Sublingual (unlabeled route): 1-2 mg; repeat dose in 3 hours then again in another 3 hours if initial and subsequent doses, respectively, are ineffective (Rosebush, 1990; Rosebush, 2010)

or

Oral, I.M., I.V.: Initial: 1 mg; may repeat in 5 minutes if necessary. If initial challenge is unsuccessful, may increase dose up to 4-8 mg per day; may continue treatment for up to 5 days (Bush, 1996)

Rapid tranquilization of agitated patient (unlabeled use): Adults: Oral, I.M.: 1-3 mg administered every 30-60 minutes; may be administered with an antipsychotic (eg, haloperidol) (Allen, 2005; Battaglia, 2005; De Fruyt, 2004). **Note:** When administering I.M., may consider a lower initial dose (eg, 0.5 mg) (Allen, 2005).

Dosage adjustment for lorazepam with concomitant medications: *Probenecid or valproic acid:* Reduce lorazepam dose by 50%

Dosage adjustment in renal impairment:

Oral: No dosage adjustment necessary (Aronoff, 2007).

I.M., I.V.: Risk of propylene glycol toxicity. Monitor closely if using for prolonged periods of time or at high doses.

Mild-to-moderate disease: Use with caution.

Severe disease or failure: Use is not recommended.

Dosage adjustment in hepatic impairment:

Oral:

Mild-to-moderate disease: No dose adjustment necessary.

Severe insufficiency and/or encephalopathy: Use with caution; may require lower doses.

I.M., I.V.:

Mild-to-moderate disease: Use with caution.

Severe disease or failure: Use is not recommended.

Administration

I.M.: Should be administered (undiluted) deep into the muscle mass.

I.V. injection: Dilute prior to use. Do not exceed 2 mg/minute or 0.05 mg/kg over 2-5 minutes. Monitor I.V. site during administration. Avoid intra-arterial administration. Avoid extravasation.

Continuous I.V. infusion (unlabeled administration mode; Barr, 2013) solutions should have an in-line filter and the solution should be checked frequently for possible precipitation (Grillo, 1996).

Oral: Lorazepam oral concentrate: Use only the provided calibrated dropper to withdraw the prescribed dose. Mix the dose with liquid (eg, water, juice, soda, soda-like beverage) or semisolid food (eg, applesauce, pudding), and stir for a few seconds to blend completely. The prepared mixture should be administered immediately.

Monitoring Parameters Respiratory and cardiovascular status, blood pressure, heart rate, symptoms of anxiety

CBC, liver function tests; clinical signs of propylene glycol toxicity (for continuous high-dose and/or long duration intravenous use) including serum creatinine, BUN, serum lactate, osmol gap

Critically-ill patients: Monitor depth of sedation with either the Richmond Agitation-Sedation Scale (RASS) or Sedation-Agitation Scale (SAS) (Barr, 2013)

Reference Range Therapeutic: 50-240 ng/mL (SI: 156-746 nmol/L)

Dosage Forms Excipient information presented when available (limited, particularly for generics); consult specific product labeling.

Concentrate, Oral:

LORazepam Intensol: 2 mg/mL (30 mL) [alcohol free, dye free, sugar free; unflavored flavor]

Generic: 2 mg/mL (30 mL)

Solution, Injection:

Ativan: 2 mg/mL (1 mL, 10 mL); 4 mg/mL (1 mL, 10 mL) [contains benzyl alcohol, polyethylene glycol, propylene glycol]

Generic: 2 mg/mL (1 mL, 10 mL); 4 mg/mL (1 mL, 10 mL)

Tablet, Oral:

Ativan: 0.5 mg

Ativan: 1 mg, 2 mg [scored]

Generic: 0.5 mg, 1 mg, 2 mg

Controlled Substance C-IV

Extemporaneous Preparations Note: Commercial oral solution is available (2 mg/mL)

Two different 1 mg/mL oral suspensions may be made from different generic lorazepam tablets (Mylan Pharmaceuticals or Watson Laboratories), sterile water, Ora-Sweet, and Ora-Plus.

Mylan tablets: Place one-hundred-eighty 2 mg tablets in a 12-ounce amber glass bottle; add 144 mL of sterile water to disperse the tablets; shake until slurry is formed. Add 108 mL Ora-Plus in incremental proportions; then add a quantity of Ora-Sweet sufficient to make 360 mL. Label "shake well" and "refrigerate". Stable for 91 days when stored in amber glass prescription bottles at room temperature or refrigerated (preferred).

Watson tablets: Place one-hundred-eighty 2 mg tablets in a 12-ounce amber glass bottle; add 48 mL sterile water to disperse the tablets; shake until slurry is formed. Add 156 mL of Ora-Plus in incremental proportions; then add a quantity of Ora-Sweet sufficient to make 360 mL. Label "shake well" and "refrigerate". Store in amber glass prescription bottles. Stable for 63 days at room temperature or 91 days refrigerated.

Lee ME, Lugo RA, Rusho WJ, et al, "Chemical Stability of Extemporaneously Prepared Lorazepam Suspension at Two Temperatures," *J Pediatr Pharmacol Ther*, 2004, 9(4):254-58.

◆ **Lorazepam Injection, USP (Can)** *see* LORazepam *on page 1242*

◆ **LORazepam Intensol** *see* LORazepam *on page 1242*

Lorcaserin (lor KA ser in)

Brand Names: U.S. Belviq

Index Terms Lorcaserin Hydrochloride

Pharmacologic Category Anorexiant; Serotonin 5-HT_{2C} Receptor Agonist

Use Chronic weight management, as an adjunct to a reduced-calorie diet and increased physical activity, in patients with either an initial body mass index (BMI) of ≥30 kg/m^2 **or** an initial BMI of ≥27 kg/m^2 and at least one weight-related comorbid condition (eg, hypertension, dyslipidemia, type 2 diabetes)

Pregnancy Risk Factor X

Pregnancy Considerations Adverse fetal effects were observed in some animal reproduction studies. Due to the fact that weight loss during pregnancy offers no clinical benefit, lorcaserin is contraindicated in pregnancy. Obese and overweight women should be encouraged to participate in weight reduction programs prior to attempting pregnancy; weight gain during pregnancy should be determined by their prepregnancy BMI and current guidelines (ADA, 2009; IOM, 2009).

Breast-Feeding Considerations Lorcaserin may alter maternal serum prolactin concentrations. It is not known if lorcaserin is excreted into breast milk. According to the manufacturer, the decision to continue or discontinue breast-feeding during therapy should take into account the risk of exposure to the infant and the benefits of treatment to the mother. Weight-loss therapy is generally not recommended for lactating women. Weight-loss programs which include physical activity and nutrition components should be discussed at the 6-week postpartum visit (ADA, 2009; IOM, 2009).

Contraindications Pregnancy

Warnings/Precautions Use may cause confusion, somnolence, fatigue, and cognitive impairment (difficulty with concentration/attention/memory); patients must be cautioned about performing tasks which require mental alertness (eg, operating machinery or driving). Agents affecting the CNS have been associated with depression and suicidal ideation; monitor patients closely during use; discontinue for suicidal thoughts or behaviors. Priapism may occur with use; men with erections >4 hours should immediately discontinue lorcaserin and seek emergency medical attention to avoid irreversible damage to erectile tissue. Use with caution in men with conditions that increase the risk for priapism (eg, sickle cell anemia, multiple myeloma, leukemia) or men with anatomical penis deformities (eg, angulation, cavernosal fibrosis, Peyronie's disease). Rare WBC and RBC count decreases (including leukopenia, lymphopenia, neutropenia, anemia, decreases in hematocrit and hemoglobin) have been observed; consider monitoring CBC periodically during use. Increased prolactin levels may occur; obtain prolactin levels if signs or symptoms of hyperprolactinemia occur (eg, galactorrhea, gynecomastia).

Primary pulmonary hypertension (PPH) is a rare and frequently fatal pulmonary disease, which has been reported in patients receiving other centrally acting, serotonergic weight loss agents. Available data from clinical trials are inadequate to determine if lorcaserin increases the risk for pulmonary hypertension (due to the low incidence of PPH occurring in the general population); however, a theoretical risk cannot be excluded. Cardiac valvular disease has been associated with the use of agents exhibiting potent 5-HT_{2B} agonist activity (eg, cabergoline, fenfluramine [not currently on the U.S. market], dexfenfluramine [not currently on the U.S. market]). Cardiac valvular disease is believed to result from activation of 5-HT_{2B} receptors in interstitial cardiac cells. Lorcaserin has greater affinity for 5-HT_{2C} receptors compared to 5-HT_{2B} receptors (at therapeutic doses). However, a slight increase in incidence of regurgitant cardiac valve disease (mitral and/or aortic) has been observed with lorcaserin compared to placebo in some clinical trials (pooled RR: 1.16; 95% CI: 0.81-1.67). The incidence observed in both groups was low, making it difficult to ascertain the risk of valvular disease with lorcaserin therapy based on available data. Evaluate patients if signs/symptoms of valvular heart disease (eg, dyspnea, dependent edema, heart failure, new onset cardiac murmur) arise during therapy; consider discontinuing therapy if present. Use has not been studied in patients with hemodynamically-significant valvular heart disease. Do not use lorcaserin in combination with potent serotonergic and dopaminergic agents that are potent

5-HT_{2B} receptor agonists (eg, cabergoline) due to the risk for cardiac valvulopathy.

Serotonin syndrome (SS)/neuroleptic malignant syndrome (NMS)-like reactions have occurred with serotonergic agents such as lorcaserin, particularly when used in combination with other serotonergic agents (eg, triptans, SNRIs, SSRIs, TCAs, bupropion, St John's wort, tryptophan), agents that impair metabolism of serotonin (eg, MAO inhibitors, dextromethorphan, tramadol, lithium), or antidopaminergic agents (eg, antipsychotics). Concurrent use with these agents should be avoided. If concomitant use cannot be avoided, coadminister with extreme caution, and closely monitor patients, particularly during treatment initiation. Discontinue treatment (and any concomitant serotonergic and/or antidopaminergic agents) immediately if signs/symptoms of SS or NMS-like reactions arise.

Use with caution in patients with bradycardia or heart block (second or third degree); bradycardia has been observed rarely with use. Use with caution in patients with heart failure (has not been studied). Effect of lorcaserin on cardiovascular morbidity and mortality has not been established. Use with caution in patients with type 2 diabetes mellitus; weight loss from therapy may result in decreased requirements of antidiabetic agents and an increased risk of hypoglycemia; monitor blood glucose. Use with caution in patients with severe hepatic impairment (not studied); lorcaserin undergoes extensive hepatic metabolism. Use is not recommended in patients with severe renal impairment or end stage renal disease. Use with caution in patients with moderate renal impairment. Serum concentrations and principal metabolite (M1 and M5) half-lives are increased in renal impairment.

In short-term studies, euphoria, hallucinations, and dissociation have been observed with lorcaserin at supratherapeutic doses. Data suggest lorcaserin may produce psychic dependence. Physical dependence or a withdrawal syndrome has not been observed. Pharmacotherapy for weight loss should be used in conjunction with a comprehensive weight management program including diet and exercise. Discontinue if significant weight loss has not occurred (ie, <5% within the first 12 weeks of treatment). Concomitant use of lorcaserin with other agents intended for weight loss (eg, phentermine, orlistat, OTC, or herbal preparations) has not been evaluated; safety and efficacy of coadministration with other weight loss agents are unknown.

Adverse Reactions

>10%:
- Central nervous system: Headache (15% to 17%)
- Endocrine & metabolic: Hypoglycemia (diabetic patients 29%; severe: 2%)
- Hematologic: Lymphocytes decreased (12%)
- Neuromuscular & skeletal: Back pain (6% to 12%)
- Respiratory: Upper respiratory tract infection (14%), nasopharyngitis (11% to 13%)

1% to 10%:
- Cardiovascular: Peripheral edema (5%), hypertension (5%), valvulopathy (at 1 year: 2.4%; placebo: 2.0%)
- Central nervous system: Dizziness (7% to 9%), fatigue (7%), anxiety (4%), insomnia (4%), depression (2% to 3%; placebo: 2%), cognitive impairment (2%), psychiatric disorders (2%)
- Dermatologic: Rash (2%)
- Endocrine & metabolic: Diabetes mellitus exacerbation (3%), prolactin increased (<2 x ULN: 7%; 2 x ULN: 2%; 5 x ULN: <1%)
- Gastrointestinal: Nausea (8% to 9%), diarrhea (7%), constipation (6%), xerostomia (5%), vomiting (4%), gastroenteritis (3%), toothache (3%), appetite decreased (2%)
- Genitourinary: Urinary tract infection (7% to 9%)
- Hematologic: Hemoglobin decreased (10%), neutrophils decreased (6%)
- Neuromuscular & skeletal: Muscle spasms (5%), musculoskeletal pain (2%)
- Ocular: Eye disorders (5%; diabetic patients 6%)
- Respiratory: Cough (4% to 8%), oropharyngeal pain (4%), sinus congestion (3%)
- Miscellaneous: Seasonal allergy (3%), stress (3%)

<1% (Limited to important or life-threatening): Bradycardia, dissociation, euphoria, serotonin syndrome, suicidal ideation

Drug Interactions

Metabolism/Transport Effects Inhibits CYP2D6 (moderate)

Avoid Concomitant Use

Avoid concomitant use of Lorcaserin with any of the following: Ergot Derivatives; Thioridazine

Increased Effect/Toxicity

Lorcaserin may increase the levels/effects of: Antipsychotics; CYP2D6 Substrates; Ergot Derivatives; Fesoterodine; Metoclopramide; Metoprolol; Nebivolol; Phosphodiesterase 5 Inhibitors; Serotonin Modulators; Thioridazine

The levels/effects of Lorcaserin may be increased by: Antipsychotics; BuPROPion; Propafenone

Decreased Effect

Lorcaserin may decrease the levels/effects of: Codeine; Tamoxifen

Storage/Stability Store at 25°C (77°F); excursions permitted to 15°C to 30°C (59°F to 86°F).

Mechanism of Action Lorcaserin is believed to activate serotonin 5-HT_{2C} receptors, which stimulate pro-opiomelanocortin (POMC) neurons in the arcuate nucleus of the hypothalamus, leading to increased alpha-melanocortin stimulating hormone release at melanocortin-4 receptors and resulting in satiety and decreased food intake. At recommended doses, lorcaserin has greater affinity for 5-HT_{2C} receptors compared to other 5-HT receptor subtypes (including 5-HT_{2A} and 5-HT_{2B}), the 5-HT receptor transporter, and 5-HT reuptake sites (Hurren, 2011).

Pharmacodynamics/Kinetics

- Distribution: Distributes to the CNS and cerebrospinal fluid
- Protein binding: ~70% to plasma proteins
- Metabolism: Extensive hepatic metabolism, via multiple enzymatic pathways, producing two major metabolites (inactive), lorcaserin sulfamate (M1) and N-carbamoyl glucuronide lorcaserin (M5), as well as minor metabolites (glucuronide and sulfate conjugates)
- Half-life elimination: ~11 hours
- Time to peak: 1.5-2 hours
- Excretion: Urine (92%, as metabolites); feces (2%, as metabolites)

Dosage Weight management: Adults: Oral: 10 mg twice daily (maximum: 10 mg twice daily); evaluate response by week 12; if patient has not lost ≥5% of baseline body weight, discontinue therapy

Dosage adjustment in renal impairment: Note: Renal function was estimated in studies using ideal body weight (IBW) with the Cockcroft-Gault formula.
- Mild impairment (Cl_{cr} >50 mL/minute): No dosage adjustment necessary.
- Moderate impairment (Cl_{cr} 30-50 mL/minute): Use with caution; serum concentrations and half-life of major metabolites are increased.
- Severe impairment (Cl_{cr} <30 mL/minute): Use is not recommended.
- ESRD: Use is not recommended; hemodialysis does not remove lorcaserin or M1 metabolite

Dosage adjustment in hepatic impairment:
- Mild-to-moderate impairment (Child-Pugh score 5-9): No dosage adjustment necessary.

Severe impairment: Use with caution (has not been studied); undergoes extensive hepatic metabolism.

Administration Administer orally with or without food.

Monitoring Parameters Weight, waist circumference; CBC (periodically during use); blood glucose (in diabetics); prolactin levels (if galactorrhea, gynecomastia or other signs/symptoms of hyperprolactinemia arise); monitor for depression or suicidal thoughts/behavior; signs/symptoms of SS/NMS-like reaction; signs/symptoms of valvular heart disease (dyspnea, dependent edema)

Additional Information *In vitro*, lorcaserin has an 18-fold and 104-fold greater affinity for $5HT_{2C}$ receptors compared to $5\text{-}HT_{2A}$ and $5HT_{2B}$ receptors, respectively (Hurren, 2011).

Dosage Forms Excipient information presented when available (limited, particularly for generics); consult specific product labeling.

Tablet, Oral:

Belviq: 10 mg [contains fd&c blue #2 aluminum lake]

Controlled Substance C-IV

◆ **Lorcaserin Hydrochloride** *see* Lorcaserin *on page 1245*

◆ **Lorcet® 10/650** *see* Hydrocodone and Acetaminophen *on page 1006*

◆ **Lorcet® Plus** *see* Hydrocodone and Acetaminophen *on page 1006*

◆ **Lortab®** *see* Hydrocodone and Acetaminophen *on page 1006*

◆ **Loryna™** *see* Ethinyl Estradiol and Drospirenone *on page 785*

◆ **Lorzone** *see* Chlorzoxazone *on page 417*

Losartan (loe SAR tan)

Brand Names: U.S. Cozaar

Brand Names: Canada Apo-Losartan; Auro-Losartan; CO Losartan; Cozaar; JAMP-Losartan; Mylan-Losartan; PMS-Losartan; RAN-Losartan; Sandoz Losartan; Teva-Losartan

Index Terms DuP 753; Losartan Potassium; MK594

Pharmacologic Category Angiotensin II Receptor Blocker; Antihypertensive

Additional Appendix Information

Angiotensin Agents *on page 2280*

Use Treatment of hypertension (HTN); treatment of diabetic nephropathy in patients with type 2 diabetes mellitus (non-insulin dependent, NIDDM) and a history of hypertension; stroke risk reduction in patients with HTN and left ventricular hypertrophy (LVH)

Unlabeled Use To slow the rate of progression of aortic-root dilation in pediatric patients with Marfan's syndrome; syndrome; heart failure patients intolerant of ACE inhibitors

Pregnancy Risk Factor C (1st trimester); D (2nd and 3rd trimesters)

Pregnancy Considerations [U.S. Boxed Warning]: Drugs that act on the renin-angiotensin system can cause injury and death to the developing fetus. Discontinue as soon as possible once pregnancy is detected. The use of drugs which act on the renin-angiotensin system are associated with oligohydramnios. Oligohydramnios, due to decreased fetal renal function, may lead to fetal lung hypoplasia and skeletal malformations. Use is also associated with anuria, hypotension, renal failure, skull hypoplasia, and death in the fetus/neonate. The exposed fetus should be monitored for fetal growth, amniotic fluid volume, and organ formation. Infants exposed *in utero* should be monitored for hyperkalemia, hypotension, and oliguria.

Untreated chronic maternal hypertension is also associated with adverse events in the fetus, infant, and mother. If treatment for hypertension during pregnancy is needed, other agents are preferred (ACOG, 2012; Chobanian, 2003). In women of reproductive potential, angiotensin II receptor blockers should be discontinued prior to conception or as soon as pregnancy is confirmed (Chobanian, 2003).

Breast-Feeding Considerations It is not known if losartan is found in breast milk. Due to the potential for serious adverse reactions in the nursing infant, the manufacturer recommends a decision be made whether to discontinue nursing or to discontinue the drug, taking into account the importance of treatment to the mother. Breast-fed infants of mothers taking medications for hypertension should be monitored for adverse effects (Chobanian, 2003).

Contraindications

Hypersensitivity to losartan or any component of the formulation; concomitant use with aliskiren in patients with diabetes mellitus

Canadian labeling: Additional contraindications (not in U.S. labeling): Concomitant use with aliskiren in patients with moderate-to-severe renal impairment (GFR <60 mL/minute/1.73 m^2)

Warnings/Precautions [U.S. Boxed Warning]: Drugs that act on the renin-angiotensin system can cause injury and death to the developing fetus. Discontinue as soon as possible once pregnancy is detected. Avoid use or use a much smaller dose in patients who are volume-depleted; correct depletion first. Use with caution in patients with significant aortic/mitral stenosis. May cause hyperkalemia; avoid potassium supplementation unless specifically required by healthcare provider. May be associated with deterioration of renal function and/or increases in serum creatinine, particularly in patients with low renal blood flow (eg, renal artery stenosis, heart failure) whose glomerular filtration rate (GFR) is dependent on efferent arteriolar vasoconstriction by angiotensin II. Use caution in patients with unstented unilateral/bilateral renal artery stenosis. When unstented bilateral renal artery stenosis is present, use is generally avoided due to the elevated risk of deterioration in renal function unless possible benefits outweigh risks. Use with caution with pre-existing renal insufficiency. AUCs of losartan (not the active metabolite) are about 50% greater in patients with Cl_{cr} <30 mL/minute and are doubled in hemodialysis patients. Potentially significant drug interactions may exist, requiring dose or frequency adjustment, additional monitoring, and/or selection of alternative therapy.

Angioedema has been reported rarely with some angiotensin II receptor antagonists (ARBs) and may occur at any time during treatment (especially following first dose). It may involve the head and neck (potentially compromising airway) or the intestine (presenting with abdominal pain). Patients with idiopathic or hereditary angioedema or previous angioedema associated with ACE-inhibitor therapy may be at an increased risk. Prolonged frequent monitoring may be required, especially if tongue, glottis, or larynx are involved, as they are associated with airway obstruction. Patients with a history of airway surgery may have a higher risk of airway obstruction. Discontinue therapy immediately if angioedema occurs. Aggressive early management is critical. Intramuscular (I.M.) administration of epinephrine may be necessary. Do not readminister to patients who have had angioedema with ARBs.

When used to reduce the risk of stroke in patients with HTN and LVH, may not be effective in African-American population. Use caution with hepatic dysfunction, dose adjustment may be needed.

Adverse Reactions Note: The incidence of some adverse reactions varied based on the underlying disease state. Notations are made, where applicable, for data derived from trials conducted in diabetic nephropathy and hypertensive patients, respectively.

>10%:

Cardiovascular: Chest pain (12% diabetic nephropathy)

Central nervous system: Fatigue (14% diabetic nephropathy)

Endocrine: Hypoglycemia (14% diabetic nephropathy)

Gastrointestinal: Diarrhea (2% hypertension to 15% diabetic nephropathy)

Genitourinary: Urinary tract infection (13% diabetic nephropathy)

Hematologic: Anemia (14% diabetic nephropathy)

Neuromuscular & skeletal: Weakness (14% diabetic nephropathy), back pain (2% hypertension to 12% diabetic nephropathy)

Respiratory: Cough (≤3% to 11%; similar to placebo; incidence higher in patients with previous cough related to ACE inhibitor therapy)

1% to 10%:

Cardiovascular: Hypotension (7% diabetic nephropathy), orthostatic hypotension (4% hypertension to 4% diabetic nephropathy), first-dose hypotension (dose related: <1% with 50 mg, 2% with 100 mg)

Central nervous system: Dizziness (4%), hypoesthesia (5% diabetic nephropathy), fever (4% diabetic nephropathy), insomnia (1%)

Dermatology: Cellulitis (7% diabetic nephropathy)

Endocrine: Hyperkalemia (<1% hypertension to 7% diabetic nephropathy)

Gastrointestinal: Gastritis (5% diabetic nephropathy), weight gain (4% diabetic nephropathy), dyspepsia (1% to 4%), abdominal pain (2%), nausea (2%)

Neuromuscular & skeletal: Muscular weakness (7% diabetic nephropathy), knee pain (5% diabetic nephropathy), leg pain (1% to 5%), muscle cramps (1%), myalgia (1%)

Respiratory: Bronchitis (10% diabetic nephropathy), upper respiratory infection (8%), nasal congestion (2%), sinusitis (1% hypertension to 6% diabetic nephropathy)

Miscellaneous: Infection (5% diabetic nephropathy), flu-like syndrome (10% diabetic nephropathy)

<1% (Limited to important or life-threatening): Acute psychosis with paranoid delusions, ageusia, allergic reaction, alopecia, anaphylactic reactions, anemia, angina, angioedema, anorexia, anxiety, arrhythmia, arthralgia, arthritis, ataxia, AV block (second degree), bilirubin increased, blurred vision, bradycardia, bronchitis, BUN increased, confusion, conjunctivitis, constipation, CVA, depression, dermatitis, dysgeusia, dyspnea, ecchymosis, epistaxis, erythroderma, erythema, facial edema, fever, flatulence, flushing, gastritis, gout, hematocrit decreased, hemoglobin decreased, Henoch-Schönlein purpura (IgA vasculitis), hepatitis, hyponatremia, hypotension, impotence, joint swelling, maculopapular rash, malaise, memory impairment, MI, migraine, muscle weakness, myositis, neoplasm, nervousness, orthostatic effects, pancreatitis, paresthesia, peripheral neuropathy, pharyngitis, photosensitivity, pruritus, rash, rhabdomyolysis, rhinitis, serum creatinine increased, sleep disorder, somnolence, syncope, tachycardia, taste perversion, thrombocytopenia, tinnitus, transaminases increased, tremor, urinary frequency, urticaria, vasculitis, ventricular arrhythmia, vertigo, visual acuity decreased, vomiting, xerostomia

Drug Interactions

Metabolism/Transport Effects Substrate of CYP2C9 (major), CYP3A4 (major); **Note:** Assignment of Major/Minor substrate status based on clinically relevant drug interaction potential; **Inhibits** CYP1A2 (weak), CYP2C19 (weak), CYP2C8 (moderate), CYP2C9 (moderate), CYP3A4 (weak)

Avoid Concomitant Use

Avoid concomitant use of Losartan with any of the following: Pimozide

Increased Effect/Toxicity

Losartan may increase the levels/effects of: ACE Inhibitors; Amifostine; Antihypertensives; ARIPiprazole; Bosentan; Carvedilol; CycloSPORINE (Systemic); CYP2C8 Substrates; CYP2C9 Substrates; Dofetilide; Hypotensive Agents; Lithium; Lomitapide; Nonsteroidal Anti-Inflammatory Agents; Obinutuzumab; Pimozide; Potassium-Sparing Diuretics; RiTUXimab; Sodium Phosphates

The levels/effects of Losartan may be increased by: Alfuzosin; Aliskiren; Antifungal Agents (Azole Derivatives, Systemic); Brimonidine (Topical); Canagliflozin; CYP2C9 Inhibitors (Moderate); CYP2C9 Inhibitors (Strong); Diazoxide; Eplerenone; Fluconazole; Heparin; Heparin (Low Molecular Weight); Herbs (Hypotensive Properties); MAO Inhibitors; Mifepristone; Milk Thistle; Pentoxifylline; Phosphodiesterase 5 Inhibitors; Potassium Salts; Prostacyclin Analogues; Tolvaptan; Trimethoprim

Decreased Effect

The levels/effects of Losartan may be decreased by: Bosentan; CYP2C9 Inducers (Strong); CYP3A4 Inducers (Strong); Dabrafenib; Deferasirox; Herbs (CYP3A4 Inducers); Herbs (Hypertensive Properties); Methylphenidate; Mitotane; Nonsteroidal Anti-Inflammatory Agents; Peginterferon Alfa-2b; Rifamycin Derivatives; Tocilizumab; Yohimbine

Ethanol/Nutrition/Herb Interactions Herb/Nutraceutical: St John's wort may decrease levels of losartan. Some herbal medications may worsen hypertension (eg, licorice); others may increase the antihypertensive effect of losartan (eg, shepherd's purse). Some herbal medications may increase the hypoglycemic effects of losartan (eg, alfalfa). Management: Avoid St John's wort. Avoid bayberry, blue cohosh, ginseng (American), kola, licorice, and yohimbe. Avoid black cohosh, California poppy, coleus, golden seal, hawthorn, mistletoe, periwinkle, quinine, and shepherd's purse. Avoid alfalfa, aloe, bilberry, bitter melon, burdock, celery, damiana, fenugreek, garcinia, garlic, ginger, ginseng (American), gymnema, marshmallow, and stinging nettle.

Storage/Stability Store at 15°C to 30°C (59°F to 86°F). Protect from light.

Mechanism of Action As a selective and competitive, nonpeptide angiotensin II receptor antagonist, losartan blocks the vasoconstrictor and aldosterone-secreting effects of angiotensin II; losartan interacts reversibly at the AT1 and AT2 receptors of many tissues and has slow dissociation kinetics; its affinity for the AT1 receptor is 1000 times greater than the AT2 receptor. Angiotensin II receptor antagonists may induce a more complete inhibition of the renin-angiotensin system than ACE inhibitors, they do not affect the response to bradykinin, and are less likely to be associated with nonrenin-angiotensin effects (eg, cough and angioedema). Losartan increases urinary flow rate and in addition to being natriuretic and kaliuretic, increases excretion of chloride, magnesium, uric acid, calcium, and phosphate.

Pharmacodynamics/Kinetics

Onset of action: 6 hours

Distribution: V_d: Losartan: 34 L; E-3174: 12 L; does not cross blood-brain barrier

Protein binding, plasma: High
Metabolism: Hepatic (14%) via CYP2C9 and 3A4 to active metabolite, E-3174 (40 times more potent than losartan); extensive first-pass effect
Bioavailability: 25% to 33%; AUC of E-3174 is four times greater than that of losartan
Half-life elimination: Losartan: 1.5-2 hours; E-3174: 6-9 hours
Time to peak, serum: Losartan: 1 hour; E-3174: 3-4 hours
Excretion: Urine (4% as unchanged drug, 6% as active metabolite)
Clearance: Plasma: Losartan: 600 mL/minute; Active metabolite: 50 mL/minute

Dosage Oral:
Hypertension:
Children 6-16 years:
U.S. labeling: 0.7 mg/kg once daily (maximum: 50 mg daily); doses >1.4 mg/kg (maximum: 100 mg) have not been studied
Canadian labeling:
≥20 kg to <50 kg: 25 mg once daily (maximum: 50 mg once daily)
≥50 kg: 50 mg once daily (maximum: 100 mg once daily)
Adults: Usual starting dose: 50 mg once daily; can be administered once or twice daily with total daily doses ranging from 25-100 mg
Patients receiving diuretics or with intravascular volume depletion: Usual initial dose: 25 mg once daily
Nephropathy in patients with type 2 diabetes and hypertension: Adults: Initial: 50 mg once daily; can be increased to 100 mg once daily based on blood pressure response
Stroke reduction (HTN with LVH): Adults: 50 mg once daily (maximum daily dose: 100 mg); may be used in combination with a thiazide diuretic
Aortic-root dilation with Marfan's syndrome (unlabeled use): Children 14 months to 16 years: Initial: 0.6 mg/kg/day; can be increased to a maximum of 1.4 mg/kg/day (not to exceed adult maximum of 100 mg daily) (Brooke, 2008)
Heart failure (unlabeled use): Adults: Initial: 12.5-25 mg once daily; target dose: 150 mg once daily (HFSA, 2010; Konstam, 2009)

Dosing adjustment in renal impairment:
Children: Use is not recommended if GFR <30 mL/minute/1.73 m^2
Adults: No dosage adjustment necessary.

Dosing adjustment in hepatic impairment:
Children 6-16 years:
U.S. labeling: No specific dosing recommendations are provided in the approved labeling, however it may be advisable to initiate therapy at a reduced dosage.
Canadian labeling: Use is not recommended.
Adults: Reduce the initial dose to 25 mg/day

Dietary Considerations May be taken without regard to meals. Some products may contain potassium.

Administration May be administered without regard to meals.

Monitoring Parameters Supine blood pressure, electrolytes, serum creatinine, BUN, urinalysis, symptomatic hypotension and tachycardia, CBC

Dosage Forms Excipient information presented when available (limited, particularly for generics); consult specific product labeling.
Tablet, Oral, as potassium:
Cozaar: 25 mg
Cozaar: 50 mg [scored]
Cozaar: 100 mg
Generic: 25 mg, 50 mg, 100 mg

Extemporaneous Preparations A 2.5 mg/mL losartan oral suspension may be made with tablets and a 1:1 mixture of Ora-Plus® and Ora-Sweet® SF. Combine 10 mL of purified water and ten losartan 50 mg tablets in an 8-ounce amber polyethylene terephthalate bottle. Shake well for at least 2 minutes. Allow concentrate to stand for 1 hour, then shake for 1 minute. Separately, prepare 190 mL of a 1:1 mixture of Ora-Plus® and Ora-Sweet® SF; add to tablet and water mixture in the bottle and shake for 1 minute. Label "shake well" and "refrigerate". Return promptly to refrigerator after each use. Stable for 4 weeks when stored in amber polyethylene terephthalate prescription bottles and refrigerated (Cozaar® prescribing information, 2008).

Cozaar® prescribing information, Merck & Co, Inc, Whitehouse Station, NJ, 2008.

Losartan and Hydrochlorothiazide

(loe SAR tan & hye droe klor oh THYE a zide)

Brand Names: U.S. Hyzaar®

Brand Names: Canada Apo-Losartan/HCTZ; CO Losartan/HCT; Hyzaar; Hyzaar DS; Losartan-HCT; Losartan-HCTZ; Mint-Losartan/HCTZ; Mint-Losartan/HCTZ DS; Mylan-Losartan/HCTZ; PMS-Losartan/HCTZ; Sandoz-Losartan HCT; Sandoz-Losartan HCT DS; Teva-Losartan/HCTZ

Index Terms Hydrochlorothiazide and Losartan

Pharmacologic Category Angiotensin II Receptor Blocker; Antihypertensive; Diuretic, Thiazide

Use Treatment of hypertension; stroke risk reduction in patients with HTN and left ventricular hypertrophy (LVH)

Pregnancy Risk Factor C/D (2nd and 3rd trimesters)

Dosage Oral: Adults: Dose is individualized (combination substituted for individual components); dose may be titrated after 2-4 weeks of therapy
Hypertension/stroke reduction in hypertension (with LVH): Usual recommended starting dose of losartan: 50 mg once daily when used as monotherapy in patients who are not volume depleted

Dosage adjustment in renal impairment: Cl_{cr} ≤30 mL/minute: Use of combination formulation not recommended

Dosage adjustment in hepatic impairment: Use is not recommended

Additional Information Complete prescribing information should be consulted for additional detail.

Dosage Forms Excipient information presented when available (limited, particularly for generics); consult specific product labeling.
Tablet, oral: 50/12.5: Losartan potassium 50 mg and hydrochlorothiazide 12.5 mg; 100/12.5: Losartan potassium 100 mg and hydrochlorothiazide 12.5 mg; 100/25: Losartan potassium 100 mg and hydrochlorothiazide 25 mg
Hyzaar® 50/12.5: Losartan potassium 50 mg and hydrochlorothiazide 12.5 mg [contains potassium 4.24 mg (0.108 mEq)]
Hyzaar® 100/12.5: Losartan potassium 100 mg and hydrochlorothiazide 12.5 mg [contains potassium 8.48 mg (0.216 mEq)]
Hyzaar® 100/25: Losartan potassium 100 mg and hydrochlorothiazide 25 mg [contains potassium 8.48 mg (0.216 mEq)]

◆ **Losartan-HCT (Can)** *see* Losartan and Hydrochlorothiazide *on page 1249*

◆ **Losartan-HCTZ (Can)** *see* Losartan and Hydrochlorothiazide *on page 1249*

◆ **Losartan Potassium** *see* Losartan *on page 1247*

◆ **LoSeasonique** *see* Ethinyl Estradiol and Levonorgestrel *on page 787*

◆ **Losec® (Can)** *see* Omeprazole *on page 1505*

◆ **Lotemax** *see* Loteprednol *on page 1250*

◆ **Lotemax® (Can)** *see* Loteprednol *on page 1250*

◆ **Lotensin** *see* Benazepril *on page 234*

◆ **Lotensin HCT®** *see* Benazepril and Hydrochlorothiazide *on page 236*

Loteprednol (loe te PRED nol)

Brand Names: U.S. Alrex; Lotemax

Brand Names: Canada Alrex®; Lotemax®

Index Terms Loteprednol Etabonate

Pharmacologic Category Corticosteroid, Ophthalmic

Use

Alrex®: Temporary relief of signs and symptoms of seasonal allergic conjunctivitis

Lotemax®: Treatment of postoperative inflammation and pain following ocular surgery; treatment of inflammatory conditions (eg, steroid-responsive inflammatory conditions of the palpebral and bulbar conjunctiva, cornea, and anterior segment of the globe such as allergic conjunctivitis, acne rosacea, superficial punctate keratitis, herpes zoster keratitis, iritis, cyclitis, selected infective conjunctivitis, when the inherent hazard of steroid use is accepted to obtain an advisable diminution in edema and inflammation)

Pregnancy Risk Factor C

Dosage

Seasonal allergic conjunctivitis: Ophthalmic: Alrex® 0.2% suspension: Instill 1 drop into affected eye(s) 4 times daily.

Inflammatory conditions: Ophthalmic: Lotemax® 0.5% suspension: Instill 1-2 drops into the conjunctival sac of the affected eye(s) 4 times daily. During the initial treatment within the first week, the dosing may be increased up to 1 drop every hour. Advise patients not to discontinue therapy prematurely. If signs and symptoms fail to improve after 2 days, re-evaluate the patient.

Postoperative inflammation: Ophthalmic:

Lotemax® 0.5% ointment: Apply ~1/2 inch ribbon into the conjunctival sac of the affected eye(s) 4 times daily beginning 24 hours after surgery and continuing throughout the first 2 weeks of the postoperative period.

Lotemax® 0.5% gel, 0.5% suspension: Instill 1-2 drops into the conjunctival sac of the affected eye(s) 4 times daily beginning 24 hours after surgery and continuing throughout the first 2 weeks of the postoperative period.

Dosage adjustment in renal impairment: No dosage adjustment provided in manufacturer's labeling. However, dosage adjustment unlikely due to low systemic absorption.

Dosage adjustment in hepatic impairment: No dosage adjustment provided in manufacturer's labeling. However, dosage adjustment unlikely due to low systemic absorption.

Additional Information Complete prescribing information should be consulted for additional detail.

Dosage Forms Excipient information presented when available (limited, particularly for generics); consult specific product labeling.

Gel, Ophthalmic, as etabonate:

Lotemax: 0.5% (5 g) [contains benzalkonium chloride, edetate disodium dihydrate, propylene glycol]

Ointment, Ophthalmic, as etabonate:

Lotemax: 0.5% (3.5 g)

Suspension, Ophthalmic, as etabonate:

Alrex: 0.2% (5 mL, 10 mL)

Lotemax: 0.5% (5 mL, 10 mL, 15 mL)

Loteprednol and Tobramycin
(loe te PRED nol & toe bra MYE sin)

Brand Names: U.S. Zylet®

Index Terms Loteprednol Etabonate and Tobramycin; Tobramycin and Loteprednol Etabonate

Pharmacologic Category Antibiotic/Corticosteroid, Ophthalmic

Use Treatment of steroid-responsive ocular inflammatory conditions where either a superficial bacterial ocular infection or the risk of a superficial bacterial ocular infection exists

Pregnancy Risk Factor C

Dosage Ophthalmic: Children and Adults: Instill 1-2 drops into the affected eye(s) every 4-6 hours; may increase frequency during the first 24-48 hours to every 1-2 hours. Interval should increase as signs and symptoms improve. Further evaluation should occur for use of greater than 20 mL.

Dosage adjustment in renal impairment: No dosage adjustment provided in manufacturer's labeling. However, dosage adjustment unlikely due to low systemic absorption.

Dosage adjustment in hepatic impairment: No dosage adjustment provided in manufacturer's labeling. However, dosage adjustment unlikely due to low systemic absorption.

Additional Information Complete prescribing information should be consulted for additional detail.

Dosage Forms Excipient information presented when available (limited, particularly for generics); consult specific product labeling.

Suspension, ophthalmic [drops]:

Zylet®: Loteprednol etabonate 0.5% and tobramycin 0.3% (2.5 mL, 5 mL, 10 mL) [contains benzalkonium chloride]

◆ **Loteprednol Etabonate** *see* Loteprednol *on page 1250*

◆ **Loteprednol Etabonate and Tobramycin** *see* Loteprednol and Tobramycin *on page 1250*

◆ **Lotrel®** *see* Amlodipine and Benazepril *on page 111*

◆ **Lotriderm® (Can)** *see* Betamethasone and Clotrimazole *on page 249*

◆ **Lotrimin AF [OTC]** *see* Clotrimazole (Topical) *on page 476*

◆ **Lotrimin AF [OTC]** *see* Miconazole (Topical) *on page 1358*

◆ **Lotrimin AF Deodorant Powder [OTC]** *see* Miconazole (Topical) *on page 1358*

◆ **Lotrimin AF For Her [OTC]** *see* Clotrimazole (Topical) *on page 476*

◆ **Lotrimin AF Jock Itch Powder [OTC]** *see* Miconazole (Topical) *on page 1358*

◆ **Lotrimin AF Powder [OTC]** *see* Miconazole (Topical) *on page 1358*

◆ **Lotrimin Ultra [OTC]** *see* Butenafine *on page 305*

◆ **Lotrisone®** *see* Betamethasone and Clotrimazole *on page 249*

Lovastatin (LOE va sta tin)

Brand Names: U.S. Altoprev; Mevacor

Brand Names: Canada Apo-Lovastatin; Ava-Lovastatin; CO Lovastatin; Dom-Lovastatin; Mevacor; Mylan-Lovastatin; PHL-Lovastatin; PMS-Lovastatin; PRO-Lovastatin; Riva-Lovastatin; Sandoz-Lovastatin; Teva-Lovastatin

Index Terms Mevinolin; Monacolin K

Pharmacologic Category Antilipemic Agent, HMG-CoA Reductase Inhibitor

Use

Adjunct to dietary therapy to decrease elevated serum total and LDL-cholesterol concentrations in primary hypercholesterolemia

Primary prevention of coronary artery disease (patients without symptomatic disease with average to moderately elevated total and LDL-cholesterol and below average HDL-cholesterol); slow progression of coronary atherosclerosis in patients with coronary heart disease and reduce the risk of myocardial infarction, unstable angina, and coronary revascularization procedures.

Adjunct to dietary therapy in adolescent patients (10-17 years of age, females >1 year postmenarche) with heterozygous familial hypercholesterolemia having LDL >189 mg/dL, **or** LDL >160 mg/dL with positive family history of premature cardiovascular disease (CVD), **or** LDL >160 mg/dL with the presence of at least two other CVD risk factors

Primary and secondary prevention of atherosclerotic cardiovascular disease (ASCVD) according to the American College of Cardiology/American Heart Association: To reduce the risk of ASCVD in patients with clinical ASCVD (eg, coronary heart disease, stroke/TIA, or peripheral arterial disease presumed to be of atherosclerotic origin) who are greater than 75 years of age or not a candidate for high-intensity statin therapy; in patients without clinical ASCVD if LDL-C is 190 mg/dL or greater and not a candidate for high-intensity statin therapy; in patients without clinical ASCVD who have type 1 or type 2 diabetes and are between 40 and 75 years of age; in patients with an estimated 10-year ASCVD risk 7.5% or greater and who are between 40 and 75 years of age (Stone, 2013).

Pregnancy Risk Factor X

Pregnancy Considerations Adverse events were observed in animal reproduction studies. There are reports of congenital anomalies following maternal use of HMG-CoA reductase inhibitors in pregnancy; however, maternal disease, differences in specific agents used, and the low rates of exposure limit the interpretation of the available data (Godfrey, 2012; Lecarpentier, 2012). Cholesterol biosynthesis may be important in fetal development; serum cholesterol and triglycerides increase normally during pregnancy. The discontinuation of lipid lowering medications temporarily during pregnancy is not expected to have significant impact on the long term outcomes of primary hypercholesterolemia treatment.

Use of lovastatin is contraindicated in pregnancy. HMG-CoA reductase inhibitors should be discontinued prior to pregnancy (ADA, 2013). If treatment of dyslipidemias is needed in pregnant women or in women of reproductive age, other agents are preferred (Berglund, 2012; Stone, 2013). The manufacturer recommends administration to women of childbearing potential only when conception is highly unlikely and patients have been informed of potential hazards.

Breast-Feeding Considerations It is not known if lovastatin is excreted into breast milk. Due to the potential for serious adverse reactions in a nursing infant, use while breast-feeding is contraindicated by the manufacturer.

Contraindications Hypersensitivity to lovastatin or any component of the formulation; active liver disease; unexplained persistent elevations of serum transaminases; concomitant use of strong CYP3A4 inhibitors (eg, clarithromycin, erythromycin, itraconazole, ketoconazole, nefazodone, posaconazole, voriconazole, protease inhibitors [including boceprevir and telaprevir], telithromycin); pregnancy; breast-feeding

Canadian labeling: Additional contraindications (not in U.S. labeling): Concomitant use of cyclosporine

Warnings/Precautions Secondary causes of hyperlipidemia should be ruled out prior to therapy. Liver enzyme tests should be obtained at baseline and as clinically indicated; routine periodic monitoring of liver enzymes is not necessary. Use with caution in patients who consume large amounts of ethanol or have a history of liver disease; use is contraindicated with active liver disease and with unexplained transaminase elevations. Rhabdomyolysis with or without acute renal failure has occurred. Risk of rhabdomyolysis is dose-related and increased with concurrent use of lipid-lowering agents which may also cause rhabdomyolysis (fibric acid derivatives or niacin at doses ≥1 g/day) or during concurrent use with potent CYP3A4 inhibitors. Use is contraindicated in patients taking strong CYP3A4 inhibitors. Concomitant use of lovastatin with some drugs may require cautious use, may not be recommended, may require dosage adjustments, or may be contraindicated. Increases in Hb A_{1c} and fasting blood glucose have been reported with HMG-CoA reductase inhibitors; however, the benefits of statin therapy far outweigh the risk of dysglycemia. Monitor closely if used with other drugs associated with myopathy (eg, colchicine). Patients should be instructed to report unexplained muscle pain or weakness; lovastatin should be discontinued if myopathy is suspected/confirmed. Immune-mediated necrotizing myopathy (IMNM), an autoimmune-mediated myopathy, has been reported (rarely) with HMG-CoA reductase inhibitor therapy. IMNM presents as proximal muscle weakness with elevated CPK levels, which persists despite discontinuation of HMG-CoA reductase inhibitor therapy; additionally, muscle biopsy may show necrotizing myopathy with limited inflammation; immunosuppressive therapy (eg, corticosteroids, azathioprine) may be used for treatment. The manufacturer recommends temporary discontinuation for elective major surgery, acute medical or surgical conditions, or in any patient experiencing an acute or serious condition predisposing to renal failure (eg, sepsis, hypotension, trauma, uncontrolled seizures). However, based upon current evidence, HMG-CoA reductase inhibitor therapy should be continued in the perioperative period unless risk outweighs cardioprotective benefit. Use with caution in patients with advanced age; these patients are predisposed to myopathy.

Adverse Reactions Percentages as reported with immediate release tablets; similar adverse reactions seen with extended release tablets.

>10%: Neuromuscular & skeletal: CPK increased (>2x normal) (11%)

1% to 10%:

- Central nervous system: Headache (2% to 3%), dizziness (≤1%)
- Dermatologic: Rash (≤1%)
- Gastrointestinal: Flatulence (4% to 5%), constipation (2% to 4%), abdominal pain (2% to 3%), diarrhea (2% to 3%), nausea (2% to 3%), dyspepsia (1% to 2%)
- Neuromuscular & skeletal: Myalgia (2% to 3%), weakness (1% to 2%), muscle cramps (≤1%)
- Ocular: Blurred vision (≤1%)

<1% (Limited to important or life-threatening): Acid regurgitation, alopecia, amnesia (reversible), arthralgia, blood glucose increased, chest pain, cognitive impairment (reversible), confusion (reversible), dermatomyositis, diabetes mellitus (new onset), eye irritation, glycosylated hemoglobin (Hb A_{1c}) increased, insomnia, leg pain, memory disturbance (reversible), memory impairment (reversible), paresthesia, pruritus, vomiting, xerostomia

Additional class-related events or case reports (not necessarily reported with lovastatin therapy): Alkaline phosphatase increased, alteration in taste, anaphylaxis, angioedema, anorexia, anxiety, arthritis, cataracts, chills, cholestatic jaundice, cirrhosis, depression, dryness of skin/mucous membranes, dyspnea, eosinophilia, erectile dysfunction, erythema multiforme, ESR increased, facial ▶

paresis, fatty liver, fever, flushing, fulminant hepatic necrosis, GGT increased, gynecomastia, hemolytic anemia, hepatic failure (fatal and nonfatal), hepatitis, hepatoma, hyperbilirubinemia, hypersensitivity reaction, immune-mediated necrotizing myopathy (IMNM), impaired extraocular muscle movement, impotence, interstitial lung disease, leukopenia, libido decreased, malaise, myopathy, nail changes, nodules, ophthalmoplegia, pancreatitis, peripheral nerve palsy, peripheral neuropathy, photosensitivity, polymyalgia rheumatica, positive ANA, psychic disturbance, purpura, renal failure (secondary to rhabdomyolysis), rhabdomyolysis, skin discoloration, Stevens-Johnson syndrome, systemic lupus erythematosus-like syndrome, thrombocytopenia, thyroid dysfunction, toxic epidermal necrolysis, transaminases increased, tremor, urticaria, vasculitis, vertigo

Drug Interactions

Metabolism/Transport Effects **Substrate** of CYP3A4 (major), P-glycoprotein; **Note:** Assignment of Major/Minor substrate status based on clinically relevant drug interaction potential; **Inhibits** CYP2C9 (weak), CYP3A4 (weak)

Avoid Concomitant Use

Avoid concomitant use of Lovastatin with any of the following: Boceprevir; Clarithromycin; CycloSPORINE (Systemic); CYP3A4 Inhibitors (Strong); Erythromycin (Systemic); Fusidic Acid (Systemic); Gemfibrozil; Lomitapide; Mifepristone; Pimozide; Protease Inhibitors; Red Yeast Rice; Telaprevir; Telithromycin

Increased Effect/Toxicity

Lovastatin may increase the levels/effects of: ARIPiprazole; DAPTOmycin; Diltiazem; Dofetilide; PAZOPanib; Pimozide; Trabectedin; Vitamin K Antagonists

The levels/effects of Lovastatin may be increased by: Amiodarone; Azithromycin (Systemic); Bezafibrate; Boceprevir; Clarithromycin; Colchicine; CycloSPORINE (Systemic); CYP3A4 Inhibitors (Moderate); CYP3A4 Inhibitors (Strong); Cyproterone; Danazol; Dasatinib; Diltiazem; Dronedarone; Erythromycin (Systemic); Fenofibrate and Derivatives; Fluconazole; Fusidic Acid (Systemic); Gemfibrozil; Grapefruit Juice; Ivacaftor; Lomitapide; Luliconazole; Mifepristone; Niacin; Niacinamide; P-glycoprotein/ABCB1 Inhibitors; Protease Inhibitors; QuiNINE; Raltegravir; Ranolazine; Red Yeast Rice; Sildenafil; Simeprevir; Telaprevir; Telithromycin; Ticagrelor; Verapamil

Decreased Effect

Lovastatin may decrease the levels/effects of: Lanthanum

The levels/effects of Lovastatin may be decreased by: Antacids; Bosentan; CYP3A4 Inducers (Strong); Dabrafenib; Deferasirox; Efavirenz; Etravirine; Fosphenytoin; Mitotane; P-glycoprotein/ABCB1 Inducers; Phenytoin; Rifamycin Derivatives; St Johns Wort; Tocilizumab

Ethanol/Nutrition/Herb Interactions

Ethanol: Excessive ethanol consumption may have harmful hepatic effects. Management: Avoid excessive ethanol consumption.

Food: Food decreases the bioavailability of lovastatin extended release tablets and increases the bioavailability of lovastatin immediate release tablets. Lovastatin serum concentrations may be increased if taken with grapefruit juice. Management: Avoid concurrent intake of large quantities (>1 quart/day) of grapefruit juice. Red yeast rice contains an estimated 2.4 mg lovastatin per 600 mg rice.

Herb/Nutraceutical: St John's wort may decrease lovastatin levels.

Storage/Stability

Tablet, immediate release: Store at 20°C to 25°C (68°F to 77°F). Protect from light

Tablet, extended release: Store at 20°C to 25°C (68°F to 77°F); excursions permitted between 15°C to 30°C (59°F to 86°F). Avoid excessive heat and humidity.

Mechanism of Action Lovastatin acts by competitively inhibiting 3-hydroxyl-3-methylglutaryl-coenzyme A (HMG-CoA) reductase, the enzyme that catalyzes the rate-limiting step in cholesterol biosynthesis

Pharmacodynamics/Kinetics

Onset of action: LDL-cholesterol reductions: 3 days

Absorption: 30%; increased with extended release tablets when taken in the fasting state

Protein binding: >95%

Metabolism: Hepatic; extensive first-pass effect; hydrolyzed to β-hydroxyacid (active)

Bioavailability: Increased with extended release tablets

Half-life elimination: 1.1-1.7 hours

Time to peak, serum: Immediate release: 2-4 hours; extended release: 12-14 hours

Excretion: Feces (~80% to 85%); urine (10%)

Dosage

Adolescents 10-17 years: Oral: Immediate release tablet:

LDL reduction <20%: Initial: 10 mg daily with evening meal

LDL reduction ≥20%: Initial: 20 mg daily with evening meal

Usual range: 10-40 mg once daily with evening meal, then adjust dose at 4-week intervals; maximum dose per manufacturer: 40 mg daily

Adults: Oral:

Immediate release: Initial: 20 mg once daily with evening meal, then adjust at 4-week intervals; maximum dose: 80 mg daily

Extended release: Initial: 20, 40, or 60 mg once daily at bedtime, then adjust at 4-week intervals; maximum dose: 60 mg daily

Note: Doses should be individualized according to the baseline LDL-cholesterol levels, the recommended goal of therapy, and patient response. For patients requiring smaller reductions in cholesterol, the use of the extended release tablet is not recommended; consider use of immediate release formulation.

ACC/AHA Blood Cholesterol Guideline recommendations to reduce the risk of atherosclerotic cardiovascular disease (ASCVD) (Stone, 2013): Adults ≥21 years: Oral:

Primary prevention:

LDL-C ≥190 mg/dL: High intensity therapy necessary; use alternate statin therapy (eg, atorvastatin or rosuvastatin)

Type 1 or 2 diabetes and age 40-75 years: Moderate intensity therapy: Immediate release: 40 mg once daily

Type 1 or 2 diabetes, age 40-75 years, and an estimated 10-year ASCVD risk ≥7.5%: High intensity therapy necessary; use alternate statin therapy (eg, atorvastatin or rosuvastatin)

Age 40-75 years and an estimated 10-year ASCVD risk ≥7.5%: Moderate to high intensity therapy: Immediate release: 40 mg once daily or consider using high intensity statin therapy (eg, atorvastatin or rosuvastatin)

Secondary prevention:

Patient has clinical ASCVD (eg, coronary heart disease, stroke/TIA, or peripheral arterial disease presumed to be of atherosclerotic origin) **and:**

Age ≤75 years: High intensity therapy necessary; use alternate statin therapy (eg, atorvastatin or rosuvastatin)

Age >75 years or not a candidate for high intensity therapy: Moderate intensity therapy: Immediate release: 40 mg once daily

Elderly: Immediate release: Refer to adult dosing; Extended release: Initial: 20 mg once daily at bedtime

Dosage adjustment for lovastatin with concomitant medications:

Amiodarone: Maximum recommended lovastatin dose (extended release and immediate release): 40 mg daily

Danazol, diltiazem, dronedarone, or verapamil: Initial lovastatin (immediate release) dose: 10 mg daily; Maximum recommended lovastatin (extended release and immediate release) dose: 20 mg daily

Lomitapide: Consider lovastatin dose reduction (per lomitapide manufacturer).

Dosage adjustment for toxicity:

Severe muscle symptoms or fatigue: Promptly discontinue use; evaluate CPK, creatinine, and urinalysis for myoglobinuria (Stone, 2013).

Mild to moderate muscle symptoms: Discontinue use until symptoms can be evaluated; evaluate patient for conditions that may increase the risk for muscle symptoms (eg, hypothyroidism, reduced renal or hepatic function, rheumatologic disorders such as polymyalgia rheumatica, steroid myopathy, vitamin D deficiency, or primary muscle diseases). Upon resolution, resume the original or lower dose of lovastatin. If muscle symptoms recur, discontinue lovastatin use. After muscle symptom resolution, may then use a low dose of a different statin; gradually increase if tolerated. In the absence of continued statin use, if muscle symptoms or elevated CPK continues after 2 months, consider other causes of muscle symptoms. If determined to be due to another condition aside from statin use, may resume statin therapy at the original dose (Stone, 2013).

Dosage adjustment in renal impairment: Cl_{cr} <30 mL/minute: Use with caution and carefully consider doses >20 mg/day.

Dosage adjustment in hepatic impairment: No dosage adjustment provided in manufacturer's labeling (has not been studied).

Dietary Considerations Before initiation of therapy, patients should be placed on a standard cholesterol-lowering diet for 6 weeks and the diet should be continued during drug therapy. Avoid intake of large quantities of grapefruit juice (≥1 quart/day); may increase toxicity. Red yeast rice contains an estimated 2.4 mg lovastatin per 600 mg rice. Immediate release tablet should be taken with the evening meal.

Administration Administer immediate release tablet with the evening meal. Administer extended release tablet at bedtime; do not crush or chew.

Monitoring Parameters

2013 ACC/AHA Blood Cholesterol Guideline recommendations (Stone, 2013):

Lipid panel (total cholesterol, HDL, LDL, triglycerides): Baseline lipid panel; fasting lipid profile within 4-12 weeks after initiation or dose adjustment and every 3-12 months (as clinically indicated) thereafter. If 2 consecutive LDL levels are <40 mg/dL, consider decreasing the dose.

Hepatic transaminase levels: Baseline measurement of hepatic transaminase levels (ie, ALT); measure hepatic function if symptoms suggest hepatotoxicity (eg, unusual fatigue or weakness, loss of appetite, abdominal pain, dark-colored urine or yellowing of skin or sclera) during therapy.

CPK: CPK should not be routinely measured. Baseline CPK measurement is reasonable for some individuals (eg, family history of statin intolerance or muscle disease, clinical presentation, concomitant drug therapy that may increase risk of myopathy). May measure CPK in any patient with symptoms suggestive of myopathy (pain, tenderness, stiffness, cramping, weakness, or generalized fatigue).

Evaluate for new-onset diabetes mellitus during therapy; if diabetes develops, continue statin therapy and encourage adherence to a heart-healthy diet, physical activity, a healthy body weight, and tobacco cessation.

If patient develops a confusional state or memory impairment, may evaluate patient for nonstatin causes (eg, exposure to other drugs), systemic and neuropsychiatric causes, and the possibility of adverse effects associated with statin therapy.

Manufacturer recommendations: Liver enzyme tests at baseline and repeated when clinically indicated. Measure CPK when myopathy is being considered or may measure CPK periodically in patients starting therapy or when dosage increase is necessary. Analyze lipid panel at intervals of 4 weeks or more.

Dosage Forms Excipient information presented when available (limited, particularly for generics); consult specific product labeling.

Tablet, Oral:
- Mevacor: 20 mg, 40 mg
- Generic: 10 mg, 20 mg, 40 mg

Tablet Extended Release 24 Hour, Oral:
- Altoprev: 20 mg, 40 mg, 60 mg [contains fd&c yellow #6 (sunset yellow)]

- ◆ **Lovastatin and Niacin** *see* Niacin and Lovastatin *on page 1450*
- ◆ **Lovaza** *see* Omega-3-Acid Ethyl Esters *on page 1504*
- ◆ **Lovenox** *see* Enoxaparin *on page 705*
- ◆ **Lovenox HP (Can)** *see* Enoxaparin *on page 705*
- ◆ **Low-Molecular-Weight Iron Dextran (INFeD)** *see* Iron Dextran Complex *on page 1119*
- ◆ **Low-Ogestrel** *see* Ethinyl Estradiol and Norgestrel *on page 797*
- ◆ **Loxapac (Can)** *see* Loxapine *on page 1253*

Loxapine (LOKS a peen)

Brand Names: U.S. Loxitane

Brand Names: Canada Apo-Loxapine; Dom-Loxapine; Loxapac; PHL-Loxapine; Xylac

Index Terms Loxapine Succinate; Oxilapine Succinate

Pharmacologic Category Antipsychotic Agent, Typical

Additional Appendix Information

Antipsychotic Agents *on page 2290*

Beers Criteria – Potentially Inappropriate Medications for Geriatrics *on page 2368*

Use

Schizophrenia: Oral: Treatment of schizophrenia.

Agitation associated with schizophrenia or bipolar I disorder: Inhalation: Acute treatment of agitation associated with schizophrenia or bipolar I disorder in adults.

Pregnancy Risk Factor C

Prescribing and Access Restrictions Adasuve is only available through a restricted program called Adasuve REMS. In order to distribute, dispense and administer Adasuve, healthcare facilities must be enrolled and comply with REMS requirements (including on-site access to equipment and personnel to provide advance airway management including intubation and mechanical ventilation). Information is available at www.adasuverems.com or 888-970-7367.

Medication Guide Available Yes

Dosage

Psychosis:

Oral:

Adults: Initial: 10 mg twice daily (up to 50 mg daily may be considered in severely disturbed patients), increase dose until psychotic symptoms are controlled; usual maintenance: 60-100 mg daily in divided doses 2-4 times daily; satisfactory response often observed with doses of 20-60 mg daily (maximum: 250 mg daily). Therapy should be maintained at lowest effective dose.

Elderly: Reduced dosing may be indicated due to risks of adverse events associated with high-dose therapy.

I.M. (Canadian availability; not available in the U.S.): Adults: 12.5-50 mg every 4-6 hours or longer; individualize dose early in therapy; some patients respond satisfactorily to twice-daily dosing

Acute treatment of agitation associated with schizophrenia or bipolar I disorder: Inhalation: 10 mg once daily; maximum dose 10 mg per 24-hour period

Dosage adjustment in renal impairment: No dosage adjustment provided in manufacturer's labeling.

Dosage adjustment in hepatic impairment: No dosage adjustment provided in manufacturer's labeling. Canadian labeling does not recommend use in severe hepatic disease.

Additional Information Complete prescribing information should be consulted for additional detail.

Product Availability Adasuve oral inhalation: FDA approved December 2012; anticipated availability is currently unknown

Dosage Forms Excipient information presented when available (limited, particularly for generics); consult specific product labeling. [DSC] = Discontinued product

Capsule, Oral:

Loxitane: 5 mg, 10 mg [DSC], 25 mg [DSC]

Generic: 5 mg, 10 mg, 25 mg, 50 mg

Dosage Forms: Canada Excipient information presented when available (limited, particularly for generics); consult specific product labeling.

Injection, solution, as hydrochloride [strength expressed as base]:

Loxapac: 50 mg/mL (1 mL) [contains polysorbate 80, propylene glycol]

Solution, oral, as hydrochloride [strength expressed as base; concentrate]:

Xylac: 25 mg/mL (100 mL) [contains propylene glycol]

Tablet, oral, as succinate [strength expressed as base]:

Xylac: 2.5 mg, 5 mg, 10 mg, 25 mg, 50 mg

- ◆ **Loxapine Succinate** *see* Loxapine *on page* 1253
- ◆ **Loxitane** *see* Loxapine *on page* 1253
- ◆ **Lozide® (Can)** *see* Indapamide *on page* 1066
- ◆ **Lozi-Flur™** *see* Fluoride *on page* 880
- ◆ **L-PAM** *see* Melphalan *on page* 1286
- ◆ **L-Phenylalanine Mustard** *see* Melphalan *on page* 1286
- ◆ **L-Sarcolysin** *see* Melphalan *on page* 1286
- ◆ **LTA 360 Kit** *see* Lidocaine (Topical) *on page* 1212
- ◆ **LTG** *see* LamoTRIgine *on page* 1165
- ◆ ***L*-Thyroxine Sodium** *see* Levothyroxine *on page* 1206
- ◆ **Lu-26-054** *see* Escitalopram *on page* 745
- ◆ **Lu AA21004** *see* Vortioxetine *on page* 2208

Lubiprostone (loo bi PROS tone)

Brand Names: U.S. Amitiza

Index Terms RU 0211; SPI 0211

Pharmacologic Category Chloride Channel Activator; Gastrointestinal Agent, Miscellaneous

Additional Appendix Information

Laxatives, Classification and Properties *on page* 2304

Use Treatment of chronic idiopathic constipation; treatment of opioid-induced constipation with chronic non-cancer pain; treatment of irritable bowel syndrome with constipation in adult women

Pregnancy Risk Factor C

Dosage

Chronic idiopathic constipation: Adults: Oral: 24 mcg twice daily

Irritable bowel syndrome with constipation: Females ≥18 years: Oral: 8 mcg twice daily

Opioid-induced constipation: Adults: Oral: 24 mcg twice daily

Dosage adjustment for renal impairment: No dosage adjustment necessary.

Dosage adjustment for hepatic impairment:

Mild hepatic impairment (Child-Pugh class A): No dosage adjustment necessary.

Moderate hepatic impairment (Child-Pugh class B):

Chronic idiopathic constipation: Initial: 16 mcg twice daily; may increase to 24 mcg twice daily if tolerated and an adequate response has not been obtained with lower dosage.

Irritable bowel syndrome with constipation: No dosage adjustment necessary.

Opioid-induced constipation: Initial: 16 mcg twice daily; may increase to 24 mcg twice daily if tolerated and an adequate response has not been obtained with lower dosage.

Severe hepatic impairment (Child-Pugh class C):

Chronic idiopathic constipation: Initial: 8 mcg twice daily; may increase to 16-24 mcg twice daily if tolerated and an adequate response has not been obtained with lower dosage.

Irritable bowel syndrome with constipation: Initial: 8 mcg once daily; may increase to 8 mcg twice daily if tolerated and an adequate response has not been obtained at lower dosage.

Opioid-induced constipation: Initial: 8 mcg twice daily; may increase to 16-24 mcg twice daily if tolerated and an adequate response has not been obtained with lower dosage.

Additional Information Complete prescribing information should be consulted for additional detail.

Dosage Forms Excipient information presented when available (limited, particularly for generics); consult specific product labeling.

Capsule, Oral:

Amitiza: 8 mcg

Amitiza: 24 mcg [contains fd&c red #40, fd&c yellow #10 (quinoline yellow)]

- ◆ **Lucentis** *see* Ranibizumab *on page* 1781
- ◆ **Lucentis® (Can)** *see* Ranibizumab *on page* 1781

Lucinactant (loo sin AK tant)

Brand Names: U.S. Surfaxin

Pharmacologic Category Lung Surfactant

Use Prevention of respiratory distress syndrome (RDS) in premature infants at high risk for RDS

Contraindications There are no contraindications listed within the FDA-approved labeling.

Warnings/Precautions For endotracheal administration only. Rapidly affects oxygenation and lung compliance; restrict use to a highly-supervised clinical setting with immediate availability of clinicians experienced in intubation and ventilatory management of premature infants. Transient episodes of bradycardia, decreased oxygen saturation, endotracheal tube blockage, or reflux of lucinactant into endotracheal tube may occur. Interrupt dosing procedure and initiate measures to stabilize infant's condition; may reinstitute after the patient is stable. Produces rapid improvements in lung oxygenation and compliance that may require frequent adjustments to oxygen delivery and ventilator settings. In clinical trials of lucinactant in adults with acute respiratory distress syndrome (ARDS), an increased incidence of sepsis, pneumothorax, pulmonary embolism, hypotension, sepsis, and death was observed; therapy is not appropriate in the treatment of ARDS in adults.

Adverse Reactions Events observed during the dosing procedure:

>10%:

Local: Endotracheal tube reflux (18% to 27%), endotracheal tube obstruction (6% to 16%)

Respiratory: Oxygen desaturation (8% to 17%)

1% to 10%: Cardiovascular: Bradycardia (3% to 5%)

Drug Interactions

Metabolism/Transport Effects None known.

Avoid Concomitant Use There are no known interactions where it is recommended to avoid concomitant use.

Increased Effect/Toxicity There are no known significant interactions involving an increase in effect.

Decreased Effect There are no known significant interactions involving a decrease in effect.

Preparation for Administration Prior to administration, warm by placing vial in a preheated dry block heater set at 44°C (111°F) for 15 minutes. After warming, shake vial vigorously until a uniform and free-flowing suspension appears. If not used immediately, may store protected from light for up to 2 hours at room temperature after warming; do not return to refrigerator. Discard vial or any unused part if not used within 2 hours.

Storage/Stability Store intact vials refrigerated at 2°C to 8°C (36°F to 46°F); do not freeze. Protect from light.

Mechanism of Action Surfactant administration replaces deficient or ineffective endogenous lung surfactant in neonates at risk of developing RDS. Surfactant prevents the alveoli from collapsing during expiration by lowering surface tension between air and alveolar surfaces. Lucinactant, a synthetic surfactant containing phospholipids, also contains sinapultide (KL4 peptide) which resembles and is believed to mimic the action of one of the human surfactant proteins (SPs), namely SP-B.

Dosage Endotracheal: Respiratory distress prophylaxis: Premature infants: 5.8 mL/kg birth weight; up to 3 subsequent doses (total of 4 doses) may be administered at ≥6-hour intervals within the first 48 hours of life

Dosage adjustment in renal impairment: No dosage adjustment provided in manufacturer's labeling.

Dosage adjustment in hepatic impairment: No dosage adjustment provided in manufacturer's labeling.

Administration For endotracheal administration only. Prior to administration, the vial containing lucinactant must be properly warmed, followed by vigorous shaking until the suspension is uniform, free-flowing, and opaque white to off-white.

Slowly draw up the appropriate amount of lucinactant into a single, appropriately sized syringe (depending on total dose volume) using a 16- or 18-gauge needle. Administer endotracheally by instillation through a 5-French end-hole catheter inserted into the infant's endotracheal tube with infant properly positioned.

Administer the dose in 4 aliquots (each aliquot to be one-fourth of total volume). Each quarter-dose is instilled as a bolus followed by a pause to evaluate infant's respiratory status. Each quarter-dose is administered with the infant in a different position; slightly downward inclination with head turned to the right, then repeat with head turned to the left; then slightly upward inclination with head turned to the right, then repeat with head turned to the left. Following administration of one full dose, withhold suctioning for 1 hour unless signs of significant airway obstruction and keep infant's bed elevated ≥10° for 1-2 hours.

Monitoring Parameters Following administration, patients should be carefully monitored so that oxygen therapy and ventilatory support can be modified in response to changes in respiratory status; frequent arterial blood gases are necessary to prevent postdosing hyperoxia and hypocarbia

Additional Information Each mL contains 30 mg phospholipids (including 22.5 mg dipalmitoylphosphatidylcholine and 7.5 mg palmitoyloleoylphosphatidylglycerol).

- **Ludiomil** *see* Maprotiline *on page 1268*
- **Lugol's Solution** *see* Potassium Iodide and Iodine *on page 1689*
- **Lumefantrine and Artemether** *see* Artemether and Lumefantrine *on page 171*
- **Lumigan** *see* Bimatoprost *on page 259*
- **Lumigan® (Can)** *see* Bimatoprost *on page 259*
- **Lumigan® RC (Can)** *see* Bimatoprost *on page 259*
- **Luminal** *see* PHENobarbital *on page 1629*
- **Luminal Sodium** *see* PHENobarbital *on page 1629*
- **Lumizyme** *see* Alglucosidase Alfa *on page 74*
- **Lunesta** *see* Eszopiclone *on page 778*
- **Lupaneta Pack** *see* Leuprolide and Norethindrone *on page 1192*
- **Lupron (Can)** *see* Leuprolide *on page 1189*
- **Lupron Depot** *see* Leuprolide *on page 1189*
- **Lupron Depot-Ped** *see* Leuprolide *on page 1189*

Lurasidone (loo RAS i done)

Brand Names: U.S. Latuda

Brand Names: Canada Latuda

Index Terms Lurasidone Hydrochloride; SM-13496

Pharmacologic Category Antipsychotic Agent, Atypical

Additional Appendix Information

Antipsychotic Agents *on page 2290*

Beers Criteria – Potentially Inappropriate Medications for Geriatrics *on page 2368*

Use Psychiatric issues:

U.S. labeling: Treatment of schizophrenia; monotherapy or adjunctive therapy of depressive episodes associated with bipolar I disorder

Canadian labeling: Treatment of schizophrenia

Pregnancy Risk Factor B

Pregnancy Considerations Adverse events were not observed in animal reproduction studies. Antipsychotic use during the third trimester of pregnancy has a risk for abnormal muscle movements (extrapyramidal symptoms [EPS]) and/or withdrawal symptoms in newborns following delivery. Symptoms in the newborn may include agitation, feeding disorder, hypertonia, hypotonia, respiratory distress, somnolence, and tremor; these effects may be self-limiting or require hospitalization. Lurasidone may cause hyperprolactinemia, which may decrease reproductive function in both males and females.

The ACOG recommends that therapy during pregnancy be individualized; treatment with psychiatric medications during pregnancy should incorporate the clinical expertise of the mental health clinician, obstetrician, primary healthcare provider, and pediatrician. Safety data related to atypical antipsychotics during pregnancy is limited and routine use is not recommended. However, if a woman is inadvertently exposed to an atypical antipsychotic while pregnant, continuing therapy may be preferable to switching to a typical antipsychotic that the fetus has not yet been exposed to; consider risk:benefit (ACOG, 2008).

Healthcare providers are encouraged to enroll women 18-45 years of age exposed to lurasidone during pregnancy in the Atypical Antipsychotics Pregnancy Registry (866-961-2388 or http://www.womensmentalhealth.org/pregnancyregistry).

Breast-Feeding Considerations It is not known if lurasidone is excreted in breast milk. Due to the potential for serious adverse reactions in the nursing infant, the manufacturer recommends a decision be made whether to discontinue nursing or to discontinue the drug, taking into account the importance of the treatment to the mother.

Contraindications Hypersensitivity to lurasidone or any component of the formulation; concomitant use with strong CYP3A4 inhibitors (eg, ketoconazole) and inducers (eg, rifampin)

Warnings/Precautions [U.S. Boxed Warning]: Antidepressants increase the risk of suicidal thinking and behavior in children, adolescents, and young adults (18-24 years of age) with major depressive disorder and other psychiatric disorders; consider risk prior to prescribing. Lurasidone is not approved in the U.S. for use in children. Short-term studies did not show an increased risk in patients >24 years of age and showed a decreased risk in patients ≥65 years. **[U.S. Boxed Warning]: Closely monitor all patients for clinical worsening, suicidality, or unusual changes in behavior,** particularly during the initial 1-2 months of therapy or during periods of dosage adjustments (increases or decreases); the patient's family or caregiver should be instructed to closely observe the patient and communicate condition with healthcare provider. A medication guide concerning the use of antidepressants should be dispensed with each prescription.

The possibility of a suicide attempt is inherent in major depression and may persist until remission occurs. Patients treated with antidepressants (for any indication) should be observed for clinical worsening and suicidality, especially during the initial few months of a course of drug therapy, or at times of dose changes (increases or decreases). Worsening depression and severe abrupt suicidality that are not part of the presenting symptoms may require discontinuation or modification of drug therapy. Use caution in high-risk patients during initiation of therapy.

Prescriptions should be written for the smallest quantity consistent with good patient care. The patient's family or caregiver should be alerted to monitor patients for the emergence of suicidality and associated behaviors such as anxiety, agitation, panic attacks, insomnia, irritability, hostility, impulsivity, akathisia, hypomania, and mania; patients should be instructed to notify their healthcare provider if any of these symptoms or worsening depression or psychosis occur.

[U.S. Boxed Warning]: Elderly patients with dementia-related psychosis treated with antipsychotics are at an increased risk of death compared to placebo. Most deaths appeared to be either cardiovascular (eg, heart failure, sudden death) or infectious (eg, pneumonia) in nature. **Lurasidone is not approved for the treatment of dementia-related psychosis.** An increased incidence of cerebrovascular effects (eg, transient ischemic attack, stroke), including fatalities, has been reported in placebo-controlled trials of antipsychotics for the unapproved use in elderly patients with dementia-related psychosis.

Leukopenia, neutropenia, and agranulocytosis (sometimes fatal) have been reported in clinical trials and postmarketing reports with antipsychotic use; presence of risk factors (eg, pre-existing low WBC or history of drug-induced leuko-/neutropenia) should prompt periodic blood count assessment. Discontinue therapy at first signs of blood dyscrasias or if absolute neutrophil count <1000/mm^3.

Low to moderately sedating, use with caution in disorders where CNS depression is a feature; patients must be cautioned about performing tasks which require mental alertness (eg, operating machinery or driving). Use with caution in Parkinson's disease. Caution in patients with predisposition to seizures, including those with a history of seizures, head trauma, brain damage, alcoholism, or concurrent therapy with medications which may lower seizure threshold. Elderly patients may be at increased risk of seizures due to an increased prevalence of predisposing factors. Use with caution in renal or hepatic dysfunction; dose reduction recommended in moderate-to-severe impairment. Esophageal dysmotility and aspiration have been associated with antipsychotic use; use with caution in patients at risk of aspiration pneumonia (ie, Alzheimer's disease). Use is associated with increased prolactin levels; clinical significance of hyperprolactinemia in patients with breast cancer or other prolactin-dependent tumors is unknown. May alter temperature regulation.

Use with caution in patients with severe cardiac disease, hemodynamic instability, prior myocardial infarction or ischemic heart disease. May cause orthostatic hypotension; use with caution in patients at risk of this effect (eg, concurrent medication use which may predispose to hypotension/bradycardia or presence of hypovolemia) or in those who would not tolerate transient hypotensive episodes. Antipsychotics may alter cardiac conduction; life-threatening arrhythmias have occurred with therapeutic doses of antipsychotics. Relative to other antipsychotics, lurasidone has minimal effects on the QT_c interval and therefore, risk for arrhythmias is low. However, Canadian labeling recommends avoiding use of lurasidone in patients with a history of cardiac arrhythmias, situations that may increase the risk of torsade de pointes and/or sudden death due to QT prolongation including bradycardia, congenital QT prolongation, electrolyte disturbances (ie, hypokalemia or hypomagnesemia), or in combination with other QT_c-prolonging agents. Increases in total cholesterol and triglyceride concentrations have been observed with atypical antipsychotic use; during clinical trials of lurasidone, there were no significant changes in total cholesterol or triglycerides observed. Potentially significant drug-drug interactions may exist, requiring dose or frequency adjustment, additional monitoring, and/or selection of alternative therapy. Consult drug interactions database for more detailed information.

May cause extrapyramidal symptoms (EPS), including pseudoparkinsonism, acute dystonic reactions, akathisia, and tardive dyskinesia (potentially irreversible). Risk of tardive dyskinesia may be increased in elderly patients, particularly elderly women. Risk of dystonia (and probably other EPS) may be greater with increased doses, use of conventional antipsychotics, males, and younger patients. Use may be associated with neuroleptic malignant syndrome (NMS); monitor for mental status changes, fever, muscle rigidity and/or autonomic instability (risk may be increased in patients with Parkinson's disease or Lewy body dementia). May cause hyperglycemia; in some cases may be extreme and associated with ketoacidosis, hyperosmolar coma, or death. Use with caution in patients with diabetes or other disorders of glucose regulation; monitor for worsening of glucose control. Significant weight gain has been observed with antipsychotic therapy; incidence varies with product. Monitor waist circumference and BMI.

Use in elderly patients with dementia is associated with an increased risk of mortality and cerebrovascular accidents; avoid antipsychotic use for behavioral problems associated with dementia unless alternative nonpharmacologic therapies have failed and patient may harm self or others. In addition, use may cause or exacerbate syndrome of inappropriate antidiuretic hormone secretion or hyponatremia; monitor sodium closely with initiation or dosage adjustments in older adults (Beers Criteria).

Adverse Reactions Frequencies reported for schizophrenia unless otherwise noted.

>10%:

Central nervous system: Drowsiness (dose-related: 8% to 27%; depressive episodes, monotherapy: 11%), extrapyramidal reaction (dose-related: 14% to 26%; depressive episodes, monotherapy: 7%), akathisia (dose-related: 6% to 22%; depressive episodes, monotherapy: 8% to 11%), parkinsonian-like syndrome (6% to 17%; depressive episodes, monotherapy: 8%)

Endocrine & metabolic: Increased serum triglycerides (10% to 14%), increased serum glucose (fasting, 10% to 14%), increased serum cholesterol (6% to 14%)

Gastrointestinal: Nausea (dose-related; 10%; depressive episodes, monotherapy: 14%)

1% to 10%:

Cardiovascular: Orthostatic hypotension (1% to 2%), tachycardia

Central nervous system: Insomnia (10%), agitation (5%; depressive episodes, monotherapy: 4%), anxiety (5%), dizziness (4%), dystonia (≤7%; depressive episodes, monotherapy: ≤2%), restlessness (1% to 3%)

Dermatologic: Pruritus, skin rash

Endocrine & metabolic: Increased serum prolactin (≥5 x ULN: females: 8%; males: ≤2%), weight gain (≥7% increase in baseline body weight: 2% to 6%)

Gastrointestinal: Vomiting (8%; depressive episodes, monotherapy: 4%), dyspepsia (6%), xerostomia (depressive episodes, monotherapy: 5%), diarrhea (≥1%; depressive episodes, monotherapy: 4%), sialorrhea (2%), abdominal pain, decreased appetite

Genitourinary: Urinary tract infection (depressive episodes, monotherapy: 2%)

Infection: Influenza (depressive episodes, monotherapy: 2%)

Neuromuscular & skeletal: Back pain (3%; depressive episodes, monotherapy: 2%), increased creatine phosphokinase

Ophthalmic: Blurred vision

Renal: Increased serum creatinine (3% to 7%; depressive episodes, monotherapy: 2% to 4%)

Respiratory: Nasopharyngitis (depressive episodes, monotherapy: 4%)

<1% (Limited to important or life-threatening): Amenorrhea, anemia, angina pectoris, angioedema, atrioventricular block, bradycardia, breast hypertrophy, cerebrovascular accident, gastritis, dysmenorrhea, erectile dysfunction, galactorrhea, hypertension, hypomania, leukopenia, mania, neuroleptic malignant syndrome, panic attack, renal failure, rhabdomyolysis, seizure, suicidal ideation, tardive dyskinesia

Drug Interactions

Metabolism/Transport Effects **Substrate** of CYP3A4 (major); **Note:** Assignment of Major/Minor substrate status based on clinically relevant drug interaction potential; **Inhibits** CYP3A4 (weak)

Avoid Concomitant Use

Avoid concomitant use of Lurasidone with any of the following: Amisulpride; Azelastine (Nasal); CYP3A4 Inducers (Strong); CYP3A4 Inhibitors (Strong); DOPamine; EPINEPHrine (Systemic, Oral Inhalation); Fusidic Acid (Systemic); Grapefruit Juice; Metoclopramide; Paraldehyde; Pimozide; St Johns Wort; Sulpiride

Increased Effect/Toxicity

Lurasidone may increase the levels/effects of: Alcohol (Ethyl); Amisulpride; ARIPiprazole; Azelastine (Nasal); Buprenorphine; CNS Depressants; Disopyramide; Dofetilide; Hydrocodone; Lomitapide; Methotrimeprazine; Methylphenidate; Paraldehyde; Pimozide; Procainamide; QuiNIDine; Serotonin Modulators; Sulpiride; Zolpidem

The levels/effects of Lurasidone may be increased by: Acetylcholinesterase Inhibitors (Central); Brimonidine (Topical); CYP3A4 Inhibitors (Moderate); CYP3A4 Inhibitors (Strong); Dasatinib; DOPamine; Doxylamine; Droperidol; EPINEPHrine (Systemic, Oral Inhalation); Fusidic Acid (Systemic); Grapefruit Juice; HydrOXYzine; Ivacaftor; Lithium formulations; Luliconazole; Magnesium Sulfate; MAO Inhibitors; Methotrimeprazine; Methylphenidate; Metoclopramide; Metyrosine; Mifepristone; Perampanel; Serotonin Modulators; Simeprevir; Sodium Oxybate; Tetrabenazine

Decreased Effect

Lurasidone may decrease the levels/effects of: Amphetamines; Anti-Parkinson's Agents (Dopamine Agonist); Quinagolide

The levels/effects of Lurasidone may be decreased by: Bosentan; CYP3A4 Inducers (Strong); Dabrafenib; Deferasirox; Lithium formulations; St Johns Wort; Tocilizumab

Ethanol/Nutrition/Herb Interactions

Ethanol: May increase CNS depression; monitor for increased effects with coadministration. Caution patients about effects.

Food: Administration with food (≥350 calories) increased C_{max} and AUC of lurasidone ~3 times and 2 times, respectively, compared to administration under fasting conditions. Lurasidone exposure was not affected by the fat content of the meal.

Storage/Stability Store at controlled room temperature of 25°C (77°F); excursions permitted to 15°C to 30°C (59°F to 86°F).

Mechanism of Action Lurasidone is a benzoisothiazol-derivative atypical antipsychotic with mixed serotonin-dopamine antagonist activity. It exhibits high affinity for D_2, 5-HT_{2A}, and 5-HT_7 receptors; moderate affinity for alpha$_{2C}$-adrenergic receptors; and is a partial agonist for 5-HT_{1A} receptors. Lurasidone has no significant affinity for muscarinic M_1 and histamine H_1 receptors. The addition of serotonin antagonism to dopamine antagonism (classic neuroleptic mechanism) is thought to improve negative symptoms of psychoses and reduce the incidence of extrapyramidal side effects as compared to typical antipsychotics.

Pharmacodynamics/Kinetics

Distribution: V_d: 6173 L

Protein binding: ~99%

Metabolism: Primarily via CYP3A4; two active metabolites (ID-14283 and ID-14326) and two major nonactive metabolites (ID-20219 and ID-20220) produced

Bioavailability: 9% to 19%

Half-life elimination: 18 hours; Main active metabolite, ID-14283 (exo-hydroxy metabolite), exhibits a half-life of 7.5-10 hours

Time to peak: 1-3 hours; steady state concentrations achieved within 7 days

Excretion: Urine (~9%); feces (~80%)

Dosage

Depressive episodes (monotherapy or as an adjunct to lithium or valproic acid): Adults: Oral: Initial: 20 mg once daily; titration is not required; maximum recommended dose: 120 mg daily. **Note:** Doses ≥80 mg daily during monotherapy studies did not provide additional efficacy compared to lower doses (eg, 20-60 mg daily).

Schizophrenia: Adults: Oral: Initial: 40 mg once daily; titration is not required; maximum recommended dose: 160 mg daily

Concomitant CYP3A4 inhibitors/inducers:

CYP3A4 inhibitors:

Concomitant administration with a **strong** CYP3A4 inhibitor (eg, ketoconazole) is contraindicated.

Concomitant administration with a **moderate** CYP3A4 inhibitor (eg, diltiazem):
U.S. labeling: Initial dose: 20 mg once daily; do not exceed 80 mg daily of lurasidone
Canadian labeling: Do not exceed 40 mg daily of lurasidone
CYP3A4 inducers:
Concomitant administration with a **strong** CYP3A4 inducer (eg, rifampin) is contraindicated.
Concomitant administration with a **moderate** CYP3A4 inducer: Lurasidone dose may need to be increased when combined with a moderate CYP3A4 inducer for ≥7 days.

Dosing adjustment in renal impairment:
U.S. labeling:
Cl_{cr} ≥50 mL/minute: No dosage adjustment necessary.
Cl_{cr} <50 mL/minute: Initial: 20 mg daily; maximum: 80 mg daily
Canadian labeling:
Cl_{cr} ≥50 mL/minute: No dosage adjustment necessary.
Cl_{cr} <50 mL/minute: Maximum: 40 mg daily

Dosing adjustment in hepatic impairment:
U.S. labeling:
Mild impairment (Child-Pugh class A): No dosage adjustment necessary.
Moderate impairment (Child-Pugh class B): Initial: 20 mg daily; maximum: 80 mg daily
Severe impairment (Child-Pugh class C): Initial: 20 mg daily; maximum: 40 mg daily
Canadian labeling:
Mild impairment (Child-Pugh class A): No dosage adjustment necessary.
Moderate and severe impairment (Child-Pugh class B and C): Maximum: 40 mg daily

Dietary Considerations Should be taken with food (≥350 calories).

Administration Administer with food (≥350 calories).

Monitoring Parameters Vital signs; fasting lipid profile and fasting blood glucose/Hgb A_{1c} (baseline and periodically); CBC frequently during first few months of therapy in patients with pre-existing low WBC or a history of drug-induced leukopenia/neutropenia; BMI, personal/family history of obesity, waist circumference; blood pressure; mental status, abnormal involuntary movement scale (AIMS), extrapyramidal symptoms; orthostatic blood pressure changes for 3-5 days after starting or increasing dose. Weight should be assessed prior to treatment and regularly throughout therapy. Consider titrating to a different antipsychotic agent for a weight gain ≥5% of the initial weight.

Dosage Forms Excipient information presented when available (limited, particularly for generics); consult specific product labeling.
Tablet, Oral, as hydrochloride:
Latuda: 20 mg, 40 mg, 60 mg
Latuda: 80 mg [contains fd&c blue #2 aluminum lake]
Latuda: 120 mg

Dosage Forms: Canada Refer to Dosage Forms. **Note:** Latuda 20 mg and 60 mg tablets are not available in Canada.

- **Lurasidone Hydrochloride** *see* Lurasidone *on page* 1255
- **Lustra** *see* Hydroquinone *on page* 1017
- **Lustra® (Can)** *see* Hydroquinone *on page* 1017
- **Lustra-AF** *see* Hydroquinone *on page* 1017
- **Lustra-Ultra** *see* Hydroquinone *on page* 1017
- **Lutera** *see* Ethinyl Estradiol and Levonorgestrel *on page* 787

Lutropin Alfa (LOO troe pin AL fa)

Index Terms r-hLH; Recombinant Human Luteinizing Hormone

Pharmacologic Category Gonadotropin; Ovulation Stimulator

Use Stimulation of follicular development in infertile hypogonadotropic hypogonadal (HH) women with profound luteinizing hormone (LH) deficiency (<1.2 units/L); to be used in combination with follitropin alfa

Pregnancy Risk Factor X

Dosage SubQ: Adults: Females: Infertility: 75 units daily until adequate follicular development is noted; maximum duration of treatment: 14 days, unless signs of imminent follicular development are present; to be used concomitantly with follitropin alfa. Once adequate follicular development is evident, administer hCG to induce final follicular maturation in preparation for oocyte retrieval. Withhold hCG if the ovaries are abnormally enlarged.

Dosage adjustment in renal impairment: No dosage adjustment provided in manufacturer's labeling (has not been studied).

Dosage adjustment in hepatic impairment: No dosage adjustment provided in manufacturer's labeling (has not been studied).

Additional Information Complete prescribing information should be consulted for additional detail.

- **Luvox** *see* FluvoxaMINE *on page* 903
- **Luvox CR** *see* FluvoxaMINE *on page* 903
- **Luxiq** *see* Betamethasone *on page* 247
- **LY139603** *see* AtoMOXetine *on page* 187
- **LY146032** *see* DAPTOmycin *on page* 541
- **LY170053** *see* OLANZapine *on page* 1493
- **LY-188011** *see* Gemcitabine *on page* 943
- **LY231514** *see* PEMEtrexed *on page* 1601
- **LY246736** *see* Alvimopan *on page* 91
- **LY248686** *see* DULoxetine *on page* 677
- **LY303366** *see* Anidulafungin *on page* 139
- **LY570310** *see* Telaprevir *on page* 1996
- **LY-640315** *see* Prasugrel *on page* 1699
- **LY2148568** *see* Exenatide *on page* 815
- **Lybrel** *see* Ethinyl Estradiol and Levonorgestrel *on page* 787
- **Lyderm® (Can)** *see* Fluocinonide *on page* 879
- **Lymphocyte Immune Globulin** *see* Antithymocyte Globulin (Equine) *on page* 149
- **Lymphocyte Mitogenic Factor** *see* Aldesleukin *on page* 63
- **Lyrica** *see* Pregabalin *on page* 1710
- **Lyrica® (Can)** *see* Pregabalin *on page* 1710
- **Lysodren** *see* Mitotane *on page* 1385
- **Lysteda** *see* Tranexamic Acid *on page* 2104
- **Lyza** *see* Norethindrone *on page* 1472
- **Maalox [OTC]** *see* Calcium Carbonate *on page* 318
- **Maalox® Advanced Maximum Strength [OTC]** *see* Aluminum Hydroxide, Magnesium Hydroxide, and Simethicone *on page* 90
- **Maalox® Advanced Regular Strength [OTC]** *see* Aluminum Hydroxide, Magnesium Hydroxide, and Simethicone *on page* 90
- **Maalox Childrens [OTC]** *see* Calcium Carbonate *on page* 318
- **MabCampath® (Can)** *see* Alemtuzumab *on page* 66
- **Macrobid** *see* Nitrofurantoin *on page* 1464

◆ **Macrobid® (Can)** *see* Nitrofurantoin *on page 1464*
◆ **Macrodantin** *see* Nitrofurantoin *on page 1464*
◆ **Macrodantin® (Can)** *see* Nitrofurantoin *on page 1464*
◆ **Macugen** *see* Pegaptanib *on page 1585*

Mafenide (MA fe nide)

Brand Names: U.S. Sulfamylon
Index Terms Mafenide Acetate
Pharmacologic Category Antibiotic, Topical
Use
Cream: Adjunctive antibacterial agent in the treatment of second- and third-degree burns
Solution: Adjunctive antibacterial agent for use under moist dressings over meshed autografts on excised burn wounds
Pregnancy Risk Factor C
Dosage Children and Adults: Topical:
Cream: Apply once or twice daily with a sterile-gloved hand; apply to a thickness of approximately 1/16 inch; the burned area should be covered with cream at all times
Solution: Cover graft area with 1 layer of fine mesh gauze. Wet an 8-ply burn dressing with mafenide solution and cover graft area. Keep dressing wet using syringe or irrigation tubing every 4 hours (or as necessary), or by moistening dressing every 6-8 hours (or as necessary). Irrigation dressing should be secured with bolster dressing and wrapped as appropriate. May leave dressings in place for up to 5 days.
Dosage adjustment for acidosis: Discontinuing treatment for 24-48 hours may aid in restoring acid-base balance
Additional Information Complete prescribing information should be consulted for additional detail.
Dosage Forms Excipient information presented when available (limited, particularly for generics); consult specific product labeling.
Cream, External, as acetate [strength expressed as base]:
Sulfamylon: 85 mg/g (56.7 g, 113.4 g, 453.6 g) [contains methylparaben, propylparaben, sodium metabisulfite]
Packet, External, as acetate:
Sulfamylon: 50 g (1 ea, 5 ea)
Generic: 50 g (1 ea, 5 ea)

◆ **Mafenide Acetate** *see* Mafenide *on page 1259*
◆ **Mag-200 [OTC]** *see* Magnesium Oxide *on page 1262*
◆ **Mag-Al [OTC]** *see* Aluminum Hydroxide and Magnesium Hydroxide *on page 90*

Magaldrate and Simethicone
(MAG al drate & sye METH i kone)

Index Terms Riopan Plus; Simethicone and Magaldrate
Pharmacologic Category Antacid; Antiflatulent
Use Relief of hyperacidity associated with peptic ulcer, gastritis, peptic esophagitis, and hiatal hernia which are accompanied by symptoms of gas
Dosage Adults: Oral: 5-10 mL (540-1080 mg magaldrate) between meals and at bedtime
Additional Information Complete prescribing information should be consulted for additional detail.
Dosage Forms Excipient information presented when available (limited, particularly for generics); consult specific product labeling.
Suspension, oral: Magaldrate 540 mg and simethicone 20 mg per 5 mL (360 mL)

◆ **Mag-Al Ultimate [OTC]** *see* Aluminum Hydroxide and Magnesium Hydroxide *on page 90*
◆ **Mag Citrate** *see* Magnesium Citrate *on page 1260*
◆ **Mag-Delay [OTC]** *see* Magnesium Chloride *on page 1259*
◆ **Mag-G [OTC]** *see* Magnesium Gluconate *on page 1260*
◆ **Magic Bullets [OTC]** *see* Bisacodyl *on page 259*
◆ **Maginex™ [OTC]** *see* Magnesium L-aspartate Hydrochloride *on page 1261*
◆ **Maginex™ DS [OTC]** *see* Magnesium L-aspartate Hydrochloride *on page 1261*
◆ **Magnacet** *see* Oxycodone and Acetaminophen *on page 1538*
◆ **Magnesia Magma** *see* Magnesium Hydroxide *on page 1260*
◆ **Magnesium L-lactate Dihydrate** *see* Magnesium L-lactate *on page 1262*
◆ **Magnesium Carbonate and Aluminum Hydroxide** *see* Aluminum Hydroxide and Magnesium Carbonate *on page 89*

Magnesium Chloride (mag NEE zhum KLOR ide)

Brand Names: U.S. Chloromag; Mag-Delay [OTC]; Mag-SR Plus Calcium [OTC]; Mag-SR [OTC]; Slow Magnesium/Calcium [OTC]; Slow-Mag [OTC]
Pharmacologic Category Electrolyte Supplement, Oral; Electrolyte Supplement, Parenteral; Magnesium Salt
Use Correction or prevention of hypomagnesemia; dietary supplement
Pregnancy Risk Factor C
Dosage Note: Serum magnesium is poor reflection of repletional status as the majority of magnesium is intracellular; serum levels may be transiently normal for a few hours after a dose is given; therefore, aim for consistently high normal serum levels in patients with normal renal function for most efficient repletion.
Dietary supplement: Adults: Oral (Mag 64®, Mag Delay™, Slow-Mag®): 2 tablets once daily
Parenteral nutrition supplementation: I.V. (elemental magnesium):
Children:
<50 kg: 0.3-0.5 mEq/kg/day
>50 kg: 10-30 mEq/day
Adults: 8-24 mEq/day

RDA (elemental magnesium) (IOM, 1997):
Children:
1-3 years: 80 mg/day
4-8 years: 130 mg/day
9-13 years: 240 mg/day
14-18 years:
Females: 360 mg/day
Pregnancy: 400 mg/day
Lactation: 360 mg/day
Males: 410 mg/day
Adults:
19-30 years:
Females: 310 mg/day
Pregnancy: 350 mg/day
Lactation: 310 mg/day
Males: 400 mg/day
≥31 years:
Females: 320 mg/day
Pregnancy: 360 mg/day
Lactation: 320 mg/day
Males: 420 mg/day

Dosage adjustment in renal impairment: Cl_{cr} <30 mL/minute: Use with caution; monitor for hypermagnesemia
Dosage adjustment in hepatic impairment: No dosage adjustment provided in manufacturer's labeling.
Additional Information Complete prescribing information should be consulted for additional detail.

Dosage Forms Considerations
1 g magnesium chloride = elemental magnesium 120 mg = magnesium 9.85 mEq = magnesium 4.93 mmol
Elemental magnesium 64 mg = magnesium 5.26 mEq = magnesium 2.62 mmol

Dosage Forms Excipient information presented when available (limited, particularly for generics); consult specific product labeling.
Solution, Injection, as hexahydrate:
Chloromag: 200 mg/mL (50 mL) [contains benzyl alcohol]
Generic: 200 mg/mL (50 mL)
Tablet Delayed Release, Oral:
Mag-SR Plus Calcium: 64-106 MG [starch free, sugar free]
Slow Magnesium/Calcium: 64-106 MG
Slow-Mag: 71.5-119 MG [contains fd&c blue #2 aluminum lake]
Tablet Extended Release, Oral:
Mag-Delay: 535 (64 Mg) MG
Mag-SR: 535 (64 Mg) MG [starch free, sugar free]

Magnesium Citrate (mag NEE zhum SIT rate)

Brand Names: U.S. Citroma [OTC]
Brand Names: Canada Citro-Mag
Index Terms Citrate of Magnesia; Mag Citrate
Pharmacologic Category Laxative, Saline; Magnesium Salt
Additional Appendix Information
Laxatives, Classification and Properties *on page 2304*
Use Relieves occasional constipation
Unlabeled Use Evacuation of bowel prior to certain surgical and diagnostic procedures or overdose situations
Dosage Laxative: Oral: Solution:
Children:
2-6 years: 60-90 mL given once or in divided doses (maximum: 90 mL/24 hours)
6-12 years: 90-210 mL given once or in divided doses
Children ≥12 years, Adolescents, and Adults: 195-300 mL given once or in divided doses

Dosage adjustment in renal impairment: No dosage adjustment provided in manufacturer's labeling; however, magnesium is renally excreted. Use caution; accumulation of magnesium in renal impairment may lead to magnesium toxicity.
Additional Information Complete prescribing information should be consulted for additional detail.
Dosage Forms Considerations
1 g magnesium citrate ≈ elemental magnesium 160 mg = magnesium 13 mEq = magnesium 6.5 mmol
Dosage Forms Excipient information presented when available (limited, particularly for generics); consult specific product labeling.
Solution, Oral:
Citroma: 1.745 g/30 mL (296 mL) [contains polyethylene glycol, saccharin sodium; lemon flavor]
Citroma: 1.745 g/30 mL (296 mL) [low sodium; lemon flavor]
Citroma: 1.745 g/30 mL (296 mL) [low sodium; contains fd&c red #40, saccharin sodium; cherry flavor]
Generic: 1.745 g/30 mL (296 mL)
Tablet, Oral:
Generic: 100 mg

Magnesium Gluconate
(mag NEE zhum GLOO koe nate)

Brand Names: U.S. Mag-G [OTC]; Magonate [OTC]
Pharmacologic Category Electrolyte Supplement, Oral; Magnesium Salt
Use Dietary supplement
Dosage RDA (elemental magnesium):
Children:
1-3 years: 80 mg/day
4-8 years: 130 mg/day
9-13 years: 240 mg/day
14-18 years:
Females: 360 mg/day
Pregnant females: 400 mg/day
Males: 410 mg/day
Adults:
19-30 years:
Females: 310 mg/day
Pregnant females: 350 mg/day
Males: 400 mg/day
≥31 years:
Females: 320 mg/day
Pregnant females: 360 mg/day
Males: 420 mg/day

Dosing in renal impairment: Cl_{cr} <30 mL/minute: Use with caution; monitor for hypermagnesemia
Additional Information Complete prescribing information should be consulted for additional detail.
Dosage Forms Considerations
1 g magnesium gluconate = elemental magnesium 54 mg = magnesium 4.5 mEq = magnesium 2.25 mmol
Dosage Forms Excipient information presented when available (limited, particularly for generics); consult specific product labeling.
Liquid, Oral:
Magonate: Magnesium carbonate equivalent to magnesium gluconate 1000 mg (54 mg elemental magnesium) per 5 mL (355 mL) [contains sodium benzoate; mixed melon flavor]
Tablet, Oral:
Mag-G: 500 mg (27 mg elemental magnesium)
Magonate: 500 mg (27 mg elemental magnesium) [scored]
Magonate: 500 mg (27 mg elemental magnesium) [scored; contains fd&c yellow #6 aluminum lake]
Generic: Elemental magnesium 27.5 mg
Tablet, Oral [preservative free]:
Generic: 500 mg (27 mg elemental magnesium)

Magnesium Hydroxide
(mag NEE zhum hye DROKS ide)

Brand Names: U.S. Dulcolax Milk of Magnesia [OTC]; Milk of Magnesia Concentrate [OTC]; Milk of Magnesia [OTC]; Pedia-Lax [OTC]
Index Terms Magnesia Magma; Milk of Magnesia; MOM
Pharmacologic Category Antacid; Laxative; Magnesium Salt
Additional Appendix Information
Laxatives, Classification and Properties *on page 2304*
Use Short-term treatment of occasional constipation and symptoms of hyperacidity, laxative
Dosage Oral:
Laxative:
Liquid:
Children: Magnesium hydroxide 400 mg/5 mL: 1-3 mL/kg/day; adjust dose to induce daily bowel movement
OTC labeling:
<2 years: Use not recommended
2-5 years: Magnesium hydroxide 400 mg/5 mL: 5-15 mL/day once daily at bedtime or in divided doses
6-11 years:
Magnesium hydroxide 400 mg/5 mL: 15-30 mL/day once daily at bedtime or in divided doses
Magnesium hydroxide 800 mg/5 mL: 7.5-15 mL/day once daily at bedtime or in divided doses

Children ≥12 years and Adults:
Magnesium hydroxide 400 mg/5 mL: 30-60 mL/day once daily at bedtime or in divided doses
Magnesium hydroxide 800 mg/5 mL: 15-30 mL/day once daily at bedtime or in divided doses
Tablet: OTC labeling:
Children:
<3 years: Use not recommended
3-5 years: Magnesium hydroxide 311 mg/tablet: 2 tablets/day once daily at bedtime or in divided doses
6-11 years: Magnesium hydroxide 311 mg/tablet: 4 tablets/day once daily at bedtime or in divided doses
Children ≥12 years and Adults: Magnesium hydroxide 311 mg/tablet: 8 tablets/day once daily at bedtime or in divided doses
Antacid: OTC labeling:
Liquid: Children ≥12 years and Adults: Magnesium hydroxide 400 mg/5 mL: 5-15 mL as needed up to 4 times/day
Tablet:
Children <12 years: Use not recommended
Children ≥12 years and Adults: Magnesium hydroxide 311 mg/tablet: 2-4 tablets every 4 hours up to 4 times/day

Dosing in renal impairment: Patients in severe renal failure should not receive magnesium due to toxicity from accumulation. Patients with a Cl_{cr} <30 mL/minute receiving magnesium should be monitored by serum magnesium levels.

Additional Information Complete prescribing information should be consulted for additional detail.

Dosage Forms Excipient information presented when available (limited, particularly for generics); consult specific product labeling.
Suspension, Oral:
Dulcolax Milk of Magnesia: 400 mg/5 mL (355 mL) [sugar free; unflavored flavor]
Dulcolax Milk of Magnesia: 400 mg/5 mL (355 mL) [sugar free; contains saccharin sodium; mint flavor]
Milk of Magnesia: 400 mg/5 mL (355 mL, 480 mL); 7.75% (360 mL, 473 mL, 480 mL)
Milk of Magnesia: 7.75% (355 mL, 473 mL) [mint flavor]
Milk of Magnesia: 7.75% (30 mL) [spearmint flavor]
Milk of Magnesia: 1200 mg/15 mL (355 mL) [gluten free, stimulant free, sugar free; contains saccharin sodium]
Milk of Magnesia: 400 mg/5 mL (355 mL, 473 mL) [low sodium, sugar free]
Milk of Magnesia: 400 mg/5 mL (473 mL, 769 mL); 1200 mg/15 mL (355 mL) [stimulant free, sugar free]
Milk of Magnesia: 1200 mg/15 mL (355 mL) [stimulant free, sugar free; contains saccharin sodium]
Milk of Magnesia: 400 mg/5 mL (473 mL) [sugar free]
Milk of Magnesia Concentrate: 2400 mg/10 mL (100 mL, 400 mL) [lemon flavor]
Tablet Chewable, Oral:
Pedia-Lax: 400 mg [scored; stimulant free; contains fd&c red #40 aluminum lake; watermelon flavor]

◆ **Magnesium Hydroxide, Aluminum Hydroxide, and Simethicone** *see* Aluminum Hydroxide, Magnesium Hydroxide, and Simethicone *on page 90*

◆ **Magnesium Hydroxide and Aluminum Hydroxide** *see* Aluminum Hydroxide and Magnesium Hydroxide *on page 90*

◆ **Magnesium Hydroxide and Calcium Carbonate** *see* Calcium Carbonate and Magnesium Hydroxide *on page 320*

Magnesium Hydroxide and Mineral Oil

(mag NEE zhum hye DROKS ide & MIN er al oyl)

Brand Names: U.S. Phillips'® M-O [OTC]

Index Terms Haley's M-O; MOM/Mineral Oil Emulsion

Pharmacologic Category Laxative

Use Short-term treatment of occasional constipation

Dosage Oral: Laxative: OTC labeling:
Children <6 years: Use not recommended
Children 6-11 years: 20-30 mL at bedtime
Children ≥12 years and Adults: 45-60 mL at bedtime

Dosage adjustment in renal impairment: Patients in severe renal failure should not receive magnesium due to toxicity from accumulation. Patients with a Cl_{cr} <30 mL/minute should be monitored by serum magnesium levels.

Additional Information Complete prescribing information should be consulted for additional detail.

Dosage Forms Excipient information presented when available (limited, particularly for generics); consult specific product labeling.
Suspension, oral:
Phillips'® M-O: Magnesium hydroxide 300 mg and mineral oil 1.25 mL per 5 mL (360 mL, 780 mL) [contains magnesium 125 mg and sodium 1.5 mg per 5 mL mint flavors]

Magnesium L-aspartate Hydrochloride

(mag NEE zhum el as PAR tate hye droe KLOR ide)

Brand Names: U.S. Maginex™ DS [OTC]; Maginex™ [OTC]

Index Terms MAH

Pharmacologic Category Electrolyte Supplement, Oral; Magnesium Salt

Use Dietary supplement

Dosage

Dietary Reference Intake for Magnesium: Dosage is in terms of elemental magnesium (IOM, 1997): Oral:
Children:
1-6 months: Adequate intake: 30 mg daily
7-12 months: Adequate intake: 75 mg daily
1-3 years: RDA: 80 mg daily
4-8 years: RDA: 130 mg daily
9-13 years: RDA: 240 mg daily
14-18 years: RDA:
Females: 360 mg daily
Pregnant females: 400 mg daily
Lactation: 360 mg daily
Males: 410 mg daily
Adults: RDA:
19-30 years:
Females: 310 mg daily
Pregnant females: 350 mg daily
Lactation: 310 mg daily
Males: 400 mg daily
≥31 years:
Females: 320 mg daily
Pregnant females: 360 mg daily
Lactation: 320 mg daily
Males: 420 mg daily

OTC labeling:

Dietary supplement (dosage in terms of magnesium-L-aspartate hydrochloride salt): Adults: Oral: One packet or 2 tablets (1230 mg) up to 3 times daily

Dosage adjustment in renal impairment: No dosage adjustment provided in manufacturer's labeling; however, magnesium is renally excreted. Use caution; accumulation of magnesium in renal impairment may lead to magnesium toxicity.

Additional Information Complete prescribing information should be consulted for additional detail.

Dosage Forms Considerations
1 g magnesium L-aspartate Hydrochloride = elemental magnesium 100 mg = magnesium 8.1 mEq = magnesium 4.05 mmol

Dosage Forms Excipient information presented when available (limited, particularly for generics); consult specific product labeling.

Granules for solution, oral [preservative free]:
Maginex™ DS: 1230 mg/packet (30s) [sugar free; lemon flavor; equivalent to elemental magnesium 122 mg]

Tablet, enteric coated, oral [preservative free]:
Maginex™: 615 mg [sugar free; equivalent to elemental magnesium 61 mg]

Magnesium L-lactate (mag NEE zhum el LAK tate)

Brand Names: U.S. Mag-Tab SR [OTC]

Index Terms Magnesium L-lactate Dihydrate

Pharmacologic Category Electrolyte Supplement; Magnesium Salt

Use Dietary supplement

Dosage

Dietary supplement: Oral: Adults: 1-2 caplets every 12 hours

RDA (elemental magnesium):

Children:
- 1-3 years: 80 mg/day
- 4-8 years: 130 mg/day
- 9-13 years: 240 mg/day
- 14-18 years:
  - Females: 360 mg/day
  - Pregnant females: 400 mg/day
  - Males: 410 mg/day

Adults:
- 19-30 years:
  - Females: 310 mg/day
  - Pregnant females: 350 mg/day
  - Males: 400 mg/day
- ≥31 years:
  - Females: 320 mg/day
  - Pregnant females: 360 mg/day
  - Males: 420 mg/day

Dosage adjustment in renal impairment: Cl_{cr} <30 mL/minute: Use with caution; monitor for hypermagnesemia

Additional Information Complete prescribing information should be consulted for additional detail.

Dosage Forms Considerations
1 g Magnesium L-lactate = elemental magnesium 120 mg = magnesium 9.8 mEq = magnesium 4.9 mmol

Dosage Forms Excipient information presented when available (limited, particularly for generics); consult specific product labeling.

Tablet Extended Release, Oral:
Mag-Tab SR: Elemental magnesium 84 mg [7 mEq]

Magnesium Oxide (mag NEE zhum OKS ide)

Brand Names: U.S. Mag-200 [OTC]; Maox [OTC]; Uro-Mag [OTC]

Index Terms Mag Oxide

Pharmacologic Category Electrolyte Supplement, Oral; Magnesium Salt

Additional Appendix Information
Laxatives, Classification and Properties *on page 2304*

Use Dietary supplement; relief of acid indigestion and upset stomach; short-term treatment of occasional constipation

Dosage

Dietary Reference Intake for Magnesium: Dosage is in terms of elemental magnesium (IOM, 1997): Oral:

Children:
- 1-6 months: Adequate intake: 30 mg daily
- 7-12 months: Adequate intake: 75 mg daily
- 1-3 years: RDA: 80 mg daily
- 4-8 years: RDA: 130 mg daily
- 9-13 years: RDA: 240 mg daily
- 14-18 years: RDA:
  - Females: 360 mg daily
  - Pregnant females: 400 mg daily
  - Lactation: 360 mg daily
  - Males: 410 mg daily

Adults: RDA:
- 19-30 years:
  - Females: 310 mg daily
  - Pregnant females: 350 mg daily
  - Lactation: 310 mg daily
  - Males: 400 mg daily
- ≥31 years:
  - Females: 320 mg daily
  - Pregnant females: 360 mg daily
  - Lactation: 320 mg daily
  - Males: 420 mg daily

OTC labeling:

Antacid (dosage in terms of magnesium oxide salt): Adults: Oral: Tablet: 1-2 tablets (400-800 mg) daily or in divided doses; maximum: 2 tablets daily

Dietary supplement (dosage in terms of magnesium oxide salt): Adults: Oral:
Mag-Ox 400®: Two tablets (800 mg) daily with food (maximum: 2 tablets/24 hours)
Uro-Mag®: 3-4 capsules (420-560 mg) daily with food

Laxative (dosage in terms of elemental magnesium): Children ≥12 years, Adolescents, and Adults: Oral: Caplet: 2-4 caplets (1000-2000 mg) at bedtime or in divided doses

Dosing in renal impairment: No dosage adjustment provided in manufacturer's labeling; however, magnesium is renally excreted. Use with caution; accumulation in renal impairment may lead to magnesium toxicity.

Additional Information Complete prescribing information should be consulted for additional detail.

Dosage Forms Considerations
400 mg magnesium oxide = elemental magnesium 240 mg = magnesium 19.9 mEq = magnesium 9.85 mmol

Dosage Forms Excipient information presented when available (limited, particularly for generics); consult specific product labeling.

Capsule, Oral:
Uro-Mag: 140 mg

Tablet, Oral:
Mag-200: 200 mg [contains para-aminobenzoic acid]
Maox: 420 mg [contains tartrazine (fd&c yellow #5)]
Generic: 250 mg, 400 mg, 420 mg, 400 (240 Mg) MG, 400 (241.3 Mg) MG

Tablet, Oral [preservative free]:
Generic: 500 mg, 400 (240 Mg) MG

◆ **Magnesium Oxide, Sodium Picosulfate, and Citric Acid** *see* Sodium Picosulfate, Magnesium Oxide, and Citric Acid *on page 1925*

Magnesium Salicylate (mag NEE zhum sa LIS i late)

Brand Names: U.S. Doans Extra Strength [OTC]; Doans Pills [OTC]; MST 600

Pharmacologic Category Salicylate

Use Mild-to-moderate pain, fever, various inflammatory conditions; relief of pain and inflammation of rheumatoid arthritis and osteoarthritis

Dosage Oral:

Children ≥12 years and Adults: Relief of mild-to-moderate pain:
Doan's® Extra Strength, Momentum®: Two caplets every 6 hours as needed (maximum: 8 caplets/24 hours)

Keygesic: One tablet every 4 hours as needed (maximum: 4 tablets/24 hours)

Additional Information Complete prescribing information should be consulted for additional detail.

Dosage Forms Excipient information presented when available (limited, particularly for generics); consult specific product labeling.

Tablet, Oral:
Doans Pills: 325 mg

Tablet, Oral, as tetrahydrate:
Doans Extra Strength: 580 mg
Doans Extra Strength: 580 mg [contains methylparaben]
MST 600: 600 mg [scored; contains fd&c yellow #10 (quinoline yellow)]

Magnesium Sulfate (mag NEE zhum SUL fate)

Brand Names: U.S. Epsom Salt [OTC]

Index Terms Epsom Salts; $MgSO_4$ (error-prone abbreviation)

Pharmacologic Category Anticonvulsant, Miscellaneous; Electrolyte Supplement, Parenteral; Magnesium Salt

Additional Appendix Information

Laxatives, Classification and Properties *on page 2304*

Use

Treatment and prevention of hypomagnesemia; prevention and treatment of seizures in severe pre-eclampsia or eclampsia, pediatric acute nephritis; torsade de pointes; treatment of cardiac arrhythmias (VT/VF) caused by hypomagnesemia

OTC labeling: Soaking aid for minor cuts and bruises; laxative for the relief of occasional constipation

Unlabeled Use Asthma exacerbation (life-threatening) unresponsive to 1 hour intensive conventional treatment

Pregnancy Risk Factor D

Pregnancy Considerations Magnesium crosses the placenta; serum concentrations in the fetus are similar to those in the mother (Idama, 1998; Osada, 2002). Continuous maternal use for >5-7 days (in doses such as those used for preterm labor, an off-label use) may cause fetal hypocalcemia and bone abnormalities, as well as fractures in the neonate. Magnesium sulfate injection is used for the prevention and treatment of seizures in pregnant women with severe pre-eclampsia or eclampsia (ACOG, 2002). Magnesium sulfate may also be used prior to early preterm delivery to reduce the risk of cerebral palsy (ACOG, 2010; Reeves, 2011). Tocolytics may be used for the short-term (48 hour) prolongation of pregnancy to allow for the administration of antenatal steroids and should not be used prior to fetal viability or when the risks of use to the fetus or mother are greater than the risk of preterm birth; maintenance therapy with tocolytics is ineffective and not recommended. Magnesium sulfate injection may be used in conjunction with tocolytics for neuroprotection (it is not preferred for use as a tocolytic); however, an increased risk of maternal complications may be observed when used in combination with some tocolytic agents (ACOG, 2012).

Breast-Feeding Considerations Magnesium is found in breast milk; concentrations remain constant during the first year of lactation and are not influenced by dietary intake under normal conditions. Magnesium requirements are the same in lactating and nonlactating females (IOM, 1997). When magnesium sulfate is used in the intrapartum management of eclampsia, breast milk concentrations are generally increased for only ~24 hours after the end of treatment (Idama, 1998). The manufacturer recommends caution be used if administered to nursing women.

Contraindications Hypersensitivity to any component of the formulation; heart block; myocardial damage; I.V. use for pre-eclampsia/eclampsia during the 2 hours prior to delivery

Warnings/Precautions Use magnesium with caution in patients with impaired renal function (accumulation of magnesium may lead to magnesium intoxication). Use with extreme caution in patients with myasthenia gravis or other neuromuscular disease. Magnesium toxicity can lead to fatal cardiovascular arrest and/or respiratory paralysis. Solution for injection may contain aluminum; toxic concentrations may occur following prolonged administration in premature neonates or patients with renal dysfunction. Concurrent hypokalemia or hypocalcemia can accompany a magnesium deficit. Unlikely to effectively terminate irregular/polymorphic VT (with normal baseline QT interval) (Neumar, 2010).

Obstetric use: Vigilant monitoring and safe administration techniques (ISMP, 2005) recommended to avoid potential for errors resulting in toxicity. Monitor mother and fetus closely. Use longer than 5-7 days may cause adverse fetal events.

Self-medication (OTC Use): When used as a soaking aid, patients should not use if there is evidence of infection or prompt relief is not obtained. When used as a laxative, patients should consult a healthcare provider prior to use if they have: kidney disease; are on a magnesium-restricted diet; have abdominal pain, nausea, or vomiting; change in bowel habits lasting >2 weeks; have already used a laxative for >1 week

Adverse Reactions Adverse effects on neuromuscular function may occur at lower concentrations in patients with neuromuscular disease (eg, myasthenia gravis).

Frequency not defined:

Cardiovascular: Flushing (I.V.; dose related), hypotension (I.V.; rate related), vasodilation (I.V.; rate related)

Endocrine & metabolic: Hypermagnesemia

Drug Interactions

Metabolism/Transport Effects None known.

Avoid Concomitant Use

Avoid concomitant use of Magnesium Sulfate with any of the following: Calcium Polystyrene Sulfonate; Raltegravir; Sodium Polystyrene Sulfonate

Increased Effect/Toxicity

Magnesium Sulfate may increase the levels/effects of: Calcium Channel Blockers; Calcium Polystyrene Sulfonate; CNS Depressants; Neuromuscular-Blocking Agents; Sodium Polystyrene Sulfonate

The levels/effects of Magnesium Sulfate may be increased by: Alfacalcidol; Calcitriol; Calcium Channel Blockers

Decreased Effect

Magnesium Sulfate may decrease the levels/effects of: Bisphosphonate Derivatives; Deferiprone; Dolutegravir; Eltrombopag; Gabapentin; Multivitamins/Fluoride (with ADE); Mycophenolate; Phosphate Supplements; Quinolone Antibiotics; Raltegravir; Tetracycline Derivatives; Trientine

The levels/effects of Magnesium Sulfate may be decreased by: Ketorolac (Nasal); Ketorolac (Systemic); Mefloquine; Orlistat; Trientine

Ethanol/Nutrition/Herb Interactions Ethanol: Increased alcohol intake can deplete magnesium stores (IOM, 1997).

Preparation for Administration

I.V.: Dilute to a ≤20% solution for I.V. infusion.

I.M.: A 25% or 50% concentration may be used for adults and dilution to a ≤20% solution is recommended for children.

Oral: Dissolve granules in 8 ounces of water prior to administration.

Topical: Dissolve 2 cups of granules per gallon of warm water to use as a soaking aid.

Storage/Stability Prior to use, store at room temperature of 20°C to 25°C (68°F to 77°F). Do not freeze.

Refrigeration of solution may result in precipitation or crystallization.

Mechanism of Action When taken orally, magnesium promotes bowel evacuation by causing osmotic retention of fluid which distends the colon with increased peristaltic activity; parenterally, magnesium decreases acetylcholine in motor nerve terminals and acts on myocardium by slowing rate of S-A node impulse formation and prolonging conduction time. Magnesium is necessary for the movement of calcium, sodium, and potassium in and out of cells, as well as stabilizing excitable membranes.

Intravenous magnesium may improve pulmonary function in patients with asthma; causes relaxation of bronchial smooth muscle independent of serum magnesium concentration.

Pharmacodynamics/Kinetics

Onset of action: Anticonvulsant: I.M.: 1 hour; I.V.: Immediate

Duration of anticonvulsant activity: I.M.: 3-4 hours; I.V.: 30 minutes

Distribution: Bone (50% to 60%); extracellular fluid (1% to 2%) (IOM, 1997)

Protein binding: 30%, to albumin

Excretion: Urine (as magnesium)

Dosage Dose represented as magnesium sulfate unless stated otherwise. **Note:** Serum magnesium is poor reflection of repletional status as the majority of magnesium is intracellular; serum concentrations may be transiently normal for a few hours after a dose is given, therefore, aim for consistently high normal serum concentrations in patients with normal renal function for most efficient repletion.

Note: 1 g of magnesium sulfate = 98.6 mg elemental magnesium = 8.12 mEq elemental magnesium

Hypomagnesemia: Note: Treatment depends on severity and clinical status. In asymptomatic patients (when oral route is available), oral replacement therapy is a better replacement method than I.V. administration.

Children: I.V., I.O.: 25-50 mg/kg/dose over 10-20 minutes (over several minutes for torsade de pointes); maximum single dose: 2000 mg (PALS, 2010)

Adults:

Mild deficiency: I.M.: Manufacturer's labeling: 1 g every 6 hours for 4 doses, or as indicated by serum magnesium concentrations

Mild-to-moderate (serum concentration 1-1.5 mg/dL): I.V.: 1-4 g (up to 0.125 g/kg), administer at ≤1 g/hour if asymptomatic; do not exceed 12 g over 12 hours (Kraft, 2005). **Note:** Additional supplementation may be required after the initial dose with replenishment occurring over several days.

Severe deficiency:

I.M.: Manufacturer's labeling: Up to 250 mg/kg within a 4-hour period

I.V.:

Severe (<1 mg/dL): 4-8 g (up to 0.1875 g/kg), administer at ≤1 g/hour if asymptomatic; in symptomatic patients, may administer ≤4 g over 4-5 minutes (Kraft, 2005)

With polymorphic VT (including torsade de pointes): I.V. push: 1-2 g (ACLS, 2010)

Obesity: Weight >130% of ideal body weight (IBW) or body mass index (BMI) ≥30 kg/m^2: When determining maximum per kg dose for replacement, some clinicians suggest using adjusted body weight (AdjBW) (Kraft, 2005).

AdjBW (men) = ([wt (kg) -IBW (kg)] x 0.3) + IBW

AdjBW (women) = ([wt (kg) -IBW (kg)] x 0.25) + IBW

Asthma (unlabeled use): I.V. (NAEPP, 2007):

Children: 25-75 mg/kg (maximum: 2 g)

Adults: 2 g

Eclampsia/pre-eclampsia (severe): Adults:

Manufacturer's labeling: I.V.: An initial total dose of 10-14 g administered as follows: 4-5 g infusion with simultaneous I.M. injections of 4-5 g in each buttock. After the initial I.V. dose, may administer a 1-2 g/hour continuous infusion or may follow with I.M. doses of 4-5 g in each buttock every 4 hours. Maximum: 40 g/24 hours. I.V. use for pre-eclampsia/eclampsia is contraindicated during the 2 hours prior to delivery.

Alternate dosing (unlabeled): I.V.: 4-6 g over 15-20 minutes followed by 2 g/hour continuous infusion (ACOG, 2002)

Torsade de pointes or VF/pulseless VT associated with torsade de pointes (unlabeled use): Adults: I.V., I.O.: 1-2 g over 15 minutes (ACLS, 2010)

Parenteral nutrition supplementation: I.V.:

Children:

<50 kg: 0.3-0.5 mEq elemental magnesium/kg/day (Mirtallo, 2004)

>50 kg: 10-30 mEq elemental magnesium daily (Mirtallo, 2004)

Adults: 8-24 mEq elemental magnesium daily

Laxative: Oral:

Children 6-12 years: 1-2 teaspoons of granules dissolved in water once daily

Children >12 years, Adolescents, and Adults: 2-6 teaspoons of granules dissolved in water once daily

Soaking aid: Topical: Adults: Dissolve 2 cupfuls of granules per gallon of warm water

RDA (IOM, 1997):

Children:

1-3 years: 80 mg elemental magnesium daily

4-8 years: 130 mg elemental magnesium daily

9-13 years: 240 mg elemental magnesium daily

14-18 years:

Females: 360 mg elemental magnesium daily

Pregnant females: 400 mg elemental magnesium daily

Breast-feeding females: 360 mg elemental magnesium daily

Males: 410 mg elemental magnesium daily

Adults:

19-30 years:

Females: 310 mg elemental magnesium daily

Pregnant females: 350 mg elemental magnesium daily

Breast-feeding females: 310 mg elemental magnesium daily

Males: 400 mg elemental magnesium daily

≥31 years:

Females: 320 mg elemental magnesium daily

Pregnant females: 360 mg elemental magnesium daily

Breast-feeding females: 320 mg elemental magnesium daily

Males: 420 mg elemental magnesium daily

Dosage adjustment in renal impairment:

Hypomagnesemia: Renal dysfunction: Reduce dose by 50% (Kraft, 2005). Use with caution; monitor for hypermagnesemia; Close monitoring is required.

Pre-eclampsia/eclampsia: Severe renal impairment: Per the manufacturer, do not exceed 20 grams during a 48 hour period.

Dosage adjustment in hepatic impairment: No dosage adjustment necessary.

Dietary Considerations Whole grains, legumes and dark-green leafy vegetables are dietary sources of magnesium (IOM, 1997).

Administration

Injection: May be administered I.M. or I.V.

I.M.: Must be diluted prior to administration for children (Adults: 25% or 50% concentration; Children: ≤20% diluted solution)

I.V.: Must be diluted to a ≤20% solution for I.V. infusion and may be administered I.V. push, IVPB, or continuous I.V. infusion. When giving I.V. push, must dilute first and should generally not be given any faster than 150 mg/minute; may administer over 1-2 minutes in patients with persistent pulseless VT or VF with known hypomagnesemia (Dager, 2006). ACLS guidelines recommend administration over 15 minutes in patients with torsade de pointes (ACLS, 2010). In patients not in cardiac arrest, hypotension and asystole may occur with rapid administration.

Maximal rate of infusion: Up to 50% of an I.V. dose may be eliminated in the urine, therefore, slower administration may improve retention. If severely symptomatic, may administer ≤4 g over 4-5 minutes. For doses <6 g, infuse over 8-12 hours and for larger doses infuse over 24 hours if patient asymptomatic (Kraft, 2005).

Oral: When used as a laxative, the patient should drink a full 8 ounces of liquid following each dose. Lemon juice may be added to the initial solution to improve the taste.

Topical: May dissolve granules to prepare a solution for use as a soaking aid or as a compress. To make a compress, use a towel to apply as a wet dressing.

Monitoring Parameters

I.V.: Rapid administration: ECG monitoring, vital signs, deep tendon reflexes; magnesium concentrations if frequent or prolonged dosing required particularly in patients with renal dysfunction, calcium, and potassium concentrations; renal function

Obstetrics: Patient status including vital signs, oxygen saturation, deep tendon reflexes, level of consciousness, fetal heart rate, maternal uterine activity.

Reference Range Serum magnesium: 1.5-2.5 mg/dL; slightly different ranges are reported by different laboratories

Dosage Forms Considerations

1 g of magnesium sulfate = elemental magnesium 98.6 mg = magnesium 8.12 mEq = magnesium 4.06 mmol

Magnesium sulfate 1% [10 mg/mL] in Dextrose 5% injection is equivalent to elemental magnesium 0.081 mEq/mL.

Magnesium sulfate 2% [20 mg/mL] in Dextrose 5% injection is equivalent to elemental magnesium 0.162 mEq/mL.

Magnesium sulfate 4% [40 mg/mL] in Water injection is equivalent to elemental magnesium 0.325 mEq/mL.

Magnesium sulfate 8% [80 mg/mL] in Water injection is equivalent to elemental magnesium 0.65 mEq/mL.

Magnesium sulfate 50% injection is equivalent to elemental magnesium 4 mEq/mL.

Dosage Forms Excipient information presented when available (limited, particularly for generics); consult specific product labeling.

Capsule, Oral:

Generic: 70 mg

Granules, Oral:

Epsom Salt: (454 g, 1810 g, 1816 g)

Solution, Injection:

Generic: 40 mg/mL (50 mL, 100 mL, 500 mL, 1000 mL); 80 mg/mL (50 mL); 50% (2 mL, 10 mL, 20 mL, 50 mL)

Solution, Intravenous:

Generic: 10 mg/mL (100 mL); 20 mg/mL (500 mL)

◆ **Magnesium Sulfate, Potassium Sulfate, and Sodium Sulfate** *see* Sodium Sulfate, Potassium Sulfate, and Magnesium Sulfate *on page 1929*

◆ **Magnesium Sulfate, Sodium Sulfate, and Potassium Sulfate** *see* Sodium Sulfate, Potassium Sulfate, and Magnesium Sulfate *on page 1929*

◆ **Magnesium Trisilicate and Aluminum Hydroxide** *see* Aluminum Hydroxide and Magnesium Trisilicate *on page 90*

◆ **Magonate [OTC]** *see* Magnesium Gluconate *on page 1260*

◆ **Mag Oxide** *see* Magnesium Oxide *on page 1262*

◆ **Mag-SR [OTC]** *see* Magnesium Chloride *on page 1259*

◆ **Mag-SR Plus Calcium [OTC]** *see* Magnesium Chloride *on page 1259*

◆ **Mag-Tab SR [OTC]** *see* Magnesium L-lactate *on page 1262*

◆ **MAH** *see* Magnesium L-aspartate Hydrochloride *on page 1261*

◆ **Makena** *see* Hydroxyprogesterone Caproate *on page 1021*

◆ **Malarone®** *see* Atovaquone and Proguanil *on page 194*

◆ **Malarone® Pediatric (Can)** *see* Atovaquone and Proguanil *on page 194*

Malathion (mal a THYE on)

Brand Names: U.S. Ovide

Pharmacologic Category Antiparasitic Agent, Topical; Pediculocide; Scabicidal Agent

Use Topical treatment of *Pediculus capitis* (head lice and their ova)

Pregnancy Risk Factor B

Dosage Topical: Children ≥6 years and Adults: Apply sufficient amount to cover and thoroughly moisten dry hair and scalp; shampoo after 8-12 hours. If required, repeat with second application in 7-9 days. Further treatment is generally not necessary.

Additional Information Complete prescribing information should be consulted for additional detail.

Dosage Forms Excipient information presented when available (limited, particularly for generics); consult specific product labeling.

Lotion, External:

Ovide: 0.5% (59 mL) [contains isopropyl alcohol]

Generic: 0.5% (59 mL)

◆ **Manda-Amlodipine (Can)** *see* AmLODIPine *on page 109*

◆ **Manda-Citalopram (Can)** *see* Citalopram *on page 440*

◆ **Mandelamine® (Can)** *see* Methenamine *on page 1319*

◆ **Mandrake** *see* Podophyllum Resin *on page 1666*

Manganese (MAN ga nees)

Brand Names: U.S. Mangimin [OTC]; MN-50 [OTC]

Index Terms Manganese Chloride; Manganese Sulfate

Pharmacologic Category Dietary Supplement; Trace Element, Parenteral

Use Trace element added to total parenteral nutrition (TPN) solution to prevent manganese deficiency; orally as a dietary supplement

Pregnancy Risk Factor C

Dosage

Oral: **Adequate intake:**

0-6 months: 0.003 mg/day

7-12 months: 0.6 mg/day

1-3 years: 1.2 mg/day

4-8 years: 1.5 mg/day

9-13 years: Males: 1.9 mg/day; Females: 1.6 mg/day

14-18 years: Males: 2.2 mg/day; Females: 1.6 mg/day

Adults: Males: 2.3 mg/day; Females: 1.8 mg/day
Pregnancy: 2 mg/day
Lactation: 2.6 mg/day

I.V.:

Children: 2-10 **mcg**/kg/day usually administered in TPN solutions

Note: Use caution in premature neonates; manganese chloride solution for injection contains aluminum

Adults: 150-800 **mcg**/day usually administered in TPN solutions

Dosage adjustment in renal impairment: Use caution; manganese chloride solution for injection contains aluminum

Dosage adjustment in hepatic impairment: Use caution; dose may need to be decreased or withheld

Additional Information Complete prescribing information should be consulted for additional detail.

Dosage Forms Excipient information presented when available (limited, particularly for generics); consult specific product labeling.

Capsule, Oral, as chelated:
MN-50: Elemental manganese 16.67 mg

Solution, Intravenous, as chloride:
Generic: Elemental manganese 0.1 mg/mL (10 mL)

Solution, Intravenous, as sulfate:
Generic: Elemental manganese 0.1 mg/mL (10 mL)

Tablet, Oral, as aspartate:
Generic: 93 mg [elemental manganese 25 mg]

Tablet, Oral, as chelated:
Mangimin: Elemental manganese 10 mg [corn free, rye free, wheat free]
Generic: Elemental manganese 15 mg, Elemental manganese 50 mg

Tablet, Oral, as gluconate:
Generic: 50 mg [elemental manganese 5.7 mg]

◆ **Manganese Chloride** *see* Manganese *on page* 1265
◆ **Manganese Sulfate** *see* Manganese *on page* 1265
◆ **Mangimin [OTC]** *see* Manganese *on page* 1265

Mannitol (MAN i tole)

Brand Names: U.S. Aridol; Osmitrol; Resectisol

Brand Names: Canada Osmitrol®

Index Terms *D*-Mannitol

Pharmacologic Category Diagnostic Agent; Diuretic, Osmotic; Genitourinary Irrigant

Use

Injection: Reduction of increased intracranial pressure associated with cerebral edema; reduction of increased intraocular pressure; promoting urinary excretion of toxic substances; genitourinary irrigant in transurethral prostatic resection or other transurethral surgical procedures

Note: Although FDA-labeled indications, the use of mannitol for the prevention of acute renal failure and/or promotion of diuresis is not routinely recommended (Kellum, 2008).

Genitourinary irrigation solution: Irrigation in transurethral prostatic resection or other transurethral surgical procedures

Powder for inhalation: Assessment of bronchial hyperresponsiveness

Unlabeled Use Improve renal transplant function

Pregnancy Risk Factor C

Pregnancy Considerations Reproduction studies have not been conducted.

Breast-Feeding Considerations It is not known if mannitol is excreted in breast milk. The manufacturer recommends that caution be exercised when administering mannitol to nursing women.

Contraindications

Injection: Hypersensitivity to mannitol or any component of the formulation; severe renal disease (anuria); severe dehydration; active intracranial bleeding except during craniotomy; progressive heart failure, pulmonary congestion, or renal dysfunction after mannitol administration; severe pulmonary edema or congestion

Genitourinary irrigation solution: Anuria

Powder for inhalation: Hypersensitivity to mannitol, gelatin, or any component of the formulation; conditions that may be compromised by induced bronchospasm or repeated spirometry (eg, aortic or cerebral aneurysm, uncontrolled hypertension, recent MI or cerebral vascular accident)

Warnings/Precautions Should not be administered until adequacy of renal function and urine flow is established; use 1-2 test doses to assess renal response. Excess amounts can lead to profound diuresis with fluid and electrolyte loss; close medical supervision and dose evaluation are required. Watch for and correct electrolyte disturbances; adjust dose to avoid dehydration. May cause renal dysfunction especially with high doses; use caution in patients taking other nephrotoxic agents, with sepsis or pre-existing renal disease. To minimize adverse renal effects, adjust to keep serum osmolality less than 320 mOsm/L. Discontinue if evidence of acute tubular necrosis.

In patients being treated for cerebral edema, mannitol may accumulate in the brain (causing rebound increases in intracranial pressure) if circulating for long periods of time as with continuous infusion; intermittent boluses preferred. Cardiovascular status should also be evaluated; do not administer electrolyte-free mannitol solutions with blood. If hypotension occurs monitor cerebral perfusion pressure to ensure adequate. Vesicant (at concentrations >5%); ensure proper catheter or needle position prior to and during I.V. infusion; avoid extravasation of I.V. infusions.

Powder for inhalation (Aridol): **[U.S. Boxed Warning] Use may result in severe bronchospasm; use only for bronchial challenge testing. Testing should only be done by trained professionals. Not for use in patients with asthma or very low baseline pulmonary function. Medications (eg, short-acting inhaled beta-agonist) and equipment for the treatment of severe bronchospasm should be readily available.** Use with caution in patients with conditions that may increase sensitivity to bronchoconstriction (eg, severe cough, ventilatory impairment, spirometry-induced bronchoconstriction, hemoptysis of unknown origin, pneumothorax, recent abdominal, thoracic, or intraocular surgery, unstable angina, active upper or lower respiratory tract infection). Patients who have ≥10% reduction in FEV_1 on administration of the 0 mg capsule, patients with a positive response to bronchial challenge testing, or patients who develop significant respiratory symptoms should receive short acting inhaled beta-agonist; monitor until full recovery to baseline. Bronchial challenge testing should not be performed in children <6 years of age as these patients are unable to provide reliable spirometric results.

Adverse Reactions

Inhalation:

1% to 10%:

Cardiovascular: Chest discomfort (1%)

Central nervous system: Headache (adults 6%; children 3%), dizziness (1%)

Gastrointestinal: Nausea (adults 2%; children 3%), throat irritation (2%), retching (1%)

Respiratory: Cough (2%), pharyngolaryngeal pain (adults 2%; children 4%), rhinorrhea (2%), dyspnea (1%), wheezing (1%)

<1% (Limited to important or life-threatening): FEV_1 decreased, gagging

Injection: Frequency not defined:

Cardiovascular: Chest pain, CHF, circulatory overload, hyper-/hypotension, peripheral edema, tachycardia

Central nervous system: Chills, convulsions, dizziness, fever, headache

Dermatologic: Bullous eruption, urticaria

Endocrine & metabolic: Fluid and electrolyte imbalance, dehydration and hypovolemia secondary to rapid diuresis, hyperglycemia, hypernatremia, hyponatremia (dilutional), hyperosmolality-induced hyperkalemia, metabolic acidosis (dilutional), osmolar gap increased, water intoxication

Gastrointestinal: Nausea, vomiting, xerostomia

Genitourinary: Dysuria, polyuria

Local: Pain, thrombophlebitis, tissue necrosis

Ocular: Blurred vision

Renal: Acute renal failure, acute tubular necrosis (adult dose >200 g/day; serum osmolality >320 mOsm/L)

Respiratory: Pulmonary edema, rhinitis

Miscellaneous: Allergic reactions

Drug Interactions

Metabolism/Transport Effects None known.

Avoid Concomitant Use There are no known interactions where it is recommended to avoid concomitant use.

Increased Effect/Toxicity

Mannitol may increase the levels/effects of: Amifostine; Antihypertensives; Hypotensive Agents; Obinutuzumab; RiTUXimab; Sodium Phosphates

The levels/effects of Mannitol may be increased by: Alfuzosin; Analgesics (Opioid); Brimonidine (Topical); Diazoxide; Herbs (Hypotensive Properties); MAO Inhibitors; Pentoxifylline; Phosphodiesterase 5 Inhibitors; Prostacyclin Analogues

Decreased Effect

The levels/effects of Mannitol may be decreased by: Herbs (Hypertensive Properties); Methylphenidate; Yohimbine

Storage/Stability

Injection: Should be stored at room temperature of 15°C to 30°C (59°F to 86°F); do not freeze. In concentrations ≥15%, crystallization may occur at low temperatures; do not use solutions that contain crystals. Heating in a hot water bath and vigorous shaking may be utilized for resolubilization. Cool solutions to body temperature before using.

Irrigation: Store at room temperature of 25°C (77°F); excursions permitted up to 40°C. Avoid excessive heat; do not warm above 150°F (66°C). Do not freeze.

Powder for inhalation: Store at <25°C (<77°F); excursions permitted between 15°C to 30°C (59°F to 86°F). Do not freeze.

Mechanism of Action Produces an osmotic diuresis by increasing the osmotic pressure of glomerular filtrate, which inhibits tubular reabsorption of water and electrolytes and increases urinary output. Mechanism of action in reduction of intracranial pressure (ICP) is controversial. However, it is thought that mannitol reduces ICP by reducing blood viscosity which transiently increases cerebral blood flow and oxygen transport. This in turn reduces cerebral blood volume and ICP. Furthermore, mannitol reduces ICP by withdrawing water from the brain parenchyma and excretes water in the urine (Allen, 2009; Bratton, 2007; Miller, 2010).

Pharmacodynamics/Kinetics

Onset of action: Diuresis: Injection: 1-3 hours; Reduction in intracranial pressure: ~15-30 minutes

Duration: Reduction in intracranial pressure: 1.5-6 hours

Distribution: 34.3 L; remains confined to extracellular space (except in extreme concentrations); does not penetrate the blood-brain barrier (generally, penetration is low)

Metabolism: Minimally hepatic to glycogen

Bioavailability: Inhaled: 59% (relative to oral administration: 96%)

Half-life elimination: Terminal: 4.7 hours

Time to peak, plasma: Inhaled: 1.5 hours

Excretion: Urine (~55% to 87% as unchanged drug)

Dosage

Children: I.V.:

Increased intracranial pressure (unlabeled dosing): 0.25-1 g/kg/dose; repeat as needed to maintain serum osmolality <300-320 mOsm/kg (Adelson, 2003; Broderick, 2007; Hegenbarth, 2008)

Reduction of intraocular pressure: 1-2 g/kg or 30-60 g/m^2 administered over 30-60 minutes 1-1.5 hours prior to surgery

Reduction of intraocular pressure (traumatic hyphema): 1.5 g/kg administered over 45 minutes twice daily for IOP >35 mm Hg; may administer every 8 hours in patients with extremely high pressure (Crouch, 1999)

Children ≥6 years and Adults: Inhalation: Assessment of bronchial hyper-responsiveness: Administer in a stepwise fashion (measuring FEV_1 in duplicate after each administration) until the patient has a positive response or 635 mg of mannitol has been administered (whichever comes first).

Positive test: 15% reduction in FEV_1 from baseline or 10% incremental reduction in FEV_1 between consecutive doses

Negative test: Administration of full dose (635 mg) without reduction in FEV_1 sufficient to meet criteria for a positive test

Administration should be as follows:

Stepwise Administration Schedule

Dose #	Dose (mg)	Cumulative Dose (mg)	Capsules/Dose
1	0	0	1
2	5	5	1
3	10	15	1
4	20	35	1
5	40	75	1
6	80	155	2 x 40 mg caps
7	160	315	4 x 40 mg caps
8	160	475	4 x 40 mg caps
9	160	635	4 x 40 mg caps

Children ≥12 years and Adults:

I.V.:

Increased intracranial pressure, cerebral edema (unlabeled dosing): 0.25-1 g/kg/dose; may repeat every 6-8 hours as needed (Adelson, 2003; Bratton, 2007); maintain serum osmolality <300-320 mOsm/kg (Adelson, 2003; Rabinstein, 2006)

Reduction of intraocular pressure: 0.25-2 g/kg administered over 30-60 minutes 1-1.5 hours prior to surgery

Reduction of intraocular pressure (traumatic hyphema): 1.5 g/kg administered over 45 minutes twice daily for IOP >35 mm Hg; may administer every 8 hours in patients with extremely high pressure (Crouch, 1999)

Severe traumatic brain injury (unlabeled use): ~1.4 g/kg as initial management prior to neurosurgery with concurrent fluid replacement (Cruz, 2001; Cruz, 2002; Cruz, 2004)

Kidney transplant:

Donor: 12.5 g (with adequate hydration) prior to nephrectomy; may repeat (Morris, 2008)

Recipient: 50 g before kidney revascularization (Sprung, 2000; Tiggeler, 1984; van Valenberg, 1987; Weimar, 1983)

Topical: Transurethral irrigation: Use 5% urogenital solution as required for irrigation

Elderly: Refer to adult dosing. Consider initiation at lower end of dosing range.

Dosage adjustment in renal impairment: Contraindicated in severe renal impairment. Use caution in patients with underlying renal disease. May be used to reduce the incidence of acute tubular necrosis when administered prior to revascularization during kidney transplantation.

Dosage adjustment in hepatic impairment: No adjustment required.

Administration

I.V.: Concentration and rate of administration depends on indication/severity, or may be adjusted to urine flow. For cerebral edema or elevated ICP, administer over 30-60 minutes. Inspect for crystals prior to administration. If crystals are present, redissolve by warming solution. Use filter-type administration set for infusion solutions containing mannitol ≥20%. Do not administer with blood. Crenation and agglutination of red blood cells may occur if administered with whole blood.

Vesicant (at concentrations >5%); ensure proper catheter or needle position prior to and during I.V. infusion. Avoid extravasation of I.V. infusions.

Extravasation management: If extravasation occurs, stop infusion immediately and disconnect (leave needle/cannula in place); gently aspirate extravasated solution (do **NOT** flush the line); initiate hyaluronidase antidote; remove needle/cannula; apply dry cold compresses (Hurst, 2004); elevate extremity.

Hyaluronidase: SubQ: Administer multiple 0.5-1 mL injections of a 15 units/mL solution around the periphery of the extravasation (Kumar, 2003).

Inhalation (Aridol): Administer using supplied single patient use inhaler; do not puncture capsule more than once; do not swallow capsules. A nose clip may be used if preferred. The patient should exhale completely, followed by a controlled rapid deep inspiration from the device; hold breath for 5 seconds and exhale through the mouth. Measure FEV_1 in duplicate 60 seconds after inhalation; repeat process until positive response or full dose (635 mg) has been administered.

Irrigation: Administer using only the appropriate transurethral urologic instrumentation.

Monitoring Parameters Renal function, daily fluid I & O, serum electrolytes, serum and urine osmolality; for treatment of elevated intracranial pressure, maintain serum osmolality in the range of 300-320 mOsm/kg (serum osmolality >320 mOsm/kg may increase the risk of acute renal tubular damage).

Bronchial challenge test: Standard spirometry prior to bronchial challenge test; FEV_1 in duplicate 60 seconds after administration of each step of test

Additional Information May autoclave or heat to redissolve crystals; mannitol 20% has an approximate osmolarity of 1100 mOsm/L and mannitol 25% has an approximate osmolarity of 1375 mOsm/L

Bronchial challenge testing: The dose of inhaled mannitol which causes a 15% reduction in FEV_1 is expressed as PD_{15}

Dosage Forms Excipient information presented when available (limited, particularly for generics); consult specific product labeling.

Kit, Inhalation:

Aridol:

Solution, Intravenous:

Osmitrol: 5% (1000 mL); 10% (500 mL); 15% (500 mL); 20% (250 mL, 500 mL)

Generic: 5% (1000 mL); 10% (1000 mL); 15% (500 mL); 20% (250 mL, 500 mL); 25% (50 mL)

Solution, Irrigation:

Resectisol: 5% (2000 mL)

◆ **Mantoux** *see* Tuberculin Tests *on page* 2134

◆ **Maox [OTC]** *see* Magnesium Oxide *on page* 1262

◆ **Mapap [OTC]** *see* Acetaminophen *on page* 28

◆ **Mapap Arthritis Pain [OTC]** *see* Acetaminophen *on page* 28

◆ **Mapap Children's [OTC]** *see* Acetaminophen *on page* 28

◆ **Mapap Extra Strength [OTC]** *see* Acetaminophen *on page* 28

◆ **Mapap Infant's [OTC]** *see* Acetaminophen *on page* 28

◆ **Mapap Junior Rapid Tabs [OTC]** *see* Acetaminophen *on page* 28

◆ **Mapap PM [OTC]** *see* Acetaminophen and Diphenhydramine *on page* 32

◆ **Mapezine® (Can)** *see* CarBAMazepine *on page* 336

Maprotiline (ma PROE ti leen)

Brand Names: Canada Novo-Maprotiline; Teva-Maprotiline

Index Terms Ludiomil; Maprotiline Hydrochloride

Pharmacologic Category Antidepressant, Tetracyclic

Additional Appendix Information

Antidepressant Agents *on page* 2284

Use Treatment of major depressive disorder (MDD) or of anxiety associated with depression

Unlabeled Use Chronic pain; panic attacks

Pregnancy Risk Factor B

Medication Guide Available Yes

Dosage Oral:

Adults:

Mild-to-moderate depression/anxiety: Initial: 75 mg/day for 2 weeks (lower doses may be considered in some patients); Maintenance: Increase by 25 mg as tolerated up to 150 mg/day; given in divided doses or in a single daily dose

Severe depression: Initial: 100-150 mg/day for 2 weeks; Maintenance: Increase by 25 mg as tolerated up to 225 mg/day; given in divided doses or in a single daily dose

Elderly: Depression/anxiety: Initial: 25 mg/day for 2 weeks; Maintenance: Increase by 25 mg as tolerated; usual dose: 50-75 mg/day, higher doses may be necessary in nonresponders

Discontinuation of therapy: Upon discontinuation of antidepressant therapy, gradually taper the dose to minimize the incidence of withdrawal symptoms and allow for the detection of re-emerging symptoms. Evidence supporting ideal taper rates is limited. APA and NICE guidelines suggest tapering therapy over at least several weeks with consideration to the half-life of the antidepressant; antidepressants with a shorter half-life may need to be tapered more conservatively. In addition for long-term treated patients, WFSBP guidelines recommend tapering over 4-6 months. If intolerable withdrawal symptoms occur following a dose reduction, consider resuming the previously prescribed dose and/or decrease dose at a more gradual rate (APA, 2010; Bauer, 2002; Haddad, 2001; NCCMH, 2010; Schatzberg, 2006; Shelton, 2001; Warner, 2006).

MAO inhibitor recommendations:

Switching to or from an MAO inhibitor intended to treat psychiatric disorders:

Allow 14 days to elapse between discontinuing an MAO inhibitor intended to treat psychiatric disorders and initiation of maprotiline.

Allow 14 days to elapse between discontinuing maprotiline and initiation of an MAO inhibitor intended to treat psychiatric disorders.

Use with other MAO inhibitors (such as linezolid or I.V. methylene blue):

Do not initiate maprotiline in patients receiving linezolid or I.V. methylene blue; consider other interventions for psychiatric condition.

If urgent treatment with linezolid or I.V. methylene blue is required in a patient already receiving maprotiline and potential benefits outweigh potential risks, discontinue maprotiline promptly and administer linezolid or I.V. methylene blue. Monitor for serotonin syndrome for 2 weeks or until 24 hours after the last dose of linezolid or I.V. methylene blue, whichever comes first. May resume maprotiline 24 hours after the last dose of linezolid or I.V. methylene blue.

Dosage adjustment in renal impairment: No dosage adjustment provided in manufacturer's labeling.

Dosage adjustment in hepatic impairment: No dosage adjustment provided in manufacturer's labeling.

Additional Information Complete prescribing information should be consulted for additional detail.

Dosage Forms Excipient information presented when available (limited, particularly for generics); consult specific product labeling.

Tablet, Oral, as hydrochloride:

Generic: 25 mg, 50 mg, 75 mg

◆ **Maprotiline Hydrochloride** *see* Maprotiline *on page 1268*

◆ **Mar-Anastrozole (Can)** *see* Anastrozole *on page 137*

Maraviroc (mah RAV er rock)

Brand Names: U.S. Selzentry

Brand Names: Canada Celsentri™

Index Terms UK-427,857

Pharmacologic Category Antiretroviral, CCR5 Antagonist (Anti-HIV)

Use Treatment of CCR5-tropic HIV-1 infection, in combination with other antiretroviral agents

Pregnancy Risk Factor B

Pregnancy Considerations Adverse fetal effects were not observed in animal reproduction studies. It is not known if maraviroc crosses the placenta. The DHHS Perinatal HIV Guidelines note there are insufficient data to recommend use in pregnancy.

Regardless of CD4 count or HIV RNA copy number, all HIV-infected pregnant women should receive a combination antepartum antiretroviral (ARV) drug regimen; this includes women who require therapy for their own health, as well as women who do not yet require therapy for their own health. ARV therapy should be started as soon as possible if required for the woman's health. Although earlier initiation may be more effective in reducing the perinatal transmission of HIV, also consider maternal conditions (eg, nausea and vomiting) and the potential risks of first trimester fetal exposure for specific agents. Plasma HIV RNA levels should be assessed at ~34-36 weeks gestation in order to help determine mode of delivery. If ARV therapy must be interrupted for <24 hours during the peripartum period, stop then restart all medications simultaneously in order to decrease the chance of developing resistance. Long-term follow-up is recommended for all infants exposed to ARV medications.

Healthcare providers are encouraged to enroll pregnant women exposed to antiretroviral medications in the Antiretroviral Pregnancy Registry (1-800-258-4263 or www.APRegistry.com). Healthcare providers caring for HIV-infected women and their infants may contact the National Perinatal HIV Hotline (888-448-8765) for clinical consultation (DHHS [perinatal], 2012).

Breast-Feeding Considerations It is not known if maraviroc is excreted into breast milk. Maternal or infant antiretroviral therapy does not completely eliminate the risk of postnatal HIV transmission. In addition, multiclass-resistant virus has been detected in breast-feeding infants despite maternal therapy. Therefore, in the United States, where formula is accessible, affordable, safe, and sustainable, and the risk of infant mortality due to diarrhea and respiratory infections is low, complete avoidance of breast-feeding by HIV-infected women is recommended to decrease potential transmission of HIV (DHHS [perinatal], 2012).

Medication Guide Available Yes

Contraindications Patients with severe renal impairment (Cl_{cr} <30 mL/minute) or end-stage renal disease (ESRD) who are taking potent CYP3A4 inhibitors or inducers

Canadian labeling: Additional contraindications (not in U.S. labeling): Hypersensitivity to maraviroc or any component of the formulation

Warnings/Precautions [U.S. Boxed Warning] Possible drug-induced hepatotoxicity with allergic type features has been reported; hepatotoxicity (usually after 1 month of treatment) may be preceded by allergic type reactions (eg, pruritic rash, eosinophilia, fever or increased IgE, excluding rash alone or Stevens-Johnson syndrome [DHHS, 2013]) and/or hepatic adverse events (transaminase increases or signs/symptoms of hepatitis); some cases have been life-threatening; immediately evaluate patients with signs and symptoms of allergic reaction or hepatitis. Use with caution in patients with pre-existing hepatic dysfunction or coinfection with HBV or HCV, however symptoms have occurred in the absence of pre-existing hepatic conditions. Monitor hepatic function at baseline and as clinically indicated during treatment. Consider discontinuation in any patient with possible hepatitis or with elevated transaminases combined with systemic allergic events.

Severe and life-threatening skin and hypersensitivity reactions, including Stevens-Johnson syndrome, toxic epidermal necrolysis and drug rash with eosinophilia with systemic symptoms (DRESS), have been reported with use, predominately in patients also receiving concomitant agents associated with these reactions. Rash and constitutional findings (eg, fever, muscle aches, conjunctivitis, oral lesions), with or without organ dysfunction, have also accompanied these reports. Discontinue maraviroc and any other suspected agent immediately if symptoms or signs of hypersensitivity occur. Monitor liver function tests and clinical status as appropriate.

Patients may develop immune reconstitution syndrome resulting in the occurrence of an inflammatory response to an indolent or residual opportunistic infection during initial HIV treatment or activation of autoimmune disorders (eg, Graves' disease, polymyositis, Guillain-Barré syndrome) later in therapy; further evaluation and treatment may be required. Monitor closely for signs/symptoms of developing infections; use associated with a small increase of certain upper respiratory tract infections and herpes virus infections during clinical trials. Use with caution in patients with cardiovascular disease or cardiac risk factors. During trials, a small increase in cardiovascular events (myocardial ischemia and/or infarction) occurred in treated patients compared to placebo, although a contributory relationship relative to therapy is unknown. Symptomatic postural hypotension has occurred; use caution in patients at risk for postural hypotension due to concomitant medication or history of condition. Adjust dose in patients with severe renal dysfunction if postural hypotension experienced.

Use caution in patients with mild-to-moderate hepatic impairment; maraviroc concentrations are increased; no dosage adjustment recommended. Maraviroc concentrations are further increased in patients with moderate hepatic impairment receiving concomitant strong CYP3A inhibitors; monitor closely for adverse events. Renal impairment may increase maraviroc concentrations. Use with caution in patients with mild-to-moderate renal impairment. Potentially significant interactions may exist, requiring dose or frequency adjustment, additional monitoring, and/or selection of alternative therapy. Prior to therapy, coreceptor tropism testing should be performed for presence of CCR5-tropic only virus HIV-1 infection. Therapy not recommended for use in patients with CXCR4- or dual/mixed tropic HIV-1 infection; efficacy not demonstrated in this population. In studies with treatment-naive patients, virologic failure and emergent lamivudine resistance was more common in maraviroc-treated patients compared to patients receiving efavirenz.

Adverse Reactions

>10%:

Central nervous system: Fever (13%)

Dermatologic: Skin rash (11%)

Respiratory: Upper respiratory tract infection (23%), cough (14%)

2% to 10%:

Cardiovascular: Vascular hypertensive disorder (3%)

Central nervous system: Dizziness (9%; including postural dizziness), insomnia (8%), paresthesia (5%), anxiety (4%), impaired consciousness (4%), depression (4%), pain (4%), peripheral neuropathy (4%), sensory disturbance (4%), amnesia (3%)

Dermatologic: Folliculitis (4%), pruritus (4%), acne vulgaris (3%), skin neoplasm (benign; 3%), alopecia (2%), erythema (2%), tinea (4%)

Endocrine & metabolic: Lipodystrophy (4%)

Gastrointestinal: Decreased gastrointestinal motility (9%), change in appetite (8%), constipation (6%)

Genitourinary: Genitourinary complaint (urinary tract/bladder symptoms, 3% to 5%), warts (genital, 2%)

Hematologic & oncologic: Neutropenia (grades 3/4: 4%)

Hepatic: Increased serum AST (grades 3/4: 5%), increased serum ALT (grades 3/4: 3%), increased serum bilirubin (grades 3/4: 6%)

Infection: Herpes infection (8%), bacterial infection (3%), *Neisseria*, (3%),

Neuromuscular & skeletal: Arthralgia (7%), myalgia (3%)

Ophthalmic: Conjunctivitis (2%), eye infection (2%)

Otic: Otitis media (2%)

Respiratory: Bronchitis (7%), sinusitis (7%), paranasal sinus disease (3% to 6%), irregular breathing (4%), nasal congestion (4%), lower respiratory tract infection (3%)

Miscellaneous: Sweat gland disturbances (5%), flu-like symptoms (2%)

<2% (Limited to important or life-threatening): Anal cancer, angina pectoris, basal cell carcinoma, bile duct neoplasm, bone marrow depression, carcinoma *in situ* of esophagus, cardiac failure, cerebrovascular accident, cholestatic jaundice, coronary artery disease, coronary artery occlusion, endocarditis, endocrine neoplasm, hepatic cirrhosis, hepatic failure, hepatotoxicity, hypoplastic anemia, immune reconstitution syndrome, increased creatine kinase, ischemic heart disease, liver metastases, lymphoma, meningitis (viral), multiorgan hypersensitivity, myocardial infarction, myositis, osteonecrosis, pneumonia, portal vein thrombosis, rhabdomyolysis, seizure, septic shock, squamous cell carcinoma, Stevens-Johnson syndrome, syncope, T-cell lymphoma, tongue neoplasm, toxic epidermal necrolysis, tremor

Drug Interactions

Metabolism/Transport Effects **Substrate** of CYP3A4 (major), P-glycoprotein; **Note:** Assignment of Major/Minor substrate status based on clinically relevant drug interaction potential

Avoid Concomitant Use

Avoid concomitant use of Maraviroc with any of the following: Fusidic Acid (Systemic); St Johns Wort

Increased Effect/Toxicity

The levels/effects of Maraviroc may be increased by: CYP3A4 Inhibitors (Moderate); CYP3A4 Inhibitors (Strong); Dasatinib; Fusidic Acid (Systemic); Ivacaftor; Luliconazole; Mifepristone; Simeprevir

Decreased Effect

The levels/effects of Maraviroc may be decreased by: Bosentan; CYP3A4 Inducers (Strong); Dabrafenib; Deferasirox; St Johns Wort; Tocilizumab

Ethanol/Nutrition/Herb Interactions Herb/Nutraceutical: St. John's wort may decrease maraviroc concentrations leading to loss of therapeutic efficacy and potentially increased risk of resistance; concomitant use not recommended.

Storage/Stability Store at 25°C (77°F); excursions permitted to 15°C to 30°C (59°F to 86°F).

Mechanism of Action Maraviroc, a CCR5 antagonist, selectively and reversibly binds to the chemokine (C-C motif receptor 5 [CCR5]) coreceptors located on human CD4 cells. CCR5 antagonism prevents interaction between the human CCR5 coreceptor and the gp120 subunit of the viral envelope glycoprotein, thereby inhibiting gp120 conformational change required for CCR5-tropic HIV-1 fusion with the CD4 cell and subsequent cell entry.

Pharmacodynamics/Kinetics

Distribution: V_d: ~194 L

Protein binding: ~76%

Metabolism: Hepatic, via CYP3A to inactive metabolites

Bioavailability: 23% to 33%

Half-life elimination: 14-18 hours

Time to peak, plasma: 0.5-4 hours

Excretion: Urine (~20%, 8% as unchanged drug); feces (76%, 25% as unchanged drug)

Dosage Oral: Adolescents ≥16 years and Adults: 300 mg twice daily

Dosage adjustment for concomitant CYP3A4 inhibitors/inducers:

CYP3A inhibitors (with or without a CYP3A4 inducer): 150 mg twice daily; dose recommended when maraviroc administered concomitantly with strong CYP3A inhibitors including (but not limited to) protease inhibitors (excluding tipranavir/ritonavir), delavirdine, ketoconazole, itraconazole, clarithromycin, nefazodone, and telithromycin.

CYP3A inducers (without a strong CYP3A4 inhibitor): 600 mg twice daily; dose recommended when maraviroc administered concomitantly with CYP3A inducers including (but not limited to) efavirenz, etravirine, rifampin, carbamazepine, phenobarbital, and phenytoin

Dosage adjustment in renal impairment:

Cl_{cr} ≥30 mL/minute:

Cl_{cr} ≥30 mL/minute and concomitant potent CYP3A4 inhibitors (with or without a CYP3A4 inducer): 150 mg twice daily

Cl_{cr} ≥30 mL/minute and concomitant potent CYP3A4 inducer (without a CYP3A4 inhibitor): 600 mg twice daily

Cl_{cr} ≥30 mL/minute and other concomitant medications (eg, tipranavir/ritonavir, nevirapine, raltegravir, all NRTIs, and enfuvirtide): 300 mg twice daily

Cl_{cr} <30 mL/minute:

Cl_{cr} <30 mL/minute and concomitant potent CYP3A inhibitors (with or without a CYP3A4 inducer) **or** concomitant potent CYP3A4 inducer (without a CYP3A4 inhibitor): Not recommended

Cl_{cr} <30 mL/minute and other concomitant medications (eg, tipranavir/ritonavir, nevirapine, raltegravir, all NRTIs, and enfuvirtide): 300 mg twice daily. If postural hypotension occurs, reduce dose to 150 mg twice daily

Cl_{cr} <30 mL/minute and experiencing postural hypotension: Reduce dose to 150 mg twice daily

ESRD requiring intermittent hemodialysis (IHD):

With concomitant potent CYP3A inhibitors (with or without a CYP3A4 inducer) or concomitant potent CYP3A4 inducer (without a CYP3A4 inhibitor): Not recommended. **Note:** Hemodialysis has minimal effect on clearance.

With other concomitant medications (eg, tipranavir/ritonavir, nevirapine, raltegravir, all NRTIs, and enfuvirtide): 300 mg twice daily. If postural hypotension occurs, reduce dose to 150 mg twice daily. **Note:** Hemodialysis has minimal effect on clearance.

Dosage adjustment in hepatic impairment:

Mild-to-moderate impairment: Use caution; maraviroc concentrations are increased although dosage adjustment is not recommended.

Moderate impairment (with concomitant strong CYP3A4 inhibitor): Use caution; maraviroc concentrations may be increased; monitor closely for adverse events.

Severe impairment: No dosage adjustment provided in manufacturer's labeling (has not been studied).

Dietary Considerations May be taken without regards to meals.

Administration Administer without regards to meals.

Monitoring Parameters Viral load, CD4 count, transaminases and bilirubin (prior to initiation and periodically during treatment); signs/symptoms of infection, rash, severe skin reactions,hepatitis and/or allergic reaction; postural hypotension; tropism testing (prior to initiation)

Additional Information Maraviroc should only be used in patients with documented CCR5-tropic only virus; if it is used in mixed tropism patients, eg, with CCR5-tropic and CXCR4-tropic, the CCR5-tropic virus will be suppressed and the CXCR4-tropic virus will continue to proliferate. A phenotypic tropism assay is generally preferred to determine HIV-1 coreceptor usage compared to genotypic testing; a genotypic tropism assay should be considered as an alternative test (DHHS, 2013).

Dosage Forms Excipient information presented when available (limited, particularly for generics); consult specific product labeling.

Tablet, Oral:

Selzentry: 150 mg, 300 mg [contains fd&c blue #2 aluminum lake, soybean lecithin]

◆ **Marcaine** *see* Bupivacaine *on page 289*

◆ **Marcaine® (Can)** *see* Bupivacaine *on page 289*

◆ **Marcaine Preservative Free** *see* Bupivacaine *on page 289*

◆ **Marcaine Spinal** *see* Bupivacaine *on page 289*

◆ **Mar-Ciprofloxacin (Can)** *see* Ciprofloxacin (Systemic) *on page 430*

◆ **Mar-Cof® CG** *see* Guaifenesin and Codeine *on page 976*

◆ **Margesic** *see* Butalbital, Acetaminophen, and Caffeine *on page 305*

◆ **Margesic® H** *see* Hydrocodone and Acetaminophen *on page 1006*

◆ **Marinol** *see* Dronabinol *on page 674*

◆ **Marinol® (Can)** *see* Dronabinol *on page 674*

◆ **Mark 1™** *see* Atropine and Pralidoxime *on page 200*

◆ **Mar-Letrozole (Can)** *see* Letrozole *on page 1185*

◆ **Marlissa** *see* Ethinyl Estradiol and Levonorgestrel *on page 787*

◆ **Mar-Metformin (Can)** *see* MetFORMIN *on page 1310*

◆ **Marqibo** *see* VinCRIStine (Liposomal) *on page 2194*

◆ **Mar-Risperidone (Can)** *see* RisperiDONE *on page 1826*

◆ **Mar-Rizatriptan (Can)** *see* Rizatriptan *on page 1844*

◆ **Mar-Tramadol/Acet (Can)** *see* Acetaminophen and Tramadol *on page 33*

◆ **Marvelon (Can)** *see* Ethinyl Estradiol and Desogestrel *on page 784*

◆ **Matulane** *see* Procarbazine *on page 1720*

◆ **Matzim LA** *see* Diltiazem *on page 613*

◆ **3M™ Avagard™ [OTC]** *see* Chlorhexidine Gluconate *on page 408*

◆ **Mavik** *see* Trandolapril *on page 2104*

◆ **Maxair Autohaler** *see* Pirbuterol *on page 1656*

◆ **Maxalt** *see* Rizatriptan *on page 1844*

◆ **Maxalt™ (Can)** *see* Rizatriptan *on page 1844*

◆ **Maxalt-MLT** *see* Rizatriptan *on page 1844*

◆ **Maxalt RPD™ (Can)** *see* Rizatriptan *on page 1844*

◆ **Maxichlor PEH [OTC]** *see* Chlorpheniramine and Phenylephrine *on page 412*

◆ **Maxichlor PEH DM [OTC] [DSC]** *see* Chlorpheniramine, Phenylephrine, and Dextromethorphan *on page 413*

◆ **Maxichlor PSE [OTC]** *see* Chlorpheniramine and Pseudoephedrine *on page 412*

◆ **Maxichlor PSE DM [OTC] [DSC]** *see* Chlorpheniramine, Pseudoephedrine, and Dextromethorphan *on page 414*

◆ **Maxidex** *see* Dexamethasone (Ophthalmic) *on page 583*

◆ **Maxidex® (Can)** *see* Dexamethasone (Ophthalmic) *on page 583*

◆ **Maxidone®** *see* Hydrocodone and Acetaminophen *on page 1006*

◆ **Maxifed [OTC]** *see* Guaifenesin and Pseudoephedrine *on page 978*

◆ **Maxifed DM [DSC]** *see* Guaifenesin, Pseudoephedrine, and Dextromethorphan *on page 979*

◆ **Maxifed DMX** *see* Guaifenesin, Pseudoephedrine, and Dextromethorphan *on page 979*

◆ **Maxifed-G [OTC] [DSC]** *see* Guaifenesin and Pseudoephedrine *on page 978*

◆ **Maxilene® (Can)** *see* Lidocaine (Topical) *on page 1212*

◆ **Maxipime** *see* Cefepime *on page 367*

◆ **Maxipime® (Can)** *see* Cefepime *on page 367*

◆ **Maxitrol®** *see* Neomycin, Polymyxin B, and Dexamethasone *on page 1439*

◆ **Maxzide** *see* Hydrochlorothiazide and Triamterene *on page 1006*

◆ **Maxzide-25** *see* Hydrochlorothiazide and Triamterene *on page 1006*

◆ **May Apple** *see* Podophyllum Resin *on page 1666*

◆ **M-Clear** *see* Guaifenesin and Codeine *on page 976*

◆ **M-Clear WC** *see* Guaifenesin and Codeine *on page 976*

◆ **MCV** *see* Meningococcal (Groups A / C / Y and W-135) Diphtheria Conjugate Vaccine *on page 1291*

◆ **MCV4** *see* Meningococcal (Groups A / C / Y and W-135) Diphtheria Conjugate Vaccine *on page 1291*

◆ **MDL 73,147EF** *see* Dolasetron *on page 647*

◆ **MDV3100** *see* Enzalutamide *on page 713*

◆ **MDX-010** *see* Ipilimumab *on page 1109*

◆ **MDX-CTLA-4** *see* Ipilimumab *on page 1109*

Measles, Mumps, and Rubella Virus Vaccine (MEE zels, mumpz & roo BEL a VYE rus vak SEEN)

Brand Names: U.S. M-M-R II

Brand Names: Canada M-M-R II; Priorix

Index Terms MMR; Mumps, Measles and Rubella Vaccines; Rubella, Measles and Mumps Vaccines

Pharmacologic Category Vaccine, Live (Viral)

Additional Appendix Information

Immunization Administration Recommendations *on page 2334*

Immunization Recommendations *on page 2339*

Use Measles, mumps, and rubella prophylaxis

The Advisory Committee on Immunization Practices (ACIP) recommends routine vaccination for the following (CDC, 2013c):

- All children (first dose given at 12-15 months of age)
- Adults born 1957 or later (without evidence of immunity or documentation of vaccination). Vaccine may be given to adults born prior to 1957 if they do not have contraindications to the MMR vaccine.
- Adults at higher risk for exposure to and transmission of measles mumps and rubella should receive special consideration for vaccination, unless an acceptable evidence of immunity exists. This includes international travelers, persons attending colleges and other post high school education, persons working in healthcare facilities.

Pregnancy Risk Factor C

Dosage SubQ: **Note:** The minimum interval between 2 doses of MMR vaccine is 28 days (CDC, 2013c).

Infants 6-11 months: 0.5 mL per dose

International travel: Children without evidence of immunity traveling internationally should receive 1 dose of MMR before departure from the United States; these children should be revaccinated with 2 doses of MMR with the first dose between 12-15 months of age (and at least 28 days after the previous dose) and the second dose at least 28 days later (CDC, 2013a; CDC, 2013c).

Measles outbreak: If there is risk of exposure to measles involving infants, one dose of MMR vaccine may be administered (CDC, 2013c).

Children ≥12 months: 0.5 mL per dose

Primary immunization is recommended at 12-15 months of age and repeated at 4-6 years of age; the second dose is recommended prior to entering kindergarten or first grade. The second dose may be administered at any time provided at least 28 days have elapsed since the first dose (CDC, 2013c).

HIV infection without evidence of MMR immunity: Children with HIV infection and without evidence of severe immunosuppression should have 2 doses of MMR. Those with perinatal HIV infection who were vaccinated prior to effective ART should have 2 doses of MMR once ART is established (CDC, 2013c).

Household/close contacts of immunocompromised persons: Two doses of MMR administered at least 28 days apart unless they have acceptable evidence of immunity (CDC, 2013c).

International travel: Children without evidence of immunity traveling internationally should receive 2 doses of MMR before departure from the United States. The first dose given ≥12 months of age and the second dose 28 days later (CDC, 2013a; 2013c).

Measles or mumps outbreak: Children ages 1-4 years who received 1 dose of MMR should be considered for a second dose if the outbreak involves preschool-aged children (CDC, 2013c).

Adults: 0.5 mL per dose; 1 or 2 doses administered at least 28 days apart based upon the following criteria (CDC, 2013c):

Adults born in or after 1957 should be vaccinated unless they have acceptable evidence of immunity.

Adults born prior to 1957 are considered immune to measles, mumps, and rubella but may be vaccinated if they do not have contraindications to the vaccine. Pregnant adults born prior to 1957 are not considered immune to rubella.

Healthcare personnel: Persons born in or after 1957 should have 2 doses of vaccine unless they have acceptable evidence of immunity. Unvaccinated persons born prior to 1957 should also consider vaccination with 2 doses unless they have laboratory evidence or laboratory confirmation of disease.

HIV infection (without severe immunosuppression): Two doses of MMR unless there is acceptable evidence of immunity.

Household/close contacts of immunocompromised persons: Two doses of MMR unless there is acceptable evidence of immunity.

International travelers: Two doses of MMR prior to travel unless there is acceptable evidence of immunity.

Measles, mumps, or rubella outbreak (community): Adults who received 1 dose of MMR should be considered for a second dose if the outbreak involves measles or mumps in adults. Vaccination should also be considered for persons born prior to 1957 without evidence of immunity who may be exposed to mumps. A single dose of a rubella-containing vaccine is considered adequate vaccination during a rubella outbreak.

Measles, mumps, or rubella outbreak (healthcare facility): Unvaccinated health care personnel without evidence of immunity regardless of birth year should receive 2 doses during a measles or mumps outbreak and one dose during a rubella outbreak.

Students: Persons entering post-high school educational facilities should receive 2 doses of MMR unless they have acceptable evidence of immunity prior to enrollment.

Women of childbearing potential: One dose of MMR unless they have acceptable evidence of immunity. Vaccination should not be given during pregnancy and pregnancy should be avoided for 28 days after vaccine administration.

Dosage adjustment in renal impairment: No dosage adjustment provided in manufacturer's labeling.

Dosage adjustment in hepatic impairment: No dosage adjustment provided in manufacturer's labeling.

Additional Information Complete prescribing information should be consulted for additional detail.

Dosage Forms Excipient information presented when available (limited, particularly for generics); consult specific product labeling.

Injection, powder for reconstitution [preservative free]:

M-M-R® II: Measles virus ≥1000 $TCID_{50}$, mumps virus ≥20,000 $TCID_{50}$, and rubella virus ≥1000 $TCID_{50}$ [contains albumin (human), bovine serum, chicken egg protein, gelatin, neomycin, sorbitol, and sucrose 1.9 mg/vial; supplied with diluent]

Measles, Mumps, Rubella, and Varicella Virus Vaccine

(MEE zels, mumpz, roo BEL a, & var i SEL a VYE rus vak SEEN)

Brand Names: U.S. ProQuad

Brand Names: Canada Priorix-Tetra

Index Terms MMRV; Mumps, Rubella, Varicella, and Measles Vaccine; Rubella, Varicella, Measles, and Mumps Vaccine; Varicella, Measles, Mumps, and Rubella Vaccine

Pharmacologic Category Vaccine, Live (Viral)

Additional Appendix Information

Immunization Administration Recommendations *on page 2334*

Immunization Recommendations *on page 2339*

Use

Measles, mumps, rubella, and varicella vaccination: To provide active immunization for the prevention of measles, mumps, rubella, and varicella in children 12 months to 12 years of age.

The Advisory Committee on Immunization Practices (ACIP) recommends routine vaccination against measles, mumps, rubella, and varicella in healthy children; the first dose should be given at 12-15 months of age and the second dose at 4-6 years of age. For children receiving their first dose at 12-47 months of age, either the MMRV combination vaccine or separate MMR and varicella vaccines can be used. (The ACIP prefers administration of separate MMR and varicella vaccines as the first dose in this age group unless the parent or caregiver expresses preference for the MMRV combination.) For children receiving the first dose at ≥48 months or their second dose at any age, use of MMRV is preferred. For children with a personal or family history of seizures, the ACIP recommends vaccination with separate MMR and varicella vaccines, as opposed to the MMRV combination vaccine (CDC, 2010).

Canadian labeling (not in U.S. labeling): MMRV combination vaccine is approved for use in healthy children 9 months to 6 years; may consider use in healthy children ≤12 years of age based upon prior experience with the separate component (live-attenuated MMR or live-attenuated varicella [OKA-strain]) vaccines.

Dosage *U.S. labeling:* SubQ: Children 12 months to 12 years: One dose (0.5 mL). The first dose is usually administered at 12-15 months of age. If a second dose of measles, mumps, rubella, and varicella vaccine is needed, ProQuad can be used with the second dose usually administered at 4-6 years of age. At least 1 month should elapse between a previous dose of a measles-containing vaccine (eg, MMR) and at least 3 months should elapse between a dose of varicella-containing vaccine.

ACIP recommendations: For children receiving their first dose at 12-47 months of age, either the MMRV combination vaccine or separate MMR and varicella vaccines can be used. (The ACIP prefers administration of separate MMR and varicella vaccines as the first dose in this age group unless the parent or caregiver expresses preference for the MMRV combination.) For children receiving the first dose at ≥48 months or their second dose at any age, use of MMRV is preferred. The ACIP recommends that children with a personal or family history of seizures be vaccinated with separate MMR and varicella vaccines, as opposed to the MMRV combination vaccine (CDC, 2010)

Canadian labeling: I.M., SubQ: Children 9 months to 6 years: Two doses (0.5 mL each dose) administered at least 4-6 weeks apart (minimum interval between doses: 4 weeks)

Dosage adjustment in renal impairment: No dosage adjustment provided in manufacturer's labeling.

Dosage adjustment in hepatic impairment: No dosage adjustment provided in manufacturer's labeling.

Additional Information Complete prescribing information should be consulted for additional detail.

Dosage Forms Excipient information presented when available (limited, particularly for generics); consult specific product labeling.

Injection, powder for reconstitution [preservative free]:

ProQuad: Measles virus ≥3.00 log_{10} $TCID_{50}$, mumps virus ≥4.3 log_{10} $TCID_{50}$, rubella virus ≥3.00 log_{10} $TCID_{50}$, and varicella virus ≥3.99 log_{10} PFU [contains albumin (human), bovine serum, chicken egg protein, gelatin, neomycin, sorbitol, and sucrose (≤21 mg/vial)]

Dosage Forms: Canada Excipient information presented when available (limited, particularly for generics); consult specific product labeling.

Injection, powder for reconstitution [preservative free]:

Priorix-Tetra (CAN): Measles virus ≥3.00 log_{10} $CCID_{50}$, mumps virus ≥4.4 log_{10} $CCID_{50}$, rubella virus ≥3.00 log_{10} $CCID_{50}$, and varicella virus ≥3.3 log_{10} PFU [contains chicken egg protein, neomycin, sorbitol, and sucrose]

Mebendazole

(me BEN da zole)

Brand Names: Canada Vermox®

Index Terms Vermox

Pharmacologic Category Anthelmintic

Use Treatment of *Ancylostoma duodenale* or *Necator amiericanus* (hookworms), *Ascaris lumbricoides* (roundworms), *Enterobius vermicularis* (pinworms), *Strongyloides stercoralis* (roundworm), *Taenia solium* (tapeworms), *Trichuris trichiura* (whipworms),

Unlabeled Use Treatment of *Ancylostoma caninum* (eosinophilic enterocolitis), *Capillaria philippinensis* (capillariasis), *Giardia duodenalis* (giardiasis), *Mansonella perstans* (filariasis), visceral larva migrans (toxocariasis)

Pregnancy Risk Factor C

Dosage Oral: Children ≥2 years; Adolescents, and Adults:

Canadian labeling:

Ancylostoma duodenale (hookworm), *Necator americanus* (hookworm), *Ascaris lumbricoides* (roundworm), *Strongyloides stercoralis* (roundworm), *Taenia solium* (tapeworms), *Trichuris trichiura* (whipworm), mixed infection: 100 mg twice daily for 3 days; repeat in 3 weeks if not cured with initial treatment

Enterobius vermicularis (pinworm): 100 mg as a single dose; repeat in 2 and 4 weeks (manufacturer's labeling); treatment should include family members in close contact with patient (*Med Lett,* 2007)

Unlabeled dosing:

Ancylostoma duodenale (hookworm), *Ascaris lumbricoides* (roundworm), *Necator americanus* (hookworm), *Trichuris trichiura* (whipworm): 500 mg as a single dose (*Med Lett*, 2007)

Unlabeled uses:

Ancylostoma caninum (eosinophilic enterocolitis): 100 mg twice daily for 3 days (*Med Lett,* 2007)

Capillaria philippinensis (capillariasis): 200 mg twice daily for 20 days (*Med Lett,* 2007)

Giardia duodenalis (giardiasis): 200 mg 3 times daily for 5 days (Canete, 2006; Chandy, 2009)

Mansonella perstans (filariasis): 100 mg twice daily for 30 days (*Med Lett,* 2007)

Visceral larva migrans (toxocariasis): 100-200 mg twice daily for 5 days (*Med Lett,* 2007)

Dosage adjustment in renal impairment: No dosage adjustment provided in manufacturer's labeling.

Dosage adjustment in hepatic impairment: No dosage adjustment provided in manufacturer's labeling; however, undergoes extensive hepatic metabolism; use with caution as systemic exposure may be increased.

Additional Information Complete prescribing information should be consulted for additional detail.

Dosage Forms: Canada Excipient information presented when available (limited, particularly for generics); consult specific product labeling.

Tablet, oral:

Vermox® 100 mg [scored]

Mechlorethamine (Systemic)

(me klor ETH a meen)

Brand Names: U.S. Mustargen

Index Terms Chlorethazine; Chlorethazine Mustard; HN_2; Mechlorethamine Hydrochloride; Mustine; Nitrogen Mustard

Pharmacologic Category Antineoplastic Agent, Alkylating Agent (Nitrogen Mustard)

Use

Hodgkin lymphoma: Palliative treatment of Hodgkin lymphoma

Malignant effusion: Palliative treatment of effusions from metastatic carcinomas

Additional approved uses (manufacturer labeling): Treatment of lymphosarcoma, chronic myelocytic or chronic lymphocytic leukemia, polycythemia vera, mycosis fungoides, and bronchogenic carcinoma

Pregnancy Risk Factor D

Pregnancy Considerations Adverse events have been observed in animal reproduction studies. Women of childbearing potential are advised not to become pregnant during treatment. **[U.S. Boxed Warning]: Avoid exposure during pregnancy.**

Breast-Feeding Considerations It is not known if mechlorethamine is excreted in human breast milk. Due to the potential for serious adverse reactions in the nursing infant, the decision to discontinue mechlorethamine or to discontinue breast-feeding should take into account the importance of treatment to the mother.

Contraindications Hypersensitivity to mechlorethamine or any component of the formulation; presence of known infection

Warnings/Precautions Hazardous agent; use appropriate precautions for handling and disposal (NIOSH, 2012). **[U.S. Boxed Warning]: Mechlorethamine is a highly toxic nitrogen mustard; avoid inhalation of vapors or dust; review and follow special handling procedures.** Avoid dust or vapor contact with skin or eyes. If accidental skin exposure occurs, wash/irrigate thoroughly with water for at least 15 minutes, followed by 2% sodium thiosulfate solution; remove and destroy any contaminated clothing. If exposure to eye(s) occurs, promptly irrigate for at least 15 minutes with copious amounts of water, normal saline, or balanced salt ophthalmic irrigating solution; obtain ophthalmology consultation. The manufacturer recommends neutralizing remaining unused mechlorethamine, empty or partial vials, gloves, tubing, glassware, etc., after mechlorethamine administration; soak in an aqueous solution containing equal volumes of sodium thiosulfate (5%) and sodium bicarbonate (5%) for 45 minutes; rinse with water; dispose of properly.

[U.S. Boxed Warning]: Mechlorethamine is a potent vesicant; extravasation results in painful inflammation with induration and sloughing. If extravasation occurs, promptly manage by infiltrating area with 1/6 molar sodium thiosulfate solution, followed by dry cold compresses for 6-12 hours. Ensure proper needle or catheter placement prior to and during infusion. Avoid extravasation.

Bone marrow suppression: May cause lymphopenia, leukopenia, granulocytopenia, thrombocytopenia and anemia. Agranulocytopenia may occur (rare); persistent pancytopenia has been reported. Monitor blood counts. Bleeding due to thrombocytopenia may occur. Use with caution in patients where neoplasm has bone marrow involvement or in those who have received prior myelosuppressive chemotherapy; marrow function may be further compromised (possibly fatal). Bone marrow function should recover after mechlorethamine administration prior to initiating radiation therapy or other chemotherapy regimens.

Hyperuricemia may occur, especially with lymphomas; ensure adequate hydration; consider antihyperuricemic therapy if appropriate. Mechlorethamine is associated with a high emetic potential (Basch, 2011); antiemetics are recommended to prevent nausea and vomiting. Hypersensitivity reactions, including anaphylaxis, have been reported. Mechlorethamine has immunosuppressant properties; may predispose patients to infections (bacterial, viral, or fungal). Alkylating agents, including mechlorethamine, are associated with in increased incidence of secondary malignancies; concurrent radiation therapy or combination chemotherapy may increase the risk. Potentially significant drug-drug interactions may exist, requiring dose or frequency adjustment, additional monitoring, and/or selection of alternative therapy.

[U.S. Boxed Warning]: Avoid exposure during pregnancy. Impaired spermatogenesis, azoospermia, and total germinal aplasia may occur in male patients treated with mechlorethamine, particularly when used in combination with other chemotherapy agents. Delayed menses, oligomenorrhea, or temporary or permanent amenorrhea may be observed in female patients treated with mechlorethamine.

Bone marrow failure and other toxicities are more common in chronic lymphocytic leukemia (CLL); in general, mechlorethamine is no longer used in the treatment of CLL. Bone and nervous system tumors typically respond poorly to treatment with mechlorethamine. The routine use of mechlorethamine in widely disseminated tumors is discouraged. **[U.S. Boxed Warning]: Should be administered under the supervision of an experienced cancer chemotherapy physician.**

Adverse Reactions Frequency not defined.

Central nervous system: Drowsiness, encephalopathy (high dose), fever, headache, lethargy, sedation, vertigo

Dermatologic: Alopecia, erythema multiforme, maculopapular rash, petechiae, rash

Endocrine & metabolic: Amenorrhea, hyperuricemia, oligomenorrhea, spermatogenesis decreased

Gastrointestinal: Anorexia, diarrhea, metallic taste, mucositis, nausea, vomiting

Hepatic: Jaundice

Hematologic: Agranulocytosis, granulocytopenia (onset 6-8 days, recovery 10-21 days), hemolytic anemia, leukopenia, lymphocytopenia, pancytopenia, secondary leukemias, thrombocytopenia

Local: Thrombophlebitis, tissue necrosis (extravasation)

Neuromuscular & skeletal: Weakness

Ocular: Lacrimation

Otic: Deafness, tinnitus

Miscellaneous: Anaphylaxis, diaphoresis, herpes zoster infection, hypersensitivity reactions

Drug Interactions

Metabolism/Transport Effects None known.

Avoid Concomitant Use

Avoid concomitant use of Mechlorethamine (Systemic) with any of the following: BCG; CloZAPine; Natalizumab; Pimecrolimus; Tacrolimus (Topical); Tofacitinib; Vaccines (Live)

Increased Effect/Toxicity

Mechlorethamine (Systemic) may increase the levels/ effects of: CloZAPine; Leflunomide; Natalizumab; Tofacitinib; Vaccines (Live)

The levels/effects of Mechlorethamine (Systemic) may be increased by: Denosumab; Pimecrolimus; Roflumilast; Tacrolimus (Topical); Trastuzumab

Decreased Effect

Mechlorethamine (Systemic) may decrease the levels/ effects of: BCG; Coccidioidin Skin Test; Sipuleucel-T; Vaccines (Inactivated); Vaccines (Live)

The levels/effects of Mechlorethamine (Systemic) may be decreased by: Echinacea

Ethanol/Nutrition/Herb Interactions Ethanol: Avoid ethanol (due to GI irritation).

Preparation for Administration Hazardous agent; use appropriate precautions for handling and disposal (NIOSH, 2012). **Must be prepared immediately before use;** degradation begins shortly after dilution. Dilute powder with 10 mL SWFI or NS to a final concentration of 1 mg/mL. May be further diluted in 50-100 mL NS for intracavitary administration.

Storage/Stability Store intact vials at room temperature of 15°C to 30°C (59°F to 86°F). Protect from light. Protect from humidity. **Must be prepared immediately before use;** degradation begins shortly after dilution.

Mechanism of Action Bifunctional alkylating agent that inhibits DNA and RNA synthesis via formation of carbonium ions; produces interstrand and intrastrand cross-links in DNA resulting in miscoding, breakage, and failure of replication. Although not cell phase-specific *per se,* mechlorethamine effect is most pronounced in the S phase, and cell proliferation is arrested in the G_2 phase.

Pharmacodynamics/Kinetics

Metabolism: Rapid hydrolysis in the plasma to active metabolites (Perry, 2012)

Half-life elimination: 15-20 minutes (Perry, 2012)

Dosage Dosage should be based on ideal dry weight (evaluate the presence of edema or ascites so that dosage is based on actual weight unaugmented by edema/ ascites). Mechlorethamine is associated with a high emetic potential (Basch, 2011); antiemetics are recommended to prevent nausea and vomiting.

Hodgkin lymphoma (unlabeled dosing): Adults: I.V.:

MOPP regimen: 6 mg/m^2 on days 1 and 8 of a 28-day cycle for 6 to 8 cycles (Canelos, 1992; DeVita, 1970)

Stanford V regimen: 6 mg/m^2 as a single dose on day 1 in weeks 1, 5, and 9 (Horning, 2000; Horning, 2002)

Malignant effusion: Intracavitary: 0.4 mg/kg as a single dose, although 0.2 mg/kg (10-20 mg) as a single dose has been used by the *intrapericardial* route

Dosage adjustment in renal impairment: No dosage adjustment provided in manufacturer's labeling.

Dosage adjustment in hepatic impairment: No dosage adjustment provided in manufacturer's labeling. The following have also been reported:

Mild-to-moderate impairment: No dosage adjustment necessary (Ecklund, 2005).

Severe liver impairment: No dosage adjustment necessary; concomitant chemotherapy may require alteration until improvement in hepatic function (Ecklund, 2005).

Dosing in obesity: *ASCO Guidelines for appropriate chemotherapy dosing in obese adults with cancer:* In general, utilize patient's actual body weight (full weight) for calculation of body surface area- or weight-based dosing, particularly when the intent of therapy is curative; manage regimen-related toxicities in the same manner as for nonobese patients; if a dose reduction is utilized due to toxicity, consider resumption of full weight-based dosing with subsequent cycles, especially if cause of toxicity (eg, hepatic or renal impairment) is resolved (Griggs, 2012). **Note:** The manufacturer recommends dosing be based on ideal dry body weight and the presence of edema or ascites should be considered so the dose will be based on unaugmented weight.

Administration

I.V.: Administer as a slow I.V. push over a few minutes into a free-flowing I.V. solution. Mechlorethamine is associated with a high emetic potential (Basch, 2011); antiemetics are recommended to prevent nausea and vomiting.

Intracavitary: May further dilute in 50-100 mL of normal saline prior to instillation; rotate patient position every 5-10 minutes for 1 hour after instillation to obtain uniform distribution.

Prepare immediately prior to administration.

Vesicant; ensure proper needle or catheter placement prior to and during infusion; avoid extravasation.

Extravasation management: If extravasation occurs, stop infusion immediately and disconnect (leave cannula/ needle in place); gently aspirate extravasated solution (do **NOT** flush the line); remove needle/cannula; elevate extremity.

Sodium thiosulfate 1/6 M solution: Inject subcutaneously into extravasation area using 2 mL for each mg of mechlorethamine suspected to have extravasated (Perez Fidalgo, 2012; Polovich, 2009). Apply ice for 6-12 hours after sodium thiosulfate administration (Mustargen prescribing information, 2013; Polovich, 2009) **or** may apply dry cold compresses for 20 minutes 4 times daily for 1-2 days (Perez Fidalgo, 2012).

Hazardous agent; use appropriate precautions for handling and disposal (NIOSH, 2012).

Monitoring Parameters CBC with differential and platelet count; renal and hepatic function; signs/symptoms of hypersensitivity reactions, infection, and extravasation

Additional Information A topical gel is commercially approved for topical treatment of cutaneous T-cell lymphoma (mycosis fungoides type), please refer to Mechlorethamine (Topical) monograph.

Product Availability Mustargen: Mustargen was acquired by Recordati Rare Diseases in 2013; availability information is currently unknown.

Dosage Forms Excipient information presented when available (limited, particularly for generics); consult specific product labeling.

Solution Reconstituted, Injection, as hydrochloride:

Mustargen: 10 mg (1 ea)

Mechlorethamine (Topical) (me klor ETH a meen)

Brand Names: U.S. Valchlor

Index Terms Mechlorethamine HCl (Topical); Mechlorethamine Topical Gel

Pharmacologic Category Antineoplastic Agent, Alkylating Agent (Nitrogen Mustard)

Use Cutaneous T-cell lymphoma: Topical treatment of stage IA and IB mycosis fungoides-type cutaneous T-cell lymphoma in patients who have received prior skin-directed therapy

Pregnancy Risk Factor D

Pregnancy Considerations Adverse events have been observed in animal reproduction studies. There have been case reports of teratogenic events following systemic use in humans. Pregnancy should be avoided if therapy is needed.

Breast-Feeding Considerations It is not known if mechlorethamine is excreted into breast milk following topical application. Due to the potential for serious adverse reactions in the nursing infant following topical or systemic exposure from the mother's skin, the manufacturer recommends a decision be made whether to discontinue nursing or to discontinue the drug, taking into account the importance of treatment to the mother.

Prescribing and Access Restrictions Valchlor is only available through a specialty pharmacy; information regarding prescribing and access may be found at www.valchlor.com.

Medication Guide Available Yes

Contraindications Known severe hypersensitivity to mechlorethamine or any component of the formulation

Warnings/Precautions Hazardous agent – use appropriate precautions for handling and disposal (NIOSH, 2012). Caregivers should wear nitrile gloves when applying to patients. Wash hands thoroughly with soap and water after handling/application. If accidental skin exposure occurs, wash thoroughly for at least 15 minutes with soap and water; remove any contaminated clothing. Eye exposure may result in pain, burning, inflammation, photophobia, and blurred vision. Blindness and severe anterior eye injury (irreversible) may occur. If exposure to eye(s) occurs, promptly irrigate for at least 15 minutes with copious amounts of water, normal saline, or balanced salt ophthalmic irrigating solution; obtain ophthalmology consultation. Exposure to mucous membranes may cause pain, redness, and ulceration; may be severe. If mucosal contact occurs, irrigate promptly for at least 15 minutes with copious amounts of water and obtain medical consultation.

Dermatitis commonly occurs; may be moderately severe or severe. Monitor for redness, swelling, itching, blistering, ulceration, and secondary skin infections. Facial, genitalia, anus and intertriginous skin areas are at increased risk for dermatitis. Dermatitis may require dosage reduction. Avoid direct contact with mechlorethamine (other than intended treatment areas for the patient). Secondary exposure risks include dermatitis, mucosal injury, and secondary malignancies. To prevent secondary exposure, follow recommended application procedures. In a clinical study, non-melanoma skin cancers developed during or within 1 year following treatment. Some instances occurred in patients who had received previous treatments that were associated with non-melanoma skin cancer. Monitor for non-melanoma skin cancers during and following treatment; may occur anywhere on the skin, including untreated areas.

Mechlorethamine gel contains alcohol and is flammable; follow recommended application procedures and avoid fire, flame, and smoking until mechlorethamine has dried.

Adverse Reactions

>10%:

- Dermatologic: Dermatitis (56%; moderately severe or severe: 23%), pruritus (20%), bacterial skin infection (11%)
- Hematologic & oncologic: Hematologic abnormality (decreased hemoglobin, neutrophils, or platelets; 13%)

1% to 10%:

- Dermatologic: Dermal ulcer (6%), skin hyperpigmentation (5%)
- Hematologic & oncologic: Malignant neoplasm (nonmelanoma skin cancer; 2%)

Postmarketing and/or case reports (Limited to important or life-threatening): Anaphylaxis, hypersensitivity reaction

Drug Interactions

Metabolism/Transport Effects None known.

Avoid Concomitant Use There are no known interactions where it is recommended to avoid concomitant use.

Increased Effect/Toxicity There are no known significant interactions involving an increase in effect.

Decreased Effect There are no known significant interactions involving a decrease in effect.

Preparation for Administration Hazardous agent – use appropriate precautions for handling and disposal (NIOSH, 2012).

Storage/Stability Prior to dispensing, store in freezer at -25°C to -15°C (-13°F to 5°F). After dispensing, refrigerate at 2°C to 8°C (36°F to 46°F); apply immediately (or within 30 minutes) after removal from refrigerator; return to refrigerator promptly after each use. Discard unused product 60 days after opening.

Mechanism of Action Mechlorethamine is a nitrogen mustard alkylating agent which forms inter- and intrastrand DNA cross-links, resulting in inhibition of DNA synthesis. Topical application allows for skin-directed treatment while minimizing systemic nitrogen mustard exposure (Lessin, 2013).

Pharmacodynamics/Kinetics

Absorption: Topical: None detected (Lessin, 2013)

Distribution: Topical: No detectable systemic exposure in a clinical study (Lessin, 2013)

Dosage

Cutaneous T-cell lymphoma (mycosis fungoides-type): Adults: Topical: Apply a thin film once daily to affected areas of skin

Note: Concurrent use of topical or systemic corticosteroids was not allowed in the clinical study (Lessin, 2013).

Dosage adjustment for toxicity: Skin ulceration (any grade), blistering, or dermatitis (moderately severe-to-severe): Withhold treatment; upon improvement, may reinitiate treatment with a reduced frequency of once every 3 days; if every 3-day application is tolerated for at least 1 week, may increase to every other day for at least 1 week, then (if tolerated) may increase to once daily.

Dosage adjustment in renal impairment: No dosage adjustment provided in the manufacturer's labeling; however, dosage adjustment is unlikely based on the lack of systemic exposure.

Dosage adjustment in hepatic impairment: No dosage adjustment provided in the manufacturer's labeling; however, dosage adjustment is unlikely based on the lack of systemic exposure.

Administration Apply a thin film topically to affected area. Apply immediately (or within 30 minutes) after removal from refrigerator; return to refrigerator promptly after each use. Apply to completely dry skin at least 4 hours before or 30 minutes after showering/washing. Allow treated area(s) to dry for 5-10 minutes after application before covering with clothing. May apply emollients (moisturizers) to treated area 2 hours before or 2 hours after mechlorethamine application. Do not use occlusive dressings over treatment areas. Avoid fire, flame, and smoking until mechlorethamine has dried.

Hazardous agent; use appropriate precautions for handling and disposal (NIOSH, 2012). Caregivers should wear nitrile gloves when applying to patients. Wash hands thoroughly with soap and water after handling/application. If accidental skin exposure occurs, wash thoroughly for at least 15 minutes with soap and water; remove any contaminated clothing.

Monitoring Parameters Monitor for dermatologic toxicity (skin ulcers, blistering, dermatitis, secondary skin infections) and signs/symptoms of non-melanoma skin cancer.

Dosage Forms Considerations Valchlor 0.016% is equivalent to 0.02% mechlorethamine hydrochloride

Dosage Forms Excipient information presented when available (limited, particularly for generics); consult specific product labeling.

Gel, External:

Valchlor: 0.016% (60 g) [contains edetate disodium, isopropyl alcohol, menthol, propylene glycol]

◆ **Mechlorethamine HCl (Topical)** *see* Mechlorethamine (Topical) *on page 1275*

◆ **Mechlorethamine Hydrochloride** *see* Mechlorethamine (Systemic) *on page 1274*

◆ **Mechlorethamine Topical Gel** *see* Mechlorethamine (Topical) *on page 1275*

Meclizine (MEK li zeen)

Brand Names: U.S. Antivert; Dramamine Less Drowsy [OTC]; Medi-Meclizine [OTC]; Travel Sickness [OTC]; UniVert; Vertin-32 [OTC]

Index Terms Meclizine Hydrochloride; Meclozine Hydrochloride

Pharmacologic Category Antiemetic; Histamine H_1 Antagonist; Histamine H_1 Antagonist, First Generation; Piperazine Derivative

Additional Appendix Information

Beers Criteria – Potentially Inappropriate Medications for Geriatrics *on page 2368*

Use Prevention and treatment of symptoms of motion sickness; management of vertigo with diseases affecting the vestibular system

Pregnancy Risk Factor B

Pregnancy Considerations Adverse events have been observed in animal reproduction studies; however, an increased risk of fetal abnormalities has not been observed following maternal use of meclizine during pregnancy.

Breast-Feeding Considerations It is not known if meclizine is excreted into breast milk.

Contraindications Hypersensitivity to meclizine or any component of the formulation

Warnings/Precautions Use with caution in patients with asthma, angle-closure glaucoma, prostatic hyperplasia, pyloric or duodenal obstruction, or bladder neck obstruction. May be inappropriate in older adults depending on comorbidities (eg, dementia, delirium, etc) due to its potent anticholinergic effects (Beers Criteria). Use with caution in the elderly; may be more sensitive to adverse effects. If vertigo does not respond in 1-2 weeks, it is advised to discontinue use. May be sedating, use with caution in disorders where CNS depression is a feature; patients must be cautioned about performing tasks which require mental alertness (eg, operating machinery or driving). Effects may be potentiated when used with other sedative drugs or ethanol.

Adverse Reactions Frequency not defined.

Central nervous system: Drowsiness, fatigue, headache

Gastrointestinal: Vomiting, xerostomia

Ocular: Blurred vision

Miscellaneous: Anaphylactoid reaction

Drug Interactions

Metabolism/Transport Effects **Substrate** of CYP2D6 (minor); **Note:** Assignment of Major/Minor substrate status based on clinically relevant drug interaction potential

Avoid Concomitant Use

Avoid concomitant use of Meclizine with any of the following: Aclidinium; Azelastine (Nasal); Ipratropium (Oral Inhalation); Paraldehyde; Tiotropium; Umeclidinium

Increased Effect/Toxicity

Meclizine may increase the levels/effects of: Alcohol (Ethyl); Analgesics (Opioid); Anticholinergics; Azelastine (Nasal); Buprenorphine; CNS Depressants; Hydrocodone; Methotrimeprazine; Metyrosine; Mirtazapine; Paraldehyde; Pramipexole; ROPINIRole; Rotigotine; Selective Serotonin Reuptake Inhibitors; Tiotropium; Zolpidem

The levels/effects of Meclizine may be increased by: Aclidinium; Brimonidine (Topical); Doxylamine; Droperidol; HydrOXYzine; Ipratropium (Oral Inhalation); Magnesium Sulfate; Methotrimeprazine; Perampanel; Pramlintide; Sodium Oxybate; Tapentadol; Umeclidinium

Decreased Effect

Meclizine may decrease the levels/effects of: Acetylcholinesterase Inhibitors (Central); Benzylpenicilloyl Polylysine; Betahistine; Hyaluronidase

The levels/effects of Meclizine may be decreased by: Acetylcholinesterase Inhibitors (Central); Amphetamines; Peginterferon Alfa-2b

Ethanol/Nutrition/Herb Interactions Ethanol: May increase CNS depression; monitor for increased effects with coadministration. Caution patients about effects.

Mechanism of Action Has central anticholinergic action by blocking chemoreceptor trigger zone; decreases excitability of the middle ear labyrinth and blocks conduction in the middle ear vestibular-cerebellar pathways

Pharmacodynamics/Kinetics

Onset of action: ~1 hour (Wang, 2012)

Duration: ~24 hours (Wang, 2012)

Distribution: V_d: 7 L/kg (Wang, 2012)

Metabolism: Hepatic to norchlorcyclizine (Wang, 2012)

Half-life elimination: 5 hours (Wang, 2011a; Wang, 2011)

Time to peak, plasma: 3 hours (Wang, 2011a; Wang, 2011)

Excretion: Urine and feces as unchanged drug and metabolites (Wang, 2012)

Dosage Children ≥12 years and Adults: Oral:

Motion sickness: 25-50 mg 1 hour before travel, repeat dose every 24 hours if needed

Vertigo: 25-100 mg daily in divided doses

Dosage adjustment in renal impairment: No dosage adjustment provided in manufacturer's labeling.

Dosage adjustment in hepatic impairment: No dosage adjustment provided in manufacturer's labeling.

Dosage Forms Excipient information presented when available (limited, particularly for generics); consult specific product labeling.

Tablet, Oral, as hydrochloride:

Antivert: 12.5 mg, 25 mg

Dramamine Less Drowsy: 25 mg [contains fd&c yellow #10 (quinoline yellow)]

Dramamine Less Drowsy: 25 mg [contains fd&c yellow #10 aluminum lake]

Medi-Meclizine: 25 mg

UniVert: 32 mg [scored; contains brilliant blue fcf (fd&c blue #1), fd&c yellow #10 (quinoline yellow)]

Vertin-32: 32 mg [contains brilliant blue fcf (fd&c blue #1), fd&c yellow #10 (quinoline yellow)]

Generic: 12.5 mg, 25 mg

Tablet Chewable, Oral, as hydrochloride:

Travel Sickness: 25 mg [scored; contains aspartame, fd&c red #40 aluminum lake; raspberry flavor]

Generic: 25 mg

◆ **Meclizine Hydrochloride** *see* Meclizine *on page 1277*

◆ **Meclozine Hydrochloride** *see* Meclizine *on page 1277*

◆ **Med-Anastrozole (Can)** *see* Anastrozole *on page 137*

◆ **Med-Baclofen (Can)** *see* Baclofen *on page 221*

◆ **Med-Derm Hydrocortisone [OTC]** *see* Hydrocortisone (Topical) *on page 1011*

◆ **Medent®-PEI [OTC]** *see* Guaifenesin and Phenylephrine *on page 978*

◆ **Med-Glybe (Can)** *see* GlyBURIDE *on page 963*

◆ **Medical Provider EZ Flu PF** *see* Influenza Virus Vaccine (Inactivated) *on page 1078*

◆ **Medicinal Carbon** *see* Charcoal, Activated *on page 401*

◆ **Medicinal Charcoal** *see* Charcoal, Activated *on page 401*

◆ **Medi-First Anti-Fungal [OTC]** *see* Tolnaftate *on page 2087*

◆ **Medi-First Hydrocortisone [OTC]** *see* Hydrocortisone (Topical) *on page 1011*

◆ **Medi-Meclizine [OTC]** *see* Meclizine *on page 1277*

◆ **Medi-Phenyl [OTC]** *see* Phenylephrine (Systemic) *on page 1636*

◆ **Mediproxen [OTC]** *see* Naproxen *on page 1425*

◆ **MED-Letrozole (Can)** *see* Letrozole *on page 1185*

◆ **Medrol** *see* MethylPREDNISolone *on page 1340*

◆ **Medrol® (Can)** *see* MethylPREDNISolone *on page 1340*

◆ **Medrol Dose Pack** *see* MethylPREDNISolone *on page 1340*

◆ **Medrol (Pak)** *see* MethylPREDNISolone *on page 1340*

◆ **Medroxy (Can)** *see* MedroxyPROGESTERone *on page 1278*

MedroxyPROGESTERone

(me DROKS ee proe JES te rone)

Brand Names: U.S. Depo-Provera; Depo-SubQ Provera 104; Provera

Brand Names: Canada Alti-MPA; Apo-Medroxy®; Depo-Prevera®; Depo-Provera®; Dom-Medroxyprogesterone; Gen-Medroxy; Medroxy; Medroxyprogesterone Acetate Injectable Suspension USP; Novo-Medrone; PMS-Medroxyprogesterone; Provera-Pak; Provera®; Teva-Medroxyprogesterone

Index Terms Acetoxymethylprogesterone; Medroxyprogesterone Acetate; Methylacetoxyprogesterone; MPA

Pharmacologic Category Contraceptive; Progestin

Use Secondary amenorrhea or abnormal uterine bleeding due to hormonal imbalance; reduction of endometrial hyperplasia in nonhysterectomized postmenopausal women receiving conjugated estrogens; prevention of pregnancy; management of endometriosis-associated pain; adjunctive therapy and palliative treatment of recurrent and metastatic endometrial carcinoma

Unlabeled Use Treatment of low-grade endometrial stromal sarcoma; treatment of paraphilia/hypersexuality

Pregnancy Risk Factor X

Pregnancy Considerations Use is contraindicated in women who are pregnant, as a diagnostic test for pregnancy, or for missed abortion. In general, there is not an increased risk of birth defects following inadvertent use of the injectable medroxyprogesterone (MPA) contraceptives early in pregnancy. Hypospadias has been reported in male babies and clitoral enlargement and labial fusion have been reported in female babies exposed to MPA during the first trimester of pregnancy. High doses impair fertility. Ectopic pregnancies have been reported with use of the MPA contraceptive injection. Median time to conception/return to ovulation following discontinuation of MPA contraceptive injection is 10 months following the last injection.

Breast-Feeding Considerations Medroxyprogesterone (MPA) is excreted into breast milk. Composition, quality, and quantity of breast milk are not affected; adverse developmental and behavioral effects have not been noted following exposure of infant to MPA while breast-feeding. The manufacturer does not recommend the use of MPA tablets in breast-feeding mothers; however, guidelines note that the injectable MPA contraceptives can be initiated immediately postpartum in women who are nursing (CDC, 2010; CDC, 2011; CDC, 2013).

Contraindications Hypersensitivity to medroxyprogesterone or any component of the formulation; history of or current thrombophlebitis or venous thromboembolic disorders (including DVT, PE); cerebral vascular disease; severe hepatic dysfunction or disease; carcinoma of the breast or other estrogen- or progesterone-dependent neoplasia; undiagnosed vaginal bleeding; missed abortion, diagnostic test for pregnancy, pregnancy

Warnings/Precautions Hazardous agent; use appropriate precautions for handling and disposal (NIOSH, 2012).

[U.S. Boxed Warning]: Prolonged use of medroxyprogesterone contraceptive injection may result in a loss of bone mineral density (BMD). It is not known if use during adolescence or early adulthood will decrease peak bone mass accretion or increase the risk for osteoporotic fractures later in life. Loss is related to the duration of use, may not be completely reversible on discontinuation of the drug, and incidence is not significantly different between the SubQ and I.M. dosage forms. The impact on peak bone mass in adolescents should be weighed against the potential for unintended pregnancies in treatment decision. Consider alternative contraceptive methods in patients at risk for osteoporosis (eg, metabolic bone disease, family history of osteoporosis, chronic use of medications associated with osteoporosis such as corticosteroids). **[U.S. Boxed Warning]: Long-term use (ie, >2 years) should be limited to situations where other birth control methods are inadequate.** Consider other methods of birth control in women with (or at risk for) osteoporosis. **[U.S. Boxed Warning]: Inform patients that injectable contraceptives do not protect against HIV infection or other sexually-transmitted diseases.** When used for contraception, the possibility of ectopic pregnancy should be considered in patients with abdominal pain. Anaphylaxis or anaphylactoid reactions have been reported with use of the injection; medication for the treatment of hypersensitivity reactions should be available for immediate use.

[U.S. Boxed Warning]: Estrogens with or without progestin should not be used to prevent cardiovascular disease. Using data from the Women's Health Initiative (WHI) studies, an increased risk of deep vein thrombosis (DVT) and stroke has been reported with CE and an increased risk of DVT, stroke, pulmonary emboli (PE) and myocardial infarction (MI) has been reported with CE with MPA in postmenopausal women. Additional risk factors include diabetes mellitus, hypercholesterolemia, hypertension, SLE, obesity, tobacco use, and/or history of venous thromboembolism (VTE). Risk factors should be managed appropriately; discontinue use if adverse cardiovascular events occur or are suspected. If thrombosis develops with contraceptive treatment, discontinue treatment (unless no other acceptable contraceptive alternative). Whenever possible, progestins in combination with estrogens should be discontinued at least 4-6 weeks prior to and for 2 weeks following elective surgery associated with an increased risk of thromboembolism or during periods of prolonged immobilization.

[U.S. Boxed Warning]: Estrogens with or without progestin should not be used to prevent dementia. In the Women's Health Initiative Memory Study (WHIMS), an increased incidence of dementia was observed in women ≥65 years of age taking CE alone or in combination with MPA.

[U.S. Boxed Warning]: Based on data from the Women's Health Initiative (WHI) studies, an increased risk of invasive breast cancer was observed in postmenopausal women using conjugated estrogens (CE) in combination with medroxyprogesterone acetate

(MPA). This risk may be associated with duration of use and declines once combined therapy is discontinued (Chlebowski, 2009). The risk of invasive breast cancer was decreased in postmenopausal women with a hysterectomy using CE only, regardless of weight. However, the risk was not significantly decreased in women at high risk for breast cancer (family history of breast cancer, personal history of benign breast disease) (Anderson, 2012). An increase in abnormal mammogram findings has also been reported with estrogen alone or in combination with progestin therapy. Use is contraindicated in patients with known or suspected breast cancer.

MPA is used to reduce the risk of endometrial hyperplasia in nonhysterectomized postmenopausal women receiving conjugated estrogens. The use of unopposed estrogen in women with an intact uterus is associated with an increased risk of endometrial cancer. The addition of a progestin to estrogen therapy may decrease the risk of endometrial hyperplasia, a precursor to endometrial cancer. Adequate diagnostic measures, including endometrial sampling if indicated, should be performed to rule out malignancy in postmenopausal women with undiagnosed abnormal vaginal bleeding. Estrogens may exacerbate endometriosis. Malignant transformation of residual endometrial implants has been reported posthysterectomy with unopposed estrogen therapy. Consider adding a progestin in women with residual endometriosis posthysterectomy. Postmenopausal estrogen therapy and combined estrogen/progesterone therapy may increase the risk of ovarian cancer; however, the absolute risk to an individual woman is small. Although results from various studies are not consistent, risk does not appear to be significantly associated with the duration, route, or dose of therapy. In one study, the risk decreased after 2 years following discontinuation of therapy (Mørch, 2009). Although the risk of ovarian cancer is rare, women who are at an increased risk (eg, family history) should be counseled about the association (NAMS, 2012).

[U.S. Boxed Warning]: Estrogens with or without progestin should be used for the shortest duration possible at the lowest effective dose consistent with treatment goals. Before prescribing estrogen therapy to postmenopausal women, the risks and benefits must be weighed for each patient. Women should be informed of these risks and benefits, as well as possible effects of progestin when added to estrogen therapy. Patients should be reevaluated as clinically appropriate to determine if treatment is still necessary. Available data related to treatment risks are from Women's Health Initiative (WHI) studies, which evaluated oral CE 0.625 mg with or without MPA 2.5 mg relative to placebo in postmenopausal women. Other combinations and dosage forms of estrogens and progestins were not studied. **Outcomes reported from clinical trials using CE with or without MPA should be assumed to be similar for other doses and other dosage forms of estrogens and progestins until comparable data becomes available.**

Discontinue pending examination in cases of sudden partial or complete vision loss, sudden onset of proptosis, diplopia, or migraine; discontinue permanently if papilledema or retinal vascular lesions are observed on examination. Use with caution in patients with diseases that may be exacerbated by fluid retention (including asthma, epilepsy, migraine, cardiac, or renal dysfunction). Contraceptive therapy with medroxyprogesterone commonly results in an average weight gain of ~2.5 kg after 1 year and ~3.7 kg after 2 years of treatment. Use caution with history of depression.

May have adverse effects on glucose tolerance; use caution in women with diabetes. MPA is extensively metabolized in the liver. Discontinue if jaundice develops or if acute or chronic hepatic disturbances occur. Use is contraindicated with severe hepatic disease. Unscheduled bleeding/spotting may occur. Presentation of irregular, unresolving vaginal bleeding following previously regular cycles warrants further evaluation including endometrial sampling, if indicated, to rule out malignancy. Not for use prior to menarche. The use of estrogens and/or progestins may change the results of some laboratory tests (eg, coagulation factors, lipids, glucose tolerance, binding proteins). The dose, route, and the specific estrogen/progestin influences these changes. In addition, personal risk factors (eg, cardiovascular disease, smoking, diabetes, age) also contribute to adverse events; use of specific products may be contraindicated in women with certain risk factors.

Adverse Reactions Adverse effects as reported with any dosage form; percent ranges presented are noted with the MPA I.M. contraceptive injection:

>5%:

Central nervous system: Dizziness, headache, nervousness

Endocrine & metabolic: Libido decreased, menstrual irregularities (includes bleeding, amenorrhea, or both)

Gastrointestinal: Abdominal pain/discomfort, weight gain (>10 lbs at 24 months: 38%)

1% to 5%:

Cardiovascular: Edema

Central nervous system: Depression, fatigue, insomnia

Dermatologic: Acne, alopecia, rash

Endocrine & metabolic: Breast pain, hot flashes

Gastrointestinal: Bloating, nausea

Genitourinary: Dysmenorrhea, leukorrhea, vaginitis

Local: Injection site reaction (SubQ administration): Atrophy, induration, pain

Neuromuscular & skeletal: Arthralgia, backache, leg cramp, weakness

<1% (Limited to important or life-threatening): Allergic reaction, anaphylaxis, anaphylactoid reactions, angioedema, asthma, blood dyscrasia, bone mineral density decreased, breast cancer, breast changes, cervical cancer, chest pain, chloasma, cholestatic jaundice, deep vein thrombosis, diaphoresis, dyspnea, facial palsy, galactorrhea, glucose tolerance decreased, hirsutism, hoarseness, injection site reactions, jaundice, lack of return to fertility, lactation decreased, melasma, nipple bleeding, optic neuritis, osteoporosis, osteoporotic fractures, paralysis, paresthesia, pulmonary embolus, rectal bleeding, retinal thrombosis, scleroderma, seizure, syncope, tachycardia, thrombophlebitis, urticaria

In addition: Depo-Provera® aqueous suspension: Residual lump, sterile abscess, or skin discoloration at the injection

Drug Interactions

Metabolism/Transport Effects Substrate of CYP3A4 (major); **Note:** Assignment of Major/Minor substrate status based on clinically relevant drug interaction potential; **Induces** CYP3A4 (weak/moderate)

Avoid Concomitant Use

Avoid concomitant use of MedroxyPROGESTERone with any of the following: Axitinib; Griseofulvin; Simeprevir; Tranexamic Acid; Ulipristal

Increased Effect/Toxicity

MedroxyPROGESTERone may increase the levels/effects of: Benzodiazepines (metabolized by oxidation); Selegiline; Tranexamic Acid; Voriconazole

The levels/effects of MedroxyPROGESTERone may be increased by: Atazanavir; Boceprevir; Cobicistat; Herbs (Progestogenic Properties); Mifepristone; Voriconazole

Decreased Effect

MedroxyPROGESTERone may decrease the levels/effects of: Anticoagulants; ARIPiprazole; Axitinib; Ibrutinib; Saxagliptin; Simeprevir; Vitamin K Antagonists

The levels/effects of MedroxyPROGESTERone may be decreased by: Acitretin; Aminoglutethimide; Aprepitant; Artemether; Barbiturates; Bexarotene (Systemic); Bile Acid Sequestrants; Bosentan; CarBAMazepine; CloBAZam; CYP3A4 Inducers (Strong); Dabrafenib; Deferasirox; Eslicarbazepine; Felbamate; Fosaprepitant; Fosphenytoin; Griseofulvin; LamoTRIgine; Mifepristone; Mitotane; Mycophenolate; Nelfinavir; Nevirapine; OXcarbazepine; Perampanel; Phenytoin; Primidone; Prucalopride; Retinoic Acid Derivatives; Rifamycin Derivatives; St Johns Wort; Sugammadex; Telaprevir; Tocilizumab; Topiramate; Ulipristal

Ethanol/Nutrition/Herb Interactions

Ethanol: Avoid ethanol (may increase risk of osteoporosis).

Food: Bioavailability of the oral tablet is increased when taken with food; half-life is unchanged.

Herb/Nutraceutical: St John's wort may diminish the therapeutic effect of progestin contraceptives (contraceptive failure is possible).

Storage/Stability Store at controlled room temperature.

Mechanism of Action Inhibits secretion of pituitary gonadotropins, which prevents follicular maturation and ovulation; causes endometrial thinning

Pharmacodynamics/Kinetics

Absorption: Oral: Well absorbed; I.M.: Slow

Protein binding: 86% to 90% primarily to albumin; does not bind to sex hormone-binding globulin

Metabolism: Extensively hepatic via hydroxylation and conjugation; forms metabolites

Half-life elimination: Oral: 12-17 hours; I.M. (Depo-Provera® Contraceptive): ~50 days; SubQ: ~40 days

Time to peak: Oral: 2-4 hours; I.M. (Depo-Provera® Contraceptive): ~3 weeks; SubQ: ~1 week

Excretion: Urine

Dosage

Adolescents and Adults:

Amenorrhea: Oral: 5-10 mg/day for 5-10 days

Abnormal uterine bleeding: Oral: 5-10 mg for 5-10 days starting on day 16 or 21 of cycle

Contraception:

Depo-Provera® Contraceptive: I.M.: 150 mg every 3 months

depo-subQ provera 104™: SubQ: 104 mg every 3 months (every 12-14 weeks)

Endometriosis (depo-subQ provera 104™): SubQ: 104 mg every 3 months (every 12-14 weeks)

Adults:

Endometrial carcinoma, recurrent or metastatic (adjunctive/palliative treatment) (Depo-Provera®): I.M.: 400-1000 mg/week

Accompanying cyclic estrogen therapy, postmenopausal: Oral: 5-10 mg for 12-14 consecutive days each month, starting on day 1 or day 16 of the cycle; lower doses may be used if given with estrogen continuously throughout the cycle

Treatment of paraphilia/hypersexuality (unlabeled use; Reilly, 2000): Males (**Note:** Avoid use if active pituitary pathology, hepatic failure or thromboembolic disease):

I.M. (Depo-Provera®): 100-600 mg weekly

Oral: 100-500 mg daily

Dosage adjustment in renal impairment: No dosage adjustment provided in manufacturer's labeling (has not been studied).

Dosage adjustment in hepatic impairment: Use is contraindicated with severe impairment. Discontinue with jaundice or if liver function disturbances occur. Consider lower dose or less frequent administration with mild-to-moderate impairment. Use of the contraceptive injection has not been studied in patients with hepatic impairment; consideration should be given to not readminister if jaundice develops

Dietary Considerations Ensure adequate calcium and vitamin D intake

Administration

I.M.: Depo-Provera® Contraceptive: Administer first dose during the first 5 days of menstrual period, or within the first 5 days postpartum if not breast-feeding, or at the sixth week postpartum if breast-feeding exclusively. Shake vigorously prior to administration. Administer by deep I.M. injection in the gluteal or deltoid muscle.

When switching from combined hormonal contraceptives (estrogen plus progestin), the first injection should be on the day after the last active tablet or (at the latest) the day after the final inactive tablet. When switching from other contraceptive methods, ensure continuous contraceptive coverage.

SubQ: depo-subQ provera 104™: Administer first dose during the first 5 days of menstrual period, or at the sixth week postpartum if breast-feeding. Shake vigorously prior to administration. Administer by SubQ injection in the anterior thigh or abdomen; avoid boney areas and the umbilicus. Administer over 5-7 seconds. Do not rub the injection area. When switching from combined hormonal contraceptives (estrogen plus progestin), the first injection should be within 7 days after the last active pill, or removal of patch or ring. If switching from the I.M. to SubQ formulation, the next dose should be given within the prescribed dosing period for the I.M. injection to assure continuous coverage.

Hazardous agent; use appropriate precautions for handling and disposal (NIOSH, 2012).

Monitoring Parameters Before starting therapy, a physical exam with reference to the breasts and pelvis are recommended, including a Papanicolaou smear. Exam may be deferred if appropriate prior to administration of MPA contraceptive injection; pregnancy should be ruled out prior to use. Monitor patient closely for loss of vision; sudden onset of proptosis, diplopia, or migraine; signs and symptoms of thromboembolic disorders; signs or symptoms of depression; glucose in patients with diabetes; or blood pressure. BMD with long-term use (per manufacturer).

Adequate diagnostic measures, including endometrial sampling, if indicated, should be performed to rule out malignancy in all cases of undiagnosed abnormal vaginal bleeding.

Treatment of paraphilia/hypersexuality (Guay, 2009; Reilly, 2000): Hepatic function test (baseline and during treatment if suspected hepatotoxicity); CBC (baseline); serum testosterone (baseline then monthly for 4 months then every 6 months); serum LH and prolactin (baseline and every 6 months); FSH (baseline); glucose; bone scan (baseline then annually) if serum testosterone significantly suppressed; gallbladder function; blood pressure; weight gain

Dosage Forms Excipient information presented when available (limited, particularly for generics); consult specific product labeling.

Suspension, Intramuscular, as acetate:

Depo-Provera: 150 mg/mL (1 mL)

Depo-Provera: 150 mg/mL (1 mL) [contains methylparaben, polyethylene glycol, polysorbate 80, propylparaben]

Depo-Provera: 400 mg/mL (2.5 mL)

Generic: 150 mg/mL (1 mL)

Suspension, Subcutaneous, as acetate:

Depo-SubQ Provera 104: 104 mg/0.65 mL (0.65 mL) [contains methylparaben, propylparaben]

Tablet, Oral, as acetate:

Provera: 2.5 mg, 5 mg, 10 mg [scored]

Generic: 2.5 mg, 5 mg, 10 mg

- ◆ **Medroxyprogesterone Acetate** *see* MedroxyPROGESTERone *on page 1278*
- ◆ **Medroxyprogesterone Acetate Injectable Suspension USP (Can)** *see* MedroxyPROGESTERone *on page 1278*
- ◆ **Med-Sotalol (Can)** *see* Sotalol *on page 1942*
- ◆ **Mefenamic-250 (Can)** *see* Mefenamic Acid *on page 1281*

Mefenamic Acid (me fe NAM ik AS id)

Brand Names: U.S. Ponstel

Brand Names: Canada Apo-Mefenamic®; Dom-Mefenamic Acid; Mefenamic-250; Nu-Mefenamic; PMS-Mefenamic Acid; Ponstan®

Pharmacologic Category Nonsteroidal Anti-inflammatory Drug (NSAID), Oral

Additional Appendix Information

Beers Criteria – Potentially Inappropriate Medications for Geriatrics *on page 2368*

Use Short-term relief of mild-to-moderate pain including primary dysmenorrhea

Pregnancy Risk Factor C

Medication Guide Available Yes

Dosage Children >14 years and Adults: Oral: 500 mg to start then 250 mg every 6 hours as needed; maximum therapy: 1 week

Dosage adjustment in renal impairment: Use is not recommended.

Dosage adjustment in hepatic impairment: No dosage adjustment provided in manufacturer's labeling (has not been studied). However, adjustment may be necessary due to extensive hepatic metabolism.

Additional Information Complete prescribing information should be consulted for additional detail.

Dosage Forms Excipient information presented when available (limited, particularly for generics); consult specific product labeling.

Capsule, Oral:

Ponstel: 250 mg

Generic: 250 mg

Mefloquine (ME floe kwin)

Index Terms Mefloquine Hydrochloride

Pharmacologic Category Antimalarial Agent

Use Treatment of mild-to-moderate acute malarial infections and prevention of malaria caused by *Plasmodium falciparum* (including chloroquine-resistant strains) or *P. vivax*

Note: Due to geographical resistance and cross-resistance, consult current CDC guidelines.

Unlabeled Use Treatment of uncomplicated, chloroquine-resistant *P. vivax* malaria

Pregnancy Risk Factor B

Pregnancy Considerations Adverse events have been observed in animal reproduction studies. Mefloquine crosses the placenta; however, clinical experience with mefloquine has not shown adverse effects in pregnant women. Use with caution during pregnancy if travel to endemic areas cannot be postponed. Malaria infection in pregnant women may be more severe than in nonpregnant women and may increase the risk of adverse pregnancy outcomes. Nonpregnant women of childbearing potential are advised to use contraception and avoid pregnancy during malaria prophylaxis and for 3 months thereafter. In case of an unplanned pregnancy, treatment with mefloquine is not considered a reason for pregnancy termination. CDC treatment guidelines are available for the use of mefloquine in the treatment of malaria during pregnancy (CDC, 2013b).

Breast-Feeding Considerations Mefloquine is excreted in breast milk in small quantities (~3% to 4% of a 250 mg dose). The manufacturer recommends that caution be exercised when administering mefloquine to nursing women. Exposure to small amounts of mefloquine from breast milk is considered safe for infants (CDC, 2014).

Medication Guide Available Yes

Contraindications Hypersensitivity to mefloquine, related compounds (eg, quinine and quinidine), or any component of the formulation; prophylactic use in patients with a history of seizures or psychiatric disorder (including active or recent history of depression, generalized anxiety disorder, psychosis, schizophrenia, or other major psychiatric disorders)

Warnings/Precautions [U.S. Boxed Warning]: May cause neuropsychiatric adverse effects that can persist after mefloquine has been discontinued. During prophylactic use, if symptoms occur, discontinue therapy and substitute an alternative medication. Should not be prescribed for prophylaxis in patients with major psychiatric disorders. Use with caution in patients with a previous history of depression. Symptoms may develop early in the course of therapy. Due to the difficulty in identifying these symptoms in children, monitor closely especially in nonverbal children. Psychiatric symptoms may include anxiety, paranoia, depression, hallucinations, and psychosis. Suicidal ideation and suicide have also been reported. Neurologic symptoms of dizziness or vertigo, tinnitus, and loss of balance may also occur and have been reported to be permanent in some cases. During prophylactic use, the occurrence of psychiatric symptoms such as acute anxiety, depression, restlessness, or confusion may be a prodrome to more serious neuropsychiatric adverse reactions. Use caution in activities requiring alertness and fine motor coordination (eg, driving, piloting planes, operating machinery) with neurologic symptoms.

Mefloquine may cause alterations in the ECG including sinus bradycardia, sinus arrhythmia, first-degree AV block, QT-interval prolongation, and abnormal T waves. Use caution or avoid concomitant use of agents known to cause QT interval prolongation (eg, halofantrine, quinine, quinidine). Use caution in patients with significant cardiac disease, hepatic impairment, or seizure disorder. If mefloquine is to be used for a prolonged period, periodic evaluations including liver function tests, evaluations for neuropsychiatric effects, and ophthalmic examinations should be performed. (Retinal abnormalities have not been observed with mefloquine in humans; however, abnormalities have been reported with long-term administration to rats.) Hypersensitivity reactions ranging from mild skin reactions to anaphylaxis have occurred. Agranulocytosis and aplastic anemia have been reported with use.

In cases of life-threatening, serious, or overwhelming malaria infections due to *Plasmodium falciparum*, patients should be treated with intravenous antimalarial drug. Mefloquine may be given orally to complete the course. In cases of acute *Plasmodium vivax* infection treated with mefloquine, patients should subsequently be treated with an 8-aminoquinoline derivative (eg, primaquine) to avoid relapse. Potentially significant drug-drug interactions may exist, requiring dose or frequency adjustment, additional monitoring, and/or selection of alternative therapy. Concurrent use with chloroquine may increase risk of seizures (WHO, 2010). Early vomiting leading to treatment failure in children has been reported in some studies; consider alternate therapy if a second dose is not tolerated.

Not recommended for the treatment of malaria acquired in Southeast Asia due to drug resistance (CDC, 2013b).

Adverse Reactions

1% to 10%:

Central nervous system: Chills, dizziness, fatigue, fever, headache

Dermatologic: Rash

Gastrointestinal: Vomiting (3%), abdominal pain, appetite decreased, diarrhea, nausea

Neuromuscular & skeletal: Myalgia

Otic: Tinnitus

<1% (Limited to important or life-threatening): Abnormal dreams, abnormal T waves, ataxia, aggressive behavior, agitation, anxiety, arrhythmia, arthralgia, AV block, cardiac arrest (with concomitant use of propranolol), chest pain, conduction abnormalities (transient), confusion, depression, diaphoresis increased, dyspepsia, dyspnea, edema, encephalopathy, erythema, erythema multiforme, exanthema, flushing, forgetfulness, hallucinations, hearing impairment, hematocrit decreased, hyper-/hypotension, insomnia, irregular pulse, leukocytosis, leukopenia, liver function tests increased, loss of balance, malaise, mood changes, muscle cramps/weakness, palpitation, panic attacks, paranoia, paresthesia, pneumonitis (allergic etiology), psychosis, QT prolongation, restlessness, somnolence, Stevens-Johnson syndrome, suicidal ideation and behavior (causal relationship not established), tachycardia, thrombocytopenia, tremor, urticaria, vertigo, visual disturbances

Drug Interactions

Metabolism/Transport Effects **Substrate** of CYP3A4 (major); **Note:** Assignment of Major/Minor substrate status based on clinically relevant drug interaction potential; **Inhibits** CYP2D6 (weak), CYP3A4 (weak), P-glycoprotein

Avoid Concomitant Use

Avoid concomitant use of Mefloquine with any of the following: Aminoquinolines (Antimalarial); Artemether; Bosutinib; Conivaptan; Fusidic Acid (Systemic); Halofantrine; Lumefantrine; PAZOPanib; Pimozide; Pomalidomide; QuiNIDine; QuiNINE; Silodosin; Topotecan; VinCRIStine (Liposomal)

Increased Effect/Toxicity

Mefloquine may increase the levels/effects of: Afatinib; Aminoquinolines (Antimalarial); Antipsychotic Agents (Phenothiazines); ARIPiprazole; Bosutinib; Colchicine; Dabigatran Etexilate; Dapsone (Systemic); Dapsone (Topical); Dofetilide; Everolimus; Halofantrine; Highest Risk QTc-Prolonging Agents; Lomitapide; Lumefantrine; Moderate Risk QTc-Prolonging Agents; PAZOPanib; P-glycoprotein/ABCB1 Substrates; Pimozide; Pomalidomide; Prucalopride; QuiNINE; Rivaroxaban; Silodosin; Topotecan; VinCRIStine (Liposomal)

The levels/effects of Mefloquine may be increased by: Aminoquinolines (Antimalarial); Artemether; Conivaptan; CYP3A4 Inhibitors (Moderate); CYP3A4 Inhibitors (Strong); Dapsone (Systemic); Dasatinib; Fusidic Acid (Systemic); Ivacaftor; Luliconazole; Mifepristone; QuiNIDine; QuiNINE; Simeprevir

Decreased Effect

Mefloquine may decrease the levels/effects of: Anticonvulsants

The levels/effects of Mefloquine may be decreased by: Bosentan; CYP3A4 Inducers (Strong); Dabrafenib; Deferasirox; Herbs (CYP3A4 Inducers); Mitotane; Tocilizumab

Ethanol/Nutrition/Herb Interactions Food: Food increases bioavailability by ~40%. Management: Take with food and at least 8 ounces of water. Maintain adequate nutrition and hydration, unless instructed to restrict fluid intake.

Storage/Stability Store at 20°C to 25°C (68°F to 77°F).

Mechanism of Action Mefloquine is a quinoline-methanol compound structurally similar to quinine; mefloquine's effectiveness in the treatment and prophylaxis of malaria is due to the destruction of the asexual blood forms of the malarial pathogens that affect humans, *Plasmodium falciparum*, *P. vivax*

Pharmacodynamics/Kinetics

Absorption: Well absorbed

Distribution: V_d: ~20 L/kg; blood, urine, CSF, tissues

Protein binding: ~98%

Metabolism: Extensively hepatic primarily by CYP3A4 to 2,8-bis-trifluoromethyl-4-quinoline carboxylic acid (inactive) and other metabolites

Bioavailability: Increased by food

Half-life elimination: ~3 weeks (range: 2-4 weeks)

Time to peak, plasma: ~17 hours (range: 6-24 hours)

Excretion: Primarily bile and feces; urine (9% of total dose as unchanged drug, 4% of total dose as primary metabolite)

Dosage Oral (dose expressed as mg of mefloquine hydrochloride):

Malaria:

Mild-to-moderate, treatment: **Note:** If clinical improvement is not seen within 48-72 hours, an alternative therapy should be used for retreatment.

Children ≥6 months: 20-25 mg/kg/day in 2 divided doses, taken 6-8 hours apart (maximum total dose: 1250 mg)

Adults: 1250 mg (5 tablets) as a single dose

Uncomplicated, treatment (unlabeled dose):

Children ≥6 months: 15 mg/kg, followed 6-12 hours later by 10 mg/kg/dose (maximum total dose: 1250 mg) (CDC, 2013b)

Adults: 750 mg (3 tablets) as initial dose, followed 6-12 hours later by 500 mg (2 tablets) (CDC, 2013b)

Uncomplicated, chloroquine-resistant *P. vivax* malaria treatment (unlabeled use):

Children ≥6 months: 15 mg/kg, followed 6-12 hours later by 10 mg/kg/dose (maximum total dose: 1250 mg) with concomitant primaquine (CDC, 2013b)

Adults: 750 mg (3 tablets) as initial dose, followed 6-12 hours later by 500 mg (2 tablets) with concomitant primaquine (CDC, 2013b)

Chemoprophylaxis:

Children ≥6 months: 5 mg/kg/dose once weekly (maximum dose: 250 mg) starting 1 week (CDC, 2014: ≥2 weeks) before arrival in endemic area, continuing weekly during travel and for 4 weeks after leaving endemic area. **Note:** Prophylaxis may begin 2-3 weeks prior to travel to ensure tolerance.

Manufacturer's labeling:

20-30 kg: 1/2 of 250 mg tablet (125 mg) once weekly

30-45 kg: 3/4 of 250 mg tablet (187.5 mg) once weekly

>45 kg: One tablet (250 mg) once weekly

Unlabeled dosing (CDC, 2014):

≤9 kg: 5 mg/kg/dose once weekly

>9-19 kg: 1/4 of 250 mg tablet (62.5 mg) once weekly

>19-30 kg: 1/2 of 250 mg tablet (125 mg) once weekly

>30-45 kg: 3/4 of 250 mg tablet (187.5 mg) once weekly

>45 kg: One tablet (250 mg) once weekly

Adults: 250 mg weekly starting 1 week (CDC, 2014: ≥2 weeks) before arrival in endemic area, continuing weekly during travel and for 4 weeks after leaving endemic area. **Note:** Prophylaxis may begin 2-3 weeks prior to travel to ensure tolerance.

Dosage adjustment in renal impairment: No dosage adjustment necessary; only a small amount of mefloquine is renally eliminated.

Dosage adjustment in hepatic impairment: No dosage adjustment provided in manufacturer's labeling; however; half-life may be prolonged and plasma levels may be higher in patients with hepatic impairment

Dietary Considerations Take with food and with at least 8 oz of water.

Administration Administer with food and with at least 8 oz of water. When used for malaria prophylaxis, dose should be taken once weekly on the same day each week. If vomiting occurs within 30 minutes after the dose, an additional full dose should be given; if it occurs within 30-60 minutes after dose, an additional half-dose should be given. Tablets may be crushed and suspended in a small amount of water, milk, or another beverage for persons unable to swallow tablets.

Monitoring Parameters When use is prolonged, periodic liver function tests, evaluations for neuropsychiatric effects, and ocular examinations

Dosage Forms Excipient information presented when available (limited, particularly for generics); consult specific product labeling.

Tablet, Oral, as hydrochloride:

Generic: 250 mg

◆ **Mefloquine Hydrochloride** *see* Mefloquine *on page 1281*

◆ **Mefoxin** *see* CefOXitin *on page 374*

◆ **Mega-C/A Plus** *see* Ascorbic Acid *on page 172*

◆ **Megace® (Can)** *see* Megestrol *on page 1283*

◆ **Megace ES** *see* Megestrol *on page 1283*

◆ **Megace Oral** *see* Megestrol *on page 1283*

◆ **Megace® OS (Can)** *see* Megestrol *on page 1283*

Megestrol (me JES trole)

Brand Names: U.S. Megace ES; Megace Oral

Brand Names: Canada Apo-Megestrol®; Megace®; Megace® OS; Nu-Megestrol

Index Terms 5071-1DL(6); Megestrol Acetate

Pharmacologic Category Antineoplastic Agent, Hormone; Appetite Stimulant; Progestin

Additional Appendix Information

Beers Criteria – Potentially Inappropriate Medications for Geriatrics *on page 2368*

Use

Tablet: Palliative treatment of advanced breast and endometrial carcinoma

Suspension: Treatment of anorexia, cachexia, or unexplained significant weight loss in patients with AIDS

Pregnancy Risk Factor D (tablet) / X (suspension)

Pregnancy Considerations Adverse events were demonstrated in animal reproduction studies. Use during pregnancy is contraindicated (suspension) and appropriate contraception is recommended in women who may become pregnant. In clinical studies, megestrol was shown to cause breakthrough vaginal bleeding in women.

Breast-Feeding Considerations Megestrol is excreted into breast milk. Information is available from five nursing women, ~8 weeks postpartum, who were administered megestrol 4 mg in combination with ethinyl estradiol 50 mcg daily for contraception. Maternal serum and milk samples were obtained over 5 days, beginning 10 days after therapy began. The highest concentrations of megestrol were found at the samples taken 3 hours after the maternal dose. Mean concentrations of megestrol were 6.5 ng/mL (maternal serum; range: 3.7-10.8 ng/mL), 4.6 ng/mL (foremilk; range: 1.1-12.7 ng/mL), and 5.6 ng/mL (hindmilk; range: 1.2-18.5 ng/mL) (Nilsson, 1977). Due to the potential for adverse reaction in the newborn, the manufacturer recommends discontinuing breast-feeding while receiving megestrol. In addition, in the United States, where formula is accessible, affordable, safe, and sustainable, and the risk of infant mortality due to diarrhea and respiratory infections is low, complete avoidance of breast-feeding by HIV-infected women is recommended to decrease potential transmission of HIV (DHHS [perinatal], 2012).

Contraindications Hypersensitivity to megestrol or any component of the formulation; known or suspected pregnancy (suspension)

Warnings/Precautions Hazardous agent - use appropriate precautions for handling and disposal (NIOSH, 2012). May suppress hypothalamic-pituitary-adrenal (HPA) axis during chronic administration; consider the possibility of adrenal suppression in any patient receiving or being withdrawn from chronic therapy when signs/symptoms suggestive of hypoadrenalism are noted (during stress or in unstressed state). Laboratory evaluation and replacement/stress doses of rapid-acting glucocorticoid should be considered. New-onset diabetes and exacerbation of preexisting diabetes have been reported with long-term use. Use with caution in patients with a history of thromboembolic disease. Avoid use in older adults due to minimal effect on weight, and an increased risk of thrombosis and possibly death (Beers Criteria). Vaginal bleeding or discharge may occur in females. Megace® ES suspension is not equivalent to other formulations on a mg per mg basis; Megace® ES suspension 625 mg/5 mL is equivalent to megestrol acetate suspension 800 mg/20 mL.

Adverse Reactions

Frequency not always defined.

Cardiovascular: Hypertension (≤8%), cardiomyopathy (1% to 3%), chest pain (1% to 3%), edema (1% to 3%), palpitation (1% to 3%), peripheral edema (1% to 3%), heart failure

Central nervous system: Headache (≤10%), insomnia (≤6%), fever (1% to 6%), pain (≤6%, similar to placebo), abnormal thinking (1% to 3%), confusion (1% to 3%), depression (1% to 3%), hypoesthesia (1% to 3%), seizure (1% to 3%), mood changes, malaise, lethargy

Dermatologic: Rash (2% to 12%), alopecia (1% to 3%), pruritus (1% to 3%), vesiculobullous rash (1% to 3%)

Endocrine & metabolic: Hyperglycemia (≤6%), gynecomastia (1% to 3%), adrenal insufficiency, amenorrhea, breakthrough bleeding, cervical erosion and secretions (changes), breast tenderness increased, Cushing's syndrome, diabetes, glucose intolerance, HPA axis suppression, hot flashes, hypercalcemia, menstrual flow changes, spotting, vaginal bleeding pattern changes

Gastrointestinal: Diarrhea (6% to 15%, similar to placebo), flatulence (≤10%), vomiting (≤6%), nausea (≤5%), dyspepsia (≤4%), abdominal pain (1% to 3%), constipation (1% to 3%), salivation increased (1% to 3%), xerostomia (1% to 3%), weight gain (not attributed to edema or fluid retention)

Genitourinary: Impotence (4% to 14%), decreased libido (≤5%), urinary incontinence (1% to 3%), urinary tract infection (1% to 3%), urinary frequency (≤2%)

Hematologic: Anemia (≤5%), leukopenia (1% to 3%)

Hepatic: Hepatomegaly (1% to 3%), LDH increased (1% to 3%), cholestatic jaundice, hepatotoxicity

Neuromuscular & skeletal: Weakness (2% to 6%), neuropathy (1% to 3%), paresthesia (1% to 3%), carpal tunnel syndrome

Ocular: Amblyopia (1% to 3%)

Renal: Albuminuria (1% to 3%)

Respiratory: Dyspnea (1% to 3%), cough (1% to 3%), pharyngitis (1% to 3%), pneumonia (≤2%), hyperpnea

Miscellaneous: Diaphoresis (1% to 3%), herpes infection (1% to 3%), infection (1% to 3%), moniliasis (1% to 3%), tumor flare

Postmarketing and/or case reports: Thromboembolic phenomena (including deep vein thrombosis, pulmonary embolism, thrombophlebitis)

Drug Interactions

Metabolism/Transport Effects None known.

Avoid Concomitant Use

Avoid concomitant use of Megestrol with any of the following: Dofetilide; Ulipristal

Increased Effect/Toxicity

Megestrol may increase the levels/effects of: Dofetilide

The levels/effects of Megestrol may be increased by: Herbs (Progestogenic Properties)

Decreased Effect

Megestrol may decrease the levels/effects of: Anticoagulants

The levels/effects of Megestrol may be decreased by: Aminoglutethimide; Ulipristal

Ethanol/Nutrition/Herb Interactions Herb/Nutraceutical: Avoid herbs with progestogenic properties (eg, bloodroot, chasteberry, damiana, oregano, and yucca); may enhance the adverse/toxic effect of megestrol.

Storage/Stability

Suspension: Store at 15°C to 25°C (59°F to 77°F); protect from heat.

Tablet: Store at 25°C (77°F); excursions permitted to 15°C to 30°C (59°F to 86°F); protect from heat (temperatures >40°C [>104°F])

Mechanism of Action A synthetic progestin with antiestrogenic properties which disrupt the estrogen receptor cycle. Megestrol interferes with the normal estrogen cycle and results in a lower LH titer. May also have a direct effect on the endometrium. Megestrol is an antineoplastic progestin thought to act through an antileutenizing effect mediated via the pituitary. May stimulate appetite by antagonizing the metabolic effects of catabolic cytokines.

Pharmacodynamics/Kinetics

Absorption: Well absorbed orally

Metabolism: Hepatic (to free steroids and glucuronide conjugates)

Half-life elimination: 13-105 hours

Time to peak, serum: 1-3 hours

Excretion: Urine (57% to 78%; 5% to 8% as metabolites); feces (8% to 30%)

Dosage Adults: Oral: **Note:** Megace® ES suspension is not equivalent to other formulations on a mg-per-mg basis:

Tablet: Females (refer to individual protocols):

Breast carcinoma: 40 mg 4 times/day

Endometrial carcinoma: 40-320 mg/day in divided doses; use for 2 months to determine efficacy; maximum doses used have been up to 800 mg/day

Suspension: Males/Females: HIV-related cachexia:

Megace®: Initial dose: 800 mg/day; daily doses of 400 and 800 mg/day were found to be clinically effective

Megace® ES: 625 mg/day

Dosage adjustment in renal impairment: No data available; however, the urinary excretion of megestrol acetate administered in doses of 4-90 mg ranged from 57% to 78% within 10 days.

Dosage adjustment in hepatic impairment: No dosage adjustment provided in manufacturer's labeling.

Administration Megestrol acetate (Megace®) oral suspension is compatible with water, orange juice, apple juice, or Sustacal H.C. for immediate consumption. Shake suspension well before use.

Hazardous agent; use appropriate precautions for handling and disposal (NIOSH, 2012).

Monitoring Parameters Observe for signs of thromboembolic events; blood pressure, weight; serum glucose

Test Interactions Altered thyroid and liver function tests

Dosage Forms Excipient information presented when available (limited, particularly for generics); consult specific product labeling.

Suspension, Oral, as acetate:

Megace ES: 625 mg/5 mL (150 mL) [contains alcohol, usp, sodium benzoate; lemon-lime flavor]

Megace Oral: 40 mg/mL (240 mL) [lemon-lime flavor]

Generic: 40 mg/mL (10 mL, 240 mL, 480 mL); 400 mg/10 mL (10 mL)

Tablet, Oral, as acetate:

Generic: 20 mg, 40 mg

◆ **Megestrol Acetate** *see* Megestrol *on page 1283*

◆ **Mekinist** *see* Trametinib *on page 2102*

◆ **Mellaril** *see* Thioridazine *on page 2047*

Meloxicam (mel OKS i kam)

Brand Names: U.S. Meloxicam Comfort Pac; Mobic

Brand Names: Canada Apo-Meloxicam®; Auro-Meloxicam; Ava-Meloxicam; CO Meloxicam; Dom-Meloxicam; Mobicox®; Mobic®; Mylan-Meloxicam; Novo-Meloxicam; PHL-Meloxicam; PMS-Meloxicam; ratio-Meloxicam; Teva-Meloxicam

Pharmacologic Category Nonsteroidal Anti-inflammatory Drug (NSAID), Oral

Additional Appendix Information

Beers Criteria – Potentially Inappropriate Medications for Geriatrics *on page 2368*

Use Relief of signs and symptoms of osteoarthritis, rheumatoid arthritis, and juvenile idiopathic arthritis (JIA)

Pregnancy Risk Factor C / D ≥30 weeks gestation

Pregnancy Considerations Adverse events were not observed in the initial animal reproduction studies; therefore, the manufacturer classifies meloxicam as pregnancy category C (category D: ≥30 weeks gestation). Meloxicam crosses the placenta. NSAID exposure during the first trimester is not strongly associated with congenital malformations; however, cardiovascular anomalies and cleft palate have been observed following NSAID exposure in some studies. The use of an NSAID close to conception may be associated with an increased risk of miscarriage. Nonteratogenic effects have been observed following NSAID administration during the third trimester including myocardial degenerative changes, prenatal constriction of the ductus arteriosus, fetal tricuspid regurgitation, failure of the ductus arteriosus to close postnatally; renal dysfunction or failure, oligohydramnios; gastrointestinal bleeding or perforation, increased risk of necrotizing enterocolitis; intracranial bleeding (including intraventricular hemorrhage), platelet dysfunction with resultant bleeding; pulmonary hypertension. Because they may cause premature closure of the ductus arteriosus, use of NSAIDs late in pregnancy should be avoided (use after 31 or 32 weeks gestation is not recommended by some clinicians). Product labeling for Mobic® specifically notes that use at ≥30 weeks gestation should be avoided and therefore classifies meloxicam as pregnancy category D at this time. The chronic use of NSAIDs in women of reproductive age may be associated with infertility that is reversible upon discontinuation of the medication.

Breast-Feeding Considerations It is not known whether meloxicam is excreted in human milk. Breast-feeding is not recommended by the manufacturer.

Medication Guide Available Yes

Contraindications Hypersensitivity (eg, asthma, urticaria, allergic-type reactions) to meloxicam, aspirin, other NSAIDs, or any component of the formulation; perioperative pain in the setting of coronary artery bypass graft (CABG) surgery

Warnings/Precautions [U.S. Boxed Warning]: NSAIDs are associated with an increased risk of adverse cardiovascular thrombotic events, including MI and stroke. Risk may be increased with duration of use or pre-existing cardiovascular risk factors or disease.

Carefully evaluate individual cardiovascular risk profiles prior to prescribing. May cause new-onset hypertension or worsening of existing hypertension. Use caution with fluid retention. Avoid use in heart failure. Concurrent administration of ibuprofen, and potentially other nonselective NSAIDs, may interfere with aspirin's cardioprotective effect. **[U.S. Boxed Warning]: Use is contraindicated for treatment of perioperative pain in the setting of coronary artery bypass graft (CABG) surgery.** Risk of MI and stroke may be increased with use within the first 10-14 days following CABG surgery.

Platelet adhesion and aggregation may be decreased; may prolong bleeding time; patients with coagulation disorders or who are receiving anticoagulants should be monitored closely. Anemia may occur; patients on long-term NSAID therapy should be monitored for anemia. Rarely, NSAID use may cause severe blood dyscrasias (eg, agranulocytosis, aplastic anemia, thrombocytopenia).

NSAID use may compromise existing renal function; dose-dependent decreases in prostaglandin synthesis may result from NSAID use, reducing renal blood flow which may cause renal decompensation. NSAID use may increase the risk for hyperkalemia. Patients with impaired renal function, dehydration, heart failure, liver dysfunction, those taking diuretics, and ACE inhibitors, and the elderly are at greater risk of renal toxicity and hyperkalemia. Rehydrate patient before starting therapy; monitor renal function closely. Not recommended for use in patients with advanced renal disease. Long-term NSAID use may result in renal papillary necrosis.

[U.S. Boxed Warning]: NSAIDs may increase risk of gastrointestinal irritation, inflammation, ulceration, bleeding, and perforation. These events may occur at any time during therapy and without warning. Use caution with a history of GI disease (bleeding or ulcers), concurrent therapy with aspirin, anticoagulants and/or corticosteroids, smoking, use of alcohol, the elderly or debilitated patients. When used concomitantly with ≤325 mg of aspirin, a substantial increase in the risk of gastrointestinal complications (eg, ulcer) occurs; concomitant gastroprotective therapy (eg, proton pump inhibitors) is recommended (Bhatt, 2008).

Use the lowest effective dose for the shortest duration of time, consistent with individual patient goals, to reduce risk of cardiovascular or GI adverse events. Alternate therapies should be considered for patients at high risk.

NSAIDs may cause serious skin adverse events including exfoliative dermatitis, Stevens-Johnson syndrome (SJS) and toxic epidermal necrolysis (TEN); discontinue use at first sign of skin rash or hypersensitivity. Anaphylactoid reactions may occur, even without prior exposure; patients with "aspirin triad" (bronchial asthma, aspirin intolerance, rhinitis) may be at increased risk. Do not use in patients who experience bronchospasm, asthma, rhinitis, or urticaria with NSAID or aspirin therapy. Use caution in other forms of asthma.

Use with caution in patients with decreased hepatic function. Closely monitor patients with any abnormal LFT. Severe hepatic reactions (eg, fulminant hepatitis, liver failure) have occurred with NSAID use, rarely; discontinue if signs or symptoms of liver disease develop, or if systemic manifestations occur.

NSAIDS may cause drowsiness, dizziness, blurred vision and other neurologic effects which may impair physical or mental abilities; patients must be cautioned about performing tasks which require mental alertness (eg, operating machinery or driving). Discontinue use with blurred or diminished vision and perform ophthalmologic exam. Monitor vision with long-term therapy.

In the elderly, avoid chronic use (unless alternative agents ineffective and patient can receive concomitant gastroprotective agent); nonselective oral NSAID use is associated with an increased risk of GI bleeding and peptic ulcer disease in older adults in high risk category (eg, >75 years or age or receiving concomitant oral/parenteral corticosteroids, anticoagulants, or antiplatelet agents) (Beers Criteria).

Oral suspension formulation may contain sorbitol. Concomitant use with sodium polystyrene sulfonate (Kayexalate®) may cause intestinal necrosis (including fatal cases); combined use should be avoided. Withhold for at least 4-6 half-lives prior to surgical or dental procedures.

Adverse Reactions Percentages reported in adult patients; abdominal pain, diarrhea, fever, headache, pyrexia, and vomiting were reported more commonly in pediatric patients

2% to 10%:

Cardiovascular: Edema (≤5%)

Central nervous system: Headache (2% to 8%), pain (1% to 5%), dizziness (≤4%), insomnia (≤4%)

Dermatologic: Pruritus (≤2%), rash (≤3%)

Gastrointestinal: Dyspepsia (4% to 10%), diarrhea (2% to 8%), nausea (2% to 7%), abdominal pain (2% to 5%), constipation (≤3%), flatulence (≤3%), vomiting (≤3%)

Genitourinary: Urinary tract infection (≤7%), micturition (≤2%)

Hematologic: Anemia (≤4%)

Neuromuscular & skeletal: Arthralgia (≤5%), back pain (≤3%)

Respiratory: Upper respiratory infection (≤8%), cough (≤2%), pharyngitis (≤3%)

Miscellaneous: Flu-like syndrome (2% to 6%), falls (≤3%)

<2% (Limited to important or life-threatening): Abnormal dreams, abnormal vision, agranulocytosis, albuminuria, allergic reaction, alopecia, anaphylactoid reactions, angina, angioedema, anxiety, appetite increased, arrhythmia, asthma, bilirubinemia, bronchospasm, bullous eruption, BUN increased, cardiac failure, colitis, confusion, conjunctivitis, creatinine increased, dehydration, depression, diaphoresis, duodenal perforation, duodenal ulcer, dyspnea, edema (facial), eructation, erythema multiforme, esophagitis, exfoliative dermatitis, fatigue, fever, gastric perforation, gastric ulcer, gastritis, gastroesophageal reflux, gastrointestinal hemorrhage, GGT increased, hematemesis, hematuria, hepatic failure, hepatitis, hot flushes, hyper-/hypotension, interstitial nephritis, intestinal perforation, jaundice, leukopenia, malaise, melena, MI, mood alterations, nervousness, palpitation, pancreatitis, paresthesia, photosensitivity reaction, pruritus, purpura, renal failure, seizure, shock, somnolence, Stevens-Johnson syndrome, syncope, tachycardia, taste perversion, thrombocytopenia, tinnitus, toxic epidermal necrolysis, transaminases increased, tremor, ulcerative stomatitis, urinary retention (acute), urticaria, vasculitis, vertigo, xerostomia, weight gain/loss

Drug Interactions

Metabolism/Transport Effects Substrate of CYP3A4 (minor); **Note:** Assignment of Major/Minor substrate status based on clinically relevant drug interaction potential; **Inhibits** CYP2C9 (weak)

Avoid Concomitant Use

Avoid concomitant use of Meloxicam with any of the following: Calcium Polystyrene Sulfonate; Floctafenine; Ketorolac (Nasal); Ketorolac (Systemic); NSAID (COX-2 Inhibitor); Omacetaxine; Sodium Polystyrene Sulfonate

Increased Effect/Toxicity

Meloxicam may increase the levels/effects of: 5-ASA Derivatives; Agents with Antiplatelet Properties; Aliskiren; Aminoglycosides; Anticoagulants; Bisphosphonate Derivatives; Calcium Polystyrene Sulfonate; Collagenase (Systemic); CycloSPORINE (Systemic); Dabigatran

Etexilate; Deferasirox; Desmopressin; Digoxin; Eplerenone; Haloperidol; Ibritumomab; Lithium; Methotrexate; Nonsteroidal Anti-Inflammatory Agents; NSAID (COX-2 Inhibitor); Omacetaxine; PEMEtrexed; Porfimer; Potassium-Sparing Diuretics; PRALAtrexate; Quinolone Antibiotics; Rivaroxaban; Salicylates; Sodium Polystyrene Sulfonate; Tenofovir; Thrombolytic Agents; Tositumomab and Iodine I 131 Tositumomab; Vancomycin; Vitamin K Antagonists

The levels/effects of Meloxicam may be increased by: ACE Inhibitors; Angiotensin II Receptor Blockers; Antidepressants (Tricyclic, Tertiary Amine); Corticosteroids (Systemic); CycloSPORINE (Systemic); Dasatinib; Floctafenine; Glucosamine; Herbs (Anticoagulant/Antiplatelet Properties); Ibrutinib; Ketorolac (Nasal); Ketorolac (Systemic); Multivitamins/Fluoride (with ADE); Multivitamins/Minerals (with ADEK, Folate, Iron); Multivitamins/Minerals (with AE, No Iron); Nonsteroidal Anti-Inflammatory Agents; Omega-3 Fatty Acids; Pentosan Polysulfate Sodium; Pentoxifylline; Probenecid; Prostacyclin Analogues; Selective Serotonin Reuptake Inhibitors; Serotonin/Norepinephrine Reuptake Inhibitors; Sodium Phosphates; Tipranavir; Treprostinil; Vitamin E; Voriconazole

Decreased Effect

Meloxicam may decrease the levels/effects of: ACE Inhibitors; Agents with Antiplatelet Properties; Aliskiren; Angiotensin II Receptor Blockers; Beta-Blockers; Eplerenone; HydrALAZINE; Loop Diuretics; Potassium-Sparing Diuretics; Prostaglandins (Ophthalmic); Salicylates; Selective Serotonin Reuptake Inhibitors; Thiazide Diuretics

The levels/effects of Meloxicam may be decreased by: Bile Acid Sequestrants; Nonsteroidal Anti-Inflammatory Agents; Salicylates

Ethanol/Nutrition/Herb Interactions

Ethanol: Avoid ethanol (may enhance gastric mucosal irritation).

Herb/Nutraceutical: Avoid alfalfa, anise, bilberry, bladderwrack, bromelain, cat's claw, celery, chamomile, coleus, cordyceps, dong quai, evening primrose, fenugreek, feverfew, garlic, ginger, ginkgo biloba, ginseng (American, Panax, Siberian), grapeseed, green tea, guggul, horse chestnut seed, horseradish, licorice, prickly ash, red clover, reishi, SAMe (S-adenosylmethionine), sweet clover, turmeric, white willow (all have additional antiplatelet activity).

Storage/Stability Store at 25°C (77°F). Protect tablets from moisture.

Mechanism of Action Reversibly inhibits cyclooxygenase-1 and 2 (COX-1 and 2) enzymes, which results in decreased formation of prostaglandin precursors; has antipyretic, analgesic, and anti-inflammatory properties

Other proposed mechanisms not fully elucidated (and possibly contributing to the anti-inflammatory effect to varying degrees), include inhibiting chemotaxis, altering lymphocyte activity, inhibiting neutrophil aggregation/activation, and decreasing proinflammatory cytokine levels.

Pharmacodynamics/Kinetics

Distribution: 10 L

Protein binding: ~99%, primarily to albumin

Metabolism: Hepatic via CYP2C9 and CYP3A4 (minor); forms 4 metabolites (inactive)

Bioavailability: 89%

Half-life elimination: Adults: 15-20 hours

Time to peak: Initial: 4-5 hours; Secondary: 12-14 hours

Excretion: Urine and feces (as inactive metabolites)

Dosage Oral:

Children ≥2 years: Juvenile idiopathic arthritis (JIA): 0.125 mg/kg/day; maximum dose: 7.5 mg/day

Adults: Osteoarthritis, rheumatoid arthritis: Initial: 7.5 mg once daily; some patients may receive additional benefit from increasing dose to 15 mg once daily; maximum dose: 15 mg/day

Elderly: Increased concentrations may occur in elderly patients (particularly in females); however, no specific dosage adjustment is recommended

Dosage adjustment in renal impairment:

Mild-to-moderate impairment: No specific dosage recommendations

Significant impairment (Cl_{cr} ≤20 mL/minute): Patients with severe renal impairment have not been adequately studied; use not recommended.

Hemodialysis: Maximum dose: 7.5 mg/day

Dosage adjustment in hepatic impairment:

Mild-to-moderate hepatic impairment (Child-Pugh class A or B): No dosage adjustment is necessary

Severe hepatic impairment: Patients with severe hepatic impairment have not been adequately studied

Dietary Considerations Should be taken with food or milk to minimize gastrointestinal irritation.

Administration May be administered with or without meals; take with food or milk to minimize gastrointestinal irritation. Oral suspension: Shake gently prior to use.

Monitoring Parameters Periodic CBC, serum chemistries, liver function, renal function (serum BUN and creatinine) with long-term use; signs and symptoms of bleeding

Dosage Forms Considerations

Meloxicam Comfort Pac is a kit containing meloxicam oral tablets 15 mg, and Duraflex topical gel.

Dosage Forms Excipient information presented when available (limited, particularly for generics); consult specific product labeling.

Kit, Combination:

Meloxicam Comfort Pac: 15 mg [contains methylparaben, trolamine (triethanolamine)]

Suspension, Oral:

Mobic: 7.5 mg/5 mL (100 mL) [contains saccharin sodium, sodium benzoate; raspberry flavor]

Generic: 7.5 mg/5 mL (100 mL)

Tablet, Oral:

Mobic: 7.5 mg, 15 mg

Generic: 7.5 mg, 15 mg

◆ **Meloxicam Comfort Pac** *see* Meloxicam *on page* 1284

◆ **Melpaque HP** *see* Hydroquinone *on page* 1017

Melphalan (MEL fa lan)

Brand Names: U.S. Alkeran

Brand Names: Canada Alkeran®

Index Terms L-PAM; L-Phenylalanine Mustard; L-Sarcolysin; Phenylalanine Mustard

Pharmacologic Category Antineoplastic Agent, Alkylating Agent

Use Palliative treatment of multiple myeloma and nonresectable epithelial ovarian carcinoma

Unlabeled Use Treatment of Hodgkin lymphoma, light chain amyloidosis; conditioning regimen for autologous hematopoietic stem cell transplantation in adults with hematologic disorders (eg, multiple myeloma) and autologous marrow or stem cell transplantation in pediatric neuroblastoma and Ewing's sarcoma

Pregnancy Risk Factor D

Pregnancy Considerations Animal studies have demonstrated embryotoxicity and teratogenicity. Therapy may suppress ovarian function leading to amenorrhea. There are no adequate and well-controlled studies in pregnant women. May cause fetal harm if administered during pregnancy. Women of childbearing potential should be advised to avoid pregnancy while on melphalan therapy.

Breast-Feeding Considerations According to the manufacturer, melphalan should not be administered if breast-feeding.

Contraindications Hypersensitivity to melphalan or any component of the formulation; patients whose disease was resistant to prior melphalan therapy

Warnings/Precautions Hazardous agent; use appropriate precautions for handling and disposal (NIOSH, 2012).

[U.S. Boxed Warning]: Bone marrow suppression is common; may be severe and result in infection or bleeding; has been demonstrated more with the I.V. formulation (compared to oral); myelosuppression is dose-related. Monitor blood counts; may require treatment delay or dose modification for thrombocytopenia or neutropenia. Use with caution in patients with prior bone marrow suppression, impaired renal function (consider dose reduction), or who have received prior (or concurrent) chemotherapy or irradiation. Myelotoxicity is generally reversible, although irreversible bone marrow failure has been reported. In patients who are candidates for autologous transplantation, avoid melphalan-containing regimens prior to transplant (due to the effects on stem cell reserve). Signs of infection, such as fever and WBC rise, may not occur; lethargy and confusion may be more prominent signs of infection.

[U.S. Boxed Warning]: Hypersensitivity reactions (including anaphylaxis) have occurred in ~2% of patients receiving I.V. melphalan, usually after multiple treatment cycles. Discontinue infusion and treat symptomatically. Hypersensitivity may also occur (rarely) with oral melphalan. Do not readminister (oral or I.V.) in patients who experience hypersensitivity to melphalan.

Gastrointestinal toxicities, including nausea, vomiting, diarrhea and mucositis, are common. When administering high-dose melphalan in autologous transplantation, cryotherapy is recommended to prevent mucositis (Keefe, 2007). Abnormal liver function tests may occur; hepatitis and jaundice have also been reported; hepatic sinusoidal obstruction syndrome (SOS; formerly called veno-occlusive disease) has been reported with I.V. melphalan. Pulmonary fibrosis (some fatal) and interstitial pneumonitis have been observed with treatment. Dosage reduction is recommended with I.V. melphalan in patients with renal impairment; reduced initial doses may also be recommended with oral melphalan. Closely monitor patients with azotemia.

[U.S. Boxed Warning]: Produces chromosomal changes and is leukemogenic and potentially mutagenic; secondary malignancies (including acute myeloid leukemia, myeloproliferative disease, and carcinoma) have been reported reported (some patients were receiving combination chemotherapy or radiation therapy); the risk is increased with increased treatment duration and cumulative doses. Suppresses ovarian function and produces amenorrhea; may also cause testicular suppression.

Extravasation may cause local tissue damage; administration by slow injection into a fast running I.V. solution into an injection port or via a central line is recommended; do not administer directly into a peripheral vein. **[U.S. Boxed Warning]: Should be administered under the supervision of an experienced cancer chemotherapy physician.** Avoid vaccination with live vaccines during treatment if immunocompromised. Toxicity may be increased in elderly; start with lowest recommended adult doses.

Adverse Reactions

>10%:

Gastrointestinal: Nausea/vomiting, diarrhea, oral ulceration

Hematologic: Myelosuppression, leukopenia (nadir: 14-21 days; recovery: 28-35 days), thrombocytopenia (nadir: 14-21 days; recovery: 28-35 days), anemia

Miscellaneous: Secondary malignancy (<2% to 20%; cumulative dose and duration dependent, includes acute myeloid leukemia, myeloproliferative syndrome, carcinoma)

1% to 10%: Miscellaneous: Hypersensitivity (I.V.: 2%; includes bronchospasm, dyspnea, edema, hypotension, pruritus, rash, tachycardia, urticaria)

Infrequent, frequency undefined, postmarketing, and/or case reports: Agranulocytosis, allergic reactions, alopecia, amenorrhea, anaphylaxis (rare), bleeding (with high-dose therapy),, bone marrow failure (irreversible), BUN increased, cardiac arrest, cardiotoxicity (angina, arrhythmia, hypertension, MI; with high-dose therapy), encephalopathy, hemolytic anemia, hemorrhagic cystitis, hepatic sinusoidal obstruction syndrome (SOS; veno-occlusive disease; high-dose I.V. melphalan), hepatitis, infection, injection site reactions (ulceration, necrosis), interstitial pneumonitis, jaundice, mucositis (with high-dose therapy), ovarian suppression, paralytic ileus (with high-dose therapy), pruritus, pulmonary fibrosis, radiation myelopathy, rash (maculopapular), renal toxicity (with high-dose therapy), seizure (with high-dose therapy), sepsis, SIADH, skin hypersensitivity, sterility, stomatitis, testicular suppression, tingling sensation, transaminases increased, vasculitis, warmth sensation

Drug Interactions

Metabolism/Transport Effects None known.

Avoid Concomitant Use

Avoid concomitant use of Melphalan with any of the following: BCG; CloZAPine; Nalidixic Acid; Natalizumab; Pimecrolimus; Tacrolimus (Topical); Tofacitinib; Vaccines (Live)

Increased Effect/Toxicity

Melphalan may increase the levels/effects of: Carmustine; CloZAPine; CycloSPORINE (Systemic); Leflunomide; Natalizumab; Tofacitinib; Vaccines (Live); Vitamin K Antagonists

The levels/effects of Melphalan may be increased by: Denosumab; Nalidixic Acid; Pimecrolimus; Roflumilast; Tacrolimus (Topical); Trastuzumab

Decreased Effect

Melphalan may decrease the levels/effects of: BCG; Cardiac Glycosides; Coccidioidin Skin Test; Sipuleucel-T; Vaccines (Inactivated); Vaccines (Live); Vitamin K Antagonists

The levels/effects of Melphalan may be decreased by: Echinacea

Ethanol/Nutrition/Herb Interactions

Ethanol: Avoid ethanol (due to GI irritation).

Food: Food interferes with oral absorption.

Preparation for Administration Hazardous agent; use appropriate precautions for handling and disposal (NIOSH, 2012).

Injection: Stability is limited; must be prepared fresh. **The time between reconstitution/dilution and administration of parenteral melphalan must be kept to a minimum (manufacturer recommends <60 minutes) because reconstituted and diluted solutions are unstable.** Dissolve powder initially with 10 mL of supplied diluent to a concentration of 5 mg/mL; shake immediately and vigorously to dissolve. **Immediately** dilute dose in NS to a concentration of ≤0.45 mg/mL (manufacturer recommended concentration). Do not refrigerate solution; precipitation occurs. The manufacturer recommends administration within 60 minutes of reconstitution.

Storage/Stability

Tablet: Store in refrigerator at 2°C to 8°C (36°F to 46°F). Protect from light.

Injection: Store at room temperature of 15°C to 30°C (59°F to 86°F). Protect from light. Stability is limited; must be prepared fresh. A 5 mg/mL concentration is chemically and physically stable for ≤90 minutes when stored at room temperature, although the manufacturer recommends administration be completed within 60 minutes of reconstitution; **immediately** dilute dose in NS. Do not refrigerate solution; precipitation occurs.

Mechanism of Action Alkylating agent which is a derivative of mechlorethamine that inhibits DNA and RNA synthesis via formation of carbonium ions; cross-links strands of DNA; acts on both resting and rapidly dividing tumor cells.

Pharmacodynamics/Kinetics Note: Pharmacokinetics listed are for FDA-approved doses.

Absorption: Oral: Variable and incomplete

Distribution: V_d: 0.5 L/kg; low penetration into CSF

Protein binding: 53% to 92%; primarily to albumin (40% to 60%), ~20% to α_1-acid glycoprotein

Metabolism: Hepatic; chemical hydrolysis to monohydroxymelphalan and dihydroxymelphalan

Bioavailability: Oral: Variable; 56% to 93%; exposure is reduced with a high-fat meal

Half-life elimination: Terminal: I.V.: 75 minutes; Oral: 1-2 hours

Time to peak, serum: Oral: ~1-2 hours

Excretion: Oral: Feces (20% to 50%); urine (~10% as unchanged drug)

Dosage Details regarding dosing in combination regimens should also be consulted.

Oral: Adults (adjust dose based on patient response and weekly blood counts):

Multiple myeloma (palliative treatment): **Note:** Response is gradual; may require repeated courses to realize benefit:

Usual dose (as described in the manufacturer's labeling):

6 mg once daily for 2-3 weeks initially, followed by up to 4 weeks rest, then a maintenance dose of 2 mg daily as hematologic recovery begins **or**

10 mg daily for 7-10 days; institute 2 mg daily maintenance dose after WBC >4000 cells/mm^3 and platelets >100,000 cells/mm^3 (~4-8 weeks); titrate maintenance dose to hematologic response **or**

0.15 mg/kg/day for 7 days, with a 2-6 week rest, followed by a maintenance dose of ≤0.05 mg/kg/day as hematologic recovery begins **or**

0.25 mg/kg/day for 4 days (or 0.2 mg/kg/day for 5 days); repeat at 4- to 6-week intervals as ANC and platelet counts return to normal

Other dosing regimens in **combination therapy** (unlabeled doses):

4 mg/m^2/day for 7 days every 4 weeks (in combination with prednisone **or** with prednisone and thalidomide) (Palumbo, 2006; Palumbo, 2008) **or**

6 mg/m^2/day for 7 days every 4 weeks (in combination with prednisone) (Palumbo, 2004) **or**

0.25 mg/kg/day for 4 days every 6 weeks (in combination with prednisone [Facon, 2006; Facon, 2007] **or** with prednisone and thalidomide [Facon, 2007]) **or**

9 mg/m^2/day for 4 days every 6 weeks (in combination with prednisone **or** with prednisone and bortezomib) (Dimopoulos, 2009; San Miguel, 2008)

Ovarian carcinoma: 0.2 mg/kg/day for 5 days, repeat every 4-5 weeks **or**

Unlabeled dosing: 7 mg/m^2/day in 2 divided doses for 5 days, repeat every 28 days (Wadler, 1996)

Amyloidosis, light chain (unlabeled use): 0.22 mg/kg/day for 4 days every 28 days (in combination with oral dexamethasone) (Palladini, 2004) **or** 10 mg/m^2/day for 4 days every month (in combination with oral dexamethasone) for 12-18 treatment cycles (Jaccard, 2007)

I.V.:

Children (unlabeled use): Conditioning regimen for autologous hematopoietic stem cell transplantation:

140 mg/m^2 2 days prior to transplantation (combined with busulfan) (Canete, 2009; Oberlin, 2006) **or**

180 mg/m^2 (with pre- and posthydration) 12-30 hours prior to transplantation (Pritchard, 2005) **or**

45 mg/m^2/day for 4 days starting 8 days prior to transplantation (combined with busulfan or etoposide and carboplatin) (Berthold, 2005)

Adults:

Multiple myeloma (palliative treatment): 16 mg/m^2 administered at 2-week intervals for 4 doses, then administer at 4-week intervals after adequate hematologic recovery.

Conditioning regimen for autologous hematopoietic stem cell transplantation (unlabeled use):

200 mg/m^2 alone 2 days prior to transplantation (Fermand, 2005; Moreau, 2002) **or**

140 mg/m^2 2 days prior to transplantation (combined with busulfan) (Fermand, 2005) **or**

140 mg/m^2 2 days prior to transplantation (combined with total body irradiation [TBI]) (Moreau, 2002) **or**

140 mg/m^2 5 days prior to transplantation (combined with TBI) (Barlogie, 2006)

Hodgkin lymphoma (unlabeled use): 30 mg/m^2 on day 6 of combination chemotherapy (mini-BEAM) regimen (Colwill, 1995; Martin, 2001)

Elderly: Refer to adult dosing; use caution and begin at the lower end of dosing range

Dosage adjustment for toxicity:

Oral:

WBC <3000/mm^3: Withhold treatment until recovery

Platelets <100,000/mm^3: Withhold treatment until recovery

I.V.: Adjust dose based on nadir blood cell counts

Dosing adjustment in renal impairment:

The FDA-approved labeling contains the following adjustment recommendations (for approved dosing levels) based on route of administration:

Oral: Moderate-to-severe renal impairment: Consider a reduced dose initially

I.V.: BUN ≥30 mg/dL: Reduce dose by up to 50%

The following guidelines have been used by some clinicians:

Aronoff, 2007 (route of administration not specified):

Adults (based on a 6 mg once-daily dose):

Cl_{cr} 10-50 mL/minute: Administer 75% of dose

Cl_{cr} <10 mL/minute: Administer 50% of dose

Hemodialysis: Administer dose after hemodialysis

Continuous ambulatory peritoneal dialysis (CAPD): Administer 50% of dose

Continuous renal replacement therapy (CRRT): Administer 75% of dose

Carlson, 2005: Oral (for melphalan-prednisone combination therapy; based on a study evaluating toxicity with melphalan dosed at 0.25 mg/kg/day for 4 days/cycle):

Cl_{cr} >10 to <30 mL/minute: Administer 75% of dose

Cl_{cr} ≤10 mL/minute: Data is insufficient for a recommendation

Kintzel, 1995:

Oral: Adjust dose in the presence of hematologic toxicity

I.V.:

Cl_{cr} 46-60 mL/minute: Administer 85% of normal dose

Cl_{cr} 31-45 mL/minute: Administer 75% of normal dose

Cl_{cr} <30 mL/minute: Administer 70% of normal dose

Badros, 2001: I.V.: Autologous stem cell transplant (single-agent conditioning regimen; no busulfan or irradiation): Serum creatinine >2 mg/dL: Reduce dose from 200 mg/m^2 over 2 days (as 100 mg/m^2/day for 2 days) to 140 mg/m^2 given as a single-dose infusion

Dosing adjustment in hepatic impairment: Melphalan is hepatically metabolized; however, dosage adjustment does not appear to be necessary (King, 2001).

Dosing in obesity: *ASCO Guidelines for appropriate chemotherapy dosing in obese adults with cancer (**Note:** Excludes HSCT dosing):* Utilize patient's actual body weight (full weight) for calculation of body surface area- or weight-based dosing, particularly when the intent of therapy is curative; manage regimen-related toxicities in the same manner as for nonobese patients; if a dose reduction is utilized due to toxicity, consider resumption of full weight-based dosing with subsequent cycles, especially if cause of toxicity (eg, hepatic or renal impairment) is resolved (Griggs, 2012).

Dietary Considerations Should be taken on an empty stomach (1 hour prior to or 2 hours after meals).

Administration

Oral: Administer on an empty stomach (1 hour prior to or 2 hours after meals)

Parenteral: Due to limited stability, complete administration of I.V. dose should occur within 60 minutes of reconstitution

I.V.: Infuse over 15-30 minutes. Extravasation may cause local tissue damage; administration by slow injection into a fast running I.V. solution into an injection port or via a central line is recommended; do not administer by direct injection into a peripheral vein.

Hazardous agent; use appropriate precautions for handling and disposal (NIOSH, 2012).

Monitoring Parameters CBC with differential and platelet count, serum electrolytes, serum uric acid

Test Interactions False-positive Coombs' test [direct]

Dosage Forms Excipient information presented when available (limited, particularly for generics); consult specific product labeling.

Solution Reconstituted, Intravenous:

Alkeran: 50 mg (1 ea) [contains alcohol, usp, propylene glycol]

Generic: 50 mg (1 ea)

Tablet, Oral:

Alkeran: 2 mg

◆ **Melquin 3** *see* Hydroquinone *on page 1017*

◆ **Melquin HP** *see* Hydroquinone *on page 1017*

Memantine (me MAN teen)

Brand Names: U.S. Namenda; Namenda Titration Pak; Namenda XR; Namenda XR Titration Pack

Brand Names: Canada Apo-Memantine; CO Memantine; Ebixa; PMS-Memantine; ratio-Memantine; Riva-Memantine; Sandoz-Memantine

Index Terms Memantine Hydrochloride

Pharmacologic Category N-Methyl-D-Aspartate Receptor Antagonist

Use Alzheimer disease: Treatment of moderate to severe dementia of the Alzheimer type.

Unlabeled Use Treatment of mild-to-moderate vascular dementia

Pregnancy Risk Factor B

Pregnancy Considerations Adverse events have been observed in some animal reproduction studies.

Breast-Feeding Considerations It is not known if memantine is excreted in breast milk. The manufacturer recommends that caution be exercised when administering memantine to nursing women.

Contraindications Hypersensitivity to memantine or any component of the formulation

Warnings/Precautions Use with caution in patients with cardiovascular disease; an increased incidence of cardiac failure, angina, bradycardia, and hypertension (compared with placebo) was observed in clinical trials. Use caution with seizure disorders or severe hepatic impairment. Use with caution in severe renal impairment; dose adjustments may be required. Worsening of corneal condition has been observed in a clinical trial; periodic ophthalmic exams during use have been recommended (Canadian labeling). Clearance is significantly reduced by alkaline urine; use caution with medications, dietary changes, or patient conditions which may alter urine pH.

Adverse Reactions Adverse reactions similar in immediate and extended release formulations except as noted.

1% to 10%:

Cardiovascular: Hypertension (4%), hypotension (extended release: 2%), cardiac failure, cerebrovascular accident, syncope, transient ischemic attacks

Central nervous system: Dizziness (5% to 7%), confusion (6%), headache (6%), anxiety (extended release: 4%), depression (extended release: 3%), hallucination (3%), pain (3%), drowsiness (3%), fatigue (2%), aggressive behavior (2%), ataxia, hypokinesia, vertigo

Dermatologic: Skin rash

Endocrine & metabolic: Weight gain (extended release: 3%), weight loss

Gastrointestinal: Constipation (3% to 5%), diarrhea (5%), vomiting (2% to 3%), abdominal pain (2%)

Genitourinary: Urinary incontinence (2%), urinary frequency

Hematologic & oncologic: Anemia

Hepatic: Increased serum alkaline phosphatase

Infection: Influenza (4%)

Neuromuscular & skeletal: Back pain (3%)

Ophthalmic: Cataract, conjunctivitis

Respiratory: Cough (4%), dyspnea (2%), pneumonia

<1% (Limited to important or life-threatening): Abnormal hepatic function tests, agranulocytosis, angina pectoris, anorexia, aphasia, apnea, arthralgia, aspiration pneumonia, atrial fibrillation, atrioventricular block, blepharitis, bone fracture, bradycardia, brain disease, bronchitis, cardiac arrest, cardiac failure, carpal tunnel syndrome, cerebral hemorrhage, cerebral infarction, chest pain, cholelithiasis, colitis, coma, complete atrioventricular block, conjunctival hemorrhage, convulsions, corneal opacity, deep vein thrombosis, delirium, diplopia, drug-induced Parkinson's disease, dyskinesia, dysphagia, dysuria, exacerbation of diabetes mellitus, extrapyramidal reaction, falling, fecal incontinence, gastroenteritis, gastroesophageal reflux disease, gastrointestinal hemorrhage, glaucoma, hearing loss, hematuria, hemiplegia, hepatic failure, hepatitis (including cytolytic and cholestatic), hyperglycemia, hyperlipidemia, hypersensitivity reaction, hypoglycemia, hyponatremia, impaired consciousness, intestinal obstruction, increased INR, intracranial hemorrhage, leukopenia, loss of consciousness, macular degeneration, muscle spasm, myocardial infarction myoclonus, myopia, neuralgia, neuropathy, neuroleptic malignant syndrome, neutropenia, orthostatic hypotension, pancreatitis, pancytopenia, peripheral edema, prolonged Q-T interval on ECG, psychosis, pulmonary edema, pulmonary embolism, renal failure, retinal detachment, retinal hemorrhage, second degree atrioventricular block, seizure, sepsis, SIADH, Stevens-Johnson syndrome, suicidal ideation, suicidal tendencies, supraventricular tachycardia, tardive dyskinesia, thrombocytopenia, thrombotic thrombocytopenic purpura, thrombophlebitis, torsades de pointes, upper respiratory tract infection, urinary tract infection

Drug Interactions

Metabolism/Transport Effects None known.

Avoid Concomitant Use There are no known interactions where it is recommended to avoid concomitant use.

Increased Effect/Toxicity

Memantine may increase the levels/effects of: Trimethoprim

The levels/effects of Memantine may be increased by: Carbonic Anhydrase Inhibitors; Sodium Bicarbonate; Trimethoprim

Decreased Effect There are no known significant interactions involving a decrease in effect.

Storage/Stability Store at 25°C (77°C); excursions permitted to 15°C to 30°C (59°F to 86°F).

Mechanism of Action Glutamate, the primary excitatory amino acid in the CNS, may contribute to the pathogenesis of Alzheimer's disease (AD) by overstimulating various glutamate receptors leading to excitotoxicity and neuronal cell death. Memantine is an uncompetitive antagonist of the N-methyl-D-aspartate (NMDA) type of glutamate receptors, located ubiquitously throughout the brain. Under normal physiologic conditions, the (unstimulated) NMDA receptor ion channel is blocked by magnesium ions, which are displaced after agonist-induced depolarization. Pathologic or excessive receptor activation, as postulated to occur during AD, prevents magnesium from reentering and blocking the channel pore resulting in a chronically open state and excessive calcium influx. Memantine binds to the intra-pore magnesium site, but with longer dwell time, and thus functions as an effective receptor blocker only under conditions of excessive stimulation; memantine does not affect normal neurotransmission.

Pharmacodynamics/Kinetics

Absorption: Well absorbed

Distribution: 9-11 L/kg

Protein binding: 45%

Metabolism: Partially hepatic, primarily independent of the CYP enzyme system; forms 3 metabolites (minimal activity)

Half-life elimination: Terminal: ~60-80 hours; severe renal impairment (Cl_{cr} 5-29 mL/minute): 117-156 hours

Time to peak, serum: Immediate release: 3-7 hours; Extended release: 9-12 hours

Excretion: Urine (74%; ~48% of the total dose as unchanged drug; undergoes active tubular secretion moderated by pH-dependent tubular reabsorption; excretion reduced by alkaline urine pH)

Dosage

Alzheimer's disease (moderate-to-severe): Adults: Oral:

Immediate release: Initial: 5 mg daily; increase dose by 5 mg daily to a target dose of 20 mg daily; wait ≥1 week between dosage changes. Doses >5 mg daily should be given in 2 divided doses. **Note:** If treatment is interrupted for longer than several days, the treatment may need to be restarted at a lower dose and retitrated.

Suggested titration: 5 mg daily for ≥1 week; 5 mg twice daily for ≥1 week; 15 mg daily given in 5 mg and 10 mg separate doses for ≥1 week; then 10 mg twice daily

Extended release: Initial: 7 mg once daily, increase dose by 7 mg daily to a target maximum dose of 28 mg once daily; wait ≥1 week between dosage changes (if previous dose well tolerated)

Note: When switching from immediate release product to the extended release product, begin the extended release product the day after the last dose of the immediate release product. Patients on immediate release 10 mg twice daily should be switched to extended release 28 mg once daily.

Mild-to-moderate vascular dementia (unlabeled use): Adults: Oral: Immediate release: Initial: 5 mg daily, titrated by 5 mg daily weekly to a target dose of 10 mg twice daily (Orgogozo, 2002)

Dosage adjustment in renal impairment: Note: Renal function may be estimated using the Cockcroft-Gault formula for dosage adjustment purposes.

Mild impairment: No dosage adjustment necessary.

Moderate impairment:

U.S. labeling: No dosage adjustment necessary.

Canadian labeling: (Cl_{cr} 30-49 mL/minute): Initial: 5 mg once daily; after at least 1 week of therapy and if tolerated, titrate up to 5 mg twice daily; based on clinical response (and if well tolerated), may further titrate dosage upward in weekly increments to 20 mg daily according to suggested titration schedule

Severe impairment:

U.S. labeling: Cl_{cr} 5-29 mL/minute: Immediate release: Initial: 5 mg once daily; after at least 1 week of therapy and if tolerated, may titrate up to a target dose of 5 mg twice daily; Extended release: Target dose of 14 mg once daily.

Note: When switching from immediate release product to the extended release product, begin the extended release product the day after the last dose of the immediate release product. Patients on immediate release 5 mg twice daily should be switched to extended release 14 mg once daily.

Canadian labeling: Cl_{cr} 15-29 mL/minute: Initial: 5 mg once daily; after at least 1 week of therapy and if tolerated, may titrate up to a target dose of 5 mg twice daily

Dosage adjustment in hepatic impairment:

Mild-to-moderate impairment: No dosage adjustment necessary.

Severe impairment:

U.S. labeling: No dosage adjustment provided in the manufacturer's labeling (has not been studied); use with caution.

Canadian labeling: No dosage adjustment provided in the manufacturer's labeling (has not been studied); avoid use.

Administration Administer without regard to meals. Extended release capsules may be swallowed whole or entire contents of capsule may be sprinkled on applesauce and swallowed immediately; do not chew, crush, or divide.

Monitoring Parameters Cognitive function; periodic ophthalmic exam (Canadian labeling)

Dosage Forms Excipient information presented when available (limited, particularly for generics); consult specific product labeling.

Capsule Extended Release 24 Hour, Oral, as hydrochloride:

Namenda XR: 7 mg, 14 mg, 21 mg, 28 mg

Namenda XR Titration Pack: 7 mg (7s), 14 mg (7s), 21 mg (7s), and 28 mg (7s)

Solution, Oral, as hydrochloride:

Namenda: 10 mg/5 mL (360 mL) [peppermint flavor]

Tablet, Oral, as hydrochloride:

Namenda: 5 mg [contains fd&c blue #2 (indigotine), fd&c yellow #6 (sunset yellow)]

Namenda: 10 mg

Namenda Titration Pak: 5 (28)-10 (21) MG [contains fd&c blue #2 (indigotine), fd&c yellow #6 (sunset yellow)]

◆ **Memantine Hydrochloride** *see* Memantine *on page 1289*

◆ **Menactra** *see* Meningococcal (Groups A / C / Y and W-135) Diphtheria Conjugate Vaccine *on page 1291*

◆ **MenACWY** *see* Meningococcal (Groups A / C / Y and W-135) Diphtheria Conjugate Vaccine *on page 1291*

◆ **MenACWY-D (Menactra)** *see* Meningococcal (Groups A / C / Y and W-135) Diphtheria Conjugate Vaccine *on page 1291*

◆ MenACWY-CRM (Menveo) *see* Meningococcal (Groups A / C / Y and W-135) Diphtheria Conjugate Vaccine *on page 1291*

◆ M-END DM [OTC] *see* Chlorpheniramine, Pseudoephedrine, and Dextromethorphan *on page 414*

◆ Menest *see* Estrogens (Esterified) *on page 775*

◆ Menest® (Can) *see* Estrogens (Esterified) *on page 775*

◆ Menhibrix *see* Meningococcal Polysaccharide (Groups C and Y) and *Haemophilus* b Tetanus Toxoid Conjugate Vaccine *on page 1293*

◆ Meningococcal Conjugate Vaccine *see* Meningococcal (Groups A / C / Y and W-135) Diphtheria Conjugate Vaccine *on page 1291*

Meningococcal (Groups A / C / Y and W-135) Diphtheria Conjugate Vaccine

(me NIN joe kok al groops aye, see, why & dubl yoo won thur tee fyve dif THEER ee a KON joo gate vak SEEN)

Brand Names: U.S. Menactra; Menveo

Brand Names: Canada Menactra; Menveo

Index Terms MCV; MCV4; MenACWY; MenACWY-CRM (Menveo); MenACWY-D (Menactra); Meningococcal Conjugate Vaccine

Pharmacologic Category Vaccine, Inactivated (Bacterial)

Additional Appendix Information

Immunization Administration Recommendations *on page 2334*

Immunization Recommendations *on page 2339*

Use Provide active immunization of children and adults against invasive meningococcal disease caused by *N. meningitidis* serogroups A, C, Y, and W-135.

The Advisory Committee on Immunization Practices (ACIP) (CDC, 62[2], 2013):

ACIP recommends routine vaccination of the following:

- Children and adolescents 11-18 years of age
- Persons ≥2 months of age who are at increased risk of meningococcal disease
- Persons (in all recommended age groups) at increased risk who are part of outbreaks caused by vaccine preventable serogroups

Those at increased risk of meningococcal disease include the following:

- Persons ≥2 months of age with medical conditions such as anatomical or functional asplenia or persistent compliment component deficiencies (eg, C_5-C_9, properdin, factor H, or factor D)
- Persons ≥9 months of age that travel to or reside in countries where meningococcal disease is hyperendemic or epidemic, especially if contact with the local population will be prolonged
- Unvaccinated or incompletely vaccinated first year college students living in residence halls
- Military recruits
- Microbiologists with occupational exposure

The Canadian National Advisory Committee on Immunization (NACI): NACI recommends a routine vaccination at ~12 years of age but no booster unless at a continued high risk of exposure. Either quadrivalent vaccine may be used; NACI does not have a preference. NACI recommends use of Menveo (unlabeled use) for high risk persons 2 months to 2 years of age if vaccination with a quadrivalent vaccine is needed; may also be considered for use in persons ≥56 years of age (NACI, 39[1], 2013). Additional recommendations may be found at www.phac-aspc.gc.ca/publicat/ccdr-rmtc/13vol39/acs-dcc-1/index-eng.php

Pregnancy Risk Factor B/C (manufacturer dependent)

Pregnancy Considerations Animal reproduction studies have not been conducted with Menactra. Patients should contact the Sanofi Pasteur Inc vaccine registry at 1-800-822-2463 if they are pregnant or become aware they were pregnant at the time of Menactra vaccination.

Adverse events were not observed in animal reproduction studies conducted with Menveo. Patients should contact the Novartis Vaccines and Diagnostics Inc. pregnancy registry at 1-877-311-8972 if they are pregnant or become aware they were pregnant at the time of Menveo vaccination.

Limited information is available following inadvertent use of meningococcal diphtheria conjugate vaccine during pregnancy. Inactivated bacterial vaccines have not been shown to cause increased risks to the fetus (CDC, 60[2], 2011). Pregnancy should not preclude vaccination if indicated (CDC, 62[2], 2013).

Breast-Feeding Considerations It is not known if this vaccine is found in breast milk. The manufacturer recommends that caution be used if administered to a nursing woman. Inactivated vaccines do not affect the safety of breast-feeding for the mother or the infant. Breast-feeding infants should be vaccinated according to the recommended schedules (CDC, 60[2], 2011).

Contraindications Hypersensitivity to other meningococcal-containing vaccines or any component of the formulation including diphtheria toxoid or CRM_{197} (a diphtheria toxin carrier protein)

Warnings/Precautions Use with caution in patients with a history of bleeding disorders (including thrombocytopenia) and/or patients on anticoagulant therapy; bleeding/hematoma may occur from I.M. administration. May consider deferring administration in patients with moderate or severe acute illness (with or without fever); may administer to patients with mild acute illness (with or without fever). Apnea has been reported following I.M. vaccine administration in premature infants; consider risk versus benefit in infants born prematurely. Vaccination may not result in effective immunity in all patients. Response depends upon multiple factors (eg, type of vaccine, age of patient) and may be improved by administering the vaccine at the recommended dose, route, and interval. Vaccines may not be effective if administered during periods of altered immune competence (CDC 60[2], 2011). Not to be used to treat meningococcal infections or to provide immunity against *N. meningitidis* serogroup B or diphtheria. Immunosuppressed patients may have a reduced response to vaccination. Syncope has been reported with use of injectable vaccines and may be accompanied by transient visual disturbances, weakness, or tonic-clonic movements. Procedures should be in place to avoid injuries from falling and to restore cerebral perfusion if syncope occurs. In general, household and close contacts of persons with altered immunocompetence may receive all age appropriate vaccines. Risk of developing Guillain-Barré syndrome (GBS) may be increased following vaccination in persons previously diagnosed with GBS. The risk of developing GBS was evaluated in a study of healthcare claims of persons 11-18 years of age (n= ~9,600,000; 15% were vaccinated with Menactra); 72 cases of GBS were confirmed and none received the vaccine within 42 days prior to symptoms; 129 reported cases of GBS could not be confirmed or excluded. Data not currently available to assess possible risk of GBS following use of Menveo. Immediate treatment for anaphylactic reactions should be available. In order to maximize vaccination rates, the ACIP recommends simultaneous administration of all age-appropriate vaccines (live or inactivated) for which a person is eligible at a single clinic visit, unless contraindications exist. Use of this vaccine for specific medical and/or other indications (eg, immunocompromising conditions, hepatic or kidney disease, diabetes) is also addressed in the ACIP Recommended Immunization Schedule (CDC, 2013a; CDC, 2013b).

Adverse Reactions All serious adverse reactions must be reported to the U.S. Department of Health and Human Services (DHHS) Vaccine Adverse Event Reporting System (VAERS) 1-800-822-7967 or online at https://vaers.hhs.gov/esub/index. In Canada, adverse reactions may be reported to local provincial/territorial health agencies or to the Vaccine Safety Section at Public Health Agency of Canada (1-866-844-0018).

Actual percentages may vary by product and age group:

>10%:

- Central nervous system: Drowsiness, excessive crying, fatigue, headache, irritability, malaise
- Gastrointestinal: Anorexia, change in appetite, diarrhea, nausea, vomiting
- Local: Erythema at injection site, induration at injection site, pain at injection site, swelling at injection site, tenderness at injection site
- Neuromuscular & skeletal: Arthralgia, myalgia
- Miscellaneous: Fever

1% to 10%:

- Central nervous system: Chills
- Dermatologic: Skin rash

<1% (Limited to important or life-threatening): Acute disseminated encephalomyelitis, anaphylactoid reaction, anaphylaxis, apnea (premature infants), appendicitis, auditory impairment, Bell's palsy, blepharoptosis, convulsions (including tonic), Cushing's syndrome, dehydration, depression, equilibrium disturbance, exfoliation of skin, facial paresis, falling, febrile seizures, gastroenteritis, Guillain-Barre syndrome, hypersensitivity, hypotension, increased serum ALT, inflammation at injection site, injection site cellulitis, Kawasaki Syndrome, ostealgia, pelvic inflammatory disease, pneumonia, pruritus at injection site, seizure, simple partial seizures, staphylococcal infection, suicidal tendencies, syncope (including vasovagal), transverse myelitis, varicella, vertebral disc disease, vestibular disturbance

Drug Interactions

Metabolism/Transport Effects None known.

Avoid Concomitant Use There are no known interactions where it is recommended to avoid concomitant use.

Increased Effect/Toxicity There are no known significant interactions involving an increase in effect.

Decreased Effect

The levels/effects of Meningococcal (Groups A / C / Y and W-135) Diphtheria Conjugate Vaccine may be decreased by: Belimumab; Fingolimod; Immunosuppressants

Preparation for Administration Menveo: Prior to use, remove liquid contents from vial of MenCYW-135 and inject into vial containing MenA powder. Invert and shake well until dissolved. The resulting solution should be clear and colorless. A small amount of liquid will remain in the vial after withdrawing the 0.5 mL dose.

Storage/Stability

Menactra: Store between 2°C to 8°C (35°F to 46°F); do not freeze. Discard product exposed to freezing. Do not mix with other vaccines in the same syringe.

Menveo: Prior to reconstitution, store between 2°C to 8°C (36°F to 46°F); do not freeze. Protect from light. Discard product exposed to freezing. Use immediately after reconstitution but may be stored at ≤25°C (77°F) for up to 8 hours. Do not mix with other vaccines in the same syringe.

Mechanism of Action Induces immunity against meningococcal disease via the formation of bactericidal antibodies directed toward the polysaccharide capsular components of *Neisseria meningitidis* serogroups A, C, Y and W-135.

Dosage I.M.:

Menactra:

- Infants ≥9 months and Children <2 years: 0.5 mL/dose given as a 2-dose series, 3 months apart
- Children ≥2 years, Adolescents, and Adults ≤55 years: 0.5 mL/dose given as a single dose

Menveo: Age at initial vaccination:

- Infants ≥2 months to <7 months: 0.5 mL/dose given as a 4-dose series at 2, 4, 6, and 12 months of age
- Infants ≥7 months and Children <2 years: 0.5 mL/dose given as a 2-dose series, with the second dose given during the second year of life and at least 3 months after the first dose
- Children ≥2 to <6 years: 0.5 mL/dose given as a single dose; for children at continued high risk of meningococcal disease, may consider an additional dose given 2 months after the first dose
- Children ≥6 years, Adolescents, and Adults ≤55 years: 0.5 mL/dose given as a single dose

ACIP recommendations (CDC, 62[2], 2013): **Note:** Use of the abbreviation, MenACWY, refers to either meningococcal quadrivalent polysaccharide vaccine. MenACWY-CRM refers specifically to Menveo; MenACWY-D refers specifically to Menactra.

Primary vaccination:

Children and Adolescents:

- <11 years: Not routinely recommended; see dosing for persons at increased risk
- 11-12 years: One 0.5 mL dose. Children not at increased risk for meningococcal disease who may have been previously vaccinated with Hib-MenCY-TT (MenHibrix) or MenACWY prior to their tenth birthday, should receive the routinely recommended doses of MenACWY at 11-12 years
- 13-18 years: One 0.5 mL dose if not previously vaccinated

Adults:

- 19-21 years: Not routinely recommended; may receive one 0.5 mL dose as a catch-up vaccination if no dose was received after the sixteenth birthday
- ≥22 years: Not routinely recommended; see dosing for persons at increased risk

Primary vaccination: Persons at increased risk for meningococcal disease:

Children 9-23 months with high-risk conditions: Two 0.5 mL doses of MenACWY-D (Menactra) given 12 weeks apart. May be given as early as 8 weeks apart if needed prior to travel. Use of MenACWY-D (Menactra) should be avoided in children with functional or anatomic asplenia prior to age of 2 to avoid interference with immune response to the pneumococcal conjugate vaccine (PCV). Infants at increased risk who are vaccinated with Hib-MenCY-TT (MenHibrix) do not need vaccinated with MenACWY until the first booster dose (3 years after the completion of the series) unless another indication is present (eg, travel to endemic area).

Children ≥2 years, Adolescents, and Adults ≤55 years not previously vaccinated and who have persistent complement deficiencies, functional or anatomic asplenia, or who have HIV infection and another indication for vaccination: Two 0.5 mL doses, given 8-12 weeks apart. If using MenACWY-D (Menactra), administer ≥4 weeks after completion of all PCV doses

Children ≥2 years, Adolescents, and Adults ≤55 years not previously vaccinated and who are either: First year college students ≤21 years of age living in residential housing, traveling to or residents of areas where meningococcal disease is endemic/hyperendemic, at risk during a community outbreak, or microbiologists routinely exposed to *Neisseria meningitidis*: One 0.5 mL dose. If using MenACWY-D (Menactra), administer ≥4 weeks after completion of all PCV doses. College students ≤21 years should have documentation of a vaccination not more than 5 years before enrollment (preferably a dose on their sixteenth birthday)

Adults ≥56 years: Meningococcal polysaccharide vaccine (MPSV4) is preferred for meningococcal vaccine-naive persons in this age group who require a single dose. If multiple doses are anticipated, see booster dosing for persons at increased risk.

Booster dose: Children ≥11 years, Adolescents, and Adults ≤21 years: One 0.5 mL dose if the first dose was given prior to the sixteenth birthday. If primary vaccination was at 11-12 years, the booster dose should be given at age 16. If the primary vaccination was given at 13-15 years, the booster dose should be given at age 16-18. Minimum interval between MenACWY doses is 8 weeks. A booster dose is not needed if the primary dose was given after the sixteenth birthday unless the person becomes at increased risk for meningococcal disease.

Booster vaccination: Persons at increased risk for meningococcal disease:

If first dose received at 2 months to 6 years of age: Repeat dose 3 years after primary vaccination, and every 5 years thereafter if the person remains at increased risk.

If first dose received at ≥7 years of age: Repeat dose 5 years after primary vaccination, and every 5 years thereafter if the person remains at increased risk.

Adults ≥56 years: Persons previously vaccinated with MenACWY and who require revaccination or for whom multiple doses are anticipated, MenACWY is preferred. Otherwise, meningococcal polysaccharide vaccine (MPSV4) is preferred for meningococcal vaccine naïve persons in this age group who require a single dose.

Dosage adjustment in renal impairment: No dosage adjustment provided in manufacturer's labeling.

Dosage adjustment in hepatic impairment: No dosage adjustment provided in manufacturer's labeling.

Administration Administer by I.M. route, preferably into the anterolateral aspect of the thigh (infants) or upper deltoid region (toddlers, adolescents, and adults). Do not administer via I.V., SubQ or I.D. route. For patients at risk of hemorrhage, the ACIP recommends "it should be administered intramuscularly if, in the opinion of a physician familiar with the patient's bleeding risk, the vaccine can be administered by this route with reasonable safety. If the patient receives antihemophilia or other similar therapy, intramuscular vaccination can be scheduled shortly after such therapy is administered. A fine needle (23 gauge or smaller) can be used for the vaccination and firm pressure applied to the site (without rubbing) for at least 2 minutes. The patient or family should be instructed concerning the risk of hematoma from the injection." Patients on anticoagulant therapy should be considered to have the same bleeding risks and treated as those with clotting factor disorders (CDC, 60[2], 2011).

For I.M. administration only. Based on limited data, inadvertent SubQ administration provides a lower serologic response, however, the response is still considered to be protective. If inadvertently administered by the SubQ route, revaccination is not necessary.

Simultaneous administration of vaccines helps ensure the patients will be fully vaccinated by the appropriate age. Simultaneous administration of vaccines is defined as administering >1 vaccine on the same day at different anatomic sites. Separate vaccines should not be combined in the same syringe unless indicated by product specific labeling. Separate needles and syringes should be used for each injection. The ACIP prefers each dose of a specific vaccine in a series come from the same manufacturer when possible. Adolescents and adults should be vaccinated while seated or lying down. In general, preterm infants should be vaccinated at the same chronological age as full-term infants (CDC, 60[2], 2011).

Antipyretics have not been shown to prevent febrile seizures. Antipyretics may be used to treat fever or discomfort following vaccination (CDC, 60[2], 2011). One study reported that routine prophylactic administration of acetaminophen to prevent fever prior to vaccination decreased the immune response of some vaccines; the clinical significance of this reduction in immune response has not been established (Prymula, 2009).

Monitoring Parameters Monitor for syncope for at least 15 minutes following administration. If seizure-like activity associated with syncope occurs, maintain patient in supine or Trendelenburg position to reestablish adequate cerebral perfusion.

Additional Information U.S. federal law requires that the name of medication, date of administration, the vaccine manufacturer, lot number of vaccine, and the administering person's name, title and address be entered into the patient's permanent medical record.

Currently, two different meningococcal (groups A/C/Y and W-135) diphtheria conjugate vaccines are available. Menveo uses oligosaccharides of the *N. meningitidis* serogroups linked to CRM_{197} (a nontoxic diphtheria toxin carrier protein). Menactra uses polysaccharides from the serogroups linked to diphtheria toxoid. Both products are administered by I.M. injection and provide active immunization against invasive meningococcal disease caused by *N. meningitidis* serogroups A, C, Y, and W-135.

Dosage Forms Excipient information presented when available (limited, particularly for generics); consult specific product labeling.

Injection, solution [preservative free]:

Menactra: 4 mcg each of polysaccharide antigen groups A, C, Y, and W-135 [bound to diphtheria toxoid 48 mcg] per 0.5 mL [MCV4 or MenACWY-D]

Menveo: MenA oligosaccharide 10 mcg, MenC oligosaccharide 5 mcg, MenY oligosaccharide 5 mcg, and MenW-135 oligosaccharide 5 mcg [bound to CRM_{197} protein 32.7-64.1 mcg] per 0.5 mL (0.5 mL) [MenACWY-CRM; supplied in two vials, one containing MenA powder and one containing MenCYW-135 liquid]

Meningococcal Polysaccharide (Groups C and Y) and *Haemophilus* b Tetanus Toxoid Conjugate Vaccine

(me NIN joe kok al pol i SAK a ride groops see & why & he MOF i lus bee TET a nus TOKS oyd KON joo gate vak SEEN)

Brand Names: U.S. Menhibrix

Index Terms Hib-MenCY-TT

Pharmacologic Category Vaccine, Inactivated (Bacterial)

Additional Appendix Information

Immunization Administration Recommendations *on page 2334*

Immunization Recommendations *on page 2339*

Use To provide active immunity to prevent invasive disease caused by meningococcal serogroups C and Y and *Haemophilus influenzae* type b

The Advisory Committee on Immunization Practices (ACIP) recommends vaccination only for infants 2-18 months of age who are at increased risk for meningococcal disease, including:
- Infants with persistent complement pathway deficiencies
- Infants with anatomic or functional asplenia, including sickle cell disease
- Infants in communities with serogroups C and Y meningococcal disease outbreaks

The ACIP does not recommend routine vaccination for infants not at increased risk for meningococcal disease. In addition, infants traveling to certain areas (eg, meningitis belt of sub-Saharan Africa) will require a meningococcal vaccine with serogroups A and W_{135}; vaccination with Hib-MenCY-TT will not be adequate (CDC, 2013).

Pregnancy Risk Factor C

Dosage Primary immunization: Infants ≥6 weeks and Children ≤18 months: I.M.: 0.5 mL/dose given as a four-dose series at 2, 4, 6, and 12-15 months of age. The first dose may be given as early as 6 weeks of age and the fourth dose may be given as late as 18 months of age.

Note: The ACIP recommends vaccination only for infants ≥2 months and children ≤18 months of age who are at an increased risk for meningococcal disease. The first dose may be given as early as 6 weeks of age and the fourth dose may be given as late as 18 months of age. If an infant at increased risk is behind on Hib vaccine doses, Hib-MenCY-TT may be used to catch up using the current Hib schedule. If the first dose of Hib-MenCY-TT is given ≥12 months of age, two doses should be given 8 weeks apart. If infants have/will receive a different Hib vaccine, a two-dose series of a quadrivalent meningococcal vaccine is recommended (Menactra® for ages 9-23 months; Menactra® or Menveo® for ages >23 months) (CDC, 2013).

Dosage adjustment in renal impairment: No dosage adjustment provided in manufacturer's labeling.

Dosage adjustment in hepatic impairment: No dosage adjustment provided in manufacturer's labeling.

Additional Information Complete prescribing information should be consulted for additional detail.

Dosage Forms Excipient information presented when available (limited, particularly for generics); consult specific product labeling.

Solution Reconstituted, Intramuscular [preservative free]:

Menhibrix: 5 mcg each of polysaccharide antigen groups C and Y, and 2.5 mcg Haemophilus b capsular polysaccharide per 0.5 mL dose (1 ea) [contains tetanus toxoid]

◆ **Meningococcal Polysaccharide Vaccine** *see* Meningococcal Polysaccharide Vaccine (Groups A / C / Y and W-135) *on page 1294*

Meningococcal Polysaccharide Vaccine (Groups A / C / Y and W-135)

(me NIN joe kok al pol i SAK a ride vak SEEN groops aye, see, why & dubl yoo won thur tee fyve)

Brand Names: U.S. Menomune®-A/C/Y/W-135

Brand Names: Canada Menomune®-A/C/Y/W-135

Index Terms Meningococcal Polysaccharide Vaccine; MPSV; MPSV4

Pharmacologic Category Vaccine, Inactivated (Bacterial)

Additional Appendix Information

Immunization Administration Recommendations *on page 2334*

Immunization Recommendations *on page 2339*

Use Provide active immunity to meningococcal serogroups contained in the vaccine

The Advisory Committee on Immunization Practices (ACIP) recommends routine vaccination for persons at increased risk for meningococcal disease. Meningococcal quadrivalent conjugate vaccine (MenACWY) is preferred; meningococcal polysaccharide vaccine (MPSV4) is preferred in meningococcal vaccine-naive adults ≥56 years of age requiring only a single vaccination (CDC, 2013).

Those at increased risk of meningococcal disease include the following:
- Persons ≥2 months of age with medical conditions such as anatomical or functional asplenia or persistent compliment component deficiencies (eg, C_5-C_9, properdin, factor H, or factor D)
- Persons ≥9 months of age that travel to or reside in countries where meningococcal disease is hyperendemic or epidemic, especially if contact with the local population will be prolonged
- Unvaccinated or incompletely vaccinated first year college students living in residence halls
- Military recruits
- Microbiologists with occupational exposure
- Persons (in all recommended age groups) at risk who are part of outbreaks caused by vaccine preventable serogroups

Pregnancy Risk Factor C

Pregnancy Considerations Animal reproduction studies have not been conducted. Inactivated bacterial vaccines have not been shown to cause increased risks to the fetus (CDC, 2011). Pregnancy should not preclude vaccination if indicated (CDC, 62[2], 2013).

Breast-Feeding Considerations It is not known if this vaccine is present in breast milk. The manufacturer recommends that caution be used if administered to a nursing woman. Inactivated vaccines do not affect the safety of breast-feeding for the mother or the infant. Breast-feeding infants should be vaccinated according to the recommended schedules (CDC, 2011).

Contraindications Hypersensitivity to any component of the formulation

Warnings/Precautions Immediate treatment (including epinephrine 1:1000) for anaphylactoid and/or hypersensitivity reactions should be available during vaccine use. Response may not be as great as desired in immunosuppressed patients. In general, household and close contacts of persons with altered immunocompetence may receive all age appropriate vaccines. Not to be used to treat meningococcal infections or to provide immunity against *N. meningitidis* serogroup B. May consider deferring administration in patients with moderate or severe acute illness (with or without fever); may administer to patients with mild acute illness (with or without fever). Vaccination may not result in effective immunity in all patients. Response depends upon multiple factors (eg, type of vaccine, age of patient) and may be improved by administering the vaccine at the recommended dose, route, and interval. Vaccines may not be effective if administered during periods of altered immune competence (CDC, 2011). Syncope has been reported with use of injectable vaccines and may be accompanied by transient visual disturbances, weakness, or tonic-clonic movements. Procedures should be in place to avoid injuries from falling and to restore cerebral perfusion if syncope occurs. Use with caution in patients with latex sensitivity; the stopper to the vial contains dry, natural latex rubber. Some dosage forms contain thimerosal. In order to maximize vaccination rates, the ACIP recommends simultaneous administration of all age-appropriate vaccines (live or inactivated) for which a person is eligible at a single clinic visit, unless contraindications exist. Use of this vaccine for specific medical and/or other indications (eg, immunocompromising conditions, hepatic or kidney disease, diabetes) is also addressed in the ACIP Recommended Immunization Schedule (CDC, 2013a; CDC, 2013b).

Adverse Reactions All serious adverse reactions must be reported to the U.S. Department of Health and Human Services (DHHS) Vaccine Adverse Event Reporting System (VAERS) 1-800-822-7967 or online at https://vaers.hhs.gov/esub/index. In Canada, adverse reactions may be reported to local provincial/territorial health agencies or to the Vaccine Safety Section at Public Health Agency of Canada (1-866-844-0018).

>10%:

Central nervous system: Headache (29% to 42%), fatigue (25% to 32%), malaise (17% to 22%), irritability (12%), drowsiness (11%)

Gastrointestinal: Diarrhea (10% to 14%)

Local: Injection site: Pain (26% to 48%), redness (6% to 16%), induration (4% to 11%)

Neuromuscular & skeletal: Arthralgia (5% to 16%)

1% to 10%:

Central nervous system: Chills (4% to 6%), fever (≤5%)

Dermatologic: Rash (≤3%)

Gastrointestinal: Anorexia (8% to 10%), vomiting (1% to 3%)

Local: Injection site: Swelling (3% to 8%)

Postmarketing and/or case reports: Dizziness, Guillain-Barré syndrome, hypersensitivity (angioedema, dyspnea, pruritus, rash, urticaria), myalgia, nausea, paresthesia, vasovagal syncope, weakness

Drug Interactions

Metabolism/Transport Effects None known.

Avoid Concomitant Use There are no known interactions where it is recommended to avoid concomitant use.

Increased Effect/Toxicity There are no known significant interactions involving an increase in effect.

Decreased Effect

The levels/effects of Meningococcal Polysaccharide Vaccine (Groups A / C / Y and W-135) may be decreased by: Belimumab; Fingolimod; Immunosuppressants

Preparation for Administration Reconstitute using provided diluent; shake well. Use single-dose vial immediately after reconstitution. Use multidose vial within 35 days of reconstitution.

Storage/Stability Prior to and following reconstitution, store vaccine and diluent at 2°C to 8°C (35°F to 46°F); do not freeze.

Mechanism of Action Induces the formation of bactericidal antibodies to meningococcal antigens; the presence of these antibodies is strongly correlated with immunity to meningococcal disease caused by *Neisseria meningitidis* groups A, C, Y and W-135.

Pharmacodynamics/Kinetics

Onset of action: Antibody levels: 7-10 days

Duration: Antibodies against group A and C polysaccharides decline markedly (to prevaccination levels) over the first 3 years following a single dose of vaccine, especially in children <4 years of age

Dosage

Immunization: Children ≥2 years and Adults: SubQ: 0.5 mL/dose

ACIP recommendations (CDC, 62[2], 2013):

Children, Adolescents, and Adults <56 years: Not routinely recommended

Adults ≥56 years: Meningococcal polysaccharide vaccine (MPSV4) is preferred for meningococcal vaccine-naive persons in this age group who are at increased risk of meningococcal infection and require a single dose (eg, travelers or during a community outbreak). Persons previously vaccinated with a quadrivalent meningococcal conjugate vaccine (MenACWY) and who require revaccination or for whom multiple doses are anticipated, MenACWY is preferred (eg, persons with asplenia or microbiologists).

Dosage adjustment in renal impairment: No dosage adjustment provided in manufacturer's labeling.

Dosage adjustment in hepatic impairment: No dosage adjustment provided in manufacturer's labeling.

Administration Administer by SubQ injection to the deltoid region; do not administer intradermally, I.M., or I.V.

Simultaneous administration of vaccines helps ensure the patients will be fully vaccinated by the appropriate age. Simultaneous administration of vaccines is defined as administering ≥1 vaccine on the same day at different anatomic sites. Separate vaccines should not be combined in the same syringe unless indicated by product specific labeling. Separate needles and syringes should be used for each injection. The ACIP prefers each dose of a specific vaccine in a series come from the same manufacturer when possible. Adolescents and adults should be vaccinated while seated or lying down. In general, preterm infants should be vaccinated at the same chronological age as full-term infants (CDC, 2011).

Antipyretics have not been shown to prevent febrile seizures. Antipyretics may be used to treat fever or discomfort following vaccination (CDC, 2011). One study reported that routine prophylactic administration of acetaminophen to prevent fever prior to vaccination decreased the immune response of some vaccines; the clinical significance of this reduction in immune response has not been established (Prymula, 2009).

Monitoring Parameters Monitor for syncope for 15 minutes following administration. If seizure-like activity associated with syncope occurs, maintain patient in supine or Trendelenburg position to reestablish adequate cerebral perfusion.

Additional Information U.S. federal law requires that the name of medication, date of administration, the vaccine manufacturer, lot number of vaccine, and the administering person's name, title and address be entered into the patient's permanent medical record.

Dosage Forms Excipient information presented when available (limited, particularly for generics); consult specific product labeling.

Injection, powder for reconstitution [MPSV4]:

Menomune®-A/C/Y/W-135: 50 mcg each of polysaccharide antigen groups A, C, Y, and W-135 per 0.5 mL dose [contains lactose 2.5-5 mg/0.5 mL, natural rubber/natural latex in packaging, thimerosal in diluent for multi-dose vial]

◆ **Menomune®-A/C/Y/W-135** *see* Meningococcal Polysaccharide Vaccine (Groups A / C / Y and W-135) *on page 1294*

◆ **Menopur®** *see* Menotropins *on page 1295*

◆ **Menostar** *see* Estradiol (Systemic) *on page 754*

Menotropins (men oh TROE pins)

Brand Names: U.S. Menopur®; Repronex®

Brand Names: Canada Menopur®; Repronex®

Index Terms hMG; Human Menopausal Gonadotropin

Pharmacologic Category Gonadotropin; Ovulation Stimulator

Use Female:

In conjunction with hCG to induce ovulation and pregnancy in infertile females experiencing oligoanovulation or anovulation when the cause of anovulation is functional and not caused by primary ovarian failure (Repronex®)

Stimulation of multiple follicle development in ovulatory patients as part of an assisted reproductive technology (ART) (Menopur®, Repronex®)

Unlabeled Use Male: Stimulation of spermatogenesis in primary or secondary hypogonadotropic hypogonadism

Pregnancy Risk Factor X

Pregnancy Considerations Ectopic pregnancy and congenital abnormalities have been reported. The incidence of congenital abnormality is similar during natural conception.

Breast-Feeding Considerations It is not known if menotropins is excreted in breast milk. The manufacturer recommends that caution be exercised when administering menotropins to nursing women.

Contraindications Hypersensitivity to menotropins or any component of the formulation; primary ovarian failure as indicated by a high follicle-stimulating hormone (FSH) level; uncontrolled thyroid and adrenal dysfunction; abnormal bleeding of undetermined origin; intracranial lesion (ie, pituitary tumor); ovarian cyst or enlargement not due to polycystic ovary syndrome; infertility due to any cause other than anovulation (except candidates for *in vitro* fertilization); sex hormone-dependent tumors of the reproductive tract and accessory organs; pregnancy

Warnings/Precautions Hazardous agent; use appropriate precautions for handling and disposal (NIOSH, 2012). These medications should only be used by physicians who are thoroughly familiar with infertility problems and their management. Advise patient of frequency and potential hazards of multiple pregnancy. May cause ovarian hyperstimulation syndrome (OHSS); if severe, treatment should be discontinued and patient should be hospitalized (may become more severe if pregnancy occurs). Monitor for ovarian enlargement; to minimize the hazard of abnormal ovarian enlargement, use the lowest possible dose. Serious pulmonary conditions (atelectasis, acute respiratory distress syndrome) and arterial thromboembolism have been reported. Safety and efficacy have not been established in renal or hepatic impairment, or in pediatric and geriatric patients. Use may lead to multiple births.

Adverse Reactions Adverse effects may vary according to specific product, route, and/or dosage.

>10%:

Central nervous system: Headache (up to 34%)
Gastrointestinal: Abdominal pain (up to 18%), nausea (up to 12%)
Genitourinary: OHSS (up to 13%, dose related)
Local: Injection site reaction (4% to 12%)

1% to 10%:

Cardiovascular: Flushing
Central nervous system: Dizziness, malaise, migraine
Endocrine & metabolic: Breast tenderness, hot flashes, menstrual irregularities
Gastrointestinal: Abdominal cramping, abdominal fullness, constipation, diarrhea, enlarged abdomen, vomiting
Genitourinary: Ectopic pregnancy, ovarian disease, vaginal hemorrhage
Local: Injection site edema/pain
Neuromuscular & skeletal: Back pain
Respiratory: Cough increased, respiratory disorder
Miscellaneous: Infection, flu-like syndrome

Frequency not defined:

Cardiovascular: Stroke, tachycardia, thrombosis (venous or arterial)
Dermatologic: Angioedema, rash, urticaria
Genitourinary: Adnexal torsion, hemoperitoneum, ovarian enlargement
Neuromuscular & skeletal: Limb necrosis
Respiratory: Acute respiratory distress syndrome, atelectasis, dyspnea, embolism, laryngeal edema, pulmonary infarction, tachypnea
Miscellaneous: Allergic reactions, anaphylaxis

Drug Interactions

Metabolism/Transport Effects None known.

Avoid Concomitant Use There are no known interactions where it is recommended to avoid concomitant use.

Increased Effect/Toxicity There are no known significant interactions involving an increase in effect.

Decreased Effect There are no known significant interactions involving a decrease in effect.

Preparation for Administration Hazardous agent; use appropriate precautions for handling and disposal (NIOSH, 2012). After reconstitution inject immediately; discard any unused portion.

Storage/Stability Lyophilized powder may be refrigerated or stored at room temperature. Protect from light.

Mechanism of Action Actions occur as a result of both follicle stimulating hormone (FSH) effects and luteinizing hormone (LH) effects; menotropins stimulate the development and maturation of the ovarian follicle (FSH), cause ovulation (LH), and stimulate the development of the corpus luteum (LH); in males it stimulates spermatogenesis (LH)

Pharmacodynamics/Kinetics Excretion: Urine (~10% as unchanged drug)

Dosage Adults:

Repronex®: I.M., SubQ:

Induction of ovulation in patients with oligoanovulation (Females): Initial: 150 units daily for the first 5 days of treatment. Adjustments should not be made more frequently than once every 2 days and should not exceed 75-150 units per adjustment. Maximum daily dose should not exceed 450 units and dosing beyond 12 days is not recommended. If patient's response is appropriate, hCG 5000-10,000 units should be given one day following the last dose of Repronex®. Hold dose if serum estradiol is >2000 pg/mL, if the ovaries are abnormally enlarged, or if abdominal pain occurs; the patient should also be advised to refrain from intercourse. May repeat process if follicular development is inadequate or if pregnancy does not occur.

Assisted reproductive technologies (Females): Initial (in patients who have received GnRH agonist or antagonist pituitary suppression): 225 units; adjustments in dose should not be made more frequently than once every 2 days and should not exceed more than 75-150 units per adjustment. The maximum daily doses of Repronex® given should not exceed 450 units and dosing beyond 12 days is not recommended. Once adequate follicular development is evident, hCG (5000-10,000 units) should be administered to induce final follicular maturation in preparation for oocyte retrieval. Withhold treatment when ovaries are abnormally enlarged on last day of therapy (to reduce chance of developing OHSS).

Menopur®: SubQ: *Assisted reproductive technologies (ART):* Initial (in patients who have received GnRH agonist for pituitary suppression): 225 units; adjustments in dose should not be made more frequently than once every 2 days and should not exceed more than 150 units per adjustment. The maximum daily dose given should not exceed 450 units and dosing beyond 20 days is not recommended. Once adequate follicular development is evident, hCG should be administered to induce final follicular maturation in preparation for oocyte retrieval. Withhold treatment when ovaries are abnormally enlarged on last day of therapy (to reduce chance of developing OHSS).

Spermatogenesis (Males) (unlabeled use): I.M.: Following pretreatment with hCG: 75 units 3 times/week and hCG 2000 units twice weekly until sperm is detected in the ejaculate (4-6 months); may then be increased to menotropins 150 units 3 times/week

Dosage adjustment in renal impairment: No dosage adjustment provided in manufacturer's labeling (has not been studied).

Dosage adjustment in hepatic impairment: No dosage adjustment provided in manufacturer's labeling (has not been studied).

Administration

Menopur®: SubQ: Administer to alternating sites of the abdomen; when administration to the lower abdomen is not possible, the injection may be given into the thigh.

Repronex®:

I.M.: Administer deep in a large muscle.

SubQ: Administer to alternating sites of the lower abdomen.

Hazardous agent; use appropriate precautions for handling and disposal (NIOSH, 2012).

Monitoring Parameters hCG levels, serum estradiol; vaginal ultrasound; in cases of suspected OHSS, monitor fluid intake and output, weight, hematocrit, serum and urinary electrolytes, urine specific gravity, BUN and creatinine, and abdominal girth

Dosage Forms Considerations

75 units of menotropins represents 75 units each of FSH activity and LH activity

Dosage Forms Excipient information presented when available (limited, particularly for generics); consult specific product labeling.

Injection, powder for reconstitution:

Menopur®: 75 units [supplied with diluent]

Repronex®: 75 units [supplied with diluent]

◆ **Mentax** *see* Butenafine *on page 305*

◆ **Menthol and Methyl Salicylate** *see* Methyl Salicylate and Menthol *on page 1344*

◆ **Menveo** *see* Meningococcal (Groups A / C / Y and W-135) Diphtheria Conjugate Vaccine *on page 1291*

Meperidine (me PER i deen)

Brand Names: U.S. Demerol; Meperitab

Brand Names: Canada Demerol®

Index Terms Isonipecaine Hydrochloride; Meperidine Hydrochloride; Pethidine Hydrochloride

Pharmacologic Category Analgesic, Opioid

Additional Appendix Information

Beers Criteria – Potentially Inappropriate Medications for Geriatrics *on page 2368*

Opioid Conversion Table *on page 2306*

Patient Information for Disposal of Unused Medications *on page 2393*

Use Management of moderate-to-severe pain; adjunct to anesthesia and preoperative sedation

Unlabeled Use Reduce postoperative shivering; reduce rigors from amphotericin B (conventional)

Pregnancy Risk Factor C

Pregnancy Considerations Animal reproduction studies have not been conducted by the manufacturer. Meperidine crosses the placenta; meperidine and its active metabolite accumulate in the fetus. Respiratory or CNS depression should be expected to occur in the newborn if maternal I.M. administration occurs within a few hours of delivery (Mattingly, 2003). When used for pain relief during labor, opioids may temporarily affect the heart rate of the fetus. Due to the prolonged half-life of the active metabolite, dose-dependant sedation in the neonate may be observed for 2-3 days following delivery. Meperidine has been used for the management of pain during labor; however, due to adverse maternal and fetal effects, other opioids may be preferred. Meperidine should also be avoided following delivery when postoperative analgesia is needed (ACOG, 2002).

If chronic opioid exposure occurs in pregnancy, adverse events in the newborn (including withdrawal) may occur; monitoring of the neonate is recommended. The minimum effective dose should be used if opioids are needed (Chou, 2009). Neonatal abstinence syndrome following opioid exposure may present with autonomic (eg, fever, temperature instability), gastrointestinal (eg, diarrhea, vomiting, poor feeding/weight gain), or neurologic (eg, high-pitched crying, increased muscle tone, irritability, seizure, tremor) symptoms (Dow, 2012; Hudak, 2012).

Breast-Feeding Considerations Meperidine is excreted in breast milk and may cause CNS and/or respiratory depression in the nursing infant. Due to the potential for serious adverse reactions in the nursing infant, the manufacturer recommends a decision be made whether to discontinue nursing or to discontinue the drug, taking into account the importance of treatment to the mother.

Small concentrations of meperidine are excreted into breast milk following single doses. With multiple doses, concentrations of meperidine and the active metabolite may increase and both are slowly eliminated by a nursing infant (Spigset, 2000). Parenteral opioids used during labor have the potential to interfere with a newborns natural reflex to nurse within the first few hours after birth. Nursing infants exposed to large doses of opioids should be monitored for apnea and sedation. If treatment for pain in nursing women is needed, other agents are preferred (Montgomery, 2012)

Contraindications Hypersensitivity to meperidine or any component of the formulation; use with or within 14 days of MAO inhibitors; severe respiratory insufficiency

Warnings/Precautions Oral meperidine is not recommended for acute/chronic pain management. Meperidine should not be used for acute/cancer pain because of the risk of neurotoxicity. Normeperidine (an active metabolite and CNS stimulant) may accumulate and precipitate anxiety, tremors, or seizures; risk increases with CNS or renal dysfunction, prolonged use (>48 hours), and cumulative dose (>600 mg/24 hours). The Institute for Safe Medication Practice recommends avoiding the use of meperidine for pain control, especially in the elderly and renally-impaired (ISMP, 2007). In the elderly; meperidine is not an effective oral analgesic at commonly used doses; may cause neurotoxicity; other agents are preferred in the elderly (Beers Criteria).

May cause CNS depression, which may impair physical or mental abilities; patients must be cautioned about performing tasks which require mental alertness (eg, operating machinery or driving). Potentially significant drug interactions may exist, requiring dose or frequency adjustment, additional monitoring, and/or selection of alternative therapy. Effects (eg, sedation, respiratory depression, hypotension) may be potentiated when used with other sedative/hypnotic drugs, general anesthetics, phenothiazines, or ethanol; consider reduced dose of meperidine if using concomitantly. Use only with extreme caution (if at all) in patients with head injury or increased intracranial pressure (ICP). Avoid use in patients with CNS depression or coma as these patients are susceptible to intracranial effects of CO_2 retention. Use caution with pulmonary, hepatic, or renal disorders, supraventricular tachycardias (including atrial flutter), acute abdominal conditions, biliary tract dysfunction, pancreatitis, delirium tremens, hypothyroidism, myxedema, toxic psychosis, kyphoscoliosis, morbid obesity, Addison's disease, seizure disorders, pheochromocytoma, BPH, or urethral stricture. May cause hypotension (including orthostatic hypotension); use with caution in patients with depleted blood volume or drugs which may exaggerate hypotensive effects (including phenothiazines or general anesthetics).

An opioid-containing analgesic regimen should be tailored to each patient's needs and based upon the type of pain being treated (acute versus chronic), the route of administration, degree of tolerance for opioids (naive versus chronic user), age, weight, and medical condition. The optimal analgesic dose varies widely among patients. ▶

Some preparations contain sulfites which may cause allergic reaction. Tolerance or drug dependence may result from extended use. Healthcare provider should be alert to problems of abuse, misuse, and diversion. Concurrent use of agonist/antagonist analgesics may precipitate withdrawal symptoms and/or reduced analgesic efficacy in patients following prolonged therapy with mu opioid agonists. Abrupt discontinuation following prolonged use may also lead to withdrawal symptoms. Avoid use in the elderly.

After chronic maternal exposure to opioids, neonatal withdrawal syndrome may occur in the newborn; monitor neonate closely. Signs and symptoms include irritability, hyperactivity and abnormal sleep pattern, high pitched cry, tremor, vomiting, diarrhea and failure to gain weight. Onset, duration and severity depend on the drug used, duration of use, maternal dose, and rate of drug elimination by the newborn. Opioid withdrawal syndrome in the neonate, unlike in adults, may be life-threatening and should be treated according to protocols developed by neonatology experts.

Adverse Reactions Frequency not defined.

Cardiovascular: Bradycardia, cardiac arrest, circulatory depression, hypotension, palpitation, shock, syncope, tachycardia

Central nervous system: Agitation, confusion, delirium, disorientation, dizziness, drowsiness, dysphoria, euphoria, fatigue, flushing, hallucinations, headache, intracranial pressure increased, lightheadedness, malaise, mental depression, nervousness, paradoxical CNS stimulation, restlessness, sedation, seizure (associated with metabolite accumulation), serotonin syndrome

Dermatologic: Pruritus, rash, urticaria

Gastrointestinal: Abdominal cramps, anorexia, biliary spasm, constipation, nausea, paralytic ileus, sphincter of Oddi spasm, vomiting, xerostomia

Genitourinary: Ureteral spasms, urinary retention

Local: Injection site reaction (including pain, wheal, and flare)

Neuromuscular & skeletal: Muscle twitching, myoclonus, tremor, weakness

Ocular: Visual disturbances

Respiratory: Dyspnea, respiratory arrest, respiratory depression

Miscellaneous: Anaphylaxis, diaphoresis, histamine release, hypersensitivity reactions, physical and psychological dependence

Drug Interactions

Metabolism/Transport Effects None known.

Avoid Concomitant Use

Avoid concomitant use of Meperidine with any of the following: Azelastine (Nasal); MAO Inhibitors; Paraldehyde

Increased Effect/Toxicity

Meperidine may increase the levels/effects of: Alcohol (Ethyl); Alvimopan; Antipsychotics; Azelastine (Nasal); CNS Depressants; Desmopressin; Diuretics; Hydrocodone; Metoclopramide; Metyrosine; Paraldehyde; Pramipexole; ROPINIRole; Rotigotine; Selective Serotonin Reuptake Inhibitors; Serotonin Modulators; Zolpidem

The levels/effects of Meperidine may be increased by: Amphetamines; Anticholinergics; Antipsychotic Agents (Phenothiazines); Antipsychotics; Barbiturates; Brimonidine (Topical); Cannabinoids; Doxylamine; HydrOXYzine; Magnesium Sulfate; MAO Inhibitors; Perampanel; Protease Inhibitors; Sodium Oxybate; Succinylcholine

Decreased Effect

Meperidine may decrease the levels/effects of: Pegvisomant

The levels/effects of Meperidine may be decreased by: Ammonium Chloride; Fosphenytoin; Mixed Agonist/Antagonist Opioids; Phenytoin; Protease Inhibitors

Ethanol/Nutrition/Herb Interactions

Ethanol: May increase CNS depression; monitor for increased effects with coadministration. Caution patients about effects.

Herb/Nutraceutical: Avoid valerian, St John's wort, kava kava, gotu kola (may increase CNS depression).

Storage/Stability

Injection solution: Store at 20°C to 25°C (68°F to 77°F); excursions permitted to 15°C to 30°C (59°F to 86°F).

Tablets: Store at 25°C (77°F); excursions permitted to 15°C to 30°C (59°F to 86°F).

Mechanism of Action Binds to opioid receptors in the CNS, causing inhibition of ascending pain pathways, altering the perception of and response to pain; produces generalized CNS depression

Pharmacodynamics/Kinetics

Onset of action: Analgesic: Oral, SubQ: 10-15 minutes; I.V.: ~5 minutes

Peak effect: SubQ.: ~1 hour; Oral: 2 hours

Duration: Oral, SubQ.: 2-4 hours

Absorption: I.M.: Erratic and highly variable

Protein binding: 65% to 75%

Metabolism: Hepatic; hydrolyzed to meperidinic acid (inactive) or undergoes N-demethylation to normeperidine (active; has 1/2 the analgesic effect and 2-3 times the CNS effects of meperidine)

Bioavailability: ~50% to 60%; increased with liver disease

Half-life elimination:

Parent drug: Terminal phase: Adults: 2.5-4 hours, Liver disease: 7-11 hours

Normeperidine (active metabolite): 15-30 hours; can accumulate with high doses (>600 mg/day) or with decreased renal function

Excretion: Urine (as metabolites)

Dosage Note: The American Pain Society (2008) and ISMP (2007) do not recommend meperidine's use as an analgesic. If use in acute pain (in patients without renal or CNS disease) cannot be avoided, treatment should be limited to ≤48 hours and doses should not exceed 600 mg/24 hours. Oral route is not recommended for treatment of acute or chronic pain. If I.V. route is required, consider a reduced dose. Patients with prior opioid exposure may require higher initial doses.

Children: Pain: Oral, I.M., SubQ: 1.1-1.8 mg/kg/dose every 3-4 hours as needed (maximum: 50-150 mg/dose)

Preoperatively: I.M., SubQ: 1.1-2.2 mg/kg given 30-90 minutes before the beginning of anesthesia (maximum: 50-150 mg/dose)

Adults:

Pain: Oral, I.M., SubQ: 50-150 mg every 3-4 hours as needed

Preoperatively: I.M., SubQ: 50-150 mg given 30-90 minutes before the beginning of anesthesia

Obstetrical analgesia: I.M., SubQ: 50-100 mg when pain becomes regular; may repeat at every 1-3 hours

Postoperative shivering (unlabeled use): I.V.: 25-50 mg once (Crowley, 2008; Kranke, 2002; Mercandante, 1994; Wang, 1999)

Elderly: Avoid use (American Pain Society, 2008; ISMP, 2007)

Dosing adjustment in renal impairment: Avoid use in renal impairment (American Pain Society, 2008; ISMP, 2007)

Dosing adjustment in hepatic impairment: Use with caution in severe hepatic impairment; consider a lower initial dose when initiating therapy. An increased opioid effect may be seen in patients with cirrhosis; dose reduction is more important for the oral than I.V. route.

Administration

Solution for injection: Meperidine may be administered I.M., SubQ, or I.V.; I.V. push should be administered slowly using a diluted solution, use of a 10 mg/mL concentration has been recommended.

Oral solution: Administer solution in 1/2 glass of water; undiluted solution may exert topical anesthetic effect on mucous membranes

Monitoring Parameters Pain relief, respiratory and mental status, blood pressure; observe patient for excessive sedation, CNS depression, seizures, respiratory depression

Test Interactions Increased amylase (S), increased BSP retention, increased CPK (I.M. injections)

Dosage Forms Excipient information presented when available (limited, particularly for generics); consult specific product labeling.

Solution, Injection, as hydrochloride:

Demerol: 25 mg/mL (1 mL); 25 mg/0.5 mL (0.5 mL); 50 mg/mL (1 mL, 30 mL); 75 mg/1.5 mL (1.5 mL); 100 mg/2 mL (2 mL); 75 mg/mL (1 mL); 100 mg/mL (1 mL, 20 mL)

Generic: 10 mg/mL (30 mL); 25 mg/mL (1 mL); 50 mg/mL (1 mL); 100 mg/mL (1 mL)

Solution, Oral, as hydrochloride:

Generic: 50 mg/5 mL (500 mL)

Tablet, Oral, as hydrochloride:

Demerol: 50 mg [scored]

Demerol: 100 mg

Meperitab: 50 mg [scored]

Meperitab: 100 mg

Generic: 50 mg, 100 mg

Controlled Substance C-II

◆ **Meperidine Hydrochloride** *see* Meperidine *on page 1297*

◆ **Meperitab** *see* Meperidine *on page 1297*

◆ **Mephyton®** *see* Phytonadione *on page 1644*

Mepivacaine (me PIV a kane)

Brand Names: U.S. Carbocaine; Carbocaine Preservative-Free; Polocaine; Polocaine-MPF

Brand Names: Canada Carbocaine®; Polocaine®

Index Terms Mepivacaine Hydrochloride

Pharmacologic Category Local Anesthetic

Use Local or regional analgesia; anesthesia by local infiltration, peripheral and central neural techniques (epidural and caudal); **not** for use in spinal anesthesia

Pregnancy Risk Factor C

Pregnancy Considerations Animal reproduction studies have not been conducted. Mepivacaine has been used in obstetrical analgesia.

Breast-Feeding Considerations It is not known if mepivacaine is excreted in breast milk. The manufacturer recommends that caution be exercised when administering mepivacaine to nursing women.

Contraindications Hypersensitivity to mepivacaine, other amide-type local anesthetics, or any component of the formulation

Warnings/Precautions Careful and constant monitoring of the patient's state of consciousness should be done following each local anesthetic injection; at such times, restlessness, anxiety, tinnitus, dizziness, blurred vision, tremors, depression, or drowsiness may be early warning signs of CNS toxicity; treatment is primarily symptomatic and supportive. Continuous intra-articular infusion of local anesthetics after arthroscopic or other surgical procedures is **not** an approved use; chondrolysis (primarily in the shoulder joint) has occurred following infusion, with some cases requiring arthroplasty or shoulder replacement. Use with caution in patients with cardiac disease, hepatic or renal disease, or hyperthyroidism. Local anesthetics have been associated with rare occurrences of sudden respiratory arrest; convulsions due to systemic toxicity leading to cardiac arrest have been reported presumably due to intravascular injection. A test dose is recommended prior to epidural administration and all reinforcing doses with continuous catheter technique. Do not use solutions containing preservatives for caudal or epidural block. Use caution in debilitated, elderly, or acutely-ill patients; dose reduction may be required. Resuscitative equipment, oxygen, and other resuscitative drugs should be available for immediate use.

Adverse Reactions Degree of adverse effects in the CNS and cardiovascular system is directly related to the blood levels of mepivacaine, route of administration, and physical status of the patient. The effects below are more likely to occur after systemic administration rather than infiltration.

Cardiovascular: Bradycardia, cardiac arrest, cardiac output decreased, heart block, hyper-/hypotension, myocardial depression, syncope, tachycardia, ventricular arrhythmias

Central nervous system: Anxiety, chills, convulsions, depression, dizziness, excitation, restlessness, tremors

Dermatologic: Angioneurotic edema, diaphoresis, erythema, pruritus, urticaria

Gastrointestinal: Fecal incontinence, nausea, vomiting

Genitourinary: Incontinence, urinary retention

Neuromuscular & skeletal: Chondrolysis (continuous intra-articular administration), paralysis

Ocular: Blurred vision, pupil constriction

Otic: Tinnitus

Respiratory: Apnea, hypoventilation, sneezing

Miscellaneous: Allergic reaction, anaphylactoid reaction

Drug Interactions

Metabolism/Transport Effects None known.

Avoid Concomitant Use There are no known interactions where it is recommended to avoid concomitant use.

Increased Effect/Toxicity

The levels/effects of Mepivacaine may be increased by: Beta-Blockers; Hyaluronidase

Decreased Effect

Mepivacaine may decrease the levels/effects of: Technetium Tc 99m Tilmanocept

Storage/Stability Store at controlled room temperature of 15°C to 30°C (59°F to 86°F). Brief exposure up to 40°C (104°F) does not adversely affect the product. Solutions may be sterilized.

Mechanism of Action Mepivacaine is an amide local anesthetic similar to lidocaine; like all local anesthetics, mepivacaine acts by preventing the generation and conduction of nerve impulses

Pharmacodynamics/Kinetics

Onset of action (route and dose dependent): Range: 3-20 minutes

Duration (route and dose dependent): 2-2.5 hours

Protein binding: ~75%

Metabolism: Primarily hepatic via N-demethylation, hydroxylation, and glucuronidation

Half-life elimination: Neonates: 8.7-9 hours; Adults: 1.9-3 hours

Excretion: Urine (90% to 95% as metabolites)

Dosage

Injectable local anesthetic: Dose varies with procedure, degree of anesthesia needed, vascularity of tissue, duration of anesthesia required, and physical condition of patient. The smallest dose and concentration required to produce the desired effect should be used.

Children: Maximum single or total dose given for one procedure: 5-6 mg/kg; only concentrations <2% should be used in children <3 years or <14 kg (30 lbs)

Adults: Maximum single or total dose given for one procedure: 400 mg; 500 mg if epinephrine has been added (Barash, 2009)

Cervical, brachial, intercostal, pudendal nerve block: 5-40 mL of a 1% solution (maximum: 400 mg) **or** 5-20 mL of a 2% solution (maximum: 400 mg). For pudendal block, inject one-half the total dose each side.

Transvaginal block (paracervical plus pudendal): Up to 30 mL (total for both sides) of a 1% solution (maximum: 300 mg). Inject one-half the total dose each side.

Paracervical block: Up to 20 mL (total for both sides) of a 1% solution (maximum: 200 mg). Inject one-half the total dose to each side. This is the maximum recommended dose per 90-minute procedure; inject slowly with 5 minutes between sides.

Caudal and epidural block (preservative free solutions only): 15-30 mL of a 1% solution (maximum: 300 mg) **or** 10-25 mL of a 1.5% solution (maximum: 375 mg) **or** 10-20 mL of a 2% solution (maximum: 400 mg)

Infiltration: Up to 40 mL of a 1% solution (maximum: 400 mg); up to 50 mL if epinephrine has been added (maximum: 500 mg) (Barash, 2009); an equivalent amount of a 0.5% solution (prepared by diluting the 1% solution with NS) may be used for large areas

Peripheral nerve block to provide a surgical level of anesthesia (Miller, 2010):

Major nerve block (blockade of two or more distinct nerves, a nerve plexus, or very large nerves at more proximal sites: 30-50 mL of a 1% or 1.5% solution (maximum: 500 mg)

Minor nerve block (blockade of a single nerve [eg, ulnar or radial]): 5-20 mL of a 1% solution (maximum: 200 mg)

Therapeutic block: 1-5 mL of 1% solution (maximum: 50 mg) **or** 1-5 mL of 2% solution (maximum: 100 mg)

Elderly: Decreased doses suggested by manufacturer's labeling; however, no dosing adjustments provided. Refer to adult dosing.

Dosage adjustment in renal impairment: No dosage adjustment provided in manufacturer's labeling; use with caution.

Dosage adjustment in hepatic impairment: No dosage adjustment provided in manufacturer's labeling; use with caution.

Administration Before injecting, withdraw syringe plunger to ensure injection is not into vein or artery.

Monitoring Parameters Vital signs, state of consciousness; signs of CNS toxicity

Dosage Forms Excipient information presented when available (limited, particularly for generics); consult specific product labeling.

Solution, Injection, as hydrochloride:

Carbocaine: 1% (50 mL); 2% (50 mL) [contains methylparaben]

Polocaine: 1% (50 mL); 2% (50 mL) [contains methylparaben]

Generic: 3% (1.8 mL)

Solution, Injection, as hydrochloride [preservative free]:

Carbocaine Preservative-Free: 1% (30 mL); 1.5% (30 mL); 2% (20 mL)

Polocaine-MPF: 1% (30 mL); 1.5% (30 mL); 2% (20 mL) [methylparaben free]

◆ **Mepivacaine Hydrochloride** *see* Mepivacaine *on page 1299*

Meprobamate (me proe BA mate)

Index Terms Equanil

Pharmacologic Category Antianxiety Agent, Miscellaneous

Additional Appendix Information

Beers Criteria – Potentially Inappropriate Medications for Geriatrics *on page 2368*

Use Management of anxiety disorders

Unlabeled Use Demonstrated value for muscle contraction, headache, external sphincter spasticity, muscle rigidity, opisthotonos-associated with tetanus; treatment of muscle spasm associated with acute temporomandibular joint (TMJ) pain

Dosage Oral:

Anxiety:

Children 6-12 years: 200-600 mg/day in 2-3 divided doses

Adults: 1200-1600 mg/day in 3-4 divided doses, up to 2400 mg/day

Muscle spasm (TMJ) pain (unlabeled use): Adults: 1200-1600 mg/day in 3-4 divided doses, up to 2400 mg/day

Dosing interval in renal impairment: No dosage adjustment provided in manufacturer's labeling; however, the following adjustments have been recommended (Aronoff, 2007): Adults:

Cl_{cr} 10-50 mL/minute: Administer every 9-12 hours.

Cl_{cr} <10 mL/minute: Administer every 12-18 hours.

Hemodialysis: No dosage adjustment necessary.

Peritoneal dialysis: Administer every 12-18 hours.

Continuous renal replacement therapy (CRRT): Administer every 9-12 hours.

Dosing adjustment in hepatic impairment: No dosage adjustment provided in manufacturer's labeling; use with caution.

Additional Information Complete prescribing information should be consulted for additional detail.

Dosage Forms Excipient information presented when available (limited, particularly for generics); consult specific product labeling.

Tablet, Oral:

Generic: 200 mg, 400 mg

Controlled Substance C-IV

◆ **Mepron** *see* Atovaquone *on page 193*

◆ **Mepron® (Can)** *see* Atovaquone *on page 193*

◆ **Mercaptoethane Sulfonate** *see* Mesna *on page 1307*

Mercaptopurine (mer kap toe PURE een)

Brand Names: U.S. Purinethol

Brand Names: Canada Purinethol®

Index Terms 6-Mercaptopurine (error-prone abbreviation); 6-MP (error-prone abbreviation)

Pharmacologic Category Antineoplastic Agent, Antimetabolite; Antineoplastic Agent, Antimetabolite (Purine Analog); Immunosuppressant Agent

Use Maintenance treatment component of acute lymphoblastic leukemia (ALL)

Unlabeled Use Steroid-sparing agent for corticosteroid-dependent Crohn's disease (CD) and ulcerative colitis (UC); maintenance of remission in CD; fistulizing Crohn's disease; maintenance treatment in acute promyelocytic leukemia (APL); treatment component for non Hodgkin lymphoma (NHL), treatment of autoimmune hepatitis

Pregnancy Risk Factor D

Pregnancy Considerations May cause fetal harm if administered during pregnancy. Case reports of fetal loss have been noted with mercaptopurine administration during the first trimester; adverse effects have also been noted with second and third trimester use. Women of child bearing potential should avoid becoming pregnant during treatment.

Breast-Feeding Considerations Mercaptopurine is the active metabolite of azathioprine. Following administration of azathioprine, mercaptopurine can be detected in breast milk (Gardiner, 2006). It is not known if/how much mercaptopurine is found in breast milk following oral administration. According to the manufacturer, the decision to discontinue mercaptopurine or discontinue breast-feeding during therapy should take into account the benefits of treatment to the mother.

Contraindications Hypersensitivity to mercaptopurine or any component of the formulation; patients whose disease showed prior resistance to mercaptopurine

Warnings/Precautions Hazardous agent - use appropriate precautions for handling and disposal (NIOSH, 2012).

Hepatotoxicity has been reported, including jaundice, ascites, hepatic necrosis (may be fatal), intrahepatic cholestasis, parenchymal cell necrosis, and/or hepatic encephalopathy; may be due to direct hepatic cell damage or hypersensitivity. While hepatotoxicity or hepatic injury may occur at any dose, dosages >2.5 mg/kg/day are associated with a higher incidence. Signs of jaundice generally appear early in treatment, after ~1-2 months (range: 1 week to 8 years) and may resolve following discontinuation; recurrence with rechallenge has been noted. Monitor liver function tests (monitor more frequently if used in combination with other hepatotoxic drugs or in patients with pre-existing hepatic impairment. Consider a reduced dose in patients with hepatic impairment. Withhold treatment for clinical signs of jaundice (hepatomegaly, anorexia, tenderness), deterioration in liver function tests, toxic hepatitis, or biliary stasis until hepatotoxicity is ruled out.

Dose-related leukopenia, thrombocytopenia, and anemia are common; however, may be indicative of disease progression. Hematologic toxicity may be delayed. Bone marrow may appear hypoplastic (could also appear normal). Monitor for bleeding (due to thrombocytopenia) or infection (due to neutropenia). Patients with homozygous genetic defect of thiopurine methyltransferase (TPMT) are more sensitive to myelosuppressive effects; generally associated with rapid myelosuppression. Significant mercaptopurine dose reductions will be necessary (possibly with continued concomitant chemotherapy at normal doses). Patients who are heterozygous for TPMT defects will have intermediate activity; may have increased toxicity (primarily myelosuppression) although will generally tolerate normal mercaptopurine doses. Consider TPMT testing for severe toxicities/excessive myelosuppression. Patients on concurrent therapy with drugs which may inhibit TPMT (eg, olsalazine) or xanthine oxidase (eg, allopurinol) may be sensitive to myelosuppressive effects.

Immunosuppressive agents, including mercaptopurine, are associated with the development of lymphoma and other malignancies including hepatosplenic T-cell lymphoma (HSTCL). Because azathioprine is metabolized to mercaptopurine, concomitant use with azathioprine may result in profound myelosuppression and should be avoided. Mercaptopurine is immunosuppressive; the risk for infection is increased; common signs of infection, such as fever and leukocytosis may not occur; lethargy and confusion may be more prominent signs of infection. Immune response to vaccines may be diminished. Consider adjusting dosage in patients with renal impairment. Some renal adverse effects may be minimized with hydration and prophylactic antihyperuricemic therapy. To avoid potentially serious dosage errors, the terms "6-mercaptopurine" or "6-MP" should be avoided; use of these terms has been associated with sixfold overdosages.

Adverse Reactions Frequency not defined.

Central nervous system: Drug fever

Dermatologic: Alopecia, hyperpigmentation, rash

Endocrine & metabolic: Hyperuricemia

Gastrointestinal: Anorexia, diarrhea, intestinal ulcers, mucositis/oral lesions (rare), nausea (minimal), pancreatitis, sprue-like symptoms, stomach pain, vomiting (minimal)

Genitourinary: Oligospermia

Hematologic: Myelosuppression (onset 7-10 days; nadir 14 days; recovery: 21 days); anemia, bleeding, granulocytopenia, leukopenia, marrow hypoplasia, thrombocytopenia

Hepatic: Hepatotoxicity, ascites, biliary stasis, hepatic damage/injury, hepatic encephalopathy, hepatic necrosis, hepatomegaly, intrahepatic cholestasis, jaundice, parenchymal cell necrosis, toxic hepatitis

Renal: Hyperuricosuria, renal toxicity

Miscellaneous: Hepatosplenic T cell lymphoma, immunosuppression, infection, secondary malignancy

Drug Interactions

Metabolism/Transport Effects None known.

Avoid Concomitant Use

Avoid concomitant use of Mercaptopurine with any of the following: AzaTHIOprine; BCG; CloZAPine; Febuxostat; Natalizumab; Pimecrolimus; Tacrolimus (Topical); Tofacitinib

Increased Effect/Toxicity

Mercaptopurine may increase the levels/effects of: CloZAPine; Leflunomide; Natalizumab; Tofacitinib; Vaccines (Live); Vitamin K Antagonists

The levels/effects of Mercaptopurine may be increased by: 5-ASA Derivatives; Allopurinol; AzaTHIOprine; Denosumab; Febuxostat; Pimecrolimus; Roflumilast; Sulfamethoxazole; Tacrolimus (Topical); Trastuzumab; Trimethoprim

Decreased Effect

Mercaptopurine may decrease the levels/effects of: BCG; Coccidioidin Skin Test; Sipuleucel-T; Vaccines (Inactivated); Vitamin K Antagonists

The levels/effects of Mercaptopurine may be decreased by: Echinacea

Ethanol/Nutrition/Herb Interactions Food: Absorption is variable with food. Management: Take on an empty stomach at the same time each day 1 hour before or 2 hours after a meal. Maintain adequate hydration, unless instructed to restrict fluid intake.

Storage/Stability Store at room temperature of 15°C to 25°C (59°F to 77°F). Protect from moisture.

Mechanism of Action Purine antagonist which inhibits DNA and RNA synthesis; acts as false metabolite and is incorporated into DNA and RNA, eventually inhibiting their synthesis; specific for the S phase of the cell cycle

Pharmacodynamics/Kinetics

Absorption: Variable and incomplete (~50%)

Distribution: V_d: > total body water; CNS penetration is poor

Protein binding: ~19%

Metabolism: Hepatic and in GI mucosa; hepatically via xanthine oxidase and methylation via TPMT to sulfate conjugates, 6-thiouric acid, and other inactive compounds; first-pass effect

Half-life elimination (age dependent): Children: 21 minutes; Adults: 47 minutes

Time to peak, serum: ~2 hours

Excretion: Urine (46% as mercaptopurine and metabolites)

Dosage Oral (also consult details concerning dosing in combination regimens):

Children:

ALL: Maintenance: 1.5-2.5 mg/kg/day **or**

Unlabeled ALL dosing (combination chemotherapy; refer to specific reference for combinations): Adolescents ≥15 years:

Consolidation phase: 60 mg/m^2/day days 0-27 days (5-week course) (Stock, 2008) **or** 60 mg/m^2/day days 0-13 and days 28-41 (9-week course) (Stock, 2008)

Early intensification (two 4-week courses): 60 mg/m^2/day days 1-14 (Larson, 1995; Larson, 1998; Stock, 2008)

Interim maintenance: 60 mg/m^2/day days 0-41 (8-week course) (Stock, 2008) **or** 60 mg/m^2/day days 1-70 (12-week course) (Larson, 1995; Larson, 1998; Stock, 2008)

Maintenance (prolonged): 50 mg 3 times/day for 2 years (Kantarjian, 2000; Thomas, 2004) **or** 60 mg/m^2/day for 2 years from diagnosis (Larson, 1995; Larson, 1998; Stock, 2008) **or** 75 mg/m^2/day for 2 years (girls) or 3 years (boys) from first interim maintenance (Stock, 2008)

APL maintenance (unlabeled use): Adolescents ≥15 years: 60 mg/m^2/day for 1 year (in combination with tretinoin and methotrexate) (Powell, 2010)

Autoimmune hepatitis (unlabeled use): 1.5 mg/kg/day (in combination with prednisone) (Manns, 2010)

Dosage adjustment with concurrent allopurinol: Reduce mercaptopurine dosage to 25% to 33% of the usual dose.

Dosage adjustment in TPMT-deficiency: Not always established; substantial reductions are generally required only in homozygous deficiency.

Adults:

ALL: Maintenance: 1.5-2.5 mg/kg/day **or**

Unlabeled ALL dosing (combination chemotherapy; refer to specific reference for combinations):

Early intensification (two 4-week courses): 60 mg/m^2/day days 1-14 (Larson, 1995; Larson, 1998)

Interim maintenance (12-week course): 60 mg/m^2/day days 1-70 (Larson, 1995; Larson, 1998)

Maintenance (prolonged): 50 mg 3 times/day for 2 years (Kantarjian, 2000; Thomas, 2004) **or** 60 mg/m^2/day for 2 years from diagnosis (Larson, 1995; Larson, 1998)

APL maintenance (unlabeled use): 60 mg/m^2/day for 1 year (in combination with tretinoin and methotrexate) (Powell, 2010)

Crohn's disease, remission maintenance or reduction of steroid use (unlabeled use): 1-1.5 mg/kg/day (Lichtenstein, 2009)

Ulcerative colitis (unlabeled use):

Initial: 50 mg once daily; titrate dose up if clinical remission not achieved or down if leukopenia occurs (Lobel, 2004) **or**

Initial: 50 mg (25 mg if heterozygous for TPMT activity) once daily; titrate up to goal of 1.5 mg/kg (0.75 mg/kg if heterozygous for TPMT activity) if WBC >4000/mm^3 (and at least 50% of baseline) and LFTs and amylase are stable (Siegel, 2005) **or**

Maintenance: 1-1.5 mg/kg/day (Carter, 2004) **or**

Remission maintenance: 1.5 mg/kg/day (Danese, 2011)

Dosage adjustment with concurrent allopurinol: Reduce mercaptopurine dosage to 25% to 33% of the usual dose.

Dosage adjustment in TPMT-deficiency: Not always established; substantial reductions are generally required only in homozygous deficiency.

Elderly: Due to renal decline with age, initiate treatment at the low end of recommended dose range

Dosing adjustment in renal impairment: The manufacturer's labeling recommends starting with reduced doses in patients with renal impairment to avoid accumulation; however, no specific dosage adjustment is provided. The following adjustments have been used by some clinicians (Aronoff, 2007): Children:

Cl_{cr} <50 mL/minute/1.73 m^2: Administer every 48 hours

Hemodialysis: Administer every 48 hours

Continuous ambulatory peritoneal dialysis (CAPD): Administer every 48 hours

Continuous renal replacement therapy (CRRT): Administer every 48 hours

Dosing adjustment in hepatic impairment: The manufacturer's labeling recommends considering a reduced dose in patients with hepatic impairment; however, no specific dosage adjustment is provided.

Dosing in obesity: *ASCO Guidelines for appropriate chemotherapy dosing in obese adults with cancer:* Utilize patient's actual body weight (full weight) for calculation of body surface area- or weight-based dosing, particularly when the intent of therapy is curative; manage regimen-related toxicities in the same manner as for nonobese patients; if a dose reduction is utilized due to toxicity, consider resumption of full weight-based dosing with subsequent cycles, especially if cause of toxicity (eg, hepatic or renal impairment) is resolved (Griggs, 2012).

Dietary Considerations Should not be administered with meals.

Administration Preferably on an empty stomach (1 hour before or 2 hours after meals)

For the treatment of ALL in children (Schmiegelow, 1997): Administration in the evening has demonstration superior outcome; administration with food did not significantly affect outcome.

Hazardous agent; use appropriate precautions for handling and disposal (NIOSH, 2012).

Monitoring Parameters CBC with differential (weekly initially, although clinical status may require increased frequency), bone marrow exam (to evaluate marrow status), liver function tests (weekly initially, then monthly; monitor more frequently if on concomitant hepatotoxic agents), renal function, urinalysis; consider TPMT genotyping to identify TPMT defect (if severe toxicity occurs)

For use as immunomodulatory therapy in CD or UC, monitor CBC with differential weekly for 1 month, then biweekly for 1 month, followed by monitoring every 1-2 months throughout the course of therapy. LFTs should be assessed every 3 months. Monitor for signs/symptoms of malignancy (eg, splenomegaly, hepatomegaly, abdominal pain, persistent fever, night sweats, weight loss).

Test Interactions TPMT testing: Recent transfusions may result in a misinterpretation of the actual TPMT activity. Concomitant drugs may influence TPMT activity in the blood.

Dosage Forms Excipient information presented when available (limited, particularly for generics); consult specific product labeling.

Tablet, Oral:

Purinethol: 50 mg [scored]

Generic: 50 mg

Extemporaneous Preparations Hazardous agent: Use appropriate precautions for handling and disposal.

A 50 mg/mL oral suspension may be prepared in a vertical flow hood with tablets and a mixture of sterile water for injection (SWFI), simple syrup, and cherry syrup. Crush thirty 50 mg tablets in a mortar and reduce to a fine powder. Add ~5 mL SWFI and mix to a uniform paste; then add ~10 mL simple syrup; mix while continuing to add cherry syrup to make a final volume of 30 mL; transfer to a calibrated bottle. Label "shake well" and "caution chemotherapy". Stable for 35 days at room temperature.

Aliabadi HM, Romanick M, Desai, S, et al, "Effect of Buffer and Antioxidant on Stability of a Mercaptopurine Suspension," *Am J Health Syst Pharm*, 2008, 65(5):441-7.

- **6-Mercaptopurine (error-prone abbreviation)** *see* Mercaptopurine *on page 1300*
- **Mercapturic Acid** *see* Acetylcysteine *on page 36*

Meropenem (mer oh PEN em)

Brand Names: U.S. Merrem

Brand Names: Canada Meropenem For Injection; Merrem

Pharmacologic Category Antibiotic, Carbapenem

Additional Appendix Information

Dosing Considerations for the Critically-Ill Patient With Morbid Obesity *on page 2379*

Use

Treatment of intra-abdominal infections (complicated appendicitis and peritonitis); treatment of bacterial meningitis in pediatric patients ≥3 months of age caused by *S. pneumoniae*, *H. influenzae*, and *N. meningitidis*; treatment of complicated skin and skin structure infections caused by susceptible organisms

Canadian labeling: Additional indications (not in U.S. labeling): Treatment of lower respiratory tract infections (community-acquired and nosocomial pneumonias), complicated urinary tract infections, gynecologic infections (excluding chlamydia), and septicemia; treatment of bacterial meningitis in adults caused by *S. pneumoniae*, *H. influenzae*, and *N. meningitidis* (use in adult meningitis based on pediatric data)

Unlabeled Use *Burkholderia pseudomallei* (melioidosis), febrile neutropenia, liver abscess, otitis externa; treatment of prosthetic joint infection

Pregnancy Risk Factor B

Pregnancy Considerations Adverse events were not observed in animal reproduction studies. Incomplete transplacental transfer of meropenem was found using an *ex vivo* human perfusion model.

Breast-Feeding Considerations Small amounts of meropenem are excreted into breast milk (case report). The manufacturer recommends that caution be exercised when administering meropenem to breast-feeding women. Nondose-related effects could include modification of bowel flora.

Contraindications Hypersensitivity to meropenem, any component of the formulation, or other carbapenems (eg, doripenem, ertapenem, imipenem); patients who have experienced anaphylactic reactions to other beta-lactams

Warnings/Precautions Serious hypersensitivity reactions, including anaphylaxis, have been reported (some without a history of previous allergic reactions to beta-lactams). Carbapenems have been associated with CNS adverse effects, including confusional states and seizures (myoclonic); use caution with CNS disorders (eg, brain lesions and history of seizures) and adjust dose in renal impairment to avoid drug accumulation, which may increase seizure risk. Outpatient use may result in paresthesias, seizures, or headaches that can impair neuromotor function and alertness; patients should not operate machinery or drive until it is established that meropenem is well tolerated. Prolonged use may result in fungal or bacterial superinfection, including *C. difficile*-associated diarrhea (CDAD) and pseudomembranous colitis; CDAD has been observed >2 months postantibiotic treatment. Use with caution in patients with renal impairment; dosage adjustment required in patients with moderate-to-severe renal dysfunction. Thrombocytopenia has been reported in patients with renal dysfunction. Lower doses (based upon renal function) are often required in the elderly. May decrease divalproex sodium/valproic acid concentrations leading to breakthrough seizures; concomitant use not recommended. Alternative antimicrobial agents should be considered; if concurrent meropenem is necessary, consider additional antiseizure medication.

Adverse Reactions

1% to 10%:

Central nervous system: Headache (2% to 8%), pain (≤5%)

Dermatologic: Rash (2% to 3%, includes diaper-area moniliasis in infants), pruritus (1%)

Endocrine & metabolic: Hypoglycemia

Gastrointestinal: Diarrhea (4% to 7%), nausea/vomiting (1% to 8%), constipation (1% to 7%), oral moniliasis (up to 2% in pediatric patients), glossitis (1%)

Hematologic: Anemia (≤6%)

Local: Inflammation at the injection site (2%), phlebitis/thrombophlebitis (1%), injection site reaction (1%)

Respiratory: Apnea (1%), pharyngitis, pneumonia

Miscellaneous: Sepsis (2%), shock (1%)

<1% (Limited to important or life-threatening): Abdominal enlargement, abdominal pain, agitation/delirium, agranulocytosis, alkaline phosphatase increased, ALT increased, AST increased, anemia (hypochromic), angioedema, anorexia, anxiety, aPTT decreased, asthma, back pain, bilirubin increased, bradycardia, BUN increased, cardiac arrest, chest pain, chills, cholestatic jaundice/jaundice, confusion, cough, creatinine increased, depression, diaphoresis, dizziness, dyspepsia, dyspnea, dysuria, eosinophilia, epistaxis, erythema multiforme, fever, flatulence, gastrointestinal hemorrhage, hallucinations, heart failure, hematuria, hemoglobin/hematocrit decreased, hemolytic anemia, hemoperitoneum, hepatic failure, hyper-/hypotension, hypervolemia, hypokalemia, hypoxia, ileus, injection site edema, injection site pain, insomnia, intestinal obstruction, LDH increased, leukocytosis, leukopenia, melena, MI, nervousness, neutropenia, paresthesia, pelvic pain, peripheral edema, platelets decreased/increased, pleural effusion, PT decreased, pulmonary edema, positive Coombs test, pulmonary embolism, renal failure, respiratory disorder, seizure, skin ulcer, somnolence, Stevens-Johnson syndrome, syncope, tachycardia, toxic epidermal necrolysis, urinary incontinence, urticaria, vaginal moniliasis, weakness, WBC decreased, whole body pain

Drug Interactions

Metabolism/Transport Effects None known.

Avoid Concomitant Use

Avoid concomitant use of Meropenem with any of the following: BCG; Probenecid

Increased Effect/Toxicity

The levels/effects of Meropenem may be increased by: Probenecid

Decreased Effect

Meropenem may decrease the levels/effects of: BCG; Sodium Picosulfate; Typhoid Vaccine; Valproic Acid and Derivatives

Preparation for Administration Meropenem infusion vials may be reconstituted with SWFI or a compatible diluent (eg, NS). The 500 mg vials should be reconstituted with 10 mL, and 1 g vials with 20 mL. May be further diluted with compatible solutions for infusion. Consult detailed reference/product labeling for compatibility.

Storage/Stability Dry powder should be stored at controlled room temperature 20°C to 25°C (68°F to 77°F).

Injection reconstitution: Stability in vial when constituted (up to 50 mg/mL) with:

SWFI: Stable for up to 2 hours at controlled room temperature of 15°C to 25°C (59°F to 77°F) or for up to 12 hours under refrigeration.

Sodium chloride: Stable for up to 2 hours at controlled room temperature of 15°C to 25°C (59°F to 77°F) or for up to 18 hours under refrigeration.

Dextrose 5% injection: Stable for 1 hour at controlled room temperature of 15°C to 25°C (59°F to 77°F) or for 8 hours under refrigeration.

Infusion admixture (1-20 mg/mL): Solution stability when diluted in NS is 4 hours at controlled room temperature of 15°C to 25°C (59°F to 77°F) or 24 hours under refrigeration. Stability in D_5W is 1 hour at controlled room temperature of 15°C to 25°C (59°F to 77°F) or for 4 hours under refrigeration. For other diluents, see prescribing information.

Mechanism of Action Inhibits bacterial cell wall synthesis by binding to several of the penicillin-binding proteins, which in turn inhibit the final transpeptidation step of peptidoglycan synthesis in bacterial cell walls, thus inhibiting cell wall biosynthesis; bacteria eventually lyse due to ongoing activity of cell wall autolytic enzymes (autolysins and murein hydrolases) while cell wall assembly is arrested

Pharmacodynamics/Kinetics

Distribution: V_d: Adults: 15-20 L, Children: 0.3-0.4 L/kg; penetrates well into most body fluids and tissues; CSF concentrations approximate those of the plasma

Protein binding: ~2%

Metabolism: Hepatic; metabolized to open beta-lactam form (inactive)

Half-life elimination:

Normal renal function: 1-1.5 hours

Cl_{cr} 30-80 mL/minute: 1.9-3.3 hours

Cl_{cr} 2-30 mL/minute: 3.82-5.7 hours

Time to peak, tissue: 1 hour following infusion

Excretion: Urine (~70% as unchanged drug)

Dosage

Usual dosage ranges:

Children ≥3 months: I.V.: 30-120 mg/kg/day divided every 8 hours (maximum dose: 6 **g** daily)

Adults: I.V.: 1.5-6 **g** daily divided every 8 hours

Extended infusion method (unlabeled dosing): I.V.: 0.5-2 **g** over 3 hours every 8 hours (Crandon, 2011; Dandekar, 2003). **Note:** Dosing used at some centers and is based on pharmacokinetic/pharmacodynamic modeling and not clinical efficacy data.

Indication-specific dosing:

Children ≥3 months (<50 kg): I.V.:

Febrile neutropenia (unlabeled use): 20 mg/kg every 8 hours (maximum dose: 1000 mg every 8 hours)

Intra-abdominal infections (complicated): 20 mg/kg every 8 hours (maximum dose: 1000 mg every 8 hours)

Meningitis: 40 mg/kg every 8 hours (maximum dose: 2000 mg every 8 hours)

Pneumonia (community-acquired): Canadian labeling (not in U.S. labeling): 10-20 mg/kg every 8 hours (maximum dose: 1000 mg every 8 hours)

Skin and skin structure infections:

Complicated: U.S. labeling: 10 mg/kg every 8 hours (maximum dose: 500 mg every 8 hours)

Uncomplicated: Canadian labeling (not in U.S. labeling): 10-20 mg/kg every 8 hours (maximum dose: 1000 mg every 8 hours)

Urinary tract infection (complicated): Canadian labeling (not in U.S. labeling): 10 mg/kg every 8 hours (maximum dose: 500 mg every 8 hours)

Children >50 kg and Adults: I.V.:

Burkholderia pseudomallei* (melioidosis) (unlabeled use), *Pseudomonas: 1 g every 8 hours

Cholangitis, intra-abdominal infections, complicated: 1 g every 8 hours. **Note:** 2010 IDSA guidelines recommend treatment duration of 4-7 days (provided source controlled). Not recommended for mild-to-moderate, community-acquired intra-abdominal infections due to risk of toxicity and the development of resistant organisms (Solomkin, 2010).

Febrile neutropenia, otitis externa, pneumonia (unlabeled uses): 1 g every 8 hours

Liver abscess (unlabeled use): 1 g every 8 hours for 2-3 weeks, then oral therapy for duration of 4-6 weeks

Meningitis: Canadian labeling (not in U.S. labeling): 2 g every 8 hours

Mild-to-moderate infection, other severe infections (unlabeled use): 1.5-3 g daily divided every 8 hours

Pneumonia (community-acquired): Canadian labeling (not in U.S. labeling): 500 mg every 8 hours

Prosthetic joint infection, *Pseudomonas aeruginosa* (unlabeled use): 1 g every 8 hours for 4-6 weeks (consider addition of aminoglycoside) (Osmon, 2013)

Skin and skin structure infections:

Complicated: U.S. labeling: 500 mg every 8 hours; diabetic foot: 1 g every 8 hours

Uncomplicated: Canadian labeling (not in U.S. labeling): 500 mg every 8 hours

Urinary tract infections (complicated): Canadian labeling (not in U.S. labeling): 500 mg every 8 hours. **Note:** Up to 1 g every 8 hours may be administered (Pallett, 2010).

Adults: Canadian labeling (not in U.S. labeling): I.V.:

Gynecologic and pelvic inflammatory disease: 500 mg every 8 hours

Pneumonia (nosocomial): 1 g every 8 hours

Septicemia: 1 g every 8 hours

Dosage adjustment in renal impairment:

Children (unlabeled dosing; Aronoff, 2007):

GFR 30-50 mL/minute: Administer 20-40 mg/kg every 12 hours

GFR 10-29 mL/minute: Administer 10-20 mg/kg every 12 hours

GFR <10 mL/minute: Administer 10-20 mg/kg every 24 hours

Intermittent hemodialysis (IHD): 10-20 mg/kg every 24 hours (administer after hemodialysis on dialysis days)

Peritoneal dialysis (PD): 10-20 mg/kg every 24 hours

Continuous renal replacement therapy (CRRT): 20-40 mg/kg every 12 hours

Adults:

Cl_{cr} >50 mL/minute: No dosage adjustment necessary.

Cl_{cr} 26-50 mL/minute: Administer recommended dose based on indication every 12 hours

Cl_{cr} 10-25 mL/minute: Administer one-half recommended dose based on indication every 12 hours

Cl_{cr} <10 mL/minute: Administer one-half recommended dose based on indication every 24 hours

Alternative dosing recommendations: (unlabeled dosing; Aronoff, 2007):

GFR 10-50 mL/minute: Administer recommended dose (based on indication) every 12 hours

GFR <10 mL/minute: Administer recommended dose (based on indication) every 24 hours

Intermittent hemodialysis (IHD) (administer after hemodialysis on dialysis days): Meropenem and its metabolite are readily dialyzable: 500 mg every 24 hours. **Note:** Dosing dependent on the assumption of 3 times weekly, complete IHD sessions.

Peritoneal dialysis (unlabeled dose): Administer recommended dose (based on indication) every 24 hours (Aronoff, 2007).

Continuous renal replacement therapy (CRRT) (Heintz, 2009; Trotman, 2005): Drug clearance is highly dependent on the method of renal replacement, filter type, and flow rate. Appropriate dosing requires close monitoring of pharmacologic response, signs of adverse reactions due to drug accumulation, as well as drug concentrations in relation to target trough (if appropriate). The following are general recommendations only (based on dialysate flow/ultrafiltration rates of 1-2 L/hour and minimal residual renal function) and should not supersede clinical judgment:

CVVH: Loading dose of 1 **g** followed by either 500 mg every 8 hours **or** 1 **g** every 12 hours

CVVHD/CVVHDF: Loading dose of 1 **g** followed by either 500 mg every 6-8 hours **or** 1 **g** every 8-12 hours

Note: Consider giving patients receiving CVVHDF dosages of 750 mg every 8 hours **or** 1.5 **g** every 12 hours (Heintz, 2009). Substantial variability exists in various published recommendations, ranging from 1-3 **g** daily in 2-3 divided doses. One gram every 12 hours achieves a target trough of ~4 mg/L.

Dosage adjustment in hepatic impairment: No dosage adjustment necessary.

Dietary Considerations Some products may contain sodium.

Administration Administer I.V. infusion over 15-30 minutes; I.V. bolus injection (5-20 mL) over 3-5 minutes

Extended infusion administration (unlabeled dosing): Administer over 3 hours (Crandon 2011; Dandekar, 2003). **Note:** Must consider meropenem's limited room temperature stability if using extended infusions

Monitoring Parameters Perform culture and sensitivity testing prior to initiating therapy. Monitor for signs of anaphylaxis during first dose. During prolonged therapy, monitor renal function, liver function, CBC.

Test Interactions Positive Coombs' [direct]

Dosage Forms Excipient information presented when available (limited, particularly for generics); consult specific product labeling.

Solution Reconstituted, Intravenous:

Merrem: 500 mg (1 ea); 1 g (1 ea)

Generic: 500 mg (1 ea); 1 g (1 ea)

◆ **Meropenem For Injection (Can)** *see* Meropenem *on page 1303*

◆ **Merrem** *see* Meropenem *on page 1303*

Mesalamine (me SAL a meen)

Brand Names: U.S. Apriso; Asacol HD; Asacol [DSC]; Canasa; Delzicol; Lialda; Pentasa; Rowasa; SfRowasa

Brand Names: Canada 5-ASA; Asacol; Asacol 800; Mesasal; Mezavant; Novo-5 ASA; Novo-5 ASA-ECT; Pentasa; Salofalk; Salofalk 5-ASA

Index Terms 5-Aminosalicylic Acid; 5-ASA; Fisalamine; Mesalazine

Pharmacologic Category 5-Aminosalicylic Acid Derivative

Use

Oral:

Asacol, Delzicol, Lialda, Mezavant, Pentasa: Treatment and maintenance of remission of mildly- to moderately-active ulcerative colitis

Apriso: Maintenance of remission of ulcerative colitis

Asacol HD: Treatment of moderately-active ulcerative colitis

Rectal: Treatment of active mild-to-moderate distal ulcerative colitis, proctosigmoiditis, or proctitis

Pregnancy Risk Factor B/C (product specific)

Pregnancy Considerations Adverse events were not observed in animal reproduction studies. Dibutyl phthalate (DBP) is an inactive ingredient in the enteric coating of Asacol and Asacol HD; adverse effects in male rats were noted at doses greater than the recommended human dose. Mesalamine is known to cross the placenta. An increased rate of congenital malformations has not been observed in human studies. Preterm birth, still birth and decreased birth weight have been observed; however, these events may also be due to maternal disease. When treatment for inflammatory bowel disease is needed during pregnancy, mesalamine may be used, although products with DBP should be avoided (Habal, 2012; Mottet, 2009).

Breast-Feeding Considerations Low concentrations of the parent drug (undetectable to 0.11 mg/L) and higher concentrations of the N-acetyl metabolite of the parent drug (5-18 mg/L) have been detected in human breast milk following oral or rectal maternal doses of 500 mg to 3 g daily. Adverse effects (diarrhea) in a nursing infant have been reported while the mother received rectal administration of mesalamine within 12 hours after the first dose (Nelis, 1989). The manufacturer recommends that caution be used if administered to a nursing woman. Other sources consider use of mesalamine to be safe while breast-feeding (Habal, 2012; Mottet, 2009).

Contraindications Hypersensitivity to mesalamine, aminosalicylates, salicylates, or any component of the formulation

Canadian labeling (Mezavant): Additional contraindications: Severe renal impairment (GFR <30 mL/minute/1.73 m^2); severe hepatic impairment

Warnings/Precautions May cause an acute intolerance syndrome (cramping, acute abdominal pain, bloody diarrhea; sometimes fever, headache, rash); discontinue if this occurs. Use caution in patients with active peptic ulcers. Patients with pyloric stenosis or other gastrointestinal obstructive disorders may have prolonged gastric retention of tablets, delaying the release of mesalamine in the colon. Pericarditis or myocarditis (mesalamine-induced cardiac hypersensitivity reactions) should be considered in patients with chest pain; use with caution in patients predisposed to these conditions. Pancreatitis should be considered in patients with new abdominal discomfort. Symptomatic worsening of colitis/IBD may occur following initiation of therapy. Oligospermia (rare, reversible) has been reported in males. Use caution in patients with sulfasalazine hypersensitivity. Use caution in patients with impaired hepatic function; hepatic failure has been reported. Renal disease (including minimal change nephropathy, acute/chronic interstitial nephritis, nephrotic syndrome, and rarely renal failure) has been reported; use caution with other medications converted to mesalamine. An evaluation of renal function is recommended prior to initiation of mesalamine products and periodically during treatment. Use caution in patients with renal impairment. Use of Mezavant (Canadian availability; not available in the U.S.) contraindicated in severe renal and/or hepatic impairment. Use caution with other medications converted to mesalamine. Postmarketing reports suggest an increased incidence of blood dyscrasias in patients >65 years of age. In addition, elderly may have difficulty administering and retaining rectal suppositories or may have decreased renal function; use with caution and monitor.

Apriso contains phenylalanine. The Asacol HD 800 mg tablet has not been shown to be bioequivalent to 2 Asacol 400 mg tablets or 2 Delzicol 400 mg capsules. Canasa suppositories contain saturated vegetable fatty acid esters (contraindicated in patients with allergy to these components). Rowasa enema contains potassium metabisulfite; may cause severe hypersensitivity reactions (ie, anaphylaxis) in patients with sulfite allergies.

Adverse Reactions Adverse effects vary depending upon dosage form. Incidence usually on lower end with enema and suppository dosage forms.

>10%:

Central nervous system: Headache (2% to 35%), pain (≤14%)

Gastrointestinal: Abdominal pain (1% to 18%), eructation (16%), nausea (3% to 13%)

Respiratory: Pharyngitis (11%)

1% to 10%:

Cardiovascular: Chest pain (3%), peripheral edema (3%), vasodilation (≥2%)

Central nervous system: Dizziness (2% to 8%), fever (1% to 6%), chills (3%), malaise (2% to 3%), fatigue (<3%), vertigo (<3%), anxiety (≥2%), migraine (≥2%), nervousness (≥2%), paresthesia (≥2%), insomnia (2%)

Dermatologic: Skin rash (1% to 6%), pruritus (1% to 3%), alopecia (<3%), acne vulgaris (1% to 2%)

Endocrine & metabolic: Increased serum triglycerides (<3%)

Gastrointestinal: Diarrhea (2% to 8%), dyspepsia (1% to 6%), flatulence (1% to 6%), constipation (5%), vomiting (1% to 5%), exacerbation of ulcerative colitis (1% to 3%), rectal hemorrhage (<3%), abdominal distention (≥2%), gastroenteritis (≥2%), gastrointestinal hemorrhage (≥2%), abnormal stools (≥2%), tenesmus (≥2%), rectal pain (1% to 2%), hemorrhoids (1%)

Genitourinary: Polyuria (≥2%)

Hematologic & oncologic: Hematocrit/hemoglobin decreased (<3%)

Hepatic: Cholestatic hepatitis (<3%), increased serum transaminases (<3%), increased serum ALT (1%)

Infection: Infection (≥2%)

Local: Pain on insertion of enema tip (1%)

Neuromuscular & skeletal: Back pain (1% to 7%), hypertonia (5%), arthralgia (≤5%), myalgia (3%), weakness (≥2%), arthritis (2%), leg/joint pain (2%)

Ophthalmic: Visual disturbance (≥2%), conjunctivitis (2%)

Otic: Tinnitus (<3%), ear pain (≥2%)

Renal: Decreased creatinine clearance (<3%), hematuria (<3%)

Respiratory: Nasopharyngitis (1% to 4%), dyspnea (<3%), bronchitis (≥2%), sinusitis (≥2%), cough (≤2%)

Miscellaneous: Flu-like symptoms (1% to 5%), diaphoresis (3%), intolerance syndrome (3%)

Postmarketing and/or case reports (Limited to important or life-threatening): Abnormal T waves on ECG, agranulocytosis, albuminuria, anxiety, anemia, angioedema, aplastic anemia, bloody diarrhea, cholestatic jaundice, cholecystitis, drug fever, dysuria, edema, eosinophilia, eosinophilic pneumonitis, erythema nodosum, exacerbation of asthma, facial edema, fibrosing alveolitis, gastrointestinal bleeding, granulocytopenia, Guillain-Barre syndrome, hepatic failure, hepatic necrosis, hepatitis, hepatocellular damage, hepatotoxicity, hypersensitivity pneumonitis, hypertension, hypotension, increased blood urea nitrogen, increased gamma-glutamyl transferase, increased lactate dehydrogenase, increased serum alkaline phosphatase, increased serum bilirubin, increased serum creatinine, interstitial nephritis, interstitial pneumonitis, irregular menses, jaundice, Kawasaki-like syndrome, leukopenia, lupus-like syndrome, lymphadenopathy, minimal change nephrotic syndrome, myocarditis, nephrotoxicity, neutropenia, oligospermia, palpitations, pancreatitis, pancytopenia, paresthesia, perforated peptic ulcer, pericardial effusion, pericarditis, peripheral neuropathy, pharyngolaryngeal pain, pleurisy, pneumonitis, pyoderma gangrenosum, rectal polyp, renal disease, renal failure, skin photosensitivity, systemic lupus erythematosus, tachycardia, tenesmus, thrombocythemia, thrombocytopenia, transverse myelitis, vasodilation

Drug Interactions

Metabolism/Transport Effects None known.

Avoid Concomitant Use There are no known interactions where it is recommended to avoid concomitant use.

Increased Effect/Toxicity

Mesalamine may increase the levels/effects of: Heparin; Heparin (Low Molecular Weight); Thiopurine Analogs; Varicella Virus-Containing Vaccines

The levels/effects of Mesalamine may be increased by: Nonsteroidal Anti-Inflammatory Agents

Decreased Effect

Mesalamine may decrease the levels/effects of: Cardiac Glycosides

The levels/effects of Mesalamine may be decreased by: Antacids; H2-Antagonists; Proton Pump Inhibitors

Storage/Stability

Capsule:

Apriso: Store at controlled room temperature of 20°C to 25°C (68°F to 77°F)

Delzicol: Store at controlled room temperature of 20°C to 25°C (68°F to 77°F); excursions permitted to 15°C to 30°C (59°F to 86°F).

Pentasa: Store at controlled room temperature of 15°C to 30°C (59°F to 86°F). Protect from light.

Enema: Store at controlled room temperature. Use promptly once foil wrap is removed. Contents may darken with time (do not use if dark brown).

Suppository: Store below 25°C (below 77°F). May store under refrigeration; do not freeze. Protect from direct heat, light, and humidity.

Tablet: Store at controlled room temperature:

Asacol, Asacol HD: 20°C to 25°C (68°F to 77°F); excursions permitted to 15°C to 30°C (59°F to 86°F).

Lialda: 15°C to 30°C (59°F to 86°F)

Mezavant: 15°C to 25°C (59°F to 77°F)

Mechanism of Action Mesalamine (5-aminosalicylic acid) is the active component of sulfasalazine; the specific mechanism of action of mesalamine is unknown; however, it is thought that it modulates local chemical mediators of the inflammatory response, especially leukotrienes, and is also postulated to be a free radical scavenger or an inhibitor of tumor necrosis factor (TNF); action appears topical rather than systemic

Pharmacodynamics/Kinetics

Absorption: Rectal: Variable and dependent upon retention time, underlying GI disease, and colonic pH; Oral: Tablet: ~20% to 28%, Capsule: ~20% to 40%

Distribution: ~18 L

Protein binding: Mesalamine (5-ASA): ~43%; N-acetyl-5-ASA: ~78%

Metabolism: Hepatic and via GI tract to N-acetyl-5-aminosalicylic acid

Half-life elimination: 5-ASA: 0.5-10 hours; N-acetyl-5-ASA: 2-15 hours

Time to peak, serum:

Capsule: Apriso: ~4 hours; Delzicol: 4-16 hours; Pentasa: 3 hours

Rectal: 4-7 hours

Tablet: Asacol: 4-12 hours; Asacol HD: 10-16 hours; Lialda: 9-12 hours; Mezavant: 8 hours

Excretion: Urine (primarily as metabolites, <8% as unchanged drug); feces (<2%)

Dosage

Children ≥5 years: Oral: Treatment of ulcerative colitis (usual course of therapy is 6 weeks): Tablet (Asacol):

17 to <33 kg: 36-71 mg/kg/day given in 2 divided doses (maximum: 1200 mg daily)

33 to <54 kg: 37-61 mg/kg/day given in 2 divided doses (maximum: 2000 mg daily)

54 to 90 kg: 27-44 mg/kg/day given in 2 divided doses (maximum: 2400 mg daily)

Adults:
Oral:
Treatment of ulcerative colitis (usual course of therapy is 3-8 weeks):
Capsule:
Delzicol: 800 mg 3 times daily for 6 weeks
Pentasa: 1 g 4 times daily
Tablet:
Asacol: 800 mg 3 times daily for 6 weeks
Asacol HD: 1.6 g 3 times daily for 6 weeks
Lialda, Mezavant: 2.4-4.8 g once daily for up to 8 weeks
Maintenance of remission of ulcerative colitis:
Capsule:
Apriso: 1.5 g once daily in the morning
Delzicol: 400 mg 4 times daily
Pentasa: 1 g 4 times daily
Tablet:
Asacol: 1.6 g daily in divided doses
Lialda, Mezavant: 2.4 g once daily
Note: Asacol HD is approved for treatment only.
Rectal:
Active mild-to-moderate distal ulcerative colitis, proctosigmoiditis, or proctitis: Retention enema: 60 mL (4 g) at bedtime, retained overnight, approximately 8 hours
Active ulcerative proctitis: Rectal suppository (Canasa): Insert one 1000 mg suppository in rectum daily at bedtime; retained for at least 1-3 hours to achieve maximum benefit
Note: Duration of rectal therapy is 3-6 weeks; some patients may require rectal and oral therapy concurrently.

Elderly: See adult dosing; use with caution

Dosage adjustment in renal impairment: No dosage adjustment provided in manufacturer's labeling; however, dosage adjustment may be necessary since mesalamine is renally eliminated. Use with caution.

Dosage adjustment in hepatic impairment: No dosage adjustment provided in manufacturer's labeling; use with caution.

Dietary Considerations Some products may contain phenylalanine.
Apriso: Do not administer with antacids.
Canasa rectal suppository contains saturated vegetable fatty acid esters.

Administration Oral:
Capsules:
Apriso: Administer with or without food; do not administer with antacids. The capsule should be swallowed whole per the manufacturer's labeling; however, opening the capsule and placing the contents (delayed release granules) on food with a pH <6 is not expected to affect the release of mesalamine once ingested (data on file, Salix Pharmaceuticals Medical Information). There is no safety/efficacy information regarding this practice. The contents of the capsules should not be chewed or crushed.
Delzicol: Administer 1 hour before or 2 hours after a meal. The capsule should be swallowed whole per the manufacturer's labeling; do not break, chew, or crush.
Pentasa: Administer with or without food. Although the manufacturer recommends swallowing the capsule whole, if a patient is unable to swallow the capsule, some clinicians support opening the capsules and placing the contents (controlled-release beads) on yogurt or peanut butter (Crohn's & Colitis Foundation of America). There are currently no published data evaluating the safety/efficacy of this practice. The contents of the capsules should not be chewed or crushed.
Tablets: Swallow whole; do not break, chew, or crush.
Asacol: Do not break outer coating; administer with or without food.
Asacol HD: Do not break outer coating; administer with or without food.
Lialda: Do not break outer coating; should be administered once daily with a meal
Mezavant: Do not break outer coating; should be administered once daily with a meal
Rectal enema: Shake bottle well. Retain enemas for 8 hours or as long as practical.
Suppository: Remove foil wrapper; avoid excessive handling. Should be retained for at least 1-3 hours to achieve maximum benefit.

Monitoring Parameters Renal function (prior to and periodically during therapy); CBC (particularly in elderly patients)

Test Interactions May cause falsely-elevated urinary normetanephrine levels when measured by liquid chromatography with electrochemical detection (due to similarity in the chromatograms of normetanephrine and mesalamine's main metabolite, N-acetylaminosalicylic acid).

Dosage Forms Excipient information presented when available (limited, particularly for generics); consult specific product labeling. [DSC] = Discontinued product
Capsule Delayed Release, Oral:
Delzicol: 400 mg
Capsule Extended Release, Oral:
Pentasa: 250 mg [contains brilliant blue fcf (fd&c blue #1), fd&c yellow #10 (quinoline yellow)]
Pentasa: 500 mg [contains brilliant blue fcf (fd&c blue #1)]
Capsule Extended Release 24 Hour, Oral:
Apriso: 0.375 g [contains aspartame]
Enema, Rectal:
SfRowasa: 4 g/60 mL (60 mL) [sulfite free; contains edetate disodium, sodium benzoate]
Generic: 4 g (60 mL)
Kit, Rectal:
Rowasa: 4 g [contains edetate disodium, potassium metabisulfite, sodium benzoate]
Generic: 4 g
Suppository, Rectal:
Canasa: 1000 mg (30 ea, 42 ea)
Tablet Delayed Release, Oral:
Asacol: 400 mg [DSC]
Asacol HD: 800 mg
Lialda: 1.2 g

Dosage Forms: Canada Excipient information presented when available (limited, particularly for generics); consult specific product labeling.
Tablet, delayed and extended release:
Mezavant: 1.2 g

◆ **Mesalazine** *see* Mesalamine *on page 1305*
◆ **Mesasal (Can)** *see* Mesalamine *on page 1305*
◆ **M-Eslon® (Can)** *see* Morphine (Systemic) *on page 1398*

Mesna (MES na)

Brand Names: U.S. Mesnex

Brand Names: Canada Mesna for injection; Uromitexan

Index Terms Mercaptoethane Sulfonate; Sodium 2-Mercaptoethane Sulfonate

Pharmacologic Category Antidote; Uroprotectant

Use Preventative agent to reduce the incidence of ifosfamide-induced hemorrhagic cystitis

Unlabeled Use Preventative agent to reduce the incidence of cyclophosphamide-induced hemorrhagic cystitis with high-dose cyclophosphamide

Pregnancy Risk Factor B

Pregnancy Considerations Teratogenic effects were not observed in animal studies. There are no adequate and well-controlled studies in pregnant women. Use during pregnancy only if clearly needed.

Breast-Feeding Considerations Due to the potential for adverse reactions in the nursing infant, breast-feeding is not recommended.

Contraindications Hypersensitivity to mesna or other thiol compounds, or any component of the formulation

Warnings/Precautions Examine morning urine specimen for hematuria prior to ifosfamide or cyclophosphamide treatment; if hematuria (>50 RBC/HPF) develops, reduce the ifosfamide/cyclophosphamide dose or discontinue the drug; will not prevent or alleviate other toxicities associated with ifosfamide or cyclophosphamide and will not prevent hemorrhagic cystitis in all patients. Mesna will not reduce the risk of thrombocytopenia-related hematuria. Allergic reactions have been reported; symptoms ranged from mild hypersensitivity to systemic anaphylactic reactions and may include fever, hypotension, and/or tachycardia; patients with autoimmune disorders receiving cyclophosphamide and mesna may be at increased risk. Patients should receive adequate hydration during treatment. I.V. formulation contains benzyl alcohol; do not use in neonates or infants (associated with "gasping syndrome").

Adverse Reactions

Mesna alone (frequency not defined):

- Cardiovascular: Flushing
- Central nervous system: Dizziness, fever, headache, hyperesthesia, somnolence
- Dermatologic: Rash
- Gastrointestinal: Anorexia, constipation, diarrhea, flatulence, nausea, taste alteration/bad taste (with oral administration), vomiting
- Local: Injection site reactions
- Neuromuscular: Arthralgia, back pain, rigors
- Ocular: Conjunctivitis
- Respiratory: Cough, pharyngitis, rhinitis
- Miscellaneous: Flu-like syndrome

Mesna alone or in combination: Postmarketing and/or case reports: Allergic reaction, anaphylactic reaction, hypersensitivity, hyper-/hypotension, injection site erythema, injection site pain, limb pain, malaise, myalgia, platelets decreased, ST-segment increased, tachycardia, tachypnea, transaminases increased

Drug Interactions

Metabolism/Transport Effects None known.

Avoid Concomitant Use There are no known interactions where it is recommended to avoid concomitant use.

Increased Effect/Toxicity There are no known significant interactions involving an increase in effect.

Decreased Effect There are no known significant interactions involving a decrease in effect.

Preparation for Administration Dilute in 50-1000 mL D_5W, NS, $D_5{}^1/_4$NS, $D_5{}^1/_3$NS, $D_5{}^1/_2$NS, or lactated Ringer's (the manufacturer recommends a final concentration of 20 mg/mL).

Storage/Stability Store intact vials and tablets at room temperature of 20°C to 25°C (68°F to 77°F). Opened multidose vials may be stored and used for use to 8 days after opening. Solutions diluted for infusion are stable for at least 24 hours at room temperature. Solutions in plastic syringes are stable for 9 days under refrigeration, or at room or body temperature. Solutions of mesna and ifosfamide in lactated Ringer's are stable for 7 days in a PVC ambulatory infusion pump reservoir. Solutions of mesna (0.5-3.2 mg/mL) and cyclophosphamide (1.8-10.8 mg/mL) in D_5W are stable for 48 hours refrigerated or 6 hours at room temperature (Menard, 2003). Mesna injection is stable for at least 7 days when diluted 1:2 or 1:5 with grape- and orange-flavored syrups or 11:1 to 1:100 in carbonated beverages for oral administration.

Mechanism of Action In blood, mesna is oxidized to dimesna which in turn is reduced in the kidney back to mesna, supplying a free thiol group which binds to and inactivates acrolein, the urotoxic metabolite of ifosfamide and cyclophosphamide

Pharmacodynamics/Kinetics

Distribution: No tissue penetration

Protein binding: 69% to 75%

Metabolism: Rapidly oxidized intravascularly to mesna disulfide (dimesna); dimesna is reduced in renal tubules back to mesna following glomerular filtration

Bioavailability: Oral: 45% to 79%

Half-life elimination:

- I.V.: Mesna: ~22 minutes; Dimesna: ~70 minutes
- I.V. followed by oral: 1-8 hours

Time to peak, plasma: 2-3 hours

Excretion: Urine (18% to 32% as mesna; 33% as dimesna)

Dosage Children and Adults: **Note:** Details concerning dosing in combination regimens should also be consulted. Mesna dosing schedule should be repeated each day ifosfamide is received. If ifosfamide dose is adjusted, the mesna dose should also be modified to maintain the mesna-to-ifosfamide ratio.

I.V.: Prevention of ifosfamide-induced hemorrhagic cystitis:

- Short infusion standard-dose ifosfamide (<2.5 g/m^2/day): Mesna dose is equal to 60% of the ifosfamide dose given in 3 divided doses (0, 4, and 8 hours after the start of ifosfamide)
- Continuous infusion standard-dose ifosfamide (<2.5 g/m^2/day): ASCO guidelines: Mesna dose (as an I.V. bolus) is equal to 20% of the ifosfamide dose, followed by a continuous infusion of mesna at 40% of the ifosfamide dose, continue mesna infusion for 12-24 hours after completion of ifosfamide infusion (Hensley, 2008)
- High-dose ifosfamide (>2.5 g/m^2/day): ASCO guidelines: Evidence for use is inadequate; more frequent and prolonged mesna administration regimens may be required.

I.V. followed by oral (for ifosfamide doses ≤2 g/m^2/day): Mesna dose is equal to 100% of the ifosfamide dose, given as 20% of the ifosfamide dose I.V. at hour 0, followed by 40% of the ifosfamide dose given orally 2- and 6 hours after start of ifosfamide

Dosage adjustment in renal impairment: No dosage adjustment provided in manufacturer's labeling (has not been studied).

Dosage adjustment in hepatic impairment: No dosage adjustment provided in manufacturer's labeling (has not been studied).

Administration

Oral: Administer orally in tablet formulation or parenteral solution diluted in water, milk, juice, or carbonated beverages; patients who vomit within 2 hours after taking oral mesna should repeat the dose or receive I.V. mesna

I.V.: Administer by short (15-30 minutes) infusion or continuous infusion (maintain continuous infusion for 12-24 after completion of ifosfamide infusion) (Hensley, 2008)

Monitoring Parameters Urinalysis

Test Interactions False-positive urinary ketones with Chemstrip®, Multistix®, or Labstix®

Additional Information Oncology Comment: Guidelines from the American Society of Clinical Oncology (ASCO) for the use of chemotherapy and radiotherapy protectants (Hensley, 2008 [update]; Schuchter, 2002) recommend mesna to decrease the incidence of ifosfamide-induced urotoxicity associated with short infusion and continuous infusion standard-dose ifosfamide (<2.5 g/m^2/day). Although evidence is inadequate regarding mesna's uroprotective effects in high-dose ifosfamide (>2.5 g/m^2/day), the guidelines suggest more frequent and prolonged mesna administration times may be required. For prevention high-dose cyclophosphamide-induced urotoxicity (associated with stem cell transplantation), the guidelines recommend mesna in conjunction with saline diuresis (or forced saline diuresis alone).

Dosage Forms Excipient information presented when available (limited, particularly for generics); consult specific product labeling.

Solution, Intravenous:

Mesnex: 100 mg/mL (10 mL) [contains benzyl alcohol, edetate disodium]

Generic: 100 mg/mL (10 mL)

Tablet, Oral:

Mesnex: 400 mg [scored]

Dosage Forms: Canada Excipient information presented when available (limited, particularly for generics); consult specific product labeling.

Injection, solution:

Mesna for injection: 100 mg/mL (10 mL)

◆ **Mesna for injection (Can)** *see* Mesna *on page* 1307

◆ **Mesnex** *see* Mesna *on page* 1307

◆ **Mestinon** *see* Pyridostigmine *on page* 1752

◆ **Mestinon® (Can)** *see* Pyridostigmine *on page* 1752

◆ **Mestinon®-SR (Can)** *see* Pyridostigmine *on page* 1752

◆ **Mestranol and Norethindrone** *see* Norethindrone and Mestranol *on page* 1474

◆ **Metadate CD** *see* Methylphenidate *on page* 1336

◆ **Metadate ER** *see* Methylphenidate *on page* 1336

◆ **Metadol™ (Can)** *see* Methadone *on page* 1313

◆ **Metadol-D™ (Can)** *see* Methadone *on page* 1313

◆ **Metafolbic Plus** *see* Methylfolate, Methylcobalamin, and Acetylcysteine *on page* 1335

◆ **Metafolbic Plus RF** *see* Methylfolate, Methylcobalamin, and Acetylcysteine *on page* 1335

◆ **Metaglip™** *see* Glipizide and Metformin *on page* 959

◆ **Metamucil® (Can)** *see* Psyllium *on page* 1748

◆ **Metamucil MultiHealth Fiber [OTC]** *see* Psyllium *on page* 1748

Metaproterenol (met a proe TER e nol)

Brand Names: Canada Apo-Orciprenaline®; ratio-Orciprenaline®; Tanta-Orciprenaline®

Index Terms Alupent; Metaproterenol Sulfate; Orciprenaline Sulfate

Pharmacologic Category $Beta_2$ Agonist

Use Bronchodilator in reversible airway obstruction due to asthma or COPD

Pregnancy Risk Factor C

Dosage Oral:

Children:

<6 years (limited experience): 1.3-2.6 mg/kg/day divided every 6-8 hours

6-9 years (or <27 kg): 10 mg/dose 3-4 times/day

Children >9 years (or ≥27 kg) and Adults: 20 mg 3-4 times/day

Elderly: Refer to adult dosing.

Dosage adjustment in renal impairment: No dosage adjustment provided in manufacturer's labeling.

Dosage adjustment in hepatic impairment: No dosage adjustment provided in manufacturer's labeling.

Additional Information Complete prescribing information should be consulted for additional detail.

Dosage Forms Excipient information presented when available (limited, particularly for generics); consult specific product labeling.

Syrup, Oral, as sulfate:

Generic: 10 mg/5 mL (473 mL)

Tablet, Oral, as sulfate:

Generic: 10 mg, 20 mg

◆ **Metaproterenol Sulfate** *see* Metaproterenol *on page* 1309

Metaxalone (me TAKS a lone)

Brand Names: U.S. Skelaxin

Brand Names: Canada Skelaxin®

Pharmacologic Category Skeletal Muscle Relaxant

Additional Appendix Information

Beers Criteria – Potentially Inappropriate Medications for Geriatrics *on page* 2368

Use Relief of discomfort associated with acute, painful musculoskeletal conditions

Pregnancy Considerations Teratogenic effects were not observed in animal studies. There are no adequate and well-controlled studies in pregnant women. Use during pregnancy (especially first trimester) only if benefits outweigh risks.

Breast-Feeding Considerations It is not known if metaxalone is excreted in breast milk. Breast-feeding is not recommended by the manufacturer.

Contraindications Hypersensitivity to metaxalone or any component of the formulation; significantly impaired hepatic or renal function, history of drug-induced hemolytic anemias or other anemias

Warnings/Precautions May cause CNS depression. CNS depressant effects may be augmented when used in conjunction with other depressants (eg, barbiturates, ethanol), when taken with food, or in the elderly. May impair mental and/or physical ability to perform hazardous tasks such as operating machinery or driving a motor vehicle. Use with caution in patients with impaired renal or hepatic function (contraindicated if significant impairment); routine monitoring of transaminases is recommended. An increase in bioavailability and half-life have been observed in female patients. Muscle relaxants are poorly tolerated by the elderly due to potent anticholinergic effects, sedation, and risk of fracture. Efficacy is questionable at dosages tolerated by elderly patients; avoid use (Beers Criteria). Safety and efficacy have not been established in children ≤12 years of age.

Adverse Reactions Frequency not defined.

Central nervous system: Dizziness, drowsiness, headache, irritability, nervousness

Dermatologic: Rash (with or without pruritus)

Gastrointestinal: Gastrointestinal upset, nausea, vomiting

Hematologic: Hemolytic anemia, leukopenia

Hepatic: Jaundice

Miscellaneous: Hypersensitivity (including rare anaphylactoid reactions)

Drug Interactions

Metabolism/Transport Effects Substrate of CYP1A2 (minor), CYP2C19 (minor), CYP2C8 (minor), CYP2C9 (minor), CYP2D6 (minor), CYP2E1 (minor), CYP3A4 (minor); **Note:** Assignment of Major/Minor substrate status based on clinically relevant drug interaction potential

Avoid Concomitant Use

Avoid concomitant use of Metaxalone with any of the following: Azelastine (Nasal); Paraldehyde

Increased Effect/Toxicity

Metaxalone may increase the levels/effects of: Alcohol (Ethyl); Azelastine (Nasal); Buprenorphine; CNS Depressants; Hydrocodone; Methotrimeprazine; Metyrosine; Mirtazapine; Paraldehyde; Pramipexole; ROPINIRole; Rotigotine; Selective Serotonin Reuptake Inhibitors; Zolpidem

The levels/effects of Metaxalone may be increased by: Brimonidine (Topical); Doxylamine; Droperidol; HydrOXYzine; Magnesium Sulfate; Methotrimeprazine; Perampanel; Sodium Oxybate; Tapentadol

Decreased Effect

The levels/effects of Metaxalone may be decreased by: Peginterferon Alfa-2b

Ethanol/Nutrition/Herb Interactions

Ethanol: May increase CNS depression; monitor for increased effects with coadministration. Caution patients about effects.

Food: Bioavailability may be increased (may increase CNS depression).

Herb/Nutraceutical: Avoid valerian, St John's wort, kava kava, gotu kola (may increase CNS depression).

Storage/Stability Store at controlled room temperature of 15°C to 30°C (59°F to 86°F).

Mechanism of Action Precise mechanism has not been established; however, efficacy appears to result from disruption of the spasm-pain-spasm cycle, probably by a general CNS depressant effect. Does not have a direct effect on skeletal muscle.

Pharmacodynamics/Kinetics

Onset of action: ~1 hour

Duration: ~4-6 hours

Distribution: V_d: ~800 L

Metabolism: Hepatic via CYP1A2, CYP2D6, CYP2E1, CYP3A4 and to lesser extent CYP2C8, CPY2C9, and CYP2C19

Bioavailability: Not established; food may increase

Half-life elimination: 4-14 hours

Time to peak: T_{max}: ~3 hours

Excretion: Urine (as metabolites)

Dosage Oral: Children >12 years and Adults: Muscle discomfort: 800 mg 3-4 times/day

Dosage adjustment in renal impairment: Use caution in patients with mild-to-moderate renal impairment; contraindicated with significant impairment. No specific recommendation are provided in approved labeling.

Dosage adjustment in hepatic impairment: Use caution in patients with mild-to-moderate hepatic impairment; contraindicated with significant impairment. No specific recommendation are provided in approved labeling.

Dietary Considerations Administration with food may increase serum concentrations.

Administration May be administered with or without food. However, serum concentrations may be increased when administered with food; clinical significance has not been established. Patients should be monitored.

Test Interactions False-positive Benedict's test

Dosage Forms Excipient information presented when available (limited, particularly for generics); consult specific product labeling.

Tablet, Oral:

Skelaxin: 800 mg [scored]

Generic: 800 mg

MetFORMIN (met FOR min)

Brand Names: U.S. Fortamet; Glucophage; Glucophage XR; Glumetza; Riomet

Brand Names: Canada Apo-Metformin®; Ava-Metformin; CO Metformin; Dom-Metformin; Glucophage®; Glumetza®; Glycon; JAMP-Metformin; JAMP-Metformin Blackberry; Mar-Metformin; Metformin FC; Mint-Metformin; Mylan-Metformin; Novo-Metformin; PHL-Metformin; PMS-Metformin; PRO-Metformin; Q-Metformin; RAN™-Metformin; ratio-Metformin; Riva-Metformin; Sandoz-Metformin FC; Septa-Metformin; Teva-Metformin

Index Terms Metformin Hydrochloride

Pharmacologic Category Antidiabetic Agent, Biguanide

Additional Appendix Information

Oral Antidiabetic Agents Comparison Table *on page 2312*

Use Management of type 2 diabetes mellitus (noninsulin dependent, NIDDM) when hyperglycemia cannot be managed with diet and exercise alone.

Note: If not contraindicated and if tolerated, metformin is the preferred initial pharmacologic agent for type 2 diabetes management (ADA, 2013).

Unlabeled Use Gestational diabetes mellitus (GDM); polycystic ovary syndrome (PCOS); prevention of type 2 diabetes mellitus

Pregnancy Risk Factor B

Pregnancy Considerations Adverse events have not been observed in animal reproduction studies. Metformin has been found to cross the placenta in concentrations which may be comparable to those found in the maternal plasma. Pharmacokinetic studies suggest that clearance of metformin may increase during pregnancy and dosing may need adjusted in some women when used during the third trimester (Charles, 2006; de Oliveira Baraldi, 2011; Eyal, 2010; Gardiner, 2003; Hughes, 2006; Vanky, 2005).

An increased risk of birth defects or adverse fetal/neonatal outcomes has not been observed following maternal use of metformin for GDM or type 2 diabetes when glycemic control is maintained (Balani, 2009; Coetzee, 1979; Coetzee, 1984; Ekpebegh, 2007; Niromanesh, 2012; Rowan, 2008; Rowan, 2010; Tertti, 2008). For women with diabetes, maternal hyperglycemia itself can be associated with adverse effects in the fetus, neonate, and mother. To prevent adverse events, prior to conception and throughout pregnancy, the maternal Hb A_{1c} should be kept close to normal but without causing significant hypoglycemia. The use of metformin in pregnant women with type 2 diabetes or GDM is under study. Until additional safety and efficacy data are obtained, use is generally not recommended for routine management of GDM or type 2 diabetes mellitus during pregnancy; insulin is the drug of choice for the control of diabetes mellitus in pregnant women (ACOG, 2005; ADA, 2013; Kitzmiller, 2008; Metzger, 2007).

Metformin is recommended to treat insulin resistance associated with PCOS; however, its use may also restore spontaneous ovulation. Women with PCOS who do not desire to become pregnant should use effective contraception. Although studied for use in women with anovulatory PCOS, there is no evidence that it improves live birth rates or decreases pregnancy complications. Routine use to treat infertility related to PCOS is not currently recommended (ACOG, 2009; ASRM, 2008; Fauser, 2012).

Breast-Feeding Considerations Low amounts of metformin (generally ≤1% of the weight-adjusted maternal dose) are excreted into breast milk. Because breast milk concentrations of metformin stay relatively constant, avoiding nursing around peak plasma concentrations in the mother would not be helpful in reducing metformin exposure to the infant (Briggs, 2005; Eyal, 2010; Gardiner, 2003; Hale, 2002). Growth and development were not affected in infants born to mothers with PCOS and who took metformin while breast-feeding (Glueck, 2006).

Breast-feeding is encouraged for all women, including those with diabetes; however, the safety of metformin during breast-feeding has not yet been established (Metzger, 2007). According to the manufacturer, due to the potential for hypoglycemia in the nursing infant, a decision should be made whether to discontinue nursing or to discontinue the drug, taking into account the importance of treatment to the mother.

Contraindications

Note: Temporarily discontinue in patients undergoing radiologic studies in which intravascular iodinated contrast media are utilized.

U.S. labeling: Hypersensitivity to metformin or any component of the formulation; renal disease or renal dysfunction (serum creatinine ≥1.5 mg/dL in males or ≥1.4 mg/dL in females) or abnormal creatinine clearance from any cause, including shock, acute myocardial infarction, or septicemia; acute or chronic metabolic acidosis with or without coma (including diabetic ketoacidosis)

Canadian labeling: Hypersensitivity to metformin or any component of the formulation; renal function unknown, renal impairment, and serum creatinine levels above the upper limit of normal range; renal disease or renal dysfunction (serum creatinine ≥136 micromol/L in males or ≥124 micromol/L in females or abnormal creatinine clearance <60 mL/minute) which may result from conditions such as cardiovascular collapse (shock), acute myocardial infarction, and septicemia; unstable and/or insulin-dependent (Type I) diabetes mellitus; history of ketoacidosis with or without coma; history of lactic acidosis (regardless of precipitating factors); excessive alcohol intake (acute or chronic); severe hepatic dysfunction or clinical or laboratory evidence of hepatic disease; cardiovascular collapse and disease states associated with hypoxemia including cardiorespiratory insufficiency, which are often associated with hyperlactacidemia; stress conditions (eg, severe infection, trauma, surgery and postoperative recovery phase); severe dehydration; pregnancy; breast-feeding

Warnings/Precautions [U.S. Boxed Warning]: Lactic acidosis is a rare, but potentially severe consequence of therapy with metformin that requires urgent care and hospitalization. The risk is increased in patients with acute congestive heart failure, dehydration, excessive alcohol intake, hepatic or renal impairment, or sepsis. Symptoms may be nonspecific (eg, abdominal distress, malaise, myalgia, respiratory distress, somnolence); low pH, increased anion gap and elevated blood lactate may be observed. Discontinue immediately if acidosis is suspected. Lactic acidosis should be suspected in any patient with diabetes receiving metformin with evidence of acidosis but without evidence of ketoacidosis. Discontinue metformin in patients with conditions associated with dehydration, sepsis, or hypoxemia. The risk of accumulation and lactic acidosis increases with the degree of impairment of renal function. Use caution in patients with congestive heart failure requiring pharmacologic management, particularly in patients with unstable or acute CHF; risk of lactic acidosis may be increased secondary to hypoperfusion.

Metformin is substantially excreted by the kidney. The risk of accumulation and lactic acidosis increases with the degree of impairment of renal function. Patients with renal function below the limit of normal for their age should not receive metformin. Metformin should be withheld in patients with prerenal azotemia. In elderly patients, renal function should be monitored regularly; should not be initiated in patients ≥80 years of age unless normal renal function is confirmed. Use of concomitant medications that may affect renal function (ie, affect tubular secretion) may also affect metformin disposition. Therapy should be suspended for any surgical procedures (Canadian labeling recommends discontinuing use 48 hours prior to surgical procedures excluding minor procedures not associated with restricted food and fluid intake). Restart only after normal oral intake resumed and normal renal function is verified. Therapy should be temporarily discontinued prior to or at the time of intravascular administration of iodinated contrast media (potential for acute alteration in renal function). Metformin should be withheld for 48 hours after the radiologic study and restarted only after renal function has been confirmed as normal. It may be necessary to discontinue metformin and administer insulin if the patient is exposed to stress (fever, trauma, infection, surgery).

Avoid use in patients with impaired liver function. Patient must be instructed to avoid excessive acute or chronic ethanol use; ethanol may potentiate metformin's effect on lactate metabolism. Administration of oral antidiabetic drugs has been reported to be associated with increased cardiovascular mortality; metformin does not appear to share this risk. Insoluble tablet shell of Glumetza® 1000 mg extended release tablet may remain intact and be visible in the stool. Other extended released tablets (Fortamet®, Glucophage® XR, Glumetza® 500 mg) may appear in the stool as a soft mass resembling the tablet.

Adverse Reactions

>10%:

Gastrointestinal: Diarrhea (IR tablet: 12% to 53%; ER tablet: 10% to 17%), nausea/vomiting (IR tablet: 7% to 26%; ER tablet: 7% to 9%), flatulence (12%)

Neuromuscular & skeletal: Weakness (9%)

1% to 10%:

Cardiovascular: Chest discomfort, flushing, palpitation

Central nervous system: Headache (6%), chills, dizziness, lightheadedness

Dermatologic: Rash

Endocrine & metabolic: Hypoglycemia

Gastrointestinal: Indigestion (7%), abdominal discomfort (6%), abdominal distention, abnormal stools, constipation, dyspepsia/ heartburn, taste disorder

Neuromuscular & skeletal: Myalgia

Respiratory: Dyspnea, upper respiratory tract infection

Miscellaneous: Decreased vitamin B_{12} levels (7%), increased diaphoresis, flu-like syndrome, nail disorder

<1% (Limited to important or life-threatening): Lactic acidosis, leukocytoclastic vasculitis, megaloblastic anemia, pneumonitis

Drug Interactions

Metabolism/Transport Effects None known.

Avoid Concomitant Use There are no known interactions where it is recommended to avoid concomitant use.

Increased Effect/Toxicity

MetFORMIN may increase the levels/effects of: Dalfampridine; Dofetilide

The levels/effects of MetFORMIN may be increased by: Carbonic Anhydrase Inhibitors; Cephalexin; Cimetidine; Dalfampridine; Dolutegravir; Glycopyrrolate; Iodinated Contrast Agents; LamoTRIgine; Pegvisomant; Ranolazine; Topiramate; Trimethoprim

Decreased Effect

MetFORMIN may decrease the levels/effects of: Trospium

The levels/effects of MetFORMIN may be decreased by: Corticosteroids (Orally Inhaled); Corticosteroids (Systemic); Luteinizing Hormone-Releasing Hormone Analogs; Somatropin; Thiazide Diuretics

Ethanol/Nutrition/Herb Interactions

Ethanol: Avoid or limit ethanol (incidence of lactic acidosis may be increased; may cause hypoglycemia).

Food: Food decreases the extent and slightly delays the absorption. May decrease absorption of vitamin B_{12} and/ or folic acid.

Herb/Nutraceutical: Caution with chromium, garlic, gymnema (may cause hypoglycemia).

Storage/Stability

Oral solution: Store at 15°C to 30°C (59°F to 86°F).

Tablets: Store at 20°C to 25°C (68°F to 77°F); excursion permitted to 15°C to 30°C (59°F to 86°F). Protect from light and moisture.

Mechanism of Action Decreases hepatic glucose production, decreasing intestinal absorption of glucose and improves insulin sensitivity (increases peripheral glucose uptake and utilization)

Pharmacodynamics/Kinetics

Onset of action: Within days; maximum effects up to 2 weeks

Distribution: V_d: 654 ± 358 L; partitions into erythrocytes

Protein binding: Negligible

Metabolism: Not metabolized by the liver

Bioavailability: Absolute: Fasting: 50% to 60%

Half-life elimination: Plasma: 4-9 hours

Time to peak, serum: Immediate release: 2-3 hours; Extended release: 7 hours (range: 4-8 hours)

Excretion: Urine (90% as unchanged drug; active secretion)

Dosage

Type 2 diabetes management: **Note:** Allow 1-2 weeks between dose titrations: Generally, clinically significant responses are not seen at doses <1500 mg daily; however, a lower recommended starting dose and gradual increased dosage is recommended to minimize gastrointestinal symptoms.

Immediate release tablet or solution: Oral:

Children 10-16 years: Initial: 500 mg twice daily; increases in daily dosage should be made in increments of 500 mg at weekly intervals, given in divided doses, up to a maximum of 2000 mg daily

Children ≥17 years and Adults: Initial: 500 mg twice daily **or** 850 mg once daily; titrate in increments of 500 mg weekly or 850 mg every other week; may also titrate from 500 mg twice a day to 850 mg twice a day after 2 weeks

If a dose >2000 mg daily is required, it may be better tolerated in 3 divided doses. Maximum recommended dose 2550 mg daily.

Extended release tablet: Oral: **Note:** If glycemic control is not achieved at maximum dose, may divide dose and administer twice daily.

Children ≥17 years and Adults:

Fortamet®: Initial: 500-1000 mg once daily; dosage may be increased by 500 mg weekly; maximum dose: 2500 mg once daily

Glucophage® XR: Initial: 500 mg once daily; dosage may be increased by 500 mg weekly; maximum dose: 2000 mg once daily

Adults: Glumetza®: Initial: 1000 mg once daily; dosage may be increased by 500 mg weekly; maximum dose: 2000 mg once daily

Elderly: The initial and maintenance dosing should be conservative, due to the potential for decreased renal function. Generally, elderly patients should not be titrated to the maximum dose of metformin. Do not use in patients ≥80 years of age unless normal renal function has been established.

Transfer from other antidiabetic agents: No transition period is generally necessary except when transferring from chlorpropamide. When transferring from chlorpropamide, care should be exercised during the first 2 weeks because of the prolonged retention of chlorpropamide in the body, leading to overlapping drug effects and possible hypoglycemia.

Concomitant metformin and oral sulfonylurea therapy: If patients have not responded to 4 weeks of the maximum dose of metformin monotherapy, consider a gradual addition of an oral sulfonylurea, even if prior primary or secondary failure to a sulfonylurea has occurred. Continue metformin at the maximum dose. If adequate response has not occurred following 3 months of metformin and sulfonylurea combination therapy, consider switching to insulin with or without metformin.

Failed sulfonylurea therapy: Patients with prior failure on glyburide may be treated by gradual addition of metformin. Initiate with glyburide 20 mg and metformin 500 mg daily. Metformin dosage may be increased by 500 mg/day at weekly intervals, up to a maximum metformin dose (dosage of glyburide maintained at 20 mg daily).

Concomitant metformin and insulin therapy: Initial: 500 mg metformin once daily, continue current insulin dose; increase by 500 mg metformin weekly until adequate glycemic control is achieved

Maximum daily dose: Immediate release and solution: 2550 mg metformin; Extended release: 2000-2500 mg (varies by product)

Decrease insulin dose 10% to 25% when FPG <120 mg/dL; monitor and make further adjustments as needed

Type 2 diabetes prevention (unlabeled use): **Immediate release tablet or solution:** Oral: Adults: Initial: 850 mg once daily; Target: 850 mg twice daily (Knowler, 2002)

Dosing adjustment/comments in renal impairment: The plasma and blood half-life of metformin is prolonged and the renal clearance is decreased in proportion to the decrease in creatinine clearance. Per the manufacturer, metformin is contraindicated in the presence of renal dysfunction defined as a serum creatinine ≥1.5 mg/dL in males, or ≥1.4 mg/dL in females and in patients with abnormal clearance.

Dosing adjustment in hepatic impairment: Avoid metformin; liver disease is a risk factor for the development of lactic acidosis during metformin therapy.

Dietary Considerations Drug may cause GI upset; take with food (to decrease GI upset). Take at the same time(s) each day. Dietary modification based on ADA recommendations is a part of therapy. Monitor for signs and symptoms of vitamin B_{12} and/or folic acid deficiency; supplementation may be required.

Administration Administer with a meal (to decrease GI upset).

Extended release: Swallow whole; do not crush, break, or chew. Administer once daily doses with the evening meal. Fortamet® should also be administered with a full glass of water.

Monitoring Parameters Urine for glucose and ketones, fasting blood glucose, hemoglobin A_{1c}, and fructosamine. Initial and periodic monitoring of hematologic parameters (eg, hemoglobin/hematocrit and red blood cell indices) and renal function should be performed, at least annually (Canadian labeling recommends monitoring renal function every 6 months or more frequently if necessary). While megaloblastic anemia has been rarely seen with metformin, if suspected, vitamin B_{12} deficiency should be excluded.

Reference Range Recommendations for glycemic control in nonpregnant adults with diabetes (ADA, 2013):

Hb A_{1c}: <7% (a more aggressive [<6.5%] or less aggressive [<8%] Hb A_{1c} goal may be targeted based on patient-specific characteristics)

Preprandial capillary plasma glucose: 70-130 mg/dL

Peak postprandial capillary blood glucose: <180 mg/dL

Dosage Forms Excipient information presented when available (limited, particularly for generics); consult specific product labeling.

Solution, Oral, as hydrochloride:

Riomet: 500 mg/5 mL (118 mL, 473 mL) [contains saccharin calcium; cherry flavor]

Tablet, Oral, as hydrochloride:

Glucophage: 500 mg, 850 mg

Glucophage: 1000 mg [scored]

Generic: 500 mg, 850 mg, 1000 mg

Tablet Extended Release 24 Hour, Oral, as hydrochloride:

Fortamet: 500 mg, 1000 mg

Glucophage XR: 500 mg, 750 mg

Glumetza: 500 mg, 1000 mg

Generic: 500 mg, 750 mg, 1000 mg

Dosage Forms: Canada Excipient information presented when available (limited, particularly for generics); consult specific product labeling.

Tablet, oral, as hydrochloride:

Glycon®: 500 mg, 850 mg

◆ **Metformin and Glipizide** *see* Glipizide and Metformin *on page 959*

◆ **Metformin and Glyburide** *see* Glyburide and Metformin *on page 965*

◆ **Metformin and Linagliptin** *see* Linagliptin and Metformin *on page 1217*

◆ **Metformin and Repaglinide** *see* Repaglinide and Metformin *on page 1799*

◆ **Metformin and Rosiglitazone** *see* Rosiglitazone and Metformin *on page 1858*

◆ **Metformin and Saxagliptin** *see* Saxagliptin and Metformin *on page 1881*

◆ **Metformin and Sitagliptin** *see* Sitagliptin and Metformin *on page 1907*

◆ **Metformin FC (Can)** *see* MetFORMIN *on page 1310*

◆ **Metformin Hydrochloride** *see* MetFORMIN *on page 1310*

◆ **Metformin Hydrochloride and Linagliptin** *see* Linagliptin and Metformin *on page 1217*

◆ **Metformin Hydrochloride and Pioglitazone Hydrochloride** *see* Pioglitazone and Metformin *on page 1652*

◆ **Metformin Hydrochloride and Rosiglitazone Maleate** *see* Rosiglitazone and Metformin *on page 1858*

◆ **Metformin Hydrochloride and Saxagliptin** *see* Saxagliptin and Metformin *on page 1881*

Methacholine (meth a KOLE leen)

Brand Names: U.S. Provocholine

Brand Names: Canada Methacholine Omega; Provocholine®

Index Terms Methacholine Chloride

Pharmacologic Category Diagnostic Agent

Use Diagnosis of bronchial airway hyperactivity

Pregnancy Risk Factor C

Dosage Note: For inhalation only: Children ≥5 years and Adults:

Before inhalation challenge, perform baseline pulmonary function tests; the patient must have an FEV_1 of at least 70% of the predicted value. The following is a suggested schedule for administration of methacholine challenge. Calculate cumulative units by multiplying number of breaths by concentration given. Total cumulative units is the sum of cumulative units for each concentration given. See table.

Methacholine

Vial	Serial Concentration (mg/mL)	No. of Breaths	Cumulative Units per Concentration	Total Cumulative Units
E	0.025	5	0.125	0.125
D	0.25	5	1.25	1.375
C	2.5	5	12.5	13.88
B	10	5	50	63.88
A	25	5	125	188.88

Determine FEV_1 within 5 minutes of challenge, a positive challenge is a 20% reduction in FEV_1

Dosage adjustment in renal impairment: No dosage adjustment provided in manufacturer's labeling.

Dosage adjustment in hepatic impairment: No dosage adjustment provided in manufacturer's labeling.

Additional Information Complete prescribing information should be consulted for additional detail.

Dosage Forms Excipient information presented when available (limited, particularly for generics); consult specific product labeling.

Solution Reconstituted, Inhalation, as chloride:
Provocholine: 100 mg (1 ea)

◆ **Methacholine Chloride** *see* Methacholine *on page 1313*

◆ **Methacholine Omega (Can)** *see* Methacholine *on page 1313*

Methadone (METH a done)

Brand Names: U.S. Dolophine; Methadone HCl Intensol; Methadose; Methadose Sugar-Free

Brand Names: Canada Metadol-D™; Metadol™

Index Terms Methadone Hydrochloride

Pharmacologic Category Analgesic, Opioid

Additional Appendix Information

Opioid Conversion Table *on page 2306*

Patient Information for Disposal of Unused Medications *on page 2393*

Use Management of moderate-to-severe pain when a continuous, around-the-clock opioid analgesic is needed for an extended period of time; detoxification and maintenance treatment of opioid addiction through a certified program

Pregnancy Risk Factor C

Pregnancy Considerations Adverse events were observed in animal reproduction studies. Methadone crosses the placenta and can be detected in cord blood, amniotic fluid, and newborn urine.

Methadone is considered the standard of care when treating opioid addition in pregnant women. Women receiving methadone for the treatment of addiction should be maintained on their daily dose of methadone in addition to receiving the same pain management options during labor and delivery as opioid-naïve women; maintenance doses of methadone will not provide adequate pain relief. Narcotic agonist-antagonists should be avoided for the treatment of labor pain in women maintained on methadone due to the risk of precipitating acute withdrawal (ACOG, 2012; Dow, 2012).

Data is available related to fetal/neonatal outcomes following maternal use of methadone during pregnancy. Information collected by the Teratogen Information System is complicated by maternal use of illicit drugs, nutrition, infection, and psychosocial circumstances. However, pregnant women in methadone treatment programs are reported to have improved fetal outcomes compared to pregnant women using illicit drugs. Fetal growth, birth weight, length, and/or head circumference may be decreased in infants born to opioid-addicted mothers treated with methadone during pregnancy. Growth deficits do not appear to persist; however, decreased performance on psychometric and behavioral tests has been found to continue into childhood. Abnormal fetal nonstress tests have also been reported. Withdrawal symptoms in the neonate may be observed up to 2-4 weeks after delivery and should be expected (ACOG, 2012). Neonatal abstinence syndrome following opioid exposure may present with autonomic (eg, fever, temperature instability), gastrointestinal (eg, diarrhea, vomiting, poor feeding/weight gain), or neurologic (eg, high-pitched crying, increased muscle tone, irritability, seizure, tremor) symptoms (Dow, 2012; Hudak, 2012).

Methadone clearance in pregnant women is increased and half-life is decreased during the 2nd and 3rd trimesters of pregnancy; the dosage of methadone may need increased or dosing interval decreased during pregnancy to avoid withdrawal symptoms in the mother. Dosage may need decreased following delivery (ACOG, 2012).

Amenorrhea may develop secondary to substance abuse; pregnancy may occur following the initiation of buprenorphine maintenance treatment. Contraception counseling is recommended to prevent unplanned pregnancies (Dow, 2012).

Breast-Feeding Considerations Methadone is excreted into breast milk; the dose to a nursing infant has been calculated to be 2% to 3% of the maternal dose (following oral doses of 10-80 mg/day). Peak methadone levels appear in breast milk 4-5 hours after an oral dose. Methadone has been detected in the plasma of some breast-fed infants whose mothers are taking methadone. Sedation and respiratory depression have been reported in nursing infants. The manufacturer recommends that women monitor their nursing infants for sedation and that they should be instructed as to when to contact their healthcare provider for emergency care. In addition, the manufacturer recommends slowly weaning to prevent withdrawal symptoms in the nursing infant.

When methadone is used to treat opioid addiction in nursing women, guidelines do not contraindicate breast-feeding as long as the infant is tolerant to the dose and other contraindications do not exist (ACOG, 2012). If additional illicit substances are being abused, women treated with methadone should pump and discard breast milk until sobriety is established (ACOG, 2012; Dow, 2012).

Prescribing and Access Restrictions When used for treatment of opioid addiction: May only be dispensed in accordance to guidelines established by the Substance Abuse and Mental Health Services Administration's (SAMHSA) Center for Substance Abuse Treatment (CSAT). Regulations regarding methadone use may vary by state and/or country. Obtain advice from appropriate regulatory agencies and/or consult with pain management/palliative care specialists.

Note: Regulatory Exceptions to the General Requirement to Provide Opioid Agonist Treatment (per manufacturer's labeling):

1. During inpatient care, when the patient was admitted for any condition other than concurrent opioid addiction, to facilitate the treatment of the primary admitting diagnosis.
2. During an emergency period of no longer than 3 days while definitive care for the addiction is being sought in an appropriately licensed facility.

Medication Guide Available Yes

Contraindications Hypersensitivity to methadone or any component of the formulation; significant respiratory depression (in the absence of resuscitative equipment or in an unmonitored setting); acute or severe bronchial asthma (in the absence of resuscitative equipment or in an unmonitored setting) or hypercarbia; known or suspected paralytic ileus; concurrent use of selegiline (Ensam® product labeling)

Methadone is not to be used on an as-needed basis; it is not for pain that is mild or not expected to persist; it is not for acute pain or postoperative pain.

Warnings/Precautions The optimal analgesic dose varies widely among patients. Doses should be titrated to pain relief/prevention. Patients maintained on stable doses of methadone may need rescue doses of a immediate release analgesic in case of acute pain (eg, postoperative pain, physical trauma). Methadone is ineffective for the relief of anxiety.

[U.S. Boxed Warning]: QT_c interval prolongation and serious arrhythmias (eg, torsade de pointes) have occurred during treatment. Patients should be informed of the potential arrhythmia risk, evaluated for any history of structural heart disease, arrhythmia, syncope, and for existence of potential drug interactions including drugs that possess QT_c interval-prolonging properties, promote hypokalemia, hypomagnesemia, or hypocalcemia, or reduce elimination of methadone (eg, CYP3A4 inhibitors). Obtain baseline ECG for all patients and risk stratify according to QT_c interval; QT_c interval prolongation and torsade de pointes may be associated with doses >200 mg/day, but have also been observed with lower doses. Potentially significant drug interactions may exist, requiring dose or frequency adjustment, additional monitoring, and/or selection of alternative therapy. May cause severe hypotension; use caution with severe volume depletion or other conditions which may compromise maintenance of normal blood pressure. Use caution with cardiovascular disease or patients predisposed to dysrhythmias.

[U.S. Boxed Warning]: Fatal respiratory depression may occur with the highest risk at initiation and with dose increases. Use caution in patients with respiratory disease or pre-existing respiratory conditions (eg, severe obesity, asthma, COPD, sleep apnea, CNS depression) and kyphoscoliosis or other skeletal disorder which may alter respiratory function. Because the respiratory effects last longer than the analgesic effects, slow titration is required. Use extreme caution during treatment initiation, dose titration and conversion from other opioid agonists. Incomplete cross tolerance may occur; patients tolerant to other mu opioid agonists may not be tolerant to methadone. Abrupt cessation may precipitate withdrawal symptoms. Gradually taper dose.

After chronic maternal exposure to opioids, neonatal withdrawal syndrome may occur in the newborn; monitor neonate closely. Signs and symptoms include irritability, hyperactivity and abnormal sleep pattern, high pitched cry, tremor, vomiting, diarrhea and failure to gain weight. Onset, duration and severity depend on the drug used, duration of use, maternal dose, and rate of drug elimination by the newborn. Opioid withdrawal syndrome in the neonate, unlike in adults, may be life-threatening and should be treated according to protocols developed by neonatology experts.

May cause CNS depression, which may impair physical or mental abilities. Patients must be cautioned about performing tasks which require mental alertness (eg, operating machinery or driving). Effects with other sedative drugs or ethanol may be potentiated. Use with caution in patients with depression or suicidal tendencies, or in patients with a history of drug or ethanol abuse. Tolerance or psychological and physical dependence may occur with prolonged use. **[U.S. Boxed Warning]: Monitor for signs of misuse, abuse and addiction during therapy.**

Avoid use of methadone in patients with CNS depression or coma as these patients are susceptible to intracranial effects of CO_2 retention. Use with caution in patients with head injury or increased intracranial pressure; reduced respiratory drive and resultant CO_2 retention may increase intracranial pressure. May obscure diagnosis or clinical course of patients with acute abdominal conditions. Avoid use in gastrointestinal obstruction.

Elderly may be more susceptible to adverse effects (eg, CNS, respiratory, gastrointestinal). Decrease initial dose and use caution in the elderly or debilitated; with hyper/hypothyroidism, morbid obesity, adrenal insufficiency, prostatic hyperplasia, or urethral stricture; or with severe renal or hepatic failure. Use with caution in patients with biliary tract dysfunction including acute pancreatitis; may cause constriction of sphincter of Oddi. **[U.S. Boxed Warning]: For oral administration only;** excipients to deter use by injection are contained in tablets.

[U.S. Boxed Warning]: When used for treatment of opioid addiction: May only be dispensed by certified opioid treatment programs. Exceptions include inpatient treatment of other conditions and emergency period (not >3 days) while definitive substance abuse treatment is being sought. **[U.S. Boxed Warning]: Accidental ingestion can result in fatal overdose, especially in children. [U.S. Boxed Warning]: Should only be prescribed by healthcare professionals who are knowledgeable in the use of potent opioids for chronic pain management.**

Adverse Reactions Frequency not defined. During prolonged administration, adverse effects may decrease over several weeks; however, constipation and sweating may persist.

Cardiovascular: Arrhythmia, bigeminal rhythms, bradycardia, cardiac arrest, cardiomyopathy, ECG changes, edema, extrasystoles, faintness, flushing, heart failure, hypotension, palpitation, peripheral vasodilation, phlebitis, orthostatic hypotension, QT interval prolonged, shock, syncope, tachycardia, torsade de pointes, T-wave inversion, ventricular fibrillation, ventricular tachycardia

Central nervous system: Agitation, confusion, disorientation, dizziness, drowsiness, dysphoria, euphoria, hallucination, headache, insomnia, lightheadedness, sedation, seizure

Dermatologic: Hemorrhagic urticaria, pruritus, rash, urticaria

Endocrine & metabolic: Antidiuretic effect, amenorrhea, hypokalemia, hypomagnesemia, libido decreased

Gastrointestinal: Abdominal pain, anorexia, biliary tract spasm, constipation, glossitis, nausea, stomach cramps, vomiting, weight gain, xerostomia

Genitourinary: Impotence, urinary retention or hesitancy

Hematologic: Thrombocytopenia (reversible, reported in patients with chronic hepatitis)

Neuromuscular & skeletal: Weakness

Local: I.M./SubQ injection: Erythema, pain, swelling; I.V. injection: Hemorrhagic urticaria (rare), pruritus, urticaria, rash

Ocular: Miosis, visual disturbances

Respiratory: Pulmonary edema, respiratory depression, respiratory arrest

Miscellaneous: Death, diaphoresis, physical and psychological dependence

Drug Interactions

Metabolism/Transport Effects Substrate of CYP2B6 (major), CYP2C19 (minor), CYP2C9 (minor), CYP2D6 (minor), CYP3A4 (major); **Note:** Assignment of Major/Minor substrate status based on clinically relevant drug interaction potential; **Inhibits** CYP2D6 (moderate), CYP3A4 (weak)

Avoid Concomitant Use

Avoid concomitant use of Methadone with any of the following: Alcohol (Ethyl); Azelastine (Nasal); Conivaptan; Fusidic Acid (Systemic); Highest Risk QTc-Prolonging Agents; Itraconazole; Ivabradine; Lopinavir; Mifepristone; Paraldehyde; Posaconazole; Thioridazine

Increased Effect/Toxicity

Methadone may increase the levels/effects of: Alvimopan; Azelastine (Nasal); CNS Depressants; CYP2D6 Substrates; Desmopressin; Diuretics; Fesoterodine; Highest Risk QTc-Prolonging Agents; Hydrocodone; Lomitapide; Lopinavir; Metoprolol; Metyrosine; Mirtazapine; Moderate Risk QTc-Prolonging Agents; Nebivolol; Paraldehyde; Pramipexole; ROPINIRole; Rotigotine; Saquinavir; Selective Serotonin Reuptake Inhibitors; Thioridazine; Zidovudine; Zolpidem

The levels/effects of Methadone may be increased by: Alcohol (Ethyl); Amphetamines; Anticholinergics; Antipsychotic Agents (Phenothiazines); Aromatase Inhibitors; Boceprevir; Brimonidine (Topical); Cannabinoids; Conivaptan; CYP2B6 Inhibitors (Moderate); CYP2B6 Inhibitors (Strong); CYP3A4 Inhibitors (Moderate); CYP3A4 Inhibitors (Strong); Dasatinib; Doxylamine; Fluconazole; Fusidic Acid (Systemic); HydrOXYzine; Interferons (Alfa); Itraconazole; Ivabradine; Ivacaftor; Ketoconazole (Systemic); Luliconazole; Magnesium Sulfate; MAO Inhibitors; Mifepristone; Perampanel; Posaconazole; QTc-Prolonging Agents (Indeterminate Risk and Risk Modifying); Quazepam; Selective Serotonin Reuptake Inhibitors; Simeprevir; Sodium Oxybate; Succinylcholine; Tapentadol; Voriconazole

Decreased Effect

Methadone may decrease the levels/effects of: Codeine; Didanosine; Fosamprenavir; Lubiprostone; Pegvisomant; Tamoxifen; TraMADol

The levels/effects of Methadone may be decreased by: Ammonium Chloride; Boceprevir; Bosentan; CarBAMazepine; CYP3A4 Inducers (Strong); Dabrafenib; Darunavir; Deferasirox; Etravirine; Fosamprenavir; Fosphenytoin; Herbs (CYP3A4 Inducers); Lopinavir; Mitotane; Mixed Agonist / Antagonist Opioids; Nelfinavir; PHENobarbital; Phenytoin; Primidone; Reverse Transcriptase Inhibitors (Non-Nucleoside); Rifamycin Derivatives; Ritonavir; Saquinavir; Telaprevir; Tipranavir; Tocilizumab

Ethanol/Nutrition/Herb Interactions

Ethanol: Ethanol may increase CNS depression. Management: Avoid ethanol.

Food: Grapefruit/grapefruit juice may increase levels of methadone. Management: Avoid concurrent use of grapefruit juice.

Herb/Nutraceutical: St John's wort may decrease methadone levels and increase CNS depression; valerian, kava kava, and gotu kola may increase CNS depression. Management: Avoid St John's wort, valerian, kava kava, and gotu kola.

Storage/Stability

Injection: Store at controlled room temperature of 15°C to 30°C (59°F to 86°F). Protect from light.

Oral concentrate, oral solution, tablet: Store at controlled room temperature of 15°C to 30°C (59°F to 86°F).

Mechanism of Action Binds to opiate receptors in the CNS, causing inhibition of ascending pain pathways, altering the perception of and response to pain; produces generalized CNS depression. Methadone has also been shown to have weak N-methyl-D-aspartate (NMDA) receptor antagonism (Callahan, 2004).

Pharmacodynamics/Kinetics

Onset of action: Oral: Analgesic: 0.5-1 hour; Parenteral: 10-20 minutes

Peak effect: Parenteral: 1-2 hours; Oral: Continuous dosing: 3-5 days

Duration of analgesia: Oral: 4-8 hours (single-dose studies), increases to 22-48 hours with repeated doses; slow release from the liver and other tissues may prolong duration of action

Distribution: Lipophilic; V_{dss}: 1-8 L/kg

Protein binding: 85% to 90% primarily to alpha-1 acid glycoprotein

Metabolism: Hepatic; N-demethylation primarily via CYP3A4, CYP2B6, and CYP2C19 to inactive metabolites

Bioavailability: Oral: 36% to 100%

Half-life elimination: Terminal: 8-59 hours; may be prolonged with alkaline pH, decreased during pregnancy

Time to peak, plasma: 1-7.5 hours

Excretion: Urine (<10% as unchanged drug); increased with urine pH <6

Dosage Regulations regarding methadone use may vary by state and/or country. Obtain advice from appropriate regulatory agencies and/or consult with pain management/ palliative care specialists. **Note:** These are guidelines and do not represent the maximum doses that may be required. Consider total daily dose, potency, prior opioid use, degree of opioid experience and tolerance, conversion from previous opioid, patient's general condition, concurrent medications, and type and severity of pain during prescribing process. Other factors to consider:

- Interpatient variability in absorption, metabolism, and relative analgesic potency.
- Population-based equianalgesic conversion ratios between methadone and other opioids may not be completely accurate.
- Duration of analgesic action is much shorter than plasma elimination half-life.
- Steady-state plasma concentrations and full analgesic effects are not attained until 3-5 days after initiation.
- Methadone has a narrow therapeutic index.

Adults: **Note:** When pain management is no longer required, do not abruptly discontinue. Reduce dose every 2-4 days to prevent signs or symptoms of withdrawal. With detoxification treatment, abrupt discontinuation may lead to relapse of illicit drug use in susceptible patients.

Chronic pain (moderate-to-severe): Opioid-naive:

Oral: Initial: 2.5-10 mg every 8-12 hours; more frequent administration may be required during initiation to maintain adequate analgesia (manufacturer's labeling)

I.V.: Initial: 2.5 mg every 8-12 hours; titrate slowly to effect; may also be administered by SubQ or I.M. injection (manufacturer's labeling)

Chronic pain (CPSO, 2000; VA/DoD, 2003): Oral:

Opioid-naive:

Gradual titration (for chronic noncancer pain and situations where frequent monitoring is unnecessary): Initial: 2.5 mg every 8 hours; may increase dosing interval to every 12 hours (in about 4-5 days); may increase dose by 2.5 mg per dose every 5-7 days

Faster titration (for cancer pain and situations where frequent monitoring is possible): Initial: 2.5 mg every 6-8 hours; may increase dosing interval to every 8-12 hours (in about 4-5 days); may increase dose by 2.5 mg per dose as often as every day over about 4 days.

Opioid-tolerant: **Conversion from oral morphine to oral methadone: Note:** 1) There is not a linear relationship when converting to methadone from oral morphine. The higher the daily morphine equivalent dose the more potent methadone is, and 2) conversion to methadone is more of a process than a calculation. In general, the starting methadone dose should not exceed 30-40 mg/day, even in patients on high doses of other opioids. Patient response to methadone needs to be monitored closely throughout the process of the conversion. There are several proposed ratios for converting from oral morphine to oral methadone (Ayonrinde, 2000; Mercadente, 2001; Ripamonti, 1998). The manufacturer of Dolophine® recommends the following conversion for chronic administration:

Daily oral morphine dose <100 mg: Estimated daily oral methadone dose: 20% to 30% of total daily morphine dose

Daily oral morphine dose 100-300 mg: Estimated daily oral methadone dose: 10% to 20% of total daily morphine dose

Daily oral morphine dose 300-600 mg: Estimated daily oral methadone dose: 8% to 12% of total daily morphine dose

Daily oral morphine dose 600-1000 mg: Estimated daily oral methadone dose: 5% to 10% of total daily morphine dose.

Daily oral morphine dose >1000 mg: Estimated daily oral methadone dose: <5% of total daily morphine dose.

Note: The estimated total daily methadone dose should then be divided to reflect the intended dosing schedule (eg, divide by 3 and administer every 8 hours).

Conversion from oral methadone to parenteral methadone dose: Initial dose: Parenteral:Oral ratio: 1:2 (eg, 5 mg parenteral methadone equals 10 mg oral methadone)

Critically-ill patients (unlabeled use; Barr, 2013): **Note:** May be used to slow development of tolerance when escalation with other opioids is required. Enteral methadone has also been used to wean prolonged continuous opioid infusions (Al Qadheeb, 2012)

Oral: 10-40 mg every 6-12 hours

I.V.: 2.5-10 mg every 8-12 hours

Detoxification: Oral:

Initial: A single dose of 20-30 mg is generally sufficient to suppress symptoms. Should not exceed 30 mg; lower doses should be considered in patients with low tolerance at initiation (eg, absence of opioids ≥5 days); an additional 5-10 mg of methadone may be provided if withdrawal symptoms have not been suppressed or if symptoms reappear after 2-4 hours; total daily dose on the first day should not exceed 40 mg. Do not increase dose without waiting for steady-state to be achieved. Levels will accumulate over the first few days. Reassure the patient that duration of effect will increase as methadone accumulates.

Maintenance: Titrate to a dosage which attenuates craving, blocks euphoric effects of other opioids, and tolerance to sedative effect of methadone. Usual range: 80-120 mg/day (titration should occur cautiously)

Withdrawal: Dose reductions should be <10% of the maintenance dose, every 10-14 days

Detoxification (short-term): Oral:

Initial: Titrate to ~40 mg/day in divided doses to achieve stabilization, may continue 40 mg dose for 2-3 days

Maintenance: Titrate to a dosage which prevents/ attenuates euphoric effects of self-administered opioids, reduces drug craving, and withdrawal symptoms are prevented for 24 hours.

Withdrawal: Requires individualization. Decrease daily or every other day, keeping withdrawal symptoms tolerable; hospitalized patients may tolerate a 20% reduction/day; ambulatory patients may require a slower reduction

Dosage adjustment during pregnancy: Methadone dose may need to be increased, or the dosing interval decreased; see Pregnancy Considerations - use should be reserved for cases where the benefits clearly outweigh the risks

Dosage adjustment for toxicity:

Excessive opioid-related adverse events: Reduce next dose. Assess and reduce both the maintenance dose and dosing interval if necessary.

QT_c prolongation (Krantz, 2009):

QT_c >450-499 msecs: Monitor QT_c more frequently

QT_c ≥500 msecs: Consider discontinuation or reducing methadone dose **or** eliminate factors promoting QT_c prolongation (eg, potassium-wasting drugs) **or** use alternative therapy (eg, buprenorphine)

Dosage adjustment in renal impairment: Unlabeled dosing (Aronoff, 2007): Adults:

Cl_{cr} ≥10 mL/minute: No dosage adjustment necessary

Cl_{cr} <10 mL/minute: Administer 50% to 75% of normal dose

Dosage adjustment in hepatic impairment: No dosage adjustment provided in manufacturer's labeling; however, undergoes hepatic metabolism and systemic exposure may be increased after repeated dosing. Avoid in severe liver disease.

Administration Oral dose for detoxification and maintenance may be administered in fruit juice or water. Dispersible tablet should not be chewed or swallowed; add to liquid and allow to dissolve before administering. May rinse if residual remains. Injectable solution can be administered I.M., SubQ, or I.V.; rate of I.V. administration not defined.

Monitoring Parameters

Assess efficacy of pain control; vital signs and mental status; signs of drug abuse, addiction, or diversion

Obtain baseline ECG (evaluate QT_c interval), within 30 days of initiation, and then annually for all patients receiving methadone. Increase ECG monitoring if patient receiving >100 mg/day or if unexplained syncope or seizure occurs while on methadone (Krantz, 2009).

If before or at anytime during therapy (Krantz, 2009):

QT_c >450-499 msecs: Discuss potential risks and benefits; monitor QT_c more frequently

QT_c ≥500 msecs: Consider discontinuation or reducing methadone dose **or** eliminate factors promoting QT_c prolongation (eg, potassium-wasting drugs) **or** use alternative therapy (eg, buprenorphine)

Reference Range Prevention of opioid withdrawal: Therapeutic: 100-400 ng/mL (SI: 0.32-1.29 micromole/L); Toxic: >2 mcg/mL (SI: >6.46 micromole/L)

Test Interactions Some quinolones may produce a false-positive urine screening result for opioids using commercially-available immunoassay kits. This has been demonstrated most consistently for levofloxacin and ofloxacin, but other quinolones have shown cross-reactivity in certain assay kits. Confirmation of positive opioid screens by more specific methods should be considered.

Dosage Forms Excipient information presented when available (limited, particularly for generics); consult specific product labeling.

Concentrate, Oral, as hydrochloride:
- Methadone HCl Intensol: 10 mg/mL (30 mL) [unflavored flavor]
- Methadose: 10 mg/mL (1000 mL) [cherry flavor]
- Methadose Sugar-Free: 10 mg/mL (1000 mL) [dye free, sugar free; unflavored flavor]
- Generic: 10 mg/mL (30 mL, 1000 mL)

Solution, Injection, as hydrochloride:
- Generic: 10 mg/mL (20 mL)

Solution, Oral, as hydrochloride:
- Generic: 5 mg/5 mL (500 mL); 10 mg/5 mL (500 mL)

Tablet, Oral, as hydrochloride:
- Dolophine: 5 mg, 10 mg [scored]
- Methadose: 10 mg [scored]
- Generic: 5 mg, 10 mg

Tablet Soluble, Oral, as hydrochloride:
- Methadose: 40 mg [scored]
- Generic: 40 mg

Controlled Substance C-II

- **Methadone HCl Intensol** *see* Methadone *on page 1313*
- **Methadone Hydrochloride** *see* Methadone *on page 1313*
- **Methadose** *see* Methadone *on page 1313*
- **Methadose Sugar-Free** *see* Methadone *on page 1313*
- **Methaminodiazepoxide Hydrochloride** *see* ChlordiazePOXIDE *on page 406*

Methamphetamine (meth am FET a meen)

Brand Names: U.S. Desoxyn

Brand Names: Canada Desoxyn

Index Terms Desoxyephedrine Hydrochloride; Methamphetamine Hydrochloride

Pharmacologic Category Anorexiant; Central Nervous System Stimulant; Sympathomimetic

Use

Attention deficit disorder with hyperactivity: For a stabilizing effect in children >6 years with a behavioral syndrome characterized by the following group of developmentally inappropriate symptoms: Moderate to severe distractibility, short attention span, hyperactivity, emotional lability, and impulsivity

Exogenous obesity: Short-term (ie, a few weeks) adjunct in a regimen of weight reduction based on caloric restriction, for patients in whom obesity is refractory to alternative therapy (eg, repeated diets, group programs, other drugs)

Unlabeled Use Narcolepsy

Pregnancy Risk Factor C

Pregnancy Considerations Adverse effects have been observed in animal reproduction studies. Methamphetamine and amphetamine were detected in newborn tissues following intermittent maternal use of Desoxyn during pregnancy (Garriott, 1973). The majority of human data is based on illicit amphetamine/methamphetamine exposure and not from therapeutic maternal use (Golub, 2005). Use of amphetamines during pregnancy may lead to an increased risk of premature birth and low birth weight; newborns may experience symptoms of withdrawal. Behavioral problems may also occur later in childhood (LaGasse, 2012).

Breast-Feeding Considerations Methamphetamine is excreted in breast milk. The majority of human data is based on illicit amphetamine/methamphetamine exposure and not from therapeutic maternal use (Golub, 2005). Amphetamines may decrease milk production. Increased irritability, agitation, and crying have been reported in nursing infants (ACOG, 2011). Due to the potential for serious adverse reactions in the nursing infant, breast-feeding is not recommended by the manufacturer.

Medication Guide Available Yes

Contraindications

During or within 14 days following MAO inhibitors; glaucoma; advanced arteriosclerosis; symptomatic cardiovascular disease; moderate to severe hypertension; hyperthyroidism; hypersensitivity or idiosyncrasy to sympathomimetic amines; agitated state; patients with a history of drug abuse

Documentation of allergenic cross-reactivity for amphetamines is limited. However, because of similarities in chemical structure and/or pharmacologic actions, the possibility of cross-sensitivity cannot be ruled out with certainty.

Warnings/Precautions CNS stimulant use has been associated with serious cardiovascular events including sudden death in patients with pre-existing structural cardiac abnormalities or other serious heart problems (sudden death in children and adolescents; sudden death, stroke and MI in adults). These products should be avoided in the patients with known serious structural cardiac abnormalities, cardiomyopathy, serious heart rhythm abnormalities, or other serious cardiac problems that could increase the risk of sudden death that these conditions alone carry. Patients should be carefully evaluated for cardiac disease prior to initiation of therapy. Patients who develop angina, unexplained syncope, or other symptoms of cardiac disease during therapy should be evaluated immediately. Use with caution in patients with hypertension and other cardiovascular conditions (heart failure, recent MI, ventricular arrhythmia) that might be exacerbated by increases in blood pressure or heart rate. Use is contraindicated in patients with moderate-to-severe hypertension. Amphetamines may impair the ability to engage in potentially hazardous activities; patients must be cautioned about performing tasks which require mental alertness (eg, operating machinery or driving). Stimulants are associated with peripheral vasculopathy, including Raynaud's phenomenon; signs/symptoms are usually mild and intermittent, and generally improve with dose reduction or discontinuation. Digital ulceration and/or soft tissue breakdown have been observed rarely; monitor for digital changes during therapy and seek further evaluation (eg, rheumatology) if necessary. Difficulty in accommodation and blurred vision has been reported with the use of stimulants.

Use with caution in patients with psychiatric disorders, diabetes, or seizure disorders. May exacerbate symptoms of behavior and thought disorder in psychotic patients. May exacerbate motor and phonic tics and Tourette's syndrome. **[U.S. Boxed Warning]: Potential for drug dependency and abuse exists.** Use is contraindicated in patients with history of drug abuse. Prescriptions should be written for the smallest quantity consistent with good patient care to minimize possibility of overdose. Recommended to be used as part of a comprehensive treatment program for attention deficit disorders. Aggression and hostility has been reported with use of medications for ADHD treatment; no evidence suggests that stimulants cause aggressive behavior, but patient should be monitored for the onset or exacerbation of these behaviors. **[U.S. Boxed Warning]: Use in weight reduction programs only when alternative therapy has been ineffective.** Avoid prolonged treatment durations due to potential for drug dependence. Abrupt discontinuation following high doses or for prolonged periods may result in symptoms for withdrawal. Discontinue if satisfactory weight loss has not occurred within the first 4 weeks of treatment, or if tolerance develops.

Therapy is not appropriate for the treatment of fatigue in normal patients. Use caution in the elderly due to the risk for causing dependence, hypertension, angina, and myocardial infarction. Use of stimulants in pediatric patients has been associated with suppression of growth; monitor growth rate during treatment.

Adverse Reactions Frequency not defined.

Cardiovascular: Hypertension, palpitation, tachycardia

Central nervous system: Dizziness, dysphoria, euphoria, exacerbation of motor and phonic tics and Tourette's syndrome, headache, insomnia, overstimulation, psychosis, restlessness

Dermatologic: Rash, urticaria

Endocrine & metabolic: Change in libido

Gastrointestinal: Anorexia, constipation, diarrhea, unpleasant taste, weight loss, xerostomia

Genitourinary: Impotence

Neuromuscular & skeletal: Tremor

Miscellaneous: Suppression of growth in children, tolerance and withdrawal with prolonged use

Drug Interactions

Metabolism/Transport Effects Substrate of CYP2D6 (major); **Note:** Assignment of Major/Minor substrate status based on clinically relevant drug interaction potential

Avoid Concomitant Use

Avoid concomitant use of Methamphetamine with any of the following: Iobenguane I 123; MAO Inhibitors

Increased Effect/Toxicity

Methamphetamine may increase the levels/effects of: Analgesics (Opioid); Sympathomimetics

The levels/effects of Methamphetamine may be increased by: Abiraterone Acetate; Alkalinizing Agents; Antacids; AtoMOXetine; Cannabinoids; Carbonic Anhydrase Inhibitors; CYP2D6 Inhibitors (Moderate); CYP2D6 Inhibitors (Strong); Darunavir; MAO Inhibitors; Proton Pump Inhibitors; Tricyclic Antidepressants

Decreased Effect

Methamphetamine may decrease the levels/effects of: Antihistamines; Ethosuximide; Iobenguane I 123; Ioflupane I 123; PHENobarbital; Phenytoin

The levels/effects of Methamphetamine may be decreased by: Ammonium Chloride; Antipsychotics; Ascorbic Acid; Gastrointestinal Acidifying Agents; Lithium; Methenamine; Multivitamins/Fluoride (with ADE); Multivitamins/Minerals (with ADEK, Folate, Iron); Multivitamins/Minerals (with AE, No Iron); Peginterferon Alfa-2b; Urinary Acidifying Agents

Ethanol/Nutrition/Herb Interactions

Ethanol: Ethanol may cause CNS depression. Management: Avoid ethanol.

Food: Amphetamine serum levels may be altered if taken with acidic food, juices, or vitamin C. Management: Avoid caffeine.

Herb/Nutraceutical: Ephedra may cause hypertension or arrhythmias. Management: Avoid ephedra.

Storage/Stability Store below 30°C (86°F).

Mechanism of Action A sympathomimetic amine related to ephedrine and amphetamine with CNS stimulant activity; causes release of catecholamines (primarily dopamine and other catecholamines) from their storage sites in the presynaptic nerve terminals. Inhibits reuptake and metabolism of catecholamines through inhibition of monoamine transporters and oxidase.

Pharmacodynamics/Kinetics

Absorption: Rapid from GI tract

Metabolism: Predominately hepatic via aromatic hydroxylation, N-dealkylation and deamination; forms ≥7 metabolites

Half-life elimination: 4-5 hours

Excretion: Urine primarily (dependent on urine pH; alkaline urine increases the half-life); 62% of dose eliminated within first 24 hours as ~33% unchanged drug with remainder as metabolites

Dosage Oral:

ADHD: Children ≥6 years: Oral: Initial: 5 mg 1-2 times daily; may increase by 5 mg increments at weekly intervals until optimum response is achieved; usual effective dose range: 20-25 mg daily in 1 or 2 divided doses

Exogenous obesity: Children ≥12 years and Adults: Oral: 5 mg given 30 minutes before each meal; treatment duration should not exceed a few weeks

Dosage adjustment in renal impairment: No dosage adjustment provided in manufacturer's labeling.

Dosage adjustment in hepatic impairment: No dosage adjustment provided in manufacturer's labeling.

Dietary Considerations Most effective when combined with a low calorie diet and behavior modification counseling.

Administration For obesity, administer 30 minutes before each meal. Late evening doses should be avoided due to potential for insomnia.

Monitoring Parameters Heart rate, respiratory rate, blood pressure, CNS activity, body weight (BMI), signs of peripheral vasculopathy (eg, digital changes); growth rate in children

When used for the treatment of ADHD, thoroughly evaluate for cardiovascular risk. Monitor heart rate, blood pressure, and consider obtaining ECG prior to initiation (Vetter, 2008). Monitor for aggression and hostility.

Reference Range

Adult classification of weight by BMI (kg/m^2):

Underweight: <18.5

Normal: 18.5-24.9

Overweight: 25-29.9
Obese, class I: 30-34.9
Obese, class II: 35-39.9
Extreme obesity (class III): ≥40

Waist circumference: In adults with a BMI of 25-34.9 kg/m^2, high-risk waist circumference is defined as:
Men >102 cm (>40 in)
Women >88 cm (>35 in)

Test Interactions Amphetamines may elevate plasma corticosteroid levels; may interfere with urinary steroid determinations.

Additional Information Illicit methamphetamine may contain lead; alkalinizing urine can result in longer methamphetamine half-life and elevated blood level; ephedrine is a precursor in the illicit manufacture of methamphetamine; ephedrine is extracted by dissolving ephedrine tablets in water or alcohol (50,000 tablets can result in 1 kg of ephedrine); conversion to methamphetamine occurs at a rate of 50% to 70% of the weight of ephedrine. 3,4-methylene dioxymethamphetamine (slang: XTC, Ecstasy, Adam) affects the serotonergic, dopaminergic, and noradrenergic pathways. As such, it can cause the serotonin syndrome associated with malignant hyperthermia and rhabdomyolysis.

Dosage Forms Excipient information presented when available (limited, particularly for generics); consult specific product labeling.

Tablet, Oral, as hydrochloride:
Desoxyn: 5 mg [contains sodium aminobenzoate]
Generic: 5 mg

Controlled Substance C-II

◆ **Methamphetamine Hydrochloride** *see* Methamphetamine *on page 1317*

Methazolamide (meth a ZOE la mide)

Brand Names: U.S. Neptazane

Brand Names: Canada Apo-Methazolamide®

Pharmacologic Category Carbonic Anhydrase Inhibitor; Diuretic, Carbonic Anhydrase Inhibitor; Ophthalmic Agent, Antiglaucoma

Use Treatment of chronic open-angle or secondary glaucoma; short-term therapy of acute angle-closure glaucoma prior to surgery

Pregnancy Risk Factor C

Dosage Adults: Oral: 50-100 mg 2-3 times/day

Dosage adjustment in renal impairment: Contraindicated in marked renal dysfunction.

Dosage adjustment in hepatic impairment: Contraindicated in marked hepatic dysfunction.

Additional Information Complete prescribing information should be consulted for additional detail.

Dosage Forms Excipient information presented when available (limited, particularly for generics); consult specific product labeling.

Tablet, Oral:
Neptazane: 25 mg
Neptazane: 50 mg [scored]
Generic: 25 mg, 50 mg

Methenamine (meth EN a meen)

Brand Names: U.S. Hiprex; Urex

Brand Names: Canada Dehydral®; Hiprex®; Mandelamine®; Urasal®

Index Terms Hexamethylenetetramine; Methenamine Hippurate; Methenamine Mandelate; Urex

Pharmacologic Category Antibiotic, Miscellaneous

Use Prophylaxis or suppression of recurrent urinary tract infections; urinary tract discomfort secondary to hypermotility

Pregnancy Risk Factor C (methenamine mandelate)

Dosage Oral:

Children:
>2-6 years: *Mandelate:* 50-75 mg/kg/day in 3-4 doses or 0.25 g/30 lb 4 times/day
6-12 years:
Hippurate: 0.5-1 g twice daily
Mandelate: 50-75 mg/kg/day in 3-4 doses or 0.5 g 4 times/day

>12 years and Adults:
Hippurate: 1 g twice daily
Mandelate: 1 g 4 times/day after meals and at bedtime

Dosage adjustment in renal impairment: Contraindicated in renal insufficiency.

Dosage adjustment in hepatic impairment: Contraindicated in severe hepatic impairment.

Additional Information Complete prescribing information should be consulted for additional detail.

Dosage Forms Excipient information presented when available (limited, particularly for generics); consult specific product labeling.

Tablet, Oral, as hippurate:
Hiprex: 1 g [scored; contains tartrazine (fd&c yellow #5)]
Urex: 1 g [scored]
Generic: 1 g

Tablet, Oral, as mandelate:
Generic: 0.5 g, 1 g

Methenamine and Sodium Acid Phosphate

(meth EN a meen & SOW dee um AS id FOS fate)

Brand Names: U.S. Uroqid-Acid® No. 2

Index Terms Methenamine Mandelate and Sodium Acid Phosphate; Sodium Acid Phosphate and Methenamine

Pharmacologic Category Antibiotic, Miscellaneous

Use Prophylaxis or suppression of bacteriuria associated with recurrent urinary tract infections

Pregnancy Risk Factor C

Dosage Oral: Adults: Initial: 2 tablets 4 times daily; maintenance: 2-4 tablets daily in divided doses

Additional Information Complete prescribing information should be consulted for additional detail.

Dosage Forms Excipient information presented when available (limited, particularly for generics); consult specific product labeling.

Tablet: Methenamine mandelate 500 mg and sodium acid phosphate 500 mg [contains 83 mg sodium]

◆ **Methenamine Hippurate** *see* Methenamine *on page 1319*

◆ **Methenamine Mandelate** *see* Methenamine *on page 1319*

◆ **Methenamine Mandelate and Sodium Acid Phosphate** *see* Methenamine and Sodium Acid Phosphate *on page 1319*

Methenamine, Phenyl Salicylate, Methylene Blue, Benzoic Acid, and Hyoscyamine

(meth EN a meen, fen nil sa LIS i late, METH i leen bloo, ben ZOE ik AS id & hye oh SYE a meen)

Brand Names: U.S. Hyophen™; Prosed®/DS

Index Terms Benzoic Acid, Hyoscyamine, Methenamine, Methylene Blue, and Phenyl Salicylate; Benzoic Acid, Methenamine, Methylene Blue, Phenyl Salicylate, and Hyoscyamine; Hyoscyamine, Methenamine, Benzoic Acid, Phenyl Salicylate, and Methylene Blue; Methylene Blue, Methenamine, Benzoic Acid, Phenyl Salicylate, and

Hyoscyamine; Phenyl Salicylate, Methenamine, Methylene Blue, Benzoic Acid, and Hyoscyamine

Pharmacologic Category Antibiotic, Miscellaneous

Use Urinary tract discomfort secondary to hypermotility resulting from infection or diagnostic procedures

Pregnancy Risk Factor C

Dosage Oral:

Children >6 years: Dosage must be individualized

Adults: One tablet 4 times/day

Dosage adjustment in renal impairment: No dosage adjustment provided in manufacturer's labeling.

Dosage adjustment in hepatic impairment: No dosage adjustment provided in manufacturer's labeling.

Additional Information Complete prescribing information should be consulted for additional detail.

Dosage Forms Excipient information presented when available (limited, particularly for generics); consult specific product labeling.

Tablet, oral:

Hyophen™: Methenamine 81.6 mg, phenyl salicylate 36.2 mg, methylene blue 10.8 mg, benzoic acid 9 mg, hyoscyamine sulfate 0.12 mg

Prosed®/DS: Methenamine 81.6 mg, phenyl salicylate 36.2 mg, methylene blue 10.8 mg, benzoic acid 9 mg, hyoscyamine sulfate 0.12 mg

Methenamine, Sodium Biphosphate, Phenyl Salicylate, Methylene Blue, and Hyoscyamine

(meth EN a meen, SOW dee um bye FOS fate, fen nil sa LIS i late, METH i leen bloo, & hye oh SYE a meen)

Brand Names: U.S. Phosphasal™; Urelle®; Uribel™; Urimar-T; Uta®

Index Terms Hyoscyamine, Methenamine, Methylene Blue, Phenyl Salicylate, and Sodium Biphosphate; Hyoscyamine, Methenamine, Sodium Biphosphate, Phenyl Salicylate, and Methylene Blue; Methylene Blue, Methenamine, Sodium Biphosphate, Phenyl Salicylate, and Hyoscyamine; Phenyl Salicylate, Methenamine, Methylene Blue, Sodium Biphosphate, and Hyoscyamine; Sodium Biphosphate, Methenamine, Methylene Blue, Phenyl Salicylate, and Hyoscyamine

Pharmacologic Category Antibiotic, Miscellaneous

Use Treatment of symptoms of irritative voiding; relief of local symptoms associated with urinary tract infections; relief of urinary tract symptoms caused by diagnostic procedures

Pregnancy Risk Factor C

Pregnancy Considerations Reproduction studies have not been conducted with this combination. Methenamine and hyoscyamine cross the placenta. Refer to individual monographs.

Breast-Feeding Considerations Methenamine and hyoscyamine are excreted in breast milk. Refer to individual monographs.

Contraindications Hypersensitivity to methenamine, hyoscyamine, methylene blue, or any component of the formulation

Warnings/Precautions Use caution in patients with a history of intolerance to belladonna alkaloids or salicylates. Use caution in patients with cardiovascular disease (cardiac arrhythmias, HF, coronary heart disease, mitral stenosis), gastrointestinal tract obstruction, glaucoma, myasthenia gravis, or obstructive uropathy (bladder neck obstruction or prostatic hyperplasia). Discontinue use immediately if tachycardia, dizziness, or blurred vision occur. May cause urinary discoloration (blue). Prolonged use may result in fungal or bacterial superinfection, including *C. difficile*-associated diarrhea and pseudomembranous colitis. Avoid use in the elderly due to potent anticholinergic effects and uncertain effectiveness (Beers Criteria). Safety and efficacy have not been established in children ≤6 years of age.

Adverse Reactions Frequency not defined.

Cardiovascular: Tachycardia, flushing

Central nervous system: Dizziness

Gastrointestinal: Xerostomia, nausea, vomiting

Genitourinary: Urinary retention (acute), micturition difficulty, discoloration of urine (blue)

Ocular: Blurred vision

Respiratory: Dyspnea

Drug Interactions

Metabolism/Transport Effects Refer to individual components.

Avoid Concomitant Use

Avoid concomitant use of Methenamine, Sodium Biphosphate, Phenyl Salicylate, Methylene Blue, and Hyoscyamine with any of the following: Aclidinium; Alpha-/Beta-Agonists (Indirect-Acting); Alpha1-Agonists; Amphetamines; Anilidopiperidine Opioids; Apraclonidine; AtoMOXetine; BCG; Bezafibrate; Buprenorphine; BuPROPion; BusPIRone; CarBAMazepine; Cyclobenzaprine; Dexmethylphenidate; Dextromethorphan; Diethylpropion; Hydrocodone; HYDROmorphone; Ipratropium (Oral Inhalation); Isometheptene; Levonordefrin; Linezolid; MAO Inhibitors; Maprotiline; Meperidine; Methyldopa; Methylphenidate; Mirtazapine; Morphine (Liposomal); Morphine (Systemic); Nefazodone; Oxymorphone; Pizotifen; Potassium Chloride; Selective Serotonin Reuptake Inhibitors; Serotonin 5-HT1D Receptor Agonists; Serotonin/Norepinephrine Reuptake Inhibitors; Sulfonamide Derivatives; Tapentadol; Tetrabenazine; Tetrahydrozoline (Nasal); Tiotropium; TraZODone; Tricyclic Antidepressants; Tryptophan; Umeclidinium

Increased Effect/Toxicity

Methenamine, Sodium Biphosphate, Phenyl Salicylate, Methylene Blue, and Hyoscyamine may increase the levels/effects of: AbobotulinumtoxinA; Alpha-/Beta-Agonists (Indirect-Acting); Alpha1-Agonists; Amphetamines; Analgesics (Opioid); Anticholinergics; Antihypertensives; Antipsychotics; Apraclonidine; AtoMOXetine; Beta2-Agonists; Betahistine; Bezafibrate; Brimonidine (Ophthalmic); Brimonidine (Topical); BuPROPion; Cannabinoids; Dexmethylphenidate; Dextromethorphan; Diethylpropion; Domperidone; Doxapram; Doxylamine; EPINEPHrine (Nasal); Epinephrine (Racemic); EPINEPHrine (Systemic, Oral Inhalation); Hydrocodone; HYDROmorphone; Hypoglycemic Agents; Isometheptene; Levonordefrin; Linezolid; Lithium; Meperidine; Methadone; Methyldopa; Methylphenidate; Metoclopramide; Mirabegron; Morphine (Liposomal); Morphine (Systemic); Norepinephrine; OnabotulinumtoxinA; Orthostatic Hypotension Producing Agents; OxyCODONE; Pizotifen; Potassium Chloride; Reserpine; RimabotulinumtoxinB; Serotonin 5-HT1D Receptor Agonists; Serotonin Modulators; Sulfonamide Derivatives; Tetrahydrozoline (Nasal); Thiazide Diuretics; Tiotropium; Topiramate

The levels/effects of Methenamine, Sodium Biphosphate, Phenyl Salicylate, Methylene Blue, and Hyoscyamine may be increased by: Aclidinium; Altretamine; Anilidopiperidine Opioids; Antipsychotics; Buprenorphine; BusPIRone; CarBAMazepine; COMT Inhibitors; Cyclobenzaprine; Ipratropium (Oral Inhalation); Levodopa; MAO Inhibitors; Maprotiline; Mirtazapine; Nefazodone; Oxymorphone; Pramlintide; Selective Serotonin Reuptake Inhibitors; Serotonin/Norepinephrine Reuptake Inhibitors; Tapentadol; Tetrabenazine; TraMADol; TraZODone; Tricyclic Antidepressants; Tryptophan; Umeclidinium

Decreased Effect

Methenamine, Sodium Biphosphate, Phenyl Salicylate, Methylene Blue, and Hyoscyamine may decrease the levels/effects of: Acetylcholinesterase Inhibitors (Central); Amphetamines; BCG; Domperidone; Secretin; Sodium Picosulfate; Typhoid Vaccine

The levels/effects of Methenamine, Sodium Biphosphate, Phenyl Salicylate, Methylene Blue, and Hyoscyamine may be decreased by: Acetylcholinesterase Inhibitors (Central); Antacids; Carbonic Anhydrase Inhibitors; Domperidone

Storage/Stability Store at controlled room temperature of 15°C to 30°C (59°F to 86°F).

Dosage Oral:

Children >6 years: Dosage must be individualized

Adults: One tablet 4 times daily (followed by liberal fluid intake)

Dosage adjustment in renal impairment: No dosage adjustment provided in manufacturer's labeling.

Dosage adjustment in hepatic impairment: No dosage adjustment provided in manufacturer's labeling.

Dosage Forms Excipient information presented when available (limited, particularly for generics); consult specific product labeling.

Capsule, oral:

Uribel™: Methenamine 118 mg, sodium biphosphate 40.8 mg, phenyl salicylate 36 mg, methylene blue 10 mg, hyoscyamine sulfate 0.12 mg

Uta®: Methenamine 120 mg, sodium biphosphate 40.8 mg, phenyl salicylate 36 mg, methylene blue 10 mg, hyoscyamine sulfate 0.12 mg

Tablet, oral:

Phosphasal™: Methenamine 81.6 mg, sodium biphosphate 40.8 mg, phenyl salicylate 36.2 mg, methylene blue 10.8 mg, hyoscyamine sulfate 0.12 mg

Urelle®: Methenamine 81 mg, sodium biphosphate 40.8 mg, phenyl salicylate 32.4 mg, methylene blue 10.8 mg, hyoscyamine sulfate 0.12 mg

Urimar-T: Methenamine 120 mg, sodium biphosphate 40.8 mg, phenyl salicylate 36.2 mg, methylene blue 10.8 mg, hyoscyamine sulfate 0.12 mg

◆ Methergine® (Can) *see* Methylergonovine *on page 1333*

Methimazole (meth IM a zole)

Brand Names: U.S. Tapazole

Brand Names: Canada Dom-Methimazole; PHL-Methimazole; Tapazole®

Index Terms Thiamazole

Pharmacologic Category Antithyroid Agent; Thioamide

Use Treatment of hyperthyroidism (including preparation for radioactive iodine therapy or thyroidectomy)

Unlabeled Use Treatment of Graves' disease

Pregnancy Risk Factor D

Pregnancy Considerations Methimazole has been found to readily cross the placenta. Congenital anomalies, including esophageal atresia, choanal atresia, aplasia cutis, and iridic and retinal coloboma, have been observed in neonates born to mothers taking methimazole during pregnancy. Nonteratogenic adverse events, including fetal and neonatal hypothyroidism, have been observed following maternal methimazole use. The transfer of thyroid-stimulating immunoglobulins can stimulate the fetal thyroid *in utero* and transiently after delivery and may increase the risk of fetal or neonatal hyperthyroidism.

Uncontrolled maternal hyperthyroidism may result in adverse neonatal outcomes (eg, prematurity, low birth weight, infants born small for gestational age) and adverse maternal outcomes (eg, pre-eclampsia, congestive heart failure). To prevent adverse fetal and maternal events, normal maternal thyroid function should be maintained prior to conception and throughout pregnancy. Antithyroid treatment is recommended for the control of hyperthyroidism during pregnancy. Due to an increased risk of congenital anomalies with methimazole, propylthiouracil is considered first-line therapy, especially during the first trimester of pregnancy. The use of methimazole is an option during the second and third trimesters of pregnancy. If drug therapy is changed, maternal thyroid function should be monitored after 2 weeks and then every 2-4 weeks.

The severity of hyperthyroidism may fluctuate throughout pregnancy and may result in decreased dose requirements or discontinuation of methimazole 2-3 weeks prior to delivery.

Breast-Feeding Considerations Methimazole is excreted into human breast milk. The thyroid function and intellectual development of breast-fed infants are not affected by exposure to maternal methimazole during breast-feeding. The American Thyroid Association considers doses of methimazole <30 mg/day to be safe during breast-feeding. Methimazole should be administered after nursing and in divided doses (Stagnaro-Green, 2011).

Contraindications Hypersensitivity to methimazole or any component of the formulation

Warnings/Precautions Antithyroid agents have been associated (rarely) with significant bone marrow depression. The most severe manifestation is agranulocytosis. Aplastic anemia, thrombocytopenia, and leukopenia may also occur. Use with extreme caution in patients receiving other drugs known to cause myelosuppression (particularly agranulocytosis) and in patients >40 years of age; avoid doses ≥40 mg/day (increased myelosuppression). Monitor patients closely; discontinue if significant bone marrow suppression occurs, particularly agranulocytosis or aplastic anemia.

May cause hypoprothrombinemia and bleeding. Rare, severe hepatic reactions (hepatic necrosis, hepatitis, encephalopathy) may occur; possibly fatal. Symptoms suggestive of hepatic dysfunction should prompt evaluation. Discontinue in the presence of hepatitis (transaminase >3 times upper limit of normal). In addition, other rare hypersensitivity reactions to antithyroid agents have been reported, including the development of ANCA-positive vasculitis, drug fever, exfoliative dermatitis, glomerulonephritis, leukocytoclastic vasculitis, and a lupus-like syndrome; prompt discontinuation is warranted in patients who develop symptoms consistent with a form of autoimmunity or other hypersensitivity during therapy. Minor dermatologic reactions may not require discontinuation, depending on severity.

Adverse Reactions Frequency not defined.

Cardiovascular: ANCA-positive vasculitis, edema, leukocytoclastic vasculitis, periarteritis

Central nervous system: Drowsiness, fever, headache, neuritis, vertigo

Dermatologic: Alopecia, exfoliative dermatitis, pruritus, skin pigmentation, skin rash, urticaria

Endocrine & metabolic: Goiter, hypoglycemic coma

Gastrointestinal: Constipation, epigastric distress, loss of taste perception, nausea, salivary gland swelling, vomiting, weight gain

Hematologic: Agranulocytosis, aplastic anemia, granulocytopenia, hypoprothrombinemia, leukopenia, thrombocytopenia

Hepatic: Hepatic necrosis, hepatitis, jaundice

Neuromuscular & skeletal: Arthralgia, myalgia, paresthesia

Renal: Nephritis

Miscellaneous: Insulin autoimmune syndrome, lymphadenopathy, SLE-like syndrome

Drug Interactions

Metabolism/Transport Effects Inhibits CYP1A2 (weak), CYP2A6 (weak), CYP2B6 (weak), CYP2C19 (weak), CYP2C9 (weak), CYP2D6 (weak), CYP2E1 (weak), CYP3A4 (weak)

Avoid Concomitant Use

Avoid concomitant use of Methimazole with any of the following: CloZAPine; Pimozide; Sodium Iodide I131

Increased Effect/Toxicity

Methimazole may increase the levels/effects of: ARIPiprazole; Cardiac Glycosides; CloZAPine; Dofetilide; Lomitapide; Pimozide; Theophylline Derivatives

Decreased Effect

Methimazole may decrease the levels/effects of: Sodium Iodide I131; Vitamin K Antagonists

Storage/Stability Store at 20°C to 25°C (68°F to 77°F); excursion permitted to 15°C to 30°C (59°F to 86°F). Protect from light.

Mechanism of Action Inhibits the synthesis of thyroid hormones by blocking the oxidation of iodine in the thyroid gland. As a result, methimazole inhibits the ability of iodine to combine with tyrosine to form thyroxine and triiodothyronine (T_3); does not inactivate circulating T_4 and T_3

Pharmacodynamics/Kinetics

Onset of action: Antithyroid: Oral: 12-18 hours (Clark, 2006)

Duration: 36-72 hours (Clark, 2006)

Distribution: Concentrated in thyroid gland

Protein binding, plasma: None (Cooper, 2005)

Metabolism: Hepatic

Bioavailability: ~93%

Half-life elimination: 4-6 hours

Time to peak, serum concentration: 1-2 hours

Excretion: Urine

Dosage Oral: Administer in equally divided doses every 8 hours

Children:

Hyperthyroidism: Initial: 0.4 mg/kg/day in 3 divided doses; maintenance: 0.2 mg/kg/day in 3 divided doses

Graves' disease (unlabeled use): 0.2-0.5 mg/kg once daily (range: 0.1-1 mg/kg/day) to restore euthyroidism, then reduce dose by 50% or more and continue for a total of 1-2 years; may then discontinue or dose reduce to assess if patient is in remission. **Note:** In severe cases, initial doses that are 50% to 100% higher may be used (Bahn, 2011).

The following dosing approach may also be used (Bahn, 2011):

Infants: 1.25 mg/day

Children 1-5 years: 2.5-5 mg/day

Children 5-10 years: 5-10 mg/day

Children 10-18 years: 10-20 mg/day

Adults:

Hyperthyroidism: Initial: 15 mg/day in 3 divided doses for mild hyperthyroidism; 30-40 mg/day in 3 divided doses for moderately-severe hyperthyroidism; 60 mg/day in 3 divided doses for severe hyperthyroidism; maintenance: 5-15 mg/day (may be given as a single daily dose in many cases)

Adjust dosage as required to achieve and maintain serum T_3, T_4, and TSH levels in the normal range. An elevated T_3 may be the sole indicator of inadequate treatment. An elevated TSH indicates excessive antithyroid treatment.

Graves' disease (unlabeled use): Initial: 10-20 mg once daily to restore euthyroidism; maintenance: 5-10 mg once daily for a total of 12-18 months, then tapered or discontinued if TSH is normal at that time (Bahn, 2011)

Iodine-induced thyrotoxicosis (unlabeled use): 20-40 mg/day given either once or twice daily (Bahn, 2011)

Thyrotoxic crisis (unlabeled use): **Note:** Recommendations vary; use in combination with other specific agents. Dosages of 20-25 mg every 6 hours have been used; once stable, dosing frequency may be reduced to once or twice daily (Nayak, 2006). The American Thyroid Association and the American Association of Clinical Endocrinologists recommend 60-80 mg/day (Bahn, 2011). Rectal administration has also been described (Nabil, 1982).

Thyrotoxicosis (type I amiodarone-induced; unlabeled use): 40 mg once daily to restore euthyroidism (generally 3-6 months). **Note:** If high doses continue to be required, dividing the dose may be more effective (Bahn, 2011).

Dosage adjustment in renal impairment: No dosage adjustment provided in manufacturer's labeling.

Dosage adjustment in hepatic impairment: No dosage adjustment provided in manufacturer's labeling.

Dietary Considerations Administer with meals.

Administration Administer consistently in relation to meals every day. In thyrotoxic crisis, rectal administration has been described (Nabil, 1982).

Monitoring Parameters Monitor for signs of hypothyroidism, hyperthyroidism, T_4, T_3; CBC with differential, liver function (baseline and as needed), serum thyroxine, free thyroxine index; prothrombin time

Additional Information A potency ratio of methimazole to propylthiouracil of at least 20-30:1 is recommended when changing from one drug to another (eg, 300 mg of propylthiouracil would be roughly equivalent to 10-15 mg of methimazole) (Bahn, 2011).

Dosage Forms Excipient information presented when available (limited, particularly for generics); consult specific product labeling.

Tablet, Oral:

Tapazole: 5 mg, 10 mg [scored]

Generic: 5 mg, 10 mg

Extemporaneous Preparations Suppositories can be made from methimazole tablets; dissolve 1200 mg methimazole in 12 mL of water and add to 52 mL cocoa butter containing 2 drops of Span 80. Stir the resulting mixture to form a water-oil emulsion and pour into 2.6 mL suppository molds to cool.

Nabil N, Miner DJ, and Amatruda JM, "Methimazole: An Alternative Route of Administration," *J Clin Endo Metab*, 1982, 54(1):180-1.

◆ **Methitest** *see* MethylTESTOSTERone *on page 1344*

Methocarbamol (meth oh KAR ba mole)

Brand Names: U.S. Robaxin; Robaxin-750

Brand Names: Canada Robaxin®

Pharmacologic Category Skeletal Muscle Relaxant

Additional Appendix Information

Beers Criteria – Potentially Inappropriate Medications for Geriatrics *on page 2368*

Use Adjunctive treatment of muscle spasm associated with acute painful musculoskeletal conditions (eg, tetanus)

Pregnancy Risk Factor C

Pregnancy Considerations Animal reproduction studies have not been conducted. The manufacturer notes that fetal and congenital abnormalities have been rarely reported following *in utero* exposure. Use during pregnancy only if clearly needed.

Breast-Feeding Considerations It is not known if methocarbamol is excreted in breast milk. The manufacturer recommends that caution be exercised when administering methocarbamol to nursing women.

Contraindications Hypersensitivity to methocarbamol or any component of the formulation; renal impairment (injection formulation)

Warnings/Precautions May cause CNS depression, which may impair physical or mental abilities; patients must be cautioned about performing tasks which require mental alertness (eg, operating machinery or driving). Effects may be potentiated when used with other sedative drugs or ethanol. Plasma protein binding and clearance are decreased and the half-life is increased in patients with hepatic impairment. Muscle relaxants are poorly tolerated by the elderly due to potent anticholinergic effects, sedation, and risk of fracture. Efficacy is questionable at dosages tolerated by elderly patients; avoid use (Beers Criteria).

Injection: Contraindicated in renal impairment. Contains polyethylene glycol. Rate of injection should not exceed 3 mL/minute; solution is hypertonic; avoid extravasation. Use with caution in patients with a history of seizures. Use caution with hepatic impairment. Vial stopper contains latex. Recommended only for the treatment of tetanus in pediatric patients.

Adverse Reactions Frequency not defined.

Cardiovascular: Bradycardia, flushing, hypotension, syncope

Central nervous system: Amnesia, confusion, coordination impaired (mild), dizziness, drowsiness, fever, headache, insomnia, lightheadedness, sedation, seizures, vertigo

Dermatologic: Angioneurotic edema, pruritus, rash, urticaria

Gastrointestinal: Dyspepsia, metallic taste, nausea, vomiting

Hematologic: Leukopenia

Hepatic: Jaundice

Local: Pain at injection site, thrombophlebitis

Ocular: Blurred vision, conjunctivitis, diplopia, nystagmus

Respiratory: Nasal congestion

Miscellaneous: Hypersensitivity reactions including anaphylaxis

Drug Interactions

Metabolism/Transport Effects None known.

Avoid Concomitant Use

Avoid concomitant use of Methocarbamol with any of the following: Azelastine (Nasal); Paraldehyde

Increased Effect/Toxicity

Methocarbamol may increase the levels/effects of: Alcohol (Ethyl); Azelastine (Nasal); Buprenorphine; CNS Depressants; Hydrocodone; Methotrimeprazine; Metyrosine; Mirtazapine; Paraldehyde; Pramipexole; ROPINIRole; Rotigotine; Selective Serotonin Reuptake Inhibitors; Zolpidem

The levels/effects of Methocarbamol may be increased by: Brimonidine (Topical); Doxylamine; Droperidol; HydrOXYzine; Magnesium Sulfate; Methotrimeprazine; Perampanel; Sodium Oxybate; Tapentadol

Decreased Effect

Methocarbamol may decrease the levels/effects of: Pyridostigmine

Ethanol/Nutrition/Herb Interactions

Ethanol: May increase CNS depression; monitor for increased effects with coadministration. Caution patients about effects.

Herb/Nutraceutical: Avoid valerian, St John's wort, kava kava, gotu kola (may increase CNS depression).

Preparation for Administration Solution for injection: May administer undiluted or diluted in D_5W or NS (1 vial/ ≤250 mL diluent).

Storage/Stability

Solution for injection: Prior to dilution, store at controlled room temperature of 20°C to 25°C (68°F to 77°F); excursions permitted to 15°C to 30°C (59°F to 86°F).

Tablet: Store at controlled room temperature of 20°C to 25°C (68°F to 77°F).

Mechanism of Action Causes skeletal muscle relaxation by general CNS depression

Pharmacodynamics/Kinetics

Onset of action: Muscle relaxation: Oral: ~30 minutes

Protein binding: 46% to 50%

Metabolism: Hepatic via dealkylation and hydroxylation

Half-life elimination: 1-2 hours

Time to peak, serum: Oral: 1-2 hours

Excretion: Urine (primarily as metabolites)

Dosage

Tetanus: I.V.:

Children: Recommended **only** for use in tetanus: 15 mg/kg/dose or 500 mg/m^2/dose, may repeat every 6 hours if needed; maximum dose: 1.8 g/m^2/day for 3 days only

Adults: Initial dose: 1-2 g by direct I.V. injection, which may be followed by an additional 1-2 g by infusion (maximum initial dose: 3 g total); followed by 1-2 g every 6 hours until oral administration by mouth or via NG tube is possible; total oral daily doses of up to 24 g may be needed; injection should not be used for more than 3 consecutive days

Muscle spasm:

Oral: Children ≥16 years and Adults: 1.5 g 4 times/day for 2-3 days (up to 8 g/day may be given in severe conditions), then decrease to 4-4.5 g/day in 3-6 divided doses

I.M., I.V.: Adults: Initial: 1 g; may repeat every 8 hours if oral administration not possible; maximum dose: 3 g/ day for no more than 3 consecutive days. If condition persists, may repeat course of therapy after a drug-free interval of 48 hours.

Dosage adjustment in renal impairment: No dosage adjustment provided in manufacturer's labeling. However, administration of the parenteral formulation is contraindicated in patients with renal dysfunction due to the presence of polyethylene glycol.

Dosage adjustment in hepatic impairment: No dosage adjustment provided in manufacturer's labeling. However, elimination may be reduced in patients with cirrhosis.

Administration

Solution for injection:

I.M.: A maximum of 5 mL can be administered into each gluteal region.

I.V.: Maximum rate: 3 mL/minute; may be administered undiluted or diluted. Monitor closely for extravasation. Administer I.V. while in recumbent position. Maintain position for at least 10-15 minutes following infusion.

Tablet: May be crushed and mixed with food or liquid if needed.

Monitoring Parameters Monitor closely for extravasation (I.V. administration).

Test Interactions May cause color interference in certain screening tests for 5-HIAA using nitrosonaphthol reagent and in screening tests for urinary VMA using the Gitlow method.

Dosage Forms Excipient information presented when available (limited, particularly for generics); consult specific product labeling.

Solution, Injection:

Robaxin: 100 mg/mL (10 mL)

Tablet, Oral:

Robaxin: 500 mg [scored; contains fd&c yellow #6 (sunset yellow), saccharin sodium]

Robaxin-750: 750 mg [contains fd&c yellow #10 (quinoline yellow), fd&c yellow #6 (sunset yellow), saccharin sodium]

Generic: 500 mg, 750 mg

Methohexital (meth oh HEKS i tal)

Brand Names: U.S. Brevital Sodium
Brand Names: Canada Brevital®
Index Terms Methohexital Sodium
Pharmacologic Category Barbiturate; General Anesthetic
Use Induction of anesthesia; procedural sedation
Unlabeled Use Wada test
Pregnancy Risk Factor B
Dosage Doses must be titrated to effect.
Infants <1 month: Safety and efficacy not established.
Infants ≥1 month and Children:
Anesthesia induction:
I.M.: 6.6-10 mg/kg of a 5% solution
Rectal: Usual: 25 mg/kg of a 1% solution
I.V. (unlabeled dose): 1-2 mg/kg/dose of a 1% solution
Procedural sedation (unlabeled dose):
I.V.: Initial: 0.5 mg/kg; may repeat 0.5 mg/kg to a maximum total dose of 2 mg/kg
Rectal: 25 mg/kg of a 10% (100 mg/mL) solution given 5-15 minutes prior to procedure; maximum dose 500 mg
Adults: I.V.:
Induction: 1-1.5 mg/kg
Procedural sedation (unlabeled dose): 0.75-1 mg/kg; can redose 0.5 mg/kg every 2-5 minutes as needed (Bahn, 2005)
Wada test (unlabeled use): 3-4 mg over 3 seconds; following signs of recovery, administer a second dose of 2 mg over 2 seconds (Buchtel, 2002)
Elderly: I.V.: Refer to adult dosing. Reduce dose or administer at the low end of the dosage range.

Dosage adjustment in renal impairment: No dosage adjustment provided in manufacturer's labeling; use with caution.

Dosage adjustment in hepatic impairment: No dosage adjustment provided in manufacturer's labeling. However, adjustment may be necessary due to hepatic metabolism. Use with caution.

Additional Information Complete prescribing information should be consulted for additional detail.

Dosage Forms Excipient information presented when available (limited, particularly for generics); consult specific product labeling.
Solution Reconstituted, Injection, as sodium:
Brevital Sodium: 200 mg (1 ea); 500 mg (1 ea); 2.5 g (1 ea)

Controlled Substance C-IV

◆ Methohexital Sodium *see* Methohexital *on page 1324*

Methotrexate (meth oh TREKS ate)

Brand Names: U.S. Otrexup; Rheumatrex; Trexall
Brand Names: Canada Apo-Methotrexate; Methotrexate Injection; Metoject; ratio-Methotrexate Sodium
Index Terms Amethopterin; Methotrexate Sodium; Methotrexatum; MTX (error-prone abbreviation)
Pharmacologic Category Antineoplastic Agent, Antimetabolite (Antifolate); Antirheumatic, Disease Modifying; Immunosuppressant Agent
Use
Oncology-related uses: Acute lymphoblastic leukemia (ALL) maintenance treatment, ALL meningeal leukemia (prophylaxis and treatment); treatment of trophoblastic neoplasms (gestational choriocarcinoma, chorioadenoma destruens and hydatidiform mole), breast cancer, head and neck cancer (epidermoid), cutaneous T-Cell lymphoma (advanced mycosis fungoides), lung cancer (squamous cell and small cell), advanced non-Hodgkin's lymphomas (NHL), osteosarcoma
Nononcology uses: Treatment of psoriasis (severe, recalcitrant, disabling), severe, active rheumatoid arthritis (RA), active polyarticular-course juvenile idiopathic arthritis (pJIA)

Unlabeled Use Treatment and maintenance of remission in Crohn disease; management of ectopic pregnancy; dermatomyositis/polymyositis; treatment of bladder cancer, central nervous system tumors (including nonleukemic meningeal cancers), acute promyelocytic leukemia (maintenance treatment), soft tissue sarcoma (desmoid tumors); acute graft-versus-host disease (GVHD) prophylaxis; medical management of abortion; systemic lupus erythematosus; Takayasu arteritis

Pregnancy Risk Factor X (psoriasis, rheumatoid arthritis)

Pregnancy Considerations [U.S. Boxed Warning]: Methotrexate may cause fetal death and/or congenital abnormalities. Studies in animals and pregnant women have shown evidence of fetal abnormalities; therefore, the manufacturer classifies methotrexate as pregnancy category X (for psoriasis or RA). A pattern of congenital malformations associated with maternal methotrexate use is referred to as the aminopterin/methotrexate syndrome. Features of the syndrome include CNS, skeletal, and cardiac abnormalities. Low birth weight and developmental delay have also been reported. The use of methotrexate may impair fertility and cause menstrual irregularities or oligospermia during treatment and following therapy. Methotrexate is approved for the treatment of trophoblastic neoplasms (gestational choriocarcinoma, chorioadenoma destruens, and hydatidiform mole) and has been used for the medical management of ectopic pregnancy and the medical management of abortion. **[U.S. Boxed Warning]: Use is contraindicated for the treatment of psoriasis or RA in pregnant women.** Pregnancy should be excluded prior to therapy in women of childbearing potential. Use for the treatment of neoplastic diseases only when the potential benefit to the mother outweighs the possible risk to the fetus. Pregnancy should be avoided for ≥3 months following treatment in male patients and ≥1 ovulatory cycle in female patients. A registry is available for pregnant women exposed to autoimmune medications including methotrexate. For additional information contact the Organization of Teratology Information Specialists, OTIS Autoimmune Diseases Study, at 877-311-8972.

Breast-Feeding Considerations Low amounts of methotrexate are excreted into breast milk. Due to the potential for serious adverse reactions in a breast-feeding infant, use is contraindicated in nursing mothers.

Contraindications Known hypersensitivity to methotrexate or any component of the formulation; breast-feeding

Additional contraindications for patients with psoriasis or rheumatoid arthritis: Pregnancy, alcoholism, alcoholic liver disease or other chronic liver disease, immunodeficiency syndrome (overt or laboratory evidence); pre-existing blood dyscrasias (eg, bone marrow hypoplasia, leukopenia, thrombocytopenia, significant anemia)

Warnings/Precautions Hazardous agent - use appropriate precautions for handling and disposal (NIOSH, 2012).

[U.S. Boxed Warning]: Methotrexate has been associated with acute (elevated transaminases) and potentially fatal chronic (fibrosis, cirrhosis) hepatotoxicity. Risk is related to cumulative dose (≥1.5 g) and prolonged exposure. Monitor closely (with liver function tests, including serum albumin) for liver toxicities. Liver enzyme elevations may be noted, but may not be predictive of hepatic disease in long term treatment for psoriasis (but generally is predictive in rheumatoid arthritis [RA] treatment). With long-term use, liver biopsy may show histologic changes, fibrosis, or cirrhosis; periodic liver biopsy is recommended with long-term use for psoriasis patients with risk factors for hepatotoxicity and for persistent abnormal liver function tests in psoriasis patients without risk factors for hepatotoxicity and in RA patients; discontinue methotrexate with moderate-to-severe change in liver biopsy. Risk factors for hepatotoxicity include history of above moderate ethanol consumption, persistent abnormal liver chemistries, history of chronic liver disease (including hepatitis B or C), family history of inheritable liver disease, diabetes, obesity, hyperlipidemia, lack of folate supplementation during methotrexate therapy, cumulative methotrexate dose exceeding 1.5 g, continuous daily methotrexate dosing and history of significant exposure to hepatotoxic drugs. Use caution with pre-existing liver impairment; may require dosage reduction. Use caution when used with other hepatotoxic agents (azathioprine, retinoids, sulfasalazine). **[U.S. Boxed Warning]: Methotrexate elimination is reduced in patients with ascites and pleural effusions;** resulting in prolonged half-life and toxicity; may require dose reduction or discontinuation. Monitor closely for toxicity.

[U.S. Boxed Warning]: May cause renal damage leading to acute renal failure, especially with high-dose methotrexate; monitor renal function and methotrexate levels closely, maintain adequate hydration and urinary alkalinization. Use caution in osteosarcoma patients treated with high-dose methotrexate in combination with nephrotoxic chemotherapy (eg, cisplatin). **[U.S. Boxed Warning]: Methotrexate elimination is reduced in patients with renal impairment;** may require dose reduction or discontinuation; monitor closely for toxicity. **[U.S. Boxed Warning]: Tumor lysis syndrome may occur in patients with high tumor burden;** use appropriate prevention and treatment.

[U.S. Boxed Warning]: May cause potentially life-threatening pneumonitis (acute or chronic); may require treatment interruption; may be irreversible. Pulmonary symptoms may occur at any time during therapy and at any dosage; monitor closely for pulmonary symptoms, particularly dry, nonproductive cough. Other potential symptoms include fever, dyspnea, hypoxemia, or pulmonary infiltrate. **[U.S. Boxed Warning]: Methotrexate elimination is reduced in patients with pleural effusions;** may require dose reduction or discontinuation. Monitor closely for toxicity.

[U.S. Boxed Warning]: Bone marrow suppression may occur (sometimes fatal); aplastic anemia has been reported; anemia, pancytopenia, leukopenia, neutropenia, and/or thrombocytopenia may occur. Use caution in patients with pre-existing bone marrow suppression. Discontinue treatment (immediately) in RA or psoriasis if a significant decrease in hematologic components is noted. **[U.S. Boxed Warning]: Use of low-dose methotrexate has been associated with the development of malignant lymphomas;** may regress upon treatment discontinuation; treat lymphoma appropriately if regression is not induced by cessation of methotrexate. Discontinue methotrexate if lymphoma does not regress. Other secondary tumors have been reported.

[U.S. Boxed Warning]: Gastrointestinal toxicity may occur; diarrhea and ulcerative stomatitis may require treatment interruption; death from hemorrhagic enteritis or intestinal perforation has been reported. Use with caution in patients with peptic ulcer disease, ulcerative colitis. Doses ≥250 mg/m^2 (I.V.) are associated with moderate emetic potential; antiemetics are recommended to prevent nausea and vomiting.

May cause neurotoxicity including seizures (usually in pediatric ALL patients receiving intermediate-dose (1 g/m^2 methotrexate), leukoencephalopathy (usually with concurrent cranial irradiation) and stroke-like encephalopathy (usually with high-dose regimens). Chemical arachnoiditis (headache, back pain, nuchal rigidity, fever) and myelopathy may result from intrathecal administration. Chronic leukoencephalopathy has been reported with high-dose and with intrathecal methotrexate; may be progressive and fatal. May cause dizziness and fatigue; may affect the ability to drive or operate heavy machinery.

[U.S. Boxed Warning]: Any dose level, route of administration, or duration of therapy may cause severe and potentially fatal dermatologic reactions, including toxic epidermal necrolysis, Stevens-Johnson syndrome, exfoliative dermatitis, skin necrosis, and erythema multiforme. Recovery has been reported with treatment discontinuation. Radiation dermatitis and sunburn may be precipitated by methotrexate administration. Psoriatic lesions may be worsened by concomitant exposure to ultraviolet radiation.

Potentially significant drug-drug interactions may exist, requiring dose or frequency adjustment, additional monitoring, and/or selection of alternative therapy. **[U.S. Boxed Warning]: Concomitant administration with NSAIDs may cause severe bone marrow suppression, aplastic anemia, and GI toxicity.** Do not administer NSAIDs prior to or during high-dose methotrexate therapy; may increase and prolong serum methotrexate levels. Doses used for psoriasis may still lead to unexpected toxicities; use caution when administering NSAIDs or salicylates with lower doses of methotrexate for RA. Methotrexate may increase the levels and effects of mercaptopurine; may require dosage adjustments. Vitamins containing folate may decrease response to systemic methotrexate; folate deficiency may increase methotrexate toxicity. Concomitant use of proton pump inhibitors with methotrexate (primarily high-dose methotrexate) may elevate and prolong serum methotrexate and metabolite (hydroxymethotrexate) levels; may lead to toxicities; use with caution. Immunization may be ineffective during methotrexate treatment. Immunization with live vaccines is not recommended; cases of disseminated vaccinia infections due to live vaccines have been reported. **[U.S. Boxed Warning]: Concomitant methotrexate administration with radiotherapy may increase the risk of soft tissue necrosis and osteonecrosis.**

[U.S. Boxed Warnings]: Should be administered under the supervision of a physician experienced in the use of antimetabolite therapy; serious and fatal toxicities have occurred at all dose levels. Immune suppression may lead to potentially fatal opportunistic infections, including *Pneumocystis jirovecii* pneumonia (PCP). Use methotrexate with extreme caution in patients with an active infection (contraindicated in patients with immunodeficiency syndrome). **[U.S. Boxed Warnings]: For rheumatoid arthritis and psoriasis, immunosuppressive therapy should only be used when disease is active, severe, recalcitrant, and disabling; and where less toxic, traditional therapy is ineffective. Methotrexate formulations and/or diluents containing preservatives should not be used for intrathecal or high-dose methotrexate therapy. May cause fetal death or congenital abnormalities; do not use for psoriasis or RA treatment in pregnant women.** May cause impairment of fertility, oligospermia, and menstrual dysfunction. Toxicity from methotrexate or any immunosuppressive is increased in the elderly. Methotrexate injection may contain benzyl alcohol and should not be used in neonates. Errors have occurred (some resulting in death) when methotrexate was administered as "daily" dose instead of a "weekly" dose intended for some indications.

When used for intrathecal administration, should not be prepared during the preparation of any other agents; after preparation, store intrathecal medications in an isolated location or container clearly marked with a label identifying as "intrathecal" use only; delivery of intrathecal medications to the patient should only be with other medications intended for administration into the central nervous system (Jacobson, 2009).

Adverse Reactions Note: Adverse reactions vary by route and dosage. Hematologic and/or gastrointestinal toxicities may be common at dosages used in chemotherapy; these reactions are much less frequent when used at typical dosages for rheumatic diseases.

>10%:

Central nervous system (with intrathecal administration or very high-dose therapy):

Arachnoiditis: Acute reaction manifested as severe headache, nuchal rigidity, vomiting, and fever; may be alleviated by reducing the dose

Central nervous system toxicity (subacute): 10% of patients treated with 12-15 mg of intrathecal methotrexate may develop this in the second or third week of therapy; consists of motor paralysis of extremities, cranial nerve palsy, seizure, or coma. This has also been seen in pediatric cases receiving very high-dose I.V. methotrexate.

Demyelinating disease of the central nervous system: Seen months or years after receiving methotrexate; usually in association with cranial irradiation or other systemic chemotherapy

Dermatologic: Erythema

Endocrine & metabolic: Hyperuricemia

Gastrointestinal: Aphthous stomatitis, gingivitis, diarrhea, glossitis, intestinal perforation, mucositis (dose dependent; appears in 3-7 days after therapy, resolving within 2 weeks), nausea, vomiting

Genitourinary: Azotemia, oligospermia

Hematologic & oncologic: Bone marrow depression (nadir: 7-10 days), leukopenia, thrombocytopenia

Hepatic: Increased liver enzymes (chronic therapy)

Immunologic: Immunosuppression

Renal: Nephropathy, renal failure

Respiratory: Pharyngitis

1% to 10%:

Cardiovascular: Vasculitis

Central nervous system: Chills, dizziness, malaise

Dermatologic: Alopecia, burning sensation of skin (psoriasis), dermatitis, hyperpigmentation, hypopigmentation, pruritus, skin photosensitivity, skin rash

Endocrine & metabolic: Diabetes mellitus

Gastrointestinal: Periportal fibrosis (chronic therapy), stomatitis

Genitourinary: Cystitis

Hematologic & oncologic: Hemorrhage, pancytopenia

Hepatic: Cirrhosis (chronic therapy)

Infection: Infection

Neuromuscular & skeletal: Arthralgia

Ophthalmic: Blurred vision

Renal: Renal insufficiency: Manifested by an abrupt rise in serum creatinine and BUN and a fall in urine output; more common with high-dose methotrexate, and may be due to precipitation of the drug.

Respiratory: Pneumonitis: Associated with fever, cough, and interstitial pulmonary infiltrates; treatment is to withhold methotrexate during the acute reaction; interstitial pneumonitis has been reported to occur with an incidence of 1% in patients with RA (dose 7.5-15 mg/week)

Miscellaneous: Fever

<1% (Limited to important or life-threatening): Adult respiratory distress syndrome, agranulocytosis, anaphylactoid reaction, anaphylaxis, anorexia, arterial thrombosis, bone fracture, cardiac arrhythmia, cerebral thrombosis, cerebrovascular accident, chronic obstructive pulmonary disease (interstitial), cognitive dysfunction (has been reported at low dosage), convulsions, cryptococcosis, cytomegalovirus disease (including cytomegaloviral pneumonia, sepsis, nocardiosis), deep vein thrombosis, dysarthria, enteritis, eosinophilia, erythema multiforme, exfoliative dermatitis, gastric ulcer, gastrointestinal hemorrhage, gynecomastia, hepatic failure, hepatitis, herpes simplex infection, herpes zoster, histoplasmosis, hypogammaglobulinemia, hypotension, impotence, infertility, intestinal perforation, ischemic bowel disease (mesenteric, acute), ischemic heart disease, leukoencephalopathy (especially following craniospinal irradiation or repeated high-dose therapy; may be chronic), lymphadenopathy, lymphoma (may regress with discontinuation), lymphoproliferative disorder, myocardial infarction, nasal septum perforation, neurological signs and symptoms (at high dosages; symptoms include confusion, hemiparesis, transient blindness, and coma), neutropenia, nodule, occlusive arterial disease (acute), osteonecrosis and soft tissue necrosis (with radiotherapy), osteoporosis (with radiotherapy), pancreatitis, pericardial effusion, pericarditis, plaque erosion (psoriasis), pneumonia, pneumonia due to *Pneumocystis carinii*, proteinuria, pulmonary alveolitis, pulmonary embolism, pulmonary fibrosis, respiratory failure, retinal thrombosis, reversible posterior leukoencephalopathy syndrome, seizure (more frequent in pediatric patients with ALL), skin abnormalities related to radiation recall, skin necrosis, skin ulceration, Stevens-Johnson syndrome, supraventricular cardiac arrhythmia, syncope, telangiectasia, thromboembolism, thrombophlebitis, tissue necrosis (with radiotherapy), toxic epidermal necrolysis, tumor lysis syndrome, upper respiratory tract infection, vaccinia (disseminated; following smallpox immunization), ventricular arrhythmia

Drug Interactions

Metabolism/Transport Effects Substrate of P-glycoprotein, SLCO1B1

Avoid Concomitant Use

Avoid concomitant use of Methotrexate with any of the following: Acitretin; BCG; CloZAPine; Natalizumab; Pimecrolimus; Tacrolimus (Topical); Tofacitinib

Increased Effect/Toxicity

Methotrexate may increase the levels/effects of: CloZAPine; CycloSPORINE (Systemic); Leflunomide; Loop Diuretics; Natalizumab; Tegafur; Theophylline Derivatives; Tofacitinib; Vaccines (Live); Vitamin K Antagonists

The levels/effects of Methotrexate may be increased by: Acitretin; Alitretinoin (Systemic); Ciprofloxacin (Systemic); CycloSPORINE (Systemic); Denosumab; Eltrombopag; Loop Diuretics; Mipomersen; Nonsteroidal Anti-Inflammatory Agents; Penicillins; P-glycoprotein/ABCB1 Inhibitors; Pimecrolimus; Probenecid; Proton Pump Inhibitors; Roflumilast; Salicylates; SulfaSALAzine; Sulfonamide Derivatives; Tacrolimus (Topical); Trastuzumab; Trimethoprim

Decreased Effect

Methotrexate may decrease the levels/effects of: BCG; Cardiac Glycosides; Coccidioidin Skin Test; Fosphenytoin-Phenytoin; Loop Diuretics; Sapropterin; Sipuleucel-T; Vaccines (Inactivated); Vitamin K Antagonists

The levels/effects of Methotrexate may be decreased by: Bile Acid Sequestrants; Echinacea; P-glycoprotein/ABCB1 Inducers

Ethanol/Nutrition/Herb Interactions

Ethanol: Ethanol may be associated with increased liver injury. Management: Avoid ethanol.

Food: Methotrexate peak serum levels may be decreased if taken with food. Milk-rich foods may decrease methotrexate absorption. Folate may decrease drug response.

Herb/Nutraceutical: Echinacea has immunostimulant properties. Management: Avoid echinacea.

Preparation for Administration Hazardous agent; use appropriate precautions for handling and disposal (NIOSH, 2012). **Use preservative-free preparations for intrathecal or high-dose methotrexate administration.**

I.V.: Dilute powder with D_5W or NS to a concentration of ≤25 mg/mL (20 mg and 50 mg vials) and 50 mg/mL (1 g vial). May further dilute in D_5W or NS.

Intrathecal: Prepare intrathecal solutions with preservative-free NS, lactated Ringer's, or Elliot's B solution to a final volume of up to 12 mL (volume generally based on institution or practitioner preference). Intrathecal methotrexate concentrations may be institution specific or based on practitioner preference, generally ranging from a final concentration of 1 mg/mL (per prescribing information; Grossman, 1993; Lin, 2008) up to ~2-4 mg/mL (de Lemos, 2009; Glantz, 1999). For triple intrathecal therapy (methotrexate 12 mg/hydrocortisone 24 mg/cytarabine 36 mg), preparation to final volume of 12 mL is reported (Lin, 2008). Intrathecal medications should **NOT** be prepared during the preparation of any other agents.

Storage/Stability

Tablets: Store at room temperature of 20°C to 25°C (68°F to 77°F); excursions are permitted between 15°C and 30°C (59°F and 86°F). Protect from light.

Injection: Store intact vials and autoinjectors at room temperature 20°C to 25°C (68°F to 77°F); excursions may be permitted between 15°C and 30°C (59°F and 86°F). Protect from light.

I.V.: Solution diluted in D_5W or NS is stable for 24 hours at room temperature (21°C to 25°C). Reconstituted solutions with a preservative may be stored under refrigeration for up to 3 months, and up to 4 weeks at room temperature.

Intrathecal: Intrathecal dilutions are preservative free and should be used as soon as possible after preparation. After preparation, store intrathecal medications (until use) in an isolated location or container clearly marked with a label identifying as "intrathecal" use only.

Mechanism of Action Methotrexate is a folate antimetabolite that inhibits DNA synthesis, repair, and cellular replication. Methotrexate irreversibly binds to and inhibits dihydrofolate reductase, inhibiting the formation of reduced folates, and thymidylate synthetase, resulting in inhibition of purine and thymidylic acid synthesis, thus interfering with DNA synthesis, repair, and cellular replication. Methotrexate is cell cycle specific for the S phase of the cycle. Actively proliferative tissues are more susceptible to the effects of methotrexate.

The MOA in the treatment of rheumatoid arthritis is unknown, but may affect immune function. In psoriasis, methotrexate is thought to target rapidly proliferating epithelial cells in the skin.

In Crohn disease, it may have immune modulator and anti-inflammatory activity.

Pharmacodynamics/Kinetics

Onset of action: Antirheumatic: 3-6 weeks; additional improvement may continue longer than 12 weeks

Absorption:

Oral: Highly variable; dose dependent

I.M. injection: Complete

Distribution: Penetrates slowly into 3rd space fluids (eg, pleural effusions, ascites), exits slowly from these compartments (slower than from plasma); sustained concentrations retained in kidney and liver

V_d: I.V.: 0.18 L/kg (initial); 0.4-0.8 L/kg (steady state)

Protein binding: ~50%

Metabolism: Partially metabolized by intestinal flora (after oral administration) to DAMPA by carboxypeptidase; hepatic aldehyde oxidase converts methotrexate to 7-hydroxy methotrexate; polyglutamates are produced intracellularly and are just as potent as methotrexate; their production is dose- and duration-dependent and they are slowly eliminated by the cell once formed. Polyglutamated forms can be converted back to methotrexate.

Bioavailability: Oral: ~20% to 95%; in general, bioavailability is dose dependent and decreases as the dose increases (especially at doses >80 mg/m^2)

Half-life elimination: Low dose: 3-10 hours; High dose: 8-15 hours; Children: 1-6 hours

Time to peak, serum: Oral: 1-2 hours; I.M.: 30-60 minutes

Excretion: Dose and route dependent; I.V.: Urine (80% to 90% as unchanged drug; 5% to 7% as 7-hydroxy methotrexate); feces (<10%)

Dosage

Note: Doses between 100-500 mg/m^2 **may require** leucovorin calcium rescue. Doses >500 mg/m^2 **require** leucovorin calcium rescue: Oral, I.M., I.V.: Leucovorin calcium 10-15 mg/m^2 every 6 hours for 8 or 10 doses, starting 24 hours after the start of methotrexate infusion. Continue until the methotrexate level is ≤0.1 micromolar (10^{-7} M). Some clinicians continue leucovorin calcium until the methotrexate level is <0.05 micromolar (5 x 10^{-8} M) or 0.01 micromolar (10^{-8} M).

If the 48-hour methotrexate level is >1 micromolar (10^{-6} M) or the 72-hour methotrexate level is >0.2 micromolar (2 x 10^{-7} M): I.V., I.M, Oral: Leucovorin calcium 100 mg/m^2 every 6 hours until the methotrexate level is ≤0.1 micromolar (10^{-7} M). Some clinicians continue leucovorin calcium until the methotrexate level is <0.05 micromolar (5 x 10^{-8} M) or 0.01 micromolar (10^{-8} M).

Children:

Polyarticular juvenile idiopathic arthritis (pJIA): Oral, I.M., SubQ: Initial: 10 mg/m^2 once weekly, adjust gradually up to 20-30 mg/m^2 once weekly

Acute lymphoblastic leukemia (ALL; intrathecal therapy is also administered [refer to specific reference]):

Consolidation/intensification phases (as part of a combination regimen): 1000 mg/m^2 I.V. over 24 hours in week 1 of intensification and 20 mg/m^2 I.M. (use 50% dose reduction if on same day as intrathecal methotrexate) on day 1 of week 2 of intensification phase; Intensification repeats every 2 weeks for a total of 12 courses (Mahoney, 2000) **or** 5000 mg/m^2 I.V. over 24 hours days 8, 22, 36, and 50 of consolidation phase (Schrappe, 2000) with leucovorin rescue

Interim maintenance (as part of a combination regimen): 15 mg/m^2 orally days 0, 7, 14, 21, 28, and 35 of interim maintenance phase (Seibel, 2008) **or** 100 mg/m^2 (escalate dose by 50 mg/m^2 each dose) I.V. days 0, 10, 20, 30, and 40 of increased intensity interim maintenance phase (Seibel, 2008)

Maintenance (as part of a combination regimen): 20 mg/m^2 I.M. weekly on day 1 of weeks 25 to 130 (Mahoney, 2000) **or** 20 mg/m^2 orally days 7, 14, 21, 28, 35, 42, 49, 56, 63, 70, and 77 (Seibel, 2008)

T-cell acute lymphoblastic leukemia (Asselin, 2011; triple intrathecal therapy is also administered [refer to specific reference]):

Induction (weeks 1 to 6; as part of a combination regimen): I.V.:

Low dose: 40 mg/m^2 day 2

High dose: 500 mg/m^2 over 30 minutes followed by 4500 mg/m^2 over 23.5 hours (with leucovorin rescue) day 22

Consolidation (weeks 7 to 33; combination chemotherapy): I.V.: High dose: 500 mg/m^2/dose over 30 minutes followed by 4500 mg/m^2/dose over 23.5 hours (with leucovorin rescue) in weeks 7, 10, and 13 with leucovorin rescue

Continuation (weeks 34 to 108; combination chemotherapy): I.V., I.M.: 30 mg/m^2 weekly until 2 years after documented complete remission

ALL, CNS prophylaxis triple intrathecal therapy (unlabeled dosing): Intrathecal: Age-based dosing (in combination with cytarabine and hydrocortisone): Days of administration vary based on risk status and protocol; refer to institutional protocols or reference for details (Matloub, 2006):

<2 years: 8 mg

2 to <3 years: 10 mg

3 to ≤8 years: 12 mg

>8 years: 15 mg

Meningeal leukemia, prophylaxis or treatment: Intrathecal: 6-12 mg/dose (based on age) every 2 to 7 days; continue for 1 dose beyond CSF cell count normalization. **Note:** Optimal intrathecal chemotherapy dosing should be based on age rather than on body surface area (BSA); CSF volume correlates with age and not to BSA (Bleyer, 1983; Kerr, 2001):

<1 year: 6 mg/dose

1 year: 8 mg/dose

2 years: 10 mg/dose

≥3 years: 12 mg/dose

Osteosarcoma: I.V.: MAP regimen: 12 g/m^2 (maximum dose: 20 g) over 4 hours (followed by leucovorin rescue) for 4 doses during induction (before surgery) at weeks 3, 4, 8, and 9, and for 8 doses during maintenance (after surgery) at weeks 15, 16, 20, 21, 25, 26, 30, and 31 (in combination with doxorubicin and cisplatin) (Meyers, 2005); other combinations, intervals, and doses (8-14 g/m^2/dose) have been described (with leucovorin rescue), refer to specific reference for details (Bacci, 2000; Bacci, 2003; Goorin, 2003; Le Deley, 2007; Meyers, 1992; Weiner, 1986; Winkler, 1988)

Dermatomyositis (unlabeled use): Oral, SubQ: 15 mg/m^2 once weekly (range: 10-20 mg/m^2 once weekly; maximum dose: 25 mg/week) in combination with prednisone (Ramanan, 2005) **or** the lesser of 15 mg/m^2 or 1 mg/kg once weekly (maximum dose: 40 mg/week) in combination with corticosteroids (Huber, 2010)

Graft-versus-host disease, acute (aGVHD) prophylaxis (unlabeled use): I.V.: Refer to adult dosing.

Adults:

Acute lymphoblastic leukemia (ALL):

Meningeal leukemia prophylaxis or treatment: Intrathecal: Manufacturer's labeling: 12 mg (maximum:15 mg/dose) every 2 to 7 days; continue for 1 dose beyond CSF cell count normalization. **Note:** Optimal intrathecal chemotherapy dosing should be based on age rather than on body surface area (BSA); CSF volume correlates with age and not to BSA (Bleyer, 1983; Kerr, 2001).

Larson regimen (Larson, 1995; combination therapy):

Early intensification: Intrathecal: 15 mg day 1 of early intensification phase, repeat in 4 weeks

CNS prophylaxis/interim maintenance phase:

Intrathecal: 15 mg days 1, 8, 15, 22, and 29

Oral: 20 mg/m^2 days 36, 43, 50, 57, and 64

Prolonged maintenance: Oral: 20 mg/m^2 days 1, 8, 15, and 22 every 4 weeks for 24 months from diagnosis

Dose-intensive regimen (Kantarjian, 2000; combination therapy):

I.V.: 200 mg/m^2 over 2 hours, followed by 800 mg/m^2 over 24 hours beginning day 1, (followed by leucovorin rescue) of even numbered cycles (in combination with cytarabine; alternates with Hyper-CVAD)

CNS prophylaxis: Intrathecal: 12 mg on day 2 of each cycle; duration depends on risk

Maintenance: I.V.: 10 mg/m^2/day for 5 days every month for 2 years (in combination with prednisone, vincristine, and mercaptopurine)

Breast cancer: I.V.: CMF regimen: 40 mg/m^2 days 1 and 8 every 4 weeks (in combination with cyclophosphamide and fluorouracil) for 6-12 cycles (Bonadonna, 1995; Levine, 1998)

Choriocarcinoma, chorioadenoma, gestational trophoblastic diseases: 15-30 mg oral or I.M. daily for a 5-day course; may repeat for 3-5 courses (manufacturer's labeling) **or** 100 mg/m^2 I.V. over 30 minutes followed by 200 mg/m^2 I.V. over 12 hours (with leucovorin 24 hours after the start of methotrexate), administer a second course if hCG levels plateau for 3 consecutive weeks (Garrett, 2002)

Head and neck cancer, advanced: I.V.: 40 mg/m^2 once weekly until disease progression or unacceptable toxicity (Forastiere, 1992; Guardiola, 2004; Stewart, 2009)

Lymphoma, non-Hodgkin: I.V.:

CODOX-M/IVAC regimen (Mead, 2008): Cycles 1 and 3 of CODOX-M (CODOX-M alternates with IVAC)

Adults ≤65 years: I.V.: 300 mg/m^2 over 1 hour (on day 10) followed by 2700 mg/m^2 over 23 hours (with leucovorin rescue)

Adults >65 years: I.V.: 100 mg/m^2 over 1 hour (on day 10) followed by 900 mg/m^2 over 23 hours (with leucovorin rescue)

Hyper-CVAD alternating with high dose methotrexate/cytarabine regimen: I.V.: 1000 mg/m^2 over 24 hours on day 1 during even courses (2, 4, 6, and 8) of 21-day treatment cycles (Thomas, 2006) **or** 200 mg/m^2 bolus day 1 followed by 800 mg/m^2 over 24 hours during even courses (2, 4, 6, and 8) of 21-day treatment cycles (Khouri, 1998) with leucovorin rescue

Mycosis fungoides (cutaneous T-cell lymphoma): 5-50 mg once weekly or 15-37.5 mg twice weekly orally or I.M. for early stages (manufacturer's labeling) **or** 25 mg orally once weekly, may increase to 50 mg once weekly (Zackheim, 2003)

Osteosarcoma: Adults ≤30 years: I.V.: MAP regimen: 12 g/m^2 (maximum dose: 20 g) over 4 hours (followed by leucovorin rescue) for 4 doses during induction (before surgery) at weeks 3, 4, 8, and 9, and for 8 doses during maintenance (after surgery) at weeks 15, 16, 20, 21, 25, 26, 30, and 31 (in combination with doxorubicin and cisplatin) (Meyers, 2005); other combinations, intervals, age ranges, and doses (8-14 g/m^2/dose) have been described (with leucovorin rescue), refer to specific reference for details (Bacci, 2000; Bacci, 2003; Goorin, 2003; Le Deley, 2007; Meyers, 1992; Weiner, 1986; Winkler, 1988)

Psoriasis: **Note:** Some experts recommend concomitant folic acid 1-5 mg daily (except the day of methotrexate) to reduce hematologic, gastrointestinal, and hepatic adverse events related to methotrexate.

Oral: 2.5-5 mg/dose every 12 hours for 3 doses given weekly **or**

Oral, I.M., SubQ: 10-25 mg/dose given once weekly; titrate to lowest effective dose

Note: An initial test dose of 2.5-5 mg is recommended in patients with risk factors for hematologic toxicity or renal impairment (Kalb, 2009).

Rheumatoid arthritis: **Note:** Some experts recommend concomitant folic acid at a dose of least 5 mg per week (except the day of methotrexate) to reduce hematologic, gastrointestinal, and hepatic adverse events related to methotrexate.

Oral (manufacturer labeling): 7.5 mg once weekly or 2.5 mg every 12 hours for 3 doses per week (dosage exceeding 20 mg per week may cause a higher incidence and severity of adverse events); *alternatively,* 10-15 mg once weekly, increased by 5 mg every 2-4 weeks to a maximum of 20-30 mg once weekly has been recommended by some experts (Visser, 2009)

I.M., SubQ: 10-25 mg once weekly (dosage varies, similar to oral) or 15 mg once weekly (Braun, 2008)

Unlabeled uses:

Bladder cancer (unlabeled use): I.V.:

Dose-dense MVAC regimen: 30 mg/m^2 day 1 every 2 weeks (in combination with vinblastine, doxorubicin, and cisplatin) (Sternberg, 2001)

CMV regimen: 30 mg/m^2 days 1 and 8 every 3 weeks for 3 cycles (in combination with cisplatin, vinblastine and leucovorin rescue) (Griffiths, 2011)

CNS Lymphoma (unlabeled use): I.V.: 8000 mg/m^2 over 4 hours (followed by leucovorin rescue) every 14 days until complete response or a maximum of 8 cycles; if complete response, follow with 2 consolidation cycles at the same dose every 14 days (with leucovorin rescue), followed by 11 maintenance cycles of 8000 mg/m^2 every 28 days with leucovorin rescue (Batchelor, 2003) **or** 2500 mg/m^2 over 2-3 hours every 14 days for 5 doses (in combination with vincristine, procarbazine, intrathecal methotrexate, leucovorin, dexamethasone, and cytarabine) (De Angelis, 2002) **or** 3500 mg/m^2 over 2 hours on day 2 every 2 weeks (in combination with rituximab, vincristine, procarbazine, and leucovorin [with intra-omaya methotrexate 12 mg between days 5 and 12 of each cycle if positive CSF cytology]) for 5 to 7 induction cycles (Shah, 2007)

Crohn disease, moderate/severe, corticosteroid-dependent or refractory (unlabeled use):

Remission induction or reduction of steroid use: I.M., SubQ: 25 mg once weekly (Lichtenstein, 2009)

Remission maintenance: I.M.: 15 mg once weekly (Feagan, 2000; Lichtenstein, 2009)

Dermatomyositis/polymyositis (unlabeled uses):

Oral: Initial: 7.5-15 mg per week, often adjunctively with high-dose corticosteroid therapy; may increase in weekly 2.5 mg increments to target dose of 10-25 mg per week (**Note:** Administration of folate 5-7 mg per week has been used to reduce side effects) (Briemberg, 2003; Newman, 1995; Wiendl, 2008).

I.V., I.M.: Doses of 20-60 mg per week have been employed if failure with oral therapy (doses >50 mg per week may require leucovorin calcium rescue) (Briemberg, 2003)

Ectopic pregnancy (unlabeled use): I.M.:

Single-dose regimen: Methotrexate 50 mg/m^2 on day 1; Measure serum hCG levels on days 4 and 7; if needed, repeat dose on day 7 (Barnhart, 2009)

Two-dose regimen: Methotrexate 50 mg/m^2 on day 1; Measure serum hCG levels on day 4 and administer a second dose of methotrexate 50 mg/m^2; Measure serum hCG levels on day 7 and if needed, administer a third dose of 50 mg/m^2 (Barnhart, 2009)

Multidose regimen: Methotrexate 1 mg/kg on day 1; leucovorin calcium 0.1 mg/kg I.M. on day 2; measure serum hCG on day 2; methotrexate 1 mg/kg on day 3; leucovorin calcium 0.1 mg/kg on day 4; measure serum hCG on day 4; continue up to a total of 4 courses based on hCG concentrations (Barnhart, 2009)

Graft-versus-host disease, acute (aGVHD), prophylaxis (unlabeled use): I.V.: 15 mg/m^2/dose on day 1 and 10 mg/m^2/dose on days 3 and 6 after allogeneic transplant (in combination with cyclosporine and prednisone) (Chao, 1993; Chao, 2000; Ross, 1999) **or** 15 mg/m^2/dose on day 1 and 10 mg/m^2/dose on days 3, 6, and 11 after allogeneic transplant (in combination with cyclosporine) (Chao, 2000) **or** 15 mg/m2/dose on day 1 and 10 mg/m^2/dose on days 3, 6, and 11 after allogeneic transplant (in combination with cyclosporine, followed by leucovorin); may omit day 11 methotrexate (Ruutu, 2013)

Nonleukemic meningeal cancer (unlabeled use): Intrathecal: 12 mg/dose twice weekly for 4 weeks, then weekly for 4 doses, then monthly for 4 doses (Glantz, 1998) **or** 10 mg twice weekly for 4 weeks, then weekly for 1 month, then every 2 weeks for 2 months (Glantz, 1999) **or** 10-15 mg twice weekly for 4 weeks, then once weekly for 4 weeks, then a maintenance regimen of once a month (Chamberlain, 2010)

Soft tissue sarcoma (desmoid tumors), advanced (unlabeled use): I.V.: 30 mg/m^2 every 7-10 days (dose usually rounded to 50 mg) in combination with vinblastine for 1 year (Azzarelli, 2001)

Systemic lupus erythematosus, moderate-to-severe (unlabeled use): Oral: Initial: 7.5 mg once weekly; may increase by 2.5 mg increments weekly (maximum: 20 mg once weekly), in combination with prednisone (Fortin, 2008)

Takayasu arteritis, refractory or relapsing disease (unlabeled use): Oral: Initial dose: 0.3 mg/kg/week (maximum: 15 mg per week), titrated by 2.5 mg increments every 1-2 weeks until reaching a maximum tolerated weekly dose of 25 mg (use in combination with a corticosteroid; Hoffman, 1994)

Elderly:

Breast cancer: Patients >60 years: I.V.: CMF regimen: 30 mg/m^2 days 1 and 8 every 4 weeks (in combination with cyclophosphamide and fluorouracil) for up to 12 cycles (Bonadonna, 1995)

Meningeal leukemia: Intrathecal: Consider a dose reduction (CSF volume and turnover may decrease with age)

Non-Hodgkin lymphoma: CODOX-M/IVAC regimen (Mead, 2008): Cycles 1 and 3 of CODOX-M (CODOX-M alternates with IVAC): I.V.: 100 mg/m^2 over 1 hour (on day 10) followed by 900 mg/m^2 over 23 hours (with leucovorin rescue)

Rheumatoid arthritis/psoriasis: Oral: Initial: 5-7.5 mg per week, not to exceed 20 mg per week

Dosage adjustment for toxicity:

Nonhematologic toxicity: Diarrhea, stomatitis, or vomiting which may lead to dehydration: Discontinue until recovery

Hematologic toxicity:

Psoriasis, rheumatoid arthritis: Significant blood count decrease: Discontinue immediately.

Oncologic uses: Profound granulocytopenia and fever: Evaluate immediately; consider broad-spectrum parenteral antimicrobial coverage

Dosage adjustment in renal impairment: No dosage adjustment provided in the manufacturer's labeling. The following adjustments have been recommended:

Aronoff, 2007:

Children:

Cl_{cr} 10-50 mL/minute/1.73 m^2: Administer 50% of dose

Cl_{cr} <10 mL/minute/1.73 m^2: Administer 30% of dose

Hemodialysis: Administer 30% of dose

Continuous ambulatory peritoneal dialysis (CAPD): Administer 30% of dose

Continuous renal replacement therapy (CRRT): Administer 50% of dose

Adults:

Cl_{cr} 10-50 mL/minute: Administer 50% of dose

Cl_{cr} <10 mL/minute: Avoid use

Hemodialysis: Administer 50% of dose
Continuous renal replacement therapy (CRRT): Administer 50% of dose

Kintzel, 1995:
Cl_{cr} 46-60 mL/minute: Administer 65% of normal dose
Cl_{cr} 31-45 mL/minute: Administer 50% of normal dose
Cl_{cr} <30 mL/minute: Avoid use

Hemodialysis patients with cancer (Janus, 2010): Administer 25% of dose after hemodialysis; monitor closely for toxicity

High-dose methotrexate, dose intensive regimen for ALL (200 mg/m^2 over 2 hours, followed by 800 mg/m^2 over 24 hours with leucovorin rescue (Kantarjian, 2000):
Serum creatinine <1.5 mg/dL: No dosage adjustment necessary
Serum creatinine 1.5-2 mg/dL: Administer 75% of dose
Serum creatinine >2 mg/dL: Administer 50% of dose

Dosage adjustment in hepatic impairment: No dosage adjustment provided in the manufacturer's labeling; use with caution in patients with impaired hepatic function or pre-existing hepatic dysfunction. The following adjustments have been recommended (Floyd, 2006):
Bilirubin 3.1-5 mg/dL **or** transaminases >3 times ULN: Administer 75% of dose
Bilirubin >5 mg/dL: Avoid use

Dosing in obesity: *ASCO Guidelines for appropriate chemotherapy dosing in obese adults with cancer:* Utilize patient's actual body weight (full weight) for calculation of body surface area- or weight-based dosing, particularly when the intent of therapy is curative; manage regimen-related toxicities in the same manner as for nonobese patients; if a dose reduction is utilized due to toxicity, consider resumption of full weight-based dosing with subsequent cycles, especially if cause of toxicity (eg, hepatic or renal impairment) is resolved (Griggs, 2012).

Dietary Considerations Some products may contain sodium.

Administration Methotrexate may be administered orally, I.M., I.V., intrathecally, or SubQ; I.V. administration may be as slow push, bolus infusion, or 24-hour continuous infusion (route and rate of administration depend on indication and/or protocol; refer to specific references). Must use preservative-free formulation for intrathecal or high-dose methotrexate administration.

Specific dosing schemes vary, but high doses should be followed by leucovorin calcium to prevent toxicity; refer to Leucovorin Calcium monograph.

Otrexup is available in an autoinjector for once weekly subcutaneous use; patient may self-administer after appropriate training on preparation and administration, and with appropriate follow-up monitoring.

Hazardous agent; use appropriate precautions for handling and disposal (NIOSH, 2012).

Monitoring Parameters

Laboratory tests should be performed on day 5 or day 6 of the weekly methotrexate cycle (eg, psoriasis, RA) to detect the leukopenia nadir and to avoid elevated LFTs 1-2 days after taking dose.

Patients with psoriasis:
CBC with differential and platelets (baseline, 7-14 days after initiating therapy or dosage increase, every 2-4 weeks for first few months, then every 1-3 months); BUN and serum creatinine (baseline and every 2-3 months); consider PPD for latent TB screening (baseline); LFTs (baseline, monthly for first 6 months, then every 1-2 months); chest x-ray (baseline if underlying lung disease); pulmonary function test (if methotrexate-induced lung disease suspected)

Liver biopsy for patients **with** risk factors for hepatotoxicity: Baseline or after 2-6 months of therapy and with each 1-1.5 g cumulative dose interval

Liver biopsy for patients **without** risk factors for hepatotoxicity: If persistent elevations in 5 of 9 AST levels during a 12-month period, or decline of serum albumin below the normal range with normal nutritional status. Consider biopsy after cumulative dose of 3.5-4 g and after each additional 1.5 g.

Patients with rheumatoid arthritis and Crohn disease:
CBC with differential and platelets, serum creatinine and LFTs (baseline then every 2-4 weeks for initial 3 months of therapy, then every 8-12 weeks for 3-6 months of therapy and then every 12 weeks after 6 months of therapy); chest x-ray (baseline); pulmonary function test (if methotrexate-induced lung disease suspected); hepatitis B or C testing (baseline)

Liver biopsy: Baseline (if persistent abnormal baseline LFTs, history of alcoholism, or chronic hepatitis B or C) or during treatment if persistent LFT elevations (6 of 12 tests abnormal over 1 year or 5 of 9 results when LFTs performed at 6-week intervals)

Patients with cancer: Baseline and frequently during treatment: CBC with differential and platelets, serum creatinine, BUN, LFTs; chest x-ray (baseline); methotrexate levels and urine pH (with high-dose therapy); pulmonary function test (if methotrexate-induced lung disease suspected)

Ectopic pregnancy (unlabeled use): Prior to therapy, measure serum hCG, CBC with differential, liver function tests, serum creatinine. Serum hCG concentrations should decrease between treatment days 4 and 7. If hCG decreases by >15%, additional courses are not needed however, continue to measure hCG weekly until no longer detectable. If <15% decrease is observed, repeat dose per regimen (Barnhart, 2009).

Reference Range Therapeutic levels: Variable; Toxic concentration: Variable; therapeutic range is dependent upon therapeutic approach.

High-dose regimens produce drug levels that are between 0.1-1 micromole/L 24-72 hours after drug infusion
Toxic: Low-dose therapy: >0.2 micromole/L; high-dose therapy: >1 micromole/L

Additional Information Oncology Comment: Methotrexate overexposure: The rescue agent, glucarpidase, is an enzyme which rapidly hydrolyzes extracellular methotrexate into inactive metabolites, resulting in a rapid reduction of methotrexate concentrations. Glucarpidase is approved for the treatment of toxic plasma methotrexate concentrations (>1 micromole/L) in patients with delayed clearance due to renal impairment. Glucarpidase has also been administered intrathecally (unlabeled use/route) for inadvertent intrathecal methotrexate overexposure. Refer to Glucarpidase monograph.

Product Availability

Otrexup: FDA approved October 2013; availability anticipated in early 2014.

Otrexup is a once-weekly subcutaneous injection indicated for adults with rheumatoid arthritis or psoriasis or children with polyarticular idiopathic arthritis.

Dosage Forms Excipient information presented when available (limited, particularly for generics); consult specific product labeling.

Solution, Injection:
Generic: 25 mg/mL (2 mL, 10 mL)

Solution, Injection [preservative free]:
Generic: 25 mg/mL (2 mL, 4 mL, 8 mL, 10 mL, 40 mL); 50 mg/2 mL (2 mL); 100 mg/4 mL (4 mL); 200 mg/8 mL (8 mL); 250 mg/10 mL (10 mL); 1 g/40 mL (40 mL)

Solution Auto-injector, Subcutaneous [preservative free]:
Otrexup: 10 mg/0.4 mL (0.4 mL); 15 mg/0.4 mL (0.4 mL); 20 mg/0.4 mL (0.4 mL); 25 mg/0.4 mL (0.4 mL)
Solution Reconstituted, Injection [preservative free]:
Generic: 1 g (1 ea)
Tablet, Oral:
Rheumatrex: 2.5 mg [scored]
Trexall: 5 mg, 7.5 mg, 10 mg, 15 mg [scored]
Generic: 2.5 mg

◆ **Methotrexate Injection (Can)** *see* Methotrexate *on page 1324*

◆ **Methotrexate Sodium** *see* Methotrexate *on page 1324*

◆ **Methotrexatum** *see* Methotrexate *on page 1324*

Methoxsalen (Systemic) (meth OKS a len)

Brand Names: U.S. 8-Mop; Oxsoralen Ultra; Uvadex

Brand Names: Canada Oxsoralen Capsule; Oxsoralen-Ultra; Ultramop

Index Terms 8-Methoxypsoralen; 8-MOP; Methoxypsoralen

Pharmacologic Category Psoralen

Use

Oral: Symptomatic control of severe, recalcitrant disabling psoriasis; repigmentation of idiopathic vitiligo; palliative treatment of skin manifestations of cutaneous T-cell lymphoma (CTCL)

Extracorporeal: Palliative treatment of skin manifestations of CTCL that is unresponsive to other forms of treatment

Pregnancy Risk Factor C/D (Uvadex)

Dosage Adults: **Note:** Refer to treatment protocols for UVA exposure guidelines.

Psoriasis: Oral:

Initial: 10-70 mg 1.5-2 hours (Oxsoralen-Ultra) or 2 hours (8-MOP) before exposure to UVA light; dose may be repeated 2-3 times per week, based on UVA exposure; doses must be given at least 48 hours apart. Dosage is based upon patient's body weight and skin type:

<30 kg: 10 mg
30-50 kg: 20 mg
51-65 kg: 30 mg
66-80 kg: 40 mg
81-90 kg: 50 mg
91-115 kg: 60 mg
>115 kg: 70 mg

Note: Dosage may be increased (one time) by 10 mg after 15th treatment if minimal or no response.

Maintenance: When 95% psoriasis clearing achieved, may begin 1 treatment every week for at least 2 treatments; followed by 1 treatment every 2 weeks for at least 2 treatments; then every 3 weeks for at least 2 treatments then as needed to maintain response while minimizing UVA exposure.

Vitiligo: Oral (8-MOP): 20 mg 2-4 hours before exposure to UVA light; dose may be repeated based on erythema and tenderness of skin; do not give on 2 consecutive days

Cutaneous T-cell lymphoma (CTCL): Extracorporeal (Uvadex): Dose is determined by treatment volume; amount of Uvadex needed for each treatment may be calculated using the following equation: Treatment volume x 0.017 = mL of Uvadex needed. Inject this amount into the recirculation bag prior to the photoactivation phase using the UVAR XTS or CELLEX photopheresis system (consult user's guide).

Treatment schedule: Two consecutive days every 4 weeks for a minimum of 7 treatment cycles, may accelerate to 2 consecutive days every 2 weeks if skin score worsens (eg, increases from baseline) after assessment during the fourth treatment cycle. If skin score improves by 25% after 4 consecutive weeks of accelerated therapy, may resume regular treatment schedule. Maximum: 20 accelerated therapy cycles. There is no clinical evidence to show that treatment with methoxsalen for more than 6 months or using a different schedule provides additional benefit.

Dosage adjustment in renal impairment: No dosage adjustment provided in manufacturer's labeling.

Dosage adjustment in hepatic impairment: No dosage adjustment provided in manufacturer's labeling; use with caution.

Additional Information Complete prescribing information should be consulted for additional detail.

Dosage Forms Excipient information presented when available (limited, particularly for generics); consult specific product labeling.

Capsule, Oral:
8-Mop: 10 mg
Oxsoralen Ultra: 10 mg
Solution, Injection:
Uvadex: 20 mcg/mL (10 mL) [contains alcohol, usp, propylene glycol]

Methoxsalen (Topical) (meth OKS a len)

Brand Names: U.S. Oxsoralen

Brand Names: Canada Oxsoralen® Lotion

Index Terms Methoxypsoralen

Pharmacologic Category Psoralen

Use Repigmentation of idiopathic vitiligo

Pregnancy Risk Factor C

Dosage Topical: **Note:** Refer to treatment protocols for UVA exposure guidelines.

Children ≥12 years and Adults: Vitiligo: Lotion is applied by healthcare provider prior to UVA light exposure, usually no more than once weekly; frequency is determined by erythema response

Additional Information Complete prescribing information should be consulted for additional detail.

Dosage Forms Excipient information presented when available (limited, particularly for generics); consult specific product labeling.

Lotion, External:
Oxsoralen: 1% (29.57 mL)

◆ **Methoxypsoralen** *see* Methoxsalen (Systemic) *on page 1331*

◆ **Methoxypsoralen** *see* Methoxsalen (Topical) *on page 1331*

◆ **8-Methoxypsoralen** *see* Methoxsalen (Systemic) *on page 1331*

Methsuximide (meth SUKS i mide)

Brand Names: U.S. Celontin

Brand Names: Canada Celontin®

Pharmacologic Category Anticonvulsant, Succinimide

Use Control of absence (petit mal) seizures that are refractory to other drugs

Unlabeled Use Partial complex (psychomotor) seizures

Medication Guide Available Yes

Dosage Oral: Adults: Anticonvulsant: 300 mg/day for the first week; may increase by 300 mg/day at weekly intervals up to 1.2 g/day in 2-4 divided doses/day

Dosage adjustment in renal impairment: No dosage adjustment provided in manufacturer's labeling; use with caution.

Dosage adjustment in hepatic impairment: No dosage adjustment provided in manufacturer's labeling; use with caution.

Additional Information Complete prescribing information should be consulted for additional detail.

Dosage Forms Excipient information presented when available (limited, particularly for generics); consult specific product labeling.

Capsule, Oral:

Celontin: 300 mg

Methyclothiazide (meth i kloe THYE a zide)

Index Terms Enduron

Pharmacologic Category Antihypertensive; Diuretic, Thiazide

Use Management of hypertension; adjunctive therapy of edema

Pregnancy Risk Factor B

Dosage Adults: Oral:

Edema: 2.5-10 mg/day

Hypertension: 2.5-5 mg/day; may add another antihypertensive if 5 mg is not adequate after a trial of 8-12 weeks of therapy

Dosage adjustment in renal impairment: No dosage adjustment provided in manufacturer's labeling. However, thiazides are usually ineffective with Cl_{cr} <30 mL/minute; use with caution.

Dosage adjustment in hepatic impairment: No dosage adjustment provided in manufacturer's labeling; use with caution.

Additional Information Complete prescribing information should be consulted for additional detail.

Dosage Forms Excipient information presented when available (limited, particularly for generics); consult specific product labeling.

Tablet, Oral:

Generic: 5 mg

◆ **Methylacetoxyprogesterone** *see* MedroxyPROGESTERone *on page 1278*

Methyl Aminolevulinate
(METH il a mee noe LEV ue lin ate)

Brand Names: U.S. Metvixia

Brand Names: Canada Metvix®

Index Terms Methyl Aminolevulinate Hydrochloride; P-1202

Pharmacologic Category Photosensitizing Agent, Topical; Topical Skin Product

Use Treatment of thin and moderately thick, nonhyperkeratotic, nonpigmented actinic keratoses of the face and scalp; to be used in conjunction with red light illumination

Pregnancy Risk Factor C

Pregnancy Considerations Animal reproduction studies have not been conducted with methyl aminolevulinate cream.

Breast-Feeding Considerations It is not known if methyl aminolevulinate is excreted in breast milk. Because many drugs are secreted in human milk, caution should be exercised when Metvixia Cream is administered to a nursing mother. If methyl aminolevulinate cream is used in a nursing mother, a decision should be made whether or not to stop nursing.

Contraindications Hypersensitivity to methyl aminolevulinate or any component of the formulation, including peanut and almond oil (has not been tested in patients with peanut allergy); individuals with cutaneous photosensitivity; allergy to porphyrins

Warnings/Precautions Treatment site will become photosensitive following application of cream and for 48 hours after. Concomitant use of other known photosensitizing agents may increase the degree of photosensitivity reaction. For external use only. Should be applied by a qualified health professional. Has not been studied for >1 course of treatment (2 application sessions separated by 1 week). Has not been tested in individuals with coagulation defects (acquired or inherited), immunosuppression, porphyria, or pigmented actinic keratosis.

Adverse Reactions Pain and burning begin during illumination and generally resolve completely within a few minutes or hours, but may last up to a few days. Erythema and other signs generally resolve within a few days up to 3 weeks.

>10%: Dermatologic: Skin burning/pain/discomfort (86%; severe: 20%), erythema (63%; severe 6%), scabbing/crusting/blister/erosions (29%), itching (22%), skin or eyelid edema (18%), skin exfoliation (14%)

1% to 10%:

Dermatologic: Skin warm (4%), hyperpigmentation (2%), skin hemorrhage (2%), skin tightness (2%)

Local: Application site discharge (2%)

Postmarketing and/or case reports: Angioedema, contact dermatitis, eczema, facial edema, infection (application site), keratitis (ocular), macular edema, squamous cell carcinoma of the skin, urticaria, vitreous detachment

Drug Interactions

Metabolism/Transport Effects None known.

Avoid Concomitant Use There are no known interactions where it is recommended to avoid concomitant use.

Increased Effect/Toxicity There are no known significant interactions involving an increase in effect.

Decreased Effect There are no known significant interactions involving a decrease in effect.

Storage/Stability Store at 2°C to 8°C (36°F to 46°F). Use contents within 1 week after opening; discard if unrefrigerated for >24 hours.

Mechanism of Action Methyl aminolevulinate (prodrug) is metabolically converted to photoactive porphyrins (PAPs), which accumulate in the skin lesions resulting in photosensitization. When exposed to light of appropriate wavelength and energy, the accumulated PAPs produce a photodynamic reaction, releasing oxygen singlets which result in local cytotoxicity.

Pharmacodynamics/Kinetics Peak fluorescence intensity: 3 hours after application

Dosage Topical: Adults: Apply up to 1 g to prepared actinic keratoses, occlude for 3 hours, followed by red light illumination; repeat in 1 week. **Note:** If multiple lesions being treated, 1 g should not be exceeded for all lesions combined.

Administration Prepare lesions using a small dermal curette to remove scales and crusts and roughen the surface of the lesion. Wearing nitrile gloves (latex and vinyl gloves do not provide enough protection) and using a spatula, apply a layer of methyl aminolevulinate cream about 1 mm thick topically to prepared lesion and the surrounding 5 mm of normal skin. Multiple lesions may be treated during the same treatment session; do not exceed a treatment field area of 80 x 180 mm; do not exceed a total of 1 g (half tube) of methyl aminolevulinate cream per treatment session. Occlude the site(s) with a nonabsorbent dressing for 3 hours (minimum 2.5 hours, maximum 4 hours), then remove. Remove excess cream with saline and illuminate with red light following lamp manufacturer's instructions. Following illumination of site, the treated area should be kept covered and away from bright indoor light and sunlight from 48 hours. If, for any reason, red light illumination is not done, the cream should be removed within 4 hours (from time of initial application) and the area protected from bright indoor light or sunlight for 48 hours.

Additional Information Use in conjunction with Atkilite® CL 128 lamp.

Dosage Forms Excipient information presented when available (limited, particularly for generics); consult specific product labeling.

Cream, External:

Metvixia: 16.8% (2 g) [contains cetostearyl alcohol, edetate disodium, methylparaben, peanut oil, propylparaben]

◆ **Methyl Aminolevulinate Hydrochloride** *see* Methyl Aminolevulinate *on page 1332*

◆ **Methylcobalamin, Acetylcysteine, and Methylfolate** *see* Methylfolate, Methylcobalamin, and Acetylcysteine *on page 1335*

Methyldopa (meth il DOE pa)

Brand Names: Canada Methyldopa; Novo-Medopa

Index Terms Aldomet; Methyldopate Hydrochloride

Pharmacologic Category Alpha$_2$-Adrenergic Agonist; Antihypertensive

Additional Appendix Information

Beers Criteria – Potentially Inappropriate Medications for Geriatrics *on page 2368*

Use Management of moderate-to-severe hypertension

Pregnancy Risk Factor B/C (injectable)

Dosage

Children:

Oral: Initial: 10 mg/kg/day in 2-4 divided doses; increase every 2 days as needed to maximum dose of 65 mg/kg/day; do not exceed 3 g/day.

I.V.: 5-10 mg/kg/dose every 6-8 hours up to a total maximum daily dose of 65 mg/kg/day or 3 g/day

Adults:

Oral: Initial: 250 mg 2-3 times/day; increase every 2 days as needed (maximum dose: 3 g/day); usual dose range (JNC 7): 250-1000 mg/day in 2 divided doses. **Note:** When administered with other antihypertensives other than thiazide diuretics, limit initial daily dose of methyldopa to 500 mg/day.

I.V.: 250-500 mg every 6-8 hours; maximum dose: 1 g every 6 hours

Elderly: Initiate at the lower end of the dosage range.

Dosing adjustment in renal impairment:

No dosage adjustment provided in manufacturer's labeling; however, the following adjustments have been recommended (Aronoff, 2007):

Cl_{cr} >50 mL/minute: Administer every 8 hours.

Cl_{cr} 10-50 mL/minute: Administer every 8-12 hours.

Cl_{cr} <10 mL/minute: Administer every 12-24 hours.

Intermittent hemodialysis (administer after hemodialysis on dialysis days): Moderately dialyzable (up to 60% with a 6-hour session) (Yeh, 1970).

Peritoneal dialysis (PD): Administer every 12-24 hours.

Continuous renal replacement therapy (CRRT): Administer every 8-12 hours. **Note:** Use of antihypertensives in patients requiring CRRT is generally not recommended since CRRT is typically employed when patient cannot tolerate intermittent hemodialysis due to hypotension.

Dosing adjustment in hepatic impairment: Use is contraindicated in patients with active hepatic disease.

Additional Information Complete prescribing information should be consulted for additional detail.

Dosage Forms Excipient information presented when available (limited, particularly for generics); consult specific product labeling.

Solution, Intravenous, as hydrochloride:

Generic: 250 mg/5 mL (5 mL)

Tablet, Oral:

Generic: 250 mg, 500 mg

Dosage Forms: Canada Note: Also refer to Dosage Forms. Excipient information presented when available (limited, particularly for generics); consult specific product labeling.

Tablet, Oral: 125 mg

◆ **Methyldopate Hydrochloride** *see* Methyldopa *on page 1333*

Methylene Blue (METH i leen bloo)

Index Terms Methylthionine Chloride; Methylthioninium Chloride

Pharmacologic Category Antidote

Use Antidote for cyanide poisoning and drug-induced methemoglobinemia, indicator dye

Unlabeled Use Treatment/prevention of ifosfamide-induced encephalopathy; topically, in conjunction with polychromatic light to photoinactivate viruses such as herpes simplex; alone or in combination with vitamin C for the management of chronic urolithiasis; vasoplegia syndrome associated with cardiac surgery

Pregnancy Risk Factor X

Dosage

Children and Adults: Methemoglobinemia: I.V.: 1-2 mg/kg or 25-50 mg/m^2 over 5-10 minutes; may be repeated in 1 hour if necessary

Adults:

Ifosfamide-induced encephalopathy (unlabeled use): **Note:** Treatment may not be necessary; encephalopathy may improve spontaneously: I.V.:

Prevention: 50 mg every 6-8 hours

Treatment: 50 mg as a single dose or every 4-8 hours until symptoms resolve

Vasoplegia syndrome associated with cardiac surgery (unlabeled use): I.V.: 1.5-2 mg/kg over 20-60 minutes administered once (Levin, 2004; Leyh, 2003). **Note:** Improvement of vasoplegia (eg, increased systemic vascular resistance, reduced vasopressor dosage) has been observed 1-2 hours following methylene blue administration.

Dosage adjustment in renal impairment: No dosage adjustment provided in manufacturer's labeling. However, use with caution in severe renal impairment.

Dosage adjustment in hepatic impairment: No dosage adjustment provided in manufacturer's labeling.

Additional Information Complete prescribing information should be consulted for additional detail.

Dosage Forms Excipient information presented when available (limited, particularly for generics); consult specific product labeling.

Solution, Injection:

Generic: 1% (1 mL, 10 mL)

◆ **Methylene Blue, Methenamine, Benzoic Acid, Phenyl Salicylate, and Hyoscyamine** *see* Methenamine, Phenyl Salicylate, Methylene Blue, Benzoic Acid, and Hyoscyamine *on page 1319*

◆ **Methylene Blue, Methenamine, Sodium Biphosphate, Phenyl Salicylate, and Hyoscyamine** *see* Methenamine, Sodium Biphosphate, Phenyl Salicylate, Methylene Blue, and Hyoscyamine *on page 1320*

◆ **Methylergometrine Maleate** *see* Methylergonovine *on page 1333*

Methylergonovine (meth il er goe NOE veen)

Brand Names: Canada Methergine®

Index Terms Methylergometrine Maleate; Methylergonovine Maleate

Pharmacologic Category Ergot Derivative

Use Management of uterine atony, hemorrhage and subinvolution of the uterus following delivery of the placenta; control of uterine hemorrhage following delivery of the anterior shoulder in the second stage of labor

Pregnancy Risk Factor C

Pregnancy Considerations Animal reproduction studies have not been conducted. Methylergonovine is intended for use after delivery of the infant; use is contraindicated during pregnancy.

Breast-Feeding Considerations At normal doses used to control postpartum uterine bleeding, small amounts are excreted in breast milk. In one study, ten women were given a single dose of methylergonovine 0.5 mg once lactation was established. Simultaneous maternal milk and plasma samples were taken 1 and 2 hours later. Maximum milk concentrations were 410-830 pg/mL, 2-3 hours after the dose and declined to 0.2 pg/mL (median) at 5 hours. The mean M/P ratios were 0.18 (at 1 hour) and 0.17 (at 2 hours) (Vogel, 2004). Methylergonovine may decrease breast milk production. Some manufacturers do not recommend breast-feeding during therapy or for 12 hours after the last dose due to adverse reactions reported in breast-feeding infants.

Contraindications Hypersensitivity to methylergonovine or any component of the formulation; hypertension; toxemia; pregnancy

Warnings/Precautions Hazardous agent - use appropriate precautions for handling and disposal (NIOSH, 2012). Use caution in patients with sepsis, obliterative vascular disease, cardiovascular disease, hepatic or renal involvement, or second stage of labor; administer with extreme caution if using intravenously. Patients with coronary artery disease (CAD) or risk factors for CAD may be more likely to develop myocardial ischemia and infarction following methylergonovine-induced vasospasm. Pleural and peritoneal fibrosis have been reported with prolonged daily use of other ergot alkaloids. Ergot alkaloid use may result in ergotism (intense vasoconstriction) resulting in peripheral vascular ischemia and possible gangrene. Concomitant use with potent inhibitors of CYP3A4 (includes protease inhibitors, azole antifungals, and some macrolide antibiotics) and ergot alkaloids has been associated with acute ergot toxicity (ergotism); concurrent use of certain ergot alkaloids (eg, ergotamine and dihydroergotamine) are not recommended by the manufacturer. Not for routine I.V. administration due to risk of inducing sudden hypertensive and cerebrovascular accidents. I.V. administration should only be considered during life-threatening situations. Inadvertent administration to newborns has been reported.

Adverse Reactions Frequency not defined.

Cardiovascular: Acute MI, angina pectoris, arterial spasm, atrioventricular block, bradycardia, cerebrovascular accident, chest pain, hyper-/hypotension, palpitation, tachycardia, vasospasm, ventricular fibrillation

Central nervous system: Dizziness, hallucinations, headache, seizure

Dermatologic: Rash

Endocrine & metabolic: Water intoxication

Gastrointestinal: Abdominal pain, diarrhea, foul taste, nausea, vomiting

Local: Thrombophlebitis

Neuromuscular & skeletal: Leg cramps, paresthesia

Otic: Tinnitus

Renal: Hematuria

Respiratory: Dyspnea, nasal congestion

Miscellaneous: Anaphylaxis, diaphoresis

Drug Interactions

Metabolism/Transport Effects Substrate of CYP3A4 (major); **Note:** Assignment of Major/Minor substrate status based on clinically relevant drug interaction potential

Avoid Concomitant Use

Avoid concomitant use of Methylergonovine with any of the following: Alpha-/Beta-Agonists; Alpha1-Agonists; Boceprevir; Cobicistat; Conivaptan; Efavirenz; Fusidic Acid (Systemic); Itraconazole; Ketoconazole (Systemic); Lorcaserin; Nitroglycerin; Posaconazole; Protease Inhibitors; Serotonin 5-HT1D Receptor Agonists; Telaprevir; Voriconazole

Increased Effect/Toxicity

Methylergonovine may increase the levels/effects of: Alpha-/Beta-Agonists; Alpha1-Agonists; Antipsychotics; Metoclopramide; Serotonin 5-HT1D Receptor Agonists; Serotonin Modulators

The levels/effects of Methylergonovine may be increased by: Antipsychotics; Beta-Blockers; Boceprevir; Cobicistat; Conivaptan; CYP3A4 Inhibitors (Moderate); CYP3A4 Inhibitors (Strong); Dasatinib; Efavirenz; Fusidic Acid (Systemic); Itraconazole; Ivacaftor; Ketoconazole (Systemic); Lorcaserin; Luliconazole; Macrolide Antibiotics; Mifepristone; Nitroglycerin; Posaconazole; Protease Inhibitors; Serotonin 5-HT1D Receptor Agonists; Simeprevir; Telaprevir; Voriconazole

Decreased Effect

Methylergonovine may decrease the levels/effects of: Nitroglycerin

Storage/Stability

Injection: Store under refrigeration at 2°C to 8°C (36°F to 46°F). Protect from light. The following stability information has also been reported: May be stored at room temperature for up to 14 days (Cohen, 2007).

Tablet: Store below 25°C (77°F).

Mechanism of Action Increases the tone, rate and amplitude of contractions on the smooth muscles of the uterus, producing sustained contractions which shortens the third stage of labor and reduces blood loss.

Pharmacodynamics/Kinetics

Onset of action: Oxytocic: Oral: 5-10 minutes; I.M.: 2-5 minutes; I.V.: Immediately

Duration: Oral: ~3 hours; I.M.: ~3 hours; I.V.: 45 minutes

Absorption: Rapid

Distribution: V_d: 39-73 L

Metabolism: Hepatic

Bioavailability: Oral: 60%; I.M.: 78%

Half-life elimination: ~3 hours (range: 1.5-12.7 hours)

Time to peak, serum: Oral: 0.3-2 hours; I.M.: 0.2-0.6 hours

Excretion: Urine and feces

Dosage Adults:

Oral: 0.2 mg 3-4 times daily in the puerperium for up to 7 days (maximum duration: 1 week)

I.M., I.V.: 0.2 mg after delivery of anterior shoulder, after delivery of placenta, or during puerperium; may be repeated every 2-4 hours as needed. **Note:** I.V. administration should only be considered during life-threatening situations.

Dosage adjustment in renal impairment: No dosage adjustment provided in manufacturer's labeling; use with caution.

Dosage adjustment in hepatic impairment: No dosage adjustment provided in manufacturer's labeling; use with caution.

Administration

I.V.: Administer over ≥60 seconds. Should not be routinely administered I.V. because of possibility of inducing sudden hypertension and cerebrovascular accident. I.V. administration should only be considered during life-threatening situations.

I.M.: May be administered intramuscularly.

Oral: Available in tablets for oral administration.

Hazardous agent; use appropriate precautions for handling and disposal (NIOSH, 2012).

Monitoring Parameters Blood pressure

Dosage Forms Excipient information presented when available (limited, particularly for generics); consult specific product labeling.

Solution, Injection, as maleate:
  Generic: 0.2 mg/mL (1 mL)
Solution, Injection, as maleate [preservative free]:
  Generic: 0.2 mg/mL (1 mL)
Tablet, Oral, as maleate:
  Generic: 0.2 mg

◆ **Methylergonovine Maleate** *see* Methylergonovine *on page 1333*

Methylfolate, Methylcobalamin, and Acetylcysteine

(meth il FO late meth il koe BAL a min & a se teel SIS teen)

Brand Names: U.S. Cerefolin® NAC; Metafolbic Plus; Metafolbic Plus RF

Index Terms Acetylcysteine, Methylcobalamin, and Methylfolate; Acetylcysteine, Methylfolate, and Methylcobalamin; L-methylfolate, Methylcobalamin, and N-acetylcysteine; Methylcobalamin, Acetylcysteine, and Methylfolate

Pharmacologic Category Dietary Supplement

Use Medicinal food for use in patients with neurovascular oxidative stress and/or hyperhomocysteinemia

Dosage Oral: Children ≥12 years and Adults: One tablet daily

Additional Information Complete prescribing information should be consulted for additional detail.

Dosage Forms Excipient information presented when available (limited, particularly for generics); consult specific product labeling.

Tablet, oral:
  Cerefolin® NAC: L-methylfolate 6 mg, methylcobalamin 2 mg, N-acetylcysteine 600 mg, and Schizochytrium algae [contains soy; gluten free, lactose free, yeast free]
  Metafolbic Plus: L-methylfolate 6 mg, methylcobalamin 2 mg, and N-acetylcysteine 600 mg [gluten free, lactose free, sugar free, yeast free]
  Metafolbic Plus RF: L-methylfolate 6 mg, methylcobalamin 2 mg, N-acetylcysteine 600 mg, and Schizochytrium algae [contains soy; gluten free, yeast free]

◆ **Methylin** *see* Methylphenidate *on page 1336*

◆ **Methylmorphine** *see* Codeine *on page 482*

Methylnaltrexone (meth il nal TREKS one)

Brand Names: U.S. Relistor

Brand Names: Canada Relistor

Index Terms Methylnaltrexone Bromide; N-methylnaltrexone Bromide

Pharmacologic Category Gastrointestinal Agent, Miscellaneous; Opioid Antagonist, Peripherally-Acting

Use **Opioid-induced constipation:** Treatment of opioid-induced constipation in patients with advanced illness (receiving palliative care) who have an inadequate response to conventional laxative regimens

Pregnancy Risk Factor B

Pregnancy Considerations Adverse effects were not observed in animal reproduction studies.

Breast-Feeding Considerations It is not known if methylnaltrexone is excreted in breast milk. The manufacturer recommends that caution be exercised when administering methylnaltrexone to nursing women.

Contraindications

Known or suspected mechanical gastrointestinal obstruction.

Canadian labeling: Additional contraindications (not in U.S. labeling): Hypersensitivity to methylnaltrexone or any component of the formulation

Warnings/Precautions Discontinue treatment for severe or persistent diarrhea. Gastrointestinal perforation of the colon, duodenum, and stomach has been reported in patients with advanced illnesses associated with impaired structural integrity of the GI wall (eg, cancer, Ogilvie's syndrome, peptic ulcer). Use caution in patients with known or history of GI tract lesions; discontinue therapy if persistent, severe, or worsening abdominal symptoms occur. Use with caution in patients with renal impairment; dosage adjustment recommended for severe renal impairment (Cl_{cr} <30 mL/minute). Has not been studied in patients with end-stage renal impairment requiring dialysis. Discontinue methylnaltrexone if opioids are discontinued. Use beyond 4 months has not been studied.

Adverse Reactions

>10%: Gastrointestinal: Abdominal pain (29%), flatulence (13%), nausea (12%)

1% to 10%:
  Central nervous system: Dizziness (7%)
  Dermatologic: Hyperhidrosis (7%)
  Gastrointestinal: Diarrhea (6%)

<1% (Limited to important or life-threatening): Abdominal cramps, gastrointestinal perforation, increased body temperature, opioid withdrawal syndrome, muscle spasm, syncope

Drug Interactions

Metabolism/Transport Effects **Substrate** of CYP2D6 (minor); **Note:** Assignment of Major/Minor substrate status based on clinically relevant drug interaction potential

Avoid Concomitant Use There are no known interactions where it is recommended to avoid concomitant use.

Increased Effect/Toxicity There are no known significant interactions involving an increase in effect.

Decreased Effect

The levels/effects of Methylnaltrexone may be decreased by: Peginterferon Alfa-2b

Storage/Stability Store intact vials and prefilled syringes between 20°C and 25°C (68°F and 77°F); excursions are permitted between 15°C and 30°C (59°F and 86°F). Do not freeze. Protect from light. Solution withdrawn from the single use vial is stable in a syringe for 24 hours at room temperature.

Mechanism of Action An opioid receptor antagonist which blocks opioid binding at the mu receptor, methylnaltrexone is a quaternary derivative of naltrexone with restricted ability to cross the blood-brain barrier. It therefore functions as a peripheral acting opioid antagonist, including actions on the gastrointestinal tract to inhibit opioid-induced decreased gastrointestinal motility and delay in gastrointestinal transit time, thereby decreasing opioid-induced constipation. Does not affect opioid analgesic effects.

Pharmacodynamics/Kinetics

Onset of action: Usually within 30-60 minutes (in responding patients)
Absorption: SubQ: Rapid
Distribution: V_{dss}: ~1.1 L/kg
Protein binding: 11% to 15%
Metabolism: Metabolized to methyl-6-naltrexol isomers, methylnaltrexone sulfate, and other minor metabolites
Half-life elimination: Terminal: ~8 hours
Time to peak, plasma: SubQ: 30 minutes
Excretion: Urine (~54%, primarily as unchanged drug); feces (~17%, primarily as unchanged drug)

Dosage Opioid-induced constipation: Adults: SubQ: Dosing is according to body weight: Administer 1 dose every other day as needed; maximum: 1 dose/24 hours

<38 kg: 0.15 mg/kg (round dose up to nearest 0.1 mL of volume)
38 to <62 kg: 8 mg
62-114 kg: 12 mg
>114 kg: 0.15 mg/kg (round dose up to nearest 0.1 mL of volume)

Dosage adjustment in renal impairment:
Mild-to-moderate renal impairment: No dosage adjustment necessary
Severe renal impairment (Cl_{cr} <30 mL/minute): Administer 50% of normal dose
End-stage renal impairment (dialysis-dependent): No dosage adjustment provided in manufacturer's labeling (has not been studied)

Dosage adjustment in hepatic impairment:
Mild-to-moderate hepatic impairment (Child-Pugh class A or B): No dosage adjustment necessary
Severe hepatic impairment: No dosage adjustment provided in manufacturer's labeling (has not been studied)

Administration SubQ: Administer subcutaneously into upper arm, abdomen, or thigh. Rotate injection site. Do not inject in tender, bruised, red, or hard areas.

Additional Information In some clinical trials, patients who received methylnaltrexone were on a palliative opioid therapy equivalent to a mean daily oral morphine dose of 172 mg, at a stable dose for ≥3 days. Constipation was defined as <3 bowel movements/week or no bowel movement for >2 days. Patients maintained their regular laxative regimen for at least 3 days prior to treatment and throughout the study.

Dosage Forms Excipient information presented when available (limited, particularly for generics); consult specific product labeling.
Kit, Subcutaneous:
Relistor: 12 mg/0.6 mL [contains edetate calcium disodium]
Solution, Subcutaneous:
Relistor: 8 mg/0.4 mL (0.4 mL); 12 mg/0.6 mL (0.6 mL) [contains edetate calcium disodium]

◆ **Methylnaltrexone Bromide** *see* Methylnaltrexone *on page 1335*

Methylphenidate (meth il FEN i date)

Brand Names: U.S. Concerta; Daytrana; Metadate CD; Metadate ER; Methylin; Quillivant XR; Ritalin; Ritalin LA; Ritalin SR

Brand Names: Canada Apo-Methylphenidate; Apo-Methylphenidate SR; Biphentin; Concerta; PHL-Methylphenidate; PMS-Methylphenidate; ratio-Methylphenidate; Ritalin; Ritalin SR; Sandoz-Methylphenidate SR; Teva-Methylphenidate ER-C

Index Terms Methylphenidate Hydrochloride

Pharmacologic Category Central Nervous System Stimulant

Additional Appendix Information
Patient Information for Disposal of Unused Medications *on page 2393*

Use
U.S. labeling: Treatment of attention-deficit/hyperactivity disorder (ADHD); symptomatic management of narcolepsy (except Concerta, Daytrana, Metadate CD, Ritalin LA, and Quillivant XR)
Canadian labeling: Treatment of attention-deficit/hyperactivity disorder (ADHD); symptomatic management of narcolepsy (except Biphentin, Concerta)

Unlabeled Use Treatment of depression in medically-ill older adults or adult patients with terminal illness and/or receiving palliative care

Pregnancy Risk Factor C

Pregnancy Considerations Adverse events were observed in animal reproduction studies. Information related to the use of methylphenidate in pregnant women with attention-deficit/hyperactivity disorder (Bolea-Akmanac, 2013; Dideriksen, 2013) or narcolepsy (Maurovich-Horvat, 2013; Thorpy, 2013) is limited.

Breast-Feeding Considerations Methylphenidate excretion into breast milk has been noted in case reports. In both cases, the authors calculated the relative infant dose to be ≤0.2% of the weight adjusted maternal dose. Adverse events were not noted in either infant, however, both were older (6 months of age and 11 months of age) and exposure was limited (Hackett, 2006; Spigset, 2007). The manufacturer recommends that caution be used if administered to a nursing woman.

Medication Guide Available Yes

Contraindications
U.S. labeling: Hypersensitivity to methylphenidate or any component of the formulation; marked anxiety, tension, and agitation; glaucoma; use during or within 14 days following MAO inhibitor therapy; family history or diagnosis of Tourette's syndrome or tics
Additional contraindications: Metadate CD and Metadate ER: Severe hypertension, heart failure, arrhythmia, hyperthyroidism, recent MI or angina; concomitant use of halogenated anesthetics
Canadian labeling: Hypersensitivity to methylphenidate or any component of the formulation; marked anxiety, tension, and agitation; glaucoma; use during or within 14 days following MAO inhibitor therapy; family history or diagnosis of Tourette's syndrome or tics, thyrotoxicosis, advanced arteriosclerosis, symptomatic cardiovascular disease, or moderate-to-severe hypertension
Additional contraindications: Ritalin and Ritalin SR: Pheochromocytoma

Warnings/Precautions CNS stimulant use has been associated with serious cardiovascular events (eg, sudden death in children and adolescents; sudden death, stroke, and MI in adults) in patients with pre-existing structural cardiac abnormalities or other serious heart problems. These products should be avoided in patients with known serious structural cardiac abnormalities, cardiomyopathy, serious heart rhythm abnormalities, or other serious cardiac problems that could further increase their risk of sudden death. Patients should be carefully evaluated for cardiac disease prior to initiation of therapy. Use of stimulants can cause an increase in blood pressure (average 2-4 mm Hg) and increases in heart rate (average 3-6 bpm), although some patients may have larger than average increases. Use caution with hypertension, hyperthyroidism, or other cardiovascular conditions that might be exacerbated by increases in blood pressure or heart rate. Some products are contraindicated in patients with heart failure, arrhythmias, severe hypertension, hyperthyroidism, angina, or recent MI. Stimulants are associated with peripheral vasculopathy, including Raynaud's phenomenon; signs/symptoms are usually mild and intermittent, and generally improve with dose reduction or discontinuation. Digital ulceration and/or soft tissue breakdown have been observed rarely; monitor for digital changes during therapy and seek further evaluation (eg, rheumatology) if necessary. Prolonged and painful erections (priapism), sometimes requiring surgical intervention, have been reported with methylphenidate use in pediatric and adult patients. Priapism has been reported to develop after some time on the drug, often subsequent to an increase in dose and also during a period of drug withdrawal (drug holidays or discontinuation). Patients who develop abnormally sustained or frequent and painful erections should seek immediate medical attention.

Has demonstrated value as part of a comprehensive treatment program for ADHD. Use with caution in patients with bipolar disorder (may induce mixed/manic episode). May exacerbate symptoms of behavior and thought disorder in psychotic patients; new-onset psychosis or mania may occur with stimulant use; observe for symptoms of aggression and/or hostility. Use caution with seizure disorders (may reduce seizure threshold). Use caution in patients with history of ethanol or drug abuse. May exacerbate symptoms of behavior and thought disorder in psychotic patients. **[U.S. Boxed Warning]: Potential for drug dependency exists - avoid abrupt discontinuation in patients who have received for prolonged periods.** Visual disturbances have been reported (rare). Not labeled for use in children <6 years of age. Use of stimulants has been associated with suppression of growth in children; monitor growth rate during treatment.

Concerta should not be used in patients with esophageal motility disorders or pre-existing severe gastrointestinal narrowing (small bowel disease, short gut syndrome, history of peritonitis, cystic fibrosis, chronic intestinal pseudo-obstruction, Meckel's diverticulum). Concomitant use of Metadate CD and Metadate ER with halogenated anesthetics is contraindicated; may cause sudden elevations in blood pressure; if surgery is planned, do not administer Metadate CD or Metadate ER on the day of surgery. Transdermal system may cause allergic contact sensitization, characterized by intense local reactions (edema, papules) that may spread beyond the patch site; sensitization may subsequently manifest systemically with other routes of methylphenidate administration; monitor closely. Avoid exposure of application site to any direct external heat sources (eg, hair dryers, heating pads, electric blankets); may increase the rate and extent of absorption and risk of overdose. Efficacy of transdermal methylphenidate therapy for >7 weeks has not been established. Potentially significant interactions may exist, requiring dose or frequency adjustment, additional monitoring, and/or selection of alternative therapy. Consult drug interactions database for more detailed information. Biphentin [Canadian product] controlled release capsules are not interchangeable with other controlled release formulations. Some dosage forms may contain lactose or sucrose; use with caution in patients intolerant to either component (some manufacturer labels recommend avoiding use in such patients).

Adverse Reactions

All dosage forms: Frequency not always defined:

Cardiovascular: Angina, cardiac arrhythmia, cerebral arteritis, cerebral hemorrhage, cerebral occlusion, cerebrovascular accidents, hyper-/hypotension, MI, murmur, palpitation, pulse increased/decreased, Raynaud's phenomenon, tachycardia, vasculitis

Central nervous system: Motion sickness (children 2%), tic (children 2%), aggression, agitation, anger, anxiety, confusional state, depression, dizziness, drowsiness, emotional lability, fatigue, fever, headache, hypervigilance, insomnia, irritability, lethargy, nervousness, neuroleptic malignant syndrome (NMS) (rare), restlessness, stroke, tension, Tourette's syndrome (rare), toxic psychosis, tremor, vertigo

Dermatologic: Excoriation (children 4%), alopecia, erythema multiforme, exfoliative dermatitis, hyperhidrosis, rash, urticaria

Endocrine & metabolic: Dysmenorrhea, growth retardation, libido decreased

Gastrointestinal: Abdominal pain, anorexia, appetite decreased, bruxism, constipation, diarrhea, dyspepsia, nausea, vomiting, weight loss, xerostomia

Genitourinary: Erectile dysfunction

Hematologic: Anemia, leukopenia, pancytopenia, thrombocytopenia, thrombocytopenic purpura

Hepatic: Bilirubin increased, hepatic coma, liver function tests abnormal, transaminases increased

Neuromuscular & skeletal: Arthralgia, dyskinesia, muscle tightness, paresthesia

Ocular: Eye pain (children 2%), blurred vision, dry eyes, mydriasis, visual accommodation disturbance

Renal: Necrotizing vasculitis

Respiratory: Cough increased, dyspnea, pharyngitis, pharyngolaryngeal pain, rhinitis, sinusitis, upper respiratory tract infection

Miscellaneous: Accidental injury, hypersensitivity reactions

Postmarketing and/or case reports (Limited to important or life-threatening): Alkaline phosphatase increased, bradycardia, disorientation, extrasystole, hallucinations; hypersensitivity reactions (eg, angioedema, anaphylactic reactions, auricular swelling, bullous conditions, exfoliative conditions, urticaria, pruritus, rash, eruptions, exanthemas); mania, migraine, obsessive-compulsive disorder, priapism, seizure, supraventricular tachycardia, ventricular extrasystole

Transdermal system: Frequency of adverse events as reported in trials of 7-week duration. Incidence of some events higher with extended use.

>10%:

Central nervous system: Headache (≤15%; long-term use in children: 28%), insomnia (6% to 13%; long-term use in children: 30%), irritability (7% to 11%)

Gastrointestinal: Appetite decreased (26%), nausea (10% to 12%)

Miscellaneous: Viral infection (long-term use in children: 28%)

1% to 10%:

Cardiovascular: Tachycardia (≤1%)

Central nervous system: Tic (7%), dizziness (adolescents 6%), emotional instability (6%)

Gastrointestinal: Vomiting (3% to 10%), weight loss (6% to 9%), abdominal pain (5% to 7%), anorexia (5%; long-term use in children: 46%)

Local: Application site reaction

Respiratory: Nasal congestion (6%) nasopharyngitis (5%)

Postmarketing and/or case reports (Limited to important or life-threatening): Allergic contact dermatitis/sensitization, anaphylaxis, angioedema, hallucinations, seizures

Drug Interactions

Metabolism/Transport Effects Inhibits CYP2D6 (weak)

Avoid Concomitant Use

Avoid concomitant use of Methylphenidate with any of the following: Alcohol (Ethyl); Inhalational Anesthetics; Iobenguane I 123; MAO Inhibitors

Increased Effect/Toxicity

Methylphenidate may increase the levels/effects of: Anti-Parkinson's Agents (Dopamine Agonist); Antipsychotics; CloNIDine; Fosphenytoin; Inhalational Anesthetics; PHEnobarbital; Phenytoin; Primidone; Sympathomimetics; Tricyclic Antidepressants; Vitamin K Antagonists

The levels/effects of Methylphenidate may be increased by: Alcohol (Ethyl); Antacids; Antipsychotics; AtoMOXetine; Cannabinoids; H2-Antagonists; MAO Inhibitors; Proton Pump Inhibitors

Decreased Effect

Methylphenidate may decrease the levels/effects of: Antihypertensives; Iobenguane I 123; Ioflupane I 123

Ethanol/Nutrition/Herb Interactions

Ethanol: Alcohol consumption increases the rate of methylphenidate release from Metadate CD and Ritalin LA (extended-release capsules), but not from Concerta (extended-release tablet); an *in vitro* study involving Metadate CD and Ritalin LA showed that an alcohol concentration of 40% resulted in 84% and 98% of the methylphenidate being released in the first hour, respectively. Alcohol may also exacerbate the CNS effects of psychoactive drugs, such as methylphenidate, regardless of dosage form. Management: Avoid consuming alcohol during therapy.

Food: Food may increase oral absorption of immediate release tablet/solution and chewable tablet. Management: Administer 30-45 minutes before meals.

Herb/Nutraceutical: Ephedra may cause hypertension or arrhythmias and yohimbe has CNS stimulatory activity. Management: Avoid ephedra and yohimbe.

Preparation for Administration

Suspension: *Extended release (Quillivant XR):* Prior to dispensing, reconstitute with an appropriate amount of water (refer to bottle).

Storage/Stability

Capsule:

Extended release (Metadate CD, Ritalin LA): Store at 25°C (77°F); excursions permitted to 15°C to 30°C (59°F to 86°F). Protect from light.

Controlled release (Biphentin [Canadian product]): Store at 15°C to 30°C (59°F to 86°F).

Solution: *Immediate release (Methylin):* Store at 20°C to 25°C (68°F to 77°F).

Suspension: *Extended release (Quillivant XR):* Store at 25°C (77°F); excursions permitted to 15°C to 30°C (59°F to 86°F), before and after reconstitution. Reconstituted bottle must be used within 4 months.

Tablet:

Chewable (Methylin): Store at 20°C to 25°C (68°F to 77°F). Protect from light and moisture.

Extended release:

Metadate ER: Store at 20°C to 25°C (68°F to 77°F); excursions permitted to 15°C to 30°C (59°F to 86°F). Protect from light and moisture.

Concerta: Store at 25°C (77°F); excursions permitted to 15°C to 30°C (59°F to 86°F). Protect from humidity.

Immediate release (Ritalin): Store at 25°C (77°F); excursions permitted to 15°C to 30°C (59°F to 86°F). Protect from light and moisture.

Sustained release (Ritalin-SR): Store at 25°C (77°F); excursions permitted to 15°C to 30°C (59°F to 86°F). Protect from light and moisture.

Transdermal system: *Daytrana:* Store at 25°C (77°F); excursions permitted to 15°C to 30°C (59°F to 86°F). Keep patches stored in protective pouch. Once tray is opened, use patches within 2 months; once an individual patch has been removed from the pouch and the protective liner removed, use immediately. Do not refrigerate or freeze.

Mechanism of Action Mild CNS stimulant; blocks the reuptake of norepinephrine and dopamine into presynaptic neurons; appears to stimulate the cerebral cortex and subcortical structures similar to amphetamines

Pharmacodynamics/Kinetics

Onset of action: Peak effect:

Immediate release tablet: Cerebral stimulation: ~2 hours

Controlled release capsule: Biphentin [Canadian product]: Initial: within 1 hour

Extended release capsule: Metadate CD, Ritalin LA: Biphasic; initial peak similar to immediate release product, followed by second rising portion (corresponding to extended release portion)

Extended release tablet: Concerta: Initial: 1-2 hours

Sustained release tablet: Ritalin-SR: 4-7 hours

Transdermal: ~2 hours; may be expedited by the application of external heat

Duration: Immediate release tablet: 3-6 hours; Sustained release tablet: Ritalin-SR: 8 hours; Extended release tablet: Metadate ER: 8 hours, Concerta: 12 hours; Controlled release capsule: Biphentin [Canadian product]: ~10-12 hours

Absorption:

Oral: Readily absorbed

Chewable tablet: Methylin: A high-fat meal delayed peak time (~1 hour) and increased AUC (~20%).

Controlled release capsule: Biphentin [Canadian product]: Food delayed initial peak slightly (~18 minutes); relative to immediate release tablets, AUC is similar in fed or fasted state (~100%)

Extended release capsule:

Metadate CD: A high-fat meal delayed the early peak (~1 hour), and increased C_{max} (~30%) and AUC (~17%).

Ritalin LA: A high-fat meal delayed absorption and peak times, but not the amount absorbed nor initial peak concentration (second peak lowered by ~25%).

Extended release suspension: Quillivant XR: A high-fat meal led to an earlier peak (~1 hour), and increased C_{max} (~28%) and AUC (~19%).

Extended release tablet: Metadate ER: Food resulted in greater C_{max} and AUC compared to fasting.

Immediate release solution: Methylin: A high-fat meal delayed peak time (~1 hour), and increased C_{max} (~13%) and AUC (~25%).

Transdermal: Absorption increased when applied to inflamed skin or exposed to heat. Absorption is continuous for 9 hours after application.

Distribution: V_d: *d*-methylphenidate: 2.65 ± 1.11 L/kg, *l*-methylphenidate: 1.80 ± 0.91 L/kg

Protein binding: 10% to 33%

Metabolism: Extensive metabolism, predominately via de-esterification by carboxylesterase CES1A1 to alpha-phenyl-piperidine acetic acid (PPAA; ritalinic acid) which has little to no pharmacologic activity.

Bioavailability: Extended release suspension: Quillivant XR: 95% (relative to immediate release oral solution)

Half-life elimination: *d*-methylphenidate: 3-6 hours; *l*-methylphenidate: 1-3 hours

Time to peak: Biphentin [Canadian product]: ~2-3 hours; Concerta: C_{max}: 6-8 hours; Daytrana: 7.5-10.5 hours; Quillivant XR: ~4 hours

Excretion: Urine (90% as metabolites and unchanged drug)

Dosage

ADHD:

Oral, immediate release (IR) products (tablets, chewable tablets, and solution): Children ≥6 years, Adolescents, and Adults: Initial: 5 mg twice daily, before breakfast and lunch; increase by 5-10 mg daily at weekly intervals; maximum dose: 60 mg daily (in 2-3 divided doses).

Oral, extended release (ER), sustained release (SR) products (capsules, tablets, and oral suspension):

Children ≥6 years and Adolescents <18 years: *Concerta:*

Patients not currently taking methylphenidate: Initial: 18 mg once daily in the morning

Patients currently taking immediate release (IR) methylphenidate: Initial: **Note:** Dosing based on current regimen and clinical judgment; suggested dosing listed below:

- Patients taking IR methylphenidate 5 mg 2-3 times daily **or** (Canadian labeling; not in U.S. labeling) methylphenidate SR 20 mg daily: 18 mg once every morning
- Patients taking IR methylphenidate 10 mg 2-3 times daily **or** (Canadian labeling; not in U.S. labeling) methylphenidate SR 40 mg daily: 36 mg once every morning
- Patients taking IR methylphenidate 15 mg 2-3 times daily **or** (Canadian labeling; not in U.S. labeling) methylphenidate SR 60 mg daily: 54 mg once every morning
- Patients taking IR methylphenidate 20 mg 2-3 times daily: 72 mg once every morning

Dose adjustment: May increase dose in increments of 18 mg at weekly intervals. A dosage strength of 27 mg is available for situations in which a dosage between 18-36 mg is desired.

Maximum dose:

U.S. labeling: 54 mg daily in children 6-12 years **or** 2 mg/kg/day (up to 72 mg daily) in adolescents <18 years

Canadian labeling: 54 mg daily in children and adolescents 6-18 years

Children ≥6 years, Adolescents, and Adults:

Biphentin [Canadian product]: Patients not currently taking methylphenidate: Initial: 10-20 mg once daily; may be adjusted in 10 mg increments at weekly intervals. Maximum: 60 mg daily (children ≥6 years, adolescents) or 80 mg daily (adults). **Note:** In some children >60 kg, a maximum dose of 1 mg/kg/daily (not to exceed 80 mg daily) may be necessary; however, close monitoring for adverse events is required. Reduce dose or discontinue if adverse events arise.

Conversion from immediate release methylphenidate formulations to Biphentin: Use equivalent total daily dose administered once daily.

Metadate ER, Ritalin-SR: May be given in place of immediate release products (duration of action ~8 hours), once the immediate release formulation daily dose is titrated and the titrated 8-hour dosage corresponds to sustained or extended release tablet size; maximum: 60 mg daily

Metadate CD, Quillivant XR: Initial: 20 mg once daily; may be adjusted in 10-20 mg increments at weekly intervals; maximum: 60 mg daily

Ritalin LA: Initial: 20 mg once daily (10 mg once daily may be considered for some patients); may be adjusted in 10 mg increments at weekly intervals; maximum: 60 mg daily

Conversion from immediate release or sustained release methylphenidate formulation to Ritalin LA: Use equivalent total daily dose administered once daily.

Adolescent ≥18 years and Adults (<65 years): *Concerta:*

Patients not currently taking methylphenidate: Initial:

U.S. labeling: 18-36 mg once every morning

Canadian labeling: 18 mg once every morning

Patients currently taking immediate release (IR) methylphenidate: Initial: **Note:** Dosing based on current regimen and clinical judgment; suggested dosing listed below:

- Patients taking IR methylphenidate 5 mg 2-3 times daily **or** (Canadian labeling; not in U.S. labeling) methylphenidate SR 20 mg daily: 18 mg once every morning
- Patients taking IR methylphenidate 10 mg 2-3 times daily **or** (Canadian labeling; not in U.S. labeling) methylphenidate SR 40 mg daily: 36 mg once every morning
- Patients taking IR methylphenidate 15 mg 2-3 times daily **or** (Canadian labeling; not in U.S. labeling) methylphenidate SR 60 mg daily: 54 mg once every morning
- Patients taking IR methylphenidate 20 mg 2-3 times daily: 72 mg once every morning

Dose adjustment: May increase dose in increments of 18 mg at weekly intervals. A dosage strength of 27 mg is available for situations in which a dosage between 18-36 mg is desired. Maximum dose: 72 mg daily.

Transdermal: (Daytrana): Children ≥6 years and Adolescents <18 years: Initial: 10 mg patch once daily; remove up to 9 hours after application. Titrate based on response and tolerability; may increase to next transdermal dose no more frequently than every week. **Note:** Application should occur 2 hours prior to desired effect. Drug absorption may continue for a period of time after patch removal. The prescribing information recommends patients converting from another formulation of methylphenidate should be initiated at 10 mg regardless of their previous dose and titrated as needed due to the differences in bioavailability of the transdermal formulation. However, some clinicians have supported higher starting patch doses for patients converting from oral methylphenidate doses of >20 mg daily; for example, the 15 mg (18.75 cm^2) patch has been investigated to have the same effect as 22.5 mg daily of the immediate release preparation, 27 mg/day of the osmotic release preparation, or 20 mg daily of the encapsulated bead preparation (Arnold, 2007).

Narcolepsy: Oral: Children ≥6 years, Adolescents, Adults:

Immediate release tablets and solution *(Methylin, Ritalin):* Initial: 5 mg twice daily before breakfast and lunch; increase by 5-10 mg daily at weekly intervals; maximum dose: 60 mg daily (in 2-3 divided doses).

Extended and sustained release tablets *(Metadate ER, Ritalin-SR):* May be given in place of immediate release products (duration of action ~8 hours), once the immediate release formulation daily dose is titrated and the titrated 8-hour dosage corresponds to sustained or extended release tablet size; maximum: 60 mg daily.

Depression in medically-ill older adults or adult patients with terminal illness and/or receiving palliative care (unlabeled use): Adults: Oral: Initial: ***Immediate release:*** 2.5-5 mg once daily before breakfast or twice daily before breakfast and lunch; increase by 2.5-5 mg daily every 1-3 days in divided doses before breakfast and lunch as tolerated; maximum dose: 20-40 mg daily (Hardy, 2009; Kerr 2012). *Do **not** use sustained release product.*

Dosage adjustment in renal impairment:

Oral: No dosage adjustment provided in manufacturer's labeling (has not been studied); undergoes extensive metabolism to a renally eliminated metabolite with little or no pharmacologic activity.

Transdermal: No dosage adjustment provided in manufacturer's labeling (has not been studied).

Dosage adjustment in hepatic impairment:

Oral: No dosage adjustment provided in manufacturer's labeling (has not been studied).

Transdermal: No dosage adjustment provided in manufacturer's labeling (has not been studied).

Dietary Considerations Administer immediate release (IR) tablet (Ritalin), IR solution (Methylin), chewable tablet (Methylin), and sustained released tablet (Ritalin-SR) 30-45 minutes before meals. Some products may contain phenylalanine.

Administration

Oral:

Controlled release capsule (Biphentin; Canadian product): Administer in the morning with breakfast. Swallow whole; do not crush or chew capsule. Alternatively, capsules may be opened and the contents sprinkled onto applesauce, ice cream, or yogurt, but the beads must not be crushed or chewed.

Immediate release (IR) tablet (Ritalin), IR solution (Methylin), chewable tablet (Methylin): Administer each dose 30-45 minutes before a meal. Ensure last daily dose is administered before 6 pm if difficulty sleeping occurs. Administer chewable tablet with at least 8 ounces of water or other fluid.

Extended release capsule (Metadate CD, Ritalin LA): Administer in the morning. May be taken with or without food. Alternatively, capsules may be opened and the contents sprinkled onto a small amount (equal to 1 tablespoon) of cold applesauce. Swallow applesauce without chewing. Do not crush or chew capsule contents.

Extended release suspension (Quillivant XR): Administer in the morning with or without food. Shake bottle ≥10 seconds prior to administration. Use the oral dosing dispenser provided; wash after each use.

Extended release tablet:

Metadate ER: May be taken with or without food. Swallow whole with water or other fluid; do not crush or chew tablet.

Concerta: Administer in the morning. May be taken with or without food, but must be taken with water or other fluid. Do not crush, chew, or divide tablet.

Sustained release tablet (Ritalin-SR): Administer 30-45 minutes before a meal. Swallow whole; do not crush or chew tablet.

Topical: Transdermal (Daytrana): Apply to clean, dry, non-oily, intact skin to the hip area, avoiding the waistline; do not premedicate the patch site with hydrocortisone or other solutions, creams, ointments, or emollients. Apply at the same time each day to alternating hips. Press firmly for 30 seconds to ensure proper adherence. Avoid exposure of application site to external heat source, which may increase the amount of drug absorbed. If difficulty is experienced when separating the patch from the liner or if any medication (sticky substance) remains on the liner after separation; discard that patch and apply a new patch. Do not use a patch that has been damaged or torn; do not cut patch. If patch should dislodge, may replace with new patch (to different site) but total wear time should not exceed 9 hours; do not reapply with dressings, tape, or common adhesives. Patch may be removed early if a shorter duration of effect is desired or if late day side effects occur. Wash hands with soap and water after handling. Avoid touching the sticky side of the patch. If patch removal is difficult, an oil-based product (eg, petroleum jelly, olive oil) may be applied to the patch edges to aid removal; never apply acetone-based products (eg, nail polish remover) to patch. Dispose of used patch by folding adhesive side onto itself, and discard in toilet or appropriate lidded container.

Monitoring Parameters Periodic CBC, differential, and platelet counts with prolonged use; blood pressure, heart rate; signs and symptoms of depression, aggression, or hostility; growth rate in children; signs of central nervous system stimulation; signs of peripheral vasculopathy (eg, digital changes)

Transdermal: Signs of worsening erythema, blistering or edema which does not improve within 48 hours of patch removal, or spreads beyond patch site.

When used for the treatment of ADHD, thoroughly evaluate for cardiovascular risk. Monitor heart rate, blood pressure, and consider obtaining ECG prior to initiation (Vetter, 2008).

Test Interactions May interfere with urine detection of amphetamines/methamphetamines (false-positive).

Additional Information Treatment with methylphenidate may include "drug holidays" or periodic discontinuation in order to assess the patient's requirements and to decrease tolerance and limit suppression of linear growth and weight. Specific patients may require 3 doses/day for treatment of ADHD (ie, additional dose at 4 PM).

Concerta is an osmotic controlled release formulation (OROS) of methylphenidate. The tablet has an immediate-release overcoat that provides an initial dose of methylphenidate within 1 hour. The overcoat covers a trilayer core. The trilayer core is composed of two layers containing the drug and excipients, and one layer of osmotic components. As water from the gastrointestinal tract enters the core, the osmotic components expand and methylphenidate is released.

Metadate CD capsules contain a mixture of immediate release and extended release beads, designed to release 30% of the dose immediately and 70% over an extended period.

Ritalin LA uses a combination of immediate release and enteric coated, delayed release beads.

Dosage Forms Excipient information presented when available (limited, particularly for generics); consult specific product labeling.

Capsule Extended Release, Oral, as hydrochloride:

Metadate CD: 10 mg, 20 mg, 30 mg [contains fd&c blue #2 (indigotine)]

Metadate CD: 40 mg

Metadate CD: 50 mg [contains fd&c blue #2 (indigotine)]

Metadate CD: 60 mg

Generic: 10 mg, 20 mg, 30 mg, 40 mg, 50 mg, 60 mg

Capsule Extended Release 24 Hour, Oral, as hydrochloride:

Ritalin LA: 10 mg, 20 mg, 30 mg, 40 mg

Generic: 20 mg, 30 mg, 40 mg

Patch, Transdermal:

Daytrana: 10 mg/9 hr (30 ea); 15 mg/9 hr (30 ea); 20 mg/9 hr (30 ea); 30 mg/9 hr (30 ea)

Solution, Oral, as hydrochloride:

Methylin: 5 mg/5 mL (500 mL); 10 mg/5 mL (500 mL) [contains polyethylene glycol]

Generic: 5 mg/5 mL (500 mL); 10 mg/5 mL (500 mL)

Suspension Reconstituted, Oral, as hydrochloride:

Quillivant XR: 25 mg/5 mL (60 mL, 120 mL, 150 mL, 180 mL) [contains sodium benzoate; banana flavor]

Tablet, Oral, as hydrochloride:

Ritalin: 5 mg

Ritalin: 10 mg, 20 mg [scored]

Generic: 5 mg, 10 mg, 20 mg

Tablet Chewable, Oral, as hydrochloride:

Methylin: 2.5 mg, 5 mg [contains aspartame; grape flavor]

Methylin: 10 mg [scored; contains aspartame; grape flavor]

Tablet Extended Release, Oral, as hydrochloride:

Concerta: 18 mg, 27 mg, 36 mg, 54 mg

Metadate ER: 20 mg

Ritalin SR: 20 mg

Generic: 10 mg, 18 mg, 20 mg, 27 mg, 36 mg, 54 mg

Dosage Forms: Canada Also refer to Dosage Forms Excipient information presented when available (limited, particularly for generics); consult specific product labeling.

Capsule, Controlled Release, Oral, as hydrochloride:

Biphentin: 10 mg, 15 mg, 20 mg, 30 mg, 40 mg, 50 mg, 60 mg, 80 mg

Controlled Substance C-II

◆ **Methylphenidate Hydrochloride** *see* Methylphenidate *on page 1336*

◆ **Methylphenoxy-Benzene Propanamine** *see* AtoMOXetine *on page 187*

◆ **Methylphenyl Isoxazolyl Penicillin** *see* Oxacillin *on page 1523*

◆ **Methylphytyl Napthoquinone** *see* Phytonadione *on page 1644*

MethylPREDNISolone (meth il pred NIS oh lone)

Brand Names: U.S. A-Methapred; Depo-Medrol; Medrol; Medrol (Pak); Solu-MEDROL

Brand Names: Canada Depo-Medrol®; Medrol®; Methylprednisolone Acetate; Solu-Medrol®

Index Terms 6-α-Methylprednisolone; A-Methapred; Medrol Dose Pack; Methylprednisolone Acetate; Methylprednisolone Sodium Succinate; Solumedrol

Pharmacologic Category Corticosteroid, Systemic

Additional Appendix Information

Contrast Media Reactions, Premedication for Prophylaxis *on page 2373*

Corticosteroids Systemic Equivalencies *on page 2297*

Use Primarily as an anti-inflammatory or immunosuppressant agent in the treatment of a variety of diseases including those of hematologic, allergic, inflammatory, neoplastic, and autoimmune origin. Prevention and treatment of graft-versus-host disease following allogeneic bone marrow transplantation.

Unlabeled Use Acute spinal cord injury

Pregnancy Risk Factor C

Pregnancy Considerations Adverse events have been observed with corticosteroids in animal reproduction studies. Methylprednisolone crosses the placenta (Anderson, 1981). Some studies have shown an association between first trimester systemic corticosteroid use and oral clefts (Park-Wyllie, 2000; Pradat, 2003). Systemic corticosteroids may also influence fetal growth (decreased birth weight); however, information is conflicting (Lunghi, 2010). Hypoadrenalism may occur in newborns following maternal use of corticosteroids in pregnancy; monitor.

When systemic corticosteroids are needed in pregnancy, it is generally recommended to use the lowest effective dose for the shortest duration of time, avoiding high doses during the first trimester (Leachman, 2006; Lunghi, 2010; Makol, 2011; Østensen, 2009). Inhaled corticosteroids are preferred for the treatment of asthma during pregnancy. Systemic corticosteroids such as methylprednisolone may be used for the treatment of severe persistent asthma if needed; the lowest dose administered on alternate days (if possible) should be used (NAEPP, 2005).

Pregnant women exposed to methylprednisolone for antirejection therapy following a transplant may contact the National Transplantation Pregnancy Registry (NTPR) at 215-955-4820. Women exposed to methylprednisolone during pregnancy for the treatment of an autoimmune disease may contact the OTIS Autoimmune Diseases Study at 877-311-8972.

Breast-Feeding Considerations Corticosteroids are excreted in human milk. The manufacturer notes that when used systemically, maternal use of corticosteroids have the potential to cause adverse events in a nursing infant (eg, growth suppression, interfere with endogenous corticosteroid production) and therefore recommends a decision be made whether to discontinue nursing or to discontinue the drug, taking into account the importance of treatment to the mother. If there is concern about exposure to the infant, some guidelines recommend waiting 4 hours after the maternal dose of an oral systemic corticosteroid before breast-feeding in order to decrease potential exposure to the nursing infant (based on a study using prednisolone) (Bae, 2011; Leachman, 2006; Makol, 2011; Ost, 1985). Other guidelines note that maternal use of systemic corticosteroids is not a contraindication to breast-feeding (NAEPP, 2005).

Contraindications Hypersensitivity to methylprednisolone or any component of the formulation; systemic fungal infection (except intra-articular injection in localized joint conditions); administration of live virus vaccines. methylprednisolone formulations containing benzyl alcohol preservative are contraindicated in premature infants; I.M. administration in idiopathic thrombocytopenia purpura; intrathecal administration

Warnings/Precautions Use with caution in patients with thyroid disease, hepatic impairment, renal impairment, cardiovascular disease, diabetes, glaucoma, cataracts, myasthenia gravis, patients at risk for osteoporosis, patients at risk for seizures, or GI diseases (diverticulitis, peptic ulcer, ulcerative colitis) due to perforation risk. Not recommended for the treatment of optic neuritis; may increase frequency of new episodes. Use caution following acute MI (corticosteroids have been associated with myocardial rupture). Cardiomegaly and congestive heart failure have been reported following concurrent use of amphotericin B and hydrocortisone for the management of fungal infections.

Because of the risk of adverse effects, systemic corticosteroids should be used cautiously in the elderly in the smallest possible effective dose for the shortest duration. May affect growth velocity; growth should be routinely monitored in pediatric patients. Withdraw therapy with gradual tapering of dose.

May cause hypercorticism or suppression of hypothalamic-pituitary-adrenal (HPA) axis, particularly in younger children or in patients receiving high doses for prolonged periods. HPA axis suppression may lead to adrenal crisis. Withdrawal and discontinuation of a corticosteroid should be done slowly and carefully. Particular care is required when patients are transferred from systemic corticosteroids to inhaled products due to possible adrenal insufficiency or withdrawal from steroids, including an increase in allergic symptoms. Patients receiving >20 mg per day of prednisone (or equivalent) may be most susceptible. Fatalities have occurred due to adrenal insufficiency in asthmatic patients during and after transfer from systemic corticosteroids to aerosol steroids; aerosol steroids do not provide the systemic steroid needed to treat patients having trauma, surgery, or infections.

Acute myopathy has been reported with high dose corticosteroids, usually in patients with neuromuscular transmission disorders; may involve ocular and/or respiratory muscles; monitor creatine kinase; recovery may be delayed. Corticosteroid use may cause psychiatric disturbances, including depression, euphoria, insomnia, mood swings, and personality changes. Pre-existing psychiatric conditions may be exacerbated by corticosteroid use. Prolonged use of corticosteroids may also increase the incidence of secondary infection, cause activation of latent infections, mask acute infection (including fungal infections), prolong or exacerbate viral or parasitic infections, or limit response to vaccines. Exposure to chickenpox or measles should be avoided; corticosteroids should not be used to treat ocular herpes simplex. Corticosteroids should not be used for cerebral malaria or viral hepatitis. Close observation is required in patients with latent tuberculosis and/or TB reactivity; restrict use in active TB (only in conjunction with antituberculosis treatment). Amebiasis should be ruled out in any patient with recent travel to tropic climates or unexplained diarrhea prior to initiation of corticosteroids. Prolonged treatment with corticosteroids has been associated with the development of Kaposi's sarcoma (case reports); discontinuation may result in clinical improvement.

High-dose corticosteroids should not be used to manage acute head injury. Rare cases of anaphylactoid reactions have been observed in patients receiving corticosteroids. Avoid injection or leakage into the dermis; dermal and/or subdermal skin depression may occur at the site of injection. Avoid deltoid muscle injection; subcutaneous atrophy may occur. Some dosage forms contain benzyl alcohol which has been associated with "gasping syndrome" in neonates.

Adverse Reactions Frequency not defined.

Cardiovascular: Arrhythmias, bradycardia, cardiac arrest, cardiomegaly, circulatory collapse, congestive heart failure, edema, fat embolism, hypertension, hypertrophic cardiomyopathy in premature infants, myocardial rupture (post MI), syncope, tachycardia, thromboembolism, vasculitis

Central nervous system: Delirium, depression, emotional instability, euphoria, hallucinations, headache, intracranial pressure increased, insomnia, malaise, mood swings, nervousness, neuritis, personality changes, psychic disorders, pseudotumor cerebri (usually following discontinuation), seizure, vertigo

Dermatologic: Acne, allergic dermatitis, alopecia, dry scaly skin, ecchymoses, edema, erythema, hirsutism, hyper-/hypopigmentation, hypertrichosis, impaired wound healing, petechiae, rash, skin atrophy, sterile abscess, skin test reaction impaired, striae, urticaria

Endocrine & metabolic: Adrenal suppression, amenorrhea, carbohydrate intolerance increased, Cushing's syndrome, diabetes mellitus, fluid retention, glucose intolerance, growth suppression (children), hyperglycemia, hyperlipidemia, hypokalemia, hypokalemic alkalosis, menstrual irregularities, negative nitrogen balance, pituitary-adrenal axis suppression, protein catabolism, sodium and water retention

Gastrointestinal: Abdominal distention, appetite increased, bowel/bladder dysfunction (after intrathecal administration), gastrointestinal hemorrhage, gastrointestinal perforation, nausea, pancreatitis, peptic ulcer, perforation of the small and large intestine, ulcerative esophagitis, vomiting, weight gain

Hematologic: Leukocytosis (transient)

Hepatic: Hepatomegaly, transaminases increased

Local: Postinjection flare (intra-articular use), thrombophlebitis

Neuromuscular & skeletal: Arthralgia, arthropathy, aseptic necrosis (femoral and humoral heads), fractures, muscle mass loss, muscle weakness, myopathy (particularly in conjunction with neuromuscular disease or neuromuscular-blocking agents), neuropathy, osteoporosis, parasthesia, tendon rupture, vertebral compression fractures, weakness

Ocular: Cataracts, exophthalmoses, glaucoma, intraocular pressure increased

Renal: Glycosuria

Respiratory: Pulmonary edema

Miscellaneous: Abnormal fat disposition, anaphylactoid reaction, anaphylaxis, angioedema, avascular necrosis, diaphoresis, hiccups, hypersensitivity reactions, infections, secondary malignancy

<1% (Limited to important or life-threatening): Venous thrombosis (Johannesdottir, 2013)

Drug Interactions

Metabolism/Transport Effects **Substrate** of CYP3A4 (minor); **Note:** Assignment of Major/Minor substrate status based on clinically relevant drug interaction potential; **Inhibits** CYP2C8 (weak), CYP3A4 (weak)

Avoid Concomitant Use

Avoid concomitant use of MethylPREDNISolone with any of the following: Aldesleukin; BCG; Mifepristone; Natalizumab; Pimecrolimus; Pimozide; Tacrolimus (Topical); Tofacitinib

Increased Effect/Toxicity

MethylPREDNISolone may increase the levels/effects of: Acetylcholinesterase Inhibitors; Amphotericin B; ARIPiprazole; CycloSPORINE (Systemic); Deferasirox; Dofetilide; Leflunomide; Lomitapide; Loop Diuretics; Natalizumab; NSAID (COX-2 Inhibitor); NSAID (Nonselective); Pimozide; Thiazide Diuretics; Tofacitinib; Vaccines (Live); Warfarin

The levels/effects of MethylPREDNISolone may be increased by: Antifungal Agents (Azole Derivatives, Systemic); Aprepitant; Calcium Channel Blockers (Nondihydropyridine); CycloSPORINE (Systemic); CYP3A4 Inhibitors (Strong); Denosumab; Estrogen Derivatives; Fluconazole; Fosaprepitant; Indacaterol; Macrolide Antibiotics; Mifepristone; Neuromuscular-Blocking Agents (Nondepolarizing); Pimecrolimus; Quinolone Antibiotics; Roflumilast; Salicylates; Tacrolimus (Topical); Telaprevir; Trastuzumab

Decreased Effect

MethylPREDNISolone may decrease the levels/effects of: Aldesleukin; Antidiabetic Agents; BCG; Calcitriol; Coccidioidin Skin Test; Corticorelin; CycloSPORINE (Systemic); Hyaluronidase; Isoniazid; Salicylates; Sipuleucel-T; Telaprevir; Urea Cycle Disorder Agents; Vaccines (Inactivated)

The levels/effects of MethylPREDNISolone may be decreased by: Aminoglutethimide; Antacids; Barbiturates; Bile Acid Sequestrants; CarBAMazepine; Echinacea; Fosphenytoin; Mifepristone; Mitotane; Phenytoin; Primidone; Rifamycin Derivatives

Ethanol/Nutrition/Herb Interactions

Ethanol: Ethanol may increase gastric mucosal irritation. Management: Avoid ethanol.

Food: Methylprednisolone interferes with calcium absorption. May cause GI upset. Management: Administer with food. Limit caffeine.

Herb/Nutraceutical: St John's wort may decrease methylprednisolone levels. Cat's claw and echinacea have immunostimulant properties. Management: Avoid St John's wort, cat's claw, and echinacea.

Preparation for Administration

Standard diluent (Solu-Medrol®): 40 mg/50 mL D_5W; 125 mg/50 mL D_5W.

Minimum volume (Solu-Medrol®): 50 mL D_5W.

Storage/Stability Intact vials of methylprednisolone sodium succinate should be stored at controlled room temperature of 20°C to 25°C (68°F to 77°F). Protect from light. Reconstituted solutions of methylprednisolone sodium succinate should be stored at room temperature of 20°C to 25°C (68°F to 77°F) and used within 48 hours. Stability of parenteral admixture at room temperature (25°C) and at refrigeration temperature (4°C) is 48 hours.

Mechanism of Action In a tissue-specific manner, corticosteroids regulate gene expression subsequent to binding specific intracellular receptors and translocation into the nucleus. Corticosteroids exert a wide array of physiologic effects including modulation of carbohydrate, protein, and lipid metabolism and maintenance of fluid and electrolyte homeostasis. Moreover cardiovascular, immunologic, musculoskeletal, endocrine, and neurologic physiology are influenced by corticosteroids. Decreases inflammation by suppression of migration of polymorphonuclear leukocytes and reversal of increased capillary permeability.

Pharmacodynamics/Kinetics

Onset of action: Peak effect (route dependent): Oral: 1-2 hours; I.M.: 4-8 days; Intra-articular: 1 week; methylprednisolone sodium succinate is highly soluble and has a rapid effect by I.M. and I.V. routes

Duration (route dependent): Oral: 30-36 hours; I.M.: 1-4 weeks; Intra-articular: 1-5 weeks; methylprednisolone acetate has a low solubility and has a sustained I.M. effect

Distribution: V_d: 0.7-1.5 L/kg

Half-life elimination: 3-3.5 hours; reduced in obese

Excretion: Clearance: Reduced in obese

Dosage Dosing should be based on the lesser of ideal body weight or actual body weight

Children: **Only sodium succinate may be given I.V.;** methylprednisolone sodium succinate is highly soluble and has a rapid effect by I.M. and I.V. routes.

Methylprednisolone acetate has a low solubility and has a sustained I.M. effect.

Acute spinal cord injury (unlabeled use): I.V. (sodium succinate): 30 mg/kg over 15 minutes, followed in 45 minutes by a continuous infusion of 5.4 mg/kg/hour for 23 hours. **Note:** Due to insufficient evidence of clinical efficacy (ie, preserving or improving spinal cord function), the routine use of methylprednisolone in the treatment of acute spinal cord injury is no longer recommended. If used in this setting, methylprednisolone should not be initiated >8 hours after the injury; not effective in penetrating trauma (eg, gunshot) (Consortium for Spinal Cord Medicine, 2008).

Anti-inflammatory or immunosuppressive: Oral, I.M., I.V. (sodium succinate): 0.5-1.7 mg/kg/day **or** 5-25 mg/m²/day in divided doses every 6-12 hours; "Pulse" therapy: 15-30 mg/kg/dose over ≥30 minutes given once daily for 3 days

Asthma exacerbations, including status asthmaticus (emergency medical care or hospital doses) (NIH Asthma Guidelines, NAEPP, 2007): Children ≤12 years: Oral, I.V.: 1-2 mg/kg/day in 2 divided doses (maximum: 60 mg/day) until peak expiratory flow is 70% of predicted or personal best

Lupus nephritis: I.V. (sodium succinate): 30 mg/kg over ≥30 minutes every other day for 6 doses

Adults: **Only sodium succinate may be given I.V.;** methylprednisolone sodium succinate is highly soluble and has a rapid effect by I.M. and I.V. routes. Methylprednisolone acetate has a low solubility and has a sustained I.M. effect.

Acute spinal cord injury (unlabeled use): I.V. (sodium succinate): 30 mg/kg over 15 minutes, followed in 45 minutes by a continuous infusion of 5.4 mg/kg/hour for 23 hours. **Note:** Due to insufficient evidence of clinical efficacy (ie, preserving or improving spinal cord function), the routine use of methylprednisolone in the treatment of acute spinal cord injury is no longer recommended. If used in this setting, methylprednisolone should not be initiated >8 hours after the injury; not effective in penetrating trauma (eg, gunshot) (Consortium for Spinal Cord Medicine, 2008).

Allergic conditions: Oral: Tapered-dosage schedule (eg, dose-pack containing 21 x 4 mg tablets):

Day 1: 24 mg on day 1 administered as 8 mg (2 tablets) before breakfast, 4 mg (1 tablet) after lunch, 4 mg (1 tablet) after supper, and 8 mg (2 tablets) at bedtime **OR** 24 mg (6 tablets) as a single dose or divided into 2 or 3 doses upon initiation (regardless of time of day)

Day 2: 20 mg on day 2 administered as 4 mg (1 tablet) before breakfast, 4 mg (1 tablet) after lunch, 4 mg (1 tablet) after supper, and 8 mg (2 tablets) at bedtime

Day 3: 16 mg on day 3 administered as 4 mg (1 tablet) before breakfast, 4 mg (1 tablet) after lunch, 4 mg (1 tablet) after supper, and 4 mg (1 tablet) at bedtime

Day 4: 12 mg on day 4 administered as 4 mg (1 tablet) before breakfast, 4 mg (1 tablet) after lunch, and 4 mg (1 tablet) at bedtime

Day 5: 8 mg on day 5 administered as 4 mg (1 tablet) before breakfast and 4 mg (1 tablet) at bedtime

Day 6: 4 mg on day 6 administered as 4 mg (1 tablet) before breakfast

Anti-inflammatory or immunosuppressive:

Oral: 2-60 mg/day in 1-4 divided doses to start, followed by gradual reduction in dosage to the lowest possible level consistent with maintaining an adequate clinical response.

I.M. (sodium succinate): 10-80 mg/day once daily

I.M. (acetate): 10-80 mg every 1-2 weeks

I.V. (sodium succinate): 10-40 mg over a period of several minutes and repeated I.V. or I.M. at intervals depending on clinical response; when high dosages are needed, give 30 mg/kg over a period ≥30 minutes and may be repeated every 4-6 hours for 48 hours.

Arthritis: Intra-articular (acetate): Administer every 1-5 weeks.

Large joints (eg, knee, ankle): 20-80 mg

Medium joints (eg, elbow, wrist): 10-40 mg

Small joints: 4-10 mg

Asthma exacerbations, including status asthmaticus (emergency medical care or hospital doses): Oral, I.V.: 40-80 mg/day in 1-2 divided doses until peak expiratory flow is 70% of predicted or personal best (NIH Asthma Guidelines, NAEPP, 2007)

Asthma, severe persistent, long-term control: Oral: 7.5-60 mg/day (or on alternate days) (NIH Asthma Guidelines, NAEPP, 2007)

Dermatitis, acute severe: I.M. (acetate): 80-120 mg as a single dose

Dermatitis, chronic: I.M. (acetate): 40-120 mg every 5-10 days

Dermatologic conditions (eg, keloids, lichen planus): Intralesional (acetate): 20-60 mg

Dermatomyositis/polymyositis: I.V. (sodium succinate): 1 g/day for 3-5 days for severe muscle weakness, followed by conversion to oral prednisone (Drake, 1996)

Lupus nephritis: High-dose "pulse" therapy: I.V. (sodium succinate): 0.5-1 g/day for 3 days (Ponticelli, 2010)

Pneumocystis pneumonia in AIDS patients: I.V.: 30 mg twice daily for 5 days, then 30 mg once daily for 5 days, then 15 mg once daily for 11 days

Dosage adjustment in renal impairment: No dosage adjustment provided in manufacturer's labeling; use with caution.

Hemodialysis effects: Slightly dialyzable (5% to 20%) Administer dose post-hemodialysis.

Dosage adjustment in hepatic impairment: No dosage adjustment provided in manufacturer's labeling.

Dietary Considerations Take with meals to decrease GI upset.; need diet rich in pyridoxine, vitamin C, vitamin D, folate, calcium, phosphorus, and protein.

Administration

Administer with meals to decrease GI upset.

Parenteral: Methylprednisolone sodium succinate may be administered I.M. or I.V.; I.V. administration may be IVP over one to several minutes or IVPB or continuous I.V. infusion. **Acetate salt should not be given I.V.** Avoid injection into the deltoid muscle due to a high incidence of subcutaneous atrophy. Avoid injection or leakage into the dermis; dermal and/or subdermal skin depression may occur at the site of injection.

I.V.: Succinate:

Low dose: ≤1.8 mg/kg or ≤125 mg/dose: I.V. push over 3-15 minutes

Moderate dose: ≥2 mg/kg or 250 mg/dose: I.V. over 15-30 minutes

High dose: 15 mg/kg or ≥500 mg/dose: I.V. over ≥30 minutes

Doses >15 mg/kg or ≥1 g: Administer over 1 hour

Do **not** administer high-dose I.V. push; hypotension, cardiac arrhythmia, and sudden death have been reported in patients given high-dose methylprednisolone I.V. push (>0.5 g over <10 minutes); intermittent infusion over 15-60 minutes; maximum concentration: I.V. push 125 mg/mL

I.M.: Avoid injection into the deltoid muscle due to a high incidence of subcutaneous atrophy. Avoid injection or leakage into the dermis; dermal and/or subdermal skin depression may occur at the site of injection. Do not inject into areas that have evidence of acute local infection.

Monitoring Parameters Blood pressure, blood glucose, electrolytes, growth in children

Test Interactions Interferes with skin tests

Additional Information Sodium content of 1 g sodium succinate injection: 2.01 mEq; 53 mg of sodium succinate salt is equivalent to 40 mg of methylprednisolone base

Methylprednisolone acetate: Depo-Medrol®

Methylprednisolone sodium succinate: Solu-Medrol®

Dosage Forms Excipient information presented when available (limited, particularly for generics); consult specific product labeling.

Solution Reconstituted, Injection, as sodium succinate [strength expressed as base]:

A-Methapred: 40 mg (1 ea); 125 mg (1 ea) [contains benzyl alcohol]

Solu-MEDROL: 500 mg (1 ea); 1000 mg (1 ea)

Solu-MEDROL: 2 g (1 ea) [contains benzyl alcohol]

Generic: 40 mg (1 ea); 125 mg (1 ea); 500 mg (1 ea); 1000 mg (1 ea); 1 g (1 ea)

Solution Reconstituted, Injection, as sodium succinate [strength expressed as base, preservative free]:

Solu-MEDROL: 40 mg (1 ea); 125 mg (1 ea); 500 mg (1 ea); 1000 mg (1 ea)

Suspension, Injection, as acetate:

Depo-Medrol: 20 mg/mL (5 mL); 40 mg/mL (5 mL, 10 mL) [contains benzyl alcohol, polyethylene glycol, polysorbate 80]

Depo-Medrol: 40 mg/mL (1 mL) [contains polyethylene glycol]

Depo-Medrol: 80 mg/mL (1 mL)

Depo-Medrol: 80 mg/mL (5 mL) [contains benzyl alcohol, polyethylene glycol, polysorbate 80]

Depo-Medrol: 80 mg/mL (1 mL) [contains polyethylene glycol]

Generic: 40 mg/mL (1 mL, 5 mL, 10 mL); 80 mg/mL (1 mL, 5 mL)

Tablet, Oral:

Medrol: 2 mg, 4 mg, 8 mg, 16 mg, 32 mg [scored]

Medrol (Pak): 4 mg [scored]

Generic: 4 mg, 8 mg, 16 mg, 32 mg

- 6-α-Methylprednisolone *see* MethylPREDNISolone *on page 1340*
- Methylprednisolone Acetate *see* MethylPREDNISolone *on page 1340*
- Methylprednisolone Sodium Succinate *see* MethylPREDNISolone *on page 1340*
- 4-Methylpyrazole *see* Fomepizole *on page 910*
- Methylrosaniline Chloride *see* Gentian Violet *on page 954*

Methyl Salicylate and Menthol

(METH il sa LIS i late & MEN thol)

Brand Names: U.S. BenGay® [OTC]; Icy Hot® [OTC]; Precise® [OTC]; Salonpas® Arthritis Pain® [OTC]; Salonpas® Jet Spray [OTC]; Salonpas® Massage Foam [OTC]; Salonpas® Pain Relief Patch® [OTC]; Thera-Gesic® Plus [OTC]; Thera-Gesic® [OTC]

Index Terms Menthol and Methyl Salicylate

Pharmacologic Category Analgesic, Topical; Salicylate; Topical Skin Product

Use Temporary relief of minor aches and pains of muscle and joints associated with arthritis, bruises, simple backache, sprains, and strains

Dosage Topical: Pain relief:

Balm, cream, foam, spray, stick: Children ≥12 years and Adults: Apply to affected area; may repeat up to 3-4 times/day

Gel: Children ≥2 years and Adults: Apply to affected area; may repeat up to 3-4 times/day for up to 7 days

Patch:

Methyl salicylate 10% and menthol 1.5%: Children ≥12 years and Adults: Apply 1 patch to affected area not more than 3-4 times daily; leave in place for no more than 8 hours

Methyl salicylate 10% and menthol 3%: Adults: Apply 1 patch to affected area and leave in place for up to 8-12 hours; do not exceed 1 patch/application. If pain still present, a second patch may be applied for up to 8-12 hours (maximum: 2 patches/24 hours; 3 days of consecutive use)

Additional Information Complete prescribing information should be consulted for additional detail.

Dosage Forms Excipient information presented when available (limited, particularly for generics); consult specific product labeling.

Aerosol, foam, topical:

Salonpas® Massage Foam: Methyl salicylate 10% and menthol 3% (118 mL)

Aerosol, spray, topical:

Salonpas® Jet Spray: Methyl salicylate 10% and menthol 3% (118 mL) [contains ethanol]

Balm, topical:

Icy Hot® Balm: Methyl salicylate 29% and menthol 7.6% (99.2 g)

Cream, topical:

BenGay® Arthritis Formula: Methyl salicylate 30% and menthol 8% (57 g, 113 g)

BenGay® Greaseless: Methyl salicylate 15% and menthol 10% (57 g, 113 g)

Icy Hot®: Methyl salicylate 30% and menthol 10% (35.4 g, 85 g)

Precise®: Methyl salicylate 30% and menthol 10% (75 g)

Thera-Gesic®: Methyl salicylate 15% and menthol 1% (85 g, 142 g)

Thera-Gesic® Plus: Methyl salicylate 15% and menthol 4% (85 g) [contains aloe]

Patch, topical:

Salonpas® Arthritis Pain®: Methyl salicylate 10% and menthol 3% (5s)

Salonpas® Pain Relief Patch®: Methyl salicylate 10% and menthol 1.5% (3s)

Salonpas® Pain Relief Patch®: Methyl salicylate 10% and menthol 3% (5s)

Stick, topical:

Icy Hot®: Methyl salicylate 30% and menthol 10% (49 g)

MethylTESTOSTERone (meth il tes TOS te rone)

Brand Names: U.S. Android; Methitest; Testred

Pharmacologic Category Androgen

Additional Appendix Information

Beers Criteria – Potentially Inappropriate Medications for Geriatrics *on page 2368*

Use

Male: Hypogonadism; delayed puberty; impotence and climacteric symptoms

Female: Palliative treatment of metastatic breast cancer

Unlabeled Use Hypogonadism (male); delayed puberty (male)

Pregnancy Risk Factor X

Dosage Oral: Adults:

Males:

Hypogonadism; delayed puberty: Individualize dose based on response and tolerability.

Androgen deficiency: 10-50 mg/day

Females: Breast cancer: 50-200 mg/day

Dosage adjustment in renal impairment: No dosage adjustment provided in manufacturer's labeling. However, patients with renal disease may be at an increased risk of fluid retention.

Dosage adjustment in hepatic impairment: No dosage adjustment provided in manufacturer's labeling. However, patients with hepatic disease may be at an increased risk of fluid retention.

Additional Information Complete prescribing information should be consulted for additional detail.

Dosage Forms Excipient information presented when available (limited, particularly for generics); consult specific product labeling.

Capsule, Oral:
Android: 10 mg
Testred: 10 mg

Tablet, Oral:
Methitest: 10 mg [scored]

Controlled Substance C-III

◆ **Methylthionine Chloride** *see* Methylene Blue *on page 1333*

◆ **Methylthioninium Chloride** *see* Methylene Blue *on page 1333*

Metipranolol (met i PRAN oh lol)

Brand Names: U.S. Optipranolol

Brand Names: Canada OptiPranolol®

Index Terms Metipranolol Hydrochloride

Pharmacologic Category Beta-Blocker, Nonselective; Ophthalmic Agent, Antiglaucoma

Use Treatment of chronic open-angle glaucoma or ocular hypertension

Pregnancy Risk Factor C

Dosage Ophthalmic: Adults: Instill 1 drop in the affected eye(s) twice daily

Dosage adjustment in renal impairment: No dosage adjustment provided in manufacturer's labeling. However, dosage adjustment unlikely due to low systemic absorption.

Dosage adjustment in hepatic impairment: No dosage adjustment provided in manufacturer's labeling. However, dosage adjustment unlikely due to low systemic absorption.

Additional Information Complete prescribing information should be consulted for additional detail.

Dosage Forms Excipient information presented when available (limited, particularly for generics); consult specific product labeling.

Solution, Ophthalmic:
Optipranolol: 0.3% (5 mL, 10 mL)
Generic: 0.3% (5 mL, 10 mL)

◆ **Metipranolol Hydrochloride** *see* Metipranolol *on page 1345*

Metoclopramide (met oh KLOE pra mide)

Brand Names: U.S. Metozolv ODT; Reglan

Brand Names: Canada Apo-Metoclop; Metoclopramide Hydrochloride Injection; Metoclopramide Omega; Metonia; Nu-Metoclopramide; PMS-Metoclopramide

Pharmacologic Category Antiemetic; Gastrointestinal Agent, Prokinetic

Additional Appendix Information

Beers Criteria – Potentially Inappropriate Medications for Geriatrics *on page 2368*

Use

Oral: Symptomatic treatment of diabetic gastroparesis; gastroesophageal reflux

I.V., I.M.: Symptomatic treatment of diabetic gastroparesis; postpyloric placement of enteral feeding tubes; prevention and/or treatment of nausea and vomiting associated with chemotherapy, or postsurgery; to stimulate gastric emptying and intestinal transit of barium during radiological examination of the stomach/small intestine

Unlabeled Use Management of gastroparesis (regardless of etiology)

Pregnancy Risk Factor B

Pregnancy Considerations Adverse events were not observed in animal reproduction studies. Metoclopramide crosses the placenta and can be detected in cord blood and amniotic fluid (Arvela, 1983; Bylsma-Howell, 1983). Available evidence suggests safe use during pregnancy (Berkovitch, 2002; Matok, 2009; Sørensen, 2000). Metoclopramide may be used for the treatment of nausea and vomiting of pregnancy (ACOG, 2004; Levichek, 2002) and prophylaxis for nausea and vomiting associated with Caesarean delivery (ASA, 2007; Mahadevan, 2006; Smith, 2011). Other agents are preferred for gastroesophageal reflux (Mahadevan, 2006).

Breast-Feeding Considerations Metoclopramide enters breast milk. Information is available from studies conducted in mothers nursing preterm infants (n=14; delivered at 23-34 weeks gestation) or term infants (n=18) and taking metoclopramide 10 mg 3 times daily. The median concentration of metoclopramide in breast milk was `45 ng/mL in the preterm infants and the mean concentration was ~48 ng/mL in the full term infants. The authors of both studies calculated the relative infant dose to be 3% to 5%, based on a therapeutic infant dose of 0.5 mg/kg/day. Metoclopramide was also detected in the serum of one nursing full term infant (Hansen, 2005; Kauppila, 1983). Metoclopramide may increase prolactin concentrations and cause galactorrhea and gynecomastia, but studies which evaluated its use to increase milk production for women who want to nurse have had mixed results. In addition, due to the potential for adverse events, nonpharmacologic measure should be considered prior to the use of medications as galactagogues (ABM, 2011). The manufacturer recommends that caution be used if administered to a nursing woman.

Medication Guide Available Yes

Contraindications Hypersensitivity to metoclopramide or any component of the formulation; GI obstruction, perforation or hemorrhage; pheochromocytoma; history of seizures or concomitant use of other agents likely to increase extrapyramidal reactions

Warnings/Precautions [U.S. Boxed Warning]: May cause tardive dyskinesia, which is often irreversible; duration of treatment and total cumulative dose are associated with an increased risk. Therapy durations >12 weeks should be avoided (except in rare cases following risk:benefit assessment). Risk appears to be increased in the elderly, women, and diabetics; however, it is not possible to predict which patients will develop tardive dyskinesia. Therapy should be discontinued in any patient if signs/symptoms of tardive dyskinesia appear.

May cause extrapyramidal symptoms, generally manifested as acute dystonic reactions within the initial 24-48 hours of use. Risk of these reactions is increased at higher doses, and in pediatric patients, and adults <30 years of age. Pseudoparkinsonism (eg, bradykinesia, tremor, rigidity) may also occur (usually within first 6 months of therapy) and is generally reversible following discontinuation. Use with caution or avoid in patients with Parkinson's disease. Avoid use in older adults (except for gastroparesis) due to risk of extrapyramidal effects, including tardive dyskinesia; risk potentially even greater in frail older adults (Beers Criteria). In addition, risk of tardive dyskinesia may be increased in older women. Neuroleptic malignant syndrome (NMS) has been reported (rarely) with metoclopramide.

May cause transient increase in serum aldosterone; use caution in patients who are at risk of fluid overload (HF, cirrhosis). Use caution in patients with hypertension or following surgical anastomosis/closure. Use caution with a history of mental illness; has been associated with depression. Abrupt discontinuation may (rarely) result in withdrawal symptoms (dizziness, headache, nervousness). Use caution and adjust dose in renal impairment. Patients with NADH-cytochrome b5 reductase deficiency are at increased risk of methemoglobinemia and/or sulfhemoglobinemia. Neonates may have an increased risk of methemoglobinemia due to decreased levels of NADH-cytochrome b5 reductase deficiency and prolonged clearance of metoclopramide.

Adverse Reactions Frequency not always defined.

Cardiovascular: Atrioventricular block, bradycardia, congestive heart failure, flushing (following high I.V. doses), hypertension, hypotension, supraventricular tachycardia

Central nervous system: Drowsiness (~10% to 70%; dose related), dystonic reaction (<1% to 25%; dose and age related), lassitude (~10%), restlessness (~10%), fatigue (2% to 10%), headache (4% to 5%), dizziness (1% to 4%), somnolence (2% to 3%), akathisia, confusion, depression, drug-induced Parkinson's disease, hallucination (rare), insomnia, neuroleptic malignant syndrome (rare), seizure, suicidal ideation, tardive dyskinesia

Dermatologic: Skin rash, urticaria

Endocrine & metabolic: Amenorrhea, fluid retention, galactorrhea, gynecomastia, hyperprolactinemia, porphyria

Gastrointestinal: Nausea (4% to 6%), vomiting (1% to 2%), diarrhea

Genitourinary: Impotence, urinary frequency, urinary incontinence

Hematologic & oncologic: Agranulocytosis, leukopenia, methemoglobinemia, neutropenia, sulfhemoglobinemia

Hepatic: Hepatotoxicity (rare)

Hypersensitivity: Angioedema (rare), hypersensitivity reaction

Neuromuscular & skeletal: Laryngospasm (rare)

Ophthalmic: Visual disturbance

Respiratory: Bronchospasm, laryngeal edema (rare)

Drug Interactions

Metabolism/Transport Effects **Substrate** of CYP1A2 (minor), CYP2D6 (minor); **Note:** Assignment of Major/Minor substrate status based on clinically relevant drug interaction potential; **Inhibits** CYP2D6 (weak)

Avoid Concomitant Use

Avoid concomitant use of Metoclopramide with any of the following: Antipsychotics; Droperidol; Promethazine; Tetrabenazine; Trimetazidine

Increased Effect/Toxicity

Metoclopramide may increase the levels/effects of: Antipsychotics; CycloSPORINE (Systemic); Prilocaine; Promethazine; Selective Serotonin Reuptake Inhibitors; Sodium Nitrite; Tetrabenazine; Tricyclic Antidepressants; Trimetazidine; Venlafaxine

The levels/effects of Metoclopramide may be increased by: Droperidol; Metyrosine; Nitric Oxide; Serotonin Modulators

Decreased Effect

Metoclopramide may decrease the levels/effects of: Anti-Parkinson's Agents (Dopamine Agonist); Atovaquone; Posaconazole; Quinagolide

The levels/effects of Metoclopramide may be decreased by: Peginterferon Alfa-2b

Ethanol/Nutrition/Herb Interactions Ethanol: Avoid ethanol (may increase CNS depression).

Preparation for Administration Injection solution: Lower doses (≤10 mg): No dilution required; Higher doses (>10 mg): Dilute in 50 mL of compatible solution (preferably NS).

Storage/Stability

Injection solution: Store intact vial at controlled room temperature; injection is photosensitive and should be protected from light during storage; parenteral admixtures in D_5W or NS are stable for at least 24 hours and do not require light protection if used within 24 hours.

Tablet: Store at controlled room temperature of 20°C to 25°C (68°F to 77°F).

Mechanism of Action Blocks dopamine receptors and (when given in higher doses) also blocks serotonin receptors in chemoreceptor trigger zone of the CNS; enhances the response to acetylcholine of tissue in upper GI tract causing enhanced motility and accelerated gastric emptying without stimulating gastric, biliary, or pancreatic secretions; increases lower esophageal sphincter tone

Pharmacodynamics/Kinetics

Onset of action: Oral: 30-60 minutes; I.V.: 1-3 minutes; I.M.: 10-15 minutes

Duration: Therapeutic: 1-2 hours, regardless of route

Absorption: Oral: Rapid

Distribution: V_d: ~3.5 L/kg

Protein binding: ~30%

Bioavailability: Oral: Range: 65% to 95%

Half-life elimination: Normal renal function: Children: ~4 hours; Adults: 5-6 hours (may be dose dependent)

Time to peak, serum: Oral: 1-2 hours

Excretion: Urine (~85%)

Dosage

Children:

Gastroesophageal reflux (unlabeled use): Oral: 0.1-0.2 mg/kg/dose 4 times daily

Antiemetic (chemotherapy-induced emesis) (unlabeled): I.V.: 1-2 mg/kg 30 minutes before chemotherapy and every 2-4 hours (maximum: 5 doses daily); pretreatment with diphenhydramine will decrease risk of extrapyramidal reactions to this dosage

Postpyloric feeding tube placement: I.V.:

<6 years: 0.1 mg/kg as a single dose

6-14 years: 2.5-5 mg as a single dose

>14 years: Refer to adult dosing.

Adults:

Gastroesophageal reflux: Oral: 10-15 mg up to 4 times daily 30 minutes before meals or food and at bedtime; single doses of 20 mg are occasionally needed prior to provoking situations. Treatment >12 weeks is not recommended.

Gastroparesis:

Manufacturer's labeling: Diabetic gastroparesis:

Oral: 10 mg up to 4 times daily 30 minutes before meals or food and at bedtime for 2-8 weeks. Treatment >12 weeks is not recommended.

I.M., I.V. (for severe symptoms): 10 mg over 1-2 minutes; 10 days of I.V. therapy may be necessary before symptoms are controlled to allow transition to oral administration

Alternative recommendations (unlabeled): Gastroparesis: Oral: Initial: 5 mg 3 times daily before meals. Dosage range: 5-10 mg 2-3 times daily before meals (maximum: 40 mg daily). Liquid formulation is preferred (to increase absorption) and the use of drug holidays or dose reductions (eg, 5 mg before the two main meals of the day) is also recommended when clinically possible (Camilleri, 2013).

Chemotherapy-induced emesis prophylaxis: I.V.: 1-2 mg/kg 30 minutes before chemotherapy and repeated every 2 hours for 2 doses, then every 3 hours for 3 doses (manufacturer labeling); pretreatment with diphenhydramine will decrease risk of extrapyramidal reactions

Alternate dosing: **Note:** Metoclopramide is considered an antiemetic with a low therapeutic index; use is generally reserved for agents with low emetogenic potential or in patients intolerant/refractory to first-line antiemetics.

Low-risk chemotherapy (unlabeled): I.V., Oral: 10-40 mg prior to chemotherapy dose, then every 4-6 hours as needed (NCCN Antiemesis guidelines, v.4.2009)

Breakthrough treatment (unlabeled): I.V., Oral: 10-40 mg every 4-6 hours (NCCN Antiemesis guidelines, v.4.2009)

Delayed-emesis prophylaxis (unlabeled): Oral: 20-40 mg (or 0.5 mg/kg/dose) 2-4 times daily for 3-4 days (in combination with dexamethasone [ASCO guidelines, 2006])

Refractory or intolerant to antiemetics with a higher therapeutic index (unlabeled; Hesketh, 2008):

I.V.: 1-2 mg/kg/dose before chemotherapy and repeat 2 hours after chemotherapy

Oral: 0.5 mg/kg every 6 hours on days 2-4

Postoperative nausea and vomiting prophylaxis: I.M., I.V. (unlabeled route): 10-20 mg near end of surgery. **Note:** Guidelines discourage use of 10 mg metoclopramide as being ineffective (Gan, 2007); comparative study indicates higher dose (20 mg) may be efficacious (Quaynor, 2002)

Postpyloric feeding tube placement, radiological exam: I.V.: 10 mg as a single dose

Elderly: Initial: Dose at the lower end of the recommended range. Refer to adult dosing.

Dosage adjustment in renal impairment: Cl_{cr} <40 mL/minute: Administer at 50% of normal dose

Hemodialysis: Not dialyzable (0% to 5%); supplemental dose is not necessary

Dosage adjustment in hepatic impairment: No dosage adjustment provided in manufacturer's labeling. However, metoclopramide has been used safely in patients with advanced liver disease with normal renal function.

Administration

Injection solution: May be given I.M., direct I.V. push, short infusion (15-30 minutes), or continuous infusion; lower doses (≤10 mg) of metoclopramide can be given I.V. push undiluted over 1-2 minutes; higher doses (>10 mg) to be diluted in 50 mL of compatible solution (preferably NS) and given IVPB over at least 15 minutes; continuous SubQ infusion and rectal administration have been reported. **Note:** Rapid I.V. administration may be associated with a transient (but intense) feeling of anxiety and restlessness, followed by drowsiness.

Orally-disintegrating tablets: Administer on an empty stomach at least 30 minutes prior to food. Do not remove from packaging until time of administration. If tablet breaks or crumbles while handling, discard and remove new tablet. Using dry hands, place tablet on tongue and allow to dissolve. Swallow with saliva.

Monitoring Parameters Dystonic reactions; signs of hypoglycemia in patients using insulin and those being treated for gastroparesis; agitation, and confusion

Dosage Forms Excipient information presented when available (limited, particularly for generics); consult specific product labeling.

Solution, Injection:

Generic: 5 mg/mL (2 mL)

Solution, Injection [preservative free]:

Generic: 5 mg/mL (2 mL)

Solution, Oral:

Generic: 5 mg/5 mL (10 mL, 473 mL); 10 mg/10 mL (10 mL)

Tablet, Oral:

Reglan: 5 mg [contains fd&c blue #1 aluminum lake, fd&c yellow #10 aluminum lake]

Reglan: 10 mg [dye free]

Generic: 5 mg, 10 mg

Tablet Dispersible, Oral:

Metozolv ODT: 5 mg

- **Metoclopramide Hydrochloride Injection (Can)** *see* Metoclopramide *on page 1345*
- **Metoclopramide Omega (Can)** *see* Metoclopramide *on page 1345*
- **Metoject (Can)** *see* Methotrexate *on page 1324*

Metolazone (me TOLE a zone)

Brand Names: U.S. Zaroxolyn

Brand Names: Canada Zaroxolyn®

Pharmacologic Category Diuretic, Thiazide-Related

Use Management of mild-to-moderate hypertension; treatment of edema in heart failure and nephrotic syndrome, impaired renal function

Pregnancy Risk Factor B

Pregnancy Considerations Teratogenic effects were not observed in animal studies. Metolazone crosses the placenta and appears in cord blood. Hypoglycemia, hypokalemia, hyponatremia, jaundice, and thrombocytopenia are reported as complications to the fetus or newborn following maternal use of thiazide diuretics.

Breast-Feeding Considerations It is not known if metolazone is excreted in breast milk. Due to the potential for serious adverse reactions in the nursing infant, a decision should be made whether to discontinue nursing or to discontinue the drug, taking into account the importance of treatment to the mother.

Contraindications Hypersensitivity to metolazone, any component of the formulation, other thiazides, and sulfonamide derivatives; anuria; hepatic coma; pregnancy (expert analysis)

Warnings/Precautions Electrolyte disturbances (hypokalemia, hypochloremic alkalosis, hyponatremia) can occur. Large or prolonged fluid and electrolyte losses may occur with concomitant furosemide administration. Use with caution in severe hepatic dysfunction; hepatic encephalopathy can be caused by electrolyte disturbances. Gout can be precipitate in certain patients with a history of gout, a familial predisposition to gout, or chronic renal failure. Cautious use in patients with prediabetes or diabetes; may see a change in glucose control. Can cause SLE exacerbation or activation. Use caution in severe renal impairment. Use with caution in patients with moderate or high cholesterol concentrations. Photosensitization may occur.

Chemical similarities are present among sulfonamides, sulfonylureas, carbonic anhydrase inhibitors, thiazides, and loop diuretics (except ethacrynic acid). Use in patients with thiazide or sulfonamide allergy is specifically contraindicated in product labeling, however, a risk of cross-reaction exists in patients with allergy to any of these compounds; avoid use when previous reaction has been severe. Discontinue if signs of hypersensitivity are noted.

Adverse Reactions Frequency not defined.

Cardiovascular: Chest pain/discomfort, necrotizing angiitis, orthostatic hypotension, palpitation, syncope, venous thrombosis, vertigo, volume depletion

Central nervous system: Chills, depression, dizziness, drowsiness, fatigue, headache, lightheadedness, restlessness

Dermatologic: Petechiae, photosensitivity, pruritus, purpura, rash, skin necrosis, Stevens-Johnson syndrome, toxic epidermal necrolysis, urticaria

Endocrine & metabolic: Gout attacks, hypercalcemia, hyperglycemia, hyperuricemia, hypochloremia, hypochloremic alkalosis, hypokalemia, hypomagnesemia, hyponatremia, hypophosphatemia

Gastrointestinal: Abdominal bloating, abdominal pain, anorexia, constipation, diarrhea, epigastric distress, nausea, pancreatitis, vomiting, xerostomia

Genitourinary: Impotence

Hematologic: Agranulocytosis, aplastic/hypoplastic anemia, hemoconcentration, leukopenia, thrombocytopenia
Hepatic: Cholestatic jaundice, hepatitis
Neuromuscular & skeletal: Joint pain, muscle cramps/spasm, neuropathy, paresthesia, weakness
Ocular: Blurred vision (transient)
Renal: BUN increased, glucosuria

Drug Interactions

Metabolism/Transport Effects None known.

Avoid Concomitant Use

Avoid concomitant use of Metolazone with any of the following: Dofetilide

Increased Effect/Toxicity

Metolazone may increase the levels/effects of: ACE Inhibitors; Allopurinol; Amifostine; Antihypertensives; Calcium Salts; CarBAMazepine; Diazoxide; Dofetilide; Hypotensive Agents; Ivabradine; Lithium; Multivitamins/Minerals (with ADEK, Folate, Iron); Multivitamins/Minerals (with AE, No Iron); Obinutuzumab; OXcarbazepine; Porfimer; RiTUXimab; Sodium Phosphates; Topiramate; Toremifene; Vitamin D Analogs

The levels/effects of Metolazone may be increased by: Alcohol (Ethyl); Alfuzosin; Analgesics (Opioid); Anticholinergic Agents; Barbiturates; Beta2-Agonists; Brimonidine (Topical); Corticosteroids (Orally Inhaled); Corticosteroids (Systemic); Herbs (Hypotensive Properties); Licorice; MAO Inhibitors; Multivitamins/Fluoride (with ADE); Pentoxifylline; Phosphodiesterase 5 Inhibitors; Prostacyclin Analogues; Selective Serotonin Reuptake Inhibitors

Decreased Effect

Metolazone may decrease the levels/effects of: Antidiabetic Agents

The levels/effects of Metolazone may be decreased by: Bile Acid Sequestrants; Herbs (Hypertensive Properties); Methylphenidate; Nonsteroidal Anti-Inflammatory Agents; Yohimbine

Ethanol/Nutrition/Herb Interactions

Ethanol: May potentiate hypotensive effect of metazolone.
Herb/Nutraceutical: Avoid herbs with *hypertensive* properties (bayberry, blue cohosh, cayenne, ephedra, ginger, ginseng [American], kola, licorice); may diminish the antihypertensive effect of metolazone. Avoid herbs with *hypotensive* properties (black cohosh, California poppy, coleus, golden seal, hawthorn, mistletoe, periwinkle, quinine, shepherd's purse); may enhance the hypotensive effect of metolazone.

Mechanism of Action Inhibits sodium reabsorption in the distal tubules causing increased excretion of sodium and water, as well as, potassium and hydrogen ions

Pharmacodynamics/Kinetics

Onset of action: Diuresis: ~60 minutes
Duration: ≥24 hours
Absorption: Incomplete
Distribution: Crosses placenta; enters breast milk
Protein binding: 95%
Half-life elimination: 20 hours
Excretion: Urine (80%); bile (10%)

Dosage Oral:

Adults:

Edema: Initial: 2.5-10 mg once daily; may increase as necessary to 20 mg once daily (ACC/AHA 2009 Heart Failure Guidelines); **Note:** Dosing frequency may be adjusted based on patient-specific diuretic needs (eg, administration every other day or weekly) (Lindenfeld, 2010).

Hypertension: 2.5-5 mg/dose every 24 hours

Elderly: Initial: 2.5 mg/day or every other day

Dosage adjustment in renal impairment: Use caution in patients with severely impaired renal function, as most of the drug is excreted by the renal route and accumulation may occur. Not dialyzable (0% to 5%) via hemo- or peritoneal dialysis; supplemental dose is not necessary.

Dosage adjustment in hepatic impairment: No dosage adjustment provided in manufacturer's labeling. However, contraindicated in hepatic coma.

Dietary Considerations Should be taken after breakfast; may require potassium supplementation

Administration May be taken with food or milk. Take early in day to avoid nocturia. Take the last dose of multiple doses no later than 6 PM unless instructed otherwise.

Monitoring Parameters Serum electrolytes (potassium, sodium, chloride, bicarbonate), renal function, blood pressure (standing, sitting/supine)

Additional Information Metolazone 5 mg is approximately equivalent to hydrochlorothiazide 50 mg.

Dosage Forms Excipient information presented when available (limited, particularly for generics); consult specific product labeling.

Tablet, Oral:
Zaroxolyn: 2.5 mg, 5 mg
Generic: 2.5 mg, 5 mg, 10 mg

Extemporaneous Preparations A 1 mg/mL oral suspension may be made by with tablets and one of three different vehicles (cherry syrup diluted 1:4 with simple syrup; a 1:1 mixture of Ora-Sweet® and Ora-Plus®; or a 1:1 mixture of Ora-Sweet® SF and Ora-Plus®). Crush twelve 10 mg tablets in a mortar and reduce to a fine powder. Add small portions of the chosen vehicle and mix to a uniform paste; mix while adding the vehicle in incremental proportions to **almost** 120 mL; transfer to a calibrated bottle, rinse mortar with vehicle, and add quantity of vehicle sufficient to make 120 mL. Label "shake well" and "refrigerate". Stable for 60 days.

A 0.25 mg/mL oral suspension may be made with tablets and a 1:1 mixture of methylcellulose 1% and simple syrup. Crush one 2.5 mg tablet in a mortar and reduce to a fine powder. Add small portions of the vehicle and mix to a uniform paste; mix while adding the vehicle in incremental proportions to **almost** 10 mL; transfer to a calibrated bottle, rinse mortar with vehicle, and add quantity of vehicle sufficient to make 10 mL. Label "shake well" and "refrigerate". Stable for 91 days refrigerated (preferred), 28 days at room temperature in plastic, and 14 days at room temperature in glass.

Nahata, MC, Pai VB, and Hipple TF, *Pediatric Drug Formulations*, 5th ed, Cincinnati, OH: Harvey Whitney Books Co, 2004.

◆ Metonia (Can) *see* Metoclopramide *on page 1345*

Metoprolol (me toe PROE lole)

Brand Names: U.S. Lopressor; Toprol XL

Brand Names: Canada Apo-Metoprolol (Type L®); Apo-Metoprolol SR®; Apo-Metoprolol®; Ava-Metoprolol; Ava-Metoprolol (Type L); Betaloc®; Dom-Metoprolol-B; Dom-Metoprolol-L; JAMP-Metoprolol-L; Lopresor SR®; Lopresor®; Metoprolol Tartrate Injection, USP; Metoprolol-25; Metoprolol-L; Mylan-Metoprolol (Type L); Nu-Metop; PMS-Metoprolol-B; PMS-Metoprolol-L; Riva-Metoprolol-L; Sandoz-Metoprolol (Type L); Sandoz-Metoprolol SR; Teva-Metoprolol

Index Terms Metoprolol Succinate; Metoprolol Tartrate

Pharmacologic Category Antianginal Agent; Antihypertensive; Beta-Blocker, Beta-1 Selective

Additional Appendix Information

Beta-Blockers *on page 2294*

Dosing Considerations for the Critically-Ill Patient With Morbid Obesity *on page 2379*

Use Treatment of angina pectoris, hypertension, or hemodynamically-stable acute myocardial infarction

Extended release: Treatment of angina pectoris or hypertension; to reduce mortality/hospitalization in patients with heart failure (stable NYHA Class II or III) already receiving ACE inhibitors, diuretics, and/or digoxin

Unlabeled Use Treatment of ventricular arrhythmias, atrial ectopy; migraine prophylaxis, essential tremor; prevention of reinfarction and sudden death after myocardial infarction; prevention and treatment of atrial fibrillation and atrial flutter; multifocal atrial tachycardia; symptomatic treatment of hypertrophic obstructive cardiomyopathy; management of thyrotoxicosis

Pregnancy Risk Factor C

Pregnancy Considerations Adverse events were observed in animal studies; therefore, the manufacturer classifies metoprolol as pregnancy category C. Metoprolol crosses the placenta and can be detected in cord blood, amniotic fluid, and the serum of newborn infants. In a cohort study, an increased risk of cardiovascular defects was observed following maternal use of beta-blockers during pregnancy. Intrauterine growth restriction (IUGR), small placentas, as well as fetal/neonatal bradycardia, hypoglycemia, and/or respiratory depression have been observed following *in utero* exposure to beta-blockers as a class. Adequate facilities for monitoring infants at birth should be available. Untreated chronic maternal hypertension and pre-eclampsia are also associated with adverse events in the fetus, infant, and mother. The clearance of metoprolol is increased and serum concentrations and AUC of metoprolol are decreased during pregnancy. Metoprolol has been evaluated for the treatment of hypertension in pregnancy, but other agents may be more appropriate for use.

Breast-Feeding Considerations Small amounts of metoprolol can be detected in breast milk. The manufacturer recommends that caution be exercised when administering metoprolol to nursing women.

Contraindications

Hypersensitivity to metoprolol, any component of the formulation, or other beta-blockers

Note: Additional contraindications are formulation and/or indication specific.

Immediate release tablets/injectable formulation:

Hypertension and angina: Sinus bradycardia; second- and third-degree heart block; cardiogenic shock; overt heart failure; sick sinus syndrome (except in patients with a functioning artificial pacemaker); severe peripheral arterial disease; pheochromocytoma (without alpha blockade)

Myocardial infarction: Severe sinus bradycardia (heart rate <45 beats/minute); significant first-degree heart block (P-R interval ≥0.24 seconds); second- and third-degree heart block; systolic blood pressure <100 mm Hg; moderate-to-severe cardiac failure

Extended release tablet: Severe bradycardia, second- and third degree heart block; cardiogenic shock; decompensated heart failure; sick sinus syndrome (except in patients with a functioning artificial pacemaker)

Warnings/Precautions [U.S. Boxed Warning]: Beta-blocker therapy should not be withdrawn abruptly (particularly in patients with CAD), but gradually tapered over 1-2 weeks to avoid acute tachycardia, hypertension, and/or ischemia. Consider pre-existing conditions such as sick sinus syndrome before initiating. Metoprolol commonly produces mild first-degree heart block (P-R interval >0.2-0.24 sec). May also produce severe first- (P-R interval ≥0.26 sec), second-, or third-degree heart block. Patients with acute MI (especially right ventricular MI) have a high risk of developing heart block of varying degrees. If severe heart block occurs, metoprolol should be discontinued and measures to increase heart rate should be employed. Symptomatic hypotension may occur with use. May precipitate or aggravate symptoms of arterial insufficiency in patients with PVD and Raynaud's disease; use with caution and monitor for progression of arterial obstruction. Potentially significant interactions may exist, requiring dose or frequency adjustment, additional monitoring, and/or selection of alternative therapy. Consult drug interactions database for more detailed information.

In general, beta-blockers should be avoided in patients with bronchospastic disease. Metoprolol, with B_1 selectivity, should be used cautiously in bronchospastic disease with close monitoring. Use cautiously in patients with diabetes because it can mask prominent hypoglycemic symptoms. May mask signs of hyperthyroidism (eg, tachycardia); if hyperthyroidism is suspected, carefully manage and monitor; abrupt withdrawal may exacerbate symptoms of hyperthyroidism or precipitate thyroid storm. Alterations in thyroid function tests may be observed. Use caution with hepatic dysfunction. Use with caution in patients with myasthenia gravis or psychiatric disease (may cause CNS depression). Although perioperative beta-blocker therapy is recommended prior to elective surgery in selected patients, use of high-dose extended release metoprolol in patients naïve to beta-blocker therapy undergoing noncardiac surgery has been associated with bradycardia, hypotension, stroke, and death. Chronic beta-blocker therapy should not be routinely withdrawn prior to major surgery. Use of beta-blockers may unmask cardiac failure in patients without a history of dysfunction. Adequate alpha-blockade is required prior to use of any beta-blocker for patients with untreated pheochromocytoma. May induce or exacerbate psoriasis. Use caution with history of severe anaphylaxis to allergens; patients taking beta-blockers may become more sensitive to repeated allergen challenges. Treatment of anaphylaxis (eg, epinephrine) in patients taking beta-blockers may be ineffective or promote undesirable effects. Bradycardia may be observed more frequently in elderly patients (>65 years of age); dosage reductions may be necessary.

Extended release: Use with caution in patients with compensated heart failure; monitor for a worsening of heart failure.

Adverse Reactions Frequency may not be defined.

Cardiovascular: Hypotension (1% to 27%), bradycardia (2% to 16%), first-degree heart block (P-R interval ≥0.26 sec; 5%), arterial insufficiency (usually Raynaud type; 1%), chest pain (1%), CHF (1%), edema (peripheral; 1%), palpitation (1%), syncope (1%)

Central nervous system: Dizziness (2% to 10%), fatigue (1% to 10%), depression (5%), confusion, hallucinations, headache, insomnia, memory loss (short-term), nightmares, sleep disturbances, somnolence, vertigo

Dermatology: Pruritus (5%), rash (5%), photosensitivity, psoriasis exacerbated

Endocrine & metabolic: Libido decreased, Peyronie's disease (<1%), diabetes exacerbated

Gastrointestinal: Diarrhea (5%), constipation (1%), flatulence (1%), gastrointestinal pain (1%), heartburn (1%), nausea (1%), xerostomia (1%), vomiting

Hematologic: Claudication

Neuromuscular & skeletal: Musculoskeletal pain

Ocular: Blurred vision, visual disturbances

Otic: Tinnitus

Respiratory: Dyspnea (1% to 3%), bronchospasm (1%), wheezing (1%), rhinitis, shortness of breath

Miscellaneous: Cold extremities (1%)

Postmarketing and/or case reports: Agranulocytosis, alkaline phosphatase increased, alopecia (reversible), anxiety, arthralgia, arthritis, cardiogenic shock, diaphoresis increased, dry eyes, gangrene, hepatitis, HDL decreased, impotence, jaundice, lactate dehydrogenase increased, nervousness, paresthesia, retroperitoneal fibrosis, second-degree heart block, taste disturbance, third-degree heart block, thrombocytopenia, transaminases increased, triglycerides increased, urticaria, vomiting, weight gain

Other events reported with beta-blockers: Catatonia, emotional lability, fever, hypersensitivity reactions, laryngospasm, nonthrombocytopenic purpura, respiratory distress, thrombocytopenic purpura

Drug Interactions

Metabolism/Transport Effects Substrate of CYP2C19 (minor), CYP2D6 (major); **Note:** Assignment of Major/ Minor substrate status based on clinically relevant drug interaction potential; **Inhibits** CYP2D6 (weak)

Avoid Concomitant Use

Avoid concomitant use of Metoprolol with any of the following: Floctafenine; Methacholine

Increased Effect/Toxicity

Metoprolol may increase the levels/effects of: Alpha-/Beta-Agonists (Direct-Acting); Alpha1-Blockers; Alpha2-Agonists; Amifostine; Antihypertensives; Antipsychotic Agents (Phenothiazines); ARIPiprazole; Bupivacaine; Cardiac Glycosides; Cholinergic Agonists; Ergot Derivatives; Fingolimod; Hypotensive Agents; Insulin; Lidocaine (Systemic); Lidocaine (Topical); Mepivacaine; Methacholine; Midodrine; Obinutuzumab; RiTUXimab; Sulfonylureas

The levels/effects of Metoprolol may be increased by: Acetylcholinesterase Inhibitors; Alpha2-Agonists; Aminoquinolines (Antimalarial); Amiodarone; Anilidopiperidine Opioids; Antipsychotic Agents (Phenothiazines); Brimonidine (Topical); Calcium Channel Blockers (Dihydropyridine); Calcium Channel Blockers (Nondihydropyridine); CYP2D6 Inhibitors; Darunavir; Diazoxide; Dipyridamole; Disopyramide; Dronedarone; Floctafenine; Herbs (Hypotensive Properties); MAO Inhibitors; Mirabegron; Pentoxifylline; Phosphodiesterase 5 Inhibitors; Propafenone; Prostacyclin Analogues; Regorafenib; Reserpine; Selective Serotonin Reuptake Inhibitors

Decreased Effect

Metoprolol may decrease the levels/effects of: Beta2-Agonists; Theophylline Derivatives

The levels/effects of Metoprolol may be decreased by: Barbiturates; Herbs (Hypertensive Properties); Methylphenidate; Mirabegron; Nonsteroidal Anti-Inflammatory Agents; Peginterferon Alfa-2b; Rifamycin Derivatives; Yohimbine

Ethanol/Nutrition/Herb Interactions

Food: Food increases absorption. Metoprolol serum levels may be increased if taken with food. Management: Take immediate release tartrate tablets with food; succinate can be taken with or without food.

Herb/Nutraceutical: Some herbal medications may worsen hypertension (eg, licorice); others may increase the antihypertensive effect of metoprolol (eg, shepherd's purse). Management: Avoid bayberry, blue cohosh, cayenne, ephedra, ginger, ginseng (American), gotu kola, licorice, and yohimbe. Avoid black cohosh, California poppy, coleus, golden seal, hawthorn, mistletoe, periwinkle, quinine, and shepherd's purse.

Storage/Stability

Injection: Store at 25°C (77°F); excursions permitted to 15°C to 30°C (59°F to 86°F). Protect from light and heat.

Tablet: Store at 25°C (77°F); excursions permitted to 15°C to 30°C (59°F to 86°F). Protect from moisture and heat.

Mechanism of Action Selective inhibitor of $beta_1$-adrenergic receptors; competitively blocks $beta_1$-receptors, with little or no effect on $beta_2$-receptors at doses <100 mg; does not exhibit any membrane stabilizing or intrinsic sympathomimetic activity

Pharmacodynamics/Kinetics

Onset of action: Peak effect: Oral: 1-2 hours (Regårdh, 1980); I.V.: 20 minutes (when infused over 10 minutes)

Duration: Oral: Immediate release: Variable (dose-related; 50% reduction in maximum heart rate after single doses of 20, 50, and 100 mg occurred at 3.3, 5, and 6.4 hours, respectively), Extended release: ~24 hours; I.V.: 5-8 hours

Absorption: Rapid and complete

Distribution: V_d: 3.2-5.6 L/kg

Protein binding: ~10% to albumin

Metabolism: Extensively hepatic via CYP2D6; significant first-pass effect (~50%)

Bioavailability: Oral: Immediate release: ~50% (Extended release: 77% relative to immediate release)

Half-life elimination: 3-4 hours (7-9 hours in poor CYP2D6 metabolizers)

Excretion: Urine (<10% as unchanged drug; increased to 30-40% in poor CYP2D6 metabolizers)

Dosage

Children: Hypertension: Oral:

1-17 years: Immediate release tablet: (National High Blood Pressure Education Program Working Group on High Blood Pressure in Children and Adolescents, 2004): Initial: 1-2 mg/kg/day; maximum 6 mg/kg/day (≤200 mg/day); administer in 2 divided doses

≥6 years: Extended release tablet: Initial: 1 mg/kg once daily (maximum initial dose: 50 mg/day). Adjust dose based on patient response (maximum: 2 mg/kg/day or 200 mg/day)

Adults:

Angina: Oral:

Immediate release: Initial: 50 mg twice daily; usual dosage range: 50-200 mg twice daily; maximum: 400 mg/day; increase dose at weekly intervals to desired effect

Extended release: Initial: 100 mg/day (maximum: 400 mg/day)

Atrial fibrillation/flutter (ventricular rate control), supraventricular tachycardia (SVT) (acute treatment; unlabeled use; Antman, 2004; Fuster, 2006; Neumar, 2010): I.V.: 2.5-5 mg every 2-5 minutes (maximum total dose: 15 mg over a 10-15 minute period). **Note:** Initiate cautiously in patients with concomitant heart failure; avoid in patients with decompensated heart failure.

Maintenance: Oral (immediate release): 25-100 mg twice daily

Heart failure: Oral (extended release): Initial: 25 mg once daily (reduce to 12.5 mg once daily in NYHA class higher than class II); may double dosage every 2 weeks as tolerated (target dose: 200 mg/day)

Hypertension: Oral:

Immediate release: Initial: 50 mg twice daily; effective dosage range: 100-450 mg/day in 2-3 divided doses; increase dose at weekly intervals to desired effect; maximum: 450 mg/day; usual dosage range (JNC 7): 50-100 mg/day

Extended release: Initial: 25-100 mg once daily; increase doses at weekly (or longer) intervals to desired effect; maximum: 400 mg/day; usual dosage range (JNC 7): 50-100 mg/day

Hypertension/ventricular rate control: I.V. (in patients having nonfunctioning GI tract): Initial: 1.25-5 mg every 6-12 hours; titrate initial dose to response. Initially, low doses may be appropriate to establish response; however, although not routine, up to 15 mg administered as frequently as every 3 hours has been employed in patients with refractory tachycardia.

Myocardial infarction:

Acute: I.V.: 5 mg every 2 minutes for 3 doses in early treatment of myocardial infarction; thereafter, give 50 mg orally every 6 hours beginning 15 minutes after last I.V. dose and continue for 48 hours; then administer a maintenance dose of 100 mg twice daily. **Note:** Do not initiate this regimen in those with signs of heart failure, a low output state, increased risk of cardiogenic shock, or other contraindications (eg, second- or third-degree heart block). If initial I.V. dosing is not tolerated, may give 25-50 mg orally (depending on degree of intolerance) every 6 hours beginning 15 minutes after the last I.V. dose or as soon as clinical condition permits.

Secondary prevention (unlabeled use; Olsson, 1992): Oral: Immediate release: 25-100 mg twice daily; optimize dose based on heart rate and blood pressure; continue indefinitely.

Thyrotoxicosis (unlabeled use): Oral: Immediate release: 25-50 mg every 6 hours; may also consider administering extended release formulation (Bahn, 2011)

Elderly: Hypertension: Initiate at the lower end of the dosage range and titrate to response

Note: Switching dosage forms:

When switching from immediate release metoprolol to extended release, the same total daily dose of metoprolol should be used.

When switching between oral and intravenous dosage forms, equivalent beta-blocking effect is achieved when doses in a 2.5:1 (Oral:I.V.) ratio is used. For example, if the patient is receiving an oral dose of 25 mg twice daily (50 mg/day), this would translate to 5 mg I.V. every 6 hours; consider reducing initial I.V. dose to evaluate patient response.

Dosage adjustment in renal impairment: No dosage adjustment necessary.

Dosage adjustment in hepatic impairment: No dosage adjustment provided in manufacturer's labeling. However, reduced dose may be necessary due to extensive hepatic metabolism.

Dietary Considerations Immediate release tablets should be taken with food. Extended release tablets may be taken without regard to meals.

Administration

Oral: Extended release tablets may be divided in half; do not crush or chew. Administer immediate release tablets with or immediately following food.

I.V.: I.V. dose is much smaller than oral dose. When administered acutely for cardiac treatment, monitor ECG and blood pressure; may administer by rapid infusion (I.V. push) over 1 minute. May also be administered by slow infusion (ie, 5-10 mg of metoprolol in 50 mL of fluid) over ~30-60 minutes during less urgent situations (eg, substitution for oral metoprolol).

Monitoring Parameters Acute cardiac treatment: Monitor ECG and blood pressure with I.V. administration; heart rate and blood pressure with oral administration. I.V. use in a nonemergency situation: Necessary monitoring for surgical patients who are unable to take oral beta-blockers (because of prolonged ileus) has not been defined. Some institutions require monitoring of baseline and postinfusion heart rate and blood pressure when a patient's response to beta-blockade has not been characterized (ie, the patient's initial dose or following a change in dose). Consult individual institutional policies and procedures.

Dosage Forms Excipient information presented when available (limited, particularly for generics); consult specific product labeling.

Solution, Intravenous, as tartrate:
Lopressor: 1 mg/mL (5 mL)
Generic: 1 mg/mL (5 mL); 5 mg/5 mL (5 mL)

Tablet, Oral, as tartrate:
Lopressor: 50 mg, 100 mg [scored]
Generic: 25 mg, 50 mg, 100 mg

Tablet Extended Release 24 Hour, Oral, as succinate:
Toprol XL: 25 mg, 50 mg, 100 mg, 200 mg [scored]
Generic: 25 mg, 50 mg, 100 mg, 200 mg

Extemporaneous Preparations A 10 mg/mL oral suspension may be made with metoprolol tartrate tablets and one of three different vehicles (cherry syrup; a 1:1 mixture of Ora-Sweet® and Ora-Plus®; or a 1:1 mixture of Ora-Sweet® SF and Ora-Plus®). Crush twelve 100 mg tablets in a mortar and reduce to a fine powder. Add 20 mL of the chosen vehicle and mix to a uniform paste; mix while adding the vehicle in incremental proportions to **almost** 120 mL; transfer to a calibrated bottle, rinse mortar with vehicle, and add quantity of vehicle sufficient to make 120 mL. Label "shake well" and "protect from light". Stable for 60 days.

Allen LV Jr and Erickson MA 3rd, "Stability of Labetalol Hydrochloride, Metoprolol Tartrate, Verapamil Hydrochloride, and Spironolactone With Hydrochlorothiazide in Extemporaneously Compounded Oral Liquids," *Am J Health Syst Pharm*, 1996, 53(19):2304-9.

- **Metoprolol-25 (Can)** *see* Metoprolol *on page 1348*
- **Metoprolol-L (Can)** *see* Metoprolol *on page 1348*
- **Metoprolol Succinate** *see* Metoprolol *on page 1348*
- **Metoprolol Tartrate** *see* Metoprolol *on page 1348*
- **Metoprolol Tartrate Injection, USP (Can)** *see* Metoprolol *on page 1348*
- **Metozolv ODT** *see* Metoclopramide *on page 1345*
- **Metro** *see* MetroNIDAZOLE (Systemic) *on page 1351*
- **MetroCream** *see* MetroNIDAZOLE (Topical) *on page 1354*
- **MetroCream® (Can)** *see* MetroNIDAZOLE (Topical) *on page 1354*
- **Metrogel** *see* MetroNIDAZOLE (Topical) *on page 1354*
- **Metrogel® (Can)** *see* MetroNIDAZOLE (Topical) *on page 1354*
- **MetroGel-Vaginal** *see* MetroNIDAZOLE (Topical) *on page 1354*
- **MetroLotion** *see* MetroNIDAZOLE (Topical) *on page 1354*
- **MetroLotion® (Can)** *see* MetroNIDAZOLE (Topical) *on page 1354*

MetroNIDAZOLE (Systemic)

(met roe NYE da zole)

Brand Names: U.S. Flagyl; Flagyl ER; Metro

Brand Names: Canada Flagyl; Novo-Nidazol; PMS-Metronidazole

Index Terms Metronidazole Hydrochloride

Pharmacologic Category Amebicide; Antibiotic, Miscellaneous; Antiprotozoal, Nitroimidazole

Use

Oral: Treatment of susceptible anaerobic bacterial and protozoal infections in the following conditions: Amebiasis, symptomatic and asymptomatic trichomoniasis, skin and skin structure infections, bone and joint infections, CNS infections, endocarditis, gynecologic infections, intra-abdominal infections (as part of combination regimen), respiratory tract infections (lower), septicemia due to anaerobes (immediate-release only); bacterial vaginosis (extended-release only); treatment of *Clostridium difficile*-associated diarrhea (CDAD)

Injection: Treatment of susceptible anaerobic bacterial infections in the following conditions: Skin and skin structure infections, bone and joint infections, CNS infections, endocarditis, gynecologic infections, intra-abdominal infections (as part of combination regimen), respiratory tract infections (lower), septicemia; surgical (preoperative) prophylaxis (colorectal surgery); treatment of CDAD

Unlabeled Use Crohn's disease; urethritis

Pregnancy Risk Factor B

Pregnancy Considerations Teratogenic effects have not been observed in animal reproduction studies. Metronidazole crosses the placenta and rapidly distributes into the fetal circulation. Although there have been a few reports of facial anomalies after *in utero* exposure, most studies have not found an increased risk of congenital abnormalities following maternal use of metronidazole during the first trimester of pregnancy. In studies that included women taking metronidazole during all trimesters of pregnancy, an increased risk of adverse fetal and neonatal outcomes has not been observed. Because metronidazole has been carcinogenic in some animal species, concern has been raised whether metronidazole should be used during pregnancy; however, a strong carcinogenic potential in humans has not been observed, including one study of prenatal exposure.

Metronidazole pharmacokinetics are similar between pregnant and nonpregnant patients. Bacterial vaginosis has been associated with adverse pregnancy outcomes (including preterm labor); metronidazole is recommended for the treatment of symptomatic bacterial vaginosis in pregnant patients. Vaginal trichomoniasis has been also associated with adverse pregnancy outcomes (including preterm labor). Treatment may relieve symptoms and prevent further sexual transmission; however, metronidazole has not resulted in reduced perinatal morbidity and should not be used solely to prevent preterm delivery. Some clinicians consider deferring therapy in asymptomatic women until >37 weeks gestation. Use of oral metronidazole is contraindicated during the first trimester (per the FDA approved labeling). Not recommended for treatment of *Clostridium difficile* infection in pregnancy (Surzwica, 2013). Consult current CDC guidelines for appropriate use in pregnant women.

Breast-Feeding Considerations Metronidazole and its active metabolite are measurable in the breast milk and infant plasma. Milk concentrations are similar to those in the maternal plasma and are highly variable. Peak concentrations of metronidazole in breast milk occur ~2-4 hours after the oral dose. In studies, the calculated relative infant doses have ranged from 0.13% to 36% of the weight-adjusted maternal dose. Use of metronidazole in a lactating patient is not recommended by the manufacturer. If metronidazole is given, breast-feeding should be withheld for 12-24 hours after the dose (CDC, 2010). Not recommended for treatment of *Clostridium difficile* infection in breast-feeding women (Surzwica, 2013).

Contraindications Hypersensitivity to metronidazole, nitroimidazole derivatives, or any component of the formulation; pregnancy (first trimester); use of disulfiram within the past 2 weeks; use of alcohol during therapy or within 3 days of therapy discontinuation

Warnings/Precautions [U.S. Boxed Warning]: Possibly carcinogenic based on animal data. Use with caution in patients with severe liver impairment and ESRD due to potential accumulation; reduce dosage in patients with severe liver impairment and consider dosage reduction in patients with severe renal impairment (Cl_{cr} <10 mL/minute) who are receiving prolonged therapy. Hemodialysis patients may need supplemental dosing. Use with caution in patients with blood dyscrasias, history of seizures, CHF or other sodium-retaining states.

Aseptic meningitis, encephalopathy, seizures, and neuropathies have been reported especially with increased doses and chronic treatment; monitor and consider discontinuation of therapy if symptoms occur. Prolonged use may result in fungal or bacterial superinfection, including *C. difficile*-associated diarrhea (CDAD) and pseudomembranous colitis; CDAD has been observed >2 months postantibiotic treatment. The Infectious Disease Society of America (IDSA) recommends the use of oral metronidazole for initial treatment of mild-to-moderate *C. difficile* infection and the use of oral vancomycin for initial treatment of severe *C. difficile* infection with or without I.V. metronidazole depending on the presence of complications. May treat recurrent mild-to-moderate infection once with oral metronidazole; avoid use beyond first reoccurrence due to potential cumulative neurotoxicity (Cohen, 2010). The American College of Gastroenterology (ACG) recommends oral vancomycin and intravenous metronidazole for severe and complicated CDI (Surawicz, 2013). Candidiasis infection (known or unknown) maybe more prominent during metronidazole treatment, antifungal treatment required. If *H. pylori* is not eradicated in patients being treated with metronidazole in a regimen, it should be assumed that metronidazole-resistance has occurred and it should not again be used.

Disulfiram-like reactions to ethanol have been reported with oral metronidazole; avoid alcoholic beverages or products containing propylene glycol during and for at least 3 days after therapy. Use with caution in the elderly; dosage adjustment may be required based on renal and/or hepatic function.

Adverse Reactions Frequency not always defined.

Cardiovascular: Flattened T-wave on ECG, flushing, local thrombophlebitis (I.V.), syncope

Central nervous system: Headache (18%), metallic taste (9%), dizziness (4%), aseptic meningitis, ataxia, brain disease, confusion, depression, disulfiram-like reaction (with alcohol), dysarthria, dyspareunia, insomnia, irritability, peripheral neuropathy, seizure, vertigo

Dermatologic: Erythematous rash, pruritus, Stevens-Johnson syndrome, toxic epidermal necrolysis, urticaria

Gastrointestinal: Nausea (10% to ~12%), abdominal pain (4%), diarrhea (4%), xerostomia (2%), abdominal cramps, anorexia, constipation, epigastric distress, glossitis, hairy tongue, pancreatitis (rare), proctitis, stomatitis, vomiting

Genitourinary: Vaginitis (15%), genital pruritus (5%), dysmenorrhea (3%), urine abnormality (3%), urinary tract infection (2%), cystitis, dark urine (rare), decreased libido, dysuria, sensation of pelvic pressure, urinary incontinence, vaginal dryness, vulvovaginal candidiasis

Hematologic & oncologic: Neutropenia (reversible), thrombocytopenia (reversible, rare)

Immunologic: Serum sickness-like reaction (joint pains)

Infection: Bacterial infection (7%), candidiasis (3%)

Neuromuscular & skeletal: Weakness

Ophthalmic: Optic neuropathy

Renal: Polyuria

Respiratory: Flu-like symptoms (6%), upper respiratory tract infection (4%), pharyngitis (3%), nasal congestion, rhinitis, sinusitis

Miscellaneous: Fever, lesion (central nervous system, reversible)

Drug Interactions

Metabolism/Transport Effects Substrate of CYP2A6 (minor); **Note:** Assignment of Major/Minor substrate status based on clinically relevant drug interaction potential; **Inhibits** CYP2C9 (weak), CYP3A4 (weak)

Avoid Concomitant Use

Avoid concomitant use of MetroNIDAZOLE (Systemic) with any of the following: Alcohol (Ethyl); BCG; Carbocisteine; Disulfiram; Pimozide

Increased Effect/Toxicity

MetroNIDAZOLE (Systemic) may increase the levels/effects of: Alcohol (Ethyl); ARIPiprazole; Busulfan; Calcineurin Inhibitors; Carbocisteine; Dofetilide; Fluorouracil

(Systemic); Fosphenytoin; Lomitapide; Phenytoin; Pimozide; Tegafur; Tipranavir; Vitamin K Antagonists

The levels/effects of MetroNIDAZOLE (Systemic) may be increased by: Disulfiram; Mebendazole

Decreased Effect

MetroNIDAZOLE (Systemic) may decrease the levels/ effects of: BCG; Mycophenolate; Sodium Picosulfate; Typhoid Vaccine

The levels/effects of MetroNIDAZOLE (Systemic) may be decreased by: Fosphenytoin; PHENobarbital; Phenytoin

Ethanol/Nutrition/Herb Interactions

Ethanol: The manufacturer recommends to avoid all ethanol or any ethanol-containing drugs (may cause disulfiram-like reaction characterized by flushing, headache, nausea, vomiting, sweating, or tachycardia) during and for 3 days after therapy.

Food: Peak antibiotic serum concentration lowered and delayed, but total drug absorbed not affected.

Storage/Stability

Oral:

Extended-release: Store at 25°C (77°F); excursions are permitted to 15°C to 30°C (59°F to 86°F).

Immediate release: Store at 15°C to 25°C (59°F to 77°F). Protect the tablets from light.

Injection: Store at 25°C (77°F). Protect from light. Brief exposure up to 40°C does not adversely affect the product. Avoid excessive heat. Do not refrigerate. Do not remove unit from overwrap until ready for use. Discard unused solution.

Mechanism of Action After diffusing into the organism, interacts with DNA to cause a loss of helical DNA structure and strand breakage resulting in inhibition of protein synthesis and cell death in susceptible organisms

Pharmacodynamics/Kinetics

Absorption: Oral: Well absorbed

Distribution: To saliva, bile, seminal fluid, bone, liver, and liver abscesses, lung and vaginal secretions; crosses blood-brain barrier

CSF:blood level ratio: Normal meninges: 16% to 43%; Inflamed meninges: 100%

Protein binding: <20%

Metabolism: Hepatic (30% to 60%) to several metabolites including an active hydroxyl metabolite which maintains activity ~30% to 65% of the parent compound (Lamp, 1999)

Half-life elimination: Neonates: 25-75 hours; Others: ~8 hours

Hepatic impairment: 18.31 hours (mean) in one study (Lau, 1987)

According to Child-Pugh classification (Muscara, 1995):

Child-Pugh class A: ~10.7 hours

Child-Pugh class B: ~13.5 hours

Child-Pugh class C: ~21.5 hours

Renal impairment (Cl_{cr} ≤65 mL/minute): Hydroxy metabolite (active): 18-32 hours (Lamp, 1999)

Time to peak, serum: Oral: Immediate release: 1-2 hours

Excretion: Urine (unchanged drug and metabolites: 60% to 80%; ~20% of total as unchanged drug); feces (6% to 15%)

Dosage

Infants and Children:

Amebiasis: Oral: 35-50 mg/kg/day in divided doses every 8 hours for 10 days

Trichomoniasis: Oral: 15-30 mg/kg/day in divided doses every 8 hours for 7 days

Anaerobic infections:

Oral: 15-35 mg/kg/day in divided doses every 8 hours

I.V.: 30 mg/kg/day in divided doses every 6 hours

Clostridium difficile (antibiotic-associated colitis): Oral: 30 mg/kg/day divided every 6 hours for 7-10 days; maximum dose: 2000 mg daily

Surgical (preoperative) prophylaxis (unlabeled use):

Infants <1200 g: I.V.: 7.5 mg/kg within 60 minutes prior to surgical incision in combination with other antibiotics (Bratzler, 2013).

Infants ≥1200 g and Children ≥1 year:

I.V.: 15 mg/kg within 60 minutes prior to surgical incision in combination with other antibiotics (maximum: 500 mg per dose) (Bratzler, 2013).

Oral (for colorectal surgical prophylaxis only): 15 mg/kg (maximum: 1000 mg) every 3-4 hours for 3 doses, starting after mechanical bowel preparation the afternoon and evening before the procedure, with or without additional oral antibiotics and with an appropriate I.V. antibiotic prophylaxis regimen (Bratzler, 2013).

Adults:

Anaerobic infections (diverticulitis, intra-abdominal, peritonitis, cholangitis, or abscess): Oral, I.V.: 500 mg every 6-8 hours, not to exceed 4 g/day; **Note:** Initial: 1 g I.V. loading dose may be administered

Amebiasis: Oral: 500-750 mg every 8 hours for 5-10 days

Clostridium difficile-associated diarrhea:

Mild-to-moderate infection: Oral: 500 mg 3 times daily for 10-14 days (Cohen, 2010; Surawicz, 2013)

Severe complicated infection (no abdominal distention): I.V.: 500 mg 3 times daily with oral vancomycin for 10-14 days (Surawicz, 2013)

Severe complicated infection (with ileus, toxic colitis, and/or abdominal distention): I.V.: 500 mg 3 times daily with oral and rectal vancomycin for 10-14 days (Surawicz, 2013)

Note: Recent guideline recommends converting to oral vancomycin therapy if the patient does not show a clear clinical response after 5-7 days of metronidazole therapy (Surawicz, 2013).

Crohn's disease (unlabeled use): I.V.: 10-20 mg/kg/day; long-term (eg, several months) safety has not been established (Lichtenstein, 2009). **Note:** Reserved for mild-to-moderate disease in patients not responsive to sulfasalazine and/or who have colonic involvement (eg, ileocolitis and colitis) (Lichtenstein, 2009; Sutherland, 1991).

Giardiasis: 500 mg twice daily for 5-7 days

Helicobacter pylori eradication: Oral: 250-500 mg with meals and at bedtime for 14 days; requires combination therapy with at least one other antibiotic and an acid-suppressing agent (proton pump inhibitor or H_2 blocker)

Intra-abdominal infection, complicated, community-acquired, mild-to-moderate (in combination with cephalosporin or fluoroquinolone): I.V.: 500 mg every 8-12 hours **or** 1.5 g every 24 hours for for 4-7 days (provided source controlled)

Bacterial vaginosis or vaginitis due to *Gardnerella*, *Mobiluncus*: Oral: 500 mg twice daily (regular release) or 750 mg once daily (extended release tablet) for 7 days

Pelvic inflammatory disease (unlabeled use): Oral: 500 mg twice daily for 14 days (in combination with a cephalosporin and doxycycline) (CDC, 2010)

Periodontitis treatment (monotherapy or combination) associated with presence of *Actinobacillus actinomycetemcomitans* (AA): Oral: 250-500 mg every 8 hours for 8-10 days used in addition to scaling and root planing (Varela, 2011)

Surgical prophylaxis:

Manufacturer's recommendation: I.V.: 15 mg/kg 1 hour prior to surgical incision; followed by 7.5 mg/kg 6 and 12 hours after initial dose

Alternative recommendation:

I.V.: 500 mg within 60 minutes prior to surgical incision in combination with other antibiotics (Bratzler, 2013).

Oral (for colorectal surgical prophylaxis only): 1 g every 3-4 hours for 3 doses, starting after mechanical bowel preparation the afternoon and evening before the procedure with or without additional oral antibiotics and with an appropriate I.V. antibiotic prophylaxis regimen (Bratzler, 2013).

Trichomoniasis: Oral: 250 mg every 8 hours for 7 days **or** 375 mg twice daily for 7 days **or** 2 g as a single dose **or** 1 g twice daily for 2 doses (on same day)

Urethritis (unlabeled use): Oral: 2 g as a single dose with azithromycin (CDC, 2010)

Elderly: Refer to adult dosing.

Dosage adjustment in renal impairment:

Manufacturer's recommendations:

Mild, moderate, or severe impairment: No dosage adjustment provided in the manufacturer's labeling.

Intermittent hemodialysis (IHD): If administration cannot be separated from hemodialysis, consider supplemental dose following hemodialysis.

Peritoneal dialysis (PD): No dosage adjustment necessary.

Alternative recommendations:

Cl_{cr} <10 mL/minute (not on dialysis): Recommendations vary: To reduce possible accumulation in patients receiving multiple doses, consider reduction to 50% of dose or administer normal dose every 12 hours; **Note:** Dosage reduction is unnecessary in short courses of therapy. Some references do not recommend reduction at any level of renal impairment (Lamp, 1999).

IHD (administer after hemodialysis on dialysis days): Dialyzable (50% to 100%): 500 mg every 8-12 hours. **Note:** Dosing regimen highly dependent on clinical indication (trichomoniasis vs *C. difficile* colitis) (Heintz, 2009). **Note:** Dosing dependent on the assumption of thrice weekly, complete IHD sessions.

PD: Dose as for Cl_{cr} <10 mL/minute

Continuous renal replacement therapy (CRRT) (Heintz, 2009; Trotman, 2005): Drug clearance is highly dependent on the method of renal replacement, filter type, and flow rate. Appropriate dosing requires close monitoring of pharmacologic response, signs of adverse reactions due to drug accumulation, as well as drug concentrations in relation to target trough (if appropriate). The following are general recommendations only (based on dialysate flow/ultrafiltration rates of 1-2 L/hour and minimal residual renal function) and should not supersede clinical judgment:

CVVH/CVVHD/CVVHDF: 500 mg every 6-12 hours (or per clinical indication; dosage reduction generally not necessary)

Dosage adjustment in hepatic impairment:

Manufacturer's recommendations:

Mild or moderate impairment (Child-Pugh A or B): No dosage adjustment is necessary; use with caution.

Severe impairment (Child-Pugh C):

Extended-release tablets: Use is not recommended.

Immediate-release capsules:

Amebiasis: 375 mg 3 times daily for 5-10 days

Trichomoniasis: 375 mg once daily for 7 days

Immediate-release tablets, injection: Reduce dose by 50%

Alternative recommendations: The pharmacokinetics of a single oral 500 mg dose were not altered in patients with cirrhosis; initial dose reduction is therefore not necessary (Daneshmend, 1982). In one study of I.V. metronidazole, patients with alcoholic liver disease (with or without cirrhosis), demonstrated a prolonged elimination half-life (eg, ~18 hours). The authors recommended the dose be reduced accordingly (clearance was reduced by ~62%) and the frequency may be prolonged (eg, every 12 hours instead of every 6 hours) (Lau, 1987). In another single I.V. dose study using metronidazole metabolism to predict hepatic function, patients classified as Child-Pugh class C demonstrated a half-life of ~21.5 hours (Muscara, 1995).

Dietary Considerations

Immediate-release tablets and capsules may be administered with food to minimize stomach upset. Extended release tablets should be taken on an empty stomach (1 hour before or 2 hours after meals).

Sodium: Injectable dosage form may contain sodium.

Alcohol: Use of alcohol is contraindicated during therapy and for 3 days after therapy discontinuation.

Administration

I.V.: Infuse intravenously over 30-60 minutes. Avoid contact of drug solution with equipment containing aluminum.

Oral: Immediate-release tablets and capsules may be administered with food to minimize stomach upset. Extended release tablets should be administered on an empty stomach (1 hour before or 2 hours after meals); do not split, crush, or chew.

Test Interactions May interfere with AST, ALT, triglycerides, glucose, and LDH testing

Dosage Forms Excipient information presented when available (limited, particularly for generics); consult specific product labeling. [DSC] = Discontinued product

Capsule, Oral:

Flagyl: 375 mg

Generic: 375 mg [DSC]

Solution, Intravenous:

Metro: 500 mg (100 mL)

Generic: 500 mg (100 mL)

Solution, Intravenous [preservative free]:

Generic: 500 mg (100 mL)

Tablet, Oral:

Flagyl: 250 mg, 500 mg

Generic: 250 mg, 500 mg

Tablet Extended Release 24 Hour, Oral:

Flagyl ER: 750 mg

Extemporaneous Preparations A 50 mg/mL oral suspension may be made with tablets and a 1:1 mixture of Ora-Sweet and Ora-Plus. Crush twenty-four 250 mg tablets in a mortar and reduce to a fine powder. Add small portions of the vehicle and mix to a uniform paste; mix while adding the vehicle in incremental portions to **almost** 120 mL; transfer to a calibrated bottle, rinse mortar with vehicle, and add quantity of vehicle sufficient to make 120 mL. Label "shake well". Stable for 60 days at room temperature or refrigerated.

Allen LV Jr and Erickson MA 3rd, "Stability of Ketoconazole, Metolazone, Metronidazole, Procainamide Hydrochloride, and Spironolactone in Extemporaneously Compounded Oral Liquids," *Am J Health Syst Pharm*, 1996, 53(17):2073-8.

MetroNIDAZOLE (Topical) (met roe NYE da zole)

Brand Names: U.S. MetroCream; Metrogel; MetroGel-Vaginal; MetroLotion; Noritate; Rosadan; Vandazole

Brand Names: Canada MetroCream®; Metrogel®; MetroLotion®; Nidagel™; Noritate®; Rosasol®

Index Terms Metronidazole Hydrochloride

Pharmacologic Category Antibiotic, Topical

Use

Topical: Treatment of inflammatory lesions and erythema of rosacea

Vaginal gel: Bacterial vaginosis

Pregnancy Risk Factor B

Dosage Adults:

Acne rosacea: Topical:

0.75%: Apply and rub a thin film twice daily, morning and evening, to entire affected areas after washing.

1%: Apply thin film to affected area once daily

Bacterial vaginosis or vaginitis due to *Gardnerella*, *Mobiluncus*: Vaginal: One applicatorful (~37.5 mg metronidazole) intravaginally once or twice daily for 5 days; apply once in morning and evening if using twice daily, if daily, use at bedtime

Additional Information Complete prescribing information should be consulted for additional detail.

Dosage Forms Excipient information presented when available (limited, particularly for generics); consult specific product labeling.

Cream, External:
- MetroCream: 0.75% (45 g) [contains benzyl alcohol]
- Noritate: 1% (60 g) [contains methylparaben, propylparaben, trolamine (triethanolamine)]
- Rosadan: 0.75% (45 g) [contains benzyl alcohol]
- Generic: 0.75% (45 g)

Gel, External:
- Metrogel: 1% (55 g, 60 g) [contains methylparaben, propylparaben]
- Rosadan: 0.75% (45 g) [contains edetate disodium, methylparaben, propylene glycol, propylparaben]
- Generic: 0.75% (45 g); 1% (55 g, 60 g)

Gel, Vaginal:
- MetroGel-Vaginal: 0.75% (70 g) [contains edetate disodium, methylparaben, propylene glycol, propylparaben]
- Vandazole: 0.75% (70 g) [contains methylparaben, propylparaben]
- Generic: 0.75% (70 g)

Kit, External:
- Rosadan: 0.75% [contains benzyl alcohol]
- Rosadan: 0.75% [contains edetate disodium, methylparaben, propylene glycol, propylparaben]

Lotion, External:
- MetroLotion: 0.75% (59 mL) [contains benzyl alcohol]
- Generic: 0.75% (59 mL)

◆ **Metronidazole Hydrochloride** *see* MetroNIDAZOLE (Systemic) *on page 1351*

◆ **Metronidazole Hydrochloride** *see* MetroNIDAZOLE (Topical) *on page 1354*

◆ **MET Tyrosine Kinase Inhibitor PF-02341066** *see* Crizotinib *on page 497*

◆ **Metvix® (Can)** *see* Methyl Aminolevulinate *on page 1332*

◆ **Metvixia** *see* Methyl Aminolevulinate *on page 1332*

Metyrosine (me TYE roe seen)

Brand Names: U.S. Demser

Index Terms AMPT; OGMT

Pharmacologic Category Tyrosine Hydroxylase Inhibitor

Use Short-term management of pheochromocytoma before surgery, long-term management when surgery is contraindicated or when chronic malignant pheochromocytoma exists

Pregnancy Risk Factor C

Dosage Oral: Children ≥12 years and Adults: Initial: 250 mg 4 times/day, increased by 250-500 mg/day up to 4 g/day in 4 divided doses; titrate hypertensive patients to achieve normal blood pressure and symptom control and titrate normotensive patients to reduce catecholamines by ≥50%. Usual maintenance: 2-3 g/day in 4 divided doses; for preoperative preparation, administer optimum effective dosage for 5-7 days.

Dosing adjustment in renal impairment: No dosage adjustment provided in manufacturer's labeling.

Dosing adjustment in hepatic impairment: No dosage adjustment provided in manufacturer's labeling.

Additional Information Complete prescribing information should be consulted for additional detail.

Dosage Forms Excipient information presented when available (limited, particularly for generics); consult specific product labeling.

Capsule, Oral:
- Demser: 250 mg [contains fd&c blue #2 (indigotine)]

◆ **Mevacor** *see* Lovastatin *on page 1250*

◆ **Mevinolin** *see* Lovastatin *on page 1250*

◆ **Mexar Wash** *see* Sulfacetamide (Topical) *on page 1957*

Mexiletine (meks IL e teen)

Brand Names: Canada Novo-Mexiletine

Pharmacologic Category Antiarrhythmic Agent, Class Ib

Use Management of serious ventricular arrhythmias; suppression of PVCs

Pregnancy Risk Factor C

Pregnancy Considerations Adverse events were observed in some animal reproduction studies. A few case reports have demonstrated safe use of mexiletine in pregnant women.

Breast-Feeding Considerations Mexiletine concentrations in breast milk are similar to those in the maternal plasma.

Contraindications Hypersensitivity to mexiletine or any component of the formulation; cardiogenic shock; second- or third-degree AV block (except in patients with a functioning artificial pacemaker)

Warnings/Precautions [U.S. Boxed Warning]: In the Cardiac Arrhythmia Suppression Trial (CAST), recent (>6 days but <2 years ago) myocardial infarction patients with asymptomatic, non-life-threatening ventricular arrhythmias did not benefit and may have been harmed by attempts to suppress the arrhythmia with flecainide or encainide. An increased mortality or nonfatal cardiac arrest rate (7.7%) was seen in the active treatment group compared with patients in the placebo group (3%). The applicability of the CAST results to other populations is unknown. Antiarrhythmic agents should be reserved for patients with life-threatening ventricular arrhythmias. Can be proarrhythmic. Electrolyte disturbances alter response; should be corrected before initiating therapy. Use cautiously in patients with first-degree block, pre-existing sinus node dysfunction, intraventricular conduction delays, significant hepatic dysfunction, hypotension, or severe HF. Alterations in urinary pH may change urinary excretion. Rare hepatic toxicity may occur; may cause acute hepatic injury.

Adverse Reactions

>10%:
- Central nervous system: Lightheadedness (11% to 25%), dizziness (20% to 25%), nervousness (5% to 10%), incoordination (10%)
- Gastrointestinal: GI distress (41%), nausea/vomiting (40%)
- Neuromuscular & skeletal: Trembling, unsteady gait, tremor (13%), ataxia (10% to 20%)

1% to 10%:
- Cardiovascular: Chest pain (3% to 8%), premature ventricular contractions (1% to 2%), palpitation (4% to 8%), angina (2%), proarrhythmia (10% to 15% in patients with malignant arrhythmia)
- Central nervous system: Confusion, headache, insomnia (5% to 7%), depression (2%)
- Dermatologic: Rash (4%)
- Gastrointestinal: Constipation or diarrhea (4% to 5%), xerostomia (3%), abdominal pain (1%)
- Neuromuscular & skeletal: Weakness (5%), numbness of fingers or toes (2% to 4%), paresthesia (2%), arthralgia (1%)
- Ocular: Blurred vision (5% to 7%), nystagmus (6%)
- Otic: Tinnitus (2% to 3%)

Respiratory: Dyspnea (3%)

<1% (Limited to important or life-threatening): Agranulocytosis, alopecia, AV block, cardiogenic shock, CHF, dysphagia, exfoliative dermatitis, hallucinations, hepatic necrosis, hepatitis, hypotension, impotence, leukopenia, myelofibrosis, pancreatitis (rare), psychosis, pulmonary fibrosis, seizure, sinus arrest, SLE syndrome, Stevens-Johnson syndrome, syncope, thrombocytopenia, torsade de pointes, upper GI bleeding, urinary retention, urticaria

Drug Interactions

Metabolism/Transport Effects Substrate of CYP1A2 (major), CYP2D6 (major); **Note:** Assignment of Major/Minor substrate status based on clinically relevant drug interaction potential; **Inhibits** CYP1A2 (strong)

Avoid Concomitant Use

Avoid concomitant use of Mexiletine with any of the following: Agomelatine; Pirfenidone; Pomalidomide

Increased Effect/Toxicity

Mexiletine may increase the levels/effects of: Agomelatine; Bendamustine; CloZAPine; CYP1A2 Substrates; Pirfenidone; Pomalidomide; Theophylline Derivatives

The levels/effects of Mexiletine may be increased by: Abiraterone Acetate; CYP1A2 Inhibitors (Moderate); CYP1A2 Inhibitors (Strong); CYP2D6 Inhibitors (Moderate); CYP2D6 Inhibitors (Strong); Darunavir; Deferasirox; Selective Serotonin Reuptake Inhibitors; Vemurafenib

Decreased Effect

The levels/effects of Mexiletine may be decreased by: CYP1A2 Inducers (Strong); Cyproterone; Etravirine; Fosphenytoin; Peginterferon Alfa-2b; Phenytoin

Ethanol/Nutrition/Herb Interactions Food: Food may decrease the rate, but not the extent of oral absorption; diets which affect urine pH can increase or decrease excretion of mexiletine. Avoid dietary changes that alter urine pH.

Mechanism of Action Class IB antiarrhythmic, structurally related to lidocaine, which inhibits inward sodium current, decreases rate of rise of phase 0, increases effective refractory period/action potential duration ratio

Pharmacodynamics/Kinetics

Absorption: Well absorbed; elderly have a slightly slower rate, but extent of absorption is the same as young adults

Distribution: V_d: 5-7 L/kg

Protein binding: 50% to 60%

Metabolism: Hepatic; low first-pass effect

Bioavailability: 80% to 95%

Half-life elimination: Adults: 10-14 hours (average: elderly: 14.4 hours, younger adults: 12 hours); prolonged with hepatic impairment or heart failure

Time to peak, serum: 2-3 hours

Excretion: Urine (10% to 15% as unchanged drug); urinary acidification increases excretion, alkalinization decreases excretion

Dosage Adults: Oral: Initial: 200 mg every 8 hours (may load with 400 mg if necessary); adjust dose every 2-3 days; usual dose: 200-300 mg every 8 hours; maximum dose: 1.2 g/day (some patients respond to every 12-hour dosing). When switching from another antiarrhythmic, initiate a 200 mg dose 6-12 hours after stopping former agents, 3-6 hours after stopping procainamide.

Dosage adjustment in renal impairment: No dosage adjustment necessary.

Dosage adjustment in hepatic impairment: Patients with hepatic impairment or hepatic congestion secondary to heart failure may require dose reduction; half-life is approximately doubled in patients with hepatic impairment.

Dietary Considerations Take with food.

Administration Administer around-the-clock rather than 3 times/day to promote less variation in peak and trough serum levels; administer with food

Monitoring Parameters Liver function tests, ECG

Reference Range Therapeutic range: 0.5-2 mcg/mL; potentially toxic: >2 mcg/mL

Test Interactions Abnormal liver function test, positive ANA, thrombocytopenia

Dosage Forms Excipient information presented when available (limited, particularly for generics); consult specific product labeling.

Capsule, Oral, as hydrochloride:

Generic: 150 mg, 200 mg, 250 mg

Extemporaneous Preparations A 10 mg/mL oral suspension may be with made with capsules and either distilled water or sorbitol USP. Empty the contents of eight 150 mg capsules in a mortar and reduce to a fine powder if necessary. Add small portions of the chosen vehicle and mix to a uniform paste; mix while adding the vehicle in incremental proportions to **almost** 120 mL; transfer to a graduated cylinder, rinse mortar with vehicle, and add quantity of vehicle sufficient to make 120 mL. Label "shake well". Sorbitol suspension is stable in plastic prescription bottles for 2 weeks at room temperature and 4 weeks refrigerated; distilled water suspension is stable in plastic prescription bottles for 7 weeks at room temperature and 13 weeks refrigerated. Extended storage under refrigeration is recommended to minimize microbial contamination.

Nahata MC, Morosco RS, and Hipple TF, "Stability of Mexiletine in Two Extemporaneous Liquid Formulations Stored Under Refrigeration and at Room Temperature," *J Am Pharm Assoc (Wash)*, 2000, 40 (2):257-9.

◆ **Mezavant (Can)** *see* Mesalamine *on page 1305*

◆ **$MgSO_4$ (error-prone abbreviation)** *see* Magnesium Sulfate *on page 1263*

◆ **Miacalcin** *see* Calcitonin *on page 312*

◆ **Miacalcin NS (Can)** *see* Calcitonin *on page 312*

◆ **Mi-Acid [OTC]** *see* Aluminum Hydroxide, Magnesium Hydroxide, and Simethicone *on page 90*

◆ **Mi-Acid™ Double Strength [OTC]** *see* Calcium Carbonate and Magnesium Hydroxide *on page 320*

◆ **Mi-Acid Maximum Strength [OTC] [DSC]** *see* Aluminum Hydroxide, Magnesium Hydroxide, and Simethicone *on page 90*

◆ **Micaderm [OTC]** *see* Miconazole (Topical) *on page 1358*

Micafungin (mi ka FUN gin)

Brand Names: U.S. Mycamine

Brand Names: Canada Mycamine

Index Terms Micafungin Sodium

Pharmacologic Category Antifungal Agent, Parenteral; Echinocandin

Additional Appendix Information

Antifungal Agents *on page 2286*

Use Treatment of esophageal candidiasis; *Candida* prophylaxis in patients undergoing hematopoietic stem cell transplant (HSCT); treatment of candidemia, acute disseminated candidiasis, and other *Candida* infections (peritonitis and abscesses)

Unlabeled Use Treatment of infections due to *Aspergillus* spp; prophylaxis of HIV-related esophageal candidiasis

Pregnancy Risk Factor C

Pregnancy Considerations Adverse events have been observed in animal reproduction studies. There are no adequate and well-controlled studies in pregnant women. Use only if benefit outweighs risk.

Breast-Feeding Considerations It is not known if micafungin is excreted in breast milk. The manufacturer recommends that caution be exercised when administering micafungin to nursing women.

Contraindications Hypersensitivity to micafungin, other echinocandins, or any component of the formulation

Warnings/Precautions Severe anaphylactic reactions, including shock, have been reported. New-onset or worsening hepatic impairment, including hepatitis and hepatic failure, has been reported. Monitor closely and evaluate appropriateness of continued use in patients who develop abnormal liver function tests during treatment. Hemolytic anemia and hemoglobinuria have been reported. Increased BUN, serum creatinine, renal dysfunction, and/or acute renal failure has been reported; use with caution in patients that develop worsening renal function during treatment; monitor closely.

Adverse Reactions Frequency of adverse events generally higher following prophylaxis of *Candida* infections in hematopoietic stem cell transplant recipients.

>10%:

Cardiovascular: Tachycardia (3% to 26%), localized phlebitis (with peripheral administration; 5% to 19%)

Central nervous system: Headache (2% to 44%), insomnia (4% to 37%), anxiety (≤23%), dizziness (13%)

Dermatologic: Pruritus (pediatric patients ages 3 days through 16 years: ≤33%; adults 6%), skin rash (2% to 30%), urticaria (pediatric patients ages 3 days through 16 years: ≤19%; adults <5%)

Endocrine & metabolic: Hypokalemia (14% to 18%), hypomagnesemia (6% to 13%)

Gastrointestinal: Diarrhea (7% to 77%), nausea (7% to 71%), vomiting (7% to 66%), abdominal pain (2% to 35%), abdominal distension (pediatric patients ages 3 days through 16 years: 2% to 19%), mucositis (14%), constipation (11%)

Genitourinary: Decreased urine output (pediatric patients ages 3 days through 16 years: ≤23%), hematuria (pediatric patients ages 3 days through 16 years: ≤23%)

Hematologic & oncologic: Neutropenia (5% to 75%), thrombocytopenia (4% to 75%), anemia (pediatric patients ages 3 days through 16 years: 13% to 51%; adults 3% to 10%), febrile neutropenia (≤16%)

Hepatic: Increased serum ALT (pediatric patients ages 3 days through 16 years: ≤16%; adults 5%), abnormal hepatic function tests (pediatric patients ages 3 days through 16 years: <15%; adults 4%), hyperbilirubinemia (pediatric patients ages 3 days through 16 years: <15%; adults <1%)

Renal: Renal failure (pediatric patients ages 3 days through 16 years: <15%)

Miscellaneous: Fever (pediatric patients ages 3 days through 16 years: 9% to 61%; adults 7% to 20%), infusion related reaction (pediatric patients ages 3 days through 16 years: ≤16%; adults <5%)

1% to 10%:

Cardiovascular: Hypotension (6% to 10%), peripheral edema (7%), edema (5%), atrial fibrillation (3% to 5%), bradycardia (3% to 5%), hypertension (3% to 5%), cardiac arrest (<5%), myocardial infarction (<5%), pericardial effusion (<5%)

Central nervous system: Rigors (9%), fatigue (6%), brain disease (<5%), convulsions (<5%), delirium (<5%), intracranial hemorrhage (<5%)

Endocrine & metabolic: Hypocalcemia (7%), hypoglycemia (6% to 7%), hyperglycemia (6%), hypernatremia (4% to 6%), hypervolemia (5%), hyperkalemia (4% to 5%)

Gastrointestinal: Anorexia (6%), dyspepsia (6%)

Hematologic & oncologic: Blood coagulation disorder (<5%), pancytopenia (<5%), thrombotic thrombocytopenic purpura (<5%)

Hepatic: Increased serum alkaline phosphatase (3% to 8%), increased serum AST (3% to 6%), hepatic failure (<5%), hepatic injury (<5%), hepatomegaly (<5%), jaundice (<5%)

Hypersensitivity: Anaphylaxis (<5%), hypersensivity reaction (<5%)

Infection: Bacteremia (5% to 9%), sepsis (5% to 6%)

Local: Venous thrombosis at injection site (<5%)

Neuromuscular & skeletal: Back pain (5%)

Respiratory: Epistaxis (≤9%), cough (8%), dyspnea (6%)

<1% (Limited to important or life-threatening) or frequency not defined: Acidosis, acute renal failure, anaphylactoid reaction, anuria, apnea, cardiac arrhythmia, cyanosis, decreased white blood cell count, deep vein thrombosis, disseminated intravascular coagulation, erythema multiforme, hemoglobinuria, hemolysis, hemolytic anemia, hepatic insufficiency, hepatitis, hiccups, hyponatremia, hypoxia, increased blood urea nitrogen, increased serum creatinine, infection, injection site reaction, oliguria, pneumonia, pulmonary embolism, renal insufficiency, renal tubular necrosis, seizure, shock, skin necrosis, Stevens-Johnson syndrome, thrombophlebitis, tissue necrosis at injection site, toxic epidermal necrolysis, vasodilatation

Drug Interactions

Metabolism/Transport Effects **Substrate** of CYP3A4 (minor); **Note:** Assignment of Major/Minor substrate status based on clinically relevant drug interaction potential; **Inhibits** CYP3A4 (weak)

Avoid Concomitant Use

Avoid concomitant use of Micafungin with any of the following: Pimozide

Increased Effect/Toxicity

Micafungin may increase the levels/effects of: ARIPiprazole; Dofetilide; Lomitapide; Pimozide

Decreased Effect

Micafungin may decrease the levels/effects of: Saccharomyces boulardii

Preparation for Administration Aseptically add 5 mL of NS (preservative free) or D_5W to each 50 or 100 mg vial. To minimize foaming, gently swirl to dissolve; do not shake. Further dilute 50-150 mg in 100 mL NS or D_5W (when used in children the final concentration should be between 0.5-4 mg/mL; concentrations >1.5 mg/mL should be administered via central catheter). Protect infusion solution from light (it is not necessary to protect the drip chamber or tubing from light).

Storage/Stability Store at 25°C (77°F); excursions permitted to 15°C to 30°C (59°F to 86°F). Reconstituted and diluted solutions are stable for 24 hours at room temperature. Protect infusion solution from light (it is not necessary to protect the drip chamber or tubing from light).

Mechanism of Action Concentration-dependent inhibition of 1,3-beta-D-glucan synthase resulting in reduced formation of 1,3-beta-D-glucan, an essential polysaccharide comprising 30% to 60% of *Candida* cell walls (absent in mammalian cells); decreased glucan content leads to osmotic instability and cellular lysis

Pharmacodynamics/Kinetics

Distribution: 0.28-0.5 L/kg

Protein binding: >99%; primarily to albumin

Metabolism: Hepatic; forms M-1 (catechol), M-2 (methoxy), and M-5 metabolites (activity unknown)

Half-life elimination: Children: 5-22 hours; Adults: 11-21 hours

Excretion: Primarily feces (71%); urine (<15%)

Dosage

Candidemia, acute disseminated candidiasis, and *Candida* peritonitis and abscesses: I.V.:

Infants ≥4 months, Children, and Adolescents: 2 mg/kg once daily; maximum: 100 mg once daily

Adults: 100 mg once daily; mean duration of therapy (from clinical trials) was 15 days (range: 10-47 days)

Esophageal candidiasis: I.V.:

Infants ≥4 months, Children, and Adolescents:

≤30 kg: 3 mg/kg once daily

>30 kg: 2.5 mg/kg once daily; maximum: 150 mg once daily

Adults: 150 mg once daily; mean duration of therapy (from clinical trials) was 15 days (range: 10-30 days)

Prophylaxis of *Candida* infection in hematopoietic stem cell transplantation: I.V.:

Infants ≥4 months, Children, and Adolescents: 1 mg/kg once daily; maximum: 50 mg once daily

Adults: 50 mg once daily; mean duration of therapy (from clinical trials) was 19 days (range: 6-51 days)

Dosing adjustment in renal impairment: No dosage adjustment necessary.

Poorly dialyzed; no supplemental dose or dosage adjustment necessary, including patients on intermittent hemodialysis.

Dosing adjustment in hepatic impairment: No dosage adjustment necessary.

Administration For intravenous use only; infuse over 1 hour. When used in children, administer infusions >1.5 mg/mL via central catheter to minimize risk of infusion reactions. Flush line with NS prior to administration.

Monitoring Parameters Liver function tests

Dosage Forms Excipient information presented when available (limited, particularly for generics); consult specific product labeling.

Solution Reconstituted, Intravenous, as sodium:

Mycamine: 50 mg (1 ea); 100 mg (1 ea)

◆ **Micafungin Sodium** *see* Micafungin *on page 1356*

◆ **Micanol® (Can)** *see* Anthralin *on page 140*

◆ **Micardis** *see* Telmisartan *on page 2002*

◆ **Micardis HCT** *see* Telmisartan and Hydrochlorothiazide *on page 2004*

◆ **Micardis Plus (Can)** *see* Telmisartan and Hydrochlorothiazide *on page 2004*

◆ **Micatin [OTC]** *see* Miconazole (Topical) *on page 1358*

◆ **Micatin® (Can)** *see* Miconazole (Topical) *on page 1358*

◆ **Miconazole 3** *see* Miconazole (Topical) *on page 1358*

◆ **Miconazole 3 Combo Pack [OTC]** *see* Miconazole (Topical) *on page 1358*

◆ **Miconazole 7 [OTC]** *see* Miconazole (Topical) *on page 1358*

Miconazole (Topical) (mi KON a zole)

Brand Names: U.S. Aloe Vesta Antifungal [OTC]; Antifungal [OTC]; Azolen Tincture [OTC]; Baza Antifungal [OTC]; Carrington Antifungal [OTC]; Critic-Aid Clear AF [OTC]; Cruex Prescription Strength [OTC]; DermaFungal [OTC]; Desenex Jock Itch [OTC]; Desenex Spray [OTC]; Desenex [OTC]; Fungoid Tincture [OTC]; Lotrimin AF Deodorant Powder [OTC]; Lotrimin AF Jock Itch Powder [OTC]; Lotrimin AF Powder [OTC]; Lotrimin AF [OTC]; Micaderm [OTC]; Micatin [OTC]; Miconazole 3; Miconazole 3 Combo Pack [OTC]; Miconazole 7 [OTC]; Micro Guard [OTC]; Miranel AF [OTC]; Mitrazol [OTC]; Podactin [OTC]; Remedy Antifungal [OTC]; Secura Antifungal Extra Thick [OTC]; Secura Antifungal [OTC]; Soothe & Cool INZO Antifungal [OTC]; Triple Paste AF [OTC]; Vagistat-3 [OTC]; Zeasorb-AF [OTC]

Brand Names: Canada Dermazole; Micatin®; Micozole; Monistat®; Monistat® 3

Index Terms Miconazole Nitrate

Pharmacologic Category Antifungal Agent, Topical; Antifungal Agent, Vaginal

Additional Appendix Information

Antifungal Agents *on page 2286*

Use Treatment of vulvovaginal candidiasis and a variety of skin and mucous membrane fungal infections

Pregnancy Considerations Following vaginal administration, small amounts are absorbed systemically (Stevens, 2002). Adverse fetal events have not been observed (Czeizel, 2004). Vaginal products (7-day therapies) may be considered for the treatment of vulvovaginal candidiasis in pregnant women. This product may weaken latex condoms and diaphragms (CDC, 2010).

Breast-Feeding Considerations It is not known if miconazole is excreted in breast milk. The manufacturer recommends that caution be exercised when administering miconazole to nursing women.

Contraindications Hypersensitivity to miconazole or any component of the formulation

Warnings/Precautions For topical use only; avoid contact with eyes. Discontinue if sensitivity or irritation develop. Petrolatum-based vaginal products may damage rubber or latex condoms or diaphragms. Separate use by 3 days. Consult with healthcare provider prior to self-medication (OTC use) of vaginal products if experiencing vaginal itching/discomfort, lower abdominal pain, back or shoulder pain, chills, nausea, vomiting, foul-smelling discharge, if this is the first vaginal yeast infection, or if exposed to HIV. Contact healthcare provider if symptoms do not begin to improve after 3 days or last longer than 7 days. Topical products are not for self-medication (OTC use) in children <2 years of age; vaginal products are not for OTC use in children <12 years of age.

Fungoid® tincture: Patients with diabetes, circulatory problems, renal or hepatic dysfunction should contact healthcare provider prior to self-medication (OTC use).

Adverse Reactions Frequency not defined.

Topical: Allergic contact dermatitis, burning, maceration

Vaginal: Abdominal cramps, burning, irritation, itching

Drug Interactions

Metabolism/Transport Effects None known.

Avoid Concomitant Use There are no known interactions where it is recommended to avoid concomitant use.

Increased Effect/Toxicity

Miconazole (Topical) may increase the levels/effects of: Vitamin K Antagonists

Decreased Effect There are no known significant interactions involving a decrease in effect.

Ethanol/Nutrition/Herb Interactions Herb/Nutraceutical: St John's wort may decrease miconazole levels.

Mechanism of Action Inhibits biosynthesis of ergosterol, damaging the fungal cell wall membrane, which increases permeability causing leaking of nutrients

Pharmacodynamics/Kinetics

Absorption: Topical: Negligible

Excretion: Feces; urine

Dosage

Topical: Children and Adults: **Note:** Not for OTC use in children <2 years:

Tinea corporis: Apply twice daily for 4 weeks

Tinea pedis: Apply twice daily for 4 weeks

Effervescent tablet: Dissolve 1 tablet in ~1 gallon of water; soak feet for 15-30 minutes; pat dry

Tinea cruris: Apply twice daily for 2 weeks

Vaginal: Children ≥12 years and Adults: Vulvovaginal candidiasis:

Cream, 2%: Insert 1 applicatorful at bedtime for 7 days

Cream, 4%: Insert 1 applicatorful at bedtime for 3 days

Suppository, 100 mg: Insert 1 suppository at bedtime for 7 days

Suppository, 200 mg: Insert 1 suppository at bedtime for 3 days

Suppository, 1200 mg: Insert 1 suppository (a one-time dose); may be used at bedtime or during the day

Note: Many products are available as a combination pack, with a suppository for vaginal instillation and cream to relieve external symptoms. External cream may be used twice daily, as needed, for up to 7 days.

Dosage Forms Excipient information presented when available (limited, particularly for generics); consult specific product labeling.

Aerosol, External, as nitrate:
- Desenex Spray: 2% (133 g)
- Lotrimin AF: 2% (150 g)

Aerosol Powder, External, as nitrate:
- Cruex Prescription Strength: 2% (85 g)
- Desenex Jock Itch: 2% (113 g)
- Desenex Spray: 2% (113 g)
- Lotrimin AF Deodorant Powder: 2% (133 g)
- Lotrimin AF Jock Itch Powder: 2% (133 g)
- Lotrimin AF Powder: 2% (133 g)

Cream, External, as nitrate:
- Antifungal: 2% (14 g, 28 g, 42.5 g) [contains benzoic acid]
- Antifungal: 2% (113 g, 198 g) [contains cetyl alcohol, methylparaben, propylene glycol, propylparaben]
- Baza Antifungal: 2% (4 g, 57 g, 142 g)
- Carrington Antifungal: 2% (141 g) [contains disodium edta, methylparaben, propylene glycol, propylparaben]
- Micaderm: 2% (30 g)
- Micatin: 2% (14 g) [contains benzoic acid]
- Micro Guard: 2% (57 g)
- Podactin: 2% (28.35 g) [contains benzoic acid]
- Remedy Antifungal: 2% (118 mL) [contains methylparaben, propylparaben, trolamine (triethanolamine)]
- Secura Antifungal: 2% (57 g) [contains cetearyl alcohol, methylparaben, propylparaben]
- Secura Antifungal Extra Thick: 2% (92 g) [contains cetearyl alcohol, methylparaben, propylparaben]
- Soothe & Cool INZO Antifungal: 2% (56.7 g, 141.7 g)
- Generic: 2% (15 g, 28.4 g, 30 g)

Cream, Vaginal, as nitrate:
- Miconazole 7: 2% (45 g) [contains benzoic acid]
- Generic: 2% (45 g)

Kit, External, as nitrate:
- Fungoid Tincture: 2% [contains benzyl alcohol]

Kit, Vaginal, as nitrate:
- Miconazole 3 Combo Pack: Cream, topical: 2% (9 g) and Suppository, vaginal: 200 mg (3s)
- Miconazole 3 Combo Pack: Cream, topical: 2% (9 g) and Suppository, vaginal: 200 mg (3s) [contains benzoic acid]
- Vagistat-3: Cream, topical: 2% (9 g) and Suppository, vaginal: 200 mg (3s) [contains benzoic acid]

Lotion, External, as nitrate:
- Zeasorb-AF: 2% (56 g) [contains alcohol, usp]

Ointment, External, as nitrate:
- Aloe Vesta Antifungal: 2% (56 g, 141 g)
- Critic-Aid Clear AF: 2% (4 g, 57 g, 142 g)
- DermaFungal: 2% (113 g)
- Triple Paste AF: 2% (56.7 g) [contains polysorbate 80]

Powder, External, as nitrate:
- Desenex: 2% (43 g, 85 g)
- Lotrimin AF: 2% (90 g)
- Micro Guard: 2% (85 g)
- Mitrazol: 2% (30 g)
- Remedy Antifungal: 2% (85 g)
- Remedy Antifungal: 2% (85 g) [talc free; contains methylparaben]
- Zeasorb-AF: 2% (71 g)
- Zeasorb-AF: 2% (71 g) [starch free]

Solution, External, as nitrate:
- Azolen Tincture: 2% (29.57 mL) [contains benzyl alcohol, isopropyl alcohol]
- Fungoid Tincture: 2% (29.57 mL) [contains benzyl alcohol]
- Miranel AF: 2% (28 g) [contains disodium edta, menthol, propylene glycol, sd alcohol 40b]

Suppository, Vaginal, as nitrate:
- Miconazole 7: 100 mg (7 ea)
- Miconazole 3: 200 mg (3 ea)
- Generic: 100 mg (7 ea)

◆ **Miconazole Nitrate** *see* Miconazole (Topical) *on page 1358*

◆ **Micozole (Can)** *see* Miconazole (Topical) *on page 1358*

◆ **MICRhoGAM Ultra-Filtered Plus** *see* Rh_0(D) Immune Globulin *on page 1801*

◆ **Microgestin 1.5/30** *see* Ethinyl Estradiol and Norethindrone *on page 793*

◆ **Microgestin 1/20** *see* Ethinyl Estradiol and Norethindrone *on page 793*

◆ **Microgestin Fe 1.5/30** *see* Ethinyl Estradiol and Norethindrone *on page 793*

◆ **Microgestin Fe 1/20** *see* Ethinyl Estradiol and Norethindrone *on page 793*

◆ **Micro Guard [OTC]** *see* Miconazole (Topical) *on page 1358*

◆ **Micro-K** *see* Potassium Chloride *on page 1684*

◆ **Micro-K Extencaps (Can)** *see* Potassium Chloride *on page 1684*

◆ **Micronase** *see* GlyBURIDE *on page 963*

◆ **Micronefrin [OTC]** *see* EPINEPHrine (Systemic, Oral Inhalation) *on page 714*

◆ **Micronized Colestipol HCl** *see* Colestipol *on page 488*

◆ **Micronor® (Can)** *see* Norethindrone *on page 1472*

◆ **Microzide** *see* Hydrochlorothiazide *on page 1004*

◆ **Midamor (Can)** *see* AMILoride *on page 99*

Midazolam (MID aye zoe lam)

Brand Names: Canada Apo-Midazolam®; Midazolam Injection

Index Terms Midazolam Hydrochloride; Versed

Pharmacologic Category Benzodiazepine

Additional Appendix Information

Benzodiazepine Comparison Table *on page 2292*

Status Epilepticus *on page 2375*

Use Preoperative sedation; moderate sedation prior to diagnostic or radiographic procedures; ICU sedation (continuous infusion); induction and maintenance of general anesthesia

Unlabeled Use Anxiety, status epilepticus, conscious sedation (intranasal route)

Pregnancy Risk Factor D

Pregnancy Considerations Adverse events were not observed in animal reproduction studies. Midazolam has been found to cross the human placenta and can be detected in the serum of the umbilical vein and artery, as well as the amniotic fluid. Teratogenic effects have been observed with some benzodiazepines; however, additional studies are needed. The incidence of premature birth and low birth weights may be increased following maternal use of benzodiazepines; hypoglycemia and respiratory problems in the neonate may occur following exposure late in pregnancy. Neonatal withdrawal symptoms may occur within days to weeks after birth and "floppy infant syndrome" (which also includes withdrawal symptoms) have been reported with some benzodiazepines (Bergman, 1992; Iqbal, 2002; Wikner, 2007).

Breast-Feeding Considerations Midazolam and hydroxymidazolam can be detected in breast milk. Based on information from two women, 2-3 months postpartum, the half-life of midazolam in breast milk is ~1 hour. Milk concentrations were below the limit of detection (<5 nmol/L) 4 hours after a single maternal dose of midazolam 15 mg. Drowsiness, lethargy, or weight loss in nursing infants have been observed in case reports following maternal use of some benzodiazepines (Iqbal, 2002; Matheson, 1990). The manufacturer recommends that caution be exercised when administering midazolam to nursing women.

Contraindications Hypersensitivity to midazolam or any component of the formulation; intrathecal or epidural injection of parenteral forms containing preservatives (ie, benzyl alcohol); acute narrow-angle glaucoma; concurrent use of potent inhibitors of CYP3A4 (amprenavir, atazanavir, or ritonavir)

Per respective protease inhibitor manufacturer's labeling: Concurrent use of oral midazolam with amprenavir, atazanavir, darunavir, indinavir, lopinavir-ritonavir, nelfinavir, ritonavir, saquinavir, tipranavir and concurrent use of oral or injectable midazolam with fosamprenavir

Warnings/Precautions **[U.S. Boxed Warning]: May cause severe respiratory depression, respiratory arrest, or apnea. Use with extreme caution, particularly in noncritical care settings.** Appropriate resuscitative equipment and qualified personnel must be available for administration and monitoring. Initial dosing must be cautiously titrated and individualized, particularly in elderly or debilitated patients, patients with hepatic impairment (including alcoholics), or in renal impairment, particularly if other CNS depressants (including opioids) are used concurrently. **[U.S. Boxed Warning]: Initial doses in elderly or debilitated patients should be conservative; as little as 1 mg, but not to exceed 2.5 mg.** Use with caution in patients with respiratory disease or impaired gag reflex. Use during upper airway procedures may increase risk of hypoventilation. Prolonged responses have been noted following extended administration by continuous infusion (possibly due to metabolite accumulation) or in the presence of drugs which inhibit midazolam metabolism.

Causes CNS depression (dose-related) resulting in sedation, dizziness, confusion, or ataxia which may impair physical and mental capabilities. Patients must be cautioned about performing tasks which require mental alertness (eg, operating machinery or driving). A minimum of 1 day should elapse after midazolam administration before attempting these tasks. Use with caution in patients receiving other CNS depressants or psychoactive agents. Effects with other sedative drugs or ethanol may be potentiated. Benzodiazepines have been associated with falls and traumatic injury and should be used with extreme caution in patients who are at risk of these events (especially the elderly).

Use with caution in patients receiving CYP3A4 inhibitors; may result in more intense and prolonged sedation; consider reducing midazolam dose and anticipate potential for prolongation and intensity of effect. The concurrent use of all protease inhibitors is contraindicated with oral midazolam per their respective manufacturer's labeling. The concurrent use of fosamprenavir is contraindicated with both oral and parenteral forms of midazolam.

May cause hypotension - hemodynamic events are more common in pediatric patients or patients with hemodynamic instability. Hypotension and/or respiratory depression may occur more frequently in patients who have received opioid analgesics. Use with caution in obese patients, chronic renal failure, and HF. Does not protect against increases in heart rate or blood pressure during intubation. Should not be used in shock, coma, or acute alcohol intoxication. **[U.S. Boxed Warning]: Do not administer by rapid I.V. injection in neonates; severe hypotension and seizures have been reported; risk may be increased with concomitant fentanyl use.**

Avoid intra-arterial administration or extravasation of parenteral formulation. Some parenteral dosage forms may contain benzyl alcohol which has been associated with "gasping syndrome" in neonates. Some formulations may contain cherry flavoring.

Midazolam causes anterograde amnesia. Paradoxical reactions, including hyperactive or aggressive behavior have been reported with benzodiazepines, particularly in adolescent/pediatric or psychiatric patients; may consider treatment with flumazenil (Massanari, 1997). Does not have analgesic, antidepressant, or antipsychotic properties.

Benzodiazepines have been associated with dependence and acute withdrawal symptoms on discontinuation or reduction in dose. Acute withdrawal, including seizures, may be precipitated after administration of flumazenil to patients receiving long-term benzodiazepine therapy.

Adverse Reactions As reported in adults unless otherwise noted:

>10%: Respiratory: Decreased tidal volume and/or respiratory rate decrease, apnea (3% children)

1% to 10%:

- Cardiovascular: Hypotension (3% children)
- Central nervous system: Drowsiness (1%), oversedation, headache (1%), seizure-like activity (1% children)
- Gastrointestinal: Nausea (3%), vomiting (3%)
- Local: Pain and local reactions at injection site (4% I.M., 5% I.V.; severity less than diazepam)
- Neuromuscular & skeletal: Myoclonic jerks (preterm infants)
- Ocular: Nystagmus (1% children)
- Respiratory: Cough (1%)
- Miscellaneous: Physical and psychological dependence with prolonged use, hiccups (4%, 1% children), paradoxical reaction (2% children)

<1% (Limited to important or life-threatening): Agitation, amnesia, bigeminy, bronchospasm, emergence delirium, euphoria, hallucinations, laryngospasm, rash

Drug Interactions

Metabolism/Transport Effects **Substrate** of CYP2B6 (minor), CYP3A4 (major); **Note:** Assignment of Major/Minor substrate status based on clinically relevant drug interaction potential; **Inhibits** CYP2C8 (weak), CYP2C9 (weak), CYP3A4 (weak)

Avoid Concomitant Use

Avoid concomitant use of Midazolam with any of the following: Azelastine (Nasal); Boceprevir; Cobicistat; Conivaptan; Efavirenz; Fusidic Acid (Systemic); Itraconazole; Ketoconazole (Systemic); OLANZapine; Paraldehyde; Pimozide; Protease Inhibitors; Sodium Oxybate; Telaprevir

Increased Effect/Toxicity

Midazolam may increase the levels/effects of: Alcohol (Ethyl); ARIPiprazole; Azelastine (Nasal); Buprenorphine; CloZAPine; CNS Depressants; Dofetilide; Fosphenytoin; Hydrocodone; Lomitapide; Methotrimeprazine; Metyrosine; Mirtazapine; Paraldehyde; Phenytoin; Pimozide; Pramipexole; Propofol; ROPINIRole; Rotigotine; Selective Serotonin Reuptake Inhibitors; Sodium Oxybate; Zolpidem

The levels/effects of Midazolam may be increased by: Antifungal Agents (Azole Derivatives, Systemic); Aprepitant; AtorvaSTATin; Boceprevir; Brimonidine (Topical); Calcium Channel Blockers (Nondihydropyridine);

Cimetidine; Cobicistat; Conivaptan; Contraceptives (Estrogens); Contraceptives (Progestins); CYP3A4 Inhibitors (Moderate); CYP3A4 Inhibitors (Strong); Dasatinib; Doxylamine; Droperidol; Efavirenz; Fosaprepitant; Fusidic Acid (Systemic); Grapefruit Juice; HydrOXYzine; Isoniazid; Itraconazole; Ivacaftor; Ketoconazole (Systemic); Luliconazole; Macrolide Antibiotics; Magnesium Sulfate; Methotrimeprazine; Mifepristone; OLANZapine; Perampanel; Propofol; Protease Inhibitors; Proton Pump Inhibitors; Selective Serotonin Reuptake Inhibitors; Simeprevir; Tapentadol; Telaprevir

Decreased Effect

The levels/effects of Midazolam may be decreased by: Bosentan; CarBAMazepine; CYP3A4 Inducers (Strong); Dabrafenib; Deferasirox; Ginkgo Biloba; Herbs (CYP3A4 Inducers); Mitotane; Rifamycin Derivatives; Theophylline Derivatives; Tocilizumab; Yohimbine

Ethanol/Nutrition/Herb Interactions

Ethanol: Ethanol may increase CNS depression. Management: Avoid ethanol.

Food: Grapefruit juice may increase serum concentrations of midazolam. Management: Avoid concurrent use of grapefruit juice with oral midazolam.

Herb/Nutraceutical: St John's wort may decrease midazolam levels and increase CNS depression; valerian, kava kava, and gotu kola may increase CNS depression. Management: Avoid concurrent use with St John's wort, valerian, kava kava, and gotu kola.

Storage/Stability The manufacturer states that midazolam, at a final concentration of 0.5 mg/mL, is stable for up to 24 hours when diluted with D_5W or NS. A final concentration of 1 mg/mL in NS has been documented to be stable for up to 10 days (McMullen, 1995). Admixtures do not require protection from light for short-term storage.

Mechanism of Action Binds to stereospecific benzodiazepine receptors on the postsynaptic GABA neuron at several sites within the central nervous system, including the limbic system, reticular formation. Enhancement of the inhibitory effect of GABA on neuronal excitability results by increased neuronal membrane permeability to chloride ions. This shift in chloride ions results in hyperpolarization (a less excitable state) and stabilization.

Pharmacodynamics/Kinetics

Onset of action: I.M.: Sedation: ~15 minutes; I.V.: 3-5 minutes; Oral: 10-20 minutes; Intranasal: Children: 4-8 minutes (Lee-Kim, 2004)

Peak effect: I.M.: 0.5-1 hour

Duration: I.M.: Up to 6 hours; Mean: 2 hours; Intranasal: Children: 18-41 minutes (Lee-Kim, 2004); I.V.: Single dose: <2 hours (dose-dependent) (Fragen, 1997); Cirrhosis: Up to 6 hours (MacGilcrhist, 1986)

Absorption: Oral: Rapid

Distribution: V_d: 1-3.1 L/kg; increased in females, elderly, and obesity

Protein binding: ~97%; in patients with cirrhosis, protein binding is reduced with a free fraction of ~5% (Trouvin, 1988)

Metabolism: Extensively hepatic CYP3A4; 60% to 70% of biotransformed midazolam is the active metabolite 1-hydroxy-midazolam (or alpha-hydroxymidazolam)

Bioavailability: Oral: 40% to 50% (Kanto, 1985), ~36% (children); I.M.: >90%

Half-life elimination: 2-6 hours; prolonged in cirrhosis, congestive heart failure, obesity, renal failure, and elderly. **Note:** In patients with renal failure, reduced elimination of active hydroxylated metabolites leads to drug accumulation and prolonged sedation.

Excretion: I.V.: Urine (primarily as glucuronide conjugates of the hydroxylated metabolites); Oral: Urine (~90% within 24 hours; primarily [60% to 70%] as glucuronide conjugates of the hydroxylated metabolites; <0.03% as unchanged drug); feces (~2% to 10% over 5 days) (Kanto, 1985; Smith, 1981)

Dosage

Children: The dose of midazolam needs to be individualized based on the patient's age, underlying diseases, and concurrent medications. Decrease dose (by ~30%) if opioids or other CNS depressants are administered concomitantly. Children <6 years may require higher doses and closer monitoring than older children; calculate dose based on ideal body weight.

Conscious sedation for procedures or preoperative sedation:

Oral, rectal: Children: 0.5-0.75 mg/kg as a single dose preprocedure (maximum: 20 mg); administer 20-30 minutes prior to procedure. Children <6 years or less cooperative patients may require as much as 1 mg/kg as a single dose; 0.25 mg/kg may suffice for children 6-16 years of age (Bozkurt, 2007).

Intranasal (unlabeled route): Children: 0.2-0.5 mg/kg (maximum total dose: 10 mg or 5 mg per nare); may be administered 10-20 minutes prior to procedure (Bozkurt, 2007; Chiaretti, 2011). **Note:** Use 5 mg/mL injectable concentrated solution to deliver dose. Due to the low pH of the solution, burning upon administration is likely to occur.

I.M.: Children: 0.1-0.15 mg/kg 30-60 minutes before surgery or procedure; range: 0.05-0.15 mg/kg; doses up to 0.5 mg/kg have been used in more anxious patients; maximum total dose: 10 mg

I.V.:

Infants <6 months: Limited information is available in nonintubated infants; dosing recommendations not clear; infants <6 months are at higher risk for airway obstruction and hypoventilation; titrate dose in small increments to desired effect

Infants 6 months to Children 5 years: Initial: 0.05-0.1 mg/kg; total dose of 0.6 mg/kg may be required; maximum total dose: 6 mg

Children 6-12 years: Initial: 0.025-0.05 mg/kg; total doses of 0.4 mg/kg may be required; maximum total dose: 10 mg

Children 12-16 years: Dose as adults; maximum total dose: 10 mg

Conscious sedation during mechanical ventilation: Children: Loading dose: 0.05-0.2 mg/kg, followed by initial continuous infusion: 0.06-0.12 mg/kg/**hour** (1-2 **mcg**/kg/minute); range in clinical trials: 0.024-0.564 mg/kg/**hour** (0.4-9.4 **mcg**/kg/minute) (Hartman, 2009)

Status epilepticus refractory to standard therapy (unlabeled use): **Note:** Intubation required; adjust dose based on hemodynamics, seizure activity, and EEG. Infants >2 months and Children: Loading dose: 0.15 mg/kg followed by a continuous infusion of 0.06 mg/kg/**hour** (1 **mcg**/kg/minute); titrate dose upward every 5 minutes until clinical seizure activity is controlled; mean infusion rate required in 24 children was 0.14 mg/kg/**hour** (2.3 **mcg**/kg/minute) with a range of 0.06-1.1 mg/kg/**hour** (1-18.3 **mcg**/kg/minute) (Rivera, 1993).

A more aggressive approach has been demonstrated to provide control of status epilepticus within 30 minutes of initiation: Loading dose: 0.5 mg/kg followed by 0.12 mg/kg/**hour** (2 **mcg**/kg/minute). If seizures persist or recur, administer 0.5 mg/kg bolus with an increase in the infusion rate to 0.24 mg/kg/**hour** (4 **mcg**/kg/minute); if seizures continue to persist/recur, administer 0.1 mg/kg bolus and increase infusion to 0.48 mg/kg/**hour** (8 **mcg**/kg/minute); continue to repeat this last incremental increase until seizure control or a maximum dose of 1.44 mg/kg/**hour** (24 **mcg**/kg/minute) is reached; do not allow >5 minutes to elapse between each dose increment while seizures persist (dose range within clinical trial: 0.12-1.92 mg/kg/**hour** or 2-32 **mcg**/kg/minute) (Morrison, 2006).

Status epilepticus, prehospital treatment (unlabeled use; Silbergleit, 2012): **Note:** Administered by paramedics when convulsions last >5 minutes **or** if convulsions are occurring after having intermittent seizures without regaining consciousness for >5 minutes. I.M.: Children and Adolescents:
13-40 kg: 5 mg once
>40 kg: Refer to adult dosing

Adults: The dose of midazolam needs to be individualized based on the patient's age, underlying diseases, and concurrent medications. Consider reducing dose by 20% to 50% in elderly, chronically ill, or debilitated patients and those receiving opioids or other CNS depressants.
Preoperative/preprocedural sedation: Healthy adults <60 years:
I.M.: 0.07-0.08 mg/kg 30-60 minutes prior to surgery/procedure; usual dose: 5 mg
I.V.: 0.02-0.04 mg/kg; repeat every 5 minutes as needed to desired effect or up to 0.1-0.2 mg/kg
Intranasal (unlabeled route): 0.1 mg/kg; administer 10-20 minutes prior to surgery/procedure (Uygur-Bayramiçli, 2002). **Note:** Use 5 mg/mL injectable solution to deliver dose. Due to the low pH of the solution, burning upon administration is likely to occur.
Conscious sedation: I.V.:
Manufacturer's labeling:
Healthy adults <60 years:
Initial: Some patients respond to doses as low as 1 mg; no more than 2.5 mg should be administered over a period of 2 minutes. Additional doses of midazolam may be administered after a 2-minute waiting period and evaluation of sedation after each dose increment. A total dose >5 mg is generally not needed.
Maintenance: 25% of dose used to reach sedative effect
Adults ≥60 years, debilitated, or chronically ill: Refer to elderly dosing.
Alternate recommendations: American Society for Gastrointestinal Endoscopy: Initial: 0.5-2 mg slow I.V. over at least 2 minutes; slowly titrate to effect by repeating doses every 2-3 minutes if needed; usual total dose: 2.5-5 mg (Waring, 2003)
Anesthesia: I.V.:
Induction: Adults <55 years:
Unpremedicated patients: 0.3-0.35 mg/kg over 20-30 seconds; after 2 minutes, may repeat if necessary at 25% of initial dose every 2 minutes, up to a total dose of 0.6 mg/kg in resistant cases
Premedicated patients: Usual dosage range: 0.05-0.2 mg/kg (Barash, 2009; Miller, 2010). Use of 0.2 mg/kg administered over 5-10 seconds has been shown to safely produce anesthesia within 30 seconds (Samuelson, 1981) and is recommended for ASA physical status P1 and P2 patients. When used with other anesthetic drugs (ie, co-induction), the dose is <0.1 mg/kg (Miller, 2010).
ASA physical status >P3 or debilitation: Reduce dose by at least 20% (Miller, 2010)
Maintenance: 0.05 mg/kg as needed (Miller, 2010), or continuous infusion 0.015-0.06 mg/kg/**hour** (0.25-1 **mcg**/kg/minute) (Barash, 2009; Miller, 2010)
Sedation in mechanically-ventilated patients: I.V.: Initial dose: 0.01-0.05 mg/kg (~0.5-4 mg); may repeat at 5- to 15-minute intervals until adequate sedation achieved; maintenance infusion: 0.02-0.1 mg/kg/**hour** (0.3-1.7 **mcg**/kg/minute). Titrate to reach desired level of sedation. Titration to maintain a light rather than a deep level of sedation is recommended unless clinically contraindicated (Barr, 2013). May consider a trial of daily awakening; if agitated after discontinuation of drip, then restart at 50% of the previous dose (Kress, 2000).
Status epilepticus refractory to standard therapy (unlabeled use): **Note:** Intubation required; adjust dose based on hemodynamics, seizure activity, and EEG. I.V.: 0.15-0.3 mg/kg (usual dose: 5-15 mg); may repeat every 10-15 minutes as needed **or** 0.2 mg/kg bolus followed by a continuous infusion of 0.05-0.6 mg/kg/**hour** (0.83-10 **mcg**/kg/minute) (Lowenstein, 2005; Meierkord, 2010)
Status epilepticus, prehospital treatment (unlabeled use): **Note:** Administered by paramedics when convulsions last >5 minutes **or** if convulsions are occurring after having intermittent seizures without regaining consciousness for >5 minutes. I.M.: 10 mg once (Silbergleit, 2012)

Elderly:
Anesthesia: I.V.: Induction: Adults >55 years:
Unpremedicated patients: Initial dose: 0.3 mg/kg
Premedicated patients: Reduce dose by at least 20% (Miller, 2010).
Conscious sedation: I.V.: Initial: 0.5 mg slow I.V.; give no more than 1.5 mg in a 2-minute period; if additional titration is needed, give no more than 1 mg over 2 minutes, waiting another 2 or more minutes to evaluate sedative effect; a total dose of >3.5 mg is rarely necessary
Preoperative/preprocedural sedation: Adults >60 years (without concomitant opioid administration): I.M.: 2-3 mg (or 0.02-0.05 mg/kg) 30-60 minutes prior to surgery/procedure; some may only require 1 mg (or 0.01 mg/kg) if anticipated intensity and duration of sedation is less critical.

Dosage adjustment in renal impairment: There are no dosage adjustments provided in manufacturer's labeling; however, patients with renal failure receiving a continuous infusion cannot adequately eliminate the active hydroxylated metabolites (eg, 1-hydroxymidazolam) contributing to prolonged sedation sometimes for days after discontinuation (Spina, 2007).
Intermittent hemodialysis: Supplemental dose is not necessary.
Continuous venovenous hemofiltration (CVVH): Unconjugated 1-hydroxymidazolam not effectively removed; 1-hydroxymidazolamglucuronide effectively removed; sieving coefficient = 0.45 (Swart, 2005).
Peritoneal dialysis: Significant drug removal is unlikely based on physiochemical characteristics.

Dosage adjustment in hepatic impairment:
Severe hepatic impairment (eg, cirrhosis): **Note:** Use with caution in patients with any degree of hepatic impairment; patients with hepatic encephalopathy likely to be more sensitive to midazolam.
Single dose (eg, induction): No dosage adjustment recommended; patients with hepatic impairment may be more sensitive compared to patients without hepatic impairment; anticipate longer duration of action (MacGilchrist, 1986; Trouvin, 1988).
Multiple dosing or continuous infusion: Expect longer duration of action and accumulation; based on patient response, dosage reduction likely to be necessary (Trouvin, 1988).

Dietary Considerations Avoid grapefruit juice with oral syrup.

Usual Infusion Concentrations: Pediatric I.V. infusion: 0.5 mg/mL **or** 1 mg/mL

Usual Infusion Concentrations: Adult I.V. infusion: 100 mg in 100 mL (concentration: 1 mg/mL) of D_5W or NS

Administration

Intranasal: **Note:** Due to the low pH of the solution, burning upon administration is likely to occur. Use of an atomizer, such as the MAD 300 Mucosal Atomizer which attaches to a tuberculin syringe, can reduce irritation. If possible, based upon dose to be administered, use higher concentration injectable solution to minimize volume administered intranasal. Smaller volume will reduce irritation and swallowing of administered dose. The maximum recommended dose volume per nare is 1 mL.

Using the 5 mg/mL injectable solution, draw up desired dose with a 1-3 mL needleless syringe; may attach a nasal mucosal atomization device prior to delivering dose. Deliver half of the total dose volume (of the 5 mg/mL concentration) into the first nare using the atomizer device or by dripping slowly into nostril, then deliver the other half of the dose into the second nare.

Oral: Do not mix with any liquid (such as grapefruit juice) prior to administration

Parenteral:

I.M.: Administer deep I.M. into large muscle.

I.V.: Administer by slow I.V. injection over at least 2-5 minutes at a concentration of 1-5 mg/mL or by I.V. infusion. For induction of anesthesia, administer I.V. bolus over 5-30 seconds. Continuous infusions should be administered via an infusion pump.

Monitoring Parameters Respiratory and cardiovascular status, blood pressure, blood pressure monitor required during I.V. administration

Critically-ill patients: Monitor depth of sedation with either the Richmond Agitation-Sedation Scale (RASS) or Sedation-Agitation Scale (SAS) (Barr, 2013)

Additional Information Abrupt discontinuation after sustained use (generally >10 days) may cause withdrawal symptoms. For neonates, since both concentrations of the injection contain 1% benzyl alcohol, use the 5 mg/mL injection and dilute to 0.5 mg/mL with SWI without preservatives to decrease the amount of benzyl alcohol delivered to the neonate; with continuous infusion, midazolam may accumulate in peripheral tissues; use lowest effective infusion rate to reduce accumulation effects; midazolam is 3-4 times as potent as diazepam; paradoxical reactions associated with midazolam use in children (eg, agitation, restlessness, combativeness) have been successfully treated with flumazenil (Massanari, 1997).

Dosage Forms Excipient information presented when available (limited, particularly for generics); consult specific product labeling.

Solution, Injection:

Generic: 2 mg/2 mL (2 mL); 5 mg/5 mL (5 mL); 10 mg/10 mL (10 mL); 5 mg/mL (1 mL, 2 mL, 5 mL, 10 mL); 10 mg/2 mL (2 mL); 25 mg/5 mL (5 mL); 50 mg/10 mL (10 mL)

Solution, Injection [preservative free]:

Generic: 2 mg/2 mL (2 mL); 5 mg/5 mL (5 mL); 5 mg/mL (1 mL); 10 mg/2 mL (2 mL)

Syrup, Oral:

Generic: 2 mg/mL (118 mL)

Controlled Substance C-IV

◆ **Midazolam Hydrochloride** *see* Midazolam *on page 1359*

◆ **Midazolam Injection (Can)** *see* Midazolam *on page 1359*

Midodrine (MI doe dreen)

Brand Names: Canada Amatine®; Apo-Midodrine®

Index Terms Midodrine Hydrochloride; ProAmatine

Pharmacologic Category Alpha$_1$ Agonist

Use Orphan drug: Treatment of symptomatic orthostatic hypotension

Unlabeled Use Management of urinary incontinence; vasovagal syncope; prevention of dialysis-induced hypotension

Pregnancy Risk Factor C

Pregnancy Considerations Adverse events were observed in animal reproduction studies. Information related to the use of midodrine in pregnancy is limited (Glatter, 2005).

Breast-Feeding Considerations It is not known if midodrine is excreted in breast milk. The manufacturer recommends that caution be exercised when administering midodrine to nursing women.

Contraindications Hypersensitivity to midodrine or any component of the formulation; severe organic heart disease; acute renal failure; urinary retention; pheochromocytoma; thyrotoxicosis; persistent and significant supine hypertension

Warnings/Precautions [U.S. Boxed Warning]: Indicated for patients for whom orthostatic hypotension significantly impairs their daily life despite standard clinical care. May cause hypertension. Use is not recommended with supine hypertension. May slow heart rate primarily due to vagal reflex. Use caution when administered concurrently with negative chronotropes (eg, digoxin, beta blockers). Use is not recommended with supine hypertension. Use cautiously in patients with renal impairment and initiate with a reduced dose; contraindicated in patients with acute renal failure. Caution should be exercised in patients with diabetes, visual problems (especially if receiving fludrocortisone), urinary retention (reduce initial dose), or hepatic dysfunction; monitor renal and hepatic function prior to and periodically during therapy.

Adverse Reactions

>10%:

Cardiovascular: Supine hypertension (7% to 13%)

Dermatologic: Piloerection (13%), pruritus (12%)

Genitourinary: Urinary urgency, retention, or polyuria, dysuria (up to 13%)

Neuromuscular & skeletal: Paresthesia (18%)

1% to 10%:

Central nervous system: Chills (5%), pain (5%)

Dermatologic: Rash (2%)

Gastrointestinal: Abdominal pain

<1% (Limited to important or life-threatening): Anxiety, backache, canker sore, confusion, dizziness, dry skin, erythema multiforme, facial flushing, flatulence, flushing, GI distress, headache, heartburn, hyperesthesia, insomnia, ICP increased, leg cramps, nausea, somnolence, visual field defect, weakness, xerostomia

Drug Interactions

Metabolism/Transport Effects None known.

Avoid Concomitant Use

Avoid concomitant use of Midodrine with any of the following: Ergot Derivatives; Iobenguane I 123; MAO Inhibitors

Increased Effect/Toxicity

Midodrine may increase the levels/effects of: Sympathomimetics

The levels/effects of Midodrine may be increased by: AtoMOXetine; Beta-Blockers; Calcium Channel Blockers (Nondihydropyridine); Cannabinoids; Cardiac Glycosides; Ergot Derivatives; Linezolid; MAO Inhibitors; Tricyclic Antidepressants

Decreased Effect

Midodrine may decrease the levels/effects of: Benzylpenicilloyl Polylysine; Iobenguane I 123

The levels/effects of Midodrine may be decreased by: Alpha1-Blockers

Mechanism of Action Midodrine forms an active metabolite, desglymidodrine, which is an alpha$_1$-agonist. This agent increases arteriolar and venous tone resulting in a rise in standing, sitting, and supine systolic and diastolic blood pressure in patients with orthostatic hypotension.

Pharmacodynamics/Kinetics
Onset of action: ~1 hour
Duration: 2-3 hours
Absorption: Rapid
Distribution: V_d (desglymidodrine): <1.6 L/kg; poorly across membrane (eg, blood-brain barrier)
Protein binding: Minimal
Metabolism: Hepatic and many other tissues; midodrine is a prodrug which undergoes rapid deglycination to desglymidodrine (active metabolite)
Bioavailability: Desglymidodrine: 93%
Half-life elimination: Desglymidodrine: ~3-4 hours; Midodrine: 25 minutes
Time to peak, serum: Desglymidodrine: 1-2 hours; Midodrine: 30 minutes
Excretion: Urine (Midodrine: Insignificant; Desglymidodrine: 80% by active renal secretion)

Dosage Adults: Oral:
Orthostatic hypotension: 10 mg 3 times/day during daytime hours (every 3-4 hours) when patient is upright (maximum: 40 mg/day)
Prevention of hemodialysis-induced hypotension (unlabeled use): 2.5-10 mg given 15-30 minutes prior to dialysis session (Cruz, 1998; KDOQI, 2005; Prakash, 2004)
Vasovagal syncope (unlabeled use): Initial: 5 mg 3 times/day during daytime hours (every 6 hours) increased up to 15 mg/dose if necessary (Perez-Lugones, 2001; Ward, 1998)

Dosage adjustment in renal impairment: Orthostatic hypotension: 2.5 mg 3 times/day, gradually increasing as tolerated
Hemodialysis: Dialyzable; dose after hemodialysis unless used for prevention of hemodialysis-induced hypotension.

Dosage adjustment in hepatic impairment: No dosage adjustment provided in manufacturer's labeling (has not been studied); use with caution.

Administration Doses may be given in approximately 3- to 4-hour intervals (eg, shortly before or upon rising in the morning, at midday, in the late afternoon not later than 6 PM). Avoid dosing after the evening meal or within 4 hours of bedtime. Continue therapy only in patients who appear to attain symptomatic improvement during initial treatment. Standing systolic blood pressure may be elevated 15-30 mm Hg at 1 hour after a 10 mg dose. Some effect may persist for 2-3 hours.

Monitoring Parameters Blood pressure; renal and hepatic function

Dosage Forms Excipient information presented when available (limited, particularly for generics); consult specific product labeling.
Tablet, Oral, as hydrochloride:
Generic: 2.5 mg, 5 mg, 10 mg

◆ **Midodrine Hydrochloride** *see* Midodrine *on page* 1363
◆ **Mifeprex** *see* Mifepristone *on page* 1364

Mifepristone (mi FE pris tone)

Brand Names: U.S. Korlym; Mifeprex
Index Terms RU-38486; RU-486
Pharmacologic Category Abortifacient; Antineoplastic Agent, Hormone Antagonist; Antiprogestin; Cortisol Receptor Blocker

Use
Korlym™: To control hyperglycemia occurring secondary to hypercortisolism in patients with endogenous Cushing's syndrome who have type 2 diabetes mellitus or glucose intolerance and who failed surgery or who are not surgical candidates
Mifeprex®: Medical termination of intrauterine pregnancy, through day 49 of pregnancy. Patients may need treatment with misoprostol and possibly surgery to complete therapy.

Unlabeled Use Treatment of unresectable meningioma; has been studied in the treatment of breast cancer and ovarian cancer; termination of pregnancy ≤63 days of pregnancy

Pregnancy Risk Factor X

Pregnancy Considerations Use of mifepristone in a pregnant woman will result in fetal loss. In addition, skull deformities were observed in rabbit reproduction studies and were most likely due to uterine contractions.
Korlym™: **[U.S. Boxed Warning]: Use of mifepristone will result in termination of pregnancy.** When used to control hyperglycemia in women with Cushing's syndrome, **pregnancy must be excluded prior to initiation of therapy. Nonhormonal contraception must be used during treatment and for 1 month after discontinuation of therapy unless the patient has had surgical sterilization. Pregnancy must be excluded if treatment is interrupted for ≥14 days.**
Mifeprex®: This medication is used to terminate pregnancy; there are no approved treatment indications for its use during pregnancy. In addition, skull defects, cranial nerve palsies, delayed growth and psychomotor development, facial malformations and limb defects have been reported following prostaglandin exposure (including misoprostol). If treatment fails, there is a risk of fetal malformation. In sexually active women, pregnancy can occur prior to the first menstrual period following treatment. Appropriate contraception can be started as soon as termination of pregnancy is confirmed or before sexual intercourse is resumed.

Breast-Feeding Considerations Mifepristone milk concentrations were evaluated in lactating women receiving a single dose for the termination of pregnancy. In women receiving mifepristone 200 mg (n=2), milk concentrations were below the limit of detection (<0.013 micromole/L) in samples collected over the following 5 days. The highest milk concentration following a single 600 mg dose (n=10) was 0.913 micromole/L on day 1 and concentrations decreased to 0.062 micromole/L by day 5. Using the highest reported milk concentration, the authors calculated the relative infant dose to be ≤1.5% of the weight adjusted maternal dose in a fully breast-fed infant (Sääv, 2010).

When using this medication for termination of pregnancy, the manufacturer recommends that breast milk be discarded for a few days following the last dose. When using for the treatment of hyperglycemia in women with Cushing's syndrome, the manufacturer recommends that the decision to continue or discontinue breast-feeding during therapy take into account the risk of exposure to the infant and the benefits of treatment to the mother.

Prescribing and Access Restrictions
Korlym™ is only available through a restricted access program. For prescriber registration and patient enrollment forms, please refer to http://www.korlym.com/hcp/how-to-prescribe-korlym.php or call 1-855-4Korlym (1-855-456-7596).

Mifeprex®: As a requirement of the REMS program, a medication guide must be given to the patient prior to receiving the medication. In addition, the manufacturer recommends distributing a patient agreement form which must be signed by the patient and prescriber confirming the patient's agreement to terminate her pregnancy. A signed copy of the patient agreement should be kept in the patient's medical record.

Mifeprex® is only available direct from Danco Laboratories' distributor. To obtain the product, please refer to, http://www.earlyoptionpill.com, or call 1-877-432-7596.

Investigators wishing to obtain the agent for use in oncology patients must apply for a patient-specific IND from the FDA.

Medication Guide Available Yes

Contraindications Hypersensitivity to mifepristone or any component of the formulation

Korlym™ (additional contraindications): Concomitant use of lovastatin, simvastatin, or CYP3A substrates with a narrow therapeutic range (eg, cyclosporine, dihydroergotamine, ergotamine, fentanyl, pimozide, quinine, sirolimus, tacrolimus); concomitant use of systemic corticosteroids for serious medical conditions (eg, immunosuppression following organ transplant); women with a history of unexplained vaginal bleeding, or endometrial hyperplasia with atypia or endometrial carcinoma; pregnancy

Mifeprex® (additional contraindications): Hypersensitivity to misoprostol; chronic adrenal failure; porphyrias; hemorrhagic disorder or concurrent anticoagulant therapy; pregnancy termination >49 days; intrauterine device (IUD) in place; ectopic pregnancy or undiagnosed adnexal mass; concurrent long-term corticosteroid therapy; inadequate or lack of access to emergency medical services; inability to understand effects and/or comply with treatment

Warnings/Precautions Hazardous agent; use appropriate precautions for handling and disposal (NIOSH, 2012).

Regardless of indication, endometrial proliferation is promoted by mifepristone resulting in endometrial thickening, cystic dilation of endometrial glands, and vaginal bleeding. **[U.S. Boxed Warning]:** When used for the termination of pregnancy, **patients should be counseled to seek medical attention in cases of excessive bleeding. Bleeding occurs and should be expected (average 9-16 days, may be ≥30 days). In some cases, bleeding may be prolonged and heavy and may be a sign of incomplete abortion or other complications,** potentially leading to hypovolemic shock; the manufacturer cites soaking through 2 thick sanitary pads per hour for 2 consecutive hours as an example of excessive bleeding. Bleeding may require blood transfusion (rare), curettage, saline infusions, and/or vasoconstrictors. Patients should be instructed to seek medical attention if prolonged heavy vaginal bleeding occurs. When used for termination of pregnancy, use is contraindicated in women with hemorrhagic disorders or those using anticoagulants; use caution in women with severe anemia, hypocoagulability or hemostatic disorders. When used for the treatment of hyperglycemia in patients with Cushing's syndrome, use caution in women with hemorrhagic disorders or women using anticoagulants and evaluate unexplained vaginal bleeding; use is contraindicated with a history of unexplained vaginal bleeding.

[U.S. Boxed Warning]: When used for the termination of pregnancy, **bacterial infections have been reported following use of this product and may have an atypical presentation. In rare cases, these infections may be serious and/or fatal,** with septic shock as a potential complication. A causal relationship has not been established. Sustained fever, abdominal pain, or pelvic tenderness should prompt evaluation; however, healthcare professionals are warned that atypical presentations of serious infection without these symptoms have also been noted. Patients presenting with nausea, vomiting, diarrhea, or weakness, with or without abdominal pain or fever, should be evaluated for serious bacterial infection when symptoms occur >24 hours after taking misoprostol. Treatment with antibiotics, including coverage for anaerobic bacteria (eg, *Clostridium sordellii*) should be initiated. Patients with Cushing's syndrome may be at risk for opportunistic infections such as *Pneumocystis jiroveci* pneumonia.

High potential for drug interactions exists when used for the treatment of hyperglycemia in patients with Cushing's syndrome. Refer to Drug Interactions for detailed information. The potential for drug interactions was not specifically studied following a single dose for the termination of pregnancy. May prolong the QT_c interval (dose related); use caution with other QT-prolonging agents. A large variability in exposure to mifepristone and its metabolites was observed at doses of 600 mg/day in patients with hepatic or renal impairment. Safety and efficacy have not been established for use in women with hepatic or impairment when used as a single dose for the termination of pregnancy; dose adjustment required when treating hyperglycemia in patients with Cushing's syndrome. Safety and efficacy have not been established for use in insulin-dependent diabetes mellitus.

Treatment of hyperglycemia in patients with Cushing's syndrome: [U.S. Boxed Warning]: Use of mifepristone will result in termination of pregnancy. Pregnancy must be excluded prior initiation of therapy. Nonhormonal contraception must be used during therapy and for 1 month after discontinuation of therapy unless the patient has had surgical sterilization. Pregnancy must be excluded if treatment is interrupted for ≥14 days. Adrenal insufficiency may occur. Serum cortisol concentrations remain elevated and may increase, and cannot be used for monitoring. If signs and symptoms of adrenal insufficiency occur (eg, fatigue, hypoglycemia, hypotension, nausea, weakness), discontinue mifepristone and administer glucocorticoids (high doses may be needed). Following resolution, treatment may be resumed at a lower dose; evaluate patient for precipitating causes (eg, infection, trauma). Hypokalemia ay occur at any time during therapy; correct hypokalemia prior to initiation of treatment. Use of mifepristone for the treatment of hyperglycemia in patients with Cushing's syndrome may antagonize the effects of steroids used for other conditions. Use is contraindicated when steroids are required for lifesaving indications. Because mifepristone does not reduce serum cortisol concentrations, mineralocorticoid receptors in cardiac tissue may be activated; use caution in patients with Cushing's syndrome who also have heart failure or coronary vascular disease.

Termination of pregnancy: [U.S. Boxed Warning]: Patients undergoing treatment with mifepristone should be instructed to bring their medication guide with them when an obtaining treatment from an emergency room or healthcare provider that did not prescribe the medication initially in order to identify that they are undergoing a medical abortion. Patient must be instructed of the treatment procedure and expected effects. A signed agreement form must be kept in the patient's file. Physicians may obtain patient agreement forms, physician enrollment forms, and medical consultation directly from Danco Laboratories at 1-877-432-7596. Prescriber should also give the patient clear instructions on whom to call and what to do in the event of an emergency following administration of therapy. Pregnancy is dated from day 1 of last menstrual period (presuming a 28-day cycle, ovulation occurring midcycle). Pregnancy duration can be determined using menstrual history and clinical examination. Ultrasound should be used if duration of pregnancy is uncertain. Confirmation of pregnancy termination by clinical exam or ultrasound must be made 14 days following treatment. Manufacturer recommends surgical termination of pregnancy when medical termination fails or is not complete. Prescriber should determine in advance whether they will provide such care themselves or through other providers. Preventative measures to prevent rhesus immunization must be taken prior to surgical abortion. Ultrasound should be used if an ectopic pregnancy is suspected or if duration of pregnancy is uncertain. Ultrasonography may not identify all ectopic pregnancies, and healthcare providers should be alert for signs and symptoms which may be related to undiagnosed ectopic pregnancy in any patient who receives mifepristone. Mifepristone is not effective in terminating ectopic pregnancies. To be administered only by physicians who can date pregnancy, diagnose ectopic pregnancies, provide access to surgical abortion (if needed), and can provide access to emergency care. Medication will be distributed directly to these physicians following signed agreement with the distributor. Must be administered under supervision by the qualified physician. Adverse effects (including blood transfusions, hospitalization, ongoing pregnancy, and other major complications) must be reported in writing to the medication distributor. Safety and efficacy have not been established for use in women with chronic cardiovascular disease, hypertension, or respiratory disease. Use with caution in patients who are heavy smokers (>10 cigarettes/day) or in women >35 years of age; these patients were excluded from clinical trials.

Adverse Reactions

Adverse events associated with treatment of hyperglycemia in patients with Cushing's syndrome:

>10%:

Cardiovascular: Peripheral edema (26%), hypertension (24%)

Central nervous system: Fatigue (48%), headache (44%), dizziness (22%), pain (14%)

Endocrine & metabolic: Hypokalemia (34% to 44%), endometrial hypertrophy (38%), thyroid function tests abnormal (18%)

Gastrointestinal: Nausea (48%), vomiting (26%), appetite decreased (20%), xerostomia (18%), diarrhea (12%)

Genitourinary: Vaginal bleeding (14%)

Neuromuscular & skeletal: Arthralgia (30%), back pain (16%), myalgia (14%), extremity pain (12%)

Respiratory: Dyspnea (16%), sinusitis (14%), nasopharyngitis (12%)

5% to 10%:

Cardiovascular: Edema, pitting edema

Central nervous system: Anxiety (10%), somnolence (10%), insomnia, malaise

Endocrine & metabolic: Hypoglycemia, triglycerides increased

Gastrointestinal: Anorexia (10%), constipation (10%), abdominal pain, GI reflux

Genitourinary: Vaginal hemorrhage, metrorrhagia

Neuromuscular & skeletal: Flank pain, malaise, musculoskeletal chest pain, weakness

Miscellaneous: Thirst

<5% or frequency not defined: Adrenal insufficiency (4%), pruritus (4%), rash (4%), HDL cholesterol decreased

Adverse events associated with treatment for termination of pregnancy: Note: Vaginal bleeding and uterine cramping are expected to occur when this medication is used to terminate a pregnancy; ~90% of women using this medication for this purpose also report adverse reactions on day 3 after the procedure. Bleeding or spotting occurs in most women for a period of 9-16 days. Up to 8% of women will experience some degree of bleeding or spotting for 30 days or more. In some cases, bleeding may be prolonged and heavy, potentially leading to hypovolemic shock.

Central nervous system: Headache (2% to 31%), dizziness (1% to 12%)

Gastrointestinal: Abdominal pain (cramping) (96%), nausea (43% to 61%), vomiting (18% to 26%), diarrhea (12% to 20%)

Genitourinary: Uterine cramping (83%)

1% to 10%:

Cardiovascular: Syncope (1%)

Central nervous system: Fatigue (10%), fever (4%), insomnia (3%), anxiety (2%), fainting (2%)

Gastrointestinal: Dyspepsia (3%)

Genitourinary: Uterine hemorrhage (5%), vaginitis (3%), pelvic pain (2%), endometriosis/salpingitis/pelvic inflammatory disease (1%)

Hematologic: Decreased hemoglobin >2 g/dL (6%), anemia (2%), leukorrhea (2%)

Neuromuscular & skeletal: Back pain (9%), rigors (3%), leg pain (2%), weakness (2%)

Respiratory: Sinusitis (2%)

Miscellaneous: Viral infection (4%)

<1% (Limited to important or life-threatening): Adult respiratory distress syndrome (ADRS), allergic reaction including urticaria and hives, bacterial infection (including an ectopic bacteria such as *Clostridium sordellii*), Crohn's disease (exacerbation), disseminated intravascular coagulopathy (DIC), dyspnea, hematometra, hypotension, lightheadedness, loss of consciousness, MI, pancreatitis (acute), pelvic infection, postabortal infection, QT prolongation, ruptured ectopic pregnancy, sepsis, septic shock, sickle cell crisis (exacerbation), tachycardia, toxic shock syndrome

Unresectable meningioma trials: Most common adverse effects included breast tenderness or gynecomastia, fatigue, hair thinning, hot flashes, and rash. In premenopausal women, vaginal bleeding may be seen shortly after beginning therapy and cessation of menses is common. Thyroiditis and effects related to antiglucocorticoid activity have also been noted.

Drug Interactions

Metabolism/Transport Effects Substrate of CYP3A4 (major); **Note:** Assignment of Major/Minor substrate status based on clinically relevant drug interaction potential; **Inhibits** BCRP, CYP1A2 (weak), CYP2A6 (weak), CYP2B6 (weak), CYP2C19 (weak), CYP2C8 (weak), CYP2C9 (weak), CYP2D6 (weak), CYP2E1 (weak), CYP3A4 (weak), P-glycoprotein

Avoid Concomitant Use

Avoid concomitant use of Mifepristone with any of the following: Corticosteroids (Systemic); CycloSPORINE (Systemic); CYP3A4 Inducers (Strong); Dihydroergotamine; Ergotamine; FentaNYL; Fusidic Acid (Systemic); Highest Risk QTc-Prolonging Agents; Ivabradine; Lovastatin; Moderate Risk QTc-Prolonging Agents; Pimozide; QuiNIDine; Simvastatin; Sirolimus; St Johns Wort; Tacrolimus (Systemic)

Increased Effect/Toxicity

Mifepristone may increase the levels/effects of: ARIPiprazole; BuPROPion; Contraceptives (Estrogens); Contraceptives (Progestins); Corticosteroids (Systemic); CycloSPORINE (Systemic); CYP2C8 Substrates; CYP2C9 Substrates; CYP3A4 Substrates; Digoxin; Dihydroergotamine; Efavirenz; Ergotamine; FentaNYL; Fluvastatin; Highest Risk QTc-Prolonging Agents; Lomitapide; Lovastatin; Moderate Risk QTc-Prolonging Agents; Pimozide; QTc-Prolonging Agents (Indeterminate Risk and Risk Modifying); QuiNIDine; Simvastatin; Sirolimus; Tacrolimus (Systemic)

The levels/effects of Mifepristone may be increased by: CYP3A4 Inhibitors (Moderate); CYP3A4 Inhibitors (Strong); Dasatinib; Fusidic Acid (Systemic); Ivabradine; Ivacaftor; Luliconazole; Moderate Risk QTc-Prolonging Agents; QTc-Prolonging Agents (Indeterminate Risk and Risk Modifying); Simeprevir

Decreased Effect

Mifepristone may decrease the levels/effects of: Contraceptives (Estrogens); Contraceptives (Progestins); Corticosteroids (Systemic)

The levels/effects of Mifepristone may be decreased by: Bosentan; CYP3A4 Inducers (Strong); Dabrafenib; Deferasirox; St Johns Wort; Tocilizumab

Ethanol/Nutrition/Herb Interactions

Food: Grapefruit juice may inhibit mifepristone metabolism, leading to increased levels. Management: Do not take with grapefruit juice.

Herb/Nutraceutical: St John's wort may induce mifepristone metabolism, leading to decreased levels. Management: Avoid St John's wort.

Storage/Stability Store at room temperature of 25°C (77°F); excursions permitted to 15°C to 30°C (59°F to 86°F).

Mechanism of Action Mifepristone is a synthetic steroid. At low doses, it competitively binds to the intracellular progesterone receptor, blocking the effects of progesterone. When used for the termination of pregnancy, this leads to contraction-inducing activity in the myometrium. In the absence of progesterone, mifepristone acts as a partial progesterone agonist. At high doses used for the treatment of hyperglycemia in patients with Cushing's syndrome, mifepristone blocks the effect of cortisol at the glucocorticoid receptor (antagonizes the effects of cortisol on glucose metabolism) while at the same time increasing circulating cortisol concentrations.

Pharmacodynamics/Kinetics

Absorption: Oral: rapid

Protein binding: 98% to albumin and α_1-acid glycoprotein

Metabolism: Hepatic via CYP3A4 to three metabolites (active)

Bioavailability: Oral: 69%

Half-life elimination: Single dose: Terminal: 18 hours following a slower phase where 50% eliminated between 12-72 hours; Multiple doses (600 mg/day): 85 hours

Time to peak: Oral: 90 minutes; Range: Single dose: 1-2 hours, Multiple doses: 1-4 hours

Excretion: Feces (83%); urine (9%)

Dosage Oral:

Adults:

Hyperglycemia in patients with Cushing's syndrome (Korlym™): Initial dose: 300 mg once daily. Dose may be increased in 300 mg increments at intervals of ≥2-4 weeks based on tolerability and symptom control. Maximum dose: 1200 mg once daily, not to exceed 20 mg/kg/day. If treatment is interrupted, reinitiate at 300 mg/day or a dose lower than the dose that caused the treatment to be stopped if interruption due to adverse reactions

Dosage adjustment with concurrent use of strong CYP450 inhibitor therapy (eg, ketoconazole): Maximum dose 300 mg/day

Termination of pregnancy (Mifeprex®): Treatment consists of 3 office visits by the patient; the patient must read medication guide and sign patient agreement prior to treatment:

Day 1 (mifepristone administration): 600 mg (three 200 mg tablets) taken as a single dose under physician supervision

Day 3 (misoprostol administration): Patient must return to the healthcare provider 2 days following administration of mifepristone; unless abortion has occurred (confirmed using ultrasound or clinical examination): Misoprostol 400 mcg (two 200 mcg tablets); **Note:** Patient may need treatment for cramps or gastrointestinal symptoms at this time

Day 14 (post-treatment exam): Patient must return to the healthcare provider ~14 days after administration of mifepristone; confirm complete termination of pregnancy by ultrasound or clinical exam. Surgical termination is recommended to manage treatment failures.

Termination of pregnancy (unlabeled dosing): Mifepristone 200 mg orally, followed by misoprostol 800 mcg vaginally 24-48 hours later (ACOG, 2005; FIGO, 2011)

Meningioma, unresectable (unlabeled use; refer to individual protocols): Mifepristone 200 mg/day, continue based on toxicity and response (Grunberg, 1991)

Elderly: Hyperglycemia in patients with Cushing's syndrome: Refer to adult dosing.

Dosage adjustment in renal impairment:

Hyperglycemia in patients with Cushing's syndrome: Maximum dose 600 mg/day; **Note:** Following doses of 1200 mg/day for 7 days in patients with severe renal impairment (Cl_{cr} <30 mL/minute), exposure to mifepristone and its metabolites was increased and a large variability in exposure was observed.

Termination of pregnancy: No dosage adjustment provided in manufacturer's labeling (has not been studied)

Dosage adjustment in hepatic impairment:

Hyperglycemia in patients with Cushing's syndrome:

Mild-to-moderate impairment: Maximum dose 600 mg/day

Severe impairment: Use is not recommended

Note: Following single and multiple doses of 600 mg/day in patients with moderate hepatic impairment (Child-Pugh class B), a large variability in exposure to mifepristone and its metabolites was observed.

Termination of pregnancy: No dosage adjustment provided in manufacturer's labeling (has not been studied); use with caution due to CYP3A4 metabolism.

Administration

Hyperglycemia in patients with Cushing's syndrome: Administer as a single daily dose with a meal. Tablets should be swallowed whole, not crushed, split, or chewed.

Termination of pregnancy: To be taken as a single dose under physician supervision

Hazardous agent; use appropriate precautions for handling and disposal (NIOSH, 2012).

Monitoring Parameters

Treatment of hyperglycemia in patients with Cushing's syndrome: Signs and symptoms of adrenal insufficiency (serum cortisol concentrations will not be accurate); thyroid function; serum potassium (1-2 weeks after initiating dose or dose increase, then periodically thereafter); serum glucose and psychiatric symptoms (may show response to therapy within 6 weeks); cushingoid appearance (acne, hirsutism, striae, weight may take >2 months of therapy to show improvement); vaginal ultrasound in women (annually)

Termination of pregnancy: Clinical exam and/or ultrasound to confirm complete termination of pregnancy; hemoglobin, hematocrit, and red blood cell count in cases of heavy bleeding. Consider CBC in any patient who reports nausea, vomiting, or diarrhea and weakness with or without abdominal pain, and without fever or other signs of infection more than 24 hours after administration of misoprostol.

Test Interactions

hCG levels will not be useful to confirm pregnancy termination until at least 10 days following mifepristone treatment

When used for the treatment of hyperglycemia in patients with Cushing's syndrome, serum cortisol concentrations remain elevated and may increase, and cannot be used for monitoring.

Additional Information Mifeprex®: Medication will be distributed directly to qualified physicians following signed agreement with the distributor, Danco Laboratories. It will not be available through pharmacies. Major adverse reactions (hospitalization, blood transfusion, ongoing pregnancy, etc) should be reported to Danco Laboratories.

Dosage Forms Excipient information presented when available (limited, particularly for generics); consult specific product labeling.

Tablet, Oral:

Korlym: 300 mg [contains fd&c yellow #10 aluminum lake, fd&c yellow #6 aluminum lake]

Mifeprex: 200 mg

Miglitol (MIG li tol)

Brand Names: U.S. Glyset

Pharmacologic Category Antidiabetic Agent, Alpha-Glucosidase Inhibitor

Additional Appendix Information

Oral Antidiabetic Agents Comparison Table *on page 2312*

Use Type 2 diabetes mellitus (noninsulin-dependent, NIDDM):

Monotherapy as an adjunct to diet to improve glycemic control in patients with type 2 diabetes mellitus (non-insulin-dependent, NIDDM) whose hyperglycemia cannot be managed with diet alone

Combination therapy with a sulfonylurea when diet plus either miglitol or a sulfonylurea alone do not result in adequate glycemic control. The effect of miglitol to enhance glycemic control is additive to that of sulfonylureas when used in combination.

Pregnancy Risk Factor B

Pregnancy Considerations Adverse events have not been reported in animal reproduction studies.

For women with diabetes, maternal hyperglycemia can be associated with adverse effects in the fetus, neonate, and mother. To prevent adverse events, prior to conception and throughout pregnancy, the maternal Hb A_{1c} should be kept close to normal but without causing significant hypoglycemia. The use of most oral antihyperglycemic agents in pregnant women is not recommended for routine management of GDM or type 2 diabetes mellitus in pregnant women; insulin is the drug of choice for the control of diabetes mellitus during pregnancy (ACOG, 2005; ADA, 2013; Kitzmiller, 2008; Metzger, 2007).

Breast-Feeding Considerations Miglitol is found in breast milk. The exposure to a nursing infant is ~0.4% of a 100 mg maternal dose. Breast-feeding is not recommended by the manufacturer.

Contraindications Hypersensitivity to miglitol or any of component of the formulation; diabetic ketoacidosis; inflammatory bowel disease; colonic ulceration; partial intestinal obstruction or predisposition to intestinal obstruction; chronic intestinal diseases associated with marked disorders of digestion or absorption or with conditions that may deteriorate as a result of increased gas formation in the intestine

Warnings/Precautions GI symptoms are the most common reactions. The incidence of abdominal pain and diarrhea tend to diminish considerably with continued treatment. Use not recommended in severe renal impairment (serum creatinine >2 mg/dL or Cl_{cr} <25 mL/minute). In combination with a sulfonylurea or insulin will cause a further lowering of blood glucose and may increase the hypoglycemic potential of the sulfonylurea or insulin. It may be necessary to discontinue miglitol and administer insulin if the patient is exposed to stress (ie, fever, trauma, infection, surgery). In patients taking miglitol, oral glucose (dextrose) should be used instead of sucrose (cane sugar) in the treatment of mild-to-moderate hypoglycemia since the hydrolysis of sucrose to glucose and fructose is inhibited by miglitol; correction of severe hypoglycemia may require the use of either glucagon or I.V. glucose.

Adverse Reactions

>10%: Gastrointestinal: Flatulence (42%), diarrhea (29%), abdominal pain (12%)

1% to 10%: Dermatologic: Rash (4%)

<1% (Limited to important or life-threatening): Abdominal distention, gastrointestinal pain, ileus, nausea, paralytic ileus, pneumatosis cystoides intestinalis, subileus

Drug Interactions

Metabolism/Transport Effects None known.

Avoid Concomitant Use There are no known interactions where it is recommended to avoid concomitant use.

Increased Effect/Toxicity

Miglitol may increase the levels/effects of: Hypoglycemic Agents

The levels/effects of Miglitol may be increased by: Herbs (Hypoglycemic Properties); MAO Inhibitors; Pegvisomant; Salicylates; Selective Serotonin Reuptake Inhibitors

Decreased Effect

The levels/effects of Miglitol may be decreased by: Corticosteroids (Orally Inhaled); Corticosteroids (Systemic); Loop Diuretics; Luteinizing Hormone-Releasing Hormone Analogs; Somatropin; Thiazide Diuretics

Storage/Stability Store at 25°C (77°F); excursions permitted to 15°C to 30°C (59°F to 86°F).

Mechanism of Action In contrast to sulfonylureas, miglitol does not enhance insulin secretion; the antihyperglycemic action of miglitol results from a reversible inhibition of membrane-bound intestinal alpha-glucosidases which hydrolyze oligosaccharides and disaccharides to glucose and other monosaccharides in the brush border of the small intestine. In patients with diabetes, this enzyme inhibition results in delayed glucose absorption and lowering of postprandial hyperglycemia.

Pharmacodynamics/Kinetics

Absorption: Saturable at high doses: 25 mg dose: Completely absorbed; 100 mg dose: 50% to 70% absorbed

Distribution: V_d: 0.18 L/kg

Protein binding: <4%

Metabolism: None

Half-life elimination: ~2 hours

Time to peak: 2-3 hours

Excretion: Urine (as unchanged drug)

Dosage Adults: Oral: Initial: 25 mg 3 times daily at the start of each meal; the dose may be increased to 50 mg 3 times daily after 4-8 weeks and continued for ~3 months; if glycosylated hemoglobin is not satisfactory, may further increase to maximum recommended dose: 100 mg 3 times daily

Dosing adjustment in renal impairment:

Cl_{cr} ≥25 mL/minute: No dosage adjustment necessary. Although miglitol is primarily excreted unchanged, the increased plasma levels in renal impairment are not expected to affect efficacy (clinical response is localized to the GI tract); however, the effects on adverse effects are unknown.

Cl_{cr} <25 mL/minute or S_{cr} >2 mg/dL: Use not recommended (not adequately studied).

Dosing adjustment in hepatic impairment: No dosage adjustment necessary.

Administration Administer orally at the start of each main meal.

Monitoring Parameters Monitor therapeutic response by periodic blood glucose tests; measurement of glycosylated hemoglobin is recommended for the monitoring of long-term glycemic control

Reference Range Recommendations for glycemic control in nonpregnant adults with diabetes (ADA, 2013):

Hb A_{1c}: <7% (a more aggressive [<6.5%] or less aggressive [<8%] Hb A_{1c} goal may be targeted based on patient-specific characteristics)

Preprandial capillary plasma glucose: 70-130 mg/dL

Peak postprandial capillary blood glucose: <180 mg/dL

Dosage Forms Excipient information presented when available (limited, particularly for generics); consult specific product labeling.

Tablet, Oral:

Glyset: 25 mg, 50 mg, 100 mg

Miglustat (MIG loo stat)

Brand Names: U.S. Zavesca

Brand Names: Canada Zavesca®

Index Terms OGT-918

Pharmacologic Category Enzyme Inhibitor

Use Treatment of mild-to-moderate type 1 Gaucher disease when enzyme replacement therapy is not a therapeutic option

Canadian labeling: Additional use (not in U.S. labeling): Treatment to delay the progression of neurological manifestations in Niemann-Pick Type C disease

Pregnancy Risk Factor X

Dosage Oral:

Type 1 Gaucher disease: Adults: 100 mg 3 times/day; dose may be reduced to 100 mg 1-2 times/day in patients with adverse effects (ie, tremor, GI distress)

Niemann-Pick Type C disease (Canadian labeling; not in U.S. labeling):

Children <12 years: **Note:** Children <4 years of age were not included in clinical trials; dose based on body surface area (BSA):

BSA >1.25 m^2: Miglustat 200 mg 3 times/day

BSA >0.88-1.25 m^2: Miglustat 200 mg 2 times/day

BSA >0.73-0.88 m^2: Miglustat 100 mg 3 times/day

BSA >0.47-0.73 m^2: Miglustat 100 mg 2 times/day

BSA ≤0.47 m^2: Miglustat 100 mg once daily

Children ≥12 and Adults: 200 mg 3 times/day

Dosage adjustment in renal impairment:

Gaucher disease: Adults:

Cl_{cr} 50-70 mL/minute/1.73 m^2: 100 mg twice daily

Cl_{cr} 30-50 mL/minute/1.73 m^2: 100 mg once daily

Cl_{cr} <30 mL/minute/1.73 m^2: Not recommended

Niemann-Pick Type C disease Canadian labeling (not in U.S. labeling):

Children <12 years:

Cl_{cr} 50-70 mL/minute/1.73 m^2: Administer two-thirds of regular dose in 2 equal doses (adjusted for BSA)

Cl_{cr} 30-50 mL/minute/1.73 m^2: Administer one-third of regular dose in 2 equal doses (adjusted for BSA)

Cl_{cr} <30 mL/minute/1.73 m^2: Not recommended

Children ≥12 years and Adults:

Cl_{cr} 50-70 mL/minute/1.73 m^2: 200 mg twice daily

Cl_{cr} 30-50 mL/minute/1.73 m^2: 100 mg twice daily

Cl_{cr} <30 mL/minute/1.73 m^2: Not recommended

Dosage adjustment in hepatic impairment: No dosage adjustment provided in manufacturer's labeling (has not been studied). However, dosage adjustment unlikely because miglustat is not metabolized by the liver.

Additional Information Complete prescribing information should be consulted for additional detail.

Dosage Forms Excipient information presented when available (limited, particularly for generics); consult specific product labeling.

Capsule, Oral:

Zavesca: 100 mg [contains soybean lecithin]

◆ **Migranal** *see* Dihydroergotamine *on page 611*

◆ **Migranal® (Can)** *see* Dihydroergotamine *on page 611*

◆ **Milk of Magnesia** *see* Magnesium Hydroxide *on page 1260*

◆ **Milk of Magnesia [OTC]** *see* Magnesium Hydroxide *on page 1260*

◆ **Milk of Magnesia Concentrate [OTC]** *see* Magnesium Hydroxide *on page 1260*

◆ **Millipred** *see* PrednisoLONE (Systemic) *on page 1704*

◆ **Millipred DP** *see* PrednisoLONE (Systemic) *on page 1704*

◆ **Millipred DP 12-Day** *see* PrednisoLONE (Systemic) *on page 1704*

Milnacipran (mil NAY ci pran)

Brand Names: U.S. Savella; Savella Titration Pack

Pharmacologic Category Antidepressant, Serotonin/Norepinephrine Reuptake Inhibitor

Additional Appendix Information

Antidepressant Agents *on page 2284*

Use Management of fibromyalgia

Pregnancy Risk Factor C

Pregnancy Considerations Adverse events were observed in some animal reproduction studies. Nonteratogenic effects in the newborn following SSRI/SNRI exposure late in the third trimester include respiratory distress, cyanosis, apnea, seizures, temperature instability, feeding difficulty, vomiting, hypoglycemia, hyper- or hypotonia, hyper-reflexia, jitteriness, irritability, constant crying, and tremor. Symptoms may be due to the toxicity of the SNRIs/SSRIs or a discontinuation syndrome and may be consistent with serotonin syndrome associated with SSRI treatment. The long-term effects of *in utero* SNRI/SSRI exposure on infant development and behavior are not known.

Women inadvertently exposed to milnacipran during pregnancy may be enrolled in the Savella Pregnancy Registry (877-643-3010 or http://www.savellapregnancyregistry.com).

Breast-Feeding Considerations Milnacipran is excreted into breast milk. The manufacturer recommends that caution be exercised when administering milnacipran to nursing women.

Medication Guide Available Yes

Contraindications Use of MAOIs intended to treat psychiatric disorders (concurrently or within 5 days of discontinuing milnacipran, or within 2 weeks of discontinuing the MAOI); initiation of milnacipran in a patient receiving linezolid or methylene blue I.V.; uncontrolled narrow-angle glaucoma

Warnings/Precautions [U.S. Boxed Warning]: Milnacipran is a serotonin/norepinephrine reuptake inhibitor (SNRI) similar to SNRIs used to treat depression and other psychiatric disorders. Antidepressants increase the risk of suicidal thinking and behavior in children, adolescents, and young adults (18-24 years of age) with major depressive disorder (MDD) and other psychiatric disorders; consider risk prior to prescribing. Short-term studies did not show an increased risk in patients >24 years of age and showed a decreased risk in patients ≥65 years. Closely monitor for clinical worsening, suicidality, or unusual changes in behavior; the patient's family or caregiver should be instructed to closely observe the patient and communicate condition with healthcare provider. A medication guide concerning the use of antidepressants in children and teenagers should be dispensed with each prescription. **Milnacipran is not FDA approved for the treatment of major depressive disorder or for use in children.**

Suicide risks should be monitored in patients treated with SNRIs regardless of the indication. The possibility of a suicide attempt is inherent in major depression and may persist until remission occurs. Patients treated with antidepressants should be observed for clinical worsening and suicidality, especially during initial few months of a course of drug therapy, or at times of dose changes, either increases or decreases. Use caution in high-risk patients. Worsening depression and severe abrupt suicidality that are not part of the presenting symptoms may require discontinuation or modification of drug therapy. Prescriptions should be written for the smallest quantity consistent with good patient care. The patient's family or caregiver should be alerted to monitor patients for the emergence of suicidality and associated behaviors (such as anxiety, agitation, panic attacks, insomnia, irritability, hostility, impulsivity, akathisia, mania, and hypomania); patients should be instructed to notify their health care provider if any of these symptoms or worsening depression or psychosis occur.

Patients with major depressive disorder were excluded from clinical trials evaluating milnacipran for fibromyalgia; however, mania has been reported in patients with mood disorders taking similar medications. May worsen psychosis in some patients or precipitate a shift to mania or hypomania in patients with bipolar disorder. Patients presenting with depressive symptoms should be screened for bipolar disorder. Monotherapy in patients with bipolar disorder should be avoided. **Milnacipran is not FDA approved for the treatment of bipolar depression.**

Potentially life-threatening serotonin syndrome (SS) has occurred with serotonergic agents (eg, SSRIs, SNRIs), particularly when used in combination with other serotonergic agents (eg, triptans, TCAs, fentanyl, lithium, tramadol, buspirone, St John's wort, tryptophan) or agents that impair metabolism of serotonin (eg, MAO inhibitors intended to treat psychiatric disorders, other MAO inhibitors [ie, linezolid and intravenous methylene blue]). Monitor patients closely for signs of SS such as mental status changes (eg, agitation, hallucinations, delirium, coma); autonomic instability (eg, tachycardia, labile blood pressure, dizziness, diaphoresis, flushing, hyperthermia, incoordination); neuromuscular changes (eg, tremor, rigidity, myoclonus, hyperreflexia, incoordination); GI symptoms (eg, nausea, vomiting, diarrhea); and/or seizures. Discontinue treatment (and any concomitant serotonergic agent) immediately if signs/symptoms arise. Potential for severe reaction when used with MAO inhibitors; autonomic instability, coma, death, delirium, diaphoresis, hyperthermia, mental status changes/agitation, muscular rigidity, myoclonus, neuroleptic malignant syndrome features, and seizures may occur; concurrent use with MAO inhibitors is contraindicated. Do not use milnacipran in combination with an MAO inhibitor or within 14 days of discontinuing an MAO inhibitor; do not start an MAO inhibitor until ≥5 days after discontinuing milnacipran. Symptoms of serotonin syndrome may occur with concomitant proserotonergic drugs (ie, SSRIs/SNRIs or triptans), agents which reduce milnacipran's metabolism, or antidopaminergic agents (including antipsychotics). Concurrent use of serotonin precursors (eg, tryptophan) is not recommended.

May increase blood pressure and heart rate. Pre-existing cardiovascular disease (including hypertension and tachyarrhythmias) should be treated prior to initiating therapy. Blood pressure and heart rate should be evaluated prior to initiating therapy and periodically thereafter; consider dose reduction or gradual discontinuation of therapy in individuals with sustained hypertension or tachycardia during therapy. Use with caution in patients with pre-existing hypertension, tachyarrhythmias (eg, atrial fibrillation), or other cardiovascular disease; and with concomitant medications known to increase blood pressure or heart rate. May impair platelet aggregation resulting in increased risk of bleeding events, particularly if used concomitantly with aspirin or NSAIDs due to ulcerogenic potential. Data are inconclusive regarding extent of bleeding risk of SNRIs in combination with warfarin or other anticoagulants. Bleeding related to SNRI use has been reported to range from relatively minor bruising and epistaxis to life-threatening hemorrhage. Avoid use in patients with substantial ethanol intake, evidence of chronic liver disease or hepatic impairment. Cases of increased liver enzymes and severe liver injury (including fulminant hepatitis) have been reported. Discontinue therapy with the presentation of jaundice or other signs of hepatic dysfunction and do not reinitiate therapy unless another source or cause is identified. Use caution in patients with a history of seizures. Use caution in patients with a history of dysuria, especially males with prostatic hypertrophy, prostatitis, or other lower urinary tract disorders. Use caution in patients with controlled narrow-angle glaucoma; use is contraindicated with uncontrolled narrow-angle glaucoma. SSRIs and SNRIs have been associated with the development of SIADH; hyponatremia has been reported rarely (including severe cases with serum sodium <110 mmol/L), predominately in the elderly. Volume depletion and/or concurrent use of diuretics likely increases risk. Bone fractures have been associated with antidepressant treatment. Use caution in elderly patients; may cause or exacerbate syndrome of inappropriate antidiuretic hormone secretion or hyponatremia. Consider the possibility of a fragility fracture if an antidepressant-treated patient presents with unexplained bone pain, point tenderness, swelling, or bruising (Rabenda, 2013; Rizzoli, 2012).

Abrupt discontinuation or interruption of antidepressant therapy has been associated with a discontinuation syndrome. Symptoms arising may vary with antidepressant however commonly include nausea, vomiting, diarrhea, headaches, light-headedness, dizziness, diminished appetite, sweating, chills, tremors, paresthesias, fatigue, somnolence, and sleep disturbances (eg, vivid dreams, insomnia). Greater risks for developing a discontinuation syndrome have been associated with antidepressants with shorter half-lives, longer durations of treatment, and abrupt discontinuation. For antidepressants of short or intermediate half-lives, symptoms may emerge within 2-5 days after treatment discontinuation and last 7-14 days (APA, 2010; Fava, 2006; Haddad, 2001; Shelton, 2001; Warner, 2006).

Adverse Reactions

>10%:

- Central nervous system: Headache (18%), insomnia (12%)
- Endocrine & metabolic: Hot flashes (12%)
- Gastrointestinal: Nausea (37%), constipation (16%)

1% to 10%:

- Cardiovascular: Palpitation (7%), heart rate increased (6%), hypertension (5%), blood pressure increased (3%), flushing (3%), tachycardia (2%), peripheral edema (≥1%)
- Central nervous system: Dizziness (10%), migraine (5%), chills (2%), tremor (2%), depression (≥1%), fatigue (≥1%), fever (≥1%), irritability (≥1%), somnolence (≥1%)
- Dermatologic: Hyperhidrosis (9%), rash (3%)
- Endocrine & metabolic: Hypercholesterolemia (≥1%)
- Gastrointestinal: Vomiting (7%), xerostomia (5%), abdominal pain (3%), appetite decreased (2%), abdominal distension (≥1%), abnormal taste (≥1%), diarrhea (≥1%), dyspepsia (≥1%), flatulence (≥1%), gastroesophageal reflux disease (≥1%), weight changes (≥1%)

Genitourinary: Dysuria (≥2%), ejaculation disorder/failure (≥2%), erectile dysfunction (≥2%), libido decreased (≥2%), prostatitis (≥2%), scrotal pain (≥2%), testicular pain (≥2%), testicular swelling (≥2%), urethral pain (≥2%), urinary hesitation (≥2%), urinary retention (≥2%), urine flow decreased (≥2%), cystitis (≥1%), urinary tract infection (≥1%)

Neuromuscular & skeletal: Falling (≥1%)

Ocular: Blurred vision (2%)

Respiratory: Dyspnea (2%)

Miscellaneous: Night sweats (≥1%)

<1% (Limited to important or life-threatening): Accommodation disorder, acute renal failure, aggressiveness, anger, anorexia, delirium, erythema multiforme, galactorrhea, hallucination, hepatitis, homicidal ideation, hyperprolactinemia, hypertensive crisis, hyponatremia, leukopenia, loss of consciousness, neuroleptic malignant syndrome, neutropenia, parkinsonism, rhabdomyolysis, seizures, serotonin syndrome, Stevens-Johnson syndrome, supraventricular tachycardia, thrombocytopenia

Drug Interactions

Metabolism/Transport Effects None known.

Avoid Concomitant Use

Avoid concomitant use of Milnacipran with any of the following: Iobenguane I 123; Linezolid; MAO Inhibitors; Methylene Blue

Increased Effect/Toxicity

Milnacipran may increase the levels/effects of: Agents with Antiplatelet Properties; Alpha-/Beta-Agonists; Anticoagulants; Antipsychotics; Aspirin; Collagenase (Systemic); Dabigatran Etexilate; Digoxin; Ibritumomab; Methylene Blue; Metoclopramide; NSAID (Nonselective); Rivaroxaban; Salicylates; Serotonin Modulators; Thrombolytic Agents; Tositumomab and Iodine I 131 Tositumomab; Vitamin K Antagonists

The levels/effects of Milnacipran may be increased by: Alcohol (Ethyl); Antipsychotics; ClomiPRAMINE; Dasatinib; Glucosamine; Herbs (Anticoagulant/Antiplatelet Properties); Ibrutinib; Linezolid; MAO Inhibitors; Multivitamins/Fluoride (with ADE); Multivitamins/Minerals (with ADEK, Folate, Iron); Multivitamins/Minerals (with AE, No Iron); Nonsteroidal Anti-Inflammatory Agents; Omega-3 Fatty Acids; Pentosan Polysulfate Sodium; Pentoxifylline; Prostacyclin Analogues; Tipranavir; Vitamin E

Decreased Effect

Milnacipran may decrease the levels/effects of: Alpha2-Agonists; Iobenguane I 123; Ioflupane I 123

The levels/effects of Milnacipran may be decreased by: Nonsteroidal Anti-Inflammatory Agents

Ethanol/Nutrition/Herb Interactions

Ethanol: Ethanol may increase CNS depression. Management: Avoid ethanol.

Herb/Nutraceutical: Some herbal medications may increase risk of serotonin syndrome and/or excessive sedation. Management: Avoid valerian, St John's wort, SAMe, kava kava, and tryptophan.

Storage/Stability Store at 25°C (77°F); excursions permitted between 15°C to 30°C (59°F to 86°F).

Mechanism of Action Potent inhibitor of norepinephrine and serotonin reuptake (3:1). Milnacipran has no significant activity for serotonergic, alpha- and beta-adrenergic, muscarinic, histaminergic, dopaminergic, opiate, benzodiazepine, and GABA receptors. It does not possess MAO-inhibitory activity.

Pharmacodynamics/Kinetics

Absorption: Well absorbed

Distribution: I.V: V_d: ~400 L

Protein binding: 13%

Metabolism: Hepatic to inactive metabolites

Bioavailability: 85% to 90%

Half-life elimination: 6-8 hours

Time to peak, plasma: Oral: 2-4 hours

Excretion: Urine (55% as unchanged drug)

Dosage Oral: Adults: 50 mg twice daily

Titration schedule: 12.5 mg once on day 1, then 12.5 mg twice daily on days 2-3, 25 mg twice daily on days 4-7, then 50 mg twice daily thereafter. Dose may be increased to 100 mg twice daily, based on individual response. Doses >200 mg daily have not been studied.

Discontinuation of therapy: Upon discontinuation of antidepressant therapy, gradually taper the dose to minimize the incidence of withdrawal symptoms and allow for the detection of re-emerging symptoms. Evidence supporting ideal taper rates is limited. APA and NICE guidelines suggest tapering therapy over at least several weeks with consideration to the half-life of the antidepressant; antidepressants with a shorter half-life may need to be tapered more conservatively. In addition for long-term treated patients, WFSBP guidelines recommend tapering over 4-6 months. If intolerable withdrawal symptoms occur following a dose reduction, consider resuming the previously prescribed dose and/or decrease dose at a more gradual rate (APA, 2010; Bauer, 2002; Haddad, 2001; NCCMH, 2010; Schatzberg, 2006; Shelton, 2001; Warner, 2006).

MAO inhibitor recommendations:

Switching to or from an MAO inhibitor intended to treat psychiatric disorders:

Allow ≥14 days to elapse between discontinuing an MAO inhibitor intended to treat psychiatric disorders and initiation of milnacipran.

Allow ≥5 days to elapse between discontinuing milnacipran and initiation of MAO inhibitor intended to treat psychiatric disorders.

Use with other MAO inhibitors (linezolid or I.V. methylene blue):

Do not initiate milnacipran in patients receiving linezolid or I.V. methylene blue; consider other interventions for psychiatric condition.

If urgent treatment with linezolid or I.V. methylene blue is required in a patient already receiving milnacipran and potential benefits outweigh potential risks, discontinue milnacipran promptly and administer linezolid or I.V. methylene blue. Monitor for serotonin syndrome for 5 days or until 24 hours after the last dose of linezolid or I.V. methylene blue, whichever comes first. May resume milnacipran 24 hours after the last dose of linezolid or I.V. methylene blue.

Dosage adjustment in renal impairment:

Mild renal impairment: No dosage adjustment necessary.

Moderate renal impairment: Use with caution

Severe renal impairment (Cl_{cr} ≤29 mL/minute): Reduce maintenance dose to 25 mg twice daily; dose may be increased to 50 mg twice daily, based on individual tolerance

End-stage renal disease (ESRD): Use not recommended

Dosage adjustment in hepatic impairment:

Mild-to-moderate hepatic impairment: No dosage adjustment necessary.

Severe hepatic impairment: No dosage adjustment necessary; use with caution.

Administration Oral: Administer with or without food; food may improve tolerability.

Monitoring Parameters Blood pressure and heart rate should be regularly monitored; renal function should be monitored for dosing purposes; mental status for suicidal ideation (especially at the beginning of therapy or when doses are increased or decreased); intraocular pressure should be monitored in those with baseline elevations or a history of glaucoma

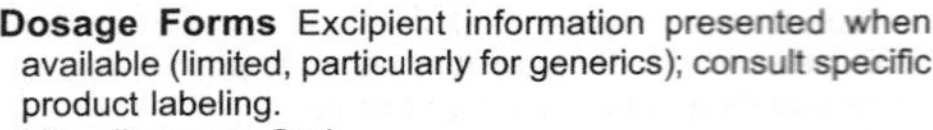

Dosage Forms Excipient information presented when available (limited, particularly for generics); consult specific product labeling.

Miscellaneous, Oral:

Savella Titration Pack: 12.5 & 25 & 50 MG (55 ea) [contains fd&c blue #2 aluminum lake]

Tablet, Oral:

Savella: 12.5 mg [contains fd&c blue #2 aluminum lake]

Savella: 25 mg, 50 mg

Savella: 100 mg [contains fd&c red #40 aluminum lake]

Milrinone (MIL ri none)

Brand Names: Canada Milrinone Lactate Injection; Primacor®

Index Terms Milrinone Lactate

Pharmacologic Category Phosphodiesterase-3 Enzyme Inhibitor

Additional Appendix Information

Vasoactive Agents, Intravenous *on page 2315*

Use Short-term I.V. therapy of acutely-decompensated heart failure

Unlabeled Use Inotropic therapy for patients unresponsive to other acute heart failure therapies (eg, dobutamine); outpatient inotropic therapy for heart transplant candidates; palliation of symptoms in end-stage heart failure patients who cannot otherwise be discharged from the hospital and are not transplant candidates

Pregnancy Risk Factor C

Pregnancy Considerations Teratogenic effects have not been observed in animal reproduction studies; however, increased resorption was reported in some studies.

Breast-Feeding Considerations It is not known if milrinone is excreted in breast milk. The manufacturer recommends that caution be exercised when administering milrinone to nursing women.

Contraindications Hypersensitivity to milrinone, inamrinone, or any component of the formulation; concurrent use of inamrinone

Warnings/Precautions Monitor closely for hypotension. Avoid in severe obstructive aortic or pulmonic valvular disease. Milrinone may aggravate outflow tract obstruction in hypertrophic subaortic stenosis. Supraventricular and ventricular arrhythmias have developed in high-risk patients. Ensure that ventricular rate controlled in atrial fibrillation/flutter prior to initiating milrinone. Not recommended for use in acute MI patients. Monitor and correct fluid and electrolyte problems. Adjust dose in renal dysfunction. Discontinue therapy if dose-related elevations in LFTs and clinical symptoms of hepatotoxicity occur.

Adverse Reactions

>10%: Cardiovascular: Ventricular arrhythmia (ectopy 9%, NSVT 3%, sustained ventricular tachycardia 1%, ventricular fibrillation <1%)

1% to 10%:

Cardiovascular: Supraventricular arrhythmia (4%), hypotension (3%), angina/chest pain (1%)

Central nervous system: Headache (3%)

<1% (Limited to important or life-threatening): Anaphylaxis, atrial fibrillation, bronchospasm, hypokalemia, injection site reaction, liver function abnormalities, MI, rash, thrombocytopenia, torsade de pointes, tremor, ventricular fibrillation

Drug Interactions

Metabolism/Transport Effects None known.

Avoid Concomitant Use

Avoid concomitant use of Milrinone with any of the following: Riociguat

Increased Effect/Toxicity

Milrinone may increase the levels/effects of: Riociguat

Decreased Effect There are no known significant interactions involving a decrease in effect.

Preparation for Administration Standard dilution: For a final concentration of 0.2 mg/mL: Dilute Primacor® 1 mg/mL (20 mL) with 80 mL diluent (final volume: 100 mL) of 1/2NS, NS or D_5W. May also dilute 1 mg/mL (10 mL) with 40 mL diluent (final volume: 50 mL).

Storage/Stability Store at 15°C to 30°C (59°F to 86°F); avoid freezing. Stable at 0.2 mg/mL in 1/2NS, NS, or D_5W for 72 hours at room temperature in normal light.

Mechanism of Action A selective phosphodiesterase inhibitor in cardiac and vascular tissue, resulting in vasodilation and inotropic effects with little chronotropic activity.

Pharmacodynamics/Kinetics

Onset of action: I.V.: 5-15 minutes

Distribution: V_{dss}: 0.32-0.45 L/kg

Protein binding, plasma: ~70%

Metabolism: Hepatic (12%)

Half-life elimination: Normal renal function: ~2.5 hours; CVVH: 20.1 hours (Taniguchi, 2000)

Excretion: Urine (85% as unchanged drug) within 24 hours; active tubular secretion is a major elimination pathway for milrinone

Dosage Adults: I.V.: Loading dose (optional; see **"Note"**): 50 mcg/kg administered over 10 minutes followed by a maintenance dose titrated according to hemodynamic and clinical response; Maintenance dose: I.V. infusion: 0.375-0.75 mcg/kg/minute; lower initial doses of 0.1 mcg/kg/minute (with final doses of 0.2-0.3 mcg/kg/minute) have also been recommended (Lindenfeld, 2010).

Note: When initiating an infusion of 0.5 mcg/kg/minute without a loading dose, significant hemodynamic changes seen at 30 minutes with similar effects on pulmonary capillary wedge pressure and cardiac index seen at 2 and 3 hours, respectively, compared to loading dose regimen (Baruch, 2011).

Dosage adjustment in renal impairment:

Manufacturer recommended adjustment:

Cl_{cr} 50 mL/minute/1.73 m^2: Administer 0.43 mcg/kg/minute

Cl_{cr} 40 mL/minute/1.73 m^2: Administer 0.38 mcg/kg/minute

Cl_{cr} 30 mL/minute/1.73 m^2: Administer 0.33 mcg/kg/minute

Cl_{cr} 20 mL/minute/ 1.73 m^2: Administer 0.28 mcg/kg/minute

Cl_{cr} 10 mL/minute/1.73 m^2: Administer 0.23 mcg/kg/minute

Cl_{cr} 5 mL/minute/1.73 m^2: Administer 0.2 mcg/kg/minute

Alternative Dosing Adjustments in Patients with Renal Impairment[1]

Cl_{cr} (mL/min)	Starting dose (mcg/kg/min)		
	0.375	**0.5**	**0.75**
50	0.25	0.375	0.5
40	0.125	0.25	0.375
30	0.0625	0.125	0.25
20	Consider alternative therapy	0.0625	0.125
10	Consider alternative therapy		0.0625
5	Consider alternative therapy		

[1]Based on expert opinion

Usual Infusion Concentrations: Pediatric Note: Premixed solutions available

I.V. infusion: 200 **mcg**/mL

Usual Infusion Concentrations: Adult Note: Premixed solutions available

I.V. infusion: 20 mg in 100 mL (total volume) (concentration: 200 **mcg**/mL) of D_5W

Administration Infuse via infusion pump

Monitoring Parameters Platelet count, CBC, electrolytes (especially potassium and magnesium), liver function and renal function tests; ECG, CVP, SBP, DBP, heart rate; infusion site

If pulmonary artery catheter is in place, monitor cardiac index, stroke volume, systemic vascular resistance, pulmonary capillary wedge pressure and pulmonary vascular resistance.

Consult individual institutional policies and procedures.

Dosage Forms Excipient information presented when available (limited, particularly for generics); consult specific product labeling. [DSC] = Discontinued product

Solution, Intravenous:

Generic: 200 mcg/mL (100 mL, 200 mL); 10 mg/10 mL (10 mL); 20 mg/20 mL (20 mL); 50 mg/50 mL (50 mL)

Solution, Intravenous [preservative free]:

Generic: 200 mcg/mL (100 mL, 200 mL); 10 mg/10 mL (10 mL [DSC]); 20 mg/20 mL (20 mL [DSC])

◆ **Milrinone Lactate** *see* Milrinone *on page 1372*

◆ **Milrinone Lactate Injection (Can)** *see* Milrinone *on page 1372*

◆ **Mimvey** *see* Estradiol and Norethindrone *on page 763*

◆ **Minastrin 24 Fe** *see* Ethinyl Estradiol and Norethindrone *on page 793*

◆ **Minestrin 1/20 (Can)** *see* Ethinyl Estradiol and Norethindrone *on page 793*

◆ **Minims Cyclopentolate (Can)** *see* Cyclopentolate *on page 504*

◆ **Minipress** *see* Prazosin *on page 1703*

◆ **Minipress® (Can)** *see* Prazosin *on page 1703*

◆ **Minirin® (Can)** *see* Desmopressin *on page 575*

◆ **Minitran** *see* Nitroglycerin *on page 1466*

◆ **Minivelle** *see* Estradiol (Systemic) *on page 754*

◆ **Minocin** *see* Minocycline *on page 1373*

◆ **Minocin® (Can)** *see* Minocycline *on page 1373*

Minocycline (mi noe SYE kleen)

Brand Names: U.S. Dynacin [DSC]; Minocin; Solodyn

Brand Names: Canada Apo-Minocycline®; Arestin Microspheres; Dom-Minocycline; Minocin®; Mylan-Minocycline; Novo-Minocycline; PHL-Minocycline; PMS-Minocycline; ratio-Minocycline; Riva-Minocycline; Sandoz-Minocycline

Index Terms Minocycline Hydrochloride; Ximino™

Pharmacologic Category Antibiotic, Tetracycline Derivative

Use Treatment of susceptible bacterial infections of both gram-negative and gram-positive organisms; treatment of anthrax (inhalational, cutaneous, and gastrointestinal); moderate-to-severe acne; meningococcal (asymptomatic) carrier state; Rickettsial diseases (including Rocky Mountain spotted fever, Q fever); nongonococcal urethritis, gonorrhea; acute intestinal amebiasis; respiratory tract infection; skin/soft tissue infections; chlamydial infections

Extended release (Solodyn®): Only indicated for treatment of inflammatory lesions of non-nodular moderate-to-severe acne

Unlabeled Use Rheumatoid arthritis (patients with low disease activity of short duration); nocardiosis; alternative treatment for community-acquired MRSA infection; chronic oral antimicrobial suppression of prosthetic joint infection

Pregnancy Risk Factor D

Pregnancy Considerations Tetracyclines cross the placenta and accumulate in developing teeth and long tubular bones. Rare spontaneous reports of congenital anomalies, including limb reduction, have been reported following maternal minocycline use. Due to limited information, a causal association cannot be established. Tetracyclines may discolor fetal teeth following maternal use during pregnancy; the specific teeth involved and the portion of the tooth affected depends on the timing and duration of exposure relative to tooth calcification. As a class, tetracyclines are generally considered second-line antibiotics in pregnant women and their use should be avoided (Mylonas, 2011). Minocycline should not be used for the treatment of acne in pregnant women, or in males or females attempting to conceive a child.

Breast-Feeding Considerations Minocycline is excreted in breast milk (Brogden, 1975). According to the manufacturer, the decision to continue or discontinue breast-feeding during therapy should take into account the risk of exposure to the infant and the benefits of treatment to the mother. Oral absorption is not affected by dairy products; therefore, oral absorption of minocycline by the breast-feeding infant would not be expected to be diminished by the calcium in the maternal milk. Nondose-related effects could include modification of bowel flora. There have been case reports of black discoloration of breast milk in women taking minocycline (Basler, 1985; Hunt, 1996).

Contraindications Hypersensitivity to minocycline, other tetracyclines, or any component of the formulation

Warnings/Precautions May be associated with increases in BUN secondary to antianabolic effects; use caution in patients with renal impairment (Cl_{cr} <80 mL/minute). Hepatotoxicity has been reported; use caution in patients with hepatic insufficiency. Autoimmune syndromes (eg, lupus-like, hepatitis, and vasculitis) have been reported; discontinue if symptoms occur. CNS effects (lightheadedness, vertigo) may occur; patients must be cautioned about performing tasks which require mental alertness (eg, operating machinery or driving). Pseudotumor cerebri has been (rarely) reported with tetracycline use; usually resolves with discontinuation. May cause photosensitivity; discontinue if skin erythema occurs. Prolonged use may result in fungal or bacterial superinfection, including *C. difficile*-associated diarrhea (CDAD) and pseudomembranous colitis; CDAD has been observed >2 months postantibiotic treatment. May cause tissue hyperpigmentation, enamel hypoplasia, or permanent tooth discoloration; use of tetracyclines should be avoided during tooth development (children <8 years of age) unless other drugs are not likely to be effective or are contraindicated. Do not use during pregnancy. In addition to affecting tooth development, tetracycline use has been associated with retardation of skeletal development and reduced bone growth. Rash, along with eosinophilia, fever, and organ failure (Drug Rash with Eosinophilia and Systemic Symptoms [DRESS] syndrome) has been reported; discontinue treatment immediately if DRESS syndrome is suspected.

Adverse Reactions Frequency not defined.

Cardiovascular: Myocarditis, pericarditis, vasculitis

Central nervous system: Bulging fontanels, dizziness, fatigue, fever, headache, hypoesthesia, malaise, mood changes, paresthesia, pseudotumor cerebri, sedation, seizure, somnolence, vertigo

Dermatologic: Alopecia, angioedema, drug rash with eosinophilia and systemic symptoms (DRESS), erythema multiforme, erythema nodosum, erythematous rash, exfoliative dermatitis, hyperpigmentation of nails, maculopapular rash, photosensitivity, pigmentation of the skin and mucous membranes, pruritus, Stevens-Johnson syndrome, toxic epidermal necrolysis, urticaria

Endocrine & metabolic: Thyroid cancer, thyroid discoloration, thyroid dysfunction

Gastrointestinal: Anorexia, diarrhea, dyspepsia, dysphagia, enamel hypoplasia, enterocolitis, esophageal ulcerations, esophagitis, glossitis, inflammatory lesions (oral/anogenital), moniliasis, nausea, oral cavity discoloration, pancreatitis, pseudomembranous colitis, stomatitis, tooth discoloration, vomiting, xerostomia

Genitourinary: Balanitis, vulvovaginitis

Hematologic: Agranulocytosis, eosinophilia, hemolytic anemia, leukopenia, neutropenia, pancytopenia, thrombocytopenia

Hepatic: Autoimmune hepatitis, hepatic cholestasis, hepatic failure, hepatitis, hyperbilirubinemia, jaundice, liver enzyme increases

Local: Injection site reaction (I.V. administration)

Neuromuscular & skeletal: Arthralgia, arthritis, bone discoloration, joint stiffness, joint swelling, myalgia

Otic: Hearing loss, tinnitus

Renal: Acute renal failure, BUN increased, interstitial nephritis

Respiratory: Asthma, bronchospasm, cough, dyspnea, pneumonitis, pulmonary infiltrate (with eosinophilia)

Miscellaneous: Anaphylaxis, hypersensitivity, lupus erythematosus, lupus-like syndrome, serum sickness

Drug Interactions

Metabolism/Transport Effects None known.

Avoid Concomitant Use

Avoid concomitant use of Minocycline with any of the following: BCG; Retinoic Acid Derivatives; Strontium Ranelate

Increased Effect/Toxicity

Minocycline may increase the levels/effects of: Mipomersen; Neuromuscular-Blocking Agents; Porfimer; Retinoic Acid Derivatives; Vitamin K Antagonists

Decreased Effect

Minocycline may decrease the levels/effects of: Atazanavir; BCG; Penicillins; Sodium Picosulfate; Typhoid Vaccine

The levels/effects of Minocycline may be decreased by: Antacids; Bile Acid Sequestrants; Bismuth; Bismuth Subsalicylate; Calcium Salts; Iron Salts; Lanthanum; Magnesium Salts; Multivitamins/Minerals (with ADEK, Folate, Iron); Multivitamins/Minerals (with AE, No Iron); Quinapril; Strontium Ranelate; Sucralfate; Sucroferric Oxyhydroxide; Zinc Salts

Ethanol/Nutrition/Herb Interactions

Food: Minocycline serum concentrations are not significantly altered if taken with food or dairy products.

Herb/Nutraceutical: Avoid dong quai, St John's wort (may also cause photosensitization).

Preparation for Administration Injection: Reconstitute with 5 mL of sterile water for injection, and further dilute in 500-1000 mL of NS, D_5W, D_5NS, Ringer's injection, or LR.

Storage/Stability

Capsule (including pellet-filled), tablet: Store at 20°C to 25°C (68°F to 77°F); protect from heat. Protect from light and moisture.

Extended release tablet: Store at 15°C to 30°C (59°F to 86°F); protect from heat. Protect from light and moisture.

Injection: Store vials at 20°C to 25°C (68°F to 77°F) prior to reconstitution. Reconstituted solution is stable at room temperature for 24 hours. Final dilutions should be administered immediately.

Mechanism of Action Inhibits bacterial protein synthesis by binding with the 30S and possibly the 50S ribosomal subunit(s) of susceptible bacteria; cell wall synthesis is not affected

Rheumatoid arthritis: The mechanism of action of minocycline in rheumatoid arthritis is not completely understood. It is thought to have antimicrobial, anti-inflammatory, immunomodulatory, and chondroprotective effects. More specifically, it is thought to be a potent inhibitor of metalloproteinases, which are active in rheumatoid arthritis joint destruction.

Pharmacodynamics/Kinetics

Absorption: Oral: Well absorbed

Protein binding: 70% to 75%

Metabolism: Hepatic to inactive metabolites

Half-life elimination: I.V.: 15-23 hours; Oral: 16 hours (range: 11-22 hours)

Time to peak: Capsule, pellet filled: 1-4 hours; Extended release tablet: 3.5-4 hours

Excretion: Urine, feces

Dosage

Usual dosage range:

I.V.:

Children >8 years: Initial: 4 mg/kg, followed by 2 mg/kg/dose every 12 hours (maximum: 400 mg daily)

Adults: Initial: 200 mg, followed by 100 mg every 12 hours (maximum: 400 mg daily)

Oral:

Capsule or immediate release tablet:

Children >8 years: Oral: Initial: 4 mg/kg, followed by 2 mg/kg/dose every 12 hours (maximum: 400 mg daily)

Adults: Oral: Initial: 200 mg, followed by 100 mg every 12 hours; more frequent dosing intervals may be used (100-200 mg initially, followed by 50 mg 4 times daily)

Extended release tablet (Solodyn®): Children ≥12 years and Adults (≥45 kg): Oral: 45-135 mg once daily (weight based)

Indication-specific dosing:

Children ≥12 years and Adults:

Acne, inflammatory, non-nodular, moderate-to-severe (Solodyn®): Oral:

45-49 kg: 45 mg once daily
50-59 kg: 55 mg once daily
60-71 kg: 65 mg once daily
72-84 kg: 80 mg once daily
85-96 kg: 90 mg once daily
97-110 kg: 105 mg once daily
111-125 kg: 115 mg once daily
126-136 kg: 135 mg once daily

Note: Therapy should be continued for 12 weeks. Higher doses do not confer greater efficacy and may be associated with more acute vestibular side effects. Safety of use beyond 12 weeks has not been established.

Cellulitis (purulent) infection due to community-acquired MRSA (unlabeled use): Oral: Children >8 years: Initial: 4 mg/kg (maximum: 200 mg); Maintenance: 2 mg/kg/dose (maximum: 100 mg) every 12 hours for 5-10 days (Liu, 2011)

Adults:

Acne: Oral: Capsule or immediate-release tablet: 50-100 mg twice daily

Cellulitis (purulent) due to community-acquired MRSA (unlabeled use): Oral: Initial: 200 mg; Maintenance: 100 mg twice daily for 5-10 days (Liu, 2011)

Chlamydial or *Ureaplasma urealyticum* infection, uncomplicated: Oral, I.V.: Urethral, endocervical, or rectal: 100 mg every 12 hours for at least 7 days

Gonococcal infection, uncomplicated (males): Oral, I.V.:

Without urethritis or anorectal infection: Initial: 200 mg, followed by 100 mg every 12 hours for at least 4 days (cultures 2-3 days post-therapy)

Urethritis: 100 mg every 12 hours for 5 days

Meningococcal carrier state (manufacturer's labeling): Oral: 100 mg every 12 hours for 5 days. **Note:** CDC recommendations do not mention use of minocycline for eradicating nasopharyngeal carriage of meningococcal

Mycobacterium marinum: Oral: 100 mg every 12 hours for 6-8 weeks

Nocardiosis, cutaneous (non-CNS) (unlabeled use): Oral: 100-200 mg every 12 hours

Prosthetic joint infection:

Staphylococci (oxacillin-sensitive or –resistant) oral phase treatment (after completion of pathogen-specific I.V. therapy) following 1-stage exchange:

Total ankle, elbow, hip, or shoulder arthroplasty: 100 mg twice daily for 3 months; **Note:** Must be used in combination with rifampin (Osmon, 2013)

Total knee arthroplasty: 100 mg twice daily for 6 months; **Note:** Must be used in combination with rifampin (Osmon, 2013)

Chronic oral antimicrobial suppression (unlabeled use): Oral:

Propionibacterium spp (alternative to penicillin or amoxicillin): 100 mg twice daily (Osmon, 2013)

Staphylococci (oxacillin-resistant): 100 mg twice daily (Osmon, 2013)

Rheumatoid arthritis (unlabeled use): Oral: 100 mg twice daily (O'Dell, 2001)

Syphilis: Oral, I.V.: Initial: 200 mg, followed by 100 mg every 12 hours for 10-15 days

Elderly: Refer to adult dosing.

Dosage adjustment in renal impairment: Use with caution; monitor BUN and creatinine clearance. Consider decreasing dose or increasing dosing interval (extended release).

Cl_{cr} <80 mL/minute: Do not exceed 200 mg daily

Dosage adjustment in hepatic impairment: No dosage adjustment provided in manufacturer's labeling; however, hepatotoxicity has been reported. Use with caution in patients with hepatic impairment.

Dietary Considerations May be taken with or without food.

Administration

I.V.: Infuse slowly; avoid rapid administration. The manufacturer's labeling does not provide a recommended administration rate. The injectable route should be used only if the oral route is not feasible or adequate. Prolonged intravenous therapy may be associated with thrombophlebitis.

Oral: May be administered with or without food. Administer with adequate fluid to decrease the risk of esophageal irritation and ulceration. Swallow pellet-filled capsule and extended release tablet whole; do not chew, crush, or split.

Monitoring Parameters LFTs, BUN, renal function with long-term treatment; if symptomatic for autoimmune disorder, include ANA, CBC

Test Interactions May cause interference with fluorescence test for urinary catecholamines (false elevations)

Product Availability Ximino™ extended-release capsules: FDA approved July 2012; anticipated availability currently unknown. Consult prescribing information for additional information.

Dosage Forms Excipient information presented when available (limited, particularly for generics); consult specific product labeling. [DSC] = Discontinued product

Capsule, Oral:

Minocin: 50 mg, 75 mg, 100 mg [contains brilliant blue fcf (fd&c blue #1), fd&c yellow #10 (quinoline yellow)]

Generic: 50 mg, 75 mg, 100 mg

Kit, Combination:

Minocin: 50 mg, 100 mg [contains brilliant blue fcf (fd&c blue #1), disodium edta, fd&c yellow #10 (quinoline yellow), sodium benzoate]

Solution Reconstituted, Intravenous:

Minocin: 100 mg (1 ea)

Tablet, Oral:

Dynacin: 50 mg [DSC], 75 mg [DSC], 100 mg [DSC]

Generic: 50 mg, 75 mg, 100 mg

Tablet Extended Release 24 Hour, Oral:

Solodyn: 55 mg [contains fd&c red #40]

Solodyn: 65 mg [contains brilliant blue fcf (fd&c blue #1), fd&c blue #2 (indigotine), fd&c yellow #10 (quinoline yellow)]

Solodyn: 80 mg [contains fd&c blue #2 (indigotine), fd&c red #40, fd&c yellow #6 (sunset yellow)]

Solodyn: 105 mg [contains brilliant blue fcf (fd&c blue #1)]

Solodyn: 115 mg [contains brilliant blue fcf (fd&c blue #1), fd&c blue #2 (indigotine), fd&c yellow #10 (quinoline yellow)]

Generic: 45 mg, 90 mg, 135 mg

◆ **Minocycline Hydrochloride** *see* Minocycline *on page 1373*

◆ **Min-Ovral (Can)** *see* Ethinyl Estradiol and Levonorgestrel *on page 787*

Minoxidil (Systemic) (mi NOKS i dil)

Brand Names: Canada Loniten®

Pharmacologic Category Antihypertensive; Vasodilator, Direct-Acting

Use Management of severe hypertension (usually in combination with a diuretic and beta-blocker)

Pregnancy Risk Factor C

Dosage Oral:

Children <12 years: Hypertension: Initial: 0.1-0.2 mg/kg once daily; maximum: 5 mg/day; increase gradually every 3 days; usual dosage range: 0.25-1 mg/kg/day in 1-2 divided doses; maximum: 50 mg/day

Children ≥12 years and Adults: Hypertension: Initial: 5 mg once daily, increase gradually every 3 days (maximum: 100 mg/day); usual dosage range (JNC 7): 2.5-80 mg/day in 1-2 divided doses

Note: Dosage adjustment is needed when added to concomitant therapy.

Elderly: Hypertension: Initial: 2.5 mg once daily; increase gradually.

Dosage adjustment in renal impairment: Patient with renal failure and/or receiving dialysis may require dosage reduction.

Supplemental dose is not necessary after hemo- or peritoneal dialysis.

Dosage adjustment in hepatic impairment: No dosage adjustment provided in manufacturer's labeling.

Additional Information Complete prescribing information should be consulted for additional detail.

Dosage Forms Excipient information presented when available (limited, particularly for generics); consult specific product labeling.

Tablet, Oral:

Generic: 2.5 mg, 10 mg

Dosage Forms: Canada Excipient information presented when available (limited, particularly for generics); consult specific product labeling.

Tablet, Oral:

Loniten: 2.5 mg, 10 mg

Minoxidil (Topical) (mi NOKS i dil)

Brand Names: U.S. Hair Regrowth Treatment Men [OTC]; Minoxidil for Men [OTC]; Rogaine Mens Extra Strength [OTC]

Brand Names: Canada Apo-Gain®; Rogaine®

Pharmacologic Category Topical Skin Product

Use Treatment of alopecia androgenetica in males and females

Dosage Topical: Adults: Alopecia: Apply twice daily; 4 months of therapy may be necessary for hair growth.

Additional Information Complete prescribing information should be consulted for additional detail.

Dosage Forms Excipient information presented when available (limited, particularly for generics); consult specific product labeling.

Foam, External:

Rogaine Mens Extra Strength: 5% (60 g) [contains sd alcohol 40b]

Solution, External:

Hair Regrowth Treatment Men: 5% (60 mL) [contains alcohol, usp, propylene glycol]

Minoxidil for Men: 2% (60 mL)

Minoxidil for Men: 2% (60 mL) [contains alcohol, usp]

Minoxidil for Men: 5% (60 mL, 120 mL) [contains alcohol, usp, propylene glycol, water, purified]

Generic: 5% (60 mL)

- ◆ Minoxidil for Men [OTC] *see* Minoxidil (Topical) *on page 1375*
- ◆ Mint-Alendronate (Can) *see* Alendronate *on page 69*
- ◆ Mint-Amlodipine (Can) *see* AmLODIPine *on page 109*
- ◆ Mint-Anastrozole (Can) *see* Anastrozole *on page 137*
- ◆ Mint-Atenolol (Can) *see* Atenolol *on page 186*
- ◆ Mint-Ciprofloxacin (Can) *see* Ciprofloxacin (Systemic) *on page 430*
- ◆ Mint-Citalopram (Can) *see* Citalopram *on page 440*
- ◆ Mint-Finasteride (Can) *see* Finasteride *on page 862*
- ◆ Mint-Fluoxetine (Can) *see* FLUoxetine *on page 885*
- ◆ Mint-Irbesartan/HCTZ (Can) *see* Irbesartan and Hydrochlorothiazide *on page 1115*
- ◆ Mint-Losartan/HCTZ (Can) *see* Losartan and Hydrochlorothiazide *on page 1249*
- ◆ Mint-Losartan/HCTZ DS (Can) *see* Losartan and Hydrochlorothiazide *on page 1249*
- ◆ Mint-Metformin (Can) *see* MetFORMIN *on page 1310*
- ◆ Mint-Ondansetron (Can) *see* Ondansetron *on page 1510*
- ◆ Mintox Plus [OTC] *see* Aluminum Hydroxide, Magnesium Hydroxide, and Simethicone *on page 90*
- ◆ Mint-Pioglitazone (Can) *see* Pioglitazone *on page 1649*
- ◆ Mint-Pravastatin (Can) *see* Pravastatin *on page 1700*
- ◆ Mint-Risperidon (Can) *see* RisperiDONE *on page 1826*
- ◆ MINT-Sertraline (Can) *see* Sertraline *on page 1889*
- ◆ Mint-Simvastatin (Can) *see* Simvastatin *on page 1899*
- ◆ Mint-Topiramate (Can) *see* Topiramate *on page 2090*
- ◆ Miochol-E *see* Acetylcholine *on page 35*
- ◆ Miochol®-E (Can) *see* Acetylcholine *on page 35*
- ◆ Miostat *see* Carbachol *on page 335*
- ◆ Miostat® (Can) *see* Carbachol *on page 335*

Mipomersen (mi poe MER sen)

Brand Names: U.S. Kynamro

Index Terms ISIS 301012; Mipomersen Sodium

Pharmacologic Category Antihyperlipidemic Agent, Apolipoprotein B Antisense Oligonucleotide

Use Adjunct to dietary therapy and other lipid-lowering treatments to reduce low-density lipoprotein cholesterol (LDL-C), total cholesterol, apolipoprotein B, and non-high-density lipoprotein cholesterol (non-HDL-C) in patients with homozygous familial hypercholesterolemia (HoFH)

Pregnancy Risk Factor B

Pregnancy Considerations Adverse events have not been observed in animal reproduction studies. There are no adequate and well-controlled studies in pregnant women. Use during pregnancy only if clearly needed.

Breast-Feeding Considerations It is not known if mipomersen is excreted in breast milk. Breast-feeding is not recommended by the manufacturer.

Prescribing and Access Restrictions As a requirement of the REMS program, access to this medication is restricted. Prescribers must enroll in the Kynamro™ REMS program and complete the prescriber training and complete, sign, and submit the Prescriber Enrollment Form to the Kynamro™ REMS program. The prescriber must then complete the Prescriber Training before activation within the Kynamro™ REMS program. Pharmacies must educate all pharmacy staff involved in the dispensing of Kynamro™ on the REMS program requirements, put processes in place to verify (prior to dispensing Kynamro™) that the prescriber is certified and the Prescription Authorization Form is received with each new prescription. Pharmacies must also agree to be audited to ensure that all processes and procedures in place are being followed in accordance with the program and be able to provide prescription data to the REMS program.

Medication Guide Available Yes

Contraindications Hypersensitivity to mipomersen or any component of the formulation; moderate or severe hepatic impairment (Child-Pugh class B or C); active liver disease; unexplained persistent elevations of hepatic transaminases

Warnings/Precautions [U.S. Boxed Warning]: As seen in clinical trials, may cause hepatic transaminase elevation and increases in hepatic steatosis (with or without concomitant increases in transaminases) which may progress to steatohepatitis and cirrhosis; measure ALT, AST, alkaline phosphatase, and total bilirubin prior to initiation, then ALT and AST on a regular basis as recommended. Withhold dose of mipomersen if ALT or AST is ≥3 x ULN. Discontinue mipomersen if clinically significant hepatotoxicity occurs. Because mipomersen has a risk of hepatotoxicity, it is only available through a restricted program under a Risk Evaluation and Mitigation Strategy (REMS) program (Kynamro™ REMS). Alcohol consumption during treatment with mipomersen should be limited to ≤1 drink/day due to potential to increase levels of hepatic fat and induce or exacerbate liver injury. Use caution when used concomitantly with other medications known to cause hepatotoxicity (eg, isotretinoin, amiodarone, acetaminophen [>4 g/day for ≥3 days/week], methotrexate, tetracyclines, and tamoxifen); consider monitoring liver function tests more frequently. Concurrent use with LDL-C lowering medications that can also increase hepatic fat is not recommended. Use is contraindicated in patients with moderate or severe hepatic impairment or active liver disease including patients with unexplained persistent elevations of hepatic transaminases. If baseline liver function tests are abnormal, consider initiation after an appropriate work up and abnormalities are explained or resolved.

Within 2 days after an injection, influenza-like symptoms (eg, fever, chills, myalgia, arthralgia, malaise, or fatigue) have been reported in 30% of patients receiving mipomersen. Injection site reactions (eg, erythema, pain, tenderness, pruritus, and local swelling) were common in patients receiving mipomersen; minimize injection site reactions by using proper subcutaneous administration technique.

Safety and efficacy in patients with hepatic impairment have not been established; use is contraindicated in patients with moderate or severe hepatic impairment

(Child-Pugh class B or C), active liver disease, or unexplained persistent elevations of hepatic transaminases. Safety and efficacy in patients with renal impairment including those who undergo hemodialysis have not been established; use is not recommended in patients with severe renal impairment, clinically significant proteinuria, or on hemodialysis.

In clinical trials, patients ≥65 years of age (n=59) experienced a higher incidence of hepatic steatosis, hypertension, and peripheral edema; use with caution in the elderly. Safety and efficacy of the treatment of hypercholesterolemia not due to homozygous familial hypercholesterolemia (HoFH) have not been established. The use of mipomersen as an adjunct to LDL-C apheresis is not recommended (use not established).

Adverse Reactions

>10%:

Central nervous system: Fatigue (15%), headache (12%)

Gastrointestinal: Nausea (14%)

Hepatic: ALT increased (≥3 x ULN to <5 x ULN: 12%; ≥5 x ULN to <10 x ULN: 3%; ≥10 x ULN: 1%)

Local: Injection site reactions: Erythema (59%), pain (56%), hematoma (32%), pruritus (29%), swelling (18%), discoloration (17%)

Miscellaneous: Antibody formation (38% to 72%), flu-like syndrome (13% to 66%)

1% to 10%:

Cardiovascular: Hypertension (7%), peripheral edema (5%), angina pectoris (4%), palpitations (3%)

Central nervous system: Fever (8%), chills (6%), insomnia (3%)

Gastrointestinal: Vomiting (4%), abdominal pain (3%)

Hepatic: Hepatic steatosis (7%), AST increased (≥3 x ULN to <5 x ULN: 7%; ≥5 x ULN to <10 x ULN: 3%)

Neuromuscular & skeletal: Limb pain (7%), musculoskeletal pain (4%)

Renal: Proteinuria (9%)

Miscellaneous: Neoplasms (4%, benign and malignant)

<1% (Limited to important or life-threatening): Angioedema, glomerular nephritis, hypersensitivity reactions

Drug Interactions

Metabolism/Transport Effects None known.

Avoid Concomitant Use There are no known interactions where it is recommended to avoid concomitant use.

Increased Effect/Toxicity

Mipomersen may increase the levels/effects of: Methotrexate

The levels/effects of Mipomersen may be increased by: Acetaminophen; Alcohol (Ethyl); Amiodarone; ISOtretinoin; Tamoxifen; Tetracycline Derivatives

Decreased Effect There are no known significant interactions involving a decrease in effect.

Ethanol/Nutrition/Herb Interactions Ethanol: Limit alcohol consumption during treatment with mipomersen to ≤1 drink/day due to potential for increased levels of hepatic fat and induced or exacerbated liver injury.

Storage/Stability Store refrigerated solution at 2°C to 8°C (36°F to 46°F) or when refrigeration is not available, may store at ≤30°C (86°F) (away from heat sources) for up to 14 days. Protect from light. Keep in original container until time of use. For single use only; discard any unused drug after removal of dose.

Mechanism of Action Mipomersen is an oligonucleotide inhibitor of apo B-100 synthesis. ApoB is the main component of LDL-C and very low density lipoprotein (VLDL), which is the precursor to LDL-C. Mipomersen binds to the messenger ribonucleic acid (mRNA) of apoB in a sequence-specific manner which results in degradation (RNase H-mediated) or disruption of the mRNA thereby reducing formation of apoB.

Pharmacodynamics/Kinetics

Protein binding: ≥90%

Metabolism: Metabolized in tissues by endonucleases to form shorter oligonucleotides available for further metabolism by exonucleases

Bioavailability: 54% to 78% (dose-dependent)

Half-life elimination: 1-2 months

Time to peak: 3-4 hours

Excretion: Mipomersen, metabolic byproducts (ie, shorter oligonucleotides): Within 24 hours after administration: Urine <4%

Dosage Homozygous familial hypercholesterolemia (HoFH): Adults: SubQ: 200 mg once weekly. **Note:** Maximal LDL-C reduction seen after ~6 months.

Dosage adjustment for toxicity:

ALT or AST ≥3 x and <5 x ULN: First, repeat measurement within 1 week to confirm elevation. Once confirmed, withhold mipomersen and obtain additional liver function tests (eg, total bilirubin, alkaline phosphatase, and INR); investigate for probable cause. If resumed when AST or ALT <3 x ULN, monitor liver function tests more frequently.

ALT or AST ≥5 x ULN: Withhold mipomersen and obtain additional liver function tests (eg, total bilirubin, alkaline phosphatase, and INR); investigate for probable cause. If resumed when AST or ALT <3 x ULN, monitor liver function tests more frequently.

Clinical symptoms of liver injury (eg, nausea, vomiting, abdominal pain, fever, jaundice, lethargy, flu-like symptoms), bilirubin increase ≥2 x ULN, or active liver disease: Discontinue mipomersen; investigate for probable cause.

Dosage adjustment in renal impairment: No dosage adjustment provided in manufacturer's labeling (has not been studied); use is not recommended in patients with severe renal impairment, clinically significant proteinuria, or receiving hemodialysis.

Dosage adjustment in hepatic impairment: No dosage adjustment provided in manufacturer's labeling (has not been studied); use is contraindicated in patients with moderate or severe hepatic impairment (Child-Pugh class B or C), active liver disease, or unexplained persistent elevations of hepatic transaminases.

Dietary Considerations

Limit alcohol consumption during treatment with mipomersen to ≤1 drink/day due to potential for increased levels of hepatic fat and induced or exacerbated liver injury.

Administration For subQ administration only. Do not administer I.M. or I.V. Remove from refrigerator, allow to reach room temperature (≥30 minutes prior to administration), and visually inspect prior to administration; do not administer if solution is cloudy or contains visible particulate matter (return to pharmacy). Administer first injection under the guidance/supervision of a qualified health care professional. Administer SubQ into the abdomen, thigh region, or outer area of upper arm; do not administer where there is active skin disease (eg, sunburns, skin rash, inflammation/infection) or into tattooed skin or scar. Administer on the same day every week. If dose is missed, administer at least 3 days before the next weekly dose.

Monitoring Parameters At baseline measure ALT, AST, total bilirubin, alkaline phosphatase, then monthly for the first year of treatment, followed by every 3 months (or more frequently if clinically indicated) after the first year; lipid levels (total cholesterol [C], LDL-C, HDL-C, triglycerides) at least every 3 months for the first year

Dosage Forms Excipient information presented when available (limited, particularly for generics); consult specific product labeling.

Solution, Subcutaneous, as sodium [preservative free]:

Kynamro: 200 mg/mL (1 mL)

◆ **Mipomersen Sodium** *see* Mipomersen *on page 1376*

Mirabegron (mir a BEG ron)

Brand Names: U.S. Myrbetriq

Brand Names: Canada Myrbetriq

Index Terms YM-178

Pharmacologic Category $Beta_3$ Agonist

Use Treatment of overactive bladder (OAB) with symptoms of urinary frequency, urgency, or urge incontinence

Pregnancy Risk Factor C

Pregnancy Considerations Adverse effects were observed in some animal reproduction studies. The Canadian labeling contraindicates use in pregnancy.

Breast-Feeding Considerations Excretion of mirabegron into breast milk is expected. According to the manufacturer, the decision to continue or discontinue breast-feeding during therapy should take into account the risk of exposure to the infant and the benefits of treatment to the mother.

Contraindications There are no contraindications listed in the manufacturer's U.S. product labeling.

Canadian labeling: Hypersensitivity to mirabegron or any component of the formulation; severe uncontrolled hypertension (systolic blood pressure ≥180 mm Hg and/or diastolic blood pressure ≥110 mm Hg); pregnancy

Warnings/Precautions Dose-related increases in blood pressure were observed in clinical trials (mean increase of ~0.5-1 mm Hg compared to placebo in overactive bladder patients treated with 50 mg); monitor blood pressure periodically during therapy. Not recommended for use in patients with severe uncontrolled hypertension (SBP ≥180 and/or DBP ≥110 mm Hg); if used in patients with controlled and less severe hypertension, use with caution and monitor blood pressure closely; exacerbation of pre-existing hypertension has been reported. Use with caution in patients with bladder outlet obstruction (BOO) or in patients taking concomitant antimuscarinic medications; the risk of urinary retention may be increased.

Mirabegron is a moderate CYP2D6 inhibitor; potentially significant drug-drug interactions may exist, requiring dose or frequency adjustment, additional monitoring, and/or selection of alternative therapy. Use with caution in patients with mild-to-moderate hepatic impairment; dosage adjustment is required in patients with moderate hepatic impairment. Use is not recommended in severe hepatic impairment. Use with caution in patients with renal impairment; dosage adjustment is required in patients with severe renal impairment. Use is not recommended in ESRD. Systemic exposure is increased in females compared to males; however, dosage adjustments are not necessary or recommended.

Adverse Reactions

>10%: Cardiovascular: Hypertension (9% to 11%)

1% to 10%:

- Cardiovascular: Tachycardia (2%)
- Central nervous system: Headache (4%), dizziness (3%)
- Gastrointestinal: Constipation (2% to 3%), xerostomia (3%), diarrhea (2%)
- Genitourinary: Urinary tract infection (3% to 6%), cystitis (2%)
- Neuromuscular & skeletal: Back pain (3%), arthralgia (2%)
- Respiratory: Nasopharyngitis (4%), sinusitis (3%)
- Miscellaneous: Flu-like syndrome (3%)

<1% (Limited to important or life-threatening): ALT/AST increased, atrial fibrillation, breast cancer, cerebrovascular accident, GGT increased, glaucoma, LDH increased, leukocytoclastic vasculitis, lung cancer, nephrolithiasis, osteoarthritis, palpitations, prostate cancer, Stevens-Johnson syndrome, urinary retention, vaginal infection, vulvovaginal pruritus

Drug Interactions

Metabolism/Transport Effects Substrate of CYP2D6 (minor), CYP3A4 (minor), P-glycoprotein; **Note:** Assignment of Major/Minor substrate status based on clinically relevant drug interaction potential; **Inhibits** CYP2D6 (moderate), CYP3A4 (weak)

Avoid Concomitant Use

Avoid concomitant use of Mirabegron with any of the following: Pimozide; Thioridazine

Increased Effect/Toxicity

Mirabegron may increase the levels/effects of: ARIPiprazole; CYP2D6 Substrates; Desipramine; Digoxin; Dofetilide; Fesoterodine; Flecainide; Lomitapide; Metoprolol; Nebivolol; Pimozide; Propafenone; Solifenacin; Thioridazine

The levels/effects of Mirabegron may be increased by: Anticholinergic Agents; Ketoconazole (Systemic)

Decreased Effect

Mirabegron may decrease the levels/effects of: Codeine; Metoprolol; Tamoxifen; TraMADol

The levels/effects of Mirabegron may be decreased by: Peginterferon Alfa-2b; Rifampin

Ethanol/Nutrition/Herb Interactions Food: Coadministration with a high-fat meal decreased C_{max} and AUC by 45% and 17%, respectively. Coadministration with a low-fat meal decreased C_{max} and AUC by 75% and 51%, respectively. However, safety and efficacy were unaffected by food intake, and mirabegron may be administered without regard to food.

Storage/Stability Store at 25°C (77°F); excursions permitted to 15°C to 30°C (59°F to 86°F).

Mechanism of Action Mirabegron, a beta-3 adrenergic receptor agonist, activates beta-3 adrenergic receptors in the bladder resulting in relaxation of the detrusor smooth muscle during the urine storage phase, thus increasing bladder capacity. At usual doses, mirabegron is believed to display selectivity for the beta-3 adrenergic receptor subtype compared to its affinity for the beta-1 and -2 adrenoceptor subtypes. Data have shown that beta-adrenoceptors, predominately the beta-3 subtype, mediate detrusor smooth muscle tone and promote the storage function of the human bladder.

Pharmacodynamics/Kinetics

Onset of action: Efficacy is seen within 8 weeks; steady state achieved within 7 days

Distribution: V_{ss}: ~1670 L (following I.V. administration)

Protein binding: ~71%; binds mainly to albumin and $alpha_1$-acid glycoprotein

Metabolism: Extensive metabolism via multiple pathways (eg, dealkylation, oxidation, glucuronidation, amide hydrolysis) via multiple enzymes (eg, UGT, esterase, CYP3A4, CYP2D6); two major pharmacologically inactive metabolites produced

Bioavailability: 29% to 35% (following 25 mg and 50 mg oral dosing, respectively); bioavailability is dose-dependent; C_{max} and AUC are higher in females compared to males

Half-life elimination: ~50 hours

Time to peak: ~3.5 hours

Excretion: Urine (radiolabeled drug: 55%; unchanged drug: ~25%); feces (radiolabeled drug: 34%; unchanged drug: 0%)

Dosage Overactive bladder (OAB): Adults: Oral: Initial: 25 mg once daily; efficacy is observed within 8 weeks for 25 mg dose. May increase to 50 mg once daily based on individual patient efficacy and tolerability.

Dosing with concomitant therapy: CYP2D6 substrates: Appropriate monitoring and possible dose adjustment of the CYP2D6 substrate (especially those with a narrow therapeutic index) may be necessary. The Canadian labeling specifically recommends limiting mirabegron to 25 mg once daily in patients receiving concomitant CYP2D6 substrates with a narrow therapeutic index (eg, flecainide, propafenone, thioridazine).

Dosing adjustment in renal impairment:

Mild-to-moderate impairment (Cl_{cr} 30-89 mL/minute or eGFR 30-89 mL/minute/1.73 m^2): No dosage adjustment necessary

Severe impairment (Cl_{cr} 15-29 mL/minute or eGFR 15-29 mL/minute/1.73 m^2): Do not exceed 25 mg once daily

ESRD (Cl_{cr} <15 mL/minute or eGFR <15 mL/minute/1.73 m^2) or patients requiring hemodialysis: Not recommended (has not been studied)

Dosing adjustment in hepatic impairment:

Mild impairment (Child-Pugh Class A): No dosage adjustment necessary

Moderate impairment (Child-Pugh Class B): Do not exceed 25 mg once daily

Severe impairment (Child-Pugh Class C): Not recommended (has not been studied)

Administration Administer orally without regard to food. Swallow the tablet whole with water; do not chew, divide, or crush.

Monitoring Parameters Monitor blood pressure at baseline and then periodically during therapy

Dosage Forms Excipient information presented when available (limited, particularly for generics); consult specific product labeling.

Tablet Extended Release 24 Hour, Oral:

Myrbetriq: 25 mg, 50 mg

◆ **MiraLax [OTC]** *see* Polyethylene Glycol 3350 *on page 1668*

◆ **Miranel AF [OTC]** *see* Miconazole (Topical) *on page 1358*

◆ **Mirapex** *see* Pramipexole *on page 1695*

◆ **Mirapex® (Can)** *see* Pramipexole *on page 1695*

◆ **Mirapex ER** *see* Pramipexole *on page 1695*

◆ **Mircette** *see* Ethinyl Estradiol and Desogestrel *on page 784*

◆ **Mirena** *see* Levonorgestrel *on page 1202*

Mirtazapine (mir TAZ a peen)

Brand Names: U.S. Remeron; Remeron SolTab

Brand Names: Canada Apo-Mirtazapine®; Auro-Mirtazapine; Ava-Mirtazapine; CO Mirtazapine; Dom-Mirtazapine; GD-Mirtazapine; Jamp-Mirtazapine; Mylan-Mirtazapine; Novo-Mirtazapine; PMS-Mirtazapine; PRO-Mirtazapine; ratio-Mirtazapine; Remeron®; Remeron® RD; Riva-Mirtazapine; Sandoz-Mirtazapine; Sandoz-Mirtazapine FC; ZYM-Mirtazapine

Pharmacologic Category Antidepressant, Alpha-2 Antagonist

Additional Appendix Information

Antidepressant Agents *on page 2284*

Beers Criteria – Potentially Inappropriate Medications for Geriatrics *on page 2368*

Use Treatment of depression

Unlabeled Use Alzheimer's dementia-related depression; post-traumatic stress disorder (PTSD)

Pregnancy Risk Factor C

Pregnancy Considerations Adverse events were observed in some animal reproduction studies. A significant increase in major teratogenic effects has not been observed in humans following exposure to mirtazapine during pregnancy; however, some nonteratogenic adverse events (similar to those observed with SSRI agents) have been reported (Djulus, 2006; Einarson, 2009; Lennestål, 2007). Mirtazapine was found to cross the placenta following a maternal overdose (Hatzidaki, 2008).

The ACOG recommends that therapy with antidepressants during pregnancy be individualized; treatment of depression during pregnancy should incorporate the clinical expertise of the mental health clinician, obstetrician, primary healthcare provider, and pediatrician. According to the American Psychiatric Association (APA), the risks of medication treatment should be weighed against other treatment options and untreated depression. Consideration should be given to using agents with safety data in pregnancy. For women who discontinue antidepressant medications during pregnancy and who may be at high risk for postpartum depression, the medications can be restarted following delivery. Treatment algorithms have been developed by the ACOG and the APA for the management of depression in women prior to conception and during pregnancy (ACOG, 2008; APA, 2010; Yonkers, 2009).

Breast-Feeding Considerations Mirtazapine and its active metabolite are found in breast milk, with higher levels in the hindmilk than foremilk. Mirtazapine can also be detected in the serum of nursing infants; adverse events have generally not been observed, although possible sedation and weight gain was noted in one case report (Kristensen, 2007; Tonn, 2009). The manufacturer recommends that caution be used if administered to a breast-feeding woman.

Medication Guide Available Yes

Contraindications Hypersensitivity to mirtazapine or any component of the formulation; use of MAO inhibitors intended to treat psychiatric disorders (concurrently or within 14 days of discontinuing either mirtazapine or the MAO inhibitor); initiation of mirtazapine in a patient receiving linezolid or intravenous methylene blue

Warnings/Precautions [U.S. Boxed Warning]: Antidepressants increase the risk of suicidal thinking and behavior in children, adolescents, and young adults (18-24 years of age) with major depressive disorder (MDD) and other psychiatric disorders; consider risk prior to prescribing. Short-term studies did not show an increased risk in patients >24 years of age and showed a decreased risk in patients ≥65 years. Closely monitor for clinical worsening, suicidality, or unusual changes in behavior; the patient's family or caregiver should be instructed to closely observe the patient and communicate condition with healthcare provider. A medication guide should be dispensed with each prescription. **Mirtazapine is not FDA approved for use in children.**

The possibility of a suicide attempt is inherent in major depression and may persist until remission occurs. Monitor for worsening of depression or suicidality, especially during initiation of therapy (generally first 1-2 months) or with dose increases or decreases. Use caution in high-risk patients. Worsening depression and severe abrupt suicidality that are not part of the presenting symptoms may require discontinuation or modification of drug therapy. The patient's family or caregiver should be alerted to monitor patients for the emergence of suicidality and associated behaviors (such as agitation, irritability, hostility, impulsivity, and hypomania) and call healthcare provider.

May worsen psychosis in some patients or precipitate a shift to mania or hypomania in patients with bipolar disorder. Patients presenting with depressive symptoms should be screened for bipolar disorder. Monotherapy in patients with bipolar disorder should be avoided. **Mirtazapine is not FDA approved for the treatment of bipolar depression.**

Potentially life-threatening serotonin syndrome (SS) has occurred with serotonergic agents (eg, SSRIs, SNRIs), particularly when used in combination with other serotonergic agents (eg, triptans, TCAs, fentanyl, lithium, tramadol, buspirone, St John's wort, tryptophan) or agents that impair metabolism of serotonin (eg, MAO inhibitors intended to treat psychiatric disorders, other MAO inhibitors such as linezolid and intravenous methylene blue). Discontinue treatment (and any concomitant serotonergic agent) immediately if signs/symptoms arise. Discontinue immediately if signs and symptoms of neutropenia/agranulocytosis occur. May cause sedation, resulting in impaired performance of tasks requiring alertness (eg, operating machinery or driving). The degree of sedation is moderate-high relative to other antidepressants. Conversely, may increase psychomotor restlessness within first few weeks of therapy. The risks of orthostatic hypotension or anticholinergic effects are low relative to other antidepressants. The incidence of sexual dysfunction with mirtazapine is generally lower than with selective serotonin reuptake inhibitors (SSRIs). May increase appetite and stimulate weight gain. In clinical trials, an increased incidence of weight gain in adults and children was observed with mirtazapine compared to placebo; up to 8% of patients discontinued therapy due to weight gain. May increase serum cholesterol and triglyceride levels. Potentially significant interactions may exist, requiring dose or frequency adjustment, additional monitoring, and/or selection of alternative therapy.

Use caution in patients with a previous seizure disorder or condition predisposing to seizures such as brain damage, alcoholism, or concurrent therapy with other drugs which lower the seizure threshold. Bone fractures have been associated with antidepressant treatment. Consider the possibility of a fragility fracture if an antidepressant-treated patient presents with unexplained bone pain, point tenderness, swelling, or bruising (Rabenda, 2013; Rizzoli, 2012). Use with caution in patients with hepatic or renal dysfunction. Use caution in elderly patients; may cause or exacerbate syndrome of inappropriate antidiuretic hormone secretion or hyponatremia; monitor sodium closely with initiation or dosage adjustments in older adults (Beers Criteria). Clinically significant transaminase elevations have been observed. SolTab® formulation contains phenylalanine.

Abrupt discontinuation or interruption of antidepressant therapy has been associated with a discontinuation syndrome. Symptoms arising may vary with antidepressant however commonly include nausea, vomiting, diarrhea, headaches, lightheadedness, dizziness, diminished appetite, sweating, chills, tremors, paresthesias, fatigue, somnolence, and sleep disturbances (eg, vivid dreams, insomnia). Greater risks for developing a discontinuation syndrome have been associated with antidepressants with shorter half-lives, longer durations of treatment, and abrupt discontinuation. For antidepressants of short or intermediate half-lives, symptoms may emerge within 2-5 days after treatment discontinuation and last 7-14 days (APA, 2010; Fava, 2006; Haddad, 2001; Shelton, 2001; Warner, 2006).

Adverse Reactions

>10%:

Central nervous system: Somnolence (54%)

Endocrine & metabolic: Cholesterol increased

Gastrointestinal: Xerostomia (25%), appetite increased (17%), constipation (13%), weight gain (12%; weight gain of >7% reported in 8% of adults, ≤49% of pediatric patients)

1% to 10%:

Cardiovascular: Peripheral edema (2%), edema (1%), hypertension, vasodilatation

Central nervous system: Dizziness (7%), abnormal dreams (4%), abnormal thoughts (3%), confusion (2%), agitation, amnesia, anxiety, apathy, depression, hyper/hypokinesia, hypoesthesia, malaise, vertigo

Dermatologic: Pruritus, rash

Endocrine & metabolic: Triglycerides increased

Gastrointestinal: Abdominal pain, anorexia, vomiting

Genitourinary: Urinary frequency (2%), urinary tract infection

Hepatic: SGPT increased (≥3 times ULN: 2%)

Neuromuscular & skeletal: Weakness (8%), back pain (2%), myalgia (2%), tremor (2%), arthralgia, myasthenia, paresthesia, twitching

Respiratory: Dyspnea (1%), cough increased, sinusitis

Miscellaneous: Flu-like syndrome (5%), thirst

<1% (Limited to important or life-threatening): Abdomen enlarged, abnormal ejaculation, accommodation abnormality, acid phosphatase increased, acne, akathisia, alopecia, ALT increased, amenorrhea, anemia, angina pectoris, aphasia, aphthous stomatitis, arthrosis, arthritis, asphyxia, AST increased, asthma, ataxia, atrial arrhythmia, bigeminy, blepharitis, bone pain, bradycardia, breast engorgement, breast enlargement, breast pain, bronchitis, bursitis, cardiomegaly, cellulitis, cerebral ischemia, chest pain, chills, cholecystitis, cirrhosis, colitis, conjunctivitis, coordination abnormal, cystitis, deafness, dehydration, delirium, delusions, dementia, depersonalization, diabetes mellitus, diplopia, drug dependence, dry skin, dysarthria, dyskinesia, dysmenorrhea, dystonia, dysuria, ear pain, emotional lability, epistaxis, eructation, euphoria, exfoliative dermatitis, extrapyramidal syndrome, eye pain, facial edema, fever, fracture, gastritis, gastroenteritis, glaucoma, glossitis, goiter, gout, grand mal seizure, gum hemorrhage, hallucinations, healing abnormalities, hematuria, herpes simplex, herpes zoster, hiccup, hostility, hyperacusis, hyponatremia, hypotension, hypothyroidism, hypotonia, impotence, intestinal obstruction, keratoconjunctivitis, kidney calculus, lacrimation disorder, laryngitis, left heart failure, leukopenia, leukorrhea, libido increased, liver function tests abnormal, lymphadenopathy, lymphocytosis, manic reaction, menorrhagia, metrorrhagia, migraine, MI, myoclonus, myositis, nausea, neck pain, neck rigidity, neurosis, nystagmus, oral moniliasis, osteoporosis, otitis media, pancreatitis, pancytopenia, paralysis, paranoid reaction, parosmia, petechia, phlebitis, photosensitivity reaction, pneumonia, pneumothorax, polyuria, psychotic depression, pulmonary embolus, reflexes increased, salivary gland enlargement, salivation increased, seborrhea, serotonin syndrome, skin hypertrophy, skin reactions (severe [including Stevens-Johnson syndrome, bullous dermatitis, erythema multiforme, toxic epidermal necrolysis]), skin ulcer, stomatitis, stupor, syncope, taste loss, tendon rupture, tenosynovitis, thrombocytopenia, tongue discoloration, tongue edema, torsade de pointes (rare), ulcer, ulcerative stomatitis, urethritis, urinary incontinence, urinary retention, urinary urgency, urticaria, vaginitis, vascular headache, ventricular extrasystoles, weight loss, withdrawal syndrome

Drug Interactions

Metabolism/Transport Effects **Substrate** of CYP1A2 (major), CYP2C9 (minor), CYP2D6 (major), CYP3A4 (major); **Note:** Assignment of Major/Minor substrate status based on clinically relevant drug interaction potential; **Inhibits** CYP1A2 (weak), CYP3A4 (weak)

Avoid Concomitant Use

Avoid concomitant use of Mirtazapine with any of the following: Alcohol (Ethyl); Azelastine (Nasal); Conivaptan; Fusidic Acid (Systemic); Linezolid; MAO Inhibitors; Methylene Blue; Paraldehyde; Tryptophan

Increased Effect/Toxicity

Mirtazapine may increase the levels/effects of: Antipsychotics; Azelastine (Nasal); Buprenorphine; Dofetilide; Highest Risk QTc-Prolonging Agents; Hydrocodone; Lomitapide; Methylene Blue; Metoclopramide; Metyrosine; Moderate Risk QTc-Prolonging Agents; Paraldehyde; Pramipexole; ROPINIRole; Rotigotine; Serotonin Modulators; Warfarin; Zolpidem

The levels/effects of Mirtazapine may be increased by: Abiraterone Acetate; Alcohol (Ethyl); Antipsychotics; Brimonidine (Topical); CNS Depressants; Conivaptan; CYP1A2 Inhibitors (Moderate); CYP1A2 Inhibitors (Strong); CYP2D6 Inhibitors (Moderate); CYP2D6 Inhibitors (Strong); CYP3A4 Inhibitors (Moderate); CYP3A4 Inhibitors (Strong); Darunavir; Dasatinib; Deferasirox; Doxylamine; Fusidic Acid (Systemic); HydrOXYzine; Ivacaftor; Linezolid; Luliconazole; Magnesium Sulfate; MAO Inhibitors; Mifepristone; Perampanel; Simeprevir; Sodium Oxybate; Tryptophan; Vemurafenib

Decreased Effect

Mirtazapine may decrease the levels/effects of: Alpha2-Agonists

The levels/effects of Mirtazapine may be decreased by: Bosentan; CYP1A2 Inducers (Strong); CYP3A4 Inducers (Strong); Cyproterone; Dabrafenib; Deferasirox; Mitotane; Peginterferon Alfa-2b; Tocilizumab

Ethanol/Nutrition/Herb Interactions

Ethanol: May increase CNS depression; monitor for increased effects with coadministration. Caution patients about effects.

Herb/Nutraceutical: Avoid St John's wort (may decrease mirtazapine levels). Avoid valerian, St John's wort, tryptophan, SAMe, kava kava (may increase CNS depression and/or increase the risk of serotonin syndrome).

Storage/Stability

Orally disintegrating tablet: Store at controlled room temperature of 25°C (77°F); excursions permitted to 15°C to 30°C (59°F to 86°F). Protect from light and moisture. Use immediately upon opening tablet blister.

Tablet: Store at controlled room temperature of 25°C (77°F); excursions permitted to 15°C to 30°C (59°F to 86°F). Protect from light and moisture.

Mechanism of Action Mirtazapine is a tetracyclic antidepressant that works by its central presynaptic $alpha_2$-adrenergic antagonist effects, which results in increased release of norepinephrine and serotonin. It is also a potent antagonist of 5-HT_2 and 5-HT_3 serotonin receptors and H1 histamine receptors and a moderate peripheral $alpha_1$-adrenergic and muscarinic antagonist; it does not inhibit the reuptake of norepinephrine or serotonin.

Pharmacodynamics/Kinetics

Absorption: Rapid and complete

Distribution: 4.5 L/kg

Protein binding: ~85%

Metabolism: Extensively hepatic via CYP1A2, 2C9, 2D6, 3A4 and via demethylation (forms demethylmirtazapine, an active metabolite) and hydroxylation (forms inactive metabolites)

Bioavailability: ~50%

Half-life elimination: 20-40 hours; increased with renal or hepatic impairment

Time to peak, serum: ~2 hours

Excretion: Urine (75%) and feces (15%) as metabolites

Dosage Oral:

Adults:

Depression: Initial: 15 mg nightly, may titrate dose up no more frequently than every 1-2 weeks to a maximum of 45 mg daily; dosage range: 15-45 mg daily; there is an inverse relationship between dose and sedation

Post-traumatic stress disorder (PTSD) (unlabeled use): 30-60 mg daily (Bandelow, 2008; Benedek, 2009)

Elderly: Use with caution. Compared to younger adults, clearance is decreased 40% in elderly males and 10% in elderly females; manufacturer's labeling does not include specific dosage adjustment

Alzheimer's dementia-related depression (unlabeled use): Initial: 7.5 mg at bedtime; may increase at 7.5-15 mg increments to 45-60 mg daily (Rabins, 2007)

Discontinuation of therapy: Upon discontinuation of antidepressant therapy, gradually taper the dose to minimize the incidence of withdrawal symptoms and allow for the detection of re-emerging symptoms. Evidence supporting ideal taper rates is limited. APA and NICE guidelines suggest tapering therapy over at least several weeks with consideration to the half-life of the antidepressant; antidepressants with a shorter half-life may need to be tapered more conservatively. In addition for long-term treated patients, WFSBP guidelines recommend tapering over 4-6 months. If intolerable withdrawal symptoms occur following a dose reduction, consider resuming the previously prescribed dose and/or decrease dose at a more gradual rate (APA, 2010; Bauer, 2002; Haddad, 2001; NCCMH, 2010; Schatzberg, 2006; Shelton, 2001; Warner, 2006).

MAO inhibitor recommendations:

Switching to or from an MAO inhibitor intended to treat psychiatric disorders:

Allow 14 days to elapse between discontinuing an MAO inhibitor intended to treat psychiatric disorders and initiation of mirtazapine.

Allow 14 days to elapse between discontinuing mirtazapine and initiation of an MAO inhibitor intended to treat psychiatric disorders.

Use with other MAO inhibitors (linezolid or I.V. methylene blue):

Do not initiate mirtazapine in patients receiving linezolid or I.V. methylene blue; consider other interventions for psychiatric condition.

If urgent treatment with linezolid or I.V. methylene blue is required in a patient already receiving mirtazapine and potential benefits outweigh potential risks, discontinue mirtazapine promptly and administer linezolid or I.V. methylene blue. Monitor for serotonin syndrome for 2 weeks or until 24 hours after the last dose of linezolid or I.V. methylene blue, whichever comes first. May resume mirtazapine 24 hours after the last dose of linezolid or I.V. methylene blue.

Dosage adjustment in renal impairment: No dosage adjustment provided in manufacturer's labeling; clearance is decreased 30% in moderate (Cl_{cr} 11-39 mL/minute/1.73 m^2) impairment and is decreased 50% in severe (Cl_{cr} <10 mL/minute/1.73 m^2) impairment. Use with caution.

Dosage adjustment in hepatic impairment: No dosage adjustment provided in manufacturer's labeling; a decrease in clearance by 30% has been observed in hepatic impairment. Use with caution.

Dietary Considerations Some products may contain phenylalanine.

Administration

Orally disintegrating tablet: Administer without regard to meals. Open blister pack and place tablet on the tongue; tablet is formulated to dissolve on the tongue without water; do not split tablet.

Tablet: Administer without regard to meals. Canadian labeling does not recommend chewing tablet.

Monitoring Parameters Patients should be monitored for signs of agranulocytosis or severe neutropenia such as sore throat, stomatitis or other signs of infection or a low WBC; renal and hepatic function; mental status for depression, suicide ideation (especially at the beginning of therapy or when doses are increased or decreased), anxiety, social functioning, mania, panic attacks; signs/symptoms of serotonin syndrome; lipid profile; weight gain

Dosage Forms Excipient information presented when available (limited, particularly for generics); consult specific product labeling.

Tablet, Oral:

Remeron: 15 mg, 30 mg [scored]

Remeron: 45 mg

Generic: 7.5 mg, 15 mg, 30 mg, 45 mg

Tablet Dispersible, Oral:

Remeron SolTab: 15 mg, 30 mg, 45 mg [contains aspartame]

Generic: 15 mg, 30 mg, 45 mg

◆ **Mirvaso** *see* Brimonidine (Topical) *on page 280*

Misoprostol (mye soe PROST ole)

Brand Names: U.S. Cytotec

Brand Names: Canada Novo-Misoprostol; PMS-Misoprostol

Pharmacologic Category Prostaglandin

Use

Prevention of NSAID-induced gastric ulcers

Medical termination of pregnancy of ≤49 days in conjunction with mifepristone (refer to Mifepristone monograph for details)

Unlabeled Use Cervical ripening and labor induction (except in women with prior cesarean delivery or major uterine surgery); prevention of postpartum hemorrhage; treatment of postpartum hemorrhage; treatment of incomplete or missed abortion in women <12 weeks gestation

Pregnancy Risk Factor X

Pregnancy Considerations Teratogenic effects were not observed in animal reproduction studies. Congenital anomalies following first trimester exposure have been reported, including skull defects, cranial nerve palsies, falcial malformations, and limb defects. Misoprostol may produce uterine contractions; fetal death, uterine perforation, and abortion may occur. **[U.S. Boxed Warning]: Use of misoprostol during pregnancy may cause abortion, birth defects, or premature birth. It is not to be used to reduce NSAID-induced ulcers in a woman of childbearing potential unless she is capable of complying with effective contraceptive measures and is at high risk of developing gastric ulcers and/or their complications.** If needed, the patient must have a negative pregnancy test within 2 weeks of starting therapy, she must use effective contraception during treatment, and therapy should begin on the second or third day of next normal menstrual period. Written and verbal warnings concerning the hazards of misoprostol should be provided.

Misoprostol is FDA approved for the medical termination of pregnancy of ≤49 days in conjunction with mifepristone.

Because misoprostol may induce or augment uterine contractions, it has been used off-label as a cervical-ripening agent for induction of labor in women who have not had a prior cesarean delivery or major uterine surgery. Hyperstimulation of the uterus, uterine rupture, or adverse events in the fetus or mother may occur with this use.

Breast-Feeding Considerations Misoprostol acid (the active metabolite of misoprostol) has been detected in breast milk. Concentrations following a single oral dose were 7.6-20.9 pg/mL after 1 hour and decreased to <1 pg/mL by 5 hours. Adverse events have not been reported in nursing infants (FIGO, 2012).

Contraindications Hypersensitivity to prostaglandins; pregnancy (when used to reduce NSAID-induced ulcers)

Warnings/Precautions [U.S. Boxed Warning]: Due to the abortifacient property of this medication, patients must be warned not to give this drug to others. [U.S. Boxed Warning]: Use of misoprostol during pregnancy may cause abortion, birth defects, or premature birth. It is not to be used to reduce NSAID-induced ulcers in a woman of childbearing potential unless she is capable of complying with effective contraceptive measures and is at high risk of developing gastric ulcers and/or their complications. If needed, the patient must have a negative pregnancy test within two weeks of starting therapy, she must use effective contraception during treatment and therapy should begin on the second or third day of next normal menstrual period. Women of childbearing potential taking this for reducing the risk of NSAID-induced gastric ulcers should be given oral and written warnings of the potential adverse events if pregnancy occurs during treatment. Adverse events have been reported when used outside of current product labeling (cervical ripening, induction of labor, postpartum hemorrhage). Uterine tachysystole may occur and progress to uterine tetany; uteroplacental blood flow may be impaired and uterine rupture or amniotic fluid embolism may occur. The risk of uterine rupture may be increased with advanced gestational age, grand multiparity, or prior uterine surgery. Uterine activity and fetal status should be monitored in a hospital setting. Misoprostol should not be used in situations where uterotonic drugs are otherwise contraindicated or inappropriate.

When used for ulcers, use only in patients at high risk of complications from gastric ulcers (eg, the elderly or patients with concomitant diseases) or patients at high risk for developing gastric ulcers (eg, those with a history of ulcers) taking NSAIDs. Misoprostol must be taken during the duration of NSAID therapy. It is not effective in preventing duodenal ulcers in patients taking NSAIDs.

Use with caution in patients with cardiovascular disease, renal impairment, and the elderly.

Adverse Reactions

>10%: Gastrointestinal: Diarrhea, abdominal pain

1% to 10%:

Central nervous system: Headache

Gastrointestinal: Constipation, dyspepsia, flatulence, nausea, vomiting

<1% (Limited to important or life-threatening): Abnormal taste, abnormal vision, alkaline phosphatase increased, alopecia, anaphylaxis, anemia, amylase increase, anxiety, arrhythmia, arterial thrombosis, arthralgia, cardiac enzymes increased, chest pain, chills, confusion, CVA, deafness, depression, diaphoresis, dizziness, drowsiness, dysphagia, dyspnea, dysuria, edema, epistaxis, ESR increased, fatigue, fever, GI bleeding, GI inflammation, gingivitis, glycosuria, gout; gynecological disorders, hematuria, hepatobiliary function abnormal, hyper-/hypotension, impotence, loss of libido, MI, muscle cramps, myalgia, neuropathy, neurosis, nitrogen increased, pallor, phlebitis, polyuria, pulmonary embolism, purpura, rash, reflux, rigors, stiffness, syncope, thirst, thrombocytopenia, tinnitus, uterine rupture, weakness, weight changes

Drug Interactions

Metabolism/Transport Effects None known.

Avoid Concomitant Use

Avoid concomitant use of Misoprostol with any of the following: Carbetocin

Increased Effect/Toxicity

Misoprostol may increase the levels/effects of: Carbetocin; Oxytocin

The levels/effects of Misoprostol may be increased by: Antacids

Decreased Effect There are no known significant interactions involving a decrease in effect.

Ethanol/Nutrition/Herb Interactions Food: Misoprostol peak serum concentrations may be decreased if taken with food (not clinically significant).

Storage/Stability Store at or below 25°C (77°F).

Mechanism of Action Misoprostol is a synthetic prostaglandin E_1 analog that replaces the protective prostaglandins consumed with prostaglandin-inhibiting therapies (eg, NSAIDs); has been shown to induce uterine contractions

Pharmacodynamics/Kinetics

Absorption: Rapid and extensive

Metabolism: Hepatic; rapidly de-esterified to misoprostol acid (active)

Protein binding: Misoprostol acid: <90%

Half-life elimination: Misoprostol acid: 20-40 minutes

Time to peak, serum: Misoprostol acid: Fasting: 6-22 minutes

Excretion: Urine (80%)

Dosage

Oral: Adults:

Prevention of NSAID-induced gastric ulcers: 200 mcg 4 times daily with food; if not tolerated, may decrease dose to 100 mcg 4 times daily with food; last dose of the day should be taken at bedtime

Medical termination of pregnancy: Refer to Mifepristone monograph.

Prevention of postpartum hemorrhage (unlabeled use): 600 mcg as a single dose administered immediately after delivery; to be used in settings where oxytocin is not available (FIGO, 2012).

Treatment of incomplete abortion (unlabeled use): 600 mcg as a single dose (ACOG, 2009a).

Sublingual: Adults:

Treatment of missed abortion (unlabeled use): 600 mcg; may repeat every 3 hours for 2 additional doses if needed (ACOG, 2009a).

Treatment of postpartum hemorrhage (unlabeled use): 800 mcg as a single dose; to be used in settings where oxytocin is not available. Use caution if a prophylactic dose was already given, especially if adverse events were observed (FIGO, 2012).

Intravaginal: Adults:

Labor induction or cervical ripening (unlabeled uses): 25 mcg (1/4 of 100 mcg tablet); may repeat at intervals no more frequent than every 3-6 hours. Do not use in patients with previous cesarean delivery or prior major uterine surgery (ACOG, 2009b).

Treatment of missed abortion (unlabeled use): 800 mcg; may repeat every 3 hours for 2 additional doses if needed (ACOG, 2009a).

Dosage adjustment in renal impairment: Dose adjustment is not routinely needed; however, the dose may be reduced if the recommended dose is not tolerated. It is not known if misoprostol is removed by dialysis.

Dosage adjustment in hepatic impairment: No dosage adjustment provided in manufacturer's labeling.

Dietary Considerations Should be taken with food.

Administration Incidence of diarrhea may be lessened by having patient take dose right after meals and avoiding magnesium-containing antacids. When used for the prevention of NSAID-induced ulcers, therapy is usually begun on the second or third day of the next normal menstrual period in women of childbearing potential.

Monitoring Parameters

Prevention of NSAID-induced gastric ulcers: Pregnancy test in women of reproductive potential prior to therapy; adequate diagnostic measures in all cases of undiagnosed abnormal vaginal bleeding

Off-label pregnancy-related uses: Uterine activity and fetal status. When used for incomplete or missed abortion, reevaluate 1-2 weeks after dosing

Dosage Forms Excipient information presented when available (limited, particularly for generics); consult specific product labeling.

Tablet, Oral:

Cytotec: 100 mcg

Cytotec: 200 mcg [scored]

Generic: 100 mcg, 200 mcg

◆ **Misoprostol and Diclofenac** *see* Diclofenac and Misoprostol *on page 600*

◆ **MITC** *see* MitoMYcin (Systemic) *on page 1383*

◆ **MITO** *see* MitoMYcin (Systemic) *on page 1383*

◆ **MITO-C** *see* MitoMYcin (Systemic) *on page 1383*

◆ **Mitomycin-X** *see* MitoMYcin (Systemic) *on page 1383*

◆ **Mitomycin-C** *see* MitoMYcin (Ophthalmic) *on page 1385*

◆ **Mitomycin-C** *see* MitoMYcin (Systemic) *on page 1383*

MitoMYcin (Systemic) (mye toe MYE sin)

Brand Names: Canada Mitomycin For Injection; Mitomycin For Injection USP; Mutamycin®

Index Terms MITC; MITO; MITO-C; Mitomycin-C; Mitomycin-X; MMC; MTC; Mutamycin

Pharmacologic Category Antineoplastic Agent, Antibiotic

Use Treatment of adenocarcinoma of stomach or pancreas

Unlabeled Use Treatment of anal carcinoma (nonmetastatic), bladder cancer, cervical cancer (recurrent or metastatic), esophageal cancer, gastric cancer, non small cell lung cancer (NSCLC)

Pregnancy Considerations Teratogenic effects have been observed in animal reproduction studies.

Breast-Feeding Considerations It is not known if mitomycin is excreted in human milk; the manufacturer recommends against breast-feeding during treatment.

Contraindications Hypersensitivity to mitomycin or any component of the formulation; thrombocytopenia; coagulation disorders, or other increased bleeding tendency

Warnings/Precautions Hazardous agent - use appropriate precautions for handling and disposal (NIOSH, 2012). **[U.S. Boxed Warning]: Bone marrow suppression (thrombocytopenia and leukopenia) is common and may be severe and/or contribute to infections.** Fatalities due to sepsis have been reported; monitor for infections. Myelosuppression is dose-limiting, delayed in onset, and cumulative; therefore, monitor blood counts closely during and for ≥8 weeks following treatment; treatment delay or dosage adjustment may be required for significant thrombocytopenia (platelets <100,000/mm^3) or leukopenia (WBC<4000/mm^3) or a progressive decline in either value. Use with caution in patients who have received radiation therapy or in the presence of hepatobiliary dysfunction; reduce dosage in patients who are receiving radiation therapy simultaneously. Monitor for renal toxicity; do not administer if serum creatinine is >1.7 mg/dL. **[U.S. Boxed Warning]: Hemolytic-uremic syndrome (HUS) has been reported (incidence not defined); condition usually involves microangiopathic hemolytic anemia (hematocrit ≤5%), thrombocytopenia (≤100,000/mm^3), and irreversible renal failure (serum creatinine ≥1.6 mg/dL). HUS may occur at any time, is generally associated with single doses ≥60 mg, and HUS symptoms may be exacerbated by blood transfusion.** Other less common effects may include pulmonary edema, neurologic abnormalities, and hypertension. High mortality from HUS development has been reported, and is largely the result of renal failure. HUS may also be associated with cumulative doses ≥50 mg/m^2. Bladder fibrosis/contraction has been reported with intravesical administration (unapproved administration route). Mitomycin is a potent vesicant; ensure proper needle or catheter placement prior to and during infusion. Avoid extravasation. May cause necrosis and tissue sloughing; delayed erythema and/or ulceration have been reported.

Cases of acute respiratory distress syndrome (ARDS) have been reported in patients receiving mitomycin in combination with other chemotherapy who were maintained at FIO_2 concentrations >50% perioperatively; use caution to provide only enough oxygen to maintain adequate arterial saturation and avoid overhydration. Pulmonary toxicity has also been reported as dyspnea with nonproductive cough and appearance of pulmonary infiltrates on radiograph; discontinue therapy if pulmonary toxicity occurs and other potential etiologies have been ruled out. Shortness of breath and bronchospasm have been reported in patients receiving vinca alkaloids in combination with mitomycin or who received mitomycin previously; this acute respiratory distress has occurred within minutes to hours following the vinca alkaloid; may be managed with bronchodilators, steroids and/or oxygen. **[U.S. Boxed Warning]: Should be administered under the supervision of an experienced cancer chemotherapy physician.**

Adverse Reactions

>10%:

Central nervous system: Fever (14%)

Gastrointestinal: Nausea, vomiting and anorexia (14%)

Hematologic: Myelosuppression (64%; onset: 4 weeks; recovery: 8-10 weeks)

Miscellaneous: Thrombotic thrombocytopenic purpura (TTP)/hemolytic uremic syndrome (HUS) (≤15%)

1% to 10%:

Dermatologic: Alopecia, mucous membrane toxicity (4%)

Gastrointestinal: Stomatitis (4%)

Renal: Serum creatinine increased (2%)

<1% (Limited to important or life-threatening): Adult respiratory distress syndrome (ARDS), bladder fibrosis/contraction (intravesical administration), dyspnea, extravasation reactions, heart failure, hepatic sinusoidal obstruction syndrome (SOS, veno-occlusive liver disease), interstitial fibrosis, nonproductive cough, pulmonary infiltrates, rash, renal failure (irreversible)

Drug Interactions

Metabolism/Transport Effects Substrate of P-glycoprotein

Avoid Concomitant Use

Avoid concomitant use of MitoMYcin (Systemic) with any of the following: BCG; CloZAPine; Natalizumab; Pimecrolimus; Tacrolimus (Topical); Tofacitinib; Vaccines (Live)

Increased Effect/Toxicity

MitoMYcin (Systemic) may increase the levels/effects of: CloZAPine; Leflunomide; Natalizumab; Tofacitinib; Vaccines (Live)

The levels/effects of MitoMYcin (Systemic) may be increased by: Antineoplastic Agents (Vinca Alkaloids); Denosumab; P-glycoprotein/ABCB1 Inhibitors; Pimecrolimus; Roflumilast; Tacrolimus (Topical); Trastuzumab

Decreased Effect

MitoMYcin (Systemic) may decrease the levels/effects of: BCG; Coccidioidin Skin Test; Sipuleucel-T; Vaccines (Inactivated); Vaccines (Live)

The levels/effects of MitoMYcin (Systemic) may be decreased by: Echinacea; P-glycoprotein/ABCB1 Inducers

Ethanol/Nutrition/Herb Interactions Herb/Nutraceutical: Avoid black cohosh, dong quai in estrogen-dependent tumors.

Preparation for Administration Hazardous agent; use appropriate precautions for handling and disposal (NIOSH, 2012). Dilute powder with SWFI to a concentration of 0.5 mg/mL. May further dilute in NS or sodium lactate to 20-40 mcg/mL.

Storage/Stability Store intact vials at controlled room temperature; avoid exposure to temperatures >40°C (104°F). Reconstituted solution is stable for 7 days at room temperature and 14 days when refrigerated. Protect reconstituted solution from light. Solution of 0.5 mg/mL in a syringe is stable for 7 days at room temperature and 28 days when refrigerated and protected from light.

Further dilution to 20-40 mcg/mL:

In normal saline: Stable for 12 hours at room temperature.

In sodium lactate: Stable for 24 hours at room temperature.

Mechanism of Action Acts like an alkylating agent and produces DNA cross-linking (primarily with guanine and cytosine pairs); cell-cycle nonspecific; inhibits DNA and RNA synthesis; degrades preformed DNA, causes nuclear lysis and formation of giant cells. While not phase-specific *per se*, mitomycin has its maximum effect against cells in late G and early S phases.

Pharmacodynamics/Kinetics

Metabolism: Hepatic

Half-life elimination: 17-78 minutes; Terminal: 50 minutes

Excretion: Urine (~10% as unchanged drug)

Dosage Details concerning dosing in combination regimens should also be consulted. Adults:

Stomach or pancreas adenocarcinoma (manufacturer's labeling): I.V.: 20 mg/m^2 every 6-8 weeks

Anal carcinoma (unlabeled use): I.V.: 10 mg/m^2 as an I.V. bolus on days 1 and 29 (maximum: 20 mg/dose) in combination with fluorouracil and radiation therapy (Ajani, 2008)

Bladder cancer, nonmuscle invasive (unlabeled use/route): Intravesicular instillation:

Low risk of recurrence (uncomplicated): 40 mg as a single dose postoperatively; retain in bladder for 2 hours (Hall, 2007)

Increased risk of recurrence: 20 mg weekly for 6 weeks, followed by 20 mg monthly for 3 years; retain in bladder for 1-2 hours (Friedrich, 2007)

Dosage adjustment based on toxicity:

Leukocytes 2000 to <3000/mm^3: Hold therapy until leukocyte count ≥4000/mm^3; reduce to 70% of dose in subsequent cycles

Leukocytes <2000/mm^3: Hold therapy until leukocyte count ≥4000/mm^3; reduce to 50% of dose in subsequent cycles

Platelets 25,000 to <75,000/mm^3: Hold therapy until platelets ≥100,000/mm^3; reduce to 70% of dose in subsequent cycles

Platelets <25,000/mm^3: Hold therapy until platelets ≥100,000 mm^3; reduce to 50% of dose in subsequent cycles

Dosage adjustment in renal impairment: The manufacturer's labeling states to avoid use in patients with serum creatine >1.7 mg/dL, but no dosage adjustments are provided. The following adjustments have been used by some clinicians (Aronoff, 2007): Adults:

Cl_{cr} <10 mL/minute: Administer 75% of dose

Continuous ambulatory peritoneal dialysis (CAPD): Administer 75% of dose

Dosage adjustment in hepatic impairment: No dosage adjustment provided in manufacturer's labeling (has not been studied).

Dosing in obesity: *ASCO Guidelines for appropriate chemotherapy dosing in obese adults with cancer:* Utilize patient's actual body weight (full weight) for calculation of body surface area- or weight-based dosing, particularly when the intent of therapy is curative; manage regimen-related toxicities in the same manner as for nonobese patients; if a dose reduction is utilized due to toxicity, consider resumption of full weight-based dosing with subsequent cycles, especially if cause of toxicity (eg, hepatic or renal impairment) is resolved (Griggs, 2012).

Administration

I.V.: Administer slow I.V. push or by slow (15-30 minute) infusion via a freely-running saline infusion. Consider using a central venous catheter.

Vesicant; ensure proper needle or catheter placement prior to and during infusion; avoid extravasation.

Extravasation management: If extravasation occurs, stop infusion immediately and disconnect (leave cannula/needle in place); gently aspirate extravasated solution (do **NOT** flush the line); remove needle/cannula; elevate extremity. Initiate dimethyl sulfate (DMSO) antidote. Apply dry cold compress for 20 minutes 4 times/day for 1-2 days (Pérez Fidalgo, 2012).

DMSO: Apply topically to a region covering twice the affected area every 8 hours for 7 days; begin within 10 minutes of extravasation; do not cover with a dressing (Perez Fidalgo, 2012).

Intravesicular (unlabeled route): Instill into bladder and retain for up to 2 hours (Friedrich, 2007; Hall, 2007); rotate patient every 15-30 minutes

Hazardous agent; use appropriate precautions for handling and disposal (NIOSH, 2012).

Monitoring Parameters Monitor CBC with differential (repeatedly during therapy and for ≥8 weeks following therapy); serum creatinine; pulmonary function tests; monitor for signs/symptoms of HUS

Dosage Forms Excipient information presented when available (limited, particularly for generics); consult specific product labeling.

Solution Reconstituted, Intravenous:

Generic: 5 mg (1 ea); 20 mg (1 ea); 40 mg (1 ea)

MitoMYcin (Ophthalmic) (mye toe MYE sin)

Brand Names: U.S. Mitosol

Index Terms Mitomycin-C; MMC

Pharmacologic Category Antineoplastic Agent, Antibiotic; Ophthalmic Agent, Miscellaneous

Use Adjunct to *ab externo* glaucoma surgery

Pregnancy Risk Factor X

Dosage Topical ophthalmic: Adults: Glaucoma surgery, adjunctive therapy: 0.2 mg solution is aseptically applied via saturated sponges to surgical site of glaucoma filtration surgery for 2 minutes

Additional Information Complete prescribing information should be consulted for additional detail.

Dosage Forms Excipient information presented when available (limited, particularly for generics); consult specific product labeling.

Kit, Ophthalmic:

Mitosol: 0.2 mg

◆ **Mitomycin For Injection (Can)** *see* MitoMYcin (Systemic) *on page 1383*

◆ **Mitomycin For Injection USP (Can)** *see* MitoMYcin (Systemic) *on page 1383*

◆ **Mitosol** *see* MitoMYcin (Ophthalmic) *on page 1385*

Mitotane (MYE toe tane)

Brand Names: U.S. Lysodren

Brand Names: Canada Lysodren

Index Terms Chloditan; Chlodithane; Khloditan; Mytotan; o,p'-DDD; Ortho,para-DDD

Pharmacologic Category Antineoplastic Agent, Miscellaneous

Use Adrenocortical carcinoma: Treatment of inoperable adrenocortical carcinoma (both functional and non-functional types)

Unlabeled Use Treatment of Cushing syndrome

Pregnancy Risk Factor D

Pregnancy Considerations Animal reproduction studies have not been conducted. May cause fetal harm if administered during pregnancy; adverse outcomes have been reported. Women of reproductive potential should use effective contraception during treatment and after treatment until plasma levels are no longer detected.

Breast-Feeding Considerations Mitotane has been detected in human breast milk. Due to the potential for serious adverse reactions in the nursing infant, breast-feeding should be discontinued until plasma levels are no longer detected.

Contraindications Hypersensitivity to mitotane or any component of the formulation

Warnings/Precautions Hazardous agent - use appropriate precautions for handling and disposal (NIOSH, 2012). Patients treated with mitotane may develop adrenal insufficiency; steroid replacement with glucocorticoid, and sometimes mineralocorticoid, is necessary. It has been recommended that steroid replacement therapy be initiated at the start of therapy, rather than waiting for evidence of adrenal insufficiency. **[U.S. Boxed Warning]: Because the primary action of mitotane is through adrenal suppression, discontinue mitotane temporarily with onset of shock or severe trauma; administer appropriate steroid coverage.** Because mitotane can increase the metabolism of exogenous steroids, higher than usual replacement steroid doses may be required. Mitotane increases hormone binding proteins; monitor free cortisol and corticotropin levels for optimal replacement. Surgically remove tumor tissues from metastatic masses prior to initiation of treatment; rapid cytotoxic effect may cause tumor hemorrhage. Long-term (>2 years) use may lead to brain damage or functional impairment; observe patients for neurotoxicity (neurologic and behavior) regularly. Plasma concentrations >20 mcg/mL are associated with an increased incidence of higher-grade neurotoxicity. Neurologic impairment may reverse upon discontinuation. Use caution with hepatic impairment (other than metastatic lesions from adrenal cortex); metabolism may be decreased. Other CNS adverse effects, including lethargy, sedation, and vertigo may occur; patients must be cautioned about performing tasks which require mental alertness (eg, operating machinery or driving). The manufacturer recommends initiating treatment within a hospital environment until a stabilized dose is achieved. Continue treatment as long as clinical benefit (maintenance of clinical status or metastatic lesion grown slowing) is observed. Clinical benefit is usually observed within 3 months at maximum tolerated dose, although 10% of patients may require more than 3 months for benefit. Continuous treatment at the maximum tolerated dose is generally the best approach. Some patients have been treated intermittently, restarting when severe symptoms reappear, although often response is no longer observed after 3 or 4 courses of intermittent treatment. Potentially significant drug-drug interactions may exist, requiring dose or frequency adjustment, additional monitoring, and/or selection of alternative therapy. Prolonged bleeding time may occur; consider bleeding possibility prior to any surgical intervention. **[U.S. Boxed Warnings]: Should be administered under the supervision of an experienced cancer chemotherapy physician.** Mitotane is associated with a moderate emetic potential; antiemetics may be needed to prevent nausea and vomiting.

Adverse Reactions The majority of adverse events are dose-dependent.

>10%:

Central nervous system: CNS depression (32%), lethargy/somnolence (25%), dizziness/vertigo (15%)

Dermatologic: Skin rash (15%)

Gastrointestinal: Anorexia (24%), nausea (39%), vomiting (37%), diarrhea (13%)

Neuromuscular & skeletal: Weakness (12%)

1% to 10%:

Central nervous system: Headache (5%), confusion (3%)

Neuromuscular & skeletal: Muscle tremor (3%)

<1% (Limited to important or life-threatening): Aches (generalized), adrenal insufficiency, albuminuria, anemia, ataxia, autoimmune hepatitis, bleeding time prolonged, blurred vision, cataract, diplopia, flushing, GGT increased, gynecomastia, hematuria, hemorrhagic cystitis, hormone binding globulins increased, hypercholesterolemia, hyperpyrexia, hypertension, hypertriglyceridemia, lens opacity, leukopenia, macular edema, memory decreased, mucositis, myalgia, neuropathy, orthostatic hypotension, primary hypogonadism, protein bound iodine decreased, thrombocytopenia, thyroid function tests altered, toxic retinopathy, transaminases increased

Drug Interactions

Metabolism/Transport Effects **Induces** CYP3A4 (strong)

Avoid Concomitant Use

Avoid concomitant use of Mitotane with any of the following: Abiraterone Acetate; Apixaban; Artemether; Axitinib; Bedaquiline; Boceprevir; Bortezomib; Bosutinib; Cabozantinib; CloZAPine; Crizotinib; Dienogest; Dronedarone; Enzalutamide; Everolimus; Ibrutinib; Itraconazole; Ivacaftor; Lapatinib; Lumefantrine; Lurasidone; Macitentan; Mifepristone; NIFEdipine; Nilotinib; Nisoldipine; PAZOPanib; Perampanel; Pomalidomide; PONATinib; Praziquantel; Ranolazine; Regorafenib; Rivaroxaban; Roflumilast; RomiDEPsin; Simeprevir; SORAfenib; Telaprevir; Ticagrelor; Tofacitinib; Tolvaptan; Toremifene; Ulipristal; Vandetanib; Vemurafenib; VinCRIStine (Liposomal)

Increased Effect/Toxicity

Mitotane may increase the levels/effects of: Clarithromycin; Ifosfamide; Vitamin K Antagonists

The levels/effects of Mitotane may be increased by: Clarithromycin; MAO Inhibitors

Decreased Effect

Mitotane may decrease the levels/effects of: Abiraterone Acetate; Apixaban; ARIPiprazole; Artemether; Axitinib; Bedaquiline; Boceprevir; Bortezomib; Bosutinib; Brentuximab Vedotin; Cabozantinib; Clarithromycin; CloZAPine; Corticosteroids (Systemic); Crizotinib; CYP3A4 Substrates; Dasatinib; Dienogest; Dronedarone; Enzalutamide; Everolimus; Exemestane; Gefitinib; GuanFACINE; Ibrutinib; Imatinib; Itraconazole; Ivacaftor; Ixabepilone; Lapatinib; Linagliptin; Lumefantrine; Lurasidone; Macitentan; Maraviroc; Mifepristone; NIFEdipine; Nilotinib; Nisoldipine; PAZOPanib; Perampanel; Pomalidomide; PONATinib; Praziquantel; QUEtiapine; Ranolazine; Regorafenib; Rivaroxaban; Roflumilast; RomiDEPsin; Saxagliptin; Simeprevir; SORAfenib; SUNItinib; Tadalafil; Telaprevir; Ticagrelor; Tofacitinib; Tolvaptan; Toremifene; Ulipristal; Vandetanib; Vemurafenib; VinCRIStine (Liposomal); Vitamin K Antagonists; Vortioxetine; Zuclopenthixol

The levels/effects of Mitotane may be decreased by: Spironolactone

Ethanol/Nutrition/Herb Interactions Ethanol: Ethanol may increase CNS depression. Management: Avoid ethanol.

Storage/Stability Store at 25°C (77°F); excursions are permitted between 15°C and 30°C (59°F and 86°F).

Mechanism of Action Adrenolytic agent which causes adrenal cortical atrophy; affects mitochondria in adrenal cortical cells and decreases production of cortisol; also alters the peripheral metabolism of steroids

Pharmacodynamics/Kinetics

Duration: Blood levels undetectable in most patients after 6-9 weeks.

Absorption: Oral: ~40%

Distribution: Stored mainly in fat tissue but is found in all body tissues

Metabolism: Hepatic and other tissues

Half-life elimination: 18-159 days

Time to peak, serum: 3-5 hours

Excretion: Urine (~10%, as metabolites); feces (1% to 17%, as metabolites)

Dosage

Adrenocortical carcinoma: Adults: Oral: Initial: 2-6 g daily in 3-4 divided doses, then increase incrementally to 9-10 g daily in 3-4 divided doses (maximum tolerated range: 2-16 g daily, usually 9-10 g daily; maximum dose studied: 18-19 g daily); continue as long as clinical benefit is demonstrated

Unlabeled dosing: Initial 1-2 g daily; increase by 1-2 g daily at 1-2 week intervals as tolerated to a maximum of 6-10 g daily; usual dose 4-5 g daily (Veytsman, 2009)

Cushing syndrome (unlabeled use): Adults: Oral: Initial dose: 500 mg 3 times daily; maximum dose: 3 g 3 times daily (Biller, 2008)

Dosage adjustment for toxicity:

Severe side effects: Reduce dose until a maximum tolerated dose is achieved

Significant neuropsychiatric adverse effects: Withhold treatment for at least 1 week and restart at a lower dose (Allolio, 2006)

Dosage adjustment in renal impairment: No dosage adjustment provided in manufacturer's labeling.

Dosage adjustment in hepatic impairment: No dosage adjustment provided in manufacturer's labeling. However, drug accumulation may occur in patients with liver disease; use with caution.

Administration Oral: Administer in 3-4 divided doses/day. Do not crush tablets. Mitotane is associated with a moderate emetic potential; antiemetics may be needed to prevent nausea and vomiting.

Hazardous agent; use appropriate precautions for handling and disposal (NIOSH, 2012). Wear impervious gloves when handling; avoid exposure to crushed or broken tablets.

Monitoring Parameters

Adrenal function; neurologic assessments (including behavioral) at regular intervals with chronic (>2 years) use.

Monitor mitotane levels (gas chromatography-flame ionization assay) every 4-8 weeks until levels at 10-14 mg/L are attained, then monitor every 3 months; urinary free cortisol levels; TSH and free thyroxine every few months (Veytsman, 2009)

Dosage Forms Excipient information presented when available (limited, particularly for generics); consult specific product labeling.

Tablet, Oral:

Lysodren: 500 mg [scored]

MitoXANtrone (mye toe ZAN trone)

Brand Names: Canada Mitoxantrone Injection®

Index Terms CL-232315; DHAD; DHAQ; Dihydroxyanthracenedione; Dihydroxyanthracenedione Dihydrochloride;

Mitoxantrone Dihydrochloride; Mitoxantrone HCl; Mitoxantrone Hydrochloride; Mitozantrone; Novantrone

Pharmacologic Category Antineoplastic Agent, Anthracenedione

Use Initial treatment of acute nonlymphocytic leukemias (ANLL [includes myelogenous, promyelocytic, monocytic and erythroid leukemias]); treatment of advanced hormone-refractory prostate cancer; secondary progressive or relapsing-remitting multiple sclerosis (MS)

Canadian labeling: Additional uses (not in U.S. labeling): Treatment of metastatic breast cancer, relapsed leukemia (adults), lymphoma, and hepatocellular carcinoma

Unlabeled Use Treatment of Hodgkin lymphoma (refractory), non-Hodgkin lymphomas (NHL), acute lymphocytic leukemia (ALL), relapsed acute myeloid leukemia (AML), breast cancer (metastatic), pediatric acute myelogenous leukemia (AML), pediatric acute promyelocytic leukemia (APL); part of a conditioning regimen for autologous hematopoietic stem cell transplantation (HSCT)

Pregnancy Risk Factor D

Pregnancy Considerations Adverse effects were noted in animal reproduction studies. May cause fetal harm if administered to a pregnant woman. Pregnancy should be avoided while on treatment. Women with multiple sclerosis who are of reproductive potential should have a pregnancy test prior to each dose.

Breast-Feeding Considerations Mitoxantrone is excreted in human milk and significant concentrations (18 ng/mL) have been reported for 28 days after the last administration. Because of the potential for serious adverse reactions in infants from mitoxantrone, breast-feeding should be discontinued before starting treatment.

Medication Guide Available Yes

Contraindications Hypersensitivity to mitoxantrone or any component of the formulation

Canadian labeling: Additional contraindications (not in U.S. labeling): Prior hypersensitivity to anthracyclines; prior substantial anthracycline exposure and abnormal cardiac function prior to initiation of mitoxantrone therapy; presence of severe myelosuppression due to prior chemo- and/or radiotherapy; severe hepatic impairment; intrathecal administration

Warnings/Precautions Hazardous agent - use appropriate precautions for handling and disposal (NIOSH, 2012).

[U.S. Boxed Warning]: Usually should not be administered if baseline neutrophil count <1500 cells/mm^3 (except for treatment of ANLL). Monitor blood counts and monitor for infection due to neutropenia. Treatment may lead to severe myelosuppression; unless the expected benefit outweighs the risk, use is generally not recommended in patients with pre-existing myelosuppression from prior chemotherapy.

[U.S. Boxed Warning]: May cause myocardial toxicity and potentially-fatal heart failure (HF); risk increases with cumulative dosing. Effects may occur during therapy or may be delayed (months or years after completion of therapy). Predisposing factors for mitoxantrone-induced cardiotoxicity include prior anthracycline or anthracenedione therapy, prior cardiovascular disease, concomitant use of cardiotoxic drugs, and mediastinal/pericardial irradiation, although may also occur in patients without risk factors. Prior to therapy initiation, evaluate all patients for cardiac-related signs/symptoms, including history, physical exam, and ECG; and evaluate baseline left ventricular ejection fraction (LVEF) with echocardiogram or multigated radionuclide angiography (MUGA) or MRI. Not recommended for use in MS patients when LVEF <50%, or baseline LVEF below the lower limit of normal (LLN). Evaluate for cardiac signs/symptoms (by history, physical exam, and ECG) and evaluate LVEF (using same method as baseline LVEF) in MS patients prior to each dose and if signs/symptoms of HF develop. Use in MS should be limited to a cumulative dose of ≤140 mg/m^2, and discontinued if LVEF falls below LLN or a significant decrease in LVEF is observed; decreases in LVEF and HF have been observed in patients with MS who have received cumulative doses <100 mg/m^2. Patients with MS should undergo annual LVEF evaluation following discontinuation of therapy to monitor for delayed cardiotoxicity.

[U.S. Boxed Warning]: For I.V. administration only, into a free-flowing I.V.; may cause severe local tissue damage if extravasation occurs; do not administer subcutaneously, intramuscularly, or intra-arterially. Do not administer intrathecally; may cause serious and permanent neurologic damage. Irritant with vesicant-like properties; extravasation resulting in burning, erythema, pain, swelling and skin discoloration (blue) has been reported; may result in tissue necrosis and require debridement for skin graft. Ensure proper needle or catheter placement prior to and during infusion. Avoid extravasation. May cause urine, saliva, tears, and sweat to turn blue-green for 24 hours postinfusion. Whites of eyes may have blue-green tinge. **[U.S. Boxed Warning]: Treatment with mitoxantrone increases the risk of developing secondary acute myelogenous leukemia (AML) in patients with cancer and in patients with MS;** acute promyelocytic leukemia (APL) has also been observed. Symptoms of acute leukemia include excessive bruising, bleeding and recurrent infections. The risk for secondary leukemia is increased in patients who are heavily pretreated, with higher doses, and with combination chemotherapy.

[U.S. Boxed Warning]: Should be administered under the supervision of a physician experienced in cancer chemotherapy agents. Dosage should be reduced in patients with impaired hepatobiliary function (clearance is reduced). Canadian labeling contraindicates use in severe hepatic impairment. Not for treatment of multiple sclerosis in patients with concurrent hepatic impairment. Not for treatment of primary progressive multiple sclerosis. Rapid lysis of tumor cells may lead to hyperuricemia.

Adverse Reactions Includes events reported with any indication; incidence varies based on treatment, dose, and/or concomitant medications

>10%:

Cardiovascular: Edema (10% to 30%), arrhythmia (3% to 18%), cardiac function changes (≤18%), ECG changes (≤11%)

Central nervous system: Fever (6% to 78%), pain (8% to 41%), fatigue (≤39%), headache (6% to 13%)

Dermatologic: Alopecia (20% to 61%), nail bed changes (≤11%), petechiae/bruising (6% to 11%)

Endocrine & metabolic: Menstrual disorder (26% to 61%), amenorrhea (28% to 53%), hyperglycemia (10% to 31%)

Gastrointestinal: Nausea (26% to 76%), vomiting (6% to 72%), diarrhea (14% to 47%), mucositis (10% to 29%; onset: ≤1 week), stomatitis (8% to 29%; onset: ≤1 week), anorexia (22% to 25%), weight gain/loss (13% to 17%), constipation (10% to 16%), GI bleeding (2% to 16%), abdominal pain (9% to 15%), dyspepsia (5% to 14%)

Genitourinary: Urinary tract infection (7% to 32%), abnormal urine (5% to 11%)

Hematologic: Neutropenia (79% to 100%; onset: ≤3 weeks; grade 4: 23% to 54%), leukopenia (9% to 100%), lymphopenia (72% to 95%), anemia/hemoglobin decreased (5% to 75%) thrombocytopenia (33% to 39%; grades 3/4: 3% to 4%), neutropenic fever (≤11%)

Hepatic: Alkaline phosphatase increased (≤37%), transaminases increased (5% to 20%), GGT increased (3% to 15%)
Neuromuscular & skeletal: Weakness (≤24%)
Renal: BUN increased (≤22%), creatinine increased (≤13%), hematuria (≤11%)
Respiratory: Upper respiratory tract infection (7% to 53%), pharyngitis (≤19%), dyspnea (6% to 18%), cough (5% to 13%)
Miscellaneous: Infection (4% to 60%), sepsis (ANLL 31% to 34%), fungal infection (9% to 15%)

1% to 10%:
Cardiovascular: CHF (≤5%), ischemia (≤5%), LVEF decreased (≤5%), hypertension (≤4%)
Central nervous system: Chills (≤5%), anxiety (5%), depression (5%), seizure (2% to 4%)
Dermatologic: Cutaneous mycosis (≤10%), skin infection (≤5%)
Endocrine & metabolic: Hypocalcemia (10%), hypokalemia (7% to 10%), hyponatremia (9%), menorrhagia (7%)
Gastrointestinal: Aphthosis (≤10%)
Genitourinary: Impotence (≤7%), sterility (≤5%)
Hematologic: Granulocytopenia (6%), hemorrhage (5% to 6%), secondary acute leukemias (≤3%; includes AML, APL)
Hepatic: Jaundice (3% to 7%)
Neuromuscular & skeletal: Back pain (6% to 8%), myalgia (≤5%), arthralgia (≤5%)
Ocular: Conjunctivitis (≤5%), blurred vision (≤3%)
Renal: Renal failure (≤8%), proteinuria (≤6%)
Respiratory: Rhinitis (10%), pneumonia (≤9%), sinusitis (≤6%)
Miscellaneous: Systemic infection (≤10%), diaphoresis (≤9%)

<1% (Limited to important or life-threatening): Allergic reaction, anaphylactoid reactions, anaphylaxis, chest pain, dehydration; extravasation at injection site (may result in burning, erythema, pain, skin discoloration, swelling, or tissue necrosis); interstitial pneumonitis (with combination chemotherapy), hyperuricemia, hypotension, phlebitis at the infusion site, rash, sclera discoloration (blue), tachycardia, urine discoloration (blue-green), urticaria

Drug Interactions

Metabolism/Transport Effects **Inhibits** CYP3A4 (weak)

Avoid Concomitant Use

Avoid concomitant use of MitoXANtrone with any of the following: BCG; CloZAPine; Natalizumab; Pimecrolimus; Pimozide; Tacrolimus (Topical); Tofacitinib; Vaccines (Live)

Increased Effect/Toxicity

MitoXANtrone may increase the levels/effects of: ARIPiprazole; CloZAPine; Dofetilide; Leflunomide; Lomitapide; Natalizumab; Pimozide; Tofacitinib; Vaccines (Live)

The levels/effects of MitoXANtrone may be increased by: CycloSPORINE (Systemic); Denosumab; Pimecrolimus; Roflumilast; Tacrolimus (Topical); Trastuzumab

Decreased Effect

MitoXANtrone may decrease the levels/effects of: BCG; Coccidioidin Skin Test; Sipuleucel-T; Vaccines (Inactivated); Vaccines (Live)

The levels/effects of MitoXANtrone may be decreased by: Echinacea

Ethanol/Nutrition/Herb Interactions Herb/Nutraceutical: Avoid echinacea (may diminish the immunosuppressant effect).

Preparation for Administration Hazardous agent; use appropriate precautions for handling and disposal (NIOSH, 2012). Dilute in at least 50 mL of NS or D_5W.

Storage/Stability Store intact vials at 15°C to 25°C (59°F to 77°F); do not freeze. Opened vials may be stored at room temperature for 7 days or under refrigeration for up to 14 days. Solutions diluted for administration are stable for 7 days at room temperature or under refrigeration, although the manufacturer recommends immediate use.

Mechanism of Action Related to the anthracyclines, mitoxantrone intercalates into DNA resulting in cross-links and strand breaks; binds to nucleic acids and inhibits DNA and RNA synthesis by template disordering and steric obstruction; replication is decreased by binding to DNA topoisomerase II and seems to inhibit the incorporation of uridine into RNA and thymidine into DNA; active throughout entire cell cycle (cell-cycle nonspecific)

Pharmacodynamics/Kinetics

Absorption: Oral: Poor
Distribution: V_d: 14 L/kg; V_{dss}: >1000 L/m^2; distributes extensively into tissue (pleural fluid, kidney, thyroid, liver, heart) and red blood cells
Protein binding: 78%
Metabolism: Hepatic; pathway not determined
Half-life elimination: Terminal: 23-215 hours (median: ~75 hours); may be prolonged with hepatic impairment
Excretion: Feces (25%); urine (6% to 11%; 65% as unchanged drug)

Dosage Details concerning dosing in combination regimens should also be consulted. I.V.:

Children: Acute nonlymphocytic leukemias:
Acute myeloid leukemia (AML) consolidation phase (second course; unlabeled use): 10 mg/m^2 once daily for 5 days (in combination with cytarabine) (Stevens, 1998)
Acute promyelocytic leukemia (APL) consolidation phase (second course; unlabeled use): 10 mg/m^2 once daily for 5 days (Ortega, 2005; Sanz, 2004)

Adults:

U.S. labeling:
Acute nonlymphocytic leukemias (ANLL):
AML induction: 12 mg/m^2 once daily for 3 days (in combination with cytarabine); for incomplete response, may repeat (7-10 days later) at 12 mg/m^2 once daily for 2 days (in combination with cytarabine) (Arlin, 1990)
AML consolidation (beginning ~6 weeks after initiation of the final induction course): 12 mg/m^2 once daily for 2 days (in combination with cytarabine), repeat in 4 weeks (Arlin, 1990)
Multiple sclerosis: 12 mg/m^2 every 3 months (maximum lifetime cumulative dose: 140 mg/m^2; discontinue use with LVEF <50% or clinically significant reduction in LVEF)
Prostate cancer (advanced, hormone-refractory): 12-14 mg/m^2 every 3 weeks (in combination with corticosteroids)

Canadian labeling:
Acute nonlymphocytic leukemias (ANLL):
AML induction: 10-12 mg/m^2 once daily for 3 days (in combination with cytarabine); for incomplete response, may repeat at 10-12 mg/m^2 once daily for 2 days (in combination with cytarabine)
AML consolidation (beginning ~6 weeks after initiation of the final induction course): 12 mg/m^2 once daily for 2 days (in combination with cytarabine), repeat in 4 weeks
Acute leukemias (relapsed): Induction: 12 mg/m^2 once daily for 5 consecutive days; may repeat once if needed (at the same dose and duration)
Breast cancer (metastatic), lymphoma: Initial: Single agent: 14 mg/m^2 every 21 days; reduce initial dose to ≤12 mg/m^2 for myelosuppression due to previous treatment or for poor general health. When used in combination with other agents, reduce initial dose to 10-12 mg/m^2.

Hepatocellular cancer: Initial: Single agent: 14 mg/m^2 every 21 days; reduce initial dose to ≤12 mg/m^2 for myelosuppression due to previous treatment or for poor general health

Adult unlabeled uses and/or dosing:

AML, refractory:

CLAG-M regimen: 10 mg/m^2 once daily for 3 days (in combination with cladribine, cytarabine, and filgrastim), may repeat once if needed (Wierzbowska, 2008)

MEC or EMA regimen: 6 mg/m^2 once daily for 6 days (in combination with cytarabine and etoposide) (Amadori, 1991)

Mitoxantrone/Etoposide: 10 mg/m^2 once daily for 5 days (in combination with etoposide) (Ho, 1988)

APL consolidation phase (second course): 10 mg/m^2 once daily for 5 days (Sanz, 2004)

Hodgkin lymphoma, refractory:

MINE-ESHAP regimen: 10 mg/m^2 on day 1 every 28 days for up to 2 cycles (MINE is combination with mesna, ifosfamide, mitoxantrone, and etoposide; MINE alternates with ESHAP for up to 2 cycles of each) (Fernandez, 2010)

VIM-D regimen: 10 mg/m^2 on day 1 every 28 days (in combination with etoposide, ifosfamide, mesna, and dexamethasone) (Phillips, 1990)

Non-Hodgkin lymphoma (as part of combination chemotherapy regimens):

CNOP regimen: 10 mg/m^2 every 21 days (Bessell, 2003)

FCMR regimen: 8 mg/m^2 every 28 days (Forstpointner, 2004)

FMR regimen: 10 mg/m^2 every 21 days (Zinzani, 2004)

FND regimen: 10 mg/m^2 every 28 days (Tsimberidou, 2002)

MINE-ESHAP regimen: 8 mg/m^2 every 21 days for 6 cycles (MINE is combination with mesna, ifosfamide, mitoxantrone, and etoposide; followed by ESHAP) (Rodriguez, 1995)

Stem cell transplantation, autologous: 60 mg/m^2 administered 4-5 days prior to autografting (as 3 divided doses over 1 hour each at 1-2 hour intervals on the same day; in combination with other chemotherapeutic agent[s]) (Oyan, 2006; Tarella, 2001)

Dosage adjustment for toxicity:

ANLL patients: Severe or life-threatening nonhematologic toxicity: Withhold treatment until toxicity resolves

MS patients:

Neutrophils <1500/mm^3: Use is not recommended

Signs/symptoms of HF: Evaluate for cardiac signs/symptoms and LVEF

LVEF <50% or baseline LVEF below the lower limit of normal (LLN): Use is not recommended

Canadian labeling (not in U.S. labeling): Hepatocellular cancer, lymphoma, or breast cancer (metastatic):

WBC nadir >1500/mm^3 **and** platelet nadir >50,000/mm^3 and recovery ≤21 days: Repeat previous dose or increase dose by 2 mg/m^2 if myelosuppression is inadequate.

WBC nadir >1500/mm^3 **and** platelet nadir >50,000/mm^3 and recovery >21 days: Withhold treatment until recovery then resume at previous dose.

WBC nadir <1500/mm^3 **or** platelet nadir <50,000/mm^3 (regardless of recovery time): Withhold treatment until recovery then decrease previous dose by 2 mg/m^2.

WBC nadir <1000/mm^3 **or** platelet nadir <25,000/mm^3 (regardless of recovery time): Withhold treatment until recovery then decrease previous dose by 4 mg/m^2.

Dosage adjustment in renal impairment: No dosage adjustment provided in manufacturer's labeling (has not been studied).

Hemodialysis: Supplemental dose is not necessary

Peritoneal dialysis: Supplemental dose is not necessary

Elderly: Clearance is decreased in elderly patients; use with caution

Dosage adjustment in hepatic impairment:

U.S. labeling: No dosage adjustment provided in the manufacturer's labeling; however, clearance is reduced in hepatic dysfunction. Patients with severe hepatic dysfunction (bilirubin >3.4 mg/dL) have an AUC of 3 times greater than patients with normal hepatic function; consider dose adjustments. **Note:** MS patients with hepatic impairment should not receive mitoxantrone.

Canadian labeling:

Mild-to-moderate impairment: No specific dosage adjustment provided; consider dose adjustments and monitor closely.

Severe impairment: Use is contraindicated.

Dosing in obesity: *ASCO Guidelines for appropriate chemotherapy dosing in obese adults with cancer:* Utilize patient's actual body weight (full weight) for calculation of body surface area- or weight-based dosing, particularly when the intent of therapy is curative; manage regimen-related toxicities in the same manner as for nonobese patients; if a dose reduction is utilized due to toxicity, consider resumption of full weight-based dosing with subsequent cycles, especially if cause of toxicity (eg, hepatic or renal impairment) is resolved (Griggs, 2012).

Administration For I.V. administration only; do not administer intrathecally, subcutaneously, intramuscularly or intra-arterially. Must be diluted prior to use. Usually administered as a short I.V. infusion over 5-15 minutes; do not infuse over <3-5 minutes.

High doses for bone marrow transplant (unlabeled use) are usually given as 3 divided doses over 1 hour each at 1-2 hour intervals on the same day (Oyan, 2006; Tarella, 2001).

Irritant with vesicant-like properties; ensure proper needle or catheter placement prior to and during infusion; avoid extravasation.

Extravasation management: If extravasation occurs, stop infusion immediately and disconnect (leave cannula/needle in place); gently aspirate extravasated solution (do **NOT** flush the line); remove needle/cannula; elevate extremity. Initiate antidote (dexrazoxane or dimethyl sulfate [DMSO]). Apply dry cold compresses for 20 minutes 4 times daily for 1-2 days (Perez Fidalgo, 2012); withhold cooling beginning 15 minutes before dexrazoxane infusion; continue withholding cooling until 15 minutes after infusion is completed. Topical DMSO should not be administered in combination with dexrazoxane; may lessen dexrazoxane efficacy.

Dexrazoxane: Adults: 1000 mg/m^2 (maximum dose: 2000 mg) I.V. (administer in a large vein remote from site of extravasation) over 1-2 hours days 1 and 2, then 500 mg/m^2 (maximum dose: 1000 mg) I.V. over 1-2 hours day 3; begin within 6 hours of extravasation. Day 2 and day 3 doses should be administered at approximately the same time (± 3 hours) as the dose on day 1 (Mouridsen, 2007; Perez Fidalgo, 2012). **Note:** Reduce dexrazoxane dose by 50% in patients with moderate to severe renal impairment (Cl_{cr} <40 mL/minute).

DMSO: Children and Adults: Apply topically to a region covering twice the affected area every 8 hours for 7 days; begin within 10 minutes of extravasation; do not cover with a dressing (Perez Fidalgo, 2012).

Hazardous agent; use appropriate precautions for handling and disposal (NIOSH, 2012).

Monitoring Parameters CBC with differential, serum uric acid (for leukemia treatment), liver function tests; for the treatment of multiple sclerosis, obtain pregnancy test; monitor injection site for extravasation

Cardiac monitoring: Prior to initiation, evaluate all patients for cardiac-related signs/symptoms, including history, physical exam, and ECG; evaluate baseline and periodic left ventricular ejection fraction (LVEF) with echocardiogram or multigated radionuclide angiography (MUGA) or MRI. In patients with MS, evaluate for cardiac signs/symptoms (by history, physical exam, and ECG) and evaluate LVEF (using same method as baseline LVEF) prior to each dose and if signs/symptoms of HF develop. Patients with MS should undergo annual LVEF evaluation following discontinuation of therapy to monitor for delayed cardiotoxicity.

Dosage Forms Excipient information presented when available (limited, particularly for generics); consult specific product labeling.

Concentrate, Intravenous:

Generic: 20 mg/10 mL (10 mL); 25 mg/12.5 mL (12.5 mL); 30 mg/15 mL (15 mL)

- **Mitoxantrone Dihydrochloride** *see* MitoXANtrone *on page* 1386
- **Mitoxantrone HCl** *see* MitoXANtrone *on page* 1386
- **Mitoxantrone Hydrochloride** *see* MitoXANtrone *on page* 1386
- **Mitoxantrone Injection® (Can)** *see* MitoXANtrone *on page* 1386
- **Mitozantrone** *see* MitoXANtrone *on page* 1386
- **Mitrazol [OTC]** *see* Miconazole (Topical) *on page* 1358
- **MK-217** *see* Alendronate *on page* 69
- **MK383** *see* Tirofiban *on page* 2072
- **MK-0431** *see* SitaGLIPtin *on page* 1906
- **MK462** *see* Rizatriptan *on page* 1844
- **MK 0517** *see* Fosaprepitant *on page* 919
- **MK-0518** *see* Raltegravir *on page* 1776
- **MK594** *see* Losartan *on page* 1247
- **MK0826** *see* Ertapenem *on page* 739
- **MK 869** *see* Aprepitant *on page* 158
- **MLN341** *see* Bortezomib *on page* 270
- **MMC** *see* MitoMYcin (Ophthalmic) *on page* 1385
- **MMC** *see* MitoMYcin (Systemic) *on page* 1383
- **MMF** *see* Mycophenolate *on page* 1407
- **MMR** *see* Measles, Mumps, and Rubella Virus Vaccine *on page* 1272
- **M-M-R II** *see* Measles, Mumps, and Rubella Virus Vaccine *on page* 1272
- **MMRV** *see* Measles, Mumps, Rubella, and Varicella Virus Vaccine *on page* 1273
- **MN-50 [OTC]** *see* Manganese *on page* 1265
- **MOAB 2C4** *see* Pertuzumab *on page* 1625
- **MOAB ABX-EGF** *see* Panitumumab *on page* 1561
- **MOAB C225** *see* Cetuximab *on page* 398
- **MoAb CD52** *see* Alemtuzumab *on page* 66
- **MOAB-CTLA-4** *see* Ipilimumab *on page* 1109
- **MOAB HER2** *see* Trastuzumab *on page* 2109
- **Mobic** *see* Meloxicam *on page* 1284
- **Mobic® (Can)** *see* Meloxicam *on page* 1284
- **Mobicox® (Can)** *see* Meloxicam *on page* 1284

Modafinil (moe DAF i nil)

Brand Names: U.S. Provigil

Brand Names: Canada Alertec®

Pharmacologic Category Central Nervous System Stimulant

Use Improve wakefulness in patients with excessive daytime sleepiness associated with narcolepsy and shift work sleep disorder (SWSD); adjunctive therapy for obstructive sleep apnea/hypopnea syndrome (OSAHS)

Unlabeled Use Attention-deficit/hyperactivity disorder (ADHD); treatment of fatigue in MS and other disorders

Pregnancy Risk Factor C

Pregnancy Considerations Adverse events were observed in some animal reproduction studies. Healthcare providers are encouraged to register pregnant patients exposed to modafinil by calling (866-404-4106).

Efficacy of steroidal contraceptives (including depot and implantable contraceptives) may be decreased; alternate means of contraception should be considered during therapy and for 1 month after modafinil is discontinued.

Breast-Feeding Considerations It is not known if modafinil is excreted into breast milk. The manufacturer recommends caution be used if administered to nursing women.

Medication Guide Available Yes

Contraindications Hypersensitivity to modafinil, armodafinil, or any component of the formulation

Canadian labeling: Additional contraindications (not in U.S. labeling): Patients in agitated states or with severe anxiety

Warnings/Precautions For use following complete evaluation of sleepiness and in conjunction with other standard treatments (eg, CPAP). The degree of sleepiness should be reassessed frequently; some patients may not return to a normal level of wakefulness. Use is not recommended with a history of angina, cardiac ischemia, recent history of myocardial infarction, left ventricular hypertrophy, or patients with mitral valve prolapse who have developed mitral valve prolapse syndrome with previous CNS stimulant use.

Serious and life-threatening rashes (including Stevens-Johnson syndrome and toxic epidermal necrolysis) have been reported with modafinil. Most cases have occurred within the first 5 weeks of therapy; however, rare cases have occurred after long-term use. No risk factors have been identified to predict occurrence or severity. Patients should be advised to discontinue at first sign of rash. The serious nature of these dermatologic adverse effects, as well reports of psychiatric events, resulted in the FDA's Pediatric Advisory Committee unanimously recommending that a specific warning against the use of modafinil in children be added to the manufacturer's labeling. Modafinil is not FDA-approved for use in pediatrics for any indication.

In addition, rare cases of multiorgan hypersensitivity reactions in association with modafinil use, and lone cases of angioedema and anaphylactoid reactions with armodafinil, have been reported. Signs and symptoms are diverse, reflecting the involvement of specific organs. Patients typically present with fever and rash associated with organ-system dysfunction. Patients should be advised to report any signs and symptoms related to these effects; discontinuation of therapy is recommended.

Caution should be exercised when modafinil is given to patients with a history of psychosis; may impair the ability to engage in potentially hazardous activities. Stimulants may unmask tics in individuals with coexisting Tourette's syndrome. Use caution with renal or hepatic impairment (dosage adjustment in severe hepatic dysfunction is recommended).

Adverse Reactions

>10%:

Central nervous system: Headache (adults 34%; children 20%; dose related)

Gastrointestinal: Appetite decreased (children 16%), abdominal pain (children 12%), nausea (11%)

1% to 10%:

Cardiovascular: Chest pain (3%), hypertension (3%), palpitation (2%), tachycardia (2%), vasodilation (2%), edema (1%)

Central nervous system: Nervousness (7%), dizziness (5%), anxiety (5%; dose related), insomnia (5%), depression (2%), somnolence (2%), chills (1%), agitation (1%), confusion (1%), emotional lability (1%), vertigo (1%)

Dermatologic: Rash (1%; includes some severe cases requiring hospitalization)

Gastrointestinal: Diarrhea (6%), dyspepsia (5%), weight loss (children 5%), xerostomia (4%), anorexia (4%), constipation (2%), flatulence (1%), mouth ulceration (1%), taste perversion (1%)

Genitourinary: Abnormal urine (1%), hematuria (1%), pyuria (1%)

Hematologic: Eosinophilia (1%)

Hepatic: LFTs abnormal (2%)

Neuromuscular & skeletal: Back pain (6%), paresthesia (2%), dyskinesia (1%), hyperkinesia (1%), hypertonia (1%), neck rigidity (1%), tremor (1%)

Ocular: Amblyopia (1%), eye pain (1%), vision abnormal (1%)

Respiratory: Rhinitis (7%), pharyngitis (4%), lung disorder (2%), asthma (1%), epistaxis (1%)

Miscellaneous: Flu-like syndrome (4%), thirst (1%), diaphoresis (1%), herpes simplex infection (1%)

Postmarketing and/or case reports: Agranulocytosis, anaphylactic reaction, angioedema, DRESS syndrome, erythema multiforme, hypersensitivity syndrome (multi-organ), mania, psychosis, Stevens-Johnson syndrome, toxic epidermal necrolysis

Drug Interactions

Metabolism/Transport Effects **Substrate** of CYP3A4 (major); **Note:** Assignment of Major/Minor substrate status based on clinically relevant drug interaction potential; **Inhibits** CYP1A2 (weak), CYP2A6 (weak), CYP2C19 (strong), CYP2C9 (weak), CYP2E1 (weak), CYP3A4 (weak); **Induces** CYP1A2 (weak/moderate), CYP2B6 (weak/moderate), CYP3A4 (weak/moderate)

Avoid Concomitant Use

Avoid concomitant use of Modafinil with any of the following: Axitinib; Bosutinib; Conivaptan; Fusidic Acid (Systemic); Iobenguane I 123; Pimozide; Simeprevir

Increased Effect/Toxicity

Modafinil may increase the levels/effects of: ARIPiprazole; Citalopram; CYP2C19 Substrates; Dofetilide; Lomitapide; Pimozide; Sympathomimetics

The levels/effects of Modafinil may be increased by: AtoMOXetine; Cannabinoids; Conivaptan; CYP3A4 Inhibitors (Moderate); CYP3A4 Inhibitors (Strong); Dasatinib; Fusidic Acid (Systemic); Ivacaftor; Linezolid; Luliconazole; Mifepristone; Simeprevir

Decreased Effect

Modafinil may decrease the levels/effects of: ARIPiprazole; Axitinib; Bosutinib; Clopidogrel; Contraceptives (Estrogens); CycloSPORINE (Systemic); Ibrutinib; Iobenguane I 123; Saxagliptin; Simeprevir

The levels/effects of Modafinil may be decreased by: Bosentan; CYP3A4 Inducers (Strong); Dabrafenib; Deferasirox; Herbs (CYP3A4 Inducers); Mitotane; Tocilizumab

Ethanol/Nutrition/Herb Interactions

Ethanol: Avoid or limit ethanol.

Food: Delays absorption, but does not affect bioavailability.

Storage/Stability

Provigil®: Store at 20°C to 25°C (68°F to 77°F).

Alertec® (Canadian availability; not available in U.S.): Store at 15°C to 30°C (59°F to 86°F).

Mechanism of Action The exact mechanism of action is unclear, it does not appear to alter the release of dopamine or norepinephrine, it may exert its stimulant effects by decreasing GABA-mediated neurotransmission, although this theory has not yet been fully evaluated; several studies also suggest that an intact central alpha-adrenergic system is required for modafinil's activity; the drug increases high-frequency alpha waves while decreasing both delta and theta wave activity, and these effects are consistent with generalized increases in mental alertness

Pharmacodynamics/Kinetics Modafinil is a racemic compound (10% *d*-isomer and 90% *l*-isomer at steady state) whose enantiomers have different pharmacokinetics

Distribution: V_d: 0.9 L/kg

Protein binding: ~60%, primarily to albumin

Metabolism: Hepatic; multiple pathways including CYP3A4

Half-life elimination: Effective half-life: 15 hours

Time to peak, serum: 2-4 hours

Excretion: Urine (as metabolites, <10% as unchanged drug)

Dosage

U.S. labeling:

Narcolepsy, obstructive sleep apnea/hypopnea syndrome (OSAHS): Adults: Oral: Initial: 200 mg as a single daily dose in the morning

Shift work sleep disorder (SWSD): Adults: Oral: Initial: 200 mg as a single dose taken ~1 hour prior to start of work shift

Note: Doses up to 400 mg daily, given as a single dose, have been well tolerated, but there is no consistent evidence that this dose confers additional benefit.

Canadian labeling:

Narcolepsy: Adults: Oral: Initial: 200 mg daily in 2 divided doses (first dose in the morning and second dose at noon [or no later than early afternoon]); may titrate dose upward in 100 mg increments as needed and tolerated (maximum single dose: <300 mg; maximum daily dose: 400 mg). Single doses ≥300 mg and daily doses >400 mg are associated with increased side effects and are not recommended.

Obstructive sleep apnea: Adults: Oral: 200 mg once daily in the morning.

Shift work sleep disorder: Adults: Oral: 200 mg as a single dose taken ~1 hour prior to start of work shift

Unlabeled use: ADHD: 100-400 mg daily (Taylor, 2000)

Elderly: Elimination of modafinil and its metabolites may be reduced as a consequence of aging and as a result, consider initiating at lower doses in this patient population.

Dosing adjustment in renal impairment: Severe impairment: No dosage adjustment provided in manufacturer's labeling (insufficient data).

Dosing adjustment in hepatic impairment: Severe hepatic impairment: Dose should be reduced to one-half of that recommended for patients with normal liver function.

Administration

U.S. labeling: For the treatment of narcolepsy and obstructive sleep apnea/hypopnea syndrome, administer dose in the morning. For the treatment of shift work sleep disorder, administer dose ~1 hour prior to start of work shift.

Canadian labeling: For the treatment of narcolepsy, administer in 2 divided doses with first dose given in the morning and the second dose given at noon (or no later than early afternoon) to avoid potential for insomnia. For treatment of obstructive sleep apnea, administer as a single dose in the morning. For the treatment of shift work sleep disorder, administer dose ~1 hour prior to start of work shift.

Monitoring Parameters Levels of sleepiness; blood pressure in patients with hypertension; body mass index and weight loss; development of severe skin reactions; development or exacerbation of psychiatric symptoms (eg, agitation, anxiety, depression)

When used for the treatment of ADHD, thoroughly evaluate for cardiovascular risk. Monitor heart rate, blood pressure, and consider obtaining ECG prior to initiation (Vetter, 2008).

Dosage Forms Excipient information presented when available (limited, particularly for generics); consult specific product labeling.

Tablet, Oral:
- Provigil: 100 mg
- Provigil: 200 mg [scored]
- Generic: 100 mg, 200 mg

Dosage Forms: Canada Excipient information presented when available (limited, particularly for generics); consult specific product labeling.

Tablet, oral: 100 mg
- Alertec®: 100 mg

Controlled Substance C-IV

◆ **Modecate® (Can)** *see* FluPHENAZine *on page 889*

◆ **Modecate® Concentrate (Can)** *see* FluPHENAZine *on page 889*

◆ **Modicon** *see* Ethinyl Estradiol and Norethindrone *on page 793*

◆ **Modified Dakin's Solution** *see* Sodium Hypochlorite Solution *on page 1918*

◆ **Modified Shohl's Solution** *see* Sodium Citrate and Citric Acid *on page 1917*

Moexipril (mo EKS i pril)

Brand Names: U.S. Univasc

Index Terms Moexipril Hydrochloride

Pharmacologic Category Angiotensin-Converting Enzyme (ACE) Inhibitor; Antihypertensive

Additional Appendix Information

Angiotensin Agents *on page 2280*

Use Treatment of hypertension, alone or in combination with thiazide diuretics

Pregnancy Risk Factor D

Dosage Adults: Oral: Initial: 7.5 mg once daily (in patients **not** receiving diuretics), 1 hour prior to a meal **or** 3.75 mg once daily (when combined with thiazide diuretics); maintenance dose: 7.5-30 mg/day in 1 or 2 divided doses 1 hour before meals

Dosage adjustment in renal impairment: Cl_{cr} ≤40 mL/minute: Patients may be cautiously placed on 3.75 mg once daily, then upwardly titrated to a maximum of 15 mg/day.

Dosage adjustment in hepatic impairment: No dosage adjustment provided in manufacturer's labeling. However, hepatic impairment increases systemic exposure.

Additional Information Complete prescribing information should be consulted for additional detail.

Dosage Forms Excipient information presented when available (limited, particularly for generics); consult specific product labeling.

Tablet, Oral, as hydrochloride:
- Univasc: 7.5 mg, 15 mg [scored]
- Generic: 7.5 mg, 15 mg

Moexipril and Hydrochlorothiazide
(mo EKS i pril & hye droe klor oh THYE a zide)

Brand Names: U.S. Uniretic®

Brand Names: Canada Uniretic®

Index Terms Hydrochlorothiazide and Moexipril

Pharmacologic Category Angiotensin-Converting Enzyme (ACE) Inhibitor; Antihypertensive; Diuretic, Thiazide

Use Treatment of hypertension; not indicated for initial treatment of hypertension

Pregnancy Risk Factor D

Dosage Adults: Oral: 7.5-30 mg of moexipril, taken either in a single or divided dose 1 hour before meals; hydrochlorothiazide dose should be ≤50 mg/day

Dosage adjustment in renal impairment:
- Cl_{cr} >40 mL/minute: No dosage adjustment necessary.
- Cl_{cr} ≤40 mL/minute: Use not recommended.

Dosage adjustment in hepatic impairment: No dosage adjustment provided in manufacturer's labeling (has not been studied). However, hepatic impairment increases systemic exposure. Use with caution.

Additional Information Complete prescribing information should be consulted for additional detail.

Dosage Forms Excipient information presented when available (limited, particularly for generics); consult specific product labeling.

Tablet, oral:
- 7.5/12.5: Moexipril hydrochloride 7.5 mg and hydrochlorothiazide 12.5 mg
- 15/12.5: Moexipril hydrochloride 15 mg and hydrochlorothiazide 12.5 mg
- 15/25: Moexipril hydrochloride 15 mg and hydrochlorothiazide 25 mg

Uniretic®:
- 7.5/12.5: Moexipril hydrochloride 7.5 mg and hydrochlorothiazide 12.5 mg [scored]
- 15/12.5: Moexipril hydrochloride 15 mg and hydrochlorothiazide 12.5 mg [scored]
- 15/25: Moexipril hydrochloride 15 mg and hydrochlorothiazide 25 mg [scored]

◆ **Moexipril Hydrochloride** *see* Moexipril *on page 1392*

◆ **MOM** *see* Magnesium Hydroxide *on page 1260*

Mometasone (Oral Inhalation)
(moe MET a sone)

Brand Names: U.S. Asmanex 120 Metered Doses; Asmanex 14 Metered Doses; Asmanex 30 Metered Doses; Asmanex 60 Metered Doses; Asmanex 7 Metered Doses

Brand Names: Canada Asmanex® Twisthaler®

Index Terms Mometasone Furoate

Pharmacologic Category Corticosteroid, Inhalant (Oral)

Additional Appendix Information

Inhaled Corticosteroids *on page 2298*

Use Maintenance treatment of asthma as prophylactic therapy

Pregnancy Risk Factor C

Pregnancy Considerations Adverse events were observed in some animal reproduction studies. Hypoadrenalism may occur in infants born to mothers receiving corticosteroids during pregnancy. Based on available data, an overall increased risk of congenital malformations or a decrease in fetal growth has not been associated with maternal use of inhaled corticosteroids during pregnancy (Bakhireva, 2005; NAEPP, 2005; Namazy, 2004).

Uncontrolled asthma is associated with adverse events in pregnancy (increased risk of perinatal mortality, pre-eclampsia, preterm birth, low birth weight infants). Inhaled corticosteroids are recommended for the treatment of asthma during pregnancy (most information available using budesonide) (ACOG, 2008; NAEPP, 2005).

Breast-Feeding Considerations Systemic corticosteroids are excreted in human milk. It is not known if sufficient quantities of mometasone are absorbed following oral inhalation to produce detectable amounts in breast milk; however, oral absorption is limited (<1%). The manufacturer recommends that caution be exercised when administering mometasone to nursing women. The use of inhaled corticosteroids is not considered a contraindication to breast-feeding (NAEPP, 2005).

Contraindications Hypersensitivity to mometasone or any component of the formulation; hypersensitivity to milk proteins; primary treatment of status asthmaticus or acute bronchospasm

Canadian labeling: Additional contraindications (not in U.S. labeling): Untreated systemic fungal, bacterial, viral, or parasitic infections; active or quiet tuberculosis infection of the respiratory tract; ocular herpes simplex

Warnings/Precautions May cause hypercorticism or suppression of hypothalamic-pituitary-adrenal (HPA) axis, particularly in younger children or in patients receiving high doses for prolonged periods. HPA axis suppression may lead to adrenal crisis. Withdrawal and discontinuation of a corticosteroid should be done slowly and carefully. Particular care is required when patients are transferred from systemic corticosteroids to inhaled products due to possible adrenal insufficiency or withdrawal from steroids, including an increase in allergic symptoms. Patients receiving >20 mg per day of prednisone (or equivalent) may be most susceptible. Fatalities have occurred due to adrenal insufficiency in asthmatic patients during and after transfer from systemic corticosteroids to aerosol steroids; aerosol steroids do not provide the systemic steroid needed to treat patients having trauma, surgery, or infections. When transferring to oral inhaler, previously-suppressed allergic conditions (rhinitis, conjunctivitis, eczema) may be unmasked.

Bronchospasm may occur with wheezing after inhalation; if this occurs, stop steroid and treat with a fast-acting bronchodilator. Supplemental steroids (oral or parenteral) may be needed during stress or severe asthma attacks. Not to be used in status asthmaticus or for the relief of acute bronchospasm. Corticosteroid use may cause psychiatric disturbances, including depression, euphoria, insomnia, mood swings, and personality changes. Pre-existing psychiatric conditions may be exacerbated by corticosteroid use. Prolonged use of corticosteroids may also increase the incidence of secondary infection, mask acute infection (including fungal infections), prolong or exacerbate viral infections, or limit response to vaccines. Exposure to chickenpox should be avoided; corticosteroids should not be used to treat ocular herpes simplex. Corticosteroids should not be used for cerebral malaria or viral hepatitis. Close observation is required in patients with latent tuberculosis and/or TB reactivity; restrict use in active TB (only in conjunction with antituberculosis treatment). Canadian labeling contraindicates use in patients with untreated systemic fungal, bacterial, viral, or parasitic infections, active or quiet tuberculosis infection of the respiratory tract and ocular herpes simplex.

Prolonged treatment with corticosteroids has been associated with the development of Kaposi's sarcoma (case reports); if noted, discontinuation of therapy should be considered. Local oropharyngeal *Candida* infections have been reported; if occurs treat appropriately while continuing mometasone therapy. Patients should be instructed to rinse mouth after each use.

Reactions including, anaphylaxis, angioedema, pruritus, and rash have been reported; if these symptoms occur discontinue use. Use with caution in patients with thyroid disease, hepatic impairment, renal impairment, cardiovascular disease, diabetes, glaucoma, cataracts, myasthenia gravis, patients with or who are at risk for osteoporosis, patients at risk for seizures, or GI diseases (diverticulitis, peptic ulcer, ulcerative colitis) due to perforation risk. Use caution following acute MI (corticosteroids have been associated with myocardial rupture). Because of the risk of adverse effects, systemic corticosteroids should be used cautiously in the elderly in the smallest possible effective dose for the shortest duration.

Orally-inhaled corticosteroids may cause a reduction in growth velocity in pediatric patients (~1 centimeter per year [range: 0.3-1.8 cm per year] and related to dose and duration of exposure). To minimize the systemic effects of orally-inhaled corticosteroids, each patient should be titrated to the lowest effective dose. Growth should be routinely monitored in pediatric patients. Prior to use, the dose and duration of treatment should be based on the risk versus benefit for each individual patient. In general, use the smallest effective dose for the shortest duration of time to minimize adverse events. A gradual tapering of dose may be required prior to discontinuing therapy. There have been reports of systemic corticosteroid withdrawal symptoms (eg, joint/muscle pain, lassitude, depression) when withdrawing inhalation therapy. May contain lactose; very rare anaphylactic reactions have been reported in patients with severe milk protein allergy.

Adverse Reactions

>10%:

- Central nervous system: Headache (17% to 22%), fatigue (1% to 13%), depression (11%)
- Neuromuscular & skeletal: Musculoskeletal pain (4% to 22%), arthralgia (13%)
- Respiratory: Sinusitis (5% to 22%), rhinitis (4% to 20%), upper respiratory infection (8% to 15%), pharyngitis (8% to 13%)
- Miscellaneous: Oral candidiasis (4% to 22%)

1% to 10%:

- Central nervous system: Fever (children 7%), pain (1% to <3%)
- Dermatologic: Bruising (children 2%)
- Gastrointestinal: Abdominal pain (2% to 6%), dyspepsia (3% to 5%), nausea (1% to 3%), vomiting (1% to ≤3%), anorexia (1% to <3%), dry throat (1% to <3%), gastroenteritis (1% to <3%)
- Genitourinary: Dysmenorrhea (4% to 9%), urinary tract infection (children 2%)
- Neuromuscular & skeletal: Back pain (3% to 6%), myalgia (2% to 3%)
- Ocular: Ocular pressure increased (3%), cataracts (1%)
- Otic: Earache (1% to <3%)
- Respiratory: Sinus congestion (9%), dysphonia (1% to <3%), epistaxis (1% to <3%), nasal irritation (1% to <3%)
- Miscellaneous: Flu-like syndrome (1% to <3%), infection (1% to <3%)

Postmarketing and/or case reports: Anaphylaxis, angioedema, asthma aggravated, bronchospasm, cough, dyspnea, growth suppression, hypersensitivity, pruritus, rash, wheezing

Drug Interactions

Metabolism/Transport Effects Substrate of CYP3A4 (minor); **Note:** Assignment of Major/Minor substrate status based on clinically relevant drug interaction potential

Avoid Concomitant Use

Avoid concomitant use of Mometasone (Oral Inhalation) with any of the following: Aldesleukin

Increased Effect/Toxicity

Mometasone (Oral Inhalation) may increase the levels/effects of: Amphotericin B; Deferasirox; Loop Diuretics; Thiazide Diuretics

The levels/effects of Mometasone (Oral Inhalation) may be increased by: CYP3A4 Inhibitors (Strong); Telaprevir

Decreased Effect

Mometasone (Oral Inhalation) may decrease the levels/effects of: Aldesleukin; Antidiabetic Agents; Corticorelin; Hyaluronidase; Telaprevir

Storage/Stability Store at 25°C (77°F); excursions permitted to 15°C to 30°C (59°F to 86°F). Discard when oral dose counter reads "00" (or 45 days [U.S. labeling] or 60 days [Canadian labeling] after opening the foil pouch).

Mechanism of Action May depress the formation, release, and activity of endogenous chemical mediators of inflammation (kinins, histamine, liposomal enzymes, prostaglandins). Leukocytes and macrophages may have to be present for the initiation of responses mediated by the above substances. Inhibits the margination and subsequent cell migration to the area of injury, and also reverses the dilatation and increased vessel permeability in the area resulting in decreased access of cells to the sites of injury.

Pharmacodynamics/Kinetics

Absorption: <1%

Protein binding: 98% to 99%

Metabolism: Hepatic via CYP3A4; forms metabolite

Half-life elimination: 5 hours

Excretion: Feces, bile, urine

Dosage Oral inhalation: **Note:** Dosage forms available in the U.S. (110 mcg and 220 mcg Twisthaler®) deliver 100 and 200 mcg mometasone furoate per actuation respectively.

U.S. labeling:

Children 4-11 years: 110 mcg once daily in the evening (maximum: 110 mcg/day)

Children ≥12 years and Adults: Previous therapy:

Bronchodilators or inhaled corticosteroids: Initial: 1 inhalation (220 mcg) daily (maximum: 2 inhalations or 440 mcg/day); may be given in the evening or in divided doses twice daily

Oral corticosteroids: Initial: 440 mcg twice daily (maximum: 880 mcg/day); prednisone should be reduced no faster than 2.5 mg/day on a weekly basis, beginning after at least 1 week of mometasone furoate use

Canadian labeling: Children ≥12 years and Adults:

Usual dose: 400 mcg once daily in the morning; maintenance: 200-400 mcg once daily in the morning. **Note:** Some patients (eg, previously receiving high-dose inhaled corticosteroids) may respond more favorably to 400 mcg daily administered in 2 divided doses.

Severe asthma and requiring oral corticosteroids: Initial: 400 mcg twice daily; taper off oral corticosteroid gradually by decreasing daily prednisone dose by 1 mg/day (or equivalent of other corticosteroid) on a weekly basis, beginning after at least 1 week of mometasone furoate use; upon successful taper off of oral steroids, titrate mometasone to lowest effective dose.

NIH Asthma Guidelines (NIH, 2007): Children ≥12 years and Adults:

"Low" dose: 200 mcg/day

"Medium" dose: 400 mcg/day

"High" dose: >400 mcg/day

Note: Maximum effects may not be evident for 1-2 weeks or longer; dose should be titrated to effect, using the lowest possible dose

Dosage adjustment in renal impairment: No dosage adjustment provided in manufacturer's labeling (has not been studied).

Dosage adjustment in hepatic impairment: No dosage adjustment provided in manufacturer's labeling (has not been studied). However, mometasone exposure is increased with hepatic impairment.

Dietary Considerations Asmanex® Twisthaler® contains lactose.

Administration Exhale fully prior to bringing the Twisthaler® up to the mouth. Place between lips and inhale quickly and deeply. Do not breathe out through the inhaler. Remove inhaler and hold breath for 10 seconds if possible. Rinse mouth after use.

Monitoring Parameters HPA axis suppression

Asthma: FEV_1, peak flow, and/or other pulmonary function tests

Dosage Forms Excipient information presented when available (limited, particularly for generics); consult specific product labeling.

Aerosol Powder Breath Activated, Inhalation, as furoate:

Asmanex 120 Metered Doses: 220 mcg/INH (1 ea) [contains milk protein]

Asmanex 14 Metered Doses: 220 mcg/INH (1 ea) [contains milk protein]

Asmanex 30 Metered Doses: 110 mcg/INH (1 ea); 220 mcg/INH (1 ea) [contains milk protein]

Asmanex 60 Metered Doses: 220 mcg/INH (1 ea) [contains milk protein]

Asmanex 7 Metered Doses: 110 mcg/INH (1 ea) [contains milk protein]

Dosage Forms: Canada Excipient information presented when available (limited, particularly for generics); consult specific product labeling.

Powder, for oral inhalation, as furoate:

Asmanex® Twisthaler®: 200 mcg (30 doses, 60 doses) [contains lactose; delivers 200 mcg/actuation]

Asmanex® Twisthaler®: 400 mcg (30 doses, 60 doses) [contains lactose; delivers 400 mcg/actuation]

Mometasone (Nasal) (moe MET a sone)

Brand Names: U.S. Nasonex

Brand Names: Canada Apo-Mometasone®; Nasonex®

Index Terms Mometasone Furoate

Pharmacologic Category Corticosteroid, Nasal

Additional Appendix Information

Inhaled Corticosteroids *on page* 2298

Use Treatment of nasal symptoms of seasonal and perennial allergic rhinitis; prevention of nasal symptoms associated with seasonal allergic rhinitis; treatment of nasal polyps in adults

Canadian labeling: Additional use (not in U.S. labeling): Treatment of mild-to-moderate uncomplicated rhinosinusitis or as adjunctive treatment (with antimicrobials) in acute rhinosinusitis

Unlabeled Use Adjunct to antibiotics in empiric treatment of acute bacterial rhinosinusitis (ABRS) (Chow, 2012)

Pregnancy Risk Factor C

Dosage Intranasal:

Allergic rhinitis (seasonal and perennial):

U.S. labeling:

Children 2-11 years: 1 spray (50 mcg) in each nostril once daily

Children ≥12 years and Adults: 2 sprays (100 mcg) in each nostril once daily; when used for the prevention of allergic rhinitis, treatment should begin 2-4 weeks prior to pollen season

Canadian labeling:

Children 3-11 years: 1 spray (50 mcg) in each nostril once daily

Children ≥12 years and Adults: Initial: 2 sprays (100 mcg) in each nostril once daily; upon symptom control, may consider dose reduction to 1 spray (50 mcg) in each nostril once daily as maintenance therapy. **Note:** If adequate symptom control is not achieved with initial dosing, may increase dose to 4 sprays (200 mcg) in each nostril once daily (total daily dose: 400 mcg). Dose reduction is recommended upon symptom control.

Nasal polyps treatment: Adults: 2 sprays (100 mcg) in each nostril twice daily; 2 sprays (100 mcg) once daily may be effective in some patients

Rhinosinusitis, adjunctive treatment (acute): Canadian labeling (not in U.S. labeling): Children ≥12 years and Adults: 2 sprays (100 mcg) in each nostril twice daily; if inadequate symptom control, may increase to 4 sprays (200 mcg) in each nostril twice daily (total daily dose: 800 mcg)

Rhinosinusitis treatment (acute, mild-to-moderate, uncomplicated): Canadian labeling (not in U.S. labeling): Children ≥12 years and Adults: 2 sprays (100 mcg) in each nostril twice daily; use beyond 15 days has not been studied.

Elderly: Refer to adult dosing.

Additional Information Complete prescribing information should be consulted for additional detail.

Dosage Forms Considerations

Nasonex 17 g bottles contain 120 sprays.

Dosage Forms Excipient information presented when available (limited, particularly for generics); consult specific product labeling.

Suspension, Nasal, as furoate:

Nasonex: 50 mcg/actuation (17 g) [contains benzalkonium chloride]

Dosage Forms: Canada Excipient information presented when available (limited, particularly for generics); consult specific product labeling.

Suspension, intranasal, as furoate [spray]:

Nasonex®: 50 mcg/spray [contains benzalkonium chloride; delivers 140 sprays]

Mometasone (Topical) (moe MET a sone)

Brand Names: U.S. Elocon

Brand Names: Canada Elocom; PMS-Mometasone; ratio-Mometasone; Taro-Mometasone

Index Terms Mometasone Furoate

Pharmacologic Category Corticosteroid, Topical

Additional Appendix Information

Topical Corticosteroids *on page 2299*

Use Relief of the inflammatory and pruritic manifestations of corticosteroid-responsive dermatoses (medium potency topical corticosteroid)

Pregnancy Risk Factor C

Dosage Topical: Apply sparingly, do not use occlusive dressings. Therapy should be discontinued when control is achieved; consider reassessment of diagnosis if no improvement is seen within 2 weeks.

Cream, ointment: Children ≥2 years, Adolescents, and Adults: Apply a thin film to affected area once daily; do not use in pediatric patients for longer than 3 weeks

Lotion: Children ≥12 years, Adolescents, and Adults: Apply a few drops to affected area once daily

Additional Information Complete prescribing information should be consulted for additional detail.

Dosage Forms Excipient information presented when available (limited, particularly for generics); consult specific product labeling.

Cream, External, as furoate:

Elocon: 0.1% (15 g, 45 g)

Elocon: 0.1% (15 g, 50 g) [contains soybean lecithin]

Generic: 0.1% (15 g, 45 g)

Lotion, External, as furoate:

Elocon: 0.1% (30 mL, 60 mL)

Ointment, External, as furoate:

Elocon: 0.1% (15 g, 45 g)

Generic: 0.1% (15 g, 45 g)

Solution, External, as furoate:

Generic: 0.1% (30 mL, 60 mL)

Mometasone and Formoterol

(moe MET a sone & for MOH te rol)

Brand Names: U.S. Dulera®

Brand Names: Canada Zenhale™

Index Terms Formoterol and Mometasone; Formoterol and Mometasone Furoate; Formoterol Fumarate Dihydrate and Mometasone

Pharmacologic Category $Beta_2$ Agonist, Long-Acting; $Beta_2$-Adrenergic Agonist, Long-Acting; Corticosteroid, Inhalant (Oral)

Use Maintenance treatment of asthma where combination therapy is indicated

Pregnancy Risk Factor C

Medication Guide Available Yes

Dosage Oral inhalation: Children ≥12 years and Adults: Asthma:

Previous therapy included inhaled low-dose corticosteroids: Canadian labeling (not in U.S. labeling): Mometasone 50 mcg/formoterol 5 mcg: Two inhalations twice daily. Maximum daily dose: 4 inhalations

Previous therapy included inhaled medium-dose corticosteroids: Mometasone 100 mcg/formoterol 5 mcg: Two inhalations twice daily. Consider the higher dose combination for patients not adequately controlled on the lower combination following 1-2 weeks of therapy. Maximum daily dose: 4 inhalations

Previous therapy included inhaled high-dose corticosteroids: Mometasone 200 mcg/formoterol 5 mcg: Two inhalations twice daily. Maximum daily dose: 4 inhalations

Dosage adjustment in renal impairment: No dosage adjustment provided in manufacturer's labeling (has not been studied).

Dosage adjustment in hepatic impairment: No dosage adjustment provided in manufacturer's labeling (has not been studied) However, mometasone exposure is increased with hepatic impairment.

Additional Information Complete prescribing information should be consulted for additional detail.

Dosage Forms Excipient information presented when available (limited, particularly for generics); consult specific product labeling.

Aerosol, for oral inhalation:

Dulera®: Mometasone furoate 100 mcg and formoterol fumarate dihydrate 5 mcg per inhalation (8.8 g) [60 metered actuations]

Dulera®: Mometasone furoate 100 mcg and formoterol fumarate dihydrate 5 mcg per inhalation (13 g) [120 metered actuations]

Dulera®: Mometasone furoate 200 mcg and formoterol fumarate dihydrate 5 mcg per inhalation (8.8 g) [60 metered actuations]

Dulera®: Mometasone furoate 200 mcg and formoterol fumarate dihydrate 5 mcg per inhalation (13 g) [120 metered actuations]

Dosage Forms: Canada Excipient information presented when available (limited, particularly for generics); consult specific product labeling.

Aerosol, for oral inhalation:

Zenhale™: Mometasone furoate 50 mcg and formoterol fumarate dihydrate 5 mcg per inhalation [120 metered actuations]

- **Mometasone Furoate** *see* Mometasone (Nasal) *on page 1394*
- **Mometasone Furoate** *see* Mometasone (Oral Inhalation) *on page 1392*
- **Mometasone Furoate** *see* Mometasone (Topical) *on page 1395*
- **MOM/Mineral Oil Emulsion** *see* Magnesium Hydroxide and Mineral Oil *on page 1261*
- **Monacolin K** *see* Lovastatin *on page 1250*
- **Monicure (Can)** *see* Fluconazole *on page 868*
- **Monistat® (Can)** *see* Miconazole (Topical) *on page 1358*
- **Monistat® 3 (Can)** *see* Miconazole (Topical) *on page 1358*
- **Monoclate-P®** *see* Antihemophilic Factor (Human) *on page 143*
- **Monoclonal Antibody 2C4** *see* Pertuzumab *on page 1625*
- **Monoclonal Antibody 5G1.1** *see* Eculizumab *on page 683*
- **Monoclonal Antibody ABX-EGF** *see* Panitumumab *on page 1561*
- **Monoclonal Antibody Anti-C5** *see* Eculizumab *on page 683*
- **Monoclonal Antibody Campath-1H** *see* Alemtuzumab *on page 66*
- **Monoclonal Antibody CD52** *see* Alemtuzumab *on page 66*
- **Monodox** *see* Doxycycline *on page 668*
- **Monoethanolamine** *see* Ethanolamine Oleate *on page 784*
- **MonoNessa** *see* Ethinyl Estradiol and Norgestimate *on page 795*
- **Mononine** *see* Factor IX (Human) *on page 825*
- **Monopril** *see* Fosinopril *on page 923*

Montelukast (mon te LOO kast)

Brand Names: U.S. Singulair

Brand Names: Canada Apo-Montelukast; Dom-Montelukast; Dom-Montelukast FC; Jamp-Montelukast; Montelukast Sodium Tablets; Mylan-Montelukast; PMS-Montelukast; PMS-Montelukast FC; Sandoz-Montelukast; Sandoz-Montelukast Granules; Singulair®; Teva-Montelukast

Index Terms Montelukast Sodium

Pharmacologic Category Leukotriene-Receptor Antagonist

Use Prophylaxis and chronic treatment of asthma; relief of symptoms of seasonal allergic rhinitis and perennial allergic rhinitis; prevention of exercise-induced bronchoconstriction

Unlabeled Use Urticaria (nonsteroidal anti-inflammatory drug–induced)

Pregnancy Risk Factor B

Pregnancy Considerations Adverse events have not been observed in animal reproduction studies. Structural defects have been reported in neonates exposed to montelukast *in utero*; however, a specific pattern and relationship to montelukast has not been established. Based on available data, an increased risk of teratogenic effects has not been observed with montelukast use in pregnancy (Bakhireva, 2007; Nelsen, 2012; Sarkar, 2009). Uncontrolled asthma is associated with adverse events on pregnancy (increased risk of perinatal mortality, pre-eclampsia, preterm birth, low birth weight infants). Montelukast may be considered for use in women who had a favorable response prior to becoming pregnant; however, initiating a leukotriene receptor antagonist during pregnancy is an alternative (but not preferred) treatment option for mild persistent asthma (NAEPP, 2005).

Breast-Feeding Considerations It is not known if montelukast is excreted into breast milk. The manufacturer recommends that caution be exercised when administering montelukast to nursing women.

Contraindications Hypersensitivity to montelukast or any component of the formulation

Warnings/Precautions Montelukast is not FDA approved for use in the reversal of bronchospasm in acute asthma attacks, including status asthmaticus; some studies, however, support its use as adjunctive therapy (Cylly, 2003; Ferreira, 2001; Harmancik, 2006). Appropriate rescue medication should be available. Montelukast treatment should continue during acute asthma exacerbation. When inhaled or systemic corticosteroid reduction is considered in patients initiating or receiving montelukast, appropriate clinical monitoring and a gradual dose reduction of the steroid are recommended.

Postmarketing reports of behavioral changes (eg, agitation, aggression, anxiety, attention deficit, depression, hallucinations, hostility, insomnia, irritability, restlessness, sleep disturbance, suicide ideation/behavior) have been noted in pediatric, adolescent, and adult patients. In a retrospective analysis performed by Merck, serious behavior-related events were rare (Philip, 2009a); assess patients for behavioral changes. Patients should be instructed to notify the prescriber if behavioral changes occur.

Potentially significant drug-drug interactions may exist, requiring dose or frequency adjustment, additional monitoring, and/or selection of alternative therapy. In rare cases, patients on therapy with montelukast may present with systemic eosinophilia, sometimes presenting with clinical features of vasculitis consistent with Churg-Strauss syndrome, a condition which is often treated with systemic corticosteroid therapy. Healthcare providers should be alert to eosinophilia, vasculitic rash, worsening pulmonary symptoms, cardiac complications, and/or neuropathy presenting in their patients. A causal association between montelukast and these underlying conditions has not been established. Montelukast will not interrupt bronchoconstrictor response to aspirin or other NSAIDs; aspirin sensitive asthmatics should continue to avoid these agents. The chewable tablet contains phenylalanine.

Adverse Reactions

Children ≥15 years and Adults:

>10%: Central nervous system: Headache (18%)

1% to 10%:

Central nervous system: Dizziness (2%), fatigue (2%), fever (2%)

Dermatologic: Skin rash (2%)

Gastrointestinal: Dyspepsia (2%), gastroenteritis (2%), toothache (2%)

Hepatic: Increased serum AST (2%), increased serum ALT (≥1%)

Neuromuscular & skeletal: Weakness (2%)

Respiratory: Nasal congestion (2%), cough (≥1%), epistaxis (≥1%), sinusitis (≥1%), upper respiratory tract infection (≥1%)

Children 2 to ≤14 years: ≥2%:

Central nervous system: Fever, headache

Dermatologic: Dermatitis, eczema, skin rash, urticaria

Gastrointestinal: Abdominal pain, diarrhea, dyspepsia, gastroenteritis, nausea

Infection: Influenza, varicella, viral infection

Ophthalmic: Conjunctivitis

Otic: Otalgia, otitis, otitis media

Respiratory: Laryngitis, pharyngitis, pneumonia, rhinorrhea, sinusitis, upper respiratory tract infection

Children 6-23 months: ≥2%: Respiratory: Cough, otitis media, pharyngitis, rhinitis, tonsillitis, upper respiratory tract infection, wheezing

Postmarketing and/or case reports (Limited to important or life-threatening): Anaphylaxis, angioedema, Churg-Strauss syndrome, depression, disorientation, eosinophilia (systemic), erythema multiforme, erythema nodosum, hallucination, hepatic eosinophilic infiltration, hepatitis (mixed pattern, hepatocellular, and cholestatic), hypersensitivity, insomnia, memory impairment, pancreatitis, paresthesia, seizure, somnambulism, Stevens-Johnson syndrome, suicidal ideation, suicidal tendencies, thrombocytopenia, toxic epidermal necrolysis, vasculitis

Drug Interactions

Metabolism/Transport Effects Substrate of CYP2C9 (major), CYP3A4 (major); **Note:** Assignment of Major/Minor substrate status based on clinically relevant drug interaction potential; **Inhibits** CYP2C8 (weak), CYP2C9 (weak)

Avoid Concomitant Use There are no known interactions where it is recommended to avoid concomitant use.

Increased Effect/Toxicity

The levels/effects of Montelukast may be increased by: CYP2C9 Inhibitors (Moderate); CYP2C9 Inhibitors (Strong); Mifepristone

Decreased Effect

The levels/effects of Montelukast may be decreased by: Bosentan; CYP2C9 Inducers (Strong); CYP3A4 Inducers (Strong); Dabrafenib; Deferasirox; Herbs (CYP3A4 Inducers); Mitotane; Peginterferon Alfa-2b; Tocilizumab

Ethanol/Nutrition/Herb Interactions Herb/Nutraceutical: St John's wort may decrease montelukast levels.

Storage/Stability Store at room temperature of 25°C (77°F); excursions permitted to 15°C to 30°C (59°F to 86°F). Store in original package. Protect from moisture and light. Granules must be used within 15 minutes of opening packet.

Mechanism of Action Selective leukotriene receptor antagonist that inhibits the cysteinyl leukotriene receptor. Cysteinyl leukotrienes and leukotriene receptor occupation have been correlated with the pathophysiology of asthma, including airway edema, smooth muscle contraction, and altered cellular activity associated with the inflammatory process, which contribute to the signs and symptoms of asthma. Cysteinyl leukotrienes are also released from the nasal mucosa following allergen exposure leading to symptoms associated with allergic rhinitis.

Pharmacodynamics/Kinetics

Duration: >24 hours

Absorption: Rapid

Distribution: V_d: 8-11 L

Protein binding, plasma: >99%

Metabolism: Extensively hepatic via CYP3A4, 2C8, and 2C9

Bioavailability: Tablet: 10 mg, Mean: 64%; Chewable tablet: 5 mg: 73% (63% when administered with a standard meal)

Half-life elimination: 2.7-5.5 hours; Mild-to-moderate hepatic impairment: 7.4 hours

Time to peak: Tablet: 10 mg: 3-4 hours; Chewable tablet: 2-2.5 hours; granules: 1-3 hours (fasting) and 3.5 to ~9 hours (with high-fat meal)

Excretion: Feces (86%); urine (<0.2%)

Dosage Note: Patients with **both** asthma and allergic rhinitis should take only one dose in the evening.

Asthma: Oral:

Children ≥1 to <2 years: 4 mg (oral granules) once daily (in the evening)

Children ≥2 to <6 years: 4 mg (chewable tablet or oral granules) once daily (in the evening)

Children ≥6 years and Adolescents <15 years: 5 mg (chewable tablet) once daily (in the evening)

Adolescents ≥15 years and Adults: 10 mg once daily (in the evening)

Bronchoconstriction, exercise-induced (prevention): Note: Additional doses should not be administered within 24 hours. Daily administration to prevent exercise-induced bronchoconstriction has not been evaluated. Patients receiving montelukast for another indication should not take an additional dose to prevent exercise-induced bronchoconstriction. Oral:

Children ≥6 years and Adolescents <15 years: 5 mg (chewable tablet) at least 2 hours prior to exercise

Adolescents ≥15 years and Adults: 10 mg once daily at least 2 hours prior to exercise

Perennial allergic rhinitis: Oral:

Children 6 months to <2 years: 4 mg (oral granules) once daily

Children ≥2 to <6 years: 4 mg (chewable tablet or oral granules) once daily

Children ≥6 years and Adolescents <15 years: 5 mg (chewable tablet) once daily

Adolescents ≥15 years and Adults: 10 mg once daily

Seasonal allergic rhinitis: Oral:

Children ≥2 to <6 years: 4 mg (chewable tablet or oral granules) once daily

Children ≥6 years and Adolescents <15 years: 5 mg (chewable tablet) once daily

Adolescents ≥15 years and Adults: 10 mg once daily

Urticaria (nonsteroidal anti-inflammatory drug–induced) (unlabeled use): Oral: Adolescents ≥15 years and Adults: 10 mg once daily (Pacor, 2001)

Dosage adjustment in renal impairment: No dosage adjustment necessary

Dosage adjustment in hepatic impairment:

Mild-to-moderate impairment: No dosage adjustment necessary.

Severe impairment: No dosage adjustment provided in manufacturer's labeling; has not been studied.

Dietary Considerations Some products may contain phenylalanine.

Administration When treating asthma, administer dose in the evening. Patients with allergic rhinitis may individualize administration time (morning or evening). Patients with **both** asthma and allergic rhinitis should take a single dose in the evening. May administer without regard to food or meals.

Granules: May be administered directly in the mouth, dissolved in 5 mL of baby formula or breast milk, or mixed with a spoonful of applesauce, carrots, rice, or ice cream; do not add to any other liquids or foods. Administer within 15 minutes of opening packet.

Monitoring Parameters Mood or behavior changes, including suicidal thinking/behavior

Dosage Forms Excipient information presented when available (limited, particularly for generics); consult specific product labeling.

Packet, Oral:
- Singulair: 4 mg (30 ea)
- Generic: 4 mg (1 ea, 30 ea)

Tablet, Oral:
- Singulair: 10 mg
- Generic: 10 mg

Tablet Chewable, Oral:
- Singulair: 4 mg [contains aspartame]
- Singulair: 4 mg [contains aspartame; cherry flavor]
- Singulair: 5 mg [contains aspartame]
- Singulair: 5 mg [contains aspartame; cherry flavor]
- Generic: 4 mg, 5 mg

◆ **Montelukast Sodium** *see* Montelukast *on page* 1396

◆ **Montelukast Sodium Tablets (Can)** *see* Montelukast *on page* 1396

◆ **Monurol** *see* Fosfomycin *on page* 922

- ◆ Monurol® (Can) *see* Fosfomycin *on page 922*
- ◆ 8-MOP *see* Methoxsalen (Systemic) *on page 1331*
- ◆ 8-Mop *see* Methoxsalen (Systemic) *on page 1331*
- ◆ Morgidox *see* Doxycycline *on page 668*
- ◆ Morning After Pill *see* Ethinyl Estradiol and Norgestrel *on page 797*

Morphine (Systemic) (MOR feen)

Brand Names: U.S. Astramorph; AVINza; Duramorph; Infumorph 200; Infumorph 500; Kadian; MS Contin

Brand Names: Canada Doloral; Kadian®; M-Eslon®; M.O.S.-SR®; M.O.S.-Sulfate®; M.O.S.® 10; M.O.S.® 20; M.O.S.® 30; Morphine Extra Forte Injection; Morphine Forte Injection; Morphine HP®; Morphine LP® Epidural; Morphine SR; Morphine-EPD; MS Contin SRT; MS Contin®; MS-IR®; Novo-Morphine SR; PMS-Morphine Sulfate SR; ratio-Morphine; ratio-Morphine SR; Sandoz-Morphine SR; Statex®; Teva-Morphine SR

Index Terms MS (error-prone abbreviation and should not be used); MSO_4 (error-prone abbreviation and should not be used); Roxanol

Pharmacologic Category Analgesic, Opioid

Additional Appendix Information

Dosing Considerations for the Critically-Ill Patient With Morbid Obesity *on page 2379*

Opioid Conversion Table *on page 2306*

Patient Information for Disposal of Unused Medications *on page 2393*

Use Relief of moderate-to-severe acute and chronic pain; relief of pain of myocardial infarction; relief of dyspnea of acute left ventricular failure and pulmonary edema; preanesthetic medication

Infumorph: Used in continuous microinfusion devices for intrathecal or epidural administration in treatment of intractable chronic pain

Extended release products: Moderate-to-severe pain when continuous, around-the-clock opioid analgesia is needed for an extended period of time

Note: Opioid tolerance: Use of morphine sulfate extended release tablets/capsules ≥90 mg, and/or the oral solution 100 mg/5 mL (20 mg/mL) should be reserved for opioid-tolerant patients (ie, already taking at least 60 mg daily of oral morphine equivalent for at least 1 week).

Pregnancy Risk Factor C

Pregnancy Considerations Adverse events have been observed in some animal reproduction studies. Morphine crosses the human placenta. The frequency of congenital malformations has not been reported to be greater than expected in children from mothers treated with morphine during pregnancy. However, following *in utero* exposure, infants may exhibit withdrawal, decreased brain volume (reversible), small size, decreased ventilatory response to CO_2, and increased risk of sudden infant death syndrome.

Morphine sulfate injection may be used for the management of pain during labor (ACOG, 2002); however, some manufacturers specifically contraindicate use of the injection during labor when a premature birth is anticipated. When used for pain relief during labor, opioids may temporarily affect the heart rate of the fetus. Morphine injection may also be used to treat pain following delivery (ACOG, 2002).

If chronic opioid exposure occurs in pregnancy, adverse events in the newborn (including withdrawal) may occur; monitoring of the neonate is recommended. The minimum effective dose should be used if opioids are needed (Chou, 2009). Neonatal abstinence syndrome following opioid exposure may present with autonomic (eg, fever, temperature instability), gastrointestinal (eg, diarrhea, vomiting, poor feeding/weight gain), or neurologic (eg, high-pitched crying, increased muscle tone, irritability, seizure, tremor) symptoms (Dow, 2012; Hudak, 2012).

Breast-Feeding Considerations Morphine concentrates in breast milk, with a milk to plasma AUC ratio of 2.5:1. Detectable serum levels of morphine can be found in infants following morphine administration to nursing mothers.

Parenteral opioids used during labor have the potential to interfere with a newborn's natural reflex to nurse within the first few hours after birth. Morphine is recommended as an analgesic in nursing women due to the limited amounts found in breast milk and poor oral bioavailability in nursing infants. Nursing infants exposed to large doses of opioids should be monitored for apnea and sedation (Montgomery, 2012).

Treatment of the mother with single doses of morphine is not expected to cause detrimental effects in nursing infants. Breast-feeding following chronic use or in neonates with hepatic or renal dysfunction may lead to higher levels of morphine in the infant and a risk of adverse effects (Spigset, 2000).

The manufacturers of extended release products note that due to the potential for serious adverse reactions in the nursing infant, a decision should be made whether to discontinue nursing or to discontinue the drug, taking into account the importance of treatment to the mother.

Medication Guide Available Yes

Contraindications Note: Some contraindications are product specific. For details, please see detailed product prescribing information.

Hypersensitivity to morphine sulfate or any component of the formulation; severe respiratory depression, acute or severe asthma (in an unmonitored setting or without resuscitative equipment); known or suspected paralytic ileus

Additional contraindication information (based on formulation):

Epidural/intrathecal:

Astramorph/PF™, Duramorph: Upper airway obstruction

Astramorph/PF™, Duramorph, Infumorph: Usual contraindications related to neuraxial analgesia apply (eg, presence of infection at infusion site, concomitant anticoagulant therapy, uncontrolled bleeding diathesis)

Extended release: GI obstruction

Immediate release tablets/solution: Hypercarbia

Injectable formulation: Heart failure due to chronic lung disease, cardiac arrhythmias; increased intracranial pressure, head injuries, brain tumors; acute alcoholism, deliriums tremens; seizure disorders; use during labor when a premature birth is anticipated

Suppository: Severe CNS depression; cardiac arrhythmias, heart failure due to chronic lung disease; increased intracranial or cerebrospinal pressure, head injuries, brain tumor; acute alcoholism, delirium tremens; seizure disorder; use after biliary tract surgery, suspected surgical abdomen, surgical anastomosis; concurrent use or within 2 weeks of MAO inhibitors

Warnings/Precautions An opioid-containing analgesic regimen should be tailored to each patient's needs and based upon the type of pain being treated (acute versus chronic), the route of administration, degree of tolerance for opioids (naive versus chronic user), age, weight, and medical condition. The optimal analgesic dose varies widely among patients. Doses should be titrated to pain relief/prevention. When used as an epidural injection, monitor for delayed sedation. **[U.S. Boxed Warning]: Healthcare provider should be alert to problems of**

abuse, misuse, and diversion. [U.S. Boxed Warning]: Extended release formulations, concentrated oral solution (100 mg/5 mL): Fatal overdose of morphine can result from accidental ingestion, especially in children.

[U.S. Boxed Warning]: Fatal respiratory depression may occur. Greatest risk during initiation and dose increases. Use with caution in patients (particularly elderly, debilitated) with impaired respiratory function (especially hypoxia or hypercapnia), COPD, other obstructive pulmonary disease, decreased respiratory reserve, kyphoscoliosis or other skeletal disorder which may alter respiratory function. Infants <3 months of age are more susceptible to respiratory depression, use with caution and generally in reduced doses in this age group.

Use caution in morbid obesity, adrenal insufficiency, prostatic hyperplasia, thyroid dysfunction, urinary stricture, renal impairment, or severe hepatic dysfunction and in patients with hypersensitivity reactions to other phenanthrene derivative opioid agonists (codeine, hydrocodone, hydromorphone, levorphanol, oxycodone, oxymorphone). Avoid use in patients with CNS depression or coma as these patients are susceptible to intracranial effects of CO_2 retention. Use with caution in patients with biliary tract dysfunction including acute pancreatitis as may cause constriction of sphincter of Oddi. May obscure diagnosis or clinical course of patients with acute abdominal conditions. Some preparations contain sulfites which may cause allergic reactions.

May cause CNS depression, which may impair physical or mental abilities; patients must be cautioned about performing tasks which require mental alertness (eg, operating machinery or driving). Potentially significant drug interactions may exist, requiring dose or frequency adjustment, additional monitoring, and/or selection of alternative therapy. Effects may be potentiated when used with other sedative drugs. **[U.S. Boxed Warning]: Do not administer Avinza® with alcoholic beverages or ethanol-containing prescription or nonprescription products, which may disrupt extended-release characteristic of product.**

May cause hypotension; use with caution in patients with hypovolemia, cardiovascular disease (including acute MI), circulatory shock, or drugs which may exaggerate hypotensive effects (including phenothiazines or general anesthetics). May cause orthostatic hypotension and syncope in ambulatory patients. Use with extreme caution in patients with head injury, intracranial lesions, or elevated intracranial pressure; exaggerated elevation of ICP may occur if respiratory drive is depressed and CO_2 retention occurs. Use with caution in patients with seizure disorders, may exacerbate pre-existing seizures. Tolerance or drug dependence may result from extended use. Concurrent use of agonist/antagonist analgesics may precipitate withdrawal symptoms and/or reduced analgesic efficacy in patients following prolonged therapy with mu opioid agonists. Abrupt discontinuation following prolonged use may also lead to withdrawal symptoms. Gradually wean dose over a short period of time. Elderly may be particularly susceptible to adverse effects. Use epidural/intrathecal formulations with extreme caution in the elderly. After chronic maternal exposure to opioids, neonatal withdrawal syndrome may occur in the newborn; monitor neonate closely. Signs and symptoms include irritability, hyperactivity and abnormal sleep pattern, high pitched cry, tremor, vomiting, diarrhea and failure to gain weight. Onset, duration and severity depend on the drug used, duration of use, maternal dose, and rate of drug elimination by the newborn. Opioid withdrawal syndrome in the neonate, unlike in adults, may be life-threatening and should be treated according to protocols developed by neonatology experts.

[U.S. Boxed Warning]: Extended release dosage forms should not be crushed, dissolved, or chewed. Extended release products are not intended for "as needed (PRN)" use. Avinza® capsules contain fumaric acid; dangerous quantities of fumaric acid may be ingested when >1600 mg/day is used; serious renal toxicity may occur above the maximum dose. **Extended release products are not interchangeable;** when determining a generic equivalent or switching from one extended release product to another, review pharmacokinetic properties.

Highly concentrated oral solutions: **[U.S. Boxed Warning]: Check doses carefully when using highly concentrated oral solutions. The 100 mg/5 mL (20 mg/mL) concentration is indicated for use in opioid-tolerant patients only.**

Injections: Products are designed for administration by specific routes (ie, I.V., intrathecal, epidural). Use caution when prescribing, dispensing, or administering to use formulations only by intended route(s).

Astramorph/PF™, Duramorph, Infumorph: **[U.S. Boxed Warning]: Due to the risk of severe and/or sustained cardiopulmonary depressant effects, must be administered in a fully equipped room for resuscitation and staffed environment.** Naloxone injection should be immediately available. Patient should remain in this environment for at least 24 hours following the initial dose. **[U.S. Boxed Warning]: Accidental dermal exposure to Astramorph/PF™, Duramorph, Infumorph should be rinsed with water. Contaminated clothing should be removed.** For patients receiving Infumorph via microinfusion device, patient may be observed, as appropriate, for the first several days after catheter implantation. Thoracic epidural administration has been shown to dramatically increase the risk of early and late respiratory depression.

[U.S. Boxed Warning]: Improper or erroneous substitution of Infumorph for regular Duramorph is likely to result in serious overdosage, leading to seizures, respiratory depression and possibly a fatal outcome. Infumorph should only be used in microinfusion devices; not for I.V., I.M., or SubQ administration or for single-dose administration. Monitor closely, especially in the first 24 hours. Inflammatory masses (eg, granulomas), some resulting in severe neurologic impairment have occurred when receiving Infumorph via indwelling intrathecal catheter; monitor carefully for new neurologic signs/symptoms. **[U.S. Boxed Warning]: Intrathecal dosage is usually 1/10 (one-tenth) that of epidural dosage.**

Adverse Reactions Note: Individual patient differences are unpredictable, and percentage may differ in acute pain (surgical) treatment. Reactions may be dose, formulation, and/or route dependent.

Frequency not defined:

- Cardiovascular: Circulatory depression, flushing, shock
- Central nervous system: Dysphonia, physical and psychological dependence, sedation
- Endocrine & metabolic: Antidiuretic hormone release, hypogonadism
- Neuromuscular & skeletal: Bone mineral density decreased

>10%:

- Cardiovascular: Bradycardia, hypotension
- Central nervous system: Drowsiness (9% to 48%; tolerance usually develops to drowsiness with regular dosing for 1-2 weeks), dizziness (6% to 20%), fever (<3% to >10%), confusion, headache (following epidural or intrathecal use)
- Dermatologic: Pruritus (may be dose related)

Gastrointestinal: Xerostomia (78%), constipation (9% to 40%; tolerance develops very slowly if at all), nausea (7% to 28%; tolerance usually develops to nausea and vomiting with chronic use), vomiting
Genitourinary: Urinary retention (16%; may be prolonged, up to 20 hours, following epidural or intrathecal use)
Hematologic: Anemia (following intrathecal use)
Local: Pain at injection site
Neuromuscular & skeletal: Weakness
Respiratory: Oxygen saturation decreased
Miscellaneous: Histamine release

1% to 10%:
Cardiovascular: Atrial fibrillation (<3%), chest pain (<3%), edema, hypertension, palpitation, peripheral edema, syncope, tachycardia, vasodilation
Central nervous system: Amnesia, agitation, anxiety, apathy, apprehension, ataxia, chills, coma, delirium, depression, dream abnormalities, euphoria, false sense of well being, hallucination, hypoesthesia, insomnia, lethargy, malaise, nervousness, restlessness, seizure, slurred speech, somnolence, vertigo
Dermatologic: Dry skin, rash, urticaria
Endocrine & metabolic: Gynecomastia (<3%), hypokalemia, hyponatremia, libido decreased
Gastrointestinal: Abdominal distension, abdominal pain, anorexia, biliary colic, diarrhea, dyspepsia, dysphagia, flatulence, gastroenteritis, GERD, GI irritation, paralytic ileus, rectal disorder, taste perversion, weight loss
Genitourinary: Bladder spasm, dysuria, ejaculation abnormal, impotence, urination decreased
Hematologic: Leukopenia (<3%), thrombocytopenia (<3%), hematocrit decreased
Hepatic: Liver function tests increased
Neuromuscular & skeletal: Arthralgia, back pain, bone pain, foot drop, gait abnormalities, paresthesia, rigors, skeletal muscle rigidity, tremor
Ocular: Amblyopia, conjunctivitis, eye pain, vision problems/disturbance
Renal: Oliguria
Respiratory: Asthma, atelectasis, dyspnea, hiccups, hypercapnia, hypoxia, pulmonary edema (noncardiogenic), respiratory depression, rhinitis
Miscellaneous: Diaphoresis, flu-like syndrome, infection, thirst, voice alteration, withdrawal syndrome

<1% (Limited to important or life-threatening): Amenorrhea, anaphylaxis, apnea, biliary tract spasm, blurred vision, bronchospasm, cardiac arrest, cough reflex decreased, dehydration, diplopia, disorientation, hemorrhagic urticaria, intestinal obstruction, intracranial pressure increased, laryngospasm, menstrual irregularities, miosis, myoclonus, nystagmus, paradoxical CNS stimulation, respiratory arrest, sepsis, urinary tract spasm, thermal dysregulation, toxic psychoses

Drug Interactions

Metabolism/Transport Effects Substrate of CYP2D6 (minor), P-glycoprotein; **Note:** Assignment of Major/Minor substrate status based on clinically relevant drug interaction potential

Avoid Concomitant Use

Avoid concomitant use of Morphine (Systemic) with any of the following: Azelastine (Nasal); MAO Inhibitors; Paraldehyde

Increased Effect/Toxicity

Morphine (Systemic) may increase the levels/effects of: Alcohol (Ethyl); Alvimopan; Azelastine (Nasal); CNS Depressants; Desmopressin; Diuretics; Hydrocodone; Metyrosine; Mirtazapine; Paraldehyde; Pramipexole; ROPINIRole; Rotigotine; Selective Serotonin Reuptake Inhibitors; Zolpidem

The levels/effects of Morphine (Systemic) may be increased by: Amphetamines; Anticholinergics; Antipsychotic Agents (Phenothiazines); Brimonidine (Topical); Cannabinoids; Doxylamine; Droperidol; HydrOXYzine; Magnesium Sulfate; MAO Inhibitors; Perampanel; P-glycoprotein/ABCB1 Inhibitors; Sodium Oxybate; Succinylcholine; Tapentadol

Decreased Effect

Morphine (Systemic) may decrease the levels/effects of: Clopidogrel; Pegvisomant

The levels/effects of Morphine (Systemic) may be decreased by: Ammonium Chloride; Mixed Agonist / Antagonist Opioids; Peginterferon Alfa-2b; P-glycoprotein/ABCB1 Inducers; Rifamycin Derivatives

Ethanol/Nutrition/Herb Interactions

Ethanol: Alcoholic beverages or ethanol-containing products may disrupt extended release formulation resulting in rapid release of entire morphine dose. Ethanol may also increase CNS depression. Management: Avoid alcohol. **Do not administer Avinza® with alcoholic beverages or ethanol-containing prescription or nonprescription products.**

Food: Administration of oral morphine solution with food may increase bioavailability (ie, a report of 34% increase in morphine AUC when morphine oral solution followed a high-fat meal). The bioavailability of Avinza®, MS Contin®, or Kadian® does not appear to be affected by food. Management: Take consistently with or without meals.

Herb/Nutraceutical: Gotu kola, valerian, and kava kava may increase CNS depression. Management: Avoid gotu kola, valerian, and kava kava.

Storage/Stability

Capsule, extended release: Store at 25°C (77°F); excursions permitted to 15°C to 30°C (59°F to 86°F). Protect from light and moisture.

Injection: Store at controlled room temperature of 20°C to 25°C (68°F to 77°F); do not freeze. Protect from light. Degradation depends on pH and presence of oxygen; relatively stable in pH ≤4; darkening of solutions indicate degradation.

Astramorph/PF™, Duramorph, Infumorph: Store in carton until use at controlled room temperature of 20°C to 25°C (68°F to 77°F); excursions permitted to 15°C to 30°C (59°F to 86°F); do not freeze; do not heat-sterilize. Contains no preservative or antioxidant. Protect from light.

Oral solution: Store at controlled room temperature of 15°C to 30°C (59°F to 86°F); do not freeze. Protect from moisture.

Suppositories: Store below controlled room temperature 25°C (77°F).

Tablet, extended release: Store at controlled room temperature of 25°C (77°F); excursions permitted to 15°C to 30°C (59°F to 86°F).

Tablet, immediate release: Store at controlled room temperature of 15°C to 30°C (59°F to 86°F). Protect from moisture.

Mechanism of Action Binds to opioid receptors in the CNS, causing inhibition of ascending pain pathways, altering the perception of and response to pain; produces generalized CNS depression

Pharmacodynamics/Kinetics

Onset of action (patient dependent; dosing must be individualized): Oral (immediate release): ~30 minutes; I.V.: 5-10 minutes

Duration (patient dependent; dosing must be individualized): Pain relief:
Immediate release formulations: 4 hours
Extended release capsule and tablet: 8-24 hours (formulation dependent)

Absorption: Variable

Distribution: V_d: 1-6 L/kg; binds to opioid receptors in the CNS and periphery (eg, GI tract)

Protein binding: 20% to 35%

Metabolism: Hepatic via conjugation with glucuronic acid primarily to morphine-6-glucuronide (active analgesic) morphine-3-glucuronide (inactive as analgesic); minor metabolites include morphine-3-6-diglucuronide; other minor metabolites include normorphine (active) and morphine 3-ethereal sulfate

Bioavailability: Oral: 17% to 33% (first-pass effect limits oral bioavailability; oral:parenteral effectiveness reportedly varies from 1:6 in opioid naive patients to 1:3 with chronic use)

Half-life elimination: Adults: Immediate release forms: 2-4 hours; Avinza® ~24 hours; Kadian®:11-13 hours

Time to peak, plasma: Avinza®: 30 minutes (maintained for 24 hours); Kadian®: ~10 hours

Excretion: Urine (primarily as morphine-3-glucuronide, ~2% to 12% excreted unchanged); feces (~7% to 10%). It has been suggested that accumulation of morphine-6-glucuronide might cause toxicity with renal insufficiency. All of the metabolites (ie, morphine-3-glucuronide, morphine-6-glucuronide, and normorphine) have been suggested as possible causes of neurotoxicity (eg, myoclonus).

Dosage These are guidelines and do not represent the doses that may be required in all patients. Doses and dosage intervals should be titrated to pain relief/prevention.

Children >6 months and <50 kg: *Acute pain (moderate-to-severe):*

Oral (immediate release formulations): 0.15-0.3 mg/kg every 3-4 hours as needed. **Note:** The American Pain Society recommends an initial dose of 0.3 mg/kg for children with severe pain (American Pain Society [APS], 2008)

I.M., SubQ: 0.1-0.2 mg/kg; **Note:** Repeated SubQ administration causes local tissue irritation, pain, and induration. The use of I.M. injections is no longer recommended especially for repeated administration due to painful administration, variable absorption and lag time to peak effect.

I.V.: 0.05-0.3 mg/kg every 3-4 hours as needed, not to exceed 10 mg per dose

Continuous infusion: Initial: 10-30 **mcg/kg/hour**; titrate as needed to control pain

Patient-controlled analgesia (PCA) (APS, 2008): **Note:** Opioid-naive: Consider lower end of dosing range:

Usual concentration: 1 mg/mL

Demand dose: Usual: 0.02 mg/kg/dose; range: 0.01-0.03 mg/kg/dose

Lockout interval: 8-10 minutes

Usual basal rate: 0-0.03 mg/kg/hour

Adults:

Acute pain (moderate-to-severe):

Oral (immediate release formulations): Opioid-naive: Initial: **Note:** Usual dosage range: 10-30 mg every 4 hours as needed. Patients with prior opioid exposure may require higher initial doses.

Solution: 10-20 mg every 4 hours as needed

Tablet: 15-30 mg every 4 hours as needed

I.M., SubQ: **Note:** Repeated SubQ administration causes local tissue irritation, pain, and induration. The use of I.M. injections is no longer recommended especially for repeated administration due to painful administration, variable absorption and lag time to peak effect; other routes are more reliable and less painful (APS, 2008).

Initial: Opioid-naive: 5-10 mg every 4 hours as needed; usual dosage range: 5-15 mg every 4 hours as needed. Patients with prior opioid exposure may require higher initial doses.

I.V.: Initial: Opioid-naive: 2.5-5 mg every 3-4 hours; patients with prior opioid exposure may require higher initial doses. **Note:** Administration of 2-3 mg every 5 minutes until pain relief or if associated sedation, oxygen saturation <95%, or serious adverse event occurs may be appropriate in treating acute moderate-to-severe pain in settings such as the immediate post-operative period or the emergency department (Aubrun, 2012; Lvovschi, 2008); dose reduction in the immediate postoperative period (postanesthesia care unit) in the elderly is usually not necessary (Aubrun, 2002). A maximum cumulative dose (eg, 10 mg) prompting reevaluation of continued morphine use and/or dose should be included as part of any medication order intended for short-term use (eg, PACU orders). Refer to institution-specific protocols as appropriate.

Acute myocardial infarction, analgesia (unlabeled use): Initial management: 4-8 mg (lower doses in the elderly); subsequently may give 2-8 mg every 5-15 minutes as needed (O'Gara, 2012)

Critically-ill patients, analgesia (unlabeled dose): 2-4 mg every 1-2 hours **or** 4-8 mg every 3-4 hours as needed (Barr, 2013)

I.V., SubQ continuous infusion: 0.8-10 mg/hour; usual range: Up to 80 mg/hour. **Note:** May administer a loading dose (amount administered should depend on severity of pain) prior to initiating the infusion. A continuous (basal) infusion is not recommended in an opioid-naive patient (ISMP, 2009)

Continuous infusion for critically-ill patients: Usual dosage range: 2-30 mg/hour (Barr, 2013)

Patient-controlled analgesia (PCA) (APS, 2008): **Note:** In opioid-naive patients, consider lower end of dosing range:

Usual concentration: 1 mg/mL

Demand dose: Usual: 1 mg; range: 0.5-2.5 mg

Lockout interval: 5-10 minutes

Epidural: Pain management: **Note: Must be preservative-free.** Administer with extreme caution and in reduced dosage to geriatric or debilitated patients. Vigilant monitoring is particularly important in these patients.

Single-dose: **Lumbar region:** Astramorph/PF™, Duramorph: 30-100 mcg/kg (optimal range: 2.5-3.75 mg; may depend upon patient comorbidities; Bujedo, 2012; Sultan, 2011)

Continuous infusion (may be combined with bupivacaine): 0.2-0.4 mg/hour (Bujedo, 2012)

Continuous microinfusion (Infumorph):

Opioid-naive: Initial: 3.5-7.5 mg over 24 hours

Opioid-tolerant: Initial: 4.5-10 mg over 24 hours, titrate to effect; usual maximum is ~30 mg per 24 hours

Intrathecal (I.T.): **Note: Must be preservative-free.** Administer with extreme caution and in reduced dosage to geriatric or debilitated patients. I.T. dose is usually 1/10 (one-tenth) that of epidural dosage.

Opioid-naive: Single dose: Lumbar region: Astramorph/PF™, Duramorph: 0.1-0.3 mg (may provide adequate relief for up to 24 hours; APS, 2008); repeat doses are **not** recommended. If pain recurs within 24 hours of administration, use of an alternate route of administration is recommended. **Note:** Although product labeling recommends doses up to 1 mg, an analgesic ceiling exists with doses >0.3 mg and the risk of respiratory depression is higher with doses >0.3 mg (Rathmell, 2005).

Continuous microinfusion (Infumorph): Lumbar region: After initial in-hospital evaluation of response to single-dose injections (Astramorph/PF™, Duramorph) the initial dose of Infumorph is 0.2-1 mg over 24 hours

Opioid-tolerant: Continuous microinfusion (Infumorph): Lumbar region: Dosage range: 1-10 mg over 24 hours, titrate to effect; usual maximum is ~20 mg over 24 hours

Rectal: 10-20 mg every 3-4 hours

Chronic pain: **Note:** Patients taking opioids chronically may become tolerant and require doses higher than the usual dosage range to maintain the desired effect. Tolerance can be managed by appropriate dose titration. There is no optimal or maximal dose for morphine in chronic pain. The appropriate dose is one that relieves pain throughout its dosing interval without causing unmanageable side effects. Consider total daily dose, potency, prior opioid use, degree of opioid experience and tolerance, conversion from previous opioid (including opioid formulation), patient's general condition, concurrent medications, and type and severity of pain during prescribing process.

Oral (extended release formulations): A patient's morphine requirement should be established using immediate release formulations. Conversion to long-acting products may be considered when chronic, continuous treatment is required. Higher dosages should be reserved for use only in opioid-tolerant patients.

Capsules, extended release (Avinza®): Daily dose administered once daily (for best results, administer at same time each day)

Opioid-naive: Initial: 30 mg once daily; adjust in increments ≤30 mg daily every 4 days

Conversion from other oral morphine formulations to Avinza®: Total daily morphine dose given as once daily. The first dose of Avinza® may be taken with the last dose of the immediate release morphine. Maximum: 1600 mg daily due to fumaric acid content.

Capsules, extended release (Kadian®): **Note:** Not intended for use as an initial opioid in the management of pain; use immediate release formulations before initiation. Total daily oral morphine dose may be either administered once daily or in 2 divided doses daily (every 12 hours). The first dose of Kadian® may be taken with the last dose of the immediate release morphine.

Tablets, extended release (MS Contin®): Daily dose divided and administered every 8 or every 12 hours

Conversion from parenteral morphine or other opioids to extended release formulations: Substantial interpatient variability exists in relative potency. Therefore, it is safer to underestimate a patient's daily oral morphine requirement and provide breakthrough pain relief with immediate release morphine than to overestimate requirements. Consider the parenteral to oral morphine ratio or other oral or parenteral opioids to oral morphine conversions.

Elderly or debilitated patients: Use with caution; may require dose reduction.

Dosing adjustment in renal impairment:

Cl_{cr} 10-50 mL/minute: Children and Adults: Administer at 75% of normal dose.

Cl_{cr} <10 mL/minute: Children and Adults: Administer at 50% of normal dose.

Intermittent HD:

Children: Administer 50% of normal dose.

Adults: No dosage adjustment necessary.

Peritoneal dialysis: Children: Administer 50% of normal dose.

CRRT: Children and Adults: Administer 75% of normal dose, titrate.

Dosing adjustment/comments in hepatic disease: No dosage adjustment provided in manufacturer's labeling. Pharmacokinetics unchanged in mild liver disease; substantial extrahepatic metabolism may occur. In cirrhosis, increases in half-life and AUC suggest dosage adjustment required.

Dietary Considerations Morphine may cause GI upset; take with food if GI upset occurs. Be consistent when taking morphine with or without meals.

Usual Infusion Concentrations: Pediatric I.V. infusion: 0.1 mg/mL, 0.5 mg/mL, **or** 1 mg/mL

Usual Infusion Concentrations: Adult I.V. infusion: 1 mg/mL

Administration

Oral: Do not crush, chew, or dissolve extended release drug product; swallow whole. Kadian® and Avinza® can be opened and sprinkled on applesauce and eaten immediately without chewing; do not crush, dissolve, or chew the beads as it can result in a rapid release of a potentially fatal dose of morphine. Ensure all pellets have been swallowed by rinsing mouth. Contents of Kadian® capsules may be opened and sprinkled over 10 mL water and flushed through prewetted 16F gastrostomy tube; do not administer Kadian® through gastric/nasogastric tubes.

I.V.: When giving morphine I.V. push, it is best to first dilute with sterile water or NS for a final concentration of 1-2 mg/mL and then administer slowly over 4-5 minutes.

Epidural, intrathecal: Use preservative-free solutions for intrathecal or epidural use. Infumorph may **only** be used as a continuous microinfusion via catheter.

Monitoring Parameters Assess efficacy of pain control, vital signs, and mental status; signs of drug abuse, addiction, or diversion

Astramorph/PF™, Duramorph, Infumorph: Patients should be observed in a fully-equipped and staffed environment for at least 24 hours following initiation, and as appropriate for the first several days after catheter implantation. Naloxone injection should be immediately available. Patient should remain in this environment for at least 24 hours following the initial dose. For patients receiving Infumorph via microinfusion device, patient may be observed, as appropriate, for the first several days after catheter implantation.

Note: Also refer to institution specific protocols as appropriate.

Test Interactions Some quinolones may produce a false-positive urine screening result for opioids using commercially-available immunoassay kits. This has been demonstrated most consistently for levofloxacin and ofloxacin, but other quinolones have shown cross-reactivity in certain assay kits. Confirmation of positive opioid screens by more specific methods should be considered.

Dosage Forms Excipient information presented when available (limited, particularly for generics); consult specific product labeling. [DSC] = Discontinued product

Capsule Extended Release 24 Hour, Oral, as sulfate:

AVINza: 30 mg [contains fd&c yellow #10 (quinoline yellow), fumaric acid]

AVINza: 45 mg [contains fd&c blue #2 (indigotine)]

AVINza: 60 mg [contains fumaric acid]

AVINza: 75 mg

AVINza: 90 mg [contains fd&c red #40, fumaric acid]

AVINza: 120 mg [contains brilliant blue fcf (fd&c blue #1), fumaric acid]

Kadian: 10 mg [contains brilliant blue fcf (fd&c blue #1)]

Kadian: 20 mg [contains fd&c yellow #10 (quinoline yellow)]

Kadian: 30 mg [contains brilliant blue fcf (fd&c blue #1)]

Kadian: 40 mg [contains brilliant blue fcf (fd&c blue #1), fd&c yellow #10 (quinoline yellow)]

Kadian: 50 mg, 60 mg [contains brilliant blue fcf (fd&c blue #1), fd&c red #40]

Kadian: 70 mg [contains brilliant blue fcf (fd&c blue #1)]

Kadian: 80 mg [contains brilliant blue fcf (fd&c blue #1), fd&c red #40, fd&c yellow #6 (sunset yellow)]

Kadian: 100 mg [contains brilliant blue fcf (fd&c blue #1), fd&c yellow #10 (quinoline yellow)]

Kadian: 130 mg [contains brilliant blue fcf (fd&c blue #1), fd&c red #40, fd&c yellow #6 (sunset yellow)]

Kadian: 150 mg [contains brilliant blue fcf (fd&c blue #1), fd&c yellow #10 (quinoline yellow)]

Kadian: 200 mg
Generic: 10 mg, 20 mg, 30 mg, 50 mg, 60 mg, 80 mg, 100 mg
Device, Intramuscular, as sulfate:
Generic: 10 mg/0.7 mL (0.7 mL)
Solution, Injection, as sulfate:
Astramorph: 1 mg/mL (10 mL)
Generic: 2 mg/mL (1 mL [DSC]); 4 mg/mL (1 mL); 5 mg/mL (1 mL); 8 mg/mL (1 mL); 10 mg/mL (1 mL, 10 mL); 15 mg/mL (1 mL, 20 mL)
Solution, Injection, as sulfate [preservative free]:
Astramorph: 0.5 mg/mL (2 mL, 10 mL); 1 mg/mL (2 mL)
Duramorph: 0.5 mg/mL (10 mL); 1 mg/mL (10 mL)
Infumorph 200: 200 MG/20ML (10 mg/mL) (20 mL) [antioxidant free]
Infumorph 500: 500 MG/20ML (25 mg/mL) (20 mL) [antioxidant free]
Generic: 0.5 mg/mL (10 mL); 1 mg/mL (10 mL)
Solution, Intravenous, as sulfate:
Generic: 1 mg/mL (10 mL, 30 mL, 250 mL); 25 mg/mL (4 mL, 10 mL); 50 mg/mL (20 mL, 50 mL)
Solution, Intravenous, as sulfate [preservative free]:
Generic: 1 mg/mL (30 mL); 2 mg/mL (1 mL); 4 mg/mL (1 mL); 150 mg/30 mL (30 mL); 8 mg/mL (1 mL); 10 mg/mL (1 mL); 15 mg/mL (1 mL); 25 mg/mL (10 mL)
Solution, Oral, as sulfate:
Generic: 10 mg/5 mL (5 mL, 100 mL, 500 mL); 20 mg/5 mL (5 mL, 100 mL, 500 mL); 20 mg/mL (15 mL, 30 mL, 120 mL, 240 mL); 100 mg/5 mL (30 mL, 120 mL)
Suppository, Rectal, as sulfate:
Generic: 5 mg (12 ea); 10 mg (12 ea); 20 mg (12 ea); 30 mg (12 ea)
Tablet, Oral, as sulfate:
Generic: 15 mg, 30 mg
Tablet Extended Release, Oral, as sulfate:
MS Contin: 15 mg, 30 mg, 60 mg, 100 mg, 200 mg
Generic: 15 mg, 30 mg, 60 mg, 100 mg, 200 mg

Dosage Forms: Canada Excipient information presented when available (limited, particularly for generics); consult specific product labeling.
Solution, oral, as hydrochloride:
Doloral: 1 mg/mL (10 mL, 250 mL, 500 mL); 5 mg/mL (10 mL, 250 mL, 500 mL)

Controlled Substance C-II

Morphine (Liposomal) (MOR feen)

Brand Names: U.S. DepoDur

Index Terms Extended Release Epidural Morphine; MS (error-prone abbreviation and should not be used); MSO_4 (error-prone abbreviation and should not be used)

Pharmacologic Category Analgesic, Opioid

Additional Appendix Information
Opioid Conversion Table *on page 2306*

Use Epidural (lumbar) single-dose management of surgical pain

Pregnancy Risk Factor C

Dosage Epidural:
Adults: Surgical anesthesia: Single-dose (extended release, DepoDur®): Lumbar epidural only; not recommended in patients <18 years of age:
Cesarean section: 10 mg (after clamping umbilical cord)
Lower abdominal/pelvic surgery: 10-15 mg
Major orthopedic surgery of lower extremity: 15 mg
To minimize the pharmacokinetic interaction resulting in higher peak serum concentrations of morphine, administer the test dose of the local anesthetic at least 15 minutes prior to administration. Use of DepoDur® with epidural local anesthetics has not been studied. Other medications should not be administered into the epidural space for at least 48 hours after administration.
Note: Some patients may benefit from a 20 mg dose; however, the incidence of adverse effects may be increased.
Elderly or debilitated patients: Use with caution; may require dose reduction

Dosage adjustment in renal impairment: No dosage adjustment necessary.

Dosage adjustment/comments in hepatic disease: No dosage adjustment necessary.

Additional Information Complete prescribing information should be consulted for additional detail.

Dosage Forms Excipient information presented when available (limited, particularly for generics); consult specific product labeling.
Suspension, Epidural, as sulfate:
DepoDur: 10 mg/mL (1 mL); 15 mg/1.5 mL (1.5 mL)

Controlled Substance C-II

- **Morphine-EPD (Can)** *see* Morphine (Systemic) *on page 1398*
- **Morphine Extra Forte Injection (Can)** *see* Morphine (Systemic) *on page 1398*
- **Morphine Forte Injection (Can)** *see* Morphine (Systemic) *on page 1398*
- **Morphine HP® (Can)** *see* Morphine (Systemic) *on page 1398*
- **Morphine LP® Epidural (Can)** *see* Morphine (Systemic) *on page 1398*
- **Morphine SR (Can)** *see* Morphine (Systemic) *on page 1398*

Morrhuate Sodium (MOR yoo ate SOW dee um)

Brand Names: U.S. Scleromate

Pharmacologic Category Sclerosing Agent

Use Treatment of small, uncomplicated varicose veins of the lower extremities

Pregnancy Risk Factor C

Dosage I.V.: Adults:
Note: A test dose of 0.25-1 mL of a 5% injection may be given (into a varicosity) 24 hours before full-dose treatment.
Full-dose treatment: 50-250 mg, depending on the size and degree of varicosity (50-100 mg for small or medium veins, 150-250 mg for large veins); may be given as multiple injections at one time or in single doses.

Dosage adjustment in renal impairment: No dosage adjustment provided in manufacturer's labeling.
Dosage adjustment in hepatic impairment: No dosage adjustment provided in manufacturer's labeling.

Additional Information Complete prescribing information should be consulted for additional detail.

Dosage Forms Excipient information presented when available (limited, particularly for generics); consult specific product labeling.
Solution, Intravenous:
Scleromate: 5% (30 mL)
Generic: 5% (30 mL)

- **M.O.S.® 10 (Can)** *see* Morphine (Systemic) *on page 1398*
- **M.O.S.® 20 (Can)** *see* Morphine (Systemic) *on page 1398*
- **M.O.S.® 30 (Can)** *see* Morphine (Systemic) *on page 1398*
- **M.O.S.-SR® (Can)** *see* Morphine (Systemic) *on page 1398*
- **M.O.S.-Sulfate® (Can)** *see* Morphine (Systemic) *on page 1398*

- ◆ Motion Sickness [OTC] *see* DimenhyDRINATE *on page 616*
- ◆ Motrin [OTC] *see* Ibuprofen *on page 1032*
- ◆ Motrin® (Children's) (Can) *see* Ibuprofen *on page 1032*
- ◆ Motrin IB [OTC] *see* Ibuprofen *on page 1032*
- ◆ Motrin® IB (Can) *see* Ibuprofen *on page 1032*
- ◆ Motrin Infants Drops [OTC] *see* Ibuprofen *on page 1032*
- ◆ Motrin Junior Strength [OTC] *see* Ibuprofen *on page 1032*
- ◆ MoviPrep *see* Polyethylene Glycol-Electrolyte Solution *on page 1669*
- ◆ Moxatag *see* Amoxicillin *on page 116*
- ◆ Moxeza *see* Moxifloxacin (Ophthalmic) *on page 1406*

Moxifloxacin (Systemic) (moxs i FLOKS a sin)

Brand Names: U.S. Avelox; Avelox ABC Pack

Brand Names: Canada Avelox; Avelox I.V.

Index Terms Moxifloxacin Hydrochloride

Pharmacologic Category Antibiotic, Fluoroquinolone; Antibiotic, Respiratory Fluoroquinolone

Additional Appendix Information

Antibiotic Treatment of Adults With Infective Endocarditis *on page 2355*

Use Treatment of mild-to-moderate community-acquired pneumonia, including multidrug-resistant *Streptococcus pneumoniae* (MDRSP); acute bacterial exacerbation of chronic bronchitis; acute bacterial rhinosinusitis (ABRS); complicated and uncomplicated skin and skin structure infections; complicated intra-abdominal infections

Unlabeled Use Treatment of *Legionella* pneumonia; treatment of mild-to-moderate community-acquired pneumonia (CAP), including multidrug-resistant *Streptococcus pneumoniae* (MDRSP) in adolescents with skeletal maturity; tuberculosis (second-line therapy); surgical (perioperative) prophylaxis

Pregnancy Risk Factor C

Pregnancy Considerations Adverse events have been observed in some animal studies; therefore, the manufacturer classifies moxifloxacin as pregnancy category C. Quinolone exposure during human pregnancy has been reported with other agents (see Ciprofloxacin [Systemic], Ofloxacin [Systemic], and Norfloxacin monographs). To date, no specific teratogenic effect or increased pregnancy risk has been identified; however, because of concerns of cartilage damage in immature animals exposed to quinolones and the limited moxifloxacin specific data, moxifloxacin should only be used during pregnancy if a safer option is not available.

Breast-Feeding Considerations It is not known if moxifloxacin is excreted into breast milk. Breast-feeding is not recommended by the manufacturer. Although there is no information on the use of moxifloxacin during breast-feeding, other quinolones are considered compatible. Non-dose-related effects could include modification of bowel flora.

Medication Guide Available Yes

Contraindications Hypersensitivity to moxifloxacin, other quinolone antibiotics, or any component of the formulation

Warnings/Precautions **[U.S. Boxed Warning]: There have been reports of tendon inflammation and/or rupture with quinolone antibiotics; risk may be increased with concurrent corticosteroids, organ transplant recipients, and in patients >60 years of age.** Rupture of the Achilles tendon sometimes requiring surgical repair has been reported most frequently; but other tendon sites (eg, rotator cuff, biceps) have also been reported. Strenuous physical activity, rheumatoid arthritis, and renal impairment may be an independent risk factor for tendonitis. Discontinue at first sign of tendon inflammation or pain. Tendon rupture may occur even after discontinuation of therapy. Use with caution in patients with rheumatoid arthritis or renal impairment; may increase risk of tendon rupture.

Use with caution in patients with significant bradycardia or acute myocardial ischemia. Moxifloxacin causes a concentration-dependent QT prolongation. Do not exceed recommended dose or infusion rate. Avoid use with uncorrected hypokalemia, with other drugs that prolong the QT interval or induce bradycardia, or with class Ia or III antiarrhythmic agents. CNS effects may occur (tremor, restlessness, confusion, and very rarely hallucinations, increased intracranial pressure [including pseudotumor cerebri] or seizures). Use with caution in patients with known or suspected CNS disorder. Potential for seizures, although very rare, may be increased with concomitant NSAID therapy. Use with caution in individuals at risk of seizures. Use with caution in patients with mild, moderate, or severe hepatic impairment or liver cirrhosis; may increase the risk of QT prolongation. Fulminant hepatitis potentially leading to liver failure (including fatalities) has been reported with use. Use with caution in diabetes; glucose regulation may be altered.

Fluoroquinolones have been associated with the development of serious, and sometimes fatal, hypoglycemia, most often in elderly diabetics, but also in patients without diabetes. This occurred most frequently with gatifloxacin (no longer available systemically) but may occur at a lower frequency with other quinolones.

Severe hypersensitivity reactions, including anaphylaxis, have occurred with quinolone therapy. Reactions may present as typical allergic symptoms after a single dose, or may manifest as severe idiosyncratic dermatologic, vascular, pulmonary, renal, hepatic, and/or hematologic events, usually after multiple doses. Prompt discontinuation of drug should occur if skin rash or other symptoms arise. Avoid excessive sunlight and take precautions to limit exposure (eg, loose fitting clothing, sunscreen); may cause moderate-to-severe phototoxicity reactions. Discontinue use if photosensitivity occurs. Prolonged use may result in fungal or bacterial superinfection, including *C. difficile*-associated diarrhea (CDAD) and pseudomembranous colitis; CDAD has been observed >2 months post-antibiotic treatment.

[U.S. Boxed Warning]: Quinolones may exacerbate myasthenia gravis; avoid use (rare, potentially life-threatening weakness of respiratory muscles may occur). Peripheral neuropathy has been reported (rare); may occur soon after initiation of therapy and may be irreversible; discontinue if symptoms of sensory or sensorimotor neuropathy occur. Hemolytic reactions may (rarely) occur with quinolone use in patients with latent or actual G6PD deficiency. Adverse effects (eg, tendon rupture, QT changes) may be increased in the elderly. Some quinolones may exacerbate myasthenia gravis, use with caution (rare, potentially life-threatening weakness of respiratory muscles may occur). Safety and efficacy of systemically administered moxifloxacin (oral, intravenous) in patients <18 years of age have not been established.

Adverse Reactions

2% to 10%:

Central nervous system: Headache (≤4%), dizziness (3%), insomnia (2%)

Endocrine & metabolic: Chloride increased (≥2%), glucose decreased (≥2%), ionized calcium increased (≥2%)

Gastrointestinal: Nausea (7%), diarrhea (6%), amylase decreased (≥2%), constipation (2%), vomiting (2%), abdominal pain (1% to 2%)

Hematologic: Decreased serum levels of the following (≥2%): Basophils, eosinophils, hemoglobin, PT, RBC, neutrophils; increased serum levels of the following (≥2%): MCH, neutrophils, PT, WBC

Hepatic: Bilirubin decreased/increased (≥2%)

Renal: Albumin increased (≥2%)

Respiratory: PO_2 decreased (≥2%)

0.1% to <2%:

Cardiovascular: Angina, atrial fibrillation, bradycardia, cardiac arrest, edema, heart failure, hypertension, hypotension, palpitation, peripheral edema, QT_c prolongation, syncope, tachycardia

Central nervous system: Fever (1%), agitation, anxiety, chills, confusion, depression, disorientation, fatigue, hallucinations, hypoesthesia, lethargy, malaise, nervousness, pain, restlessness, somnolence, vertigo

Dermatologic: Allergic dermatitis, erythema, hyperhidrosis, pruritus, rash, urticaria

Endocrine & metabolic: Hypokalemia (1%), dehydration, hyperglycemia, hyperlipidemia, triglycerides increased, uric acid increased

Gastrointestinal: Dyspepsia (1%), abdominal discomfort, abdominal distension, amylase increased, anorexia, appetite decreased, flatulence, gastritis, gastroenteritis, gastroesophageal reflux disease, lactic dehydrogenase increased, lipase increased, taste perversion, xerostomia

Genitourinary: Dysuria, vaginitis, vulvovaginal candidiasis, vulvovaginal mycotic infection, vulvovaginal pruritus

Hematologic: Anemia (1%), eosinophilia, hematocrit decreased, leukocytosis, leukopenia, aPTT increased, thrombocythemia, thrombocytopenia

Hepatic: ALT increased (1%), AST increased, alkaline phosphatase increased, GGTP increased, liver function test abnormal

Local: Injection site extravasation, phlebitis

Neuromuscular & skeletal: Arthralgia, back pain, chest pain (noncardiac), facial pain, limb pain, muscle spasms, musculoskeletal pain, myalgia, paresthesia, tremor, weakness

Ocular: Blurred vision

Otic: Tinnitus

Renal: BUN increased, creatinine increased, renal failure

Respiratory: Asthma, bronchospasm, dyspnea, wheezing

Miscellaneous: Allergic reaction, candidiasis, fungal infection, night sweats, oral candidiasis

<0.1% (Limited to important or life-threatening): Agranulocytosis, anaphylactic reaction, anaphylactic shock, angioedema, aplastic anemia, *C. difficile*-positive diarrhea, cholestasis, deafness (reversible), ECG abnormalities, hearing impairment, hemolytic anemia, hepatic failure, hepatic necrosis, hepatitis, hypersensitivity reactions, INR decreased, interstitial nephritis, intracranial pressure increased, jaundice (cholestatic), myasthenia gravis exacerbation, nightmares, pancytopenia, peripheral neuropathy, photosensitivity/toxicity, pneumonitis (allergic), polyneuropathy, pseudomembranous colitis, pseudotumor cerebri, psychotic reaction, renal dysfunction, seizure, Stevens-Johnson syndrome, suicidal behavior/ideation, tendonitis, tendon rupture, thrombotic thrombocytopenic purpura, toxic epidermal necrolysis, ventricular tachyarrhythmias (including torsade de pointes and cardiac arrest [usually in patients with concurrent, severe proarrhythmic conditions]), vasculitis, vision loss (transient)

Drug Interactions

Metabolism/Transport Effects None known.

Avoid Concomitant Use

Avoid concomitant use of Moxifloxacin (Systemic) with any of the following: BCG; Highest Risk QTc-Prolonging Agents; Ivabradine; Mifepristone; Strontium Ranelate

Increased Effect/Toxicity

Moxifloxacin (Systemic) may increase the levels/effects of: Corticosteroids (Systemic); Highest Risk QTc-Prolonging Agents; Moderate Risk QTc-Prolonging Agents; Porfimer; Sulfonylureas; Varenicline; Vitamin K Antagonists

The levels/effects of Moxifloxacin (Systemic) may be increased by: Insulin; Ivabradine; Mifepristone; Nonsteroidal Anti-Inflammatory Agents; Probenecid; QTc-Prolonging Agents (Indeterminate Risk and Risk Modifying)

Decreased Effect

Moxifloxacin (Systemic) may decrease the levels/effects of: BCG; Didanosine; Mycophenolate; Sodium Picosulfate; Sulfonylureas; Typhoid Vaccine

The levels/effects of Moxifloxacin (Systemic) may be decreased by: Antacids; Didanosine; Iron Salts; Lanthanum; Magnesium Salts; Multivitamins/Minerals (with ADEK, Folate, Iron); Multivitamins/Minerals (with AE, No Iron); Quinapril; Sevelamer; Strontium Ranelate; Sucralfate; Zinc Salts

Ethanol/Nutrition/Herb Interactions Food: Absorption is not affected by administration with a high-fat meal or yogurt.

Storage/Stability Store at controlled room temperature of 25°C (77°F). Do not refrigerate infusion solution.

Mechanism of Action Moxifloxacin is a DNA gyrase inhibitor, and also inhibits topoisomerase IV. DNA gyrase (topoisomerase II) is an essential bacterial enzyme that maintains the superhelical structure of DNA. DNA gyrase is required for DNA replication and transcription, DNA repair, recombination, and transposition; inhibition is bactericidal.

Pharmacodynamics/Kinetics

Absorption: Well absorbed; not affected by high-fat meal or yogurt

Distribution: V_d: 1.7 to 2.7 L/kg; tissue concentrations often exceed plasma concentrations in respiratory tissues, alveolar macrophages, abdominal tissues/fluids, uterine tissue (endometrium, myometrium), and sinus tissues

Protein binding: ~30% to 50%

Metabolism: Hepatic (~52% of dose) via glucuronide (~14%) and sulfate (~38%) conjugation

Bioavailability: ~90%

Half-life elimination: Single dose: Oral: 12-16 hours; I.V.: 8-15 hours

Excretion: Urine (as unchanged drug [20%] and glucuronide conjugates); feces (as unchanged drug [25%] and sulfate conjugates)

Dosage

Children ≥1 year (unlabeled use): **Surgical (perioperative) prophylaxis (unlabeled use):** I.V.: 10 mg/kg within 120 minutes prior to surgical incision (maximum dose: 400 mg) (Bratzler, 2013).

Adolescents (unlabeled use): **Community-acquired pneumonia (CAP) due to atypical pathogens (*M. pneumoniae, C. trachomatis, or C. pneumoniae*), mild infection or step-down therapy in adolescents with skeletal maturity, (alternative to azithromycin) (IDSA/PIDS, 2011):** Oral: 400 mg once daily

Adults: Oral, I.V.: Usual dosage range: 400 mg every 24 hours

Indication-specific dosing:

Acute bacterial rhinosinusitis: 400 mg every 24 hours for 10 days or 5-7 days (Chow, 2012). **Note:** Recommended in patients with beta-lactam allergy; may also be used if initial therapy fails, in areas with high endemic rates of penicillin nonsusceptible *S. pneumoniae*, those with severe infections, age >65 years, recent hospitalization, antibiotic use within the past month, or who are immunocompromised.

Chronic bronchitis, acute bacterial exacerbation: 400 mg every 24 hours for 5 days

Community-acquired pneumonia (CAP) (including MDRSP): 400 mg every 24 hours for 7-14 days

Intra-abdominal infections, complicated: 400 mg every 24 hours for 5-14 days (initiate with I.V.); **Note:** 2010 IDSA guidelines recommend a treatment duration of 4-7 days (provided source controlled) for community-acquired, mild-to-moderate IAI

***M. genitalium* infections** (including confirmed cases or clinically significant persistent cervicitis, pelvic inflammatory disease or urethritis in patients who previously received azithromycin or doxycycline; unlabeled use): Oral, I.V.: 400 mg every 24 hours for 7-10 days (Manhart, 2011)

Skin and skin structure infections:

Complicated: 400 mg every 24 hours for 7-21 days

Uncomplicated: 400 mg every 24 hours for 7 days

Surgical (perioperative) prophylaxis (unlabeled use): I.V.: 400 mg within 120 minutes prior to surgical incision (Bratzler, 2013).

Tuberculosis, drug-resistant tuberculosis, or intolerance to first-line agents (unlabeled use): Oral: 400 mg every 24 hours (*MMWR*, 2003)

Elderly: No dosage adjustments are required based on age

Dosage adjustment in renal impairment: No dosage adjustment required in renal impairment.

Poorly dialyzed; no supplemental dose or dosage adjustment necessary, including patients on intermittent hemodialysis, peritoneal dialysis, or continuous renal replacement therapy (eg, CVVHD).

Dosage adjustment in hepatic impairment: No dosage adjustment is required in mild, moderate, or severe hepatic insufficiency (Child-Pugh class A, B, or C); however, use with caution in this patient population secondary to the risk of QT prolongation.

Dietary Considerations May be taken without regard to meals. Take 4 hours before or 8 hours after multiple vitamins, antacids, or other products containing magnesium, aluminum, iron, or zinc.

Avelox® I.V. infusion (premixed in sodium chloride 0.8%) contains sodium 34.2 mEq (~787 mg)/250 mL.

Administration Administer without regard to meals.

I.V.: Infuse over 60 minutes; do not infuse by rapid or bolus intravenous infusion

Monitoring Parameters WBC, signs of infection

Test Interactions Some quinolones may produce a false-positive urine screening result for opioids using commercially-available immunoassay kits. This has been demonstrated most consistently for levofloxacin and ofloxacin, but other quinolones have shown cross-reactivity in certain assay kits. Confirmation of positive opioid screens by more specific methods should be considered.

Dosage Forms Excipient information presented when available (limited, particularly for generics); consult specific product labeling.

Solution, Intravenous [preservative free]:

Avelox: 400 mg/250 mL (250 mL) [latex free]

Tablet, Oral:

Avelox: 400 mg

Avelox ABC Pack: 400 mg

Extemporaneous Preparations A 20 mg/mL oral suspension may be made using tablets. Crush three 400 mg tablets and reduce to a fine powder. Carefully sieve powder from enteric-coating remnants to improve pharmaceutical elegance. Add a small amount of a 1:1 mixture of Ora-Plus® and Ora-Sweet® or Ora-Sweet® SF and mix to a uniform paste; mix while adding the vehicle in geometric proportions to **almost** 60 mL; transfer to a calibrated bottle, rinse mortar with vehicle, and add quantity of vehicle sufficient to make 60 mL. Label "shake well". Stable 90 days at room temperature.

Hutchinson DJ, Johnson CE, and Klein KC, "Stability of Extemporaneously Prepared Moxifloxacin Oral Suspensions," *Am J Health Syst Pharm*, 2009, 66(7):665-7.

Moxifloxacin (Ophthalmic) (moxs i FLOKS a sin)

Brand Names: U.S. Moxeza; Vigamox

Brand Names: Canada Vigamox®

Index Terms Moxifloxacin Hydrochloride

Pharmacologic Category Antibiotic, Fluoroquinolone; Antibiotic, Ophthalmic

Use Treatment of bacterial conjunctivitis caused by susceptible organisms

Pregnancy Risk Factor C

Dosage Ophthalmic: Bacterial conjunctivitis:

Children ≥4 months and Adults (Moxeza™): Instill 1 drop into affected eye(s) 2 times/day for 7 days

Children ≥1 year and Adults (Vigamox®): Instill 1 drop into affected eye(s) 3 times/day for 7 days

Dosage adjustment in renal impairment: No dosage adjustment provided in manufacturer's labeling. However, dosage adjustment unlikely due to low systemic absorption.

Dosage adjustment in hepatic impairment: No dosage adjustment provided in manufacturer's labeling. However, dosage adjustment unlikely due to low systemic absorption.

Additional Information Complete prescribing information should be consulted for additional detail.

Dosage Forms Excipient information presented when available (limited, particularly for generics); consult specific product labeling.

Solution, Ophthalmic:

Moxeza: 0.5% (3 mL)

Vigamox: 0.5% (3 mL)

- **Moxifloxacin Hydrochloride** *see* Moxifloxacin (Ophthalmic) *on page 1406*
- **Moxifloxacin Hydrochloride** *see* Moxifloxacin (Systemic) *on page 1404*
- **Mozobil** *see* Plerixafor *on page 1657*
- **4-MP** *see* Fomepizole *on page 910*
- **MP-424** *see* Telaprevir *on page 1996*
- **MPA** *see* MedroxyPROGESTERone *on page 1278*
- **MPA** *see* Mycophenolate *on page 1407*
- **6-MP (error-prone abbreviation)** *see* Mercaptopurine *on page 1300*
- **MPSV** *see* Meningococcal Polysaccharide Vaccine (Groups A / C / Y and W-135) *on page 1294*
- **MPSV4** *see* Meningococcal Polysaccharide Vaccine (Groups A / C / Y and W-135) *on page 1294*
- **MRA** *see* Tocilizumab *on page 2080*
- **MS Contin** *see* Morphine (Systemic) *on page 1398*
- **MS Contin® (Can)** *see* Morphine (Systemic) *on page 1398*
- **MS Contin SRT (Can)** *see* Morphine (Systemic) *on page 1398*
- **MS (error-prone abbreviation and should not be used)** *see* Morphine (Liposomal) *on page 1403*
- **MS (error-prone abbreviation and should not be used)** *see* Morphine (Systemic) *on page 1398*
- **MS-IR® (Can)** *see* Morphine (Systemic) *on page 1398*
- **MSO_4 (error-prone abbreviation and should not be used)** *see* Morphine (Liposomal) *on page 1403*
- **MSO_4 (error-prone abbreviation and should not be used)** *see* Morphine (Systemic) *on page 1398*
- **MST 600** *see* Magnesium Salicylate *on page 1262*
- **MTC** *see* MitoMYcin (Systemic) *on page 1383*
- **MTX (error-prone abbreviation)** *see* Methotrexate *on page 1324*

- ◆ **Mucinex [OTC]** *see* GuaiFENesin *on page 974*
- ◆ **Mucinex® D [OTC]** *see* Guaifenesin and Pseudoephedrine *on page 978*
- ◆ **Mucinex® D Maximum Strength [OTC]** *see* Guaifenesin and Pseudoephedrine *on page 978*
- ◆ **Mucinex Chest Congestion Child [OTC]** *see* GuaiFENesin *on page 974*
- ◆ **Mucinex® Cold [OTC]** *see* Guaifenesin and Phenylephrine *on page 978*
- ◆ **Mucinex DM [OTC]** *see* Guaifenesin and Dextromethorphan *on page 976*
- ◆ **Mucinex DM Maximum Strength [OTC]** *see* Guaifenesin and Dextromethorphan *on page 976*
- ◆ **Mucinex For Kids [OTC]** *see* GuaiFENesin *on page 974*
- ◆ **Mucinex Kid's Cough [OTC]** *see* Guaifenesin and Dextromethorphan *on page 976*
- ◆ **Mucinex Kid's Cough Mini-Melts [OTC]** *see* Guaifenesin and Dextromethorphan *on page 976*
- ◆ **Mucinex Maximum Strength [OTC]** *see* GuaiFENesin *on page 974*
- ◆ **Mucomyst** *see* Acetylcysteine *on page 36*
- ◆ **Mucomyst® (Can)** *see* Acetylcysteine *on page 36*
- ◆ **Mucosa [OTC]** *see* GuaiFENesin *on page 974*
- ◆ **Mucus-ER [OTC]** *see* GuaiFENesin *on page 974*
- ◆ **Mucus Relief [OTC]** *see* GuaiFENesin *on page 974*
- ◆ **Mucus Relief Childrens [OTC]** *see* GuaiFENesin *on page 974*
- ◆ **Mucus Relief Sinus [OTC]** *see* Guaifenesin and Phenylephrine *on page 978*
- ◆ **Multaq** *see* Dronedarone *on page 675*
- ◆ **Multaq® (Can)** *see* Dronedarone *on page 675*
- ◆ **Mumps, Measles and Rubella Vaccines** *see* Measles, Mumps, and Rubella Virus Vaccine *on page 1272*
- ◆ **Mumps, Rubella, Varicella, and Measles Vaccine** *see* Measles, Mumps, Rubella, and Varicella Virus Vaccine *on page 1273*

Mupirocin (myoo PEER oh sin)

Brand Names: U.S. Bactroban; Bactroban Nasal; Centany; Centany AT

Brand Names: Canada Bactroban®

Index Terms Mupirocin Calcium; Pseudomonic Acid A

Pharmacologic Category Antibiotic, Topical

Use

Intranasal: Eradication of nasal colonization with MRSA in adult patients and healthcare workers

Topical: Treatment of impetigo or secondary infected traumatic skin lesions due to *S. aureus* and *S. pyogenes*

Unlabeled Use Intranasal: Surgical prophylaxis to prevent wound infections

Pregnancy Risk Factor B

Dosage

Intranasal: Children ≥12 years and Adults: Eradication of nasal MRSA: Approximately one-half of the ointment from the single-use tube should be applied into one nostril and the other half into the other nostril twice daily for 5 days

Topical:

Children ≥2 months and Adults: Impetigo: Ointment: Apply to affected area 3 times/day; re-evaluate after 3-5 days if no clinical response

Children ≥3 months and Adults: Secondary skin infections: Cream: Apply to affected area 3 times/day for 10 days; re-evaluate after 3-5 days if no clinical response

Additional Information Complete prescribing information should be consulted for additional detail.

Dosage Forms Excipient information presented when available (limited, particularly for generics); consult specific product labeling.

Cream, External, as calcium [strength expressed as base]:
- Bactroban: 2% (15 g, 30 g)
- Generic: 2% (15 g, 30 g)

Kit, External:
- Centany AT: 2% [contains propylene glycol monostearate]

Ointment, External:
- Bactroban: 2% (22 g)
- Centany: 2% (30 g) [contains propylene glycol monostearate]
- Generic: 2% (22 g)

Ointment, Nasal, as calcium [strength expressed as base]:
- Bactroban Nasal: 2% (1 g)

- ◆ **Mupirocin Calcium** *see* Mupirocin *on page 1407*
- ◆ **Muro 128 [OTC]** *see* Sodium Chloride *on page 1914*
- ◆ **Muse** *see* Alprostadil *on page 83*
- ◆ **Muse® Pellet (Can)** *see* Alprostadil *on page 83*
- ◆ **Mustargen** *see* Mechlorethamine (Systemic) *on page 1274*
- ◆ **Mustine** *see* Mechlorethamine (Systemic) *on page 1274*
- ◆ **Mutamycin** *see* MitoMYcin (Systemic) *on page 1383*
- ◆ **Mutamycin® (Can)** *see* MitoMYcin (Systemic) *on page 1383*
- ◆ **Myambutol** *see* Ethambutol *on page 782*
- ◆ **Mycamine** *see* Micafungin *on page 1356*
- ◆ **Mycelex** *see* Clotrimazole (Oral) *on page 476*
- ◆ **Mycobutin** *see* Rifabutin *on page 1809*
- ◆ **Mycobutin® (Can)** *see* Rifabutin *on page 1809*
- ◆ **Mycocide CX Callus Exfoliator [OTC]** *see* Urea *on page 2140*
- ◆ **Mycocide Clinical NS [OTC]** *see* Tolnaftate *on page 2087*

Mycophenolate (mye koe FEN oh late)

Brand Names: U.S. CellCept; CellCept Intravenous; Myfortic

Brand Names: Canada Apo-Mycophenolate; CellCept; CO Mycophenolate; JAMP-Mycophenolate; Myfortic; Mylan-Mycophenolate; Novo-Mycophenolate; Sandoz-Mycophenolate; Sandoz-Mycophenolate Mofetil

Index Terms MMF; MPA; Mycophenolate Mofetil; Mycophenolate Sodium; Mycophenolic Acid

Pharmacologic Category Immunosuppressant Agent

Use Prophylaxis of organ rejection concomitantly with cyclosporine and corticosteroids in patients receiving allogeneic renal (CellCept, Myfortic), cardiac (CellCept), or hepatic (CellCept) transplants

Unlabeled Use Treatment of rejection in liver transplant patients unable to tolerate tacrolimus or cyclosporine due to toxicity; treatment of recurrent or persistent rejection in heart transplant patients; treatment of moderate-severe psoriasis; treatment of lupus nephritis; treatment of myasthenia gravis; prevention of graft-versus-host disease (GVHD); treatment of refractory acute GVHD and chronic GVHD; treatment of refractory autoimmune hepatitis

Pregnancy Risk Factor D

Pregnancy Considerations [U.S. Boxed Warning]: Mycophenolate is associated with an increased risk of congenital malformations and first trimester pregnancy loss when used by pregnant women. Females of reproductive potential must be counseled about pregnancy prevention and planning. Alternative agents should be considered for women planning a pregnancy. Adverse events have been reported in animal reproduction studies. In humans, the following congenital malformations have been reported: external ear abnormalities, cleft lip and palate, anomalies of the distal limbs, heart, esophagus and kidney. Spontaneous abortions have also been noted. Females of reproductive potential (girls who have entered puberty, women with a uterus who have not passed through clinically confirmed menopause) should have a negative pregnancy test with a sensitivity of ≥25 mIU/mL immediately before therapy and the test should be repeated 8-10 days later. Pregnancy tests should be repeated during routine follow-up visits. Acceptable forms of contraception should be used during treatment and for 6 weeks after therapy is discontinued. The effectiveness of hormonal contraceptive agents may be affected by mycophenolate. For women with lupus nephritis taking mycophenolate and who are planning a pregnancy, mycophenolate should be discontinued at least 6 weeks prior to trying to conceive (Hahn, 2012).

Healthcare providers should report female exposures to mycophenolate during pregnancy or within 6 weeks of discontinuing therapy to the Mycophenolate Pregnancy Registry (800-617-8191). The National Transplantation Pregnancy Registry (NTPR, Temple University) is a registry for pregnant women taking immunosuppressants following any solid organ transplant. The NTPR encourages reporting of all immunosuppressant exposures during pregnancy in transplant recipients at 877-955-6877.

Breast-Feeding Considerations It is unknown if mycophenolate is excreted in human milk. Due to potentially serious adverse reactions, the decision to discontinue the drug or discontinue breast-feeding should be considered. Breast-feeding is not recommended during therapy or for 6 weeks after treatment is complete.

Medication Guide Available Yes

Contraindications Hypersensitivity to mycophenolate mofetil, mycophenolic acid, mycophenolate sodium, or any component of the formulation

Cellcept: Intravenous formulation is also contraindicated in patients who are allergic to polysorbate 80

Warnings/Precautions Hazardous agent - use appropriate precautions for handling and disposal (NIOSH, 2012). **[U.S. Boxed Warning]: Risk for bacterial, viral, fungal, and protozoal infections, including opportunistic infections, is increased with immunosuppressant therapy**; infections may be serious and potentially fatal. Due to the risk of oversuppression of the immune system, which may increase susceptibility to infection, combination immunosuppressant therapy should be used with caution. Polyomavirus associated nephropathy (PVAN), JC virus-associated progressive multifocal leukoencephalopathy (PML), cytomegalovirus (CMV) infections, reactivation of hepatitis B (HBV) or hepatitis C (HCV), have been reported with use. A reduction in immunosuppression should be considered for patients with new or reactivated viral infections; however, in transplant recipients, the risk that reduced immunosuppression presents to the functioning graft should also be considered. PVAN, primarily from activation of BK virus, may lead to the deterioration of renal function and/or renal graft loss. PML, a potentially fatal condition, commonly presents with hemiparesis, apathy, ataxia, cognitive deficiencies, confusion, and hemiparesis. Risk factors for development of PML include treatment with immunosuppressants and immune function impairment; consultation with a neurologist should be considered in any patient with neurological symptoms receiving immunosuppressants. Risk of CMV viremia or disease is increased in transplant recipients CMV seronegative at the time of transplant who receive a graft from a CMV seropositive donor. In patients infected with HBV or HCV, viral reactivation may occur; these patients should be monitored for signs of active HBV or HCV. **[U.S. Boxed Warning]: Risk of development of lymphoma and skin malignancy is increased.** The risk for malignancies is related to intensity/duration of therapy. Patients should be monitored appropriately, instructed to limit exposure to sunlight/UV light to decrease the risk of skin cancer, and given supportive treatment should these conditions occur. Post-transplant lymphoproliferative disorder related to EBV infection has been reported in immunosuppressed organ transplant patients; risk is highest in EBV seronegative patients (including many young children). Neutropenia (including severe neutropenia) may occur, requiring dose reduction or interruption of treatment (risk greater from day 31-180 post-transplant). Use may rarely be associated with gastric or duodenal ulcers, GI bleeding and/or perforation. Use caution in patients with active serious digestive system disease; patients with active peptic ulcers were not included in clinical studies. Use caution in renal impairment as toxicity may be increased; may require dosage adjustment in severe impairment.

[U.S. Boxed Warning]: Mycophenolate is associated with an increased risk of congenital malformations and first trimester pregnancy loss when used by pregnant women. Females of reproductive potential must be counseled about pregnancy prevention and planning. Alternative agents should be considered for women planning a pregnancy. Females of reproductive potential should have a negative pregnancy test with a sensitivity of ≥25 mIU/mL immediately before therapy and the test should be repeated 8-10 days later. Pregnancy tests should be repeated during routine follow-up visits. Acceptable forms of contraception should be used during treatment and for 6 weeks after therapy is discontinued. Females of childbearing potential should have a negative pregnancy test within 1 week prior to beginning therapy. Two reliable forms of contraception should be used beginning 4 weeks prior to, during, and for 6 weeks after therapy. Because mycophenolate mofetil has demonstrated teratogenic effects in rats and rabbits, tablets should not be crushed, and capsules should not be opened or crushed. Avoid inhalation or direct contact with skin or mucous membranes of the powder contained in the capsules and the powder for oral suspension. Caution should be exercised in the handling and preparation of solutions of intravenous mycophenolate. Avoid skin contact with the intravenous solution and reconstituted suspension. If such contact occurs, wash thoroughly with soap and water, rinse eyes with plain water.

Theoretically, use should be avoided in patients with the rare hereditary deficiency of hypoxanthine-guanine phosphoribosyltransferase (such as Lesch-Nyhan or Kelley-Seegmiller syndrome). Intravenous solutions should be given over at least 2 hours; never administer intravenous solution by rapid or bolus injection. Live attenuated vaccines should be avoided during use; vaccinations may be less effective during therapy. **[U.S. Boxed Warning]: Should be administered under the supervision of a physician experienced in immunosuppressive therapy.**

Note: CellCept and Myfortic dosage forms should not be used interchangeably due to differences in absorption. Some dosage forms may contain phenylalanine. The intravenous formulation contains polysorbate 80.

Adverse Reactions Data for incidence >20% as reported in adults following oral dosing of CellCept alone in renal, cardiac, and hepatic allograft rejection studies. Profile in 3% to <20% range reflects use in combination with cyclosporine and corticosteroids. In general, lower doses used in renal rejection patients had less adverse effects than higher doses. Rates of adverse effects were similar for each indication, except for those unique to the specific organ involved. The type of adverse effects observed in pediatric patients was similar to those seen in adults, with the exception of abdominal pain, anemia, diarrhea, fever, hypertension, infection, pharyngitis, respiratory tract infection, sepsis, and vomiting; lymphoproliferative disorder was the only type of malignancy observed. Percentages of adverse reactions were similar in studies comparing CellCept to Myfortic in patients following renal transplant.

>20%:

Cardiovascular: Hypertension (28% to 78%), hypotension (33%), peripheral edema (27% to 64%), edema (27% to 28%), chest pain (26%), tachycardia (20% to 22%)

Central nervous system: Pain (31% to 76%), headache (16% to 54%), insomnia (41% to 52%), fever (21% to 52%), dizziness (29%), anxiety (28%)

Dermatologic: Rash (22%)

Endocrine & metabolic: Hyperglycemia (44% to 47%), hypercholesterolemia (41%), hypomagnesemia (39%), hypokalemia (32% to 37%), hypocalcemia (30%), hyperkalemia (22%)

Gastrointestinal: Abdominal pain (25% to 63%), nausea (20% to 55%), diarrhea (31% to 51%), constipation (19% to 41%), vomiting (33% to 34%), anorexia (25%), dyspepsia (22%)

Genitourinary: Urinary tract infection (37%)

Hematologic: Leukopenia (23% to 46%), anemia (26% to 43%; hypochromic 25%), leukocytosis (22% to 41%), thrombocytopenia (24% to 38%)

Hepatic: Liver function tests abnormal (25%), ascites (24%)

Neuromuscular & skeletal: Back pain (35% to 47%), weakness (35% to 43%), tremor (24% to 34%), paresthesia (21%)

Renal: Creatinine increased (39%), BUN increased (35%), kidney function abnormal (22% to 26%)

Respiratory: Dyspnea (31% to 37%), respiratory tract infection (22% to 37%), pleural effusion (34%), cough (31%), lung disorder (22% to 30%), sinusitis (26%)

Miscellaneous: Infection (18% to 27%), sepsis (27%), lactate dehydrogenase increased (23%), *Candida* (17% to 22%), herpes simplex (10% to 21%)

3% to <20%:

Cardiovascular: Angina, arrhythmia, arterial thrombosis, atrial fibrillation, atrial flutter, bradycardia, cardiac arrest, cardiac failure, CHF, extrasystole, facial edema, hyper-/hypovolemia, orthostatic hypotension, pallor, palpitation, pericardial effusion, peripheral vascular disorder, supraventricular extrasystoles, supraventricular tachycardia, syncope, thrombosis, vasodilation, vasospasm, venous pressure increased, ventricular extrasystole, ventricular tachycardia

Central nervous system: Agitation, chills with fever, confusion, delirium, depression, emotional lability, hallucinations, hypoesthesia, malaise, nervousness, psychosis, seizure, somnolence, thinking abnormal, vertigo

Dermatologic: Acne, alopecia, bruising, cellulitis, fungal dermatitis, hirsutism, petechia, pruritus, skin carcinoma, skin hypertrophy, skin ulcer, vesiculobullous rash

Endocrine & metabolic: Acidosis, alkalosis, Cushing's syndrome, dehydration, diabetes mellitus, gout, hypercalcemia, hyper-hypophosphatemia, hyperlipemia, hyperuricemia, hypochloremia, hypoglycemia, hyponatremia, hypoproteinemia, hypothyroidism, parathyroid disorder

Gastrointestinal: Abdomen enlarged, dysphagia, esophagitis, flatulence, gastritis, gastroenteritis, gastrointestinal hemorrhage, gastrointestinal moniliasis, gingivitis, gum hyperplasia, ileus, melena, mouth ulceration, oral moniliasis, stomach disorder, stomach ulcer, stomatitis, xerostomia, weight gain/loss

Genitourinary: Impotence, nocturia, pelvic pain, prostatic disorder, scrotal edema, urinary frequency, urinary incontinence, urinary retention, urinary tract disorder

Hematologic: Coagulation disorder, hemorrhage, neutropenia, pancytopenia, polycythemia, prothrombin time increased, thromboplastin time increased

Hepatic: Alkaline phosphatase increased, bilirubinemia, cholangitis, cholestatic jaundice, GGT increased, hepatitis, jaundice, liver damage, transaminases increased

Local: Abscess

Neuromuscular & skeletal: Arthralgia, hypertonia, joint disorder, leg cramps, myalgia, myasthenia, neck pain, neuropathy, osteoporosis

Ocular: Amblyopia, cataract, conjunctivitis, eye hemorrhage, lacrimation disorder, vision abnormal

Otic: Deafness, ear disorder, ear pain, tinnitus

Renal: Albuminuria, creatinine increased, dysuria, hematuria, hydronephrosis, oliguria, pyelonephritis, renal failure, renal tubular necrosis

Respiratory: Apnea, asthma, atelectasis, bronchitis, epistaxis, hemoptysis, hiccup, hyperventilation, hypoxia, respiratory acidosis, pharyngitis, pneumonia, pneumothorax, pulmonary edema, pulmonary hypertension, respiratory moniliasis, rhinitis, sputum increased, voice alteration

Miscellaneous: *Candida* (mucocutaneous 16% to 18%), CMV viremia/syndrome (12% to 14%), CMV tissue invasive disease (6% to 12%), herpes zoster cutaneous disease (4% to 10%), cyst, diaphoresis, flu-like syndrome, healing abnormal, hernia, ileus infection, neoplasm, peritonitis, thirst

Postmarketing and/or case reports: Atypical mycobacterial infection, BK virus-associated nephropathy, colitis, gastrointestinal perforation, infectious endocarditis, interstitial lung disorder, intestinal villous atrophy, lymphoma, lymphoproliferative disease, malignancy, meningitis, pancreatitis, progressive multifocal leukoencephalopathy (sometimes fatal), pulmonary fibrosis (fatal), pure red cell aplasia, tuberculosis

Drug Interactions

Metabolism/Transport Effects None known.

Avoid Concomitant Use

Avoid concomitant use of Mycophenolate with any of the following: BCG; Cholestyramine Resin; Natalizumab; Pimecrolimus; Rifamycin Derivatives; Tacrolimus (Topical); Tofacitinib; Vaccines (Live)

Increased Effect/Toxicity

Mycophenolate may increase the levels/effects of: Acyclovir-Valacyclovir; Ganciclovir-Valganciclovir; Leflunomide; Natalizumab; Tofacitinib; Vaccines (Live)

The levels/effects of Mycophenolate may be increased by: Acyclovir-Valacyclovir; Belatacept; Denosumab; Ganciclovir-Valganciclovir; Pimecrolimus; Probenecid; Roflumilast; Tacrolimus (Topical); Trastuzumab

Decreased Effect

Mycophenolate may decrease the levels/effects of: BCG; Coccidioidin Skin Test; Contraceptives (Estrogens); Contraceptives (Progestins); Sipuleucel-T; Vaccines (Inactivated); Vaccines (Live)

The levels/effects of Mycophenolate may be decreased by: Antacids; Cholestyramine Resin; CycloSPORINE (Systemic); Echinacea; Magnesium Salts; MetroNIDAZOLE (Systemic); Penicillins; Proton Pump Inhibitors; Quinolone Antibiotics; Rifamycin Derivatives; Sevelamer

Ethanol/Nutrition/Herb Interactions

Food: Food decreases C_{max} of MPA by 40% following CellCept administration and 33% following Myfortic use; the extent of absorption is not changed. Management: Take CellCept or Myfortic on an empty stomach to decrease variability; however, Cellcept may be taken with food if necessary in stable renal transplant patients.

Herb/Nutraceutical: Cat's claw and echinacea have immunostimulant properties. Management: Avoid cat's claw and echinacea.

Preparation for Administration Hazardous agent; use appropriate precautions for handling and disposal (NIOSH, 2012).

Oral suspension: Should be constituted prior to dispensing to the patient and **not** mixed with any other medication. Add 47 mL of water to the bottle and shake well for ~1 minute. Add another 47 mL of water to the bottle and shake well for an additional minute. Final concentration is 200 mg/mL of mycophenolate mofetil.

I.V.: Reconstitute the contents of each vial with 14 mL of 5% dextrose injection; dilute the contents of a vial with 5% dextrose in water to a final concentration of 6 mg mycophenolate mofetil per mL. **Note:** Vial is vacuum-sealed; if a lack of vacuum is noted during preparation, the vial should not be used.

Storage/Stability

Capsules: Store at 25°C (77°F); excursions permitted to 15°C to 30°C (59°F to 86°F).

Tablets: Store at 25°C (77°F); excursions permitted to 15°C to 30°C (59°F to 86°F). Protect from moisture and light.

Oral suspension: Store powder for oral suspension at 25°C (77°F); excursions permitted to 15°C to 30°C (59°F to 86°F). Once reconstituted, the oral solution may be stored at room temperature or under refrigeration. Do not freeze. The mixed suspension is stable for 60 days.

Injection: Store intact vials and diluted solutions at 25°C (77°F); excursions permitted to 15°C to 30°C (59°F to 86°F). Begin infusion within 4 hours of reconstitution.

Mechanism of Action MPA exhibits a cytostatic effect on T and B lymphocytes. It is an inhibitor of inosine monophosphate dehydrogenase (IMPDH) which inhibits *de novo* guanosine nucleotide synthesis. T and B lymphocytes are dependent on this pathway for proliferation.

Pharmacodynamics/Kinetics

Onset of action: Peak effect: Correlation of toxicity or efficacy is still being developed, however, one study indicated that 12-hour AUCs >40 mcg/mL/hour were correlated with efficacy and decreased episodes of rejection

Absorption: AUC values for MPA are lower in the early post-transplant period versus later (>3 months) post-transplant period. The extent of absorption in pediatrics is similar to that seen in adults, although there was wide variability reported.

Oral: Myfortic: 93%

Distribution:

CellCept: MPA: Oral: 4 L/kg; I.V.: 3.6 L/kg

Myfortic: MPA: Oral: 54 L (at steady state); 112 L (elimination phase)

Protein binding: MPA: >97%, MPAG 82%

Metabolism: Hepatic and via GI tract; CellCept is completely hydrolyzed in the liver to mycophenolic acid (MPA; active metabolite); enterohepatic recirculation of MPA may occur; MPA is glucuronidated to MPAG (inactive metabolite)

Bioavailability: Oral: CellCept: 94%; Myfortic: 72%

Half-life elimination:

CellCept: MPA: Oral: 18 hours; I.V.: 17 hours

Myfortic: MPA: Oral: 8-16 hours; MPAG: 13-17 hours

Time to peak, plasma: Oral: MPA:

CellCept: 1-1.5 hours

Myfortic: 1.5-2.75 hours

Excretion:

CellCept: MPA: Urine (<1%), feces (6%); MPAG: Urine (87%)

Myfortic: MPA: Urine (3%), feces; MPAG: Urine (>60%)

Dosage

Infants ≥3 months, Children, and Adolescents: Renal transplant: Oral:

CellCept suspension: 600 mg/m^2/dose twice daily; maximum dose: 1 g twice daily

Alternatively, may use Cellcept solid dosage forms according to BSA as follows:

BSA 1.25-1.5 m^2: 750 mg capsule twice daily

BSA >1.5 m^2: 1 g capsule or tablet twice daily

Children≥5 years and Adolescents: Renal transplant: Oral:

Myfortic: Usual dosage: 400 mg/m^2/dose twice daily; maximum dose: 720 mg twice daily

BSA <1.19 m^2: Use of this formulation is not recommended

BSA 1.19-1.58 m^2: 540 mg twice daily (maximum: 1080 mg/day)

BSA >1.58 m^2: 720 mg twice daily (maximum: 1440 mg/day)

Adults: **Note:** May be used I.V. for up to 14 days; transition to oral therapy as soon as tolerated.

Renal transplant:

CellCept:

Oral: 1 g twice daily. Doses >2 g/day are not recommended.

I.V.: 1 g twice daily

Myfortic: Oral: 720 mg twice daily (total daily dose: 1440 mg)

Cardiac transplantation: CellCept:

Oral: 1.5 g twice daily

I.V.: 1.5 g twice daily

Hepatic transplantation: CellCept:

Oral: 1.5 g twice daily

I.V.: 1 g twice daily

Autoimmune hepatitis, refractory (unlabeled use): CellCept: Oral: 2 g/day (Manns, 2010)

Lupus nephritis (unlabeled use): CellCept: Oral:

Induction: 1 g twice daily for 6 months in combination with a glucocorticoid (Ong, 2005) **or** 2-3 g daily for 6 months in combination with glucocorticoids (Hahn, 2012)

Maintenance: 0.5-3 g daily (Contreras, 2004) **or** 1 g twice daily (Dooley, 2011) **or** 1-2 g daily (Hahn, 2012)

Myasthenia gravis (unlabeled use): CellCept: Oral: 1 g twice daily (range: 1-3 g daily) (Cahoon, 2006; Ciafaloni, 2001; Merriggioli, 2003)

Psoriasis, moderate-to-severe (unlabeled use): CellCept: Oral: 2-3 g daily (Menter, 2009)

Elderly: Dosage is the same as younger patients, however, dosing should be cautious due to possibility of increased hepatic, renal or cardiac dysfunction; elderly patients may be at an increased risk of certain infections, gastrointestinal hemorrhage, and pulmonary edema, as compared to younger patients

Dosing adjustment for toxicity (neutropenia): Neutropenia (ANC <1.3 x 10^3/µL): Dosing should be interrupted or the dose reduced, appropriate diagnostic tests performed and patients managed appropriately

Dosing adjustment in renal impairment:

Renal transplant: GFR <25 mL/minute/1.73 m^2 in patients outside the immediate post-transplant period:

CellCept: Doses of >1 g administered twice daily should be avoided; patients should also be carefully observed; no dose adjustments are needed in renal transplant patients experiencing delayed graft function postoperatively

Myfortic: No dose adjustments are needed in renal transplant patients experiencing delayed graft function postoperatively; however, monitor carefully for potential concentration dependent adverse events

Cardiac or liver transplant: No data available; mycophenolate may be used in cardiac or hepatic transplant patients with severe chronic renal impairment if the potential benefit outweighs the potential risk

Hemodialysis: Not removed; supplemental dose is not necessary

Peritoneal dialysis: Supplemental dose is not necessary

Dosage adjustment in hepatic impairment: No dosage adjustment is recommended for renal patients with severe hepatic parenchymal disease; however, it is not currently known whether dosage adjustments are necessary for hepatic disease with other etiologies

Dietary Considerations Oral dosage formulations should be taken on an empty stomach to avoid variability in MPA absorption. However, in stable renal transplant patients, Cellcept may be administered with food if necessary. Some products may contain phenylalanine.

Administration

Oral dosage formulations (tablet, capsule, suspension) should be administered on an empty stomach (1 hour before or 2 hours after meals) to avoid variability in MPA absorption. The oral solution may be administered via a nasogastric tube (minimum 8 French, 1.7 mm interior diameter); oral suspension should not be mixed with other medications. Delayed release tablets should not be crushed, cut, or chewed. Cellcept may be administered with food in stable renal transplant patients when necessary. If a dose is missed, administer as soon as it is remembered. If it is close to the next scheduled dose, skip the missed dose and resume at next regularly scheduled time; do not double a dose to make up for a missed dose.

Intravenous solutions should be administered over at least 2 hours (either peripheral or central vein); do **not** administer intravenous solution by rapid or bolus injection.

Hazardous agent; use appropriate precautions for handling and disposal (NIOSH, 2012).

Monitoring Parameters Complete blood count (weekly for first month, twice monthly during months 2 and 3, then monthly thereafter through the first year); renal and liver function; signs and symptoms of organ rejection; signs and symptoms of bacterial, fungal, protozoal, new or reactivated viral, or opportunistic infections; neurological symptoms (eg, hemiparesis, confusion, cognitive deficiencies, ataxia) suggestive of PML, pregnancy test (immediately prior to initiation and 8-10 days later in females of childbearing potential, followed by repeat tests during therapy); monitor skin (for lesions suspicious of skin cancer); monitor for signs of lymphoma

Additional Information Females of reproductive potential are required to have contraceptive counseling and use acceptable birth control unless heterosexual intercourse is completely avoided. Use of an intrauterine device (IUD), tubal sterilization, or vasectomy of the female patient's partner are acceptable contraceptive methods that can be used alone. If a hormonal contraceptive is used (eg, combination oral contraceptive pills, transdermal patches, vaginal rings, or progestin only products), then one barrier method must also be used (eg, diaphragm or cervical cap with spermicide, contraceptive sponge, male or female condom). Alternatively, the use of two barrier methods is also acceptable (eg, diaphragm or cervical cap with spermicide, or contraceptive sponge **PLUS** male or female condom). Refer to manufacturer's labeling for full details.

Dosage Forms Excipient information presented when available (limited, particularly for generics); consult specific product labeling.

Capsule, Oral, as mofetil:

CellCept: 250 mg [contains fd&c blue #2 (indigotine)]

Generic: 250 mg

Solution Reconstituted, Intravenous, as mofetil hydrochloride:

CellCept Intravenous: 500 mg (1 ea)

Suspension Reconstituted, Oral, as mofetil:

CellCept: 200 mg/mL (160 mL) [contains aspartame, methylparaben, soybean lecithin; mixed fruit flavor]

Tablet, Oral, as mofetil:

CellCept: 500 mg [contains fd&c blue #2 aluminum lake]

Generic: 500 mg

Tablet, Oral, as mycophenolic acid:

Generic: 500 mg

Tablet Delayed Release, Oral, as mycophenolic acid:

Myfortic: 180 mg [contains fd&c blue #2 (indigotine)]

Myfortic: 360 mg

Generic: 180 mg, 360 mg

Extemporaneous Preparations Hazardous agent: Use appropriate precautions for handling and disposal.

A 50 mg/mL oral suspension may be made with mycophenolate mofetil capsules, Ora-Plus, and cherry syrup. In a vertical flow hood, empty six 250 mg capsules into a mortar; add 7.5 mL Ora-Plus and mix to a uniform paste. Mix while adding 15 mL of cherry syrup in incremental proportions; transfer to a calibrated bottle, rinse mortar with cherry syrup, and add sufficient quantity of cherry syrup to make 30 mL. Label "shake well". Stable for 210 days at 5°C, for 28 days at 25°C to 37°C, and for 11 days at 45°C.

Venkataramanan R, McCombs JR, Zuckerman S, et al, "Stability of Mycophenolate Mofetil as an Extemporaneous Suspension," *Ann Pharmacother*, 1998, 32(7-8):755-7.

- **Mycophenolate Mofetil** *see* Mycophenolate *on page 1407*
- **Mycophenolate Sodium** *see* Mycophenolate *on page 1407*
- **Mycophenolic Acid** *see* Mycophenolate *on page 1407*
- **Mydral** *see* Tropicamide *on page 2132*
- **Mydriacyl** *see* Tropicamide *on page 2132*
- **Mydriacyl® (Can)** *see* Tropicamide *on page 2132*
- **Myferon 150 [OTC]** *see* Polysaccharide-Iron Complex *on page 1673*
- **Myfortic** *see* Mycophenolate *on page 1407*
- **Mylan-Acebutolol (Can)** *see* Acebutolol *on page 28*
- **Mylan-Acebutolol (Type S) (Can)** *see* Acebutolol *on page 28*
- **Mylan-Acyclovir (Can)** *see* Acyclovir (Systemic) *on page 42*
- **Mylan-Alendronate (Can)** *see* Alendronate *on page 69*
- **Mylan-Almotriptan (Can)** *see* Almotriptan *on page 79*
- **Mylan-Alprazolam (Can)** *see* ALPRAZolam *on page 81*
- **Mylan-Amantadine (Can)** *see* Amantadine *on page 92*
- **Mylan-Amiodarone (Can)** *see* Amiodarone *on page 101*
- **Mylan-Amlodipine (Can)** *see* AmLODIPine *on page 109*
- **Mylan-Amoxicillin (Can)** *see* Amoxicillin *on page 116*
- **Mylan-Anagrelide (Can)** *see* Anagrelide *on page 136*
- **Mylan-Anastrozole (Can)** *see* Anastrozole *on page 137*
- **Mylan-Atenolol (Can)** *see* Atenolol *on page 186*
- **Mylan-Atomoxetine (Can)** *see* AtoMOXetine *on page 187*
- **Mylan-Atorvastatin (Can)** *see* AtorvaSTATin *on page 190*
- **Mylan-Azathioprine (Can)** *see* AzaTHIOprine *on page 208*
- **Mylan-Azithromycin (Can)** *see* Azithromycin (Systemic) *on page 214*
- **Mylan-Baclofen (Can)** *see* Baclofen *on page 221*

- ◆ **Mylan-Rizatriptan ODT (Can)** *see* Rizatriptan *on page* *1844*
- ◆ **Mylan-Rosuvastatin (Can)** *see* Rosuvastatin *on page* *1858*
- ◆ **Mylan-Salbutamol Respirator Solution (Can)** *see* Albuterol *on page* *61*
- ◆ **Mylan-Salbutamol Sterinebs P.F. (Can)** *see* Albuterol *on page* *61*
- ◆ **Mylan-Selegiline (Can)** *see* Selegiline *on page* *1884*
- ◆ **Mylan-Sertraline (Can)** *see* Sertraline *on page* *1889*
- ◆ **Mylan-Simvastatin (Can)** *see* Simvastatin *on page* *1899*
- ◆ **Mylan-Sotalol (Can)** *see* Sotalol *on page* *1942*
- ◆ **Mylan-Sumatriptan (Can)** *see* SUMAtriptan *on page* *1969*
- ◆ **Mylanta™ (Can)** *see* Aluminum Hydroxide and Magnesium Hydroxide *on page* *90*
- ◆ **Mylanta® Classic Maximum Strength Liquid [OTC]** *see* Aluminum Hydroxide, Magnesium Hydroxide, and Simethicone *on page* *90*
- ◆ **Mylanta® Classic Regular Strength Liquid [OTC]** *see* Aluminum Hydroxide, Magnesium Hydroxide, and Simethicone *on page* *90*
- ◆ **Mylanta® Double Strength (Can)** *see* Aluminum Hydroxide, Magnesium Hydroxide, and Simethicone *on page* *90*
- ◆ **Mylanta® Extra Strength (Can)** *see* Aluminum Hydroxide, Magnesium Hydroxide, and Simethicone *on page* *90*
- ◆ **Mylan-Tamoxifen (Can)** *see* Tamoxifen *on page* *1987*
- ◆ **Mylan-Tamsulosin (Can)** *see* Tamsulosin *on page* *1990*
- ◆ **Mylanta® Regular Strength (Can)** *see* Aluminum Hydroxide, Magnesium Hydroxide, and Simethicone *on page* *90*
- ◆ **Mylanta® Supreme [OTC]** *see* Calcium Carbonate and Magnesium Hydroxide *on page* *320*
- ◆ **Mylanta® Ultra [OTC]** *see* Calcium Carbonate and Magnesium Hydroxide *on page* *320*
- ◆ **Mylan-Telmisartan (Can)** *see* Telmisartan *on page* *2002*
- ◆ **Mylan-Telmisartan HCTZ (Can)** *see* Telmisartan and Hydrochlorothiazide *on page* *2004*
- ◆ **Mylan-Terbinafine (Can)** *see* Terbinafine (Systemic) *on page* *2017*
- ◆ **Mylan-Ticlopidine (Can)** *see* Ticlopidine *on page* *2059*
- ◆ **Mylan-Timolol (Can)** *see* Timolol (Ophthalmic) *on page* *2064*
- ◆ **Mylan-Tizanidine (Can)** *see* TiZANidine *on page* *2074*
- ◆ **Mylan-Topiramate (Can)** *see* Topiramate *on page* *2090*
- ◆ **Mylan-Trazodone (Can)** *see* TraZODone *on page* *2112*
- ◆ **Mylan-Triazolam (Can)** *see* Triazolam *on page* *2124*
- ◆ **Mylan-Valacyclovir (Can)** *see* ValACYclovir *on page* *2145*
- ◆ **Mylan-Valproic (Can)** *see* Valproic Acid and Derivatives *on page* *2149*
- ◆ **Mylan-Valsartan (Can)** *see* Valsartan *on page* *2154*
- ◆ **Mylan-Valsartan HCTZ (Can)** *see* Valsartan and Hydrochlorothiazide *on page* *2156*
- ◆ **Mylan-Venlafaxine XR (Can)** *see* Venlafaxine *on page* *2178*
- ◆ **Mylan-Verapamil (Can)** *see* Verapamil *on page* *2182*
- ◆ **Mylan-Verapamil SR (Can)** *see* Verapamil *on page* *2182*
- ◆ **Mylan-Warfarin (Can)** *see* Warfarin *on page* *2211*
- ◆ **Mylan-Zolmitriptan (Can)** *see* ZOLMitriptan *on page* *2240*
- ◆ **Mylan-Zolmitriptan ODT (Can)** *see* ZOLMitriptan *on page* *2240*
- ◆ **Myleran** *see* Busulfan *on page* *301*
- ◆ **Myleran® (Can)** *see* Busulfan *on page* *301*
- ◆ **Myl-Letrozole (Can)** *see* Letrozole *on page* *1185*
- ◆ **Mylotarg** *see* Gemtuzumab Ozogamicin *on page* *950*
- ◆ **Myl-Ranitidine (Can)** *see* Ranitidine *on page* *1782*
- ◆ **Myobloc** *see* RimabotulinumtoxinB *on page* *1820*
- ◆ **Myocet (Can)** *see* DOXOrubicin (Liposomal) *on page* *663*
- ◆ **Myorisan** *see* ISOtretinoin *on page* *1129*
- ◆ **Myozyme** *see* Alglucosidase Alfa *on page* *74*
- ◆ **Myozyme® (Can)** *see* Alglucosidase Alfa *on page* *74*
- ◆ **Myrbetriq** *see* Mirabegron *on page* *1378*
- ◆ **Mysoline** *see* Primidone *on page* *1715*
- ◆ **Mytotan** *see* Mitotane *on page* *1385*
- ◆ **Mytussin® DAC** *see* Guaifenesin, Pseudoephedrine, and Codeine *on page* *979*
- ◆ **My Way** *see* Levonorgestrel *on page* *1202*
- ◆ **Myzilra** *see* Ethinyl Estradiol and Levonorgestrel *on page* *787*
- ◆ **N-9** *see* Nonoxynol 9 *on page* *1471*
- ◆ **N-0923** *see* Rotigotine *on page* *1863*
- ◆ **NAAK** *see* Atropine and Pralidoxime *on page* *200*
- ◆ **Nabi-HB** *see* Hepatitis B Immune Globulin (Human) *on page* *993*
- ◆ **nab-Paclitaxel** *see* PACLitaxel (Protein Bound) *on page* *1546*

Nabumetone (na BYOO me tone)

Brand Names: Canada Apo-Nabumetone®; Gen-Nabumetone; Mylan-Nabumetone; Novo-Nabumetone; Relafen®; Rhoxal-nabumetone; Sandoz-Nabumetone

Index Terms Relafen

Pharmacologic Category Nonsteroidal Anti-inflammatory Drug (NSAID), Oral

Additional Appendix Information

Beers Criteria − Potentially Inappropriate Medications for Geriatrics *on page* *2368*

Use Management of osteoarthritis and rheumatoid arthritis

Unlabeled Use Moderate pain

Pregnancy Risk Factor C

Pregnancy Considerations Adverse events were not observed in the initial animal reproduction studies; therefore, the manufacturer classifies nabumetone as pregnancy category C. NSAID exposure during the first trimester is not strongly associated with congenital malformations; however, cardiovascular anomalies and cleft palate have been observed following NSAID exposure in some studies. The use of an NSAID close to conception may be associated with an increased risk of miscarriage. Nonteratogenic effects have been observed following NSAID administration during the third trimester including myocardial degenerative changes, prenatal constriction of the ductus arteriosus, fetal tricuspid regurgitation, failure of the ductus arteriosus to close postnatally; renal dysfunction or failure, oligohydramnios; gastrointestinal bleeding or perforation, increased risk of necrotizing enterocolitis; intracranial bleeding (including intraventricular hemorrhage), platelet dysfunction with resultant bleeding; pulmonary hypertension. Because they may cause premature closure of the ductus arteriosus, use of NSAIDs late in pregnancy should be avoided (use after 31 or 32 weeks gestation is not recommended by some clinicians). The chronic use of NSAIDs in women of reproductive age may be associated with infertility that is reversible upon discontinuation of the medication. A registry is available for pregnant women exposed to autoimmune medications including nabumetone. For additional information contact the Organization of Teratology Information Specialists, OTIS Autoimmune Diseases Study, at 877-311-8972.

Breast-Feeding Considerations It is not known if nabumetone or 6MNA are excreted into breast milk. Breast-feeding is not recommended by the manufacturer.

Medication Guide Available Yes

Contraindications Hypersensitivity to nabumetone, aspirin, other NSAIDs, or any component of the formulation; perioperative pain in the setting of coronary artery bypass graft (CABG) surgery

Warnings/Precautions [U.S. Boxed Warning]: NSAIDs are associated with an increased risk of adverse cardiovascular thrombotic events, including MI and stroke. Risk may be increased with duration of use or pre-existing cardiovascular risk factors or disease. Carefully evaluate individual cardiovascular risk profiles prior to prescribing. May cause new-onset hypertension or worsening of existing hypertension. Use caution with fluid retention. Avoid use in heart failure. Concurrent administration of ibuprofen, and potentially other nonselective NSAIDs, may interfere with aspirin's cardioprotective effect. **[U.S. Boxed Warning]: Use is contraindicated for treatment of perioperative pain in the setting of coronary artery bypass graft (CABG) surgery.** Risk of MI and stroke may be increased with use following CABG surgery.

Platelet adhesion and aggregation may be decreased; may prolong bleeding time; patients with coagulation disorders or who are receiving anticoagulants should be monitored closely. Anemia may occur; patients on long-term NSAID therapy should be monitored for anemia. Rarely, NSAID use may cause severe blood dyscrasias (eg, agranulocytosis, aplastic anemia, thrombocytopenia).

NSAID use may compromise existing renal function; dose-dependent decreases in prostaglandin synthesis may result from NSAID use, reducing renal blood flow which may cause renal decompensation. NSAID use may increase the risk for hyperkalemia. Patients with impaired renal function, dehydration, heart failure, liver dysfunction, those taking diuretics, and ACE inhibitors, and the elderly are at greater risk of renal toxicity and hyperkalemia. Rehydrate patient before starting therapy; monitor renal function closely. Not recommended for use in patients with advanced renal disease. Long-term NSAID use may result in renal papillary necrosis.

[U.S. Boxed Warning]: NSAIDs may increase risk of gastrointestinal irritation, inflammation, ulceration, bleeding, and perforation. These events may occur at any time during therapy and without warning. Use caution with a history of GI disease (bleeding or ulcers), concurrent therapy with aspirin, anticoagulants and/or corticosteroids, smoking, use of alcohol, the elderly or debilitated patients. When used concomitantly with ≤325 mg of aspirin, a substantial increase in the risk of gastrointestinal complications (eg, ulcer) occurs; concomitant gastroprotective therapy (eg, proton pump inhibitors) is recommended (Bhatt, 2008).

Use the lowest effective dose for the shortest duration of time, consistent with individual patient goals, to reduce risk of cardiovascular or GI adverse events. Alternate therapies should be considered for patients at high risk.

NSAIDs may cause serious skin adverse events including exfoliative dermatitis, Stevens-Johnson syndrome (SJS) and toxic epidermal necrolysis (TEN); discontinue use at first sign of skin rash or hypersensitivity. Anaphylactoid reactions may occur, even without prior exposure; patients with "aspirin triad" (bronchial asthma, aspirin intolerance, rhinitis) may be at increased risk. Do not use in patients who experience bronchospasm, asthma, rhinitis, or urticaria with NSAID or aspirin therapy. Use caution in other forms of asthma.

Use with caution in patients with decreased hepatic function. Closely monitor patients with any abnormal LFT. Severe hepatic reactions (eg, fulminant hepatitis, liver failure) have occurred with NSAID use, rarely; discontinue if signs or symptoms of liver disease develop, or if systemic manifestations occur.

NSAIDS may cause drowsiness, dizziness, blurred vision and other neurologic effects which may impair physical or mental abilities; patients must be cautioned about performing tasks which require mental alertness (eg, operating machinery or driving). Discontinue use with blurred or diminished vision and perform ophthalmologic exam. Monitor vision with long-term therapy.

In the elderly, avoid chronic use (unless alternative agents ineffective and patient can receive concomitant gastroprotective agent); nonselective oral NSAID use is associated with an increased risk of GI bleeding and peptic ulcer disease in older adults in high risk category (eg, >75 years or age or receiving concomitant oral/parenteral corticosteroids, anticoagulants, or antiplatelet agents) (Beers Criteria).

Withhold for at least 4-6 half-lives prior to surgical or dental procedures. May cause photosensitivity reactions.

Adverse Reactions

>10%: Gastrointestinal: Diarrhea (14%), dyspepsia (13%), abdominal pain (12%)

1% to 10%:

Cardiovascular: Edema (3% to 9%)

Central nervous system: Dizziness (3% to 9%), headache (3% to 9%), fatigue (1% to 3%), insomnia (1% to 3%), nervousness (1% to 3%), somnolence (1% to 3%)

Dermatologic: Pruritus (3% to 9%), rash (3% to 9%)

Gastrointestinal: Constipation (3% to 9%), flatulence (3% to 9%), guaiac positive (3% to 9%), nausea (3% to 9%), gastritis (1% to 3%), stomatitis (1% to 3%), vomiting (1% to 3%), xerostomia (1% to 3%)

Otic: Tinnitus

Miscellaneous: Diaphoresis (1% to 3%)

<1% (Limited to important or life-threatening): Abnormal vision, acne, agitation, albuminuria, alopecia, anaphylactoid reaction, anaphylaxis, anemia, angina, angioneurotic edema, anorexia, anxiety, arrhythmia, asthma, azotemia, bilirubinemia duodenitis, bullous eruptions, CHF, chills, confusion, cough, depression, duodenal ulcer, dysphagia, dyspnea, dysuria, eosinophilic pneumonia, eructation, erythema multiforme, fever, gallstones, gastric ulcer, gastroenteritis, gingivitis, GI bleeding, glossitis, granulocytopenia, hematuria, hepatic failure, hyperglycemia, hypersensitivity pneumonitis, hypertension, hyperuricemia, hypokalemia, impotence, interstitial nephritis, interstitial pneumonitis, jaundice, leukopenia, liver function abnormalities, malaise, melena, MI, nephrotic syndrome, nightmares, palpitation, pancreatitis, paresthesia, photosensitivity, pseudoporphyria cutanea tarda, rectal bleeding, renal failure, renal stones, Stevens-Johnson syndrome, syncope, taste disorder, thrombocytopenia, thrombophlebitis, toxic epidermal necrolysis, tremor, urticaria, vasculitis, vertigo, weakness, weight gain/loss

Drug Interactions

Metabolism/Transport Effects None known.

Avoid Concomitant Use

Avoid concomitant use of Nabumetone with any of the following: Floctafenine; Ketorolac (Nasal); Ketorolac (Systemic); NSAID (COX-2 Inhibitor); Omacetaxine

Increased Effect/Toxicity

Nabumetone may increase the levels/effects of: 5-ASA Derivatives; Agents with Antiplatelet Properties; Aliskiren; Aminoglycosides; Anticoagulants; Bisphosphonate Derivatives; Collagenase (Systemic); CycloSPORINE

(Systemic); Dabigatran Etexilate; Deferasirox; Desmopressin; Digoxin; Eplerenone; Haloperidol; Ibritumomab; Lithium; Methotrexate; Nonsteroidal Anti-Inflammatory Agents; NSAID (COX-2 Inhibitor); Omacetaxine; PEMEtrexed; Porfimer; Potassium-Sparing Diuretics; PRALAtrexate; Quinolone Antibiotics; Rivaroxaban; Salicylates; Tenofovir; Thrombolytic Agents; Tositumomab and Iodine I 131 Tositumomab; Vancomycin; Vitamin K Antagonists

The levels/effects of Nabumetone may be increased by: ACE Inhibitors; Angiotensin II Receptor Blockers; Antidepressants (Tricyclic, Tertiary Amine); Corticosteroids (Systemic); CycloSPORINE (Systemic); Dasatinib; Floctafenine; Glucosamine; Herbs (Anticoagulant/Antiplatelet Properties); Ibrutinib; Ketorolac (Nasal); Ketorolac (Systemic); Multivitamins/Fluoride (with ADE); Multivitamins/Minerals (with ADEK, Folate, Iron); Multivitamins/Minerals (with AE, No Iron); Nonsteroidal Anti-Inflammatory Agents; Omega-3 Fatty Acids; Pentosan Polysulfate Sodium; Pentoxifylline; Probenecid; Prostacyclin Analogues; Selective Serotonin Reuptake Inhibitors; Serotonin/Norepinephrine Reuptake Inhibitors; Sodium Phosphates; Tipranavir; Treprostinil; Vitamin E

Decreased Effect

Nabumetone may decrease the levels/effects of: ACE Inhibitors; Agents with Antiplatelet Properties; Aliskiren; Angiotensin II Receptor Blockers; Beta-Blockers; Eplerenone; HydrALAZINE; Loop Diuretics; Potassium-Sparing Diuretics; Prostaglandins (Ophthalmic); Salicylates; Selective Serotonin Reuptake Inhibitors; Thiazide Diuretics

The levels/effects of Nabumetone may be decreased by: Bile Acid Sequestrants; Nonsteroidal Anti-Inflammatory Agents; Salicylates

Ethanol/Nutrition/Herb Interactions

Ethanol: Avoid ethanol (may enhance gastric mucosal irritation).

Food: Nabumetone peak serum concentrations may be increased if taken with food or dairy products.

Herb/Nutraceutical: Avoid alfalfa, anise, bilberry, bladderwrack, bromelain, cat's claw, celery, chamomile, coleus, cordyceps, dong quai, evening primrose, fenugreek, feverfew, garlic, ginger, ginkgo biloba, ginseng (American, Panax, Siberian), grapeseed, green tea, guggul, horse chestnut seed, horseradish, licorice, prickly ash, red clover, reishi, SAMe (S-adenosylmethionine), sweet clover, turmeric, white willow (all have additional antiplatelet activity).

Mechanism of Action Reversibly inhibits cyclooxygenase-1 and 2 (COX-1 and 2) enzymes, which results in decreased formation of prostaglandin precursors; has antipyretic, analgesic, and anti-inflammatory properties

Other proposed mechanisms not fully elucidated (and possibly contributing to the anti-inflammatory effect to varying degrees), include inhibiting chemotaxis, altering lymphocyte activity, inhibiting neutrophil aggregation/activation, and decreasing proinflammatory cytokine levels.

Pharmacodynamics/Kinetics

Onset of action: Several days

Distribution: Diffusion occurs readily into synovial fluid

V_d: 6MNA: 29-82 L

Protein binding: 6MNA: >99%

Metabolism: Prodrug, rapidly metabolized in the liver to an active metabolite [6-methoxy-2-naphthylacetic acid (6MNA)] and inactive metabolites; extensive first-pass effect

Half-life elimination: 6MNA: ~24 hours

Time to peak, serum: 6MNA: Oral: 2.5-4 hours; Synovial fluid: 4-12 hours

Excretion: 6MNA: Urine (80%) and feces (9%)

Dosage Adults: Oral: 1000 mg/day; an additional 500-1000 mg may be needed in some patients to obtain more symptomatic relief; may be administered once or twice daily (maximum dose: 2000 mg/day)

Note: Patients <50 kg are less likely to require doses >1000 mg/day.

Dosage adjustment in renal impairment: In general, NSAIDs are not recommended for use in patients with advanced renal disease, but the manufacturer of nabumetone does provide some guidelines for adjustment in renal dysfunction:

Moderate impairment (Cl_{cr} 30-49 mL/minute): Initial dose: 750 mg/day; maximum dose: 1500 mg/day

Severe impairment (Cl_{cr} <30 mL/minute): Initial dose: 500 mg/day; maximum dose: 1000 mg/day

Dosage adjustment in hepatic impairment: No dosage adjustment provided in manufacturer's labeling (has not been studied). Prodrug activation and metabolism are hepatic function dependent and may be reduced in severe hepatic impairment.

Monitoring Parameters Patients with renal insufficiency: Baseline renal function followed by repeat test within weeks (to determine if renal function has deteriorated)

Dosage Forms Excipient information presented when available (limited, particularly for generics); consult specific product labeling.

Tablet, Oral:

Generic: 500 mg, 750 mg

◆ **NAC** *see* Acetylcysteine *on page 36*

◆ ***N*-Acetyl-L-cysteine** *see* Acetylcysteine *on page 36*

◆ ***N* Acetylcysteine** *see* Acetylcysteine *on page 36*

◆ **N-Acetyl-P-Aminophenol** *see* Acetaminophen *on page 28*

◆ **NaCl** *see* Sodium Chloride *on page 1914*

Nadolol (NAY doe lol)

Brand Names: U.S. Corgard

Brand Names: Canada Apo-Nadol; Teva-Nadolol

Pharmacologic Category Antianginal Agent; Antihypertensive; Beta-Blocker, Nonselective

Additional Appendix Information

Beta-Blockers *on page 2294*

Use Treatment of hypertension and angina pectoris

Unlabeled Use Migraine headache prophylaxis; primary and secondary prophylaxis of variceal hemorrhage; management of thyrotoxicosis

Pregnancy Risk Factor C

Pregnancy Considerations Adverse events were observed in some animal reproduction studies; therefore, the manufacturer classifies nadolol as pregnancy category C. Nadolol crosses the placenta and is measurable in infant serum after birth. In a cohort study, an increased risk of cardiovascular defects was observed following maternal use of beta-blockers during pregnancy. Intrauterine growth restriction (IUGR), small placentas, as well as fetal/neonatal bradycardia, hypoglycemia, and/or respiratory depression have been observed following *in utero* exposure to beta-blockers as a class. Adequate facilities for monitoring infants at birth should be available. Untreated chronic maternal hypertension and pre-eclampsia are also associated with adverse events in the fetus, infant, and mother. Nadolol is indicated for the treatment of hypertension, but due to its long half-life and potential effects to the fetus, other agents may be more appropriate for use during pregnancy.

Breast-Feeding Considerations Nadolol is excreted into breast milk in concentrations higher than the maternal serum. According to the manufacturer, the decision to continue or discontinue breast-feeding during therapy should take into account the risk of exposure to the infant and the benefits of treatment to the mother. The time to peak milk concentration is 6 hours after the oral dose, the half-life of nadolol in breast milk is similar to that in the maternal serum, and nadolol can still be detected in breast milk for several days after the last maternal dose.

Contraindications

U.S. labeling: Hypersensitivity to nadolol or any component of the formulation; bronchial asthma; sinus bradycardia; sinus node dysfunction; heart block greater than first degree (except in patients with a functioning artificial pacemaker); cardiogenic shock; uncompensated cardiac failure

Canadian labeling: Hypersensitivity to nadolol or any component of the formulation; bronchial asthma; sinus bradycardia; sinus node dysfunction; heart block greater than first degree (except in patients with a functioning artificial pacemaker); cardiogenic shock; uncompensated cardiac failure; anesthesia with agents that produce myocardial depression; allergic rhinitis; severe chronic obstructive pulmonary disease (COPD)

Warnings/Precautions Consider pre-existing conditions such as sick sinus syndrome before initiating. Administer only with extreme caution in patients with compensated heart failure, monitor for a worsening of the condition. Efficacy in heart failure has not been established for nadolol. **[U.S. Boxed Warning]: Beta-blocker therapy should not be withdrawn abruptly (particularly in patients with CAD), but gradually tapered to avoid acute tachycardia, hypertension, and/or ischemia.** Chronic beta-blocker therapy should not be routinely withdrawn prior to major surgery. In general, patients with bronchospastic disease should not receive beta-blockers. Nadolol, if used at all, should be used cautiously in bronchospastic disease with close monitoring. Use cautiously in diabetics because it can mask prominent hypoglycemic symptoms. May mask signs of hyperthyroidism (eg, tachycardia); if hyperthyroidism is suspected, carefully manage and monitor; abrupt withdrawal may exacerbate symptoms of hyperthyroidism or precipitate thyroid storm. Use cautiously in the renally impaired (dosage adjustments are required). Use with caution in patients with myasthenia gravis, peripheral vascular disease, or psychiatric disease (may cause CNS depression). Bradycardia may be observed more frequently in elderly patients (>65 years of age); dosage reductions may be necessary. Potentially significant drug-drug interactions may exist, requiring dose or frequency adjustment, additional monitoring, and/or selection of alternative therapy. Adequate alpha-blockade is required prior to use of any beta-blocker for patients with untreated pheochromocytoma. May induce or exacerbate psoriasis. Use caution with history of severe anaphylaxis to allergens; patients taking beta-blockers may become more sensitive to repeated challenges. Treatment of anaphylaxis (eg, epinephrine) in patients taking beta-blockers may be ineffective or promote undesirable effects.

Adverse Reactions

>10%: Central nervous system: Drowsiness, insomnia

1% to 10%:

Cardiovascular: Atrioventricular block, bradycardia, cardiac conduction disturbance, cardiac failure, cold extremities, edema, hypotension, palpitations, peripheral vascular insufficiency, Raynaud's phenomenon

Central nervous system: Depression, dizziness, fatigue, sedation

<1% (Limited to important or life-threatening): Anorexia, bloating, bronchospasm, cardiac arrhythmia, confusion (especially in the elderly), cough, decreased libido, diarrhea, dyspepsia, facial edema, hallucination, headache, impotence, nasal congestion, nausea, paresthesia, pruritus, sedation, skin rash, slurred speech, thrombocytopenia, transient alopecia, weight gain, xeroderma, xerophthalmia

Drug Interactions

Metabolism/Transport Effects **Substrate** of P-glycoprotein

Avoid Concomitant Use

Avoid concomitant use of Nadolol with any of the following: Beta2-Agonists; Floctafenine; Methacholine

Increased Effect/Toxicity

Nadolol may increase the levels/effects of: Alpha-/Beta-Agonists (Direct-Acting); Alpha1-Blockers; Alpha2-Agonists; Amifostine; Antihypertensives; Bupivacaine; Cardiac Glycosides; Cholinergic Agonists; Ergot Derivatives; Fingolimod; Hypotensive Agents; Insulin; Lidocaine (Systemic); Lidocaine (Topical); Mepivacaine; Methacholine; Midodrine; Obinutuzumab; RiTUXimab; Sulfonylureas

The levels/effects of Nadolol may be increased by: Acetylcholinesterase Inhibitors; Alpha2-Agonists; Amiodarone; Anilidopiperidine Opioids; Brimonidine (Topical); Calcium Channel Blockers (Dihydropyridine); Calcium Channel Blockers (Nondihydropyridine); Diazoxide; Dipyridamole; Disopyramide; Dronedarone; Floctafenine; Herbs (Hypotensive Properties); MAO Inhibitors; Pentoxifylline; P-glycoprotein/ABCB1 Inhibitors; Phosphodiesterase 5 Inhibitors; Prostacyclin Analogues; Regorafenib; Reserpine

Decreased Effect

Nadolol may decrease the levels/effects of: Beta2-Agonists; Theophylline Derivatives

The levels/effects of Nadolol may be decreased by: Herbs (Hypertensive Properties); Methylphenidate; Nonsteroidal Anti-Inflammatory Agents; P-glycoprotein/ABCB1 Inducers; Yohimbine

Ethanol/Nutrition/Herb Interactions Herb/Nutraceutical: Avoid dong quai if using for hypertension (has estrogenic activity). Avoid ephedra, garlic, yohimbe, ginseng (may worsen hypertension). Avoid natural licorice (causes sodium and water retention and increases potassium loss).

Mechanism of Action Competitively blocks response to $beta_1$- and $beta_2$-adrenergic stimulation; does not exhibit any membrane stabilizing or intrinsic sympathomimetic activity. Nonselective beta-adrenergic blockers (propranolol, nadolol) reduce portal pressure by producing splanchnic vasoconstriction ($beta_2$ effect) thereby reducing portal blood flow.

Pharmacodynamics/Kinetics

Duration: 17-24 hours

Absorption: ~30%

Distribution: V_d: ~2 L/kg

Protein binding: 30%

Metabolism: Not metabolized

Half-life elimination: Adults: 20-24 hours; prolonged with renal impairment; (up to 45 hours in severe impairment) (Herrera, 1979)

Time to peak, serum: 3-4 hours

Excretion: Urine (as unchanged drug)

Dosage

U.S. labeling: Adults: Oral:

Angina: Initial: 40 mg once daily, increase dosage gradually by 40-80 mg increments at 3- to 7-day intervals until optimum clinical response is obtained usual dose: 40-80 mg daily; maximum dose: 240 mg daily

Hypertension: Initial: 40 mg once daily, increase dosage gradually by 40-80 mg increments until optimum blood pressure reduction achieved. Usual dosage range (JNC 7): 40-120 mg once daily. Doses up to 240-320 mg once daily in hypertension may be necessary

Canadian labeling: Adults: Oral:

Angina: Initial: 80 mg once daily, increase dosage gradually by 80 mg increments at 7-day intervals until optimum clinical response is obtained; may consider dose reduction to 40 mg once daily for patients stable on 80 mg daily; maximum dose: 240 mg daily

Hypertension: Initial: 80 mg once daily; increase dosage gradually by 80 mg increments at 7-day intervals until optimum blood pressure reduction achieved. Doses ≤240 mg daily are typically effective; maximum dose: 320 mg once daily

Unlabeled uses: Adults: Oral:

Variceal hemorrhage prophylaxis (Garcia-Tsao, 2007):

Primary prophylaxis: Initial: 40 mg once daily; adjust to maximal tolerated dose. **Note:** Risk factors for hemorrhage include Child-Pugh class B/C or variceal red wale markings on endoscopy.

Secondary prophylaxis: Initial: 40 mg once daily; adjust to maximal tolerated dose

Thyrotoxicosis: 40-160 mg once daily (Bahn, 2011)

Elderly: Hypertension: Consider lower initial doses (eg, 20 mg/day) and titrate to response (Aronow, 2011)

Dosing adjustment in renal impairment:

Cl_{cr} >50 mL/minute/1.73 m^2: Administer every 24 hours

Cl_{cr} 31-50 mL/minute/1.73 m^2: Administer every 24-36 hours

Cl_{cr} 10-30 mL/minute/1.73 m^2: Administer every 24-48 hours

Cl_{cr} <10 mL/minute/1.73 m^2: Administer every 40-60 hours

Dosage adjustments for dialysis are not provided in the manufacturer's labeling; however, the following guidelines have been used by some clinicians (Aronoff, 2007):

ESRD requiring hemodialysis: Administer dose post-dialysis.

Peritoneal dialysis: Administer every 40-60 hours

Dosing adjustment in hepatic impairment: There are no dosage adjustments provided in the manufacturer's labeling.

Dietary Considerations May be taken without regard to meals.

Administration May be administered without regard to meals.

Monitoring Parameters Heart rate, blood pressure, signs/symptom of angina exacerbation when discontinued

Dosage Forms Excipient information presented when available (limited, particularly for generics); consult specific product labeling.

Tablet, Oral:

Corgard: 20 mg, 40 mg, 80 mg [scored]

Generic: 20 mg, 40 mg, 80 mg

Nafarelin (naf a REL in)

Brand Names: U.S. Synarel

Brand Names: Canada Synarel®

Index Terms Nafarelin Acetate

Pharmacologic Category Gonadotropin Releasing Hormone Agonist

Use Treatment of endometriosis, including pain and reduction of lesions; treatment of central precocious puberty (CPP; gonadotropin-dependent precocious puberty) in children of both sexes

Pregnancy Risk Factor X

Dosage Intranasal:

Endometriosis: Adults: Females: 1 spray (200 mcg) in 1 nostril each morning and the other nostril each evening starting on days 2-4 of menstrual cycle (total: 2 sprays/day). Dose may be increased to 2 sprays (400 mcg; 1 spray in each nostril) in the morning and evening if amenorrhea is not achieved (total: 4 sprays [800 mcg]/day). Total duration of therapy should not exceed 6 months due to decreases in bone mineral density; retreatment is not recommended by the manufacturer.

Central precocious puberty: Children: Males/Females: 2 sprays (400 mcg) into each nostril in the morning and 2 sprays (400 mcg) into each nostril in the evening (total: 8 sprays [1600 mcg]/day). If inadequate suppression, may increase dose to 3 sprays (600 mcg) into alternating nostrils 3 times/day (total: 9 sprays [1800 mcg]/day).

Dosage adjustment in renal impairment: No dosage adjustment provided in manufacturer's labeling (has not been studied).

Dosage adjustment in hepatic impairment: No dosage adjustment provided in manufacturer's labeling (has not been studied).

Additional Information Complete prescribing information should be consulted for additional detail.

Dosage Forms Excipient information presented when available (limited, particularly for generics); consult specific product labeling.

Solution, Nasal:

Synarel: 2 mg/mL (8 mL)

◆ **Nafarelin Acetate** *see* Nafarelin *on page 1417*

Nafcillin (naf SIL in)

Brand Names: U.S. Nallpen in Dextrose

Index Terms Ethoxynaphthamido Penicillin Sodium; Nafcillin Sodium; Nallpen; Sodium Nafcillin

Pharmacologic Category Antibiotic, Penicillin

Additional Appendix Information

Antibiotic Treatment of Adults With Infective Endocarditis *on page 2355*

Desensitization Protocols *on page 2325*

Use Treatment of infections such as osteomyelitis, bacteremia, septicemia, endocarditis, and CNS infections caused by susceptible strains of *Staphylococcus* species

Pregnancy Risk Factor B

Pregnancy Considerations Adverse events have not been observed in animal reproduction studies. Information specific to nafcillin use in pregnancy is limited. Maternal use of penicillins has generally not resulted in an increased risk of birth defects.

Breast-Feeding Considerations Penicillins are excreted into breast milk. The manufacturer recommends that caution be exercised when administering nafcillin to nursing women. Nondose-related effects could include modification of bowel flora.

Contraindications Hypersensitivity to nafcillin, or any component of the formulation, or penicillins

Warnings/Precautions Serious and occasionally severe or fatal hypersensitivity (anaphylactoid) reactions have been reported in patients on penicillin therapy, especially with a history of beta-lactam hypersensitivity, history of sensitivity to multiple allergens, or previous IgE-mediated reactions (eg, anaphylaxis, angioedema, urticaria). Use with caution in asthmatic patients. Contains sodium; use with caution in patients with heart failure. Vesicant; ensure proper catheter or needle position prior to and during I.V. infusion; avoid extravasation of I.V. infusions. Large I.V. or intraventricular doses have been associated with neurotoxicity. Modification of dosage is necessary in patients with both severe renal and hepatic impairment. Elimination may be decreased in pediatric patients. Prolonged use ▶

may result in fungal or bacterial superinfection, including *C. difficile*-associated diarrhea (CDAD) and pseudomembranous colitis; CDAD has been observed >2 months postantibiotic treatment. Potentially significant drug-drug interactions may exist, requiring dose or frequency adjustment, additional monitoring, and/or selection of alternative therapy.

Adverse Reactions Frequency not always defined.

Central nervous system: Neurotoxicity (high doses)

Gastrointestinal: *C. difficile*-associated diarrhea

Hematologic: Agranulocytosis, bone marrow depression, neutropenia

Local: Inflammation, pain, phlebitis, skin sloughing, swelling, and thrombophlebitis at the injection site; tissue necrosis with sloughing (SubQ extravasation)

Renal: Interstitial nephritis (rare), renal tubular damage (rare)

Miscellaneous: Anaphylaxis, hypersensitivity reactions (immediate and delayed; general incidence of 1% to 10% for penicillins), serum sickness

<1% (Limited to important or life-threatening): ALT increased, AST increased, bilirubin increased, cholestatic hepatitis, diarrhea, drug-induced lupus erythematosus, fever, hypokalemia, itching, nausea, rash (including bullous skin eruptions), vomiting

Drug Interactions

Metabolism/Transport Effects Induces CYP3A4 (strong)

Avoid Concomitant Use

Avoid concomitant use of Nafcillin with any of the following: Abiraterone Acetate; Apixaban; Artemether; Axitinib; BCG; Bedaquiline; Boceprevir; Bortezomib; Bosutinib; Cabozantinib; CloZAPine; Crizotinib; Dienogest; Dronedarone; Enzalutamide; Everolimus; Ibrutinib; Itraconazole; Ivacaftor; Lapatinib; Lumefantrine; Lurasidone; Macitentan; Mifepristone; NIFEdipine; Nilotinib; Nisoldipine; PAZOPanib; Perampanel; Pomalidomide; PONATinib; Praziquantel; Ranolazine; Regorafenib; Rivaroxaban; Roflumilast; RomiDEPsin; Simeprevir; SORAfenib; Telaprevir; Ticagrelor; Tofacitinib; Tolvaptan; Toremifene; Ulipristal; Vandetanib; Vemurafenib; VinCRIStine (Liposomal)

Increased Effect/Toxicity

Nafcillin may increase the levels/effects of: Clarithromycin; Ifosfamide; Methotrexate; Vitamin K Antagonists

The levels/effects of Nafcillin may be increased by: Clarithromycin; Probenecid

Decreased Effect

Nafcillin may decrease the levels/effects of: Abiraterone Acetate; Apixaban; ARIPiprazole; Artemether; Axitinib; BCG; Bedaquiline; Boceprevir; Bortezomib; Bosutinib; Brentuximab Vedotin; Cabozantinib; Calcium Channel Blockers; Clarithromycin; CloZAPine; Contraceptives (Estrogens); Crizotinib; CycloSPORINE (Systemic); CYP3A4 Substrates; Dasatinib; Dienogest; Dronedarone; Enzalutamide; Everolimus; Exemestane; Gefitinib; GuanFACINE; Ibrutinib; Imatinib; Itraconazole; Ivacaftor; Ixabepilone; Lapatinib; Linagliptin; Lumefantrine; Lurasidone; Macitentan; Maraviroc; Mifepristone; Mycophenolate; NIFEdipine; Nilotinib; Nisoldipine; PAZOPanib; Perampanel; Pomalidomide; PONATinib; Praziquantel; QUEtiapine; Ranolazine; Regorafenib; Rivaroxaban; Roflumilast; RomiDEPsin; Saxagliptin; Simeprevir; Sodium Picosulfate; SORAfenib; SUNItinib; Tadalafil; Telaprevir; Ticagrelor; Tofacitinib; Tolvaptan; Toremifene; Typhoid Vaccine; Ulipristal; Vandetanib; Vemurafenib; VinCRIStine (Liposomal); Vitamin K Antagonists; Vortioxetine; Zuclopenthixol

The levels/effects of Nafcillin may be decreased by: Tetracycline Derivatives

Storage/Stability

Premixed infusions: Store in a freezer at -20°C (-4°F). Thaw at room temperature or under refrigeration only. Thawed bags are stable for 21 days under refrigeration or 72 hours at room temperature. Do not refreeze.

Vials: Reconstituted parenteral solution is stable for 3 days at room temperature and 7 days when refrigerated. For I.V. infusion in NS or D_5W, solution is stable for 24 hours at room temperature and 7 days when refrigerated.

Mechanism of Action Interferes with bacterial cell wall synthesis during active multiplication, causing cell wall destruction and resultant bactericidal activity against susceptible bacteria; resistant to inactivation by staphylococcal penicillinase

Pharmacodynamics/Kinetics

Distribution: Widely distributed; CSF penetration is poor but enhanced by meningeal inflammation

Protein binding: ~90%; primarily to albumin

Metabolism: Primarily hepatic; undergoes enterohepatic recirculation

Half-life elimination:

Neonates: <3 weeks: 2.2-5.5 hours; 4-9 weeks: 1.2-2.3 hours

Children 1 month to 14 years: 0.75-1.9 hours

Adults: Normal renal/hepatic function: 30-60 minutes

Time to peak, serum: I.M.: 30-60 minutes

Excretion: Primarily feces; urine (~30% as unchanged drug)

Dosage

Indication-specific dosing:

Children:

Mild-to-moderate infections: I.M., I.V.: 100-150 mg/kg/day in divided doses every 6 hours (maximum dose: 4000 mg daily)

Severe infections: I.M., I.V.: 150-200 mg/kg/day in divided doses every 4-6 hours; for life-threatening infection (eg, meningitis) daily doses up to 200 mg/kg are used (maximum dose: 12 g daily)

Adults: I.V.:

Endocarditis: Methicillin-susceptible *Staphylococcus aureus* (MSSA):

Native valve: 12 g/24 hours in 4-6 divided doses (ie, 2 g every 4 hours or 3 g every 6 hours) for 6 weeks. **Note:** Dosing intended for ***complicated*** right-sided infective endocarditis (IE) or left-sided IE. For ***uncomplicated*** right-sided IE, 2 weeks of therapy may be adequate (Baddour, 2005). The British Society for Antimicrobial Chemotherapy (BSAC) recommends 4 weeks of therapy with a penicillinase-resistant penicillin for all patients with native valve IE due to MSSA unless patient has intracardiac prostheses, secondary lung abscesses, or osteomyelitis, then extend treatment to ≥6 weeks (Gould, 2012).

Prosthetic valve: 12 g/24 hours in 6 divided doses (ie, 2 g every 4 hours) for ≥6 weeks (use with rifampin for entire course and gentamicin for first 2 weeks) (Baddour, 2005)

Prosthetic joint infections: *Staphylococci (oxacillin-susceptible):* 1500-2000 mg every 4-6 hours for 4-6 weeks (2-6 weeks if in combination with rifampin), followed by oral antibiotic treatment and suppressive regimens (Osmon, 2013)

Skin and soft tissue infections: *Methicillin-susceptible Staphylococcus aureus (including necrotizing infection of fascia, muscle, skin):* 1000-2000 mg every 4 hours (Stevens, 2005)

Dosing adjustment in renal impairment: No dosage adjustment is necessary unless in the setting of concomitant hepatic impairment; however, manufacturer labeling does not provide specific dosage adjustments.

Poorly dialyzed. No supplemental dose or dosage adjustment necessary, including patients on intermittent hemodialysis, peritoneal dialysis, or continuous renal replacement therapy (eg, CVVHD) (Aronoff, 2007; Heintz, 2009).

Dosing adjustment in hepatic impairment: No specific dosage adjustments provided in manufacturer's labeling; however, dosage adjustment may be necessary particularly in the setting of concomitant renal impairment; nafcillin primarily undergoes hepatic metabolism. In patients with both hepatic and renal impairment, monitoring of serum drug levels and modification of dosage may be necessary.

Dietary Considerations Some products may contain sodium.

Administration

I.M.: Administer as a deep intragluteal injection; rotate injection sites.

I.V.: Infuse over 30-60 minutes. Vesicant; ensure proper needle or catheter placement prior to and during I.V. infusion. Avoid extravasation.

Extravasation management: If extravasation occurs, stop infusion immediately and disconnect (leave needle/cannula in place); gently aspirate extravasated solution (do **NOT** flush the line); initiate hyaluronidase antidote; remove needle/cannula (if not using I.V. hyaluronidase antidote), apply dry cold compresses (Hurst, 2004); elevate extremity.

Hyaluronidase: Intradermal or SubQ: Inject a total of 1 mL (15 units/mL) as five separate 0.2 mL injections (using a 25-gauge needle) into area of extravasation at the leading edge in a clockwise manner (MacCara, 1983; Zenk, 1981).

Monitoring Parameters Baseline and periodic CBC with differential; periodic urinalysis, BUN, serum creatinine, AST and ALT; observe for signs and symptoms of anaphylaxis during first dose

Test Interactions Positive Coombs' test (direct), false-positive urinary and serum proteins; may inactivate aminoglycosides *in vitro*

Dosage Forms Excipient information presented when available (limited, particularly for generics); consult specific product labeling.

Solution, Intravenous:

Nallpen in Dextrose: 1 g/50 mL (50 mL); 2 g/100 mL (100 mL)

Solution Reconstituted, Injection:

Generic: 1 g (1 ea); 2 g (1 ea); 10 g (1 ea)

Solution Reconstituted, Injection [preservative free]:

Generic: 1 g (1 ea); 2 g (1 ea); 10 g (1 ea)

Solution Reconstituted, Intravenous:

Generic: 1 g (1 ea); 2 g (1 ea)

◆ **Nafcillin Sodium** *see* Nafcillin *on page 1417*

Naftifine (NAF ti feen)

Brand Names: U.S. Naftin

Index Terms Naftifine Hydrochloride

Pharmacologic Category Antifungal Agent, Topical

Use

Tineal infections: Cream 1% and 2%, Gel 1%: Topical treatment of tinea cruris (jock itch), tinea corporis (ringworm), and tinea pedis (athlete's foot).

Tinea pedis: Gel 2%: Topical treatment of tinea pedis (athlete's foot).

Pregnancy Risk Factor B

Dosage Topical: Adults:

Cream: Apply once daily to affected area and surrounding skin for up to 2 weeks (2%) or up to 4 weeks (1%)

Gel: Apply once daily (2%) or twice daily (1%) (morning and evening) to affected area and healthy surrounding skin (1/2 inch margin) for up to 2 weeks (2%) or 4 weeks (1%)

Additional Information Complete prescribing information should be consulted for additional detail.

Dosage Forms Excipient information presented when available (limited, particularly for generics); consult specific product labeling.

Cream, External, as hydrochloride:

Naftin: 1% (60 g, 90 g); 2% (45 g) [contains benzyl alcohol, cetyl alcohol]

Gel, External, as hydrochloride:

Naftin: 1% (40 g, 60 g, 90 g) [contains alcohol, usp, edetate disodium, polysorbate 80]

Naftin: 2% (45 g) [contains alcohol, usp, benzyl alcohol, edetate disodium, propylene glycol, trolamine (triethanolamine)]

◆ **Naftifine Hydrochloride** *see* Naftifine *on page 1419*

◆ **Naftin** *see* Naftifine *on page 1419*

◆ **$NaHCO_3$** *see* Sodium Bicarbonate *on page 1912*

Nalbuphine (NAL byoo feen)

Index Terms Nalbuphine Hydrochloride; Nubain

Pharmacologic Category Analgesic, Opioid; Analgesic, Opioid Partial Agonist

Additional Appendix Information

Opioid Conversion Table *on page 2306*

Use Relief of moderate-to-severe pain; preoperative analgesia, postoperative and surgical anesthesia, and obstetrical analgesia during labor and delivery

Unlabeled Use Opioid-induced pruritus

Pregnancy Risk Factor C

Pregnancy Considerations Adverse events were observed in some animal reproduction studies. Nalbuphine crosses the placenta. Nalbuphine is approved for use in obstetrical analgesia during labor and delivery. When used for pain relief during labor, opioids may temporarily affect the heart rate of the fetus (ACOG, 2002) and severe fetal bradycardia has been reported following use of nalbuphine in labor/delivery. Fetal bradycardia may occur when administered earlier in pregnancy (not documented). Use only if clearly needed, with monitoring to detect and manage possible adverse fetal effects. Naloxone has been reported to reverse bradycardia. Newborn should be monitored for respiratory depression or bradycardia following nalbuphine use in labor.

If chronic opioid exposure occurs in pregnancy, adverse events in the newborn (including withdrawal) may occur; monitoring of the neonate is recommended. The minimum effective dose should be used if opioids are needed (Chou, 2009). Neonatal abstinence syndrome following opioid exposure may present with autonomic (eg, fever, temperature instability), gastrointestinal (eg, diarrhea, vomiting, poor feeding/weight gain), or neurologic (eg, high-pitched crying, increased muscle tone, irritability, seizure, tremor) symptoms (Dow, 2012; Hudak, 2012).

Breast-Feeding Considerations Small amounts (<1% of maternal dose) of nalbuphine are excreted in breast milk. The manufacturer recommends that caution be exercised when administering nalbuphine to nursing women.

Parenteral opioids used during labor have the potential to interfere with a newborns natural reflex to nurse within the first few hours after birth. If nalbuphine is administered to a nursing woman, it is recommended to monitor both the mother and baby for psychotomimetic reactions. Nursing infants exposed to large doses of opioids should also be monitored for apnea and sedation (Montgomery, 2012).

Contraindications Hypersensitivity to nalbuphine or any component of the formulation

Warnings/Precautions Use caution in CNS depression. Sedation and psychomotor impairment are likely, and are additive with other CNS depressants or ethanol. May cause respiratory depression. Ambulatory patients must be cautioned about performing tasks which require mental alertness (eg, operating machinery or driving). Potentially significant drug interactions may exist, requiring dose or frequency adjustment, additional monitoring, and/or selection of alternative therapy. Effects may be potentiated when used with other sedative drugs or ethanol. Use with caution in patients with recent myocardial infarction, biliary tract impairment, pancreatitis, morbid obesity, thyroid dysfunction, head trauma, or increased intracranial pressure. Avoid use in patients with CNS depression or coma as these patients are susceptible to intracranial effects of CO_2 retention. Use caution in patients with prostatic hyperplasia and/or urinary stricture, adrenal insufficiency, decreased hepatic or renal function. Use with caution in patients with pre-existing respiratory compromise (hypoxia and/or hypercapnia), COPD or other obstructive pulmonary disease; critical respiratory depression may occur, even at therapeutic dosages. May cause hypotension; use with caution in patients with hypovolemia, cardiovascular disease (including acute MI), or drugs which may exaggerate hypotensive effects (including phenothiazines or general anesthetics). May obscure diagnosis or clinical course of patients with acute abdominal conditions. May result in tolerance and/or drug dependence with chronic use; use with caution in patients with a history of drug dependence. Abrupt discontinuation following prolonged use may lead to withdrawal symptoms. May precipitate withdrawal symptoms in patients following prolonged therapy with mu opioid agonists.

Use with caution in pregnancy (close neonatal monitoring required when used in labor and delivery). After chronic maternal exposure to opioids, neonatal withdrawal syndrome may occur in the newborn; monitor neonate closely. Signs and symptoms include irritability, hyperactivity and abnormal sleep pattern, high pitched cry, tremor, vomiting, diarrhea and failure to gain weight. Onset, duration and severity depend on the drug used, duration of use, maternal dose, and rate of drug elimination by the newborn. Opioid withdrawal syndrome in the neonate, unlike in adults, may be life-threatening and should be treated according to protocols developed by neonatology experts. Use with caution in the elderly and debilitated patients; may be more sensitive to adverse effects. Safety and efficacy in children have not been established.

Adverse Reactions

>10%: Central nervous system: Sedation (36%)

1% to 10%:

Central nervous system: Dizziness (5%), headache (3%)
Gastrointestinal: Nausea/vomiting (6%), xerostomia (4%)
Miscellaneous: Clamminess (9%)

<1% (Limited to important or life-threatening): Abdominal pain, agitation, allergic reaction, anaphylaxis, anaphylactoid reaction, anxiety, asthma, bitter taste, blurred vision, bradycardia, cardiac arrest, confusion, crying, delusion, depersonalization, depression, diaphoresis, dreams (abnormal), dyspepsia, dysphoria, dyspnea, euphoria, faintness, fever, floating sensation, flushing, gastrointestinal cramps, hallucinations, hostility, hypertension, hypotension, injection site reactions (pain, swelling, redness, burning); laryngeal edema, loss of consciousness, nervousness, numbness, pruritus, pulmonary edema, rash, respiratory depression, respiratory distress, restlessness, seizure, sensation of warmth/burning, somnolence, speech disorder, stridor, tachycardia, tingling, tremor, unreality, urinary urgency, urticaria

Drug Interactions

Metabolism/Transport Effects None known.

Avoid Concomitant Use

Avoid concomitant use of Nalbuphine with any of the following: Azelastine (Nasal); Paraldehyde

Increased Effect/Toxicity

Nalbuphine may increase the levels/effects of: Alcohol (Ethyl); Alvimopan; Azelastine (Nasal); CNS Depressants; Desmopressin; Diuretics; Metyrosine; Mirtazapine; Paraldehyde; Pramipexole; ROPINIRole; Rotigotine; Selective Serotonin Reuptake Inhibitors; Zolpidem

The levels/effects of Nalbuphine may be increased by: Amphetamines; Anticholinergics; Antipsychotic Agents (Phenothiazines); Brimonidine (Topical); Cannabinoids; Doxylamine; Droperidol; HydrOXYzine; Magnesium Sulfate; Perampanel; Sodium Oxybate; Succinylcholine

Decreased Effect

Nalbuphine may decrease the levels/effects of: Analgesics (Opioid); Pegvisomant

The levels/effects of Nalbuphine may be decreased by: Ammonium Chloride; Mixed Agonist / Antagonist Opioids

Ethanol/Nutrition/Herb Interactions

Ethanol: May increase CNS depression; monitor for increased effects with coadministration. Caution patients about effects.

Herb/Nutraceutical: Avoid valerian, St John's wort, kava kava, gotu kola (may increase CNS depression).

Storage/Stability Store at room temperature of 15°C to 30°C (59°F to 86°F). Protect from light.

Mechanism of Action Agonist of kappa opiate receptors and partial antagonist of mu opiate receptors in the CNS, causing inhibition of ascending pain pathways, altering the perception of and response to pain; produces generalized CNS depression

Pharmacodynamics/Kinetics

Onset of action: Peak effect: SubQ, I.M.: <15 minutes; I.V.: 2-3 minutes
Metabolism: Hepatic
Half-life elimination: 5 hours
Excretion: Feces; urine (~7% as metabolites)

Dosage

Children ≥1 year (unlabeled use): Pain management: I.M., I.V., SubQ: 0.1-0.2 mg/kg every 3-4 hours as needed; maximum: 20 mg/dose and/or 160 mg/day

Adults:

Pain management: I.M., I.V., SubQ: 10 mg/70 kg every 3-6 hours; maximum single dose in nonopioid-tolerant patients: 20 mg; maximum daily dose: 160 mg

Surgical anesthesia supplement: I.V.: Induction: 0.3-3 mg/kg over 10-15 minutes; maintenance doses of 0.25-0.5 mg/kg may be given as required

Opioid-induced pruritus (unlabeled use): I.V. 2.5-5 mg; may repeat dose

Dosing adjustment in renal impairment: Use with caution and reduce dose; monitor.

Dosing adjustment in hepatic impairment: Use with caution and reduce dose.

Administration Administer I.M., SubQ, or I.V.

Monitoring Parameters Relief of pain, respiratory and mental status, blood pressure

Test Interactions May interfere with certain enzymatic methods used to detect opioids, depending on sensitivity and specificity of the test (refer to test manufacturer for details)

Dosage Forms Excipient information presented when available (limited, particularly for generics); consult specific product labeling.

Solution, Injection, as hydrochloride:

Generic: 10 mg/mL (1 mL, 10 mL); 20 mg/mL (1 mL, 10 mL)

◆ **Nalbuphine Hydrochloride** *see* Nalbuphine *on page 1419*

◆ **Nalfon** *see* Fenoprofen *on page 842*

◆ **Nalfon® (Can)** *see* Fenoprofen *on page 842*

◆ **Nallpen** *see* Nafcillin *on page 1417*

◆ **Nallpen in Dextrose** *see* Nafcillin *on page 1417*

◆ ***N*-allylnoroxymorphine Hydrochloride** *see* Naloxone *on page 1421*

Naloxone (nal OKS one)

Brand Names: Canada Naloxone Hydrochloride Injection®; Naloxone Hydrochloride Injection® USP

Index Terms *N*-allylnoroxymorphine Hydrochloride; Naloxone Hydrochloride; Narcan

Pharmacologic Category Antidote; Opioid Antagonist

Use Complete or partial reversal of opioid drug effects, including respiratory depression; management of known or suspected opioid overdose; diagnosis of suspected opioid dependence or acute opioid overdose

Unlabeled Use Opioid-induced pruritus

Pregnancy Risk Factor C

Pregnancy Considerations Adverse events were not observed in animal reproduction studies. Naloxone crosses the placenta. Consider the benefit to the mother and the risk to the fetus before administering to a pregnant woman who is known or suspected to be opioid dependent; may precipitate withdrawal in both the mother and fetus. In general, medications used as antidotes should take into consideration the health and prognosis of the mother; antidotes should be administered to pregnant women if there is a clear indication for use and should not be withheld because of fears of teratogenicity (Bailey, 2003). Use caution in pregnant women with mild-to-moderate hypertension during labor; severe hypertension may occur.

Breast-Feeding Considerations It is not known if naloxone is excreted into breast milk, however, systemic absorption following oral administration is low (Smith, 2012) and any exposure of naloxone to a nursing infant would therefore be limited. Since naloxone is used for opioid reversal, the opioid concentrations in the milk of a breast-feeding mother and potential transfer of the opioid to the infant should be considered.

Contraindications Hypersensitivity to naloxone or any component of the formulation

Warnings/Precautions Due to an association between naloxone and acute pulmonary edema, use with caution in patients with cardiovascular disease or in patients receiving medications with potential adverse cardiovascular effects (eg, hypotension, pulmonary edema, or arrhythmias). Administration of naloxone causes the release of catecholamines; may precipitate acute withdrawal or unmask pain in those who regularly take opioids. Excessive dosages should be avoided after use of opioids in surgery. Abrupt postoperative reversal may result in nausea, vomiting, sweating, tachycardia, hypertension, seizures, and other cardiovascular events (including pulmonary edema and arrhythmias). May precipitate withdrawal symptoms in patients addicted to opioids, including pain, hypertension, sweating, agitation, irritability; in neonates, symptoms may include shrill cry, failure to feed; carefully titrate dose to reverse hypoventilation; do not fully awaken patient or reverse analgesic effect (postoperative patient). Use caution in patients with history of seizures; avoid use in treatment of meperidine-induced seizures. Recurrence of respiratory depression is possible if the opioid involved is long-acting; observe patients until there is no reasonable risk of recurrent respiratory depression.

To prevent overdose deaths, there are initiatives to dispense naloxone for self- or buddy-administration to patients at risk of opioid overdose (eg, recipients of high-dose opioids, suspected or confirmed history of illicit opioid use) and individuals likely to be present in an overdose situation (eg, family members of illicit drug users) (Albert, 2011; Bennett, 2011). Needleless administration via nebulization and the intranasal route by first responders and bystanders has also been described (Doe-Simkins, 2009; Weber, 2012). Needleless administration provides an alternative route of administration in patients with venous scarring due to illicit drug use (eg, heroin). There is a low incidence of death following naloxone reversal of opioid toxicity in patients who refuse transport to a healthcare facility (Wampler, 2011).

Adverse Reactions Adverse reactions are related to reversing dependency and precipitating withdrawal. Withdrawal symptoms are the result of sympathetic excess. Adverse events occur secondarily to reversal (withdrawal) of opioid analgesia and sedation.

Cardiovascular: Cardiac arrest, fever, flushing, hypertension, hypotension, tachycardia, ventricular fibrillation ventricular tachycardia

Central nervous system: Agitation, coma, crying (excessive [neonates]), encephalopathy, hallucination, irritability, nervousness, restlessness, seizure (neonates), tremulousness

Gastrointestinal: Abdominal cramps, diarrhea, nausea, vomiting

Local: Injection site reaction

Neuromuscular & skeletal: Ache, hyperreflexia (neonates), paresthesia, piloerection, tremor, weakness

Respiratory: Dyspnea, hypoxia, pulmonary edema, respiratory depression, rhinorrhea, sneezing

Miscellaneous: Diaphoresis, hot flashes, shivering, yawning

Drug Interactions

Metabolism/Transport Effects None known.

Avoid Concomitant Use There are no known interactions where it is recommended to avoid concomitant use.

Increased Effect/Toxicity There are no known significant interactions involving an increase in effect.

Decreased Effect There are no known significant interactions involving a decrease in effect.

Preparation for Administration

I.V. push: Dilute naloxone 0.4 mg (1 mL ampul) with 9 mL of NS for a total volume of 10 mL to achieve a concentration of 0.04 mg/mL (APS, 2008)

I.V. infusion: Dilute naloxone 2 mg in 500 mL of NS or D_5W to make a final concentration of 4 **mcg**/mL; use within 24 hours

Inhalation via nebulization (unlabeled route): Dilute 2 mg of naloxone with 3 mL of normal saline (Mycyk, 2003; Weber, 2012)

Storage/Stability Store at 20°C to 25°C (68°F to 77°F). Protect from light.

Mechanism of Action Pure opioid antagonist that competes and displaces opioids at opioid receptor sites

Pharmacodynamics/Kinetics

Onset of action: Endotracheal, I.M., SubQ: 2-5 minutes; Inhalation via nebulization: ~5 minutes (Mycyk, 2003); Intranasal: ~8-13 minutes (Kelley, 2005; Robertson, 2009); I.V.: ~2 minutes

Duration: ~30-120 minutes depending on route of administration; I.V. has a shorter duration of action than I.M. administration; since naloxone's action is shorter than that of most opioids, repeated doses are usually needed

Metabolism: Primarily hepatic via glucuronidation

Half-life elimination: Neonates: 3-4 hours; Adults: 0.5-1.5 hours

Excretion: Urine (as metabolites)

Dosage Note: Available routes of administration include I.V. (preferred), I.M., and SubQ; other available routes (unlabeled) include endotracheal, inhalation via nebulization (adults only), intranasal (adults only), and intraosseous (I.O.). Endotracheal administration is the least desirable and is supported by only anecdotal evidence (case report) (Neumar, 2010); nebulized naloxone has been shown to be an effective alternative to parenteral administration when needleless administration is desired (Weber, 2012):

Infants, Children, and Adolescents:

Opioid overdose (with standard PALS protocols): I.V., intraosseous (I.O.) (unlabeled route), endotracheal (unlabeled route): **Note:** I.V. administration is preferred; I.O. and endotracheal routes are alternative routes recommended by the PALS guidelines (Kleinman, 2010)

<5 years or ≤20 kg (unlabeled dose): 0.1 mg/kg/dose (maximum dose: 2 mg); repeat every 2-3 minutes if needed (Hegenbarth, 2008; Kleinman, 2010)

≥5 years or >20 kg: 2 mg; if no response, repeat every 2-3 minutes. If no response is observed after 10 mg total, consider other causes of respiratory depression (Hegenbarth, 2008; Kleinman, 2010).

Continuous infusion (unlabeled dosing): I.V.: If continuous infusion is required, calculate dosage/hour based on effective intermittent dose used and duration of adequate response seen (Tenenbein, 1984) **or** use two-thirds ($^2/_3$) of the initial effective naloxone bolus on an hourly basis; titrate dose (typically 0.04-0.16 mg/kg/hour for 2-5 days in children); one-half ($^1/_2$) of the initial bolus dose should be readministered 15 minutes after initiation of the continuous infusion to prevent a drop in naloxone levels; increase infusion rate as needed to assure adequate ventilation and prevent withdrawal symptoms (Goldfrank, 1986). **Note:** The infusion should be discontinued by reducing the infusion in decrements of 25%; closely monitor the patient (eg, pulse oximetry) after each adjustment and after discontinuation of the infusion for recurrence of opioid-induced respiratory depression (Perry, 1996).

Reversal of respiratory depression with therapeutic opioid dosing: I.V.: 0.001-0.015 mg/kg/dose; dose may be repeated as needed (Hegenbarth, 2008; Kleinman, 2010)

Postoperative reversal: I.V.: 0.005-0.01 mg/kg (Fischer, 1974); may repeat every 2-3 minutes as needed based on response (adequate ventilation without significant pain)

Adults:

Opioid overdose (with standard ACLS protocols):

I.V., I.M., SubQ: Initial: 0.4-2 mg; may need to repeat doses every 2-3 minutes; after reversal, may need to readminister dose(s) at a later interval (ie, 20-60 minutes) depending on type/duration of opioid. If no response is observed after 10 mg total, consider other causes of respiratory depression. **Note:** May be given endotracheally (unlabeled route) as 2-2.5 times the initial I.V. dose (ie, 0.8-5 mg) (Neumar, 2010).

Continuous infusion (unlabeled dosing): I.V.: **Note:** For use with exposures to long-acting opioids (eg, methadone), sustained release product, and symptomatic body packers after initial naloxone response. Calculate dosage/hour based on effective intermittent dose used and duration of adequate response seen (Tenenbein, 1984) **or** use two-thirds ($^2/_3$) of the initial effective naloxone bolus on an hourly basis (typically 0.25-6.25 mg/hour); one-half ($^1/_2$) of the initial bolus dose should be readministered 15 minutes after initiation of the continuous infusion to prevent a drop in naloxone levels; adjust infusion rate as needed to assure adequate ventilation and prevent withdrawal symptoms (Goldfrank, 1986).

Inhalation via nebulization (unlabeled route): 2 mg; may repeat. Switch to I.V. or I.M. administration when possible (Weber, 2012).

Intranasal administration (unlabeled route): 2 mg (1 mg per nostril); may repeat in 5 minutes if respiratory depression persists. **Note:** Onset of action is slightly delayed compared to I.M. or I.V. routes (Kelly, 2005; Robertson, 2009; Vanden Hoek, 2010).

Reversal of respiratory depression with therapeutic opioid doses: I.V., I.M., SubQ.: Initial: 0.04-0.4 mg; may repeat until desired response achieved. If desired response is not observed after 0.8 mg total, consider other causes of respiratory depression. **Note:** May be given endotracheally (unlabeled route) as 2-2.5 times the initial I.V. dose (ie, 0.08-1 mg) (Neumar, 2010).

Continuous infusion (unlabeled dosing): I.V.: **Note:** For use with exposures to long-acting opioids (eg, methadone) or sustained release products. Calculate dosage/hour based on effective intermittent dose used and duration of adequate response seen (Tenenbein, 1984) **or** use two-thirds ($^2/_3$) of the initial effective naloxone bolus on an hourly basis (typically 0.2-0.6 mg/hour); one-half ($^1/_2$) of the initial bolus dose should be readministered 15 minutes after initiation of the continuous infusion to prevent a drop in naloxone levels; adjust infusion rate as needed to assure adequate ventilation and prevent withdrawal symptoms (Goldfrank, 1986).

Opioid-dependent patients being treated for cancer pain (NCCN guidelines, v.2.2011): I.V.: 0.04-0.08 mg (40-80 **mcg**) slow I.V. push; administer every 30-60 seconds until improvement in symptoms; if no response is observed after total naloxone dose 1 mg, consider other causes of respiratory depression. **Note:** May dilute 0.4 mg/mL (1 mL) ampul into 9 mL of normal saline for a total volume of 10 mL to achieve a 0.04 mg/mL (40 **mcg**/mL) concentration.

Postoperative reversal: I.V.: 0.1-0.2 mg every 2-3 minutes until desired response (adequate ventilation and alertness without significant pain). **Note:** Repeat doses may be needed within 1-2 hour intervals depending on type, dose, and timing of the last dose of opioid administered.

Opioid-induced pruritus (unlabeled use): I.V. infusion: 0.25 **mcg/kg/hour**; **Note:** Monitor pain control; verify that the naloxone is not reversing analgesia (Gan, 1997)

Dosage adjustment in renal impairment: No dosage adjustment provided in manufacturer's labeling.

Dosage adjustment in hepatic impairment: No dosage adjustment provided in manufacturer's labeling.

Administration

I.V. push: Administer over 30 seconds as undiluted preparation **or** administer as diluted preparation slow I.V. push by diluting 0.4 mg (1 mL) ampul with 9 mL of normal saline for a total volume of 10 mL to achieve a concentration of 0.04 mg/mL (APS, 2008)

I.V. continuous infusion: Dilute to 4 **mcg**/mL in D_5W or normal saline

I.M., SubQ: May administer I.M. or SubQ if unable to obtain I.V. access

Endotracheal (unlabeled route): There is only anecdotal support for this route of administration. May require a slightly higher dose than used in other routes. Dilute to 1-2 mL with normal saline; flush with 5 mL of saline and then administer 5 ventilations.

Inhalation via nebulization (unlabeled route): Dilute 2 mg of naloxone with 3 mL of normal saline and administer via nebulizer face mask (Mycyk, 2003; Weber, 2012).

Intranasal (unlabeled route): Administer total dose equally divided into each nostril using a mucosal atomizer device (MAD) (Kelly, 2005; Robertson, 2009; Vanden Hoek, 2010).

Monitoring Parameters Respiratory rate, heart rate, blood pressure, temperature, level of consciousness, ABGs or pulse oximetry

Additional Information May contain methyl and propylparabens

Dosage Forms Excipient information presented when available (limited, particularly for generics); consult specific product labeling.

Solution, Injection, as hydrochloride:
Generic: 0.4 mg/mL (1 mL, 10 mL)

Solution, Injection, as hydrochloride [preservative free]:
Generic: 1 mg/mL (2 mL)

◆ **Naloxone and Buprenorphine** *see* Buprenorphine and Naloxone *on page 295*

◆ **Naloxone Hydrochloride** *see* Naloxone *on page 1421*

◆ **Naloxone Hydrochloride Dihydrate and Buprenorphine Hydrochloride** *see* Buprenorphine and Naloxone *on page 295*

◆ **Naloxone Hydrochloride Injection® (Can)** *see* Naloxone *on page 1421*

◆ **Naloxone Hydrochloride Injection® USP (Can)** *see* Naloxone *on page 1421*

Naltrexone (nal TREKS one)

Brand Names: U.S. ReVia; Vivitrol

Brand Names: Canada ReVia

Index Terms Naltrexone Hydrochloride

Pharmacologic Category Antidote; Opioid Antagonist

Use

Alcohol dependence: Treatment of alcohol dependence.

Opioid dependence: For the blockade of the effects of exogenously administered opioids.

Pregnancy Risk Factor C

Pregnancy Considerations Adverse events were observed in animal reproduction studies.

Breast-Feeding Considerations Naltrexone is excreted into breast milk. Due to the potential for serious adverse reactions in the nursing infant, the manufacturer recommends a decision be made whether to discontinue nursing or to discontinue the drug, taking into account the importance of treatment to the mother.

Medication Guide Available Yes

Contraindications Hypersensitivity to naltrexone or any component of the formulation; opioid dependence or current use of opioid analgesics (including partial opioid agonists); acute opioid withdrawal; failure to pass naloxone challenge or positive urine screen for opioids

Warnings/Precautions Dose-related hepatocellular injury is possible; the margin of separation between the apparent safe and hepatotoxic doses appears to be ≤5-fold. Discontinue therapy if signs/symptoms of acute hepatitis develop. Clinicians should note that elevated transaminases may be a result of pre-existing alcoholic liver disease, hepatitis B and/or C infection, or concomitant use of other hepatotoxic drugs; abrupt opioid withdrawal may also lead to acute liver injury. Therapy may precipitate withdrawal symptoms in patients addicted to opioids; patients should be opioid-free (including tramadol) for a minimum of 7-10 days; a naloxone challenge test may help to confirm patient is opioid-free prior to therapy if there is any suspicion since urinary opioid screen may not be sufficient proof. Patients transitioning from buprenorphine or methadone may be vulnerable to precipitation of withdrawal symptoms for as long as 2 weeks. Use of naltrexone does not eliminate or diminish withdrawal symptoms. Patients who had been treated with naltrexone may respond to lower opioid doses than previously used. This could result in potentially life-threatening opioid intoxication. Patients should be aware that they may be more sensitive to lower doses of opioids after naltrexone treatment is discontinued, after a missed dose, or near the end of the dosing interval. Warn patients that any attempt to overcome opioid blockade during naltrexone therapy, could potentially lead to fatal opioid overdose; the opioid competitive receptor blockade produced by naltrexone is potentially surmountable in the presence of large amounts of opioids. In naltrexone-treated patients requiring emergency pain management, consider alternatives to opioid therapy (eg, regional analgesia, nonopioid analgesics, general anesthesia). If opioid therapy is required for pain therapy, patients should be under the direct care of a trained anesthesia provider.

Suicidal thoughts, attempted suicide, and depression have been reported postmarketing; monitor closely. Hypersensitivity, including anaphylaxis, has been reported. Cases of eosinophilic pneumonia have been reported and should be considered in patients presenting with progressive hypoxia and dyspnea. Use with caution in patients with severe hepatic impairment (has not been studied; if coagulopathy presents, I.M. injection may cause hematoma formation). Use with caution in patients with moderate-to-severe renal impairment (has not been studied). Use I.M. injection with caution in patients with thrombocytopenia or any bleeding disorder (hemophilia and severe hepatic failure), and patients on anticoagulant therapy; bleeding/hematoma may occur from I.M. administration. Serious injection site reactions (eg, cellulitis, induration, hematoma, abscess, necrosis) have been reported with use, including severe cases requiring surgical debridement. Females appear to be at a higher risk. Patients should report any injection site pain, swelling, bruising, pruritus, or redness that does not improve (or worsens). For I.M. use only in the gluteal muscle; do **not** administer I.V., SubQ, or into fatty tissue; incorrect administration may increase the risk of injection site reactions. Vehicle used in the injectable naltrexone formulation (polylactide-co-glycolide microspheres) has rarely been associated with retinal artery occlusion in patients with abnormal arteriovenous anastomosis following injection of other drug products that also use the polylactide-co-glycolide microspheres vehicle.

Adverse Reactions Combined reporting of adverse events from oral and injectable formulations:

>10%:

Cardiovascular: Syncope (13%)

Central nervous system: Headache (3% to 25%), insomnia (3% to 14%), dizziness (4% to 13%), anxiety (2% to 12%), nervousness (4% to >10%)

Gastrointestinal: Nausea (10% to 33%), vomiting (3% to 14%), appetite decreased (14%), diarrhea (13%), abdominal pain (11%), abdominal cramping

Hepatic: ALT increased (13%)

Local: Injection site reaction (≤69%; includes bruising, induration, nodules, pain, pruritus, swelling, tenderness)

Neuromuscular & skeletal: Arthralgia (12%), CPK increased (11% to 39%)

Respiratory: Pharyngitis (7% to 11%)

1% to 10%:

Cardiovascular: Hypertension (5%)

Central nervous system: Suicidal thoughts (≤10%), depression (8%), somnolence (2% to 4%), fatigue (4%), chills, energy increased, feeling down, irritability

Dermatologic: Rash (6%)

Endocrine & metabolic: Polydipsia

Gastrointestinal: Dry mouth (5%), toothache (4%)

Genitourinary: Delayed ejaculation, impotency

Hepatic: AST increased (2% to 10%), GGT increased (7%)

Neuromuscular & skeletal: Muscle cramps (8%), back pain (6%)

Miscellaneous: Influenza (5%)

<1% (Limited to important or life-threatening): Angina, atrial fibrillation, blood pressure increased, cerebral aneurysm, chest pain, chest tightness, cholecystitis, cholelithiasis, colitis, COPD, dehydration, delirium, diaphoresis, DVT, dyspnea, ECG changes, eosinophilia (transient), eosinophilic pneumonia, GI hemorrhage, HF, hypercholesterolemia, hypersensitivity reaction (includes anaphylaxis, angioedema, and urticaria), ischemic stroke, leukocytosis, lymphadenopathy, MI, opioid withdrawal, palpitation, pancreatitis, paralytic ileus, paranoia, PE, perirectal abscess, pneumonia, rigors, seizure, shortness of breath, suicide, tachycardia, thrombocytopenia

Drug Interactions

Metabolism/Transport Effects None known.

Avoid Concomitant Use There are no known interactions where it is recommended to avoid concomitant use.

Increased Effect/Toxicity There are no known significant interactions involving an increase in effect.

Decreased Effect There are no known significant interactions involving a decrease in effect.

Preparation for Administration Injection: Prior to reconstitution, allow drug vial and provided diluent to reach room temperature (~45 minutes). Using the provided 1-inch *preparation* needle, reconstitute with 3.4 mL of the diluent and allow to dissolve by vigorously shaking the vial for ~1 minute. Mixed suspension will be milky white, free of clumps, and will move freely down the walls of the vial. Immediately after suspension, withdraw 4.2 mL of the suspension using the same preparation needle.

Prior to administration, replace the preparation needle with the appropriate size provided *administration* needle (use the 2-inch needle with the needle protection device for patients with a larger amount of subcutaneous tissue overlying the gluteal muscle; for very lean patients, the 1.5-inch needle may be appropriate; either needle may be used for patients with average body habitus). Prior to injection, remove any air bubbles and push on the plunger until 4 mL of the suspension remains in the syringe. Following reconstitution of the suspension, administer immediately.

Storage/Stability

Injection: Store unopened kit at 2°C to 8°C (36°F to 46°F). Kit may be kept at room temperature of ≤25°C (77°F) for ≤7 days prior to use; do not freeze. Following reconstitution of the suspension, administer immediately.

Tablet: Store at 20°C to 25°C (68°F to 77°F).

Mechanism of Action Naltrexone (a pure opioid antagonist) is a cyclopropyl derivative of oxymorphone similar in structure to naloxone and nalorphine (a morphine derivative); it acts as a competitive antagonist at opioid receptor sites, showing the highest affinity for mu receptors.

Pharmacodynamics/Kinetics

Duration: Oral: 50 mg: 24 hours; 100 mg: 48 hours; 150 mg: 72 hours; I.M.: 4 weeks

Absorption: Oral: Almost complete

Distribution: V_d: ~1350 L; widely throughout the body but considerable interindividual variation exists

Metabolism: Extensively metabolized via noncytochrome-mediated dehydrogenase conversion to 6-beta-naltrexol (primary metabolite) and related minor metabolites; glucuronide conjugates are also formed from naltrexone and its metabolites

Oral: Extensive first-pass effect

Protein binding: 21%

Bioavailability: Oral: Variable range (5% to 40%)

Half-life elimination: Oral: 4 hours; 6-beta-naltrexol: 13 hours; I.M.: naltrexone and 6-beta-naltrexol: 5-10 days (dependent upon erosion of polymer)

Time to peak, serum: Oral: ~60 minutes; I.M.: Biphasic: ~2 hours (first peak), ~2-3 days (second peak)

Excretion: Primarily urine (as metabolites and small amounts of unchanged drug)

Dosage Adults: **Note:** Do not initiate therapy until patient is opioid-free (including tramadol) for at least 7-10 days as determined by urinalysis; consider naloxone challenge test to confirm patient is opioid-free if there is any suspicion since urinary opioid screen may not be sufficient proof.

Alcohol dependence:

Oral: 50 mg daily; alternative maintenance regimens may be used and include: 50 mg on weekdays with a 100 mg dose on Saturday; 100 mg every other day; or 150 mg every 3 days (degree of blockade may be reduced with extended dosing interval regimens and doses >50 mg may increase risk of hepatocellular injury)

I.M.: 380 mg once every 4 weeks

Opioid dependence:

Oral: Initial: 25 mg; if no withdrawal signs occur, administer 50 mg daily thereafter; alternative maintenance regimens may be used and include: 50 mg on weekdays with a 100 mg dose on Saturday; 100 mg every other day; or 150 mg every 3 days (degree of blockade may be reduced with extended dosing interval regimens and doses >50 mg may increase risk of hepatocellular injury)

I.M.: 380 mg once every 4 weeks

Dosage adjustment in renal impairment:

Mild impairment: No dosage adjustment necessary.

Moderate-to-severe impairment: No dosage adjustment provided in manufacturer's labeling (has not been studied); use with caution since naltrexone and its primary metabolite are primarily excreted in urine.

Dosage adjustment in hepatic impairment:

Mild-to-moderate impairment: No dosage adjustment necessary.

Severe impairment: No dosage adjustment provided in manufacturer's labeling (has not been studied); naltrexone AUC increased ~5- and 10-fold in patients with compensated or decompensated hepatic cirrhosis respectively.

Administration

Oral: May be administered with or without food. Administration with food or after meals may minimize adverse gastrointestinal effects. Advise patient not to self-administer opioids while receiving naltrexone therapy.

I.M.: Vivitrol: Administer I.M. into the upper outer quadrant of the gluteal area; must inject dose using one of the provided needles for administration. Use either the 1.5-inch needle (for very lean patients) or the 2-inch needle (for patients with a larger amount of subcutaneous tissue overlying the gluteal muscle). Either needle may be used for patients with average body habitus. Avoid inadvertent injection into a blood vessel; do not administer I.V., SubQ, or into fatty tissue (the risk of serious injection site reaction is increased if given incorrectly as a SubQ injection or into fatty tissue instead of the gluteal muscle). Injection should alternate between the 2 buttocks. Do not substitute any components of the dose-pack.

Monitoring Parameters Liver function tests (baseline and periodic); monitor for opioid withdrawal, injection site reactions with I.M. administration, and depression and/or suicidal thinking

Test Interactions May cause cross-reactivity with some opioid immunoassay methods.

Dosage Forms Excipient information presented when available (limited, particularly for generics); consult specific product labeling.

Suspension Reconstituted, Intramuscular:

Vivitrol: 380 mg (1 ea)

Tablet, Oral, as hydrochloride:

ReVia: 50 mg [scored]

Generic: 50 mg

◆ **Naltrexone Hydrochloride** *see* Naltrexone *on page 1423*

◆ **Namenda** *see* Memantine *on page 1289*

◆ **Namenda Titration Pak** *see* Memantine *on page 1289*

◆ **Namenda XR** *see* Memantine *on page 1289*

◆ **Namenda XR Titration Pack** *see* Memantine *on page 1289*

◆ **Nanoparticle Albumin-Bound Paclitaxel** *see* PACLitaxel (Protein Bound) *on page 1546*

◆ **NAPA and NABZ** *see* Sodium Phenylacetate and Sodium Benzoate *on page 1922*

Naphazoline (Nasal) (naf AZ oh leen)

Brand Names: U.S. Privine® [OTC]

Index Terms Naphazoline Hydrochloride

Pharmacologic Category Alpha$_1$ Agonist; Imidazoline Derivative

Use Temporary relief of nasal congestion associated with the common cold, upper respiratory allergies, or sinusitis

Dosage Intranasal: Children ≥12 years and Adults: 0.05% instill 1-2 drops or sprays every 6 hours if needed; therapy should not exceed 3 days

Additional Information Complete prescribing information should be consulted for additional detail.

Dosage Forms Excipient information presented when available (limited, particularly for generics); consult specific product labeling.

Solution, intranasal, as hydrochloride [drops]:

Privine®: 0.05% (25 mL) [contains benzalkonium chloride]

Solution, intranasal, as hydrochloride [spray]:

Privine®: 0.05% (20 mL) [contains benzalkonium chloride]

Naphazoline (Ophthalmic) (naf AZ oh leen)

Brand Names: U.S. Clear Eyes Redness Relief [OTC]; VasoClear [OTC]; VasoClear-A [OTC]

Brand Names: Canada Naphcon Forte®; Vasocon®

Index Terms Naphazoline Hydrochloride

Pharmacologic Category Alpha$_1$ Agonist; Imidazoline Derivative; Ophthalmic Agent, Vasoconstrictor

Use Topical ocular vasoconstrictor; relief of redness of the eye due to minor irritation

Pregnancy Risk Factor C

Dosage Ophthalmic: Adults:

0.1% solution (prescription): 1-2 drops into conjunctival sac every 3-4 hours as needed

0.012% or 0.025% solution (OTC): 1-2 drops into affected eye(s) up to 4 times/day; therapy should not exceed 3 days

Dosage adjustment in renal impairment: No dosage adjustment provided in manufacturer's labeling.

Dosage adjustment in hepatic impairment: No dosage adjustment provided in manufacturer's labeling.

Additional Information Complete prescribing information should be consulted for additional detail.

Dosage Forms Excipient information presented when available (limited, particularly for generics); consult specific product labeling.

Solution, Ophthalmic, as hydrochloride:

Clear Eyes Redness Relief: 0.012% (6 mL) [contains benzalkonium chloride]

VasoClear: 0.02% (15 mL)

VasoClear-A: 0.02% (15 mL)

Generic: 0.1% (15 mL)

Naphazoline and Pheniramine

(naf AZ oh leen & fen NIR a meen)

Brand Names: U.S. Naphcon-A [OTC]; Opcon-A [OTC]; Visine-A [OTC]

Brand Names: Canada Naphcon-A; Visine Advanced Allergy

Index Terms Pheniramine and Naphazoline

Pharmacologic Category Alkylamine Derivative; Alpha$_1$ Agonist; Histamine H$_1$ Antagonist; Histamine H$_1$ Antagonist, First Generation; Imidazoline Derivative; Ophthalmic Agent, Vasoconstrictor

Use Treatment of ocular congestion, irritation, and itching

Dosage Ophthalmic: Children ≥6 years and Adults: 1-2 drops into the affected eye(s) up to 4 times/day

Additional Information Complete prescribing information should be consulted for additional detail.

Dosage Forms Excipient information presented when available (limited, particularly for generics); consult specific product labeling.

Solution, ophthalmic:

Naphcon-A: Naphazoline hydrochloride 0.025% and pheniramine maleate 0.3% (5 mL) [contains benzalkonium chloride; 2 bottles/box], (15 mL) [contains benzalkonium chloride]

Opcon-A: Naphazoline hydrochloride 0.027% and pheniramine maleate 0.3% (15 mL) [contains benzalkonium chloride]

Visine-A: Naphazoline hydrochloride 0.025% and pheniramine maleate 0.3% (15 mL) [contains benzalkonium chloride]

Generic: Naphazoline hydrochloride 0.027% and pheniramine maleate 0.315% (15 mL)

◆ **Naphazoline Hydrochloride** *see* Naphazoline (Nasal) *on page 1425*

◆ **Naphazoline Hydrochloride** *see* Naphazoline (Ophthalmic) *on page 1425*

◆ **Naphcon-A [OTC]** *see* Naphazoline and Pheniramine *on page 1425*

◆ **Naphcon-A (Can)** *see* Naphazoline and Pheniramine *on page 1425*

◆ **Naphcon Forte® (Can)** *see* Naphazoline (Ophthalmic) *on page 1425*

◆ **Naprelan** *see* Naproxen *on page 1425*

◆ **Naproderm [DSC]** *see* Naproxen *on page 1425*

◆ **Naprosyn** *see* Naproxen *on page 1425*

◆ **Naprosyn E (Can)** *see* Naproxen *on page 1425*

◆ **Naprosy SR (Can)** *see* Naproxen *on page 1425*

Naproxen (na PROKS en)

Brand Names: U.S. Aleve [OTC]; All Day Pain Relief [OTC]; All Day Relief [OTC]; Anaprox; Anaprox DS; EC-Naprosyn; Flanax Pain Relief [OTC]; Mediproxen [OTC]; Naprelan; Naproderm [DSC]; Naprosyn; Naproxen Comfort Pac; Naproxen DR

Brand Names: Canada Anaprox; Anaprox DS; Apo-Napro-Na; Apo-Napro-Na DS; Apo-Naproxen; Apo-Naproxen EC; Apo-Naproxen SR; Ava-Naproxen EC; Mylan-Naproxen EC; Naprelan; Naprosy SR; Naprosyn; Naprosyn E; Naproxen Sodium DS; Naproxen-NA; Naproxen-NA DF; PMS-Naproxen; PMS-Naproxen EC; PRO-Naproxen EC; Teva-Naproxen; Teva-Naproxen EC; Teva-Naproxen Sodium; Teva-Naproxen Sodium DS; Teva-Naproxen SR

Index Terms Naproxen Sodium

Pharmacologic Category Nonsteroidal Anti-inflammatory Drug (NSAID), Oral

Additional Appendix Information

Beers Criteria – Potentially Inappropriate Medications for Geriatrics *on page 2368*

Use

Acute gout/Ankylosing spondylitis/Bursitis/Juvenile arthritis/Juvenile rheumatoid arthritis/Osteoarthritis/Rheumatoid arthritis/Tendonitis (Rx products only): For the relief of the signs and symptoms of acute gout, ankylosing spondylitis, bursitis, juvenile arthritis (excluding ER tablets), juvenile rheumatoid arthritis (oral suspension only), osteoarthritis, rheumatoid arthritis, and tendonitis. Delayed-release naproxen is not recommended for initial treatment of acute pain.

Pain/Primary dysmenorrhea (Rx and OTC products): For the relief of mild-to-moderate pain and the treatment of primary dysmenorrhea. Delayed-release naproxen is not recommended for initial treatment of acute pain.

Unlabeled Use Migraine prophylaxis

Pregnancy Risk Factor C

Pregnancy Considerations Adverse events were not observed in the initial animal reproduction studies; therefore, the manufacturer classifies naproxen as pregnancy category C. Naproxen crosses the placenta and can be detected in fetal tissue and the serum of newborn infants following *in utero* exposure. NSAID exposure during the first trimester is not strongly associated with congenital malformations; however, cardiovascular anomalies and cleft palate have been observed following NSAID exposure in some studies. The use of a NSAID close to conception may be associated with an increased risk of miscarriage. Nonteratogenic effects have been observed following NSAID administration during the third trimester including: Myocardial degenerative changes, prenatal constriction of the ductus arteriosus, fetal tricuspid regurgitation, failure of the ductus arteriosus to close postnatally; renal dysfunction or failure, oligohydramnios; gastrointestinal bleeding or perforation, increased risk of necrotizing enterocolitis; intracranial bleeding (including intraventricular hemorrhage), platelet dysfunction with resultant bleeding; pulmonary hypertension. Because they may cause premature closure of the ductus arteriosus, use of NSAIDs late in pregnancy should be avoided (use after 31 or 32 weeks gestation is not recommended by some clinicians). The chronic use of NSAIDs in women of reproductive age may be associated with infertility that is reversible upon discontinuation of the medication. A registry is available for pregnant women exposed to autoimmune medications including naproxen. For additional information contact the Organization of Teratology Information Specialists, OTIS Autoimmune Diseases Study, at (877) 311-8972.

Breast-Feeding Considerations Small amounts of naproxen are excreted into breast milk. Naproxen has been detected in the urine of a breast-feeding infant. Breast-feeding is not recommended by the manufacturer. In a study which included 20 mother-infant pairs, there were two cases of drowsiness and one case of vomiting in the breast-fed infants. Maternal naproxen dose, duration, and relationship to breast-feeding were not provided.

Medication Guide Available Yes

Contraindications Hypersensitivity to naproxen, aspirin, other NSAIDs, or any component of the formulation; treatment of perioperative pain in the setting of coronary artery bypass graft (CABG) surgery

Warnings/Precautions **[U.S. Boxed Warning]: NSAIDs are associated with an increased risk of adverse cardiovascular thrombotic events, including MI and stroke.** Risk may be increased with duration of use or pre-existing cardiovascular risk factors or disease. Carefully evaluate individual cardiovascular risk profiles prior to prescribing. May cause new-onset hypertension or worsening of existing hypertension. Monitor blood pressure closely with initiation and during therapy. Use caution with fluid retention. Avoid use in heart failure. Use the lowest effective dose for the shortest duration of time, consistent with individual patient goals, to reduce risk of cardiovascular or GI adverse events. Alternate therapies should be considered for patients at high risk. Concurrent administration of ibuprofen, and potentially other nonselective NSAIDs, may interfere with aspirin's cardioprotective effect. **[U.S. Boxed Warning]: Use is contraindicated for treatment of perioperative pain in the setting of coronary artery bypass graft (CABG) surgery.** Risk of MI and stroke may be increased with use following CABG surgery.

[U.S. Boxed Warning]: NSAIDs may increase risk of gastrointestinal irritation, inflammation, ulceration, bleeding, and perforation. These events may occur at any time during therapy and without warning. Risk for serious events is greater in elderly patients. Use caution with a history of GI disease (bleeding or ulcers), concurrent therapy with aspirin, anticoagulants and/or corticosteroids, smoking, use of alcohol, the elderly or debilitated patients. When used concomitantly with ≤325 mg of aspirin, a substantial increase in the risk of gastrointestinal complications (eg, ulcer) occurs; concomitant gastroprotective therapy (eg, proton pump inhibitors) is recommended (Bhatt, 2008).

May increase the risk of aseptic meningitis, especially in patients with systemic lupus erythematosus (SLE) and mixed connective tissue disorders. Platelet adhesion and aggregation may be decreased; may prolong bleeding time; patients with coagulation disorders or who are receiving anticoagulants should be monitored closely. Anemia may occur; patients on long-term NSAID therapy should be monitored for anemia. Rarely, NSAID use may cause severe blood dyscrasias (eg, agranulocytosis, aplastic anemia, thrombocytopenia).

NSAID use may compromise existing renal function; dose-dependent decreases in prostaglandin synthesis may result from NSAID use, reducing renal blood flow which may cause renal decompensation. NSAID use may increase the risk for hyperkalemia. Patients with impaired renal function, dehydration, heart failure, liver dysfunction, those taking diuretics, and ACE inhibitors, and the elderly are at greater risk of renal toxicity and hyperkalemia. Rehydrate patient before starting therapy; monitor renal function closely. Not recommended for use in patients with advanced renal disease. Long-term NSAID use may result in renal papillary necrosis.

NSAIDs may cause serious skin adverse events including exfoliative dermatitis, Stevens-Johnson Syndrome (SJS) and toxic epidermal necrolysis (TEN); discontinue use at first sign of skin rash or hypersensitivity. Anaphylactoid reactions may occur, even without prior exposure; patients with "aspirin triad" (bronchial asthma, aspirin intolerance, rhinitis) may be at increased risk. Do not use in patients who experience bronchospasm, asthma, rhinitis, or urticaria with NSAID or aspirin therapy. Use caution in other forms of asthma.

Use with caution in patients with decreased hepatic function. Closely monitor patients with any abnormal LFT. Severe hepatic reactions (eg, fulminant hepatitis, liver failure) have occurred with NSAID use, rarely; discontinue if signs or symptoms of liver disease develop, or if systemic manifestations occur.

NSAIDS may cause drowsiness, dizziness, blurred vision and other neurologic effects which may impair physical or mental abilities; patients must be cautioned about performing tasks which require mental alertness (eg, operating machinery or driving). Discontinue use with blurred or diminished vision and perform ophthalmologic exam.

Monitor vision with long-term therapy. Withhold for at least 4-6 half-lives prior to surgical or dental procedures.

Use with caution in the elderly, particularly at higher doses; unbound plasma fraction increased. Dose adjustments may be necessary; avoid chronic use (unless alternative agents ineffective and patient can receive concomitant gastroprotective agent); nonselective oral NSAID use is associated with an increased risk of GI bleeding and peptic ulcer disease in older adults in high risk category (eg, >75 years or age or receiving concomitant oral/parenteral corticosteroids, anticoagulants, or antiplatelet agents) (Beers Criteria).

OTC labeling: Prior to self-medication, patients should contact healthcare provider if they have had recurring stomach pain or upset, ulcers, bleeding problems, asthma, high blood pressure, heart or kidney disease, other serious medical problems, are currently taking a diuretic, anticoagulant, other NSAIDs, or are ≥60 years of age. Recommended dosages and duration should not be exceeded, due to an increased risk of GI bleeding, MI, and stroke. Patients should stop use and consult a healthcare provider if symptoms get worse, newly appear, or continue; if an allergic reaction occurs; if feeling faint, vomit blood or have bloody/black stools; if having difficulty swallowing or heartburn, or if fever lasts for >3 days or pain >10 days. Consuming ≥3 alcoholic beverages/day or taking longer than recommended may increase the risk of GI bleeding. Not for self-medication (OTC use) in children <12 years of age.

Adverse Reactions

1% to 10%:

- Cardiovascular: Edema (3% to 9%), palpitations (<3%)
- Central nervous system: Dizziness (3% to 9%), drowsiness (3% to 9%), headache (3% to 9%), lightheadedness (<3%), vertigo (<3%)
- Dermatologic: Pruritus (3% to 9%), skin eruption (3% to 9%), ecchymosis (3% to 9%), purpura (<3%), rash
- Endocrine & metabolic: Fluid retention (3% to 9%)
- Gastrointestinal: Abdominal pain (3% to 9%), constipation (3% to 9%), nausea (3% to 9%), heartburn (3% to 9%), diarrhea (<3%), dyspepsia (<3%), stomatitis (<3%), flatulence, gross bleeding/perforation, indigestion, ulcers, vomiting
- Genitourinary: Abnormal renal function
- Hematologic: Hemolysis (3% to 9%), ecchymosis (3% to 9%), anemia, bleeding time increased
- Hepatic: LFTs increased
- Ocular: Visual disturbances (<3%)
- Otic: Tinnitus (3% to 9%), hearing disturbances (<3%)
- Respiratory: Dyspnea (3% to 9%)
- Miscellaneous: Diaphoresis (<3%), thirst (<3%)

<1% (Limited to important or life-threatening): Agranulocytosis, alopecia, anaphylactic/anaphylactoid reaction, angioneurotic edema, arrhythmia, aseptic meningitis, asthma, blurred vision, cognitive dysfunction, colitis, coma, confusion, CHF, conjunctivitis, cystitis, depression, dream abnormalities, dysuria, eosinophilia, eosinophilic pneumonitis, erythema multiforme, exfoliative dermatitis, glossitis, granulocytopenia, hallucinations, hematemesis, hepatitis, hyper-/hypoglycemia, hyper-/hypotension, infection, interstitial nephritis, melena, jaundice, leukopenia, liver failure, lymphadenopathy, menstrual disorders, malaise, MI, muscle weakness, myalgia, oliguria, pancreatitis, pancytopenia, paresthesia, photosensitivity, pneumonia, polyuria, proteinuria, pyrexia, rectal bleeding, renal failure, renal papillary necrosis, respiratory depression, sepsis, Stevens-Johnson syndrome, tachycardia, seizure, syncope, thrombocytopenia, toxic epidermal necrolysis ulcerative stomatitis, vasculitis

Drug Interactions

Metabolism/Transport Effects Substrate of CYP1A2 (minor), CYP2C9 (minor); **Note:** Assignment of Major/Minor substrate status based on clinically relevant drug interaction potential

Avoid Concomitant Use

Avoid concomitant use of Naproxen with any of the following: Floctafenine; Ketorolac (Nasal); Ketorolac (Systemic); NSAID (COX-2 Inhibitor); Omacetaxine

Increased Effect/Toxicity

Naproxen may increase the levels/effects of: 5-ASA Derivatives; Agents with Antiplatelet Properties; Aliskiren; Aminoglycosides; Anticoagulants; Bisphosphonate Derivatives; Collagenase (Systemic); CycloSPORINE (Systemic); Dabigatran Etexilate; Deferasirox; Desmopressin; Digoxin; Eplerenone; Haloperidol; Ibritumomab; Lithium; Methotrexate; Nonsteroidal Anti-Inflammatory Agents; NSAID (COX-2 Inhibitor); Omacetaxine; PEMEtrexed; Porfimer; Potassium-Sparing Diuretics; PRALAtrexate; Quinolone Antibiotics; Rivaroxaban; Salicylates; Tenofovir; Thrombolytic Agents; Tositumomab and Iodine I 131 Tositumomab; Vancomycin; Vitamin K Antagonists

The levels/effects of Naproxen may be increased by: ACE Inhibitors; Angiotensin II Receptor Blockers; Antidepressants (Tricyclic, Tertiary Amine); Corticosteroids (Systemic); CycloSPORINE (Systemic); Dasatinib; Floctafenine; Glucosamine; Herbs (Anticoagulant/Antiplatelet Properties); Ibrutinib; Ketorolac (Nasal); Ketorolac (Systemic); Multivitamins/Fluoride (with ADE); Multivitamins/Minerals (with ADEK, Folate, Iron); Multivitamins/Minerals (with AE, No Iron); Nonsteroidal Anti-Inflammatory Agents; Omega-3 Fatty Acids; Pentosan Polysulfate Sodium; Pentoxifylline; Probenecid; Prostacyclin Analogues; Selective Serotonin Reuptake Inhibitors; Serotonin/Norepinephrine Reuptake Inhibitors; Sodium Phosphates; Tipranavir; Treprostinil; Vitamin E

Decreased Effect

Naproxen may decrease the levels/effects of: ACE Inhibitors; Agents with Antiplatelet Properties; Aliskiren; Angiotensin II Receptor Blockers; Beta-Blockers; Eplerenone; HydrALAZINE; Loop Diuretics; Potassium-Sparing Diuretics; Prostaglandins (Ophthalmic); Salicylates; Selective Serotonin Reuptake Inhibitors; Thiazide Diuretics

The levels/effects of Naproxen may be decreased by: Bile Acid Sequestrants; Nonsteroidal Anti-Inflammatory Agents; Salicylates

Ethanol/Nutrition/Herb Interactions

Ethanol: Avoid ethanol (may enhance gastric mucosal irritation).

Food: Naproxen absorption rate/levels may be decreased if taken with food.

Herb/Nutraceutical: Avoid alfalfa, anise, bilberry, bladderwrack, bromelain, cat's claw, celery, chamomile, coleus, cordyceps, dong quai, evening primrose, fenugreek, feverfew, garlic, ginger, ginkgo biloba, ginseng (American, Panax, Siberian), grapeseed, green tea, guggul, horse chestnut seed, horseradish, licorice, prickly ash, red clover, reishi, SAMe (S-adenosylmethionine), sweet clover, turmeric, white willow (all have additional antiplatelet activity).

Storage/Stability Store at 15° to 30°C (59° to 86°F); suspension should not be exposed to excessive heat (>40°C [104°F]).

Mechanism of Action Reversibly inhibits cyclooxygenase-1 and 2 (COX-1 and 2) enzymes, which results in decreased formation of prostaglandin precursors; has antipyretic, analgesic, and anti-inflammatory properties

Other proposed mechanisms not fully elucidated (and possibly contributing to the anti-inflammatory effect to varying degrees), include inhibiting chemotaxis, altering lymphocyte activity, inhibiting neutrophil aggregation/activation, and decreasing proinflammatory cytokine levels.

Pharmacodynamics/Kinetics

Onset of action: Analgesic: 30-60 minutes

Duration: Analgesic: <12 hours

Absorption: Almost 100%

Distribution: 0.16 L/kg

Protein binding: >99% to albumin; increased free fraction in elderly

Metabolism: Hepatic to metabolites

Bioavailability: 95%

Half-life elimination: Normal renal function: 12-17 hours; Moderate-to-severe renal impairment: ~15-21 hours (Anttila, 1980)

Time to peak, serum:

- Tablets, naproxen: 2-4 hours
- Tablets, naproxen sodium: 1-2 hours
- Tablets, delayed-release (empty stomach): 4-6 hours; range: 2-12 hours
- Tablets, delayed-release (with food): 12 hours; range: 4-24 hours
- Suspension: 1-4 hours

Excretion: Urine (95%; primarily as metabolites); feces (≤3%)

Dosage Oral: **Note:** Dosage expressed as naproxen base; 200 mg naproxen base is equivalent to 220 mg naproxen sodium.

Children >2 years: Juvenile idiopathic arthritis: **Note:** Oral suspension is recommended: 10 mg/kg/day in 2 divided doses (up to 15 mg/kg/day has been tolerated). Do not exceed 15 mg/kg/day.

Adults: **Note:** For relief of acute pain, naproxen sodium may be preferred due to more rapid absorption and onset; naproxen base may also be used, however, EC-Naprosyn® is not recommended.

Ankylosing spondylitis, osteoarthritis, rheumatoid arthritis: 500-1000 mg daily in 2 divided doses; if tolerating well and clinically indicated, may increase to 1500 mg daily of naproxen base for limited time period (<6 months)

Naproxen extended-release tablets: Initial: 750-1000 mg once daily; may temporarily increase to 1500 mg daily of naproxen base if tolerating well and clinically indicated

Gout, acute: Initial: 750 mg, followed by 250 mg every 8 hours until attack subsides

Naproxen extended-release tablets: Initial: 1000-1500 mg once daily followed by 1000 mg once daily until attack subsides

Pain (mild-to-moderate), dysmenorrhea, acute tendonitis, bursitis: Initial: 500 mg, followed by 500 mg every 12 hours **or** 250 mg every 6-8 hours; maximum daily dose: Day 1: 1250 mg naproxen base; subsequent daily doses should not exceed 1000 mg naproxen base

Naproxen extended-release tablets: Initial: 1000 mg once daily; may temporarily increase to 1500 mg once daily if greater pain relief is needed. Dose should be subsequently reduced to a maximum of 1000 mg daily.

Migraine, acute (unlabeled use): Initial: 750 mg; an additional 250-500 mg may be given if needed (maximum: 1250 mg in 24 hours) (Andersson, 1989; Nestvold, 1985).

Elderly: Use with caution; dosage adjustment may be required. Refer to adult dosing.

OTC labeling: Pain, fever: Children ≥12 years, Adolescents, and Adults: 200 mg naproxen base every 8-12 hours; if needed, may take 400 mg naproxen base for the initial dose; maximum: 400 mg naproxen base in any 8- to 12-hour period or 600 mg naproxen base/24 hours

Dosage adjustment in renal impairment: Cl_{cr} <30 mL/minute: Use is not recommended

Dosage adjustment in hepatic impairment: Manufacturer's labeling suggests that a reduced dose should be considered; use with caution in chronic disease (eg, alcoholic liver disease), particularly at higher doses; dose adjustment may be required.

Dietary Considerations Drug may cause GI upset, bleeding, ulceration, perforation; take with food or milk to minimize GI upset.

Administration Administer with food, milk, or antacids to decrease GI adverse effects

Suspension: Shake suspension well before administration.

Tablet, delayed or extended release: Swallow tablet whole; do not break, crush, or chew.

Monitoring Parameters Occult blood loss, periodic liver function test, CBC, BUN, serum creatinine; urine output; blood pressure (hypertensive patients); ophthalmic exam (for vision changes/disturbances)

Test Interactions Naproxen may interfere with 5-HIAA urinary assays; due to an interaction with m-dinitrobenzene, naproxen should be discontinued 72 hours before adrenal function testing if the Porter-Silber test is used. May interfere with urine detection of cannabinoids and barbiturates (false-positives).

Dosage Forms Excipient information presented when available (limited, particularly for generics); consult specific product labeling. [DSC] = Discontinued product

Capsule, Oral, as sodium:

- Aleve: 220 mg [contains brilliant blue fcf (fd&c blue #1)]

Cream, Transdermal:

- Naproderm: 15% (60 g [DSC])

Kit, Combination:

- Naproxen Comfort Pac: 500 mg [contains methylparaben, trolamine (triethanolamine)]

Suspension, Oral:

- Naprosyn: 125 mg/5 mL (480 mL)
- Generic: 125 mg/5 mL (500 mL)

Tablet, Oral:

- Naprosyn: 250 mg [scored]
- Naprosyn: 375 mg
- Naprosyn: 500 mg [scored]
- Generic: 250 mg, 375 mg, 500 mg

Tablet, Oral, as sodium:

- Aleve: 220 mg [contains fd&c blue #2 aluminum lake]
- All Day Pain Relief: 220 mg [contains fd&c blue #2 aluminum lake]
- All Day Pain Relief: 220 mg [gluten free; contains fd&c blue #2 aluminum lake]
- All Day Relief: 220 mg
- Anaprox: 275 mg
- Anaprox DS: 550 mg [scored]
- Flanax Pain Relief: 220 mg [contains fd&c blue #2 (indigotine)]
- Mediproxen: 220 mg
- Generic: 220 mg, 275 mg, 550 mg

Tablet Delayed Release, Oral:

- EC-Naprosyn: 375 mg, 500 mg
- Naproxen DR: 375 mg, 500 mg

Tablet Extended Release 24 Hour, Oral, as sodium [strength expressed as base]:

- Naprelan: 375 mg, 500 mg, 750 mg, 500 & 750 MG [DSC]

◆ **Naproxen and Sumatriptan** *see* Sumatriptan and Naproxen *on page* 1972

◆ **Naproxen Comfort Pac** *see* Naproxen *on page* 1425

◆ **Naproxen DR** *see* Naproxen *on page 1425*
◆ **Naproxen-NA (Can)** *see* Naproxen *on page 1425*
◆ **Naproxen-NA DF (Can)** *see* Naproxen *on page 1425*
◆ **Naproxen Sodium** *see* Naproxen *on page 1425*
◆ **Naproxen Sodium and Sumatriptan** *see* Sumatriptan and Naproxen *on page 1972*
◆ **Naproxen Sodium and Sumatriptan Succinate** *see* Sumatriptan and Naproxen *on page 1972*
◆ **Naproxen Sodium DS (Can)** *see* Naproxen *on page 1425*

Naratriptan (NAR a trip tan)

Brand Names: U.S. Amerge

Brand Names: Canada Amerge; Sandoz-Naratriptan; Teva-Naratriptan

Index Terms Naratriptan Hydrochloride

Pharmacologic Category Antimigraine Agent; Serotonin 5-$HT_{1B, 1D}$ Receptor Agonist

Additional Appendix Information

Antimigraine Drugs: 5-HT_1 Receptor Agonists *on page 2288*

Use Migraines: Acute treatment of migraine attacks with or without aura in adults.

Unlabeled Use Short-term prevention of menstrually associated migraines (MAMs)

Pregnancy Risk Factor C

Pregnancy Considerations Adverse events were observed in animal reproduction studies. Pregnancy outcome information for naratriptan is available from a pregnancy registry sponsored by GlaxoSmithKline. As of October 2008, data was available for 55 infants/fetuses exposed to naratriptan, and seven exposed to both naratriptan and sumatriptan. Following naratriptan exposure, there was one infant born with a birth defect; this infant was also exposed to sumatriptan during the first trimester of pregnancy (Cunnington, 2009). The pregnancy registry was closed in January, 2012 and additional information may be obtained from the manufacturer (800-336-2176). Additional information related to the use of naratriptan in pregnancy is limited (Källén, 2011; Nezvalová-Henriksen, 2010; Nezvalová-Henriksen, 2012). Until additional information is available, other agents are preferred for the initial treatment of migraine in pregnancy (Da Silva, 2012; MacGregor, 2012; Williams, 2012).

Breast-Feeding Considerations It is not known if naratriptan is excreted in breast milk. Due to the potential for serious adverse reactions in the nursing infant, the manufacturer recommends a decision be made whether to discontinue nursing or to discontinue the drug, taking into account the importance of treatment to the mother.

Contraindications

Ischemic coronary artery disease (CAD) (angina pectoris, history of myocardial infarction [MI], or documented silent ischemia); coronary artery vasospasm, including Prinzmetal's angina; Wolff-Parkinson-White syndrome or arrhythmias associated with other cardiac accessory conduction pathway disorders; history of stroke, transient ischemic attack (TIA), or history of hemiplegic or basilar migraine; peripheral vascular disease; ischemic bowel disease; uncontrolled hypertension; recent use (within 24 hours) of another 5-HT_1 agonist, ergotamine-containing medication, or ergot-type medication (eg, dihydroergotamine or methysergide); severe renal impairment (Cl_{cr} <15 mL/minute) or severe hepatic impairment; hypersensitivity to naratriptan or any component of the formulation

Canadian labeling: Additional contraindications (not in U.S. labeling): Cardiac arrhythmias (especially tachycardias); valvular heart disease, congenital heart disease, atherosclerotic disease; management of ophthalmoplegic migraine; Raynaud's syndrome

Documentation of allergenic cross-reactivity for triptans is limited. However, because of similarities in chemical structure and/or pharmacologic actions, the possibility of cross-sensitivity cannot be ruled out with certainty.

Warnings/Precautions Use only if there is a clear diagnosis of migraine. Use is contraindicated in patients with severe hepatic or renal impairment. Do not give to patients with risk factors for CAD until a cardiovascular evaluation has been performed; if evaluation is satisfactory, the healthcare provider should administer the first dose (consider ECG monitoring) and cardiovascular status should be periodically re-evaluated. Cardiac events (coronary artery vasospasm, transient ischemia, myocardial infarction, ventricular tachycardia/fibrillation, cardiac arrest, and death), cerebral/subarachnoid hemorrhage, stroke (some fatal), peripheral vascular ischemia, gastrointestinal vascular ischemia/infarction, splenic infarction, and Raynaud's syndrome have been reported with 5-HT_1 agonist administration. Partial vision loss and blindness (transient and permanent) have been reported with use of 5-HT_1 agonists; a causal relationship between these events and 5-HT_1 agonist administration has not been clearly determined. Patients who experience sensations of chest pain/pressure/tightness or symptoms suggestive of angina following dosing should be evaluated for coronary artery disease or Prinzmetal's angina before receiving additional doses; if dosing is resumed and similar symptoms recur, monitor with ECG. Significant elevation in blood pressure, including hypertensive crisis with acute impairment of organ systems, has been reported on rare occasions in patients with and without a history of hypertension; monitor blood pressure. Blood pressure increases may be more pronounced in the elderly. May cause CNS depression, such as dizziness, weakness, or drowsiness, which may impair physical or mental abilities; patients must be cautioned about performing tasks which require mental alertness (eg, operating machinery or driving). Only indicated for the acute treatment of migraine; not indicated for migraine prophylaxis, or for the treatment of cluster headache, hemiplegic or basilar migraine. Acute migraine agents (eg, triptans, opioids, ergotamine, or a combination of the agents) used for 10 or more days per month may lead to worsening of headaches (medication overuse headache); withdrawal treatment may be necessary in the setting of overuse. If a patient does not respond to the first dose, the diagnosis of migraine should be reconsidered; rule out underlying neurologic disease in patients with atypical headache and in patients with no prior history of migraine.

Potentially significant drug-drug interactions may exist, requiring dose or frequency adjustment, additional monitoring, and/or selection of alternative therapy. Symptoms of agitation, confusion, hallucinations, hyper-reflexia, myoclonus, shivering, and tachycardia may occur with concomitant proserotonergic drugs (ie, SSRIs/SNRIs or triptans) or agents which reduce naratriptan's metabolism. Concurrent use of serotonin precursors (eg, tryptophan) is not recommended. If concomitant administration with SSRIs is warranted, monitor closely, especially at initiation and with dose increases. Discontinue naratriptan if serotonin syndrome is suspected. Anaphylaxis, anaphylactoid, and hypersensitivity reactions (including angioedema) have occurred; may be life-threatening or fatal.

Adverse Reactions

1% to 10%:

Central nervous system: Pain/pressure (2% to 4%), malaise/fatigue (2%), dizziness (1% to 2%), drowsiness (1% to 2%), vertigo (1%)

Gastrointestinal: Nausea (4% to 5%), hyposalivation (1%), vomiting (1%)

Neuromuscular & skeletal: Paresthesia (1% to 2%)
Ocular: Photophobia (1%)
Miscellaneous: Ear/nose/throat infection (1%), pressure/tightness/heaviness sensations (1%), warm/cold temperature sensations (1%)

<1% (Limited to important or life-threatening): Abnormal bilirubin tests, abnormal liver function tests, anaphylactoid reaction, anaphylaxis, anemia, bradycardia, cerebral infarction, colonic ischemia, coronary artery vasospasm, depression, dyspnea, ECG changes (atrial fibrillation, atrial flutter, premature ventricular contractions, PR prolongation, or QT_c prolongation), eye hemorrhage, glycosuria, hallucinations, heart murmurs, hypercholesterolemia, hyperglycemia, hyper-/hypotension, hyperlipidemia, hypothyroidism, hypersensitivity reaction, ketonuria, MI, palpitation, panic, rash, seizure, serotonin syndrome, syncope, subarachnoid hemorrhage, thrombocytopenia, TIA, transient myocardial ischemia, ventricular fibrillation, ventricular tachycardia

Drug Interactions

Metabolism/Transport Effects None known.

Avoid Concomitant Use

Avoid concomitant use of Naratriptan with any of the following: Ergot Derivatives

Increased Effect/Toxicity

Naratriptan may increase the levels/effects of: Antipsychotics; Ergot Derivatives; Metoclopramide; Serotonin Modulators

The levels/effects of Naratriptan may be increased by: Antipsychotics; Ergot Derivatives

Decreased Effect There are no known significant interactions involving a decrease in effect.

Storage/Stability Store at 20°C to 25°C (68°F to 77°F).

Mechanism of Action Selective agonist for serotonin ($5\text{-}HT_{1B}$ and $5\text{-}HT_{1D}$ receptors) in cranial arteries; causes vasoconstriction and reduces sterile inflammation associated with antidromic neuronal transmission correlating with relief of migraine

Pharmacodynamics/Kinetics

Onset of action: ~1-2 hours (Bomhof, 1999; Tfelt-Hansen, 2000)
Absorption: Well absorbed
Distribution: V_{dss}: 170 L
Protein binding, plasma: 28% to 31%
Metabolism: Hepatic via CYP
Bioavailability: ~70%
Half-life, elimination: 6 hours; increased in renal impairment (moderate impairment; mean: 11 hours; range: 7-20 hours); increased in hepatic impairment (moderate impairment: 8-16 hours)
Time to peak: 2-3 hours
Excretion: Urine (50% of total dose as unchanged drug; 30% of total dose as metabolites)

Dosage Note: If the first dose is ineffective, diagnosis needs to be re-evaluated. The safety of treating >4 migraines/month has not been established.

Acute migraine: Adults: Oral: Initial: 1-2.5 mg; if headache recurs or does not fully resolve, a second dose may be administered after 4 hours (maximum: 5 mg daily).

Elderly:
U.S. labeling: Refer to adult dosing. Dosing should generally start at the lower end of the dosing range due to possible increased incidence of hepatic, renal, and cardiac impairment.
Canadian labeling: Use is not recommended

Dosing in renal impairment:

Mild-to-moderate renal impairment:
U.S. labeling: Initial: 1 mg; do not exceed 2.5 mg in 24 hours
Canadian labeling: Initial: 1 mg; do not exceed 2 mg in 24 hours

Severe renal impairment (Cl_{cr} <15 mL/minute): Use is contraindicated

Dosing in hepatic impairment:

Mild-to-moderate hepatic impairment (Child-Pugh grade A or B):
U.S. labeling: Initial: 1 mg; do not exceed 2.5 mg in 24 hours
Canadian labeling: Initial: 1 mg; do not exceed 2 mg in 24 hours

Severe hepatic impairment (Child-Pugh grade C): Use is contraindicated

Administration Administer orally as soon as symptoms appear; may take with or without food. Do **not** crush or chew tablet; swallow whole with water.

Monitoring Parameters Headache severity, blood pressure, signs/symptoms suggestive of angina; perform a cardiovascular evaluation in triptan-naïve patients who have multiple cardiovascular risk factors (eg, increased age, diabetes, hypertension, smoking, obesity, strong family history of CAD), monitor ECG with first dose in patients with multiple cardiovascular risk factors who have a negative cardiovascular evaluation and consider periodic cardiovascular evaluation in such patients if they are intermittent long-term users; signs/symptoms of serotonin syndrome and hypersensitivity reactions.

Dosage Forms Excipient information presented when available (limited, particularly for generics); consult specific product labeling.

Tablet, Oral:
Amerge: 1 mg, 2.5 mg
Generic: 1 mg, 2.5 mg

Extemporaneous Preparations A 0.5 mg/mL oral suspension may be made using tablets. Crush fifty 2.5 mg tablets and reduce to a fine powder. In small amounts, add 125 mL of Ora-Plus® and mix well after each addition. Transfer to a calibrated bottle, rinse mortar with vehicle, then add quantity of Ora-Sweet® or Ora-Sweet® SF sufficient to make 250 mL. Label "shake well" and "refrigerate". Stable 90 days refrigerated.

Nahata MC, Pai VB, and Hipple TF, *Pediatric Drug Formulations*, 5th ed, Cincinnati, OH: Harvey Whitney Books Co, 2004.

◆ **Naratriptan Hydrochloride** *see* Naratriptan *on page 1429*
◆ **Narcan** *see* Naloxone *on page 1421*
◆ **Nardil** *see* Phenelzine *on page 1627*
◆ **Nardil® (Can)** *see* Phenelzine *on page 1627*
◆ **Naropin** *see* Ropivacaine *on page 1854*
◆ **Naropin® (Can)** *see* Ropivacaine *on page 1854*
◆ **Nasacort Allergy 24HR [OTC]** *see* Triamcinolone (Nasal) *on page 2123*
◆ **Nasacort AQ** *see* Triamcinolone (Nasal) *on page 2123*
◆ **NasalCrom [OTC]** *see* Cromolyn (Nasal) *on page 500*
◆ **Nasal Decongestant [OTC]** *see* Phenylephrine (Systemic) *on page 1636*
◆ **Nasal Decongestant [OTC]** *see* Pseudoephedrine *on page 1746*
◆ **Nasal Decongestant PE Max St [OTC]** *see* Phenylephrine (Systemic) *on page 1636*
◆ **Nasalide® (Can)** *see* Flunisolide (Nasal) *on page 878*
◆ **Nasal Moist [OTC]** *see* Sodium Chloride *on page 1914*
◆ **Nascobal** *see* Cyanocobalamin *on page 501*
◆ **nasohist™ [OTC]** *see* Chlorpheniramine and Phenylephrine *on page 412*
◆ **nasohist™ DM pediatric [OTC]** *see* Chlorpheniramine, Phenylephrine, and Dextromethorphan *on page 413*
◆ **Nasonex** *see* Mometasone (Nasal) *on page 1394*

◆ **Nasonex® (Can)** *see* Mometasone (Nasal) *on page 1394*

◆ **Natacyn** *see* Natamycin *on page 1431*

◆ **Natacyn® (Can)** *see* Natamycin *on page 1431*

Natalizumab (na ta LIZ u mab)

Brand Names: U.S. Tysabri

Brand Names: Canada Tysabri®

Index Terms AN100226; Anti-4 Alpha Integrin; IgG4-Kappa Monoclonal Antibody

Pharmacologic Category Gastrointestinal Agent, Miscellaneous; Monoclonal Antibody, Selective Adhesion-Molecule Inhibitor

Use Monotherapy for the treatment of relapsing forms of multiple sclerosis; treatment of moderately- to severely-active Crohn's disease

Canada labeling: Treatment of relapsing forms of multiple sclerosis

Pregnancy Risk Factor C

Prescribing and Access Restrictions

U.S.: Tysabri® is deemed to have an approved REMS program. As a requirement of the REMS program, access to this medication is restricted. Patients must be enrolled in the Tysabri® Outreach Unified Commitment to Health (TOUCH™) Prescribing Program (800-456-2255) to receive natalizumab (MS-TOUCH™ for multiple sclerosis or CD-TOUCH™ for Crohn's disease). Healthcare providers must also register with the program in order to prescribe, dispense or administer natalizumab. Treatment must be reauthorized every 6 months. Natalizumab is available only through infusion centers registered with the TOUCH™ program; infusion center information is available at 1-800-456-2255.

Canada: Patients receiving natalizumab therapy for multiple sclerosis are to be enrolled in the Tysabri Care Program™ (888-827-2827). This program is associated with the prescribing, administration, and monitoring of Canadian patients receiving natalizumab. Clinicians are educated on the appropriate use of natalizumab and are expected to discuss the benefits/risks of therapy. Clinicians should evaluate patients every 6 months during treatment.

Medication Guide Available Yes

Dosage I.V.: Adults:

Multiple sclerosis: 300 mg infused over 1 hour every 4 weeks

Crohn's disease: 300 mg infused over 1 hour every 4 weeks; discontinue if therapeutic benefit is not observed within initial 12 weeks of therapy

Concomitant use with corticosteroids: For patients who begin treatment while on chronic oral corticosteroids, begin tapering oral steroids when the onset of natalizumab therapeutic benefit is observed; discontinue use if patient cannot be tapered off of oral corticosteroids within 6 months of therapy initiation. If additional concomitant corticosteroids are required and exceed 3 months/year (in addition to initial corticosteroid taper), consider discontinuing therapy.

Dosage adjustment in renal impairment: No dosage adjustment provided in manufacturer's labeling (has not been studied).

Dosage adjustment in hepatic impairment: No dosage adjustment provided in manufacturer's labeling (has not been studied). Discontinue use with jaundice or signs/symptoms of hepatic injury.

Additional Information Complete prescribing information should be consulted for additional detail.

Dosage Forms Excipient information presented when available (limited, particularly for generics); consult specific product labeling.

Concentrate, Intravenous [preservative free]:

Tysabri: 300 mg/15 mL (15 mL) [contains polysorbate 80]

Natamycin (na ta MYE sin)

Brand Names: U.S. Natacyn

Brand Names: Canada Natacyn®

Index Terms Pimaricin

Pharmacologic Category Antifungal Agent, Ophthalmic

Use Treatment of blepharitis, conjunctivitis, and keratitis caused by susceptible fungi (*Aspergillus*, *Candida*, *Cephalosporium*, *Fusarium*, and *Penicillium*)

Pregnancy Risk Factor C

Dosage Adults: Ophthalmic:

Fungal keratitis: Instill 1 drop in conjunctival sac every 1-2 hours, after 3-4 days reduce to one drop 6-8 times/day; usual course of therapy is 2-3 weeks or until resolution of active fungal keratitis (may be useful to gradually reduce dosage at 4-7 day intervals to assure elimination of organism)

Fungal blepharitis or conjunctivitis: Instill 1 drop in conjunctival sac every 4-6 hours

Dosage adjustment in renal impairment: No dosage adjustment provided in manufacturer's labeling. However, dosage adjustment unlikely due to low systemic absorption.

Dosage adjustment in hepatic impairment: No dosage adjustment provided in manufacturer's labeling. However, dosage adjustment unlikely due to low systemic absorption.

Additional Information Complete prescribing information should be consulted for additional detail.

Dosage Forms Excipient information presented when available (limited, particularly for generics); consult specific product labeling.

Suspension, Ophthalmic:

Natacyn: 5% (15 mL)

◆ **Natazia®** *see* Estradiol and Dienogest *on page 762*

Nateglinide (na te GLYE nide)

Brand Names: U.S. Starlix

Brand Names: Canada Starlix

Pharmacologic Category Antidiabetic Agent, Meglitinide Derivative

Additional Appendix Information

Oral Antidiabetic Agents Comparison Table *on page 2312*

Use Type 2 diabetes mellitus: For the treatment of adults with type 2 diabetes mellitus as an adjunct to diet and exercise to improve glycemic control.

Pregnancy Risk Factor C

Pregnancy Considerations Adverse events have been observed in animal reproduction studies. Information describing the effects of nateglinide on pregnancy outcomes is limited.

For women with diabetes, maternal hyperglycemia can be associated with adverse effects in the fetus, neonate, and mother. To prevent adverse fetal/neonatal events, prior to conception and throughout pregnancy, the maternal Hb A_{1c} should be kept close to normal but without causing significant hypoglycemia. The use of meglitinide derivatives in pregnant women is not recommended; insulin is the drug of choice for the control of diabetes mellitus during pregnancy (ACOG, 2005; ADA, 2013; Kitzmiller, 2008; Metzger, 2007).

Breast-Feeding Considerations It is not known if nateglinide is excreted in breast milk. Breast-feeding is not recommended by the manufacturer.

Contraindications Hypersensitivity to nateglinide or any component of the formulation; type 1 diabetes; diabetic ketoacidosis (this condition should be treated with insulin)

Warnings/Precautions Use with caution in patients with moderate-to-severe hepatic impairment. Use caution in severe renal dysfunction, elderly, malnourished, or patients with adrenal/pituitary dysfunction; may be more susceptible to glucose-lowering effects. All oral hypoglycemic agents are capable of producing hypoglycemia. Proper patient selection, dosage, and instructions to the patients are important to avoid hypoglycemic episodes. It may be necessary to discontinue nateglinide and administer insulin if the patient is exposed to stress (eg, fever, trauma, infection, surgery). Indicated for adjunctive therapy with metformin; not to be used as a substitute for metformin monotherapy. Combination treatment with sulfonylureas is not recommended (no additional benefit). Patients not adequately controlled on oral agents which stimulate insulin release (eg, glyburide) should not be switched to nateglinide or have nateglinide added to therapy.

Adverse Reactions As reported with nateglinide monotherapy:

>10%: Respiratory: Upper respiratory infection (11%)

1% to 10%:

Central nervous system: Dizziness (4%)

Endocrine & metabolic: Hypoglycemia (2%), uric acid increased

Gastrointestinal: Diarrhea (3%), weight gain

Neuromuscular & skeletal: Back pain, (4%), arthropathy (3%)

Respiratory: Bronchitis (3%), cough (2%)

Miscellaneous: Flu-like syndrome (4%)

Postmarketing and/or case reports: Cholestatic hepatitis, hypersensitivity reactions (including pruritus, rash, urticaria), jaundice, liver enzymes increased

Drug Interactions

Metabolism/Transport Effects **Substrate** of CYP2C9 (major), CYP3A4 (major), SLCO1B1; **Note:** Assignment of Major/Minor substrate status based on clinically relevant drug interaction potential; **Inhibits** CYP2C9 (weak)

Avoid Concomitant Use

Avoid concomitant use of Nateglinide with any of the following: Conivaptan; Fusidic Acid (Systemic)

Increased Effect/Toxicity

Nateglinide may increase the levels/effects of: Hypoglycemic Agents

The levels/effects of Nateglinide may be increased by: Conivaptan; CYP2C9 Inhibitors (Moderate); CYP2C9 Inhibitors (Strong); CYP3A4 Inhibitors (Moderate); CYP3A4 Inhibitors (Strong); Dasatinib; Eltrombopag; Fusidic Acid (Systemic); Herbs (Hypoglycemic Properties); Ivacaftor; Luliconazole; MAO Inhibitors; Mifepristone; Pegvisomant; Salicylates; Selective Serotonin Reuptake Inhibitors; Simeprevir

Decreased Effect

The levels/effects of Nateglinide may be decreased by: Bosentan; Corticosteroids (Orally Inhaled); Corticosteroids (Systemic); CYP2C9 Inducers (Strong); CYP3A4 Inducers (Strong); Dabrafenib; Deferasirox; Herbs (CYP3A4 Inducers); Loop Diuretics; Luteinizing Hormone-Releasing Hormone Analogs; Mitotane; Peginterferon Alfa-2b; Somatropin; Thiazide Diuretics; Tocilizumab

Ethanol/Nutrition/Herb Interactions

Ethanol: Ethanol may increase the risk of hypoglycemia. Management: Avoid ethanol.

Food: Rate of absorption is decreased and T_{max} is delayed when taken with food. Food does not affect AUC. Multiple peak plasma concentrations may be observed if fasting. Not affected by composition of meal.

Herb/Nutraceutical: Alfalfa, aloe, bilberry, bitter melon, burdock, celery, damiana, fenugreek, garcinia, garlic, ginger, ginseng (American), gymnema, marshmallow, and stinging nettle may enhance the hypoglycemic effects of antidiabetic agents. St. John's wort may decrease the levels/effect of nateglinide. Management: Avoid alfalfa, aloe, bilberry, bitter melon, burdock, celery, damiana, fenugreek, garcinia, garlic, ginger, ginseng (American), gymnema, marshmallow, and stinging nettle. Avoid St John's wort.

Storage/Stability Store at 25°C (77°F); excursions are permitted between 15°C and 30°C (59°F and 86°F).

Mechanism of Action Nonsulfonylurea hypoglycemic agent which blocks ATP-dependent potassium channels, depolarizing the membrane and facilitating calcium entry through calcium channels. Increased intracellular calcium stimulates insulin release from the pancreatic beta cells. Nateglinide-induced insulin release is glucose-dependent.

Pharmacodynamics/Kinetics

Onset of action: Insulin secretion: ~20 minutes

Peak effect: 1 hour

Duration: 4 hours

Absorption: Rapid

Distribution: 10 L

Protein binding: 98%, primarily to albumin

Metabolism: Hepatic via hydroxylation followed by glucuronide conjugation via CYP2C9 (70%) and CYP3A4 (30%) to metabolites

Bioavailability: 73%

Half-life elimination: 1.5 hours

Time to peak: ≤1 hour

Excretion: Urine (83%, 16% as unchanged drug); feces (10%)

Dosage

Adults: Management of type 2 diabetes mellitus: Oral: Initial and maintenance dose: 120 mg 3 times daily; may be given alone or in combination with metformin or a thiazolidinedione. Patients close to Hb A_{1c} goal at initiation of therapy may be started at 60 mg 3 times daily

Elderly: Refer to adult dosing

Dosage adjustment in renal impairment:

Mild to moderate impairment: No dosage adjustment necessary.

Severe impairment: No dosage adjustment necessary. Use with caution; may be more susceptible to glucose-lowering effects.

Dosage adjustment in hepatic impairment:

Mild impairment (Child-Pugh class A): No dosage adjustment necessary.

Moderate to severe impairment (Child-Pugh class B or C): No dosage adjustment provided in manufacturer's labeling. Use with caution; has not been studied.

Dietary Considerations Nateglinide should be taken 1-30 minutes prior to meals. Scheduled dose should not be taken if meal is missed to avoid hypoglycemia. Dietary modification based on ADA recommendations is a part of therapy. Decreases blood glucose concentration. Hypoglycemia may occur. Must be able to recognize symptoms of hypoglycemia (sweating, dizziness, palpitations, increased appetite, trembling).

Administration Administer 1-30 minutes prior to meals. Scheduled dose should not be administered if a meal is missed to avoid hypoglycemia.

Monitoring Parameters Monitor weight and lipid profile. Monitor fasting blood glucose (periodically) and glycosylated hemoglobin (Hb A_{1c}) levels (every 3 months) with a goal of decreasing these levels towards the normal range. During dose adjustment, fasting glucose can be used to determine response.

Reference Range Recommendations for glycemic control in nonpregnant adults with diabetes (ADA, 2013):

Hb A_{1c}: <7% (a more aggressive [<6.5%] or less aggressive [<8%] Hb A_{1c} goal may be targeted based on patient-specific characteristics)

Preprandial capillary plasma glucose: 70-130 mg/dL

Peak postprandial capillary blood glucose: <180 mg/dL

Additional Information An increase in weight was seen in nateglinide monotherapy, which was not seen when used in combination with metformin.

Dosage Forms Excipient information presented when available (limited, particularly for generics); consult specific product labeling.

Tablet, Oral:

Starlix: 60 mg, 120 mg

Generic: 60 mg, 120 mg

- **Natrecor** *see* Nesiritide *on page 1443*
- **Natriuretic Peptide** *see* Nesiritide *on page 1443*
- **Natroba** *see* Spinosad *on page 1946*
- **NatrOVA** *see* Spinosad *on page 1946*
- **Natulan (Can)** *see* Procarbazine *on page 1720*
- **Natural Fiber Therapy [OTC]** *see* Psyllium *on page 1748*
- **Natural Lung Surfactant** *see* Beractant *on page 245*
- **Natural Psyllium Seed [OTC]** *see* Psyllium *on page 1748*
- **Natural Vegetable Fiber [OTC]** *see* Psyllium *on page 1748*
- **Natural Vitamin E [OTC]** *see* Vitamin E *on page 2202*
- **Nature-Throid** *see* Thyroid, Desiccated *on page 2052*
- **Nauseatol [OTC] (Can)** *see* DimenhyDRINATE *on page 616*
- **Navane** *see* Thiothixene *on page 2051*
- **NAVA-SC** *see* Hydroquinone *on page 1017*
- **Navelbine** *see* Vinorelbine *on page 2196*
- **Navelbine® (Can)** *see* Vinorelbine *on page 2196*
- **Na-Zone [OTC]** *see* Sodium Chloride *on page 1914*
- **N-Carbamoyl-L-Glutamic Acid** *see* Carglumic Acid *on page 350*
- **N-Carbamylglutamate** *see* Carglumic Acid *on page 350*
- ***n*-Docosanol** *see* Docosanol *on page 644*

Nebivolol (ne BIV oh lole)

Brand Names: U.S. Bystolic

Brand Names: Canada Bystolic®

Index Terms Nebivolol Hydrochloride

Pharmacologic Category Antihypertensive; Beta-Blocker, Beta-1 Selective

Additional Appendix Information

Beta-Blockers *on page 2294*

Use Treatment of hypertension, alone or in combination with other agents

Unlabeled Use Heart failure

Pregnancy Risk Factor C

Dosage

Adults: Oral:

U.S. labeling: Hypertension: Initial: 5 mg once daily; if initial response is inadequate, may be increased at 2-week intervals to a maximum dose of 40 mg once daily

Canadian labeling: Hypertension: Initial: 5 mg once daily; if initial response is inadequate, may be increased at 2-week intervals to a maximum dose of 20 mg once daily

Unlabeled use: Heart failure: Adults ≥70 years: Initial: 1.25 mg once daily; if tolerated, may increase by 2.5 mg at 1- to 2-week intervals to a maximum dose of 10 mg once daily (Flather, 2005). **Note:** Nebivolol has not been shown to reduce mortality in the general HF population.

Elderly: Refer to adult dosing.

Dosing adjustment in renal impairment: Severe impairment (Cl_{cr} <30 mL/minute): Initial: 2.5 mg daily; if initial response is inadequate, may increase cautiously.

Dosage adjustment in hepatic impairment:

Moderate impairment (Child-Pugh class B): Initial: 2.5 mg daily; if initial response is inadequate, may increase cautiously

Severe impairment (Child-Pugh class C): Use is contraindicated.

Additional Information Complete prescribing information should be consulted for additional detail.

Dosage Forms Excipient information presented when available (limited, particularly for generics); consult specific product labeling.

Tablet, Oral:

Bystolic: 2.5 mg, 5 mg, 10 mg, 20 mg [contains fd&c blue #2 aluminum lake, fd&c yellow #6 aluminum lake, polysorbate 80]

- **Nebivolol Hydrochloride** *see* Nebivolol *on page 1433*
- **Nebupent** *see* Pentamidine *on page 1613*
- **Nebusal** *see* Sodium Chloride *on page 1914*
- **Necon 0.5/35** *see* Ethinyl Estradiol and Norethindrone *on page 793*
- **Necon 1/35** *see* Ethinyl Estradiol and Norethindrone *on page 793*
- **Necon® 1/50** *see* Norethindrone and Mestranol *on page 1474*
- **Necon 7/7/7** *see* Ethinyl Estradiol and Norethindrone *on page 793*
- **Necon 10/11** *see* Ethinyl Estradiol and Norethindrone *on page 793*

Nedocromil (ne doe KROE mil)

Brand Names: U.S. Alocril

Brand Names: Canada Alocril®

Index Terms Nedocromil Sodium

Pharmacologic Category Mast Cell Stabilizer

Use Treatment of itching associated with allergic conjunctivitis

Pregnancy Risk Factor B

Dosage Ophthalmic: Children ≥3 years and Adults: 1-2 drops in each eye twice daily daily throughout the period of exposure to allergen

Dosage adjustment in renal impairment: No dosage adjustment provided in manufacturer's labeling. However, dosage adjustment unlikely due to low systemic absorption.

Dosage adjustment in hepatic impairment: No dosage adjustment provided in manufacturer's labeling. However, dosage adjustment unlikely due to low systemic absorption.

Additional Information Complete prescribing information should be consulted for additional detail.

Dosage Forms Excipient information presented when available (limited, particularly for generics); consult specific product labeling.

Solution, Ophthalmic, as sodium:

Alocril: 2% (5 mL) [contains benzalkonium chloride]

- **Nedocromil Sodium** *see* Nedocromil *on page 1433*

Nefazodone (nef AY zoe done)

Index Terms Nefazodone Hydrochloride; Serzone
Pharmacologic Category Antidepressant, Serotonin Reuptake Inhibitor/Antagonist
Additional Appendix Information
Antidepressant Agents *on page 2284*
Use Treatment of depression
Unlabeled Use Post-traumatic stress disorder (PTSD)
Pregnancy Risk Factor C
Medication Guide Available Yes
Dosage Oral:
Adults:
Depression: 200 mg/day, administered in 2 divided doses initially, with a range of 300-600 mg/day in 2 divided doses thereafter
Post-traumatic stress disorder (PTSD) (unlabeled use): Initial: 100 mg twice daily; target dose: 600 mg/day (average daily dose: 463 mg)
Elderly: Initial: 50 mg twice daily; increase dose to 100 mg twice daily in 2 weeks; usual maintenance dose: 200-400 mg/day

Discontinuation of therapy: Upon discontinuation of antidepressant therapy, gradually taper the dose to minimize the incidence of withdrawal symptoms and allow for the detection of re-emerging symptoms. Evidence supporting ideal taper rates is limited. APA and NICE guidelines suggest tapering therapy over at least several weeks with consideration to the half-life of the antidepressant; antidepressants with a shorter half-life may need to be tapered more conservatively. In addition for long-term treated patients, WFSBP guidelines recommend tapering over 4-6 months. If intolerable withdrawal symptoms occur following a dose reduction, consider resuming the previously prescribed dose and/or decrease dose at a more gradual rate (APA, 2010; Bauer, 2002; Haddad, 2001; NCCMH, 2010; Schatzberg, 2006; Shelton, 2001; Warner, 2006).

MAO inhibitor recommendations:
Switching to or from an MAO inhibitor intended to treat psychiatric disorders:
Allow 14 days to elapse between discontinuing an MAO inhibitor intended to treat psychiatric disorders and initiation of nefazodone.
Allow 14 days to elapse between discontinuing nefazodone and initiation of an MAO inhibitor intended to treat psychiatric disorders.
Use with other MAO inhibitors (such as linezolid or I.V. methylene blue):
Do not initiate nefazodone in patients receiving linezolid or I.V. methylene blue; consider other interventions for psychiatric condition.
If urgent treatment with linezolid or I.V. methylene blue is required in a patient already receiving nefazodone and potential benefits outweigh potential risks, discontinue nefazodone promptly and administer linezolid or I.V. methylene blue. Monitor for serotonin syndrome for 2 weeks or until 24 hours after the last dose of linezolid or I.V. methylene blue, whichever comes first. May resume nefazodone 24 hours after the last dose of linezolid or I.V. methylene blue.

Dosage adjustment in renal impairment: No dosage adjustment provided in manufacturer's labeling. However, adjustment unlikely since renal impairment does not alter steady state nefazodone plasma concentrations.
Dosage adjustment in hepatic impairment: No dosage adjustment provided in manufacturer's labeling. However, use with caution since the AUC of nefazodone and its metabolites were ~25% greater in patients with cirrhosis

Additional Information Complete prescribing information should be consulted for additional detail.
Dosage Forms Excipient information presented when available (limited, particularly for generics); consult specific product labeling.
Tablet, Oral, as hydrochloride:
Generic: 50 mg, 100 mg, 150 mg, 200 mg, 250 mg

◆ Nefazodone Hydrochloride *see* Nefazodone *on page 1434*

Nelarabine (nel AY re been)

Brand Names: U.S. Arranon
Brand Names: Canada Atriance™
Index Terms 2-Amino-6-Methoxypurine Arabinoside; 506U78; GW506U78
Pharmacologic Category Antineoplastic Agent, Antimetabolite; Antineoplastic Agent, Antimetabolite (Purine Analog)
Use Treatment of relapsed or refractory T-cell acute lymphoblastic leukemia (ALL) and T-cell lymphoblastic lymphoma
Pregnancy Risk Factor D
Pregnancy Considerations Teratogenic effects were observed in animal reproduction studies. May cause fetal harm if administered during pregnancy. Women of childbearing potential should be advised to use effective contraception and avoid becoming pregnant during therapy.
Breast-Feeding Considerations Due to the potential for serious adverse reactions in the nursing infant, the decision to discontinue breast-feeding or discontinue nelarabine should take into account the benefits of treatment to the mother.
Contraindications There are no contraindications listed within the manufacturer's labeling.
Warnings/Precautions Hazardous agent - use appropriate precautions for handling and disposal (NIOSH, 2012). **[U.S. Boxed Warning]: Severe neurotoxicity, including mental status changes, severe somnolence, seizure, and peripheral neuropathy (ranging from numbness to motor weakness or paralysis), has been reported. Observe closely for signs and symptoms of neurotoxicity; discontinue if ≥ grade 2. Adverse effects associated with demyelination or similar to Guillain-Barré syndrome (ascending peripheral neuropathies) have also been reported. Neurologic toxicities may not fully return to baseline after treatment cessation.** Neurologic toxicity is dose-limiting. Risk of neurotoxicity may increase in patients with concurrent or previous intrathecal chemotherapy or history of craniospinal irradiation. Tumor lysis syndrome (TLS) may occur as a consequence of leukemia treatment. May lead to life threatening acute renal failure; adequate hydration and prophylactic allopurinol should be instituted prior to treatment to prevent hyperuricemia and TLS; monitor closely. Bone marrow suppression, including leukopenia, thrombocytopenia, anemia, neutropenia and febrile neutropenia are associated with treatment; monitor blood counts regularly. Avoid administration of live vaccines. Use caution in patients with renal impairment; ara-G clearance may be reduced with renal dysfunction. Use caution with severe hepatic impairment; risk of adverse reactions may be higher with hepatic dysfunction.
Adverse Reactions Note: Pediatric adverse reactions fell within a range similar to adults except where noted.
>10%:
Cardiovascular: Peripheral edema (15%), edema (11%)

Central nervous system: Fatigue (50%), fever (23%), somnolence (7% to 23%; grades 2-4: 1% to 6%), dizziness (21%; grade 2: 8% adults), headache (15% to 17%; grades 2-4: 4% to 8%), hypoesthesia (6% to 17%; grades 2/3: children 5%, adults 12%), pain (11%)

Dermatologic: Petechiae (12%)

Endocrine & metabolic: Hypokalemia (11%)

Gastrointestinal: Nausea (41%), diarrhea (22%), vomiting (10% to 22%), constipation (21%)

Hematologic: Anemia (95% to 99%; grade 4: 10% to 14%), neutropenia (81% to 94%; grade 4: children 62%, adults 49%), thrombocytopenia (86% to 88%; grade 4: 22% to 32%), leukopenia (38%; grade 4: 7%), neutropenic fever (12%; grade 4: 1%)

Hepatic: Transaminases increased (12%; grade 3: 4%)

Neuromuscular & skeletal: Peripheral neuropathy (12% to 21%; grades 2/3: 11% to 14%), weakness (6% to 17%; grade 4: 1%), paresthesia (4% to 15%; grades 2/3: 3% to 4%), myalgia (13%)

Respiratory: Cough (25%), dyspnea (7% to 20%)

1% to 10%:

Cardiovascular: Hypotension (8%), sinus tachycardia (8%), chest pain (5%)

Central nervous system: Ataxia (2% to 9%; grades 2/3: children 1%, adults 8%), confusion (8%), insomnia (7%), depressed level of consciousness (6%; grades 2-4: 2%), depression (6%), seizure (grade 3: 1% adults; grade 4: 6% children), motor dysfunction (4%; grades 2/3: 2%), amnesia (3%; grade 2: 1%), balance disorder (2%; grade 2: 1%), sensory loss (1% to 2%), aphasia (grade 3: 1%), attention disturbance (1%), cerebral hemorrhage (grade 4: 1%), coma (grade 4: 1%), encephalopathy (grade 4: 1%), hemiparesis (grade 3: 1%), hydrocephalus (1%), intracranial hemorrhage (grade 4: 1%), lethargy (1%), leukoencephalopathy (grade 4: 1%), loss of consciousness (grade 3: 1%), mental impairment (1%), nerve paralysis (1%), neuropathic pain (1%), nerve palsy (1%), paralysis (1%), sciatica (1%), sensory disturbance (1%), speech disorder (1%)

Endocrine & Metabolic: Hypocalcemia (8%), dehydration (7%), hyper-/hypoglycemia (6%), hypomagnesemia (6%)

Gastrointestinal: Abdominal pain (9%), anorexia (9%), stomatitis (8%), abdominal distension (6%), taste perversion (3%)

Hepatic: Albumin decreased (10%), bilirubin increased (10%; grade 3: 7%, grade 4: 2%), AST increased (6%)

Neuromuscular & skeletal: Arthralgia (9%), back pain (8%), muscle weakness (8%), rigors (8%), limb pain (7%), abnormal gait (6%), noncardiac chest pain (5%), tremor (4% to 5%; grade 2: 2% to 3%), dysarthria (1%), hyporeflexia (1%), hypertonia (1%), incoordination (1%)

Ocular: Blurred vision (4%), nystagmus (1%)

Renal: Creatinine increased (6%)

Respiratory: Pleural effusion (10%), epistaxis (8%), pneumonia (8%), sinusitis (7%), wheezing (5%), sinus headache (1%)

Miscellaneous: Infection (5% to 9%)

<1% (Limited to important or life-threatening): Craniospinal demyelination, neuropathy (peripheral) (similar to Guillain-Barré syndrome), opportunistic infection, pneumothorax, progressive multifocal leukoencephalopathy (PML), respiratory arrest, rhabdomyolysis, tumor lysis syndrome

Drug Interactions

Metabolism/Transport Effects None known.

Avoid Concomitant Use

Avoid concomitant use of Nelarabine with any of the following: BCG; CloZAPine; Natalizumab; Pentostatin; Pimecrolimus; Tacrolimus (Topical); Tofacitinib; Vaccines (Live)

Increased Effect/Toxicity

Nelarabine may increase the levels/effects of: CloZAPine; Leflunomide; Natalizumab; Tofacitinib; Vaccines (Live)

The levels/effects of Nelarabine may be increased by: Denosumab; Pimecrolimus; Roflumilast; Tacrolimus (Topical); Trastuzumab

Decreased Effect

Nelarabine may decrease the levels/effects of: BCG; Coccidioidin Skin Test; Sipuleucel-T; Vaccines (Inactivated); Vaccines (Live)

The levels/effects of Nelarabine may be decreased by: Echinacea; Pentostatin

Preparation for Administration Hazardous agent; use appropriate precautions for handling and disposal (NIOSH, 2012). Reconstitution is not required; do not dilute; the appropriate dose should be added to empty plastic (PVC) bag or glass container.

Storage/Stability Store unopened vials at 25°C (77°F); excursions permitted to 15°C to 30°C (59°F to 86°F). Stable in plastic (PVC) or glass containers for up to 8 hours at room temperature.

Mechanism of Action Nelarabine, a prodrug of ara-G, is demethylated by adenosine deaminase to ara-G and then converted to ara-GTP. Ara-GTP is incorporated into the DNA of the leukemic blasts, leading to inhibition of DNA synthesis and inducing apoptosis. Ara-GTP appears to accumulate at higher levels in T-cells, which correlates to clinical response.

Pharmacodynamics/Kinetics

Distribution: V_{ss}:

Nelarabine: Children: ~213 L/m^2; Adults: ~197 L/m^2

Ara-G: Children: ~33 L/m^2; Adults: ~50 L/m^2

Protein binding: Nelarabine and ara-G: <25%

Metabolism: Hepatic; demethylated by adenosine deaminase to form ara-G (active); also hydrolyzed to form methylguanine. Both ara-G and methylguanine metabolized to guanine. Guanine is deaminated into xanthine, which is further oxidized to form uric acid, which is then oxidized to form allantoin.

Half-life elimination: Children: Nelarabine: 13 minutes, Ara-G: 2 hours; Adults: Nelarabine: 18 minutes, Ara-G: 3 hours

Time to peak: Ara-G: Adults: 3-25 hours (of day 1)

Excretion: Urine (nelarabine 5% to 10%, ara-G 20% to 30%)

Dosage I.V.: T-cell ALL, T-cell lymphoblastic lymphoma:

Children: 650 mg/m^2/dose on days 1 through 5; repeat every 21 days until transplant, disease progression, or unacceptable toxicity

Adults: 1500 mg/m^2/dose on days 1, 3, and 5; repeat every 21 days until transplant, disease progression, or unacceptable toxicity

Dosage adjustment for toxicity:

Neurologic toxicity ≥ grade 2: Discontinue treatment.

Hematologic or other (non-neurologic) toxicity: Consider treatment delay.

Dosage adjustment in renal impairment:

Cl_{cr} ≥50 mL/minute: No dosage adjustment necessary.

Cl_{cr} <50 mL/minute: No dosage adjustment provided in manufacturer's labeling, (although ARA-G clearance is decreased as renal function declines, data is insufficient for a dosing recommendation); monitor closely.

Dosage adjustment in hepatic impairment: No dosage adjustment provided in manufacturer's labeling (has not been studied); closely monitor with severe impairment (total bilirubin >3 times ULN)

Dosing in obesity: *ASCO Guidelines for appropriate chemotherapy dosing in obese adults with cancer:* Utilize patient's actual body weight (full weight) for calculation of body surface area- or weight-based dosing, particularly when the intent of therapy is curative; manage regimen-related toxicities in the same manner as for nonobese patients; if a dose reduction is utilized due to toxicity, consider resumption of full weight-based dosing with subsequent cycles, especially if cause of toxicity (eg, hepatic or renal impairment) is resolved (Griggs, 2012).

Administration Adequate I.V. hydration recommended to prevent tumor lysis syndrome; allopurinol may be used if hyperuricemia is anticipated.

Children: Infuse over 1 hour daily for 5 consecutive days

Adults: Infuse over 2 hours on days 1, 3, and 5

Hazardous agent; use appropriate precautions for handling and disposal (NIOSH, 2012).

Monitoring Parameters Closely monitor for neurologic toxicity (severe somnolence, seizure, peripheral neuropathy, confusion, ataxia, paresthesia, hypoesthesia, coma, or craniospinal demyelination); signs and symptoms of tumor lysis syndrome; hydration status; CBC with differential, liver and kidney function

Dosage Forms Excipient information presented when available (limited, particularly for generics); consult specific product labeling.

Solution, Intravenous:

Arranon: 5 mg/mL (50 mL)

Dosage Forms: Canada Excipient information presented when available (limited, particularly for generics); consult specific product labeling.

Injection, solution:

Atriance™: 5 mg/mL (50 mL)

Nelfinavir (nel FIN a veer)

Brand Names: U.S. Viracept

Brand Names: Canada Viracept

Index Terms NFV

Pharmacologic Category Antiretroviral, Protease Inhibitor (Anti-HIV)

Additional Appendix Information

Desensitization Protocols *on page 2325*

Use In combination with other antiretroviral therapy in the treatment of HIV infection

Pregnancy Risk Factor B

Pregnancy Considerations Adverse events were not observed in animal reproduction studies. Nelfinavir crosses the placenta. A modest increased risk of overall birth defects has been observed following first trimester exposure in humans according to data collected by the antiretroviral pregnancy registry. However, no pattern of defects has been detected. The DHHS Perinatal HIV Guidelines recommend nelfinavir to be used only in special circumstances during pregnancy for the prophylaxis of perinatal transmission in antiretroviral-naive women when alternative agents cannot be tolerated. A dose of 1250 mg twice daily has been shown to provide adequate plasma concentrations although lower and variable levels may occur late in pregnancy. A small increased risk of preterm birth has been associated with maternal use of protease inhibitor-based combination antiretroviral (ARV) therapy during pregnancy; however, the benefits of use generally outweigh this risk and protease inhibitors (PIs) should not be withheld if otherwise recommended. Hyperglycemia, new onset of diabetes mellitus, or diabetic ketoacidosis have been reported with PIs; it is not clear if pregnancy increases this risk.

Regardless of CD4 count or HIV RNA copy number, all HIV-infected pregnant women should receive a combination antepartum ARV drug regimen; this includes women who require therapy for their own health, as well as women who do not yet require therapy for their own health. ARV therapy should be started as soon as possible if required for the woman's health. Although earlier initiation may be more effective in reducing the perinatal transmission of HIV, also consider maternal conditions (eg, nausea and vomiting) and the potential risks of first trimester fetal exposure for specific agents. Plasma HIV RNA levels should be assessed at ~34-36 weeks gestation in order to help determine mode of delivery. If ARV therapy must be interrupted for <24 hours during the peripartum period, stop then restart all medications simultaneously in order to decrease the chance of developing resistance. Long-term follow-up is recommended for all infants exposed to ARV medications.

Healthcare providers are encouraged to enroll pregnant women exposed to antiretroviral medications in the Antiretroviral Pregnancy Registry (1-800-258-4263 or www.-APRegistry.com). Healthcare providers caring for HIV-infected women and their infants may contact the National Perinatal HIV Hotline (888-448-8765) for clinical consultation (DHHS [perinatal], 2012).

Breast-Feeding Considerations Maternal or infant antiretroviral therapy does not completely eliminate the risk of postnatal HIV transmission. In addition, multiclass-resistant virus has been detected in breast-feeding infants despite maternal therapy. Therefore, in the United States, where formula is accessible, affordable, safe, and sustainable, and the risk of infant mortality due to diarrhea and respiratory infections is low, complete avoidance of breast-feeding by HIV-infected women is recommended to decrease potential transmission of HIV (DHHS [perinatal], 2012).

Contraindications Hypersensitivity to nelfinavir or any component of the formulation; concurrent therapy with alfuzosin, amiodarone, cisapride, dihydroergotamine, ergotamine, lovastatin, methylergonovine, midazolam (oral), pimozide, quinidine, rifampin, sildenafil (when used for pulmonary artery hypertension [eg, Revatio®]), simvastatin, St John's wort, triazolam

Warnings/Precautions High potential for drug interactions; concomitant use of nelfinavir with some drugs may require cautious use, may not be recommended, may require dosage adjustments, or may be contraindicated.

Use caution with hepatic impairment; use not recommended with moderate-to-severe impairment. Warn patients that redistribution of body fat can occur. New-onset diabetes mellitus, exacerbation of diabetes, and hyperglycemia have been reported in HIV-infected patients receiving protease inhibitors. Use with caution in patients with hemophilia A or B; increased bleeding during protease inhibitor therapy has been reported. Patients may develop immune reconstitution syndrome resulting in the occurrence of an inflammatory response to an indolent or residual opportunistic infection during initial HIV treatment or activation of autoimmune disorders (eg, Graves' disease, polymyositis, Guillain-Barré syndrome) later in therapy; further evaluation and treatment may be required.

Adverse Reactions Data presented on experience in adults, unless otherwise noted.

>10%: Gastrointestinal: Diarrhea (14% to 20%; children: 39% to 47%)

2% to 10%:

Dermatologic: Rash (1% to 3%)

Gastrointestinal: Nausea (3% to 7%), flatulence (1% to 5%)

Hematologic: Lymphocytes decreased (1% to 6%), neutrophils decreased (1% to 5%)

<2% (Limited to important or life-threatening): Abdominal pain, acute iritis, alkaline phosphatase increased, allergic reaction, amylase increased, anemia, anorexia, anxiety, arthralgia, arthritis, back pain, bilirubinemia, body fat redistribution/accumulation, cramps, creatine phosphokinase increased, dehydration, depression, dermatitis, diaphoresis, dizziness, dyspepsia, dyspnea, emotional lability, epigastric pain, eye disorder, fever, folliculitis, fungal dermatitis, gastrointestinal bleeding, GGTP increased, headache, hepatitis, hyperkinesia, hyper-/hypoglycemia, hyperlipemia; hypersensitivity reaction (bronchospasm, rash, edema); hyperuricemia, immune reconstitution syndrome, insomnia, jaundice, kidney calculus, lactic dehydrogenase increased, leukopenia, lipoatrophy, lipodystrophy, liver function tests abnormal, maculopapular rash, malaise, metabolic acidosis, migraine, mouth ulceration, myalgia, myasthenia, myopathy, pain, pancreatitis, paresthesia, pharyngitis, pruritus, QT_c prolongation, rhinitis, seizure, sexual dysfunction, sinusitis, sleep disorder, somnolence, suicidal ideation, thrombocytopenia, torsade de pointes, transaminases increased, urine abnormality, urticaria, vomiting, weakness

Drug Interactions

Metabolism/Transport Effects Substrate of CYP2C19 (major), CYP2C9 (minor), CYP2D6 (minor), CYP3A4 (major), P-glycoprotein; **Note:** Assignment of Major/Minor substrate status based on clinically relevant drug interaction potential; **Inhibits** CYP1A2 (weak), CYP2B6 (weak), CYP2C19 (weak), CYP2C9 (weak), CYP2D6 (weak), CYP3A4 (strong), P-glycoprotein

Avoid Concomitant Use

Avoid concomitant use of Nelfinavir with any of the following: Ado-Trastuzumab Emtansine; Alfuzosin; Amiodarone; Apixaban; Avanafil; Axitinib; Bosutinib; Cabozantinib; Cisapride; Conivaptan; Crizotinib; Dronedarone; Eplerenone; Ergot Derivatives; Everolimus; Halofantrine; Ibrutinib; Imatinib; Ivabradine; Lapatinib; Lomitapide; Lovastatin; Lurasidone; Macitentan; Midazolam; Nilotinib; Nisoldipine; Pimozide; Pomalidomide; Proton Pump Inhibitors; QuiNIDine; Ranolazine; Red Yeast Rice; Regorafenib; Rifampin; Rivaroxaban; Salmeterol; Silodosin; Simeprevir; Simvastatin; St Johns Wort; Tamsulosin; Ticagrelor; Tolvaptan; Topotecan; Toremifene; Triazolam; Ulipristal; Vemurafenib; VinCRIStine (Liposomal)

Increased Effect/Toxicity

Nelfinavir may increase the levels/effects of: Ado-Trastuzumab Emtansine; Afatinib; Alfuzosin; Almotriptan; Alosetron; ALPRAZolam; Amiodarone; Apixaban; ARIPiprazole; AtorvaSTATin; Avanafil; Axitinib; Azithromycin (Systemic); Bedaquiline; Bortezomib; Bosentan; Bosutinib; Brentuximab Vedotin; Brinzolamide; Budesonide (Nasal); Budesonide (Systemic, Oral Inhalation); Cabozantinib; Calcium Channel Blockers (Dihydropyridine); Calcium Channel Blockers (Nondihydropyridine); CarBAMazepine; Cisapride; Clarithromycin; Colchicine; Conivaptan; Corticosteroids (Orally Inhaled); Crizotinib; CycloSPORINE (Systemic); CYP3A4 Substrates; Dabigatran Etexilate; Dienogest; Digoxin; Dofetilide; Dronedarone; Dutasteride; Enfuvirtide; Enzalutamide; Eplerenone; Ergot Derivatives; Everolimus; FentaNYL; Fesoterodine; Fluticasone (Nasal); Fluticasone (Oral Inhalation); GuanFACINE; Halofantrine; Ibrutinib; Iloperidone; Imatinib; Ivabradine; Ivacaftor; Ixabepilone; Lacosamide; Lapatinib; Levomilnacipran; Lomitapide; Lovastatin; Lumefantrine; Lurasidone; Macitentan; Maraviroc; Meperidine; MethylPREDNISolone; Midazolam; Mifepristone; Nefazodone; Nilotinib; Nisoldipine; Ospemifene; OxyCODONE; Paricalcitol; PAZOPanib; P-glycoprotein/ABCB1 Substrates; Pimecrolimus; Pimozide; Pomalidomide; PONATinib; Propafenone; Protease Inhibitors; Prucalopride; QUEtiapine; QuiNIDine; Ranolazine; Red Yeast Rice; Regorafenib; Repaglinide; Rifabutin; Rilpivirine; Riociguat; Rivaroxaban; RomiDEPsin; Rosuvastatin; Ruxolitinib; Salmeterol; Saxagliptin; Sildenafil; Silodosin; Simeprevir; Simvastatin; Sirolimus; SORAfenib; Tacrolimus (Systemic); Tacrolimus (Topical); Tadalafil; Tamsulosin; Temsirolimus; Ticagrelor; Tofacitinib; Tolterodine; Tolvaptan; Topotecan; Toremifene; TraZODone; Triazolam; Tricyclic Antidepressants; Ulipristal; Vardenafil; Vemurafenib; Vilazodone; VinCRIStine (Liposomal); Warfarin; Zuclopenthixol

The levels/effects of Nelfinavir may be increased by: Clarithromycin; CycloSPORINE (Systemic); Delavirdine; Enfuvirtide; Etravirine; Lopinavir; P-glycoprotein/ABCB1 Inhibitors; Simeprevir; Voriconazole

Decreased Effect

Nelfinavir may decrease the levels/effects of: Abacavir; Boceprevir; Clarithromycin; Contraceptives (Estrogens); Contraceptives (Progestins); Delavirdine; Etravirine; Fosphenytoin; Ifosfamide; Lopinavir; Meperidine; Methadone; Phenytoin; Prasugrel; Pravastatin; Theophylline Derivatives; Ticagrelor; Valproic Acid and Derivatives; Warfarin; Zidovudine

The levels/effects of Nelfinavir may be decreased by: Antacids; Boceprevir; Bosentan; CarBAMazepine; CYP2C19 Inducers (Strong); CYP3A4 Inducers (Strong); Dabrafenib; Deferasirox; Fosphenytoin; Garlic; H2-Antagonists; Mitotane; Nevirapine; Peginterferon Alfa-2b; P-glycoprotein/ABCB1 Inducers; Phenytoin; Proton Pump Inhibitors; Rifabutin; Rifampin; St Johns Wort; Tocilizumab

Ethanol/Nutrition/Herb Interactions

Food: Nelfinavir taken with food increases plasma concentration time curve (AUC) by two- to threefold. Do not administer with acidic food or juice (orange juice, apple juice, or applesauce) since the combination may have a bitter taste.

Herb/Nutraceutical: St John's wort may decrease the levels/effects of protease inhibitors; concurrent use should probably be avoided.

Storage/Stability Store at room temperature of 15°C to 30°C (59°F to 86°F). Oral powder (or dissolved tablets) diluted in nonacidic liquid is stable for 6 hours under refrigeration.

Mechanism of Action Binds to the site of HIV-1 protease activity and inhibits cleavage of viral Gag-Pol polyprotein precursors into individual functional proteins required for infectious HIV. This results in the formation of immature, noninfectious viral particles.

Pharmacodynamics/Kinetics

Absorption: Food increases AUC of nelfinavir by two- to fivefold

Distribution: V_d: 2-7 L/kg

Protein binding: >98%

Metabolism: Hepatic via CYP2C19 and 3A4; major metabolite has activity comparable to parent drug

Half-life elimination: 3.5-5 hours

Time to peak, serum: 2-4 hours

Excretion: Feces (98% to 99%, 78% as metabolites, 22% as unchanged drug); urine (1% to 2%)

Dosage Oral:

Children 2-13 years: 45-55 mg/kg twice daily **or** 25-35 mg/kg 3 times daily (maximum: 2500 mg daily).

Adolescents and Adults: 750 mg 3 times daily or 1250 mg twice daily with meals in combination with other antiretroviral therapies. **Note:** The DHHS Perinatal HIV Guidelines do not recommend the 3 times/day dosing in pregnant women (DHHS [perinatal], 2012).

Dosage adjustment in renal impairment: No dosage adjustment provided in manufacturer's labeling (has not been studied). However, since <2% excreted in urine a dosage reduction would not be expected

Dosage adjustment in hepatic impairment:

Mild impairment (Child-Pugh class A): No dosage adjustment necessary.

Moderate to severe impairment (Child-Pugh class B or C): Use not recommended.

Dietary Considerations Should be taken as scheduled with a meal.

Administration Tablets: Administer with a meal. If unable to swallow tablets, may dissolve tablets in a small amount of water; mix cloudy liquid well and consume immediately. Rinse glass with water to ensure receiving full dose.

Monitoring Parameters Liver function tests, viral load, CD4 count, triglycerides, cholesterol, blood glucose, CBC with differential

Additional Information Nelfinavir (alone or in combination) is not recommended as initial therapy in the treatment of HIV infection due to inferior virologic efficacy and a high incidence of diarrhea (DHHS, 2013).

Dosage Forms Excipient information presented when available (limited, particularly for generics); consult specific product labeling.

Tablet, Oral:

Viracept: 250 mg, 625 mg

◆ Nembutal *see* PENTobarbital *on page 1615*

◆ Nembutal® Sodium (Can) *see* PENTobarbital *on page 1615*

◆ NeoCeuticals Post-Acne Fade [OTC] *see* Hydroquinone *on page 1017*

◆ Neo DM [OTC] [DSC] *see* Chlorpheniramine, Phenylephrine, and Dextromethorphan *on page 413*

◆ Neo-Fradin *see* Neomycin *on page 1438*

Neomycin (nee oh MYE sin)

Brand Names: U.S. Neo-Fradin

Index Terms Neomycin Sulfate

Pharmacologic Category Ammonium Detoxicant; Antibiotic, Aminoglycoside; Antibiotic, Topical

Use Surgical (perioperative) prophylaxis for GI surgery; treatment of diarrhea caused by *E. coli*; adjunct in the treatment of hepatic encephalopathy

Pregnancy Risk Factor D

Pregnancy Considerations Aminoglycosides cross the placenta; however, neomycin has limited maternal absorption. Therefore the portion of an orally administered maternal dose available to cross the placenta is very low. Teratogenic effects have not been observed following maternal use of neomycin. Because of several reports of total irreversible bilateral congenital deafness in children whose mothers received another aminoglycoside (streptomycin) during pregnancy, the manufacturer classifies neomycin as pregnancy category D.

Breast-Feeding Considerations It is not known if neomycin is excreted into breast milk; however, limited oral absorption by both the mother and infant would minimize exposure to the nursing infant. Nondose-related effects could include modification of bowel flora. Breast-feeding is not recommended by the manufacturer.

Contraindications Hypersensitivity to neomycin or any component of the formulation, or other aminoglycosides; intestinal obstruction, inflammatory or ulcerative gastrointestinal disease

Warnings/Precautions **[U.S. Boxed Warning]: May cause neurotoxicity, nephrotoxicity, and/or neuromuscular blockade and respiratory paralysis;** usual risk factors include pre-existing renal impairment, concomitant neuro-/nephrotoxic medications, advanced age and dehydration. The drug's neurotoxicity can result in respiratory paralysis from neuromuscular blockade, especially when the drug is given soon after anesthesia or muscle relaxants. Use with caution in patients with renal impairment, pre-existing hearing impairment, neuromuscular disorders; neomycin is more toxic than other aminoglycosides when given parenterally; **do not administer parenterally**; **do not use as peritoneal lavage** due to significant systemic adsorption of the drug. Prolonged use may result in fungal or bacterial superinfection, including *C. difficile*-associated diarrhea (CDAD) and pseudomembranous colitis; CDAD has been observed >2 months postantibiotic treatment.

Adverse Reactions

>10%: Gastrointestinal: Nausea, diarrhea, vomiting, irritation or soreness of the mouth or rectal area

<1% (Limited to important or life-threatening): Dyspnea, eosinophilia, nephrotoxicity, neurotoxicity, ototoxicity (auditory), ototoxicity (vestibular)

Drug Interactions

Metabolism/Transport Effects None known.

Avoid Concomitant Use

Avoid concomitant use of Neomycin with any of the following: BCG; Gallium Nitrate

Increased Effect/Toxicity

Neomycin may increase the levels/effects of: AbobotulinumtoxinA; Acarbose; Bisphosphonate Derivatives; CARBOplatin; Colistimethate; CycloSPORINE (Systemic); Gallium Nitrate; Neuromuscular-Blocking Agents; OnabotulinumtoxinA; RimabotulinumtoxinB; Tenofovir; Vitamin K Antagonists

The levels/effects of Neomycin may be increased by: Amphotericin B; Capreomycin; Cephalosporins (2nd Generation); Cephalosporins (3rd Generation); Cephalosporins (4th Generation); CISplatin; Loop Diuretics; Nonsteroidal Anti-Inflammatory Agents; Tenofovir; Vancomycin

Decreased Effect

Neomycin may decrease the levels/effects of: BCG; Cardiac Glycosides; Sodium Picosulfate; SORAfenib

The levels/effects of Neomycin may be decreased by: Penicillins

Mechanism of Action Interferes with bacterial protein synthesis by binding to 30S ribosomal subunits

Pharmacodynamics/Kinetics

Absorption: Oral, percutaneous: Poor (3%)

Distribution: 97% of an orally administered dose remains in the GI tract. Absorbed neomycin distributes to tissues and concentrates in the renal cortex. With repeated doses, accumulation also occurs in the inner ear.

V_d: 0.36 L/kg

Protein binding: 0% to 30%

Metabolism: Slightly hepatic

Half-life elimination (age and renal function dependent): 3 hours

Time to peak, serum: Oral: 1-4 hours

Excretion: Feces (97% of oral dose as unchanged drug); urine (30% to 50% of absorbed drug as unchanged drug)

Dosage

Children: Oral:

Surgical (perioperative) prophylaxis: Oral: 15 mg/kg/dose for 3 doses administered over 10 hours (eg, at 1 PM, 2 PM, and 11 PM) on the day preceding surgery; maximum dose: 1000 mg; (Bratzler, 2013); used as an adjunct to mechanical cleansing of the intestine and in combination with erythromycin base and perioperative I.V. antibiotics

Hepatic encephalopathy: 50-100 mg/kg/day in divided doses every 6-8 hours or 2.5-7 g/m^2/day divided every 4-6 hours for 5-6 days not to exceed 12 g daily

Adults: Oral:

Surgical (perioperative) prophylaxis:

Manufacturer's recommendations: 1 g at 1 PM, 2 PM, and 11 PM on the day preceding 8 AM surgery as an adjunct to mechanical cleansing of the bowel and oral erythromycin

Alternative recommendation: 1 g at 1 PM, 2 PM, and 11 PM on the day preceding 8 AM surgery combined with mechanical cleansing of the large intestine and oral erythromycin or metronidazole, and I.V. antibiotics on the day of surgery (Bratzler, 2013)

Hepatic encephalopathy: 500-2000 mg every 6-8 hours or 4-12 g daily divided every 4-6 hours for 5-6 days

Chronic hepatic insufficiency: 4 g daily for an indefinite period

Dosage adjustment in renal impairment: No specific dosage adjustment provided in manufacturer's labeling; however, dosage reduction or discontinuation of therapy should be considered if a patient develops renal insufficiency. The risk of nephro- and/or ototoxicity is increased in patients with renal impairment.

Dosage adjustment in hepatic impairment: No dosage adjustment provided in manufacturer's labeling.

Monitoring Parameters Renal function tests, audiometry in symptomatic patients

Dosage Forms Excipient information presented when available (limited, particularly for generics); consult specific product labeling.

Solution, Oral, as sulfate:

Neo-Fradin: 25 mg/mL (480 mL) [cherry flavor]

Tablet, Oral, as sulfate:

Generic: 500 mg

Neomycin and Polymyxin B

(nee oh MYE sin & pol i MIKS in bee)

Brand Names: U.S. Neosporin® G.U. Irrigant

Brand Names: Canada Neosporin® Irrigating Solution

Index Terms Polymyxin B and Neomycin

Pharmacologic Category Antibiotic, Topical; Genitourinary Irrigant

Use Short-term as a continuous irrigant or rinse in the urinary bladder to prevent bacteriuria and gram-negative rod septicemia associated with the use of indwelling catheters

Pregnancy Risk Factor D

Dosage Children and Adults: Bladder irrigation: **Not for injection**; add 1 mL irrigant to 1 L isotonic saline solution and connect container to the inflow of lumen of 3-way catheter. Continuous irrigant or rinse in the urinary bladder for up to a maximum of 10 days with administration rate adjusted to patient's urine output; usually no more than 1 L of irrigant is used per day.

Additional Information Complete prescribing information should be consulted for additional detail.

Dosage Forms Excipient information presented when available (limited, particularly for generics); consult specific product labeling.

Solution, irrigation: Neomycin 40 mg and polymyxin B sulfate 200,000 units per 1 mL (1 mL, 20 mL)

Neosporin® G.U. Irrigant: Neomycin 40 mg and polymyxin sulfate B 200,000 units per 1 mL (1 mL, 20 mL)

◆ **Neomycin, Bacitracin, and Polymyxin B** *see* Bacitracin, Neomycin, and Polymyxin B *on page 221*

◆ **Neomycin, Bacitracin, Polymyxin B, and Hydrocortisone** *see* Bacitracin, Neomycin, Polymyxin B, and Hydrocortisone *on page 221*

Neomycin, Colistin, Hydrocortisone, and Thonzonium

(nee oh MYE sin, koe LIS tin, hye droe KOR ti sone, & thon ZOE nee um)

Brand Names: U.S. Coly-Mycin® S; Cortisporin®-TC

Index Terms Colistin, Hydrocortisone, Neomycin, and Thonzonium; Hydrocortisone, Neomycin, Colistin, and Thonzonium; Thonzonium, Neomycin, Colistin, and Hydrocortisone

Pharmacologic Category Antibiotic, Otic; Antibiotic/Corticosteroid, Otic; Corticosteroid, Otic

Use Treatment of superficial and susceptible bacterial infections of the external auditory canal; for treatment of susceptible bacterial infections of mastoidectomy and fenestration cavities

Pregnancy Risk Factor C

Dosage Otic:

Calibrated dropper:

Children: 4 drops in affected ear 3-4 times/day

Adults: 5 drops in affected ear 3-4 times/day

Dropper bottle:

Children: 3 drops in affected ear 3-4 times/day

Adults: 4 drops in affected ear 3-4 times/day

Note: Alternatively, a cotton wick may be inserted in the ear canal and saturated with suspension every 4 hours; wick should be replaced at least every 24 hours

Dosage adjustment in renal impairment: No dosage adjustment provided in manufacturer's labeling. However, dosage adjustment unlikely due to low systemic absorption.

Dosage adjustment in hepatic impairment: No dosage adjustment provided in manufacturer's labeling. However, dosage adjustment unlikely due to low systemic absorption.

Additional Information Complete prescribing information should be consulted for additional detail.

Dosage Forms Excipient information presented when available (limited, particularly for generics); consult specific product labeling.

Suspension, otic [drops]:

Coly-Mycin® S: Neomycin 0.33%, colistin 0.3%, hydrocortisone acetate 1%, and thonzonium bromide 0.05% (5 mL) [contains thimerosal]

Cortisporin®-TC: Neomycin 0.33%, colistin 0.3%, hydrocortisone acetate 1%, and thonzonium bromide 0.05% (10 mL) [contains thimerosal]

Neomycin, Polymyxin B, and Dexamethasone

(nee oh MYE sin, pol i MIKS in bee, & deks a METH a sone)

Brand Names: U.S. Maxitrol®

Brand Names: Canada Dioptrol®; Maxitrol®

Index Terms Dexamethasone, Neomycin, and Polymyxin B; Polymyxin B, Neomycin, and Dexamethasone

Pharmacologic Category Antibiotic/Corticosteroid, Ophthalmic

Use Steroid-responsive inflammatory ocular conditions in which a corticosteroid is indicated and where bacterial infection or a risk of bacterial infection exists

Pregnancy Risk Factor C

Dosage Ophthalmic:

Children ≥2 years and Adults: Suspension: Instill 1-2 drops into the conjunctival sac of the affected eye(s) 4-6 times/day; in severe disease, drops may be used hourly and tapered to discontinuation

Adults: Ointment: Place ~1/2" ribbon in the conjunctival sac of the affected eye(s) 3-4 times/day or apply at bedtime as an adjunct with suspension

Note: If signs and symptoms do not improve after 2 days of treatment, the patient should be re-evaluated.

Additional Information Complete prescribing information should be consulted for additional detail.

Dosage Forms Excipient information presented when available (limited, particularly for generics); consult specific product labeling.

Ointment, ophthalmic: Neomycin 3.5 mg, polymyxin B sulfate 10,000 units, and dexamethasone 0.1% per g (3.5 g)

Maxitrol®: Neomycin 3.5 mg, polymyxin B sulfate 10,000 units, and dexamethasone 0.1% per g (3.5 g)

Suspension, ophthalmic [drops]: Neomycin 3.5 mg, polymyxin B sulfate 10,000 units, and dexamethasone 0.1% per 1 mL (5 mL)

Maxitrol®: Neomycin 3.5 mg, polymyxin B sulfate 10,000 units, and dexamethasone 0.1% per 1 mL (5 mL) [contains benzalkonium chloride]

Neomycin, Polymyxin B, and Gramicidin

(nee oh MYE sin, pol i MIKS in bee, & gram i SYE din)

Brand Names: U.S. Neosporin® Ophthalmic Solution

Brand Names: Canada Neosporin®; Optimyxin Plus®

Index Terms Gramicidin, Neomycin, and Polymyxin B; Polymyxin B, Neomycin, and Gramicidin

Pharmacologic Category Antibiotic, Ophthalmic

Use Treatment of superficial ocular infection

Pregnancy Risk Factor C

Dosage Children and Adults: Ophthalmic: Instill 1-2 drops 4-6 times/day or more frequently as required for severe infections

Additional Information Complete prescribing information should be consulted for additional detail.

Dosage Forms Excipient information presented when available (limited, particularly for generics); consult specific product labeling.

Solution, ophthalmic [drops]: Neomycin 1.75 mg, polymyxin B 10,000 units, and gramicidin 0.025 mg per 1 mL (10 mL)

Neosporin® Ophthalmic Solution: Neomycin 1.75 mg, polymyxin B 10,000 units, and gramicidin 0.025 mg per 1 mL (10 mL)

Neomycin, Polymyxin B, and Hydrocortisone

(nee oh MYE sin, pol i MIKS in bee, & hye droe KOR ti sone)

Brand Names: U.S. Cortisporin®; Cortomycin

Brand Names: Canada Cortimyxin®; Cortisporin® Otic

Index Terms Hydrocortisone, Neomycin, and Polymyxin B; Polymyxin B, Neomycin, and Hydrocortisone

Pharmacologic Category Antibiotic, Ophthalmic; Antibiotic, Otic; Antibiotic, Topical; Antibiotic/Corticosteroid, Otic; Corticosteroid, Ophthalmic; Corticosteroid, Otic; Corticosteroid, Topical

Use Steroid-responsive inflammatory condition for which a corticosteroid is indicated and where bacterial infection or a risk of bacterial infection exists

Pregnancy Risk Factor C

Dosage Note: Duration of use of ophthalmic and otic preparations should be limited to 10 days unless otherwise directed by the healthcare provider.

Ophthalmic:

Children (unlabeled use): Instill 1-2 drops 2-4 times/day, or more frequently as required for severe infections

Adults: Instill 1-2 drops 2-4 times/day, or more frequently as required for severe infections

Otic: Otic solution is used **only** for bacterial infections of external auditory canal (eg, swimmer's ear).

Children 6 months to 2 years (unlabeled use): Instill 3 drops into affected ear 3-4 times/day

Children ≥2 years: Instill 3 drops into affected ear 3-4 times/day

Adults: Instill 4 drops into affected ear 3-4 times/day; otic suspension is the preferred otic preparation

Topical:

Children (unlabeled use): Apply a thin layer 1-4 times/day. Therapy should be discontinued when control is achieved; if no improvement is seen, reassessment of diagnosis may be necessary.

Adults: Apply a thin layer 1-4 times/day. Therapy should be discontinued when control is achieved; if no improvement is seen, reassessment of diagnosis may be necessary.

Dosage adjustment in renal impairment: No dosage adjustment provided in manufacturer's labeling. However, dosage adjustment unlikely due to low systemic absorption.

Dosage adjustment in hepatic impairment: No dosage adjustment provided in manufacturer's labeling. However, dosage adjustment unlikely due to low systemic absorption.

Additional Information Complete prescribing information should be consulted for additional detail.

Dosage Forms Excipient information presented when available (limited, particularly for generics); consult specific product labeling.

Cream, topical:

Cortisporin®: Neomycin 3.5 mg, polymyxin B 10,000 units, and hydrocortisone acetate 5 mg per g (7.5 g)

Solution, otic: Neomycin 3.5 mg, polymyxin B 10,000 units, and hydrocortisone 10 mg per 1 mL (10 mL)

Cortisporin®: Neomycin 3.5 mg, polymyxin B 10,000 units, and hydrocortisone 10 mg per 1 mL (10 mL) [contains potassium metabisulfite]

Cortomycin: Neomycin 3.5 mg, polymyxin B 10,000 units, and hydrocortisone 10 mg per 1 mL (10 mL) [contains potassium metabisulfate]

Suspension, ophthalmic [drops]: Neomycin 3.5 mg, polymyxin B 10,000 units, and hydrocortisone 10 mg per 1 mL (7.5 mL)

Suspension, otic: Neomycin 3.5 mg, polymyxin B 10,000 units, and hydrocortisone 10 mg per 1 mL (10 mL)

Cortomycin: Neomycin 3.5 mg, polymyxin B 10,000 units, and hydrocortisone 10 mg per 1 mL (10 mL) [contains thimerosal]

- ◆ **Neomycin Sulfate** *see* Neomycin *on page* 1438
- ◆ **Neo-Polycin™** *see* Bacitracin, Neomycin, and Polymyxin B *on page* 221
- ◆ **Neo-Polycin™ HC** *see* Bacitracin, Neomycin, Polymyxin B, and Hydrocortisone *on page* 221
- ◆ **NeoProfen** *see* Ibuprofen *on page* 1032
- ◆ **Neoral** *see* CycloSPORINE (Systemic) *on page* 508
- ◆ **Neosar** *see* Cyclophosphamide *on page* 504
- ◆ **Neosporin® (Can)** *see* Neomycin, Polymyxin B, and Gramicidin *on page* 1440
- ◆ **Neosporin® G.U. Irrigant** *see* Neomycin and Polymyxin B *on page* 1439
- ◆ **Neosporin® Irrigating Solution (Can)** *see* Neomycin and Polymyxin B *on page* 1439
- ◆ **Neosporin® Neo To Go® [OTC]** *see* Bacitracin, Neomycin, and Polymyxin B *on page* 221
- ◆ **Neosporin® Ophthalmic Solution** *see* Neomycin, Polymyxin B, and Gramicidin *on page* 1440
- ◆ **Neosporin® Topical [OTC]** *see* Bacitracin, Neomycin, and Polymyxin B *on page* 221

Neostigmine (nee oh STIG meen)

Brand Names: U.S. Bloxiverz; Prostigmin

Brand Names: Canada Prostigmin

Index Terms Neostigmine Bromide; Neostigmine Methylsulfate

Pharmacologic Category Acetylcholinesterase Inhibitor

Use

Myasthenia gravis (excluding Bloxiverz): Symptomatic control of myasthenia gravis

Postoperative bladder distention/Urinary retention (excluding Bloxiverz and Prostigmin tablets): Prevention and treatment of postoperative bladder distention and urinary retention after mechanical obstruction has been excluded.

Reversal of nondepolarizing muscle relaxants (excluding Prostigmin tablets): Reversal of effects of nondepolarizing neuromuscular blocking agents (eg, tubocurarine, or pancuronium) after surgery.

Pregnancy Risk Factor C

Pregnancy Considerations Animal reproduction studies have not been conducted; anticholinesterases have caused uterine irritability and induced premature labor with I.V. use in near-term pregnant women. When used as adjunct to analgesia in labor, adverse events to the fetus and mother are dose- and route-dependent (Habib, 2006). Neostigmine may be used to treat myasthenia gravis in pregnant women; however, if an acetylcholinesterase inhibitor is needed during pregnancy, another agent may be preferred (Norwood, 2013; Silvestri, 2012).

Breast-Feeding Considerations It is not known if neostigmine is excreted into breast milk. The manufacturer recommends caution be used if administered to nursing women. Babies born to women with myasthenia gravis may have feeding difficulties due to transient myasthenia gravis of the newborn (Norwood, 2013).

Contraindications

Hypersensitivity to neostigmine or any component of the formulation; history of reaction to bromides (tablets only); peritonitis or mechanical obstruction of the intestinal or urinary tract

Documentation of allergenic cross-reactivity for cholinesterase inhibitors is limited. However, because of similarities in chemical structure and/or pharmacologic actions, the possibility of cross-sensitivity cannot be ruled out with certainty.

Warnings/Precautions Bradycardia, hypotension, and dysrhythmias may occur, particularly with IV use; cardiovascular complications may also be increased in patients with myasthenia gravis. Use with caution in patients with epilepsy, asthma, bradycardia, hypotension, hyperthyroidism, cardiac arrhythmias, coronary artery disease, recent acute coronary syndrome, vagotonia, or peptic ulcer. Cardiovascular complications may also be increased in patients with myasthenia gravis. When I.V. neostigmine is administered for the reversal of nondepolarizing neuromuscular-blocking agents, atropine or glycopyrrolate should be administered concurrently or prior to neostigmine to lessen the risk of bradycardia. Adequate facilities should be available for cardiopulmonary resuscitation when testing and adjusting dose for myasthenia gravis. Symptoms of hypersensitivity have included urticaria, angioedema, erythema multiforme, generalized rash, facial swelling, peripheral edema, pyrexia, flushing, hypotension, bronchospasm, bradycardia, and anaphylaxis. Have atropine and epinephrine ready to treat hypersensitivity reactions. Overdosage may result in cholinergic crisis, this must be distinguished from myasthenic crisis. Large doses of I.V. neostigmine administered for the reversal of nondepolarizing neuromuscular blocking-agents when neuromuscular blockade is minimal can result in neuromuscular dysfunction. Reduce the dose of neostigmine if recovery from neuromuscular blockade is nearly complete.

Infants and small children may be at greater risk of complications from incomplete reversal of neuromuscular blockade due to decreased respiratory drive; observe the effects of an anticholinergic agent (eg, atropine) prior to administration of neostigmine to lessen the probability of bradycardia and hypotension. Use with caution in the elderly and monitor for a longer period in the elderly; may experience slower spontaneous recovery from neuromuscular blocking agents. Use with caution in the elderly and monitor for a longer period in the elderly; may experience slower spontaneous recovery from neuromuscular blocking agents.

Adverse Reactions Frequency not defined.

Cardiovascular: Arrhythmias (especially bradycardia), AV block, cardiac arrest, flushing, hypotension, nodal rhythm, nonspecific ECG changes, syncope, tachycardia

Central nervous system: Convulsions, dizziness, drowsiness, dysarthria, dysphonia, headache, loss of consciousness

Dermatologic: Skin rash, thrombophlebitis (I.V.), urticaria

Gastrointestinal: Diarrhea, dysphagia, flatulence, hyperperistalsis, nausea, salivation, stomach cramps, vomiting

Genitourinary: Urinary urgency

Neuromuscular & skeletal: Arthralgias, fasciculations, muscle cramps, spasms, weakness

Ocular: Lacrimation, small pupils

Respiratory: Bronchiolar constriction, bronchospasm, dyspnea, increased bronchial secretions, laryngospasm, respiratory arrest, respiratory depression, respiratory muscle paralysis

Miscellaneous: Allergic reactions, anaphylaxis, diaphoresis increased

Drug Interactions

Metabolism/Transport Effects None known.

Avoid Concomitant Use There are no known interactions where it is recommended to avoid concomitant use.

Increased Effect/Toxicity

Neostigmine may increase the levels/effects of: Beta-Blockers; Cholinergic Agonists; Succinylcholine

The levels/effects of Neostigmine may be increased by: Corticosteroids (Systemic)

Decreased Effect

Neostigmine may decrease the levels/effects of: Neuromuscular-Blocking Agents (Nondepolarizing)

The levels/effects of Neostigmine may be decreased by: Dipyridamole

Storage/Stability

Injection: Store between 20°C and 25°C (68°F and 77°F); excursions permitted to 15°C to 30°C (59°F to 86°F). Protect from light. Store in carton until time of use.

Tablets: Store at 25°C (77°F); excursions permitted to 15°C to 30°C (59°F to 86°F).

Mechanism of Action Inhibits destruction of acetylcholine by acetylcholinesterase which facilitates transmission of impulses across myoneural junction; direct cholinomimetic effect on skeletal muscle and possible on autonomic ganglion cells and neurons of the CNS

Pharmacodynamics/Kinetics

Onset of action: I.M.: 20-30 minutes; Oral: 1-2 hours

Duration: I.M.: 2.5-4 hours

Absorption: Oral: Poor

Distribution: V_d: I.V.: 0.12-1.4 L/kg

Protein binding: 15% to 25%

Metabolism: Hepatic

Half-life elimination: I.M.: 51-90 minutes; I.V.: 24-113 minutes; Oral: 42-60 minutes

Excretion: Urine (50% as unchanged drug)

Dosage
Myasthenia gravis: Diagnosis (unlabeled use): I.M.:
Children: 0.025-0.04 mg/kg as a single dose
Adults: 0.02 mg/kg as a single dose
Myasthenia gravis: Treatment:
Children (unlabeled use):
Oral: 2 mg/kg/day, not to exceed 375 mg daily
I.M., I.V., SubQ: 0.01-0.04 mg/kg every 2-4 hours as needed
Adults:
Manufacturer's labeling:
Oral: Usual dose: 150 mg administered over a 24-hour period; interval between doses is of paramount importance and therapy is frequently required day and night. Dosage range: 15-375 mg daily in divided doses.
I.M, SubQ: 0.5 mg; subsequent dosing based on individual patient response
Alternative recommendations (unlabeled dosing):
Oral: Initial: 15 mg every 8 hours; may increase every 1-2 days up to 375 mg daily maximum; interval between doses must be individualized to maximal response
I.M., I.V., SubQ: 0.5-2.5 mg every 1-3 hours as needed up to 10 mg/24 hours maximum
Reversal of nondepolarizing neuromuscular-blocking agents (NMBAs) after surgery:
Bloxiverz: I.V.: **Note:** An anticholinergic agent (atropine or glycopyrrolate) should be given prior to or in conjunction with neostigmine; in the presence of bradycardia, administer the anticholinergic prior to neostigmine. Peripheral nerve stimulation delivering train-of-four (TOF) stimulus must also be used to determine time of neostigmine initiation and need for additional doses.
Infants, Children, Adolescents, and Adults: Usual dose: 0.03-0.07 mg/kg generally achieves a TOF twitch ratio of 90% within 10-20 minutes of administration; maximum total dose: 0.07 mg/kg or 5 mg (whichever is less)
Dose selection guide:
The 0.03 mg/kg dose is recommended for reversal of NMBAs with shorter half-lives (eg, rocuronium); **or** when the first twitch response to the TOF stimulus is substantially >10% of baseline or when a second twitch is present.
The 0.07 mg/kg dose is recommended for NMBAs with longer half-lives (eg, vecuronium, pancuronium); **or** when the first twitch response is relatively weak (ie, not substantially >10% of baseline); or rapid recovery is needed.
Generic products: I.V.: **Note:** Administer with atropine 0.6-1.2 mg in a separate syringe several minutes before neostigmine.
Adults: 0.5-2 mg; repeat as required. Only in exceptional cases should the total dose exceed 5 mg.
Postoperative urinary retention: Adults: I.M., SubQ:
Prevention: 0.25 mg as soon as possible after operation; repeat every 4-6 hours for 2-3 days
Treatment: 0.5 mg; if urination does not occur within an hour, patient should be catheterized. After the bladder has emptied or patient has voided, continue 0.5 mg every 3 hours for at least 5 doses.
Postoperative bladder distention: Adults: I.M., SubQ:
Prevention: 0.25 mg as soon as possible after operation; repeat every 4-6 hours for 2-3 days
Treatment: 0.5 mg as needed

Dosage adjustment in renal impairment:
No dosage adjustment provided in manufacturer's labeling; however, the following adjustments have been recommended (Aronoff, 2007): Adults: Oral:
Cl_{cr} >50 mL/minute: No dosage adjustment necessary
Cl_{cr} 10-50 mL/minute: Administer 50% of normal dose
Cl_{cr} <10 mL/minute: Administer 25% of normal dose
Hemodialysis: No dosage adjustment necessary
Peritoneal dialysis: No dosage adjustment necessary
Continuous renal replacement therapy (CRRT): Administer 50% of normal dose

Dosage adjustment in hepatic impairment: No dosage adjustment provided in manufacturer's labeling.

Administration Tablets (neostigmine bromide): Administer without regard to food. Consider giving larger portions of the daily dose around fatigue prone times (eg, mealtimes, afternoons).
Injectable (neostigmine methylsulfate): Administer I.M., SubQ, or by slow I.V. injection over at least 1 minute.

Monitoring Parameters ECG, blood pressure, and heart rate especially with I.V. use; consult individual institutional policies and procedures

Additional Information Due to poor absorption of tablets in the GI tract, neostigmine bromide 15 mg administered orally is generally considered to be equivalent to neostigmine methylsulfate 0.5 mg administered parenterally.

Dosage Forms Excipient information presented when available (limited, particularly for generics); consult specific product labeling.
Solution, Injection, as methylsulfate:
Prostigmin: 0.5 mg/mL (1 mL, 10 mL)
Generic: 0.5 mg/mL (10 mL); 1 mg/mL (10 mL)
Solution, Intravenous, as methylsulfate:
Bloxiverz: 5 mg/10 mL (10 mL); 10 mg/10 mL (10 mL) [contains phenol]
Tablet, Oral, as bromide:
Prostigmin: 15 mg [scored]

◆ **Neostigmine Bromide** *see* Neostigmine *on page 1441*

◆ **Neostigmine Methylsulfate** *see* Neostigmine *on page 1441*

◆ **NeoStrata® HQ (Can)** *see* Hydroquinone *on page 1017*

◆ **NeoStrata HQ Skin Lightening [OTC]** *see* Hydroquinone *on page 1017*

◆ **Neo-Synephrine [DSC]** *see* Phenylephrine (Systemic) *on page 1636*

Nepafenac (ne pa FEN ak)

Brand Names: U.S. Ilevro; Nevanac
Brand Names: Canada Nevanac®
Pharmacologic Category Nonsteroidal Anti-inflammatory Drug (NSAID), Ophthalmic
Use Treatment of pain and inflammation associated with cataract surgery
Pregnancy Risk Factor C
Dosage
Ophthalmic: Children ≥10 years, Adolescents, and Adults:
Ilevro™: Instill 1 drop into affected eye(s) once daily, beginning 1 day prior to surgery, the day of surgery, and through the first 2 weeks of the postoperative period. Instill 1 additional drop 30-120 minutes prior to surgery.
Nevanac®: Instill 1 drop into affected eye(s) 3 times/day, beginning 1 day prior to surgery, the day of surgery, and through the first 2 weeks of the postoperative period.

Dosage adjustment in renal impairment: No dosage adjustment provided in manufacturer's labeling.
Dosage adjustment in hepatic impairment: No dosage adjustment provided in manufacturer's labeling.

Additional Information Complete prescribing information should be consulted for additional detail.

Dosage Forms Excipient information presented when available (limited, particularly for generics); consult specific product labeling.

Suspension, Ophthalmic:

Ilevro: 0.3% (1.7 mL) [contains benzalkonium chloride, edetate disodium, propylene glycol]

Nevanac: 0.1% (3 mL) [contains edentate disodium benzalkonium chloride]

◆ **Neptazane** *see* Methazolamide *on page 1319*

◆ **Nerve Agent Antidote Kit** *see* Atropine and Pralidoxime *on page 200*

◆ **Nesacaine** *see* Chloroprocaine *on page 409*

◆ **Nesacaine®-CE (Can)** *see* Chloroprocaine *on page 409*

◆ **Nesacaine-MPF** *see* Chloroprocaine *on page 409*

Nesiritide (ni SIR i tide)

Brand Names: U.S. Natrecor

Index Terms B-type Natriuretic Peptide (Human); hBNP; Natriuretic Peptide

Pharmacologic Category Natriuretic Peptide, B-Type, Human

Additional Appendix Information

Vasoactive Agents, Intravenous *on page 2315*

Use Treatment of acutely decompensated heart failure (HF) with dyspnea at rest or with minimal activity

Pregnancy Risk Factor C

Pregnancy Considerations Adverse events were not observed in an animal reproduction study. Nesiritide is a recombinant B-type natriuretic peptide (rhBNP). BNP and NT-proBNP (which has been used as a marker of BNP), are endogenous peptides and NT-proBNP is measurable in the umbilical cord serum of normal pregnancies. Information related to the administration of nesiritide during pregnancy has not been located.

Breast-Feeding Considerations It is not known if nesiritide is excreted in breast milk.

Contraindications Hypersensitivity to natriuretic peptide or any component of the formulation; cardiogenic shock (when used as primary therapy); hypotension (persistent systolic blood pressure <100 mm Hg) prior to therapy

Warnings/Precautions May cause hypotension; administer in clinical situations when blood pressure may be closely monitored. Effects may be additive with other agents capable of causing hypotension. Hypotensive effects may last for several hours.

Should not be used in patients with low cardiac filling pressures, or in patients with conditions which depend on venous return including significant valvular stenosis, restrictive or obstructive cardiomyopathy, constrictive pericarditis, and pericardial tamponade. May be associated with development of azotemia; use caution in patients with renal impairment or in patients where renal perfusion is dependent on renin-angiotensin-aldosterone system; avoid initiation at doses higher than recommended.

Monitor for allergic or anaphylactic reactions; use caution in patients with history of hypersensitivity to other recombinant peptides. Use caution with prolonged infusions; limited experience with infusions >96 hours.

Adverse Reactions Note: Frequencies cited below were recorded in VMAC trial, unless otherwise noted, at dosages similar to approved labeling. Higher frequencies have been observed in trials using higher dosages of nesiritide. The percentages marked with an asterisk (*) indicate frequency less than or equal to placebo or other standard therapy.

>10%:

Cardiovascular: Hypotension (total: 11% [27% in ASCEND-HF trial]; symptomatic: 4% [7% in ASCEND-HF trial] at recommended dose, up to 17% at higher doses)

Renal: Increased serum creatinine (28% with >0.5 mg/dL increase over baseline)

1% to 10%:

Cardiovascular: Ventricular tachycardia (3%)*, ventricular extrasystoles (3%)*, angina (2%)*, bradycardia (1%), tachycardia, atrial fibrillation, AV node conduction abnormalities

Central nervous system: Headache (8%)*, dizziness (3%), insomnia (2%)*, anxiety (3%), confusion, fever, paresthesia, somnolence, tremor

Dermatologic: Pruritus, rash

Gastrointestinal: Nausea (4%)*, abdominal pain (1%)*, vomiting (1%)*

Hematologic: Anemia

Local: Injection site reaction, catheter pain

Neuromuscular & skeletal: Back pain (4%), leg cramps

Ocular: Amblyopia

Respiratory: Apnea, cough increased, hemoptysis

Miscellaneous: Diaphoresis

Postmarketing and/or case reports: Extravasation, hypersensitivity reactions (rare)

Drug Interactions

Metabolism/Transport Effects None known.

Avoid Concomitant Use There are no known interactions where it is recommended to avoid concomitant use.

Increased Effect/Toxicity

Nesiritide may increase the levels/effects of: Hypotensive Agents

Decreased Effect There are no known significant interactions involving a decrease in effect.

Ethanol/Nutrition/Herb Interactions Herb/Nutraceutical: Avoid bayberry, blue cohosh, cayenne, ephedra, ginger, ginseng (American), kola, and licorice (may increase blood pressure). Avoid black cohosh, California poppy, coleus, golden seal, hawthorn, mistletoe, periwinkle, quinine, and shepherd's purse (may enhance decreased blood pressure).

Preparation for Administration Reconstitute 1.5 mg vial with 5 mL of diluent removed from a prefilled 250 mL plastic I.V. bag (compatible with D_5W, $D_5{}^1/_2NS$, $D_5{}^1/_4NS$, NS). Do not shake vial to dissolve (roll gently). Withdraw entire contents of vial and add to 250 mL I.V. bag. Invert several times to mix. Resultant concentration of solution is ~6 mcg/mL.

Storage/Stability Vials may be stored below 25°C (77°F); do not freeze. Protect from light. Following reconstitution, vials are stable at 2°C to 25°C (36°F to 77°F) for up to 24 hours. Use reconstituted solution within 24 hours.

Mechanism of Action Binds to guanylate cyclase receptor on vascular smooth muscle and endothelial cells, increasing intracellular cyclic GMP, resulting in smooth muscle cell relaxation. Has been shown to produce dose-dependent reductions in pulmonary capillary wedge pressure (PCWP) and systemic arterial pressure.

Pharmacodynamics/Kinetics

Onset of action: PCWP reduction: 15 minutes (60% of 3-hour effect achieved within this time period)

Peak effect: Within 1 hour

Duration: >60 minutes (up to several hours) for systolic blood pressure; hemodynamic effects persist longer than serum half-life would predict

Distribution: V_{ss}: 0.19 L/kg

Metabolism: Proteolytic cleavage by vascular endopeptidases and proteolysis following binding to the membrane bound natriuretic peptide (NPR-C) and cellular internalization

Half-life elimination: Initial (distribution) ~2 minutes; Terminal: ~18 minutes

Excretion: Primarily eliminated by metabolism; also excreted in the urine

Dosage Adults: I.V.: Initial: 2 mcg/kg (bolus optional); followed by continuous infusion at 0.01 mcg/kg/minute. **Note:** Should not be initiated at a dosage higher than initial recommended dose. There is limited experience with increasing the dose >0.01 mcg/kg/minute; in one trial, a limited number of patients received higher doses that were increased no faster than every 3 hours by 0.005 mcg/kg/minute (preceded by a bolus of 1 mcg/kg), up to a maximum of 0.03 mcg/kg/minute. Increases beyond the initial infusion rate should be limited to selected patients and accompanied by close hemodynamic and renal function monitoring.

Patients experiencing hypotension during the infusion: Infusion dose should be reduced or discontinued. Other measures to support blood pressure should be initiated (eg, I.V. fluids, Trendelenburg position). Hypotension may be prolonged (up to hours); once patient is stabilized, may attempt to restart at a lower dose (reduce previous infusion dose by 30% and omit bolus).

Maximum dosing weight: According to the manufacturer, the PRECEDENT Trial capped dosing weight at 160 kg and the VMAC Trial capped dosing weight at 175 kg. There are no specific guidelines on maximum dosing weight and clinical judgment should be used.

Dosage adjustment in renal impairment: No dosage adjustment necessary. Use cautiously in patients with renal impairment or those patients who rely on the renin-angiotensin-aldosterone system for renal perfusion. Monitor renal function closely.

Dosage adjustment in hepatic impairment: No dosage adjustment provided in manufacturer's labeling.

Usual Infusion Concentrations: Adult I.V. infusion: 1.5 mg in 250 mL (concentration: 6 **mcg**/mL) of D_5W or NS

Administration Do not administer through a heparin-coated catheter (concurrent administration of heparin via a separate catheter is acceptable, per manufacturer).

Prime I.V. tubing with 5 mL of infusion prior to connection with vascular access port and prior to administering bolus or starting the infusion. Withdraw bolus from the prepared infusion bag and administer over 60 seconds. Begin infusion immediately following administration of the bolus.

Monitoring Parameters Blood pressure, hemodynamic responses (PCWP, RAP, CI), BUN, creatinine; urine output; consult individual institutional policies and procedures

Additional Information The duration of symptomatic improvement with nesiritide following discontinuation of the infusion has been limited (generally lasting several days). Atrial natriuretic peptide, which is related to nesiritide, has been associated with increased vascular permeability. This has not been observed in clinical trials with nesiritide, but patients should be monitored for this effect.

Dosage Forms Excipient information presented when available (limited, particularly for generics); consult specific product labeling.

Solution Reconstituted, Intravenous:

Natrecor: 1.5 mg (1 ea)

- **NESP** *see* Darbepoetin Alfa *on page 543*
- **Neulasta** *see* Pegfilgrastim *on page 1588*
- **Neulasta® (Can)** *see* Pegfilgrastim *on page 1588*
- **Neumega** *see* Oprelvekin *on page 1514*
- **Neupogen** *see* Filgrastim *on page 859*
- **Neupro** *see* Rotigotine *on page 1863*
- **Neuro-K-50 [OTC]** *see* Pyridoxine *on page 1753*
- **Neuro-K-250 T.D. [OTC]** *see* Pyridoxine *on page 1753*
- **Neuro-K-250 Vitamin B6 [OTC]** *see* Pyridoxine *on page 1753*
- **Neuro-K-500 [OTC]** *see* Pyridoxine *on page 1753*
- **Neurontin** *see* Gabapentin *on page 933*
- **Neut** *see* Sodium Bicarbonate *on page 1912*
- **NeutraCare®** *see* Fluoride *on page 880*
- **NeutraGard® Advanced** *see* Fluoride *on page 880*
- **Neutrahist PDX [OTC] [DSC]** *see* Chlorpheniramine, Pseudoephedrine, and Dextromethorphan *on page 414*
- **Neutrahist Pediatric [OTC]** *see* Chlorpheniramine and Pseudoephedrine *on page 412*
- **Neutra-Phos** *see* Potassium Phosphate and Sodium Phosphate *on page 1691*
- **Neutra-Phos®-K [OTC] [DSC]** *see* Potassium Phosphate *on page 1690*
- **Nevanac** *see* Nepafenac *on page 1442*
- **Nevanac® (Can)** *see* Nepafenac *on page 1442*

Nevirapine (ne VYE ra peen)

Brand Names: U.S. Viramune; Viramune XR

Brand Names: Canada Auro-Nevirapine; Mylan-Nevirapine; Teva-Nevirapine; Viramune XR®; Viramune®

Index Terms NVP

Pharmacologic Category Antiretroviral, Reverse Transcriptase Inhibitor, Non-nucleoside (Anti-HIV)

Use In combination therapy with other antiretroviral agents for the treatment of HIV-1

Pregnancy Risk Factor B

Pregnancy Considerations Teratogenic effects were not observed in animal reproduction studies. Nevirapine crosses the placenta. No increased risk of overall birth defects has been observed following first trimester exposure according to data collected by the antiretroviral pregnancy registry. Pharmacokinetics are not altered during pregnancy and dose adjustment is not needed. The DHHS Perinatal HIV Guidelines recommend nevirapine as the preferred NNRTI for use during pregnancy. Nevirapine may be initiated in pregnant women with a $CD4^+$ lymphocyte count <250/mm^3 or continued in women who are virologically suppressed and tolerating therapy once pregnancy is detected (regardless of $CD4^+$ lymphocyte count); however, **do not** initiate therapy in pregnant women with a $CD4^+$ lymphocyte count >250/mm^3 unless the benefit of therapy clearly outweighs the risk. Elevated transaminase concentrations at baseline may increase the risk of toxicity; the monitoring recommendation for transaminase levels is generally the same as in nonpregnant women. Hypersensitivity reactions (including hepatic toxicity and rash) are more common in women on NNRTI.

Regardless of CD4 count or HIV RNA copy number, all HIV-infected pregnant women should receive a combination antepartum antiretroviral (ARV) drug regimen; this includes women who require therapy for their own health, as well as women who do not yet require therapy for their own health. ARV therapy should be started as soon as possible if required for the woman's health. Although earlier initiation may be more effective in reducing the perinatal transmission of HIV), also consider maternal conditions (eg, nausea and vomiting) and the potential risks of first trimester fetal exposure for specific agents. Plasma HIV RNA levels should be assessed at ~34-36 weeks gestation in order to help determine mode of delivery. If ARV therapy must be interrupted for <24 hours during the peripartum period, stop then restart all medications simultaneously in order to decrease the chance of developing resistance. Long-term follow-up is recommended for all infants exposed to ARV medications.

Healthcare providers are encouraged to enroll pregnant women exposed to antiretroviral medications in the Antiretroviral Pregnancy Registry (1-800-258-4263 or www.-APRegistry.com). Healthcare providers caring for HIV-infected women and their infants may contact the National Perinatal HIV Hotline (888-448-8765) for clinical consultation (DHHS [perinatal], 2012).

Breast-Feeding Considerations Although breast-feeding is not recommended, nevirapine is excreted into breast milk and measurable in the serum of nursing infants. Maternal or infant antiretroviral therapy does not completely eliminate the risk of postnatal HIV transmission. In addition, multiclass resistant virus has been detected in breast-feeding infants despite maternal therapy. Therefore, in the United States, where formula is accessible, affordable, safe, and sustainable, and the risk of infant mortality due to diarrhea and respiratory infections is low, complete avoidance of breast-feeding by HIV-infected women is recommended to decrease potential transmission of HIV (DHHS [perinatal], 2012).

Medication Guide Available Yes

Contraindications Moderate-to-severe hepatic impairment (Child-Pugh class B or C); use in occupational or nonoccupational postexposure prophylaxis (PEP) regimens

Canadian labeling: Additional contraindications (not in U.S. labeling): Clinically significant hypersensitivity to nevirapine or any component of the formulation; therapy rechallenge in patients with prior hypersensitivity reactions, severe rash, rash accompanied by constitutional symptoms, or clinical hepatitis due to nevirapine; severe hepatic dysfunction or AST or ALT >5 times ULN (pretreatment or during prior use of nevirapine); hereditary conditions of galactose intolerance (eg, galactosemia, Lapp lactase deficiency, glucose-galactose malabsorption); concomitant use of herbal products containing St John's wort

Warnings/Precautions [U.S. Boxed Warning]: Severe hepatotoxic reactions may occur (fulminant and cholestatic hepatitis, hepatic necrosis) and, in some cases, have resulted in hepatic failure and death. The greatest risk of these reactions is within the initial 6 weeks of treatment. Patients with a history of chronic hepatitis (B or C) or increased baseline transaminase levels may be at increased risk of hepatotoxic reactions. Female gender and patients with increased $CD4^+$-cell counts may be at substantially greater risk of hepatic events (often associated with rash). Therapy in antiretroviral naive patients should not be started with elevated $CD4^+$-cell counts unless the benefit of therapy outweighs the risk of serious hepatotoxicity (adult/postpubertal females: $CD4^+$-cell counts >250 cells/mm^3; adult males: $CD4^+$-cell counts >400 cells/mm^3). Use with caution in patients with preexisting dysfunction; monitor closely for drug-induced hepatotoxicity. U.S. labeling contraindicates use in patients with moderate-to-severe impairment (Child-Pugh class B or C). Canadian labeling contraindicates use in severe impairment.

[U.S. Boxed Warning]: Severe life-threatening skin reactions (eg, Stevens-Johnson syndrome, toxic epidermal necrolysis, hypersensitivity reactions with rash and organ dysfunction), including fatal cases, have occurred. The greatest risk of these reactions is within the initial 6 weeks of treatment; intensive monitoring is required during the initial 18 weeks of therapy to detect potentially life-threatening dermatologic, hypersensitivity, and hepatic reactions. Risk is greatest in African-Americans, Asian, or Hispanic race/ethnicity or in females. A 14-day lead-in dosing period with immediate release formulation must be initiated to decrease the incidence of adverse effects. The lead-in dosing can be extended up to 28 days if necessary, but an alternative regimen is necessary if >28 days is required. If a severe dermatologic or hypersensitivity reaction occurs, or if signs and symptoms of hepatitis occur, nevirapine should be permanently discontinued. These events may include a severe rash, or a rash associated with fever, blisters, oral lesions, conjunctivitis, facial edema, muscle or joint aches, transaminase elevations, general malaise, hepatitis, eosinophilia, granulocytopenia, lymphadenopathy, or renal dysfunction. Coadministration of prednisone during the first 6 weeks of therapy increases incidence and severity of rash; concomitant prednisone is not recommended to prevent rash.

May cause redistribution of fat (eg, buffalo hump, peripheral wasting with increased abdominal girth, cushingoid appearance). Patients may develop immune reconstitution syndrome resulting in the occurrence of an inflammatory response to an indolent or residual opportunistic infection during initial HIV treatment or activation of autoimmune disorders (eg, Graves' disease, polymyositis, Guillain-Barré syndrome) later in therapy; further evaluation and treatment may be required. Rhabdomyolysis has been observed in conjunction with skin and/or hepatic adverse events during postmarketing surveillance. Termination of therapy is warranted with evidence of severe skin or liver toxicity.

Use with caution in patients taking strong CYP3A4 inhibitors, moderate or strong CYP3A4 inducers and major CYP3A4 substrates (see Drug Interactions); consider alternative agents that avoid or lessen the potential for CYP-mediated interactions. Concurrent use of St John's wort or efavirenz is not recommended; may decrease the therapeutic efficacy (St John's wort) or increase adverse effects (efavirenz). Canadian labeling contraindicates concurrent use with products containing St John's wort.

Nevirapine-based initial regimens should not be used in children <3 years of age if previously exposed to nevirapine during prevention of maternal-to-child transmission of HIV due to increased risk of resistance and treatment failure. Protease inhibitor-based initial regimens preferred in this population.

Due to rapid emergence of resistance, nevirapine should not be used as monotherapy or the only agent added to a failing regimen for the treatment of HIV. Consider alteration of antiretroviral therapies if disease progression occurs while patients are receiving nevirapine. Use care when timing discontinuation of regimens containing nevirapine; levels are sustained after levels of other medications decrease, leading to nevirapine resistance. Cross-resistance may be conferred to other non-nucleoside reverse transcriptase inhibitors (DHHS, 2012).

Adverse Reactions Note: Potentially life-threatening nevirapine-associated adverse effects may present with the following symptoms: Abrupt onset of flu-like symptoms, abdominal pain, jaundice, or fever with or without rash; may progress to hepatic failure with encephalopathy. Skin rash is present in ~50% of cases.

>10%:

- Dermatologic: Rash (1% to 7%; grade 1/2: 13%; grade 3/4: 2%)
- Endocrine & metabolic: Cholesterol increased (240-300 mg/dL: 18% to 19%; >300 mg/dL: 3% to 4%), LDL increased (160-190 mg/dL: 15%; >190 mg/dL: 5%)
- Hematologic: Neutropenia (4% to 13%; grades 3/4: 1% to 2%)
- Hepatic: ALT increased (2.6-5 x ULN: 10% to 13%; ≥5.1 x ULN: 6% to 7%), symptomatic hepatic events (including hepatitis and hepatic failure: 2% to 11%; risk higher in ARV-naive women with CD4 counts >250 cells/mm^3 and ARV-naive men with CD4 counts >400 cells/mm^3)

1% to 10%:

Central nervous system: Fatigue (≤5%), headache (1% to 4%), fever (1% to 2%)

Gastrointestinal: Nausea (<1% to 9%), amylase increased (1.6-5 x ULN: 7% to 8%; ≥5.1 x ULN: <1%), abdominal pain (≤2%), diarrhea (≤2%)

Hepatic: AST increased (≥5.1 x ULN: 4% to 5%)

Neuromuscular & skeletal: Arthralgia (2%)

<1% (Limited to important or life-threatening): Allergic reactions, anaphylaxis, anemia, angioedema, bullous eruptions, cholestatic hepatitis, conjunctivitis, eosinophilia, fulminant hepatitis, granulocytopenia, hepatic necrosis, hypersensitivity syndrome, hypophosphatemia, immune reconstitution syndrome, jaundice, lymphadenopathy, oral lesions, redistribution/accumulation of body fat, renal dysfunction, rhabdomyolysis, Stevens-Johnson syndrome, toxic epidermal necrolysis, ulcerative stomatitis

Drug Interactions

Metabolism/Transport Effects Substrate of CYP2B6 (minor), CYP2D6 (minor), CYP3A4 (major); **Note:** Assignment of Major/Minor substrate status based on clinically relevant drug interaction potential; **Inhibits** CYP1A2 (weak), CYP2D6 (weak), CYP3A4 (weak); **Induces** CYP2B6 (strong), CYP3A4 (strong)

Avoid Concomitant Use

Avoid concomitant use of Nevirapine with any of the following: Abiraterone Acetate; Apixaban; Artemether; Atazanavir; Axitinib; Bedaquiline; Boceprevir; Bortezomib; Bosutinib; Cabozantinib; CarBAMazepine; CloZAPine; Crizotinib; Dienogest; Dolutegravir; Dronedarone; Efavirenz; Enzalutamide; Etravirine; Everolimus; Ibrutinib; Itraconazole; Ivacaftor; Ketoconazole (Systemic); Lapatinib; Lumefantrine; Lurasidone; Macitentan; Mifepristone; NIFEdipine; Nilotinib; Nisoldipine; PAZOPanib; Perampanel; Pimozide; Pomalidomide; PONATinib; Praziquantel; Ranolazine; Regorafenib; Rilpivirine; Rivaroxaban; Roflumilast; RomiDEPsin; Simeprevir; SORAfenib; St Johns Wort; Telaprevir; Ticagrelor; Tofacitinib; Tolvaptan; Toremifene; Ulipristal; Vandetanib; Vemurafenib; VinCRIStine (Liposomal)

Increased Effect/Toxicity

Nevirapine may increase the levels/effects of: ARIPiprazole; Clarithromycin; Dofetilide; Efavirenz; Etravirine; Ifosfamide; Lomitapide; Pimozide; Rifabutin; Rilpivirine

The levels/effects of Nevirapine may be increased by: Atazanavir; Clarithromycin; Efavirenz; Fluconazole; Voriconazole

Decreased Effect

Nevirapine may decrease the levels/effects of: Abiraterone Acetate; Apixaban; ARIPiprazole; Artemether; Atazanavir; Axitinib; Bedaquiline; Boceprevir; Bortezomib; Bosutinib; Brentuximab Vedotin; Cabozantinib; CarBAMazepine; Caspofungin; Clarithromycin; CloZAPine; Contraceptives (Estrogens); Contraceptives (Progestins); Crizotinib; CYP2B6 Substrates; CYP3A4 Substrates; Dasatinib; Dienogest; Dolutegravir; Dronedarone; Efavirenz; Enzalutamide; Etravirine; Everolimus; Exemestane; Fosamprenavir; Gefitinib; GuanFACINE; Ibrutinib; Imatinib; Indinavir; Itraconazole; Ivacaftor; Ixabepilone; Ketoconazole (Systemic); Lapatinib; Linagliptin; Lopinavir; Lumefantrine; Lurasidone; Macitentan; Maraviroc; Methadone; Mifepristone; Nelfinavir; NIFEdipine; Nilotinib; Nisoldipine; PAZOPanib; Perampanel; Pomalidomide; PONATinib; Praziquantel; QUEtiapine; Ranolazine; Regorafenib; Rifabutin; Rilpivirine; Rivaroxaban; Roflumilast; RomiDEPsin; Saquinavir; Saxagliptin; Simeprevir; SORAfenib; SUNItinib; Tadalafil; Telaprevir; Ticagrelor; Tofacitinib; Tolvaptan; Toremifene; Ulipristal; Vandetanib; Vemurafenib; VinCRIStine (Liposomal); Voriconazole; Vortioxetine; Zuclopenthixol

The levels/effects of Nevirapine may be decreased by: Bosentan; CarBAMazepine; CYP3A4 Inducers (Strong); Dabrafenib; Deferasirox; Mitotane; Peginterferon Alfa-2b; Rifabutin; Rifampin; St Johns Wort; Tocilizumab

Ethanol/Nutrition/Herb Interactions Herb/Nutraceutical: Nevirapine serum concentration may be decreased by St John's wort; avoid concurrent use.

Storage/Stability Store at 25°C (77°F); excursion permitted to 15°C to 30°C (59°F to 86°F).

Mechanism of Action As a non-nucleoside reverse transcriptase inhibitor, nevirapine has activity against HIV-1 by binding to reverse transcriptase. It consequently blocks the RNA-dependent and DNA-dependent DNA polymerase activities including HIV-1 replication. It does not require intracellular phosphorylation for antiviral activity.

Pharmacodynamics/Kinetics

Absorption: >90%

Distribution: Widely; V_d: 1.2 L/kg; CSF penetration approximates 40% to 50% of plasma

Protein binding, plasma: ~60%

Metabolism: Extensively hepatic via CYP3A4 and CYP2B6 (hydroxylation to inactive compounds); may undergo enterohepatic recycling

Bioavailability: 93% (immediate release tablet); ~75% (extended release tablet [relative to immediate release]); 91% (oral solution)

Half-life elimination: Decreases over 2- to 4-week time with chronic dosing due to autoinduction (ie, half-life = 45 hours initially and decreases to 25-30 hours)

Time to peak, serum: Immediate release: 4 hours; Extended release: ~24 hours

Excretion: Urine (~81%, primarily as metabolites, <3% as unchanged drug); feces (~10%)

Dosage Oral:

HIV infection:

Note: If patient experiences a rash during the 14-day lead-in period, dose should not be increased until the rash has resolved. A lead-in period must always be done with immediate release formulation and regimen should not exceed 28 days; alternative treatment should be considered at that point. If a rash occurs within the first 18 weeks of therapy, immediately check serum transaminases. Discontinue if severe rash, rash with constitutional symptoms, or rash with elevated hepatic transaminases is noted. Coadministration of prednisone during the first 6 weeks of therapy increases incidence and severity of rash; concomitant prednisone is not recommended to prevent rash. Permanently discontinue if symptomatic hepatic events occur. If therapy with any formulation is interrupted for >7 days, restart with initial dose of immediate release formulation for 14 days. Use of nevirapine in children <15 years of age is not approved in the Canadian labeling.

Infants and Children: *Immediate release:* 150 mg/m²/dose once daily for first 14 days (maximum: 200 mg daily); increase dose to 150 mg/m²/dose twice daily if no rash or untoward effects (maximum: 400 mg daily).

Children 6 to <18 years: *Extended release:* Dose based on body surface area (Mosteller formula); maintenance therapy using the extended release must follow a 14-day initial dosing period (lead-in) using the immediate release formulation unless patient is already maintained on a nevirapine immediate release regimen.

0.58 m^2 to 0.83 m^2: 200 mg once daily

0.84 m^2 to 1.16 m^2: 300 mg once daily

≥1.17 m^2: 400 mg once daily (do not exceed 400 mg daily)

DHHS pediatric guidelines:

Note: Children <3 years of age: Nevirapine-based initial regimens should not be used in children previously exposed to nevirapine during prevention of maternal-to-child transmission of HIV

Children <8 years: *Immediate release:* 200 mg/m^2/dose once daily for first 14 days (maximum dose: 200 mg); increase dose to 200 mg/m^2/dose twice daily if no rash or untoward effects (maximum: 400 mg daily)

Children ≥8 years: *Immediate release:* 120-150 mg/m^2/dose once daily for 14 days (maximum dose: 200 mg); increase dose to 120-150 mg/m^2/dose twice daily if no rash or untoward effects (maximum: 400 mg daily)

Adolescents and Adults: **Note:** Therapy should not be initiated in patients with elevated CD4$^+$-cell counts unless the benefit of therapy outweighs the risk of serious hepatotoxicity (adult/post-pubertal females: CD4$^+$-cell counts >250 cells/mm^3; adult males: CD4$^+$-cell counts >400 cells/mm^3)

Immediate release:

Initial: 200 mg once daily for first 14 days

Maintenance: 200 mg twice daily (in combination with additional antiretroviral agents) if there is no rash or untoward effects during initial dosing period

Adults: *Extended release:* Maintenance: 400 mg once daily; maintenance therapy using the extended release must follow a 14-day initial dosing period (lead-in) using the immediate release formulation unless patient is already maintained on a nevirapine immediate release regimen.

Prevention of maternal-fetal HIV transmission (DHHS [perinatal], 2012): Note: Nevirapine is used in combination with zidovudine in select situations (eg, infants born to mothers with only intrapartum therapy or no therapy). Use is not recommended in women receiving standard recommended antenatal antiretroviral prophylaxis.

Dosage adjustment in renal impairment:

Immediate release:

Cl_{cr} ≥20 mL/minute: No dosage adjustment necessary.

Cl_{cr} <20 mL/minute: No dosage adjustment provided in manufacturer's labeling (has not been studied).

Extended release: No dosage adjustment provided in manufacturer's labeling (has not been studied).

Hemodialysis: An additional 200 mg *immediate release* dose is recommended following dialysis.

Dosage adjustment in hepatic impairment: Permanently discontinue if symptomatic hepatic events occur.

U.S. labeling:

Mild impairment (Child-Pugh class A):

Immediate release: No dosage adjustment provided in manufacturer's labeling; use with caution.

Extended release: Not studied.

Moderate-to-severe impairment (Child-Pugh class B or C): Use is contraindicated.

Canadian labeling:

Mild impairment (Child-Pugh class A): No dosage adjustment is necessary.

Moderate impairment (Child-Pugh class B): No dosage adjustment provided in manufacturer's labeling. Use with caution.

Severe impairment (Child-Pugh class C): Use is contraindicated.

Administration Oral: May be administered with or without food; may be administered with an antacid or didanosine. Shake suspension gently prior to administration; the use of an oral dosing syringe is recommended, especially if the dose is ≤5 mL; if using a dosing cup, after administration, rinse cup with water and also administer rinse. Extended release tablets must be swallowed whole and not crushed, chewed, or divided.

Monitoring Parameters Monitor CBC and viral load. Baseline liver function tests should be obtained prior to nevirapine's initiation. DHHS adult guidelines recommend serum transaminase monitoring every 2 weeks for the first 4 weeks of therapy, monthly for the first 18 weeks, then frequently thereafter. Patients receiving maintenance immediate release nevirapine who change to the extended release formulation should adhere to their regular monitoring schedule. DHHS adult guidelines recommend serum transaminase monitoring every 2 weeks for the first 4 weeks of therapy, then monthly for 3 months, followed by every 3-4 months. DHHS pediatric guidelines recommend serum transaminase monitoring every 2 weeks for the first 4 weeks of therapy, followed by every 4 months. Assess/evaluate AST/ALT immediately in any patients with a rash. Permanently discontinue if patient experiences severe rash, constitutional symptoms associated with rash, rash with elevated AST/ALT, or clinical hepatitis. Mild-to-moderate rash without AST/ALT elevation may continue treatment per discretion of prescriber. If mild-to-moderate urticarial rash, do not restart if treatment is interrupted.

Additional Information Patients should never be taking more than one form (ie, immediate release or extended release) of nevirapine concomitantly. Potential compliance problems, frequency of administration, and adverse effects should be discussed with patients before initiating therapy to help prevent the emergence of resistance. Early virologic failure was observed with tenofovir and didanosine delayed release capsules, plus either efavirenz or nevirapine; use caution in treatment-naive patients with high baseline viral loads. Due to rapid emergence of resistance, nevirapine should not be used as monotherapy or as the only agent added to a failing regimen for the treatment of HIV. Use care when timing discontinuation of regimens containing nevirapine; levels of nevirapine are sustained after levels of other medications decrease, potentially leading to nevirapine resistance. Cross-resistance may be conferred to other non-nucleoside reverse transcriptase inhibitors.

Dosage Forms Excipient information presented when available (limited, particularly for generics); consult specific product labeling.

Suspension, Oral:

Viramune: 50 mg/5 mL (240 mL) [contains methylparaben, propylparaben]

Generic: 50 mg/5 mL (240 mL)

Tablet, Oral:

Viramune: 200 mg [scored]

Generic: 200 mg

Tablet Extended Release 24 Hour, Oral:

Viramune XR: 100 mg, 400 mg

◆ New-Fill® *see* Poly-L-Lactic Acid *on page 1671*
◆ Nexafed [OTC] *see* Pseudoephedrine *on page 1746*
◆ NexAVAR *see* SORAfenib *on page 1938*
◆ Nexavar (Can) *see* SORAfenib *on page 1938*
◆ NexIUM *see* Esomeprazole *on page 750*
◆ Nexium (Can) *see* Esomeprazole *on page 750*
◆ NexIUM I.V. *see* Esomeprazole *on page 750*
◆ Next Choice [DSC] *see* Levonorgestrel *on page 1202*
◆ Next Choice (Can) *see* Levonorgestrel *on page 1202*
◆ Next Choice One Dose *see* Levonorgestrel *on page 1202*
◆ Nexterone *see* Amiodarone *on page 101*
◆ NFV *see* Nelfinavir *on page 1436*

Niacin (NYE a sin)

Brand Names: U.S. Niacin-50 [OTC]; Niacor; Niaspan; Slo-Niacin [OTC]

Brand Names: Canada Niaspan; Niaspan FCT; Niodan

Index Terms Nicotinic Acid; Vitamin B_3

Pharmacologic Category Antilipemic Agent, Miscellaneous; Vitamin, Water Soluble

Use Treatment of dyslipidemias (Fredrickson types IIa and IIb or primary hypercholesterolemia) as mono- or adjunctive therapy; to lower the risk of recurrent MI in patients with a history of MI and hyperlipidemia; to slow progression or promote regression of coronary artery disease; treatment of hypertriglyceridemia in patients at risk of pancreatitis; dietary supplement

Unlabeled Use Treatment of pellagra

Pregnancy Risk Factor C

Pregnancy Considerations Animal reproduction studies have not been conducted. Water soluble vitamins cross the placenta. When used as a dietary supplement, niacin requirements may be increased in pregnant women compared to nonpregnant women (IOM, 1998). It is not known if niacin at lipid-lowering doses is harmful to the developing fetus. If a woman becomes pregnant while receiving niacin for primary hypercholesterolemia, niacin should be discontinued. If a woman becomes pregnant while receiving niacin for hypertriglyceridemia, the benefits and risks of continuing niacin should be assessed on an individual basis.

Breast-Feeding Considerations Niacin is excreted in human breast milk. When used as a dietary supplement, niacin requirements may be increased in nursing women compared to non-nursing women (IOM, 1998). Because lipid-lowering doses of niacin may cause serious adverse reactions in nursing infants, a decision should be made whether to discontinue nursing or discontinue the drug, taking into account the importance of the drug to the mother.

Contraindications Hypersensitivity to niacin, niacinamide, or any component of the formulation; active hepatic disease or significant or unexplained persistent elevations in hepatic transaminases; active peptic ulcer; arterial hemorrhage

Warnings/Precautions Prior to initiation, secondary causes for hypercholesterolemia (eg, poorly controlled diabetes mellitus, hypothyroidism) should be excluded; management with diet and other nonpharmacologic measures (eg, exercise or weight reduction) should be attempted prior to initiation. Use has not been evaluated in Fredrickson type I or III dyslipidemias. Use with caution in patients with unstable angina or MI, renal disease, active gallbladder disease (can exacerbate), or with anticoagulants (may slightly increase prothrombin time). In patients with pre-existing coronary artery disease, the incidence of atrial fibrillation was observed more frequently in those receiving immediate release (crystalline) niacin as compared to placebo (Coronary Drug Project Research Group, 1975). Niacin should not be used if patient experiences new-onset atrial fibrillation during therapy (Stone, 2013). Use with caution in patients with diabetes (may interfere with glucose control); niacin should not be used if patient experiences persistent hyperglycemia during therapy (Stone, 2013). Use with caution in patients with gout; niacin should not be used if patient experiences acute gout during therapy (Stone, 2013).

Use with caution in patients with a past history of hepatic impairment and/or who consume substantial amounts of ethanol; contraindicated with active liver disease or unexplained persistent transaminase elevation. Niacin should not be used if hepatic transaminase elevations >2-3 times upper limit of normal occur during therapy (Stone, 2013). Rare cases of rhabdomyolysis have occurred during concomitant use with HMG-CoA reductase inhibitors. With concurrent use or if symptoms suggestive of myopathy occur, monitor creatine phosphokinase (CPK) and potassium; use with caution in patients with renal impairment, inadequately treated hypothyroidism, patients with diabetes or the elderly; risk for myopathy and rhabdomyolysis may be increased. May cause gastrointestinal distress, vomiting, diarrhea, or aggravate peptic ulcer. Use is contraindicated in patients with active peptic ulcer disease. Niacin should not be used if patient experiences unexplained abdominal pain or gastrointestinal symptoms or unexplained weight loss during therapy (Stone, 2013).

Immediate and extended or sustained release products are not interchangeable. Cases of severe hepatotoxicity have occurred when immediate release (crystalline) niacin products have been substituted with sustained-release (modified release, timed-release) niacin products at equivalent doses. Patients should be initiated with low doses (eg, 500 mg at bedtime) with titration to achieve desired response. Flushing and pruritus, common adverse effects of niacin, may be attenuated with a gradual increase in dose, and/or by taking aspirin (adults: 325 mg) or an NSAID 30 minutes before dosing (Stone, 2013). May also use other NSAIDs according to the manufacturer. Flushing associated with extended-release preparation is significantly reduced (Guyton, 2007). Compliance is enhanced with twice-daily dosing (extended-release product excluded). Niacin should not be used if patient experiences persistent severe cutaneous symptoms during therapy (Stone, 2013).

Adverse Reactions Frequency not defined.

Cardiovascular: Arrhythmias, atrial fibrillation, edema, flushing, hypotension, orthostasis, palpitation, syncope (rare), tachycardia

Central nervous system: Chills, dizziness, headache, insomnia, migraine, nervousness, pain

Dermatologic: Acanthosis nigricans, burning skin, dry skin, hyperpigmentation, maculopapular rash, pruritus, rash, skin discoloration, urticaria

Endocrine & metabolic: Glucose tolerance decreased, gout, phosphorous levels decreased, hyperuricemia

Gastrointestinal: Abdominal pain, amylase increased, diarrhea, dyspepsia, eructation, flatulence, nausea, peptic ulcers, vomiting

Hematologic: Platelet counts decreased

Hepatic: Hepatic necrosis (rare), hepatitis, jaundice, transaminases increased (dose-related), prothrombin time increased, total bilirubin increased

Neuromuscular & skeletal: CPK increased, leg cramps, myalgia, myasthenia, myopathy (with concurrent HMG-CoA reductase inhibitor), paresthesia, rhabdomyolysis (with concurrent HMG-CoA reductase inhibitor; rare), weakness

Ocular: Blurred vision, cystoid macular edema, toxic amblyopia

Respiratory: Cough, dyspnea

Miscellaneous: Diaphoresis, hypersensitivity reactions (rare; includes anaphylaxis, angioedema, laryngismus, vesiculobullous rash), LDH increased

Drug Interactions

Metabolism/Transport Effects None known.

Avoid Concomitant Use There are no known interactions where it is recommended to avoid concomitant use.

Increased Effect/Toxicity

Niacin may increase the levels/effects of: HMG-CoA Reductase Inhibitors

The levels/effects of Niacin may be increased by: Alcohol (Ethyl)

Decreased Effect

The levels/effects of Niacin may be decreased by: Bile Acid Sequestrants

Ethanol/Nutrition/Herb Interactions Ethanol: Avoid heavy use; avoid use around niacin dose.

Storage/Stability

Niaspan: Store at room temperature of 20°C to 25°C (68°F to 77°F).

Niacor: Store at controlled room temperature of 15°C to 30°C (59°F to 86°F).

Mechanism of Action Niacin (nicotinic acid) is bioconverted to nicotinamide which is further converted to nicotinamide adenine dinucleotide (NAD+) and the hydride equivalent (NADH) which are coenzymes necessary for tissue metabolism, lipid metabolism, and glycogenolysis (Belenky, 2006; Suave, 2008). The mechanism by which niacin (in gram doses) affects plasma lipoproteins is not fully understood. It may involve several actions including partial inhibition of release of free fatty acids from adipose tissue, and increased lipoprotein lipase activity, which may increase the rate of chylomicron triglyceride removal from plasma. Ultimately, niacin reduces total cholesterol, apolipoprotein (apo) B, triglycerides, VLDL, LDL, lipoprotein (a), and increases HDL and other important components and subfractions (eg, LPA-I) (Kamanna, 2000)

Pharmacodynamics/Kinetics

Absorption: Rapid and extensive (60% to 76%)

Distribution: Mainly to hepatic, renal, and adipose tissue

Metabolism: Extensive first-pass effects; converted to nicotinamide adenine dinucleotide, nicotinuric acid, and other metabolites

Half-life elimination: 20-45 minutes

Time to peak, serum: Immediate release formulation: 30-60 minutes; extended release formulation: 4-5 hours

Excretion: Urine 60% to 88% (unchanged drug [up to 12% recovered after multiple dosing] and metabolites)

Dosage Oral: **Note:** Formulations of niacin (regular release versus extended release) are not interchangeable.

Children:

Pellagra (unlabeled use): 50-100 mg/dose 3 times daily (some experts prefer niacinamide for treatment due to more favorable side effect profile)

Adequate intake (National Academy of Sciences, 1998):

0-5 months: 2 mg daily

6-11 months: 3 mg daily

Recommended daily allowances (National Academy of Sciences, 1998):

1-3 years: 6 mg daily

4-8 years: 8 mg daily

9-13 years: 12 mg daily

14-18 years: Females: 14 mg daily; Males: 16 mg daily

≥19 years: Refer to adult dosing

Adults:

Recommended daily allowances (National Academy of Sciences, 1998):

≥19 years: Females: 14 mg daily; Males: 16 mg daily

Pregnancy (all ages): 18 mg daily

Lactation (all ages): 17 mg daily

Dietary supplement (OTC labeling): 50 mg twice daily or 100 mg once daily. **Note:** Many over-the-counter formulations exist.

Hyperlipidemia:

Regular release formulation (Niacor): Initial: 250 mg once daily (with evening meal); increase frequency and/or dose every 4-7 days to desired response or first-level therapeutic dose (1.5-2 g daily in 2-3 divided doses); after 2 months, may increase at 2- to 4-week intervals to 3 g daily in 3 divided doses (maximum dose: 6 g daily in 3 divided doses). **Note:** Many over-the-counter formulations exist.

ACC/AHA Blood Cholesterol Guideline recommendations: Initial: 100 mg administered 3 times daily; increase dose gradually as tolerated to 3 g daily divided in 2-3 doses (Stone, 2013)

Sustained release (or controlled release) formulations: **Note:** Several over-the-counter formulations exist. Slo-Niacin: Usual dosage is 250-750 mg once daily, taken morning or evening, or as directed. Before using more than 500 mg daily, patient should consult health care provider.

Extended release formulation (Niaspan): Initial: 500 mg at bedtime for 4 weeks, then 1 g at bedtime for 4 weeks; adjust dose to response and tolerance; may increase dose every 4 weeks by 500 mg daily to a maximum of 2 g daily.

If additional LDL-lowering is necessary with lovastatin or simvastatin: Recommended initial lovastatin or simvastatin dose: 20 mg daily (maximum lovastatin or simvastatin dose: 40 mg daily); **Note:** Lovastatin prescribing information recommends a maximum dose of 20 mg daily with concurrent use of niacin (>1 g daily).

ACC/AHA Blood Cholesterol Guideline recommendations: Initial: 500 mg once daily; increase dose gradually (ie, no sooner than at weekly intervals) over 4-8 weeks as tolerated to a maximum dose of 2 g once daily (Stone, 2013)

Pellagra (unlabeled use): 50-100 mg 3-4 times daily; maximum: 500 mg daily (some experts prefer niacinamide for treatment due to more favorable side effect profile)

Dosage adjustment in renal impairment: No dosage adjustment provided in manufacturer's labeling (has not been studied); use with caution.

Dosage adjustment in hepatic impairment: No dosage adjustment provided in manufacturer's labeling (has not been studied). However, contraindicated in patients with significant or unexplained hepatic dysfunction, active liver disease or unexplained persistent transaminase elevations.

Dosage adjustment for hepatic toxicity: Transaminases rise ≥3 times ULN, either persistent or if symptoms of nausea, fever, and/or malaise occur: Discontinue therapy.

Dietary Considerations Should be taken with meal; low-fat meal if treating hyperlipidemia. Avoid hot drinks around the time of niacin dose.

Administration Administer with food. To attenuate flushing symptoms, may premedicate with aspirin 325 mg administered 30 minutes before dose; avoid ingestion of hot liquids or alcohol concurrently with niacin (Stone, 2013). May also use other NSAIDs to prevent flushing according to the manufacturer.

Niaspan: Administer at bedtime. Tablet strengths are not interchangeable. When switching from immediate release tablet, initiate Niaspan at lower dose and titrate. If therapy is interrupted for an extended period, dose should be retitrated.

Long-acting forms should not be crushed, broken, or chewed. Slo-Niacin may be broken along the score line. Do not substitute long-acting forms for immediate release ones.

Monitoring Parameters

2013 ACC/AHA Blood Cholesterol Guideline recommendations (Stone, 2013): Baseline hepatic transaminases, fasting blood glucose or hemoglobin A1c, and uric acid before initiation and repeat during uptitration to maintenance dose and every 6 months thereafter.

Manufacturer recommendations: Blood glucose (in diabetic patients); if on concurrent HMG-CoA reductase inhibitor, may periodically check CPK and serum potassium; liver function tests pretreatment, every 6-12 weeks for first year, then periodically (approximately every 6 months), monitor liver function more frequently if history of transaminase elevation with prior use; lipid profile; platelets (if on anticoagulants); PT (if on anticoagulants); uric acid (if predisposed to gout); phosphorus (if predisposed to hypophosphatemia)

Test Interactions False elevations in some fluorometric determinations of plasma or urinary catecholamines; false-positive urine glucose (Benedict's reagent)

Dosage Forms Excipient information presented when available (limited, particularly for generics); consult specific product labeling.
Capsule Extended Release, Oral:
Generic: 250 mg, 500 mg
Capsule Extended Release, Oral [preservative free]:
Generic: 250 mg, 500 mg
Tablet, Oral:
Niacin-50: 50 mg [starch free, sugar free, wheat free]
Niacor: 500 mg [scored]
Generic: 50 mg, 100 mg, 250 mg, 500 mg
Tablet, Oral [preservative free]:
Generic: 50 mg, 100 mg, 500 mg
Tablet Extended Release, Oral:
Niaspan: 500 mg, 750 mg, 1000 mg [contains fd&c yellow #6 aluminum lake]
Slo-Niacin: 250 mg [scored]
Slo-Niacin: 500 mg, 750 mg [scored; contains fd&c red #40]
Generic: 500 mg, 750 mg, 1000 mg
Tablet Extended Release, Oral [preservative free]:
Generic: 250 mg, 500 mg, 1000 mg

◆ **Niacin-50 [OTC]** *see* Niacin *on page 1447*

Niacinamide (nye a SIN a mide)

Index Terms Nicomide-T; Nicotinamide; Nicotinic Acid Amide; Vitamin B_3
Pharmacologic Category Vitamin, Water Soluble
Use Dietary supplement
Unlabeled Use Prophylaxis and treatment of pellagra
Dosage Pellagra (unlabeled use): Oral:
Children: 10-50 mg every 6 hours until resolution of signs and symptoms (Hegyi, 2004)
Adults: 100 mg every 6 hours for several days (or until resolution of major signs and symptoms), followed by 50 mg every 8-12 hours until skin lesions heal (Hegyi, 2004)
Additional Information Complete prescribing information should be consulted for additional detail.
Dosage Forms Excipient information presented when available (limited, particularly for generics); consult specific product labeling.
Tablet, Oral:
Generic: 100 mg, 500 mg
Tablet, Oral [preservative free]:
Generic: 100 mg, 500 mg

Niacin and Lovastatin (NYE a sin & LOE va sta tin)

Brand Names: U.S. Advicor®
Brand Names: Canada Advicor®
Index Terms Lovastatin and Niacin
Pharmacologic Category Antilipemic Agent, HMG-CoA Reductase Inhibitor; Antilipemic Agent, Miscellaneous
Use For use when treatment with both extended-release niacin and lovastatin is appropriate in combination with a standard cholesterol-lowering diet:
Extended-release niacin: Adjunctive treatment of dyslipidemias (types IIa and IIb or primary hypercholesterolemia) to lower the risk of recurrent MI and/or slow progression of coronary artery disease, including combination therapy with other antidyslipidemic agents when additional triglyceride-lowering or HDL-increasing effects are desired; treatment of hypertriglyceridemia in patients at risk of pancreatitis
Lovastatin: Treatment of primary hypercholesterolemia (Frederickson types IIa and IIb); primary and secondary prevention of cardiovascular disease
Pregnancy Risk Factor X
Dosage Dosage forms are a fixed combination of niacin and lovastatin.
Oral: Adults: Lowest dose: Niacin 500 mg/lovastatin 20 mg; may increase by not more than 500 mg (niacin) at 4-week intervals (maximum dose: Niacin 2000 mg/lovastatin 40 mg daily); should be taken at bedtime with a low-fat snack. **Note:** If therapy is interrupted for >7 days, reinstitution of therapy should begin with the lowest dose followed by retitration as needed.
Not for use as initial therapy of dyslipidemias. May be substituted for equivalent dose of Niaspan®; however, manufacturer does not recommend direct substitution with other niacin products.
Dosage adjustment for lovastatin component with concomitant medications:
Amiodarone: Maximum recommended lovastatin dose: 40 mg daily
Danazol, diltiazem, dronedarone, or verapamil: Initial lovastatin dose: 10 mg daily (dosage unavailable with combination product; use separate components); Maximum recommended lovastatin dose: 20 mg daily
Dosage adjustment in renal impairment:
Mild-to-moderate impairment: No dosage adjustment required
Cl_{cr} <30 mL/minute: Use doses of lovastatin >20 mg daily with caution
Dosage adjustment in hepatic impairment: Do not use in active liver disease or unexplained persistent elevations of serum transaminases.
Additional Information Complete prescribing information should be consulted for additional detail.
Dosage Forms Excipient information presented when available (limited, particularly for generics); consult specific product labeling.
Tablet, variable release, oral (Advicor®):
500/20: Niacin 500 mg [extended release] and lovastatin 20 mg [immediate release]
750/20: Niacin 750 mg [extended release] and lovastatin 20 mg [immediate release]
1000/20: Niacin 1000 mg [extended release] and lovastatin 20 mg [immediate release]
1000/40: Niacin 1000 mg [extended release] and lovastatin 40 mg [immediate release]

◆ **Niacor** *see* Niacin *on page 1447*
◆ **Niaspan** *see* Niacin *on page 1447*
◆ **Niaspan FCT (Can)** *see* Niacin *on page 1447*
◆ **Niastase® (Can)** *see* Factor VIIa (Recombinant) *on page 821*
◆ **Niastase® RT (Can)** *see* Factor VIIa (Recombinant) *on page 821*

NiCARdipine (nye KAR de peen)

Brand Names: U.S. Cardene IV; Cardene SR
Index Terms Nicardipine Hydrochloride
Pharmacologic Category Antianginal Agent; Antihypertensive; Calcium Channel Blocker; Calcium Channel Blocker, Dihydropyridine
Additional Appendix Information
Calcium Channel Blockers – Comparative Pharmacokinetics *on page 2296*
Use Chronic stable angina (immediate-release product only); management of hypertension (immediate and sustained release products); parenteral only for short-term use when oral treatment is not feasible

Unlabeled Use Control of blood pressure in acute ischemic stroke and spontaneous intracranial hemorrhage, postoperative hypertension associated with carotid endarterectomy, perioperative hypertension, prevention of migraine headaches, subarachnoid hemorrhage associated cerebral vasospasm

Pregnancy Risk Factor C

Pregnancy Considerations Adverse events were observed in some animal reproduction studies. Nicardipine has been used for the treatment of severe hypertension in pregnancy and preterm labor. Nicardipine crosses the placenta; changes in fetal heart rate, neonatal hypotension and neonatal acidosis have been observed following maternal use (rare; based on limited data). Adverse effects reported in pregnant women are generally similar to those reported in nonpregnant patients; however, pulmonary edema has been observed (Nij, 2010). Untreated chronic maternal hypertension is also associated with adverse events in the fetus, infant, and mother. If treatment for hypertension during pregnancy is needed, other agents are preferred (ACOG, 2012; Chobanian, 2003).

Breast-Feeding Considerations Nicardipine is minimally excreted into breast milk. Per the manufacturer, the possibility of infant exposure should be considered. In one study, peak milk concentrations ranged from 1.9-18.8 mcg/mL following oral maternal doses of 40-150 mg/day. The estimated exposure to the breast-feeding infant was calculated to be 0.073% of the weight-adjusted maternal oral dose or 0.14% of the weight-adjusted maternal I.V. dose. Adverse events were not noted in the infants. Breast-fed infants of mothers taking medications for hypertension should be monitored for adverse effects (Chobanian, 2003).

Contraindications Hypersensitivity to nicardipine or any component of the formulation; advanced aortic stenosis

Warnings/Precautions Symptomatic hypotension with or without syncope can rarely occur; blood pressure must be lowered at a rate appropriate for the patient's clinical condition. Close monitoring of blood pressure and heart rate is required. Reflex tachycardia may occur resulting in angina and/or MI in patients with obstructive coronary disease especially in the absence of concurrent beta blockade. The most common side effect is peripheral edema (dose-dependent); occurs within 2-3 weeks of starting therapy. Use with caution in CAD (can cause increase in angina), HF (can worsen heart failure symptoms), aortic stenosis (may reduce coronary perfusion resulting in ischemia; use is contraindicated in patients with advanced aortic stenosis), and hypertrophic cardiomyopathy with outflow tract obstruction. To minimize infusion site reactions, peripheral infusion sites (for I.V. therapy) should be changed every 12 hours; use of small peripheral veins should be avoided. Titrate I.V. dose cautiously in patients with HF, renal or hepatic dysfunction. Use the I.V. form cautiously in patients with portal hypertension (can cause increase in hepatic pressure gradient). Initiate at the low end of the dosage range in the elderly.

Adverse Reactions

1% to 10%:

Cardiovascular: Cardiovascular: Flushing (6% to 10%), peripheral edema (dose related; 6% to 8%), hypotension (I.V. 6%), increased angina (dose related; 6%), palpitation (3% to 4%), tachycardia (1% to 4%), vasodilation (1% to 5%), chest pain (I.V. 1%), ECG abnormal (I.V. 1%), extrasystoles (I.V. 1%), hemopericardium (I.V. 1%), hypertension (I.V. 1%), orthostasis (1%), supraventricular tachycardia (I.V. 1%), syncope (1%), ventricular extrasystoles (I.V. 1%), ventricular tachycardia (I.V. 1%)

Central nervous system: Headache (6% to 15%), dizziness (1% to 7%), hypoesthesia (1%), intracranial hemorrhage (1%) pain (1%), somnolence (1%)

Dermatologic: Rash (1%)

Endocrine & metabolic: Hypokalemia (I.V. 1%)

Gastrointestinal: Nausea (2% to 5%), vomiting (I.V. 5%), dyspepsia (oral 2%), abdominal pain (I.V. 1%), dry mouth (1%)

Genitourinary: Polyuria (1%)

Local: Injection site pain (I.V. 1%), injection site reaction (I.V. 1%)

Neuromuscular & skeletal: Weakness (1% to 6%), myalgia (1%), paresthesia (1%)

Renal: Hematuria (1%)

Respiratory: Dyspnea (1%)

Miscellaneous: Diaphoresis (1%)

<1% (Limited to important or life-threatening): Allergic reaction, confusion, constipation, deep vein thrombophlebitis; ECG effects (AV block, inverted T wave, ST segment depression); gingival hyperplasia, hypertonia, hypophosphatemia, insomnia, malaise, nervousness, nocturia, parotitis, thrombocytopenia, tinnitus, tremor

Drug Interactions

Metabolism/Transport Effects Substrate of CYP1A2 (minor), CYP2C9 (minor), CYP2D6 (minor), CYP2E1 (minor), CYP3A4 (major), P-glycoprotein; **Note:** Assignment of Major/Minor substrate status based on clinically relevant drug interaction potential; **Inhibits** CYP2C19 (moderate), CYP2C9 (strong), CYP2D6 (moderate), CYP3A4 (strong), P-glycoprotein

Avoid Concomitant Use

Avoid concomitant use of NiCARdipine with any of the following: Ado-Trastuzumab Emtansine; Alfuzosin; Apixaban; Avanafil; Axitinib; Bosutinib; Cabozantinib; Conivaptan; Crizotinib; Dronedarone; Eplerenone; Everolimus; Fusidic Acid (Systemic); Halofantrine; Ibrutinib; Imatinib; Ivabradine; Lapatinib; Lomitapide; Lovastatin; Lurasidone; Macitentan; Nilotinib; Nisoldipine; Pimozide; Pomalidomide; Ranolazine; Red Yeast Rice; Regorafenib; Rivaroxaban; Salmeterol; Silodosin; Simeprevir; Simvastatin; Tamsulosin; Thioridazine; Ticagrelor; Tolvaptan; Topotecan; Toremifene; Ulipristal; Vemurafenib; VinCRIStine (Liposomal)

Increased Effect/Toxicity

NiCARdipine may increase the levels/effects of: Ado-Trastuzumab Emtansine; Afatinib; Alfuzosin; Almotriptan; Alosetron; Amifostine; Antihypertensives; Apixaban; ARIPiprazole; Atosiban; Avanafil; Axitinib; Bedaquiline; Beta-Blockers; Bortezomib; Bosentan; Bosutinib; Brentuximab Vedotin; Brinzolamide; Budesonide (Nasal); Budesonide (Systemic, Oral Inhalation); Cabozantinib; Calcium Channel Blockers (Nondihydropyridine); Carvedilol; Citalopram; Colchicine; Conivaptan; Corticosteroids (Orally Inhaled); Crizotinib; CYP2C19 Substrates; CYP2C9 Substrates; CYP2D6 Substrates; CYP3A4 Substrates; Dabigatran Etexilate; Diclofenac (Systemic); Dienogest; Dofetilide; Dronedarone; Dutasteride; Enzalutamide; Eplerenone; Everolimus; FentaNYL; Fesoterodine; Fluticasone (Nasal); Fluticasone (Oral Inhalation); Fosphenytoin; GuanFACINE; Halofantrine; Highest Risk QTc-Prolonging Agents; Hypotensive Agents; Ibrutinib; Iloperidone; Imatinib; Ivabradine; Ivacaftor; Ixabepilone; Lacosamide; Lapatinib; Levomilnacipran; Lomitapide; Lovastatin; Lumefantrine; Lurasidone; Macitentan; Magnesium Salts; Maraviroc; MethylPREDNISolone; Metoprolol; Mifepristone; Moderate Risk QTc-Prolonging Agents; Neuromuscular-Blocking Agents (Nondepolarizing); Nilotinib; Nisoldipine; Nitroprusside; Obinutuzumab; Ospemifene; OxyCODONE; Paricalcitol; PAZOPanib; P-glycoprotein/ABCB1 Substrates; Phenytoin; Pimecrolimus; Pimozide; Pomalidomide; PONATinib; Propafenone; Propranolol; Prucalopride; QUEtiapine; QuiNIDine; Ranolazine; Red Yeast Rice; Regorafenib; Repaglinide; Rilpivirine; RiTUXimab; Rivaroxaban; RomiDEPsin; Ruxolitinib; Salmeterol; Saxagliptin; Sildenafil; Silodosin; Simeprevir; Simvastatin; SORAfenib; Tacrolimus (Systemic); Tadalafil; Tamsulosin; Thioridazine;

Ticagrelor; Tofacitinib; Tolterodine; Tolvaptan; Topotecan; Toremifene; Ulipristal; Vardenafil; Vemurafenib; Vilazodone; VinCRIStine (Liposomal); Zuclopenthixol

The levels/effects of NiCARdipine may be increased by: Alpha1-Blockers; Antifungal Agents (Azole Derivatives, Systemic); Brimonidine (Topical); Calcium Channel Blockers (Nondihydropyridine); CycloSPORINE (Systemic); CYP3A4 Inhibitors (Moderate); CYP3A4 Inhibitors (Strong); Dasatinib; Diazoxide; Fluconazole; Fusidic Acid (Systemic); Grapefruit Juice; Herbs (Hypotensive Properties); Luliconazole; Macrolide Antibiotics; Magnesium Salts; MAO Inhibitors; Pentoxifylline; P-glycoprotein/ABCB1 Inhibitors; Prostacyclin Analogues; Protease Inhibitors; QuiNIDine

Decreased Effect

NiCARdipine may decrease the levels/effects of: Clopidogrel; Codeine; Ifosfamide; Prasugrel; QuiNIDine; Tamoxifen; Ticagrelor; TraMADol

The levels/effects of NiCARdipine may be decreased by: Barbiturates; Calcium Salts; CarBAMazepine; CYP3A4 Inducers (Strong); Dabrafenib; Deferasirox; Herbs (CYP3A4 Inducers); Herbs (Hypertensive Properties); Melatonin; Methylphenidate; Mitotane; Nafcillin; Peginterferon Alfa-2b; P-glycoprotein/ABCB1 Inducers; Rifamycin Derivatives; Tocilizumab; Yohimbine

Ethanol/Nutrition/Herb Interactions

Ethanol: Ethanol may increase CNS depression. Management: Avoid ethanol.

Food: Nicardipine average peak concentrations may be decreased if taken with food. Serum concentrations/toxicity of nicardipine may be increased by grapefruit juice. Management: Avoid grapefruit juice.

Herb/Nutraceutical: St John's wort may decrease levels. Some herbal medications may worsen hypertension (eg, licorice); others may increase the antihypertensive effect of nicardipine (eg, shepherd's purse). Management: Avoid St John's wort. Avoid bayberry, blue cohosh, cayenne, ephedra, ginger, ginseng (American), kola, licorice, and yohimbe. Avoid black cohosh, California poppy, coleus, golden seal, hawthorn, mistletoe, periwinkle, quinine, and shepherd's purse.

Preparation for Administration I.V.: Vial: Dilute 25 mg vial with 240 mL of compatible solution to provide a 250 mL total volume solution and a final concentration of 0.1 mg/mL.

Storage/Stability

I.V.:

Premixed bags: Store at controlled room temperature of 20°C to 25°C (68°F to 77°F). Protect from light and excessive heat. Do not freeze.

Vials: Store at controlled room temperature of 20°C to 25°C (68°F to 77°F). Protect from light. Diluted solution (0.1 mg/mL) is stable at room temperature for 24 hours in glass or PVC containers. Stability has also been demonstrated at room temperature at concentrations up to 0.5 mg/mL in PVC containers for 24 hours or in glass containers for up to 7 days (Baaske, 1996).

Oral (Cardene®, Cardene SR®): Store at 15°C to 30°C (59°F to 86°F). Protect from light. Freezing does not affect stability.

Mechanism of Action Inhibits calcium ion from entering the "slow channels" or select voltage-sensitive areas of vascular smooth muscle and myocardium during depolarization, producing a relaxation of coronary vascular smooth muscle and coronary vasodilation; increases myocardial oxygen delivery in patients with vasospastic angina

Pharmacodynamics/Kinetics

Onset of action: Oral: 0.5-2 hours; I.V.: 10 minutes; Hypotension: ~20 minutes

Duration:

I.V.: ≤8 hours

Oral: Immediate release capsules: ≤8 hours; Sustained release capsules: 8-12 hours

Absorption: Oral: ~100%

Protein binding: >95%

Metabolism: Hepatic; CYP3A4 substrate (major); extensive first-pass effect (saturable)

Bioavailability: 35%

Half-life elimination: 2-4 hours

Time to peak, serum: Oral: Immediate release: 30-120 minutes; Sustained release: 60-240 minutes

Excretion: Urine (49% to 60% as metabolites); feces (43% as metabolites)

Dosage

Adults:

Oral:

Immediate release: Initial: 20 mg 3 times/day; usual: 20-40 mg 3 times/day (allow 3 days between dose increases)

Sustained release: Initial: 30 mg twice daily, titrate up to 60 mg twice daily

Note: The total daily dose of immediate-release product may not automatically be equivalent to the daily sustained-release dose; use caution in converting.

I.V.:

Acute hypertension: Initial: 5 mg/hour increased by 2.5 mg/hour every 5 minutes (for rapid titration) to every 15 minutes (for gradual titration) up to a maximum of 15 mg/hour; in rapidly titrated patients, consider reduction to 3 mg/hour after response is achieved.

Arterial hypertension in acute ischemic stroke (unlabeled use [Jauch, 2013]):

Patient otherwise eligible for reperfusion treatment (eg, alteplase) except blood pressure (BP) >185/110 mm Hg: Initiate 5 mg/hour; titrate by 2.5 mg/hour at 5- to 15-minute intervals (maximum dose: 15 mg/hour). When goal BP obtained, adjust dose to maintain proper BP limits. If BP does not decline and remains >185/110 mm Hg, alteplase should not be administered.

Management of BP during and after reperfusion treatment (eg, alteplase) to maintain BP ≤180/105 mm Hg: If systolic BP >180-230 mm Hg or diastolic >105-120 mm Hg: Initiate 5 mg/hour; titrate by 2.5 mg/hour at 5- to 15-minute intervals (maximum dose: 15 mg/hour). If hypertension is refractory or diastolic BP >140 mm Hg, consider other I.V. antihypertensives (eg, nitroprusside).

Substitution for oral therapy (approximate equivalents):

20 mg every 8 hours oral, equivalent to 0.5 mg/hour I.V. infusion

30 mg every 8 hours oral, equivalent to 1.2 mg/hour I.V. infusion

40 mg every 8 hours oral, equivalent to 2.2 mg/hour I.V. infusion

Conversion to oral antihypertensive agent: Initiate oral antihypertensive at the same time that I.V. nicardipine is discontinued, if transitioning to oral nicardipine, start oral nicardipine 1 hour prior to I.V. discontinuation.

Elderly: Initiate at the low end of the dosage range. Specific guidelines for adjustment of nicardipine are not available, but careful monitoring is warranted and adjustment may be necessary.

Dosing adjustment in renal impairment:

Oral: Per the manufacturer: Titrate dose beginning with 20 mg 3 times/day (immediate release capsule) or 30 mg twice daily (sustained release capsule).

I.V.: Specific guidelines for adjustment of nicardipine are not available, but careful monitoring is warranted and adjustment may be necessary.

Dosing adjustment in hepatic impairment:

Oral: Per the manufacturer: Starting dose: 20 mg twice daily (immediate release) with titration. Refer to **"Note"** in adult dosing.

I.V.: Specific guidelines for adjustment of nicardipine are not available, but careful monitoring is warranted and adjustment may be necessary.

Dietary Considerations Avoid grapefruit juice.

Usual Infusion Concentrations: Pediatric Note: Premixed solutions available

I.V. infusion: 100 **mcg**/mL **or** 500 **mcg**/mL

Usual Infusion Concentrations: Adult Note: Premixed solutions available

I.V. infusion: 25 mg in 250 mL (total volume) (concentration: 0.1 mg/mL) **or** 25 mg in 50 mL (total volume) (concentration: 0.5 mg/mL) of D_5W or NS

Administration

Oral: The total daily dose of immediate-release product may not automatically be equivalent to the daily sustained-release dose; use caution in converting. Do not chew or crush the sustained release formulation, swallow whole. Do not open or cut capsules.

I.V.:

Vials must be diluted before use. Administer as a slow continuous infusion at a concentration of 0.1 mg/mL or 0.2 mg/mL. Peripheral venous irritation may be minimized by changing the site of infusion every 12 hours. Concentrations of 0.5 mg/mL may be administered via a central line only.

Premixed bags: No further dilution needed. For single use only, discard any unused portion. Use only if solution is clear; the manufacturer recommends not to admix or run in the same line as other medications.

Monitoring Parameters Blood pressure, heart rate; consult individual institutional policies and procedures

Dosage Forms Excipient information presented when available (limited, particularly for generics); consult specific product labeling.

Capsule, Oral, as hydrochloride:
Generic: 20 mg, 30 mg

Capsule Extended Release 12 Hour, Oral, as hydrochloride:
Cardene SR: 30 mg [contains fd&c red #40]
Cardene SR: 60 mg [contains fd&c blue #2 (indigotine)]

Solution, Intravenous, as hydrochloride:
Cardene IV: 20 mg (200 mL); 40 mg (200 mL); 2.5 mg/mL (10 mL)
Generic: 2.5 mg/mL (10 mL)

- **Nicardipine Hydrochloride** *see* NiCARdipine *on page 1450*
- **NicAzelDoxy 30** *see* Doxycycline *on page 668*
- **NicAzelDoxy 60** *see* Doxycycline *on page 668*
- **Nicoderm® (Can)** *see* Nicotine *on page 1453*
- **Nicoderm CQ [OTC]** *see* Nicotine *on page 1453*
- **Nicomide-T** *see* Niacinamide *on page 1450*
- **Nicorelief [OTC]** *see* Nicotine *on page 1453*
- **Nicorette [OTC]** *see* Nicotine *on page 1453*
- **Nicorette® (Can)** *see* Nicotine *on page 1453*
- **Nicorette Mini [OTC]** *see* Nicotine *on page 1453*
- **Nicorette® Plus (Can)** *see* Nicotine *on page 1453*
- **Nicorette Starter Kit [OTC]** *see* Nicotine *on page 1453*
- **Nicotinamide** *see* Niacinamide *on page 1450*

Nicotine (nik oh TEEN)

Brand Names: U.S. Nicoderm CQ [OTC]; Nicorelief [OTC]; NICOrelief [OTC] [DSC]; Nicorette Mini [OTC]; Nicorette Starter Kit [OTC]; Nicorette [OTC]; Nicotrol; Nicotrol NS; Thrive [OTC]

Brand Names: Canada Habitrol®; Nicoderm®; Nicorette®; Nicorette® Plus; Nicotrol®

Index Terms Habitrol; Nicotine Patch

Pharmacologic Category Smoking Cessation Aid

Use Treatment to aid smoking cessation for the relief of nicotine withdrawal symptoms (including nicotine craving)

Unlabeled Use Management of ulcerative colitis (transdermal)

Pregnancy Risk Factor D (nasal)

Pregnancy Considerations Nicotine is teratogenic in animal studies. Nicotine exposure via cigarette smoke may cause increased ectopic pregnancy, low birth weight, increased risk of spontaneous abortion, increased perinatal mortality; increased aortic blood flow, increased heart rate, decreased uterine blood flow, and decreased breathing have been reported in the fetus. Smoking during pregnancy is associated with sudden infant death syndrome (SIDS), an increased risk of asthma, infantile colic, and childhood obesity. Women who are pregnant should be encouraged not to smoke. The use of nicotine replacement products to aid in smoking cessation has not been adequately studied in pregnant women (amount of nicotine exposure is varied). Nonpharmacologic treatments are recommended. If the benefits of nicotine replacement therapy outweigh the unknown risks, products with intermittent dosing are suggested to be tried first. If a patch is used, it is suggested to remove it overnight while sleeping to decrease fetal exposure.

Breast-Feeding Considerations Nicotine from cigarette smoke is found in breast milk at 1.5-3 times the maternal plasma concentrations. The amount from nicotine replacement products is not known. Women who are breastfeeding are encouraged not to smoke.

Contraindications Hypersensitivity to nicotine or any component of the formulation; patients who are smoking during the postmyocardial infarction period; patients with life-threatening arrhythmias, or severe or worsening angina pectoris; active temporomandibular joint disease (gum); pregnancy; not for use in nonsmokers

Warnings/Precautions Hazardous agent - use appropriate precautions for handling and disposal (EPA, P-listed). Use caution in patients with hyperthyroidism, pheochromocytoma, or insulin-dependent diabetes. Use with caution in oropharyngeal inflammation and in patients with history of esophagitis, peptic ulcer, coronary artery disease, recent MI, serious cardiac arrhythmias, vasospastic disease, angina, hypertension, hyperthyroidism, pheochromocytoma, diabetes, severe renal dysfunction, and hepatic dysfunction. The oral inhaler and nasal spray should be used with caution in patients with bronchospastic disease (other forms of nicotine replacement may be preferred). Use of nasal product is not recommended with chronic nasal disorders (eg, allergy, rhinitis, nasal polyps, and sinusitis). Transdermal patch may contain conducting metal (eg, aluminum); remove patch prior to MRI. Cautious use of topical nicotine in patients with certain skin diseases. Hypersensitivity to the topical products can occur. Dental problems may be worsened by chewing the gum. Urge patients to stop smoking completely when initiating therapy.

Adverse Reactions

Nasal spray/inhaler:

>10%:
Central nervous system: Headache (18% to 26%)
Gastrointestinal: Inhaler: Mouth/throat irritation (66%), dyspepsia (18%)
Respiratory: Inhaler: Cough (32%), rhinitis (23%)

1% to 10%:
Dermatologic: Acne (3%)
Endocrine & metabolic: Dysmenorrhea (3%)

Gastrointestinal: Flatulence (4%), gum problems (4%), diarrhea, hiccup, nausea, taste disturbance, tooth abrasions

Neuromuscular & skeletal: Back pain (6%), arthralgia (5%), jaw/neck pain

Respiratory: Nasal burning (nasal spray), sinusitis

Miscellaneous: Withdrawal symptoms

<1% (Limited to important or life-threatening): Allergy, amnesia, aphasia, bronchitis, bronchospasm, edema, migraine, numbness, pain, purpura, rash, sputum increased, vision abnormalities, xerostomia

Adverse events previously reported in prescription labeling for chewing gum, lozenge, and/or transdermal systems. Frequency not defined; may be product or dose specific:

Central nervous system: Concentration impaired, depression, dizziness, headache, insomnia, nervousness, pain

Gastrointestinal: Aphthous stomatitis, constipation, cough, diarrhea, dyspepsia, flatulence, gingival bleeding, glossitis, hiccups, jaw pain, nausea, salivation increased, stomatitis, taste perversion, tooth abrasions, ulcerative stomatitis, xerostomia

Dermatologic: Rash

Local: Application site reaction, local edema, local erythema

Neuromuscular & skeletal: Arthralgia, myalgia, paresthesia

Respiratory: Cough, sinusitis

Miscellaneous: Allergic reaction, diaphoresis

Drug Interactions

Metabolism/Transport Effects **Substrate** of CYP1A2 (minor), CYP2A6 (minor), CYP2B6 (minor), CYP2C19 (minor), CYP2C9 (minor), CYP2D6 (minor), CYP2E1 (minor), CYP3A4 (minor); **Note:** Assignment of Major/Minor substrate status based on clinically relevant drug interaction potential; **Inhibits** CYP2A6 (weak), CYP2E1 (weak)

Avoid Concomitant Use There are no known interactions where it is recommended to avoid concomitant use.

Increased Effect/Toxicity

Nicotine may increase the levels/effects of: Adenosine

The levels/effects of Nicotine may be increased by: Cimetidine

Decreased Effect

The levels/effects of Nicotine may be decreased by: Peginterferon Alfa-2b

Ethanol/Nutrition/Herb Interactions Food: Lozenge: Acidic foods/beverages decrease absorption of nicotine.

Storage/Stability

Nicotrol®: Store inhaler cartridge at room temperature not to exceed 30°C (86°F). Protect cartridges from light.

Nicotrol® NS: Store at room temperature not to exceed 30°C (86°F).

Mechanism of Action Nicotine is one of two naturally-occurring alkaloids which exhibit their primary effects via autonomic ganglia stimulation. The other alkaloid is lobeline which has many actions similar to those of nicotine but is less potent. Nicotine is a potent ganglionic and central nervous system stimulant, the actions of which are mediated via nicotine-specific receptors. Biphasic actions are observed depending upon the dose administered. The main effect of nicotine in small doses is stimulation of all autonomic ganglia; with larger doses, initial stimulation is followed by blockade of transmission. Biphasic effects are also evident in the adrenal medulla; discharge of catecholamines occurs with small doses, whereas prevention of catecholamines release is seen with higher doses as a response to splanchnic nerve stimulation. Stimulation of the central nervous system (CNS) is characterized by tremors and respiratory excitation. However, convulsions may occur with higher doses, along with respiratory failure secondary to both central paralysis and peripheral blockade to respiratory muscles.

Pharmacodynamics/Kinetics

Onset of action: Intranasal: More closely approximate the time course of plasma nicotine levels observed after cigarette smoking than other dosage forms

Duration: Transdermal: 24 hours

Absorption: Transdermal: Slow

Metabolism: Hepatic, primarily to cotinine ($^1/_5$ as active)

Half-life elimination: 4 hours; Nasal spray: 1-2 hours

Time to peak, serum: Transdermal: 8-9 hours; Nasal spray: 10-20 minutes

Excretion: Urine

Clearance: Renal: pH dependent

Dosage

Smoking deterrent: Patients should be advised to completely stop smoking upon initiation of therapy.

Oral:

Gum: Chew 1 piece of gum when urge to smoke, up to 24 pieces/day. Patients who smoke <25 cigarettes/day should start with 2-mg strength; patients smoking ≥25 cigarettes/day should start with the 4-mg strength. Use according to the following 12-week dosing schedule:

Weeks 1-6: Chew 1 piece of gum every 1-2 hours; to increase chances of quitting, chew at least 9 pieces/day during the first 6 weeks

Weeks 7-9: Chew 1 piece of gum every 2-4 hours

Weeks 10-12: Chew 1 piece of gum every 4-8 hours

Inhaler: Usually 6 to 16 cartridges per day; best effect was achieved by frequent continuous puffing (20 minutes); recommended duration of treatment is 3 months, after which patients may be weaned from the inhaler by gradual reduction of the daily dose over 6-12 weeks

Lozenge: Patients who smoke their first cigarette within 30 minutes of waking should use the 4 mg strength; otherwise the 2 mg strength is recommended. Use according to the following 12-week dosing schedule:

Weeks 1-6: One lozenge every 1-2 hours

Weeks 7-9: One lozenge every 2-4 hours

Weeks 10-12: One lozenge every 4-8 hours

Note: Use at least 9 lozenges/day during first 6 weeks to improve chances of quitting; do not use more than one lozenge at a time (maximum: 5 lozenges every 6 hours, 20 lozenges/day)

Topical:

Transdermal patch: Apply new patch every 24 hours to nonhairy, clean, dry skin on the upper body or upper outer arm; each patch should be applied to a different site. **Note:** Adjustment may be required during initial treatment (move to higher dose if experiencing withdrawal symptoms; lower dose if side effects are experienced).

NicoDerm CQ®:

Patients smoking >10 cigarettes/day: Begin with **step 1** (21 mg/day) for 6 weeks, followed by **step 2** (14 mg/day) for 2 weeks; finish with **step 3** (7 mg/day) for 2 weeks

Patients smoking ≤10 cigarettes/day: Begin with **step 2** (14 mg/day) for 6 weeks, followed by **step 3** (7 mg/day) for 2 weeks

Note: Patients receiving >600 mg/day of cimetidine: Decrease to the next lower patch size

Note: Benefits of use of nicotine transdermal patches beyond 3 months have not been demonstrated.

Nasal: Spray: 1-2 sprays/hour; do not exceed more than 5 doses (10 sprays) per hour [maximum: 40 doses/day (80 sprays); each dose (2 sprays) contains 1 mg of nicotine]

Dietary Considerations Some products may contain phenylalanine and/or sodium.

Administration

Gum: Should be chewed slowly to avoid jaw ache and to maximize benefit. Chew slowly until it tingles, then park gum between cheek and gum until tingle is gone; repeat process until most of tingle is gone (~30 minutes).

Lozenge: Should not be chewed or swallowed; allow to dissolve slowly (~20-30 minutes)

Nasal spray: Prime pump prior to first use (pump 6-8 times until fine spray appears) or if it has not been used for 24 hours (pump 1-2 times). Blow nose prior to use. Tilt head back slightly and insert tip of bottle into nostril. Breathe through mouth and spray once in each nostril. Do not sniff, swallow, or inhale through the nose during administration. After administration, wait 2-3 minutes before blowing nose.

Oral Inhalant: Insert cartridge into inhaler and push hard until it pops into place. Replace mouthpiece and twist the top and bottom so that markings do not line up. Inhale deeply into the back of the throat or puff in short breaths. Nicotine in cartridge is used up after about 20 minutes of active puffing.

Transdermal patch: Do not cut patch; causes rapid evaporation, rendering the patch useless

Hazardous agent; use appropriate precautions for handling and disposal (EPA, P-listed).

Monitoring Parameters Heart rate and blood pressure periodically during therapy; discontinue therapy if signs of nicotine toxicity occur (eg, severe headache, dizziness, mental confusion, disturbed hearing and vision, abdominal pain; rapid, weak and irregular pulse; salivation, nausea, vomiting, diarrhea, cold sweat, weakness); therapy should be discontinued if rash develops; discontinuation may be considered if other adverse effects of patch occur such as myalgia, arthralgia, abnormal dreams, insomnia, nervousness, dry mouth, sweating

Additional Information A cigarette has 10-25 mg nicotine.

Dosage Forms Excipient information presented when available (limited, particularly for generics); consult specific product labeling. [DSC] = Discontinued product

Gum, Mouth/Throat, as polacrilex:

- Nicorelief: 2 mg (50 ea, 110 ea)
- Nicorelief: 2 mg (50 ea, 110 ea) [mint flavor]
- Nicorelief: 4 mg (50 ea, 110 ea) [contains fd&c yellow #10 (quinoline yellow)]
- Nicorelief: 4 mg (50 ea, 110 ea) [contains fd&c yellow #10 (quinoline yellow); mint flavor]
- Nicorette: 2 mg (170 ea, 200 ea)
- Nicorette: 2 mg (190 ea) [contains menthol; fresh mint flavor]
- Nicorette: 2 mg (20 ea, 40 ea, 100 ea, 190 ea) [contains menthol; fruit flavor]
- Nicorette: 2 mg (110 ea, 170 ea) [contains menthol; mint flavor]
- Nicorette: 2 mg (20 ea, 100 ea, 190 ea) [contains menthol, polysorbate 80; cinnamon flavor]
- Nicorette: 2 mg (20 ea, 100 ea, 160 ea, 190 ea) [contains menthol, polysorbate 80; ice mint flavor]
- Nicorette: 4 mg (60 ea [DSC], 170 ea, 200 ea) [contains fd&c yellow #10 (quinoline yellow)]
- Nicorette: 4 mg (100 ea, 160 ea, 190 ea) [contains fd&c yellow #10 (quinoline yellow), menthol, polysorbate 80; cinnamon flavor]
- Nicorette: 4 mg (100 ea, 190 ea) [contains fd&c yellow #10 aluminum lake, menthol; fresh mint flavor]
- Nicorette: 4 mg (20 ea, 40 ea, 100 ea, 190 ea) [contains fd&c yellow #10 aluminum lake, menthol; fruit flavor]
- Nicorette: 4 mg (110 ea, 170 ea) [contains fd&c yellow #10 aluminum lake, menthol; mint flavor]
- Nicorette: 4 mg (20 ea, 100 ea, 190 ea) [contains fd&c yellow #10 aluminum lake, menthol, polysorbate 80; mint flavor]
- Nicorette Starter Kit: 2 mg (110 ea)
- Nicorette Starter Kit: 2 mg (100 ea) [contains menthol]
- Nicorette Starter Kit: 4 mg (110 ea) [contains fd&c yellow #10 aluminum lake]
- Thrive: 2 mg (100 ea, 110 ea) [contains saccharin sodium]
- Thrive: 4 mg (100 ea, 110 ea) [contains fd&c blue #2 (indigotine), saccharin sodium]
- Generic: 2 mg (20 ea, 40 ea, 50 ea, 100 ea, 110 ea); 4 mg (20 ea, 40 ea, 50 ea, 100 ea, 110 ea)

Inhaler, Inhalation:

- Nicotrol: 10 mg (168 ea) [contains menthol]

Kit, Transdermal:

- Generic: 21-14-7 MG/24HR

Lozenge, Mouth/Throat, as polacrilex:

- NICOrelief: 2 mg (72 ea [DSC]); 4 mg (72 ea [DSC]) [contains aspartame; mint flavor]
- Nicorette: 2 mg (72 ea, 81 ea) [cherry flavor]
- Nicorette: 2 mg (108 ea) [contains aspartame]
- Nicorette: 2 mg (72 ea, 81 ea, 168 ea) [contains aspartame, soy protein; mint flavor]
- Nicorette: 4 mg (72 ea, 81 ea) [cherry flavor]
- Nicorette: 4 mg (108 ea) [contains aspartame]
- Nicorette: 4 mg (72 ea, 81 ea, 168 ea) [contains aspartame, soy protein; mint flavor]
- Nicorette Mini: 2 mg (81 ea, 135 ea); 4 mg (81 ea, 135 ea)
- Generic: 2 mg (72 ea); 4 mg (72 ea)

Patch 24 Hour, Transdermal:

- Nicoderm CQ: 7 mg/24 hr (14 ea); 14 mg/24 hr (14 ea, 21 ea); 21 mg/24 hr (7 ea, 14 ea, 21 ea)
- Generic: 7 mg/24 hr (7 ea, 14 ea); 14 mg/24 hr (7 ea, 14 ea); 21 mg/24 hr (7 ea, 14 ea, 28 ea)

Solution, Nasal:

- Nicotrol NS: 10 mg/mL (10 mL)

- ◆ **Nicotine Patch** *see* Nicotine *on page* 1453
- ◆ **Nicotinic Acid** *see* Niacin *on page* 1447
- ◆ **Nicotinic Acid Amide** *see* Niacinamide *on page* 1450
- ◆ **Nicotrol** *see* Nicotine *on page* 1453
- ◆ **Nicotrol® (Can)** *see* Nicotine *on page* 1453
- ◆ **Nicotrol NS** *see* Nicotine *on page* 1453
- ◆ **Nidagel™ (Can)** *see* MetroNIDAZOLE (Topical) *on page* 1354
- ◆ **Nifediac CC** *see* NIFEdipine *on page* 1455
- ◆ **Nifedical XL** *see* NIFEdipine *on page* 1455

NIFEdipine (nye FED i peen)

Brand Names: U.S. Adalat CC; Afeditab CR; Nifediac CC; Nifedical XL; Procardia; Procardia XL

Brand Names: Canada Adalat® XL®; Apo-Nifed PA®; Mylan-Nifedipine Extended Release; Nu-Nifed; Nu-Nifedipine-PA; PMS-Nifedipine

Pharmacologic Category Antianginal Agent; Antihypertensive; Calcium Channel Blocker; Calcium Channel Blocker, Dihydropyridine

Additional Appendix Information

Beers Criteria – Potentially Inappropriate Medications for Geriatrics *on page* 2368

Calcium Channel Blockers – Comparative Pharmacokinetics *on page* 2296

Use Management of chronic stable or vasospastic angina; treatment of hypertension (sustained release products only)

Unlabeled Use Management of pulmonary hypertension, preterm labor, and Raynaud's phenomenon; prevention and treatment of high altitude pulmonary edema

Pregnancy Risk Factor C

Pregnancy Considerations Adverse events were observed in animal reproduction studies. Nifedipine crosses the placenta and small amounts can be detected in the urine of newborn infants (Manninen, 1991; Silberschmidt, 2008). An increase in perinatal asphyxia, cesarean delivery, prematurity, and intrauterine growth retardation have been reported following maternal use. Untreated chronic maternal hypertension is also associated with adverse events in the fetus, infant, and mother. If treatment for hypertension during pregnancy is needed, nifedipine is one of the preferred agents (ACOG, 2012; Chobanian, 2003).

Nifedipine has also been evaluated for the treatment of preterm labor. Tocolytics may be used for the short-term (48 hour) prolongation of pregnancy to allow for the administration of antenatal steroids and should not be used prior to fetal viability or when the risks of use to the fetus or mother are greater than the risk of preterm birth (ACOG, 2012). Nifedipine is ineffective for maintenance tocolytic therapy (ACOG, 2012; Roos, 2013).

Breast-Feeding Considerations

Nifedipine is excreted into breast milk. Reported concentrations are low and similar to those in the maternal serum (Ehrenkranz, 1989; Manninen, 1991; Penny, 1989). Breast-feeding is not recommended by the manufacturer. Breast-fed infants of mothers taking medications for hypertension should be monitored for adverse effects (Chobanian, 2003). Nifedipine has been used for the treatment of Raynaud's phenomenon of the nipple in breast-feeding mothers (Barrett, 2013; Wu, 2012).

Contraindications Hypersensitivity to nifedipine or any component of the formulation; concomitant use with strong CYP3A4 inducers (eg, rifampin); cardiogenic shock; immediate release preparation for treatment of urgent or emergent hypertension (Chobanian, 2003); acute MI (Antman, 2004)

Warnings/Precautions Symptomatic hypotension with or without syncope can rarely occur; blood pressure must be lowered at a rate appropriate for the patient's clinical condition. **The use of immediate release nifedipine (sublingually or orally) in hypertensive emergencies and urgencies is neither safe nor effective.** Serious adverse events (eg, death, cerebrovascular ischemia, syncope, stroke, acute myocardial infarction, and fetal distress) have been reported. **Immediate release nifedipine should not be used for acute blood pressure reduction.**

Blood pressure lowering should be done at a rate appropriate for the patient's condition. Rapid drops in blood pressure can lead to arterial insufficiency. Increased angina and/or MI have occurred with initiation or dosage titration of dihydropyridine calcium channel blockers; use with caution in patients with obstructive coronary disease especially in the absence of concurrent beta-blockade. Use with caution before major surgery. Cardiopulmonary bypass, intraoperative blood loss or vasodilating anesthesia may result in severe hypotension and/or increased fluid requirements. Consider withdrawing nifedipine (>36 hours) before surgery if possible.

The most common side effect is peripheral edema; occurs within 2-3 weeks of starting therapy. Reflex tachycardia may occur with use. Use with caution in HF or severe aortic stenosis (especially with concomitant beta-adrenergic blocker), severe left ventricular dysfunction, renal impairment, hypertrophic cardiomyopathy (especially obstructive), concomitant therapy with beta-blockers or digoxin, and edema. Use caution in patients with severe hepatic impairment. Clearance of nifedipine is reduced in cirrhotic patients leading to increased systemic exposure; monitor closely for adverse effects/toxicity and consider dose adjustments. Mild and transient elevations in liver function enzymes may be apparent within 8 weeks of therapy initiation. Abrupt withdrawal may cause rebound angina in patients with CAD. In the elderly, immediate release nifedipine should be avoided in due to potential to cause hypotension and risk of precipitating myocardial ischemia (Beers Criteria). Immediate release formulations should not be used to manage primary hypertension, adequate studies to evaluate outcomes have not been conducted. Avoid use of extended release tablets (Procardia XL®) in patients with known stricture/narrowing of the GI tract. Adalat® CC tablets contain lactose; do not use with galactose intolerance, Lapp lactase deficiency, or glucose-galactose malabsorption syndromes.

Use with caution in patients taking CYP3A4 inhibitors; may result in increased nifedipine concentrations; monitor for adverse effects/toxicity and consider dose adjustments. Use with strong CYP3A4 inducers (eg, rifampin, rifabutin, phenobarbital, phenytoin, carbamazepine, St John's wort) is contraindicated due to reduced bioavailability and efficacy.

Adverse Reactions

>10%:

Cardiovascular: Flushing (10% to 25%; extended release products 3% to 4%), peripheral edema (dose related 7% to 30%)

Central nervous system: Dizziness/lightheadedness/giddiness (10% to 27%), headache (10% to 23%)

Gastrointestinal: Nausea/heartburn (10% to 11%)

≥1% to 10%:

Cardiovascular: Palpitation (≤2% to 7%), transient hypotension (dose related 5%), CHF (2%)

Central nervous system: Nervousness/mood changes (≤2% to 7%), fatigue (6%), shakiness (≤2%), jitteriness (≤2%), sleep disturbances (≤2%), difficulties in balance (≤2%), fever (≤2%), chills (≤2%)

Dermatologic: Dermatitis (≤2%), pruritus (≤2%), urticaria (≤2%)

Endocrine & metabolic: Sexual difficulties (≤2%)

Gastrointestinal: Diarrhea (≤2%), constipation (≤2%), cramps (≤2%), flatulence (≤2%), gingival hyperplasia (≤10%)

Neuromuscular & skeletal: Muscle cramps/tremor (≤2% to 8%), weakness (<3%), inflammation (≤2%), joint stiffness (≤2%)

Ocular: Blurred vision (≤2%)

Respiratory: Cough/wheezing (6%), nasal congestion/sore throat (≤2% to 6%), chest congestion (≤2%), dyspnea (≤2%)

Miscellaneous: Diaphoresis (≤2%)

<1% (Limited to important or life-threatening): Agranulocytosis, allergic hepatitis, alopecia, anemia, angina, angioedema, aplastic anemia, arrhythmia, arthritis with positive ANA, bezoars (Procardia XL®), cerebral ischemia, depression, dysosmia, epistaxis, EPS, erectile dysfunction, erythema multiforme, erythromelalgia, exanthematous pustulosis, exfoliative dermatitis, facial edema, gastroesophageal reflux, gastrointestinal obstruction (Procardia XL®), gastrointestinal ulceration (Procardia XL®), gynecomastia, hematuria, ischemia, leukopenia, lip cancer (Friedman, 2012), memory dysfunction, migraine, myalgia, myoclonus, nocturia, paranoid syndrome, parotitis, periorbital edema, photosensitivity, polyuria, purpura, Stevens-Johnson syndrome, syncope, tachycardia, taste perversion, thrombocytopenia, tinnitus, toxic epidermal necrolysis, transient blindness, ventricular arrhythmia

Reported with use of sublingual short-acting nifedipine: Acute MI, cerebrovascular ischemia, ECG changes, fetal distress, heart block, severe hypotension, sinus arrest, stroke, syncope

Drug Interactions

Metabolism/Transport Effects Substrate of CYP2D6 (minor), CYP3A4 (major); **Note:** Assignment of Major/Minor substrate status based on clinically relevant drug interaction potential; **Inhibits** CYP1A2 (weak), CYP2C9 (weak), CYP2D6 (weak), CYP3A4 (weak)

Avoid Concomitant Use

Avoid concomitant use of NIFEdipine with any of the following: Conivaptan; CYP3A4 Inducers (Strong); Fusidic Acid (Systemic); Grapefruit Juice; Pimozide

Increased Effect/Toxicity

NIFEdipine may increase the levels/effects of: Amifostine; Antihypertensives; ARIPiprazole; Atosiban; Beta-Blockers; Calcium Channel Blockers (Nondihydropyridine); Digoxin; Dofetilide; Fosphenytoin; Hypotensive Agents; Lomitapide; Magnesium Salts; Neuromuscular-Blocking Agents (Nondepolarizing); Nitroprusside; Obinutuzumab; Phenytoin; Pimozide; QuiNIDine; RiTUXimab; Tacrolimus (Systemic); VinCRIStine; VinCRIStine (Liposomal)

The levels/effects of NIFEdipine may be increased by: Alcohol (Ethyl); Alpha1-Blockers; Antifungal Agents (Azole Derivatives, Systemic); Brimonidine (Topical); Calcium Channel Blockers (Nondihydropyridine); Cimetidine; Cisapride; Conivaptan; CycloSPORINE (Systemic); CYP3A4 Inhibitors (Moderate); CYP3A4 Inhibitors (Strong); Dasatinib; Diazoxide; Fluconazole; FLUoxetine; Fusidic Acid (Systemic); Grapefruit Juice; Herbs (Hypotensive Properties); Ivacaftor; Luliconazole; Macrolide Antibiotics; Magnesium Salts; MAO Inhibitors; Mifepristone; Pentoxifylline; Phosphodiesterase 5 Inhibitors; Prostacyclin Analogues; Protease Inhibitors; QuiNIDine; Simeprevir

Decreased Effect

NIFEdipine may decrease the levels/effects of: Clopidogrel; QuiNIDine

The levels/effects of NIFEdipine may be decreased by: Barbiturates; Bosentan; Calcium Salts; CarBAMazepine; CYP3A4 Inducers (Strong); Dabrafenib; Deferasirox; Herbs (CYP3A4 Inducers); Herbs (Hypertensive Properties); Melatonin; Methylphenidate; Nafcillin; Peginterferon Alfa-2b; Rifamycin Derivatives; Tocilizumab; Yohimbine

Ethanol/Nutrition/Herb Interactions

Ethanol: Ethanol may increase CNS depression and may increase the effects of nifedipine. Management: Avoid ethanol.

Food: Nifedipine serum levels may be decreased if taken with food. Food may decrease the rate but not the extent of absorption of Procardia XL®. Increased nifedipine concentrations resulting in therapeutic and vasodilator side effects, including severe hypotension and myocardial ischemia, may occur if nifedipine is taken by patients ingesting grapefruit. Management: Avoid grapefruit/grapefruit juice. Avoid caffeine.

Herb/Nutraceutical: St John's wort may decrease nifedipine levels. Some herbal medications (eg, licorice) may worsen hypertension; others may increase the antihypertensive effect of nifedipine (eg, shepherd's purse). Management: Avoid bayberry, blue cohosh, cayenne, ephedra, ginger, ginseng (American), kola, licorice, and yohimbe. Avoid black cohosh, California poppy, coleus, golden seal, hawthorn, mistletoe, periwinkle, quinine, and shepherd's purse.

Mechanism of Action Inhibits calcium ion from entering the "slow channels" or select voltage-sensitive areas of vascular smooth muscle and myocardium during depolarization, producing a relaxation of coronary vascular smooth muscle and coronary vasodilation; increases myocardial oxygen delivery in patients with vasospastic angina; also reduces peripheral vascular resistance, producing a reduction in arterial blood pressure.

Pharmacodynamics/Kinetics

Onset of action: Immediate release: ~20 minutes

Protein binding (concentration dependent): 92% to 98%

Metabolism: Hepatic via CYP3A4 to inactive metabolites

Bioavailability: Capsule: 40% to 77%; Sustained release: 65% to 89% relative to immediate release capsules; bioavailability increased with significant hepatic disease

Half-life elimination: Adults: Healthy: 2-5 hours; Cirrhosis: 7 hours; Elderly: 7 hours (extended release tablet)

Excretion: Urine (60% to 80% as inactive metabolites); feces

Dosage Oral:

Children 1-17 years:

High altitude pulmonary edema (unlabeled use; Pollard, 2001): **Note:** Treatment with nifedipine is only necessary if response to oxygen and/or descent is unsatisfactory; extended release preparation is preferred at equivalent dose with proper frequency adjustment:

Immediate release: 0.5 mg/kg/dose (maximum: 20 mg/dose) every 8 hours

Hypertension (unlabeled use): Extended release tablet: Initial: 0.25-0.5 mg/kg/day once daily or in 2 divided doses; maximum: 3 mg/kg/day up to 120 mg/day

Adults: **Note:** Dosage adjustments should occur at 7- to 14-day intervals, to allow for adequate assessment of new dose; when switching from immediate release to sustained release formulations, use same total daily dose.

Chronic stable or vasospastic angina:

Immediate release: Initial: 10 mg 3 times/day; usual dose: 10-20 mg 3 times/day; coronary artery spasm may require up to 20-30 mg 3-4 times/day; single doses >30 mg and total daily doses >120 mg are rarely needed; maximum: 180 mg/day; **Note:** Do not use for acute anginal episodes; may precipitate myocardial infarction

Extended release: Initial: 30 or 60 mg once daily; maximum: 120-180 mg/day

Hypertension: Extended release: Initial: 30 or 60 mg once daily; maximum: 90-120 mg/day

High altitude pulmonary edema (unlabeled use; Luks, 2010):

Prevention: Extended release: 30 mg every 12 hours starting the day before ascent and may be discontinued after staying at the same elevation for 5 days or if descent initiated

Treatment: Extended release: 30 mg every 12 hours

Pulmonary hypertension (unlabeled use; Galie, 2004): Extended release: Initial: 30 mg twice daily; may increase cautiously to 120-240 mg/day

Raynaud's phenomenon (unlabeled use; Wigley, 2002): Extended release: Dosage range: 30-120 mg once daily

Elderly: Hypertension: Consider lower initial doses and titrate to response (Aronow, 2011)

Dosage adjustment in renal impairment: No dosage adjustment provided in manufacturer's labeling (has not been studied); use with caution.

Hemodialysis: Supplemental dose is not necessary

Peritoneal dialysis effects: Supplemental dose is not necessary

Dosage adjustment in hepatic impairment: No dosage adjustment provided in manufacturer's labeling (has not been studied); use with caution. Clearance of nifedipine is reduced in cirrhotic patients, which may lead to increased systemic exposure; monitor closely for adverse effects/toxicity and consider dose adjustments.

Dietary Considerations Avoid grapefruit juice with all products.

Immediate release: Capsule is rapidly absorbed orally if it is administered without food, but may result in vasodilator side effects; if flushing is problematic, administration with low-fat meals may decrease. In general, can take with or without food.

Extended release: Adalat® CC, Afeditab® CR, Nifediac CC®: Take on an empty stomach (manufacturer recommendation). Other extended release products may not have this recommendation; consult product labeling.

Administration

Immediate release: In general, may be administered with or without food.

Extended release: Tablets should be swallowed whole; do not crush, split, or chew.

Adalat® CC, Afeditab® CR, Nifediac CC®: Administer on an empty stomach (per manufacturer). Other extended release products may not have this recommendation; consult product labeling.

Monitoring Parameters Heart rate, blood pressure, signs and symptoms of CHF, peripheral edema

Additional Information When measuring smaller doses from the liquid-filled capsules, consider the following concentrations (for Procardia®) 10 mg capsule = 10 mg/0.34 mL; 20 mg capsule = 20 mg/0.45 mL; may be used preoperative to treat hypertensive urgency.

Considerable attention has been directed to potential increases in mortality and morbidity when short-acting nifedipine is used in treating hypertension. The rapid reduction in blood pressure may precipitate adverse cardiovascular events.

Short-acting nifedipine should not be used for acute anginal episodes since this may precipitate myocardial infarction. Extended-release formulations are preferred for the management of chronic or vasospastic angina (Poole-Wilson, 2004).

Equivalency of extended release formulation (Adalat® CC): The manufacturer states that it is acceptable to interchange two 30 mg tablets with one 60 mg tablet to effectively deliver a 60 mg dose. However, it is not recommended to substitute one 90 mg tablet with three 30 mg tablets, since the resulting C_{max} is 29% higher compared to giving the single 90 mg tablet.

Dosage Forms Excipient information presented when available (limited, particularly for generics); consult specific product labeling.

Capsule, Oral:
- Procardia: 10 mg
- Generic: 10 mg, 20 mg

Tablet Extended Release 24 Hour, Oral:
- Adalat CC: 30 mg, 60 mg, 90 mg
- Afeditab CR: 30 mg, 60 mg
- Nifediac CC: 30 mg, 60 mg
- Nifediac CC: 90 mg [contains tartrazine (fd&c yellow #5)]
- Nifedical XL: 30 mg, 60 mg
- Procardia XL: 30 mg, 60 mg, 90 mg
- Generic: 30 mg, 60 mg, 90 mg

Extemporaneous Preparations A 4 mg/mL oral suspension may be made with liquid capsules (**Note:** Concentration inside capsule may vary depending on manufacturer. Procardia®: 10 mg capsule contains a concentration of 10 mg/0.34 mL [29.4 mg/mL]). Puncture the top of twelve 10 mg liquid capsules with one needle to create a vent. Insert a second needle attached to a syringe and extract the liquid; transfer to a calibrated bottle and add sufficient quantity of a 1:1 mixture of Ora-Sweet® and Ora-Plus® to make 30 mL. Label "shake well". Stable 90 days under refrigeration or at room temperature.

Nahata MC, Morosco RS, and Willhite EA, "Stability of Nifedipine in Two Oral Suspensions Stored at Two Temperatures," *J Am Pharm Assoc*, 2002, 42(6):865-7.

◆ **Niftolid** *see* Flutamide *on page 892*

◆ **Nighttime Sleep Aid [OTC]** *see* DiphenhydrAMINE (Systemic) *on page 622*

◆ **Nilandron** *see* Nilutamide *on page 1459*

Nilotinib (nye LOE ti nib)

Brand Names: U.S. Tasigna

Brand Names: Canada Tasigna

Index Terms AMN107; Nilotinib Hydrochloride Monohydrate

Pharmacologic Category Antineoplastic Agent, Tyrosine Kinase Inhibitor

Use Chronic myeloid leukemia (CML): Treatment of newly-diagnosed Philadelphia chromosome-positive CML (Ph+ CML) in chronic phase; treatment of chronic and accelerated phase Ph+ CML refractory or intolerant to prior therapy (including imatinib)

Unlabeled Use Treatment of refractory gastrointestinal stromal tumor (GIST)

Pregnancy Risk Factor D

Medication Guide Available Yes

Dosage

Chronic myeloid leukemia (CML), Ph+, newly-diagnosed in chronic phase: Adults: Oral: 300 mg twice daily

CML, Ph+, resistant or intolerant in chronic or accelerated phase: Adults: Oral: 400 mg twice daily

Gastrointestinal stromal tumor (GIST), refractory (unlabeled use): Adults: Oral: 400 mg twice daily until disease progression or unacceptable toxicity (Reichardt, 2012)

Missed doses: If a dose is missed, do not make up, resume with next scheduled dose.

Dosage adjustment for concomitant CYP3A4 inhibitors/inducers:

CYP3A4 inhibitors: Avoid the concomitant use of a strong CYP3A4 inhibitor with nilotinib. If a strong CYP3A4 inhibitor is required, interruption of nilotinib treatment is recommended; if therapy cannot be interrupted and concurrent use cannot be avoided, consider reducing the nilotinib dose to 300 mg once daily in patients with resistant or intolerant Ph+ CML (chronic or accelerated phase) or to 200 mg once daily in newly-diagnosed chronic phase Ph+ CML, with careful monitoring, especially of the QT interval. When a strong CYP3A4 inhibitor is discontinued, allow a washout period prior to adjusting nilotinib dose upward.

CYP3A4 inducers: Avoid the concomitant use of a strong CYP3A4 inducer with nilotinib (based on pharmacokinetic parameters, an increased nilotinib dose is not likely to compensate for decreased exposure).

Dosage adjustment in renal impairment: Not studied in patients with serum creatinine >1.5 times ULN, however, nilotinib and its metabolites have minimal renal excretion; dosage adjustments for renal dysfunction may not be necessary.

Dosage adjustment in hepatic impairment: Note: Dosage adjustment for impairment at treatment initiation (if possible, consider alternative therapies first); recommendations vary by indication.

Newly-diagnosed Ph+ CML in chronic phase: Mild-to-severe impairment (Child-Pugh class A, B, or C): Initial: 200 mg twice daily; may increase to 300 mg twice daily based on patient tolerability

Resistant or intolerant Ph+ CML in chronic or accelerated phase:

Mild-to-moderate impairment (Child-Pugh class A or B): Initial: 300 mg twice daily; may increase to 400 mg twice daily based on patient tolerability

Severe impairment (Child-Pugh class C): Initial: 200 mg twice daily; may increase to 300 mg twice daily and then further increased to 400 mg twice daily based on patient tolerability

For hepatotoxicity during treatment:

If bilirubin >3 times ULN (≥grade 3): Withhold treatment, monitor bilirubin, resume treatment at 400 mg once daily when bilirubin returns to ≤1.5 times ULN (≤grade 1)

If ALT or AST >5 times ULN (≥grade 3): Withhold treatment, monitor transaminases, resume treatment at 400 mg once daily when ALT or AST returns to ≤2.5 times ULN (≤grade 1)

Dosage adjustment for hematologic toxicity:

ANC <1000/mm^3 and/or platelets <50,000/mm^3: Withhold treatment, monitor blood counts

If ANC >1000/mm^3 and platelets >50,000/mm^3 within 2 weeks: Resume at prior dose

If ANC <1000/mm^3 and/or platelets <50,000/mm^3 for >2 weeks: Reduce dose to 400 mg once daily

Dosage adjustment for nonhematologic toxicity:

Amylase or lipase >2 times ULN (≥grade 3): Withhold treatment, monitor serum amylase or lipase, resume treatment at 400 mg once daily when lipase or amylase returns to ≤1.5 times ULN (≤grade 1)

Lipase increases in conjunction with abdominal symptoms: Withhold treatment and consider diagnostics to exclude pancreatitis

Clinically-significant moderate or severe nonhematologic toxicity: Withhold treatment, upon resolution of toxicity, resume at 400 mg once daily; may escalate back to initial dose (300 mg twice daily or 400 mg twice daily depending on indication) if clinically appropriate.

Dosage adjustment for QT prolongation: Note: Repeat ECG ~7 days after any dosage adjustment.

QT_c >480 msec: Withhold treatment, monitor and correct potassium and magnesium levels; review concurrent medications.

If QT_cF returns to <450 msec and to within 20 msec of baseline within 2 weeks: Resume at prior dose

If QT_cF returns to 450-480 msec after 2 weeks: Reduce dose to 400 mg once daily

If QT_cF >480 msec after dosage reduction to 400 mg once daily: Discontinue treatment

Additional Information Complete prescribing information should be consulted for additional detail.

Dosage Forms Excipient information presented when available (limited, particularly for generics); consult specific product labeling.

Capsule, Oral:

Tasigna: 150 mg

Tasigna: 200 mg [contains lactose]

◆ **Nilotinib Hydrochloride Monohydrate** *see* Nilotinib *on page 1458*

Nilutamide (ni LOO ta mide)

Brand Names: U.S. Nilandron

Brand Names: Canada Anandron®

Index Terms RU-23908

Pharmacologic Category Antiandrogen; Antineoplastic Agent, Antiandrogen

Use Treatment of metastatic prostate cancer (in combination with surgical castration)

Pregnancy Risk Factor C

Pregnancy Considerations Animal reproduction studies have not been conducted. Not indicated for use in women.

Breast-Feeding Considerations Not indicated for use in women.

Contraindications Hypersensitivity to nilutamide or any component of the formulation; severe hepatic impairment; severe respiratory insufficiency

Warnings/Precautions Hazardous agent - use appropriate precautions for handling and disposal (NIOSH, 2012). **[U.S. Boxed Warning]: Interstitial pneumonitis has been reported in 2% of patients exposed to nilutamide.** Symptoms typically include exertional dyspnea, cough, chest pain and fever; interstitial changes (including pulmonary fibrosis) leading to hospitalization and fatalities have been reported (rarely). The suggestive signs of pneumonitis most often occurred within the first 3 months of treatment. X-rays showed interstitial or alveolo-interstitial changes; pulmonary function tests revealed a restrictive pattern with decreased DLco. Consider baseline pulmonary function testing. Discontinue if signs and/or symptoms of interstitial pneumonitis are noted.

Hepatitis or marked increases in liver enzymes leading to drug discontinuation occurred in 1% of nilutamide patients; rare cases of hospitalization or deaths due to severe liver injury have been reported. Discontinue treatment for jaundice or ALT >2 times the upper limit of normal (ULN).

A delay in adaptation to dark has been reported; in clinical studies, this was reported by 13% to 57% of patients; the delay ranged from seconds to a few minutes after passing from a light to a dark area (this may not abate with continued treatment although may be alleviated by wearing tinted sunglasses); caution patients who experience adaptation delay about driving at night or through tunnels. Not indicated for use in women. Patients with disease progression while receiving antiandrogen therapy may experience clinical improvement with discontinuation of the antiandrogen.

Adverse Reactions

>10%:

Central nervous system: Insomnia (16%), headache (14%)

Endocrine & metabolic: Hot flashes (28% to 67%)

Gastrointestinal: Nausea (10% to 24%), constipation (7% to 20%), anorexia (11%), abdominal pain (10%)

Genitourinary: Testicular atrophy (16%), libido decreased (11%)

Hepatic: AST increased (8% to 13%), ALT increased (8% to 9%)

Ocular: Impaired dark adaptation (13% to 57%)

Respiratory: Dyspnea (6% to 11%)

1% to 10%:

Cardiovascular: Hypertension (5% to 9%), chest pain (7%), heart failure (3%), angina (2%), edema (2%), syncope (2%)

Central nervous system: Dizziness (7% to 10%), depression (9%), hypoesthesia (5%), malaise (2%), nervousness (2%)

Dermatologic: Alopecia (6%), dry skin (5%), rash (5%), pruritus (2%)

Endocrine & metabolic: Alcohol intolerance (5%), hyperglycemia (4%)

Gastrointestinal: Vomiting (6%), diarrhea (2%), GI hemorrhage (2%), melena (2%), weight loss (2%), xerostomia (2%), dyspepsia

Genitourinary: Nocturia (7%)

Hematologic: Anemia (7%), haptoglobin increased (2%), leukopenia (2%)

Hepatic: Alkaline phosphatase increased (3%)

Neuromuscular & skeletal: Bone pain (6%), arthritis (2%), paresthesia (2%)

Ocular: Chromatopsia (9%), impaired light adaptation (8%), abnormal vision (6% to 7%), cataract (2%), photophobia (2%)

Renal: Hematuria (8%), BUN increased (2%), creatinine increased (2%)

Respiratory: Pneumonia (5%), cough (2%), interstitial pneumonitis (2%), rhinitis (2%)

Miscellaneous: Flu-like syndrome (7%), diaphoresis (6%)

<1% (Limited to important or life-threatening): Aplastic anemia, hepatitis

Drug Interactions

Metabolism/Transport Effects Substrate of CYP2C19 (major); **Note:** Assignment of Major/Minor substrate status based on clinically relevant drug interaction potential; **Inhibits** CYP2C19 (weak)

Avoid Concomitant Use There are no known interactions where it is recommended to avoid concomitant use.

Increased Effect/Toxicity

The levels/effects of Nilutamide may be increased by: CYP2C19 Inhibitors (Moderate); CYP2C19 Inhibitors (Strong); Luliconazole

Decreased Effect

The levels/effects of Nilutamide may be decreased by: CYP2C19 Inducers (Strong); Dabrafenib

Ethanol/Nutrition/Herb Interactions Ethanol: Approximately 5% of patients experience an intolerance (facial flushing, hypotension, malaise) when ethanol is combined with nilutamide. Management: Avoid ethanol.

Storage/Stability Store at room temperature of 25°C (77°F); excursions permitted between 15°C to 30°C (59°F to 86°F). Protect from light.

Mechanism of Action Nonsteroidal antiandrogen which blocks testosterone effects at the androgen receptor level, preventing androgen response.

Pharmacodynamics/Kinetics

Absorption: Rapid and complete

Metabolism: Hepatic (extensive), forms active metabolites

Half-life elimination: Terminal: 38-59 hours; Metabolites: 59-126 hours

Excretion: Urine (62%; <2% as unchanged drug); feces (1% to 7%)

Dosage Oral: Adults: Prostate cancer, metastatic: 300 mg once daily (starting the same day or day after surgical castration) for 30 days, followed by 150 mg once daily

Dosage adjustment in renal impairment: No dosage adjustment provided in manufacturer's labeling.

Dosage adjustment in hepatic impairment:

No dosage adjustment provided in manufacturer's labeling. However, use is contraindicated in severe hepatic impairment.

During treatment: ALT >2 times ULN or jaundice: Discontinue treatment.

Dietary Considerations May be taken without regard to meals.

Administration Administer without regard to meals.

Hazardous agent; use appropriate precautions for handling and disposal (NIOSH, 2012).

Monitoring Parameters Hepatic enzymes (at baseline, regularly during the first 4 months of treatment, periodically thereafter); chest x-ray (at baseline); consider pulmonary function testing (at baseline)

Dosage Forms Excipient information presented when available (limited, particularly for generics); consult specific product labeling.

Tablet, Oral:

Nilandron: 150 mg

◆ Nimbex *see* Cisatracurium *on page* 436

NiMODipine (nye MOE di peen)

Brand Names: U.S. Nymalize

Brand Names: Canada Nimotop

Index Terms Nymalize

Pharmacologic Category Calcium Channel Blocker; Calcium Channel Blocker, Dihydropyridine

Additional Appendix Information

Calcium Channel Blockers - Comparative Pharmacokinetics *on page* 2296

Use Subarachnoid hemorrhage: For the improvement of neurological outcome by reducing the incidence and severity of ischemic deficits in adult patients with subarachnoid hemorrhage (SAH) from ruptured intracranial berry aneurysms regardless of their postictus neurological condition (ie, Hunt and Hess grades I to V)

Pregnancy Risk Factor C

Pregnancy Considerations Adverse events have been observed in animal reproduction studies. Nimodipine crosses the placenta (Belfort, 1994). Nimodipine has been evaluated for the management of pre-eclampsia (Belfort, 1994; Belfort, 2003), but it is not one of the agents currently recommended for this condition (ACOG, 2011).

Breast-Feeding Considerations Nimodipine is excreted into breast milk; two case reports note concentrations to be <1% of the weight-adjusted maternal dose (Carcas, 1996; Tonks, 1995). Breast-feeding is not recommended by the manufacturer.

Contraindications There are no contraindications listed in the manufacturer's labeling.

Warnings/Precautions [U.S. Boxed Warning]: Nimodipine has inadvertently been administered I.V. when withdrawn from capsules into a syringe for subsequent nasogastric administration. Severe cardiovascular adverse events, including fatalities, have resulted; precautions (eg, adequate labeling, use of oral syringes) should be employed against such an event.

Increased angina and/or MI have occurred with initiation or dosage titration of calcium channel blockers. Reflex tachycardia may occur resulting in angina and/or MI in patients with obstructive coronary disease, especially in the absence of concurrent beta-blockade. Peripheral edema is a common adverse event; occurs within 2-3 weeks of starting therapy. Symptomatic hypotension with or without syncope can occur; blood pressure must be lowered at a rate appropriate for the patient's clinical condition. Monitor blood pressure closely during treatment. Use with caution in patients with cirrhosis due to the increased plasma concentrations of nimodipine and an increased risk of adverse reactions; a lower dose and close monitoring of blood pressure and heart rate is required. Intestinal pseudo-obstruction and ileus have been reported (rarely) during therapy.

Potentially significant drug-drug interactions may exist, requiring dose or frequency adjustment, additional monitoring, and/or selection of alternative therapy.

Adverse Reactions

1% to 10%:

Cardiovascular: Decreased blood pressure (4% to 5%), bradycardia (1%)

Central nervous system: Headache (1%)

Gastrointestinal: Nausea (1%)

<1% (Limited to important or life-threatening): Anemia, decreased platelet count, disseminated intravascular coagulation, edema, gastrointestinal hemorrhage, gastrointestinal pseudo-obstruction, hematoma, hepatitis, hypertension, increased lactate dehydrogenase, increased serum alkaline phosphatase, increased serum ALT, increased serum glucose, intestinal obstruction, jaundice, rebound vasospasm, thrombocytopenia

Drug Interactions

Metabolism/Transport Effects Substrate of CYP3A4 (major); **Note:** Assignment of Major/Minor substrate status based on clinically relevant drug interaction potential

Avoid Concomitant Use

Avoid concomitant use of NiMODipine with any of the following: Conivaptan; Fusidic Acid (Systemic); Grapefruit Juice

Increased Effect/Toxicity

NiMODipine may increase the levels/effects of: Amifostine; Antihypertensives; Atosiban; Beta-Blockers; Calcium Channel Blockers (Nondihydropyridine); Fosphenytoin; Hypotensive Agents; Magnesium Salts; Neuromuscular-Blocking Agents (Nondepolarizing); Nitroprusside; Obinutuzumab; Phenytoin; QuiNIDine; RiTUXimab; Tacrolimus (Systemic)

The levels/effects of NiMODipine may be increased by: Alpha1-Blockers; Antifungal Agents (Azole Derivatives, Systemic); Brimonidine (Topical); Calcium Channel Blockers (Nondihydropyridine); Cimetidine; Conivaptan; CycloSPORINE (Systemic); CYP3A4 Inhibitors (Moderate); CYP3A4 Inhibitors (Strong); Dasatinib; Diazoxide; Fluconazole; FLUoxetine; Fusidic Acid (Systemic); Grapefruit Juice; Herbs (Hypotensive Properties); Ivacaftor; Luliconazole; Macrolide Antibiotics; Magnesium Salts; MAO Inhibitors; Mifepristone; Pentoxifylline; Phosphodiesterase 5 Inhibitors; Prostacyclin Analogues; Protease Inhibitors; QuiNIDine; Simeprevir

Decreased Effect

NiMODipine may decrease the levels/effects of: Clopidogrel; QuiNIDine

The levels/effects of NiMODipine may be decreased by: Barbiturates; Bosentan; Calcium Salts; CarBAMazepine; CYP3A4 Inducers (Strong); Dabrafenib; Deferasirox; Herbs (CYP3A4 Inducers); Herbs (Hypertensive Properties); Melatonin; Methylphenidate; Mitotane; Nafcillin; Rifamycin Derivatives; Tocilizumab; Yohimbine

Ethanol/Nutrition/Herb Interactions Food: Administration with a standard breakfast results in a 68% lower maximum plasma concentration and 38% lower bioavailability as compared to administration under fasted conditions. In addition, AUC and maximum plasma concentration were increased by an average of 51% and 24%, respectively, following administration of nimodipine with grapefruit juice (Fuhr, 1998). Management: Administer on an empty stomach, at least 1 hour before or 2 hours after meals. Avoid concurrent use of grapefruit juice and nimodipine.

Storage/Stability Store at 25°C (77°F); excursions are permitted to 15°C to 30°C (59°F to 86°F). Protect from capsules light and freezing. Protect solution from light and do not refrigerate.

Mechanism of Action Nimodipine shares the pharmacology of other calcium channel blockers; animal studies indicate that nimodipine has a greater effect on cerebral arterials than other arterials; this increased specificity may be due to the drug's increased lipophilicity and cerebral distribution as compared to nifedipine; inhibits calcium ion from entering the "slow channels" or select voltage sensitive areas of vascular smooth muscle and myocardium during depolarization

Pharmacodynamics/Kinetics

Protein binding: >95%

Metabolism: Extensively hepatic via CYP3A4; undergoes first-pass metabolism

Bioavailability: 13%

Half-life elimination: 1-2 hours; prolonged with renal impairment

Time to peak, serum: ~1 hour

Excretion: Urine (<1% as unchanged drug); feces

Dosage Note: For oral administration **ONLY.**

Adults: Oral: 60 mg every 4 hours for 21 consecutive days. **Note:** Start therapy within 96 hours of the onset of subarachnoid hemorrhage.

Dosage adjustment in renal impairment: No dosage adjustment provided in manufacturer's labeling. However, nimodipine undergoes minimal renal elimination and dose adjustment may not be necessary. Not removed by hemo- or peritoneal dialysis; supplemental dose is not necessary.

Dosage adjustment in hepatic impairment: Reduce dosage to 30 mg every 4 hours in patients with cirrhosis.

Administration For enteral administration ONLY. Life-threatening adverse events have occurred when administered parenterally. Administer on an empty stomach at least 1 hour before or 2 hours after meals.

Nasogastric (NG) or gastric tube administration:

Oral solution (Nymalzine): Administer using the supplied oral syringe labeled **"ORAL USE ONLY"**. Following administration, refill the oral syringe with 20 mL of NS and flush any remaining contents from NG or gastric tube into the stomach.

Capsules: If the capsules cannot be swallowed, the liquid may be removed by making a hole in each end of the capsule with an 18-gauge needle and extracting the contents into a syringe; transfer these contents into an oral syringe (amber-colored oral syringe preferred). It is strongly recommended that preparation be done in the pharmacy. Label oral syringe with **"WARNING: For ORAL use only"** or **"Not for I.V. use."** Follow with a flush of 30 mL NS.

Dosage Forms Excipient information presented when available (limited, particularly for generics); consult specific product labeling.

Capsule, Oral:

Generic: 30 mg

Solution, Oral:

Nymalize: 60 mg/20 mL (20 mL, 473 mL) [contains alcohol, usp, methylparaben, polyethylene glycol]

- ◆ **Nimotop (Can)** *see* NiMODipine *on page* 1460
- ◆ **Niodan (Can)** *see* Niacin *on page* 1447
- ◆ **Nipent** *see* Pentostatin *on page* 1617
- ◆ **Nipent® (Can)** *see* Pentostatin *on page* 1617
- ◆ **Nipride® (Can)** *see* Nitroprusside *on page* 1469
- ◆ **Niravam** *see* ALPRAZolam *on page* 81

Nisoldipine (nye SOL di peen)

Brand Names: U.S. Sular

Pharmacologic Category Antihypertensive; Calcium Channel Blocker; Calcium Channel Blocker, Dihydropyridine

Additional Appendix Information

Calcium Channel Blockers – Comparative Pharmacokinetics *on page* 2296

Use Management of hypertension, alone or in combination with other antihypertensive agents

Pregnancy Risk Factor C

Pregnancy Considerations Adverse events were not observed in animal reproduction studies when using doses that were not maternally toxic. Untreated chronic maternal hypertension is associated with adverse events in the fetus, infant, and mother. If treatment for hypertension during pregnancy is needed, other agents are preferred (ACOG, 2012; Chobanian, 2003).

Breast-Feeding Considerations It is not known if nisoldipine is excreted into breast milk. The manufacturer recommends a decision be made whether to discontinue nursing or to discontinue the drug, taking into account the importance of treatment to the mother. Breast-fed infants of mothers taking medications for hypertension should be monitored for adverse effects (Chobanian, 2003.)

Contraindications Hypersensitivity to nisoldipine, any component of the formulation, or other dihydropyridine calcium channel blockers

Warnings/Precautions With initiation or dosage titration of dihydropyridine calcium channel blockers, reflex tachycardia may occur resulting in angina and/or MI in patients with obstructive coronary disease especially in the absence of concurrent beta-blockade. Use with caution in patients with severe aortic stenosis, HF, and hypertrophic cardiomyopathy with outflow tract obstruction. Use with caution in hepatic impairment; lower starting dose required. The most common side effect is peripheral edema; occurs within 2-3 weeks of starting therapy. Symptomatic hypotension with or without syncope can rarely occur; blood pressure must be lowered at a rate appropriate for the patient's clinical condition. Some dosage forms contain tartrazine, which may cause allergic reactions in certain individuals (eg, aspirin hypersensitivity). Use with caution in patients >65 years of age; lower starting dose recommended.

Adverse Reactions

>10%:

Cardiovascular: Peripheral edema (dose related; 7% to 29%)

Central nervous system: Headache (22%)

1% to 10%:

Cardiovascular: Vasodilation (4%), palpitation (3%), angina exacerbation (2%), chest pain (2%)

Central nervous system: Dizziness (3% to 10%)

Dermatologic: Rash (2%)

Gastrointestinal: Nausea (2%)

Respiratory: Pharyngitis (5%), sinusitis (3%)

<1% (Limited to important or life-threatening): Alopecia, amblyopia, amnesia, anemia, anorexia, anxiety, appetite increased, arthralgia, arthritis, asthma, ataxia, atrial fibrillation, blepharitis, BUN increased, bruising, cellulitis, cerebral ischemia, colitis, conjunctivitis, creatinine increased, creatine kinase increased, CVA, depression, diabetes mellitus, diaphoresis, diarrhea, dreams abnormal, dyspepsia, dysphagia, dyspnea, dysuria, end inspiratory wheeze, epistaxis, exfoliative dermatitis, facial edema, fever, first-degree AV block, flu-like syndrome, gastritis, gastrointestinal hemorrhage, gingival hyperplasia, glaucoma, glossitis, gout, gynecomastia, heart failure (decompensated), hematuria, hepatomegaly, herpes simplex, herpes zoster; hypersensitivity reaction (eg, angioedema, shortness of breath, tachycardia, chest tightness, hypotension, and rash); hyper-/hypotension, hypertonia, hypoesthesia, hypokalemia, insomnia, jugular venous distention, keratoconjunctivitis, leukopenia, libido decreased, liver function tests abnormal, maculopapular rash, malaise, melena, migraine, mouth ulceration, myalgia, myasthenia, MI, myositis, nocturia, nonprotein nitrogen increased, orthostatic hypotension, paresthesia, petechiae, photosensitivity, pleural effusion, pruritus, pustular rash, rales, retinal detachment, skin discoloration, skin ulcer, somnolence, supraventricular tachycardia, syncope, systolic ejection murmur, taste disturbance, temporary unilateral loss of vision, tenosynovitis, thyroiditis, tremor; T-wave abnormalities on ECG (flattening, inversion, nonspecific changes); urinary frequency, urticaria, vaginal hemorrhage, venous insufficiency, ventricular extrasystoles, vertigo, vitreous floater, weight gain/loss, xerostomia

Drug Interactions

Metabolism/Transport Effects Substrate of CYP3A4 (major); **Note:** Assignment of Major/Minor substrate status based on clinically relevant drug interaction potential; **Inhibits** CYP1A2 (weak), CYP3A4 (weak)

Avoid Concomitant Use

Avoid concomitant use of Nisoldipine with any of the following: CYP3A4 Inducers (Strong); CYP3A4 Inhibitors (Strong); Fusidic Acid (Systemic); Grapefruit Juice; Pimozide

Increased Effect/Toxicity

Nisoldipine may increase the levels/effects of: Amifostine; Antihypertensives; ARIPiprazole; Atosiban; Beta-Blockers; Calcium Channel Blockers (Nondihydropyridine); Dofetilide; Fosphenytoin; Hypotensive Agents; Lomitapide; Magnesium Salts; Neuromuscular-Blocking Agents (Nondepolarizing); Nitroprusside; Obinutuzumab; Phenytoin; Pimozide; RiTUXimab; Tacrolimus (Systemic)

The levels/effects of Nisoldipine may be increased by: Alpha1-Blockers; Antifungal Agents (Azole Derivatives, Systemic); Brimonidine (Topical); Calcium Channel Blockers (Nondihydropyridine); Cimetidine; CycloSPORINE (Systemic); CYP3A4 Inhibitors (Moderate); CYP3A4 Inhibitors (Strong); Dasatinib; Diazoxide; Fluconazole; Fusidic Acid (Systemic); Grapefruit Juice; Herbs (Hypotensive Properties); Ivacaftor; Luliconazole; Macrolide Antibiotics; Magnesium Salts; MAO Inhibitors; Mifepristone; Pentoxifylline; Phosphodiesterase 5 Inhibitors; Prostacyclin Analogues; Protease Inhibitors; Simeprevir

Decreased Effect

Nisoldipine may decrease the levels/effects of: Clopidogrel

The levels/effects of Nisoldipine may be decreased by: Barbiturates; Bosentan; Calcium Salts; CarBAMazepine; CYP3A4 Inducers (Strong); Dabrafenib; Deferasirox; Herbs (CYP3A4 Inducers); Herbs (Hypertensive Properties); Melatonin; Methylphenidate; Nafcillin; Rifamycin Derivatives; Tocilizumab; Yohimbine

Ethanol/Nutrition/Herb Interactions

Food: Peak concentrations of nisoldipine may be significantly increased if taken with high-lipid foods; however, total exposure (AUC) may be reduced. Grapefruit juice has been shown to significantly increase the bioavailability of nisoldipine. Management: Take on an empty stomach 1 hour before or 2 hours after a meal. Avoid a high-fat diet. Avoid grapefruit products before and after dosing.

Herb/Nutraceutical: St John's wort may decrease nisoldipine levels. Some herbal medications may worsen hypertension (eg, licorice); others may increase the antihypertensive effect of nisoldipine (eg, shepherd's purse). Management: Avoid St John's wort. Avoid bayberry, blue cohosh, cayenne, ephedra, ginger, ginseng (American), kola, licorice, and yohimbe. Avoid black cohosh, California poppy, coleus, golden seal, hawthorn, mistletoe, periwinkle, quinine, and shepherd's purse.

Storage/Stability Store at controlled room temperature of 20°C to 25°C (68°F to 77°F). Protect from light; protect from moisture.

Mechanism of Action As a dihydropyridine calcium channel blocker, structurally similar to nifedipine, nisoldipine impedes the movement of calcium ions into vascular smooth muscle and cardiac muscle. Dihydropyridines are potent vasodilators and are not as likely to suppress cardiac contractility and slow cardiac conduction as other calcium antagonists such as verapamil and diltiazem; nisoldipine is 5-10 times as potent a vasodilator as nifedipine.

Pharmacodynamics/Kinetics

Duration: >24 hours

Absorption: Well absorbed. Peak concentrations significantly increased with high-lipid meals; however, AUC is reduced.
Protein binding: >99%
Metabolism: Extensively hepatic; 1 active metabolite (10% of activity of parent); first-pass effect
Bioavailability: ~5%
Half-life elimination: 9-18 hours
Time to peak: 4-14 hours
Excretion: Urine (60% to 80% as inactive metabolites); feces

Dosage Oral:

Sular® (Geomatrix® delivery system):

Adults: Initial: 17 mg once daily, then increase by 8.5 mg/week (or longer intervals) to attain adequate control of blood pressure

Usual dose range: 17-34 mg once daily; doses >34 mg once daily are not recommended

Elderly: Initial dose: 8.5 mg once daily, increase by 8.5 mg/week (or longer intervals) to attain adequate blood pressure control

Nisoldipine extended-release tablet (original formulation):

Adults: Oral: Initial: 20 mg once daily, then increase by 10 mg/week (or longer intervals) to attain adequate control of blood pressure

Usual dose range (JNC 7): 10-40 mg once daily; doses >60 mg once daily are not recommended

Elderly: Initial dose: 10 mg once daily, increase by 10 mg/week (or longer intervals) to attain adequate blood pressure control

Conversion from nisoldipine extended-release (original formulation) to Sular® Geomatrix® delivery system:

Nisoldipine Extended Release Dosing Equivalency

Original Extended Release Formulation	Sular® Extended Release (Geomatrix® delivery system)
10 mg	8.5 mg
20 mg	17 mg
30 mg	25.5 mg
40 mg	34 mg

Dosage adjustment in renal impairment:

Mild to moderate impairment: No dosage adjustment necessary.

Severe impairment: No dosage adjustment provided in manufacturer's labeling.

Dosage adjustment in hepatic impairment:

Sular® (Geomatrix® delivery system): An initial dose exceeding 8.5 mg once daily is not recommended for patients with hepatic impairment.

Nisoldipine extended-release (original formulation): An initial dose exceeding 10 mg once daily is not recommended for patients with hepatic impairment.

Dietary Considerations Take on an empty stomach (1 hour before or 2 hours after a meal). Avoid grapefruit juice before and after dosing. Avoid grapefuit juice; avoid high-fat diet.

Administration Administer at the same time each day to ensure minimal fluctuation of serum levels. Avoid high-fat diet. Administer on an empty stomach (1 hour before or 2 hours after a meal). Swallow whole; do not crush, break, split, or chew.

Monitoring Parameters Blood pressure, heart rate

Dosage Forms Excipient information presented when available (limited, particularly for generics); consult specific product labeling.

Tablet Extended Release 24 Hour, Oral:
Sular: 8.5 mg
Sular: 17 mg [contains tartrazine (fd&c yellow #5)]
Sular: 34 mg
Generic: 8.5 mg, 17 mg, 20 mg, 25.5 mg, 30 mg, 34 mg, 40 mg

◆ **Nitalapram** *see* Citalopram *on page 440*

Nitazoxanide (nye ta ZOX a nide)

Brand Names: U.S. Alinia

Index Terms NTZ

Pharmacologic Category Antiprotozoal

Use Treatment of diarrhea caused by *Cryptosporidium parvum* or *Giardia lamblia*

Unlabeled Use Alternative treatment for *Clostridium difficile*-associated diarrhea (CDAD)

Pregnancy Risk Factor B

Pregnancy Considerations Teratogenic effects were not observed in animal reproduction studies.

Breast-Feeding Considerations It is not known if nitazoxanide is excreted in breast milk. The manufacturer recommends that caution be exercised when administering nitazoxanide to nursing women.

Contraindications Hypersensitivity to nitazoxanide or any component of the formulation

Warnings/Precautions Use caution with renal or hepatic impairment. Safety and efficacy have not been established in patients with HIV infection or immunodeficiency. Oral suspension contains sucrose; use caution in patients with diabetes mellitus.

Adverse Reactions Rates of adverse effects were similar to those reported with placebo.

1% to 10%:

Central nervous system: Headache (1% to 3%)

Gastrointestinal: Abdominal pain (7% to 8%), diarrhea (2% to 4%), nausea (3%), vomiting (1%)

<1% (Limited to important or life-threatening): Allergic reaction, ALT increased, anemia, anorexia, appetite increased, creatinine increased, diaphoresis, dizziness, eye discoloration (pale yellow), fever, flatulence, hypertension, infection, malaise, pruritus, rhinitis, salivary glands enlarged, tachycardia, urine discoloration

Drug Interactions

Metabolism/Transport Effects None known.

Avoid Concomitant Use There are no known interactions where it is recommended to avoid concomitant use.

Increased Effect/Toxicity There are no known significant interactions involving an increase in effect.

Decreased Effect There are no known significant interactions involving a decrease in effect.

Ethanol/Nutrition/Herb Interactions Food: Food increases AUC. Management: Take with food.

Preparation for Administration For preparation at time of dispensing, add 48 mL incrementally to 60 mL bottle; shake vigorously. Resulting suspension is 20 mg/mL (100 mg per 5 mL).

Storage/Stability

Suspension: Prior to and following reconstitution, store at 25°C (77°F); excursions permitted to 15°C to 30°C (59°F to 86°F). For preparation at time of dispensing, add 48 mL incrementally to 60 mL bottle; shake vigorously. Resulting suspension is 20 mg/mL (100 mg per 5 mL). Following reconstitution, discard unused portion of suspension after 7 days.

Tablet: Store at 25°C (77°F); excursions permitted to 15°C to 30°C (59°F to 86°F).

Mechanism of Action Nitazoxanide is rapidly metabolized to the active metabolite tizoxanide *in vivo*. Activity may be due to interference with the pyruvate:ferredoxin oxidoreductase (PFOR) enzyme-dependent electron transfer reaction which is essential to anaerobic metabolism. *In vitro*, nitazoxanide and tizoxanide inhibit the growth of sporozoites and oocysts of *Cryptosporidium parvum* and trophozoites of *Giardia lamblia*.

Pharmacodynamics/Kinetics

Protein binding: Tizoxanide: >99%

Bioavailability: Relative bioavailability of suspension compared to tablet: 70%

Metabolism: Hepatic, to an active metabolite, tizoxanide. Tizoxanide undergoes conjugation to form tizoxanide glucuronide. Nitazoxanide is not detectable in the serum following oral administration.

Time to peak, plasma: Tizoxanide and tizoxanide glucuronide: 1-4 hours

Excretion: Tizoxanide: Urine, bile, and feces; Tizoxanide glucuronide: Urine and bile

Dosage Oral:

Children: Diarrhea caused by *Cryptosporidium parvum* or *Giardia lamblia*:

Children 1-3 years: Oral suspension: 100 mg every 12 hours for 3 days; may consider increasing duration up to 14 days in HIV-exposed/-infected pediatric patients with cryptosporidiosis (CDC, 2009)

Children 4-11 years: Oral suspension: 200 mg every 12 hours for 3 days; may consider increasing duration up to 14 days in HIV-exposed/-infected pediatric patients with cryptosporidiosis (CDC, 2009)

Children ≥12 years: Refer to adult dosing.

Adults:

Diarrhea caused by *Cryptosporidium parvum* or *Giardia lamblia*: Oral suspension or tablets: 500 mg every 12 hours for 3 days

Clostridium difficile-associated diarrhea (unlabeled use): Oral suspension or tablets: 500 mg every 12 hours for 10 days (Musher, 2009)

Dosage adjustment in renal impairment: No dosage adjustment provided in manufacturer's labeling (has not been studied); use with caution.

Dosage adjustment in hepatic impairment: No dosage adjustment provided in manufacturer's labeling (has not been studied); use with caution.

Dietary Considerations Should be taken with food.

Administration Administer with food. Shake suspension well prior to administration.

Dosage Forms Excipient information presented when available (limited, particularly for generics); consult specific product labeling.

Suspension Reconstituted, Oral:

Alinia: 100 mg/5 mL (60 mL) [contains fd&c red #40, sodium benzoate; strawberry flavor]

Tablet, Oral:

Alinia: 500 mg [contains fd&c blue #2 aluminum lake, fd&c yellow #10 aluminum lake, fd&c yellow #6 aluminum lake, soybean lecithin]

◆ **Nithiodote** *see* Sodium Nitrite and Sodium Thiosulfate *on page 1920*

Nitisinone (ni TIS i known)

Brand Names: U.S. Orfadin

Index Terms NTBC

Pharmacologic Category 4-Hydroxyphenylpyruvate Dioxygenase Inhibitor

Use Treatment of hereditary tyrosinemia type 1 (HT-1) as an adjunct to dietary restriction of tyrosine and phenylalanine

Pregnancy Risk Factor C

Prescribing and Access Restrictions Distributed by Rare Disease Therapeutics, Inc; for information regarding acquisition of product, call Accredo Health Group, Inc at 1-888-454-8860

Dosage Oral: HT-1; **Note:** Must be used in conjunction with a diet restricted in tyrosine and phenylalanine.

Infants: Initial: 1 mg/kg/day in 2 divided doses

Children and Adults: Initial: 1 mg/kg/day in 2 divided doses

Dosage adjustment for inadequate response: Note: Inadequate response is defined as continued abnormal biological parameters (erythrocyte PBG-synthase activity, urine 5-ALA, and urine succinylacetone) despite treatment. If the aforementioned parameters are not available, may use urine succinylacetone, liver function tests, alpha-fetoprotein, serum tyrosine, and serum phenylalanine to evaluate response (exceptions may include during initiation of therapy and exacerbations).

Abnormal biological parameters at 1 month: Increase dose to 1.5 mg/kg/day

Abnormal biological parameters at 3 months: Further increase to maximum dose of 2 mg/kg/day

Dosage adjustment in renal impairment: No dosage adjustment provided in manufacturer's labeling (has not been studied).

Dosage adjustment in hepatic impairment: No dosage adjustment provided in manufacturer's labeling (has not been studied).

Additional Information Complete prescribing information should be consulted for additional detail.

Dosage Forms Excipient information presented when available (limited, particularly for generics); consult specific product labeling.

Capsule, Oral:

Orfadin: 2 mg, 5 mg, 10 mg

◆ **Nitoman (Can)** *see* Tetrabenazine *on page 2033*

◆ **Nitro-Bid** *see* Nitroglycerin *on page 1466*

◆ **Nitro-Dur** *see* Nitroglycerin *on page 1466*

Nitrofurantoin (nye troe fyoor AN toyn)

Brand Names: U.S. Furadantin; Macrobid; Macrodantin

Brand Names: Canada Apo-Nitrofurantoin®; Macrobid®; Macrodantin®; Novo-Furantoin; Teva-Nitrofurantoin

Pharmacologic Category Antibiotic, Miscellaneous

Additional Appendix Information

Beers Criteria – Potentially Inappropriate Medications for Geriatrics *on page 2368*

Use Prevention and treatment of urinary tract infections caused by susceptible strains of *E. coli*, *S. aureus*, *Enterococcus*, *Klebsiella*, and *Enterobacter*

Pregnancy Risk Factor B (contraindicated at term)

Pregnancy Considerations Adverse effects have not been observed in animal reproduction studies. Nitrofurantoin crosses the placenta (Perry, 1967) and maternal serum concentrations may be lower in pregnancy (Philipson, 1979). Current studies evaluating maternal use of nitrofurantoin during pregnancy and the development of birth defects have had mixed results (ACOG, 2011). An increased risk of neonatal jaundice was observed following maternal nitrofurantoin use during the last 30 days of pregnancy (Nordeng, 2013). Nitrofurantoin may be used to treat infections in pregnant women; use during the first trimester should be limited to situations where no alternative therapies are available. Prescriptions should be written when clinically appropriate and for the shortest effective duration for confirmed infections (ACOG, 2011). Nitrofurantoin is contraindicated in pregnant patients at term (38-42 weeks gestation), during labor and delivery, or when the onset of labor is imminent due to the possibility of hemolytic anemia in the neonate. Alternative antibiotics should be considered in pregnant women with G-6-PD deficiency (Nordeng, 2013).

Breast-Feeding Considerations Trace amounts of nitrofurantoin can be detected in breast milk. Due to the potential for serious adverse reactions in the nursing infant, the manufacturer recommends a decision be made whether to discontinue nursing or to discontinue the drug, taking into account the importance of treatment to the mother. The therapeutic use of nitrofurantoin is contraindicated in neonates (<1 month of age) due to the possibility of hemolytic anemia caused by immature erythrocyte enzyme systems. In case reports, diarrhea was reported in two nursing infants and decreased milk volume was reported by one mother (dose, duration, relationship to breast-feeding not provided) (Ito, 1993).

Contraindications Hypersensitivity to nitrofurantoin or any component of the formulation; infants <1 month (due to the possibility of hemolytic anemia); pregnancy at term (38-42 weeks gestation), during labor and delivery, or when the onset of labor is imminent; use in patients with a history of cholestatic jaundice or hepatic impairment with previous nitrofurantoin therapy; anuria, oliguria or significant renal impairment (clinically significant elevated serum creatinine or Cl_{cr} <60 mL/minute). **Note:** The manufacturer's contraindication in patients with Cl_{cr} <60 mL/minute has been challenged in the literature; limited data suggest that an alternative creatinine clearance threshold may be considered (Oplinger, 2013).

Warnings/Precautions Use with caution in patients with G6PD deficiency (increased risk of hemolytic anemia). Urinary nitrofurantoin concentrations are variable in patients with impaired renal function. The manufacturer contraindicates use in Cl_{cr} <60 mL/minute; however, limited data suggest clinicians may consider using a lower threshold of Cl_{cr} <40 mL/minute when treatment is short term (≤1 week) for an uncomplicated UTI (Oplinger, 2013).

Use with caution if prolonged therapy is anticipated due to possible pulmonary toxicity. Acute, subacute, or chronic (usually after 6 months of therapy) pulmonary reactions (possibly fatal) have been observed in patients treated with nitrofurantoin; if these occur, discontinue therapy immediately; monitor closely for malaise, dyspnea, cough, fever, radiologic evidence of diffuse interstitial pneumonitis or fibrosis. Rare, but severe and sometimes fatal hepatic reactions (eg, cholestatic jaundice, hepatitis, hepatic necrosis) have been associated with nitrofurantoin (onset may be insidious); discontinue immediately if hepatitis occurs. Monitor liver function test periodically. Has been associated with peripheral neuropathy (rare); risk may be increased in patients with anemia, renal impairment, diabetes, vitamin B deficiency, debilitating disease, or electrolyte imbalance; use caution. Potentially significant drug-drug interactions may exist, requiring dose or frequency adjustment, additional monitoring, and/or selection of alternative therapy. Use in the elderly, particularly females receiving long-term prophylaxis for recurrent UTIs, has been associated with an increased risk of hepatic and pulmonary toxicity, and peripheral neuropathy. In the elderly, avoid use for long-term suppression due to potential for pulmonary toxicity and availability of safer alternative agents (Beers Criteria). Use in the elderly, particularly females receiving long-term prophylaxis for recurrent UTIs, has also been associated with an increased risk of hepatic toxicity and peripheral neuropathy; monitor closely for toxicities during use. Prolonged use may result in fungal or bacterial superinfection, including *C. difficile*-associated diarrhea (CDAD) and pseudomembranous colitis; CDAD has been observed >2 months postantibiotic treatment. Use is contraindicated in children <1 month of age (at increased risk for hemolytic anemia). Not indicated for the treatment of pyelonephritis or perinephric abscesses.

Adverse Reactions Frequency not defined.

Cardiovascular: Cyanosis, ECG changes (nonspecific ST/T wave changes, bundle branch block)

Central nervous system: Bulging fontanels (infants), chills, confusion, depression, dizziness, drowsiness, fever, headache, malaise, pseudotumor cerebri, psychotic reaction, vertigo

Dermatologic: Alopecia, angioedema, erythema multiforme, exfoliative dermatitis, pruritus, rash (eczematous, erythematous, maculopapular), Stevens-Johnson syndrome, urticaria

Endocrine & metabolic: Hyperphosphatemia

Gastrointestinal: Abdominal pain, anorexia, *C. difficile* colitis, constipation, diarrhea, dyspepsia, flatulence, nausea, pancreatitis, pseudomembranous colitis, sialadenitis, vomiting

Genitourinary: Urine discoloration (brown)

Hematologic: Agranulocytosis, aplastic anemia, eosinophilia, glucose-6-phosphate dehydrogenase deficiency anemia, granulocytopenia, hemoglobin decreased, hemolytic anemia, leukopenia, megaloblastic anemia, thrombocytopenia

Hepatic: Hepatitis, hepatic necrosis, transaminases increased, jaundice (cholestatic)

Neuromuscular & skeletal: Arthralgia, myalgia, numbness, paresthesia, peripheral neuropathy, weakness

Ocular: Amblyopia, nystagmus, optic neuritis

Respiratory: Cough, dyspnea, pneumonitis, pulmonary fibrosis (with long-term use), pulmonary infiltration

Miscellaneous: Acute pulmonary reaction (symptoms include chills, chest pain, cough, dyspnea, fever, and eosinophilia), anaphylaxis, hypersensitivity (including acute pulmonary hypersensitivity), lupus-like syndrome, superinfections (eg, *Pseudomonas* or *Candida*)

Drug Interactions

Metabolism/Transport Effects None known.

Avoid Concomitant Use

Avoid concomitant use of Nitrofurantoin with any of the following: BCG; Magnesium Trisilicate; Norfloxacin

Increased Effect/Toxicity

Nitrofurantoin may increase the levels/effects of: Eplerenone; Prilocaine; Sodium Nitrite; Spironolactone

The levels/effects of Nitrofurantoin may be increased by: Nitric Oxide; Probenecid

Decreased Effect

Nitrofurantoin may decrease the levels/effects of: BCG; Norfloxacin; Sodium Picosulfate; Typhoid Vaccine

The levels/effects of Nitrofurantoin may be decreased by: Magnesium Trisilicate

Ethanol/Nutrition/Herb Interactions

Ethanol: Avoid ethanol (may increase CNS depression).

Food: Nitrofurantoin serum concentrations may be increased if taken with food.

Storage/Stability Store at 20°C to 25°C (68°F to 77°F); excursions permitted to 15°C to 30°C (59°F to 86°F). Protect oral suspension from light.

Mechanism of Action Inhibits several bacterial enzyme systems including acetyl coenzyme A interfering with metabolism and possibly cell wall synthesis

Pharmacodynamics/Kinetics

Absorption: Well absorbed; macrocrystalline form absorbed more slowly due to slower dissolution (causes less GI distress)

Distribution: V_d: 0.8 L/kg

Protein binding: 60% to 90%

Metabolism: Body tissues (except plasma) metabolize 60% of drug to inactive metabolites

Bioavailability: Increased with food

Half-life elimination: 20-60 minutes; prolonged with renal impairment

Excretion:
Suspension: Urine (~40%) and feces (small amounts) as metabolites and unchanged drug
Macrocrystals: Urine (20% to 25% as unchanged drug)

Dosage Oral:
Children >1 month:
UTI treatment (Furadantin®, Macrodantin®): 5-7 mg/kg/day in divided doses every 6 hours; maximum: 400 mg/day. Administer for 7 days or at least 3 days after obtaining sterile urine
UTI prophylaxis (Furadantin®, Macrodantin®): 1-2 mg/kg/day in divided doses every 12-24 hours; maximum: 100 mg/day
Children >12 years: UTI treatment (Macrobid®): 100 mg twice daily for 7 days
Adults:
UTI treatment:
Furadantin®, Macrodantin®: 50-100 mg/dose every 6 hours; administer for 7 days or at least 3 days after obtaining sterile urine
Macrobid®: 100 mg twice daily for 7 days
UTI prophylaxis (Furadantin®, Macrodantin®): 50-100 mg/dose at bedtime
Elderly: Avoid use; alternative agents preferred.

Dosage adjustment in renal impairment:
Cl_{cr} ≥60 mL/minute: No dosage adjustment provided in manufacturer's labeling.
Cl_{cr} <60 mL/minute: Use is contraindicated. **Note:** Although more evidence is needed, limited data suggest clinicians consider use in patients with Cl_{cr} ≥40 mL/minute when treatment is short term (≤1 week) for an uncomplicated UTI (Oplinger, 2013).

Dosage adjustment in hepatic impairment: No dosage adjustment provided in manufacturer's labeling. Contraindicated in patients with a previous history of cholestatic jaundice or hepatic dysfunction associated with nitrofurantoin.

Dietary Considerations Take with meals to improve absorption and decrease adverse effects.

Administration Administer with meals to improve absorption and decrease adverse effects; suspension may be mixed with water, milk, fruit juice, or infant formula. Shake suspension well before use.

Monitoring Parameters Signs of pulmonary reaction; signs of numbness or tingling of the extremities; CBC, periodic liver function tests, periodic renal function tests with long-term use

Test Interactions False-positive urine glucose (Benedict's and Fehling's methods); no false positives with enzymatic tests

Dosage Forms Excipient information presented when available (limited, particularly for generics); consult specific product labeling.
Capsule, Oral:
Macrobid: 100 mg [contains brilliant blue fcf (fd&c blue #1), fd&c red #40, fd&c yellow #10 (quinoline yellow)]
Macrodantin: 25 mg
Macrodantin: 50 mg, 100 mg [contains fd&c yellow #10 (quinoline yellow), fd&c yellow #6 (sunset yellow)]
Generic: 50 mg, 100 mg
Suspension, Oral:
Furadantin: 25 mg/5 mL (230 mL)
Generic: 25 mg/5 mL (230 mL, 240 mL)

◆ Nitrogen Mustard *see* Mechlorethamine (Systemic) *on page 1274*

Nitroglycerin (nye troe GLI ser in)

Brand Names: U.S. Minitran; Nitro-Bid; Nitro-Dur; Nitro-Time; Nitrolingual; NitroMist; Nitrostat; Rectiv

Brand Names: Canada Minitran; Mylan-Nitro Sublingual Spray; Nitro-Dur; Nitroglycerin Injection, USP; Nitrol; Nitrostat; Rho-Nitro Pump Spray; Transderm-Nitro; Trinipatch

Index Terms Glyceryl Trinitrate; Nitroglycerol; NTG; Tridil

Pharmacologic Category Antianginal Agent; Antidote, Extravasation; Vasodilator

Additional Appendix Information
Nitrates *on page 2305*
Vasoactive Agents, Intravenous *on page 2315*

Use Treatment or prevention of angina pectoris
Intravenous (I.V.) administration: Treatment or prevention of angina pectoris; acute decompensated heart failure (especially when associated with acute myocardial infarction); perioperative hypertension (especially during cardiovascular surgery); induction of intraoperative hypotension
Intra-anal administration (Rectiv ointment): Treatment of moderate-to-severe pain associated with chronic anal fissure

Unlabeled Use Short-term management of pulmonary hypertension (I.V.); esophageal spastic disorders; uterine relaxation; treatment of sympathomimetic vasopressor extravasation injury (alternative to phentolamine)

Pregnancy Risk Factor C

Pregnancy Considerations Adverse events were not observed in animal reproduction studies conducted using the ointment. Nitroglycerin crosses the placenta (David, 2000). Concentrations following application of a transdermal patch 0.4 mg/hour were low but detectable in the fetal serum (fetal/maternal ratio: 0.23) (Bustard, 2003). Nitroglycerin may be used in pregnancy when immediate relaxation of the uterus is needed (ACOG, 2006; Axemo, 1998; Chandraharan, 2005). Intravenous nitroglycerin may be used to treat pre-eclampsia with pulmonary edema (ESG, 2011).

Breast-Feeding Considerations It is not known if nitroglycerin is excreted in breast milk. The manufacturer recommends that caution be exercised when administering nitroglycerin to nursing women. Information related to the use of nitroglycerin and breast-feeding is limited (Böttiger, 2010; O'Sullivan, 2011).

Contraindications Hypersensitivity to organic nitrates or any component of the formulation (includes adhesives for transdermal product); concurrent use with phosphodiesterase-5 (PDE-5) inhibitors (sildenafil, tadalafil, or vardenafil); increased intracranial pressure; severe anemia

Additional contraindications for I.V. product: Constrictive pericarditis; pericardial tamponade; restrictive cardiomyopathy

Note: According to the 2010 American Heart Association guidelines for the treatment of acute coronary syndromes, nitrates are considered contraindicated in the following conditions: Hypotension (SBP <90 mm Hg or ≥30 mm Hg below baseline), extreme bradycardia (<50 bpm), tachycardia in the absence of heart failure (>100 bpm), and right ventricular infarction (O'Connor, 2010).

Warnings/Precautions Severe hypotension can occur. Use with caution in volume depletion, moderate hypotension, and extreme caution with inferior wall MI and suspected right ventricular involvement. Use considered contraindicated in patients with severe hypotension (SBP <90 mm Hg or ≥30 mm Hg below baseline), extreme bradycardia (<50 bpm), and right ventricular MI (O'Connor, 2010). Avoid use in patients with hypertrophic cardiomyopathy (HCM) with outflow tract obstruction; nitrates may reduce preload, exacerbating obstruction and cause hypotension or syncope and/or worsening of heart failure (Gersh, 2011).

Paradoxical bradycardia and increased angina pectoris can accompany hypotension. Orthostatic hypotension can also occur. Ethanol can accentuate this. Tolerance does develop to nitrates and appropriate dosing is needed to minimize this (drug-free interval). Avoid use of long-acting agents in acute MI or acute HF; cannot easily reverse effects. Nitrates may aggravate angina caused by hypertrophic cardiomyopathy. Nitroglycerin may precipitate or aggravate increased intracranial pressure and subsequently may worsen clinical outcomes in patients with neurologic injury (eg, intracranial hemorrhage, traumatic brain injury). Nitroglycerin transdermal patches may contain conducting metal (eg, aluminum); remove patch prior to MRI. Potentially significant drug-drug interactions may exist, requiring dose or frequency adjustment, additional monitoring, and/or selection of alternative therapy. Avoid concurrent use with PDE-5 inhibitors (eg, sildenafil, tadalafil, vardenafil). When nitrate administration becomes medically necessary, may administer nitrates only if 24 hours have elapsed after use of sildenafil or vardenafil (48 hours after tadalafil use) (Trujillo, 2007).

Use caution when treating rectal anal fissures with nitroglycerin ointment formulation in patients with suspected or known significant cardiovascular disorders (eg, cardiomyopathies, heart failure, acute MI); intra-anal nitroglycerin administration may decrease systolic blood pressure and decrease arterial vascular resistance.

Adverse Reactions

Frequency not defined:

Cardiovascular: Flushing, hypotension, orthostatic hypotension, peripheral edema, syncope, tachycardia

Central nervous system: Headache (common), dizziness, lightheadedness

Gastrointestinal: Nausea, vomiting, xerostomia

Neuromuscular & skeletal: Paresthesia, weakness

Respiratory: Dyspnea, pharyngitis, rhinitis

Miscellaneous: Diaphoresis

<1% (Limited to important or life-threatening): Allergic reactions, anaphylactoid reaction, application site irritation (patch), blurred vision, cardiovascular collapse, contact dermatitis (ointment, patch), crescendo angina, exfoliative dermatitis, fixed drug eruption (ointment, patch), methemoglobinemia (rare; overdose), pallor, palpitation, rash, rebound hypertension, restlessness, shock, vertigo

Drug Interactions

Metabolism/Transport Effects None known.

Avoid Concomitant Use

Avoid concomitant use of Nitroglycerin with any of the following: Ergot Derivatives; Phosphodiesterase 5 Inhibitors; Riociguat

Increased Effect/Toxicity

Nitroglycerin may increase the levels/effects of: Ergot Derivatives; Hypotensive Agents; Prilocaine; Riociguat; Rosiglitazone; Sodium Nitrite

The levels/effects of Nitroglycerin may be increased by: Alfuzosin; Nitric Oxide; Phosphodiesterase 5 Inhibitors

Decreased Effect

Nitroglycerin may decrease the levels/effects of: Alteplase; Heparin

The levels/effects of Nitroglycerin may be decreased by: Ergot Derivatives

Ethanol/Nutrition/Herb Interactions

Ethanol: Avoid ethanol (may increase the hypotensive effects of nitroglycerin). Monitor.

Herb/Nutraceutical: Avoid bayberry, blue cohosh, cayenne, ephedra, ginger, ginseng (American), kola, licorice (may worsen hypertension). Avoid black cohosh, California poppy, coleus, golden seal, hawthorn, mistletoe, periwinkle, quinine, shepherd's purse (may cause hypotension).

Storage/Stability

I.V. solution: Doses should be made in glass bottles, EXCEL® or PAB® containers. Adsorption occurs to soft plastic (eg, PVC). Nitroglycerin diluted in D_5W or NS in glass containers is physically and chemically stable for 48 hours at room temperature and 7 days under refrigeration. In D_5W or NS in EXCEL®/PAB® containers it is physically and chemically stable for 24 hours at room temperature.

Store sublingual tablets, topical ointment, and rectal ointment in tightly closed containers at 20°C to 25°C (68°F to 77°F); slow release capsules at 20°C to 25°C (68°F to 77°F); translingual spray and transdermal patch at 15°C to 30°C (59°F to 86°F).

Mechanism of Action Nitroglycerin forms free radical nitric oxide. In smooth muscle, nitric oxide activates guanylate cyclase which increases guanosine 3'5' monophosphate (cGMP) leading to dephosphorylation of myosin light chains and smooth muscle relaxation. Produces a vasodilator effect on the peripheral veins and arteries with more prominent effects on the veins. Primarily reduces cardiac oxygen demand by decreasing preload (left ventricular end-diastolic pressure); may modestly reduce afterload; dilates coronary arteries and improves collateral flow to ischemic regions. For use in rectal fissures, intra-anal administration results in decreased sphincter tone and intra-anal pressure.

Pharmacodynamics/Kinetics

Onset of action: Sublingual tablet: 1-3 minutes; Translingual spray: Similar to sublingual tablet; Extended release: ~60 minutes; Topical: 15-30 minutes; Transdermal: ~30 minutes; I.V.: Immediate

Peak effect: Sublingual tablet: 5 minutes; Translingual spray: 4-10 minutes; Extended release: 2.5-4 hours; Topical: ~60 minutes; Transdermal: 120 minutes; I.V.: Immediate

Duration: Sublingual tablet: At least 25 minutes; Translingual spray: Similar to sublingual tablet; Extended release: 4-8 hours (Gibbons, 2002); Topical: 7 hours; Transdermal: 10-12 hours; I.V.: 3-5 minutes

Distribution: V_d: ~3 L/kg

Protein binding: 60%

Metabolism: Extensive first-pass effect; metabolized hepatically to glycerol di- and mononitrate metabolites via liver reductase enzyme; subsequent metabolism to glycerol and organic nitrate; nonhepatic metabolism via red blood cells and vascular walls also occurs

Half-life elimination: ~1-4 minutes

Excretion: Urine (as inactive metabolites)

Dosage Note: Hemodynamic and antianginal tolerance often develop within 24-48 hours of continuous nitrate administration. Nitrate-free interval (10-12 hours/day) is recommended to avoid tolerance development; gradually decrease dose in patients receiving NTG for prolonged period to avoid withdrawal reaction.

Extravasation (sympathomimetic vasopressors), treatment (alternative to phentolamine; unlabeled use): **Based on limited data in neonates; optimal dosing has not been established:** Pediatrics and Adults: Topical 2% ointment: 4 mm/kg applied as a thin ribbon to the affected area has been reported in a case series; after 8 hours, if no improvement, the dose may be reapplied to the affected site (Wong, 1992). Application of a 1-inch strip on the affected site has also been described to be successful (Denkler, 1989); may also be considered for adults as an alternative to phentolamine (Hurst, 2004).

Angina/coronary artery disease: Adults:

Oral: Initial: 2.5-6.5 mg 3-4 times/day; may titrate up to 26 mg 4 times/day

I.V.: 5 mcg/minute, increase by 5 mcg/minute every 3-5 minutes to 20 mcg/minute; if no response at 20 mcg/minute, may increase by 10-20 mcg/minute every 3-5 minutes (generally accepted maximum dose: 400 mcg/minute)

Sublingual: 0.3-0.6 mg every 5 minutes for maximum of 3 doses in 15 minutes; may also use prophylactically 5-10 minutes prior to activities which may provoke an attack

Topical 2% ointment: 1/2" upon rising and 1/2" 6 hours later; if necessary, the dose may be doubled to 1" and subsequently doubled again to 2" if response is inadequate. Doses of 1/2" to 2" were used in clinical trials. Recommended maximum: 2 doses/day; include a nitrate free-interval ~10-12 hours/day.

Topical patch, transdermal: Initial: 0.2-0.4 mg/hour, titrate to 0.4-0.8 mg/hour; tolerance is minimized by using a patch-on period of 12-14 hours and patch-off period of 10-12 hours

Translingual: 1-2 sprays onto or under tongue every 3-5 minutes for maximum of 3 doses in 15 minutes, may also be used prophylactically 5-10 minutes prior to activities which may provoke an angina attack

Anal fissure, chronic (0.4% ointment): Adults: Intra-anal: 1 inch (equals 1.5 mg of nitroglycerin) every 12 hours for up to 3 weeks

Esophageal spastic disorders (unlabeled use): Adults: Sublingual: 0.3-0.6 mg (Swamy, 1977)

Uterine relaxation (unlabeled use): Adults: I.V. bolus: 100-200 mcg; may repeat dose every 2 minutes as necessary (Axemo, 1998; Chandraharan, 2005)

Elderly: In general, dose selection should be cautious, usually starting at the low end of the dosing range

Dosage adjustment in renal impairment: No dosage adjustment provided in manufacturer's labeling.

Dosage adjustment in hepatic impairment: No dosage adjustment provided in manufacturer's labeling.

Usual Infusion Concentrations: Pediatric Note: Premixed solutions available

I.V. infusion: 100 **mcg**/mL, 200 **mcg**/mL, or 400 **mcg**/mL

Usual Infusion Concentrations: Adult Note: Premixed solutions available

I.V. infusion: 50 mg in 250 mL (concentration: 200 **mcg**/mL) **or** 100 mg in 250 mL (concentration: 400 **mcg**/mL) of D_5W

Administration

I.V.: Prepare in glass bottles, EXCEL® or PAB® containers. Adsorption occurs to soft plastic (eg, PVC); use administration sets intended for nitroglycerin. Administer via infusion pump.

Intra-anal ointment: Using a finger covering (eg, plastic wrap, surgical glove, finger cot), place finger beside 1 inch measuring guide on the box and squeeze ointment the length of the measuring line directly onto covered finger. Insert ointment into the anal canal using the covered finger up to first finger joint (do not insert further than the first finger joint) and apply ointment around the side of the anal canal. If intra-anal application is too painful, may apply the ointment to the outside of the anus. Wash hands following application.

Oral (extended release capsule): Swallow whole. Do not chew, break, or crush. Take with a full glass of water.

Sublingual: Do not crush sublingual product (tablet). Place under tongue and allow to dissolve.

Topical ointment: Wash hands prior to and after use. Application site should be clean, dry, and hair-free. Apply to chest or back with the applicator or dose-measuring paper. Spread in a thin layer over a 2.25 x 3.5 inch area. Do not rub into skin. Tape applicator into place.

Drug extravasation management, (treatment), sympathomimetic vasopressors (alternative to phentolamine) (unlabeled use): Stop vesicant infusion immediately and disconnect I.V. line (leave needle/cannula in place); gently aspirate extravasated solution from the I.V. line (do **NOT** flush the line); remove needle/cannula; elevate extremity. Apply nitroglycerin ointment as a thin ribbon to the affected area (Wong, 1992). May also apply dry warm compresses (Hurst, 2004).

Topical patch, transdermal: Application site should be clean, dry and hair-free. Remove patch after 12-14 hours. Rotate patch sites.

Translingual spray: Do not shake container. Prior to initial use, the pump must be primed by spraying 5 times (Nitrolingual®) or 10 times (Nitromist®) into the air. Priming sprays should be directed away from patient and others. Release spray onto or under tongue. Close mouth after administration. Do not rinse the mouth for at least 5-10 minutes. The end of the pump should be covered by the fluid in the bottle. If pump is unused for 6 weeks, a single priming spray (Nitrolingual®) or 2 priming sprays (Nitromist®) should be completed.

Monitoring Parameters Blood pressure, heart rate; consult individual institutional policies and procedures

Test Interactions I.V. formulation: Due to propylene glycol content, triglyceride assays dependent on glycerol oxidase may be falsely elevated.

Additional Information I.V. preparations contain alcohol and/or propylene glycol; may need to use nitrate-free interval (10-12 hours/day) to avoid tolerance development. Tolerance may possibly be reversed with acetylcysteine; gradually decrease dose in patients receiving NTG for prolonged period to avoid withdrawal reaction.

Concomitant use of sildenafil (Viagra®) or other phosphodiesterase-5 enzyme inhibitors (PDE-5) may precipitate acute hypotension, myocardial infarction, or death. Nitrates used in right ventricular infarction may induce acute hypotension. Nitrate use in severe pericardial effusion may reduce cardiac filling pressure and precipitate cardiac tamponade. In the management of heart failure, the combination of isosorbide dinitrate and hydralazine confers beneficial effects on disease progression and cardiac outcomes.

Dosage Forms Excipient information presented when available (limited, particularly for generics); consult specific product labeling.

Aerosol Solution, Translingual:

NitroMist: 400 mcg/spray (4.1 g, 8.5 g) [contains menthol]

Generic: 400 mcg/spray (4.1 g, 8.5 g)

Capsule Extended Release, Oral:

Nitro-Time: 2.5 mg [contains brilliant blue fcf (fd&c blue #1), fd&c red #40, fd&c yellow #10 (quinoline yellow)]

Nitro-Time: 6.5 mg [contains brilliant blue fcf (fd&c blue #1), fd&c yellow #10 (quinoline yellow), fd&c yellow #6 (sunset yellow)]

Nitro-Time: 9 mg [contains fd&c yellow #10 (quinoline yellow), fd&c yellow #6 (sunset yellow)]

Generic: 2.5 mg, 6.5 mg, 9 mg

Ointment, Rectal:

Rectiv: 0.4% (30 g) [contains propylene glycol]

Ointment, Transdermal:

Nitro-Bid: 2% (1 g, 30 g, 60 g)

Patch 24 Hour, Transdermal:

Minitran: 0.1 mg/hr (30 ea); 0.2 mg/hr (30 ea); 0.4 mg/hr (30 ea); 0.6 mg/hr (30 ea)

Nitro-Dur: 0.1 mg/hr (30 ea, 100 ea); 0.2 mg/hr (30 ea, 100 ea); 0.3 mg/hr (30 ea, 100 ea); 0.4 mg/hr (30 ea, 100 ea); 0.6 mg/hr (30 ea, 100 ea); 0.8 mg/hr (30 ea, 100 ea)

Generic: 0.1 mg/hr (30 ea, 4350 ea); 0.2 mg/hr (30 ea, 4350 ea); 0.4 mg/hr (30 ea, 4350 ea); 0.6 mg/hr (30 ea, 4350 ea)

Solution, Intravenous:

Generic: 25 mg (250 mL); 50 mg (250 mL, 500 mL); 100 mg (250 mL); 200 mg (500 mL); 5 mg/mL (10 mL)

Solution, Translingual:
Nitrolingual: 0.4 mg/spray (4.9 g, 12 g) [contains alcohol, usp]
Generic: 0.4 mg/spray (4.9 g, 12 g)
Tablet Sublingual, Sublingual:
Nitrostat: 0.3 mg, 0.4 mg, 0.6 mg

- **Nitroglycerin Injection, USP (Can)** *see* Nitroglycerin *on page 1466*
- **Nitroglycerol** *see* Nitroglycerin *on page 1466*
- **Nitrol (Can)** *see* Nitroglycerin *on page 1466*
- **Nitrolingual** *see* Nitroglycerin *on page 1466*
- **NitroMist** *see* Nitroglycerin *on page 1466*
- **Nitropress** *see* Nitroprusside *on page 1469*

Nitroprusside (nye troe PRUS ide)

Brand Names: U.S. Nitropress
Brand Names: Canada Nipride®
Index Terms Nitroprusside Sodium; Sodium Nitroferricyanide; Sodium Nitroprusside
Pharmacologic Category Antihypertensive; Vasodilator
Additional Appendix Information
Vasoactive Agents, Intravenous *on page 2315*
Use Management of hypertensive crises; acute decompensated heart failure (HF); used for controlled hypotension to reduce bleeding during surgery
Unlabeled Use Management of hypertension during acute ischemic stroke
Pregnancy Risk Factor C
Pregnancy Considerations Animal studies have shown that nitroprusside may cross the placental barrier and result in fetal cyanide levels that are dose-related to maternal nitroprusside levels. However, information related to use in pregnancy is limited.
Breast-Feeding Considerations It is not known if nitroprusside is excreted in breast milk. Due to the potential for serious adverse reactions in the nursing infant, a decision should be made whether to discontinue nursing or to discontinue the drug, taking into account the importance of treatment to the mother.
Contraindications Treatment of compensatory hypertension (aortic coarctation, arteriovenous shunting); to produce controlled hypotension during surgery in patients with known inadequate cerebral circulation or in moribund patients requiring emergency surgery; high output heart failure associated with reduced systemic vascular resistance (eg, septic shock); congenital optic atrophy or tobacco amblyopia
Warnings/Precautions [U.S. Boxed Warning] Excessive hypotension resulting in compromised perfusion of vital organs may occur; continuous blood pressure monitoring by experienced personnel is required. Except when used briefly or at low (<2 mcg/kg/minute) infusion rates, nitroprusside gives rise to large cyanide quantities. Do not use the maximum dose for more than 10 minutes; if blood pressure is not controlled by the maximum rate (ie, 10 mcg/kg/minute) after 10 minutes, discontinue infusion. Monitor for cyanide toxicity via acid-base balance and venous oxygen concentration; however, clinicians should note that these indicators may not always reliably indicate cyanide toxicity. Patients at risk of cyanide toxicity include those who are malnourished, have hepatic impairment, or those undergoing cardiopulmonary bypass, or therapeutic hypothermia (Rindone, 1992). Discontinue use of nitroprusside if signs and/or symptoms of cyanide toxicity (eg, metabolic acidosis, decreased oxygen saturation, bradycardia, confusion, convulsions) occur. Although not routinely done, sodium thiosulfate has been co-administered with nitroprusside using a 10:1 ratio of sodium thiosulfate to nitroprusside when higher doses of nitroprusside are used (eg, 4-10 mcg/kg/minute) for extended periods of time in order to prevent cyanide toxicity (Varon, 2008; Shulz, 2010); thiocyanate toxicity may still occur with this approach (Rindone, 1992). The use of other agents (eg, clevidipine, labetalol, nicardipine) should be considered if blood pressure is not controlled with nitroprusside. Use the lowest end of the dosage range with renal impairment. Cyanide toxicity may occur in patients with decreased liver function. Thiocyanate toxicity occurs in patients with renal impairment or those on prolonged infusions.

When nitroprusside is used for controlled hypotension during surgery, correct pre-existing anemia and hypovolemia prior to use when possible. Use with extreme caution in patients with elevated intracranial pressure (head trauma, cerebral hemorrhage), severe renal impairment, hepatic failure, hypothyroidism. **[U.S. Boxed Warning]: Solution must be further diluted with 5% dextrose in water. Do not administer by direct injection.**

Adverse Reactions Frequency not defined.
Cardiovascular: Bradycardia, ECG changes, flushing, hypotension (excessive), palpitation, substernal distress, tachycardia
Central nervous system: Apprehension, dizziness, headache, intracranial pressure increased, restlessness
Dermatologic: Rash
Endocrine & metabolic: Metabolic acidosis (secondary to cyanide toxicity), hypothyroidism
Gastrointestinal: Abdominal pain, ileus, nausea, retching, vomiting
Hematologic: Methemoglobinemia, platelet aggregation decreased
Local: Injection site irritation
Neuromuscular & skeletal: Hyperreflexia (secondary to thiocyanate toxicity), muscle twitching
Ocular: Miosis (secondary to thiocyanate toxicity)
Otic: Tinnitus (secondary to thiocyanate toxicity)
Respiratory: Hyperoxemia (secondary to cyanide toxicity)
Miscellaneous: Cyanide toxicity, diaphoresis, thiocyanate toxicity

Drug Interactions
Metabolism/Transport Effects None known.
Avoid Concomitant Use There are no known interactions where it is recommended to avoid concomitant use.
Increased Effect/Toxicity
Nitroprusside may increase the levels/effects of: Amifostine; Antihypertensives; Hypotensive Agents; Obinutuzumab; Prilocaine; RiTUXimab; Sodium Nitrite

The levels/effects of Nitroprusside may be increased by: Alfuzosin; Brimonidine (Topical); Calcium Channel Blockers; Diazoxide; Herbs (Hypotensive Properties); MAO Inhibitors; Nitric Oxide; Pentoxifylline; Phosphodiesterase 5 Inhibitors; Prostacyclin Analogues
Decreased Effect
The levels/effects of Nitroprusside may be decreased by: Herbs (Hypertensive Properties); Methylphenidate; Yohimbine

Preparation for Administration
Prior to administration, nitroprusside sodium should be further diluted by diluting 50 mg in 250-1000 mL of D_5W (preferred), LR, or NS.
Use only clear solutions; solutions of nitroprusside exhibit a color described as brownish, brown, brownish-pink, light orange, and straw. Solutions are highly sensitive to light. Exposure to light causes decomposition, resulting in a highly colored solution of orange, dark brown or blue. **A blue color indicates almost complete decomposition.** Do not use discolored solutions (eg, blue, green, red) or solutions in which particulate matter is visible.

Prepared solutions should be wrapped with aluminum foil or other opaque material to protect from light (do as soon as possible).

Storage/Stability Store the intact vial at 20°C to 25°C (68°F to 77°F). Protect from light.

Stability of parenteral admixture at room temperature (25°C) and at refrigeration temperature (4°C) is 24 hours.

Mechanism of Action Causes peripheral vasodilation by direct action on venous and arteriolar smooth muscle, thus reducing peripheral resistance; will increase cardiac output by decreasing afterload; reduces aortal and left ventricular impedance

Pharmacodynamics/Kinetics

Onset of action: Hypotensive effect: <2 minutes

Duration: Hypotensive effect: 1-10 minutes

Metabolism: Nitroprusside combines with hemoglobin to produce cyanide and cyanmethemoglobin. Cyanide detoxification occurs via rhodanase-mediated conversion of cyanide to thiocyanate; rhodanase couples cyanide molecules to sulfane sulfur groups from a sulfur donor (eg, thiosulfate, cystine, cysteine). This process has limited capacity and may become overwhelmed with large exposures once sulfur donor supplies are exhausted resulting in toxicity.

Half-life elimination: Nitroprusside, circulatory: ~2 minutes; Thiocyanate, elimination: ~3 days (may be doubled or tripled in renal failure)

Excretion: Urine (as thiocyanate)

Dosage I.V.:

Children: Acute hypertension: Initial: 0.3-0.5 mcg/kg/minute; may be titrated every few minutes to achieve desired hemodynamic effect; maximum dose: 10 mcg/kg/minute (Hegenbarth, 2008; NHBPEP, 2005). Doses ≥1.8 mcg/kg/minute are associated with increased cyanide concentration in pediatric patients (Moffett, 2008); monitor cyanide levels with prolonged use (eg, >72 hours) (NHBPEP, 2005).

Adults:

Acute hypertension: Initial: 0.25-0.3 mcg/kg/minute; may be titrated by 0.5 mcg/kg/minute every few minutes to achieve desired hemodynamic effect (JNC 7; Rhoney, 2009); usual dose: 3 mcg/kg/minute; maximum dose: 10 mcg/kg/minute. When administered in doses >3 mcg/kg/minute for prolonged periods of time (eg, 3-4 days), thiocyanate levels should be monitored daily.

Acute decompensated heart failure: Initial: 5-10 **mcg/minute**; may be titrated rapidly (eg, up to every 5 minutes) to achieve desired hemodynamic effect; usual dosage range: 5-300 **mcg/minute**. Doses >400 **mcg/minute** are not recommended due to minimal added benefit and increased risk for thiocyanate toxicity (HFSA, 2010).

Dosage adjustment in renal impairment: No dosage adjustment provided in manufacturer's labeling. However, use in patients with renal impairment may lead to the accumulation of thiocyanate and subsequent toxicity; limit use.

Dosage adjustment in hepatic impairment: No dosage adjustment provided in manufacturer's labeling; due to the risk of cyanide toxicity, use with caution.

Usual Infusion Concentrations: Pediatric I.V. infusion: 100 **mcg**/mL **or** 200 **mcg**/mL

Usual Infusion Concentrations: Adult I.V. infusion: 50 mg in 250 mL (concentration: 200 **mcg**/mL) **or** 100 mg in 250 mL (concentration: 400 **mcg**/mL) of D_5W

Administration I.V. infusion only; infusion pump required; must be diluted prior to administration; not for direct injection. Due to potential for excessive hypotension, continuously monitor patient's blood pressure during therapy.

Monitoring Parameters Blood pressure, heart rate (cardiac monitor and blood pressure monitor required); monitor for cyanide and thiocyanate toxicity; monitor venous oxygen saturation; monitor acid-base status as acidosis can be the earliest sign of cyanide toxicity; monitor thiocyanate levels if requiring prolonged infusion (>3 days) or dose >3 mcg/kg/minute or patient has renal dysfunction; monitor cyanide blood levels (if available with appropriate turnaround time) in patients with decreased hepatic function

Consult individual institutional policies and procedures.

Reference Range Serum thiocyanate levels are not helpful in detecting toxicity. A level may be confirmatory if a patient is exhibiting signs and symptoms of thiocyanate toxicity. Initial signs of toxicity (eg, tinnitus) may be observed at levels >35 mcg/mL (manufacturer suggests 60 mcg/mL), but serious toxicity typically may not occur with levels <100 mcg/mL.

Dosage Forms Excipient information presented when available (limited, particularly for generics); consult specific product labeling.

Solution, Intravenous, as sodium:

Nitropress: 25 mg/mL (2 mL)

- **Nitroprusside Sodium** *see* Nitroprusside *on page 1469*
- **Nitrostat** *see* Nitroglycerin *on page 1466*
- **Nitro-Time** *see* Nitroglycerin *on page 1466*
- **Nix® (Can)** *see* Permethrin *on page 1624*

Nizatidine (ni ZA ti deen)

Brand Names: U.S. Axid; Axid AR [OTC]

Brand Names: Canada Apo-Nizatidine®; Axid®; Gen-Nizatidine; Novo-Nizatidine; Nu-Nizatidine; PMS-Nizatidine

Pharmacologic Category Histamine H_2 Antagonist

Use Treatment and maintenance of duodenal ulcer; treatment of benign gastric ulcer; treatment of gastroesophageal reflux disease (GERD)

Unlabeled Use Part of a multidrug regimen for *H. pylori* eradication to reduce the risk of duodenal ulcer recurrence

Pregnancy Risk Factor B

Dosage Oral:

Children:

<12 years: GERD (unlabeled use): 10 mg/kg/day in divided doses given twice daily; may not be as effective in children <12 years

≥12 years:

GERD: Refer to adult dosing

Adults:

Duodenal ulcer:

Treatment of active ulcer: 300 mg at bedtime or 150 mg twice daily

Maintenance of healed ulcer: 150 mg/day at bedtime

Gastric ulcer: 150 mg twice daily or 300 mg at bedtime

GERD: 150 mg twice daily

Helicobacter pylori eradication (unlabeled use): 150 mg twice daily; requires combination therapy

Dosage adjustment in renal impairment:

Active treatment:

Cl_{cr} 20-50 mL/minute: 150 mg/day

Cl_{cr} <20 mL/minute: 150 mg every other day

Maintenance treatment:

Cl_{cr} 20-50 mL/minute: 150 mg every other day

Cl_{cr} <20 mL/minute: 150 mg every 3 days

Dosage adjustment in hepatic impairment: No dosage adjustment provided in manufacturer's labeling.

Additional Information Complete prescribing information should be consulted for additional detail.

Dosage Forms Excipient information presented when available (limited, particularly for generics); consult specific product labeling.

Capsule, Oral:

Axid: 300 mg

Generic: 150 mg, 300 mg

Solution, Oral:

Axid: 15 mg/mL (480 mL) [contains methylparaben, propylparaben, saccharin sodium; bubble-gum flavor]

Generic: 15 mg/mL (473 mL, 480 mL)

Tablet, Oral:

Axid AR: 75 mg

◆ **Nizoral** *see* Ketoconazole (Systemic) *on page 1147*

◆ **Nizoral** *see* Ketoconazole (Topical) *on page 1149*

◆ **Nizoral A-D [OTC]** *see* Ketoconazole (Topical) *on page 1149*

◆ **N-Methylhydrazine** *see* Procarbazine *on page 1720*

◆ **N-methylnaltrexone Bromide** *see* Methylnaltrexone *on page 1335*

◆ **NN2211** *see* Liraglutide *on page 1223*

◆ **No Doz® Maximum Strength [OTC]** *see* Caffeine *on page 309*

◆ **NoHist DM [OTC]** *see* Chlorpheniramine, Phenylephrine, and Dextromethorphan *on page 413*

◆ **NoHist LQ [OTC]** *see* Chlorpheniramine and Phenylephrine *on page 412*

◆ **Nolvadex** *see* Tamoxifen *on page 1987*

◆ **Nolvadex®-D (Can)** *see* Tamoxifen *on page 1987*

◆ **Non-Aspirin Pain Reliever [OTC]** *see* Acetaminophen *on page 28*

Nonoxynol 9 (non OKS i nole nine)

Brand Names: U.S. Shur-Seal Contraceptive [OTC]; VCF Vaginal Contraceptive [OTC]

Index Terms N-9

Pharmacologic Category Contraceptive; Spermicide

Use Prevention of pregnancy

Dosage Adolescents and Adults: **Note:** Prior to use, refer to specific product labeling for complete instructions.

Prevention of pregnancy: Vaginal:

Encare®: Unwrap and insert 1 suppository vaginally at least 10 minutes prior to intercourse; effective for 1 hour

Today®: Insert 1 sponge vaginally prior to intercourse; allow to remain in place for 6 hours after intercourse before removing; effective for use up to 24 continuous hours. Do not leave in place for >30 hours.

VCF®:

Film: Insert 1 film vaginally at least 15 minutes, but no more than 3 hours, prior to intercourse. Insert new film for each act of intercourse or if more than 3 hours have elapsed.

Foam: Insert 1 applicatorful at least 15 minutes prior to intercourse; effective for up to 1 hour

Additional Information Complete prescribing information should be consulted for additional detail.

Dosage Forms Excipient information presented when available (limited, particularly for generics); consult specific product labeling.

Film, Vaginal:

VCF Vaginal Contraceptive: 28% (3 ea, 6 ea, 9 ea) [contains glycerin, polyvinyl alcohol]

Foam, Vaginal:

VCF Vaginal Contraceptive: 12.5% (17 g) [hormone free; contains benzoic acid, cetyl alcohol, methylparaben, propylene glycol]

Gel, Vaginal:

Shur-Seal Contraceptive: 2% (24 ea)

◆ **Non-Pseudo Sinus Decongestant [OTC]** *see* Phenylephrine (Systemic) *on page 1636*

◆ **Nora-BE** *see* Norethindrone *on page 1472*

◆ **Noradrenaline** *see* Norepinephrine *on page 1471*

◆ **Noradrenaline Acid Tartrate** *see* Norepinephrine *on page 1471*

◆ **Norco®** *see* Hydrocodone and Acetaminophen *on page 1006*

◆ **Norcuron** *see* Vecuronium *on page 2174*

◆ **Norcuron® (Can)** *see* Vecuronium *on page 2174*

◆ **Nordeoxyguanosine** *see* Ganciclovir (Systemic) *on page 939*

◆ **Nordette 28 [DSC]** *see* Ethinyl Estradiol and Levonorgestrel *on page 787*

◆ **Norditropin FlexPro** *see* Somatropin *on page 1934*

◆ **Norditropin NordiFlex Pen** *see* Somatropin *on page 1934*

◆ **Norditropin Simplexx (Can)** *see* Somatropin *on page 1934*

◆ **Norelgestromin and Ethinyl Estradiol** *see* Ethinyl Estradiol and Norelgestromin *on page 792*

Norepinephrine (nor ep i NEF rin)

Brand Names: U.S. Levophed

Brand Names: Canada Levophed®

Index Terms Levarterenol Bitartrate; Noradrenaline; Noradrenaline Acid Tartrate; Norepinephrine Bitartrate

Pharmacologic Category Alpha/Beta Agonist

Additional Appendix Information

Vasoactive Agents, Intravenous *on page 2315*

Use Treatment of shock which persists after adequate fluid volume replacement; severe hypotension

Note: Recommended as the first-choice vasopressor for the treatment of sepsis and septic shock in adult patients (Dellinger, 2013)

Pregnancy Risk Factor C

Pregnancy Considerations Animal reproduction studies have not been conducted. Norepinephrine is an endogenous catecholamine and crosses the placenta (Minzter, 2010; Wang, 1999).

Breast-Feeding Considerations It is not known if norepinephrine is excreted in breast milk. The manufacturer recommends that caution be exercised when administering norepinephrine to nursing women.

Contraindications Hypersensitivity to norepinephrine, bisulfites (contains metabisulfite), or any component of the formulation; hypotension from hypovolemia except as an emergency measure to maintain coronary and cerebral perfusion until volume could be replaced; mesenteric or peripheral vascular thrombosis unless it is a lifesaving procedure; during anesthesia with cyclopropane (not available in U.S.) or halothane (not available in U.S.) anesthesia (risk of ventricular arrhythmias)

Warnings/Precautions Assure adequate circulatory volume to minimize need for vasoconstrictors. Avoid hypertension; monitor blood pressure closely and adjust infusion rate. Use with extreme caution in patients taking MAO-Inhibitors. Vesicant; ensure proper needle or catheter placement prior to and during infusion. Avoid extravasation; infuse into a large vein if possible. Avoid infusion into leg veins. Montior I.V. site closely. **[U.S. Boxed Warning]: If extravasation occurs, infiltrate the area with diluted phentolamine (5-10 mg in 10-15 mL of saline) with a fine hypodermic needle. Phentolamine should be administered as soon as possible after extravasation is noted to prevent sloughing/necrosis**. Product may contain sodium metabisulfite.

Adverse Reactions Frequency not defined.
Cardiovascular: Arrhythmias, bradycardia, peripheral (digital) ischemia
Central nervous system: Anxiety, headache (transient)
Local: Skin necrosis (with extravasation)
Respiratory: Dyspnea, respiratory difficulty

Drug Interactions

Metabolism/Transport Effects Substrate of COMT

Avoid Concomitant Use

Avoid concomitant use of Norepinephrine with any of the following: Ergot Derivatives; Inhalational Anesthetics; Iobenguane I 123

Increased Effect/Toxicity

Norepinephrine may increase the levels/effects of: Sympathomimetics

The levels/effects of Norepinephrine may be increased by: Antacids; AtoMOXetine; Beta-Blockers; Cannabinoids; Carbonic Anhydrase Inhibitors; COMT Inhibitors; Ergot Derivatives; Hyaluronidase; Inhalational Anesthetics; MAO Inhibitors; Serotonin/Norepinephrine Reuptake Inhibitors; Tricyclic Antidepressants

Decreased Effect

Norepinephrine may decrease the levels/effects of: Benzylpenicilloyl Polylysine; Iobenguane I 123; Ioflupane I 123

The levels/effects of Norepinephrine may be decreased by: Alpha1-Blockers; Spironolactone

Preparation for Administration Dilute with D_5W, D_5NS, or NS; dilution in NS is not recommended by the manufacturer; however, stability in NS has been demonstrated (Tremblay, 2008).

Storage/Stability Readily oxidized. Protect from light. Do not use if brown coloration. Stability of parenteral admixture at room temperature (25°C) is 24 hours.

Mechanism of Action Stimulates $beta_1$-adrenergic receptors and alpha-adrenergic receptors causing increased contractility and heart rate as well as vasoconstriction, thereby increasing systemic blood pressure and coronary blood flow; clinically, alpha effects (vasoconstriction) are greater than beta effects (inotropic and chronotropic effects)

Pharmacodynamics/Kinetics
Onset of action: I.V.: Very rapid-acting
Duration: vasopressor: 1-2 minutes
Metabolism: Via catechol-o-methyltransferase (COMT) and monoamine oxidase (MAO)
Excretion: Urine (84% to 96% as inactive metabolites)

Dosage Administration requires the use of an infusion pump.

Note: Norepinephrine dosage is stated in terms of norepinephrine base.

Continuous I.V. infusion:

Children: Initial: 0.05-0.1 mcg/kg/minute; titrate to desired effect; maximum dose: 2 mcg/kg/minute (AHA, 2010; Kleinman, 2007)

Adults: Initial: 8-12 mcg/minute; titrate to desired response. Usual maintenance range: 2-4 mcg/minute; dosage range varies greatly depending on clinical situation. If patient remains hypotensive despite large doses, evaluate for occult hypovolemia and provide fluid resuscitation as appropriate.

ACLS dosing range (weight-based dosing): Post cardiac arrest care: Initial: 0.1-0.5 mcg/**kg**/minute (7-35 mcg/minute in a 70 kg patient); titrate to desired response (AHA, 2010)

Sepsis and septic shock (weight-based dosing): Range from clinical trials: 0.01-3 mcg/**kg**/minute (0.7-210 mcg/minute in a 70 kg patient) (Hollenberg, 2004)

Dosage adjustment in renal impairment: No dosage adjustment provided in manufacturer's labeling.

Dosage adjustment in hepatic impairment: No dosage adjustment provided in manufacturer's labeling.

Usual Infusion Concentrations: Pediatric I.V. infusion: 8 **mcg**/mL **or** 16 **mcg**/mL

Usual Infusion Concentrations: Adult I.V. infusion: 4 mg in 250 mL (concentration: 16 **mcg**/mL) **or** 8 mg in 250 mL (concentration: 32 **mcg**/mL) of D_5W or NS

Administration Administer as a continuous infusion with the use of an infusion pump. Dilute prior to use. Administration via central line recommended (may cause severe ischemic necrosis if extravasated). Do not administer sodium bicarbonate (or any alkaline solution) through an I.V. line containing norepinephrine; inactivation of norepinephrine may occur.

Vesicant; ensure proper needle or catheter placement prior to and during infusion; avoid extravasation.

Extravasation management: If extravasation occurs, stop infusion immediately and disconnect (leave cannula/needle in place); gently aspirate extravasated solution (do **NOT** flush the line); remove needle/cannula; elevate extremity. Initiate phentolamine (or alternative) antidote. Apply dry warm compresses (Hurst, 2004).

Phentolamine: Dilute 5-10 mg in 10-15 mL NS and administer into extravasation site as soon as possible after extravasation (Peberdy, 2010) **or** dilute 5-10 mg in 10 mL NS and administer into extravasation area (within 12 hours of extravasation).

Alternatives to phentolamine (due to shortage):

Nitroglycerin topical 2% ointment (based on limited case reports in neonates/infants): Apply 4 mm/kg as a thin ribbon to the affected areas; may repeat after 8 hours if needed (Wong, 1992) **or** apply a 1-inch strip on the affected site (Denkler, 1989).

Terbutaline (based on limited case reports): Infiltrate extravasation area using a solution of terbutaline 1 mg diluted to 10 mL in NS (large extravasation site; administration volume varied from 3-10 mL) **or** 1 mg diluted in 1 mL NS (small/distal extravasation site; administration volume varied from 0.5-1 mL) (Stier, 1999).

Monitoring Parameters Blood pressure (or mean arterial pressure), heart rate; cardiac output (as appropriate), intravascular volume status, pulmonary capillary wedge pressure (as appropriate); monitor infusion site closely

Consult individual institutional policies and procedures.

Additional Information Norepinephrine dosage is stated in terms of norepinephrine base. Although the intravenous product vial designates the contents as norepinephrine bitartrate, the actual concentration shown is in terms of norepinephrine base 1 mg/mL.

Dosage Forms Excipient information presented when available (limited, particularly for generics); consult specific product labeling.

Solution, Injection [strength expressed as base]:
Levophed: 1 mg/mL (4 mL) [contains sodium metabisulfite]
Generic: 1 mg/mL (4 mL)

Solution, Injection [strength expressed as base, preservative free]:
Generic: 1 mg/mL (4 mL)

◆ **Norepinephrine Bitartrate** *see* Norepinephrine *on page 1471*

Norethindrone (nor ETH in drone)

Brand Names: U.S. Aygestin; Camila; Errin; Heather; Jencycla; Jolivette; Lyza; Nor-QD; Nora-BE; Ortho Micronor

Brand Names: Canada Micronor®; Norlutate®

Index Terms Norethindrone Acetate; Norethisterone

Pharmacologic Category Contraceptive; Progestin

Use Treatment of amenorrhea; abnormal uterine bleeding; endometriosis; prevention of pregnancy

Pregnancy Risk Factor X

Pregnancy Considerations First trimester exposure may cause genital abnormalities including hypospadias in male infants and mild virilization of external female genitalia. Significant adverse events related to growth and development have not been observed (limited studies). Use is contraindicated during pregnancy. May be started immediately postpartum if not breast-feeding.

Breast-Feeding Considerations Small amounts of progestins are found in breast milk (1% to 6% of maternal serum concentration). Norethindrone can cause changes in milk production in the mother. When used for contraception, may start 3 weeks after delivery in women who are partially breast-feeding, or 6 weeks after delivery in women who are fully breast-feeding.

Contraindications Hypersensitivity to norethindrone or any component of the formulation; history of or current thrombophlebitis or venous thromboembolic disorders (including DVT, PE); hepatic dysfunction or tumor; known or suspected breast carcinoma; undiagnosed vaginal bleeding; pregnancy; missed abortion or as a diagnostic test for pregnancy

Warnings/Precautions Hazardous agent - use appropriate precautions for handling and disposal (NIOSH, 2012). Progestin only contraceptives do not protect against HIV infection or other sexually-transmitted diseases. Irregular menstrual bleeding patterns are common with progestin-only contraceptives; nonpharmacologic causes of abnormal bleeding should be ruled out. Progestin use has been associated with retinal vascular lesions; discontinue pending examination in case of sudden vision loss, complete loss of vision, sudden onset of proptosis, diplopia or migraine. May have adverse effects on glucose tolerance; use caution in women with diabetes. May have adverse effects on lipid metabolism; use caution in women with hyperlipidemias. Use with caution in patients with depression.

Use with caution in patients with diseases which may be exacerbated by fluid retention, including asthma, epilepsy, migraine, cardiac or renal dysfunction. Use caution in patients at increased risk of thromboembolism; includes elective surgery associated with an increased risk of thromboembolism or during periods of prolonged immobilization. The use of combination hormonal contraceptives has been associated with a slight increase in the frequency of breast cancer, however studies are not consistent. Data is insufficient to determine if progestin-only contraceptives also increase this risk. The risk of cardiovascular side effects increases in women using estrogen containing combined hormonal contraceptives and who smoke cigarettes, especially those who are >35 years of age. This risk relative to progestin-only contraceptives has not been established. Extremely rare hepatic adenomas and focal nodular hyperplasia resulting in fatal intra-abdominal hemorrhage have been reported in association with long-term combination oral contraceptive use. Data is insufficient to determine if progestin-only contraceptives also increase this risk. Not for use prior to menarche.

The use of estrogens and/or progestins may change the results of some laboratory tests (eg, coagulation factors, lipids, glucose tolerance, binding proteins). The dose, route, and the specific estrogen/progestin influences these changes. In addition, personal risk factors (eg, cardiovascular disease, smoking, diabetes, age) also contribute to adverse events; use of specific products may be contraindicated in women with certain risk factors.

Adverse Reactions Frequency not defined.

Cardiovascular: Cerebral embolism, cerebral thrombosis, DVT, edema

Central nervous system: Depression, dizziness, headache, insomnia, migraine, mood swings

Dermatologic: Acne, chloasma, hirsutism, melasma, pruritus, rash, urticaria

Endocrine & metabolic: Amenorrhea, breakthrough bleeding, breast enlargement/tenderness, menstrual flow changes, spotting

Gastrointestinal: Nausea, weight gain/loss

Genitourinary: Cervical erosion changes, cervical secretion changes

Hepatic: Cholestatic jaundice, liver function test abnormalities

Ocular: Optic neuritis (with or without vision loss), retinal vascular thrombosis

Respiratory: Pulmonary embolism

Miscellaneous: Anaphylactic/anaphylactoid reactions

Drug Interactions

Metabolism/Transport Effects Substrate of CYP3A4 (major); **Note:** Assignment of Major/Minor substrate status based on clinically relevant drug interaction potential; **Induces** CYP2C19 (weak/moderate)

Avoid Concomitant Use

Avoid concomitant use of Norethindrone with any of the following: Griseofulvin; Tranexamic Acid; Ulipristal

Increased Effect/Toxicity

Norethindrone may increase the levels/effects of: Benzodiazepines (metabolized by oxidation); Selegiline; Tranexamic Acid; Voriconazole

The levels/effects of Norethindrone may be increased by: Atazanavir; Boceprevir; Cobicistat; Herbs (Progestogenic Properties); Mifepristone; Voriconazole

Decreased Effect

Norethindrone may decrease the levels/effects of: Anticoagulants; Vitamin K Antagonists

The levels/effects of Norethindrone may be decreased by: Acitretin; Aminoglutethimide; Aprepitant; Artemether; Barbiturates; Bexarotene (Systemic); Bile Acid Sequestrants; Bosentan; CarBAMazepine; CloBAZam; Colesevelam; CYP3A4 Inducers (Strong); Dabrafenib; Darunavir; Deferasirox; Eslicarbazepine; Exenatide; Felbamate; Fosaprepitant; Fosphenytoin; Griseofulvin; LamoTRIgine; Mifepristone; Mitotane; Mycophenolate; Nelfinavir; Nevirapine; OXcarbazepine; Perampanel; Phenytoin; Primidone; Prucalopride; Retinoic Acid Derivatives; Rifamycin Derivatives; Rufinamide; St Johns Wort; Sugammadex; Telaprevir; Tocilizumab; Topiramate; Ulipristal

Ethanol/Nutrition/Herb Interactions Herb/Nutraceutical: Avoid bloodroot, chasteberry, damiana, oregano, and yucca; may enhance the adverse/toxic effect of progestins. Avoid St John's wort; may diminish the therapeutic effect of progestin contraceptives; contraceptive failure is possible.

Storage/Stability Store at controlled room temperature of 25°C (77°F).

Mechanism of Action Inhibits secretion of pituitary gonadotropin (LH) which prevents follicular maturation and ovulation

Pharmacodynamics/Kinetics

Absorption: Oral: Rapidly absorbed

Distribution: V_d: 4 L/kg

Protein binding: 61% to albumin; 36% to sex hormone-binding globulin (SHBG); SHBG capacity affected by plasma ethinyl estradiol levels

Metabolism: Oral: Hepatic via reduction and conjugation; first-pass effect

Bioavailability: 64%

Half-life elimination: ~8 hours

Time to peak: 1-2 hours

Excretion: Urine (>50% as metabolites); feces (20% to 40% as metabolites)

Dosage Oral: Adolescents and Adults: Females:

Contraception: Progesterone only: Norethindrone 0.35 mg every day (no missed days)

Initial dose: Start on first day of menstrual period or the day after a miscarriage or abortion. If switching from a combined oral contraceptive, begin the day after finishing the last active combined tablet.

Missed dose: Take as soon as remembered. A back up method of contraception should be used for 48 hours if dose is taken ≥3 hours late.

Amenorrhea and abnormal uterine bleeding: Norethindrone acetate: 2.5-10 mg/day for 5-10 days during the second half of the menstrual cycle

Endometriosis: Norethindrone acetate: 5 mg/day for 14 days; increase at increments of 2.5 mg/day every 2 weeks to reach 15 mg/day; continue for 6-9 months or until breakthrough bleeding demands temporary termination

Dosage adjustment in renal impairment: No dosage adjustment provided in manufacturer's labeling.

Dosage adjustment in hepatic impairment: No dosage adjustment provided in manufacturer's labeling. However, contraindicated in patients with hepatic tumors or impairment.

Dietary Considerations Should be taken at same time each day.

Administration Administer at the same time each day. When used for the prevention of pregnancy, a back up method of contraception should be used for 48 hours if dose is missed or taken ≥3 hours late.

Hazardous agent; use appropriate precautions for handling and disposal (NIOSH, 2012).

Monitoring Parameters Contraception: Before starting therapy, a physical exam with reference to the breasts and pelvis are recommended, including a Papanicolaou smear. Exam may be deferred if appropriate; pregnancy should be ruled out prior to use. Monitor patient closely for loss of vision, sudden onset of proptosis, diplopia, migraine; blood pressure; signs and symptoms of thromboembolic disorders; signs or symptoms of depression; glycemic control in patients with diabetes; lipid profiles in patients being treated for hyperlipidemias. Adequate diagnostic measures, including endometrial sampling, if indicated, should be performed to rule out malignancy in all cases of undiagnosed abnormal vaginal bleeding.

Dosage Forms Excipient information presented when available (limited, particularly for generics); consult specific product labeling.

Tablet, Oral:

- Camila: 0.35 mg
- Errin: 0.35 mg
- Heather: 0.35 mg [contains fd&c yellow #10 aluminum lake, fd&c yellow #6 aluminum lake]
- Jencycla: 0.35 mg [contains brilliant blue fcf (fd&c blue #1), fd&c yellow #10 (quinoline yellow)]
- Jolivette: 0.35 mg
- Lyza: 0.35 mg [contains fd&c yellow #10 (quinoline yellow)]
- Nor-QD: 0.35 mg
- Nora-BE: 0.35 mg
- Ortho Micronor: 0.35 mg [contains fd&c yellow #10 (quinoline yellow)]
- Generic: 0.35 mg

Tablet, Oral, as acetate:

- Aygestin: 5 mg [scored]
- Generic: 5 mg

◆ **Norethindrone Acetate** *see* Norethindrone *on page 1472*

◆ **Norethindrone Acetate and Ethinyl Estradiol** *see* Ethinyl Estradiol and Norethindrone *on page 793*

◆ **Norethindrone and Estradiol** *see* Estradiol and Norethindrone *on page 763*

◆ **Norethindrone and Leuprolide** *see* Leuprolide and Norethindrone *on page 1192*

Norethindrone and Mestranol

(nor eth IN drone & MES tra nole)

Brand Names: U.S. Necon® 1/50; Norinyl® 1+50

Brand Names: Canada Ortho-Novum® 1/50

Index Terms Mestranol and Norethindrone; Ortho Novum 1/50

Pharmacologic Category Contraceptive; Estrogen and Progestin Combination

Use Prevention of pregnancy

Unlabeled Use Treatment of hypermenorrhea (menorrhagia); pain associated with endometriosis; dysmenorrhea; dysfunctional uterine bleeding

Pregnancy Risk Factor X

Dosage Oral: Adults: Females: Contraception:

Schedule 1 (Sunday starter): Dose begins on first Sunday after onset of menstruation; if the menstrual period starts on Sunday, take first tablet that very same day. **With a Sunday start, an additional method of contraception should be used until after the first 7 days of consecutive administration.**

For 21-tablet package: Dosage is 1 tablet daily for 21 consecutive days, followed by 7 days off of the medication; a new course begins on the 8th day after the last tablet is taken.

For 28-tablet package: Dosage is 1 tablet daily without interruption.

Schedule 2 (Day 1 starter): Dose starts on first day of menstrual cycle taking 1 tablet daily.

For 21-tablet package: Dosage is 1 tablet daily for 21 consecutive days, followed by 7 days off of the medication; a new course begins on the 8th day after the last tablet is taken.

For 28-tablet package: Dosage is 1 tablet daily without interruption.

If all doses have been taken on schedule and one menstrual period is missed, continue dosing cycle. If two consecutive menstrual periods are missed, pregnancy test is required before new dosing cycle is started.

Missed doses **monophasic formulations** (refer to package insert for complete information):

One dose missed: Take as soon as remembered or take 2 tablets next day

Two consecutive doses missed in the first 2 weeks: Take 2 tablets as soon as remembered or 2 tablets next 2 days. **An additional method of contraception should be used for 7 days after missed dose.**

Two consecutive doses missed in week 3 or three consecutive doses missed at any time: **An additional method of contraception must be used for 7 days after a missed dose:**

Schedule 1 (Sunday starter): Continue dose of 1 tablet daily until Sunday, then discard the rest of the pack, and a new pack should be started that same day.

Schedule 2 (Day 1 starter): Current pack should be discarded, and a new pack should be started that same day.

Dosage adjustment in renal impairment: No dosage adjustment provided in manufacturer's labeling. Use with caution and monitor blood pressure closely. Consider other forms of contraception.

Dosage adjustment in hepatic impairment: No dosage adjustment provided in manufacturer's labeling.

However, contraindicated in patients with hepatic tumors or impairment.

Additional Information Complete prescribing information should be consulted for additional detail.

Dosage Forms Excipient information presented when available (limited, particularly for generics); consult specific product labeling.

Tablet, monophasic formulations:

Necon® 1/50: Norethindrone 1 mg and mestranol 0.05 mg [21 light blue tablets and 7 white inactive tablets] (28s)

Norinyl® 1+50: Norethindrone 1 mg and mestranol 0.05 mg [21 white tablets and 7 orange inactive tablets] (28s)

◆ **Norethisterone** *see* Norethindrone *on page* 1472
◆ **Norflex** *see* Orphenadrine *on page* 1517
◆ **Norflex™ (Can)** *see* Orphenadrine *on page* 1517

Norfloxacin (nor FLOKS a sin)

Brand Names: U.S. Noroxin

Brand Names: Canada Apo-Norflox®; CO Norfloxacin; Norfloxacine®; Novo-Norfloxacin; PMS-Norfloxacin; Riva-Norfloxacin

Pharmacologic Category Antibiotic, Fluoroquinolone

Use Uncomplicated and complicated urinary tract infections caused by susceptible gram-negative and gram-positive bacteria; sexually-transmitted disease (eg, uncomplicated urethral and cervical gonorrhea) caused by *N. gonorrhoeae*; prostatitis due to *E. coli*

Note: As of April 2007, the CDC no longer recommends the use of fluoroquinolones for the treatment of gonococcal disease.

Unlabeled Use Shigella dysentery type 1

Pregnancy Risk Factor C

Medication Guide Available Yes

Dosage

Usual dosage range:

Adults: Oral: 400 mg every 12 hours (maximum: 800 mg/day)

Indication-specific dosing:

Adults: Oral:

Dysenteric enterocolitis *(Shigella)* (unlabeled use): 400 mg twice daily for 3 days (IDSA, 2001)

Prostatitis: 400 mg every 12 hours for 4-6 weeks

Traveler's diarrhea (unlabeled use): 400 mg twice daily for 3 days (Mattila, 1993), single dose may also be effective

Uncomplicated gonorrhea: 800 mg as a single dose. **Note:** As of April 2007, the CDC no longer recommends the use of fluoroquinolones for the treatment of uncomplicated gonococcal disease.

Urinary tract infections:

Uncomplicated due to *E. coli, K. pneumoniae, P. mirabilis*: 400 mg twice daily for 3 days

Uncomplicated due to other organisms: 400 mg twice daily for 7-10 days

Complicated: 400 mg twice daily for 10-21 days

Dosage adjustment in renal impairment: Cl_{cr} ≤30 mL/minute/1.73 m^2: 400 mg once daily

Dosage adjustment in hepatic impairment: No dosage adjustment provided in manufacturer's labeling.

Additional Information Complete prescribing information should be consulted for additional detail.

Dosage Forms Excipient information presented when available (limited, particularly for generics); consult specific product labeling.

Tablet, Oral:

Noroxin: 400 mg

◆ **Norfloxacine® (Can)** *see* Norfloxacin *on page* 1475
◆ **Norgesic** *see* Orphenadrine, Aspirin, and Caffeine *on page* 1517
◆ **Norgestimate and Ethinyl Estradiol** *see* Ethinyl Estradiol and Norgestimate *on page* 795
◆ **Norgestrel and Ethinyl Estradiol** *see* Ethinyl Estradiol and Norgestrel *on page* 797
◆ **Norinyl 1+35** *see* Ethinyl Estradiol and Norethindrone *on page* 793
◆ **Norinyl® 1+50** *see* Norethindrone and Mestranol *on page* 1474
◆ **Noritate** *see* MetroNIDAZOLE (Topical) *on page* 1354
◆ **Noritate® (Can)** *see* MetroNIDAZOLE (Topical) *on page* 1354
◆ **NorLevo (Can)** *see* Levonorgestrel *on page* 1202
◆ **Norlutate® (Can)** *see* Norethindrone *on page* 1472
◆ **Normal Human Serum Albumin** *see* Albumin *on page* 59
◆ **Normal Saline** *see* Sodium Chloride *on page* 1914
◆ **Normal Serum Albumin (Human)** *see* Albumin *on page* 59
◆ **Normocarb HF® 25** *see* Electrolyte Solution, Renal Replacement *on page* 691
◆ **Normocarb HF® 35** *see* Electrolyte Solution, Renal Replacement *on page* 691
◆ **Normodyne® (Can)** *see* Labetalol *on page* 1156
◆ **Noroxin** *see* Norfloxacin *on page* 1475
◆ **Norpace** *see* Disopyramide *on page* 636
◆ **Norpace® (Can)** *see* Disopyramide *on page* 636
◆ **Norpace CR** *see* Disopyramide *on page* 636
◆ **Norpramin** *see* Desipramine *on page* 572
◆ **Nor-QD** *see* Norethindrone *on page* 1472
◆ **Nortemp Children's [OTC]** *see* Acetaminophen *on page* 28
◆ **Nortrel 0.5/35** *see* Ethinyl Estradiol and Norethindrone *on page* 793
◆ **Nortrel 1/35** *see* Ethinyl Estradiol and Norethindrone *on page* 793
◆ **Nortrel 7/7/7** *see* Ethinyl Estradiol and Norethindrone *on page* 793

Nortriptyline (nor TRIP ti leen)

Brand Names: U.S. Pamelor

Brand Names: Canada Apo-Nortriptyline®; Ava-Nortriptyline; Aventyl®; Dom-Nortriptyline; Norventyl; Nu-Nortriptyline; PMS-Nortriptyline; Teva-Nortriptyline

Index Terms Nortriptyline Hydrochloride

Pharmacologic Category Antidepressant, Tricyclic (Secondary Amine)

Additional Appendix Information

Antidepressant Agents *on page* 2284

Beers Criteria – Potentially Inappropriate Medications for Geriatrics *on page* 2368

Use Treatment of symptoms of depression

Unlabeled Use Chronic pain (including neuropathic pain), myofascial pain, burning mouth sydrome, anxiety disorders, attention-deficit/hyperactivity disorder (ADHD); enuresis; adjunctive therapy for smoking cessation

Pregnancy Considerations Animal reproduction studies are inconclusive. Nortriptyline and its metabolites cross the human placenta and can be detected in cord blood (Loughhead, 2006). Tricyclic antidepressants may be associated with irritability, jitteriness, and convulsions (rare) in the neonate (Yonkers, 2009).

The ACOG recommends that therapy for depression during pregnancy be individualized; treatment should incorporate the clinical expertise of the mental health clinician, obstetrician, primary healthcare provider, and pediatrician (ACOG, 2008). According to the American Psychiatric Association (APA), the risks of medication treatment should be weighed against other treatment options and untreated depression. For women who discontinue antidepressant medications during pregnancy and who may be at high risk for postpartum depression, the medications can be restarted following delivery (APA, 2010). Treatment algorithms have been developed by the ACOG and the APA for the management of depression in women prior to conception and during pregnancy (Yonkers, 2009).

Breast-Feeding Considerations Nortriptyline is excreted into breast milk and the M/P ratio ranged from 0.87 to 3.71 in one case report (Matheson, 1988). Based on available information, nortriptyline has not been detected in the serum of nursing infants; however, low levels of the active metabolite E-10-hydroxynortriptyline have been detected in the serum of newborns following breast-feeding (Wisner, 1991). Based on information from one mother-infant pair, following maternal use of nortriptyline 125 mg/day, the estimated exposure to the breast-feeding infant would be 0.6% to 3% of the weight-adjusted maternal dose. Adverse events have not been reported in nursing infants. Infants should be monitored for signs of adverse events; routine monitoring of infant serum concentrations is not recommended (Fortinguerra, 2009).

Medication Guide Available Yes

Contraindications Hypersensitivity to nortriptyline and similar chemical class, or any component of the formulation; use in a patient during the acute recovery phase of MI; use of MAO inhibitors intended to treat psychiatric disorders (concurrently or within 14 days of discontinuing either nortriptyline or the MAO inhibitor); initiation of nortriptyline in a patient receiving linezolid or intravenous methylene blue

Warnings/Precautions [U.S. Boxed Warning]: Antidepressants increase the risk of suicidal thinking and behavior in children, adolescents, and young adults (18-24 years of age) with major depressive disorder (MDD) and other psychiatric disorders; consider risk prior to prescribing. Short-term studies did not show an increased risk in patients >24 years of age and showed a decreased risk in patients ≥65 years. Closely monitor for clinical worsening, suicidality, or unusual changes in behavior; the patient's family or caregiver should be instructed to closely observe the patient and communicate condition with healthcare provider. A medication guide should be dispensed with each prescription. **Nortriptyline is not FDA approved for use in children.**

The possibility of a suicide attempt is inherent in major depression and may persist until remission occurs. Monitor for worsening of depression or suicidality, especially during initiation of therapy (generally first 1-2 months) or with dose increases or decreases. Use caution in high-risk patients. Worsening depression and severe abrupt suicidality that are not part of the presenting symptoms may require discontinuation or modification of drug therapy. The patient's family or caregiver should be alerted to monitor patients for the emergence of suicidality and associated behaviors (such as agitation, irritability, hostility, impulsivity, and hypomania) and call healthcare provider.

May worsen psychosis in some patients or precipitate a shift to mania or hypomania in patients with bipolar disorder. Patients presenting with depressive symptoms should be screened for bipolar disorder. Monotherapy in patients with bipolar disorder should be avoided. **Nortriptyline is not FDA approved for the treatment of bipolar depression.**

Potentially life-threatening serotonin syndrome (SS) has occurred with serotonergic agents (eg, SSRIs, SNRIs), particularly when used in combination with other serotonergic agents (eg, triptans, TCAs, fentanyl, lithium, tramadol, buspirone, St John's wort, tryptophan) or agents that impair metabolism of serotonin (eg, MAO inhibitors intended to treat psychiatric disorders, other MAO inhibitors [ie, linezolid and intravenous methylene blue]). Discontinue treatment (and any concomitant serotonergic agent) immediately if signs/symptoms arise. TCAs may rarely cause bone marrow suppression; monitor for any signs of infection and obtain CBC if symptoms (eg, fever, sore throat) evident. The risk of sedation and orthostatic effects are low relative to other antidepressants. However, nortriptyline may result in impaired performance of tasks requiring alertness (eg, operating machinery or driving). The degree of anticholinergic blockade produced by this agent is moderate relative to other cyclic antidepressants, however, caution should still be used in patients with urinary retention, benign prostatic hyperplasia, narrow-angle glaucoma, xerostomia, visual problems, constipation, or history of bowel obstruction. May cause orthostatic hypotension (risk is low relative to other antidepressants) or conduction disturbances. Use with caution in patients with a history of cardiovascular disease (including previous MI, stroke, tachycardia, or conduction abnormalities). The risk conduction abnormalities with this agent is moderate relative to other antidepressants.

Recommended by the manufacturer to discontinue prior to elective surgery; risks exist for drug interactions with anesthesia and for cardiac arrhythmias. However, definitive drug interactions have not been widely reported in the literature and continuation of tricyclic antidepressants is generally recommended as long as precautions are taken to reduce the significance of any adverse events that may occur (Pass, 2004). May alter glucose regulation - use caution in patients with diabetes. Use caution in patients with a previous seizure disorder or condition predisposing to seizures such as brain damage, alcoholism, or concurrent therapy with other drugs which lower the seizure threshold. May increase the risks associated with electroconvulsive therapy. Bone fractures have been associated with antidepressant treatment. Consider the possibility of a fragility fracture if an antidepressant-treated patient presents with unexplained bone pain, point tenderness, swelling, or bruising (Rabenda, 2013; Rizzoli, 2012). Use with caution in hyperthyroid patients or those receiving thyroid supplementation. Use with caution in patients with hepatic or renal dysfunction.

Use caution in elderly patients; may cause or exacerbate syndrome of inappropriate antidiuretic hormone secretion or hyponatremia; monitor sodium closely with initiation or dosage adjustments in older adults. May be inappropriate in older adults depending on comorbidities (eg, dementia, delirium) due to its potent anticholinergic effects (Beers Criteria).

Abrupt discontinuation or interruption of antidepressant therapy has been associated with a discontinuation syndrome. Symptoms arising may vary with antidepressant however commonly include nausea, vomiting, diarrhea, headaches, lightheadedness, dizziness, diminished appetite, sweating, chills, tremors, paresthesias, fatigue, somnolence, and sleep disturbances (eg, vivid dreams, insomnia). Greater risks for developing a discontinuation syndrome have been associated with antidepressants with shorter half-lives, longer durations of treatment, and abrupt discontinuation. For antidepressants of short or intermediate half-lives, symptoms may emerge within 2-5 days after treatment discontinuation and last 7-14 days (APA, 2010; Fava, 2006; Haddad, 2001; Shelton, 2001; Warner, 2006).

Adverse Reactions Frequency not defined.

Cardiovascular: Arrhythmia, flushing, heart block, hypertension, MI, orthostatic hypotension, palpitation, tachycardia

Central nervous system: Agitation, anxiety, ataxia, confusion, delirium, delusions, disorientation, dizziness, drowsiness, EEG changes, exacerbation of psychosis, extrapyramidal symptoms, fatigue, hallucinations, headache, hypomania, incoordination, insomnia, nightmares, panic, restlessness, seizure

Dermatologic: Alopecia, itching, petechiae, photosensitivity, rash, urticaria

Endocrine & metabolic: Blood sugar increased/decreased, breast enlargement, galactorrhea, gynecomastia, libido increased/decreased, sexual dysfunction, SIADH

Gastrointestinal: Abdominal cramps, anorexia, black tongue, constipation, diarrhea, epigastric distress, nausea, paralytic ileus, stomatitis, taste disturbance, vomiting, weight gain/loss, xerostomia

Genitourinary: Delayed micturition, impotence, nocturia, polyuria, testicular edema, urinary retention

Hematologic: Agranulocytosis (rare), eosinophilia, purpura, thrombocytopenia

Hepatic: Cholestatic jaundice, transaminases increased

Neuromuscular & skeletal: Numbness, paresthesia, peripheral neuropathy, tingling, tremor, weakness

Ocular: Blurred vision, disturbances in accommodation, eye pain, mydriasis

Otic: Tinnitus

Miscellaneous: Allergic reactions (eg, general edema or of the face/tongue), diaphoresis (excessive), withdrawal symptoms

Drug Interactions

Metabolism/Transport Effects **Substrate** of CYP1A2 (minor), CYP2C19 (minor), CYP2D6 (major), CYP3A4 (minor); **Note:** Assignment of Major/Minor substrate status based on clinically relevant drug interaction potential; **Inhibits** CYP2D6 (weak), CYP2E1 (weak)

Avoid Concomitant Use

Avoid concomitant use of Nortriptyline with any of the following: Aclidinium; Iobenguane I 123; Ipratropium (Oral Inhalation); Linezolid; MAO Inhibitors; Methylene Blue; Moxonidine; Tiotropium; Umeclidinium

Increased Effect/Toxicity

Nortriptyline may increase the levels/effects of: Alpha-/Beta-Agonists (Direct-Acting); Alpha1-Agonists; Amphetamines; Analgesics (Opioid); Anticholinergics; Antipsychotics; Beta2-Agonists; Citalopram; Desmopressin; Escitalopram; Highest Risk QTc-Prolonging Agents; Methylene Blue; Metoclopramide; Moderate Risk QTc-Prolonging Agents; QuiNIDine; Serotonin Modulators; Sodium Phosphates; Sulfonylureas; Tiotropium; TraMADol; Vitamin K Antagonists; Yohimbine

The levels/effects of Nortriptyline may be increased by: Abiraterone Acetate; Aclidinium; Altretamine; Antipsychotics; BuPROPion; Cimetidine; Cinacalcet; Citalopram; Cobicistat; CYP2D6 Inhibitors (Moderate); CYP2D6 Inhibitors (Strong); Dexmethylphenidate; DULoxetine; Escitalopram; FLUoxetine; FluvoxaMINE; Ipratropium (Oral Inhalation); Linezolid; Lithium; MAO Inhibitors; Methylphenidate; Metoclopramide; Metyrosine; Mifepristone; PARoxetine; Pramlintide; Protease Inhibitors; QuiNIDine; Sertraline; Terbinafine (Systemic); Thyroid Products; TraMADol; Umeclidinium; Valproic Acid and Derivatives

Decreased Effect

Nortriptyline may decrease the levels/effects of: Acetylcholinesterase Inhibitors (Central); Alpha2-Agonists; Alpha2-Agonists (Ophthalmic); Iobenguane I 123; Moxonidine

The levels/effects of Nortriptyline may be decreased by: Acetylcholinesterase Inhibitors (Central); Barbiturates; CarBAMazepine; Peginterferon Alfa-2b; St Johns Wort

Ethanol/Nutrition/Herb Interactions

Ethanol: May increase CNS depression; monitor for increased effects with coadministration. Caution patients about effects.

Herb/Nutraceutical: Avoid valerian, St John's wort, tryptophan, SAMe, kava kava (may increase risk of serotonin syndrome and/or excessive sedation).

Storage/Stability Store at 20°C to 25°C (68°F to 77°F). Protect from light.

Mechanism of Action Traditionally believed to increase the synaptic concentration of serotonin and/or norepinephrine in the central nervous system by inhibition of their reuptake by the presynaptic neuronal membrane. However, additional receptor effects have been found including desensitization of adenyl cyclase, down regulation of beta-adrenergic receptors, and down regulation of serotonin receptors.

Pharmacodynamics/Kinetics

Onset of action: Therapeutic: 1-3 weeks

Distribution: V_d: 21 L/kg

Protein binding: 93% to 95%

Metabolism: Primarily hepatic; extensive first-pass effect

Half-life elimination: 28-31 hours

Time to peak, serum: 7-8.5 hours

Excretion: Urine (as metabolites and small amounts of unchanged drug); feces (small amounts)

Dosage Oral:

Nocturnal enuresis: Children (unlabeled use): 10-20 mg/day; titrate to a maximum of 40 mg/day

Depression: Children (unlabeled use): 1-3 mg/kg/day

Depression:

Adults: 25 mg 3-4 times/day up to 150 mg/day; doses may be given once daily

Elderly: Initial: 30-50 mg/day, given as a single daily dose or in divided doses. **Note:** Nortriptyline is one of the best tolerated TCAs in the elderly.

Myofascial pain, neuralgia, burning mouth syndrome (unlabeled uses): Adults: Initial: 10-25 mg at bedtime; dosage may be increased by 25 mg/day weekly, if tolerated; usual maintenance dose: 75 mg as a single bedtime dose or 2 divided doses

Chronic urticaria, angioedema, nocturnal pruritus (unlabeled use): Adults: Oral: 75 mg/day

Smoking cessation (unlabeled use; Fiore, 2008): Adults: Initial: 25 mg/day; titrate dose to 75-100 mg/day 10-28 days prior to selected "quit" date; continue therapy for ≥12 weeks after "quit" day

Discontinuation of therapy: Upon discontinuation of antidepressant therapy, gradually taper the dose to minimize the incidence of withdrawal symptoms and allow for the detection of re-emerging symptoms. Evidence supporting ideal taper rates is limited. APA and NICE guidelines suggest tapering therapy over at least several weeks with consideration to the half-life of the antidepressant; antidepressants with a shorter half-life may need to be tapered more conservatively. In addition for long-term treated patients, WFSBP guidelines recommend tapering over 4-6 months. If intolerable withdrawal symptoms occur following a dose reduction, consider resuming the previously prescribed dose and/or decrease dose at a more gradual rate (APA, 2010; Bauer, 2002; Haddad, 2001; NCCMH, 2010; Schatzberg, 2006; Shelton, 2001; Warner, 2006).

MAO inhibitor recommendations:

Switching to or from an MAO inhibitor intended to treat psychiatric disorders:

Allow 14 days to elapse between discontinuing an MAO inhibitor intended to treat psychiatric disorders and initiation of nortriptyline.

Allow 14 days to elapse between discontinuing nortriptyline and initiation of an MAO inhibitor intended to treat psychiatric disorders.

Use with other MAO inhibitors (linezolid or I.V. methylene blue):

Do not initiate nortriptyline in patients receiving linezolid or I.V. methylene blue; consider other interventions for psychiatric condition.

If urgent treatment with linezolid or I.V. methylene blue is required in a patient already receiving nortriptyline and potential benefits outweigh potential risks, discontinue nortriptyline promptly and administer linezolid or I.V. methylene blue. Monitor for serotonin syndrome for 2 weeks or until 24 hours after the last dose of linezolid or I.V. methylene blue, whichever comes first. May resume nortriptyline 24 hours after the last dose of linezolid or I.V. methylene blue.

Dosage adjustment in renal impairment: No dosage adjustment provided in manufacturer's labeling.

Dosage adjustment in hepatic impairment: Lower doses and slower titration dependent on individualization of dosage is recommended

Monitoring Parameters Blood pressure and pulse rate (ECG, cardiac monitoring) prior to and during initial therapy in older adults; weight; blood levels are useful for therapeutic monitoring; suicide ideation (especially at the beginning of therapy or when doses are increased or decreased); signs/symptoms of serotonin syndrome

Reference Range

Plasma levels do not always correlate with clinical effectiveness

Therapeutic: 50-150 ng/mL (SI: 190-570 nmol/L)

Toxic: >500 ng/mL (SI: >1900 nmol/L)

Additional Information The maximum antidepressant effect of nortriptyline may not be seen for ≥2 weeks after initiation of therapy.

Dosage Forms Excipient information presented when available (limited, particularly for generics); consult specific product labeling.

Capsule, Oral:

Pamelor: 10 mg, 25 mg [contains fd&c yellow #10 (quinoline yellow), fd&c yellow #6 (sunset yellow)]

Pamelor: 50 mg

Pamelor: 75 mg [contains fd&c yellow #10 (quinoline yellow), fd&c yellow #6 (sunset yellow)]

Generic: 10 mg, 25 mg, 50 mg, 75 mg

Solution, Oral:

Generic: 10 mg/5 mL (473 mL)

- **Nortriptyline Hydrochloride** *see* Nortriptyline *on page 1475*
- **Norvasc** *see* AmLODIPine *on page 109*
- **Norvasc® (Can)** *see* AmLODIPine *on page 109*
- **Norventyl (Can)** *see* Nortriptyline *on page 1475*
- **Norvir** *see* Ritonavir *on page 1830*
- **Norvir® (Can)** *see* Ritonavir *on page 1830*
- **Norvir® SEC (Can)** *see* Ritonavir *on page 1830*
- **NovaFerrum 50 [OTC]** *see* Polysaccharide-Iron Complex *on page 1673*
- **NovaFerrum Pediatric Drops [OTC]** *see* Polysaccharide-Iron Complex *on page 1673*
- **Novahistex® DM Decongestant (Can)** *see* Pseudoephedrine and Dextromethorphan *on page 1748*
- **Novahistex® Expectorant with Decongestant (Can)** *see* Guaifenesin and Pseudoephedrine *on page 978*
- **Novahistine DH** *see* Dihydrocodeine, Chlorpheniramine, and Phenylephrine *on page 611*
- **Novahistine® DM Decongestant (Can)** *see* Pseudoephedrine and Dextromethorphan *on page 1748*
- **Novamoxin® (Can)** *see* Amoxicillin *on page 116*
- **Novantrone** *see* MitoXANtrone *on page 1386*
- **Novarel** *see* Chorionic Gonadotropin (Human) *on page 419*
- **Novasen (Can)** *see* Aspirin *on page 177*
- **Novel Erythropoiesis-Stimulating Protein** *see* Darbepoetin Alfa *on page 543*
- **Novo-5 ASA (Can)** *see* Mesalamine *on page 1305*
- **Novo-5 ASA-ECT (Can)** *see* Mesalamine *on page 1305*
- **Novo-Ampicillin (Can)** *see* Ampicillin *on page 130*
- **Novo-Atorvastatin (Can)** *see* AtorvaSTATin *on page 190*
- **Novo-Azithromycin (Can)** *see* Azithromycin (Systemic) *on page 214*
- **Novo-AZT (Can)** *see* Zidovudine *on page 2226*
- **Novo-Baclofen (Can)** *see* Baclofen *on page 221*
- **Novo-Bicalutamide (Can)** *see* Bicalutamide *on page 258*
- **Novo-Bisoprolol (Can)** *see* Bisoprolol *on page 261*
- **Novo-Bupropion SR (Can)** *see* BuPROPion *on page 296*
- **Novo-Buspirone (Can)** *see* BusPIRone *on page 300*
- **Novo-Carvedilol (Can)** *see* Carvedilol *on page 355*
- **Novo-Cefaclor (Can)** *see* Cefaclor *on page 360*
- **Novo-Chloroquine (Can)** *see* Chloroquine *on page 409*
- **Novo-Cholamine (Can)** *see* Cholestyramine Resin *on page 418*
- **Novo-Cholamine Light (Can)** *see* Cholestyramine Resin *on page 418*
- **Novo-Cimetidine (Can)** *see* Cimetidine *on page 427*
- **Novo-Ciprofloxacin (Can)** *see* Ciprofloxacin (Systemic) *on page 430*
- **Novo-Clavamoxin (Can)** *see* Amoxicillin and Clavulanate *on page 119*
- **Novo-Clobazam (Can)** *see* CloBAZam *on page 455*
- **Novo-Clobetasol (Can)** *see* Clobetasol *on page 457*
- **Novo-Clomipramine (Can)** *see* ClomiPRAMINE *on page 462*
- **Novo-Clonidine (Can)** *see* CloNIDine *on page 468*
- **Novo-Clopate (Can)** *see* Clorazepate *on page 475*
- **Novo-Cycloprine (Can)** *see* Cyclobenzaprine *on page 502*
- **Novo-Desipramine (Can)** *see* Desipramine *on page 572*
- **Novo-Desmopressin (Can)** *see* Desmopressin *on page 575*
- **Novo-Diflunisal (Can)** *see* Diflunisal *on page 605*
- **Novo-Dimenate [OTC] (Can)** *see* DimenhyDRINATE *on page 616*
- **Novo-Dipam (Can)** *see* Diazepam *on page 594*
- **Novo-Divalproex (Can)** *see* Valproic Acid and Derivatives *on page 2149*
- **Novo-Docusate Calcium (Can)** *see* Docusate *on page 644*
- **Novo-Docusate Sodium (Can)** *see* Docusate *on page 644*
- **Novo-Doxazosin (Can)** *see* Doxazosin *on page 656*
- **Novo-Doxepin (Can)** *see* Doxepin (Systemic) *on page 658*
- **Novo-Doxylin (Can)** *see* Doxycycline *on page 668*
- **Novoeight** *see* Antihemophilic Factor (Recombinant) *on page 144*

- ◆ **NovoSeven RT** *see* Factor VIIa (Recombinant) *on page* 821
- ◆ **Novo-Sorbide (Can)** *see* Isosorbide Dinitrate *on page* 1126
- ◆ **Novo-Sotalol (Can)** *see* Sotalol *on page* 1942
- ◆ **Novo-Sucralate (Can)** *see* Sucralfate *on page* 1955
- ◆ **Novo-Sundac (Can)** *see* Sulindac *on page* 1967
- ◆ **Novo-Temazepam (Can)** *see* Temazepam *on page* 2005
- ◆ **Novo-Theophyl SR (Can)** *see* Theophylline *on page* 2042
- ◆ **Novo-Ticlopidine (Can)** *see* Ticlopidine *on page* 2059
- ◆ **Novo-Timol (Can)** *see* Timolol (Ophthalmic) *on page* 2064
- ◆ **Novo-Topiramate (Can)** *see* Topiramate *on page* 2090
- ◆ **Novo-Trazodone (Can)** *see* TraZODone *on page* 2112
- ◆ **Novo-Trifluzine (Can)** *see* Trifluoperazine *on page* 2125
- ◆ **Novo-Trimel (Can)** *see* Sulfamethoxazole and Trimethoprim *on page* 1959
- ◆ **Novo-Trimel D.S. (Can)** *see* Sulfamethoxazole and Trimethoprim *on page* 1959
- ◆ **Novo-Triptyn (Can)** *see* Amitriptyline *on page* 105
- ◆ **Novo-Veramil (Can)** *see* Verapamil *on page* 2182
- ◆ **Novo-Veramil SR (Can)** *see* Verapamil *on page* 2182
- ◆ **Novo-Warfarin (Can)** *see* Warfarin *on page* 2211
- ◆ **Novoxapram® (Can)** *see* Oxazepam *on page* 1529
- ◆ **Noxafil** *see* Posaconazole *on page* 1679
- ◆ **NPH Insulin** *see* Insulin NPH *on page* 1092
- ◆ **NPH Insulin and Regular Insulin** *see* Insulin NPH and Insulin Regular *on page* 1093
- ◆ **Nplate** *see* RomiPLOStim *on page* 1850
- ◆ **Nplate® (Can)** *see* RomiPLOStim *on page* 1850
- ◆ **NP Thyroid** *see* Thyroid, Desiccated *on page* 2052
- ◆ **NRP104** *see* Lisdexamfetamine *on page* 1225
- ◆ **NTBC** *see* Nitisinone *on page* 1464
- ◆ **NTG** *see* Nitroglycerin *on page* 1466
- ◆ **NTP-Alprazolam (Can)** *see* ALPRAZolam *on page* 81
- ◆ **NTP-Amoxicillin (Can)** *see* Amoxicillin *on page* 116
- ◆ **NTP-Diclofenac (Can)** *see* Diclofenac (Systemic) *on page* 597
- ◆ **NTP-Diclofenac SR (Can)** *see* Diclofenac (Systemic) *on page* 597
- ◆ **NTP-Furosemide (Can)** *see* Furosemide *on page* 931
- ◆ ***N*-trifluoroacetyladriamycin-14-valerate** *see* Valrubicin *on page* 2153
- ◆ **NTZ** *see* Nitazoxanide *on page* 1463
- ◆ **Nu-Acebutolol (Can)** *see* Acebutolol *on page* 28
- ◆ **Nu-Acyclovir (Can)** *see* Acyclovir (Systemic) *on page* 42
- ◆ **Nu-Alpraz (Can)** *see* ALPRAZolam *on page* 81
- ◆ **Nu-Amoxi (Can)** *see* Amoxicillin *on page* 116
- ◆ **Nu-Ampi (Can)** *see* Ampicillin *on page* 130
- ◆ **Nuartez™** *see* Artesunate *on page* 171
- ◆ **Nu-Atenol (Can)** *see* Atenolol *on page* 186
- ◆ **Nu-Baclo (Can)** *see* Baclofen *on page* 221
- ◆ **Nubain** *see* Nalbuphine *on page* 1419
- ◆ **Nu-Beclomethasone (Can)** *see* Beclomethasone (Nasal) *on page* 229
- ◆ **Nu-Capto (Can)** *see* Captopril *on page* 333
- ◆ **Nu-Carbamazepine (Can)** *see* CarBAMazepine *on page* 336
- ◆ **Nu-Cefaclor (Can)** *see* Cefaclor *on page* 360
- ◆ **Nu-Cephalex (Can)** *see* Cephalexin *on page* 391
- ◆ **Nu-Cimet (Can)** *see* Cimetidine *on page* 427
- ◆ **Nu-COPD [OTC]** *see* Guaifenesin and Phenylephrine *on page* 978
- ◆ **NuCort** *see* Hydrocortisone (Topical) *on page* 1011
- ◆ **Nu-Cotrimox (Can)** *see* Sulfamethoxazole and Trimethoprim *on page* 1959
- ◆ **Nucynta** *see* Tapentadol *on page* 1992
- ◆ **Nucynta CR (Can)** *see* Tapentadol *on page* 1992
- ◆ **Nucynta ER** *see* Tapentadol *on page* 1992
- ◆ **Nucynta IR (Can)** *see* Tapentadol *on page* 1992
- ◆ **Nu-Desipramine (Can)** *see* Desipramine *on page* 572
- ◆ **Nu-Diclo (Can)** *see* Diclofenac (Systemic) *on page* 597
- ◆ **Nu-Diclo-SR (Can)** *see* Diclofenac (Systemic) *on page* 597
- ◆ **Nu-Diflunisal (Can)** *see* Diflunisal *on page* 605
- ◆ **Nu-Diltiaz (Can)** *see* Diltiazem *on page* 613
- ◆ **Nu-Diltiaz-CD (Can)** *see* Diltiazem *on page* 613
- ◆ **Nuedexta™** *see* Dextromethorphan and Quinidine *on page* 592
- ◆ **Nu-Erythromycin-S (Can)** *see* Erythromycin (Systemic) *on page* 741
- ◆ **Nu-Famotidine (Can)** *see* Famotidine *on page* 832
- ◆ **Nu-Fluoxetine (Can)** *see* FLUoxetine *on page* 885
- ◆ **Nu-Flurprofen (Can)** *see* Flurbiprofen (Systemic) *on page* 892
- ◆ **Nu-Furosemide (Can)** *see* Furosemide *on page* 931
- ◆ **Nu-Gemfibrozil (Can)** *see* Gemfibrozil *on page* 947
- ◆ **Nu-Glyburide (Can)** *see* GlyBURIDE *on page* 963
- ◆ **Nu-Hydral (Can)** *see* HydrALAZINE *on page* 1002
- ◆ **Nu-Hydro (Can)** *see* Hydrochlorothiazide *on page* 1004
- ◆ **Nu-Hydroxyzine (Can)** *see* HydrOXYzine *on page* 1025
- ◆ **Nu-Ibuprofen (Can)** *see* Ibuprofen *on page* 1032
- ◆ **Nu-Indapamide (Can)** *see* Indapamide *on page* 1066
- ◆ **Nu-Indo (Can)** *see* Indomethacin *on page* 1070
- ◆ **Nu-Ipratropium (Can)** *see* Ipratropium (Systemic) *on page* 1111
- ◆ **Nu-Iron [OTC]** *see* Polysaccharide-Iron Complex *on page* 1673
- ◆ **Nu-Ketoprofen (Can)** *see* Ketoprofen *on page* 1150
- ◆ **Nu-Ketoprofen-E (Can)** *see* Ketoprofen *on page* 1150
- ◆ **NuLev** *see* Hyoscyamine *on page* 1026
- ◆ **Nu-Levocarb (Can)** *see* Carbidopa and Levodopa *on page* 340
- ◆ **Nulojix** *see* Belatacept *on page* 231
- ◆ **Nu-Loraz (Can)** *see* LORazepam *on page* 1242
- ◆ **NuLYTELY** *see* Polyethylene Glycol-Electrolyte Solution *on page* 1669
- ◆ **Nu-Mefenamic (Can)** *see* Mefenamic Acid *on page* 1281
- ◆ **Nu-Megestrol (Can)** *see* Megestrol *on page* 1283
- ◆ **Nu-Metoclopramide (Can)** *see* Metoclopramide *on page* 1345
- ◆ **Nu-Metop (Can)** *see* Metoprolol *on page* 1348
- ◆ **Nu-Nifed (Can)** *see* NIFEdipine *on page* 1455
- ◆ **Nu-Nifedipine-PA (Can)** *see* NIFEdipine *on page* 1455
- ◆ **Nu-Nizatidine (Can)** *see* Nizatidine *on page* 1470
- ◆ **Nu-Nortriptyline (Can)** *see* Nortriptyline *on page* 1475
- ◆ **Nu-Oxybutyn (Can)** *see* Oxybutynin *on page* 1533
- ◆ **Nu-Pen-VK (Can)** *see* Penicillin V Potassium *on page* 1611

Nystatin (Oral) (nye STAT in)

Brand Names: U.S. Bio-Statin

Brand Names: Canada PMS-Nystatin

Pharmacologic Category Antifungal Agent, Oral Non-absorbed

Use Treatment of susceptible cutaneous, mucocutaneous, and oral cavity fungal infections normally caused by the *Candida* species

Pregnancy Risk Factor C

Pregnancy Considerations Animal reproduction studies have not been conducted. Adverse events in the fetus or newborn have not been reported following maternal use of vaginal nystatin during pregnancy. Absorption following oral use is poor.

Breast-Feeding Considerations Excretion into breast milk is not known; however, absorption following oral use is poor.

Contraindications Hypersensitivity to nystatin or any component of the formulation

Adverse Reactions

1% to 10%: Gastrointestinal: Diarrhea, nausea, stomach pain, vomiting

<1% (Limited to important or life-threatening): Hypersensitivity reactions

Drug Interactions

Metabolism/Transport Effects None known.

Avoid Concomitant Use There are no known interactions where it is recommended to avoid concomitant use.

Increased Effect/Toxicity There are no known significant interactions involving an increase in effect.

Decreased Effect

Nystatin (Oral) may decrease the levels/effects of: Saccharomyces boulardii

Storage/Stability

Tablet and suspension: Store at controlled room temperature of 15°C to 25°C (59°F to 77°F).

Powder for suspension: Store under refrigeration at 2°C to 8°C (36°F to 46°F).

Mechanism of Action Binds to sterols in fungal cell membrane, changing the cell wall permeability allowing for leakage of cellular contents

Pharmacodynamics/Kinetics

Onset of action: Symptomatic relief from candidiasis: 24-72 hours

Absorption: Poorly absorbed

Excretion: Feces (as unchanged drug)

Dosage Oral:

Oral candidiasis:

Suspension:

Premature infants: 100,000 units 4 times/day; paint suspension into recesses of the mouth

Infants: 200,000 units 4 times/day or 100,000 units to each side of mouth 4 times/day; paint suspension into recesses of the mouth

Children and Adults: 400,000-600,000 units 4 times/day; swish in the mouth and retain for as long as possible (several minutes) before swallowing

Powder for compounding: Children and Adults: 1/8 teaspoon (500,000 units) to equal approximately 1/2 cup of water; give 4 times/day

Intestinal infections: Adults: 500,000-1,000,000 units every 8 hours

Dosage adjustment in renal impairment: No dosage adjustment provided in manufacturer's labeling.

Dosage adjustment in hepatic impairment: No dosage adjustment provided in manufacturer's labeling.

Administration Suspension: Shake well before using. Should be swished about the mouth and retained in the mouth for as long as possible (several minutes) before swallowing. For neonates and infants, paint nystatin suspension into recesses of the mouth.

Dosage Forms Excipient information presented when available (limited, particularly for generics); consult specific product labeling.

Capsule, Oral [preservative free]:

Bio-Statin: 500,000 units, 1,000,000 units [dye free]

Powder, Oral:

Bio-Statin: (1 ea)

Generic: (1 ea)

Suspension, Mouth/Throat:

Generic: 100,000 units/mL (5 mL, 60 mL, 473 mL, 480 mL)

Tablet, Oral:

Generic: 500,000 units

Nystatin (Topical) (nye STAT in)

Brand Names: U.S. Nyamyc; Nystop; Pedi-Dri; Pediaderm AF Complete
Brand Names: Canada Candistatin; Nyaderm
Pharmacologic Category Antifungal Agent, Topical
Additional Appendix Information
Antifungal Agents *on page 2286*
Use Treatment of susceptible cutaneous and mucocutaneous fungal infections normally caused by the *Candida* species
Pregnancy Risk Factor C
Dosage Mucocutaneous infections: Children and Adults: Topical: Apply 2-3 times/day to affected areas; very moist topical lesions are treated best with powder
Additional Information Complete prescribing information should be consulted for additional detail.
Dosage Forms Excipient information presented when available (limited, particularly for generics); consult specific product labeling.
Cream, External:
Generic: 100,000 units/g (15 g, 30 g)
Kit, External:
Pediaderm AF Complete: 100,000 units/g [contains methylparaben, propylene glycol, propylparaben]
Ointment, External:
Generic: 100,000 units/g (15 g, 30 g)
Powder, External:
Nyamyc: 100,000 units/g (15 g, 30 g, 60 g)
Nystop: 100,000 units/g (15 g, 30 g, 60 g)
Pedi-Dri: 100,000 units/g (56.7 g)
Generic: 100,000 units/g (15 g, 30 g, 60 g)

Nystatin and Triamcinolone
(nye STAT in & trye am SIN oh lone)

Index Terms Triamcinolone and Nystatin
Pharmacologic Category Antifungal Agent, Topical; Corticosteroid, Topical
Use Treatment of cutaneous candidiasis
Pregnancy Risk Factor C
Dosage Children and Adults: Topical: Apply sparingly to affected area(s) twice daily. Therapy should be discontinued when control is achieved or if symptoms persist for >25 days of therapy.
Additional Information Complete prescribing information should be consulted for additional detail.
Dosage Forms Excipient information presented when available (limited, particularly for generics); consult specific product labeling.
Cream: Nystatin 100,000 units and triamcinolone acetonide 0.1% (15 g, 30 g, 60 g)
Ointment: Nystatin 100,000 units and triamcinolone acetonide 0.1% (15 g, 30 g, 60 g)

- ◆ Nystop *see* Nystatin (Topical) *on page 1482*
- ◆ Nytol [OTC] *see* DiphenhydrAMINE (Systemic) *on page 622*
- ◆ Nytol® (Can) *see* DiphenhydrAMINE (Systemic) *on page 622*
- ◆ Nytol® Extra Strength (Can) *see* DiphenhydrAMINE (Systemic) *on page 622*
- ◆ Nytol Maximum Strength [OTC] *see* DiphenhydrAMINE (Systemic) *on page 622*

Obinutuzumab (oh bi nue TOOZ ue mab)

Brand Names: U.S. Gazyva
Index Terms GA101; R05072759; R7159
Pharmacologic Category Antineoplastic Agent, Monoclonal Antibody; Monoclonal Antibody
Use Chronic lymphocytic leukemia: Treatment of patients with previously untreated chronic lymphocytic leukemia (CLL) in combination with chlorambucil
Pregnancy Risk Factor C
Pregnancy Considerations Teratogenic effects were not observed in animal reproduction studies. However based on animal data, if exposure occurs during pregnancy, B-cell counts and immunologic function may be affected in the neonate after birth. Women of child bearing potential should use effective contraception during therapy and for 12 months after treatment.
Breast-Feeding Considerations It is not known if obinutuzumab is excreted into breast milk. However, human immunoglobulin can be detected in milk. Due to the potential for serious adverse reactions in the nursing infant, the manufacturer recommends a decision be made whether to discontinue nursing or to discontinue the drug, taking into account the importance of treatment to the mother.
Contraindications There are no contraindications listed in the manufacturer's labeling.
Warnings/Precautions [U.S. Boxed Warning]: Hepatitis B virus (HBV) reactivation may occur with use of CD20-directed cytolytic antibodies (including obinutuzumab) and may result in fulminant hepatitis, hepatic failure, and death. Screen all patients for HBV infection by measuring hepatitis B surface antigen (HBsAg) and hepatitis B core antibody (anti-HBc) prior to therapy initiation; monitor patients for clinical and laboratory signs of hepatitis or HBV during and for several months after treatment. Discontinue obinutuzumab (and concomitant chemotherapy) if viral hepatitis develops and initiate appropriate antiviral therapy. Reactivation has occurred in patients who are HBsAg positive as well as in those who are HBsAg negative but are anti-HBc positive; HBV reactivation has also been observed in patients who had previously resolved HBV infection. HBV reactivation has been reported for other CD20-directed antibodies after therapy discontinuation. Reactivation of HBV replication is often followed by hepatitis. Use cautiously in patients who show evidence of prior HBV infection (eg, HBsAg positive [regardless of antibody status] or HBsAG negative but anti-HBc positive); consult with appropriate clinicians regarding monitoring and consideration of antiviral therapy before and/or during obinutuzumab treatment. The safety of resuming obinutuzumab treatment following HBV reactivation is not known; discuss reinitiation of therapy in patients with resolved HBV reactivation with physicians experienced in HBV management. **[U.S. Boxed Warning]: Progressive multifocal leukoencephalopathy (PML) resulting in death may occur with treatment.** PML is due to JC virus infection. Consider PML in any patient with new onset or worsening neurological symptoms and if PML is suspected, discontinue obinutuzumab (consider discontinuation or dose reduction of any concomitant chemotherapy or immunosuppressive therapy) and evaluate promptly.

May cause severe and life-threatening infusion reactions; reactions may include bronchospasm, dyspnea, tachycardia, larynx and throat irritation, wheezing, laryngeal edema, flushing, hypertension, hypotension, fever, nausea, vomiting, diarrhea, headache and/or chills. Infusion reactions occur more frequently with the first 1000 mg infused. Delayed reactions (up to 24 hours later) have occurred. Premedicate with acetaminophen, an antihistamine, and a glucocorticoid prior to infusion; may require rate reduction, interruption of therapy, or treatment discontinuation. Monitor during the entire infusion; monitor patients with pre-existing cardiac or pulmonary conditions closely. Due to the risk for hypotension, consider temporarily withholding antihypertensive therapies for 12 hours prior to, during, and for 1 hour after administration. Administer in a facility with immediate access to resuscitative measures (eg, glucocorticoids, epinephrine, bronchodilators, and/or oxygen).

In clinical trials, grade 3 and 4 neutropenia and thrombocytopenia occurred when used in combination with chlorambucil. Neutropenia may have a late onset (>28 days after therapy completion) and/or be prolonged (duration >28 days). Monitor for signs/symptoms of infection; antimicrobial prophylaxis is recommended in neutropenic patients. Antiviral and/or antifungal prophylaxis may also be considered. In a small percentage of patients, thrombocytopenia occurred acutely (within 24 hours) after obinutuzumab administration; platelet transfusions may be necessary. Leukopenia and lymphopenia commonly occur. Monitor blood counts frequently throughout therapy. Bacterial, fungal, and new or reactivated viral infections may occur during and/or following therapy; do not administer to patients with an active infection. Patients with a history of recurrent or chronic infections may be at increased risk. Tumor lysis syndrome may occur within 12-24 hours following the first dose. Acute renal failure, hyperkalemia, hypocalcemia, hyperuricemia, and/or hyperphosphatemia may occur. Administer prophylaxis (antihyperuricemic therapy, hydration) in patients at high risk (high numbers of circulating malignant cells ≥25,000/mm^3 or high tumor burden). Correct electrolyte abnormalities; monitor renal function and hydration status. Administration of live virus vaccines during treatment (and until B-cell recovery) is not recommended; the safety and efficacy of immunization with live or attenuated viral vaccines during or after obinutuzumab therapy has not been determined.

Adverse Reactions Adverse reactions reported in combination with chlorambucil.

>10%:

Endocrine & metabolic: Hypocalcemia (32%), hyperkalemia (31%), hyponatremia (29%), hypoalbuminemia (22%), hypokalemia (13%)

Hematologic & oncologic: Leukopenia (7% to 84%; grades 3/4: 5% to 36%), lymphocytopenia (80%; grades 3/4: 40%), neutropenia (40% to 77%; grades 3/4: 34% to 46%; onset ≥28 days after completion of treatment: 16%), thrombocytopenia (15% to 47%; grades 3/4: 11% to 14%; onset within 24 hours of infusion: 5%), anemia (12%; grades 3/4: 4%)

Hepatic: Increased serum AST (28%), increased serum ALT (25%), increased serum alkaline phosphatase (16%)

Immunologic: Antibody development (13%)

Infection: Infection (38%)

Neuromuscular & skeletal: Musculoskeletal signs and symptoms (17%)

Renal: Increased serum creatinine (28%)

Miscellaneous: Infusion related reaction: Initial infusion: 69%; grades 3/4: 21%; second infusion: 3%; subsequent infusions: <1%)

1% to 10%:

Hematologic & oncologic: Tumor lysis syndrome (grades 3/4: 2%)

Respiratory: Cough (10%)

Miscellaneous: Fever (10%)

Frequency not defined: Exacerbation of cardiac disease, progressive multifocal leukoencephalopathy, reactivation of HBV

Drug Interactions

Metabolism/Transport Effects None known.

Avoid Concomitant Use

Avoid concomitant use of Obinutuzumab with any of the following: BCG; Belimumab; CloZAPine; Natalizumab; Pimecrolimus; Tacrolimus (Topical); Tofacitinib; Vaccines (Live)

Increased Effect/Toxicity

Obinutuzumab may increase the levels/effects of: Belimumab; CloZAPine; Leflunomide; Natalizumab; Tofacitinib; Vaccines (Live); Vitamin K Antagonists

The levels/effects of Obinutuzumab may be increased by: Abciximab; Antihypertensives; Denosumab; Pimecrolimus; Roflumilast; Tacrolimus (Topical); Trastuzumab

Decreased Effect

Obinutuzumab may decrease the levels/effects of: BCG; Cardiac Glycosides; Coccidioidin Skin Test; Sipuleucel-T; Vaccines (Inactivated); Vaccines (Live); Vitamin K Antagonists

The levels/effects of Obinutuzumab may be decreased by: Echinacea

Preparation for Administration

Cycle 1, day 1 and 2 doses (100 mg and 900 mg, respectively): Withdraw 40 mL of obinutuzumab solution from vial. Dilute 4 mL into a 100 mL infusion bag of NS (100 mg dose; use immediately). Dilute remaining 36 mL into a 250 mL NS infusion bag (900 mg dose, for use on day 2); store at 2°C to 8°C (36°F to 46°F) for up to 24 hours; use immediately after reaching room temperature. Gently invert to mix; do not shake or freeze.

Cycle 1 (day 8 and 15 doses) and cycles 2-6 (1000 mg): Withdraw 40 mL of obinutuzumab solution from vial. Dilute into a 250 mL NS infusion bag. Gently invert to mix; do not shake or freeze.

Do not use other diluents (eg, dextrose) to prepare the infusion. Final concentration for administration should be 0.4-4 mg/mL. May use PVC or non-PVC infusion bags.

Storage/Stability Store intact vials at 2°C to 8°C (36°F to 46°F); do not freeze or shake. Protect from light. Diluted solutions for infusion should be used immediately. If not used immediately, the diluted solutions may be stored up to 24 hours at 2°C to 8°C (36°F to 46°F) followed by 48 hours (including infusion time) at room temperature of ≤30°C (≤86°F).

Mechanism of Action Obinutuzumab is a glycoengineered type II anti-CD20 monoclonal antibody. The CD20 antigen is expressed on the surface of pre B- and mature B-lymphocytes; upon binding to CD20, obinutuzumab activates complement-dependent cytotoxicity, antibody-dependent cellular cytotoxicity and antibody-dependent cellular phagocytosis, resulting in cell death (Sehn, 2012).

Pharmacodynamics/Kinetics

Distribution: V_d: ~3.8 L

Half-life elimination: ~28.4 days

Dosage Note: Premedication with acetaminophen, an antihistamine, and a glucocorticoid 30-60 minutes prior to treatment may be necessary (see Administration). Antihyperuricemic prophylaxis and adequate hydration are recommended for patients with a high tumor burden and/or high circulating absolute lymphocyte count. Antimicrobial, antiviral, and antifungal prophylaxis may be considered in certain patients.

Chronic lymphocytic leukemia (CLL): Adults: I.V.:

Cycle 1: 100 mg on day 1, followed by 900 mg on day 2, followed by 1000 mg weekly for 2 doses (days 8 and 15)

Cycles 2-6: 1000 mg on day 1 every 28 days for 5 doses

Missed doses: Administer the missed dose as soon as possible; adjust dosing schedule accordingly. In some cases, patients who do not complete the day 1 cycle 1 dose may proceed to the day 2 cycle 1 treatment (if appropriate).

Dosage adjustment for toxicity:

Hematologic: Grade 3 or 4 cytopenias: Consider treatment interruption

Infusion reactions:

Mild-to-moderate (Grades 1 and 2): Reduce infusion rate or interrupt infusion and manage symptoms as appropriate. Upon symptom resolution, continue or resume infusion. If no further infusion reaction symptoms occur, may resume infusion rate escalation as appropriate for the treatment cycle dose.

Severe (Grade 3): Interrupt therapy; manage symptoms as appropriate. Upon symptom resolution, may reinitiate infusion at no more than 50% of the rate at which the reaction occurred. If no further infusion reaction symptoms occur, may resume infusion rate escalation as appropriate for the treatment cycle dose. Permanently discontinue if ≥ grade 3 toxicity occurs upon rechallenge.

Life-threatening (Grade 4): Discontinue infusion immediately; permanently discontinue therapy.

Infection: Consider treatment interruption.

Other toxicity: Consider treatment interruption for ≥ grade 2 nonhematologic toxicity.

Dosage adjustment for renal impairment:

Cl_{cr} ≥30 mL/minute: No dosage adjustment provided in manufacturer's labeling; however, pharmacokinetics are not affected (based on pharmacokinetic analysis).

Cl_{cr} <30 mL/minute: No dosage adjustment provided in manufacturer's labeling (has not been studied).

Dosage adjustment for hepatic impairment: No dosage adjustment provided in manufacturer's labeling (has not been studied).

Administration For I.V. infusion only. Do not administer I.V. push or as a bolus. Premedication with acetaminophen, an antihistamine, and a glucocorticoid (eg, dexamethasone or methylprednisolone) may be required (see below). Do not mix with or infuse with other medications. May use PVC or non-PVC administration sets.

Premedication:

Cycle 1 (days 1 and 2): All patients should receive acetaminophen (650-1000 mg) and an antihistamine (eg, diphenhydramine 50 mg) at least 30 minutes prior to infusion. In addition, an I.V. glucocorticoid (eg, dexamethasone 20 mg or methylprednisolone 80 mg) should be administered at least 1 hour prior to infusion.

Cycle 1 (days 8 and 15), and cycles 2-6: All patients should receive acetaminophen 650-1000 mg at least 30 minutes prior to infusion.

If patients experienced grade 1 or higher infusion-related reaction with previous infusion: Administer an antihistamine (eg, diphenhydramine 50 mg) in addition to acetaminophen at least 30 minutes prior to infusion.

If patients experienced ≥ grade 3 infusion-related reaction with previous infusion **or** have a lymphocyte count >25,000 cells/mm^3 prior to next treatment: Administer an I.V. glucocorticoid (eg, dexamethasone 20 mg or methylprednisolone 80 mg) at least 1 hour prior to infusion, in addition to acetaminophen and an antihistamine at least 30 minutes prior to infusion.

Infusion rate:

Cycle 1 (day 1): Infuse at 25 mg/hour over 4 hours; do not increase the infusion rate

Cycle 1 (day 2): Initiate infusion at 50 mg/hour for 30 minutes; if tolerated, may escalate rate in increments of 50 mg/hour every 30 minutes to a maximum rate of 400 mg/hour.

Cycle 1 (days 8 and 15), and cycles 2-6: Initiate infusion at 100 mg/hour for 30 minutes; if tolerated, may escalate infusion rate in increments of 100 mg/hour every 30 minutes to a maximum rate of 400 mg/hour.

Monitoring Parameters CBC with differential (at regular intervals), hepatitis B screening in all patients (HBsAG and anti-HBc measurements) prior to therapy initiation; renal function, electrolytes; signs of active hepatitis B infection (during and for several months after therapy completion); signs or symptoms of infusion reaction; signs of infection; fluid status; signs/symptoms of progressive multifocal leukoencephalopathy (PML; focal neurologic deficits, which may present as hemiparesis, visual field deficits, cognitive impairment, aphasia, ataxia, and/or cranial nerve deficits); evaluate for PML with brain MRI, lumbar puncture, and neurologist consultation.

Dosage Forms Excipient information presented when available (limited, particularly for generics); consult specific product labeling.

Solution, Intravenous [preservative free]:

Gazyva: 1000 mg/40 mL (40 mL)

- ◆ **OCBZ** *see* OXcarbazepine *on page 1530*
- ◆ **Ocean Complete Sinus Rinse [OTC]** *see* Sodium Chloride *on page 1914*
- ◆ **Ocean for Kids [OTC]** *see* Sodium Chloride *on page 1914*
- ◆ **Oceanic Selenium [OTC]** *see* Selenium *on page 1888*
- ◆ **Ocean Nasal Spray [OTC]** *see* Sodium Chloride *on page 1914*
- ◆ **Ocean Ultra Saline Mist [OTC]** *see* Sodium Chloride *on page 1914*
- ◆ **Ocella™** *see* Ethinyl Estradiol and Drospirenone *on page 785*

Ocriplasmin (ok ri PLAZ min)

Brand Names: U.S. Jetrea

Pharmacologic Category Ophthalmic Agent; Vitreolytic

Use Treatment of symptomatic vitreomacular adhesion (VMA)

Pregnancy Risk Factor C

Pregnancy Considerations Animal reproduction studies have not been conducted. Systemic exposure following a single intravitreal injection is expected to be low.

Breast-Feeding Considerations Systemic exposure following a single intravitreal injection is expected to be low. It is not known if ocriplasmin is excreted in breast milk. The manufacturer recommends that caution be exercised when administering ocriplasmin to nursing women.

Contraindications There are no contraindications listed in the manufacturer's labeling.

Warnings/Precautions May cause decreased visual acuity as a result of condition progression with traction, which may require surgical intervention. Monitor visual acuity appropriately. Administration of higher than recommended doses may result in lens subluxation (1 case report). May cause dyschromatopsia, described as yellowish vision, following injection. Intraocular inflammation, infection, hemorrhage, or increased intraocular pressure may result after intravitreal injection. In clinical trials, intraocular inflammation occurred at a higher rate with ocriplasmin when compared to placebo; intraocular inflammation events were typically mild and transient. After ocriplasmin administration, retinal detachment or retinal tear (with or without retinal detachment) may occur before, during, or after future vitrectomy.

Adverse Reactions

>10%: Ocular: Blurred vision (5% to 20%), conjunctival hemorrhage (5% to 20%), eye pain (5% to 20%), macular hole (5% to 20%), photopsia (5% to 20%), retinal edema (5% to 20%), visual acuity decreased (5% to 20%; ≥3-line decrease 6%), visual impairment (5% to 20%), vitreous floaters (5% to 20%)

1% to 10%: Ocular: Intraocular inflammation (7%), anterior chamber cell (2% to 5%), cataract (2% to 5%), conjunctival hyperemia (2% to 5%), dry eyes (2% to 5%), intraocular pressure increased (2% to 5%), iritis (2% to 5%), macular edema (2% to 5%), metamorphopsia (2% to 5%), ocular discomfort (2% to 5%), photophobia (2% to 5%), retinal degeneration (2% to 5%), vitreous detachment (2% to 5%), dyschromatopsia (2%), a-wave and b-wave amplitude decreased (1%)

<1% (Limited to important or life-threatening): Lens subluxation (high dose; 0.175 mg), retinal detachment

Drug Interactions

Metabolism/Transport Effects None known.

Avoid Concomitant Use There are no known interactions where it is recommended to avoid concomitant use.

Increased Effect/Toxicity There are no known significant interactions involving an increase in effect.

Decreased Effect There are no known significant interactions involving a decrease in effect.

Preparation for Administration Ocriplasmin should thaw at room temperature (within a few minutes) prior to reconstitution. Using aseptic technique, add 0.2 mL of preservative free NS to the vial and gently swirl to mix. Visually inspect solution for particulate matter and ensure a clear, colorless solution is present. Use immediately after reconstitution and discard any unused portion of diluted solution.

Storage/Stability Store frozen at or below -4°F (-20°C). Protect from light.

Mechanism of Action Ocriplasmin is a recombinant form of human plasmin that acts as a proteolytic within the vitreous body and vitreoretinal interface. Protein matrix components responsible for the vitreomacular adhesion (eg, laminin, fibronectin, and collagen) are lysed by ocriplasmin.

Pharmacodynamics/Kinetics

Absorption: Detectable levels in systemic circulation are not expected

Metabolism: Endogenous protein catabolism pathway; rapidly inactivated by protease inhibitor alpha-2-antiplasmin or alpha-2-macroglobulin

Note: <3% of the administered dose is detected in vitreous fluid 24 hours after administration.

Dosage Symptomatic vitreomacular adhesion: Adults: Intravitreal: 0.125 mg once (as a single dose to the affected eye)

Dosage adjustment in renal impairment: No dosage adjustment provided in manufacturer's labeling. However, dosage adjustment unlikely due to low systemic absorption.

Dosage adjustment in hepatic impairment: No dosage adjustment provided in manufacturer's labeling. However, dosage adjustment unlikely due to low systemic absorption.

Administration Intravitreal: For intravitreal injection only. Must be diluted prior to use. Controlled aseptic conditions should be established prior to administration. After reconstitution, remove contents from vial using a syringe with a sterile, 19-gauge needle. Discard 19-gauge needle and replace with a sterile 30-gauge needle for intravitreal injection procedure (do not use 19-gauge needle for intravitreal injection). Depress plunger to expel excess air and medication (plunger tip should align with the 0.1 mL marking on syringe). Insert the injection needle 3.5-4 mm posterior to the limbus aiming toward the center of the vitreous cavity, avoiding the horizontal meridian, then deliver the 0.1 mL injection (corresponds to 0.125 mg ocriplasmin) into the mid-vitreous. Adequate anesthesia and a broad-spectrum antimicrobial agent should be administered prior to the procedure. Only one eye should be treated with each vial. Treatment of a patient's contralateral eye requires a new vial and administration supplies and is not recommended within 7 days of the first injection. Repeated administration to the same eye is not recommended. Each vial should only be used as a single injection for the treatment of one eye.

Monitoring Parameters Following intravitreal injection, monitor for elevation in intraocular pressure, signs of endophthalmitis, retinal detachment, or decreased vision.

Dosage Forms Excipient information presented when available (limited, particularly for generics); consult specific product labeling.

Solution, Intraocular [preservative free]:

Jetrea: 0.5 mg/0.2 mL (0.2 mL)

◆ **Octagam** *see* Immune Globulin *on page 1059*

◆ **Octagam 10% (Can)** *see* Immune Globulin *on page 1059*

◆ **Octaplex (Can)** *see* Prothrombin Complex Concentrate (Human) [(Factors II, VII, IX, X), Protein C, and Protein S] *on page 1743*

◆ **Octostim® (Can)** *see* Desmopressin *on page 575*

Octreotide (ok TREE oh tide)

Brand Names: U.S. SandoSTATIN; SandoSTATIN LAR Depot

Brand Names: Canada Octreotide Acetate Injection; Octreotide Acetate Omega; Sandostatin LAR; Sandostatin®

Index Terms Longastatin; Octreotide Acetate

Pharmacologic Category Antidiarrheal; Antidote; Somatostatin Analog

Use Control of symptoms (diarrhea and flushing) in patients with metastatic carcinoid tumors; treatment of watery diarrhea associated with vasoactive intestinal peptide-secreting tumors (VIPomas); treatment of acromegaly

Unlabeled Use Treatment of AIDS-associated diarrhea (including *Cryptosporidiosis*), chemotherapy-induced diarrhea, graft-versus-host disease (GVHD) associated diarrhea, postgastrectomy dumping syndrome; control of bleeding of esophageal varices; second-line treatment for thymic malignancies; Cushing's syndrome (ectopic); insulinomas; small bowel fistulas; islet cell tumors; Zollinger-Ellison syndrome; congenital hyperinsulinism; hypothalamic obesity; treatment of hypoglycemia secondary to sulfonylurea poisoning; treatment of malignant bowel obstruction

Pregnancy Risk Factor B

Pregnancy Considerations Adverse effects were not observed in animal reproduction studies. Octreotide crosses the placenta and can be detected in the newborn at delivery (Caron, 1995; Fassnacht, 2001; Maffei, 2010); data concerning use in pregnancy is limited. In case reports of acromegalic women who received normal doses of octreotide during pregnancy, no congenital malformations were reported. Because normalization of IGF-1 and GH may restore fertility in women with acromegaly, women of childbearing potential should use adequate contraception during treatment. Long-acting formulations should be discontinued 2-3 months prior to a planned pregnancy when possible; however, octreotide therapy may be resumed in pregnant women with worsening symptoms if needed (Katznelson, 2011).

Breast-Feeding Considerations Octreotide is excreted in breast milk. In a case report, a woman was taking octreotide SubQ in doses up to 2400 mcg/day prior to and throughout pregnancy. Octreotide was measurable in the colostrum in concentrations similar to those in the maternal serum (Maffei, 2010); however, oral absorption of octreotide is considered to be poor (Battershill, 1989). The manufacturer recommends that caution be exercised when administering octreotide to nursing women.

Contraindications Hypersensitivity to octreotide or any component of the formulation

Warnings/Precautions May impair gallbladder function; monitor patients for cholelithiasis. The incidence of gallbladder stone or biliary sludge increases with a duration of therapy of ≥12 months. In patients with neuroendocrine tumors, the NCCN guidelines (v.1.2011) recommend considering prophylactic cholecystectomy in patients undergoing abdominal surgery if octreotide treatment is planned. Use with caution in patients with renal and/or hepatic impairment; dosage adjustment may be required in patients receiving dialysis and in patients with established cirrhosis. Somatostatin analogs may affect glucose regulation. In type I diabetes, severe hypoglycemia may occur; in type II diabetes or patients without diabetes, hyperglycemia may occur. Insulin and other hypoglycemic medication requirements may change. Octreotide may worsen hypoglycemia in patients with insulinomas; use with caution. Do not use depot formulation for the treatment of sulfonylurea-induced hypoglycemia. Bradycardia, conduction abnormalities, and arrhythmia have been observed in acromegalic and carcinoid syndrome patients; use caution with CHF or concomitant medications that alter heart rate or rhythm. Cardiovascular medication requirements may change. Octreotide may enhance the adverse/toxic effects of other QT_c-prolonging agents. May alter absorption of dietary fats; monitor for pancreatitis. May reduce excessive fluid loss in patients with conditions that cause such loss; monitor for elevations in zinc levels in such patients that are maintained on total parenteral nutrition (TPN). Chronic treatment has been associated with abnormal Schillings test; monitor vitamin B_{12} levels. Suppresses secretion of TSH; monitor for hypothyroidism.

Postmarketing cases of serious and fatal events, including hypoxia and necrotizing enterocolitis, have been reported with octreotide use in children (usually with serious underlying conditions), particularly in children <2 years of age. In studies with octreotide depot, the incidence of cholelithiasis in children is higher than the reported incidences for adults and efficacy was not demonstrated. Therapy may restore fertility; females of childbearing potential should use adequate contraception. Dosage adjustment may be necessary in the elderly; significant increases in elimination half-life have been observed in older adults. Vehicle used in depot injection (polylactide-co-glycolide microspheres) has rarely been associated with retinal artery occlusion in patients with abnormal arteriovenous anastomosis.

Adverse Reactions Adverse reactions vary by route of administration and dosage form. Frequency of cardiac, endocrine, and gastrointestinal adverse reactions was generally higher in acromegalics.

>16%:

- Cardiovascular: Sinus bradycardia (19% to 25%), chest pain (≤20%; non-depot formulations)
- Central nervous system: Fatigue (1% to 32%), headache (6% to 30%), malaise (16% to 20%), fever (16% to 20%), dizziness (5% to 20%)
- Dermatologic: Pruritus (≤18%)
- Endocrine & metabolic: Hyperglycemia (2% to 27%)
- Gastrointestinal: Abdominal pain (5% to 61%), loose stools (5% to 61%), nausea (5% to 61%), diarrhea (34% to 61%), flatulence (≤38%), cholelithiasis (13% to 38%; length of therapy dependent), biliary sludge (24%; length of therapy dependent), constipation (9% to 21%), vomiting (4% to 21%), biliary duct dilatation (12%)
- Local: Injection site pain (2% to 50%; dose and formulation related)
- Neuromuscular & skeletal: Back pain (1% to 27%), arthropathy (8% to 19%), myalgia (≤18%)
- Respiratory: Upper respiratory infection (10% to 23%), dyspnea (≤20%; non-depot formulations)
- Miscellaneous: Antibodies to octreotide (up to 25%; no efficacy change), flu symptoms (1% to 20%)

5% to 15%:

- Cardiovascular: Hypertension (≤13%), conduction abnormalities (9% to 10%), arrhythmia (3% to 9%), palpitation, peripheral edema
- Central nervous system: Pain (4% to 15%), anxiety, confusion, hypoesthesia, insomnia
- Dermatologic: Rash (15%; depot formulation), alopecia (≤13%)
- Endocrine & metabolic: Hypothyroidism (≤12%; non-depot formulations), goiter (≤8%; non-depot formulations)
- Gastrointestinal: Dyspepsia (4% to 6%), feces discoloration (4% to 6%), steatorrhea (4% to 6%), tenesmus (4% to 6%), anorexia, cramping
- Hematologic: Anemia (≤15%; non-depot formulations: <1%)
- Neuromuscular & skeletal: Arthralgia, myalgia, paresthesia, rigors, weakness
- Otic: Earache
- Renal: Renal calculus
- Respiratory: Cough, pharyngitis, rhinitis, sinusitis
- Miscellaneous: Allergy, diaphoresis

1% to 4%:

- Cardiovascular: Angina, cardiac failure, edema, flushing, hematoma, phlebitis
- Central nervous system: Abnormal gait, amnesia, depression, dysphonia, hallucinations, nervousness, neuralgia, somnolence, vertigo
- Dermatologic: Acne, bruising, cellulitis
- Endocrine & metabolic: Hypoglycemia (2% to 4%), hypokalemia, hypoproteinemia, gout, cachexia, breast pain, impotence
- Gastrointestinal: Colitis, diverticulitis, dysphagia, fat malabsorption, gastritis, gastroenteritis, gingivitis, glossitis, melena, stomatitis, taste perversion, xerostomia
- Genitourinary: Incontinence, pollakiuria (non-depot formulations), urinary tract infection
- Local: Injection site hematoma
- Neuromuscular & skeletal: Hyperkinesia, hypertonia, joint pain, neuropathy, tremor
- Ocular: Blurred vision, visual disturbance
- Otic: Tinnitus
- Renal: Albuminuria, renal abscess
- Respiratory: Bronchitis, epistaxis
- Miscellaneous: Bacterial infection, cold symptoms, moniliasis

<1% (Limited to important or life-threatening): Amenorrhea, anaphylactic shock, anaphylactoid reactions, aneurysm, aphasia, appendicitis, arthritis, ascending cholangitis, ascites, atrial fibrillation, basal cell carcinoma, Bell's palsy, biliary obstruction, breast carcinoma, cardiac arrest, cerebral vascular disorder, CHF, cholecystitis, cholestatic hepatitis, CK increased, deafness, diabetes insipidus, diabetes mellitus, fatty liver, galactorrhea, gallbladder polyp, GI bleeding, GI hemorrhage, GI ulcer, glaucoma, gynecomastia, hematuria, hepatitis, hypoadrenalism, hypoxia (children), intestinal obstruction, intracranial hemorrhage, intraocular pressure increased, ischemia, joint effusion, malignant hyperpyrexia, MI, migraine, necrotizing enterocolitis (neonates), nephrolithiasis, neuritis, oligomenorrhea, orthostatic hypotension, pancreatitis, pancytopenia, paresis, pituitary apoplexy, pleural effusion, pneumonia, pneumothorax, polymenorrhea, pulmonary embolism, pulmonary hypertension, pulmonary nodule, Raynaud's syndrome, renal failure, renal insufficiency, retinal vein thrombosis, seizures, status asthmaticus, suicide attempt, syncope, tachycardia, thrombocytopenia, thrombophlebitis, thrombosis, weight loss

Drug Interactions

Metabolism/Transport Effects None known.

Avoid Concomitant Use There are no known interactions where it is recommended to avoid concomitant use.

Increased Effect/Toxicity

Octreotide may increase the levels/effects of: Codeine; Highest Risk QTc-Prolonging Agents; Hypoglycemic Agents; Moderate Risk QTc-Prolonging Agents; Pegvisomant

The levels/effects of Octreotide may be increased by: Herbs (Hypoglycemic Properties); MAO Inhibitors; Mifepristone; Salicylates; Selective Serotonin Reuptake Inhibitors

Decreased Effect

Octreotide may decrease the levels/effects of: CycloSPORINE (Systemic)

The levels/effects of Octreotide may be decreased by: Loop Diuretics

Ethanol/Nutrition/Herb Interactions

Food: Octreotide may alter absorption of dietary fats. Management: Administer injections between meals to decrease GI effects.

Herb/Nutraceutical: Some herbal medications may enhance the hypoglycemic effect of octreotide. Management: Avoid hypoglycemic herbs, including alfalfa, aloe, bilberry, bitter melon, burdock, celery, damiana, fenugreek, garcinia, garlic, ginger, ginseng (American), gymnema, marshmallow, and stinging nettle.

Storage/Stability

Solution: Octreotide is a clear solution and should be stored at refrigerated temperatures between 2°C and 8°C (36°F and 46°F). Protect from light. May be stored at room temperature of 20°C to 30°C (68°F and 86°F) for up to 14 days when protected from light. Stable as a parenteral admixture in NS for 96 hours at room temperature (25°C) and in D_5W for 24 hours. Stable for up to 7 days in a polypropylene syringe. Discard multidose vials within 14 days after initial entry.

Suspension: Prior to dilution, store at refrigerated temperatures between 2°C and 8°C (36°F and 46°F). Protect from light. Additionally, the manufacturer reports that octreotide suspension may be stored at room temperature of 20°C to 25°C (68°F and 77°F) for up to 10 days when protected from light (data on file [Novartis, 2011]). Depot drug product kit may be at room temperature for 30-60 minutes prior to use. Use suspension immediately after preparation.

Mechanism of Action Mimics natural somatostatin by inhibiting serotonin release, and the secretion of gastrin, VIP, insulin, glucagon, secretin, motilin, and pancreatic polypeptide. Decreases growth hormone and IGF-1 in acromegaly. Octreotide provides more potent inhibition of growth hormone, glucagon, and insulin as compared to endogenous somatostatin. Also suppresses LH response to GnRH, secretion of thyroid-stimulating hormone and decreases splanchnic blood flow.

Pharmacodynamics/Kinetics

Duration: SubQ: 6-12 hours

Absorption: SubQ: Rapid and complete; I.M. (depot formulation): Released slowly (via microsphere degradation in the muscle)

Distribution: V_d: 14 L (13-30 L in acromegaly)

Protein binding: 65%, primarily to lipoprotein (41% in acromegaly)

Metabolism: Extensively hepatic

Bioavailability: SubQ: 100%; I.M: 60% to 63% of SubQ dose

Half-life elimination: 1.7-1.9 hours; Increased in elderly patients; Cirrhosis: Up to 3.7 hours; Fatty liver disease: Up to 3.4 hours; Renal impairment: Up to 3.1 hours

Time to peak, plasma: SubQ: 0.4 hours (0.7 hours acromegaly); I.M.: 1 hour

Excretion: Urine (32% as unchanged drug)

Dosage

Acromegaly: Adults:

SubQ, I.V.: Initial: 50 mcg 3 times/day; titrate to achieve growth hormone levels <5 ng/mL or IGF-I (somatomedin C) levels <1.9 units/mL in males and <2.2 units/mL in females. Usual effective dose 100-200 mcg 3 times/day; range: 300-1500 mcg/day. **Note:** Should be withdrawn yearly for a 4-week interval (8 weeks for depot injection) in patients who have received irradiation. Resume if levels increase and signs/symptoms recur.

I.M. depot injection: Patients must be stabilized on subcutaneous octreotide for at least 2 weeks before switching to the long-acting depot. Upon switch: 20 mg I.M. intragluteally every 4 weeks for 3 months, then the dose may be modified based upon response.

Dosage adjustment for acromegaly: After 3 months of depot injections, the dosage may be continued or modified as follows:

GH ≤1 ng/mL, IGF-1 normal, and symptoms controlled: Reduce octreotide depot to 10 mg I.M. every 4 weeks

GH ≤2.5 ng/mL, IGF-1 normal, and symptoms controlled: Maintain octreotide depot at 20 mg I.M. every 4 weeks

GH >2.5 ng/mL, IGF-1 elevated, and/or symptoms uncontrolled: Increase octreotide depot to 30 mg I.M. every 4 weeks

Note: Patients not adequately controlled at a dose of 30 mg may increase dose to 40 mg every 4 weeks. Dosages >40 mg are not recommended.

Carcinoid tumors: Adults:

Manufacturer labeling:

SubQ, I.V.: Initial 2 weeks: 100-600 mcg/day in 2-4 divided doses; usual range: 50-750 mcg/day (some patients may require up to 1500 mcg/day)

I.M. depot injection: Patients must be stabilized on subcutaneous octreotide for at least 2 weeks before switching to the long-acting depot. Upon switch: 20 mg I.M. intragluteally every 4 weeks for 2 months, then the dose may be modified based upon response.

NCCN guidelines (Neuroendocrine Tumor, v.1.2011):

SubQ: 150-250 mcg 3 times/day; dose and frequency may be increased if needed for symptom control

I.M. depot injection: 20-30 mg every 4 weeks; dose and frequency may be increased if needed for symptom control; SubQ octreotide may be used for breakthrough symptoms

Note: Patients should continue to receive their SubQ injections for the first 2 weeks at the same dose in order to maintain therapeutic levels (some patients may require 3-4 weeks of continued SubQ injections). Patients who experience periodic exacerbations of symptoms may require temporary SubQ injections in addition to depot injections (at their previous SubQ dosing regimen) until symptoms have resolved.

Dosage adjustment for carcinoid tumors: After 2 months of depot injections, the dosage may be continued or modified as follows:

Increase to 30 mg I.M. every 4 weeks if symptoms are inadequately controlled

Decrease to 10 mg I.M. every 4 weeks, for a trial period, if initially responsive to 20 mg dose

Dosage >30 mg is not recommended

VIPomas:

Manufacturer labeling:

SubQ, I.V.: Initial 2 weeks: 200-300 mcg/day in 2-4 divided doses; titrate dose based on response/tolerance. Range: 150-750 mcg/day (doses >450 mcg/day are rarely required)

I.M. depot injection: Patients must be stabilized on subcutaneous octreotide for at least 2 weeks before switching to the long-acting depot. Upon switch: 20 mg I.M. intragluteally every 4 weeks for 2 months, then the dose may be modified based upon response.

NCCN guidelines (Neuroendocrine Tumor, v.1.2011):
SubQ: 150-250 mcg 3 times/day; dose and frequency may be increased if needed for symptom control
I.M. depot injection: 20-30 mg every 4 weeks dose and frequency may be increased if needed for symptom control; SubQ octreotide may be used for breakthrough symptoms

Note: Patients receiving depot injection should continue to receive their SubQ injections for the first 2 weeks at the same dose in order to maintain therapeutic levels (some patients may require 3-4 weeks of continued SubQ injections). Patients who experience periodic exacerbations of symptoms may require temporary SubQ injections in addition to depot injections (at their previous SubQ dosing regimen) until symptoms have resolved.

Dosage adjustment for VIPomas: After 2 months of depot injections, the dosage may be continued or modified as follows:
Increase to 30 mg I.M. every 4 weeks if symptoms are inadequately controlled
Decrease to 10 mg I.M. every 4 weeks, for a trial period, if initially responsive to 20 mg dose
Dosage >30 mg is not recommended

Congenital hyperinsulinism (unlabeled use): Infants and Children: SubQ: Initial: 2-10 mcg/kg/day; up to 40 mcg/kg/day have been used (Stanley, 1997)

Diarrhea (unlabeled use):
Infants and Children: I.V., SubQ: Doses of 1-10 mcg/kg every 12 hours have been used in children beginning at the low end of the range and increasing by 0.3 mcg/kg/dose at 3-day intervals. Suppression of growth hormone (animal data) is of concern when used as long-term therapy.
Adults: I.V.: Initial: 50-100 mcg every 8 hours; increase by 100 mcg/dose at 48-hour intervals; maximum dose: 500 mcg every 8 hours

Diarrhea associated with chemotherapy (unlabeled use):
Low grade or uncomplicated: SubQ: 100-150 mcg every 8 hours (Benson, 2004; Kornblau, 2000)
Severe: Initial: SubQ: 100-150 mcg every 8 hours; may increase to 500-1500 mcg I.V. or SubQ every 8 hours (Kornblau, 2000)
Complicated: I.V., SubQ: Initial: 100-150 mcg 3 times/day or I.V. Infusion: 25-50 mcg/hour; may escalate to 500 mcg 3 times/day until controlled (Benson, 2004)

Diarrhea associated with GVHD (unlabeled use): I.V.: 500 mcg every 8 hours; discontinue within 24 hours of resolution; Maximum duration of therapy if diarrhea is not resolved: 7 days (Kornblau, 2000)

Esophageal varices bleeding (unlabeled use): Adults: I.V. bolus: 25-100 mcg (usual bolus dose: 50 mcg) followed by continuous I.V. infusion of 25-50 mcg/hour for 2-5 days; may repeat bolus in first hour if hemorrhage not controlled (Corley, 2001; Erstad, 2001; Garcia-Tsao, 2010)

Hypoglycemia in sulfonylurea poisoning (unlabeled use): Note: SubQ is the preferred route of administration; repeat dosing, dose escalation, or initiation of a continuous infusion may be required in patients who experience recurrent hypoglycemia. Duration of treatment may exceed 24 hours. Optimal care decisions should be made based upon patient-specific details:
Children: SubQ: 1-1.5 mcg/kg; repeat in 6-12 hours as needed based upon blood glucose concentrations (Calello, 2005; Glatstein, 2009)
Adults:
SubQ: 50-100 mcg; repeat in 6-12 hours as needed based upon blood glucose concentrations (Braatvedt, 1997; Carr, 2002; Graudins, 1997; Hung, 1997)
I.V.: Doses up to 100-125 mcg/hour have been used successfully (McLaughlin, 2000)

Islet cell tumors (unlabeled use): SubQ: 150-250 mcg 3 times/day or I.M. (depot): 20-30 mg every 4 weeks dose and frequency may be increased if needed for symptom control; SubQ octreotide may be used for breakthrough symptoms (NCCN Neuroendocrine Tumor guidelines v.1.2011)

Malignant bowel obstruction (unlabeled use):
SubQ: 100-300 mcg 2-3 times/day (Mercadante, 2007; NCCN Palliative Care guidelines v.2.2011)
Continuous SubQ/I.V. infusion: 10-40 mcg/hour (NCCN Palliative Care guidelines v.2.2011)

Elderly: Elimination half-life is increased by 46% and clearance is decreased by 26%; dose adjustment may be required. Dosing should generally begin at the lower end of dosing range.

Dosage adjustment in renal impairment:
Regular injection:
Mild to severe impairment: No dosage adjustment provided in manufacturer's labeling.
Dialysis-dependent impairment: No specific dosage adjustment provided in manufacturer's labeling; however, a dosage adjustment may be needed since clearance is reduced by ~50%.
Depot injection:
Mild to severe impairment: No dosage adjustment necessary.
Dialysis-dependent impairment: Initial dose: 10 mg I.M. every 4 weeks; titrate based upon response (clearance is reduced by ~50%).

Dosage adjustment in hepatic impairment:
Regular injection: No dosage adjustment provided in manufacturer's labeling. Half-life is prolonged and total body clearance is decreased in patients with cirrhosis and fatty liver disease.
Depot injection: Patients with established cirrhosis of the liver: Initial dose: 10 mg I.M. every 4 weeks; titrate based upon response.

Dietary Considerations Schedule injections between meals to decrease GI effects. May alter absorption of dietary fats.

Usual Infusion Concentrations: Adult I.V. infusion: 500 mcg in 250 mL (concentration: 2 **mcg**/mL) of D_5W or NS

Administration
Regular injection formulation (do not use if solution contains particles or is discolored): Administer SubQ or I.V.; I.V. administration may be I.V. push (undiluted over 3 minutes), intermittent I.V. infusion (over 15-30 minutes), or continuous I.V. infusion (unlabeled route).
SubQ: Use the concentration with smallest volume to deliver dose to reduce injection site pain. Rotate injection site; may bring to room temperature prior to injection.
Depot formulation: Administer I.M. intragluteal (avoid deltoid administration); alternate gluteal injection sites to avoid irritation. **Do not** administer Sandostatin LAR® intravenously or subcutaneously; must be administered immediately after mixing.

Monitoring Parameters
Acromegaly: Growth hormone, somatomedin C (IGF-1)
Carcinoid: 5-HIAA, plasma serotonin and plasma substance P
VIPomas: Vasoactive intestinal peptide
Chronic therapy: Thyroid function (baseline and periodic), vitamin B_{12} level, blood glucose, glycemic control and antidiabetic regimen (patients with diabetes mellitus), cardiac function (heart rate, ECG), zinc level (patients with excessive fluid loss maintained on TPN)

Reference Range Vasoactive intestinal peptide: <75 ng/L; levels vary considerably between laboratories

Dosage Forms Excipient information presented when available (limited, particularly for generics); consult specific product labeling.

Kit, Intramuscular:
SandoSTATIN LAR Depot: 10 mg, 20 mg, 30 mg

Solution, Injection:
SandoSTATIN: 50 mcg/mL (1 mL); 100 mcg/mL (1 mL)
SandoSTATIN: 200 mcg/mL (5 mL) [contains phenol]
SandoSTATIN: 500 mcg/mL (1 mL)
SandoSTATIN: 1000 mcg/mL (5 mL) [contains phenol]
Generic: 50 mcg/mL (1 mL); 100 mcg/mL (1 mL); 200 mcg/mL (5 mL); 1000 mcg/5 mL (5 mL); 500 mcg/mL (1 mL); 1000 mcg/mL (5 mL)

Solution, Injection [preservative free]:
Generic: 100 mcg/mL (1 mL); 500 mcg/mL (1 mL)

◆ **Octreotide Acetate** *see* Octreotide *on page 1485*
◆ **Octreotide Acetate Injection (Can)** *see* Octreotide *on page 1485*
◆ **Octreotide Acetate Omega (Can)** *see* Octreotide *on page 1485*
◆ **Ocudox** *see* Doxycycline *on page 668*
◆ **Ocufen** *see* Flurbiprofen (Ophthalmic) *on page 892*
◆ **Ocuflox** *see* Ofloxacin (Ophthalmic) *on page 1492*
◆ **Ocuflox® (Can)** *see* Ofloxacin (Ophthalmic) *on page 1492*
◆ **O-desmethylvenlafaxine** *see* Desvenlafaxine *on page 579*
◆ **ODV** *see* Desvenlafaxine *on page 579*
◆ **Oesclim (Can)** *see* Estradiol (Systemic) *on page 754*

Ofatumumab (oh fa TOOM yoo mab)

Brand Names: U.S. Arzerra

Brand Names: Canada Arzerra

Index Terms HuMax-CD20

Pharmacologic Category Antineoplastic Agent, Monoclonal Antibody; Monoclonal Antibody

Use Chronic lymphocytic leukemia: Treatment of refractory chronic lymphocytic leukemia (CLL)

Pregnancy Risk Factor C

Pregnancy Considerations Teratogenicity was not observed in animal reproduction studies, although prolonged depletion of circulating B cells was observed in animal offspring. Use in pregnancy only if the potential benefit to the mother outweighs the potential risk to the fetus.

Breast-Feeding Considerations It is not known if ofatumumab is excreted in human milk. However, human IgG is excreted in breast milk, and therefore, ofatumumab may also be excreted in milk. The effects of local GI and systemic exposure are unknown, therefore caution should be used in nursing women receiving ofatumumab.

Contraindications There are no contraindications listed within the manufacturer's labeling.

Warnings/Precautions [U.S. Boxed Warning]: Hepatitis B virus (HBV) reactivation may occur with use and may result in fulminant hepatitis, hepatic failure, and death. Fatal cases of HBV have also occurred in patients not previously infected with HBV. Prior to initiating therapy, obtain hepatitis B surface antigen (HBsAg) and hepatitis B core antibody (anti-HBc) measurements in all patients; monitor for clinical and laboratory signs of hepatitis or HBV during and for several months after treatment. HBV reactivation has been reported up to 12 months after therapy discontinuation. Discontinue ofatumumab (and concomitant medications) if viral hepatitis develops and initiate appropriate antiviral therapy. Reactivation has occurred in patients who are HBsAg positive as well as in those who are HBsAg negative but are anti-HBc positive; HBV reactivation has also been observed in patients who had previously resolved HBV infection. Use cautiously in patients who show evidence of prior HBV infection (eg, HBsAg positive [regardless of antibody status] or HBsAG negative but anti-HBc positive); consult with appropriate clinicians regarding monitoring and consideration of antiviral therapy before and/or during ofatumumab treatment. The safety of resuming ofatumumab treatment following HBV reactivation is not known; discuss reinitiation of therapy in patients with resolved HBV reactivation with physicians experienced in HBV management.

May cause serious infusion reaction; reactions may include bronchospasm, dyspnea, laryngeal edema, pulmonary edema, flushing, hypertension, hypotension, syncope, cardiac ischemia/infarction, back pain, abdominal pain, fever, rash, urticaria, and/or angioedema. Infusion reactions occur more frequently with the first 2 infusions. Premedicate with acetaminophen, an antihistamine, and a corticosteroid prior to infusion; interrupt infusion for reaction (and institute appropriate treatment) for reaction; may require subsequent rate modification.

[U.S. Boxed Warning]: Progressive multifocal leukoencephalopathy (PML) resulting in death may occur with treatment. Consider PML in any patient with new onset or worsening neurological symptoms, and if suspected, discontinue ofatumumab and evaluate promptly. Severe and prolonged (≥1 week) cytopenias (neutropenia and thrombocytopenia) may occur. Monitor blood counts during treatment; more frequently if grade 3 or 4 cytopenias develop. Small intestine obstruction may occur with treatment; evaluate if suspected (eg, abdominal pain or repeated vomiting). Tumor lysis syndrome has occurred in patients receiving ofatumumab; administer prophylactic antihyperuricemic therapy and aggressive hydration. Correct electrolyte abnormalities; monitor renal function and hydration status.

Live vaccines should not be given concurrently with ofatumumab; there is no data concerning secondary transmission; the ability to generate an immune response to any vaccine following treatment is unknown.

Adverse Reactions

>10%:
Central nervous system: Fatigue (15%)
Dermatologic: Skin rash (14%)
Gastrointestinal: Diarrhea (18%), nausea (11%)
Hematologic & oncologic: Neutropenia (≥grade 3: 42%; grade 4: 18%; may be prolonged >2 weeks), anemia (16%; grades 3/4: 5%)
Infection: Infection (70%; includes bacterial, fungal, or viral; ≥grade 3: 29%)
Respiratory: Pneumonia (23%), cough (19%), dyspnea (14%), bronchitis (11%), upper respiratory tract infection (11%)
Miscellaneous: Infusion related reaction (first infusion [300 mg]: 44%; second infusion [2000 mg]: 29%), fever (20%)

1% to 10%:
Cardiovascular: Peripheral edema (9%), hypertension (5%), hypotension (5%), tachycardia (5%)
Central nervous system: Chills (8%), insomnia (7%), headache (6%)
Dermatologic: Urticaria (8%), hyperhidrosis (5%)
Infection: Sepsis (8%), herpes zoster (6%)
Neuromuscular & skeletal: Back pain (8%), muscle spasm (5%)
Respiratory: Nasopharyngitis (8%), sinusitis (5%)

<1% (Limited to important or life-threatening): Angina pectoris, bacteremia, hemolytic anemia, hepatitis B (new onset or reactivation), hepatitis (cytolytic), hypoxia, interstitial pulmonary disease (infectious), intestinal obstruction, peritonitis, progressive multifocal

leukoencephalopathy (PML), rigors, sepsis (neutropenic), septic shock, thrombocytopenia

Drug Interactions

Metabolism/Transport Effects None known.

Avoid Concomitant Use

Avoid concomitant use of Ofatumumab with any of the following: BCG; Belimumab; Natalizumab; Pimecrolimus; Tacrolimus (Topical); Tofacitinib; Vaccines (Live)

Increased Effect/Toxicity

Ofatumumab may increase the levels/effects of: Belimumab; Leflunomide; Natalizumab; Tofacitinib; Vaccines (Live); Vitamin K Antagonists

The levels/effects of Ofatumumab may be increased by: Abciximab; Denosumab; Pimecrolimus; Roflumilast; Tacrolimus (Topical); Trastuzumab

Decreased Effect

Ofatumumab may decrease the levels/effects of: BCG; Cardiac Glycosides; Coccidioidin Skin Test; Sipuleucel-T; Vaccines (Inactivated); Vaccines (Live); Vitamin K Antagonists

The levels/effects of Ofatumumab may be decreased by: Echinacea

Preparation for Administration

300 mg dose: Withdraw 15 mL from a 1000 mL NS bag. Add contents of three ofatumumab 100 mg vials (total volume = 15 mL) to NS bag (final concentration of 0.3 mg/mL). Gently invert to mix; do not shake. Begin infusion within 12 hours of preparation.

2000 mg dose: Withdraw 100 mL from a 1000 mL NS bag. Add contents of two ofatumumab 1000 mg vials (total volume = 100 mL) to NS bag (final concentration of 2 mg/mL). Gently invert to mix; do not shake. Begin infusion within 12 hours of preparation.

Storage/Stability Store intact vials at 2°C to 8°C (36°F to 46°F); do not freeze. Protect from light. Diluted solutions for infusion must be started within 12 hours of preparation (may store at 2°C to 8°C [36°F to 46°F] if not used immediately); discard any remaining solution 24 hours after preparation.

Mechanism of Action Ofatumumab is a monoclonal antibody which binds specifically the extracellular (large and small) loops of the CD20 molecule (which is expressed on normal B lymphocytes and in B-cell CLL) resulting in potent complement-dependent cell lysis and antibody-dependent cell-mediated toxicity in cells that overexpress CD20.

Pharmacodynamics/Kinetics

Distribution: V_{dss}: 1.7-5.1 L

Half-life elimination: Between dose 4 and dose 12: ~14 days (range: 2-62 days)

Dosage Note: Premedicate with acetaminophen, an antihistamine, and a corticosteroid 30-120 minutes prior to treatment (see Administration).

Chronic lymphocytic leukemia (CLL): Adults: I.V.: Initial dose: 300 mg week 1, followed 1 week later by 2000 mg once weekly for 7 doses (doses 2-8), followed 4 weeks later by 2000 mg once every 4 weeks for 4 doses (doses 9-12; for a total of 12 doses)

Dosage adjustment for toxicity: Infusion reaction: Interrupt infusion for infusion reaction (any severity).

Grade 1 or 2 infusion reaction: Resume at one-half of the previous rate; may increase (see Administration) based on patient tolerance

Grade 3: Resume infusion at 12 mL/hour; may increase (see Administration) based on patient tolerance

Grade 4: Do not resume

Dosage adjustment in renal impairment: No dosage adjustment provided in manufacturer's labeling. However, there were no clinically relevant pharmacokinetic effects observed in patients with baseline Cl_{cr} >33 mL/minute.

Dosage adjustment in hepatic impairment: No dosage adjustment provided in manufacturer's labeling (has not been studied).

Administration Do not administer I.V. push or as a bolus. Premedicate with acetaminophen, an antihistamine, and a corticosteroid 30-120 minutes prior to administration. Administer with an in-line filter (supplied). Do not mix with or infuse with other medications. Flush line before and after infusion with NS. Begin infusion within 12 hours of preparation. The final concentration of dose 1 is 0.3 mg/mL and final concentration of doses 2-12 is 2 mg/mL.

Premedication: Premedicate with oral acetaminophen (1000 mg), an oral or I.V. antihistamine (eg, cetirizine 10 mg orally or equivalent), and an I.V. corticosteroid. Full dose corticosteroid is recommended for doses 1, 2, and 9; in the absence of infusion reaction ≥grade 3, may gradually reduce corticosteroid dose for doses 3-8; administer full or half corticosteroid dose with doses 10-12 if ≥grade 3 did not occur with dose 9.

Doses 1 and 2: Initiate infusion at 12 mL/hour for 30 minutes, if tolerated (no infusion reaction) increase to 25 mL/hour for 30 minutes, if tolerated, increase to 50 mL/hour for 30 minutes, if tolerated, increase to 100 mL/hour for 30 minutes, if tolerated, increase to 200 mL/hour for duration of infusion.

Doses 3-12: Initiate infusion at 25 mL/hour for 30 minutes, if tolerated (no infusion reaction) increase to 50 mL/hour for 30 minutes, if tolerated, increase to 100 mL/hour for 30 minutes, if tolerated, increase to 200 mL/hour for 30 minutes, if tolerated, increase to 400 mL/hour for remainder of infusion.

Monitoring Parameters CBC with differential, hepatitis B screening in all patients (HBsAG and anti-HBc measurements) prior to therapy initiation; renal function, electrolytes; signs of active hepatitis B infection (during and for up to 12 months after therapy completion); signs or symptoms of infusion reaction; signs of infection; fluid status; signs/symptoms of intestinal obstruction (eg, abdominal pain, repeated vomiting); signs/symptoms of progressive multifocal leukoencephalopathy (focal neurologic deficits, which may present as hemiparesis, visual field deficits, cognitive impairment, aphasia, ataxia, and/or cranial nerve deficits).

Dosage Forms Excipient information presented when available (limited, particularly for generics); consult specific product labeling.

Concentrate, Intravenous [preservative free]:

Arzerra: 100 mg/5 mL (5 mL); 1000 mg/50 mL (50 mL) [contains edetate disodium, mouse protein (murine) (hamster), polysorbate 80]

◆ **Ofirmev** *see* Acetaminophen *on page* 28

Ofloxacin (Systemic) (oh FLOKS a sin)

Brand Names: Canada Apo-Oflox®; Novo-Ofloxacin

Pharmacologic Category Antibiotic, Fluoroquinolone

Use Quinolone antibiotic for the treatment of acute exacerbations of chronic bronchitis, community-acquired pneumonia, skin and skin structure infections (uncomplicated), urethral and cervical gonorrhea (acute, uncomplicated), urethritis and cervicitis (nongonococcal), mixed infections of the urethra and cervix, pelvic inflammatory disease (acute), cystitis (uncomplicated), urinary tract infections (complicated), prostatitis

Note: As of April 2007, the CDC no longer recommends the use of fluoroquinolones for the treatment of gonococcal disease.

Unlabeled Use Epididymitis (nongonococcal), leprosy, Traveler's diarrhea

Pregnancy Risk Factor C

Pregnancy Considerations Adverse events have been observed in some animal studies; therefore, the manufacturer classifies ofloxacin as pregnancy category C. Ofloxacin crosses the placenta and produces measurable concentrations in the amniotic fluid. An increased risk of teratogenic effects has not been observed in animals or humans following ofloxacin use during pregnancy; however, because of concerns of cartilage damage in immature animals, ofloxacin should only be used during pregnancy if a safer option is not available. Serum concentrations of ofloxacin may be lower during pregnancy than in nonpregnant patients.

Breast-Feeding Considerations Ofloxacin is excreted in breast milk. Breast-feeding is not recommended by the manufacturer. Due to the low concentrations in human milk, minimal toxicity would be expected in the nursing infant. Nondose-related effects could include modification of bowel flora.

Medication Guide Available Yes

Contraindications Hypersensitivity to ofloxacin or other members of the quinolone group, such as oxolinic acid, cinoxacin, norfloxacin, and ciprofloxacin; hypersensitivity to any component of the formulation

Warnings/Precautions **[U.S. Boxed Warning]: There have been reports of tendon inflammation and/or rupture with quinolone antibiotics; risk may be increased with concurrent corticosteroids, organ transplant recipients, and in patients >60 years of age.** Rupture of the Achilles tendon sometimes requiring surgical repair has been reported most frequently; but other tendon sites (eg, rotator cuff, biceps) have also been reported. Strenuous physical activity, rheumatoid arthritis, and renal impairment may be an independent risk factor for tendonitis. Discontinue at first sign of tendon inflammation or pain. May occur even after discontinuation of therapy. Use with caution in patients with rheumatoid arthritis; may increase risk of tendon rupture. CNS effects may occur (tremor, restlessness, confusion, and very rarely hallucinations, increased intracranial pressure [including pseudotumor cerebri] or seizures). Use with caution in patients with known or suspected CNS disorder. Potential for seizures, although very rare, may be increased with concomitant NSAID therapy. Use with caution in individuals at risk of seizures. Use with caution in patients with renal or hepatic impairment. Peripheral neuropathy has been reported (rare); may occur soon after initiation of therapy and may be irreversible; discontinue if symptoms of sensory or sensorimotor neuropathy occur.

Fluoroquinolones have been associated with the development of serious, and sometimes fatal, hypoglycemia, most often in elderly diabetics, but also in patients without diabetes. This occurred most frequently with gatifloxacin (no longer available systemically) but may occur at a lower frequency with other quinolones.

Rare cases of torsade de pointes have been reported in patients receiving ofloxacin and other quinolones. Risk may be minimized by avoiding use in patients with known prolongation of the QT interval, bradycardia, hypokalemia, hypomagnesemia, cardiomyopathy, or in those receiving concurrent therapy with Class Ia or Class III antiarrhythmics.

Severe hypersensitivity reactions, including anaphylaxis, have occurred with quinolone therapy. Reactions may present as typical allergic symptoms after a single dose, or may manifest as severe idiosyncratic dermatologic, vascular, pulmonary, renal, hepatic, and/or hematologic events, usually after multiple doses. Prompt discontinuation of drug should occur if skin rash or other symptoms arise. Prolonged use may result in fungal or bacterial superinfection, including *C. difficile*-associated diarrhea (CDAD) and pseudomembranous colitis; CDAD has been observed >2 months postantibiotic treatment. **[U.S. Boxed Warning]: Quinolones may exacerbate myasthenia gravis; avoid use (rare, potentially life-threatening weakness of respiratory muscles may occur).** Avoid excessive sunlight and take precautions to limit exposure (eg, loose fitting clothing, sunscreen); may cause moderate-to-severe phototoxicity reactions. Discontinue use if photosensitivity occurs. Since ofloxacin is ineffective in the treatment of syphilis and may mask symptoms, all patients should be tested for syphilis at the time of gonorrheal diagnosis and 3 months later. Hemolytic reactions may (rarely) occur with quinolone use in patients with latent or actual G6PD deficiency. Safety and efficacy have not been established in children.

Adverse Reactions

1% to 10%:

Cardiovascular: Chest pain (1% to 3%)

Central nervous system: Headache (1% to 9%), insomnia (3% to 7%), dizziness (1% to 5%), fatigue (1% to 3%), somnolence (1% to 3%), sleep disorders (1% to 3%), nervousness (1% to 3%), pyrexia (1% to 3%)

Dermatologic: Rash/pruritus (1% to 3%)

Gastrointestinal: Diarrhea (1% to 4%), vomiting (1% to 4%), GI distress (1% to 3%), abdominal cramps (1% to 3%), flatulence (1% to 3%), abnormal taste (1% to 3%), xerostomia (1% to 3%), appetite decreased (1% to 3%), nausea (3% to 10%), constipation (1% to 3%)

Genitourinary: Vaginitis (1% to 5%), external genital pruritus in women (1% to 3%)

Ocular: Visual disturbances (1% to 3%)

Respiratory: Pharyngitis (1% to 3%)

Miscellaneous: Trunk pain

<1%, postmarketing, and/or case reports (limited to important or life-threatening): Anaphylaxis reactions, anxiety, blurred vision, chills, cognitive change, cough, depression, dream abnormality, ecchymosis, edema, erythema nodosum, euphoria, extremity pain, hallucinations, hearing acuity decreased, hepatic dysfunction, hepatic failure (some fatal), hepatitis, hyper-/hypoglycemia, hypertension, interstitial nephritis, intracranial pressure increased, lightheadedness, malaise, myasthenia gravis exacerbation, palpitation, paresthesia, peripheral neuropathy, photophobia, photosensitivity, pneumonitis, pseudotumor cerebri, psychotic reactions, rhabdomyolysis, seizure, Stevens-Johnson syndrome, syncope, tendonitis and tendon rupture, thirst, tinnitus, torsade de pointes, Tourette's syndrome, toxic epidermal necrolysis, vasculitis, vasodilation, vertigo, weakness, weight loss

Drug Interactions

Metabolism/Transport Effects Inhibits CYP1A2 (strong)

Avoid Concomitant Use

Avoid concomitant use of Ofloxacin (Systemic) with any of the following: Agomelatine; BCG; Highest Risk QTc-Prolonging Agents; Ivabradine; Mifepristone; Pirfenidone; Pomalidomide; Strontium Ranelate

Increased Effect/Toxicity

Ofloxacin (Systemic) may increase the levels/effects of: Agomelatine; Bendamustine; CloZAPine; Corticosteroids (Systemic); CYP1A2 Substrates; Highest Risk QTc-Prolonging Agents; Moderate Risk QTc-Prolonging Agents; Pirfenidone; Pomalidomide; Porfimer; Sulfonylureas; Theophylline Derivatives; Varenicline; Vitamin K Antagonists

The levels/effects of Ofloxacin (Systemic) may be increased by: Insulin; Ivabradine; Mifepristone; Nonsteroidal Anti-Inflammatory Agents; Probenecid; QTc-Prolonging Agents (Indeterminate Risk and Risk Modifying)

Decreased Effect

Ofloxacin (Systemic) may decrease the levels/effects of: BCG; Didanosine; Mycophenolate; Sodium Picosulfate; Sulfonylureas; Typhoid Vaccine

The levels/effects of Ofloxacin (Systemic) may be decreased by: Antacids; Calcium Salts; Didanosine; Iron Salts; Lanthanum; Magnesium Salts; Multivitamins/Minerals (with ADEK, Folate, Iron); Multivitamins/Minerals (with AE, No Iron); Quinapril; Sevelamer; Strontium Ranelate; Sucralfate; Zinc Salts

Ethanol/Nutrition/Herb Interactions

Food: Ofloxacin average peak serum concentrations may be decreased by 20% if taken with food.

Herb/Nutraceutical: Avoid dong quai, St John's wort (may also cause photosensitization).

Storage/Stability Store at 25°C (77°F); excursions permitted to 15°C to 30°C (59°F to 86°F).

Mechanism of Action Ofloxacin is a DNA gyrase inhibitor. DNA gyrase is an essential bacterial enzyme that maintains the superhelical structure of DNA. DNA gyrase is required for DNA replication and transcription, DNA repair, recombination, and transposition; bactericidal

Pharmacodynamics/Kinetics

Absorption: Well absorbed; food causes only minor alterations

Distribution: V_d: 2.4-3.5 L/kg

Protein binding: 32%

Bioavailability: 98%

Half-life elimination: Biphasic: 4-5 hours and 20-25 hours (accounts for <5%); prolonged with renal impairment

Excretion: Primarily urine (as unchanged drug)

Dosage

Usual dosage range: Adults: Oral: 200-400 mg every 12 hours

Indication-specific dosing: Adults: Oral:

Cervicitis/urethritis:

Nongonococcal: 300 mg every 12 hours for 7 days

Gonococcal (acute, uncomplicated): 400 mg as a single dose; **Note:** As of April 2007, the CDC no longer recommends the use of fluoroquinolones for the treatment of uncomplicated gonococcal disease.

Chronic bronchitis (acute exacerbation), community-acquired pneumonia, skin and skin structure infections (uncomplicated): 400 mg every 12 hours for 10 days

Epididymitis, nongonococcal (unlabeled use): 300 mg twice daily for 10 days (CDC, 2010); 200 mg twice daily for 14 days (Canadian STI Guidelines, 2008)

Leprosy (unlabeled use): 400 mg once daily

Pelvic inflammatory disease (acute): 400 mg every 12 hours for 10-14 days with or without metronidazole; **Note:** The CDC recommends use only if standard cephalosporin therapy is not feasible and community prevalence of quinolone-resistant gonococcal organisms is low. Culture sensitivity must be confirmed.

Prostatitis:

Acute: 400 mg for 1 dose, then 300 mg twice daily for 10 days

Chronic: 200 mg every 12 hours for 6 weeks

Traveler's diarrhea (unlabeled use): 300 mg twice daily for 3 days

UTI:

Uncomplicated: 200 mg every 12 hours for 3-7 days

Complicated: 200 mg every 12 hours for 10 days

Dosing adjustment/interval in renal impairment: Adults: Oral: After a normal initial dose, adjust as follows:

Cl_{cr} 20-50 mL/minute: Administer usual dose every 24 hours

Cl_{cr} <20 mL/minute: Administer half the usual dose every 24 hours

Continuous arteriovenous or venovenous hemodiafiltration effects: Administer 300 mg every 24 hours

Dosing adjustment in hepatic impairment: Severe impairment: Maximum dose: 400 mg/day

Administration Do not take within 2 hours of food or any antacids which contain zinc, magnesium, or aluminum.

Monitoring Parameters Monitor CBC, renal and hepatic function periodically if therapy is prolonged.

Test Interactions Some quinolones may produce a false-positive urine screening result for opioids using commercially-available immunoassay kits. This has been demonstrated most consistently for levofloxacin and ofloxacin, but other quinolones have shown cross-reactivity in certain assay kits. Confirmation of positive opioid screens by more specific methods should be considered.

Dosage Forms Excipient information presented when available (limited, particularly for generics); consult specific product labeling.

Tablet, Oral:

Generic: 200 mg, 300 mg, 400 mg

Ofloxacin (Ophthalmic) (oh FLOKS a sin)

Brand Names: U.S. Ocuflox

Brand Names: Canada Ocuflox®

Pharmacologic Category Antibiotic, Fluoroquinolone; Antibiotic, Ophthalmic

Use Treatment of superficial ocular infections involving the conjunctiva or cornea due to strains of susceptible organisms

Pregnancy Risk Factor C

Dosage

Usual dosage range: Ophthalmic:

Children >1 year: 1-2 drops every 30 minutes to 4 hours initially, decreasing to every 4-6 hours

Adults: 1-2 drops every 30 minutes to 4 hours initially, decreasing to every 4-6 hours

Indication-specific dosing: Children >1 year and Adults: Ophthalmic:

Conjunctivitis: Instill 1-2 drops in affected eye(s) every 2-4 hours for the first 2 days, then use 4 times/day for an additional 5 days

Corneal ulcer: Instill 1-2 drops every 30 minutes while awake and every 4-6 hours after retiring for the first 2 days; beginning on day 3, instill 1-2 drops every hour while awake for 4-6 additional days; thereafter, 1-2 drops 4 times/day until clinical cure.

Dosage adjustment in renal impairment: No dosage adjustment provided in manufacturer's labeling. However, dosage adjustment unlikely due to low systemic absorption.

Dosage adjustment in hepatic impairment: No dosage adjustment provided in manufacturer's labeling. However, dosage adjustment unlikely due to low systemic absorption.

Additional Information Complete prescribing information should be consulted for additional detail.

Dosage Forms Excipient information presented when available (limited, particularly for generics); consult specific product labeling.

Solution, Ophthalmic:

Ocuflox: 0.3% (5 mL) [contains benzalkonium chloride]

Generic: 0.3% (5 mL, 10 mL)

Ofloxacin (Otic) (oh FLOKS a sin)

Index Terms Floxin Otic Singles

Pharmacologic Category Antibiotic, Fluoroquinolone; Antibiotic, Otic

Use Otitis externa, chronic suppurative otitis media, acute otitis media

Pregnancy Risk Factor C

Dosage

Usual dosage range: Otic:

Children ≥6 months: 5 drops daily

Children >12 years: 10 drops once or twice daily

Adults: 10 drops once or twice daily

Indication-specific dosing: Otic:

Children 6 months to 13 years: **Otitis externa:** Instill 5 drops (or the contents of 1 single-dose container) into affected ear(s) once daily for 7 days

Children 1-12 years: **Acute otitis media with tympanostomy tubes:** Instill 5 drops (or the contents of 1 single-dose container) into affected ear(s) twice daily for 10 days

Children >12 years and Adults: **Otitis media, chronic suppurative with perforated tympanic membranes:** Instill 10 drops (or the contents of 2 single-dose containers) into affected ear twice daily for 14 days

Children ≥13 years and Adults: **Otitis externa:** Instill 10 drops (or the contents of 2 single-dose containers) into affected ear(s) once daily for 7 days

Dosage adjustment in renal impairment: No dosage adjustment provided in manufacturer's labeling. However, dosage adjustment unlikely due to low systemic absorption.

Dosage adjustment in hepatic impairment: No dosage adjustment provided in manufacturer's labeling. However, dosage adjustment unlikely due to low systemic absorption.

Additional Information Complete prescribing information should be consulted for additional detail.

Dosage Forms Excipient information presented when available (limited, particularly for generics); consult specific product labeling.

Solution, Otic:

Generic: 0.3% (5 mL, 10 mL)

◆ **Ogen® (Can)** *see* Estropipate *on page 778*

◆ **Ogestrel** *see* Ethinyl Estradiol and Norgestrel *on page 797*

◆ **OGMT** *see* Metyrosine *on page 1355*

◆ **OGT-918** *see* Miglustat *on page 1369*

◆ **17OHPC** *see* Hydroxyprogesterone Caproate *on page 1021*

◆ **9-OH-risperidone** *see* Paliperidone *on page 1549*

OLANZapine (oh LAN za peen)

Brand Names: U.S. ZyPREXA; ZyPREXA Relprevv; ZyPREXA Zydis

Brand Names: Canada Apo-Olanzapine; Apo-Olanzapine ODT; Ava-Olanzapine; CO Olanzapine; CO Olanzapine ODT; Mylan-Olanzapine; Olanzapine ODT; PHL-Olanzapine; PHL-Olanzapine ODT; PMS-Olanzapine; PMS-Olanzapine ODT; Riva-Olanzapine; Riva-Olanzapine ODT; Sandoz-Olanzapine; Sandoz-Olanzapine ODT; Teva-Olanzapine; Teva-Olanzapine OD; Zyprexa; Zyprexa Intramuscular; Zyprexa Zydis

Index Terms LY170053; Olanzapine Pamoate; Zyprexa Zydis

Pharmacologic Category Antimanic Agent; Antipsychotic Agent, Atypical

Additional Appendix Information

Antipsychotic Agents *on page 2290*

Beers Criteria – Potentially Inappropriate Medications for Geriatrics *on page 2368*

Use

Oral: Treatment of the manifestations of schizophrenia; treatment of acute or mixed mania episodes associated with bipolar I disorder (as monotherapy or in combination with lithium or valproate); maintenance treatment of bipolar disorder; in combination with fluoxetine for treatment-resistant or bipolar I depression

I.M., extended-release (Zyprexa Relprevv): Treatment of schizophrenia

I.M., short-acting (Zyprexa IntraMuscular): Treatment of acute agitation associated with schizophrenia and bipolar I mania

Unlabeled Use Treatment of psychosis/schizophrenia in children; chronic pain; prevention of chemotherapy-associated delayed nausea or vomiting; psychosis/agitation related to Alzheimer's dementia; acute treatment of delirium

Pregnancy Risk Factor C

Pregnancy Considerations Adverse events were observed in animal reproduction studies. Olanzapine crosses the placenta and can be detected in cord blood at birth (Newport, 2007). Information related to olanzapine use in pregnancy is limited (Goldstein, 2000). Antipsychotic use during the third trimester of pregnancy has a risk for abnormal muscle movements (extrapyramidal symptoms [EPS]) and/or withdrawal symptoms in newborns following delivery. Symptoms in the newborn may include agitation, feeding disorder, hypertonia, hypotonia, respiratory distress, somnolence, and tremor; these effects may be self-limiting or require hospitalization. Olanzapine may cause hyperprolactinemia, which may decrease reproductive function in both males and females.

The ACOG recommends that therapy during pregnancy be individualized; treatment with psychiatric medications during pregnancy should incorporate the clinical expertise of the mental health clinician, obstetrician, primary healthcare provider, and pediatrician. Safety data related to atypical antipsychotics during pregnancy is limited and routine use is not recommended. However, if a woman is inadvertently exposed to an atypical antipsychotic while pregnant, continuing therapy may be preferable to switching to a typical antipsychotic that the fetus has not yet been exposed to; consider risk:benefit (ACOG, 2008). Evaluate risk factors for gestational diabetes and weight gain if considering use of olanzapine in a pregnant woman (NICE, 2007).

Healthcare providers are encouraged to enroll women 18-45 years of age exposed to olanzapine during pregnancy in the Atypical Antipsychotics Pregnancy Registry (1-866-961-2388 or http://www.womensmentalhealth.org/pregnancyregistry).

Breast-Feeding Considerations Olanzapine is excreted into breast milk. At steady-state concentrations, it is estimated that a breast-fed infant may be exposed to ~2% of the maternal dose. In one study, the median time to peak milk concentration was ~5 hours after the maternal dose and serum concentrations in the nursing infants were low (<5 ng/mL; n=5) (Gardiner, 2003). An increased risk of adverse events in nursing infants has not been reported (Gardiner, 2003; Gilad, 2011). Breast-feeding is not recommended by the manufacturer.

Prescribing and Access Restrictions As a requirement of the REMS program, only prescribers, healthcare facilities, and pharmacies registered with the Zyprexa Relprevv Patient Care Program are able to prescribe, distribute, or dispense Zyprexa Relprevv for patients who are enrolled in and meet all conditions of the program. Zyprexa Relprevv must be administered at a registered healthcare facility. Prescribers will need to be recertified every 3 years. Contact the Zyprexa Relprevv Patient Care Program at 1-877-772-9390.

Medication Guide Available Yes

Contraindications There are no contraindications listed in the manufacturer's labeling.

Canadian labeling: Hypersensitivity to olanzapine or any component of the formulation

Warnings/Precautions [U.S. Boxed Warning]: Elderly patients with dementia-related psychosis treated with antipsychotics are at an increased risk of death compared to placebo. Most deaths appeared to be either cardiovascular (eg, heart failure, sudden death) or infectious (eg, pneumonia) in nature. In addition, an increased incidence of cerebrovascular effects (eg, transient ischemic attack, stroke) has been reported in studies of placebo-controlled trials of olanzapine in elderly patients with dementia-related psychosis. Olanzapine is not approved for the treatment of dementia-related psychosis.

Moderate to highly sedating, use with caution in disorders where CNS depression is a feature; patients must be cautioned about performing tasks which require mental alertness (eg, operating machinery or driving). Use caution in patients with cardiac disease. Use with caution in Parkinson's disease, predisposition to seizures, or severe hepatic or renal disease. Life-threatening arrhythmias have occurred with therapeutic doses of some neuroleptics. May induce orthostatic hypotension; use caution with history of cardiovascular disease, hemodynamic instability, prior myocardial infarction, or ischemic heart disease. Increases in cholesterol and triglycerides have been noted. Use with caution in patients with pre-existing abnormal lipid profile. Esophageal dysmotility and aspiration have been associated with antipsychotic use; use with caution in patients at risk of aspiration pneumonia. May increase prolactin levels; clinical significance of hyperprolactinemia in patients with breast cancer or other prolactin-dependent tumors is unknown. Significant weight gain (>7% of baseline weight) may occur; monitor waist circumference and BMI. Impaired core body temperature regulation may occur; caution with strenuous exercise, heat exposure, dehydration, and concomitant medication possessing anticholinergic effects.

Leukopenia, neutropenia, and agranulocytosis (sometimes fatal) have been reported in clinical trials and postmarketing reports with antipsychotic use; presence of risk factors (eg, pre-existing low WBC or history of drug-induced leuko-/neutropenia) should prompt periodic blood count assessment. Discontinue therapy at first signs of blood dyscrasias or if absolute neutrophil count $<1000/mm^3$.

May cause anticholinergic effects; use with caution in patients with decreased gastrointestinal motility, urinary retention, BPH, xerostomia, or narrow-angle glaucoma. Relative to other neuroleptics, olanzapine has a moderate potency of cholinergic blockade. May cause extrapyramidal symptoms (EPS), although risk of these reactions is lower relative to other neuroleptics. Risk of dystonia (and probably other EPS) may be greater with increased doses, use of conventional antipsychotics, males, and younger patients. May be associated with neuroleptic malignant syndrome (NMS). May cause extreme and life-threatening hyperglycemia; use with caution in patients with diabetes or other disorders of glucose regulation; monitor. Olanzapine levels may be lower in patients who smoke; the manufacturer does not require dosage adjustments, although dosage adjustments may be considered. Use in adolescent patients ≥13 years of age may result in increased weight gain and sedation, as well as greater increases in LDL cholesterol, total cholesterol, triglycerides, prolactin, and liver transaminase levels when compared to adults. Adolescent patients should be maintained on the lowest dose necessary.

Use in elderly patients with dementia is associated with an increased risk of mortality and cerebrovascular accidents; avoid antipsychotic use for behavioral problems associated with dementia unless alternative nonpharmacologic therapies have failed and patient may harm self or others. In addition, use may cause or exacerbate syndrome of inappropriate antidiuretic hormone secretion or hyponatremia; monitor sodium closely with initiation or dosage adjustments in older adults. May also be inappropriate in older adults depending on comorbidities (eg, dementia, delirium) due to its potent anticholinergic effects (Beers Criteria).

The possibility of a suicide attempt is inherent in psychotic illness or bipolar disorder; use caution in high-risk patients during initiation of therapy. Prescriptions should be written for the smallest quantity consistent with good patient care.

There are two Zyprexa formulations for intramuscular injection: Zyprexa Relprevv is an extended-release formulation and Zyprexa Intramuscular is short-acting:

Extended-release I.M. injection (Zyprexa Relprevv): Monitor for post injection delirium/sedation syndrome; patients should be continuously watched (≥3 hours) for symptoms of olanzapine overdose. Only available through a restricted drug distribution program.

Short-acting I.M. injection (Zyprexa IntraMuscular): Patients should remain recumbent if drowsy/dizzy until hypotension, bradycardia, and/or hypoventilation have been ruled out. Concurrent use of I.M./I.V. benzodiazepines is not recommended (fatalities have been reported, though causality not determined).

Adverse Reactions

Oral: Unless otherwise noted, adverse events are reported for placebo-controlled trials in adult patients on monotherapy:

>10%:

Central nervous system: Somnolence (dose dependent; 20% to 39%; adolescents 39% to 48%), extrapyramidal symptoms (dose dependent; ≤32%), dizziness (11% to 18%), headache (adolescents 17%), fatigue (adolescents 3% to 14%), insomnia (12%)

Endocrine & metabolic: Prolactin increased (30%; adolescents 47%)

Gastrointestinal: Weight gain (5% to 6%, has been reported as high as 40%; adolescents 29% to 31%), appetite increased (3% to 6%; adolescents 17% to 29%), xerostomia (dose dependent; 3% to 22%), constipation (9% to 11%), dyspepsia (7% to 11%)

Hepatic: ALT increased ≥3 x ULN (adolescents 12%; adults 5%)

Neuromuscular & skeletal: Weakness (dose dependent; 8% to 20%)

Miscellaneous: Accidental injury (12%)

1% to 10%:

Cardiovascular: Chest pain, hypertension, orthostatic hypotension, peripheral edema, tachycardia

Central nervous system: Fever, personality changes, restlessness (adolescents)

Dermatologic: Bruising

Endocrine & metabolic: Breast-related events ([adolescents] discharge, enlargement, galactorrhea, gynecomastia, lactation disorder); menstrual-related events (amenorrhea, hypomenorrhea, menstruation delayed, oligomenorrhea); sexual function-related events (anorgasmia, ejaculation delayed, erectile dysfunction, changes in libido, abnormal orgasm, sexual dysfunction)

Gastrointestinal: Abdominal pain (adolescents), diarrhea (adolescents), flatulence, nausea (dose dependent), vomiting

Genitourinary: Incontinence, UTI

Hepatic: Hepatic enzymes increased

Neuromuscular & skeletal: Abnormal gait, akathisia, articulation impairment, back pain, falling, hypertonia, joint/extremity pain, muscle stiffness (adolescents), tremor (dose dependent)

Ocular: Amblyopia

Respiratory: Cough, epistaxis (adolescents), pharyngitis, respiratory tract infection (adolescents), rhinitis, sinusitis (adolescents)

<1% (Limited to important or life-threatening): Acidosis, agranulocytosis, anaphylactoid reaction, angioedema, apnea, atelectasis, atrial fibrillation, cerebrovascular accident, congestive heart failure, deafness, diabetes mellitus, diabetic ketoacidosis, diabetic coma, dystonia,

encephalopathy, facial paralysis, glaucoma, heart arrest, heart failure, hemorrhage (eye, rectal, subarachnoid, vaginal), hepatitis, hypercholesterolemia, hyper-/hypoglycemia, hyper-/hypokalemia, hyperlipemia, hyper-/hyponatremia, hypertriglyceridemia, hyperuricemia, hyper-/hypoventilation, hypoproteinemia, hypoxia, jaundice, ileus, ketosis, leukocytosis (eosinophilia), leukopenia, liver damage (cholestatic or mixed), liver fatty deposit, lung edema, lymphadenopathy, myasthenia, myopathy, neuralgia, neuroleptic malignant syndrome, neutropenia, pancreatitis, paralysis, pulmonary embolus, rash, rhabdomyolysis, seizure, sudden death, suicide attempt, syncope, tardive dyskinesia, thrombocythemia, thrombocytopenia, transient ischemic attack, venous thrombotic events

Injection: Unless otherwise noted, adverse events are reported for placebo-controlled trials in adult patients on extended-release I.M. injection (Zyprexa Relprevv). Also refer to adverse reactions noted with oral therapy.

>10%: Central nervous system: Headache (13% to 18%), sedation (8% to 13%)

1% to 10%:

Cardiovascular: Hypertension, hypotension (short-acting), orthostatic hypotension (short-acting), QT prolongation

Central nervous system: Abnormal dreams, abnormal thinking, auditory hallucination, dizziness, dysarthria, extrapyramidal symptoms, fatigue, fever, pain, restlessness, somnolence

Dermatologic: Acne

Gastrointestinal: Abdominal pain, appetite increased, diarrhea, flatulence, nausea, vomiting, weight gain, xerostomia

Genitourinary: Vaginal discharge

Hepatic: Liver enzymes increased

Local: Injection site pain

Neuromuscular & skeletal: Arthralgia, back pain, muscle spasms, stiffness, tremor, weakness (short-acting)

Otic: Ear pain

Respiratory: Cough, nasal congestion, nasopharyngitis, pharyngolaryngeal pain, sneezing, upper respiratory tract infection

Miscellaneous: Toothache, tooth infection, viral infection

<1% (Limited to important or life-threatening): CPK increased, post-injection delirium/sedation syndrome, syncope (short-acting)

Drug Interactions

Metabolism/Transport Effects **Substrate** of CYP1A2 (major), CYP2D6 (minor); **Note:** Assignment of Major/Minor substrate status based on clinically relevant drug interaction potential; **Inhibits** CYP1A2 (weak), CYP2C19 (weak), CYP2C9 (weak), CYP2D6 (weak), CYP3A4 (weak)

Avoid Concomitant Use

Avoid concomitant use of OLANZapine with any of the following: Aclidinium; Amisulpride; Azelastine (Nasal); Benzodiazepines; Ipratropium (Oral Inhalation); Metoclopramide; Paraldehyde; Pimozide; Sulpiride; Tiotropium; Umeclidinium

Increased Effect/Toxicity

OLANZapine may increase the levels/effects of: Alcohol (Ethyl); Amisulpride; Analgesics (Opioid); Anticholinergics; ARIPiprazole; Azelastine (Nasal); Benzodiazepines; Buprenorphine; CNS Depressants; Dofetilide; Highest Risk QTc-Prolonging Agents; Hydrocodone; Lomitapide; Methotrimeprazine; Methylphenidate; Moderate Risk QTc-Prolonging Agents; Paraldehyde; Pimozide; Serotonin Modulators; Sulpiride; Tiotropium; Zolpidem

The levels/effects of OLANZapine may be increased by: Abiraterone Acetate; Acetylcholinesterase Inhibitors (Central); Aclidinium; Brimonidine (Topical); CYP1A2 Inhibitors (Moderate); CYP1A2 Inhibitors (Strong); Deferasirox; Doxylamine; Droperidol; FluvoxaMINE; HydrOXYzine; Ipratropium (Oral Inhalation); LamoTRIgine; Lithium formulations; Magnesium Sulfate; Methotrimeprazine; Methylphenidate; Metoclopramide; Metyrosine; Mifepristone; Perampanel; Pramlintide; Serotonin Modulators; Sodium Oxybate; Tetrabenazine; Umeclidinium; Vemurafenib

Decreased Effect

OLANZapine may decrease the levels/effects of: Amphetamines; Anti-Parkinson's Agents (Dopamine Agonist); Quinagolide

The levels/effects of OLANZapine may be decreased by: CYP1A2 Inducers (Strong); Cyproterone; Lithium formulations; Peginterferon Alfa-2b; Valproic Acid and Derivatives

Ethanol/Nutrition/Herb Interactions

Ethanol: May increase CNS depression; monitor for increased effects with coadministration. Caution patients about effects.

Herb/Nutraceutical: Avoid dong quai, St John's wort (may also cause photosensitization). Avoid kava kava, gotu kola, valerian, St John's wort (may increase CNS depression).

Preparation for Administration

Injection, extended-release: Dilute as directed to final concentration of 150 mg/mL. Shake vigorously to mix; will form yellow, opaque suspension. Following reconstitution, suspension may be stored at room temperature and used within 24 hours. Shake vigorously to resuspend prior to administration. Use immediately once suspension is in syringe. Suspension may be irritating to skin; wear gloves during reconstitution.

Injection, short-acting: Reconstitute 10 mg vial with 2.1 mL SWFI. Resulting solution is ~5 mg/mL. Use immediately (within 1 hour) following reconstitution. Discard any unused portion.

Storage/Stability

Injection, extended-release: Store at 20°C to 25°C (68°F to 77°F); excursions permitted to 15°C to 30°C (59°F to 86°F).

Injection, short-acting: Store at 20°C to 25°C (68°F to 77°F); excursions permitted to 15°C to 30°C (59°F to 86°F); do not freeze. Protect from light.

Tablet and orally-disintegrating tablet: Store at 20°C to 25°C (68°F to 77°F); excursions permitted to 15°C to 30°C (59°F to 86°F). Protect from light and moisture.

Mechanism of Action Olanzapine is a second generation thienobenzodiazepine antipsychotic which displays potent antagonism of serotonin 5-HT_{2A} and 5-HT_{2C}, dopamine D_{1-4}, histamine H_1, and alpha$_1$-adrenergic receptors. Olanzapine shows moderate antagonism of 5-HT_3 and muscarinic M_{1-5} receptors, and weak binding to GABA-A, BZD, and beta-adrenergic receptors. Although the precise mechanism of action in schizophrenia and bipolar disorder is not known, the efficacy of olanzapine is thought to be mediated through combined antagonism of dopamine and serotonin type 2 receptor sites.

Pharmacodynamics/Kinetics

Absorption:

Oral: Well absorbed; not affected by food; tablets and orally-disintegrating tablets are bioequivalent

Short-acting injection: Rapidly absorbed

Distribution: V_d: Extensive, 1000 L

Protein binding, plasma: 93% bound to albumin and alpha$_1$-glycoprotein

Metabolism: Highly metabolized via direct glucuronidation and cytochrome P450 mediated oxidation (CYP1A2, CYP2D6); 40% removed via first pass metabolism

Half-life elimination: 21-54 hours; ~1.5 times greater in elderly; Extended-release injection: ~30 days

Time to peak, plasma: Maximum plasma concentrations after I.M. administration are 5 times higher than maximum plasma concentrations produced by an oral dose.
Extended-release injection: ~7 days
Short-acting injection: 15-45 minutes
Oral: ~6 hours

Excretion: Urine (57%, 7% as unchanged drug); feces (30%)
Clearance: 40% increase in olanzapine clearance in smokers; 30% decrease in females

Dosage

Children and Adolescents 10-17 years: Depression associated with bipolar I disorder (in combination with fluoxetine): Oral: Initial: 2.5 mg once daily in the evening (in combination with fluoxetine); adjust dose, if needed, as tolerated; safety of doses >12 mg of olanzapine in combination with fluoxetine doses >50 mg has not been studied in pediatrics. See **"Note"** below for olanzapine/fluoxetine combination (Symbyax).

Adolescents ≥13 years:
Bipolar I acute mixed or manic episodes: Oral: Initial: 2.5-5 mg once daily; adjust by 2.5-5 mg daily to target dose of 10 mg daily; dosing range: 2.5-20 mg daily
Schizophrenia: Oral: Initial: 2.5-5 mg once daily; adjust by 2.5-5 mg daily to target dose of 10 mg daily; dosing range: 2.5-20 mg daily

Adults:
Agitation (acute, associated with bipolar I mania or schizophrenia): Short-acting I.M. injection: Initial dose: 10 mg (a lower dose of 5-7.5 mg may be considered when clinical factors warrant); additional doses (up to 10 mg) may be considered, however, 2-4 hours should be allowed between doses to evaluate response (maximum total daily dose: 30 mg, per manufacturer's recommendation)
Bipolar I acute mixed or manic episodes: Oral:
Monotherapy: Initial: 10-15 mg once daily; increase by 5 mg daily at intervals of not less than 24 hours. Maintenance: 5-20 mg daily; recommended maximum dose: 20 mg daily.
Combination therapy (with lithium or valproate): Initial: 10 mg once daily; dosing range: 5-20 mg daily; recommended maximum dose: 20 mg daily.
Depression:
Depression associated with bipolar disorder (in combination with fluoxetine): Oral: Initial: 5 mg in the evening; adjust as tolerated to usual range of 5-12.5 mg daily. See **"Note."**
Treatment-resistant depression (in combination with fluoxetine): Oral: Initial: 5 mg in the evening; adjust as tolerated to range of 5-20 mg daily. See **"Note."**
Note (Olanzapine/fluoxetine combination [Symbyax]): When using individual components of fluoxetine with olanzapine rather than fixed dose combination product (Symbyax), approximate dosage correspondence is as follows:
Olanzapine 2.5 mg + fluoxetine 20 mg = Symbyax 3/25
Olanzapine 5 mg + fluoxetine 20 mg = Symbyax 6/25
Olanzapine 12.5 mg + fluoxetine 20 mg = Symbyax 12/25
Olanzapine 5 mg + fluoxetine 50 mg = Symbyax 6/50
Olanzapine 12.5 mg + fluoxetine 50 mg = Symbyax 12/50
Schizophrenia:
Oral: Initial: 5-10 mg once daily (increase to 10 mg once daily within 5-7 days); thereafter, adjust by 5 mg daily at 1-week intervals, up to a recommended maximum of 20 mg daily. Maintenance: 10-20 mg once daily. Doses of 30-50 mg daily have been used; however, doses >10 mg daily have not demonstrated better efficacy, and safety and efficacy of doses >20 mg daily have not been evaluated.
Extended-release I.M. injection: **Note:** Establish tolerance to oral olanzapine prior to changing to extended-release I.M. injection. Maximum dose: 300 mg/2 weeks or 405 mg/4 weeks
Patients established on oral olanzapine 10 mg daily: Initial dose: 210 mg every 2 weeks for 4 doses or 405 mg every 4 weeks for 2 doses; Maintenance dose: 150 mg every 2 weeks or 300 mg every 4 weeks
Patients established on oral olanzapine 15 mg daily: Initial dose: 300 mg every 2 weeks for 4 doses; Maintenance dose: 210 mg every 2 weeks or 405 mg every 4 weeks
Patients established on oral olanzapine 20 mg daily: Initial and maintenance dose: 300 mg every 2 weeks
Delirium (unlabeled use): Oral: 5 mg daily for up to 5 days (NICE, 2010)
Prevention of chemotherapy-associated delayed nausea or vomiting (unlabeled use; in combination with a corticosteroid and serotonin [5-HT_3] antagonist): Oral: 10 mg once daily for 3-5 days, beginning on day 1 of chemotherapy **or** 5 mg once daily for 2 days before chemotherapy, followed by 10 mg once daily (beginning on the day of chemotherapy) for 3-8 days

Elderly:
Short-acting I.M., Oral: Consider lower starting dose of 2.5-5 mg daily for elderly or debilitated patients; may increase as clinically indicated and tolerated with close monitoring of orthostatic blood pressure
Extended release I.M.: Consider lower starting dose of 150 mg every 4 weeks for elderly or debilitated patients; increase dose with caution as clinically indicated.
Delirium (unlabeled use): Patients >60 years: 2.5 mg daily for up to 5 days (NICE, 2010)
Psychosis/agitation related to Alzheimer's dementia (unlabeled use): Oral: Initial: 2.5-5 mg daily (Sultzer, 2008)

Dosage adjustment in renal impairment: No dosage adjustment necessary. Not removed by dialysis.

Dosage adjustment in hepatic impairment: No dosage adjustment provided in manufacturer's labeling except when used in combination with fluoxetine (as separate components) the initial olanzapine dose should be limited to 2.5-5 mg daily. Use with caution (cases of hepatitis and liver injury have been reported with olanzapine use).

Dietary Considerations Tablets may be taken without regard to meals. Some products may contain phenylalanine.

Administration

Short-acting I.M. injection: **For I.M. administration only**; do not administer injection intravenously or subcutaneously; inject slowly, deep into muscle. If dizziness and/or drowsiness are noted, patient should remain recumbent until examination indicates postural hypotension and/or bradycardia are not a problem.

Extended-release I.M. injection: **For I.M. gluteal injection only**; do not administer I.V. or subcutaneously. After needle insertion into muscle, aspirate to verify that no blood appears. Do not massage injection site. Use diluent, syringes, and needles provided in convenience kit; obtain a new kit if aspiration of blood occurs.

Tablet: May be administered without regard to meals.

Orally-disintegrating: Remove from foil blister by peeling back (do not push tablet through the foil); place tablet in mouth immediately upon removal; tablet dissolves rapidly in saliva and may be swallowed with or without liquid. May be administered with or without food/meals.

Monitoring Parameters Vital signs; fasting lipid profile and fasting blood glucose/Hgb A_{1c} (prior to treatment, at 3 months, then annually); periodic assessment of hepatic transaminases (in patients with hepatic disease); BMI, waist circumference; orthostatic blood pressure; mental status, abnormal involuntary movement scale (AIMS), extrapyramidal symptoms (EPS). Weight should be assessed prior to treatment, at 4 weeks, 8 weeks, 12 weeks, and then at quarterly intervals. Consider titrating to a different antipsychotic agent for a weight gain ≥5% of the initial weight.

Extended-release I.M. injection: Sedation/delirium for 3 hours after each dose

Dosage Forms Excipient information presented when available (limited, particularly for generics); consult specific product labeling.

Solution Reconstituted, Intramuscular:
- ZyPREXA: 10 mg (1 ea) [contains tartaric acid]
- Generic: 10 mg (1 ea)

Suspension Reconstituted, Intramuscular:
- ZyPREXA Relprevv: 210 mg (1 ea); 300 mg (1 ea); 405 mg (1 ea) [contains polysorbate 80]

Tablet, Oral:
- ZyPREXA: 2.5 mg, 5 mg, 7.5 mg, 10 mg
- ZyPREXA: 15 mg [contains fd&c blue #2 aluminum lake]
- ZyPREXA: 20 mg
- Generic: 2.5 mg, 5 mg, 7.5 mg, 10 mg, 15 mg, 20 mg

Tablet Dispersible, Oral:
- ZyPREXA Zydis: 5 mg, 10 mg, 15 mg, 20 mg [contains aspartame, methylparaben sodium, propylparaben sodium]
- Generic: 5 mg, 10 mg, 15 mg, 20 mg

◆ **Olanzapine ODT (Can)** *see* OLANZapine *on page 1493*
◆ **Olanzapine Pamoate** *see* OLANZapine *on page 1493*
◆ **Oleovitamin A** *see* Vitamin A *on page 2201*
◆ **Oleptro [DSC]** *see* TraZODone *on page 2112*
◆ **Oleptro™ (Can)** *see* TraZODone *on page 2112*
◆ **Olestyr (Can)** *see* Cholestyramine Resin *on page 418*

Olmesartan (ole me SAR tan)

Brand Names: U.S. Benicar

Brand Names: Canada Olmetec

Index Terms Olmesartan Medoxomil

Pharmacologic Category Angiotensin II Receptor Blocker; Antihypertensive

Additional Appendix Information

Angiotensin Agents *on page 2280*

Use Treatment of hypertension with or without concurrent use of other antihypertensive agents

Pregnancy Risk Factor D

Pregnancy Considerations [U.S. Boxed Warning]: Drugs that act on the renin-angiotensin system can cause injury and death to the developing fetus. Discontinue as soon as possible once pregnancy is detected. The use of drugs which act on the renin-angiotensin system are associated with oligohydramnios. Oligohydramnios, due to decreased fetal renal function, may lead to fetal lung hypoplasia and skeletal malformations. Use is also associated with anuria, hypotension, renal failure, skull hypoplasia, and death in the fetus/neonate. The exposed fetus should be monitored for fetal growth, amniotic fluid volume, and organ formation. Infants exposed *in utero* should be monitored for hyperkalemia, hypotension, and oliguria.

Untreated chronic maternal hypertension is also associated with adverse events in the fetus, infant, and mother. If treatment for hypertension during pregnancy is needed, other agents are preferred (ACOG, 2012; Chobanian, 2003). In women of reproductive potential, angiotensin II receptor blockers should be discontinued prior to conception or as soon as pregnancy is confirmed (Chobanian, 2003).

Breast-Feeding Considerations It is not known if olmesartan is excreted into breast milk. Due to the potential for serious adverse reactions in the nursing infant, the manufacturer recommends a decision be made whether to discontinue nursing or to discontinue the drug, taking into account the importance of treatment to the mother. Breastfed infants of mothers taking medications for hypertension should be monitored for adverse effects (Chobanian, 2003).

Contraindications Concomitant use with aliskiren in patients with diabetes mellitus

Canadian labeling: Additional contraindications (not in U.S. labeling): Hypersensitivity to olmesartan or any component of the formulation; concomitant use with aliskiren in patients with moderate to severe renal impairment (GFR <60 mL/minute/1.73m^2)

Warnings/Precautions [U.S. Boxed Warning]: Drugs that act on the renin-angiotensin system can cause injury and death to the developing fetus. Discontinue as soon as possible once pregnancy is detected. May cause hyperkalemia; avoid potassium supplementation unless specifically required by healthcare provider. Avoid use or use a smaller dose in patients who are volume depleted; correct depletion first. May be associated with deterioration of renal function and/or increases in serum creatinine, particularly in patients with low renal blood flow (eg, renal artery stenosis, heart failure) whose glomerular filtration rate (GFR) is dependent on efferent arteriolar vasoconstriction by angiotensin II. Use with caution in unstented unilateral/bilateral renal artery stenosis. When unstented bilateral renal artery stenosis is present, use is generally avoided due to the elevated risk of deterioration in renal function unless possible benefits outweigh risks. Use with caution with pre-existing renal insufficiency; significant aortic/mitral stenosis. Potentially significant drug-drug interactions may exist, requiring dose or frequency adjustment, additional monitoring, and/or selection of alternative therapy.

Symptoms of sprue-like enteropathy (ie, severe, chronic diarrhea with significant weight loss) has been reported; may develop years after treatment initiation with villous atrophy commonly found on intestinal biopsy. Once other etiologies have been excluded, discontinue treatment and consider other antihypertensive treatment. Clinical and histologic improvement was noted after treatment was discontinued in a case series of 22 patients (Rubio-Tapia, 2012).

Angioedema has been reported rarely with some angiotensin II receptor antagonists (ARBs) and may occur at any time during treatment (especially following first dose). It may involve the head and neck (potentially compromising airway) or the intestine (presenting with abdominal pain). Patients with idiopathic or hereditary angioedema or previous angioedema associated with ACE-inhibitor therapy may be at an increased risk. Prolonged frequent monitoring may be required, especially if tongue, glottis, or larynx are involved, as they are associated with airway obstruction. Patients with a history of airway surgery may have a higher risk of airway obstruction. Discontinue therapy immediately if angioedema occurs. Aggressive early management is critical. Intramuscular (I.M.) administration of epinephrine may be necessary. Do not readminister to patients who have had angioedema with ARBs.

Adverse Reactions

1% to 10%:
- Central nervous system: Dizziness (3%), headache
- Endocrine & metabolic: Hyperglycemia, hypertriglyceridemia
- Gastrointestinal: Diarrhea
- Neuromuscular & skeletal: Back pain, CPK increased
- Renal: Hematuria
- Respiratory: Bronchitis, pharyngitis, rhinitis, sinusitis

Miscellaneous: Flu-like syndrome

<1% (Limited to important or life-threatening): Acute renal failure, alopecia, anaphylaxis, angioedema, arthritis, gastroenteritis, hypercholesterolemia, hyperkalemia, hyperlipidemia, hyperuricemia, liver enzymes increased, peripheral edema, rhabdomyolysis, serum creatinine increased, sprue-like symptoms, tachycardia

Drug Interactions

Metabolism/Transport Effects Substrate of SLCO1B1

Avoid Concomitant Use There are no known interactions where it is recommended to avoid concomitant use.

Increased Effect/Toxicity

Olmesartan may increase the levels/effects of: ACE Inhibitors; Amifostine; Antihypertensives; CycloSPORINE (Systemic); Hypotensive Agents; Lithium; Nonsteroidal Anti-Inflammatory Agents; Obinutuzumab; Potassium-Sparing Diuretics; RiTUXimab; Sodium Phosphates

The levels/effects of Olmesartan may be increased by: Alfuzosin; Aliskiren; Brimonidine (Topical); Canagliflozin; Diazoxide; Eltrombopag; Eplerenone; Heparin; Heparin (Low Molecular Weight); Herbs (Hypotensive Properties); MAO Inhibitors; Pentoxifylline; Phosphodiesterase 5 Inhibitors; Potassium Salts; Prostacyclin Analogues; Tolvaptan; Trimethoprim

Decreased Effect

The levels/effects of Olmesartan may be decreased by: Colesevelam; Herbs (Hypertensive Properties); Methylphenidate; Nonsteroidal Anti-Inflammatory Agents; Yohimbine

Ethanol/Nutrition/Herb Interactions

Food: Does not affect olmesartan bioavailability. Potassium supplements and/or potassium-containing salts may cause or worsen hyperkalemia. Management: Consult prescriber before consuming a potassium-rich diet, potassium supplements, or salt substitutes.

Herb/Nutraceutical: Some herbal medications may worsen hypertension (eg, licorice); others may increase the antihypertensive effect of olmesartan (eg, shepherd's purse). Management: Avoid bayberry, blue cohosh, cayenne, ephedra, ginger, ginseng (American), kola, licorice, and yohimbe. Avoid black cohosh, California poppy, coleus, golden seal, hawthorn, mistletoe, periwinkle, quinine, and shepherd's purse.

Storage/Stability Store at 20°C to 25°C (68°F to 77°F).

Mechanism of Action As a selective and competitive, nonpeptide angiotensin II receptor antagonist, olmesartan blocks the vasoconstrictor and aldosterone-secreting effects of angiotensin II; olmesartan interacts reversibly at the AT1 and AT2 receptors of many tissues and has slow dissociation kinetics; its affinity for the AT1 receptor is 12,500 times greater than the AT2 receptor. Angiotensin II receptor antagonists may induce a more complete inhibition of the renin-angiotensin system than ACE inhibitors, they do not affect the response to bradykinin, and are less likely to be associated with nonrenin-angiotensin effects (eg, cough and angioedema). Olmesartan increases urinary flow rate and, in addition to being natriuretic and kaliuretic, increases excretion of chloride, magnesium, uric acid, calcium, and phosphate.

Pharmacodynamics/Kinetics

Distribution: 17 L; does not cross the blood-brain barrier (animal studies)

Protein binding: 99%

Metabolism: Olmesartan medoxomil is hydrolyzed in the GI tract to active olmesartan. No further metabolism occurs.

Bioavailability: 26%

Half-life elimination: Terminal: 13 hours

Time to peak: 1-2 hours

Excretion: All as unchanged drug: Feces (50% to 65%); urine (35% to 50%)

Dosage Oral:

Children 6-16 years:

20 kg to <35 kg: Initial: 10 mg once daily; if initial response inadequate after 2 weeks, dose may be increased (maximum: 20 mg/day)

≥35 kg: Initial: 20 mg once daily; if initial response inadequate after 2 weeks, dose may be increased (maximum: 40 mg/day)

Adults: Initial: Usual starting dose is 20 mg once daily; if initial response is inadequate, may be increased to 40 mg once daily after 2 weeks. May administer with other antihypertensive agents if blood pressure inadequately controlled with olmesartan. Consider lower starting dose in patients with possible depletion of intravascular volume (eg, patients receiving diuretics).

Elderly: No initial dosage adjustment necessary per labeling; however, may consider starting at 5-10 mg/day (due to concomitant disease or age changes).

Dosage adjustment in renal impairment: Initial: No dosage adjustment necessary. However, AUC increased three-fold in patients with Cl_{cr} <20 mL/minute; use with caution.

Dosage adjustment in hepatic impairment: Initial: No dosage adjustment necessary. Total drug exposure increased (60%) in patients with moderate impairment.

Dietary Considerations May be taken with or without food.

Administration May be administered with or without food.

Monitoring Parameters Blood pressure, serum potassium

Dosage Forms Excipient information presented when available (limited, particularly for generics); consult specific product labeling.

Tablet, Oral, as medoxomil:

Benicar: 5 mg, 20 mg, 40 mg

Extemporaneous Preparations A 2 mg/mL oral suspension may be made with olmesartan tablets. Combine 50 mL purified water and twenty 20 mg tablets in an 8-ounce amber bottle and allow to stand for ≥5 minutes. Shake well for ≥1 minute, then allow to stand for ≥1 minute. Repeat shaking and standing process four additional times. Add 100 mL Ora-Sweet® and 50 mL Ora-Plus® to the suspension and shake well for ≥1 minute. Label "shake well" and "refrigerate". Stable for 28 days refrigerated.

Benicar® prescribing information, Daiichi Sankyo, Inc, Parsippany, NJ, 2010.

Olmesartan, Amlodipine, and Hydrochlorothiazide

(ole me SAR tan, am LOE di peen, & hye droe klor oh THYE a zide)

Brand Names: U.S. Tribenzor™

Index Terms Amlodipine Besylate, Olmesartan Medoxomil, and Hydrochlorothiazide; Amlodipine, Hydrochlorothiazide, and Olmesartan; Hydrochlorothiazide, Olmesartan, and Amlodipine; Olmesartan, Hydrochlorothiazide, and Amlodipine

Pharmacologic Category Angiotensin II Receptor Blocker; Antianginal Agent; Antihypertensive; Calcium Channel Blocker; Calcium Channel Blocker, Dihydropyridine; Diuretic, Thiazide

Use Treatment of hypertension (not for initial therapy)

Pregnancy Risk Factor D

Dosage Oral: **Note:** Not for initial therapy. Dose is individualized; combination product may be substituted for individual components in patients currently maintained on all 3 agents separately or in patients not adequately controlled with any 2 of the following antihypertensive classes: Calcium channel blockers, angiotensin II receptor blockers, and diuretics.

Adults: Hypertension: Add-on/switch/replacement therapy: Amlodipine 5-10 mg, olmesartan 20-40 mg, and hydrochlorothiazide 12.5-25 mg once daily; dose may be titrated after 2 weeks of therapy. Maximum recommended daily dose: Amlodipine 10 mg/olmesartan 40 mg/hydrochlorothiazide 25 mg

Elderly: Patients ≥75 years of age should start amlodipine at 2.5 mg (combination product dosage form not available in this strength)

Dosage adjustment in renal impairment:

Cl_{cr} >30 mL/minute: No dosage adjustment necessary.

Cl_{cr} ≤30 mL/minute: Use of combination not recommended; contraindicated in patients with anuria

Dosage adjustment in hepatic impairment:

Mild-to-moderate hepatic impairment: No dosage adjustment provided in manufacturer's labeling. Use with caution.

Severe hepatic impairment: Use not recommended; initial daily dose of amlodipine is 2.5 mg (this dose of amlodipine is not available as a combination product).

Additional Information Complete prescribing information should be consulted for additional detail.

Dosage Forms Excipient information presented when available (limited, particularly for generics); consult specific product labeling.

Tablet, oral:

Tribenzor™: Olmesartan medoxomil 20 mg, amlodipine 5 mg, and hydrochlorothiazide 12.5 mg

Tribenzor™: Olmesartan medoxomil 40 mg, amlodipine 5 mg, and hydrochlorothiazide 12.5 mg

Tribenzor™: Olmesartan medoxomil 40 mg, amlodipine 5 mg, and hydrochlorothiazide 25 mg

Tribenzor™: Olmesartan medoxomil 40 mg, amlodipine 10 mg, and hydrochlorothiazide 12.5 mg

Tribenzor™: Olmesartan medoxomil 40 mg, amlodipine 10 mg, and hydrochlorothiazide 25 mg

◆ **Olmesartan and Amlodipine** *see* Amlodipine and Olmesartan *on page 112*

Olmesartan and Hydrochlorothiazide

(ole me SAR tan & hye droe klor oh THYE a zide)

Brand Names: U.S. Benicar HCT

Brand Names: Canada Olmetec Plus

Index Terms Hydrochlorothiazide and Olmesartan Medoxomil; Olmesartan Medoxomil and Hydrochlorothiazide

Pharmacologic Category Angiotensin II Receptor Blocker; Diuretic, Thiazide

Use Treatment of hypertension (not recommended for initial treatment)

Pregnancy Risk Factor D

Dosage Hypertension: Adults: Oral: One tablet daily; dosage must be individualized. May be titrated at 2- to 4-week intervals.

Replacement therapy: May be substituted for previously titrated dosages of the individual components.

Patients not controlled with single-agent therapy: Initiate by adding the lowest available dose of the alternative component (hydrochlorothiazide 12.5 mg or olmesartan 20 mg). Titrate to effect (maximum daily hydrochlorothiazide dose: 25 mg; maximum daily olmesartan dose: 40 mg).

Dosage adjustment in renal impairment:

Cl_{cr} >30 mL/minute: No dosage adjustment necessary.

Cl_{cr} ≤30 mL/minute: Use not recommended.

Dosage adjustment in hepatic impairment: No dosage adjustment necessary.

Additional Information Complete prescribing information should be consulted for additional detail.

Dosage Forms Excipient information presented when available (limited, particularly for generics); consult specific product labeling.

Tablet:

20/12.5: Olmesartan medoxomil 20 mg and hydrochlorothiazide 12.5 mg

40/12.5: Olmesartan medoxomil 40 mg and hydrochlorothiazide 12.5 mg

40/25: Olmesartan medoxomil 40 mg and hydrochlorothiazide 25 mg

◆ **Olmesartan, Hydrochlorothiazide, and Amlodipine** *see* Olmesartan, Amlodipine, and Hydrochlorothiazide *on page 1498*

◆ **Olmesartan Medoxomil** *see* Olmesartan *on page 1497*

◆ **Olmesartan Medoxomil and Hydrochlorothiazide** *see* Olmesartan and Hydrochlorothiazide *on page 1499*

◆ **Olmetec (Can)** *see* Olmesartan *on page 1497*

◆ **Olmetec Plus (Can)** *see* Olmesartan and Hydrochlorothiazide *on page 1499*

Olopatadine (Nasal) (oh la PAT a deen)

Brand Names: U.S. Patanase

Index Terms Olopatadine Hydrochloride

Pharmacologic Category Histamine H_1 Antagonist; Histamine H_1 Antagonist, Second Generation; Piperidine Derivative

Use Treatment of the symptoms of seasonal allergic rhinitis

Pregnancy Risk Factor C

Dosage Intranasal:

Children 6-11 years: 1 spray into each nostril twice daily

Children ≥12 years, Adolescents, and Adults: 2 sprays into each nostril twice daily

Dosage adjustment in renal impairment: No dosage adjustment necessary.

Dosage adjustment in hepatic impairment: No dosage adjustment necessary.

Additional Information Complete prescribing information should be consulted for additional detail.

Dosage Forms Considerations

Patanase 30.5 g bottles contain 240 sprays.

Dosage Forms Excipient information presented when available (limited, particularly for generics); consult specific product labeling.

Solution, Nasal:

Patanase: 0.6% (30.5 g) [contains benzalkonium chloride, edetate disodium]

Olopatadine (Ophthalmic) (oh la PAT a deen)

Brand Names: U.S. Pataday; Patanol

Brand Names: Canada Pataday™; Patanol®

Index Terms Olopatadine Hydrochloride

Pharmacologic Category Histamine H_1 Antagonist; Histamine H_1 Antagonist, Second Generation; Piperidine Derivative

Use Treatment of the signs and symptoms of allergic conjunctivitis

Pregnancy Risk Factor C

Pregnancy Considerations Adverse effects were observed in animal reproduction studies when using doses greater than the equivalent maximum recommended ocular human dose.

Breast-Feeding Considerations It is not known if olopatadine (ophthalmic) is excreted in breast milk. The manufacturer recommends that caution be exercised when administering olopatadine (ophthalmic) to nursing women.

Contraindications Hypersensitivity to olopatadine hydrochloride or any component of the formulation

Warnings/Precautions Not for use to treat contact lens-related irritation. Solution contains benzalkonium chloride; remove lens prior to administration and wait at least 10 minutes before reinserting. Do not use contact lenses if eyes are red.

Adverse Reactions

>5%:

Central nervous system: Cold syndrome (up to 10%), headache (up to 7%)

Respiratory: Pharyngitis (up to 10%)

≤5%:

Gastrointestinal: Nausea, taste perversion

Neuromuscular & skeletal: Back pain, weakness

Ocular: Blurred vision, burning, conjunctivitis, dry eyes, eye pain, eyelid edema, foreign body sensation, hyperemia, keratitis, ocular pruritus, stinging

Respiratory: Cough, rhinitis, sinusitis

Miscellaneous: Flu-like syndrome, hypersensitivity, infection

Drug Interactions

Metabolism/Transport Effects None known.

Avoid Concomitant Use There are no known interactions where it is recommended to avoid concomitant use.

Increased Effect/Toxicity There are no known significant interactions involving an increase in effect.

Decreased Effect There are no known significant interactions involving a decrease in effect.

Storage/Stability Store at 2°C to 25°C (36°F to 77°F).

Mechanism of Action Selective histamine H_1-antagonist; inhibits release of histamine from mast cells. Inhibits histamine induced effects on conjunctival epithelial cells.

Pharmacodynamics/Kinetics

Absorption: Low systemic absorption

Protein binding: ~55% (primarily albumin)

Metabolism: Not extensively metabolized

Half-life elimination: ~3 hours

Excretion: Urine (60% to 70%, mostly as unchanged drug); feces (17%)

Dosage Ophthalmic:

Children ≥3 years, Adolescents, and Adults: Patanol®: Instill 1 drop into each affected eye twice daily (allowing 6-8 hours between doses); results from an environmental study demonstrated that olopatadine was effective when dosed twice daily for up to 6 weeks

Children ≥2 years, Adolescents, and Adults: Pataday™: Instill 1 drop into each affected eye once daily

Dosage adjustment in renal impairment: No dosage adjustment provided in manufacturer's labeling. However, dosage adjustment unlikely due to low systemic absorption.

Dosage adjustment in hepatic impairment: No dosage adjustment provided in manufacturer's labeling. However, dosage adjustment unlikely due to low systemic absorption.

Administration For topical ophthalmic use only. Wash hands prior to use. Do not touch tip of container to eye. After instilling drops, wait at least 10 minutes before inserting contact lenses. Do not insert contacts if eyes are red.

Dosage Forms Excipient information presented when available (limited, particularly for generics); consult specific product labeling.

Solution, Ophthalmic:

Pataday: 0.2% (2.5 mL) [contains benzalkonium chloride, edetate disodium]

Patanol: 0.1% (5 mL) [contains benzalkonium chloride]

◆ **Olopatadine Hydrochloride** *see* Olopatadine (Nasal) *on page 1499*

◆ **Olopatadine Hydrochloride** *see* Olopatadine (Ophthalmic) *on page 1499*

Olsalazine (ole SAL a zeen)

Brand Names: U.S. Dipentum

Brand Names: Canada Dipentum®

Index Terms Olsalazine Sodium

Pharmacologic Category 5-Aminosalicylic Acid Derivative

Use Maintenance of remission of ulcerative colitis in patients intolerant to sulfasalazine

Pregnancy Risk Factor C

Pregnancy Considerations Animal studies have demonstrated fetal developmental toxicities. There are no well-controlled studies in pregnant women. Use during pregnancy only if clearly necessary.

Breast-Feeding Considerations The active metabolite, 5-aminosalicylic acid may pass into breast milk. Diarrhea has been reported in breast-fed infants whose mothers took olsalazine.

Contraindications Hypersensitivity to olsalazine, salicylates, or any component of the formulation

Warnings/Precautions Diarrhea is a common adverse effect of olsalazine. May exacerbate symptoms of colitis. Use with caution in patients with renal or hepatic impairment. Use with caution in elderly patients. Use with caution in patients with severe allergies or asthma.

Adverse Reactions

>10%: Gastrointestinal: Diarrhea (11% to 17%; dose related)

1% to 10%:

Central nervous system: Depression (2%), dizziness/vertigo (1%)

Dermatologic: Rash (2%), pruritus (1%)

Gastrointestinal: Abdominal pain/cramps (10%), nausea (5%), bloating (2%), stomatitis (1%), vomiting (1%)

Neuromuscular & skeletal: Arthralgia (4%)

Respiratory: Upper respiratory infection (2%)

<1% (Limited to important or life-threatening): Alkaline phosphatase increased, Alopecia, ALT increased, anemia, angioedema, aplastic anemia, AST increased, bilirubin increased, blood in stool, blurred vision, bronchospasm, cholestatic hepatitis, cholestatic jaundice, chest pain, chills, cirrhosis, dehydration, dry eyes, dyspnea, dysuria, eosinophilia, epigastric discomfort, erythema, erythema nodosum, fever, flare of symptoms, flatulence, GGT increased, heart block (second degree), hematuria, hemolytic anemia, hepatitis, hepatic failure, hepatic necrosis, hot flashes, hypertension, impotence, insomnia, interstitial nephritis, interstitial pneumonia, irritability, jaundice, Kawasaki-like syndrome, LDH increased, leukopenia, lymphopenia, menorrhagia, mood swings, muscle cramps, myalgia, myocarditis, nephrotic syndrome, neutropenia, orthostatic hypotension, palpitation, pancreatitis, pancytopenia, paresthesia, pericarditis, peripheral edema, peripheral neuropathy, photosensitivity, proteinuria, rectal bleeding, rectal discomfort, reticulocytosis, rigors, tachycardia, thrombocytopenia, tinnitus, tremor, urinary frequency, watery eyes, xerostomia

Drug Interactions

Metabolism/Transport Effects None known.

Avoid Concomitant Use There are no known interactions where it is recommended to avoid concomitant use.

Increased Effect/Toxicity

Olsalazine may increase the levels/effects of: Heparin; Heparin (Low Molecular Weight); Thiopurine Analogs; Varicella Virus-Containing Vaccines

The levels/effects of Olsalazine may be increased by: Nonsteroidal Anti-Inflammatory Agents

Decreased Effect

Olsalazine may decrease the levels/effects of: Cardiac Glycosides

Storage/Stability Store at 20°C to 25°C (77°F); excursions permitted to 15°C to 30°C (59°F to 86°F).

Mechanism of Action Mesalamine (5-aminosalicylic acid) is the active component of olsalazine; the specific mechanism of action of mesalamine is unknown; however, it is thought that it modulates local chemical mediators of the inflammatory response, especially leukotrienes, and is also postulated to be a free radical scavenger or an inhibitor of tumor necrosis factor (TNF); action appears topical rather than systemic.

Pharmacodynamics/Kinetics

Absorption: <3%; very little intact olsalazine is systemically absorbed

Protein binding, plasma: >99%

Metabolism: Primarily via colonic bacteria to active drug, 5-aminosalicylic acid (5-ASA)

Half-life elimination: 54 minutes

Time to peak: ~1 hour

Excretion: Primarily feces; urine (<1%)

Dosage Adults: Oral: 1 g/day in 2 divided doses

Dosage adjustment in renal impairment: No dosage adjustment provided in manufacturer's labeling. Monitor patients with impaired renal function.

Dosage adjustment in hepatic impairment: No dosage adjustment provided in manufacturer's labeling. Monitor patients with impaired hepatic function.

Dietary Considerations Take with food.

Administration Administer with food in evenly divided doses.

Monitoring Parameters CBC, hepatic function, renal function; stool frequency

Dosage Forms Excipient information presented when available (limited, particularly for generics); consult specific product labeling.

Capsule, Oral, as sodium:

Dipentum: 250 mg

◆ **Olsalazine Sodium** *see* Olsalazine *on page 1500*

◆ **Olux** *see* Clobetasol *on page 457*

◆ **Olux-E** *see* Clobetasol *on page 457*

◆ **Olysio** *see* Simeprevir *on page 1897*

Omacetaxine (oh ma se TAX een)

Brand Names: U.S. Synribo

Index Terms CGX-625; HHT; Homoharringtonine; Omacetaxine Mepesuccinate

Pharmacologic Category Antineoplastic Agent, Cephalotaxine; Antineoplastic Agent, Protein Synthesis Inhibitor

Use Treatment of chronic or accelerated phase chronic myelogenous leukemia (CML) in patients resistant and/or intolerant to ≥2 tyrosine kinase inhibitors

Pregnancy Risk Factor D

Pregnancy Considerations Adverse events were observed in animal reproduction studies at doses less than the equivalent human dose (based on BSA). Based on the mechanism of action, omacetaxine may cause fetal harm if administered during pregnancy. Women of reproductive potential should avoid pregnancy during therapy.

Breast-Feeding Considerations It is not known if omacetaxine is excreted in breast milk. Due to the potential for serious adverse reactions in the nursing infant, the decision to discontinue omacetaxine or to discontinue breast-feeding should take into account the importance of treatment to the mother.

Contraindications There are no contraindications listed in the manufacturer's labeling.

Warnings/Precautions Hazardous agent: Use appropriate precautions for handling and disposal (meets NIOSH, 2012 criteria). Grade 3/4 neutropenia, thrombocytopenia, and anemia commonly occur; generally reversible, although may require treatment delay and/or a reduction in the number of treatment days with future cycles. Myelosuppression may rarely be fatal. Monitor blood counts (in induction and maintenance cycles). Neutropenia may increase the risk for infection. Thrombocytopenia may increase the risk of bleeding; cerebrovascular hemorrhages have been reported (some fatal); gastrointestinal hemorrhages have occurred. Due to the increased risk of bleeding, avoid the use of anticoagulants, aspirin, and NSAIDs when the platelet count is <50,000/mm^3. Patients ≥65 years of age are more likely to experience hematologic toxicity. Omacetaxine may induce glucose intolerance; hyperglycemia has been observed; hyperosmolar nonketotic hyperglycemia has been reported (case report). Monitor blood glucose frequently, especially in patients with diabetes or with risk factors for diabetes. Avoid use in patients with poorly controlled diabetes; may initiate after glycemic control has been established.

Adverse Reactions

>10%:

Cardiovascular: Peripheral edema (13%)

Central nervous system: Fatigue (26% to 31%), fever (24% to 29%), headache (13% to 19%), chills (13%)

Dermatologic: Alopecia (15%)

Endocrine & metabolic: Uric acid increased (grades 3/4: 56% to 57%), hyperglycemia (grades 3/4: 10% to 15%; hyperosmolar nonketotic hyperglycemia: <1%)

Gastrointestinal: Diarrhea (35% to 42%), nausea (27% to 32%), constipation (15%), vomiting (12% to 15%), abdominal pain (13% to 14%), anorexia (13%)

Hematologic: Thrombocytopenia (grades 3/4: 49% to 88%), neutropenia (grades 3/4: 18% to 81%), anemia (grades 3/4: 36% to 80%), leukocytes decreased (grades 3/4: 61% to 72%), neutropenic fever (10% to 20%; grades 3/4: 10% to 16%), lymphopenia (17%; grades 3/4: 16%)

Local: Injection site reactions (22% to 34%)

Neuromuscular & skeletal: Weakness (23% to 24%), arthralgia (19%), limb pain (11% to 13%), back pain (11%)

Renal: Creatinine increased (grades 3/4: 9% to 16%)

Respiratory: Cough (≤16%), epistaxis (11% to 15%), dyspnea (11%)

Miscellaneous: Infection (46% to 56%; grades 3/4: 11% to 20%)

1% to 10%:

Cardiovascular: Acute coronary syndrome, angina pectoris, arrhythmia, bradycardia, cerebral hemorrhage, chest pain, edema, hyper-/hypotension, palpitations, tachycardia, ventricular extrasystoles

Central nervous system: Insomnia (10%), anxiety, agitation, confusion, depression, dizziness, dysphonia, hyperthermia, hypoesthesia, lethargy, malaise, mental status change, pain, seizures

Dermatologic: Bruising, burning sensation, dry skin, erythema, hyperhidrosis, hyperpigmentation, petechiae, pruritus, purpura, rash, skin exfoliation, skin lesions, skin ulceration

Endocrine & metabolic: Glucose decreased (grades 3/4: 6% to 8%), dehydration, diabetes mellitus, gout, hot flashes

Gastrointestinal: Abdominal distension, abnormal taste, anal fissure, aphthous stomatitis, appetite decreased, dyspepsia, dysphagia, gastritis, gastroesophageal reflux disease, GI bleeding, gingival bleeding, gingival pain, gingivitis, hemorrhoids, melena, mouth ulceration, mouth hemorrhage, mucosal inflammation, oral pain, stomatitis, xerostomia

Genitourinary: Dysuria

Hematologic: Bone marrow failure (10%; grades 3/4: 10%), hematoma

Hepatic: Bilirubin increased (grades 3/4: 6% to 9%), ALT increased (grades 3/4: 2% to 6%)

Neuromuscular & skeletal: Bone pain, muscle spasms, muscle weakness, musculoskeletal chest pain, musculoskeletal discomfort, musculoskeletal pain myalgia, paresthesia, sciatica, stiffness, tremor

Ocular: Blurred vision, cataract, conjunctival hemorrhage, conjunctivitis, diplopia, dry eyes, eye pain, eyelid edema, lacrimation increased

Otic: Ear hemorrhage, ear pain, tinnitus

Respiratory: Hemoptysis, nasal congestion, pharyngolaryngeal pain, rales, rhinorrhea, sinus congestion

Miscellaneous: Flu-like syndrome, hypersensitivity reactions, night sweats, transfusion reaction

Drug Interactions

Metabolism/Transport Effects Substrate of P-glycoprotein

Avoid Concomitant Use

Avoid concomitant use of Omacetaxine with any of the following: Anticoagulants; Aspirin; BCG; Natalizumab; Nonsteroidal Anti-Inflammatory Agents; Pimecrolimus; Tacrolimus (Topical); Tofacitinib; Vaccines (Live)

Increased Effect/Toxicity

Omacetaxine may increase the levels/effects of: Leflunomide; Natalizumab; Tofacitinib; Vaccines (Live); Vitamin K Antagonists

The levels/effects of Omacetaxine may be increased by: Anticoagulants; Aspirin; Denosumab; Nonsteroidal Anti-Inflammatory Agents; Pimecrolimus; Roflumilast; Tacrolimus (Topical); Trastuzumab

Decreased Effect

Omacetaxine may decrease the levels/effects of: BCG; Cardiac Glycosides; Coccidioidin Skin Test; Sipuleucel-T; Vaccines (Inactivated); Vaccines (Live); Vitamin K Antagonists

The levels/effects of Omacetaxine may be decreased by: Echinacea

Preparation for Administration Hazardous agent: Use appropriate precautions for handling and disposal (meets NIOSH, 2012 criteria). Reconstitute each 3.5 mg vial with sodium chloride 0.9% (NS) 1 mL, resulting in a concentration of 3.5 mg/mL. Gently swirl until solution is clear (lyophilized powder dissolves completely in <1 minute).

Storage/Stability Store intact vials at 20°C to 25°C (68°F to 77°F); excursions permitted between 15°C to 30°C (59°F to 86°F). Protect from light (intact vial and reconstituted solutions). Reconstituted solution should be used within 12 hours if stored at room temperature or within 24 hours if refrigerated at 2°C to 8°C (36°F to 46°F).

Mechanism of Action Omacetaxine is a reversible protein synthesis inhibitor which binds to the A-site cleft of the ribosomal subunit to interfere with chain elongation and inhibit protein synthesis. It acts independently of BCR-ABL1 kinase-binding activity, and has demonstrated activity against tyrosine kinase inhibitor-resistant BCR-ABL mutations.

Pharmacodynamics/Kinetics

Onset:

Chronic phase CML: Mean time to major cytogenetic response: 3.5 months

Accelerated phase CML: Mean time to response: 2.3 months

Duration:

Chronic phase CML: Median duration of major cytogenetic response: 12.5 months

Accelerated phase CML: Median duration of complete hematologic response: 4.7 months

Absorption: SubQ: Rapid (Nemunaitis, 2013)

Distribution: V_{dss}: 141 ± 93 L

Protein binding: ≤50%

Metabolism: Hydrolyzed by plasma esterases to 4'-DMHHT; minimal hepatic metabolism

Half-life elimination: ~6 hours

Time to peak: SubQ: ~30 minutes

Excretion: Urine (<15%)

Dosage Chronic myelogenous leukemia (CML), chronic or accelerated phase: Adults: SubQ:

Induction: 1.25 mg/m^2 twice daily for 14 consecutive days of a 28-day treatment cycle; continue until hematologic response is achieved

Maintenance: 1.25 mg/m^2 twice daily for 7 consecutive days of a 28-day treatment cycle; continue until no longer achieving clinical treatment benefit

Dosing adjustment for toxicity:

Hematologic toxicity: May delay treatment cycles and/or reduce the number of treatment days during a cycle for hematologic toxicities.

Neutropenia grade 4 (ANC <500/mm^3) or thrombocytopenia ≥ grade 3 (platelets <50,000/mm^3) during a cycle: Delay the start of the next cycle until ANC ≥1000/mm^3 and platelets ≥50,000/mm^3 **AND** reduce the number of treatment days by 2 days (eg, reduce from 14 days to 12 days or reduce from 7 days to 5 days)

Nonhematologic toxicity: Manage symptomatically; interrupt and/or delay treatment until toxicity resolves.

Dosage adjustment in renal impairment: No dosage adjustment provided in the manufacturer's labeling (has not been studied). Based on the minimal amount of unchanged drug excreted in the urine, dosage adjustment is not likely necessary (Nemunaitis, 2013).

Dosage adjustment in hepatic impairment: No dosage adjustment provided in the manufacturer's labeling (has not been studied).

Dosing in obesity: *ASCO Guidelines for appropriate chemotherapy dosing in obese adults with cancer:* Utilize patient's actual body weight (full weight) for calculation of body surface area- or weight-based dosing, particularly when the intent of therapy is curative; manage regimen-related toxicities in the same manner as for nonobese patients; if a dose reduction is utilized due to toxicity, consider resumption of full weight-based dosing with subsequent cycles, especially if cause of toxicity (eg, hepatic or renal impairment) is resolved (Griggs, 2012).

Administration Administer subcutaneously.

Hazardous agent: Use appropriate precautions for handling and disposal (meets NIOSH, 2012 criteria).

Monitoring Parameters CBC with differential (weekly during induction and initial maintenance cycles, then every 2 weeks or as clinically indicated after initial maintenance cycles); blood glucose (frequently); signs/symptoms of infection; signs of bleeding

Dosage Forms Excipient information presented when available (limited, particularly for generics); consult specific product labeling.

Solution Reconstituted, Subcutaneous, as mepesuccinate [preservative free]:

Synribo: 3.5 mg (1 ea)

◆ **Omacetaxine Mepesuccinate** *see* Omacetaxine *on page 1501*

Omalizumab (oh mah lye ZOO mab)

Brand Names: U.S. Xolair

Brand Names: Canada Xolair®

Index Terms rhuMAb-E25

Pharmacologic Category Monoclonal Antibody, Anti-Asthmatic

Use Treatment of moderate-to-severe, persistent allergic asthma in patients with a positive skin test or *in vitro* reactivity to a perennial aeroallergen and not adequately controlled with inhaled corticosteroids

Pregnancy Risk Factor B

Pregnancy Considerations Teratogenic effects were not observed in animal studies. There are no adequate and well-controlled studies in pregnant women. IgG molecules are known to cross the placenta; use during pregnancy only if clearly needed. A registry has been established to monitor outcomes of women exposed to omalizumab during pregnancy or within 8 weeks prior to pregnancy (866-496-5247).

Breast-Feeding Considerations It is not known if omalizumab is excreted in breast milk; however, IgG is excreted in human milk and excretion of omalizumab is expected. Effects to nursing infant are not known; use with caution.

Medication Guide Available Yes

Contraindications Severe hypersensitivity to omalizumab or any component of the formulation

Warnings/Precautions [U.S. Boxed Warning]: Anaphylaxis, including delayed-onset anaphylaxis, has been reported following administration; anaphylaxis may present as bronchospasm, hypotension, syncope, urticaria, and/or angioedema of the throat or tongue. Anaphylaxis has occurred after the first dose and in some cases >1 year after initiation of regular treatment. Due to the risk, patients should be observed closely for an appropriate time period after administration and should receive treatment only under direct medical supervision. Healthcare providers should be prepared to administer appropriate therapy for managing potentially life-threatening anaphylaxis. Patients should be instructed on identifying signs/symptoms of anaphylaxis and to seek immediate care if they arise. In postmarketing reports, anaphylaxis usually occurred with the first or second dose and with a time to onset of ≤60 minutes; however, reactions have been reported with subsequent doses (after 39 doses) and with a time to onset of up to 4 days after administration. Discontinue therapy following any severe reaction.

In rare cases, patients may present with systemic eosinophilia, sometimes presenting with clinical features of vasculitis consistent with Churg-Strauss syndrome, a condition which is often treated with systemic corticosteroid therapy. Healthcare providers should be alert to eosinophilia, vasculitic rash, worsening pulmonary symptoms, cardiac complications, and/or neuropathy presenting in their patients. A causal association between omalizumab and these underlying conditions has not been established. Reports of a constellation of symptoms including fever, arthritis or arthralgia, rash, and lymphadenopathy have been reported with postmarketing use (symptoms resemble those seen in patients experiencing serum sickness, although circulating immune complexes or a skin biopsy consistent with a Type III hypersensitivity reaction were not been observed with these cases). Onset of symptoms generally occurred 1-5 days following the first or subsequent doses. Discontinue therapy in any patient reporting this constellation of signs/symptoms. Malignant neoplasms have been reported rarely with use in short-term studies; impact of long-term use is not known. Use caution with and monitor patients at high risk for parasitic (helminth) infections (risk of infection may be increased).

Therapy has not been shown to alleviate acute asthma exacerbations; do not use to treat acute bronchospasm or status asthmaticus. Dosing is based on body weight and pretreatment total IgE serum levels. IgE levels remain elevated up to 1 year following treatment, therefore, levels taken during treatment cannot and should not be used as a dosage guide. Gradually taper systemic or inhaled corticosteroid therapy; do not discontinue corticosteroids abruptly following initiation of omalizumab therapy.

Adverse Reactions

>10%: Local: Injection site reaction (45%; placebo 43%; severe 12%). Most reactions occurred within 1 hour, lasted <8 days, and decreased in frequency with additional dosing.

1% to 10%:

Central nervous system: Pain (7%), dizziness (3%), fatigue (3%)

Dermatologic: Dermatitis (2%), pruritus (2%)

Neuromuscular & skeletal: Arthralgia (8%), leg pain (4%), arm pain (2%), bone fracture (2%)

Otic: Otalgia (2%)

<1% (Limited to important or life-threatening): Alopecia, anaphylaxis, antibody development, arthritis, bronchospasm, chest tightness, cough, eosinophilia, hypotension, local pruritus, lymphadenopathy, malignant neoplasm (0.5%; placebo 0.2%), pharyngeal edema, skin edema, skin rash, swollen tongue, syncope, thrombocytopenia, urticaria

Drug Interactions

Metabolism/Transport Effects None known.

Avoid Concomitant Use

Avoid concomitant use of Omalizumab with any of the following: BCG; Natalizumab; Pimecrolimus; Tacrolimus (Topical); Tofacitinib; Vaccines (Live)

Increased Effect/Toxicity

Omalizumab may increase the levels/effects of: Leflunomide; Natalizumab; Tofacitinib; Vaccines (Live)

The levels/effects of Omalizumab may be increased by: Denosumab; Pimecrolimus; Roflumilast; Tacrolimus (Topical); Trastuzumab

Decreased Effect

Omalizumab may decrease the levels/effects of: BCG; Coccidioidin Skin Test; Sipuleucel-T; Vaccines (Inactivated); Vaccines (Live)

The levels/effects of Omalizumab may be decreased by: Echinacea

Preparation for Administration Reconstitute using SWFI, USP only; add SWFI 1.4 mL to upright vial using a 1-inch, 18-gauge needle on a 3 mL syringe and swirl gently for ~1 minute to evenly wet the powder; do not shake. Then gently swirl the upright vial for 5-10 seconds approximately every 5 minutes until dissolved; generally takes 15-20 minutes to dissolve completely. If it takes >20 minutes to dissolve completely, continue to swirl the upright vial for 5-10 seconds every 5 minutes until no gel-like particles are visible in the solution; do not use if contents are not completely dissolved after 40 minutes. Resulting solution is 150 mg/1.2 mL. Invert the vial for 15 seconds so the solution drains toward the stopper. Remove all of the solution by inserting a new 3 mL syringe with a 1-inch, 18-gauge needle into the inverted vial. Replace the 18-gauge needle with a 25-gauge needle for subcutaneous injection, and expel any air, bubbles, or excess solution to obtain the 1.2 mL dose.

Storage/Stability Prior to reconstitution, store under refrigeration at 2°C to 8°C (36°F to 46°F); product may be shipped at room temperature. Following reconstitution, protect from direct sunlight. May be stored for up to 8 hours if refrigerated or 4 hours if stored at room temperature.

Mechanism of Action Omalizumab is an IgG monoclonal antibody (recombinant DNA derived) which inhibits IgE binding to the high-affinity IgE receptor on mast cells and basophils. By decreasing bound IgE, the activation and release of mediators in the allergic response (early and late phase) is limited. Serum free IgE levels and the number of high-affinity IgE receptors are decreased. Long-term treatment in patients with allergic asthma showed a decrease in asthma exacerbations and corticosteroid usage.

Pharmacodynamics/Kinetics

Absorption: Slow following SubQ injection

Distribution: V_d: 78 ± 32 mL/kg

Metabolism: Degradation of IgG and omalizumab: IgE complexes by reticuloendothelial system and endothelial cells in the liver

Bioavailability: 62%

Half-life elimination: 26 days (asthma patients)

Time to peak: 7-8 days

Excretion: Primarily via hepatic degradation; intact IgG may be secreted in bile

Dosage Asthma: Children ≥12 years and Adults: SubQ: Dose and frequency based on body weight and **pretreatment** total IgE serum levels. Dosing should be adjusted during therapy for significant changes in body weight. Dosing should **not** be adjusted based on total IgE levels taken during treatment or <1 year following interruption of therapy. If therapy has been interrupted for ≥1 year, total IgE levels may be re-evaluated for dosage determination.

Pretreatment serum IgE ≥30-100 units/mL:
- U.S. labeling:
  - 30-90 kg: 150 mg every 4 weeks
  - >90-150 kg: 300 mg every 4 weeks
- Canadian labeling:
  - >20-90 kg: 150 mg every 4 weeks
  - >90-150 kg: 300 mg every 4 weeks

Pretreatment serum IgE >100-200 units/mL:
- U.S. labeling:
  - 30-90 kg: 300 mg every 4 weeks
  - >90-150 kg: 225 mg every 2 weeks
- Canadian labeling:
  - >20-40 kg: 150 mg every 4 weeks
  - >40-90 kg: 300 mg every 4 weeks
  - >90-125 kg: 225 mg every 2 weeks
  - >125-150 kg: 300 mg every 2 weeks

Pretreatment serum IgE >200-300 units/mL:
- U.S. labeling:
  - 30-60 kg: 300 mg every 4 weeks
  - >60-90 kg: 225 mg every 2 weeks
  - >90-150 kg: 300 mg every 2 weeks
- Canadian labeling:
  - >20-30 kg: 150 mg every 4 weeks
  - >30-60 kg: 300 mg every 4 weeks
  - >60-90 kg: 225 mg every 2 weeks
  - >90-125 kg: 300 mg every 2 weeks
  - >125-150 kg: 375 mg every 2 weeks

Pretreatment serum IgE >300-400 units/mL:
- U.S. labeling:
  - 30-70 kg: 225 mg every 2 weeks
  - >70-90 kg: 300 mg every 2 weeks
  - >90 kg: Do not administer dose
- Canadian labeling:
  - >20-40 kg: 300 mg every 4 weeks
  - >40-70 kg: 225 mg every 2 weeks
  - >70-90 kg: 300 mg every 2 weeks
  - >90 kg: Do not administer dose

Pretreatment serum IgE >400-500 units/mL:
- U.S. labeling:
  - 30-70 kg: 300 mg every 2 weeks
  - >70-90 kg: 375 mg every 2 weeks
  - >90 kg: Do not administer dose
- Canadian labeling:
  - >20-30 kg: 300 mg every 4 weeks
  - >30-50 kg: 225 mg every 2 weeks
  - >50-70 kg: 300 mg every 2 weeks
  - >70-90 kg: 375 mg every 2 weeks
  - >90 kg: Do not administer dose

Pretreatment serum IgE >500-600 units/mL:
- U.S. labeling:
  - 30-60 kg: 300 mg every 2 weeks
  - >60-70 kg: 375 mg every 2 weeks
  - >70 kg: Do not administer dose
- Canadian labeling:
  - >20-30 kg: 300 mg every 4 weeks
  - >30-40 kg: 225 mg every 2 weeks
  - >40-60 kg: 300 mg every 2 weeks
  - >60-70 kg: 375 mg every 2 weeks
  - >70 kg: Do not administer dose

Pretreatment serum IgE >600-700 units/mL:
- U.S. labeling:
  - 30-60 kg: 375 mg every 2 weeks
  - >60 kg: Do not administer dose
- Canadian labeling:
  - >20-40 kg: 225 mg every 2 weeks
  - >40-50 kg: 300 mg every 2 weeks
  - >50-60 kg: 375 mg every 2 weeks
  - >60 kg: Do not administer dose

Dosage adjustment for toxicity:

Severe hypersensitivity reaction or anaphylaxis: Discontinue treatment.

Fever, arthralgia, and rash: Discontinue treatment if this constellation of symptoms occurs.

Dosage adjustment in renal impairment: No dosage adjustment provided in manufacturer's labeling.

Dosage adjustment in hepatic impairment: No dosage adjustment provided in manufacturer's labeling.

Administration For SubQ injection only; doses >150 mg should be divided over more than one injection site (eg, 225 mg or 300 mg administered as two injections, 375 mg administered as three injections). Injections may take 5-10 seconds to administer (solution is slightly viscous). Administer only under direct medical supervision and observe patient for a minimum of 2 hours following administration of any dose given.

Monitoring Parameters Anaphylactic/hypersensitivity reactions, baseline serum total IgE; FEV_1, peak flow, and/or other pulmonary function tests; monitor for signs of infection

Test Interactions Total IgE levels are elevated for up to 1 year following treatment. Total serum IgE may be retested after interruption of therapy for 1 year or more.

Dosage Forms Excipient information presented when available (limited, particularly for generics); consult specific product labeling.

Solution Reconstituted, Subcutaneous [preservative free]:

Xolair: 150 mg (1 ea)

◆ **Omeclamox-Pak®** *see* Omeprazole, Clarithromycin, and Amoxicillin *on page 1508*

◆ **Omega 3** *see* Omega-3-Acid Ethyl Esters *on page 1504*

Omega-3-Acid Ethyl Esters

(oh MEG a three AS id ETH il ES ters)

Brand Names: U.S. Lovaza

Index Terms Docosahexaenoic Acid; Eicosapentaenoic Acid; Ethyl Esters of Omega-3 Fatty Acids; Fish Oil; Omega 3; P-OM3

Pharmacologic Category Antilipemic Agent, Omega-3 Fatty Acids

Use Lovaza: Adjunct to diet therapy in the treatment of hypertriglyceridemia (≥500 mg/dL)

Note: The Endocrine Society recommends that omega-3 fatty acids such as Lovaza may be considered for triglyceride levels >1000 mg/dL and may be used alone or in combination with HMG-CoA reductase inhibitors (Berglund, 2012). A number of OTC formulations containing omega-3 fatty acids are marketed as nutritional supplements; these do not have FDA-approved indications and may not contain the same amounts of the active ingredient.

Unlabeled Use Lovaza: Treatment of IgA nephropathy

Pregnancy Risk Factor C

Dosage Oral: Adults:

Hypertriglyceridemia: 4 g/day as a single daily dose or in 2 divided doses

Treatment of IgA nephropathy (unlabeled use): 4 g/day (Donadio, 2001)

Dosage adjustment in renal impairment: No dosage adjustment provided in manufacturer's labeling (has not been studied).

Dosage adjustment in hepatic impairment: No dosage adjustment provided in manufacturer's labeling (has not been studied).

Additional Information Complete prescribing information should be consulted for additional detail.

Dosage Forms Excipient information presented when available (limited, particularly for generics); consult specific product labeling.

Capsule, liquid gel, oral:

Lovaza: 1 g [contains DHA ~375 mg/capsule, EPA ~465 mg/capsule, soybean oil]

Omeprazole (oh MEP ra zole)

Brand Names: U.S. First-Omeprazole; Omeprazole+Syrspend SF Alka; PriLOSEC; PriLOSEC OTC [OTC]

Brand Names: Canada Apo-Omeprazole®; Ava-Omeprazole; Dom-Omeprazole DR; Losec®; Mylan-Omeprazole; PMS-Omeprazole; PMS-Omeprazole DR; Q-Omeprazole; RAN™-Omeprazole; ratio-Omeprazole; Sandoz-Omeprazole; Teva-Omeprazole

Index Terms Omeprazole Magnesium

Pharmacologic Category Proton Pump Inhibitor; Substituted Benzimidazole

Use Short-term (4-8 weeks) treatment of active duodenal ulcer disease or active benign gastric ulcer; treatment of heartburn and other symptoms associated with gastroesophageal reflux disease (GERD); short-term (4-8 weeks) treatment of endoscopically-diagnosed erosive esophagitis; maintenance healing of erosive esophagitis; long-term treatment of pathological hypersecretory conditions (eg, Zollinger-Ellison syndrome); as part of a multidrug regimen for *H. pylori* eradication to reduce the risk of duodenal ulcer recurrence

OTC labeling: Short-term treatment of frequent, uncomplicated heartburn occurring ≥2 days/week

Unlabeled Use Healing NSAID-induced ulcers; prevention of NSAID-induced ulcer; stress ulcer prophylaxis in the critically-ill

Pregnancy Risk Factor C

Pregnancy Considerations Adverse events were observed in some animal reproduction studies. An increased risk of hypospadias was reported following maternal use of proton pump inhibitors (PPIs) during pregnancy (Anderka, 2012), but this was based on a small number of exposures and the same association was not found in another study (Erichsen, 2012). Most available studies have not shown an increased risk of major birth defects following maternal use of omeprazole during pregnancy (Diav-Citrin, 2005; Källén, 2001; Lalkin, 1998; Matok, 2012; Pasternak, 2010). When treating GERD in pregnancy, PPIs may be used when clinically indicated (Katz, 2013).

Breast-Feeding Considerations Omeprazole is excreted into breast milk. Milk concentrations of omeprazole were studied in a breast-feeding woman at 3 weeks postpartum. The mother had taken omeprazole 20 mg daily starting her 29th week of gestation and continued after delivery. Following administration of omeprazole 20 mg, peak concentrations in the maternal serum occurred 240 minutes after the dose and peak concentrations in the breast milk were 180 minutes after the dose. The concentrations of omeprazole detected in the breast milk were <7% of the highest maternal serum concentration (Marshall, 1998).The manufacturer recommends caution be used if administered to a nursing woman. The acidic content of the nursing infants' stomach may potentially inactivate any ingested omeprazole (Marshall, 1998).

Medication Guide Available Yes

Contraindications Hypersensitivity to omeprazole, other substituted benzimidazole proton pump inhibitors, or any component of the formulation

Warnings/Precautions Use of proton pump inhibitors (PPIs) may increase the risk of gastrointestinal infections (eg, *Salmonella, Campylobacter*). Relief of symptoms does not preclude the presence of a gastric malignancy. Atrophic gastritis (by biopsy) has been noted with long-term omeprazole therapy. In long-term (2-year) studies in rats, omeprazole produced a dose-related increase in gastric carcinoid tumors. While available endoscopic evaluations and histologic examinations of biopsy specimens from human stomachs have not detected a risk from short-term exposure to omeprazole, further human data on the effect of sustained hypochlorhydria and hypergastrinemia are needed to rule out the possibility of an increased risk for the development of tumors in humans receiving long-term therapy. Use of PPIs may increase risk of *Clostridium difficile*-associated diarrhea (CDAD), especially in hospitalized patients; consider CDAD diagnosis in patients with persistent diarrhea that does not improve. Use the lowest dose and shortest duration of PPI therapy appropriate for the condition being treated.

PPIs may diminish the therapeutic effect of clopidogrel, thought to be due to reduced formation of the active metabolite of clopidogrel. The manufacturer of clopidogrel recommends either avoidance both omeprazole (even when scheduled 12 hours apart) and esomeprazole or use of a PPI with comparatively less effect on the active metabolite of clopidogrel (eg, pantoprazole). In contrast to these warnings, others have recommended the continued use of PPIs, regardless of the degree of inhibition, in patients with a history of GI bleeding or multiple risk factors for GI bleeding who are also receiving clopidogrel since no evidence has established clinically meaningful differences in outcome; however, a clinically-significant interaction cannot be excluded in those who are poor metabolizers of clopidogrel (Abraham, 2010; Levine, 2011). Additionally, concomitant use of omeprazole with some drugs may require cautious use, may not be recommended, or may require dosage adjustments.

Increased incidence of osteoporosis-related bone fractures of the hip, spine, or wrist may occur with PPI therapy. Patients on high-dose (multiple daily doses) or long-term (≥1 year) therapy should be monitored. Use the lowest effective dose for the shortest duration of time, use vitamin D and calcium supplementation, and follow appropriate guidelines to reduce risk of fractures in patients at risk.

Hypomagnesemia, reported rarely, usually with prolonged PPI use of >3 months (most cases >1 year of therapy); may be symptomatic or asymptomatic; severe cases may cause tetany, seizures, and cardiac arrhythmias. Consider obtaining serum magnesium concentrations prior to beginning long-term therapy, especially if taking concomitant digoxin, diuretics, or other drugs known to cause hypomagnesemia; and periodically thereafter. Hypomagnesemia may be corrected by magnesium supplementation, although discontinuation of omeprazole may be necessary; magnesium levels typically return to normal within 1 week of stopping. Serum chromogranin A levels may be increased if assessed while patient on omeprazole; may lead to diagnostic errors related to neuroendocrine tumors.

Decreased *H. pylori* eradication rates have been observed with short-term (≤7 days) combination therapy. The American College of Gastroenterology recommends 10-14 days of therapy (triple or quadruple) for eradication of *H. pylori* (Chey, 2007). Bioavailability may be increased in Asian populations and patients with hepatic dysfunction; consider dosage reductions, especially for maintenance healing of erosive esophagitis. Bioavailability may be increased in the elderly. When used for self-medication (OTC), do not use for >14 days.

Adverse Reactions

1% to 10%:

Central nervous system: Headache (7%), dizziness (2%)

Dermatologic: Rash (2%)

Gastrointestinal: Abdominal pain (5%), diarrhea (4%), nausea (4%), vomiting (3%), flatulence (3%), acid regurgitation (2%), constipation (2%)

Neuromuscular & skeletal: Back pain (1%), weakness (1%)

Respiratory: Upper respiratory infection (2%), cough (1%)

≤1% (Limited to important or life-threatening; adverse event occurrence may vary based on formulation): Abdominal swelling, abnormal dreams, aggression, agitation, agranulocytosis, alkaline phosphatase increased, allergic reactions, alopecia, ALT increased, anaphylaxis, anemia, angina, angioedema, anorexia, anxiety, apathy, AST increased, atrophic gastritis, benign gastric polyps, bilirubin increased, blurred vision, bradycardia, bronchospasm, chest pain, cholestatic hepatitis, *Clostridium difficile*-associated diarrhea (CDAD), confusion, creatinine increased, depression, double vision, dry skin, epistaxis, erythema multiforme, esophageal candidiasis, fatigue, fecal discoloration, fever, fracture, gastroduodenal carcinoids, GGT increased, glycosuria, gynecomastia, hallucinations, hematuria, hemolytic anemia, hepatic encephalopathy, hepatic failure, hepatic necrosis, hepatitis, hepatocellular hepatitis, hyperhidrosis, hypersensitivity, hypertension, hypoglycemia, hypomagnesemia, hyponatremia, insomnia, interstitial nephritis, irritable colon, jaundice, joint pain, leg pain, leukocytosis, leukopenia, liver disease (hepatocellular, cholestatic, mixed), malaise, microscopic colitis, microscopic pyuria, mucosal atrophy (tongue), muscle cramps, muscle weakness, myalgia, nervousness, neutropenia, ocular irritation, optic atrophy, optic neuritis, optic neuropathy (anterior ischemic), osteoporosis-related fracture, pain, palpitation, pancreatitis, pancytopenia, paresthesia, peripheral edema, petechiae, pharyngeal pain, photosensitivity, pneumonia, proteinuria, pruritus, psychiatric disturbance, purpura, skin inflammation, sleep disturbance, somnolence, Stevens-Johnson syndrome, stomatitis, tachycardia, taste perversion, testicular pain, thrombocytopenia, tinnitus, toxic epidermal necrolysis, tremor, urinary frequency, urinary tract infection, urticaria, vertigo, weight gain, xerophthalmia, xerostomia

Drug Interactions

Metabolism/Transport Effects **Substrate** of CYP2A6 (minor), CYP2C19 (major), CYP2C9 (minor), CYP2D6 (minor), CYP3A4 (minor); **Note:** Assignment of Major/Minor substrate status based on clinically relevant drug interaction potential; **Inhibits** CYP1A2 (weak), CYP2C19 (moderate), CYP2C9 (moderate), CYP2D6 (weak), CYP3A4 (weak); **Induces** CYP1A2 (weak/moderate)

Avoid Concomitant Use

Avoid concomitant use of Omeprazole with any of the following: Clopidogrel; Dasatinib; Delavirdine; Erlotinib; Nelfinavir; Pimozide; PONATinib; Rifampin; Rilpivirine; Risedronate; St Johns Wort

Increased Effect/Toxicity

Omeprazole may increase the levels/effects of: Amphetamines; ARIPiprazole; Benzodiazepines (metabolized by oxidation); Bosentan; Carvedilol; Cilostazol; Citalopram; CloZAPine; CycloSPORINE (Systemic); CYP2C19 Substrates; CYP2C9 Substrates; Dexmethylphenidate; Dofetilide; Escitalopram; Fosphenytoin; Lomitapide; Methotrexate; Methylphenidate; Phenytoin; Pimozide; Raltegravir; Risedronate; Saquinavir; Tacrolimus (Systemic); Vitamin K Antagonists; Voriconazole

The levels/effects of Omeprazole may be increased by: Fluconazole; Ketoconazole (Systemic); Voriconazole

Decreased Effect

Omeprazole may decrease the levels/effects of: Atazanavir; Bisphosphonate Derivatives; Bosutinib; Cefditoren; Clopidogrel; CloZAPine; Dabigatran Etexilate; Dabrafenib; Dasatinib; Delavirdine; Erlotinib; Gefitinib; Indinavir; Iron Salts; Itraconazole; Ketoconazole (Systemic); Mesalamine; Multivitamins/Minerals (with ADEK, Folate, Iron); Mycophenolate; Nelfinavir; Nilotinib; PONATinib; Posaconazole; Rilpivirine; Riociguat; Risedronate; Vismodegib

The levels/effects of Omeprazole may be decreased by: CYP2C19 Inducers (Strong); Dabrafenib; Fosphenytoin; Peginterferon Alfa-2b; Phenytoin; Rifampin; St Johns Wort; Tipranavir

Ethanol/Nutrition/Herb Interactions

Ethanol: Avoid ethanol (may cause gastric mucosal irritation).

Food: Food delays absorption.

Herb/Nutraceutical: Avoid use of St John's wort (may decrease efficacy of omeprazole).

Preparation for Administration Granules for oral suspension: For oral administration, empty the contents of the 2.5 mg packet into 5 mL of water (10 mg packet into 15 mL of water); stir. For NG administration, add 5 mL of water into a catheter-tipped syringe, and then add the contents of a 2.5 mg packet (15 mL water for the 10 mg packet); shake. **Note:** Regardless of the route of administration, the suspension should be left to thicken for 2-3 minutes prior to administration.

Storage/Stability

Capsules, tablets: Store at 15°C to 30°C (59°F to 86°F). Protect from light and moisture.

Granules for oral suspension: Store at 25°C (77°F); excursions permitted to 15°C to 30°C (59°F to 86°F).

Mechanism of Action Proton pump inhibitor; suppresses gastric basal and stimulated acid secretion by inhibiting the parietal cell H+/K+ ATP pump

Pharmacodynamics/Kinetics

Onset of action: Antisecretory: ~1 hour

Peak effect: Within 2 hours

Duration: Up to 72 hours; 50% of maximum effect at 24 hours; after stopping treatment, secretory activity gradually returns over 3-5 days

Absorption: Rapid

Protein binding: ~95%

Metabolism: Hepatic via CYP2C19 primarily and (to a lesser extent) via 3A4 to hydroxy, desmethyl, and sulfone metabolites (all inactive); saturable first-pass effect

Bioavailability: Oral: ~30% to 40%; Hepatic dysfunction: ~100%; Asians: AUC increased up to fourfold compared to Caucasians

Half-life elimination: 0.5-1 hour; hepatic impairment: ~3 hours

Time to peak, plasma: 0.5-3.5 hours

Excretion: Urine (~77% as metabolites, very small amount as unchanged drug); feces

Dosage

Children 1-16 years: Oral: GERD or other acid-related disorders:

5 kg to <10 kg: 5 mg once daily

10 kg to <20 kg: 10 mg once daily

≥20 kg: 20 mg once daily

Adults: Oral:

Active duodenal ulcer: 20 mg once daily for 4-8 weeks

Gastric ulcers: 40 mg once daily for 4-8 weeks

Symptomatic GERD (without esophageal lesions): 20 mg once daily for up to 4 weeks

Erosive esophagitis: 20 mg once daily for 4-8 weeks; maintenance of healing: 20 mg once daily for up to 12 months total therapy (including treatment period of 4-8 weeks)

Helicobacter pylori eradication: Dose varies with regimen:

Manufacturer labeling: 40 mg once daily administered with clarithromycin 500 mg 3 times daily for 14 days **or** 20 mg twice daily administered with amoxicillin 1000 mg *and* clarithromycin 500 mg twice daily for 10 days. **Note:** Presence of ulcer at time of therapy initiation may necessitate an additional 14-18 days of omeprazole 20 mg daily (monotherapy) after completion of combination therapy.

American College of Gastroenterology guidelines (Chey, 2007):

Nonpenicillin allergy: 20 mg twice daily administered with amoxicillin 1000 mg *and* clarithromycin 500 mg twice daily for 10-14 days

Penicillin allergy: 20 mg twice daily administered with clarithromycin 500 mg *and* metronidazole 500 mg twice daily for 10-14 days **or** 20 mg once or twice daily administered with bismuth subsalicylate 525 mg *and* metronidazole 250 mg *plus* tetracycline 500 mg 4 times daily for 10-14 days

Pathological hypersecretory conditions: Initial: 60 mg once daily; doses up to 120 mg 3 times daily have been administered; administer daily doses >80 mg in divided doses

NSAID-induced ulcer treatment (unlabeled use): 20 mg once daily for 4-8 weeks; Maintenance: 20 mg once daily for up to 6 months (Hawkey, 1998)

NSAID-induced ulcer prophylaxis (unlabeled use): 20 mg once daily for up to 6 months (Cullen, 1998)

Stress ulcer prophylaxis, ICU patients (unlabeled use): 40 mg once daily (Levy, 1997) or may administer 40 mg loading dose followed by 20-40 mg once daily (ASHP, 1999). **Note:** Intended for patients with associated risk factors (eg, coagulopathy, mechanical ventilation for ≥48 hours, severe sepsis); discontinue use once risk factors have resolved (Dellinger, 2013). Omeprazole 20 mg via NG tube once daily may be less effective in some critically ill populations compared to 40 mg via NG tube once daily (Balaban, 1997).

Frequent heartburn (OTC labeling): 20 mg once daily for 14 days; treatment may be repeated after 4 months if needed

Dosage adjustment in renal impairment: No dosage adjustment necessary.

Dosage adjustment in hepatic impairment: No dosage adjustment provided in manufacturer's labeling. However, based on increased bioavailability, a dosage reduction should be considered, especially for maintenance of healing of erosive esophagitis.

Dietary Considerations Should be taken on an empty stomach; best if taken before breakfast.

Administration

Oral: Best if administered before breakfast.

Capsule: Should be swallowed whole; do not chew or crush. Delayed release capsule may be opened and contents added to 1 tablespoon of applesauce (use immediately after adding to applesauce); mixture should not be chewed or warmed.

Oral suspension: Following reconstitution, the suspension should be left to thicken for 2-3 minutes and administered within 30 minutes. If any material remains after administration, add more water, stir, and administer immediately.

Tablet: Should be swallowed whole; do not crush or chew.

Nasogastric/orogastric (NG/OG) tube administration:

Oral suspension (using packets): After removing a catheter-tip syringe plunger, add 5 mL of water to the syringe and the contents of a 2.5 mg packet (or 15 mL of water for the 10 mg packet). Immediately shake syringe and leave to thicken for 2-3 minutes; shake syringe again and within 30 minutes administer via NG or gastric tube (French size 6 or larger). Refill syringe with an equal amount of water, shake, and flush remaining contents through NG or gastric tube

Oral suspension (using capsules): The manufacturer of Prilosec® does not give recommendations for extemporaneous preparation of omeprazole capsules for NG/OG administration. Consider using the packets for oral suspension. If packets are unavailable, methods of preparation of capsules for NG/OG administration have been described (Balaban, 1997; Phillips, 1996). An extemporaneously prepared suspension with extended stability may also be used (DiGiacinto, 2000; Quercia, 1997; Sharma, 1999).

Monitoring Parameters Susceptibility testing is recommended in patients who fail *H. pylori*-eradication regimen.

Test Interactions Omeprazole may falsely elevate serum chromogranin A (CgA) levels. The increased CgA level may cause false-positive results in the diagnosis of a neuroendocrine tumor. Temporarily stop omeprazole if assessing CgA level; repeat level if initially elevated; use the same laboratory for all testing of CgA levels.

Dosage Forms Excipient information presented when available (limited, particularly for generics); consult specific product labeling.

Capsule Delayed Release, Oral:

PriLOSEC: 10 mg, 20 mg, 40 mg

Generic: 10 mg, 20 mg, 40 mg, 20 mg

Packet, Oral:

PriLOSEC: 2.5 mg (30 ea); 10 mg (30 ea)

Suspension, Oral:

First-Omeprazole: 2 mg/mL (90 mL, 150 mL, 300 mL) [contains benzyl alcohol, fd&c red #40, saccharin sodium; strawberry flavor]

Omeprazole+Syrspend SF Alka: 2 mg/mL (100 mL)

Tablet Delayed Release, Oral:

PriLOSEC OTC: 20 mg

Generic: 20 mg

Extemporaneous Preparations Note: More palatable omeprazole (2 mg/mL) suspensions are commercially available as compounding kits (First-Omeprazole, Omeprazole+Syrspend SF Alka Cherry Kit).

A 2 mg/mL oral omeprazole solution (Simplified Omeprazole Solution) may be made with five omeprazole 20 mg delayed release capsules and 50 mL sodium bicarbonate 8.4%. Empty capsules into beaker. Add sodium bicarbonate solution. Gently stir (about 15 minutes) until a white suspension forms. Transfer to amber-colored syringe or bottle. Stable for 14 days at room temperature or for 30 days refrigerated.

DiGiacinto JL, Olsen KM, Bergman KL, et al, "Stability of Suspension Formulations of Lansoprazole and Omeprazole Stored in Amber-Colored Plastic Oral Syringes," *Ann Pharmacother*, 2000, 34 (5):600-5.

Quercia R, Fan C, Liu X, et al, "Stability of Omeprazole in an Extemporaneously Prepared Oral Liquid," *Am J Health Syst Pharm*, 1997, 54(16):1833-6.

Sharma V, "Comparison of 24-hour Intragastric pH Using Four Liquid Formulations of Lansoprazole and Omeprazole," *Am J Health Syst Pharm*, 1999, 56(23 Suppl 4):18-21.

◆ **Omeprazole, Amoxicillin, and Clarithromycin** *see* Omeprazole, Clarithromycin, and Amoxicillin *on page 1508*

Omeprazole and Sodium Bicarbonate

(oh MEP ra zole & SOW dee um bye KAR bun ate)

Brand Names: U.S. Zegerid OTC™ [OTC]; Zegerid®

Index Terms Sodium Bicarbonate and Omeprazole

Pharmacologic Category Proton Pump Inhibitor; Substituted Benzimidazole

Use Short-term (4-8 weeks) treatment of active duodenal ulcer or active benign gastric ulcer; treatment of heartburn and other symptoms associated with gastroesophageal reflux disease (GERD); short-term (4-8 weeks) treatment of endoscopically-diagnosed erosive esophagitis; maintenance healing of erosive esophagitis; reduction of risk of upper gastrointestinal bleeding in critically-ill patients

OTC labeling: Short-term (2 weeks) treatment of frequent (2 days/week), uncomplicated heartburn

Pregnancy Risk Factor C

Medication Guide Available Yes

Dosage Note: Both strengths of Zegerid® capsule and powder for oral suspension have identical sodium bicarbonate content, respectively. Do not substitute two 20 mg capsules/packets for one 40 mg dose.

Oral: Adults:

Active duodenal ulcer: 20 mg once daily for 4-8 weeks

Gastric ulcers: 40 mg once daily for 4-8 weeks

Symptomatic GERD: 20 mg once daily for up to 4 weeks

Erosive esophagitis: 20 mg once daily for 4-8 weeks; maintenance of healing: 20 mg once daily for up to 12 months total therapy (including treatment period of 4-8 weeks)

Heartburn (OTC labeling): 20 mg once daily for 14 days. Do not take for >14 days or more often than every 4 months, unless instructed by healthcare provider.

Risk reduction of upper GI bleeding in critically-ill patients (Zegerid® powder for oral suspension):

Loading dose: Day 1: 40 mg every 6-8 hours for two doses

Maintenance dose: 40 mg daily for up to 14 days; therapy >14 days has not been evaluated

Dosage adjustment in renal impairment: No dosage adjustment necessary.

Dosage adjustment in hepatic impairment: No dosage adjustment provided in manufacturer's labeling. However, based on increased bioavailability, a dosage reduction should be considered, especially for maintenance of healing of erosive esophagitis.

Additional Information Complete prescribing information should be consulted for additional detail.

Dosage Forms Excipient information presented when available (limited, particularly for generics); consult specific product labeling.

Capsule, oral: Omeprazole 20 mg [immediate release] and sodium bicarbonate 1100 mg; omeprazole 40 mg [immediate release] and sodium bicarbonate 1100 mg

Zegerid®: Omeprazole 20 mg [immediate release] and sodium bicarbonate 1100 mg [contains sodium 304 mg (13 mEq) per capsule]

Zegerid®: Omeprazole 40 mg [immediate release] and sodium bicarbonate 1100 mg [contains sodium 304 mg (13 mEq) per capsule]

Zegerid OTC™: Omeprazole 20 mg [immediate release] and sodium bicarbonate 1100 mg [contains sodium 303 mg (13 mEq) per capsule]

Powder for suspension, oral:

Zegerid®: Omeprazole 20 mg and sodium bicarbonate 1680 mg per packet (30s) [contains sodium 460 mg (20 mEq) per packet]

Zegerid®: Omeprazole 40 mg and sodium bicarbonate 1680 mg per packet (30s) [contains sodium 460 mg (20 mEq) per packet]

Omeprazole, Clarithromycin, and Amoxicillin

(oh MEP ra zole, kla RITH roe mye sin, & a moks i SIL in)

Brand Names: U.S. Omeclamox-Pak®

Index Terms Amoxicillin, Clarithromycin, and Omeprazole; Clarithromycin, Amoxicillin, and Omeprazole; Omeprazole, Amoxicillin, and Clarithromycin

Pharmacologic Category Antibiotic, Macrolide Combination; Antibiotic, Penicillin; Gastrointestinal Agent, Miscellaneous; Proton Pump Inhibitor; Substituted Benzimidazole

Use Eradication of *H. pylori* infection in patients with duodenal ulcer disease (active or a history of up to 1 year)

Pregnancy Risk Factor C

Dosage Oral: Adults: Omeprazole 20 mg (one capsule), clarithromycin 500 mg (one tablet), and amoxicillin 1000 mg (two capsules) twice daily for 10 days. **Note:** If patient has an active duodenal ulcer at therapy initiation, an additional 18 days of omeprazole 20 mg once daily is recommended.

Dosage adjustment in renal impairment: Amoxicillin and clarithromycin pharmacokinetics are altered in renal impairment. The manufacturer's labeling suggests that prolonged dosing intervals for clarithromycin may be appropriate in severe renal impairment, but provides no recommendation in regards to amoxicillin.

Dosage adjustment in hepatic impairment: Avoid use in hepatic impairment.

Additional Information Complete prescribing information should be consulted for additional detail.

Dosage Forms Excipient information presented when available (limited, particularly for generics); consult specific product labeling.

Combination package, oral [each administration card contains]:

Omeclamox-Pak™:

Capsule, delayed release: Omeprazole: 20 mg (2s)

Tablet: Clarithromycin: 500 mg (2s)

Capsule: Amoxicillin: 500 mg (4s) [contains sodium ≤0.0052 mEq (0.119 mg)/capsule]

- **Omeprazole Magnesium** *see* Omeprazole *on page* 1505
- **Omeprazole+Syrspend SF Alka** *see* Omeprazole *on page* 1505
- **Omnaris** *see* Ciclesonide (Nasal) *on page* 423
- **Omnicef** *see* Cefdinir *on page* 365
- **Omni Gel™ [OTC]** *see* Fluoride *on page* 880
- **Omnipred** *see* PrednisoLONE (Ophthalmic) *on page* 1706
- **Omnitarg** *see* Pertuzumab *on page* 1625
- **Omnitrope** *see* Somatropin *on page* 1934
- **Omontys®** *see* Peginesatide *on page* 1589
- **Omontys** *see* Peginesatide *on page* 1589

OnabotulinumtoxinA

(oh nuh BOT yoo lin num TOKS in aye)

Brand Names: U.S. Botox; Botox Cosmetic

Brand Names: Canada Botox; Botox Cosmetic

Index Terms Botulinum Toxin Type A; BTX-A

Pharmacologic Category Neuromuscular Blocker Agent, Toxin; Ophthalmic Agent, Toxin

Use Treatment of strabismus and blepharospasm associated with dystonia (including benign essential blepharospasm or VII nerve disorders) in patients ≥12 years of age; treatment of cervical dystonia (spasmodic torticollis) in patients ≥16 years of age; temporary improvement in the appearance of lines/wrinkles of the face (moderate-to-severe glabellar lines associated with corrugator and/or procerus muscle activity) in adult patients ≤65 years of age; treatment of severe primary axillary hyperhidrosis in adults not adequately controlled with topical treatments; treatment of focal spasticity (specifically upper limb spasticity) in adults; prophylaxis of chronic migraine headache (≥15 days/month with ≥4 hours/day headache duration) in adults; treatment of urinary incontinence due to detrusor overactivity associated with neurologic conditions in adults; treatment of overactive bladder (with symptoms of urge urinary incontinence, urgency, and frequency) in adults with an inadequate response or intolerance to anticholinergic medication.

Canadian labeling: Additional use (not in U.S. labeling): Dynamic equinus foot deformity in pediatric cerebral palsy patients; treatment of forehead, lateral canthus, and glabellar lines in adults >65 years of age

Unlabeled Use Treatment of oromandibular dystonia, spasmodic dysphonia (laryngeal dystonia) and other dystonias (ie, writer's cramp, focal task-specific dystonias); treatment of dynamic muscle contracture in pediatric cerebral palsy patients

Pregnancy Risk Factor C

Medication Guide Available Yes

Dosage Note: The lowest recommended dose should be used when initiating treatment (regardless of indication). In adults treated for more than one indication, the maximum cumulative dose should be ≤360 units/3 months. Canadian labeling recommends a maximum cumulative dose of 6 units/kg (adults up to 360 units; children up to 200 units) over 3 months in patients receiving additional treatment for noncosmetic indications.

Bladder dysfunction: Adults: Intradetrusor: **Note:** Prophylactic antimicrobial therapy (excluding aminoglycosides) should be administered 1-3 days prior to, on the day of, and for 1-3 days following onabotulinumtoxinA administration to decrease risk of UTI. Discontinue antiplatelet therapy at least 3 days prior to administration.

Detrusor overactivity associated with neurologic condition: 30 injections of 1 mL (recommended concentration: ~6.7 units/mL) for a total dose of 200 units/30 mL (maximum: 200 units); for the final injection, ~1 mL of sterile NS should be injected to ensure that the remaining medication in the needle is delivered to the bladder; may consider retreatment with diminishing effect but no sooner than 12 weeks from previous administration (median time until second treatment in studies: 42-48 weeks).

Overactive bladder: 20 injections of 0.5 mL (recommended concentration: 10 units/mL) for a total dose of 100 units/10 mL (maximum: 100 units); for the final injection, ~1 mL of sterile NS should be injected to ensure that the remaining medication in the needle is delivered to the bladder; may consider retreatment with diminishing effect but no sooner than 12 weeks from the previous administration (median time until second treatment in studies: ~24 weeks)

Blepharospasm:

Botox®: Children ≥12 years and Adults: I.M.: Initial dose: 1.25-2.5 units injected into the medial and lateral pretarsal orbicularis oculi of the upper lid and lateral pretarsal orbicularis oculi of lower lid

Dose may be increased up to twice the previous dose if the response from the initial dose lasted ≤2 months; maximum dose per site: 5 units. Tolerance may occur if treatments are given more often than every 3 months, but the effect is not usually permanent. Cumulative dose:

U.S. labeling: ≤200 units in 30-day period

Canadian labeling (not in U.S. labeling): Botox®: ≤200 units in 2-month period

Cervical dystonia:

Children ≥16 years and Adults: I.M.: For dosing guidance, the mean dose is 236 units (25th to 75th percentile range 198-300 units) divided among the affected muscles in patients previously treated with botulinum toxin (maximum: ≤50 units/site). Initial dose in previously untreated patients should be lower. Sequential dosing should be based on the patient's head and neck position, localization of pain, muscle hypertrophy, patient response, and previous adverse reactions. The total dose injected into the sternocleidomastoid muscles should be ≤100 units to decrease the occurrence of dysphagia.

Canadian labeling (not in U.S. labeling): Botox®: Children ≥16 years and Adults: I.M.: Effective range of 200-360 units has been used in clinical practice; administer no more frequently than every 2 months

Chronic migraine: Adults: I.M.: Administer 5 units/0.1 mL per site. Recommended total dose is 155 units once every 12 weeks. Each 155 unit dose should be equally divided and administered bilaterally, into 31 total sites as described below (refer to prescribing information for specific diagrams of recommended injection sites):

Corrugator: 5 units to each side (2 sites)

Procerus: 5 units (1 site only)

Frontalis: 10 units to each side (divided into 2 sites/side)

Temporalis: 20 units to each side (divided into 4 sites/side)

Occipitalis: 15 units to each side (divided into 3 sites/side)

Cervical paraspinal: 10 units to each side (divided into 2 sites/side)

Trapezius: 15 units to each side (divided into 3 sites/side)

Strabismus: Children ≥12 years and Adults: I.M.: **Note:** Several minutes prior to injection, administration of local anesthetic and ocular decongestant drops are recommended.

Initial dose:

Vertical muscles and for horizontal strabismus <20 prism diopters: 1.25-2.5 units in any one muscle

Horizontal strabismus of 20-50 prism diopters: 2.5-5 units in any one muscle

Persistent VI nerve palsy ≥1 month: 1.25-2.5 units in the medial rectus muscle

Re-examine patients 7-14 days after each injection to assess the effect of that dose. Subsequent doses for patients experiencing incomplete paralysis of the target may be increased up to twice the previous administered dose. The maximum recommended dose as a single injection for any one muscle is 25 units. Do not administer subsequent injections until the effects of the previous dose are gone.

Primary axillary hyperhidrosis: Adults ≥18 years: Intradermal: 50 units/axilla. Injection area should be defined by standard staining techniques. Injections should be evenly distributed into multiple sites (10-15), administered in 0.1-0.2 mL aliquots, ~1-2 cm apart. May repeat when clinical effect diminishes.

Spasticity (cerebral palsy related [dynamic equinus foot deformity]: Canadian labeling [not approved in U.S. labeling]): Children ≥2 years: I.M.: 4 units/kg (total dose) divided into two injections into medial and lateral heads of the gastrocnemius of affected leg; if clinically indicated, may repeat every 2 months (maximum dose: 200 units); in diplegia, the recommended dose is 6 units/kg (total dose) divided between affected limbs

Spasticity (focal): Adults ≥18 years: I.M.: Individualize dose based on patient size, extent, and location of muscle involvement, degree of spasticity, local muscle weakness, and response to prior treatment. In clinical trials, total doses up to 360 units (Botox®) were administered as separate injections typically divided among selected muscles; may repeat therapy at ≥3 months with appropriate dosage based upon the clinical condition of patient at time of retreatment.

Suggested guidelines for the treatment of upper limb spasticity. The lowest recommended starting dose should be used and ≤50 units/site should be administered. **Note:** Dose listed is total dose administered as individual or separate intramuscular injection(s):

Biceps brachii: 100-200 units (divided into 4 sites)
Flexor digitorum profundus: 30-50 units (1 site)
Flexor digitorum sublimes: 30-50 units (1 site)
Flexor carpi radialis: 12.5-50 units (1 site)
Flexor carpi ulnaris: 12.5-50 units (1 site)

Suggested guidelines for the treatment of stroke-related upper limb spasticity: Canadian labeling: **Note:** Dose listed is total dose administered as individual or separate intramuscular injection(s):

Biceps brachii: 100-200 units (up to 4 sites)
Flexor digitorum profundus: 15-50 units (1-2 sites)
Flexor digitorum sublimes: 15-50 units (1-2 sites)
Flexor carpi radialis: 15-60 units (1-2 sites)
Flexor carpi ulnaris: 10-50 units (1-2 sites)
Adductor pollicis: 20 units (1-2 sites)
Flexor pollicis longus: 20 units (1-2 sites)

Cosmetic uses:

Reduction of glabellar lines: Adults ≤65 years: I.M.: An effective dose is determined by gross observation of the patient's ability to activate the superficial muscles injected. The location, size and use of muscles may vary markedly among individuals. Inject 0.1 mL (4 units) dose into each of five sites, two in each corrugator muscle and one in the procerus muscle for a total dose 0.5 mL (20 units) administered no more frequently than every 3-4 months. **Note:** Treatment of adults >65 years is approved in the Canadian labeling.

Reduction of forehead lines (Canadian labeling; not in U.S. labeling): Adults: I.M.: Inject 2-6 units into each of four sites in the frontalis muscle every 1-2 cm along either side of forehead crease and 2-3 cm above eyebrows for total dose of 24 units.

Reduction of lateral canthus lines (Canadian labeling; not in U.S. labeling): Adults: I.M.: Inject 2-6 units into each of 1-3 injection sites, lateral to the lateral orbital rim.

Elderly: No specific adjustment recommended; initiate therapy at lowest recommended dose

Dosage adjustment in renal impairment: No dosage adjustment provided in manufacturer's labeling.

Dosage adjustment in hepatic impairment: No dosage adjustment provided in manufacturer's labeling.

Additional Information Complete prescribing information should be consulted for additional detail.

Dosage Forms Excipient information presented when available (limited, particularly for generics); consult specific product labeling.

Solution Reconstituted, Injection:
Botox: 100 units (1 ea)
Solution Reconstituted, Injection [preservative free]:
Botox: 200 units (1 ea)
Solution Reconstituted, Intramuscular:
Botox Cosmetic: 100 units (1 ea) [contains albumin human]
Solution Reconstituted, Intramuscular [preservative free]:
Botox Cosmetic: 50 units (1 ea) [contains albumin human]

Dosage Forms: Canada Excipient information presented when available (limited, particularly for generics); consult specific product labeling.

Injection, powder for reconstitution [preservative free]:
Botox: Botulinum toxin A 50 units [contains albumin (human)], 100 units [contains albumin (human)], 200 units [contains albumin (human)]
Botox Cosmetic: Botulinum toxin A 50 units [contains albumin (human)], 100 units [contains albumin (human)], 200 units [contains albumin (human)]

◆ **Onbrez® Breezhaler® (Can)** *see* Indacaterol *on page 1065*
◆ **Oncaspar** *see* Pegaspargase *on page 1586*
◆ **Oncotice™ (Can)** *see* BCG *on page 226*
◆ **Oncovin** *see* VinCRIStine *on page 2191*

Ondansetron (on DAN se tron)

Brand Names: U.S. Zofran; Zofran ODT; Zuplenz

Brand Names: Canada Apo-Ondansetron®; CO Ondansetron; Dom-Ondansetron; JAMP-Ondansetron; Mint-Ondansetron; Mylan-Ondansetron; Ondansetron Injection; Ondansetron Injection USP; Ondansetron-Odan; Ondansetron-Omega; PHL-Ondansetron; PMS-Ondansetron; RAN™-Ondansetron; ratio-Ondansetron; Sandoz-Ondansetron; Teva-Ondansetron; Zofran®; Zofran® ODT; ZYM-Ondansetron

Index Terms GR38032R; Ondansetron Hydrochloride; Zuplenz®

Pharmacologic Category Antiemetic; Selective 5-HT_3 Receptor Antagonist

Use

I.V.: Prevention of nausea and vomiting associated with initial and repeat courses of emetogenic cancer chemotherapy (including high-dose cisplatin); prevention of postoperative nausea and/or vomiting (PONV); treatment of PONV if no prophylactic dose of ondansetron received

Oral: Prevention of nausea and vomiting associated with highly emetogenic cancer chemotherapy (including high-dose cisplatin); prevention of nausea and vomiting associated with initial and repeat courses of moderately emetogenic cancer chemotherapy; prevention of nausea and vomiting associated with radiotherapy (either total body irradiation, single high-dose fraction to the abdomen, or daily fractions to the abdomen); prevention of PONV

Unlabeled Use Hyperemesis gravidarum (severe or refractory); breakthrough treatment of nausea and vomiting associated with chemotherapy

Pregnancy Risk Factor B

Pregnancy Considerations Teratogenic effects were not observed in animal reproduction studies. Ondansetron readily crosses the human placenta in the first trimester of pregnancy and can be detected in fetal tissue (Siu, 2006). The use of ondansetron for the treatment of nausea and vomiting of pregnancy (NVP) has been evaluated. Although a significant increase in birth defects has not been described in case reports and some studies (Ferreira, 2012; Pasternak, 2013), other studies have shown a possible association with ondansetron exposure and adverse fetal events (Anderka, 2012; Einarson, 2004). Additional studies are needed to determine safety to the fetus, particularly during the first trimester. Based on available data, use is generally reserved for severe NVP (hyperemesis gravidarum) or when conventional treatments are not effective (ACOG, 2004; Koren, 2012; Levicheck, 2002; Tan, 2011). Because a dose-dependent QT-interval prolongation occurs with use, the manufacturer recommends ECG monitoring in patients with electrolyte abnormalities (which can be associated with some cases of NVP; Koren, 2012).

Breast-Feeding Considerations It is not known if ondansetron is excreted into breast milk. The manufacturer recommends caution be used if administered to nursing women.

Contraindications Hypersensitivity to ondansetron or any component of the formulation; concomitant use of apomorphine

Warnings/Precautions Ondansetron should be used on a scheduled basis, not on an "as needed" (PRN) basis, since data support the use of this drug only in the prevention of nausea and vomiting (due to antineoplastic therapy) and not in the rescue of nausea and vomiting. Ondansetron should only be used in the first 24-48 hours of chemotherapy. Data do not support any increased efficacy of ondansetron in delayed nausea and vomiting. Does not stimulate gastric or intestinal peristalsis; may mask progressive ileus and/or gastric distension. Use with caution in patients allergic to other 5-HT_3 receptor antagonists; cross-reactivity has been reported.

Dose-dependent QT interval prolongation occurs with ondansetron use. Cases of torsade de pointes have also been reported to the manufacturer. Selective 5-HT_3 antagonists, including ondansetron, have been associated with a number of dose-dependent increases in ECG intervals (eg, PR, QRS duration, QT/QT_c, JT), usually occurring 1-2 hours after I.V. administration. Single doses >16 mg ondansetron I.V. are no longer recommended due to the potential for an increased risk of QT prolongation. In most patients, these changes are not clinically relevant; however, when used in conjunction with other agents that prolong these intervals or in those at risk for QT prolongation, arrhythmia may occur. When used with agents that prolong the QT interval (eg, Class I and III antiarrhythmics) or in patients with cardiovascular disease, clinically relevant QT interval prolongation may occur resulting in torsade de pointes. Avoid ondansetron use in patients with congenital long QT syndrome. Use caution and monitor ECG in patients with other risk factors for QT prolongation (eg, medications known to prolong QT interval, electrolyte abnormalities [hypokalemia or hypomagnesemia], heart failure, bradyarrhythmias, and cumulative high-dose anthracycline therapy). I.V. formulations of 5-HT_3 antagonists have more association with ECG interval changes, compared to oral formulations. Dose limitations are recommended for patients with severe hepatic impairment (Child-Pugh class C); use with caution in mild-moderate hepatic impairment; clearance is decreased and half-life increased in hepatic impairment.

Orally-disintegrating tablets contain phenylalanine.

Adverse Reactions Note: Percentages reported in adult patients.

>10%:

- Central nervous system: Headache (9% to 27%), malaise/fatigue (9% to 13%)
- Gastrointestinal: Constipation (6% to 11%)

1% to 10%:

- Central nervous system: Drowsiness (8%), fever (2% to 8%), dizziness (7%), anxiety (6%), cold sensation (2%)
- Dermatologic: Pruritus (2% to 5%), rash (1%)
- Gastrointestinal: Diarrhea (2% to 7%)
- Genitourinary: Gynecological disorder (7%), urinary retention (5%)
- Hepatic: ALT increased (>2 times ULN: 1% to 5%), AST increased (>2 times ULN: 1% to 5%)
- Local: Injection site reaction (4%; pain, redness, burning)
- Neuromuscular & skeletal: Paresthesia (2%)
- Respiratory: Hypoxia (9%)

<1% (Limited to important or life-threatening): Abnormal hepatic function, anaphylactoid reactions, anaphylaxis, angina, angioedema, arrhythmia, atrial fibrillation, AV block, blindness (transient/following infusion; lasting ≤48 hours), blurred vision (transient/following infusion), bradycardia, cardiopulmonary arrest, dystonic reaction, electrocardiographic alterations (second-degree heart block and ST-segment depression), extrapyramidal symptoms, hepatic failure, hepatic necrosis, hepatitis, hypersensitivity reaction, hypokalemia, hypotension, oculogyric crisis, premature ventricular contractions (PVC), QT interval increased, seizure, shock, supraventricular tachycardia, syncope, tachycardia, torsade de pointes, vascular occlusive events, ventricular arrhythmia, ventricular fibrillation, ventricular tachycardia

Drug Interactions

Metabolism/Transport Effects Substrate of CYP1A2 (minor), CYP2C9 (minor), CYP2D6 (minor), CYP2E1 (minor), CYP3A4 (major), P-glycoprotein; **Note:** Assignment of Major/Minor substrate status based on clinically relevant drug interaction potential; **Inhibits** CYP1A2 (weak), CYP2C9 (weak), CYP2D6 (weak)

Avoid Concomitant Use

Avoid concomitant use of Ondansetron with any of the following: Apomorphine; Highest Risk QTc-Prolonging Agents; Ivabradine; Mifepristone

Increased Effect/Toxicity

Ondansetron may increase the levels/effects of: Apomorphine; ARIPiprazole; Highest Risk QTc-Prolonging Agents; Moderate Risk QTc-Prolonging Agents

The levels/effects of Ondansetron may be increased by: Ivabradine; Mifepristone; P-glycoprotein/ABCB1 Inhibitors; QTc-Prolonging Agents (Indeterminate Risk and Risk Modifying)

Decreased Effect

Ondansetron may decrease the levels/effects of: Tapentadol; TraMADol

The levels/effects of Ondansetron may be decreased by: Bosentan; CYP3A4 Inducers (Strong); Dabrafenib; Deferasirox; Herbs (CYP3A4 Inducers); Mitotane; Peginterferon Alfa-2b; P-glycoprotein/ABCB1 Inducers; Rifamycin Derivatives; Tocilizumab

Ethanol/Nutrition/Herb Interactions

Food: Tablet: Food slightly increases the extent of absorption.

Herb/Nutraceutical: St John's wort may decrease ondansetron levels.

Preparation for Administration Prior to I.V. infusion, dilute in 50 mL D_5W or NS.

Storage/Stability

Oral soluble film: Store between 20°C and 25°C (68°F and 77°F). Store pouches in cartons; keep film in individual pouch until ready to use.

Oral solution: Store between 15°C and 30°C (59°F and 86°F). Protect from light.

Tablet: Store between 2°C and 30°C (36°F and 86°F).

Vial: Store between 2°C and 30°C (36°F and 86°F). Protect from light. Stable when mixed in D_5W or NS for 48 hours at room temperature.

Mechanism of Action Selective 5-HT_3-receptor antagonist, blocking serotonin, both peripherally on vagal nerve terminals and centrally in the chemoreceptor trigger zone

Pharmacodynamics/Kinetics

Onset of action: ~30 minutes

Absorption: Oral: Well absorbed from GI tract

Distribution: V_d: Children: 1.7-3.7 L/kg; Adults: 2.2-2.5 L/kg

Protein binding, plasma: 70% to 76%

Metabolism: Extensively hepatic via hydroxylation, followed by glucuronide or sulfate conjugation; CYP1A2, CYP2D6, and CYP3A4 substrate; some demethylation occurs

Bioavailability: Oral: 56% to 71% (some first pass metabolism); Rectal: 58% to 74%

Half-life elimination: Children <15 years: 2-7 hours; Adults: 3-6 hours

- Mild-to-moderate hepatic impairment (Child-Pugh classes A and B): Adults: 12 hours
- Severe hepatic impairment (Child-Pugh class C): Adults: 20 hours

Time to peak: Oral: ~2 hours; Oral soluble film: ~1 hour

Excretion: Urine (44% to 60% as metabolites, ~5% as unchanged drug); feces (~25%)

Dosage

Children:

I.V.:

Prevention of nausea and vomiting associated with emetogenic chemotherapy: 6 months to 18 years: 0.15 mg/kg/dose (maximum: 16 mg/dose) over 15 minutes for 3 doses, beginning with the first dose administered 30 minutes prior to chemotherapy, followed by subsequent doses administered 4 and 8 hours after the first dose

Prevention of postoperative nausea and vomiting: 1 month to 12 years:

≤40 kg: 0.1 mg/kg as a single dose over 2-5 minutes

>40 kg: 4 mg as a single dose over 2-5 minutes

Oral: Prevention of nausea and vomiting associated with moderately-emetogenic chemotherapy:

4-11 years: 4 mg 30 minutes before chemotherapy; repeat 4 and 8 hours after initial dose, then 4 mg every 8 hours for 1-2 days after chemotherapy completed

≥12 years: Refer to adult dosing.

Adults:

I.V.:

Prevention of nausea and vomiting associated with emetogenic chemotherapy:

Manufacturer's labeling: 0.15 mg/kg/dose (maximum: 16 mg/dose) over 15 minutes for 3 doses, beginning with the first dose administered 30 minutes prior to chemotherapy, followed by subsequent doses administered 4 and 8 hours after the first dose

American Society of Clinical Oncology Antiemetic Guideline recommendations (Basch, 2011): High emetic risk: Day(s) chemotherapy is administered: 8 mg or 0.15 mg/kg. **Note:** Single I.V. doses >16 mg are no longer recommended by the manufacturer due to the potential for QT prolongation.

Prevention of nausea and vomiting associated with radiation therapy (unlabeled route/dosing): American Society of Clinical Oncology Antiemetic Guideline recommendations (Basch, 2011): 8 mg or 0.15 mg/kg. Give before each fraction throughout radiation therapy for high emetic risk (continue for at least 24 hours after completion) and for moderate emetic risk; for low emetic risk, may give either as prevention or rescue; for minimal emetic risk, give as rescue (if rescue used for either low or minimal emetic risk, then prophylaxis should be given until the end of radiation therapy).

Note: Single I.V. doses >16 mg are no longer recommended by the manufacturer due to the potential for QT prolongation.

Treatment of severe or refractory hyperemesis gravidum (unlabeled use): 8 mg administered over 15 minutes every 12 hours (ACOG, 2004)

I.M., I.V.: Postoperative nausea and vomiting (PONV): 4 mg as a single dose (over 2-5 minutes if giving I.V.) administered ~30 minutes before the end of anesthesia (see **"Note"** below) or as treatment if vomiting occurs after surgery (Gan, 2007).

Note: The manufacturer recommends administration immediately before induction of anesthesia; however, this has been shown not to be as effective as administration at the end of surgery (Sun, 1997). Repeat doses given in response to inadequate control of nausea/vomiting from preoperative doses are generally ineffective.

Oral:

Prevention of nausea and vomiting associated with emetogenic chemotherapy:

Highly-emetogenic agents/single-day therapy:

Manufacturer's labeling: 24 mg given as three 8 mg tablets 30 minutes prior to the start of therapy

American Society of Clinical Oncology Antiemetic Guideline recommendations (Basch, 2011): High emetic risk: Day(s) chemotherapy is administered: 8 mg twice daily

Moderately-emetogenic agents: 8 mg beginning 30 minutes before chemotherapy; repeat dose 8 hours after initial dose, then 8 mg every 12 hours for 1-2 days after chemotherapy completed

Prevention of nausea and vomiting associated with radiation therapy:

Manufacturer's labeling:

Total body irradiation: 8 mg 1-2 hours before each daily fraction of radiotherapy

Single high-dose fraction radiotherapy to abdomen: 8 mg 1-2 hours before irradiation, then 8 mg every 8 hours after first dose for 1-2 days after completion of radiotherapy

Daily fractionated radiotherapy to abdomen: 8 mg 1-2 hours before irradiation, then 8 mg every 8 hours after first dose for each day of radiotherapy

American Society of Clinical Oncology Antiemetic Guideline recommendations (Basch, 2011): 8 mg twice daily. Give before each fraction throughout radiation therapy for high emetic risk (continue for at least 24 hours after completion) and for moderate emetic risk; for low emetic risk, may give either as prevention or rescue; for minimal emetic risk, give as rescue (if rescue used for either low or minimal emetic risk, then prophylaxis should be given until the end of radiation therapy).

Postoperative nausea and vomiting: 16 mg given 1 hour prior to induction of anesthesia

Treatment of severe or refractory hyperemesis gravidum (unlabeled use): 8 mg every 12 hours (Levichek, 2002)

Elderly: No dosing adjustment required

Dosage adjustment in renal impairment: No dosage adjustment necessary (there is no experience for oral ondansetron beyond day 1)

Dosage adjustment in hepatic impairment: Severe liver impairment (Child-Pugh C):

I.V.: Day 1: Maximum dose: 8 mg (there is no experience beyond day 1)

Oral: Maximum daily dose: 8 mg

Dietary Considerations Take without regard to meals. Some products may contain phenylalanine.

Administration

Oral: Oral dosage forms should be administered 30 minutes prior to chemotherapy; 1-2 hours before radiotherapy; 1 hour prior to the induction of anesthesia

Orally-disintegrating tablets: Do not remove from blister until needed. Peel backing off the blister, do not push tablet through. Using dry hands, place tablet on tongue and allow to dissolve. Swallow with saliva.

Oral soluble film: Do not remove from pouch until immediately before use. Using dry hands, place film on top of tongue and allow to dissolve (4-20 seconds). Swallow with or without liquid. If using more than one film, each film should be allowed to dissolve completely before administering the next film.

I.M.: Should be administered undiluted.

I.V.:

IVPB: Infuse diluted solution over 15-30 minutes; 24-hour continuous infusions have been reported, but are rarely used.

Chemotherapy-induced nausea and vomiting: Give first dose 30 minutes prior to beginning chemotherapy.

I.V. push: Prevention of postoperative nausea and vomiting: Single doses may be administered I.V. injection over 2-5 minutes as undiluted solution.

Monitoring Parameters ECG (if applicable in high risk patients); potassium, magnesium

Dosage Forms Excipient information presented when available (limited, particularly for generics); consult specific product labeling.

Film, Oral:

Zuplenz: 4 mg (1 ea, 10 ea); 8 mg (1 ea, 10 ea)

Solution, Injection:

Zofran: 40 mg/20 mL (20 mL) [contains methylparaben, propylparaben]

Generic: 4 mg/2 mL (2 mL); 40 mg/20 mL (20 mL)

Solution, Injection [preservative free]:

Generic: 4 mg/2 mL (2 mL)

Solution, Oral:

Zofran: 4 mg/5 mL (50 mL) [strawberry flavor]

Generic: 4 mg/5 mL (50 mL)

Tablet, Oral:

Zofran: 4 mg, 8 mg

Generic: 4 mg, 8 mg, 24 mg

Tablet Dispersible, Oral:

Zofran ODT: 4 mg, 8 mg [contains aspartame, methylparaben sodium, propylparaben sodium; strawberry flavor]

Generic: 4 mg, 8 mg

Extemporaneous Preparations Note: Commercial oral solution is available (0.8 mg/mL)

If commercial oral solution is unavailable, a 0.8 mg/mL syrup may be made with ondansetron tablets, Ora-Plus® (Paddock), and any of the the following syrups: Cherry syrup USP, Syrpalta® (HUMCO), Ora-Sweet® (Paddock), or Ora-Sweet® Sugar-Free (Paddock). Crush ten 8 mg tablets in a mortar and reduce to a fine powder (flaking of the tablet coating occurs). Add 50 mL Ora-Plus® in 5 mL increments, mixing thoroughly; mix while adding the chosen syrup in incremental proportions to **almost** 100 mL; transfer to a calibrated bottle, rinse mortar with syrup, and add sufficient quantity of syrup to make 100 mL. Label "shake well" and "refrigerate". Stable for 42 days refrigerated (Trissel, 1996).

Rectal suppositories: Calibrate a suppository mold for the base being used. Determine the displacement factor (DF) for ondansetron for the base being used (Fattibase® = 1.1; Polybase® = 0.6). Weigh the ondansetron tablet(s). Divide the tablet weight by the DF; this result is the weight of base displaced by the drug. Subtract the weight of base displaced from the calculated weight of base required for each suppository. Grind the ondansetron tablets in a mortar and reduce to a fine powder. Weigh out the appropriate weight of suppository base. Melt the base over a water bath (<55°C). Add the ondansetron powder to the suppository base and mix well. Pour the mixture into the suppository mold and cool. Stable for at least 30 days refrigerated (Tenjarla, 1998).

Tenjarla SN, Ward ES, and Fox JL, "Ondansetron Suppositories: Extemporaneous Preparation, Drug Release, Stability and Flux Through Rabbit Rectal Membrane," *Int J Pharm Compound*, 1998, 2(1):83-8.

Trissel LA, *Trissel's Stability of Compounded Formulations*, Washington, DC: American Pharmaceutical Association, 1996.

◆ **Ondansetron Hydrochloride** *see* Ondansetron *on page* 1510

◆ **Ondansetron Injection (Can)** *see* Ondansetron *on page* 1510

◆ **Ondansetron Injection USP (Can)** *see* Ondansetron *on page* 1510

◆ **Ondansetron-Odan (Can)** *see* Ondansetron *on page* 1510

◆ **Ondansetron-Omega (Can)** *see* Ondansetron *on page* 1510

◆ **OneTab™ Congestion & Cold [OTC]** *see* Guaifenesin and Phenylephrine *on page* 978

◆ **Onfi** *see* CloBAZam *on page* 455

◆ **Onglyza** *see* Saxagliptin *on page* 1879

◆ **Onglyza™ (Can)** *see* Saxagliptin *on page* 1879

◆ **Onmel** *see* Itraconazole *on page* 1132

◆ **Onsolis** *see* FentaNYL *on page* 842

◆ **Opana** *see* Oxymorphone *on page* 1540

◆ **Opana ER** *see* Oxymorphone *on page* 1540

◆ **OPC-13013** *see* Cilostazol *on page* 425

◆ **OPC-14597** *see* ARIPiprazole *on page* 163

◆ **OPC-41061** *see* Tolvaptan *on page* 2089

◆ **Opcon-A [OTC]** *see* Naphazoline and Pheniramine *on page* 1425

◆ **o,p'-DDD** *see* Mitotane *on page* 1385

◆ **Ophtho-Dipivefrin™ (Can)** *see* Dipivefrin *on page* 634

◆ **Ophtho-Tate® (Can)** *see* PrednisoLONE (Ophthalmic) *on page* 1706

◆ **Opium and Belladonna** *see* Belladonna and Opium *on page* 234

Opium Tincture (OH pee um TING chur)

Index Terms Deodorized Tincture of Opium (error-prone synonym); DTO (error-prone abbreviation); Opium Tincture, Deodorized; Tincture of Opium

Pharmacologic Category Analgesic, Opioid; Antidiarrheal

Use Treatment of diarrhea in adults

Pregnancy Risk Factor C

Pregnancy Considerations Animal reproduction studies have not been conducted. Opium tincture contains morphine; refer to the Morphine (Systemic) monograph for additional information. In addition, this preparation contains large amounts of alcohol (19%).

Breast-Feeding Considerations Opium tincture contains morphine, which is excreted into breast milk; refer to the Morphine (Systemic) monograph for additional information. In addition, this preparation contains large amounts of alcohol (19%). The manufacturer recommends that caution be used if administered to a nursing woman.

Contraindications Hypersensitivity to opium, morphine sulfate, or any component of the formulation; diarrhea caused by poisoning prior to the toxic material being removed from the GI tract

Note: Manufacturer does not recommend use in children.

Warnings/Precautions May cause CNS depression, which may impair physical or mental abilities; patients must be cautioned about performing tasks which require mental alertness (eg, operating machinery or driving). Effects may be potentiated when used with other sedative drugs or ethanol. Opium shares the toxic potential of opioid agonists, and usual precautions of opioid agonist therapy should be observed; use with caution in patients with morbid obesity, adrenal insufficiency, hepatic impairment, biliary tract impairment, pancreatitis, head trauma, GI hemorrhage, thyroid dysfunction, prostatic hyperplasia/urinary stricture, respiratory disease, or a history of drug abuse. Avoid use in patients with CNS depression or coma as these patients are susceptible to intracranial effects of CO_2 retention. May cause hypotension; use with caution in patients with hypovolemia, cardiovascular disease (including acute MI), or with drugs which may exaggerate hypotensive effects (including phenothiazines or general anesthetics). May obscure diagnosis or clinical course of patients with acute abdominal conditions. Concurrent use of agonist/antagonist analgesics may precipitate withdrawal symptoms and/or reduced analgesic efficacy in patients following prolonged therapy with mu opioid agonists. Abrupt discontinuation following prolonged use may also lead to withdrawal symptoms. Use with caution in the elderly and debilitated patients; may be more sensitive to adverse effects. Some preparations contain sulfites which may cause allergic reactions. Infants <3 months of age are more susceptible to respiratory depression; if used, diluted doses are recommended and use with caution. Manufacturer does not recommend use in children.

Do not confuse opium tincture with paregoric; opium tincture is 25 times more potent than paregoric; opium shares the toxic potential of opioid agonists, usual precautions of opioid agonist therapy should be observed; opium may mask dehydration by producing fluid retention in the bowel; monitor patients with prolonged or severe diarrhea carefully; abrupt discontinuation after prolonged use may result in withdrawal symptoms. Opium tincture is no longer recommended as a source of morphine to treat neonatal abstinence syndrome in infants exposed to chronic opioids *in utero*. In addition, use for this purpose may increase the risk of drug error and morphine overdose in the infant (Dow, 2012; Hudack, 2012).

Adverse Reactions Frequency not defined.

Cardiovascular: Palpitation, hypotension, bradycardia, peripheral vasodilation

Central nervous system: Drowsiness, dizziness, restlessness, headache, malaise, CNS depression, intracranial pressure increased, insomnia, mental depression

Gastrointestinal: Nausea, vomiting, constipation, anorexia, stomach cramps, biliary tract spasm

Genitourinary: Urination decreased, urinary tract spasm

Neuromuscular & skeletal: Weakness

Ocular: Miosis

Respiratory: Respiratory depression

Miscellaneous: Histamine release, physical and psychological dependence

Drug Interactions

Metabolism/Transport Effects None known.

Avoid Concomitant Use

Avoid concomitant use of Opium Tincture with any of the following: Azelastine (Nasal); Paraldehyde

Increased Effect/Toxicity

Opium Tincture may increase the levels/effects of: Alcohol (Ethyl); Alvimopan; Azelastine (Nasal); CNS Depressants; Desmopressin; Diuretics; Hydrocodone; Metyrosine; Mirtazapine; Paraldehyde; Pramipexole; ROPINIRole; Rotigotine; Selective Serotonin Reuptake Inhibitors; Zolpidem

The levels/effects of Opium Tincture may be increased by: Amphetamines; Anticholinergics; Antipsychotic Agents (Phenothiazines); Brimonidine (Topical); Cannabinoids; Doxylamine; Droperidol; HydrOXYzine; Magnesium Sulfate; Perampanel; Sodium Oxybate; Succinylcholine; Tapentadol

Decreased Effect

Opium Tincture may decrease the levels/effects of: Pegvisomant

The levels/effects of Opium Tincture may be decreased by: Ammonium Chloride; Mixed Agonist / Antagonist Opioids

Ethanol/Nutrition/Herb Interactions Ethanol: May increase CNS depression; monitor for increased effects with coadministration. Caution patients about effects.

Storage/Stability Store at 68° to 77°F (20° to 25°C). Protect from light.

Mechanism of Action Contains many opioid alkaloids including morphine; its mechanism for gastric motility inhibition is primarily due to this morphine content; it results in a decrease in digestive secretions, an increase in GI muscle tone, and therefore a reduction in GI propulsion

Pharmacodynamics/Kinetics

Duration: 4-5 hours

Absorption: Variable

Metabolism: Hepatic

Excretion: Urine

Dosage Oral: **Note:** Opium tincture contains morphine 10 mg/mL. Use caution in ordering, dispensing, and/or administering. The following doses are expressed in **mg** (milligram) dosing units of morphine.

Adults: Diarrhea: Usual: 6 **mg** of undiluted opium tincture (10 mg/mL) 4 times daily

Dosage adjustment in renal impairment: No dosage adjustment provided in manufacturer's labeling.

Dosage adjustment in hepatic impairment: No dosage adjustment provided in manufacturer's labeling; use with caution.

Administration May administer with food to decrease GI upset.

Monitoring Parameters Observe patient for excessive sedation, respiratory depression, implement safety measures, assist with ambulation

Test Interactions Increased aminotransferase [ALT/AST] (S)

Dosage Forms Excipient information presented when available (limited, particularly for generics); consult specific product labeling.

Tincture, Oral:

Generic: 10 mg/mL (1%) (118 mL, 473 mL)

Controlled Substance C-II

◆ **Opium Tincture, Deodorized** *see* Opium Tincture *on page 1513*

Oprelvekin (oh PREL ve kin)

Brand Names: U.S. Neumega

Index Terms IL-11; Interleukin-11; Recombinant Human Interleukin-11; Recombinant Interleukin-11; rhIL-11

Pharmacologic Category Biological Response Modulator; Human Growth Factor

Use Prevention of severe thrombocytopenia; reduce the need for platelet transfusions following myelosuppressive chemotherapy for nonmyeloid malignancy

Pregnancy Risk Factor C

Pregnancy Considerations Animal studies have demonstrated adverse fetal effects. There are no adequate and well-controlled studies in pregnant women. Use during pregnancy only if the potential benefits outweigh the potential risk to the fetus.

Breast-Feeding Considerations Due to the potential for serious adverse reactions in the nursing infant, breastfeeding is not recommended.

Contraindications Hypersensitivity to oprelvekin or any component of the formulation

Warnings/Precautions [U.S. Boxed Warning]: Allergic or hypersensitivity reactions, including anaphylaxis have been reported. Permanently discontinue in any patient developing an allergic or hypersensitivity reaction. May occur with the first or with subsequent doses. May cause serious fluid retention (reversible) which may result in peripheral edema, capillary leak syndrome, arrhythmias, or exacerbation of pleural effusion. Use cautiously in patients with conditions where expansion of plasma volume should be avoided (eg, left ventricular dysfunction, HF, hypertension). Monitor fluid balance. Closely monitor fluid and electrolytes in patient on chronic diuretic therapy; severe hypokalemia contributing to sudden death have been reported in these patients. Reversible dilutional anemia may occur due to increased plasma volume; generally appears within 3-5 days of initiation of therapy and resolves over ~1 week following discontinuation. Atrial arrhythmias, pulmonary edema, and cardiac arrest have been reported; use in patients with a history of atrial arrhythmia only if the potential benefit exceeds possible risks. Patients experiencing arrhythmia may be at risk for stroke; use caution in patients with a history of transient ischemic attack or stroke. Ventricular arrhythmia has also been reported, occurring within 2-7 days of treatment initiation. Use caution in patients with conduction defects; history of thromboembolic problems; pre-existing pericardial effusions or ascites. May cause exacerbation of effusion; consider drainage if indicated. Use with caution in renal dysfunction; dosage adjustment required in severe renal impairment; monitor fluid balance.

Not indicated following myeloablative chemotherapy; increased toxicities were reported when used following myeloablative therapy. A higher incidence of adverse events has been reported when used following bone marrow transplantation. Begin 6-24 hours following completion of chemotherapy; use has not been adequately studied immediately before or during chemotherapy. Efficacy has not been established with chemotherapy regimens >5 days duration or with regimens associated with delayed myelosuppression (eg, nitrosoureas, mitomycin). Safety and efficacy have not been established with chronic administration. Papilledema, more frequently associated with use in children, has occurred (usually following repeated cycles); use caution in patients with pre-existing papilledema or with tumors involving the central nervous system; may worsen pre-existing papilledema. Papilledema is dose limiting. Patients experiencing oprelvekin-related papilledema may be at risk for visual acuity changes, including blurred vision or blindness. Although used in children in clinical trials, safety and efficacy have not been established in pediatric patients. The incidence of certain adverse events may be higher in children. Use in children, especially <12 years of age, should be as part of a clinical trial.

Adverse Reactions

>10%:

Cardiovascular: Tachycardia (children 84%; adults 20%), edema (59%), cardiomegaly (children 21%), vasodilation (19%), atrial arrhythmia (12% to 15%), palpitation (14%), syncope (13%)

Central nervous system: Neutropenic fever (48%), headache (41%), dizziness (38%), fever (36%), insomnia (33%)

Dermatologic: Rash (25%)

Endocrine & metabolic: Fluid retention

Gastrointestinal: Nausea/vomiting (77%), diarrhea (43%), mucositis (43%), oral moniliasis (14%), weight gain (due to fluid retention)

Hematologic: Anemia (dilutional; onset: 3-5 days; duration: ≤1 week)

Neuromuscular & skeletal: Weakness (severe 14%), periostitis (children 11%), arthralgia

Ocular: Conjunctival injection/redness/swelling (children 57%; adults 19%), papilledema (children 16%; adults 1%)

Respiratory: Dyspnea (48%), rhinitis (42%), cough (29%), pharyngitis (25%)

1% to 10%: Respiratory: Pleural effusion (10%)

<1% (Limited to important or life-threatening): Allergic reaction, amblyopia, anaphylaxis/anaphylactoid reactions, blindness, blurred vision, capillary leak syndrome, cardiac arrest, chest pain, dehydration, dysarthria, exfoliative dermatitis, eye hemorrhage, facial edema, fibrinogen increased, fluid overload, HF, hypoalbuminemia, hypocalcemia, hypokalemia, hypotension, injection site reactions (dermatitis, pain, discoloration), loss of consciousness, mental status changes, optic neuropathy, paresthesia, pericardial effusion, peripheral edema, pneumonia, pulmonary edema, renal failure, shock, skin discoloration, stroke, urticaria, ventricular arrhythmia, visual acuity changes, visual field defect, von Willebrand factor concentration increased, wheezing

Drug Interactions

Metabolism/Transport Effects None known.

Avoid Concomitant Use There are no known interactions where it is recommended to avoid concomitant use.

Increased Effect/Toxicity There are no known significant interactions involving an increase in effect.

Decreased Effect There are no known significant interactions involving a decrease in effect.

Preparation for Administration Reconstitute to a final concentration of 5 mg/mL with SWFI; direct diluent down side of vial, swirl gently, do not shake.

Storage/Stability Store vials under refrigeration between 2°C to 8°C (36°F to 46°F); do not freeze. Protect from light. Use reconstituted oprelvekin within 3 hours of reconstitution; store reconstituted solution in the vial at either 2°C to 8°C (36°F to 46°F) or room temperature of ≤25°C (77°F). Do not freeze or shake reconstituted solution.

Mechanism of Action Oprelvekin is a thrombopoietic growth factor which stimulates multiple stages of megakaryocytopoiesis and thrombopoiesis, resulting in proliferation of megakaryocyte progenitors and megakaryocyte maturation, thereby increasing platelet production.

Pharmacodynamics/Kinetics

Bioavailability: >80%

Half-life elimination: Terminal: 5-9 hours

Time to peak, serum: 1-6 hours

Excretion: Urine (primarily as metabolites)

Dosage SubQ: Administer first dose ~6-24 hours after the end of chemotherapy. Discontinue at least 48 hours before beginning the next cycle of chemotherapy.

Adults: 50 mcg/kg once daily for ~10-21 days (until postnadir platelet count ≥50,000/mm^3)

Dosage adjustment in renal impairment:

Cl_{cr} ≥30 mL/minute: No dosage adjustment necessary.

Cl_{cr} <30 mL/minute: 25 mcg/kg once daily for ~10-21 days (until postnadir platelet count ≥50,000/mm^3)

Dosage adjustment in hepatic impairment: No dosage adjustment provided in manufacturer's labeling.

Administration Subcutaneously in the abdomen, thigh, hip, or upper arm.

Monitoring Parameters Monitor electrolytes and fluid balance during therapy; obtain a CBC at regular intervals during therapy; monitor platelet counts until adequate recovery has occurred; renal function (at baseline)

Dosage Forms Excipient information presented when available (limited, particularly for generics); consult specific product labeling.

Solution Reconstituted, Subcutaneous [preservative free]:
Neumega: 5 mg (1 ea)

◆ **OPT-80** *see* Fidaxomicin *on page* 859

◆ **Opticrom® (Can)** *see* Cromolyn (Ophthalmic) *on page* 501

◆ **Optics Eye Wash [OTC]** *see* Sodium Chloride *on page* 1914

◆ **Optimyxin® (Can)** *see* Bacitracin and Polymyxin B *on page* 220

◆ **Optimyxin Plus® (Can)** *see* Neomycin, Polymyxin B, and Gramicidin *on page* 1440

◆ **Optipranolol** *see* Metipranolol *on page* 1345

◆ **OptiPranolol® (Can)** *see* Metipranolol *on page* 1345

◆ **Optivar** *see* Azelastine (Ophthalmic) *on page* 211

◆ **Oracea** *see* Doxycycline *on page* 668

◆ **Oracit®** *see* Sodium Citrate and Citric Acid *on page* 1917

◆ **Oracort (Can)** *see* Triamcinolone (Topical) *on page* 2123

◆ **Ora-film [OTC]** *see* Benzocaine *on page* 240

◆ **Oralone** *see* Triamcinolone (Topical) *on page* 2123

◆ **Oral Pain Relief Max St [OTC]** *see* Benzocaine *on page* 240

- Oral Purgative (Can) *see* Sodium Picosulfate, Magnesium Oxide, and Citric Acid *on page 1925*
- Orap *see* Pimozide *on page 1648*
- Orap® (Can) *see* Pimozide *on page 1648*
- Orapred *see* PrednisoLONE (Systemic) *on page 1704*
- Orapred ODT *see* PrednisoLONE (Systemic) *on page 1704*
- Oraqix® *see* Lidocaine and Prilocaine *on page 1213*
- Ora-Sweet SF [OTC] *see* Sorbitol *on page 1942*
- OraVerse *see* Phentolamine *on page 1634*
- Oraxyl [DSC] *see* Doxycycline *on page 668*
- Orazinc [OTC] *see* Zinc Sulfate *on page 2230*
- Orbivan [DSC] *see* Butalbital, Acetaminophen, and Caffeine *on page 305*
- Orciprenaline Sulfate *see* Metaproterenol *on page 1309*
- Orencia *see* Abatacept *on page 20*
- Orenitram *see* Treprostinil *on page 2115*
- Orfadin *see* Nitisinone *on page 1464*
- ORG 9426 *see* Rocuronium *on page 1846*
- Orgalutran® (Can) *see* Ganirelix *on page 940*
- Organ-I NR [OTC] *see* GuaiFENesin *on page 974*
- ORG NC 45 *see* Vecuronium *on page 2174*
- Orinase *see* TOLBUTamide *on page 2085*

Orlistat (OR li stat)

Brand Names: U.S. Alli [OTC]; Xenical

Brand Names: Canada Xenical

Pharmacologic Category Lipase Inhibitor

Use Management of obesity, including weight loss and weight management, when used in conjunction with a reduced-calorie and low-fat diet; reduce the risk of weight regain after prior weight loss; indicated for obese patients with an initial body mass index (BMI) ≥30 kg/m^2 or ≥27 kg/m^2 in the presence of other risk factors (eg, diabetes, dyslipidemia, hypertension)

Pregnancy Risk Factor X

Pregnancy Considerations Adverse events were not observed in animal reproduction studies. Although orlistat is minimally absorbed, weight-loss therapy is not recommended for pregnant women. Obese and overweight women should be encouraged to participate in weight reduction programs prior to attempting pregnancy; weight gain during pregnancy should be determined by their prepregnancy BMI and current guidelines (ADA, 2009; IOM, 2009). Use of orlistat is contraindicated in pregnant women.

Breast-Feeding Considerations Weight-loss therapy is generally not recommended for lactating women. Weight-loss programs which include physical activity and nutrition components should be discussed at the 6-week postpartum visit (ADA, 2009; IOM, 2009).

Contraindications Hypersensitivity to orlistat or any component of the formulation; chronic malabsorption syndrome or cholestasis; pregnancy

Warnings/Precautions Prior to use other causes for obesity (eg, hypothyroidism) should be ruled out. Cases of severe liver injury (some fatal) with hepatocellular necrosis or acute hepatic failure have been reported (rare); liver transplantation has been required in some patients. Patients should be instructed to report any symptoms of hepatic dysfunction (eg, anorexia, pruritus, jaundice, dark urine, light colored stools, right upper quadrant pain); discontinue orlistat and obtain liver function test immediately if symptoms occur. Advise patients to adhere to dietary guidelines; if taken with a diet high in fat (>30% total daily calories from fat) gastrointestinal adverse events may increase. Distribute daily fat intake over 3 main meals. If taken with any 1 meal very high in fat, the possibility of gastrointestinal effects increases. Counsel patients to take a multivitamin supplement that contains fat-soluble vitamins ≥2 hours before or after orlistat administration to ensure adequate nutrition; orlistat has been shown to reduce the absorption of some fat-soluble vitamins and beta-carotene. Increased levels of urinary oxalate following treatment may occur in some patients; monitor renal function in patients at risk for renal failure; use with caution in patients with a history of hyperoxaluria or calcium oxalate nephrolithiasis. Orlistat may decrease cyclosporine plasma concentrations; administer cyclosporine ≥3 hours before or after orlistat and monitor frequently. The potential exists for misuse in inappropriate patient populations (eg, patients with anorexia nervosa or bulimia) similar to any weight loss agent. In general, substantial weight loss may increase the risk of cholelithiasis.

Self-medication (OTC use): Prior to use, patients should contact their healthcare provider if they have ever had kidney stones, gall bladder disease, or pancreatitis. Patients taking medications for diabetes or thyroid disease, anticoagulants, or other weight-loss products should consult their healthcare provider or pharmacist. Patients who have had an organ transplant should not use orlistat. If severe and/or continuous abdominal pain, itching, yellowing of the eyes or skin, dark urine, or loss of appetite occurs, use should be discontinued and healthcare provider consulted.

Adverse Reactions Note: The frequency of most adverse reactions (especially gastrointestinal effects) decreases over time.

>10%:

Central nervous system: Headache (≤31%)

Gastrointestinal: Oily spotting (4% to 27%), abdominal pain/discomfort (≤26%), flatus with discharge (2% to 24%), fecal urgency (3% to 22%), fatty/oily stool (6% to 20%), oily evacuation (2% to 12%), defecation increased (3% to 11%)

Neuromuscular & skeletal: Back pain (≤14%)

Respiratory: Upper respiratory infection (26% to 38%)

Miscellaneous: Influenza (≤40%)

1% to 10%:

Cardiovascular: Pedal edema (≤3%)

Central nervous system: Fatigue (3% to 7%), anxiety (3% to 5%), sleep disorder (≤4%)

Dermatologic: Dry skin (≤2%)

Endocrine & metabolic: Menstrual irregularities (≤10%)

Gastrointestinal: Nausea (4% to 8%), fecal incontinence (2% to 8%), infectious diarrhea (≤5%), rectal pain/discomfort (3% to 5%), tooth disorder (3% to 4%), gingival disorder (2% to 4%)

Genitourinary: Urinary tract infection (6% to 8%), vaginitis (3% to 4%)

Neuromuscular & skeletal: Myalgia (≤4%)

Otic: Otitis (3% to 4%)

Respiratory: Lower respiratory infection (≤8%)

<1% (Limited to important or life-threatening): Abdominal distension (in patients with diabetes), alkaline phosphatase increased, anaphylaxis, angioedema, bronchospasm, bullous eruption, cholelithiasis (may be caused by weight loss), coagulation parameters altered (concurrent use with warfarin), hepatic failure, hepatitis, hypersensitivity, hypoglycemia (in patients with diabetes), hypothyroidism (concurrent use with levothyroxine), kidney injury (acute), pancreatitis, pruritus, rash, transaminases increased, urinary oxalate levels increased, urticaria

Drug Interactions

Metabolism/Transport Effects None known.

Avoid Concomitant Use There are no known interactions where it is recommended to avoid concomitant use.

Increased Effect/Toxicity
Orlistat may increase the levels/effects of: Warfarin

Decreased Effect
Orlistat may decrease the levels/effects of: Amiodarone; Anticonvulsants; CycloSPORINE (Systemic); Levothyroxine; Multivitamins/Fluoride (with ADE); Multivitamins/Minerals (with ADEK, Folate, Iron); Multivitamins/Minerals (with AE, No Iron); Paricalcitol; Propafenone; Vitamin D Analogs; Vitamins (Fat Soluble)

Ethanol/Nutrition/Herb Interactions Fat-soluble vitamins: Absorption of vitamins A, D, E, and K may be decreased by orlistat. A multivitamin containing the fat-soluble vitamins (A, D, E, and K) should be administered once daily at least 2 hours before or after orlistat.

Storage/Stability Store at 25°C (77°F); excursions permitted to 15°C to 30°C (59°F to 86°F).

Mechanism of Action A reversible inhibitor of gastric and pancreatic lipases, thus inhibiting absorption of dietary fats by 30% (at doses of 120 mg 3 times/day).

Pharmacodynamics/Kinetics
Onset of action: 24-48 hours
Duration: 48-72 hours
Absorption: Minimal
Protein binding: >99% (lipoproteins and albumin)
Metabolism: Metabolized within the gastrointestinal wall; forms inactive metabolites
Half-life elimination: 1-2 hours
Time to peak, serum: ~8 hours
Excretion: Feces (~97%, 83% as unchanged drug); urine (<2%)

Dosage Oral:
Children ≥12 years and Adults (Xenical®): 120 mg 3 times/day with each main meal containing fat (during or up to 1 hour after the meal); omit dose if meal is occasionally missed or contains no fat.
Adults (Alli™): OTC labeling: 60 mg 3 times/day with each main meal containing fat

Dosage adjustment in renal impairment: No dosage adjustment provided in manufacturer's labeling (has not been studied). However, dosage adjustment unlikely due to low systemic absorption.

Dosage adjustment in hepatic impairment: No dosage adjustment provided in manufacturer's labeling (has not been studied). However, dosage adjustment unlikely due to low systemic absorption.

Dietary Considerations Multivitamin supplements that contain fat-soluble vitamins should be taken once daily at least 2 hours before or after the administration of orlistat (ie, bedtime). Gastrointestinal effects of orlistat may increase if taken with any one meal very high in fat. Distribute daily intake of carbohydrates, fat (~30% of daily calories), and protein over three main meals.

Administration Administer during or up to 1 hour after each main meal containing fat.

Monitoring Parameters BMI; diet (calorie and fat intake); serum glucose in patients with diabetes; thyroid function in patient with thyroid disease; liver function tests in patients exhibiting symptoms of hepatic dysfunction

Dosage Forms Excipient information presented when available (limited, particularly for generics); consult specific product labeling.
Capsule, Oral:
Alli: 60 mg [contains fd&c blue #2 (indigotine)]
Xenical: 120 mg [contains fd&c blue #2 (indigotine)]

◆ **Ornex® [OTC]** *see* Acetaminophen and Pseudoephedrine *on page* 33

◆ **Ornex® Maximum Strength [OTC]** *see* Acetaminophen and Pseudoephedrine *on page* 33

◆ **ORO-Clense (Can)** *see* Chlorhexidine Gluconate *on page* 408

◆ **Orphenace® (Can)** *see* Orphenadrine *on page* 1517

Orphenadrine (or FEN a dreen)

Brand Names: U.S. Norflex

Brand Names: Canada Norflex™; Orphenace®; Rhoxal-orphendrine

Index Terms Orphenadrine Citrate

Pharmacologic Category Skeletal Muscle Relaxant

Additional Appendix Information
Beers Criteria – Potentially Inappropriate Medications for Geriatrics *on page* 2368

Use Treatment of muscle spasm associated with acute painful musculoskeletal conditions

Pregnancy Risk Factor C

Dosage
Adults:
Oral: 100 mg twice daily
I.M., I.V.: 60 mg every 12 hours
Elderly: Use caution; generally not recommended for use in the elderly

Dosage adjustment in renal impairment: No dosage adjustment provided in manufacturer's labeling.

Dosage adjustment in hepatic impairment: No dosage adjustment provided in manufacturer's labeling.

Additional Information Complete prescribing information should be consulted for additional detail.

Dosage Forms Excipient information presented when available (limited, particularly for generics); consult specific product labeling.
Solution, Injection, as citrate:
Norflex: 30 mg/mL (2 mL) [contains sodium metabisulfite]
Generic: 30 mg/mL (2 mL)
Solution, Injection, as citrate [preservative free]:
Generic: 30 mg/mL (2 mL)
Tablet Extended Release 12 Hour, Oral, as citrate:
Generic: 100 mg

Orphenadrine, Aspirin, and Caffeine
(or FEN a dreen, AS pir in, & KAF een)

Index Terms Aspirin, Caffeine, and Orphenadrine; Aspirin, Orphenadrine, and Caffeine; Caffeine, Orphenadrine, and Aspirin; Norgesic

Pharmacologic Category Skeletal Muscle Relaxant

Use Relief of discomfort associated with skeletal muscular conditions

Dosage Oral: 1-2 tablets 3-4 times/day

Dosage adjustment in renal impairment: No dosage adjustment provided in manufacturer's labeling.

Dosage adjustment in hepatic impairment: No dosage adjustment provided in manufacturer's labeling.

Additional Information Complete prescribing information should be consulted for additional detail.

Dosage Forms Excipient information presented when available (limited, particularly for generics); consult specific product labeling.
Tablet: Orphenadrine citrate 25 mg, aspirin 385 mg, and caffeine 30 mg; orphenadrine citrate 50 mg, aspirin 770 mg, and caffeine 60 mg

◆ **Orphenadrine Citrate** *see* Orphenadrine *on page* 1517

◆ **Orsythia** *see* Ethinyl Estradiol and Levonorgestrel *on page* 787

◆ **Ortho 0.5/35 (Can)** *see* Ethinyl Estradiol and Norethindrone *on page* 793

◆ **Ortho 1/35 (Can)** *see* Ethinyl Estradiol and Norethindrone *on page* 793

◆ **Ortho 7/7/7 (Can)** *see* Ethinyl Estradiol and Norethindrone *on page* 793

◆ **Ortho Cept** *see* Ethinyl Estradiol and Desogestrel *on page 784*

◆ **Ortho-Cept** *see* Ethinyl Estradiol and Desogestrel *on page 784*

◆ **Ortho Cyclen** *see* Ethinyl Estradiol and Norgestimate *on page 795*

◆ **Ortho-Cyclen** *see* Ethinyl Estradiol and Norgestimate *on page 795*

◆ **Ortho Est** *see* Estropipate *on page 778*

◆ **Ortho-Est 0.625** *see* Estropipate *on page 778*

◆ **Ortho-Est 1.25** *see* Estropipate *on page 778*

◆ **Ortho-Evra** *see* Ethinyl Estradiol and Norelgestromin *on page 792*

◆ **Ortho Evra®** *see* Ethinyl Estradiol and Norelgestromin *on page 792*

◆ **Ortho Micronor** *see* Norethindrone *on page 1472*

◆ **Ortho Novum** *see* Ethinyl Estradiol and Norethindrone *on page 793*

◆ **Ortho-Novum 1/35** *see* Ethinyl Estradiol and Norethindrone *on page 793*

◆ **Ortho Novum 1/50** *see* Norethindrone and Mestranol *on page 1474*

◆ **Ortho-Novum® 1/50 (Can)** *see* Norethindrone and Mestranol *on page 1474*

◆ **Ortho-Novum 7/7/7** *see* Ethinyl Estradiol and Norethindrone *on page 793*

◆ **Ortho,para-DDD** *see* Mitotane *on page 1385*

◆ **Ortho Tri Cyclen** *see* Ethinyl Estradiol and Norgestimate *on page 795*

◆ **Ortho Tri-Cyclen** *see* Ethinyl Estradiol and Norgestimate *on page 795*

◆ **Ortho Tri-Cyclen Lo** *see* Ethinyl Estradiol and Norgestimate *on page 795*

◆ **Orthovisc** *see* Hyaluronate and Derivatives *on page 1000*

◆ **OrthoVisc (Can)** *see* Hyaluronate and Derivatives *on page 1000*

◆ **OrthoWash™** *see* Fluoride *on page 880*

◆ **Orviban CF** *see* Butalbital and Acetaminophen *on page 305*

◆ **Oscal** *see* Calcium Carbonate *on page 318*

◆ **Os-Cal [OTC] [DSC]** *see* Calcium Carbonate *on page 318*

◆ **Os-Cal® (Can)** *see* Calcium Carbonate *on page 318*

◆ **Os-Cal 500+D [OTC]** *see* Calcium and Vitamin D *on page 318*

◆ **Oscimin** *see* Hyoscyamine *on page 1026*

◆ **Oscimin SR** *see* Hyoscyamine *on page 1026*

Oseltamivir (oh sel TAM i vir)

Brand Names: U.S. Tamiflu

Brand Names: Canada Tamiflu

Pharmacologic Category Antiviral Agent; Neuraminidase Inhibitor

Use Treatment of uncomplicated acute illness due to influenza (A or B) infection in children ≥2 weeks and adults who have been symptomatic for no more than 2 days; prophylaxis against influenza (A or B) infection in children ≥1 year of age and adults

The Advisory Committee on Immunization Practices (ACIP) recommends that **treatment** be considered for the following:

- Persons with severe, complicated or progressive illness
- Hospitalized persons
- Persons at higher risk for influenza complications:
  - Children <2 years of age (highest risk in children <6 months of age)
  - Adults ≥65 years of age
  - Persons with chronic disorders of the pulmonary (including asthma) or cardiovascular systems (except hypertension)
  - Persons with chronic metabolic diseases (including diabetes mellitus), hepatic disease, renal dysfunction, hematologic disorders (including sickle cell disease), or immunosuppression (including immunosuppression caused by medications or HIV)
  - Persons with neurologic/neuromuscular conditions (including conditions such as spinal cord injuries, seizure disorders, cerebral palsy, stroke, mental retardation, moderate to severe developmental delay, or muscular dystrophy) which may compromise respiratory function, the handling of respiratory secretions, or that can increase the risk of aspiration
  - Pregnant or postpartum women (≤2 weeks after delivery)
  - Persons <19 years of age on long-term aspirin therapy
  - American Indians and Alaskan Natives
  - Persons who are morbidly obese (BMI ≥40)
  - Residents of nursing homes or other chronic care facilities
- Use may also be considered for previously healthy, nonhigh-risk outpatients with confirmed or suspected influenza based on clinical judgment when treatment can be started within 48 hours of illness onset.

The ACIP recommends that **prophylaxis** be considered for the following:

- Postexposure prophylaxis may be considered for family or close contacts of suspected or confirmed cases, who are at higher risk of influenza complications, and who have not been vaccinated against the circulating strain at the time of the exposure.
- Postexposure prophylaxis may be considered for unvaccinated healthcare workers who had occupational exposure without protective equipment.
- Pre-exposure prophylaxis should only be used for persons at very high risk of influenza complications who cannot be otherwise protected at times of high risk for exposure.
- Prophylaxis should also be administered to all eligible residents of institutions that house patients at high risk when needed to control outbreaks.

The ACIP recommends that treatment and prophylaxis be given to children <1 year of age when indicated.

Pregnancy Risk Factor C

Pregnancy Considerations In animal reproduction studies, a dose-dependent increase in the rates of minor skeleton abnormalities was found in exposed offspring. The rate of each abnormality remained within the background rate of occurrence in the species studied. Oseltamivir phosphate and its active metabolite oseltamivir carboxylate cross the placenta (*in vitro* data). An increased risk of adverse neonatal outcomes has generally not been observed following maternal use of oseltamivir during pregnancy. Untreated influenza infection is associated with an increased risk of adverse events to the fetus and an increased risk of complications or death to the mother. Oseltamivir and zanamivir are currently recommended for the treatment or prophylaxis of influenza in pregnant women and women up to 2 weeks postpartum. Oseltamivir and zanamivir are currently recommended as an adjunct to vaccination and should not be used as a substitute for vaccination in pregnant women (consult current CDC guidelines).

Breast-Feeding Considerations Small amounts of oseltamivir and oseltamivir carboxylate have been detected in breast milk. Breast-feeding is not recommended by the manufacturer. According to the CDC, breast-feeding while taking oseltamivir can be continued. The CDC recommends that women infected with the influenza virus follow general precautions (eg, frequent hand washing) to decrease viral transmission to the child. Mothers with influenza-like illnesses at delivery should consider avoiding close contact with the infant until they have received 48 hours of antiviral medication, fever has resolved, and cough and secretions can be controlled. These measures may help decrease (but not eliminate) the risk of transmitting influenza to the newborn. During this time, breast milk can be expressed and bottle-fed to the infant by another person who is well. Protective measures, such as wearing a face mask, changing into a clean gown or clothing, and strict hand hygiene should be continued by the mother for ≥7 days after the onset of symptoms or until symptom-free for 24 hours. Infant care should be performed by a noninfected person when possible (consult current CDC guidelines). Influenza may cause serious illness in postpartum women and prompt evaluation for febrile respiratory illnesses is recommended.

Contraindications Hypersensitivity to oseltamivir or any component of the formulation

Warnings/Precautions Oseltamivir is not a substitute for the influenza virus vaccine. It has not been shown to prevent primary or concomitant bacterial infections that may occur with influenza virus. Use caution with renal impairment; dosage adjustment is required for creatinine clearance <30 mL/minute. Safety and efficacy for use in patients with chronic cardiac and/or kidney disease, severe hepatic impairment, or for treatment or prophylaxis in immunocompromised patients have not been established. Rare but severe hypersensitivity reactions (anaphylaxis, severe dermatologic reactions) have been associated with use. Rare occurrences of neuropsychiatric events (including confusion, delirium, hallucinations, and/or self-injury) have been reported from postmarketing surveillance (primarily in pediatric patients); direct causation is difficult to establish (influenza infection may also be associated with behavioral and neurologic changes). Monitor closely for signs of any unusual behavior.

Antiviral treatment should begin within 48 hours of symptom onset. However, the CDC recommends that treatment may still be beneficial and should be started in hospitalized patients with severe, complicated or progressive illness if >48 hours. Treatment should not be delayed while awaiting results of laboratory tests for influenza. Nonhospitalized persons who are not at high risk for developing severe or complicated illness and who have a mild disease are not likely to benefit if treatment is started >48 hours after symptom onset. Nonhospitalized persons who are already beginning to recover do not need treatment.

Adverse Reactions

>10%: Gastrointestinal: Vomiting (2% to 15%)

1% to 10%:

Gastrointestinal: Nausea (4% to 10%), abdominal pain (2% to 5%), diarrhea (1% to 3%)

Ocular: Conjunctivitis (1%)

Respiratory: Epistaxis (1%)

<1% (Limited to important or life-threatening): Allergy, anaphylactic/anaphylactoid reaction, angina, arrhythmia, confusion, erythema multiforme, fracture, gastrointestinal bleeding, hemorrhagic colitis, hepatitis, liver function tests abnormal, neuropsychiatric events, pseudomembranous colitis, pyrexia, seizure, Stevens-Johnson syndrome, swelling of face or tongue, toxic epidermal necrolysis

Drug Interactions

Metabolism/Transport Effects None known.

Avoid Concomitant Use There are no known interactions where it is recommended to avoid concomitant use.

Increased Effect/Toxicity

The levels/effects of Oseltamivir may be increased by: Probenecid

Decreased Effect

Oseltamivir may decrease the levels/effects of: Influenza Virus Vaccine (Live/Attenuated)

Preparation for Administration Oral suspension: Reconstitute with 55 mL of water to a final concentration of 6 mg/mL (to make 60 mL total suspension).

Storage/Stability

Capsules: Store at 25°C (77°F); excursions permitted to 15°C to 30°C (59°F to 86°F).

Oral suspension: Store powder for suspension at 25°C (77°F); excursions permitted to 15°C to 30°C (59°F to 86°F). Once reconstituted, store suspension under refrigeration at 2°C to 8°C (36°F to 46°F) or at room temperature; do not freeze. Use within 10 days of preparation if stored at room temperature or within 17 days of preparation if stored under refrigeration.

Mechanism of Action Oseltamivir, a prodrug, is hydrolyzed to the active form, oseltamivir carboxylate (OC). OC inhibits influenza virus neuraminidase, an enzyme known to cleave the budding viral progeny from its cellular envelope attachment point (neuraminic acid) just prior to release.

Pharmacodynamics/Kinetics Note: Concurrent use of extracorporeal membrane oxygenation (ECMO): When used alone, ECMO has been shown not to impact oseltamivir carboxylate C_{max} and AUC in 2 small studies (Lemaitre, 2012; Mulla, 2013).

Absorption: Well absorbed

Distribution: V_d: 23-26 L (oseltamivir carboxylate); may be significantly increased in patients receiving ECMO (Lemaitre, 2012; Mulla, 2013)

Protein binding, plasma: Oseltamivir carboxylate: 3%; Oseltamivir: 42%

Metabolism: Hepatic (90%) to oseltamivir carboxylate; neither the parent drug nor active metabolite has any effect on the cytochrome P450 system

Bioavailability: 75% as oseltamivir carboxylate

Half-life elimination: Oseltamivir: 1-3 hours; Oseltamivir carboxylate: 6-10 hours

Excretion: Urine (>90% as oseltamivir carboxylate); feces

Dosage Oral:

Influenza prophylaxis: Initiate prophylaxis within 48 hours of contact with an infected individual

Manufacturer's recommendation:

Children: 1-12 years:

- ≤15 kg: 30 mg once daily
- >15 kg to ≤23 kg: 45 mg once daily
- >23 kg to ≤40 kg: 60 mg once daily
- >40 kg: 75 mg once daily

Adolescents ≥13 years and Adults: 75 mg once daily

Alternate recommendations:

Children 3-11 months (unlabeled dosing; AAP, 2010): **Note:** Dosing based on age (use only if weight not available)

- 3-5 months: 20 mg once daily
- 6-11 months: 25 mg once daily

Children <12 months (unlabeled dosing, CDC, 2012): **Note:** Prophylaxis is not recommended for infants <3 months of age unless clinically critical; weight-based dosing recommendations are not intended for premature neonates: 3 mg/kg/dose once daily

Children 3-23 months (unlabeled dosing, IDSA/PIDS, 2011):
3-8 months: 3 mg/kg/dose once daily (do not exceed maximum dose of weight-based dosing)
9-23 months: 3.5 mg/kg/dose once daily (do not exceed maximum dose of weight-based dosing)

Prophylaxis duration:
Individual/household exposure:
Manufacturer recommendation: 10 days
Alternate recommendations: 7 days (CDC, 2012)
Community/institutional outbreak:
Manufacturer recommendation: May be used for up to 6 weeks
Alternate recommendations: Continue for ≥2 weeks and until ~7 days after identification of illness onset in the last patient (CDC, 2012) or until influenza activity in community subsides or immunity obtained from immunization (IDSA/PIDS, 2011). During community outbreaks, duration of protection lasts for length of dosing period; safety and efficacy have been demonstrated for use up to 6 weeks in immunocompetent patients and safety has been demonstrated for use up to 12 weeks in patients who are immunocompromised.

Influenza treatment: Initiate treatment within 48 hours of onset of symptoms; duration of treatment: 5 days unless severely ill and hospitalized. **Note:** Hospitalized patients may require longer (eg, ≥10 days) treatment courses. Some experts also recommend empirically doubling the treatment dose (CDC, 2009). Doubling the dose in adult outpatients was not associated with increased adverse events. As no double-dose studies have been published in children, use caution. Initiate as early as possible in any hospitalized patient with suspected/confirmed influenza regardless of the time of presentation from symptom onset (CDC, 2011); may be administered via naso- or orogastric tube in mechanically-ventilated patients (Taylor, 2008).
Manufacturer's recommendation: **Note:** The following dosing is also supported by some clinicians (IDSA/PIDS, 2011):
Infants ≥2 weeks: 3 mg/kg/dose twice daily
Children: 1-12 years:
≤15 kg: 30 mg twice daily
>15 kg to ≤23 kg: 45 mg twice daily
>23 kg to ≤40 kg: 60 mg twice daily
>40 kg: 75 mg twice daily
Adolescents ≥13 years and Adults: 75 mg twice daily
Critically ill: Concurrent use of extracorporeal membrane oxygenation (ECMO) alone: No dosage adjustment necessary (Lemaitre, 2012; Mulla, 2013).
Alternate recommendations:
Infants <2 weeks (unlabeled dosing, CDC, 2012): **Note:** Weight-based dosing recommendations are not intended for premature neonates: 3 mg/kg/dose twice daily.
Infants <12 months (unlabeled dosing; AAP, 2010): **Note:** Dosing based on age (use only if weight not available):
<3 months: 12 mg twice daily
3-5 months: 20 mg twice daily
6-11 months: 25 mg twice daily
Infants and Children <24 months (unlabeled dosing; IDSA/PIDS, 2011): **Note:** Do not exceed maximum dose of weight-based dosing.
Infants, premature: 1 mg/kg/dose twice daily
0-8 months: 3 mg/kg/dose twice daily
9-23 months: 3.5 mg/kg/dose twice daily

Dosage adjustment in renal impairment:
Treatment: Adults:
U.S. labeling: Cl_{cr} 10-30 mL/minute: 75 mg once daily for 5 days
Canadian labeling:
Cl_{cr} >30-60 mL/minute: 30 mg twice daily for 5 days
Cl_{cr} 10-30 mL/minute: 30 mg once daily for 5 days
High-dose treatment (unlabeled [eg, severely-ill hospitalized patients with 2009 H1N1 influenza]): Currently no data are available; consider 150 mg once daily
Prophylaxis: Adults:
U.S. labeling: Cl_{cr} 10-30 mL/minute: 75 mg every other day or 30 mg once daily
Canadian labeling:
Cl_{cr} >30-60 mL/minute: 30 mg once daily for 10-14 days
Cl_{cr} 10-30 mL/minute: 30 mg every other day for 10-14 days
CAPD: Adults:
Unlabeled dose: 30 mg once weekly (Robson, 2006)
Canadian labeling (not in U.S. labeling):
Treatment: 30 mg prior to start of dialysis
Prophylaxis: 30 mg prior to start of dialysis, then 30 mg every 7 days for 10-14 days
Continuous veno-venous hemodialysis (CVVHD): Adults: **Note:** Limited information available; optimal dosing has not been established: 150 mg twice daily administered via nasogastric or postpyloric feeding tube demonstrated supratherapeutic oseltamivir carboxylate concentrations at effluent rates of 3300 ± 919 mL/hour; the authors determined that the manufacturer recommended dosage of 75 mg once daily for patients with Cl_{cr} 10-30 mL/minute will likely achieve concentrations necessary to inhibit viral neuraminidase activity at these effluent rates; however, doses greater than 75 mg once daily may be required when using higher effluent rates (Eyler, 2012).
CVVHD and concurrent use of ECMO: Lower oseltamivir carboxylate concentrations (~981 ng/mL) were observed as compared to those with the use of CVVHD alone (~2760 ng/mL) when patients were administered 150 mg twice daily (n=4; Eyler, 2012).
Intermittent hemodialysis:
Children >1 year (unlabeled dose; Schreuder, 2010):
≤15 kg: 7.5 mg after each hemodialysis session
>15 kg to ≤23 kg: 10 mg after each hemodialysis session
>23 kg to ≤40 kg: 15 mg after each hemodialysis session
>40 kg: 30 mg after each hemodialysis session
Adults:
Unlabeled dose: 30 mg after every other session (Robson, 2006) **or** 75 mg every 48 hours (Ariano, 2010)
Canadian labeling (not in U.S. labeling):
Treatment: 30 mg prior to dialysis; if symptomatic between dialysis sessions, then administer 30 mg after each dialysis session over period of 5 days
Prophylaxis: 30 mg prior to dialysis, then 30 mg after every other dialysis session for period of 10-14 days

Dosage adjustment in hepatic impairment:
Mild-to-moderate impairment: No dosage adjustment necessary.
Severe impairment: No dosage adjustment provided in manufacturer's labeling (has not been studied).

Dosing in obesity: In adult morbidly-obese patients (BMI >40 kg/m^2), systemic exposure of oseltamivir carboxylate was not reduced; therefore, no dosage adjustment is necessary (Thorne-Humphrey, 2011).

Dietary Considerations Take without regard to meals; take with food to improve tolerance.

Administration May be administered without regard to meals; take with food to improve tolerance.

Capsules may be opened and mixed with sweetened liquid (eg, chocolate syrup). Administer oral suspension using the supplied oral syringe (exception: for children <1 year, a smaller volume [ie, <10 mL] oral syringe should be used in place of the supplied oral syringe to ensure accurate dosing); shake well.

Mechanically-ventilated critically-ill patients: May administer via naso- or orogastric (NG/OG) tube. For a 150 mg dose, dissolve powder from two 75 mg capsules in 20 mL of sterile water and inject down the NG/OG tube; follow with a 10 mL sterile water flush (Taylor, 2008).

Monitoring Parameters Signs or symptoms of unusual behavior, including attempts at self-injury, confusion, and/or delirium

Critically-ill patients: Repeat rRT-PCR or viral culture may help to determine on-going viral replication

Additional Information In clinical studies of the influenza virus, 1.3% of post-treatment isolates in adults and adolescents and 8.6% of isolates in children had decreased neuraminidase susceptibility *in vitro* to oseltamivir carboxylate.

The absence of symptoms does not rule out viral influenza infection and clinical judgment should guide the decision for therapy. Treatment should not be delayed while waiting for the results of diagnostic tests. Treatment should be considered for high-risk patients with symptoms despite a negative rapid influenza test when the illness cannot be contributed to another cause. Use of oseltamivir is not a substitute for vaccination (when available); susceptibility to influenza infection returns once therapy is discontinued.

Dosage Forms Excipient information presented when available (limited, particularly for generics); consult specific product labeling.

Capsule, Oral, as phosphate:

Tamiflu: 30 mg, 45 mg, 75 mg

Suspension Reconstituted, Oral, as base:

Tamiflu: 6 mg/mL (60 mL) [contains saccharin sodium, sodium benzoate; tutti-frutti flavor]

Extemporaneous Preparations

If the commercially prepared oral suspension is not available, the manufacturer provides the following compounding information to prepare a **6 mg/mL** suspension in emergency situations.

1. Place the specified amount of water into a polyethyleneterephthalate (PET) or glass bottle.
2. Carefully separate the capsule body and cap and pour the contents of the required number of 75 mg capsules into the PET or glass bottle.
3. Gently swirl the suspension to ensure adequate wetting of the powder for at least 2 minutes.
4. Slowly add the specified amount of vehicle to the bottle.
5. Close the bottle using a child-resistant cap and shake well for 30 seconds to completely dissolve the active drug.
6. Label "Shake Well Before Use."

Stable for 35 days refrigerated or 5 days at room temperature. Shake gently prior to use. Do **not** dispense with dosing device provided with commercially-available product.

Preparation of Oseltamivir 6 mg/mL Suspension

Body Weight	Total Volume per Patient[1]	# of 75 mg Capsules[2]	Required Volume of Water	Required Volume of Vehicle[2,3]	Treatment Dose (wt based)[4]	Prophylactic Dose (wt based)[4]
≤15 kg	75 mL	6	5 mL	69 mL	5 mL (30 mg) twice daily for 5 days	5 mL (30 mg) once daily for 10 days
16-23 kg	100 mL	8	7 mL	91 mL	7.5 mL (45 mg) twice daily for 5 days	7.5 mL (45 mg) once daily for 10 days
24-40 kg	125 mL	10	8 mL	115 mL	10 mL (60 mg) twice daily for 5 days	10 mL (60 mg) once daily for 10 days
≥41 kg	150 mL	12	10 mL	137 mL	12.5 mL (75 mg) twice daily for 5 days	12.5 mL (75 mg) once daily for 10 days

[1]Entire course of therapy.

[2]Based on total volume per patient.

[3]Acceptable vehicles are cherry syrup, Ora-Sweet® SF, or simple syrup.

[4]Using 6 mg/mL suspension.

◆ **OSI-774** *see* Erlotinib *on page* 735

◆ **Osmitrol** *see* Mannitol *on page* 1266

◆ **Osmitrol® (Can)** *see* Mannitol *on page* 1266

◆ **OsmoPrep** *see* Sodium Phosphates *on page* 1923

Ospemifene (os PEM i feen)

Brand Names: U.S. Osphena

Index Terms FC1271a

Pharmacologic Category Selective Estrogen Receptor Modulator (SERM)

Use Treatment of moderate-to-severe dyspareunia due to vulvar and vaginal atrophy (VVA) of menopause

Pregnancy Risk Factor X

Pregnancy Considerations Adverse events were observed in animal reproduction studies. Use is contraindicated in women who are or may become pregnant. Ospemifene is currently approved only for the treatment of moderate-to-severe dyspareunia due to vulvar and vaginal atrophy (VVA) of menopause.

Breast-Feeding Considerations It is not known if ospemifene is excreted into breast milk.

Contraindications Undiagnosed abnormal vaginal bleeding; DVT or PE (current or history of); active or history of arterial thromboembolic disease (eg, stroke, MI); estrogen-dependent tumor (known or suspected); women who are or may become pregnant

Warnings/Precautions [U.S. Boxed Warning]: The use of unopposed estrogen in women with an intact uterus is associated with an increased risk of endometrial cancer. The addition of a progestin to estrogen therapy may decrease the risk of endometrial hyperplasia, a precursor to endometrial cancer. Adequate diagnostic measures, including endometrial sampling if indicated, should be performed to rule out malignancy in postmenopausal women with undiagnosed abnormal vaginal bleeding. Ospemifene is an estrogen agonist/antagonist with agonistic effects on the endometrium. For women with an intact uterus using an estrogen without a progestin, the risk of endometrial cancer is dependent upon dose and duration of therapy. Endometrial cancer was not reported in clinical studies of ospemifene (duration ≤52 weeks) and the use of progestins was not evaluated. Ospemifene was not studied in women with breast cancer. Use is not currently recommended in women with carcinoma of the breast (known, suspected or history of) and use is contraindicated with an estrogen-dependent tumor.

[U.S. Boxed Warning]: Using data from the Women's Health Initiative (WHI) studies, an increased risk of deep vein thrombosis (DVT) and stroke has been reported with oral conjugated estrogens. The following were reported with ospemifene in clinical trials lasting ≤15 months duration: thromboembolic stroke 0.72/1000 women (placebo 1.04/1000 women); hemorrhagic stroke 1.45/1000 women (placebo 0/1000 women); DVT 1.45/1000 women (placebo 1.04/1000 women). Risk factors for cardiovascular disorders, arterial vascular disorders and /or venous thromboembolism (VTE) should be managed appropriately. Risk factors include diabetes mellitus, hypercholesterolemia, hypertension, SLE, obesity, tobacco use, and/or history of VTE. Discontinue immediately if a VTE, thromboembolic or hemorrhagic stroke occur or are suspected.

[U.S. Boxed Warning]: Ospemifene should be used for the shortest duration possible consistent with treatment goals and risks for the individual woman.

Ospemifene has not been studied in patients with severe hepatic impairment; use is not recommended. Potentially significant interactions may exist, requiring dose or frequency adjustment, additional monitoring, and/or selection of alternative therapy. Consult drug interactions database for more detailed information. Whenever possible, discontinue at least 4-6 weeks prior to elective surgery associated with an increased risk of thromboembolism or during periods of prolonged immobilization.

Hazardous agent: Use appropriate precautions for handling and disposal (meets NIOSH, 2012 criteria).

Adverse Reactions

1% to 10%:

Dermatologic: Hyperhidrosis (2%)

Endocrine & metabolic: Hot flashes (8%)

Genitourinary: Vaginal discharge (4%), genital discharge (1%)

Neuromuscular & skeletal: Muscle spasm (3%)

<1% (Limited to important or life-threatening: DVT, hemorrhagic stroke, thromboembolic stroke

Drug Interactions

Metabolism/Transport Effects Substrate of CYP2C19 (minor), CYP2C9 (major), CYP3A4 (major); **Note:** Assignment of Major/Minor substrate status based on clinically relevant drug interaction potential; **Inhibits** CYP2B6 (weak), CYP2C19 (weak), CYP2C8 (weak), CYP2C9 (weak), CYP2D6 (weak), CYP3A4 (weak)

Avoid Concomitant Use

Avoid concomitant use of Ospemifene with any of the following: Estrogen Derivatives; Fluconazole; Pimozide; Selective Estrogen Receptor Modulators

Increased Effect/Toxicity

Ospemifene may increase the levels/effects of: ARIPiprazole; Dofetilide; Lomitapide; Pimozide

The levels/effects of Ospemifene may be increased by: CYP2C9 Inhibitors (Strong); CYP3A4 Inhibitors (Strong); Estrogen Derivatives; Fluconazole; Selective Estrogen Receptor Modulators

Decreased Effect

The levels/effects of Ospemifene may be decreased by: Bosentan; CYP2C9 Inducers (Strong); CYP3A4 Inducers (Strong); Dabrafenib; Deferasirox; Estrogen Derivatives; Herbs (CYP3A4 Inducers); Mitotane; Peginterferon Alfa-2b; Selective Estrogen Receptor Modulators; Tocilizumab

Storage/Stability Store at controlled room temperature of 20°C to 25°C (68°F to 77°F); excursions permitted to 15°C to 30°C (59°F to 86°F).

Mechanism of Action Ospemifene is a selective estrogen receptor modulator (SERM); it activates estrogen pathways in some tissues and blocks estrogen pathways in others, and specifically has agonistic effects on the endometrium. In women with VVA, ospemifene was shown to improve vaginal changes associated with the decrease in natural estrogen production associated with menopause (improves vaginal maturation index, decreases vaginal pH) and significantly decreased the most bothersome moderate-to-severe subjective findings reported by women (vaginal dryness and dyspareunia) after 12 weeks of therapy (Bachmann, 2010).

Pharmacodynamics/Kinetics

Onset of action: A significant decrease in vaginal dryness and dyspareunia were observed after 12 weeks of therapy (Bachmann, 2010).

Distribution: V_d: 448 L

Protein binding: >99% bound to serum proteins

Metabolism: Hepatic via CYP3A4, 2C9, and 2C19; forms a metabolite (4-hydroxyospemifene)

Bioavailability: Increased approximately two- to threefold by food

Half-life elimination: ~26 hours

Time to peak: ~2 hours (range: 1-8 hours)

Excretion: Feces (75%); urine (7%; <0.2% as unchanged drug)

Dosage Dyspareunia, moderate-to-severe: Postmenopausal females: Oral: 60 mg once daily

Dosage adjustment in renal impairment: No dosage adjustment necessary.

Dosage adjustment in hepatic impairment:

Mild or moderate impairment (Child-Pugh class A or B): No dosage adjustment necessary.

Severe impairment (Child-Pugh class C): No dosage adjustment provided in manufacturer's labeling (has not been studied). Use is not recommended.

Administration Administer with food.

Hazardous agent: Use appropriate precautions for handling and disposal (meets NIOSH, 2012 criteria).

Monitoring Parameters Monitor for signs of endometrial cancer in female patients with uterus. Adequate diagnostic measures, including endometrial sampling, if indicated, should be performed to rule out malignancy in all cases of undiagnosed abnormal vaginal bleeding. Assess need for therapy at regular intervals. Monitor for signs/symptoms of stroke and VTE.

Dosage Forms Excipient information presented when available (limited, particularly for generics); consult specific product labeling.

Tablet, Oral:

Osphena: 60 mg

◆ **Osphena** *see* Ospemifene *on page* 1521

◆ **Osteocit® (Can)** *see* Calcium Citrate *on page* 321

◆ **Ostoforte® (Can)** *see* Ergocalciferol *on page* 733

◆ **OTFC (Oral Transmucosal Fentanyl Citrate)** *see* FentaNYL *on page* 842

◆ **Otrexup** *see* Methotrexate *on page* 1324

◆ **Ovace Plus** *see* Sulfacetamide (Topical) *on page* 1957

◆ **Ovace Plus Wash** *see* Sulfacetamide (Topical) *on page* 1957

◆ **Ovace Wash** *see* Sulfacetamide (Topical) *on page* 1957

◆ **Ovcon 35** *see* Ethinyl Estradiol and Norethindrone *on page* 793

◆ **Ovide** *see* Malathion *on page* 1265

◆ **Ovidrel** *see* Chorionic Gonadotropin (Recombinant) *on page 420*

◆ **Ovidrel® (Can)** *see* Chorionic Gonadotropin (Recombinant) *on page 420*

◆ **Ovine Corticotrophin-Releasing Hormone (oCRH)** *see* Corticorelin *on page 493*

◆ **Ovral® (Can)** *see* Ethinyl Estradiol and Norgestrel *on page 797*

Oxacillin (oks a SIL in)

Brand Names: U.S. Bactocill in Dextrose

Index Terms Methylphenyl Isoxazolyl Penicillin; Oxacillin Sodium

Pharmacologic Category Antibiotic, Penicillin

Additional Appendix Information

Antibiotic Treatment of Adults With Infective Endocarditis *on page 2355*

Use

Staphylococcal infections: In the treatment of infections caused by penicillinase-producing staphylococci that have demonstrated susceptibility to the drug; to initiate therapy in suspected cases of resistant staphylococcal infections prior to the availability of laboratory test results.

Oxacillin should not be used in infections caused by organisms susceptible to penicillin G. Oxacillin should be used only to treat or prevent infections that are proven or strongly suspected to be caused by susceptible bacteria. If the susceptibility test results indicate a non–penicillinase-producing staphylococcus, discontinue treatment. In the absence of such data, local epidemiology and susceptibility patterns may contribute to the empiric selection of therapy.

Pregnancy Risk Factor B

Pregnancy Considerations Adverse events have not been observed in animal reproduction studies. Oxacillin is distributed into the amniotic fluid and is detected in cord blood. Maternal use of penicillins has generally not resulted in an increased risk of adverse fetal effects.

Breast-Feeding Considerations Oxacillin is excreted in breast milk. The manufacturer recommends that caution be exercised when administering oxacillin to nursing women. Nondose-related effects could include modification of bowel flora.

Contraindications History of hypersensitivity (anaphylactic) reaction to any penicillin

Warnings/Precautions Elimination rate will be slow in neonates. Modify dosage in patients with renal impairment and in the elderly. Serious and occasionally severe or fatal hypersensitivity (anaphylactoid) reactions have been reported in patients on penicillin therapy, especially with a history of beta-lactam hypersensitivity, history of sensitivity to multiple allergens, or previous IgE-mediated reactions (eg, anaphylaxis, angioedema, urticaria). Acute hepatitis and reversible elevations of serum transaminases have been reported, including rash and leukopenia; onset after 2-3 weeks of therapy; monitor periodically throughout therapy (Dahlgren 1997; Faden 2009; Maraqa, 2002). Oxacillin contains 57.3 mg (2.5 mEq) of sodium per gram. The elderly population may respond with a blunted natriuresis to salt loading. This may be clinically important in diseases such as congestive heart failure. Use with caution in asthmatic patients. Prolonged use may result in fungal or bacterial superinfection, including *C. difficile*-associated diarrhea (CDAD) and pseudomembranous colitis; CDAD has been observed >2 months postantibiotic treatment.

Adverse Reactions Frequency not defined.

Central nervous system: Fever

Dermatologic: Rash

Gastrointestinal: Nausea, diarrhea, vomiting

Hematologic: Eosinophilia, leukopenia, neutropenia, thrombocytopenia, agranulocytosis

Hepatic: Hepatotoxicity, AST increased

Renal: Acute interstitial nephritis, hematuria

Miscellaneous: Serum sickness-like reactions

Drug Interactions

Metabolism/Transport Effects None known.

Avoid Concomitant Use

Avoid concomitant use of Oxacillin with any of the following: BCG

Increased Effect/Toxicity

Oxacillin may increase the levels/effects of: Methotrexate; Vitamin K Antagonists

The levels/effects of Oxacillin may be increased by: Probenecid

Decreased Effect

Oxacillin may decrease the levels/effects of: BCG; Mycophenolate; Sodium Picosulfate; Typhoid Vaccine

The levels/effects of Oxacillin may be decreased by: Tetracycline Derivatives

Preparation for Administration

I.M.: After reconstitution, vials will contain oxacillin 250 mg/1.5 mL.

1 gram vial: Add sterile water for injection 5.7 mL; shake well.

2 gram vial: Add sterile water for injection 11.5 mL; shake well.

I.V.:

1 gram vial: Add sterile water for injection or NS 10 mL; shake well.

2 gram vial: Add sterile water for injection or NS 20 mL; shake well.

10 gram vial: Add sterile water for injection or NS 93 mL; shake well. The resulting solution will contain oxacillin 100 mg/mL and requires further dilution prior to administration.

Storage/Stability

Premixed infusions: Store in a freezer at -20°C (4°F). Thaw at room temperature or under refrigeration only. Thawed bags are stable for 21 days under refrigeration or 48 hours at room temperature. Do not refreeze.

Vials: Store dry powder at 20°C to 25°C (68°F to 77°F); reconstituted parenteral solution (250 mg/1.5 mL) is stable for 3 days at room temperature and 7 days when refrigerated or 30 days when frozen. For I.V. infusion, oxacillin in D_5W is stable for 48 hours at room temperature and 10 days when refrigerated; oxacillin in NS is stable for 7 days at room temperature and 10 days when refrigerated. The reconstituted hospital bulk package is stable for 24 hours at room temperature. Reconstituted ADD-Vantage vials are stable for 24 hours in D_5W and 3 days in NS.

Mechanism of Action Inhibits bacterial cell wall synthesis by binding to one or more of the penicillin-binding proteins (PBPs); which in turn inhibits the final transpeptidation step of peptidoglycan synthesis in bacterial cell walls, thus inhibiting cell wall biosynthesis. Bacteria eventually lyse due to ongoing activity of cell wall autolytic enzymes (autolysins and murein hydrolases) while cell wall assembly is arrested.

Pharmacodynamics/Kinetics

Distribution: Into bile, amniotic, and pleural fluids; insignificant concentrations in CSF and aqueous humor

Protein binding: ~94% (mainly albumin)

Metabolism: Hepatic

Half-life elimination: Adults: 20-60 minutes; prolonged in neonates and with renal impairment

Time to peak, serum: I.M.: 30-60 minutes; I.V.: 5 minutes

Excretion: Urine and bile (unchanged drug)

Dosage Note: Oxacillin contains 57.3 mg (2.5 mEq) of sodium per gram.

Usual dosage range:

Infants and Children: I.M., I.V.: 50-200 mg/kg/day in divided doses every 6 hours (maximum: 12 g daily)

Adults: I.M., I.V.: 250-2000 mg every 4-6 hours

Indication-specific dosing:

Infants >3 months and Children:

Community-acquired pneumonia (CAP) (IDSA/PIDS, 2011), moderate-to-severe infection, *S. aureus* (methicillin-susceptible) (preferred): I.V.: 150-200 mg/kg/day divided every 6-8 hours

Children:

Mild-to-moderate infections: I.M., I.V.: 50 mg/kg/day in divided doses every 6 hours (maximum: 4 g daily)

Severe infections: Infants and Children: I.M., I.V.: 100 mg/kg/day in divided doses every 4-6 hours (maximum: 12 g daily)

Adults:

Endocarditis: I.V.: 2 g every 4 hours with gentamicin

Mild-to-moderate infections: I.M., I.V.: 250-500 mg every 4-6 hours

Prosthetic joint infection: I.V.: 2 g every 4 hours with rifampin

Severe infections: I.M., I.V.: 1 g every 4-6 hours

***Staphylococcus aureus*, methicillin-susceptible infections, including brain abscess, bursitis, erysipelas, mastitis, mastoiditis, osteomyelitis, perinephric abscess, pneumonia, pyomyositis, scalded skin syndrome, toxic shock syndrome:** I.V.: 2 g every 4 hours

Dosage adjustment in renal impairment: No dosage adjustment provided in manufacturer's labeling.

Intermittent hemodialysis: Not dialyzable (0% to 5%)

Dosage adjustment in hepatic impairment: No dosage adjustment provided in manufacturer's labeling.

Dietary Considerations Some products may contain sodium.

Administration Administer I.V. or I.M. around-the-clock to promote less variation in peak and trough serum levels. Administer IVP over 10 minutes. Administer IVPB over 30 minutes. Rapid administration may result in seizures.

Monitoring Parameters Observe for signs and symptoms of anaphylaxis during first dose; monitor periodic CBC, urinalysis, BUN, serum creatinine, AST and ALT

Test Interactions May interfere with urinary glucose tests using cupric sulfate (Benedict's solution, Clinitest®); may inactivate aminoglycosides *in vitro*; false-positive urinary and serum proteins

Dosage Forms Excipient information presented when available (limited, particularly for generics); consult specific product labeling.

Solution, Intravenous:

Bactocill in Dextrose: 1 g/50 mL (50 mL); 2 g/50 mL (50 mL)

Solution Reconstituted, Injection:

Generic: 1 g (1 ea); 2 g (1 ea); 10 g (1 ea)

Solution Reconstituted, Injection [preservative free]:

Generic: 1 g (1 ea); 2 g (1 ea); 10 g (1 ea)

◆ **Oxacillin Sodium** *see* Oxacillin *on page* 1523

◆ **Oxalatoplatin** *see* Oxaliplatin *on page* 1524

◆ **Oxalatoplatinum** *see* Oxaliplatin *on page* 1524

Oxaliplatin (ox AL i pla tin)

Brand Names: U.S. Eloxatin

Brand Names: Canada Eloxatin

Index Terms Diaminocyclohexane Oxalatoplatinum; L-OHP; Oxalatoplatin; Oxalatoplatinum

Pharmacologic Category Antineoplastic Agent, Alkylating Agent; Antineoplastic Agent, Platinum Analog

Use Treatment of stage III colon cancer (adjuvant) after complete resection of primary tumor; treatment of advanced colorectal cancer

Unlabeled Use Treatment of esophageal cancer, gastric cancer, hepatobiliary cancer (advanced), non-Hodgkin's lymphoma (refractory), ovarian cancer (advanced, platinum-pretreated), pancreatic cancer (advanced), testicular cancer (refractory)

Pregnancy Risk Factor D

Pregnancy Considerations Adverse events were observed in animal reproduction studies at one-tenth the equivalent human dose. Women of childbearing potential should be advised to avoid pregnancy and use effective contraception during treatment.

Canadian labeling: Use in pregnant women is contraindicated in the Canadian labeling. Males should be advised not to father children during and for up to 6 months following therapy. May cause permanent infertility in males. Prior to initiating therapy, advise males desiring to father children, to seek counseling on sperm storage.

Breast-Feeding Considerations It is not known if oxaliplatin is excreted in breast milk. Due to the potential for serious adverse reactions in the nursing infant, the decision to discontinue breast-feeding or to discontinue oxaliplatin should take into account the benefits of treatment to the mother.

Contraindications Hypersensitivity to oxaliplatin, other platinum-containing compounds, or any component of the formulation

Canadian labeling: Additional contraindications (not in U.S. labeling): Pregnancy, breast-feeding; severe renal impairment (Cl_{cr} <30 mL/minute)

Warnings/Precautions Hazardous agent - use appropriate precautions for handling and disposal (NIOSH, 2012). **[U.S. Boxed Warning]: Anaphylactic/anaphylactoid reactions have been reported with oxaliplatin (may occur within minutes of administration); symptoms may be managed with epinephrine, corticosteroids, antihistamines,** and discontinuation; oxygen and bronchodilators have also been used (Kim, 2009). Grade 3 or 4 hypersensitivity has been observed. Allergic reactions are similar to reactions reported with other platinum analogs, and may occur with any cycle. Reactions typically occur after multiple cycles; in retrospective reviews, reaction occurred at a median of 7-9 cycles, with an onset of 5-70 minutes (Kim, 2009; Polyzos, 2009). Symptoms may include bronchospasm (rare), erythema, hypotension (rare), pruritus, rash, and/or urticaria; previously-untreated patients have also experienced flushing, diaphoresis, diarrhea, shortness of breath, chest pain, hypotension, syncope, and disorientation. According to the manufacturer, rechallenge is contraindicated (deaths due to anaphylaxis have been associated with platinum derivatives). In patients rechallenged after mild hypersensitivity, reaction recurred at a higher level of severity; for patients with severe hypersensitivity, rechallenge (with 2-3 days of antihistamine and corticosteroid premedication, and prolongation of infusion time) allowed for 2-4 additional oxaliplatin cycles; however, rechallenge was not feasible in nearly two-thirds of patients due to the severity of the initial reaction (Polyzos, 2009).

Two different types of peripheral sensory neuropathy may occur: First, an acute (within hours to 1-2 days), reversible (resolves within 14 days), with primarily peripheral symptoms that are often exacerbated by cold (may include pharyngolaryngeal dysesthesia); commonly recur with subsequent doses; avoid mucositis prophylaxis with ice chips during oxaliplatin infusion. Secondly, a more persistent (>14 days) presentation that often interferes with daily activities (eg, writing, buttoning, swallowing), these symptoms may improve in some patients upon discontinuing treatment. In a retrospective evaluation of patients treated with oxaliplatin for colorectal cancer, the incidence of peripheral sensory neuropathy was similar between diabetic and nondiabetic patients (Ramanathan, 2010). Several retrospective studies (as well as a small, underpowered randomized trial) have suggested calcium and magnesium infusions before and after oxaliplatin administration may reduce incidence of cumulative sensory neuropathy; however, a recent abstract of an ongoing randomized, placebo-controlled, double-blind study in patients with colorectal cancer suggests there is no benefit of calcium and magnesium in preventing sensory neuropathy or in decreasing oxaliplatin discontinuation rates (Loprinzi, 2013).

Oxaliplatin is associated with a moderate emetic potential; antiemetics are recommended to prevent nausea and vomiting. Cases of reversible posterior leukoencephalopathy syndrome (RPLS) have been reported. Signs/symptoms include headache, mental status changes, seizure, blurred vision, blindness and/or other vision changes; may be associated with hypertension; diagnosis is confirmed with brain imaging. May cause pulmonary fibrosis; withhold treatment for unexplained pulmonary symptoms (eg, crackles, dyspnea, nonproductive cough, pulmonary infiltrates) until interstitial lung disease or pulmonary fibrosis are excluded. Hepatotoxicity (including rare cases of hepatitis and hepatic failure) has been reported. Liver biopsy has revealed peliosis, nodular regenerative hyperplasia, sinusoidal alterations, perisinusoidal fibrosis, and veno-occlusive lesions; the presence of hepatic vascular disorders (including veno-occlusive disease) should be considered, especially in individuals developing portal hypertension or who present with increased liver function tests. Use caution with renal dysfunction; increased toxicity may occur; reduce initial dose in severe impairment. Potentially significant drug-drug interactions may exist, requiring dose or frequency adjustment, additional monitoring, and/or selection of alternative therapy. Elderly patients are more sensitive to some adverse events including diarrhea, dehydration, hypokalemia, leukopenia, fatigue and syncope. Oxaliplatin is an irritant with vesicant-like properties; ensure proper needle or catheter placement prior to and during infusion; avoid extravasation.

Adverse Reactions Percentages reported with monotherapy.

>10%:

Central nervous system: Peripheral neuropathy (may be dose limiting; 76% to 92%; acute 65%; grades 3/4: 5%; persistent 43%; grades 3/4: 3%), fatigue (61%), pain (14%), headache (13%), insomnia (11%)

Gastrointestinal: Nausea (64%), diarrhea (46%), vomiting (37%), abdominal pain (31%), constipation (31%), anorexia (20%), stomatitis (14%)

Hematologic & oncologic: Anemia (64%; grades 3/4: 1%), thrombocytopenia (30%; grades 3/4: 3%), leukopenia (13%)

Hepatic: Increased serum AST (54%; grades 3/4: 4%), increased serum ALT (36%; grades 3/4: 1%), increased serum bilirubin (13%; grades 3/4: 5%)

Neuromuscular & skeletal: Back pain (11%)

Respiratory: Dyspnea (13%), cough (11%)

Miscellaneous: Fever (25%)

1% to 10%:

Cardiovascular: Edema (10%), chest pain (5%), peripheral edema (5%), flushing (3%), thromboembolism (2%)

Central nervous system: Rigors (9%), dizziness (7%)

Dermatologic: Skin rash (5%), alopecia (3%), palmar-plantar erythrodysesthesia (1%)

Endocrine & metabolic: Dehydration (5%), hypokalemia (3%)

Gastrointestinal: Dyspepsia (7%), dysgeusia (5%), flatulence (3%), hiccups (2%), mucositis (2%), gastroesophageal reflux disease (1%), dysphagia (acute 1% to 2%)

Genitourinary: Dysuria (1%)

Hematologic & oncologic: Neutropenia (7%)

Hypersensitivity: Hypersensitivity reaction (3%; includes urticaria, pruritus, facial flushing, shortness of breath, bronchospasm, diaphoresis, hypotension, syncope: grades 3/4: 2% to 3%)

Local: Injection site reaction (9%; redness/swelling/pain)

Neuromuscular & skeletal: Arthralgia (7%)

Ocular: Abnormal lacrimation (1%)

Renal: Increased serum creatinine (5% to 10%)

Respiratory: Upper respiratory tract infection (7%), rhinitis (6%), epistaxis (2%), pharyngitis (2%), pharyngolaryngeal dysesthesia (grades 3/4: 1% to 2%)

<1% (Limited to important or life-threatening; reported with mono- and combination therapy): Abnormal gait, acute renal failure, anaphylaxis, anaphylactic shock, anaphylactoid reaction, angioedema, aphonia, ataxia, blepharoptosis, cerebral hemorrhage, colitis, cranial nerve palsy, decreased deep tendon reflex, deafness, decreased visual acuity, diplopia, dysarthria, eosinophilic pneumonitis, fasciculations, febrile neutropenia,hematuria, hemolysis, hemolytic anemia (immuno-allergic), hemolytic-uremic syndrome, hemorrhage, hepatic failure, hepatic sinusoidal obstruction syndrome (SOS; veno-occlusive disease), hepatitis, hepatotoxicity, hypertension, hypomagnesemia, hypoxia, idiopathic noncirrhotic portal hypertension (nodular regenerative hyperplasia), increased INR, increased serum alkaline phosphatase, infusion related reaction (extravasation [including necrosis]), interstitial nephritis (acute), interstitial pulmonary disease, intestinal obstruction, laryngospasm, Lhermittes' sign, metabolic acidosis, muscle spasm, myoclonus, neutropenic enterocolitis, neutropenic infection (sepsis), optic neuritis, pancreatitis, prolonged prothrombin time, purpura, rectal hemorrhage, renal tubular necrosis, reversible posterior leukoencephalopathy syndrome (RPLS), rhabdomyolysis, seizure, sepsis, temporary vision loss, thrombocytopenia (immuno-allergic), trigeminal neuralgia, visual field loss, voice disorder

Drug Interactions

Metabolism/Transport Effects None known.

Avoid Concomitant Use

Avoid concomitant use of Oxaliplatin with any of the following: BCG; CloZAPine; Natalizumab; Pimecrolimus; Tacrolimus (Topical); Tofacitinib; Vaccines (Live)

Increased Effect/Toxicity

Oxaliplatin may increase the levels/effects of: CloZAPine; Leflunomide; Natalizumab; Taxane Derivatives; Tofacitinib; Topotecan; Vaccines (Live); Vitamin K Antagonists

The levels/effects of Oxaliplatin may be increased by: Denosumab; Pimecrolimus; Roflumilast; Tacrolimus (Topical); Trastuzumab

Decreased Effect

Oxaliplatin may decrease the levels/effects of: BCG; Cardiac Glycosides; Coccidioidin Skin Test; Fosphenytoin-Phenytoin; Sipuleucel-T; Vaccines (Inactivated); Vaccines (Live); Vitamin K Antagonists

The levels/effects of Oxaliplatin may be decreased by: Echinacea

Preparation for Administration

Hazardous agent; use appropriate precautions for handling and disposal (NIOSH, 2012).

Do not prepare using a chloride-containing solution such as NaCl due to rapid conversion to monochloroplatinum, dichloroplatinum, and diaquoplatinum; all highly reactive in sodium chloride (Takimoto, 2007). Do not use needles or administration sets containing aluminum during preparation.

Aqueous solution: Dilution with D_5W (250 or 500 mL) is required prior to administration.

Lyophilized powder: Use only SWFI or D_5W to reconstitute powder. To obtain final concentration of 5 mg/mL add 10 mL of diluent to 50 mg vial or 20 mL diluent to 100 mg vial. Gently swirl vial to dissolve powder. Dilution with D_5W (250 or 500 mL) is required prior to administration. Discard unused portion of vial.

Storage/Stability Store intact vials at room temperature of 25°C (77°F); excursions permitted to 15°C to 30°C (59°F to 86°F); do not freeze. Protect concentrated solution from light (store in original outer carton). According to the manufacturer, solutions diluted for infusion are stable up to 6 hours at room temperature of 20°C to 25°C (68°F to 77°F) or up to 24 hours under refrigeration at 2°C to 8°C (36°F to 46°F). Oxaliplatin solution diluted with D_5W to a final concentration of 0.7 mg/mL (polyolefin container) has been shown to retain >90% of the original concentration for up to 30 days when stored at room temperature or refrigerated; artificial light did not affect the concentration (Andre, 2007). As this study did not examine sterility, refrigeration would be preferred to limit microbial growth. Solutions diluted for infusion do not require protection from light.

Mechanism of Action Oxaliplatin, a platinum derivative, is an alkylating agent. Following intracellular hydrolysis, the platinum compound binds to DNA forming cross-links which inhibit DNA replication and transcription, resulting in cell death. Cytotoxicity is cell-cycle nonspecific.

Pharmacodynamics/Kinetics

Distribution: V_d: 440 L

Protein binding: >90% primarily albumin and gamma globulin (irreversible binding to platinum)

Metabolism: Nonenzymatic (rapid and extensive), forms active and inactive derivatives

Half-life elimination: Terminal: 391 hours

Excretion: Urine (~54%); feces (~2%)

Dosage Note: Oxaliplatin is associated with a moderate emetic potential; antiemetics are recommended to prevent nausea and vomiting. Details concerning dosing in combination regimens should also be consulted.

Advanced colorectal cancer: Adults: I.V.: 85 mg/m^2 every 2 weeks until disease progression or unacceptable toxicity (in combination with fluorouracil/leucovorin)

Stage III colon cancer (adjuvant): Adults: I.V.: 85 mg/m^2 every 2 weeks for a total of 6 months (12 cycles; in combination with fluorouracil/leucovorin)

Colon/colorectal cancer (unlabeled doses or combinations): Adults: I.V.: 85 mg/m^2/dose on days 1, 15, and 29 of an 8-week treatment cycle in combination with fluorouracil/leucovorin (Kuebler, 2007) **or** 85 mg/m^2 every 2 weeks in combination with fluorouracil/leucovorin/irinotecan (Falcone, 2007) **or** 130 mg/m^2 every 3 weeks in combination with capecitabine (Cassidy, 2008; Haller, 2011)

Esophageal/gastric cancers (unlabeled use; as part of a combination chemotherapy regimen): Adults: I.V.: 85 mg/m^2 every 2 weeks in combination with docetaxel, leucovorin, and fluorouracil (Al-Batran, 2008) **or** 85 mg/m^2 every 2 weeks in combination with leucovorin and fluorouracil (Conroy, 2010) **or** 130 mg/m^2 every 3 weeks in combination with epirubicin and either capecitabine or fluorouracil (Cunningham, 2008)

or

Gastric cancer: Adults: I.V: 100 mg/m^2 every 2 weeks in combination with leucovorin and fluorouracil (Louvet, 2002) **or** 130 mg/m^2 every 3 weeks in combination with capecitabine (Bang, 2012)

Hepatobiliary cancer, advanced (unlabeled use; as part of a combination chemotherapy regimen): Adults: I.V.: 100 mg/m^2 every 2 weeks (Andre, 2004) **or** 130 mg/m^2 every 3 weeks (Nehls, 2008)

Non-Hodgkin's lymphoma, refractory (unlabeled use; as part of a combination chemotherapy regimen): Adults: I.V.: 25 mg/m^2/day for 4 days every 4 weeks (Tsimberidou, 2008) **or** 100 mg/m^2 every 3 weeks (Lopez, 2008; Rodriguez, 2007) **or** 130 mg/m^2 every 3 weeks (Chau, 2001)

Ovarian cancer, advanced (unlabeled use): Adults: I.V.: 130 mg/m^2 every 3 weeks (Dieras, 2002; Piccart, 2000)

Pancreatic cancer, advanced (unlabeled use; as part of a combination chemotherapy regimen): Adults: I.V.: 85 mg/m^2 every 2 weeks (Conroy, 2005; Conroy, 2011; Pelzer, 2011) **or** 100 mg/m^2 every 2 weeks (Louvet, 2005) **or** 110-130 mg/m^2 every 3 weeks (Xiong, 2008)

Testicular cancer, refractory (unlabeled use): Adults: I.V.: 130 mg/m^2 every 3 weeks in combination with gemcitabine (De Georgi, 2006; Kollmannsberger, 2004; Pectasides, 2004) **or** 130 mg/m^2 every 3 weeks in combination with gemcitabine and paclitaxel) (Bokemeyer, 2008)

Elderly: No dosage adjustment recommended; refer to adult dosing.

Dosage adjustments for toxicity: Acute toxicities: Longer infusion time (6 hours) may mitigate acute toxicities (eg, pharyngolaryngeal dysesthesia).

Neurosensory events:

Persistent (>7 days) grade 2 neurosensory events:

Adjuvant treatment of stage III colon cancer: Reduce dose to 75 mg/m^2

Advanced colorectal cancer: Reduce dose to 65 mg/m^2

Consider withholding oxaliplatin for grade 2 neuropathy lasting >7 days despite dose reduction.

Persistent (>7 days) grade 3 neurosensory events:

U.S. labeling: Consider discontinuing oxaliplatin.

Canadian labeling:

Adjuvant treatment of stage III colon cancer: Discontinue oxaliplatin.

Advanced colorectal cancer: Reduce dose to 65 mg/m^2; if not resolved prior to next cycle, then discontinue.

Gastrointestinal toxicity (grade 3/4):

Adjuvant treatment of stage III colon cancer: Delay next dose until recovery from toxicity, then reduce dose to 75 mg/m^2.

Advanced colorectal cancer: Delay next dose until recovery from toxicity, then reduce dose to 65 mg/m^2.

Hematologic toxicity (grade 4 neutropenia or grade 3/4 thrombocytopenia):

Adjuvant treatment of stage III colon cancer: Delay next dose until neutrophils recover to ≥1500/mm^3 and platelets recover to ≥75,000/mm^3, then reduce dose to 75 mg/m^2.

Advanced colorectal cancer: Delay next dose until neutrophils recover to ≥1500/mm^3 and platelets recover to ≥75,000/mm^3, then reduce dose to 65 mg/m^2.

Pulmonary toxicity (unexplained respiratory symptoms including nonproductive cough, dyspnea, crackles, pulmonary infiltrates): Discontinue until interstitial lung disease or pulmonary fibrosis have been excluded.

Dosage adjustment in renal impairment:

Manufacturer's recommendations:

U.S. labeling:

Cl_{cr} ≥30 mL/minute: No dosage adjustment necessary.

Cl_{cr} <30 mL/minute: Reduce dose from 85 mg/m^2 to 65 mg/m^2.

Canadian labeling: Cl_{cr} <30 mL/minute: Use is contraindicated.

Alternate recommendations: Cl_{cr} ≥20 mL/minute: In a study with a limited number of patients with mild-to-moderate impairment, defined by the authors as Cl_{cr} 20-59 mL/minute (determined using 24-hour urine collection), oxaliplatin was well-tolerated, suggesting a dose reduction may not be necessary in patients with Cl_{cr} ≥20 mL/minute receiving every-3-week dosing (dose range: 80-130 mg/m^2 every 3 weeks) (Takimoto, 2003).

Dosage adjustment in hepatic impairment: Mild, moderate, or severe impairment: No dosage adjustment necessary (Doroshow, 2003; Synold, 2007).

Dosing in obesity: *ASCO Guidelines for appropriate chemotherapy dosing in obese adults with cancer:* Utilize patient's actual body weight (full weight) for calculation of body surface area- or weight-based dosing, particularly when the intent of therapy is curative; manage regimen-related toxicities in the same manner as for nonobese patients; if a dose reduction is utilized due to toxicity, consider resumption of full weight-based dosing with subsequent cycles, especially if cause of toxicity (eg, hepatic or renal impairment) is resolved (Griggs, 2012).

Administration Administer as I.V. infusion over 2 hours; extend infusion time to 6 hours for acute toxicities. Flush infusion line with D_5W prior to administration of any concomitant medication. Patients should receive an antiemetic premedication regimen. Avoid mucositis prophylaxis with ice chips during oxaliplatin infusion (may exacerbate acute neurological symptoms). Do not use needles or administration sets containing aluminum.

Oxaliplatin is associated with a moderate emetic potential; antiemetics are recommended to prevent nausea and vomiting.

Irritant with vesicant-like properties; ensure proper needle or catheter placement prior to and during infusion. Avoid extravasation; monitor I.V. site for redness, swelling, or pain.

Extravasation management: If extravasation occurs, stop infusion immediately and disconnect (leave cannula/needle in place); gently aspirate extravasated solution (do **NOT** flush the line); remove needle/cannula; elevate extremity. Information conflicts regarding use of warm or cold compresses. Cold compresses could potentially precipitate or exacerbate peripheral neuropathy (de Lemos, 2005).

Hazardous agent; use appropriate precautions for handling and disposal (NIOSH, 2012).

Monitoring Parameters CBC with differential, blood chemistries (including serum creatinine, ALT, AST, and bilirubin); INR and prothrombin time (in patients on oral anticoagulant therapy); signs of neuropathy, hypersensitivity, respiratory effects, and/or RPLS

Dosage Forms Excipient information presented when available (limited, particularly for generics); consult specific product labeling.

Solution, Intravenous [preservative free]:
- Eloxatin: 50 mg/10 mL (10 mL); 100 mg/20 mL (20 mL); 200 mg/40 mL (40 mL)
- Generic: 50 mg/10 mL (10 mL); 100 mg/20 mL (20 mL)

Solution Reconstituted, Intravenous [preservative free]:
- Generic: 50 mg (1 ea); 100 mg (1 ea)

◆ **Oxandrin** *see* Oxandrolone *on page 1527*

Oxandrolone (oks AN droe lone)

Brand Names: U.S. Oxandrin

Pharmacologic Category Androgen

Use Adjunctive therapy to promote weight gain after weight loss following extensive surgery, chronic infections, or severe trauma, and in some patients who, without definite pathophysiologic reasons, fail to gain or to maintain normal weight; to offset protein catabolism with prolonged corticosteroid administration; relief of bone pain associated with osteoporosis

Pregnancy Risk Factor X

Dosage

Children: Total daily dose: ≤0.1 mg/kg; may be repeated intermittently as needed

Adults: 2.5-20 mg in divided doses 2-4 times daily based on individual response; a course of therapy of 2-4 weeks is usually adequate. This may be repeated intermittently as needed.

Elderly: 5 mg twice daily

Dosing adjustment in renal impairment: No dosage adjustment provided in manufacturer's labeling; use with caution due to propensity to cause edema.

Dosing adjustment in hepatic impairment: No dosage adjustment provided in manufacturer's labeling; use with caution.

Additional Information Complete prescribing information should be consulted for additional detail.

Dosage Forms Excipient information presented when available (limited, particularly for generics); consult specific product labeling.

Tablet, Oral:
- Oxandrin: 2.5 mg [scored]
- Oxandrin: 10 mg
- Generic: 2.5 mg, 10 mg

Controlled Substance C-III

Oxaprozin (oks a PROE zin)

Brand Names: U.S. Daypro

Brand Names: Canada Apo-Oxaprozin®; Daypro®

Pharmacologic Category Nonsteroidal Anti-inflammatory Drug (NSAID), Oral

Additional Appendix Information

Beers Criteria – Potentially Inappropriate Medications for Geriatrics *on page 2368*

Use Management of signs and symptoms of osteoarthritis, rheumatoid arthritis, and juvenile idiopathic arthritis (JIA)

Pregnancy Risk Factor C

Pregnancy Considerations Adverse events were not observed in the initial animal reproduction studies; therefore, the manufacturer classifies oxaprozin as pregnancy category C. NSAID exposure during the first trimester is not strongly associated with congenital malformations; however, cardiovascular anomalies and cleft palate have been observed following NSAID exposure in some studies. The use of an NSAID close to conception may be associated with an increased risk of miscarriage. Nonteratogenic effects have been observed following NSAID administration during the third trimester including myocardial degenerative changes, prenatal constriction of the ductus arteriosus, fetal tricuspid regurgitation, failure of the ductus arteriosus to close postnatally; renal dysfunction or failure, oligohydramnios; gastrointestinal bleeding or perforation, increased risk of necrotizing enterocolitis; intracranial bleeding (including intraventricular hemorrhage), platelet dysfunction with resultant bleeding; pulmonary hypertension. Because they may cause premature closure of the ductus arteriosus, use of NSAIDs late in pregnancy should be avoided (use after 31 or 32 weeks gestation is not recommended by some clinicians). The chronic use of NSAIDs in women of reproductive age may be associated with infertility that is reversible upon discontinuation of the medication. A registry is available for pregnant women exposed to autoimmune medications ▶

including oxaprozin. For additional information, contact the Organization of Teratology Information Specialists, OTIS Autoimmune Diseases Study, at 877-311-8972.

Breast-Feeding Considerations The amount of oxaprozin found in breast milk is not known; however, distribution into breast milk would be expected. Breast-feeding is not recommended by the manufacturer.

Medication Guide Available Yes

Contraindications Hypersensitivity to oxaprozin, aspirin, other NSAIDs, or any component of the formulation; perioperative pain in the setting of coronary artery bypass graft (CABG) surgery

Warnings/Precautions [U.S. Boxed Warning]: NSAIDs are associated with an increased risk of adverse cardiovascular thrombotic events, including MI and stroke. Risk may be increased with duration of use or pre-existing cardiovascular risk factors or disease. Carefully evaluate individual cardiovascular risk profiles prior to prescribing. May cause new onset hypertension or worsening of existing hypertension. Use caution with fluid retention. Avoid use in heart failure. Concurrent administration of ibuprofen, and potentially other nonselective NSAIDs, may interfere with aspirin' s cardioprotective effect. **[U.S. Boxed Warning]: Use is contraindicated for treatment of perioperative pain in the setting of coronary artery bypass graft (CABG) surgery.** Risk of MI and stroke may be increased with use following CABG surgery.

Platelet adhesion and aggregation may be decreased; may prolong bleeding time; patients with coagulation disorders or who are receiving anticoagulants should be monitored closely. Anemia may occur; patients on long-term NSAID therapy should be monitored for anemia. Rarely, NSAID use may cause severe blood dyscrasias (eg, agranulocytosis, aplastic anemia, thrombocytopenia).

NSAID use may compromise existing renal function; dose-dependent decreases in prostaglandin synthesis may result from NSAID use, reducing renal blood flow which may cause renal decompensation. NSAID use may increase the risk for hyperkalemia. Patients with impaired renal function, dehydration, heart failure, liver dysfunction, those taking diuretics, and ACE inhibitors, and the elderly are at greater risk of renal toxicity and hyperkalemia. In the elderly, may be inappropriate for long-term use due to potential for GI bleeding, hypertension, heart failure, and renal failure (Beers Criteria). Rehydrate patient before starting therapy; monitor renal function closely. Not recommended for use in patients with advanced renal disease. Long-term NSAID use may result in renal papillary necrosis.

[U.S. Boxed Warning]: NSAIDs may increase risk of gastrointestinal irritation, inflammation, ulceration, bleeding, and perforation. These events may occur at any time during therapy and without warning. Use caution with a history of GI disease (bleeding or ulcers); concurrent therapy with aspirin, anticoagulants, and/or corticosteroids; smoking; use of alcohol; and the elderly or debilitated patients. When used concomitantly with ≤325 mg of aspirin, a substantial increase in the risk of gastrointestinal complications (eg, ulcer) occurs; concomitant gastroprotective therapy (eg, proton pump inhibitors) is recommended (Bhatt, 2008).

Use the lowest effective dose for the shortest duration of time, consistent with individual patient goals, to reduce risk of cardiovascular or GI adverse events. Alternate therapies should be considered for patients at high risk.

NSAIDs may cause serious skin adverse events including exfoliative dermatitis, Stevens-Johnson syndrome (SJS), and toxic epidermal necrolysis (TEN); discontinue use at first sign of skin rash or hypersensitivity. Anaphylactoid reactions may occur, even without prior exposure; patients with "aspirin triad" (bronchial asthma, aspirin intolerance, rhinitis) may be at increased risk. Do not use in patients who experience bronchospasm, asthma, rhinitis, or urticaria with NSAID or aspirin therapy. Use caution in other forms of asthma.

Use with caution in patients with decreased hepatic function. Closely monitor patients with any abnormal LFT. Severe hepatic reactions (eg, fulminant hepatitis, liver failure) have occurred with NSAID use, rarely; discontinue if signs or symptoms of liver disease develop, or if systemic manifestations occur.

NSAIDS may cause drowsiness, dizziness, blurred vision and other neurologic effects which may impair physical or mental abilities; patients must be cautioned about performing tasks which require mental alertness (eg, operating machinery or driving). Discontinue use with blurred or diminished vision and perform ophthalmologic exam. Monitor vision with long-term therapy.

In the elderly, avoid chronic use (unless alternative agents ineffective and patient can receive concomitant gastroprotective agent); nonselective oral NSAID use is associated with an increased risk of GI bleeding and peptic ulcer disease in older adults in high risk category (eg, >75 years or age or receiving concomitant oral/parenteral corticosteroids, anticoagulants, or antiplatelet agents) (Beers Criteria).

Withhold for at least 4-6 half-lives prior to surgical or dental procedures. May cause mild photosensitivity reactions.

Adverse Reactions

1% to 10%:

Cardiovascular: Edema

Central nervous system: Confusion, depression, dizziness, headache, sedation, sleep disturbance, somnolence

Dermatologic: Pruritus, rash

Gastrointestinal: Abdominal distress, abdominal pain, anorexia, constipation, diarrhea, dyspepsia, flatulence, gastrointestinal ulcer, gross bleeding with perforation, heartburn, nausea, vomiting

Hematologic: Anemia, bleeding time increased

Hepatic: Liver enzymes increased

Otic: Tinnitus

Renal: Dysuria, renal function abnormal, urinary frequency

<1% (Limited to important or life-threatening; effects reported with oxaprozin or other NSAIDs): Acute interstitial nephritis, acute renal failure, agranulocytosis, alopecia, anaphylaxis, angioedema, anxiety, aplastic anemia, appetite changes, arrhythmia, asthma, blurred vision, bruising, coma, conjunctivitis, cystitis, death, diaphoresis, dream abnormalities, drowsiness, dyspnea, eosinophilia, eructation, erythema multiforme, esophagitis, exfoliative dermatitis, fever, gastritis, GI bleeding, glossitis, hallucinations, hearing decreased, heart failure, hematemesis, hematuria, hemolytic anemia, hemorrhoidal bleeding, hepatitis, hyperglycemia, hypersensitivity reaction, hyper-/hypotension, infection, insomnia, jaundice, leukopenia, liver failure, liver function abnormalities, lymphadenopathy, malaise, melena, meningitis, menstrual flow increased/decreased, myocardial infarction, nephrotic syndrome, nervousness, oliguria, palpitation, pancreatitis, pancytopenia, paresthesia, peptic ulcer, photosensitivity, pneumonia, polyuria, proteinuria, pseudoporphyria, pulmonary infection, purpura, rectal bleeding, renal insufficiency, respiratory depression, seizures, sepsis, serum sickness, sinusitis, Stevens-Johnson syndrome, stomatitis, syncope, tachycardia, taste alteration, thrombocytopenia, toxic epidermal necrolysis, tremor, upper respiratory tract infection, urticaria, vasculitis, vertigo, weakness, weight changes, xerostomia

Drug Interactions

Metabolism/Transport Effects None known.

Avoid Concomitant Use

Avoid concomitant use of Oxaprozin with any of the following: Floctafenine; Ketorolac (Nasal); Ketorolac (Systemic); NSAID (COX-2 Inhibitor); Omacetaxine

Increased Effect/Toxicity

Oxaprozin may increase the levels/effects of: 5-ASA Derivatives; Agents with Antiplatelet Properties; Aliskiren; Aminoglycosides; Anticoagulants; Bisphosphonate Derivatives; Collagenase (Systemic); CycloSPORINE (Systemic); Dabigatran Etexilate; Deferasirox; Desmopressin; Digoxin; Eplerenone; Haloperidol; Ibritumomab; Lithium; Methotrexate; Nonsteroidal Anti-Inflammatory Agents; NSAID (COX-2 Inhibitor); Omacetaxine; PEMEtrexed; Porfimer; Potassium-Sparing Diuretics; PRALAtrexate; Quinolone Antibiotics; Rivaroxaban; Salicylates; Tenofovir; Thrombolytic Agents; Tositumomab and Iodine I 131 Tositumomab; Vancomycin; Vitamin K Antagonists

The levels/effects of Oxaprozin may be increased by: ACE Inhibitors; Angiotensin II Receptor Blockers; Antidepressants (Tricyclic, Tertiary Amine); Corticosteroids (Systemic); CycloSPORINE (Systemic); Dasatinib; Floctafenine; Glucosamine; Herbs (Anticoagulant/Antiplatelet Properties); Ibrutinib; Ketorolac (Nasal); Ketorolac (Systemic); Multivitamins/Fluoride (with ADE); Multivitamins/Minerals (with ADEK, Folate, Iron); Multivitamins/Minerals (with AE, No Iron); Nonsteroidal Anti-Inflammatory Agents; Omega-3 Fatty Acids; Pentosan Polysulfate Sodium; Pentoxifylline; Probenecid; Prostacyclin Analogues; Selective Serotonin Reuptake Inhibitors; Serotonin/Norepinephrine Reuptake Inhibitors; Sodium Phosphates; Tipranavir; Treprostinil; Vitamin E

Decreased Effect

Oxaprozin may decrease the levels/effects of: ACE Inhibitors; Agents with Antiplatelet Properties; Aliskiren; Angiotensin II Receptor Blockers; Beta-Blockers; Eplerenone; HydrALAZINE; Loop Diuretics; Potassium-Sparing Diuretics; Prostaglandins (Ophthalmic); Salicylates; Selective Serotonin Reuptake Inhibitors; Thiazide Diuretics

The levels/effects of Oxaprozin may be decreased by: Bile Acid Sequestrants; Nonsteroidal Anti-Inflammatory Agents; Salicylates

Ethanol/Nutrition/Herb Interactions

Ethanol: Avoid ethanol (may enhance gastric mucosal irritation).

Herb/Nutraceutical: Avoid alfalfa, anise, bilberry, bladderwrack, bromelain, cat's claw, celery, chamomile, coleus, cordyceps, dong quai, evening primrose, fenugreek, feverfew, garlic, ginger, ginkgo biloba, ginseng (American, Panax, Siberian), grapeseed, green tea, guggul, horse chestnut seed, horseradish, licorice, prickly ash, red clover, reishi, SAMe (S-adenosylmethionine), sweet clover, turmeric, white willow (all have additional antiplatelet activity).

Storage/Stability Store at 25°C (77°F); excursions permitted to 15°C to 30°C (59°F to 86°C). Protect from light; keep bottle tightly closed.

Mechanism of Action Reversibly inhibits cyclooxygenase-1 and 2 (COX-1 and 2) enzymes, which results in decreased formation of prostaglandin precursors; has antipyretic, analgesic, and anti-inflammatory properties.

Other proposed mechanisms not fully elucidated (and possibly contributing to the anti-inflammatory effect to varying degrees) include inhibiting chemotaxis, altering lymphocyte activity, inhibiting neutrophil aggregation/activation, and decreasing proinflammatory cytokine levels.

Pharmacodynamics/Kinetics

Absorption: Oral: 95%

Distribution: V_d: 11-17 L/70 kg

Protein binding: 99% primarily to albumin

Metabolism: Hepatic via oxidation and glucuronidation; no active metabolites

Half-life elimination: 41-55 hours

Time to peak: 2-3 hours

Excretion: Urine (5% unchanged, 65% as metabolites); feces (35% as metabolites)

Dosage Oral: **Note:** Individualize dosage to lowest effective dose for the shortest duration to minimize adverse effects.

Children 6-16 years: Juvenile idiopathic arthritis (JIA):
- 22-31 kg: 600 mg once daily
- 32-54 kg: 900 mg once daily
- ≥55 kg: 1200 mg once daily

Adults: Osteoarthritis, rheumatoid arthritis: 1200 mg once daily. **Note:** Patients with low body weight should start with 600 mg daily. A one-time loading dose of 1200-1800 mg (≤26 mg/kg) may be used when a quick onset of action is desired.

Maximum doses:
- Patient <50 kg: Maximum: 1200 mg daily
- Patient >50 kg with normal renal/hepatic function and low risk of peptic ulcer: Maximum: 1800 mg daily or 26 mg/kg/day (whichever is lower) in divided doses

Dosing adjustment in renal impairment: In general, NSAIDs are not recommended for use in patients with advanced renal disease but the manufacturer of oxaprozin does provide some guidelines for adjustment in renal dysfunction.

Severe renal impairment or on dialysis: 600 mg once daily; may increase cautiously to 1200 mg daily with close monitoring

Dosing adjustment in hepatic impairment: Use caution in patients with severe hepatic impairment.

Monitoring Parameters Blood pressure; CBC; signs/symptoms of GI bleeding; hepatic and renal function

Test Interactions False-positive urine immunoassay screening tests for benzodiazepines have been reported and may occur several days after discontinuing oxaprozin.

Dosage Forms Excipient information presented when available (limited, particularly for generics); consult specific product labeling.

Tablet, Oral:
- Daypro: 600 mg [scored]
- Generic: 600 mg

Oxazepam (oks A ze pam)

Brand Names: Canada Apo-Oxazepam®; Bio-Oxazepam; Novoxapram®; Oxpam®; Oxpram®; PMS-Oxazepam; Riva-Oxazepam

Index Terms Serax

Pharmacologic Category Benzodiazepine

Additional Appendix Information

Beers Criteria – Potentially Inappropriate Medications for Geriatrics *on page 2368*

Benzodiazepine Comparison Table *on page 2292*

Use Management of anxiety disorders, including anxiety associated with depression; management of ethanol withdrawal

Dosage Oral:

Children >12 years, Adolescents, and Adults:
- Anxiety, mild-to-moderate: 10-15 mg 3-4 times daily
- Anxiety, severe or associated with depression: 15-30 mg 3-4 times daily
- Ethanol withdrawal: 15-30 mg 3-4 times daily

Elderly: Anxiety: Initial: 10 mg 3 times daily. If necessary, increase cautiously to 15 mg 3-4 times daily. Dose titration should be slow to evaluate sensitivity.

Dosage adjustment in renal impairment: No dosage adjustment provided in manufacturer's labeling

Hemodialysis: Not dialyzable (0% to 5%) (Greenblatt, 1981; Mokhlesi, 2003)

Dosage adjustment in hepatic impairment: No dosage adjustment provided in manufacturer's labeling; however, pharmacokinetic studies have shown that hepatic dysfunction is not expected to significantly decrease clearance (Furlan, 1999; Greenblatt, 1981).

Additional Information Complete prescribing information should be consulted for additional detail.

Dosage Forms Excipient information presented when available (limited, particularly for generics); consult specific product labeling.

Capsule, Oral:

Generic: 10 mg, 15 mg, 30 mg

Controlled Substance C-IV

OXcarbazepine (ox car BAZ e peen)

Brand Names: U.S. Oxtellar XR; Trileptal

Brand Names: Canada Apo-Oxcarbazepine®; Trileptal®

Index Terms GP 47680; OCBZ

Pharmacologic Category Anticonvulsant, Miscellaneous

Use

Oxtellar XR™: Adjunctive therapy in the treatment of partial seizures in patients with epilepsy

Trileptal®: Monotherapy or adjunctive therapy in the treatment of partial seizures in patients with epilepsy

Unlabeled Use Bipolar disorder; treatment of neuropathic pain

Pregnancy Risk Factor C

Pregnancy Considerations Adverse events have been observed in animal reproduction studies; therefore, the manufacturer classifies oxcarbazepine as pregnancy category C. Oxcarbazepine, the active metabolite MHD and the inactive metabolite DHD, crosses the placenta and can be detected in the newborn. An increased risk in the overall rate of major congenital malformations has not been observed following maternal use of oxcarbazepine. Available studies have not been large enough to determine if there is an increased risk of specific defects. In general, the risk of teratogenic effects is higher with AED polytherapy than monotherapy. Plasma concentrations of MHD gradually decrease due to physiologic changes which occur during pregnancy; patients should be monitored during pregnancy and postpartum. Oxcarbazepine may decrease plasma concentrations of hormonal contraceptives.

Patients exposed to oxcarbazepine during pregnancy are encouraged to enroll themselves into the AED Pregnancy Registry by calling 1-888-233-2334. Additional information is available at www.aedpregnancyregistry.org.

Breast-Feeding Considerations Oxcarbazepine and the active 10-hydroxy metabolite (MHD) are found in breast milk (small amounts). According to the manufacturer, the decision to continue or discontinue breast-feeding during therapy should take into account the risk of exposure to the infant and the benefits of treatment to the mother.

Medication Guide Available Yes

Contraindications Hypersensitivity to oxcarbazepine or any component of the formulation

Warnings/Precautions Hazardous agent - use appropriate precautions for handling and disposal (NIOSH, 2012). Antiepileptics are associated with an increased risk of suicidal behavior/thoughts with use (regardless of indication); patients should be monitored for signs/symptoms of depression, suicidal tendencies, and other unusual behavior changes during therapy and instructed to inform their healthcare provider immediately if symptoms occur.

Clinically-significant hyponatremia (serum sodium <125 mmol/L) may develop during oxcarbazepine use. Rare cases of anaphylaxis and angioedema have been reported, even after initial dosing; permanently discontinue should symptoms occur. Use caution in patients with previous hypersensitivity to carbamazepine (cross-sensitivity occurs in 25% to 30% of patients). Potentially serious, sometimes fatal, dermatologic reactions (eg, Stevens-Johnson, toxic epidermal necrolysis) and multiorgan hypersensitivity reactions have been reported in adults and children; monitor for signs and symptoms of skin reactions and possible disparate manifestations associated with lymphatic, hepatic, renal, and/or hematologic organ systems; discontinuation and conversion to alternate therapy may be required. As with all antiepileptic drugs, oxcarbazepine should be withdrawn gradually to minimize the potential of increased seizure frequency. Use of oxcarbazepine has been associated with CNS-related adverse events, most significant of these were cognitive symptoms including psychomotor slowing, difficulty with concentration, speech or language problems, somnolence or fatigue, and coordination abnormalities, including ataxia and gait disturbances. Effects with other sedative drugs or ethanol may be potentiated. Single-dose studies show that half-life of the primary active metabolite is prolonged three- to fourfold and AUC is doubled in patients with Cl_{cr} <30 mL/minute; dose adjustment required in these patients. May reduce the efficacy of oral contraceptives (nonhormonal contraceptive measures are recommended). Agranulocytosis, leukopenia, and pancytopenia have been reported with use (rare). Discontinuation and conversion to alternate therapy may be required.

Adverse Reactions Incidence in children was similar.

>10%:

Central nervous system: Dizziness (22% to 49%), drowsiness (20% to 36%), headache (13% to 32%), ataxia (1% to 31%), fatigue (12% to 15%), vertigo (6% to 15%)

Gastrointestinal: Vomiting (7% to 36%), nausea (15% to 29%), abdominal pain (10% to 13%)

Neuromuscular & skeletal: Abnormal gait (5% to 17%), tremor (3% to 16%)

Ophthalmic: Diplopia (14% to 40%), nystagmus (7% to 26%), visual disturbance (4% to 14%)

1% to 10%:

Cardiovascular: Hypotension (≤2%), lower extremity edema (1% to 2%)

Central nervous system: Nervousness (2% to 5%), amnesia (4%), abnormality in thinking (≤4%), insomnia (2% to 4%), fever (3%), dysmetria (1% to 3%), speech disorder (1% to 3%), feeling abnormal (≤2%), abnormal electroencephalogram (≤2%), agitation (1% to 2%), confusion (1% to 2%)

Dermatologic: Skin rash (4%), acne vulgaris (1% to 2%)

Endocrine & metabolic: Hyponatremia (1% to 3%)

Gastrointestinal: Diarrhea (5% to 7%), dyspepsia (5% to 6%), constipation (2% to 6%), dysgeusia (5%), xerostomia (3%), gastritis (1% to 2%), weight gain (1% to 2%)

Genitourinary: Urinary frequency (2%)

Neuromuscular & skeletal: Weakness (3% to 6%), back pain (4%), falling (4%), sprain (≤2%), myasthenia (1% to 2%)

Ophthalmic: Accommodation disturbance (≤2%)

Respiratory: Upper respiratory tract infection (7%), rhinitis (2% to 5%), pulmonary infection (4%), epistaxis (4%), sinusitis (4%)

Postmarketing and/or case reports (Limited to important or life-threatening): Aggressive behavior, alopecia, anaphylaxis, angioedema, anxiety, aphasia, aphthous stomatitis, aplastic anemia, biliary colic, blepharoptosis, bradycardia, bruise, cardiac failure, cerebral hemorrhage, chest pain, cholelithiasis, colitis, conjunctival hemorrhage, delirium, delusion, dysphagia, dyspnea, dystonia, dysuria, emotional lability, enteritis, erythema multiforme, erythematosus rash, esophagitis, extrapyramidal reaction, gingival hemorrhage, gingival hyperplasia, hematuria, hemianopia, hemiplegia, hematemesis, hypersensitivity reaction, hypertension, hypocalcemia, hypoesthesia, hypokalemia, hypothyroidism, hysteria, impaired consciousness, increased gamma-glutamyl transferase, increased liver enzymes, increased serum amylase, increased serum lipase, laryngismus, leukopenia, leukorrhea, maculopapular rash, manic behavior, multiorgan hypersensitivity (eosinophilia, arthralgia, rash, fever, lymphadenopathy), muscle spasm, mydriasis, nephrolithiasis, neuralgia, nightmares, ocular edema, oculogyric crisis, orthostatic hypotension, palpitations, pancreatitis, pancytopenia, panic disorder, paralysis, photophobia, pleurisy, priapism, purpura, psychosis, renal pain, right hypochondrium pain, rigors, scotoma, seizure (aggravated), sialoadenitis, skin photosensitivity, Stevens-Johnson syndrome, stupor, suicidal ideation, suicidal tendencies, syncope, systemic lupus erythematosus, tachycardia, tetany, thrombocytopenia, toxic epidermal necrolysis, urinary tract pain, urticaria, vitiligo, voice disorder, weight loss, xerophthalmia

Drug Interactions

Metabolism/Transport Effects **Induces** CYP3A4 (strong)

Avoid Concomitant Use

Avoid concomitant use of OXcarbazepine with any of the following: Abiraterone Acetate; Apixaban; Artemether; Axitinib; Bedaquiline; Boceprevir; Bortezomib; Bosutinib; Cabozantinib; CloZAPine; Crizotinib; Dienogest; Dolutegravir; Dronedarone; Enzalutamide; Everolimus; Ibrutinib; Itraconazole; Ivacaftor; Lapatinib; Lumefantrine; Lurasidone; Macitentan; Mifepristone; NIFEdipine; Nilotinib; Nisoldipine; PAZOPanib; Pomalidomide; PONATinib; Praziquantel; Ranolazine; Regorafenib; Rilpivirine; Rivaroxaban; Roflumilast; RomiDEPsin; Selegiline; Simeprevir; Sofosbuvir; SORAfenib; Telaprevir; Ticagrelor; Tofacitinib; Tolvaptan; Toremifene; Ulipristal; Vandetanib; Vemurafenib; VinCRIStine (Liposomal)

Increased Effect/Toxicity

OXcarbazepine may increase the levels/effects of: Clarithromycin; Fosphenytoin-Phenytoin; Ifosfamide; PHENobarbital; Selegiline

The levels/effects of OXcarbazepine may be increased by: Clarithromycin; Perampanel; Thiazide Diuretics

Decreased Effect

OXcarbazepine may decrease the levels/effects of: Abiraterone Acetate; Apixaban; ARIPiprazole; Artemether; Axitinib; Bedaquiline; Boceprevir; Bortezomib; Bosutinib; Brentuximab Vedotin; Cabozantinib; Clarithromycin; CloZAPine; Cobicistat; Contraceptives (Estrogens); Contraceptives (Progestins); Crizotinib; CYP3A4 Substrates; Dasatinib; Dienogest; Dolutegravir; Dronedarone; Elvitegravir; Enzalutamide; Everolimus; Exemestane; Gefitinib; GuanFACINE; Ibrutinib; Imatinib; Itraconazole; Ivacaftor; Ixabepilone; Lapatinib; Linagliptin; Lumefantrine; Lurasidone; Macitentan; Maraviroc; Mifepristone; NIFEdipine; Nilotinib; Nisoldipine; PAZOPanib; Perampanel; Pomalidomide; PONATinib; Praziquantel; QUEtiapine; Ranolazine; Regorafenib; Rilpivirine; Rivaroxaban; Roflumilast; RomiDEPsin; Saxagliptin; Simeprevir; Sofosbuvir; SORAfenib; SUNItinib; Tadalafil; Telaprevir; Ticagrelor; Tofacitinib; Tolvaptan; Toremifene; Ulipristal; Vandetanib; Vemurafenib; VinCRIStine (Liposomal); Vortioxetine; Zuclopenthixol

The levels/effects of OXcarbazepine may be decreased by: CarBAMazepine; Fosphenytoin-Phenytoin; Ketorolac (Nasal); Ketorolac (Systemic); Mefloquine; Orlistat; PHENobarbital; Valproic Acid and Derivatives

Ethanol/Nutrition/Herb Interactions

Ethanol: Avoid ethanol (may increase CNS depression).

Herb/Nutraceutical: St John's wort may decrease oxcarbazepine levels. Avoid evening primrose (seizure threshold decreased). Avoid valerian, St John's wort, kava kava, gotu kola.

Storage/Stability Store tablets and suspension at 25°C (77°F); excursions permitted to 15°C to 30°C (59°F to 86°F). Use suspension within 7 weeks of first opening container.

Mechanism of Action Pharmacological activity results from both oxcarbazepine and its monohydroxy metabolite (MHD). Precise mechanism of anticonvulsant effect has not been defined. Oxcarbazepine and MHD block voltage-sensitive sodium channels, stabilizing hyperexcited neuronal membranes, inhibiting repetitive firing, and decreasing the propagation of synaptic impulses. These actions are believed to prevent the spread of seizures. Oxcarbazepine and MHD also increase potassium conductance and modulate the activity of high-voltage activated calcium channels.

Pharmacodynamics/Kinetics

Absorption: Complete

Distribution: MHD: V_d: 49 L

Protein binding, serum: MHD: ~40% (primarily to albumin)

Metabolism: Extensive to 10-monohydroxy metabolite (MHD; active); MHD is further glucuronidated or oxidized to a 10,11-dihydroxy metabolite (DHD; inactive)

Bioavailability: Immediate release: Decreased in children <8 years; increased in elderly >60 years

Half-life elimination: Immediate release: Parent drug: 2 hours; MHD: 9 hours; renal impairment (Cl_{cr} 30 mL/minute): MHD: 19 hours; Extended release: Parent drug: 7-11 hours; MHD: 9-11 hours

Clearance of MHD is increased in younger children (~80% in children 2-4 years of age) and approaches that of adults by ~13 years of age

Time to peak, serum (median): Immediate release: Tablets: 4.5 hours; Oral suspension: 6 hours

Excretion: Urine (95%, <1% as unchanged oxcarbazepine, 27% as unchanged MHD, 49% as MHD glucuronides); feces (<4%)

Dosage Adjunctive therapy, partial seizures (epilepsy): Oral:

Children 2-3 years: Immediate release (Trileptal®):

Initial: 8-10 mg/kg/day, not to exceed 600 mg daily, given in 2 divided daily doses

Maintenance: The target maintenance dose should be achieved over 2-4 weeks, and is dependent upon patient weight (should not exceed 60 mg/kg/day given in 2 divided daily doses).

<20 kg: Consider initiating dose at 16-20 mg/kg/day; maximum maintenance dose should be achieved over 2-4 weeks and should not exceed 60 mg/kg/day

Children 4-16 years: Immediate release (Trileptal®):

Initial: 8-10 mg/kg/day, not to exceed 600 mg daily, given in 2 divided daily doses

Maintenance: The target maintenance dose should be achieved over 2 weeks, and is dependent upon patient weight, according to the following:

20-29 kg: 900 mg daily in 2 divided doses

29.1-39 kg: 1200 mg daily in 2 divided doses

>39 kg: 1800 mg daily in 2 divided doses

Children 6-17 years: Extended release (Oxtellar XR™):

Initial: 8-10 mg/kg once daily (not to exceed 600 mg daily in the first week)

Maintenance: The target maintenance dose should be achieved over 2-3 weeks with dose increases of 8-10 mg/kg/day increments at weekly intervals. Target maintenance dose depends on weight:

20-29 kg: 900 mg once daily

29.1-39 kg: 1200 mg once daily

>39 kg: 1800 mg once daily

Adults:

Immediate release (Trileptal®): Initial: 600 mg daily in 2 divided doses; dose may be increased by as much as 600 mg/day increments at weekly intervals; recommended daily dose: 1200 mg daily in 2 divided doses. Although daily doses >1200 mg daily were somewhat more efficacious, most patients were unable to tolerate 2400 mg daily (due to CNS effects).

Extended release (Oxtellar XR™): Initial: 600 mg once daily; dosage may be increased by 600 mg/day increments at weekly intervals. Recommended daily dose is 1200-2400 mg once daily. Although daily doses >1200 mg daily were somewhat more efficacious, most patients were unable to tolerate 2400 mg daily (due to CNS effects).

Elderly: Extended release (Oxtellar XR™): Initial: 300 mg or 450 mg once daily should be considered; dosage may be increased by 300-450 mg daily increments at weekly intervals to desired clinical response; do not exceed 2400 mg daily.

Conversion to monotherapy, partial seizures (epilepsy): Patients receiving concomitant antiepileptic drugs (AEDs):

Children 4-16 years: Immediate release (Trileptal®): Initial: 8-10 mg/kg/day in twice daily divided doses, while simultaneously initiating the dose reduction of concomitant antiepileptic drugs; the concomitant drugs should be withdrawn over 3-6 weeks. Oxcarbazepine dose may be increased by a maximum of 10 mg/kg/day at weekly intervals. See below for recommended total daily dose by weight.

Adults: Immediate release (Trileptal®): Initial: 600 mg daily in 2 divided doses while simultaneously reducing the dose of concomitant AEDs. Withdraw concomitant AEDs completely over 3-6 weeks, while increasing the oxcarbazine dose in increments of 600 mg daily at weekly intervals, reaching the maximum oxcarbazine dose (2400 mg daily) in about 2-4 weeks (lower doses have been effective in patients in whom monotherapy has been initiated).

Initiation of monotherapy, partial seizures (epilepsy): Patients not receiving prior AEDs:

Children 4-16 years: Immediate release (Trileptal®): Initial: 8-10 mg/kg/day in twice daily divided doses; doses may be titrated by 5 mg/kg/day every third day. See below for recommended total daily dose by weight.

Range of maintenance doses by weight during monotherapy:

20 kg: 600-900 mg daily
25-30 kg: 900-1200 mg daily
35-40 kg: 900-1500 mg daily
45 kg: 1200-1500 mg daily
50-55 kg: 1200-1800 mg daily
60-65 kg: 1200-2100 mg daily
70 kg: 1500-2100 mg daily

Adults: Immediate release (Trileptal®): Initial: 600 mg daily in 2 divided doses. Increase dose by 300 mg daily every third day to a dose of 1200 mg daily. Higher dosages (2400 mg daily) have been shown to be effective in patients converted to monotherapy from other AEDs.

Conversion from immediate release (Trileptal®) to extended release (Oxtellar XR™): Children ≥6 years, Adolescents, and Adults: Higher doses of Oxtellar XR™ may be necessary.

Dosage adjustment with concomitant antiepileptic drugs (AEDs): Children ≥6 years, Adolescents, and Adults: Extended release (Oxtellar XR™): Concomitant use with enzyme-inducing antiepileptic drugs (eg, carbamazepine, phenobarbital, phenytoin): Consider initiating dose at 900 mg once daily.

Dosing adjustment in renal impairment:

Severe impairment (Cl_{cr} <30 mL/minute): Immediate release (Trileptal®), Extended release (Oxtellar XR™): Therapy should be initiated at one-half the usual starting dose (300 mg daily in adults) and increased slowly to achieve desired clinical response (eg, 300-450 mg daily at weekly intervals).

ESRD (on dialysis): Immediate release formulations should be used instead of extended release formulation.

Dosing adjustment in hepatic impairment:

Mild-to-moderate impairment: No dosage adjustment necessary.

Severe impairment:

Immediate release (Trileptal®): Use caution (not studied).

Extended release (Oxtellar XR™): Not recommended (not studied).

Administration

Immediate release: Administer twice daily without regard to meals.

Suspension: Prior to using for the first time, firmly insert the plastic adapter provided with the bottle. Cover adapter with child-resistant cap when not in use. Shake bottle for at least 10 seconds, remove child-resistant cap, and insert the oral dosing syringe provided to withdraw appropriate dose. Dose may be taken directly from oral syringe or may be mixed in a small glass of water immediately prior to swallowing. Rinse syringe with warm water after use and allow to dry thoroughly. Discard any unused portion after 7 weeks of first opening bottle.

Extended release: Administer once daily on an empty stomach at least 1 hour before or 2 hours after food. Swallow whole; do not cut, crush, or chew the tablets.

Hazardous agent; use appropriate precautions for handling and disposal (NIOSH, 2012).

Monitoring Parameters Seizure frequency; serum sodium as deemed necessary (particularly during first 3 months of therapy); symptoms of CNS depression (dizziness, headache, somnolence); hypersensitivity reactions. Additional serum sodium monitoring recommended during maintenance treatment in patients receiving other medications known to decrease sodium levels, in patients with signs/symptoms of hyponatremia, and in patients with an increase in seizure frequency or severity. Monitor for suicidality (eg, suicidal thoughts, depression, behavioral changes). Serum levels of concomitant antiepileptic drugs during titration as necessary.

Test Interactions Thyroid function tests; may depress serum T_4 without affecting T_3 levels or TSH

Additional Information At steady state, the extended release product administered once daily is not bioequivalent to the same daily dose of the immediate release formulation administered twice daily.

Dosage Forms Excipient information presented when available (limited, particularly for generics); consult specific product labeling.

Suspension, Oral:

Trileptal: 300 mg/5 mL (250 mL) [contains alcohol, usp, methyl hydroxybenzoate, propyl hydroxybenzoate, propylene glycol, saccharin sodium; lemon flavor]

Generic: 300 mg/5 mL (250 mL)

Tablet, Oral:

Trileptal: 150 mg, 300 mg, 600 mg [scored]

Generic: 150 mg, 300 mg, 600 mg

Tablet Extended Release 24 Hour, Oral:

Oxtellar XR: 150 mg, 300 mg, 600 mg

◆ **Oxecta** *see* OxyCODONE *on page* 1535

◆ **Oxeze® Turbuhaler® (Can)** *see* Formoterol *on page* 914

Oxiconazole (oks i KON a zole)

Brand Names: U.S. Oxistat

Brand Names: Canada Oxistat®

Index Terms Oxiconazole Nitrate

Pharmacologic Category Antifungal Agent, Topical

Use

Cream: Treatment of tinea pedis (athlete's foot), tinea cruris (jock itch), tinea corporis (ringworm), and tinea (pityriasis) versicolor

Lotion: Treatment of tinea pedis (athlete's foot), tinea cruris (jock itch), tinea corporis (ringworm)

Pregnancy Risk Factor B

Dosage Topical: Children ≥12 years, Adolescents, and Adults:

Tinea corporis/tinea cruris: Cream, lotion: Apply to affected areas 1-2 times daily for 2 weeks

Tinea pedis: Cream, lotion: Apply to affected areas 1-2 times daily for 1 month

Tinea versicolor: Cream: Apply to affected areas once daily for 2 weeks

Additional Information Complete prescribing information should be consulted for additional detail.

Dosage Forms Excipient information presented when available (limited, particularly for generics); consult specific product labeling.

Cream, External:

Oxistat: 1% (30 g, 60 g, 90 g) [contains benzoic acid, cetyl alcohol, propylene glycol]

Lotion, External:

Oxistat: 1% (30 mL, 60 mL) [contains benzoic acid, cetyl alcohol, propylene glycol]

◆ **Oxiconazole Nitrate** *see* Oxiconazole *on page 1533*

◆ **Oxilapine Succinate** *see* Loxapine *on page 1253*

◆ **Oxistat** *see* Oxiconazole *on page 1533*

◆ **Oxistat® (Can)** *see* Oxiconazole *on page 1533*

◆ **Oxpam® (Can)** *see* Oxazepam *on page 1529*

◆ **Oxpentifylline** *see* Pentoxifylline *on page 1619*

◆ **Oxpram® (Can)** *see* Oxazepam *on page 1529*

◆ **Oxsoralen** *see* Methoxsalen (Topical) *on page 1331*

◆ **Oxsoralen Capsule (Can)** *see* Methoxsalen (Systemic) *on page 1331*

◆ **Oxsoralen® Lotion (Can)** *see* Methoxsalen (Topical) *on page 1331*

◆ **Oxsoralen Ultra** *see* Methoxsalen (Systemic) *on page 1331*

◆ **Oxsoralen-Ultra (Can)** *see* Methoxsalen (Systemic) *on page 1331*

◆ **Oxtellar XR** *see* OXcarbazepine *on page 1530*

◆ **Oxybate** *see* Sodium Oxybate *on page 1922*

◆ **Oxybutyn (Can)** *see* Oxybutynin *on page 1533*

Oxybutynin (oks i BYOO ti nin)

Brand Names: U.S. Ditropan XL; Gelnique; Oxytrol; Oxytrol For Women [OTC]

Brand Names: Canada Apo-Oxybutynin; Ditropan XL; Dom-Oxybutynin; Gelnique; Mylan-Oxybutynin; Novo-Oxybutynin; Nu-Oxybutyn; Oxybutyn; Oxybutynine; Oxytrol; PHL-Oxybutynin; PMS-Oxybutynin; Riva-Oxybutynin; Uromax

Index Terms Ditropan; Oxybutynin Chloride; Oxytrol for Women

Pharmacologic Category Antispasmodic Agent, Urinary

Additional Appendix Information

Beers Criteria – Potentially Inappropriate Medications for Geriatrics *on page 2368*

Use Treatment of symptoms associated with overactive uninhibited neurogenic or reflex neurogenic bladder (eg, urgency, frequency, leakage, urge incontinence, dysuria); treatment of symptoms associated with detrusor overactivity due to a neurological condition (eg, spina bifida) (extended release tablet only)

Pregnancy Risk Factor B

Pregnancy Considerations Adverse events were not observed in animal reproduction studies.

Breast-Feeding Considerations It is not known if oxybutynin is excreted into breast milk. The manufacturer recommends that caution be used if administered to a nursing woman. Suppression of lactation has been reported.

Contraindications Hypersensitivity to oxybutynin or any component of the formulation; patients with or at risk for uncontrolled narrow-angle glaucoma, urinary retention, gastric retention or conditions with severely decreased GI motility

OTC labeling: When used for self-medication, do not use if you have pain or burning when urinating, blood in urine, unexplained lower back or side pain, cloudy or foul-smelling urine; in males; age <18 years; only experience accidental urine loss when cough, sneeze, or laugh; diagnosis of urinary or gastric retention; glaucoma; hypersensitivity to oxybutynin.

Warnings/Precautions Cases of angioedema involving the face, lips, tongue, and/or larynx have been reported with oral oxybutynin; some cases have occurred after a single dose. Discontinue immediately if tongue, hypopharynx, or larynx is involved; promptly initiate appropriate management. Use with caution in patients with bladder outflow obstruction (may increase the risk of urinary retention), treated angle-closure glaucoma (use is contraindicated in uncontrolled narrow-angle glaucoma), hyperthyroidism, coronary artery disease, heart failure, hypertension, cardiac arrhythmias, hepatic or renal impairment, prostatic hyperplasia (may cause urinary retention), hiatal hernia, myasthenia gravis, dementia. Use with caution in patients with decreased GI motility or gastrointestinal obstructive disorders (eg, ulcerative colitis, intestinal atony, pyloric stenosis); may increase the risk of gastric retention. In patients with ulcerative colitis, use may decrease gastric motility to the point of increasing the risk of paralytic ileus or toxic megacolon. Use with caution in patients with gastroesophageal reflux or with medications that may exacerbate esophagitis (eg, bisphosphonates). May increase the risk of heat prostration. Anticholinergics may cause agitation, confusion, drowsiness, dizziness, hallucinations, headache, and/or blurred vision, which may impair physical or mental abilities; patients must be cautioned about performing tasks which require mental alertness (eg, operating machinery or driving). Dose reduction or discontinuation should be considered if CNS effects occur.

Potentially significant drug-drug interactions may exist, requiring dose or frequency adjustment, additional monitoring, and/or selection of alternative therapy. This medication is associated with potent anticholinergic properties which may be inappropriate in older adults depending on comorbidities (eg, dementia, delirium) (Beers Criteria).

The extended release formulation consists of drug within a nondeformable matrix; following drug release/absorption, the matrix/shell is expelled in the stool. The use of nondeformable products in patients with known stricture/narrowing of the GI tract has been associated with symptoms of obstruction. Transdermal patch may contain conducting metal (eg, aluminum); remove patch prior to MRI. When using the topical gel, cover treatment area with clothing after gel has dried to minimize transferring medication to others. Discontinue gel if skin irritation occurs. Gel contains ethanol; do not expose to open flame or smoking until gel has dried.

When used for self-medication (OTC), other causes of frequent urination (UTI, diabetes, early pregnancy, other serious conditions) may need to be considered prior to use. Patients should contact a health care provider if symptoms do not improve within 2 weeks of initial use or for new or worsening symptoms.

Adverse Reactions

Oral:

>10%:

Central nervous system: Dizziness (4% to 17%), drowsiness (2% to 14%)

Gastrointestinal: Xerostomia (29% to 71%; dose related), constipation (7% to 15%), nausea (2% to 12%)

1% to 10%:

Cardiovascular: Cardiac arrhythmia (sinus; 1% to <5%), chest pain (1% to <5%), decreased blood pressure (1% to <5%), edema (1% to <5%), flushing (1% to <5%), hypertension (1% to <5%), palpitations (1% to <5%), peripheral edema (1% to <5%)

Central nervous system: Headache (6% to 10%), nervousness (1% to 7%), pain (1% to 7%), insomnia (1% to 6%), confusion (1% to <5%), depression (1% to <5%), fatigue (1% to <5%)

Dermatologic: Pruritus (1% to <5%), xeroderma (1% to <5%)

Endocrine & metabolic: Fluid retention (1% to <5%), hyperglycemia (1% to <5%)

Gastrointestinal: Diarrhea (1% to 9%), dyspepsia (5% to 7%), abdominal pain (1% to <5%), dry throat (1% to <5%), dysphagia (1% to <5%), eructation (1% to <5%), flatulence (1% to <5%), gastroesophageal reflux disease (1% to <5%), unpleasant taste (1% to <5%), vomiting (1% to <5%)

Genitourinary: Urinary hesitancy (1% to 9%), urinary tract infection (5% to 7%), urinary retention (1% to 6%), cystitis (1% to <5%), dysuria (1% to <5%), pollakiuria (1% to <5%)

Infection: Fungal infection (1% to <5%)

Neuromuscular & skeletal: Weakness (1% to 7%), arthralgia (1% to <5%), back pain (1% to <5%), flank pain (1% to <5%), limb pain (1% to <5%)

Ophthalmic: Blurred vision (1% to 10%), xerophthalmia (3% to 6%), eye irritation (1% to <5%), keratoconjunctivitis sicca (1% to <5%)

Respiratory: Asthma (1% to <5%), bronchitis (1% to <5%), cough (1% to <5%), dry throat (1% to <5%), hoarseness (1% to <5%), nasal congestion (1% to <5%), dry nose (1% to <5%), nasopharyngitis (1% to <5%), pharyngolaryngeal pain (1% to <5%), sinus congestion (1% to <5%), upper respiratory tract infection (1% to <5%)

Miscellaneous: Increased thirst (1% to <5%)

<1% (Limited to important or life-threatening): Anaphylaxis, anorexia, cycloplegia, decreased gastrointestinal motility, glaucoma, hallucination, hypersensitivity reaction, impotence, suppressed lactation, memory impairment, mydriasis, psychotic reaction, prolonged Q-T interval on ECG, seizure, tachycardia

Topical gel:

>10%:

Gastrointestinal: Xerostomia (2% to 12%)

Local: Application site reaction (4% to 14%; includes erythema [4%], pruritus [3%], dermatitis [2%], anesthesia, irritation, pain, papules, rash [3%])

1% to 10%:

Central nervous system: Dizziness (2% to 3%), fatigue (2%), headache (2%)

Dermatologic: Pruritus (1%)

Gastrointestinal: Gastroenteritis (2%), constipation (1%)

Genitourinary: Urinary tract infection (5% to 7%)

Ophthalmic: Conjunctivitis (4%), blurred vision (<2%), xerophthalmia (<2%)

Respiratory: Nasopharyngitis (3% to 5%), upper respiratory tract infection (5%)

Transdermal:

>10%: Local: Pruritus (14% to 17%)

1% to 10%:

Gastrointestinal: Xerostomia (4% to 10%), constipation (3%), diarrhea (3%)

Genitourinary: Dysuria (2%)

Local: Erythema (6% to 8%), localized vesiculation (3%), macular eruption (3%), skin rash (3%)

Ophthalmic: Visual disturbance (3%)

Postmarketing and/or case reports (Limited to important or life-threatening): Dizziness, drowsiness

Drug Interactions

Metabolism/Transport Effects Substrate of CYP3A4 (minor); **Note:** Assignment of Major/Minor substrate status based on clinically relevant drug interaction potential; **Inhibits** CYP2C8 (weak), CYP2D6 (weak), CYP3A4 (weak)

Avoid Concomitant Use

Avoid concomitant use of Oxybutynin with any of the following: Aclidinium; Ipratropium (Oral Inhalation); Pimozide; Potassium Chloride; Tiotropium; Umeclidinium

Increased Effect/Toxicity

Oxybutynin may increase the levels/effects of: AbobotulinumtoxinA; Analgesics (Opioid); Anticholinergics; ARIPiprazole; Cannabinoids; Dofetilide; Lomitapide; Mirabegron; OnabotulinumtoxinA; Pimozide; Potassium Chloride; RimabotulinumtoxinB; Thiazide Diuretics; Tiotropium; Topiramate

The levels/effects of Oxybutynin may be increased by: Aclidinium; Ipratropium (Oral Inhalation); Pramlintide; Umeclidinium

Decreased Effect

Oxybutynin may decrease the levels/effects of: Acetylcholinesterase Inhibitors (Central); Secretin

The levels/effects of Oxybutynin may be decreased by: Acetylcholinesterase Inhibitors (Central)

Ethanol/Nutrition/Herb Interactions Ethanol: Use ethanol with caution (may increase CNS depression and toxicity). Watch for sedation.

Storage/Stability

Immediate release tablet and syrup: Store at 20°C to 25°C (68°F to 77°F). Protect from light.

Extended release tablet: Store at 25°C (77°F); excursions permitted to 15°C to 30°C (59°F to 86°F). Protect from moisture and humidity.

Topical gel (pump or sachets): Store at 25°C (77°F); excursions permitted to 15°C to 30°C (59°F to 86°F). Protect from moisture and humidity. Keep gel away from open flame. Do not store sachets outside the sealed pouch; apply immediately after removal from the protective pouch. Discard used sachets such that accidental application or ingestion by children, pets, or others is avoided.

Transdermal patch: Store at 20°C to 25°C (68°F to 77°F). Protect from moisture and humidity. Do not store outside the sealed pouch; apply immediately after removal from the protective pouch. Discard used patches such that accidental application or ingestion by children, pets, or others is avoided.

Mechanism of Action Direct antispasmodic effect on smooth muscle, also inhibits the action of acetylcholine on smooth muscle (exhibits 1/5 the anticholinergic activity of atropine, but has 4-10 times the antispasmodic activity); does not block effects at skeletal muscle or at autonomic ganglia; increases bladder capacity, decreases uninhibited contractions, and delays desire to void, therefore, decreases urgency and frequency

Pharmacodynamics/Kinetics

Onset of action: Oral: Immediate release: 30-60 minutes
Peak effect: 3-6 hours

Duration: Oral: Immediate release: 6-10 hours; Extended release: Up to 24 hours

Absorption: Oral: Rapid and well absorbed; Transdermal: High

Distribution: I.V.: V_d: 193 L

Protein binding: >99% primarily to alpha$_1$-acid glycoprotein

Metabolism: Hepatic via CYP3A4; Oral: High first-pass metabolism; forms active and inactive metabolites

Bioavailability: Oral: ~6%

Half-life elimination: I.V.: ~2 hours (parent drug), 7-8 hours (metabolites); Oral: Immediate release: ~2-3 hours; Extended release: ~13 hours; Transdermal: 30-64 hours

Time to peak, serum: Oral: Immediate release: ~60 minutes; Extended release: 4-6 hours; Transdermal: 24-48 hours

Excretion: Urine, as metabolites and unchanged drug (<0.1%)

Dosage Overactive bladder:

Oral:

Children: >5 years: Immediate release: 5 mg twice daily; maximum: 5 mg 3 times daily

Children ≥6 years: Extended release: 5 mg once daily; adjust dose in 5 mg increments; maximum: 20 mg once daily

Adults:

Immediate release: 5 mg 2-3 times daily; maximum: 5 mg 4 times daily

Extended release: Initial: 5-10 mg once daily, adjust dose in 5 mg increments at weekly intervals; maximum: 30 mg once daily

Elderly: Immediate release: Initial: 2.5 mg 2-3 times daily; increase cautiously

Topical gel: Adults:

Gelnique 3%: Apply 3 pumps (84 mg) once daily

Gelnique 10%: Apply contents of 1 sachet (100 mg/g) once daily

Transdermal: Adults: Apply one 3.9 mg/day patch twice weekly (every 3-4 days)

Dosage adjustment in renal impairment: No dosage adjustment provided in the manufacturer's labeling (not studied); use with caution.

Dosage adjustment in hepatic impairment: No dosage adjustment provided in the manufacturer's labeling (not studied); use with caution.

Dietary Considerations Food causes a slight delay in the absorption of the oral solution and bioavailability is increased by ~25%. Absorption of the extended release tablet is not affected by food. May be taken without regard to meals.

Administration

Oral: Administer without regard to meals. Extended release tablets must be swallowed whole with liquid; do not crush, divide, or chew; take at approximately the same time each day.

Topical gel: For topical use only. Apply to clean, dry, intact skin on abdomen, thighs, or upper arms/shoulders. Wash hands after use. Cover treated area with clothing after gel has dried to prevent transfer of medication to others. Do not bathe, shower, or swim until 1 hour after gel applied. Do not apply to recently shaved skin.

Gelnique 3%: Prior to initial use, press pump 4 times to prime pump; discard any gel dispensed from pump during priming. Rotate application sites to avoid skin irritation.

Gelnique 10%: Rotate site; do not apply to same site on consecutive days.

Transdermal: Apply to clean, dry skin on abdomen, hip, or buttock. Select a new site for each new system (avoid reapplication to same site within 7 days). Wear patch under clothing; do not expose to sunlight.

Monitoring Parameters Incontinence episodes, postvoid residual (PVR)

Test Interactions May suppress the wheal and flare reactions to skin test antigens.

Product Availability Oxytrol for Women: FDA approved January 2013; availability anticipated in the fall of 2013. Oxytrol for Women is an over-the-counter (OTC) transdermal patch indicated for the treatment of overactive bladder.

Dosage Forms Excipient information presented when available (limited, particularly for generics); consult specific product labeling. [DSC] = Discontinued product

Gel, Transdermal:

Gelnique: 3% (92 g) [contains propylene glycol]

Gel, Transdermal, as chloride:

Gelnique: 10% (1 g) [contains alcohol, usp]

Patch Biweekly, Transdermal:

Oxytrol: 3.9 mg/24 hr (1 ea, 2 ea, 4 ea, 8 ea)

Oxytrol For Women: 3.9 mg/24 hr (8 ea); 3.9 mg/24hr (4 ea)

Syrup, Oral, as chloride:

Generic: 5 mg/5 mL (5 mL [DSC], 473 mL)

Tablet, Oral, as chloride:

Generic: 5 mg

Tablet Extended Release 24 Hour, Oral, as chloride:

Ditropan XL: 5 mg, 10 mg, 15 mg [contains polysorbate 80]

Generic: 5 mg, 10 mg, 15 mg

◆ **Oxybutynin Chloride** *see* Oxybutynin *on page 1533*

◆ **Oxybutynine (Can)** *see* Oxybutynin *on page 1533*

◆ **Oxycodan® (Can)** *see* Oxycodone and Aspirin *on page 1539*

OxyCODONE (oks i KOE done)

Brand Names: U.S. Oxecta; OxyCONTIN; Roxicodone

Brand Names: Canada Apo-Oxycodone CR; CO Oxycodone CR; Oxy.IR; OxyContin; OxyNEO; PMS-Oxycodone; PMS-Oxycodone CR; Supeudol

Index Terms Dihydrohydroxycodeinone; Oxecta; Oxycodone Hydrochloride

Pharmacologic Category Analgesic, Opioid

Additional Appendix Information

Opioid Conversion Table *on page 2306*

Patient Information for Disposal of Unused Medications *on page 2393*

Use Management of moderate-to-severe pain, normally used in combination with nonopioid analgesics

OxyContin is indicated for around-the-clock management of moderate-to-severe pain when a continuous analgesic is needed for an extended period of time.

Pregnancy Risk Factor B

Pregnancy Considerations Adverse events were not observed in animal reproduction studies. Opioids cross the placenta. Oxycodone should not be used immediately prior to or during labor.

If chronic opioid exposure occurs in pregnancy, adverse events in the newborn (including withdrawal) may occur; monitoring of the neonate is recommended. The minimum effective dose should be used if opioids are needed (Chou, 2009). Neonatal abstinence syndrome following opioid exposure may present with autonomic (eg, fever, temperature instability), gastrointestinal (eg, diarrhea, vomiting, poor feeding/weight gain), or neurologic (eg, high-pitched crying, increased muscle tone, irritability, seizure, tremor) symptoms (Dow, 2012; Hudak, 2012).

Breast-Feeding Considerations Oxycodone is excreted into breast milk. Breast-feeding is not recommended by the manufacturer. Sedation and/or respiratory depression may occur in the infant; symptoms of opioid withdrawal may occur following the cessation of breast-feeding. Nursing infants exposed to large doses of opioids should be monitored for apnea and sedation. Use caution in a woman who may be an ultrarapid metabolizer; oxycodone is a substrate for CYP2D6 and their nursing infants may be at higher risk for adverse events (Montgomery, 2012).

Prescribing and Access Restrictions As a requirement of the REMS program, healthcare providers who prescribe OxyContin need to receive training on the proper use and potential risks of OxyContin. For training, please refer to http://www.oxycontinrems.com. Prescribers will need retraining every 2 years or following any significant changes to the OxyContin REMS program.

Medication Guide Available Yes

Contraindications Hypersensitivity to oxycodone or any component of the formulation; significant respiratory depression; hypercarbia; acute or severe bronchial asthma; paralytic ileus (known or suspected); GI obstruction

Warnings/Precautions May cause CNS depression, which may impair physical or mental abilities; patients must be cautioned about performing tasks which require mental alertness (eg, operating machinery or driving). Potentially significant drug interactions may exist, requiring dose or frequency adjustment, additional monitoring, and/or selection of alternative therapy. Effects may be potentiated when used with other sedative drugs or ethanol. Use with caution in patients with hypersensitivity reactions to other phenanthrene derivative opioid agonists (morphine, hydrocodone, hydromorphone, levorphanol, oxymorphone), respiratory diseases including asthma, emphysema, or COPD. Use with caution in pancreatitis or biliary tract disease, acute alcoholism (including delirium tremens), morbid obesity, adrenocortical insufficiency, history of seizure disorders, kyphoscoliosis (or other skeletal disorder which may alter respiratory function), hypothyroidism (including myxedema), prostatic hyperplasia, urethral stricture, and toxic psychosis. May obscure diagnosis or clinical course of patients with acute abdominal conditions. Avoid use in patients with CNS depression/coma as these patients are susceptible to intracranial effects of CO_2 retention.

Use with caution in the elderly, debilitated, or cachectic patients, and hepatic or renal dysfunction. Hemodynamic effects (hypotension, orthostasis) may be exaggerated in patients with hypovolemia, concurrent vasodilating drugs, or in patients with head injury. Monitor for symptoms of hypotension following initiation or dose titration. Respiratory depressant effects and capacity to elevate CSF pressure may be exaggerated in presence of head injury, other intracranial lesion, or pre-existing intracranial pressure.

Concomitant use with CYP3A4 inhibitors may result in increased effects and potentially fatal respiratory depression. Concurrent use of agonist/antagonist analgesics may precipitate withdrawal symptoms and/or reduced analgesic efficacy in patients following prolonged therapy with mu opioid agonists. Abrupt discontinuation following prolonged use may also lead to withdrawal symptoms. Healthcare provider should be alert to problems of abuse, misuse, and diversion; abuse of products by crushing, chewing, snorting, or injecting may result in severe overdose, adverse effects, or death.

After chronic maternal exposure to opioids, neonatal withdrawal syndrome may occur in the newborn; monitor neonate closely. Signs and symptoms include irritability, hyperactivity and abnormal sleep pattern, high pitched cry, tremor, vomiting, diarrhea and failure to gain weight. Onset, duration and severity depend on the drug used, duration of use, maternal dose, and rate of drug elimination by the newborn. Opioid withdrawal syndrome in the neonate, unlike in adults, may be life-threatening and should be treated according to protocols developed by neonatology experts.

Controlled-release tablets: OxyContin is not intended for use as an "as needed" analgesic or for the treatment of mild pain, acute pain, or postoperative pain requiring short-term analgesia (should be used postoperatively only if the patient has received it prior to surgery or if severe, persistent pain is anticipated). **[U.S. Boxed Warning]: May cause potentially life-threatening respiratory depression even with therapeutic use. Ensure proper dosing and titration; monitor for respiratory depression especially within the first 24-72 hours of initiation or dose escalation. Oxycodone controlled-release tablets should only be prescribed by healthcare professionals familiar with the use of potent opioids for chronic pain. Do NOT crush, break, chew or dissolve controlled-release tablets (may result in a potentially fatal overdose);** 60 mg and 80 mg strengths, a single dose >40 mg, or a total dose of >80 mg/day are for use only in opioid-tolerant patients. Tablets may be difficult to swallow and could become lodged in throat; patients with swallowing difficulties may be at increased risk. Cases of intestinal obstruction or diverticulitis exacerbation have also been reported, including cases requiring medical intervention to remove the tablet; patients with an underlying GI disease (eg, esophageal cancer, colon cancer) may be at increased risk. **[U.S. Boxed Warning]: Accidental exposure may result in fatal overdose of oxycodone, especially in children. [U.S. Boxed Warning]: Healthcare provider should be alert to problems of abuse, misuse, and diversion. Tolerance or drug dependence may result from extended use. Patients should be assessed for risk of abuse or addiction prior to therapy and all patients should be monitored for signs of misuse, abuse, and addiction. Risk of opioid abuse is increased in patients with a history or family history of alcohol or drug abuse or mental illness.**

Oral solutions: **[U.S. Boxed Warning]: Highly concentrated oral solution (20 mg/mL) should only be used in opioid tolerant patients (taking ≥30 mg/day of oxycodone or equivalent for ≥1 week). [U.S. Boxed Warning]: Orders for oxycodone oral solutions (20 mg/mL or 5 mg/5 mL) should be clearly written to include the intended dose (in mg vs mL) and the intended product concentration to be dispensed to avoid potential dosing errors. Products should be stored out of reach of children; seek immediate medical care in the event of accidental ingestion.**

Adverse Reactions Note: Percentages as reported with OxyContin

>10%:

Central nervous system: Somnolence (23%), dizziness (13%)

Dermatologic: Pruritus (13%)

Gastrointestinal: Constipation (23%), nausea (23%), vomiting (12%)

1% to 10%:

Cardiovascular: Orthostatic hypotension (1% to 5%)

Central nervous system: Headache (7%), abnormal dreams (1% to 5%), anxiety (1% to 5%), chills (1% to 5%), confusion (1% to 5%), dysphoria (1% to 5%), euphoria (1% to 5%), fever (1% to 5%), insomnia (1% to 5%), nervousness (1% to 5%), thought abnormalities (1% to 5%)

Dermatologic: Rash (1% to 5%)

Gastrointestinal: Xerostomia (6%), abdominal pain (1% to 5%), anorexia (1% to 5%), diarrhea (1% to 5%), dyspepsia (1% to 5%), gastritis (1% to 5%)

Neuromuscular & skeletal: Weakness (6%), twitching (1% to 5%)

Respiratory: Dyspnea (1% to 5%), hiccups (1% to 5%)

Miscellaneous: Diaphoresis (5%)

<1% (Limited to important or life-threatening): Agitation, amnesia, anaphylactoid reaction, anaphylaxis, chest pain, dehydration, depression, diverticulitis exacerbation, dysphagia, dysuria, edema, emotional lability, eructation, hallucinations, hematuria, histamine release, hyperalgesia, hyperkinesia, hypoesthesia, hyponatremia, hypotonia, ileus, intestinal obstruction, intracranial pressure increased, malaise, paralytic ileus, paresthesia, seizures, SIADH, speech disorder, ST segment depression, stomatitis, stupor, syncope, tablet in stool (some controlled release dosage forms), tremor, urinary retention, vertigo, withdrawal syndrome

Drug Interactions

Metabolism/Transport Effects Substrate of CYP2D6 (minor), CYP3A4 (major); **Note:** Assignment of Major/Minor substrate status based on clinically relevant drug interaction potential

Avoid Concomitant Use

Avoid concomitant use of OxyCODONE with any of the following: Azelastine (Nasal); Fusidic Acid (Systemic); Paraldehyde

Increased Effect/Toxicity

OxyCODONE may increase the levels/effects of: Alcohol (Ethyl); Alvimopan; Azelastine (Nasal); CNS Depressants; Desmopressin; Diuretics; Hydrocodone; Metyrosine; Mirtazapine; Paraldehyde; Pramipexole; ROPINIRole; Rotigotine; Selective Serotonin Reuptake Inhibitors; Zolpidem

The levels/effects of OxyCODONE may be increased by: Amphetamines; Anticholinergics; Antipsychotic Agents (Phenothiazines); Brimonidine (Topical); Cannabinoids; CYP3A4 Inhibitors (Moderate); CYP3A4 Inhibitors (Strong); Dasatinib; Doxylamine; Droperidol; Fusidic Acid (Systemic); HydrOXYzine; Ivacaftor; Luliconazole; Magnesium Sulfate; MAO Inhibitors; Mifepristone; Perampanel; Simeprevir; Sodium Oxybate; Succinylcholine; Tapentadol; Voriconazole

Decreased Effect

OxyCODONE may decrease the levels/effects of: Pegvisomant

The levels/effects of OxyCODONE may be decreased by: Ammonium Chloride; Bosentan; CYP3A4 Inducers (Strong); Dabrafenib; Deferasirox; Mitotane; Mixed Agonist / Antagonist Opioids; Rifampin; St Johns Wort; Tocilizumab

Ethanol/Nutrition/Herb Interactions

Ethanol: May increase CNS depression; monitor for increased effects with coadministration. Caution patients about effects.

Herb/Nutraceutical: Avoid valerian, St John's wort, kava kava, gotu kola (may increase CNS depression).

Storage/Stability Store at 25°C (77°F); excursions permitted between 15°C to 30°C (59°F to 86°F). Protect from light.

Mechanism of Action Binds to opiate receptors in the CNS, causing inhibition of ascending pain pathways, altering the perception of and response to pain; produces generalized CNS depression

Pharmacodynamics/Kinetics

Onset of action: Pain relief: Immediate release: 10-15 minutes

Peak effect: Immediate release: 0.5-1 hour

Duration: Immediate release: 3-6 hours; Controlled release: ≤12 hours

Distribution: V_d: 2.6 L/kg; distributed to skeletal muscle, liver, intestinal tract, lungs, spleen, and brain

Protein binding: ~45%

Metabolism: Hepatically via CYP3A4 to noroxycodone (has weak analgesic), noroxymorphone, and alpha- and beta-noroxycodol. CYP2D6 mediated metabolism produces oxymorphone (has analgesic activity; low plasma concentrations), alpha- and beta-oxymorphol.

Bioavailability: Controlled release, immediate release: 60% to 87%

Half-life elimination: Immediate release: 2-4 hours; controlled release: ~5 hours

Time to peak, plasma: Immediate release: 1.2-1.9 hours; Controlled release: 4-5 hours

Excretion: Urine (~19% as parent; >64% as metabolites)

Dosage Oral: **Note:** All doses should be titrated to appropriate effect:

Children (unlabeled use): Immediate release, initial dose: 0.1-0.2 mg/kg/dose (moderate pain) or 0.2 mg/kg/dose (severe pain) (APS 6th edition). For severe chronic pain, administer on a regularly scheduled basis, every 4-6 hours, at the lowest dose that will achieve adequate analgesia.

Adults:

Immediate release: Initial: 5-15 mg every 4-6 hours as needed; dosing range: 5-20 mg per dose (APS 6th edition). For severe chronic pain, administer on a regularly scheduled basis, every 4-6 hours, at the lowest dose that will achieve adequate analgesia.

Controlled release: **Note:** 60 mg and 80 mg strengths, a single dose >40 mg, or a total dose of >80 mg daily are for use only in opioid-tolerant patients.

Opioid naive: Initial: 10 mg every 12 hours

Concurrent CNS depressants: Reduce usual initial oxycodone dose by one-third (1/3) to one-half (1/2)

Conversion from transdermal fentanyl: For each 25 mcg/hour transdermal dose, substitute 10 mg controlled release oxycodone every 12 hours; should be initiated 18 hours after the removal of the transdermal fentanyl patch

Currently on opioids: Initiate controlled release oxycodone with one-half (1/2) the estimated oxycodone daily dose (mg/day) and provide rescue medication in the form of immediate release oxycodone. Divide the initial controlled release oxycodone daily dose in 2 (for twice-daily dosing, usually every 12 hours) and round down to nearest dosage form.

Dose adjustment: Doses may be adjusted by changing the total daily dose (not by changing the dosing interval). Doses may be adjusted every 1-2 days and may be increased by 25% to 50%. Dose should be gradually tapered when no longer required in order to prevent withdrawal.

Dosage adjustment in renal impairment: Serum concentrations are increased ~50% in patients with Cl_{cr} <60 mL/minute; adjust dose based on clinical situation.

Dosage adjustment in hepatic impairment:

Immediate release: Reduced initial doses may be necessary (use a conservative approach to initial dosing); adjust dose based on clinical situation.

Controlled release: Decrease initial dose to one-third (1/3) to one-half (1/2) the usual starting dose; titrate carefully.

Dietary Considerations Instruct patient to avoid high-fat meals when taking some products (food has no effect on the reformulated OxyContin).

Administration

Controlled release: Swallow tablet whole. Do not moisten, dissolve, cut, crush, break, or chew controlled release tablets. Controlled release tablets are not indicated for rectal administration; increased risk of adverse events due to better rectal absorption. Controlled release tablets should be administered one at a time and each followed with water immediately after placing in the mouth.

Immediate release (Oxecta): Must be swallowed whole with enough water to ensure complete swallowing immediately after placing in the mouth. The tablet should not be wet prior to placing in the mouth. Do not crush, chew, or dissolve the tablets. Do not administer via feeding tubes (eg, gastric, NG) due to potential for obstruction. The formulation uses technology designed to discourage common methods of tampering to prevent misuse/abuse.

Appropriate laxatives should be administered to avoid the constipating side effects associated with use. Antiemetics may be needed for persistent nausea.

Monitoring Parameters Pain relief, respiratory and mental status, blood pressure; signs of misuse, abuse, and addiction

Test Interactions Some quinolones may produce a false-positive urine screening result for opioids using commercially-available immunoassay kits. This has been demonstrated most consistently for levofloxacin and ofloxacin, but other quinolones have shown cross-reactivity in certain assay kits. Confirmation of positive opioid screens by more specific methods should be considered.

Additional Information Oxecta utilizes Acura Pharmaceutical's Aversion® technology which may help discourage misuse and abuse potential. Reduced abuse potential of Oxecta compared to other immediate-release oxycodone tablet formulations has not been proven; the FDA is requiring Pfizer to complete a post-approval epidemiological study to determine whether the formulation actually results in a decrease of misuse/abuse. In one clinical trial in nondependent recreational opioid users, the "drug-liking" responses and safety of crushed Oxecta tablets were compared to crushed immediate-release oxycodone tablets following the self-administered intranasal use. A small difference in "drug-liking" scores was observed, with lower scores reported in the crushed Oxecta group. In regards to safety, there was an increased incidence of nasopharyngeal and facial adverse events in the Oxecta group. In addition, there was decreased ability in the Oxecta group to completely administer the two crushed Oxecta tablets intranasally within a set time period. However, whether these differences translate into a significant clinical difference is unknown. Of note, pharmacokinetic studies showed that Oxecta is bioequivalent with oxycodone immediate-release tablets with no differences in T_{max} and half-life when administered in the fasted state.

Dosage Forms Excipient information presented when available (limited, particularly for generics); consult specific product labeling.

Capsule, Oral, as hydrochloride:
- Generic: 5 mg

Concentrate, Oral, as hydrochloride:
- Generic: 20 mg/mL (30 mL)

Solution, Oral, as hydrochloride:
- Generic: 5 mg/5 mL (5 mL, 15 mL, 500 mL)

Tablet, Oral:
- Generic: 5 mg, 15 mg, 30 mg

Tablet, Oral, as hydrochloride:
- Roxicodone: 5 mg [scored]
- Roxicodone: 15 mg [scored; contains fd&c blue #2 (indigotine), fd&c yellow #10 (quinoline yellow)]
- Roxicodone: 30 mg [scored]
- Generic: 5 mg, 10 mg, 15 mg, 20 mg, 30 mg

Tablet Abuse-Deterrent, Oral, as hydrochloride:
- Oxecta: 5 mg, 7.5 mg

Tablet ER 12 Hour Abuse-Deterrent, Oral, as hydrochloride:
- OxyCONTIN: 10 mg, 15 mg, 20 mg, 30 mg, 40 mg, 60 mg
- OxyCONTIN: 80 mg [contains fd&c blue #2 aluminum lake]

Controlled Substance C-II

Oxycodone and Acetaminophen

(oks i KOE done & a seet a MIN oh fen)

Brand Names: U.S. Endocet; Magnacet; Percocet; Primlev; Roxicet; Roxicet 5/500

Brand Names: Canada Apo-Oxycodone/Acet; Endocet; Percocet; Percocet-Demi; PMS-Oxycodone-Acetaminophen; Ratio-Oxycocet; Sandoz-Oxycodone/Acetaminophen

Index Terms Acetaminophen and Oxycodone; Tylox

Pharmacologic Category Analgesic Combination (Opioid)

Use Moderate to moderately severe pain: Management of moderate to moderately-severe pain

Pregnancy Risk Factor C

Dosage Oral: Doses should be titrated to appropriate analgesic effects. **Note:** Initial dose is based on the **oxycodone** content; however, the maximum daily dose is based on the **acetaminophen** content.

Children and Adolescents (unlabeled; American Pain Society [APS], 2008):

Moderate pain: Initial dose,**based on oxycodone content**: 0.1-0.2 mg/kg/dose. Doses typically given every 4-6 hours as needed; manufacturer's labeling recommends every 6 hours as needed; maxi mum initial oxycodone dose: 5 mg/dose. Do not exceed maximum daily acetaminophen dose: Children <45 kg: 90 mg/kg/day; Children ≥45 kg: 4000 mg daily

Severe pain: Initial dose, **based on oxycodone content**: 0.2 mg/kg/dose. Doses typically given every 4-6 hours as needed; manufacturer's labeling recommends every 6 hours as needed; maximum initial oxycodone dose: 10 mg. Do not exceed maximum daily acetaminophen dose: Children <45 kg: 90 mg/kg/day; Children ≥45 kg: 4000 mg daily

Adults:

Manufacturer's labeling: Moderate to moderately severe pain: Initial dose, **based on oxycodone content**: 2.5-10 mg every 6 hours as needed. Titrate according to pain severity and individual response. Do not exceed acetaminophen 4 g daily.

Alternate recommendations (APS, 2008):

Moderate pain (unlabeled): Initial dose, **based on oxycodone content**: 5 mg. Doses typically given every 4-6 hours as needed; manufacturer's labeling recommends every 6 hours as needed. Do not exceed acetaminophen 4 g daily.

Severe pain (unlabeled): Initial dose, **based on oxycodone content**: 10-20 mg. Doses typically given every 4-6 hours as needed; manufacturer's labeling recommends every 6 hours as needed. Do not exceed acetaminophen 4 g daily.

Elderly: No dosage adjustment provided in manufacturer's labeling; however, use with caution and consider decreasing the initial dose and/or increasing the frequency.

Severe pain (unlabeled dosing): Elderly >70 years: Consider decreasing the initial dose **(based on oxycodone content)** by 25% to 50%, then titrating the dose upward or downward as needed; monitor frequently during titration. Do not exceed acetaminophen 4 g daily (APS, 2008).

Dosage adjustment in renal impairment: No dosage adjustment provided in manufacturer's labeling. Use with caution; reduced clearance in severe impairment may require dosage adjustment.

Dosage adjustment in hepatic impairment: No dosage adjustment provided in manufacturer's labeling. Use with caution; reduced clearance in severe impairment may require dosage adjustment.

Additional Information Complete prescribing information should be consulted for additional detail.

Dosage Forms Excipient information presented when available (limited, particularly for generics); consult specific product labeling. [DSC] = Discontinued product

Caplet, oral:

Roxicet 5/500: Oxycodone hydrochloride 5 mg and acetaminophen 500 mg

Capsule, oral: 5/500: Oxycodone hydrochloride 5 mg and acetaminophen 500 mg

Solution, oral:

Roxicet: Oxycodone hydrochloride 5 mg and acetaminophen 325 mg per 5 mL (5 mL, 500 mL) [contains ethanol <0.5%; mint flavor]

Tablet, oral: 2.5/325: Oxycodone hydrochloride 2.5 mg and acetaminophen 325 mg; 5/325: Oxycodone hydrochloride 5 mg and acetaminophen 325 mg; 7.5/325: Oxycodone hydrochloride 7.5 mg and acetaminophen 325 mg; 7.5/500: Oxycodone hydrochloride 7.5 mg and acetaminophen 500 mg; 10/325: Oxycodone hydrochloride 10 mg and acetaminophen 325 mg; 10/650: Oxycodone hydrochloride 10 mg and acetaminophen 650 mg

Endocet 5/325 [scored]: Oxycodone hydrochloride 5 mg and acetaminophen 325 mg

Endocet 7.5/325: Oxycodone hydrochloride 7.5 mg and acetaminophen 325 mg

Endocet 7.5/500: Oxycodone hydrochloride 7.5 mg and acetaminophen 500 mg [DSC]

Endocet 10/325: Oxycodone hydrochloride 10 mg and acetaminophen 325 mg

Endocet 10/650: Oxycodone hydrochloride 10 mg and acetaminophen 650 mg [DSC]

Magnacet 5/400: Oxycodone hydrochloride 5 mg and acetaminophen 400 mg

Magnacet 10/400: Oxycodone hydrochloride 10 mg and acetaminophen 400 mg

Percocet 2.5/325: Oxycodone hydrochloride 2.5 mg and acetaminophen 325 mg

Percocet 5/325 [scored]: Oxycodone hydrochloride 5 mg and acetaminophen 325 mg

Percocet 7.5/325: Oxycodone hydrochloride 7.5 mg and acetaminophen 325 mg

Percocet 7.5/500: Oxycodone hydrochloride 7.5 mg and acetaminophen 500 mg

Percocet 10/325: Oxycodone hydrochloride 10 mg and acetaminophen 325 mg

Percocet 10/650: Oxycodone hydrochloride 10 mg and acetaminophen 650 mg

Primlev 5/300: Oxycodone hydrochloride 5 mg and acetaminophen 300 mg

Primlev 7.5/300: Oxycodone hydrochloride 7.5 mg and acetaminophen 300 mg

Primlev 10/300: Oxycodone hydrochloride 10 mg and acetaminophen 300 mg

Roxicet 5/325 [scored]: Oxycodone hydrochloride 5 mg and acetaminophen 325 mg

Controlled Substance C-II

Oxycodone and Aspirin (oks i KOE done & AS pir in)

Brand Names: U.S. Endodan®; Percodan®

Brand Names: Canada Endodan®; Oxycodan®; Percodan®

Index Terms Aspirin and Oxycodone

Pharmacologic Category Analgesic Combination (Opioid)

Use Management of moderate- to moderately-severe pain

Pregnancy Risk Factor B (oxycodone); D (aspirin)

Dosage Oral:

Children (dose based on total oxycodone content): Oxycodone 0.1-0.2 mg/kg/dose (maximum oxycodone: 5 mg/dose; maximum aspirin: 4 g/day). Doses should be given every 4-6 hours as needed (American Pain Society, 2008)

Adults: One tablet every 6 hours as needed for pain; maximum aspirin dose should not exceed 4 g/day

Dosing adjustment in renal impairment: Use with caution. Avoid use of aspirin in patients with Cl_{cr} <10 mL/minute.

Dosing adjustment in hepatic impairment: Use with caution. Avoid use of aspirin-containing products in severe impairment.

Additional Information Complete prescribing information should be consulted for additional detail.

Dosage Forms Excipient information presented when available (limited, particularly for generics); consult specific product labeling.

Tablet: Oxycodone hydrochloride 4.8355 mg and aspirin 325 mg

Endodan®, Percodan®: Oxycodone hydrochloride 4.8355 mg and aspirin 325 mg

Controlled Substance C-II

Oxycodone and Ibuprofen
(oks i KOE done & eye byoo PROE fen)

Index Terms Ibuprofen and Oxycodone

Pharmacologic Category Analgesic Combination (Opioid); Nonsteroidal Anti-inflammatory Drug (NSAID), Oral

Use Short-term (≤7 days) management of acute, moderate-to-severe pain

Pregnancy Risk Factor C/D ≥30 weeks gestation

Medication Guide Available Yes

Dosage Oral: Adults: Pain: Take 1 tablet as needed (maximum: 4 tablets/24 hours); do not take for longer than 7 days

Dosage adjustment in renal impairment: No dosage adjustment provided in manufacturer's labeling (has not been studied).

Dosage adjustment in hepatic impairment: No dosage adjustment provided in manufacturer's labeling (has not been studied).

Additional Information Complete prescribing information should be consulted for additional detail.

Dosage Forms Excipient information presented when available (limited, particularly for generics); consult specific product labeling.

Tablet: Oxycodone hydrochloride 5 mg and ibuprofen 400 mg

Controlled Substance C-II

◆ **Oxycodone Hydrochloride** *see* OxyCODONE *on page 1535*

◆ **OxyCONTIN** *see* OxyCODONE *on page 1535*

◆ **OxyContin (Can)** *see* OxyCODONE *on page 1535*

◆ **Oxy.IR (Can)** *see* OxyCODONE *on page 1535*

Oxymetholone (oks i METH oh lone)

Brand Names: U.S. Anadrol-50

Pharmacologic Category Anabolic Steroid

Use Treatment of anemias caused by deficient red cell production

Pregnancy Risk Factor X

Dosage Note: The National Kidney Foundation does not recommend the use of androgens as an adjuvant to ESA treatment in anemic patients with chronic kidney disease (KDOQI, 2006).

Oral: Children and Adults: Erythropoietic effects: 1-5 mg/kg/day once daily; usual effective dose: 1-2 mg/kg/day; give for a minimum trial of 3-6 months because response may be delayed

Dosage adjustment in renal impairment: No dosage adjustment provided in manufacturer's labeling. Use with caution due to risk of edema in patients with renal impairment.

Dosage adjustment in hepatic impairment:

Mild to moderate impairment: There are no dosage adjustments provided in the manufacturer's labeling.

Severe impairment: Use is contraindicated.

Additional Information Complete prescribing information should be consulted for additional detail.

Dosage Forms Excipient information presented when available (limited, particularly for generics); consult specific product labeling.

Tablet, Oral:

Anadrol-50: 50 mg [scored]

Controlled Substance C-III

Oxymorphone (oks i MOR fone)

Brand Names: U.S. Opana; Opana ER

Index Terms Oxymorphone Hydrochloride

Pharmacologic Category Analgesic, Opioid

Additional Appendix Information

Opioid Conversion Table *on page 2306*

Patient Information for Disposal of Unused Medications *on page 2393*

Use

Parenteral: Management of moderate-to-severe acute pain; analgesia during labor; preoperative medication; anesthesia support; relief of anxiety in patients with dyspnea associated with pulmonary edema secondary to acute left ventricular failure

Oral, regular release: Management of moderate-to-severe acute pain

Oral, extended release: Management of moderate-to-severe pain in patients requiring around-the-clock opioid treatment for an extended period of time

Pregnancy Risk Factor C

Pregnancy Considerations Adverse events were observed in some animal reproduction studies. Opioids cross the placenta. When used for pain relief during labor, opioids may temporarily affect the heart rate of the fetus (ACOG, 2002). Oxymorphone injection is indicated for analgesia during labor. Neonates should be monitored for respiratory depression.

If chronic opioid exposure occurs in pregnancy, adverse events in the newborn (including withdrawal) may occur; monitoring of the neonate is recommended. The minimum effective dose should be used if opioids are needed (Chou, 2009). Neonatal abstinence syndrome following opioid exposure may present with autonomic (eg, fever, temperature instability), gastrointestinal (eg, diarrhea, vomiting, poor feeding/weight gain), or neurologic (eg, high-pitched crying, increased muscle tone, irritability, seizure, tremor) symptoms (Dow, 2012; Hudak, 2012).

Breast-Feeding Considerations Some opioids can be found in breast milk. Withdrawal symptoms may be observed in breast-feeding infants when opioid analgesics are discontinued. The manufacturer recommends that caution be used if administered to a nursing woman. Nursing infants exposed to large doses of opioids should be monitored for apnea and sedation (Montgomery, 2012).

Medication Guide Available Yes

Contraindications Hypersensitivity to oxymorphone, other morphine analogs (phenanthrene derivatives), or any component of the formulation; paralytic ileus (known or suspected); moderate-to-severe hepatic impairment; severe respiratory depression (unless using immediate release or parenteral formulation in monitored setting with resuscitative equipment); acute/severe bronchial asthma; hypercarbia

Note: Parenteral formulation is also contraindicated in the treatment of upper airway obstruction and pulmonary edema due to a chemical respiratory irritant.

Warnings/Precautions An opioid-containing analgesic regimen should be tailored to each patient's needs and based upon the type of pain being treated (acute versus chronic), the route of administration, degree of tolerance for opioids (naive versus chronic user), age, weight, and patient comorbidities. The optimal analgesic dose varies widely among patients. Doses should be titrated to pain relief/prevention.

May cause CNS depression, which may impair physical or mental abilities; patients must be cautioned about performing tasks which require mental alertness (eg, operating machinery or driving). Potentially significant drug interactions may exist, requiring dose or frequency adjustment, additional monitoring, and/or selection of alternative therapy. Effects may be potentiated when used with other sedative drugs or ethanol. Use not recommended within 14 days of MAO inhibitors. Due to structural similarities, hypersensitivity to other phenanthrene-derivative opioid agonists (codeine, hydrocodone, hydromorphone, levorphanol, morphine) may result in similar hypersensitivity reaction if oxymorphone is used; therefore, the use of oxymorphone is contraindicated in patients with previous hypersensitivity to other phenanthrene derivatives. May cause respiratory depression. Use extreme caution in patients with COPD or other chronic respiratory conditions characterized by hypoxia, hypercapnia, or diminished respiratory reserve (myxedema, cor pulmonale, kyphoscoliosis, obstructive sleep apnea, severe obesity). Use with caution in patients (particularly elderly or debilitated) with impaired respiratory function, adrenal disease, morbid obesity, seizure disorders, toxic psychosis, thyroid dysfunction, prostatic hyperplasia, or renal impairment. Use caution in mild hepatic dysfunction; use is contraindicated in moderate-to-severe hepatic impairment. Avoid use in patients with CNS depression or coma as these patients are susceptible to intracranial effects of CO_2 retention. Use only with extreme caution (if at all) in patients with head injury or increased intracranial pressure (ICP); potential to elevate ICP and/or blunt papillary response may be greatly exaggerated in these patients. Use with caution in patients with biliary tract dysfunction including acute pancreatitis; may cause constriction of sphincter of Oddi. May obscure diagnosis or clinical course of patients with acute abdominal conditions.

Oxymorphone shares the toxic potential of opioid agonists and usual precautions of opioid agonist therapy should be observed; may cause hypotension in patients with acute myocardial infarction, volume depletion, or concurrent drug therapy which may exaggerate vasodilation. The elderly may be particularly susceptible to adverse effects of opioids.

[U.S. Boxed Warning]: Healthcare provider should be alert to problems of abuse, misuse, and diversion. Tolerance or drug dependence may result from extended use. Use caution in patients with a history of drug dependence or abuse. Abrupt discontinuation may precipitate withdrawal syndrome. After chronic maternal exposure to opioids, neonatal withdrawal syndrome may occur in the newborn; monitor neonate closely. Signs and symptoms include irritability, hyperactivity and abnormal sleep pattern, high pitched cry, tremor, vomiting, diarrhea and failure to gain weight. Onset, duration and severity depend on the drug used, duration of use, maternal dose, and rate of drug elimination by the newborn. Opioid withdrawal syndrome in the neonate, unlike in adults, may be life-threatening and should be treated according to protocols developed by neonatology experts.

Extended release formulation:

[U.S. Boxed Warnings]: Opana® ER is an extended release oral formulation of oxymorphone and is not suitable for use as an "as needed" analgesic. Tablets should not be broken, chewed, dissolved, or crushed; tablets should be swallowed whole. Opana® ER is intended for use in long-term, continuous management of moderate-to-severe chronic pain. It is not indicated for use in the immediate postoperative period (12-24 hours). Cases of thrombotic thrombocytopenic purpura (TTP) resulting in kidney failure (requiring dialysis) and death have been reported as a result of misuse by drug abusers injecting the extended-release tablets intravenously; tablets are intended for oral administration only. **[U.S. Boxed Warning]: The coingestion of ethanol or ethanol-containing medications with Opana® ER may result in accelerated release of drug from the dosage form, abruptly increasing plasma levels, which may have fatal consequences.**

Adverse Reactions Incidence usually on higher end with extended release (ER) tablet.

>10%:

Central nervous system: Somnolence (9% to 19%), dizziness (7% to 18%), fever (1% to 14%), headache (7% to 12%)

Dermatologic: Pruritus (8% to 15%)

Gastrointestinal: Nausea (19% to 33%), constipation (4% to 28%), vomiting (9% to 16%)

1% to 10%:

Cardiovascular: Hypotension (<10%), tachycardia (<10%), edema (<10%), flushing (<10%), hypertension (<10%)

Central nervous system: Anxiety (1% to <10%), sedation (1% to <10%), depression (<10%), disorientation (<10%), lethargy (<10%), nervousness (<10%), restlessness (<10%), fatigue (≤4%), insomnia (≤4%), confusion (3%)

Endocrine & metabolic: Dehydration (<10%)

Gastrointestinal: Abdominal distension (<10%), flatulence (1% to <10%), xerostomia (1% to <10%), dyspepsia (<10%), weight loss (<10%), diarrhea (≤4%), abdominal pain (≤3%), appetite decreased (≤3%)

Neuromuscular & skeletal: Weakness (<10%)

Ocular: Blurred vision (<10%)

Respiratory: Hypoxia (<10%), dyspnea (<10%)

Miscellaneous: Diaphoresis (1% to <10%)

<1% (Limited to important or life-threatening): Agitation, allergic reaction, apnea (injection), atelectasis (injection), biliary colic, bradycardia, bronchospasm (injection), clamminess, dermatitis, diplopia (injection), dysphoria, euphoric mood, hallucination, hot flashes, hypersensitivity, ileus, injection site reaction, micturition difficulty, miosis, oliguria (injection), orthostatic hypotension, palpitation, physical and psychological dependence, respiratory depression, syncope, TTP (inappropriate injection of ER tablet); ureteral spasm (injection), urinary retention, urticaria

Drug Interactions

Metabolism/Transport Effects None known.

Avoid Concomitant Use

Avoid concomitant use of Oxymorphone with any of the following: Azelastine (Nasal); MAO Inhibitors; Paraldehyde

Increased Effect/Toxicity

Oxymorphone may increase the levels/effects of: Alcohol (Ethyl); Alvimopan; Azelastine (Nasal); CNS Depressants; Desmopressin; Diuretics; Hydrocodone; MAO Inhibitors; Metyrosine; Mirtazapine; Paraldehyde; Pramipexole; ROPINIRole; Rotigotine; Selective Serotonin Reuptake Inhibitors; Zolpidem

The levels/effects of Oxymorphone may be increased by: Amphetamines; Anticholinergics; Antipsychotic Agents (Phenothiazines); Brimonidine (Topical); Cannabinoids; Doxylamine; Droperidol; HydrOXYzine; Magnesium Sulfate; Perampanel; Sodium Oxybate; Succinylcholine; Tapentadol

Decreased Effect

Oxymorphone may decrease the levels/effects of: Pegvisomant

The levels/effects of Oxymorphone may be decreased by: Ammonium Chloride; Mixed Agonist / Antagonist Opioids

Ethanol/Nutrition/Herb Interactions

Ethanol: Ethanol ingestion with extended-release tablets is specifically contraindicated due to possible accelerated release and potentially fatal overdose. Ethanol may also increase CNS depression; monitor for increased effects with coadministration. Caution patients about effects.

Food: When taken orally with a high-fat meal, peak concentration is 38% to 50% greater. Both immediate-release and extended-release tablets should be taken 1 hour before or 2 hours after eating.

Herb/Nutraceutical: Avoid valerian, St John's wort, kava kava, gotu kola (may increase CNS depression).

Storage/Stability Injection solution, tablet: Store at 25°C (77°F); excursions permitted to 15°C to 30°C (59°F to 86°F). Protect injection from light.

Mechanism of Action Oxymorphone hydrochloride is a potent opioid analgesic with uses similar to those of morphine. The drug is a semisynthetic derivative of morphine (phenanthrene derivative) and is closely related to hydromorphone chemically (Dilaudid®).

Pharmacodynamics/Kinetics

Onset of action: Parenteral: 5-10 minutes

Duration: Analgesic: Parenteral: 3-6 hours

Distribution: V_d: I.V.: 1.94-4.22 L/kg

Protein binding: 10% to 12%

Metabolism: Hepatic via glucuronidation to active and inactive metabolites

Bioavailability: Oral: ~10%

Half-life elimination: Oral: Immediate release: 7-9 hours; Extended release: 9-11 hours

Excretion: Urine (<1% as unchanged drug); feces

Dosage Adults: **Note:** Dosage must be individualized.

I.M., SubQ: Initial: 1-1.5 mg; may repeat every 4-6 hours as needed

Labor analgesia: I.M.: 0.5-1 mg

I.V.: Initial: 0.5 mg

Oral:

Immediate release: Acute pain:

Opioid-naive: Initial: 5-10 mg every 4-6 hours as needed (American Pain Society, 2008). Dosage adjustment should be based on level of analgesia, side effects, pain intensity, and patient comorbidities.

Currently on stable dose of parenteral oxymorphone: Approximately 10 times the total daily parenteral requirement. The calculated total oral daily amount should be given in 4-6 equally divided doses.

Currently on other opioids: Use standard conversion chart to convert total daily dose of current opioid to oxymorphone equivalent. Generally start with one-half (1/2) the calculated total daily oxymorphone dosage and administer in divided doses every 4-6 hours.

Extended release (Opana® ER): Chronic pain:

Opioid-naive: Initial: 5 mg every 12 hours. Supplemental doses of immediate-release oxymorphone may be used as "rescue" medication as dosage is titrated.

Note: Continued requirement for supplemental dosing may be used to titrate the dose of extended-release continuous therapy. Adjust therapy incrementally, by 5-10 mg every 12 hours at intervals of every 3-7 days. Ideally, scheduled (basal) dosage may be titrated to generally mild pain or no pain with the regular use of fewer than 2 supplemental doses per 24 hours.

Currently on stable dose of parenteral oxymorphone: Approximately 10 times the total daily parenteral requirement. The calculated total oral daily amount should be given in 2 divided doses (for every 12-hour oxymorphone extended release dosing).

Currently on opioids: Use conversion chart (see **"Note"**) to convert daily dose of current opioid to oxymorphone equivalent. Generally start with one-half (1/2) the calculated daily oxymorphone dosage. Divide daily dose in 2 (for every 12-hour oxymorphone extended release dosing) and round down to nearest dosage strength. **Note:** Per manufacturer, the following approximate oral dosages are equivalent to a daily dose of oxymorphone 10 mg:

Hydrocodone 20 mg

Oxycodone 20 mg

Methadone 20 mg (methadone has a long half-life and accumulates; ratio can vary widely)

Morphine 30 mg

Conversion of stable dose of immediate-release oxymorphone to extended-release oxymorphone: Use same total daily dose. Administer one-half (1/2) of the daily dose of immediate-release oxymorphone (Opana®) as the extended-release formulation (Opana® ER) every 12 hours

Elderly: Initiate dosing at the lower end of the dosage range

Dosing adjustment in renal impairment: Cl_{cr} <50 mL/minute: Reduce initial dosage of oral and parenteral formulations (bioavailability increased 57% to 65%). Begin therapy at lowest dose and titrate slowly with careful monitoring.

Dosing adjustment in hepatic impairment:

Mild impairment: Initiate with lowest possible dose and titrate slowly with careful monitoring.

Moderate-to-severe impairment: Use is contraindicated.

Dietary Considerations Immediate release and extended release tablets should be taken 1 hour before or 2 hours after eating.

Administration Oral: Administer immediate release and extended release tablets 1 hour before or 2 hours after eating. Opana® ER tablet should be swallowed whole; do not break, crush, dissolve, or chew.

Monitoring Parameters Respiratory rate, heart rate, blood pressure, CNS activity

Test Interactions Some quinolones may produce a false-positive urine screening result for opioids using commercially-available immunoassay kits. This has been demonstrated most consistently for levofloxacin and ofloxacin, but other quinolones have shown cross-reactivity in certain assay kits. Confirmation of positive opioid screens by more specific methods should be considered. May cause elevation in amylase (due to constriction of the sphincter of Oddi).

Dosage Forms Excipient information presented when available (limited, particularly for generics); consult specific product labeling.

Solution, Injection, as hydrochloride:

Opana: 1 mg/mL (1 mL)

Tablet, Oral, as hydrochloride:

Opana: 5 mg [contains fd&c blue #2 aluminum lake]

Opana: 10 mg [contains d&c red #30 aluminum lake]

Generic: 5 mg, 10 mg

Tablet ER 12 Hour Abuse-Deterrent, Oral, as hydrochloride:

Opana ER: 5 mg, 7.5 mg

Opana ER: 10 mg [contains fd&c yellow #6 (sunset yellow)]

Opana ER: 15 mg

Opana ER: 20 mg [contains brilliant blue fcf (fd&c blue #1), fd&c yellow #10 (quinoline yellow), fd&c yellow #6 (sunset yellow)]

Opana ER: 30 mg

Opana ER: 40 mg [contains fd&c yellow #10 (quinoline yellow), fd&c yellow #6 (sunset yellow)]

Tablet Extended Release 12 Hour, Oral, as hydrochloride:

Generic: 5 mg, 7.5 mg, 10 mg, 15 mg, 20 mg, 30 mg, 40 mg

Controlled Substance C-II

◆ Oxymorphone Hydrochloride *see* Oxymorphone *on page 1540*

◆ OxyNEO (Can) *see* OxyCODONE *on page 1535*

Oxytocin (oks i TOE sin)

Brand Names: U.S. Pitocin

Brand Names: Canada Oxytocin for injection

Index Terms Pit

Pharmacologic Category Oxytocic Agent

Use Induction of labor in patients with a medical indication; stimulation or reinforcement of labor; adjunctive therapy in management of abortion; to produce uterine contractions during the third stage of labor; control of postpartum bleeding

Pregnancy Risk Factor C (manufacturer specific)

Pregnancy Considerations [U.S. Boxed Warning]: To be used for medical rather than elective induction of labor. Animal reproduction studies have not been conducted. When used as indicated, teratogenic effects would not be expected. Nonteratogenic adverse reactions are reported in the neonate as well as the mother.

Breast-Feeding Considerations Endogenous levels of oxytocin naturally increase during breast-feeding.

Contraindications Hypersensitivity to oxytocin or any component of the formulation; significant cephalopelvic disproportion; unfavorable fetal positions; fetal distress when delivery is not imminent; hypertonic or hyperactive uterus; contraindicated vaginal delivery (invasive cervical cancer, active genital herpes, prolapse of the cord, cord presentation, total placenta previa, or vasa previa); obstetrical emergencies where surgical intervention is favored; where adequate uterine activity fails to achieve satisfactory progress

Warnings/Precautions Hazardous agent - use appropriate precautions for handling and disposal (NIOSH, 2012). **[U.S. Boxed Warning]: To be used for medical rather than elective induction of labor.** Medical indications for labor induction may include Rh problems, maternal diabetes, preeclampsia at or near term, when delivery is in the best interest of mother or fetus, or premature rupture of membranes when delivery is indicated. Use is generally not recommended in the following conditions: Fetal distress, hydramnios, partial placenta previa, prematurity, borderline cephalopelvic disproportion, or conditions where there is a predisposition for uterine rupture. May produce antidiuretic effect (ie, water intoxication). Severe water intoxication with convulsions, coma, and death is associated with a slow oxytocin infusion over 24 hours. High doses or hypersensitivity to oxytocin may cause uterine hypertonicity, spasm, tetanic contraction, or rupture of the uterus. Intravenous preparations should be administered by adequately trained individuals familiar with its use and able to identify complications.

Adverse Reactions Frequency not defined.

Fetus or neonate:

Cardiovascular: Arrhythmias (including premature ventricular contractions), bradycardia

Central nervous system: Brain or CNS damage (permanent), neonatal seizure

Hepatic: Neonatal jaundice

Ocular: Neonatal retinal hemorrhage

Miscellaneous: Fetal death, low Apgar score (5 minute)

Mother:

Cardiovascular: Arrhythmias (including premature ventricular contractions), hypertensive episodes

Gastrointestinal: Nausea, vomiting

Genitourinary: Pelvic hematoma, postpartum hemorrhage, uterine hypertonicity, tetanic contraction of the uterus, uterine rupture, uterine spasm

Hematologic: Afibrinogenemia (fatal)

Miscellaneous: Anaphylactic reaction, subarachnoid hemorrhage; severe water intoxication with convulsions, coma, and death is associated with a slow oxytocin infusion over 24 hours

Drug Interactions

Metabolism/Transport Effects None known.

Avoid Concomitant Use There are no known interactions where it is recommended to avoid concomitant use.

Increased Effect/Toxicity

Oxytocin may increase the levels/effects of: Highest Risk QTc-Prolonging Agents; Moderate Risk QTc-Prolonging Agents

The levels/effects of Oxytocin may be increased by: Dinoprostone; Mifepristone; Misoprostol

Decreased Effect There are no known significant interactions involving a decrease in effect.

Preparation for Administration Hazardous agent; use appropriate precautions for handling and disposal (NIOSH, 2012).

I.V.:

Induction or stimulation of labor: Add oxytocin 10 units to NS or LR 1000 mL to yield a solution containing oxytocin 10 milliunits/mL. Rotate solution to mix.

Postpartum uterine bleeding: Add oxytocin 10-40 units to running I.V. infusion; maximum: 40 units/1000 mL.

Adjunctive management of abortion: Add oxytocin 10 units to 500 mL of a physiologic saline solution or D_5W.

Storage/Stability Store at 20°C to 25°C (68°F to 77°F); excursions permitted to 15°C to 30°C (59°F to 86°F); do not freeze.

Mechanism of Action Oxytocin stimulates uterine contraction by activating G-protein-coupled receptors that trigger increases in intracellular calcium levels in uterine myofibrils. Oxytocin also increases local prostaglandin production, further stimulating uterine contraction.

Pharmacodynamics/Kinetics

Onset of action: Uterine contractions: I.M.: 3-5 minutes; I.V.: ~1 minute

Duration: I.M.: 2-3 hour; I.V.: 1 hour

Metabolism: Rapidly hepatic and via plasma (by oxytocinase) and to a smaller degree the mammary gland

Half-life elimination: 1-6 minutes; decreased in late pregnancy and during lactation

Excretion: Urine

Dosage I.V. administration requires the use of an infusion pump. Adults:

Induction of labor: Manufacturer's labeling: I.V.: 0.5-1 milliunits/minute; gradually increase dose in 30-60 minute intervals by increments of 1-2 milliunits/minute until desired contraction pattern is established; dose may be decreased after desired frequency of contractions is reached and labor has progressed to 5-6 cm dilation. Infusion rates of 6 milliunits/minute provide oxytocin levels similar to those at spontaneous labor; rates >9-10 milliunits/minute are rarely required. Higher dose regimens (example, initial dose 2-6 milliunits/minute) with larger incremental dose increases (example, 1-6 milliunits/minute) have also been proposed; decrease or discontinue dose for abnormal or excessive uterine contractions (ACOG, 2009).

Postpartum bleeding:

I.M.: Total dose of 10 units after delivery of the placenta

I.V.: 10-40 units by I.V. infusion in 1000 mL of intravenous fluid at a rate sufficient to control uterine atony

Adjunctive treatment of abortion: I.V.: 10-20 milliunits/minute; maximum total dose: 30 units/12 hours

Dosage adjustment in renal impairment: No dosage adjustment provided in manufacturer's labeling.

Dosage adjustment in hepatic impairment: No dosage adjustment provided in manufacturer's labeling.

Administration I.V.: An infusion pump is required for administration

Hazardous agent; use appropriate precautions for handling and disposal (NIOSH, 2012).

Monitoring Parameters Fluid intake and output during administration, uterine activity, blood pressure; fetal monitoring

Dosage Forms Excipient information presented when available (limited, particularly for generics); consult specific product labeling.

Solution, Injection:

Pitocin: 10 units/mL (1 mL, 10 mL, 50 mL) [contains chlorobutanol (chlorobutol)]

Generic: 10 units/mL (1 mL, 10 mL, 30 mL)

- ◆ **Oxytocin for injection (Can)** *see* Oxytocin *on page* 1542
- ◆ **Oxytrol** *see* Oxybutynin *on page* 1533
- ◆ **Oxytrol for Women** *see* Oxybutynin *on page* 1533
- ◆ **Oxytrol For Women [OTC]** *see* Oxybutynin *on page* 1533
- ◆ **Oysco D [OTC]** *see* Calcium and Vitamin D *on page* 318
- ◆ **Oysco 500 [OTC]** *see* Calcium Carbonate *on page* 318
- ◆ **Oysco 500+D [OTC]** *see* Calcium and Vitamin D *on page* 318
- ◆ **Ozurdex** *see* Dexamethasone (Ophthalmic) *on page* 583
- ◆ **Ozurdex® (Can)** *see* Dexamethasone (Ophthalmic) *on page* 583
- ◆ **P01BE03** *see* Artesunate *on page* 171
- ◆ **P-071** *see* Cetirizine *on page* 396
- ◆ **P-1202** *see* Methyl Aminolevulinate *on page* 1332
- ◆ **Pacerone** *see* Amiodarone *on page* 101

PACLitaxel (pac li TAKS el)

Brand Names: Canada Apo-Paclitaxel®; Paclitaxel for Injection; Paclitaxel Injection USP

Index Terms Conventional Paclitaxel; Paclitaxel (Conventional); Taxol

Pharmacologic Category Antineoplastic Agent, Antimicrotubular; Antineoplastic Agent, Natural Source (Plant) Derivative; Antineoplastic Agent, Taxane Derivative

Use Treatment of breast, nonsmall cell lung, and ovarian cancers; treatment of AIDS-related Kaposi's sarcoma (KS)

Unlabeled Use Treatment of bladder, cervical, small cell lung, and head and neck cancers; treatment of (unknown primary) adenocarcinoma

Pregnancy Risk Factor D

Pregnancy Considerations Adverse events (embryotoxicity, fetal toxicity, and maternal toxicity) have been observed in animal reproduction studies at doses less than the recommended human dose. An *ex vivo* human placenta perfusion model illustrated that paclitaxel crossed the placenta at term. Placental transfer was low and affected by the presence of albumin; higher albumin concentrations resulted in lower paclitaxel placental transfer (Berveiller, 2012). Women of childbearing potential should be advised to avoid becoming pregnant. A pregnancy registry is available for all cancers diagnosed during pregnancy at Cooper Health (877-635-4499).

Breast-Feeding Considerations Paclitaxel is excreted in breast milk (case report). The mother (3 months postpartum) was treated with paclitaxel 30 mg/m^2 (56.1 mg) and carboplatin once weekly for papillary thyroid cancer. Milk samples were obtained 4-316 hours after the infusion given at the sixth and final week of therapy. The average paclitaxel milk concentration over the testing interval was 0.78 mg/L. Although maternal serum concentrations were not noted in the report, the relative infant dose to a nursing infant was calculated to be ~17% of the maternal dose. Paclitaxel continued to be detected in breast milk when sampled at 172 hours after the dose and was below the limit of detection when sampled at 316 hours after the infusion (Griffin, 2012). Due to the potential for serious adverse reactions in a nursing infant, breast-feeding is not recommended.

Contraindications Hypersensitivity to paclitaxel, Cremophor® EL (polyoxyethylated castor oil), or any component of the formulation

Warnings/Precautions Hazardous agent - use appropriate precautions for handling and disposal (NIOSH, 2012). **[U.S. Boxed Warning]: Anaphylaxis and severe hypersensitivity reactions (dyspnea requiring bronchodilators, hypotension requiring treatment, angioedema, and/or urticaria) have been reported; premedicate with corticosteroids, diphenhydramine, and H_2 antagonists prior to infusion. Some reactions have been fatal despite premedication. If severe hypersensitivity occurs, stop infusion and do not rechallenge.** Minor hypersensitivity reactions (flushing, skin reactions, dyspnea, hypotension, or tachycardia) do not require interruption of treatment. **[U.S. Boxed Warning]: Bone marrow suppression (primarily neutropenia; may be severe or result in infection) is the dose-limiting toxicity; do not administer if baseline absolute neutrophil count (ANC) is <1500 cells/mm^3 (for solid tumors) or <1000 cells/mm^3 (for patients with AIDS-related KS). Monitor blood counts frequently.** Reduce future doses by 20% for severe neutropenia (<500 cells/mm^3 for 7 days or more) and consider the use of supportive therapy, including growth factor treatment.

Use extreme caution with hepatic dysfunction (myelotoxicity may be worsened); dose reductions are recommended. Peripheral neuropathy may occur; patients with pre-existing neuropathies from chemotherapy or coexisting conditions (eg, diabetes mellitus) may be at a higher risk; reduce dose by 20% for severe neuropathy. Paclitaxel formulations contain dehydrated alcohol; may cause adverse CNS effects. Infusion-related hypotension, bradycardia, and/or hypertension may occur; frequent monitoring of vital signs is recommended, especially during the first hour of the infusion. Rare but severe conduction abnormalities have been reported; conduct cardiac monitoring during subsequent infusions for these patients. Elderly patients have an increased risk of toxicity (neutropenia, neuropathy). **[U.S. Boxed Warning]: Should be administered under the supervision of an experienced cancer chemotherapy physician; administer in a facility sufficient to appropriately diagnose and manage complications.** Paclitaxel is an irritant with vesicant-like properties; ensure proper needle or catheter placement prior to and during infusion; avoid extravasation.

Adverse Reactions Percentages reported with single-agent therapy. **Note:** Myelosuppression is dose related, schedule related, and infusion-rate dependent (increased incidences with higher doses, more frequent doses, and longer infusion times) and, in general, rapidly reversible upon discontinuation.

>10%:

Cardiovascular: Flushing (28%), ECG abnormal (14% to 23%), edema (21%), hypotension (4% to 12%)

Dermatologic: Alopecia (87%), rash (12%)

Gastrointestinal: Nausea/vomiting (52%), diarrhea (38%), mucositis (17% to 35%; grades 3/4: up to 3%), stomatitis (15%; most common at doses >390 mg/m^2), abdominal pain (with intraperitoneal paclitaxel)

Hematologic: Neutropenia (78% to 98%; grade 4: 14% to 75%; onset 8-10 days, median nadir 11 days, recovery 15-21 days), leukopenia (90%; grade 4: 17%), anemia (47% to 90%; grades 3/4: 2% to 16%), thrombocytopenia (4% to 20%; grades 3/4: 1% to 7%), bleeding (14%)

Hepatic: Alkaline phosphatase increased (22%), AST increased (19%)

Local: Injection site reaction (erythema, tenderness, skin discoloration, swelling: 13%)

Neuromuscular & skeletal: Peripheral neuropathy (42% to 70%; grades 3/4: up to 7%), arthralgia/myalgia (60%), weakness (17%)

Renal: Creatinine increased (observed in KS patients only: 18% to 34%; severe: 5% to 7%)

Miscellaneous: Hypersensitivity reaction (31% to 45%; grades 3/4: up to 2%), infection (15% to 30%)

1% to 10%:

Cardiovascular: Bradycardia (3%), tachycardia (2%), hypertension (1%), rhythm abnormalities (1%), syncope (1%), venous thrombosis (1%)

Dermatologic: Nail changes (2%)

Hematologic: Febrile neutropenia (2%)

Hepatic: Bilirubin increased (7%)

Respiratory: Dyspnea (2%)

<1% (Limited to important or life-threatening): Anaphylaxis, arrhythmia, ataxia, atrial fibrillation, AV block, back pain, cardiac conduction abnormalities, cellulitis, CHF, chills, conjunctivitis, dehydration, enterocolitis, extravasation recall, hepatic encephalopathy, hepatic necrosis, induration, intestinal obstruction, intestinal perforation, interstitial pneumonia, ischemic colitis, lacrimation increased, maculopapular rash, malaise, MI, myocardial ischemia, necrotic changes and ulceration following extravasation, neuroencephalopathy, neutropenic enterocolitis, neutropenic typhlitis, ototoxicity (tinnitus and hearing loss), pancreatitis, paralytic ileus, phlebitis, pneumonitis, pruritus, pulmonary embolism, pulmonary fibrosis, radiation recall, radiation pneumonitis, renal insufficiency, seizure, skin exfoliation, skin fibrosis, skin necrosis, Stevens-Johnson syndrome, supraventricular tachycardia, toxic epidermal necrolysis, ventricular tachycardia (asymptomatic), visual disturbances (scintillating scotomata)

Drug Interactions

Metabolism/Transport Effects **Substrate** of CYP2C8 (major), CYP3A4 (major), P-glycoprotein; **Note:** Assignment of Major/Minor substrate status based on clinically relevant drug interaction potential; **Induces** CYP3A4 (weak/moderate)

Avoid Concomitant Use

Avoid concomitant use of PACLitaxel with any of the following: Axitinib; BCG; CloZAPine; Conivaptan; Fusidic Acid (Systemic); Natalizumab; Pimecrolimus; Simeprevir; SORAfenib; Tacrolimus (Topical); Tofacitinib; Vaccines (Live)

Increased Effect/Toxicity

PACLitaxel may increase the levels/effects of: Antineoplastic Agents (Anthracycline, Systemic); Bexarotene (Systemic); CloZAPine; DOXOrubicin; Leflunomide; Natalizumab; Tofacitinib; Trastuzumab; Vaccines (Live); Vinorelbine

The levels/effects of PACLitaxel may be increased by: Conivaptan; CYP2C8 Inhibitors (Moderate); CYP2C8 Inhibitors (Strong); CYP3A4 Inhibitors (Moderate); CYP3A4 Inhibitors (Strong); Dasatinib; Deferasirox; Denosumab; Fusidic Acid (Systemic); Ivacaftor; Luliconazole; Mifepristone; P-glycoprotein/ABCB1 Inhibitors; Pimecrolimus; Platinum Derivatives; Roflumilast; Simeprevir; SORAfenib; Tacrolimus (Topical)

Decreased Effect

PACLitaxel may decrease the levels/effects of: ARIPiprazole; Axitinib; BCG; Coccidioidin Skin Test; Ibrutinib; Saxagliptin; Simeprevir; Sipuleucel-T; Vaccines (Inactivated); Vaccines (Live)

The levels/effects of PACLitaxel may be decreased by: Bexarotene (Systemic); Bosentan; CYP2C8 Inducers (Strong); CYP3A4 Inducers (Strong); Dabrafenib; Deferasirox; Echinacea; Herbs (CYP3A4 Inducers); Mitotane; P-glycoprotein/ABCB1 Inducers; Tocilizumab; Trastuzumab

Ethanol/Nutrition/Herb Interactions Herb/Nutraceutical: Avoid black cohosh, dong quai in estrogen-dependent tumors. Avoid valerian, St John's wort (may decrease paclitaxel levels), kava kava, gotu kola (may increase CNS depression).

Preparation for Administration Hazardous agent; use appropriate precautions for handling and disposal (NIOSH, 2012). Dilute for infusion in 250-1000 mL D_5W, D_5LR, D_5NS, or NS to a concentration of 0.3-1.2 mg/mL, use a non-PVC container (glass or polyethylene). Chemotherapy dispensing devices (eg, Chemo Dispensing Pin™) should not be used to withdraw paclitaxel from the vial.

Storage/Stability Store intact vials at room temperature of 20°C to 25°C (68°F to 77°F). Protect from light. Solutions diluted for infusion in D_5W and NS are stable for up to 3 days at room temperature (25°C).

Paclitaxel should be dispensed in either glass or non-PVC containers (eg, Excel™/PAB™). Use **nonpolyvinyl** (non-PVC) tubing (eg, polyethylene) to minimize leaching. Formulated in a vehicle known as Cremophor® EL (polyoxyethylated castor oil). Cremophor® EL has been found to leach the plasticizer DEHP from polyvinyl chloride infusion bags or administration sets. Contact of the undiluted concentrate with plasticized polyvinyl chloride (PVC) equipment or devices is not recommended.

Mechanism of Action Paclitaxel promotes microtubule assembly by enhancing the action of tubulin dimers, stabilizing existing microtubules, and inhibiting their disassembly, interfering with the late G_2 mitotic phase, and inhibiting cell replication. In addition, the drug can distort mitotic spindles, resulting in the breakage of chromosomes. Paclitaxel may also suppress cell proliferation and modulate immune response.

Pharmacodynamics/Kinetics

Distribution:

V_d: Widely distributed into body fluids and tissues; affected by dose and duration of infusion

V_{dss}:

1- to 6-hour infusion: 67.1 L/m^2

24-hour infusion: 227-688 L/m^2

Protein binding: 89% to 98%

Metabolism: Hepatic via CYP2C8 and 3A4; forms metabolites (primarily 6α-hydroxypaclitaxel)

Half-life elimination:

1- to 6-hour infusion: Mean (beta): 6.4 hours

3-hour infusion: Mean (terminal): 13.1-20.2 hours

24-hour infusion: Mean (terminal): 15.7-52.7 hours

Excretion: Feces (~70%, 5% as unchanged drug); urine (14%)

Clearance: Mean: Total body: After 1- and 6-hour infusions: 5.8-16.3 L/hour/m^2; After 24-hour infusions: 14.2-17.2 L/hour/m^2

Dosage Premedication with dexamethasone (20 mg orally or I.V. at 12 and 6 hours **or** 14 and 7 hours before the dose; reduce dexamethasone dose to 10 mg orally with advanced HIV disease), diphenhydramine (50 mg I.V. 30-60 minutes prior to the dose), and cimetidine, famotidine, or ranitidine (I.V. 30-60 minutes prior to the dose) is recommended.

Adults: I.V.: Refer to individual protocols

Ovarian carcinoma: 135-175 mg/m^2 over 3 hours every 3 weeks **or**

135 mg/m^2 over 24 hours every 3 weeks **or**

50-80 mg/m^2 over 1-3 hours weekly **or**

1.4-4 mg/m^2/day continuous infusion for 14 days every 4 weeks

Metastatic breast cancer: 175-250 mg/m^2 over 3 hours every 3 weeks **or**

50-80 mg/m^2 weekly **or**

1.4-4 mg/m^2/day continuous infusion for 14 days every 4 weeks

Nonsmall cell lung carcinoma: 135 mg/m^2 over 24 hours every 3 weeks

AIDS-related Kaposi's sarcoma: 135 mg/m^2 over 3 hours every 3 weeks **or**

100 mg/m^2 over 3 hours every 2 weeks

Intraperitoneal (unlabeled route): Ovarian carcinoma: 60 mg/m^2 on day 8 of a 21-day treatment cycle for 6 cycles, in combination with I.V. paclitaxel and intraperitoneal cisplatin. **Note:** Administration of intraperitoneal paclitaxel should include the standard paclitaxel premedication regimen.

Dosage modification for toxicity (solid tumors, including ovary, breast, and lung carcinoma): Courses of paclitaxel should not be repeated until the neutrophil count is ≥1500 cells/mm^3 and the platelet count is ≥100,000 cells/mm^3; reduce dosage by 20% for patients experiencing severe peripheral neuropathy or severe neutropenia (neutrophil <500 cells/mm^3 for a week or longer)

Dosage modification for immunosuppression in advanced HIV disease: Paclitaxel should not be given to patients with HIV if the baseline or subsequent neutrophil count is <1000 cells/mm^3. Additional modifications include: Reduce dosage of dexamethasone in premedication to 10 mg orally; reduce dosage by 20% in patients experiencing severe peripheral neuropathy or severe neutropenia (neutrophil <500 cells/mm^3 for a week or longer); initiate concurrent hematopoietic growth factor (G-CSF) as clinically indicated

Dosage adjustment in renal impairment: No dosage adjustment provided in manufacturer's labeling. Aronoff (2007) recommends no dosage adjustment necessary for adults with Cl_{cr} <50 mL/minute.

Dosage adjustment in hepatic impairment: Note: The FDA-approved labeling recommendations are based upon the patient's first course of therapy where the usual dose would be 135 mg/m^2 dose over 24 hours or the 175 mg/m^2 dose over 3 hours in patients with normal hepatic function. Dosage in subsequent courses should be based upon individual tolerance. Adjustments for other regimens are not available.

24-hour infusion:

Transaminases <2 times upper limit of normal (ULN) and bilirubin level ≤1.5 mg/dL: 135 mg/m^2

Transaminases 2-<10 times ULN and bilirubin level ≤1.5 mg/dL: 100 mg/m^2

Transaminases <10 times ULN and bilirubin level 1.6-7.5 mg/dL: 50 mg/m^2
Transaminases ≥10 times ULN **or** bilirubin level >7.5 mg/dL: Avoid use
3-hour infusion:
Transaminases <10 times ULN and bilirubin level ≤1.25 times ULN: 175 mg/m^2
Transaminases <10 times ULN and bilirubin level 1.26-2 times ULN: 135 mg/m^2
Transaminases <10 times ULN and bilirubin level 2.01-5 times ULN: 90 mg/m^2
Transaminases ≥10 times ULN **or** bilirubin level >5 times ULN: Avoid use

Dosing in obesity: *ASCO Guidelines for appropriate chemotherapy dosing in obese adults with cancer:* Utilize patient's actual body weight (full weight) for calculation of body surface area- or weight-based dosing, particularly when the intent of therapy is curative; manage regimen-related toxicities in the same manner as for nonobese patients; if a dose reduction is utilized due to toxicity, consider resumption of full weight-based dosing with subsequent cycles, especially if cause of toxicity (eg, hepatic or renal impairment) is resolved (Griggs, 2012).

Administration

I.V.: Infuse over 1-96 hours. When administered as a part of a combination chemotherapy regimen, sequence of administration may vary by regimen; refer to specific protocol for sequence recommendation.

Premedication with dexamethasone (20 mg orally or I.V. at 12 and 6 hours **or** 14 and 7 hours before the dose; reduce to 10 mg with advanced HIV disease), diphenhydramine (50 mg I.V. 30-60 minutes prior to the dose), and cimetidine 300 mg, famotidine 20 mg, or ranitidine 50 mg (I.V. 30-60 minutes prior to the dose) is recommended.

Administer I.V. infusion over 1-24 hours; infuse through a 0.22 micron in-line filter and nonsorbing administration set.

Irritant with vesicant-like properties; avoid extravasation. Ensure proper needle or catheter position prior to administration.

Extravasation management: If extravasation occurs, stop infusion immediately and disconnect (leave cannula/ needle in place); gently aspirate extravasated solution (do **NOT** flush the line); remove needle/cannula; initiate antidote (hyaluronidase); remove needle/cannula; elevate extremity. Information conflicts regarding the use of warm or cold compresses (Perez Fidalgo, 2012; Polovich, 2009).

Hyaluronidase: If needle/cannula still in place: Administer 1-6 mL (150 units/mL) into existing I.V. line; usual dose is 1 mL for each 1 mL of extravasated drug; if needle/ cannula has been removed, inject subcutaneously in a clockwise manner around area of extravasation; may repeat several times over the next 3-4 hours (Ener, 2004).

Intraperitoneal: 1- to 2-hour infusion

Hazardous agent; use appropriate precautions for handling and disposal (NIOSH, 2012).

Monitoring Parameters CBC with differential and platelet count, liver and kidney function; monitor for hypersensitivity reactions, vital signs (frequently during the first hour of infusion), continuous cardiac monitoring (patients with conduction abnormalities)

Reference Range Mean maximum serum concentrations: 435-802 ng/mL following 24-hour infusions of 200-275 mg/m^2 and were approximately 10% to 30% of those following 6-hour infusions of equivalent doses

Additional Information Sensory neuropathy is almost universal at doses >250 mg/m^2; motor neuropathy is uncommon at doses <250 mg/m^2. Myopathic effects are common with doses >200 mg/m^2, generally occur within 2-3 days of treatment, and resolve over 5-6 days. Intraperitoneal administration of paclitaxel is associated with a higher incidence of chemotherapy related toxicity.

Dosage Forms Excipient information presented when available (limited, particularly for generics); consult specific product labeling.

Concentrate, Intravenous:
Generic: 100 mg/16.7 mL (16.7 mL); 30 mg/5 mL (5 mL); 150 mg/25 mL (25 mL); 300 mg/50 mL (50 mL)

Concentrate, Intravenous [preservative free]:
Generic: 100 mg/16.7 mL (16.7 mL); 30 mg/5 mL (5 mL); 300 mg/50 mL (50 mL)

- **Paclitaxel, Albumin-Bound** *see* PACLitaxel (Protein Bound) *on page 1546*
- **Paclitaxel (Conventional)** *see* PACLitaxel *on page 1543*
- **Paclitaxel for Injection (Can)** *see* PACLitaxel *on page 1543*
- **Paclitaxel Injection USP (Can)** *see* PACLitaxel *on page 1543*
- **Paclitaxel (Nanoparticle Albumin Bound)** *see* PACLitaxel (Protein Bound) *on page 1546*

PACLitaxel (Protein Bound)

(pac li TAKS el PROE teen bownd)

Brand Names: U.S. Abraxane

Brand Names: Canada Abraxane for Injectable Suspension

Index Terms ABI-007; Albumin-Bound Paclitaxel; Albumin-Stabilized Nanoparticle Paclitaxel; nab-Paclitaxel; Nanoparticle Albumin-Bound Paclitaxel; Paclitaxel (Nanoparticle Albumin Bound); Paclitaxel, Albumin-Bound; Protein-Bound Paclitaxel

Pharmacologic Category Antineoplastic Agent, Antimicrotubular; Antineoplastic Agent, Natural Source (Plant) Derivative; Antineoplastic Agent, Taxane Derivative

Use

Breast cancer: Treatment of refractory (metastatic) or relapsed (within 6 months of adjuvant therapy) breast cancer after failure of combination chemotherapy (including anthracycline-based therapy unless clinically contraindicated)

Nonsmall cell lung cancer (NSCLC): First-line treatment of locally advanced or metastatic NSCLC (in combination with carboplatin) in patients ineligible for curative surgery or radiation therapy

Pancreatic cancer: First-line treatment of patients with metastatic adenocarcinoma of the pancreas (in combination with gemcitabine)

Unlabeled Use Treatment of recurrent or persistent ovarian, fallopian tube, or primary peritoneal cancers

Pregnancy Risk Factor D

Dosage Note: When administered as part of a combination chemotherapy regimen, sequence of administration may vary by regimen; refer to specific protocol for sequence of administration. Premedication is not generally necessary prior to paclitaxel (protein bound), but may be needed in patients with prior mild-to-moderate hypersensitivity reactions.

Breast cancer, metastatic: Adults: I.V.: 260 mg/m^2 every 3 weeks (Gradishar, 2005)

Nonsmall cell lung cancer (NSCLC), locally advanced or metastatic: Adults: I.V.: 100 mg/m^2 on days 1, 8, and 15 of each 21-day cycle (in combination with carboplatin) (Socinski, 2012)

Pancreatic cancer, metastatic: Adults: I.V.: 125 mg/m^2 on days 1, 8, and 15 of a 28-day cycle (in combination with gemcitabine) (Von Hoff, 2013)

Breast cancer (unlabeled dosing): Adults: I.V.: 100-150 mg/m^2 on days 1, 8, and 15 of a 28-day cycle (Gradishar, 2009)

Ovarian, fallopian tube, or primary peritoneal cancer (recurrent; unlabeled use): Adults: I.V.: 260 mg/m^2 on day 1 of a 21-day cycle for 6-8 cycles (Teneriello, 2009) **or** 100 mg/m^2 on days 1, 8, and 15 of a 28-day cycle until disease progression or unacceptable toxicity (Coleman, 2011)

Dosage adjustment for toxicity:

Breast cancer (every 3 week regimen):

Severe neutropenia (<500 cells/mm^3) ≥1 week: Reduce dose to 220 mg/m^2 for subsequent courses

Recurrent severe neutropenia: Reduce dose to 180 mg/m^2 for subsequent courses

Sensory neuropathy

Grade 1 or 2: Dosage adjustment generally not required

Grade 3: Hold treatment until resolved to grade 1 or 2, then resume with reduced dose for all subsequent cycles

Severe sensory neuropathy: Reduce dose to 220 mg/m^2 for subsequent courses

Recurrent severe sensory neuropathy: Reduce dose to 180 mg/m^2 for subsequent courses

Nonsmall cell lung cancer (NSCLC):

Neutropenia: ANC <1500 cells/mm^3: Withhold therapy until ANC is ≥1500 cells/mm^3 on day 1 or ≥500 cells/mm^3 on days 8 or 15. Reduce dose upon therapy reinitiation if:

Neutropenic fever (ANC <500 cells/mm^3 with fever >38°C) **or** delay of next cycle by >7 days due to ANC <1500 cells/mm^3 **or** ANC <500 cells/mm^3 for >7 days:

First occurrence: Permanently reduce dose to 75 mg/m^2

Second occurrence: Permanently reduce dose to 50 mg/m^2

Third occurrence: Discontinue therapy.

Thrombocytopenia: Platelet count <100,000 cells/mm^3: Withhold therapy until platelet count is ≥100,000 cells/mm^3 on day 1 or ≥50,000 cells/mm^3 on days 8 or 15. Reduce dose upon therapy reinitiation if:

Platelet count <50,000 cells/mm^3:

First occurrence: Permanently reduce dose to 75 mg/m^2

Second occurrence: Discontinue therapy.

Sensory neuropathy: Withhold therapy for grade 3-4 peripheral neuropathy. Resume therapy at reduced doses when neuropathy completely resolves or improves to grade 1:

First occurrence: Permanently reduce dose to 75 mg/m^2

Second occurrence: Permanently reduce dose to 50 mg/m^2

Third occurrence: Discontinue therapy.

Pancreatic adenocarcinoma:

Note: Dose level reductions for toxicity:

Full dose: 125 mg/m^2

First dose reduction: 100 mg/m^2

Second dose reduction: 75 mg/m^2

If additional dose reduction is necessary: Discontinue.

Hematologic toxicity (neutropenia and/or thrombocytopenia):

Day 1: If ANC is <1500 cells/mm^3 **or** platelet count is <100,000 cells/mm^3: Withhold therapy until ANC is ≥1500 cells/mm^3 and platelet count is ≥100,000 cells/mm^3

Day 8:

If ANC is 500 to <1000 cells/mm^3 **or** platelet count is 50,000 to <75,000 cells/mm^3: Reduce 1 dose level

If ANC is <500 cells/mm^3 **or** platelet count is <50,000 cells/mm^3: Withhold day 8 dose

Day 15 (if day 8 doses were reduced or given without modification):

If ANC is 500 to <1000 cells/mm^3 **or** platelet count is 50,000 to <75,000 cells/mm^3: Reduce 1 dose level from day 8

If ANC is <500 cells/mm^3 **or** platelet count is <50,000 cells/mm^3: Withhold day 15 dose

Day 15 (if day 8 doses were withheld):

If ANC is ≥1000 cells/mm^3 or platelet count is ≥75,000 cells/mm^3: Reduce 1 dose level from day 1

If ANC is 500 to <1000 cells/mm^3 or platelet count is 50,000 to <75,000 cells/mm^3: Reduce 2 dose levels from day 1

If ANC is <500 cells/mm^3 **or** platelet count is <50,000 cells/mm^3: Withhold day 15 dose

Neutropenic fever: Withhold therapy for grade 3-4 fever. Resume therapy at next lower dose level when fever resolves and ANC is ≥1500 cells/mm^3.

Peripheral neuropathy: Withhold therapy for grade 3-4 peripheral neuropathy. Resume therapy at next lower dose level when neuropathy improves to ≤ grade 1.

Dermatologic toxicity: For grade 2-3 toxicity, reduce dose to next lower dose level; if toxicity persists, discontinue.

Gastrointestinal toxicity: Withhold therapy for grade 3 mucositis or diarrhea. Resume therapy at next lower dose level when improves to ≤ grade 1.

Dosage adjustment in renal impairment: No dosage adjustment provided in manufacturer's labeling (has not been studied).

Dosage adjustment in hepatic impairment:

Dosage adjustment for hepatic impairment at treatment initiation:

Breast cancer (every 3 week regimen):

Mild impairment (AST <10 times ULN and bilirubin ≤1.25 times ULN): No adjustment required.

Moderate impairment (AST <10 times ULN and bilirubin 1.26-2 times ULN): Reduce dose to 200 mg/m^2

Severe impairment:

AST <10 times ULN and bilirubin 2.01-5 times ULN: Reduce dose to 130 mg/m^2; may increase up to 200 mg/m^2 in subsequent cycles (based on individual tolerance)

AST >10 times ULN or bilirubin >5 times ULN: Use is not recommended

Nonsmall cell lung cancer (NSCLC) regimen:

Mild impairment (AST <10 times ULN and bilirubin ≤1.25 times ULN): No dosage adjustment necessary.

Moderate impairment (AST <10 times ULN and bilirubin 1.26-2 times ULN): Reduce dose to 75 mg/m^2

Severe impairment:

AST <10 times ULN and bilirubin 2.01-5 times ULN: Reduce dose to 50 mg/m^2; may increase up to 75 mg/m^2 in subsequent cycles (based on individual tolerance)

AST >10 times ULN or bilirubin >5 times ULN: Use is not recommended.

Pancreatic adenocarcinoma:

Mild impairment (AST <10 times ULN and bilirubin ≤1.25 times ULN): No dosage adjustment necessary.

Moderate impairment (AST <10 times ULN and bilirubin 1.26-2 times ULN): Use is not recommended.

Severe impairment:

AST <10 times ULN and bilirubin 2.01-5 times ULN: Use is not recommended.

AST >10 times ULN or bilirubin >5 times ULN: Use is not recommended.

Dosage adjustment for hepatic impairment during treatment: AST >10 times ULN or bilirubin >5 times ULN: Withhold treatment

Dosing in obesity: *ASCO Guidelines for appropriate chemotherapy dosing in obese adults with cancer:* Utilize patient's actual body weight (full weight) for calculation of body surface area- or weight-based dosing, particularly when the intent of therapy is curative; manage regimen-related toxicities in the same manner as for nonobese patients; if a dose reduction is utilized due to toxicity, consider resumption of full weight-based dosing with subsequent cycles, especially if cause of toxicity (eg, hepatic or renal impairment) is resolved (Griggs, 2012).

Additional Information Complete prescribing information should be consulted for additional detail.

Dosage Forms Excipient information presented when available (limited, particularly for generics); consult specific product labeling.

Suspension Reconstituted, Intravenous:
Abraxane: 100 mg (1 ea)

◆ **Pain Eze [OTC]** *see* Acetaminophen *on page 28*

◆ **Pain & Fever Children's [OTC]** *see* Acetaminophen *on page 28*

◆ **Pain-Off [OTC]** *see* Acetaminophen, Aspirin, and Caffeine *on page 33*

◆ **Palafer® (Can)** *see* Ferrous Fumarate *on page 854*

◆ **Palgic** *see* Carbinoxamine *on page 343*

Palifermin (pal ee FER min)

Brand Names: U.S. Kepivance

Brand Names: Canada Kepivance®

Index Terms AMJ 9701; Keratinocyte Growth Factor, Recombinant Human; rhKGF; rhu Keratinocyte Growth Factor; rHu-KGF

Pharmacologic Category Keratinocyte Growth Factor

Use Decrease the incidence and duration of severe oral mucositis associated with hematologic malignancies in patients receiving myelotoxic therapy requiring hematopoietic stem cell support (when the preparative regimen is expected to result in mucositis ≥grade 3 in most patients)

Note: Use (safety and efficacy) is not established for nonhematologic malignancies; use is not recommended with conditioning regimens containing melphalan 200 mg/m^2

Pregnancy Risk Factor C

Pregnancy Considerations Palifermin has been shown to be embryotoxic in animal reproduction studies at doses also associated with maternal toxicity. Use in pregnancy only if the potential benefit outweighs the potential risk for the fetus.

Breast-Feeding Considerations According to the manufacturer labeling, the decision to discontinue palifermin or discontinue breast-feeding during treatment should take into account the benefits of treatment to the mother.

Contraindications There are no contraindications listed within the manufacturer's U.S. product labeling.

Canadian labeling: Hypersensitivity to palifermin, *E. coli*-derived proteins, or any component of the formulation

Warnings/Precautions Hazardous agent - use appropriate precautions for handling and disposal (NIOSH, 2012). Edema, erythema, pruritus, rash, oral/perioral dysesthesia, taste alteration, tongue discoloration, and tongue thickening may occur (median onset of cutaneous toxicities following initial dose is 6 days; median duration is 5 days); instruct patients to report mucocutaneous effects. Safety and efficacy have not been established with nonhematologic malignancies; effect on the growth of keratinocyte growth factor (KGF) receptor expressing, nonhematopoietic human tumors is not known. Palifermin has been shown to enhance epithelial tumor cell lines *in vitro*. Do not administer within 24 hours before, during, or after myelotoxic chemotherapy. If administered during or within 24 hours of (before or after) chemotherapy, palifermin may increase the severity and duration of mucositis due to the increased sensitivity of rapidly-dividing epithelial cells.

Adverse Reactions

>10%:

Cardiovascular: Edema (28%)

Central nervous system: Fever (39%); pain (16%); dysesthesia (oral hyperesthesia, hypoesthesia, and paresthesia 12%)

Dermatologic: Rash (62%; grade 3: 3%), pruritus (35%), erythema (32%)

Gastrointestinal: Serum amylase increased (62%, grades 3/4: 38%), serum lipase increased (28%, grades 3/4: 11%), mouth/tongue discoloration or thickness (17%), taste alteration (16%)

1% to 10%:

Neuromuscular & skeletal: Arthralgia (10%)

Miscellaneous: Antibody formation (2%)

<1% (Limited to important or life-threatening): Cataracts, cough, flexural hyperpigmentation, palmar-plantar erythrodysesthesia syndrome (hand-foot syndrome), perianal pain, rhinitis, vaginal edema, vaginal erythema

Drug Interactions

Metabolism/Transport Effects None known.

Avoid Concomitant Use

Avoid concomitant use of Palifermin with any of the following: Heparin

Increased Effect/Toxicity

The levels/effects of Palifermin may be increased by: Heparin; Heparin (Low Molecular Weight)

Decreased Effect There are no known significant interactions involving a decrease in effect.

Preparation for Administration Hazardous agent; use appropriate precautions for handling and disposal (NIOSH, 2012). To reconstitute, slowly add 1.2 mL SWFI, to a final concentration of 5 mg/mL. Swirl gently; do not shake or vigorously agitate. May take up to 3 minutes to dissolve; reconstituted solution should be clear and colorless. Do not filter during preparation or administration.

Storage/Stability Store intact vials under refrigeration at 2°C to 8°C (36°F to 46°F). Protect from light. Although the manufacturer recommends immediate use, reconstituted vials are stable for up to 24 hours refrigerated. Bring to room temperature for up to 1 hour prior to administration; however, do not use if left at room temperature >1 hour. Protect reconstituted solution from light. Do not freeze reconstituted product.

Mechanism of Action Palifermin is a recombinant keratinocyte growth factor (KGF) produced in *E. coli*. Endogenous KGF is produced by mesenchymal cells in response to epithelial tissue injury. KGF binds to the KGF receptor resulting in proliferation, differentiation and migration of epithelial cells in multiple tissues, including (but not limited to) the tongue, buccal mucosa, esophagus, and salivary gland.

Pharmacodynamics/Kinetics

Onset of action: Epithelial cell proliferation (dose-dependent): 48 hours

Half-life elimination: 4.5 hours (range: 3.3-5.7 hours)

Dosage I.V.: Adults: Oral mucositis associated with hematopoietic stem cell transplant (HSCT) conditioning regimens: 60 mcg/kg/day for 3 consecutive days before and 3 consecutive days after myelotoxic therapy; total of 6 doses (Spielberger, 2004)

Note: Administer first 3 doses prior to myelotoxic therapy, with the 3rd dose given 24-48 hours before beginning the myelotoxic conditioning regimen. Administer the last 3 doses after completion of the conditioning regimen, with the first of these doses after but on the same day as HSCT infusion and at least 4 days after the most recent dose of palifermin.

Dosage adjustment in renal impairment: No dosage adjustment necessary.

Dosage adjustment in hepatic impairment: No dosage adjustment provided in the manufacturer's labeling (has not been studied).

Administration Administer by I.V. bolus. If heparin is used to maintain the patency of the I.V. line, flush line with saline prior to and after palifermin administration. Do not administer palifermin during or within 24 hours before or after chemotherapy. Allow solution to reach room temperature prior to administration; do not use if at room temperature >1 hour. Do not filter.

Hazardous agent; use appropriate precautions for handling and disposal (NIOSH, 2012).

Monitoring Parameters Monitor for oral mucositis

Additional Information Oncology Comment: The Multinational Association of Supportive Care in Cancer and the International Society for Oral Oncology (MASCC/ISOO) guidelines for the prevention and treatment of mucositis recommend palifermin (at the FDA-approved dose) for the prevention of oral mucositis in patients with hematologic malignancies who are receiving high-dose chemotherapy and total body irradiation with autologous stem cell transplantation (Keefe, 2007).

Guidelines from the American Society of Clinical Oncology (ASCO) for the use of chemotherapy and radiotherapy protectants (Hensley, 2008) recommend the use of palifermin to decrease the incidence of severe mucositis in patients undergoing autologous stem-cell transplantation with a total body irradiation (TBI) conditioning regimen. According to the ASCO guidelines, data are insufficient to recommend palifermin when the conditioning regimen is chemotherapy only. Palifermin may be considered in patients undergoing myeloablative allogeneic stem-cell transplantation with a TBI conditioning regimen, however data are again insufficient to recommend palifermin when the conditioning regimen is chemotherapy only. Due to a lack of appropriate data, the guidelines also do not recommend palifermin use in non-stem-cell transplantation treatment regimens or for use when treating solid tumors.

Dosage Forms Excipient information presented when available (limited, particularly for generics); consult specific product labeling.

Solution Reconstituted, Intravenous [preservative free]:
Kepivance: 6.25 mg (1 ea)

Paliperidone (pal ee PER i done)

Brand Names: U.S. Invega; Invega Sustenna

Brand Names: Canada Invega; Invega Sustenna

Index Terms 9-hydroxy-risperidone; 9-OH-risperidone; Paliperidone Palmitate

Pharmacologic Category Antipsychotic Agent, Atypical

Additional Appendix Information

Antipsychotic Agents *on page 2290*

Beers Criteria – Potentially Inappropriate Medications for Geriatrics *on page 2368*

Use

Oral: Treatment of schizophrenia; acute treatment of schizoaffective disorder (monotherapy or adjunctive therapy to mood stabilizers and/or antidepressants)

Injection: Treatment of schizophrenia

Unlabeled Use Psychosis/agitation related to Alzheimer's dementia

Pregnancy Risk Factor C

Pregnancy Considerations Adverse events were not observed in animal reproduction studies. Antipsychotic use during the third trimester of pregnancy has a risk for extrapyramidal symptoms (EPS) and/or withdrawal symptoms in newborns following delivery. Symptoms in the newborn may include agitation, feeding disorder, hypertonia, hypotonia, respiratory distress, somnolence, and tremor. These effects may be self-limiting and allow recovery within hours or days with no specific treatment, or they may be severe requiring prolonged hospitalization.

Paliperidone may cause hyperprolactinemia, which may decrease reproductive function in both males and females. Paliperidone is the active metabolite of risperidone; refer to Risperidone monograph for additional information.

The ACOG recommends that therapy during pregnancy be individualized; treatment with psychiatric medications during pregnancy should incorporate the clinical expertise of the mental health clinician, obstetrician, primary healthcare provider, and pediatrician. Safety data related to atypical antipsychotics during pregnancy is limited and routine use is not recommended. However, if a woman is inadvertently exposed to an atypical antipsychotic while pregnant, continuing therapy may be preferable to switching to a typical antipsychotic that the fetus has not yet been exposed to; consider risk:benefit (ACOG, 2008).

Healthcare providers are encouraged to enroll women 18-45 years of age exposed to paliperidone during pregnancy in the Atypical Antipsychotics Pregnancy Registry (1-866-961-2388 or http://www.womensmentalhealth.org/pregnancyregistry).

Breast-Feeding Considerations Paliperidone is excreted into breast milk. According to the manufacturer, the decision to continue or discontinue breast-feeding during therapy should take into account the risk of exposure to the infant and the benefits of treatment to the mother.

Contraindications Hypersensitivity to paliperidone, risperidone, or any component of the formulation

Warnings/Precautions [U.S. Boxed Warning]: Elderly patients with dementia-related psychosis treated with antipsychotics are at an increased risk of death compared to placebo. Most deaths appeared to be either cardiovascular (eg, heart failure, sudden death) or infectious (eg, pneumonia) in nature. In addition, an increased incidence of cerebrovascular adverse effects (eg, transient ischemic attack, cerebrovascular accidents) has been reported in studies of placebo-controlled trials of risperidone (paliperidone is the primary active metabolite of risperidone) in elderly patients with dementia-related psychosis. Paliperidone is not approved for the treatment of dementia-related psychosis. In addition, patients with Lewy body dementia (LBD) may be more sensitive to CNS-related and extrapyramidal effects.

Compared with risperidone, paliperidone is low to moderately sedating; use with caution in disorders where CNS depression is a feature. Use caution in patients with predisposition to seizures. Use with caution in mild renal dysfunction; dose reduction recommended. Not recommended in patients with moderate-to-severe impairment. Esophageal dysmotility and aspiration have been associated with antipsychotic use; use with caution in patients at risk of aspiration pneumonia (eg, Alzheimer's disease).

Leukopenia, neutropenia, and agranulocytosis (sometimes fatal) have been reported in clinical trials and postmarketing reports with antipsychotic use; presence of risk factors (eg, pre-existing low WBC or history of drug-induced leuko-/neutropenia) should prompt periodic blood count assessment. Discontinue therapy at first signs of blood dyscrasias or if absolute neutrophil count <1000/mm^3.

Paliperidone is associated with increased prolactin levels; clinical significance of hyperprolactinemia in patients with breast cancer or other prolactin-dependent tumors is unknown. May alter temperature regulation. May mask toxicity of other drugs or conditions (eg, intestinal obstruction, Reye's syndrome, brain tumor) due to antiemetic effects. Priapism has been reported rarely with use.

May cause orthostasis and syncope. Use with caution in patients with cardiovascular diseases (eg, heart failure, history of myocardial infarction or ischemia, cerebrovascular disease, conduction abnormalities). Use caution in patients receiving medications for hypertension (orthostatic effects may be exacerbated) or in patients with hypovolemia or dehydration. May alter cardiac conduction; life-threatening arrhythmias have occurred with therapeutic doses of neuroleptics. Avoid use in combination with QT_c-prolonging drugs. Avoid use in patients with congenital long QT syndrome and in patients with history of cardiac arrhythmia.

May cause extrapyramidal symptoms (EPS), including pseudoparkinsonism, acute dystonic reactions, akathisia, and tardive dyskinesia (risk of these reactions is low relative to other neuroleptics, and is dose dependent). Risk of dystonia (and probably other EPS) may be greater with increased doses, use of conventional antipsychotics, males, and younger patients. Risk of neuroleptic malignant syndrome (NMS) may be increased in patients with Parkinson's disease or Lewy body dementia; monitor for symptoms of confusion, obtundation, postural instability and extrapyramidal symptoms. May cause hyperglycemia; in some cases may be extreme and associated with ketoacidosis, hyperosmolar coma, or death. Use with caution in patients with diabetes (or risk factors) or other disorders of glucose regulation; monitor for worsening of glucose control. Significant weight gain has been observed with antipsychotic therapy; incidence varies with product. Monitor waist circumference and BMI. May cause lipid abnormalities (LDL and triglycerides increased; HDL decreased). Few case reports describe intraoperative floppy iris syndrome (IFIS) in patients receiving risperidone and undergoing cataract surgery (Ford, 2011). IFIS has not been reported with paliperidone but caution is advised since it is the active metabolite of risperidone. Prior to cataract surgery, evaluate for prior or current paliperidone or risperidone use. The benefits or risks of interrupting paliperidone or risperidone prior to surgery have not been established; clinicians are advised to proceed with surgery cautiously.

The possibility of a suicide attempt is inherent in psychotic illness or bipolar disorder; use caution in high-risk patients during initiation of therapy. Prescriptions should be written for the smallest quantity consistent with good patient care.

Use in elderly patients with dementia is associated with an increased risk of mortality and cerebrovascular accidents; avoid antipsychotic use for behavioral problems associated with dementia unless alternative nonpharmacologic therapies have failed and patient may harm self or others. In addition, use may cause or exacerbate syndrome of inappropriate antidiuretic hormone secretion or hyponatremia; monitor sodium closely with initiation or dosage adjustments in older adults (Beers Criteria).

The tablet formulation consists of drug within a nonabsorbable shell that is expelled and may be visible in the stool. Use is not recommended in patients with pre-existing severe gastrointestinal narrowing disorders. Patients with upper GI tract alterations in transit time may have increased or decreased bioavailability of paliperidone. Do not use in patients unable to swallow the tablet whole.

Adverse Reactions Unless otherwise noted, frequency of adverse effects is reported for the oral/I.M. formulation in adults.

>10%:

Cardiovascular: Tachycardia (1% to 14%)

Central nervous system: EPS (≤26%; dose dependent), insomnia (10% to 15%), headache (6% to 15%), parkinsonism (3% to 14%; dose dependent), somnolence (adolescents 9% to 26%; adults 1% to 12%; dose dependent)

Neuromuscular & skeletal: Tremor (2% to 12%)

3% to 10%:

Cardiovascular: Orthostatic hypotension (1% to 4%; dose dependent), bundle branch block (≤3%)

Central nervous system: Agitation (4% to 10%), akathisia (adolescents 4% to 17%; adults 1% to 10%; dose dependent), anxiety (adolescents ≤9%; adults 3% to 8%), dizziness (1% to 6%), dystonia (1% to 5%; dose dependent), dysarthria (1% to 4%; dose dependent), fatigue (adolescents ≤4%), sleep disorder (≤3%), lethargy (adolescents ≤3%)

Endocrine and metabolic: Amenorrhea (adolescents ≤6%), galactorrhea (adolescents ≤4%), gynecomastia (adolescents ≤3%)

Gastrointestinal: Weight gain (1% to 9%; dose dependent), nausea (2% to 8%), dyspepsia (5% to 6%), vomiting (adolescents ≤11%; adults 2% to 5%), constipation (1% to 5%), salivation increased (adolescents ≤6%; adults ≤4%; dose dependent), appetite increased (2% to 3%), toothache (1% to 3%), abdominal pain (≤3%), diarrhea (≤3%), xerostomia (≤3%); tongue swelling (adolescents ≤3%), tongue paralysis (adolescents ≤3%)

Local: I.M. formulation: Injection site reaction (≤10%)

Neuromuscular & skeletal: Hyperkinesia (2% to 10% dose dependent), dyskinesia (1% to 9%), weakness (≤4%), myalgia (≤4% dose dependent), back pain (1% to 3%), extremity pain (≤3%)

Ocular: Blurred vision (adolescents ≤3%)

Respiratory: Nasopharyngitis (≤5%; dose dependent), upper respiratory tract infection (1% to 4%), cough (≤3%; dose dependent), rhinitis (1% to 3%; dose dependent)

≤2% (Limited to important or life-threatening): Agranulocytosis, ALT increased, amenorrhea, appetite decreased, anaphylactic reaction, angioedema, arrhythmia, arthralgia, aspiration pneumonia, AV block (first degree), blurred vision, bradycardia, breast abnormalities (includes discharge, engorgement, pain, tenderness), cerebrovascular accident, drooling, edema, erectile dysfunction, epistaxis (adolescents), fatigue, flatulence, galactorrhea, gynecomastia, hyper-/hypotension, hyperprolactinemia, hypertonia, intestinal obstruction, ischemia, lethargy, leukopenia, menstrual irregularities, nasal congestion, neuroleptic malignant syndrome, neutropenia, nightmares, oculogyric crisis, palpitation, peripheral edema, pharyngolaryngeal pain (dose dependent), postural dizziness, postural orthostatic tachycardia syndrome, priapism, pruritus, psychomotor hyperactivity, QT_c-interval prolongation, rash, restlessness, retrograde ejaculation, seizure, sexual dysfunction, stiffness, suicidal ideation, syncope, thrombotic thrombocytopenic purpura (TTP), tongue swelling, transient ischemic attack, urinary incontinence, urinary retention, urinary tract infection, vertigo

Drug Interactions

Metabolism/Transport Effects Substrate of P-glycoprotein

Avoid Concomitant Use

Avoid concomitant use of Paliperidone with any of the following: Amisulpride; Azelastine (Nasal); Highest Risk QTc-Prolonging Agents; Ivabradine; Metoclopramide; Mifepristone; Moderate Risk QTc-Prolonging Agents; Paraldehyde; Sulpiride

Increased Effect/Toxicity

Paliperidone may increase the levels/effects of: Alcohol (Ethyl); Amisulpride; Azelastine (Nasal); Buprenorphine; CNS Depressants; Highest Risk QTc-Prolonging Agents; Hydrocodone; Methotrimeprazine; Methylphenidate; Paraldehyde; Serotonin Modulators; Sulpiride; Zolpidem

The levels/effects of Paliperidone may be increased by: Acetylcholinesterase Inhibitors (Central); Brimonidine (Topical); Doxylamine; HydrOXYzine; Itraconazole;

Ivabradine; Lithium formulations; Magnesium Sulfate; Methotrimeprazine; Methylphenidate; Metoclopramide; Metyrosine; Mifepristone; Moderate Risk QTc-Prolonging Agents; Perampanel; P-glycoprotein/ABCB1 Inhibitors; QTc-Prolonging Agents (Indeterminate Risk and Risk Modifying); RisperiDONE; Serotonin Modulators; Sodium Oxybate; Tetrabenazine; Valproic Acid and Derivatives

Decreased Effect

Paliperidone may decrease the levels/effects of: Amphetamines; Anti-Parkinson's Agents (Dopamine Agonist); Quinagolide

The levels/effects of Paliperidone may be decreased by: CarBAMazepine; Lithium formulations; P-glycoprotein/ABCB1 Inducers

Ethanol/Nutrition/Herb Interactions

Ethanol: May increase CNS depression; monitor for increased effects with coadministration. Caution patients about effects.

Herb/Nutraceutical: Paliperidone may increase the serotonergic effect of St John's wort; use caution and monitor for serotonin toxicity or NMS during concomitant use. St John's wort is also a strong CYP3A4 inducer; dose of paliperidone may need to be increased when St John's wort is coadministered and decreased when St. John's wort is discontinued.

Storage/Stability Store at controlled room temperature of ≤25°C (77°F); excursions permitted to 15°C to 30°C (59°F to 86°F). Protect tablets from moisture.

Mechanism of Action Paliperidone is considered a benzisoxazole atypical antipsychotic as it is the primary active metabolite of risperidone. As with other atypical antipsychotics, its therapeutic efficacy is believed to result from mixed central serotonergic and dopaminergic antagonism. The addition of serotonin antagonism to dopamine antagonism (classic neuroleptic mechanism) is thought to improve negative symptoms of psychoses and reduce the incidence of extrapyramidal side effects. Similar to risperidone, paliperidone demonstrates high affinity to α_1, D_2, H_1, and 5-HT_{2C} receptors, and low affinity for muscarinic and 5-HT_{1A} receptors. In contrast to risperidone, paliperidone displays nearly 10-fold lower affinity for α_2 and 5-HT_{2A} receptors, and nearly three- to fivefold less affinity for 5-HT_{1A} and 5-HT_{1D}, respectively.

Pharmacodynamics/Kinetics

Absorption: I.M.: Slow release (begins on day 1 and continues up to 126 days)

Distribution: V_d: 391-487 L

Protein binding: 74%

Metabolism: Hepatic via CYP2D6 and 3A4 (limited role in elimination); minor metabolism (<10% each) via dealkylation, hydroxylation, dehydrogenation, and benzisoxazole scission

Bioavailability: 28%

Half-life elimination:

- Oral: 23 hours; 24-51 hours with renal impairment (Cl_{cr} <80 mL/minute)
- I.M. (following a single-dose administration): Range: 25-49 days

Time to peak, plasma: Oral: ~24 hours; I.M.: 13 days

Excretion: Urine (80%); feces (11%)

Dosage

U.S. labeling:

Schizoaffective disorder: Adults: Oral: Usual: 6 mg once daily in the morning; titration not required, though some may benefit from lower or higher doses (range: 3-12 mg daily). If exceeding 6 mg daily, increases of 3 mg daily are recommended no more frequently than every 4 days, up to a maximum of 12 mg daily.

Schizophrenia:

Adolescents 12-17 years: Oral: Initial: 3 mg once daily; titration not required (no known benefit to efficacy from higher doses [ie, 6 mg daily for patients <51 kg and 12 mg daily for patients ≥51 kg]). If exceeding 3 mg daily, increases of 3 mg daily are recommended no more frequently than every 5 days.

Adults:

Oral: Usual: 6 mg once daily in the morning; titration not required, though some may benefit from lower or higher doses (range: 3-12 mg daily). If exceeding 6 mg daily, increases of 3 mg daily are recommended no more frequently than every 5 days, up to a maximum of 12 mg daily.

I.M.: **Note:** Prior to initiation of I.M therapy, tolerability should be established with oral paliperidone or oral risperidone. Previous oral antipsychotics can be discontinued at the time of initiation of I.M. therapy.

Dosing based on paliperidone palmitate.

Initiation of therapy:

Initial: 234 mg on treatment day 1 followed by 156 mg 1 week later with both doses administered in the deltoid muscle. The second dose may be administered 4 days before or after the weekly time point.

Maintenance: Following the 1-week initiation regimen, begin a maintenance dose of 117 mg every month administered in either the deltoid or gluteal muscle. Some patients may benefit from higher or lower monthly maintenance doses (monthly maintenance dosage range: 39-234 mg). The monthly maintenance dose may be administered 7 days before or after the monthly time point.

Conversion from oral paliperidone to I.M paliperidone: Initiate I.M. therapy as described using the 1-week initiation regimen. Patients previously stabilized on oral doses can expect similar steady state exposure during maintenance treatment with I.M. therapy using the following conversion:

- Oral extended release dose of 12 mg daily, then I.M. maintenance dose of 234 mg monthly
- Oral extended release dose of 6 mg daily, then I.M. maintenance dose of 117 mg monthly
- Oral extended release dose of 3 mg daily, then I.M. maintenance dose of 39-78 mg monthly

Switching from other long-acting injectable antipsychotics to I.M. paliperidone: Initiate I.M. paliperidone in the place of the next scheduled injection and continue at monthly intervals. The 1-week initiation regimen is not required in these patients.

Dosage adjustments: Adjustments may be made monthly (full effect from adjustments may not be seen for several months)

Missed second initiation dose:

If <4 weeks have elapsed since the first injection: Administer the missed dose (156 mg) in the deltoid as soon as possible, followed by a third dose of 117 mg in either the deltoid or gluteal muscle 5 weeks after the first injection (regardless of when the second injection was administered), then begin normal monthly maintenance dosing.

If >4 weeks and ≤7 weeks have elapsed since the first injection: Administer a dose of 156 mg in the deltoid as soon as possible, followed by another 156 mg dose in the deltoid 1 week later, then begin normal monthly maintenance dosing.

If >7 weeks has elapsed since the first injection: Therapy must be reinitiated following dosing recommendations for initiation of therapy.

Missed maintenance dose:

If <6 weeks have elapsed since the last monthly injection: Administer the missed dose as soon as possible and continue therapy at monthly intervals.

If >6 weeks and ≤6 months have elapsed since the last monthly injection:
If the maintenance dose was <234 mg: Administer the same dose the patient was previously stabilized on in the deltoid as soon as possible, followed by a second equivalent dose in the deltoid 1 week later, then resume maintenance dose at monthly intervals.
If the maintenance dose was 234 mg: Administer a 156 mg dose in the deltoid as soon as possible, followed by a second dose of 156 mg in the deltoid 1 week later, then resume maintenance dose at monthly intervals.
If >6 months have elapsed since last monthly maintenance injection: Therapy must be reinitiated following dosing recommendations for initiation of therapy.

Canadian labeling:
Schizophrenia: Adults:
Oral: Usual: 6 mg once daily in the morning; titration not required, though some may benefit from lower or higher doses (range: 3-12 mg daily). If exceeding 6 mg daily, increases of 3 mg daily are recommended no more frequently than every 5 days in schizophrenia, up to a maximum of 12 mg daily.
I.M.: **Note:** Prior to initiation of I.M therapy, tolerability should be established with oral paliperidone or oral risperidone. Previous oral antipsychotics can be discontinued at the time of initiation of I.M. therapy. **Dosing based on paliperidone.**
Initiation of therapy:
Initial: 150 mg on treatment day 1 followed by 100 mg 1 week later (day 8) with both doses administered in the deltoid. The second dose may be administered 2 days before or after the weekly time point.
Maintenance: Following the 1-week initiation regimen, begin a maintenance dose of 75 mg every month administered in either the deltoid or gluteal muscle. Some patients may benefit from higher or lower monthly maintenance doses (monthly maintenance dosage range: 50-150 mg). The monthly maintenance dose may be administered 7 days before or after the monthly time point.
Conversion from oral paliperidone to I.M paliperidone: Initiate I.M. therapy as described using the 1-week initiation regimen. Patients previously stabilized on oral doses can expect similar steady state exposure during maintenance treatment with I.M. therapy using the following conversion:
Oral extended release dose of 12 mg daily, then I.M. maintenance dose of 150 mg monthly
Oral extended release dose of 6 mg daily, then I.M. maintenance dose of 75 mg monthly
Oral extended release dose of 3 mg daily, then I.M. maintenance dose of 50 mg monthly
Switching from other long-acting injectable antipsychotics (eg, Risperdal® Consta®) to I.M. paliperidone: Initiate I.M. paliperidone in the place of the next scheduled injection and continue at monthly intervals. The 1-week initiation regimen is not required in these patients.
Switching from injectable risperidone (Risperdal® Consta®) to I.M. paliperidone:
Risperdal® Consta® dose of 25 mg every 2 weeks, then I.M. paliperidone maintenance dose of 50 mg monthly
Risperdal® Consta® dose of 37.5 mg every 2 weeks, then I.M. paliperidone maintenance dose of 75 mg monthly
Risperdal® Consta® dose of 50 mg every 2 weeks, then I.M. paliperidone maintenance dose of 100 mg monthly

Dosage adjustments: Adjustments may be made monthly (full effect from adjustments may not be seen for several months)
Missed second initiation dose:
If <4 weeks has elapsed since first injection: Administer the missed dose (100 mg) in the deltoid as soon as possible followed by a third dose of 75 mg in either the deltoid or gluteal muscle 5 weeks after the first injection (regardless of the when the second injection was administered), then begin normal monthly maintenance dosing.
If 4-7 weeks have elapsed since first injection: Administer a dose of 100 mg in the deltoid as soon as possible, followed by another 100 mg dose in the deltoid 1 week later, then begin normal monthly maintenance dosing.
If >7 weeks has elapsed since the first injection: Therapy must be reinitiated following dosing recommendations for initiation of therapy.
Missed maintenance dose:
If <6 weeks have elapsed since the last monthly injection: Administer the missed dose as soon as possible and continue therapy at monthly intervals.
If >6 weeks and ≤6 months have elapsed since the last monthly injection: Therapy may be resumed at same dose (50-100 mg) the patient was previously stabilized on and then repeated 1 week later (day 8) with both doses administered in the deltoid. Resume usual monthly maintenance dosing cycle thereafter. If the dose was 150 mg, administer a 100 mg dose as soon as possible and repeat 1 week later (day 8) with both doses administered in the deltoid, then resume usual monthly maintenance dosing cycle 50-150 mg.
If >6 months have elapsed since last monthly maintenance injection: Therapy must be reinitiated following dosing recommendations for initiation of therapy.

Dosage adjustment in renal impairment: Clearance is decreased in renal impairment; adjust dose according to renal function:
Oral:
Mild impairment (Cl_{cr} 50-79 mL/minute): Initial dose: 3 mg once daily; maximum dose: 6 mg once daily
Moderate-to-severe impairment (Cl_{cr} 10-49 mL/minute): Initial dose: 1.5 mg once daily; maximum dose: 3 mg once daily
Severe impairment (Cl_{cr} <10 mL/minute): Use not recommended (has not been studied).
I.M., U.S. labeling:
Mild impairment (Cl_{cr} 50-79 mL/minute): Initiation of therapy: 156 mg on treatment day 1, followed by 117 mg 1 week later with both doses administered in the deltoid, followed by a maintenance dose of 78 mg every month (administered in the deltoid or gluteal muscle)
Moderate-to-severe impairment (Cl_{cr} <50 mL/minute): Use not recommended
I.M., Canadian labeling:
Mild impairment (Cl_{cr} 50-79 mL/minute): Initiation of therapy: 100 mg on treatment day 1, followed by 75 mg 1 week later with both doses administered in the deltoid, followed by a maintenance dose of 50 mg every month (administered in the deltoid or gluteal muscle). Based on tolerability and/or response, maintenance dose may be adjusted within range of 50-100 mg.
Moderate-to-severe impairment (Cl_{cr} <50 mL/minute): Use not recommended

Dosage adjustment in hepatic impairment: Oral, I.M.:
Mild to moderate impairment (Child-Pugh class A or B): No dosage adjustment necessary.

Severe impairment: No dosage adjustment provided in manufacturer's labeling (has not been studied).

Dietary Considerations May be taken without regard to meals.

Administration

Oral: Administer in the morning without regard to meals. Extended release tablets should be swallowed whole with liquids; do not crush, chew, or divide.

Injection: Invega® Sustenna™ should be administered by I.M. route only as a single injection (do not divide); do not administer I.V. or subcutaneously. Avoid inadvertent injection into vasculature. Prior to injection, shake syringe for at least 10 seconds to ensure a homogenous suspension. The 2 initial injections should be administered in the deltoid muscle using a 1½ inch, 22-gauge needle for patients ≥90 kg, and a 1 inch, 23-gauge needle for patients <90 kg. The 2 initial deltoid intramuscular injections help attain therapeutic concentrations rapidly. Alternate deltoid injections (right and left deltoid muscle). The second dose may be administered 4 days before or after the weekly time point (Canadian labeling suggests the second dose may be administered 2 days before or after the weekly time point). Monthly maintenance doses can be administered in either the deltoid or gluteal muscle. Administer injections in the gluteal muscle using a 1 ½ inch, 22-gauge needle in the upper-outer quadrant of the gluteal area. Alternate gluteal injections (right and left gluteal muscle). The monthly maintenance dose may be administered 7 days before or after the monthly time point.

Monitoring Parameters Vital signs; fasting lipid profile and fasting blood glucose/Hgb A_{1c} (prior to treatment, at 3 months, then annually), prolactin levels, CBC frequently during first few months of therapy in patients with preexisting low WBC or a history of drug-induced leukopenia/neutropenia; BMI, personal/family history of obesity, diabetes, waist circumference; blood pressure; mental status, abnormal involuntary movement scale (AIMS), extrapyramidal symptoms; orthostatic blood pressure changes for 3-5 days after starting or increasing dose. Weight should be assessed prior to treatment, at 4 weeks, 8 weeks, 12 weeks, and then at quarterly intervals. Consider titrating to a different antipsychotic agent for a weight gain ≥5% of the initial weight.

Additional Information Invega® is an extended release tablet based on the OROS® osmotic delivery system. Water from the GI tract enters through a semipermeable membrane coating the tablet, solubilizing the drug into a gelatinous form which, through hydrophilic expansion, is then expelled through laser-drilled holes in the coating.

Dosage Forms Excipient information presented when available (limited, particularly for generics); consult specific product labeling.

Suspension, Intramuscular, as palmitate:

Invega Sustenna: 39 mg/0.25 mL (0.25 mL); 78 mg/0.5 mL (0.5 mL); 117 mg/0.75 mL (0.75 mL); 156 mg/mL (1 mL); 234 mg/1.5 mL (1.5 mL) [contains polyethylene glycol]

Tablet Extended Release 24 Hour, Oral:

Invega: 1.5 mg, 3 mg, 6 mg, 9 mg

Dosage Forms: Canada Excipient information presented when available (limited, particularly for generics); consult specific product labeling.

Injection, suspension, extended release:

Invega Sustenna: 25 mg/0.25 mL (0.25 mL), 50 mg/0.5 mL (0.5 mL), 75 mg/0.75 mL (0.75 mL), 100 mg/1 mL (1 mL), 150 mg/1.5 mL (1.5 mL)

◆ **Paliperidone Palmitate** *see* Paliperidone *on page 1549*

Palivizumab (pah li VIZ u mab)

Brand Names: U.S. Synagis

Brand Names: Canada Synagis®

Pharmacologic Category Monoclonal Antibody

Use Prevention of serious lower respiratory tract disease caused by respiratory syncytial virus (RSV) in infants and children at high risk of RSV disease

The American Academy of Pediatrics recommends RSV prophylaxis with palivizumab during RSV season for:

- Infants <3 months of age who were born between 32 and 34 6/7 weeks gestational age and have one of the following:
  - Day care attendance
  - One or more siblings <5 years of age living in the same household
- Infants <6 months of age who were born between 29 and 31 6/7 weeks gestational age
- Infants <12 months of age who were born <28 weeks gestational age
- Infants <12 months of age with congenital airway abnormality or neuromuscular disorder that decreases the ability to manage airway secretions
- Infants and children <24 months of age with chronic lung disease (CLD) necessitating medical therapy within 6 month prior to the beginning of RSV season
- Infants and children ≤24 months of age with congenital heart disease and one of the following:
  - Receiving medication to treat congestive heart failure
  - Moderate-to-severe pulmonary hypertension
  - Cyanotic heart disease

Pregnancy Risk Factor C

Pregnancy Considerations Not for adult use; reproduction studies have not been conducted

Contraindications History of severe prior reaction to palivizumab or any component of the formulation

Warnings/Precautions Very rare cases of anaphylaxis have been observed following palivizumab. Rare cases of severe acute hypersensitivity reactions have also been reported. Use with caution after mild hypersensitivity reaction; permanently discontinue for severe hypersensitivity reaction. Safety and efficacy of palivizumab have not been demonstrated in the treatment of established RSV disease. Use with caution in patients with thrombocytopenia or any coagulation disorder; bleeding/hematoma may occur from I.M. administration.

Adverse Reactions

>10%:

Central nervous system: Fever (27%)

Dermatologic: Rash (12%)

1% to 10%: Miscellaneous: Antibody formation (1% to 2%)

<1% (Limited to important or life-threatening): Anaphylaxis (very rare - includes angioedema, dyspnea, hypotonia, pruritus, respiratory failure, unresponsiveness, urticaria); hypersensitivity reactions, injection site reactions, thrombocytopenia

Drug Interactions

Metabolism/Transport Effects None known.

Avoid Concomitant Use

Avoid concomitant use of Palivizumab with any of the following: Belimumab

Increased Effect/Toxicity

Palivizumab may increase the levels/effects of: Belimumab

The levels/effects of Palivizumab may be increased by: Abciximab

Decreased Effect There are no known significant interactions involving a decrease in effect.

Storage/Stability Store in refrigerator at a temperature between 2°C to 8°C (36°F to 46°F) in original container; do not freeze. Intact vials may be exposed to room temperature for a cumulative 14 days (data on file [MedImmune, 2011]). Do not shake, vigorously agitate or dilute the solution.

Mechanism of Action Exhibits neutralizing and fusion-inhibitory activity against RSV; these activities inhibit RSV replication in laboratory and clinical studies

Pharmacodynamics/Kinetics Half-life elimination: Children <24 months: 20 days

Dosage I.M.: Infants and Children <2 years:

Prevention of RSV: 15 mg/kg of body weight, monthly throughout RSV season (first dose administered prior to commencement of RSV season)

Note: The AAP recommends a maximum of 3 doses for patients born 32-34 6/7 weeks without significant congenital heart disease or chronic lung disease; maximum of 5 doses for all others (AAP, 2009).

Cardiopulmonary bypass patients: Administer a dose as soon as possible after cardiopulmonary bypass procedure, even if <1 month from previous dose.

Dosage adjustment in renal impairment: No dosage adjustment provided in manufacturer's labeling.

Dosage adjustment in hepatic impairment: No dosage adjustment provided in manufacturer's labeling.

Administration Injection should (preferably) be in the anterolateral aspect of the thigh; gluteal muscle should not be used routinely; injection volume over 1 mL should be administered as divided doses

Monitoring Parameters Monitor for anaphylaxis or acute hypersensitivity reactions

Test Interactions May interfere (false negatives) with immunological-based RSV diagnostic tests (antigen detection) and viral culture assays; rely on reverse-transcriptase-polymerase chain reaction-based assays and clinical findings.

Additional Information RSV prophylaxis should be initiated no earlier than July 1 in Southeast Florida, September 15 in North-central and Southwest Florida and November 1 in most other areas of the United States.

Dosage Forms Excipient information presented when available (limited, particularly for generics); consult specific product labeling.

Solution, Intramuscular [preservative free]:

Synagis: 50 mg/0.5 mL (0.5 mL); 100 mg/mL (1 mL) [contains glycine, histidine]

Palonosetron (pal oh NOE se tron)

Brand Names: U.S. Aloxi

Index Terms Palonosetron Hydrochloride; RS-25259; RS-25259-197

Pharmacologic Category Antiemetic; Selective 5-HT_3 Receptor Antagonist

Use Prevention of chemotherapy-associated nausea and vomiting; indicated for prevention of acute (highly-emetogenic therapy) as well as acute and delayed (moderately-emetogenic therapy) nausea and vomiting; prevention of postoperative nausea and vomiting (PONV)

Pregnancy Risk Factor B

Pregnancy Considerations Teratogenic effects were not observed in animal studies. There are no adequate and well-controlled studies in pregnant women; use during pregnancy only if clearly needed.

Breast-Feeding Considerations The extent to which palonosetron is excreted in breast milk, if at all, is unknown. Due to the potential for adverse effects in the nursing infant, breast-feeding is not recommended.

Contraindications Hypersensitivity to palonosetron or any component of the formulation

Warnings/Precautions Hypersensitivity has been observed rarely with I.V. palonosetron. Use caution in patients allergic to other 5-HT_3 receptor antagonists; cross-reactivity is possible. Some selective 5-HT_3 receptor antagonists have been associated with dose-dependent increases in ECG intervals (eg, PR, QRS duration, QT/QT_c, JT), usually occurring 1-2 hours after I.V. administration. In general, these changes are not clinically relevant, however, when these agents are used in conjunction with other agents that prolong these intervals, arrhythmia may occur. When used with agents that prolong the QT interval (eg, Class I and III antiarrhythmics), clinically relevant QT interval prolongation could result in torsade de pointes. A number of trials have shown that 5-HT_3 antagonists produce QT interval prolongation to variable degrees. Use with caution in patients at risk of QT prolongation and/or ventricular arrhythmia. Reduction in heart rate may also occur with the 5-HT_3 antagonists. Use with caution in patients with congenital long QT syndrome or other risk factors for QT prolongation (eg, medications known to prolong QT interval, electrolyte abnormalities, and cumulative high dose anthracycline therapy).

Not intended for treatment of nausea and vomiting or for chronic continuous therapy. **For chemotherapy, should be used on a scheduled basis, not on an "as needed" (PRN) basis,** since data support the use of this drug only in the prevention of nausea and vomiting (due to antineoplastic therapy) and not in the rescue of nausea and vomiting. For PONV, may use for low expectation of PONV if it is essential to avoid nausea and vomiting in the postoperative period; use is not recommended if there is little expectation of nausea and vomiting.

Adverse Reactions Adverse events may vary according to indication.

1% to 10%:

Cardiovascular: QT prolongation (chemotherapy-associated <1%; PONV 1% to 5%), bradycardia (chemotherapy-associated 1%; PONV 4%), hypotension (≤1%), sinus bradycardia (≤1%), tachycardia (nonsustained) (≤1%)

Central nervous system: Headache (chemotherapy-associated 5% to 9%; PONV 3%), anxiety (1%), dizziness (≤1%)

Dermatologic: Pruritus (≤1%)

Endocrine & metabolic: Hyperkalemia (1%)

Gastrointestinal: Constipation (2% to 5%), diarrhea (≤1%), flatulence (≤1%)

Genitourinary: Urinary retention (≤1%)

Hepatic: ALT increased (≤1%; transient), AST increased (≤1%; transient)

Neuromuscular & skeletal: Weakness (1%)

<1% (Limited to important or life-threatening): Abdominal pain, allergic dermatitis, amblyopia, anemia, anorexia, appetite decreased, arrhythmia, arthralgia, bilirubin increased (transient), chills, dyspepsia, edema (generalized), electrolyte fluctuations, epistaxis, erythema, euphoric mood, extrasystoles, eye irritation, fatigue, fever, flu-like syndrome, glycosuria, hiccups, hot flash, hyperglycemia, hypersensitivity (rare), hypersomnia, hypertension, hypokalemia, hypoventilation, injection site reactions (burning/discomfort/induration/pain; rare), insomnia, intestinal hypomotility, laryngospasm, metabolic acidosis, motion sickness, myocardial ischemia, pain in extremities, paresthesia, platelets decreased, rash, salivation increased, seizure, sinus arrhythmia, sinus tachycardia, somnolence, supraventricular extrasystoles, tinnitus, T-wave amplitude decreased, vein discoloration, vein distention, ventricular extrasystoles, xerostomia

Drug Interactions

Metabolism/Transport Effects Substrate of CYP1A2 (minor), CYP2D6 (minor), CYP3A4 (minor); **Note:** Assignment of Major/Minor substrate status based on clinically relevant drug interaction potential

Avoid Concomitant Use

Avoid concomitant use of Palonosetron with any of the following: Apomorphine

Increased Effect/Toxicity

Palonosetron may increase the levels/effects of: Apomorphine

Decreased Effect

Palonosetron may decrease the levels/effects of: Tapentadol; TraMADol

The levels/effects of Palonosetron may be decreased by: Peginterferon Alfa-2b

Storage/Stability Store intact vials at room temperature of 20°C to 25°C (68°F to 77°F); excursions permitted to 15°C to 30°C (59°F to 86°F); do not freeze. Protect from light. Solutions of 5 mcg/mL and 30 mcg/mL in NS, D_5W, $D_5{}^1/_2NS$, and D_5LR injection are stable for 48 hours at room temperature and 14 days under refrigeration (Trissel, 2004).

Mechanism of Action Selective 5-HT_3 receptor antagonist, blocking serotonin, both on vagal nerve terminals in the periphery and centrally in the chemoreceptor trigger zone

Pharmacodynamics/Kinetics

Distribution: V_d: 8.3 ± 2.5 L/kg

Protein binding: ~62%

Metabolism: ~50% metabolized via CYP enzymes (and likely other pathways) to relatively inactive metabolites (N-oxide-palonosetron and 6-S-hydroxy-palonosetron); CYP1A2, 2D6, and 3A4 contribute to its metabolism

Half-life elimination: I.V.: Terminal: ~40 hours

Excretion: Urine (80% to 93%, 40% as unchanged drug); feces (5% to 8%)

Dosage I.V.: Adults:

Chemotherapy-associated nausea and vomiting: 0.25 mg 30 minutes prior to the start of chemotherapy administration

Breakthrough: Palonosetron has not been shown to be effective in terminating nausea or vomiting once it occurs and should not be used for this purpose.

PONV: 0.075 mg immediately prior to anesthesia induction

Elderly: No dosage adjustment necessary

Dosage adjustment in renal/hepatic impairment: No dosage adjustment necessary

Administration Flush I.V. line with NS prior to and following administration.

Chemotherapy-associated nausea and vomiting: Infuse over 30 seconds, 30 minutes prior to the start of chemotherapy

PONV: Infuse over 10 seconds immediately prior to anesthesia induction

Dosage Forms Excipient information presented when available (limited, particularly for generics); consult specific product labeling.

Solution, Intravenous:

Aloxi: 0.25 mg/5 mL (5 mL) [contains edetate disodium]

◆ **Palonosetron Hydrochloride** *see* Palonosetron *on page 1554*

◆ **Pal-Tizanidine (Can)** *see* TiZANidine *on page 2074*

◆ **2-PAM** *see* Pralidoxime *on page 1694*

Pamabrom (PAM a brom)

Pharmacologic Category Diuretic

Use Temporary relief of symptoms associated with premenstrual and menstrual periods (eg, bloating, water-weight gain, swelling, full feeling)

Dosage Oral: Adults: 50 mg after breakfast and then every 6 hours as needed (maximum: 200 mg/24 hours); should be taken 5-6 days prior to onset of menstrual period and continued until desired relief or end of period

Additional Information Complete prescribing information should be consulted for additional detail.

◆ **Pamelor** *see* Nortriptyline *on page 1475*

Pamidronate (pa mi DROE nate)

Brand Names: Canada Aredia®; Pamidronate Disodium Omega; Pamidronate Disodium®; PMS-Pamidronate

Index Terms Pamidronate Disodium

Pharmacologic Category Antidote; Bisphosphonate Derivative

Use Treatment of moderate or severe hypercalcemia associated with malignancy (in conjunction with adequate hydration) with or without bone metastases; treatment of osteolytic bone lesions associated with multiple myeloma or metastatic breast cancer; moderate-to-severe Paget's disease of bone

Unlabeled Use Treatment of osteogenesis imperfecta; treatment of symptomatic bone metastases of thyroid cancer; prevention of bone loss associated with androgen deprivation treatment in prostate cancer

Pregnancy Risk Factor D

Pregnancy Considerations Adverse events were observed in animal reproduction studies. It is not known if bisphosphonates cross the placenta, but fetal exposure is expected (Djokanovic, 2008; Stathopoulos, 2011). Bisphosphonates are incorporated into the bone matrix and gradually released over time. The amount available in the systemic circulation varies by dose and duration of therapy. Theoretically, there may be a risk of fetal harm when pregnancy follows the completion of therapy; however, available data have not shown that exposure to bisphosphonates during pregnancy significantly increases the risk of adverse fetal events (Djokanovic, 2008; Levy, 2009; Stathopoulos, 2011). Until additional data is available, most sources recommend discontinuing bisphosphonate therapy in women of reproductive potential as early as possible prior to a planned pregnancy; use in premenopausal women should be reserved for special circumstances when rapid bone loss is occurring (Bhalla, 2010; Pereira, 2012; Stathopoulos, 2011). Because hypocalcemia has been described following *in utero* bisphosphonate exposure, exposed infants should be monitored for hypocalcemia after birth (Djokanovic, 2008; Stathopoulos, 2011).

Breast-Feeding Considerations It is not known if pamidronate is excreted into breast milk. Pamidronate was not detected in the milk of a nursing woman receiving pamidronate 30 mg I.V. monthly (therapy started ~6 months postpartum). Following the first infusion, milk was pumped and collected for 0-24 hours and 25-48 hours, and each day pooled for analysis. Pamidronate readings were below the limit of quantification (<0.4 micromole/L). During therapy, breast milk was pumped and discarded for the first 48 hours following each infusion prior to resuming nursing. The infant was breast-fed >80% of the time; adverse events were not observed in the nursing infant (Simonoski, 2000). Monitoring the serum calcium concentrations of nursing infants is recommended (Stathopoulos, 2011). Due to the potential for serious adverse reactions in the nursing infant, the manufacturer recommends a decision be made whether to discontinue nursing or to discontinue the drug, taking into account the importance of treatment to the mother.

Contraindications Hypersensitivity to pamidronate, other bisphosphonates, or any component of the formulation

Warnings/Precautions Hazardous agent - use appropriate precautions for handling and disposal (meets NIOSH, 2012 criteria). Osteonecrosis of the jaw (ONJ) has been reported in patients receiving bisphosphonates. Risk factors include invasive dental procedures (eg, tooth extraction, dental implants, boney surgery); a diagnosis of cancer, with concomitant chemotherapy, radiotherapy, or corticosteroids; poor oral hygiene, ill-fitting dentures; and comorbid disorders (anemia, coagulopathy, infection, preexisting dental disease). Most reported cases occurred after I.V. bisphosphonate therapy; however, cases have been reported following oral therapy. A dental exam and preventative dentistry should be performed prior to placing patients with risk factors on chronic bisphosphonate therapy. There is no evidence that discontinuing therapy reduces the risk of developing ONJ (Assael, 2009). The benefit/risk must be assessed by the treating physician and/or dentist/surgeon prior to any invasive dental procedure. Patients developing ONJ while on bisphosphonates should receive care by an oral surgeon.

Atypical femur fractures (after minimal or no trauma) have been reported. The fractures include subtrochanteric femur (bone just below the hip joint) and diaphyseal femur (long segment of the thigh bone). Some patients experience prodromal pain weeks or months before the fracture occurs. It is unclear if bisphosphonate therapy is the cause for these fractures. Patients receiving long-term (>3-5 years) bisphosphonate therapy may be at an increased risk. Consider discontinuing pamidronate in patients with a suspected femoral shaft fracture. Patients who present with thigh or groin pain in the absence of trauma should be evaluated. Infrequently, severe (and occasionally debilitating) musculoskeletal (bone, joint, and/or muscle) pain have been reported during bisphosphonate treatment. The onset of pain ranged from a single day to several months. Consider discontinuing therapy in patients who experience severe symptoms; symptoms usually resolve upon discontinuation. Some patients experienced recurrence when rechallenged with same drug or another bisphosphonate; avoid use in patients with a history of these symptoms in association with bisphosphonate therapy.

Initial or single doses have been associated with renal deterioration, progressing to renal failure and dialysis. Withhold pamidronate treatment (until renal function returns to baseline) in patients with evidence of renal deterioration. Glomerulosclerosis (focal segmental) with or without nephrotic syndrome has also been reported. Longer infusion times (>2 hours) may reduce the risk for renal toxicity, especially in patients with pre-existing renal insufficiency. Single pamidronate doses should not exceed 90 mg. Patients with serum creatinine >3 mg/dL were not studied in clinical trials; limited data are available in patients with Cl_{cr} <30 mL/minute. Evaluate serum creatinine prior to each treatment. For the treatment of bone metastases, use is not recommended in patients with severe renal impairment; for renal impairment in indications other than bone metastases, use clinical judgment to determine if benefits outweigh potential risks.

Use has been associated with asymptomatic electrolyte abnormalities (including hypophosphatemia, hypokalemia, hypomagnesemia, and hypocalcemia). Rare cases of symptomatic hypocalcemia, including tetany have been reported. Patients with a history of thyroid surgery may have relative hypoparathyroidism; predisposing them to pamidronate-related hypocalcemia. Patients with pre-existing anemia, leukopenia, or thrombocytopenia should be closely monitored during the first 2 weeks of treatment.

Multiple myeloma: According to the American Society of Clinical Oncology (ASCO) guidelines for bisphosphonates in multiple myeloma, treatment with pamidronate is not recommended for asymptomatic (smoldering) or indolent myeloma or with solitary plasmacytoma (Kyle, 2007). The National Comprehensive Cancer Network® (NCCN) multiple myeloma guidelines (v.2.2013) recommend bisphosphonates for all patients receiving treatment for symptomatic disease; the use of bisphosphonates in stage 1 or smoldering disease may be considered, although preferably as part of a clinical trial. Patients with Bence-Jones proteinuria and dehydration should be adequately hydrated prior to therapy.

Hypercalcemia of malignancy (HCM): Adequate hydration is required during treatment (urine output ~2 L/day); avoid overhydration, especially in patients with heart failure.

Adverse Reactions Note: Actual percentages may vary by indication; treatment for multiple myeloma is associated with higher percentage.

>10%:

Central nervous system: Fever (18% to 39%; transient), fatigue (≤37%), headache (≤26%), insomnia (≤22%)
Endocrine & metabolic: Hypophosphatemia (≤18%), hypokalemia (4% to 18%), hypomagnesemia (4% to 12%), hypocalcemia (≤12%)
Gastrointestinal: Nausea (≤54%), vomiting (≤36%), anorexia (≤26%), abdominal pain (≤23%), dyspepsia (≤23%)
Genitourinary: Urinary tract infection (≤19%)
Hematologic: Anemia (≤43%), granulocytopenia (≤20%)
Local: Infusion site reaction (≤18%; includes induration, pain, redness and swelling)
Neuromuscular & skeletal: Myalgia (≤26%), weakness (≤22%), arthralgia (≤14%), osteonecrosis of the jaw (cancer patients: 1% to 11%)
Renal: Serum creatinine increased (≤19%)
Respiratory: Dyspnea (≤30%), cough (≤26%), upper respiratory tract infection (≤24%), sinusitis (≤16%), pleural effusion (≤11%)

1% to 10%:

Cardiovascular: Atrial fibrillation (≤6%), hypertension (≤6%), syncope (≤6%), tachycardia (≤6%), atrial flutter (≤1%), cardiac failure (≤1%), edema (≤1%)
Central nervous system: Somnolence (≤6%), psychosis (≤4%), seizure (≤2%)
Endocrine & metabolic: Hypothyroidism (≤6%)
Gastrointestinal: Constipation (≤6%), gastrointestinal hemorrhage (≤6%), diarrhea (≤1%), stomatitis (≤1%)
Hematologic: Leukopenia (≤4%), neutropenia (≤1%), thrombocytopenia (≤1%)
Neuromuscular & skeletal: Back pain, bone pain
Renal: Uremia (≤4%)
Respiratory: Rales (≤6%), rhinitis (≤6%)
Miscellaneous: Moniliasis (≤6%)

<1% (Limited to important or life-threatening): Acute renal failure, adult respiratory distress syndrome, allergic reaction, anaphylactic shock, angioedema, bone/joint/muscle pain (severe and occasionally incapacitating), bronchospasm, CHF, confusion, conjunctivitis, electrolyte/mineral abnormality, episcleritis, femoral fractures (atypical subtrochanteric, diaphyseal femoral), fluid overload, flu-like syndrome, focal segmental glomerulosclerosis (including collapsing variant), glomerulonephropathies, hallucinations (visual), hematuria, herpes virus reactivation, hyperkalemia, hypernatremia, hypotension, injection site phlebitis/thrombophlebitis, interstitial pneumonitis, iridocyclitis, iritis, joint and/or muscle pain (sometimes severe and/or incapacitating), left ventricular failure, lymphocytopenia, malaise, nephrotic syndrome, orbital inflammation, osteonecrosis (other than jaw), paresthesia, pruritus, rash, renal deterioration, renal failure, renal tubular disorders, scleritis, tetany, tubulointerstitial nephritis, uveitis, xanthopsia

Drug Interactions

Metabolism/Transport Effects None known.

Avoid Concomitant Use There are no known interactions where it is recommended to avoid concomitant use.

Increased Effect/Toxicity

Pamidronate may increase the levels/effects of: Deferasirox; Phosphate Supplements

The levels/effects of Pamidronate may be increased by: Aminoglycosides; Nonsteroidal Anti-Inflammatory Agents; Systemic Angiogenesis Inhibitors; Thalidomide

Decreased Effect

The levels/effects of Pamidronate may be decreased by: Proton Pump Inhibitors

Preparation for Administration Hazardous agent; use appropriate precautions for handling and disposal (meets NIOSH, 2012 criteria).

Powder for injection: Reconstitute by adding 10 mL of SWFI to each vial of lyophilized pamidronate disodium powder, the resulting solution will be 30 mg/10 mL or 90 mg/10 mL.

Pamidronate may be further diluted in 250-1000 mL of 0.45% or 0.9% sodium chloride or 5% dextrose. (The manufacturer recommends dilution in 1000 mL for hypercalcemia of malignancy, 500 mL for Paget's disease and bone metastases of myeloma, and 250 mL for bone metastases of breast cancer.)

Storage/Stability

Powder for reconstitution: Store at or below 30°C (86°F). The reconstituted solution is stable for 24 hours stored under refrigeration at 2°C to 8°C (36°F to 46°F).

Solution for injection: Store at 20°C to 25°C (68°F to 77°F).

Pamidronate solution for infusion is stable at room temperature for up to 24 hours.

Mechanism of Action Nitrogen-containing bisphosphonate; inhibits bone resorption and decreases mineralization by disrupting osteoclast activity (Gralow, 2009; Rogers, 2011)

Pharmacodynamics/Kinetics

Onset of action:

Hypercalcemia of malignancy (HCM): ≤24 hours for decrease in albumin-corrected serum calcium; maximum effect: ≤7 days

Paget's disease: ~1 month for ≥50% decrease in serum alkaline phosphatase

Duration: HCM: 7-14 days; Paget's disease: 1-372 days

Absorption: Oral: Poor

Metabolism: Not metabolized

Half-life elimination: 21-35 hours

Excretion: Biphasic; urine (30% to 62% as unchanged drug; lower in patients with renal dysfunction) within 120 hours

Dosage Note: Single doses should not exceed 90 mg.

Hypercalcemia of malignancy: Adults: I.V.:

Moderate cancer-related hypercalcemia (corrected serum calcium: 12-13.5 mg/dL): 60-90 mg, as a single dose over 2-24 hours

Severe cancer-related hypercalcemia (corrected serum calcium: >13.5 mg/dL): 90 mg, as a single dose over 2-24 hours

Retreatment in patients who show an initial complete or partial response (allow at least 7 days to elapse prior to retreatment): May retreat at the same dose if serum calcium does not return to normal or does not remain normal after initial treatment.

Multiple myeloma, osteolytic bone lesions: Adults: I.V.: 90 mg over 4 hours once monthly:

Lytic disease: American Society of Clinical Oncology (ASCO) guidelines: 90 mg over at least 2 hours once every 3-4 weeks for 2 years; discontinue after 2 years in patients with responsive and/or stable disease; resume therapy with new-onset skeletal-related events (Kyle, 2007)

Newly-diagnosed, symptomatic (unlabeled dose): 30 mg over 2.5 hours once monthly for at least 3 years (Gimsing, 2010)

Breast cancer, osteolytic bone metastases: Adults: I.V.: 90 mg over 2 hours once every 3-4 weeks

Paget's disease (moderate-to-severe): Adults: I.V.: 30 mg over 4 hours once daily for 3 consecutive days (total dose = 90 mg); may retreat at initial dose if clinically indicated

Prevention of androgen deprivation-induced osteoporosis (unlabeled use): Adults: Males: I.V.: 60 mg over 2 hours once every 3 months (Smith, 2001)

Elderly: Begin at lower end of adult dosing range.

Dosing adjustment in renal impairment: Patients with serum creatinine >3 mg/dL were excluded from clinical trials; there are only limited pharmacokinetic data in patients with Cl_{cr} <30 mL/minute.

Manufacturer recommends the following guidelines:

Treatment of bone metastases: Use is not recommended in patients with severe renal impairment.

Renal impairment in indications other than bone metastases: Use clinical judgment to determine if benefits outweigh potential risks.

Multiple myeloma: American Society of Clinical Oncology (ASCO) guidelines (Kyle, 2007):

Severe renal impairment (serum creatinine >3 mg/dL **or** Cl_{cr} <30 mL/minute) and extensive bone disease: 90 mg over 4-6 hours. However, a reduced initial dose should be considered if renal impairment was pre-existing.

Albuminuria >500 mg/24 hours (unexplained): Withhold dose until returns to baseline, then recheck every 3-4 weeks; consider reinitiating at a dose not to exceed 90 mg every 4 weeks and with a longer infusion time of at least 4 hours

Dosing adjustment in renal toxicity: In patients with bone metastases, treatment should be withheld for deterioration in renal function (increase of serum creatinine ≥0.5 mg/dL in patients with normal baseline or ≥1 mg/dL in patients with abnormal baseline). Resumption of therapy may be considered when serum creatinine returns to within 10% of baseline.

Dosage adjustment in hepatic impairment:

Mild to moderate impairment: No dosage adjustment necessary.

Severe impairment: No dosage adjustment provided in manufacturer's labeling (has not been studied).

Dietary Considerations Multiple myeloma or metastatic bone lesions from solid tumors or Paget's disease: Take adequate daily calcium and vitamin D supplement (if patient is not hypercalcemic).

Administration I.V.: Infusion rate varies by indication. Longer infusion times (>2 hours) may reduce the risk for renal toxicity, especially in patients with pre-existing renal insufficiency. The manufacturer recommends infusing over 2-24 hours for hypercalcemia of malignancy; over 2 hours for osteolytic bone lesions with metastatic breast cancer; and over 4 hours for Paget's disease and for osteolytic bone lesions with multiple myeloma. The ASCO guidelines for bisphosphonate use in multiple myeloma recommend infusing pamidronate over at least 2 hours; if therapy is withheld due to renal toxicity, infuse over at least 4 hours upon reintroduction of treatment after renal recovery (Kyle, 2007).

Hazardous agent; use appropriate precautions for handling and disposal (meets NIOSH, 2012 criteria).

Monitoring Parameters Serum creatinine (prior to each treatment); serum electrolytes, including calcium, phosphate, magnesium, and potassium; CBC with differential; monitor for hypocalcemia for at least 2 weeks after therapy; dental exam and preventative dentistry prior to therapy for patients at risk of osteonecrosis, including all cancer patients; patients with pre-existing anemia, leukopenia, or thrombocytopenia should be closely monitored during the first 2 weeks of treatment; in addition, monitor urine albumin every 3-6 months in multiple myeloma patients

Reference Range Calcium (total): Adults: 9-11 mg/dL (SI: 2.05-2.54 mmol/L), may slightly decrease with aging; Phosphorus: 2.5-4.5 mg/dL (SI: 0.81-1.45 mmol/L)

Test Interactions Bisphosphonates may interfere with diagnostic imaging agents such as technetium-99m-diphosphonate in bone scans.

Additional Information

Oncology Comment:

Metastatic breast cancer: The American Society of Clinical Oncology (ASCO) updated guidelines on the role of bone-modifying agents (BMAs) in the prevention and treatment of skeletal-related events for metastatic breast cancer patients (Van Poznak, 2011). The guidelines recommend initiating a BMA (denosumab, pamidronate, zoledronic acid) in patients with metastatic breast cancer to the bone. There is currently no literature indicating the superiority of one particular BMA. Optimal duration is not defined; however, the guidelines recommend continuing therapy until substantial decline in patient's performance status. In patients with normal Cl_{cr} (>60 mL/minute), no dosage/interval/infusion rate changes for pamidronate or zoledronic acid are necessary. For patients with Cl_{cr} <30 mL/minute, pamidronate and zoledronic acid are not recommended. While no renal dose adjustments are recommended for denosumab, close monitoring is advised for risk of hypocalcemia in patients with Cl_{cr} <30 mL/minute or on dialysis. The ASCO guidelines are in alignment with package insert guidelines for dosing, renal dose adjustments, infusion times, prevention and management of osteonecrosis of the jaw, and monitoring of laboratory parameter recommendations. BMAs are not the first-line therapy for pain. BMAs are to be used as adjunctive therapy for cancer-related bone pain associated with bone metastasis, demonstrating a modest pain control benefit. BMAs should be used in conjunction with agents such as NSAIDs, opioid and nonopioid analgesics, corticosteroids, radiation/surgery, and interventional procedures.

Multiple myeloma: The American Society of Clinical Oncology (ASCO) has also published guidelines on the use of bisphosphonates for prevention and treatment of bone disease in multiple myeloma (Kyle, 2007). Pamidronate or zoledronic acid use is recommended in multiple myeloma patients with lytic bone destruction or compression spine fracture from osteopenia. Clodronate (not available in the U.S.; available in Canada), administered orally or I.V., is an alternative treatment. The use of the bisphosphonates pamidronate and zoledronic acid may be considered in patients with pain secondary to osteolytic disease, adjunct therapy to stabilize fractures or impending fractures, and I.V. bisphosphonates for multiple myeloma patients with osteopenia but no radiographic evidence of lytic bone disease. Bisphosphonates are not recommended in patients with solitary plasmacytoma, smoldering (asymptomatic) or indolent myeloma, or monoclonal gammopathy of undetermined significance. The guidelines recommend monthly treatment for a period of 2 years. At that time, physicians need to consider discontinuing in responsive and stable patients, and reinitiate if a new-onset skeletal-related event occurs. The ASCO guidelines are in alignment with package insert guidelines for dosing, renal dose adjustments, infusion times, prevention and management of osteonecrosis of the jaw, and monitoring of laboratory parameter recommendations. The guidelines also recommend in patients with extensive bone disease with existing severe renal disease (a serum creatinine >3 mg/dL or Cl_{cr} <30 mL/minute) pamidronate at a dose of 90 mg over 4-6 hours (unless pre-existing renal disease in which a reduced initial dose should be considered). ASCO also recommends monitoring for albuminuria every 3-6 months. In patients with unexplained albuminuria >500 mg/24 hours, withhold the dose until level returns to baseline, then recheck every 3-4 weeks. Pamidronate may be reinitiated at a dose not to exceed 90 mg every 4 weeks with a longer infusion time of at least 4 hours.

Dosage Forms Excipient information presented when available (limited, particularly for generics); consult specific product labeling.

Solution, Intravenous, as disodium:
Generic: 30 mg/10 mL (10 mL); 90 mg/10 mL (10 mL)

Solution, Intravenous, as disodium [preservative free]:
Generic: 30 mg/10 mL (10 mL); 6 mg/mL (10 mL); 90 mg/10 mL (10 mL)

Solution Reconstituted, Intravenous, as disodium:
Generic: 30 mg (1 ea); 90 mg (1 ea)

- Pamidronate Disodium *see* Pamidronate *on page 1555*
- Pamidronate Disodium® (Can) *see* Pamidronate *on page 1555*
- Pamidronate Disodium Omega (Can) *see* Pamidronate *on page 1555*
- p-amino-benzenesulfonamide *see* Sulfanilamide *on page 1963*
- p-Aminoclonidine *see* Apraclonidine *on page 158*
- Pamix [OTC] *see* Pyrantel Pamoate *on page 1750*
- Pancrease MT (Can) *see* Pancrelipase *on page 1558*
- Pancreatic Enzymes *see* Pancrelipase *on page 1558*
- Pancreaze *see* Pancrelipase *on page 1558*

Pancrelipase (pan kre LYE pase)

Brand Names: U.S. Creon; Pancreaze; Pancrelipase (Lip-Prot-Amyl); Pertzye; Ultresa; Viokace; Zenpep

Brand Names: Canada Cotazym; Creon; Pancrease MT; Ultrase; Ultrase MT; Viokase

Index Terms Amylase, Lipase, and Protease; Lipancreatin; Lipase, Protease, and Amylase; Pancreatic Enzymes; Protease, Lipase, and Amylase

Pharmacologic Category Enzyme

Use Treatment of exocrine pancreatic insufficiency (EPI) due to conditions such as cystic fibrosis (Creon, Pancreaze, Pertzye, Ultresa, Zenpep); chronic pancreatitis (Creon, Viokace); or pancreatectomy (Creon, Viokace)

Note: Viokace must be administered with a proton pump inhibitor (PPI) since it is not enteric coated.

Pregnancy Risk Factor C

Pregnancy Considerations Reproduction studies have not been conducted. Nutrition should be optimized in pregnancy; in cystic fibrosis patients with malabsorption, pancreatic enzyme replacement is not considered to cause a risk to the pregnancy.

Breast-Feeding Considerations Systemic absorption and concentration into the breast milk is unlikely, but unknown.

Medication Guide Available Yes

Contraindications There are no contraindications listed in the manufacturer's labeling.

Warnings/Precautions Fibrosing colonopathy advancing to colonic strictures have been reported with doses of lipase >6000 units/kg/meal over long periods of time in children <12 years of age. Patients taking doses of lipase >6000 units/kg/meal should be examined and the dose decreased. Doses of lipase >2500 units/kg/meal (or lipase >10,000 units/kg/day) should be used with caution and only with documentation of 3-day fecal fat measures. Crushing or chewing the contents of the capsules or tablets, or mixing the capsule contents with foods outside of product labeling, may cause early release of the enzymes, causing irritation of the oral mucosa and/or loss of enzyme activity. When mixing the contents of capsules with food, the mixture should be swallowed immediately and followed with water or juice to ensure complete ingestion. Use caution in patients with gout, hyperuricemia, or renal impairment; products contain purines which may increase uric acid concentrations. Products are derived from porcine pancreatic glands. Severe, allergic reactions (rare) have been observed; use with caution in patients hypersensitive to pork proteins. Transmission of porcine viruses is theoretically a risk; however, testing and/or inactivation or removal of certain viruses, reduces the risk. There have been no cases of transmission of an infectious illness reported. Available brand products are **not** interchangeable.

Adverse Reactions The following adverse reactions were reported in a short-term safety studies; actual frequency varies with different products; adverse events, particularly gastrointestinal events, were often greater with placebo:

>10%:

Central nervous system: Headache (3% to 15%)
Gastrointestinal: Abdominal pain (3% to 18%)
Neuromuscular & skeletal: Neck pain (14%)
Otic: Ear pain (11%)
Respiratory: Nasal congestion (14%), beta-hemolytic streptococcal infection (11%)
Miscellaneous: Lymphadenopathy (11%)

1% to 10%:

Cardiovascular: Peripheral edema (3%)
Central nervous system: Dizziness (4% to 6%)
Dermatologic: Rash (3%)
Endocrine & metabolic: Hyperglycemia (4% to 8%), diabetes mellitus exacerbation (4%), hypoglycemia (4%)
Gastrointestinal: Dyspepsia (10%), diarrhea (≤10%), flatulence (3% to 9%), anal itching (7%), biliary tract stones (7%), early satiety (6%), vomiting (6%), weight loss (3% to 6%), upper abdominal pain (≤5%), feces abnormal (≤4%)
Hematologic: Anemia (3%)
Hepatic: Ascites (3%), hydrocholecystis (3%)
Renal: Renal cyst (3%)
Respiratory: Cough (4% to 10%), epistaxis (7%), pharyngolaryngeal pain (7%), nasopharyngitis (4%)
Miscellaneous: Viral infection (3%)

<1% (Limited to important or life-threatening; reported with various formulations of pancrelipase): Allergic reactions (severe), anaphylaxis, asthma, carcinoma recurrence, constipation, distal intestinal obstruction syndrome (DIOS), duodenitis, fibrosing colonopathy, gastritis, hives, hyperuricemia, muscle spasm, myalgia, nausea, neutropenia (transient), pruritus, transaminases increased (asymptomatic), urticaria, vision blurred

Drug Interactions

Metabolism/Transport Effects None known.

Avoid Concomitant Use There are no known interactions where it is recommended to avoid concomitant use.

Increased Effect/Toxicity There are no known significant interactions involving an increase in effect.

Decreased Effect

Pancrelipase may decrease the levels/effects of: Iron Salts; Multivitamins/Minerals (with ADEK, Folate, Iron)

Ethanol/Nutrition/Herb Interactions

Food: Delayed release capsules: Enteric coated contents of delayed release capsules opened and sprinkled on alkaline foods may result in early release of pancrelipase followed by enzyme inactivation by gastric acid in the stomach after swallowing. Management: Avoid placing contents of opened capsules on alkaline food (soft acidic foods with a pH of ≤4.5 are recommended for patients who cannot swallow capsules).

Herb/Nutraceutical: Pancrelipase may impair absorption of oral iron. Management: Monitor response to iron replacement.

Storage/Stability

Creon: Store at 25°C (77°F); excursions permitted between 25°C to 40°C (77°F to 104°F) for ≤30 days. Protect from moisture, and discard if moisture conditions are >70%. Keep bottle tightly closed.

Pancreaze: Store at ≤25°C (77°F). Protect from moisture; keep bottle tightly closed.

Pertzye: Store at 20°C to 25°C (68°F to 77°F); excursions permitted between 15°C to 40°C (59°F to 104°F). Protect from moisture; keep bottle tightly closed after opening.

Ultresa: Store at 20°C to 25°C (68°F to 77°F). Protect from moisture; keep bottle tightly closed after opening.

Viokace: Store at 20°C to 25°C (68°F to 77°F); excursions permitted up to 40°C (104°F) for up to 24 hours. Protect from moisture; keep bottle tightly closed after opening.

Zenpep:

Original glass container: Store at 20°C to 25°C (68°F to 77°F); excursions permitted between 15°C to 40°C (59°F to 104°F). Protect from moisture; keep bottle tightly closed after opening.

Repackaged HDPE container: Store at ≤30°C (86°F) for up to 6 months; excursions permitted between 15°C to 40°C (59°F to 104°F) for ≤30 days. Protect from moisture; keep bottle tightly closed after opening.

Mechanism of Action Pancrelipase is a natural product harvested from the porcine pancreatic glands. It contains a combination of lipase, amylase, and protease. Products are formulated to dissolve in the more basic pH of the duodenum so that they may act locally to break down fats, protein, and starch.

Pharmacodynamics/Kinetics

Absorption: None; acts locally in GI tract
Excretion: Feces

Dosage Oral: **Note:** Adjust dose based on body weight, clinical symptoms, and stool fat content. Allow several days between dose adjustments. Total daily dose reflects ~3 meals/day and 2-3 snacks/day, with half the mealtime dose given with a snack. Doses of lipase >2500 units/kg/meal (or lipase >10,000 units/kg/**day**) should be used with caution and only with documentation of 3-day fecal fat measures. Doses of lipase >6000 units/kg/meal are associated with colonic stricture and should be decreased.

Pancreatic insufficiency due to conditions such as cystic fibrosis:

Infants, Children, and Adolescents:

≤1 year (Creon, Pancreaze, Zenpep): Lipase 2000-4000 units per 120 mL of formula or per breast-feeding

>1 and <4 years (Creon, Pancreaze, Zenpep, Pertzye [and weight ≥8 kg], Ultresa [and weight ≥14 kg]): Initial: Lipase 1000 units/kg/meal. Dosage range: Lipase 1000-2500 units/kg/meal. Maximum: Lipase ≤2500 units/kg/**meal or** lipase ≤10,000 units/kg/**day or** lipase <4000 units/g of fat daily

≥4 years (Creon, Pancreaze, Zenpep, Pertzye [and weight ≥16 kg], Ultresa [and weight ≥28 kg]): Refer to adult dosing.

Adults (Creon, Pancreaze, Pertzye, Ultresa, Zenpep): Initial: Lipase 500 units/kg/meal. Dosage range: Lipase 500-2500 units/kg/meal. Maximum: Lipase ≤2500 units/kg/**meal or** lipase ≤10,000 units/kg/**day or** lipase <4000 units/g of fat daily

Pancreatic insufficiency due to chronic pancreatitis or pancreatectomy: Adults:

Creon: Lipase 72,000 units/meal while consuming ≥100 g of fat daily; alternatively, lower initial doses of lipase 500 units/kg/meal with individualized dosage titrations have also been used

Viokace (administer in combination with a proton pump inhibitor): Initial: Lipase 500 units/kg/meal. Dosage range: Lipase 500-2500 units/kg/meal. Maximum: Lipase ≤2500 units/kg/**meal or** lipase ≤10,000 units/kg/**day or** lipase <4000 units/g of fat daily

Dosage adjustment in renal impairment: No dosage adjustment provided in manufacturer's labeling. Use with caution.

Dosage adjustment in hepatic impairment: No dosage adjustment provided in manufacturer's labeling.

Dietary Considerations Take with meals or snacks and swallow whole with a generous amount of liquid. Vitamin supplementation should be per current guidelines for patients with cystic fibrosis.

Administration Oral: Administer with meals or snacks and swallow whole with a generous amount of liquid. Do not crush or chew; retention in the mouth before swallowing may cause mucosal irritation and stomatitis.

Capsules, delayed release: If necessary, capsules may also be opened and contents added to a small amount of an acidic food (pH ≤4.5), such as applesauce. The food should be at room temperature and swallowed immediately after mixing. The contents of the capsule should not be crushed or chewed. Follow with water or juice to ensure complete ingestion and that no medication remains in the mouth.

When administering to infants <1 year of age, do not mix with breast milk or infant formula. Open capsule and place the contents directly into the mouth or mix with a small amount of acidic soft food (pH ≤4.5), such as applesauce or other acidic commercially prepared baby food (pears or bananas) at room temperature. Administer immediately after mixing (or within 15 minutes of mixing using Pancreaze). Follow with infant formula or breast milk to ensure complete ingestion and that no medication remains in the mouth.

Tablets: Viokace: Tablets are not enteric coated and should be taken with a proton pump inhibitor.

Administration via gastrostomy (G) tube: An *in vitro* study demonstrated that Creon delayed-release capsules sprinkled onto a small amount of baby food (pH <4.5; applesauce or bananas manufactured by both Gerber and Beech-Nut) stirred gently and after 15 minutes was administered through the following G-tubes without significant loss of lipase activity: Kimberly-Clark MIC Bolus size 18 Fr, Kimberly-Clark MIC-KEY size 16 Fr, Bard Tri-Funnel size 18 Fr, and Bard Button size 18 Fr (Shlieout, 2011).

Monitoring Parameters Abdominal symptoms, nutritional intake, weight, growth (in children), stool character, fecal fat

Additional Information Unapproved PEPs are no longer allowed to be distributed in the U.S. There are six PEPs with FDA approval commercially available in the U.S.: Creon, Pancreaze, Pertzye, Ultresa, Viokace, and Zenpep. PEPs are **not** interchangeable, and patients will require new prescriptions when changing from one product to another. However, Pancrelipase lipase 5000 units strength (manufactured by Eurand Pharmaceuticals and distributed by X-Gen Pharmaceuticals) is an authorized generic which may be used interchangeably with the Zenpep lipase 5000 units product (manufactured by Eurand Pharmaceuticals).

Creon: Capsules contain enteric coated microspheres which are 0.71-1.6 mm in diameter.

Pancreaze: Capsules contain enteric coated microtablets which are ~2 mm in diameter.

Pertzye: Capsules contain enteric coated microspheres which are 0.8-2.2 mm in diameter.

Ultresa: Capsules contain enteric coated minitablets which are ~2 mm in diameter.

Zenpep: Capsules contain enteric coated beads which are 1.8-2.5 mm in diameter.

Dosage Forms Excipient information presented when available (limited, particularly for generics); consult specific product labeling.

Capsule, delayed release, bicarbonate buffered enteric coated microspheres, oral [porcine derived]:
- Pertzye: Lipase 8,000 USP units, protease 28,750 USP units, and amylase 30,250 USP units
- Pertzye: Lipase 16,000 USP units, protease 57,500 USP units, and amylase 60,500 USP units

Capsule, delayed release, enteric coated beads, oral [porcine derived]:
- Pancrelipase (Lip-Prot-Amyl): Lipase 5000 USP units, protease 17,000 USP units, amylase 27,000 USP units
- Zenpep: Lipase 3000 USP units, protease 10,000 USP units, and amylase 16,000 USP units
- Zenpep: Lipase 5000 USP units, protease 17,000 USP units, and amylase 27,000 USP units
- Zenpep: Lipase 10,000 USP units, protease 34,000 USP units, and amylase 55,000 USP units
- Zenpep: Lipase 15,000 USP units, protease 51,000 USP units, and amylase 82,000 USP units
- Zenpep: Lipase 20,000 USP units, protease 68,000 USP units, and amylase 109,000 USP units
- Zenpep: Lipase 25,000 USP units, protease 85,000 USP units, and amylase 136,000 USP units

Capsule, delayed release, enteric coated microspheres, oral [porcine derived]:
- Creon: Lipase 3000 USP units, protease 9500 USP units, and amylase 15,000 USP units
- Creon: Lipase 6000 USP units, protease 19,000 USP units, and amylase 30,000 USP units
- Creon: Lipase 12,000 USP units, protease 38,000 USP units, and amylase 60,000 USP units
- Creon: Lipase 24,000 USP units, protease 76,000 USP units, and amylase 120,000 USP units
- Creon: Lipase 36,000 USP units, protease 114,000 USP units, and amylase 180,000 USP units

Capsule, delayed release, enteric coated microtablets, oral [porcine derived]:
- Pancreaze: Lipase 4200 USP units, protease 10,000 USP units, and amylase 17,500 USP units
- Pancreaze: Lipase 10,500 USP units, protease 25,000 USP units, and amylase 43,750 USP units
- Pancreaze: Lipase 16,800 USP units, protease 40,000 USP units, and amylase 70,000 USP units
- Pancreaze: Lipase 21,000 USP units, protease 37,000 USP units, and amylase 61,000 USP units

Capsule, delayed release, enteric coated minitablets, oral [porcine derived]:
- Ultresa: Lipase 13,800 USP units, protease 27,600 USP units, and amylase 27,600 USP units
- Ultresa: Lipase 20,700 USP units, protease 41,400 USP units, and amylase 41,400 USP units
- Ultresa: Lipase 23,000 USP units, protease 46,000 USP units, and amylase 46,000 USP units

Tablet, oral [porcine derived]:
- Viokace: Lipase 10,440 USP units, protease 39,150 USP units, and amylase 39,150 USP units
- Viokace: Lipase 20,880 USP units, protease 78,300 USP units, and amylase 78,300 USP units

◆ **Pancrelipase (Lip-Prot-Amyl)** *see* Pancrelipase *on page 1558*

Pancuronium (pan kyoo ROE nee um)

Brand Names: Canada Pancuronium Bromide®

Index Terms Pancuronium Bromide; Pavulon [DSC]

Pharmacologic Category Neuromuscular Blocker Agent, Nondepolarizing

Use Facilitation of endotracheal intubation and relaxation of skeletal muscles during surgery; facilitation of mechanical ventilation in ICU patients; does not relieve pain or produce sedation

Pregnancy Risk Factor C

Pregnancy Considerations Animal reproduction studies have not been conducted. Small amounts of pancuronium cross the placenta (Daily, 1984). May be used short-term in cesarean section; reduced doses recommended in patients also receiving magnesium sulfate due to enhanced effects.

Contraindications Hypersensitivity to pancuronium, bromide, or any component of the formulation

Warnings/Precautions Ventilation must be supported during neuromuscular blockade; use with caution in patients with renal and/or hepatic impairment (adjust dose appropriately); certain clinical conditions may result in potentiation or antagonism of neuromuscular blockade:

Potentiation: Electrolyte abnormalities, severe hyponatremia, severe hypocalcemia, severe hypokalemia, hypermagnesemia, neuromuscular diseases, acidosis, acute intermittent porphyria, renal failure, hepatic failure

Antagonism: Alkalosis, hypercalcemia, demyelinating lesions, peripheral neuropathies, diabetes mellitus

Increased sensitivity in patients with myasthenia gravis, Eaton-Lambert syndrome; resistance in burn patients (>30% of body) for period of 5-70 days postinjury; resistance in patients with muscle trauma, denervation, immobilization, infection. Cross-sensitivity with other neuromuscular-blocking agents may occur; use extreme caution in patients with previous anaphylactic reactions. Use caution in the elderly. **[U.S. Boxed Warning]: Should be administered by adequately trained individuals familiar with its use.** Some dosage forms may contain benzyl alcohol which has been associated with "gasping syndrome" in neonates.

Adverse Reactions Frequency not defined.

Cardiovascular: Elevation in pulse rate, elevated blood pressure and cardiac output, tachycardia, edema, skin flushing, circulatory collapse

Dermatologic: Rash, itching, erythema, burning sensation along the vein

Gastrointestinal: Excessive salivation

Neuromuscular & skeletal: Profound muscle weakness

Respiratory: Wheezing, bronchospasm

Miscellaneous: Hypersensitivity reaction

Postmarketing and/or case reports: Acute quadriplegic myopathy syndrome (prolonged use), anaphylactoid reactions, anaphylaxis, myositis ossificans (prolonged use)

Drug Interactions

Metabolism/Transport Effects None known.

Avoid Concomitant Use

Avoid concomitant use of Pancuronium with any of the following: QuiNINE

Increased Effect/Toxicity

Pancuronium may increase the levels/effects of: Cardiac Glycosides; Corticosteroids (Systemic); OnabotulinumtoxinA; RimabotulinumtoxinB

The levels/effects of Pancuronium may be increased by: AbobotulinumtoxinA; Aminoglycosides; Calcium Channel Blockers; Capreomycin; Colistimethate; CycloSPORINE (Systemic); Fosphenytoin-Phenytoin; Inhalational Anesthetics; Ketorolac (Nasal); Ketorolac (Systemic); Lincosamide Antibiotics; Lithium; Loop Diuretics; Magnesium Salts; Polymyxin B; Procainamide; QuiNIDine; QuiNINE; Spironolactone; Tetracycline Derivatives; Theophylline Derivatives; Vancomycin

Decreased Effect

The levels/effects of Pancuronium may be decreased by: Acetylcholinesterase Inhibitors; Fosphenytoin-Phenytoin; Loop Diuretics; Theophylline Derivatives

Storage/Stability Refrigerate; however, stable for up to 6 months at room temperature.

Mechanism of Action Blocks neural transmission at the myoneural junction by binding with cholinergic receptor sites

Pharmacodynamics/Kinetics

Onset of effect: Peak effect: I.V.: 2-3 minutes

Duration (dose dependent): 60-100 minutes

Metabolism: Hepatic (30% to 45%); active metabolite 3-hydroxypancuronium (1/3 to 1/2 the activity of parent drug)

Half-life elimination: 110 minutes

Excretion: Urine (55% to 70% as unchanged drug)

Dosage Administer I.V.; dose to effect; doses will vary due to interpatient variability

Surgery:

Infants >1 month, Children, and Adults: Initial: 0.06-0.1 mg/kg or 0.05 mg/kg after initial dose of succinylcholine for intubation; maintenance dose: 0.01 mg/kg administered 60-100 minutes after initial dose and then 0.01 mg/kg every 25-60 minutes

Pretreatment/priming: 10% of intubating dose given 3-5 minutes before intubating dose

ICU paralysis (eg, facilitate mechanical ventilation) in select adequately sedated patients: 0.06-0.1 mg/kg bolus followed by either:

Continuous infusion: 1-2 **mcg**/kg/**minute** (0.06-0.12 **mg**/kg/**hour**) (Murray, 2002) **or** 0.8-1.7 **mcg**/kg/**minute** (0.048-0.102 **mg**/kg/**hour**) (Greenberg, 2013)

or

Intermittent bolus: 0.1-0.2 mg/kg every 1-3 hours

Dosage adjustment in renal impairment: Elimination half-life is doubled, plasma clearance is reduced and rate of recovery is sometimes much slower. No dosage adjustment provided in manufacturer's labeling; however, the following adjustments have been recommended (Aronoff 2007):

Cl_{cr} >50 mL/minute: No dosage adjustment necessary.

Cl_{cr} 10-50 mL/minute: Administer 50% of normal dose

Cl_{cr} <10 mL/minute: Avoid use.

Hemodialysis/peritoneal dialysis: Avoid use.

CRRT: Administer 50% of normal dose.

Dosage adjustment in hepatic impairment: Elimination half-life is doubled, plasma clearance is reduced, recovery time is prolonged, volume of distribution is increased (50%) and results in a slower onset, higher total initial dosage, and prolongation of neuromuscular blockade. Patients with liver disease may develop slow resistance to nondepolarizing muscle relaxant. Large doses may be required and problems may arise in antagonism

Dosing in obesity: Use ideal body weight for obese patients.

Administration May be administered undiluted by rapid I.V. injection

Monitoring Parameters Heart rate, blood pressure, assisted ventilation status; cardiac monitor, blood pressure monitor, and ventilator required

Additional Information Pancuronium is classified as a long-duration neuromuscular-blocking agent. Neuromuscular blockade will be prolonged in patients with decreased renal function. Pancuronium does not relieve pain or produce sedation. It may produce cumulative effect on duration of blockade. It produces tachycardia secondary to vagolytic activity and sympathetic stimulation.

Dosage Forms Excipient information presented when available (limited, particularly for generics); consult specific product labeling.

Solution, Intravenous, as bromide:

Generic: 1 mg/mL (10 mL); 2 mg/mL (2 mL, 5 mL)

◆ **Pancuronium Bromide** *see* Pancuronium *on page 1560*

◆ **Pancuronium Bromide® (Can)** *see* Pancuronium *on page 1560*

◆ **Pandel** *see* Hydrocortisone (Topical) *on page 1011*

◆ **Panglobulin** *see* Immune Globulin *on page 1059*

Panitumumab (pan i TOOM yoo mab)

Brand Names: U.S. Vectibix

Brand Names: Canada Vectibix

Index Terms ABX-EGF; MOAB ABX-EGF; Monoclonal Antibody ABX-EGF; rHuMAb-EGFr

Pharmacologic Category Antineoplastic Agent, Monoclonal Antibody; Epidermal Growth Factor Receptor (EGFR) Inhibitor

Use

Colorectal cancer: As a single agent for the treatment of EGFR-expressing metastatic colorectal carcinoma (mCRC) with disease progression on or following fluoropyrimidine-, oxaliplatin-, and irinotecan-containing chemotherapy regimens.

Limitations of use: Panitumumab is not indicated for the treatment of patients with *KRAS* mutation-positive mCRC or for whom *KRAS* mCRC status is unknown. Retrospective subset analyses of mCRC trials have not shown a treatment benefit for panitumumab in patients whose tumors had *KRAS* mutations in codon 12 or 13. Panitumumab in combination with oxaliplatin-based chemotherapy is not indicated for the treatment of patients with *RAS* (*KRAS* or *NRAS*) mutation-positive mCRC or for whom *RAS* status is unknown.

Unlabeled Use Treatment of metastatic colorectal cancer (KRAS wild-type) in combination with other chemotherapy agents

Pregnancy Risk Factor C

Pregnancy Considerations Animal reproduction studies have demonstrated adverse fetal effects. Based on animal studies, panitumumab may disrupt normal menstrual cycles. IgG is known to cross the placenta; therefore, it is possible the developing fetus may be exposed to panitumumab. Because panitumumab inhibits epidermal growth factor (EGF), a component of fetal development, adverse effects on pregnancy would be expected. Panitumumab should only be given to a pregnant woman if the potential benefit justifies the potential risk to the fetus. Women of childbearing potential should use effective contraception during and for 6 months after treatment. Women who become pregnant during panitumumab treatment are encouraged to enroll in Amgen's Pregnancy Surveillance Program (1-800-772-6436).

Breast-Feeding Considerations It is not known if panitumumab is excreted in breast milk. The decision to discontinue panitumumab or discontinue breast-feeding should take into account the benefits of treatment to the mother. If breast-feeding is interrupted for panitumumab treatment, based on the half-life, breast-feeding should not be resumed for at least 2 months following the last dose.

Contraindications There are no contraindications listed in the manufacturer's labeling.

Warnings/Precautions [U.S. Boxed Warning]: Dermatologic toxicities have been reported in ~90% of patients receiving single agent panitumumab and were severe (grade 3 or higher) in ~12% of patients); may include dermatitis acneiform, pruritus, erythema, rash, skin exfoliation, paronychia, dry skin and skin fissures. Severe skin toxicities may be complicated by infection, sepsis, or abscesses. The median time to development of skin (or ocular) toxicity was 2 weeks, with resolution ~12 weeks after discontinuation. Monitor all dermatologic toxicities for development of inflammation or infection. Withhold treatment for severe or life-threatening dermatologic toxicities; may require dose reduction or permanent discontinuation. The severity of dermatologic toxicity is predictive for response; grades 2-4 skin toxicity correlates with improved progression free survival and overall survival, compared to grade 1 skin toxicity (Peeters, 2009; Van Cutsem, 2007). Patients should minimize sunlight exposure; may exacerbate skin reactions. Keratitis and ulcerative keratitis (known risk factors for corneal perforation) have occurred. Monitor for evidence of ocular toxicity; interrupt or discontinue treatment for acute or worsening keratitis. Gastric mucosal and nail toxicities have also been reported.

[U.S. Boxed Warning]: Severe infusion reactions (anaphylactic reaction, bronchospasm, fever, chills, and hypotension) have been reported in ~1% of patients; fatal infusion reactions have been reported with postmarketing surveillance. Discontinue infusion for severe reactions; permanently discontinue in patients with persistent severe infusion reactions. Appropriate medical support for the management of infusion reactions should be readily available. Mild-to-moderate infusion reactions are managed by slowing the infusion rate.

Pulmonary fibrosis has been observed (rarely) in clinical trials; fatalities have been reported. Interrupt treatment for acute onset or worsening of pulmonary symptoms; permanently discontinue treatment if interstitial lung disease is confirmed. Patients with a history of or evidence of interstitial pneumonitis or pulmonary fibrosis were excluded from most clinical trials. May cause diarrhea; the incidence and severity of chemotherapy-induced diarrhea and other toxicities (rash, electrolyte abnormalities, stomatitis) is increased with combination chemotherapy; severe diarrhea and dehydration (which may lead to acute renal failure) has been observed with panitumumab in combination with chemotherapy. In a study of bevacizumab with combination chemotherapy ± panitumumab, the use of panitumumab resulted in decreased progression-free survival and significantly increased toxicity compared to regimens without panitumumab (Hecht, 2009). Toxicities included rash, diarrhea/dehydration, electrolyte disturbances, stomatitis, infection, and an increased incidence of pulmonary embolism. Magnesium and/or calcium depletion may occur during treatment (may be delayed; hypomagnesemia occurred ≥6 weeks after panitumumab initiation) and after treatment is discontinued; electrolyte repletion may be necessary; monitor for hypomagnesemia and hypocalcemia during treatment and for at least 8 weeks after completion.

Patients with colorectal cancer with tumors with a codon 12 or 13 *KRAS* mutation are unlikely to benefit from EGFR inhibitor therapy. Panitumumab is not indicated patients with *KRAS* mutation-positive metastatic colorectal cancer or patients in which *KRAS* mutation status is unknown. In a study of FOLFOX4 (fluorouracil, leucovorin and oxaliplatin) ± panitumumab, patients with a *KRAS* mutation who received panitumumab with FOLFOX4 experienced a significantly shortened progression-free survival (Douillard, 2010). In addition, a subset analysis of patients with wild-type *KRAS* identified additional *RAS* (*KRAS* [exons 3 and 4] or *NRAS* [exons 2, 3, 4]) mutations; progression-free survival and overall survival were significantly shortened in patients with *RAS* mutations who received FOLFOX4 in combination with panitumumab (Douillard, 2013). Panitumumab should not be used in combination with oxaliplatin-based regimens in patients with *RAS* (*KRAS* or *NRAS*) mutations or if mutation status is unknown. Panitumumab is also reported to be ineffective in patients with BRAF V600E mutation (Di Nicolantonio, 2008). According to the manufacturer, evidence of EGFR expression is necessary to determine patient selection (the Dako EGFR pharmDX® kit has been used).

Adverse Reactions

>10%:

Cardiovascular: Peripheral edema (12%)

Central nervous system: Fatigue (26%)

Dermatologic: Skin toxicity (90%; grades 3/4: 14% to 16%), erythema (65%; grades 3/4: 5%), acneiform rash (57%; grades 3/4: 7%), pruritus (57%; grades 3/4: 2%), nail toxicity (29%; grades 3/4: 2%), exfoliation (25%; grades 3/4: 2%), paronychia (25%), rash (22%; grades 3/4: 1%), fissures (20%; grades 3/4: 1%), acne (13%; grades 3/4: 1%)

Endocrine & metabolic: Hypomagnesemia (38%; grades 3/4: 4%)

Gastrointestinal: Abdominal pain (25%), nausea (23%), diarrhea (21%; grades 3/4: 2%), constipation (21%), vomiting (19%)
Ocular: Ocular toxicity (15%)
Respiratory: Cough (14%)

1% to 10%:
Dermatologic: Dry skin (10%)
Gastrointestinal: Stomatitis (7%), mucositis (6%)
Ocular: Eyelash growth (6%), conjunctivitis (4%), ocular hyperemia (3%), lacrimation increased (2%), eye/eye lid irritation (1%)
Miscellaneous: Antibody formation (≤5%), infusion reactions (3%; grades 3/4: 1%)

<1% (Limited to important or life-threatening): Abscess, allergic reaction, anaphylactoid reaction, angioedema, chills, dyspnea, fever, hypocalcemia, hypoxia, keratitis, keratitis ulcerative, pulmonary embolism, pulmonary fibrosis, pulmonary infiltrate, sepsis, septic death, skin necrosis

Drug Interactions

Metabolism/Transport Effects None known.

Avoid Concomitant Use There are no known interactions where it is recommended to avoid concomitant use.

Increased Effect/Toxicity There are no known significant interactions involving an increase in effect.

Decreased Effect There are no known significant interactions involving a decrease in effect.

Preparation for Administration Dilute in 100 mL (for doses ≤1000 mg) or 150 mL (doses >1000 mg) of normal saline to a final concentration of ≤10 mg/mL. Gently invert to mix; do not shake. Discard any unused portion remaining in the vial.

Storage/Stability Store vials in the original cartons under refrigeration at 2°C to 8°C (36°F to 46°F) until the time of use. Do not freeze; do not shake; protect from direct sunlight. Solution diluted for infusion should be used within 6 hours of preparation if stored at room temperature or within 24 hours of dilution if stored at 2°C to 8°C (36°F to 46°F); do not freeze.

Mechanism of Action Recombinant human IgG2 monoclonal antibody which binds specifically to the epidermal growth factor receptor (EGFR, HER1, c-ErbB-1) and competitively inhibits the binding of epidermal growth factor (EGF) and other ligands. Binding to the EGFR blocks phosphorylation and activation of intracellular tyrosine kinases, resulting in inhibition of cell survival, growth, proliferation and transformation. EGFR signal transduction results in *KRAS* wild-type activation; cells with *KRAS* mutations appear to be unaffected by EGFR inhibition.

Pharmacodynamics/Kinetics Half-life elimination: ~7.5 days (range: 4-11 days)

Dosage

Colorectal cancer, metastatic, *KRAS* mutation-negative: Adults: I.V.: 6 mg/kg every 14 days as a single agent

Colorectal cancer, metastatic (*KRAS* wild-type), in combination with FOLFIRI (unlabeled use): Adults: I.V.: 6 mg/kg every 14 days in combination with fluorouracil, leucovorin, and irinotecan (Peeters, 2010)

Colorectal cancer, metastatic (*RAS* wild-type), in combination with FOLFOX (unlabeled use): Adults: I.V.: 6 mg/kg every 14 days in combination with fluorouracil, leucovorin, and oxaliplatin (Douillard, 2010; Douillard, 2013)

Dosing adjustment for toxicity:

Infusion reactions, mild-to-moderate (grade 1 or 2): Reduce the infusion rate by 50% for the duration of infusion.

Infusion reactions, severe (grade 3 or 4): Stop infusion; consider permanent discontinuation (depending on severity or persistence of reaction).

Dermatologic toxicity (≥grade 3, or intolerable): Withhold treatment; if skin toxicity does not improve to ≤grade 2 within 1 month, permanently discontinue. If skin toxicity improves to ≤grade 2 within 1 month (with patient missing ≤2 doses), resume treatment at 50% of the original dose. Dose may be increased in increments of 25% of the original dose (up to 6 mg/kg) if skin toxicities do not recur. For recurrent skin toxicity, permanently discontinue.

Ocular toxicity (acute or worsening keratitis): Interrupt or discontinue treatment.

Pulmonary toxicity:

Acute onset or worsening pulmonary symptoms: Interrupt treatment.

Interstitial lung disease: Permanently discontinue treatment.

Dosage adjustment in renal impairment: No dosage adjustment provided in the manufacturer's labeling (has not been studied).

Dosage adjustment in hepatic impairment: No dosage adjustment provided in the manufacturer's labeling (has not been studied).

Administration I.V.: Doses ≤1000 mg, infuse over 1 hour; doses >1000 mg, infuse over 90 minutes (via infusion pump); do not administer I.V. push or as a bolus. Administer through a low protein-binding 0.2 or 0.22 micrometer in-line filter. Flush line with NS before and after infusion. Reduce infusion rate by 50% for mild-to-moderate infusion reactions (grades 1 and 2); stop infusion for severe infusion reactions (grades 3 and 4) and consider permanent discontinuation.

Monitoring Parameters *KRAS* genotyping of tumor tissue. Monitor serum electrolytes, including magnesium and calcium (periodically during and for at least 8 weeks after therapy). Monitor vital signs and temperature before, during, and after infusion. Monitor for skin toxicity, for evidence of ocular toxicity, and for acute onset or worsening pulmonary symptoms.

Additional Information Oncology Comment: The American Society of Clinical Oncology (ASCO) provisional clinical opinion (Allegra, 2009) recommends genotyping tumor tissue for *KRAS* mutation in all patients with metastatic colorectal cancer (genotyping may be done on archived specimens). Patients with known codon 12 or 13 *KRAS* gene mutations are unlikely to respond to EGFR inhibitors and should not receive panitumumab. Favorable progression-free survival and higher response rates have been demonstrated with panitumumab in patients with *KRAS* wild-type; patients with the *KRAS* mutation did not respond to panitumumab (Amado, 2008). Panitumumab is also reported to be ineffective in patients with BRAF V600E mutation (Di Nicolantonio, 2008). Severity of dermatologic toxicity associated with panitumumab is predictive for response; grades 2-4 skin toxicity correlates with improved progression free survival and overall survival, compared to patients with grade 1 skin toxicity (Peeters, 2009; Van Cutsem, 2007). The association between dermatologic toxicity and progression free survival was not noted in patients with *KRAS* mutation (Peeters, 2009).

Dosage Forms Excipient information presented when available (limited, particularly for generics); consult specific product labeling.

Solution, Intravenous [preservative free]:
Vectibix: 100 mg/5 mL (5 mL); 400 mg/20 mL (20 mL)

◆ **Panto™ I.V. (Can)** *see* Pantoprazole *on page* 1563

◆ **Pantoloc® (Can)** *see* Pantoprazole *on page* 1563

Pantoprazole (pan TOE pra zole)

Brand Names: U.S. Protonix

Brand Names: Canada Apo-Pantoprazole®; Ava-Pantoprazole; CO Pantoprazole; Mylan-Pantoprazole; Pantoloc®; Pantoprazole for Injection; Panto™ I.V.; PMS-Pantoprazole; Q-Pantoprazole; RAN™-Pantoprazole;

ratio-Pantoprazole; Riva-Pantoprazole; Sandoz-Pantoprazole; Tecta®; Teva-Pantoprazole

Index Terms Pantoprazole Magnesium; Pantoprazole Sodium

Pharmacologic Category Proton Pump Inhibitor; Substituted Benzimidazole

Use

Oral: Short-term (up to 8 weeks) treatment and maintenance of healing of erosive esophagitis associated with GERD; reduction in relapse rates of daytime and nighttime heartburn symptoms in GERD; hypersecretory disorders associated with Zollinger-Ellison syndrome or other GI hypersecretory disorders

I.V.: Short-term treatment (7-10 days) of patients with gastroesophageal reflux disease (GERD) and a history of erosive esophagitis; hypersecretory disorders associated with Zollinger-Ellison syndrome or other GI hypersecretory disorders

Canadian labeling: Additional use (not in U.S. labeling): Oral: Peptic ulcer disease (eg, duodenal or gastric ulcer); adjunct treatment with antibiotics for *Helicobacter pylori* eradication; prevention of GI lesions in patients receiving prolonged NSAID therapy

Unlabeled Use Peptic ulcer disease, active ulcer bleeding (parenteral formulation); adjunct treatment with antibiotics for *Helicobacter pylori* eradication; stress ulcer prophylaxis in the critically-ill (parenteral formulation)

Pregnancy Risk Factor B

Pregnancy Considerations Adverse events were not observed in animal reproduction studies. Most available studies have not shown an increased risk of major birth defects following maternal use of proton pump inhibitors during pregnancy (Diav-Citrin, 2005; Erichsen, 2012; Matok, 2012; Pasternak, 2010). When treating GERD in pregnancy, PPIs may be used when clinically indicated (Katz, 2013).

Breast-Feeding Considerations Pantoprazole is excreted into breast milk. The excretion of pantoprazole into breast milk was studied in a nursing woman, 10 months postpartum. Following a single dose of pantoprazole 40 mg, maternal milk and serum samples were obtained over 24 hours. Peak concentrations appeared in both the plasma and milk 2 hours after the dose. Pantoprazole concentrations in breast milk were below the limits of detection during most of the study period. Based on this single dose study, the authors calculated the expected exposure to a nursing infant to be 0.14% of the weight-adjusted maternal dose (Plante, 2004). Due to the potential for serious adverse reactions in the nursing infant, the manufacturer recommends a decision be made whether to discontinue nursing or to discontinue the drug, taking into account the importance of treatment to the mother; however, the acidic content of the nursing infants' stomach may potentially inactivate any ingested pantoprazole (Plante, 2004).

Medication Guide Available Yes

Contraindications Hypersensitivity to pantoprazole, substituted benzimidazole proton pump inhibitors, or any component of the formulation

Warnings/Precautions Use of proton pump inhibitors (PPIs) may increase the risk of gastrointestinal infections (eg, *Salmonella, Campylobacter*). Relief of symptoms does not preclude the presence of a gastric malignancy. Long-term pantoprazole therapy (especially in patients who were *H. pylori* positive) has caused biopsy-proven atrophic gastritis. Benign and malignant neoplasia has been observed in long-term rodent studies; while not reported in humans, the relevance of these findings in regards to tumorigenicity in humans is not known. Use of PPIs may increase risk of *Clostridium difficile*-associated diarrhea (CDAD), especially in hospitalized patients; consider CDAD diagnosis in patients with persistent diarrhea that does not improve. Use the lowest dose and shortest duration of PPI therapy appropriate for the condition being treated. Prolonged treatment (typically >3 years) may lead to vitamin B_{12} malabsorption and subsequent deficiency. Intravenous preparation contains edetate sodium (EDTA); use caution in patients who are at risk for zinc deficiency if other EDTA-containing solutions are coadministered. Decreased *H. pylori* eradication rates have been observed with short-term (≤7 days) combination therapy. The American College of Gastroenterology recommends 10-14 days of therapy (triple or quadruple) for eradication of *H. pylori* (Chey, 2007).

PPIs may diminish the therapeutic effect of clopidogrel, thought to be due to reduced formation of the active metabolite of clopidogrel. The manufacturer of clopidogrel recommends either avoidance of both omeprazole (even when scheduled 12 hours apart) and esomeprazole or use of a PPI with comparatively less effect on the active metabolite of clopidogrel. Of the PPIs, pantoprazole has the lowest degree of CYP2C19 inhibition *in vitro* (Li, 2004) and has been shown to have less effect on conversion of clopidogrel to its active metabolite compared to omeprazole (Angiolillo, 2011). In contrast to these warnings, others have recommended the continued use of PPIs, regardless of the degree of inhibition, in patients with a history of GI bleeding or multiple risk factors for GI bleeding who are also receiving clopidogrel since no evidence has established clinically meaningful differences in outcome; however, a clinically-significant interaction cannot be excluded in those who are poor metabolizers of clopidogrel (Abraham, 2010; Levine, 2011). Concomitant use of pantoprazole with some drugs may require cautious use, may not be recommended, or may require dosage adjustments.

Increased incidence of osteoporosis-related bone fractures of the hip, spine, or wrist may occur with PPI therapy. Patients on high-dose or long-term therapy (≥1 year) should be monitored. Use the lowest effective dose for the shortest duration of time, use vitamin D and calcium supplementation, and follow appropriate guidelines to reduce risk of fractures in patients at risk. Thrombophlebitis and hypersensitivity reactions including anaphylaxis, Stevens-Johnson syndrome, and toxic epidermal necrolysis have been reported with IV administration.

Hypomagnesemia, reported rarely, usually with prolonged PPI use of >3 months (most cases >1 year of therapy); may be symptomatic or asymptomatic; severe cases may cause tetany, seizures, and cardiac arrhythmias. Consider obtaining serum magnesium concentrations prior to beginning long-term therapy, especially if taking concomitant digoxin, diuretics, or other drugs known to cause hypomagnesemia; and periodically thereafter. Hypomagnesemia may be corrected by magnesium supplementation, although discontinuation of pantoprazole may be necessary; magnesium levels typically return to normal within 2 weeks of stopping.

Adverse Reactions

>10%: Central nervous system: Headache (adults 12%; children >4%)

1% to 10%:

Cardiovascular: Facial edema (≤4%), generalized edema (≤2%)

Central nervous system: Dizziness (≤4%), vertigo (≤4%), depression (≤2%), fever (adults ≤2%; children >4%)

Dermatologic: Rash (adults ≤2%; children >4%), urticaria (≤4%), photosensitivity (≤2%), pruritus (≤2%)

Endocrine & metabolic: Triglycerides increased (≤4%)

Gastrointestinal: Diarrhea (≤9%), abdominal pain (children >4%), vomiting (≥4%), constipation (≤4%), flatulence (children ≤4%), nausea (children ≤4%), xerostomia (≤2%)
Hematologic: Leukopenia (≤2%), thrombocytopenia (≤2%)
Hepatic: Liver function tests abnormal (≤4%), hepatitis (≤2%)
Local: Injection site reaction (thrombophlebitis ≤2%)
Neuromuscular & skeletal: Arthralgia (≤4%), myalgia (≤4%), CPK increased (≤4%)
Ocular: Blurred vision (≤2%)
Respiratory: Upper respiratory tract infection (children >4%)
Miscellaneous: Allergic reaction (≤4%)

<1% (Limited to important or life-threatening): Albuminuria, alkaline phosphatase increased, anaphylaxis (including anaphylactic shock), anemia, angioedema, angina pectoris, aphthous stomatitis, arrhythmia, asthma exacerbation, atrial fibrillation/flutter, atrophic gastritis, biliary pain, bone pain, breast pain, bursitis, cataract, CHF, cholecystitis, cholelithiasis, *Clostridium difficile*-associate diarrhea (CDAD), colitis, contact dermatitis, creatinine increased, cystitis, deafness, dehydration, diabetes mellitus, diplopia, duodenitis, dysarthria, dysmenorrhea, dysphagia, dysuria, ecchymosis, ECG abnormality, eosinophilia, epididymitis, epistaxis, erythema multiforme, esophagitis, extraocular palsy, fatigue, fracture, fungal dermatitis, gastrointestinal carcinoma, gastrointestinal hemorrhage, gastrointestinal moniliasis, GGT increased, gingivitis, glaucoma, glossitis, glycosuria, goiter, gout, hallucinations, hematemesis, hematuria, hemorrhage, hepatic failure, hernia, hyperbilirubinemia, hyperesthesia, hyper-/hypotension, hyperkinesia, hyperuricemia, hypokinesia, hypomagnesemia, hyponatremia, impotence, interstitial nephritis, jaundice, kidney calculus, kidney pain, leukocytosis, lichenoid dermatitis, maculopapular rash, melena, mouth ulceration, myocardial infarction, myocardial ischemia, neoplasm, neuralgia, neuritis, optic neuropathy (including anterior ischemic), palpitation, pancreatitis, pancytopenia, paresthesia, periodontitis, pneumonia, pyelonephritis, rectal hemorrhage, retinal vascular disorder, rhabdomyolysis, scrotal edema, seizure, Stevens-Johnson syndrome, stomach ulcer, stomatitis, syncope, tachycardia, tenosynovitis, thrombosis, tinnitus, tongue discoloration, toxic epidermal necrolysis, tremor, urethritis, vision abnormal

Drug Interactions

Metabolism/Transport Effects Substrate of CYP2C19 (major), CYP2D6 (minor), CYP3A4 (minor); **Note:** Assignment of Major/Minor substrate status based on clinically relevant drug interaction potential; **Inhibits** BCRP, CYP2C19 (weak); **Induces** CYP1A2 (weak/moderate)

Avoid Concomitant Use

Avoid concomitant use of Pantoprazole with any of the following: Dasatinib; Delavirdine; Erlotinib; Nelfinavir; PAZOPanib; PONATinib; Rilpivirine; Risedronate

Increased Effect/Toxicity

Pantoprazole may increase the levels/effects of: Amphetamines; Dexmethylphenidate; Methotrexate; Methylphenidate; PAZOPanib; Raltegravir; Risedronate; Saquinavir; Topotecan; Voriconazole

The levels/effects of Pantoprazole may be increased by: Fluconazole; Ketoconazole (Systemic); Voriconazole

Decreased Effect

Pantoprazole may decrease the levels/effects of: Atazanavir; Bisphosphonate Derivatives; Bosutinib; Cefditoren; Clopidogrel; Dabigatran Etexilate; Dabrafenib; Dasatinib; Delavirdine; Erlotinib; Gefitinib; Indinavir; Iron Salts; Itraconazole; Ketoconazole (Systemic); Mesalamine; Multivitamins/Minerals (with ADEK, Folate, Iron); Mycophenolate; Nelfinavir; Nilotinib; PONATinib; Posaconazole; Rilpivirine; Riociguat; Risedronate; Vismodegib

The levels/effects of Pantoprazole may be decreased by: CYP2C19 Inducers (Strong); Dabrafenib; Peginterferon Alfa-2b; Tipranavir

Ethanol/Nutrition/Herb Interactions

Ethanol: Avoid ethanol (may cause gastric mucosal irritation).

Herb/Nutraceutical: Prolonged treatment (typically >3 years) may lead to vitamin B_{12} malabsorption and subsequent deficiency.

Preparation for Administration Reconstitute with 10 mL NS (final concentration 4 mg/mL). When administering by I.V. infusion, reconstituted solution may be added to 100 mL D_5W, NS, or LR.

Storage/Stability

Oral: Store tablet and oral suspension at controlled room temperature of 20°C to 25°C (68°F to 77°F); excursions permitted to 15°C to 30°C (59°F to 86°F).

I.V.: Prior to reconstitution, store at controlled room temperature of 20°C to 25°C (68°F to 77°F); excursions permitted to 15°C to 30°C (59°F to 86°F). Do not freeze. Protect from light prior to reconstitution; upon reconstitution, protection from light is not required. Per manufacturer's labeling, reconstituted solution is stable at room temperature for 6 hours; further diluted (admixed) solution should be stored at room temperature and used within 24 hours from the time of initial reconstitution. However, studies have shown that reconstituted solution (4 mg/mL) in polypropylene syringes is stable up to 96 hours at room temperature (Johnson, 2005). Upon further dilution, the admixed solution should be used within 96 hours from the time of initial reconstitution. The preparation should be stored at 3°C to 5°C (37°F to 41°F) if it is stored beyond 48 hours to minimize discoloration.

Mechanism of Action Suppresses gastric acid secretion by inhibiting the parietal cell H^+/K^+ ATP pump

Pharmacodynamics/Kinetics

Absorption: Rapid, well absorbed
Distribution: V_d: 11-24 L
Protein binding: 98%, primarily to albumin
Metabolism: Extensively hepatic; CYP2C19 (demethylation), CYP3A4; no evidence that metabolites have pharmacologic activity
Bioavailability: ~77%
Half-life elimination: 1 hour; increased to 3.5-10 hours with CYP2C19 deficiency
Time to peak: Oral: 2.5 hours
Excretion: Urine (71%); feces (18%)

Dosage

Oral:

Children ≥5 years: Erosive esophagitis associated with GERD:
≥15 to <40 kg: 20 mg once daily for up to 8 weeks
≥40 kg: 40 mg once daily for up to 8 weeks

Adults:

Erosive esophagitis associated with GERD:

Treatment: 40 mg once daily for up to 8 weeks; an additional 8 weeks may be used in patients who have not healed after an 8-week course. **Note:** Canadian labeling recommends initial treatment for up to 4 weeks and an additional 4 weeks in patients who have not healed after the initial 4-week course. Lower doses (20 mg once daily) have been used successfully in mild GERD treatment (Dettmer, 1998).

Maintenance of healing: 40 mg once daily (U.S. labeling) or 20-40 mg once daily (Canadian labeling); 20 mg once daily has been used successfully in maintenance of healing (Escourrou, 1999). **Note:** Has not been studied beyond 12 months.

Hypersecretory disorders (including Zollinger-Ellison): Initial: 40 mg twice daily; adjust dose based on patient needs; doses up to 240 mg daily have been administered

Helicobacter pylori eradication (unlabeled use in U.S.):

American College of Gastroenterology guidelines (Chey, 2007):

Nonpenicillin allergy: 40 mg twice daily administered with amoxicillin 1000 mg *and* clarithromycin 500 mg twice daily for 10-14 days

Penicillin allergy: 40 mg twice daily administered with clarithromycin 500 mg *and* metronidazole 500 mg twice daily for 10-14 days **or** 40 mg once or twice daily administered with bismuth subsalicylate 525 mg *and* metronidazole 250 mg *plus* tetracycline 500 mg 4 times daily for 10-14 days

Canadian labeling: 40 mg twice daily administered with clarithromycin 500 mg twice daily *and* either metronidazole 500 mg **or** amoxicillin 1000 mg twice daily for 7 days

Peptic ulcer disease (Canadian labeling): Treatment: 40 mg once daily for 2 weeks (duodenal ulcer) or 4 weeks (gastric ulcer); may extend therapy for an additional 2 or 4 weeks (based on indication) for inadequate healing

Prevention of GI lesions associated with NSAID use (Canadian labeling): 20 mg once daily

Symptomatic GERD (Canadian labeling): Treatment: 40 mg once daily for up to 4 weeks; failure to achieve adequate symptom relief after the initial 4 weeks of therapy warrants further evaluation

I.V.:

Erosive esophagitis associated with GERD: 40 mg once daily for 7-10 days

Hypersecretory disorders: 80 mg every 12 hours; adjust dose based on acid output measurements; 160-240 mg daily in divided doses has been used for a limited period (up to 7 days)

Prevention of rebleeding in peptic ulcer bleed (unlabeled use) (Barkun, 2010; Zargar, 2006): 80 mg, followed by 8 mg/hour infusion for 72 hours. **Note:** A daily infusion of 40 mg does not raise gastric pH sufficiently to enhance coagulation in active GI bleeds.

Elderly: Dosage adjustment not required

Dosage adjustment in renal impairment: No dosage adjustment necessary; pantoprazole is not removed by hemodialysis

Dosage adjustment in hepatic impairment:

U.S. labeling: No dosage adjustment necessary; doses >40 mg daily have not been evaluated in patients with hepatic impairment.

Canadian labeling:

Mild-moderate impairment: No dosage adjustment necessary.

Severe impairment: I.V., Oral: Manufacturer labeling suggests a maximum dose of 20 mg daily.

Dietary Considerations

Oral: May be taken with or without food; best if taken before breakfast.

I.V.: Due to EDTA in preparation, zinc supplementation may be needed in patients prone to zinc deficiency.

Usual Infusion Concentrations: Adult I.V. infusion: 80 mg in 100 mL (concentration: 0.8 mg/mL) of D_5W or NS

Administration

I.V.: Flush I.V. line before and after administration. In-line filter not required.

2-minute infusion: The volume of reconstituted solution (4 mg/mL) to be injected may be administered intravenously over at least 2 minutes.

15-minute infusion: Infuse over 15 minutes at a rate not to exceed 7 mL/minute (3 mg/minute).

Oral:

Tablet: Should be swallowed whole, do not crush or chew. Best if taken before breakfast.

Delayed-release oral suspension: Should only be administered in apple juice or applesauce and taken ~30 minutes before a meal. Do not administer with any other liquid (eg, water) or foods.

Oral administration in **applesauce**: Sprinkle intact granules on 1 tablespoon of applesauce and swallow within 10 minutes of preparation.

Oral administration in **apple juice**: Empty intact granules into 5 mL of apple juice, stir for 5 seconds, and swallow immediately after preparation. Rinse container once or twice with apple juice and swallow immediately.

Nasogastric tube administration: Separate the plunger from the barrel of a 60 mL catheter tip syringe and connect to a ≥16 French nasogastric tube. Holding the syringe attached to the tubing as high as possible, empty the contents of the packet into barrel of the syringe, add 10 mL of apple juice and gently tap/shake the barrel of the syringe to help empty the syringe. Add an additional 10 mL of apple juice and gently tap/shake the barrel to help rinse. Repeat rinse with at least 2-10 mL aliquots of apple juice. No granules should remain in the syringe.

Monitoring Parameters Hypersecretory disorders: Acid output measurements, target level <10 mEq/hour (<5 mEq/hour if prior gastric acid-reducing surgery)

Test Interactions False-positive urine screening tests for tetrahydrocannabinol (THC) have been noted in patients receiving proton pump inhibitors, including pantoprazole.

Dosage Forms Excipient information presented when available (limited, particularly for generics); consult specific product labeling.

Packet, Oral:

Protonix: 40 mg (1 ea, 30 ea) [contains polysorbate 80]

Solution Reconstituted, Intravenous:

Protonix: 40 mg (1 ea) [contains edetate disodium]

Generic: 40 mg (1 ea)

Tablet Delayed Release, Oral:

Protonix: 20 mg, 40 mg

Generic: 20 mg, 40 mg

Dosage Forms: Canada Excipient information presented when available (limited, particularly for generics); consult specific product labeling.

Note: Strength expressed as base

Tablet, enteric coated, as magnesium:

Tecta®: 40 mg

Extemporaneous Preparations A 2 mg/mL pantoprazole oral suspension may be made with pantoprazole tablets, sterile water, and sodium bicarbonate powder. Remove the Protonix® imprint from twenty 40 mg tablets with a paper towel dampened with ethanol (improves the look of product). Let tablets air dry. Crush the tablets in a mortar and reduce to a fine powder. Transfer to a 600 mL beaker, and add 340 mL sterile water. Place beaker on a magnetic stirrer. Add 16.8 g of sodium bicarbonate powder and stir for about 20 minutes until the tablet remnants have disintegrated. While stirring, add another 16.8 g of sodium bicarbonate powder and stir for about 5 minutes until powder has dissolved. Add enough sterile water for irrigation to bring the final volume to 400 mL. Mix well. Transfer to amber-colored bottle. Label "shake well" and "refrigerate". Stable for 62 days refrigerated.

Dentinger PJ, Swenson CF, and Anaizi NH, "Stability of Pantoprazole in an Extemporaneously Compounded Oral Liquid," *Am J Health Syst Pharm*, 2002, 59(10):953-6.

◆ **Pantoprazole for Injection (Can)** *see* Pantoprazole *on page 1563*

◆ **Pantoprazole Magnesium** *see* Pantoprazole *on page 1563*

◆ Pantoprazole Sodium *see* Pantoprazole *on page 1563*

◆ Pantothenyl Alcohol *see* Dexpanthenol *on page 587*

Papaverine (pa PAV er een)

Index Terms Papaverine Hydrochloride; Pavabid

Pharmacologic Category Vasodilator

Use Various vascular spasms associated with smooth muscle spasms as in myocardial infarction, angina, peripheral and pulmonary embolism, peripheral vascular disease; cerebral angiospastic states; visceral spasms (ureteral, biliary, and GI colic). **Note:** Labeled uses have fallen out of favor; safer and more effective alternatives are available.

Unlabeled Use Prevention of vasospasm during harvesting mammary arteries for coronary artery bypass graft surgery

Pregnancy Risk Factor C

Dosage Note: Labeled uses have fallen out of favor; safer and more effective alternatives are available. The manufacturer's labeling recommends the following dosing:

Arterial spasm: Adults: I.M., I.V.: 30-120 mg; may repeat dose every 3 hours; if cardiac extrasystole occurs during use, may administer 2 doses 10 minutes apart

Dosage adjustment in renal impairment: No dosage adjustment provided in the manufacturer's labeling.

Dosage adjustment in hepatic impairment: No dosage adjustment provided in the manufacturer's labeling.

Additional Information Complete prescribing information should be consulted for additional detail.

Dosage Forms Excipient information presented when available (limited, particularly for generics); consult specific product labeling.

Solution, Injection, as hydrochloride:

Generic: 30 mg/mL (2 mL, 10 mL)

◆ Papaverine Hydrochloride *see* Papaverine *on page 1567*

Papillomavirus (Types 6, 11, 16, 18) Vaccine (Human, Recombinant)

(pap ih LO ma VYE rus typs six e LEV en SIX teen AYE teen vak SEEN YU man ree KOM be nant)

Brand Names: U.S. Gardasil

Brand Names: Canada Gardasil

Index Terms HPV Vaccine (Quadrivalent); HPV4; Human Papillomavirus Vaccine (Quadrivalent); Papillomavirus Vaccine, Recombinant; Quadrivalent Human Papillomavirus Vaccine

Pharmacologic Category Vaccine, Inactivated (Viral)

Additional Appendix Information

Immunization Administration Recommendations *on page 2334*

Immunization Recommendations *on page 2339*

Use

U.S. labeling:

Females 9 to 26 years of age:

For the prevention of the following diseases: cervical, vulvar, vaginal, and anal cancer caused by HPV types 16 and 18; genital warts (condyloma acuminatum) caused by HPV types 6 and 11;

For the prevention of the following precancerous or dysplastic lesions caused by HPV types 6, 11, 16, and 18: cervical intraepithelial neoplasia (CIN) grade 2/3 and cervical adenocarcinoma in situ; CIN grade 1; vulvar intraepithelial neoplasia grade 2 and 3; vaginal intraepithelial neoplasia grade 2 and 3; and anal intraepithelial neoplasia grades 1, 2, and 3.

Males 9 through 26 years of age:

For the prevention of the following diseases: anal cancer caused by HPV types 16 and 18; genital warts (condyloma acuminata) caused by HPV types 6 and 11;

For the prevention of anal intraepithelial neoplasia grades 1, 2, and 3 caused by HPV types 6, 11, 16, and 18.

Limitations of use: Does not provide protection against vaccine HPV types to which a person has already been previously exposed, or HPV types not contained in the vaccine; does not prevent CIN grade 2/3 or worse in women >26 years of age.

Canadian labeling:

Females ≥9 years and ≤26 years of age: Prevention of anal cancer caused by HPV types 16 and 18; anal intraepithelial neoplasia caused by HPV types 6, 11, 16, and 18

Females ≥9 years and ≤45 years of age: Prevention of cervical, vulvar, and vaginal cancer caused by HPV types 16 and 18; genital warts caused by HPV types 6 and 11; cervical adenocarcinoma *in situ*, vulvar, vaginal, or cervical intraepithelial neoplasia caused by HPV types 6, 11, 16, and 18

Males ≥9 years and ≤26 years of age: Prevention of anal cancer caused by HPV types 16 and 18; anal intraepithelial neoplasia caused by HPV types 6, 11, 16, and 18; genital warts caused by HPV types 6 and 11

The Advisory Committee on Immunization Practices (ACIP) recommends routine vaccination for females and males 11-12 years of age; catch-up vaccination is recommended for females 13-26 years of age and males 13-21 years of age. Males 22-26 years may also be vaccinated. The ACIP also recommends routine vaccination for men who have sex with men (MSM) through 26 years of age (CDC, 2007; CDC, 59[20], 2010; CDC, 60[50], 2011). Vaccination is also recommended for immunocompromised persons or MSM through 26 years of age who were not previously vaccinated when they were younger. Although not specifically recommended for their profession, health care providers within the recommended age groups should also receive the HPV vaccine (CDC, 2013a).

Pregnancy Risk Factor B

Pregnancy Considerations Teratogenic effects were not observed in animal reproduction studies. In clinical trials, women who were found to be pregnant before the completion of the 3-dose regimen were instructed to defer any remaining dose until pregnancy resolution. Pregnancies detected within 30 days of vaccination had a higher rate of congenital anomalies (pyloric stenosis, congenital megacolon, congenital hydronephrosis, hip dysplasia, club foot) than the placebo group. Pregnancies with onset beyond 30 days of vaccination had a rate of congenital anomalies consistent with the general population. Overall, the type of teratogenic events were the same as those generally observed for this age group. Administration of the vaccine in pregnancy is not recommended; until additional information is available, the vaccine series (or completion of the series) should be delayed until pregnancy is completed (CDC, 2007). Pregnancy testing is not required prior to administration of the vaccine (CDC, 2013a).

A registry has been established for women exposed to the HPV vaccine during pregnancy (1-877-888-4231).

Breast-Feeding Considerations It is not known if this vaccine is excreted into breast milk. Infants had a higher incidence of acute respiratory illness when breast-fed by mothers within 30 days postvaccination. The manufacturer recommends that caution be exercised when administering papilloma virus vaccine to nursing women. Lactating women may receive vaccine (CDC, 2007; CDC, 59[20], 2010).

Contraindications Hypersensitivity, including severe allergic reactions to yeast (a vaccine component), or a previous dose of the vaccine

Warnings/Precautions Immediate treatment for anaphylactoid reaction should be available during vaccine use. Patients who develop hypersensitivity after administration should not receive further dosing. There is no evidence that individuals already infected with HPV will be protected; those already infected with 1 or more HPV types were protected from disease in the remaining HPV types. Not for the treatment of active disease; will not protect against diseases not caused by human papillomavirus (HPV) vaccine types 6, 11, 16, and 18. May administer with mild concurrent febrile illness; consider deferring vaccination with serious illness. Vaccination may not result in effective immunity in all patients. Response depends upon multiple factors (eg, type of vaccine, age of patient) and may be improved by administering the vaccine at the recommended dose, route, and interval. Vaccines may not be effective if administered during periods of altered immune competence. May be administered to those who are immunosuppressed. Immunocompromised patients may have a reduced response to vaccination. In general, household and close contacts of persons with altered immunocompetence may receive all age appropriate vaccines. Administered I.M., therefore use caution in patients at risk for bleeding. The entire 3-dose regimen should be completed for maximum efficacy. Not recommended for use during pregnancy. Syncope has been reported with use of injectable vaccines and may be accompanied by transient visual disturbances, weakness, or tonic-clonic movements. Procedures should be in place to avoid injuries from falling and to restore cerebral perfusion if syncope occurs. Safety and efficacy in children <9 years of age have not been established. Product may contain yeast. In order to maximize vaccination rates, the ACIP recommends simultaneous administration of all age-appropriate vaccines (live or inactivated) for which a person is eligible at a single clinic visit, unless contraindications exist. Use of this vaccine for specific medical and/or other indications (eg, immunocompromising conditions, hepatic or kidney disease, diabetes) is also addressed in the ACIP Recommended Immunization Schedule (CDC, 2007; CDC, 59[20], 2010; CDC 60[2], 2011; CDC, 2013a; CDC, 2013b).

Adverse Reactions All serious adverse reactions must be reported to the U.S. Department of Health and Human Services (DHHS) Vaccine Adverse Event Reporting System (VAERS) 1-800-822-7967 or online at https://vaers.hhs.gov/esub/index. In Canada, adverse reactions may be reported to local provincial/territorial health agencies or to the Vaccine Safety Section at Public Health Agency of Canada (1-866-844-0018).

>10%:

- Central nervous system: Headache (12% to 28%), fever (8% to 13%)
- Local: Injection site: Pain (61% to 84%), erythema (17% to 25%), swelling (14% to 25%)

1% to 10%:

- Central nervous system: Dizziness (1% to 4%), malaise (1%), insomnia (1%)
- Gastrointestinal: Nausea (2% to 7%), diarrhea (3% to 4%), vomiting (1% to 2%), toothache (2%)
- Local: Injection site: Bruising (3%), pruritus (3%), hematoma (1%)
- Neuromuscular & skeletal: Arthralgia (1%), myalgia (≤1%)
- Respiratory: Pharyngolaryngeal pain (3%), cough (2%), nasal congestion (1%)

<1% (Limited to important or life-threatening): Acute disseminated encephalomyelitis, alopecia areata, anaphylactic/anaphylactoid reaction, appendicitis, arrhythmia, arthritis, asthma, autoimmune hemolytic anemia and other autoimmune diseases, bronchospasm, cellulitis, cerebrovascular accident, chills, DVT, fatigue, gastroenteritis, Guillain-Barré syndrome, hypersensitivity reaction, hyper-/hypothyroidism, injection site joint movement impairment, ITP, JIA, lymphadenopathy, motor neuron disease, pancreatitis, paralysis, pelvic inflammatory disease, pulmonary embolus, RA, renal failure (acute), seizure, sepsis, syncope (may result in falls with injury or be associated with tonic-clonic movements), transverse myelitis, urticaria, weakness

Drug Interactions

Metabolism/Transport Effects None known.

Avoid Concomitant Use There are no known interactions where it is recommended to avoid concomitant use.

Increased Effect/Toxicity There are no known significant interactions involving an increase in effect.

Decreased Effect

The levels/effects of Papillomavirus (Types 6, 11, 16, 18) Vaccine (Human, Recombinant) may be decreased by: Belimumab; Fingolimod; Immunosuppressants

Storage/Stability Store refrigerated at 2°C to 8°C (36°F to 46°F). Do not freeze. Protect from light. Administer as soon as possible after removing it from refrigeration; can be out of refrigeration (at temperatures at or below 25°C [77°F]) for a total time of not more than 72 hours.

Mechanism of Action Contains inactive human papillomavirus (HPV) proteins HPV 6 L1, HPV 11 L1, HPV 16 L1, and HPV 18 L1 which produce neutralizing antibodies to prevent cervical cancer, cervical adenocarcinoma, cervical, vaginal and vulvar neoplasia, and genital warts caused by HPV. The vaccine has not been shown to provide cross protective efficacy to HPV types not contained in the vaccine. Immunogenicity has been measured by the percentage of persons who became seropositive for antibodies contained in the vaccine; the minimum anti-HPV antibody concentration needed to protect against disease has not been determined. The population benefit to vaccination is influenced by the prevalence of HPV within the geographic area and subject characteristics (eg, lifetime sexual partners).

Pharmacodynamics/Kinetics

Onset: Peak seroconversion was observed 1 month following the last dose of vaccine

Duration: Not well defined; at least 5 years

Dosage

U.S. labeling: I.M.: Children ≥9 years, Adolescents, and Adults ≤26 years: 0.5 mL followed by 0.5 mL at 2 and 6 months after initial dose

Canadian labeling: I.M. Children ≥9 years, Adolescents, and Adults ≤45 years: 0.5 mL followed by 0.5 mL at 2 and 6 months after initial dose

CDC recommended immunization schedule: Administer first dose at age 11-12 years; begin series in females aged 13-26 years or males 13-21 years if not previously vaccinated. Males may also be vaccinated through 26 years of age. Minimum interval between first and second doses is 4 weeks; the minimum interval between first and third doses is 24 weeks. Inadequate doses or doses received following a shorter than recommended dosing interval should be repeated. The HPV vaccine series should be completed with the same product whenever possible (CDC, 2007; CDC, 59[20], 2010; CDC, 60 [50] 2011).

Dosage adjustment in renal impairment: No dosage adjustment provided in the manufacturer's labeling.

Dosage adjustment in hepatic impairment: No dosage adjustment provided in the manufacturer's labeling.

Administration Shake suspension well before use. Inject the entire dose I.M. into the deltoid region of the upper arm or higher anterolateral thigh area. Observe for syncope for 15 minutes following administration. If the vaccine series is interrupted and only one dose was given, administer the second dose as soon as possible and give the third dose ≥12 weeks later. If the vaccine series is interrupted and the first two doses were given, administer the third dose as soon as possible (CDC, 2007). Minimum interval between first and second doses is 4 weeks; the minimum interval between first and third doses is 24 weeks (CDC, 59[20], 2010; CDC, 2013a). Inadequate doses or doses received following a shorter than recommended dosing interval should be repeated (CDC, 2007). The HPV vaccine series should be completed with the same product whenever possible (CDC, 59[20], 2010).

For patients at risk of hemorrhage following intramuscular injection, the ACIP recommends "it should be administered intramuscularly if, in the opinion of the physician familiar with the patient's bleeding risk, the vaccine can be administered by this route with reasonable safety. If the patient receives antihemophilia or other similar therapy, intramuscular vaccination can be scheduled shortly after such therapy is administered. A fine needle (23 gauge or smaller) can be used for the vaccination and firm pressure applied to the site (without rubbing) for at least 2 minutes. The patient should be instructed concerning the risk of hematoma from the injection." Patients on anticoagulant therapy should be considered to have the same bleeding risks and treated as those with clotting factor disorders (CDC 60[2], 2011).

Simultaneous administration of vaccines helps ensure the patients will be fully vaccinated by the appropriate age. Simultaneous administration of vaccines is defined as administering >1 vaccine on the same day at different anatomic sites. Separate vaccines should not be combined in the same syringe unless indicated by product specific labeling. Separate needles and syringes should be used for each injection. The ACIP prefers each dose of a specific vaccine in a series come from the same manufacturer when possible. Adolescents and adults should be vaccinated while seated or lying down. In general, preterm infants should be vaccinated at the same chronological age as full-term infants (CDC 60[2], 2011).

Antipyretics have not been shown to prevent febrile seizures. Antipyretics may be used to treat fever or discomfort following vaccination (CDC 60[2], 2011). One study reported that routine prophylactic administration of acetaminophen to prevent fever prior to vaccination decreased the immune response of some vaccines; the clinical significance of this reduction in immune response has not been established (Prymula, 2009).

Monitoring Parameters Screening for HPV is not required prior to vaccination. Monitor for syncope for 15 minutes following administration. If seizure-like activity associated with syncope occurs, maintain patient in supine or Trendelenburg position to reestablish adequate cerebral perfusion (CDC 60[2], 2011).

Females: Gynecologic screening exam, papillomavirus test; screening for cervical cancer should continue per current guidelines following vaccination

Additional Information U.S. federal law requires that the name of medication, date of administration, the vaccine manufacturer, lot number of vaccine, and the administering person's name, title and address be entered into the patient's permanent medical record. Ideally, administration of vaccine should occur prior to potential HPV exposure. Benefits of vaccine decrease once infected with ≥1 of the HPV vaccine types, although patients are protected from precancerous cervical lesions and external genital lesions caused by other HPV vaccine types.

Comparison of HPV vaccines: Cervarix and Gardasil are both vaccines formulated to protect against infection with the human papillomavirus. Both are inactive vaccines which contain proteins HPV16 L1 and HPV 18 L1, the cause of >70% of invasive cervical cancer. The vaccines differ in that Gardasil also contains HPV 6 L1 and HPV 11 L1 proteins which protect against 75% to 90% of genital warts. The vaccines also differ in their preparation and adjuvants used. The viral proteins in Cervarix are prepared using *Trichoplusia ni* (insect cells) which are adsorbed on to an aluminum salt which is also combined with a monophosphoryl lipid. The viral proteins in Gardasil are prepared using *S. cerevisiae* (baker's yeast) which are then adsorbed onto an aluminum salt. Results from a short term study (measurements obtained 1 month following the third vaccination in the series) have shown that the immune response to HPV 16 and HPV 18 may be greater with Cervarix; although the clinical significance of this differences is not known, local adverse events may also occur more frequently with this preparation. Both vaccines were effective and results from long term studies are pending (Einstein, 2009).

Dosage Forms Excipient information presented when available (limited, particularly for generics); consult specific product labeling.

Injection, suspension [preservative free]:

Gardasil: HPV 6 L1 protein 20 mcg, HPV 11 L1 protein 40 mcg, HPV 16 L1 protein 40 mcg, and HPV 18 L1 protein 20 mcg per 0.5 mL (0.5 mL) [contains aluminum, polysorbate 80; manufactured using *S. cerevisiae* (baker's yeast)]

Papillomavirus (Types 16, 18) Vaccine (Human, Recombinant)

(pap ih LO ma VYE rus typs SIX teen AYE teen vak SEEN YU man ree KOM be nant)

Brand Names: U.S. Cervarix®

Brand Names: Canada Cervarix®

Index Terms Bivalent Human Papillomavirus Vaccine; GSK-580299; HPV 16/18 L1 VLP/AS04 VAC; HPV Vaccine (Bivalent); HPV2; Human Papillomavirus Vaccine (Bivalent); Papillomavirus Vaccine, Recombinant

Pharmacologic Category Vaccine, Inactivated (Viral)

Additional Appendix Information

Immunization Administration Recommendations *on page 2334*

Immunization Recommendations *on page 2339*

Use

U.S. labeling: Females 9 through 25 years of age: Prevention of cervical cancer, cervical adenocarcinoma *in situ*, and cervical intraepithelial neoplasia caused by human papillomavirus (HPV) types 16, 18

The Advisory Committee on Immunization Practices (ACIP) recommends routine vaccination for females 11-12 years of age; catch-up vaccination is recommended for females 13-25 years of age (CDC, 59[20], 2010). Vaccination is also recommended for immunocompromised females through 26 years of age who were not previously vaccinated when they were younger. Although not specifically recommended for their profession, female health care providers within the recommended age groups should also receive the HPV vaccine (CDC, 2013).

Canadian labeling: Females 9 through 45 years of age: Prevention of cervical cancer, cervical adenocarcinoma *in situ*, and cervical intraepithelial neoplasia caused by human papillomavirus (HPV) types 16, 18

The National Advisory Committee on Immunization (NACI) recommends routine vaccination for females between 9 and 26 years of age. It should not be administered in females <9 years but may be administered to females >26 years (CCDR, 2012).

Pregnancy Risk Factor B

Pregnancy Considerations Adverse events were not observed in animal reproduction studies. Vaccination with papilloma virus vaccine is not recommended in pregnant women. In clinical trials, pregnancy testing was conducted prior to each vaccine administration and vaccination was discontinued if the woman was found to be pregnant; women were also instructed to avoid pregnancy for 2 months after receiving the vaccine. Pregnancies detected within 30 days prior or 45 days after vaccination had a higher rate of spontaneous abortions. A registry has been established for women exposed to Cervarix® during pregnancy (888-452-9622).

Administration of the vaccine in pregnancy is not recommended; until additional information is available, the vaccine series (or completion of the series) should be delayed until pregnancy is completed. Pregnancy testing is not required prior to administration of the vaccine (CDC, 2013).

Breast-Feeding Considerations It is not known if this vaccine is excreted into breast milk. The manufacturer recommends that caution be exercised when administering papilloma virus vaccine to nursing women. Lactating women may receive vaccine (CDC, 2010).

Contraindications Hypersensitivity to papillomavirus recombinant vaccine or any component of the formulation

Warnings/Precautions Immediate treatment (including epinephrine 1:1000) for anaphylactoid and/or hypersensitivity reactions should be available during vaccine use. May consider deferring administration in patients with moderate or severe acute illness (with or without fever); may administer to patients with mild acute illness (with or without fever). Vaccination may not result in effective immunity in all patients. Response depends upon multiple factors (eg, type of vaccine, age of patient) and may be improved by administering the vaccine at the recommended dose, route, and interval. Vaccines may not be effective if administered during periods of altered immune competence (CDC, 2011). Use with caution in patients with a history of bleeding disorders (including thrombocytopenia) and/or patients on anticoagulant therapy; bleeding/hematoma may occur from I.M. administration. There is no evidence that individuals already exposed to or infected with HPV will be protected; those already infected with 1 or more HPV types were protected from disease in the remaining HPV types. Not for the treatment of active disease; will not protect against diseases not caused by HPV vaccine types 16 and 18. Use with caution in severely immunocompromised patients (eg, patients receiving chemo/radiation therapy or other immunosuppressive therapy [including high-dose corticosteroids]); may have a reduced response to vaccination. In general, household and close contacts of persons with altered immunocompetence may receive all age appropriate vaccines. Syncope has been reported with use of injectable vaccines and may be accompanied by transient visual disturbances, weakness, or tonic-clonic movements. Procedures should be in place to avoid injuries from falling and to restore cerebral perfusion if syncope occurs.

Packaging may contain natural rubber/natural latex. Safety and efficacy have not been established in males or in females <9 years of age. Not recommended for use during pregnancy. The entire 3-dose regimen should be completed for maximum efficacy. In order to maximize vaccination rates, the ACIP recommends simultaneous administration of all age-appropriate vaccines (live or inactivated) for which a person is eligible at a single clinic visit, unless contraindications exist. Use of this vaccine for specific medical and/or other indications (eg, immunocompromising conditions, hepatic or kidney disease, diabetes) is also addressed in the ACIP Recommended Immunization Schedule (CDC, 2013a; CDC, 2013b).

Adverse Reactions All serious adverse reactions must be reported to the U.S. Department of Health and Human Services (DHHS) Vaccine Adverse Event Reporting System (VAERS) 1-800-822-7967 or online at https://vaers.hhs.gov/esub/index. In Canada, adverse reactions may be reported to local provincial/territorial health agencies or to the Vaccine Safety Section at Public Health Agency of Canada (1-866-844-0018).

>10%:

Central nervous system: Fatigue (55%)

Local: Injection site reactions: Pain (92%), redness (48%), swelling (44%)

Neuromuscular & skeletal: Myalgia (49%), arthralgia (21%)

1% to 10%:

Dermatologic: Urticaria (7%)

Local: Injection site: Pruritus (1%)

Respiratory: Nasopharyngitis (4%), pharyngolaryngeal pain (3%), upper respiratory tract infection (2%), pharyngitis (1%)

Miscellaneous: Influenza (3%), chlamydia infection (2%), vaginal infection (1%)

<1%, postmarketing, and/or case reports: Allergic reactions, anaphylactic/anaphylactoid reactions, angioedema, erythema multiforme, lymphadenopathy, syncope (may be associated with tonic-clonic movements), vasovagal response

Drug Interactions

Metabolism/Transport Effects None known.

Avoid Concomitant Use There are no known interactions where it is recommended to avoid concomitant use.

Increased Effect/Toxicity There are no known significant interactions involving an increase in effect.

Decreased Effect

The levels/effects of Papillomavirus (Types 16, 18) Vaccine (Human, Recombinant) may be decreased by: Belimumab; Fingolimod; Immunosuppressants

Storage/Stability

U.S. labeling: Store under refrigeration at 2°C to 8°C (36°F to 46°F); do not freeze; discard if frozen. May develop a fine, white deposit with a clear, colorless supernatant during storage (not a sign of deterioration).

Canadian labeling: Store under refrigeration at 2°C to 8°C (36°F to 46°F); do not freeze; discard if frozen. Vaccine can be administered if stored between 8°C and 25°C (46°F to 77°F) for up to 3 days or stored between 25°C and 37°C (77°F to 98.6°F) for up to 1 day. Discard vaccine if exposed to temperatures >37°C (98.6°F). Protect from light.

Mechanism of Action Contains inactive human papillomavirus (HPV) proteins HPV 16 L1, and HPV 18 L1 which produce neutralizing antibodies to prevent cervical cancer, cervical adenocarcinoma, and cervical neoplasia cause by HPV.

Pharmacodynamics/Kinetics

Onset: Peak seroconversion was observed 1 month following the last dose of vaccine

Duration: Not well defined; >5 years

Dosage Immunization: I.M.:

U.S. labeling: Children ≥9 years, Adolescents, and Adults ≤25 years: Females: 0.5 mL followed by 0.5 mL at 1 and 6 months after initial dose

CDC recommended immunization schedule: Administer first dose to females at age 11-12 years; begin series in females aged 13-25 years if not previously vaccinated. Minimum interval between first and second doses is 4 weeks; the minimum interval between first and third doses is 24 weeks. Inadequate doses or doses received following a shorter than recommended dosing interval should be repeated. The HPV vaccine series should be completed with the same product whenever possible.

Canadian labeling: Children ≥9 years, Adolescents, and Adults ≤45 years: Females: 0.5 mL followed by 0.5 mL at 1 and 6 months after initial dose; if necessary, may administer the second and third doses at 1-2.5 months and 5-12 months respectively after the initial dose.

Dosage adjustment in renal impairment: No dosage adjustment provided in the manufacturer's labeling.

Dosage adjustment in hepatic impairment: No dosage adjustment provided in the manufacturer's labeling.

Administration Shake well prior to use. Do not use if discolored or if containing particulate matter, or if vial or syringe is cracked. Inject I.M. into the deltoid region of the upper arm. Do not administer I.V., SubQ, or intradermally.

For patients at risk of hemorrhage following intramuscular injection, the ACIP recommends "it should be administered intramuscularly if, in the opinion of the physician familiar with the patient's bleeding risk, the vaccine can be administered by this route with reasonable safety. If the patient receives antihemophilia or other similar therapy, intramuscular vaccination can be scheduled shortly after such therapy is administered. A fine needle (23 gauge or smaller) can be used for the vaccination and firm pressure applied to the site (without rubbing) for at least 2 minutes. The patient should be instructed concerning the risk of hematoma from the injection." Patients on anticoagulant therapy should be considered to have the same bleeding risks and treated as those with clotting factor disorders (CDC, 2011).

Simultaneous administration of vaccines helps ensure the patients will be fully vaccinated by the appropriate age. Simultaneous administration of vaccines is defined as administering >1 vaccine on the same day at different anatomic sites. Separate vaccines should not be combined in the same syringe unless indicated by product specific labeling. Separate needles and syringes should be used for each injection. The ACIP prefers each dose of a specific vaccine in a series come from the same manufacturer when possible. Adolescents and adults should be vaccinated while seated or lying down. In general, preterm infants should be vaccinated at the same chronological age as full-term infants (CDC, 2011).

Antipyretics have not been shown to prevent febrile seizures. Antipyretics may be used to treat fever or discomfort following vaccination (CDC, 2011). One study reported that routine prophylactic administration of acetaminophen to prevent fever prior to vaccination decreased the immune response of some vaccines; the clinical significance of this reduction in immune response has not been established (Prymula, 2009).

Monitoring Parameters Gynecologic screening exam, papillomavirus test as per current guidelines; screening for HPV is not required prior to vaccination and screening for cervical cancer should continue as recommended following vaccination. Monitor for syncope for 15 minutes following administration. If seizure-like activity associated with syncope occurs, maintain patient in supine or Trendelenburg position to reestablish adequate cerebral perfusion.

Additional Information U.S. federal law requires that the name of medication, date of administration, the vaccine manufacturer, lot number of vaccine, and the administering person's name, title and address be entered into the patient's permanent medical record. Ideally, administration of vaccine should occur prior to potential HPV exposure.

Comparison of HPV vaccines: Cervarix® and Gardasil® are both vaccines formulated to protect against infection with the human papillomavirus. Both are inactive vaccines which contain proteins HPV16 L1 and HPV 18 L1, the cause of >70% of invasive cervical cancer. The vaccines differ in that Gardasil® also contains HPV 6 L1 and HPV 11 L1 proteins which protect against 75% to 90% of genital warts. The vaccines also differ in their preparation and adjuvants used. The viral proteins in Cervarix® are prepared using *Trichoplusia ni* (insect cells) which are adsorbed on to an aluminum salt which is also combined with a monophosphoryl lipid. The viral proteins in Gardasil® are prepared using *S. cerevisiae* (baker's yeast) which are then adsorbed onto an aluminum salt. Results from a short-term study (measurements obtained 1 month following the third vaccination in the series) have shown that the immune response to HPV 16 and HPV 18 may be greater with Cervarix®; although the clinical significance of this differences is not known, local adverse events may also occur more frequently with this preparation. Both vaccines were effective and results from long-term studies are pending.

Dosage Forms Excipient information presented when available (limited, particularly for generics); consult specific product labeling. [DSC] = Discontinued product

Injection, suspension [preservative free]:

Cervarix®: HPV 16 L1 protein 20 mcg and HPV 18 L1 protein 20 mcg per 0.5 mL (0.5 mL [DSC]) [contains aluminum; manufactured using *Trichoplusia ni* (insect cells)]

Cervarix®: HPV 16 L1 protein 20 mcg and HPV 18 L1 protein 20 mcg per 0.5 mL (0.5 mL) [contains aluminum, natural rubber/natural latex in prefilled syringe; manufactured using *Trichoplusia ni* (insect cells)]

- **Papillomavirus Vaccine, Recombinant** *see* Papillomavirus (Types 6, 11, 16, 18) Vaccine (Human, Recombinant) *on page 1567*
- **Papillomavirus Vaccine, Recombinant** *see* Papillomavirus (Types 16, 18) Vaccine (Human, Recombinant) *on page 1569*
- **PAR-101** *see* Fidaxomicin *on page 859*
- **Paracetamol** *see* Acetaminophen *on page 28*
- **Parafon Forte DSC** *see* Chlorzoxazone *on page 417*
- **Paraplatin** *see* CARBOplatin *on page 344*
- **Parathyroid Hormone (1-34)** *see* Teriparatide *on page 2023*
- **Parcaine** *see* Proparacaine *on page 1733*
- **Parcopa®** *see* Carbidopa and Levodopa *on page 340*

Paregoric (par e GOR ik)

Index Terms Camphorated Tincture of Opium (error-prone synonym)

Pharmacologic Category Analgesic, Opioid

Use Treatment of diarrhea

Pregnancy Risk Factor C

Pregnancy Considerations Animal reproduction studies have not been conducted. Paregoric contains morphine; refer to the Morphine (Systemic) monograph for additional information. In addition, this preparation contains large amounts of alcohol (47%).

Breast-Feeding Considerations Paregoric contains morphine, which is excreted into breast milk; refer to the Morphine (Systemic) monograph for additional information. In addition, this preparation contains large amounts of alcohol (47%). The manufacturer recommends that caution be used if administered to a nursing woman.

Contraindications Hypersensitivity to opium or any component of the formulation; diarrhea caused by poisoning until the toxic material has been removed from the gastrointestinal tract; convulsive states (eg, status epilepticus, tetanus, strychnine poisoning) since morphine stimulates the spinal cord

Warnings/Precautions May cause CNS depression, which may impair physical or mental abilities; patients must be cautioned about performing tasks which require mental alertness (eg, operating machinery or driving). Effects may be potentiated when used with other sedative drugs or ethanol. May cause hypotension; use with caution in patients with hypovolemia, cardiovascular disease (including acute MI), or drugs which may exaggerate hypotensive effects (including phenothiazines or general anesthetics). Use with caution in patients with atrial flutter or other supraventricular tachycardias, respiratory compromise, hepatic or renal dysfunction, adrenal insufficiency, morbid obesity, severe prostatic hyperplasia, urinary stricture, head trauma, thyroid dysfunction, seizure disorder, or history of drug abuse or acute alcoholism. Avoid use in patients with CNS depression or coma as these patients are susceptible to intracranial effects of CO_2 retention. Use with caution in patients with biliary tract dysfunction including acute pancreatitis; use may cause constriction of sphincter of Oddi. May obscure diagnosis or clinical course of patients with acute abdominal conditions. Opium shares the toxic potential of opioid agonists, and usual precautions of opioid agonist therapy should be observed; tolerance or drug dependence may result from extended use. Concurrent use of agonist/antagonist analgesics may precipitate withdrawal symptoms and/or reduced analgesic efficacy in patients following prolonged therapy with mu opioid agonists. Abrupt discontinuation following prolonged use may also lead to withdrawal symptoms. Additives in paregoric (eg, alcohol, benzoic acid, noscapine, and papaverine) may be harmful to neonates. Paregoric is no longer recommended as a source of morphine to treat neonatal abstinence syndrome in infants exposed to chronic opioids *in utero* (Dow, 2012; Hudack, 2012). Infants <3 months of age are more susceptible to respiratory depression; use with caution and generally in reduced doses in this age group. Use with caution in the elderly and debilitated patients; may be more sensitive to adverse effects. Do not confuse paregoric with opium tincture which is 25 times **more** potent. Some preparations contain sulfites which may cause allergic reactions; contains ≤47% alcohol.

Adverse Reactions Frequency not defined.

Cardiovascular: Hypotension, peripheral vasodilation

Central nervous system: Central nervous system depression, depression, dizziness, drowsiness, drug dependence (physical and psychological), dysphoria, euphoria, headache, increased intracranial pressure, insomnia, malaise, restlessness, sedation

Dermatologic: Pruritus

Gastrointestinal: Anorexia, biliary tract spasm, constipation, nausea, stomach cramps, vomiting

Genitourinary: Decreased urine output, ureteral spasm

Hepatic: Increased liver enzymes

Hypersensitivity: Histamine release

Neuromuscular & skeletal: Weakness

Ophthalmic: Miosis

Respiratory: Respiratory depression

Drug Interactions

Metabolism/Transport Effects None known.

Avoid Concomitant Use

Avoid concomitant use of Paregoric with any of the following: Azelastine (Nasal); Paraldehyde

Increased Effect/Toxicity

Paregoric may increase the levels/effects of: Alcohol (Ethyl); Alvimopan; Azelastine (Nasal); CNS Depressants; Desmopressin; Diuretics; Hydrocodone; Metyrosine; Mirtazapine; Paraldehyde; Pramipexole; ROPINIRole; Rotigotine; Selective Serotonin Reuptake Inhibitors; Zolpidem

The levels/effects of Paregoric may be increased by: Amphetamines; Anticholinergics; Antipsychotic Agents (Phenothiazines); Brimonidine (Topical); Cannabinoids; Doxylamine; Droperidol; HydrOXYzine; Magnesium Sulfate; Perampanel; Sodium Oxybate; Succinylcholine; Tapentadol

Decreased Effect

Paregoric may decrease the levels/effects of: Pegvisomant

The levels/effects of Paregoric may be decreased by: Ammonium Chloride; Mixed Agonist / Antagonist Opioids

Ethanol/Nutrition/Herb Interactions Ethanol: May increase CNS depression; monitor for increased effects with coadministration. Caution patients about effects.

Storage/Stability Store at room temperature 15°C to 30°C (59°F to 86°F). Store in light-resistant, tightly closed container; protect from heat.

Mechanism of Action Increases smooth muscle tone in GI tract, decreases motility and peristalsis, diminishes digestive secretions

Pharmacodynamics/Kinetics In terms of opium:

Metabolism: Hepatic

Excretion: Urine (primarily as morphine glucuronide conjugates and unchanged drug - morphine, codeine, papaverine, etc)

Dosage Diarrhea: Oral: **Note:** Paregoric oral liquid contains morphine 2 mg/5 mL (0.4 mg/mL)

Children: 0.25-0.5 mL/kg 1-4 times daily

Adults: 5-10 mL 1-4 times daily

Dosage adjustment in renal impairment: No dosage adjustment provided in the manufacturer's labeling. Use with caution in severe impairment.

Dosage adjustment in hepatic impairment: No dosage adjustment provided in the manufacturer's labeling. Use with caution in severe impairment.

Additional Information Contains morphine 0.4 mg/mL and alcohol ≤47%. Do **not** confuse this product with opium tincture which is 25 times **more** potent; each 5 mL of paregoric contains 2 mg morphine equivalent, 0.02 mL anise oil, 20 mg benzoic acid, 20 mg camphor, 0.2 mL glycerin and alcohol; final alcohol content ≤47%; paregoric also contains papaverine and noscapine; because all of these additives may be harmful to neonates, **a 25-fold dilution of opium tincture** is often preferred for treatment of neonatal abstinence syndrome (opioid withdrawal).

Dosage Forms Excipient information presented when available (limited, particularly for generics); consult specific product labeling.

Tincture, Oral:

Generic: 2 mg/5 mL (473 mL)

Controlled Substance C-III

◆ Parenteral Nutrition *see* Total Parenteral Nutrition *on page 2098*

Paricalcitol (pah ri KAL si tole)

Brand Names: U.S. Zemplar

Brand Names: Canada Zemplar

Pharmacologic Category Vitamin D Analog

Use

I.V.: Prevention and treatment of secondary hyperparathyroidism associated with stage 5 chronic kidney disease (CKD)

Oral: Prevention and treatment of secondary hyperparathyroidism associated with stage 3 and 4 CKD and stage 5 CKD patients on hemodialysis or peritoneal dialysis

Pregnancy Risk Factor C

Pregnancy Considerations Adverse events were observed in some animal reproduction studies.

Breast-Feeding Considerations It is not known if paricalcitol is excreted in breast milk. Due to the potential for serious adverse reactions in the nursing infant, a decision should be made whether to discontinue nursing or to discontinue the drug, taking into account the importance of treatment to the mother.

Contraindications Hypersensitivity to paricalcitol or any component of the formulation; patients with evidence of vitamin D toxicity; hypercalcemia

Warnings/Precautions Excessive administration may lead to over suppression of PTH, hypercalcemia, hypercalciuria, hyperphosphatemia and adynamic bone disease. Acute hypercalcemia may increase risk of cardiac arrhythmias and seizures; use caution with cardiac glycosides as digitalis toxicity may be increased. Chronic hypercalcemia may lead to generalized vascular and other soft-tissue calcification. Phosphate and vitamin D (and its derivatives) should be withheld during therapy to avoid hypercalcemia. Risk of hypercalcemia may be increased by concomitant use of calcium-containing supplements and/or medications that increase serum calcium (eg, thiazide diuretics). Avoid regular administration to prevent aluminum overload and toxicity. Dialysate concentration of aluminum should be maintained at <10 mcg/L.

Adverse Reactions

>10%:

Gastrointestinal: Nausea (5% to 13%), diarrhea (7% to 12%)

Miscellaneous: Infection (bacterial, fungal, viral: 3% to 15%)

2% to 10%:

Cardiovascular: Edema (7%), hypertension (7%), hypervolemia (5%), hypotension (5%), palpitation (3%), chest pain (3%), peripheral edema (3%), syncope (3%)

Central nervous system: Pain (8%), dizziness (5% to 7%), chills (5%), insomnia (5%), lightheadedness (5%), vertigo (5%), fever (3% to 5%), headache (3% to 5%), anxiety (3%), depression (3%)

Dermatologic: Rash (6%), bruising (3%), skin ulcer (3%)

Endocrine & metabolic: Dehydration (3%), hypoglycemia (3%)

Gastrointestinal: Vomiting (5% to 8%), GI bleeding (5%), constipation (4% to 5%), abdominal pain (4%), dyspepsia (3%), xerostomia (3%)

Genitourinary: Urinary tract infection (3%)

Neuromuscular & skeletal: Arthritis (5%), weakness (3% to 5%), back pain (4%), leg cramps (3%)

Renal: Uremia (3%)

Respiratory: Pneumonia (5%), rhinitis (5%), oropharyngeal pain (4%), bronchitis (3%), cough (3%), sinusitis (3%)

Miscellaneous: Allergic reaction (6%), flu-like syndrome (5%), peritonitis (5%), sepsis (5%)

<2% (Limited to important or life-threatening): Agitation, anemia, angioedema (including laryngeal edema), arrhythmia, atrial flutter, bleeding time prolonged, breast cancer, cardiac arrest, cerebrovascular accident, chest discomfort, confusional state, conjunctivitis, delirium, dysphagia, dyspnea, erectile dysfunction, gait disturbance, gastritis, gastroesophageal reflux, glaucoma, hepatic enzyme (abnormal), hirsutism, hypercalciuria, hyper-/hypocalcemia, hyper-/hypoparathyroidism, hyperkalemia, hyperphosphatemia, injection site extravasation, injection site pain, intestinal ischemia, lymphadenopathy, myalgia, myoclonus, nasopharyngitis, night sweats, ocular hyperemia, oral edema, orthopnea, paresthesia, pruritus, pulmonary edema, rectal hemorrhage, skin burning sensation, taste perversion (metallic), upper respiratory tract infection, urticaria, vaginal infection, weight loss, wheezing

Drug Interactions

Metabolism/Transport Effects Substrate of CYP3A4 (minor); **Note:** Assignment of Major/Minor substrate status based on clinically relevant drug interaction potential

Avoid Concomitant Use

Avoid concomitant use of Paricalcitol with any of the following: Aluminum Hydroxide; Multivitamins/Fluoride (with ADE); Multivitamins/Minerals (with ADEK, Folate, Iron); Sucralfate; Sucroferric Oxyhydroxide; Vitamin D Analogs

Increased Effect/Toxicity

Paricalcitol may increase the levels/effects of: Aluminum Hydroxide; Cardiac Glycosides; Digoxin; Sucralfate; Vitamin D Analogs

The levels/effects of Paricalcitol may be increased by: Calcium Salts; CYP3A4 Inhibitors (Strong); Danazol; Multivitamins/Fluoride (with ADE); Multivitamins/Minerals (with ADEK, Folate, Iron); Thiazide Diuretics

Decreased Effect

The levels/effects of Paricalcitol may be decreased by: Bile Acid Sequestrants; Mineral Oil; Orlistat; Sucroferric Oxyhydroxide

Storage/Stability Store at 25°C (77°F); excursions permitted between 15°C to 30°C (59°F to 86°F).

Mechanism of Action Decreased renal conversion of vitamin D to its primary active metabolite (1,25-hydroxyvitamin D) in chronic renal failure leads to reduced activation of vitamin D receptor (VDR), which subsequently removes inhibitory suppression of parathyroid hormone (PTH) release; increased serum PTH (secondary hyperparathyroidism) reduces calcium excretion and enhances bone resorption. Paricalcitol is a synthetic vitamin D analog which binds to and activates the VDR in kidney, parathyroid gland, intestine and bone, thus reducing PTH levels and improving calcium and phosphate homeostasis.

Pharmacodynamics/Kinetics

Distribution: V_d:

Healthy subjects: Oral: 34 L; I.V.: 24 L

Stage 3 and 4 CKD: Oral: 44-46 L

Stage 5 CKD: Oral: 38-49 L; I.V.: 31-35 L

Protein binding: >99%

Metabolism: Hydroxylation and glucuronidation via hepatic and nonhepatic enzymes, including CYP24, CYP3A4, UGT1A4; forms metabolites (at least one active)

Bioavailability: Oral: 72% to 86% in healthy subjects

Half-life elimination:

Healthy subjects: Oral: 4-6 hours; I.V.: 5-7 hours

Stage 3 and 4 CKD: Oral: 14-20 hours

Stage 5 CKD: Oral: 14-20 hours; I.V.: 14-15 hours

Time to peak, plasma: 3 hours: Delayed by food

Excretion: Healthy subjects: Feces (oral: 70%; I.V.: 63%); urine (oral: 18%, I.V.: 19%)

Dosage Note: In stage 3-5 CKD maintain calcium phosphorus product (Ca x P) <55 mg^2/dL^2, reduce or interrupt dosing if recommended Ca x P is exceeded or hypercalcemia is observed (K/DOQI Clinical Practice Guidelines, 2003).

Secondary hyperparathyroidism associated with chronic renal failure (stage 5 CKD):

Children ≥5 years and Adults: I.V.: 0.04-0.1 mcg/kg (2.8-7 mcg) given as a bolus dose no more frequently than every other day at any time during dialysis; dose may be increased by 2-4 mcg every 2-4 weeks; doses as high as 0.24 mcg/kg (16.8 mcg) have been administered safely; the dose of paricalcitol should be adjusted based on serum intact PTH (iPTH) levels, as follows:

Same or increasing iPTH level: Increase paricalcitol dose

iPTH level decreased by <30%: Increase paricalcitol dose

iPTH level decreased by >30% and <60%: Maintain paricalcitol dose iPTH level decrease by >60%: Decrease paricalcitol dose

iPTH level 1.5-3 times upper limit of normal: Maintain paricalcitol dose

Adults: Oral: Initial dose, in mcg, based on baseline iPTH level divided by 80. Administered 3 times weekly, no more frequently than every other day. **Note:** To reduce the risk of hypercalcemia initiate only after baseline serum calcium has been adjusted to ≤9.5 mg/dL.

Dose titration:

Titration dose (mcg) = Most recent iPTH level (pg/mL) divided by 80

Note: In situations where monitoring of iPTH, calcium, and phosphorus occurs less frequently than once per week, a more modest initial and dose titration rate may be warranted:

Modest titration dose (mcg) = Most recent iPTH level (pg/mL) divided by 100

Dosage adjustment for hypercalcemia or elevated Ca x P: Decrease calculated dose by 2-4 mcg. If further adjustment is required, dose should be reduced or interrupted until these parameters are normalized. If applicable, phosphate binder dosing may also be adjusted or withheld, or switch to a noncalcium-based phosphate binder

Secondary hyperparathyroidism associated with stage 3 and 4 CKD: Adults: Oral: Initial dose based on baseline serum iPTH:

iPTH ≤500 pg/mL: 1 mcg/day or 2 mcg 3 times/week

iPTH >500 pg/mL: 2 mcg/day or 4 mcg 3 times/week

Dosage adjustment based on iPTH level relative to baseline, adjust dose at 2-4 week intervals:

iPTH same or increased: Increase paricalcitol dose by 1 mcg/day or 2 mcg 3 times/week

iPTH decreased by <30%: Increase paricalcitol dose by 1 mcg/day or 2 mcg 3 times/week

iPTH decreased by ≥30% and ≤60%: Maintain paricalcitol dose

iPTH decreased by >60%: Decrease paricalcitol dose by 1 mcg/day* or 2 mcg 3 times/week

iPTH <60 pg/mL: Decrease paricalcitol dose by 1 mcg/day* or 2 mcg 3 times/week

*If patient is taking the lowest dose on a once-daily regimen, but further dose reduction is needed, decrease dose to 1 mcg 3 times/week. If further dose reduction is required, withhold drug as needed and restart at a lower dose. If applicable, calcium-phosphate binder dosing may also be adjusted or withheld, or switch to noncalcium-based binder.

Dosage adjustment in renal impairment: No dosage adjustment necessary.

Dosage adjustment in hepatic impairment:

Mild to moderate impairment: No dosage adjustment necessary.

Severe impairment: No dosage adjustment provided in manufacturer's labeling (has not been studied).

Dietary Considerations May be taken with or without food. Some products may contain coconut or palm kernel oil.

Administration

Oral: May be administered with or without food. With the 3 times/week dosing schedule, doses should not be given more frequently than every other day.

I.V.: Administered as a bolus dose at anytime during dialysis. Doses should not be administered more often than every other day.

Monitoring Parameters

Signs and symptoms of vitamin D intoxication

Serum calcium and phosphorus (closely monitor levels during dosage titration and after initiation of a strong CYP3A4 inhibitor):

I.V.: Twice weekly during initial phase, then at least monthly once dose established

Oral: At least every 2 weeks for 3 months or following dose adjustment, then monthly for 3 months, then every 3 months

Serum or plasma intact PTH (iPTH):

I.V.: Every 3 months

Oral: At least every 2 weeks for 3 months or following dose adjustment, then monthly for 3 months, then every 3 months

Reference Range

Corrected total serum calcium (K/DOQI, 2003): CKD stages 3 and 4: 8.4-10.2 mg/dL (2.1-2.6 mmol/L); CKD stage 5: 8.4-9.5 mg/dL (2.1-2.37 mmol/L); KDIGO guidelines recommend maintaining normal ranges for all stages of CKD (3-5D) (KDIGO, 2009)

Phosphorus (K/DOQI, 2003):

CKD stages 3 and 4: 2.7-4.6 mg/dL (0.87-1.48 mmol/L) (adults); maintain within age-appropriate limits (children)

CKD stage 5 (including those treated with dialysis): 3.5-5.5 mg/dL (1.13-1.78 mmol/L) (children >12 years and adults); 4-6 mg/dL (1.29-1.94 mmol/L) (children 1-12 years)

KDIGO guidelines recommend maintaining normal ranges for CKD stages 3-5 and lowering elevated phosphorus levels toward the normal range for CKD stage 5D (KDIGO, 2009)

Serum calcium-phosphorus product (K/DOQI, 2003): CKD stage 3-5: <55 mg^2/dL^2 (children >12 years and adults); <65 mg^2/dL^2 (children ≤12 years)

PTH: Whole molecule, immunochemiluminometric assay (ICMA): 1.0-5.2 pmol/L; whole molecule, radioimmunoassay (RIA): 10.0-65.0 pg/mL; whole molecule, immunoradiometric, double antibody (IRMA): 1.0-6.0 pmol/L

Target ranges by stage of chronic kidney disease (KDIGO, 2009): CKD stage 3-5: Optimal iPTH is unknown; maintain normal range (assay-dependent); CKD stage 5D: Maintain iPTH within 2-9 times the upper limit of normal for the assay used

Dosage Forms Excipient information presented when available (limited, particularly for generics); consult specific product labeling.

Capsule, Oral:

Zemplar: 1 mcg, 2 mcg, 4 mcg [contains alcohol, usp]

Generic: 1 mcg, 2 mcg, 4 mcg

Solution, Intravenous:

Zemplar: 2 mcg/mL (1 mL); 5 mcg/mL (1 mL, 2 mL) [contains alcohol, usp, propylene glycol]

◆ Pariet (Can) *see* RABEprazole *on page* 1769

◆ Pariprazole *see* RABEprazole *on page* 1769

◆ Parlodel *see* Bromocriptine *on page* 281

◆ Parnate *see* Tranylcypromine *on page* 2106

◆ Parnate® (Can) *see* Tranylcypromine *on page* 2106

Paromomycin (par oh moe MYE sin)

Brand Names: Canada Humatin®

Index Terms Paromomycin Sulfate

Pharmacologic Category Amebicide

Use Treatment of acute and chronic intestinal amebiasis; hepatic coma

Unlabeled Use Treatment of cryptosporidiosis

Pregnancy Considerations Paromomycin is poorly absorbed when given orally. Because it does not reach the maternal serum, it would not be expected to adversely affect the fetus. No adverse effects were observed in two infants whose mothers took paromomycin during pregnancy.

Breast-Feeding Considerations Paromomycin is poorly absorbed when given orally. Because it does not reach the maternal serum, it would not be expected to distribute into human milk.

Contraindications Hypersensitivity to paromomycin or any component of the formulation; intestinal obstruction

Warnings/Precautions Use with caution in patients with impaired renal function or possible or proven ulcerative bowel lesions. Prolonged use may result in fungal or bacterial superinfection, including *C. difficile*-associated diarrhea (CDAD) and pseudomembranous colitis; CDAD has been observed >2 months postantibiotic treatment.

Adverse Reactions

1% to 10%: Gastrointestinal: Diarrhea, abdominal cramps, nausea, vomiting, heartburn

<1% (Limited to important or life-threatening): Eosinophilia, exanthema, headache, ototoxicity, pruritus, rash, secondary enterocolitis, steatorrhea, vertigo

Drug Interactions

Metabolism/Transport Effects None known.

Avoid Concomitant Use There are no known interactions where it is recommended to avoid concomitant use.

Increased Effect/Toxicity There are no known significant interactions involving an increase in effect.

Decreased Effect There are no known significant interactions involving a decrease in effect.

Ethanol/Nutrition/Herb Interactions Food: Paromomycin may cause malabsorption of xylose, sucrose, and fats.

Mechanism of Action Acts directly on ameba; has antibacterial activity against normal and pathogenic organisms in the GI tract; interferes with bacterial protein synthesis by binding to 30S ribosomal subunits

Pharmacodynamics/Kinetics

Absorption: Poor oral absorption

Excretion: Feces (100% as unchanged drug)

Dosage Oral:

Intestinal amebiasis: Children and Adults: 25-35 mg/kg/day in 3 divided doses for 5-10 days

Dientamoeba fragilis: Children and Adults: 25-30 mg/kg/day in 3 divided doses for 7 days

Cryptosporidium (unlabeled use): Adults with AIDS: 1.5-2.25 g/day in 3-6 divided doses for 10-14 days (occasionally courses of up to 4-8 weeks may be needed)

Tapeworm (fish, dog, bovine, porcine):

Children: 11 mg/kg every 15 minutes for 4 doses

Adults: 1 g every 15 minutes for 4 doses

Hepatic coma: Adults: 4 g/day in 2-4 divided doses for 5-6 days

Dwarf tapeworm: Children and Adults: 45 mg/kg/dose every day for 5-7 days

Dosage adjustment in renal impairment: No dosage adjustment provided in the manufacturer's labeling (has not been studied).

Dosage adjustment in hepatic impairment: No dosage adjustment provided in the manufacturer's labeling (has not been studied).

Dosage Forms Excipient information presented when available (limited, particularly for generics); consult specific product labeling.

Capsule, Oral:

Generic: 250 mg

◆ **Paromomycin Sulfate** *see* Paromomycin *on page 1574*

PARoxetine (pa ROKS e teen)

Brand Names: U.S. Brisdelle; Paxil; Paxil CR; Pexeva

Brand Names: Canada Apo-Paroxetine; Auro-Paroxetine; CO Paroxetine; Dom-Paroxetine; JAMP-Paroxetine; Mylan-Paroxetine; Novo-Paroxetine; Paxil; Paxil CR; PHL-Paroxetine; PMS-Paroxetine; Q-Paroxetine; ratio-Paroxetine; Riva-Paroxetine; Sandoz-Paroxetine; Teva-Paroxetine

Index Terms Brisdelle; Paroxetine Hydrochloride; Paroxetine Mesylate

Pharmacologic Category Antidepressant, Selective Serotonin Reuptake Inhibitor

Additional Appendix Information

Antidepressant Agents *on page 2284*

Beers Criteria – Potentially Inappropriate Medications for Geriatrics *on page 2368*

Selective Serotonin Reuptake Inhibitors (SSRIs) Pharmacokinetics *on page 2314*

Use

Generalized anxiety disorder (immediate release): For the treatment of generalized anxiety disorder (GAD)

Major depressive disorder (immediate and controlled release): For the treatment of major depressive disorder (MDD)

Obsessive-compulsive disorder (immediate release): For the treatment of obsessions and compulsions in patients with obsessive-compulsive disorder (OCD)

Panic disorder (immediate and controlled release): For the treatment of panic disorder, with or without agoraphobia

Post-traumatic stress disorder (immediate release): For the treatment of posttraumatic stress disorder (PTSD)

Premenstrual dysphoric disorder (controlled release): For the treatment of premenstrual dysphoric disorder (PMDD)

Social anxiety disorder (immediate and controlled release): For the treatment of social anxiety disorder, also known as social phobia

Vasomotor symptoms of menopause (Brisdelle only): For the treatment of moderate to severe vasomotor symptoms associated with menopause

Unlabeled Use May be useful in eating disorders, impulse control disorders; treatment of obsessive-compulsive disorder (OCD) in children; treatment of mild dementia-associated agitation in nonpsychotic patients; treatment of paraphilia/hypersexuality

Pregnancy Risk Factor D//X (product specific)

Pregnancy Considerations Studies in pregnant women have demonstrated a risk to the fetus. Paroxetine crosses the placenta. An increased risk of teratogenic effects, including cardiovascular defects, may be associated with maternal use of paroxetine or other SSRIs; however, available information is conflicting. Nonteratogenic effects in the newborn following SSRI/SNRI exposure late in the third trimester include respiratory distress, cyanosis, apnea, seizures, temperature instability, feeding difficulty, vomiting, hypoglycemia, hypo- or hypertonia, hyperreflexia, jitteriness, irritability, constant crying, and tremor. Symptoms may be due to the toxicity of the SSRIs/SNRIs or a discontinuation syndrome and may be consistent with serotonin syndrome associated with SSRI treatment. Persistent pulmonary hypertension of the newborn (PPHN) has also been reported with SSRI exposure. The long-term effects of *in utero* SSRI exposure on infant development and behavior are not known.

Due to pregnancy-induced physiologic changes, some pharmacokinetic parameters of paroxetine may be altered. The maternal CYP2D6 genotype also influences paroxetine plasma concentrations during pregnancy.

The manufacturer suggests discontinuing paroxetine or switching to another antidepressant unless the benefits of therapy justify continuing treatment during pregnancy; consider other treatment options for women who are planning to become pregnant. The ACOG recommends that therapy with SSRIs or SNRIs during pregnancy be individualized; treatment of depression during pregnancy should incorporate the clinical expertise of the mental health clinician, obstetrician, primary healthcare provider, and pediatrician. The ACOG also recommends that therapy with paroxetine be avoided during pregnancy if possible and that fetuses exposed in early pregnancy be assessed with a fetal echocardiography. According to the American Psychiatric Association (APA), the risks of medication treatment should be weighed against other treatment options and untreated depression. The use of paroxetine is not recommended as first line therapy during pregnancy. For women who discontinue antidepressant medications during pregnancy and who may be at high risk for postpartum depression, the medications can be restarted following delivery. Treatment algorithms have been developed by the ACOG and the APA for the management of depression in women prior to conception and during pregnancy. Menopausal vasomotor symptoms do not occur during pregnancy; therefore, the use of paroxetine for the treatment of menopausal vasomotor symptoms is contraindicated in pregnant women.

Breast-Feeding Considerations Paroxetine is excreted in breast milk and concentrations in the hindmilk are higher than in foremilk. Paroxetine has not been detected in the serum of nursing infants. Adverse reactions have been reported in nursing infants exposed to some SSRIs. The manufacturer recommends that caution be exercised when administering paroxetine to nursing women. Maternal use of an SSRI during pregnancy may cause delayed milk secretion. The American Academy of Breast-feeding Medicine suggests that paroxetine may be considered for the treatment of postpartum depression in appropriately selected women who are nursing. Mothers should be monitored for changes in symptoms and infants should be monitored for growth. The long-term effects on development and behavior have not been studied.

Medication Guide Available Yes

Contraindications Concurrent use with or within 14 days of MAOIs intended to treat psychiatric disorders; initiation in patients being treated with linezolid or methylene blue I.V.; concomitant use with pimozide or thioridazine; hypersensitivity to paroxetine or any of its inactive ingredients; pregnancy (Brisdelle only).

Warnings/Precautions Hazardous agent - use appropriate precautions for handling and disposal (NIOSH, 2012). **[U.S. Boxed Warning]: Antidepressants increase the risk of suicidal thinking and behavior in children, adolescents, and young adults (18-24 years of age) with major depressive disorder (MDD) and other psychiatric disorders;** consider risk prior to prescribing. Short-term studies did not show an increased risk in patients >24 years of age and showed a decreased risk in patients ≥65 years. Closely monitor patients for clinical worsening, suicidality, or unusual changes in behavior, particularly during the initial 1-2 months of therapy or during periods of dosage adjustments (increases or decreases); the patient's family or caregiver should be instructed to closely observe the patient and communicate condition with healthcare provider. A medication guide concerning the use of antidepressants should be dispensed with each prescription. **Paroxetine is not FDA approved for use in children.**

The possibility of a suicide attempt is inherent in major depression and may persist until remission occurs. Patients treated with antidepressants (for any indication) should be observed for clinical worsening and suicidality, especially during the initial few months of a course of drug therapy, or at times of dose changes, either increases or decreases. Use caution in high-risk patients. Worsening depression and severe abrupt suicidality that are not part of the presenting symptoms may require discontinuation or modification of drug therapy. The patient's family or caregiver should be alerted to monitor patients for the emergence of suicidality and associated behaviors (such as agitation, irritability, hostility, impulsivity, and hypomania) and call healthcare provider.

May worsen psychosis in some patients or precipitate a shift to mania or hypomania in patients with bipolar disorder. Patients presenting with depressive symptoms should be screened for bipolar disorder. Monotherapy in patients with bipolar disorder should be avoided. **Paroxetine is not FDA approved for the treatment of bipolar depression.**

Potentially life-threatening serotonin syndrome (SS) has occurred with serotonergic agents (eg, SSRIs, SNRIs), particularly when used in combination with other serotonergic agents (eg, triptans, TCAs, fentanyl, lithium, tramadol, buspirone, St John's wort, tryptophan) or agents that impair metabolism of serotonin (eg, MAO inhibitors intended to treat psychiatric disorders, other MAO inhibitors [ie, linezolid and intravenous methylene blue]). Discontinue treatment (and any concomitant serotonergic agent) immediately if signs/symptoms arise.

Paroxetine may increase the risks associated with electroconvulsive therapy. Has a low potential to impair cognitive or motor performance - use caution when operating hazardous machinery or driving. Symptoms of agitation and/or restlessness may occur during initial few weeks of therapy. Low potential for sedation or anticholinergic effects relative to cyclic antidepressants. Bone fractures have been associated with SSRI treatment. Consider the possibility of a fragility fracture if an SSRI-treated patient presents with unexplained bone pain, point tenderness, swelling, or bruising.

Use caution in elderly patients; may cause or exacerbate syndrome of inappropriate antidiuretic hormone secretion or hyponatremia; monitor sodium closely with initiation or dosage adjustments in older adults. Medication associated with potent anticholinergic properties which may be inappropriate in older adults depending on comorbidities (eg, dementia, delirium) (Beers Criteria).

Use caution in patients with a previous seizure disorder or condition predisposing to seizures such as brain damage, alcoholism, or concurrent therapy with other drugs which lower the seizure threshold. Use with caution in patients with hepatic dysfunction. May cause SIADH; volume depletion and/or diuretics may increase risk. Potentially significant drug-drug interactions may exist, requiring dose or frequency adjustment, additional monitoring, and/or selection of alternative therapy. Use with caution in patients with renal insufficiency or other concurrent illness (due to limited experience); dose reduction recommended with severe renal impairment. May cause or exacerbate sexual dysfunction. Use caution in patients with narrow-angle glaucoma. Avoid use in the first trimester of pregnancy. Menopausal vasomotor symptoms do not occur during pregnancy; therefore, the use of paroxetine for the treatment of menopausal vasomotor symptoms is contraindicated in pregnant women.

Brisdelle contains a lower dose than what is required for the treatment of psychiatric conditions. Patients who require paroxetine for the treatment of psychiatric conditions should discontinue Brisdelle and begin treatment with a paroxetine-containing medication which provides an adequate dosage.

Abrupt discontinuation or interruption of antidepressant therapy has been associated with a discontinuation syndrome. Symptoms arising may vary with antidepressant however commonly include nausea, vomiting, diarrhea, headaches, lightheadedness, dizziness, diminished appetite, sweating, chills, tremors, paresthesias, fatigue, somnolence, and sleep disturbances (eg, vivid dreams, insomnia). Greater risks for developing a discontinuation syndrome have been associated with antidepressants with shorter half-lives, longer durations of treatment, and abrupt discontinuation. For antidepressants of short or intermediate half-lives, symptoms may emerge within 2-5 days after treatment discontinuation and last 7-14 days (APA, 2010; Fava, 2006; Haddod, 2001; Shelton, 2001; Warner, 2006).

Adverse Reactions Frequency varies by dose and indication. Adverse reactions reported as a composite of all indications.

>10%:

Central nervous system: Drowsiness (15% to 24%), insomnia (11% to 24%), headache (6% to 18%), dizziness (6% to 14%)

Dermatologic: Diaphoresis (5% to 14%)

Endocrine & metabolic: Decreased libido (3% to 15%)

Gastrointestinal: Nausea (19% to 26%), xerostomia (9% to 18%), constipation (5% to 16%), diarrhea (9% to 12%)

Genitourinary: Ejaculatory disorder (13% to 28%)

Neuromuscular & skeletal: Weakness (12% to 22%), tremor (4% to 11%)

1% to 10%:

Cardiovascular: Vasodilatation (2% to 4%), chest pain (3%), palpitations (2% to 3%), hypertension (≥1%), tachycardia (≥1%)

Central nervous system: Nervousness (4% to 9%), anxiety (5%), fatigue (5%), agitation (3% to 5%), paresthesia (4%), abnormal dreams (3% to 4%), lack of concentration (3% to 4%), yawning (2% to 4%), depersonalization (≤3%), myoclonus (2% to 3%), amnesia (2%), chills (2%), emotional lability (≥1%), vertigo (≥1%), confusion (1%), myasthenia (1%)

Dermatologic: Skin rash (2% to 3%), pruritus (≥1%)

Endocrine & metabolic: Orgasm disturbance (2% to 9%), dysmenorrhea (5%), weight gain (≥1%)

Gastrointestinal: Decreased appetite (5% to 9%), dyspepsia (2% to 5%), flatulence (4%), abdominal pain (4%), nausea and vomiting (4%), increased appetite (2% to 4%), vomiting (2% to 3%), dysgeusia (2%)

Genitourinary: Male genital disease (10%), female genital tract disease (2% to 9%), impotence (2% to 9%), urinary frequency (2% to 3%), urinary tract infection (2%)

Infection: Infection (5% to 6%)

Neuromuscular & skeletal: Myalgia (2% to 4%), back pain (3%), myopathy (2%), arthralgia (≥1%)

Ophthalmic: Blurred vision (4%), visual disturbance (2% to 4%)

Otic: Tinnitus (≥1%)

Respiratory: Dyspnea (≤7%), pharyngitis (4%), sinusitis (≤4%), rhinitis (3%)

<1% (Limited to important or life-threatening): Abnormal hepatic function tests, acute angle-closure glaucoma, acute renal failure, adrenergic syndrome, agranulocytosis, akathisia, akinesia, anaphylactoid reaction, anaphylaxis, anemia (various), angina pectoris, angioedema, aphasia, aphthous stomatitis, aplastic anemia, asthma, atrial arrhythmia, atrial fibrillation, bilirubinemia, bloody diarrhea, bone marrow aplasia, bradycardia, bronchitis, bulimia nervosa, bundle branch block, cardiac failure, cataract, cellulitis, cerebral ischemia, cerebrovascular accident, change in platelet count, cholelithiasis, colitis, deafness, dehydration, delirium, depression, diabetes mellitus, disorientation, drug dependence, dyskinesia, dysphagia, dystonia, eclampsia, electrolyte disturbance, emphysema, esophageal achalasia, exfoliative dermatitis, extrapyramidal reaction, fecal impaction, fungal skin infection, gastroenteritis, glaucoma, goiter, Guillain-Barre syndrome, hallucination, hematemesis, hematologic abnormality, hematologic disease, hematoma, hemoptysis, hemorrhage, hemorrhagic pancreatitis, hepatic failure, hepatic necrosis, hepatitis, hepatotoxicity, homicidal ideation, hypercholesteremia, hypergammaglobulinemia, hyperglycemia, hyperhidrosis, hypersensitivity reaction, hyperthyroidism, hypoglycemia, hypotension, hypothyroidism, immune thrombocytopenia, increased blood urea nitrogen, increased creatine phosphokinase, increased lactate dehydrogenase, increased serum alkaline phosphatase, intestinal obstruction, ischemic heart disease, jaundice, ketosis, low cardiac output, lymphadenopathy, meningitis, migraine, mydriasis, myelitis, myocardial infarction, neuroleptic malignant syndrome, neuropathy, osteoarthritis, osteoporosis, pancreatitis, pancytopenia, paralytic ileus, peptic ulcer, peritonitis, phlebitis, pneumonia, prolonged bleeding time, pulmonary edema, pulmonary embolism, pulmonary fibrosis, pulmonary hypertension, restlessness, seizure, sepsis, serotonin syndrome, spermatozoa disorder (activity altered, DNA fragmentation [abnormal] increased), status epilepticus, Stevens-Johnson syndrome, suicidal ideation, suicidal tendencies, syncope, tetany, thrombophlebitis, thrombosis, torsades de pointes, toxic epidermal necrolysis, uncontrolled diabetes mellitus, vasculitis, ventricular arrhythmia, ventricular fibrillation, ventricular tachycardia, withdrawal syndrome (including increased dreaming/nightmares, muscle cramps/spasms/twitching, headache, nervousness/anxiety, fatigue/tiredness, restless feeling in legs, and trouble sleeping/insomnia)

Drug Interactions

Metabolism/Transport Effects Substrate of CYP2D6 (major); **Note:** Assignment of Major/Minor substrate status based on clinically relevant drug interaction potential; **Inhibits** CYP1A2 (weak), CYP2B6 (moderate), CYP2C19 (weak), CYP2C9 (weak), CYP2D6 (strong), CYP3A4 (weak)

Avoid Concomitant Use

Avoid concomitant use of PARoxetine with any of the following: Dosulepin; Iobenguane I 123; Linezolid; MAO Inhibitors; Methylene Blue; Pimozide; Tamoxifen; Thioridazine; Tryptophan

Increased Effect/Toxicity

PARoxetine may increase the levels/effects of: Agents with Antiplatelet Properties; Anticoagulants; Antidepressants (Serotonin Reuptake Inhibitor/Antagonist); Antipsychotics; ARIPiprazole; Asenapine; Aspirin; AtoMOXetine; Beta-Blockers; BusPIRone; CarBAMazepine; CloZAPine; Collagenase (Systemic); CYP2B6 Substrates; CYP2D6 Substrates; Dabigatran Etexilate; Desmopressin; Dextromethorphan; Dofetilide; Dosulepin; DULoxetine; Fesoterodine; Galantamine; Highest Risk QTc-Prolonging Agents; Hypoglycemic Agents; Ibritumomab; Iloperidone; Lomitapide; Methadone; Methylene Blue; Metoclopramide; Metoprolol; Mexiletine; Moderate Risk QTc-Prolonging Agents; Nebivolol; NSAID (COX-2 Inhibitor); NSAID (Nonselective); Pimozide; Propafenone; RisperiDONE; Rivaroxaban; Salicylates; Serotonin Modulators; Tetrabenazine; Thiazide Diuretics; Thioridazine; Thrombolytic Agents; Tositumomab and Iodine I 131 Tositumomab; TraMADol; Tricyclic Antidepressants; Vitamin K Antagonists; Vortioxetine

The levels/effects of PARoxetine may be increased by: Abiraterone Acetate; Alcohol (Ethyl); Analgesics (Opioid); Antipsychotics; ARIPiprazole; Asenapine; BuPROPion; BusPIRone; Cimetidine; CNS Depressants; Cobicistat; CYP2D6 Inhibitors (Moderate); CYP2D6 Inhibitors (Strong); Dasatinib; DULoxetine; Glucosamine; Herbs (Anticoagulant/Antiplatelet Properties); Ibrutinib;

Linezolid; Lithium; MAO Inhibitors; Metoclopramide; Metyrosine; Mifepristone; Multivitamins/Fluoride (with ADE); Multivitamins/Minerals (with ADEK, Folate, Iron); Multivitamins/Minerals (with AE, No Iron); Omega-3 Fatty Acids; Pentosan Polysulfate Sodium; Pentoxifylline; Pravastatin; Prostacyclin Analogues; Tipranavir; TraMADol; Tryptophan; Vitamin E

Decreased Effect

PARoxetine may decrease the levels/effects of: Aprepitant; Codeine; Fosaprepitant; Iloperidone; Iobenguane I 123; Ioflupane I 123; Tamoxifen; Thyroid Products; TraMADol

The levels/effects of PARoxetine may be decreased by: Aprepitant; CarBAMazepine; Cyproheptadine; Darunavir; Fosamprenavir; Fosaprepitant; NSAID (COX-2 Inhibitor); NSAID (Nonselective); Peginterferon Alfa-2b

Ethanol/Nutrition/Herb Interactions

Ethanol: May increase CNS depression; monitor for increased effects with coadministration. Caution patients about effects.

Food: Peak concentration is increased, but bioavailability is not significantly altered by food.

Herb/Nutraceutical: Avoid valerian, St John's wort, tryptophan, SAMe, kava kava.

Storage/Stability

Capsules: Store between 20°C and 25°C (68°F and 77°F); excursions permitted between 15°C and 30°C (59°F and 86°F). Protect from light and humidity.

Tablets: Store immediate-release tablets between 15°C and 30°C (59°F and 86°F) and controlled-release tablets at or below 25°C (77°F).

Suspension: Store at or below 25°C (77°F).

Mechanism of Action Paroxetine is a selective serotonin reuptake inhibitor, chemically unrelated to tricyclic, tetracyclic, or other antidepressants; presumably, the inhibition of serotonin reuptake from brain synapse stimulated serotonin activity in the brain

Pharmacodynamics/Kinetics

Onset of action: Depression: The onset of action is within a week; however, individual response varies greatly and full response may not be seen until 8-12 weeks after initiation of treatment.

Absorption: Completely absorbed following oral administration

Distribution: V_d: 8.7 L/kg (3-28 L/kg)

Protein binding: 93% to 95%

Metabolism: Extensively hepatic via CYP2D6 enzymes; primary metabolites are formed via oxidation and methylation of parent drug, with subsequent glucuronide/sulfate conjugation; nonlinear pharmacokinetics (via 2D6 saturation) may be seen with higher doses and longer duration of therapy. Metabolites exhibit ~2% potency of parent compound. C_{min} concentrations are 70% to 80% greater in the elderly compared to nonelderly patients; clearance is also decreased.

Half-life elimination: 21 hours (3-65 hours)

Time to peak:

- Capsules: 3-8 hours
- Tablets, oral suspension: Immediate release: 5.2-8.1 hours
- Tablets: Controlled release: 6-10 hours

Excretion: Urine (64%, 2% as unchanged drug); feces (36% primarily via bile, <1% as unchanged drug)

Dosage Oral:

Children ≥8 years:

Obsessive-compulsive disorder (OCD) unlabeled use): Initial: 10 mg/day; titrate every 7-14 days in 10 mg/day increments as necessary to a maximum 60 mg/day; trials have typically continued for a 10- to 12-week treatment course (Geller, 2004; Rosenberg, 1999)

Social anxiety disorder (unlabeled use): Initial: 2.5-10 mg/day; titrate every ≥7 days in 5-10 mg/day increments to a maximum of 50 mg/day; trials have typically continued for a 16-week treatment course (Mancini, 1999; Wagner, 2004)

Adults:

Major depressive disorder (MDD):

Paxil, Pexeva: Initial: 20 mg once daily, preferably in the morning; increase if needed by 10 mg/day increments at intervals of at least 1 week; maximum dose: 50 mg/day

Paxil CR: Initial: 25 mg once daily; increase if needed by 12.5 mg/day increments at intervals of at least 1 week; maximum dose: 62.5 mg/day

Generalized anxiety disorder (GAD) (Paxil, Pexeva): Initial: 20 mg once daily, preferably in the morning (if dose is increased, adjust in increments of 10 mg/day at 1-week intervals); doses of 20-50 mg/day were used in clinical trials, however, no greater benefit was seen with doses >20 mg.

Obsessive-compulsive disorder (OCD) (Paxil, Pexeva): Initial: 20 mg once daily, preferably in the morning; increase if needed by 10 mg/day increments at intervals of at least 1 week; recommended dose: 40 mg/day; range: 20-60 mg/day; maximum dose: 60 mg/day

Panic disorder:

Paxil, Pexeva: Initial: 10 mg once daily, preferably in the morning; increase if needed by 10 mg/day increments at intervals of at least 1 week; recommended dose: 40 mg/day; range: 10-60 mg/day; maximum dose: 60 mg/day

Paxil CR: Initial: 12.5 mg once daily; increase if needed by 12.5 mg/day at intervals of at least 1 week; maximum dose: 75 mg/day

Premenstrual dysphoric disorder (PMDD) (Paxil CR): Initial: 12.5 mg once daily in the morning; may be increased to 25 mg/day; dosing changes should occur at intervals of at least 1 week. May be given daily throughout the menstrual cycle or limited to the luteal phase.

Post-traumatic stress disorder (PTSD) (Paxil): Initial: 20 mg once daily, preferably in the morning; increase if needed by 10 mg/day increments at intervals of at least 1 week; range: 20-50 mg. Limited data suggest doses of 40 mg/day were not more efficacious than 20 mg/day.

Social anxiety disorder:

Paxil: Initial: 20 mg once daily, preferably in the morning; recommended dose: 20 mg/day; range: 20-60 mg/day; doses >20 mg may not have additional benefit

Paxil CR: Initial: 12.5 mg once daily, preferably in the morning; may be increased by 12.5 mg/day at intervals of at least 1 week; maximum dose: 37.5 mg/day

Vasomotor symptoms of menopause:

Brisdelle: 7.5 mg once daily at bedtime

Paxil CR (unlabeled use): 12.5-25 mg once daily (Stearns, 2003)

Elderly:

Paxil, Pexeva: Initial: 10 mg/day; increase if needed by 10 mg/day increments at intervals of at least 1 week; maximum dose: 40 mg/day

Paxil CR: Initial: 12.5 mg/day; increase if needed by 12.5 mg/day increments at intervals of at least 1 week; maximum dose: 50 mg/day

Discontinuation of therapy: Upon discontinuation of antidepressant therapy, gradually taper the dose to minimize the incidence of withdrawal symptoms and allow for the detection of re-emerging symptoms. Evidence supporting ideal taper rates is limited. APA and NICE guidelines suggest tapering therapy over at least several weeks with consideration to the half-life of the antidepressant; antidepressants with a shorter half-life may need to be tapered more conservatively. In addition for long-term treated patients, WFSBP guidelines recommend tapering over 4-6 months. If intolerable withdrawal symptoms occur following a dose reduction, consider resuming the previously prescribed dose and/or decrease dose at a more gradual rate (APA, 2010; Bauer, 2002; Haddod, 2001; NCCMH, 2010; Schatzberg, 2006; Shelton, 2001; Warner, 2006).

MAO inhibitor recommendations:

Switching to or from an MAO inhibitor intended to treat psychiatric disorders:

Allow 14 days to elapse between discontinuing an MAO inhibitor intended to treat psychiatric disorders and initiation of paroxetine.

Allow 14 days to elapse between discontinuing paroxetine and initiation of an MAO inhibitor intended to treat psychiatric disorders.

Use with other MAO inhibitors (linezolid or I.V. methylene blue):

Do not initiate paroxetine in patients receiving linezolid or I.V. methylene blue; consider other interventions for psychiatric condition.

If urgent treatment with linezolid or I.V. methylene blue is required in a patient already receiving paroxetine and potential benefits outweigh potential risks, discontinue paroxetine promptly and administer linezolid or I.V. methylene blue. Monitor for serotonin syndrome for 2 weeks or until 24 hours after the last dose of linezolid or I.V. methylene blue, whichever comes first. May resume paroxetine 24 hours after the last dose of linezolid or I.V. methylene blue.

Dosage adjustment in renal impairment: Adults:

Brisdelle: No dosage adjustment necessary.

Paxil, Paxil CR, Pexeva:

Cl_{cr} 30-60 mL/minute: Plasma concentration is 2 times that seen in normal function. There are no dosage adjustments provided in manufacturer's labeling.

Severe impairment (Cl_{cr} <30 mL/minute): Mean plasma concentration is ~4 times that seen in normal function.

Paxil, Pexeva: Initial: 10 mg/day; increase if needed by 10 mg/day increments at intervals of at least 1 week; maximum dose: 40 mg/day

Paxil CR: Initial: 12.5 mg/day; increase if needed by 12.5 mg/day increments at intervals of at least 1 week; maximum dose: 50 mg/day

Dosage adjustment in hepatic impairment: Adults: In hepatic dysfunction, plasma concentration is 2 times that seen in normal function.

Brisdelle: No dosage adjustment necessary.

Paxil, Paxil CR, Pexeva:

Mild-to-moderate impairment: There are no dosage adjustments provided in manufacturer's labeling.

Severe impairment:

Paxil, Pexeva: Initial: 10 mg/day; increase if needed by 10 mg/day increments at intervals of at least 1 week; maximum dose: 40 mg/day

Paxil CR: Initial: 12.5 mg/day; increase if needed by 12.5 mg/day increments at intervals of at least 1 week; maximum dose: 50 mg/day

Dietary Considerations May be taken without regard to meals.

Administration May be administered without regard to meals. Paxil, Paxil CR, and Pexeva should preferentially be administered in the morning; whereas Brisdelle is recommended to be administered at bedtime. Do not crush, break, or chew controlled-release tablets.

Hazardous agent; use appropriate precautions for handling and disposal (NIOSH, 2012).

Monitoring Parameters Mental status for depression, suicide ideation (especially at the beginning of therapy or when doses are increased or decreased), anxiety, social functioning, mania, panic attacks; signs/symptoms of serotonin syndrome; akathisia

Additional Information Paxil CR incorporates a degradable polymeric matrix (Geomatrix) to control dissolution rate over a period of 4-5 hours. An enteric coating delays the start of drug release until tablets have left the stomach.

Dosage Forms Excipient information presented when available (limited, particularly for generics); consult specific product labeling.

Capsule, Oral, as mesylate [strength expressed as base]:

Brisdelle: 7.5 mg [contains fd&c red #40, fd&c yellow #6 (sunset yellow)]

Suspension, Oral, as hydrochloride [strength expressed as base]:

Paxil: 10 mg/5 mL (250 mL) [contains fd&c yellow #6 aluminum lake, methylparaben, propylene glycol, propylparaben, saccharin sodium; orange flavor]

Tablet, Oral, as hydrochloride [strength expressed as base]:

Paxil: 10 mg, 20 mg [scored]

Paxil: 30 mg, 40 mg

Generic: 10 mg, 20 mg, 30 mg, 40 mg

Tablet, Oral, as mesylate [strength expressed as base]:

Pexeva: 10 mg

Pexeva: 20 mg [scored]

Pexeva: 30 mg, 40 mg

Tablet Extended Release 24 Hour, Oral, as hydrochloride [strength expressed as base]:

Paxil CR: 12.5 mg [contains fd&c yellow #10 aluminum lake, fd&c yellow #6 aluminum lake]

Paxil CR: 25 mg

Paxil CR: 37.5 mg [contains fd&c blue #2 aluminum lake]

Generic: 12.5 mg, 25 mg, 37.5 mg

◆ **Paroxetine Hydrochloride** *see* PARoxetine *on page 1575*

◆ **Paroxetine Mesylate** *see* PARoxetine *on page 1575*

◆ **Parvolex® (Can)** *see* Acetylcysteine *on page 36*

Pasireotide (pas i REE oh tide)

Brand Names: U.S. Signifor

Brand Names: Canada Signifor

Index Terms Pasireotide Diaspartate; SOM230

Pharmacologic Category Somatostatin Analog

Use Treatment of Cushing's disease in patients for whom pituitary surgery is not an option or has not been curative

Pregnancy Risk Factor C

Pregnancy Considerations Adverse events were observed in animal reproduction studies.

Breast-Feeding Considerations It is not known if pasireotide is excreted into breast milk. The manufacturer recommends that caution be exercised when administering pasireotide to nursing women.

Prescribing and Access Restrictions In Canada, patients must be enrolled in the Access Program for Signifor (Novartis Canada).

Medication Guide Available Yes

Contraindications

There are no contraindications listed in the manufacturer's labeling.

Canadian labeling: Hypersensitivity to pasireotide or any component of the formulation; moderate or severe hepatic impairment (Child-Pugh B or C); uncontrolled diabetes (Hb A_{1c} ≥8%); NYHA Class III to IV heart failure; cardiogenic shock; second- or third-degree atrioventricular (AV) block, sinoatrial block, sick sinus syndrome (unless patient has a functioning pacemaker); severe bradycardia; congenital long QT syndrome or baseline QTc interval ≥500 ms.

Warnings/Precautions Bradycardia and QT prolongation have been observed with therapy. Use with caution in patients with pre-existing cardiac disease, patients with risk factors for bradycardia (eg, heart block, history of significant bradycardia, receiving concomitant drugs known to cause bradycardia), and patients at risk for QT prolongation (eg, congenital long QT, recent MI, heart failure, hypokalemia, hypomagnesemia, receiving concomitant drugs known to cause QT prolongation). The Canadian labeling contraindicates use in several of these disorders (refer to Contraindications). Obtain baseline ECG prior to therapy and consider continued monitoring during therapy for an effect on the QT_c interval. Correct hypokalemia, hypomagnesemia, or hypocalcemia prior to therapy and monitor during therapy. May impair gallbladder, leading to gallstone formation; monitor patients for cholelithiasis with ultrasound prior to therapy and at 6-12 month intervals during therapy. Increased liver enzymes have been reported; ALT, AST, and bilirubin should be monitored per recommendations in manufacturer's labeling. May require dosage interruption to investigate probable cause of confirmed or rising liver enzyme values; patients with significant elevations in liver function tests (≥5 times baseline values) require more frequent monitoring and extensive monitoring (ALT, AST, alkaline phosphatase, total bilirubin). Use with caution in patients with hepatic impairment; lower doses are recommended at therapy initiation in patients with moderate impairment (Child-Pugh class B). Use is not recommended in patients with severe impairment (Child-Pugh class C). Canadian labeling contraindicates use in moderate or severe impairment. Inhibition of insulin and glucagon secretion may affect glucose regulation, leading to hyperglycemia. Exacerbation of glycemia occurred in almost all patients during the initial 2 weeks of therapy, including patients with normal glucose levels at baseline; diabetes and prediabetes has also been observed. Assess fasting blood glucose (FBG) levels or hemoglobin A1c (Hb A_{1c}) prior to initiation of therapy. Patients should also do self-monitoring and/or FBG weekly for the first 2-3 months, then periodically during use. If hyperglycemia occurs, initiation or dosage adjustment of antidiabetic therapy is recommended; if uncontrolled hyperglycemia persists despite antidiabetic therapy, consider dosage reduction or discontinuation of pasireotide. Prior to initiation, patients with poorly controlled or uncontrolled diabetes should have antidiabetic therapy optimized; exacerbation of glycemia commonly occurs with pasireotide use. Suppression of the adrenocorticotropic hormone (ACTH) from therapy may lead to hypocortisolism. Monitor patients for signs or symptoms of hypocortisolism (eg, anorexia, fatigue, hypoglycemia, hyponatremia, hypotension, nausea, vomiting, weakness). If symptoms occur, consider stopping or reducing the dose until symptoms improve. Glucocorticoid replacement therapy may also be needed temporarily. Decreases (slight) in thyroid function have been observed during therapy; monitor thyroid function tests prior to initiation of therapy and periodically during therapy. Evaluate for treatment response with 24-hour urinary free cortisol levels and/or improvement in symptoms. Maximum reduction in urinary free cortisol levels is usually seen by 2 months of therapy. Therapy may cause inhibition of additional pituitary hormones (other than ACTH); additional monitoring for pituitary deficiency is advised (eg, TSH, free T4, GH, IGF-1), particularly in patients who have undergone transsphenoidal surgery and pituitary irradiation who are at an increased risk for deficiency. Potentially significant drug-drug interactions may exist, requiring dose or frequency adjustment, additional monitoring, and/or selection of alternative therapy.

Adverse Reactions

>10%:

Central nervous system: Headache (28%), fatigue (19%)

Dermatologic: Alopecia (12%)

Endocrine & metabolic: Hyperglycemia (40%), diabetes mellitus (18%), Hb A_{1c} increased (11%)

Gastrointestinal: Diarrhea (58%), nausea (52%), cholelithiasis (30%), abdominal pain (24%)

Hepatic: Prothrombin time increased (2% to 33%)

Local: Injection site reactions (17%; including pain, erythema, hematoma, hemorrhage, pruritus)

Neuromuscular & skeletal: Weakness (11%)

Respiratory: Nasopharyngitis (13%)

1% to 10%:

Cardiovascular: Hypertension (10%), peripheral edema (10%), hypotension (7%), bradycardia (6%), QT prolongation (6%; >480 msec 2%)

Central nervous system: Anxiety (9%), dizziness (9%), insomnia (9%), vertigo (6%)

Dermatologic: Pruritus (8%), dry skin (6%)

Endocrine & metabolic: Hypercholesterolemia (10%), hypoglycemia (9%), type 2 diabetes mellitus (9%), adrenal insufficiency (6%), hypokalemia (6%), hypothyroidism (4%)

Gastrointestinal: Appetite decreased (10%), constipation (7%), lipase increased (7%), vomiting (7%), abdominal distension (6%), amylase increased (2%)

Hematologic: Anemia (4%)

Hepatic: ALT increased (10%), GGT increased (10%), AST increased (6%), bilirubin increased (2%)

Neuromuscular & skeletal: Myalgia (9%), arthralgia (8%), back pain (6%), limb pain (6%)

Miscellaneous: Flu-like syndrome (9%)

Drug Interactions

Metabolism/Transport Effects None known.

Avoid Concomitant Use

Avoid concomitant use of Pasireotide with any of the following: Highest Risk QTc-Prolonging Agents; Ivabradine; Mifepristone

Increased Effect/Toxicity

Pasireotide may increase the levels/effects of: Codeine; Highest Risk QTc-Prolonging Agents; Moderate Risk QTc-Prolonging Agents; Pegvisomant

The levels/effects of Pasireotide may be increased by: Ivabradine; Mifepristone; QTc-Prolonging Agents (Indeterminate Risk and Risk Modifying)

Decreased Effect

Pasireotide may decrease the levels/effects of: CycloSPORINE (Systemic)

Storage/Stability Store at 25°C (77°F); excursions permitted to 15°C to 30°C (59°F to 86°F). Protect from light.

Mechanism of Action Synthetic cyclohexapeptide analogue of somatostatin which is a peptide inhibitor of multiple endocrine, neuroendocrine, and exocrine mechanisms. Binds to somatostatin receptor (sst_{1-5}), with high affinity for the sst_1, sst_2, sst_3 subtypes, and highest affinity for the sst_5 subtype, resulting in inhibition of ACTH secretion which leads to decreased cortisol secretion.

Pharmacodynamics/Kinetics

Distribution: V_d: >100 L

Protein binding: 88%

Metabolism: Primarily eliminated as unchanged drug hepatically (via biliary excretion)

Half-life elimination: ~12 hours

Time to peak, plasma: 0.25-0.5 hours

Excretion: Feces (~40% to 56%, primarily as unchanged drug); urine (~6% to 10%, primarily as unchanged drug)

Dosage Cushing's disease: Adults: SubQ:

Initial:

U.S. labeling: 0.6 mg or 0.9 mg twice daily.

Canadian labeling: 0.6 mg twice daily.

Titrate based on response and tolerability. If adverse reactions occur, temporarily decrease dose by 0.3 mg increments. Recommended dosage range: 0.3-0.9 mg twice daily. **Note:** Maximum urinary free cortisol reductions are usually observed by 2 months of treatment. The Canadian labeling recommends to consider discontinuation if clinical improvement is not observed after 2 months of therapy.

Dosage adjustment in renal impairment: No dosage adjustment necessary.

Dosage adjustment in hepatic impairment:

Prior to initiation:

U.S. labeling:

Mild impairment (Child-Pugh class A): No dosage adjustment necessary.

Moderate impairment (Child-Pugh class B): Initial: 0.3 mg twice daily (maximum: 0.6 mg twice daily)

Severe impairment (Child-Pugh class C): Use not recommended.

Canadian labeling:

Mild impairment (Child-Pugh class A): No dosage adjustment necessary.

Moderate or severe impairment (Child-Pugh class B or C): Use is contraindicated.

During therapy:

U.S. labeling:

If ALT increases >3 times ULN or baseline value: Recheck ALT during recommended timeframe per recommendations in manufacturer's labeling for confirmation. If ALT level confirmed or increasing, interrupt therapy and investigate potential cause.

If any liver test ≥5 times ULN (with a normal baseline) **OR** >5 times the baseline value (with an abnormal baseline): Interrupt therapy and monitor liver tests more frequently per recommendations in manufacturer's labeling. If values return to normal or near normal, therapy may be reinitiated with extreme caution/monitoring only if another likely cause for hepatic effects discovered.

Canadian labeling:

If ALT increases >3 times ULN <5 times ULN: Recheck ALT in 48 hours and if value remains <5 times ULN continue monitoring ALT every 48 hours. If levels increase >5 times ULN discontinue therapy and do not reinitiate.

If ALT increases >5 times ULN or if ALT or AST increase >3 times ULN concurrently with an increased bilirubin >2 times ULN or if jaundice or other signs of clinically significant hepatic impairment: Discontinue therapy and investigate potential cause. Do not reinitiate therapy.

Administration Administer by subcutaneous injection into the top of the thigh or abdomen (excluding the navel and waistline). Do not inject into inflamed or irritated skin. Alternate the injection site. Do not use if vial contains particulates or solution is discolored.

Monitoring Parameters Urinary free cortisol (24-hour); fasting plasma glucose (FBG) or hemoglobin A1c (Hb A_{1c}) (prior to initiation); FBG and/or self-monitoring glucose (weekly for first 2-3 months then periodically during therapy; Canadian labeling recommends resuming weekly monitoring with dose increases), and FBG or Hb A_{1c} (following discontinuation as clinically appropriate); serum GH and IGF-1 (baseline then periodically); thyroid function (baseline then periodically); potassium and magnesium (prior to therapy then periodically during therapy); ECG (baseline and consider continued monitoring during treatment); gall bladder ultrasonography (baseline, then every 6-12 months during therapy); signs and symptoms of hypocortisolism (eg, weakness, fatigue, nausea, vomiting); heart rate. Additional Canadian labeling recommendations include calcium and lipase prior to therapy and then periodically during therapy.

Liver function tests:

U.S. labeling: 1-2 weeks after initiation, then monthly for 3 months, then every 6 months thereafter; more frequent testing may be necessary:

If ALT ***normal at baseline*** *and ALT increases 3-5 times ULN on therapy:* Repeat ALT within 1 week

If ALT ***normal at baseline*** *and ALT increases >5 times ULN on therapy:* Repeat ALT within 48 hours

If ALT ***abnormal at baseline*** *and ALT increases 3-5 times baseline values on therapy:* Repeat ALT within 1 week

If ALT ***abnormal at baseline*** *and ALT increases >5 times ULN on therapy:* Repeat ALT <1 week

Note: ALT levels should be done in a laboratory capable of same-day results; if ALT levels are confirmed or rising, interrupt therapy and investigate cause.

During therapy, if any liver test ≥5 times ULN (with a normal baseline) **OR** >5 times the baseline value (with an abnormal baseline), interrupt therapy and monitor ALT, AST, alkaline phosphatase, and total bilirubin weekly or more frequently. If values return to normal or near normal, therapy may be reinitiated with extreme caution/monitoring only if another likely cause for hepatic effects discovered.

Canadian labeling: Baseline, weekly for the first month, then every 2 weeks for the next 3 months, then every 3 months thereafter. More frequent testing may be necessary with dose increase or:

If ALT increases >3 times ULN <5 times ULN: Recheck ALT in 48 hours and if value remains <5 times ULN continue monitoring ALT every 48 hours. If levels increase >5 times ULN or if ALT or AST increase >3 times ULN concurrently with an increased bilirubin >2 times ULN or if jaundice or other signs of clinically significant hepatic impairment occur, discontinue therapy and monitor until resolution of hepatic function. Do not reinitiate therapy.

Dosage Forms Excipient information presented when available (limited, particularly for generics); consult specific product labeling.

Solution, Subcutaneous:

Signifor: 0.3 mg/mL (1 mL); 0.6 mg/mL (1 mL); 0.9 mg/mL (1 mL)

- Pasireotide Diaspartate *see* Pasireotide *on page 1579*
- Pataday *see* Olopatadine (Ophthalmic) *on page 1499*
- Pataday™ (Can) *see* Olopatadine (Ophthalmic) *on page 1499*
- Patanase *see* Olopatadine (Nasal) *on page 1499*
- Patanol *see* Olopatadine (Ophthalmic) *on page 1499*
- Patanol® (Can) *see* Olopatadine (Ophthalmic) *on page 1499*
- PAT-Galantamine ER (Can) *see* Galantamine *on page 937*
- Pat-Rabeprazole (Can) *see* RABEprazole *on page 1769*
- Pat-Tramadol/Acet (Can) *see* Acetaminophen and Tramadol *on page 33*
- Pavabid *see* Papaverine *on page 1567*
- Pavulon [DSC] *see* Pancuronium *on page 1560*
- Paxil *see* PARoxetine *on page 1575*
- Paxil CR *see* PARoxetine *on page 1575*

PAZOPanib (paz OH pa nib)

Brand Names: U.S. Votrient

Brand Names: Canada Votrient

Index Terms GW786034; Pazopanib Hydrochloride

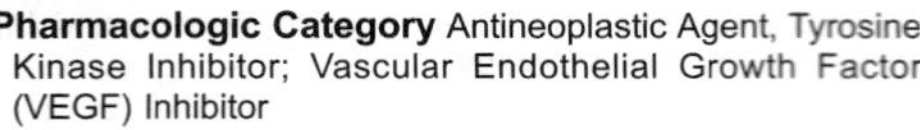

Pharmacologic Category Antineoplastic Agent, Tyrosine Kinase Inhibitor; Vascular Endothelial Growth Factor (VEGF) Inhibitor

Use

Renal cell cancer (RCC): Treatment of advanced RCC

Soft tissue sarcoma (STS): Treatment of advanced STS (in patients previously treated with chemotherapy)

Note: Efficacy for adipocytic STS or gastrointestinal stromal tumor (GIST) has not been demonstrated

Unlabeled Use Treatment of advanced, differentiated thyroid cancer

Pregnancy Risk Factor D

Pregnancy Considerations Adverse effects were observed in animal reproduction studies. Based on its mechanism of action, pazopanib would be expected to cause fetal harm if administered to a pregnant woman. Women of childbearing potential should avoid becoming pregnant during treatment.

Breast-Feeding Considerations It is not known if pazopanib is excreted in breast milk. According to the manufacturer, the decision to continue or discontinue breastfeeding during therapy should take into account the risk of exposure to the infant and the benefits of treatment to the mother.

Medication Guide Available Yes

Contraindications There are no contraindications listed within the manufacturer's U.S. labeling.

Canadian labeling: Hypersensitivity to pazopanib or any component of the formulation

Warnings/Precautions Hazardous agent - use appropriate precautions for handling and disposal (NIOSH, 2012). **[U.S. Boxed Warning]: Severe and fatal hepatotoxicity (transaminase and bilirubin elevations) has been reported with use; monitor hepatic function at baseline, at weeks 3, 5, 7, and 9, at months 3 and 4, and as clinically necessary, then periodically (after month 4); may require dosage interruption, reduction, or discontinuation.** Transaminase elevations usually occur early in the treatment course. Use is not recommended in patients with pre-existing severe hepatic impairment (bilirubin >3 times ULN with any ALT level); dosage reductions is recommended for pre-existing moderate hepatic impairment (bilirubin >1.5-3 times ULN). Patients >60 years of age may be at higher risk for ALT >3 times ULN. Mild indirect (unconjugated) hyperbilirubinemia may occur in patients with Gilbert's syndrome; for patients with known Gilbert's syndrome (only a mild indirect bilirubin elevation) and ALT >3 times ULN, follow isolated ALT elevation dosage modification recommendations.

Venous and arterial thromboembolism have been reported. DVT, pulmonary embolism, angina, transient ischemic attack, MI, and ischemic stroke were observed more frequently in the pazopanib group (versus placebo) in clinical trials. Fatalities were observed. Use with caution in patients with a history of or an increased risk for these events. Use in patients with recent arteriothrombotic event (within 6 months) has not been studied and is not recommended. Thrombotic microangiopathy (TMA), including thrombotic thrombocytopenic purpura (TTP) and hemolytic uremic syndrome (HUS), has been observed in clinical studies. TMA has occurred with pazopanib monotherapy or when used in combination with bevacizumab or topotecan (unlabeled use); it typically occurs within 90 days of treatment initiation. Monitor for signs/symptoms and permanently discontinue in patients who develop TMA. Hemorrhagic events (including fatal) have been reported. In clinical studies, the most common events in renal cell carcinoma patients were hematuria, epistaxis, hemoptysis, and rectal hemorrhage. Epistaxis, mouth hemorrhage, and anal hemorrhage were most common in soft tissue sarcoma patients. Use is not recommended in patients with a history of hemoptysis, cerebral hemorrhage or clinically significant gastrointestinal hemorrhage within 6 months (these populations were excluded from clinical trials).

May cause and/or worsen hypertension (hypertensive crisis has been observed); monitor frequently; blood pressure should be controlled prior to treatment initiation; antihypertensive therapy should be used if needed. Hypertension usually occurs early in the treatment course. Dosage reduction may be necessary for persistent hypertension (despite antihypertensive therapy); discontinue for hypertensive crisis, or for severe and persistent hypertension which is refractory to dose reduction and antihypertensive therapy. May cause new-onset or worsening of existing heart failure; baseline and periodic LVEF monitoring is recommended in patients at increased risk of heart failure (eg, prior anthracycline treatment). Concurrent hypertension may increase the risk for cardiac dysfunction. QT_c prolongation, including torsade de pointes, has been observed; use caution in patients with a history of QT_c prolongation, with medications known to prolong the QT interval, or with pre-existing cardiac disease. Obtain baseline and periodic ECGs; correct electrolyte (potassium, calcium, and magnesium) abnormalities prior to and during treatment.

Gastrointestinal perforation and fistula (including fatal) have been reported; monitor for symptoms of gastrointestinal perforation and fistula. Proteinuria has been reported with use. Obtain baseline and periodic urinalysis and 24-hour urine protein when clinically indicated. Dosage reduction may be necessary for significant proteinuria (≥3 g/24 hours); discontinue for recurrent proteinuria. Hypothyroidism has been reported with use; monitor thyroid function tests. Vascular endothelial growth factor (VEGF) receptor inhibitors are associated with impaired wound healing. Discontinue treatment at least 7 days prior to scheduled surgery; treatment reinitiation should be guided by clinical judgment. Discontinue if wound dehiscence occurs.

Patients with mild-to-moderate renal impairment (Cl_{cr} ≥30 mL/minute) were included in trials. There are no pharmacokinetic data in patients with severe renal impairment undergoing dialysis (peritoneal and hemodialysis); however, renal impairment is not expected to significantly influence pazopanib pharmacokinetics or exposure. Potentially significant drug-drug interactions may exist, requiring dose or frequency adjustment, additional monitoring, and/or selection of alternative therapy. Avoid use with strong CYP3A4 inhibitors or inducers. If pazopanib must be administered concomitantly with a potent enzyme inhibitor, dose reductions are recommended. Use is not recommended in situations where the chronic use of a strong CYP3A4 inducer is required. Pazopanib inhibits UGT1A1 and OATP1B1; pazopanib may increase concentration of drugs eliminated by UGT1A1 and OATP1B1. Pazopanib is a P-glycoprotein (P-gp) and breast cancer resistance protein (BCRP) substrate. Avoid concomitant administration with strong P-gp or BCRP inhibitors; may increase exposure to pazopanib. Increased toxicity and mortality has been observed in trials evaluating concurrent use of pazopanib with other chemotherapeutic agents (pemetrexed, lapatinib). Pazopanib is not approved for use in combination with other chemotherapy.

Reversible posterior leukoencephalopathy syndrome (RPLS) has been reported (rarely); may be fatal. Monitor for neurological changes or symptoms (blindness, confusion, headache, lethargy, seizure, visual or neurologic disturbances); permanently discontinue pazopanib in patients who develop RPLS. Serious, including fatal, infections have been reported; monitor for signs and symptoms of infection. Temporarily or permanently discontinue therapy for serious infections as clinically indicated. Patients ≥65 years of age may be at higher risk of fatigue (grade 3 or 4), hypertension, and decreased appetite. Pazopanib is not approved for use in pediatric patients. Based on its mechanism of action, organ growth, and maturation during early postnatal development may be severely affected, particularly if used in children <2 years of age.

Adverse Reactions

>10%:

Cardiovascular: Hypertension (40% to 42%; grade 3: 4% to 7%), bradycardia (2% to 19%), peripheral edema (14%)

Central nervous system: Fatigue (19% to 65%), headache (10% to 23%), dizziness (11%)

Dermatologic: Hair discoloration (38% to 39%), skin rash (8% to 18%), alopecia (8% to 12%), palmar-plantar erythrodysesthesia (6% to 11%), skin depigmentation (3% to 11%)

Endocrine & metabolic: Hyperglycemia (41% to 45%), hypophosphatemia (34%), hyponatremia (31%), increased thyroid-stimulating hormone (TSH) (27%), hypomagnesemia (26%), hypoglycemia (17%), hyperkalemia (16%)

Gastrointestinal: Diarrhea (52% to 59%; grade 3: 3% to 5%; grade 4: <1%), nausea (26% to 56%), weight loss (9% to 48%), anorexia (22% to 40%), vomiting (21% to 33%), dysgeusia (8% to 28%), increased serum lipase (4% to 27%), abdominal pain (11% to 23%), mucositis (12%), stomatitis (11%)

Hematologic: Leukopenia (37% to 44%; grade 3: ≤1%), lymphocytopenia (31% to 43%; grade 3: 4% to 10%; grade 4: <1%), thrombocytopenia (32% to 36%; grade 3: ≤3%; grade 4: ≤1%), neutropenia (33% to 34%; grade 3: 1% to 4%; grade 4: <1%)

Hepatic: Increased serum AST (51% to 53%; grade 3: 5% to 7%; grade 4: <3%), increased serum ALT (46% to 53%; grade 3: 8% to 10%; grade 4: 2%), increased serum bilirubin (29% to 36%; grade 3: ≤3%; grade 4: <1%), decreased serum albumin (34%), increased serum alkaline phosphatase (32%)

Neuromuscular & skeletal: Musculoskeletal pain (23%), myalgia (23%), weakness (14%)

Respiratory: Dyspnea (20%), cough (17%)

Miscellaneous: Tumor pain (29%)

1% to 10%:

Cardiovascular: Chest pain (5% to 10%), left ventricular systolic dysfunction (≤8%), venous thrombosis (≤5%), ischemic heart disease or myocardial infarction (2%), prolonged QT interval on ECG (≤1% to 2%), facial edema (1%), transient ischemic attacks (≤1%)

Central nervous system: Insomnia (9%), voice disorder (4% to 8%), chills (5%)

Dermatologic: Xeroderma (6%), nail disease (5%)

Endocrine & metabolic: Hypothyroidism (4% to 8%)

Gastrointestinal: Dyspepsia (5% to 7%), oral hemorrhage (3%), rectal hemorrhage (1% to 2%)

Ocular: Blurred vision (5%)

Renal: Proteinuria (1% to 9%), hematuria (4%)

Respiratory: Epistaxis (2% to 8%), pneumothorax (≤3%), hemoptysis (2%), pulmonary embolism (fatal; 1%)

<1% (Limited to important or life-threatening): Cardiac disease, cerebral hemorrhage, cerebrovascular accident, congestive heart failure, gastrointestinal fistula, gastrointestinal perforation (including fistulas), hemolytic-uremic syndrome, hepatotoxicity, hypertensive crisis, intracranial hemorrhage, nephrotic syndrome, pancreatitis, reversible posterior leukoencephalopathy syndrome (RPLS), thrombotic thrombocytopenic purpura, torsade de pointes

Drug Interactions

Metabolism/Transport Effects Substrate of CYP1A2 (minor), CYP2C8 (minor), CYP3A4 (major), P-glycoprotein; **Note:** Assignment of Major/Minor substrate status based on clinically relevant drug interaction potential; **Inhibits** CYP2C8 (weak), CYP2D6 (weak), CYP3A4 (weak), SLCO1B1, UGT1A1

Avoid Concomitant Use

Avoid concomitant use of PAZOPanib with any of the following: BCG; BCRP/ABCG2 Inhibitors; CYP3A4 Inducers (Strong); Fusidic Acid (Systemic); Grapefruit Juice; Highest Risk QTc-Prolonging Agents; Ivabradine; Lapatinib; Mifepristone; Natalizumab; P-glycoprotein/ABCB1 Inhibitors; Pimecrolimus; Tacrolimus (Topical); Tofacitinib; Vaccines (Live)

Increased Effect/Toxicity

PAZOPanib may increase the levels/effects of: ARIPiprazole; Bisphosphonate Derivatives; Highest Risk QTc-Prolonging Agents; Leflunomide; Lomitapide; Moderate Risk QTc-Prolonging Agents; Natalizumab; Tofacitinib; Vaccines (Live); Vitamin K Antagonists

The levels/effects of PAZOPanib may be increased by: BCRP/ABCG2 Inhibitors; CYP3A4 Inhibitors (Moderate); CYP3A4 Inhibitors (Strong); Dasatinib; Denosumab; Fusidic Acid (Systemic); Grapefruit Juice; HMG-CoA Reductase Inhibitors; Ivabradine; Ivacaftor; Lapatinib; Luliconazole; Mifepristone; P-glycoprotein/ABCB1 Inhibitors; Pimecrolimus; QTc-Prolonging Agents (Indeterminate Risk and Risk Modifying); Roflumilast; Simeprevir; Tacrolimus (Topical); Trastuzumab

Decreased Effect

PAZOPanib may decrease the levels/effects of: BCG; Cardiac Glycosides; Coccidioidin Skin Test; Sipuleucel-T; Vaccines (Inactivated); Vaccines (Live); Vitamin K Antagonists

The levels/effects of PAZOPanib may be decreased by: Bosentan; CYP3A4 Inducers (Strong); Deferasirox; Echinacea; Herbs (CYP3A4 Inducers); P-glycoprotein/ABCB1 Inducers; Tocilizumab

Ethanol/Nutrition/Herb Interactions

Food: Systemic exposure of pazopanib is increased when administered with food (AUC twofold higher with a meal). Take on an empty stomach 1 hour before or 2 hours after a meal. Maintain adequate nutrition and hydration, unless instructed to restrict fluid intake. Grapefruit juice may increase the levels/effects of pazopanib. Management: Avoid grapefruit/grapefruit juice.

Herb/Nutraceutical: St John's wort may increase metabolism and decrease pazopanib concentrations. Echinacea may diminish the therapeutic effect. Management: Avoid St John's wort. Consider avoiding echinacea.

Storage/Stability Store at room temperature, 20°C to 25°C (68°F to 77°F); excursions permitted between 15°C and 30°C (59°F and 86°F).

Mechanism of Action Tyrosine kinase (multikinase) inhibitor; limits tumor growth via inhibition of angiogenesis by inhibiting cell surface vascular endothelial growth factor receptors (VEGFR-1, VEGFR-2, VEGFR-3), platelet-derived growth factor receptors (PDGFR-alpha and -beta), fibroblast growth factor receptor (FGFR-1 and -3), cytokine receptor (cKIT), interleukin-2 receptor inducible T-cell kinase, leukocyte-specific protein tyrosine kinase (Lck), and transmembrane glycoprotein receptor tyrosine kinase (c-Fms)

Pharmacodynamics/Kinetics

Protein binding: >99%

Metabolism: Hepatic; primarily via CYP3A4, minor metabolism via CYP1A2 and CYP2C8

Bioavailability: Rate and extent of bioavailability are increased with food and increased if tablets are crushed (do not crush tablets)

Half-life elimination: ~31 hours

Time to peak, plasma: 2-4 hours

Excretion: Feces (primarily); urine (<4%)

Dosage

Renal cell cancer (RCC): Adults: Oral: 800 mg once daily (Sternberg, 2010)

Soft tissue sarcoma (STS), advanced refractory: Adults: Oral: 800 mg once daily (Van Der Graaf, 2012)

Thyroid cancer, advanced differentiated (unlabeled use): Adults: Oral: 800 mg once daily until disease progression or unacceptable toxicity (Bible, 2010)

Missed doses: If a dose is missed, do not take if <12 hours until the next dose.

Dosage adjustment for toxicity:

Initial dosage reduction: **Note:** Prior to dose reduction, temporarily discontinue therapy if 24-hour urine protein ≥3 g or for other toxicities when clinically indicated.

RCC: Reduce to 400 mg once daily

STS: Reduce to 600 mg once daily

Further modification: RCC, STS: Adjust dose in 200 mg increments or decrements based on individual tolerance; maximum dose: 800 mg

Proteinuria (recurrent 24-hour urine protein ≥3 g refractory to dose reduction), hypertension (severe, persistent, and refractory to antihypertensives and dose reduction) or evidence of hypertensive crisis, wound dehiscence: Discontinue treatment.

Infection, serious: Consider treatment interruption or discontinuation.

Reversible posterior leukoencephalopathy syndrome (RPLS), thrombotic microangiopathy (TMA): Permanently discontinue.

Concomitant CYP3A4 inhibitors/inducers:

CYP3A4 inhibitors: Avoid concomitant strong CYP3A4 inhibitors (may increase pazopanib concentrations). If pazopanib must be administered concomitantly with a potent enzyme inhibitor, reduce pazopanib to 400 mg once daily with careful monitoring; further dosage reductions may be needed if adverse events occur.

CYP3A4 inducers: Avoid concomitant strong CYP3A4 inducers (may decrease pazopanib concentrations); use of pazopanib is not recommended in situations where the chronic use of a strong CYP3A4 inducer is required.

Dosage adjustment in renal impairment: No dosage adjustment necessary.

Dosage adjustment in hepatic impairment:

Pre-existing impairment:

Mild (bilirubin ≤1.5 times ULN or ALT >ULN): No dosage adjustment required (Shibata, 2010).

Moderate (bilirubin >1.5-3 times ULN): Consider alternative therapy or reduce to 200 mg once daily (maximum tolerated dose in patients with moderate hepatic impairment) (Shibata, 2010).

Severe (bilirubin >3 times ULN with any ALT level): Use is not recommended.

During treatment:

Isolated ALT elevations 3-8 times ULN: Continue treatment, monitor liver function weekly until ALT returns to grade 1 or baseline.

Isolated ALT elevations >8 times ULN: Interrupt treatment until ALT returns to grade 1 or baseline. If therapy benefit is greater than the risk of hepatotoxicity, may reinitiate treatment at ≤400 mg once daily (with liver function monitored weekly for 8 weeks); permanently discontinue if ALT >3 times ULN occurs with reinitiation.

ALT >3 times ULN concurrently with bilirubin >2 times ULN: Permanently discontinue; monitor until resolution.

Gilbert's syndrome with mild indirect bilirubin elevation and ALT >3 times ULN: Refer to isolated ALT elevations dosage recommendations above.

Dietary Considerations Take on an empty stomach, 1 hour before or 2 hours after a meal. Avoid grapefruit juice.

Administration Administer on an empty stomach, 1 hour before or 2 hours after a meal. Do not crush tablet (rate of absorption may be increased; may affect systemic exposure).

Hazardous agent; use appropriate precautions for handling and disposal (NIOSH, 2012).

Monitoring Parameters Monitor liver function tests at baseline, at weeks 3, 5, 7, and 9, at months 3 and 4, and as clinically necessary, then periodically after month 4 (U.S. labeling) or at weeks 2, 4, 6, and 8 (Canadian labeling); months 3 and 4, and periodically thereafter (monitor more frequently if clinically indicated); serum electrolytes (eg, calcium, magnesium, potassium); urinalysis (for proteinuria; baseline and periodic), 24-hour urine protein (if clinically indicated); thyroid function (TSH and T_4 at baseline and TSH every 6-8 weeks during treatment [Appleby, 2011]); blood pressure; ECG (baseline and periodic); LVEF (if at risk for cardiac dysfunction; baseline and periodic); signs/symptoms of gastrointestinal perforation or fistula, infection, heart failure, or neurological changes.

Additional Information Hand-foot skin reaction (Appleby, 2011): Hand-foot skin reaction (HFSR) observed with tyrosine kinase inhibitors (TKIs) is distinct from hand-foot syndrome (palmar-plantar erythrodysesthesia) associated with traditional chemotherapy agents. HFSR due to TKIs is localized with defined hyperkeratotic lesions; symptoms include burning, dysesthesia, paresthesia, or tingling of the palms/soles, and generally occur within the first 2-4 weeks of treatment. Pressure and flexor areas may develop blisters (callus-like), dry/cracked skin, edema, erythema, desquamation, or hyperkeratosis. The incidence of hand-foot skin reaction (HFSR) is lower with pazopanib (compared to other tyrosine kinase inhibitors). Examine skin at baseline (remove calluses with pedicure prior to treatment) and with each visit; apply an emollient based moisturizer twice daily during treatment. If HSFR develops, consider changing moisturizer to a urea-based product; topical steroids may be utilized for the anti-inflammatory effect; avoid excessive friction or pressure to affected areas and avoid restrictive footwear. Temporary dose reduction or treatment interruption may be necessary.

Dosage Forms Excipient information presented when available (limited, particularly for generics); consult specific product labeling.

Tablet, Oral:

Votrient: 200 mg

- **Pazopanib Hydrochloride** *see* PAZOPanib *on page 1581*
- **PCA (error-prone abbreviation)** *see* Procainamide *on page 1718*
- **PCB** *see* Procarbazine *on page 1720*
- **PCC (Caution: Confusion-prone synonym)** *see* Factor IX Complex (Human) [(Factors II, IX, X)] *on page 822*
- **PCC (Caution: Confusion-prone synonym)** *see* Prothrombin Complex Concentrate (Human) [(Factors II, VII, IX, X), Protein C, and Protein S] *on page 1743*
- **PCE** *see* Erythromycin (Systemic) *on page 741*
- **PCEC** *see* Rabies Vaccine *on page 1772*
- **PCI-32765** *see* Ibrutinib *on page 1030*
- **PCV13** *see* Pneumococcal Conjugate Vaccine (13-Valent) *on page 1661*
- **PCZ** *see* Procarbazine *on page 1720*
- **PDX** *see* PRALAtrexate *on page 1692*
- **PediaCare Childrens Allergy [OTC]** *see* DiphenhydrAMINE (Systemic) *on page 622*

- **PediaCare® Children's Multi-Symptom Cold [OTC]** *see* Dextromethorphan and Phenylephrine *on page 591*
- **Pediacel® (Can)** *see* Diphtheria and Tetanus Toxoids, Acellular Pertussis, Poliovirus and *Haemophilus* b Conjugate Vaccine *on page 629*
- **Pediaderm AF Complete** *see* Nystatin (Topical) *on page 1482*
- **Pediaderm HC** *see* Hydrocortisone (Topical) *on page 1011*
- **Pediaderm TA** *see* Triamcinolone (Topical) *on page 2123*
- **Pedia-Lax [OTC]** *see* Docusate *on page 644*
- **Pedia-Lax [OTC]** *see* Magnesium Hydroxide *on page 1260*
- **Pediapred** *see* PrednisoLONE (Systemic) *on page 1704*
- **Pediapred® (Can)** *see* PrednisoLONE (Systemic) *on page 1704*
- **Pedia Relief Cough and Cold [OTC]** *see* Pseudoephedrine and Dextromethorphan *on page 1748*
- **Pedia Relief™ Cough-Cold [OTC]** *see* Chlorpheniramine, Pseudoephedrine, and Dextromethorphan *on page 414*
- **Pediarix®** *see* Diphtheria, Tetanus Toxoids, Acellular Pertussis, Hepatitis B (Recombinant), and Poliovirus (Inactivated) Vaccine *on page 634*
- **Pediatex® TD** *see* Triprolidine and Pseudoephedrine *on page 2131*
- **Pediatric Cough & Cold [OTC]** *see* Chlorpheniramine, Pseudoephedrine, and Dextromethorphan *on page 414*
- **Pediatric Digoxin CSD (Can)** *see* Digoxin *on page 605*
- **Pediatrix (Can)** *see* Acetaminophen *on page 28*
- **Pediazole® (Can)** *see* Erythromycin and Sulfisoxazole *on page 744*
- **Pedi-Boro® [OTC]** *see* Aluminum Sulfate and Calcium Acetate *on page 91*
- **Pedi-Dri** *see* Nystatin (Topical) *on page 1482*
- **Pedipirox-4 Nail** *see* Ciclopirox *on page 423*
- **PedvaxHIB®** *see* *Haemophilus* b Conjugate Vaccine *on page 981*
- **PEG** *see* Polyethylene Glycol 3350 *on page 1668*
- **PEG-L-asparaginase** *see* Pegaspargase *on page 1586*
- **Peg 3350 (Can)** *see* Polyethylene Glycol 3350 *on page 1668*

Pegademase Bovine (peg A de mase BOE vine)

Brand Names: U.S. Adagen

Brand Names: Canada Adagen®

Pharmacologic Category Enzyme

Use Enzyme replacement therapy for adenosine deaminase (ADA) deficiency in patients with severe combined immunodeficiency disease (SCID) who are not candidates for or who have failed bone marrow transplant

Pregnancy Risk Factor C

Dosage Note: Dose should be individualized based on monitoring of plasma ADA activity levels and dATP content.

Infants and Children: I.M.: Dose given every 7 days, 10 units/kg the first dose, 15 units/kg the second dose, and 20 units/kg the third dose; maintenance dose: 20 units/kg/week is recommended depending on patient's ADA level; maximum single dose: 30 units/kg

Dosage adjustment in renal impairment: No dosage adjustment provided in the manufacturer's labeling.

Dosage adjustment in hepatic impairment: No dosage adjustment provided in the manufacturer's labeling.

Additional Information Complete prescribing information should be consulted for additional detail.

Dosage Forms Excipient information presented when available (limited, particularly for generics); consult specific product labeling.

Solution, Intramuscular:

Adagen: 250 units/mL (1.5 mL)

- **Pegalax (Can)** *see* Polyethylene Glycol 3350 *on page 1668*

Pegaptanib (peg AP ta nib)

Brand Names: U.S. Macugen

Brand Names: Canada Macugen

Index Terms EYE001; Pegaptanib Sodium

Pharmacologic Category Ophthalmic Agent; Vascular Endothelial Growth Factor (VEGF) Inhibitor

Use Macular degeneration: Treatment of neovascular (wet) age-related macular degeneration (AMD)

Pregnancy Risk Factor B

Pregnancy Considerations Adverse events have not been observed in animal reproduction studies.

Breast-Feeding Considerations It is not known if pegaptanib is excreted in breast milk. The manufacturer recommends that caution be exercised when administering pegaptanib to nursing women.

Contraindications Hypersensitivity to pegaptanib or any component of the formulation; ocular or periocular infection

Warnings/Precautions Intravitreous injections are associated with endophthalmitis. Proper aseptic injection techniques should be used and patients should be instructed to report any signs of infection immediately. Retinal detachment and iatrogenic traumatic cataract have been reported. Intraocular pressure may increase within 30 minutes following intravitreal injection. Monitor intraocular pressure and optic nerve perfusion. Safety and efficacy for administration into both eyes concurrently have not been studied. Rare hypersensitivity reactions (including anaphylaxis/anaphylactoid reactions and angioedema) have been associated with pegaptanib, occurring within several hours of use; monitor closely. Equipment and appropriate personnel should be available for monitoring and treatment of anaphylaxis. Thromboembolic events (eg, nonfatal stroke/MI, vascular death) have been reported following intravitreal administration of other VEGF inhibitors.

Adverse Reactions

10% to 40%:

Cardiovascular: Hypertension

Ophthalmic: Anterior chamber inflammation, blurred vision, cataract, conjunctival hemorrhage, corneal edema, eye discharge, eye irritation, eye pain, intraocular pressure increased, ocular discomfort, punctate keratitis, visual acuity decreased, visual disturbance, vitreous floaters, vitreous opacities

1% to 10%:

Cardiovascular: Carotid artery occlusion (1% to 5%), cerebrovascular accident (1% to 5%), chest pain (1% to 5%), transient ischemic attack (1% to 5%)

Central nervous system: Dizziness (6% to 10%), headache (6% to 10%), vertigo (1% to 5%)

Dermatologic: Contact dermatitis (1% to 5%)

Endocrine & metabolic: Diabetes mellitus (1% to 5%)

Gastrointestinal: Diarrhea (6% to 10%), nausea (6% to 10%), dyspepsia (1% to 5%), vomiting (1% to 5%)

Genitourinary: Urinary retention (1% to 5%)

Neuromuscular & skeletal: Arthritis (1% to 5%), bone spur (1% to 5%)

Ophthalmic: Blepharitis (6% to 10%), conjunctivitis (6% to 10%), photopsia (6% to 10%), vitreous disorder (6% to 10%), allergic conjunctivitis (1% to 5%), conjunctival edema (1% to 5%), corneal abrasion (1% to 5%), corneal deposits (1% to 5%), corneal epithelium disorder (1% to 5%), endophthalmitis (1% to 5%), eye inflammation (1% to 5%), eye swelling (1% to 5%), eyelid irritation (1% to 5%), meibomianitis (1% to 5%), mydriasis (1% to 5%), periorbital hematoma (1% to 5%), retinal edema (1% to 5%), vitreous hemorrhage (1% to 5%)

Otic: Hearing loss (1% to 5%)

Renal: Urinary tract infection (6% to 10%)

Respiratory: Bronchitis (6% to 10%), pleural effusion (1% to 5%)

Miscellaneous: Contusion (1% to 5%)

<1% (Limited to important or life-threatening): Anaphylactoid reaction, anaphylaxis, angioedema, blindness, choroidal detachment, colonic polyps, decreased white blood cell count, dysphagia, giant-cell arteritis, hematochezia, hemoptysis, hemorrhage, hypersensitivity, iatrogenic traumatic cataract, immune thrombocytopenia, intracranial hemorrhage, iridocyclitis, iritis, loss of consciousness, mass (pulmonary), neuritis, non-small-cell lung carcinoma (adenocarcinoma), obstructive pulmonary disease, ocular hyperemia, prolonged partial thromboplastin time, pulmonary hemorrhage, retinal detachment, retinal hole without detachment, sprue-like symptoms, subretinal neovascularization, syncope, uveitis (intermediate)

Drug Interactions

Metabolism/Transport Effects None known.

Avoid Concomitant Use There are no known interactions where it is recommended to avoid concomitant use.

Increased Effect/Toxicity There are no known significant interactions involving an increase in effect.

Decreased Effect

The levels/effects of Pegaptanib may be decreased by: Pegloticase

Storage/Stability Store refrigerated at 2°C to 8°C (36°F to 46°F); do not freeze. Do not shake vigorously.

Mechanism of Action Pegaptanib is an apatamer, an oligonucleotide covalently bound to polyethylene glycol, which can adopt a three-dimensional shape and bind to vascular endothelial growth factor (VEGF). Pegaptanib binds to extracellular VEGF, selectively inhibiting VEGF from binding to its receptors and thereby suppressing neovascularization and slowing vision loss.

Pharmacodynamics/Kinetics

Absorption: Slow systemic absorption following intravitreous injection

Metabolism: Metabolized by endo- and exonucleases

Half-life elimination: Plasma: 6-14 days

Dosage Age-related macular degeneration (AMD): Adults: Intravitreous injection: 0.3 mg into affected eye once every 6 weeks

Dosage adjustment in renal impairment:

U.S. labeling: No dosage adjustment provided in manufacturer's labeling.

Canadian labeling:

Cl_{cr} ≥30 mL/minute: No dosage adjustment necessary.

Cl_{cr} <20 mL/minute: No dosage adjustment provided in manufacturer's labeling (has not been studied).

ESRD requiring hemodialysis: No dosage adjustment provided in manufacturer's labeling (has not been studied).

Dosage adjustment in hepatic impairment:

U.S. labeling: No dosage adjustment provided in manufacturer's labeling.

Canadian labeling: Use has not been studied in patients with hepatic impairment.

Administration For ophthalmic intravitreal injection only. Attach a 30 gauge 1/2 inch needle to the medication syringe. Slowly depress plunger to expel excess air and medication (refer to product labeling for detailed instructions). Adequate anesthesia and a topical broad spectrum antibiotic should be administered prior to the procedure.

Monitoring Parameters Intraocular pressure (within 30 minutes and during the week after injection); signs of infection/inflammation (for first week following injection); retinal perfusion, endophthalmitis, visual acuity

Dosage Forms Excipient information presented when available (limited, particularly for generics); consult specific product labeling.

Solution, Intraocular [preservative free]:

Macugen: 0.3 mg (0.09 mL)

◆ **Pegaptanib Sodium** *see* Pegaptanib *on page 1585*

◆ **PEG-ASP** *see* Pegaspargase *on page 1586*

◆ **PEG-asparaginase** *see* Pegaspargase *on page 1586*

Pegaspargase (peg AS par jase)

Brand Names: U.S. Oncaspar

Index Terms L-asparaginase with Polyethylene Glycol; PEG-ASP; PEG-asparaginase; PEG-L-asparaginase; PEGLA; Polyethylene Glycol-L-asparaginase

Pharmacologic Category Antineoplastic Agent, Miscellaneous; Enzyme

Use Treatment of acute lymphocytic leukemia (ALL); treatment of ALL with previous hypersensitivity to native L-asparaginase

Pregnancy Risk Factor C

Pregnancy Considerations Reproduction studies have not been conducted with pegaspargase.

Breast-Feeding Considerations Due to the potential for serious adverse reactions in the nursing infant, breast-feeding is not recommended.

Contraindications History of serious allergic reactions to pegaspargase; history of any of the following with prior L-asparaginase treatment: pancreatitis, serious hemorrhagic events, serious thrombosis

Warnings/Precautions Hazardous agent - use appropriate precautions for handling and disposal (NIOSH, 2012). Serious allergic reactions may occur; discontinue in patients with serious allergic reaction. Observe patients for at least 1 hour after administration; immediate treatment for hypersensitivity reactions should be available during administration. Pegaspargase is indicated for use in patients who have had hypersensitivity reactions to native L-asparaginase; however, in one study, 32% of patients with a history of allergic reaction to *E. coli* asparaginase products also experienced allergic reaction to pegaspargase.

Serious thrombotic events, including sagittal sinus thrombosis may occur; discontinue with serious thrombotic event. Pancreatitis may occur; promptly evaluate patients with abdominal pain; discontinue if pancreatitis occurs during treatment. May cause glucose intolerance; irreversible in some cases; use with caution in patients with hyperglycemia, or diabetes. Coagulopathy has been reported; monitor coagulation parameters; severe or symptomatic coagulopathy may require treatment with fresh-frozen plasma; use with caution in patients with underlying coagulopathy. Reversible hepatotoxicity (hyperbilirubinemia and liver enzyme elevation) may occur; use with caution in patients with hepatic dysfunction or concomitant hepatotoxic medications. Use cautiously in patients with previous hematologic complications from asparaginase.

Adverse Reactions

>5%:

Cardiovascular: Edema

Central nervous system: Fever, malaise

Dermatologic: Rash

Gastrointestinal: Nausea, vomiting

Hematologic: Coagulopathy (7%; grades 3/4: 2%)

Hepatic: Transaminases increased (11%; grades 3/4: 3%)

Miscellaneous: Allergic reactions (including bronchospasm, chills, dyspnea, edema, erythema, hypotension, rash, swelling, urticaria; no prior asparaginase hypersensitivity: 1% to 10%; grades 3/4: 2%; prior asparaginase hypersensitivity: 32%; grades 3/4: 8%)

1% to 5%:

Cardiovascular: Hypotension, peripheral edema, tachycardia, thrombosis (4%)

Central nervous system: Chills, CNS thrombosis (2% to 4%; grades 3/4: 3%), CNS hemorrhage (2%), headache, seizure

Dermatologic: Lip edema, urticaria

Endocrine & metabolic: Hyperglycemia (3% to 5%; grades 3/4: ≤5%), hyperuricemia, hypoglycemia, hypoproteinemia

Gastrointestinal: Abdominal pain, anorexia, diarrhea, pancreatitis (1% to 2%; grades 3/4: 2%)

Hematologic: Anticoagulant effect decreased, disseminated intravascular coagulation (DIC), fibrinogen decreased, hemolytic anemia, leukopenia, pancytopenia, thrombocytopenia, thromboplastin increased, myelosuppression

Hepatic: Liver function tests abnormal (grades 3/4: 5%), hyperbilirubinemia (grades 3/4: 2%), jaundice

Local: Injection site hypersensitivity, pain or reaction

Neuromuscular & skeletal: Arthralgia, limb pain, myalgia, paresthesia

Respiratory: Dyspnea

Miscellaneous: Anaphylactic reactions, night sweats

<1% (Limited to important or life-threatening): Abnormal renal function, alopecia, amylase increased, anemia, antithrombin III decreased, ascites, bacteremia, bone pain, bronchospasm, bruising, BUN increased, chest pain, coagulation time increased, colitis, coma, confusion, constipation, cough, creatinine increased, dizziness, DVT, emotional lability, endocarditis, epistaxis, excessive thirst, face edema, fatigue, fatty liver deposits, gastrointestinal pain, hematuria, hemorrhagic cystitis, hepatomegaly, hyperammonemia, hypertension, hypoalbuminemia, hyponatremia, lipase increased, liver failure, metabolic acidosis, mucositis, petechial rash, proteinuria, prothrombin time increased, purpura, renal failure, sagittal sinus thrombosis, sepsis, septic shock, subacute bacterial endocarditis, superficial venous thrombosis, uric acid nephropathy

Drug Interactions

Metabolism/Transport Effects None known.

Avoid Concomitant Use

Avoid concomitant use of Pegaspargase with any of the following: BCG; Natalizumab; Pimecrolimus; Tacrolimus (Topical); Tofacitinib; Vaccines (Live)

Increased Effect/Toxicity

Pegaspargase may increase the levels/effects of: Leflunomide; Natalizumab; Tofacitinib; Vaccines (Live)

The levels/effects of Pegaspargase may be increased by: Denosumab; Pimecrolimus; Roflumilast; Tacrolimus (Topical); Trastuzumab

Decreased Effect

Pegaspargase may decrease the levels/effects of: BCG; Coccidioidin Skin Test; Sipuleucel-T; Vaccines (Inactivated); Vaccines (Live)

The levels/effects of Pegaspargase may be decreased by: Echinacea; Pegloticase

Preparation for Administration Hazardous agent; use appropriate precautions for handling and disposal (NIOSH, 2012).

I.V.: Dilute in 100 mL NS or D_5W.

Storage/Stability Refrigerate unused vials at 2°C to 8°C (36°F to 46°F); do not freeze. Do not shake; protect from light. Discard vial if previously frozen, stored at room temperature for >48 hours, excessively shaken/agitated, or if cloudy, discolored, or if precipitate is present. If not used immediately, solutions for infusion should be refrigerated at 2°C to 8°C (36°F to 46°F) and used within 48 hours (including administration time).

Mechanism of Action Pegaspargase is a modified version of asparaginase. Leukemic cells, especially lymphoblasts, require exogenous asparagine; normal cells can synthesize asparagine. Asparaginase contains L-asparaginase amidohydrolase type EC-2 which inhibits protein synthesis by deaminating asparagine to aspartic acid and ammonia in the plasma and extracellular fluid and therefore deprives tumor cells of the amino acid for protein synthesis. Asparaginase is cycle-specific for the G_1 phase of the cell cycle.

Pharmacodynamics/Kinetics

Onset: Asparagine depletion: I.M.: Within 4 days

Duration: Asparagine depletion: I.M.: ~21 days; I.V. (in asparaginase naive adults): 2-4 weeks

Absorption: I.M.: Slow

Distribution: I.M.: Children: 1.5 L/m^2; I.V.: Adults (asparaginase naive): 2.4 L/m^2

Metabolism: Systemically degraded

Half-life elimination: I.M.: ~5.5-6 days; unaffected by age, renal or hepatic function; half life decreased to 1.8-3.2 days in patients with previous hypersensitivity to native L-asparaginase; I.V.: Adults (asparaginase naive): 7 days

Time to peak: I.M.: 3-4 days

Excretion: Urine (trace amounts)

Dosage Details concerning dosing in combinations regimens should also be consulted.

Children and Adults: I.M., I.V.: 2500 units/m^2 (as part of a combination chemotherapy regimen), do not administer more frequently than every 14 days

Dosage adjustment in renal impairment: No dosage adjustment provided in manufacturer's labeling.

Hemodialysis, peritoneal dialysis: Significant drug removal is unlikely based on physiochemical characteristics.

Dosage adjustment in hepatic impairment: No dosage adjustment provided in manufacturer's labeling.

Dosing in obesity: *ASCO Guidelines for appropriate chemotherapy dosing in obese adults with cancer:* Utilize patient's actual body weight (full weight) for calculation of body surface area- or weight-based dosing, particularly when the intent of therapy is curative; manage regimen-related toxicities in the same manner as for nonobese patients; if a dose reduction is utilized due to toxicity, consider resumption of full weight-based dosing with subsequent cycles, especially if cause of toxicity (eg, hepatic or renal impairment) is resolved (Griggs, 2012).

Administration Have available appropriate agents for maintenance of an adequate airway and treatment of a hypersensitivity reaction (antihistamine, epinephrine, oxygen, I.V. corticosteroids). Be prepared to treat anaphylaxis at each administration.

I.M.: Must only be administered as a deep intramuscular injection into a large muscle. Do not exceed 2 mL per injection site; use multiple injection sites for I.M. injection volume >2 mL.

I.V.: Administer over 1-2 hours through a running I.V. infusion line; **do not administer I.V. push.**

Hazardous agent; use appropriate precautions for handling and disposal (NIOSH, 2012).

Monitoring Parameters Vital signs during administration, CBC with differential, platelets, amylase, liver enzymes, fibrinogen, PT, PTT (coagulation parameters [baseline and periodic]), renal function tests, urine glucose, blood glucose; monitor for onset of abdominal pain; observe for allergic reaction (for 1 hour after administration)

Dosage Forms Excipient information presented when available (limited, particularly for generics); consult specific product labeling.

Solution, Injection [preservative free]:

Oncaspar: 750 units/mL (5 mL)

◆ Pegasys *see* Peginterferon Alfa-2a *on page 1590*

◆ Pegasys® (Can) *see* Peginterferon Alfa-2a *on page 1590*

◆ Pegasys ProClick *see* Peginterferon Alfa-2a *on page 1590*

Pegfilgrastim (peg fil GRA stim)

Brand Names: U.S. Neulasta

Brand Names: Canada Neulasta®

Index Terms G-CSF (PEG Conjugate); Granulocyte Colony Stimulating Factor (PEG Conjugate); Pegylated G-CSF; SD/01

Pharmacologic Category Colony Stimulating Factor

Use To decrease the incidence of infection, by stimulation of granulocyte production, in patients with nonmyeloid malignancies receiving myelosuppressive therapy associated with a significant risk of febrile neutropenia

Pregnancy Risk Factor C

Pregnancy Considerations Adverse events were observed in some animal reproduction studies.

Women who are exposed to Neulasta during pregnancy are encouraged to enroll in the Amgen Pregnancy Surveillance Program (800-772-6436).

Breast-Feeding Considerations It is not known if pegfilgrastim is excreted in breast milk. The manufacturer recommends that caution be exercised when administering pegfilgrastim to nursing women.

Contraindications Hypersensitivity to pegfilgrastim, filgrastim, or any component of the formulation

Warnings/Precautions Do not use pegfilgrastim in the period 14 days before to 24 hours after administration of cytotoxic chemotherapy because of the potential sensitivity of rapidly dividing myeloid cells to cytotoxic chemotherapy. Benefit has not been demonstrated with regimens under a two-week duration. Administration on the same day as chemotherapy is not recommended (NCCN Myeloid Growth Factor Guidelines, v.1.2011). Pegfilgrastim can potentially act as a growth factor for any tumor type, particularly myeloid malignancies. Caution should be exercised in the usage of pegfilgrastim in any malignancy with myeloid characteristics. Tumors of nonhematopoietic origin may have surface receptors for pegfilgrastim. Pegfilgrastim has not been evaluated with patients receiving radiation therapy, or with chemotherapy associated with delayed myelosuppression (nitrosoureas, mitomycin). Safety and efficacy have not been evaluated for peripheral blood progenitor cell (PBPC) mobilization.

Allergic-type reactions (anaphylaxis, angioedema, erythema, skin rash, urticaria) have occurred primarily with the initial dose and may recur (possibly delayed) after discontinuation; close follow up for several days and permanent discontinuation are recommended for severe reactions. Rare cases of splenic rupture have been reported; patients must be instructed to report left upper quadrant pain or shoulder tip pain. Acute respiratory distress syndrome (ARDS) has been associated with use; evaluate patients with pulmonary symptoms such as fever, lung infiltrates, or respiratory distress; discontinue or withhold pegfilgrastim if ARDS occurs. May precipitate sickle cell crises in patients with sickle cell disease; carefully evaluate potential risks and benefits. The packaging (needle cover) contains latex. The 6 mg fixed dose should not be used in infants, children, and adolescents weighing <45 kg.

Adverse Reactions

>10%:

Cardiovascular: Peripheral edema (12%)

Central nervous system: Headache (16%)

Gastrointestinal: Vomiting (13%)

Neuromuscular & skeletal: Bone pain (31% to 57%), myalgia (21%), arthralgia (16%), weakness (13%)

1% to 10%:

Gastrointestinal: Constipation (10%)

Miscellaneous: Antibody formation (1% to 6%)

<1% (Limited to important or life-threatening): Acute respiratory distress syndrome (ARDS), allergic reaction, anaphylaxis, cutaneous vasculitis, erythema, fever, flushing, hyperleukocytosis, hypoxia, injection site reactions (erythema, induration, pain), leukocytosis, rash, sickle cell crisis, splenic rupture, Sweet's syndrome (acute febrile dermatosis), urticaria. Cytopenias resulting from an antibody response to exogenous growth factors have been reported on rare occasions in patients treated with other recombinant growth factors.

Drug Interactions

Metabolism/Transport Effects None known.

Avoid Concomitant Use There are no known interactions where it is recommended to avoid concomitant use.

Increased Effect/Toxicity There are no known significant interactions involving an increase in effect.

Decreased Effect

The levels/effects of Pegfilgrastim may be decreased by: Pegloticase

Storage/Stability Store under refrigeration 2°C to 8°C (36°F to 46°F); do not freeze. If inadvertently frozen, allow to thaw in refrigerator; discard if frozen more than one time. Protect from light. Do not shake. Allow to reach room temperature prior to injection. May be kept at room temperature for up to 48 hours.

Mechanism of Action Stimulates the production, maturation, and activation of neutrophils, pegfilgrastim activates neutrophils to increase both their migration and cytotoxicity. Pegfilgrastim has a prolonged duration of effect relative to filgrastim and a reduced renal clearance.

Pharmacodynamics/Kinetics Half-life elimination: SubQ: Adults: 15-80 hours; Children (100 mcg/kg dose): ~20-30 hours (range: up to 68 hours)

Dosage SubQ: **Note:** Do not administer in the period between 14 days before and 24 hours after administration of cytotoxic chemotherapy. According to the NCCN guidelines, efficacy has been demonstrated with every-2-week chemotherapy regimens, however, benefit has not been demonstrated with regimens under a 2-week duration (NCCN Myeloid Growth Factor Guidelines, v.1.2011)

Children (unlabeled dose): 100 mcg/kg (maximum dose: 6 mg) once per chemotherapy cycle, beginning 24-72 hours after completion of chemotherapy

Adolescents >45 kg and Adults: 6 mg once per chemotherapy cycle, beginning 24-72 hours after completion of chemotherapy

Dosage adjustment in renal impairment: No dosage adjustment necessary.

Dosage adjustment in hepatic impairment: No dosage adjustment provided in manufacturer's labeling (has not been studied).

Administration Administer subcutaneously. Do not use 6 mg fixed dose in infants, children, or adolescents <45 kg. Engage/activate needle guard following use to prevent accidental needlesticks.

Monitoring Parameters Complete blood count (with differential) and platelet count should be obtained prior to chemotherapy. Leukocytosis (white blood cell counts 100,000/mm^3) has been observed in <1% of patients receiving pegfilgrastim. Monitor platelets and hematocrit regularly. Evaluate fever, pulmonary infiltrates, and respiratory distress; evaluate for left upper abdominal pain, shoulder tip pain, or splenomegaly. Monitor for sickle cell crisis (in patients with sickle cell anemia).

Test Interactions May interfere with bone imaging studies; increased hematopoietic activity of the bone marrow may appear as transient positive bone imaging changes

Dosage Forms Excipient information presented when available (limited, particularly for generics); consult specific product labeling.

Solution, Subcutaneous [preservative free]:

Neulasta: 6 mg/0.6 mL (0.6 mL)

◆ PEG-IFN Alfa-2a *see* Peginterferon Alfa-2a *on page 1590*

◆ PEG-IFN Alfa-2b *see* Peginterferon Alfa-2b *on page 1594*

Peginesatide (peg in ESS a tide)

Brand Names: U.S. Omontys

Index Terms Erythropoiesis-Stimulating Agent (ESA); Hematide; Omontys®

Pharmacologic Category Colony Stimulating Factor; Erythropoiesis-Stimulating Agent (ESA); Growth Factor

Use Treatment of anemia due to chronic kidney disease (CKD) in patients receiving dialysis

Note: Peginesatide is **not** indicated for use under the following conditions:

- CKD patients not receiving dialysis
- Cancer patients with anemia that is not due to CKD
- As a substitute for RBC transfusion in patients requiring immediate correction of anemia

Note: Peginesatide has not demonstrated improved symptoms, physical functioning, or health-related quality of life.

Pregnancy Risk Factor C

Pregnancy Considerations Adverse events were observed in animal reproduction studies with maternal exposure similar to that observed with human doses.

Breast-Feeding Considerations It is not known if peginesatide is excreted in breast milk. The manufacturer recommends that caution be exercised when administering peginesatide to nursing women.

Medication Guide Available Yes

Contraindications Serious hypersensitivity to peginesatide or any component of the formulation; uncontrolled hypertension

Warnings/Precautions [U.S. Boxed Warning]: An increased risk of death, serious cardiovascular events, and stroke was reported in chronic kidney disease (CKD) patients administered ESAs to target hemoglobin levels >11 g/dL; use the lowest dose sufficient to reduce the need for RBC transfusions. An optimal target hemoglobin level, dose, or dosing strategy to reduce these risks have not been identified in clinical trials. Hemoglobin rising >1 g/dL in a 2-week period may contribute to the risk (dosage reduction recommended). CKD patients who exhibit an inadequate hemoglobin response to ESA therapy may be at a higher risk for cardiovascular events and mortality compared to other patients. Adjustments in dialysis parameters may be needed after initiation of peginesatide. Patients treated with peginesatide may require increased heparinization during dialysis to prevent clotting of the extracorporeal circuit. Therapy is not appropriate for anemia treatment in CKD patients *not* receiving dialysis.

Use with caution in patients with a history of hypertension (contraindicated in uncontrolled hypertension) or cardiovascular disease (history or active) and stroke. Blood pressure should be controlled prior to start of (and during) therapy; monitor closely throughout treatment and reduce or withhold peginesatide if blood pressure becomes difficult to control. In clinical trials involving ESAs, an increased risk of death was observed in patients undergoing coronary artery bypass surgery (CABG) and an increased risk of deep vein thrombosis (DVT) was seen in those undergoing orthopedic procedures. Clinical trials involving ESAs in cancer patients have shown an increased risk of death, MI, and stroke. Peginesatide is not indicated in cancer patients with anemia who do not have chronic kidney disease. Due to the delayed onset of erythropoiesis, peginesatide is not recommended for acute correction of severe anemia or as a substitute for emergency transfusion.

Allergic reactions, including anaphylactic reactions, hypotension, bronchospasm, angioedema, and generalized pruritus, have been reported (rarely). Discontinue immediately and treat symptoms appropriately in patients who experience serious allergic/anaphylactic reactions. Seizures have been observed in clinical studies with use; use with caution in patients with a history of seizures. Monitor closely for neurologic symptoms during the first several months of therapy. Prior to and periodically during therapy, iron stores must be evaluated. Supplemental iron is recommended if serum ferritin <100 mcg/L or serum transferrin saturation <20%. Most patients with CKD will require iron supplementation.

Prior to treatment, correct or exclude deficiencies of iron, vitamin B_{12}, and/or folate, as well as other factors which may impair erythropoiesis (inflammatory conditions, infections, bleeding). Patients with a sudden loss of hemoglobin response should also be evaluated for potential causes of decreased response. If common causes are excluded, patient should be evaluated for the presence of peginesatide antibodies. During trials, peginesatide-specific binding antibodies were detected rarely (with a higher incidence noted in patients receiving subcutaneous compared to I.V. administration); however, no cases of pure red cell aplasia (PRCA) were observed in studies. Peginesatide is a synthetic, peptide-based ESA agent and cross-reactivity of the immune response against either endogenous or recombinant protein-based erythropoietin agents (eg, epoetin, darbepoetin) to peginesatide is unlikely due to the difference in amino acid sequence (Macdougall, 2011).

Adverse Reactions

>10%:

Cardiovascular: Hypotension (14%), hypertension (13%), procedural hypotension (11%)

Central nervous system: Headache (15%), fever (12%)

Endocrine & metabolic: Hyperkalemia (11%)

Gastrointestinal: Diarrhea (18%), nausea (17%), vomiting (15%)

Neuromuscular & skeletal: Muscle spasms (15%), arthralgia (11%), back pain (11%), extremity pain (11%)

Respiratory: Dyspnea (18%), cough (16%), upper respiratory tract infection (11%)

Miscellaneous: Arteriovenous fistula site complication (16%)

1% to 10%: Miscellaneous: Peginesatide-specific binding antibodies (1%)

<1% (Limited to important or life-threatening): Allergic reaction, infusion-related reactions, seizures

Drug Interactions

Metabolism/Transport Effects None known.

Avoid Concomitant Use There are no known interactions where it is recommended to avoid concomitant use.

Increased Effect/Toxicity There are no known significant interactions involving an increase in effect.

Decreased Effect There are no known significant interactions involving a decrease in effect.

Preparation for Administration Do not dilute prior to administration.

Storage/Stability Store refrigerated at 2°C to 8°C (36°F to 46°F). Protect from light. If necessary, may store at temperatures ≤25°C (77°F) for ≤30 days. After initial entry, store multidose vials at 2°C to 8°C (36°F to 46°F); discard after 28 days.

Mechanism of Action Peginesatide, a pegylated synthetic peptide, binds to the human erythropoietin receptor to induce erythropoiesis by stimulating the division and differentiation of committed erythroid progenitor cells; induces the release of reticulocytes from the bone marrow into the bloodstream, where they mature to erythrocytes. There is a dose response relationship with this effect. This results in an increase in reticulocyte counts followed by a rise in hemoglobin levels.

Pharmacodynamics/Kinetics

Distribution: I.V.: Dialysis patients: V_d: 34.9 mL/kg

Bioavailability: SubQ: ~46%

Half-life elimination: I.V.: Healthy subjects: 25 hours, Dialysis patients: 47.9 hours; SubQ: Healthy patients: 53 hours

Time to peak: SubQ: ~48 hours

Dosage I.V., SubQ: Adults: Anemia associated with chronic kidney disease in patients receiving dialysis: Individualize dosing and use the lowest dose necessary to reduce the need for RBC transfusions.

Patients not currently receiving an erythropoiesis-stimulating agent (ESA) (initiate when hemoglobin is <10 g/dL): Initial dose: 0.04 mg/kg once monthly

Conversion from another ESA (epoetin or darbepoetin) to peginesatide: **Note:** The initial monthly peginesatide dose can be estimated based on the weekly dose of epoetin or darbepoetin at the time of substitution (see table); the same route of administration (SubQ or I.V.) of the previous ESA should be maintained after conversion to peginesatide. If previous ESA was epoetin, the first dose of peginesatide should be 1 week after the last epoetin dose. If previous ESA was darbepoetin, the first dose of peginesatide should be given in the place of darbepoetin at the next scheduled dose.

Conversion from Another ESA (Epoetin or Darbepoetin) to Peginesatide

Previous *Epoetin Alfa* Total WEEKLY Dose (units/wk)	Previous *Darbepoetin Alfa* WEEKLY Dose (mcg/wk)	Initial *Peginesatide* MONTHLY Dose (mg/mo)
<2500	<12	2
2500 to <4300	12 to <18	3
4300 to <6500	18 to <25	4
6500 to <8900	25 to <35	5
8900 to <13,000	35 to <45	6
13,000 to <19,000	45 to <60	8
19,000 to <33,000	60 to <95	10
33,000 to <68,000	95 to <175	15
≥68,000	≥175	20

Dosage adjustments:

If hemoglobin does not increase by >1 g/dL after 4 weeks: Increase dose by 25%; do not increase the dose more frequently than once every 4 weeks

If hemoglobin increases >1 g/dL in the 2-week period prior to the dose or >2 g/dL in 4 weeks: Reduce dose by 25% (or more) as needed to reduce rapid response

If hemoglobin approaches or exceeds 11 g/dL: Reduce or interrupt dose; after dose has been withheld and once the hemoglobin begins to decrease, may resume dose at ~25% below the previous dose

Inadequate or lack of response over a 12-week escalation period: Further increases are unlikely to improve response and may increase risks; use the minimum effective dose that will maintain a Hgb level sufficient to avoid RBC transfusions and evaluate patient for other causes of anemia. Discontinue therapy if responsiveness does not improve.

Missed doses: Administer a missed dose as soon as possible and restart peginesatide at the prescribed once monthly dosing frequency.

Dosing adjustment in renal impairment: No dosage adjustment provided in manufacturer's labeling.

Dosing adjustment in hepatic impairment: No dosage adjustment provided in manufacturer's labeling (has not been studied).

Administration May be administered as an I.V. injection or SubQ injection. The I.V. route is generally used for hemodialysis patients; medication is injected via a special access port on the dialysis tubing during the dialysis procedure. Peritoneal dialysis patients should only administer therapy via the SubQ route. For SubQ injections, may inject in either the outer area of the upper arms, the front of the middle thighs, the abdomen (excluding the 2-inch area around the navel), or the upper outer buttocks area. Do not inject in skin that is tender, red, hard, scarred, or bruised.

Monitoring Parameters Transferrin saturation and serum ferritin (prior to initiation and during therapy); hemoglobin (every 2 weeks after initiation and following dose adjustments until stable and sufficient to minimize need for RBC transfusion, then at least monthly following hemoglobin stability); blood pressure; seizures (following initiation for first few months, includes new-onset or change in seizure frequency or premonitory symptoms); allergic reaction; presence of antibodies (if common causes of lack or loss of response are ruled out)

Additional Information For information regarding evaluating patients for the presence of binding and neutralizing antibodies to peginesatide, contact Affymax, Inc (1-855-466-6689).

Dosage Forms Excipient information presented when available (limited, particularly for generics); consult specific product labeling.

Solution, Injection:

Omontys: 10 mg/mL (1 mL); 20 mg/2 mL (2 mL) [contains phenol]

Peginterferon Alfa-2a

(peg in ter FEER on AL fa too aye)

Brand Names: U.S. Pegasys; Pegasys ProClick

Brand Names: Canada Pegasys®

Index Terms Interferon Alfa-2a (PEG Conjugate); PEG-IFN Alfa-2a; Pegylated Interferon Alfa-2a

Pharmacologic Category Interferon

Use

Chronic hepatitis B: Treatment of adults with hepatitis B e antigen (HBeAg)-positive and HBeAG-negative chronic hepatitis B virus (HBV) infection who have compensated liver disease and evidence of viral replication and liver inflammation

Chronic hepatitis C:

Treatment of patients with chronic hepatitis C virus (HCV) infection who have compensated liver disease and have not been previously treated with interferon alfa, alone or in combination with ribavirin (monotherapy with peginterferon alfa-2a is not recommended for treatment of chronic hepatitis C infection unless a patient has a contraindication to or significant intolerance of ribavirin). Efficacy was demonstrated in patients with compensated liver disease and histological evidence of cirrhosis (Child-Pugh class A), and adult patients with clinically stable HIV disease (CD4 count >100 cells/mm^3).

Combination with ribavirin and an HCV NS3/4A protease inhibitor is indicated in adults with HCV genotype 1.

Combination with ribavirin is indicated in patients with HCV genotypes other than 1, children ≥5 years of age and adolescents, or patients with HCV genotype 1 where use of an HCV NS3/4A protease inhibitor is not warranted based on tolerability, contraindications or other clinical factors.

Pregnancy Risk Factor C / X in combination with ribavirin

Pregnancy Considerations Reproduction studies with pegylated interferon alfa have not been conducted. Animal studies with nonpegylated interferon alfa-2b have demonstrated abortifacient effects. Disruption of the normal menstrual cycle was also observed in animal studies; therefore, the manufacturer recommends that reliable contraception is used in women of childbearing potential. Alfa interferon is endogenous to normal amniotic fluid. *In vitro* administration studies have reported that when administered to the mother, it does not cross the placenta. Case reports of use in pregnant women are limited. The Perinatal HIV Guidelines Working Group does not recommend that peginterferon-alfa be used during pregnancy. Peginterferon monotherapy should only be used in pregnancy when the potential benefit to the mother justifies the possible risk to the fetus. **[U.S. Boxed Warning]: Combination therapy with ribavirin may cause birth defects; avoid pregnancy in females and female partners of male patients;** combination therapy with ribavirin is contraindicated in pregnancy (refer to Ribavirin monograph); a pregnancy registry has been established for women inadvertently exposed to ribavirin while pregnant (800-593-2214).

Breast-Feeding Considerations Breast milk samples obtained from a lactating mother prior to and after administration of interferon alfa-2b showed that interferon alfa is present in breast milk and administration of the medication did not significantly affect endogenous levels. Breast-feeding is not linked to the spread of hepatitis C virus; however, if nipples are cracked or bleeding, breast-feeding is not recommended. Mothers coinfected with HIV are discouraged from breast-feeding to decrease potential transmission of HIV.

Medication Guide Available Yes

Contraindications Hypersensitivity to polyethylene glycol (PEG), interferon alfa, or any component of the formulation; autoimmune hepatitis; decompensated liver disease in cirrhotic patients (Child-Pugh score >6); decompensated liver disease (Child-Pugh score ≥6, class B and C) in CHC coinfected with HIV; neonates and infants

Warnings/Precautions **[U.S. Boxed Warning]: May cause or exacerbate life-threatening neuropsychiatric disorders; monitor closely; discontinue treatment with worsening or persistently severe signs/symptoms of neuropsychiatric disorders. In most cases these effects were reversible following discontinuation, but not all cases.** Neuropsychiatric adverse effects include depression, suicidal ideation, suicide attempt, homicidal ideation, drug overdose, and relapse of drug addiction, and may occur in patients with or without a prior history of psychiatric disorder. Avoid use in severe psychiatric disorders; use with extreme caution in patients with a history of depression. Patients who experience dizziness, confusion, somnolence or fatigue should use caution when performing tasks which require mental alertness (eg, operating machinery or driving).

[U.S. Boxed Warning]: May cause or exacerbate autoimmune disorders; monitor closely; discontinue treatment in patients with worsening or persistently severe signs/symptoms of autoimmune disease. Thyroiditis, thrombotic thrombocytopenic purpura, immune thrombocytopenia (ITP), rheumatoid arthritis, interstitial nephritis, systemic lupus erythematosus, and psoriasis have been reported with interferon therapy; use with caution in patients with autoimmune disorders.

[U.S. Boxed Warning]: May cause or aggravate infectious disorders; monitor closely; discontinue treatment in patients with worsening or persistently severe signs/symptoms of infectious disorders. Serious and severe infections (bacterial, viral, and fungal) have been reported with treatment. Interferon therapy is commonly associated with flu-like symptoms, including fever; however, rule out other causes/infection with persistent or high fever.

[U.S. Boxed Warning]: May cause or aggravate ischemic disorders and hemorrhagic cerebrovascular events; monitor closely; discontinue treatment in patients with worsening or persistent ischemia. Has been reported in patients without risk factors for stroke.

[U.S. Boxed Warning]: Combination treatment with ribavirin may cause birth defects and/or fetal mortality (avoid pregnancy in females and female partners of male patients); hemolytic anemia (which may worsen cardiac disease), genotoxicity, mutagenicity, and may possibly be carcinogenic.

May cause myelosuppression (including neutropenia, thrombocytopenia, lymphopenia, aplastic anemia). Use caution with baseline neutrophil count <1500/mm^3, platelet count <90,000/mm^3 or hemoglobin <10 g/dL. Discontinue therapy (at least temporarily) if ANC <500/mm^3 or platelet count <25,000/mm^3.

Hepatic decompensation and death have been associated with the use of alpha interferons including Pegasys®, in cirrhotic chronic hepatitis C patients; patients coinfected with HIV and receiving highly active antiretroviral therapy have shown an increased risk. Monitor hepatic function closely during use; discontinue if decompensation occurs (Child-Pugh score >6) in monoinfected patients and (Child-Pugh score ≥6, class B and C) in patients coinfected with HIV. In hepatitis B patients, flares (transient and potentially severe increases in serum ALT) may occur during or after treatment; more frequent monitoring of LFTs and a dose reduction are recommended. Discontinue if ALT elevation continues despite dose reduction or if increased bilirubin or hepatic decompensation occur.

Gastrointestinal hemorrhage, ulcerative and hemorrhagic/ischemic colitis have been observed with interferon alfa treatment; may be severe and/or life-threatening; discontinue if symptoms of colitis (eg, abdominal pain, bloody diarrhea, and/or fever) develop. Colitis generally resolves within 1-3 weeks of discontinuation. Discontinue therapy if known or suspected pancreatitis develops.

Use with caution in patients with diabetes mellitus; hyper- or hypoglycemia have been reported which may require adjustments in medications. Use with caution in patients with pre-existing thyroid disease; thyroid disorders (hyper- or hypothyroidism) or exacerbations have been reported. Use with caution in patients with prior cardiovascular disease; hypertension, arrhythmia, chest pain, and MI have been observed with treatment.

Severe acute hypersensitivity reactions (including anaphylaxis) have occurred rarely; prompt discontinuation is advised. Serious cutaneous reactions, including vesiculobullous eruptions, Stevens-Johnson syndrome and exfoliative dermatitis, have been reported (rarely) with use, with or without ribavirin therapy; discontinue with signs or symptoms of severe skin reactions.

Discontinue if new or worsening ophthalmologic disorders occur including decreased vision, retinal hemorrhages, retinal detachment (serous), cotton wool spots, and retinal artery or vein obstruction; if any ocular symptoms occur during use, a complete eye exam should be performed promptly. Prior to use, all patients should have a visual exam and patients with pre-existing disorders (eg, diabetic or hypertensive retinopathy) should have exams periodically during therapy.

May cause or aggravate dyspnea, pulmonary infiltrates, pneumonia, bronchiolitis obliterans, interstitial pneumonia, and sarcoidosis, resulting in potentially fatal respiratory failure; may recur upon rechallenge with interferons. Discontinue with unexplained pulmonary infiltrates or evidence of impaired pulmonary function. Use caution in patients with a history of pulmonary disease. Use with caution in patients with renal dysfunction (Cl_{cr} <30 mL/minute); monitor for signs/symptoms of toxicity (dosage adjustment required if toxicity occurs).

Safety and efficacy have not been established in patients who have failed other alpha interferon therapy, have received liver or other organ transplants, have been coinfected with HBV **and** HCV or HIV, have been coinfected with HCV **and** HBV or HIV with a $CD4^+$ cell count <100 cells/mm^3, or been treated for >48 weeks.

Due to differences in dosage, patients should not change brands of interferon without the concurrence of their healthcare provider.

Delay in weight and height increases have been noted in children treated with interferon alfa and concomitant ribavirin for 48 weeks. At two-year follow up after treatment, most children had returned to their baseline growth curve percentiles. Use with caution in the elderly; certain adverse effects (eg, neuropsychiatric, cardiac, flu-like reactions) may be more severe. Pretreatment hematological and biochemical tests are recommended for all patients; pregnancy screening (if woman of childbearing age) and ECG (if pre-existing cardiac abnormalities) are also recommended.

Adverse Reactions Note: Percentages are reported for peginterferon alfa-2a in chronic hepatitis C (CHC) patients. Other percentages indicated as "with ribavirin" or "in HIV/CHC" are those which significantly exceed incidence reported for peginterferon monotherapy in CHC patients.

>10%:

- Central nervous system: Headache (54%), fatigue (56%), fever (37%; 41% with ribavirin; 54% in hepatitis B), insomnia (19%; 30% with ribavirin), depression (18%), dizziness (16%), irritability/anxiety/nervousness (19%; 33% with ribavirin), pain (11%)
- Dermatologic: Alopecia (23%; 28% with ribavirin), pruritus (12%; 19% with ribavirin), dermatitis (16% with ribavirin)
- Endocrine & metabolic: Growth suppression (children) percentile decrease (≥15 percentiles), weight (43%), height (25%)
- Gastrointestinal: Nausea/vomiting (24%), anorexia (17%; 24% with ribavirin), diarrhea (16%), weight loss (16% in HIV/CHC), abdominal pain (15%)
- Hematologic: Neutropenia (21%; 27% with ribavirin; 40% in HIV/CHC), lymphopenia (14% with ribavirin), anemia (11% with ribavirin; 14% in HIV/CHC)
- Hepatic: ALT increases 5-10 x ULN during treatment (25% to 27% in hepatitis B); ALT increases >10 x ULN during treatment (12% to 18% in hepatitis B); ALT increases 5-10 x ULN after treatment (13% to 16% in hepatitis B); ALT increases >10 x ULN after treatment (7% to 12% in hepatitis B)
- Local: Injection site reaction (22%)
- Neuromuscular & skeletal: Weakness (56%; 65% with ribavirin), myalgia (37%), rigors (35%; 25% to 27% in hepatitis B), arthralgia (28%)
- Respiratory: Dyspnea (13% with ribavirin)

1% to 10%:

- Central nervous system: Concentration impaired (8%), memory impaired (5%), mood alteration (3%; 9% in HIV/CHC)
- Dermatologic: Dermatitis (8%), rash (5%), dry skin (4%; 10% with ribavirin), eczema (1%; 5% with ribavirin)
- Endocrine & metabolic: Hypothyroidism (3% to 4%), hyperthyroidism (≤1%)
- Gastrointestinal: Xerostomia (6%), dyspepsia (<1%; 6% with ribavirin), weight loss (4%; 10% with ribavirin)
- Hematologic: Thrombocytopenia (5%; 8% in HIV/CHC), lymphopenia (3%), anemia (2%)
- Hepatic: Hepatic decompensation (2% in CHC/HIV)
- Neuromuscular & skeletal: Back pain (9%)
- Ocular: Blurred vision (4%)
- Respiratory: Cough (4%; 10% with ribavirin), dyspnea (4%), exertional dyspnea (4% with ribavirin)
- Miscellaneous: Diaphoresis (6%), bacterial infection (3%; 5% in HIV/CHC)

≤1% (Limited to important or life-threatening): Aggression, anaphylaxis, angioedema, angina, aplastic anemia, arrhythmia, autoimmune disorders, bronchiolitis obliterans, bronchoconstriction, cerebral hemorrhage, chest pain, cholangitis, colitis, coma, corneal ulcer, cotton wool spots, dehydration, diabetes mellitus, endocarditis, erythema multiforme major, exertional dyspnea, exfoliative dermatitis, fatty liver, gastrointestinal bleeding, hallucination, hearing impairment, hearing loss, hemoglobin decreased, hematocrit decreased, hepatic dysfunction, hepatic graft rejection, hepatitis B flares, hyper-/hypoglycemia, hypersensitivity reactions, hypertension, influenza, interstitial pneumonitis, macular edema, MI, myositis, optic neuritis, papilledema, pancreatitis, peptic ulcer, peripheral neuropathy, pneumonia, psychiatric disorder, psychosis, pulmonary embolism, pulmonary infiltrates, pure red cell aplasia, renal graft rejection, retinal artery/vein thrombosis, retinal detachment, retinal hemorrhage, retinopathy, rheumatoid arthritis, sarcoidosis, seizures, Stevens-Johnson syndrome, substance overdose, suicidal ideation, suicide, supraventricular arrhythmia, systemic lupus erythematosus, thrombotic thrombocytopenic purpura, triglycerides (increased), urticaria, vesiculobullous eruptions, vision decreased/loss

Drug Interactions

Metabolism/Transport Effects Inhibits CYP1A2 (weak)

Avoid Concomitant Use

Avoid concomitant use of Peginterferon Alfa-2a with any of the following: CloZAPine; Telbivudine

Increased Effect/Toxicity

Peginterferon Alfa-2a may increase the levels/effects of: Aldesleukin; CloZAPine; Methadone; Ribavirin; Telbivudine; Theophylline Derivatives; Zidovudine

Decreased Effect

The levels/effects of Peginterferon Alfa-2a may be decreased by: Pegloticase

Ethanol/Nutrition/Herb Interactions Ethanol: Avoid use in patients with hepatitis C virus.

Storage/Stability Store in refrigerator at 2°C to 8°C (36°F to 46°F). Do not freeze or shake. Protect from light. The following stability information has also been reported:

- Intact vial: May be stored at room temperature for up to 14 days (Cohen, 2007).
- Prefilled syringe: May be stored at room temperature for up to 6 days (Cohen, 2007).

Mechanism of Action Alpha interferons are a family of proteins, produced by nucleated cells that have antiviral, antiproliferative, and immune-regulating activity. There are 16 known subtypes of alpha interferons. Interferons interact with cells through high affinity cell surface receptors. Following activation, multiple effects can be detected including induction of gene transcription. Interferons inhibit cellular growth, alter the state of cellular differentiation, interfere with oncogene expression, alter cell surface antigen expression, increase phagocytic activity of macrophages, and augment cytotoxicity of lymphocytes for target cells.

Pharmacodynamics/Kinetics

Half-life elimination: Terminal: 50-160 hours; increased with renal dysfunction

Time to peak, serum: 72-96 hours

Dosage

Chronic hepatitis C: Children ≥5 years and Adolescents: SubQ: 180 mcg/1.73 m^2 x body surface area (BSA) once weekly (maximum dose: 180 mcg) with ribavirin (Copegus®)

Duration of therapy (based on genotype):

Genotypes 1,4,5,6: 48 weeks

Genotypes 2,3: 24 weeks

Chronic hepatitis C (monoinfection or coinfection with HIV): Adults: SubQ: 180 mcg once weekly for 48 weeks as monotherapy or in combination with ribavirin (Copegus®)

Duration of combination therapy: Monoinfection (based on genotype):

Genotypes 1,4: 48 weeks

Genotypes 2,3: 24 weeks

Genotypes 5,6: No dosing recommendations provided; data insufficient

Duration of therapy: Coinfection with HIV: 48 weeks

Note: *American Association for the Study of Liver Diseases (AASLD) guidelines recommendation:* Adults with chronic HCV infection (Ghany, 2009): Treatment of choice: Ribavirin plus **peginterferon**; clinical condition and ability of patient to tolerate therapy should be evaluated to determine length and/or likely benefit of therapy. Recommended treatment duration (AASLD guidelines): Genotypes 1,4: 48 weeks; Genotypes 2,3: 24 weeks; Coinfection with HIV: 48 weeks.

Chronic hepatitis B: Adults: SubQ: 180 mcg once weekly for 48 weeks

Dose modifications for adverse reactions/toxicity:

Children ≥5 years: HCV:

For moderate-to-severe adverse reactions: Decrease to 135 mcg/1.73 m^2 x BSA once weekly for initial dose reduction; further dose reductions to 90 mcg/1.73 m^2 x BSA once weekly or 45 mcg/1.73 m^2 x BSA once weekly may be necessary in some cases if reaction persists or recurs. Up to 3 dosing adjustments for toxicity may be made before discontinuation is considered.

Based on hematologic parameters:

ANC 750-999/mm^3: Week 1-2: 135 mcg/1.73 m^2 x BSA once weekly; Weeks 3-48: No modification

ANC 500-749/mm^3: Week 1-2: Hold dose until ANC >750/mm^3 then resume dose with 135 mcg/1.73 m^2 x BSA once weekly. Assess WBC weekly for 3 weeks to verify ANC >750/mm^3; Weeks 3-48: 135 mcg/1.73 m^2 x BSA once weekly

ANC 250-499/mm^3: Week 1-2: Hold dose until ANC >750/mm^3 then resume dose with 90 mcg/1.73 m^2 x BSA once weekly; Weeks 3-48: Hold dose until ANC >750/mm^3 then resume dose with 135 mcg/1.73 m^2 x BSA once weekly

ANC <250/mm^3 (or febrile neutropenia): Discontinue treatment.

Platelet count <50,000/mm^3: 90 mcg/1.73 m^2 x BSA once weekly

Depression (severity based on DSM-IV criteria [similar to adult dosing adjustment recommendations]):

Mild depression: No dosage adjustment required; evaluate once weekly by visit/phone call. If depression remains stable, continue weekly visits. If depression improves, resume normal visit schedule

Moderate depression: Decrease interferon dose to 135 mcg/1.73 m^2 x BSA once weekly (or to 90 mcg/1.73 m^2 x BSA once weekly **or** 45 mcg/1.73 m^2 x BSA once weekly); evaluate once weekly with an office visit at least every other week. If depression remains stable, consider psychiatric evaluation and continue reduced dosing. If symptoms improve and remain stable for 4 weeks, resume normal visit schedule; continue reduced dosing or return to normal dose.

Severe depression: Discontinue interferon permanently. Obtain immediate psychiatric consultation. Discontinue ribavirin.

Adults: HCV, HBV:

For moderate-to-severe adverse reactions: Decrease to 135 mcg weekly for initial dose reduction; further dose reductions to 90 mcg weekly may be necessary in some cases if reaction persists or recurs.

Based on hematologic parameters:

ANC <750/mm^3: 135 mcg weekly

ANC <500/mm^3: Suspend therapy until >1000/mm^3, then restart at 90 mcg weekly; monitor ANC

Platelet count <50,000/mm^3: 90 mcg weekly

Platelet count <25,000/mm^3: Discontinue therapy

Depression (severity based on DSM-IV criteria):

Mild depression: No dosage adjustment required; evaluate once weekly by visit/phone call. If depression remains stable, continue weekly visits. If depression improves, resume normal visit schedule

Moderate depression: Decrease interferon dose to 135 mcg once weekly (or to 90 mcg once weekly); evaluate once weekly with an office visit at least every other week. If depression remains stable, consider psychiatric evaluation and continue with reduced dosing. If symptoms improve and remain stable for 4 weeks, resume normal visit schedule; continue reduced dosing or return to normal dose.

Severe depression: Discontinue interferon permanently. Obtain immediate psychiatric consultation.

Dosage adjustment in renal impairment:

Children: No dosage adjustment provided in manufacturer's labeling (has not been studied).

Adults:

Cl_{cr} ≥30 mL/minute: No adjustment required.

Cl_{cr} <30 mL/minute: 135 mcg weekly; monitor for toxicity

End-stage renal disease (ESRD) requiring hemodialysis: 135 mcg weekly; monitor for toxicity

Dosage adjustment in hepatic impairment:

Children: HCV:

ALT ≥5 but <10 x ULN: Decrease interferon dose to 135 mcg/1.73 m^2 x BSA once weekly. Monitor weekly; further modify dose if needed until ALT stabilizes or decreases.

ALT ≥10 x ULN (persistent): Discontinue interferon.

Adults:

HCV: ALT progressively rising above baseline: Decrease dose to 135 mcg weekly **and** monitor LFTs more frequently. If ALT continues to rise despite dose reduction or ALT increase is accompanied by increased bilirubin or hepatic decompensation, discontinue therapy immediately. Therapy may resume after ALT flare subsides.

HBV:

ALT >5 x ULN: Consider decreasing dose to 135 mcg weekly or temporarily discontinuing (may resume after ALT flare subsides) **and** monitor LFTs more frequently. If ALT continues to rise despite dose reduction or ALT increase is accompanied by increased bilirubin or hepatic decompensation, discontinue therapy immediately.

ALT >10 x ULN: Consider discontinuing.

Dietary Considerations Avoid ethanol use in patients with hepatitis C virus.

Administration SubQ: Administer in the abdomen or thigh. Rotate injection site. Do not use if solution contains particulate matter or is discolored. Discard unused solution. Administration should be done on the same day and at approximately the same time each week.

Monitoring Parameters

Clinical studies tested as follows:

Children: Hematologic and biochemical assessments were made at weeks 1, 3, 5, and 8, and then every 4 weeks thereafter; TSH measured every 12 weeks

Adults: CBC (including hemoglobin, WBC, and platelets) and chemistries (including liver function tests and uric acid) measured at weeks 1, 2, 4, 6, and 8, and then every 4-6 weeks (more frequently if abnormal); TSH measured every 12 weeks.

In addition, the following baseline values were used as entrance criteria in adults:

Platelet count ≥90,000/mm^3 (as low as 75,000/mm^3 in patients with cirrhosis or 70,000/mm^3 in patients with CHC coinfected with HIV)

ANC ≥1500/mm^3

Serum creatinine <1.5 times ULN

TSH and T_4 within normal limits or adequately controlled

CD4$^+$ cell count ≥200 cells/mm^3 or CD4$^+$ cell count ≥100 cells/mm^3, but <200 cells/mm^3 **and** HIV-1 RNA <5000 copies/mL in CHC patients coinfected with HIV

Hemoglobin ≥12 g/dL for women and ≥13 g/dL for men in CHC monoinfected patients

Hemoglobin ≥11 g/dL for women and ≥12 g/dL for men in CHC patients coinfected with HIV

Serum HCV RNA levels (pretreatment, 12- and 24 weeks after therapy initiation, 24 weeks after completion of therapy). **Note:** Discontinuation of therapy may be considered after 12 weeks in patients with HCV (genotype 1) who fail to achieve an early virologic response (EVR) (defined as ≥2-log decrease in HCV RNA compared to pretreatment) or after 24 weeks with detectable HCV RNA. Treat patients with HCV (genotypes 2,3) for 24 weeks (if tolerated) and then evaluate HCV RNA levels (Ghany, 2009).

Prior to treatment, pregnancy screening should occur for women of childbearing age who are receiving treatment or who have male partners who are receiving treatment. In combination therapy with ribavirin, pregnancy tests should continue monthly up to 6 months after discontinuation of therapy. Evaluate for depression and other psychiatric symptoms before and during therapy; baseline eye examination and periodically in patients with baseline disorders; baseline echocardiogram in patients with cardiac disease.

Dosage Forms Excipient information presented when available (limited, particularly for generics); consult specific product labeling.

Kit, Subcutaneous [preservative free]:

Pegasys: 180 mcg/0.5 mL [contains benzyl alcohol]

Solution, Subcutaneous [preservative free]:

Pegasys: 180 mcg/mL (1 mL) [contains benzyl alcohol]

Pegasys: 180 mcg/0.5 mL (0.5 mL) [contains benzyl alcohol, polysorbate 80]

Pegasys ProClick: 135 mcg/0.5 mL (0.5 mL) [contains benzyl alcohol, polysorbate 80]

Pegasys ProClick: 180 mcg/0.5 mL (0.5 mL) [contains benzyl alcohol]

Peginterferon Alfa-2b

(peg in ter FEER on AL fa too bee)

Brand Names: U.S. Peg-Intron; Peg-Intron Redipen; Peg-Intron Redipen Pak 4; Sylatron

Brand Names: Canada PegIntron

Index Terms Interferon Alfa-2b (PEG Conjugate); PEG-IFN Alfa-2b; Pegylated Interferon Alfa-2b; Polyethylene Glycol Interferon Alfa-2b

Pharmacologic Category Interferon

Use

PegIntron: Treatment of chronic hepatitis C (CHC; in combination with ribavirin) in patients who have compensated liver disease; treatment of chronic hepatitis C (as monotherapy) in adult patients with compensated liver disease who have never received alfa interferons and are intolerant to ribavirin or have contraindications to ribavirin. **Note:** Combination therapy with ribavirin provides better response rates than peginterferon monotherapy

Sylatron: Adjuvant treatment of melanoma (with microscopic or gross nodal involvement within 84 days of definitive surgical resection, including complete lymphadenectomy)

Pregnancy Risk Factor C / X in combination with ribavirin

Pregnancy Considerations Reproduction studies with pegylated interferon alfa have not been conducted. Animal reproduction studies with nonpegylated interferon alfa-2b have demonstrated abortifacient effects. Disruption of the normal menstrual cycle was also observed in animal studies; therefore, the manufacturer recommends that reliable contraception is used in women of childbearing potential. Alfa interferon is endogenous to normal amniotic fluid (Lebon, 1982). *In vitro* administration studies have reported that when administered to the mother, it does not cross the placenta (Waysbort, 1993). Case reports of use in pregnant women are limited. The DHHS Perinatal HIV Guidelines do not recommend that peginterferon alfa be used during pregnancy (DHHS [perinatal], 2012). **[U.S. Boxed Warning]: Combination therapy with ribavirin may cause birth defects and/or fetal mortality; avoid pregnancy in females and female partners of male patients;** combination therapy with ribavirin is contraindicated in pregnancy. Two forms of contraception should be used along with monthly pregnancy tests during combination therapy and for 6 months after therapy has been discontinued.

A pregnancy registry has been established for women inadvertently exposed to ribavirin while pregnant (800-593-2214).

Breast-Feeding Considerations Breast milk samples obtained from a lactating mother prior to and after administration of interferon alfa-2b showed that interferon alfa is present in breast milk and administration of the medication did not significantly affect endogenous levels (Kumar, 2000). Breast-feeding is not linked to the spread of hepatitis C virus (ACOG, 2007); however, if nipples are cracked or bleeding, breast-feeding is not recommended (CDC, 2010). Mothers coinfected with HIV are discouraged from breast-feeding to decrease potential transmission of HIV (DHHS [perinatal], 2012).

Medication Guide Available Yes

Contraindications Hypersensitivity (including urticaria, angioedema, bronchoconstriction, anaphylaxis, Stevens Johnson syndrome and toxic epidermal necrolysis) to peginterferon alfa-2b, interferon alfa-2b, other alfa interferons, or any component of the formulation; autoimmune hepatitis; decompensated liver disease (Child-Pugh score >6, classes B and C)

Combination therapy with peginterferon alfa-2b and ribavirin is also contraindicated in pregnancy, women who may become pregnant, males with pregnant partners; hemoglobinopathies (eg, thalassemia major, sickle-cell anemia); renal dysfunction (Cl_{cr} <50 mL/minute)

Warnings/Precautions [U.S. Boxed Warnings]: May cause or aggravate severe depression or other neuropsychiatric adverse events (including suicide and suicidal ideation) in patients with and without a history of psychiatric disorder; monitor closely with clinical evaluations (periodic); discontinue treatment with worsening or persistently severe signs/symptoms of neuropsychiatric disorders (eg, depression, encephalopathy, psychosis). Many cases resolve upon discontinuation, although some cases may persist. May cause or aggravate fatal or life-threatening autoimmune disorders, infectious disorders, ischemic disorders; monitor closely with clinical evaluations (periodic); discontinue treatment in patients with worsening or persistently severe signs/symptoms of infectious disorders; may resolve with discontinuation. May also cause hemorrhagic cerebrovascular events.

Neuropsychiatric disorders: Neuropsychiatric effects may occur in patients with and without a history of psychiatric disorder; addiction relapse, aggression, depression, homicidal ideation and suicidal behavior/ideation have been observed with peginterferon alfa-2b; bipolar disorder, encephalopathy, hallucinations, mania, and psychosis have been observed with other alfa interferons. Onset may be delayed (up to 6 months after discontinuation). Higher doses may be associated with the development of encephalopathy (higher risk in elderly patients). Use with caution in patients with a history of psychiatric disorders, including depression or substance abuse history. New or exacerbated neuropsychiatric or substance abuse disorders are best managed with early intervention. Drug screening and periodic health evaluation (including monitoring of psychiatric symptoms) is recommended if initiating treatment in patients with coexisting psychiatric condition or substance abuse disorders. Monitor all patients for evidence of depression and other psychiatric symptoms; patients being treated for melanoma should be monitored for depression and psychiatric symptoms every 3 weeks during the first 8 weeks of treatment and every 6 months thereafter; permanently discontinue treatment if psychiatric symptoms persist, worsen or if suicidal behavior develops. Patients should continue to be monitored for 6 months after completion of therapy.

Bone marrow suppression: Causes bone marrow suppression, including potentially severe cytopenias; alfa interferons may (rarely) cause aplastic anemia. Use with caution in patients who are chronically immunosuppressed, with low peripheral blood counts or myelosuppression, including concurrent use of myelosuppressive therapy. Dosage modification may be necessary for hematologic toxicity. Combination therapy with ribavirin may potentiate the neutropenic effects of alfa interferons. When used in combination with ribavirin, an increased incidence of anemia was observed when using ribavirin weight-based dosing, as compared to flat-dose ribavirin.

Hepatic disease: Use is contraindicated in patients with hepatic decompensation or autoimmune hepatitis. Discontinue treatment immediately with hepatic decompensation (Child Pugh score >6) or evidence of severe hepatic injury. Patients with chronic hepatitis C (CHC) with cirrhosis receiving peginterferon alfa-2b are at risk for hepatic decompensation. CHC patients coinfected with human immunodeficiency virus (HIV) are at increased risk for hepatic decompensation when receiving highly active antiretroviral therapy (HAART); monitor closely. A transient increase in ALT (2-5 times above baseline) which is not associated with deterioration of liver function may occur with peginterferon alfa-2b use (for the treatment of chronic hepatitis C); therapy generally may continue with monitoring.

Gastrointestinal disorders: Pancreatitis (including fatal cases) has been observed with alfa interferon therapy; discontinue therapy if known or suspected pancreatitis develops. Ulcerative or hemorrhagic/ischemic colitis has been observed with alfa interferons (within 12 weeks of initiation); withhold treatment for suspected pancreatitis; discontinue therapy for known pancreatitis. Ulcerative or hemorrhagic/ischemic colitis has been observed with alfa interferons; discontinue therapy if signs of colitis (abdominal pain, bloody diarrhea, fever) develop; symptoms typically resolve within 1-3 weeks.

Autoimmune disorders: Thyroiditis, thrombotic thrombocytopenic purpura, immune thrombocytopenia (ITP), rheumatoid arthritis, interstitial nephritis, systemic lupus erythematosus, and psoriasis have been reported with therapy; use with caution in patients with autoimmune disorders.

Cardiovascular disease: Use with caution in patients with cardiovascular disease or a history of cardiovascular disease; hypotension, arrhythmia, bundle branch block, tachycardia, cardiomyopathy, angina pectoris and MI have been observed with treatment. Patients with pre-existing cardiac abnormalities should have baseline ECGs prior to combination treatment with ribavirin; closely monitor patients with a history of MI or arrhythmia. Patients with a history of significant or unstable cardiac disease should not receive combination treatment with ribavirin. Discontinue treatment (permanently) for new-onset ventricular arrhythmia or cardiovascular decompensation.

Endocrine disorders: Diabetes mellitus (including new-onset type I diabetes), hyperglycemia, and thyroid disorders have been reported; discontinue peginterferon alfa-2b if cannot be effectively managed with medication. Use caution in patients with a history of diabetes mellitus, particularly if prone to DKA. Use with caution in patients with thyroid disorders; may cause or aggravate hyper- or hypothyroidism.

Pulmonary disease: May cause or aggravate dyspnea, pulmonary infiltrates, pneumonia, bronchiolitis obliterans, interstitial pneumonitis, pulmonary hypertension, and sarcoidosis which may result in respiratory failure; may recur upon rechallenge with treatment; monitor closely. Use with caution in patients with existing pulmonary disease (eg, chronic obstructive pulmonary disease). Withhold combination therapy with ribavirin for development of pulmonary infiltrate or pulmonary function impairment.

Ophthalmic disorders: Ophthalmologic disorders (including decreased visual acuity, blindness, macular edema, retinal hemorrhages, optic neuritis, papilledema, cotton wool spots, retinal detachment [serous], and retinal artery or vein thrombosis) have occurred with peginterferon alfa-2b and/or with other alfa interferons. Prior to start of therapy, ophthalmic exams are recommended for all patients; patients with diabetic or hypertensive retinopathy should have periodic ophthalmic exams during treatment; a complete eye exam should be done promptly in patients who develop ocular symptoms. Permanently discontinue treatment with new or worsening ophthalmic disorder.

[U.S. Boxed Warning]: Combination treatment with ribavirin may cause birth defects and/or fetal mortality (avoid pregnancy in females and female partners of male patients); hemolytic anemia (which may worsen cardiac disease), genotoxicity, mutagenicity, and may possibly be carcinogenic. Interferon therapy is commonly associated with flu-like symptoms, including fever; rule out other causes/infection with persistent or high fever. Acute hypersensitivity reactions (eg, urticaria, angioedema, bronchoconstriction, anaphylaxis) and cutaneous reactions (eg, Stevens-Johnson syndrome, toxic epidermal necrolysis) have been reported (rarely) with alfa interferons; prompt discontinuation is recommended; transient rashes do not require interruption of therapy. Hypertriglyceridemia has been reported (may result in pancreatitis); periodically monitor and manage with appropriate treatment; consider discontinuing peginterferon if persistent and severe (triglycerides >1000 mg/dL), particularly if combined with symptoms of pancreatitis. Interferons are commonly associated with flu-like symptoms. Use with caution in patients with debilitating conditions. Use with caution in patients with renal impairment (Cl_{cr} <50 mL/minute); monitor closely for signs of interferon toxicity. For the treatment of chronic hepatitis C, dosage adjustments are recommended with monotherapy in patients with moderate-to-severe impairment; do not use combination therapy with ribavirin in adult patients renal dysfunction (Cl_{cr} <50 mL/minute); discontinue if serum creatinine >2 mg/dL in children. Has not been studied in melanoma patients with renal impairment. Serum creatinine increases have been reported in patients with renal insufficiency. Use with caution in the elderly; the potential adverse effects (eg, neuropsychiatric events, cardiac events, systemic effects) may be more pronounced. Encephalopathy has also been observed in primarily elderly patients treated with higher doses of peginterferon alfa-2b. For the treatment of hepatitis, elderly patients generally do not respond to interferon treatment as well as younger patients. When used in combination with ribavirin, closely monitor adults >50 years of age for the development of anemia. Dental/periodontal disorders have been reported with combination therapy; dry mouth may affect teeth and mucous membranes; instruct patients to brush teeth twice daily; encourage regular dental exams; rinse mouth thoroughly after vomiting.

Combination therapy with ribavirin is preferred over monotherapy for the treatment of chronic hepatitis C. Safety and efficacy have not been established in patients who have received organ transplants or are coinfected with HIV or hepatitis B. Patients with significant bridging fibrosis or cirrhosis, genotype 1 infection or who have not responded to prior therapy, including previous pegylated interferon treatment are less likely to benefit from combination therapy with peginterferon alfa-2b and ribavirin. Growth velocity (height and weight) was decreased in children on combination treatment with ribavirin during the length of treatment. Long-term data indicate that combination therapy may inhibit growth, resulting in reduced adult height. Growth should be closely monitored in pediatric patients during therapy and posttreatment. **[U.S. Boxed Warning]: Combination therapy with ribavirin is contraindicated in pregnancy.** Due to differences in dosage, patients should not change brands of interferon.

Adverse Reactions Note: Percentages reported for adults receiving monotherapy unless noted:

>10%:

Central nervous system: Fatigue (52% to 94%), fever (22% to 75%), headache (56% to 70%), chills (≤63%), depression (29% to 59%; may be severe), dizziness (12% to 35%), anxiety/emotional liability/irritability (28%), insomnia (23%), olfactory nerve disorder (≤23%)

Dermatologic: Rash (6% to 36%), alopecia (22% to 34%), pruritus (12%), dry skin (11%)

Gastrointestinal: Anorexia (20% to 69%), nausea (26% to 64%), taste perversion (≤38%), diarrhea (18% to 37%), vomiting (7% to 26%), abdominal pain (8% to 15%), weight loss (11%)

Hematologic: Neutropenia (6% to 70%; grade 4: 1%), thrombocytopenia (7% to 20%; grades 3/4: <4%), anemia (6%; in combination with ribavirin: 12% to 47%)

Hepatic: ALT/AST increased (10% to 77%), alkaline phosphatase increased (≤23%)

Local: Injection site inflammation/reaction (23% to 62%)

Neuromuscular & skeletal: Myalgia (54% to 68%), weakness (52%), arthralgia (23% to 51%), musculoskeletal pain (28%), rigors (23%), paresthesia (21%)

Miscellaneous: Binding antibodies (melanoma patients 35%), viral infection (11%)

1% to 10%:

Cardiovascular: Chest pain (6%), flushing (6%), bundle branch block (4%), myocardial infarction (4%), supraventricular arrhythmia (4%), ventricular tachycardia (4%)

Central nervous system: Concentration impaired (10%), malaise (7%), nervousness (4%), agitation (2%), suicidal behavior (ideation/attempt/suicide ≤2%)

Endocrine & metabolic: Hypothyroidism (5%), menstrual disorder (4%), hyperthyroidism (3%)

Gastrointestinal: Dyspepsia (6%), xerostomia (6%), constipation (1%)

Hepatic: GGT increased (8%), hepatomegaly (6%)

Local: Injection site pain (2% to 3%)

Ocular: Conjunctivitis (4%), blurred vision (2%)

Renal: Proteinuria (≤7%)

Respiratory: Pharyngitis (10%), cough (5% to 8%), sinusitis (7%), dyspnea (4% to 6%), rhinitis (2%)

Miscellaneous: Diaphoresis (6%), neutralizing antibodies (≤2%)

<1% (Limited to important and life-threatening): Addiction (drug) relapse, anaphylaxis, angina, angioedema, aphthous stomatitis, aplastic anemia, arrhythmia, autoimmune thrombocytopenia (with or without purpura), bacterial infection, bipolar disorders, blindness, bronchiolitis obliterans, cardiac arrest, cardiomyopathy, cellulitis, colitis, cotton wool spots, cytopenia, diabetes mellitus, diabetic ketoacidosis, drug overdose, emphysema, encephalopathy, erythema multiforme, fungal infection, gastroenteritis, gout, hallucinations, hearing impairment/loss, hemorrhagic colitis, homicidal ideation, hyperglycemia, hyper-/hypotension, hypersensitivity reactions, hypertriglyceridemia, injection site necrosis, interstitial nephritis, interstitial pneumonitis, ischemic colitis, leukopenia, loss of consciousness, lupus-like syndrome, macular edema, mania, memory loss, migraine, myositis, nerve palsy (facial/oculomotor), optic neuritis, palpitation, pancreatitis, papilledema, pericardial effusion, peripheral neuropathy, phototoxicity, pleural effusion, pneumonia, psoriasis, psychosis, pulmonary hypertension, pulmonary infiltrates, pure red cell aplasia, renal failure, renal insufficiency, retinal artery or vein thrombosis, retinal detachment (serous), retinal hemorrhage, retinal ischemia, retinopathy, rhabdomyolysis, rheumatoid arthritis, sarcoidosis, seizure, sepsis, serum creatinine increased, Stevens-Johnson syndrome, stroke, systemic lupus erythematosus, tachycardia, thrombotic thrombocytopenic purpura, thyroiditis, toxic epidermal necrolysis, transient ischemic attack, ulcerative colitis, vasculitis, vision decrease/loss, Vogt-Koyanagi-Harada syndrome

Drug Interactions

Metabolism/Transport Effects Inhibits CYP1A2 (weak)

Avoid Concomitant Use

Avoid concomitant use of Peginterferon Alfa-2b with any of the following: CloZAPine; Telbivudine

Increased Effect/Toxicity

Peginterferon Alfa-2b may increase the levels/effects of: Aldesleukin; CloZAPine; Methadone; Ribavirin; Telbivudine; Theophylline Derivatives; Zidovudine

Decreased Effect

Peginterferon Alfa-2b may decrease the levels/effects of: CYP2C9 Substrates; CYP2D6 Substrates; FLUoxetine

The levels/effects of Peginterferon Alfa-2b may be decreased by: Pegloticase

Ethanol/Nutrition/Herb Interactions Ethanol: Avoid use in patients with hepatitis C virus.

Preparation for Administration

Redipen: Hold cartridge upright and press the two halves together until there is a "click". Gently invert to mix; do not shake; do not reuse (single use).

PegIntron (vial): Add 0.7 mL sterile water for injection, USP (supplied single-use diluent) to the vial. Gently swirl. Do not re-enter vial after dose removed.

Sylatron (vial): Add 0.7 mL sterile water for injection and swirl gently (do not withdraw more than 0.5 mL), resulting in the following concentrations:

296 mcg vial: 40 mcg/0.1 mL
444 mcg vial: 60 mcg/0.1 mL
888 mcg vial: 120 mcg/0.1 mL

Storage/Stability Prior to reconstitution, store Redipen at 2°C to 8°C (36°F to 46°F). Store intact vials at 25°C (77°F); excursions permitted to 15°C to 30°C (59°F to 86°F). Do not freeze. Once reconstituted each product should be used immediately or may be stored for ≤24 hours at 2°C to 8°C (36°F to 46°F); do not freeze. Do not shake. Keep away from heat. Products do not contain preservative (single use; do not reuse).

Mechanism of Action Alpha interferons are a family of proteins, produced by nucleated cells, that have antiviral, antiproliferative, and immune-regulating activity. There are 16 known subtypes of alpha interferons. Interferons interact with cells through high affinity cell surface receptors. Following activation, multiple effects can be detected including induction of gene transcription. Inhibits cellular growth, alters the state of cellular differentiation, interferes with oncogene expression, alters cell surface antigen expression, increases phagocytic activity of macrophages, and augments cytotoxicity of lymphocytes for target cells.

Pharmacodynamics/Kinetics

Bioavailability: Increases with chronic dosing

Half-life elimination: CHC: ~40 hours (range: 22-60 hours); Melanoma: ~43-51 hours

Time to peak: CHC: 15-44 hours

Excretion: Urine (~30%)

Dosage SubQ:

Children ≥3 years: CHC:

Manufacturer labeling: Combination therapy with ribavirin: 60 mcg/m^2 once weekly; **Note:** Children who reach their 18th birthday during treatment should remain on the pediatric regimen. Treatment duration is 48 weeks for genotype 1, 24 weeks for genotypes 2 and 3. Discontinue combination therapy in patients with HCV (genotype 1) at 12 weeks if HCV-RNA does not decrease by at least 2 log (compared to pretreatment) or if detectable HCV-RNA present at 24 weeks.

American Association for the Study of Liver Diseases (AASLD) guideline recommendations (Ghany, 2009): Children 2-17 years: Treatment of choice: **Peginterferon alfa-2b** 60 mcg/m^2 once weekly in combination with oral ribavirin 15 mg/kg/day for 48 weeks

Adults:

Melanoma: 6 mcg/kg/week for 8 doses, followed by 3 mcg/kg/week for up to 5 years. **Note:** Premedicate with acetaminophen (500-1000 mg orally) 30 minutes prior to the first dose and as needed for subsequent doses thereafter.

CHC: Administer dose once weekly; **Note:** Discontinue in patients with HCV (genotype 1) after 12 weeks if HCV RNA does not decrease by at least 2 log (compared to pretreatment) or if detectable HCV RNA present at 24 weeks. Discontinuation is also recommended in patients who previously failed therapy (regardless of genotype) if detectable HCV RNA present at 12 or 24 weeks.

Monotherapy (duration of treatment is 1 year): Initial dose (based on average weekly dose of 1 mcg/kg):

≤45 kg: 40 mcg once weekly
46-56 kg: 50 mcg once weekly
57-72 kg: 64 mcg once weekly
73-88 kg: 80 mcg once weekly
89-106 kg: 96 mcg once weekly
107-136 kg: 120 mcg once weekly
137-160 kg: 150 mcg once weekly

Combination therapy with ribavirin(treatment duration is 48 weeks for genotype 1, 24 weeks for genotypes 2 and 3, or 48 weeks for patients who previously failed therapy [regardless of genotype]): Initial dose (based on an average weekly dose of 1.5 mcg/kg):

<40 kg: 50 mcg once weekly (with ribavirin 800 mg/day)
40-50 kg: 64 mcg once weekly (with ribavirin 800 mg/day)
51-60 kg: 80 mcg once weekly (with ribavirin 800 mg/day)
61-65 kg: 96 mcg once weekly (with ribavirin 800 mg/day)
66-75 kg: 96 mcg once weekly (with ribavirin 1000 mg/day)
76-80 kg: 120 mcg once weekly (with ribavirin 1000 mg/day)
81-85 kg: 120 mcg once weekly (with ribavirin 1200 mg/day)
86-105 kg: 150 mcg once weekly (with ribavirin 1200 mg/day)
>105 kg: 1.5 mcg/kg once weekly (with ribavirin 1400 mg/day)

Note: *American Association for the Study of Liver Diseases (AASLD) guidelines recommendation:* Adults with chronic HCV infection: Treatment of choice: Ribavirin plus **peginterferon**; clinical condition and ability of patient to tolerate therapy should be evaluated to determine length and/or likely benefit of therapy. Recommended treatment duration (AASLD guidelines; Ghany, 2009): Genotypes 1,4: 48 weeks; Genotypes 2,3: 24 weeks; Coinfection with HIV: 48 weeks.

Elderly: Refer to adult dosing.

Dosage adjustment for toxicity:

Melanoma:

Discontinue for any of the following: Persistent or worsening severe neuropsychiatric disorders (depression, psychosis, encephalopathy), grade 4 nonhematologic toxicity, new or worsening retinopathy, new-onset ventricular arrhythmia or cardiovascular decompensation, evidence of hepatic injury (severe) or hepatic decompensation (Child-Pugh score >6 [Class B or C]), development of hyper- or hypothyroidism or diabetes that cannot be effectively managed with medication, or inability to tolerate a dose of 1 mcg/kg/week

Temporarily withhold for any of the following: ANC <500/mm^3, platelets <50,000/mm^3, ECOG performance status (PS) ≥2, nonhematologic toxicity ≥ grade 3. May reinitiate at a reduced dose once ANC ≥500/mm^3, platelets ≥50,000/mm^3, ECOG PS at 0-1, and nonhematologic toxicity completely resolved or improved to grade 1.

Reduced dose schedule, Weeks 1-8:
First dose reduction (if prior dose 6 mcg/kg/week): 3 mcg/kg/week
Second dose reduction (if prior dose 3 mcg/kg/week): 2 mcg/kg/week
Third dose reduction (if prior dose 2 mcg/kg/week): 1 mcg/kg/week
Discontinue permanently if unable to tolerate 1 mcg/kg/week
Reduced dose schedule, Weeks 9-260:
First dose reduction (if prior dose 3 mcg/kg/week): 2 mcg/kg/week
Second dose reduction (if prior dose 2 mcg/kg/week): 1 mcg/kg/week
Discontinue permanently if unable to tolerate 1 mcg/kg/week

***Chronic hepatitis C:* Dosage adjustment for depression (severity based upon DSM-IV criteria):**
Mild depression: No dosage adjustment required; evaluate once weekly by visit/phone call. If depression remains stable, continue weekly visits. If depression improves, resume normal visit schedule. For worsening depression, see "Moderate depression" or "Severe depression" below.
Moderate depression: **Note:** Evaluate once weekly (visit or phone) with an office visit at least every other week. If depression remains stable, consider psychiatric evaluation and continue with reduced dosing. If symptoms improve and remain stable for 4 weeks, resume normal visit schedule; continue reduced dosing or return to normal dose. For worsening depression, see "Severe depression" below.
Children: Decrease peginterferon alfa-2b dose to 40 mcg/m^2/week, may further decrease to 20 mcg/m^2/week if needed
Adults:
Peginterferon alfa-2b monotherapy: Refer to adult weight-based dosage reduction with monotherapy for depression below
Peginterferon alfa-2b combination therapy: Refer to adult weight-based dosage reduction with combination therapy for depression below
Severe depression: Discontinue peginterferon alfa-2b and ribavirin permanently. Obtain immediate psychiatric consultation. Utilize follow-up psychiatric therapy as needed.

***Chronic hepatitis C:* Dosage adjustment in hematologic toxicity:**
Children:
Hemoglobin decrease ≥2 g/dL in any 4-week period and stable cardiac disease: Decrease peginterferon alfa-2b dose by 50%; decrease ribavirin dose by 200 mg daily (regardless of the patient's initial dose); monitor and evaluate weekly. If hemoglobin <8.5 g/dL any time after dose reduction or <12 g/dL after 4 weeks of dose reduction, permanently discontinue both peginterferon alfa-2b and ribavirin.
Hemoglobin 8.5 to <10 g/dL and no history of cardiac disease: Decrease ribavirin dose to 12 mg/kg/day; may further reduce to 8 mg/kg/day; no dosage adjustment necessary for peginterferon alfa-2b.
WBC 1000 to <1500/mm^3, neutrophils 500 to <750/mm^3, or platelets 50,000 to <70,000/mm^3: Reduce peginterferon alfa-2b dose to 40 mcg/m^2/week; may further reduce to 20 mcg/m^2/week
Hemoglobin <8.5 g/dL, WBC <1000/mm^3, neutrophils <500/mm^3, or platelets <50,000/mm^3: Permanently discontinue peginterferon alfa-2b and ribavirin.
Adults:
Hemoglobin decrease ≥2 g/dL in any 4-week period and stable cardiac disease: Decrease peginterferon alfa-2b dose by 50%; decrease ribavirin dose by 200 mg daily. If hemoglobin <8.5 g/dL any time after dose reduction or <12 g/dL after 4 weeks of dose reduction, permanently discontinue both peginterferon alfa-2b and ribavirin.
Hemoglobin 8.5 to <10 g/dL and no history of cardiac disease: Decrease ribavirin dose by 200 mg daily (patients receiving 1400 mg daily should decrease dose by 400 mg daily [ie, first dose reduction to 1000 mg daily]); may further reduce ribavirin dose by additional 200 mg daily if needed. No dosage adjustment necessary for peginterferon alfa-2b.
WBC 1000 to <1500/mm^3, neutrophils 500 to <750/mm^3, or platelets 25,000 to <50,000/mm^3:
Peginterferon alfa-2b monotherapy: Refer to adult weight-based dosage reduction monotherapy for hematologic toxicity below.
Peginterferon alfa-2b combination therapy: Refer to adult weight-based dosage reduction with combination therapy for hematologic toxicity below.
Hemoglobin <8.5 g/dL, WBC <1000/mm^3, neutrophils <500/mm^3, or platelets <25,000/mm^3: Permanently discontinue peginterferon alfa-2b and ribavirin.

***Chronic hepatitis C:* Adult weight-based dosage reduction for depression or hematologic toxicity:**
Peginterferon alfa-2b monotherapy: Reduce to average weekly dose of 0.5 mcg/kg as follows:
≤45 kg: 20 mcg once weekly
46-56 kg: 25 mcg once weekly
57-72 kg: 30 mcg once weekly
73-88 kg: 40 mcg once weekly
89-106 kg: 50 mcg once weekly
107-136 kg: 64 mcg once weekly
≥137 kg: 80 mcg once weekly
Peginterferon alfa-2b combination therapy: Initially reduce to average weekly dose of 1 mcg/kg; may further reduce to average weekly dose of 0.5 mcg/kg if needed as follows:
<40 kg: 35 mcg once weekly; may further reduce to 20 mcg once weekly if needed
40-50 kg: 45 mcg once weekly; may further reduce to 25 mcg once weekly if needed
51-60 kg: 50 mcg once weekly; may further reduce to 30 mcg once weekly if needed
61-75 kg: 64 mcg once weekly; may further reduce to 35 mcg once weekly if needed
76-85 kg: 80 mcg once weekly; may further reduce to 45 mcg once weekly if needed
86-104 kg: 96 mcg once weekly; may further reduce to 50 mcg once weekly if needed
105-125 kg: 108 mcg once weekly; may further reduce to 64 mcg once weekly if needed
>125 kg: 135 mcg once weekly; may further reduce to 72 mcg once weekly if needed

Dosage adjustment in renal impairment: Chronic hepatitis C:
Peginterferon alfa-2b monotherapy:
Cl_{cr} 30-50 mL/minute: Reduce dose by 25%
Cl_{cr} 10-29 mL/minute: Reduce dose by 50%
Hemodialysis: Reduce dose by 50%
Discontinue use if renal function declines during treatment.
Peginterferon alfa-2b combination with ribavirin:
Children: Serum creatinine >2 mg/dL: Discontinue treatment
Adults: Cl_{cr} <50 mL/minute: Combination therapy with ribavirin is not recommended

Dosage adjustment in hepatic impairment:

Decompensated liver disease or autoimmune hepatitis: Use is contraindicated.

Hepatic decompensation or severe hepatic injury during treatment (Child-Pugh score >6 [class B or C]): Discontinue immediately.

Administration For SubQ administration; rotate injection site; thigh, outer surface of upper arm, and abdomen are preferred injection sites; do not inject near navel or waistline; patients who are thin should only use thigh or upper arm. Do not inject into bruised, infected, irritated, red, or scarred skin. The weekly dose may be administered at bedtime to reduce flu-like symptoms. For the treatment of CHC, the administration volume depends on the patient's weight and the peginterferon concentration used.

Monitoring Parameters Baseline and periodic TSH (for patients being treated for melanoma, obtain baseline within 4 weeks prior to treatment initiation, and then at 3 and 6 months, and every 6 months thereafter during treatment); CBC with differential and platelets; serum chemistries, liver function tests (for patients with melanoma, monitor serum bilirubin, ALT, AST, alkaline phosphatase, and LDH at 2 and 8 weeks, and 2 and 3 months following initiation, then every 6 months during therapy), renal function, triglycerides; serum glucose or Hb A_{1c} (for patients with diabetes mellitus). Clinical studies (for combination therapy) tested as follows: CBC (including hemoglobin, WBC, and platelets) and chemistries (including liver function tests and uric acid) measured at weeks 2, 4, 8, and 12, and then every 6 weeks; TSH measured every 12 weeks during treatment. ECG at baseline for patients with pre-existing cardiac abnormalities (for combination therapy with ribavirin).

Hepatitic C: Serum HCV RNA levels (pretreatment, 12 and 24 weeks after therapy initiation, 24 weeks after completion of therapy). **Note:** Discontinuation of therapy may be considered after 12 weeks in patients with HCV (genotype 1) who fail to achieve an early virologic response (EVR) (defined as ≥2-log decrease in HCV RNA compared to pretreatment) or after 24 weeks with detectable HCV RNA. Treat patients with HCV (genotypes 2,3) for 24 weeks (if tolerated) and then evaluate HCV RNA levels (Ghany, 2009).

Evaluate for depression and other psychiatric symptoms before and after initiation of therapy; patients being treated for melanoma should be monitored for depression and psychiatric symptoms every 3 weeks during the first eight weeks of treatment and every 6 months thereafter, and continued monitoring for 6 months after the last dose; baseline ophthalmic eye examination; periodic ophthalmic exam in patients with diabetic or hypertensive retinopathy; baseline ECG in patients with cardiac disease; serum glucose or Hb A_{1c} (for patients with diabetes mellitus). In combination therapy with ribavirin, pregnancy tests (for women of childbearing age who are receiving treatment or who have male partners who are receiving treatment), continue monthly up to 6 months after discontinuation of therapy. In pediatric patients, growth velocity and weight should also be monitored during and periodically after treatment discontinuation.

Dosage Forms Excipient information presented when available (limited, particularly for generics); consult specific product labeling.

Kit, Subcutaneous:

Peg-Intron: 50 mcg/0.5 mL, 80 mcg/0.5 mL, 120 mcg/0.5 mL, 150 mcg/0.5 mL

Peg-Intron Redipen: 50 mcg/0.5 mL, 80 mcg/0.5 mL, 120 mcg/0.5 mL, 150 mcg/0.5 mL

Sylatron: 296 mcg, 444 mcg, 888 mcg, 4 X 296 MCG, 4 X 444 MCG, 4 X 888 MCG [contains polysorbate 80]

Kit, Subcutaneous [preservative free]:

Peg-Intron Redipen Pak 4: 50 mcg/0.5 mL, 80 mcg/0.5 mL, 120 mcg/0.5 mL, 150 mcg/0.5 mL

◆ **Peg-Intron** *see* Peginterferon Alfa-2b *on page 1594*

◆ **PegIntron (Can)** *see* Peginterferon Alfa-2b *on page 1594*

◆ **Peg-Intron Redipen** *see* Peginterferon Alfa-2b *on page 1594*

◆ **Peg-Intron Redipen Pak 4** *see* Peginterferon Alfa-2b *on page 1594*

◆ **PEGLA** *see* Pegaspargase *on page 1586*

Pegloticase (peg LOE ti kase)

Brand Names: U.S. Krystexxa

Index Terms PEG-Uricase; Pegylated Urate Oxidase; Polyethylene Glycol-Conjugated Uricase; Recombinant Urate Oxidase, Pegylated; Urate Oxidase, Pegylated

Pharmacologic Category Enzyme; Enzyme, Urate-Oxidase (Recombinant)

Use Treatment of chronic gout refractory to conventional therapy

Pregnancy Risk Factor C

Pregnancy Considerations Adequate animal reproduction studies have not been conducted. There are no adequate and well-controlled studies in pregnant women. Use during pregnancy only if the benefit to the mother outweigh the potential risk to the fetus.

Breast-Feeding Considerations Due to the potential for serious adverse reactions in the nursing infant, breastfeeding is not recommended.

Medication Guide Available Yes

Contraindications Glucose-6-phosphate dehydrogenase (G6PD) deficiency

Warnings/Precautions [U.S. Boxed Warning]: Anaphylaxis and infusion reactions have been reported during and after administration; patients should be closely monitored during infusion and for an appropriate period of time after the infusion. Therapy should be administered in a healthcare facility by skilled medical personnel prepared for the immediate treatment of anaphylaxis. All patients should be premedicated with antihistamines and corticosteroids. Anaphylaxis may occur at any time during treatment (including the initial dose). **Reactions generally occur within 2 hours of administration; however, delayed hypersensitivity reactions have also been reported.** Infusion reactions are varied; symptoms range from chest pain, pruritus/urticaria, or dyspnea to a clinical presentation of anaphylaxis (eg, hemodynamic instability, perioral or lingual edema). If a less severe (nonanaphylactic) infusion reaction occurs, the infusion may be slowed, or stopped and restarted at a slower rate, at the physician's discretion. **Risk of an infusion reaction is increased in patients whose uric acid is >6 mg/dL; therefore, monitor serum uric acid concentrations prior to infusion and consider discontinuing treatment if concentrations exceed 6 mg/dL, particularly in the event of 2 consecutive concentrations >6 mg/dL.** Concurrent use with oral antihyperuricemic agents may delay interpretations of ineffective pegloticase treatment (ie, serum uric acid >6 mg/dL) and ultimately increase risk for anaphylactoid and/or infusion reactions. Discontinue use of oral antihyperuricemic agents prior to and do not initiate during the course of pegloticase therapy.

Therapy with antihyperuricemic agents commonly results in gout flare, particularly upon initiation due to rapid lowering of urate concentrations; gout flare-ups during treatment do not warrant discontinuation of therapy. Gout flare prophylaxis is recommended, using nonsteroidal anti-inflammatory agents (NSAID) or colchicines, unless ▶

contraindicated, beginning ≥1 week before initiation of pegloticase and continuing for at least 6 months. Exacerbation of heart failure has been observed in clinical trials; use caution in patients with pre-existing heart failure. Due to the risk for hemolysis and methemoglobinemia, pegloticase is contraindicated in patients with G6PD deficiency. Patients at higher risk for G6PD deficiency (eg, African, Mediterranean) should be screened prior to therapy. Therapy is not appropriate for the treatment of asymptomatic hyperuricemia. Potential for immunogenicity exists with the use of therapeutic proteins. Antipegloticase antibodies and antiPEG antibodies commonly occurred during clinical trials in pegloticase-treated patients. High antipegloticase antibody titers were associated with failure to maintain uric acid normalization and were also associated with a higher incidence of infusion reactions. Due to potential for immunogenicity, closely monitor patients who reinitiate therapy after discontinuing treatment for >4 weeks; patients may be at increased risk for anaphylaxis and infusion reactions.

Adverse Reactions

>10%:

Dermatologic: Bruising (11%), urticaria (11%)

Gastrointestinal: Nausea (12%)

Miscellaneous: Antibody formation (antipegloticase antibodies: 92%; antiPEG antibodies: 42%), gout flare (74% within the first 3 months), infusion reactions (26%)

1% to 10%:

Cardiovascular: Chest pain (6% to 10%)

Dermatologic: Erythema (10%), pruritus (10%)

Gastrointestinal: Constipation (6%), vomiting (5%)

Respiratory: Dyspnea (7%), nasopharyngitis (7%)

Miscellaneous: Anaphylaxis (≤7%)

Frequency not defined: Anemia, diarrhea, headache, muscle spasms, nephrolithiasis

Drug Interactions

Metabolism/Transport Effects None known.

Avoid Concomitant Use

Avoid concomitant use of Pegloticase with any of the following: Allopurinol; Febuxostat; Probenecid

Increased Effect/Toxicity

The levels/effects of Pegloticase may be increased by: Allopurinol; Febuxostat; Probenecid

Decreased Effect

Pegloticase may decrease the levels/effects of: Certolizumab Pegol; Pegademase Bovine; Pegaptanib; Pegaspargase; Pegfilgrastim; Peginterferon Alfa-2a; Peginterferon Alfa-2b; Pegvisomant

Preparation for Administration To prepare solution for administration, withdraw 1 mL (8 mg) and add to a 250 mL bag of NS or 1/2NS; invert bag several times to mix thoroughly (do **not** shake). Do not use vial if particulate matter is present or if solution is discolored (solution should be a clear and colorless). After withdrawal, discard any unused portion of the product remaining in the vial.

Storage/Stability Prior to use, vials must be stored in the carton to protect from light and kept under refrigeration between 2°C to 8°C (36°F to 46°F) at all times. Do **not** shake or freeze.

Diluted solution may be stored up to 4 hours at 2°C to 8°C (36°F to 46°F). Diluted solution is also stable for 4 hours at room temperature of 20°C to 25°C (68°F to 77°F); however, refrigeration is preferred. The diluted solution should be protected from light, not frozen, and used within 4 hours of dilution. Prior to administration, allow the diluted solution to reach room temperature; do not warm to room temperature using any form of artificial heating such as a microwave or warm water bath.

Mechanism of Action Pegloticase is a pegylated recombinant form of urate-oxidase enzyme, also known as uricase (an enzyme normally absent in humans and high primates), which converts uric acid to allantoin (an inactive and water soluble metabolite of uric acid); it does not inhibit the formation of uric acid.

Pharmacodynamics/Kinetics

Onset of action: ~24 hours following the first dose, serum uric acid concentrations decreased

Duration: >300 hours (12.5 days)

Half-life elimination: Median: ~14 days

Dosage Note: Discontinue use of oral antihyperuricemic agents prior to initiating pegloticase and do not initiate during the course of therapy. Premedicate with antihistamines and corticosteroids. Gout flare prophylaxis with either NSAIDs or colchicine is also recommended, beginning at least 1 week prior to initiation and continuing for at least 6 months.

I.V.: Adults: Refractory gout: 8 mg every 2 weeks

Dosage adjustment in renal impairment: No dosage adjustment necessary.

Dosage adjustment in hepatic impairment: No dosage adjustment provided in manufacturer's labeling (has not been studied).

Administration Administer diluted solution by I.V. infusion over ≥120 minutes via gravity feed or an infusion pump or syringe-type pump. Do **not** administer by I.V. push or bolus. Administer in a healthcare setting by healthcare providers prepared to manage potential anaphylaxis. Monitor closely for infusion reactions during infusion and for an appropriate period of time after the infusion (anaphylaxis has been reported within 2 hours of the infusion). In the event or a less severe infusion reaction, infusion may be slowed, or stopped and restarted at a slower rate, based on the discretion of the physician.

Reference Range

Uric acid, serum: An increase occurs during childhood

Adults:

Males: 3.4-7 mg/dL or slightly more

Females: 2.4-6 mg/dL or slightly more

Values >7 mg/dL are sometimes arbitrarily regarded as hyperuricemia, but there is no sharp line between normals on the one hand, and the serum uric acid of those with clinical gout. Normal ranges cannot be adjusted for purine ingestion, but high purine diet increases uric acid. Uric acid may be increased with body size, exercise, and stress.

Dosage Forms Excipient information presented when available (limited, particularly for generics); consult specific product labeling.

Solution, Intravenous:

Krystexxa: 8 mg/mL (1 mL)

◆ PegLyte (Can) *see* Polyethylene Glycol-Electrolyte Solution *on page 1669*

◆ PEG-Uricase *see* Pegloticase *on page 1599*

Pegvisomant (peg VI soe mant)

Brand Names: U.S. Somavert

Brand Names: Canada Somavert®

Index Terms B2036-PEG

Pharmacologic Category Growth Hormone Receptor Antagonist

Use Treatment of acromegaly in patients resistant to or unable to tolerate other therapies

Pregnancy Risk Factor B

Dosage SubQ: Adults: Initial loading dose: 40 mg; maintenance dose: 10 mg once daily; doses may be adjusted by 5 mg increments in 4- to 6-week intervals based on IGF-I concentrations (maximum maintenance dose: 30 mg/day)

Dosage adjustment in renal impairment: No dosage adjustment provided in manufacturer's labeling (has not been studied).

Dosage adjustment in hepatic impairment:

At initiation of therapy:

Normal liver function test (LFT): Initiate therapy; monitor LFT monthly for first 6 months, quarterly for next 6 months, then biannually the following year.

Baseline LFT elevated but ≤3 x ULN: May initiate therapy with monthly evaluation of LFT for 1 year then biannually the following year.

Baseline LFT >3 x ULN: Do not initiate treatment without comprehensive work-up to determine cause; monitor closely if treatment is started.

With ongoing therapy:

LFT ≥3 x but <5 x ULN without signs/symptoms of hepatitis, hepatic injury, or increase in total bilirubin: Continue treatment, but monitor LFT weekly for further increases; perform comprehensive hepatic work-up to rule out alternative cause of hepatic dysfunction

LFT ≥5 x ULN or transaminase ≥3 x ULN associated with any increase in total bilirubin: Discontinue immediately and perform comprehensive hepatic work-up. If LFTs return to normal, may cautiously consider restarting therapy with frequent LFT monitoring.

Signs or symptoms of hepatitis or hepatic injury: Discontinue therapy immediately and perform comprehensive hepatic work-up; discontinue permanently if liver injury is confirmed.

Additional Information Complete prescribing information should be consulted for additional detail.

Dosage Forms Excipient information presented when available (limited, particularly for generics); consult specific product labeling.

Solution Reconstituted, Subcutaneous:

Somavert: 10 mg (1 ea); 15 mg (1 ea); 20 mg (1 ea)

- **Pegylated DOXOrubicin Liposomal** *see* DOXOrubicin (Liposomal) *on page 663*
- **Pegylated G-CSF** *see* Pegfilgrastim *on page 1588*
- **Pegylated Interferon Alfa-2a** *see* Peginterferon Alfa-2a *on page 1590*
- **Pegylated Interferon Alfa-2b** *see* Peginterferon Alfa-2b *on page 1594*
- **Pegylated Liposomal DOXOrubicin** *see* DOXOrubicin (Liposomal) *on page 663*
- **Pegylated Liposomal DOXOrubicin Hydrochloride (Doxil®, Caelyx®)** *see* DOXOrubicin (Liposomal) *on page 663*
- **Pegylated Urate Oxidase** *see* Pegloticase *on page 1599*
- **PEGyLAX** *see* Polyethylene Glycol 3350 *on page 1668*
- **PE-Hist-DM [OTC]** *see* Chlorpheniramine, Phenylephrine, and Dextromethorphan *on page 413*

PEMEtrexed (pem e TREKS ed)

Brand Names: U.S. Alimta

Brand Names: Canada Alimta

Index Terms LY231514; Pemetrexed Disodium

Pharmacologic Category Antineoplastic Agent, Antimetabolite; Antineoplastic Agent, Antimetabolite (Antifolate)

Use Treatment of unresectable malignant pleural mesothelioma (in combination with cisplatin); treatment of locally advanced or metastatic **non**squamous nonsmall cell lung cancer (NSCLC; as initial treatment in combination with cisplatin, as single-agent maintenance treatment after 4 cycles of initial platinum-based double therapy, and single-agent treatment after prior chemotherapy)

Note: Not indicated for the treatment of **squamous** cell NSCLC

Unlabeled Use Treatment of bladder cancer (metastatic), cervical cancer (recurrent or metastatic), ovarian cancer (recurrent or persistent), thymic malignancies; treatment of malignant pleural mesothelioma (either as a single agent or in combination with carboplatin)

Pregnancy Risk Factor D

Pregnancy Considerations Adverse effects (embryotoxicity, fetotoxicity and teratogenicity) were observed in animal reproduction studies. Based on the mechanism of action, may cause fetal harm if administered to a pregnant woman. Women of childbearing potential should have a negative serum pregnancy test prior to treatment and should use effective contraceptive measures to avoid becoming pregnant during treatment. Irreversible infertility has been reported in males; prior to receiving treatment, males should be counseled on sperm storage. The Canadian labeling recommends that males receiving therapy use effective contraceptive measures and not father a child during, and for up to 6 months after therapy.

Breast-Feeding Considerations According to the manufacturer, the decision to continue or discontinue breast-feeding during therapy should take into account the risk of exposure to the infant and the benefits of treatment to the mother.

Contraindications Severe hypersensitivity to pemetrexed or any component of the formulation

Canadian labeling (additional contraindications; not in U.S. labeling): Concomitant yellow fever vaccine

Warnings/Precautions Hazardous agent - use appropriate precautions for handling and disposal (NIOSH, 2012). Hypersensitivity (including anaphylaxis) has been reported with use. May cause bone marrow suppression (anemia, neutropenia, thrombocytopenia and/or pancytopenia); frequent laboratory monitoring is necessary (myelosuppression is often dose-limiting). Dose reductions in subsequent cycles may be required. Prophylactic folic acid and vitamin B_{12} supplements are necessary to reduce hematologic and gastrointestinal toxicity and infection; initiate supplementation 1 week before the first dose of pemetrexed. Pretreatment with dexamethasone is necessary to reduce the incidence and severity of cutaneous reactions. Rarely, Stevens-Johnson syndrome and toxic epidermal necrolysis have been reported. Although the effect of third space fluid is not fully defined, studies have determined pemetrexed concentrations in patients with mild-to-moderate ascites/pleural effusions were similar to concentrations in trials of patients without third space fluid accumulation. Drainage of fluid from ascites/effusions may be considered, but is not likely necessary. Use caution with hepatic dysfunction not due to metastases; may require dose adjustment. Interstitial pneumonitis with respiratory insufficiency has been observed with use; interrupt therapy and evaluate promptly with progressive dyspnea and cough.

The manufacturer does not recommend use in patients with Cl_{cr} <45 mL/minute. Decreased renal function results in increased toxicity. Use caution in patients receiving concurrent nephrotoxins; may result in delayed pemetrexed clearance. NSAIDs may reduce the clearance of pemetrexed. In patients with Cl_{cr} 45-79 mL/minute, interruption of NSAID therapy may be necessary prior to, during, and immediately after pemetrexed therapy. Not indicated for use in patients with squamous cell NSCLC.

Adverse Reactions

>10%:

Central nervous system: Fatigue (18% to 34%; dose-limiting)

Dermatologic: Rash/desquamation (10% to 14%)

Gastrointestinal: Nausea (12% to 31%), anorexia (19% to 22%), vomiting (6% to 16%), stomatitis (5% to 15%), diarrhea (5% to 13%)

Hematologic: Anemia (15% to 19%; grades 3/4: 3% to 5%), leukopenia (6% to 12%; grades 3/4: 2% to 4%), neutropenia (6% to 11%; grades 3/4: 3% to 5%; dose-limiting; nadir: 8-10 days; recovery: 4-8 days after nadir)

Respiratory: Pharyngitis (15%)

1% to 10%:
- Cardiovascular: Edema (1% to 5%)
- Central nervous system: Fever (1% to 8%)
- Dermatologic: Pruritus (1% to 7%), alopecia (1% to 6%), erythema multiforme (≤5%)
- Gastrointestinal: Constipation (1% to 6%), weight loss (1%), abdominal pain (≤5%)
- Hematologic: Thrombocytopenia (1% to 8%; grades 3/4: 2%; dose-limiting), febrile neutropenia (grades 3/4: 2%)
- Hepatic: ALT increased (8% to 10%; grades 3/4: ≤2%), AST increased (7% to 8%; grades 3/4: ≤1%)
- Neuromuscular & skeletal: Sensory neuropathy (≤9%), motor neuropathy (≤5%)
- Ocular: Conjunctivitis (≤5%), lacrimation increased (≤5%)
- Renal: Creatinine increased/creatinine clearance decreased (1% to 5%)
- Miscellaneous: Allergic reaction/hypersensitivity (≤5%), infection (≤5%), sepsis (1%)

<1% (Limited to important or life-threatening): Arrhythmia, colitis, dehydration, esophagitis, gastrointestinal obstruction, hemolytic anemia, hepatobiliary failure, hypertension, interstitial pneumonitis, pancreatitis, pancytopenia, peripheral ischemia, pulmonary embolism, radiation recall (median onset: 6 days; range: 1-35 days), renal failure, Stevens-Johnson syndrome, supraventricular arrhythmia, syncope, thrombosis/embolism, toxic epidermal necrolysis, ventricular tachycardia

Drug Interactions

Metabolism/Transport Effects None known.

Avoid Concomitant Use

Avoid concomitant use of PEMEtrexed with any of the following: BCG; CloZAPine; Natalizumab; Pimecrolimus; Tacrolimus (Topical); Tofacitinib; Vaccines (Live)

Increased Effect/Toxicity

PEMEtrexed may increase the levels/effects of: CloZAPine; Leflunomide; Natalizumab; Tofacitinib; Vaccines (Live)

The levels/effects of PEMEtrexed may be increased by: Denosumab; NSAID (Nonselective); Pimecrolimus; Roflumilast; Tacrolimus (Topical); Trastuzumab

Decreased Effect

PEMEtrexed may decrease the levels/effects of: BCG; Coccidioidin Skin Test; Sipuleucel-T; Vaccines (Inactivated); Vaccines (Live)

The levels/effects of PEMEtrexed may be decreased by: Echinacea

Ethanol/Nutrition/Herb Interactions Lower ANC nadirs occur in patients with elevated baseline cystathionine or homocysteine concentrations. Levels of these substances can be reduced by folic acid and vitamin B_{12} supplementation.

Preparation for Administration Hazardous agent; use appropriate precautions for handling and disposal (NIOSH, 2012). Reconstitute with NS (preservative free); add 4.2 mL to the 100 mg vial and 20 mL to the 500 mg vial, resulting in a 25 mg/mL concentration. Gently swirl. Solution may be colorless to green-yellow. Further dilute in 100 mL NS for infusion; may also dilute in D_5W (Zhang, 2006), although the manufacturer recommends NS.

Storage/Stability Store intact vials at room temperature of 25°C (77°F); excursions permitted to 15°C to 30°C (59°F to 86°F). Reconstituted solution in NS and infusion solutions (in D_5W or NS) are stable for 24 hours when refrigerated at 2°C to 8°C (36°F to 46°F). Concentrations at 25 mg/mL are stable in polypropylene syringes for 2 days at room temperature (23°C) (Zhang, 2005).

Mechanism of Action Antifolate; disrupts folate-dependent metabolic processes essential for cell replication. Inhibits thymidylate synthase (TS), dihydrofolate reductase (DHFR), glycinamide ribonucleotide formyltransferase (GARFT), and aminoimidazole carboxamide ribonucleotide formyltransferase (AICARFT), the enzymes involved in folate metabolism and DNA synthesis, resulting in inhibition of purine and thymidine nucleotide and protein synthesis.

Pharmacodynamics/Kinetics

Distribution: V_{dss}: 16.1 L

Protein binding: ~73% to 81%

Metabolism: Minimal

Half-life elimination: Normal renal function: 3.5 hours; Cl_{cr} 40-59 mL/minute: 5.3-5.8 hours

Excretion: Urine (70% to 90% as unchanged drug)

Dosage Details concerning dosing in combination regimens should also be consulted. **Note:** Start vitamin supplements 1 week before initial pemetrexed dose: Folic acid 400-1000 mcg daily orally (begin 7 days prior to treatment initiation; continue daily during treatment and for 21 days after last pemetrexed dose) and vitamin B_{12} 1000 mcg I.M. 7 days prior to treatment initiation and then every 3 cycles. Give dexamethasone 4 mg orally twice daily for 3 days, beginning the day before treatment to minimize cutaneous reactions. New treatment cycles should not begin unless ANC ≥1500/mm³, platelets ≥100,000/mm³, and Cl_{cr} ≥45 mL/minute.

I.V.: Adults:
- Malignant pleural mesothelioma: 500 mg/m² on day 1 of each 21-day cycle (in combination with cisplatin) **or** (unlabeled) in combination with carboplatin (Castagneto, 2008; Ceresoli, 2006) **or** (unlabeled) as single-agent therapy (Jassem, 2008; Taylor, 2008)
- Nonsmall cell lung cancer:
  - *Initial treatment:* 500 mg/m² on day 1 of each 21-day cycle (in combination with cisplatin)
  - *Maintenance or second-line treatment:* 500 mg/m² on day 1 of each 21-day cycle (as a single-agent)
- Bladder cancer (unlabeled use): 500 mg/m² on day 1 of each 21-day cycle (Sweeney, 2006)
- Cervical cancer, persistent or recurrent (unlabeled use): 500 mg/m² on day 1 of each 21-day cycle until disease progression or unacceptable toxicity occurs (Lorusso, 2010) **or** 900 mg/m² on day 1 of each 21-day cycle (Miller, 2008)
- Ovarian cancer, platinum-resistant (unlabeled use): 500 mg/m² on day 1 of each 21-day cycle (Vergote, 2009)
- Thymic malignancies, metastatic (unlabeled use): 500 mg/m² on day 1 of each 21-day cycle for 6 cycles or until disease progression or unacceptable toxicity occurs (Loehrer, 2006)

Dosage adjustments for toxicities:
- *Toxicity:* Discontinue if patient develops grade 3 or 4 toxicity after two dose reductions or immediately if grade 3 or 4 neurotoxicity develops
- *Hematologic toxicity:* Upon recovery, reinitiate therapy
  - Nadir ANC <500/mm³ and nadir platelets ≥50,000/mm³: Reduce dose to 75% of previous dose of pemetrexed (and cisplatin)
  - Nadir platelets <50,000/mm³ **without bleeding** (regardless of nadir ANC): Reduce dose to 75% of previous dose of pemetrexed (and cisplatin)
  - Nadir platelets <50,000/mm³ **with bleeding** (regardless of nadir ANC): Reduce dose to 50% of previous dose of pemetrexed (and cisplatin)
- *Nonhematologic toxicity ≥grade 3 (excluding neurotoxicity):* Withhold treatment until recovery to baseline; upon recovery, reinitiate therapy as follows:
  - Grade 3 or 4 toxicity (excluding mucositis): Reduce dose to 75% of previous dose of pemetrexed (and cisplatin)
  - Grade 3 or 4 diarrhea or any diarrhea requiring hospitalization: Reduce dose to 75% of previous dose of pemetrexed (and cisplatin)

Grade 3 or 4 mucositis: Reduce pemetrexed dose to 50% of previous dose (continue cisplatin at 100% of previous dose)

Neurotoxicity:

Grade 0-1: Continue pemetrexed at 100% of previous dose (and cisplatin)

Grade 2: Continue pemetrexed at 100% of previous dose; reduce cisplatin dose to 50% of previous dose

Dosage adjustment in renal impairment: Renal function may be estimated using the Cockcroft-Gault formula (using actual body weight) or glomerular filtration rate (GFR) measured by Tc99m-DPTA serum clearance.

Cl_{cr} ≥45 mL/minute: No dosage adjustment necessary.

Cl_{cr} <45 mL/minute: Use not recommended (an insufficient number of patients have been studied for dosage recommendations).

Concomitant NSAID use with renal dysfunction:

Cl_{cr} ≥80 mL/minute: No dosage adjustment necessary.

Cl_{cr} 45 to 79 mL/minute and NSAIDs with short half-lives (eg, ibuprofen, indomethacin, ketoprofen, ketorolac): Avoid NSAID for 2 days before, the day of, and for 2 days following a dose of pemetrexed

Any creatinine clearance and NSAIDs with long half-lives (eg, nabumetone, naproxen, oxaprozin, piroxicam): Avoid NSAID for 5 days before, the day of, and 2 days following a dose of pemetrexed

Dosage adjustment in hepatic impairment: Grade 3 (5.1-20 times ULN) **or** 4 (>20 times ULN) transaminase elevation during treatment: Reduce pemetrexed dose to 75% of previous dose (and cisplatin)

Dosing in obesity: *ASCO Guidelines for appropriate chemotherapy dosing in obese adults with cancer:* Utilize patient's actual body weight (full weight) for calculation of body surface area- or weight-based dosing, particularly when the intent of therapy is curative; manage regimen-related toxicities in the same manner as for nonobese patients; if a dose reduction is utilized due to toxicity, consider resumption of full weight-based dosing with subsequent cycles, especially if cause of toxicity (eg, hepatic or renal impairment) is resolved (Griggs, 2012).

Dietary Considerations Initiate folic acid supplementation 1 week before first dose of pemetrexed, continue for full course of therapy, and for 21 days after last dose. Institute vitamin B_{12} 1 week before the first dose; administer every 9 weeks thereafter.

Administration I.V.: Infuse over 10 minutes.

Hazardous agent; use appropriate precautions for handling and disposal (NIOSH, 2012).

Monitoring Parameters CBC with differential and platelets (before each dose; monitor for nadir and recovery); serum creatinine, creatinine clearance, BUN, total bilirubin, ALT, AST (periodic); signs/symptoms of mucositis and diarrhea

Dosage Forms Excipient information presented when available (limited, particularly for generics); consult specific product labeling.

Solution Reconstituted, Intravenous:

Alimta: 100 mg (1 ea); 500 mg (1 ea)

◆ **Pemetrexed Disodium** *see* PEMEtrexed *on page 1601*

Penciclovir (pen SYE kloe veer)

Brand Names: U.S. Denavir

Pharmacologic Category Antiviral Agent

Use Topical treatment of recurrent herpes simplex labialis (cold sores)

Pregnancy Risk Factor B

Dosage Children ≥12 years and Adults: Topical: Apply cream at the first sign or symptom of cold sore (eg, tingling, swelling); apply every 2 hours during waking hours for 4 days

Additional Information Complete prescribing information should be consulted for additional detail.

Dosage Forms Excipient information presented when available (limited, particularly for generics); consult specific product labeling.

Cream, External:

Denavir: 1% (1.5 g, 5 g) [contains cetostearyl alcohol, propylene glycol]

PenicillAMINE (pen i SIL a meen)

Brand Names: U.S. Cuprimine; Depen Titratabs

Brand Names: Canada Cuprimine®

Index Terms D-3-Mercaptovaline; D-Penicillamine; β,β-Dimethylcysteine

Pharmacologic Category Chelating Agent

Use Treatment of Wilson's disease, cystinuria; adjunctive treatment of severe, active rheumatoid arthritis

Canadian labeling: Additional use (not in U.S. labeling): Treatment of chronic lead poisoning

Pregnancy Risk Factor D

Pregnancy Considerations Birth defects, including congenital cutix laxa and associated defects, have been reported in infants following penicillamine exposure during pregnancy. Use for the treatment of rheumatoid arthritis during pregnancy is contraindicated. Use for the treatment of cystinuria only if the possible benefits to the mother outweigh the potential risks to the fetus. Continued treatment of Wilson's disease during pregnancy protects the mother against relapse. Discontinuation has detrimental maternal and fetal effects. Daily dosage should be limited to 750 mg. For planned cesarean section, reduce dose to 250 mg/day for the last 6 weeks of pregnancy, and continue at this dosage until wound healing is complete.

Breast-Feeding Considerations It is not known if penicillamine is excreted in breast milk. Use while breast-feeding is contraindicated by the manufacturer.

Contraindications Renal insufficiency (in patients with rheumatoid arthritis); patients with previous penicillamine-related aplastic anemia or agranulocytosis; breast-feeding; pregnancy (in patients with rheumatoid arthritis)

Canadian labeling: Additional contraindications (not in U.S. labeling): Hypersensitivity to penicillamine or any component of the formulation; use in patients with chronic lead poisoning who have radiographic evidence of lead-containing substances in the GI tract; pregnancy (in patients with chronic lead poisoning); concomitant use with gold therapy, antimalarial or cytotoxic drugs, oxyphenbutazone or phenylbutazone

Warnings/Precautions Approximately 33% of patients will experience an allergic reaction; toxicity may be dose related; use caution in the elderly. Once instituted for Wilson's disease or cystinuria, continue treatment on a daily basis; interruptions of even a few days have been followed by hypersensitivity with reinstitution of therapy. Rash may occur early (more commonly) or late in therapy; early-onset rash typically resolves within days of discontinuation of therapy and does not recur upon rechallenge with reduced dose; discontinue therapy for late-onset rash (eg, after >6 months) and do not rechallenge; rash typically recurs with rechallenge. Drug fever sometimes in conjunction with macular cutaneous eruptions may be observed usually 2-3 weeks after therapy initiation. Discontinue use in patients with rheumatoid arthritis, Wilson's disease or cystinuria who develop a marked febrile response. Consider alternative therapy for patients with rheumatoid arthritis due to high incidence of fever reoccurrence with penicillamine rechallenge. May resume therapy at a reduced dose in Wilson's disease or cystinuria upon resolution of fever. Discontinue therapy for skin reactions accompanied by lymphadenopathy, fever, arthralgia, or other allergic reactions. Patients with a penicillin allergy may theoretically have cross-sensitivity to penicillamine; however, the possibility has been eliminated now that penicillamine is produced synthetically and no longer contains trace amounts of penicillin.

[U.S. Boxed Warning]: Patients should be warned to report promptly any symptoms suggesting toxicity (fever, sore throat, chills, bruising, or bleeding); penicillamine has been associated with fatalities due to agranulocytosis, aplastic anemia, and thrombocytopenia. Use caution with other hematopoietic-depressant drugs (eg, gold, immunosuppressants, antimalarials, phenylbutazone; Canadian labeling contraindicates concomitant use with these agents). Discontinue therapy for WBC <3500/mm^3. Withhold therapy at least temporarily for platelet counts <100,000/mm^3 or a progressive fall in WBC or platelets in 3 successive determinations, even though values may remain within the normal range. Proteinuria or hematuria may develop; monitor for membranous glomerulopathy which can lead to nephrotic syndrome. In rheumatoid arthritis patients, discontinue if gross hematuria or persistent microscopic hematuria develop and discontinue therapy or reduce dose for proteinuria that is either >1 g/day or progressively increasing. Dose reduction may lead to resolution of proteinuria.

[U.S. Boxed Warning]: Should be administered under the close supervision of a physician familiar with the toxicity and dosage considerations. Monitor liver function tests periodically due to rare reports of intrahepatic cholestasis or toxic hepatitis. Has been associated with myasthenic syndrome which in some cases progressed to myasthenia gravis. Resolution of symptoms has been observed in most cases following discontinuation of therapy. Bronchiolitis obliterans has been reported rarely with use. Pemphigus may occur early or late in therapy; discontinue use with suspicion of pemphigus. Lupus erythematosus-like syndrome may be observed in some patients; Taste alteration may occur (rare in Wilson's disease); usually self-limited with continued therapy, however may last ≥2 months and result in total loss of taste. Oral ulceration (eg, stomatitis) may occur; typically recurs on rechallenge, but often resolves with dose reduction. Other dose-related lesions (eg, glossitis, gingivostomatitis) have been observed with use and may require therapy discontinuation. Pyridoxine supplementation (25-50 mg/day) is recommended in Wilson's disease (Roberts, 2008) or 25 mg/day in cystinuria or in rheumatoid arthritis patients with impaired nutrition.

Penicillamine increases the amount of soluble collagen; may increase skin friability, particularly at sites subject to pressure or trauma (eg, knees, elbows shoulders). Purpuric areas with localized bleeding (if skin is broken) or vesicles with dark blood may be observed. Effects are considered localized and do not necessitate discontinuation of therapy; may not recur with dose reduction. Dose reduction may be considered prior to surgical procedures. May resume normal recommended dosing postoperatively once wound healing is complete.

Lead poisoning: Investigate, identify, and remove sources of lead exposure and confirm lead-containing substances are absent from the GI tract prior to initiating therapy. Do not permit patients to re-enter the contaminated environment until lead abatement has been completed. Penicillamine is considered to be a third-line agent for the treatment of lead poisoning in children due to the overall toxicity associated with its use (AAP, 2005; Chandran, 2010); penicillamine should only be used when unacceptable reactions have occurred with edetate CALCIUM disodium and succimer. Primary care providers should consult experts in the chemotherapy of lead toxicity before using chelation drug therapy.

Adverse Reactions Frequency not always defined and may vary by indication.

Cardiovascular: Vasculitis

Central nervous system: Anxiety, agitation, fever, Guillain-Barré syndrome, hyperpyrexia, psychiatric disturbances, worsening neurologic symptoms

Dermatologic: Alopecia, cheilosis, dermatomyositis, drug eruptions, exfoliative dermatitis, lichen planus, pemphigus, pruritus, rash (early and late: 5%), skin friability increased, toxic epidermal necrolysis, urticaria, wrinkling (excessive), yellow nail syndrome

Endocrine & metabolic: Hypoglycemia, thyroiditis

Gastrointestinal: Diarrhea (17%), taste alteration (12%), anorexia, epigastric pain, gingivostomatitis, glossitis, nausea, oral ulcerations, pancreatitis, peptic ulcer reactivation, vomiting

Hematologic: Thrombocytopenia (4%), leukopenia (2%), agranulocytosis, aplastic anemia, eosinophilia, hemolytic anemia, leukocytosis, monocytosis, red cell aplasia, sideroblastic anemia, thrombotic thrombocytopenia purpura, thrombocytosis

Hepatic: Alkaline phosphatase increased, hepatic failure, intrahepatic cholestasis, toxic hepatitis

Local: Thrombophlebitis, white papules at venipuncture and surgical sites

Neuromuscular & skeletal: Arthralgia, dystonia, myasthenia gravis, muscle weakness, neuropathies, polyarthralgia (migratory, often with objective synovitis), polymyositis

Ocular: Diplopia, extraocular muscle weakness, optic neuritis, ptosis, visual disturbances

Otic: Tinnitus

Renal: Proteinuria (6%), Goodpasture's syndrome, hematuria, nephrotic syndrome, renal failure, renal vasculitis

Respiratory: Asthma, interstitial pneumonitis, pulmonary fibrosis, obliterative bronchiolitis

Miscellaneous: Allergic alveolitis, anetoderma, elastosis perforans serpiginosa, lupus-like syndrome, lactic dehydrogenase increased, lymphadenopathy, mammary hyperplasia, positive ANA test

Drug Interactions

Metabolism/Transport Effects None known.

Avoid Concomitant Use There are no known interactions where it is recommended to avoid concomitant use.

Increased Effect/Toxicity

The levels/effects of PenicillAMINE may be increased by: Multivitamins/Minerals (with ADEK, Folate, Iron)

Decreased Effect

PenicillAMINE may decrease the levels/effects of: Digoxin

The levels/effects of PenicillAMINE may be decreased by: Antacids; Iron Salts

Ethanol/Nutrition/Herb Interactions

Ethanol: Management: Avoid or limit ethanol.

Food: Penicillamine serum levels may be decreased if taken with food. Management: Administer on an empty stomach 1 hour before or 2 hours after meals and at least 1 hour apart from other drugs, milk, antacids, and zinc- or iron-containing products. Certain disease states require further diet adjustment. Limit intake of vitamin A.

Storage/Stability Store in tight, well-closed containers.

Mechanism of Action Chelates with lead, copper, mercury and other heavy metals to form stable, soluble complexes that are excreted in urine; depresses circulating IgM rheumatoid factor, depresses T-cell but not B-cell activity; combines with cystine to form a compound which is more soluble, thus cystine calculi are prevented

Pharmacodynamics/Kinetics

Onset of action: Rheumatoid arthritis: 2-3 months; Wilson's disease: 1-3 months

Absorption: Rapid but incomplete

Protein binding: >80% to albumin and ceruloplasmin

Metabolism: Hepatic (small amounts metabolized to s-methyl-d-penicillamine)

Bioavailability: 40% to 70%; reduced by food, antacids, and iron

Half-life elimination: 1.7-7 hours (Roberts, 2008)

Time to peak, serum: 1-3 hours

Excretion: Urine (primarily as disulfides)

Dosage Oral: **Note:** Dose reduction to 250 mg/day may be considered prior to surgical procedures. May resume normal recommended dosing postoperatively once wound healing is complete.

Cystinuria: **Note:** Adjust dose to limit cystine excretion to 100-200 mg/day (<100 mg/day with history of stone formation)

Children: 30 mg/kg/day in 4 divided doses

Adults: 1-4 g/day in 4 divided doses; usual dose: 2 g/day; initiation of therapy at 250 mg/day with gradual upward titration may reduce the risk of unwanted effects

Lead poisoning:

Canadian labeling:

Children: 30-40 mg/kg/day or 600-750 mg/m^2/day in 1-2 divided doses (maximum dose: 750 mg/day); treat until blood lead concentrations <40 mcg/dL for 2 consecutive months and at least 1 of the following: Decrease in erythrocyte protoporphyrin level to <3-5 times the average normal level or the excretion of coproporphyrin or delta-aminolevulinic acid decreases to the upper limit of normal. **Note:** Manufacturer labeling recommends initiating therapy only in children who meet the following criteria: Asymptomatic, blood lead concentrations of 50-80 mcg/dL, erythrocyte protoporphyrin level >400-500 mcg/dL erythrocytes, excessive excretion of delta-aminolevulinic acid and/or coproporphyrin.

Adults: 900-1500 mg/day in 3 divided doses for 1-2 weeks, then 750 mg/day in divided doses until blood lead concentrations <60 mcg/dL or urinary lead excretion <500 mcg/L for 2 consecutive months

Alternate recommendations (unlabeled dosing): **Note:** The American Academy of Pediatrics (AAP) considers penicillamine a third-line agent for the management of lead poisoning (AAP, 2005; Chandran, 2010): Children: 10-15 mg/kg/day for 4-12 weeks (Chandran, 2010). **Note:** The CDC recommends chelation treatment when blood lead concentrations are >45 mcg/dL (CDC, 2002). Children with blood lead concentrations >70 mcg/dL or symptomatic lead poisoning should be treated with parenteral agents (AAP, 2005).

Rheumatoid arthritis:

Children (unlabeled use): Initial: 3 mg/kg/day (≤250 mg/day) for 3 months, then 6 mg/kg/day (≤500 mg/day) in divided doses twice daily for 3 months to a maximum of 10 mg/kg/day in 3-4 divided doses; maximum dose: 750 mg/day (Rosenberg, 1989)

Adults: Initial: 125-250 mg/day, may increase dose by 125-250 mg/day at 1- to 3-month intervals up to 1-1.5 g/day; discontinue in patients failing to improve after 3-4 months at these doses

Elderly: Therapy should be initiated at low end of dosing range and titrated upward cautiously.

Wilson's disease: **Note:** Dose that results in an initial 24-hour urinary copper excretion >2 mg/day should be continued for ~3 months; maintenance dose defined by amount resulting in <10 mcg serum free copper/dL.

Manufacturer labeling recommendations:

Adults: 750-1500 mg/day in divided doses; maximum dose: 2000 mg/day. **Note:** Limit daily dose to 750 mg/day (U.S. labeling) or 1000 mg/day (Canadian labeling) in pregnant women; if planned caesarian, limit dose to 250 mg/day during the last 6 weeks of pregnancy and postoperatively until wound healing is complete.

Elderly: Therapy should be initiated at low end of dosing range and titrated upward cautiously.

Alternate recommendations (unlabeled dosing): American Association for the Study of Liver Diseases (AASLD) guidelines (Roberts, 2008):

Children: 20 mg/kg/day in 2-3 divided doses, round off to the nearest 250 mg dose

Adults: To increase tolerability, therapy may be initiated at 250-500 mg/day then titrated upward in 250 mg increments every 4-7 days; usual maintenance dose: 750-1000 mg/day in 2 divided doses; maximum: 1000-1500 mg/day in 2-4 divided doses

Dosing adjustment in renal impairment:

Manufacturer labeling recommendations: No dosage adjustment provided in manufacturer's labeling; however, the manufacturer labeling does suggest a cautious approach to dosing as this drug undergoes mainly renal elimination.

Alternate recommendations:

Cl_{cr} <50 mL/minute: Avoid use (Aronoff, 2007)

Hemodialysis: Dialyzable; Administer 33% of usual dose (Aronoff, 2007); a dosing decrease from 250 mg/day to 250 mg 3 times/week after dialysis has been suggested in the treatment of rheumatoid arthritis (Swarup, 2004).

Dosage adjustment in hepatic impairment: No dosage adjustment provided in manufacturer's labeling; however, only a small fraction is metabolized hepatically.

Dietary Considerations Should be taken at least 1 hour before or 2 hours after meals on an empty stomach (Note: Canadian labeling recommends administration at least 2 hours before meals in patients with lead poisoning). Pyridoxine supplementation is recommended. Patients with Wilson's disease should receive 25-50 mg/day of pyridoxine (Roberts, 2008); a multivitamin (without copper) may also be considered. Patients with cystinuria or patients with rheumatoid arthritis and impaired nutritional intake should receive 25 mg/day of pyridoxine. For Wilson's disease, decrease copper in diet to <1-2 mg/day and omit chocolate, nuts, shellfish, mushrooms, liver, raisins, broccoli, copper-enriched cereal, multivitamins with copper, and molasses. May consider short courses of iron supplementation if dietary modifications (eg, low copper diet in Wilson's disease, low methionine diet in cystinuria) results in iron deficiency; pediatric patients and menstruating women may be particularly susceptible to iron deficiency. Allow 2 hours between administration of iron supplementation and penicillamine as iron may decrease drug absorption. For cystinuria, increase daily fluid intake including 1 pint (~500 mL) of fluid prior to bedtime and 1 additional pint during the night. For lead poisoning, decrease calcium in diet.

Administration Doses ≤500 mg may be administered as single dose; doses >500 mg should be administered in divided doses. For patients who cannot swallow, contents of capsules may be administered in 15-30 mL of chilled puréed fruit or fruit juice within 5 minutes of administration. Administer on an empty stomach (1 hour before or 2 hours after meals) and at least 1 hour apart from other drugs, milk, antacids, and zinc or iron-containing products. Canadian labeling recommends administering at least 2 hours before meals in patients with lead poisoning.

Cystinuria: If administering 4 equal doses is not feasible, administer the larger dose at bedtime.

Monitoring Parameters Urinalysis, CBC with differential, platelet count, skin, lymph nodes, and body temperature twice weekly during the first month of therapy, then every 2 weeks for 5 months, then monthly; LFTs every 6 months; signs/symptoms of hypersensitivity

Cystinuria: Urinary cystine, annual X-ray for renal stones

Lead poisoning: Serum lead concentration (baseline and 7-21 days after completing chelation therapy); hemoglobin or hematocrit, iron status, free erythrocyte protoporphyrin or zinc protoporphyrin; neurodevelopmental changes

Wilson's disease: Serum non-ceruloplasmin bound copper, 24-hour urinary copper excretion, LFTs every 3 months (at least) during the first year of treatment; periodic ophthalmic exam

Urinalysis: Monitor for proteinuria and hematuria. A quantitative 24-hour urine protein at 1- to 2-week intervals initially (first 2-3 months) is recommended if proteinuria develops.

Reference Range Wilson's disease: 24-hour urinary copper excretion: 200-500 mcg (3-8 micromoles)/day

Dosage Forms Excipient information presented when available (limited, particularly for generics); consult specific product labeling.

Capsule, Oral:

Cuprimine: 250 mg [contains fd&c yellow #10 (quinoline yellow)]

Tablet, Oral:

Depen Titratabs: 250 mg [scored]

Extemporaneous Preparations A 50 mg/mL oral suspension may be made with capsules. Mix the contents of sixty 250 mg capsules with 3 g carboxymethylcellulose, 150 g sucrose, 300 mg citric acid, and parabens (methylparaben 120 mg, propylparaben 12 mg). Add quantity of propylene glycol sufficient to make 100 mL, then add quantity of purified water sufficient to make 300 mL. Cherry flavor may be added. Label "shake well" and "refrigerate". Stable for 30 days refrigerated.

DeCastro FJ, Jaeger RQ, and Rolfe UT, "An Extemporaneously Prepared Penicillamine Suspension Used to Treat Lead Intoxication," *Hosp Pharm*, 1977, 2:446-8.

Penicillin G Benzathine

(pen i SIL in jee BENZ a theen)

Brand Names: U.S. Bicillin L-A

Brand Names: Canada Bicillin® L-A

Index Terms Benzathine Benzylpenicillin; Benzathine Penicillin G; Benzylpenicillin Benzathine

Pharmacologic Category Antibiotic, Penicillin

Use Active against some gram-positive organisms, few gram-negative organisms such as *Neisseria gonorrhoeae*, and some anaerobes and spirochetes; used in the treatment of syphilis; used only for the treatment of mild to moderately-severe upper respiratory tract infections caused by organisms susceptible to low concentrations of penicillin G or for prophylaxis of infections caused by these organisms; primary and secondary prevention of rheumatic fever

Pregnancy Risk Factor B

Pregnancy Considerations Adverse events have not been observed in animal reproduction studies. Penicillin crosses the placenta and distributes into amniotic fluid. Maternal use of penicillins has generally not resulted in an increased risk of adverse fetal effects. Penicillin G is the drug of choice for treatment of syphilis during pregnancy.

Breast-Feeding Considerations Penicillins are excreted in breast milk. The manufacturer recommends that caution be exercised when administering penicillin to nursing women. Nondose-related effects could include modification of bowel flora and allergic sensitization.

Contraindications Hypersensitivity to penicillin(s) or any component of the formulation

Warnings/Precautions Use with caution in patients with impaired renal function, seizure disorder, or history of hypersensitivity to other beta-lactams; CDC and AAP do not currently recommend the use of penicillin G benzathine to treat congenital syphilis or neurosyphilis due to reported treatment failures and lack of published clinical data on its efficacy. Prolonged use may result in fungal or bacterial superinfection, including *C. difficile*-associated diarrhea (CDAD) and pseudomembranous colitis; CDAD has been observed >2 months postantibiotic treatment. **[U.S. Boxed Warning]: Not for intravenous use; cardiopulmonary arrest and death have occurred from inadvertent I.V. administration;** administer by deep I.M. injection only; injection into or near an artery or nerve could result in severe neurovascular damage or permanent neurological damage. Extended duration of therapy or use associated with high serum concentrations may be associated with an increased risk for some adverse reactions.

Adverse Reactions Frequency not defined.

Cardiovascular: Cardiac arrest, cerebral vascular accident, cyanosis, gangrene, hypotension, pallor, palpitations, syncope, tachycardia, vasodilation, vasospasm, vasovagal reaction

Central nervous system: Anxiety, coma, confusion, dizziness, euphoria, fatigue, headache, nervousness, pain, seizure, somnolence

In addition, a syndrome of CNS symptoms has been reported which includes: Severe agitation with confusion, hallucinations (auditory and visual), and fear of death (Hoigne's syndrome); other symptoms include cyanosis, dizziness, palpitations, psychosis, seizures, tachycardia, taste disturbance, tinnitus

Gastrointestinal: Bloody stool, intestinal necrosis, nausea, vomiting

Genitourinary: Impotence, priapism

Hepatic: AST increased

Local: Injection site reactions: Abscess, atrophy, bruising, cellulitis, edema, hemorrhage, inflammation, lump, necrosis, pain, skin ulcer

Neuromuscular & skeletal: Arthritis exacerbation, joint disorder, neurovascular damage, numbness, periostitis, rhabdomyolysis, transverse myelitis, tremor, weakness

Ocular: Blindness, blurred vision

Renal: BUN increased, creatinine increased, hematuria, myoglobinuria, neurogenic bladder, proteinuria, renal failure

Miscellaneous: Diaphoresis, hypersensitivity reactions, Jarisch-Herxheimer reaction, lymphadenopathy, mottling, warmth

Drug Interactions

Metabolism/Transport Effects None known.

Avoid Concomitant Use

Avoid concomitant use of Penicillin G Benzathine with any of the following: BCG

Increased Effect/Toxicity

Penicillin G Benzathine may increase the levels/effects of: Methotrexate; Vitamin K Antagonists

The levels/effects of Penicillin G Benzathine may be increased by: Probenecid

Decreased Effect

Penicillin G Benzathine may decrease the levels/effects of: BCG; Mycophenolate; Sodium Picosulfate; Typhoid Vaccine

The levels/effects of Penicillin G Benzathine may be decreased by: Tetracycline Derivatives

Storage/Stability Refrigerate at 2°C to 8°C (36°F to 46°F); do not freeze. The following stability information has also been reported: May be stored at 25°C (77°F) for 7 days (Cohen, 2007).

Mechanism of Action Interferes with bacterial cell wall synthesis during active multiplication, causing cell wall death and resultant bactericidal activity against susceptible bacteria

Pharmacodynamics/Kinetics

Duration: 1-4 weeks (dose dependent); larger doses result in more sustained levels

Distribution: Highest levels in the kidney; lesser amounts in liver, skin, intestines

Protein Binding: ~60%

Absorption: I.M.: Slow

Time to peak, serum: 12-24 hours

Dosage Note: Administer undiluted injection; higher doses result in more sustained rather than higher levels. Use a penicillin G benzathine-penicillin G procaine combination to achieve early peak levels in acute infections.

Usual dosage range:

Children: I.M.: 25,000-50,000 units/kg as a single dose (maximum: 2.4 million units)

Adults: I.M.: 1.2-2.4 million units as a single dose

Indication-specific dosing:

Infants and Children: I.M.:

Upper respiratory infection, group A streptococci:

Primary prevention of rheumatic fever (Gerber, 2009): ≤27 kg: 600,000 units as a single dose; >27 kg: 1.2 million units as a single dose

Secondary prevention of rheumatic fever (Gerber, 2009): ≤27 kg: 600,000 units every 3-4 weeks; >27 kg: 1.2 million units every 3-4 weeks

Pharyngitis, group A streptococci (IDSA guidelines):

Acute treatment: <27 kg: 600,000 units as a single dose; ≥27 kg: 1.2 million units as a single dose (Shulman, 2012)

Chronic carrier treatment: <27 kg: 600,000 units as a single dose (in combination with oral rifampin); ≥27 kg: 1.2 million units as a single dose (in combination with oral rifampin) (Shulman, 2012)

Syphilis (CDC, 2010):

Primary, Secondary, Early Latent (<1 year duration): Infants and Children: I.M.: 50,000 units/kg as a single injection (maximum: 2.4 million units)

Late Latent, Latent with unknown duration: Children: I.M.: 50,000 units/kg every week for 3 doses (maximum: 2.4 million units/dose)

Adults: I.M.:

Upper respiratory infection, group A streptococci: 1.2 million units as a single dose

Secondary prevention of glomerulonephritis: 1.2 million units every 4 weeks or 600,000 units twice monthly

Secondary prevention of rheumatic fever: 1.2 million units every 3-4 weeks or 600,000 units twice monthly

Pharyngitis, group A streptococci (IDSA guidelines):

Acute treatment: 1.2 million units as a single dose (Shulman, 2012)

Chronic carrier treatment: 1.2 million units as a single dose in combination with oral rifampin (Shulman, 2012)

Syphilis (CDC, 2010):

Primary, Secondary, Early Latent (<1 year duration): 2.4 million units as a single dose

Late Latent, Latent with unknown duration: 2.4 million units once weekly for 3 doses

Neurosyphilis: Not indicated as single-drug therapy, but may be given once weekly for 3 weeks following I.V. treatment; refer to Penicillin G (Parenteral/Aqueous) monograph for dosing

Dosage adjustment in renal impairment: No dosage adjustment provided in manufacturer's labeling.

Dosage adjustment in hepatic impairment: No dosage adjustment provided in manufacturer's labeling.

Administration Warm to room temperature before administration to lessen the pain associated with injection. Administer by deep I.M. injection in the upper outer quadrant of the buttock; in children <2 years of age, I.M. injections should be made into the midlateral muscle of the thigh, not the gluteal region. Do not inject near an artery or a nerve; permanent neurological damage or gangrene may result. When doses are repeated, rotate the injection site. **Do not administer I.V., intra-arterially, or SubQ.**

Monitoring Parameters Observe for signs and symptoms of anaphylaxis during first dose

Test Interactions Positive Coombs' [direct], false-positive urinary and/or serum proteins; false-positive or negative urinary glucose using Clinitest®

Dosage Forms Excipient information presented when available (limited, particularly for generics); consult specific product labeling.

Suspension, Intramuscular:

Bicillin L-A: 600,000 units/mL (1 mL); 1,200,000 units/2 mL (2 mL); 2,400,000 units/4 mL (4 mL) [contains methylparaben, propylparaben]

Penicillin G Benzathine and Penicillin G Procaine

(pen i SIL in jee BENZ a theen & pen i SIL in jee PROE kane)

Brand Names: U.S. Bicillin® C-R; Bicillin® C-R 900/300

Index Terms Penicillin G Procaine and Benzathine Combined

Pharmacologic Category Antibiotic, Penicillin

Use May be used in specific situations in the treatment of streptococcal infections; primary prevention of rheumatic fever

Pregnancy Risk Factor B

Dosage

Usual dosage range and indication-specific dosing:

Streptococcal infections:

Children: I.M.:

<14 kg: 600,000 units in a single dose

14-27 kg: 900,000 units to 1.2 million units in a single dose

Children >27 kg and Adults: 2.4 million units in a single dose

Rheumatic fever, primary prevention (Bicillin® C-R 900/300): Children 6 months to 12 years: 1.2 million units as a single dose (Bass, 1976; Gerber, 2009). **Note:** The efficacy of this regimen for heavier patients is unknown.

Dosage adjustment in renal impairment: No dosage adjustment provided in manufacturer's labeling.

Dosage adjustment in hepatic impairment: No dosage adjustment provided in manufacturer's labeling.

Additional Information Complete prescribing information should be consulted for additional detail.

Dosage Forms Excipient information presented when available (limited, particularly for generics); consult specific product labeling. [DSC] = Discontinued product

Injection, suspension [prefilled syringe]:

Bicillin® C-R:

600,000 units: Penicillin G benzathine 300,000 units and penicillin G procaine 300,000 units per 1 mL (1 mL) [DSC]

1,200,000 units: Penicillin G benzathine 600,000 units and penicillin G procaine 600,000 units per 2 mL (2 mL)

2,400,000 units: Penicillin G benzathine 1,200,000 units and penicillin G procaine 1,200,000 units per 4 mL (4 mL) [DSC]

Bicillin® C-R 900/300: 1,200,000 units: Penicillin G benzathine 900,000 units and penicillin G procaine 300,000 units per 2 mL (2 mL)

Penicillin G (Parenteral/Aqueous)

(pen i SIL in jee, pa REN ter al, AYE kwee us)

Brand Names: U.S. Pfizerpen-G

Brand Names: Canada Crystapen®

Index Terms Benzylpenicillin Potassium; Benzylpenicillin Sodium; Crystalline Penicillin; Penicillin G Potassium; Penicillin G Sodium

Pharmacologic Category Antibiotic, Penicillin

Additional Appendix Information

Antibiotic Treatment of Adults With Infective Endocarditis *on page 2355*

Desensitization Protocols *on page 2325*

Use Treatment of infections (including sepsis, pneumonia, pericarditis, endocarditis, meningitis, anthrax) caused by susceptible organisms; active against some gram-positive organisms, generally not *Staphylococcus aureus*; some gram-negative organisms such as *Neisseria gonorrhoeae*, and some anaerobes and spirochetes

Pregnancy Risk Factor B

Pregnancy Considerations Adverse events have not been observed in animal reproduction studies. Penicillin crosses the placenta and distributes into amniotic fluid. Maternal use of penicillins has generally not resulted in an increased risk of adverse fetal effects. Penicillin G is the drug of choice for treatment of syphilis during pregnancy and penicillin G (parenteral/aqueous) is the drug of choice for the prevention of early-onset Group B Streptococcal (GBS) disease in newborns (consult current guidelines).

Breast-Feeding Considerations Very small amounts of penicillin G transfer into breast milk. Peak milk concentrations occur at approximately 1 hour after an IM dose and are higher if multiple doses are given. The manufacturer recommends that caution be exercised when administering penicillin to nursing women. Nondose-related effects could include modification of bowel flora and allergic sensitization.

Contraindications Hypersensitivity to penicillin or any component of the formulation

Warnings/Precautions Avoid intra-arterial administration or injection into or near major peripheral nerves or blood vessels since such injections may cause severe and/or permanent neurovascular damage; use with caution in patients with renal impairment (dosage reduction required), concomitant renal and hepatic impairment (further dosage adjustment may be required), pre-existing seizure disorders, or with a history of hypersensitivity to cephalosporins. Prolonged use may result in fungal or bacterial superinfection, including *C. difficile*-associated diarrhea (CDAD) and pseudomembranous colitis; CDAD has been observed >2 months postantibiotic treatment. Serious and occasionally severe or fatal hypersensitivity (anaphylactoid) reactions have been reported in patients on penicillin therapy, especially with a history of beta-lactam hypersensitivity, history of sensitivity to multiple allergens, or previous IgE-mediated reactions (eg, anaphylaxis, angioedema, urticaria). Use with caution in asthmatic patients. Extended duration of therapy or use associated with high serum concentrations may be associated with an increased risk for some adverse reactions. Neonates may have decreased renal clearance of penicillin and require frequent dosage adjustments depending on age. Product contains sodium and potassium; high doses of I.V. therapy may alter serum levels.

Adverse Reactions Frequency not defined.

Cardiovascular: Localized phlebitis, local thrombophlebitis

Central nervous system: Coma (high doses), hyperreflexia (high doses), myoclonus (high doses), seizure (high doses)

Dermatologic: Contact dermatitis, skin rash

Endocrine & metabolic: Electrolyte disturbance (high doses)

Gastrointestinal: Pseudomembranous colitis

Hematologic & oncologic: Neutropenia, positive direct Coombs test (rare, high doses)

Hypersensitivity: Anaphylaxis, hypersensitivity reaction (immediate and delayed), serum sickness

Immunologic: Jarisch-Herxheimer reaction

Local: Injection site reaction

Renal: Acute interstitial nephritis (high doses), renal tubular disease (high doses)

Drug Interactions

Metabolism/Transport Effects None known.

Avoid Concomitant Use

Avoid concomitant use of Penicillin G (Parenteral/Aqueous) with any of the following: BCG

Increased Effect/Toxicity

Penicillin G (Parenteral/Aqueous) may increase the levels/effects of: Methotrexate; Vitamin K Antagonists

The levels/effects of Penicillin G (Parenteral/Aqueous) may be increased by: Probenecid

Decreased Effect

Penicillin G (Parenteral/Aqueous) may decrease the levels/effects of: BCG; Mycophenolate; Sodium Picosulfate; Typhoid Vaccine

The levels/effects of Penicillin G (Parenteral/Aqueous) may be decreased by: Tetracycline Derivatives

Preparation for Administration

Intermittent I.V.: 5 million unit vial: Add 8.2 mL for a final concentration of 500,000 units/mL; add 3.2 mL for a final concentration of 1,000,000 units/mL. Dilute further to 50,000-145,000 units/mL prior to infusion.

Continuous I.V. infusion: 20 million unit vial: Add 11.5 mL for a final concentration of 1,000,000 units/mL. Dilute further in 1-2 L of infusion solution and administer over a 24-hour period.

Storage/Stability

Penicillin G potassium powder for injection should be stored below 86°F (30°C). Following reconstitution, solution may be stored for up to 7 days under refrigeration. Premixed bags for infusion should be stored in the freezer (-20°C or -4°F); frozen bags may be thawed at room temperature or in refrigerator. Once thawed, solution is stable for 14 days if stored in refrigerator or for 24 hours when stored at room temperature. Do not refreeze once thawed.

Penicillin G sodium powder for injection should be stored at controlled room temperature. Reconstituted solution may be stored under refrigeration for up to 3 days.

Mechanism of Action Interferes with bacterial cell wall synthesis during active multiplication, causing cell wall death and resultant bactericidal activity against susceptible bacteria

Pharmacodynamics/Kinetics

Distribution: Poor penetration across blood-brain barrier, despite inflamed meninges

Relative diffusion from blood into CSF: Poor unless meninges inflamed (exceeds usual MICs)

CSF:blood level ratio: Normal meninges: <1%; Inflamed meninges: 2% to 6%

Protein binding: 65%

Metabolism: Hepatic (30%) to penicilloic acid

Half-life elimination:

Neonates: <6 days old: 3.2-3.4 hours; 7-13 days old: 1.2-2.2 hours; >14 days old: 0.9-1.9 hours

Children and Adults: Normal renal function: 30-50 minutes

End-stage renal disease: 3.3-5.1 hours
Time to peak, serum: I.M.: ~30 minutes; I.V.: ~1 hour
Excretion: Urine (58% to 85% as unchanged drug)

Dosage

Usual dosage range:

Infants ≥1 month and Children: I.M., I.V.: 100,000-400,000 units/kg/day in divided doses every 4-6 hours (maximum dose: 24 million units/day)

Adults: I.M., I.V.: 2-30 million units/day in divided doses every 4-6 hours depending on sensitivity of the organism and severity of the infection

Indication-specific dosing:

Infants ≥1 month and Children:

Community-acquired pneumonia (CAP) (IDSA/PIDS, 2011): I.V.: Infants >3 months and Children: **Note:** May consider addition of vancomycin or clindamycin to empiric therapy if community-acquired MRSA suspected. In children ≥5 years, a macrolide antibiotic should be added if atypical pneumonia cannot be ruled out.

Empiric treatment or *S. pneumoniae* (moderate-to-severe; MICs to penicillin ≤2.0 mcg/mL) (preferred): 200,000-250,000 units/kg/day divided every 4-6 hours

Group A *Streptococcus* (moderate-to-severe) (preferred): 100,000-250,000 units/kg/day divided every 4-6 hours

***Meningitis* (gonococcal):** I.V.: 250,000 units/kg/day in 4 divided doses

Moderate infections: I.M., I.V.: 100,000-250,000 units/kg/day in 4 divided doses

Neurosyphilis: I.V.: 200,000-300,000 units/kg/day divided every 4-6 hours for 10-14 days (maximum dose: 24 million units/day)

Severe infections: I.M., I.V.: 250,000-400,000 units/kg/day in divided doses every 4-6 hours (maximum dose: 24 million units/day)

Syphilis (congenital): I.V.:

Infants: 50,000 units/kg every 12 hours for first 7 days of life, then every 8 hours for a total of 10 days (CDC, 2010)

Children: 50,000 units/kg every 4-6 hours for 10 days (CDC, 2010)

Adults:

***Actinomyces* species:** I.V.: 10-20 million units/day in divided doses every 4-6 hours for 4-6 weeks

Clostridium perfringens: I.V.: 24 million units/day in divided doses every 4-6 hours with clindamycin

Corynebacterium diphtheriae: I.V.: 2-3 million units/day in divided doses every 4-6 hours for 10-12 days

Erysipelas: I.V.: 1-2 million units every 4-6 hours

Erysipelothrix: I.V.: 2-4 million units every 4 hours

Fascial space infections: I.V.: 2-4 million units every 4-6 hours with metronidazole

Leptospirosis: I.V.: 1.5 million units every 6 hours for 7 days

Listeria: I.V.: 15-20 million units/day in divided doses every 4-6 hours for 2 weeks (meningitis) or 4 weeks (endocarditis)

Lyme disease (meningitis): I.V.: 20 million units/day in divided doses

Neurosyphilis: I.V.: 18-24 million units/day in divided doses every 4 hours (or by continuous infusion) for 10-14 days (CDC, 2006; CDC, 2009; CDC, 2010)

Prosthetic joint infection: I.V.:

Enterococcus spp (penicillin-susceptible), streptococci (beta-hemolytic): 20-24 million units daily continuous infusion every 24 hours or in divided doses every 4 hours for 4-6 weeks (Osmon, 2013); **Note:** For penicillin-susceptible *Enterococcus* spp, consider addition of aminoglycoside.

Propionibacterium acnes: 20 million units daily continuous infusion every 24 hours or in divided doses every 4 hours for 4-6 weeks (Osmon, 2013)

Streptococcus:

Brain abscess: I.V.: 18-24 million units/day in divided doses every 4 hours with metronidazole

Endocarditis or osteomyelitis: I.V.: 3-4 million units every 4 hours for at least 4 weeks

Group B streptococcus (neonatal prophylaxis): I.V.: 5 million units x 1 dose, then 2.5-3.0 million units every 4 hours until delivery (CDC, 2010)

Skin and soft tissue: I.V.: 3-4 million units every 4 hours for 10 days

Toxic shock: I.V.: 24 million units/day in divided doses with clindamycin

Streptococcal pneumonia: I.V.: 2-3 million units every 4 hours

Whipple's disease: I.V.: 2 million units every 4 hours for 2 weeks, followed by oral trimethoprim/sulfamethoxazole or doxycycline for 1 year

Relapse or CNS involvement: 4 million units every 4 hours for 4 weeks

Dosing adjustment in renal impairment:

Manufacturer's recommendation:

Uremic patients with Cl_{cr} >10 mL/minute/1.73 m^2: Administer a normal dose followed by 50% of the normal dose every 4-5 hours

Cl_{cr} <10 mL/minute/1.73 m^2: Administer a normal dose followed by 50% of the normal dose every 8-10 hours

Alternate recommendation:

GFR >50 mL/minute: No dosage adjustments are necessary (Aronoff, 2007).

GFR 10-50 mL/minute: Administer 75% of the normal dose (Aronoff, 2007).

GFR <10 mL/minute: Administer 20% to 50% of the normal dose (Aronoff, 2007).

Intermittent hemodialysis (IHD) (administer after hemodialysis on dialysis days) (Heintz, 2009): Administer a normal dose followed by either 25% to 50% of normal dose every 4-6 hours **or** 50% to 100% of normal dose every 8-12 hours. For *mild-to-moderate* infections, administer 0.5-1 million units every 4-6 hours **or** 1-2 million units every 8-12 hours. For *neurosyphilis, endocarditis, or serious infections*, administer up to 2 million units every 4-6 hours; administer after dialysis on dialysis days **or** supplement with 500,000 units after dialysis. **Note:** Dosing dependent on the assumption of 3 times weekly, complete IHD sessions.

Continuous renal replacement therapy (CRRT) (Heintz, 2009; Trotman, 2005): Drug clearance is highly dependent on the method of renal replacement, filter type, and flow rate. Appropriate dosing requires close monitoring of pharmacologic response, signs of adverse reactions due to drug accumulation, as well as drug concentrations in relation to target trough (if appropriate). The following are general recommendations only (based on dialysate flow/ultrafiltration rates of 1-2 L/hour and minimal residual renal function) and should not supersede clinical judgment:

CVVH: Loading dose of 4 million units, followed by 2 million units every 4-6 hours

CVVHD: Loading dose of 4 million units, followed by 2-3 million units every 4-6 hours

CVVHDF: Loading dose of 4 million units, followed by 2-4 million units every 4-6 hours

Dosing adjustment in hepatic impairment: No dosage adjustment provided in manufacturer's labeling. However, the manufacturer's labeling recommends further adjustment of doses adjusted for renal impairment in patients with both renal and hepatic impairment.

Dietary Considerations Some products may contain potassium and/or sodium.

Administration

I.M.; Administer I.M. by deep injection in the upper outer quadrant of the buttock

I.V.: **Note:** The 20 million unit dosage form may be administered by continuous I.V. infusion only.

Intermittent I.V.: May be dissolved in small amounts of SWFI, NS, D_5W and administered peripherally as a 50,000-100,000 unit/mL solution. In fluid-restricted patients, 146,000 units/mL in SW results in a maximum recommended osmolality for peripheral infusion. Infuse over 15-30 minutes.

Continuous I.V. infusion: Determine the volume of fluid and rate of its administration required by the patient in a 24-hour period. Add the appropriate daily dosage of penicillin to this fluid. For example, if the daily dose is 10 million units and 2 L of fluid/day is required, add 5 million units to 1 L and adjust the rate of flow so the liter will be infused over 12 hours (83 mL/hour). Repeat steps (5 million units/L at 83 mL/hour) for the remaining 12 hours.

Monitoring Parameters Periodic electrolyte, hepatic, renal, cardiac and hematologic function tests during prolonged/high-dose therapy; observe for signs and symptoms of anaphylaxis during first dose

Test Interactions False-positive or negative urinary glucose determination using Clinitest®; positive Coombs' [direct]; false-positive urinary and/or serum proteins

Additional Information 1 million units is approximately equal to 625 mg.

Dosage Forms Excipient information presented when available (limited, particularly for generics); consult specific product labeling.

Solution, Intravenous, as potassium:
- Generic: 20,000 units/mL (50 mL); 40,000 units/mL (50 mL); 60,000 units/mL (50 mL)

Solution Reconstituted, Injection:
- Pfizerpen-G: 5,000,000 units (1 ea)

Solution Reconstituted, Injection, as potassium:
- Pfizerpen-G: 5,000,000 units (1 ea); 20,000,000 units (1 ea)
- Pfizerpen-G: 5,000,000 units (1 ea); 20,000,000 units (1 ea) [pyrogen free]
- Generic: 5,000,000 units (1 ea); 20,000,000 units (1 ea)

Solution Reconstituted, Injection, as potassium [preservative free]:
- Generic: 20,000,000 units (1 ea)

Solution Reconstituted, Injection, as sodium:
- Generic: 5,000,000 units (1 ea)

◆ **Penicillin G Potassium** *see* Penicillin G (Parenteral/Aqueous) *on page 1608*

Penicillin G Procaine (pen i SIL in jee PROE kane)

Brand Names: Canada Pfizerpen-AS®; Wycillin®

Index Terms APPG; Aqueous Procaine Penicillin G; Procaine Benzylpenicillin; Procaine Penicillin G; Wycillin

Pharmacologic Category Antibiotic, Penicillin

Use Treatment of moderately-severe infections due to *Treponema pallidum* and other penicillin G-sensitive microorganisms that are susceptible to low, but prolonged serum penicillin concentrations; anthrax due to *Bacillus anthracis* (postexposure) to reduce the incidence or progression of disease following exposure to aerolized *Bacillus anthracis*

Pregnancy Risk Factor B

Pregnancy Considerations Adverse events have not been observed in animal reproduction studies. Penicillin crosses the placenta and distributes into amniotic fluid. Maternal use of penicillins has generally not resulted in an increased risk of adverse fetal effects.

Breast-Feeding Considerations Penicillins are excreted in breast milk. The manufacturer recommends that caution be used when administering penicillin to nursing women. Nondose-related effects could include modification of bowel flora and allergic sensitization.

Contraindications Hypersensitivity to penicillin, procaine, or any component of the formulation

Warnings/Precautions May need to modify dosage in patients with severe renal impairment or seizure disorders; avoid I.V., intravascular, or intra-arterial administration of penicillin G procaine since severe and/or permanent neurovascular damage may occur. Serious and occasionally severe or fatal hypersensitivity (anaphylactoid) reactions have been reported in patients on penicillin therapy, especially with a history of beta-lactam hypersensitivity, history of sensitivity to multiple allergens, or previous IgE-mediated reactions (eg, anaphylaxis, angioedema, urticaria). Use with caution in asthmatic patients. Extended duration of therapy or use associated with high serum concentrations may be associated with an increased risk for some adverse reactions. Prolonged use may result in fungal or bacterial superinfection, including *C. difficile*-associated diarrhea (CDAD) and pseudomembranous colitis; CDAD has been observed >2 months postantibiotic treatment.

Adverse Reactions Frequency not defined.

Cardiovascular: Conduction disturbances, myocardial depression, vasodilation

Central nervous system: CNS stimulation, confusion, drowsiness, myoclonus, seizure

Hematologic: Hemolytic anemia, neutropenia, positive Coombs' reaction

Local: Pain at injection site, sterile abscess at injection site, thrombophlebitis

Renal: Interstitial nephritis

Miscellaneous: Hypersensitivity reactions, Jarisch-Herxheimer reaction, pseudoanaphylactic reactions, serum sickness

Drug Interactions

Metabolism/Transport Effects None known.

Avoid Concomitant Use

Avoid concomitant use of Penicillin G Procaine with any of the following: BCG

Increased Effect/Toxicity

Penicillin G Procaine may increase the levels/effects of: Methotrexate; Vitamin K Antagonists

The levels/effects of Penicillin G Procaine may be increased by: Probenecid

Decreased Effect

Penicillin G Procaine may decrease the levels/effects of: BCG; Mycophenolate; Sodium Picosulfate; Typhoid Vaccine

The levels/effects of Penicillin G Procaine may be decreased by: Tetracycline Derivatives

Storage/Stability Refrigerate

Mechanism of Action Inhibits bacterial cell wall synthesis by binding to one or more of the penicillin-binding proteins (PBPs); which in turn inhibits the final transpeptidation step of peptidoglycan synthesis in bacterial cell walls, thus inhibiting cell wall biosynthesis. Bacteria eventually lyse due to ongoing activity of cell wall autolytic enzymes (autolysins and murein hydrolases) while cell wall assembly is arrested.

Pharmacodynamics/Kinetics

Duration: Therapeutic: 15-24 hours

Absorption: I.M.: Slow

Distribution: Penetration across the blood-brain barrier is poor, despite inflamed meninges

Protein binding: 65%

Metabolism: ~30% hepatically inactivated

Time to peak, serum: 1-4 hours

Excretion: Urine (60% to 90% as unchanged drug)

Clearance: Renal: Delayed in neonates, young infants, and with impaired renal function

Dosage

Usual dosage range:

Infants and Children: I.M.: 25,000-50,000 units/kg/day in divided doses 1-2 times/day (maximum: 4.8 million units/day)

Adults: I.M.: 0.6-4.8 million units/day in divided doses every 12-24 hours

Indication-specific dosing:

Children: I.M.:

Anthrax, inhalational (postexposure prophylaxis): 25,000 units/kg every 12 hours (maximum: 1,200,000 units every 12 hours); see **"Note"** in adult dosing

Syphilis (congenital): 50,000 units/kg/day for 10 days; if more than 1 day of therapy is missed, the entire course should be restarted

Adults: I.M.:

Anthrax:

Inhalational (postexposure prophylaxis): 1,200,000 units every 12 hours

Note: Overall treatment duration should be 60 days. Available safety data suggest continued administration of penicillin G procaine for longer than 2 weeks may incur additional risk for adverse reactions. Clinicians may consider switching to effective alternative treatment for completion of therapy beyond 2 weeks.

Cutaneous (treatment): 600,000-1,200,000 units/day; alternative therapy is recommended in severe cutaneous or other forms of anthrax infection

Endocarditis caused by susceptible viridans *Streptococcus* (when used in conjunction with an aminoglycoside): 1.2 million units every 6 hours for 2-4 weeks

Neurosyphilis: 2.4 million units/day with 500 mg probenecid by mouth 4 times/day for 10-14 days; **Note: Penicillin G aqueous I.V. is the preferred agent**

Whipple's disease: 1.2 million units/day (with streptomycin) for 10-14 days, followed by oral trimethoprim/sulfamethoxazole or doxycycline for 1 year

Dosage adjustment in renal impairment:

Cl_{cr} 10-30 mL/minute: Administer every 8-12 hours.

Cl_{cr} <10 mL/minute: Administer every 12-18 hours.

Hemodialysis: Moderately dialyzable (20% to 50%)

Dosage adjustment in hepatic impairment: No dosage adjustment provided in manufacturer's labeling.

Administration Procaine suspension for deep I.M. injection only; do not inject in gluteal muscle in children <2 years of age; rotate the injection site; avoid I.V., intravascular, or intra-arterial administration of penicillin G procaine since severe and/or permanent neurovascular damage may occur

Monitoring Parameters Periodic renal and hematologic function tests with prolonged therapy; fever, mental status, WBC count

Test Interactions Positive Coombs' [direct], false-positive urinary and/or serum proteins

Dosage Forms Excipient information presented when available (limited, particularly for generics); consult specific product labeling.

Suspension, Intramuscular:

Generic: 600,000 units/mL (1 mL, 2 mL)

◆ **Penicillin G Procaine and Benzathine Combined** *see* Penicillin G Benzathine and Penicillin G Procaine *on page 1607*

◆ **Penicillin G Sodium** *see* Penicillin G (Parenteral/Aqueous) *on page 1608*

Penicillin V Potassium

(pen i SIL in vee poe TASS ee um)

Brand Names: Canada Apo-Pen VK; Novo-Pen-VK; Nu-Pen-VK

Index Terms Pen VK; Phenoxymethyl Penicillin

Pharmacologic Category Antibiotic, Penicillin

Additional Appendix Information

Desensitization Protocols *on page 2325*

Use Treatment of infections caused by susceptible organisms involving the respiratory tract, otitis media, sinusitis, skin, and soft tissues; prophylaxis in rheumatic fever

Unlabeled Use Chronic antimicrobial suppression of prosthetic joint infection; community-acquired cutaneous anthrax; cutaneous erysipeloid; group A streptococcal chronic carrier eradication; pneumococcal prophylaxis in patients with sickle cell disease or asplenia

Pregnancy Considerations Penicillin crosses the placenta and distributes into amniotic fluid. Maternal use of penicillins has generally not resulted in an increased risk of adverse fetal effects. Due to pregnancy-induced physiologic changes, some pharmacokinetic parameters of penicillin V may be altered in the second and third trimester. Higher doses or increased dosing frequency may be required.

Breast-Feeding Considerations Penicillin V is excreted into breast milk (low concentrations) and may be detected in the urine of some breast-feeding infants. Loose stools and rash have been reported in nursing infants.

Contraindications Hypersensitivity to penicillin or any component of the formulation

Warnings/Precautions Use with caution in patients with severe renal impairment or history of seizures. Serious and occasionally severe or fatal hypersensitivity (anaphylactoid) reactions have been reported in patients on penicillin therapy, especially with a history of beta-lactam hypersensitivity, history of sensitivity to multiple allergens, or previous IgE-mediated reactions (eg, anaphylaxis, angioedema, urticaria). Use with caution in asthmatic patients. Extended duration of therapy or use associated with high serum concentrations may be associated with an increased risk for some adverse reactions. Prolonged use may result in fungal or bacterial superinfection, including *C. difficile*-associated diarrhea (CDAD) and pseudomembranous colitis; CDAD has been observed >2 months postantibiotic treatment.

Adverse Reactions

>10%: Gastrointestinal: Mild diarrhea, vomiting, nausea, oral candidiasis

<1% (Limited to important or life-threatening): Acute interstitial nephritis, convulsions, hemolytic anemia, positive Coombs' reaction

Drug Interactions

Metabolism/Transport Effects None known.

Avoid Concomitant Use

Avoid concomitant use of Penicillin V Potassium with any of the following: BCG

Increased Effect/Toxicity

Penicillin V Potassium may increase the levels/effects of: Methotrexate; Vitamin K Antagonists

The levels/effects of Penicillin V Potassium may be increased by: Probenecid

Decreased Effect

Penicillin V Potassium may decrease the levels/effects of: BCG; Mycophenolate; Sodium Picosulfate; Typhoid Vaccine

The levels/effects of Penicillin V Potassium may be decreased by: Tetracycline Derivatives

Ethanol/Nutrition/Herb Interactions Food: Decreases drug absorption rate; decreases drug serum concentration.

Management: Take on an empty stomach 1 hour before or 2 hours after meals around-the-clock to promote less variation in peak and trough serum levels.

Storage/Stability Refrigerate suspension after reconstitution; discard after 14 days.

Mechanism of Action Inhibits bacterial cell wall synthesis by binding to one or more of the penicillin-binding proteins (PBPs); which in turn inhibits the final transpeptidation step of peptidoglycan synthesis in bacterial cell walls, thus inhibiting cell wall biosynthesis. Bacteria eventually lyse due to ongoing activity of cell wall autolytic enzymes (autolysins and murein hydrolases) while cell wall assembly is arrested.

Pharmacodynamics/Kinetics

Absorption: 60% to 73%

Distribution: Widely distributed to kidneys, liver, skin, tonsils, and into synovial, pleural, and pericardial fluids

Protein binding, plasma: 80%

Half-life elimination: 30 minutes; prolonged with renal impairment

Time to peak, serum: 0.5-1 hour

Excretion: Urine (as unchanged drug and metabolites)

Dosage

Usual dosage range:

Children <12 years: Oral: 25-50 mg/kg/day in divided doses every 6-8 hours (maximum dose: 3000 mg daily)

Children ≥12 years and Adults: Oral: 125-500 mg every 6-8 hours

Indication-specific dosing:

Infants >3 months and Children: Oral: **Community-acquired pneumonia (CAP) due to group A *Streptococcus*, mild infection or step-down therapy (preferred) (IDSA/PIDS, 2011):** 50-75 mg/kg/day in 3-4 divided doses

Infants and Children: Oral: **Pneumococcal infection prophylaxis for anatomic or functional asplenia (eg, sickle cell disease [SCD]) (AAP, 2000; AAP, 2002; Kavanagh, 2011; NHLBI, 2002):**

Before 2 months of age (or as soon as SCD diagnosed or asplenia occurs) to 3 years of age: 125 mg twice daily

>3 years: 250 mg twice daily; the decision to discontinue penicillin prophylaxis after 5 years of age in children who have not experienced invasive pneumococcal infection and have received recommended pneumococcal immunizations is patient and clinician dependent; **Note:** Some clinicians recommend in patients <5 years, a lower dose of 125 mg twice daily (*Red Book*, 2012)

Children: Oral:

Community-acquired cutaneous anthrax (unlabeled use): 25-50 mg/kg/day in divided doses 2-4 times daily (maximum single dose 500 mg) for 5-9 days (Stevens, 2005)

Pharyngitis (streptococcal) (IDSA guidelines):

Acute treatment: 250 mg 2-3 times daily for 10 days

Chronic carrier treatment, group A streptococci: 50 mg/kg/day in 4 divided doses (maximum: 2000 mg daily) for 10 days in combination with oral rifampin (Shulman, 2012)

Prophylaxis of recurrent rheumatic fever: Refer to adult dosing.

Children ≥12 years and Adolescents: Oral:

Fusospirochetosis (Vincent infection): Refer to adult dosing.

Adolescents: Oral:

Pharyngitis (streptococcal), acute treatment (IDSA guidelines): Refer to adult dosing.

Adults: Oral:

Actinomycosis:

Mild: 2000-4000 mg daily in 4 divided doses for 8 weeks

Surgical: 2000-4000 mg in 4 divided doses for 6-12 months (after I.V. penicillin G therapy of 4-6 weeks)

Erysipelas: 500 mg 4 times daily

Fusospirochetosis (Vincent infection): 250-500 mg 3-4 times daily

Cutaneous anthrax, community-acquired (unlabeled use): 250-500 mg 4 times daily for 5-9 days (Stevens, 2005)

Cutaneous erysipeloid (unlabeled use): 500 mg 4 times daily for 7-10 days (Stevens, 2005)

Periodontal infections: 250-500 mg every 6 hours for 5-7 days

Note: Efficacy of antimicrobial therapy in periapical abscess is questionable; the American Academy of Periodontology recommends use of antibiotic therapy only when systemic symptoms (eg, fever, lymphadenopathy) are present or in immunocompromised patients.

Pharyngitis (streptococcal):

Manufacturer's labeling: 500 mg 3-4 times daily for 10 days

Acute treatment, group A streptococci (IDSA guidelines): 250 mg 4 times daily or 500 mg twice daily for 10 days (Shulman, 2012)

Chronic carrier treatment, group A streptococcal (IDSA guidelines): 500 mg 4 times daily (maximum: 2000 mg daily) for 10 days in combination with oral rifampin (Shulman, 2012)

Prophylaxis of recurrent rheumatic fever infections: 250 mg twice daily (Gerber, 2009)

Prosthetic joint infection (unlabeled use): *Chronic oral antimicrobial suppression (Enterococcus spp [penicillin-susceptible], streptococci [beta-hemolytic], Propionibacterium spp):* 500 mg 2-4 times daily (Osmon, 2013)

Dosage adjustment in renal impairment: No dosage adjustment provided in manufacturer's labeling. Use with caution; excretion is prolonged in patients with renal impairment.

Dosage adjustment in hepatic impairment: No dosage adjustment provided in manufacturer's labeling.

Dietary Considerations Take on an empty stomach 1 hour before or 2 hours after meals.

Administration Administer on an empty stomach to increase oral absorption

Monitoring Parameters Periodic renal and hematologic function tests during prolonged therapy; monitor for signs of anaphylaxis during first dose

Test Interactions False-positive or negative urinary glucose determination using Clinitest®; positive Coombs' [direct]; false-positive urinary and/or serum proteins

Additional Information 0.7 mEq of potassium per 250 mg penicillin V; 250 mg equals 400,000 units of penicillin

Dosage Forms Excipient information presented when available (limited, particularly for generics); consult specific product labeling.

Solution Reconstituted, Oral:

Generic: 125 mg/5 mL (100 mL, 200 mL); 250 mg/5 mL (100 mL, 200 mL)

Tablet, Oral:

Generic: 250 mg, 500 mg

◆ **Penlac** *see* Ciclopirox *on page 423*

◆ **Pentacel®** *see* Diphtheria and Tetanus Toxoids, Acellular Pertussis, Poliovirus and *Haemophilus* b Conjugate Vaccine *on page 629*

◆ **Pentahydrate** *see* Sodium Thiosulfate *on page 1931*

◆ **Pentam** *see* Pentamidine *on page 1613*

Pentamidine (pen TAM i deen)

Brand Names: U.S. Nebupent; Pentam

Index Terms Pentamidine Isethionate

Pharmacologic Category Antifungal Agent; Antiprotozoal

Use

I.M., I.V.: Treatment of pneumonia caused by *Pneumocystis jirovecii* pneumonia (PCP)

Inhalation: Prevention of PCP in high-risk, HIV-infected patients either with a history of PCP or with a CD4+ count ≤200/mm^3

Unlabeled Use Prevention of PCP in nonHIV-infected patients; treatment of African trypanosomiasis, cutaneous leishmaniasis, and amebic meningoencephalitis

Pregnancy Risk Factor C

Pregnancy Considerations Animal reproduction studies were not conducted by the manufacturer; therefore, pentamidine is classified pregnancy category C. In postmarketing studies, pentamidine was embryocidal but not teratogenic when administered to animals. Pentamidine crosses the human placenta. Administration via the aerosolized route may minimize maternal serum concentrations. Concern regarding occupational exposure of pregnant healthcare workers has been discussed in the literature. Pregnant healthcare workers should avoid aerolized exposure if possible. If avoidance is not possible, they should wear a mask and gloves and ensure proper ventilation. Pentamidine may be used in pregnancy for prophylaxis or treatment of PCP if the patient is unable to take first line medications.

Breast-Feeding Considerations It is not known if pentamidine is excreted in human milk and use of pentamidine during breast-feeding is not recommended by the manufacturer. In the United States where formula is accessible, affordable, safe, and sustainable, complete avoidance of breast-feeding by HIV-infected women is recommended by the AAP and the CDC to decrease potential transmission of HIV.

Contraindications Hypersensitivity to pentamidine isethionate or any component of the formulation

Warnings/Precautions Hazardous agent - use appropriate precautions for handling and disposal (NIOSH, 2012). Severe hypotension (some fatalities) has been observed (even after a single dose); may occur with either I.V. or I.M administration, although more common with rapid I.V. administration; monitor blood pressure during (and after) infusion. May cause QT prolongation and subsequent torsade de pointes; avoid use in patients with diagnosed or suspected congenital long QT syndrome. Use with caution in patients with pre-existing cardiovascular disease; hyper-/hypotension and arrhythmia, including ventricular tachycardia (eg, torsade de pointes) have been reported.

Use with caution in patients with diabetes mellitus or hypocalcemia; hyper-/hypoglycemia and pancreatic islet cell necrosis with hyperinsulinemia has been reported. Symptoms may occur months after therapy; monitor blood glucose daily on therapy and periodically thereafter. Use with caution in patients with a history of pancreatic disease or elevated amylase/lipase levels; acute pancreatitis (with fatality) has been reported. Discontinue if signs/symptoms of acute pancreatitis occur. Concurrent use with other bone marrow suppressants may increase the risk for myelotoxicity; use with caution in patients with current evidence and/or prior history of hematologic disorders; anemia, leukopenia and/or thrombocytopenia have been reported. Use with caution in patients with hepatic or renal disease. Concurrent use with other nephrotoxic drugs may increase the risk for nephrotoxicity. Avoid concurrent use with other drugs known to prolong QT_c interval. Stevens-Johnson syndrome has been reported with use. Avoid extravasation; may cause tissue ulceration, necrosis, and/or sloughing; if extravasation occurs, treat symptomatically. Assess catheter position before and during infusion.

Aerosolized pentamidine may induce bronchospasm or cough, especially in patients with a smoking or asthma history (an inhaled bronchodilator prior to pentamidine may ameliorate symptoms). Use appropriate precautions to minimize exposure to healthcare personnel; refer to individual institutional policy. Acute PCP may develop despite aerosolized pentamidine prophylaxis. Although rare, extrapulmonary PCP disease may occur and has been associated with aerosolized pentamidine.

Adverse Reactions

Aerosol:

>10%:

Central nervous system: Fatigue (66%), fever (51%), dizziness/lightheadedness (45%)

Gastrointestinal: Appetite decreased (50%)

Respiratory: Cough (1% to 63%), dyspnea (48%), wheezing (32%)

Miscellaneous: Infection (15%)

1% to 10%:

Central nervous system: Headache

Gastrointestinal: Diarrhea, nausea, oral candida, taste alteration

Hematologic: Anemia

Respiratory: Bronchitis, chest pain, pharyngitis, sinusitis, upper respiratory tract infection

Miscellaneous: Herpes infection, influenza, night sweats

Injection:

>10%:

Local: Local reactions at I.M. injection site (11%; includes sterile abscess, necrosis, pain, induration)

Renal: Renal function impaired (29%), creatinine increased (24%)

1% to 10%:

Cardiovascular: Hypotension (5%)

Central nervous system: Confusion/hallucinations (2%)

Dermatologic: Rash (3%)

Endocrine & metabolic: Hypoglycemia (6%)

Gastrointestinal: Nausea/anorexia (6%), taste alteration (2%)

Hematologic: Leukopenia (10%), thrombocytopenia (3%), anemia (1%)

Hepatic: Liver function tests increased (9%)

Renal: Azotemia (9%), BUN increased (7%)

Aerosol or injection: <1% (Limited to important or life-threatening): Abdominal pain, allergic reaction, anaphylaxis, anxiety, arthralgia, asthma, blepharitis, blurred vision, bronchitis, bronchospasm, cardiac arrhythmia, central venous line related sepsis, cerebrovascular accident, chest tightness, chills, clotting time prolonged, CMV infection, colitis, confusion, congestion (chest, nasal), conjunctivitis, cough, cryptococcal meningitis, cyanosis, defibrination, depression, dermatitis, desquamation, diabetes mellitus, diabetic ketoacidosis, diarrhea, dizziness, drowsiness, dyspepsia, dyspnea, emotional lability, eosinophilia, erythema, esophagitis, extrapulmonary pneumocystosis, extravasation (tissue ulceration, necrosis, and/or sloughing), facial edema, flank pain, gait unsteady, gagging, gingivitis, headache, hearing loss, hematochezia, hematuria, hemoptysis, hepatic dysfunction, hepatitis, hepatomegaly, histoplasmosis, hyperglycemia, hyperkalemia, hypersalivation, hypertension, hyperventilation, hypesthesia, hypocalcemia, hypomagnesemia, incontinence, insomnia, laryngitis, laryngospasm, leg edema, melena, memory loss, nephritis, nervousness, neuralgia, neuropathy, neutropenia, night sweats, palpitation, pancreatitis, pancytopenia, paranoia, paresthesia, peripheral neuropathy, phlebitis, pleuritis, pneumonitis (eosinophilic or interstitial), pneumothorax, pruritus, rales, renal dysfunction, renal failure, rhinitis, seizure, splenomegaly, Stevens-Johnson syndrome, ST segment abnormal, syncope, syndrome of inappropriate antidiuretic hormone (SIADH), tachycardia, tachypnea, temperature abnormal, torsade de pointes, tremor, vasodilation, vasculitis, ventricular tachycardia, vertigo, vomiting, urticaria, xerostomia

Drug Interactions

Metabolism/Transport Effects Substrate of CYP2C19 (major); **Note:** Assignment of Major/Minor substrate status based on clinically relevant drug interaction potential; **Inhibits** CYP2C19 (weak), CYP2C9 (weak), CYP2D6 (weak), CYP3A4 (weak)

Avoid Concomitant Use

Avoid concomitant use of Pentamidine with any of the following: BCG; Highest Risk QTc-Prolonging Agents; Ivabradine; Mifepristone

Increased Effect/Toxicity

Pentamidine may increase the levels/effects of: ARIPiprazole; Foscarnet; Highest Risk QTc-Prolonging Agents; Lomitapide; Moderate Risk QTc-Prolonging Agents

The levels/effects of Pentamidine may be increased by: CYP2C19 Inhibitors (Moderate); CYP2C19 Inhibitors (Strong); Ivabradine; Luliconazole; Mifepristone; QTc-Prolonging Agents (Indeterminate Risk and Risk Modifying)

Decreased Effect

Pentamidine may decrease the levels/effects of: BCG; Sodium Picosulfate; Typhoid Vaccine

The levels/effects of Pentamidine may be decreased by: CYP2C19 Inducers (Strong); Dabrafenib

Ethanol/Nutrition/Herb Interactions Ethanol: Avoid ethanol (may increase CNS depression or aggravate hypoglycemia).

Preparation for Administration Hazardous agent; use appropriate precautions for handling and disposal (NIOSH, 2012). Do not use sodium chloride for initial reconstitution (sodium chloride will cause precipitation).

Aerosol: Reconstitute with 6 mL SWFI. Do not mix with other nebulizer solutions.

Injection: I.M.: Reconstitute with 3 mL SWFI; I.V.: Reconstitute with 3-5 mL SWFI or D_5W; the manufacturer recommends further dilution in 50-250 mL D_5W; however, stability with further dilution in NS has also been documented.

Storage/Stability Store intact vials at 20°C to 25°C (68°F to 77°F); protect from light. Do not use sodium chloride for initial reconstitution (sodium chloride will cause precipitation).

Aerosol: The manufacturer recommends the use of freshly prepared solutions for inhalation; however, may be stored for up to 48 hours in the vial at room temperature if protected from light.

Injection: Reconstituted solution is stable for 48 hours in the vial at room temperature and protected from light. Solutions for injection (1-2.5 mg/mL) in D_5W are stable for at least 24 hours at room temperature. Store at room temperature to avoid crystallization.

Mechanism of Action Interferes with microbial RNA/DNA, phospholipids and protein synthesis, through inhibition of oxidative phosphorylation and/or interference with incorporation of nucleotides and nucleic acids into RNA and DNA

Pharmacodynamics/Kinetics

Absorption: I.M.: Well absorbed; Inhalation: Limited systemic absorption

Distribution: V_{dss}: I.V.: 286-1356 L; I.M.: 1658-3790 L

Half-life elimination: I.V.: 5-8 hours; I.M.: 7-11 hours; may be prolonged with severe renal impairment

Excretion: Urine (I.V.: ≤12% as unchanged drug)

Dosage

Children:

PCP:

FDA-approved labeling: Children >4 months: Treatment: I.M., I.V.: 4 mg/kg once daily for 14-21 days

CDC recommendation:

Prevention (children ≥5 years): Inhalation: 300 mg/dose monthly via Respirgard® II nebulizer

Treatment: I.V.: 3-4 mg/kg once daily for 21 days

AIDS*info* guidelines (2009):

Prevention: Children ≥5 years: Inhalation: 300 mg/dose monthly via Respirgard® II nebulizer

Treatment: I.V.: 4 mg/kg once daily, if clinical improvement may change to atovaquone after 7-10 days

PCP prevention in pediatric oncology patients (age <5 years, intolerant to trimethoprim-sulfamethoxazole; unlabeled use): 4 mg/kg I.V. once monthly (Kim, 2008; Prasad, 2007)

Cutaneous leishmaniasis (unlabeled use; CDC recommendation): I.M., I.V.: 2-3 mg/kg once daily or every second day for 4-7 doses

Trypanosomiasis (unlabeled use; CDC recommendation): I.M.: 4 mg/kg once daily for 7 days

Adults:

PCP:

FDA-approved labeling:

Prevention: Inhalation: 300 mg every 4 weeks via Respirgard® II nebulizer

Treatment: I.M., I.V.: 4 mg/kg once daily for 14-21 days

CDC recommendation:

Prevention: Inhalation: 300 mg monthly via Respirgard® II nebulizer

Treatment: I.V.: 3-4 mg/kg once daily for 21 days

AIDS*info* guidelines (2009):

Prevention: Inhalation: 300 mg/dose monthly via Respirgard® II nebulizer

Treatment: I.V.: 4 mg/kg once daily, 3 mg/kg may be used by some clinicians

Cutaneous leishmaniasis (unlabeled use; CDC recommendation): I.M., I.V.: 2-3 mg/kg once daily or every second day for 4-7 doses

Trypanosomiasis (unlabeled use; CDC recommendation): I.M.: 4 mg/kg once daily for 7 days

Dosing adjustment in renal impairment: I.V.: The FDA-approved labeling recommends that caution should be used in patients with renal impairment; however, no specific dosage adjustment guidelines are available. The following guidelines have been used by some clinicians (Aronoff, 2007):

Children:

Cl_{cr} >30 mL/minute: No dosage adjustment necessary.

Cl_{cr} 10-30 mL/minute: Administer 4 mg/kg every 36 hours

Cl_{cr} <10 mL/minute and peritoneal dialysis: Administer 4 mg/kg every 48 hours

Hemodialysis: Administer 4 mg/kg every 48 hours, after dialysis on dialysis days

Adults:

Cl_{cr} ≥10 mL/minute: No dosage adjustment necessary.

Cl_{cr} <10 mL/minute: Administer 4 mg/kg every 24-36 hours

Dosage adjustment in hepatic impairment: No dosage adjustment provided in manufacturer's labeling (has not been studied). Use with caution.

Administration Do not use NS to reconstitute.

Inhalation: Deliver via Respirgard® II nebulizer until nebulizer is emptied (30-45 minutes). Administer at a flow rate of 5-7 L/minute from a 40-50 pound-per-square inch (PSI) oxygen or air source. A 40-50 PSI air compressor can be used alternatively, with a set flow rate at 5-7 L/minute or a set pressure of 22-25 PSI. Air compressors <20 PSI should not be used. Use appropriate precautions to minimize exposure to healthcare personnel; refer to individual institutional policy.

I.V.: Infuse slowly over 60-120 minutes. Avoid extravasation; assess catheter position before and during infusion.

I.M.: Administer deep I.M.

Hazardous agent; use appropriate precautions for handling and disposal (NIOSH, 2012).

Monitoring Parameters Liver function tests, renal function tests, blood glucose, serum potassium and calcium, CBC and platelets; ECG, blood pressure

Dosage Forms Excipient information presented when available (limited, particularly for generics); consult specific product labeling.

Solution Reconstituted, Inhalation, as isethionate:
Nebupent: 300 mg (1 ea)

Solution Reconstituted, Injection, as isethionate:
Pentam: 300 mg (1 ea)

◆ **Pentamidine Isethionate** *see* Pentamidine *on page 1613*

◆ **Pentamycetin® (Can)** *see* Chloramphenicol *on page 405*

◆ **Pentasa** *see* Mesalamine *on page 1305*

◆ **Pentasodium Colistin Methanesulfonate** *see* Colistimethate *on page 488*

◆ **Pentavalent Human-Bovine Reassortant Rotavirus Vaccine (PRV)** *see* Rotavirus Vaccine *on page 1861*

Pentazocine (pen TAZ oh seen)

Brand Names: U.S. Talwin

Brand Names: Canada Talwin®

Index Terms Pentazocine Lactate

Pharmacologic Category Analgesic, Opioid; Analgesic, Opioid Partial Agonist

Additional Appendix Information

Beers Criteria – Potentially Inappropriate Medications for Geriatrics *on page 2368*

Opioid Conversion Table *on page 2306*

Use Relief of moderate-to-severe pain; has also been used as a sedative prior to surgery and as a supplement to surgical anesthesia

Pregnancy Risk Factor C

Dosage

Preoperative/preanesthetic: Children 1-16 years: I.M.: 0.5 mg/kg

Analgesia:
- Children (unlabeled use): I.M.:
  - 5-8 years: 15 mg
  - 9-14 years: 30 mg
- Adults:
  - I.M., SubQ: 30-60 mg every 3-4 hours; do not exceed 60 mg/dose (maximum: 360 mg/day)
  - I.V.: 30 mg every 3-4 hours; do not exceed 30 mg/dose (maximum: 360 mg/day)

Labor pain: Adults:
- I.M.: 30 mg once
- I.V.: 20 mg every 2-3 hours as needed (maximum total dose: 60 mg)

Elderly: Elderly patients may be more sensitive to the analgesic and sedating effects. The elderly may also have impaired renal function. If needed, dosing should be started at the lower end of dosing range and adjust dose for renal function.

Dosing adjustment in renal impairment: No dosage adjustment provided in manufacturer's labeling. Use with caution. The following guidelines have been used by some clinicians (Aronoff, 2007):
- Cl_{cr} ≥50 mL/minute: No dosage adjustment necessary.
- Cl_{cr} 10-50 mL/minute: Administer 75% of normal dose.
- Cl_{cr} <10 mL/minute: Administer 50% of normal dose.

Dosing adjustment in hepatic impairment: No dosage adjustment provided in manufacturer's labeling. However, dosage adjustment may be necessary due to decreased metabolism and predisposition to adverse effects. Use with caution.

Additional Information Complete prescribing information should be consulted for additional detail.

Dosage Forms Excipient information presented when available (limited, particularly for generics); consult specific product labeling.

Solution, Injection:
- Talwin: 30 mg/mL (1 mL)
- Talwin: 30 mg/mL (10 mL) [contains methylparaben, sodium bisulfite]

Controlled Substance C-IV

◆ **Pentazocine Lactate** *see* Pentazocine *on page 1615*

PENTobarbital (pen toe BAR bi tal)

Brand Names: U.S. Nembutal

Brand Names: Canada Nembutal® Sodium

Index Terms Pentobarbital Sodium

Pharmacologic Category Anticonvulsant, Barbiturate; Barbiturate

Additional Appendix Information

Beers Criteria – Potentially Inappropriate Medications for Geriatrics *on page 2368*

Status Epilepticus *on page 2375*

Use Sedative/hypnotic; refractory status epilepticus

Unlabeled Use Barbiturate coma in patients with severe brain injury (eg, hemorrhagic stroke, traumatic brain injury) and increased intracranial pressure

Pregnancy Risk Factor D

Pregnancy Considerations Barbiturates can be detected in the placenta, fetal liver and fetal brain. Fetal and maternal blood concentrations may be similar following parenteral administration. An increased incidence of fetal abnormalities may occur following maternal use. When used during the third trimester of pregnancy, withdrawal symptoms may occur in the neonate including seizures and hyperirritability; symptoms may be delayed up to 14 days. Use during labor does not impair uterine activity; however, respiratory depression may occur in the newborn; resuscitation equipment should be available, especially for premature infants.

Breast-Feeding Considerations Small amounts of barbiturates are found in breast milk.

Contraindications Hypersensitivity to barbiturates or any component of the formulation; porphyria

Warnings/Precautions May cause hypotension particularly when administered intravenously; use with caution in hemodynamically unstable patients (hypotension or shock). High doses used to induce pentobarbital coma cause hypotension requiring vasopressor therapy. May cause respiratory depression particularly when administered intravenously; use with caution in patients with respiratory disease. Intubation is typically required prior to treatment for status epilepticus or traumatic brain injury. Anticonvulsants should not be discontinued abruptly because of the possibility of increasing seizure frequency; therapy should be withdrawn gradually to minimize the potential of increased seizure frequency, unless safety concerns require a more rapid withdrawal. Do not administer to patients in acute pain; may heighten/worsen sense of pain.

Use with caution in patients with hepatic or renal impairment; reduce dose as appropriate. Do not use in patients with premonitory signs of hepatic coma. Use with caution in patients with a history of drug abuse; potential for drug dependency exists. Tolerance, psychological and physical dependence may occur with prolonged use. Use with caution in patients with depression or suicidal tendencies. Avoid use in the elderly due to risk of overdose with low dosages, tolerance to sleep effects, and increased risk of physical dependence (Beers Criteria). May cause CNS depression, which may impair physical or mental abilities; patients must be cautioned about performing tasks which require mental alertness (eg, operating machinery or driving). Effects with other sedative drugs or ethanol may be potentiated.

Solution for injection is highly alkaline and extravasation may cause local tissue damage. Intravenous solution may contain propylene glycol (PG). One case report has described a patient who developed lactic acidosis possibly secondary to PG accumulation following a continuous infusion of pentobarbital (Miller, 2008). Consider monitoring for signs of PG toxicity (eg, lactic acidosis, acute renal failure, osmol gap) in patients who require a continuous infusion of pentobarbital.

Adverse Reactions Frequency not defined.

Cardiovascular: Bradycardia, hypotension, syncope

Central nervous system: Abnormal thinking, agitation, anxiety, ataxia, CNS excitation, confusion, depression, dizziness, drowsiness, fever, hallucinations, headache, hyperkinesia, insomnia, nervousness, nightmares, psychiatric disturbances, somnolence

Dermatologic: Angioedema, exfoliative dermatitis, rash

Gastrointestinal: Constipation, nausea, vomiting

Hematologic: Megaloblastic anemia

Hepatic: Hepatotoxicity

Local: Injection site reactions

Respiratory: Apnea (especially with rapid I.V. use), hypoventilation, laryngospasm, respiratory depression

Miscellaneous: Gangrene with inadvertent intra-arterial injection, hypersensitivity reactions

Drug Interactions

Metabolism/Transport Effects Induces CYP2A6 (strong), CYP3A4 (strong)

Avoid Concomitant Use

Avoid concomitant use of PENTobarbital with any of the following: Abiraterone Acetate; Apixaban; Artemether; Axitinib; Azelastine (Nasal); Bedaquiline; Boceprevir; Bortezomib; Bosutinib; Cabozantinib; CloZAPine; Crizotinib; Dienogest; Dronedarone; Enzalutamide; Everolimus; Ibrutinib; Itraconazole; Ivacaftor; Lapatinib; Lumefantrine; Lurasidone; Macitentan; Mifepristone; NIFEdipine; Nilotinib; Nisoldipine; Paraldehyde; PAZOPanib; Perampanel; Pomalidomide; PONATinib; Praziquantel; Ranolazine; Regorafenib; Rivaroxaban; Roflumilast; RomiDEPsin; Simeprevir; SORAfenib; Telaprevir; Ticagrelor; Tofacitinib; Tolvaptan; Toremifene; Ulipristal; Vandetanib; Vemurafenib; VinCRIStine (Liposomal)

Increased Effect/Toxicity

PENTobarbital may increase the levels/effects of: Alcohol (Ethyl); Azelastine (Nasal); Buprenorphine; Clarithromycin; CNS Depressants; Hydrocodone; Ifosfamide; Meperidine; Methotrimeprazine; Metyrosine; Mirtazapine; Paraldehyde; Pramipexole; ROPINIRole; Rotigotine; Selective Serotonin Reuptake Inhibitors; Thiazide Diuretics; Zolpidem

The levels/effects of PENTobarbital may be increased by: Brimonidine (Topical); Carbonic Anhydrase Inhibitors; Chloramphenicol; Clarithromycin; Doxylamine; Droperidol; Felbamate; HydrOXYzine; Magnesium Sulfate; Methotrimeprazine; Primidone; Sodium Oxybate; Tapentadol; Valproic Acid and Derivatives

Decreased Effect

PENTobarbital may decrease the levels/effects of: Abiraterone Acetate; Acetaminophen; Apixaban; ARIPiprazole; Artemether; Axitinib; Bedaquiline; Beta-Blockers; Boceprevir; Bortezomib; Bosutinib; Brentuximab Vedotin; Cabozantinib; Calcium Channel Blockers; Chloramphenicol; Clarithromycin; CloZAPine; Contraceptives (Estrogens); Contraceptives (Progestins); Corticosteroids (Systemic); Crizotinib; CycloSPORINE (Systemic); CYP2A6 Substrates; CYP3A4 Substrates; Dasatinib; Dienogest; Doxycycline; Dronedarone; Enzalutamide; Etoposide; Etoposide Phosphate; Everolimus; Exemestane; Felbamate; Gefitinib; Griseofulvin; GuanFACINE; Ibrutinib; Imatinib; Itraconazole; Ivacaftor; Ixabepilone; LamoTRIgine; Lapatinib; Linagliptin; Lumefantrine; Lurasidone; Macitentan; Maraviroc; Mifepristone; NIFEdipine; Nilotinib; Nisoldipine; PAZOPanib; Perampanel; Pomalidomide; PONATinib; Praziquantel; Propafenone; QUEtiapine; Ranolazine; Regorafenib; Rivaroxaban; Roflumilast; RomiDEPsin; Saxagliptin; Simeprevir; SORAfenib; SUNItinib; Tadalafil; Telaprevir; Teniposide; Theophylline Derivatives; Ticagrelor; Tofacitinib; Tolvaptan; Toremifene; Tricyclic Antidepressants; Ulipristal; Valproic Acid and Derivatives; Vandetanib; Vemurafenib; VinCRIStine (Liposomal); Vitamin K Antagonists; Vortioxetine; Zuclopenthixol

The levels/effects of PENTobarbital may be decreased by: Ketorolac (Nasal); Ketorolac (Systemic); Mefloquine; Multivitamins/Minerals (with ADEK, Folate, Iron); Orlistat; Pyridoxine; Rifamycin Derivatives

Ethanol/Nutrition/Herb Interactions Ethanol: May increase CNS depression; monitor for increased effects with coadministration. Caution patients about effects.

Storage/Stability Store at controlled room temperature of 15°C to 30°C (68°F to 77°F); protect from freezing and avoid excessive heat. When mixed with an acidic solution, precipitate may form. Use only clear solution.

Mechanism of Action Barbiturate with sedative, hypnotic, and anticonvulsant properties. Barbiturates depress the sensory cortex, decrease motor activity, alter cerebellar function, and produce drowsiness, sedation, and hypnosis. In high doses, barbiturates exhibit anticonvulsant activity; barbiturates produce dose-dependent respiratory depression; reduce brain metabolism and cerebral blood flow in order to decrease intracranial pressure

Pharmacodynamics/Kinetics

Onset of action: I.M.: 10-15 minutes (Krauss, 2006); I.V.: Almost immediate, within 3-5 minutes (Krauss, 2006)

Duration: I.V.: Variable

Distribution: V_d: Children: 0.8 L/kg (Schaible, 1982); Adults: 1 L/kg (Ehrnebo, 1974)

Protein binding: 45% to 70%

Metabolism: Hepatic via hydroxylation and glucuronidation (Wermeling, 1985)

Half-life elimination: Terminal: Children: 26 ± 16 hours (Schaible, 1982); Adults: Healthy: 22 hours (average; Ehrnebo, 1974); (range: 15-50 hours; dose dependent)

Excretion: Urine

Dosage Note: Adjust dose based on patients age, weight, and condition.

Children:

Hypnotic/sedative:

I.M.: 2-6 mg/kg; maximum: 100 mg/dose

I.V.: 1-6 mg/kg titrated in 1-2 mg/kg increments every 3-5 minutes to desired effect (Krauss, 2006)

Refractory status epilepticus: I.V.: **Note:** Intubation required; adjust dose based on hemodynamics, seizure activity, and EEG. Various regimens available (Abend, 2008; Hanhan, 2001; Holmes, 1999; Kim, 2001):

Loading dose: 5-15 mg/kg given slowly over 1 hour; maintenance infusion: 0.5-5 mg/kg/hour to maintain burst suppression; continue for 12-48 hours of no seizure activity; may taper infusion rate by 0.5 mg/kg/hour every 12 hours

Adults:
Hypnotic/sedative:
I.M.: 150-200 mg
I.V.: Initial: 100 mg; decrease dose for elderly or debilitated patients. If needed, may administer additional increments after at least 1 minute, up to a total dose of 200-500 mg
Barbiturate coma in severe brain injury patients/elevated intracranial pressure (unlabeled use; Bratton, 2007): I.V.: Loading dose: 10 mg/kg given over 30 minutes (or ≤25 mg/minute), followed by 5 mg/kg every hour for 3 doses; monitor blood pressure and respiratory rate. Maintenance infusion: Initial: 1 mg/kg/hour; may increase to 2-4 mg/kg/hour; maintain burst suppression on EEG.
Refractory status epilepticus: I.V.: **Note:** Intubation required; adjust dose based on hemodynamics, seizure activity, and EEG. Various regimens available (Abou Khaled, 2008; Millikan, 2009; Mirski, 2008; Yaffe, 1993): Loading dose: 10-15 mg/kg (5-10 mg/kg in patients with pre-existing hypotension) administer slowly over 1 hour; initial maintenance infusion: 0.5-1 mg/kg/hour; adjust to maintain burst suppression pattern on EEG; maintenance infusion dose range: 0.5-10 mg/kg/hour
Note: During active seizure activity when increasing maintenance infusion rate, some experts suggest administration of an additional 5 mg/kg bolus given the long half-life of pentobarbital.
Elderly: Not recommended for use in the elderly; decrease dose if use becomes necessary

Dosing adjustment in renal impairment: No dosage adjustment provided in manufacturer's labeling. However, a reduced dosage in patients with renal dysfunction is recommended.

Dosing adjustment in hepatic impairment: No dosage adjustment provided in manufacturer's labeling. However, a reduced dosage in patients with liver dysfunction is recommended.

Administration Pentobarbital may be administered by deep I.M. or slow I.V. injection.
I.M.: Inject into a large muscle. No more than 5 mL (250 mg) should be injected at any one site because of possible tissue irritation.
I.V.: Do not exceed 50 mg/minute; I.V. push doses may be given undiluted. Parenteral solutions are highly alkaline; avoid extravasation; avoid intra-arterial injection.

Monitoring Parameters Respiratory status (for conscious sedation, includes pulse oximetry), cardiovascular status, CNS status; cardiac monitor and blood pressure monitor required; temperature with high doses (eg, barbiturate coma)

Elevated ICP: Monitor ICP, CPP, EEG

Reference Range
Therapeutic:
Sedation: 1-5 mcg/mL (SI: 4-22 micromole/L)
Coma or intracranial pressure therapy: Target: 30-40 mcg/mL (SI: 132-176 micromole/L) (Bratton, 2007)
Potentially toxic: >10 mcg/mL (SI: >44 micromole/L); dependent on reason for use and patient condition

Dosage Forms Excipient information presented when available (limited, particularly for generics); consult specific product labeling.
Solution, Injection, as sodium:
Nembutal: 50 mg/mL (20 mL, 50 mL) [latex free; contains alcohol, usp, propylene glycol]

Controlled Substance C-II

◆ **Pentobarbital Sodium** *see* PENTobarbital *on page* 1615

Pentosan Polysulfate Sodium

(PEN toe san pol i SUL fate SOW dee um)

Brand Names: U.S. Elmiron
Brand Names: Canada Elmiron®
Index Terms PPS
Pharmacologic Category Analgesic, Urinary
Use Relief of bladder pain or discomfort due to interstitial cystitis
Pregnancy Risk Factor B
Dosage Children ≥16 years and Adults: Oral: 100 mg 3 times/day taken with water 1 hour before or 2 hours after meals

Note: Patients should be evaluated at 3 months and may be continued an additional 3 months if there has been no improvement and if there are no therapy-limiting side effects. **The risks and benefits of continued use beyond 6 months in patients who have not responded is not yet known.**

Dosing adjustment in renal impairment: No dosage adjustment provided in manufacturer's labeling (has not been studied).
Dosing adjustment in hepatic impairment: No dosage adjustment provided in manufacturer's labeling (has not been studied). However, dosage adjustment may be necessary due to hepatic impairment impact on pharmacokinetics. Use with caution.

Additional Information Complete prescribing information should be consulted for additional detail.
Dosage Forms Excipient information presented when available (limited, particularly for generics); consult specific product labeling.
Capsule, Oral:
Elmiron: 100 mg [contains fd&c blue #1 aluminum lake, fd&c blue #2 aluminum lake, fd&c red #40 aluminum lake, fd&c yellow #10 aluminum lake]

Pentostatin (pen toe STAT in)

Brand Names: U.S. Nipent
Brand Names: Canada Nipent®
Index Terms 2′-Deoxycoformycin; Co-Vidarabine; dCF; Deoxycoformycin
Pharmacologic Category Antineoplastic Agent, Antibiotic; Antineoplastic Agent, Antimetabolite (Purine Analog)
Use Treatment of hairy cell leukemia
Unlabeled Use Treatment of cutaneous T-cell lymphoma, chronic lymphocytic leukemia (CLL), and acute and chronic graft-versus-host-disease (GVHD)
Pregnancy Risk Factor D
Pregnancy Considerations Animal studies have demonstrated teratogenicity, maternal toxicity, and fetal loss. There are no adequate and well-controlled studies in pregnant women. Women of childbearing potential should be advised to avoid becoming pregnant.
Breast-Feeding Considerations Due to the potential for serious adverse reactions in nursing the infant, breast-feeding is not recommended.
Contraindications Hypersensitivity to pentostatin or any component of the formulation
Warnings/Precautions Hazardous agent - use appropriate precautions for handling and disposal (NIOSH, 2012). **[U.S. Boxed Warnings]: Severe renal, liver, pulmonary and CNS toxicities have occurred with doses higher than recommended; do not exceed the recommended dose. Do not administer concurrently with fludarabine; concomitant use has resulted in serious or fatal pulmonary toxicity.** Bone marrow suppression may occur, primarily early in treatment; if neutropenia persists beyond early cycles, evaluate for disease status. In patients who

present with infections prior to treatment, infections should be resolved, if possible, prior to initiation of treatment; treatment should be temporarily withheld for active infections during therapy. Use cautiously in patients with renal dysfunction (the half-life is prolonged); appropriate dosing guidelines in renal insufficiency have not been determined. May cause elevations (reversible) in liver function tests. Withhold treatment for CNS toxicity or severe rash. Fatal pulmonary edema and hypotension have been reported in patients treated with pentostatin in combination with carmustine, etoposide, or high-dose cyclophosphamide as part of a myeloablative regimen for bone marrow transplant. **[U.S. Boxed Warning]: Should be administered under the supervision of an experienced cancer chemotherapy physician.** Safety and efficacy in children have not been established.

Adverse Reactions

>10%:

Central nervous system: Fever (42% to 46%), fatigue (29% to 42%), pain (8% to 20%), chills (11% to 19%), headache (13% to 17%), CNS toxicity (1% to 11%)

Dermatologic: Rash (26% to 43%), pruritus (10% to 21%), skin disorder (4% to 17%)

Gastrointestinal: Nausea/vomiting (22% to 63%), diarrhea (15% to 17%), anorexia (13% to 16%), abdominal pain (4% to 16%), stomatitis (5% to 12%)

Hematologic: Myelosuppression (nadir: 7 days; recovery: 10-14 days), leukopenia (22% to 60%), anemia (8% to 35%), thrombocytopenia (6% to 32%)

Hepatic: Transaminases increased (2% to 19%)

Neuromuscular & skeletal: Myalgia (11% to 19%), weakness (10% to 12%)

Respiratory: Cough (17% to 20%), upper respiratory infection (13% to 16%), rhinitis (10% to 11%), dyspnea (8% to 11%)

Miscellaneous: Infection (7% to 36%), allergic reaction (2% to 11%)

1% to 10%:

Cardiovascular: Chest pain (3% to 10%), facial edema (3% to 10%), hypotension (3% to 10%), peripheral edema (3% to 10%), angina (<3%), arrhythmia (<3%), AV block (<3%), bradycardia (<3%), cardiac arrest (<3%), deep thrombophlebitis (<3%), heart failure (<3%), hypertension (<3%), pericardial effusion (<3%), sinus arrest (<3%), syncope (<3%), tachycardia (<3%), vasculitis (<3%), ventricular extrasystoles (<3%)

Central nervous system: Anxiety (3% to 10%), confusion (3% to 10%), depression (3% to 10%), dizziness (3% to 10%), insomnia (3% to 10%), nervousness (3% to 10%), somnolence (3% to 10%), abnormal dreams/thinking (<3%), amnesia (<3%), ataxia (<3%), emotional lability (<3%), encephalitis (<3%), hallucination (<3%), hostility (<3%), meningism (<3%), neuritis (<3%), neurosis (<3%), seizure (<3%), vertigo (<3%)

Dermatologic: Cellulitis (6%), furunculosis (4%), dry skin (3% to 10%), urticaria (3% to 10%), acne (<3%), alopecia (<3%), eczema (<3%), petechial rash (<3%), photosensitivity (<3%), abscess (2%)

Endocrine & metabolic: Amenorrhea (<3%), hypercalcemia (<3%), hyponatremia (<3%), gout (<3%), libido decreased/loss (<3%)

Gastrointestinal: Dyspepsia (3% to 10%) flatulence (3% to 10%), gingivitis (3% to 10%), constipation (<3%), dysphagia (<3%), glossitis (<3%), ileus (<3%), taste perversion (<3%), oral moniliasis (2%)

Genitourinary: Urinary tract infection (3%), impotence (<3%)

Hematologic: Agranulocytosis (3% to 10%), hemorrhage (3% to 10%), acute leukemia (<3%), aplastic anemia (<3%), hemolytic anemia (<3%)

Local: Phlebitis (<3%)

Neuromuscular & skeletal: Arthralgia (3% to 10%), paresthesia (3% to 10%), arthritis (<3%), dysarthria (<3%), hyperkinesia (<3%), neuralgia (<3%), neuropathy (<3%), paralysis (<3%), twitching (<3%), osteomyelitis (1%)

Ocular: Conjunctivitis (4%), amblyopia (<3%), eyes nonreactive (<3%), lacrimation disorder (<3%), photophobia (<3%), retinopathy (<3%), vision abnormal (<3%), watery eyes (<3%), xerophthalmia (<3%)

Otic: Deafness (<3%), earache (<3%), labyrinthitis (<3%), tinnitus (<3%)

Renal: Creatinine increased (3% to 10%), nephropathy (<3%), renal failure (<3%), renal insufficiency (<3%), renal function abnormal (<3%), renal stone (<3%)

Respiratory: Pharyngitis (8% to 10%), sinusitis (6%), pneumonia (5%), asthma (3% to 10%), bronchitis (3%), bronchospasm (<3%), laryngeal edema (<3%), pulmonary embolus (<3%)

Miscellaneous: Diaphoresis (8% to 10%), herpes zoster (8%), viral infection (≤8%), bacterial infection (5%), herpes simplex (4%), sepsis (3%), flu-like syndrome (<3%)

<1% (Limited to important or life-threatening): Dysuria, fungal infection (skin), hematuria, lethargy, pulmonary edema, pulmonary toxicity (fatal; in combination with fludarabine), uveitis/vision loss

Drug Interactions

Metabolism/Transport Effects None known.

Avoid Concomitant Use

Avoid concomitant use of Pentostatin with any of the following: BCG; CloZAPine; Fludarabine; Natalizumab; Nelarabine; Pegademase Bovine; Pimecrolimus; Tacrolimus (Topical); Tofacitinib; Vaccines (Live)

Increased Effect/Toxicity

Pentostatin may increase the levels/effects of: CloZAPine; Cyclophosphamide; Fludarabine; Leflunomide; Natalizumab; Tofacitinib; Vaccines (Live)

The levels/effects of Pentostatin may be increased by: Denosumab; Fludarabine; Pimecrolimus; Roflumilast; Tacrolimus (Topical); Trastuzumab

Decreased Effect

Pentostatin may decrease the levels/effects of: BCG; Coccidioidin Skin Test; Nelarabine; Pegademase Bovine; Sipuleucel-T; Vaccines (Inactivated); Vaccines (Live)

The levels/effects of Pentostatin may be decreased by: Echinacea; Pegademase Bovine

Preparation for Administration Hazardous agent; use appropriate precautions for handling and disposal (NIOSH, 2012). Reconstitute with 5 mL SWFI to a concentration of 2 mg/mL. The solution may be further diluted in 25-50 mL NS or D_5W for infusion.

Storage/Stability Store intact vials under refrigeration at 2°C to 8°C (36°F to 46°F); reconstituted vials, or further dilutions, are stable at room temperature for 8 hours in D_5W or 48 hours in NS.

Mechanism of Action Pentostatin is a purine antimetabolite that inhibits adenosine deaminase, preventing the deamination of adenosine to inosine. Accumulation of deoxyadenosine (dAdo) and deoxyadenosine 5'-triphosphate (dATP) results in a reduction of purine metabolism and DNA synthesis and cell death.

Pharmacodynamics/Kinetics

Distribution: I.V.: V_d: 36.1 L (20.1 L/m^2); rapidly to body tissues

Protein binding: ~4%

Half-life elimination:

Distribution half-life: 11-85 minutes

Terminal: 3-7 hours

Renal impairment (Cl_{cr} <50 mL/minute): 4-18 hours

Excretion: Urine (~50% to 96%) within 24 hours (30% to 90% as unchanged drug)

Dosage I.V.: Adults (refer to individual protocols):

Hairy cell leukemia: 4 mg/m^2 every 2 weeks

CLL (unlabeled use): 4 mg/m^2 weekly for 3 weeks, then every 2 weeks

Cutaneous T-cell lymphoma (unlabeled use): 3.75-5 mg/m^2 daily for 3 days every 3 weeks

Acute GVHD (unlabeled use): 1.5 mg/m^2 daily for 3 days; may repeat after 2 weeks if needed

Chronic GVHD (unlabeled use): 4 mg/m^2 every 2 weeks for 12 doses; then 4 mg/m^2 every 3-4 weeks (if still improving)

Dosage adjustment in renal impairment: No dosage adjustment provided in manufacturer's labeling; use with caution in patients with Cl_{cr} <60 mL/minute. Two patients with Cl_{cr} 50-60 mL/minute achieved responses when treated with 2 mg/m^2/dose. The following guidelines have been used by some clinicians:

Kintzel, 1995:

Cl_{cr} 46-60 mL/minute: Administer 70% of dose

Cl_{cr} 31-45 mL/minute: Administer 60% of dose

Cl_{cr} <30 mL/minute: Consider use of alternative drug

Lathia, 2002:

Cl_{cr} 40-59 mL/minute: Administer 3 mg/m^2/dose

Cl_{cr} 20-39 mL/minute: Administer 2 mg/m^2/dose

Dosage adjustment in hepatic impairment: No dosage adjustment provided in manufacturer's labeling.

Dosing in obesity: *ASCO Guidelines for appropriate chemotherapy dosing in obese adults with cancer:* Utilize patient's actual body weight (full weight) for calculation of body surface area- or weight-based dosing, particularly when the intent of therapy is curative; manage regimen-related toxicities in the same manner as for nonobese patients; if a dose reduction is utilized due to toxicity, consider resumption of full weight-based dosing with subsequent cycles, especially if cause of toxicity (eg, hepatic or renal impairment) is resolved (Griggs, 2012).

Administration Administer I.V. 20- to 30-minute infusion or I.V. bolus over 5 minutes. Hydrate with 500-1000 mL fluid prior to infusion and 500 mL after infusion.

Hazardous agent; use appropriate precautions for handling and disposal (NIOSH, 2012).

Monitoring Parameters CBC with differential, platelet count, liver function, serum uric acid, renal function (creatinine clearance), bone marrow evaluation

Dosage Forms Excipient information presented when available (limited, particularly for generics); consult specific product labeling.

Solution Reconstituted, Intravenous:

Nipent: 10 mg (1 ea)

Generic: 10 mg (1 ea)

Pentoxifylline (pen toks IF i lin)

Brand Names: U.S. TRENtal [DSC]

Brand Names: Canada Pentoxifylline SR

Index Terms Oxpentifylline

Pharmacologic Category Blood Viscosity Reducer Agent

Use Treatment of intermittent claudication on the basis of chronic occlusive arterial disease of the limbs; may improve function and symptoms, but not intended to replace more definitive therapy

Note: The American College of Chest Physicians (ACCP) discourages the use of pentoxifylline for the treatment of intermittent claudication refractory to exercise therapy (and smoking cessation) (Guyatt, 2012).

Unlabeled Use Severe alcoholic hepatitis; venous leg ulcers (with compression therapy)

Pregnancy Risk Factor C

Pregnancy Considerations Adverse events were observed in animal reproduction studies. Information related to use in pregnant women has not been located. Pentoxifylline may be used to test sperm viability when evaluating nonfertile males (ASRM, 2012). It has also been evaluated for the treatment of infertility due to endometriosis, but use for this purpose is not currently recommended (Lu, 2012).

Breast-Feeding Considerations Pentoxifylline and its metabolites are excreted into breast milk. Five nursing women (~6 weeks postpartum) were given a single dose of pentoxifylline 400 mg and maternal milk and serum samples were measured 2 and 4 hours later. The mean M/P ratio of pentoxifylline was 0.87 at 4 hours; actual milk concentrations ranged from below the limit of detection to 67.4 ng/mL. Three metabolites were also measured in breast milk, with mean M/P ratios ranging from 0.54-1.13 at 4 hours (Witter, 1985). Due to the potential for serious adverse reactions in the nursing infant, the manufacturer recommends a decision be made whether to discontinue nursing or to discontinue the drug, taking into account the importance of treatment to the mother.

Contraindications Hypersensitivity to pentoxifylline, xanthines (eg, caffeine, theophylline), or any component of the formulation; recent cerebral and/or retinal hemorrhage

Warnings/Precautions Use with caution in renal impairment; active metabolite may accumulate in renal impairment leading to increased risk of adverse effects. Use caution in the elderly and assess renal function before initiating.

Adverse Reactions

1% to 10%: Gastrointestinal: Nausea (2%), vomiting (1%)

<1% (Limited to important or life-threatening): Anaphylactic shock, anaphylactoid reaction, anaphylaxis, angioedema, angina, anorexia, aplastic anemia, arrhythmia, aseptic meningitis, blurred vision, chest pain, cholecystitis, conjunctivitis, depression, fibrinogen decreased (serum), hallucinations, hepatitis, hypotension, leukemia, leukopenia, liver enzymes increased, pancytopenia, scotoma, seizure, tachycardia, thrombocytopenia

Drug Interactions

Metabolism/Transport Effects Inhibits CYP1A2 (weak)

Avoid Concomitant Use

Avoid concomitant use of Pentoxifylline with any of the following: Ketorolac (Nasal); Ketorolac (Systemic)

Increased Effect/Toxicity

Pentoxifylline may increase the levels/effects of: Agents with Antiplatelet Properties; Antihypertensives; Heparin; Heparin (Low Molecular Weight); Theophylline Derivatives; Vitamin K Antagonists

The levels/effects of Pentoxifylline may be increased by: Cimetidine; Ciprofloxacin (Systemic); Ketorolac (Nasal); Ketorolac (Systemic)

Decreased Effect There are no known significant interactions involving a decrease in effect.

Ethanol/Nutrition/Herb Interactions Food: Food may decrease rate but not extent of absorption. Pentoxifylline peak serum levels may be decreased if taken with food.

Storage/Stability Store between 15°C to 30°C (59°F to 86°F).

Mechanism of Action Reduces blood viscosity via increased leukocyte and erythrocyte deformability and decreased neutrophil adhesion/activation; improves peripheral tissue oxygenation presumably through enhanced blood flow.

Pharmacodynamics/Kinetics

Absorption: Well absorbed

Metabolism: Hepatic to 3-carboxybutyl (M-IV, inactive) and 3-carboxypropyl (M-V, active) and via erythrocytes to 5-hydroxyhexyl (M-I, active); extensive first-pass effect; M-I is further metabolized in the liver

Half-life elimination: Parent drug: 24-48 minutes; Metabolites: 60-96 minutes
Time to peak, serum: 2-4 hours
Excretion: Primarily urine (50% to 80% as M-V, 20% as other metabolites); feces (<4%)

Dosage Oral:
Adults:
Intermittent claudication: 400 mg 3 times/day; maximal therapeutic benefit may take 2-4 weeks to develop; recommended to maintain therapy for at least 8 weeks. May reduce to 400 mg twice daily if GI or CNS side effects occur.
Note: Use for the treatment of intermittent claudication refractory to exercise therapy (and smoking cessation) has been discouraged by The American College of Chest Physicians (ACCP) (Guyatt, 2012).
Severe alcoholic hepatitis (Maddrey Discriminant Function [MDF] score ≥32, especially when corticosteroids contraindicated) (unlabeled use): 400 mg 3 times/day for 4 weeks (O'Shea, 2010)
Venous leg ulcer (unlabeled use): 400 mg 3 times/day (with compression therapy) (Jull, 2002; Robson, 2006)
Elderly: Dosage adjustment based on creatinine clearance can be considered.

Dosage adjustment in renal impairment: No dosage adjustments provided in the manufacturer's labeling; however, the following guidelines have been used by some clinicians:
Aronoff, 2007: Adults:
Cl_{cr} >50 mL/minute: 400 mg every 8-12 hours
Cl_{cr} 10-50 mL/minute: 400 mg every 12-24 hours
Cl_{cr} <10 mL minute: 400 mg every 24 hours
Hemodialysis: supplemental postdialysis dose is not necessary
Peritoneal dialysis: 400 mg every 24 hours
Paap, 1996: Adults:
Moderate renal impairment (Cl_{cr} ~60 mL/minute): 400 mg twice daily
Severe renal impairment (Cl_{cr} ~20 mL/minute): 400 mg once daily; further reduction may be required; Paap suggests 200 mg once daily, but with current products (extended or controlled release; unscored) may require adaptation to 400 mg once every other day

Dosage adjustment in hepatic impairment: No dosage adjustment provided in manufacturer's labeling (has not been studied).

Dietary Considerations May be taken with meals.

Administration Tablets should be swallowed whole; do not chew, break, or crush. May be administered with food.

Test Interactions False-positive theophylline levels

Dosage Forms Excipient information presented when available (limited, particularly for generics); consult specific product labeling. [DSC] = Discontinued product
Tablet Extended Release, Oral:
TRENtal: 400 mg [DSC] [contains benzyl alcohol]
Generic: 400 mg

Extemporaneous Preparations A 20 mg/mL oral suspension may be made using tablets. Crush ten 400 mg tablets and reduce to a fine powder. Add a small amount of purified water and mix to a uniform paste; mix while adding purified water to **almost** 200 mL; transfer to a calibrated bottle, rinse mortar with vehicle, and add quantity of vehicle sufficient to make 200 mL. Label "shake well" and "refrigerate". Stable 91 days.

Nahata MC, Pai VB, and Hipple TF, *Pediatric Drug Formulations*, 5th ed, Cincinnati, OH: Harvey Whitney Books Co, 2004.

◆ **Pentoxifylline SR (Can)** *see* Pentoxifylline *on page 1619*
◆ **Pen VK** *see* Penicillin V Potassium *on page 1611*
◆ **PEP005** *see* Ingenol Mebutate *on page 1085*
◆ **Pepcid** *see* Famotidine *on page 832*
◆ **Pepcid® (Can)** *see* Famotidine *on page 832*
◆ **Pepcid® AC (Can)** *see* Famotidine *on page 832*
◆ **Pepcid® I.V. (Can)** *see* Famotidine *on page 832*
◆ **Peptic Relief [OTC]** *see* Bismuth *on page 260*
◆ **Pepto-Bismol [OTC]** *see* Bismuth *on page 260*
◆ **Pepto-Bismol To-Go [OTC]** *see* Bismuth *on page 260*

Perampanel (per AM pa nel)

Brand Names: U.S. Fycompa

Pharmacologic Category AMPA Glutamate Receptor Antagonist; Anticonvulsant, Miscellaneous

Use Adjunctive therapy in the treatment of partial-onset seizures (with or without generalized seizures)

Pregnancy Risk Factor C

Pregnancy Considerations Adverse events were observed in animal reproduction studies at doses equivalent to the human dose (based on BSA). Contraceptives containing levonorgestrel may be less effective; additional nonhormonal forms of contraception are recommended during perampanel therapy.

Patients exposed to perampanel during pregnancy are encouraged to enroll in the North American Antiepileptic Drug (NAAED) Pregnancy Registry by calling 1-888-233-2334. Additional information is available at www.aedpregnancyregistry.org.

Breast-Feeding Considerations It is not known if perampanel is excreted in breast milk. The manufacturer recommends that caution be exercised when administering perampanel to nursing women.

Medication Guide Available Yes

Contraindications There are no contraindications listed in manufacturer's labeling.

Warnings/Precautions [U.S. Boxed Warning]: Dose-related serious and/or life-threatening neuropsychiatric events (including aggression, anger, homicidal thoughts, hostility, and irritability) have been reported most often occurring in first 6 weeks of therapy in patients with or without pre-existing psychiatric disease; monitor patients closely especially during dosage adjustments and when receiving higher doses. Adjust dose or immediately discontinue use if severe or worsening symptoms occur. Inform patients and caregivers to contact their healthcare provider immediately if they experience any atypical behavioral and/or mood changes. Pooled analysis of trials involving various antiepileptics (regardless of indication) showed an increased risk of suicidal thoughts/behavior (incidence rate: 0.43% treated patients compared to 0.24% of patients receiving placebo); risk observed as early as 1 week after initiation and continued through duration of trials (most trials ≤24 weeks). Monitor all patients for notable changes in behavior that might indicate suicidal thoughts or depression; notify healthcare provider immediately if symptoms occur. Dizziness, fatigue (including lethargy and weakness), gait disturbances (including abnormal coordination, ataxia, and balance disorder), and somnolence may occur during therapy; patients should be cautioned about performing tasks which require alertness (eg, operating machinery or driving). Concomitant use with CNS depressant (including alcohol) may increase the risk of CNS depression. Use caution if a CNS depressant must be used concurrently with perampanel. Not recommended for use in patients with severe hepatic impairment, renal impairment, or on hemodialysis; dosage adjustment recommended for mild-to-moderate hepatic impairment. Use with extreme caution in patients who are at risk of falls; perampanel has been associated with falls and traumatic injury. Anticonvulsants should not be discontinued abruptly because of the possibility of increasing seizure frequency; therapy should be withdrawn gradually (≥1 week) to minimize the potential of increased seizure frequency, unless safety concerns require a more rapid withdrawal.

Adverse Reactions

>10%: Central nervous system: Dizziness (16% to 43%), somnolence (9% to 18%), headache (13%), fatigue (8% to 12%), irritability (4% to 12%)

1% to 10%:

Cardiovascular: Peripheral edema (2%)

Central nervous system: Ataxia (1% to 8%), vertigo (3% to 5%), balance impaired (≤5%), gait disturbance (4%), anxiety (2% to 4%), aggression (2% to 3%), hypersomnia (1% to 3%), anger (≤3%), hypoesthesia (≤3%), confusion (2%), coordination impaired (≤2%), euphoria (≤2%), memory impaired (≤2%), mood changes (1% to 2%)

Dermatologic: Bruising (≤2%), skin laceration (≤2%)

Endocrine & metabolic: Hyponatremia (≤2%)

Gastrointestinal: Weight gain (4% to 9%), nausea (6% to 8%), vomiting (4%), constipation (3%)

Neuromuscular & skeletal: Falling (5% to 10%), back pain (5%), dysarthria (1% to 4%), myalgia (3%), arthralgia (≤3%), limb pain (≤3%), limb injury (2%), musculoskeletal pain (2%), weakness (2%), paresthesia (≤2%)

Ocular: Blurred vision (3% to 4%), diplopia (3%)

Respiratory: Cough (4%), upper respiratory tract infection (4%), oropharyngeal pain (2%)

Miscellaneous: Head injury (3%)

Drug Interactions

Metabolism/Transport Effects **Substrate** of CYP3A4 (major); **Note:** Assignment of Major/Minor substrate status based on clinically relevant drug interaction potential; **Induces** CYP3A4 (weak/moderate)

Avoid Concomitant Use

Avoid concomitant use of Perampanel with any of the following: Alcohol (Ethyl); Axitinib; Azelastine (Nasal); CYP3A4 Inducers (Strong); Paraldehyde; Simeprevir; St Johns Wort

Increased Effect/Toxicity

Perampanel may increase the levels/effects of: Alcohol (Ethyl); Azelastine (Nasal); Buprenorphine; CNS Depressants; Hydrocodone; Methotrimeprazine; Metyrosine; Mirtazapine; OXcarbazepine; Paraldehyde; Pramipexole; ROPINIRole; Rotigotine; Selective Serotonin Reuptake Inhibitors; Zolpidem

The levels/effects of Perampanel may be increased by: Brimonidine (Topical); Doxylamine; Droperidol; HydrOXYzine; Magnesium Sulfate; Methotrimeprazine; Sodium Oxybate; Tapentadol

Decreased Effect

Perampanel may decrease the levels/effects of: ARIPiprazole; Axitinib; Contraceptives (Progestins); Ibrutinib; Saxagliptin; Simeprevir

The levels/effects of Perampanel may be decreased by: Bosentan; CarBAMazepine; CYP3A4 Inducers (Strong); Dabrafenib; Deferasirox; Fosphenytoin; Ketorolac (Nasal); Ketorolac (Systemic); Mefloquine; Orlistat; OXcarbazepine; Phenytoin; St Johns Wort; Tocilizumab

Ethanol/Nutrition/Herb Interactions

Ethanol: Avoid ethanol (may increase CNS depression).

Herb/Nutraceutical: St John's wort may decrease perampanel levels. Avoid valerian, St John's wort, kava kava, gotu kola (may increase CNS depression).

Storage/Stability Store at 25°C (77°F); excursions permitted between 15°C to 30°C (59°F to 86°F).

Mechanism of Action The exact mechanism by which perampanel exerts antiseizure activity is not definitively known; it is a noncompetitive antagonist of the ionotropic alpha-amino-3-hydroxy-5-methyl-4-isoxazolepropionic acid (AMPA) glutamate receptor on postsynaptic neurons. Glutamate is a primary excitatory neurotransmitter in the central nervous center causing many neurological disorders from neuronal over excitation.

Pharmacodynamics/Kinetics

Absorption: Rapid and complete

Protein binding: 95% to 96%; primarily albumin and alpha$_1$-acid glycoprotein

Metabolism: Extensive via primary oxidation mediated by CYP3A4 and/or CYP3A5 and sequential glucuronidation

Half-life elimination: 105 hours

Time to peak: 0.5-2.5 hours

Excretion: Feces (48%); urine (22%)

Dosage Children ≥12 years, Adolescents, and Adults: Oral: Partial seizures (adjunct):

Patients **not** receiving enzyme-inducing AED regimens: Initial: 2 mg once daily at bedtime; may increase daily dose by 2 mg at weekly intervals based on response and tolerability. Recommended dose: 8-12 mg once daily at bedtime.

Patients receiving enzyme-inducing AED regimens (eg, phenytoin, carbamazepine, oxcarbazepine): Initial: 4 mg once daily at bedtime; may increase daily dose by 2 mg at weekly intervals based on response and tolerability. Recommended dose: 8-12 mg once daily at bedtime.

Elderly: Refer to adult dosing. Increase dose no more frequently than every 2 weeks.

Dosage adjustment in renal impairment:

Cl_{cr} ≥50 mL/minute: No dosage adjustment necessary.

Cl_{cr} 30-49 mL/minute: No dosage adjustment necessary; monitor closely and consider slower titration based on response and tolerability.

Cl_{cr} <30 mL/minute: Use not recommended (has not been studied).

Hemodialysis: Use not recommended (has not been studied).

Dosage adjustment in hepatic impairment:

Mild impairment (Child-Pugh class A): Initial: 2 mg once daily; may increase daily dose by 2 mg every 2 weeks based on response and tolerability. Maximum: 6 mg once daily

Moderate impairment (Child-Pugh class B): Initial: 2 mg once daily; may increase daily dose by 2 mg every 2 weeks based on response and tolerability. Maximum: 4 mg once daily

Severe impairment (Child-Pugh class C): Use not recommended (has not been studied).

Dietary Considerations May be taken without regard to meals.

Administration Administer at bedtime. May be administered without regard to meals.

Monitoring Parameters Seizure frequency/duration; suicidality (eg, suicidal thoughts, depression, behavioral changes); weight

Dosage Forms Excipient information presented when available (limited, particularly for generics); consult specific product labeling.

Tablet, Oral:

Fycompa: 2 mg, 4 mg, 6 mg, 8 mg

Controlled Substance C-III

- ◆ **Percocet** *see* Oxycodone and Acetaminophen *on page 1538*
- ◆ **Percocet-Demi (Can)** *see* Oxycodone and Acetaminophen *on page 1538*
- ◆ **Percodan®** *see* Oxycodone and Aspirin *on page 1539*
- ◆ **Percogesic® Extra Strength [OTC]** *see* Acetaminophen and Diphenhydramine *on page 32*
- ◆ **Perforomist** *see* Formoterol *on page 914*
- ◆ **Periactin** *see* Cyproheptadine *on page 515*
- ◆ **Peri-Colace® [OTC]** *see* Docusate and Senna *on page 645*

◆ Peridex *see* Chlorhexidine Gluconate *on page 408*

◆ Peridex® Oral Rinse (Can) *see* Chlorhexidine Gluconate *on page 408*

Perindopril Erbumine (per IN doe pril er BYOO meen)

Brand Names: U.S. Aceon

Brand Names: Canada Coversyl

Pharmacologic Category Angiotensin-Converting Enzyme (ACE) Inhibitor; Antihypertensive

Additional Appendix Information

Angiotensin Agents *on page 2280*

Use Treatment of hypertension; reduction of cardiovascular mortality or nonfatal myocardial infarction in patients with stable coronary artery disease

Canadian labeling: Additional use (unlabeled use in U.S.): Treatment of mild-moderate (NYHA I-III) heart failure

Unlabeled Use To delay the progression of nephropathy and reduce risks of cardiovascular events in hypertensive patients with type 1 or 2 diabetes mellitus

Pregnancy Risk Factor D

Pregnancy Considerations [U.S. Boxed Warning]: Drugs that act on the renin-angiotensin system can cause injury and death to the developing fetus. Discontinue as soon as possible once pregnancy is detected. Perindopril crosses the placenta; teratogenic effects may occur following maternal use during pregnancy. Drugs that act on the renin-angiotensin system are associated with oligohydramnios. Oligohydramnios, due to decreased fetal renal function, may lead to fetal lung hypoplasia and skeletal malformations. Their use in pregnancy is also associated with anuria, hypotension, renal failure, skull hypoplasia, and death in the fetus/neonate. Chronic maternal hypertension itself is also associated with adverse events in the fetus/infant. ACE inhibitors are not recommended during pregnancy to treat maternal hypertension or heart failure. Use of an ACE inhibitor should also be avoided in any woman of reproductive age. Women who are planning a pregnancy should be considered for other medication options if an ACE inhibitor is currently prescribed or the ACE inhibitor should be discontinued as soon as possible once pregnancy is detected. The exposed fetus should be monitored for fetal growth, amniotic fluid volume, and organ formation. Infants exposed to an ACE inhibitor *in utero* should be monitored for hyperkalemia, hypotension, and oliguria.

Breast-Feeding Considerations It is not known if perindopril is excreted in human breast milk. The U.S. labeling recommends that caution be exercised when administering perindopril to nursing women. The Canadian labeling contraindicates use in nursing women.

Contraindications

Hypersensitivity to perindopril, any other ACE inhibitor, or any component of the formulation; angioedema related to previous treatment with an ACE inhibitor; history of hereditary/idiopathic angioedema; concomitant use with aliskiren in patients with diabetes mellitus

Canadian labeling: Additional contraindications (not in U.S. labeling): Concomitant use with aliskiren in patients with moderate-to-severe renal impairment (GFR <60 mL/minute/1.73 m^2); women who are pregnant, planning to become pregnant, or nursing; hereditary problems of galactose intolerance, glucose-galactose malabsorption, or the Lapp lactase deficiency (formulation contains lactose)

Warnings/Precautions Anaphylactic reactions may occur rarely with ACE inhibitors. At any time during treatment (especially following first dose), angioedema may occur rarely with ACE inhibitors; it may involve the head and neck (potentially compromising airway) or the intestine (presenting with abdominal pain). African-Americans and patients with idiopathic or hereditary angioedema may be at an increased risk. Prolonged frequent monitoring may be required especially if tongue, glottis, or larynx are involved as they are associated with airway obstruction. Patients with a history of airway surgery may have a higher risk of airway obstruction. Aggressive early and appropriate management is critical. Use in patients with previous angioedema associated with ACE inhibitor therapy is contraindicated. Severe anaphylactoid reactions may be seen during hemodialysis (eg, CVVHD) with high-flux dialysis membranes (eg, AN69), and rarely, during low density lipoprotein apheresis with dextran sulfate cellulose. Rare cases of anaphylactoid reactions have been reported in patients undergoing sensitization treatment with hymenoptera (bee, wasp) venom while receiving ACE inhibitors.

Symptomatic hypotension with or without syncope can occur with ACE inhibitors (usually with the first several doses); effects are most often observed in volume-depleted patients; correct volume depletion prior to initiation; close monitoring of patient is required especially with initial dosing and dosing increases; blood pressure must be lowered at a rate appropriate for the patient's clinical condition. Initiation of therapy in patients with ischemic heart disease or cerebrovascular disease warrants close observation due to the potential consequences posed by falling blood pressure (eg, MI, stroke). Use with caution in hypertrophic cardiomyopathy with outflow tract obstruction, severe aortic stenosis, or before, during, or immediately after major surgery. **[U.S. Boxed Warning]: Drugs that act on the renin-angiotensin system can cause injury and death to the developing fetus. Discontinue as soon as possible once pregnancy is detected.**

Hyperkalemia may occur with ACE inhibitors; risk factors include renal dysfunction, diabetes mellitus, concomitant use of potassium-sparing diuretics, potassium supplements, and/or potassium-containing salts. Use cautiously, if at all, with these agents and monitor potassium closely. Cough may occur with ACE inhibitors. Other causes of cough should be considered (eg, pulmonary congestion in patients with heart failure) and excluded prior to discontinuation.

May be associated with deterioration of renal function and/or increases in serum creatinine, particularly in patients with low renal blood flow (eg, renal artery stenosis, heart failure) whose glomerular filtration rate (GFR) is dependent on efferent arteriolar vasoconstriction by angiotensin II; deterioration may result in oliguria, acute renal failure, and progressive azotemia. Small increases in serum creatinine may occur following initiation; consider discontinuation only in patients with progressive and/or significant deterioration in renal function. Use with caution in patients with unstented unilateral/bilateral renal artery stenosis. When unstented bilateral renal artery stenosis is present, use is generally avoided due to the elevated risk of deterioration in renal function unless possible benefits outweigh risks. Potentially significant drug-drug interactions may exist, requiring dose or frequency adjustment, additional monitoring, and/or selection of alternative therapy.

Rare toxicities associated with ACE inhibitors include cholestatic jaundice (which may progress to fulminant hepatic necrosis), agranulocytosis, neutropenia or leukopenia with myeloid hypoplasia. Patients with collagen vascular diseases (especially with concomitant renal impairment) or renal impairment alone may be at increased risk for hematologic toxicity; periodically monitor CBC with differential in these patients.

Adverse Reactions

>10%:

Central nervous system: Headache (24%)

Respiratory: Cough (incidence is higher in women, 3:1) (12%)

1% to 10%:

Cardiovascular: Edema (4%), chest pain (2%), ECG abnormal (2%), palpitation (1%)

Central nervous system: Dizziness (8%, less than placebo), sleep disorders (3%), depression (2%), fever (2%), nervousness (1%), somnolence (1%)

Dermatologic: Rash (2%)

Endocrine & metabolic: Hyperkalemia (1%, less than placebo), triglycerides increased (1%), menstrual disorder (1%)

Gastrointestinal: Diarrhea (4%), abdominal pain (3%), nausea (2%), vomiting (2%), dyspepsia (2%), flatulence (1%)

Genitourinary: Urinary tract infection (3%), sexual dysfunction (male 1%)

Hepatic: ALT increased (2%)

Neuromuscular & skeletal: Weakness (8%), back pain (6%), lower extremity pain (5%), upper extremity pain (3%), hypertonia (3%), paresthesia (2%), joint pain (1%), myalgia (1%), arthritis (1%), neck pain (1%)

Renal: Proteinuria (2%)

Respiratory: Upper respiratory tract infection (9%), sinusitis (5%), rhinitis (5%), pharyngitis (3%)

Otic: Tinnitus (2%), ear infection (1%)

Miscellaneous: Viral infection (3%), seasonal allergy (2%)

Note: Some reactions occurred at an incidence >1% but ≤ placebo.

<1% (Limited to important or life-threatening): Amnesia, anaphylaxis, angioedema, anxiety, AST increased, dyspnea, erythema, fluid retention, gout, leukopenia, migraine, MI, nephrolithiasis, neutropenia, orthostatic hypotension, pruritus, psychosocial disorder, pulmonary fibrosis, purpura, stroke, syncope, urinary retention, vertigo, visual hallucinations (Doane, 2013)

Additional adverse effects that have been reported with **ACE inhibitors** include agranulocytosis (especially in patients with renal impairment or collagen vascular disease), neutropenia, anemia, bullous pemphigoid, cardiac arrest, eosinophilic pneumonitis, exfoliative dermatitis, falls, hepatic failure, hyponatremia, jaundice, pancreatitis (acute), pancytopenia, pemphigus, psoriasis, thrombocytopenia; decreases in creatinine clearance in some elderly hypertensive patients or those with chronic renal failure, and worsening of renal function in patients with bilateral renal artery stenosis or hypovolemic patients (diuretic therapy). In addition, a syndrome which may include fever, myalgia, arthralgia, interstitial nephritis, vasculitis, rash, eosinophilia and positive ANA, and elevated ESR has been reported with ACE inhibitors.

Drug Interactions

Metabolism/Transport Effects None known.

Avoid Concomitant Use There are no known interactions where it is recommended to avoid concomitant use.

Increased Effect/Toxicity

Perindopril Erbumine may increase the levels/effects of: Allopurinol; Amifostine; Antihypertensives; AzaTHIOprine; CycloSPORINE (Systemic); Ferric Gluconate; Gold Sodium Thiomalate; Hypotensive Agents; Iron Dextran Complex; Lithium; Nonsteroidal Anti-Inflammatory Agents; Obinutuzumab; RiTUXimab; Sodium Phosphates

The levels/effects of Perindopril Erbumine may be increased by: Alfuzosin; Aliskiren; Angiotensin II Receptor Blockers; Brimonidine (Topical); Canagliflozin; Diazoxide; DPP-IV Inhibitors; Eplerenone; Everolimus; Heparin; Heparin (Low Molecular Weight); Herbs (Hypotensive Properties); Loop Diuretics; MAO Inhibitors; Pentoxifylline; Phosphodiesterase 5 Inhibitors; Potassium Salts; Potassium-Sparing Diuretics; Prostacyclin Analogues; Sirolimus; Temsirolimus; Thiazide Diuretics; TiZANidine; Tolvaptan; Trimethoprim

Decreased Effect

The levels/effects of Perindopril Erbumine may be decreased by: Antacids; Aprotinin; Herbs (Hypertensive Properties); Icatibant; Lanthanum; Methylphenidate; Nonsteroidal Anti-Inflammatory Agents; Salicylates; Yohimbine

Ethanol/Nutrition/Herb Interactions

Food: Perindopril active metabolite concentrations may be lowered if taken with food. Potassium supplements and/or potassium-containing salts may cause or worsen hyperkalemia. Management: Consult prescriber before consuming a potassium-rich diet, potassium supplements, or salt substitutes.

Herb/Nutraceutical: Some herbal medications may worsen hypertension (eg, licorice); others may increase the antihypertensive effect of perindopril (eg, shepherd's purse). Avoid bayberry, blue cohosh, cayenne, ephedra, ginger, ginseng (American), kola, licorice, and yohimbe. Avoid black cohosh, California poppy, coleus, golden seal, hawthorn, mistletoe, periwinkle, quinine, and shepherd's purse.

Storage/Stability Store at room temperature of 20°C to 25°C (68°F to 77°F). Protect from moisture.

Mechanism of Action Perindopril is a prodrug for perindoprilat, which acts as a competitive inhibitor of angiotensin-converting enzyme (ACE); prevents conversion of angiotensin I to angiotensin II, a potent vasoconstrictor; results in lower levels of angiotensin II which, in turn, causes an increase in plasma renin activity and a reduction in aldosterone secretion

Pharmacodynamics/Kinetics

Onset of action: Peak effect: 1-2 hours

Protein binding: Perindopril: 60%; Perindoprilat: 10% to 20%

Metabolism: Hepatically hydrolyzed to active metabolite, perindoprilat (~17% to 20% of a dose) and other inactive metabolites

Bioavailability: Perindopril: 75%; Perindoprilat ~25% (~16% with food)

Half-life elimination: Parent drug: 1.5-3 hours; Metabolite: Effective: 3-10 hours, Terminal: 30-120 hours

Time to peak: Chronic therapy: Perindopril: 1 hour; Perindoprilat: 3-7 hours (maximum perindoprilat serum levels are 2-3 times higher and T_{max} is shorter following chronic therapy); CHF: Perindoprilat: 6 hours

Excretion: Urine (75%, 4% to 12% as unchanged drug)

Dosage Oral:

Adults:

Heart failure (Canadian labeling; unlabeled use in U.S.): Initial: 2 mg once daily; if necessary, may titrate over 2-4 weeks to 4 mg once daily. The American College of Cardiology/ American Heart Association (ACC/AHA) 2009 Heart Failure Guidelines recommend an initial dose of 2 mg once daily with dose titration at 1- to 2-week intervals to a target dose of 8-16 mg once daily.

Hypertension: Initial: 4 mg/day but may be titrated to response; usual range: 4-8 mg/day (may be given in 2 divided doses); increase at 1- to 2-week intervals (maximum: 16 mg/day). **Note:** The Canadian labeling recommended maximum dose is 8 mg/day.

Concomitant therapy with diuretics: To reduce the risk of hypotension, discontinue diuretic, if possible, 2-3 days prior to initiating perindopril. If unable to stop diuretic, initiate perindopril at 2-4 mg/day (given in 1-2 divided doses) and monitor blood pressure closely for the first 2 weeks of therapy, and after any dose adjustment of perindopril or diuretic.

Stable coronary artery disease: Initial: 4 mg once daily for 2 weeks; then increase as tolerated to 8 mg once daily.

Elderly:
Hypertension: >65 years:
U.S. labeling: Initial: 4 mg/day; maintenance: 8 mg/day; experience with doses >8 mg/day is limited; may be given in 1-2 divided doses
Canadian labeling: Initial: 2 mg/day; if necessary may increase dose after 4 weeks to 4 mg/day; then to 8 mg/day (based on renal function); may be given in 1 or 2 divided doses.
ACCF/AHA Expert Consensus recommendations: Consider lower initial doses and titrating to response (Aronow, 2011)
Stable coronary artery disease: >70 years: Initial: 2 mg/day for 1 week; then increase as tolerated to 4 mg/day for 1 week; then increase as tolerated to 8 mg/day.

Dosage adjustment in renal impairment:
U.S. labeling:
Cl_{cr} >30 mL/minute: Initial: 2 mg/day; maintenance dosing not to exceed 8 mg/day.
Cl_{cr} <30 mL/minute: Safety and efficacy not established.
Hemodialysis: Perindopril and its metabolites are dialyzable.
Canadian labeling:
Cl_{cr} ≥60 mL/minute: Initial: 4 mg/day; maintenance dosing not to exceed 8 mg/day
Cl_{cr} 30-60 mL/minute: 2 mg/day
Cl_{cr} 15-30 mL/minute: 2 mg every other day
Hemodialysis (Cl_{cr} <15 mL/minute): 2 mg on dialysis days (given after dialysis)
Dosage adjustment in hepatic impairment: No dosage adjustment provided in manufacturer's labeling. However, perindoprilat bioavailability is increased with hepatic impairment.

Administration Administer prior to a meal.

Monitoring Parameters Blood pressure; serum creatinine and potassium; if patient has collagen vascular disease and/or renal impairment, periodically monitor CBC with differential

Dosage Forms Excipient information presented when available (limited, particularly for generics); consult specific product labeling.
Tablet, Oral:
Aceon: 4 mg, 8 mg [scored]
Generic: 2 mg, 4 mg, 8 mg

Dosage Forms: Canada Excipient information presented when available (limited, particularly for generics); consult specific product labeling.
Tablet, Oral:
Coversyl: 2 mg, 4 mg, 8 mg

- ◆ **Periogard** *see* Chlorhexidine Gluconate *on page 408*
- ◆ **PerioMed™** *see* Fluoride *on page 880*
- ◆ **Periostat® (Can)** *see* Doxycycline *on page 668*
- ◆ **Perjeta** *see* Pertuzumab *on page 1625*
- ◆ **Perlane** *see* Hyaluronate and Derivatives *on page 1000*
- ◆ **Perlane-L** *see* Hyaluronate and Derivatives *on page 1000*

Permethrin (per METH rin)

Brand Names: U.S. Acticin; Elimite
Brand Names: Canada Kwellada-P™; Nix®
Index Terms Elimite
Pharmacologic Category Antiparasitic Agent, Topical; Pediculocide; Scabicidal Agent
Use Single-application treatment of infestation with *Pediculus humanus capitis* (head louse) and its nits or *Sarcoptes scabiei* (scabies); indicated for prophylactic use during epidemics of lice
Pregnancy Risk Factor B
Dosage Topical:
Head lice: Children >2 months and Adults: After hair has been washed with shampoo, rinsed with water, and towel dried, apply a sufficient volume of topical liquid (lotion or cream rinse) to saturate the hair and scalp. Leave on hair for 10 minutes before rinsing off with water; remove remaining nits; may repeat in 1 week if lice or nits still present.
Scabies: Apply cream from head to toe; leave on for 8-14 hours before washing off with water; for infants, also apply on the hairline, neck, scalp, temple, and forehead; may reapply in 1 week if live mites appear
Additional Information Complete prescribing information should be consulted for additional detail.
Dosage Forms Excipient information presented when available (limited, particularly for generics); consult specific product labeling.
Cream, External:
Acticin: 5% (60 g)
Elimite: 5% (60 g) [contains formaldehyde solution]
Generic: 5% (60 g)
Lotion, External:
Generic: 1% (59 mL)

Perphenazine (per FEN a zeen)

Brand Names: Canada Apo-Perphenazine®
Index Terms Trilafon
Pharmacologic Category Antiemetic; Antipsychotic Agent, Typical, Phenothiazine
Additional Appendix Information
Antipsychotic Agents *on page 2290*
Beers Criteria – Potentially Inappropriate Medications for Geriatrics *on page 2368*
Use Treatment of schizophrenia; severe nausea and vomiting
Unlabeled Use Psychosis; psychosis/agitation related to Alzheimer's dementia (risks vs benefits)
Dosage Oral:
Adults:
Schizophrenia:
Nonhospitalized: Initial: 4-8 mg 3 times/day; reduce dose as soon as possible to minimum effective dosage (maximum: 24 mg/day)
Hospitalized: 8-16 mg 2-4 times/day (maximum: 64 mg/day)
Nausea/vomiting: 8-16 mg/day in divided doses; reduce dose as soon as possible to minimum effective dosage (maximum: 24 mg/day)
Elderly: No dosage adjustment provided in manufacturer's labeling; however, initiate dosing at the lower end of the dosing range. Refer to adult dosing.

Dosing adjustment in renal impairment: 0% to 5% removed by hemodialysis (HD); no dosage adjustment provided in manufacturer's labeling.
Dosing adjustment in hepatic impairment: No dosage adjustment provided in manufacturer's labeling.

Additional Information Complete prescribing information should be consulted for additional detail.
Dosage Forms Excipient information presented when available (limited, particularly for generics); consult specific product labeling.
Tablet, Oral:
Generic: 2 mg, 4 mg, 8 mg, 16 mg

- ◆ **Perphenazine and Amitriptyline Hydrochloride** *see* Amitriptyline and Perphenazine *on page 108*
- ◆ **Persantine** *see* Dipyridamole *on page 635*
- ◆ **Persantine® (Can)** *see* Dipyridamole *on page 635*

◆ **Pertussis, Acellular (Adsorbed)** *see* Diphtheria and Tetanus Toxoids, Acellular Pertussis, Poliovirus and *Haemophilus* b Conjugate Vaccine *on page 629*

Pertuzumab (per TU zoo mab)

Brand Names: U.S. Perjeta

Brand Names: Canada Perjeta

Index Terms 2C4 Antibody; MOAB 2C4; Monoclonal Antibody 2C4; Omnitarg; rhuMAb-2C4

Pharmacologic Category Antineoplastic Agent, Anti-HER2; Antineoplastic Agent, Monoclonal Antibody

Use

Breast cancer, metastatic: Treatment of human epidermal growth factor receptor 2 (HER2)-positive metastatic breast cancer (in combination with trastuzumab and docetaxel) in patients who have not received prior anti-HER2 therapy or chemotherapy to treat metastatic disease

Breast cancer, neoadjuvant treatment: Neoadjuvant treatment of locally advanced, inflammatory, or early stage HER2-positive, breast cancer (either greater than 2 cm in diameter or node positive) in combination with trastuzumab and docetaxel (as part of a complete treatment regimen for early breast cancer).

Pregnancy Risk Factor D

Pregnancy Considerations May cause fetal harm if administered during pregnancy. **[U.S. Boxed Warning]: Pertuzumab exposure during pregnancy may result in embryo-fetal mortality and birth defects. Oligohydramnios, delayed fetal kidney development, and embryo-fetal death have been observed in animal reproduction studies. Advise patients of the risks and the need for effective contraception.** Verify pregnancy status prior to treatment initiation. Effective contraception should be used during therapy and for 6 months after treatment. Advise patients to immediately report to healthcare provider if pregnancy is suspected during treatment. Effects during pregnancy are likely to occur in all 3 trimesters. If administered during pregnancy, monitor for oligohydramnios (if oligohydramnios occurs, fetal testing is indicated). Report pregnancies exposed to pertuzumab to the Genentech Adverse Event Line (1-888-835-2555). Women exposed to pertuzumab during pregnancy are encouraged to enroll in MotHER (the Pregnancy Registry; 1-800-690-6720).

Breast-Feeding Considerations It is not known if pertuzumab is excreted in human milk. Because many immunoglobulins are excreted in human milk, and the potential for serious adverse reactions in the nursing infant exists, the decision to discontinue breast-feeding or to discontinue pertuzumab should take into account the benefits of treatment to the mother. The extended half-life should be considered for decisions regarding breast-feeding after treatment is completed.

Contraindications Hypersensitivity to pertuzumab or any component of the formulation

Warnings/Precautions Hazardous agent - use appropriate precautions for handling and disposal (meets NIOSH, 2012 criteria). **[U.S. Boxed Warning]: May result in cardiac failure (clinical and subclinical). Assess left ventricular ejection fraction (LVEF) in all patients at baseline and during treatment. Discontinue for confirmed clinically significant decline in left ventricular function.** Decreases in LVEF are associated with HER-2 inhibitors, including pertuzumab. Patients who received prior anthracycline therapy or chest irradiation may be at an increased risk for cardiotoxicity. In studies of pertuzumab (versus placebo) in combination with trastuzumab and docetaxel for the treatment of metastatic breast cancer, the rate of cardiotoxicity (LVEF decline or symptomatic LV systolic dysfunction) was not increased in the pertuzumab group when compared to placebo. In the neoadjuvant setting, the incidence of LV dysfunction was higher in patients treated with pertuzumab. In a study of pertuzumab, trastuzumab and docetaxel, compared with trastuzumab and docetaxel, the incidence of LVEF decline (of >10% decrease from baseline or to <50%) was 8.4% and 1.9%., respectively; LVEF recovered to ≥50% in all patients. In another neoadjuvant study, LVEF declines (of >10% decrease from baseline or to <50%) were noted in 6.9% to 16% of patients receiving various combinations and sequences of pertuzumab plus trastuzumab with FEC (fluorouracil, epirubicin, and cyclophosphamide), docetaxel, and/or carboplatin; LVEF recovered to ≥50% in most patients. Of note, patients with pretreatment LVEF ≤50%, CHF, LVEF decreases to <50% during prior trastuzumab treatment, or conditions which could impair LV function (eg, uncontrolled hypertension, recent MI, serious arrhythmia requiring treatment, or cumulative lifetime anthracycline exposure >360 mg/m^2 doxorubicin or its equivalent) were excluded from studies. Assess LVEF at baseline, every 3 months during treatment (metastatic patients) or every 6 weeks during treatment (neoadjuvant setting), and every 6 months after therapy discontinuation up to 24 months after the last dose of pertuzumab and/or trastuzumab. Withhold pertuzumab and trastuzumab if LVEF <45% **or** 45% to 49% with a ≥10% absolute decline from baseline; repeat LVEF assessment in ~3 weeks; discontinue if LVEF has not improved or has declined further (unless potential benefits outweigh risks).

Infusion reactions (either during or on the day of infusion) have been associated with pertuzumab; commonly described as fever, chills, fatigue, headache, weakness, myalgia, hypersensitivity, abnormal taste or vomiting. The incidence of hypersensitivity/anaphylaxis was slightly higher in the group receiving pertuzumab (compared to placebo) in combination with trastuzumab and docetaxel. Monitor for 1 hour after the first infusion and for 30 minutes after subsequent infusions. For significant infusion reactions, interrupt or slow infusion rate; for severe infusion reactions, consider permanently discontinuing. Medications and equipment for the treatment of hypersensitivity should be available for immediate use during infusion. May cause fetal harm is administered during pregnancy. **[U.S. Boxed Warning]: Pertuzumab exposure during pregnancy may result in embryo-fetal mortality and birth defects. Oligohydramnios, delayed fetal kidney development, and embryo-fetal death have been observed in animal reproduction studies. Advise patients of the risks and the need for effective contraception.** Verify pregnancy status prior to treatment initiation. Effective contraception should be used by all patients receiving pertuzumab during therapy and for 6 months after treatment. Effects during pregnancy are likely to occur in any trimester.

Establish HER2 status prior to treatment; has only been studied in patients with evidence of HER2 overexpression, either as 3+ IHC (Dako Herceptest™) or FISH amplification ratio ≥2 (Dako *HER*2 FISH pharmDx™ test). Safety of combination therapy with doxorubicin-containing regimens has not been established. For early breast cancer, the safety of treatment beyond 6 cycles has not been determined.

Adverse Reactions Note: Reactions reported in combination therapy with trastuzumab and docetaxel unless otherwise noted.

>10%:

Central nervous system: Fatigue (38%), headache (21%), fever (19%; grades 3/4: 1%), dizziness (13%)

Dermatologic: Rash (34%; grades 3/4: <1%), pruritus (14%), dry skin (11%)

Gastrointestinal: Diarrhea (67%; grades 3/4: 8%), appetite decreased (29%), mucosal inflammation (28%), nausea (monotherapy 24%), stomatitis (19%), abnormal taste (18%), vomiting (monotherapy 15%), abdominal pain (monotherapy 12%)
Hematologic: Neutropenia (53%; grades 3/4: 49%), anemia (23%; grades 3/4: 3%), neutropenic fever (14%; grades 3/4: 13%)
Respiratory: Upper respiratory tract infection (17%; grades 3/4: <1%)
Miscellaneous: Infusion reactions (13%; grades 3/4: <1%), hypersensitivity reactions (10% to 11%; grades 3/4: 2%)

1% to 10%:
Dermatologic: Paronychia (7%)
Gastrointestinal: Anorexia (monotherapy 5%)

<1% and/or case reports with combination therapy (Limited to important or life-threatening): Alopecia, arthralgia, dyspnea, heart failure, insomnia, left ventricular ejection fraction decreased, myalgia, peripheral edema, leukopenia, peripheral neuropathy, pleural effusion, sepsis

Drug Interactions

Metabolism/Transport Effects None known.

Avoid Concomitant Use

Avoid concomitant use of Pertuzumab with any of the following: Belimumab

Increased Effect/Toxicity

Pertuzumab may increase the levels/effects of: Belimumab

The levels/effects of Pertuzumab may be increased by: Abciximab

Decreased Effect There are no known significant interactions involving a decrease in effect.

Preparation for Administration Hazardous agent; use appropriate precautions for handling and disposal (meets NIOSH, 2012 criteria). Dilute in 250 mL NS only (do not use dextrose 5% solutions) in PVC or non-PVC (polyolefin) bags. Gently invert to mix; do not shake. Do not mix with other medications.

Storage/Stability Store intact vials at 2°C to 8°C (36°F to 46°F) until time of use. Protect from light. Do not freeze. Do not shake. Solutions diluted for infusion should be used immediately; if not used immediately, maybe stored at 2°C to 8°C (36°F to 46°F) for up to 24 hours.

Mechanism of Action Pertuzumab is a recombinant humanized monoclonal antibody which targets the extracellular human epidermal growth factor receptor 2 protein (HER2) dimerization domain. Inhibits HER2 dimerization and blocks HER downstream signaling halting cell growth and initiating apoptosis. Pertuzumab binds to a different HER2 epitope than trastuzumab so that when pertuzumab is combined with trastuzumab, a more complete inhibition of HER2 signaling occurs (Baselga, 2012).

Pharmacodynamics/Kinetics

Distribution: V_d: 5.12 L (Gianni, 2010)
Half-life elimination: Terminal: 18 days

Dosage Note: Pertuzumab and trastuzumab may be administered in any order. However, for docetaxel-containing regimens, docetaxel should be given after pertuzumab and trastuzumab. Before subsequent infusions of trastuzumab or docetaxel, observe patients for 30-60 minutes after each pertuzumab infusion.

Breast cancer, metastatic HER2+: Adults: I.V.: 840 mg over 60 minutes followed by a maintenance dose of 420 mg over 30-60 minutes every 3 weeks until disease progression or unacceptable toxicity (in combination with trastuzumab and docetaxel) (Baselga, 2012).

Breast cancer, neoadjuvant treatment HER2+: Adults: I.V.: 840 mg over 60 minutes followed by a maintenance dose of 420 mg over 30-60 minutes every 3 weeks for 3-6 cycles; may be administered as one of the regimens below. Post-operatively, continue trastuzumab to complete 1 year of treatment.

Four preoperative cycles of pertuzumab, trastuzumab, and docetaxel, followed by 3 postoperative cycles of fluorouracil, epirubicin, and cyclophosphamide (FEC) (Gianni, 2012) **or**

Three preoperative cycles of FEC (alone) followed by 3 preoperative cycles of pertuzumab, trastuzumab, and docetaxel (Schneeweiss, 2013) **or**

Six preoperative cycles of pertuzumab, trastuzumab, docetaxel, and carboplatin (Schneeweiss, 2013)

Missed doses or delays: If <6 weeks has elapsed, administer the 420 mg maintenance dose; do not wait until the next planned dose. If ≥6 weeks has elapsed, readminister the 840 mg initial dose (over 60 minutes), and then follow with a maintenance dose of 420 mg (over 30-60 minutes) every 3 weeks.

Dosage adjustment for toxicity: Note: Dose reductions are not recommended for pertuzumab; if trastuzumab is withheld, pertuzumab should also be withheld; if trastuzumab is discontinued, pertuzumab should be discontinued; pertuzumab and trastuzumab may be continued if docetaxel is discontinued.

Infusion-related reaction: Slow or interrupt the infusion
Serious hypersensitivity: Discontinue immediately
Cardiotoxicity: Left ventricular ejection fraction (LVEF) declines to <45% **or** LVEF between 45% to 49% with ≥10% absolute decrease below pretreatment values: Withhold treatment (pertuzumab and trastuzumab) for at least 3 weeks; may resume if LVEF returns to >49% **or** to 45% to 49% with <10% absolute decrease below pretreatment values. If after a repeat assessment within ~3 weeks, LVEF has not improved (or has declined further), discontinue pertuzumab and trastuzumab (unless the benefit of treatment outweighs risks).

Dosage adjustment in renal impairment:

Cl_{cr} ≥30 mL/minute: No dosage adjustment necessary.
Cl_{cr} <30 mL/minute: No dosage adjustment provided in the manufacturer's labeling (has not been studied).

Dosage adjustment in hepatic impairment: No dosage adjustment provided in the manufacturer's labeling (has not been studied).

Administration For I.V. infusion only, as a short infusion; infuse initial dose (840 mg) over 60 minutes; infuse maintenance dose (420 mg) over 30-60 minutes. Do not administer I.V. push or as a rapid bolus. Do not mix with other medications. When administered with trastuzumab and docetaxel, pertuzumab and trastuzumab may be administered in any order. However, for docetaxel-containing regimens, docetaxel should be given after pertuzumab and trastuzumab. Before subsequent infusions of trastuzumab or docetaxel, observe patients for 30-60 minutes after each pertuzumab infusion.

Hazardous agent; use appropriate precautions for handling and disposal (meets NIOSH, 2012 criteria).

Monitoring Parameters HER2 expression (either as 3+ IHC [Dako Herceptest™] or FISH amplification ratio ≥2 [Dako *HER*2 FISH pharmDx™ test]); pregnancy test; assess LVEF at baseline, every 3 months during treatment (more frequently for declines) in metastatic treatment and every 6 weeks for neoadjuvant treatment, and every 6 months following discontinuation for up to 24 months from the last dose of pertuzumab and/or trastuzumab); monitor for infusion reaction and hypersensitivity

Dosage Forms Excipient information presented when available (limited, particularly for generics); consult specific product labeling.

Solution, Intravenous [preservative free]:
Perjeta: 420 mg/14 mL (14 mL) [contains mouse protein (murine) (hamster)]

◆ **Pertzye** *see* Pancrelipase *on page* 1558

◆ **Pethidine Hydrochloride** *see* Meperidine *on page 1297*
◆ **Pexeva** *see* PARoxetine *on page 1575*
◆ **PF-02341066** *see* Crizotinib *on page 497*
◆ **PFA** *see* Foscarnet *on page 920*
◆ **Pfizerpen-AS® (Can)** *see* Penicillin G Procaine *on page 1610*
◆ **Pfizerpen-G** *see* Penicillin G (Parenteral/Aqueous) *on page 1608*
◆ **PGE_1** *see* Alprostadil *on page 83*
◆ **PGE_2** *see* Dinoprostone *on page 619*
◆ **PGI_2** *see* Epoprostenol *on page 727*
◆ **PGX** *see* Epoprostenol *on page 727*
◆ **Pharbedryl [OTC]** *see* DiphenhydrAMINE (Systemic) *on page 622*
◆ **Pharmorubicin® (Can)** *see* Epirubicin *on page 718*
◆ **Phenadoz** *see* Promethazine *on page 1728*
◆ **Phenagil [OTC]** *see* Chlorpheniramine and Phenylephrine *on page 412*

Phenazopyridine (fen az oh PEER i deen)

Brand Names: U.S. Azo-Gesic [OTC]; Baridium [OTC]; Pyridium; Urinary Pain Relief [OTC]

Index Terms Phenazopyridine Hydrochloride; Phenylazo Diamino Pyridine Hydrochloride

Pharmacologic Category Analgesic, Urinary

Use Symptomatic relief of urinary burning, itching, frequency, and urgency in association with urinary tract infection or following urologic procedures

Pregnancy Risk Factor B

Dosage Oral:

Children: 12 mg/kg/day in 3 divided doses administered after meals for 2 days

Adults: 100-200 mg 3 times/day after meals for 2 days when used concomitantly with an antibacterial agent

Dosage adjustment in renal impairment: Use is contraindicated in renal impairment.

Dosage adjustment in hepatic impairment: No dosage adjustment provided in manufacturer's labeling.

Additional Information Complete prescribing information should be consulted for additional detail.

Dosage Forms Excipient information presented when available (limited, particularly for generics); consult specific product labeling.

Tablet, Oral, as hydrochloride:
- Azo-Gesic: 95 mg
- Baridium: 97.2 mg
- Pyridium: 100 mg, 200 mg
- Urinary Pain Relief: 95 mg
- Generic: 95 mg, 100 mg, 200 mg

◆ **Phenazopyridine Hydrochloride** *see* Phenazopyridine *on page 1627*

Phenelzine (FEN el zeen)

Brand Names: U.S. Nardil

Brand Names: Canada Nardil®

Index Terms Phenelzine Sulfate

Pharmacologic Category Antidepressant, Monoamine Oxidase Inhibitor

Additional Appendix Information

Antidepressant Agents *on page 2284*

Tyramine Content of Foods *on page 2394*

Use Symptomatic treatment of atypical, nonendogenous, or neurotic depression

Pregnancy Risk Factor C

Pregnancy Considerations Safe use during pregnancy has not been established; use only if benefits outweigh the risks.

Breast-Feeding Considerations Safe use during breast-feeding has not been established; use only if benefits outweigh the risks.

Medication Guide Available Yes

Contraindications Hypersensitivity to phenelzine or any component of the formulation; congestive heart failure; pheochromocytoma; abnormal liver function tests or history of hepatic disease; renal disease or severe renal disease/impairment

Concurrent use of sympathomimetics (including amphetamines, cocaine, dopamine, epinephrine, methylphenidate, norepinephrine, or phenylephrine) and related compounds (methyldopa, levodopa, phenylalanine, tryptophan, or tyrosine), ophthalmic $alpha_2$-agonists (apraclonidine, brimonidine), CNS depressants, cyclobenzaprine, dextromethorphan, ethanol, meperidine, bupropion, or buspirone

At least 2 weeks should elapse between the discontinuation of serotoninergic agents (including SNRIs, SSRIs, and tricyclics) and other MAO inhibitors and the initiation of phenelzine. At least 5 weeks should elapse between the discontinuation of fluoxetine and the initiation of phenelzine. In all cases, a sufficient amount of time must be allowed for the clearance of the serotoninergic agent and any active metabolites prior to the initiation of phenelzine.

At least 2 weeks should elapse between the discontinuation of phenelzine and the initiation of the following agents: Serotoninergic agents (including SNRIs, SSRIs, fluoxetine, and tricyclics), bupropion, buspirone, and other antidepressants.

General anesthesia, spinal anesthesia (hypotension may be exaggerated). Use caution with local anesthetics containing sympathomimetic agents. Phenelzine should be discontinued ≥10 days prior to elective surgery.

Foods high in tyramine or dopamine content; foods and/or supplements containing tyrosine, phenylalanine, tryptophan, or caffeine

Warnings/Precautions [U.S. Boxed Warning]: Antidepressants increase the risk of suicidal thinking and behavior in children, adolescents, and young adults (18-24 years of age) with major depressive disorder (MDD) and other psychiatric disorders; consider risk prior to prescribing. Short-term studies did not show an increased risk in patients >24 years of age and showed a decreased risk in patients ≥65 years. Closely monitor for clinical worsening, suicidality, or unusual changes in behavior; the patient's family or caregiver should be instructed to closely observe the patient and communicate condition with healthcare provider. Such observation would generally include at least weekly face-to-face contact with patients or their family members or caregivers during the first 4 weeks of treatment, then every other week visits for the next 4 weeks, then at 12 weeks, and as clinically indicated beyond 12 weeks. Additional contact by telephone may be appropriate between face-to-face visits. Adults treated with antidepressants should be observed similarly for clinical worsening and suicidality, especially during the initial few months of a course of drug therapy, or at times of dose changes, either increases or decreases. A medication guide should be dispensed with each prescription. Phenelzine is not generally considered a first-line agent for the treatment of depression; phenelzine is typically used in patients who have failed to respond to other treatments. **Phenelzine is not FDA approved for the treatment of depression in children ≤16 years of age.**

The possibility of a suicide attempt is inherent in major depression and may persist until remission occurs. Monitor for worsening of depression or suicidality, especially during initiation of therapy (generally first 1-2 months) or with dose increases or decreases. Worsening depression and severe abrupt suicidality that are not part of the presenting symptoms may require discontinuation or modification of drug therapy. Use caution in high-risk patients during initiation of therapy. Prescriptions should be written for the smallest quantity consistent with good patient care. The patient's family or caregiver should be alerted to monitor patients for the emergence of suicidality and associated behaviors such as anxiety, agitation, panic attacks, insomnia, irritability, hostility, impulsivity, akathisia, hypomania, and mania; patients should be instructed to notify their healthcare provider if any of these symptoms or worsening depression occur.

May worsen psychosis in some patients or precipitate a shift to mania or hypomania in patients with bipolar disorder. Monotherapy in patients with bipolar disorder should be avoided. Patients presenting with depressive symptoms should be screened for bipolar disorder. Phenelzine is not FDA approved for the treatment of bipolar depression.

Sensitization to the effects of insulin may occur; monitor blood glucose closely in patients with diabetes. Use with caution in patients who have glaucoma, or hyperthyroidism. Cases of hypertensive crisis (sometimes fatal) have occurred; symptoms include: severe headache, nausea/vomiting, neck stiffness/soreness, photophobia, and sweating. Monitor blood pressure closely in all patients. Hypertensive crisis may occur with tyramine-, tryptophan-, or dopamine-containing foods. Phentolamine is recommended for the treatment of hypertensive crisis. Do not use with other MAO inhibitors or antidepressants. Do not use within 5 weeks of fluoxetine discontinuation or 2 weeks of other antidepressant discontinuation. Avoid products containing sympathomimetic stimulants or dextromethorphan. Concurrent use with antihypertensive agents may lead to exaggeration of hypotensive effects. May cause orthostatic hypotension; use with caution in patients with hypotension or patients who would not tolerate transient hypotensive episodes (cardiovascular or cerebrovascular disease); effects may be additive with other agents which cause orthostasis. Use with caution in patients at risk of seizures, or in patients receiving other drugs which may lower seizure threshold. Discontinue at least 48 hours prior to myelography. May increase the risks associated with electroconvulsive therapy. Pyridoxine deficiency has occurred; symptoms include numbness and edema of hands; may respond to supplementation.

Abrupt discontinuation or interruption of antidepressant therapy has been associated with a discontinuation syndrome. Symptoms arising may vary with antidepressant however commonly include nausea, vomiting, diarrhea, headaches, lightheadedness, dizziness, diminished appetite, sweating, chills, tremors, paresthesias, fatigue, somnolence, and sleep disturbances (eg, vivid dreams, insomnia). Greater risks for developing a discontinuation syndrome have been associated with antidepressants with shorter half-lives, longer durations of treatment, and abrupt discontinuation. More severe symptoms have also been associated with MAO inhibitors. For antidepressants of short or intermediate half-lives, symptoms may emerge within 2-5 days after treatment discontinuation and last 7-14 days (APA, 2010; Fava, 2006; Haddad, 2001; Shelton, 2001; Warner, 2006).

Adverse Reactions Frequency not defined.

Cardiovascular: Edema, orthostatic hypotension

Central nervous system: Anxiety (acute), ataxia, coma, delirium, dizziness, drowsiness, euphoria, fatigue, fever, headache, hyper-reflexia, hypersomnia, insomnia, mania, schizophrenia, seizure, twitching

Dermatologic: Pruritus, rash

Endocrine & metabolic: Decreased sexual ability (anorgasmia, ejaculatory disturbances, impotence), hypermetabolic syndrome, hypernatremia

Gastrointestinal: Constipation, weight gain, xerostomia

Genitourinary: Urinary retention

Hematologic: Leukopenia

Hepatic: Jaundice, necrotizing hepatocellular necrosis (rare), transaminases increased

Neuromuscular & skeletal: Myoclonia, paresthesia, tremor, weakness

Ocular: Blurred vision, glaucoma, nystagmus

Respiratory: Edema (glottis)

Miscellaneous: Diaphoresis, lupus-like syndrome, transient cardiac or respiratory depression (following ECT), withdrawal syndrome (nausea, vomiting, malaise)

Drug Interactions

Metabolism/Transport Effects Inhibits Monoamine Oxidase

Avoid Concomitant Use

Avoid concomitant use of Phenelzine with any of the following: Aclidinium; Alpha-/Beta-Agonists (Indirect-Acting); Alpha1-Agonists; Amphetamines; Anilidopiperidine Opioids; Antidepressants (Serotonin Reuptake Inhibitor/Antagonist); Apraclonidine; AtoMOXetine; Bezafibrate; Buprenorphine; BuPROPion; BusPIRone; CarBAMazepine; Cyclobenzaprine; Dexmethylphenidate; Dextromethorphan; Diethylpropion; Hydrocodone; HYDROmorphone; Ipratropium (Oral Inhalation); Isometheptene; Levonordefrin; Linezolid; Maprotiline; Meperidine; Methyldopa; Methylene Blue; Methylphenidate; Mirtazapine; Morphine (Liposomal); Morphine (Systemic); Oxymorphone; Pizotifen; Selective Serotonin Reuptake Inhibitors; Serotonin 5-HT1D Receptor Agonists; Serotonin/Norepinephrine Reuptake Inhibitors; Tapentadol; Tetrabenazine; Tetrahydrozoline (Nasal); Tiotropium; Tricyclic Antidepressants; Tryptophan; Umeclidinium

Increased Effect/Toxicity

Phenelzine may increase the levels/effects of: Alpha-/Beta-Agonists (Indirect-Acting); Alpha1-Agonists; Amphetamines; Analgesics (Opioid); Anticholinergics; Antidepressants (Serotonin Reuptake Inhibitor/Antagonist); Antihypertensives; Antipsychotics; Apraclonidine; AtoMOXetine; Beta2-Agonists; Betahistine; Bezafibrate; Brimonidine (Ophthalmic); Brimonidine (Topical); BuPROPion; Dexmethylphenidate; Dextromethorphan; Diethylpropion; Domperidone; Doxapram; Doxylamine; EPINEPHrine (Nasal); Epinephrine (Racemic); EPINEPHrine (Systemic, Oral Inhalation); Hydrocodone; HYDROmorphone; Hypoglycemic Agents; Isometheptene; Levonordefrin; Linezolid; Lithium; Meperidine; Methadone; Methyldopa; Methylene Blue; Methylphenidate; Metoclopramide; Mirtazapine; Morphine (Liposomal); Morphine (Systemic); Norepinephrine; Orthostatic Hypotension Producing Agents; OxyCODONE; Pizotifen; Reserpine; Selective Serotonin Reuptake Inhibitors; Serotonin 5-HT1D Receptor Agonists; Serotonin Modulators; Serotonin/Norepinephrine Reuptake Inhibitors; Succinylcholine; Tetrahydrozoline (Nasal); Tiotropium; Tricyclic Antidepressants

The levels/effects of Phenelzine may be increased by: Aclidinium; Altretamine; Anilidopiperidine Opioids; Antipsychotics; Buprenorphine; BusPIRone; CarBAMazepine; COMT Inhibitors; Cyclobenzaprine; Ipratropium (Oral Inhalation); Levodopa; MAO Inhibitors; Maprotiline; Oxymorphone; Pramlintide; Tapentadol; Tetrabenazine; TraMADol; Tryptophan; Umeclidinium

Decreased Effect

Phenelzine may decrease the levels/effects of: Acetylcholinesterase Inhibitors (Central); Domperidone

The levels/effects of Phenelzine may be decreased by: Acetylcholinesterase Inhibitors (Central); Domperidone

Ethanol/Nutrition/Herb Interactions

Ethanol: Ethanol may increase CNS depression. Beverages containing tyramine (eg, hearty red wine and beer) may increase toxic effects. Management: Avoid ethanol and beverages containing tyramine.

Food: Concurrent ingestion of foods rich in tyramine, dopamine, tyrosine, phenylalanine, tryptophan, or caffeine may cause sudden and severe high blood pressure (hypertensive crisis or serotonin syndrome). Management: Avoid tyramine-containing foods (aged or matured cheese, air-dried or cured meats including sausages and salamis; fava or broad bean pods, tap/draft beers, Marmite concentrate, sauerkraut, soy sauce, and other soybean condiments). Food's freshness is also an important concern; improperly stored or spoiled food can create an environment in which tyramine concentrations may increase. Avoid foods containing dopamine, tyrosine, phenylalanine, tryptophan, or caffeine.

Herb/Nutraceutical: Kava kava, valerian, St John's wort, and SAMe may increase risk of serotonin syndrome and/or excessive sedation. Supplements containing caffeine, tyrosine, tryptophan, or phenylalanine may increase the risk of severe side effects like hypertensive reactions or serotonin syndrome. Management: Avoid kava kava, valerian, St John's wort, SAMe, and supplements containing caffeine, tyrosine, tryptophan, or phenylalanine.

Storage/Stability Store at 20°C to 25°C (68°F to 77°F). Protect from heat and light.

Mechanism of Action Thought to act by increasing endogenous concentrations of norepinephrine, dopamine, and serotonin through inhibition of the enzyme (monoamine oxidase) responsible for the breakdown of these neurotransmitters

Pharmacodynamics/Kinetics

Onset of action: Therapeutic: 2-4 weeks; geriatric patients receiving an average of 55 mg/day developed a mean platelet MAO activity inhibition of about 85%.

Duration: May continue to have a therapeutic effect and interactions 2 weeks after discontinuing therapy

Absorption: Well absorbed

Metabolism: Oxidized via monoamine oxidase (primary pathway) and acetylation (minor pathway)

Half-life elimination: 12 hours

Excretion: Urine (73% as metabolites)

Dosage Oral:

Adults: Depression: Initial: 15 mg 3 times/day

Early phase: Increase rapidly, based on patient tolerance, to 60-90 mg/day (may take 4 weeks of 60 mg/day therapy before clinical response)

Maintenance: After maximum benefit is obtained, slowly reduce dose over several weeks; dose may be as low as 15 mg/day to 15 mg every other day

Elderly: Depression: Select dose with caution; generally initiating at the lower end of the dosing range; some clinicians recommend an initial dose of 7.5 mg, with dose increases of 7.5 mg/day every 4-8 days as tolerated to a usual therapeutic dose of 22.5-60 mg/day in older adults (Alexopoulos, 2004).

Discontinuation of therapy: Upon discontinuation of antidepressant therapy, gradually taper the dose to minimize the incidence of withdrawal symptoms and allow for the detection of re-emerging symptoms. Evidence supporting ideal taper rates is limited. APA and NICE guidelines suggest tapering therapy over at least several weeks with consideration to the half-life of the antidepressant; antidepressants with a shorter half-life and MAO inhibitors may need to be tapered more conservatively. In addition for long-term treated patients, WFSBP guidelines recommend tapering over 4-6 months. If intolerable withdrawal symptoms occur following a dose reduction, consider resuming the previously prescribed dose and/or decrease dose at a more gradual rate (APA, 2010; Bauer, 2002; Haddad, 2001; NCCMH, 2010; Schatzberg, 2006; Shelton, 2001; Warner, 2006).

MAO inhibitor recommendations:

Switching to or from an MAO inhibitor intended to treat psychiatric disorders:

Allow 14 days to elapse between discontinuing an alternative antidepressant without long half-life metabolites (eg, TCAs, paroxetine, fluvoxamine, venlafaxine) or MAO inhibitor intended to treat psychiatric disorders and initiation of phenelzine.

Allow 5 weeks to elapse between discontinuing fluoxetine (with long half-life metabolites) intended to treat psychiatric disorders and initiation of phenelzine.

Allow 14 days to elapse between discontinuing phenelzine and initiation of an alternative antidepressant or MAO inhibitor intended to treat psychiatric disorders.

Use with other MAO inhibitors (such as linezolid or I.V. methylene blue):

Do not initiate phenelzine in patients receiving linezolid or I.V. methylene blue; consider other interventions for psychiatric condition.

If urgent treatment with linezolid or I.V. methylene blue is required in a patient already receiving phenelzine and potential benefits outweigh potential risks, discontinue phenelzine promptly and administer linezolid or I.V. methylene blue. Monitor for serotonin syndrome for 2 weeks or until 24 hours after the last dose of linezolid or I.V. methylene blue, whichever comes first. May resume phenelzine 24 hours after the last dose of linezolid or I.V. methylene blue.

Dosage adjustment in renal impairment:

Mild to moderate impairment: No dosage adjustment provided in manufacturer's labeling.

Severe impairment: Use is contraindicated.

Dosage adjustment in hepatic impairment: Use is contraindicated.

Dietary Considerations Avoid tyramine-containing foods/beverages. Some examples include aged or matured cheese, air-dried or cured meats (including sausages and salamis), fava or broad bean pods, tap/draft beers, Marmite concentrate, sauerkraut, soy sauce and other soybean condiments. Food's freshness is also an important concern; improperly stored or spoiled food can create an environment where tyramine concentrations may increase.

Monitoring Parameters Blood pressure, heart rate; diet, weight; mood (if depressive symptoms), suicide ideation (especially during the initial months of therapy or when doses are increased or decreased)

Dosage Forms Excipient information presented when available (limited, particularly for generics); consult specific product labeling.

Tablet, Oral:

Nardil: 15 mg

Generic: 15 mg

◆ **Phenelzine Sulfate** *see* Phenelzine *on page 1627*

◆ **Phenergan** *see* Promethazine *on page 1728*

◆ **Pheniramine and Naphazoline** *see* Naphazoline and Pheniramine *on page 1425*

PHENobarbital (fee noe BAR bi tal)

Brand Names: U.S. Luminal

Brand Names: Canada PMS-Phenobarbital

Index Terms Luminal Sodium; Phenobarbital Sodium; Phenobarbitone; Phenylethylmalonylurea

Pharmacologic Category Anticonvulsant, Barbiturate; Barbiturate

Additional Appendix Information

Beers Criteria – Potentially Inappropriate Medications for Geriatrics *on page 2368*

Status Epilepticus *on page 2375*

Use Management of generalized tonic-clonic (grand mal), status epilepticus, and partial seizures; sedative/hypnotic

Note: Use to treat insomnia is not recommended (Schutte-Rodin, 2008)

Unlabeled Use Prevention and treatment of neonatal hyperbilirubinemia and lowering of bilirubin in chronic cholestasis; neonatal seizures

Pregnancy Risk Factor B/D (manufacturer dependent)

Pregnancy Considerations Barbiturates can be detected in the placenta, fetal liver, and fetal brain. Fetal and maternal blood concentrations may be similar following parenteral administration. An increased incidence of fetal abnormalities may occur following maternal use. The use of folic acid throughout pregnancy and vitamin K during the last month of pregnancy is recommended; epilepsy itself, number of medications, genetic factors, or a combination of these probably influence the teratogenicity of anticonvulsant therapy. When used during the third trimester of pregnancy, withdrawal symptoms may occur in the neonate, including seizures and hyperirritability; symptoms of withdrawal may be delayed in the neonate up to 14 days after birth. Use during labor does not impair uterine activity; however, respiratory depression may occur in the newborn; resuscitation equipment should be available, especially for premature infants.

Breast-Feeding Considerations Phenobarbital is excreted into breast milk. Infantile spasms and other withdrawal symptoms have been reported following the abrupt discontinuation of breast-feeding.

Contraindications Hypersensitivity to barbiturates or any component of the formulation; marked hepatic impairment; dyspnea or airway obstruction; porphyria (manifest and latent); intra-arterial administration, subcutaneous administration (not recommended); use in patients with a history of sedative/hypnotic addiction is not recommended; nephritic patients (large doses)

Warnings/Precautions Potential for drug dependency exists, abrupt cessation may precipitate withdrawal, including status epilepticus in epileptic patients. Do not administer to patients in acute pain. Use caution in debilitated, renal or hepatic dysfunction, and pediatric patients. May cause paradoxical responses, including agitation and hyperactivity, particularly in acute pain and pediatric patients. Avoid use in the eldely due to risk of overdose with low dosages, tolerance to sleep effects, and increased risk of physical dependence (Beers Criteria). Use with caution in patients with depression or suicidal tendencies, or in patients with a history of drug abuse. Tolerance, psychological and physical dependence may occur with prolonged use. May cause CNS depression, which may impair physical or mental abilities. Effects with other sedative drugs or ethanol may be potentiated. May cause respiratory depression or hypotension, particularly when administered intravenously. Use with caution in hemodynamically unstable patients (hypovolemic shock, CHF) or patients with respiratory disease. Due to its long half-life and risk of dependence, phenobarbital is not recommended as a sedative in the elderly. Use has been associated with cognitive deficits in children. Use with caution in patients with hypoadrenalism. Intra-arterial administration may cause reactions ranging from transient pain to gangrene and is contraindicated. Subcutaneous administration may cause tissue irritation (eg, redness, tenderness, necrosis) and is not recommended.

Adverse Reactions Frequency not defined.

Cardiovascular: Bradycardia, hypotension, syncope

Central nervous system: Agitation, anxiety, ataxia, CNS excitation or depression, confusion, dizziness drowsiness, hallucinations, "hangover" effect, headache, hyperkinesia, impaired judgment, insomnia, lethargy, nervousness, nightmares, somnolence

Dermatologic: Exfoliative dermatitis, rash, Stevens-Johnson syndrome

Gastrointestinal: Nausea, vomiting, constipation

Hematologic: Agranulocytosis, thrombocytopenia, megaloblastic anemia

Local: Pain at injection site, thrombophlebitis with I.V. use

Renal: Oliguria

Respiratory: Laryngospasm, respiratory depression, apnea (especially with rapid I.V. use), hypoventilation

Miscellaneous: Gangrene with inadvertent intra-arterial injection

Drug Interactions

Metabolism/Transport Effects Substrate of CYP2C19 (major), CYP2C9 (minor), CYP2E1 (minor); **Note:** Assignment of Major/Minor substrate status based on clinically relevant drug interaction potential; **Induces** CYP1A2 (strong), CYP2A6 (strong), CYP2B6 (strong), CYP2C8 (strong), CYP2C9 (strong), CYP3A4 (strong), P-glycoprotein

Avoid Concomitant Use

Avoid concomitant use of PHENobarbital with any of the following: Abiraterone Acetate; Apixaban; Artemether; Axitinib; Azelastine (Nasal); Bedaquiline; Boceprevir; Bortezomib; Bosutinib; Cabozantinib; CloZAPine; Crizotinib; Dabigatran Etexilate; Darunavir; Dienogest; Dolutegravir; Dronedarone; Enzalutamide; Etravirine; Everolimus; Ibrutinib; Itraconazole; Ivacaftor; Lapatinib; Lumefantrine; Lurasidone; Macitentan; Mifepristone; NIFEdipine; Nilotinib; Nisoldipine; Paraldehyde; PAZOPanib; Perampanel; Pirfenidone; Pomalidomide; PONATinib; Praziquantel; Ranolazine; Regorafenib; Rilpivirine; Rivaroxaban; Roflumilast; RomiDEPsin; Simeprevir; Sofosbuvir; SORAfenib; Telaprevir; Ticagrelor; Tofacitinib; Tolvaptan; Toremifene; Ulipristal; Vandetanib; Vemurafenib; VinCRIStine (Liposomal); Voriconazole

Increased Effect/Toxicity

PHENobarbital may increase the levels/effects of: Alcohol (Ethyl); Azelastine (Nasal); Buprenorphine; Clarithromycin; CNS Depressants; Hydrocodone; Ifosfamide; Meperidine; Methotrimeprazine; Metyrosine; Mirtazapine; Paraldehyde; Pramipexole; Prilocaine; QuiNIDine; ROPINIRole; Rotigotine; Selective Serotonin Reuptake Inhibitors; Sodium Nitrite; Thiazide Diuretics; Zolpidem

The levels/effects of PHENobarbital may be increased by: Brimonidine (Topical); Carbonic Anhydrase Inhibitors; Chloramphenicol; Clarithromycin; Cosyntropin; CYP2C19 Inhibitors (Moderate); CYP2C19 Inhibitors (Strong); Dexmethylphenidate; Doxylamine; Droperidol; Felbamate; Fosphenytoin; HydrOXYzine; Luliconazole; Magnesium Sulfate; Methotrimeprazine; Methylphenidate; Nitric Oxide; OXcarbazepine; Phenytoin; Primidone; QuiNINE; Rufinamide; Sodium Oxybate; Tapentadol; Valproic Acid and Derivatives

Decreased Effect

PHENobarbital may decrease the levels/effects of: Abiraterone Acetate; Acetaminophen; Afatinib; Apixaban; ARIPiprazole; Artemether; Axitinib; Bazedoxifene; Bedaquiline; Bendamustine; Beta-Blockers; Boceprevir; Bortezomib; Bosutinib; Brentuximab Vedotin; Cabozantinib; Calcium Channel Blockers; Canagliflozin; Chloramphenicol; Clarithromycin; CloZAPine; Cobicistat; Contraceptives (Estrogens); Contraceptives (Progestins); Corticosteroids (Systemic); Crizotinib; CycloSPORINE (Systemic); CYP1A2 Substrates; CYP2A6 Substrates; CYP2B6 Substrates; CYP2C8 Substrates; CYP2C9

Substrates; CYP3A4 Substrates; Dabigatran Etexilate; Darunavir; Dasatinib; Deferasirox; Diclofenac (Systemic); Dienogest; Disopyramide; Dolutegravir; Doxycycline; Dronedarone; Elvitegravir; Enzalutamide; Eslicarbazepine; Etoposide; Etoposide Phosphate; Etravirine; Everolimus; Exemestane; Felbamate; Fosphenytoin; Gefitinib; Griseofulvin; GuanFACINE; Ibrutinib; Imatinib; Irinotecan; Itraconazole; Ivacaftor; Ixabepilone; Lacosamide; LamoTRIgine; Lapatinib; Linagliptin; Lopinavir; Lumefantrine; Lurasidone; Macitentan; Maraviroc; Methadone; MetroNIDAZOLE (Systemic); Mifepristone; NIFEdipine; Nilotinib; Nisoldipine; OXcarbazepine; PAZOPanib; Perampanel; P-glycoprotein/ABCB1 Substrates; Phenytoin; Pirfenidone; Pomalidomide; PONATinib; Praziquantel; Propafenone; QUEtiapine; QuiNIDine; QuiNINE; Ranolazine; Regorafenib; Rilpivirine; Rivaroxaban; Roflumilast; RomiDEPsin; Rufinamide; Saxagliptin; Simeprevir; Sofosbuvir; SORAfenib; SUNItinib; Tadalafil; Telaprevir; Teniposide; Theophylline Derivatives; Ticagrelor; Tipranavir; Tofacitinib; Tolvaptan; Toremifene; Treprostinil; Tricyclic Antidepressants; Ulipristal; Valproic Acid and Derivatives; Vandetanib; Vemurafenib; VinCRIStine (Liposomal); Vitamin K Antagonists; Voriconazole; Vortioxetine; Zonisamide; Zuclopenthixol

The levels/effects of PHENobarbital may be decreased by: Amphetamines; Cholestyramine Resin; CYP2C19 Inducers (Strong); Dabrafenib; Folic Acid; Ketorolac (Nasal); Ketorolac (Systemic); Leucovorin Calcium-Levoleucovorin; Levomefolate; Mefloquine; Methylfolate; Multivitamins/Minerals (with ADEK, Folate, Iron); Orlistat; Pyridoxine; Rifamycin Derivatives; Tipranavir

Ethanol/Nutrition/Herb Interactions

Ethanol: May increase CNS depression; monitor for increased effects with coadministration. Caution patients about effects.

Food: May cause decrease in vitamin D and calcium.

Herb/Nutraceutical: Avoid evening primrose (seizure threshold decreased). Avoid valerian, St John's wort, kava kava, gotu kola (may increase CNS depression).

Storage/Stability Protect elixir from light. Not stable in aqueous solutions; use only clear solutions. Do not add to acidic solutions; precipitation may occur.

Mechanism of Action Long-acting barbiturate with sedative, hypnotic, and anticonvulsant properties. Barbiturates depress the sensory cortex, decrease motor activity, alter cerebellar function, and produce drowsiness, sedation, and hypnosis. In high doses, barbiturates exhibit anticonvulsant activity; barbiturates produce dose-dependent respiratory depression.

Pharmacodynamics/Kinetics

Onset of action: Oral: Hypnosis: 20-60 minutes; I.V.: ~5 minutes

Peak effect: I.V.: ~30 minutes

Duration: Oral: 6-10 hours; I.V.: 4-10 hours

Absorption: Oral: 70% to 90%

Protein binding: 20% to 45%; decreased in neonates

Metabolism: Hepatic via hydroxylation and glucuronide conjugation

Half-life elimination: Neonates: 45-500 hours; Infants: 20-133 hours; Children: 37-73 hours; Adults: 53-140 hours

Time to peak, serum: Oral: 1-6 hours

Excretion: Urine (20% to 50% as unchanged drug)

Dosage

Children:

Sedation: Oral: 2 mg/kg 3 times/day

Preoperative sedation: Oral, I.M., I.V.: 1-3 mg/kg 1-1.5 hours before procedure

Adults:

Sedation: Oral, I.M.: 30-120 mg/day in 2-3 divided doses

Preoperative sedation: I.M.: 100-200 mg 1-1.5 hours before procedure

Anticonvulsant: Status epilepticus: **Loading dose:** I.V.:

Infants and Children: 15-20 mg/kg (maximum: 1000 mg/dose, maximum rate ≤30 mg/minute in children <60 kg); may repeat dose after 15 minutes as needed (maximum total dose: 40 mg/kg)

Adults: 10-20 mg/kg (maximum rate ≤60 mg/minute in patients ≥60 kg); may repeat dose in 20-minute intervals as needed (maximum total dose: 30 mg/kg)

Anticonvulsant maintenance dose: Oral, I.V.:

Infants: 5-8 mg/kg/day in 1-2 divided doses

Children:

1-5 years: 6-8 mg/kg/day in 1-2 divided doses

5-12 years: 4-6 mg/kg/day in 1-2 divided doses

Children >12 years and Adults: 1-3 mg/kg/day in divided doses or 50-100 mg 2-3 times/day

Sedative/hypnotic withdrawal (unlabeled use): Initial daily requirement is determined by substituting phenobarbital 30 mg for every 100 mg pentobarbital used during tolerance testing; then daily requirement is decreased by 10% of initial dose

Elderly or debilitated: Initiate at the lowest recommended dose.

Dosage adjustment in renal impairment: Adults: No dosage adjustment provided in manufacturer's labeling. However, the following guidelines have been used by some clinicians (Aronoff, 2007):

Cl_{cr} ≥10 mL/minute: No dosage adjustment necessary.

Cl_{cr} <10 mL/minute: Administer every 12-16 hours.

Hemodialysis (moderately dialyzable [20% to 50%]): Administer dose before dialysis and 50% of dose after dialysis.

Peritoneal dialysis: Administer 50% of normal dose.

CRRT: Administer normal dose and monitor levels.

Dosage adjustment in hepatic impairment: No dosage adjustment provided in manufacturer's labeling. However, phenobarital exposure is increased with hepatic impairment. Use with caution.

Dietary Considerations Vitamin D: Loss in vitamin D due to malabsorption; increase intake of foods rich in vitamin D. Supplementation of vitamin D and/or calcium may be necessary. Injection may contain sodium.

Administration May be administered I.V., I.M. or orally. Avoid rapid I.V. administration >60 mg/minute in adults and >30 mg/minute in children; intra-arterial injection is contraindicated; avoid subcutaneous administration; parenteral solutions are highly alkaline; avoid extravasation. For I.M. administration, inject deep into muscle. Do not exceed 5 mL per injection site due to potential for tissue irritation

Monitoring Parameters Phenobarbital serum concentrations, mental status, CBC, LFTs, seizure activity

Reference Range

Therapeutic:

Infants and Children: 15-30 mcg/mL (SI: 65-129 micromole/L)

Adults: 20-40 mcg/mL (SI: 86-172 micromole/L)

Toxic: >40 mcg/mL (SI: >172 micromole/L)

Toxic concentration: Slowness, ataxia, nystagmus: 35-80 mcg/mL (SI: 150-344 micromole/L)

Coma with reflexes: 65-117 mcg/mL (SI: 279-502 micromole/L)

Coma without reflexes: >100 mcg/mL (SI: >430 micromole/L)

Test Interactions Assay interference of LDH

Additional Information Injectable solutions contain propylene glycol.

Phenobarbital tablets are also available from some generic manufacturers in strengths that are exactly equivalent to fractional grain strengths: 16.2 mg (1/4 grain), 32.4 mg (1/2 grain), 64.8 mg (1 grain). To avoid medication errors, do not prescribe phenobarbital in grains.

Dosage Forms Excipient information presented when available (limited, particularly for generics); consult specific product labeling.

Elixir, Oral:
 Generic: 20 mg/5 mL (473 mL)
Solution, Oral:
 Generic: 20 mg/5 mL (473 mL)
Solution, Injection, as sodium:
 Luminal: 130 mg/mL (1 mL) [contains alcohol, usp]
 Generic: 65 mg/mL (1 mL); 130 mg/mL (1 mL)
Tablet, Oral:
 Generic: 15 mg, 16.2 mg, 30 mg, 32.4 mg, 60 mg, 64.8 mg, 97.2 mg, 100 mg

Controlled Substance C-IV

Extemporaneous Preparations An alcohol-free 10 mg/mL phenobarbital oral suspension may be made from tablets and one of two different vehicles (a 1:1 mixture of Ora-Plus® and Ora-Sweet® or a 1:1 mixture of Ora-Plus® and Ora-Sweet® SF). Crush ten phenobarbital 60 mg tablets in a glass mortar and reduce to a fine powder. Mix 30 mL of Ora-Plus® and 30 mL of either Ora-Sweet® or Ora-Sweet® SF; stir vigorously. Add 15 mL of the vehicle to the powder and mix to a uniform paste. Transfer the mixture to a 2 ounce amber plastic prescription bottle. Rinse mortar and pestle with 15 mL of the vehicle; transfer to bottle. Repeat, then add quantity of vehicle sufficient to make 60 mL. Label "shake well." May mix dose with chocolate syrup (1:1 volume) immediately before administration to mask the bitter aftertaste. Stable for 115 days when stored in amber plastic prescription bottles at room temperature.

Cober M and Johnson CE, "Stability of an Extemporaneously Prepared Alcohol-Free Phenobarbital Suspension," *Am J Health Syst Pharm*, 2007, 64(6):644-6.

- **Phenobarbital, Hyoscyamine, Atropine, and Scopolamine** *see* Hyoscyamine, Atropine, Scopolamine, and Phenobarbital *on page 1028*
- **Phenobarbital Sodium** *see* PHENobarbital *on page 1629*
- **Phenobarbitone** *see* PHENobarbital *on page 1629*
- **Phenoptin** *see* Sapropterin *on page 1875*

Phenoxybenzamine (fen oks ee BEN za meen)

Brand Names: U.S. Dibenzyline

Index Terms Phenoxybenzamine Hydrochloride

Pharmacologic Category Alpha$_1$ Blocker; Antidote

Use Symptomatic management of pheochromocytoma

Unlabeled Use Micturition problems associated with neurogenic bladder, functional outlet obstruction, and partial prostate obstruction; treatment of hypertensive crisis caused by sympathomimetic amines

Pregnancy Risk Factor C

Dosage Oral:

Children (unlabeled use): Initial: 0.25-1 mg/kg/day (maximum: 10 mg); increase slowly to blood pressure control

Adults:

 Pheochromocytoma, hypertension: Initial: 10 mg twice daily; increase by 10 mg every other day until optimal blood pressure response is achieved; usual range: 20-40 mg 2-3 times/day. Doses up to 240 mg/day have been reported (Kinney, 2000).

 Micturition disorders (unlabeled use): 10-20 mg 1-2 times/day

Dosage adjustment in renal impairment: No dosage adjustment provided in manufacturer's labeling. Use with caution.

Dosage adjustment in hepatic impairment: No dosage adjustment provided in manufacturer's labeling.

Additional Information Complete prescribing information should be consulted for additional detail.

Dosage Forms Excipient information presented when available (limited, particularly for generics); consult specific product labeling.

Capsule, Oral, as hydrochloride:
 Dibenzyline: 10 mg [contains benzyl alcohol]

- **Phenoxybenzamine Hydrochloride** *see* Phenoxybenzamine *on page 1632*
- **Phenoxymethyl Penicillin** *see* Penicillin V Potassium *on page 1611*

Phentermine (FEN ter meen)

Brand Names: U.S. Adipex-P; Suprenza

Index Terms Phentermine Hydrochloride

Pharmacologic Category Anorexiant; Central Nervous System Stimulant; Sympathomimetic

Use Short-term (few weeks) adjunct therapy in obese patients with an initial body mass index (BMI) ≥30 kg/m^2 or ≥27 kg/m^2 in the presence of other risk factors (eg, diabetes, hyperlipidemia, controlled hypertension); therapy should be used in conjunction with a comprehensive weight management program.

Pregnancy Risk Factor X

Pregnancy Considerations Animal reproduction studies have not been conducted. Use is contraindicated during pregnancy. The risks of using appetite suppressing drugs in pregnant women are not known and limited information is available about the use of phentermine in pregnancy. Weight loss therapy is generally not recommended for pregnant women. Obese and overweight women should be encouraged to participate in weight reduction programs prior to attempting pregnancy; weight gain during pregnancy should be determined by their prepregnancy BMI and current guidelines.

Breast-Feeding Considerations It is unknown if phentermine is excreted in breast milk; however, other amphetamines have been detected in breast milk. Use is contraindicated in breast-feeding women. Weight loss therapy is generally not recommended for lactating women. Weight loss programs which include physical activity and nutrition components should be discussed at the 6-week postpartum visit.

Contraindications Hypersensitivity or idiosyncrasy to phentermine or other sympathomimetic amines or any component of the formulation; history of cardiovascular disease (arrhythmias, congestive heart failure, coronary artery disease, stroke, uncontrolled hypertension); hyperthyroidism, glaucoma, agitated states, history of drug abuse; use during or within 14 days following MAO inhibitor therapy; pregnancy, breast-feeding

Warnings/Precautions Primary pulmonary hypertension (PPH), a rare and frequently fatal pulmonary disease, has been reported to occur in patients receiving a combination of phentermine and fenfluramine or dexfenfluramine. The possibility of an association between PPH and the use of phentermine alone cannot be ruled out; rare cases of PPH have been reported in patients taking phentermine alone. Discontinue in patients experiencing new-onset dyspnea, chest pain, syncope or lower extremity edema. Serious regurgitant cardiac valvular disease (primarily affecting the mitral, aortic, and/or tricuspid valves) has been reported to occur in patients receiving a combination of phentermine and fenfluramine or dexfenfluramine. The possibility of an association between valvular heart disease and the use of phentermine alone cannot be ruled out; rare cases of valvular heart disease have been reported in patients taking phentermine alone. Avoid stimulants in patients with known serious structural cardiac abnormalities, cardiomyopathy, serious heart rhythm abnormalities, or other serious cardiac problems that could increase the risk of sudden death that these conditions alone carry. Caution should be used in patients with mild hypertension and other cardiovascular conditions that might be exacerbated by increases in blood pressure or heart rate.

Use caution with diabetes; antidiabetic agent requirements may be decreased with anorexigens and concomitant dietary restrictions. Stimulants may unmask tics in individuals with coexisting Tourette's syndrome. Use caution with seizure disorders. Phentermine is pharmacologically related to the amphetamines, which have a high abuse potential; prolonged use may lead to dependency. Prescriptions should be written for the smallest quantity consistent with good patient care to minimize possibility of overdose. Amphetamines may impair the ability to engage in potentially hazardous activities (eg, operating machinery or driving). Use caution in patients with renal impairment; use has not been studied; however, an increase in exposure is expected in renal impairment. Use caution in the elderly due to the risk for causing dependence, hypertension, angina, and myocardial infarction.

Discontinue if weight loss ≥4 pounds (1.82 kg) has not occurred within the first 4 weeks of treatment (NHLBI, 1998). Tolerance to the anorectic effect usually develops within a few weeks; discontinue use when tolerance develops, do not exceed recommended dosage in an attempt to overcome tolerance. Potentially significant drug-drug interactions may exist, requiring dose or frequency adjustment, additional monitoring, and/or selection of alternative therapy. Consult drug interactions database for more detailed information. Some products may contain tartrazine which may cause allergic reactions in patients with sensitivity (caution in patients with asthma or aspirin hypersensitivity).

Adverse Reactions Frequency not defined.

Cardiovascular: Hypertension, ischemic events, palpitation, primary pulmonary hypertension and/or regurgitant cardiac valvular disease, tachycardia

Central nervous system: Dizziness, dysphoria, euphoria, headache, insomnia, overstimulation, psychosis, restlessness

Dermatologic: Urticaria

Endocrine & metabolic: Changes in libido

Gastrointestinal: Constipation, diarrhea, unpleasant taste, xerostomia

Genitourinary: Impotence

Neuromuscular & skeletal: Tremor

Drug Interactions

Metabolism/Transport Effects **Substrate** of CYP3A4 (minor); **Note:** Assignment of Major/Minor substrate status based on clinically relevant drug interaction potential

Avoid Concomitant Use

Avoid concomitant use of Phentermine with any of the following: Iobenguane I 123; MAO Inhibitors

Increased Effect/Toxicity

Phentermine may increase the levels/effects of: Analgesics (Opioid); Sympathomimetics

The levels/effects of Phentermine may be increased by: Alcohol (Ethyl); Alkalinizing Agents; Antacids; AtoMOXetine; Cannabinoids; Carbonic Anhydrase Inhibitors; MAO Inhibitors; Proton Pump Inhibitors; Tricyclic Antidepressants

Decreased Effect

Phentermine may decrease the levels/effects of: Antihistamines; Ethosuximide; Iobenguane I 123; Ioflupane I 123; PHENobarbital; Phenytoin

The levels/effects of Phentermine may be decreased by: Ammonium Chloride; Antipsychotics; Ascorbic Acid; Gastrointestinal Acidifying Agents; Lithium; Methenamine; Multivitamins/Fluoride (with ADE); Multivitamins/Minerals (with ADEK, Folate, Iron); Multivitamins/Minerals (with AE, No Iron); Urinary Acidifying Agents

Ethanol/Nutrition/Herb Interactions Ethanol: Concurrent use of phentermine with ethanol may result in adverse effects.

Storage/Stability Store at controlled room temperature of 20°C to 25°C (68°F to 77°F).

Mechanism of Action Phentermine is a sympathomimetic amine with pharmacologic properties similar to the amphetamines. The mechanism of action in reducing appetite appears to be secondary to CNS effects, including stimulation of the hypothalamus to release norepinephrine.

Pharmacodynamics/Kinetics

Absorption: Well absorbed

Time to peak: Orally disintegrating tablet: 3-4.4 hours

Excretion: Primarily urine

Dosage Note: Dosing is presented in terms of the salt, phentermine hydrochloride (not as phentermine base).

Oral: Children >16 years and Adults: Obesity:

Capsule, tablet: 15-37.5 mg daily given in 1-2 divided doses. Individualize to achieve adequate response with lowest effective dose.

Orally disintegrating tablet (ODT): One tablet (15-37.5 mg daily) every morning. Individualize to achieve adequate response with lowest effective dose.

Dosing adjustment in renal impairment: No dosage adjustment provided in manufacturer's labeling (has not been studied). Phentermine is excreted in the urine and systemic exposure may be increased in renal impairment; use with caution.

Dosing adjustment in hepatic impairment: No dosage adjustment provided in manufacturer's labeling (has not been studied).

Dietary Considerations Capsules, tablets: Should be taken before breakfast or 1-2 hours after breakfast; avoid taking in the late evening. Most effective when combined with a low-calorie diet and behavior modification counseling.

Administration Avoid late evening administration.

Capsules, tablets: Administer before breakfast or 1-2 hours after breakfast. Tablets may be divided in half and dose may be given in 2 divided doses.

Orally disintegrating tablets (Suprenza): With dry hands, place tablet on the tongue and allow to dissolve, then swallow with or without water. May administer with or without food.

Monitoring Parameters Weight, waist circumference; blood pressure

Reference Range

Adult classification of weight by BMI (kg/m^2):

Underweight: <18.5

Normal: 18.5-24.9

Overweight: 25-29.9

Obese, class I: 30-34.9

Obese, class II: 35-39.9

Extreme obesity (class III): ≥40

Waist circumference: In adults with a BMI of 25-34.9 kg/m^2, high-risk waist circumference is defined as:

Men >102 cm (>40 in)

Women >88 cm (>35 in)

Test Interactions May interfere with urine detection of amphetamines/methamphetamines (false-positive).

Dosage Forms Excipient information presented when available (limited, particularly for generics); consult specific product labeling.

Capsule, Oral, as hydrochloride:

Adipex-P: 37.5 mg

Generic: 15 mg, 30 mg, 37.5 mg

Tablet, Oral, as hydrochloride:

Adipex-P: 37.5 mg [scored]

Generic: 37.5 mg

Tablet Dispersible, Oral, as hydrochloride:
- Suprenza: 15 mg [contains fd&c blue #1 aluminum lake, fd&c yellow #5 aluminum lake]
- Suprenza: 30 mg [contains fd&c yellow #5 aluminum lake]
- Suprenza: 37.5 mg [contains fd&c blue #1 aluminum lake]

Controlled Substance C-IV

◆ **Phentermine Hydrochloride** *see* Phentermine *on page 1632*

Phentolamine (fen TOLE a meen)

Brand Names: U.S. OraVerse
Brand Names: Canada Rogitine®
Index Terms Phentolamine Mesylate; Regitine [DSC]
Pharmacologic Category $Alpha_1$ Blocker; Antidote, Extravasation; Antihypertensive
Use Diagnosis of pheochromocytoma via the phentolamine-blocking test (see **"Note"**); prevention and management of hypertensive episodes associated with pheochromocytoma resulting from stress or manipulation during the perioperative period; prevention and treatment of dermal necrosis/sloughing after extravasation of norepinephrine

OraVerse™: Reversal of soft tissue anesthesia and the associated functional deficits resulting from a local dental anesthetic containing a vasoconstrictor

Note: The phentolamine-blocking test for the diagnosis of pheochromocytoma has largely been supplanted by the measurement of catecholamine concentrations and catecholamine metabolites (eg, metanephrine) in the plasma and urine; reserve phentolamine for cases when additional confirmation is necessary to determine diagnosis.

Unlabeled Use Management of extravasations of sympathomimetic vasopressors (in addition to norepinephrine) including dopamine, epinephrine and phenylephrine; treatment of hypertensive crisis
Pregnancy Risk Factor C
Pregnancy Considerations Adverse events were observed in some oral animal reproduction studies. Diagnosing and treating pheochromocytoma is critical for favorable maternal and fetal outcomes (Schenker, 1971; Schenker, 1982).
Breast-Feeding Considerations It is not known if phentolamine is excreted in breast milk. Due to the potential for serious adverse reaction in the nursing infant, the decision to discontinue phentolamine or discontinue breast-feeding during treatment should take in account the benefits of treatment to the mother.
Contraindications Hypersensitivity to phentolamine, any component of the formulation, or related compounds; MI (or history of MI), coronary insufficiency, angina, or other evidence suggestive of coronary artery disease

Canadian labeling: Additional contraindications (not in U.S. labeling): Hypotension

OraVerse™: There are no contraindications listed in the manufacturer's labeling.

Warnings/Precautions MI, cerebrovascular spasm, and cerebrovascular occlusion have been reported following administration, usually associated with hypotensive episodes. Tachycardia and cardiac arrhythmias may occur. Discontinue if symptoms of angina occur or worsen. The use of phentolamine as a blocking agent in the screening of patients with hypertension has predominantly been replaced with urinary/biochemical assays; phentolamine use should be reserved for situations where additional confirmation is necessary and after risks associated with use have been considered. Use with caution in patients with gastritis or peptic ulcer disease. Use with caution in patients with renal impairment; primarily eliminated by the kidneys. Potentially significant drug-drug interactions may exist, requiring dose or frequency adjustment, additional monitoring, and/or selection of alternative therapy. The efficacy of OraVerse™ has not been established in children <6 years of age or <15 kg (33 pounds).
Adverse Reactions Frequency not always defined.
- Cardiovascular: Tachycardia (OraVerse ≤6%), bradycardia (OraVerse ≤4%), hypertension (OraVerse <3%), cerebrovascular occlusion, hypotension, myocardial infarction
- Central nervous system: Headache (OraVerse ≤6%), mouth pain (OraVerse <3%) paresthesia (OraVerse <3%; mild, transient), cerebrovascular spasm
- Dermatologic: Facial swelling (OraVerse <3%), pruritus (OraVerse <3%)
- Gastrointestinal: Diarrhea (OraVerse <3%), upper abdominal pain (OraVerse <3%), vomiting (OraVerse <3%), nausea
- Local: Pain at injection site (OraVerse 4% to 6%)
- Neuromuscular & skeletal: Jaw pain (OraVerse <3%)
- Postmarketing and/or case reports (Limited to important or life-threatening): Cardiac arrhythmia, orthostatic hypotension

Drug Interactions
Metabolism/Transport Effects None known.
Avoid Concomitant Use
Avoid concomitant use of Phentolamine with any of the following: Alpha1-Blockers
Increased Effect/Toxicity
Phentolamine may increase the levels/effects of: Alpha1-Blockers; Amifostine; Antihypertensives; Calcium Channel Blockers; Obinutuzumab; RiTUXimab

The levels/effects of Phentolamine may be increased by: Beta-Blockers; Brimonidine (Topical); Diazoxide; Herbs (Hypotensive Properties); MAO Inhibitors; Pentoxifylline; Phosphodiesterase 5 Inhibitors; Prostacyclin Analogues
Decreased Effect
Phentolamine may decrease the levels/effects of: Alpha-/Beta-Agonists; Alpha1-Agonists

The levels/effects of Phentolamine may be decreased by: Herbs (Hypertensive Properties); Methylphenidate; Yohimbine

Preparation for Administration Powder for injection: Reconstitute 5 mg vial with 1 mL sterile water for injection. For treatment of extravasation, further dilute 5-10 mg in 10 mL of normal saline (manufacturer's recommendation) or in 10-15 mL of saline (Peberdy, 2010).
Storage/Stability
- Powder for injection: Store intact vials at room temperature of 15°C to 30°C (59°F to 86°F). Reconstituted solution should be used immediately after preparation (per manufacturer).
- Solution for injection (OraVerse™): Store at 20°C to 25°C (68°F to 77°F); brief excursions permitted between 15°C to 30°C (59°F to 86°F). Protect from heat and light. Do not freeze.

Mechanism of Action Competitively blocks alpha-adrenergic receptors (nonselective) to produce brief antagonism of circulating epinephrine and norepinephrine to reduce hypertension caused by alpha effects of these catecholamines and minimizes tissue injury due to extravasation of these and other sympathomimetic vasoconstrictors (eg, dopamine, phenylephrine); also has a positive inotropic and chronotropic effect on the heart thought to be due to presynaptic alpha-2 receptor blockade which results in release of presynaptic norepinephrine (Hoffman, 1980)

OraVerse™: Causes vasodilation and increased blood flow in injection area via alpha-adrenergic blockade to accelerate reversal of soft tissue anesthesia

Pharmacodynamics/Kinetics

Onset of action: I.M.: 15-20 minutes; I.V.: 1-2 minutes (Chobanian, 2003)

Peak effect: OraVerse™: 10-20 minutes

Duration: I.M.: 30-45 minutes; I.V.: 10-30 minutes (Chobanian, 2003)

Metabolism: Hepatic

Half-life elimination: I.V.: 19 minutes

Excretion: Urine (~13% as unchanged drug)

Dosage

Extravasation of norepinephrine, management: Children and Adults (manufacturer's labeling): Local infiltration: Inject 5-10 mg (diluted in 10 mL 0.9% sodium chloride) into extravasation area (as soon as extravasation is noted but within 12 hours of extravasation)

Extravasation of sympathomimetic vasopressors, management (unlabeled use): Infiltrate extravasation site with 5-10 mg diluted in 10-15 mL 0.9% sodium chloride as soon as possible after extravasation (Peberdy, 2010).

Diagnosis of pheochromocytoma (phentolamine-blocking test): **Note:** The phentolamine-blocking test for the diagnosis of pheochromocytoma has largely been supplanted by the measurement of catecholamine concentrations and catecholamine metabolites (eg, metanephrine) in the plasma and urine; reserve phentolamine for cases when additional confirmation is necessary to determine diagnosis.

Children:

I.M.: 3 mg

I.V.: 1 mg

Adults: I.M., I.V.: 5 mg

Hypertensive episodes associated with pheochromocytoma, prevention and management: **Note:** In the perioperative period, the use of other agents may be preferred due to slow onset of action and prolonged duration of phentolamine in comparison to the other agents (eg, nitroprusside) (Miller, 2010)

Children:

Preoperative: I.M., I.V.: 1 mg given 1-2 hours before surgery and repeat if needed

Intraoperative: I.V.: Administer 1 mg as indicated to prevent or control paroxysms of hypertension, tachycardia, respiratory depression, seizure, or other effects associated with epinephrine intoxication resulting from tumor manipulation or other stressor (eg, intubation) (Miller, 2010).

Adults:

Preoperative: I.M., I.V.: 5 mg given 1-2 hours before surgery and repeat if needed

Intraoperative: I.V.: Administer 5 mg as indicated to prevent or control paroxysms of hypertension, tachycardia, respiratory depression, seizure, or other effects associated with epinephrine intoxication resulting from tumor manipulation or other stressor (eg, intubation) (Miller, 2010).

Hypertensive crisis (unlabeled use): Adults: **Note:** Generally used in the setting of catecholamine excess (eg, pheochromocytoma) (Rhoney, 2009): I.V.: 5-15 mg (Chobanian, 2003)

Reversal of oral soft tissue (lip, tongue) anesthesia (OraVerse™): Infiltration or block technique: Submucosal oral injection:

Children: 15-30 kg: 0.2 mg maximum dose

Children >30 kg and <12 years: 0.4 mg maximum dose

Adults: **Note:** Dose is based upon the number of cartridges of local anesthetic administered. Infiltration or block injection:

0.2 mg if one-half cartridge of anesthesia was administered

0.4 mg if 1 cartridge of anesthesia was administered

0.8 mg if 2 cartridges of anesthesia were administered

Dosage adjustment in renal impairment: No dosage adjustment provided in manufacturer's labeling.

Dosage adjustment in hepatic impairment: No dosage adjustment provided in manufacturer's labeling.

Administration

Extravasation management (treatment), sympathomimetic vasopressors: Stop vesicant infusion immediately and disconnect I.V. line (leave needle/cannula in place); gently aspirate extravasated solution from the I.V. line (do **NOT** flush the line); remove needle/cannula; elevate extremity. Inject phentolamine 5-10 mg/10 mL saline into extravasation site (as soon as possible but within 12 hours of extravasation). AHA recommends diluting 5-10 mg in 10-15 mL saline and administering into the site (Peberdy, 2010).

Pheochromocytoma diagnosis: Patient should be supine throughout test, preferable in a quiet, dark room. Blood pressure should be monitored every 10 minutes for at least 30 minutes, delay phentolamine administration until after blood pressure is stable (at an untreated, hypertensive level). A drop in blood pressure >35 mm Hg (systolic) and >25 mm Hg (diastolic) is considered a positive response. If blood pressure is elevated, unchanged, or decrease is <35 mm Hg (systolic) and <25 mm Hg (diastolic), then response is negative. Confirm positive response with other diagnostic measure. Negative responses do not exclude a pheochromocytoma diagnosis, particularly in patients with paroxysmal hypertension where an incidence of false negatives is high.

I.M.: After I.M. injection, monitor blood pressure every 5 minutes for 35-40 minutes. Blood pressure drops to above parameters within 20 minutes are considered positive.

I.V.: Inject rapidly (after venous response to venipuncture has subsided); then monitor blood pressure immediately after injection, every 30 seconds for 3 minutes, then every minute for 7 minutes. Maximum response is generally achieved within 2 minutes; duration may last 15-30 minutes (although return to prior blood pressure may be sooner).

Pheochromocytoma-associated hypertensive episode: Administer I.M. or I.V. 1-2 hours prior to surgery and repeat during surgery (I.V.) if necessary.

Reversal of oral soft tissue (lip, tongue) anesthesia (OraVerse™): Submucosal oral injection: Use the same location and dental technique employed for administration of the local anesthetic.

Hypertensive crisis (unlabeled use): Administer as an I.V. bolus (Chobanian, 2003).

Monitoring Parameters Blood pressure, heart rate; monitor and document extravasation site; monitor patient for orthostasis; assist patient with ambulation

Dosage Forms Excipient information presented when available (limited, particularly for generics); consult specific product labeling.

Solution, Injection, as mesylate:

OraVerse™: 0.4 mg/1.7 mL (1.7 mL) [contains edetate disodium; dental cartridge]

Generic: 5 mg/mL (1 mL)

Solution Reconstituted, Injection, as mesylate:

Generic: 5 mg (1 ea)

◆ **Phentolamine Mesylate** *see* Phentolamine *on page 1634*

◆ **Phenylalanine Mustard** *see* Melphalan *on page 1286*

◆ **Phenylazo Diamino Pyridine Hydrochloride** *see* Phenazopyridine *on page 1627*

Phenylephrine (Systemic) (fen il EF rin)

Brand Names: U.S. Little Colds Decongestant [OTC]; Medi-Phenyl [OTC]; Nasal Decongestant PE Max St [OTC]; Nasal Decongestant [OTC]; Neo-Synephrine [DSC]; Non-Pseudo Sinus Decongestant [OTC]; Sudafed PE Childrens [OTC]; Sudafed PE Maximum Strength [OTC]; Sudogest PE [OTC]

Index Terms Phenylephrine Hydrochloride

Pharmacologic Category Alpha-Adrenergic Agonist

Additional Appendix Information

Vasoactive Agents, Intravenous *on page 2315*

Use Treatment of hypotension, vascular failure in shock (see **"Note"**); as a vasoconstrictor in regional analgesia; supraventricular tachycardia (see **"Note"**); as a decongestant [OTC]

Note: Not recommended for routine use in the treatment of septic shock or supraventricular tachycardias.

Pregnancy Risk Factor C

Pregnancy Considerations Animal reproduction studies have not been conducted; therefore, the manufacturer classifies phenylephrine as pregnancy category C. Phenylephrine crosses the placenta at term. Maternal use of phenylephrine during the first trimester of pregnancy is not strongly associated with an increased risk of fetal malformations; maternal dose and duration of therapy were not reported in available publications. Phenylephrine is available over-the-counter (OTC) for the symptomatic relief of nasal congestion. Decongestants are not the preferred agents for the treatment of rhinitis during pregnancy. Oral phenylephrine should be avoided during the first trimester of pregnancy; short-term use (<3 days) of intranasal phenylephrine may be beneficial to some patients although its safety during pregnancy has not been studied. Phenylephrine injection is used at delivery for the prevention and/or treatment of maternal hypotension associated with spinal anesthesia in women undergoing cesarean section. Phenylephrine may be associated with a more favorable fetal acid base status than ephedrine; however, overall fetal outcomes appear to be similar. Nausea or vomiting may be less with phenylephrine than ephedrine but is also dependent upon blood pressure control. Phenylephrine may be preferred in the absence of maternal bradycardia.

Breast-Feeding Considerations It is not known if phenylephrine is excreted into breast milk. The manufacturer recommends that caution be exercised when administering phenylephrine to nursing women.

Contraindications Hypersensitivity to phenylephrine or any component of the formulation

Injection: Severe hypertension; ventricular tachycardia

Oral: Use with or within 14 days of MAO inhibitor therapy

Warnings/Precautions Some products contain sulfites which may cause allergic reactions in susceptible individuals. Use with extreme caution in patients taking MAO inhibitors.

Intravenous: Use with caution in the elderly, patients with hyperthyroidism, bradycardia, partial heart block, myocardial disease, or severe CAD. Avoid or use with extreme caution in patients with heart failure or cardiogenic shock; increased systemic vascular resistance may significantly reduce cardiac output. Assure adequate circulatory volume to minimize need for vasoconstrictors. Avoid use in patients with hypertension (contraindicated in severe hypertension); monitor blood pressure closely and adjust infusion rate. Vesicant; ensure proper needle or catheter placement prior to and during infusion; avoid extravasation. **[U.S. Boxed Warning]: Should be administered by adequately trained individuals familiar with its use.**

Oral: When used for self-medication (OTC), use caution with asthma, bowel obstruction/narrowing, hyperthyroidism, diabetes mellitus, cardiovascular disease, ischemic heart disease, hypertension, increased intraocular pressure, prostatic hyperplasia or in the elderly. Notify healthcare provider if symptoms do not improve within 7 days or are accompanied by fever. Discontinue and contact healthcare provider if nervousness, dizziness, or sleeplessness occur.

Adverse Reactions Frequency not defined.

Injection:

Cardiovascular: Arrhythmia (rare), decreased cardiac output, hypertension, pallor, precordial pain or discomfort, reflex bradycardia, severe peripheral and visceral vasoconstriction

Central nervous system: Anxiety, dizziness, excitability, giddiness, headache, insomnia, nervousness, restlessness

Endocrine & metabolic: Metabolic acidosis

Gastrointestinal: Gastric irritation, nausea

Local: I.V.: Extravasation which may lead to necrosis and sloughing of surrounding tissue, blanching of skin

Neuromuscular & skeletal: Paresthesia, pilomotor response, tremor, weakness

Renal: Decreased renal perfusion, reduced urine output

Respiratory: Respiratory distress

Miscellaneous: Hypersensitivity reactions (including rash, urticaria, leukopenia, agranulocytosis, thrombocytopenia)

Oral: Central nervous system: Anxiety, dizziness, excitability, giddiness, headache, insomnia, nervousness, restlessness

Drug Interactions

Metabolism/Transport Effects None known.

Avoid Concomitant Use

Avoid concomitant use of Phenylephrine (Systemic) with any of the following: Ergot Derivatives; Hyaluronidase; Iobenguane I 123; MAO Inhibitors

Increased Effect/Toxicity

Phenylephrine (Systemic) may increase the levels/effects of: Sympathomimetics

The levels/effects of Phenylephrine (Systemic) may be increased by: AtoMOXetine; Cannabinoids; Ergot Derivatives; Hyaluronidase; Linezolid; MAO Inhibitors; Tricyclic Antidepressants

Decreased Effect

Phenylephrine (Systemic) may decrease the levels/effects of: Benzylpenicilloyl Polylysine; FentaNYL; Iobenguane I 123

The levels/effects of Phenylephrine (Systemic) may be decreased by: Alpha1-Blockers

Ethanol/Nutrition/Herb Interactions Herb/Nutraceutical: Avoid ephedra, yohimbe (may cause CNS stimulation).

Preparation for Administration Solution for injection:

I.V. infusion: May dilute 10 mg in 500 mL NS or D_5W. May also dilute 50 mg in 500 mL NS or 100 mg in 500 mL NS; both concentrations are stable for at least 14 days at room temperature of 25°C (77°F) (Gupta, 2004). Dilution of 1250 mg in 500 mL NS retained potency for at least 24 hours at 22°C (Weber, 1970).

I.V. injection: May dilute with SWFI to a concentration of 1 mg/mL.

Stability in syringes (Kiser, 2007): Concentration of 0.1 mg/mL in NS (polypropylene syringes) is stable for at least 30 days at -20°C (-4°F), 3°C to 5°C (37°F to 41°F), or 23°C to 25°C (73.4°F to 77°F).

Storage/Stability

Solution for injection: Store vials at controlled room temperature of 15°C to 25°C (59°F to 77°F). Protect from light. Do not use solution if brown or contains a precipitate.

Oral: Store at controlled room temperature of 15°C to 25°C (59°F to 77°F). Protect from light.

Mechanism of Action Potent, direct-acting alpha-adrenergic agonist with virtually no beta-adrenergic activity; produces systemic arterial vasoconstriction. Such increases in systemic vascular resistance result in dose dependent increases in systolic and diastolic blood pressure and reductions in heart rate and cardiac output especially in patients with heart failure.

Pharmacodynamics/Kinetics

Onset of action:

Blood pressure increase/vasoconstriction: I.M., SubQ: 10-15 minutes; I.V.: Immediate

Nasal decongestant: Oral: 15-30 minutes (Kollar, 2007)

Duration:

Blood pressure increase/vasoconstriction: I.M.: 1-2 hours; I.V.: ~15-20 minutes; SubQ: 50 minutes

Nasal decongestant: Oral: ≤4 hours (Kollar, 2007)

Absorption: Oral: Rapid and complete (Kanfer, 1993)

Distribution: V_d: Initial: 26-61 L; V_{dss}: 184-543 L (mean: 340 L) (Hengstmann, 1982)

Metabolism: Hepatic via oxidative deamination (Oral: 24%; I.V.: 50%); Undergoes sulfation (Oral [mostly within gut wall]: 46%; I.V.: 8%) and some glucuronidation; forms inactive metabolites (Kanfer, 1993)

Bioavailability: Oral: ≤38% (Hengstmann, 1982; Kanfer, 1993)

Half-life elimination: Alpha phase: ~5 minutes; Terminal phase: 2-3 hours (Hengstmann, 1982; Kanfer, 1993)

Time to peak: Oral: 0.75-2 hours (Kanfer, 1993)

Excretion: Urine (mostly as inactive metabolites)

Dosage

Hypotension/shock: **Note:** Phenylephrine is not recommended for septic shock except in the following circumstances: Norepinephrine (preferred first-line agent) is associated with serious arrhythmias, cardiac output is known to be high and blood pressure persistently low, or when the combination of inotrope/vasopressor and low-dose vasopressin failed to achieve target mean arterial pressure and phenylephrine is used as salvage therapy (Dellinger, 2013).

Children:

I.V. bolus: 5-20 mcg/kg/dose every 10-15 minutes as needed

I.V. infusion: 0.1-0.5 mcg/kg/minute

Adults:

I.V. bolus: 100-500 mcg/dose every 10-15 minutes as needed (initial dose should not exceed 500 mcg)

I.V. infusion: Initial dose: 100-180 mcg/minute, **or alternatively**, 0.5 mcg/kg/minute; titrate to desired response. Dosing ranges between 0.4-9.1 mcg/kg/minute have been reported when treating septic shock (Gregory, 1991).

Nasal decongestant: Oral: OTC labeling:

Children:

4 to <6 years: 2.5 mg every 4 hours as needed for ≤7 days (maximum: 15 mg/24 hours)

6 to <12 years: 5 mg every 4 hours as needed for ≤7 days (maximum: 30 mg/24 hours)

Children ≥12 years and Adults: 10 mg every 4 hours as needed for ≤7 days (maximum: 60 mg/24 hours)

Paroxysmal supraventricular tachycardia (**Note:** Not recommended for routine use in treatment of supraventricular tachycardias): I.V.:

Children: 5-10 mcg/kg/dose over 20-30 seconds

Adults: 250-500 mcg/dose over 20-30 seconds

Dietary Considerations Some products may contain phenylalanine and/or sodium.

Usual Infusion Concentrations: Pediatric I.V. infusion: 20 **mcg**/mL, 40 **mcg**/mL, or 60 **mcg**/mL

Usual Infusion Concentrations: Adult I.V. infusion: 10 mg in 500 mL (concentration: 20 **mcg**/mL) of D_5W or NS, 50 mg in 500 mL (concentration: 100 **mcg**/mL) of NS, **or** 100 mg in 500 mL (concentration: 200 **mcg**/mL) of NS

Other institutions may use concentrations of 40 **mcg**/mL **or** 160 **mcg**/mL; however, stability information is not available for these concentrations.

Administration I.V.: Administer by slow injection or as a continuous infusion (after diluting); when administering as a continuous infusion, central line administration is preferred. I.V. infusions require an infusion pump.

Vesicant; ensure proper needle or catheter placement prior to and during infusion; avoid extravasation.

Extravasation management: If extravasation occurs, stop infusion immediately and disconnect (leave cannula/needle in place); gently aspirate extravasated solution (do **NOT** flush the line); remove needle/cannula; elevate extremity. Initiate phentolamine (or alternative antidote). Apply dry warm compresses (Hurst, 2004).

Phentolamine: Dilute 5-10 mg in 10-15 mL NS and administer into extravasation site as soon as possible after extravasation (Peberdy, 2010).

Alternatives to phentolamine (due to shortage):

Nitroglycerin topical 2% ointment (based on limited case reports in neonates/infants): Apply 4 mm/kg as a thin ribbon to the affected areas; may repeat after 8 hours if needed (Wong, 1992) **or** apply a 1-inch strip on the affected site (Denkler, 1989).

Terbutaline (based on limited case reports): Infiltrate extravasation area using a solution of terbutaline 1 mg diluted to 10 mL in NS (large extravasation site; administration volume varied from 3-10 mL) **or** 1 mg diluted in 1 mL NS (small/distal extravasation site; administration volume varied from 0.5-1 mL) (Stier, 1999).

Monitoring Parameters Blood pressure (or mean arterial pressure), heart rate; cardiac output (as appropriate), intravascular volume status, pulmonary capillary wedge pressure (as appropriate); monitor infusion site closely

Consult individual institutional policies and procedures.

Dosage Forms Excipient information presented when available (limited, particularly for generics); consult specific product labeling. [DSC] = Discontinued product

Liquid, Oral, as hydrochloride:

Little Colds Decongestant: 2.5 mg/mL (30 mL) [alcohol free, dye free, saccharin free; contains sodium benzoate; grape flavor]

Solution, Injection, as hydrochloride:

Neo-Synephrine: 10 mg/mL (1 mL [DSC]) [contains sodium metabisulfite]

Generic: 10 mg/mL (1 mL, 5 mL, 10 mL)

Solution, Oral, as hydrochloride:

Sudafed PE Childrens: 2.5 mg/5 mL (118 mL) [alcohol free, sugar free; contains edetate disodium, fd&c red #40, sodium benzoate]

Tablet, Oral, as hydrochloride:

Medi-Phenyl: 5 mg

Nasal Decongestant: 10 mg [contains fd&c blue #2 (indigotine), fd&c red #40, fd&c yellow #6 aluminum lake]

Nasal Decongestant PE Max St: 10 mg [pseudoephedrine free; contains fd&c red #40 aluminum lake]

Non-Pseudo Sinus Decongestant: 10 mg [contains fd&c red #40 aluminum lake, fd&c yellow #6 aluminum lake]

Sudafed PE Maximum Strength: 10 mg [contains fd&c red #40 aluminum lake, fd&c yellow #10 aluminum lake, fd&c yellow #6 aluminum lake]

Sudafed PE Maximum Strength: 10 mg [contains fd&c red #40 aluminum lake, fd&c yellow #6 aluminum lake]

Sudafed PE Maximum Strength: 10 mg [pseudoephedrine free; contains fd&c red #40 aluminum lake, fd&c yellow #10 aluminum lake, fd&c yellow #6 aluminum lake]
Sudogest PE: 10 mg [contains fd&c red #40]

- **Phenylephrine and Chlorpheniramine** *see* Chlorpheniramine and Phenylephrine *on page 412*
- **Phenylephrine and Cyclopentolate** *see* Cyclopentolate and Phenylephrine *on page 504*
- **Phenylephrine and Dextromethorphan** *see* Dextromethorphan and Phenylephrine *on page 591*
- **Phenylephrine and Diphenhydramine** *see* Diphenhydramine and Phenylephrine *on page 625*
- **Phenylephrine, Chlorpheniramine, and Dextromethorphan** *see* Chlorpheniramine, Phenylephrine, and Dextromethorphan *on page 413*
- **Phenylephrine, Chlorpheniramine, and Dihydrocodeine** *see* Dihydrocodeine, Chlorpheniramine, and Phenylephrine *on page 611*
- **Phenylephrine Hydrochloride** *see* Phenylephrine (Systemic) *on page 1636*
- **Phenylephrine Hydrochloride and Diphenhydramine Hydrochloride** *see* Diphenhydramine and Phenylephrine *on page 625*
- **Phenylephrine Hydrochloride and Guaifenesin** *see* Guaifenesin and Phenylephrine *on page 978*
- **Phenylephrine Tannate and Diphenhydramine Tannate** *see* Diphenhydramine and Phenylephrine *on page 625*
- **Phenylethylmalonylurea** *see* PHENobarbital *on page 1629*
- **Phenyl Salicylate, Methenamine, Methylene Blue, Benzoic Acid, and Hyoscyamine** *see* Methenamine, Phenyl Salicylate, Methylene Blue, Benzoic Acid, and Hyoscyamine *on page 1319*
- **Phenyl Salicylate, Methenamine, Methylene Blue, Sodium Biphosphate, and Hyoscyamine** *see* Methenamine, Sodium Biphosphate, Phenyl Salicylate, Methylene Blue, and Hyoscyamine *on page 1320*
- **Phenytek** *see* Phenytoin *on page 1638*

Phenytoin (FEN i toyn)

Brand Names: U.S. Dilantin; Dilantin Infatabs; Phenytek; Phenytoin Infatabs

Brand Names: Canada Dilantin; Novo-Phenytoin; Taro-Phenytoin; Tremytoine Inj

Index Terms Diphenylhydantoin; DPH; Phenytoin Sodium; Phenytoin Sodium, Extended; Phenytoin Sodium, Prompt

Pharmacologic Category Anticonvulsant, Hydantoin

Additional Appendix Information

Dosing Considerations for the Critically-Ill Patient With Morbid Obesity *on page 2379*
Status Epilepticus *on page 2375*

Use Management of generalized tonic-clonic (grand mal), complex partial seizures; prevention of seizures following neurosurgery

Unlabeled Use Prevention of early (within 1 week) post-traumatic seizures (PTS) following traumatic brain injury

Pregnancy Risk Factor D

Pregnancy Considerations Phenytoin crosses the placenta (Harden and Pennell, 2009). An increased risk of congenital malformations and adverse outcomes may occur following *in utero* phenytoin exposure. Reported malformations include orofacial clefts, cardiac defects, dysmorphic facial features, nail/digit hypoplasia, growth abnormalities including microcephaly, and mental deficiency. Isolated cases of malignancies (including neuroblastoma) and coagulation defects in the neonate (may be life threatening) following delivery have also been reported. Maternal use of phenytoin should be avoided when possible to decrease the risk of cleft palate and poor cognitive outcomes. Polytherapy may also increase the risk of congenital malformations; monotherapy is recommended (Harden and Meader, 2009). The maternal use of folic acid throughout pregnancy is recommended to reduce the risk of major congenital malformations (Harden and Pennell, 2009).

Total plasma concentrations of phenytoin are decreased in the mother during pregnancy; unbound plasma (free) concentrations are also decreased and plasma clearance is increased. Due to pregnancy-induced physiologic changes, women who are pregnant may require dose adjustments of phenytoin in order to maintain clinical response; monitoring during pregnancy should be considered (Harden and Pennell, 2009). For women with epilepsy who are planning a pregnancy in advance, baseline serum concentrations should be measured once or twice prior to pregnancy during a period when seizure control is optimal. Monitoring can then be continued once each trimester during pregnancy and postpartum; more frequent monitoring may be needed in some patients. Monitoring of unbound plasma concentrations is recommended (Patsalos, 2008). In women taking phenytoin who are trying to avoid pregnancy, potentially significant interactions may exist with hormone-containing contraceptives; consult drug interactions database for more detailed information.

Patients exposed to phenytoin during pregnancy are encouraged to enroll themselves into the North American Antiepileptic Drug (NAAED) Pregnancy Registry by calling 1-888-233-2334. Additional information is available at https:\\aedpregnancyregistry.org.

Breast-Feeding Considerations Phenytoin is excreted in breast milk; however, the amount to which the infant is exposed is considered small. The manufacturers of phenytoin do not recommend breast-feeding during therapy.

Medication Guide Available Yes

Contraindications Hypersensitivity to phenytoin, other hydantoins, or any component of the formulation; concurrent use of delavirdine (due to loss of virologic response and possible resistance to delavirdine or other non-nucleoside reverse transcriptase inhibitors [NNRTIs])

I.V.: Sinus bradycardia, sinoatrial block, second- and third-degree heart block, Adams-Stokes syndrome

Warnings/Precautions Antiepileptics are associated with an increased risk of suicidal behavior/thoughts with use (regardless of indication); patients should be monitored for signs/symptoms of depression, suicidal tendencies, and other unusual behavior changes during therapy and instructed to inform their healthcare provider immediately if symptoms occur.

[U.S. Boxed Warning]: Phenytoin must be administered slowly. Intravenous administration should not exceed 50 mg/minute in adult patients. In pediatric patients, intravenous administration rate should not exceed 1-3 mg/kg/minute or 50 mg/minute whichever is slower. Hypotension and severe cardiac arrhythmias (eg, heart block, ventricular tachycardia, ventricular fibrillation) may occur with rapid administration; adverse cardiac events have been reported at or below the recommended infusion rate. Cardiac monitoring is necessary during and after administration of intravenous phenytoin; reduction in rate of administration or discontinuation of infusion may be necessary. For nonemergency use, intravenous phenytoin should be administered more slowly; the use of oral phenytoin should be used whenever possible. Vesicant (intravenous administration); ensure proper catheter or needle position prior to and during infusion; avoid extravasation; I.V. form may cause soft tissue irritation and inflammation, and skin necrosis at I.V. site; avoid I.V. administration in small veins. The "purple glove syndrome" (ie, discoloration with edema and pain of distal limb) may occur following peripheral I.V. administration of phenytoin; may or may not be associated with drug extravasation; symptoms may resolve spontaneously; however, skin necrosis and limb ischemia may occur; interventions such as fasciotomies, skin grafts, and amputation (rare) may be required. May increase frequency of petit mal seizures; use with caution in patients with porphyria; discontinue if rash or lymphadenopathy occurs; a spectrum of hematologic effects have been reported with use (eg, agranulocytosis, neutropenia, leukopenia, thrombocytopenia, pancytopenia, and anemias); use with caution in patients with hepatic dysfunction, hypothyroidism, or underlying cardiac disease; I.V. use is contraindicated in patients with sinus bradycardia, sinoatrial block, or second- and third-degree heart block; use with caution in elderly or debilitated patients, or in any condition associated with low serum albumin levels, which will increase the free fraction of phenytoin in the serum and, therefore, the pharmacologic response. Sedation, confusional states, or cerebellar dysfunction (loss of motor coordination) may occur at higher total serum concentrations, or at lower total serum concentrations when the free fraction of phenytoin is increased. Effects with other sedative drugs or ethanol may be potentiated. Abrupt withdrawal may precipitate status epilepticus. Severe reactions, including toxic epidermal necrolysis and Stevens-Johnson syndromes, although rarely reported, have resulted in fatalities; drug should be discontinued if there are any signs of rash and evaluate for signs and symptoms of drug reaction with eosinophilia and systemic symptoms (DRESS). Patients of Asian descent with the variant *HLA-B*1502* may be at an increased risk of developing Stevens-Johnson syndrome and/or toxic epidermal necrolysis. Chronic use of phenytoin has been associated with decreased bone mineral density (osteopenia, osteoporosis, and osteomalacia) and bone fractures. Chronic use may result in decreased vitamin D concentrations due to hepatic enzyme induction and may lead to hypocalcemia and hypophosphatemia; monitor as appropriate and consider implementing vitamin D and calcium supplementation.

Adverse Reactions I.V. effects: Hypotension, bradycardia, cardiac arrhythmia, cardiovascular collapse (especially with rapid I.V. use), venous irritation and pain, thrombophlebitis

Effects not related to plasma phenytoin concentrations: Hypertrichosis, gingival hypertrophy, thickening of facial features, carbohydrate intolerance, folic acid deficiency, peripheral neuropathy, vitamin D deficiency, osteomalacia, systemic lupus erythematosus

Concentration-related effects: Nystagmus, blurred vision, diplopia, ataxia, slurred speech, dizziness, drowsiness, lethargy, coma, rash, fever, nausea, vomiting, gum tenderness, confusion, mood changes, folic acid depletion, osteomalacia, hyperglycemia

Related to elevated concentrations:

>20 mcg/mL: Far lateral nystagmus
>30 mcg/mL: 45° lateral gaze nystagmus and ataxia
>40 mcg/mL: Decreased mentation
>100 mcg/mL: Death

Cardiovascular: Bradycardia, cardiac arrhythmia, cardiovascular collapse, hypotension
Central nervous system: Dizziness, drowsiness, headache, insomnia, psychiatric changes, slurred speech
Dermatologic: Rash
Gastrointestinal: Constipation, gingival hyperplasia, enlargement of lips, nausea, taste disturbance, vomiting
Genitourinary: Peyronie's disease
Hematologic: Agranulocytosis, granulocytopenia, leukopenia, pancytopenia, thrombocytopenia
Hepatic: Hepatitis
Local: I.V. administration: Inflammation, irritation, necrosis, sloughing, tenderness, thrombophlebitis
Neuromuscular & skeletal: Paresthesia, peripheral neuropathy, tremor
Ocular: Blurred vision, diplopia, nystagmus
Rarely seen effects: Anaphylaxis, blood dyscrasias, coarsening of facial features, DRESS, dyskinesias, hepatitis, Hodgkin lymphoma,, hypertrichosis, immunoglobulin abnormalities, lymphadenopathy, lymphoma, macrocytosis, megaloblastic anemia, periarteritis nodosa, pseudolymphoma, SLE-like syndrome, Stevens-Johnson syndrome, toxic epidermal necrolysis, venous irritation and pain

Drug Interactions

Metabolism/Transport Effects Substrate of CYP2C19 (major), CYP2C9 (major), CYP3A4 (minor); **Note:** Assignment of Major/Minor substrate status based on clinically relevant drug interaction potential; **Induces** CYP2B6 (strong), CYP2C19 (strong), CYP2C8 (strong), CYP2C9 (strong), CYP3A4 (strong), P-glycoprotein

Avoid Concomitant Use

Avoid concomitant use of Phenytoin with any of the following: Abiraterone Acetate; Apixaban; Artemether; Axitinib; Azelastine (Nasal); Bedaquiline; Boceprevir; Bortezomib; Bosutinib; Cabozantinib; CloZAPine; Crizotinib; Dabigatran Etexilate; Darunavir; Delavirdine; Dienogest; Dolutegravir; Dronedarone; Enzalutamide; Etravirine; Everolimus; Ibrutinib; Itraconazole; Ivacaftor; Lapatinib; Lumefantrine; Lurasidone; Macitentan; Mifepristone; NIFEdipine; Nilotinib; Nisoldipine; Paraldehyde; PAZOPanib; Pomalidomide; PONATinib; Praziquantel; Ranolazine; Regorafenib; Rilpivirine; Rivaroxaban; Roflumilast; RomiDEPsin; Simeprevir; Sofosbuvir; SORAfenib; Telaprevir; Ticagrelor; Tofacitinib; Tolvaptan; Toremifene; Ulipristal; Vandetanib; Vemurafenib; VinCRIStine (Liposomal)

Increased Effect/Toxicity

Phenytoin may increase the levels/effects of: Azelastine (Nasal); Buprenorphine; Clarithromycin; CNS Depressants; Fosamprenavir; Hydrocodone; Ifosfamide; Lithium; Methotrimeprazine; Metyrosine; Mirtazapine; Neuromuscular-Blocking Agents (Nondepolarizing); Paraldehyde; PHENobarbital; Pramipexole; Prilocaine; ROPINIRole; Rotigotine; Selective Serotonin Reuptake Inhibitors; Sodium Nitrite; Vitamin K Antagonists; Zolpidem

The levels/effects of Phenytoin may be increased by: Alcohol (Ethyl); Allopurinol; Amiodarone; Antifungal Agents (Azole Derivatives, Systemic); Benzodiazepines; Brimonidine (Topical); Calcium Channel Blockers; Capecitabine; CarBAMazepine; Carbonic Anhydrase Inhibitors; CeFAZolin; Chloramphenicol; Cimetidine; Clarithromycin; Cosyntropin; CYP2C19 Inhibitors (Moderate); CYP2C19 Inhibitors (Strong); CYP2C9 Inhibitors (Moderate); CYP2C9 Inhibitors (Strong); Delavirdine; Dexmethylphenidate; Disulfiram; Doxylamine; Droperidol; Efavirenz; Eslicarbazepine; Ethosuximide; Felbamate; Floxuridine; Fluconazole; Fluorouracil (Systemic); Fluorouracil (Topical); FLUoxetine; FluvoxaMINE; Halothane; HydrOXYzine; Isoniazid; Luliconazole; Magnesium Sulfate; Methotrimeprazine; Methylphenidate; MetroNIDAZOLE (Systemic); Nitric Oxide; Omeprazole; OXcarbazepine; Rufinamide; Sertraline; Sodium Oxybate; Tacrolimus (Systemic); Tapentadol; Tegafur; Telaprevir; Ticlopidine; Topiramate; TraZODone; Trimethoprim; Vitamin K Antagonists

Decreased Effect

Phenytoin may decrease the levels/effects of: Abiraterone Acetate; Acetaminophen; Afatinib; Amiodarone; Antifungal Agents (Azole Derivatives, Systemic); Apixaban; ARIPiprazole; Artemether; Axitinib; Bedaquiline; Boceprevir; Bortezomib; Bosutinib; Brentuximab Vedotin;

Busulfan; Cabozantinib; Canagliflozin; CarBAMazepine; Caspofungin; Chloramphenicol; Clarithromycin; CloZAPine; Cobicistat; Contraceptives (Estrogens); Contraceptives (Progestins); Crizotinib; CycloSPORINE (Systemic); CYP2B6 Substrates; CYP2C19 Substrates; CYP2C8 Substrates; CYP2C9 Substrates; CYP3A4 Substrates; Dabigatran Etexilate; Darunavir; Dasatinib; Deferasirox; Delavirdine; Diclofenac (Systemic); Dienogest; Disopyramide; Dolutegravir; Doxycycline; Dronedarone; Efavirenz; Elvitegravir; Enzalutamide; Eslicarbazepine; Ethosuximide; Etoposide; Etoposide Phosphate; Etravirine; Everolimus; Exemestane; Ezogabine; Felbamate; Flunarizine; Gefitinib; GuanFACINE; HMG-CoA Reductase Inhibitors; Ibrutinib; Imatinib; Irinotecan; Itraconazole; Ivacaftor; Ixabepilone; Lacosamide; LamoTRIgine; Lapatinib; Levodopa; Linagliptin; Loop Diuretics; Lopinavir; Lumefantrine; Lurasidone; Macitentan; Maraviroc; Mebendazole; Meperidine; Methadone; MethylPREDNISolone; MetroNIDAZOLE (Systemic); Metyrapone; Mexiletine; Mifepristone; Nelfinavir; Neuromuscular-Blocking Agents (Nondepolarizing); NIFEdipine; Nilotinib; Nisoldipine; Omeprazole; OXcarbazepine; PAZOPanib; Perampanel; P-glycoprotein/ABCB1 Substrates; Pomalidomide; PONATinib; Praziquantel; PrednisoLONE (Systemic); PredniSONE; Primidone; QUEtiapine; QuiNIDine; QuiNINE; Ranolazine; Regorafenib; Rilpivirine; Ritonavir; Rivaroxaban; Roflumilast; RomiDEPsin; Rufinamide; Saxagliptin; Sertraline; Simeprevir; Sirolimus; Sofosbuvir; SORAfenib; SUNItinib; Tacrolimus (Systemic); Tadalafil; Telaprevir; Temsirolimus; Teniposide; Theophylline Derivatives; Thyroid Products; Ticagrelor; Tipranavir; Tofacitinib; Tolvaptan; Topiramate; Topotecan; Toremifene; TraZODone; Treprostinil; Trimethoprim; Ulipristal; Valproic Acid and Derivatives; Vandetanib; Vemurafenib; VinCRIStine; VinCRIStine (Liposomal); Vortioxetine; Zonisamide; Zuclopenthixol

The levels/effects of Phenytoin may be decreased by: Alcohol (Ethyl); Amphetamines; Antacids; Bleomycin; CarBAMazepine; Ciprofloxacin (Systemic); Colesevelam; CYP2C19 Inducers (Strong); CYP2C9 Inducers (Strong); Dabrafenib; Diazoxide; Enzalutamide; Folic Acid; Fosamprenavir; Ketorolac (Nasal); Ketorolac (Systemic); Leucovorin Calcium-Levoleucovorin; Levomefolate; Lopinavir; Mefloquine; Methotrexate; Methylfolate; Multivitamins/Minerals (with ADEK, Folate, Iron); Nelfinavir; Orlistat; Peginterferon Alfa-2b; PHENobarbital; Platinum Derivatives; Pyridoxine; Rifampin; Ritonavir; Theophylline Derivatives; Tipranavir; Valproic Acid and Derivatives; Vigabatrin; VinCRIStine

Ethanol/Nutrition/Herb Interactions

Ethanol:

Acute use: Ethanol inhibits metabolism of phenytoin and may also increase CNS depression. Management: Avoid or limit ethanol. Caution patients about effects.

Chronic use: Ethanol stimulates metabolism of phenytoin. Management: Avoid or limit ethanol.

Food: Phenytoin serum concentrations may be altered if taken with food. If taken with enteral nutrition, phenytoin serum concentrations may be decreased. Tube feedings decrease bioavailability. Phenytoin may decrease calcium, folic acid, and vitamin D levels. Supplementing folic acid may lower the seizure threshold. Management: Hold tube feedings 1-2 hours before and 1-2 hours after phenytoin administration. Do not supplement folic acid. Consider vitamin D supplementation. Take preferably on an empty stomach.

Herb/Nutraceutical: Evening primrose may decrease the seizure threshold; other herbal medications may increase CNS depression. Management: Avoid evening primrose, valerian, St John's wort, kava kava, and gotu kola.

Preparation for Administration I.V.: May be further diluted in NS to a final concentration ≥5 mg/mL; infusion must be completed within 4 hours after preparation. Do not refrigerate.

Storage/Stability

Capsule, tablet: Store at 20°C to 25°C (68°F to 77°F). Protect capsules from light. Protect capsules and tablets from moisture.

Oral suspension: Store at room temperature of 20°C to 25°C (68°F to 77°F); do not freeze. Protect from light.

Solution for injection: Store at room temperature of 15°C to 30°C (59°F to 86°F). Use only clear solutions free of precipitate and haziness; slightly yellow solutions may be used. Precipitation may occur if solution is refrigerated and may dissolve at room temperature.

Mechanism of Action Stabilizes neuronal membranes and decreases seizure activity by increasing efflux or decreasing influx of sodium ions across cell membranes in the motor cortex during generation of nerve impulses; prolongs effective refractory period and suppresses ventricular pacemaker automaticity, shortens action potential in the heart

Pharmacodynamics/Kinetics

Onset of action: I.V.: ~0.5-1 hour

Absorption: Oral: Slow

Distribution: V_d:

- Neonates: Premature: 1-1.2 L/kg; Full-term: 0.8-0.9 L/kg
- Infants: 0.7-0.8 L/kg
- Children: 0.7 L/kg
- Adults: 0.6-0.7 L/kg

Protein binding:

- Neonates: ≥80% (≤20% free)
- Infants: ≥85% (≤15% free)
- Adults: 90% to 95%
- Others: Decreased protein binding
  - **Disease states resulting in a decrease in serum albumin concentration**: Burns, hepatic cirrhosis, nephrotic syndrome, pregnancy, cystic fibrosis
  - **Disease states resulting in an apparent decrease in affinity of phenytoin for serum albumin**: Renal failure, jaundice (severe), other drugs (displacers), hyperbilirubinemia (total bilirubin >15 mg/dL), Cl_{cr} <25 mL/minute (unbound fraction is increased two- to threefold in uremia)

Metabolism: Follows dose-dependent capacity-limited (Michaelis-Menten) pharmacokinetics with increased V_{max} (ie, metabolic capacity) in infants >6 months of age and children versus adults; major metabolite (via oxidation), HPPA, undergoes enterohepatic recirculation

Bioavailability: Formulation dependent

Half-life elimination: Range: 7-42 hours; **Note:** Elimination is not first-order (ie, follows Michaelis-Menten pharmacokinetics); half-life increases with increasing phenytoin concentrations; best described using parameters such as V_{max} (metabolic capacity) and Km (constant equal to the concentration at which the rate of metabolism is 1/2 of V_{max}).

Time to peak, serum (formulation dependent): Oral: Extended-release capsule: 4-12 hours; Immediate release preparation: 2-3 hours

Excretion: Urine (<5% as unchanged drug); as glucuronides

Clearance: Highly variable, dependent upon intrinsic hepatic function and dose administered; increased clearance and decreased serum concentrations with febrile illness

Dosage Note: Phenytoin base (eg, oral suspension, chewable tablets) contains ~8% more drug than phenytoin sodium (~92 mg base is equivalent to 100 mg phenytoin sodium). Dosage adjustments and closer serum monitoring may be necessary when switching dosage forms.

Status epilepticus: I.V.:

Infants and Children: Loading dose: 15-20 mg/kg, then begin maintenance therapy usually 12 hours after loading dose

Adolescents and Adults: Loading dose: Manufacturer recommends 10-15 mg/kg; however, 15-20 mg/kg at a maximum rate of 50 mg/minute is generally recommended (Kalvianines, 2007; Lowenstein, 2005); initial maintenance dose: I.V. or Oral: 100 mg every 6-8 hours

Anticonvulsant (nonemergent use): Oral:

Loading dose: Children, Adolescents, and Adults: 15-20 mg/kg; consider prior phenytoin serum concentrations and/or recent dosing history if available; administer oral loading dose in 3 divided doses given every 2-4 hours to decrease GI adverse effects and to ensure complete oral absorption

Maintenance dose:

Infants and Children: Initial maintenance dose: 5 mg/kg/day in 2-3 divided doses; usual maintenance dose range: 4-8 mg/kg/day; maximum daily dose: 300 mg. Some experts suggest higher maintenance doses may be necessary in infant and young children (range: 8-10 mg/kg/day in divided doses).

Adolescents and Adults: Initial maintenance dose: 300 mg daily in 3 divided doses; may also administer in 1-2 divided doses using extended release formulation; adjust dosage based on individual requirements; usual maintenance dose range: 300-600 mg daily

Dosing adjustment in renal impairment: No dosage adjustment provided in manufacturer's labeling; <5% excreted as unchanged drug. Serum concentration may be difficult to interpret in renal failure. Monitoring of free (unbound) concentrations or adjustment to allow interpretation is recommended.

Dosage adjustment in hepatic impairment: No dosage adjustment provided in manufacturer's labeling; undergoes hepatic metabolism and clearance may be decreased. Monitor free phenytoin levels closely. Dosage adjustments may be necessary.

Dosage in obesity: Adults: Loading dose: Use adjusted body weight (AdjBW) correction based on a pharmacokinetic study of phenytoin loading doses in obese patients (Abernethy, 1985). The larger correction factor (ie, 1.33) is due to a doubling of V_d estimated in these obese patients.

AdjBW = [(Actual body weight – IBW) x 1.33] + IBW

Maintenance doses should be based on ideal body weight, conventional daily doses with adjustments based upon therapeutic drug monitoring and clinical effectiveness. (Abernethy, 1985; Erstad, 2002; Erstad, 2004)

Dietary Considerations

Folic acid: Phenytoin may decrease mucosal uptake of folic acid; to avoid folic acid deficiency and megaloblastic anemia, some clinicians recommend giving patients on anticonvulsants prophylactic doses of folic acid and cyanocobalamin. Folic acid 0.5 mg/day has been shown to reduce the incidence of phenytoin-induced gingival overgrowth in children (Arya, 2011). However, folate supplementation may increase seizures in some patients (dose dependent). Discuss with healthcare provider prior to using any supplements.

Calcium: Hypocalcemia has been reported in patients taking prolonged high-dose therapy with an anticonvulsant. Some clinicians have given an additional 4000 units/week of vitamin D (especially in those receiving poor nutrition and getting no sun exposure) to prevent hypocalcemia.

Vitamin D: Phenytoin interferes with vitamin D metabolism and osteomalacia may result; may need to supplement with vitamin D

Tube feedings: Tube feedings decrease phenytoin absorption. To avoid decreased serum levels with continuous NG feeds, hold feedings for 1-2 hours prior to and 1-2 hours after phenytoin administration, if possible. There is a variety of opinions on how to administer phenytoin with enteral feedings. Be **consistent** throughout therapy.

Injection may contain sodium.

Administration

Oral: Suspension: Shake well prior to use. Absorption is impaired when phenytoin suspension is given concurrently to patients who are receiving continuous nasogastric feedings. A method to resolve this interaction is to divide the daily dose of phenytoin and withhold the administration of nutritional supplements for 1-2 hours before and after each phenytoin dose.

I.M.: **Avoid** I.M. administration due to severe risk of local tissue destruction and necrosis; use **fos**phenytoin if I.M. administration necessary (Boucher, 1996; Meek, 1999). The manufacturer's labeling includes I.M. administration; however, in general the I.M. route should be avoided and should **NOT** be used for status epilepticus.

I.V.: Fosphenytoin may be considered for loading in patients who are in status epilepticus, hemodynamically unstable, or develop hypotension/bradycardia with I.V. administration of phenytoin. Although, phenytoin may be administered by direct I.V. injection, it is preferable that phenytoin be administered via infusion pump either undiluted or diluted in normal saline as an I.V. piggyback (IVPB) to prevent exceeding the maximum infusion rate (monitor closely for extravasation during infusion). The maximum rate of I.V. administration is 50 mg/minute in adults. Highly sensitive patients (eg, elderly, patients with pre-existing cardiovascular conditions) should receive phenytoin more slowly (eg, 20 mg/minute) (Meek, 1999). In neonates, the manufacturer recommends a maximum rate of 1-3 mg/kg/minute; however, a lower maximum rate of 0.5-1 mg/kg/minute is used clinically (Sankar, 2010; Shields, 1989). An in-line 0.22-0.55 micron filter is recommended for IVPB solutions due to the potential for precipitation of the solution. Following I.V. administration, NS should be injected through the same needle or I.V. catheter to prevent irritation.

Vesicant; ensure proper needle or catheter placement prior to and during I.V. infusion. Avoid extravasation.

Extravasation management: If extravasation occurs, stop infusion immediately and disconnect (leave needle/cannula in place); gently aspirate extravasated solution (do **NOT** flush the line); remove needle/cannula; elevate extremity. There is conflicting information regarding an antidote; some sources recommend not to use an antidote (Montgomery, 1999 [pediatric reference]), while other sources recommend hyaluronidase.

Hyaluronidase (if appropriate): SubQ: Administer four separate 0.2 mL injections of a 15 units/mL solution (using a 25-gauge needle) into area of extravasation (Sokol, 1998)

SubQ: SubQ administration is not recommended because of the possibility of local tissue damage (due to high pH).

Monitoring Parameters CBC, liver function; suicidality (eg, suicidal thoughts, depression, behavioral changes); plasma phenytoin concentrations (if available, free phenytoin concentrations should be obtained in patients with renal impairment and/or hypoalbuminemia; if free phenytoin concentrations are unavailable, the adjusted total concentration may be determined based upon equations in adult patients). Trough concentrations are generally recommended for routine monitoring.

Additional monitoring with I.V. use: Continuous cardiac monitoring (rate, rhythm, blood pressure) and observation during administration recommended; blood pressure and pulse should be monitored every 15 minutes for 1 hour after administration (Meek, 1999); infusion site reactions

Consult individual institutional policies and procedures.

Reference Range Timing of serum samples: Because it is slowly absorbed, peak blood levels may occur 4-8 hours after ingestion of an oral dose. The serum half-life varies with the dosage and the drug follows Michaelis-Menten kinetics. The average adult half-life is about 24 hours. Steady-state concentrations are reached in 5-10 days.

Children and Adults: Toxicity is measured clinically, and some patients require levels outside the suggested therapeutic range

Therapeutic range:

Total phenytoin: 10-20 mcg/mL (children and adults), 8-15 mcg/mL (neonates)

Concentrations of 5-10 mcg/mL may be therapeutic for some patients but concentrations <5 mcg/mL are not likely to be effective

50% of patients show decreased frequency of seizures at concentrations >10 mcg/mL

86% of patients show decreased frequency of seizures at concentrations >15 mcg/mL

Add another anticonvulsant if satisfactory therapeutic response is not achieved with a phenytoin concentration of 20 mcg/mL

Free phenytoin: 1-2.5 mcg/mL

Total phenytoin:

Toxic: >30 mcg/mL (SI: >119 micromole/L)

Lethal: >100 mcg/mL (SI: >400 micromole/L)

When to draw levels (Winter, 2010):

Key points: Time of sampling is dependent on the disease state being treated and the clinical condition of the patient. Trough concentrations are generally recommended for routine monitoring. However, timing of sampling is not as critical in patients receiving the extended-release dosage form because the slow absorption minimizes the fluctuations between peak and trough concentrations.

After a loading dose:

First concentration: It is prudent to draw within 2-3 days of therapy initiation to ensure that the patient's metabolism is not remarkably altered. Alternatively, if rapid therapeutic levels are needed, a level may be drawn 2 hours after completion of an I.V. loading dose (Meek, 1999) or 24 hours after administration of an oral loading dose (Osborn, 1987) to aid in determining maintenance dose or need to reload.

Second concentration: Draw within 5-8 days of therapy initiation with subsequent doses of phenytoin adjusted accordingly

If plasma concentrations have not changed over a 3- to 5-day period, monitoring interval may be increased to once weekly in the acute clinical setting. In stable patients requiring long-term therapy, generally monitor levels at 3- to 12-month intervals

Adjustment of serum concentration: See tables.

Note: Although it is ideal to obtain free phenytoin concentrations to assess serum concentrations in patients with hypoalbuminemia or renal failure (Cl_{cr} ≤10 mL/minute), it may not always be possible. If free phenytoin concentrations are unavailable, the following equations may be utilized in adult patients.

Adjustment of Serum Concentration in Adults With Low Serum Albumin

Measured Total Phenytoin Concentration (mcg/mL)	Patient's Serum Albumin (g/dL)			
	3.5	3	2.5	2
	Adjusted Total Phenytoin Concentration (mcg/mL)[1]			
5	6	7	8	10
10	13	14	17	20
15	19	21	25	30

[1]Adjusted concentration = measured total concentration divided by [(0.2 x albumin) + 0.1].

Adjustment of Serum Concentration in Adults With Renal Failure (Cl_{cr} ≤10 mL/min)

Measured Total Phenytoin Concentration (mcg/mL)	Patient's Serum Albumin (g/dL)				
	4	3.5	3	2.5	2
	Adjusted Total Phenytoin Concentration (mcg/mL)[1]				
5	10	11	13	14	17
10	20	22	25	29	33
15	30	33	38	43	50

[1]Adjusted concentration = measured total concentration divided by [(0.1 x albumin) + 0.1].

Dosage Forms Excipient information presented when available (limited, particularly for generics); consult specific product labeling.

Capsule, Oral, as sodium:

Dilantin: 30 mg [contains fd&c yellow #10 (quinoline yellow)]

Dilantin: 100 mg

Phenytek: 200 mg, 300 mg [contains brilliant blue fcf (fd&c blue #1), fd&c blue #1 aluminum lake, fd&c blue #2 aluminum lake, fd&c red #40 aluminum lake, fd&c yellow #10 aluminum lake]

Generic: 100 mg, 200 mg, 300 mg

Solution, Injection, as sodium:

Generic: 50 mg/mL (2 mL, 5 mL)

Suspension, Oral:

Dilantin: 125 mg/5 mL (237 mL) [orange-vanilla flavor]

Generic: 125 mg/5 mL (4 mL, 237 mL)

Tablet Chewable, Oral:

Dilantin Infatabs: 50 mg [scored]

Phenytoin Infatabs: 50 mg [scored; contains fd&c yellow #10 aluminum lake, fd&c yellow #6 aluminum lake, saccharin sodium]

Generic: 50 mg

◆ **Phenytoin Infatabs** *see* Phenytoin *on page 1638*

◆ **Phenytoin Sodium** *see* Phenytoin *on page 1638*

◆ **Phenytoin Sodium, Extended** *see* Phenytoin *on page 1638*

◆ **Phenytoin Sodium, Prompt** *see* Phenytoin *on page 1638*

◆ **Philith** *see* Ethinyl Estradiol and Norethindrone *on page 793*

◆ **Phillips'® M-O [OTC]** *see* Magnesium Hydroxide and Mineral Oil *on page 1261*

◆ **PHL-Alendronate (Can)** *see* Alendronate *on page 69*

◆ **PHL-Amantadine (Can)** *see* Amantadine *on page 92*

◆ **PHL-Amiodarone (Can)** *see* Amiodarone *on page 101*

◆ **PHL-Amlodipine (Can)** *see* AmLODIPine *on page 109*

- PHL-Amoxicillin (Can) *see* Amoxicillin *on page 116*
- PHL-Azithromycin (Can) *see* Azithromycin (Systemic) *on page 214*
- PHL-Baclofen (Can) *see* Baclofen *on page 221*
- PHL-Bethanechol (Can) *see* Bethanechol *on page 250*
- PHL-Bicalutamide (Can) *see* Bicalutamide *on page 258*
- PHL-Bisoprolol (Can) *see* Bisoprolol *on page 261*
- PHL-Ciprofloxacin (Can) *see* Ciprofloxacin (Systemic) *on page 430*
- PHL-Citalopram (Can) *see* Citalopram *on page 440*
- PHL-Clonazepam (Can) *see* ClonazePAM *on page 465*
- PHL-Clonazepam-R (Can) *see* ClonazePAM *on page 465*
- PHL-Cyclobenzaprine (Can) *see* Cyclobenzaprine *on page 502*
- PHL-Dexamethasone (Can) *see* Dexamethasone (Systemic) *on page 580*
- PHL-Divalproex (Can) *see* Valproic Acid and Derivatives *on page 2149*
- PHL-Doxycycline (Can) *see* Doxycycline *on page 668*
- PHL-Fenofibrate Micro (Can) *see* Fenofibrate and Derivatives *on page 837*
- PHL-Fluconazole (Can) *see* Fluconazole *on page 868*
- PHL-Fluoxetine (Can) *see* FLUoxetine *on page 885*
- PHL-Fluvoxamine (Can) *see* FluvoxaMINE *on page 903*
- PHL-Gabapentin (Can) *see* Gabapentin *on page 933*
- PHL-Indapamide (Can) *see* Indapamide *on page 1066*
- PHL-Leflunomide (Can) *see* Leflunomide *on page 1178*
- PHL-Levetiracetam (Can) *see* LevETIRAcetam *on page 1194*
- PHL-Lithium Carbonate (Can) *see* Lithium *on page 1229*
- PHL-Lorazepam (Can) *see* LORazepam *on page 1242*
- PHL-Lovastatin (Can) *see* Lovastatin *on page 1250*
- PHL-Loxapine (Can) *see* Loxapine *on page 1253*
- PHL-Meloxicam (Can) *see* Meloxicam *on page 1284*
- PHL-Metformin (Can) *see* MetFORMIN *on page 1310*
- PHL-Methimazole (Can) *see* Methimazole *on page 1321*
- PHL-Methylphenidate (Can) *see* Methylphenidate *on page 1336*
- PHL-Minocycline (Can) *see* Minocycline *on page 1373*
- PHL-Olanzapine (Can) *see* OLANZapine *on page 1493*
- PHL-Olanzapine ODT (Can) *see* OLANZapine *on page 1493*
- PHL-Ondansetron (Can) *see* Ondansetron *on page 1510*
- PHL-Oxybutynin (Can) *see* Oxybutynin *on page 1533*
- PHL-Paroxetine (Can) *see* PARoxetine *on page 1575*
- PHL-Pioglitazone (Can) *see* Pioglitazone *on page 1649*
- PHL-Pravastatin (Can) *see* Pravastatin *on page 1700*
- PHL-Quetiapine (Can) *see* QUEtiapine *on page 1757*
- PHL-Ranitidine (Can) *see* Ranitidine *on page 1782*
- PHL-Risperidone (Can) *see* RisperiDONE *on page 1826*
- PHL-Salbutamol (Can) *see* Albuterol *on page 61*
- PHL-Sertraline (Can) *see* Sertraline *on page 1889*
- PHL-Simvastatin (Can) *see* Simvastatin *on page 1899*
- PHL-Sotalol (Can) *see* Sotalol *on page 1942*
- PHL-Sumatriptan (Can) *see* SUMAtriptan *on page 1969*
- PHL-Temazepam (Can) *see* Temazepam *on page 2005*
- PHL-Terazosin (Can) *see* Terazosin *on page 2015*
- PHL-Terbinafine (Can) *see* Terbinafine (Systemic) *on page 2017*
- PHL-Topiramate (Can) *see* Topiramate *on page 2090*
- PHL-Trazodone (Can) *see* TraZODone *on page 2112*
- PHL-Ursodiol C (Can) *see* Ursodiol *on page 2142*
- PHL-Valacyclovir (Can) *see* ValACYclovir *on page 2145*
- PHL-Valproic Acid (Can) *see* Valproic Acid and Derivatives *on page 2149*
- PHL-Valproic Acid E.C. (Can) *see* Valproic Acid and Derivatives *on page 2149*
- PHL-Verapamil SR (Can) *see* Verapamil *on page 2182*
- Phos-Flur® *see* Fluoride *on page 880*
- Phos-Flur® Rinse [OTC] *see* Fluoride *on page 880*
- PhosLo *see* Calcium Acetate *on page 317*
- PhosLo® (Can) *see* Calcium Acetate *on page 317*
- Phoslyra *see* Calcium Acetate *on page 317*
- Phos-NaK *see* Potassium Phosphate and Sodium Phosphate *on page 1691*
- Phospha 250™ Neutral *see* Potassium Phosphate and Sodium Phosphate *on page 1691*
- Phosphasal™ *see* Methenamine, Sodium Biphosphate, Phenyl Salicylate, Methylene Blue, and Hyoscyamine *on page 1320*
- Phosphate, Potassium *see* Potassium Phosphate *on page 1690*
- Phosphates, Sodium *see* Sodium Phosphates *on page 1923*
- Phospholine Iodide *see* Echothiophate Iodide *on page 682*
- Phosphonoformate *see* Foscarnet *on page 920*
- Phosphonoformic Acid *see* Foscarnet *on page 920*
- Photofrin *see* Porfimer *on page 1679*
- Photofrin® (Can) *see* Porfimer *on page 1679*
- Phrenilin Forte *see* Butalbital and Acetaminophen *on page 305*
- *p*-Hydroxyampicillin *see* Amoxicillin *on page 116*
- Phylloquinone *see* Phytonadione *on page 1644*
- Physicians EZ Use B-12 *see* Cyanocobalamin *on page 501*
- Physicians EZ Use Flu *see* Influenza Virus Vaccine (Inactivated) *on page 1078*

Physostigmine (fye zoe STIG meen)

Index Terms Eserine Salicylate; Physostigmine Salicylate; Physostigmine Sulfate

Pharmacologic Category Acetylcholinesterase Inhibitor; Antidote

Use Reversal of central nervous system anticholinergic syndrome

Note: Physostigmine should only be used to reverse toxic, life-threatening delirium caused by pure anticholinergic agents (ie, atropine, diphenhydramine, dimenhydrinate, *Atropa belladonna* [deadly nightshade], or jimson weed [*Datura* spp]). Consultation with a clinical toxicologist or poison control center is recommended in patients who require physostigmine administration.

Pregnancy Considerations In general, medications used as antidotes should take into consideration the health and prognosis of the mother; antidotes should be administered to pregnant women if there is a clear indication for use and should not be withheld because of fears of teratogenicity (Bailey, 2003).

Breast-Feeding Considerations It is not known if physostigmine is excreted in breast milk. According to the manufacturer, the decision to continue or discontinue breast-feeding during therapy should take into account the risk of exposure to the infant and the benefits of treatment to the mother.

Contraindications Gastrointestinal or genitourinary obstruction; asthma; gangrene; diabetes; cardiovascular disease; any vagotonic state; coadministration of choline esters and depolarizing neuromuscular-blocking agents (eg, succinylcholine)

Warnings/Precautions Hazardous agent - use appropriate precautions for handling and disposal (EPA, P-listed). Patient must have a normal QRS interval, as measured by ECG, in order to receive; use caution in poisoning with agents known to prolong intraventricular conduction (Howland, 2011). Discontinue if symptoms of excessive cholinergic activity occur (eg, salivation, urinary incontinence, defecation, vomiting); overdosage may result in cholinergic crisis, which must be distinguished from myasthenic crisis. If excessive diaphoresis or nausea occurs, reduce subsequent doses. Due to the possibility of hypersensitivity or overdose/cholinergic crisis, atropine should be readily available. When administering by I.V. injection, administer no faster than 1 mg/minute in adults or 0.5 mg/minute in children to prevent bradycardia, respiratory distress, and seizures from too rapid administration. Although the use of continuous infusions of physostigmine have been described in the literature (Eyer, 2008; Hail, 2013), experts do not recommend the routine use of continuous infusions. It is preferable to titrate physostigmine to patient needs through the use of intermittent administration; intermittent administration will minimize the risk of cholinergic toxicity, which can be associated with considerable morbidity. Asystole and seizures have been reported when physostigmine was administered to TCA poisoned patients. Physostigmine is not recommended in patients with known or suspected TCA intoxication. Products may contain benzyl alcohol which has been associated with "gasping syndrome" in neonates. Products may contain sodium metabisulfite which may cause allergic reactions in some individuals. Hazardous agent; use appropriate precautions for handling and disposal (EPA, P-listed).

Adverse Reactions Frequency not defined.

Cardiovascular: Asystole, bradycardia, palpitation

Central nervous system: Hallucinations, nervousness, restlessness, seizure

Gastrointestinal: Defecation, diarrhea, nausea, salivation, stomach pain, vomiting

Genitourinary: Urinary frequency

Neuromuscular & skeletal: Twitching

Ocular: Lacrimation, miosis

Respiratory: Bronchospasm, dyspnea, pulmonary edema, respiratory distress, respiratory paralysis

Miscellaneous: Diaphoresis, hypersensitivity

Drug Interactions

Metabolism/Transport Effects None known.

Avoid Concomitant Use There are no known interactions where it is recommended to avoid concomitant use.

Increased Effect/Toxicity

Physostigmine may increase the levels/effects of: Beta-Blockers; Cholinergic Agonists; Succinylcholine

The levels/effects of Physostigmine may be increased by: Corticosteroids (Systemic)

Decreased Effect

Physostigmine may decrease the levels/effects of: Neuromuscular-Blocking Agents (Nondepolarizing)

The levels/effects of Physostigmine may be decreased by: Dipyridamole

Ethanol/Nutrition/Herb Interactions Herb/Nutraceutical: Ginkgo biloba may enhance the adverse/toxic effect of physostigmine; monitor.

Preparation for Administration Hazardous agent; use appropriate precautions for handling and disposal (EPA, P-listed).

Storage/Stability Store at 20°C to 25°C (68°F to 77°F).

Mechanism of Action Physostigmine is a carbamate which inhibits the enzyme acetylcholinesterase and prolongs the central and peripheral effects of acetylcholine

Pharmacodynamics/Kinetics

Onset of action: Approximately several minutes

Duration: 45-60 minutes

Absorption: I.M.: Readily absorbed

Distribution: Crosses blood-brain barrier readily and reverses both central and peripheral anticholinergic effects

Metabolism: Via hydrolysis by cholinesterases

Dosage Reversal of toxic anticholinergic effects:

Children: **Note:** Reserve for life-threatening situations only. When administering by I.V. injection, administer no faster than 0.5 mg/minute to prevent bradycardia, respiratory distress, and seizures from too rapid administration.

I.M., I.V.: Initial: 0.02 mg/kg; may repeat every 5-10 minutes until response occurs (maximum total dose: 2 mg)

Adults: **Note:** When administering by I.V. injection, administer no faster than 1 mg/minute to prevent bradycardia, respiratory distress, and seizures from too rapid administration.

I.M., I.V.: Initial: 0.5-2 mg; may repeat every 10-30 minutes until response occurs. Subsequent doses may be required to manage life-threatening anticholinergic effects (Krenzelok, 2010).

Dosage adjustment in renal impairment: No dosage adjustment provided in manufacturer's labeling.

Dosage adjustment in hepatic impairment: No dosage adjustment provided in manufacturer's labeling.

Administration I.V.: Infuse no faster than 1 mg/minute in adults or 0.5 mg/minute in children. Too rapid administration can cause bradycardia, respiratory distress, and seizures. May also be administered I.M. (according to the manufacturer's labeling).

Hazardous agent; use appropriate precautions for handling and disposal (EPA, P-listed).

Monitoring Parameters ECG, vital signs; consult individual institutional policies and procedures

Test Interactions Increased aminotransferase [ALT/AST] (S), increased amylase (S)

Dosage Forms Excipient information presented when available (limited, particularly for generics); consult specific product labeling.

Solution, Injection, as salicylate:

Generic: 1 mg/mL (2 mL)

◆ Physostigmine Salicylate *see* Physostigmine *on page 1643*

◆ Physostigmine Sulfate *see* Physostigmine *on page 1643*

◆ Phytomenadione *see* Phytonadione *on page 1644*

Phytonadione (fye toe na DYE one)

Brand Names: U.S. Mephyton®

Brand Names: Canada AquaMEPHYTON®; Konakion; Mephyton®

Index Terms Methylphytyl Napthoquinone; Phylloquinone; Phytomenadione; Vitamin K; Vitamin K_1

Pharmacologic Category Vitamin, Fat Soluble

Additional Appendix Information

Reversal of Oral Anticoagulants *on page 2308*

Use Prevention and treatment of hypoprothrombinemia caused by vitamin K antagonist (VKA)-induced (eg, warfarin-induced) or other drug-induced vitamin K deficiency, altered activity, or altered metabolism; hypoprothrombinemia caused by malabsorption or inability to synthesize vitamin K; prophylaxis and treatment of hemorrhagic disease of the newborn

Unlabeled Use Treatment of hypoprothrombinemia caused by long-acting anticoagulant rodenticides (LAARs)

Pregnancy Risk Factor C

Pregnancy Considerations Animal reproduction studies have not been conducted. Phytonadione crosses the placenta in limited concentrations (Kazzi, 1990). The dietary requirements of vitamin K are the same in pregnant and nonpregnant women (IOM, 2000). In general, medications used as antidotes should take into consideration the health and prognosis of the mother; antidotes should be administered to pregnant women if there is a clear indication for use and should not be withheld because of fears of teratogenicity (Bailey, 2003).

Breast-Feeding Considerations Small amounts of dietary vitamin K can be detected in breast milk and the dietary requirements of vitamin K are the same in nursing and non-nursing women (IOM, 2000). Information following the use of phytonadione has not been located. The manufacturer recommends caution be used if phytonadione is administered to a nursing woman.

Contraindications Hypersensitivity to phytonadione or any component of the formulation

Warnings/Precautions [U.S. Boxed Warning]: Severe reactions resembling hypersensitivity reactions (eg, anaphylaxis) have occurred rarely during or immediately after I.V. administration (even with proper dilution and rate of administration); some patients had no previous exposure to phytonadione. Anaphylactoid reactions typically occurred when patients received large I.V. doses administered rapidly with formulations containing polyethoxylated castor oil; proper dosing, dilution, and administration will minimize risk (Ageno, 2012; Riegert-Johnson, 2002). Limit I.V. administration to situations where an alternative route of administration is not feasible and the benefit of therapy outweighs the risk of hypersensitivity reactions. Allergic reactions have also occurred with I.M. and SubQ injections, albeit less frequently. In obstructive jaundice or with biliary fistulas concurrent administration of bile salts is necessary. Manufacturers recommend the SubQ route over other parenteral routes. SubQ is less predictable when compared to the oral route. The American College of Chest Physicians recommends the I.V. route in patients with major bleeding secondary to warfarin. The I.V. route should be restricted to emergency situations where oral phytonadione cannot be used. Efficacy is delayed regardless of route of administration; patient management may require other treatments in the interim. In patients receiving a therapeutic vitamin K antagonist (VKA) (eg, warfarin), administer a dose of phytonadione that will quickly lower the INR into a safe range without causing resistance to warfarin. High phytonadione doses may lead to warfarin resistance for at least one week. Patients with LAAR-induced coagulopathy require much larger doses and longer treatment durations (up to months) after exposure compared to that needed to reverse VKA-induced coagulopathy. Use caution in newborns especially premature infants; hemolysis, jaundice and hyperbilirubinemia have been reported with larger than recommended doses. Some dosage forms contain benzyl alcohol which has been associated with "gasping syndrome" in premature infants. In liver disease, if initial doses do not reverse coagulopathy then higher doses are unlikely to have any effect. Ineffective in hereditary hypoprothrombinemia. Injectable products may contain aluminum; may result in toxic levels following prolonged administration. Product may contain polysorbate 80. Some dosage forms contain Cremophor® EL which has been associated with anaphylactoid reactions; use these formulations with caution.

Adverse Reactions Frequency not defined.

Cardiovascular: Cyanosis, flushing, hyper-/hypotension

Central nervous system: Dizziness

Dermatologic: Erythematous skin eruptions, pruritus, scleroderma-like lesions

Endocrine & metabolic: Hyperbilirubinemia (newborn; greater than recommended doses)

Gastrointestinal: Abnormal taste

Local: Injection site reactions

Respiratory: Dyspnea

Miscellaneous: Diaphoresis, hypersensitivity reactions, nonimmunologic anaphylaxis (formerly known as anaphylactoid reaction), sweating

Drug Interactions

Metabolism/Transport Effects None known.

Avoid Concomitant Use There are no known interactions where it is recommended to avoid concomitant use.

Increased Effect/Toxicity There are no known significant interactions involving an increase in effect.

Decreased Effect

Phytonadione may decrease the levels/effects of: Vitamin K Antagonists

The levels/effects of Phytonadione may be decreased by: Mineral Oil; Orlistat

Preparation for Administration Dilute injection solution in preservative-free NS, D_5W, or D_5NS. To reduce the incidence of anaphylactoid reaction upon I.V. administration, dilute dose in a minimum of 50 mL of compatible solution and administer using an infusion pump over at least 20 minutes (Ageno, 2012).

Storage/Stability

Injection: Store at 15°C to 30°C (59°F to 86°F). Protect from light. **Note:** Store Hospira product at 20°C to 25°C (68°F to 77°F).

Oral: Store tablets at 15°C to 30°C (59°F to 86°F). Protect from light.

Mechanism of Action Promotes liver synthesis of clotting factors (II, VII, IX, X); however, the exact mechanism as to this stimulation is unknown. Menadiol is a water soluble form of vitamin K; phytonadione has a more rapid and prolonged effect than menadione; menadiol sodium diphosphate (K_4) is half as potent as menadione (K_3).

Pharmacodynamics/Kinetics

Onset of action: Increased coagulation factors: Oral: 6-10 hours; I.V.: 1-2 hours

Peak effect: INR values return to normal: Oral: 24-48 hours; I.V.: 12-14 hours

Absorption: Oral: From intestines in presence of bile; SubQ: Variable

Metabolism: Rapidly hepatic

Excretion: Urine and feces

Dosage Note: According to the manufacturer, SubQ is the preferred parenteral route; I.M. route should be avoided due to the risk of hematoma formation; I.V. route should be restricted for emergency use only. The American College of Chest Physicians (ACCP) recommends the I.V. route in patients with major bleeding secondary to use of vitamin K antagonists (VKAs).

Adequate intake (AI): Oral:

Infants:

- 0-6 months: 2 **mcg**/day
- 7-12 months: 2.5 **mcg**/day

Children:

- 1-3 years: 30 **mcg**/day
- 4-8 years: 55 **mcg**/day
- 9-13 years: 60 **mcg**/day
- 14-18 years: 75 **mcg**/day

Adults: Males: 120 **mcg**/day; Females: 90 **mcg**/day

Hemorrhagic disease of the newborn:

Prophylaxis: I.M.: 0.5-1 mg within 1 hour of birth

Treatment: I.M., SubQ: 1 mg/dose/day; higher doses may be necessary if mother has been receiving oral anticoagulants

Hypoprothrombinemia due to drugs (other than coumarin derivatives) or factors limiting absorption or synthesis: Adults: Oral, SubQ, I.M., I.V.: Initial: 2.5-25 mg (rarely up to 50 mg)

Vitamin K deficiency (supratherapeutic INR) secondary to VKAs (eg, warfarin):

Infants and Children (unlabeled use): ***Excessively prolonged INR (usually INR >8; no significant bleeding):*** **Note:** Limited data available: I.V.: 0.03 mg/kg/dose; maximum dose: 1 mg (Bolton-Maggs, 2002); if significant bleeding, consider use of fresh frozen plasma, prothrombin complex concentrates, or recombinant factor VIIa (Monagle, 2012).

Adults (unlabeled dose):

If INR above therapeutic range to <4.5 (no evidence of bleeding): Lower or hold next VKA dose and monitor frequently; when INR approaches desired range, resume VKA dosing with a lower dose (Patriquin, 2011).

If INR 4.5-10 (no evidence of bleeding): The 2012 ACCP guidelines recommend against routine phytonadione (aka, vitamin K) administration in this setting (Guyatt, 2012). Previously, the 2008 ACCP guidelines recommended if no risk factors for bleeding exist, to omit next 1 or 2 VKA doses, monitor INR more frequently, and resume with an appropriately adjusted VKA dose when INR in desired range; may consider administering vitamin K orally 1-2.5 mg if other risk factors for bleeding exist (Hirsh, 2008). Others have recommended consideration of vitamin K 1 mg orally or 0.5 mg I.V. (Patriquin, 2011).

If INR >10 (no evidence of bleeding): The 2012 ACCP guidelines recommend administration of oral vitamin K (dose not specified) in this setting (Guyatt, 2012). Previously, the 2008 ACCP guidelines recommended to hold warfarin, administer vitamin K orally 2.5-5 mg, expect INR to be reduced within 24-48 hours, monitor INR more frequently and give additional vitamin K at an appropriate dose if necessary; resume warfarin at an appropriately adjusted dose when INR is in desired range (Hirsh, 2008). Others have recommended consideration of vitamin K 2-2.5 mg orally or 0.5-1 mg I.V. (Patriquin, 2011).

If minor bleeding at any INR elevation: Hold warfarin, may administer vitamin K orally 2.5-5 mg, monitor INR more frequently, may repeat dose after 24 hours if INR correction incomplete; resume warfarin at an appropriately adjusted dose when INR is in desired range (Patriquin, 2011).

If major bleeding at any INR elevation: The 2012 ACCP guidelines recommend administration of four-factor prothrombin complex concentrate (PCC) and I.V. vitamin K 5-10 mg in this setting (Guyatt, 2012). The only available four-factor PCC in the U.S. is Kcentra. Other four-factor PCCs **not** available in the U.S. include Beriplex P/N, Cofact, Konyne, and Octaplex. Bebulin VH and Profilnine SD **do not** contain adequate levels of factor VII and are considered **three**-factor PCCs. Previously, the 2008 ACCP guidelines recommended to hold warfarin, administer vitamin K 10 mg by slow I.V. infusion and supplement with PCC depending on the urgency of the situation; I.V. vitamin K may be repeated every 12 hours (Hirsh, 2008).

Note: Use of high doses of vitamin K (eg, 10-15 mg) may cause warfarin resistance for ≥1 week. During this period of resistance, heparin or low-molecular-weight heparin (LMWH) may be given until INR responds (Ansell, 2008).

Preprocedural/surgical INR normalization in patients receiving warfarin (routine use): Adults: Oral: 1-2.5 mg once administered on the day before surgery; recheck INR on day of procedure/surgery (Douketis, 2012). Others have recommended the use of vitamin K 1 mg orally for mild INR elevations (ie, INR 3.0-4.5) (Patriquin, 2011).

Dosage adjustment in renal impairment: No dosage adjustment provided in manufacturer's labeling.

Dosage adjustment in hepatic impairment: No dosage adjustment provided in manufacturer's labeling.

Administration

I.V. administration: Infuse slowly; rate of infusion should not exceed 1 mg/minute (3 mg/m^2/minute in children and infants). Alternatively, dilute dose in a minimum of 50 mL of compatible solution and administer using an infusion pump over at least 20 minutes (Ageno, 2012). The injectable route should be used only if the oral route is not feasible or there is a greater urgency to reverse anticoagulation.

Oral: The parenteral formulation may also be used for small oral doses (eg, 1 mg) or situations in which tablets cannot be swallowed (Crowther, 2000; O'Connor, 1986).

Monitoring Parameters PT, INR

Dosage Forms Excipient information presented when available (limited, particularly for generics); consult specific product labeling.

Injection, aqueous colloidal: 1 mg/0.5 mL (0.5 mL) [contains benzyl alcohol, polyoxyethylated castor oil]; 10 mg/mL (1 mL) [contains benzyl alcohol, polyoxyethylated castor oil]

Injection, aqueous colloidal [preservative free]: 1 mg/0.5 mL (0.5 mL) [contains polysorbate 80, propylene glycol 10.4 mg/0.5 mL]

Tablet, oral: 100 mcg

Mephyton®: 5 mg [scored]

Extemporaneous Preparations A 1 mg/mL oral suspension may be made with tablets. Crush six 5 mg tablets in a mortar and reduce to a fine powder. Add 5 mL each of water and methylcellulose 1% and mix to a uniform paste. Mix while adding sorbitol in incremental proportions to **almost** 30 mL; transfer to a calibrated bottle, rinse mortar with sorbitol, and add quantity of sorbitol sufficient to make 30 mL. Label "shake well" and "refrigerate". Stable for 3 days.

Nahata MC and Hipple TF, *Pediatric Drug Formulations*, 3rd ed, Cincinnati, OH: Harvey Whitney Books Co, 1997.

Note: The parenteral formulation may also be used for small oral doses (eg, 1 mg) or situations in which tablets cannot be swallowed (Crowther, 2000; O'Connor, 1986).

◆ **PIC 200 [OTC]** *see* Polysaccharide-Iron Complex *on page 1673*

◆ **Picato** *see* Ingenol Mebutate *on page 1085*

◆ **Picodan (Can)** *see* Sodium Picosulfate, Magnesium Oxide, and Citric Acid *on page 1925*

◆ **Picoflo (Can)** *see* Sodium Picosulfate, Magnesium Oxide, and Citric Acid *on page 1925*

◆ **Pico-Salax® (Can)** *see* Sodium Picosulfate, Magnesium Oxide, and Citric Acid *on page 1925*

◆ **Pidorubicin** *see* Epirubicin *on page 718*

◆ **Pidorubicin Hydrochloride** *see* Epirubicin *on page 718*

Pilocarpine (Systemic) (pye loe KAR peen)

Brand Names: U.S. Salagen

Brand Names: Canada Salagen®

Index Terms Pilocarpine Hydrochloride

Pharmacologic Category Cholinergic Agonist

Use Symptomatic treatment of xerostomia caused by salivary gland hypofunction resulting from radiotherapy for cancer of the head and neck or Sjögren's syndrome

Pregnancy Risk Factor C

Dosage Oral: Adults: Xerostomia:

Following head and neck cancer: 5 mg 3 times daily, titration up to 10 mg 3 times daily may be considered for patients who have not responded adequately; do not exceed 2 tablets per dose

Sjögren's syndrome: 5 mg 4 times daily

Dosage adjustment in renal impairment: No dosage adjustment necessary.

Dosage adjustment in hepatic impairment:

Mild impairment (Child-Pugh score 5-6): No dosage adjustment necessary.

Moderate impairment (Child-Pugh score 7-9): 5 mg twice daily regardless of indication; adjust dose based on response and tolerability

Severe impairment (Child-Pugh score >10): Not recommended.

Additional Information Complete prescribing information should be consulted for additional detail.

Dosage Forms Excipient information presented when available (limited, particularly for generics); consult specific product labeling.

Tablet, Oral, as hydrochloride:

Salagen: 5 mg

Salagen: 7.5 mg [contains fd&c blue #2 aluminum lake]

Generic: 5 mg, 7.5 mg

Pilocarpine (Ophthalmic) (pye loe KAR peen)

Brand Names: U.S. Isopto Carpine; Pilopine HS

Brand Names: Canada Diocarpine; Isopto® Carpine; Pilopine HS®

Index Terms Pilocarpine Hydrochloride

Pharmacologic Category Ophthalmic Agent, Antiglaucoma; Ophthalmic Agent, Miotic

Use Management of chronic simple glaucoma, chronic and acute angle-closure glaucoma

Unlabeled Use Counter effects of cycloplegics

Pregnancy Risk Factor C

Dosage Ophthalmic: Adults:

Glaucoma:

Solution: Instill 1-2 drops up to 6 times/day; adjust the concentration and frequency as required to control elevated intraocular pressure

Gel: Instill 0.5" ribbon into lower conjunctival sac once daily at bedtime

To counteract the mydriatic effects of sympathomimetic agents (unlabeled use): Solution: Instill 1 drop of a 1% solution in the affected eye

Dosage adjustment in renal impairment: No dosage adjustment provided in manufacturer's labeling.

Dosage adjustment in hepatic impairment: No dosage adjustment provided in manufacturer's labeling.

Additional Information Complete prescribing information should be consulted for additional detail.

Dosage Forms Excipient information presented when available (limited, particularly for generics); consult specific product labeling.

Gel, Ophthalmic, as hydrochloride:

Pilopine HS: 4% (4 g) [contains benzalkonium chloride, edetate disodium]

Solution, Ophthalmic, as hydrochloride:

Isopto Carpine: 1% (15 mL); 2% (15 mL); 4% (15 mL)

Generic: 1% (15 mL); 2% (15 mL); 4% (15 mL)

◆ **Pilocarpine Hydrochloride** *see* Pilocarpine (Ophthalmic) *on page 1647*

◆ **Pilocarpine Hydrochloride** *see* Pilocarpine (Systemic) *on page 1646*

◆ **Pilopine HS** *see* Pilocarpine (Ophthalmic) *on page 1647*

◆ **Pilopine HS® (Can)** *see* Pilocarpine (Ophthalmic) *on page 1647*

◆ **Pimaricin** *see* Natamycin *on page 1431*

Pimecrolimus (pim e KROE li mus)

Brand Names: U.S. Elidel

Brand Names: Canada Elidel®

Pharmacologic Category Calcineurin Inhibitor; Immunosuppressant Agent; Topical Skin Product

Use Short-term and intermittent long-term treatment of mild-to-moderate atopic dermatitis in patients not responsive to conventional therapy or when conventional therapy is not appropriate

Unlabeled Use Second-line treatment of oral lichen planus; treatment of intertriginous and facial psoriasis

Pregnancy Risk Factor C

Pregnancy Considerations Adverse events were not observed in animal reproduction studies following topical application. Experience with pimecrolimus use in pregnant women is limited.

Breast-Feeding Considerations It is not known if pimecrolimus is excreted in breast milk. Due to the potential for serious adverse reactions in the nursing infant, breast-feeding is not recommended.

Medication Guide Available Yes

Contraindications Hypersensitivity to pimecrolimus or any component of the formulation

Warnings/Precautions **[U.S. Boxed Warning]: Topical calcineurin inhibitors (including pimecrolimus) have been associated with rare cases of lymphoma and skin malignancy.** Avoid use on malignant or premalignant skin conditions (eg, cutaneous T-cell lymphoma). Topical calcineurin agents are considered second-line therapies in the treatment of atopic dermatitis/eczema, and should be limited to use in patients who have failed treatment with other therapies. **[U.S. Boxed Warning]: They should be used for short-term and intermittent treatment using the minimum amount necessary for the control of symptoms should be used.** Application should be limited to involved areas. Diagnosis should be reconfirmed if sign/symptoms do not improve within 6 weeks of treatment. Safety of intermittent use for >1 year has not been established.

May cause local symptoms (eg, burning, soreness, stinging) during first few days of treatment; usually self-resolving. Should not be used in immunocompromised patients. Do not apply to areas of active bacterial or viral infection; local infections at the treatment site should be resolved prior to therapy. Patients with atopic dermatitis are predisposed to skin infections, and pimecrolimus therapy has been associated with risk of developing eczema herpeticum, varicella zoster, and herpes simplex. Papilloma/warts have been observed with use; discontinue pimecrolimus until resolution if worsening or do not respond to conventional treatment. Pimecrolimus may be associated with development of lymphadenopathy; possible infectious causes should be investigated. Discontinue use in patients with unknown cause of lymphadenopathy or acute infectious mononucleosis. Not recommended for use in patients with skin disease which may increase the potential for systemic absorption (eg, Netherton's syndrome). Avoid artificial or natural sunlight exposure, even when pimecrolimus is not on the skin. Safety not established in patients with generalized erythroderma. **[U.S. Boxed Warning]: The use of pimecrolimus in children <2 years of age is not recommended,** particularly since the effect on immune system development is unknown.

Adverse Reactions

>10%:

Central nervous system: Headache (children and adolescents 11% to 25%; adults 7%), fever (children and adolescents 13%; adults 1%)

Infection: Influenza (3% to 13%)

Local: Local burning (adults 26%; children and adolescents 2% to 8%; tends to resolve/improve as lesions resolve), application site reaction (adults 15%; children and adolescents 2%)

Respiratory: Nasopharyngitis (infants, children, and adolescents 10% to 27%; adults 8%), upper respiratory tract infection (children and adolescents 14% to 19%; adults 4%), cough (children and adolescents 9% to 16%; adults 2%), bronchitis (children and adolescents ≤11%; adults ≤2%)

1% to 10%:

Dermatologic: Folliculitis (adults 6%; children and adolescents 1%), skin infection (5% to 6%), impetigo (4%), warts (children and adolescents ≤3%), acne vulgaris (≤2%), herpes simplex dermatitis (≤2%), molluscum contagiosum (children and adolescents ≤2%), urticaria (≤1%)

Gastrointestinal: Diarrhea (children and adolescents 1% to 8%; adults ≤2%), gastroenteritis (children and adolescents ≤7%; adults 2%), vomiting (1% to 4%), constipation (children and adolescents ≤4%), abdominal pain (≤3%), toothache (≤3%), nausea (1% to 2%)

Genitourinary: Dysmenorrhea (1% to 2%)

Hypersensitivity: Hypersensitivity (3% to 5%)

Infection: Viral infection (children and adolescents ≤7%), herpes simplex infection (≤4%), bacterial infection (1% to 2%), staphylococcal infection (1% to 2%), varicella (≤1%)

Local: Local irritation (adults ≤6%; children and adolescents ≤1%), local pruritus (1% to 6%), localized erythema (≤2%)

Neuromuscular & skeletal: Arthralgia (≤2%), back pain (≤2%)

Ocular: Conjunctivitis (≤2% to 3%), eye infection (≤1%)

Otic: Otic infection (1% to 6%), otitis media (1% to 3%)

Respiratory: Sore throat (4% to 8%), pharyngitis (children and adolescents 1% to 8%; adults 1%), tonsillitis (children and adolescents ≤6%; adults <1%), asthma (3% to 4%), asthma aggravated (children and adolescents ≤4%), streptococcal pharyngitis (children and adolescents 3%), nasal congestion (1% to 3%), sinusitis (1% to 3%), epistaxis (≤3%), dyspnea (≤2%), flu-like symptoms (≤2%), pneumonia (≤2%), rhinitis (≤2%), rhinorrhea (children and adolescents ≤2%), viral upper respiratory tract infection (≤2%), wheezing (children and adolescents ≤1%)

Miscellaneous: Laceration (children and adolescents ≤2%)

<1% (Limited to important or life-threatening): Anaphylaxis, angioedema, eczema (herpeticum), lymphadenopathy, malignant neoplasm (basal cell carcinoma, squamous cell carcinoma, malignant melanoma, malignant lymphoma), skin discoloration

Drug Interactions

Metabolism/Transport Effects Substrate of CYP3A4 (minor); **Note:** Assignment of Major/Minor substrate status based on clinically relevant drug interaction potential

Avoid Concomitant Use

Avoid concomitant use of Pimecrolimus with any of the following: Immunosuppressants

Increased Effect/Toxicity

Pimecrolimus may increase the levels/effects of: Immunosuppressants

The levels/effects of Pimecrolimus may be increased by: CYP3A4 Inhibitors (Moderate); CYP3A4 Inhibitors (Strong)

Decreased Effect There are no known significant interactions involving a decrease in effect.

Ethanol/Nutrition/Herb Interactions Ethanol: Avoid ethanol (topical pimecrolimus may increase the potential for experiencing facial flushing following the consumption of alcoholic beverages).

Storage/Stability Store at 25°C (77°F); excursions permitted to 15°C to 30°C (59°F to 86°F); do not freeze.

Mechanism of Action Penetrates inflamed epidermis to inhibit T cell activation by blocking transcription of proinflammatory cytokine genes such as interleukin-2, interferon gamma (Th1-type), interleukin-4, and interleukin-10 (Th2-type). Pimecrolimus binds to the intracellular protein FKBP-12, inhibiting calcineurin, which blocks cytokine transcription and inhibits T-cell activation. Prevents release of inflammatory cytokines and mediators from mast cells *in vitro* after stimulation by antigen/IgE.

Pharmacodynamics/Kinetics Absorption: Poor when applied to 13% to 62% body surface area in adults treated for atopic dermatitis for up to a year; detectable blood levels were observed in a higher proportion of children, as compared to adults. Does not penetrate psoriatic plaque (Menter, 2009)

Dosage

Atopic dermatitis (mild-to-moderate): Children ≥2 years, Adolescents, and Adults: Topical: Apply thin layer to affected area twice daily; rub in gently and completely. **Note:** Limit application to involved areas. Continue as long as signs and symptoms persist; discontinue if resolution occurs; re-evaluate if symptoms persist >6 weeks.

Oral lichen planus (unlabeled use): Adults: Topical: Apply twice daily for 1 month (Passeron, 2007; Volz, 2008)

Psoriasis (unlabeled use): Adults: Topical: Apply twice daily (Gribetz, 2004; Menter, 2009)

Administration Apply a thin layer to affected skin. Do not use with occlusive dressings. Burning at the application site is most common in first few days; improves as atopic dermatitis improves. Limit application to areas of involvement. Continue as long as signs and symptoms persist; discontinue if resolution occurs; re-evaluate if symptoms persist >6 weeks.

Oral lichen planus (unlabeled use): Apply to affected oral mucosa, cover with a thin layer of gauze to delay dilution with saliva (Volz, 2008). Eating, drinking or chewing gum was not allowed for 30 minutes after application (Passeron, 2007).

Dosage Forms Excipient information presented when available (limited, particularly for generics); consult specific product labeling.

Cream, External:

Elidel: 1% (30 g, 60 g, 100 g) [contains benzyl alcohol, cetyl alcohol, propylene glycol]

Pimozide (PI moe zide)

Brand Names: U.S. Orap

Brand Names: Canada Apo-Pimozide®; Orap®; PMS-Pimozide

Pharmacologic Category Antipsychotic Agent, Typical

Additional Appendix Information

Antipsychotic Agents *on page 2290*

Beers Criteria – Potentially Inappropriate Medications for Geriatrics *on page 2368*

Use Suppression of severe motor and phonic tics in patients with Tourette's disorder who have failed to respond satisfactorily to standard treatment

Unlabeled Use Psychosis; reported use in individuals with delusions focused on physical symptoms (ie, preoccupation with parasitic infestation); Huntington's chorea

Pregnancy Risk Factor C

Dosage Oral: **Note:** An ECG should be performed baseline and periodically thereafter, especially during dosage adjustment:

Children 2-12 years: Tourette's disorder: Initial: 0.05 mg/kg preferably once at bedtime; may be increased every third day to a maximum of 0.2 mg/kg/day (do not exceed 10 mg/day); usual range: 2-4 mg/day. **Note:** If therapy requires exceeding dose of 0.05 mg/kg/day, CYP2D6 geno-/phenotyping should be performed; CYP2D6 poor metabolizers should be dose titrated in ≥14-day increments and should not receive doses in excess of 0.05 mg/kg/day.

Children >12 years and Adults: Tourette's disorder: Initial: 1-2 mg/day in divided doses, then increase dosage as needed every other day; maximum dose: 10 mg/day or 0.2 mg/kg/day (whichever is less); **Note:** If therapy requires exceeding dose of 4 mg/day, CYP2D6 geno-/phenotyping should be performed; CYP2D6 poor metabolizers should be dose titrated in ≥14-day increments and should not receive doses in excess of 4 mg/day.

Elderly: Recommend initial dose of 1 mg/day; periodically attempt gradual reduction of dose to determine if tic persists; follow up for 1-2 weeks before concluding the tic is a persistent disease phenomenon and not a manifestation of drug withdrawal. **Note:** An ECG should be performed baseline and periodically thereafter, especially during dosage adjustment.

Dosage adjustment for toxicity:

ECG changes:

Children: QT_c prolongation >0.47 seconds or >25% above baseline: Decrease dose

Adults: QT_c prolongation >0.52 seconds or >25% above baseline: Decrease dose

NMS syndrome: Discontinue (monitor carefully if therapy is reinitiated)

Tardive dyskinesia signs/symptoms: Consider discontinuing.

Dosage adjustment in renal impairment: No dosage adjustment provided in manufacturer's labeling. Use with caution.

Dosage adjustment in hepatic impairment: No dosage adjustment provided in manufacturer's labeling. Use with caution.

Additional Information Complete prescribing information should be consulted for additional detail.

Dosage Forms Excipient information presented when available (limited, particularly for generics); consult specific product labeling.

Tablet, Oral:

Orap: 1 mg, 2 mg [scored]

◆ **Pimtrea** *see* Ethinyl Estradiol and Desogestrel *on page 784*

◆ **Pin-X [OTC]** *see* Pyrantel Pamoate *on page 1750*

Pindolol (PIN doe lole)

Brand Names: Canada Apo-Pindol; Dom-Pindolol; PMS-Pindolol; Sandoz-Pindolol; Teva-Pindolol; Visken

Pharmacologic Category Antihypertensive; Beta-Blocker With Intrinsic Sympathomimetic Activity

Additional Appendix Information

Beta-Blockers *on page 2294*

Use

U.S. labeling: Treatment of hypertension, alone or in combination with other agents

Canadian labeling: Treatment of hypertension, alone or in combination with other agents; prophylaxis of angina pectoris

Unlabeled Use Potential augmenting agent for antidepressants; ventricular arrhythmias/tachycardia, antipsychotic-induced akathisia, situational anxiety; aggressive behavior associated with dementia

Pregnancy Risk Factor B

Dosage

U.S. labeling: Hypertension: Adults: Oral: Initial: 5 mg twice daily; increase as necessary by 10 mg daily every 3-4 weeks (maximum daily dose: 60 mg). Usual dose range (JNC 7): 10-40 mg twice daily.

Canadian labeling:

Angina pectoris: Adults: Oral: Initial: 5 mg 3 times daily; increase as necessary every 1-2 weeks. Usual maintenance dose: 15-40 mg daily in 3 or 4 divided doses (maximum daily dose: 40 mg)

Hypertension: Adults: Oral: Initial: 5 mg twice daily; increase as necessary by 10 mg daily every 1-2 weeks. Usual maintenance dose: 15-45 mg daily (maximum daily dose: 45 mg). If daily maintenance dose is ≤20 mg daily, may give as single dose in the morning; if >30 mg daily, administer in 3 divided doses.

Unlabeled use: Antidepressant augmentation: 2.5 mg 3 times daily (Geretsegger, 2008)

Elderly: Refer to adult dosing. Use with caution.

Dosage adjustment in renal impairment: No dosage adjustment provided in manufacturer's labeling. In uremic patients, use with caution due to significantly decreased clearance.

Dosage adjustment in hepatic impairment: No dosage adjustment provided in manufacturer's labeling. In cirrhotic patients, use with caution due to significantly prolonged elimination half-life (may be 10 times as long compared to normal patients).

Additional Information Complete prescribing information should be consulted for additional detail.

Dosage Forms Excipient information presented when available (limited, particularly for generics); consult specific product labeling.

Tablet, Oral:

Generic: 5 mg, 10 mg

Dosage Forms: Canada Excipient information presented when available (limited, particularly for generics); consult specific product labeling.

Tablet, Oral:

Generic: 5 mg, 10 mg, 15 mg

◆ **Pink Bismuth** *see* Bismuth *on page 260*

◆ **Pink Bismuth [OTC]** *see* Bismuth *on page 260*

◆ **Pinnacaine Otic** *see* Benzocaine *on page 240*

Pioglitazone (pye oh GLI ta zone)

Brand Names: U.S. Actos

Brand Names: Canada Accel-Pioglitazone; Actos®; Apo-Pioglitazone®; Auro-Pioglitazone; Ava-Pioglitazone; CO Pioglitazone; Dom-Pioglitazone; JAMP-Pioglitazone; Mint-Pioglitazone; Mylan-Pioglitazone; Novo-Pioglitazone; PHL-Pioglitazone; PMS-Pioglitazone; PRO-Pioglitazone; RAN™-Pioglitazone; ratio-Pioglitazone; Sandoz-Pioglitazone; Teva-Pioglitazone; ZYM-Pioglitazone

Pharmacologic Category Antidiabetic Agent, Thiazolidinedione

Additional Appendix Information

Oral Antidiabetic Agents Comparison Table *on page 2312*

Use Type 2 diabetes mellitus (noninsulin dependent, NIDDM), monotherapy or combination therapy: Adjunct to diet and exercise, to improve glycemic control

Pregnancy Risk Factor C

Pregnancy Considerations Adverse effects were observed in animal reproduction studies. The use of pioglitazone in pregnant women is limited to very few case reports in which pregnancy occurred during treatment for polycystic ovarian syndrome (PCOS); details concerning fetal outcomes are limited (Glueck, 2003; Ortega-Gonzalez, 2005; Ota, 2008). Thiazolidinediones may cause ovulation in anovulatory premenopausal women, increasing the risk of pregnancy; adequate contraception in premenopausal women is recommended. Insulin sensitizing agents, including pioglitazone, have been evaluated for the treatment of polycystic ovary syndrome (ASRM, 2008). However, due to long-term safety concerns associated with their use, thiazolidinediones should be avoided in women of reproductive age (Fauser, 2012).

For women with diabetes, maternal hyperglycemia itself can be associated with adverse effects in the fetus, neonate, and mother. To prevent adverse events, prior to conception and throughout pregnancy, the maternal HbA_{1c} should be kept close to normal but without causing significant hypoglycemia. Maternal hyperglycemia can be associated with adverse effects in the mother. The use of thiazolidinediones in pregnant women is not recommended; insulin is the drug of choice for the control of diabetes mellitus during pregnancy (ACOG, 2005; ADA, 2013; Kitzmiller, 2008; Metzger, 2007).

Breast-Feeding Considerations It is not known if pioglitazone is excreted in breast milk. Although breast-feeding is encouraged for all women, including those with diabetes, the safety of pioglitazone during breast-feeding has not yet been established (Metzger, 2007). According to the manufacturer, due to the potential for adverse events in the nursing infant, a decision should be made whether to discontinue nursing or to discontinue the drug, taking into account the importance of treatment to the mother.

Medication Guide Available Yes

Contraindications Hypersensitivity to pioglitazone or any component of the formulation; NYHA Class III/IV heart failure (initiation of therapy)

Canadian labeling: Additional contraindications (not is U.S. labeling): Any stage of heart failure (eg, NYHA Class I, II, III, IV); serious hepatic impairment; active bladder cancer; history of bladder cancer; uninvestigated macroscopic hematuria; pregnancy

Warnings/Precautions [U.S. Boxed Warning]: Thiazolidinediones, including pioglitazone, may cause or exacerbate heart failure; closely monitor for signs and symptoms of heart failure (eg, rapid weight gain, dyspnea, edema), particularly after initiation or dose increases; if heart failure develops, treat accordingly and consider dose reduction or discontinuation of pioglitazone. Not recommended for use in any patient with symptomatic heart failure. Initiation of therapy is contraindicated in patients with NYHA class III or IV heart failure. If used in patients with NYHA class I or II (systolic heart failure), initiate at lowest dosage and monitor closely. In Canada, use in any stage of heart failure (NYHA I, II, III, IV) is contraindicated. Dose reduction or discontinuation is recommended if heart failure suspected. Dose-related edema and weight gain observed with use; use with caution in patients with edema; monitor for signs/symptoms of heart failure.

Should not be used in diabetic ketoacidosis. Mechanism requires the presence of insulin; therefore use in type 1 diabetes is not recommended. Use with caution in premenopausal, anovulatory women - may result in a resumption of ovulation, increasing the risk of pregnancy. Use with caution in patients with anemia (may reduce hemoglobin and hematocrit). Increased incidence of bone fractures in females treated with pioglitazone; majority of fractures occurred in the lower limb and distal upper limb. Clinical trial data suggest an increased risk of bladder cancer in patients exposed to pioglitazone; risk may be increased with duration of use. Avoid use in patients with active bladder cancer and consider risks vs. benefits prior to initiating therapy in patients with a history of bladder cancer. In Canada, use is contraindicated in patients with active or a history of bladder cancer.

Hepatic failure, including fatalities, has been reported. Monitor for signs/symptoms of liver injury closely during therapy; discontinuation of therapy may be necessary. Due to this risk, serum liver function tests (ALT, AST, alkaline phosphatase, and total bilirubin) should be obtained prior to initiation in all patients. In patients with abnormal hepatic tests, therapy should be initiated with caution (Canadian labeling recommends avoiding use in patients with baseline ALT >3 x ULN). During therapy, if signs/symptoms of liver injury (eg, fatigue, anorexia, jaundice, dark urine, right upper abdominal discomfort) arise, interrupt pioglitazone therapy, obtain liver tests immediately, and evaluate alternative etiologies. Depending on the results of the liver tests and whether an alternative etiology is identified, discontinuation of therapy may be recommended. U.S. labeling states that routine periodic monitoring of serum liver tests during therapy is not necessary unless patient has liver disease or signs/symptoms of liver injury arise during use (Canadian labeling recommends periodic monitoring of liver enzymes in all patients per clinical judgment). Macular edema has been reported with thiazolidinedione use, including pioglitazone. Patients should be seen by an ophthalmologist if any visual symptoms arise during therapy and all diabetic patients should have regular eye exams.

Concomitant administration of pioglitazone with a strong CYP2C8 inhibitor increases pioglitazone exposure 3-fold; dosage adjustments are recommended if pioglitazone is coadministered with a strong CYP2C8 inhibitor (eg, gemfibrozil). Risk of hypoglycemia is increased when pioglitazone is combined with insulin or other diabetic medications; dosage adjustment of concomitant hypoglycemic agents may be necessary. Canadian labeling (not in U.S. labeling) states use with insulin **or** as part of triple therapy (pioglitazone in combination with a sulfonylurea and metformin) is not indicated. Use in pediatrics is not recommended; risks and adverse effects have not been evaluated in this population and there is a lack of long-term safety data.

Adverse Reactions Adverse reactions and incidences reported are associated with monotherapy unless otherwise stated.

>10%:

- Cardiovascular: Edema (combination trials: ≤27%)
- Endocrine and metabolic: Hypoglycemia (combination trials: ≤27%)
- Respiratory: Upper respiratory tract infection (13%)

1% to 10%:

- Cardiovascular: Heart failure (combination trials: ≤8%)
- Central nervous system: Headache (9%)
- Neuromuscular & skeletal: Fractures (females: ≤5%), myalgia (5%)
- Respiratory: Sinusitis (6%), pharyngitis (5%)

Frequency not defined: HDL-cholesterol increased, hematocrit/hemoglobin decreased, serum triglycerides decreased, weight gain/loss

<1% (Limited to important or life-threatening): Bladder cancer, blurred vision, CPK increased, dyspnea (associated with weight gain and/or edema), hepatic failure (very rare), hepatitis, macular edema (new onset or worsening), transaminases increased, pulmonary edema, rhabdomyolysis, visual acuity decreased

Drug Interactions

Metabolism/Transport Effects Substrate of CYP2C8 (major), CYP3A4 (minor); **Note:** Assignment of Major/Minor substrate status based on clinically relevant drug interaction potential; **Inhibits** CYP2C19 (weak), CYP2C8 (moderate), CYP2C9 (weak); **Induces** CYP3A4 (weak/moderate)

Avoid Concomitant Use

Avoid concomitant use of Pioglitazone with any of the following: Axitinib; Simeprevir

Increased Effect/Toxicity

Pioglitazone may increase the levels/effects of: CYP2C8 Substrates; Hypoglycemic Agents

The levels/effects of Pioglitazone may be increased by: CYP2C8 Inhibitors (Moderate); CYP2C8 Inhibitors (Strong); Deferasirox; Gemfibrozil; Herbs (Hypoglycemic Properties); Insulin; MAO Inhibitors; Mifepristone; Pegvisomant; Pregabalin; Salicylates; Selective Serotonin Reuptake Inhibitors; Trimethoprim

Decreased Effect

Pioglitazone may decrease the levels/effects of: ARIPiprazole; Axitinib; Ibrutinib; Saxagliptin; Simeprevir

The levels/effects of Pioglitazone may be decreased by: Bile Acid Sequestrants; Corticosteroids (Orally Inhaled); Corticosteroids (Systemic); CYP2C8 Inducers (Strong); Dabrafenib; Loop Diuretics; Luteinizing Hormone-Releasing Hormone Analogs; Rifampin; Somatropin; Thiazide Diuretics

Ethanol/Nutrition/Herb Interactions

Ethanol: Caution with ethanol (may cause hypoglycemia).

Food: Peak concentrations are delayed when administered with food, but the extent of absorption is not affected. Pioglitazone may be taken without regard to meals.

Herb/Nutraceutical: Caution with alfalfa, aloe, bilberry, bitter melon, burdock, celery, damiana, fenugreek, garcinia, garlic, ginger, ginseng (American), gymnema, marshmallow, and stinging nettle (may cause hypoglycemia).

Mechanism of Action Thiazolidinedione antidiabetic agent that lowers blood glucose by improving target cell response to insulin, without increasing pancreatic insulin secretion. It has a mechanism of action that is dependent on the presence of insulin for activity. Pioglitazone is a potent and selective agonist for peroxisome proliferator-activated receptor-gamma (PPARgamma). Activation of nuclear PPARgamma receptors influences the production of a number of gene products involved in glucose and lipid metabolism. PPARgamma is abundant in the cells within the renal collecting tubules; fluid retention results from stimulation by thiazolidinediones which increases sodium reabsorption.

Pharmacodynamics/Kinetics

Onset of action: Delayed

Peak effect: Glucose control: Several weeks

Distribution: V_{ss} (apparent): 0.63 L/kg

Protein binding: Pioglitazone >99% and active metabolites >98%; primarily to albumin

Metabolism: Hepatic (99%) via CYP2C8 and 3A4 to both active and inactive metabolites

Half-life elimination: Parent drug: 3-7 hours; Total: 16-24 hours

Time to peak: ~2 hours; delayed with food

Excretion: Urine (15% to 30%) and feces as metabolites

Dosage Type 2 diabetes: Adults: Oral:

Initial:

U.S. labeling: Monotherapy or combination therapy: 15-30 mg once daily

Patients with heart failure (NYHA Class I or II): Monotherapy or combination therapy: 15 mg once daily

Note: Not recommended in patients with symptomatic heart failure

Canadian labeling: Monotherapy or combination therapy (with a sulfonylurea or metformin): 15-30 mg once daily

Dosage titration: If response is inadequate based on Hb A_{1c}, the dosage may be increased in 15 mg increments with careful monitoring of adverse effects (eg, weight gain, edema, signs/symptoms of heart failure); maximum recommended dose: 45 mg once daily

Dosage adjustment for hypoglycemia with combination therapy:

With an insulin secretagogue (eg, sulfonylurea): Decrease the insulin secretagogue dose.

With insulin: Decrease insulin dose by 10% to 25%

Dosage adjustment with strong CYP2C8 inhibitors (eg, gemfibrozil): Maximum recommended dose: 15 mg once daily

Dosage adjustment in renal impairment: No dosage adjustment necessary.

Dosage adjustment in hepatic impairment: No dosage adjustment necessary (mean AUC values are unaffected in Child-Pugh grade B/C compared to healthy subjects); however, liver injury has been associated with use.

U.S. labeling:

Prior to initiation: Evaluate liver tests (ALT, AST, alkaline phosphatase, total bilirubin) and if abnormal, initiate with caution.

During therapy: If liver injury is suspected (eg, fatigue, jaundice, dark urine): Interrupt therapy, measure serum liver tests, and investigate possible etiologies:

If ALT >3 x ULN **and** without alternative etiologies: Do not reinitiate therapy.

If ALT >3 x ULN **and** total bilirubin >2 x ULN **and** without alternative etiologies: Do not reinitiate therapy (these patients are at increased risk for severe drug-induced hepatotoxicity).

If ALT elevated (but <3 x ULN) **or** total bilirubin elevated (but <2 x ULN) **and** with an alternative etiology: May reinitiate with caution.

Canadian labeling:

Severe hepatic impairment: Use is contraindicated.

Prior to initiation:

If ALT >2.5 x ULN or clinical evidence of active liver disease: Do not initiate therapy.

If ALT 1-2.5 x ULN: Initiate therapy with caution and investigate etiology of liver enzyme elevation.

During therapy:

If ALT levels >3 x ULN: Recheck levels immediately and if ALT elevation >3 x ULN persists, discontinue therapy.

If ALT 1-2.5 x ULN: Continue therapy with caution and investigate etiology of liver enzyme elevation.

Dietary Considerations Dietary modification based on ADA recommendations is a part of therapy.

Administration May be administered without regard to meals

Monitoring Parameters Hemoglobin A_{1c}, serum glucose; signs and symptoms of heart failure; liver enzymes (ALT, AST, alkaline phosphatase, and total bilirubin) prior to initiation in all patients (with or without liver disease); continue routine periodic monitoring during treatment only in patients with liver disease or suspected liver disease (Canadian labeling recommends continued periodic monitoring per clinician judgment in all patients). Routine ophthalmic exams are recommended; patients reporting visual deterioration should have a prompt referral to an ophthalmologist and consideration should be given to discontinuing pioglitazone. Signs/symptoms of bladder cancer (dysuria, macroscopic hematuria, dysuria, urinary urgency).

Reference Range Recommendations for glycemic control in nonpregnant adults with diabetes (ADA, 2013):

Hb A_{1c}: <7% (a more aggressive [<6.5%] or less aggressive [<8%] Hb A_{1c} goal may be targeted based on patient-specific characteristics)

Preprandial capillary plasma glucose: 70-130 mg/dL

Peak postprandial capillary blood glucose: <180 mg/dL

Dosage Forms Excipient information presented when available (limited, particularly for generics); consult specific product labeling.

Tablet, Oral:

Actos: 15 mg, 30 mg, 45 mg

Generic: 15 mg, 30 mg, 45 mg

Pioglitazone and Glimepiride

(pye oh GLI ta zone & GLYE me pye ride)

Brand Names: U.S. Duetact™

Index Terms Glimepiride and Pioglitazone; Glimepiride and Pioglitazone Hydrochloride

Pharmacologic Category Antidiabetic Agent, Sulfonylurea; Antidiabetic Agent, Thiazolidinedione; Hypoglycemic Agent, Oral

Use Management of type 2 diabetes mellitus (noninsulin dependent, NIDDM) as an adjunct to diet and exercise in patients already treated with a thiazolidinedione and a sulfonylurea or who have inadequate control on either agent alone

Pregnancy Risk Factor C

Medication Guide Available Yes

Dosage Oral: Type 2 diabetes mellitus:

Adults: Initial dose should be based on current dose of pioglitazone and/or sulfonylurea.

Patients inadequately controlled on **glimepiride** alone: Initial dose: 30 mg/2 mg or 30 mg/4 mg once daily

Patients inadequately controlled on **pioglitazone** alone: Initial dose: 30 mg/2 mg once daily

Patients with systolic dysfunction (eg, NYHA Class I and II): Initiate only after patient has been safely titrated to 30 mg of pioglitazone. Initial dose: 30 mg/2 mg or 30 mg/4 mg once daily.

Note: No exact dosing relationship exists between glimepiride and other sulfonlyureas. Dosing should be limited to less than or equal to the maximum initial dose of glimepiride (2 mg). When converting patients from other sulfonylureas with longer half-lives (eg, chlorpropamide) to glimepiride, observe patient carefully for 1-2 weeks due to overlapping hypoglycemic effects.

Dosing adjustment: Dosage may be increased up to max dose and formulation strengths available; tablet should not be given more than once daily; see individual agents for frequency of adjustments. Dosage adjustments in patients with systolic dysfunction should be done carefully and patient monitored for symptoms of worsening heart failure.

Maximum dose: Pioglitazone 45 mg/glimepiride 8 mg daily

Elderly: Initial: Glimepiride 1 mg/day prior to initiating Duetact™; dose titration and maintenance dosing should be conservative to avoid hypoglycemia

Dosage adjustment in renal impairment: Cl_{cr} <22 mL/minute: Initial dose should be 1 mg of glimepiride and dosage increments should be based on fasting blood glucose levels

Dosage adjustment in hepatic impairment: Do not initiate treatment with active liver disease or ALT >2.5 times ULN. During treatment, if ALT levels elevate >3 times ULN, the test should be repeated as soon as possible. If ALT levels remain >3 times ULN or if the patient is jaundiced, Duetact™ should be discontinued.

Additional Information Complete prescribing information should be consulted for additional detail.

Dosage Forms Excipient information presented when available (limited, particularly for generics); consult specific product labeling.

Tablet: 30/2: Pioglitazone 30 mg and glimepiride 2 mg; 30/4: Pioglitazone 30 mg and glimepiride 4 mg

Duetact™:

30 mg/2 mg: Pioglitazone 30 mg and glimepiride 2 mg

30 mg/4 mg: Pioglitazone 30 mg and glimepiride 4 mg

Pioglitazone and Metformin

(pye oh GLI ta zone & met FOR min)

Brand Names: U.S. Actoplus Met®; Actoplus Met® XR

Index Terms Metformin Hydrochloride and Pioglitazone Hydrochloride

Pharmacologic Category Antidiabetic Agent, Biguanide; Antidiabetic Agent, Thiazolidinedione

Use Management of type 2 diabetes mellitus (noninsulin dependent, NIDDM) in patients already receiving a thiazolidinedione and metformin or who have inadequate control on either agent

Pregnancy Risk Factor C

Medication Guide Available Yes

Dosage Type 2 diabetes mellitus:

Adults: Oral: Initial dose should be based on current dose of pioglitazone and/or metformin

Immediate release tablet:

Initial: Pioglitazone 15 mg plus metformin 500 mg twice daily **or** pioglitazone 15 mg plus metformin 850 mg tablets once or twice daily

Patients with heart failure (NYHA Class I or II): Initial: Pioglitazone 15 mg plus metformin 500 mg once daily **or** pioglitazone 15 mg plus metformin 850 mg once daily. **Note:** Not recommended in patients with symptomatic heart failure.

Dose titration: If necessary, may titrate gradually with careful monitoring of adverse effects (eg, weight gain, edema, signs/symptoms of heart failure). Maximum daily dose: Pioglitazone 45 mg/metformin 2550 mg. **Note:** Metformin daily doses >2000 mg may be better tolerated if given 3 times daily.

Variable release tablet: Initial: Pioglitazone 15-30 mg plus metformin 1000 mg once daily with evening meal. If necessary, titrate gradually with careful monitoring of adverse effects (eg, weight gain, edema, signs/symptoms of heart failure). Maximum daily dose: Pioglitazone 45 mg/metformin 2000 mg.

Elderly: *Immediate release or variable release tablet:* The initial and maintenance dosing should be conservative, due to the potential for decreased renal function (monitor). Generally, elderly patients should not be titrated to the maximum; do not use in patients ≥80 years of age unless normal renal function has been established.

Dosage adjustment for hypoglycemia with combination therapy:

With an insulin secretagogue (eg, sulfonylurea): Decrease the insulin secretagogue dose.

With insulin: Decrease insulin dose by 10% to 25%.

Dosage adjustment with strong CYP2C8 inhibitors (eg, gemfibrozil): Maximum recommended dose: Pioglitazone 15 mg plus metformin 850 mg daily

Dosage adjustment in renal impairment: *Immediate release or variable release tablet:* Contraindicated in patients with renal disease or renal dysfunction (serum creatinine ≥1.5 mg/dL in males or ≥1.4 mg/dL in females or abnormal clearance).

Dosage adjustment in hepatic impairment: *Immediate release or variable release:* Not recommended in hepatic impairment due to potential for lactic acidosis associated with metformin component.

Additional Information Complete prescribing information should be consulted for additional detail.

Dosage Forms Excipient information presented when available (limited, particularly for generics); consult specific product labeling.

Tablet, oral: 15/500: Pioglitazone 15 mg and metformin hydrochloride 500 mg; 15/850: Pioglitazone 15 mg and metformin hydrochloride 850 mg

Actoplus Met®:

15/500: Pioglitazone 15 mg and metformin hydrochloride 500 mg

15/850: Pioglitazone 15 mg and metformin hydrochloride 850 mg

Tablet, variable release, oral:

Actoplus Met® XR:

15/1000: Pioglitazone 15 mg [immediate release] and metformin hydrochloride 1000 mg [extended release]

30/1000: Pioglitazone 30 mg [immediate release] and metformin hydrochloride 1000 mg [extended release]

Piperacillin and Tazobactam

(pi PER a sil in & ta zoe BAK tam)

Brand Names: U.S. Zosyn

Brand Names: Canada AJ-PIP/TAZ; Piperacillin and Tazobactam for Injection; Tazocin

Index Terms Piperacillin and Tazobactam Sodium; Piperacillin Sodium and Tazobactam Sodium; Tazobactam and Piperacillin

Pharmacologic Category Antibiotic, Penicillin

Additional Appendix Information

Desensitization Protocols *on page 2325*

Use

Moderate to severe bacterial infections: For the treatment of patients with moderate to severe infections caused by susceptible isolates of the designated bacteria in the following conditions.

Community-acquired pneumonia: Treatment of moderate severity community-acquired pneumonia (CAP) caused by beta-lactamase-producing strains of *Haemophilus influenzae.* IDSA/ATS guidelines only recommend piperacillin/tazobactam for CAP caused by *P. aeruginosa* or due to aspiration (Mandell, 2007).

Intra-abdominal infections: Treatment of appendicitis complicated by rupture or abscess and peritonitis caused by beta-lactamase-producing strains of *Escherichia coli*, *Bacteroides fragilis*, *Bacteroides ovatus*, *Bacteroides thetaiotaomicron*, or *Bacteroides vulgatus*.

Nosocomial pneumonia: Treatment of moderate to severe nosocomial pneumonia caused by beta-lactamase-producing strains of *Staphylococcus aureus* and by piperacillin/tazobactam-susceptible *Acinetobacter baumanii*, *H. influenzae*, *Klebsiella pneumoniae*, and *Pseudomonas aeruginosa* (nosocomial pneumonia caused by *P. aeruginosa* should be treated in combination with an aminoglycoside).

Pelvic infections: Treatment of postpartum endometriosis or pelvic inflammatory disease caused by beta-lactamase-producing strains of *E. coli*.

Skin and skin structure infections: Treatment of skin and skin structure infections, including cellulitis, cutaneous abscesses, and ischemic/diabetic foot infections caused by beta-lactamase-producing strains of *S. aureus*.

Unlabeled Use Treatment of moderate-to-severe infections caused by susceptible organisms, including urinary tract infections, bone and joint infections, septicemia, endocarditis, and cystic fibrosis exacerbations; surgical (perioperative) prophylaxis

Pregnancy Risk Factor B

Pregnancy Considerations Adverse events have not been observed in animal reproduction studies. Piperacillin and tazobactam both cross the placenta and are found in the fetal serum, placenta, amniotic fluid, and fetal urine. When used during pregnancy, the clearance and volume of distribution of piperacillin/tazobactam are increased; half-life and AUC are decreased (Bourget, 1998). Piperacillin/tazobactam is approved for the treatment of postpartum gynecologic infections, including endometritis or pelvic inflammatory disease, caused by susceptible organisms.

Breast-Feeding Considerations Low concentrations of piperacillin are excreted in breast milk; information for tazobactam is not available. The manufacturer recommends that caution be used when administering piperacillin/tazobactam to nursing women. Nondose-related effects could include modification of bowel flora.

Contraindications Hypersensitivity to penicillins, cephalosporins, beta-lactamase inhibitors, or any component of the formulation

Warnings/Precautions Serious and occasionally severe or fatal hypersensitivity (anaphylactic/anaphylactoid) reactions have been reported in patients on penicillin therapy, especially with a history of beta-lactam hypersensitivity, history of sensitivity to multiple allergens, or previous IgE-mediated reactions (eg, anaphylaxis, angioedema, urticaria). Serious skin reactions, including toxic epidermal necrolysis (TEN) and Stevens-Johnson syndrome (SJS), have been reported. If a skin rash develops, monitor closely. Discontinue if lesions progress.

Bleeding disorders have been observed, particularly in patients with renal impairment; discontinue if thrombocytopenia or bleeding occurs. Leukopenia/neutropenia may occur; appears to be reversible and most frequently associated with prolonged administration. Assess hematologic parameters periodically, especially with prolonged (≥21 days) use.

Assess electrolytes periodically in patients with low potassium reserves, especially those receiving cytotoxic therapy or diuretics. Due to sodium load and to the adverse effects of high serum concentrations of penicillins, dosage modification is required in patients with impaired or underdeveloped renal function; use with caution in patients with seizures or in patients with history of beta-lactam allergy; associated with an increased incidence of rash and fever in cystic fibrosis patients. Use may result in fungal or bacterial superinfection, including *C. difficile*-associated diarrhea (CDAD) and pseudomembranous colitis; CDAD has been observed >2 months postantibiotic treatment.

Potentially significant drug-drug interactions may exist, requiring dose or frequency adjustment, additional monitoring, and/or selection of alternative therapy.

Adverse Reactions

>10%: Gastrointestinal: Diarrhea (7% to 11%)

1% to 10%:

Cardiovascular: Hypertension (2%), chest pain (1%), edema (1%)

Central nervous system: Insomnia (7%), headache (8%), fever (2% to 5%), agitation (2%), pain (2%), anxiety (1% to 2%), dizziness (1% to 2%)

Dermatologic: Rash (4%), pruritus (3%)

Gastrointestinal: Constipation (1% to 8%), nausea (7%), vomiting (3% to 4%), dyspepsia (3%), stool changes (2%), abdominal pain (1% to 2%)

Hepatic: AST increased (1%)

Local: Local reaction (3%), abscess (2%), phlebitis (1%)
Respiratory: Pharyngitis (2%), dyspnea (1%), rhinitis (1%)
Miscellaneous: Moniliasis (2%), sepsis (2%), infection (2%)

<1%, postmarketing, and/or case reports (Limited to important and life-threatening): Agranulocytosis, anaphylaxis/anaphylactoid reaction, anemia, anxiety, arrhythmia, arthralgia, atrial fibrillation, back pain, bradycardia, bronchospasm, *C. difficile*-associated diarrhea (CDAD), candidiasis, cardiac arrest, cardiac failure, cholestatic jaundice, circulatory failure, confusion, convulsions, coughing, depression, diaphoresis, dysuria, epistaxis, erythema multiforme, flatulence, flushing, gastritis, genital pruritus, hallucination, hematuria, hemolytic anemia, hemorrhage, hepatitis, hiccough, hypoglycemia, hypokalemia, hypotension, ileus, incontinence, inflammation, injection site reaction, interstitial nephritis, leukorrhea, malaise, melena, mesenteric embolism, myalgia, myocardial infarction, oliguria, pancytopenia, photophobia, pulmonary edema, pulmonary embolism, purpura, renal failure, rigors, Stevens-Johnson syndrome, syncope, tachycardia (supraventricular and ventricular), taste perversion, thirst, thrombocytopenia, thrombocytosis, thrombophlebitis, tinnitus, toxic epidermal necrolysis, tremor, ulcerative stomatitis, urinary retention, vaginitis, ventricular fibrillation, vertigo

Drug Interactions

Metabolism/Transport Effects None known.

Avoid Concomitant Use

Avoid concomitant use of Piperacillin and Tazobactam with any of the following: BCG

Increased Effect/Toxicity

Piperacillin and Tazobactam may increase the levels/effects of: Floxacillin; Methotrexate; Vecuronium; Vitamin K Antagonists

The levels/effects of Piperacillin and Tazobactam may be increased by: Probenecid

Decreased Effect

Piperacillin and Tazobactam may decrease the levels/effects of: Aminoglycosides; BCG; Mycophenolate; Sodium Picosulfate; Typhoid Vaccine

The levels/effects of Piperacillin and Tazobactam may be decreased by: Tetracycline Derivatives

Preparation for Administration Reconstitute single-dose vials with 5 mL of diluent per 1 g of piperacillin and then further dilute to a volume of 50-150 mL. Reconstitute pharmacy bulk vials with 152 mL of diluent to yield a concentration of piperacillin 200 mg/mL and tazobactam 25 mg/mL; transfer reconstituted solution and further dilute to a volume of 50-150 mL for administration.

Storage/Stability

Vials: Store at 20°C to 25°C (68°F to 77°F) prior to reconstitution. Use single-dose or bulk vials immediately after reconstitution. Discard any unused portion after 24 hours if stored at 20°C to 25°C (68°F to 77°F) or after 48 hours if stored refrigerated (2°C to 8°C [36°F to 46°F]). Do not freeze vials after reconstitution. Stability in I.V. bags has been demonstrated for up to 24 hours at room temperature and up to 1 week at refrigerated temperature. Stability in an ambulatory I.V. infusion pump has been demonstrated for a period of 12 hours at room temperature.

Galaxy containers: Store at or below -20°C (-4°F). The thawed solution is stable for 14 days under refrigeration (2°C to 8°C [36°F to 46°F]) or 24 hours at 20°C to 25°C (68°F to 77°F). Do not refreeze.

Mechanism of Action Piperacillin inhibits bacterial cell wall synthesis by binding to one or more of the penicillin-binding proteins (PBPs); which in turn inhibits the final transpeptidation step of peptidoglycan synthesis in bacterial cell walls, thus inhibiting cell wall biosynthesis. Bacteria eventually lyse due to ongoing activity of cell wall autolytic enzymes (autolysins and murein hydrolases) while cell wall assembly is arrested. Piperacillin exhibits time-dependent killing. Tazobactam inhibits many beta-lactamases, including staphylococcal penicillinase and Richmond-Sykes types 2, 3, 4, and 5, including extended spectrum enzymes; it has only limited activity against class 1 beta-lactamases other than class 1C types.

Pharmacodynamics/Kinetics

Distribution: Well into lungs, intestinal mucosa, uterus, ovary, fallopian tube, interstitial fluid, gallbladder, and bile; penetration into CSF is low in subjects with noninflamed meninges

Protein binding: Piperacillin and tazobactam: ~30%

Metabolism:

Piperacillin: Desethyl metabolite (weak activity)
Tazobactam: Inactive metabolite

Half-life elimination: Piperacillin and tazobactam: 0.7-1.2 hours (unaffected by dose or duration of infusion)

Time to peak, plasma: Immediately following completion of 30-minute infusion

Excretion: Clearance of both piperacillin and tazobactam are directly proportional to renal function

Piperacillin: Urine (68% as unchanged drug); feces (10% to 20%)
Tazobactam: Urine (80% as unchanged drug; remainder as inactive metabolite)
Dialysis: Hemodialysis removes 30% to 40% of a piperacillin/tazobactam dose; peritoneal dialysis removes 6% of piperacillin and 21% of tazobactam

Dosage Note: Dosing presented is based on traditional infusion method (I.V. infusion over 30 minutes) unless otherwise specified as the extended infusion method (I.V. infusion over 4 hours [unlabeled method]).

Usual dosage range: I.V.:

Infants 2-8 months: 80 mg of piperacillin component/kg every 8 hours
Infants and Children ≥9 months and ≤40 kg: 100 mg of piperacillin component/kg every 8 hours
Children and Adolescents >40 kg: Refer to adult dosing.
Adults: I.V.: 3.375 g every 6 hours **or** 4.5 g every 6 hours; maximum: 18 g daily
Extended infusion method (unlabeled dosing): 3.375-4.5 g I.V. over 4 hours every 8 hours (Kim, 2007; Shea, 2009); an alternative regimen of 4.5 g I.V. over 3 hours every 6 hours has also been described (Kim, 2007).

Indication-specific dosing: I.V.:

Children:

Appendicitis, peritonitis:
Infants 2-8 months: 80 mg/kg of piperacillin component every 8 hours
Infants and Children ≥9 months and ≤40 kg: 100 mg/kg of piperacillin component every 8 hours
Children and Adolescents >40 kg: Refer to adult dosing.

Cystic fibrosis, pseudomonal infections (unlabeled use): I.V.: 240-400 mg/kg/day of piperacillin component divided every 8 hours; in some cases, higher doses may be necessary: 450-600 mg/kg/day divided every 4-6 hours (Zobell, 2013)

Intra-abdominal infection, complicated (unlabeled use): 200-300 mg/kg/day of piperacillin component divided every 6-8 hours (Solomkin, 2010).

Surgical (perioperative) prophylaxis (unlabeled use): Note: Doses may be repeated in 2 hours if procedure is lengthy or if there is excessive blood loss (Bratzler, 2013):
Infants 2-9 months: 80 mg/kg of piperacillin component within 60 minutes prior to surgical incision (maximum: 3.375 g).

Infants and Children >9 months and ≤40 kg: 100 mg/kg of piperacillin component within 60 minutes prior to surgical incision (maximum: 3.375 g).

Children and Adolescents >40 kg: Refer to adult dosing.

Adults:

Diverticulitis, intra-abdominal abscess, peritonitis: I.V.: 3.375 g every 6 hours for 7-10 days.

Pneumonia:

Community-acquired pneumonia (CAP): I.V.: 3.375 g every 6 hours for 7-10 days. **Note:** IDSA/ATS guidelines only recommend piperacillin/tazobactam for CAP caused by *P. aeruginosa* or due to aspiration (Mandell, 2007).

Nosocomial pneumonia: I.V.: 4.5 g every 6 hours for 7-14 days (when used empirically, combination with an aminoglycoside or antipseudomonal fluoroquinolone is recommended; consider discontinuation of additional agent if *P. aeruginosa* is not isolated) (ATS, 2005).

Skin and soft tissue infection: I.V.: 3.375 g every 6-8 hours for 7-14 days. **Notes:** When used for necrotizing infection of skin, fascia, or muscle, combination with clindamycin and ciprofloxacin is recommended (Stevens, 2005); for severe diabetic foot infections, recommended treatment duration is up to 4 weeks depending on severity of infection and response to therapy (Lipsky, 2012).

Surgical (perioperative) prophylaxis (unlabeled use): I.V.: 3.375 g within 60 minutes prior to surgical incision. Doses may be repeated in 2 hours if procedure is lengthy or if there is excessive blood loss (Bratzler, 2013).

Intra-abdominal infection, complicated (unlabeled use): I.V.: 3.375 g every 6 hours for 4-7 days (provided source controlled). **Note:** Increase to 3.375 g every 4 hours or 4.5 g every 6 hours if *P. aeruginosa* is suspected. Not recommended for mild-to-moderate, community-acquired intra-abdominal infections due to risk of toxicity and the development of resistant organisms (Solomkin, 2010).

Dosing interval in renal impairment:

Traditional infusion method (ie, I.V. infusion over 30 minutes): Manufacturer's labeling:

Cl_{cr} >40 mL/minute: No dosage adjustment required

Cl_{cr} 20-40 mL/minute: Administer 2.25 g every 6 hours (3.375 g every 6 hours for nosocomial pneumonia)

Cl_{cr} <20 mL/minute: Administer 2.25 g every 8 hours (2.25 g every 6 hours for nosocomial pneumonia)

Note: Some clinicians suggest adjusting the dose at Cl_{cr} ≤20 mL/minute (rather than Cl_{cr} <40 mL/minute) in patients receiving either traditional or extended-infusion methods, particularly if treating serious gram-negative infections (empirically or definitively) (Patel, 2010).

Extended infusion method (unlabeled dosing): Cl_{cr} ≤20 mL/minute: 3.375 g I.V. over 4 hours every 12 hours (Patel, 2010)

Intermittent hemodialysis (IHD)/peritoneal dialysis (PD): 2.25 g every 12 hours (2.25 g every 8 hours for nosocomial pneumonia). **Note:** Dosing dependent on the assumption of 3 times/week, complete IHD sessions. Administer scheduled doses after hemodialysis on dialysis days; if next regularly scheduled dose is not due right after dialysis session, administer an additional dose of 0.75 g after the dialysis session.

Continuous renal replacement therapy (CRRT) (Heintz, 2009; Trotman, 2005): Drug clearance is highly dependent on the method of renal replacement, filter type, and flow rate. Appropriate dosing requires close monitoring of pharmacologic response, signs of adverse reactions due to drug accumulation, as well as drug concentrations in relation to target trough (if appropriate). The following are general recommendations only (based on dialysate flow/ultrafiltration rates of 1-2 L/hour and minimal residual renal function) and should not supersede clinical judgment (Trotman, 2005):

CVVH: 2.25-3.375 g every 6-8 hours

CVVHD: 2.25-3.375 g every 6 hours

CVVHDF: 3.375 g every 6 hours

Note: Higher dose of 3.375 g should be considered when treating resistant pathogens (especially *Pseudomonas* spp); alternative recommendations suggest dosing of 4.5 g every 8 hours (Valtonen, 2001); regardless of regimen, there is some concern of tazobactam (TAZ) accumulation, given its lower clearance relative to piperacillin (PIP). Some clinicians advocate dosing with PIP to alternate with PIP/TAZ, particularly in CVVH-dependent patients, to lessen this concern.

Dosage adjustment in hepatic impairment: No dosage adjustment necessary.

Dietary Considerations Some products may contain sodium.

Administration Administer by I.V. infusion over 30 minutes. For extended infusion administration (unlabeled dosing), administer over 3-4 hours (Kim 2007; Shea, 2009).

Some penicillins (eg, carbenicillin, ticarcillin, and piperacillin) have been shown to inactivate aminoglycosides *in vitro*. This has been observed to a greater extent with tobramycin and gentamicin, while amikacin has shown greater stability against inactivation. Concurrent use of these agents may pose a risk of reduced antibacterial efficacy *in vivo*, particularly in the setting of profound renal impairment. However, definitive clinical evidence is lacking. If combination penicillin/aminoglycoside therapy is desired in a patient with renal dysfunction, separation of doses (if feasible), and routine monitoring of aminoglycoside levels, CBC, and clinical response should be considered. **Note:** Reformulated Zosyn® containing EDTA has been shown to be compatible *in vitro* for Y-site infusion with amikacin and gentamicin diluted in NS or D_5W (applies **only** to specific concentrations and varies by product; consult manufacturer's labeling). Reformulated Zosyn® containing EDTA is **not** compatible with tobramycin.

Monitoring Parameters Creatinine, BUN, CBC with differential, PT, PTT, serum electrolytes, LFTs, urinalysis; signs of bleeding; monitor for signs of anaphylaxis during first dose

Test Interactions Positive Coombs' [direct] test; false positive reaction for urine glucose using copper-reduction method (Clinitest®); may result in false positive results with the Platelia® *Aspergillus* enzyme immunoassay (EIA)

Some penicillin derivatives may accelerate the degradation of aminoglycosides *in vitro*, leading to a potential underestimation of aminoglycoside serum concentration. **Note:** Reformulated Zosyn® containing EDTA has been shown to be compatible *in vitro* for Y-site infusion with amikacin and gentamicin diluted in NS or D_5W (applies **only** to specific concentrations and varies by product; consult manufacturer's labeling). Reformulated Zosyn® containing EDTA is **not** compatible with tobramycin.

Dosage Forms Excipient information presented when available (limited, particularly for generics); consult specific product labeling.

Note: 8:1 ratio of piperacillin sodium/tazobactam sodium

Infusion [premixed iso-osmotic solution]:

Zosyn®: 2.25 g: Piperacillin 2 g and tazobactam 0.25 g (50 mL) [contains edetate disodium, sodium 128 mg (5.58 mEq)]

Zosyn®: 3.375 g: Piperacillin 3 g and tazobactam 0.375 g (50 mL) [contains edetate disodium, sodium 192 mg (8.38 mEq)]

Zosyn®: 4.5 g: Piperacillin 4 g and tazobactam 0.5 g (100 mL) [contains edetate disodium, sodium 256 mg (11.17 mEq)]

Injection, powder for reconstitution: 2.25 g: Piperacillin 2 g and tazobactam 0.25 g; 3.375 g: Piperacillin 3 g and tazobactam 0.375 g; 4.5 g: Piperacillin 4 g and tazobactam 0.5 g; 40.5 g: Piperacillin 36 g and tazobactam 4.5 g

Zosyn®: 2.25 g: Piperacillin 2 g and tazobactam 0.25 g [contains edetate disodium, sodium 128 mg (5.58 mEq)]

Zosyn®: 3.375 g: Piperacillin 3 g and tazobactam 0.375 g [contains edetate disodium, sodium 192 mg (8.38 mEq)]

Zosyn®: 4.5 g: Piperacillin 4 g and tazobactam 0.5 g [contains edetate disodium, sodium 256 mg (11.17 mEq)]

Zosyn®: 40.5 g: Piperacillin 36 g and tazobactam 4.5 g [contains edetate disodium, sodium 2304 mg (100.4 mEq); bulk pharmacy vial]

◆ **Piperacillin and Tazobactam for Injection (Can)** *see* Piperacillin and Tazobactam *on page 1653*

◆ **Piperacillin and Tazobactam Sodium** *see* Piperacillin and Tazobactam *on page 1653*

◆ **Piperacillin Sodium and Tazobactam Sodium** *see* Piperacillin and Tazobactam *on page 1653*

◆ **Piperazine Estrone Sulfate** *see* Estropipate *on page 778*

◆ **Piperonyl Butoxide and Pyrethrins** *see* Pyrethrins and Piperonyl Butoxide *on page 1752*

Pirbuterol (peer BYOO ter ole)

Brand Names: U.S. Maxair Autohaler

Index Terms Pirbuterol Acetate

Pharmacologic Category $Beta_2$ Agonist

Use Prevention and treatment of reversible bronchospasm including asthma

Pregnancy Risk Factor C

Dosage Bronchospasm, prevention and treatment: Children ≥12 years, Adolescents, and Adults: Inhalation: 1-2 inhalations every 4-6 hours; not to exceed 12 inhalations daily. Patients should be advised to promptly consult healthcare provider or seek medical attention if no relief from acute treatment

Dosage adjustment in renal impairment: No dosage adjustment provided in manufacturer's labeling. However, dosage adjustment unlikely due to low systemic absorption.

Dosage adjustment in hepatic impairment: No dosage adjustment provided in manufacturer's labeling. However, dosage adjustment unlikely due to low systemic absorption.

Additional Information Complete prescribing information should be consulted for additional detail.

Dosage Forms Considerations

Maxair Autohaler 14 g canisters contain 400 inhalations.

Dosage Forms Excipient information presented when available (limited, particularly for generics); consult specific product labeling.

Aerosol Breath Activated, Inhalation, as acetate:

Maxair Autohaler: 200 mcg/INH (14 g)

◆ **Pirbuterol Acetate** *see* Pirbuterol *on page 1656*

◆ **Pirmella 1/35** *see* Ethinyl Estradiol and Norethindrone *on page 793*

Piroxicam (peer OKS i kam)

Brand Names: U.S. Feldene

Brand Names: Canada Apo-Piroxicam®; Dom-Piroxicam; Novo-Pirocam; Nu-Pirox; PMS-Piroxicam

Pharmacologic Category Nonsteroidal Anti-inflammatory Drug (NSAID), Oral

Additional Appendix Information

Beers Criteria – Potentially Inappropriate Medications for Geriatrics *on page 2368*

Use Symptomatic treatment of acute and chronic rheumatoid arthritis and osteoarthritis

Canadian labeling: Additional use (not in U.S. labeling): Symptomatic treatment of ankylosing spondylitis

Pregnancy Risk Factor C

Medication Guide Available Yes

Dosage Osteoarthritis, rheumatoid arthritis: Adults: Oral: 10-20 mg daily in 1-2 divided doses (maximum dose: 20 mg daily)

Ankylosing spondylitis (Canadian labeling; not an approved use in U.S. labeling): Adults: Oral: 10-20 mg daily in 1-2 divided doses (maximum dose: 20 mg daily)

Elderly: Refer to adult dosing. Initiate therapy cautiously at low end of dosing range.

Dosing adjustment in renal impairment:

Mild-to-moderate impairment:

U.S. labeling: No dosage adjustment provided in manufacturer's labeling.

Canadian labeling: No specific dosage adjustment provided in manufacturer's labeling; however, a dosage reduction is recommended. Caution and close monitoring is advised for patients with Cl_{cr} <60 mL/minute. Use is contraindicated in patients with deteriorating renal disease.

Severe impairment:

U.S. labeling: Use is not recommended (has not been studied); if therapy must be initiated, close monitoring is recommended.

Canadian labeling: Use is contraindicated in severe impairment (Cl_{cr} <30 mL/minute) or in patients with deteriorating renal disease.

Dosing adjustment in hepatic impairment: No specific dosage adjustment provided in manufacturer's labeling; however, a dosage reduction is recommended. **Note:** Canadian labeling contraindicates use in severe impairment or in patients with active liver disease.

Additional Information Complete prescribing information should be consulted for additional detail.

Dosage Forms Excipient information presented when available (limited, particularly for generics); consult specific product labeling.

Capsule, Oral:

Feldene: 10 mg, 20 mg

Generic: 10 mg, 20 mg

◆ ***p*-Isobutylhydratropic Acid** *see* Ibuprofen *on page 1032*

◆ **Pit** *see* Oxytocin *on page 1542*

Pitavastatin (pi TA va sta tin)

Brand Names: U.S. Livalo

Index Terms Pitavastatin Calcium

Pharmacologic Category Antilipemic Agent, HMG-CoA Reductase Inhibitor

Use Adjunct to dietary therapy to reduce elevations in total cholesterol (TC), LDL-C, apolipoprotein B (Apo B), and triglycerides (TG), and to increase low HDL-C in patients with primary hyperlipidemia and mixed dyslipidemia

Unlabeled Use Primary and secondary prevention of atherosclerotic cardiovascular disease (ASCVD) according to the American College of Cardiology/American Heart Association: To reduce the risk of ASCVD in patients with clinical ASCVD (eg, coronary heart disease, stroke/TIA, or peripheral arterial disease presumed to be of atherosclerotic origin) who are greater than 75 years of age or not a candidate for high-intensity statin therapy; in patients without clinical ASCVD if LDL-C is 190 mg/dL or greater and not a candidate for high-intensity statin therapy; in patients without clinical ASCVD who have type 1 or type 2 diabetes and are between 40 and 75 years of age; in patients with an estimated 10-year ASCVD risk 7.5% or greater and who are between 40 and 75 years of age (Stone, 2013).

Pregnancy Risk Factor X

Dosage Note: Doses should be individualized according to the baseline LDL-cholesterol levels, the recommended goal of therapy, and patient response; adjustments should be made at intervals of 4 weeks.

Primary hyperlipidemia and mixed dyslipidemia: Adults: Oral: Initial: 2 mg once daily; may be increased to maximum 4 mg once daily

ACC/AHA Blood Cholesterol Guideline recommendations to reduce the risk of atherosclerotic cardiovascular disease (ASCVD) (unlabeled use; Stone, 2013): Adults ≥21 years: Oral:

Primary prevention:

LDL-C ≥190 mg/dL: High intensity therapy necessary; use alternate statin therapy (eg, atorvastatin or rosuvastatin)

Type 1 or 2 diabetes and age 40-75 years: Moderate intensity therapy: 2-4 mg once daily

Type 1 or 2 diabetes, age 40-75 years, and an estimated 10-year ASCVD risk ≥7.5%: High intensity therapy necessary; use alternate statin therapy (eg, atorvastatin or rosuvastatin)

Age 40-75 years and an estimated 10-year ASCVD risk ≥7.5%: Moderate to high intensity therapy: 2-4 mg once daily or consider using high intensity statin therapy (eg, atorvastatin or rosuvastatin)

Secondary prevention:

Patient has clinical ASCVD (eg, coronary heart disease, stroke/TIA, or peripheral arterial disease presumed to be of atherosclerotic origin) **and:**

Age ≤75 years: High intensity therapy necessary; use alternate statin therapy (eg, atorvastatin or rosuvastatin)

Age >75 years or not a candidate for high intensity therapy: Moderate intensity therapy: 2-4 mg once daily

Dosage adjustment with concomitant medications:

Erythromycin: Pitavastatin dose should not exceed 1 mg once daily

Rifampin: Pitavastatin dose should not exceed 2 mg once daily

Dosing adjustment for toxicity:

Severe muscle symptoms or fatigue: Promptly discontinue use; evaluate CPK, creatinine, and urinalysis for myoglobinuria (Stone, 2013).

Mild to moderate muscle symptoms: Discontinue use until symptoms can be evaluated; evaluate patient for conditions that may increase the risk for muscle symptoms (eg, hypothyroidism, reduced renal or hepatic function, rheumatologic disorders such as polymyalgia rheumatica, steroid myopathy, vitamin D deficiency, or primary muscle diseases). Upon resolution, resume the original or lower dose of atorvastatin. If muscle symptoms recur, discontinue atorvastatin use. After muscle symptom resolution, may then use a low dose of a different statin; gradually increase if tolerated. In the absence of continued statin use, if muscle symptoms or elevated CPK continues after 2 months, consider other causes of muscle symptoms. If determined to be due to another condition aside from statin use, may resume statin therapy at the original dose (Stone, 2013).

Dosage adjustment in renal impairment:

Cl_{cr} 15-60 mL/minute/1.73 m^2 (not receiving hemodialysis): Initial: 1 mg once daily; maximum: 2 mg once daily

ESRD: Initial: 1 mg once daily; maximum: 2 mg once daily

Dosage adjustment in hepatic impairment: Contraindicated in active liver disease or in patients with unexplained persistent elevations of serum transaminases

Additional Information Complete prescribing information should be consulted for additional detail.

Dosage Forms Excipient information presented when available (limited, particularly for generics); consult specific product labeling.

Tablet, Oral:

Livalo: 1 mg, 2 mg, 4 mg

- ◆ **Pitavastatin Calcium** *see* Pitavastatin *on page* 1657
- ◆ **Pitocin** *see* Oxytocin *on page* 1542
- ◆ **Pitressin Synthetic** *see* Vasopressin *on page* 2172
- ◆ **Pitrex (Can)** *see* Tolnaftate *on page* 2087
- ◆ **PLA** *see* Poly-L-Lactic Acid *on page* 1671
- ◆ **Plan B** *see* Levonorgestrel *on page* 1202
- ◆ **Plan B One-Step** *see* Levonorgestrel *on page* 1202
- ◆ **Plantago Seed** *see* Psyllium *on page* 1748
- ◆ **Plantain Seed** *see* Psyllium *on page* 1748
- ◆ **Plaquenil** *see* Hydroxychloroquine *on page* 1019
- ◆ **Plasbumin-5** *see* Albumin *on page* 59
- ◆ **Plasbumin®-5 (Can)** *see* Albumin *on page* 59
- ◆ **Plasbumin-25** *see* Albumin *on page* 59
- ◆ **Plasbumin®-25 (Can)** *see* Albumin *on page* 59
- ◆ **Platinol** *see* CISplatin *on page* 437
- ◆ **Platinol-AQ** *see* CISplatin *on page* 437
- ◆ **Plavix** *see* Clopidogrel *on page* 471
- ◆ **Plendil** *see* Felodipine *on page* 836
- ◆ **Plendil® (Can)** *see* Felodipine *on page* 836

Plerixafor (pler IX a fore)

Brand Names: U.S. Mozobil

Brand Names: Canada Mozobil

Index Terms AMD3100; LM3100

Pharmacologic Category Hematopoietic Stem Cell Mobilizer

Use Peripheral stem cell mobilization: Mobilization of hematopoietic stem cells (HSC) for collection and subsequent autologous transplantation (in combination with filgrastim) in patients with non-Hodgkin lymphoma (NHL) and multiple myeloma (MM)

Pregnancy Risk Factor D

Pregnancy Considerations Adverse effects (including fetal mortality, decreased fetal weights, and teratogenicity) have been reported in animal studies. May cause fetal harm if administered to pregnant women. Women of child-bearing potential should use effective contraceptive measures to avoid becoming pregnant during treatment.

Breast-Feeding Considerations It is not known if plerixafor is excreted in breast milk. Due to the potential for serious adverse reactions in the nursing infant, the decision to discontinue plerixafor or to discontinue breast feeding should take in to account the importance of treatment to the mother.

Contraindications Hypersensitivity to plerixafor or any component of the formulation (anaphylactic shock has occurred).

Warnings/Precautions Hazardous agent - use appropriate precautions for handling and disposal (NIOSH, 2012). Serious hypersensitivity reactions, including anaphylactic-type reactions (may be life-threatening with serious hypotension and shock) have been reported. Observe patients for hypersensitivity symptoms during, for 30 minutes after administration, and until clinically stable. Medication, personnel, and equipment for hypersensitivity management should be available. Mild-to-moderate allergic reactions may also occur, usually within 30 minutes of administration. Increases circulating leukocytes when used in conjunction with filgrastim; monitor WBC counts. Thrombocytopenia has been observed; monitor platelet counts. Not intended for mobilization in patients with leukemia; may contaminate apheresis product by mobilizing leukemic cells. When used in combination with filgrastim, tumor cells released from marrow could be collected in leukapheresis product; potential effect of tumor cell reinfusion is unknown. Splenomegaly and splenic rupture have been reported (rarely) with filgrastim use; instruct patients to report left upper quadrant pain or scapular/shoulder tip pain; promptly evaluate in any patient who report these symptoms.

Primary route of elimination is renal; dosage reduction is recommended in patients with moderate-to-severe renal impairment (Cl_{cr} ≤50 mL/minute). Medications that may reduce renal function or compete for active tubular secretion may increase serum concentrations of plerixafor. Use has not been studied in patients weighing >175% of ideal body weight.

Adverse Reactions Adverse reactions reported with filgrastim combination therapy.

>10%:

Central nervous system: Fatigue (27%), headache (22%), dizziness (11%)

Gastrointestinal: Diarrhea (37%), nausea (34%)

Local: Injection site reaction (34%, including erythema, hematoma, hemorrhage, induration, inflammation, irritation, pain, paresthesia, pruritus, skin rash, edema, urticaria)

Neuromuscular & skeletal: Arthralgia (13%)

5% to 10%:

Central nervous system: Insomnia (7%)

Gastrointestinal: Vomiting (10%), flatulence (7%)

<5% (Limited to important or life-threatening): Abdominal distension, abdominal pain, anaphylaxis, dyspepsia, hypesthesia (oral), hypoxia, leukocytosis, musculoskeletal pain, orthostatic hypotension, periorbital swelling, syncope, thrombocytopenia

Drug Interactions

Metabolism/Transport Effects None known.

Avoid Concomitant Use There are no known interactions where it is recommended to avoid concomitant use.

Increased Effect/Toxicity There are no known significant interactions involving an increase in effect.

Decreased Effect There are no known significant interactions involving a decrease in effect.

Storage/Stability Use appropriate precautions for handling and disposal (NIOSH, 2012). Store at 25°C (77°F); excursions permitted to 15°C to 30°C (59°F to 86°F). Discard unused drug remaining in the vial after use (per manufacturer).

Mechanism of Action Reversibly inhibits binding of stromal cell-derived factor-1-alpha (SDF-1α), expressed on bone marrow stromal cells, to the CXC chemokine receptor 4 (CXCR4), resulting in mobilization of hematopoietic stem and progenitor cells from bone marrow into peripheral blood. Plerixafor used in combination with filgrastim results in synergistic increase in CD34+ cell mobilization. Mobilized CD34+ cells are capable of engrafting with extended repopulating capacity.

Pharmacodynamics/Kinetics

Onset of action: Peak CD34+ mobilization (healthy volunteers): Plerixafor monotherapy: 6-9 hours after administration; Plerixafor + filgrastim: 10-14 hours

Duration: Sustained elevation in CD34+ cells (healthy volunteers): 4-18 hours after administration

Absorption: SubQ: Rapid

Distribution: 0.3 L/kg; primarily to extravascular fluid space

Protein binding: ≤58%

Metabolism: Not metabolized

Half-life elimination: Terminal: 3-6 hours

Time to peak, plasma: SubQ: 30-60 minutes

Excretion: Urine (~70%; as parent drug)

Dosage Note: Dosing is based on actual body weight. Begin plerixafor after patient has received filgrastim (10 mcg/kg once daily) for 4 days; plerixafor, filgrastim, and apheresis should be continued daily until sufficient cell collection up to a maximum of 4 days.

Hematopoietic stem cell mobilization (in non-Hodgkin lymphoma and multiple myeloma): Adults: SubQ: 0.24 mg/kg once daily (~11 hours prior to apheresis) for up to 4 consecutive days; maximum dose: 40 mg daily

Dosage adjustment in renal impairment: Note: Creatinine clearance estimate based on Cockcroft-Gault formula:

Cl_{cr} >50 mL/minute: No dosage adjustment necessary.

Cl_{cr} ≤50 mL/minute: 0.16 mg/kg; maximum dose: 27 mg daily

Hemodialysis: No dosage adjustment provided in manufacturer's labeling (has not been studied).

Dosage adjustment in hepatic impairment: No dosage adjustment provided in manufacturer's labeling.

Dosing in obesity: The manufacturer recommends calculating the dose based on actual weight for patients weighing up to 175% of ideal body weight (maximum dose: 40 mg daily). Dosing in patients >175% of ideal body weight has not been studied.

Administration Administer subcutaneously, ~11 hours prior to initiation of apheresis. In some clinical trials, plerixafor administration began in the evening prior to apheresis; filgrastim was begun on day 1, plerixafor initiated in the evening on day 4 and apheresis in the morning on day 5; with filgrastim, plerixafor, and apheresis then continued daily until sufficient cell collection for autologous transplant (DiPersio, 2009a; DiPersio, 2009b).

Hazardous agent; use appropriate precautions for handling and disposal (NIOSH, 2012).

Monitoring Parameters CBC with differential and platelets; signs/symptoms of hypersensitivity (during, for 30 minutes after administration, and until clinically stable); signs/symptoms of splenomegaly

Dosage Forms Excipient information presented when available (limited, particularly for generics); consult specific product labeling.

Solution, Subcutaneous [preservative free]:

Mozobil: 24 mg/1.2 mL (1.2 mL)

◆ **PMS-Quetiapine (Can)** *see* QUEtiapine *on page 1757*
◆ **PMS-Rabeprazole EC (Can)** *see* RABEprazole *on page 1769*
◆ **PMS-Ramipril (Can)** *see* Ramipril *on page 1778*
◆ **PMS-Ranitidine (Can)** *see* Ranitidine *on page 1782*
◆ **PMS-Repaglinide (Can)** *see* Repaglinide *on page 1797*
◆ **PMS-Risedronate (Can)** *see* Risedronate *on page 1824*
◆ **PMS-Risperidone (Can)** *see* RisperiDONE *on page 1826*
◆ **PMS-Risperidone ODT (Can)** *see* RisperiDONE *on page 1826*
◆ **PMS-Rivastigmine (Can)** *see* Rivastigmine *on page 1841*
◆ **PMS-Ropinirole (Can)** *see* ROPINIRole *on page 1851*
◆ **PMS-Rosuvastatin (Can)** *see* Rosuvastatin *on page 1858*
◆ **PMS-Salbutamol (Can)** *see* Albuterol *on page 61*
◆ **PMS-Sertraline (Can)** *see* Sertraline *on page 1889*
◆ **PMS-Sildenafil (Can)** *see* Sildenafil *on page 1894*
◆ **PMS-Simvastatin (Can)** *see* Simvastatin *on page 1899*
◆ **PMS-Sodium Polystyrene Sulfonate (Can)** *see* Sodium Polystyrene Sulfonate *on page 1927*
◆ **PMS-Sotalol (Can)** *see* Sotalol *on page 1942*
◆ **PMS-Sucralate (Can)** *see* Sucralfate *on page 1955*
◆ **PMS-Sulfacetamide (Can)** *see* Sulfacetamide (Ophthalmic) *on page 1956*
◆ **PMS-Sulfasalazine (Can)** *see* SulfaSALAzine *on page 1964*
◆ **PMS-Sumatriptan (Can)** *see* SUMAtriptan *on page 1969*
◆ **PMS-Tamoxifen (Can)** *see* Tamoxifen *on page 1987*
◆ **PMS-Telmisartan (Can)** *see* Telmisartan *on page 2002*
◆ **PMS-Telmisartan HCTZ (Can)** *see* Telmisartan and Hydrochlorothiazide *on page 2004*
◆ **PMS-Temazepam (Can)** *see* Temazepam *on page 2005*
◆ **PMS-Terazosin (Can)** *see* Terazosin *on page 2015*
◆ **PMS-Terbinafine (Can)** *see* Terbinafine (Systemic) *on page 2017*
◆ **PMS-Testosterone (Can)** *see* Testosterone *on page 2026*
◆ **PMS-Tetrabenazine (Can)** *see* Tetrabenazine *on page 2033*
◆ **PMS-Theophylline (Can)** *see* Theophylline *on page 2042*
◆ **PMS-Ticlopidine (Can)** *see* Ticlopidine *on page 2059*
◆ **PMS-Timolol (Can)** *see* Timolol (Ophthalmic) *on page 2064*
◆ **PMS-Tobramycin (Can)** *see* Tobramycin (Ophthalmic) *on page 2079*
◆ **PMS-Topiramate (Can)** *see* Topiramate *on page 2090*
◆ **PMS-Trazodone (Can)** *see* TraZODone *on page 2112*
◆ **PMS-Trifluoperazine (Can)** *see* Trifluoperazine *on page 2125*
◆ **PMS-Trihexyphenidyl (Can)** *see* Trihexyphenidyl *on page 2127*
◆ **PMS-Ursodiol C (Can)** *see* Ursodiol *on page 2142*
◆ **PMS-Valacyclovir (Can)** *see* ValACYclovir *on page 2145*
◆ **PMS-Valproic Acid (Can)** *see* Valproic Acid and Derivatives *on page 2149*
◆ **PMS-Valproic Acid E.C. (Can)** *see* Valproic Acid and Derivatives *on page 2149*
◆ **PMS-Valsartan (Can)** *see* Valsartan *on page 2154*
◆ **PMS-Vancomycin (Can)** *see* Vancomycin *on page 2157*
◆ **PMS-Venlafaxine XR (Can)** *see* Venlafaxine *on page 2178*
◆ **PMS-Verapamil SR (Can)** *see* Verapamil *on page 2182*
◆ **PMS-Zolmitriptan (Can)** *see* ZOLMitriptan *on page 2240*
◆ **PMS-Zolmitriptan ODT (Can)** *see* ZOLMitriptan *on page 2240*
◆ **PN** *see* Total Parenteral Nutrition *on page 2098*
◆ **PN401** *see* Uridine Triacetate *on page 2141*
◆ **Pneumo 23™ (Can)** *see* Pneumococcal Polysaccharide Vaccine (Polyvalent) *on page 1664*

Pneumococcal Conjugate Vaccine (13-Valent)

(noo moe KOK al KON ju gate vak SEEN, thur TEEN vay lent)

Brand Names: U.S. Prevnar 13
Brand Names: Canada Prevnar 13
Index Terms PCV13; Pneumococcal 13-Valent Conjugate Vaccine
Pharmacologic Category Vaccine, Inactivated (Bacterial)
Additional Appendix Information
Immunization Administration Recommendations *on page 2334*
Immunization Recommendations *on page 2339*

Use

U.S. labeling:

Immunization of children 6 weeks through 17 years of age against *Streptococcus pneumoniae* infection caused by serotypes included in the vaccine

Immunization of children 6 weeks through 5 years of age against otitis media caused by *Streptococcus pneumoniae* serotypes 4, 6B, 9V, 14, 18C, 19F, and 23F

Immunization of adults ≥50 years against pneumococcal pneumonia and invasive disease caused by *Streptococcus pneumoniae* serotypes included in the vaccine

Canadian labeling:

Immunization of children 6 weeks through 17 years of age against *Streptococcus pneumoniae* infection caused by serotypes included in the vaccine

Immunization of adults ≥50 years against pneumococcal pneumonia and invasive disease caused by *Streptococcus pneumoniae* serotypes included in the vaccine

The Advisory Committee on Immunization Practices (ACIP) recommends routine vaccination for the following (CDC 59[RR-11], 2010):

All children age 2-59 months

Children 60-71 months with underlying medical conditions including:

Immunocompetent children with chronic heart disease (particularly cyanotic congenital heart disease and heart failure), chronic lung disease (including asthma if treated with high dose corticosteroids), diabetes, cerebrospinal fluid leaks, or cochlear implants

Children with functional or anatomic asplenia, including sickle cell disease or other hemoglobinopathies, congenital or acquired asplenia, or splenic dysfunction.

Children with immunocompromising conditions including congenital immunodeficiency (includes B or T cell deficiency, compliment deficiencies and phagocytic disorders; excludes chronic granulomatous disease), HIV infection, chronic renal failure, nephrotic syndrome, leukemia, lymphoma, Hodgkin disease, generalized malignancies, solid organ transplant, or other diseases requiring immunosuppressive drugs (including long term systemic corticosteroids and radiation therapy)

Children who received ≥1 dose of PCV7

Note: Routine use is not recommended for healthy children ≥5 years of age.

Children ≥6 years and Adolescents ≤18 years of age (CDC, 2013c), and Adults ≥19 years of age (CDC, 2012): The ACIP also recommends routine vaccination for persons with the following underlying medical conditions:

Immunocompetent persons with cerebrospinal fluid leaks or cochlear implants

Persons with functional or anatomic asplenia, including sickle cell disease or other hemoglobinopathies, congenital or acquired asplenia

Persons with immunocompromising conditions including congenital or acquired immunodeficiency (includes B or T cell deficiency, compliment deficiencies and phagocytic disorders; excludes chronic granulomatous disease), HIV infection, chronic renal failure, nephrotic syndrome, leukemia, lymphoma, Hodgkin disease, generalized malignancies, solid organ transplant, multiple myeloma, or other diseases requiring immunosuppressive drugs (including long term systemic corticosteroids and radiation therapy)

Pregnancy Risk Factor B

Pregnancy Considerations Animal reproduction studies have not shown adverse fetal effects. Inactivated vaccines have not been shown to cause increased risks to the fetus (CDC, 2011).

Breast-Feeding Considerations

It is not known if this vaccine is excreted into breast milk. The manufacturer recommends that caution be exercised when administering this vaccine to nursing women. Inactivated vaccines do not affect the safety of breast-feeding for the mother or the infant. Breast-feeding infants should be vaccinated according to the recommended schedules (CDC, 2011).

Contraindications Severe allergic reaction (eg, anaphylaxis) to pneumococcal vaccine or any component of the formulation, including diphtheria toxoid

Warnings/Precautions Immediate treatment (including epinephrine 1:1000) for anaphylactoid and/or hypersensitivity reactions should be available during vaccine use. Use with caution in patients with a history of bleeding disorders (including thrombocytopenia) and/or patients on anticoagulant therapy; bleeding/hematoma may occur from I.M. administration. Use with caution in severely immunocompromised patients (eg, patients receiving chemo/radiation therapy or other immunosuppressive therapy including high-dose corticosteroids); may have a reduced response to vaccination. In general, household and close contacts of persons with altered immunocompetence may receive all age appropriate vaccines (CDC, 2011). Syncope has been reported with use of injectable vaccines and may be accompanied by transient visual disturbances, weakness, or tonic-clonic movements. Procedures should be in place to avoid injuries from falling and to restore cerebral perfusion if syncope occurs (CDC, 2008).

The decision to administer or delay vaccination because of current or recent febrile illness depends on the severity of symptoms and the etiology of the disease. Immunization should be delayed during the course of an acute severe febrile illness; may administer to patients with mild acute illness (with or without fever). In order to maximize vaccination rates, the ACIP recommends simultaneous administration of all age-appropriate vaccines (live or inactivated) for which a person is eligible at a single clinic visit, unless contraindications exist. Vaccination may not result in effective immunity in all patients. Response depends upon multiple factors (eg, type of vaccine, age of patient) and may be improved by administering the vaccine at the recommended dose, route, and interval. Vaccines may not be effective if administered during periods of altered immune competence (CDC, 2011).

Use of pneumococcal conjugate vaccine does not replace use of the 23-valent pneumococcal polysaccharide vaccine in children ≥24 months of age with chronic illness, asplenia, sickle cell disease or are immunocompromised or have HIV infection (CDC 59[RR-11], 2010). Antibody responses were lower in older adults >65 years of age compared to adults 50-59 years of age. Apnea has been reported following I.M. vaccine administration in premature infants; consider risk versus benefit in infants born prematurely. Not to be used to treat pneumococcal infections or to provide immunity against diphtheria. Use of this vaccine for specific medical and/or other indications (eg, immunocompromising conditions, hepatic or kidney disease, diabetes) is also addressed in the ACIP Recommended Immunization Schedule (CDC, 2013a; CDC, 2013b).

Adverse Reactions All serious adverse reactions must be reported to the U.S. Department of Health and Human Services (DHHS) Vaccine Adverse Event Reporting System (VAERS) 1-800-822-7967 or online at https://vaers.hhs.gov/esub/index.

>10%:

Central nervous system: Chills, drowsiness, fatigue, fever, headache, insomnia, irritability

Dermatologic: Rash

Gastrointestinal: Appetite decreased

Local: Erythema, limitation of arm motion, pain, swelling, tenderness

Neuromuscular & skeletal: Arthralgia, myalgia

1% to 10%:

Dermatological: Hives

Gastrointestinal: Diarrhea, vomiting

<1% (Limited to important or life-threatening): Abnormal crying, erythema multiforme, febrile seizures, hypersensitivity reaction (bronchospasm, dyspnea, facial edema), seizure, urticaria, urticaria-like rash

Adverse reactions observed with PCV7 which may also be seen with PCV-13: Anaphylactic reaction, angioneurotic edema, apnea, breath holding, edema, hypotonic hyporesponsive episode, injection site reaction (dermatitis, pruritus), lymphadenopathy (localized), shock

Drug Interactions

Metabolism/Transport Effects None known.

Avoid Concomitant Use There are no known interactions where it is recommended to avoid concomitant use.

Increased Effect/Toxicity There are no known significant interactions involving an increase in effect.

Decreased Effect

Pneumococcal Conjugate Vaccine (13-Valent) may decrease the levels/effects of: Influenza Virus Vaccine (Inactivated)

The levels/effects of Pneumococcal Conjugate Vaccine (13-Valent) may be decreased by: Belimumab; Fingolimod; Immunosuppressants; Influenza Virus Vaccine (Inactivated)

Storage/Stability Store under refrigeration at 2°C to 8°C (36°F to 46°F); do not freeze; discard if frozen. **Note:** The Canadian labeling suggests that the vaccine is stable at temperatures up to 25°C (77°F) for 4 days.

Mechanism of Action Promotes active immunization against invasive disease caused by *S. pneumoniae* capsular serotypes 1, 3, 4, 5, 6A, 6B, 7F, 9V, 14, 18C, 19A, 19F, and 23F, all which are individually conjugated to CRM197 protein

Dosage I.M.:

Infants, Children, and Adolescents:

Primary immunization: *Infants and Children 6 weeks to 59 months:* 0.5 mL/dose for a total of 4 doses. The first dose may be given as young as 6 weeks of age, but is typically given at 8 weeks (2 months of age). The 3 remaining doses are usually given at 4, 6, and 12-15 months of age. The recommended dosing interval is 4-8 weeks. The minimum interval between doses in children <1 year of age is 1 month. The minimum interval between the third and fourth dose is 8 weeks.

Immunization: *Older Infants, Children, and Adolescents:*

Children 7-11 months (previously unvaccinated): 0.5 mL for a total of 3 doses; 2 doses at least 4 weeks apart, followed by a third dose after the 1-year birthday (12-15 months), separated from the second dose by at least 8 weeks

Children 12-23 months (previously unvaccinated): 0.5 mL for a total of 2 doses, separated by at least 8 weeks

Healthy Children 24-59 months (previously unvaccinated): 0.5 mL as a single dose

Children 24-71 months with an underlying medical condition (previously unvaccinated): 0.5 mL for a total of 2 doses, separated by 8 weeks (CDC 59[RR-11], 2010)

Children 6 through 17 years: 0.5 mL as a single dose. If PCV7 was previously administered, give PCV13 ≥8 weeks after that dose

Previously vaccinated with PCV7 and/or PCV13, and with a lapse in vaccine administration (CDC 59[RR-11], 2010):

Children 7-11 months: Previously received 1 or 2 doses: 0.5 mL dose at 7-11 months of age, followed by a second dose ≥8 weeks later at 12-15 months of age

Children 12-23 months:

Previously received 1 dose <12 months of age: 0.5 mL dose, followed by a second dose ≥8 weeks later

Previously received 1 dose at ≥12 months of age: 0.5 mL dose ≥8 weeks after the most recent dose

Previously received 2 or 3 doses before age 12 months: 0.5 mL dose ≥8 weeks after the most recent dose

Healthy Children 24-59 months with any incomplete schedule: 0.5 mL dose ≥8 weeks after the most recent dose

Children 24-71 months with an underlying medical condition:

Previously received <3 doses: 0.5 mL dose ≥8 weeks after the most recent dose, followed by a second dose ≥8 weeks later

Previously received 3 doses: 0.5 mL as a single dose ≥8 weeks after the most recent dose

Children ≥6 years and Adolescents ≤18 years with specified underlying medical conditions (CDC, 2013c):

Pneumococcal vaccine-naive (no previous PCV13 or PPSV23 vaccine): Administer PCV13 0.5 mL as a single dose, followed by 1 dose of PPSV23 ≥8-weeks later.

Previously vaccinated with PPSV23: If PCV13 has never been administered, give PCV13 0.5 mL as a single dose ≥8 weeks after the last dose of PPSV23. PCV13 should be administered even if the child had received PCV7.

Adults: **Immunization: Note:** Efficacy of PCV13 administered <5 years after PPSV23 is unknown.

Adults ≥50 years (manufacturers labeling): 0.5 mL as a single dose

Adults ≥19 years with specified underlying medical conditions (CDC, 2012): Eligible adults should be vaccinated at their next pneumococcal vaccination opportunity

Pneumococcal vaccine naive (no previous PCV13 or PPSV23 vaccine): Administer PCV13 0.5 mL as a single dose followed by 1 dose of PPSV23 8-weeks later.

Previously vaccinated with PPSV23: PCV13 0.5 mL as a single dose ≥1 year after the last dose of PPSV23.

Dosage adjustment in renal impairment: No dosage adjustment provided in manufacturer's labeling.

Dosage adjustment in hepatic impairment: No dosage adjustment provided in manufacturer's labeling.

Administration Shake well prior to use. Do not use if a homogenous white suspension does not form. Administer I.M. (deltoid muscle for toddlers, young children, and adults or lateral midthigh in infants). Do not inject I.V. or SubQ; avoid intradermal route. Concurrent administration of PCV13 and PPV23 has not been studied and is not recommended (CDC, 2010).

For patients at risk of hemorrhage following intramuscular injection, the ACIP recommends "it should be administered intramuscularly if, in the opinion of the physician familiar with the patient's bleeding risk, the vaccine can be administered by this route with reasonable safety. If the patient receives antihemophilia or other similar therapy, intramuscular vaccination can be scheduled shortly after such therapy is administered. A fine needle (23 gauge or smaller) can be used for the vaccination and firm pressure applied to the site (without rubbing) for at least 2 minutes. The patient should be instructed concerning the risk of hematoma from the injection." Patients on anticoagulant therapy should be considered to have the same bleeding risks and treated as those with clotting factor disorders (CDC, 2011).

Antipyretics have not been shown to prevent febrile seizures. Antipyretics may be used to treat fever or discomfort following vaccination (CDC, 2011). One study reported that routine prophylactic administration of acetaminophen to prevent fever prior to vaccination decreased the immune response of some vaccines; the clinical significance of this reduction in immune response has not been established (Prymula, 2009).

Simultaneous administration of vaccines helps ensure the patients will be fully vaccinated by the appropriate age. Simultaneous administration of vaccines is defined as administering >1 vaccine on the same day at different anatomic sites. Separate vaccines should not be combined in the same syringe unless indicated by product specific labeling. Separate needles and syringes should be used for each injection. The ACIP prefers each dose of a specific vaccine in a series come from the same manufacturer when possible. Adolescents and adults should be vaccinated while seated or lying down. In general, preterm infants should be vaccinated at the same chronological age as full-term infants (CDC, 2011).

Monitoring Parameters Monitor for syncope for 15 minutes following administration. If seizure-like activity associated with syncope occurs, maintain patient in supine or Trendelenburg position to reestablish adequate cerebral perfusion (CDC, 2008).

Additional Information U.S. federal law requires that the name of medication, date of administration, the vaccine manufacturer, lot number of vaccine, and the administering person's name, title and address be entered into the patient's permanent medical record.

Pneumococcal 13-valent conjugate vaccine (PCV13; Prevnar 13) is the successor to the previously-marketed pneumococcal 7-valent conjugate vaccine (PCV7; Prevnar). Prevnar 13 contains an additional 6 serotypes of *Streptococcus pneumoniae*, compared to the 7 serotypes provided in the original Prevnar formulation.

Dosage Forms Excipient information presented when available (limited, particularly for generics); consult specific product labeling.

Injection, suspension:

Prevnar 13: 2 mcg of each capsular saccharide for serotypes 1, 3, 4, 5, 6A, 7F, 9V, 14, 18C, 19A, 19F, and 23F, and 4 mcg of serotype 6B [bound to diphtheria CRM_{197} protein ~34 mcg] per 0.5 mL (0.5 mL) [contains aluminum, polysorbate 80, and yeast]

Pneumococcal Polysaccharide Vaccine (Polyvalent)

(noo moe KOK al pol i SAK a ride vak SEEN, pol i VAY lent)

Brand Names: U.S. Pneumovax® 23

Brand Names: Canada Pneumo 23™; Pneumovax® 23

Index Terms 23-Valent Pneumococcal Polysaccharide Vaccine; 23PS; PPSV; PPSV23; PPV23

Pharmacologic Category Vaccine, Inactivated (Bacterial)

Additional Appendix Information

Immunization Administration Recommendations *on page 2334*

Immunization Recommendations *on page 2339*

Use Immunization against pneumococcal disease caused by serotypes included in the vaccine. Routine vaccination is recommended for persons ≥50 years of age and persons ≥2 years in certain situations.

The Advisory Committee on Immunization Practices (ACIP) recommends routine vaccination for patients with the following underlying medical conditions (CDC, 59[34], 2010; CDC, 59[11], 2010; CDC, 2012):

Children ≥2 years of age and adults 19-64 years with functional or anatomic asplenia, including sickle cell disease or other hemoglobinopathies, congenital or acquired asplenia, splenic dysfunction, or splenectomy

Immunocompetent children ≥2 years of age with chronic heart disease (particularly cyanotic congenital heart disease and heart failure), chronic lung disease (including asthma if treated with high dose corticosteroids), diabetes, cerebrospinal fluid leaks, or cochlear implants

Immunocompetent adults 19-64 years with chronic heart disease (including heart failure and cardiomyopathies; excluding hypertension), chronic lung disease (including COPD, emphysema, and asthma), diabetes, cerebrospinal fluid leaks, cochlear implants, alcoholism, chronic liver disease, cirrhosis, and cigarette smokers

Immunocompromised children ≥2 years of age and adults 19-64 years with congenital or acquired immunodeficiency (includes B or T cell deficiency, compliment deficiencies and phagocytic disorders; excludes chronic granulomatous disease), HIV infection, chronic renal failure, nephrotic syndrome, leukemia, lymphoma, Hodgkin disease, generalized malignancies, solid organ transplant, multiple myeloma, or other diseases requiring immunosuppressive drugs (including long-term systemic corticosteroids and radiation therapy)

All adults ≥65 years of age

Pregnancy Risk Factor C

Pregnancy Considerations Animal reproduction studies have not been conducted. Vaccination should be considered in pregnant women at high risk for infection. Inactivated vaccines have not been shown to cause increased risks to the fetus (CDC, 2011)

Breast-Feeding Considerations Inactivated vaccines do not affect the safety of breast-feeding for the mother or the infant. Breast-feeding infants should be vaccinated according to the recommended schedules (CDC, 2011).

Contraindications Hypersensitivity to pneumococcal vaccine or any component of the formulation

Warnings/Precautions Use caution in patients with severely compromised cardiovascular function or pulmonary disease where a systemic reaction may pose a significant risk. May cause relapse in patients with stable idiopathic thrombocytopenia purpura. Epinephrine injection (1:1000) must be immediately available in the case of anaphylaxis. Syncope has been reported with use of injectable vaccines and may be accompanied by transient visual disturbances, weakness, or tonic-clonic movements. Procedures should be in place to avoid injuries from falling and to restore cerebral perfusion if syncope occurs.

Patients who will be receiving immunosuppressive therapy (including Hodgkin's disease, cancer chemotherapy, or transplantation) should be vaccinated at least 2 weeks prior to the initiation of therapy. Immune responses may be impaired for several months following intensive immunosuppressive therapy (up to 2 years in Hodgkin's disease patients). Vaccination may not result in effective immunity in all patients. Response depends upon multiple factors (eg, type of vaccine, age of patient) and may be improved by administering the vaccine at the recommended dose, route, and interval. Vaccines may not be effective if administered during periods of altered immune competence (CDC, 2011). Patients who will undergo splenectomy or who will undergo cochlear implant placement should also be vaccinated at least 2 weeks prior to surgery, if possible. In general, household and close contacts of persons with altered immunocompetence may receive all age appropriate vaccines. Patients with HIV should be vaccinated as soon as possible (following confirmation of the diagnosis). The decision to administer or delay vaccination because of current or recent febrile illness depends on the severity of symptoms and the etiology of the disease. Immunization should be delayed during the course of an acute febrile illness or other active infection. In order to maximize vaccination rates, the ACIP recommends simultaneous administration of all age-appropriate vaccines (live or inactivated) for which a person is eligible at a single clinic visit, unless contraindications exist. If a person has not received any pneumococcal vaccine or if pneumococcal vaccination status is unknown, PPSV23 should be administered as indicated. Postmarketing reports of adverse effects in the elderly, especially those with comorbidities, have been significant enough to require hospitalization. Use of this vaccine for specific medical and/or other indications (eg, immunocompromising conditions, hepatic or kidney disease, diabetes) is also addressed in the ACIP Recommended Immunization Schedule (CDC, 2013a; CDC, 2013b).

Adverse Reactions All serious adverse reactions must be reported to the U.S. Department of Health and Human Services (DHHS) Vaccine Adverse Event Reporting System (VAERS) 1-800-822-7967 or online at https://vaers.hhs.gov/esub/index. In Canada, adverse reactions may be reported to local provincial/territorial health agencies or to the Vaccine Safety Section at Public Health Agency of Canada (1-866-844-0018).

Frequency not defined.

Central nervous system: Chills, Guillain-Barré syndrome, fever ≤102°F*, fever >102°F, headache, malaise, pain, radiculoneuropathy, seizure (febrile)

Dermatologic: Angioneurotic edema, cellulitis, rash, urticaria

Gastrointestinal: Nausea, vomiting

Hematologic: Hemolytic anemia (in patients with other hematologic disorders), leukocytosis, thrombocytopenia (in patients with stabilized ITP)

Local: Injection site reaction* (erythema, induration, swelling, soreness, warmth); peripheral edema in injected extremity

Neuromuscular & skeletal: Arthralgia, arthritis, limb mobility decreased, myalgia, paresthesia, weakness

Miscellaneous: Anaphylactoid reaction, C-reactive protein increased, lymphadenitis, lymphadenopathy, serum sickness

*Reactions most commonly reported in clinical trials.

Drug Interactions

Metabolism/Transport Effects None known.

Avoid Concomitant Use There are no known interactions where it is recommended to avoid concomitant use.

Increased Effect/Toxicity There are no known significant interactions involving an increase in effect.

Decreased Effect

Pneumococcal Polysaccharide Vaccine (Polyvalent) may decrease the levels/effects of: Zoster Vaccine

The levels/effects of Pneumococcal Polysaccharide Vaccine (Polyvalent) may be decreased by: Belimumab; Fingolimod; Immunosuppressants

Storage/Stability Store under refrigeration at 2°C to 8°C (36°F to 46°F).

Mechanism of Action Although there are more than 80 known pneumococcal capsular types, pneumococcal disease is mainly caused by only a few types of pneumococci. Pneumococcal vaccine contains capsular polysaccharides of 23 pneumococcal types of *Streptococcal pneumoniae* which represent at least 85% to 90% of pneumococcal disease isolates in the United States. The 23 capsular pneumococcal vaccine contains purified capsular polysaccharides of pneumococcal types 1, 2, 3, 4, 5, 6B, 7F, 8, 9N, 9V, 10A, 11A, 12F, 14, 15B, 17F, 18C, 19F, 19A, 20, 22F, 23F, and 33F.

Dosage I.M., SubQ:

Children ≥2 years: 0.5 mL as a single dose

Primary vaccination: Children with specified underlying medical conditions: One dose of PPSV23 should be given at ≥2 years of age. Immunization with PCV13 should be completed prior to PPSV23 as recommended. The minimum interval between the last dose of PCV13 and PPSV23 is 8 weeks (CDC, 59[11] 2010).

Revaccination: Children with functional or anatomic asplenia, or who are immunocompromised: One revaccination dose ≥5 years after the first dose of PPSV23. Revaccination of immunocompetent individuals is generally not recommended (CDC, 59[11] 2010).

Adults: 0.5 mL as a single dose

Primary vaccination: Adults 19-64 years with specified underlying medical conditions and all patients at 65 years of age without previous PPSV23 vaccination should receive one dose of PPSV23 (CDC, 59[34], 2010). In patients who are pneumococcal vaccine naïve (no previous PCV13 or PPSV23 vaccine), administer a single dose of PCV13 followed by 1 dose of PPSV23 8-weeks later (CDC, 2012).

Revaccination:

Adults 19-64 years with functional or anatomic asplenia, or who are immunocompromised: One revaccination dose ≥5 years after first dose of PPSV23 (CDC, 59 [34], 2010) and ≥8 weeks after PCV13 (CDC, 2012)

Adults ≥65 years: One revaccination dose if ≥5 years after first dose of PPSV23 and if <65 years of age at the time of the initial vaccination (for any indication). Immunocompetent adults who received primary vaccination at ≥65 years do not need to be revaccinated (CDC, 59[34], 2010; CDC 2012).

Dosage adjustment in renal impairment: No dosage adjustment provided in manufacturer's labeling.

Dosage adjustment in hepatic impairment: No dosage adjustment provided in manufacturer's labeling.

Administration Do not inject I.V.; avoid intradermal administration (may cause severe local reactions); administer SubQ or I.M. (deltoid muscle or lateral midthigh)

For patients at risk of hemorrhage following intramuscular injection, the ACIP recommends "it should be administered intramuscularly if, in the opinion of the physician familiar with the patient's bleeding risk, the vaccine can be administered by this route with reasonable safety. If the patient receives antihemophilia or other similar therapy, intramuscular vaccination can be scheduled shortly after such therapy is administered. A fine needle (23 gauge or smaller) can be used for the vaccination and firm pressure applied to the site (without rubbing) for at least 2 minutes. The patient should be instructed concerning the risk of hematoma from the injection." Patients on anticoagulant therapy should be considered to have the same bleeding risks and treated as those with clotting factor disorders (CDC, 2011).

Antipyretics have not been shown to prevent febrile seizures. Antipyretics may be used to treat fever or discomfort following vaccination (CDC, 2011). One study reported that routine prophylactic administration of acetaminophen to prevent fever prior to vaccination decreased the immune response of some vaccines; the clinical significance of this reduction in immune response has not been established (Prymula, 2009).

Simultaneous administration of vaccines helps ensure the patients will be fully vaccinated by the appropriate age. Simultaneous administration of vaccines is defined as administering >1 vaccine on the same day at different anatomic sites. Separate vaccines should not be combined in the same syringe unless indicated by product specific labeling. Separate needles and syringes should be used for each injection. The ACIP prefers each dose of a specific vaccine in a series come from the same manufacturer when possible. Adolescents and adults should be vaccinated while seated or lying down. In general, preterm infants should be vaccinated at the same chronological age as full-term infants (CDC, 2011).

Monitoring Parameters Monitor for syncope for 15 minutes following administration. If seizure-like activity associated with syncope occurs, maintain patient in supine or Trendelenburg position to reestablish adequate cerebral perfusion.

Additional Information U.S. federal law requires that the name of medication, date of administration, the vaccine manufacturer, lot number of vaccine, and the administering person's name, title, and address be entered into the patient's permanent medical record.

Dosage Forms Excipient information presented when available (limited, particularly for generics); consult specific product labeling.

Injection, solution:

Pneumovax® 23: 25 mcg each of 23 capsular polysaccharide isolates/0.5 mL (0.5 mL, 2.5 mL)

◆ **Pneumococcal 13-Valent Conjugate Vaccine** *see* Pneumococcal Conjugate Vaccine (13-Valent) *on page 1661*

◆ **Pneumovax® 23** *see* Pneumococcal Polysaccharide Vaccine (Polyvalent) *on page 1664*

◆ **PNU-140690E** *see* Tipranavir *on page 2070*

◆ **Podactin [OTC]** *see* Miconazole (Topical) *on page 1358*

◆ **Podactin [OTC]** *see* Tolnaftate *on page 2087*

◆ **Podocon** *see* Podophyllum Resin *on page 1666*

◆ **Podofilm® (Can)** *see* Podophyllum Resin *on page 1666*

◆ **Podophyllin** *see* Podophyllum Resin *on page 1666*

Podophyllum Resin (po DOF fil um REZ in)

Brand Names: U.S. Podocon
Brand Names: Canada Podofilm®
Index Terms Mandrake; May Apple; Podophyllin
Pharmacologic Category Keratolytic Agent
Use Topical treatment of soft external genital (venereal) warts (condylomata acuminata); compound benzoin tincture generally is used as the medium for topical application
Dosage Topical: Children and Adults: Condylomata acuminatum: Applied by physician only.
Additional Information Complete prescribing information should be consulted for additional detail.
Dosage Forms Excipient information presented when available (limited, particularly for generics); consult specific product labeling.
Solution, External:
Podocon: 25% (15 mL)

Polidocanol (pol i DOE kuh nol)

Brand Names: U.S. Asclera
Index Terms Varithena
Pharmacologic Category Sclerosing Agent
Use Treatment of small, uncomplicated varicose veins of the lower extremities
Pregnancy Risk Factor C
Pregnancy Considerations Adverse events were observed in animal reproduction studies.
Breast-Feeding Considerations It is not known if polidocanol is excreted in breast milk. Due to the potential for adverse reactions in a nursing infant, the manufacturer recommends avoiding use in nursing women.
Contraindications Hypersensitivity to polidocanol or any component of the formulation; acute thromboembolic diseases
Warnings/Precautions Severe allergic reactions, including anaphylaxis and fatal anaphylactoid reactions have been reported with polidocanol; more frequent with larger volumes (>3 mL), therefore, dose should be minimized. Observe 15-20 minutes following injection to monitor for hypersensitivity/anaphylactic reaction; emergency resuscitation equipment should be available. Necrosis of the tissue may occur; pain may occur with inadvertent perivascular injection and may be resolved with a local anesthetic (without epinephrine). Severe necrosis, ischemia, or gangrene can occur with accidental intra-arterial injection; consult vascular surgeon immediately.

After injection is complete, apply compression/bandage, and have patient walk for 15-20 minutes.

Adverse Reactions
>10%: Local: Hematoma (42%), irritation (41%), discoloration (38%), pain (24%), pruritus (19%), warmth (16%)
1% to 10%: Local: Neovascularization (8%), injection site thrombosis (6%)
Postmarketing and/or case reports: Allergic dermatitis, anaphylactic shock, angioedema, asthma, cardiac arrest, cerebrovascular accident, circulatory collapse, confusion, deep vein thrombosis, dizziness, dyspnea, hot flush, hypertrichosis, injection site necrosis, loss of consciousness, migraine, nerve injury, palpitation, paresthesia, pulmonary embolism, pyrexia, skin hyperpigmentation, syncope (vasovagal), urticaria, vasculitis

Drug Interactions
Metabolism/Transport Effects None known.
Avoid Concomitant Use There are no known interactions where it is recommended to avoid concomitant use.
Increased Effect/Toxicity There are no known significant interactions involving an increase in effect.
Decreased Effect There are no known significant interactions involving a decrease in effect.

Storage/Stability Store at 15°C to 30°C (59°F to 86°F). Each ampul is intended for immediate use.
Mechanism of Action Acts by irritation of the vein intimal endothelium and causes thrombosis formation leading to occlusion of the injected vein
Pharmacodynamics/Kinetics Half-life elimination: 1.5 hours
Dosage I.V.: Adults: Varicose veins:
Reticular veins (1-3 mm diameter): 0.1-0.3 mL of 1% solution per injection (maximum: 10 mL per session); may repeat in 7-14 days
Spider veins (≤1 mm diameter): 0.1-0.3 mL of 0.5% solution per injection (maximum: 10 mL per session); may repeat in 7-14 days

Dosage adjustment in renal impairment: No dosage adjustment provided in manufacturer's labeling.
Dosage adjustment in hepatic impairment: No dosage adjustment provided in manufacturer's labeling.

Administration For intravenous use only. Avoid extravasation. After injection, apply compression in the form of a stocking or bandage (maintain for 2-3 days [spider veins] and 5-7 days [reticular veins]). After applying compression, patient should walk for 15-20 minutes and be observed for anaphylactic or allergic reaction.
Monitoring Parameters Monitor patient for anaphylactic or allergic reaction after injection, and for signs/symptoms of DVT or PE.
Product Availability
Varithena (polidocanol injectable foam): FDA approved November 2013; availability anticipated in the second quarter of 2014.
Varithena is a sclerosing agent indicated for the treatment of incompetent great saphenous veins, accessory saphenous veins and visible varicosities of the great saphenous vein system above and below the knee.
Dosage Forms Excipient information presented when available (limited, particularly for generics); consult specific product labeling.
Solution, Intravenous [preservative free]:
Asclera: 0.5% (2 mL); 1% (2 mL) [contains alcohol, usp]

◆ **Polio Vaccine** *see* Poliovirus Vaccine (Inactivated) *on page 1666*

◆ **Poliovirus, Inactivated (IPV)** *see* Diphtheria and Tetanus Toxoids, Acellular Pertussis, and Poliovirus Vaccine *on page 629*

◆ **Poliovirus, Inactivated (IPV)** *see* Diphtheria and Tetanus Toxoids, Acellular Pertussis, Poliovirus and *Haemophilus* b Conjugate Vaccine *on page 629*

Poliovirus Vaccine (Inactivated)
(POE lee oh VYE rus vak SEEN, in ak ti VAY ted)

Brand Names: U.S. IPOL®
Brand Names: Canada Imovax® Polio
Index Terms Enhanced-Potency Inactivated Poliovirus Vaccine; IPV; Polio Vaccine; Salk Vaccine
Pharmacologic Category Vaccine, Inactivated (Viral)
Additional Appendix Information
Immunization Administration Recommendations *on page 2334*
Immunization Recommendations *on page 2339*
Use Active immunization against poliomyelitis caused by poliovirus types 1, 2, and 3. **Note:** Combination products containing polio vaccine are also available and may be preferred in certain age groups if recipients are likely to be susceptible to the agents contained within each vaccine.

The Advisory Committee on Immunization Practices (ACIP) recommends routine vaccination for the following:
- All children (first dose given at 2 months of age)

Routine immunization of adults in the United States is generally not recommended. Adults with previous wild poliovirus disease, who have never been immunized, or those who are incompletely immunized may receive inactivated poliovirus vaccine if they fall into one of the following categories:
- Travelers to regions or countries where poliomyelitis is endemic or epidemic
- Healthcare workers in close contact with patients who may be excreting poliovirus
- Laboratory workers handling specimens that may contain poliovirus
- Members of communities or specific population groups with diseases caused by wild poliovirus
- Incompletely vaccinated or unvaccinated adults in a household or with other close contact with children receiving oral poliovirus (may be at increased risk of vaccine associated paralytic poliomyelitis)

Pregnancy Risk Factor C

Pregnancy Considerations Animal reproduction studies have not been conducted. Although adverse effects of IPV have not been documented in pregnant women or their fetuses, vaccination of pregnant women should be avoided on theoretical grounds. Pregnant women at increased risk for infection and requiring immediate protection against polio may be administered the vaccine.

Breast-Feeding Considerations Inactivated virus vaccines do not affect the safety of breast-feeding for the mother or the infant. Breast-feeding infants should be vaccinated according to the recommended schedules (CDC, 2011).

Contraindications Hypersensitivity to any component of the vaccine

Warnings/Precautions Patients with prior clinical poliomyelitis, incomplete immunization with oral poliovirus vaccine (OPV), HIV infection, severe combined immunodeficiency, hypogammaglobulinemia, agammaglobulinemia, or altered immunity (due to corticosteroids, alkylating agents, antimetabolites or radiation) may receive inactivated poliovirus vaccine (IPV). In general, household and close contacts of persons with altered immunocompetence may receive all age appropriate vaccines. Immune response may be decreased in patients receiving immune globulin. Vaccination may be deferred with an acute febrile illness; minor illnesses with or without a low-grade fever are not reasons to postpone vaccination. Vaccination may not result in effective immunity in all patients. Response depends upon multiple factors (eg, type of vaccine, age of patient) and may be improved by administering the vaccine at the recommended dose, route, and interval. Vaccines may not be effective if administered during periods of altered immune competence (CDC, 2011). Immediate treatment for anaphylactic/anaphylactoid reaction should be available during vaccine use. In order to maximize vaccination rates, the ACIP recommends simultaneous administration of all age-appropriate vaccines (live or inactivated) for which a person is eligible at a single clinic visit, unless contraindications exist. The use of combination vaccines is generally preferred over separate injections, taking into consideration provider assessment, patient preference, and adverse events. Syncope has been reported with use of injectable vaccines and may be accompanied by transient visual disturbances, weakness, or tonic-clonic movements. Procedures should be in place to avoid injuries from falling and to restore cerebral perfusion if syncope occurs.

The injection contains 2-phenoxyethanol, calf serum protein, formaldehyde, neomycin, streptomycin, and polymyxin B. Use of the minimum age and minimum intervals during the first 6 months of life should only be done when the vaccine recipient is at risk for imminent exposure to circulating poliovirus (shorter intervals and earlier start dates may lead to lower seroconversion).

Adverse Reactions All serious adverse reactions must be reported to the U.S. Department of Health and Human Services (DHHS) Vaccine Adverse Event Reporting System (VAERS) 1-800-822-7967 or online at https://vaers.hhs.gov/esub/index. In Canada, adverse reactions may be reported to local provincial/territorial health agencies or to the Vaccine Safety Section at Public Health Agency of Canada (1-866-844-0018).

Percentages noted with concomitant administration of DTP or DTaP vaccine and observed within 48 hours of injection.

>10%:

Central nervous system: Irritability (7% to 65%; most common in infants 2 months of age), tiredness (4% to 61%)

Gastrointestinal: Anorexia (1% to 17%)

Local: Injection Site: Tenderness (≤29%), swelling (≤11%)

1% to 10%:

Central nervous system: Fever >39°C (≤4%)

Gastrointestinal: Vomiting (1% to 3%)

Local: Injection site: Erythema (≤3%)

Miscellaneous: Persistent crying (≤1% reported within 72 hours)

Postmarketing and/or case reports (Limited to important or life-threatening): Allergic reaction, anaphylactic shock, anaphylaxis, febrile seizures, hypersensitivity reactions, lymphadenopathy, seizures; Guillain-Barré syndrome has been temporally related to another inactivated poliovirus vaccine

Drug Interactions

Metabolism/Transport Effects None known.

Avoid Concomitant Use There are no known interactions where it is recommended to avoid concomitant use.

Increased Effect/Toxicity There are no known significant interactions involving an increase in effect.

Decreased Effect

The levels/effects of Poliovirus Vaccine (Inactivated) may be decreased by: Belimumab; Fingolimod; Immunosuppressants

Storage/Stability Store under refrigeration 2°C to 8°C (35°F to 46°F); do not freeze. Protect from light

Dosage I.M., SubQ:

Children:

Primary immunization: Administer three 0.5 mL doses, at 2, 4, and 6-18 months of age; do not administer more frequently than 4 weeks apart (preferably given more than 8 weeks apart)

Booster dose: 0.5 mL at 4-6 years of age; Minimum interval between booster and previous dose is 6 months. The final (booster) dose should be given at ≥4 years of age, regardless of the number of previous doses. If the final dose is not given at 4-6 years of age, it should be given as soon as feasible.

Note: Use of the minimum age and minimum intervals during the first 6 months of life should only be done when the vaccine recipient is at risk for imminent exposure to circulating poliovirus (shorter intervals and earlier start dates may lead to lower seroconversion).

Adults:

Previously unvaccinated: Two 0.5 mL doses administered at 1- to 2-month intervals, followed by a third dose 6-12 months later. If <3 months, but at least 2 months are available before protection is needed, 3 doses may be administered at least 1 month apart. If administration must be completed within 1-2 months, give 2 doses at least 1 month apart. If <1 month is available, give 1 dose.

Incompletely vaccinated: Adults with at least 1 previous dose of OPV, <3 doses of IPV, or a combination of OPV and IPV equaling <3 doses, administer at least one 0.5 mL dose of IPV. Additional doses to complete the series may be given if time permits.

Completely vaccinated and at increased risk of exposure: One 0.5 mL dose

Dosage adjustment in renal impairment: No dosage adjustment provided in manufacturer's labeling.

Dosage adjustment in hepatic impairment: No dosage adjustment provided in manufacturer's labeling.

Administration Do not administer I.V.; for I.M. or SubQ administration. Administer to midlateral aspect of the thigh in infants and small children. Administer in the deltoid area to adults or older children.

Simultaneous administration of vaccines helps ensure the patients will be fully vaccinated by the appropriate age. Simultaneous administration of vaccines is defined as administering >1 vaccine on the same day at different anatomic sites. The use of licensed combination vaccines is generally preferred over separate injections of the equivalent components. Separate vaccines should not be combined in the same syringe unless indicated by product specific labeling. Separate needles and syringes should be used for each injection. The ACIP prefers each dose of a specific vaccine in a series come from the same manufacturer when possible. Adolescents and adults should be vaccinated while seated or lying down. In general, preterm infants should be vaccinated at the same chronological age as full-term infants (CDC, 2011).

Antipyretics have not been shown to prevent febrile seizures. Antipyretics may be used to treat fever or discomfort following vaccination (CDC, 2011). One study reported that routine prophylactic administration of acetaminophen to prevent fever prior to vaccination decreased the immune response of some vaccines; the clinical significance of this reduction in immune response has not been established (Prymula, 2009).

Monitoring Parameters Monitor for syncope for 15 minutes following administration. If seizure-like activity associated with syncope occurs, maintain patient in supine or Trendelenburg position to reestablish adequate cerebral perfusion.

Test Interactions May temporarily suppress tuberculin skin test sensitivity (4-6 weeks)

Additional Information U.S. federal law requires that the name of medication, date of administration, the vaccine manufacturer, lot number of vaccine, and the administering person's name, title, and address be entered into the patient's permanent medical record.

As the global eradication of poliomyelitis continues, the risk for importation of wild-type poliovirus into the United States decreases dramatically. To eliminate the risk for vaccine-associated paralytic poliomyelitis (VAPP), an all-IPV schedule is recommended for routine childhood vaccination in the United States. Oral poliovirus vaccine (OPV), is not commercially available in the United States, but has been stockpiled for use in the following special circumstances:

Mass vaccination campaigns to control outbreaks of paralytic polio

Unvaccinated children who will be traveling within 4 weeks to areas where polio is endemic or epidemic

Children of parents who do not accept the recommended number of vaccine injections; these children may receive OPV only for the third or fourth dose or both. In this situation, healthcare providers should administer OPV only after discussing the risk for VAPP with parents or caregivers.

Currently, the primary risk for paralytic polio in U.S. residents is through travel to countries where polio remains endemic or where polio outbreaks are occurring. Unvaccinated persons traveling to countries that use OPV should be aware of the risk caused by OPV and should consider polio vaccination prior to travel.

Dosage Forms Excipient information presented when available (limited, particularly for generics); consult specific product labeling.

Injection, suspension:

IPOL®: Type 1 poliovirus 40 D-antigen units, type 2 poliovirus 8 D-antigen units, and type 3 poliovirus 32 D-antigen units per 0.5 mL (0.5 mL, 5 mL) [contains 2-phenoxyethanol, formaldehyde, calf serum protein, neomycin (may have trace amounts), streptomycin (may have trace amounts), and polymyxin B (may have trace amounts)]

- ◆ **Polocaine** *see* Mepivacaine *on page* *1299*
- ◆ **Polocaine® (Can)** *see* Mepivacaine *on page* *1299*
- ◆ **Polocaine-MPF** *see* Mepivacaine *on page* *1299*
- ◆ **Polycin™** *see* Bacitracin and Polymyxin B *on page* *220*
- ◆ **Polycitra** *see* Citric Acid, Sodium Citrate, and Potassium Citrate *on page* *443*
- ◆ **Polycitra K** *see* Potassium Citrate and Citric Acid *on page* *1686*
- ◆ **Polyethylene Glycol-L-asparaginase** *see* Pegaspargase *on page* *1586*

Polyethylene Glycol 3350

(pol i ETH i leen GLY kol 3350)

Brand Names: U.S. GaviLAX [OTC]; GlycoLax [OTC]; HealthyLax [OTC]; MiraLax [OTC]; PEGyLAX

Brand Names: Canada Peg 3350; Pegalax; Relaxa

Index Terms PEG

Pharmacologic Category Laxative, Osmotic

Additional Appendix Information

Laxatives, Classification and Properties *on page* *2304*

Use Treatment of occasional constipation in adults

Unlabeled Use Treatment of constipation in children; bowel preparation before colonoscopy

Dosage Oral:

Children ≥6 months: Occasional constipation (unlabeled use): 0.5-1.5 g/kg daily (initial dose: 0.5-1 g/kg; titrate to effect); not to exceed 17 g/day; do not use for >2 weeks (Bell, 2004; Loening-Baucke, 2005; Michail, 2004; Voskuijl, 2004)

Adults:

Occasional constipation: 17 g of powder (~1 heaping tablespoon) dissolved in 4-8 ounces of beverage, once daily; do not use for >1 week unless directed by healthcare provider

Bowel preparation before colonoscopy (unlabeled use): Mix 17 g of powder (~1 heaping tablespoon) in 8 ounces of clear liquid and administer the entire mixture every 10 minutes until 2 L are consumed (start within 6 hours after administering 20 mg bisacodyl delayed-release tablets) (Wexner, 2006)

Additional Information Complete prescribing information should be consulted for additional detail.

Dosage Forms Excipient information presented when available (limited, particularly for generics); consult specific product labeling.

Packet, Oral:
- HealthyLax: (1 ea, 14 ea)
- MiraLax: (1 ea, 10 ea, 12 ea, 24 ea)
- Generic: (1 ea, 14 ea, 30 ea, 100 ea)

Powder, Oral:
- GaviLAX: (238 g, 510 g)
- GlycoLax: (119 g, 255 g, 527 g)
- MiraLax: (119 g, 238 g, 510 g)
- PEGyLAX: (527 g)
- Generic: 17 g/dose (119 g, 238 g, 510 g); (119 g, 238 g, 250 g, 255 g, 500 g, 510 g, 527 g, 850 g)

Dosage Forms: Canada

Excipient information presented when available (limited, particularly for generics); consult specific product labeling.

Powder, Oral: 17 g/dose (238 g, 510 g)

Sachet, Oral: (4 ea, 14 ea)

◆ **Polyethylene Glycol-Conjugated Uricase** *see* Pegloticase *on page 1599*

Polyethylene Glycol-Electrolyte Solution

(pol i ETH i leen GLY kol ee LEK troe lite soe LOO shun)

Brand Names: U.S. Colyte; GaviLyte-C; GaviLyte-G; GaviLyte-N; GoLYTELY; MoviPrep; NuLYTELY; TriLyte

Brand Names: Canada Colyte; Klean-Prep; PegLyte

Index Terms Electrolyte Lavage Solution

Pharmacologic Category Laxative, Osmotic

Additional Appendix Information

Laxatives, Classification and Properties *on page 2304*

Use Bowel cleansing prior to colonoscopy or barium enema X-ray examination

Unlabeled Use Whole bowel irrigation (WBI) in the following toxic ingestions: Packets of illicit drugs (body packers, body stuffers), potentially toxic sustained-release or enteric-coated agents, substantial amounts of iron (AACT, 2004)

Pregnancy Risk Factor C

Pregnancy Considerations Animal reproduction studies have not been conducted. Information related to the use of polyethylene glycol-electrolyte solution in pregnancy is limited (Neri, 2004). Colonoscopy in pregnant women is generally reserved for strong indications or life-threatening emergencies; until additional safety data for polyethylene glycol-electrolyte solution is available, other agents may be preferred for this purpose (Siddiqui, 2006; Wexner, 2006).

Breast-Feeding Considerations It is not known if polyethylene glycol-electrolyte solution is excreted into breast milk. Significant changes in the mother's fluid or electrolyte balance would not be expected with most products.

Medication Guide Available Yes

Contraindications Hypersensitivity to polyethylene glycol or any component of the formulation; ileus, gastrointestinal obstruction, gastric retention, bowel perforation, toxic colitis, toxic megacolon

Warnings/Precautions Evaluate patients with symptoms of bowel obstruction or perforation (nausea, vomiting, abdominal pain or distension) prior to use; if a patient develops severe bloating, distention or abdominal pain during administration, slow the rate of administration or temporarily discontinue use until the symptoms subside. Correct electrolyte abnormalities in patients prior to use. No additional ingredients or flavors (other than the flavor packets provided) should be added to the polyethylene glycol-electrolyte solution.

Fluid and electrolyte disturbances can lead to arrhythmias, seizures, and renal impairment. Advise patients to maintain adequate hydration before, during, and after treatment. If patient becomes dehydrated or experiences significant vomiting after treatment, consider post-colonoscopy lab tests (electrolytes, creatinine, and BUN). Serious arrhythmias have been reported (rarely) with the use of ionic osmotic laxative products. Use with caution in patients who may be at risk of cardiac arrhythmias (eg, patients with a history of prolonged QT, uncontrolled arrhythmias, recent MI, unstable angina, CHF, or cardiomyopathy). Consider pre-dose and post-colonoscopy ECGs in these patients. Generalized tonic-clonic seizures and/or loss of consciousness have occurred rarely in patients with no prior history of seizures. Seizures resolved with the correction of fluid and electrolyte abnormalities. Use with caution in patients with a history of seizures or who are at an increased risk of seizures (eg, concomitant administration of medications that lower the seizures threshold, patients withdrawing from alcohol or benzodiazepines) and in patients with known or suspected hyponatremia or low serum osmolality.

Cases of ischemic colitis have been reported; concomitant use of stimulant laxatives may increase the risk and is not recommended. The potential for mucosal aphthous ulcerations as a result of the bowel preparation should be considered, especially when evaluating colonoscopy results in patients with known or suspected inflammatory bowel disease. Use with caution in patients with severe ulcerative colitis. Use with caution in patients with renal impairment and/or in patients taking medications that may adversely affect renal function (eg, diuretics, NSAIDs, ACE inhibitors, ARBs). Patients with impaired renal function should be instructed to remain adequately hydrated; consider pre-dose and post-colonoscopy lab tests (electrolytes, creatinine, BUN) in these patients. Observe unconscious or semiconscious patients with impaired gag reflex or those who are otherwise prone to regurgitation or aspiration during administration; use with caution.

MoviPrep: Use with caution in patients with G6PD deficiency (especially patients with an active infection, history of hemolysis, or taking concomitant medications known to precipitate hemolytic reactions) due to the presence of sodium ascorbate and ascorbic acid in the formulation. Contains phenylalanine.

Use in patients <2 years of age may result in hypoglycemia, dehydration, and hypokalemia. Use with caution in patients >60 years of age; serious adverse events have been reported (eg, asystole, esophageal perforation, chest infiltration following vomiting and aspiration, Mallory-Weiss tear with GI bleeding, pulmonary edema with sudden dyspnea).

Adverse Reactions

>10%:

Central nervous system: Sleep disorder (35%; evening prep vs oral sodium phosphate solution [90 mL]), rigors (34%; evening prep vs oral sodium phosphate solution [90 mL]), malaise (18% to 27%; MoviPrep split dose vs 4 L PEG with electrolytes [18%]; evening dose vs oral sodium phosphate solution [90 mL] [53%])

Endocrine & metabolic: Increased thirst (<47%)

Gastrointestinal: Abdominal distention (<60%; evening prep vs oral sodium phosphate solution [90 mL]), anorectal pain (<52%; evening prep vs oral sodium phosphate solution [90 mL]), bloating (≤50%), nausea (14% to ≤50%; split dose vs 4 L PEG with electrolytes [20%]; evening prep vs oral sodium phosphate solution [90 mL] [47%]), abdominal pain (6% to 39%; evening prep vs oral sodium phosphate solution [90 mL] [32%]; split dose vs PEG with electrolytes [6%]), vomiting (7% to 12%; evening MoviPrep vs oral sodium phosphate solution (90 mL) [8%]; split dose vs PEG with electrolytes [13%])

1% to 10%:

Central nervous system: Dizziness (3% to 7%; evening prep vs oral sodium phosphate solution [90 mL]), headache (2%; evening prep vs oral sodium phosphate solution [90 mL])

Endocrine & metabolic: Hypokalemia (children 0%; evening prep vs oral sodium phosphate solution [90 mL] [6%])

Gastrointestinal: Dyspepsia (1% to 3%)

Frequency not defined, postmarketing, and/or case reports: Abdominal cramps, anaphylaxis, angioedema, aspiration, asystole (older adults >60 years), chest tightness, chills, dehydration, dermatitis, dyspnea, epigastric fullness, esophageal perforation (older adults >60 years), facial edema, fever, flatulence, hypersensitivity reaction, ischemic colitis, lip edema, Mallory-Weiss syndrome (older adults >60 years), pruritus, pulmonary edema (older adults >60 years), rhinorrhea, seizure, shock, skin rash, tightness in chest and throat, tongue edema, upper gastrointestinal hemorrhage (older adults >60 years), urticaria

Drug Interactions

Metabolism/Transport Effects None known.

Avoid Concomitant Use There are no known interactions where it is recommended to avoid concomitant use.

Increased Effect/Toxicity There are no known significant interactions involving an increase in effect.

Decreased Effect There are no known significant interactions involving a decrease in effect.

Preparation for Administration

CoLyte, GaviLyte-C, GaviLyte-G, GaviLyte-N, GoLYTELY, NuLYTELY, TriLyte: Using the container provided, add lukewarm water (may use tap water) up to the 4 L water mark; shake vigorously several times to ensure dissolution of the powder. No additional ingredients or flavors should be added to the solution (other than the flavor packets provided).

MoviPrep: Mix the contents of pouch A and pouch B (one each) in container provided. Add lukewarm water to fill line (~1 L); mix the solution until dissolved. No additional ingredients or flavors should be added to the solution.

Concentrations for reconstituted solutions:

CoLyte, GaviLyte-C: When dissolved in sufficient water to make 4 L, the final solution contains PEG-3350 18 mmol/L, sodium 125 mmol/L, sulfate 80 mmol/L, chloride 35 mmol/L, bicarbonate 20 mmol/L, and potassium 10 mmol/L

GaviLyte-G, GoLYTELY: When dissolved in sufficient water to make 4 L, the final solution contains PEG-3350 17.6 mmol/L, sodium 125 mmol/L, sulfate 40 mmol/L, chloride 35 mmol/L, bicarbonate 20 mmol/L, and potassium 10 mmol/L

GaviLyte-N, NuLYTELY, TriLyte: When dissolved in sufficient water to make 4 L, the final solution contains PEG-3350 31.3 mmol/L, sodium 65 mmol/L, chloride 53 mmol/L, bicarbonate 17 mmol/L, and potassium 5 mmol/L.

Storage/Stability

CoLyte, GaviLyte-C, GaviLyte-G, GaviLyte-N, GoLYTELY, NuLYTELY, TriLyte: Prior to reconstitution, store at 25°C (77°F); excursions permitted to 15°C to 30°C (59°F to 86°F). Refrigerate reconstituted solution. Use within 48 hours of preparation; discard any unused portion.

MoviPrep: Prior to reconstitution, store at 20°C to 25°C (68°F to 77°F); excursions permitted to 15°C to 30°C (59°F to 86°F). Refrigerate reconstituted solution in an upright position. Use within 24 hours of preparation; discard any unused portion.

Mechanism of Action Induces catharsis by strong electrolyte and osmotic effects

Pharmacodynamics/Kinetics Onset of effect: Oral: ~1 hour

Dosage

Bowel cleansing:

Infants ≥6 months, Children, and Adolescents: GaviLyte-N, NuLYTELY, TriLyte: Oral, Nasogastric: 25 mL/kg/hour until the rectal effluent is clear (maximum total dose: 4 L)

Adults:

CoLyte, GaviLyte-C, GaviLyte-G, GaviLyte-N, GoLYTELY, NuLYTELY, TriLyte:

Oral: 240 mL (8 oz) every 10 minutes until 4 L are consumed or the rectal effluent is clear; rapid drinking of each portion is preferred to drinking small amounts continuously

Nasogastric: 20-30 mL/minute until 4 L are administered or the rectal effluent is clear

MoviPrep: Oral: Administer 2 L total with an additional 1 L of clear fluid prior to colonoscopy as follows:

Split dose (2 day regimen) (preferred method):

Dose 1: Evening before colonoscopy (10-12 hours before dose 2): 240 mL (8 oz) every 15 minutes until 1 L (entire contents of container) is consumed. Then fill container with 480 mL (16 oz) of clear liquid and consume prior to going to bed.

Dose 2: On the morning of the colonoscopy (beginning at least 3.5 hours prior to procedure): 240 mL (8 oz) every 15 minutes until 1 L (entire contents of container) is consumed. Then fill container with 480 mL (16 oz) of clear liquid and consume at least 2 hours before the procedure.

Evening only dose (1 day regimen) (alternate method):

Dose 1: Evening before colonoscopy (at least 3.5 hours before bedtime): 240 mL (8 oz) every 15 minutes until 1 L (entire contents of container) is consumed

Dose 2: ~90 minutes after starting dose 1: 240 mL (8 oz) every 15 minutes until 1 L (entire contents of container) is consumed. Then fill container with 1 L (32 oz) of clear liquid and consume all of the liquid prior to going to bed.

Whole bowel irrigation (unlabeled use; AACT, 2004):

Nasogastric:

Infants ≥9 months and Children <6 years: 500 mL/hour until the rectal effluent is clear

Children ≥6 years: 1000 mL/hour until the rectal effluent is clear

Adolescents and Adults: 1500-2000 mL/hour until the rectal effluent is clear

Note: Continue treatment at least until the rectal effluent is clear; treatment duration may be extended based on corroborative evidence of continued presence of poisons in the GI tract as determined by radiographic means or the presence of the poison in the effluent.

Dosage adjustment in renal impairment: No dosage adjustment provided in manufacturer's labeling. Use with caution due to risks of fluid and electrolyte abnormalities.

Dosage adjustment in hepatic impairment: No dosage adjustment provided in manufacturer's labeling (has not been studied).

Dietary Considerations

CoLyte, GaviLyte-C, GaviLyte-G, GaviLyte-N, GoLYTELY, NuLYTELY, TriLyte: Ideally, the patient should fast for ~3-4 hours prior to administration, but in no case should solid food be given for at least 2 hours before the solution is given. Some products contain aspartame which is metabolized to phenylalanine.

MoviPrep: Patient should not eat solid food from start of solution administration until after colonoscopy. Patient may have clear liquid soup/plain yogurt for dinner; finish at least 1 hour before start of colon prep. MoviPrep contains phenylalanine.

Administration

Oral: Rapid drinking of each portion is preferred to drinking small amounts continuously. No additional ingredients or flavors (other than the flavor packets provided) should be added to the polyethylene glycol-electrolyte solution. Chilling the solution may improve palatability; administration of a chilled solution is **not** recommended in infants. Oral medications should not be administered within 1 hour of start of therapy.

Nasogastric administration: CoLyte, GaviLyte-C, GaviLyte-G, GaviLyte-N, GoLYTELY, NuLYTELY, TriLyte: The solution may be administered via nasogastric tube for bowel cleansing and whole bowel irrigation (preferred route; unlabeled use) in patients who are unwilling or unable to drink the solution.

Monitoring Parameters Electrolytes, serum glucose, BUN, urine osmolality; children <2 years of age should be monitored for hypoglycemia, dehydration, hypokalemia

Whole bowel irrigation (unlabeled use; AACT, 2004): Rectal effluent (continue until clear or the poison is completely removed)

Dosage Forms Excipient information presented when available (limited, particularly for generics); consult specific product labeling.

Powder, for solution, oral: PEG 3350 240 g, sodium sulfate 22.72 g, sodium bicarbonate 6.72 g, sodium chloride 5.84 g, and potassium chloride 2.98 g (4000 mL); PEG 3350 236 g, sodium sulfate 22.74 g, sodium bicarbonate 6.74 g, sodium chloride 5.86 g, and potassium chloride 2.97 g (4000 mL); PEG 3350 240 g, sodium bicarbonate 5.72 g, sodium chloride 11.2 g, and potassium chloride 1.48 g (4000 mL)

Colyte: PEG 3350 227.1 g, sodium sulfate 21.5 g, sodium bicarbonate 6.36 g, sodium chloride 5.53 g, and potassium chloride 2.82 g (3785 mL) [supplied with cherry, lemon lime, and orange flavor packs]

Colyte: PEG 3350 240 g, sodium sulfate 22.72 g, sodium bicarbonate 6.72 g, sodium chloride 5.84 g, and potassium chloride 2.98 g (4000 mL) [supplied with cherry, citrus berry, lemon lime, orange, and pineapple flavor packs]

GaviLyte-C: PEG 3350 240 g, sodium sulfate 22.72 g, sodium bicarbonate 6.72 g, sodium chloride 5.84 g, and potassium chloride 2.98 g (4000 mL) [supplied with lemon flavor packet]

GaviLyte-G: PEG 3350 236 g, sodium sulfate 22.74 g, sodium bicarbonate 6.74 g, sodium chloride 5.86 g, and potassium chloride 2.97 g (4000 mL) [supplied with lemon flavor packet]

GaviLyte-N: PEG 3350 420 g, sodium bicarbonate 5.72 g, sodium chloride 11.2 g, and potassium chloride 1.48 g (4000 mL) [supplied with lemon flavor packet]

GoLYTELY: PEG 3350 227.1 g, sodium sulfate 21.5 g, sodium bicarbonate 6.36 g, sodium chloride 5.53 g, and potassium chloride 2.82 g per packet (1s) [regular flavor; makes 1 gallon of solution after mixing]

GoLYTELY: PEG 3350 236 g, sodium sulfate 22.74 g, sodium bicarbonate 6.74 g, sodium chloride 5.86 g, and potassium chloride 2.97 g (4000 mL) [regular and pineapple flavor]

MoviPrep: Pouch A: PEG 3350 100g, sodium sulfate 7.5 g, sodium chloride 2.69 g, potassium chloride 1.02 g; Pouch B: Ascorbic acid 4.7 g, sodium ascorbate 5.9 g (1000 mL) [contains phenylalanine 131 mg/treatment; lemon flavor; packaged with 2 of Pouch A and 2 of Pouch B in carton and a disposable reconstitution container]

NuLYTELY: PEG 3350 420 g, sodium bicarbonate 5.72 g, sodium chloride 11.2 g, and potassium chloride 1.48 g (4000 mL) [supplied with cherry, lemon-lime, orange, and pineapple flavor packs]

TriLyte: PEG 3350 420 g, sodium bicarbonate 5.72 g, sodium chloride 11.2 g, and potassium chloride 1.48 g (4000 mL) [supplied with cherry, citrus berry, lemon lime, orange, and pineapple flavor packs]

- **Polyethylene Glycol Interferon Alfa-2b** *see* Peginterferon Alfa-2b *on page 1594*
- **Poly-Iron 150 [OTC]** *see* Polysaccharide-Iron Complex *on page 1673*

Poly-L-Lactic Acid (POL i el LAK tik AS id)

Brand Names: U.S. Sculptra®; Sculptra® Aesthetic

Index Terms New-Fill®; PLA

Pharmacologic Category Cosmetic Agent, Implant

Use Restoration and/or correction of facial lipoatrophy in patients with HIV; correction of shallow to deep nasolabial fold contour deficiencies and other facial wrinkles in immunocompetent patients

Dosage Adults:

Facial wrinkles (Sculptra® Aesthetic): Intradermal: 0.1-0.2 mL per individual injection to a maximum of 2.5 mL per nasolabial fold as a single treatment; may repeat treatment at ≥3 week intervals up to 4 times

Lipoatrophy (Sculptra®): Intradermal or SubQ: ~0.05-0.2 mL per individual injection depending on technique used; ~20 injections may be needed per cheek. Treatment should be individualized. Separate treatments by ≥2 weeks. Typical course involves 3-6 treatments. Supplemental injections may be needed. Do not overfill contour deficiency. For patients with severe facial fat loss, the average treatment requires ~1 vial per cheek area per treatment.

Additional Information Complete prescribing information should be consulted for additional detail.

Dosage Forms Excipient information presented when available (limited, particularly for generics); consult specific product labeling.

Injection, powder for suspension:

Sculptra®, Sculptra® Aesthetic: Poly-L-lactic acid USP

Polymyxin B (pol i MIKS in bee)

Index Terms Polymyxin B Sulfate

Pharmacologic Category Antibiotic, Irrigation; Antibiotic, Miscellaneous

Use Treatment of acute infections caused by susceptible strains of *Pseudomonas aeruginosa*; parenteral use of polymyxin B has mainly been replaced by less toxic antibiotics, reserved for life-threatening infections caused by organisms resistant to the preferred drugs (eg, pseudomonal meningitis - intrathecal administration)

Unlabeled Use Selective gastrointestinal tract decontamination

Pregnancy Considerations [U.S. Boxed Warning]: Safety in pregnant women has not been established. Animal reproduction studies are lacking. A teratogenic potential has not been identified for polymyxin b, but very limited data is available (Heinonen, 1977; Kazy, 2005). Based on the relative toxicity compared to other antibiotics, systemic use in pregnancy is not recommended (Knothe, 1985). Due to poor tissue diffusion, topical use would be expected to have only minimal risk to the mother or fetus (Leachman, 2006).

Breast-Feeding Considerations It is not known if polymyxin b is excreted in human milk. If present in breast milk, polymyxin b is not absorbed well from a normal gastrointestinal tract. Nondose-related effects could include modification of the bowel flora.

Contraindications Hypersensitivity to polymyxin B or any component of the formulation; concurrent use of neuromuscular blockers

Warnings/Precautions [U.S. Boxed Warning]: May cause neurotoxicity, nephrotoxicity, and/or neuromuscular blockade and respiratory paralysis; usual risk factors include pre-existing renal impairment, concomitant neuro-/nephrotoxic medications, advanced age and dehydration. Use with caution in patients with impaired renal function (modify dosage); polymyxin B-induced nephrotoxicity may be manifested by albuminuria, cellular casts, and azotemia. Discontinue therapy with decreasing urinary output and increasing BUN; neurotoxic reactions are usually associated with high serum levels, often in patients with renal dysfunction. Avoid concurrent or sequential use of other nephrotoxic and neurotoxic drugs (eg, aminoglycosides). The drug's neurotoxicity can result in respiratory paralysis from neuromuscular blockade, especially when the drug is given soon after anesthesia or muscle relaxants. Polymyxin B sulfate is most toxic when given parenterally; avoid parenteral use whenever possible. Prolonged use may result in fungal or bacterial superinfection, including *C. difficile*-associated diarrhea (CDAD) and pseudomembranous colitis; CDAD has been observed >2 months postantibiotic treatment. **[U.S. Boxed Warnings]: Safety in pregnant women not established; intramuscular/intrathecal administration only to hospitalized patients.**

Adverse Reactions Frequency not defined.

Cardiovascular: Facial flushing

Central nervous system: Neurotoxicity (irritability, drowsiness, ataxia, perioral paresthesia, numbness of the extremities, and blurred vision); dizziness, drug fever, meningeal irritation with intrathecal administration

Dermatologic: Urticarial rash

Endocrine & metabolic: Hypocalcemia, hyponatremia, hypokalemia, hypochloremia

Local: Pain at injection site

Neuromuscular & skeletal: Neuromuscular blockade, weakness

Renal: Nephrotoxicity

Respiratory: Respiratory arrest

Miscellaneous: Anaphylactoid reaction

Drug Interactions

Metabolism/Transport Effects None known.

Avoid Concomitant Use

Avoid concomitant use of Polymyxin B with any of the following: BCG

Increased Effect/Toxicity

Polymyxin B may increase the levels/effects of: Colistimethate; Neuromuscular-Blocking Agents

The levels/effects of Polymyxin B may be increased by: Capreomycin

Decreased Effect

Polymyxin B may decrease the levels/effects of: BCG; Sodium Picosulfate

Storage/Stability Prior to reconstitution, store at room temperature of 15°C to 30°C (59°F to 86°F) and protect from light. After reconstitution, store under refrigeration at 2°C to 8°C (36°F to 46°F). Discard any unused solution after 72 hours.

Mechanism of Action Binds to phospholipids, alters permeability, and damages the bacterial cytoplasmic membrane permitting leakage of intracellular constituents

Pharmacodynamics/Kinetics

Absorption: Well absorbed from peritoneum; minimal from GI tract (except in neonates) from mucous membranes or intact skin. Clinically insignificant amounts are absorbed following irrigation of an intact urinary bladder; systemic absorption may occur from a denuded bladder. Small amounts are systemically absorbed following ophthalmic installation.

Distribution: Minimal into CSF; V_d: 71-194 mL/kg

Protein binding: ~56%; 79% to 92% (critically ill patients) (Zavascki, 2008)

Half-life elimination: 6 hours

Time to peak, serum: I.M.: ~2 hours

Excretion: Urine (<1% as unchanged drug)

Dosage

Infants and Children <2 years:

- I.M.: Up to 40,000 units/kg/day divided every 6 hours (not routinely recommended due to pain at injection sites)
- I.V.: Up to 40,000 units/kg/day divided every 12 hours
- Intrathecal: 20,000 units daily for 3-4 days, then 25,000 units every other day for at least 2 weeks after CSF cultures are negative and CSF (glucose) has returned to within normal limits

Children ≥2 years, Adolescents, and Adults:

- I.M.: 25,000-30,000 units/kg/day divided every 4-6 hours (not routinely recommended due to pain at injection sites)
- I.V.: 15,000-25,000 units/kg/day divided every 12 hours
- Intrathecal: 50,000 units daily for 3-4 days, then every other day for at least 2 weeks after CSF cultures are negative and CSF (glucose) has returned to within normal limits
- Total daily dose should not exceed 2,000,000 units
- Irrigation:
  - Bladder irrigation: Continuous irrigant or rinse in the urinary bladder for up to 10 days using 20 mg (equal to 200,000 units) added to 1 L of normal saline; usually no more than 1 L of irrigant is used per day unless urine flow rate is high; administration rate is adjusted to patient's urine output
  - Topical irrigation or topical solution: 500,000 units/L of normal saline; maximum total daily dose should not exceed 2 million units in adults
- Ophthalmic: A concentration of 0.1% to 0.25% is administered as 1-3 drops to the affected eye(s) every hour, then increasing the interval as response indicates to 1-3 drops 4-6 times daily
- Oral: Selective gastrointestinal tract decontamination (unlabeled use): 1,000,000 units orally 4 times daily, starting 2 days prior to surgery through post-operative day 3 in combination with tobramycin and amphotericin B (Roos, 2011).
- Otic (in combination with other drugs): 1-2 drops, 3-4 times daily; should be used sparingly to avoid accumulation of excess debris

Dosage adjustment in renal impairment:

For individuals with renal impairment, the manufacturer's labeling recommends a dosage reduction so that the dose does not exceed 15,000 units/kg/day.

The following adjustments have been used by some clinicians (modified from Hoeprich, 1970): I.V., I.M.:

- Loading dose (first day of therapy): Cl_{cr} <80 mL/minute: 25,000 units/kg in 2 equally divided doses every 12 hours
- Subsequent dosage:
  - Cl_{cr} 30-80 mL/minute: 10,000-15,000 units/kg in 2 equally divided doses every 12 hours
  - Cl_{cr} <30 mL/minute: 10,000-15,000 units/kg every 2-3 days
  - Anuric patients: 10,000 units/kg every 5-7 days

Hemodialysis, peritoneal dialysis (Cunha, 1988): Adults: I.M.: 250,000 units every 24 hours; no supplemental dose necessary.

Note: Some data suggest that renal adjustment may not be necessary since total body clearance of polymyxin B is not altered in the setting of renal impairment and non-renal pathways are primarily responsible for elimination (Zavascki, 2008). These authors suggest that renal dosage adjustment recommendations should await further data from larger clinical trials.

Dosage adjustment in hepatic impairment: No dosage adjustment provided in manufacturer's labeling.

Administration Dissolve 500,000 units in 300-500 mL D_5W for continuous I.V. drip; dissolve 500,000 units in 2 mL water for injection, saline, or 1% procaine solution for I.M. injection; dissolve 500,000 units in 10 mL physiologic solution for intrathecal administration

Extravasation management: Monitor I.V. site closely; extravasation may cause serious injury with possible necrosis and tissue sloughing. Rotate infusion site frequently.

Monitoring Parameters Neurologic symptoms and signs of superinfection; renal function (decreasing urine output and increasing BUN may require discontinuance of therapy)

Reference Range Serum concentrations >5 mcg/mL are toxic in adults

Additional Information 1 mg = 10,000 units

Some data suggests that dosage adjustments may not be necessary in patients with renal impairment. Total body clearance of polymyxin B is not altered in the setting of renal impairment and nonrenal pathways are primarily responsible for elimination. In critically ill patients, <1% of unchanged drug was recovered in urine, and plasma protein binding appeared to increase (79% to 92%). Previous renal function dosing adjustment recommendations were based on less precise methods and assumptions made decades ago. The authors suggest that renal dosage adjustment recommendations should await further data from larger clinical trials (Zavascki, 2008).

Dosage Forms Excipient information presented when available (limited, particularly for generics); consult specific product labeling.

Solution Reconstituted, Injection:
- Generic: 500,000 units (1 ea)

Solution Reconstituted, Injection [preservative free]:
- Generic: 500,000 units (1 ea)

- ◆ **Polymyxin B and Bacitracin** *see* Bacitracin and Polymyxin B *on page 220*
- ◆ **Polymyxin B and Neomycin** *see* Neomycin and Polymyxin B *on page 1439*
- ◆ **Polymyxin B and Trimethoprim** *see* Trimethoprim and Polymyxin B *on page 2130*
- ◆ **Polymyxin B, Bacitracin, and Neomycin** *see* Bacitracin, Neomycin, and Polymyxin B *on page 221*
- ◆ **Polymyxin B, Bacitracin, Neomycin, and Hydrocortisone** *see* Bacitracin, Neomycin, Polymyxin B, and Hydrocortisone *on page 221*
- ◆ **Polymyxin B, Neomycin, and Dexamethasone** *see* Neomycin, Polymyxin B, and Dexamethasone *on page 1439*
- ◆ **Polymyxin B, Neomycin, and Gramicidin** *see* Neomycin, Polymyxin B, and Gramicidin *on page 1440*
- ◆ **Polymyxin B, Neomycin, and Hydrocortisone** *see* Neomycin, Polymyxin B, and Hydrocortisone *on page 1440*
- ◆ **Polymyxin B Sulfate** *see* Polymyxin B *on page 1671*
- ◆ **Polymyxin E** *see* Colistimethate *on page 488*

Polysaccharide-Iron Complex

(pol i SAK a ride-EYE ern KOM pleks)

Brand Names: U.S. EZFE 200 [OTC]; Ferrex 150 Plus [OTC]; Ferrex 150 [OTC]; FerUS [OTC]; iFerex 150 [OTC]; Myferon 150 [OTC]; NovaFerrum 50 [OTC]; NovaFerrum Pediatric Drops [OTC]; Nu-Iron [OTC]; PIC 200 [OTC]; Poly-Iron 150 [OTC]

Index Terms Iron-Polysaccharide Complex

Pharmacologic Category Iron Salt

Use Prevention and treatment of iron-deficiency anemias

Dosage

Dietary Reference Intake: Dose is RDA presented as elemental iron unless otherwise noted:

0-6 months: 0.27 mg/day (adequate intake)
7-12 months: 11 mg/day
1-3 years: 7 mg/day
4-8 years: 10 mg/day
9-13 years: 8 mg/day
14-18 years: Males: 11 mg/day; Females: 15 mg/day; Pregnant females: 27 mg/day; Lactating females: 10 mg/day
19-50 years: Males: 8 mg/day; Females: 18 mg/day; Pregnant females: 27 mg/day; Lactating females: 9 mg/day
≥50 years: 8 mg/day

Iron deficiency: Oral:

Children ≥6 years: 50-100 mg/day; may be given in divided doses
Adults: 150-300 mg/day

Additional Information Complete prescribing information should be consulted for additional detail.

Dosage Forms Excipient information presented when available (limited, particularly for generics); consult specific product labeling.

Capsule, Oral:
- EZFE 200: 434.8 (200 Fe) MG [non-toxic; contains brilliant blue fcf (fd&c blue #1), fd&c red #40, fd&c yellow #10 (quinoline yellow)]
- Ferrex 150: 150 mg [contains fd&c blue #1 aluminum lake, fd&c red #40 aluminum lake, fd&c yellow #5 aluminum lake]
- Ferrex 150 Plus: 150-50-50 MG [contains fd&c red #40 aluminum lake, fd&c yellow #6 aluminum lake]
- FerUS: 150 mg
- iFerex 150: 150 mg [contains brilliant blue fcf (fd&c blue #1), fd&c red #40, fd&c yellow #10 (quinoline yellow)]
- Myferon 150: 150 mg
- NovaFerrum 50: 50 mg
- Nu-Iron: 150 mg [contains brilliant blue fcf (fd&c blue #1), fd&c red #40]
- PIC 200: 434.8 (200 Fe) MG
- Poly-Iron 150: 150 mg

Liquid, Oral:
- NovaFerrum Pediatric Drops: 15 mg/mL (120 mL) [alcohol free, dye free, gluten free, lactose free, sodium free, sugar free; contains sodium benzoate; raspberry-grape flavor]

- ◆ **Polysporin® [OTC]** *see* Bacitracin and Polymyxin B *on page 220*
- ◆ **Polytrim®** *see* Trimethoprim and Polymyxin B *on page 2130*
- ◆ **Polytrim™ (Can)** *see* Trimethoprim and Polymyxin B *on page 2130*
- ◆ **P-OM3** *see* Omega-3-Acid Ethyl Esters *on page 1504*

Pomalidomide (poe ma LID oh mide)

Brand Names: U.S. Pomalyst

Index Terms CC-4047

Pharmacologic Category Angiogenesis Inhibitor; Antineoplastic Agent; Immunomodulator, Systemic

Use Treatment of multiple myeloma in patients who have received at least two prior therapies (including lenalidomide and bortezomib) and have continued disease progression on or within 60 days of completion of the last therapy

Pregnancy Risk Factor X

Pregnancy Considerations [U.S. Boxed Warning]: Pomalidomide is an analogue of thalidomide (a known human teratogen) and may cause severe birth defects or embryo-fetal death if taken during pregnancy. Pomalidomide cannot be used in women who are pregnant or may become pregnant during therapy. Obtain 2 negative pregnancy tests prior to initiation of treatment; 2 forms of contraception (or abstain from heterosexual intercourse) must be used at least 4 weeks prior to, during, and for ≥4 weeks after pomalidomide treatment (and during treatment interruptions) in females of reproductive potential. Distribution is restricted; physicians, pharmacists, and patients must be registered with the Pomalyst® REMS ™ Program. Studies in animals have shown evidence of fetal abnormalities and use is contraindicated in women who are or may become pregnant. Women of childbearing potential should be treated only if they are able to comply with the conditions of the Pomalyst® REMS ™ Program. Reliable contraception is required even with a history of infertility (unless due to hysterectomy or if ≥24 consecutive months postmenopausal (natural). Pregnancy tests should be performed 10-14 days and 24 hours prior to beginning therapy; weekly for the first 4 weeks and then every 4 weeks (every 2 weeks if menstrual cycle irregular) thereafter and during therapy interruptions. Pomalidomide must be immediately discontinued for a missed period, abnormal pregnancy test or abnormal menstrual bleeding; refer patient to a reproductive toxicity specialist if pregnancy occurs during treatment. Pomalidomide is present in the semen of males taking this medication. Males (including those vasectomized) should use a latex or synthetic condom during any sexual contact with women of childbearing age during treatment, during treatment interruptions, and for 28 days after discontinuation. Male patients should not donate sperm. Any suspected fetal exposure should be reported to the FDA via the MedWatch program (1-800-332-1088) and to Celgene Corporation (1-888-423-5436).

Breast-Feeding Considerations It is not known if pomalidomide is excreted into breast milk. Due to the potential for serious adverse reactions in the nursing infant, a decision should be made to discontinue nursing or to discontinue treatment with pomalidomide, taking into account the importance of treatment to the mother.

Prescribing and Access Restrictions As a requirement of the REMS program, access to this medication is restricted. Pomalidomide is approved for marketing in the U.S. only under a Food and Drug Administration (FDA) approved, restricted distribution program called Pomalyst REMS™ (celgeneriskmanagement.com or 1-888-423-5436). Physicians, pharmacies, and patients must be registered; a maximum 28-day supply may be dispensed; a new prescription is required each time it is filled; pregnancy testing is required for women of childbearing potential.

Medication Guide Available Yes

Contraindications Pregnancy

Warnings/Precautions Hazardous agent - use appropriate precautions for handling and disposal (meets NIOSH, 2012 criteria). **[U.S. Boxed Warning]: Pomalidomide is only available through the restricted Pomalyst REMS™ program.** Pomalidomide should only be prescribed to patients who can understand and comply with the conditions of the Pomalyst REMS program. Prescribers and pharmacies must be certified with the REMS program. **[U.S. Boxed Warning]: Pomalidomide is a thalidomide (human teratogen) analog and may cause severe life-threatening birth defects or embryo-fetal deaths; use is contraindicated in pregnancy. Pregnancy must be excluded prior to therapy initiation with 2 negative pregnancy tests; prevent pregnancy during therapy with 2 reliable forms of contraception (or abstain from heterosexual intercourse) beginning 4 weeks prior to, during and for 4 weeks after pomalidomide therapy (and during treatment interruptions) in females of reproductive potential.** Males taking pomalidomide must use a latex or synthetic condom during any sexual contact with a woman of childbearing potential during therapy and for up to 28 days after treatment discontinuation, even if successfully vasectomized. Patients should not donate blood during pomalidomide treatment and for 1 month after therapy discontinuation; male patients receiving pomalidomide must not donate sperm.

Neutropenia, anemia, and thrombocytopenia were frequently reported in clinical trials. Monitor complete blood counts weekly for the first 8 weeks of therapy and monthly or as clinically indicated thereafter; may require therapy interruption, reduction and/or discontinuation. Acute myelogenous leukemia (AML) as a secondary malignancy has been reported in patients receiving pomalidomide in the investigational treatment of condition(s) other than multiple myeloma. **[U.S. Boxed Warning]: Venous thromboembolic events such as deep vein thrombosis (DVT) and pulmonary embolism (PE) have occurred during pomalidomide therapy. Consider individualized anticoagulation prophylaxis based on patient risk factors.** Monitor for signs/symptoms of thromboembolism (shortness of breath, chest pain, or arm or leg swelling) and advise patients to promptly seek medical attention should symptoms occur. May cause dizziness and/or confusion; caution patients about performing tasks that require mental alertness (eg, operating machinery or driving). Avoid concomitant medications which may exacerbate dizziness and confusion. Use with caution in patients with a prior history of serious hypersensitivity reactions to thalidomide or lenalidomide; such patients were excluded from pomalidomide clinical trials and may therefore be at risk for hypersensitivity reactions when administered pomalidomide. Peripheral and sensory neuropathy occurred in clinical trials, but no cases of grade 3 or higher neuropathy were observed. Monitor closely for signs/symptoms of neuropathy; may require therapy interruption, dose modification and/or discontinuation.

Safety and efficacy have not been evaluated in patients with renal or hepatic impairment. Pomalidomide is hepatically metabolized; avoid use in patients with serum bilirubin >2 mg/dL and AST/ALT >3 times ULN (has not been studied). Pomalidomide and its metabolites are excreted by the kidneys; avoid use in patients with serum creatinine >3 mg/dL (has not been studied). Potentially significant drug-drug interactions may exist, requiring dose or frequency adjustment, additional monitoring, and/or selection of alternative therapy. Cigarette smoking may induce CYP1A2 mediated metabolism of pomalidomide, potentially reducing its systemic exposure and efficacy.

Adverse Reactions

>10%:

Cardiovascular: Peripheral edema (23%)

Central nervous system: Fatigue (55%), dizziness (18% to 20%), fever (19%), neuropathy (18%), headache (13%), confusion (10% to 12%), anxiety (11%)

Dermatologic: Skin rash (22%), pruritus (15%)

Endocrine & metabolic: Hypercalcemia (21%), hyperglycemia (12%)

Gastrointestinal: Constipation (36%), nausea (36%), diarrhea (34%), decreased appetite (22%), vomiting (14%), weight loss (14%)

Hematologic & oncologic: Neutropenia (50% to 52%; grades 3/4: 43% to 47%), anemia (38%; grades 3/4: 22%), thrombocytopenia (25%; grades 3/4: 22%), leukopenia (11%; grades 3/4: 6%)

Neuromuscular & skeletal: Back pain (32%), musculoskeletal chest pain (22%), muscle spasm (19%), arthralgia (16%), ostealgia (12%), myasthenia (12%), musculoskeletal pain (11%)
Renal: Increased serum creatinine (15%), renal failure (15%)
Respiratory: Dyspnea (34%), upper respiratory tract infection (32%), pneumonia (23%), epistaxis (15%), cough (14%)

1% to 10%:
Cardiovascular: Thrombosis (venous thrombosis, pulmonary embolism, 3%), atrial fibrillation (2%)
Central nervous system: Peripheral neuropathy (10%), chills (9%), insomnia (7%), pain (6%)
Dermatologic: Xeroderma (9%), hyperhidrosis (6%)
Endocrine & metabolic: Hypokalemia (10%), hyponatremia (10%), hypocalcemia (6%), dehydration (5%)
Gastrointestinal: Weight gain (1%)
Genitourinary: Urinary tract infection (8%)
Hematologic & oncologic: Lymphocytopenia (4%; grades 3/4: 2%), febrile neutropenia (3% to 5%)
Infection: Sepsis (6%)
Neuromuscular & skeletal: Tremor (9%), limb pain (5%)
Miscellaneous: Night sweats (5%)

Frequency not defined: Acute myelocytic leukemia, hyperbilirubinemia, hyperkalemia, increased serum ALT, interstitial pulmonary disease, neutropenic sepsis, pelvic pain, *Pneumocystis jiroveci* pneumonia, respiratory syncytial virus infection, urinary retention, vertigo

Drug Interactions

Metabolism/Transport Effects Substrate of CYP1A2 (major), CYP2C19 (minor), CYP2D6 (minor), CYP3A4 (major), P-glycoprotein; **Note:** Assignment of Major/Minor substrate status based on clinically relevant drug interaction potential

Avoid Concomitant Use

Avoid concomitant use of Pomalidomide with any of the following: Abatacept; Anakinra; Azelastine (Nasal); BCG; Canakinumab; Certolizumab Pegol; CloZAPine; CYP1A2 Inducers (Strong); CYP1A2 Inhibitors (Strong); CYP3A4 Inducers (Strong); CYP3A4 Inhibitors (Strong); Fusidic Acid (Systemic); Natalizumab; Paraldehyde; P-glycoprotein/ABCB1 Inducers; P-glycoprotein/ABCB1 Inhibitors; Pimecrolimus; Rilonacept; Tacrolimus (Topical); Tocilizumab; Tofacitinib; Vaccines (Live)

Increased Effect/Toxicity

Pomalidomide may increase the levels/effects of: Abatacept; Alcohol (Ethyl); Anakinra; Azelastine (Nasal); Bisphosphonate Derivatives; Buprenorphine; Canakinumab; Certolizumab Pegol; CloZAPine; CNS Depressants; Hydrocodone; Leflunomide; Methotrimeprazine; Metyrosine; Mirtazapine; Natalizumab; Paraldehyde; Pramipexole; Rilonacept; ROPINIRole; Rotigotine; Selective Serotonin Reuptake Inhibitors; Tofacitinib; Vaccines (Live); Zolpidem

The levels/effects of Pomalidomide may be increased by: Abiraterone Acetate; Brimonidine (Topical); CYP1A2 Inhibitors (Moderate); CYP1A2 Inhibitors (Strong); CYP3A4 Inhibitors (Moderate); CYP3A4 Inhibitors (Strong); Dasatinib; Deferasirox; Denosumab; Doxylamine; Droperidol; Fusidic Acid (Systemic); HydrOXYzine; Ivacaftor; Luliconazole; Magnesium Sulfate; Methotrimeprazine; Mifepristone; Perampanel; P-glycoprotein/ABCB1 Inhibitors; Pimecrolimus; Roflumilast; Simeprevir; Sodium Oxybate; Tacrolimus (Topical); Tapentadol; Tocilizumab; Trastuzumab; Vemurafenib

Decreased Effect

Pomalidomide may decrease the levels/effects of: BCG; Coccidioidin Skin Test; Sipuleucel-T; Vaccines (Inactivated); Vaccines (Live)

The levels/effects of Pomalidomide may be decreased by: Bosentan; CYP1A2 Inducers (Strong); CYP3A4 Inducers (Strong); Cyproterone; Dabrafenib; Deferasirox; Echinacea; Herbs (CYP3A4 Inducers); Peginterferon Alfa-2b; P-glycoprotein/ABCB1 Inducers

Storage/Stability Store at 20°C to 25°C (68°F to 77°F); excursions permitted to 15°C to 30°C (59°F to 86°F).

Mechanism of Action Induces cell cycle arrest and apoptosis directly in multiple myeloma cells; enhances T cell- and natural killer (NK) cell-mediated cytotoxicity; inhibits production of proinflammatory cytokines tumor necrosis factor-α (TNF-α), IL-1, IL-6, and IL-12; inhibits angiogenesis (Zhu, 2013)

Pharmacodynamics/Kinetics

Absorption: Rapid
Distribution: V_{dss}: 62-138L; semen distribution is ~67% of plasma levels
Protein binding: 12% to 44%
Metabolism: Hepatic via CYP1A2 and CYP3A4 (major); CYP2C19 and CYP2D6 (minor)
Half-life elimination: ~9.5 hours (healthy subjects); ~7.5 hours (multiple myeloma patients)
Time to peak: 2-3 hours
Excretion: Urine (73%; 2% as unchanged drug); feces (15%; 8% as unchanged drug)

Dosage Note: ANC should be ≥500 cells/mm³ and platelets ≥50,000 cells/mm³ prior to initiating new cycles of therapy.

Multiple myeloma, relapsed/refractory: Adults: Oral: 4 mg once daily on days 1-21 of 28-day cycles (may be given in combination with dexamethasone); continue until disease progression or unacceptable toxicity

Dosage adjustment for toxicity:

Hematologic:

If ANC <500 cells/mm³ (or ANC <1000 cells/mm³ with fever ≥38.5°C) and/or platelets <25,000 cells/mm³: Interrupt therapy and follow weekly CBCs. When ANC ≥500 cells/mm³ and/or platelets ≥50,000 cells/mm³: Resume dosing at 3 mg once daily.

For each subsequent drop of ANC <500 cells/mm³ and/or platelets <25,000 cells/mm³: Interrupt therapy. When ANC ≥500 cells/mm³ and/or platelets ≥50,000 cells/mm³: Resume dosing at 1 mg less than the previous dose. If toxicities occur at 1 mg daily dose, discontinue treatment.

Nonhematologic: If grade 3 or 4 toxicity occurs, interrupt therapy until resolved to ≤ grade 2; if appropriate, may restart therapy at 1 mg less than the previous dose. If toxicities occur at 1 mg daily dose, discontinue treatment.

Dosage adjustment for renal impairment: Serum creatinine >3 mg/dL: Avoid use (has not been studied).

Dosage adjustment for hepatic impairment: Bilirubin >2 mg/dL and AST/ALT >3 times ULN: Avoid use (has not been studied).

Dietary Considerations Must be taken on an empty stomach (at least 2 hours before or 2 hours after a meal)

Administration Administer on an empty stomach with water (at least 2 hours before or 2 hours after a meal). Should be swallowed whole; do not break, chew, or open the capsules. May administer a missed dose if within 12 hours of usual dosing time. If >12 hours, skip the dose for that day and resume usual dosing the following day. Do not take 2 doses to make up for a skipped dose.

Hazardous agent; use appropriate precautions for handling and disposal (meets NIOSH, 2012 criteria).

Monitoring Parameters CBC with differential and platelets weekly for the first 8 weeks and monthly or as clinically necessary thereafter; serum creatinine; liver function tests; monitor for signs/symptoms of thromboembolism and neuropathy. Consider thyroid function tests (TSH recommended at baseline and every 2-3 months during treatment for structurally similar medications [Hamnvik, 2011]).

Women of childbearing potential: Pregnancy test 10-14 days **and** 24 hours prior to initiating therapy, weekly during the first month, then monthly thereafter in women with regular menstrual cycles or every 2 weeks in women with irregular menstrual cycles

Dosage Forms Excipient information presented when available (limited, particularly for generics); consult specific product labeling.

Capsule, Oral:

Pomalyst: 1 mg, 2 mg, 3 mg [contains fd&c blue #2 (indigotine)]

Pomalyst: 4 mg [contains brilliant blue fcf (fd&c blue #1), fd&c blue #2 (indigotine)]

◆ **Pomalyst** *see* Pomalidomide *on page 1673*

PONATinib (poe NA ti nib)

Brand Names: U.S. Iclusig

Index Terms AP24534; Ponatinib Hydrochloride

Pharmacologic Category Antineoplastic Agent, Tyrosine Kinase Inhibitor

Use

Acute lymphoblastic leukemia: Treatment of Philadelphia chromosome-positive acute lymphoblastic leukemia (Ph+ ALL) for whom no other tyrosine kinase inhibitor therapy is indicated or who are T315I positive

Chronic myeloid leukemia: Treatment of chronic myeloid leukemia (CML) in chronic, accelerated, or blast phase for whom no other tyrosine kinase inhibitor therapy is indicated or who are T315I positive

Pregnancy Risk Factor D

Pregnancy Considerations Adverse events were observed in animal reproduction studies when administered in doses lower than or equivalent to the normal human dose. Based on its mechanism of action, adverse effects on pregnancy would be expected. Women of childbearing potential should be advised to avoid pregnancy during therapy.

Breast-Feeding Considerations It is not known if ponatinib is excreted in breast milk. Due to the potential for serious adverse reactions in the nursing infant, a decision should be made whether to discontinue nursing or to discontinue the drug, taking into account the importance of treatment to the mother.

Prescribing and Access Restrictions Patient access and support is available through the ARIAD PASS program. Information regarding program enrollment may be found at http://www.ariadpass.com or by calling 1-855-447-PASS (7277).

Medication Guide Available Yes

Contraindications There are no contraindications listed in the manufacturer's labeling.

Warnings/Precautions Hazardous agent - use appropriate precautions for handling and disposal (meets NIOSH, 2012 criteria). **[U.S. Boxed Warning]: Arterial and venous thrombosis and occlusions have occurred in ponatinib-treated patients. Events included fatal myocardial infarction (MI), stroke, stenosis of large arterial vessels of the brain, severe peripheral vascular disease, and the need for urgent revascularization procedures; incidents were observed in patients with and without cardiovascular risk factors (including patients ≤50 years of age). Monitor closely for thromboembolism/vascular occlusion; interrupt or discontinue therapy immediately for vascular occlusion. Consider benefit/risk ratio when deciding to restart therapy.** Fatal and life-threatening vascular occlusion may occur within 2 weeks of therapy initiation and is not dose dependent (events have occurred at doses as low as 15 mg daily), and may cause recurrent or multisite occlusion. Increasing age and a prior history of ischemia, hypertension, diabetes, or hyperlipidemia are risk factors for development of ponatinib-associated vascular occlusion. Many patients required a revascularization procedure (cerebrovascular, coronary, and peripheral arterial) due to serious arterial thrombosis/occlusion. MI and coronary artery occlusion may result in heart failure due to myocardial ischemia. Peripheral arterial occlusive events, including fatal mesenteric artery occlusion and life-threatening peripheral arterial disease, have occurred. Some patients have required amputation due to digital or distal extremity necrosis. Venous thromboembolism, including deep vein thrombosis, pulmonary embolism, superficial thrombophlebitis, and retinal vein thrombosis, have been reported. May require dosage adjustment or discontinuation. Monitor for signs/symptoms of arterial or venous thromboembolism.

[U.S. Boxed Warning]: Serious heart failure (HF) or left ventricular dysfunction, including fatalities, were reported in clinical trials. Monitor for signs/symptoms of HF; interrupt or discontinue ponatinib therapy for new or worsening HF. Treat as clinically warranted if HF develops. Consider ponatinib discontinuation in the event of serious HF. Cardiac arrhythmias (bradyarrhythmias and tachyarrhythmias) have also been reported. Symptomatic bradyarrhythmia which required pacemaker implantation occurred in a few patients; other rhythms identified were complete heart block, sick sinus syndrome, and atrial fibrillation with bradycardia and pauses. Tachyarrhythmias reported include atrial fibrillation (most common), atrial flutter, supraventricular tachycardia, and atrial tachycardia; some events required hospitalization. Monitor for sign/symptoms of bradycardia (fainting, dizziness, chest pain) and tachycardia (palpitations, dizziness). May require therapy interruption. Treatment-emergent hypertension developed in over half of ponatinib-treated patients; symptomatic hypertension or hypertensive crisis were reported in several patients, requiring urgent intervention. Blood pressure may worsen in patients with pre-existing hypertension. Monitor blood pressure closely, and manage elevated pressures as clinically indicated. May require therapy interruption, dosage reduction, or discontinuation if hypertension is resistant to medical management.

[U.S. Boxed Warning]: Liver failure and death resulting from ponatinib-induced hepatotoxicity were observed; monitor liver function prior to and at least monthly (or as clinically indicated) during treatment. Hepatotoxicity may require treatment interruption (followed by dose reduction) or discontinuation. One case of fulminant hepatic failure leading to death occurred within 1 week of therapy initiation; acute liver failure has also occurred. Treatment may result in ALT and/or AST elevations, and may be irreversible. While ponatinib has not been studied in patients with hepatic impairment, it is metabolized and eliminated primarily through hepatic mechanisms; increased drug exposure (and increased adverse reactions) would be expected in patients with hepatic dysfunction. Avoid use in patients with moderate to severe (Child Pugh class B or C) impairment unless the benefit of therapy outweighs the risk of toxicity.

Severe myelosuppression (grade 3 or 4) was commonly observed in clinical trials, and the incidence was greater in patients with accelerated or blast phase CML and Ph+ ALL. Monitor blood counts closely; may require therapy interruption and/or dosage reduction. Hemorrhagic events occurred commonly in ponatinib-treated patients, including serious events such as cerebral and gastrointestinal hemorrhages; fatalities were reported. Serious bleeding episodes occurred more frequently in patients with accelerated or blast phase CML, and Ph+ ALL; most patients had grade 4 thrombocytopenia. Monitor platelet levels closely and for signs/symptoms of bleeding, and interrupt therapy if necessary.

Treatment-related lipase elevations and clinical pancreatitis occurred in clinical studies; the majority of cases resolved within 2 weeks of therapy interruption or dose reduction. Monitor serum lipase every 2 weeks for the first 2 months and monthly thereafter or as clinically indicated; more frequent monitoring may be considered in patients with a history of pancreatitis or alcohol abuse. Monitor for clinical signs of pancreatitis, such as abdominal symptoms; interrupt therapy if necessary. Do not reinitiate treatment until complete resolution of symptoms and lipase level is <1.5 times ULN. Serious gastrointestinal perforation (fistula) occurred very rarely; monitor for signs/symptoms of perforation and/or fistula. Serious fluid retention events, including fatality due to brain edema (very rare), were observed in ponatinib-treated patients. Peripheral edema, pleural effusions, and pericardial effusions were commonly seen; effusions and ascites were less common. Monitor patients for fluid retention; may require therapy interruption, dosage reduction, or discontinuation.

Peripheral and cranial neuropathy have been reported. Peripheral neuropathy, paresthesia, hypoesthesia, and hyperesthesia occurred most frequently; cranial neuropathy occurred rarely. In one-third of patients who experienced symptoms, neuropathy developed during the first month of therapy. Monitor for signs/symptoms of neuropathy; consider interrupting treatment if neuropathy develops. Serious ocular events such as blindness and blurred vision have occurred with ponatinib use. Macular edema, retinal vein occlusion, and retinal hemorrhage have been reported in a small percentage of patients; conjunctival or corneal irritation, dry eye, or eye pain occurred more frequently. Other toxicities include cataracts, glaucoma, iritis, iridocyclitis, and ulcerative keratitis. Perform comprehensive ophthalmic exams prior to therapy initiation and periodically during treatment.

Hyperuricemia and serious tumor lysis syndrome (rare) were reported. Patients should receive adequate hydration and be monitored for elevated uric acid levels and/or the development of tumor lysis syndrome. Correct elevated uric acid levels prior to initiating therapy. As ponatinib inhibits VEGF activity, therapy may impair wound healing. Hold therapy for at least 1 week prior to major surgery; resume therapy post procedure based on clinical judgment of appropriate wound healing. Potentially significant drug-drug interactions may exist, requiring dose or frequency adjustment, additional monitoring, and/or selection of alternative therapy. Elevated gastric pH may reduce ponatinib bioavailability; if possible, avoid concomitant use with proton pump inhibitors, H_2 blockers, or antacids. Patients ≥65 years of age may be more likely to experience weakness, decreased appetite, dyspnea, increased lipase, muscle spasms, peripheral edema, and thrombocytopenia; monitor closely. Cautious dose selection is recommended based on greater frequency of decreased hepatic, renal, or cardiac function, and of concomitant disease or other drug therapy.

Adverse Reactions

>10%:

Cardiovascular: Hypertension (53% to 71%), peripheral edema (13% to 22%; grades 3/4: ≤1%), heart failure (6% to 15%; including ejection fraction decreased, pulmonary edema, cardiogenic shock, cardiopulmonary failure), arterial ischemia (3% to 13%; grades 3/4: ≤7%; including cardiac, cerebro-, and peripheral-vascular events)

Central nervous system: Fatigue or weakness (31% to 39%), headache (25% to 39%), fever (23% to 32%), pain (6% to 16%), chills (7% to 13%), insomnia (7% to 12%), dizziness (3% to 11%)

Dermatologic: Rash (34% to 54%), dry skin (24% to 39%), cellulitis (≤11%)

Endocrine & metabolic: Glucose increased (58%), phosphorus decreased (57%), calcium decreased (52%), sodium decreased (29%), glucose decreased (24%), potassium decreased (16%), potassium increased (15%), bicarbonate decreased (11%)

Gastrointestinal: Abdominal pain (34% to 49%), constipation (24% to 47%), lipase increased (41%; grades 3/4: 15%), nausea (22% to 32%), appetite decreased (8% to 31%), diarrhea (13% to 26%), vomiting (13% to 24%), oral mucositis (9% to 23%), weight loss (5% to 13%), gastrointestinal hemorrhage (2% to 11%; grades 3/4: ≤6%)

Genitourinary: Urinary tract infection (≤12%)

Hematologic: Neutropenia (grades 3/4: 24% to 63%), leukopenia (grades 3/4: 14% to 63%), thrombocytopenia (grades 3/4: 36% to 57%), anemia (grades 3/4: 9% to 55%), lymphopenia (grades 3/4: 10% to 37%), neutropenic fever (1% to 25%), hemorrhage (24%; grades 3/4: 4% to 5%; including cerebral and gastrointestinal)

Hepatic: ALT increased (53%; grades 3/4: 8%), AST increased (41%; grades 3/4: 4%), alkaline phosphatase increased (37%), albumin decreased (28%), bilirubin increased (19%)

Neuromuscular & skeletal: Arthralgia (13% to 31%), myalgia (6% to 22%), limb pain (9% to 17%), back pain (11% to 16%), peripheral neuropathy (6% to 13%), muscle spasm (5% to 13%), bone pain (9% to 12%)

Respiratory: Dyspnea (6% to 21%), pleural effusion (3% to 19%; grades 3/4: ≤3%), cough (6% to 18%), pneumonia (3% to 13%), nasopharyngitis (3% to 12%), upper respiratory tract infection (≤11%)

Miscellaneous: Sepsis (1% to 22%)

1% to 10%:

Cardiovascular: Myocardial infarction or other cardiac ischemic event (5%), supraventricular tachyarrhythmia (5%), atrial fibrillation (4%), venous thromboembolism (3%; including deep vein thrombosis, pulmonary embolism, portal vein thrombosis, and retinal vein thrombosis), pericardial effusion (1% to 3%), cerebral hemorrhage (2%), peripheral ischemia (2%), stroke or TIA (2%), bradyarrhythmia (1%; symptomatic)

Endocrine & metabolic: Sodium increased (10%), hyperuricemia (7%), calcium increased (5%), triglycerides increased (3%)

Gastrointestinal: Pancreatitis (6%; grade 3: 5%), amylase increased (3%)

Renal: Creatinine increased (7%)

<1% (Limited to important or life-threatening): Ascites, atrial flutter, atrial tachycardia, cerebral edema, gastrointestinal fistula, gastrointestinal perforation, heart block (complete), hepatic failure, sick sinus syndrome, supraventricular tachycardia, tumor lysis syndrome

Drug Interactions

Metabolism/Transport Effects Substrate of BCRP, CYP2C8 (minor), CYP2D6 (minor), CYP3A4 (minor), P-glycoprotein; **Note:** Assignment of Major/Minor substrate status based on clinically relevant drug interaction potential; **Inhibits** BCRP, P-glycoprotein

Avoid Concomitant Use

Avoid concomitant use of PONATinib with any of the following: Antacids; CloZAPine; CYP3A4 Inducers (Strong); H2-Antagonists; Proton Pump Inhibitors; St Johns Wort

Increased Effect/Toxicity

PONATinib may increase the levels/effects of: CloZAPine; Vitamin K Antagonists

The levels/effects of PONATinib may be increased by: CYP3A4 Inhibitors (Strong); Grapefruit Juice

Decreased Effect

PONATinib may decrease the levels/effects of: Cardiac Glycosides; Vitamin K Antagonists

The levels/effects of PONATinib may be decreased by: Antacids; CYP3A4 Inducers (Strong); H2-Antagonists; Peginterferon Alfa-2b; Proton Pump Inhibitors; St Johns Wort

Storage/Stability Store at 20°C to 25°C (68°F to 77°F); excursions permitted between 15°C to 30°C (59°F to 86°F).

Mechanism of Action Ponatinib is a pan-BCR-ABL tyrosine kinase inhibitor with *in vitro* activity against cells expressing native or mutant BCR-ABL (including T315I); it also inhibits VEGFR, FGFR, PDGFR, EPH, and SRC kinases, as well as KIT, RET, TIE2, and FLT3.

Pharmacodynamics/Kinetics

Absorption: Plasma concentrations not affected by food

Distribution: V_d: 1223 L

Protein binding: >99% to plasma proteins

Metabolism: Primarily hepatic through CYP3A4; CYP2C8, CYP2D6, and CYP3A5 are also involved in metabolism. Phase II metabolism occurs via esterases and/or amidases.

Bioavailability: May be reduced with a higher gastric pH

Half-life elimination: ~24 hours (range: 12-66 hours)

Time to peak: ≤6 hours

Excretion: Feces (~87%); urine (~5%)

Dosage Note: The optimal ponatinib dose has not been identified. Consider discontinuing therapy if no response has occurred by 3 months of therapy.

Acute lymphoblastic leukemia (ALL), Philadelphia chromosome-positive (Ph+), in patients for whom no other tyrosine kinase inhibitor therapy is indicated or who are T315I-positive: Adults: Oral: 45 mg once daily

Chronic myeloid leukemia (CML; chronic, accelerated, or blast phase), in patients for whom no other tyrosine kinase inhibitor therapy is indicated or who are T315I-positive: Adults: Oral: 45 mg once daily; consider reducing the dose for patients in chronic or accelerated phase who have achieved a major cytogenetic response

Dosage adjustment for strong CYP3A inhibitors: Reduce ponatinib dose to 30 mg once daily when administered with concomitant strong CYP3A inhibitors (eg, boceprevir, clarithromycin, conivaptan, grapefruit juice, indinavir, itraconazole, ketoconazole, lopinavir/ritonavir, nefazodone, nelfinavir, posaconazole, ritonavir, saquinavir, telaprevir, telithromycin, voriconazole).

Dosage adjustment for toxicity:

Hematologic: ANC <1000/mm^3 or platelets <50,000/mm^3:

First occurrence: Interrupt therapy; upon recovery of ANC to ≥1500/mm^3 and platelets to ≥75,000/mm^3, resume therapy at 45 mg daily.

Second occurrence: Interrupt therapy; upon recovery of ANC to ≥1500/mm^3 and platelets to ≥75,000/mm^3, resume therapy at a reduced dose of 30 mg daily.

Third occurrence: Interrupt therapy; upon recovery of ANC to ≥1500/mm^3 and platelets to ≥75,000/mm^3, resume therapy at a reduced dose of 15 mg daily.

Nonhematologic toxicity:

Arterial or venous occlusive reactions: Interrupt therapy; do not resume ponatinib in the event of serious occlusive events unless the potential benefit of therapy outweighs the risk of recurrent occlusions and other treatment options are not available.

Pancreatitis and lipase elevations:

Asymptomatic grade 1 or 2 serum lipase elevation: Consider interrupting therapy or dose reduction.

Asymptomatic grade 3 or 4 serum lipase elevation (>2 times ULN) or asymptomatic radiologic pancreatitis (grade 2): If toxicity occurs at dose of 45 mg daily, interrupt therapy; upon recovery to ≤grade 1 (<1.5 times ULN), resume therapy at a reduced dose of 30 mg daily. If toxicity occurs at dose of 30 mg daily, interrupt therapy; upon recovery to ≤grade 1, resume therapy at a reduced dose of 15 mg daily. If toxicity occurs at dose 15 mg daily, discontinue therapy.

Symptomatic grade 3 pancreatitis: If toxicity occurs at dose of 45 mg daily, interrupt therapy; upon recovery of serum lipase elevation to ≤grade 1 and complete symptom resolution, resume therapy at a reduced dose of 30 mg daily. If toxicity occurs at dose of 30 mg daily, interrupt therapy; upon recovery of serum lipase elevation to ≤grade 1 and complete symptom resolution, resume therapy at a reduced dose of 15 mg daily. If toxicity occurs at dose of 15 mg daily, discontinue therapy.

Grade 4 pancreatitis: Discontinue therapy.

Other nonhematologic toxicities: For serious reactions (other than arterial or venous occlusion), do not restart therapy until symptom resolution or unless the benefit of therapy outweighs the risk of recurrent toxicity.

Dosage adjustment for renal impairment: No dosage adjustment provided in manufacturer's labeling (has not been studied); although renal excretion is not a major excretion route for ponatinib.

Dosage adjustment for hepatic impairment:

Pre-existing impairment:

Mild impairment (Child-Pugh class A): No dosage adjustment provided in manufacturer's labeling (has not been studied); however, hepatic elimination is the major route of ponatinib excretion.

Moderate to severe impairment (Child-Pugh class B or C): Avoid use (unless potential benefit outweighs potential risk of overexposure).

Hepatotoxicity during treatment:

AST or ALT >3 times ULN (≥ Grade 2): If toxicity occurs at dose of 45 mg daily, interrupt therapy; upon recovery to ≤ grade 1 (<3 times ULN), resume therapy at 30 mg daily. If toxicity occurs at dose of 30 mg daily, interrupt therapy; upon recovery to ≤ grade 1, resume therapy at 15 mg daily. If toxicity occurs at dose of 15 mg daily, discontinue therapy.

ALT or AST ≥3 times ULN with bilirubin >2 times ULN and alkaline phosphatase <2 times ULN: Discontinue therapy.

Dietary Considerations May be taken without regard to food. Avoid grapefruit juice.

Administration Administer with or without food. Swallow tablets whole (do not crush or dissolve).

Hazardous agent; use appropriate precautions for handling and disposal (meets NIOSH, 2012 criteria).

Monitoring Parameters CBC with differential and platelets every 2 weeks for the first 3 months, then monthly or as clinically needed; liver function tests at baseline and at least monthly thereafter or more frequently if clinically warranted; serum lipase every 2 weeks for the first 2 months and monthly thereafter (more frequently in patients with a history of pancreatitis or alcohol abuse); serum electrolytes and uric acid; monitor cardiac function, blood pressure, signs/symptoms of arterial/venous occlusion or thromboembolism, hemorrhage, fluid retention, pancreatitis (clinical signs), gastrointestinal perforation/fistula

Dosage Forms Excipient information presented when available (limited, particularly for generics); consult specific product labeling.

Tablet, Oral:

Iclusig: 15 mg, 45 mg

◆ **Ponatinib Hydrochloride** *see* PONATinib *on page 1676*

◆ **Ponstan® (Can)** *see* Mefenamic Acid *on page 1281*

◆ **Ponstel** *see* Mefenamic Acid *on page 1281*

◆ **Pontocaine** *see* Tetracaine (Systemic) *on page 2033*

◆ **Pontocaine** *see* Tetracaine (Topical) *on page 2034*

◆ **Pontocaine® (Can)** *see* Tetracaine (Ophthalmic) *on page 2034*

◆ **Pontocaine® (Can)** *see* Tetracaine (Systemic) *on page 2033*

◆ **Pontocaine® (Can)** *see* Tetracaine (Topical) *on page 2034*

Porfimer (POR fi mer)

Brand Names: U.S. Photofrin

Brand Names: Canada Photofrin®

Index Terms CL-184116; Dihematoporphyrin Ether; Porfimer Sodium

Pharmacologic Category Antineoplastic Agent, Miscellaneous

Use Palliation in patients with obstructing (partial or complete) esophageal cancer; treatment of microinvasive endobronchial nonsmall cell lung cancer (NSCLC); reduction of obstruction and palliation in patients with obstructing (partial or complete) NSCLC; ablation of high-grade dysplasia in Barrett's esophagus

Canadian labeling: Additional use (not in U.S. labeling): Second-line treatment of recurrent, superficial papillary bladder cancer

Unlabeled Use Treatment of actinic keratoses and low-risk basal and squamous cell skin cancers

Pregnancy Risk Factor C

Dosage I.V.: Adults:

Photodynamic therapy in esophageal cancer or endobronchial nonsmall cell lung cancer: 2 mg/kg, followed by endoscopic exposure to the appropriate laser light and debridement; repeat courses must be separated by at least 30 days (delay subsequent treatment for insufficient healing) for a maximum of 3 courses

Photodynamic therapy in Barrett's esophagus dysplasia: 2 mg/kg, followed by endoscopic exposure to the appropriate laser light; repeat courses must be separated by at least 90 days (delay subsequent treatment for insufficient healing) for a maximum of 3 courses

Photodynamic therapy in papillary bladder cancer (Canadian labeling; not in U.S. labeling): 2 mg/kg, followed by cystoscopic exposure to the appropriate laser light. **Note:** Repeat dosing is not recommended due to increased risk of bladder contracture.

Dosage adjustment in renal impairment: No dosage adjustment provided in manufacturer's labeling.

Dosage adjustment in hepatic impairment: No dosage adjustment provided in manufacturer's labeling (has not been studied).

Additional Information Complete prescribing information should be consulted for additional detail.

Dosage Forms Excipient information presented when available (limited, particularly for generics); consult specific product labeling.

Solution Reconstituted, Intravenous, as sodium [preservative free]:

Photofrin: 75 mg (1 ea)

Dosage Forms: Canada Excipient information presented when available (limited, particularly for generics); consult specific product labeling.

Injection, powder for reconstitution, as sodium:

Photofrin®: 15 mg

◆ **Porfimer Sodium** *see* Porfimer *on page 1679*

◆ **Portia** *see* Ethinyl Estradiol and Levonorgestrel *on page 787*

Posaconazole (poe sa KON a zole)

Brand Names: U.S. Noxafil

Brand Names: Canada Posanol Suspension

Index Terms SCH 56592

Pharmacologic Category Antifungal Agent, Oral

Additional Appendix Information

Antifungal Agents *on page 2286*

Use

U.S. labeling:

Invasive *Aspergillus* and *Candida* infections: Suspension and delayed release tablets: Prophylaxis of invasive *Aspergillus* and *Candida* infections in severely-immunocompromised patients (eg, hematopoietic stem cell transplant [HSCT] recipients with graft-versus-host disease [GVHD] or those with prolonged neutropenia secondary to chemotherapy for hematologic malignancies)

Oropharyngeal candidiasis: Suspension: Treatment of oropharyngeal candidiasis (including patients refractory to itraconazole and/or fluconazole)

Canadian labeling:

Invasive *Aspergillus* and *Candida* infections: Prophylaxis of invasive *Aspergillus* and *Candida* infections in severely-immunocompromised patients (eg, hematopoietic stem cell transplant [HSCT] recipients with graft-versus-host disease [GVHD] or those with prolonged neutropenia); treatment of invasive aspergillosis in patients refractory to or intolerant of itraconazole or amphotericin B; treatment of oropharyngeal candidiasis

Unlabeled Use Salvage therapy of refractory or relapsed invasive fungal infections; mucormycosis; pulmonary infection (nonimmunosuppressed)

Pregnancy Risk Factor C

Pregnancy Considerations Posaconazole has been shown to be teratogenic in animal studies. There are no adequate and well-controlled studies in pregnant women. Use only if the benefit to the mother justifies potential risk to the fetus.

Breast-Feeding Considerations Excretion in breast milk has not been investigated; use only if the benefit to the mother justifies potential risk to the fetus.

Contraindications Coadministration with sirolimus, ergot alkaloids (eg, ergotamine, dihydroergotamine), HMG-CoA reductase inhibitors that are primarily metabolized through CYP3A4 (eg, atorvastatin, lovastatin, simvastatin), or CYP3A4 substrates that prolong the QT interval (eg, pimozide, quinidine); hypersensitivity to posaconazole, other azole antifungal agents, or any component of the formulation.

Warnings/Precautions Hepatic dysfunction has occurred, ranging from mild/moderate increases of ALT, AST, alkaline phosphatase, total bilirubin, and/or clinical hepatitis to severe reactions (cholestasis, hepatic failure including death). Consider discontinuation of therapy in patients who develop clinical evidence of liver disease that may be secondary to posaconazole. Elevations in liver function tests have been generally reversible after posaconazole has been discontinued; some cases resolved without drug interruption. More severe reactions have been observed in patients with underlying serious medical conditions (eg, hematologic malignancy) and primarily with suspension total daily doses of 800 mg. Monitor liver function tests at baseline and periodically during therapy. If increases occur, monitor for severe hepatic injury development. Use caution in patients with an increased risk of arrhythmia (long QT syndrome, concurrent QT_c-prolonging drugs, drugs metabolized through CYP3A4, hypokalemia). Correct electrolyte abnormalities (eg, potassium, magnesium, and calcium) before initiating therapy. Concurrent use with cyclosporine or tacrolimus may significantly increase cyclosporine/tacrolimus concentrations and may result in rare serious adverse events (eg, nephrotoxicity, leukoencephalopathy, and death); dose reduction and close monitoring are recommended with initiation of posaconazole therapy. Concurrent use with midazolam may increase midazolam concentrations and potentiate midazolam-related adverse effects. Potentially significant drug-drug interactions may exist, requiring dose or frequency adjustment, additional monitoring, and/or selection of alternative therapy.

U.S. labeling contraindicates use in patients with hypersensitivity to other azole antifungal agents; Canadian labeling does not contraindicate use, but recommends using caution in hypersensitivity with other azole antifungal agents; cross-reaction may occur, but has not been established. Consider alternative therapy or closely monitor for breakthrough fungal infections in patients receiving drugs that decrease absorption or increase the metabolism of posaconazole or in any patient unable to eat or tolerate an oral liquid nutritional supplement. Use caution in severe renal impairment; monitor for breakthrough fungal infections. Patients weighing ≥120 kg may have lower plasma drug exposure; monitor closely for breakthrough fungal infections.

Adverse Reactions Note: Percentages reflect data from use in comparator trials with multiple concomitant conditions and medications; some adverse reactions may be due to underlying condition(s).

>10%:

Cardiovascular: Hypertension (11% to 18%), peripheral edema (16%), edema (9% to 15%), hypotension (14%), tachycardia (12%)

Central nervous system: Headache (8% to 28%), rigors (≤20%), fatigue (3% to 17%), insomnia (1% to 17%), dizziness (11%), pain (1% to 11%)

Dermatologic: Skin rash (16%), pruritus (11%)

Endocrine & metabolic: Hypokalemia (≤30%), hypomagnesemia (10% to 18%), weight loss (1% to 14%), hyperglycemia (11%), dehydration (1% to 11%)

Gastrointestinal: Diarrhea (10% to 42%), nausea (2% to 38%), vomiting (7% to 29%), abdominal pain (5% to 27%), constipation (10% to 21%), anorexia (2% to 19%), mucositis (17%), oral candidiasis (1% to 12%)

Hematologic & oncologic: Thrombocytopenia (14% to 29%), anemia (2% to 25%), neutropenia (4% to 23%), febrile neutropenia (20%), petechia (11%)

Hepatic: Increased serum ALT (6% to 17%)

Infection: Bacteremia (18%), herpes simplex infection (3% to 15%), cytomegalovirus disease (14%)

Neuromuscular & skeletal: Musculoskeletal pain (16%), weakness (2% to 13%), arthralgia (11%)

Respiratory: Cough (3% to 25%), dyspnea (1% to 20%), epistaxis (14%), stomatitis (14%), pharyngitis (12%)

Miscellaneous: Fever (6% to 45%)

1% to 10%:

Central nervous system: Chills (10%), anxiety (9%)

Dermatologic: Diaphoresis (2% to 10%)

Endocrine & metabolic: Hypocalcemia (9%)

Gastrointestinal: Dyspepsia (10%)

Genitourinary: Vaginal hemorrhage (10%)

Hepatic: Hyperbilirubinemia (7% to 10%), increased serum AST (3% to 4%), increased serum alkaline phosphatase (1% to 3%)

Neuromuscular & skeletal: Back pain (10%)

Respiratory: Pneumonia (3% to 10%), upper respiratory tract infection (7%)

<1% (Limited to important or life-threatening): Acute renal failure, adrenocortical insufficiency, atrial fibrillation, cholestasis, hemolytic-uremic syndrome, hepatic failure, hepatitis, hepatomegaly, hypersensitivity, hypersensitivity reaction, jaundice, paresthesia, prolonged Q-T interval on ECG, pulmonary embolism, reduced ejection fraction, syncope, thrombotic thrombocytopenic purpura, torsades de pointes

Drug Interactions

Metabolism/Transport Effects Inhibits CYP3A4 (strong)

Avoid Concomitant Use

Avoid concomitant use of Posaconazole with any of the following: Ado-Trastuzumab Emtansine; Alfuzosin; Apixaban; AtorvaSTATin; Avanafil; Axitinib; Bosutinib; Cabozantinib; Cisapride; Conivaptan; Crizotinib; Dihydroergotamine; Dofetilide; Dronedarone; Efavirenz; Eletriptan; Eplerenone; Ergoloid Mesylates; Ergonovine; Ergotamine; Everolimus; Halofantrine; Ibrutinib; Imatinib; Ivabradine; Lapatinib; Lomitapide; Lovastatin; Lurasidone; Macitentan; Methadone; Methylergonovine; Nilotinib; Nisoldipine; Pimozide; Pomalidomide; QuiNIDine; Ranolazine; Red Yeast Rice; Regorafenib; Rivaroxaban; Salmeterol; Silodosin; Simeprevir; Simvastatin; Sirolimus; Tamsulosin; Ticagrelor; Tolvaptan; Toremifene; Ulipristal; Vemurafenib; VinCRIStine (Liposomal)

Increased Effect/Toxicity

Posaconazole may increase the levels/effects of: Ado-Trastuzumab Emtansine; Alfentanil; Alfuzosin; Almotriptan; Alosetron; Antineoplastic Agents (Vinca Alkaloids); Apixaban; ARIPiprazole; Atazanavir; AtorvaSTATin; Avanafil; Axitinib; Bedaquiline; Benzodiazepines (metabolized by oxidation); Boceprevir; Bortezomib; Bosentan; Bosutinib; Brentuximab Vedotin; Brinzolamide; Budesonide (Nasal); Budesonide (Systemic, Oral Inhalation); BusPIRone; Busulfan; Cabozantinib; Calcium Channel Blockers; Cilostazol; Cisapride; Colchicine; Conivaptan; Corticosteroids (Orally Inhaled); Corticosteroids (Systemic); Crizotinib; CycloSPORINE (Systemic); CYP3A4 Substrates; Dienogest; Digoxin; Dihydroergotamine; DOCEtaxel; Dofetilide; Dronedarone; Dutasteride; Eletriptan; Enzalutamide; Eplerenone; Ergoloid Mesylates; Ergonovine; Ergotamine; Etravirine; Everolimus; FentaNYL; Fesoterodine; Fluticasone (Nasal); Fluticasone (Oral Inhalation); Fosamprenavir; Fosphenytoin; GlipiZIDE; GuanFACINE; Halofantrine; Highest Risk QTc-Prolonging Agents; Ibrutinib; Iloperidone; Imatinib; Irinotecan; Ivabradine; Ivacaftor; Ixabepilone; Lacosamide; Lapatinib; Levomilnacipran; Lomitapide; Losartan; Lovastatin; Lumefantrine; Lurasidone; Macitentan; Macrolide Antibiotics; Maraviroc; Methadone; Methylergonovine; MethylPREDNISolone; Mifepristone; Moderate Risk QTc-Prolonging Agents; Nilotinib; Nisoldipine; Ospemifene; OxyCODONE; Paricalcitol; PAZOPanib; Phenytoin; Pimecrolimus; Pimozide; Pomalidomide; PONATinib; Propafenone; QUEtiapine; QuiNIDine; Ranolazine; Red Yeast Rice; Regorafenib; Repaglinide; Rifamycin Derivatives; Rilpivirine; Ritonavir; Rivaroxaban; RomiDEPsin; Ruxolitinib; Salmeterol; Saxagliptin; Sildenafil; Silodosin; Simeprevir; Simvastatin; Sirolimus; Solifenacin; SORAfenib; SUNItinib; Tacrolimus (Systemic); Tacrolimus (Topical); Tadalafil; Tamsulosin; Telaprevir; Temsirolimus; Ticagrelor; Tofacitinib; Tolterodine; Tolvaptan; Toremifene; Ulipristal; Vardenafil; Vemurafenib; Vilazodone; VinCRIStine (Liposomal); Vitamin K Antagonists; Zolpidem; Zuclopenthixol

The levels/effects of Posaconazole may be increased by: Boceprevir; Etravirine; Macrolide Antibiotics; Telaprevir

Decreased Effect

Posaconazole may decrease the levels/effects of: Amphotericin B; Ifosfamide; Prasugrel; Saccharomyces boulardii; Ticagrelor

The levels/effects of Posaconazole may be decreased by: Didanosine; Efavirenz; Etravirine; Fosamprenavir; Fosphenytoin; H2-Antagonists; Metoclopramide; Phenytoin; Proton Pump Inhibitors; Rifamycin Derivatives; Sucralfate

Ethanol/Nutrition/Herb Interactions Food: Bioavailability increased ~3 times when posaconazole is administered with a nonfat meal or an oral liquid nutritional supplement; increased ~4 times when administered with a high-fat meal. Management: Suspension must be administered with or within 20 minutes of a full meal or an oral liquid nutritional supplement, or may be administered with an acidic carbonated beverage (eg, ginger ale). Take tablet with food. Consider alternative antifungal therapy in patients with inadequate oral intake or severe diarrhea/vomiting.

Storage/Stability Suspension: Store at 25°C (77°F); excursions are permitted between 15°C and 30°C (59°F and 86°F). Do not freeze.

Tablets: Store between 20°C and 25°C (68°F and 77°F); excursions are permitted between 15°C and 30°C (59°F and 86°F).

Mechanism of Action Interferes with fungal cytochrome P450 (latosterol-14α-demethylase) activity, decreasing ergosterol synthesis (principal sterol in fungal cell membrane) and inhibiting fungal cell membrane formation.

Pharmacodynamics/Kinetics

Absorption: Coadministration with food, liquid nutritional supplements, and/or acidic carbonated beverages (eg, ginger ale) increases absorption; fasting states do not provide sufficient absorption to ensure adequate plasma concentrations.

Distribution: V_d: 287 L

Protein binding: >98%; predominantly bound to albumin

Metabolism: Not significantly metabolized; ~15% to 17% undergoes non-CYP-mediated metabolism, primarily via hepatic glucuronidation into metabolites

Half-life elimination: Suspension: 35 hours (range: 20-66 hours); Tablets: 26-31 hours

Time to peak, plasma: Suspension: ~3-5 hours; Tablets: ~4-5 hours

Excretion: Feces 71% to 77% (~66% of the total dose as unchanged drug); urine 13% to 14% (<0.2% of the total dose as unchanged drug)

Dosage

Aspergillosis, invasive:

Prophylaxis: Children ≥13 years, Adolescents, and Adults: Oral:

Tablets (delayed release): Initial: 300 mg twice daily for 1 day; Maintenance dose: 300 mg once daily. Duration is based on recovery from neutropenia or immunosuppression; initiate posaconazole in patients with acute myelogenous leukemia (AML) or myelodysplastic syndromes (MDS) several days before the anticipated onset of neutropenia (eg, at the time of chemotherapy initiation) and discontinue once neutropenia is resolved (Cornely, 2007; NCCN, 2009).

Missed doses: Take as soon as remembered. If it is <12 hours until the next dose, skip the missed does and return to the regular schedule. Do not double doses.

Suspension: 200 mg 3 times daily; duration of therapy is based on recovery from neutropenia or immunosuppression; initiate posaconazole in patients with acute myelogenous leukemia (AML) or myelodysplastic syndromes (MDS) several days before the anticipated onset of neutropenia (eg, at the time of chemotherapy initiation) and discontinue once neutropenia is resolved (Cornely, 2007; NCCN, 2009).

Treatment (refractory to or intolerant of conventional therapy):

U.S. unlabeled use: Adults: Oral: Suspension: 200 mg 4 times daily initially; after disease stabilization, may decrease frequency to 400 mg twice daily (Walsh, 2007). **Note:** Duration of therapy should be a minimum of 6-12 weeks or throughout period of immunosuppression and until lesions have resolved (Walsh, 2008).

Canadian labeling: Children ≥13 years, Adolescents, and Adults: Oral: 400 mg twice daily; in patients unable to tolerate food or nutritional supplement, administer 200 mg 4 times daily; duration of therapy is based on severity of underlying disease, recovery from immunosuppression, and clinical response.

Candidal infections: Children ≥13 years, Adolescents, and Adults: Oral:

U.S. labeling:

Prophylaxis:

Tablets (delayed release): Initial: 300 mg twice daily for 1 day; Maintenance dose: 300 mg once daily; duration of therapy is based on recovery from neutropenia or immunosuppression.

Missed doses: Take as soon as remembered. If it is <12 hours until the next dose, skip the missed does and return to the regular schedule. Do not double doses.

Suspension: 200 mg 3 times daily; duration of therapy is based on recovery from neutropenia or immunosuppression

Treatment: Suspension:

Oropharyngeal infection: Initial: 100 mg twice daily for 1 day; maintenance: 100 mg once daily for 13 days

Refractory oropharyngeal infection: 400 mg twice daily; duration of therapy is based on underlying disease and clinical response

Canadian labeling:

Prophylaxis: 200 mg 3 times daily; duration of therapy is based on recovery from neutropenia or immunosuppression

Treatment: Oropharyngeal infection: Initial: 100 mg twice daily for 1 day; maintenance: 100 mg once daily for 13 days

Mucormycosis (unlabeled use): Adults: Oral: Suspension: 800 mg daily in 2 or 4 divided doses; duration of therapy is based on response and risk of relapse due to immunosuppression (Greenburg, 2006)

Cryptococcal infections: Adults: Oral: Suspension:

Pulmonary, nonimmunosuppressed (unlabeled use): 400 mg twice daily. **Note:** Fluconazole is considered first-line treatment (Perfect, 2010).

Salvage treatment of relapsed infection (unlabeled use): 400 mg twice daily (or 200 mg 4 times daily) for 10-12 weeks. **Note:** Salvage treatment should only be started after an appropriate course of an induction regimen (Perfect, 2010).

Dosage adjustment in renal impairment:

Mild-to-moderate insufficiency (Cl_{cr} 20-80 mL/minute/1.73 m^2): No dosage adjustment necessary.

Severe insufficiency (Cl_{cr} <20 mL/minute/1.73 m^2): No dosage adjustment necessary; however, monitor for breakthrough fungal infections due to variability in posaconazole exposure.

Dosage adjustment in hepatic impairment: Mild-to-severe insufficiency (Child-Pugh class A, B, or C): No dosage adjustment necessary. **Note:** if patient shows clinical signs and symptoms of liver disease due to posaconazole, consider discontinuing therapy.

Dietary Considerations

Tablets (delayed release): Take with food.

Suspension: Give during or within 20 minutes following a full meal or liquid nutritional supplement; alternatively, posaconazole may be administered with an acidic carbonated beverage (eg, ginger ale).

Consider alternative antifungal therapy in patients with inadequate oral intake or severe diarrhea/vomiting; if alternative therapy is not an option, closely monitoring for breakthrough fungal infections.

Adequate posaconazole absorption from GI tract and subsequent plasma concentrations are dependent on food for efficacy. Lower average plasma concentrations have been associated with an increased risk of treatment failure.

Administration

Suspension: Oral: Shake well before use. Must be administered during or within 20 minutes following a full meal or an oral liquid nutritional supplement; alternatively, posaconazole may be administered with an acidic carbonated beverage (eg, ginger ale). In patients able to swallow, administer oral suspension using dosing spoon provided by the manufacturer; spoon should be rinsed clean with water after each use and before storage.

Tablets (delayed release): Oral: Swallow tablets whole; do not divide, crush, or chew. Administer with food.

Consider alternative antifungal therapy in patients with inadequate oral intake or severe diarrhea/vomiting; if alternative therapy is not an option, closely monitoring for breakthrough fungal infections. Adequate posaconazole absorption from GI tract and subsequent plasma concentrations are dependent on food for efficacy. Lower average plasma concentrations have been associated with an increased risk of treatment failure.

Monitoring Parameters Hepatic function (eg, AST/ALT, alkaline phosphatase and bilirubin) prior to initiation and during treatment; renal function; electrolyte disturbances (eg, calcium, magnesium, potassium); CBC; breakthrough fungal infections; adequate oral intake

Dosage Forms Excipient information presented when available (limited, particularly for generics); consult specific product labeling.

Suspension, Oral:

Noxafil: 40 mg/mL (105 mL) [contains polysorbate 80, sodium benzoate; cherry flavor]

Tablet Delayed Release, Oral:

Noxafil: 100 mg

◆ **Posanol Suspension (Can)** *see* Posaconazole *on page 1679*

Potassium Acetate (poe TASS ee um AS e tate)

Pharmacologic Category Electrolyte Supplement, Parenteral

Use Potassium deficiency; to avoid chloride when high concentration of potassium is needed, source of bicarbonate

Pregnancy Risk Factor C

Pregnancy Considerations Animal reproduction studies have not been conducted. Potassium requirements are the same in pregnant and nonpregnant women. Adverse events have not been observed following use of potassium supplements in healthy women with normal pregnancies. Use caution in pregnant women with other medical conditions (eg, pre-eclampsia; may be more likely to develop hyperkalemia) (IOM, 2004).

Breast-Feeding Considerations Potassium is excreted into breast milk (IOM, 2004).

Contraindications Severe renal impairment or adrenal insufficiency; hyperkalemia

Warnings/Precautions Close monitoring of serum potassium concentrations is needed to avoid hyperkalemia. Use with caution in patients with renal impairment (contraindicated in severe renal insufficiency), cardiac disease, acid/base disorders, or potassium-altering conditions/disorders. Use with caution in digitalized patients or patients receiving concomitant medications or therapies that increase potassium (eg, ACEIs, potassium-sparing diuretics, potassium containing salt substitutes). Do **NOT** administer undiluted or I.V. push; inappropriate parenteral administration may be fatal. Always administer potassium further diluted; refer to appropriate dilution and administration rate recommendations. Vesicant/irritant (at concentrations >0.1 mEq/mL); ensure proper catheter or needle position prior to and during infusion; avoid extravasation. Pain and phlebitis may occur during parenteral infusion requiring a decrease in infusion rate or potassium concentration. Potassium acetate solution for injection contains aluminum; use caution with impaired renal function and in premature infants.

Adverse Reactions Frequency not defined.

Cardiovascular: Arrhythmias, EEG abnormalities, heart block, hypotension

Central nervous system: Confusion, listlessness

Neuromuscular & skeletal: Paralysis, paresthesia, weakness

Local: Local tissue necrosis with extravasation

Drug Interactions

Metabolism/Transport Effects None known.

Avoid Concomitant Use There are no known interactions where it is recommended to avoid concomitant use.

Increased Effect/Toxicity

Potassium Acetate may increase the levels/effects of: ACE Inhibitors; Angiotensin II Receptor Blockers; Potassium-Sparing Diuretics

The levels/effects of Potassium Acetate may be increased by: Eplerenone; Heparin; Heparin (Low Molecular Weight)

Decreased Effect There are no known significant interactions involving a decrease in effect.

Preparation for Administration Parenteral: Potassium must be diluted prior to parenteral administration. The concentration of infusion may be dependent on patient condition and specific institution policy. Some clinicians recommend that the maximum concentration for peripheral infusion is 10 mEq/100 mL and 20-40 mEq/100 mL for central infusions.

Mechanism of Action Potassium is the major cation of intracellular fluid and is essential for the conduction of nerve impulses in heart, brain, and skeletal muscle; contraction of cardiac, skeletal and smooth muscles; maintenance of normal renal function, acid-base balance, carbohydrate metabolism, and gastric secretion

Pharmacodynamics/Kinetics

Distribution: Enters cells via active transport from extracellular fluid

Excretion: Primarily urine; skin and feces (small amounts); most intestinal potassium reabsorbed

Dosage I.V. doses should be incorporated into the patient's maintenance I.V. fluids, intermittent I.V. potassium administration should be reserved for severe depletion situations and requires ECG monitoring; doses listed as mEq of potassium

Children:

Treatment of hypokalemia: I.V.: 2-5 mEq/kg/day

I.V. intermittent infusion (must be diluted prior to administration): 0.5-1 mEq/kg/dose (maximum: 30 mEq/dose) to infuse at 0.3-0.5 mEq/kg/hour (maximum: 1 mEq/kg/hour)

Note: Use caution in premature neonates; potassium acetate for injection contains aluminum.

Adults:

Treatment of hypokalemia: I.V.: 40-100 mEq/day

I.V. intermittent infusion (must be diluted prior to administration): 5-10 mEq/dose (maximum: 40 mEq/dose) to infuse over 2-3 hours (maximum: 40 mEq over 1 hour)

Note: Continuous cardiac monitor recommended for rates >0.5 mEq/kg/hour

Potassium dosage/rate of infusion guidelines:

Serum potassium >2.5 mEq/L: Maximum infusion rate: 10 mEq/hour; maximum concentration: 40 mEq/L; maximum 24-hour dose: 200 mEq

Serum potassium <2.5 mEq/L: Maximum infusion rate: 40 mEq/hour; maximum concentration: 80 mEq/L; maximum 24-hour dose: 400 mEq

Dosage adjustment in renal impairment: No dosage adjustment provided in manufacturer's labeling. Use caution; potassium acetate injection may increase serum aluminum and/or potassium.

Dosage adjustment in hepatic impairment: No dosage adjustment provided in manufacturer's labeling. Use with caution.

Administration Potassium must be diluted prior to parenteral administration; maximum recommended concentration (peripheral line): 80-100 mEq/L; maximum recommended concentration (central line): 150 mEq/L or 15 mEq/100 mL; in severely fluid-restricted patients (with central lines): 200 mEq/L or 20 mEq/100 mL has been used; maximum rate of infusion, see Dosage, I.V. intermittent infusion

Vesicant/irritant (at concentrations >0.1 mEq/mL); ensure proper needle or catheter placement prior to and during I.V. infusion. Avoid extravasation.

Extravasation management: If extravasation occurs, stop infusion immediately and disconnect (leave needle/cannula in place); gently aspirate extravasated solution (do **NOT** flush the line); initiate hyaluronidase antidote; remove needle/cannula; apply dry cold compresses (Hurst, 2004); elevate extremity.

Hyaluronidase: Intradermal or SubQ: Inject a total of 1 mL (15 units/mL) as five separate 0.2 mL injections (using a 25-gauge needle) into area of extravasation at the leading edge in a clockwise manner (MacCara, 1983; Zenk, 1981).

Monitoring Parameters Serum potassium, magnesium (to facilitate potassium repletion), and bicarbonate; cardiac monitor (if intermittent infusion or potassium infusion rates 0.5 mEq/kg/hour in children or >10 mEq/hour in adults); to assess adequate replacement, repeat serum potassium level 2-4 hours after dose

Reference Range Note: Reference ranges may vary depending on the laboratory

Serum potassium: 3.5-5.2 mEq/L

Additional Information 1 mEq of acetate is equivalent to the alkalinizing effect of 1 mEq of bicarbonate.

Dosage Forms Excipient information presented when available (limited, particularly for generics); consult specific product labeling.

Solution, Intravenous:

Generic: 2 mEq/mL (20 mL, 50 mL, 100 mL); 4 mEq/mL (50 mL)

Potassium Acid Phosphate

(poe TASS ee um AS id FOS fate)

Brand Names: U.S. K-Phos

Index Terms Potassium Phosphate Monobasic

Pharmacologic Category Urinary Acidifying Agent

Use To acidify the urine to lower urinary calcium concentrations; reduce odor and rash caused by ammonia in urine; to increase the antibacterial activity of methenamine

Pregnancy Risk Factor C

Pregnancy Considerations Animal reproduction studies have not been conducted.

Breast-Feeding Considerations Potassium is excreted into breast milk (IOM, 2004).

Contraindications Severe renal impairment; hyperkalemia, hyperphosphatemia; infected phosphate stones

Warnings/Precautions May cause hyperkalemia; use with caution in patients who require regulation of serum potassium concentrations. A mild laxative effect may occur within the first few days of therapy; if the laxative effect persists to a self-limiting degree, consider reducing the dose or discontinue use until diarrhea improves. Use with caution in patients with severe adrenal insufficiency (eg, Addison's disease), renal impairment or chronic renal disease (contraindicated in severe renal impairment), cardiac disease (including heart failure [especially patients receiving digoxin] and hypertension), myotonia congenita, hypoparathyroidism, rickets (may increase the risk of extraskeletal calcification), acute dehydration, acute pancreatitis, or extensive tissue breakdown (eg, severe burns). Patients with renal calculi may pass old stones when phosphate therapy is initiated. Patients with renal calculi may pass old stones when phosphate therapy is initiated.

Tablets should be dissolved completely in water prior to administration to avoid GI injury due to administration of a concentrated potassium salt preparation.

Adverse Reactions Frequency not defined.

Cardiovascular: Bradycardia, cardiac arrhythmia, chest pain, confusion, edema, paralysis, paresthesia, phlebitis,

Central nervous system: Dizziness, fatigue

Endocrine & metabolic: Alkalosis, hyperkalemia, hyperphosphatemia, hypocalcemia, increased thirst, weight gain

Gastrointestinal: Abdominal pain, diarrhea, nausea, stomach pain, flatulence, sore throat, vomiting

Genitourinary: Decreased urine output

Local: Local tissue necrosis with extravasation

Neuromuscular & skeletal: Arthralgia, limb pain, muscle cramps, ostealgia, tetany, weakness

Respiratory: Dyspnea

Drug Interactions

Metabolism/Transport Effects None known.

Avoid Concomitant Use There are no known interactions where it is recommended to avoid concomitant use.

Increased Effect/Toxicity

Potassium Acid Phosphate may increase the levels/effects of: ACE Inhibitors; Angiotensin II Receptor Blockers; Potassium-Sparing Diuretics; Salicylates

The levels/effects of Potassium Acid Phosphate may be increased by: Eplerenone; Heparin; Heparin (Low Molecular Weight)

Decreased Effect

Potassium Acid Phosphate may decrease the levels/effects of: Amphetamines

The levels/effects of Potassium Acid Phosphate may be decreased by: Antacids

Storage/Stability Store at 20°C to 25°C (68°F to 77°F).

Mechanism of Action The principal intracellular cation; involved in transmission of nerve impulses, muscle contractions, enzyme activity, and glucose utilization

Pharmacodynamics/Kinetics

Absorption: Well absorbed from upper GI tract

Distribution: Enters cells via active transport from extracellular fluid

Excretion: Primarily urine; skin and feces (small amounts); most intestinal potassium reabsorbed

Dosage Adults: Oral: 1000 mg 4 times daily

Dosage adjustment in renal impairment: No dosage adjustment provided in manufacturer's labeling. Use with caution. Contraindicated in patients with severe impairment (<30% of normal function) or with hyperphosphatemia or hyperkalemia.

Dosage adjustment in hepatic impairment: No dosage adjustment provided in manufacturer's labeling. Use with caution.

Dietary Considerations Take with meals.

Administration

Oral: Administer at mealtime and at bedtime. Dissolve tablets in 6-8 oz of water prior to administration to avoid GI injury. For best results, soak tablets in water for 2-5 minutes and stir. If any tablet particles remain undissolved, crush and stir vigorously to speed dissolution.

Monitoring Parameters Serum potassium, phosphorus, and calcium; renal function; serum salicylate concentration (in patients taking concomitant salicylates)

Reference Range Note: Reference ranges may vary depending on the laboratory

Serum phosphorus: Both low and high ends of the normal range are higher in children than in adults.

Infants: 4.5-7.5 mg/dL (1.45-2.42 mmol/L)

Children: ~4-6 mg/dL (1.29-1.94 mmol/L)

Adults: 2.5-4.5 mg/dL (0.81-1.45 mmol/L)

Urinary pH: 4.6-8.0

Test Interactions Decreased ammonia (B)

Additional Information Each mmol of phosphate contains 31 mg elemental phosphorus

Additional terminology for the potassium and sodium salts:

Sodium phosphate monobasic = Sodium acid phosphate

Sodium phosphate dibasic = Disodium phosphate

Potassium phosphate monobasic = Potassium acid phosphate

Potassium phosphate dibasic = Dipotassium phosphate

Dosage Forms Considerations

500 mg of potassium acid phosphate = elemental potassium 144 mg = potassium 3.7 mEq = potassium 3.7 mmol

500 mg of potassium acid phosphate = elemental phosphorus 114 mg = phosphorus 3.7 mmol

Dosage Forms Excipient information presented when available (limited, particularly for generics); consult specific product labeling.

Tablet, Oral:

K-Phos: 500 mg [scored]

Potassium Bicarbonate and Potassium Chloride

(poe TASS ee um bye KAR bun ate & poe TASS ee um KLOR ide)

Index Terms K-Lyte/Cl; Potassium Bicarbonate and Potassium Chloride (Effervescent)

Pharmacologic Category Electrolyte Supplement, Oral

Use Treatment or prevention of hypokalemia

Pregnancy Risk Factor C

Dosage Oral:

Children: 1-4 mEq/kg/24 hours in divided doses as required to maintain normal serum potassium

Adults:

Prevention: 16-24 mEq/day in 2-4 divided doses

Treatment: 40-100 mEq/day in 2-4 divided doses

Dosage adjustment in renal impairment: No dosage adjustment provided in manufacturer's labeling. However, patients with chronic renal failure require serum potassium monitoring and appropriate dosage adjustment.

Dosage adjustment in hepatic impairment: No dosage adjustment provided in manufacturer's labeling.

Additional Information Complete prescribing information should be consulted for additional detail.

Dosage Forms Excipient information presented when available (limited, particularly for generics); consult specific product labeling.

Tablet for solution, oral [effervescent]: Potassium chloride 25 mEq [potassium bicarbonate 0.5 g and potassium chloride 1.5 g]

◆ **Potassium Bicarbonate and Potassium Chloride (Effervescent)** *see* Potassium Bicarbonate and Potassium Chloride *on page 1684*

Potassium Bicarbonate and Potassium Citrate

(poe TASS ee um bye KAR bun ate & poe TASS ee um SIT rate)

Brand Names: U.S. Effer-K®; Klor-Con®/EF

Index Terms Potassium Bicarbonate and Potassium Citrate (Effervescent)

Pharmacologic Category Electrolyte Supplement, Oral

Use Treatment or prevention of hypokalemia, particularly when it is necessary to avoid chloride or the acid/base status requires bicarbonate

Pregnancy Risk Factor C

Dosage Note: Doses expressed as mEq of potassium.

Normal daily requirement: Adults: 40-100 mEq/day or 1-2 mEq/kg/day (unlabeled dose; Mirtallo, 2004)

Hypokalemia: Adults: Oral:

Prevention: 10-80 mEq/day in 1-4 divided doses

Treatment: 40-100 mEq/day in 2-4 divided doses. **Note:** For asymptomatic mild hypokalemia, generally recommended to limit doses to 20-25 mEq/dose to avoid GI discomfort.

Dosage adjustment in renal impairment: No dosage adjustment provided in manufacturer's labeling. However, patients with chronic renal failure require serum potassium monitoring and appropriate dosage adjustment.

Dosage adjustment in hepatic impairment: No dosage adjustment provided in manufacturer's labeling.

Additional Information Complete prescribing information should be consulted for additional detail.

Dosage Forms Excipient information presented when available (limited, particularly for generics); consult specific product labeling.

Tablet for solution, oral [effervescent]:

Effer-K®: Potassium 10 mEq [unflavored and cherry vanilla flavor]

Effer-K®: Potassium 20 mEq [unflavored and orange cream flavor]

Effer-K®: Potassium 25 mEq [unflavored, orange, lemon citrus, and cherry berry flavor]

Klor-Con®/EF: Potassium 25 mEq [sugar free; orange flavor]

◆ **Potassium Bicarbonate and Potassium Citrate (Effervescent)** *see* Potassium Bicarbonate and Potassium Citrate *on page 1684*

Potassium Chloride (poe TASS ee um KLOR ide)

Brand Names: U.S. K-Lor; K-Tabs; K-Vescent; Klor-Con; Klor-Con 10; Klor-Con M10; Klor-Con M15; Klor-Con M20; Micro-K

Brand Names: Canada Apo-K; K-10; K-Dur; Micro-K Extencaps; Roychlor; Slo-Pot; Slow-K

Index Terms KCl; Kdur

Pharmacologic Category Electrolyte Supplement, Oral; Electrolyte Supplement, Parenteral

Use Treatment or prevention of hypokalemia

Pregnancy Risk Factor C

Pregnancy Considerations Reproduction studies have not been conducted. Potassium requirements are the same in pregnant and nonpregnant women. Adverse events have not been observed following use of potassium supplements in healthy women with normal pregnancies. Use caution in pregnant women with other medical conditions (eg, pre-eclampsia; may be more likely to develop hyperkalemia) (IOM, 2004). Potassium supplementation (that does not cause maternal hyperkalemia) would not be expected to cause adverse fetal events.

Breast-Feeding Considerations Potassium is excreted into breast milk (IOM, 2004). The normal content of potassium in human milk is ~13 mEq/L. Supplementation (that does not cause maternal hyperkalemia) would not be expected to affect normal concentrations.

Contraindications Hypersensitivity to any component of the formulation; hyperkalemia. In addition, solid oral dosage forms are contraindicated in patients in whom there is a structural, pathological, and/or pharmacologic cause for delay or arrest in passage through the GI tract.

Warnings/Precautions Close monitoring of serum potassium concentrations is needed to avoid hyperkalemia. Use with caution in patients with renal impairment, cardiac disease, acid/base disorders, or potassium-altering conditions/disorders. Use with caution in digitalized patients or patients receiving concomitant medications or therapies that increase potassium (eg, ACEI, potassium-sparing diuretics, potassium containing salt substitutes). Do **NOT** administer undiluted or I.V. push; inappropriate parenteral administration may be fatal. Always administer potassium further diluted; refer to appropriate dilution and administration rate recommendations. Vesicant/irritant (at concentrations >0.1 mEq/mL); ensure proper catheter or needle position prior to and during infusion; avoid extravasation. Pain and phlebitis may occur during parenteral infusion requiring a decrease in infusion rate or potassium concentration. Avoid administering potassium diluted in dextrose solutions during initial therapy; potential for transient decreases in serum potassium due to intracellular shift of potassium from dextrose-stimulated insulin release. May cause GI upset (eg, nausea, vomiting, diarrhea, abdominal pain, discomfort) and lead to GI ulceration, bleeding, perforation, and/or obstruction. Oral liquid preparations (not solid) should be used in patients with esophageal compression or delayed gastric emptying.

Adverse Reactions Frequency not defined.

Dermatologic: Rash

Endocrine & metabolic: Hyperkalemia

Gastrointestinal: Abdominal pain/discomfort, diarrhea, flatulence, GI bleeding (oral), GI obstruction (oral), GI perforation (oral), nausea, vomiting

Drug Interactions

Metabolism/Transport Effects None known.

Avoid Concomitant Use

Avoid concomitant use of Potassium Chloride with any of the following: Anticholinergic Agents; Glycopyrrolate

Increased Effect/Toxicity

Potassium Chloride may increase the levels/effects of: ACE Inhibitors; Angiotensin II Receptor Blockers; Potassium-Sparing Diuretics

The levels/effects of Potassium Chloride may be increased by: Anticholinergic Agents; Eplerenone; Glycopyrrolate; Heparin; Heparin (Low Molecular Weight)

Decreased Effect There are no known significant interactions involving a decrease in effect.

Preparation for Administration Parenteral: Potassium must be diluted prior to parenteral administration. The concentration of infusion may be dependent on patient condition and specific institution policy. Some clinicians recommend that the maximum concentration for peripheral infusion is 10 mEq/100 mL and 20-40 mEq/100 mL for central infusions.

Storage/Stability

Capsule: MicroK®: Store between 20°C to 25°C (68°F to 77°F).

Powder for oral solution: Klor-Con®: Store at room temperature of 15°C to 30°C (59°F to 86°F).

Solution for injection: Store at room temperature; do not freeze. Use only clear solutions. Use admixtures within 24 hours.

Tablet: K-Tab®: Store below 30°C (86°F).

Mechanism of Action Potassium is the major cation of intracellular fluid and is essential for the conduction of nerve impulses in heart, brain, and skeletal muscle; contraction of cardiac, skeletal and smooth muscles; maintenance of normal renal function, acid-base balance, carbohydrate metabolism, and gastric secretion

Pharmacodynamics/Kinetics

Absorption: Well absorbed from upper GI tract

Distribution: Enters cells via active transport from extracellular fluid

Excretion: Primarily urine; skin and feces (small amounts); most intestinal potassium reabsorbed

Dosage I.V. doses should be incorporated into the patient's maintenance I.V. fluids; intermittent I.V. potassium administration should be reserved for severe depletion situations in patients undergoing ECG monitoring. Doses expressed as mEq of potassium.

Normal daily requirements: Oral, I.V.:
- Children: 1-2 mEq/kg/day
- Adults: 40-80 mEq/day

Prevention of hypokalemia: Oral:
- Children: 1-2 mEq/kg/day in 1-2 divided doses
- Adults: 20-40 mEq/day in 1-2 divided doses

Treatment of hypokalemia: Children:
- Oral: 1-2 mEq/kg initially, then as needed based on frequently obtained lab values. If deficits are severe or ongoing losses are great, I.V. route should be considered.
- I.V. intermittent infusion: 0.5-1 mEq/kg/dose (maximum dose: 40 mEq). If infusion exceeds 0.5 mEq/kg/hour, physician should be at bedside and patient should have continuous ECG monitoring; repeat as needed based on frequently obtained lab values.

Treatment of hypokalemia: Adults:
- Oral:
  - Asymptomatic, mild hypokalemia: Usual dosage range: 40-100 mEq/day divided in 2-5 doses; generally recommended to limit doses to 20-25 mEq/dose to avoid GI discomfort.
  - Mild-to-moderate hypokalemia: Some clinicians may administer up to 120-240 mEq/day divided in 3-4 doses; generally recommended to limit doses to 40-60 mEq/dose. If deficits are severe or ongoing losses are great, I.V. route should be considered.
- I.V. intermittent infusion: Peripheral or central line: ≤10 mEq/hour; repeat as needed based on frequently obtained lab values; central line infusion and continuous ECG monitoring highly recommended for infusions >10 mEq/hour.
  - Potassium dosage/rate of infusion general guidelines (per product labeling): **Note:** High variability exists in dosing/infusion rate recommendations; therapy guided by patient condition and specific institutional guidelines.
    - Serum potassium >2.5-3.5 mEq/L: Maximum infusion rate: 10 mEq/hour; maximum concentration: 40 mEq/L; maximum 24-hour dose: 200 mEq
    - Serum potassium <2.5 mEq/L or symptomatic hypokalemia (excluding emergency treatment of cardiac arrest): Maximum infusion rate (central line only): 40 mEq/hour in presence of continuous ECG monitoring and frequent lab monitoring; In selected situations, patients may require up to 400 mEq/24 hours.

Dosage adjustment in renal impairment: No dosage adjustment provided in manufacturer's labeling. Use caution; potassium acetate injection may increase serum aluminum and/or potassium.

Dosage adjustment in hepatic impairment: No dosage adjustment provided in manufacturer's labeling.

Dietary Considerations Administer with plenty of fluid to decrease stomach irritation and discomfort. Some dietary sources of potassium include leafy green vegetables (eg, spinach, cabbage), tomatoes, cucumbers, zucchini, fruits (eg, apples, oranges, and bananas), root vegetables (eg, carrots, radishes), beans, and peas.

Administration

Parenteral: Potassium must be diluted prior to parenteral administration. Do not administer I.V. push. In general, the dose, concentration of infusion and rate of administration may be dependent on patient condition and specific institution policy. Some clinicians recommend that the maximum concentration for peripheral infusion is 10 mEq/100 mL and maximum rate of administration for peripheral infusion is 10 mEq/hour. ECG monitoring is recommended for peripheral or central infusions >10 mEq/hour in adults. Concentrations and rates of infusion may be greater with central line administration. Some clinicians recommend that the maximum concentration for central infusion is 20-40 mEq/100 mL and maximum rate of administration for central infusion is 40 mEq/hour.

Vesicant/irritant (at concentrations >0.1 mEq/mL); ensure proper needle or catheter placement prior to and during I.V. infusion. Avoid extravasation.

Extravasation management: If extravasation occurs, stop infusion immediately and disconnect (leave needle/cannula in place); gently aspirate extravasated solution (do **NOT** flush the line); initiate hyaluronidase antidote; remove needle/cannula; apply dry cold compresses (Hurst, 2004); elevate extremity.

Hyaluronidase: Intradermal or SubQ: Inject a total of 1 mL (15 units/mL) as five separate 0.2 mL injections (using a 25-gauge needle) into area of extravasation at the leading edge in a clockwise manner (MacCara, 1983; Zenk, 1981).

Oral: Oral dosage forms should be taken with meals and a full glass of water or other liquid to minimize the risk of GI irritation. Prescribing information for the various oral preparations recommend that no more than 20 mEq or 25 mEq should be given as single dose.

Capsule: MicroK®: Swallow whole, do not chew. Capsules may also be opened and contents sprinkled on a spoonful of applesauce or pudding and should be swallowed immediately without chewing.

Powder: Klor-Con®: Dissolve one packet in 4-5 ounces of water or other beverage prior to administration.

Tablet:

K-Tab®, Kaon-Cl®, Klor-Con®: Swallow tablets whole; do not crush, chew, or suck on tablet.

Klor-Con® M: Swallow tablets whole; do not crush, chew, or suck on tablet. Tablet may also be broken in half and each half swallowed separately; the whole tablet may be dissolved in ~4 ounces of water (allow ~2 minutes to dissolve, stir well and drink immediately)

Monitoring Parameters Serum potassium, chloride, magnesium (to facilitate potassium repletion), cardiac monitor (if intermittent infusion or potassium infusion rates 0.5 mEq/kg/hour in children or >10 mEq/hour in adults); to assess adequate replacement, repeat serum potassium level 2-4 hours after dose

Reference Range Note: Reference ranges may vary depending on the laboratory

Serum potassium: 3.5-5.2 mEq/L

Dosage Forms Considerations

750 mg potassium chloride = elemental potassium 390 mg = potassium 10 mEq = potassium 10 mmol

Dosage Forms Excipient information presented when available (limited, particularly for generics); consult specific product labeling.

Capsule Extended Release, Oral:
- Micro-K: 8 mEq, 10 mEq
- Generic: 8 mEq, 10 mEq

Liquid, Oral:
- Generic: 20 MEQ/15ML (10%) (473 mL); 40 MEQ/15ML (20%) (473 mL)

Packet, Oral:
- K-Lor: 20 mEq (30 ea, 100 ea)
- K-Vescent: 20 mEq (100 ea)
- Klor-Con: 20 mEq (1 ea, 30 ea, 100 ea); 25 mEq (30 ea, 100 ea) [sugar free; contains fd&c yellow #6 (sunset yellow); fruit flavor]
- Generic: 20 mEq (30 ea, 100 ea)

Solution, Intravenous:
- Generic: 5 mEq (250 mL); 10 mEq (500 mL, 1000 mL); 20 mEq (1000 mL); 30 mEq (1000 mL); 40 mEq (1000 mL); 0.4 mEq/mL (50 mL); 10 mEq/100 mL (100 mL); 10 mEq/50 mL (50 mL); 20 mEq/100 mL (100 mL); 20 mEq/50 mL (50 mL); 30 mEq/100 mL (100 mL); 40 mEq/100 mL (100 mL); 2 mEq/mL (5 mL, 10 mL, 15 mL, 20 mL, 30 mL, 250 mL); 20 mEq/L (1000 mL); 40 mEq/L (1000 mL)

Solution, Oral:
- Generic: 20 MEQ/15ML (10%) (15 mL, 30 mL, 473 mL)

Tablet Extended Release, Oral:
- K-Tabs: 10 mEq [contains fd&c yellow #10 (quinoline yellow)]
- Klor-Con: 8 mEq [contains fd&c blue #1 aluminum lake, fd&c blue #2 aluminum lake]
- Klor-Con 10: 10 mEq [contains fd&c yellow #10 aluminum lake, fd&c yellow #6 aluminum lake]
- Klor-Con M10: 10 mEq
- Klor-Con M15: 15 mEq [scored]
- Klor-Con M20: 20 mEq [scored]
- Generic: 8 mEq, 10 mEq, 20 mEq

Potassium Citrate and Citric Acid

(poe TASS ee um SIT rate & SI trik AS id)

Brand Names: U.S. Cytra-K

Index Terms Citric Acid and Potassium Citrate; Polycitra K

Pharmacologic Category Alkalinizing Agent, Oral

Use Treatment of metabolic acidosis; alkalinizing agent in conditions where long-term maintenance of an alkaline urine is desirable

Dosage Urine alkalizing agent:

Children: Solution: 5-15 mL after meals and at bedtime; adjust dose based on urinary pH

Adults:

Powder: One packet dissolved in water after meals and at bedtime; adjust dose to urinary pH

Solution: 15-30 mL after meals and at bedtime; adjust dose based on urinary pH

Dosage adjustment in renal impairment: No dosage adjustment provided in manufacturer's labeling. Use is contraindicated in patients with severe renal impairment with oliguria or azotemia.

Dosage adjustment in hepatic impairment: No dosage adjustment provided in manufacturer's labeling.

Additional Information Complete prescribing information should be consulted for additional detail.

Dosage Forms Excipient information presented when available (limited, particularly for generics); consult specific product labeling. [DSC] = Discontinued product

Powder for solution, oral:
- Cytra-K: Potassium citrate monohydrate 3300 mg and citric acid monohydrate 1002 mg per packet (100s) [sugar free; fruit-punch flavor; each packet contains potassium 30 mEq equivalent to bicarbonate 30 mEq]

Solution, oral: Potassium citrate monohydrate 1100 mg and citric acid monohydrate 334 mg per 5 mL (473 mL) [DSC]
- Cytra-K: Potassium citrate monohydrate 1100 mg and citric acid monohydrate 334 mg per 5 mL (480 mL) [ethanol free, sugar free; contains propylene glycol; cherry flavor; contains potassium 2 mEq/mL equivalent to bicarbonate 2 mEq /mL]

◆ **Potassium Citrate, Citric Acid, and Sodium Citrate** *see* Citric Acid, Sodium Citrate, and Potassium Citrate *on page 443*

Potassium Gluconate

(poe TASS ee um GLOO coe nate)

Brand Names: U.S. K-99 [OTC]

Pharmacologic Category Electrolyte Supplement, Oral

Use Dietary supplement

Pregnancy Considerations Potassium requirements are the same in pregnant and non-pregnant women. Adverse events have not been observed following use of potassium supplements in healthy women with normal pregnancies. Use caution in pregnant women with other medical conditions (eg, pre-eclampsia; may be more likely to develop hyperkalemia) (IOM, 2004).

Breast-Feeding Considerations Potassium is excreted into breast milk (IOM, 2004).

Contraindications Hyperkalemia

Warnings/Precautions Use caution in patients with acid/base disorders, cardiovascular disease, potassium-altering conditions/disorders, or renal impairment. Use with caution in patients receiving concomitant medications or therapies that increase potassium (eg, ACEI, potassium-sparing diuretics, potassium containing salt substitutes). Close monitoring of serum potassium concentrations is needed to avoid hyperkalemia. May cause GI upset (eg, nausea, vomiting, diarrhea, abdominal pain, discomfort) and lead to GI ulceration, bleeding, perforation and/or obstruction. Oral liquid preparations (not solid) should be used in patients with esophageal compression or delayed gastric emptying.

Drug Interactions

Metabolism/Transport Effects None known.

Avoid Concomitant Use There are no known interactions where it is recommended to avoid concomitant use.

Increased Effect/Toxicity

Potassium Gluconate may increase the levels/effects of: ACE Inhibitors; Angiotensin II Receptor Blockers; Potassium-Sparing Diuretics

The levels/effects of Potassium Gluconate may be increased by: Eplerenone; Heparin; Heparin (Low Molecular Weight)

Decreased Effect There are no known significant interactions involving a decrease in effect.

Storage/Stability Store at room temperature.

Mechanism of Action Potassium is the major cation of intracellular fluid and is essential for the conduction of nerve impulses in heart, brain, and skeletal muscle; contraction of cardiac, skeletal and smooth muscles; maintenance of normal renal function, acid-base balance, carbohydrate metabolism, and gastric secretion

Pharmacodynamics/Kinetics

Absorption: Well absorbed from upper GI tract

Distribution: Enters cells via active transport from extracellular fluid

Excretion: Primarily urine; skin and feces (small amounts); most intestinal potassium reabsorbed

Dosage Oral: Adults: One tablet daily as dietary supplement

Dosage adjustment in renal impairment: No dosage adjustment provided in manufacturer's labeling.

Dosage adjustment in hepatic impairment: No dosage adjustment provided in manufacturer's labeling.

Monitoring Parameters Serum potassium and magnesium (to facilitate potassium repletion)

Reference Range Note: Reference ranges may vary depending on the laboratory

Serum potassium: 3.5-5.2 mEq/L

Test Interactions Decreased ammonia (B)

Additional Information 9.4 g potassium gluconate is approximately equal to 40 mEq potassium (4.3 mEq potassium/g potassium gluconate).

Dosage Forms Considerations

1 g potassium gluconate = elemental potassium 167 mg = potassium 4.3 mEq = potassium 4.3 mmol

Dosage Forms Excipient information presented when available (limited, particularly for generics); consult specific product labeling.

Capsule, Oral [preservative free]:

K-99: 595 mg [dye free, sugar free, yeast free]

Tablet, Oral:

Generic: 2 mEq, 2.5 mEq

Tablet, Oral [strength expressed as base]:

Generic: 80 mg

Potassium Iodide (poe TASS ee um EYE oh dide)

Brand Names: U.S. SSKI; ThyroShield [OTC]

Index Terms KI; Saturated Potassium Iodide Solution; Saturated Solution of Potassium Iodide

Pharmacologic Category Antidote; Antithyroid Agent; Expectorant

Use Expectorant for the symptomatic treatment of chronic pulmonary diseases complicated by mucous; block thyroidal uptake of radioactive isotopes of iodine in a nuclear radiation emergency

Unlabeled Use Lymphocutaneous and cutaneous sporotrichosis; reduce thyroid vascularity prior to thyroidectomy; management of thyrotoxic crisis; block thyroidal uptake of radioactive isotopes of iodine after therapeutic or diagnostic exposure to radioactive iodine

Pregnancy Risk Factor D

Pregnancy Considerations Iodide crosses the placenta (may cause hypothyroidism and goiter in fetus/newborn). Use as an expectorant during pregnancy is contraindicated by the AAP. Use for protection against thyroid cancer secondary to radioactive iodine exposure is considered acceptable based upon risk:benefit, keeping in mind the dose and duration. Repeat dosing should be avoided if possible.

Breast-Feeding Considerations Potassium iodide is excreted in breast milk. May cause skin rash in nursing infant. Nursing mothers should take as instructed by public officials and contact their physician.

Contraindications Hypersensitivity to iodide, iodine, or any component of the formulation; dermatitis herpetiformis; hypocomplementemic vasculitis, nodular thyroid condition with heart disease

Warnings/Precautions Prolonged use can lead to hypothyroidism; iodide may cause underactive or overactive thyroid; thyroid enlargement may also occur; use with caution in patients with a history of hyperthyroidism; use is contraindicated in patients with nodular thyroid condition (goiter) with heart disease. Iodism or chronic iodide poisoning may occur with high doses or prolonged treatment; symptoms include burning of mouth/throat, sore teeth/gums, severe headache, metallic taste, eye irritation/eye lid swelling, increased salivation, acneform skin lesions, and (rarely) severe skin lesions; withhold potassium iodide treatment and manage with supportive care.

May cause acne flare-ups, can cause dermatitis; use with caution in patients with a history of renal impairment, Addison's disease, cardiac disease, myotonia congenita, tuberculosis, and/or acute bronchitis. Iodide hypersensitivity may occur, manifesting as angioedema, cutaneous/mucosal hemorrhage, and serum sickness-like symptoms (fever, arthralgia, lymph node enlargement, and eosinophilia). Potentially significant drug-drug interactions may exist, requiring dose or frequency adjustment, additional monitoring, and/or selection of alternative therapy. For thyroid gland protection (radiopharmaceutical use), potassium iodide must be administered prior to receiving radiopharmaceuticals that require thyroid gland protection. For nuclear radiation emergency, take only when instructed by public health officials; do not take more or more often than instructed; follow other emergency measures recommended by officials. In a nuclear radiation emergency, infants and children are more likely to experience thyroid damage. Infants <1 month are at higher risk for hypothyroidism with potassium iodide use; evaluate thyroid function if repeat dosing is required in this patient population.

Adverse Reactions Frequency not defined.

Cardiovascular: Cardiac arrhythmia

Central nervous system: Confusion, fatigue, fever, numbness, tingling sensation

Dermatologic: Skin rash, urticaria

Endocrine & metabolic: Goiter, hyperthyroidism (prolonged use), hypothyroidism (prolonged use), myxedema

Gastrointestinal: Diarrhea, enlargement of salivary glands, gastric distress, gastrointestinal hemorrhage, metallic taste, nausea, stomach pain, vomiting

Hematologic & oncologic: Lymphedema, thyroid adenoma

Hypersensitivity: Hypersensitivity reaction (angioedema, cutaneous and mucosal hemorrhage, serum sickness-like symptoms)

Neuromuscular & skeletal: Weakness

Respiratory: Dyspnea, wheezing

Miscellaneous: Iodine poisoning (with prolonged treatment/high doses)

Drug Interactions

Metabolism/Transport Effects None known.

Avoid Concomitant Use

Avoid concomitant use of Potassium Iodide with any of the following: Sodium Iodide I131

Increased Effect/Toxicity

Potassium Iodide may increase the levels/effects of: ACE Inhibitors; Angiotensin II Receptor Blockers; Cardiac Glycosides; Lithium; Potassium-Sparing Diuretics; Theophylline Derivatives

The levels/effects of Potassium Iodide may be increased by: Eplerenone; Heparin; Heparin (Low Molecular Weight)

Decreased Effect

Potassium Iodide may decrease the levels/effects of: Sodium Iodide I131; Vitamin K Antagonists

Preparation for Administration SSKI®: Mix in water, fruit juice, or milk.

Storage/Stability Store at room temperature of 25°C (77°F); excursions permitted to 15°C to 30°C (59°F to 86°F). Protect from light. Keep tightly closed.

SSKI®: If exposed to cold, crystallization may occur. Warm and shake to redissolve. If solution becomes brown/yellow, it should be discarded.

iOSAT™, Thyrosafe®: Keep dry and keep intact in foil.

Mechanism of Action Reduces viscosity of mucus by increasing respiratory tract secretions; inhibits secretion of thyroid hormone, fosters colloid accumulation in thyroid follicles. Following radioactive iodine exposure, potassium iodide blocks the uptake of radioactive iodine by the thyroid, reducing the risk of thyroid cancer.

Pharmacodynamics/Kinetics

Onset of action: Hyperthyroidism: 24-48 hours

Peak effect: 10-15 days after continuous therapy

Duration: Radioactive iodine exposure: Each dose has a duration of ~24 hours

Dosage

RDA: Adults: 150 mcg (iodine)

Expectorant (SSKI®): Adults: Oral: 300-600 mg (0.3-0.6 mL) 3-4 times daily

Thyroid block following nuclear radiation emergency (iOSAT™, ThyroSafe®, ThyroShield®): Dosing should continue for 10-14 days or as directed by public officials (until risk of exposure has passed or other measures are implemented): Oral:

Infants ≤1 month: 16.25 mg once daily

Infants >1 month to Children ≤3 years: 32.5 mg once daily

Children >3 to ≤12 years: 65 mg once daily

Children >12-18 years weighing <68 kg: 65 mg once daily

Children >12-18 years weighing ≥68 kg and Adults (including pregnant/lactating women): 130 mg once daily

Thyroidectomy preparation (unlabeled use): Oral:

Children: 150-350 mg (3-7 drops **or** 0.15-0.35 mL SSKI®) 3 times daily; administer for 10 days before surgery; if not euthyroid prior to surgery, consider concurrent beta-blockade (eg, propranolol) in the immediate preoperative period to reduce the risk of thyroid storm (Bahn, 2011)

Adults: 50-100 mg (1-2 drops **or** 0.05-0.1 mL SSKI®) 3 times daily; administer for 10 days before surgery; if not euthyroid prior to surgery, consider concurrent beta-blockade (eg, propranolol) in the immediate preoperative period to reduce the risk of thyroid storm (Bahn, 2011)

Thyroid gland protection during radiopharmaceutical use (unlabeled use): Oral:

Note: Begin at 1-48 hours prior to exposure. Continue potassium iodide after radiopharmaceutical administration until risk of exposure has diminished (treatment duration and time of initiation is dependent on the radiopharmaceutical, consult specific protocol).

Children (Giammarile, 2008; Olivier, 2003):

Infants <5 kg: 16 mg once daily

1 month to 3 years or 5-15 kg: 32 mg once daily

3-13 years or 15-50 kg: 65 mg once daily

>13 years or >50 kg: 130 mg once daily

Adults: Tablet: 130 mg once daily **or** Solution (SSKI®): 4 drops 3 times daily (Bexxar® prescribing information, 2012)

Thyrotoxic crisis/thyroid storm (unlabeled use): Oral: **Note:** Administer at least 1-2 hours after antithyroid drug administration:

Infants: 100 mg (2 drops **or** 0.1 mL SSKI®) 4 times daily (Eyal, 2008)

Children: 250 mg (5 drops **or** 0.25 mL SSKI®) 2-4 times daily (Eyal, 2008)

Adults: 250 mg (5 drops **or** 0.25 mL SSKI®) every 6 hours (Bahn, 2011)

Sporotrichosis (cutaneous, lymphocutaneous; unlabeled use) (SSKI®): Adults: Oral: Initial: 5 drops 3 times daily; increase to 40-50 drops 3 times daily as tolerated until 2-4 weeks after lesions have resolved (usual duration 3-6 months) (Kauffman, 2007)

Dosage adjustment in renal impairment: No dosage adjustment provided in the manufacturer's labeling.

Dosage adjustment in hepatic impairment: No dosage adjustment provided in the manufacturer's labeling.

Dietary Considerations SSKI®: Take with food or milk to decrease gastric irritation.

Administration

SSKI®: Dilute in a glassful of water, fruit juice, or milk. Take with food or milk to decrease gastric irritation.

iOSAT™, Thyrosafe®, Thyroshield®: Take as soon as possible after instructed to do so by public officials. Take every 24 hours; do not take more than 1 dose in 24 hours. Tablets may be crushed and mixed with water, low fat milk (white or chocolate), orange juice, soda (flat), raspberry syrup, or infant formula.

Monitoring Parameters Thyroid function tests, signs/symptoms of hyperthyroidism; thyroid function should be monitored in pregnant or breast-feeding women, neonates, and young infants if repeat doses are required following radioactive iodine exposure

Test Interactions Iodide may alter thyroid function tests.

Additional Information 10 drops of SSKI® = potassium iodide 500 mg

Dosage Forms Excipient information presented when available (limited, particularly for generics); consult specific product labeling.

Solution, Oral:

SSKI: 1 g/mL (30 mL, 237 mL)

ThyroShield: 65 mg/mL (30 mL) [contains brilliant blue fcf (fd&c blue #1), fd&c red #40, methylparaben, propylene glycol, propylparaben, saccharin sodium; black raspberry flavor]

Extemporaneous Preparations A 16.25 mg/5 mL oral solution may be made with tablets. Crush one 130 mg tablet and reduce to a fine powder. Add 20 mL of water and mix until powder is dissolved. Add an additional 20 mL of low-fat milk (white or chocolate), orange juice, flat soda, raspberry syrup, or infant formula. Stable for 7 days under refrigeration.

To prepare an 8.125 mg/5 mL oral solution, crush one 65 mg tablet and reduce to a fine powder. Add 20 mL of water and mix until powder is dissolved. Add an additional 20 mL of low-fat milk (white or chocolate), orange juice, flat soda, raspberry syrup, or infant formula. Stable for 7 days under refrigeration.

Potassium Iodide and Iodine

(poe TASS ee um EYE oh dide & EYE oh dine)

Index Terms Iodine and Potassium Iodide; Lugol's Solution; Strong Iodine Solution

Pharmacologic Category Antithyroid Agent

Use Topical antiseptic

Unlabeled Use Reduce thyroid vascularity prior to thyroidectomy and management of thyrotoxic crisis; block thyroidal uptake of radioactive isotopes of iodine in a radiation emergency or after therapeutic/diagnostic use of radioactive iodine

Pregnancy Risk Factor D (potassium iodide)

Pregnancy Considerations Iodide crosses the placenta (may cause hypothyroidism and goiter in fetus/newborn). Use for protection against thyroid cancer secondary to radioactive iodine exposure is considered acceptable based upon risk/benefit, keeping in mind the dose and duration. Repeat dosing should be avoided if possible.

Breast-Feeding Considerations Skin rash in the nursing infant has been reported with maternal intake of potassium iodide.

Contraindications Hypersensitivity to iodine or any component of the formulation; iodine-induced goiter; dermatitis herpetiformis; hypocomplementemic vasculitis; nodular thyroid disease with heart disease

Warnings/Precautions Prolonged use can lead to hypothyroidism; can cause acne flare-ups and/or dermatitis; use with caution in patients with a history of renal impairment, hyperthyroidism, Addison's disease, cardiac disease, myotonia congenita, tuberculosis, acute bronchitis. Potentially significant interactions may exist, requiring dose or frequency adjustment, additional monitoring, and/or selection of alternative therapy. Potassium iodide and iodine solution must be administered prior to receiving radiopharmaceuticals that require thyroid gland protection.

Adverse Reactions Frequency not defined.

Cardiovascular: Irregular heart beat

Central nervous system: Confusion, tiredness, fever

Dermatologic: Skin rash

Endocrine & metabolic: Goiter, salivary gland swelling/tenderness, thyroid adenoma, swelling of neck/throat, myxedema, lymph node swelling, hyper-/hypothyroidism

Gastrointestinal: Diarrhea, gastrointestinal bleeding, metallic taste, nausea, stomach pain, stomach upset, vomiting

Neuromuscular & skeletal: Numbness, tingling, weakness, joint pain

Miscellaneous: Chronic iodine poisoning (with prolonged treatment/high doses); iodism, hypersensitivity reactions (angioedema, cutaneous and mucosal hemorrhage, serum sickness-like symptoms)

Drug Interactions

Metabolism/Transport Effects None known.

Avoid Concomitant Use

Avoid concomitant use of Potassium Iodide and Iodine with any of the following: Sodium Iodide I131

Increased Effect/Toxicity

Potassium Iodide and Iodine may increase the levels/effects of: ACE Inhibitors; Angiotensin II Receptor Blockers; Cardiac Glycosides; Lithium; Potassium-Sparing Diuretics; Theophylline Derivatives

The levels/effects of Potassium Iodide and Iodine may be increased by: Eplerenone; Heparin; Heparin (Low Molecular Weight)

Decreased Effect

Potassium Iodide and Iodine may decrease the levels/effects of: Sodium Iodide I131; Vitamin K Antagonists

Storage/Stability Store at room temperature of 15°C to 30°C (59°F to 86°F). Protect from light and keep container tightly closed.

Mechanism of Action In hyperthyroidism, iodine temporarily inhibits thyroid hormone synthesis and secretion into the circulation; use also decreases thyroid gland size and vascularity. Serum T_4 and T_3 concentrations can be reduced for several weeks with use but effect will not be maintained.

Following radioactive iodine exposure, potassium iodide blocks uptake of radioiodine by the thyroid, reducing the risk of thyroid cancer.

Pharmacodynamics/Kinetics

Onset of action: Hyperthyroidism: 24-48 hours

Peak effect: 10-15 days after continuous therapy

Dosage

Topical: Adults: Antiseptic: Apply directly to area(s) requiring antiseptic.

Oral:

Children and Adults:

Thyrotoxic crisis (unlabeled use):

Children: 4-8 drops 3 times daily; begin therapy preferably 2 hours following the initial dose of propylthiouracil or alternatively, methimazole (Eyal, 2008)

Adults: 4-8 drops every 6-8 hours; begin administration ≥1 hour following the initial dose of either propylthiouracil or methimazole (Nayak, 2006)

Adults:

RDA: 150 mcg (iodine)

Preparation for thyroidectomy (unlabeled use): 5-7 drops (0.25-0.35 mL) 3 times daily; administer for 10 days before surgery; if not euthyroid prior to surgery, consider concurrent beta-blockade (eg, propranolol) in the immediate preoperative period to reduce the risk of thyroid storm (Bahn, 2011)

Thyroid gland protection during radiopharmaceutical use (unlabeled use): 20 drops 3 times daily has been recommended (Bexxar® prescribing information, 2012)

Note: Initiate 1-48 hours prior to radiopharmaceutical exposure and continue after radiopharmaceutical administration until risk of exposure has diminished (treatment initiation time and duration is dependent on the radiopharmaceutical agent used, consult specific protocol or labeling.

Dosage adjustment in renal impairment: No dosage adjustment provided in manufacturer's labeling.

Dosage adjustment in hepatic impairment: No dosage adjustment provided in manufacturer's labeling.

Administration Apply topically directly to area(s) requiring antiseptic. Has also been used orally (unlabeled route).

Monitoring Parameters Thyroid function tests, signs/symptoms of hyperthyroidism; thyroid function should be monitored in pregnant women, neonates, and young infants if repeat doses are required following radioactive iodine exposure

Test Interactions Iodide may alter thyroid function tests.

Dosage Forms Excipient information presented when available (limited, particularly for generics); consult specific product labeling.

Solution, oral: Potassium iodide 100 mg/mL and iodine 50 mg/mL (473 mL)

Solution, topical: Potassium iodide 100 mg/mL and iodine 50 mg/mL (8 mL)

Potassium Phosphate (poe TASS ee um FOS fate)

Brand Names: U.S. Neutra-Phos®-K [OTC] [DSC]

Index Terms Phosphate, Potassium

Pharmacologic Category Electrolyte Supplement, Parenteral

Use Treatment and prevention of hypophosphatemia; **Note:** The concomitant amount of potassium must be calculated into the total electrolyte content. For each 1 mmol of phosphate, ~1.5 mEq of potassium will be administered. Therefore, if ordering 30 mmol of potassium phosphate, the patient will receive ~45 mEq of potassium.

Pregnancy Risk Factor C

Pregnancy Considerations Reproduction studies have not been conducted. Phosphorus requirements are the same in pregnant and nonpregnant women (IOM, 1997). Although this product is not used for potassium supplementation, adverse events have not been observed following use of potassium supplements in healthy women with normal pregnancies. Use caution in pregnant women with other medical conditions (eg, pre-eclampsia; may be more likely to develop hyperkalemia) (IOM, 2004).

Breast-Feeding Considerations Phosphorus, sodium, and potassium are normal constituents of human milk.

Contraindications Hyperphosphatemia, hyperkalemia, hypocalcemia

Warnings/Precautions Close monitoring of serum potassium concentrations is needed to avoid hyperkalemia. Use with caution in patients with renal insufficiency, cardiac disease, metabolic alkalosis. Use with caution in digitalized patients and patients receiving concomitant potassium-altering therapies. Parenteral potassium may cause pain and phlebitis, requiring a decrease in infusion rate or potassium concentration. Solutions for injection may contain aluminum; toxic levels may occur following prolonged administration in premature neonates or patients with renal impairment.

Adverse Reactions Frequency not defined.

Cardiovascular: Arrhythmia, bradycardia, chest pain, ECG changes, edema, heart block, hypotension

Central nervous system: Listlessness, mental confusion, tetany (with large doses of phosphate)

Endocrine & metabolic: Hyperkalemia

Gastrointestinal: Diarrhea, nausea, stomach pain, vomiting

Genitourinary: Urine output decreased

Local: Phlebitis

Neuromuscular & skeletal: Paralysis, paresthesia, weakness

Renal: Acute renal failure

Respiratory: Dyspnea

Drug Interactions

Metabolism/Transport Effects None known.

Avoid Concomitant Use There are no known interactions where it is recommended to avoid concomitant use.

Increased Effect/Toxicity

Potassium Phosphate may increase the levels/effects of: ACE Inhibitors; Angiotensin II Receptor Blockers; Potassium-Sparing Diuretics

The levels/effects of Potassium Phosphate may be increased by: Bisphosphonate Derivatives; Eplerenone; Heparin; Heparin (Low Molecular Weight)

Decreased Effect

The levels/effects of Potassium Phosphate may be decreased by: Antacids; Calcium Salts; Iron Salts; Magnesium Salts; Multivitamins/Minerals (with ADEK, Folate, Iron); Sucralfate

Ethanol/Nutrition/Herb Interactions Food: Avoid administering with oxalate (berries, nuts, chocolate, beans, celery, tomato) or phytate-containing foods (bran, whole wheat).

Preparation for Administration In general, the dose, concentration of infusion, and rate of administration may be dependent on patient condition and specific institution policy. Intermittent infusion doses of potassium phosphate are typically prepared in 100-250 mL of NS or D_5W (usual phosphate concentration range: 0.15-0.6 mmol/mL) (Charron, 2003; Rosen, 1995). Suggested maximum concentrations:

Central line administration: 26.8 mmoL potassium phosphate/100 mL (40 mEq potassium/100 mL)

Peripheral line administration: 6.7 mmoL potassium phosphate/100 mL (10 mEq potassium/100 mL)

Observe the vial for the presence of translucent visible particles. Do not use vial if particles are present. Dilute in a compatible I.V. fluid. **Note:** Due to the potential presence of particulates, American Regent, Inc recommends the use of a 5 micron filter when preparing I.V. sodium phosphate-containing solutions (Important Drug Administration Information, American Regent, 2013); a similar recommendation has not been noted by other manufacturers.

Storage/Stability Store intact vials at 20°C to 25°C (68°F to 77°F); excursions permitted between 15°C and 30°C (59°F and 86°F).

Mechanism of Action

Phosphorus in the form of organic and inorganic phosphate has a variety of important biochemical functions in the body and is involved in many significant metabolic and enzymatic reactions in almost all organs and tissues. It exerts a modifying influence on the steady state of calcium levels, a buffering effect on acid-base equilibrium and a primary role in the renal excretion of hydrogen ion.

Potassium is the major cation of intracellular fluid and is essential for the conduction of nerve impulses in heart, brain, and skeletal muscle; contraction of cardiac, skeletal and smooth muscles; maintenance of normal renal function, acid-base balance, carbohydrate metabolism, and gastric secretion.

Dosage Note: If phosphate repletion is required and a phosphate product is not available at your institution, consider the use of sodium glycerophosphate pentahydrate (Glycophos) as a suitable substitute. Concentration and dosing are different from FDA-approved products; use caution when switching between products. Refer to Sodium Glycerophosphate Pentahydrate monograph.

I.V.: **Caution: The concomitant amount of potassium must be calculated into the total electrolyte content. For each 1 mmol of phosphate, ~1.5 mEq of potassium will be administered. Therefore, if ordering 30 mmol of potassium phosphate, the patient will receive ~45 mEq of potassium. With orders for I.V. phosphate, there is considerable confusion associated with the use of millimoles (mmol) versus milliequivalents (mEq) to express the phosphate requirement.** The most reliable method of ordering I.V. phosphate is by millimoles, then specifying the potassium or sodium salt. Doses listed as mmol of phosphate.

Acute treatment of hypophosphatemia: Repletion of severe hypophosphatemia should be done I.V. because large doses of oral phosphate may cause diarrhea and intestinal absorption may be unreliable. Reserve intermittent I.V. infusion for severe depletion situations; may require continuous cardiac monitoring depending on potassium administration rate. Guidelines differ based on degree of illness, need/use of parenteral nutrition, and severity of hypophosphatemia. If potassium >4.0 mEq/L consider phosphate replacement strategy without potassium (eg, sodium phosphates). Patients with severe renal impairment were excluded from phosphate supplement trials. **Note:** 1 mmol phosphate = 31 mg phosphorus; 1 mg phosphorus = 0.032 mmol phosphate.

Children and Adults: **Note:** There are no prospective studies of parenteral phosphate replacement in children. The following weight-based guidelines for adult dosing may be cautiously employed in pediatric patients.

General replacement guidelines (Lentz, 1978):

Low dose, if serum phosphate losses are recent and uncomplicated: Initial: 0.08 mmol/kg over 6 hours

Intermediate dose, if serum phosphorus level <1 mg/dL (<0.32 mmol/L): Initial: 0.16 mmol/kg per dose over 6 hours

Note: The initial dose may be increased by 25% to 50% if the patient is symptomatic secondary to hypophosphatemia and lowered by 25% to 50% if the patient is hypercalcemic. Do not exceed the maximum dose of 0.24 mmol/kg/dose (or 16.9 mmol for a 70-kg patient).

Critically-ill adult patients receiving concurrent enteral/parenteral nutrition (Brown, 2006; Clark, 1995): Note: Round doses to the nearest 7.5 mmol for ease of preparation. If administering with phosphate-containing parenteral nutrition, do not exceed 15 mmol/L within parenteral nutrition.

Low dose, serum phosphorus level 2.3-3 mg/dL (0.74-0.96 mmol/L): 0.16-0.32 mmol/kg over 4-6 hours

Intermediate dose, serum phosphorus level 1.6-2.2 mg/dL (0.51-0.71 mmol/L): 0.32-0.64 mmol/kg over 4-6 hours

High dose, serum phosphorus <1.5 mg/dL (<0.5 mmol/L): 0.64-1 mmol/kg over 8-12 hours

Obesity: May use adjusted body weight for patients weighing >130% of ideal body weight (and BMI <40 kg/m^2) by using [IBW + 0.25 (actual body weight - IBW)].

Parenteral nutrition:

Infants and Children: 0.5-2 mmol/kg/24 hours (Mirtallo, 2004 [ASPEN guidelines])

Children >50 kg and Adolescents: 10-40 mmol/24 hours (Mirtallo, 2004 [ASPEN guidelines])

Adults: 10-15 mmol/1000 kcal (Hicks, 2001) **or** 20-40 mmol/24 hours (Mirtallo, 2004 [ASPEN guidelines])

Administration Injection must be diluted in appropriate I.V. solution and volume prior to administration. In general, the dose, concentration of infusion, and rate of administration may be dependent on patient condition and specific institution policy. Must consider administration precautions for phosphate and potassium when prescribing. **Note:** Due to the potential presence of translucent visible particles, American Regent, Inc recommends the use of a 0.22 micron in-line filter for I.V. administration (1.2 micron filter if admixture contains lipids) (Important Drug Administration Information, American Regent, 2013); a similar recommendation has not been noted by other manufacturers.

For adult patients with severe symptomatic hypophosphatemia (ie, <1.5 mg/dL), may administer at rates up to 15 mmol phosphate/hour (this rate will deliver potassium at 22.5 mEq/hour) (Charron, 2003; Rosen, 1995). Potassium infusion rates >10 mEq/hour should be administered via central line (minimizes burning and phlebitis). ECG monitoring is recommended for potassium infusions >10 mEq/hour in adults or >0.5 mEq/kg/hour in children. In patients with renal dysfunction and/or less severe hypophosphatemia, slower administration rates (eg, over 4-6 hours) or oral repletion is recommended.

Monitoring Parameters Serum potassium, calcium, phosphorus, magnesium (to facilitate potassium repletion); cardiac monitor (if intermittent infusion or potassium infusion rates >0.5 mEq/kg/hour in children or >10 mEq/hour in adults); to assess adequate replacement, repeat serum potassium and phosphorus levels 2-4 hours after dose

Reference Range Note: Reference ranges may vary depending on the laboratory

Serum calcium: 8.4-10.2 mg/dL

Serum phosphorus: Both low and high ends of the normal range are higher in children than in adults.

Infants: 4.5-7.5 mg/dL (1.45-2.42 mmol/L)

Children: ~4-6 mg/dL (1.29-1.94 mmol/L)

Adults: 2.5-4.5 mg/dL (0.81-1.45 mmol/L)

Serum potassium: 3.5-5.2 mEq/L

Dosage Forms Considerations

Potassium 4.4 mEq is equivalent to potassium 170 mg

Phosphorous 3 mmol is equivalent to phosphorus 93 mg

Dosage Forms Excipient information presented when available (limited, particularly for generics); consult specific product labeling.

Injection, solution: Potassium 4.4 mEq and phosphorus 3 mmol per mL (5 mL, 15 mL, 50 mL) [equivalent to potassium 170 mg and elemental phosphorus 93 mg per mL]

Potassium Phosphate and Sodium Phosphate

(poe TASS ee um FOS fate & SOW dee um FOS fate)

Brand Names: U.S. K-Phos® Neutral; K-Phos® No. 2; Phos-NaK; Phospha 250™ Neutral

Index Terms Neutra-Phos; Sodium Phosphate and Potassium Phosphate

Pharmacologic Category Electrolyte Supplement, Oral

Use Phosphorus supplement; to increase urinary phosphate and pyrophosphate; to acidify the urine to lower calcium concentrations; to increase the antibacterial activity of methenamine; reduce odor and rash caused by ammonia in urine

Pregnancy Risk Factor C

Dosage Oral: **Note:** Dosage expressed in terms of **elemental phosphorus**.

Children ≥4 years and Adolescents: Phosphate supplement: 250 mg 4 times daily

Adults:

Phosphate supplement: 250-500 mg 4 times daily

Urinary acidification: 250 mg 4 times daily; may be increased to 250 mg every 2 hours when the urine is difficult to acidify (maximum daily dose: 2000 mg)

Dosage adjustment in renal impairment: No dosage adjustment provided in manufacturer's labeling. Use with caution. Contraindicated in patients with severe impairment (<30% of normal function).

Dosage adjustment in hepatic impairment: No dosage adjustment provided in manufacturer's labeling. Use with caution.

Additional Information Complete prescribing information should be consulted for additional detail.

Dosage Forms Excipient information presented when available (limited, particularly for generics); consult specific product labeling.

Powder for solution, oral:

Phos-NaK: Dibasic potassium phosphate, monobasic potassium phosphate, dibasic sodium phosphate, and monobasic sodium phosphate per packet (100s) [sugar free; equivalent to elemental phosphorus 250 mg (8 mmol), sodium 160 mg (6.9 mEq), and potassium 280 mg (7.1 mEq) per packet; fruit flavor]

Tablet, oral:

K-Phos® Neutral: Monobasic potassium phosphate 155 mg, dibasic sodium phosphate 852 mg, and monobasic sodium phosphate 130 mg [equivalent to elemental phosphorus 250 mg (8 mmol), sodium 298 mg (13 mEq), and potassium 45 mg (1.1 mEq)]

K-Phos® No. 2: Potassium acid phosphate 305 mg and sodium acid phosphate 700 mg [equivalent to elemental phosphorus 250 mg (8 mmol), sodium 134 mg (5.8 mEq), and potassium 88 mg (2.3 mEq)]

Phospha 250™ Neutral: Monobasic potassium phosphate 155 mg, dibasic sodium phosphate 852 mg, and monobasic sodium phosphate 130 mg [equivalent to elemental phosphorus 250 mg (8 mmol), sodium 298 mg (13 mEq), and potassium 45 mg (1.1 mEq)]

- ◆ **Potassium Phosphate Monobasic** *see* Potassium Acid Phosphate *on page 1683*
- ◆ **Potassium Sulfate, Magnesium Sulfate, and Sodium Sulfate** *see* Sodium Sulfate, Potassium Sulfate, and Magnesium Sulfate *on page 1929*
- ◆ **Potassium Sulfate, Sodium Sulfate, and Magnesium Sulfate** *see* Sodium Sulfate, Potassium Sulfate, and Magnesium Sulfate *on page 1929*
- ◆ **Potiga** *see* Ezogabine *on page 819*
- ◆ **PPD** *see* Tuberculin Tests *on page 2134*
- ◆ **PPI-0903** *see* Ceftaroline Fosamil *on page 378*
- ◆ **PPI-0903M** *see* Ceftaroline Fosamil *on page 378*
- ◆ **PPS** *see* Pentosan Polysulfate Sodium *on page 1617*
- ◆ **PPSV** *see* Pneumococcal Polysaccharide Vaccine (Polyvalent) *on page 1664*
- ◆ **PPSV23** *see* Pneumococcal Polysaccharide Vaccine (Polyvalent) *on page 1664*
- ◆ **PPV23** *see* Pneumococcal Polysaccharide Vaccine (Polyvalent) *on page 1664*
- ◆ **PR-171** *see* Carfilzomib *on page 348*
- ◆ **Pradaxa** *see* Dabigatran Etexilate *on page 525*
- ◆ **Pradaxa® (Can)** *see* Dabigatran Etexilate *on page 525*

PRALAtrexate (pral a TREX ate)

Brand Names: U.S. Folotyn

Index Terms PDX

Pharmacologic Category Antineoplastic Agent, Antimetabolite (Antifolate)

Use Treatment of relapsed or refractory peripheral T-cell lymphoma (PTCL)

Unlabeled Use Treatment of relapsed or refractory cutaneous T-cell lymphomas (mycosis fungoides [MF] and Sézary syndrome [SS])

Pregnancy Risk Factor D

Pregnancy Considerations Adverse effects were observed in animal reproduction studies. May cause fetal harm if administered to a pregnant woman.

Breast-Feeding Considerations Due to the potential for serious adverse reactions in the nursing infant, the decision to discontinue breast-feeding or to discontinue pralatrexate should take into account the benefits of treatment to the mother.

Contraindications There are no contraindications listed within the manufacturer's labeling.

Warnings/Precautions Hazardous agent - use appropriate precautions for handling and disposal (NIOSH, 2012). May cause bone marrow suppression (thrombocytopenia, neutropenia and anemia); may require dosage modification; monitor blood counts. Mucositis, including stomatitis or mucosal inflammation of gastrointestinal and genitourinary tracts, may occur; monitor weekly; may require dosage modification. Prophylactic folic acid and vitamin B_{12} supplements are necessary to reduce hematologic toxicity and treatment-related mucositis. Severe and potentially fatal dermatologic reactions, including skin exfoliation, ulceration, and toxic epidermal necrolysis (TEN) have been reported. Skin reaction may be progressive; severity may increase with continued treatment; may also involve skin and subcutaneous tissues which are affected by lymphoma; monitor all dermatologic reactions closely; withhold or discontinue treatment for severe dermatologic reaction.

Pralatrexate may cause tumor lysis syndrome (TLS); monitor closely, if TLS develops, treat for associated complications. Use with caution in patients with moderate-to-severe renal impairment (has not been studied in patients with renal impairment); monitor renal function and for systemic toxicity due to increased exposure. Concurrent use with drugs with substantial renal clearance (eg, NSAIDs, sulfamethoxazole/trimethoprim) may result in delayed pralatrexate clearance. Liver function test abnormalities have been observed with use; monitor liver function; persistent abnormalities may indicate hepatotoxicity and may require dosage modification.

Patients with moderate-to-severe renal impairment are at risk for increased exposure and toxicity. Avoid use in patients with end-stage renal disease (ESRD), including patients undergoing dialysis (unless the potential benefit outweighs potential risks); serious adverse reactions, including toxic epidermal necrolysis and mucositis were reported in patients with ESRD undergoing dialysis. Monitor renal function and for systemic toxicity due to increased exposure.

Adverse Reactions

>10%:

Cardiovascular: Edema (30%)

Central nervous system: Fatigue (36%), fever (32%)

Dermatologic: Rash (15%; grades 3/4: 0%), pruritus (14%; grade 3: 2%; grade 4: 0%)

Endocrine & metabolic: Hypokalemia (15%)

Gastrointestinal: Mucositis (70%; grade 3: 17%; grade 4: 4%), nausea (40%), constipation (33%), vomiting (25%), diarrhea (21%), anorexia (15%), abdominal pain (12%)

Hematologic: Thrombocytopenia (41%; grade 3: 14%; grade 4: 19%), anemia (34%; grade 3: 15%; grade 4: 2%), neutropenia (24%; grade 3: 13%; grade 4: 7%), leukopenia (11%; grade 3: 3%; grade 4: 4%)

Hepatic: Transaminases increased (13%; grade 3: 5%; grade 4: 0%)

Neuromuscular & skeletal: Limb pain (12%), back pain (11%)

Respiratory: Cough (28%), epistaxis (26%), dyspnea (19%), pharyngolaryngeal pain (14%)

Miscellaneous: Night sweats (11%), infection

1% to 10%:

Cardiovascular: Tachycardia (10%)

Endocrine & metabolic: Dehydration (serious >3%)

Hematologic: Neutropenic fever (serious >3%)

Neuromuscular & skeletal: Weakness (10%)

Respiratory: Upper respiratory infection (10%)

Miscellaneous: Sepsis (serious >3%)

<1% (Limited to important or life-threatening): Bowel obstruction, cardiopulmonary arrest, lymphopenia, odynophagia, pancytopenia, skin exfoliation, skin ulceration, toxic epidermal necrolysis (TEN), tumor lysis syndrome (TLS)

Drug Interactions

Metabolism/Transport Effects Substrate of BCRP

Avoid Concomitant Use

Avoid concomitant use of PRALAtrexate with any of the following: BCG; Natalizumab; Pimecrolimus; Tacrolimus (Topical); Tofacitinib; Vaccines (Live)

Increased Effect/Toxicity

PRALAtrexate may increase the levels/effects of: Leflunomide; Natalizumab; Tofacitinib; Vaccines (Live); Vitamin K Antagonists

The levels/effects of PRALAtrexate may be increased by: Denosumab; Nonsteroidal Anti-Inflammatory Agents; Pimecrolimus; Probenecid; Roflumilast; Salicylates; Sulfamethoxazole; Tacrolimus (Topical); Trastuzumab; Trimethoprim

Decreased Effect

PRALAtrexate may decrease the levels/effects of: BCG; Cardiac Glycosides; Coccidioidin Skin Test; Sapropterin; Sipuleucel-T; Vaccines (Inactivated); Vaccines (Live); Vitamin K Antagonists

The levels/effects of PRALAtrexate may be decreased by: Echinacea

Preparation for Administration Hazardous agent; use appropriate precautions for handling and disposal (NIOSH, 2012). Withdraw into syringe for administration; do not dilute (manufacturer recommends immediate use after placing in syringe). Discard unused portion in the vial.

Storage/Stability Store intact vials refrigerated at 2°C to 8°C (36°F to 46°F). Store in original carton to protect from light until use. Unopened vials (stored in the original carton) are stable for up to 72 hours at room temperature (discard after 72 hours).

Mechanism of Action Antifolate analog; inhibits DNA, RNA, and protein synthesis by selectively entering cells expressing reduced folate carrier (RFC-1), is polyglutamylated by folylpolyglutamate synthetase (FPGS) and then competes for the DHFR-folate binding site to inhibit dihydrofolate reductase (DHFR)

Pharmacodynamics/Kinetics

Distribution: *S*-diastereomer: 105 L; *R*-diastereomer: 37 L

Protein binding: ~67%

Half-life elimination: 12-18 hours

Excretion: Urine (~34% as unchanged drug)

Dosage Note: Initite vitamin supplements before initial pralatrexate dose: Folic acid 1-1.25 mg/day orally beginning 10 days prior to initial pralatrexate dose; continue during treatment and for 30 days after last pralatrexate dose; vitamin B_{12} 1000 mcg I.M. within 10 weeks prior to initial pralatrexate dose and every 8-10 weeks thereafter (after initial dose, B_{12} may be administered on the same day as pralatrexate).

Prior to administering any dose, mucositis should be ≤grade 1 and absolute neutrophil count (ANC) should be ≥1000/mm^3; platelets should be ≥100,000/mm^3 for the first dose and ≥50,000/mm^3 for subsequent doses

I.V.: Adults:

Peripheral T-cell lymphoma (PTCL), relapsed or refractory: 30 mg/m^2 once weekly for 6 weeks of a 7-week treatment cycle; continue until disease progression or unacceptable toxicity (O'Connor, 2011)

Cutaneous T-cell lymphoma, relapsed or refractory (unlabeled use): 15 mg/m^2 once weekly for 3 weeks of a 4-week treatment cycle (Horwitz, 2012)

Dosage adjustment for toxicity: Severe or intolerable adverse events may require dose omission, reduction or interruption. Do not make up omitted doses at the end of a cycle; do not re-escalate dose after a reduction due to toxicity.

Hematologic toxicity:

Platelets:

<50,000/mm^3 (for 1-week duration): Omit dose; continue at previous dose if platelets recover within 1 week

<50,000/mm^3 (for 2-week duration): Omit dose; decrease to 20 mg/m^2 if platelets recover within 2 weeks

<50,000/mm^3 (for 3-week duration): Discontinue treatment

ANC:

500-1000/mm^3 without fever (for 1-week duration): Omit dose; continue at previous dose if ANC recovers within 1 week

500-1000/mm^3 with fever **or** ANC <500/mm^3 (for 1-week duration): Omit dose, give filgrastim or sargramostim support; continue at previous dose (with growth factor support) if ANC recovers within 1 week

500-1000/mm^3 with fever **or** ANC <500/mm^3 (recurrent or for 2-week duration): Omit dose and give filgrastim or sargramostim support; decrease to 20 mg/m^2 (with growth factor support) if ANC recovers within 2 weeks

500-1000/mm^3 with fever **or** ANC <500/mm^3 (second recurrence or for 3-week duration): Discontinue treatment

Nonhematologic toxicity: Mucositis (on day of treatment):

Grade 2: Omit dose; continue at previous dose when recovers to ≤grade 1

Grade 3 or recurrent grade 2: Omit dose and decrease to 20 mg/m^2 when recovers to ≤grade 1

Grade 4: Discontinue treatment

Nonhematologic toxicity (other than mucositis):

Grade 3: Omit dose; decrease to 20 mg/m^2 when recovers to ≤grade 2

Grade 4: Discontinue treatment

Dosage adjustment in renal impairment:

Moderate-to-severe renal impairment: Exposure and toxicities may be increased; monitor for toxicities and adjust dose accordingly.

End-stage renal disease (ESRD), including dialysis-dependent: Avoid use (unless the potential benefit outweighs risks).

Dosage adjustment in hepatic impairment: Patients with total bilirubin >1.5 mg/dL, AST or ALT >2.5 times the upper limit of normal (ULN), or ALT or AST >5 times ULN if documented hepatic lymphoma involvement were excluded from clinical trials. Persistent abnormalities may indicate hepatotoxicity requiring dosage modification:

Grade 3 (AST or ALT >5-20 times ULN or bilirubin >3-10 times ULN): Omit dose; decrease to 20 mg/m^2 when recovers to ≤grade 2

Grade 4 (AST or ALT >20 times ULN or bilirubin >10 times ULN): Discontinue treatment.

Dosing in obesity: *ASCO Guidelines for appropriate chemotherapy dosing in obese adults with cancer:* Utilize patient's actual body weight (full weight) for calculation of body surface area- or weight-based dosing, particularly when the intent of therapy is curative; manage regimen-related toxicities in the same manner as for nonobese patients; if a dose reduction is utilized due to toxicity, consider resumption of full weight-based dosing with subsequent cycles, especially if cause of toxicity (eg, hepatic or renal impairment) is resolved (Griggs, 2012).

Administration Administer I.V. push (undiluted) over 3-5 minutes into the line of a free-flowing normal saline I.V.

Hazardous agent; use appropriate precautions for handling and disposal (NIOSH, 2012).

Monitoring Parameters CBC with differential (baseline and weekly), serum chemistries, including renal and liver function tests (prior to the first and fourth doses in each cycle); mucositis severity (baseline and weekly); monitor for signs of tumor lysis syndrome

Dosage Forms Excipient information presented when available (limited, particularly for generics); consult specific product labeling.

Solution, Intravenous [preservative free]:

Folotyn: 20 mg/mL (1 mL); 40 mg/2 mL (2 mL)

Pralidoxime (pra li DOKS eem)

Brand Names: U.S. Protopam Chloride

Index Terms 2-PAM; 2-Pyridine Aldoxime Methochloride; 2PAM; Pralidoxime Chloride

Pharmacologic Category Antidote

Use Treatment of muscle weakness and/or respiratory depression secondary to poisoning due to organophosphate anticholinesterase pesticides and chemicals (eg, nerve agents); control of overdose of anticholinesterase medications used to treat myasthenia gravis (ambenonium, neostigmine, pyridostigmine)

Pregnancy Risk Factor C

Pregnancy Considerations Animal reproduction studies have not been conducted. A case report did not show evidence of adverse events after pralidoxime administration during the second trimester (Kamha, 2005). In general, medications used as antidotes should take into consideration the health and prognosis of the mother; antidotes should be administered to pregnant women if there is a clear indication for use and should not be withheld because of fears of teratogenicity (Bailey, 2003).

Breast-Feeding Considerations It is not known if pralidoxime is excreted in breast milk. The manufacturer recommends that caution be exercised when administering pralidoxime to nursing women.

Contraindications There are no absolute contraindications listed within the manufacturer's labeling. **Note:** According to the manufacturer, relative contraindications include hypersensitivity to pralidoxime or any component of the formulation and other situations where the risk of administration clearly outweighs possible benefit.

Warnings/Precautions Pralidoxime is not indicated for the treatment of poisoning due to phosphorus, inorganic phosphates, organophosphates without anticholinesterase activity, or carbamate pesticides (acetylcholinesterase is weakly, but not permanently, affected by carbamates). Use with caution in patients with myasthenia gravis (may precipitate a myasthenic crisis); dosage modification required in patients with impaired renal function. Clinical symptoms that are consistent with suspected organophosphate poisoning (eg, organophosphate anticholinesterase pesticides and nerve agents) should be treated with the antidote immediately; administration should not be delayed for confirmatory laboratory tests. Treatment should include proper evacuation and decontamination procedures as indicated; medical personnel should protect themselves from inadvertent contamination. Antidote administration is intended only for initial management; definitive and more intensive medical care is required following administration. Individuals should not rely solely on antidote for treatment; the concomitant use of atropine will be necessary and other supportive measures (eg, artificial respiration) may still be required.

Adverse Reactions Frequency not defined.

Cardiovascular: Cardiac arrest, hypertension, tachycardia

Central nervous system: Dizziness, drowsiness, headache, paralysis, seizure

Dermatologic: Skin rash

Gastrointestinal: Nausea

Hepatic: Increased serum ALT (transient), increased serum AST (transient)

Local: Pain at injection site (I.M.)

Neuromuscular & skeletal: Fasciculations, increased creatine phosphokinase, laryngospasm, muscle rigidity, weakness

Ophthalmic: Accommodation disturbance, blurred vision, diplopia

Renal: Renal insufficiency

Respiratory: Apnea, hyperventilation

Drug Interactions

Metabolism/Transport Effects None known.

Avoid Concomitant Use There are no known interactions where it is recommended to avoid concomitant use.

Increased Effect/Toxicity There are no known significant interactions involving an increase in effect.

Decreased Effect There are no known significant interactions involving a decrease in effect.

Preparation for Administration Powder for solution:

I.V. administration: Dilute 1000 mg with 20 mL SWFI to make a concentration of 50 mg/mL; this concentration may be administered in fluid-restricted patients or in situations where a more rapid administration is required. For administration in all other patients, the reconstituted solution should be further diluted with NS to a final concentration of 10-20 mg/mL. Discard any unused portion of vial.

I.M. administration: Dilute 1000 mg with 3.3 mL SWFI to a final concentration of ~300 mg/mL; discard any unused portion of vial.

Storage/Stability Store at 20°C to 25°C (68°F to 77°F); excursions permitted to 15°C to 30°C (59°F to 86°F).

Mechanism of Action Reactivates cholinesterase that had been inactivated by phosphorylation due to exposure to organophosphate pesticides and cholinesterase-inhibiting nerve agents (eg, terrorism and chemical warfare agents such as sarin) by displacing the enzyme from its receptor sites; removes the phosphoryl group from the active site of the inactivated enzyme

Pharmacodynamics/Kinetics

Distribution: V_{dss}: 0.6-2.7 L/kg; may increase with increasing severity of organophosphate intoxication (~9 L/kg in a severely poisoned pediatric patients; Schexnayder, 1998)

Protein binding: None

Metabolism: Hepatic

Half-life elimination: Apparent: 74-77 minutes; Poisoned patients (I.M., I.V.): 3-4 hours

Time to peak, serum: I.V.: 5-15 minutes; I.M.: ~35 minutes

Excretion: Urine (as metabolites and unchanged drug)

Dosage

I.V.:

Anticholinesterase overdose (eg, neostigmine, pyridostigmine): Adults: 1000-2000 mg; followed by increments of 250 mg every 5 minutes as needed

Organophosphate poisoning: **Note:** Use in conjunction with atropine; a response to atropine should be established before pralidoxime is administered. I.M. or SubQ administration should be considered when I.V. administration is not feasible:

Children and Adolescents ≤16 years: Loading dose: 20-50 mg/kg (maximum: 2000 mg/dose); Maintenance infusion: 10-20 mg/kg/hour; alternatively, a repeat bolus of 20-50 mg/kg (maximum: 2000 mg/dose) may be administered after 1 hour and repeated every 10-12 hours thereafter, as needed

Adolescents >16 years and Adults: Loading dose: 1000-2000 mg; Maintenance: Repeat bolus of 1000-2000 mg after 1 hour and repeated every 10-12 hours thereafter, as needed. Alternatively, administer a loading dose of 30 mg/kg followed by a maintenance infusion of 8 mg/kg/hour (unlabeled dose; Roberts, 2007).

I.M.: Organophosphate poisoning: **Note:** Use in conjunction with atropine; a response to atropine should be established before pralidoxime is administered. I.M. or SubQ administration should be considered when I.V. administration is not feasible:

Children <40 kg:

Mild symptoms: 15 mg/kg; repeat as needed for persistent mild symptoms every 15 minutes to a maximum total dose of 45 mg/kg; may administer doses in rapid succession if severe symptoms develop

Severe symptoms: 15 mg/kg; repeat twice in rapid succession to deliver a total dose of 45 mg/kg

Persistent symptoms: May repeat the entire series (45 mg/kg) beginning ~1 hour after administration of the last injection

Children ≥40 kg, Adolescents, and Adults:

Mild symptoms: 600 mg; repeat as needed for persistent mild symptoms every 15 minutes to a maximum total dose of 1800 mg; may administer doses in rapid succession if severe symptoms develop

Severe symptoms: 600 mg; repeat twice in rapid succession to deliver a total dose of 1800 mg

Persistent symptoms: May repeat the entire series (1800 mg) beginning ~1 hour after administration of the last injection

Elderly: Refer to adult dosing.

Dosing adjustment in renal impairment: No specific dosage adjustment provided in manufacturer's labeling; however, because pralidoxime is excreted in the urine, dosage reduction is recommended in patients with renal impairment.

Dosage adjustment in hepatic impairment: No dosage adjustment provided in the manufacturer's labeling; undergoes hepatic metabolism.

Administration

I.V.:

Loading dose: Infuse as a 10-20 mg/mL solution over 15-30 minutes. Alternatively, if this is not practical or if pulmonary edema is present and/or fluid restriction is necessary, may administer as a 50 mg/mL solution by slow I.V. injection over ≥5 minutes.

Maintenance dose: Administer as a continuous or intermittent infusion at a rate not to exceed 200 mg/minute.

I.M., SubQ: May administer I.M. or SubQ if I.V. administration is not feasible. For pediatric patients, I.M. injection should be into the anterolateral aspect of the thigh. If using the auto-injector (solution for I.M. injection), remove gray safety cap and place black end against outer thigh. Push hard until injector administers, hold in place for 10 seconds, then remove and massage area of injection. Auto-injector is intended for use by military personnel for self or buddy administration; may also be administered by qualified civilian emergency responders who have received adequate training on the recognition and treatment of nerve agent intoxication.

Monitoring Parameters Heart rate, respiratory rate, muscle fasciculations and strength, pulse oximetry; cardiac monitor and blood pressure monitor required for I.V. administration

Dosage Forms Excipient information presented when available (limited, particularly for generics); consult specific product labeling.

Device, Intramuscular, as chloride:

Generic: 600 mg/2 mL (2 mL)

Solution Reconstituted, Intravenous, as chloride:

Protopam Chloride: 1 g (1 ea)

◆ **Pralidoxime and Atropine** *see* Atropine and Pralidoxime *on page 200*

◆ **Pralidoxime Chloride** *see* Pralidoxime *on page 1694*

◆ **PramCort** *see* Pramoxine and Hydrocortisone *on page 1699*

Pramipexole (pra mi PEKS ole)

Brand Names: U.S. Mirapex; Mirapex ER

Brand Names: Canada Apo-Pramipexole®; Ava-Pramipexole; CO Pramipexole; Mirapex®; PMS-Pramipexole; Sandoz-Pramipexole; Teva-Pramipexole

Index Terms Pramipexole Dihydrochloride Monohydrate

Pharmacologic Category Anti-Parkinson's Agent, Dopamine Agonist

Additional Appendix Information

Antiparkinsonian Agents *on page 2289*

Use

Immediate release: Treatment of the signs and symptoms of idiopathic Parkinson's disease; treatment of moderate-to-severe primary Restless Legs Syndrome (RLS)

Extended release: Treatment of the signs and symptoms of idiopathic Parkinson's disease

Unlabeled Use Treatment of depression in bipolar disorder; treatment of fibromyalgia

Pregnancy Risk Factor C

Pregnancy Considerations Adverse events were observed in animal reproduction studies. Information related to the use of pramipexole for the treatment of Parkinson's disease (Benbir, 2013; Mucchiut 2004) or restless legs syndrome (RLS) (Dostal, 2013) in pregnant women is limited. Current guidelines note that the available information is insufficient to make a recommendation for the treatment of RLS in pregnant women (Aurora, 2012).

Breast-Feeding Considerations It is not known if pramipexole is excreted into breast milk; however, pramipexole inhibits prolactin secretion in humans and may potentially inhibit lactation. Due to the potential for serious adverse reactions in the nursing infant, the manufacturer recommends a decision be made whether to discontinue nursing or to discontinue the drug, taking into account the importance of treatment to the mother.

Contraindications There are no contraindications listed in the manufacturer's labeling.

Warnings/Precautions Caution should be taken in patients with renal insufficiency; dose adjustment may be necessary. May cause or exacerbate dyskinesias; use caution in patients with pre-existing dyskinesias. May cause orthostatic hypotension; Parkinson's disease patients appear to have an impaired capacity to respond to a postural challenge. Use with caution in patients at risk of hypotension or where transient hypotensive episodes would be poorly tolerated. Parkinson's patients being treated with dopaminergic agonists ordinarily require careful monitoring for signs and symptoms of postural hypotension, especially during dose escalation. May cause hallucinations.

Dopamine agonists have been associated with compulsive behaviors and/or loss of impulse control, which has manifested as pathological gambling, libido increases (hypersexuality), and/or binge eating. Causality has not been established, and controversy exists as to whether this phenomenon is related to the underlying disease, prior behaviors/addictions and/or drug therapy. Dose reduction or discontinuation of therapy has been reported to reverse these behaviors in some, but not all cases. Risk for melanoma development is increased in Parkinson's disease patients; drug causation or factors contributing to risk ▶

have not been established. Patients should be monitored closely and periodic skin examinations should be performed.

Taper gradually when discontinuing therapy in Parkinson's disease; dopaminergic agents have been associated with a syndrome resembling neuroleptic malignant syndrome on abrupt withdrawal or significant dosage reduction after long-term use. Ergot-derived dopamine agonists have been associated with fibrotic complications (eg, retroperitoneal fibrosis, pleural thickening, and pulmonary infiltrates). Although pramipexole is not an ergot, there have been postmarketing reports of possible fibrotic complications (peritoneal, pleural, pulmonary) with pramipexole; monitor closely for signs and symptoms of fibrosis.

Pramipexole has been associated with somnolence, particularly at higher dosages (>1.5 mg/day). In addition, patients have been reported to fall asleep during activities of daily living, including driving, while taking this medication. Whether these patients exhibited somnolence prior to these events is not clear. Patients should be advised of this issue and factors which may increase risk (sleep disorders, other sedating medications, or concomitant medications which increase pramipexole concentrations) and instructed to report daytime somnolence or sleepiness to the prescriber. Patients should use caution in performing activities which require alertness (driving or operating machinery), and to avoid other medications which may cause CNS depression, including ethanol. Use caution in the elderly as they may be more sensitive to these adverse drug reactions.

Pathologic degenerative changes were observed in the retinas of albino rats during studies with this agent, but were not observed in the retinas of albino mice or in other species. The significance of these data for humans remains uncertain. Augmentation (earlier onset of symptoms in the evening/afternoon, increase and/or spread of symptoms to other extremities) or rebound (shifting of symptoms to early morning hours) may occur in some RLS patients.

Adverse Reactions

Parkinson's disease: Actual frequency may be dependent on dose and/or formulation:

>10%:

Cardiovascular: Orthostatic hypotension (dose related; ≤53%)

Central nervous system: Somnolence (dose related; 9% to 36%), extrapyramidal syndrome (28%), insomnia (4% to 27%), dizziness (2% to 26%), hallucinations (5% to 17%), abnormal dreams (11%), headache (4% to 7%)

Gastrointestinal: Nausea (dose related; 11% to 28%), constipation (dose related; 6% to 14%)

Neuromuscular & skeletal: Dyskinesia (17% to 47%), weakness (1% to 14%)

Miscellaneous: Accidental injury (17%)

1% to 10%:

Cardiovascular: Edema (2% to 8%), chest pain (3%)

Central nervous system: Confusion (4% to 10%), dystonia (2% to 8%), fatigue (6%), amnesia (dose related; 4% to 6%), sudden onset of sleep (3% to 6%), vertigo (2% to 4%), hypesthesia (3%), abnormal thinking (2% to 3%), akathisia (2% to 3%), malaise (2% to 3%), paranoia (2%), sleep disorder (1% to 3%), depression (≤2%), delusions (1%), fever (1%), myoclonus (1%)

Endocrine & metabolic: Libido decreased (1%)

Gastrointestinal: Xerostomia (4% to 7%), anorexia (1% to 5%), vomiting (4%), abdominal discomfort/pain (1% to 4%), dyspepsia (3%), appetite increased (2% to 3%), dysphagia (2%), weight loss (2%), salivary hypersecretion (≤2%), diarrhea (1% to 2%)

Genitourinary: Urinary frequency (6%), urinary tract infection (4%), impotence (2%), urinary incontinence (2%)

Neuromuscular & skeletal: Gait abnormalities (7%), hypertonia (7%), muscle spasm (3% to 5%), falls (4%), arthritis (3%), tremor (3%), back pain (2% to 3%), bursitis (2%), muscle twitching (2%), balance abnormalities (≤2%), CPK increased (1%), myasthenia (1%)

Ocular: Accommodation abnormalities (4%), vision abnormalities (3%), diplopia (1%)

Respiratory: Dyspnea (4%), cough (3%), rhinitis (3%), pneumonia (2%)

Postmarketing and/or case reports (Limited to important or life-threatening): Blackouts, heart failure, impulsive/compulsive behaviors (eg, binge eating, hypersexuality, pathological gambling, shopping), libido increased, pruritus, rhabdomyolysis, SIADH, syncope

Restless legs syndrome: Actual frequency may be dependent on dose:

>10%:

Central nervous system: Headache (16%), insomnia (9% to 13%)

Gastrointestinal: Nausea (11% to 27%)

1% to 10%:

Central nervous system: Fatigue (3% to 9%), abnormal dreams (1% to 8%), somnolence (6%)

Gastrointestinal: Diarrhea (1% to 7%), constipation (4%), xerostomia (3%)

Neuromuscular & skeletal: Limb pain (3% to 7%)

Respiratory: Nasal congestion (≤6%)

Miscellaneous: Influenza (1% to 7%)

Postmarketing and/or case reports (Limited to important or life-threatening): Augmentation (~20% but similar to placebo), blackouts, hallucinations, hypotension, impulsive/compulsive behaviors (eg, binge eating, hypersexuality, pathological gambling, shopping), libido changes, pruritus, rebound, tolerance, syncope

Drug Interactions

Metabolism/Transport Effects None known.

Avoid Concomitant Use

Avoid concomitant use of Pramipexole with any of the following: Amisulpride; Sulpiride

Increased Effect/Toxicity

The levels/effects of Pramipexole may be increased by: Alcohol (Ethyl); Cimetidine; CNS Depressants; MAO Inhibitors; Methylphenidate

Decreased Effect

Pramipexole may decrease the levels/effects of: Amisulpride; Antipsychotics (Typical); Sulpiride

The levels/effects of Pramipexole may be decreased by: Amisulpride; Antipsychotics (Atypical); Antipsychotics (Typical); Metoclopramide; Sulpiride

Ethanol/Nutrition/Herb Interactions

Ethanol: May increase CNS depression; monitor for increased effects with coadministration. Caution patients about effects.

Food: Food intake does not affect the extent of drug absorption although the time to maximal plasma concentration is delayed when taken with a meal.

Herb/Nutraceutical: Avoid valerian, St John's wort, SAMe, kava kava (may increase risk of serotonin syndrome and/or excessive sedation).

Storage/Stability Store at 25°C (77°F); excursions permitted to 15°C to 30°C (59°F to 86°F). Protect from light and high humidity.

Mechanism of Action Pramipexole is a nonergot dopamine agonist with specificity for the D_2 subfamily dopamine receptor, and has also been shown to bind to D_3 and D_4 receptors. By binding to these receptors, it is thought that pramipexole can stimulate dopamine activity on the nerves of the striatum and substantia nigra.

Pharmacodynamics/Kinetics

Absorption: Rapid

Distribution: V_d: 500 L

Protein binding: ~15%
Metabolism: Negligible (<10%)
Bioavailability: Immediate release: >90%; Extended release (as compared to immediate release): 100%
Half-life elimination: 8.5 hours; Elderly: 12 hours
Time to peak, serum: Immediate release: ~2 hours; Extended release: 6 hours
Excretion: Urine (90% as unchanged drug)

Dosage Oral: Adults: **Note:** Retitration of dose should be considered for any significant interruption in therapy.

Immediate release formulation:

Parkinson's disease: Initial: 0.125 mg 3 times daily, increase gradually every 5-7 days; maintenance (usual): 0.5-1.5 mg 3 times daily

Discontinuation of therapy: Reduce dose by 0.75 mg daily until daily dose is equivalent to 0.75 mg once daily, then reduce by 0.375 mg daily thereafter

Restless legs syndrome: Initial: 0.125 mg once daily 2-3 hours before bedtime. Dose may be doubled every 4-7 days up to 0.5 mg once daily. Maximum: 0.5 mg once daily (manufacturer's recommendation).

Discontinuation of therapy: No gradual dose reduction recommended in manufacturer's labeling; however, worsening of symptoms may occur with abrupt discontinuation.

Note: Most patients require <0.5 mg daily, but higher doses have been used (2 mg daily). If augmentation occurs, dose earlier in the day.

Depression (unlabeled use): Initial: 0.25-0.375 mg daily given in 2-3 divided doses with a gradual titration; mean dose: 1.6-1.7 mg daily (Aiken, 2007; Goldberg, 2004)

Fibromyalgia (unlabeled use): Initial: 0.25 mg once daily at bedtime; may be increased weekly by 0.25 mg/day increments up to 4.5 mg daily (Holman, 2005)

Extended release formulation: Parkinson's disease: Initial: 0.375 mg once daily; increase gradually to 0.75 mg once daily. If necessary, may increase by 0.75 mg per dose not more frequently than every 5-7 days; maximum recommended dose 4.5 mg once daily.

Discontinuation of therapy: Taper gradually over a period of 1 week

Converting from immediate release to extended release: May initiate extended release preparation the morning after the last immediate release evening tablet is taken. The total daily dose should remain the same.

Dosage adjustment in renal impairment:

Parkinson's disease: Immediate release formulation:

Cl_{cr} >50 mL/minute: No dosage adjustment necessary.

Cl_{cr} 30-50 mL/minute: Initial: 0.125 mg twice daily (maximum: 0.75 mg 3 times daily)

Cl_{cr} 15-29 mL/minute: 0.125 mg once daily (maximum: 1.5 mg once daily)

Cl_{cr} <15 mL/minute: No dosage adjustment provided in manufacturer's labeling (has not been studied); use not recommended.

ESRD requiring hemodialysis: No dosage adjustment provided in manufacturer's labeling (has not been studied); use not recommended; a negligible amount of pramipexole is removed by dialysis.

Parkinson's disease: Extended release formulation:

Cl_{cr} >50 mL/minute: No dosage adjustment necessary.

Cl_{cr} 30-50 mL/minute: Initial: 0.375 mg every other day; may increase to 0.375 mg once daily no sooner than 1 week after initiation. If necessary, may increase by 0.375 mg per dose not more frequently than every 7 days; maximum recommended dose: 2.25 mg once daily

Cl_{cr} <30 mL/minute: No dosage adjustment provided in manufacturer's labeling (has not been studied); use not recommended.

ESRD requiring hemodialysis: No dosage adjustment provided in manufacturer's labeling (has not been studied); use not recommended; a negligible amount of pramipexole is removed by dialysis.

Restless legs syndrome: Immediate release formulation:

Cl_{cr} >60 mL/minute: No dosage adjustment necessary.

Cl_{cr} 20-60 mL/minute: No dosage adjustment necessary; however, duration between titration should be increased to 14 days.

Cl_{cr} <20 mL/minute: No dosage adjustment provided in manufacturer's labeling (has not been studied).

Dosage adjustment in hepatic impairment: Immediate release and extended release: No dosage adjustment provided in manufacturer's labeling (has not been studied); however, no adjustment expected since undergoes minimal hepatic metabolism.

Dietary Considerations May be taken with or without food. May be taken with food to decrease nausea.

Administration Doses should be titrated gradually in all patients to avoid the onset of intolerable side effects. The dosage should be increased to achieve a maximum therapeutic effect, balanced against the side effects of dyskinesia, hallucinations, somnolence, and dry mouth. May be administered with or without food; may be administered with food to decrease nausea. Extended release tablets should be swallowed whole and not chewed, crushed, or divided.

Monitoring Parameters Blood pressure, heart rate; body weight changes; CNS depression, fall risk, skin changes, behavior changes (eg, compulsive behaviors)

Dosage Forms Excipient information presented when available (limited, particularly for generics); consult specific product labeling.

Tablet, Oral, as dihydrochloride monohydrate:
- Mirapex: 0.125 mg
- Mirapex: 0.25 mg, 0.5 mg [scored]
- Mirapex: 0.75 mg
- Mirapex: 1 mg, 1.5 mg [scored]
- Generic: 0.125 mg, 0.25 mg, 0.5 mg, 0.75 mg, 1 mg, 1.5 mg

Tablet Extended Release 24 Hour, Oral, as dihydrochloride monohydrate:
- Mirapex ER: 0.375 mg, 0.75 mg, 1.5 mg, 2.25 mg, 3 mg, 3.75 mg, 4.5 mg

◆ **Pramipexole Dihydrochloride Monohydrate** *see* Pramipexole *on page 1695*

Pramlintide (PRAM lin tide)

Brand Names: U.S. SymlinPen 120; SymlinPen 60

Index Terms Pramlintide Acetate

Pharmacologic Category Amylinomimetic; Antidiabetic Agent

Additional Appendix Information

Injectable Agents (Non-Insulin) for Type 2 Diabetes *on page 2302*

Use

Adjunctive treatment with mealtime insulin in type 1 diabetes mellitus (insulin dependent, IDDM) patients who have failed to achieve desired glucose control despite optimal insulin therapy

Adjunctive treatment with mealtime insulin in type 2 diabetes mellitus (noninsulin dependent, NIDDM) patients who have failed to achieve desired glucose control despite optimal insulin therapy, with or without concurrent sulfonylurea and/or metformin

Pregnancy Risk Factor C

Pregnancy Considerations Adverse events have been observed in animal reproduction studies. Based on *in vitro* data, pramlintide has a low potential to cross the placenta. Maternal hyperglycemia can be associated with adverse effects in the fetus, including macrosomia, neonatal hyperglycemia, and hyperbilirubinemia; the risk of congenital malformations is increased when the Hb A_{1c} is above the normal range. Diabetes can also be associated with adverse effects in the mother. Poorly-treated diabetes may cause end-organ damage that may in turn negatively affect obstetric outcomes. Physiologic glucose levels should be maintained prior to and during pregnancy to decrease the risk of adverse events in the mother and the fetus. Until additional safety and efficacy data are obtained, the use of pramlintide is generally not recommended in the routine management of diabetes mellitus during pregnancy. Insulin is the drug of choice for the control of diabetes mellitus during pregnancy.

Breast-Feeding Considerations It is not known if pramlintide is present in breast milk. The manufacturer recommends that pramlintide be used in nursing women only when the potential benefit to the mother outweighs the possible risk to the infant.

Medication Guide Available Yes

Contraindications Hypersensitivity to pramlintide or any component of the formulation; confirmed diagnosis of gastroparesis; hypoglycemia unawareness

Warnings/Precautions [U.S. Boxed Warning]: Coadministration with insulin may induce severe hypoglycemia (usually within 3 hours following administration); coadministration with insulin therapy is an approved indication but does require an initial dosage reduction of insulin and frequent pre and post blood glucose monitoring to reduce risk of severe hypoglycemia. Concurrent use of other glucose-lowering agents may increase risk of hypoglycemia. Avoid use in patients with poor compliance with their insulin regimen and/or blood glucose monitoring. Do not use in patients with Hb A_{1c} levels >9% or recent, recurrent episodes of hypoglycemia; obtain detailed history of glucose control (eg, Hb A_{1c}, incidence of hypoglycemia, glucose monitoring, and medication compliance) and body weight before initiating therapy. Use caution in patients with visual or dexterity impairment. Use caution when driving or operating heavy machinery until effects on blood sugar are known. Use caution with certain antihypertensive agents (eg, beta-adrenergic blockers) which may mask signs/symptoms of hypoglycemia. Avoid use in patients with conditions or concurrent medications likely to impair gastric motility (eg, anticholinergics); do not use in patients requiring medication(s) to stimulate gastric emptying. According to the Centers for Disease Control and Prevention (CDC), pen-shaped injection devices should never be used for more than one person (even when the needle is changed) because of the risk of infection. The injection device should be clearly labeled with individual patient information to ensure that the correct pen is used (CDC, 2012).

Adverse Reactions

>10%:

Central nervous system: Headache (5% to 13%)

Gastrointestinal: Nausea (28% to 48%), vomiting (7% to 11%), anorexia (≤17%)

Endocrine & metabolic: Severe hypoglycemia (type 1 diabetes ≤17%)

Miscellaneous: Inflicted injury (8% to 14%)

1% to 10%:

Central nervous system: Fatigue (3% to 7%), dizziness (2% to 6%)

Endocrine & metabolic: Severe hypoglycemia (type 2 diabetes ≤8%)

Gastrointestinal: Abdominal pain (2% to 8%)

Respiratory: Pharyngitis (3% to 5%), cough (2% to 6%)

Neuromuscular & skeletal: Arthralgia (2% to 7%)

Miscellaneous: Allergic reaction (≤6%)

Postmarketing and/or case reports: Injection site reactions

Drug Interactions

Metabolism/Transport Effects None known.

Avoid Concomitant Use There are no known interactions where it is recommended to avoid concomitant use.

Increased Effect/Toxicity

Pramlintide may increase the levels/effects of: Anticholinergics

Decreased Effect There are no known significant interactions involving a decrease in effect.

Ethanol/Nutrition/Herb Interactions

Ethanol: Use caution with ethanol (may increase hypoglycemia).

Herb/Nutraceutical: Use caution with garlic, chromium, gymnema (may increase hypoglycemia).

Storage/Stability Store at 2°C to 8°C (36°F to 46°F); do not freeze. After initial use, may be kept refrigerated or at room temperature ≤30°C (≤86°F); discard after 30 days. Protect from light.

Mechanism of Action Synthetic analog of human amylin cosecreted with insulin by pancreatic beta cells; reduces postprandial glucose increases via the following mechanisms: 1) prolongation of gastric emptying time, 2) reduction of postprandial glucagon secretion, and 3) reduction of caloric intake through centrally-mediated appetite suppression

Pharmacodynamics/Kinetics

Duration: 3 hours

Protein binding: ~60%

Metabolism: Primarily renal to des-lys[1] pramlintide (active metabolite)

Bioavailability: ~30% to 40%

Half-life elimination: ~48 minutes

Time to peak, plasma: 20 minutes

Excretion: Primarily urine

Dosage SubQ: Adults: **Note:** When initiating pramlintide, reduce current insulin dose (including rapidly- and mixed-acting preparations) by 50% to avoid hypoglycemia. If pramlintide is discontinued for any reason, restart therapy with same initial titration protocol.

Type 1 diabetes mellitus (insulin dependent, IDDM): Initial: 15 mcg immediately prior to meals; titrate in 15 mcg increments every 3 days (if no significant nausea occurs) to target dose of 30-60 mcg (consider discontinuation if intolerant of 30 mcg dose)

Type 2 diabetes mellitus (noninsulin dependent, NIDDM): Initial: 60 mcg immediately prior to meals; after 3-7 days, increase to 120 mcg prior to meals if no significant nausea occurs (if nausea occurs at 120 mcg dose, reduce to 60 mcg)

Dosage adjustment in renal impairment:

Cl_{cr} >20 mL/minute: No dosage adjustment necessary.

Cl_{cr} ≤20 mL/minute: No dosage adjustment provided in manufacturer's labeling (has not been studied).

Dialysis: No dosage adjustment provided in manufacturer's labeling (has not been studied).

Dosage adjustment in hepatic impairment: No dosage adjustment provided in manufacturer's labeling (has not been studied); however, need for adjustment not likely since undergoes minimal hepatic metabolism.

Dietary Considerations Dietary modification based on ADA recommendations is a part of therapy; pramlintide to be administered prior to major meals consisting of ≥250 Kcal or ≥30 g carbohydrates

Administration Do not mix with insulins; administer subcutaneously into abdominal or thigh areas at sites distinct from concomitant insulin injections (do not administer into arm due to variable absorption); rotate injection sites frequently. Allow solution to reach room temperature before administering; may reduce injection site reactions. For oral medications in which a rapid onset of action is desired, administer 1 hour before, or 2 hours after pramlintide, if possible. Do not transfer drug from the pen injector to a syringe; dosing errors could occur.

Monitoring Parameters Prior to initiating therapy: Hb A_{1c}, hypoglycemic history, body weight. During therapy: Pre- and postprandial and bedtime serum glucose, Hb A_{1c}

Reference Range Recommendations for glycemic control in nonpregnant adults with diabetes (ADA, 2013):

Hb A_{1c}: <7% (a more aggressive [<6.5%] or less aggressive [<8%] Hb A_{1c} goal may be targeted based on patient-specific characteristics)

Preprandial capillary plasma glucose: 70-130 mg/dL

Peak postprandial capillary blood glucose: <180 mg/dL

Dosage Forms Excipient information presented when available (limited, particularly for generics); consult specific product labeling.

Solution, Subcutaneous, as acetate:

SymlinPen 60: 1500 mcg/1.5 mL (1.5 mL) [contains metacresol]

SymlinPen 120: 2700 mcg/2.7 mL (2.7 mL) [contains metacresol]

◆ **Pramlintide Acetate** *see* Pramlintide *on page 1697*

◆ **Pramosone®** *see* Pramoxine and Hydrocortisone *on page 1699*

◆ **Pramosone E™** *see* Pramoxine and Hydrocortisone *on page 1699*

◆ **Pramox® HC (Can)** *see* Pramoxine and Hydrocortisone *on page 1699*

Pramoxine and Hydrocortisone

(pra MOKS een & hye droe KOR ti sone)

Brand Names: U.S. Analpram E™; Analpram HC®; Epifoam®; PramCort; Pramosone E™; Pramosone®; ProCort®; ProctoFoam® HC; Zypram™

Brand Names: Canada Pramox® HC; Proctofoam™-HC

Index Terms Hydrocortisone and Pramoxine; Pramoxine Hydrochloride and Hydrocortisone Acetate

Pharmacologic Category Anesthetic/Corticosteroid

Use Relief of inflammatory and pruritic manifestations of corticosteroid-responsive dermatoses

Pregnancy Risk Factor C

Dosage Topical/rectal: Apply to affected areas 3-4 times/day. If clinical improvement is not seen within 2-3 weeks after initiating treatment or if condition worsens, product should be discontinued.

Additional Information Complete prescribing information should be consulted for additional detail.

Dosage Forms Excipient information presented when available (limited, particularly for generics); consult specific product labeling.

Aerosol, foam, rectal:

ProctoFoam® HC: Pramoxine hydrochloride 1% and hydrocortisone acetate 1% (10 g)

Aerosol, foam, topical:

Epifoam®: Pramoxine hydrochloride 1% and hydrocortisone acetate 1% (10 g)

Cream, topical: Pramoxine hydrochloride 1% and hydrocortisone acetate 1% (30 g); pramoxine hydrochloride 1% and hydrocortisone acetate 2.5% (30 g)

Analpram Advanced™ Kit: Pramoxine hydrochloride 1% and hydrocortisone acetate 2.5% (1s) [kit includes Analpram HC® cream (4 g x 30), diosmiplex (Vasculera™) tablets, AloeClean™ wipes, and applicators]

Analpram Advanced™ Kit: Pramoxine hydrochloride 1% and hydrocortisone acetate 2.5% (1s) [kit includes Analpram HC® cream (30 g), diosmiplex (Vasculera™) tablets, AloeClean™ wipes, and applicator]

Analpram E™: Pramoxine hydrochloride 1% and hydrocortisone acetate 2.5% (4 g, 30 g)

Analpram HC®: Pramoxine hydrochloride 1% and hydrocortisone acetate 1% (4 g, 30 g); pramoxine hydrochloride 1% and hydrocortisone acetate 2.5% (4 g, 30 g)

PramCort: Pramoxine hydrochloride 1% and hydrocortisone acetate 1% (30 g) [contains propylene glycol]

Pramosone®: Pramoxine hydrochloride 1% and hydrocortisone acetate 1% (30 g, 60 g); pramoxine hydrochloride 1% and hydrocortisone acetate 2.5% (30 g, 60 g)

Pramosone E™: Pramoxine hydrochloride 1% and hydrocortisone acetate 2.5% (30 g, 60 g)

ProCort®: Pramoxine hydrochloride 1.15% and hydrocortisone acetate 1.85% (60 g)

Zypram™: Pramoxine hydrochloride 1% and hydrocortisone acetate 2.35% (30 g) [contains benzyl alcohol, propylene glycol]

Lotion, topical:

Analpram-HC®: Pramoxine hydrochloride 1% and hydrocortisone acetate 2.5% (60 mL)

Pramosone®: Pramoxine hydrochloride 1% and hydrocortisone acetate 1% (60 mL, 120 mL, 240 mL); pramoxine hydrochloride 1% and hydrocortisone acetate 2.5% (60 mL, 120 mL)

Ointment, topical:

Pramosone®: Pramoxine hydrochloride 1% and hydrocortisone acetate 1% (30 g); pramoxine hydrochloride 1% and hydrocortisone acetate 2.5% (30 g)

◆ **Pramoxine Hydrochloride and Hydrocortisone Acetate** *see* Pramoxine and Hydrocortisone *on page 1699*

◆ **PrandiMet®** *see* Repaglinide and Metformin *on page 1799*

◆ **Prandin** *see* Repaglinide *on page 1797*

◆ **Prascion** *see* Sulfur and Sulfacetamide *on page 1966*

◆ **Prascion FC** *see* Sulfur and Sulfacetamide *on page 1966*

◆ **Prascion RA** *see* Sulfur and Sulfacetamide *on page 1966*

Prasugrel (PRA soo grel)

Brand Names: U.S. Effient

Brand Names: Canada Effient®

Index Terms CS-747; LY-640315; Prasugrel Hydrochloride

Pharmacologic Category Antiplatelet Agent; Antiplatelet Agent, Thienopyridine

Additional Appendix Information

Beers Criteria – Potentially Inappropriate Medications for Geriatrics *on page 2368*

Oral Antiplatelet Comparison Chart *on page 2313*

Use Reduces rate of thrombotic cardiovascular events (including stent thrombosis) in patients who are to be managed with percutaneous coronary intervention (PCI) for unstable angina (UA), non-ST-segment elevation MI (NSTEMI), or ST-elevation MI (STEMI)

Unlabeled Use Initial treatment of UA/NSTEMI in patients undergoing PCI with allergy or major gastrointestinal intolerance to aspirin (**Note:** Dual antiplatelet therapy with another P2Y12 receptor inhibitor is not recommended in this situation [Jneid, 2012].)

Pregnancy Risk Factor B

Medication Guide Available Yes

Dosage Oral:

Adults: Acute coronary syndrome (ACS): Oral:

Percutaneous coronary intervention (PCI) for ACS: Loading dose: 60 mg administered promptly (as soon as coronary anatomy is known or before if risk for bleeding is low and need for CABG considered unlikely) and no later than 1 hour after PCI; Maintenance dose: 10 mg once daily (in combination with aspirin 81-325 mg/day day; 81 mg/day recommended [Levine, 2011]). For patients with STEMI, a loading dose may also be administered if PCI is performed >24 hours after treatment with a fibrin-specific thrombolytic (ie, alteplase, reteplase, tenecteplase) (O'Gara, 2013).

Duration of prasugrel (in combination with aspirin) after stent placement: **Premature interruption of therapy may result in stent thrombosis with subsequent fatal or nonfatal MI.** Those with ACS receiving either stent type (bare metal [BMS] or drug-eluting stent [DES]) or those receiving a DES for a non-ACS indication, prasugrel for at least 12 months is recommended. Those receiving a BMS for a non-ACS indication should be given at least 1 month and ideally up to 12 months; if patient is at increased risk of bleeding, give for a minimum of 2 weeks. A duration >12 months, regardless of indication, may be considered in patients with DES placement (Jneid, 2012; Levine, 2011).

Maintenance dosing in low body weight (ie, <60 kg) individuals: Due to a higher incidence of bleeding in patients weighing <60 kg, a maintenance dose of 5 mg once daily may be considered. In aspirin-treated patients weighing <60 kg (mean: 56.4 ± 3.7 kg) with stable coronary artery disease, the use of prasugrel 5 mg once daily was shown to reduce platelet reactivity to a similar extent as prasugrel 10 mg administered once daily to patients >60 kg (mean: 84.7 ± 14.9 kg); clinical events were not evaluated (Erlinge, 2012). In patients with ACS (medically managed) treated with aspirin, a 5 mg daily maintenance dose (after a 30 mg loading dose) in patients <60 kg did not demonstrate a significant difference in the composite primary end point of death from cardiovascular causes, MI, or stroke compared to patients >60 kg treated with a 10 mg maintenance dose; bleeding risk was not increased (Roe, 2012).

Elderly: Refer to adult dosing. Patients ≥75 years: Use not recommended; may be considered in high-risk situations (eg, patients with diabetes or history of MI)

Dosing adjustment in renal impairment: No dosage adjustment necessary

Dosing adjustment in hepatic impairment: No dosage adjustment necessary for mild-to-moderate hepatic impairment; use in severe hepatic impairment has not been evaluated

Additional Information Complete prescribing information should be consulted for additional detail.

Dosage Forms Excipient information presented when available (limited, particularly for generics); consult specific product labeling.

Tablet, Oral:

Effient: 5 mg, 10 mg

◆ Prasugrel Hydrochloride *see* Prasugrel *on page 1699*

◆ Pravachol *see* Pravastatin *on page 1700*

Pravastatin (prav a STAT in)

Brand Names: U.S. Pravachol

Brand Names: Canada Apo-Pravastatin®; CO Pravastatin; Dom-Pravastatin; JAMP-Pravastatin; Mint-Pravastatin; Mylan-Pravastatin; Novo-Pravastatin; Nu-Pravastatin; PHL-Pravastatin; PMS-Pravastatin; Pravachol; RAN-Pravastatin; ratio-Pravastatin; Riva-Pravastatin; Sandoz-Pravastatin; Teva-Pravastatin; ZYM-Pravastatin

Index Terms Pravastatin Sodium

Pharmacologic Category Antilipemic Agent, HMG-CoA Reductase Inhibitor

Use Use with dietary therapy for the following:

Primary prevention of coronary events: In hypercholesterolemic patients without established coronary heart disease to reduce cardiovascular morbidity (myocardial infarction, coronary revascularization procedures) and mortality.

Secondary prevention of cardiovascular events in patients with established coronary heart disease: To slow the progression of coronary atherosclerosis; to reduce cardiovascular morbidity (myocardial infarction, coronary vascular procedures) and to reduce mortality; to reduce the risk of stroke and transient ischemic attacks

Primary and secondary prevention of atherosclerotic cardiovascular disease (ASCVD) according to the American College of Cardiology/American Heart Association: To reduce the risk of ASCVD in patients with clinical ASCVD (eg, coronary heart disease, stroke/TIA, or peripheral arterial disease presumed to be of atherosclerotic origin) who are greater than 75 years of age or not a candidate for high-intensity statin therapy; in patients without clinical ASCVD if LDL-C is 190 mg/dL or greater and not a candidate for high-intensity statin therapy; in patients without clinical ASCVD who have type 1 or type 2 diabetes and are between 40 and 75 years of age; in patients with an estimated 10-year ASCVD risk 7.5% or greater and who are between 40 and 75 years of age.

Hyperlipidemias: Reduce elevations in total cholesterol, LDL-C, apolipoprotein B, and triglycerides (elevations of 1 or more components are present in Fredrickson type IIa, IIb, III, and IV hyperlipidemias)

Heterozygous familial hypercholesterolemia (HeFH): In pediatric patients, 8-18 years of age, with HeFH having LDL-C ≥190 mg/dL **or** LDL ≥160 mg/dL with positive family history of premature cardiovascular disease (CVD) or 2 or more CVD risk factors in the pediatric patient

Pregnancy Risk Factor X

Pregnancy Considerations Adverse events were observed in some animal reproduction studies. Pravastatin was found to cross the placenta in an *ex vivo* study using term human placentas (Nanovskaya, 2013). There are reports of congenital anomalies following maternal use of HMG-CoA reductase Inhibitors in pregnancy; however, maternal disease, differences in specific agents used, and the low rates of exposure limit the interpretation of the available data (Godfrey, 2012; Lecarpentier, 2012). Cholesterol biosynthesis may be important in fetal development; serum cholesterol and triglycerides increase normally during pregnancy. The discontinuation of lipid lowering medications temporarily during pregnancy is not expected to have significant impact on the long term outcomes of primary hypercholesterolemia treatment.

Use of pravastatin is contraindicated in pregnancy. HMG-CoA reductase Inhibitors should be discontinued prior to pregnancy (ADA, 2013). If treatment of dyslipidemias is needed in pregnant women or in women of reproductive age, other agents are preferred (Berglund, 2012; Stone, 2013). The manufacturer recommends administration to women of childbearing potential only when conception is highly unlikely and patients have been informed of potential hazards.

Breast-Feeding Considerations A small amount of pravastatin is excreted into breast milk. Data is available from eight lactating females administered pravastatin 20 mg twice daily for 2.5 days. After the fifth dose, maximum maternal serum concentrations were ~40 ng/mL (pravastatin) and ~26 ng/mL (metabolite) and maximum milk concentrations were ~3.9 ng/mL (pravastatin) and ~2.1 ng/mL (metabolite). Maximum milk concentrations were detected ~3 hours after the dose (Pan, 1988). Due to the potential for serious adverse reactions in a nursing infant, use while breast-feeding is contraindicated by the manufacturer.

Contraindications Hypersensitivity to pravastatin or any component of the formulation; active liver disease; unexplained persistent elevations of serum transaminases; pregnancy; breast-feeding

Warnings/Precautions Secondary causes of hyperlipidemia should be ruled out prior to therapy. Liver function must be monitored by periodic laboratory assessment. Rhabdomyolysis with acute renal failure has occurred. Risk may be increased with concurrent use of other drugs which may cause rhabdomyolysis (including colchicine, gemfibrozil, fibric acid derivatives, or niacin at doses ≥1 g/day). Discontinue in any patient in which CPK levels are markedly elevated (>10 times ULN) or if myopathy is suspected/diagnosed. Immune-mediated necrotizing myopathy (IMNM), an autoimmune-mediated myopathy, has been reported (rarely) with HMG-CoA reductase inhibitor therapy. IMNM presents as proximal muscle weakness with elevated CPK levels, which persists despite discontinuation of HMG-CoA reductase inhibitor therapy; additionally, muscle biopsy may show necrotizing myopathy with limited inflammation; immunosuppressive therapy (eg, corticosteroids, azathioprine) may be used for treatment. The manufacturer recommends temporary discontinuation for elective major surgery, acute medical or surgical conditions, or in any patient experiencing an acute or serious condition predisposing to renal failure (eg, sepsis, hypotension, trauma, uncontrolled seizures). However, based upon current evidence, HMG-CoA reductase inhibitor therapy should be continued in the perioperative period unless risk outweighs cardioprotective benefit. Use with caution in patients with advanced age, these patients are predisposed to myopathy. Use caution in patients with previous liver disease or heavy ethanol use. If serious hepatotoxicity with clinical symptoms and/or hyperbilirubinemia or jaundice occurs during treatment, interrupt therapy. If an alternate etiology is not identified, do not restart pravastatin. Liver enzyme tests should be obtained at baseline and as clinically indicated; routine periodic monitoring of liver enzymes is not necessary. Increases in Hb A_{1c} and fasting blood glucose have been reported with HMG-CoA reductase inhibitors; however, the benefits of statin therapy far outweigh the risk of dysglycemia. Treatment in patients <8 years of age is not recommended.

Adverse Reactions As reported in short-term trials; safety and tolerability with long-term use were similar to placebo

1% to 10%:

- Cardiovascular: Chest pain (4%)
- Central nervous system: Headache (2% to 6%), fatigue (4%), dizziness (1% to 3%)
- Dermatologic: Rash (4%)
- Gastrointestinal: Nausea/vomiting (7%), diarrhea (6%), heartburn (3%)
- Hepatic: Transaminases increased (>3x normal on two occasions: 1%)
- Neuromuscular & skeletal: Myalgia (2%)
- Respiratory: Cough (3%)
- Miscellaneous: Influenza (2%)

<1% (Limited to important or life-threatening): Allergy, amnesia (reversible), anaphylaxis, angioedema, cholestatic jaundice, cirrhosis, cognitive impairment (reversible), confusion (reversible), cranial nerve dysfunction, dermatomyositis, erythema multiforme, ESR increase, fulminant hepatic necrosis, gynecomastia, hemolytic anemia, hepatitis, hepatoma, lens opacity, libido change, lupus erythematosus-like syndrome, memory disturbance (reversible), memory impairment (reversible), muscle weakness, myopathy, neuropathy, pancreatitis, paresthesia, peripheral nerve palsy, polymyalgia rheumatica, positive ANA, purpura, rhabdomyolysis, Stevens-Johnson syndrome, taste disturbance, tremor, vasculitis, vertigo

Additional class-related events or case reports (not necessarily reported with pravastatin therapy): Angioedema, blood glucose increased, cataracts, depression, diabetes mellitus (new onset), dyspnea, eosinophilia, erectile dysfunction, facial paresis, glycosylated hemoglobin (Hb A_{1c}) increased, hypersensitivity reaction, immune-mediated necrotizing myopathy (IMNM), impaired extraocular muscle movement, impotence, interstitial lung disease, leukopenia, malaise, memory loss, ophthalmoplegia, paresthesia, peripheral neuropathy, photosensitivity, psychic disturbance, skin discoloration, thrombocytopenia, thyroid dysfunction, toxic epidermal necrolysis, transaminases increased, vomiting

Drug Interactions

Metabolism/Transport Effects **Substrate** of CYP3A4 (minor), P-glycoprotein, SLCO1B1; **Note:** Assignment of Major/Minor substrate status based on clinically relevant drug interaction potential; **Inhibits** CYP2C9 (weak), CYP2D6 (weak), CYP3A4 (weak)

Avoid Concomitant Use

Avoid concomitant use of Pravastatin with any of the following: Fusidic Acid (Systemic); Gemfibrozil; Pimozide; Red Yeast Rice

Increased Effect/Toxicity

Pravastatin may increase the levels/effects of: ARIPiprazole; CycloSPORINE (Systemic); DAPTOmycin; Dofetilide; Lomitapide; PARoxetine; PAZOPanib; Pimozide; Trabectedin; Vitamin K Antagonists

The levels/effects of Pravastatin may be increased by: Bezafibrate; Boceprevir; Clarithromycin; Colchicine; CycloSPORINE (Systemic); Darunavir; Eltrombopag; Erythromycin (Systemic); Fenofibrate and Derivatives; Fusidic Acid (Systemic); Gemfibrozil; Itraconazole; Niacin; Niacinamide; P-glycoprotein/ABCB1 Inhibitors; Raltegravir; Red Yeast Rice; Simeprevir; Telaprevir; Telithromycin

Decreased Effect

Pravastatin may decrease the levels/effects of: Lanthanum

The levels/effects of Pravastatin may be decreased by: Antacids; Bile Acid Sequestrants; Efavirenz; Fosphenytoin; Nelfinavir; P-glycoprotein/ABCB1 Inducers; Phenytoin; Rifamycin Derivatives; Saquinavir

Ethanol/Nutrition/Herb Interactions

Ethanol: Consumption of large amounts of ethanol may increase the risk of liver damage with HMG-CoA reductase inhibitors.

Food: Red yeast rice contains an estimated 2.4 mg lovastatin per 600 mg rice.

Herb/Nutraceutical: St John's wort may decrease pravastatin levels.

Storage/Stability Store at 25°C (77°F); excursions permitted to 15°C to 30°C (59°F to 86°F). Protect from moisture and light.

Mechanism of Action Pravastatin is a competitive inhibitor of 3-hydroxy-3-methylglutaryl coenzyme A (HMG-CoA) reductase, which is the rate-limiting enzyme involved in *de novo* cholesterol synthesis.

Pharmacodynamics/Kinetics

Onset of action: Several days

Peak effect: 4 weeks

Absorption: Rapidly absorbed; average absorption 34%

Protein binding: 50%

Metabolism: Hepatic multiple metabolites; primary metabolite is 3α-hydroxy-iso-pravastatin (2.5% to 10% activity of parent drug)

Bioavailability: 17%

Half-life elimination: 77 hours (including all metabolites); pravastatin: ~2-3 hours (Pan, 1990); 3α-hydroxy-iso-pravastatin: ~1.5 hours (Gustavson, 2005)

Time to peak, serum: 1-1.5 hours

Excretion: Feces (70%); urine (≤20%, 8% as unchanged drug)

Dosage Note: Doses should be individualized according to the baseline LDL-cholesterol levels, the recommended goal of therapy, and patient response; adjustments should be made at intervals of 4 weeks or more; doses may need adjusted based on concomitant medications

Heterozygous familial hypercholesterolemia (HeFH): Oral:

Children 8-13 years: 20 mg/day

Adolescents 14-18 years: 40 mg/day

Dosage adjustment for pravastatin with concomitant medications (clarithromycin, cyclosporine): Refer to adult dosing.

Hyperlipidemias, primary prevention of coronary events, secondary prevention of cardiovascular events (also see ACC/AHA Blood Cholesterol Guideline recommendations): Adults: Oral: Initial: 40 mg once daily; titrate dosage to response; usual range: 10-80 mg; (maximum dose: 80 mg once daily)

ACC/AHA Blood Cholesterol Guideline recommendations to reduce the risk of atherosclerotic cardiovascular disease (ASCVD) (Stone, 2013): Adults ≥21 years: Oral:

Primary prevention:

LDL-C ≥190 mg/dL: High intensity therapy necessary; use alternate statin therapy (eg, atorvastatin or rosuvastatin)

Type 1 or 2 diabetes and age 40-75 years: Moderate intensity therapy: 40-80 mg once daily

Type 1 or 2 diabetes, age 40-75 years, and an estimated 10-year ASCVD risk ≥7.5%: High intensity therapy necessary; use alternate statin therapy (eg, atorvastatin or rosuvastatin)

Age 40-75 years and an estimated 10-year ASCVD risk ≥7.5%: Moderate to high intensity therapy: 40-80 mg once daily or consider using high intensity statin therapy (eg, atorvastatin or rosuvastatin)

Secondary prevention:

Patient has clinical ASCVD (eg, coronary heart disease, stroke/TIA, or peripheral arterial disease presumed to be of atherosclerotic origin) **and**:

Age ≤75 years: High intensity therapy necessary; use alternate statin therapy (eg, atorvastatin or rosuvastatin)

Age >75 years or not a candidate for high intensity therapy: Moderate intensity therapy: 40-80 mg once daily

Dosage adjustment for pravastatin with concomitant medications:

Clarithromycin: Limit daily pravastatin dose to 40 mg/day

Cyclosporine: Initial: 10 mg pravastatin daily, titrate with caution (maximum dose: 20 mg/day)

Elderly: No specific dosage recommendations. Clearance is reduced in the elderly, resulting in an increase in AUC between 25% to 50%. However, substantial accumulation is not expected.

Dosing adjustment for toxicity:

Severe muscle symptoms or fatigue: Promptly discontinue use; evaluate CPK, creatinine, and urinalysis for myoglobinuria (Stone, 2013).

Mild to moderate muscle symptoms: Discontinue use until symptoms can be evaluated; evaluate patient for conditions that may increase the risk for muscle symptoms (eg, hypothyroidism, reduced renal or hepatic function, rheumatologic disorders such as polymyalgia rheumatica, steroid myopathy, vitamin D deficiency, primary muscle diseases). Upon resolution, resume the original or lower dose of pravastatin. If muscle symptoms recur, discontinue pravastatin use. After muscle symptom resolution, may then use a low dose of a different statin; gradually increase if tolerated. In the absence of continued statin use, if muscle symptoms or elevated CPK continues after 2 months, consider other causes of muscle symptoms. If determined to be due to another condition aside from statin use, may resume statin therapy at the original dose (Stone, 2013).

Dosage adjustment in renal impairment: Significant impairment: Initial dose: 10 mg/day

Dosage adjustment in hepatic impairment: Contraindicated in active liver disease or in patients with unexplained persistent elevations of serum transaminases

Dietary Considerations May be taken without regard to meals. Before initiation of therapy, patients should be placed on a standard cholesterol-lowering diet for 6 weeks and the diet should be continued during drug therapy. Red yeast rice contains an estimated 2.4 mg lovastatin per 600 mg rice.

Administration May be administered without regard to meals.

Monitoring Parameters

2013 ACC/AHA Blood Cholesterol Guideline recommendations (Stone, 2013):

Lipid panel (total cholesterol, HDL, LDL, triglycerides): Baseline lipid panel; fasting lipid profile within 4-12 weeks after initiation or dose adjustment and every 3-12 months (as clinically indicated) thereafter. If 2 consecutive LDL levels are <40 mg/dL, consider decreasing the dose.

Hepatic transaminase levels: Baseline measurement of hepatic transaminase levels (ie, ALT); measure hepatic function if symptoms suggest hepatotoxicity (eg, unusual fatigue or weakness, loss of appetite, abdominal pain, dark-colored urine or yellowing of skin or sclera) during therapy.

CPK: CPK should not be routinely measured. Baseline CPK measurement is reasonable for some individuals (eg, family history of statin intolerance or muscle disease, clinical presentation, concomitant drug therapy that may increase risk of myopathy). May measure CPK in any patient with symptoms suggestive of myopathy (pain, tenderness, stiffness, cramping, weakness, or generalized fatigue).

Evaluate for new-onset diabetes mellitus during therapy; if diabetes develops, continue statin therapy and encourage adherence to a heart-healthy diet, physical activity, a healthy body weight, and tobacco cessation.

If patient develops a confusional state or memory impairment, may evaluate patient for nonstatin causes (eg, exposure to other drugs), systemic and neuropsychiatric causes, and the possibility of adverse effects associated with statin therapy.

Manufacturer recommendations: Liver enzyme tests at baseline and repeated when clinically indicated. **Upon initiation or titration, lipid panel should be analyzed at intervals of 4 weeks or more.**

Dosage Forms Excipient information presented when available (limited, particularly for generics); consult specific product labeling.

Tablet, Oral, as sodium:

Pravachol: 20 mg, 40 mg, 80 mg

Generic: 10 mg, 20 mg, 40 mg, 80 mg

◆ **Pravastatin Sodium** *see* Pravastatin *on page 1700*

◆ **Praxis ASA EC 81 Mg Daily Dose (Can)** *see* Aspirin *on page 177*

Praziquantel (pray zi KWON tel)

Brand Names: U.S. Biltricide

Brand Names: Canada Biltricide®

Pharmacologic Category Anthelmintic

Use Treatment of all stages of schistosomiasis caused by all *Schistosoma* species; treatment of infection (clonorchiasis and opisthorchiasis) due to liver flukes

Unlabeled Use Cysticercosis and many intestinal tapeworms

Pregnancy Risk Factor B

Pregnancy Considerations Adverse effects have not been observed in animal reproduction studies. There are no adequate and well-controlled studies in pregnant women. Use in pregnant women only if clearly needed.

Breast-Feeding Considerations Appears in breast milk at a concentration of ¼ that of maternal serum. Women should be advised to not breast-feed on the day of treatment and for 72 hours after treatment.

Contraindications Hypersensitivity to praziquantel or any component of the formulation; ocular cysticercosis; concurrent use with strong CYP3A4 inducers, particularly rifampin

Warnings/Precautions Use caution in patients with moderate-to-severe hepatic disease or patients with cardiac abnormalities; patients with cerebral cysticercosis require hospitalization. Use not recommended in patients with a history of seizures or signs of central nervous system involvement (eg, subcutaneous nodules suggestive of cysticercosis); may exacerbate condition. Therapeutic levels of praziquantel may not be achieved with concurrent administration of strong inducers of cytochrome P450 (eg, rifampin); concurrent use is contraindicated. Patients should be instructed to not drive or operate machinery on the day of treatment and the day after treatment.

Adverse Reactions Frequency not defined.

Central nervous system: Dizziness, fever, headache, malaise

Dermatologic: Urticaria (rare)

Gastrointestinal: Abdominal discomfort, nausea

Postmarketing and/or case reports: Allergic reaction, anorexia, arrhythmia, AV block, bloody diarrhea, bradycardia, ectopic rhythms, eosinophilia, hypersensitivity, liver enzymes increased, myalgia, polyserositis, pruritus, seizure, somnolence, ventricular fibrillation, vertigo, vomiting, weakness

Drug Interactions

Metabolism/Transport Effects **Substrate** of CYP3A4 (major); **Note:** Assignment of Major/Minor substrate status based on clinically relevant drug interaction potential; **Inhibits** CYP2D6 (weak)

Avoid Concomitant Use

Avoid concomitant use of Praziquantel with any of the following: Conivaptan; CYP3A4 Inducers (Strong); Fusidic Acid (Systemic)

Increased Effect/Toxicity

Praziquantel may increase the levels/effects of: ARIPiprazole

The levels/effects of Praziquantel may be increased by: Cimetidine; Conivaptan; CYP3A4 Inhibitors (Moderate); CYP3A4 Inhibitors (Strong); Dasatinib; Fusidic Acid (Systemic); Ivacaftor; Ketoconazole (Systemic); Luliconazole; Mifepristone; Simeprevir

Decreased Effect

The levels/effects of Praziquantel may be decreased by: Aminoquinolines (Antimalarial); Bosentan; CYP3A4 Inducers (Strong); Dabrafenib; Deferasirox; Herbs (CYP3A4 Inducers); Tocilizumab

Storage/Stability Store below 30°C (86°F).

Mechanism of Action Increases the cell permeability to calcium in schistosomes, causing strong contractions and paralysis of worm musculature leading to detachment of suckers from the blood vessel walls and to dislodgment

Pharmacodynamics/Kinetics

Absorption: Oral: 80%

Protein binding: ~80%

Metabolism: Extensive first-pass effect

Half-life elimination: Parent drug: 0.8-1.5 hours; Metabolites: 4.5 hours

Time to peak, serum: 1-3 hours

Excretion: Urine ~80% (>99% as metabolites)

Dosage Oral: Children ≥4 years and Adults:

Schistosomiasis: 20 mg/kg/dose 3 times/day for 1 day at 4- to 6-hour intervals

Clonorchiasis/opisthorchiasis: 25 mg/kg/dose 3 times/day for 1 day at 4- to 6-hour intervals

Cysticercosis (unlabeled use): 50 mg/kg/day divided every 8 hours for 14 days (Takayanagui, 2004)

Tapeworms (unlabeled use): 5-10 mg/kg as a single dose (25 mg/kg for *Hymenolepis nana*) (Liu, 1996)

Dosage adjustment in renal impairment: No dosage adjustment necessary.

Dosage adjustment in hepatic impairment: No dosage adjustment provided in manufacturer's labeling. However, total drug exposure in moderate-to-severe impairment is increased.

Administration Administer tablets with water during meals. Tablets should be promptly swallowed to avoid bitter taste that may cause gagging or vomiting. Tablets may be halved or quartered; do not chew.

Monitoring Parameters Culture urine or feces for ova prior to instituting therapy

Dosage Forms Excipient information presented when available (limited, particularly for generics); consult specific product labeling.

Tablet, Oral:

Biltricide: 600 mg [scored]

Prazosin (PRAZ oh sin)

Brand Names: U.S. Minipress

Brand Names: Canada Apo-Prazo®; Minipress®; Novo-Prazin; Nu-Prazo; Teva-Prazosin

Index Terms Furazosin; Prazosin Hydrochloride

Pharmacologic Category Alpha$_1$ Blocker; Antihypertensive

Additional Appendix Information

Beers Criteria – Potentially Inappropriate Medications for Geriatrics *on page 2368*

Use Treatment of hypertension

Unlabeled Use Post-traumatic stress disorder (PTSD) related nightmares and sleep disruption; benign prostatic hyperplasia; Raynaud's syndrome

Pregnancy Risk Factor C

Dosage Oral:

Children: Hypertension (unlabeled use): Initial: 0.05-0.1 mg/kg/day in 3 divided doses; maximum: 0.5 mg/kg/day (not to exceed 20 mg) (NHBPEP, Fourth Report)

Adults:

Hypertension: Initial: 1 mg/dose 2-3 times/day; usual maintenance dose: 2-20 mg/day in divided doses 2-3 times/day (JNC 7); maximum daily dose: 20 mg

PTSD-related nightmares and sleep disruption (unlabeled use): Initial: 1 mg at bedtime (Raskind, 2002; Raskind, 2007); titrate as tolerated to 2-15 mg at bedtime (Benedek, 2009)

Raynaud's (unlabeled use): Dosage range: 1-5 mg twice daily (Bakst, 2008)

Benign prostatic hyperplasia (unlabeled use): Initial: 0.5 mg twice daily; titrate as tolerated to 2 mg twice daily (Moran, 2001)

Elderly: Hypertension: Consider lower initial doses and titrate to response (Aronow, 2011)

Dosage adjustment in renal impairment: No dosage adjustment provided in manufacturer's labeling.

Dosage adjustment in hepatic impairment: No dosage adjustment provided in manufacturer's labeling.

Additional Information Complete prescribing information should be consulted for additional detail.

Dosage Forms Excipient information presented when available (limited, particularly for generics); consult specific product labeling.

Capsule, Oral:

Minipress: 1 mg, 2 mg, 5 mg

Generic: 1 mg, 2 mg, 5 mg

◆ **Prazosin Hydrochloride** *see* Prazosin *on page 1703*

◆ **Precedex** *see* Dexmedetomidine *on page 584*

◆ **Precise® [OTC]** *see* Methyl Salicylate and Menthol *on page 1344*

◆ **Precose** *see* Acarbose *on page 26*

◆ **Predator [OTC]** *see* Lidocaine (Topical) *on page 1212*

◆ **Pred Forte** *see* PrednisoLONE (Ophthalmic) *on page 1706*

◆ **Pred Forte® (Can)** *see* PrednisoLONE (Ophthalmic) *on page 1706*

◆ **Pred-G®** *see* Prednisolone and Gentamicin *on page 1707*

◆ **Pred Mild** *see* PrednisoLONE (Ophthalmic) *on page 1706*

◆ **Pred Mild® (Can)** *see* PrednisoLONE (Ophthalmic) *on page 1706*

Prednicarbate (pred ni KAR bate)

Brand Names: U.S. Dermatop

Brand Names: Canada Dermatop®

Pharmacologic Category Corticosteroid, Topical

Additional Appendix Information

Topical Corticosteroids *on page 2299*

Use Relief of the inflammatory and pruritic manifestations of corticosteroid-responsive dermatoses (medium potency topical corticosteroid)

Pregnancy Risk Factor C

Dosage Note: Therapy should be discontinued when control is achieved; if no improvement is seen within 2 weeks, reassessment of diagnosis may be necessary.

Cream: Children ≥1 year and Adults: Topical: Apply a thin film to affected area twice daily

Ointment: Children ≥10 year and Adults: Topical: Apply a thin film to affected area twice daily

Additional Information Complete prescribing information should be consulted for additional detail.

Dosage Forms Excipient information presented when available (limited, particularly for generics); consult specific product labeling.

Cream, External:

Dermatop: 0.1% (60 g)

Generic: 0.1% (15 g, 60 g)

Ointment, External:

Dermatop: 0.1% (60 g)

Generic: 0.1% (15 g, 60 g)

PrednisoLONE (Systemic) (pred NISS oh lone)

Brand Names: U.S. Flo-Pred; Millipred; Millipred DP; Millipred DP 12-Day; Orapred; Orapred ODT; Pediapred; Prelone; Veripred 20

Brand Names: Canada Hydeltra T.B.A.®; Novo-Prednisolone; Pediapred®

Index Terms Prednisolone Sodium Phosphate

Pharmacologic Category Corticosteroid, Systemic

Additional Appendix Information

Corticosteroids Systemic Equivalencies *on page 2297*

Use Treatment of endocrine disorders, rheumatic disorders, collagen diseases, allergic states, respiratory diseases, hematologic disorders, neoplastic diseases, edematous states, and gastrointestinal diseases; resolution of acute exacerbations of multiple sclerosis; management of fulminating or disseminated tuberculosis and trichinosis; acute or chronic solid organ rejection

Unlabeled Use Severe alcoholic hepatitis; Bell's palsy; acute exacerbations of chronic obstructive pulmonary disease (COPD)

Pregnancy Risk Factor C/D (manufacturer specific)

Pregnancy Considerations Adverse events have been observed with corticosteroids in animal reproduction studies. Prednisolone crosses the placenta; prior to reaching the fetus, prednisolone is converted by placental enzymes to prednisone. As a result, the amount of prednisolone reaching the fetus is ~8-10 times lower than the maternal serum concentration (healthy women at term; similar results observed with preterm pregnancies complicated by HELLP syndrome) (Beitins, 1972; van Runnard Heimel, 2005). Some studies have shown an association between first trimester systemic corticosteroid use and oral clefts (Park-Wyllie, 2000; Pradat, 2003). Systemic corticosteroids may also influence fetal growth (decreased birth weight); however, information is conflicting (Lunghi, 2010). Hypoadrenalism may occur in newborns following maternal use of corticosteroids in pregnancy; monitor.

When systemic corticosteroids are needed in pregnancy, it is generally recommended to use the lowest effective dose for the shortest duration of time, avoiding high doses during the first trimester (Leachman, 2006; Lunghi, 2010; Makol, 2011; Østensen, 2009). Inhaled corticosteroids are preferred for the treatment of asthma during pregnancy. Oral corticosteroids, such as prednisolone, may be used for the treatment of severe persistent asthma if needed; the lowest dose administered on alternate days (if possible) should be used (NAEPP, 2005). Prednisolone may be used to treat women during pregnancy who require therapy for congenital adrenal hyperplasia (Speiser, 2010). Topical agents are preferred for managing atopic dermatitis in pregnancy; for severe symptomatic or recalcitrant atopic dermatitis, a short course of prednisolone may be used during the third trimester (Koutroulis, 2011).

Women exposed to prednisolone during pregnancy for the treatment of an autoimmune disease may contact the OTIS Autoimmune Diseases Study at 877-311-8972.

Breast-Feeding Considerations Prednisolone is excreted into breast milk. In one study (n=6), milk concentrations were 5% to 25% of the maternal serum concentration with peak concentrations occurring ~1 hour after the maternal dose. The milk/plasma ratio was found to be 0.2 with doses ≥30 mg/day and 0.1 with doses <30 mg/day. Following a maternal dose of prednisolone 80 mg/day, it was calculated that a breast-feeding infant would ingest <0.1% of the maternal dose (Ost, 1985). One manufacturer notes that when used systemically, maternal use of corticosteroids have the potential to cause adverse events in a nursing infant (eg, growth suppression, interfere with endogenous corticosteroid production) and therefore caution should be used when administered to nursing women. In order to decrease potential exposure to a nursing infant, one manufacturer recommends administering the dose after nursing, at the time of day with the longest interval between feeds. Other sources recommend waiting 4 hours after the maternal dose before breast-feeding (Bae, 2012; Leachman, 2006; Makol, 2011; Ost, 1985). Other guidelines note that maternal use of systemic corticosteroids is not a contraindication to breast-feeding (NAEPP, 2005).

Contraindications Hypersensitivity to prednisolone or any component of the formulation; acute superficial herpes simplex keratitis; live or attenuated virus vaccines (with immunosuppressive doses of corticosteroids); systemic fungal infections; varicella

Warnings/Precautions May cause hypercorticism or suppression of hypothalamic-pituitary-adrenal (HPA) axis, particularly in younger children or in patients receiving high doses for prolonged periods. HPA axis suppression may lead to adrenal crisis. Withdrawal and discontinuation of a corticosteroid should be done slowly and carefully. Particular care is required when patients are transferred from systemic corticosteroids to inhaled products due to possible adrenal insufficiency or withdrawal from steroids, including an increase in allergic symptoms. Patients receiving >20 mg per day of prednisone (or equivalent) may be most susceptible. Fatalities have occurred due to adrenal insufficiency in asthmatic patients during and after transfer from systemic corticosteroids to aerosol steroids; aerosol steroids do **not** provide the systemic steroid needed to treat patients having trauma, surgery, or infections.

Acute myopathy has been reported with high dose corticosteroids, usually in patients with neuromuscular transmission disorders; may involve ocular and/or respiratory muscles; monitor creatine kinase; recovery may be delayed. Corticosteroid use may cause psychiatric disturbances, including depression, euphoria, insomnia, mood swings, and personality changes. Pre-existing psychiatric conditions may be exacerbated by corticosteroid use. Prolonged use of corticosteroids may also increase the incidence of secondary infection, mask acute infection (including fungal infections), prolong or exacerbate viral infections, or limit response to vaccines. Exposure to chickenpox should be avoided; corticosteroids should not be used to treat ocular herpes simplex. Corticosteroids should not be used for cerebral malaria or viral hepatitis. Close observation is required in patients with latent tuberculosis and/or TB reactivity; restrict use in active TB (only in conjunction with antituberculosis treatment). Prolonged use of corticosteroids may result in glaucoma; cataract formation may occur. Prolonged treatment with corticosteroids has been associated with the development of Kaposi's sarcoma (case reports); if noted, discontinuation of therapy should be considered.

Use with caution in patients with thyroid disease, hepatic impairment, renal impairment, cardiovascular disease, diabetes, glaucoma, cataracts, myasthenia gravis, patients at risk for osteoporosis, patients at risk for seizures, or GI diseases (diverticulitis, peptic ulcer, ulcerative colitis) due to perforation risk. Use caution following acute MI (corticosteroids have been associated with myocardial rupture). Because of the risk of adverse effects, systemic corticosteroids should be used cautiously in the elderly in the smallest possible effective dose for the shortest duration. Withdraw therapy with gradual tapering of dose. May affect growth velocity; growth should be routinely monitored in pediatric patients. Potentially significant drug-drug interactions may exist, requiring dose or frequency adjustment, additional monitoring, and/or selection of alternative therapy.

Adverse Reactions Frequency not defined.

Cardiovascular: Cardiomyopathy, CHF, edema, facial edema, hypertension

Central nervous system: Headache, insomnia, malaise, nervousness, pseudotumor cerebri, psychic disorders, seizure, vertigo

Dermatologic: Bruising, facial erythema, hirsutism, petechiae, skin test reaction suppression, thin fragile skin, urticaria

Endocrine & metabolic: Carbohydrate tolerance decreased, Cushing's syndrome, diabetes mellitus, growth suppression, hyperglycemia, hypernatremia, hypokalemia, hypokalemic alkalosis, menstrual irregularities, negative nitrogen balance, pituitary adrenal axis suppression

Gastrointestinal: Abdominal distention, increased appetite, indigestion, nausea, pancreatitis, peptic ulcer, ulcerative esophagitis, weight gain

Hepatic: LFTs increased (usually reversible)

Neuromuscular & skeletal: Arthralgia, aseptic necrosis (humeral/femoral heads), fractures, muscle mass decreased, muscle weakness, osteoporosis, steroid myopathy, tendon rupture, weakness

Ocular: Cataracts, exophthalmus, eyelid edema, glaucoma, intraocular pressure increased, irritation

Respiratory: Epistaxis

Miscellaneous: Diaphoresis increased, impaired wound healing

<1% (Limited to important or life-threatening): Venous thrombosis (Johannesdottir, 2013)

Drug Interactions

Metabolism/Transport Effects Substrate of CYP3A4 (minor); **Note:** Assignment of Major/Minor substrate status based on clinically relevant drug interaction potential; **Inhibits** CYP3A4 (weak)

Avoid Concomitant Use

Avoid concomitant use of PrednisoLONE (Systemic) with any of the following: Aldesleukin; BCG; Mifepristone; Natalizumab; Pimecrolimus; Pimozide; Tacrolimus (Topical); Tofacitinib

Increased Effect/Toxicity

PrednisoLONE (Systemic) may increase the levels/effects of: Acetylcholinesterase Inhibitors; Amphotericin B; ARIPiprazole; CycloSPORINE (Systemic); Deferasirox; Dofetilide; Leflunomide; Lomitapide; Loop Diuretics; Natalizumab; NSAID (COX-2 Inhibitor); NSAID (Nonselective); Pimozide; Thiazide Diuretics; Tofacitinib; Vaccines (Live); Warfarin

The levels/effects of PrednisoLONE (Systemic) may be increased by: Antifungal Agents (Azole Derivatives, Systemic); Aprepitant; Boceprevir; Calcium Channel Blockers (Nondihydropyridine); CycloSPORINE (Systemic); Denosumab; Estrogen Derivatives; Fluconazole; Fosaprepitant; Indacaterol; Macrolide Antibiotics; Mifepristone; Neuromuscular-Blocking Agents (Nondepolarizing); Pimecrolimus; Quinolone Antibiotics; Ritonavir; Roflumilast; Salicylates; Tacrolimus (Topical); Telaprevir; Trastuzumab

Decreased Effect

PrednisoLONE (Systemic) may decrease the levels/effects of: Aldesleukin; Antidiabetic Agents; BCG; Calcitriol; Coccidioidin Skin Test; Corticorelin; CycloSPORINE (Systemic); Hyaluronidase; Isoniazid; Salicylates; Sipuleucel-T; Telaprevir; Urea Cycle Disorder Agents; Vaccines (Inactivated)

The levels/effects of PrednisoLONE (Systemic) may be decreased by: Aminoglutethimide; Antacids; Barbiturates; Bile Acid Sequestrants; Echinacea; Fosphenytoin; Mifepristone; Mitotane; Phenytoin; Primidone; Rifamycin Derivatives

Ethanol/Nutrition/Herb Interactions

Ethanol: Avoid ethanol (may increase gastric mucosal irritation).

Food: Prednisolone interferes with calcium absorption. Limit caffeine.

Herb/Nutraceutical: St John's wort may decrease prednisolone levels. Avoid cat's claw, echinacea (have immunostimulant properties).

Storage/Stability

Flo-Pred™: Store at 20°C to 25°C (68°F to 77°F). Flo-Pred™ should be dispensed in the original container (to avoid loss of formulation during transfer).

Millipred™: Store at 20°C to 25°C (68°F to 77°F).

Orapred ODT®: Store at 20°C to 25°C (68°F to 77°F) in blister pack. Protect from moisture.

Orapred®, Veripred™ 20: 2°C to 8°C (36°F to 46°F).

Pediapred®: 4°C to 25°C (39°F to 77°F); may be refrigerated.

Mechanism of Action Decreases inflammation by suppression of migration of polymorphonuclear leukocytes and reversal of increased capillary permeability; suppresses the immune system by reducing activity and volume of the lymphatic system

Pharmacodynamics/Kinetics

Duration: 18-36 hours

Protein binding (concentration dependent): 65% to 91%; decreased in elderly

Metabolism: Primarily hepatic, but also metabolized in most tissues, to inactive compounds

Half-life elimination: 3.6 hours; End-stage renal disease: 3-5 hours

Excretion: Primarily urine (as glucuronides, sulfates, and unconjugated metabolites)

Dosage Dose depends upon condition being treated and response of patient; dosage for infants and children should be based on severity of the disease and response of the patient rather than on strict adherence to dosage indicated by age, weight, or body surface area. Oral dosage expressed in terms of prednisolone base. Consider alternate day therapy for long-term therapy. Discontinuation of long-term therapy requires gradual withdrawal by tapering the dose. Patients undergoing unusual stress while receiving corticosteroids should receive increased doses prior to, during, and after the stressful situation.

Children: Oral:

Acute asthma: 1-2 mg/kg/day in divided doses 1-2 times daily for 3-5 days

Anti-inflammatory or immunosuppressive dose: 0.1-2 mg/kg/day in divided doses 1-4 times daily

Nephrotic syndrome:

Initial (first 3 episodes): 2 mg/kg/day **or** 60 mg/m^2/day (maximum: 80 mg daily) in divided doses 3-4 times daily until urine is protein free for 3 consecutive days (maximum: 28 days); followed by 1-1.5 mg/kg/dose **or** 40 mg/m^2/dose given every other day for 4 weeks

Maintenance (long-term maintenance dose for frequent relapses): 0.5-1 mg/kg/dose given every other day for 3-6 months

Adults: Oral:

Usual range: 5-60 mg daily

Multiple sclerosis: 200 mg daily for 1 week followed by 80 mg every other day for 1 month

Rheumatoid arthritis: Initial: 5-7.5 mg daily; adjust dose as necessary

Acute exacerbations of chronic obstructive pulmonary disease (COPD) (unlabeled use): 30-40 mg daily for 10-14 days (GOLD guidelines, 2013)

Bell's palsy (unlabeled use): 60 mg once daily for 5 days, then taper dose downward by 10 mg daily for 5 days (total treatment duration: 10 days) (Engstrom, 2008; Berg, 2012)

Severe alcoholic hepatitis (Maddrey Discriminant Function [MDF] score ≥32) (unlabeled use): 40 mg daily for 28 days, followed by a 2-week taper (O'Shea, 2010)

Elderly: Use lowest effective dose

Dosing adjustment in hyperthyroidism: Prednisolone dose may need to be increased to achieve adequate therapeutic effects

Dosage adjustment in renal impairment: No dosage adjustment provided in manufacturer's labeling. Use with caution.

Hemodialysis: Slightly dialyzable (5% to 20%); administer dose posthemodialysis

Peritoneal dialysis: Supplemental dose is not necessary

Dosage adjustment in hepatic impairment: No dosage adjustment provided in manufacturer's labeling.

Dietary Considerations Should be taken after meals or with food or milk to decrease GI effects; increase dietary intake of pyridoxine, vitamin C, vitamin D, folate, calcium, and phosphorus.

Administration Administer oral formulation with food or milk to decrease GI effects.

Flo-Pred™: Administer using the provided calibrated syringe (supplied by manufacturer) to accurately measure the dose. Syringe should be washed prior to next use.

Orapred ODT®: Do not break or use partial tablet. Remove tablet from blister pack just prior to use. May swallow whole or allow to dissolve on tongue.

Monitoring Parameters Blood pressure; blood glucose, electrolytes; intraocular pressure (use >6 weeks); bone mineral density; growth in children

Test Interactions Response to skin tests

Dosage Forms Excipient information presented when available (limited, particularly for generics); consult specific product labeling. [DSC] = Discontinued product

Solution, Oral, as base:

Generic: 15 mg/5 mL (240 mL, 480 mL)

Solution, Oral, as sodium phosphate [strength expressed as base]:

Millipred: 10 mg/5 mL (237 mL) [dye free; contains edetate disodium, methylparaben, saccharin sodium; grape flavor]

Orapred: 15 mg/5 mL (20 mL, 237 mL) [dye free; contains alcohol, usp, sodium benzoate; grape flavor]

Pediapred: 5 mg/5 mL (120 mL) [alcohol free, dye free, sugar free; contains edetate disodium, methylparaben; raspberry flavor]

Veripred 20: 20 mg/5 mL (237 mL) [alcohol free, dye free; contains edetate disodium, methylparaben, saccharin sodium; grape flavor]

Generic: 15 mg/5 mL (237 mL, 473 mL [DSC]); 25 mg/5 mL (237 mL); 5 mg/5 mL (120 mL)

Suspension, Oral, as acetate [strength expressed as base]:

Flo-Pred: 15 mg/5 mL (30 mL) [contains butylparaben, disodium edta, propylene glycol; cherry flavor]

Syrup, Oral, as base:

Prelone: 15 mg/5 mL (240 mL) [contains alcohol, usp, benzoic acid, brilliant blue fcf (fd&c blue #1), fd&c red #40, propylene glycol, saccharin sodium; cherry flavor]

Generic: 15 mg/5 mL (240 mL, 480 mL)

Tablet, Oral, as base:

Millipred: 5 mg [scored; contains fd&c yellow #10 (quinoline yellow), fd&c yellow #6 (sunset yellow), sodium benzoate]

Millipred DP: 5 mg [scored; contains fd&c yellow #10 (quinoline yellow), fd&c yellow #6 (sunset yellow), sodium benzoate]

Millipred DP 12-Day: 5 mg [scored; contains fd&c yellow #10 (quinoline yellow), fd&c yellow #6 (sunset yellow), sodium benzoate]

Tablet Dispersible, Oral, as sodium phosphate [strength expressed as base]:

Orapred ODT: 10 mg

Orapred ODT: 15 mg [grape flavor]

Orapred ODT: 30 mg

PrednisoLONE (Ophthalmic) (pred NISS oh lone)

Brand Names: U.S. Omnipred; Pred Forte; Pred Mild

Brand Names: Canada Diopred®; Ophtho-Tate®; Pred Forte®; Pred Mild®

Index Terms Econopred; Prednisolone Acetate, Ophthalmic; Prednisolone Sodium Phosphate, Ophthalmic

Pharmacologic Category Corticosteroid, Ophthalmic

Use Treatment of palpebral and bulbar conjunctivitis; corneal injury from chemical, radiation, thermal burns, or foreign body penetration; steroid-responsive inflammatory ophthalmic diseases

Pregnancy Risk Factor C

Dosage Ophthalmic suspension/solution: Children and Adults: Instill 1-2 drops in the eye 2-4 times daily

Dosage adjustment in renal impairment: No dosage adjustment provided in manufacturer's labeling.

Dosage adjustment in hepatic impairment: No dosage adjustment provided in manufacturer's labeling.

Additional Information Complete prescribing information should be consulted for additional detail.

Dosage Forms Excipient information presented when available (limited, particularly for generics); consult specific product labeling.

Solution, Ophthalmic, as sodium phosphate:
- Generic: 1% (10 mL)

Suspension, Ophthalmic, as acetate:
- Omnipred: 1% (5 mL, 10 mL) [contains benzalkonium chloride, edetate disodium, polysorbate 80]
- Pred Forte: 1% (1 mL, 5 mL, 10 mL, 15 mL)
- Pred Mild: 0.12% (5 mL, 10 mL)
- Generic: 1% (5 mL, 10 mL, 15 mL)

◆ **Prednisolone Acetate, Ophthalmic** *see* PrednisoLONE (Ophthalmic) *on page 1706*

Prednisolone and Gentamicin

(pred NIS oh lone & jen ta MYE sin)

Brand Names: U.S. Pred-G®

Index Terms Gentamicin and Prednisolone

Pharmacologic Category Antibiotic/Corticosteroid, Ophthalmic

Use Treatment of steroid responsive inflammatory conditions where either a superficial bacterial ocular infection or the risk of bacterial ocular infection exists

Pregnancy Risk Factor C

Dosage Ophthalmic: Adults:

Ointment: Apply 1/2 inch ribbon into the conjunctival sac of the affected eye(s) 1-3 times/day

Suspension: Instill 1 drop into the conjunctival sac of the affected eye(s) 2-4 times/day; during the initial 24-48 hours, the dosing frequency may be increased if necessary up to 1 drop every hour

Note: If signs and symptoms do not improve after 2 days of treatment, the patient should be re-evaluated.

Additional Information Complete prescribing information should be consulted for additional detail.

Dosage Forms Excipient information presented when available (limited, particularly for generics); consult specific product labeling. [DSC] = Discontinued product

Ointment, ophthalmic:
- Pred-G®: Prednisolone acetate 0.6% and gentamicin sulfate 0.3% (3.5 g)

Suspension, ophthalmic:
- Pred-G®: Prednisolone acetate 1% and gentamicin sulfate 0.3% (5 mL, 10 mL [DSC]) [contains benzalkonium chloride]

◆ **Prednisolone and Sulfacetamide** *see* Sulfacetamide and Prednisolone *on page 1957*

◆ **Prednisolone Sodium Phosphate** *see* PrednisoLONE (Systemic) *on page 1704*

◆ **Prednisolone Sodium Phosphate, Ophthalmic** *see* PrednisoLONE (Ophthalmic) *on page 1706*

PredniSONE (PRED ni sone)

Brand Names: U.S. PredniSONE Intensol; Rayos

Brand Names: Canada Apo-Prednisone®; Novo-Prednisone; Winpred™

Index Terms Deltacortisone; Deltadehydrocortisone; Rayos®

Pharmacologic Category Corticosteroid, Systemic

Additional Appendix Information

Contrast Media Reactions, Premedication for Prophylaxis *on page 2373*

Corticosteroids Systemic Equivalencies *on page 2297*

Use Treatment of a variety of diseases, including:

Allergic conditions: Atopic dermatitis, drug hypersensitivity reactions, allergic rhinitis, serum sickness, adjunctive treatment of anaphylaxis

Dermatologic diseases: Bullous dermatitis herpetiformis, contact dermatitis, exfoliative erythroderma, mycosis fungoides, pemphigus, severe erythema multiforme (Stevens-Johnson syndrome), severe seborrheic dermatitis (immediate release only)

Endocrine conditions: Congenital adrenal hyperplasia, hypercalcemia of malignancy, nonsuppurative thyroiditis, adrenocortical insufficiency

Gastrointestinal diseases: Crohn's disease, ulcerative colitis

Hematologic diseases: Acquired (autoimmune) hemolytic anemia, Diamond-Blackfan anemia, immune thrombocytopenia (ITP), pure red cell aplasia, secondary thrombocytopenia

Infectious diseases: Trichinosis with neurologic or myocardial involvement, tuberculosis meningitis with subarachnoid block or impending block

Neoplastic conditions: Acute leukemia, aggressive lymphomas

Nervous system conditions (delayed release only): Acute exacerbations of multiple sclerosis, cerebral edema associated with primary or metastatic brain tumor, craniotomy or head injury

Ophthalmic conditions:

Immediate release only: Allergic conjunctivitis, keratitis, allergic corneal marginal ulcers, herpes zoster ophthalmicus, iritis and iridocyclitis, chorioretinitis, anterior segment inflammation, diffuse posterior uveitis and choroiditis, optic neuritis

Delayed release only: Uveitis, and ocular inflammatory conditions

Organ transplantation-related conditions (delayed release only): Solid organ rejection

Pulmonary diseases: Aspiration pneumonitis, asthma, pulmonary tuberculosis, symptomatic sarcoidosis

Immediate release only: Loeffler's syndrome not manageable by other means, berylliosis

Delayed release only: Acute exacerbations of chronic obstructive pulmonary disease (COPD), allergic bronchopulmonary aspergillosis, hypersensitivity pneumonitis, idiopathic bronchiolitis obliterans with organizing pneumonia, idiopathic eosinophilic pneumonias, idiopathic pulmonary fibrosis, *Pneumocystis jiroveci* (formerly *carinii*) pneumonia (PCP)

Renal conditions: Nephrotic syndrome (idiopathic or related to lupus erythematosus), without uremia

Rheumatologic conditions, short-term therapy: Psoriatic arthritis, rheumatoid and juvenile arthritis, ankylosing spondylitis, acute gouty arthritis, systemic lupus erythematosus, dermatomyositis/polymyositis

Immediate release only: Bursitis, tenosynovitis, posttraumatic osteoarthritis, synovitis of osteoarthritis, epicondylitis acute rheumatic carditis

Delayed release only: Polymyalgia rheumatica, relapsing polychondritis, Sjogren's syndrome, vasculitis

Rheumatologic conditions, maintenance therapy: Rheumatoid and juvenile arthritis, systemic lupus erythematosus, dermatomyositis/polymyositis

Immediate release only: Acute rheumatic carditis

Delayed release only: Ankylosing spondylitis, polymyalgia rheumatic, psoriatic arthritis, relapsing polychondritis, Sjogren's syndrome, vasculitis

Unlabeled Use Autoimmune hepatitis; adjunctive therapy for pain management in immunocompetent patients with herpes zoster; Takayasu arteritis; giant cell arteritis; Grave's ophthalmopathy prophylaxis; subacute thyroiditis; thyrotoxicosis (type II amiodarone-induced); acute exacerbation of chronic obstructive pulmonary disease (COPD) (immediate release products)

Pregnancy Risk Factor C

Pregnancy Considerations Adverse events have been observed with corticosteroids in animal reproduction studies. Prednisone and its metabolite, prednisolone, cross the human placenta. In the mother, prednisone is converted to the active metabolite prednisolone by the liver. Prior to reaching the fetus, prednisolone is converted by placental enzymes back to prednisone. As a result, the level of prednisone remaining in the maternal serum and reaching the fetus are similar; however, the amount of prednisolone reaching the fetus is ~8-10 times lower than the maternal serum concentration (healthy women at term) (Beitins, 1972). Some studies have shown an association between first trimester systemic corticosteroid use and oral clefts (Park-Wyllie, 2000; Pradat, 2003). Systemic corticosteroids may also influence fetal growth (decreased birth weight); however, information is conflicting (Lunghi, 2010). Hypoadrenalism may occur in newborns following maternal use of corticosteroids in pregnancy; monitor.

When systemic corticosteroids are needed in pregnancy, it is generally recommended to use the lowest effective dose for the shortest duration of time, avoiding high doses during the first trimester (Leachman, 2006; Lunghi, 2010; Makol, 2011; Østensen, 2009). Inhaled corticosteroids are preferred for the treatment of asthma during pregnancy. Oral corticosteroids, such as prednisone, may be used for the treatment of severe persistent asthma if needed; the lowest dose administered on alternate days (if possible) should be used (NAEPP, 2005). Prednisone may be used to treat lupus nephritis in pregnant women who have active nephritis or substantial extrarenal disease activity (Hahn, 2012).

Pregnant women exposed to prednisone for antirejection therapy following a transplant may contact the National Transplantation Pregnancy Registry (NTPR) at 215-955-4820. Women exposed to prednisone during pregnancy for the treatment of an autoimmune disease (eg, rheumatoid arthritis) may contact the OTIS Autoimmune Diseases Study at 877-311-8972.

Breast-Feeding Considerations Prednisone and its metabolite, prednisolone, are found in low concentrations in breast milk. Following a maternal dose of 10 mg (n=1), milk concentrations were measured ~2 hours after the maternal dose (prednisone 0.0016 mcg/mL; prednisolone 0.0267 mcg/mL) (Katz, 1975). In a study which included six mother/infant pairs, adverse events were not observed in nursing infants (maternal prednisone dose not provided) (Ito, 1993).

The manufacturer notes that when used systemically, maternal use of corticosteroids have the potential to cause adverse events in a nursing infant (eg, growth suppression, interfere with endogenous corticosteroid production) and therefore, a decision should be made whether to discontinue nursing or to discontinue the drug, taking into account the importance of treatment to the mother. If there is concern about exposure to the infant, some guidelines recommend waiting 4 hours after the maternal dose of an oral systemic corticosteroid before breast-feeding in order to decrease potential exposure to the nursing infant (based on a study using prednisolone) (Bae, 2011; Leachman, 2006; Makol, 2011; Ost, 1985). Other guidelines note that maternal use of prednisone is not a contraindication to breast-feeding (NAEPP, 2005).

Contraindications Hypersensitivity to any component of the formulation; systemic fungal infections; administration of live or live attenuated vaccines with immunosuppressive doses of prednisone

Warnings/Precautions May cause hypercorticism or suppression of hypothalamic-pituitary-adrenal (HPA) axis, particularly in younger children or in patients receiving high doses for prolonged periods. HPA axis suppression may lead to adrenal crisis. Withdrawal and discontinuation of a corticosteroid should be done slowly and carefully. Particular care is required when patients are transferred from systemic corticosteroids to inhaled products due to possible adrenal insufficiency or withdrawal from steroids, including an increase in allergic symptoms. Patients receiving >20 mg per day of prednisone (or equivalent) may be most susceptible. Fatalities have occurred due to adrenal insufficiency in asthmatic patients during and after transfer from systemic corticosteroids to aerosol steroids; aerosol steroids do **not** provide the systemic steroid needed to treat patients having trauma, surgery, or infections.

Acute myopathy has been reported with high dose corticosteroids, usually in patients with neuromuscular transmission disorders; may involve ocular and/or respiratory muscles; monitor creatine kinase; recovery may be delayed. Prolonged use of corticosteroids may increase the incidence of secondary infection, mask acute infection (including fungal infections), prolong or exacerbate viral infections, or limit response to vaccines. Exposure to chickenpox should be avoided. Corticosteroids should not be used to treat ocular herpes simplex or cerebral malaria. Close observation is required in patients with latent tuberculosis and/or TB reactivity; restrict use in active TB (only in conjunction with antituberculosis treatment). Prolonged treatment with corticosteroids has been associated with the development of Kaposi's sarcoma (case reports); if noted, discontinuation of therapy should be considered. Prolonged use may cause posterior subcapsular cataracts, glaucoma (with possible nerve damage) and may increase the risk for ocular infections. Corticosteroid use may cause psychiatric disturbances, including depression, euphoria, insomnia, mood swings, and personality changes. Pre-existing psychiatric conditions may be exacerbated by corticosteroid use.

Use with caution in patients with HF, diabetes, GI diseases (diverticulitis, peptic ulcer, ulcerative colitis; due to risk of perforation), hepatic impairment, myasthenia gravis, MI, patients with or who are at risk for osteoporosis, seizure disorders or thyroid disease. May affect growth velocity; growth should be routinely monitored in pediatric patients.

Prior to use, the dose and duration of treatment should be based on the risk versus benefit for each individual patient. In general, use the smallest effective dose for the shortest duration of time to minimize adverse events. A gradual tapering of dose may be required prior to discontinuing therapy.

Adverse Reactions Frequency not defined.

Cardiovascular: Congestive heart failure (in susceptible patients), hypertension

Central nervous system: Emotional instability, headache, intracranial pressure increased (with papilledema), psychic derangements (including euphoria, insomnia, mood swings, personality changes, severe depression), seizure, vertigo

Dermatologic: Bruising, facial erythema, petechiae, thin fragile skin, urticaria, wound healing impaired

Endocrine & metabolic: Adrenocortical and pituitary unresponsiveness (in times of stress), carbohydrate intolerance, Cushing's syndrome, diabetes mellitus, fluid retention, growth suppression (in children), hypokalemic alkalosis, hypothyroidism enhanced, menstrual irregularities, negative nitrogen balance due to protein catabolism, potassium loss, sodium retention

Gastrointestinal: Abdominal distension, pancreatitis, peptic ulcer (with possible perforation and hemorrhage), ulcerative esophagitis

Hepatic: ALT increased, AST increased, alkaline phosphatase increased

Neuromuscular & skeletal: Aseptic necrosis of femoral and humeral heads, muscle mass loss, muscle weakness, osteoporosis, pathologic fracture of long bones, steroid myopathy, tendon rupture (particularly Achilles tendon), vertebral compression fractures

Ocular: Exophthalmos, glaucoma, intraocular pressure increased, posterior subcapsular cataracts

Miscellaneous: Allergic reactions, anaphylactic reactions, diaphoresis, hypersensitivity reactions, infections, Kaposi's sarcoma

<1% (Limited to important or life-threatening): Venous thrombosis (Johannesdottir, 2013)

Drug Interactions

Metabolism/Transport Effects Substrate of CYP3A4 (minor); **Note:** Assignment of Major/Minor substrate status based on clinically relevant drug interaction potential; **Induces** CYP2C19 (weak/moderate), CYP3A4 (weak/moderate)

Avoid Concomitant Use

Avoid concomitant use of PredniSONE with any of the following: Aldesleukin; Axitinib; BCG; Mifepristone; Natalizumab; Pimecrolimus; Simeprevir; Tacrolimus (Topical); Tofacitinib

Increased Effect/Toxicity

PredniSONE may increase the levels/effects of: Acetylcholinesterase Inhibitors; Amphotericin B; CycloSPORINE (Systemic); Deferasirox; Leflunomide; Loop Diuretics; Natalizumab; NSAID (COX-2 Inhibitor); NSAID (Nonselective); Thiazide Diuretics; Tofacitinib; Vaccines (Live); Warfarin

The levels/effects of PredniSONE may be increased by: Antifungal Agents (Azole Derivatives, Systemic); Aprepitant; Boceprevir; Calcium Channel Blockers (Nondihydropyridine); CycloSPORINE (Systemic); Denosumab; Estrogen Derivatives; Fluconazole; Fosaprepitant; Indacaterol; Macrolide Antibiotics; Mifepristone; Neuromuscular-Blocking Agents (Nondepolarizing); Pimecrolimus; Quinolone Antibiotics; Ritonavir; Roflumilast; Salicylates; Tacrolimus (Topical); Telaprevir; Trastuzumab

Decreased Effect

PredniSONE may decrease the levels/effects of: Aldesleukin; Antidiabetic Agents; ARIPiprazole; Axitinib; BCG; Calcitriol; Coccidioidin Skin Test; Corticorelin; CycloSPORINE (Systemic); Hyaluronidase; Ibrutinib; Isoniazid; Salicylates; Simeprevir; Sipuleucel-T; Telaprevir; Urea Cycle Disorder Agents; Vaccines (Inactivated)

The levels/effects of PredniSONE may be decreased by: Aminoglutethimide; Antacids; Barbiturates; Bile Acid Sequestrants; Echinacea; Fosphenytoin; Mifepristone; Mitotane; Phenytoin; Primidone; Rifamycin Derivatives; Somatropin; Tesamorelin

Ethanol/Nutrition/Herb Interactions

Ethanol: Avoid ethanol (may increase gastric mucosal irritation)

Food: Prednisone interferes with calcium absorption. Limit caffeine.

Herb/Nutraceutical: St John's wort may decrease prednisone levels. Avoid cat's claw, echinacea (have immunostimulant properties).

Mechanism of Action Decreases inflammation by suppression of migration of polymorphonuclear leukocytes and reversal of increased capillary permeability; suppresses the immune system by reducing activity and volume of the lymphatic system; suppresses adrenal function at high doses. Antitumor effects may be related to inhibition of glucose transport, phosphorylation, or induction of cell death in immature lymphocytes. Antiemetic effects are thought to occur due to blockade of cerebral innervation of the emetic center via inhibition of prostaglandin synthesis.

Pharmacodynamics/Kinetics

Absorption: 50% to 90% (may be altered in IBS or hyperthyroidism)

Protein binding (concentration dependent): 65% to 91%

Metabolism: Hepatically converted from prednisone (inactive) to prednisolone (active); may be impaired with hepatic dysfunction

Half-life elimination: Normal renal function: ~3.5 hours

Time to peak: Oral:

Immediate release tablet: 2 hours; Delayed release tablet (Rayos®): 6-6.5 hours

Excretion: Urine (small portion)

Dosage Oral:

General dosing range: Children and Adults: Initial: 5-60 mg daily: **Note:** Dose depends upon condition being treated and response of patient; dosage for infants and children should be based on severity of the disease and response of the patient rather than on strict adherence to dosage indicated by age, weight, or body surface area. Consider alternate day therapy for long-term therapy. Discontinuation of long-term therapy requires gradual withdrawal by tapering the dose.

Prednisone taper (other regimens also available):

Day 1: 30 mg divided as 10 mg before breakfast, 5 mg at lunch, 5 mg at dinner, 10 mg at bedtime

Day 2: 5 mg at breakfast, 5 mg at lunch, 5 mg at dinner, 10 mg at bedtime

Day 3: 5 mg 4 times daily (with meals and at bedtime)

Day 4: 5 mg 3 times daily (breakfast, lunch, bedtime)

Day 5: 5 mg 2 times daily (breakfast, bedtime)

Day 6: 5 mg before breakfast

Indication-specific dosing:

Children:

Acute asthma (NIH guidelines, 2007):

0-11 years 1-2 mg/kg/day for 3-10 days (maximum: 60 mg daily)

≥12 years: Refer to Adults dosing

Autoimmune hepatitis (unlabeled use; Czaja, 2002): Initial treatment: 2 mg/kg/day for 2 weeks (maximum: 60 mg daily), followed by a taper over 6-8 weeks to a dose of 0.1-0.2 mg/kg/day or 5 mg daily

Nephrotic syndrome (Pediatric Nephrology Panel recommendations [Hogg, 2000]): Initial: 2 mg/kg/day or 60 mg/m^2/day given every day in 1-3 divided doses (maximum: 80 mg daily) until urine is protein free or for 4-6 weeks; followed by maintenance dose: 2 mg/kg/dose or 40 mg/m^2/dose given every other day in the morning; gradually taper and discontinue after 4-6 weeks. **Note:** No definitive treatment guidelines exist. Dosing is dependent on institution protocols and individual response.

PCP pneumonia (AIDS*info* guidelines, 2008): 1 mg/kg twice daily for 5 days, *followed by* 0.5-1 mg/kg twice daily for 5 days, *followed by* 0.5 mg/kg once daily for 11-21 days

Adolescents and Adults:

PCP pneumonia (AIDS*info* guidelines, 2008): Note: Begin within 72 hours of PCP therapy: 40 mg twice daily for 5 days, *followed by* 40 mg once daily for 5 days, *followed by* 20 mg once daily for 11 days or until antimicrobial regimen is completed

Adults:

Acute asthma (NIH guidelines, 2007): 40-60 mg daily for 3-10 days; administer as single or 2 divided doses

Acute exacerbations of chronic obstructive pulmonary disease (COPD) (unlabeled use for immediate release products; unlabeled dose): 30-40 mg once daily (based on prednisolone equivalency) for 10-14 days (GOLD guidelines, 2013).

Anaphylaxis, adjunctive treatment (Lieberman, 2005): 0.5 mg/kg

Antineoplastic: Usual range: 10 mg daily to 100 mg/m^2/day (depending on indication). **Note:** Details concerning dosing in combination regimens should also be consulted.

Autoimmune hepatitis (unlabeled use; Czaja, 2002): Initial treatment: 60 mg daily for 1 week, *followed by* 40 mg daily for 1 week, *then* 30 mg daily for 2 weeks, *then* 20 mg daily. Half this dose should be given when used in combination with azathioprine

Crohn's disease, moderate/severe (unlabeled use): 40-60 mg daily until resolution of symptoms and resumption of weight gain (usual duration: 7-28 days) (Lichtenstein, 2009)

Dermatomyositis/polymyositis: Oral: 1 mg/kg daily (range: 0.5-1.5 mg/kg/day), often in conjunction with steroid-sparing therapies; depending on response/tolerance, consider slow tapering after 2-8 weeks depending on response; taper regimens vary widely, but often involve 5-10 mg decrements per week and may require 6-12 months to reach a low once-daily or every-other-day dose to prevent disease flare (Briemberg, 2003; Hengstman, 2009; Iorizzo, 2008; Wiendl, 2008)

Giant cell arteritis (unlabeled use): Oral: Initial: 40-60 mg daily; typically requires 1-2 years of treatment, but may begin to taper after 2-3 months; alternative dosing of 30-40 mg daily has demonstrated similar efficacy (Hiratzka, 2010)

Graves' ophthalmopathy prophylaxis (unlabeled use): 0.4-0.5 mg/kg/day, starting 1-3 days after radioactive iodine treatment, and continued for 1 month, then gradually taper over 2 months (Bahn, 2011)

Herpes zoster (unlabeled use; Dworkin, 2007): 60 mg daily for 7 days, *followed by* 30 mg daily for 7 days, *then* 15 mg daily for 7 days

Immune thrombocytopenia (ITP) (American Society of Hematology, 1997): 1-2 mg/kg/day

Lupus nephritis, induction (Hahn, 2012): Oral:

Class III-IV lupus nephritis: 0.5-1 mg/kg/day (after glucocorticoid pulse) tapered after a few weeks to lowest effective dose, in combination with an immunosuppressive agent

Class V lupus nephritis: 0.5 mg/kg/day for 6 months in combination mycophenolate mofetil; if not improved after 6 months, use 0.5-1 mg/kg/day (after a glucocorticoid pulse) for an additional 6 months in combination with cyclophosphamide

Rheumatoid arthritis (American College of Rheumatology, 2002): ≤10 mg daily

Subacute thyroiditis (unlabeled use): 40 mg daily for 1-2 weeks; gradually taper over 2-4 weeks or longer depending on clinical response. **Note:** NSAIDs should be considered first-line therapy in such patients (Bahn, 2011).

Takayasu arteritis (unlabeled use): Oral: Initial: 40-60 mg daily; taper to lowest effective dose when ESR and CRP levels are normal; usual duration: 1-2 years (Hiratzka, 2010)

Thyrotoxicosis (type II amiodarone-induced; unlabeled use): 40 mg daily for 14-28 days; gradually taper over 2-3 months depending on clinical response (Bahn, 2011)

Tuberculosis, severe, paradoxical reactions (unlabeled dose, AIDS*info* guidelines, 2008): 1 mg/kg/day, gradually reduce after 1-2 weeks

Elderly: Use the lowest effective dose

Dosing adjustment in renal impairment: No dosage adjustment provided in manufacturer's labeling. Use with caution.

Hemodialysis effects: Supplemental dose is not necessary.

Dosing adjustment in hepatic impairment: No dosage adjustment provided in manufacturer's labeling. Prednisone is inactive and must be metabolized by the liver to prednisolone. This conversion may be impaired in patients with liver disease, however, prednisolone levels are observed to be higher in patients with severe liver failure than in normal patients. Therefore, compensation for the inadequate conversion of prednisone to prednisolone occurs.

Dosing adjustment in hyperthyroidism: Prednisone dose may need to be increased to achieve adequate therapeutic effects.

Dietary Considerations Should be taken after meals or with food or milk; may require increased dietary intake of pyridoxine, vitamin C, vitamin D, folate, calcium, and phosphorus; may require decreased dietary intake of sodium

Administration Administer with food to decrease GI upset. Delayed release tablet (Rayos®) should be swallowed whole; do not crush or chew.

Monitoring Parameters Blood pressure, blood glucose, electrolytes

Following prolonged use: Bone mass density, growth in children, signs and symptoms of infection, cataract formation, intraocular pressure (use >6 weeks)

Test Interactions Decreased response to skin tests

Additional Information Tapering of corticosteroids after a short course of therapy (<7-10 days) is generally not required unless the disease/inflammatory process is slow to respond. Tapering after prolonged exposure is dependent upon the individual patient, duration of corticosteroid treatments, and size of steroid dose. Recovery of the HPA axis may require several months. Subtle but important HPA axis suppression may be present for as long as several months after a course of as few as 10-14 days duration. Testing of HPA axis (cosyntropin) may be required, and signs/symptoms of adrenal insufficiency should be monitored in patients with a history of use.

Dosage Forms Excipient information presented when available (limited, particularly for generics); consult specific product labeling.

Concentrate, Oral:

PredniSONE Intensol: 5 mg/mL (30 mL) [contains alcohol, usp; unflavored flavor]

Solution, Oral:

Generic: 5 mg/5 mL (5 mL, 120 mL, 500 mL)

Tablet, Oral:

Generic: 1 mg, 2.5 mg, 5 mg, 10 mg, 20 mg, 50 mg

Tablet Delayed Release, Oral:

Rayos: 1 mg, 2 mg, 5 mg

◆ **PredniSONE Intensol** *see* PredniSONE *on page* 1707

Pregabalin (pre GAB a lin)

Brand Names: U.S. Lyrica

Brand Names: Canada GD-Pregabalin; Lyrica®; PMS-Pregabalin; RAN™-Pregabalin; Riva-Pregabalin; Teva-Pregabalin

Index Terms CI-1008; S-(+)-3-isobutylgaba

Pharmacologic Category Analgesic, Miscellaneous; Anticonvulsant, Miscellaneous

Use Management of neuropathic pain associated with diabetic peripheral neuropathy or with spinal cord injury; management of postherpetic neuralgia; adjunctive therapy for partial-onset seizure disorder; management of fibromyalgia

Pregnancy Risk Factor C

Pregnancy Considerations Adverse events were observed in animal reproduction studies. In addition, male-mediated teratogenicity has been observed in animal reproduction studies; implications in humans are not defined. Impaired male and female fertility has been noted in animal studies.

Patients exposed to pregabalin during pregnancy are encouraged to enroll themselves into the North American Antiepileptic Drug (NAAED) Pregnancy Registry by calling 1-888-233-2334. Additional information is available at www.aedpregnancyregistry.org.

Breast-Feeding Considerations It is not known if pregabalin is excreted in breast milk. Due to the potential for serious adverse reactions in the nursing infant, a decision should be made whether to discontinue nursing or to discontinue the drug, taking into account the importance of treatment to the mother.

Medication Guide Available Yes

Contraindications Hypersensitivity to pregabalin or any component of the formulation

Warnings/Precautions Antiepileptics are associated with an increased risk of suicidal behavior/thoughts with use (regardless of indication); patients should be monitored for signs/symptoms of depression, suicidal tendencies, and other unusual behavior changes during therapy and instructed to inform their healthcare provider immediately if symptoms occur.

Angioedema has been reported; may be life threatening; use with caution in patients with a history of angioedema episodes. Concurrent use with other drugs known to cause angioedema (eg, ACE inhibitors) may increase risk. Hypersensitivity reactions, including skin redness, blistering, hives, rash, dyspnea, and wheezing have been reported; discontinue treatment of hypersensitivity occurs. Dizziness and somnolence are commonly reported; effects generally occur shortly after initiation and occur more frequently at higher doses. Patients must be cautioned about performing tasks which require mental alertness (eg, operating machinery or driving). Visual disturbances (blurred vision, decreased acuity and visual field changes) have been associated with pregabalin therapy; patients should be instructed to notify their physician if these effects are noted.

Pregabalin has been associated with increases in CPK and rare cases of rhabdomyolysis. Patients should be instructed to notify their prescriber if unexplained muscle pain, tenderness, or weakness, particularly if fever and/or malaise are associated with these symptoms. Use may cause peripheral edema or weight gain; use with caution in patients with heart failure (NYHA Class III or IV) due to limited data in this patient population. In addition, effect on weight gain/edema may be additive with the thiazolidinedione class of antidiabetic agents; use caution when coadministering these agents, particularly in patients with prior cardiovascular disease. May decrease platelet count or prolong PR interval.

Has been noted to be tumorigenic (increased incidence of hemangiosarcoma) in animal studies; significance of these findings in humans is unknown. Pregabalin has been associated with discontinuation symptoms following abrupt cessation, and increases in seizure frequency (when used as an antiepileptic) may occur. Should not be discontinued abruptly; dosage tapering over at least 1 week is recommended. Use caution in renal impairment; dosage adjustment required.

Adverse Reactions Note: Frequency of adverse effects may be influenced by dose or concurrent therapy. In add-on trials in epilepsy, frequency of CNS and adverse effects were higher than those reported in pain management trials. Range noted below is inclusive of all trials.

>10%:

Cardiovascular: Peripheral edema (≤16%)

Central nervous system: Dizziness (8% to 45%), somnolence (4% to 36%), ataxia (1% to 20%), headache (5% to 14%), fatigue (5% to 11%)

Gastrointestinal: Weight gain (≤16%), xerostomia (1% to 15%)

Neuromuscular & skeletal: Tremor (≤11%)

Ocular: Blurred vision (1% to 12%), diplopia (≤12%)

Miscellaneous: Infection (3% to 14%), accidental injury (2% to 11%)

1% to 10%:

Cardiovascular: Edema (≤8%), chest pain (1% to 4%), hypertension (2%), hypotension (2%)

Central nervous system: Neuropathy (2% to 9%), thinking abnormal (≤9%), confusion (≤7%), euphoria (≤7%), speech disorder (≤7%), attention disturbance (4% to 6%), amnesia (≤6%), incoordination (≤6%), pain (2% to 5%), insomnia (4%), memory impaired (1% to 4%), vertigo (1% to 4%), hypoesthesia (2% to 3%), feeling abnormal (1% to 3%), anxiety (2%), lethargy (1% to 2%), drunk feeling (1% to 2%), disorientation (≤2%), depersonalization (≥1%), fever (≥1%), hypertonia (≥1%), sedation (≥1%), stupor (≥1%), nervousness (≤1%)

Dermatologic: Decubitus ulcer (3%), facial edema (≤3%), bruising (≥1%), pruritus (≥1%)

Endocrine & metabolic: Fluid retention (2% to 3%), hypoglycemia (1% to 3%), libido decreased (≥1%)

Gastrointestinal: Constipation (≤10%), appetite increased (2% to 7%), nausea (5%), flatulence (≤3%), vomiting (1% to 3%), abdominal distension (2%), abdominal pain (≥1%), gastroenteritis (≥1%)

Genitourinary: Incontinence (≤3%), anorgasmia (≥1%), impotence (≥1%), urinary frequency (≥1%)

Hematologic: Thrombocytopenia (≥1%)

Neuromuscular & skeletal: Balance disorder (2% to 9%), abnormal gait (≤8%), weakness (2% to 7%), arthralgia (3% to 6%), twitching (≤5%), muscle spasm (2% to 4%), back pain (≤4%), myoclonus (≤4%), CPK increased (3%), neck pain (3%), pain in extremity (3%), joint swelling (2%), paresthesia (2%), leg cramps (≥1%), myalgia (≥1%), myasthenia (1%)

Ocular: Visual abnormalities (≤5%), eye disorder (≤2%), conjunctivitis (≥1%), nystagmus (≥1%)

Otic: Otitis media (≥1%), tinnitus (≥1%)

Respiratory: Nasopharyngitis (8%), sinusitis (4% to 7%), pharyngolaryngeal pain (1% to 3%), bronchitis (≤3%), dyspnea (≤3%)

Miscellaneous: Flu-like syndrome (1% to 2%), allergic reaction (≥1%)

<1% (Limited to important or life-threatening): Abnormal ejaculation, abscess, acute renal failure, addiction, agitation, albuminuria, alopecia, amenorrhea, anaphylactoid reaction, anemia, angioedema, anisocoria, apathy, aphasia, aphthous stomatitis, apnea, arthrosis, ascites, atelectasis, bladder cancer, blepharitis, blindness, bronchiolitis, cellulitis, cerebellar syndrome, cervicitis, chills, cholecystitis, cholelithiasis, chondrodystrophy, circumoral paresthesia, cogwheel rigidity, colitis, coma, corneal ulcer, crystalluria (urate), delirium, delusions, diarrhea, dry eyes, dysarthria, dysautonomia, dyskinesia, dysmenorrhea, dysphagia, dyspareunia, dystonia, dysuria, eczema, encephalopathy, eosinophilia, epididymitis,

esophageal ulcer, esophagitis, exfoliative dermatitis, exophthalmos, extraocular palsy, extrapyramidal syndrome, eye hemorrhage, female lactation, gastritis, GI hemorrhage, glomerulitis, glucose tolerance decreased, granuloma, Guillain-Barré syndrome, gynecomastia, hallucinations, heart failure, hematuria, hirsutism, hostility, hyperacusis, hyperalgesia, hyperesthesia, hyper-/hypokinesia; hypersensitivity (including skin redness, blistering, hives, rash, dyspnea, and wheezing); hypotonia, intracranial hypertension, iritis, keratitis, keratoconjunctivitis, libido increased, laryngismus, leukopenia, leukorrhea, leukocytosis, lichenoid dermatitis, lung edema, lung fibrosis, lymphadenopathy, malaise, manic reaction, melanosis, melena, miosis, mouth ulcer, mydriasis, myelofibrosis, neck rigidity, nephritis, neuralgia, night blindness, ocular hemorrhage, oliguria, ophthalmoplegia, optic atrophy, pancreatitis, papilledema, paranoid reaction, parosmia, pelvic pain, periodontal abscess, peripheral neuritis, personality disorder, photophobia, photosensitivity, polycythemia, postural hypotension, prothrombin decreased, psychotic depression, ptosis, pulmonary edema, pulmonary fibrosis, purpura, pyelonephritis, rash (vesiculobullous, petechial, purpuric, pustular); rectal hemorrhage, renal calculus, retinal edema, retinal vascular disorder, retroperitoneal fibrosis, rhabdomyolysis, schizophrenic reaction, shock, skin atrophy, skin necrosis, skin nodule, skin ulcer, ST depression, Stevens-Johnson syndrome, subcutaneous nodule, suicide, suicide attempt, syncope, taste loss, taste perversion, thrombocythemia, thrombophlebitis, tongue edema, torticollis, trismus, urinary retention, urticaria, uveitis, ventricular fibrillation

Drug Interactions

Metabolism/Transport Effects None known.

Avoid Concomitant Use

Avoid concomitant use of Pregabalin with any of the following: Azelastine (Nasal); Paraldehyde

Increased Effect/Toxicity

Pregabalin may increase the levels/effects of: Alcohol (Ethyl); Antidiabetic Agents (Thiazolidinedione); Azelastine (Nasal); Buprenorphine; CNS Depressants; Hydrocodone; Methotrimeprazine; Metyrosine; Mirtazapine; Paraldehyde; Pramipexole; ROPINIRole; Rotigotine; Selective Serotonin Reuptake Inhibitors; Zolpidem

The levels/effects of Pregabalin may be increased by: Brimonidine (Topical); Doxylamine; Droperidol; HydrOXYzine; Magnesium Sulfate; Methotrimeprazine; Perampanel; Sodium Oxybate; Tapentadol

Decreased Effect

The levels/effects of Pregabalin may be decreased by: Ketorolac (Nasal); Ketorolac (Systemic); Mefloquine; Orlistat

Ethanol/Nutrition/Herb Interactions

Ethanol: May increase CNS depression; monitor for increased effects with coadministration. Caution patients about effects.

Herb/Nutraceutical: Avoid valerian, St John's wort, kava kava, gotu kola (may increase CNS depression).

Storage/Stability Store at 25°C (77°F); excursions permitted to15°C to 30°C (59°F to 86°F).

Mechanism of Action Binds to alpha$_2$-delta subunit of voltage-gated calcium channels within the CNS and modulates calcium influx at the nerve terminals, thereby inhibiting excitatory neurotransmitter release including glutamate, norepinephrine (noradrenaline), serotonin, dopamine, substance P, and calcitonin gene-related peptide (Gajraj, 2007; McKeage, 2009). Although structurally related to GABA, it does not bind to GABA or benzodiazepine receptors. Exerts antinociceptive and anticonvulsant activity. Pregabalin may also affect descending noradrenergic and serotonergic pain transmission pathways from the brainstem to the spinal cord.

Pharmacodynamics/Kinetics

Onset of action: Pain management: Effects may be noted as early as the first week of therapy.

Distribution: V_d: 0.5 L/kg

Protein binding: 0%

Metabolism: Negligible

Bioavailability: >90%

Half-life elimination: 6.3 hours

Time to peak, plasma: 1.5 hours (3 hours with food)

Excretion: Urine (90% as unchanged drug; minor metabolites)

Dosage Oral: Adults: **Note:** When discontinuing, taper off gradually over at least 1 week.

Fibromyalgia:

U.S. labeling: Initial: 150 mg daily in divided doses (75 mg twice daily); may be increased to 300 mg daily (150 mg twice daily) within 1 week based on tolerability and effect; may be further increased to 450 mg daily (225 mg twice daily). Maximum dose: 450 mg daily (dosages up to 600 mg daily were evaluated with no significant additional benefit and an increase in adverse effects)

Canadian labeling: Initial: 150 mg daily in divided doses (75 mg twice daily); may be increased to 300 mg daily (150 mg twice daily) after 1 week based on tolerability and effect; may be further increased to 450 mg daily (225 mg twice daily). The manufacturer labeling suggests that patients with severe ongoing symptoms may receive up to a maximum of 600 mg daily (300 mg twice daily). However, dosages up to 600 mg daily have been evaluated with no significant additional benefit and an increase in adverse effects.

Neuropathic pain, diabetes-associated:

U.S. labeling: Initial: 150 mg daily in divided doses (50 mg 3 times daily); may be increased within 1 week based on tolerability and effect; maximum dose: 300 mg daily in 3 divided doses (dosages up to 600 mg daily were evaluated with no significant additional benefit and an increase in adverse effects)

Canadian labeling: Initial: 150 mg daily in divided doses (50 mg 3 times daily or 75 mg twice daily); may be increased after 1 week based on tolerability and effect to 300 mg daily (150 mg twice daily). The manufacturer labeling suggests that patients with severe ongoing symptoms may receive up to a maximum of 600 mg daily (300 mg twice daily). However, dosages up to 600 mg daily have been evaluated with no significant additional benefit and an increase in adverse effects.

Neuropathic pain, spinal cord injury associated: Initial: 150 mg daily in divided doses (75 mg twice daily); may be increased to 300 mg daily (150 mg twice daily) within 1 week based on tolerability and effect; further titration to 600 mg daily (300 mg twice daily) after 2-3 weeks may be considered in patients who do not experience sufficient relief of pain provided they are able to tolerate pregabalin. Maximum dose: 600 mg daily

Partial-onset seizures (adjunctive therapy): Initial: 150 mg daily in divided doses (75 mg twice daily or 50 mg 3 times daily); may be increased based on tolerability and effect (optimal titration schedule has not been defined). Maximum dose: 600 mg daily

Postherpetic neuralgia: Initial: 150 mg daily in divided doses (75 mg twice daily or 50 mg 3 times daily); may be increased to 300 mg daily within 1 week based on tolerability and effect; further titration (to 600 mg daily) after 2-4 weeks may be considered in patients who do not experience sufficient relief of pain provided they are able to tolerate pregabalin. Maximum dose: 600 mg daily

Dosage adjustment in renal impairment: Renal function may be estimated using the Cockcroft-Gault formula. Then determine recommended dosage regimen based on the indication-specific total daily dose for normal renal function (Cl_{cr} ≥60 mL/minute). For example, if the indication-specific daily dose is 450 mg daily for normal renal function, the daily dose should be reduced to 225 mg daily (in 2-3 divided doses) for a creatinine clearance of 30-60 mL/minute (see table).

Pregabalin Renal Impairment Dosing

Cl_{cr} (mL/minute)	Total Pregabalin Daily Dose (mg/day)				Dosing Frequency
≥60 (normal renal function)	150	300	450	600	2-3 divided doses
30-60	75	150	225	300	2-3 divided doses
15-30	25-50	75	100-150	150	1-2 divided doses
<15	25	25-50	50-75	75	Single daily dose

Posthemodialysis supplementary dosage (as a single additional dose):
25 mg/day schedule: Single supplementary dose of 25 mg **or** 50 mg
25-50 mg/day schedule: Single supplementary dose of 50 mg **or** 75 mg
50-75 mg/day schedule: Single supplementary dose of 75 mg **or** 100 mg
75 mg/day schedule: Single supplementary dose of 100 mg **or** 150 mg

Dosage adjustment in hepatic impairment: No dosage adjustment provided in manufacturer's labeling. However, no adjustment expected since undergoes minimal hepatic metabolism.

Dietary Considerations May be taken with or without food.

Administration May be administered with or without food.

Monitoring Parameters Measures of efficacy (pain intensity/seizure frequency); degree of sedation; symptoms of myopathy or ocular disturbance; weight gain/edema; skin integrity (in patients with diabetes); suicidality (eg, suicidal thoughts, depression, behavioral changes)

Dosage Forms Excipient information presented when available (limited, particularly for generics); consult specific product labeling.

Capsule, Oral:

Lyrica: 25 mg, 50 mg, 75 mg, 100 mg, 150 mg, 200 mg, 225 mg, 300 mg

Solution, Oral:

Lyrica: 20 mg/mL (473 mL) [contains methylparaben, propylparaben]

Controlled Substance C-V

- **Pregnenedione** *see* Progesterone *on page 1725*
- **Pregnyl** *see* Chorionic Gonadotropin (Human) *on page 419*
- **Pregnyl® (Can)** *see* Chorionic Gonadotropin (Human) *on page 419*
- **Prelone** *see* PrednisoLONE (Systemic) *on page 1704*
- **Premarin** *see* Estrogens (Conjugated/Equine, Systemic) *on page 770*
- **Premarin** *see* Estrogens (Conjugated/Equine, Topical) *on page 773*
- **Premarin® (Can)** *see* Estrogens (Conjugated/Equine, Systemic) *on page 770*
- **Premarin® (Can)** *see* Estrogens (Conjugated/Equine, Topical) *on page 773*
- **Premium Activated Charcoal [OTC] (Can)** *see* Charcoal, Activated *on page 401*
- **Preparation H Hydrocortisone [OTC]** *see* Hydrocortisone (Topical) *on page 1011*
- **Prepidil** *see* Dinoprostone *on page 619*
- **Prepidil® (Can)** *see* Dinoprostone *on page 619*
- **Prepopik™** *see* Sodium Picosulfate, Magnesium Oxide, and Citric Acid *on page 1925*
- **Pressyn® (Can)** *see* Vasopressin *on page 2172*
- **Pressyn® AR (Can)** *see* Vasopressin *on page 2172*
- **Pretz [OTC]** *see* Sodium Chloride *on page 1914*
- **Pretz Irrigation [OTC]** *see* Sodium Chloride *on page 1914*
- **Prevacid** *see* Lansoprazole *on page 1170*
- **Prevacid® (Can)** *see* Lansoprazole *on page 1170*
- **Prevacid 24HR [OTC]** *see* Lansoprazole *on page 1170*
- **Prevacid® FasTab (Can)** *see* Lansoprazole *on page 1170*
- **Prevacid SoluTab** *see* Lansoprazole *on page 1170*
- **Prevalite** *see* Cholestyramine Resin *on page 418*
- **Prevex® B (Can)** *see* Betamethasone *on page 247*
- **Prevex® HC (Can)** *see* Hydrocortisone (Topical) *on page 1011*
- **PreviDent®** *see* Fluoride *on page 880*
- **PreviDent® 5000 Booster** *see* Fluoride *on page 880*
- **PreviDent® 5000 Booster Plus** *see* Fluoride *on page 880*
- **PreviDent® 5000 Dry Mouth** *see* Fluoride *on page 880*
- **PreviDent® 5000 Plus®** *see* Fluoride *on page 880*
- **PreviDent® 5000 Sensitive** *see* Fluoride *on page 880*
- **Previfem** *see* Ethinyl Estradiol and Norgestimate *on page 795*
- **Prevnar 13** *see* Pneumococcal Conjugate Vaccine (13-Valent) *on page 1661*
- **Prevpac®** *see* Lansoprazole, Amoxicillin, and Clarithromycin *on page 1173*
- **Prezista** *see* Darunavir *on page 547*
- **Prezista® (Can)** *see* Darunavir *on page 547*
- **Prialt** *see* Ziconotide *on page 2224*
- **Priftin** *see* Rifapentine *on page 1813*
- **Priftin® (Can)** *see* Rifapentine *on page 1813*
- **Prilocaine and Lidocaine** *see* Lidocaine and Prilocaine *on page 1213*
- **PriLOSEC** *see* Omeprazole *on page 1505*
- **PriLOSEC OTC [OTC]** *see* Omeprazole *on page 1505*
- **Primaclone** *see* Primidone *on page 1715*
- **Primacor® (Can)** *see* Milrinone *on page 1372*

Primaquine (PRIM a kween)

Index Terms Primaquine Phosphate; Prymaccone

Pharmacologic Category Aminoquinoline (Antimalarial)

Use Prevention of relapse of *P. vivax* malaria

Unlabeled Use Prevention of relapse of *P. ovale* malaria; prevention of malaria; treatment of uncomplicated *P. vivax* and *P. ovale* malaria; treatment of *Pneumocystis jirovecii* pneumonia (PCP); prevention of malaria

Pregnancy Considerations Animal reproduction studies have not been conducted. Primaquine use is not recommended in pregnant women per CDC Guidelines. Consult current CDC guidelines for the treatment of malaria during pregnancy.

Breast-Feeding Considerations It is not known if primaquine is excreted in breast milk. If therapy is needed, the mother and infant should be tested for G6PD deficiency; primaquine before primaquine is given to a woman who is breast-feeding. It may be used in breast-feeding mothers and infants with normal G6PD levelsconcentrations (CDC, 2012).

Contraindications Use in acutely-ill patients who have a tendency to develop granulocytopenia (eg, rheumatoid arthritis, SLE); concurrent use with other medications causing hemolytic anemia or myeloid bone marrow suppression; concurrent use with or recent use of quinacrine

Warnings/Precautions Use with caution in patients with G6PD deficiency (hemolytic anemia may occur), NADH methemoglobin reductase deficiency (methemoglobinemia may occur); do not exceed recommended dosage and duration. Moderate-to-severe hemolytic reactions may occur in individuals with G6PD deficiency and personal or familial history of favism. Geographic regions with a high prevalence of G6PD deficiency (eg, Africa, southern Europe, Mediterranean region, Middle East, southeast Asia, Oceania) are associated with a higher incidence of hemolytic anemia. Promptly discontinue with signs of hemolytic anemia (darkening of urine, marked fall in hemoglobin or erythrocyte count). The CDC recommends screening for G6PD deficiency prior to therapy initiation. Anemia, methemoglobinemia, and leukopenia have been associated with primaquine use; monitor during treatment. **[U.S. Boxed Warning]: Should be prescribed only by physicians familiar with its use.**

Adverse Reactions Frequency not defined.

Cardiovascular: Arrhythmias (rare)

Central nervous system: Headache

Dermatologic: Pruritus

Gastrointestinal: Abdominal cramps, dyspepsia, nausea, vomiting

Hematologic: Agranulocytosis, anemia, hemolytic anemia (in patients with G6PD deficiency), leukopenia, leukocytosis, methemoglobinemia (in NADH-methemoglobin reductase-deficient individuals)

Ocular: Interference with visual accommodation

Drug Interactions

Metabolism/Transport Effects Substrate of CYP2D6 (major), CYP3A4 (major); **Note:** Assignment of Major/Minor substrate status based on clinically relevant drug interaction potential; **Inhibits** CYP1A2 (strong), CYP2D6 (weak), CYP3A4 (weak); **Induces** CYP1A2 (weak/moderate)

Avoid Concomitant Use

Avoid concomitant use of Primaquine with any of the following: Agomelatine; Artemether; Lumefantrine; Mefloquine; Pimozide; Pirfenidone; Pomalidomide

Increased Effect/Toxicity

Primaquine may increase the levels/effects of: Agomelatine; Antipsychotic Agents (Phenothiazines); ARIPiprazole; Bendamustine; Beta-Blockers; Cardiac Glycosides; CloZAPine; CYP1A2 Substrates; Dapsone (Systemic); Dapsone (Topical); Dofetilide; Lomitapide; Lumefantrine; Mefloquine; Pimozide; Pirfenidone; Pomalidomide; Prilocaine; Sodium Nitrite

The levels/effects of Primaquine may be increased by: Abiraterone Acetate; Artemether; CYP2D6 Inhibitors (Moderate); CYP2D6 Inhibitors (Strong); Dapsone (Systemic); Darunavir; Mefloquine; Nitric Oxide

Decreased Effect

Primaquine may decrease the levels/effects of: Anthelmintics

The levels/effects of Primaquine may be decreased by: Bosentan; CYP3A4 Inducers (Strong); Dabrafenib; Deferasirox; Herbs (CYP3A4 Inducers); Mitotane; Peginterferon Alfa-2b; Tocilizumab

Ethanol/Nutrition/Herb Interactions Ethanol: Avoid ethanol (due to GI irritation).

Mechanism of Action Eliminates the primary tissue exoerythrocytic forms of *P. ovale* and *P. vivax*; disrupts mitochondria and binds to DNA

Pharmacodynamics/Kinetics

Absorption: Well absorbed

Metabolism: Hepatic to carboxyprimaquine (active)

Half-life elimination: 3.7-9.6 hours

Time to peak, serum: 1-2 hours

Excretion: Urine (small amounts as unchanged drug)

Dosage Oral: Dosage expressed as mg of base (15 mg base = 26.3 mg primaquine phosphate). **Note:** The CDC requires screening for G6PD deficiency prior to initiating treatment with primaquine.

Malaria:

Treatment or prevention of relapse of *P. vivax* malaria:

Adults: 30 mg once daily for 14 days

Treatment of uncomplicated *P. vivax* and *P. ovale* malaria (unlabeled use):

Children: 0.5 mg /kg (maximum: 30 mg/day) daily for 14 days with chloroquine or hydroxychloroquine (CDC, 2011)

Adults: 30 mg once daily for 14 days with chloroquine or hydroxychloroquine; alternative regimen (for mild G6PD deficiency or as an alternative to daily regimen): 45 mg once weekly for 8 weeks (use only after consultation with an infectious disease/tropical medicine expert) (CDC, 2011)

Chemoprophylaxis (unlabeled use):

Children: 0.5 mg/kg once daily (maximum dose: 30 mg/day); start 1-2 days prior to travel and continue for 7 days after departure from malaria-endemic area (CDC, 2012)

Adults: 30 mg once daily; start 1-2 days prior to travel and continue for 7 days after departure from malaria-endemic area (CDC, 2012)

Presumptive antirelapse therapy for *P. vivax* and *P. ovale* malaria (unlabeled use):

Children: 0.5 mg/kg (maximum dose: 30 mg/day) once daily for 14 days after departure from malaria-endemic area (CDC, 2012)

Adults: 30 mg once daily for 14 days after departure from malaria-endemic area (CDC, 2012)

Pneumocystis jirovecii **pneumonia treatment (unlabeled use):** CDC recommendation (as alternative):

Children: 0.3 mg/kg once daily for 21 days (in combination with clindamycin)

Adults: 30 mg once daily for 21 days (in combination with clindamycin)

Dosage adjustment in renal impairment: No dosage adjustment provided in manufacturer's labeling.

Dosage adjustment in hepatic impairment: No dosage adjustment provided in manufacturer's labeling.

Administration Take with meals to decrease adverse GI effects. Drug has a bitter taste.

Monitoring Parameters Periodic CBC, visual color check of urine, glucose, electrolytes; if hemolysis suspected, monitor CBC, haptoglobin, peripheral smear, urinalysis dipstick for occult blood, G6PD deficiency screening (prior to initiating treatment; CDC recommendation)

Dosage Forms Excipient information presented when available (limited, particularly for generics); consult specific product labeling.

Tablet, Oral, as phosphate:

Generic: 26.3 mg

Extemporaneous Preparations A 6 mg base/5 mL oral suspension may be made using tablets. Crush ten 15 mg base tablets and reduce to a fine powder. In small amounts, add a total of 10 mL Carboxymethylcellulose 1.5% and mix to a uniform paste; mix while adding Simple Syrup, NF to **almost** 125 mL; transfer to a calibrated bottle, rinse mortar with vehicle, and add quantity of vehicle sufficient to make 125 mL. Label "shake well" and "refrigerate". Stable 7 days.

Nahata MC, Pai VB, and Hipple TF, *Pediatric Drug Formulations*, 5th ed, Cincinnati, OH: Harvey Whitney Books Co, 2004.

◆ **Primaquine Phosphate** *see* Primaquine *on page 1713*

◆ **Primaxin® I.M. [DSC]** *see* Imipenem and Cilastatin *on page 1052*

◆ **Primaxin® I.V.** *see* Imipenem and Cilastatin *on page 1052*

◆ **Primaxin® I.V. Infusion (Can)** *see* Imipenem and Cilastatin *on page 1052*

Primidone (PRI mi done)

Brand Names: U.S. Mysoline

Brand Names: Canada Apo-Primidone®

Index Terms Desoxyphenobarbital; Primaclone

Pharmacologic Category Anticonvulsant, Miscellaneous; Barbiturate

Use Management of grand mal, psychomotor, and focal seizures

Unlabeled Use Benign familial tremor (essential tremor)

Pregnancy Considerations Primidone and its metabolites (PEMA, phenobarbital, and p-hydroxyphenobarbital) cross the placenta; neonatal serum concentrations at birth are similar to those in the mother. Withdrawal symptoms may occur in the neonate and may be delayed due to the long half-life of primidone and its metabolites. Use may be associated with birth defects and adverse events; the use of folic acid throughout pregnancy and vitamin K during the last month of pregnancy is recommended. Epilepsy itself, number of medications, genetic factors, or a combination of these probably influence the teratogenicity of anticonvulsant therapy.

Patients exposed to primidone during pregnancy are encouraged to enroll themselves into the NAAED Pregnancy Registry by calling 1-888-233-2334. Additional information is available at www.aedpregnancyregistry.org.

Breast-Feeding Considerations Primidone and its metabolites (PEMA, phenobarbital, and p-hydroxyphenobarbital) are found in breast milk (variable concentrations). The manufacturer recommends discontinuing breast-feeding if undue drowsiness and somnolence occur in the newborn.

Medication Guide Available Yes

Contraindications Hypersensitivity to phenobarbital; porphyria

Warnings/Precautions Antiepileptics are associated with an increased risk of suicidal behavior/thoughts with use (regardless of indication); patients should be monitored for signs/symptoms of depression, suicidal tendencies, and other unusual behavior changes during therapy and instructed to inform their healthcare provider immediately if symptoms occur.

Use with caution in patients with renal or hepatic impairment, pulmonary insufficiency; abrupt withdrawal may precipitate status epilepticus. Potential for drug dependency exists. Do not administer to patients in acute pain. Use caution in elderly, debilitated, or pediatric patients - may cause paradoxical responses. May cause CNS depression, which may impair physical or mental abilities. Patients must cautioned about performing tasks which require mental alertness (eg, operating machinery or driving). Effects with other sedative drugs or ethanol may be potentiated. Use with caution in patients with depression or suicidal tendencies, or in patients with a history of drug abuse. Tolerance or psychological and physical dependence may occur with prolonged use. Primidone's metabolite, phenobarbital, has been associated with cognitive deficits in children. Use with caution in patients with hypoadrenalism.

Adverse Reactions Frequency not defined.

Central nervous system: Ataxia, drowsiness, emotional disturbances, fatigue, hyperirritability, suicidal ideation, vertigo

Dermatologic: Morbilliform skin eruptions

Gastrointestinal: Anorexia, nausea, vomiting

Genitourinary: Impotence

Hematologic: Agranulocytosis, granulocytopenia, megaloblastic anemia (idiosyncratic), red cell aplasia/hypoplasia

Ocular: Diplopia, nystagmus

Drug Interactions

Metabolism/Transport Effects **Induces** CYP1A2 (strong), CYP2B6 (strong), CYP2C8 (strong), CYP2C9 (strong), CYP3A4 (strong), P-glycoprotein

Avoid Concomitant Use

Avoid concomitant use of Primidone with any of the following: Abiraterone Acetate; Apixaban; Artemether; Axitinib; Azelastine (Nasal); Bedaquiline; Boceprevir; Bortezomib; Bosutinib; Cabozantinib; CloZAPine; Crizotinib; Dabigatran Etexilate; Dienogest; Dolutegravir; Dronedarone; Enzalutamide; Etravirine; Everolimus; Ibrutinib; Itraconazole; Ivacaftor; Lapatinib; Lumefantrine; Lurasidone; Macitentan; Mifepristone; NIFEdipine; Nilotinib; Nisoldipine; Paraldehyde; PAZOPanib; Perampanel; Pirfenidone; Pomalidomide; PONATinib; Praziquantel; Ranolazine; Regorafenib; Rilpivirine; Rivaroxaban; Roflumilast; RomiDEPsin; Simeprevir; Sofosbuvir; SORAfenib; Telaprevir; Ticagrelor; Tofacitinib; Tolvaptan; Toremifene; Ulipristal; Vandetanib; Vemurafenib; VinCRIStine (Liposomal)

Increased Effect/Toxicity

Primidone may increase the levels/effects of: Alcohol (Ethyl); Azelastine (Nasal); Barbiturates; Buprenorphine; Clarithromycin; CNS Depressants; Hydrocodone; Ifosfamide; Methotrimeprazine; Metyrosine; Mirtazapine; Paraldehyde; Pramipexole; ROPINIRole; Rotigotine; Selective Serotonin Reuptake Inhibitors; Valproic Acid and Derivatives; Zolpidem

The levels/effects of Primidone may be increased by: Brimonidine (Topical); Carbonic Anhydrase Inhibitors; Clarithromycin; Cosyntropin; Dexmethylphenidate; Doxylamine; Droperidol; Felbamate; HydrOXYzine; Magnesium Sulfate; Methotrimeprazine; Methylphenidate; Sodium Oxybate; Tapentadol; Valproic Acid and Derivatives

Decreased Effect

Primidone may decrease the levels/effects of: Abiraterone Acetate; Afatinib; Apixaban; ARIPiprazole; Artemether; Axitinib; Bazedoxifene; Bedaquiline; Bendamustine; Boceprevir; Bortezomib; Bosutinib; Brentuximab Vedotin; Cabozantinib; Canagliflozin; Clarithromycin; CloZAPine; Contraceptives (Progestins); Corticosteroids (Systemic); Crizotinib; CYP1A2 Substrates; CYP2B6 Substrates; CYP2C8 Substrates; CYP2C9 Substrates; CYP3A4 Substrates; Dabigatran Etexilate; Dasatinib; Diclofenac (Systemic); Dienogest; Dolutegravir; Dronedarone; Enzalutamide; Eslicarbazepine; Etravirine; Everolimus; Exemestane; Felbamate; Gefitinib; GuanFACINE; Ibrutinib; Imatinib; Itraconazole; Ivacaftor; Ixabepilone; LamoTRIgine; Lapatinib; Linagliptin; Lumefantrine; Lurasidone; Macitentan; Maraviroc; Methadone; Mifepristone; NIFEdipine; Nilotinib; Nisoldipine; PAZOPanib; Perampanel; P-glycoprotein/ABCB1 Substrates; Pirfenidone; Pomalidomide; PONATinib;

Praziquantel; QUEtiapine; QuiNIDine; Ranolazine; Regorafenib; Rilpivirine; Rivaroxaban; Roflumilast; RomiDEPsin; Rufinamide; Saxagliptin; Simeprevir; Sofosbuvir; SORAfenib; SUNItinib; Tadalafil; Telaprevir; Ticagrelor; Tofacitinib; Tolvaptan; Toremifene; Treprostinil; Ulipristal; Vandetanib; Vemurafenib; VinCRIStine (Liposomal); Vortioxetine; Zuclopenthixol

The levels/effects of Primidone may be decreased by: Carbonic Anhydrase Inhibitors; Folic Acid; Fosphenytoin; Ketorolac (Nasal); Ketorolac (Systemic); Leucovorin Calcium-Levoleucovorin; Levomefolate; Mefloquine; Methylfolate; Orlistat; Phenytoin

Ethanol/Nutrition/Herb Interactions

Ethanol: May increase CNS depression; monitor for increased effects with coadministration. Caution patients about effects.

Food: Protein-deficient diets increase duration of action of primidone.

Herb/Nutraceutical: Avoid valerian, St John's wort, kava kava, gotu kola (may increase CNS depression).

Storage/Stability Store at 20°C to 25°C (68°F to 77°F).

Mechanism of Action Decreases neuron excitability, raises seizure threshold similar to phenobarbital; primidone has two active metabolites, phenobarbital and phenylethylmalonamide (PEMA); PEMA may enhance the activity of phenobarbital

Pharmacodynamics/Kinetics

Absorption: 60% to 80%

Distribution: Adults: V_d: 0.6 L/kg

Protein binding: 30%

Metabolism: Hepatic to phenobarbital (active) by oxidation and to phenylethylmalonamide (PEMA; active) by scission of the heterocyclic ring

Half-life elimination (age dependent): Primidone: Mean: 5-15 hours (variable); PEMA: 16 hours (variable)

Time to peak, serum: ~3 hours (variable)

Excretion: Urine (40% as unchanged drug; the remainder is unconjugated PEMA, phenobarbital and its metabolites)

Dosage Oral:

Seizure disorders:

Children <8 years: Initial: Days 1-3: 50 mg/day given at bedtime; days 4-6: 50 mg twice daily; days 7-9: 100 mg twice daily; usual dose: 375-750 mg/day in 3-4 divided doses (10-25 mg/kg/day)

Children ≥8 years and Adults: Days 1-3: 100-125 mg/day at bedtime; days 4-6: 100-125 twice daily; days 7-9: 100-125 mg 3 times daily; usual dose: 750-1500 mg/day in divided doses 3-4 times/day with maximum dosage of 2 g/day

Patients already receiving other anticonvulsants: Initial: 100-125 mg at bedtime; gradually increase to maintenance dose as other drug is gradually decreased, continue until desired level obtained or other drug completely withdrawn. If goal is monotherapy, conversion should be completed over ≥2 weeks.

Essential tremor (unlabeled use): Adults: Initial 12.5-25 mg/day at bedtime; titrate up to 250 mg/day in 1-2 divided doses; doses up to 750 mg/day may be beneficial

Dosage adjustment in renal impairment: Adults: No dosage adjustment provided in manufacturer's labeling. However, the following guidelines have been used by some clinicians (Aronoff, 2007): **Note:** Avoid in renal failure if possible; due to active metabolites with long half-lives and complex kinetics:

Cl_{cr} ≥50 mL/minute: Administer every 12 hours

Cl_{cr} 10-50 mL/minute: Administer every 12-24 hours

Cl_{cr} <10 mL/minute: Administer every 24 hours

Hemodialysis: Administer dose postdialysis

Dosage adjustment in hepatic impairment: No dosage adjustment provided in manufacturer's labeling. However, increased side effects may occur in severe liver disease; monitor plasma levels and adjust dose accordingly.

Dietary Considerations Folic acid: Low erythrocyte and CSF folate concentrations. Megaloblastic anemia has been reported. To avoid folic acid deficiency and megaloblastic anemia, some clinicians recommend giving patients on anticonvulsants prophylactic doses of folic acid and cyanocobalamin.

Monitoring Parameters Serum primidone and phenobarbital concentration, neurological status. Due to CNS effects, monitor closely when initiating drug in elderly. Monitor CBC and sequential multiple analysis-12 (SMA-12) at 6-month intervals to compare with baseline obtained at start of therapy. Monitor for suicidality (eg, suicidal thoughts, depression, behavioral changes). Since elderly metabolize phenobarbital at a slower rate than younger adults, it is suggested to measure both primidone and phenobarbital levels together.

Reference Range Therapeutic: Children <5 years: 7-10 mcg/mL (SI: 32-46 micromole/L); Adults: 5-12 mcg/mL (SI: 23-55 micromole/L); toxic effects rarely present with levels <10 mcg/mL (SI: 46 micromole/L) if phenobarbital concentrations are low. Dosage of primidone is adjusted with reference mostly to the phenobarbital level; Toxic: >15 mcg/mL (SI: >69 micromole/L)

Dosage Forms Excipient information presented when available (limited, particularly for generics); consult specific product labeling.

Tablet, Oral:

Mysoline: 50 mg, 250 mg [scored]

Generic: 50 mg, 250 mg

Dosage Forms: Canada Excipient information presented when available (limited, particularly for generics); consult specific product labeling.

Tablet, oral:

Apo-Primidone®: 125 mg, 250 mg

◆ **Primlev** *see* Oxycodone and Acetaminophen *on page* 1538

◆ **Primsol** *see* Trimethoprim *on page* 2129

◆ **Prinivil** *see* Lisinopril *on page* 1226

◆ **Prinzide** *see* Lisinopril and Hydrochlorothiazide *on page* 1229

◆ **Priorix (Can)** *see* Measles, Mumps, and Rubella Virus Vaccine *on page* 1272

◆ **Priorix-Tetra (Can)** *see* Measles, Mumps, Rubella, and Varicella Virus Vaccine *on page* 1273

◆ **PrismaSol** *see* Electrolyte Solution, Renal Replacement *on page* 691

◆ **Pristiq** *see* Desvenlafaxine *on page* 579

◆ **Privigen** *see* Immune Globulin *on page* 1059

◆ **Privine® [OTC]** *see* Naphazoline (Nasal) *on page* 1425

◆ **ProAir HFA** *see* Albuterol *on page* 61

◆ **ProAmatine** *see* Midodrine *on page* 1363

◆ **PRO-Amiodarone (Can)** *see* Amiodarone *on page* 101

◆ **Pro-Amox-250 (Can)** *see* Amoxicillin *on page* 116

◆ **Pro-Amox-500 (Can)** *see* Amoxicillin *on page* 116

◆ **PRO-Azithromycin (Can)** *see* Azithromycin (Systemic) *on page* 214

Probenecid (proe BEN e sid)

Brand Names: Canada Benuryl™

Index Terms Benemid [DSC]

Pharmacologic Category Uricosuric Agent

Use Treatment of hyperuricemia associated with gout or gouty arthritis; prolongation and elevation of beta-lactam plasma levels (eg, uncomplicated gonococcal infection)

Unlabeled Use Prolongation and elevation of beta-lactam plasma levels (eg, neurosyphilis, pelvic inflammatory disease)

Pregnancy Considerations Probenecid crosses the placenta. Based on available data, an increased risk of adverse fetal events have not been reported (Gutman, 2012).

Contraindications Hypersensitivity to probenecid or any component of the formulation; small- or large-dose aspirin therapy; blood dyscrasias; uric acid kidney stones; children <2 years of age; initiation during an acute gout attack

Warnings/Precautions Use with caution in patients with peptic ulcer. Salicylates may diminish the therapeutic effect of probenecid. This effect may be more pronounced with high, chronic doses, however, the manufacturer recommends the use of an alternative analgesic even in place of small doses of aspirin. Use of probenecid with penicillin in patients with renal insufficiency is not recommended. Probenecid monotherapy may not be effective in patients with a creatinine clearance <30 mL/minute. Probenecid may increase the serum concentration of methotrexate. Avoid concomitant use of probenecid and methotrexate if possible. If used together, consider lower methotrexate doses and monitor for methotrexate toxicity. May cause exacerbation of acute gouty attack. If hypersensitivity reaction or anaphylaxis occurs, discontinue medication. Use caution in patients with G6PD deficiency; may increase risk for hemolytic anemia.

Adverse Reactions Frequency not defined.

Cardiovascular: Flushing

Central nervous system: Dizziness, fever, headache

Dermatologic: Alopecia, dermatitis, pruritus, rash

Gastrointestinal: Anorexia, dyspepsia, gastroesophageal reflux, nausea, sore gums, vomiting

Genitourinary: Hematuria, polyuria

Hematologic: Anemia, aplastic anemia, hemolytic anemia (in G6PD deficiency), leukopenia

Hepatic: Hepatic necrosis

Neuromuscular & skeletal: Costovertebral pain, gouty arthritis (acute)

Renal: Nephrotic syndrome, renal colic

Miscellaneous: Anaphylaxis, hypersensitivity

Drug Interactions

Metabolism/Transport Effects **Inhibits** CYP2C19 (weak), UGT1A6

Avoid Concomitant Use

Avoid concomitant use of Probenecid with any of the following: Doripenem; Ketorolac (Nasal); Ketorolac (Systemic); Meropenem; Pegloticase

Increased Effect/Toxicity

Probenecid may increase the levels/effects of: Acetaminophen; Cefotaxime; Cephalosporins; Dapsone (Systemic); Deferiprone; Doripenem; Ertapenem; Ganciclovir-Valganciclovir; Gemifloxacin; Imipenem; Ketoprofen; Ketorolac (Nasal); Ketorolac (Systemic); Loop Diuretics; LORazepam; Meropenem; Methotrexate; Mycophenolate; Nitrofurantoin; Nonsteroidal Anti-Inflammatory Agents; Oseltamivir; Pegloticase; Penicillins; PRALAtrexate; Quinolone Antibiotics; Sodium Benzoate; Sodium Phenylacetate; Sulfonylureas; Theophylline Derivatives; Urea Cycle Disorder Agents; Zidovudine

Decreased Effect

Probenecid may decrease the levels/effects of: Loop Diuretics

The levels/effects of Probenecid may be decreased by: Salicylates

Storage/Stability Store at 20°C to 25°C (68°F to 77°F). Protect from light.

Mechanism of Action Competitively inhibits the reabsorption of uric acid at the proximal convoluted tubule, thereby promoting its excretion and reducing serum uric acid levels; increases plasma levels of weak organic acids (penicillins, cephalosporins, or other beta-lactam antibiotics) by competitively inhibiting their renal tubular secretion

Pharmacodynamics/Kinetics

Onset of action: Effect on penicillin levels: 2 hours

Absorption: Rapid and complete

Metabolism: Hepatic

Half-life elimination (dose dependent): Normal renal function: 6-12 hours

Time to peak, serum: 2-4 hours

Excretion: Urine

Dosage Oral:

Children:

<2 years: Contraindicated

2-14 years: Prolong penicillin serum levels: Initial: 25 mg/kg, then 40 mg/kg/day in 4 divided doses (maximum: 500 mg/dose)

Gonorrhea: >50 kg: Refer to adult dosing.

Adults:

Hyperuricemia with gout: 250 mg twice daily for 1 week; may increase to 500 mg twice daily; if needed, may increase to a maximum of 2 g/day (increase dosage in 500 mg increments every 4 weeks). If serum uric acid levels are within normal limits and gout attacks have been absent for 6 months, daily dosage may be reduced by 500 mg every 6 months.

Prolong penicillin serum levels: 500 mg 4 times/day. **Note:** Dosing per manufacturer, see indication-specific dosing.

Gonorrhea, uncomplicated infections of cervix, urethra, and rectum: Oral: 1 g once with cefoxitin 2 g I.M. (CDC, 2010)

Pelvic inflammatory disease (unlabeled use): Oral: 1 g once with cefoxitin 2 g I.M. plus doxycycline (CDC, 2010)

Neurosyphilis (unlabeled use): Oral: 500 mg 4 times/day with procaine penicillin 2.4 million units/day I.M for 10-14 days (CDC, 2010). **Note:** Penicillin G aqueous I.V. is the preferred agent.

Dosing adjustment in renal impairment: Cl_{cr} <30 mL/minute: Avoid use.

Dosing adjustment in hepatic impairment: No dosage adjustment provided in manufacturer's labeling.

Dietary Considerations Drug may cause GI upset; take with food if GI upset. Drink plenty of fluids.

Administration Administer with food or antacids to minimize GI effects.

Monitoring Parameters Uric acid, renal function, CBC

Reference Range

Uric acid, serum: An increase occurs during childhood

Adults:

Males: 3.4-7 mg/dL or slightly more

Females: 2.4-6 mg/dL or slightly more

Target: <6 mg/dL

Values >7 mg/dL are sometimes arbitrarily regarded as hyperuricemia, but there is no sharp line between normals and the serum uric acid of those with clinical gout. Normal ranges cannot be adjusted for purine ingestion, but high-purine diet increases uric acid. Uric acid may be increased with body size, exercise, and stress.

Test Interactions False-positive glucosuria with Clinitest®, a falsely high determination of theophylline has occurred and the renal excretion of phenolsulfonphthalein 17-ketosteroids and bromsulfophthalein (BSP) may be inhibited

Additional Information Avoid fluctuation in uric acid (increase or decrease); may precipitate gout attack. The manufacturer recommends the use of sodium bicarbonate (3-7.5 g daily) or potassium citrate (7.5 g daily) is suggested until serum uric acid normalizes and tophaceous deposits disappear.

Dosage Forms Excipient information presented when available (limited, particularly for generics); consult specific product labeling.

Tablet, Oral:

Generic: 500 mg

◆ **Probenecid and Colchicine** *see* Colchicine and Probenecid *on page 487*

◆ **PRO-Bicalutamide (Can)** *see* Bicalutamide *on page 258*

◆ **PRO-Bisoprolol (Can)** *see* Bisoprolol *on page 261*

Procainamide (pro KANE a mide)

Brand Names: Canada Apo-Procainamide®; Procainamide Hydrochloride Injection, USP; Procan SR®

Index Terms PCA (error-prone abbreviation); Procainamide Hydrochloride; Procaine Amide Hydrochloride; Procanbid; Pronestyl

Pharmacologic Category Antiarrhythmic Agent, Class Ia

Additional Appendix Information

Adult ACLS Algorithms *on page 2363*

Beers Criteria – Potentially Inappropriate Medications for Geriatrics *on page 2368*

Dosing Considerations for the Critically-Ill Patient With Morbid Obesity *on page 2379*

Pediatric ALS (PALS) Algorithms *on page 2359*

Use

Intravenous: Treatment of life-threatening ventricular arrhythmias

Oral (Canadian labeling; not available in U.S.): Treatment of supraventricular arrhythmias. **Note:** In the treatment of atrial fibrillation, use only when preferred treatment is ineffective or cannot be used. Use in paroxysmal atrial tachycardia when reflex stimulation or other measures are ineffective.

Unlabeled Use

Paroxysmal supraventricular tachycardia (PSVT); prevent recurrence of ventricular tachycardia; symptomatic premature ventricular contractions

ACLS guidelines: I.V.: Treatment of the following arrhythmias in patients with preserved left ventricular function: Stable monomorphic VT; pre-excited atrial fibrillation; stable wide complex regular tachycardia (likely VT)

PALS guidelines: I.V.: Tachycardia with pulses and poor perfusion (probable SVT [unresponsive to vagal maneuvers and adenosine or synchronized cardioversion]; probable VT [unresponsive to synchronized cardioversion or adenosine])

Pregnancy Risk Factor C

Pregnancy Considerations Animal reproduction studies have not been conducted. Procainamide crosses the placenta; procainamide and its active metabolite (N-acetyl procainamide) can be detected in the cord blood and neonatal serum.

Breast-Feeding Considerations Procainamide and its metabolite are found in breast milk and concentrations may be higher than in the maternal serum. In a case report, procainamide was used throughout pregnancy with a dose of 2 g/day prior to delivery. After birth (39 weeks gestation) milk and maternal serum concentrations were obtained over 15 hours of a dosing interval. Mean maternal serum concentrations were procainamide 1.1 mcg/mL and N-acetyl procainamide 1.6 mcg/mL. Mean milk concentrations were procainamide 5.4 mcg/mL and N-acetyl procainamide 3.5 mcg/mL. Due to the potential for adverse events in the nursing infant, breast-feeding is not recommended by the manufacturer.

Contraindications Hypersensitivity to procainamide, procaine, other ester-type local anesthetics, or any component of the formulation; complete heart block; second-degree AV block or various types of hemiblock (without a functional artificial pacemaker); SLE; torsade de pointes

Warnings/Precautions Monitor and adjust dose to prevent QT_c prolongation. Watch for proarrhythmic effects. Avoid use in patients with QT prolongation (ACLS, 2010). May precipitate or exacerbate HF due to negative inotropic actions; use with caution or avoid (ACLS, 2010) in patients with HF. Correct electrolyte disturbances, especially hypokalemia or hypomagnesemia, prior to use and throughout therapy. Reduce dosage in renal impairment. May increase ventricular response rate in patients with atrial fibrillation or flutter; control AV conduction before initiating. Correct hypokalemia before initiating therapy; hypokalemia may worsen toxicity. Reduce dose if first-degree heart block occurs. Use caution with concurrent use of other antiarrhythmics; may exacerbate or increase the risk of conduction disturbances. Avoid concurrent use with other drugs known to prolong QT_c interval. Avoid use in myasthenia gravis (may worsen condition).

Use caution and dose cautiously in older adults; renal clearance of procainamide/NAPA declines in patients ≥50 years of age (independent of creatinine clearance reductions) and in the presence of concomitant renal impairment. In the treatment of atrial fibrillation, avoid antiarrhythmics as first-line treatment. In older adults, data suggests rate control may provide more benefits than risks compared to rhythm control for most patients (Beers Criteria).

This product contains sodium metabisulfite which may cause allergic-type reactions, including anaphylactic symptoms and life-threatening asthmatic episodes in susceptible people; this is seen more frequently in asthmatics.

[U.S. Boxed Warning]: Potentially fatal blood dyscrasias (eg, agranulocytosis) have occurred with therapeutic doses; weekly monitoring is recommended during the first 3 months of therapy and periodically thereafter. Discontinue procainamide if this occurs.

[U.S. Boxed Warning]: Long-term administration leads to the development of a positive antinuclear antibody (ANA) test in 50% of patients which may result in a drug-induced lupus erythematosus-like syndrome (in 20% to 30% of patients); discontinue procainamide with rising ANA titers or with SLE symptoms and choose an alternative agent.

[U.S. Boxed Warning] In the Cardiac Arrhythmia Suppression Trial (CAST), recent (>6 days but <2 years ago) myocardial infarction patients with asymptomatic, non-life-threatening ventricular arrhythmias did not benefit and may have been harmed by attempts to suppress the arrhythmia with flecainide or encainide. An increased mortality or nonfatal cardiac arrest rate (7.7%) was seen in the active treatment group compared with patients in the placebo group (3%). The applicability of the CAST results to other populations is unknown. Procainamide should be reserved for patients with life-threatening ventricular arrhythmias.

Adverse Reactions

>1%:

Cardiovascular: Hypotension (I.V. up to 5%)

Dermatologic: Rash

Gastrointestinal: Diarrhea (oral: 3% to 4%), nausea (oral: 3% to 4%), taste disorder (oral: 3% to 4%), vomiting (oral: 3% to 4%)

Miscellaneous: Positive ANA (≤50%), SLE-like syndrome (≤30%, increased incidence with long-term therapy or slow acetylators; syndrome may include abdominal pain, arthralgia, arthritis, chills, fever, hepatomegaly, myalgia, pericarditis, pleural effusion, pulmonary infiltrates, rash)

<1% (Limited to important or life-threatening): Agranulocytosis, alkaline phosphatase increased, angioedema, anorexia, aplastic anemia, arrhythmia exacerbated, arthralgia, asystole, bone marrow suppression, cerebellar ataxia, confusion, demyelinating polyradiculoneuropathy, disorientation, dizziness, drug fever, fever, first degree heart block, flushing, granulomatous hepatitis, hallucinations, hemolytic anemia, hepatic failure, hyperbilirubinemia, hypoplastic anemia, intrahepatic cholestasis, leukopenia, lightheadedness, maculopapular rash, mania, mental depression, myasthenia gravis worsened, myocardial contractility depressed, myocarditis, myopathy, neuromuscular blockade, neutropenia, pancreatitis, pancytopenia, paradoxical increase in ventricular rate in atrial fibrillation/flutter, peripheral/polyneuropathy, pleural effusion, positive Coombs' test, proarrhythmia, pseudo-obstruction, psychosis, pulmonary embolism, QT_c-interval prolongation, pruritus, rash, respiratory failure due to myopathy, second-degree heart block, tachycardia, thrombocytopenia, torsade de pointes, transaminases increased, urticaria, vasculitis, ventricular fibrillation, weakness

Drug Interactions

Metabolism/Transport Effects Substrate of CYP2D6 (major); **Note:** Assignment of Major/Minor substrate status based on clinically relevant drug interaction potential

Avoid Concomitant Use

Avoid concomitant use of Procainamide with any of the following: Amiodarone; Fingolimod; Highest Risk QTc-Prolonging Agents; Ivabradine; Mifepristone; Moderate Risk QTc-Prolonging Agents; Propafenone

Increased Effect/Toxicity

Procainamide may increase the levels/effects of: Highest Risk QTc-Prolonging Agents; Neuromuscular-Blocking Agents

The levels/effects of Procainamide may be increased by: Abiraterone Acetate; Amiodarone; Cimetidine; CYP2D6 Inhibitors (Moderate); CYP2D6 Inhibitors (Strong); Darunavir; Fingolimod; Ivabradine; LamoTRIgine; Lurasidone; Mifepristone; Moderate Risk QTc-Prolonging Agents; Propafenone; QTc-Prolonging Agents (Indeterminate Risk and Risk Modifying); Ranitidine; Trimethoprim

Decreased Effect

The levels/effects of Procainamide may be decreased by: Peginterferon Alfa-2b

Ethanol/Nutrition/Herb Interactions

Ethanol: Avoid ethanol (acute ethanol administration reduces procainamide serum concentrations).

Herb/Nutraceutical: Avoid ephedra (may worsen arrhythmia).

Preparation for Administration I.V.: Dilute loading dose to a maximum concentration of 20 mg/mL.

Storage/Stability Store undiluted vials at room temperature of 15°C to 30°C (59°F to 86°F). The solution is initially colorless but may turn slightly yellow on standing. Injection of air into the vial causes solution to darken. Discard solutions darker than light amber. Color formation may occur upon refrigeration. When admixed in NS or D_5W to a final concentration of 2-4 mg/mL, solution is stable at room temperature for 24 hours and for 7 days under refrigeration.

Mechanism of Action Decreases myocardial excitability and conduction velocity and may depress myocardial contractility, by increasing the electrical stimulation threshold of ventricle, His-Purkinje system and through direct cardiac effects

Pharmacodynamics/Kinetics

Onset of action: I.M. 10-30 minutes

Distribution: V_d: Children: 2.2 L/kg; Adults: 2 L/kg; decreased with congestive heart failure or shock

Protein binding: 15% to 20%

Metabolism: Hepatic via acetylation to produce N-acetyl procainamide (NAPA) (active metabolite)

Half-life elimination:

Procainamide (hepatic acetylator, phenotype, cardiac and renal function dependent): Children: 1.7 hours; Adults: 2.5-4.7 hours; Anephric: 11 hours

NAPA (dependent upon renal function): Children: 6 hours; Adults: 6-8 hours; Anephric: 42 hours

Time to peak, serum: I.M.: 15-60 minutes

Excretion: Urine (30% to 60% unchanged procainamide; 6% to 52% as NAPA); feces (<5% unchanged procainamide. **Note:** >80% of formed NAPA is renally eliminated in contrast to procainamide which is ~50% renally eliminated (Gibson, 1977).

Dosage Must be titrated to patient's response

Children:

I.M.: 20-30 mg/kg/day divided every 4-6 hours; maximum: 4 g/day

I.V.:

Load: 3-6 mg/kg/dose over 5 minutes not to exceed 100 mg/dose; may repeat every 5-10 minutes to maximum of 15 mg/kg/load

Maintenance as continuous I.V. infusion: 20-80 mcg/kg/minute; maximum: 2 g/24 hours

Possible VT (PALS, 2010): I.V.; I.O.: 15 mg/kg over 30-60 minutes

Adults:

I.M.: 50 mg/kg/day divided every 3-6 hours **or** 0.5-1 g every 4-8 hours (Koch-Weser, 1971)

I.V.:

Loading dose: 15-18 mg/kg administered as slow infusion over 25-30 minutes **or** 100 mg/dose at a rate not to exceed 50 mg/minute repeated every 5 minutes as needed to a total dose of 1 g.

Hemodynamically stable monomorphic VT or pre-excited atrial fibrillation (ACLS, 2010): Loading dose: Infuse 20-50 mg/minute **or** 100 mg every 5 minutes until arrhythmia controlled, hypotension occurs, QRS complex widens by 50% of its original width, or total of 17 mg/kg is given. Follow with a continuous infusion of 1-4 mg/minute. **Note:** Not recommended for use in ongoing ventricular fibrillation (VF) or pulseless ventricular tachycardia (VT) due to prolonged administration time and uncertain efficacy.

Maintenance dose: 1-4 mg/minute by continuous infusion. Maintenance infusions should be reduced by one-third in patients with moderate renal or cardiac impairment and by two-thirds in patients with severe renal or cardiac impairment.

Oral (not available in the U.S.; Canadian labeling): Sustained release formulation (Procan SR®): Maintenance: 50 mg/kg/24 hours given in divided doses every 6 hours

Suggested Procan SR® maintenance dose:

<55 kg: 500 mg every 6 hours

55-91 kg: 750 mg every 6 hours

>91 kg: 1000 mg every 6 hours

Elderly: Initiate doses at lower end of dosage range.

Dosing interval in renal impairment:
Oral:
Cl_{cr} 10-50 mL/minute: Administer every 6-12 hours.
Cl_{cr} <10 mL/minute: Administer every 8-24 hours.
I.V.:
Loading dose: Reduce dose to 12 mg/kg in severe renal impairment.
Maintenance infusion: Reduce dose by one-third in patients with mild renal impairment. Reduce dose by two-thirds in patients with severe renal impairment.
Dialysis:
Procainamide: Moderately hemodialyzable (20% to 50%): Monitor procainamide/N-acetylprocainamide (NAPA) concentrations; supplementation may be necessary.
NAPA: Not dialyzable (0% to 5%)
Procainamide/NAPA: Not peritoneal dialyzable (0% to 5%)
Procainamide/NAPA: Replace according to blood concentration monitoring during continuous arteriovenous or venovenous hemofiltration.
Dosing adjustment in hepatic impairment: Reduce dose by 50%.

Usual Infusion Concentrations: Adult I.V. infusion: 1000 mg in 500 mL (concentration: 2 mg/mL), 1000 mg in 250 mL (concentration: 4 mg/mL), **or** 2000 mg in 250 mL (concentration: 8 mg/mL) of D_5W or NS

Administration
Oral: Do **not** crush or chew sustained release drug products (not available in the U.S.).
I.V.: Must dilute prior to I.V. administration. Dilute loading dose to a maximum concentration of 20 mg/mL; administer loading dose at a maximum rate of 50 mg/minute

Monitoring Parameters ECG, blood pressure, renal function; with prolonged use monitor CBC with differential, platelet count; procainamide and NAPA blood concentrations in patients with hepatic impairment, renal impairment, or receiving constant infusion >3 mg/minute for longer than 24 hours; ANA titers

Consult individual institutional policies and procedures.

Reference Range
Timing of serum samples: Draw 6-12 hours after I.V. infusion has started; half-life is 2.5-5 hours
Therapeutic concentrations: Procainamide: 4-10 mcg/mL; NAPA 15-25 mcg/mL; Combined: 10-30 mcg/mL
Toxic concentration: Procainamide: >10-12 mcg/mL

Test Interactions In the presence of propranolol or suprapharmacologic concentrations of lidocaine or meprobamate, tests which depend on fluorescence to measure procainamide/NAPA concentrations may be affected.

Dosage Forms Excipient information presented when available (limited, particularly for generics); consult specific product labeling.
Solution, Injection, as hydrochloride:
Generic: 100 mg/mL (10 mL); 500 mg/mL (2 mL)

Dosage Forms: Canada Excipient information presented when available (limited, particularly for generics); consult specific product labeling.
Tablet, sustained release, oral, as hydrochloride:
Procan SR®: 250 mg, 500 mg, 750 mg

◆ **Procainamide Hydrochloride** *see* Procainamide *on page 1718*

◆ **Procainamide Hydrochloride Injection, USP (Can)** *see* Procainamide *on page 1718*

◆ **Procaine Amide Hydrochloride** *see* Procainamide *on page 1718*

◆ **Procaine Benzylpenicillin** *see* Penicillin G Procaine *on page 1610*

◆ **Procaine Penicillin G** *see* Penicillin G Procaine *on page 1610*

◆ **PRO-Calcitonin (Can)** *see* Calcitonin *on page 312*

◆ **Procanbid** *see* Procainamide *on page 1718*

◆ **Procan SR® (Can)** *see* Procainamide *on page 1718*

Procarbazine (proe KAR ba zeen)

Brand Names: U.S. Matulane
Brand Names: Canada Matulane; Natulan
Index Terms Benzmethyzin; Ibenzmethyzin; N-Methylhydrazine; PCB; PCZ; Procarbazine Hydrochloride
Pharmacologic Category Antineoplastic Agent, Alkylating Agent
Additional Appendix Information
Tyramine Content of Foods *on page 2394*
Use Treatment of Hodgkin lymphoma
Unlabeled Use Treatment of CNS tumors (anaplastic oligodendroglioma/oligoastrocytoma), non-Hodgkin lymphomas, and primary CNS lymphomas
Pregnancy Risk Factor D
Pregnancy Considerations Adverse events were observed in animal reproduction studies. There are case reports of fetal malformations in the offspring of pregnant women exposed to procarbazine as part of a combination chemotherapy regimen. Women of reproductive potential should avoid becoming pregnant during treatment.
Breast-Feeding Considerations It is not known if procarbazine is excreted in breast milk. Due to the potential for serious adverse reactions in the nursing infant, nursing is not recommended during treatment with procarbazine.
Contraindications Hypersensitivity to procarbazine or any component of the formulation; inadequate bone marrow reserve
Warnings/Precautions Hazardous agent - use appropriate precautions for handling and disposal (NIOSH, 2012). Hematologic toxicity (leukopenia and thrombocytopenia) may occur 2-8 weeks after treatment initiation. Allow ≥1 month interval between radiation therapy or myelosuppressive chemotherapy and initiation of procarbazine treatment. Withhold treatment for leukopenia (WBC <4000/mm^3) or thrombocytopenia (platelets <100,000/mm^3). Monitor for infections due to neutropenia. May cause hemolysis and/or presence of Heinz inclusion bodies in erythrocytes. Procarbazine is associated with a high emetic potential; antiemetics are recommended to prevent nausea and vomiting. May cause diarrhea and stomatitis; withhold treatment for diarrhea or stomatitis. Withhold treatment for CNS toxicity, hemorrhage, or hypersensitivity. Azoospermia and infertility have been reported with procarbazine when used in combination with other chemotherapy agents. Possibly carcinogenic; acute myeloid leukemia and lung cancer have been reported following use.

Use with caution in patients with hepatic or renal impairment. Potentially significant drug-drug interactions may exist, requiring dose or frequency adjustment, additional monitoring, and/or selection of alternative therapy. Possesses MAO inhibitor activity and has potential for severe drug and food interactions; follow MAOI diet (avoid tyramine-containing foods). Avoid ethanol consumption, may cause disulfiram-like reaction. **[U.S. Boxed Warning]: Should be administered under the supervision of an experienced cancer chemotherapy physician.**

Adverse Reactions Frequency not always defined.
Cardiovascular: Edema, flushing, hypotension, syncope, tachycardia
Central nervous system: Apprehension, ataxia, chills, coma, confusion, depression, dizziness, drowsiness, falling, fatigue, hallucination, headache, hyporeflexia, insomnia, lethargy, nervousness, neuropathy, nightmares, pain, paresthesia, seizure, slurred speech, unsteadiness

Dermatologic: Alopecia, dermatitis, diaphoresis, hyperpigmentation, pruritus, skin rash, urticaria
Endocrine & metabolic: Gynecomastia (in prepubertal and early pubertal males)
Gastrointestinal: Nausea and vomiting (60% to 90%; increasing the dose in a stepwise fashion over several days may minimize), abdominal pain, anorexia, constipation, diarrhea, dysphagia, hematemesis, melena, stomatitis, xerostomia
Genitourinary: Reduced fertility (>10%), azoospermia (reported with combination chemotherapy), hematuria, nocturia
Hematologic & oncologic: Malignant neoplasm (2% to 15%; secondary; nonlymphoid; reported with combination therapy), anemia, bone marrow depression, eosinophilia, hemolysis (in patients with G6PD deficiency), hemolytic anemia, pancytopenia, petechia, purpura, thrombocytopenia
Hepatic: Hepatic insufficiency, jaundice
Hypersensitivity: Hypersensitivity reaction
Infection: Herpes virus infection, increased susceptibility to infection
Neuromuscular & skeletal: Arthralgia, foot-drop, myalgia, tremor, weakness
Ophthalmic: Accommodation disturbance, diplopia, nystagmus, papilledema, photophobia, retinal hemorrhage
Otic: Hearing loss
Renal: Polyuria
Respiratory: Cough, epistaxis, hemoptysis, hoarseness, pleural effusion, pneumonitis, pulmonary toxicity (<1%)
Miscellaneous: Fever

Drug Interactions

Metabolism/Transport Effects Inhibits Monoamine Oxidase

Avoid Concomitant Use

Avoid concomitant use of Procarbazine with any of the following: Alpha-/Beta-Agonists (Indirect-Acting); Alpha1-Agonists; Amphetamines; Anilidopiperidine Opioids; Antidepressants (Serotonin Reuptake Inhibitor/Antagonist); Apraclonidine; AtoMOXetine; BCG; Bezafibrate; Buprenorphine; BuPROPion; BusPIRone; CarBAMazepine; CloZAPine; Cyclobenzaprine; Dexmethylphenidate; Dextromethorphan; Diethylpropion; Hydrocodone; HYDROmorphone; Isometheptene; Levonordefrin; Linezolid; Maprotiline; Meperidine; Methyldopa; Methylene Blue; Methylphenidate; Mirtazapine; Morphine (Liposomal); Morphine (Systemic); Natalizumab; Oxymorphone; Pimecrolimus; Pizotifen; Selective Serotonin Reuptake Inhibitors; Serotonin 5-HT1D Receptor Agonists; Serotonin/Norepinephrine Reuptake Inhibitors; Tacrolimus (Topical); Tapentadol; Tetrabenazine; Tetrahydrozoline (Nasal); Tofacitinib; Tricyclic Antidepressants; Tryptophan; Vaccines (Live)

Increased Effect/Toxicity

Procarbazine may increase the levels/effects of: Alpha-/Beta-Agonists (Indirect-Acting); Alpha1-Agonists; Amphetamines; Antidepressants (Serotonin Reuptake Inhibitor/Antagonist); Antihypertensives; Antipsychotics; Apraclonidine; AtoMOXetine; Beta2-Agonists; Betahistine; Bezafibrate; Brimonidine (Ophthalmic); Brimonidine (Topical); BuPROPion; CloZAPine; Dexmethylphenidate; Dextromethorphan; Diethylpropion; Domperidone; Doxapram; Doxylamine; EPINEPHrine (Nasal); Epinephrine (Racemic); EPINEPHrine (Systemic, Oral Inhalation); Hydrocodone; HYDROmorphone; Hypoglycemic Agents; Isometheptene; Leflunomide; Levonordefrin; Linezolid; Lithium; Meperidine; Methadone; Methyldopa; Methylene Blue; Methylphenidate; Metoclopramide; Mirtazapine; Morphine (Liposomal); Morphine (Systemic); Natalizumab; Norepinephrine; Orthostatic Hypotension Producing Agents; OxyCODONE; Pizotifen; Reserpine; Selective Serotonin Reuptake Inhibitors; Serotonin 5-HT1D Receptor Agonists; Serotonin Modulators; Serotonin/Norepinephrine Reuptake Inhibitors; Tetrahydrozoline (Nasal); Tofacitinib; Tricyclic Antidepressants; Vaccines (Live); Vitamin K Antagonists

The levels/effects of Procarbazine may be increased by: Altretamine; Anilidopiperidine Opioids; Antipsychotics; Buprenorphine; BusPIRone; CarBAMazepine; COMT Inhibitors; Cyclobenzaprine; Denosumab; Levodopa; MAO Inhibitors; Maprotiline; Oxymorphone; Pimecrolimus; Roflumilast; Tacrolimus (Topical); Tapentadol; Tetrabenazine; TraMADol; Trastuzumab; Tryptophan

Decreased Effect

Procarbazine may decrease the levels/effects of: BCG; Cardiac Glycosides; Coccidioidin Skin Test; Domperidone; Sipuleucel-T; Vaccines (Inactivated); Vaccines (Live); Vitamin K Antagonists

The levels/effects of Procarbazine may be decreased by: Domperidone; Echinacea

Ethanol/Nutrition/Herb Interactions

Ethanol: Ethanol may enhance the adverse/toxic effects of procarbazine or cause a disulfiram reaction. Management: Avoid ethanol.
Food: Concurrent ingestion of foods rich in tyramine may cause sudden and severe high blood pressure (hypertensive crisis or serotonin syndrome). Management: Avoid tyramine-containing foods (aged or matured cheese, air-dried or cured meats including sausages and salamis; fava or broad bean pods, tap/draft beers, Marmite concentrate, sauerkraut, soy sauce, and other soybean condiments). Food's freshness is also an important concern; improperly stored or spoiled food can create an environment in which tyramine concentrations may increase.
Herb/Nutraceutical: Supplements containing caffeine, tyrosine, tryptophan, or phenylalanine may increase the risk of severe side effects (eg, hypertensive reactions, serotonin syndrome). Echinacea may diminish the therapeutic effect of immunosuppressants. Management: Avoid supplements containing caffeine, tyrosine, tryptophan, or phenylalanine. Consider avoiding echinacea.

Storage/Stability Protect from light.

Mechanism of Action Inhibits DNA, RNA, and protein synthesis by inhibiting transmethylation of methionine into transfer RNA; may also damage DNA directly through alkylation.

Pharmacodynamics/Kinetics

Absorption: Rapid and complete
Distribution: Crosses blood-brain barrier; equilibrates between plasma and CSF
Metabolism: Oxidized to active metabolites methylazoxy-procarbazine and benzylazoxy-procarbazine, then further metabolized to inactive metabolites (Kintzel, 1995)
Half-life elimination: ~1 hour
Time to peak, plasma: ≤1 hour
Excretion: Urine (70% as inactive metabolites [Kintzel, 1995])

Dosage Note: Procarbazine is associated with a high emetic potential; antiemetics are recommended to prevent nausea and vomiting. The manufacturer suggests that an estimated lean body mass be used in obese patients and patients with rapid weight gain due to edema, ascites, or abnormal fluid retention.

Hodgkin lymphoma:

Children and Adults: MOPP regimen: While procarbazine is approved as part of the MOPP regimen, the MOPP regimen is generally no longer used due to improved toxicity profiles with other combination regimens used in the treatment of Hodgkin lymphoma.

Children: BEACOPP regimen (unlabeled dosing): Oral: 100 mg/m² days 0-6 of a 21-day treatment cycle (in combination with bleomycin, etoposide, doxorubicin, cyclophosphamide, vincristine, and prednisone) for 4 cycles (Kelley, 2011).

Adults: BEACOPP, standard or escalated regimen (unlabeled dosing): Oral: 100 mg/m² days 1-7 every 21 days (in combination with bleomycin, etoposide, doxorubicin, cyclophosphamide, vincristine, and prednisone) for 8 cycles (Diehl, 2003)

Non-Hodgkin lymphomas (NHL; unlabeled use): Adults:

CEPP regimen: Oral: 60 mg/m² days 1-10 every 28 days (in combination with cyclophosphamide, etoposide and prednisone) (Chao, 1990)

PEP-C regimen: Oral: 50 mg daily at bedtime (length of induction cycle depends on phase of treatment and blood counts; frequency may vary based on tolerance in maintenance cycle; in combination with prednisone, etoposide, and cyclophosphamide) (Coleman, 2008)

CNS tumors, anaplastic oligodendroglioma/oligoastrocytoma (unlabeled use): Adults: PCV regimen: Oral: 60 mg/m² days 8-21 every 6 weeks (in combination with lomustine and vincristine) for 6 cycles (van den Bent, 2006) **or** 75 mg/m² days 8-21 every 6 weeks (in combination with lomustine and vincristine) for up to 4 cycles (Cairncross, 2006).

Primary CNS lymphoma (unlabeled use): Adults: Oral: 100 mg/m² for 7 days in cycles 1, 3, and 5 (in combination with methotrexate [high-dose], vincristine, methotrexate [intrathecal], leucovorin, dexamethasone, cytarabine [high-dose], and whole brain radiation) (DeAngelis, 2002).

Dosage adjustment for toxicity: Withhold treatment (promptly) for any of the following: CNS toxicity (eg, paresthesia, confusion, neuropathy), hematologic toxicity (WBC <4000/mm³ or platelets <100,000/mm³), hypersensitivity, gastrointestinal toxicities (stomatisis, diarrhea), and hemorrhage or bleeding.

Dosage adjustment in renal impairment: No dosage adjustment provided in manufacturer's labeling; use with caution; may result in increased toxicity. However, because predominantly inactive metabolites are excreted via the kidneys, dosage adjustment is not necessary (Kintzel, 1995).

Dosage adjustment in hepatic impairment: No dosage adjustment provided in manufacturer's labeling; use with caution; may result in increased toxicity. The following adjustments have been reported in literature:

Floyd, 2006:

Transaminases 1.6-6 times ULN: Administer 75% of dose

Transaminases >6 times ULN: Use clinical judgment

Serum bilirubin >5 mg/dL or transaminases >3 times ULN: Avoid use

King, 2001: Serum bilirubin >5 mg/dL or transaminases >180 units/L: Avoid use

Dosing in obesity: *ASCO Guidelines for appropriate chemotherapy dosing in obese adults with cancer:* Utilize patient's actual body weight (full weight) for calculation of body surface area- or weight-based dosing, particularly when the intent of therapy is curative; manage regimen-related toxicities in the same manner as for nonobese patients; if a dose reduction is utilized due to toxicity, consider resumption of full weight-based dosing with subsequent cycles, especially if cause of toxicity (eg, hepatic or renal impairment) is resolved (Griggs, 2012). **Note:** The manufacturer suggests that an estimated lean body mass be used in obese patients and patients with rapid weight gain due to edema, ascites, or abnormal fluid retention.

Dietary Considerations Avoid tyramine-containing foods/beverages. Some examples include aged or matured cheese, air-dried or cured meats (including sausages and salamis), fava or broad bean pods, tap/draft beers, Marmite concentrate, sauerkraut, soy sauce and other soybean condiments.

Administration Oral: May be given as a single daily dose or in 2-3 divided doses. Procarbazine is associated with a high emetic potential; antiemetics are recommended to prevent nausea and vomiting.

Hazardous agent; use appropriate precautions for handling and disposal (NIOSH, 2012).

Monitoring Parameters CBC with differential, platelet and reticulocyte count, urinalysis, liver function test, renal function test. Monitor for infections, CNS toxicity, and gastrointestinal toxicities.

Dosage Forms Excipient information presented when available (limited, particularly for generics); consult specific product labeling.

Capsule, Oral, as hydrochloride:

Matulane: 50 mg

Extemporaneous Preparations Hazardous agent: Use appropriate precautions for handling and disposal.

A 10 mg/mL oral suspension may be prepared using capsules, glycerin, and strawberry syrup. Empty the contents of ten 50 mg capsules into a mortar. Add 2 mL glycerin and mix to a thick uniform paste. Add 10 mL strawberry syrup in incremental proportions; mix until uniform. Transfer the mixture to an amber glass bottle and rinse mortar with small amounts of strawberry syrup; add rinses to the bottle in sufficient quantity to make 50 mL. Label "shake well" and "protect from light". Stable for 7 days at room temperature.

Matulane® data on file, Sigma Tau Pharmaceuticals, Inc.

- **Procarbazine Hydrochloride** *see* Procarbazine *on page 1720*
- **Procardia** *see* NIFEdipine *on page 1455*
- **Procardia XL** *see* NIFEdipine *on page 1455*
- **PRO-Cefadroxil (Can)** *see* Cefadroxil *on page 361*
- **PRO-Cefuroxime (Can)** *see* Cefuroxime *on page 386*
- **ProCentra** *see* Dextroamphetamine *on page 588*
- **Procetofene** *see* Fenofibrate and Derivatives *on page 837*

Prochlorperazine (proe klor PER a zeen)

Brand Names: U.S. Compazine; Compro

Brand Names: Canada Apo-Prochlorperazine; Nu-Prochlor; PMS-Prochlorperazine; Sandoz-Prochlorperazine

Index Terms Chlormeprazine; Prochlorperazine Edisylate; Prochlorperazine Maleate; Prochlorperazine Mesylate

Pharmacologic Category Antiemetic; Antipsychotic Agent, Typical, Phenothiazine

Additional Appendix Information

Beers Criteria – Potentially Inappropriate Medications for Geriatrics *on page 2368*

Use Management of nausea and vomiting; psychotic disorders, including schizophrenia and anxiety; nonpsychotic anxiety

Unlabeled Use Behavioral syndromes in dementia; psychosis/agitation related to Alzheimer's dementia

Pregnancy Considerations Jaundice or hyper-/hyporeflexia have been reported in newborn infants following maternal use of phenothiazines. Antipsychotic use during the third trimester of pregnancy has a risk for abnormal muscle movements (extrapyramidal symptoms [EPS]) and withdrawal symptoms in newborns following delivery. Symptoms in the newborn may include agitation, feeding disorder, hypertonia, hypotonia, respiratory distress, somnolence, and tremor; these effects may be self-limiting or require hospitalization. Use may interfere with pregnancy tests, causing false positive results. Prochlorperazine has been used for the treatment of nausea and vomiting associated with pregnancy (Levicheck, 2002; Mahadevan, 2006); however, other agents may be preferred (ACOG, 2004).

Breast-Feeding Considerations Other phenothiazines are excreted in human milk; excretion of prochlorperazine is not known.

Contraindications Hypersensitivity to prochlorperazine or any component of the formulation (cross-reactivity between phenothiazines may occur); coma or presence of large amounts of CNS depressants (eg, alcohol, opioids, barbiturates); pediatric surgery; children <2 years of age or <9 kg

Canadian labeling: Additional contraindications (not in U.S. labeling): Presence of circulatory collapse; severe cardiovascular disorders; altered state of consciousness; concomitant use of high dose hypnotics; severe depression; presence of blood dyscrasias, hepatic or renal impairment, or pheochromocytoma; suspected or established subcortical brain damage with or without hypothalamic damage

Warnings/Precautions [U.S. Boxed Warning]: Elderly patients with dementia-related psychosis treated with antipsychotics are at an increased risk of death compared to placebo. Most deaths appeared to be either cardiovascular (eg, heart failure, sudden death) or infectious (eg, pneumonia) in nature. Prochlorperazine is not approved for the treatment of dementia-related psychosis. May cause extrapyramidal symptoms (EPS), including pseudoparkinsonism, acute dystonic reactions, akathisia, and tardive dyskinesia. Risk of dystonia (and possibly other EPS) may be greater with increased doses, use of conventional antipsychotics, males, and younger patients. Risk of tardive dyskinesia and potential for irreversibility often associated with total cumulative dose and therapy duration and may also be increased in elderly patients (particularly elderly women); antipsychotics may also mask signs/symptoms of tardive dyskinesia. Consider therapy discontinuation with signs/symptoms of tardive dyskinesia. Antipsychotic use has been associated with esophageal dysmotility and aspiration; use with caution in patients at risk of pneumonia (ie, Alzheimer's disease).

May be sedating and impair physical or mental abilities; use with caution in disorders where CNS depression is a feature. Effects with other sedative drugs or ethanol may be potentiated. Use with caution in Parkinson's disease; hemodynamic instability; predisposition to seizures; subcortical brain damage; and in severe cardiac, hepatic, or renal disease. Canadian labeling contraindicates use in patients with severe cardiac disease, hepatic or renal impairment, subcortical brain damage, and circulatory collapse. May alter temperature regulation, obscure intestinal obstruction or brain tumor or mask toxicity of other drugs. May alter cardiac conduction. Hypotension may occur following administration, particularly when parenteral form is used or in high dosages. May cause orthostatic hypotension; use with caution in patients at risk of this effect or in those who would not tolerate transient hypotensive episodes (cerebrovascular disease, cardiovascular disease, hypovolemia, or concurrent medication use which may predispose to hypotension/bradycardia).

Leukopenia, neutropenia, and agranulocytosis (sometimes fatal) have been reported in clinical trials and postmarketing reports with antipsychotic use; presence of risk factors (eg, pre-existing low WBC or history of drug-induced leuko-/neutropenia) should prompt periodic blood count assessment. Discontinue therapy at first signs of blood dyscrasias or if absolute neutrophil count <1000/mm^3.

Due to its potent anticholinergic effects, may be inappropriate in older adults depending on comorbidities (eg, dementia, delirium) (Beers Criteria). Use with caution in patients with decreased gastrointestinal motility, urinary retention, BPH, xerostomia, visual problems, or narrow-angle glaucoma (screening is recommended). Use caution with exposure to heat. May cause pigmentary retinopathy, and lenticular and corneal deposits, particularly with prolonged therapy. Use associated with increased prolactin levels; clinical significance of hyperprolactinemia in patients with breast cancer or other prolactin-dependent tumors is unknown. Avoid use in patients with signs/symptoms suggestive of Reye's syndrome. Children with acute illness or dehydration are more susceptible to neuromuscular reactions; use cautiously. May be associated with neuroleptic malignant syndrome (NMS). Some dosage forms may contain benzyl alcohol which has been associated with "gasping syndrome" in neonates. Some dosage forms may contain sodium sulfite.

Adverse Reactions Reported with prochlorperazine or other phenothiazines. Frequency not defined.

Cardiovascular: Cardiac arrest, cerebral edema, hypotension, peripheral edema, Q-wave distortions, sudden death, T-wave distortions

Central nervous system: Agitation, altered cerebrospinal fluid proteins, catatonia, coma, cough reflex suppressed, dizziness, drowsiness, fever (mild [I.M.]), headache, hyperpyrexia, impairment of temperature regulation, insomnia, neuroleptic malignant syndrome (NMS), oculogyric crisis, opisthotonos, restlessness, seizure, somnolence, tremulousness

Dermatologic: Angioedema, contact dermatitis, epithelial keratopathy, erythema, eczema, exfoliative dermatitis, itching, photosensitivity, skin pigmentation, urticaria

Endocrine & metabolic: Amenorrhea, galactorrhea, gynecomastia, glucosuria, hyper-/hypoglycemia, lactation, libido (changes in), menstrual irregularity

Gastrointestinal: Appetite increased, atonic colon, constipation, ileus, nausea, obstipation, vomiting, weight gain, xerostomia

Genitourinary: Ejaculating dysfunction, ejaculatory disturbances, impotence, priapism, urinary retention

Hematologic: Agranulocytosis, aplastic anemia, eosinophilia, hemolytic anemia, leukopenia, pancytopenia, thrombocytopenic purpura

Hepatic: Biliary stasis, cholestatic jaundice, hepatotoxicity

Neuromuscular & skeletal: Dystonias (torticollis, carpopedal spasm, trismus, protrusion of tongue); extrapyramidal symptoms (pseudoparkinsonism, akathisia, dystonias, tardive dyskinesia, hyperreflexia); SLE-like syndrome, tremor

Ocular: Blurred vision, lenticular/corneal deposits, miosis, mydriasis, pigmentary retinopathy

Respiratory: Asthma, laryngeal edema, nasal congestion

Miscellaneous: Allergic reactions, asphyxia, diaphoresis

Drug Interactions

Metabolism/Transport Effects None known.

Avoid Concomitant Use

Avoid concomitant use of Prochlorperazine with any of the following: Aclidinium; Amisulpride; Azelastine (Nasal); Dofetilide; Ipratropium (Oral Inhalation); Metoclopramide; Paraldehyde; Sulpiride; Tiotropium; Umeclidinium

Increased Effect/Toxicity

Prochlorperazine may increase the levels/effects of: Alcohol (Ethyl); Amisulpride; Analgesics (Opioid); Anticholinergics; Antidepressants (Serotonin Reuptake Inhibitor/Antagonist); Azelastine (Nasal); Beta-Blockers; CNS Depressants; Dofetilide; Methotrimeprazine; Methylphenidate; Paraldehyde; Porfimer; Serotonin Modulators; Sulpiride; Tiotropium; Zolpidem

The levels/effects of Prochlorperazine may be increased by: Acetylcholinesterase Inhibitors (Central); Aclidinium; Antidepressants (Serotonin Reuptake Inhibitor/Antagonist); Antimalarial Agents; Beta-Blockers; Brimonidine (Topical); Deferoxamine; Doxylamine; Droperidol; HydrOXYzine; Ipratropium (Oral Inhalation); Lithium formulations; Magnesium Sulfate; Methotrimeprazine; Methylphenidate; Metoclopramide; Metyrosine; Perampanel; Pramlintide; Serotonin Modulators; Sodium Oxybate; Tetrabenazine; Umeclidinium

Decreased Effect

Prochlorperazine may decrease the levels/effects of: Amphetamines; Anti-Parkinson's Agents (Dopamine Agonist); Quinagolide

The levels/effects of Prochlorperazine may be decreased by: Antacids; Anti-Parkinson's Agents (Dopamine Agonist); Lithium formulations

Ethanol/Nutrition/Herb Interactions

Ethanol: May increase CNS depression; monitor for increased effects with coadministration. Caution patients about effects.

Herb/Nutraceutical: Avoid dong quai, St John's wort (may also cause photosensitization). Avoid kava kava, gotu kola, valerian, St John's wort (may increase CNS depression).

Storage/Stability

Injection:

Edisylate: Store at 20°C to 25°C (68°F to 77°F); do not freeze. Protect from light. Clear or slightly yellow solutions may be used.

Mesylate (Canadian availability; not available in U.S.): Store at 15°C to 30°C (59°F to 86°F). Protect from light. Do not use if solution is discolored or hazy.

I.V. infusion: Injection may be diluted in 50-100 mL NS or D_5W.

Suppository: Store at 20°C to 25°C (68°F to 77°F). Protect from light.

Tablet: Store at 20°C to 25°C (68°F to 77°F). Protect from light.

Mechanism of Action Prochlorperazine is a piperazine phenothiazine antipsychotic which blocks postsynaptic mesolimbic dopaminergic D_1 and D_2 receptors in the brain, including the chemoreceptor trigger zone; exhibits a strong alpha-adrenergic and anticholinergic blocking effect and depresses the release of hypothalamic and hypophyseal hormones; believed to depress the reticular activating system, thus affecting basal metabolism, body temperature, wakefulness, vasomotor tone and emesis

Pharmacodynamics/Kinetics

Onset of action: Oral: 30-40 minutes; I.M.: 10-20 minutes; Rectal: ~60 minutes

Peak antiemetic effect: I.V.: 30-60 minutes

Duration: Rectal: 3-12 hours; I.M., Oral: 3-4 hours

Distribution: V_d: 1400-1548 L (Taylor, 1987)

Metabolism: Primarily hepatic; N-desmethyl prochlorperazine (major active metabolite)

Bioavailability: Oral: 12.5% (Isah, 1991)

Half-life elimination: Oral: 6-10 hours (single dose), 14-22 hours (repeated dosing) (Isah, 1991); I.V.: 6-10 hours (Isah, 1991; Taylor, 1987)

Excretion: Mainly in feces

Dosage Note: Injection solution mesylate formulation has Canadian availability (not available in U.S.).

Antiemetic: Children (therapy >1 day usually not required): **Note:** Use is contraindicated in children <9 kg or <2 years:

Oral, rectal:

9-13 kg: 2.5 mg 1-2 times/day as needed (maximum: 7.5 mg/day)

>13-18 kg: 2.5 mg 2-3 times/day as needed (maximum: 10 mg/day)

>18-39 kg: 2.5 mg 3 times/day or 5 mg 2 times/day as needed (maximum: 15 mg/day)

I.M. (as edisylate): 0.13 mg/kg/dose; convert to oral therapy as soon as possible\

I.M. (as mesylate): 0.14 mg/kg/dose; convert to oral therapy at equivalent or greater dose (if necessary) as soon as possible

Antiemetic: Adults:

Oral (tablet): 5-10 mg 3-4 times/day; usual maximum: 40 mg/day; larger doses may rarely be required

I.M. (as edisylate): 5-10 mg every 3-4 hours; usual maximum: 40 mg/day

I.M. (as mesylate): 5-10 mg 2-3 times/day; usual maximum: 40 mg/day

I.V. (as edisylate): 2.5-10 mg; maximum: 10 mg/dose or 40 mg/day; may repeat dose every 3-4 hours as needed

Rectal:

U.S. labeling: 25 mg twice daily

Canadian labeling: 5-10 mg 3-4 times/day

Surgical nausea/vomiting: Adults: **Note:** Should not exceed 40 mg/day

I.M. (as edisylate): 5-10 mg 1-2 hours before anesthesia induction or to control symptoms during or after surgery; may repeat once if necessary

I.M. (as mesylate): 5-10 mg 1-2 hours before anesthesia induction; may repeat once if needed during surgery; postoperatively: 5-10 mg every 3-4 hours as needed up to maximum of 40 mg daily

I.V. (as edisylate): 5-10 mg 15-30 minutes before anesthesia induction or to control symptoms during or after surgery; may repeat once if necessary

I.V. (as mesylate): 20 mg/L of I.V. solution during surgery or postoperatively; usual maximum: 30 mg daily

Rectal (unlabeled use; Golembiewski, 2005): 25 mg

Antipsychotic:

Children 2-12 years (contraindicated in children <9 kg or <2 years):

Oral, rectal: 2.5 mg 2-3 times/day; do not give more than 10 mg the first day; increase dosage as needed to maximum daily dose of 20 mg for 2-5 years and 25 mg for 6-12 years

I.M. (as edisylate): 0.13 mg/kg/dose; convert to oral therapy as soon as possible

I.M. (as mesylate): 0.14 mg/kg/dose; convert to oral therapy at equivalent or greater dose (if necessary) as soon as possible

Adults:

Oral: 5-10 mg 3-4 times/day; titrate dose slowly every 2-3 days; doses up to 150 mg/day may be required in some patients for treatment of severe disturbances

I.M. (as edisylate): Initial: 10-20 mg; if necessary repeat initial dose every 2-4 hours to gain control; more than 3-4 doses are rarely needed. If parenteral administration is still required; give 10-20 mg every 4-6 hours; convert to oral therapy as soon as possible

I.M. (as mesylate): Initial: 10-20 mg; if necessary repeat initial dose every 2-4 hours to gain control; more than 3-4 doses are rarely needed; convert to oral therapy as soon as possible

Nonpsychotic anxiety: Oral (tablet): Adults: Usual dose: 5 mg 3-4 times/day; do not exceed 20 mg/day or administer >12 weeks

Elderly: Initiate at lower end of dosage range; titrate slowly and cautiously. Refer to adult dosing.

Dosage adjustment in renal impairment:

U.S. labeling: No dosage adjustment provided in manufacturer's labeling.

Canadian labeling: Use is contraindicated.

Dosage adjustment in hepatic impairment:

U.S. labeling: No dosage adjustment provided in manufacturer's labeling; systemic exposure may be increased as drug undergoes hepatic metabolism.

Canadian labeling: Use is contraindicated.

Dietary Considerations Increase dietary intake of riboflavin; should be administered with food or water. Rectal suppositories may contain coconut and palm oil.

Administration

I.M.: Inject by deep I.M. into outer quadrant of buttocks.

I.V.: May be administered by slow I.V. push at a rate not exceeding 5 mg/minute or by I.V. infusion. Do not administer as a bolus injection. To reduce the risk of hypotension, patients receiving I.V. prochlorperazine must remain lying down and be observed for at least 30 minutes following administration. Avoid skin contact with injection solution, contact dermatitis has occurred. Do not dilute with any diluent containing parabens as a preservative.

Oral: Administer tablet without regard to meals.

Monitoring Parameters Vital signs; CBC (baseline, frequently during first few months of therapy, periodically thereafter); lipid profile; fasting blood glucose/Hgb A_{1c}; BMI; mental status; abnormal involuntary movement scale (AIMS); periodic ophthalmic exams (if chronically used); extrapyramidal symptoms (EPS)

Test Interactions False-positives for phenylketonuria, pregnancy

Additional Information Not recommended as an antipsychotic due to inferior efficacy compared to other phenothiazines.

Dosage Forms Excipient information presented when available (limited, particularly for generics); consult specific product labeling.

Solution, Injection, as edisylate [strength expressed as base]:
Generic: 5 mg/mL (2 mL, 10 mL)

Suppository, Rectal:
Compazine: 25 mg (12 ea)
Compro: 25 mg (12 ea)
Generic: 25 mg (12 ea, 1000 ea)

Tablet, Oral, as maleate [strength expressed as base]:
Generic: 5 mg, 10 mg

Dosage Forms: Canada Excipient information presented when available (limited, particularly for generics); consult specific product labeling.

Injection, solution, as mesylate [strength expressed as base]: 5 mg/mL (2 mL)

Suppository, rectal: 10 mg (10s)

- **Prochlorperazine Edisylate** *see* Prochlorperazine *on page 1722*
- **Prochlorperazine Maleate** *see* Prochlorperazine *on page 1722*
- **Prochlorperazine Mesylate** *see* Prochlorperazine *on page 1722*
- **PRO-Ciprofloxacin (Can)** *see* Ciprofloxacin (Systemic) *on page 430*
- **PRO-Clonazepam (Can)** *see* ClonazePAM *on page 465*
- **ProCort®** *see* Pramoxine and Hydrocortisone *on page 1699*
- **Procrit** *see* Epoetin Alfa *on page 723*
- **Proctocort** *see* Hydrocortisone (Topical) *on page 1011*
- **Proctocream HC [DSC]** *see* Hydrocortisone (Topical) *on page 1011*
- **Proctofene** *see* Fenofibrate and Derivatives *on page 837*
- **ProctoFoam® HC** *see* Pramoxine and Hydrocortisone *on page 1699*
- **Proctofoam™-HC (Can)** *see* Pramoxine and Hydrocortisone *on page 1699*
- **Procto-Pak** *see* Hydrocortisone (Topical) *on page 1011*
- **Proctosol HC** *see* Hydrocortisone (Topical) *on page 1011*
- **Proctozone-HC** *see* Hydrocortisone (Topical) *on page 1011*
- **Procysbi™** *see* Cysteamine (Systemic) *on page 516*
- **Procysbi** *see* Cysteamine (Systemic) *on page 516*
- **Procytox® (Can)** *see* Cyclophosphamide *on page 504*
- **PRO-Dexamethasone (Can)** *see* Dexamethasone (Systemic) *on page 580*
- **PRO-Diclo-Rapide (Can)** *see* Diclofenac (Systemic) *on page 597*
- **PRO-Enalapril (Can)** *see* Enalapril *on page 701*
- **PRO-Feno-Super (Can)** *see* Fenofibrate and Derivatives *on page 837*
- **Profilnine SD** *see* Factor IX Complex (Human) [(Factors II, IX, X)] *on page 822*
- **Proflavanol C™ (Can)** *see* Ascorbic Acid *on page 172*
- **PRO-Fluconazole (Can)** *see* Fluconazole *on page 868*
- **PRO-Fluoxetine (Can)** *see* FLUoxetine *on page 885*
- **PRO-Gabapentin (Can)** *see* Gabapentin *on page 933*

Progesterone (proe JES ter one)

Brand Names: U.S. Crinone; Endometrin; First-Progesterone VGS 100; First-Progesterone VGS 200; First-Progesterone VGS 25; First-Progesterone VGS 400; First-Progesterone VGS 50; Prometrium

Brand Names: Canada Crinone; Endometrin; Prometrium

Index Terms Pregnenedione; Progestin

Pharmacologic Category Progestin

Use

Oral: Prevention of endometrial hyperplasia in nonhysterectomized, postmenopausal women who are receiving conjugated estrogen tablets; secondary amenorrhea

I.M.: Amenorrhea; abnormal uterine bleeding due to hormonal imbalance

Intravaginal gel: Part of assisted reproductive technology (ART) for infertile women with progesterone deficiency; secondary amenorrhea

Vaginal tablet: Part of ART for infertile women with progesterone deficiency

Unlabeled Use Reduce the risk of recurrent spontaneous preterm birth in appropriately selected women

Pregnancy Risk Factor B (Prometrium®; none established for vaginal gel, vaginal tablet, or injection

Pregnancy Considerations Adverse events were not observed following oral administration in animal reproduction studies. There is an increased risk of minor birth defects in children whose mothers take progesterones during the first 4 months of pregnancy. Hypospadias has been reported in male and mild masculinization of the external genitalia has been reported in female babies exposed during the first trimester. Cleft lip, cleft palate, congenital heart disease, patent ductus arteriosus, ventricular septal defect, intrauterine death, and spontaneous abortion have been noted in case reports following use of oral progesterone during pregnancy. High doses of progesterone would be expected to impair fertility. Use of vaginal progesterone may be considered to decrease the risk of recurrent spontaneous preterm birth in women with a singleton pregnancy and prior spontaneous preterm singleton birth; use is not recommended as an intervention for women with multiple gestations (ACOG, 2012). The vaginal gel and tablet are indicated for use in ART. The oral capsules are contraindicated for use during pregnancy.

Breast-Feeding Considerations Progesterone is excreted into breast milk. The manufacturer recommends caution be used if progesterone is administered to a nursing woman.

Contraindications Hypersensitivity to progesterone or any component of the formulation; undiagnosed abnormal vaginal bleeding; history of or current thrombophlebitis or venous thromboembolic disorders (including DVT, PE); active or history of arterial thromboembolic disease (eg, stroke, MI); history of or known or suspected carcinoma of the breast or genital organs; hepatic dysfunction or disease; missed abortion or ectopic pregnancy; diagnostic test for pregnancy; capsules are also contraindicated for use during pregnancy

Warnings/Precautions Hazardous agent - use appropriate precautions for handling and disposal (NIOSH, 2012).

[U.S. Boxed Warning]: Estrogens with or without progestin should not be used to prevent cardiovascular disease. Using data from the Women's Health Initiative (WHI) studies, an increased risk of deep vein thrombosis (DVT) and stroke has been reported with CE and an increased risk of DVT, stroke, pulmonary emboli (PE) and myocardial infarction (MI) has been reported with CE with MPA in postmenopausal women. Additional risk factors include diabetes mellitus, hypercholesterolemia, hypertension, SLE, obesity, tobacco use, and/or history of venous thromboembolism (VTE). Risk factors should be managed appropriately; discontinue use if adverse cardiovascular events occur or are suspected.

[U.S. Boxed Warning]: Estrogens with or without progestin should not be used to prevent dementia. In the Women's Health Initiative Memory Study (WHIMS), an increased incidence of dementia was observed in women ≥65 years of age taking CE alone or in combination with MPA.

[U.S. Boxed Warning]: Based on data from the Women's Health Initiative (WHI) studies, an increased risk of invasive breast cancer was observed in postmenopausal women using conjugated estrogens (CE) in combination with medroxyprogesterone acetate (MPA). This risk may be associated with duration of use and declines once combined therapy is discontinued (Chlebowski, 2009). The risk of invasive breast cancer was decreased in postmenopausal women with a hysterectomy using CE only, regardless of weight. However, the risk was not significantly decreased in women at high risk for breast cancer (family history of breast cancer, personal history of benign breast disease) (Anderson, 2012). An increase in abnormal mammogram findings has also been reported with estrogen alone or in combination with progestin therapy. Use is contraindicated in patients with known or suspected breast cancer.

Progesterone is used to reduce the risk of endometrial hyperplasia in nonhysterectomized postmenopausal women receiving conjugated estrogens. The use of unopposed estrogen in women with an intact uterus is associated with an increased risk of endometrial cancer. The addition of a progestin to estrogen therapy may decrease the risk of endometrial hyperplasia, a precursor to endometrial cancer. Adequate diagnostic measures, including endometrial sampling if indicated, should be performed to rule out malignancy in postmenopausal women with undiagnosed abnormal vaginal bleeding.

Estrogens may exacerbate endometriosis. Malignant transformation of residual endometrial implants has been reported posthysterectomy with unopposed estrogen therapy. Consider adding a progestin in women with residual endometriosis posthysterectomy. Postmenopausal estrogen therapy and combined estrogen/progesterone therapy may increase the risk of ovarian cancer; however, the absolute risk to an individual woman is small. Although results from various studies are not consistent, risk does not appear to be significantly associated with the duration, route, or dose of therapy. In one study, the risk decreased after 2 years following discontinuation of therapy (Mørch, 2009). Although the risk of ovarian cancer is rare, women who are at an increased risk (eg, family history) should be counseled about the association (NAMS, 2012).

Discontinue pending examination in cases of sudden partial or complete vision loss, sudden onset of proptosis, diplopia, or migraine; discontinue permanently if papilledema or retinal vascular lesions are observed on examination. Use with caution in patients with diseases that may be exacerbated by fluid retention, including asthma, epilepsy, migraine, diabetes or renal dysfunction. Use caution with history of depression. Patients should be warned that progesterone might cause transient dizziness or drowsiness during initial therapy. Whenever possible, progestins in combination with estrogens should be discontinued at least 4-6 weeks prior to surgeries associated with an increased risk of thromboembolism or during periods of prolonged immobilization.

[U.S. Boxed Warning]: Estrogens with or without progestin should be used for the shortest duration possible at the lowest effective dose consistent with treatment goals. Before prescribing estrogen therapy to postmenopausal women, the risks and benefits must be weighed for each patient. Women should be informed of these risks and benefits, as well as possible effects of progestin when added to estrogen therapy. Patients should be reevaluated as clinically appropriate to determine if treatment is still necessary. Available data related to treatment risks are from Women's Health Initiative (WHI) studies, which evaluated oral CE 0.625 mg with or without MPA 2.5 mg relative to placebo in postmenopausal women. Other combinations and dosage forms of estrogens and progestins were not studied. **Outcomes reported from clinical trials using CE with or without MPA should be assumed to be similar for other doses and other dosage forms of estrogens and progestins until comparable data becomes available.**

Products may contain palm oil, peanut oil, sesame oil, or benzyl alcohol. Not for use prior to menarche.

Adverse Reactions

Injection (I.M.):

Cardiovascular: Cerebral edema, cerebral thrombosis, edema

Central nervous system: Depression, fever, insomnia, somnolence

Dermatologic: Acne, allergic rash (rare), alopecia, hirsutism, pruritus, rash, urticaria

Endocrine & metabolic: Amenorrhea, breakthrough bleeding, breast tenderness, galactorrhea, menstrual flow changes, spotting

Gastrointestinal: Nausea, weight gain/loss

Genitourinary: Cervical erosion changes, cervical secretion changes

Hepatic: Cholestatic jaundice

Local: Injection site: Irritation, pain, redness

Ocular: Optic neuritis, retinal thrombosis

Respiratory: Pulmonary embolism

Miscellaneous: Anaphylactoid reactions

Oral capsule (percentages reported when used in combination with or cycled with conjugated estrogens):

>10%:

Central nervous system: Headache (16% to 31%), dizziness (15% to 24%), depression (19%)

Endocrine & metabolic: Breast tenderness (27%), breast pain (6% to 16%)

Gastrointestinal: Abdominal pain (10% to 20%), abdominal bloating (8% to 12%)

Genitourinary: Urinary problems (11%)

Neuromuscular & skeletal: Joint pain (20%), musculoskeletal pain (12%)

Miscellaneous: Viral infection (12%)

5% to 10%:
- Cardiovascular: Chest pain (7%)
- Central nervous system: Fatigue (8%), irritability (8%), worry (8%)
- Gastrointestinal: Nausea/vomiting (8%), diarrhea (7% to 8%)
- Genitourinary: Vaginal discharge (10%)
- Respiratory: Cough (8%)

<5%: Breast biopsy, breast cancer, cholecystectomy, constipation

Postmarketing and/or case reports: Aggression, alopecia, anaphylactic reaction, arthralgia, asthma, blurred vision, choking, cholestasis, cholestatic hepatitis, circulatory collapse, confusion, consciousness depressed/loss, convulsion, depersonalization, diplopia, disorientation, drunk feeling, dysarthria, dysphagia, dyspnea, endometrial carcinoma, facial edema, feeling abnormal, gait abnormal, hepatic enzymes increased, hepatic failure, hepatic necrosis, hepatitis, hyperglycemia, hyper-/hypotension, hypersensitivity, jaundice, liver function tests increased, menorrhagia, menstrual disorder, metrorrhagia, muscle cramps, ovarian cyst, pancreatitis (acute), paresthesia, pruritus, sedation, slurred speech, stupor, suicidal ideation, syncope, tachycardia, throat tightness, TIA, tinnitus, tongue swelling, urticaria, vertigo, visual disturbance, walking difficulty, weight gain/loss

Vaginal gel (percentages reported with ART); also refer to oral capsule reactions listing for additional effects noted with progesterone:

>10%:
- Central nervous system: Somnolence (27%), headache (13% to 17%), nervousness (16%), depression (11%)
- Endocrine & metabolic: Breast enlargement (40%), breast pain (13%), libido decreased (11%)
- Gastrointestinal: Constipation (27%), nausea (7% to 22%), cramps (15%), abdominal pain (12%)
- Genitourinary: Perineal pain (17%), nocturia (13%)

5% to 10%:
- Central nervous system: Pain (8%), dizziness (5%)
- Gastrointestinal: Diarrhea (8%), bloating (7%), vomiting (5%)
- Genitourinary: Vaginal discharge (7%), dyspareunia (6%), genital moniliasis (5%), genital pruritus (5%)
- Neuromuscular & skeletal: Arthralgia (8%)

Vaginal tablet (percentages reported with ART); also refer to oral capsule reactions listing for additional effects noted with progesterone:

>10%:
- Gastrointestinal: Abdominal pain (12%)
- Miscellaneous: Post-oocyte retrieval pain (25% to 28%)

1% to 10%:
- Central nervous system: Headache (3% to 4%), fatigue (2% to 3%)
- Endocrine & metabolic: Ovarian hyperstimulation syndrome (7%)
- Gastrointestinal: Nausea (7% to 8%), abdominal distension (4%), constipation (2% to 3%), vomiting (2% to 3%)
- Genitourinary: Uterine spasm (3% to 4%), vaginal bleeding (3%), urinary tract infection (1% to 2%)

<1%: Burning, discomfort, itching, peripheral edema, urticaria, vaginal irritation

Drug Interactions

Metabolism/Transport Effects **Substrate** of CYP1A2 (minor), CYP2A6 (minor), CYP2C19 (major), CYP2C9 (minor), CYP2D6 (minor), CYP3A4 (major); **Note:** Assignment of Major/Minor substrate status based on clinically relevant drug interaction potential; **Inhibits** CYP2C19 (weak), CYP2C9 (weak), CYP3A4 (weak), P-glycoprotein

Avoid Concomitant Use

Avoid concomitant use of Progesterone with any of the following: Bosutinib; PAZOPanib; Pimozide; Pomalidomide; Silodosin; Topotecan; Ulipristal; VinCRIStine (Liposomal)

Increased Effect/Toxicity

Progesterone may increase the levels/effects of: Afatinib; ARIPiprazole; Bosutinib; Colchicine; Dabigatran Etexilate; Dofetilide; Everolimus; Lomitapide; PAZOPanib; P-glycoprotein/ABCB1 Substrates; Pimozide; Pomalidomide; Prucalopride; Rivaroxaban; Silodosin; Topotecan; VinCRIStine (Liposomal)

The levels/effects of Progesterone may be increased by: Herbs (Progestogenic Properties)

Decreased Effect

Progesterone may decrease the levels/effects of: Anticoagulants

The levels/effects of Progesterone may be decreased by: Aminoglutethimide; Bosentan; CYP2C19 Inducers (Strong); CYP3A4 Inducers (Strong); Dabrafenib; Deferasirox; Herbs (CYP3A4 Inducers); Mitotane; Peginterferon Alfa-2b; Tocilizumab; Ulipristal

Ethanol/Nutrition/Herb Interactions

Food: Food increases oral bioavailability.

Herb/Nutraceutical: St John's wort may decrease progesterone levels. Herbs with progestogenic properties may enhance the adverse/toxic effects of progestin; example herbs include bloodroot, chasteberry, damiana, oregano, yucca.

Storage/Stability Store at controlled room temperature. Protect capsules from excessive moisture.

Mechanism of Action Natural steroid hormone that induces secretory changes in the endometrium, promotes mammary gland development, relaxes uterine smooth muscle, blocks follicular maturation and ovulation, and maintains pregnancy. When used as part of an ART program in the luteal phase, progesterone supports embryo implantation.

Pharmacodynamics/Kinetics

Absorption: Vaginal gel: Prolonged
- Absorption half-life: 25-50 hours

Protein binding: Albumin (50% to 54%) and cortisol-binding protein (43% to 48%)

Metabolism: Hepatic to metabolites

Half-life elimination: Vaginal gel: 5-20 minutes

Time to peak: Oral: Within 3 hours; I.M.: ~8 hours; Vaginal tablet: ~17-24 hours

Excretion: Urine, bile, feces

Dosage Adults:

I.M.: Females:
- Amenorrhea: 5-10 mg/day for 6-8 consecutive days
- Functional uterine bleeding: 5-10 mg/day for 6 doses

Oral: Females:
- Prevention of endometrial hyperplasia (in postmenopausal women with a uterus who are receiving daily conjugated estrogen tablets): 200 mg as a single daily dose every evening for 12 days sequentially per 28-day cycle
- Amenorrhea: 400 mg every evening for 10 days

Intravaginal gel: Females:
- ART in women who require progesterone supplementation: 90 mg (8% gel) once daily; if pregnancy occurs, may continue treatment for up to 10-12 weeks
- ART in women with partial or complete ovarian failure: 90 mg (8% gel) intravaginally twice daily; if pregnancy occurs, may continue up to 10-12 weeks
- Secondary amenorrhea: 45 mg (4% gel) intravaginally every other day for up to 6 doses; women who fail to respond may be increased to 90 mg (8% gel) every other day for up to 6 doses

Intravaginal tablet: Females: ART: 100 mg 2-3 times daily starting at oocyte retrieval and continuing for up to 10 weeks.

Dosage adjustment in renal impairment:

Injection, oral: No dosage adjustment provided in manufacturer's labeling (has not been studied). Use with caution.

Intravaginal gel, insert: No dosage adjustment provided in manufacturer's labeling.

Dosage adjustment in hepatic impairment: Use is contraindicated in liver dysfunction or disease.

Administration

I.M.: Administer deep I.M. only

Intravaginal:

Vaginal gel: (A small amount of gel will remain in the applicator following insertion): Administer into the vagina directly from sealed applicator. Remove applicator from wrapper; holding applicator by thickest end, shake down to move contents to thin end; while holding applicator by flat section of thick end, twist off tab; gently insert into vagina and squeeze thick end of applicator.

For use at altitudes above 2500 feet: Remove applicator from wrapper; hold applicator on both sides of bubble in the thick end; using a lancet, make a single puncture in the bubble to relieve air pressure; holding applicator by thickest end, shake down to move contents to thin end; while holding applicator by flat section of thick end, twist off tab; gently insert into vagina and squeeze thick end of applicator.

Vaginal tablet: Insert tablet in vagina using disposable applicator provided.

Oral capsule: For patients who experience difficulty swallowing the capsules, taking with a full glass of water in the standing position may be beneficial.

Hazardous agent; use appropriate precautions for handling and disposal (NIOSH, 2012).

Monitoring Parameters Routine physical examination that includes blood pressure and Papanicolaou smear, breast exam, mammogram. Adequate diagnostic measures, including endometrial sampling, if indicated, should be performed to rule out malignancy in all cases of undiagnosed abnormal vaginal bleeding. Signs and symptoms of thromboembolic disorders, vision changes

Test Interactions Thyroid function, metyrapone, liver function, coagulation tests, endocrine function tests

Dosage Forms Excipient information presented when available (limited, particularly for generics); consult specific product labeling.

Capsule, Oral:

Prometrium: 100 mg, 200 mg [contains peanut oil]

Generic: 100 mg, 200 mg

Gel, Vaginal:

Crinone: 4% (1.125 g); 8% (1.125 g)

Insert, Vaginal:

Endometrin: 100 mg (21 ea)

Oil, Intramuscular:

Generic: 50 mg/mL (10 mL)

Suppository, Vaginal:

First-Progesterone VGS 25: 25 mg (30 ea)

First-Progesterone VGS 50: 50 mg (30 ea)

First-Progesterone VGS 100: 100 mg (30 ea)

First-Progesterone VGS 200: 200 mg (30 ea)

First-Progesterone VGS 400: 400 mg (30 ea)

- ◆ **Progestin** *see* Progesterone *on page 1725*
- ◆ **PRO-Glyburide (Can)** *see* GlyBURIDE *on page 963*
- ◆ **Proglycem** *see* Diazoxide *on page 597*
- ◆ **Proglycem® (Can)** *see* Diazoxide *on page 597*
- ◆ **Prograf** *see* Tacrolimus (Systemic) *on page 1976*
- ◆ **Proguanil and Atovaquone** *see* Atovaquone and Proguanil *on page 194*
- ◆ **Proguanil Hydrochloride and Atovaquone** *see* Atovaquone and Proguanil *on page 194*
- ◆ **PRO-Hydroxyquine (Can)** *see* Hydroxychloroquine *on page 1019*
- ◆ **PRO-Indapamide (Can)** *see* Indapamide *on page 1066*
- ◆ **Pro-Indo (Can)** *see* Indomethacin *on page 1070*
- ◆ **PRO-ISMN (Can)** *see* Isosorbide Mononitrate *on page 1128*
- ◆ **Prokine** *see* Sargramostim *on page 1877*
- ◆ **Prolensa** *see* Bromfenac *on page 281*
- ◆ **Proleukin** *see* Aldesleukin *on page 63*
- ◆ **Proleukin® (Can)** *see* Aldesleukin *on page 63*
- ◆ **PRO-Levetiracetam (Can)** *see* LevETIRAcetam *on page 1194*
- ◆ **PRO-Levocarb (Can)** *see* Carbidopa and Levodopa *on page 340*
- ◆ **Prolia** *see* Denosumab *on page 568*
- ◆ **PRO-Lisinopril (Can)** *see* Lisinopril *on page 1226*
- ◆ **PRO-Lorazepam (Can)** *see* LORazepam *on page 1242*
- ◆ **PRO-Lovastatin (Can)** *see* Lovastatin *on page 1250*
- ◆ **Promacet** *see* Butalbital and Acetaminophen *on page 305*
- ◆ **Promacta** *see* Eltrombopag *on page 693*
- ◆ **PRO-Metformin (Can)** *see* MetFORMIN *on page 1310*

Promethazine (proe METH a zeen)

Brand Names: U.S. Phenadoz; Phenergan; Promethegan

Brand Names: Canada Bioniche Promethazine; Histantil; Phenergan; PMS-Promethazine

Index Terms Promethazine Hydrochloride

Pharmacologic Category Antiemetic; Histamine H_1 Antagonist; Histamine H_1 Antagonist, First Generation; Phenothiazine Derivative

Additional Appendix Information

Beers Criteria – Potentially Inappropriate Medications for Geriatrics *on page 2368*

Use Symptomatic treatment of various allergic conditions; antiemetic; motion sickness; sedative; adjunct to postoperative analgesia and anesthesia

Unlabeled Use Treatment of nausea and vomiting of pregnancy (NVP)

Pregnancy Risk Factor C

Pregnancy Considerations Teratogenic effects were not observed in animal reproduction studies. Promethazine crosses the placenta. Maternal promethazine use has generally not resulted in an increased risk of birth defects. Platelet aggregation may be inhibited in newborns following maternal use of promethazine within 2 weeks of delivery. Promethazine is used for the treatment of nausea and vomiting of pregnancy (refer to current guidelines). Promethazine is also indicated for use during labor for obstetric sedation and may be used alone or as an adjunct to opioid analgesics.

Breast-Feeding Considerations It is not known if promethazine is excreted in breast milk. According to the manufacturer, the decision to continue or discontinue breast-feeding during therapy should take into account the risk of exposure to the infant and the benefits of treatment to the mother. Antihistamines may decrease maternal serum prolactin concentrations when administered prior to the establishment of nursing.

Contraindications Hypersensitivity to promethazine or any component of the formulation (cross-reactivity between phenothiazines may occur); coma; treatment of lower respiratory tract symptoms, including asthma; children <2 years of age; intra-arterial or subcutaneous administration

Warnings/Precautions [U.S. Boxed Warning]: Respiratory fatalities have been reported in children <2 years of age. Contraindicated in children <2 years of age. In children ≥2 years, use the lowest possible dose; other drugs with respiratory depressant effects should be avoided.

[U.S. Boxed Warning]: Promethazine injection can cause severe tissue injury (including gangrene) regardless of the route of administration. Tissue irritation and damage may result from perivascular extravasation, unintentional intra-arterial administration, and intraneuronal or perineuronal infiltration. In addition to gangrene, adverse events reported include tissue necrosis, abscesses, burning, pain, erythema, edema, paralysis, severe spasm of distal vessels, phlebitis, thrombophlebitis, venous thrombosis, sensory loss, paralysis, and palsies. Surgical intervention including fasciotomy, skin graft, and/or amputation have been necessary in some cases. The preferred route of administration is by deep intramuscular (I.M.) injection. Subcutaneous administration is contraindicated. Discontinue intravenous injection immediately with onset of pain and evaluate for arterial injection or perivascular extravasation. Although there is no proven successful management of unintentional intra-arterial injection or perivascular extravasation, sympathetic block and heparinization have been used in the acute management of unintentional intra-arterial injection based on results from animal studies. Vesicant; for I.V. administration (**not** the preferred route of administration), ensure proper needle or catheter placement prior to and during administration; avoid extravasation.

May be sedating; use with caution in disorders where CNS depression is a feature. May impair physical or mental abilities; patients must be cautioned about performing tasks which require mental alertness. Use with caution in hemodynamic instability; bone marrow suppression; subcortical brain damage; and in severe cardiac, hepatic or respiratory disease. Avoid use in Reye's syndrome. May lower seizure threshold; use caution in persons with seizure disorders or in persons using opioids or local anesthetics which may also affect seizure threshold. May alter temperature regulation or mask toxicity of other drugs due to antiemetic effects. May alter cardiac conduction (life-threatening arrhythmias have occurred with therapeutic doses of phenothiazines). May cause orthostatic hypotension; use with caution in patients at risk of hypotension or where transient hypotensive episodes would be poorly tolerated (cardiovascular disease or cerebrovascular disease).

Phenothiazines may cause anticholinergic effects; therefore, they should be used with caution in patients with decreased gastrointestinal motility, GI or GU obstruction, urinary retention, BPH, xerostomia, or visual problems. Conditions which also may be exacerbated by cholinergic blockade include narrow-angle glaucoma (screening is recommended) and worsening of myasthenia gravis. Use with caution in Parkinson's disease. May cause extrapyramidal symptoms, including pseudoparkinsonism, acute dystonic reactions, akathisia, and tardive dyskinesia. May be associated with neuroleptic malignant syndrome (NMS). May cause photosensitivity. In the elderly, avoid use of this potent anticholinergic agent due to increased risk of confusion, dry mouth, constipation, and other anticholinergic effects; clearance decreases in patients of advanced age (Beers Criteria). Injection may contain sodium metabisulfite.

Adverse Reactions Frequency not defined.

Cardiovascular: Bradycardia, hyper-/hypotension, nonspecific QT changes, orthostatic hypotension, tachycardia,

Central nervous system: Agitation akathisia, catatonic states, confusion, delirium, disorientation, dizziness, drowsiness, dystonias, euphoria, excitation, extrapyramidal symptoms, faintness, fatigue, hallucinations, hysteria, insomnia, lassitude, pseudoparkinsonism, tardive dyskinesia, nervousness, neuroleptic malignant syndrome, nightmares, sedation, seizure, somnolence

Dermatologic: Angioneurotic edema, dermatitis, photosensitivity, skin pigmentation (slate gray), urticaria

Endocrine & metabolic: Amenorrhea, breast engorgement, gynecomastia, hyperglycemia, lactation

Gastrointestinal: Constipation, nausea, vomiting, xerostomia

Genitourinary: Ejaculatory disorder, impotence, urinary retention

Hematologic: Agranulocytosis, leukopenia, thrombocytopenia, thrombocytopenic purpura

Hepatic: Jaundice

Local: Abscess, distal vessel spasm, gangrene, injection site reactions (burning, edema, erythema, pain), palsies, paralysis, phlebitis, sensory loss, thrombophlebitis, tissue necrosis, venous thrombosis

Neuromuscular & skeletal: Incoordination, tremor

Ocular: Blurred vision, corneal and lenticular changes, diplopia, epithelial keratopathy, pigmentary retinopathy

Otic: Tinnitus

Respiratory: Apnea, asthma, nasal congestion, respiratory depression

Drug Interactions

Metabolism/Transport Effects Substrate of CYP2B6 (major), CYP2D6 (major); **Note:** Assignment of Major/Minor substrate status based on clinically relevant drug interaction potential; **Inhibits** CYP2D6 (weak)

Avoid Concomitant Use

Avoid concomitant use of Promethazine with any of the following: Aclidinium; Azelastine (Nasal); Ipratropium (Oral Inhalation); Metoclopramide; Paraldehyde; Tiotropium; Umeclidinium

Increased Effect/Toxicity

Promethazine may increase the levels/effects of: Alcohol (Ethyl); Analgesics (Opioid); Anticholinergics; Antipsychotics; Azelastine (Nasal); Buprenorphine; CNS Depressants; Highest Risk QTc-Prolonging Agents; Hydrocodone; Moderate Risk QTc-Prolonging Agents; Paraldehyde; Pramipexole; ROPINIRole; Rotigotine; Serotonin Modulators; Tiotropium; Zolpidem

The levels/effects of Promethazine may be increased by: Abiraterone Acetate; Aclidinium; Antipsychotics; Brimonidine (Topical); CYP2B6 Inhibitors (Moderate); CYP2B6 Inhibitors (Strong); CYP2D6 Inhibitors (Moderate); CYP2D6 Inhibitors (Strong); Darunavir; Doxylamine; HydrOXYzine; Ipratropium (Oral Inhalation); Magnesium Sulfate; MAO Inhibitors; Metoclopramide; Metyrosine; Mifepristone; Perampanel; Pramlintide; Quazepam; Sodium Oxybate; Umeclidinium

Decreased Effect

Promethazine may decrease the levels/effects of: Acetylcholinesterase Inhibitors (Central); EPINEPHrine (Nasal); Epinephrine (Racemic); EPINEPHrine (Systemic, Oral Inhalation)

The levels/effects of Promethazine may be decreased by: Acetylcholinesterase Inhibitors (Central); CYP2B6 Inducers (Strong); Dabrafenib; Peginterferon Alfa-2b

Ethanol/Nutrition/Herb Interactions
Ethanol: Avoid ethanol (may increase CNS depression).
Herb/Nutraceutical: Avoid valerian, St John's wort, kava kava, gotu kola (may increase CNS depression).

Storage/Stability
Injection: Prior to dilution, store at 20°C to 25°C (68°F to 77°F). Protect from light. Solutions in NS or D_5W are stable for 24 hours at room temperature.
Oral solution: Store at 15°C to 25°C (59°F to 77°F). Protect from light.
Suppositories: Store refrigerated at 2°C to 8°C (36°F to 46°F).
Tablets: Store at 20°C to 25°C (68°F to 77°F). Protect from light.

Mechanism of Action Phenothiazine derivative; blocks postsynaptic mesolimbic dopaminergic receptors in the brain; exhibits a strong alpha-adrenergic blocking effect and depresses the release of hypothalamic and hypophyseal hormones; competes with histamine for the H_1-receptor; muscarinic-blocking effect may be responsible for antiemetic activity; reduces stimuli to the brainstem reticular system

Pharmacodynamics/Kinetics
Onset of action: Oral, I.M.: ~20 minutes; I.V.: ~5 minutes
Duration: Usually 4-6 hours (up to 12 hours)
Absorption: Oral: Rapid and complete; large first pass effect limits systemic bioavailability (Sharma, 2003)
Distribution: V_d: Syrup: 98 L/kg (range: 17-277 L/kg) (Strenkoski-Nox, 2000)
Metabolism: Hepatic; hydroxylation via CYP2D6 and N-demethylation via CYP2B6; significant first-pass effect (Sharma, 2003)
Bioavailability: Oral: ~25% (Sharma, 2003)
Half-life elimination: I.M.: ~10 hours; I.V.: 9-16 hours; Suppositories, syrup: 16-19 hours (range: 4-34 hours) (Strenkoski-Nox, 2000)
Time to maximum serum concentration: Suppositories: 6.7-8.6 hours; Syrup: 4.4 hours (Strenkoski-Nox, 2000)
Excretion: Urine

Dosage
Children ≥2 years:
Allergic conditions: Oral, rectal: 0.1 mg/kg/dose (maximum: 12.5 mg) every 6 hours during the day and 0.5 mg/kg/dose (maximum: 25 mg) at bedtime as needed
Antiemetic: Oral, I.M., I.V., rectal: 0.25-1 mg/kg 4-6 times/day as needed (maximum: 25 mg/dose)
Motion sickness: Oral, rectal: 0.5 mg/kg/dose 30 minutes to 1 hour before departure, then every 12 hours as needed (maximum dose: 25 mg twice daily)
Preoperative analgesia/hypnotic adjunct: I.M., I.V.: 1.1 mg/kg in combination with an analgesic or hypnotic (at reduced doses) and an atropine-like agent. **Note:** Dose should not exceed half of suggested adult dose.
Sedation: Oral, I.M., I.V., rectal: 12.5-25 mg at bedtime or preoperatively (maximum: 25 mg/dose)
Adults:
Allergic conditions (including allergic reactions to blood or plasma):
Oral, rectal: 25 mg at bedtime **or** 12.5 mg before meals and at bedtime (range: 6.25-12.5 mg 3 times/day)
I.M., I.V.: 25 mg, may repeat in 2 hours when necessary; switch to oral route as soon as feasible
Antiemetic: Oral, I.M., I.V., rectal: 12.5-25 mg every 4-6 hours as needed
Motion sickness: Oral, rectal: 25 mg 30-60 minutes before departure, then every 12 hours as needed
Obstetrics (labor) as adjunct to analgesia: I.M., I.V.: Early labor: 50 mg; Established labor: 25-75 mg; may repeat every 4 hours for up to 2 additional doses (maximum: 100 mg/day while in labor). **Note:** Dosage of concomitant analgesic should be reduced.
Pre-/postoperative analgesia/hypnotic adjunct: I.M., I.V.: 25-50 mg in combination with analgesic or hypnotic (at reduced dosage)
Sedation: Oral, I.M., I.V., rectal: 12.5-50 mg/dose

Dosage adjustment in renal impairment: No dosage adjustment provided in manufacturer's labeling.

Dosage adjustment in hepatic impairment:
Children ≥2 years: No dosage adjustment provided in manufacturer's labeling; however, avoid use in patients with signs of hepatic disease (adverse reactions caused by promethazine may be confused with signs of hepatic disease).
Adults: No dosage adjustment provided in manufacturer's labeling; use with caution (cholestatic jaundice has been reported with use).

Dietary Considerations Increase dietary intake of riboflavin.

Administration Formulations available for oral, rectal, I.M./I.V.; not for SubQ administration. Administer I.M. into deep muscle (preferred route of administration). I.V. administration is **not** the preferred route; severe tissue damage may occur. Solution for injection should be administered in a maximum concentration of 25 mg/mL (more dilute solutions are recommended). Administer via running I.V. line at port farthest from patient's vein, or through a large bore vein (not hand or wrist). Consider administering over 10-15 minutes (maximum: 25 mg/minute).

Vesicant; ensure proper needle or catheter placement prior to and during infusion; avoid extravasation. Discontinue immediately if burning or pain occurs with administration; evaluate for inadvertent arterial injection or extravasation.

Extravasation management: If extravasation occurs, stop infusion immediately and disconnect (leave cannula/needle in place); gently aspirate extravasated solution (do **NOT** flush the line); remove needle/cannula; elevate extremity. Apply dry cold compresses (Hurst, 2004).

Monitoring Parameters Relief of symptoms, mental status; signs and symptoms of tissue injury (burning or pain at injection site, phlebitis, edema) with I.V. administration

Test Interactions May interfere with urine detection of amphetamine/methamphetamine (false-positive); alters the flare response in intradermal allergen tests; hCG-based pregnancy tests may result in false-negatives or false-positives

Dosage Forms Excipient information presented when available (limited, particularly for generics); consult specific product labeling.
Solution, Injection, as hydrochloride:
Phenergan: 50 mg/mL (1 mL) [contains edetate disodium, phenol, sodium metabisulfite]
Phenergan: 25 mg/mL (1 mL) [pyrogen free; contains edetate disodium, phenol, sodium metabisulfite]
Generic: 25 mg/mL (1 mL); 50 mg/mL (1 mL)
Solution, Oral, as hydrochloride:
Generic: 6.25 mg/5 mL (118 mL, 473 mL)
Suppository, Rectal, as hydrochloride:
Phenadoz: 12.5 mg (12 ea); 25 mg (12 ea)
Promethegan: 12.5 mg (12 ea); 25 mg (12 ea, 1000 ea); 50 mg (12 ea)
Generic: 12.5 mg (1 ea, 12 ea); 25 mg (1 ea, 12 ea)
Syrup, Oral, as hydrochloride:
Generic: 6.25 mg/5 mL (118 mL, 473 mL)
Tablet, Oral, as hydrochloride:
Generic: 12.5 mg, 25 mg, 50 mg

Promethazine and Codeine
(proe METH a zeen & KOE deen)

Index Terms Codeine and Promethazine

Pharmacologic Category Analgesic, Opioid; Antitussive; Histamine H_1 Antagonist; Histamine H_1 Antagonist, First Generation; Phenothiazine Derivative

Use Temporary relief of coughs and upper respiratory symptoms associated with allergy or the common cold

Pregnancy Risk Factor C

Dosage Oral:

Children:

<6 years: **Note:** Use of promethazine/codeine combination is contraindicated in children <6 years of age

6-11 years: 2.5-5 mL every 4-6 hours (maximum: 30 mL per 24 hours)

Children ≥12 years and Adults: 5 mL every 4-6 hours (maximum: 30 mL per 24 hours)

Elderly: Use with caution; consider decreased dose

Dosage adjustment in renal/hepatic impairment: Use with caution; consider decreased dose

Additional Information Complete prescribing information should be consulted for additional detail.

Dosage Forms Excipient information presented when available (limited, particularly for generics); consult specific product labeling.

Syrup: Promethazine hydrochloride 6.25 mg and codeine phosphate 10 mg per 5 mL (5 mL, 118 mL, 473 mL)

Controlled Substance C-V

Promethazine and Dextromethorphan

(proe METH a zeen & deks troe meth OR fan)

Index Terms Dextromethorphan and Promethazine

Pharmacologic Category Antitussive; Histamine H_1 Antagonist; Histamine H_1 Antagonist, First Generation; Phenothiazine Derivative

Use Temporary relief of coughs and upper respiratory symptoms associated with allergy or the common cold

Pregnancy Risk Factor C

Dosage Oral:

Children:

<2 years: Use of promethazine is contraindicated

2-6 years: 1.25-2.5 mL every 4-6 hours up to 10 mL in 24 hours

6-12 years: 2.5-5 mL every 4-6 hours up to 20 mL in 24 hours

Adults: 5 mL every 4-6 hours up to 30 mL in 24 hours

Dosage adjustment in renal impairment: No dosage adjustment provided in manufacturer's labeling.

Dosage adjustment in hepatic impairment:

Children: No dosage adjustment provided in manufacturer's labeling; however, avoid use in patients with signs of hepatic disease (adverse reactions caused by promethazine may be confused with signs of hepatic disease).

Adults: No dosage adjustment provided in manufacturer's labeling; use with caution.

Additional Information Complete prescribing information should be consulted for additional detail.

Dosage Forms Excipient information presented when available (limited, particularly for generics); consult specific product labeling.

Syrup: Promethazine hydrochloride 6.25 mg and dextromethorphan hydrobromide 15 mg per 5 mL (120 mL, 480 mL)

◆ **Promethazine Hydrochloride** *see* Promethazine *on page* 1728

◆ **Promethegan** *see* Promethazine *on page* 1728

◆ **Prometrium** *see* Progesterone *on page* 1725

◆ **PRO-Mirtazapine (Can)** *see* Mirtazapine *on page* 1379

◆ **Promolaxin [OTC]** *see* Docusate *on page* 644

◆ **PRO-Naproxen EC (Can)** *see* Naproxen *on page* 1425

◆ **Pronestyl** *see* Procainamide *on page* 1718

◆ **Pronto® Complete Lice Removal System [OTC]** *see* Pyrethrins and Piperonyl Butoxide *on page* 1752

◆ **Pronto® Lice Control (Can)** *see* Pyrethrins and Piperonyl Butoxide *on page* 1752

◆ **Pronto® Plus Lice Killing Mousse Plus Vitamin E [OTC]** *see* Pyrethrins and Piperonyl Butoxide *on page* 1752

◆ **Pronto® Plus Lice Killing Mousse Shampoo Plus Natural Extracts and Oils [OTC]** *see* Pyrethrins and Piperonyl Butoxide *on page* 1752

◆ **Pronto® Plus Warm Oil Treatment and Conditioner [OTC]** *see* Pyrethrins and Piperonyl Butoxide *on page* 1752

Propafenone (pro PAF en one)

Brand Names: U.S. Rythmol; Rythmol SR

Brand Names: Canada Apo-Propafenone®; Mylan-Propafenone; PMS-Propafenone; Rythmol® Gen-Propafenone

Index Terms Propafenone Hydrochloride

Pharmacologic Category Antiarrhythmic Agent, Class Ic

Additional Appendix Information

Beers Criteria – Potentially Inappropriate Medications for Geriatrics *on page* 2368

Use Treatment of life-threatening ventricular arrhythmias; treatment of paroxysmal atrial fibrillation/flutter (PAF) or paroxysmal supraventricular tachycardia (PSVT) in patients with disabling symptoms and without structural heart disease

Extended release capsule: Prolong the time to recurrence of symptomatic atrial fibrillation in patients without structural heart disease

Unlabeled Use Cardioversion of recent-onset atrial fibrillation (single dose); supraventricular tachycardia in patients with Wolff-Parkinson-White syndrome

Pregnancy Risk Factor C

Pregnancy Considerations Adverse events were observed in some animal reproduction studies.

Breast-Feeding Considerations Propafenone is excreted in breast milk. Due to the potential for serious adverse reactions in the nursing infant, the manufacturer recommends a decision be made whether to discontinue nursing or to discontinue the drug, taking into account the importance of treatment to the mother.

Contraindications Hypersensitivity to propafenone or any component of the formulation; sinoatrial, AV, and intraventricular disorders of impulse generation and/or conduction (except in patients with a functioning artificial pacemaker); Brugada syndrome, sinus bradycardia; cardiogenic shock; uncompensated cardiac failure; marked hypotension; bronchospastic disorders or severe obstructive pulmonary disease; uncorrected electrolyte abnormalities

Warnings/Precautions **[U.S. Boxed Warning]: In the Cardiac Arrhythmia Suppression Trial (CAST), recent (>6 days but <2 years ago) myocardial infarction patients with asymptomatic, non-life-threatening ventricular arrhythmias did not benefit and may have been harmed by attempts to suppress the arrhythmia with flecainide or encainide.** An increased mortality or non-fatal cardiac arrest rate (7.7%) was seen in the active treatment group compared with patients in the placebo group (3%). The applicability of the CAST results to other populations is unknown. Antiarrhythmic agents should be reserved for patients with life-threatening ventricular arrhythmias.

Can cause life-threatening drug-induced arrhythmias, including ventricular fibrillation, ventricular tachycardia, asystole, and torsade de pointes (Hii, 1991). The manufacturer notes that propafenone may increase the QT interval; however, due to QRS prolongation; changes in the QT interval are difficult to interpret. In an evaluation of propafenone (450 mg/day) in healthy individuals compared to other selected antiarrhythmic agents, propafenone did not affect repolarization time (eg, QT, QTc, JT, JTc) only depolarization time (ie, QRS interval) (Sarubbi, 1998). Monitor for proarrhythmic effects, and when necessary, adjust dose to prevent QT_c prolongation. Initiation of propafenone may unmask Brugada syndrome; obtain ECG after treatment initiation and discontinue if ECG indicative of Brugada syndrome.

In the treatment of atrial fibrillation in the elderly, avoid antiarrhythmics as first-line treatment. In older adults, data suggests rate control may provide more benefits than risks compared to rhythm control for most patients (Beers Criteria).

Concurrent use of propafenone with QT-prolonging agents has not been extensively evaluated. The manufacturer recommends withholding Class Ia or Class III antiarrhythmics for at least 5 half-lives prior to starting propafenone. Slows atrioventricular conduction, potentially leading to first degree AV block; degree of PR interval prolongation and increased QRS duration are dose and concentration related. Avoid in patients with conduction disturbances (unless functioning pacemaker present).

May alter pacing and sensing thresholds of artificial pacemakers. The use of propafenone is not recommended in patients with obstructive lung disease (eg, chronic bronchitis, COPD, emphysema) (Fuster, 2006). Use in patients with bronchospastic disease or severe obstructive lung disease is contraindicated.

Avoid use in patients with heart failure; similar agents have been shown to increase mortality in this population; may precipitate or exacerbate condition. Correct electrolyte disturbances, especially hypokalemia or hypomagnesemia, prior to use and throughout therapy. Administer cautiously in significant hepatic or renal dysfunction. Use with caution in patients with myasthenia gravis; may exacerbate condition. Avoid the concurrent use of a CYP2D6 inhibitor and CYP3A4 inhibitor; may result in an increased risk of proarrhythmia or exaggerated beta-adrenergic blocking activity Agranulocytosis has been reported; generally occurring within the first 2 months of therapy. Upon therapy discontinuation, WBC usually normalized by 14 days. Positive ANA titers have been reported. Titers have decreased with and without propafenone discontinuation. Positive titers have not usually been associated with clinical symptoms, although at least one case of drug induced lupus erythematosus has been reported. Consider therapy discontinuation in symptomatic patients with positive ANA titers.

Adverse Reactions

1% to 10%:

Cardiovascular: New or worsened arrhythmia (proarrhythmic effect) (2% to 10%), angina (2% to 5%), CHF (1% to 4%), ventricular tachycardia (1% to 3%), palpitation (1% to 3%), AV block (first-degree) (1% to 3%), syncope (1% to 2%), increased QRS interval (1% to 2%), chest pain (1% to 2%), PVCs (1% to 2%), bradycardia (1% to 2%), edema (0% to 1%), bundle branch block (0% to 1%), atrial fibrillation (1%), hypotension (0% to 1%), intraventricular conduction delay (0% to 1%)

Central nervous system: Dizziness (4% to 15%), fatigue (2% to 6%), headache (2% to 5%), ataxia (0% to 2%), insomnia (0% to 2%), anxiety (1% to 2%), drowsiness (1%)

Dermatologic: Rash (1% to 3%)

Gastrointestinal: Nausea/vomiting (2% to 11%), unusual taste (3% to 23%), constipation (2% to 7%), dyspepsia (1% to 3%), diarrhea (1% to 3%), xerostomia (1% to 2%), anorexia (1% to 2%), abdominal pain (1% to 2%), flatulence (0% to 1%)

Neuromuscular & skeletal: Tremor (0% to 1%), arthralgia (0% to 1%), weakness (1% to 2%)

Ocular: Blurred vision (1% to 6%)

Respiratory: Dyspnea (2% to 5%)

Miscellaneous: Diaphoresis (1%)

<1% (Limited to important or life-threatening): Agranulocytosis, alopecia, amnesia, anemia, apnea, AV block (second or third degree), asystole, AV dissociation, cardiac arrest, cholestasis (0.1%), coma, confusion, CHF, depression, granulocytopenia, hepatitis (0.03%), hyperglycemia, impotence, increased bleeding time, leukopenia, lupus erythematosus, mania, memory loss, nephrotic syndrome, paresthesia, peripheral neuropathy, pruritus, psychosis, purpura, renal failure, seizure (0.3%), SIADH, sinus node dysfunction, thrombocytopenia, tinnitus, torsade de pointes, ventricular fibrillation, vertigo

Drug Interactions

Metabolism/Transport Effects Substrate of CYP1A2 (minor), CYP2D6 (minor), CYP3A4 (minor); **Note:** Assignment of Major/Minor substrate status based on clinically relevant drug interaction potential; **Inhibits** CYP1A2 (weak), CYP2D6 (weak)

Avoid Concomitant Use

Avoid concomitant use of Propafenone with any of the following: Amiodarone; Antiarrhythmic Agents (Class Ia); Antiarrhythmic Agents (Class III); FLUoxetine; Fosamprenavir; Highest Risk QTc-Prolonging Agents; Ivabradine; Mifepristone; QuiNIDine; Ritonavir; Saquinavir; Tipranavir

Increased Effect/Toxicity

Propafenone may increase the levels/effects of: Antiarrhythmic Agents (Class Ia); Antiarrhythmic Agents (Class III); ARIPiprazole; Beta-Blockers; Cardiac Glycosides; CYP2D6 Inhibitors (Moderate); FLUoxetine; Highest Risk QTc-Prolonging Agents; Moderate Risk QTc-Prolonging Agents; Propranolol; Theophylline Derivatives; Venlafaxine; Vitamin K Antagonists

The levels/effects of Propafenone may be increased by: Amiodarone; Boceprevir; Cimetidine; CYP2D6 Inhibitors (Strong); CYP3A4 Inhibitors (Moderate); CYP3A4 Inhibitors (Strong); FLUoxetine; FluvoxaMINE; Fosamprenavir; Ivabradine; Mifepristone; Mirabegron; PARoxetine; QTc-Prolonging Agents (Indeterminate Risk and Risk Modifying); QuiNIDine; Ritonavir; Saquinavir; Sertraline; Telaprevir; Tipranavir

Decreased Effect

The levels/effects of Propafenone may be decreased by: Barbiturates; Etravirine; Orlistat; Peginterferon Alfa-2b; Rifamycin Derivatives

Ethanol/Nutrition/Herb Interactions

Food: Propafenone serum concentrations may be increased if taken with food.

Herb/Nutraceutical: St John's wort may decrease propafenone levels. Avoid ephedra (may worsen arrhythmia).

Storage/Stability Store at 25°C (77°F); excursions permitted to 15°C to 30°C (59°F to 86°F).

Mechanism of Action Propafenone is a class 1c antiarrhythmic agent which possesses local anesthetic properties, blocks the fast inward sodium current, and slows the rate of increase of the action potential. Prolongs conduction and refractoriness in all areas of the myocardium, with a slightly more pronounced effect on intraventricular conduction; it prolongs effective refractory period, reduces spontaneous automaticity and exhibits some beta-blockade activity.

Pharmacodynamics/Kinetics

Absorption: Well absorbed

Distribution: V_d: Adults: 252 L

Protein binding: 95% to alpha$_1$-acid glycoprotein

Metabolism: Hepatic via CYP2D6, CYP3A4 and CYP1A2 to two active metabolites (5-hydroxypropafenone and N-depropylpropafenone) then ultimately to glucuronide or sulfate conjugates. Two genetically determined metabolism groups exist (extensive and poor metabolizers); 10% of Caucasians are poor metabolizers. Exhibits nonlinear pharmacokinetics; when dose is increased from 300-900 mg/day, serum concentrations increase tenfold; this nonlinearity is thought to be due to saturable first-pass effect.

Bioavailability: Immediate release (IR): 150 mg: 3.4%; 300 mg: 10.6%; relative bioavailability of extended release (ER) capsule is less than IR tablet; the bioavailability of an ER capsule regimen of 325 mg twice-daily regimen approximates an IR tablet regimen of 150 mg 3 times/day.

Half-life elimination: Extensive metabolizers: 2-10 hours; Poor metabolizers: 10-32 hours

Time to peak, serum: IR: 3.5 hours; ER: 3-8 hours

Excretion: Urine (<1% unchanged; remainder as glucuronide or sulfate conjugates); feces

Dosage Oral: Adults: **Note:** Patients who exhibit significant widening of QRS complex or second- or third-degree AV block may need dose reduction.

Atrial fibrillation (to prevent recurrence): Extended release capsule: Initial: 225 mg every 12 hours; dosage increase may be made at a minimum of 5-day intervals; may increase to 325 mg every 12 hours; if further increase is necessary, may increase to 425 mg every 12 hours

Paroxysmal atrial fibrillation/flutter, paroxysmal supraventricular tachycardia, ventricular arrhythmias: Immediate release tablet: Initial: 150 mg every 8 hours; dosage increase may be made at minimum of 3- to 4-day intervals, may increase to 225 mg every 8 hours; if further increase is necessary, may increase to 300 mg every 8 hours

Atrial fibrillation, pharmacologic cardioversion (unlabeled use): **Note:** To prevent rapid AV conduction, start an AV nodal-blocking agent (eg, beta-blocker, nondihydropyridine calcium channel blocker) prior to pharmacologic cardioversion. Effect occurs between 2-6 hours after administration.

Immediate release tablet: 600 mg as single dose (Fuster, 2006)

Dosage adjustment in renal impairment: No dosage adjustments provided in manufacturer's labeling; however, 50% of propafenone metabolites (some active) are excreted in the urine; some data suggest that no dosage adjustment is necessary (Burgess, 1989; Fromm, 1994); however, use with caution.

Hemodialysis/CVVH: Minimally dialyzable (Burgess, 1989; Seto, 1999); supplemental dose not necessary

Dosing adjustment in hepatic impairment: No dosage adjustment provided in manufacturer's labeling; however, dosage reduction should be considered as drug undergoes hepatic metabolism. Use with caution.

Dietary Considerations Capsule: May be taken without regard to meals.

Administration Capsules should be swallowed whole; do not crush or chew; may be taken without regard to meals.

Monitoring Parameters ECG, blood pressure, pulse (particularly at initiation of therapy)

Dosage Forms Excipient information presented when available (limited, particularly for generics); consult specific product labeling.

Capsule Extended Release 12 Hour, Oral, as hydrochloride:

Rythmol SR: 225 mg, 325 mg, 425 mg [contains soybean lecithin]

Generic: 225 mg, 325 mg, 425 mg

Tablet, Oral, as hydrochloride:

Rythmol: 150 mg, 225 mg [scored]

Generic: 150 mg, 225 mg, 300 mg

◆ **Propafenone Hydrochloride** *see* Propafenone *on page 1731*

Propantheline (proe PAN the leen)

Index Terms Propantheline Bromide

Pharmacologic Category Anticholinergic Agent

Additional Appendix Information

Beers Criteria – Potentially Inappropriate Medications for Geriatrics *on page 2368*

Use Adjunctive treatment of peptic ulcer

Unlabeled Use Decreased salivation and drooling

Pregnancy Risk Factor C

Dosage Oral:

Antisecretory (unlabeled use):

Children: 1-2 mg/kg/day in 3-4 divided doses

Adults: 15 mg 3 times/day before meals or food and 30 mg at bedtime

Elderly: 7.5 mg 3 times/day before meals and at bedtime

Antispasmodic:

Children: 2-3 mg/kg/day in divided doses every 4-6 hours and at bedtime

Adults: 15 mg 3 times/day before meals or food and 30 mg at bedtime

Dosage adjustment in renal impairment: No dosage adjustment provided in manufacturer's labeling.

Dosage adjustment in hepatic impairment: No dosage adjustment provided in manufacturer's labeling.

Additional Information Complete prescribing information should be consulted for additional detail.

Dosage Forms Excipient information presented when available (limited, particularly for generics); consult specific product labeling.

Tablet, Oral, as bromide:

Generic: 15 mg

◆ **Propantheline Bromide** *see* Propantheline *on page 1733*

Proparacaine (proe PAR a kane)

Brand Names: U.S. Alcaine; Parcaine

Brand Names: Canada Alcaine®; Diocaine®

Index Terms Proparacaine Hydrochloride; Proxymetacaine

Pharmacologic Category Local Anesthetic, Ophthalmic

Use Topical anesthesia for tonometry, gonioscopy; suture removal from cornea; removal of corneal foreign body; short operative procedure involving the cornea and conjunctiva

Pregnancy Risk Factor C

Dosage Ophthalmic: Children, Adolescents, and Adults:

Short corneal and conjunctival procedures: Instill 1 drop in eye(s) every 5-10 minutes for 5-7 doses

Tonometry, gonioscopy, suture removal: Instill 1-2 drops in eye(s) just prior to procedure

Dosage adjustment in renal impairment: No dosage adjustment provided in manufacturer's labeling.

Dosage adjustment in hepatic impairment: No dosage adjustment provided in manufacturer's labeling.

Additional Information Complete prescribing information should be consulted for additional detail.

Dosage Forms Excipient information presented when available (limited, particularly for generics); consult specific product labeling.

Solution, Ophthalmic, as hydrochloride:
- Alcaine: 0.5% (15 mL)
- Parcaine: 0.5% (15 mL)
- Generic: 0.5% (15 mL)

Proparacaine and Fluorescein
(proe PAR a kane & FLURE e seen)

Brand Names: U.S. Flucaine

Index Terms Fluorescein and Proparacaine

Pharmacologic Category Diagnostic Agent; Local Anesthetic

Use For use in ophthalmic procedures when a topical disclosing agent is needed along with an anesthetic

Dosage

Short corneal and conjunctival surgical procedures requiring deep ophthalmic anesthesia: Adults: Ophthalmic: Instill 1 drop in each eye every 5-10 minutes for 5-7 doses

Tonometry, gonioscopy, foreign body or suture removal: Adults: Ophthalmic: Instill 1-2 drops in each eye just prior to procedure

Dosage adjustment in renal impairment: No dosage adjustment provided in manufacturer's labeling.

Dosage adjustment in hepatic impairment: No dosage adjustment provided in manufacturer's labeling.

Additional Information Complete prescribing information should be consulted for additional detail.

Dosage Forms Excipient information presented when available (limited, particularly for generics); consult specific product labeling. [DSC] = Discontinued product

Solution, ophthalmic: Proparacaine hydrochloride 0.5% and fluorescein sodium 0.25% (5 mL)
- Flucaine: Proparacaine hydrochloride 0.5% and fluorescein sodium 0.25% (5 mL)

◆ **Proparacaine Hydrochloride** *see* Proparacaine *on page 1733*

◆ **Propecia** *see* Finasteride *on page 862*

◆ **Propecia® (Can)** *see* Finasteride *on page 862*

◆ **Propine® (Can)** *see* Dipivefrin *on page 634*

◆ **PRO-Pioglitazone (Can)** *see* Pioglitazone *on page 1649*

Propofol (PROE po fole)

Brand Names: U.S. Diprivan; Fresenius Propoven

Brand Names: Canada Diprivan; PMS-Propofol; Propofol Injection

Pharmacologic Category General Anesthetic

Additional Appendix Information

Dosing Considerations for the Critically-Ill Patient With Morbid Obesity *on page 2379*

Status Epilepticus *on page 2375*

Use Induction of anesthesia in patients ≥3 years of age; maintenance of anesthesia in patients >2 months of age; in adults, for monitored anesthesia care sedation during procedures; sedation in intubated, mechanically-ventilated ICU patients

Unlabeled Use Postoperative antiemetic; refractory delirium tremens (case reports)

Pregnancy Risk Factor B

Pregnancy Considerations Propofol crosses the placenta and may be associated with neonatal CNS and respiratory depression. Propofol is not recommended by the manufacturer for obstetrics, including cesarean section deliveries.

Breast-Feeding Considerations Propofol is excreted in breast milk. Breast-feeding is not recommended by the manufacturer. A green discoloration to the breast milk was noted in a woman following administration of propofol during surgery for removal of an ectopic pregnancy. Although other medications were also administered, propofol was detected in the milk and assumed to be the cause; resolution of this effect occurred within 48 hours after surgery (Birkholz, 2009).

Contraindications Hypersensitivity to propofol or any component of the formulation; hypersensitivity to eggs, egg products, soybeans, or soy products; when general anesthesia or sedation is contraindicated

Note: Fresenius Propoven is also contraindicated in patients who are hypersensitive to peanuts. In July 2012, the FDA initiated temporary importation of Fresenius Propoven 1% (propofol) injection into the U.S. market to address a propofol shortage.

Warnings/Precautions May rarely cause hypersensitivity, anaphylaxis, anaphylactoid reactions, angioedema, bronchospasm, and erythema; medications for the treatment of hypersensitivity reactions should be available for immediate use. Use with caution in patients with history of hypersensitivity/anaphylactic reaction to peanuts; a low risk of crossreactivity between soy and peanuts may exist. Use is contraindicated in patients who are hypersensitive to eggs, egg products, soybeans, or soy products. The major cardiovascular effect of propofol is hypotension especially if patient is hypovolemic or if bolus dosing is used; use with caution in patients who are hemodynamically unstable, hypovolemic, or have abnormally low vascular tone (eg, sepsis). Use requires careful patient monitoring, should only be used by experienced personnel who are not actively engaged in the procedure or surgery. If used in a nonintubated and/or nonmechanically-ventilated patient, qualified personnel and appropriate equipment for rapid institution of respiratory and/or cardiovascular support must be immediately available. Use to induce moderate (conscious) sedation in patients warrants monitoring equivalent to that seen with deep anesthesia.

Use a lower induction dose, a slower maintenance rate of administration, and avoid rapidly administered boluses in the elderly, debilitated, or ASA-PS (American Society of Anesthesiologists - Physical Status) 3/4 patients to reduce the incidence of unwanted cardiorespiratory depressive events. Use caution in patients with severe cardiac disease (ejection fraction <50%) or respiratory disease; may have more profound adverse cardiovascular responses to propofol. Use caution in patients with a history of epilepsy or seizures; seizure may occur during recovery phase. Use caution in patients with increased intracranial pressure or impaired cerebral circulation; substantial decreases in mean arterial pressure and subsequent decreases in cerebral perfusion pressure may occur; consider continuous infusion or administer as a slow bolus.

Propofol-related infusion syndrome (PRIS) is a serious side effect with a high mortality rate (up to 33%) characterized by dysrhythmia (eg, bradycardia or tachycardia), heart failure, hyperkalemia, lipemia, metabolic acidosis, and/or rhabdomyolysis or myoglobinuria with subsequent renal failure. Risk factors include poor oxygen delivery, sepsis, serious cerebral injury, and the administration of high doses of propofol (usually doses >83 mcg/kg/minute or >5 mg/kg/hour for >48 hours), but has also been reported following large dose, short term infusions during surgical anesthesia. PRIS has also been reported with lower-dose infusions (Chukwuemeka, 2006; Merz, 2006). The onset of the syndrome is rapid, occurring within 4 days of initiation. Alternate sedative therapy should be considered for patients with escalating doses of vasopressors or inotropes, when cardiac failure occurs during high-dose propofol infusion, when metabolic acidosis is observed, or in whom lengthy and/or high-dose sedation is needed (Barr, 2013; Corbett, 2008).

Because propofol is formulated within a 10% fat emulsion, hypertriglyceridemia is an expected side effect. Patients who develop hypertriglyceridemia (eg, >500 mg/dL) are at risk of developing pancreatitis. An alternative sedative agent should be employed if significant hypertriglyceridemia occurs. Use with caution in patients with pre-existing pancreatitis; use of propofol may exacerbate this condition. Use caution in patients with pre-existing hyperlipidemia as evidenced by increased serum triglyceride levels or serum turbidity. Transient local pain may occur during I.V. injection; perioperative myoclonia has occurred. Propofol should only be used in pregnancy if clearly needed. Not recommended for use in obstetrics, including cesarean section deliveries. Safety and efficacy in pediatric intensive care unit patients have not been established. Concurrent use of fentanyl and propofol in pediatric patients may result in bradycardia.

Concomitant use with opioids may lead to increased sedative or anesthetic effects of propofol, more pronounced decreases in systolic, diastolic, and mean arterial pressures and cardiac output; lower doses of propofol may be needed. In addition, fentanyl may cause serious bradycardia when used with propofol in pediatric patients. Alfentanil use with propofol has precipitated seizure activity in patients without any history of epilepsy. Discontinue opioids and paralytic agents prior to weaning. Avoid abrupt discontinuation prior to weaning or daily wake up assessments. Abrupt discontinuation can result in rapid awakening, anxiety, agitation, and resistance to mechanical ventilation; wean the infusion rate so the patient awakens slowly. Propofol lacks analgesic properties; pain management requires specific use of analgesic agents, at effective dosages, propofol must be titrated separately from the analgesic agent.

Propofol vials and prefilled syringes have the potential to support the growth of various microorganisms despite product additives intended to suppress microbial growth. To limit the potential for contamination, recommendations in product labeling for handling and administering propofol should be strictly adhered to. Some formulations may contain edetate disodium which may lead to decreased zinc levels in patients with prolonged therapy (>5 days) or a predisposition to zinc deficiency (eg, burns, diarrhea, or sepsis). A holiday from propofol infusion should take place after 5 days of therapy to allow for evaluation and necessary replacement of zinc. Some formulations may contain sulfites. Some products may contain benzyl alcohol; benzyl alcohol has been associated with the "gasping syndrome" in neonates and low-birth-weight infants.

Adverse Reactions

>10%:

Cardiovascular: Hypotension (children 17%; adults 3% to 26%)

Central nervous system: Movement (children 17%; adults 3% to 10%)

Local: Injection site burning, stinging, or pain (children 10%; adults 18%)

Respiratory: Apnea lasting 30-60 seconds (children 10%; adults 24%), apnea lasting >60 seconds (children 5%; adults 12%)

1% to 10%:

Cardiovascular: Hypertension (children 8%), arrhythmia (1% to 3%), bradycardia (1% to 3%), cardiac output decreased (1% to 3%; concurrent opioid use increases incidence), tachycardia (1% to 3%)

Dermatologic: Pruritus (1% to 3%), rash (children 5%; adults 1% to 3%)

Endocrine & metabolic: Hypertriglyceridemia (3% to 10%)

Respiratory: Respiratory acidosis during weaning (3% to 10%)

<1% (Limited to important or life-threatening): Agitation, amblyopia, anaphylaxis, anaphylactoid reaction, anticholinergic syndrome, asystole, atrial arrhythmia, bigeminy, cardiac arrest, chills, cough, dizziness, delirium, discoloration (green [urine, hair, or nailbeds]), extremity pain, fever, flushing, hemorrhage, hypersalivation, hypertonia, hypomagnesemia, hypoxia, infusion site reactions (including pain, swelling, blisters and/or tissue necrosis following accidental extravasation); laryngospasm, leukocytosis, lung function decreased, myalgia, myoclonia (rarely including convulsions and opisthotonos), nausea, pancreatitis, paresthesia, phlebitis, postoperative unconsciousness with or without increase in muscle tone, premature atrial contractions, premature ventricular contractions, pulmonary edema, propofol-related infusion syndrome, rhabdomyolysis, somnolence, syncope, thrombosis, urine cloudy, vision abnormality, wheezing

Drug Interactions

Metabolism/Transport Effects **Substrate** of CYP1A2 (minor), CYP2A6 (minor), CYP2B6 (major), CYP2C19 (minor), CYP2C9 (minor), CYP2D6 (minor), CYP2E1 (minor), CYP3A4 (minor); **Note:** Assignment of Major/Minor substrate status based on clinically relevant drug interaction potential; **Inhibits** CYP1A2 (weak), CYP2C9 (weak), CYP2D6 (weak), CYP2E1 (weak), CYP3A4 (weak)

Avoid Concomitant Use

Avoid concomitant use of Propofol with any of the following: Pimozide

Increased Effect/Toxicity

Propofol may increase the levels/effects of: ARIPiprazole; Dofetilide; Lomitapide; Midazolam; Pimozide; Ropivacaine

The levels/effects of Propofol may be increased by: Alfentanil; CYP2B6 Inhibitors (Moderate); CYP2B6 Inhibitors (Strong); Midazolam; Quazepam; Rifampin

Decreased Effect

The levels/effects of Propofol may be decreased by: Peginterferon Alfa-2b

Ethanol/Nutrition/Herb Interactions Food: Edetate disodium, an ingredient of propofol emulsion, may lead to decreased zinc levels in patients on prolonged therapy (>5 days) or those predisposed to deficiency (burns, diarrhea, and/or major sepsis).

Preparation for Administration Does not need to be diluted; however, propofol may be further diluted in 5% dextrose in water to a concentration of ≥2 mg/mL and is stable for 8 hours at room temperature.

Storage/Stability Store between 4°C to 22°C (40°F to 72°F); refrigeration is not required. Do not freeze. If transferred to a syringe or other container prior to administration, use within 6 hours. If used directly from vial/prefilled syringe, use within 12 hours. Shake well before use. Do not use if there is evidence of separation of phases of emulsion.

Mechanism of Action Propofol is a short-acting, lipophilic intravenous general anesthetic. The drug is unrelated to any of the currently used barbiturate, opioid, benzodiazepine, arylcyclohexylamine, or imidazole intravenous anesthetic agents. Propofol causes global CNS depression, presumably through agonism of $GABA_A$ receptors and perhaps reduced glutamatergic activity through NMDA receptor blockade.

Pharmacodynamics/Kinetics

Onset of action: Anesthetic: Bolus infusion (dose dependent): 9-51 seconds (average 30 seconds)

Duration (dose and rate dependent): 3-10 minutes

Distribution: V_d: 2-10 L/kg; after a 10-day infusion, V_d approaches 60 L/kg; decreased in the elderly

Protein binding: 97% to 99%

Metabolism: Hepatic to water-soluble sulfate and glucuronide conjugates (~50%)

Half-life elimination: Biphasic: Initial: 40 minutes; Terminal: 4-7 hours (after 10-day infusion, may be up to 1-3 days)

Excretion: Urine (~88% as metabolites, 40% as glucuronide metabolite); feces (<2%)

Dosage Dosage must be individualized based on total body weight and titrated to the desired clinical effect; wait at least 3-5 minutes between dosage adjustments to clinically assess drug effects; smaller doses are required when used with opioids; the following are general dosing guidelines:

General anesthesia: Note: Increase dose in patients with chronic alcoholism (Fassoulaki, 1993); decrease dose with acutely intoxicated (alcoholic) patients.

Induction: I.V.:

Children (healthy) 3-16 years, ASA-PS 1 or 2: 2.5-3.5 mg/kg over 20-30 seconds; use a lower dose for children ASA-PS 3 or 4

Adults (healthy), ASA-PS 1 or 2, <55 years: 2-2.5 mg/kg (~40 mg every 10 seconds until onset of induction)

Elderly, debilitated, or ASA-PS 3 or 4: 1-1.5 mg/kg (~20 mg every 10 seconds until onset of induction)

Maintenance: I.V. infusion:

Children (healthy) 2 months to 16 years, ASA-PS 1 or 2: 125-300 mcg/kg/minute (or 7.5-18 mg/kg/**hour**); after 30 minutes, if clinical signs of light anesthesia are absent, decrease the infusion rate. Children ≤5 years may require larger infusion rates compared to older children.

Adults (healthy), ASA-PS 1 or 2, <55 years: Initial: 100-200 mcg/kg/minute (or 6-12 mg/kg/**hour**) for 10-15 minutes; usual maintenance infusion rate: 50-100 mcg/kg/minute (or 3-6 mg/kg/**hour**) to optimize recovery time

Elderly, debilitated, ASA-PS 3 or 4: 50-100 mcg/kg/minute (or 3-6 mg/kg/**hour**)

Maintenance: I.V. intermittent bolus: Adults (healthy), ASA-PS 1 or 2, <55 years: 25-50 mg increments as needed

Monitored anesthesia care sedation:

Adults (healthy), ASA-PS 1 or 2, <55 years: Slow I.V. infusion: 100-150 mcg/kg/minute (or 6-9 mg/kg/**hour**) for 3-5 minutes **or** slow injection: 0.5 mg/kg over 3-5 minutes followed by I.V. infusion of 25-75 mcg/kg/minute (or 1.5-4.5 mg/kg/**hour**) **or** incremental bolus doses: 10 mg or 20 mg

Elderly, debilitated, or ASA-PS 3 or 4 patients: Use 80% of healthy adult dose

ICU sedation in intubated mechanically-ventilated patients: Avoid rapid bolus injection; individualize dose and titrate to response. Adults: Continuous infusion: Initial: 5 mcg/kg/minute (or 0.3 mg/kg/**hour**); increase by 5-10 mcg/kg/minute (or 0.3-0.6 mg/kg/**hour**) every 5-10 minutes until desired sedation level is achieved; usual maintenance: 5-50 mcg/kg/minute (or 0.3-3 mg/kg/**hour**); reduce dose after adequate sedation established and adjust to response (eg, evaluate frequently to use minimum dose for sedation). Daily interruption with retitration or a light target level of sedation is recommended to minimize prolonged sedative effects (Barr, 2013).

Postoperative nausea and vomiting (PONV), rescue therapy (unlabeled use; Gan, 2007; Unlugenc, 2004): Adults: I.V.: 20 mg, may be repeated

Refractory status epilepticus (unlabeled use): Adults: 1-2 mg/kg bolus (optional), then 33-167 mcg/kg/minute (or 2-10 mg/kg/**hour**) (Claassen, 2002; Kälviäinen, 2007; Meierkord, 2010; Rossetti, 2004); titrate to desired effect (eg, burst suppression on EEG). **Note:** Doses >83 mcg/kg/minute (or >5 mg/kg/**hour**) may increase the risk of hypotension and propofol-related infusion syndrome (PRIS) especially if used for >48 hours; consider alternative therapies to avoid the risk of PRIS in longer term propofol infusions.

Dosing adjustment in renal impairment: No dosage adjustment necessary.

Dosing adjustment in hepatic impairment: No dosage adjustment necessary.

Dietary Considerations Propofol is formulated in an oil-in-water emulsion. If on parenteral nutrition, may need to adjust the amount of lipid infused. Propofol emulsion contains 1.1 kcal/mL. Soybean fat emulsion is used as a vehicle for propofol. Formulations also contain egg phosphatide and glycerol.

Administration Strict aseptic technique must be maintained in handling although a preservative has been added. Do not use if contamination is suspected. Do not administer through the same I.V. catheter with blood or plasma. Tubing and any unused portions of propofol vials should be discarded after 12 hours.

To reduce pain associated with injection, use larger veins of forearm or antecubital fossa; lidocaine I.V. (1 mL of a 1% solution) may also be used prior to administration or it may be added to propofol immediately before administration in a quantity not to exceed 20 mg lidocaine per 200 mg propofol. Do not use filter <5 micron for administration.

Monitoring Parameters Cardiac monitor, blood pressure, oxygen saturation (during monitored anesthesia care sedation), arterial blood gas (with prolonged infusions). With prolonged infusions (eg, ICU sedation), monitor for metabolic acidosis, hyperkalemia, rhabdomyolysis or elevated CPK, hepatomegaly, and progression of cardiac and renal failure.

ICU sedation: Assess and adjust sedation according to scoring system (Richmond Agitation-Sedation Scale [RASS] or Sedation-Agitation Scale [SAS]) (Barr, 2013); assess CNS function daily. Serum triglyceride levels should be obtained prior to initiation of therapy and every 3-7 days thereafter, especially if receiving for >48 hours with doses exceeding 50 mcg/kg/minute (Devlin, 2005); use intravenous port opposite propofol infusion or temporarily suspend infusion and flush port prior to blood draw.

Diprivan®: Monitor zinc levels in patients predisposed to deficiency (burns, diarrhea, major sepsis) or after 5 days of treatment.

Dosage Forms Excipient information presented when available (limited, particularly for generics); consult specific product labeling.

Emulsion, Intravenous:

Diprivan: 10 mg/mL (20 mL, 50 mL, 100 mL) [contains edetate disodium, egg phospholipids (egg lecithin), glycerin, soybean oil]

Generic: 10 mg/mL (20 mL, 50 mL, 100 mL)

Emulsion, Intravenous [preservative free]:

Fresenius Propoven: 10 mg/mL (20 mL, 50 mL, 100 mL) [contains egg phosphatides, soybean oil]

Generic: 10 mg/mL (20 mL, 50 mL, 100 mL)

◆ **Propofol Injection (Can)** *see* Propofol *on page 1734*

Propranolol (proe PRAN oh lole)

Brand Names: U.S. Inderal LA; InnoPran XL

Brand Names: Canada Apo-Propranolol; Dom-Propranolol; Inderal; Inderal LA; Novo-Pranol; Nu-Propranolol; PMS-Propranolol; Propranolol Hydrochloride Injection, USP; Teva-Propranolol

Index Terms Propranolol Hydrochloride

Pharmacologic Category Antianginal Agent; Antiarrhythmic Agent, Class II; Antihypertensive; Beta-Adrenergic Blocker, Nonselective

Additional Appendix Information

Beta-Blockers *on page 2294*

Use Management of hypertension; angina pectoris; pheochromocytoma; essential tremor; supraventricular arrhythmias (such as atrial fibrillation and flutter, AV nodal re-entrant tachycardias), ventricular tachycardias (catecholamine-induced arrhythmias, digoxin toxicity); prevention of myocardial infarction; migraine headache prophylaxis; symptomatic treatment of hypertrophic subaortic stenosis (hypertrophic obstructive cardiomyopathy)

Unlabeled Use Tremor due to Parkinson's disease; aggressive behavior (not recommended for dementia-associated aggression), anxiety, schizophrenia; antipsychotic-induced akathisia; primary and secondary prophylaxis of variceal hemorrhage; acute panic; thyrotoxicosis; tetralogy of Fallot (TOF) hypercyanotic spells

Pregnancy Risk Factor C

Pregnancy Considerations Adverse events have been observed in some animal reproduction studies; therefore, the manufacturer classifies propranolol as pregnancy category C. Propranolol crosses the placenta and is measurable in the newborn serum following maternal use during pregnancy. In a cohort study, an increased risk of cardiovascular defects was observed following maternal use of beta-blockers during pregnancy. Intrauterine growth restriction (IUGR), small placentas, as well as fetal/neonatal bradycardia, hypoglycemia, and/or respiratory depression have been observed following *in utero* exposure to beta-blockers as a class. Adequate facilities for monitoring infants at birth should be available. Untreated chronic maternal hypertension and pre-eclampsia are also associated with adverse events in the fetus, infant, and mother. The peak maternal serum concentrations of propranolol and the active metabolite 4-hydroxypropranolol do not change during pregnancy; peak serum concentrations of naphthoxylactic acid are lower in the third trimester when compared to postpartum. Propranolol is recommended for use in the management of thyrotoxicosis in pregnancy. Propranolol has been evaluated for the treatment of hypertension in pregnancy, but other agents may be more appropriate for use. Propranolol has also been used in the management of hypertrophic obstructive cardiomyopathy in pregnancy and has been studied for use as an adjunctive agent in the management of dysfunctional labor (dystocia).

Breast-Feeding Considerations Propranolol is excreted into breast milk with peak concentrations occurring ~2-3 hours after an oral dose. The inactive metabolites of propranolol have also been detected in breast milk. The manufacturer recommends that caution be exercised when administering propranolol to nursing women. Due to immature hepatic metabolism in newborns, breast-feeding infants should be monitored for adverse events.

Contraindications Hypersensitivity to propranolol, beta-blockers, or any component of the formulation; uncompensated congestive heart failure (unless the failure is due to tachyarrhythmias being treated with propranolol), cardiogenic shock; severe sinus bradycardia, sick sinus syndrome, or heart block greater than first-degree (except in patients with a functioning artificial pacemaker); severe hyperactive airway disease (asthma or COPD)

Warnings/Precautions Consider pre-existing conditions such as sick sinus syndrome before initiating. Administer cautiously in compensated heart failure and monitor for a worsening of the condition (efficacy of propranolol in HF has not been demonstrated). **[U.S. Boxed Warning]: Beta-blocker therapy should not be withdrawn abruptly (particularly in patients with CAD), but gradually tapered to avoid acute tachycardia, hypertension, and/or ischemia.** Chronic beta-blocker therapy should not be routinely withdrawn prior to major surgery. May precipitate or aggravate symptoms of arterial insufficiency in patients with PVD and Raynaud's disease; use with caution and monitor for progression of arterial obstruction. Bradycardia may be observed more frequently in elderly patients (>65 years of age); dosage reductions may be necessary. Potentially significant drug-drug interactions may exist, requiring dose or frequency adjustment, additional monitoring, and/or selection of alternative therapy.

Use cautiously in patients with diabetes because it can mask prominent hypoglycemic symptoms. May mask signs of hyperthyroidism (eg, tachycardia); if hyperthyroidism is suspected, carefully manage and monitor; abrupt withdrawal may exacerbate symptoms of hyperthyroidism or precipitate thyroid storm. May alter thyroid-function tests. Use with caution in myasthenia gravis or psychiatric disease (may cause CNS depression). Use cautiously in renal and hepatic dysfunction; dosage adjustment required in hepatic impairment. In general, patients with bronchospastic disease should not receive beta-blockers; if used at all, should be used cautiously with close monitoring. Adequate alpha-blockade is required prior to use of any beta-blocker for patients with untreated pheochromocytoma. May induce or exacerbate psoriasis. Use caution with history of severe anaphylaxis to allergens; patients taking beta-blockers may become more sensitive to repeated challenges. Treatment of anaphylaxis (eg, epinephrine) in patients taking beta-blockers may be ineffective or promote undesirable effects.

Adverse Reactions Frequency not defined.

Cardiovascular: Angina, arterial insufficiency, AV conduction disturbance increased, bradycardia, cardiogenic shock, CHF, hypotension, impaired myocardial contractility, mesenteric arterial thrombosis (rare), Raynaud's syndrome, syncope

Central nervous system: Amnesia, catatonia, cognitive dysfunction, confusion, depression, dizziness, emotional lability, fatigue, hallucinations, hypersomnolence, insomnia, lethargy, lightheadedness, psychosis, vertigo, vivid dreams

Dermatologic: Alopecia, contact dermatitis, cutaneous ulcers, eczematous eruptions, erythema multiforme, exfoliative dermatitis, hyperkeratosis, nail changes, oculomucocutaneous reactions, pruritus, psoriasiform eruptions, rash, Stevens-Johnson syndrome, toxic epidermal necrolysis, ulcers, ulcerative lichenoid, urticaria

Endocrine & metabolic: Hyper-/hypoglycemia, hyperkalemia, hyperlipidemia

Gastrointestinal: Anorexia, cramping, constipation, diarrhea, ischemic colitis, nausea, stomach discomfort, vomiting

Genitourinary: Impotence, interstitial nephritis (rare), oliguria (rare), Peyronie's disease, proteinuria (rare)

Hematologic: Agranulocytosis, nonthrombocytopenic purpura, thrombocytopenia, thrombocytopenic purpura

Hepatic: Alkaline phosphatase increased, transaminases increased

Neuromuscular & skeletal: Arthropathy, carpal tunnel syndrome (rare), myotonus, paresthesia, polyarthritis, weakness

Ocular: Hyperemia of the conjunctiva, mydriasis, visual acuity decreased, visual disturbances, xerophthalmia

Renal: BUN increased

Respiratory: Bronchospasm, dyspnea, laryngospasm, pharyngitis, pulmonary edema, respiratory distress, wheezing

Miscellaneous: Anaphylactic/anaphylactoid allergic reaction, cold extremities, lupus-like syndrome (rare)

Drug Interactions

Metabolism/Transport Effects **Substrate** of CYP1A2 (major), CYP2C19 (minor), CYP2D6 (major), CYP3A4 (minor); **Note:** Assignment of Major/Minor substrate status based on clinically relevant drug interaction potential; **Inhibits** CYP1A2 (weak), CYP2D6 (weak), P-glycoprotein

Avoid Concomitant Use

Avoid concomitant use of Propranolol with any of the following: Beta2-Agonists; Bosutinib; Floctafenine; Methacholine; PAZOPanib; Pomalidomide; Topotecan; VinCRIStine (Liposomal)

Increased Effect/Toxicity

Propranolol may increase the levels/effects of: Afatinib; Alpha-/Beta-Agonists (Direct-Acting); Alpha1-Blockers; Alpha2-Agonists; Amifostine; Antihypertensives; Antipsychotic Agents (Phenothiazines); ARIPiprazole; Bosutinib; Bupivacaine; Cardiac Glycosides; Cholinergic Agonists; Colchicine; Dabigatran Etexilate; Ergot Derivatives; Everolimus; Fingolimod; Hypotensive Agents; Insulin; Lidocaine (Systemic); Lidocaine (Topical); Mepivacaine; Methacholine; Midodrine; Obinutuzumab; PAZOPanib; P-glycoprotein/ABCB1 Substrates; Pomalidomide; Prucalopride; RiTUXimab; Rivaroxaban; Rizatriptan; Sulfonylureas; Topotecan; VinCRIStine (Liposomal); ZOLMitriptan

The levels/effects of Propranolol may be increased by: Abiraterone Acetate; Acetylcholinesterase Inhibitors; Alcohol (Ethyl); Alpha2-Agonists; Aminoquinolines (Antimalarial); Amiodarone; Anilidopiperidine Opioids; Antipsychotic Agents (Phenothiazines); Brimonidine (Topical); Calcium Channel Blockers (Dihydropyridine); Calcium Channel Blockers (Nondihydropyridine); CYP1A2 Inhibitors (Moderate); CYP1A2 Inhibitors (Strong); CYP2D6 Inhibitors (Moderate); CYP2D6 Inhibitors (Strong); Darunavir; Deferasirox; Diazoxide; Dipyridamole; Disopyramide; Dronedarone; Floctafenine; FluvoxaMINE; Herbs (Hypotensive Properties); Lacidipine; MAO Inhibitors; NiCARdipine; Pentoxifylline; Phosphodiesterase 5 Inhibitors; Propafenone; Prostacyclin Analogues; QuiNIDine; Regorafenib; Reserpine; Selective Serotonin Reuptake Inhibitors; Vemurafenib; Zileuton

Decreased Effect

Propranolol may decrease the levels/effects of: Beta2-Agonists; Lacidipine; Theophylline Derivatives

The levels/effects of Propranolol may be decreased by: Alcohol (Ethyl); Barbiturates; Bile Acid Sequestrants; CYP1A2 Inducers (Strong); Cyproterone; Herbs (Hypertensive Properties); Methylphenidate; Nonsteroidal Anti-Inflammatory Agents; Peginterferon Alfa-2b; Rifamycin Derivatives; Yohimbine

Ethanol/Nutrition/Herb Interactions

Cigarette: Smoking may decrease plasma levels of propranolol by increasing metabolism. Management: Avoid smoking.

Ethanol: Ethanol may increase or decrease plasma levels of propranolol. Reports are variable and have shown both enhanced as well as inhibited hepatic metabolism (of propranolol). Management: Caution advised with consumption of ethanol and monitor for heart rate and/or blood pressure changes.

Food: Propranolol serum levels may be increased if taken with food. Protein-rich foods may increase bioavailability; a change in diet from high carbohydrate/low protein to low carbohydrate/high protein may result in increased oral clearance. Management: Tablets (immediate release) should be taken on an empty stomach. Capsules (extended release) may be taken with or without food, but be consistent with regard to food.

Herb/Nutraceutical: Dong quai has estrogenic activity. Some herbal medications may worsen hypertension (eg, licorice); others may enhance the antihypertensive effect of propranolol (eg, shepherd's purse). Management: Avoid dong quai if using for hypertension. Avoid bayberry, blue cohosh, cayenne, ephedra, ginger, ginseng (American), gotu kola, licorice, and yohimbe. Avoid black cohosh, california poppy, coleus, garlic, golden seal, hawthorn, mistletoe, periwinkle, quinine, and shepherd's purse.

Storage/Stability

Injection: Store at 20°C to 25°C (68°F to 77°F); protect from freezing or excessive heat. Once diluted, propranolol is stable for 24 hours at room temperature in D_5W or NS. Protect from light. Solution has a maximum stability at pH of 3 and decomposes rapidly in alkaline pH.

Capsule, tablet: Store at 20°C to 25°C (68°F to 77°F); protect from freezing or excessive heat. Protect from light and moisture.

Mechanism of Action Nonselective beta-adrenergic blocker (class II antiarrhythmic); competitively blocks response to $beta_1$- and $beta_2$-adrenergic stimulation which results in decreases in heart rate, myocardial contractility, blood pressure, and myocardial oxygen demand. Nonselective beta-adrenergic blockers (propranolol, nadolol) reduce portal pressure by producing splanchnic vasoconstriction ($beta_2$ effect) thereby reducing portal blood flow.

Pharmacodynamics/Kinetics

Onset of action: Beta-blockade: Oral: 1-2 hours

Duration: Immediate release: 6-12 hours; Extended-release formulations: ~24-27 hours

Absorption: Oral: Rapid and complete

Distribution: V_d: 4 L/kg in adults

Protein binding: Newborns: 68%; Adults: ~90% (S-isomer primarily to $alpha_1$-acid glycoprotein; R-isomer primarily to albumin)

Metabolism: Hepatic via CYP2D6, and CYP1A2 to 4-hydroxypropranolol (active) and inactive compounds; extensive first-pass effect

Bioavailability: ~25% reaches systemic circulation due to high first-pass metabolism; protein-rich foods increase bioavailability by ~50%

Half-life elimination: Neonates and Infants: Possible increased half-life; Children: 3.9-6.4 hours; Adults: Immediate release formulation: 3-6 hours; Extended-release formulations: 8-10 hours

Time to peak: Immediate release: 1-4 hours; Extended-release formulations: ~6-14 hours

Excretion: Metabolites are excreted primarily in urine (96% to 99%); <1% excreted in urine as unchanged drug

Dosage

Akathisia (unlabeled use): Oral: Adults: 30-120 mg/day in 2-3 divided doses

Essential tremor: Oral: Adults: 40 mg twice daily initially; maintenance doses: Usually 120-320 mg/day

Hypertension:

Oral:

Children (unlabeled use): Initial: 0.5-1 mg/kg/day in divided doses every 6-12 hours; increase gradually every 5-7 days; maximum: 16 mg/kg/24 hours

Adults: Initial: 40 mg twice daily; increase dosage every 3-7 days; usual dose: 120-240 mg divided in 2-3 doses/day; maximum daily dose: 640 mg; usual dosage range (JNC 7): 40-160 mg/day in 2 divided doses

Extended release formulations:

Inderal LA: Initial: 80 mg once daily; usual maintenance: 120-160 mg once daily; maximum daily dose: 640 mg; usual dosage range (JNC 7): 60-180 mg/day once daily

InnoPran XL: Initial: 80 mg once daily at bedtime; if initial response is inadequate, may be increased at 2-3 week intervals to a maximum dose of 120 mg

Elderly: Consider lower initial doses and titrate to response (Aronow, 2011)

Hypertrophic subaortic stenosis: Oral: Adults: 20-40 mg 3-4 times/day

Inderal LA: 80-160 mg once daily

Migraine headache prophylaxis: Oral:

Children (unlabeled use): Initial: 2-4 mg/kg/day **or**

≤35 kg: 10-20 mg 3 times/day

>35 kg: 20-40 mg 3 times/day

Adults: Initial: 80 mg/day divided every 6-8 hours; increase by 20-40 mg/dose every 3-4 weeks to a maximum of 160-240 mg/day given in divided doses every 6-8 hours; if satisfactory response not achieved within 6 weeks of starting therapy, drug should be withdrawn gradually over several weeks

Inderal LA: Initial: 80 mg once daily; effective dose range: 160-240 mg once daily

Post-MI mortality reduction: Oral: Adults: Initial: 40 mg 3 times/day; usual dosage range: 180-240 mg/day in 3-4 divided doses

Pheochromocytoma: Oral: Adults: 30-60 mg/day in divided doses

Stable angina: Oral: Adults: 80-320 mg/day in doses divided 2-4 times/day

Inderal LA: Initial: 80 mg once daily; maximum dose: 320 mg once daily

Tachyarrhythmias:

Oral:

Children (unlabeled use): Initial: 0.5-1 mg/kg/day in divided doses every 6-8 hours; titrate dosage upward every 3-7 days; usual dose: 2-6 mg/kg/day; higher doses may be needed; do not exceed 16 mg/kg/day or 60 mg/day

Adults: 10-30 mg/dose every 6-8 hours

Elderly: Initial: 10 mg twice daily; increase dosage every 3-7 days; usual dosage range: 10-320 mg given in 2 divided doses

I.V.:

Children (unlabeled use): 0.01-0.1 mg/kg/dose slow IVP over 10 minutes; maximum dose: 1 mg for infants; 3 mg for children

Adults: 1-3 mg/dose slow IVP; repeat every 2-5 minutes up to a total of 5 mg; titrate initial dose to desired response

or

0.5-1 mg over 1 minute; may repeat, if necessary, up to a total maximum dose of 0.1 mg/kg (ACLS guidelines, 2010)

Note: Once response achieved or maximum dose administered, additional doses should not be given for at least 4 hours.

Elderly: Use caution; initiate at lower end of the dosing range.

Hypercyanotic spells (TOF) (unlabeled use): Children:

Oral: Palliation: Initial: 1 mg/kg/day every 6 hours; if ineffective, may increase dose after 1 week by 1 mg/kg/day to a maximum of 5 mg/kg/day; if patient becomes refractory, may increase slowly to a maximum of 10-15 mg/kg/day. Allow 24 hours between dosing changes.

I.V.: 0.01-0.2 mg/kg/dose infused over 10 minutes; maximum dose: 5 mg

Thyroid storm (unlabeled use):

Children: 0.5 mg/kg/dose every 4-8 hours; titrate to effective dose (Eyal, 2008)

Adults:

Oral: 60-80 mg every 4 hours; may consider the use of an intravenous shorter-acting beta-blocker (ie, esmolol) (Bahn, 2011)

I.V.: 0.5-1 mg administered over 10 minutes every 3 hours (Gardner, 2011)

Thyrotoxicosis (unlabeled use): Oral:

Children: 10-40 mg every 6 hours; titrate to effective dose (Eyal, 2008)

Adolescents and Adults: Oral: 10-40 mg/dose every 6-8 hours; may also consider administering extended or sustained release formulations (Bahn, 2011)

Variceal hemorrhage prophylaxis (unlabeled use; Garcia-Tsao, 2007): Oral: Adults:

Primary prophylaxis: Initial: 20 mg twice daily; adjust to maximal tolerated dose. **Note:** Risk factors for hemorrhage include Child-Pugh class B/C or variceal red wale markings on endoscopy.

Secondary prophylaxis: Initial: 20 mg twice daily; adjust to maximal tolerated dose

Dosage adjustment in renal impairment: No dosage adjustment provided in manufacturer's labeling. However, renal impairment increases systemic exposure to propranolol. Use with caution.

Not dialyzable (0% to 5%); supplemental dose is not necessary.

Peritoneal dialysis effects: Supplemental dose is not necessary.

Dosage adjustment in hepatic disease: No dosage adjustment provided in manufacturer's labeling. However, hepatic impairment increases systemic exposure to propranolol. Use with caution.

Dietary Considerations Tablets (immediate release) should be taken on an empty stomach; capsules (extended release) may be taken with or without food, but should always be taken consistently (with food or on an empty stomach)

Administration I.V. dose is much smaller than oral dose. When administered acutely for cardiac treatment, monitor ECG and blood pressure. May administer by rapid infusion (I.V. push) at a rate of 1 mg/minute or by slow infusion over ~30 minutes. Necessary monitoring for surgical patients who are unable to take oral beta-blockers (prolonged ileus) has not been defined. Some institutions require monitoring of baseline and postinfusion heart rate and blood pressure when a patient's response to beta-blockade has not been characterized (ie, the patient's initial dose or following a change in dose). Consult individual institutional policies and procedures. Do not crush long-acting oral forms.

Monitoring Parameters Acute cardiac treatment: Monitor ECG, heart rate, and blood pressure with I.V. administration; heart rate and blood pressure with oral administration

Consult individual institutional policies and procedures.

Reference Range Therapeutic: 50-100 ng/mL (SI: 190-390 nmol/L) at end of dose interval

Dosage Forms Excipient information presented when available (limited, particularly for generics); consult specific product labeling.

Capsule Extended Release 24 Hour, Oral, as hydrochloride:

Inderal LA: 60 mg, 80 mg, 120 mg, 160 mg [contains brilliant blue fcf (fd&c blue #1)]

InnoPran XL: 80 mg, 120 mg

Generic: 60 mg, 80 mg, 120 mg, 160 mg

Solution, Intravenous, as hydrochloride:

Generic: 1 mg/mL (1 mL)

Solution, Oral, as hydrochloride:

Generic: 20 mg/5 mL (500 mL); 40 mg/5 mL (500 mL)

Tablet, Oral, as hydrochloride:

Generic: 10 mg, 20 mg, 40 mg, 60 mg, 80 mg

◆ **Propranolol Hydrochloride** *see* Propranolol *on page 1737*

◆ **Propranolol Hydrochloride Injection, USP (Can)** *see* Propranolol *on page 1737*

◆ **Proprinal® Cold and Sinus [OTC]** *see* Pseudoephedrine and Ibuprofen *on page 1748*

◆ **Propylene Glycol Diacetate, Acetic Acid, and Hydrocortisone** *see* Acetic Acid, Propylene Glycol Diacetate, and Hydrocortisone *on page 35*

◆ **2-Propylpentanoic Acid** *see* Valproic Acid and Derivatives *on page 2149*

Propylthiouracil (proe pil thye oh YOOR a sil)

Brand Names: Canada Propyl-Thyracil®

Index Terms PTU (error-prone abbreviation)

Pharmacologic Category Antithyroid Agent; Thioamide

Use Adjunctive therapy in patients intolerant of methimazole to ameliorate hyperthyroidism symptoms in preparation for surgical treatment or radioactive iodine therapy; treatment of hyperthyroidism in patients intolerant of methimazole and not candidates for surgical/radiotherapy

Unlabeled Use Management of Graves' disease, thyrotoxic crisis, or thyroid storm

Pregnancy Risk Factor D

Pregnancy Considerations Propylthiouracil has been found to readily cross the placenta. Teratogenic effects have not been observed; however, nonteratogenic adverse effects, including fetal and neonatal hypothyroidism, goiter, and hyperthyroidism, have been reported following maternal propylthiouracil use. The transfer of thyroid-stimulating immunoglobulins can stimulate the fetal thyroid *in utero* and transiently after delivery and may increase the risk of fetal or neonatal hyperthyroidism.

Uncontrolled maternal hyperthyroidism may result in adverse neonatal outcomes (eg, prematurity, low birth weight) and adverse maternal outcomes (eg, pre-eclampsia, congestive heart failure, stillbirth, and abortion). To prevent adverse fetal and maternal events, normal maternal thyroid function should be maintained prior to conception and throughout pregnancy. Antithyroid treatment is recommended for the control of hyperthyroidism during pregnancy. Propylthiouracil is considered first-line therapy, especially during the first trimester. Due to an increased risk of liver toxicity, use of methimazole may be preferred during the second and third trimesters. If drug therapy is changed, maternal thyroid function should be monitored after 2 weeks and then every 2-4 weeks. Propylthiouracil, along with other medications, is used for the treatment of thyroid storm in pregnant women; alternative therapy is recommended if oral administration is not possible.

The pharmacokinetics of propylthiouracil are not significantly changed during pregnancy; however, the severity of hyperthyroidism may fluctuate throughout pregnancy. Doses of propylthiouracil may be decreased as pregnancy progresses and discontinued weeks to months prior to delivery.

Breast-Feeding Considerations Propylthiouracil is excreted in human breast milk; however, the infant dose is considered low and unlikely to affect infant thyroid hormones. The American Thyroid Association considers doses <300 mg/day to be safe during breast-feeding (Stagnaro-Green, 2011).

Medication Guide Available Yes

Contraindications Hypersensitivity to propylthiouracil or any component of the formulation

Warnings/Precautions [U.S. Boxed Warning]: Severe liver injury (some fatal) and acute liver failure (some cases requiring transplantation) have been reported. Patients should be counseled to recognize and report symptoms suggestive of hepatic dysfunction (especially in first 6 months of treatment), which should prompt immediate discontinuation. Routine liver function test monitoring may not reduce risk due to unpredictable and rapid onset.

Has been associated with significant bone marrow depression. The most severe manifestation is agranulocytosis (commonly within first 3 months of therapy). Aplastic anemia, thrombocytopenia, and leukopenia may also occur. Use with caution in patients receiving other drugs known to cause myelosuppression particularly agranulocytosis. Discontinue if significant bone marrow suppression occurs, particularly agranulocytosis or aplastic anemia.

Rare hypersensitivity reactions have been reported, including the development of ANCA-positive vasculitis, drug fever, interstitial pneumonitis, exfoliative dermatitis, glomerulonephritis, leukocytoclastic vasculitis, and a lupus-like syndrome; prompt discontinuation is warranted in patients who develop symptoms consistent with a form of autoimmunity or other hypersensitivity during therapy. May cause hypoprothrombinemia and bleeding.

Adverse Reactions Frequency not defined.

Cardiovascular: Periarteritis, vasculitis (ANCA-positive, cutaneous, leukocytoclastic)

Central nervous system: Drowsiness, drug fever, fever, headache, neuritis, vertigo

Dermatologic: Alopecia, erythema nodosum, exfoliative dermatitis, pruritus, skin pigmentation, skin rash, skin ulcers, urticaria

Endocrine & metabolic: Goiter, weight gain

Gastrointestinal: Constipation, loss of taste, nausea, sialoadenopathy, splenomegaly, stomach pain, taste perversion, vomiting

Hematologic: Agranulocytosis, aplastic anemia, bleeding, granulopenia, hypoprothrombinemia, leukopenia, thrombocytopenia

Hepatic: Acute liver failure, cholestatic jaundice, hepatitis

Neuromuscular & skeletal: Arthralgia, myalgia, paresthesia

Renal: Acute renal failure, glomerulonephritis, nephritis

Respiratory: Alveolar hemorrhage, interstitial pneumonitis

Miscellaneous: Lymphadenopathy, SLE-like syndrome

Drug Interactions

Metabolism/Transport Effects None known.

Avoid Concomitant Use

Avoid concomitant use of Propylthiouracil with any of the following: CloZAPine; Sodium Iodide I131

Increased Effect/Toxicity

Propylthiouracil may increase the levels/effects of: Cardiac Glycosides; CloZAPine; Theophylline Derivatives

Decreased Effect

Propylthiouracil may decrease the levels/effects of: Sodium Iodide I131; Vitamin K Antagonists

Ethanol/Nutrition/Herb Interactions Food: Propylthiouracil serum levels may be altered if taken with food.

Storage/Stability Store at 25°C (77°F); excursions permitted to 15°C to 30°C (59°F to 86°F).

Mechanism of Action Inhibits the synthesis of thyroid hormones by blocking the oxidation of iodine in the thyroid gland; blocks synthesis of thyroxine and triiodothyronine

Pharmacodynamics/Kinetics

Duration: 12-24 hours

Distribution: Concentrated in the thyroid gland

Protein binding: 80% to 85%

Metabolism: Hepatic

Bioavailability: 53% to 88%

Half-life elimination: ~1 hour

Time to peak, serum: 1-2 hours

Excretion: Urine (35%; primarily as metabolites)

Dosage Oral: Administer in equally divided doses every 8 hours. Adjust dosage to maintain T_3, T_4, and TSH levels in normal range; elevated T_3 may be sole indicator of inadequate treatment. Elevated TSH indicates excessive antithyroid treatment.

Children: Initial: 5-7 mg/kg/day **or** 150-200 mg/m^2/day in divided doses every 8 hours

or

Manufacturer's recommendations:

6-10 years: 50-150 mg/day

>10 years: 150-300 mg/day

Adults:

Hyperthyroidism: Initial: 300 mg/day in 3 divided doses; 400 mg/day in patients with severe hyperthyroidism and/or very large goiters; an occasional patient will require 600-900 mg/day; usual maintenance: 100-150 mg/day

Graves' disease (unlabeled use): Initial: 50-150 mg (depending on severity) 3 times daily to restore euthyroidism; maintenance: 50 mg 2-3 times daily for a total of 12-18 months, then tapered or discontinued if TSH is normal at that time (Bahn, 2011)

Thyrotoxic crisis/thyroid storm (unlabeled use): **Note:** Recommendations vary widely and have not been evaluated in comparative trials. Typical dosing is 800-1200 mg/day given as 200-300 mg every 4-6 hours; some clinicians advocate an initial loading dose of 600-1000 mg. After initial response, dose may be reduced gradually to a maintenance dosage (100-600 mg/day in divided doses) (Goldberg, 2003; Nayak, 2006). The American Thyroid Association and the American Association of Clinical Endocrinologists recommend 500-1000 mg loading dose followed by 250 mg every 4 hours (Bahn, 2011).

Duration of therapy: Clinical improvement generally occurs in 1-3 months, after which dosage reduction may be employed (to prevent hypothyroidism), with discontinuation considered after 12-18 months of therapy. Thyroid function should be monitored every 2 months thereafter for 6 months until remission is confirmed, followed by annual evaluations (Cooper, 2005).

Dosage adjustment in renal impairment: No dosage adjustment provided in manufacturer's labeling.

Dosage adjustment in hepatic impairment: No dosage adjustment provided in manufacturer's labeling.

Dietary Considerations Take at the same time in relation to meals each day, either always with meals or always between meals.

Administration Administer at the same time in relation to meals each day, either always with meals or always between meals.

Monitoring Parameters CBC with differential, prothrombin time, liver function tests (bilirubin, alkaline phosphatase, transaminases), and thyroid function tests (TSH, T_3, T_4) every 4-6 weeks until euthyroid; periodic blood counts are recommended for chronic therapy

Reference Range Normal laboratory values:

Total T_4: 5-12 mcg/dL

Serum T_3: 90-185 ng/dL

Free thyroxine index (FT_4 I): 6-10.5

TSH: 0.5-4.0 microunits/mL

Additional Information Preferred over methimazole in thyroid storm due to inhibition of peripheral conversion as well as synthesis of thyroid hormone.

Graves' hyperthyroidism: Elevated T_3 may be the sole indicator of inadequate treatment. Elevated TSH indicates excessive antithyroid treatment. Monitoring of TSH is a poor indicator of treatment effectiveness, as levels may remain suppressed for months, despite euthyroid state (Cooper, 2005).

A potency ratio of methimazole to propylthiouracil of at least 20-30:1 is recommended when changing from one drug to another (eg, 300 mg of propylthiouracil would be roughly equivalent to 10-15 mg of methimazole) (Bahn, 2011).

Dosage Forms Excipient information presented when available (limited, particularly for generics); consult specific product labeling.

Tablet, Oral:

Generic: 50 mg

Extemporaneous Preparations A 5 mg/mL oral suspension may be made with tablets and a 1:1 mixture of Ora-Plus® and Ora-Sweet®. Crush twenty 50 mg propylthiouracil tablets in a mortar and reduce to a fine powder. Add small portions of vehicle and mix to a uniform paste; mix while adding vehicle in incremental proportions to **almost** 200 mL; transfer to a calibrated bottle, rinse mortar with vehicle, and add quantity of vehicle sufficient to make 200 mL. Label "shake well" and "refrigerate". Stable for 91 days refrigerated (preferred) and 70 days at room temperature.

Nahata MC, Pai VB, and Hipple TF, *Pediatric Drug Formulations*, 5th ed, Cincinnati, OH: Harvey Whitney Books Co, 2004.

◆ **Propyl-Thyracil® (Can)** *see* Propylthiouracil *on page 1740*

◆ **2-Propylvaleric Acid** *see* Valproic Acid and Derivatives *on page 2149*

◆ **ProQuad** *see* Measles, Mumps, Rubella, and Varicella Virus Vaccine *on page 1273*

◆ **PRO-Quetiapine (Can)** *see* QUEtiapine *on page 1757*

◆ **PRO-Rabeprazole (Can)** *see* RABEprazole *on page 1769*

◆ **Pro-Ramipril (Can)** *see* Ramipril *on page 1778*

◆ **PRO-Risperidone (Can)** *see* RisperiDONE *on page 1826*

◆ **Proscar** *see* Finasteride *on page 862*

◆ **Proscar® (Can)** *see* Finasteride *on page 862*

◆ **Prosed®/DS** *see* Methenamine, Phenyl Salicylate, Methylene Blue, Benzoic Acid, and Hyoscyamine *on page 1319*

◆ **ProSom** *see* Estazolam *on page 754*

◆ **PRO-Sotalol (Can)** *see* Sotalol *on page 1942*

◆ **Prostacyclin** *see* Epoprostenol *on page 727*

◆ **Prostacyclin PGI_2** *see* Iloprost *on page 1047*

◆ **Prostaglandin E_1** *see* Alprostadil *on page 83*

◆ **Prostaglandin E_2** *see* Dinoprostone *on page 619*

◆ **Prostaglandin F_2 Alpha Analog** *see* Carboprost Tromethamine *on page 347*

◆ **Prostaglandin F_2 Analog** *see* Carboprost Tromethamine *on page 347*

◆ **Prostate Cancer Vaccine, Cell-Based** *see* Sipuleucel-T *on page 1902*

◆ **Prostigmin** *see* Neostigmine *on page 1441*

◆ **Prostin E2** *see* Dinoprostone *on page 619*

◆ **Prostin E_2® (Can)** *see* Dinoprostone *on page 619*

◆ **Prostin VR** *see* Alprostadil *on page 83*

◆ **Prostin® VR (Can)** *see* Alprostadil *on page 83*

Protamine (PROE ta meen)

Index Terms Protamine Sulfate

Pharmacologic Category Antidote

Additional Appendix Information

Reversal of Oral Anticoagulants *on page 2308*

Use Treatment of heparin overdosage; neutralize heparin during surgery or dialysis procedures

Unlabeled Use Treatment of low molecular weight heparin (LMWH) overdose

Pregnancy Risk Factor C

Pregnancy Considerations Animal reproduction studies have not been conducted. In general, medications used as antidotes should take into consideration the health and prognosis of the mother; antidotes should be administered to pregnant women if there is a clear indication for use and should not be withheld because of fears of teratogenicity (Bailey, 2003). Protamine sulfate may be used during delivery to reduce the risk of bleeding following maternal use of heparin or low molecular weight heparin (LMWH) (Bates, 2012).

Breast-Feeding Considerations It is not known if protamine is excreted in breast milk. The manufacturer recommends that caution be exercised when administering protamine to nursing women.

Contraindications Hypersensitivity to protamine or any component of the formulation

Warnings/Precautions May not be totally effective in some patients following cardiac surgery despite adequate doses. May cause hypersensitivity reaction in patients (have epinephrine 1:1000 and resuscitation equipment available). **[U.S. Boxed Warning]: Hypotension, cardiovascular collapse, noncardiogenic pulmonary edema, pulmonary vasoconstriction, and pulmonary hypertension may occur. Risk factors for such events include: use of high doses or overdose, repeated doses, previous protamine administration (including protamine-containing drugs), fish allergy, vasectomy, severe left ventricular dysfunction, abnormal preoperative pulmonary hemodynamics.** Too rapid administration can cause severe hypotensive and anaphylactoid-like reactions. Heparin rebound associated with anticoagulation and bleeding has been reported to occur occasionally; symptoms typically occur 8-9 hours after protamine administration, but may occur as long as 18 hours later.

Adverse Reactions Frequency not defined.

Cardiovascular: Sudden fall in blood pressure, bradycardia, flushing, hypotension

Central nervous system: Lassitude

Gastrointestinal: Nausea, vomiting

Hematologic: Hemorrhage

Respiratory: Dyspnea, pulmonary hypertension

Miscellaneous: Hypersensitivity reactions

Drug Interactions

Metabolism/Transport Effects None known.

Avoid Concomitant Use There are no known interactions where it is recommended to avoid concomitant use.

Increased Effect/Toxicity There are no known significant interactions involving an increase in effect.

Decreased Effect There are no known significant interactions involving a decrease in effect.

Storage/Stability Refrigerate; do not freeze. Stable for at least 2 weeks at room temperature. Preservative-free formulation does not require refrigeration.

Mechanism of Action Combines with strongly acidic heparin to form a stable complex (salt) neutralizing the anticoagulant activity of both drugs

Pharmacodynamics/Kinetics

Onset of action: I.V.: Heparin neutralization: ~5 minutes

Half-life elimination: ~7 minutes

Dosage

Heparin neutralization: I.V.: Protamine dosage is determined by the dosage of heparin; 1 mg of protamine neutralizes ~100 units of heparin; maximum dose: 50 mg

Note: When heparin is given as a continuous I.V. infusion, only heparin given in the preceding several hours should be considered when administering protamine. For example, a patient receiving heparin at 1250 units/hour will require ~30 mg of protamine for reversal of heparin given in the last 2-2.5 hours (Garcia, 2012).

Heparin overdosage, following intravenous administration: I.V.: Since blood heparin concentrations decrease rapidly **after** administration, adjust the protamine dosage depending upon the duration of time since heparin administration as follows: See table.

Time Elapsed	Dose of Protamine (mg) to Neutralize 100 units of Heparin
Immediate	1-1.5
30-60 min	0.5-0.75
>2 h	0.25-0.375

Heparin overdosage, following SubQ injection: I.V.: 1-1.5 mg protamine per 100 units heparin; this may be done by a portion of the dose (eg, 25-50 mg) given slowly I.V. followed by the remaining portion as a continuous infusion over 8-16 hours (the expected absorption time of the SubQ heparin dose)

LMWH overdose (unlabeled use): I.V.: **Note:** Anti-Xa activity is never completely neutralized (maximum: ~60% to 75%). Excessive protamine doses may worsen bleeding potential.

Enoxaparin (Lovenox® prescribing information, 2011):

Enoxaparin administered in ≤8 hours: Dose of protamine should equal the dose of enoxaparin administered. Therefore, 1 mg of protamine sulfate neutralizes 1 mg of enoxaparin.

Enoxaparin administered in >8 hours or if it has been determined that a second dose of protamine is required (eg, if aPTT measured 2-4 hours after the first dose remains prolonged or if bleeding continues): 0.5 mg of protamine sulfate for every 1 mg of enoxaparin administered

Dalteparin or tinzaparin (Fragmin ® prescribing information, 2010; Innohep® prescribing information, 2010): 1 mg protamine for each 100 anti-Xa units of dalteparin or tinzaparin; if PTT prolonged 2-4 hours after first dose (or if bleeding continues), consider additional dose of 0.5 mg for each 100 anti-Xa units of dalteparin or tinzaparin.

Dosage adjustment in renal impairment: No dosage adjustment provided in manufacturer's labeling.

Dosage adjustment in hepatic impairment: No dosage adjustment provided in manufacturer's labeling.

Administration For I.V. use only; **incompatible** with cephalosporins and penicillins; administer slow IVP (50 mg over 10 minutes); rapid I.V. infusion causes hypotension; inject without further dilution over 1-3 minutes; maximum of 50 mg in any 10-minute period

Monitoring Parameters Coagulation test, aPTT or ACT, cardiac monitor and blood pressure monitor required during administration

Dosage Forms Excipient information presented when available (limited, particularly for generics); consult specific product labeling.

Solution, Intravenous, as sulfate:

Generic: 10 mg/mL (5 mL, 25 mL)

Solution, Intravenous, as sulfate [preservative free]:

Generic: 10 mg/mL (5 mL, 25 mL)

◆ **Protamine Sulfate** *see* Protamine *on page* 1741

◆ **Protease, Lipase, and Amylase** *see* Pancrelipase *on page* 1558

◆ **Protein C** *see* Protein C Concentrate (Human) *on page* 1743

◆ **Protein-Bound Paclitaxel** *see* PACLitaxel (Protein Bound) *on page* 1546

Protein C Concentrate (Human)

(PROE teen cee KON suhn trate HYU man)

Brand Names: U.S. Ceprotin

Index Terms Protein C

Pharmacologic Category Anticoagulant; Blood Product Derivative; Enzyme; Protein C

Use Replacement therapy for severe congenital protein C deficiency for the prevention and/or treatment of venous thromboembolism and purpura fulminans

Pregnancy Risk Factor C

Dosage Patient variables (including age, clinical condition, and plasma levels of protein C) will influence dosing and duration of therapy. Individualize dosing based on protein C activity and patient pharmacokinetic profile. Dosing is dependent on the severity of protein C deficiency, age of patient, clinical condition, and patient's level of protein C. The frequency, duration, and dose should be individualized.

I.V.: Children and Adults: Severe congenital protein C deficiency:

Acute episode/short-term prophylaxis: Initial dose: 100-120 units/kg (for determination of recovery and half-life)

Subsequent 3 doses: 60-80 units/kg every 6 hours (adjust to maintain peak protein C activity of 100%)

Maintenance dose: 45-60 units/kg every 6 or 12 hours (adjust to maintain recommended maintenance trough protein C activity levels >25%)

Long-term prophylaxis: Maintenance dose: 45-60 units/kg every 12 hours (recommended maintenance trough protein C activity levels >25%)

Note: Maintain target peak protein C activity of 100% during acute episodes and short-term prophylaxis. Maintain trough levels of protein C activity >25%. Higher peak levels of protein C may be necessary in prophylactic therapy of patients at increased risk for thrombosis (eg, infection, trauma, surgical intervention).

Dosage adjustment in renal impairment: No dosage adjustment provided in manufacturer's labeling (has not been studied). Patients with renal impairment should be monitored more closely for sodium overload.

Dosage adjustment in hepatic impairment: No dosage adjustment provided in manufacturer's labeling (has not been studied).

Additional Information Complete prescribing information should be consulted for additional detail.

Dosage Forms Excipient information presented when available (limited, particularly for generics); consult specific product labeling.

Solution Reconstituted, Intravenous [preservative free]:

Ceprotin: 500 units (1 ea); 1000 units (1 ea) [contains albumin human, heparin, mouse protein (murine) (hamster)]

◆ **Prothrombin Complex Concentrate (Caution: Confusion-prone synonym)** *see* Factor IX Complex (Human) [(Factors II, IX, X)] *on page 822*

◆ **Prothrombin Complex Concentrate (Caution: Confusion-prone synonym)** *see* Prothrombin Complex Concentrate (Human) [(Factors II, VII, IX, X), Protein C, and Protein S] *on page 1743*

Prothrombin Complex Concentrate (Human) [(Factors II, VII, IX, X), Protein C, and Protein S]

(PRO throm bin KOM pleks KON cen trate HYU man FAK ters too SEV en nyne ten PROE teen cee & PROE teen ess)

Brand Names: U.S. Kcentra

Brand Names: Canada Octaplex

Index Terms 4 Factor PCC; 4-Factor PCC; Beriplex P/N; Confidex; Four-Factor PCC; PCC (Caution: Confusion-prone synonym); Prothrombin Complex Concentrate (Caution: Confusion-prone synonym)

Pharmacologic Category Blood Product Derivative; Hemostatic Agent; Prothrombin Complex Concentrate (PCC)

Additional Appendix Information

Reversal of Oral Anticoagulants *on page 2308*

Use

Kcentra: Urgent reversal of acquired coagulation factor deficiency induced by vitamin K antagonist (VKA, eg, warfarin) therapy in patients with acute major bleeding

Octaplex (Canadian availability; not available in the U.S.): Prophylaxis (perioperative) and treatment of bleeding due to acquired deficiency (eg, treatment or overdose of VKA) of one or more of the prothrombin complex coagulation factors II, VII, IX, and X, when rapid correction of factor deficiency is necessary

Pregnancy Risk Factor C

Pregnancy Considerations Animal reproduction studies have not been conducted. Parvovirus B19 or hepatitis A, which may be present in plasma-derived products, may affect a pregnant woman more seriously than a nonpregnant woman.

Breast-Feeding Considerations It is not known if prothrombin complex concentrate is excreted in breast milk. The manufacturer recommends that PCC be administered only if clearly needed when treating a nursing woman.

Contraindications

Kcentra: Hypersensitivity (ie, anaphylaxis or severe systemic reaction) to prothrombin complex concentrate (PCC) or any component of the formulation including factors II, VII, IX, X, protein C and S, antithrombin III and human albumin; disseminated intravascular coagulation (DIC); known heparin-induced thrombocytopenia (product contains heparin).

Octaplex (Canadian availability; not available in the U.S.): Hypersensitivity to prothrombin complex concentrate (PCC) or any component of the formulation; heparin-induced thrombocytopenia type II or known allergy to heparin (product contains heparin); non-life-threatening bleeding episodes in individuals with recent myocardial infarction, high risk of thrombosis, or angina pectoris; non-life-threatening bleeding episodes in individuals with untreated disseminated intravascular coagulation (DIC) who can be given fresh frozen plasma (FFP); coagulation disorders due to chronic liver disease or liver transplantation; bleeding associated with hepatic parenchyme disorders, esophageal varices, or major hepatic surgery; immunoglobulin A (IgA) deficiency, with known antibodies against IgA

Warnings/Precautions [U.S. Boxed Warning]: Because patients being treated with vitamin K antagonist (VKA) therapy have an underlying risk of or a diagnosed thromboembolic disease state, administration of prothrombin complex concentrate (PCC) may predispose the patient to a thromboembolic complication. Benefits of reversing VKA therapy should be weighed against the potential risk of a thromboembolic event. Resumption of anticoagulation should occur once the risk of thromboembolism outweighs the risk of acute bleeding. Fatal and nonfatal arterial and venous thromboembolic complications have been reported; closely monitor for thromboembolic events during and after administration. Use has not be evaluated in patients who have experienced a thromboembolic event, MI, DIC, CVA, TIA, unstable angina, or severe peripheral vascular disease within the prior 3 months. Administration of PCC may exacerbate underlying hypercoagulable states in recipients of vitamin K antagonists.

Prothrombin complex concentrate (Human) [(Factors II, VII, IX, X), Protein C, Protein S] (Kcentra, Octaplex) contains therapeutic levels of factor VII component and should not be confused with Factor IX complex (Human) [Factors II, IX, X] (Bebulin, Profilnine) which contains low or nontherapeutic levels of factor VII. Hypersensitivity reaction (eg, angioedema, bronchospasm, dyspnea, flushing, hypotension, nausea/vomiting, pulmonary edema, urticaria, tachycardia, tachypnea) may occur; if serious reaction occurs, discontinue administration and begin appropriate treatment. Since severe hypersensitivity and anaphylactic reactions may rarely occur with use; immediate medical treatment (including epinephrine 1:1000) should be readily available in the event of a severe reaction. May consider prophylactic treatment (eg, antihistamines, glucocorticoids) in patients predisposed to allergies. Formulations contain heparin.

Product of human plasma; may potentially contain infectious agents which could transmit disease. Screening of donors, as well as testing and/or inactivation or removal of certain viruses, reduces the risk. Infections thought to be transmitted by this product should be reported to the manufacturer. Octaplex (Canadian availability; not available in the U.S.) labeling recommends hepatitis B vaccination for all patients and hepatitis A vaccination for seronegative patients.

Hepatic synthesis of the prothrombin complex (Factors II, VII, IX and X) coagulation factors is vitamin K dependent. Severe hepatic dysfunction, inadequate absorption of vitamin K (eg, pancreatic disorders, diarrhea) or vitamin K antagonist therapy or overdose may lead to coagulation factor deficiencies. In patients with an acquired deficiency of the vitamin K-dependent coagulation factors, administer PCC only if a rapid correction (eg, emergency surgery, major bleeding) is necessary. If not indicated and caused by Vitamin K antagonist therapy, coagulation factor deficiencies may be managed by reducing or discontinuing therapy of the vitamin K antagonist and/or administration of vitamin K.

Octaplex (Canadian labeling): Development of antibodies to one or more of the human prothrombin factors may occur rarely, resulting in an inadequate clinical response; monitor for signs of antibody formation. Product labeling recommends monitoring antithrombin (AT) levels in patients being treated for bleeding as a result of chronic liver disease or liver transplantation. If AT levels are deficient, AT should be administered concomitantly with PCC. No clinical data are available for use of PCC to treat bleeding due to liver parenchyme disorders, major liver surgery, or esophageal varices; use of PCC for these indications is contraindicated and the preferred method of treatment is fresh frozen plasma (FFP).

Adverse Reactions

1% to 10%:

Cardiovascular: Hypotension (5%), hypertension (1% to 3%), tachycardia (3%), pulmonary embolism (≤2%), arteriovenous fistula site complication (clot, 1%), cerebrovascular accident (1%), chest pain (1%), deep vein thrombosis (1%), venous thrombosis (calf, 1%)

Central nervous system: Headache (1% to 8%), intracranial hemorrhage (3%), mental status changes (3%), insomnia (1%)

Endocrine & metabolic: Hypervolemia (1% to 6%), hypokalemia (2%)

Gastrointestinal: Nausea and vomiting (4%), constipation (2%)

Hepatic: Increased serum transaminases (1%)

Immunologic: Antibody development (parvovirus B19 seropositive, 3%)

Local: Burning sensation at injection site (1%)

Neuromuscular & skeletal: Arthralgia (4%)

Respiratory: Respiratory distress (2%), rales (1%)

Postmarketing and/or case reports (Limited to important or life-threatening): Angioedema, arterial thrombosis, bronchospasm, disseminated intravascular coagulation, hypersensitivity reaction, myocardial infarction, peripheral ischemia, pulmonary edema, thromboembolic complications, thrombosis, transient ischemic attacks, venous insufficiency

Preparation for Administration Kcentra or Octaplex: Store at 2°C to 25°C (36°F to 77°F); do not freeze. Protect from light. Prior to reconstitution, allow diluent (SWFI) and prothrombin complex concentrate (PCC) vials to warm to room temperature. Aseptically push the plastic spike at the blue end of the Mix2Vial transfer set through the center of the stopper of the diluent vial. After carefully removing only the clear package from the Mix2Vial transfer set, invert the diluent vial with the transfer set still attached and push the plastic spike through the center of the stopper of PCC vial; diluent will automatically transfer. While still attached, gently swirl PCC vial to ensure product is dissolved; do not shake. Disconnect the 2 vials; contents of PCC vial are now available for removal by screwing a syringe onto the transfer set. Inject appropriate amount of air into vial, invert vial, and withdraw amount needed. Remove syringe from transfer set and attach an administration set to the syringe.

Storage/Stability

Kcentra: Store at 2°C to 25°C (35°F to 77°F); do not freeze. Protect from light. Reconstituted product may be stored at 2°C to 25°C (35°F to 77°F) and used within 4 hours following reconstitution. If cooled, warm to 20°C to 25°C (68°F to 77°F) prior to administration.

Octaplex (Canadian product labeling): Store at 2°C to 25°C (36°F to 77°F); do not freeze. Protect from light. Reconstituted solution should be administered immediately, but may be stored for up to 8 hours at 2°C to 25°C (36°F to 77°F) if sterility is maintained.

Mechanism of Action Prothrombin complex concentrate provides an increase in the levels of the vitamin K-dependent coagulation factors (II, VII, IX, and X) with the addition of protein C and protein S. Coagulation factors II, IX, and X are part of the intrinsic coagulation pathway, while factor VII is part of the extrinsic coagulation pathway. In the *extrinsic* pathway, damaged blood vessels release endothelial tissue factor (TF) which complexes with factor VII to form TF-factor VIIa. Within the *intrinsic* pathway, factor IX is converted to IXa. Factor IXa (as well as TF-factor VIIa) converts factor X to factor Xa in the final common pathway of coagulation. Factor Xa activates prothrombin (factor II) into thrombin (IIa) which converts fibrinogen into fibrin resulting in clot formation. Proteins C and S are vitamin K-dependent inhibiting enzymes involved in regulating the coagulation process. Protein S serves as a cofactor for protein C which is converted to activated protein C (APC). APC is a serine protease which inactivates factors Va and VIIIa, limiting thrombotic formation.

Pharmacodynamics/Kinetics

Onset of action: Rapid; significant INR decline within 10 minutes

Duration: ~6-8 hours

Distribution: V_{dss}: Factor II: 71 mL/kg; Factor VII: 41.8 mL/kg; Factor IX: 92.4 mL/kg; Factor X: 56.1 mL/kg; Protein C: 62.9 mL/kg; Protein S: 76.6 mL/kg

Half-life elimination: Factor II: 48–60 hours; Factor VII: 1.5-6 hours; Factor IX: 20-24 hours; Factor X: 24-48 hours; Protein C: 1.5–6 hours; Protein S: 24-48 hours

Note: Half-lives may be significantly reduced in severe hepatocellular damage, DIC, or extended catabolic metabolism.

Dosage Note: Prothrombin complex concentrate (Human) [(Factors II, VII, IX, X), Protein C, Protein S] (Kcentra, Octaplex) contains therapeutic levels of factor VII component and should not be confused with Factor IX complex (Human) [Factors II, IX, X] (Bebulin, Profilnine) which contains low or nontherapeutic levels of factor VII.

Kcentra: Vitamin K antagonist (VKA) reversal in patients with acute major bleeding: Adults: I.V.: Individualize dosing based on current pre-dose INR. Dosage is expressed in units of factor IX activity. Administer with vitamin K concurrently. Repeat dosing is not recommended (has not been studied).

Pretreatment INR: 2 to <4: Administer 25 units/kg (maximum dose: 2500 units)

Pretreatment INR: 4-6: Administer 35 units/kg (maximum dose: 3500 units)

Pretreatment INR: >6: Administer 50 units/kg (maximum dose: 5000 units)

Octaplex (Canadian product labeling): Bleeding/perioperative prophylaxis of bleeding during vitamin K antagonist therapy: Individualize dosing based on severity of disorder, extent and location of bleeding, and clinical status of patient. Adolescents ≥17 years and Adults: I.V.: Approximate doses required for normalization of INR (≤1.2 within 1 hour):

Pretreatment INR: 2-2.5: Administer 22.5-32.5 units/kg (or 0.9-1.3 **mL**/kg)

Pretreatment INR: 2.5-3: Administer 32.5-40 units/kg (or 1.3-1.6 **mL**/kg)

Pretreatment INR: 3-3.5: Administer 40-47.5 units/kg (or 1.6-1.9 **mL**/kg)

Pretreatment INR: >3.5: Administer >47.5 units/kg (or >1.9 **mL**/kg)

Maximum dose: 3000 units (or 120 mL)

With the correction of vitamin K antagonist-induced impairment of hemostasis in patients who have been treated concomitantly with an appropriate vitamin K dose, repeat dosing with PCC is usually not necessary.

Dosing in obesity: Kcentra: In patients weighing >100 kg, do not exceed maximum dose.

Dosage adjustment in renal impairment: No dosage adjustment provided in manufacturer's labeling.

Dosage adjustment in hepatic impairment: No dosage adjustment provided in manufacturer's labeling.

Administration

Kcentra: I.V.: Administer at room temperature at a rate of 0.12 mL/kg/minute (~3 **units**/kg/minute); do **not** exceed 8.4 mL/minute (~210 **units**/minute). Do not allow blood to enter into syringe; since fibrin clot formation may occur.

Octaplex (Canadian product labeling): I.V.: Administer at a rate of 1 mL/minute initially, followed by 2-3 mL/minute. Reduce infusion rate or interrupt infusion if patient's pulse rate increases significantly.

Monitoring Parameters

Kcentra: INR (baseline and at 30 minutes post dose); clinical response during and after treatment

Octaplex (Canadian product labeling): Coagulation factor assays, protein C, protein S, aPTT, PT, INR, CBC, AT, D-dimer, fibrinogen; transaminases; development of circulating coagulation factor antibodies (inhibitors); heart rate (before and during administration)

Test Interactions aPTT (formulation contains heparin)

Additional Information

Kcentra: Composition per 500-unit vial (exact potency of active and inactive components is listed on each container):

Factor II: 380-800 units
Factor VII: 200-500 units
Factor IX: 400-620 units
Factor X: 500-1020 units
Protein C: 420-820 units
Protein S: 240-680 units

Octaplex Composition per 500-unit vial (exact potency of active and inactive components is listed on each container):

Factor II: 280-760 units
Factor VII: 180-480 units
Factor IX: 500 units
Factor X: 360-600 units
Protein C: 140-620 units
Protein S: 140-640 units

Dosage Forms Excipient information presented when available (limited, particularly for generics); consult specific product labeling.

Injection, powder for reconstitution [preservative free]:

Kcentra: 500 units [contains albumin (human); packaged with diluent]

Dosage Forms: Canada Excipient information presented when available (limited, particularly for generics); consult specific product labeling.

Injection, powder for reconstitution:

Octaplex: Human coagulation factor II: 11-38 units/mL; factor VII: 9-24 units/mL; factor IX: 20-31 units/mL; factor X: 18-30 units/mL: protein C: 7-31 units/mL; protein S: 7-32 units/mL (20 mL) [contains heparin 4-15.5 units/mL, polysorbate 80 ≤50 mcg/mL, sodium citrate 17-27 mmoL/L; packaged with diluent]

◆ **Protonix** *see* Pantoprazole *on page 1563*

◆ **Protopam Chloride** *see* Pralidoxime *on page 1694*

◆ **Protopic** *see* Tacrolimus (Topical) *on page 1981*

◆ **Protopic® (Can)** *see* Tacrolimus (Topical) *on page 1981*

◆ **PRO-Topiramate (Can)** *see* Topiramate *on page 2090*

◆ **Pro-Triazide (Can)** *see* Hydrochlorothiazide and Triamterene *on page 1006*

Protriptyline (proe TRIP ti leen)

Brand Names: U.S. Vivactil

Index Terms Protriptyline Hydrochloride

Pharmacologic Category Antidepressant, Tricyclic (Secondary Amine)

Additional Appendix Information

Antidepressant Agents *on page 2284*

Beers Criteria – Potentially Inappropriate Medications for Geriatrics *on page 2368*

Use Treatment of depression

Medication Guide Available Yes

Dosage Oral:

Adolescents: 15-20 mg/day

Adults: 15-60 mg/day in 3-4 divided doses

Elderly: Initial: 5-10 mg/day; increase every 3-7 days by 5-10 mg; usual dose: 15-20 mg/day

Discontinuation of therapy: Upon discontinuation of antidepressant therapy, gradually taper the dose to minimize the incidence of withdrawal symptoms and allow for the detection of re-emerging symptoms. Evidence supporting ideal taper rates is limited. APA and NICE guidelines suggest tapering therapy over at least several weeks with consideration to the half-life of the antidepressant; antidepressants with a shorter half-life may need to be tapered more conservatively. In addition for long-term treated patients, WFSBP guidelines recommend tapering over 4-6 months. If intolerable withdrawal symptoms occur following a dose reduction, consider resuming the previously prescribed dose and/or decrease dose at a more gradual rate (APA, 2010; Bauer, 2002; Haddad, 2001; NCCMH, 2010; Schatzberg, 2006; Shelton, 2001; Warner, 2006).

MAO inhibitor recommendations:

Switching to or from an MAO inhibitor intended to treat psychiatric disorders:

Allow 14 days to elapse between discontinuing an MAO inhibitor intended to treat psychiatric disorders and initiation of protriptyline.

Allow 14 days to elapse between discontinuing protriptyline and initiation of an MAO inhibitor intended to treat psychiatric disorders.

Use with other MAO inhibitors (such as linezolid or I.V. methylene blue):

Do not initiate protriptyline in patients receiving linezolid or I.V. methylene blue; consider other interventions for psychiatric condition.

If urgent treatment with linezolid or I.V. methylene blue is required in a patient already receiving protriptyline and potential benefits outweigh potential risks, discontinue protriptyline promptly and administer linezolid or I.V. methylene blue. Monitor for serotonin syndrome for 2 weeks or until 24 hours after the last dose of linezolid or I.V. methylene blue, whichever comes first. May resume protriptyline 24 hours after the last dose of linezolid or I.V. methylene blue.

Dosage adjustment in renal impairment: No dosage adjustment provided in manufacturer's labeling.

Dosage adjustment in hepatic impairment: No dosage adjustment provided in manufacturer's labeling.

Additional Information Complete prescribing information should be consulted for additional detail.

Dosage Forms Excipient information presented when available (limited, particularly for generics); consult specific product labeling.

Tablet, Oral, as hydrochloride:

Vivactil: 5 mg [contains fd&c red #40, fd&c yellow #6 (sunset yellow)]

Vivactil: 10 mg [contains fd&c yellow #10 (quinoline yellow)]

Generic: 5 mg, 10 mg

◆ **Protriptyline Hydrochloride** *see* Protriptyline *on page 1745*

◆ **Protylol (Can)** *see* Dicyclomine *on page 601*

◆ **PRO-Valacyclovir (Can)** *see* ValACYclovir *on page 2145*

◆ **Provenge** *see* Sipuleucel-T *on page 1902*

◆ **Proventil HFA** *see* Albuterol *on page 61*

◆ **Provera** *see* MedroxyPROGESTERone *on page 1278*

◆ **Provera® (Can)** *see* MedroxyPROGESTERone *on page 1278*

◆ **Provera-Pak (Can)** *see* MedroxyPROGESTERone *on page 1278*

◆ **PRO-Verapamil SR (Can)** *see* Verapamil *on page 2182*

◆ **Provigil** *see* Modafinil *on page 1390*

◆ **Provil [OTC]** *see* Ibuprofen *on page 1032*

◆ **Provir** *see* Crofelemer *on page 500*

◆ **Provisc** *see* Hyaluronate and Derivatives *on page 1000*

◆ **Provocholine** *see* Methacholine *on page 1313*

◆ **Provocholine® (Can)** *see* Methacholine *on page 1313*

◆ **Proxymetacaine** *see* Proparacaine *on page 1733*

◆ **PROzac** *see* FLUoxetine *on page 885*

◆ **Prozac (Can)** *see* FLUoxetine *on page 885*

◆ **PROzac Weekly** *see* FLUoxetine *on page 885*

◆ **PRP-OMP** *see Haemophilus* b Conjugate Vaccine *on page 981*

◆ **PRP-T** *see Haemophilus* b Conjugate Vaccine *on page 981*

◆ **Prudoxin** *see* Doxepin (Topical) *on page 660*

◆ **Prussian Blue** *see* Ferric Hexacyanoferrate *on page 853*

◆ **Prymaccone** *see* Primaquine *on page 1713*

◆ **23PS** *see* Pneumococcal Polysaccharide Vaccine (Polyvalent) *on page 1664*

◆ **PS-341** *see* Bortezomib *on page 270*

Pseudoephedrine (soo doe e FED rin)

Brand Names: U.S. Childrens Silfedrine [OTC]; Decongestant 12Hour Max St [OTC]; Decongestant [OTC]; Elix-Sure Congestion [OTC]; Genaphed [OTC]; Nasal Decongestant [OTC]; Nexafed [OTC]; Psudatabs [OTC]; Simply Stuffy [OTC]; Sudafed 12 Hour [OTC]; Sudafed 24 Hour [OTC]; Sudafed Childrens [OTC]; Sudafed [OTC]; Sudanyl [OTC]; SudoGest 12 Hour [OTC]; SudoGest [OTC]; Suphedrine [OTC]; Unifed [OTC]; Zephrex-D [OTC]

Brand Names: Canada Balminil Decongestant; Benylin® D for Infants; Contac® Cold 12 Hour Relief Non Drowsy; Drixoral® ND; Eltor®; PMS-Pseudoephedrine; Pseudofrin; Robidrine®; Sudafed® Decongestant

Index Terms *d*-Isoephedrine Hydrochloride; Pseudoephedrine Hydrochloride; Pseudoephedrine Sulfate; Sudafed

Pharmacologic Category Alpha/Beta Agonist; Decongestant

Use Temporary symptomatic relief of nasal congestion due to common cold, upper respiratory allergies, and sinusitis; also promotes nasal or sinus drainage

Pregnancy Considerations Use of pseudoephedrine during the first trimester may be associated with a possible risk of gastroschisis, small intestinal atresia, and hemifacial microsomia due to pseudoephedrine's vasoconstrictive effects; additional studies are needed to define the magnitude of risk. Single doses of pseudoephedrine were not found to adversely affect the fetus during the third trimester of pregnancy (limited data); however, fetal tachycardia was noted in a case report following maternal use of an extended release product for multiple days. Decongestants are not the preferred agents for the treatment of rhinitis during pregnancy. Oral pseudoephedrine should be avoided during the first trimester.

Breast-Feeding Considerations Pseudoephedrine is excreted into breast milk in concentrations that are ~4% of the weight adjusted maternal dose. The time to maximum milk concentration is ~1-2 hours after the maternal dose. Irritability has been reported in nursing infants (limited data; dose, duration, relationship to breast-feeding not provided). Milk production may be decreased in some women.

Contraindications Hypersensitivity to pseudoephedrine or any component of the formulation; with or within 14 days of MAO inhibitor therapy

Warnings/Precautions Use with caution in the elderly; may be more sensitive to adverse effects; administer with caution to patients with hypertension, hyperthyroidism, diabetes mellitus, cardiovascular disease, ischemic heart disease, increased intraocular pressure, prostatic hyperplasia, seizure disorders, or renal impairment. When used for self-medication (OTC), notify healthcare provider if symptoms do not improve within 7 days or are accompanied by fever. Discontinue and contact healthcare provider if nervousness, dizziness, or sleeplessness occur. Some products may contain sodium. Not for OTC use in children <4 years of age.

Adverse Reactions Frequency not defined.

Cardiovascular: Arrhythmia, cardiovascular collapse with hypotension, hypertension, palpitation, tachycardia

Central nervous system: Chills, confusion, coordination impaired, dizziness, drowsiness, excitability, fatigue, hallucination, headache, insomnia, nervousness, neuritis, restlessness, seizure, transient stimulation, vertigo

Dermatologic: Photosensitivity, rash, urticaria

Gastrointestinal: Anorexia, constipation, diarrhea, dry throat, ischemic colitis, nausea, vomiting, xerostomia

Genitourinary: Difficult urination, dysuria, polyuria, urinary retention

Hematologic: Agranulocytosis, hemolytic anemia, thrombocytopenia

Neuromuscular & skeletal: Tremor, weakness

Ocular: Blurred vision, diplopia

Otic: Tinnitus

Respiratory: Chest/throat tightness, dry nose, dyspnea, nasal congestion, thickening of bronchial secretions, wheezing

Miscellaneous: Anaphylaxis, diaphoresis

Drug Interactions

Metabolism/Transport Effects None known.

Avoid Concomitant Use

Avoid concomitant use of Pseudoephedrine with any of the following: Ergot Derivatives; Iobenguane I 123; MAO Inhibitors

Increased Effect/Toxicity

Pseudoephedrine may increase the levels/effects of: Sympathomimetics

The levels/effects of Pseudoephedrine may be increased by: Antacids; AtoMOXetine; Cannabinoids; Carbonic Anhydrase Inhibitors; Ergot Derivatives; Linezolid; MAO Inhibitors; Serotonin/Norepinephrine Reuptake Inhibitors

Decreased Effect

Pseudoephedrine may decrease the levels/effects of: Benzylpenicilloyl Polylysine; FentaNYL; Iobenguane I 123

The levels/effects of Pseudoephedrine may be decreased by: Alpha1-Blockers; Spironolactone

Ethanol/Nutrition/Herb Interactions

Food: Onset of effect may be delayed if pseudoephedrine is taken with food.

Herb/Nutraceutical: Avoid ephedra, yohimbe (may cause hypertension).

Mechanism of Action Directly stimulates alpha-adrenergic receptors of respiratory mucosa causing vasoconstriction; directly stimulates beta-adrenergic receptors causing bronchial relaxation, increased heart rate and contractility

Pharmacodynamics/Kinetics

Onset of action: Decongestant: Oral: 30 minutes (Chua, 1989)

Peak effect: Decongestant: Oral: ~1-2 hours (Chua, 1989)

Duration: Immediate release tablet: 3-8 hours (Chua, 1989)

Absorption: Rapid (Simons, 1996)

Distribution: Children: ~2.5 L/kg (Simons, 1996); Adults: 2.64-3.51 L/kg (Kanfer, 1993)

Metabolism: Undergoes n-demethylation to norpseudoephedrine (active) (Chua, 1989; Kanfer, 1993); Hepatic (<1%) (Kanfer, 1993)

Half-life elimination: Varies by urine pH and flow rate; alkaline urine decreases renal elimination of pseudoephedrine (Kanfer, 1993)

Children: ~3 hours (urine pH ~6.5) (Simons, 1996)

Adults: 9-16 hours (pH 8); 3-6 hours (pH 5) (Chua, 1989)

Time to peak:

Children (immediate release) ~2 hours (Simons, 1996)

Adults (immediate release): 1-3 hours (dose dependent) (Kanfer, 1993)

Excretion: Urine (43% to 96% as unchanged drug, 1% to 6% as active norpseudoephedrine); dependent on urine pH and flow rate; alkaline urine decreases renal elimination of pseudoephedrine (Kanfer, 1993)

Dosage Oral: General dosing guidelines:

Children:

4-5 years: 15 mg every 4-6 hours: maximum: 60 mg/24 hours

6-12 years: 30 mg every 4-6 hours; maximum: 120 mg/24 hours

Children >12 years and Adults: Immediate release: 60 mg every 4-6 hours; Extended release: 120 mg every 12 hours **or** 240 mg every 24 hours; maximum: 240 mg/24 hours

Dosage adjustment in renal impairment: No dosage adjustment provided in manufacturer's labeling.

Dosage adjustment in hepatic impairment: No dosage adjustment provided in manufacturer's labeling.

Dietary Considerations Some products may contain sodium. May be taken with or without food.

Administration Do not crush extended release drug product, swallow whole. May administer with or without food. Sudafed® 24 Hour tablet may not completely dissolve and appear in stool

Test Interactions Interferes with urine detection of amphetamine (false-positive)

Dosage Forms Excipient information presented when available (limited, particularly for generics); consult specific product labeling.

Gel, Oral, as hydrochloride:

ElixSure Congestion: 15 mg/5 mL (120 mL) [alcohol free; contains brilliant blue fcf (fd&c blue #1), carbomer 934p, propylene glycol, propylparaben; grape bubblegum flavor]

Liquid, Oral, as hydrochloride:

Childrens Silfedrine: 15 mg/5 mL (118 mL, 237 mL) [grape flavor]

Nasal Decongestant: 30 mg/5 mL (118 mL) [contains fd&c red #40, methylparaben, saccharin sodium, sodium benzoate; raspberry flavor]

Sudafed Childrens: 15 mg/5 mL (118 mL) [alcohol free, sugar free; contains brilliant blue fcf (fd&c blue #1), edetate disodium, fd&c red #40, menthol, polyethylene glycol, saccharin sodium, sodium benzoate; grape flavor]

Unifed: 30 mg/5 mL (120 mL, 480 mL, 3840 mL)

Syrup, Oral, as hydrochloride:

Nasal Decongestant: 30 mg/5 mL (473 mL) [contains fd&c red #40, methylparaben, saccharin sodium, sodium benzoate; raspberry flavor]

Tablet, Oral, as hydrochloride:

Decongestant: 30 mg

Genaphed: 30 mg

Nasal Decongestant: 30 mg [contains fd&c red #40 aluminum lake, fd&c yellow #6 aluminum lake]

Nasal Decongestant: 30 mg [contains fd&c red #40 aluminum lake, polysorbate 80]

Psudatabs: 30 mg [contains fd&c red #40, fd&c yellow #10 (quinoline yellow), fd&c yellow #6 (sunset yellow)]

Simply Stuffy: 30 mg

Sudafed: 30 mg

Sudafed: 30 mg [contains fd&c red #40 aluminum lake, fd&c yellow #10 aluminum lake, fd&c yellow #6 aluminum lake]

Sudanyl: 30 mg

SudoGest: 30 mg [contains fd&c red #40 aluminum lake, fd&c yellow #6 aluminum lake]

SudoGest: 60 mg [scored]

Suphedrine: 30 mg

Generic: 30 mg, 60 mg

Tablet Abuse-Deterrent, Oral, as hydrochloride:

Nexafed: 30 mg

Zephrex-D: 30 mg

Tablet Extended Release 12 Hour, Oral, as hydrochloride:
Decongestant 12Hour Max St: 120 mg [contains polysorbate 80]
Sudafed 12 Hour: 120 mg
Sudafed 12 Hour: 120 mg [contains fd&c blue #1 aluminum lake]
SudoGest 12 Hour: 120 mg
Generic: 120 mg
Tablet Extended Release 24 Hour, Oral, as hydrochloride:
Sudafed 24 Hour: 240 mg

◆ **Pseudoephedrine and Acetaminophen** *see* Acetaminophen and Pseudoephedrine *on page* *33*

◆ **Pseudoephedrine and Chlorpheniramine** *see* Chlorpheniramine and Pseudoephedrine *on page* *412*

◆ **Pseudoephedrine and Desloratadine** *see* Desloratadine and Pseudoephedrine *on page* *575*

Pseudoephedrine and Dextromethorphan

(soo doe e FED rin & deks troe meth OR fan)

Brand Names: U.S. Pedia Relief Cough and Cold [OTC]; Sudafed® Children's Cold & Cough [OTC]

Brand Names: Canada Balminil DM D; Benylin® DM-D; Koffex DM-D; Novahistex® DM Decongestant; Novahistine® DM Decongestant; Robitussin® Childrens Cough & Cold

Index Terms Dextromethorphan and Pseudoephedrine

Pharmacologic Category Antitussive/Decongestant

Use Temporary symptomatic relief of nasal congestion and cough due to common cold, hay fever, upper respiratory allergies

Dosage Relief of nasal congestion and cough: Oral:

General dosing guidelines base on pseudoephedrine component:

Children 2-6 years: 15 mg every 4-6 hours (maximum: 60 mg/24 hours)

Children 6-12 years: 30 mg every 4-6 hours (maximum: 120 mg/24 hours)

Children ≥12 years and Adults: 60 mg every 4-6 hours (maximum: 240 mg/24 hours)

Product-specific dosing:

Children 2-6 years (Sudafed® Children's Cold & Cough): 5 mL every 4 hours (maximum: 20 mL/24 hours)

Children 6-12 years (Sudafed® Children's Cold & Cough): 10 mL every 4 hours (maximum: 40 mL/24 hours)

Children ≥12 years and Adults (Sudafed® Children's Cold & Cough): 20 mL every 4 hours (maximum: 80 mL/24 hours)

Additional Information Complete prescribing information should be consulted for additional detail.

Dosage Forms Excipient information presented when available (limited, particularly for generics); consult specific product labeling.

Liquid:

Sudafed® Children's Cold & Cough: Pseudoephedrine hydrochloride 15 mg and dextromethorphan hydrobromide 5 mg per 5 mL (120 mL) [alcohol free, sugar free; contains sodium benzoate; cherry berry flavor]

Syrup:

Pedia Relief Cough and Cold: Pseudoephedrine hydrochloride 15 mg and dextromethorphan hydrobromide 7.5 mg per 5 mL (120 mL) [cherry flavor]

◆ **Pseudoephedrine and Fexofenadine** *see* Fexofenadine and Pseudoephedrine *on page* *858*

◆ **Pseudoephedrine and Guaifenesin** *see* Guaifenesin and Pseudoephedrine *on page* *978*

Pseudoephedrine and Ibuprofen

(soo doe e FED rin & eye byoo PROE fen)

Brand Names: U.S. Advil® Cold & Sinus [OTC]; Proprinal® Cold and Sinus [OTC]

Brand Names: Canada Advil® Cold & Sinus; Advil® Cold & Sinus Daytime; Children's Advil® Cold; Sudafed® Sinus Advance

Index Terms Ibuprofen and Pseudoephedrine

Pharmacologic Category Decongestant/Analgesic

Use For temporary relief of cold, sinus, and flu symptoms (including nasal congestion, sinus pressure, headache, minor body aches and pains, and fever)

Dosage OTC labeling: Oral: Children ≥12 years and Adults: Ibuprofen 200 mg and pseudoephedrine 30 mg per dose: One dose every 4-6 hours as needed; may increase to 2 doses if necessary (maximum: 6 doses/24 hours). Contact healthcare provider if symptoms have not improved within 7 days when treating cold symptoms or within 3 days when treating fever.

Additional Information Complete prescribing information should be consulted for additional detail.

Dosage Forms Excipient information presented when available (limited, particularly for generics); consult specific product labeling.

Caplet:

Advil® Cold & Sinus, Proprinal® Cold and Sinus: Pseudoephedrine hydrochloride 30 mg and ibuprofen 200 mg

Capsule, liquid filled:

Advil® Cold & Sinus: Pseudoephedrine hydrochloride 30 mg and ibuprofen 200 mg [solubilized ibuprofen as free acid and potassium salt; contains potassium 20 mg/capsule and coconut oil]

◆ **Pseudoephedrine and Loratadine** *see* Loratadine and Pseudoephedrine *on page* *1242*

◆ **Pseudoephedrine and Triprolidine** *see* Triprolidine and Pseudoephedrine *on page* *2131*

◆ **Pseudoephedrine, Chlorpheniramine, and Dextromethorphan** *see* Chlorpheniramine, Pseudoephedrine, and Dextromethorphan *on page* *414*

◆ **Pseudoephedrine, Dextromethorphan, and Guaifenesin** *see* Guaifenesin, Pseudoephedrine, and Dextromethorphan *on page* *979*

◆ **Pseudoephedrine, Guaifenesin, and Codeine** *see* Guaifenesin, Pseudoephedrine, and Codeine *on page* *979*

◆ **Pseudoephedrine Hydrochloride** *see* Pseudoephedrine *on page* *1746*

◆ **Pseudoephedrine Hydrochloride and Acetaminophen** *see* Acetaminophen and Pseudoephedrine *on page* *33*

◆ **Pseudoephedrine Hydrochloride and Acrivastine** *see* Acrivastine and Pseudoephedrine *on page* *41*

◆ **Pseudoephedrine Sulfate** *see* Pseudoephedrine *on page* *1746*

◆ **Pseudofrin (Can)** *see* Pseudoephedrine *on page* *1746*

◆ **Pseudomonic Acid A** *see* Mupirocin *on page* *1407*

◆ **Psudatabs [OTC]** *see* Pseudoephedrine *on page* *1746*

Psyllium (SIL i yum)

Brand Names: U.S. Dietary Fiber Laxative [OTC]; Evac [OTC]; Fiber Therapy [OTC]; Geri-Mucil [OTC]; Konsyl [OTC]; Konsyl-D [OTC]; Laxmar Natural Vegetable Laxat [OTC]; Metamucil MultiHealth Fiber [OTC]; Natural Fiber Therapy [OTC]; Natural Psyllium Seed [OTC]; Natural Vegetable Fiber [OTC]; Reguloid [OTC]; Sorbulax [OTC]

Brand Names: Canada Metamucil®

Index Terms Plantago Seed; Plantain Seed; Psyllium Husk; Psyllium Hydrophilic Mucilloid

Pharmacologic Category Antidiarrheal; Fiber Supplement; Laxative, Bulk-Producing

Additional Appendix Information

Laxatives, Classification and Properties *on page 2304*

Use OTC labeling: Dietary fiber supplement; treatment of occasional constipation; reduce risk of coronary heart disease (CHD)

Unlabeled Use Treatment of diarrhea, chronic constipation, irritable bowel syndrome, inflammatory bowel disease, colon cancer, or diabetes

Pregnancy Considerations Psyllium is not absorbed systemically. When administered with adequate fluids, use is considered safe for the treatment of occasional constipation during pregnancy (Wald, 2003).

Contraindications Hypersensitivity to psyllium or any component of the formulation; fecal impaction; GI obstruction

Warnings/Precautions Use with caution in patients with esophageal strictures, ulcers, stenosis, intestinal adhesions, or difficulty swallowing. Use with caution in the elderly; may have insufficient fluid intake which may predispose them to fecal impaction and bowel obstruction. Products must be taken with at least 8 ounces of fluid in order to prevent choking. To reduce the risk of CHD, the soluble fiber from psyllium should be used in conjunction with a diet low in saturated fat and cholesterol. Some products may contain calcium, potassium, sodium, soy lecithin, or phenylalanine.

When used for self-medication (OTC), do not use in the presence of abdominal pain, nausea, or vomiting. Notify healthcare provider in case of sudden changes of bowel habits which last >2 weeks or in case of rectal bleeding. Not for self-treatment of constipation lasting >1 week

Adverse Reactions Frequency not defined.

Gastrointestinal: Abdominal cramps, constipation, diarrhea, esophageal or bowel obstruction

Respiratory: Bronchospasm

Miscellaneous: Anaphylaxis upon inhalation in susceptible individuals, rhinoconjunctivitis

Drug Interactions

Metabolism/Transport Effects None known.

Avoid Concomitant Use There are no known interactions where it is recommended to avoid concomitant use.

Increased Effect/Toxicity There are no known significant interactions involving an increase in effect.

Decreased Effect There are no known significant interactions involving a decrease in effect.

Mechanism of Action Psyllium is a soluble fiber. It absorbs water in the intestine to form a viscous liquid which promotes peristalsis and reduces transit time.

Pharmacodynamics/Kinetics

Onset of action: Relief of constipation: 12-72 hours

Absorption: None; small amounts of grain extracts present in the preparation have been reportedly absorbed following colonic hydrolysis

Dosage Oral: General dosing guidelines; consult specific product labeling.

Adequate intake for total fiber: Note: The definition of "fiber" varies; however, the soluble fiber in psyllium is only one type of fiber which makes up the daily recommended intake of total fiber.

Children 1-3 years: 19 g/day

Children 4-8 years: 25 g/day

Children 9-13 years: Males: 31 g/day; Females: 26 g/day

Children 14-18 years: Males: 38 g/day; Females: 26 g/day

Adults 19-50 years: Males: 38 g/day; Females: 25 g/day

Adults ≥51 years: Males: 30 g/day; Females: 21 g/day

Pregnancy: 28 g/day

Lactation: 29 g/day

Constipation:

Children 6-11 years: Psyllium: 1.25-15 g per day in divided doses

Children ≥12 years and Adults: Psyllium: 2.5-30 g per day in divided doses

Reduce risk of CHD: Children ≥12 years and Adults: Soluble fiber ≥7 g (psyllium seed husk ≥10.2 g) per day (DHHS, 1998)

Dietary Considerations Products should be taken with at least 8 ounces of fluids. Some products may contain phenylalanine, potassium, sodium, as well as additional ingredients. Check individual product information for caloric and nutritional value.

When used to reduce the risk of CHD, the amount of **soluble fiber** from psyllium should be ≥7 g/day and it should be used in conjunction with a diet low in saturated fat and cholesterol.

Administration Inhalation of psyllium dust may cause sensitivity to psyllium (eg, runny nose, watery eyes, wheezing). Drink at least 8 ounces of liquid with each dose. Powder must be mixed in a glass of water or juice. Capsules should be swallowed one at a time. When more than one dose is required, they should be divided throughout the day. Separate dose by at least 2 hours from other drug therapies.

Dosage Forms Considerations

Psyllium hydrophilic mucilloid 3.4 g is equivalent to 2 g Soluble fiber

Dosage Forms Excipient information presented when available (limited, particularly for generics); consult specific product labeling. [DSC] = Discontinued product

Capsule, Oral:

Konsyl: 520 mg [gluten free, sugar free]

Reguloid: 0.52 g [contains fd&c yellow #6 aluminum lake]

Packet, Oral:

Konsyl: 28.3% (30 ea) [gluten free, kosher certified; contains fd&c yellow #10 (quinoline yellow), fd&c yellow #6 (sunset yellow); orange flavor]

Konsyl: 60.3% (30 ea) [gluten free, kosher certified, sugar free; contains aspartame, fd&c yellow #6 (sunset yellow)]

Konsyl: 60.3% (1 ea, 30 ea) [gluten free, kosher certified, sugar free; contains aspartame, fd&c yellow #6 (sunset yellow); orange flavor]

Konsyl: 100% (30 ea, 100 ea) [gluten free, kosher certified, sugar free; bland flavor]

Powder, Oral:

Dietary Fiber Laxative: 28.3% (283 g, 300 g, 425 g, 660 g) [contains fd&c yellow #6 (sunset yellow)]

Fiber Therapy: 58.6% (283 g) [sugar free; contains aspartame, fd&c yellow #6 (sunset yellow)]

Geri-Mucil: 68% (368 g)

Geri-Mucil: 68% (368 g) [contains fd&c yellow #6 aluminum lake]

Geri-Mucil: 68% (284 g) [sugar free]

Geri-Mucil: 68% (283 g) [sugar free; contains aspartame, fd&c yellow #6 aluminum lake]

Konsyl: 28.3% (538 g) [gluten free, kosher certified; contains fd&c yellow #10 (quinoline yellow), fd&c yellow #6 (sunset yellow)]

Konsyl: 28.3% (538 g) [gluten free, kosher certified; contains fd&c yellow #10 (quinoline yellow), fd&c yellow #6 (sunset yellow); orange flavor]

Konsyl: 30.9% (397 g) [gluten free, kosher certified; contains fd&c yellow #6 (sunset yellow)]

Konsyl: 30.9% (397 g) [gluten free, kosher certified; contains fd&c yellow #6 (sunset yellow); orange flavor]

Konsyl: 60.3% (450 g) [gluten free, kosher certified, sugar free; contains aspartame, fd&c yellow #6 (sunset yellow)]

Konsyl: 60.3% (450 g) [gluten free, kosher certified, sugar free; contains aspartame, fd&c yellow #6 (sunset yellow); orange flavor]
Konsyl: 71.67% (300 g) [gluten free, kosher certified, sugar free]
Konsyl: 71.67% (300 g) [gluten free, kosher certified, sugar free; bland flavor]
Konsyl: 100% (450 g) [gluten free, kosher certified, sugar free]
Konsyl: 100% (300 g, 450 g) [gluten free, kosher certified, sugar free; bland flavor]
Konsyl: 60.3% (283 g) [sugar free; contains aspartame, fd&c yellow #6 (sunset yellow)]
Konsyl: 60.3% (283 g) [sugar free; contains aspartame, fd&c yellow #6 (sunset yellow); orange flavor]
Konsyl-D: 52.3% (397 g) [flavor free]
Konsyl-D: 52.3% (397 g, 500 g [DSC]) [flavor free; sweet flavor]
Laxmar Natural Vegetable Laxat: 58.6% (397 g) [sugar free]
Metamucil MultiHealth Fiber: 58.6% (425 g) [gluten free, sugar free; contains aspartame, brilliant blue fcf (fd&c blue #1), fd&c red #40]
Metamucil MultiHealth Fiber: 63% (660 g) [gluten free, sugar free]
Natural Fiber Therapy: 30.9% (368 g, 539 g); 48.57% (368 g, 538 g)
Natural Psyllium Seed: 100% (480 g) [animal products free, gelatin free, gluten free, kosher certified, lactose free, no artificial color(s), no artificial flavor(s), starch free, sugar free, yeast free]
Natural Vegetable Fiber: 48.57% (368 g)
Reguloid: 48.57% (369 g, 540 g)
Reguloid: 28.3% (369 g, 540 g) [contains fd&c yellow #6 (sunset yellow), fd&c yellow #6 aluminum lake; orange flavor]
Reguloid: 58.6% (284 g, 426 g) [sugar free; natural flavor]
Reguloid: 58.6% (284 g, 426 g) [sugar free; contains aspartame, fd&c yellow #6 (sunset yellow), fd&c yellow #6 aluminum lake]
Sorbulax: 100% (420 g)

Powder, Oral [preservative free]:
Evac: (480 g) [dye free]

- **Psyllium Husk** *see* Psyllium *on page 1748*
- **Psyllium Hydrophilic Mucilloid** *see* Psyllium *on page 1748*
- **Pteroylglutamic Acid** *see* Folic Acid *on page 907*
- **PTG** *see* Teniposide *on page 2012*
- **PTU (error-prone abbreviation)** *see* Propylthiouracil *on page 1740*
- **Pulmicort** *see* Budesonide (Systemic) *on page 282*
- **Pulmicort Flexhaler** *see* Budesonide (Systemic) *on page 282*
- **Pulmicort® Turbuhaler® (Can)** *see* Budesonide (Systemic) *on page 282*
- **Pulmophylline (Can)** *see* Theophylline *on page 2042*
- **Pulmozyme** *see* Dornase Alfa *on page 654*
- **Pulmozyme® (Can)** *see* Dornase Alfa *on page 654*
- **Puregon® (Can)** *see* Follitropin Beta *on page 909*
- **Purg-Odan™ (Can)** *see* Sodium Picosulfate, Magnesium Oxide, and Citric Acid *on page 1925*
- **Purified Chick Embryo Cell** *see* Rabies Vaccine *on page 1772*
- **Purinethol** *see* Mercaptopurine *on page 1300*
- **Purinethol® (Can)** *see* Mercaptopurine *on page 1300*

Pyrantel Pamoate (pi RAN tel PAM oh ate)

Brand Names: U.S. Pamix [OTC]; Pin-X [OTC]; Reeses Pinworm Medicine [OTC]

Brand Names: Canada Combantrin™

Pharmacologic Category Anthelmintic

Use Treatment of pinworms caused by *Enterobius vermicularis* (alternative agent; not preferred therapy)

Unlabeled Use Treatment of hookworms caused by *Ancylostoma caninum, Ancylostoma duodenale,* and *Necator americanus*); *Moniliformis;* roundworms caused by *Ascaris lumbricoides*; *Trichostrongylus*

Pregnancy Considerations Pyrantel pamoate has minimal systemic absorption. Systemic absorption would be required in order for pyrantel pamoate to cross the placenta and reach the fetus.

Contraindications Hypersensitivity to pyrantel pamoate or any component of the formulation

Warnings/Precautions Use with caution in patients with liver impairment. Since pinworm infections are easily spread to others, treat all family members in close contact with the patient. When used for self-medication, patients should be instructed to contact healthcare provider if symptoms or pinworm infection persists after treatment or if any worms other than pinworms are present before or after treatment. Patients should not repeat dose unless directed to by their healthcare provider. Some products may contain aspartame or sodium benzoate.

Adverse Reactions Frequency not defined.

Central nervous system: Dizziness, headache
Gastrointestinal: Abdominal cramps, diarrhea, nausea, vomiting

Drug Interactions

Metabolism/Transport Effects Substrate of CYP2D6 (minor); **Note:** Assignment of Major/Minor substrate status based on clinically relevant drug interaction potential

Avoid Concomitant Use There are no known interactions where it is recommended to avoid concomitant use.

Increased Effect/Toxicity There are no known significant interactions involving an increase in effect.

Decreased Effect

The levels/effects of Pyrantel Pamoate may be decreased by: Aminoquinolines (Antimalarial); Peginterferon Alfa-2b

Storage/Stability Store at 15°C to 30°C (59°F to 86°F).

Mechanism of Action Causes the release of acetylcholine and inhibits cholinesterase; acts as a depolarizing neuromuscular blocker, paralyzing the helminths

Pharmacodynamics/Kinetics

Absorption: Oral: Poor
Metabolism: Partially hepatic
Time to peak, serum: 1-3 hours
Excretion: Feces (>50% as unchanged drug); urine (7% as unchanged drug and metabolites)

Dosage Oral: Children ≥2 years and Adults: **Note:** Dose is expressed as pyrantel base; not preferred therapy since newer treatments are available.

Enterobius vermicularis (pinworm): 11 mg/kg administered as a single dose; maximum: 1 g/dose

Ancylostoma caninum (hookworm) (unlabeled use): 11 mg/kg (maximum: 1 g/dose) administered once daily for 3 days

Ancylostoma duodenale (hookworm), *Ascariasis lumbricoides* (roundworm), *Necator americanus* (hookworm) (unlabeled use): 11 mg/kg (maximum: 1 g/dose) administered once daily for 3 days (Kappagoda, 2011)

Moniliformis (unlabeled use): 11 mg/kg administered as a single dose; repeat twice 2 weeks apart

Trichostrongylus (unlabeled use): 11 mg/kg administered as a single dose; maximum: 1 g/dose

Dietary Considerations May take without regard to meals.

Administration May be mixed with milk or fruit juice. May be administered without regard to meals. Purgation is not required prior to, during, or after use.

Suspension: Shake well before use.

Tablet: Chewable tablet must be chewed thoroughly before swallowing

Monitoring Parameters Stool for presence of eggs, worms, and occult blood

Dosage Forms Excipient information presented when available (limited, particularly for generics); consult specific product labeling.

Suspension, Oral, as pamoate:

Pamix: 50 mg/mL (30 mL, 60 mL, 240 mL)

Pin-X: 50 mg/mL (30 mL, 60 mL) [sugar free; contains methylparaben, propylene glycol, propylparaben, saccharin sodium, sodium benzoate; caramel flavor]

Reeses Pinworm Medicine: 144 mg/mL (30 mL) [contains saccharin sodium, sodium benzoate]

Tablet, Oral, as pamoate:

Reeses Pinworm Medicine: 180 mg [scored]

Tablet Chewable, Oral, as pamoate:

Pin-X: 720.5 mg [scored; contains aspartame, fd&c yellow #6 aluminum lake; orange flavor]

Pyrazinamide (peer a ZIN a mide)

Brand Names: Canada Tebrazid™

Index Terms Pyrazinoic Acid Amide

Pharmacologic Category Antitubercular Agent

Use Adjunctive treatment of tuberculosis in combination with other antituberculosis agents

Pregnancy Risk Factor C

Pregnancy Considerations Teratogenic effects have not been observed in animal reproduction studies. Due to the risk of tuberculosis to the fetus, treatment is recommended when the probability of maternal disease is moderate to high. Although not recommended as the initial treatment regimen, the use of pyrazinamide during pregnancy is recommended by The World Health Organization (Blumberg, 2003).

Breast-Feeding Considerations Low concentrations of pyrazinamide have been detected in breast milk; concentrations are less than maternal plasma concentration (Holdiness, 1984). The amount of drug in breast milk is considered insufficient for the treatment of tuberculosis in breast-fed infants.

Contraindications Hypersensitivity to pyrazinamide or any component of the formulation; acute gout; severe hepatic damage

Warnings/Precautions Use with caution in patients with a history of alcoholism, renal failure, chronic gout, diabetes mellitus, or porphyria. Dose-related hepatotoxicity ranging from transient ALT/AST elevations to jaundice, hepatitis and/or liver atrophy (rare) has occurred. Use with caution in patients receiving concurrent medications associated with hepatotoxicity (particularly with rifampin).

Adverse Reactions

1% to 10%:

Central nervous system: Malaise

Gastrointestinal: Anorexia, nausea, vomiting

Neuromuscular & skeletal: Arthralgia, myalgia

<1% (Limited to important or life-threatening): Acne, angioedema (rare), anticoagulant effect, dysuria, fever, gout, hepatotoxicity, interstitial nephritis, itching, photosensitivity, porphyria, rash, sideroblastic anemia, thrombocytopenia, urticaria

Drug Interactions

Metabolism/Transport Effects None known.

Avoid Concomitant Use There are no known interactions where it is recommended to avoid concomitant use.

Increased Effect/Toxicity

Pyrazinamide may increase the levels/effects of: CycloSPORINE (Systemic); Rifampin

Decreased Effect There are no known significant interactions involving a decrease in effect.

Storage/Stability Store at controlled room temperature of 15°C to 30°C (59°F to 86°F).

Mechanism of Action Converted to pyrazinoic acid in susceptible strains of *Mycobacterium* which lowers the pH of the environment; exact mechanism of action has not been elucidated

Pharmacodynamics/Kinetics Bacteriostatic or bactericidal depending on drug's concentration at infection site

Absorption: Well absorbed

Distribution: Widely into body tissues and fluids including liver, lung, and CSF

Relative diffusion from blood into CSF: Adequate with or without inflammation (exceeds usual MICs)

CSF:blood level ratio: Inflamed meninges: 100%

Protein binding: 50%

Metabolism: Hepatic

Half-life elimination: 9-10 hours

Time to peak, serum: Within 2 hours

Excretion: Urine (4% as unchanged drug)

Dosage Oral: Treatment of tuberculosis:

Note: Used as part of a multidrug regimen. Treatment regimens consist of an initial 2-month phase, followed by a continuation phase of 4 or 7 additional months; pyrazinamide is administered in the initial phase of treatment.

Children:

HIV negative (CDC, 2003):

Daily therapy: 15-30 mg/kg/day (maximum: 2 g/day)

Twice weekly directly observed therapy (DOT): 50 mg/kg/dose (maximum: 2 g/dose)

HIV-exposed/-infected: Daily therapy: 20-40 mg/kg/dose once daily (maximum: 2 g/day) (CDC, 2009)

Adults: Suggested dosing based on lean body weight (Blumberg, 2003; CDC, 2003):

Daily therapy:

40-55 kg: 1000 mg

56-75 kg: 1500 mg

76-90 kg: 2000 mg (maximum dose regardless of weight)

Twice weekly directly observed therapy (DOT):

40-55 kg: 2000 mg

56-75 kg: 3000 mg

76-90 kg: 4000 mg (maximum dose regardless of weight)

Three times/week DOT:

40-55 kg: 1500 mg

56-75 kg: 2500 mg

76-90 kg: 3000 mg (maximum dose regardless of weight)

Dosage adjustment in renal impairment: Adults: Cl_{cr} <30 mL/minute or receiving hemodialysis: Treatment of TB: 25-35 mg/kg/dose 3 times per week administered after dialysis (Blumberg, 2003; CDC, 2003)

Dosage adjustment in hepatic impairment: No dosage adjustment provided in manufacturer's labeling. Use is contraindicated in cases of severe hepatic impairment.

Monitoring Parameters Periodic liver function tests, serum uric acid, sputum culture, chest x-ray 2-3 months into treatment and at completion

Test Interactions Reacts with Acetest® and Ketostix® to produce pinkish-brown color

Dosage Forms Excipient information presented when available (limited, particularly for generics); consult specific product labeling.

Tablet, Oral:

Generic: 500 mg

Extemporaneous Preparations A 100 mg/mL oral suspension may be made with tablets. Crush two-hundred pyrazinamide 500 mg tablets and mix with a suspension containing 500 mL methylcellulose 1% and 500 mL simple syrup. Add to this a suspension containing one-hundred forty crushed pyrazinamide tablets in 350 mL methylcellulose 1% and 350 mL simple syrup to make 1.7 L suspension. Label "shake well" and "refrigerate". Stable for 60 days refrigerated (preferred) and 45 days at room temperature.

Nahata MC, Morosco RS, and Peritre SP, "Stability of Pyrazinamide in Two Suspensions," *Am J Health Syst Pharm*, 1995, 52(14):1558-60.

◆ Pyrazinoic Acid Amide *see* Pyrazinamide *on page* 1751

Pyrethrins and Piperonyl Butoxide

(pye RE thrins & pi PER oh nil byo TOKS ide)

Brand Names: U.S. A-200® Lice Treatment Kit [OTC]; A-200® Maximum Strength [OTC]; Licide® [OTC]; Pronto® Complete Lice Removal System [OTC]; Pronto® Plus Lice Killing Mousse Plus Vitamin E [OTC]; Pronto® Plus Lice Killing Mousse Shampoo Plus Natural Extracts and Oils [OTC]; Pronto® Plus Warm Oil Treatment and Conditioner [OTC]; RID® Maximum Strength [OTC]

Brand Names: Canada Pronto® Lice Control; R & C™ II; R & C™ Shampoo/Conditioner; RID® Mousse

Index Terms Piperonyl Butoxide and Pyrethrins

Pharmacologic Category Antiparasitic Agent, Topical; Pediculocide; Shampoo, Pediculocide

Use Treatment of *Pediculus humanus* infestations (head lice, body lice, pubic lice, and their eggs)

Pregnancy Risk Factor C

Dosage Application of pyrethrins: Topical products:

Apply enough solution to completely wet infested area, including hair

Allow to remain on area for 10 minutes

Wash and rinse with large amounts of warm water.

Use fine-toothed comb to remove lice and eggs from hair

Shampoo hair to restore body and luster

Treatment may be repeated if necessary once in a 24-hour period

Repeat treatment in 7-10 days to kill newly hatched lice

Note: Keep out of eyes when rinsing hair; protect eyes with a wash cloth or towel

Additional Information Complete prescribing information should be consulted for additional detail.

Dosage Forms Excipient information presented when available (limited, particularly for generics); consult specific product labeling.

Kit:

A-200® Lice Treatment Kit:

Shampoo: Pyrethrins 0.33% and piperonyl butoxide 4% (120 mL)

Solution [spray; for bedding; not for human or animal use]: Permethrin 0.5% (180 mL)

[packaged with nit removal comb]

Pronto® Complete Lice Removal System:

Shampoo: Pyrethrins 0.33% and piperonyl butoxide 4% (60 mL)

Solution, topical: Benzalkonium chloride 0.1% (60 mL) [lice egg remover antiseptic]

[packaged with household furniture spray and nit removal comb]

Oil, topical:

Pronto® Plus Warm Oil Treatment and Conditioner: Pyrethrins 0.33% and piperonyl butoxide 4% (36 mL) [fruity herbal scent; packaged with nit removal comb]

Shampoo:

A-200® Maximum Strength: Pyrethrins 0.33% and piperonyl butoxide 4% (60 mL, 120 mL) [contains benzyl alcohol; packaged with nit removal comb]

Licide®: Pyrethrins 0.33% and piperonyl butoxide 4% (120 mL) [packaged with nit removal comb; also available in a kit containing shampoo, household spray, and nit removal comb]

Pronto® Plus Lice Killing Mousse Shampoo Plus Natural Extracts and Oils: Pyrethrins 0.33% and piperonyl butoxide 4% (60 mL) [packaged with nit removal comb]

Pronto® Plus Lice Killing Mousse Shampoo Plus Vitamin E: Pyrethrins 0.33% and piperonyl butoxide 4% (120 mL) [blue mousse shampoo; contains vitamin E; packaged with nit removal comb]

RID® Maximum Strength: Pyrethrins 0.33% and piperonyl butoxide 4% (60 mL, 120 mL, 180 mL, 240 mL) [packaged with nit removal comb; also available in a kit containing shampoo, gel, and furniture spray]

◆ Pyri 500 [OTC] *see* Pyridoxine *on page* 1753

◆ 2-Pyridine Aldoxime Methochloride *see* Pralidoxime *on page* 1694

◆ Pyridium *see* Phenazopyridine *on page* 1627

Pyridostigmine (peer id oh STIG meen)

Brand Names: U.S. Mestinon; Regonol

Brand Names: Canada Mestinon®; Mestinon®-SR

Index Terms Pyridostigmine Bromide

Pharmacologic Category Acetylcholinesterase Inhibitor

Use Symptomatic treatment of myasthenia gravis; antagonism of nondepolarizing neuromuscular blockers

Military use: Pretreatment for Soman nerve gas exposure

Pregnancy Risk Factor B

Pregnancy Considerations Safety has not been established for use during pregnancy. The potential benefit to the mother should outweigh the potential risk to the fetus. When pyridostigmine is needed in myasthenic mothers, giving dose parenterally 1 hour before completion of the second stage of labor may facilitate delivery and protect the neonate during the immediate postnatal state.

Breast-Feeding Considerations Neonates of myasthenia gravis mothers may have difficulty in sucking and swallowing (as well as breathing). Neonatal pyridostigmine may be indicated by symptoms (confirmed by edrophonium test).

Contraindications Hypersensitivity to pyridostigmine, bromides, or any component of the formulation; GI or GU obstruction

Warnings/Precautions Use with caution in patients with epilepsy, bradycardia, hyperthyroidism, cardiac arrhythmias, or peptic ulcer; use with extreme caution in patients with asthma or bronchospastic disease; adequate facilities should be available for cardiopulmonary resuscitation when testing and adjusting dose for myasthenia gravis; have atropine and epinephrine ready to treat hypersensitivity reactions; overdosage may result in cholinergic crisis, this must be distinguished from myasthenic crisis; anticholinesterase insensitivity can develop for brief or prolonged periods. Regonol® injection contains 1% benzyl alcohol as the preservative (not intended for use in newborns). **[U.S. Boxed Warning]: Regonol® injection must be administered by trained personnel.**

Adverse Reactions Frequency not defined.

Cardiovascular: Arrhythmias (especially bradycardia), AV block, cardiac arrest, decreased carbon monoxide, flushing, hypotension, nodal rhythm, nonspecific ECG changes, syncope, tachycardia

Central nervous system: Convulsions, dizziness, drowsiness, dysphonia, headache, loss of consciousness

Dermatologic: Skin rash, thrombophlebitis (I.V.), urticaria

Gastrointestinal: Abdominal pain, diarrhea, dysphagia, flatulence, hyperperistalsis, nausea, salivation, stomach cramps, vomiting
Genitourinary: Urinary urgency
Neuromuscular & skeletal: Arthralgia, dysarthria, fasciculations, muscle cramps, myalgia, spasms, weakness
Ocular: Amblyopia, lacrimation, small pupils
Respiratory: Bronchial secretions increased, bronchiolar constriction, bronchospasm, dyspnea, laryngospasm, respiratory arrest, respiratory depression, respiratory muscle paralysis
Miscellaneous: Allergic reactions, anaphylaxis, diaphoresis increased

Drug Interactions

Metabolism/Transport Effects None known.

Avoid Concomitant Use There are no known interactions where it is recommended to avoid concomitant use.

Increased Effect/Toxicity

Pyridostigmine may increase the levels/effects of: Beta-Blockers; Cholinergic Agonists; Succinylcholine

The levels/effects of Pyridostigmine may be increased by: Corticosteroids (Systemic)

Decreased Effect

Pyridostigmine may decrease the levels/effects of: Neuromuscular-Blocking Agents (Nondepolarizing)

The levels/effects of Pyridostigmine may be decreased by: Dipyridamole; Methocarbamol

Storage/Stability
Injection: Protect from light.
Tablet:
30 mg: Store under refrigeration at 2°C to 8°C (36°F to 46°F). Protect from light. Stable at room temperature for up to 3 months.
Mestinon®: Store at 25°C (77°F). Protect from moisture.

Mechanism of Action Inhibits destruction of acetylcholine by acetylcholinesterase which facilitates transmission of impulses across myoneural junction

Pharmacodynamics/Kinetics
Onset of action: Oral, I.M.: 15-30 minutes; I.V. injection: 2-5 minutes
Duration: Oral: Up to 6-8 hours (due to slow absorption); I.V.: 2-3 hours
Absorption: Oral: Very poor
Distribution: 19 ± 12 L
Metabolism: Hepatic
Bioavailability: 10% to 20%
Half-life elimination: 1-2 hours; Renal failure: ≤6 hours
Excretion: Urine (80% to 90% as unchanged drug)

Dosage
Myasthenia gravis:
Oral:
Children: 7 mg/kg/24 hours divided into 5-6 doses
Adults: Highly individualized dosing ranges: 60-1500 mg/day, usually 600 mg/day divided into 5-6 doses, spaced to provide maximum relief
Sustained release formulation: Highly individualized dosing ranges: 180-540 mg once or twice daily (doses separated by at least 6 hours); **Note:** Most clinicians reserve sustained release dosage form for bedtime dose only.
I.M., slow I.V. push:
Children: 0.05-0.15 mg/kg/dose
Adults: To supplement oral dosage pre- and postoperatively during labor and postpartum, during myasthenic crisis, or when oral therapy is impractical: ~1/30th of oral dose; observe patient closely for cholinergic reactions
or
I.V. infusion: Initial: 2 mg/hour with gradual titration in increments of 0.5-1 mg/hour, up to a maximum rate of 4 mg/hour

Reversal of nondepolarizing muscle relaxants: **Note:** Atropine sulfate (0.6-1.2 mg) I.V. immediately prior to pyridostigmine to minimize side effects: I.V.:
Children: Dosing range: 0.1-0.25 mg/kg/dose*
Adults: 0.1-0.25 mg/kg/dose; 10-20 mg is usually sufficient*
*Full recovery usually occurs ≤15 minutes, but ≥30 minutes may be required

Pretreatment for Soman nerve gas exposure (military use):
Oral: Adults: 30 mg every 8 hours beginning several hours prior to exposure; discontinue at first sign of nerve agent exposure, then begin atropine and pralidoxime

Dosage adjustment in renal impairment: No dosage adjustment provided in manufacturer's labeling. However, lower dosages may be required due to prolonged elimination in renal impairment.

Dosage adjustment in hepatic impairment: No dosage adjustment provided in manufacturer's labeling.

Administration Do **not** crush sustained release tablet.

Monitoring Parameters Observe for cholinergic reactions, particularly when administered I.V.; consult individual institutional policies and procedures

Dosage Forms Excipient information presented when available (limited, particularly for generics); consult specific product labeling.
Solution, Injection, as bromide:
Regonol: 5 mg/mL (2 mL) [contains benzyl alcohol]
Syrup, Oral, as bromide:
Mestinon: 60 mg/5 mL (473 mL) [contains alcohol, usp, brilliant blue fcf (fd&c blue #1), fd&c red #40, sodium benzoate; raspberry flavor]
Tablet, Oral, as bromide:
Mestinon: 60 mg [scored]
Generic: 60 mg
Tablet Extended Release, Oral, as bromide:
Mestinon: 180 mg [scored]

◆ **Pyridostigmine Bromide** *see* Pyridostigmine *on page 1752*

Pyridoxine (peer i DOKS een)

Brand Names: U.S. Neuro-K-250 T.D. [OTC]; Neuro-K-250 Vitamin B6 [OTC]; Neuro-K-50 [OTC]; Neuro-K-500 [OTC]; Pyri 500 [OTC]

Index Terms B6; B_6; Pyridoxine Hydrochloride; Vitamin B_6

Pharmacologic Category Vitamin, Water Soluble

Use Prevention and treatment of vitamin B_6 deficiency

Unlabeled Use Treatment and prophylaxis of neurological toxicities (ie, seizures, coma) associated with isoniazid and Gyromitrin-containing mushroom (false morel) overdose/toxicity; nausea and vomiting of pregnancy; prevention of peripheral neuropathy associated with isoniazid therapy for *Mycobacterium tuberculosis*

Pregnancy Risk Factor A

Pregnancy Considerations Water soluble vitamins cross the placenta. Maternal pyridoxine plasma concentrations may decrease as pregnancy progresses and requirements may be increased in pregnant women (IOM, 1998). Pyridoxine is used to treat nausea and vomiting of pregnancy (Neibyl, 2010). In general, medications used as antidotes should take into consideration the health and prognosis of the mother; antidotes should be administered to pregnant women if there is a clear indication for use and should not be withheld because of fears of teratogenicity (Bailey, 2003).

Breast-Feeding Considerations Pyridoxine is found in breast milk and concentrations vary by maternal intake. Pyridoxine requirements are increased in nursing women compared to non-nursing women (IOM, 1998). Possible inhibition of lactation at doses >600 mg/day when taken immediately postpartum (Foukas, 1973).

Contraindications Hypersensitivity to pyridoxine or any component of the formulation

Warnings/Precautions Severe, permanent peripheral neuropathies have been reported; neurotoxicity is more common with long-term administration of large doses (>2 g/day). Dependence and withdrawal may occur with doses >200 mg/day. Single vitamin deficiency is rare; evaluate for other deficiencies. Some parenteral products contain aluminum; use caution in patients with impaired renal function and neonates.

Pharmacy supply of emergency antidotes: Guidelines suggest that at least 8-24 g be stocked. This is enough to treat 1 patient weighing 100 kg for an initial 8- to 24-hour period. In areas where tuberculosis is common, hospitals should consider stocking 24 g. This is enough to treat 1 patient for 24 hours (Dart, 2009).

Adverse Reactions Frequency not defined.

Central nervous system: Headache, seizure (following very large I.V. doses), somnolence
Endocrine & metabolic: Acidosis, folic acid decreased
Gastrointestinal: Nausea
Hepatic: AST increased
Neuromuscular & skeletal: Neuropathy, paresthesia
Miscellaneous: Allergic reactions

Drug Interactions

Metabolism/Transport Effects None known.

Avoid Concomitant Use There are no known interactions where it is recommended to avoid concomitant use.

Increased Effect/Toxicity There are no known significant interactions involving an increase in effect.

Decreased Effect

Pyridoxine may decrease the levels/effects of: Altretamine; Barbiturates; Fosphenytoin; Levodopa; Phenytoin

Storage/Stability Injection: Store at 20°C to 25°C (68°F to 77°F). Protect from light.

Mechanism of Action Precursor to pyridoxal, which functions in the metabolism of proteins, carbohydrates, and fats; pyridoxal also aids in the release of liver and muscle-stored glycogen and in the synthesis of GABA (within the central nervous system) and heme

Pharmacodynamics/Kinetics

Absorption: Enteral, parenteral: Well absorbed
Metabolism: Hepatic to pyridoxal phosphate and pyridoxamine phosphate (active forms)
Half-life elimination: Biologic: 15-20 days
Excretion: Urine

Dosage

Oral:

Adequate intake (AI) (IOM, 1998):
Infants:
1-6 months: 0.1 mg/day
7-12 months: 0.3 mg/day

Recommended daily allowance (RDA) (IOM, 1998):
Children:
1-3 years: 0.5 mg
4-8 years: 0.6 mg
9-13 years: 1 mg
14-18 years:
Females: 1.2 mg
Males: 1.3 mg
Adults:
19-50 years: 1.3 mg
≥51 years:
Females: 1.5 mg
Males: 1.7 mg
Pregnancy: 1.9 mg
Lactation: 2 mg

Prevention of peripheral neuropathy associated with isoniazid therapy for *Mycobacterium tuberculosis:*
Adults: 25-50 mg/day (CDC, 2009)

Treatment of nausea and vomiting of pregnancy (unlabeled use): 10 to 25 mg every 8 hours (Neibyl, 2010)

I.M., I.V.: Dietary deficiency: Adults: 10-20 mg/day for 3 weeks, followed by oral therapy. Doses up to 600 mg/day may be needed with pyridoxine dependency syndrome.

I.V.:

Treatment of isoniazid-induced seizures and/or coma (unlabeled use):

Children:

Acute ingestion of known amount: Initial: A total dose of pyridoxine equal to the amount of isoniazid ingested (maximum dose: 70 mg/kg, up to 5 g); administer at a rate of 0.5-1 g/minute until seizures stop or the maximum initial dose has been administered; may repeat every 5-10 minutes as needed to control persistent seizure activity and/or CNS toxicity. If seizures stop prior to the administration of the calculated initial dose, infuse the remaining pyridoxine over 4-6 hours (Howland, 2006; Morrow, 2006).

Acute ingestion of unknown amount: Initial: 70 mg/kg (maximum dose: 5 g); administer at a rate of 0.5-1 g/minute; may repeat every 5-10 minutes as needed to control persistent seizure activity and/or CNS toxicity (Howland, 2006; Morrow, 2006; Santucci, 1999)

Adults:

Acute ingestion of known amount: Initial: A total dose of pyridoxine equal to the amount of isoniazid ingested (maximum dose: 5 g); administer at a rate of 0.5-1 g/minute until seizures stop or the maximum initial dose has been administered; may repeat every 5-10 minutes as needed to control persistent seizure activity and/or CNS toxicity. If seizures stop prior to the administration of the calculated initial dose, infuse the remaining pyridoxine over 4-6 hours (Howland, 2006; Morrow, 2006).

Acute ingestion of unknown amount: Initial: 5 g; administer at a rate of 0.5-1 g/minute; may repeat every 5-10 minutes as needed to control persistent seizure activity and/or CNS toxicity (Howland, 2006; Morrow, 2006)

Prevention of isoniazid-induced seizures and/or coma (unlabeled use): Children and Adults: Asymptomatic patients who present within 2 hours of ingesting a potentially toxic amount of isoniazid should receive a prophylactic dose of pyridoxine (Boyer, 2006). Dosing recommendations are the same as for the treatment of symptomatic patients.

Treatment of seizures from acute Gyromitrin-containing mushroom toxicity (unlabeled use): Children and Adults: 25 mg/kg over 15-30 minutes; repeat dose as needed to control seizures (Diaz, 2005)

Administration Burning may occur at the injection site after I.M. or SubQ administration; seizures have occurred following I.V. administration of very large doses.

Isoniazid toxicity (unlabeled use): Initial doses should be administered at a rate of 0.5-1 g/minute. If the parenteral formulation is not available, anecdotal reports suggest that pyridoxine tablets may be crushed and made into a slurry and given at the same dose orally or via nasogastric (NG) tube (Boyer, 2006). Oral administration is not recommended for acutely poisoned patients with seizure activity.

Monitoring Parameters For treatment of isoniazid or Gyromitrin-containing mushroom toxicity: Anion gap, arterial blood gases, electrolytes, neurological exam, seizure activity

Reference Range Over 50 ng/mL (SI: 243 nmol/L) (varies considerably with method). A broad range is ~25-80 ng/mL (SI: 122-389 nmol/L). HPLC method for pyridoxal phosphate has normal range of 3.5-18 ng/mL (SI: 17-88 nmol/L).

Test Interactions False positive urobilinogen spot test using Ehrlich's reagent

Dosage Forms Excipient information presented when available (limited, particularly for generics); consult specific product labeling.

Capsule, Oral, as hydrochloride:
- Neuro-K-250 T.D.: 250 mg [corn free, rye free, starch free, sugar free, wheat free]

Solution, Injection, as hydrochloride:
- Generic: 100 mg/mL (1 mL)

Tablet, Oral, as hydrochloride:
- Neuro-K-50: 50 mg
- Neuro-K-500: 500 mg
- Neuro-K-250 Vitamin B6: 250 mg
- Pyri 500: 500 mg
- Generic: 25 mg, 50 mg, 100 mg, 250 mg

Tablet, Oral, as hydrochloride [preservative free]:
- Generic: 25 mg, 50 mg, 100 mg

Tablet Extended Release, Oral, as hydrochloride:
- Generic: 200 mg

Extemporaneous Preparations A 1 mg/mL oral solution may be made using pyridoxine injection. Withdraw 100 mg (1 mL of a 100 mg/mL injection) from a vial with a needle and syringe; add to 99 mL simple syrup in an amber bottle. Label "refrigerate". Stable for 30 days refrigerated.

Nahata MC, Pai VB, and Hipple TF, *Pediatric Drug Formulations*, 5th ed, Cincinnati, OH: Harvey Whitney Books Co, 2004.

◆ **Pyridoxine and Doxylamine** *see* Doxylamine and Pyridoxine *on page 673*

◆ **Pyridoxine, Folic Acid, and Cyanocobalamin** *see* Folic Acid, Cyanocobalamin, and Pyridoxine *on page 908*

◆ **Pyridoxine Hydrochloride** *see* Pyridoxine *on page 1753*

Pyrimethamine (peer i METH a meen)

Brand Names: U.S. Daraprim

Brand Names: Canada Daraprim®

Pharmacologic Category Antimalarial Agent

Use Prophylaxis of malaria due to susceptible strains of plasmodia; used in conjunction with a sulfonamide for the treatment of uncomplicated malaria due to susceptible strains of plasmodia (alternative agent; not preferred therapy); synergistic combination with sulfonamide in treatment of toxoplasmosis

Pregnancy Risk Factor C

Pregnancy Considerations Teratogenic effects have been observed in animal reproduction studies. If administered during pregnancy (ie, for toxoplasmosis), supplementation of folate is strongly recommended. Pregnancy should be avoided during therapy.

Breast-Feeding Considerations Pyrimethamine enters breast milk and may result in significant systemic concentrations in breast-fed infants. The effect of concurrent therapy with sulfonamide or dapsone (frequently used with pyrimethamine as combination treatment) must be considered.

Contraindications Hypersensitivity to pyrimethamine or any component of the formulation; megaloblastic anemia secondary to folate deficiency

Warnings/Precautions When used for more than 3-4 days, it may be advisable to administer leucovorin calcium to prevent hematologic complications; monitor CBC and platelet counts every 2 weeks in patients receiving high-dose therapy (eg, when used for toxoplasmosis treatment); use with caution in patients with impaired renal or hepatic function or with possible G6PD. Use caution in patients with seizure disorders or possible folate deficiency (eg, malabsorption syndrome, pregnancy, alcoholism).

Adverse Reactions Frequency not defined.

Cardiovascular: Arrhythmias (large doses)

Dermatologic: Erythema multiforme, rash, Stevens-Johnson syndrome, toxic epidermal necrolysis

Gastrointestinal: Anorexia, atrophic glossitis, vomiting

Hematologic: Leukopenia, megaloblastic anemia, pancytopenia, pulmonary eosinophilia, thrombocytopenia

Genitourinary: Hematuria

Miscellaneous: Anaphylaxis

Drug Interactions

Metabolism/Transport Effects Inhibits CYP2C9 (moderate)

Avoid Concomitant Use

Avoid concomitant use of Pyrimethamine with any of the following: Artemether; Lumefantrine

Increased Effect/Toxicity

Pyrimethamine may increase the levels/effects of: Antipsychotic Agents (Phenothiazines); Bosentan; Carvedilol; CYP2C9 Substrates; Dapsone (Systemic); Dapsone (Topical); Lumefantrine

The levels/effects of Pyrimethamine may be increased by: Artemether; Dapsone (Systemic)

Decreased Effect

The levels/effects of Pyrimethamine may be decreased by: Methylfolate

Storage/Stability Store at 15°C to 25°C (59°F to 77°F). Protect from light.

Mechanism of Action Inhibits parasitic dihydrofolate reductase, resulting in inhibition of vital tetrahydrofolic acid synthesis

Pharmacodynamics/Kinetics

Onset of action: ~1 hour

Absorption: Well absorbed

Distribution: Widely, mainly in blood cells, kidneys, lungs, liver, and spleen; crosses into CSF

Protein binding: 80% to 87%

Metabolism: Hepatic

Half-life elimination: 80-95 hours

Time to peak, serum: 1.5-8 hours

Excretion: Urine (20% to 30% as unchanged drug)

Dosage Oral:

Isosporiasis (*Isospora belli* infection) in HIV-positive patients (unlabeled use; CDC, 2009): Adults:

Treatment (alternative to trimethoprim-sulfamethoxazole): 50-75 mg once daily in combination with leucovorin calcium

Chronic maintenance (secondary prophylaxis): 25 mg once daily in combination with leucovorin calcium

Malaria chemoprophylaxis: Begin prophylaxis before entering endemic area: **Note:** Current CDC recommendations for malaria prophylaxis do not include the use of pyrimethamine; resistance to pyrimethamine is prevalent worldwide.

Manufacturer's labeling:

Children <4 years: 6.25 mg once weekly

Children 4-10 years: 12.5 mg once weekly

Children >10 years and Adults: 25 mg once weekly

Malaria treatment (non-*falciparum* malaria; use in conjunction with a sulfonamide [eg, sulfadoxine]): Note: Current CDC recommendations for the malaria treatment do not include the use of pyrimethamine; resistance to pyrimethamine is prevalent worldwide.

Manufacturer's labeling:

Children 4-10 years: 25 mg daily for 2 days; following clinical cure, administer a once weekly chemoprophylaxis regimen for ≥10 weeks

Children >10 years and Adults: 25 mg daily for 2 days; following clinical cure, administer a once weekly chemoprophylaxis regimen for ≥10 weeks

Note: Pyrimethamine use alone is **not** recommended; if circumstances arise where it must be used alone in semi-immune patients, give adults 50 mg daily for 2 days (children receive 25 mg daily for 2 days), then (following clinical cure) administer a once-weekly chemoprophylaxis regimen for ≥10 weeks.

***Pneumocystis jirovecii* pneumonia (PCP) in HIV-positive patients (unlabeled use; CDC, 2009):** Adults:

Prophylaxis (alternative to trimethoprim-sulfamethoxazole): 50 mg once weekly in combination with dapsone and leucovorin calcium; **or** 25 mg once daily with atovaquone in combination with oral leucovorin calcium

Chronic maintenance (secondary prophylaxis; alternative to trimethoprim-sulfamethoxazole): 50-75 mg once weekly in combination with dapsone and leucovorin calcium; **or** 25 mg once daily with atovaquone in combination with leucovorin calcium

Toxoplasmosis treatment: *Manufacturer's labeling:*

Children: Loading dose: 1 mg/kg/day divided into 2 equal daily doses for 2-4 days, then may decrease dose to 0.5 mg/kg/day divided into 2 doses for 4 weeks; use with a sulfonamide in combination with leucovorin calcium

Adults: 50-75 mg/day for 1-3 weeks depending on patient's tolerance and response, then may reduce dose by 50% and continue for 4-5 weeks; use with a sulfonamide in combination with leucovorin calcium

Toxoplasmosis prophylaxis and treatment in HIV-positive patients (unlabeled; CDC, 2009):

Prophylaxis for first episode of Toxoplasma gondii:

Children ≥1 month of age: 1 mg/kg/day (or 15 mg/m^2) once daily (maximum: 25 mg), with dapsone or atovaquone in combination with leucovorin calcium

Adolescents and Adults (alternative to trimethoprim sulfamethoxazole): 50 mg or 75 mg once weekly with dapsone in combination with leucovorin calcium; **or** 25 mg once daily with atovaquone in combination with leucovorin calcium

Prophylaxis to prevent recurrence of Toxoplasma gondii:

Children ≥1 month of age: 1 mg/kg/day (or 15 mg/m^2) once daily (maximum: 25 mg) given with sulfadiazine (or atovaquone or clindamycin) in combination with leucovorin calcium

Adolescents and Adults: 25-50 mg once daily with sulfadiazine in combination with leucovorin calcium (preferred); **or** 25-50 mg once daily with clindamycin in combination with leucovorin calcium; **or** 25 mg once daily with atovaquone in combination with leucovorin calcium

Treatment of congenital toxoplasmosis: Infants and Children: Loading dose: 2 mg/kg/day once daily for 2 days, then 1 mg/kg/day once daily for 2-6 months, followed by 1 mg/kg administered 3 times weekly, with sulfadiazine or clindamycin in combination with leucovorin calcium (treatment duration: 12 months)

Treatment of acquired toxoplasmosis: Infants and Children: Acute induction: Loading dose: 2 mg/kg once daily (maximum: 50 mg/day) for 3 days, then 1 mg/kg/day once daily (maximum: 25 mg/day), with sulfadiazine or clindamycin in combination with leucovorin calcium (treatment duration: ≥6 weeks)

Treatment of Toxoplasma gondii encephalitis: Adolescents and Adults: 200 mg as a single dose, followed by 50 mg (<60 kg) or 75 mg (≥60 kg) daily, with sulfadiazine in combination with leucovorin calcium for at least 6 weeks (preferred); **or** 200 mg as a single dose, followed by 50 mg (<60 kg) or 75 mg (≥60 kg) daily, with clindamycin, atovaquone, or azithromycin in combination with leucovorin calcium

Dosage adjustment in renal impairment: No dosage adjustment provided in manufacturer's labeling. Use with caution.

Dosage adjustment in hepatic impairment: No dosage adjustment provided in manufacturer's labeling. Use with caution.

Dietary Considerations Take with meals to minimize GI distress.

Administration Administer with meals to minimize GI distress.

Monitoring Parameters CBC, including platelet counts twice weekly with high-dose therapy (eg, when used for toxoplasmosis treatment; frequency not defined for lower doses); liver and renal function

Dosage Forms Excipient information presented when available (limited, particularly for generics); consult specific product labeling.

Tablet, Oral:

Daraprim: 25 mg [scored]

Extemporaneous Preparations A 2 mg/mL oral suspension may be made with tablets and a 1:1 mixture of Simple Syrup, NF and methylcellulose 1%. Crush forty 25 mg tablets in a mortar and reduce to a fine powder. Add small portions of vehicle and mix to a uniform paste; mix while adding vehicle in incremental proportions to **almost** 500 mL; transfer to a calibrated bottle, rinse mortar with vehicle, and add quantity of vehicle sufficient to make 500 mL. Label "shake well" and "refrigerate". Stable for 91 days.

Nahata MC, Pai VB, and Hipple TF, *Pediatric Drug Formulations*, 5th ed, Cincinnati, OH: Harvey Whitney Books Co, 2004.

- ◆ **Pyrimethamine and Sulfadoxine** *see* Sulfadoxine and Pyrimethamine *on page 1959*
- ◆ **QAB149** *see* Indacaterol *on page 1065*
- ◆ **Q-Alendronate (Can)** *see* Alendronate *on page 69*
- ◆ **Q-Amlodipine (Can)** *see* AmLODIPine *on page 109*
- ◆ **Q-Citalopram (Can)** *see* Citalopram *on page 440*
- ◆ **Q-Cyclobenzaprine (Can)** *see* Cyclobenzaprine *on page 502*
- ◆ **Q-Dryl [OTC]** *see* DiphenhydrAMINE (Systemic) *on page 622*
- ◆ **Q-Fenofibrate Micro (Can)** *see* Fenofibrate and Derivatives *on page 837*
- ◆ **Q-Fluoxetine (Can)** *see* FLUoxetine *on page 885*
- ◆ **Qinghao Derivative** *see* Artesunate *on page 171*
- ◆ **Qinghaosu Derivative** *see* Artesunate *on page 171*
- ◆ **Q-Metformin (Can)** *see* MetFORMIN *on page 1310*
- ◆ **Qnasl** *see* Beclomethasone (Nasal) *on page 229*
- ◆ **Q-Omeprazole (Can)** *see* Omeprazole *on page 1505*
- ◆ **Q-Pan H5N1 Influenza Vaccine** *see* Influenza Virus Vaccine (H5N1) *on page 1076*
- ◆ **Q-Pantoprazole (Can)** *see* Pantoprazole *on page 1563*
- ◆ **Q-Pap [OTC]** *see* Acetaminophen *on page 28*
- ◆ **Q-Pap Children's [OTC]** *see* Acetaminophen *on page 28*
- ◆ **Q-Pap Extra Strength [OTC]** *see* Acetaminophen *on page 28*
- ◆ **Q-Pap Infant's [OTC]** *see* Acetaminophen *on page 28*
- ◆ **Q-Paroxetine (Can)** *see* PARoxetine *on page 1575*
- ◆ **Q-Sertraline (Can)** *see* Sertraline *on page 1889*
- ◆ **Q-Simvastatin (Can)** *see* Simvastatin *on page 1899*
- ◆ **Q-Terbinafine (Can)** *see* Terbinafine (Systemic) *on page 2017*
- ◆ **Q-Tussin [OTC]** *see* GuaiFENesin *on page 974*
- ◆ **Q-Tussin DM [OTC]** *see* Guaifenesin and Dextromethorphan *on page 976*
- ◆ **Quad Pill** *see* Elvitegravir, Cobicistat, Emtricitabine, and Tenofovir *on page 696*

- **Quadrivalent Human Papillomavirus Vaccine** *see* Papillomavirus (Types 6, 11, 16, 18) Vaccine (Human, Recombinant) *on page 1567*
- **Qualaquin** *see* QuiNINE *on page 1766*
- **Quartette** *see* Ethinyl Estradiol and Levonorgestrel *on page 787*
- **Quasense** *see* Ethinyl Estradiol and Levonorgestrel *on page 787*
- **Quaternium-18 Bentonite** *see* Bentoquatam *on page 240*

Quazepam (KWAZ e pam)

Brand Names: U.S. Doral

Brand Names: Canada Doral

Pharmacologic Category Benzodiazepine

Additional Appendix Information

Beers Criteria – Potentially Inappropriate Medications for Geriatrics *on page 2368*

Benzodiazepine Comparison Table *on page 2292*

Use Insomnia: For the treatment of insomnia characterized by difficulty in falling asleep, frequent nocturnal awakenings, and/or early morning

Pregnancy Risk Factor C

Medication Guide Available Yes

Dosage

Adults: Oral: Initial: 7.5 mg at bedtime; in some patients, the dose may be increased to 15 mg if necessary for efficacy.

Elderly: Dosing should be cautious; begin at lower end of dosing range (ie, 7.5 mg)

Dosing adjustment in renal impairment: No dosage adjustment provided in manufacturer's labeling.

Dosing adjustment in hepatic impairment: No dosage adjustment provided in manufacturer's labeling.

Additional Information Complete prescribing information should be consulted for additional detail.

Dosage Forms Excipient information presented when available (limited, particularly for generics); consult specific product labeling.

Tablet, Oral:

Doral: 15 mg [contains fd&c yellow #6 aluminum lake]

Generic: 15 mg

Controlled Substance C-IV

- **Quelicin** *see* Succinylcholine *on page 1954*
- **Quelicin® (Can)** *see* Succinylcholine *on page 1954*
- **Quelicin-1000** *see* Succinylcholine *on page 1954*
- **Quenalin [OTC]** *see* DiphenhydrAMINE (Systemic) *on page 622*
- **Questran** *see* Cholestyramine Resin *on page 418*
- **Questran Light** *see* Cholestyramine Resin *on page 418*
- **Questran Light Sugar Free (Can)** *see* Cholestyramine Resin *on page 418*

QUEtiapine (kwe TYE a peen)

Brand Names: U.S. SEROquel; SEROquel XR

Brand Names: Canada Apo-Quetiapine; Auro-Quetiapine; Ava-Quetiapine; CO Quetiapine; Dom-Quetiapine; JAMP-Quetiapine; Mylan-Quetiapine; PHL-Quetiapine; PMS-Quetiapine; PRO-Quetiapine; ratio-Quetiapine; Riva-Quetiapine; Sandoz-Quetiapine; Seroquel; Seroquel XR; Teva-Quetiapine; Teva-Quetiapine XR

Index Terms Quetiapine Fumarate

Pharmacologic Category Antipsychotic Agent, Atypical

Additional Appendix Information

Antipsychotic Agents *on page 2290*

Beers Criteria – Potentially Inappropriate Medications for Geriatrics *on page 2368*

Use

Bipolar disorder: Treatment of bipolar disorder (immediate release and extended release), which includes the following: Acute treatment of manic episodes associated with bipolar I disorder (as monotherapy or as an adjunct to lithium or divalproex); acute treatment of depressive episodes associated with bipolar I and II; maintenance treatment of bipolar I (as an adjunct to lithium or divalproex

Major depressive disorder: Treatment of major depressive disorder (as adjunctive treatment) (extended release)

Schizophrenia: Treatment of schizophrenia (immediate release and extended release)

Unlabeled Use Delirium in the critically-ill patient; psychosis/agitation related to Alzheimer's dementia

Pregnancy Risk Factor C

Pregnancy Considerations Adverse events were observed in animal reproduction studies. Quetiapine crosses the placenta and can be detected in cord blood (Newport, 2007). Congenital malformations have not been observed in humans (based on limited data). Antipsychotic use during the third trimester of pregnancy has a risk for abnormal muscle movements (extrapyramidal symptoms [EPS]) and/or withdrawal symptoms in newborns following delivery. Symptoms in the newborn may include agitation, feeding disorder, hypertonia, hypotonia, respiratory distress, somnolence, and tremor; these effects may be self-limiting or require hospitalization. Quetiapine may cause hyperprolactinemia, which may decrease reproductive function in both males and females.

Treatment algorithms have been developed by the ACOG and the APA for the management of depression in women prior to conception and during pregnancy (Yonkers, 2009). The ACOG recommends that therapy during pregnancy be individualized; treatment with psychiatric medications during pregnancy should incorporate the clinical expertise of the mental health clinician, obstetrician, primary healthcare provider, and pediatrician. Safety data related to atypical antipsychotics during pregnancy is limited and routine use is not recommended. However, if a woman is inadvertently exposed to an atypical antipsychotic while pregnant, continuing therapy may be preferable to switching to a typical antipsychotic that the fetus has not yet been exposed to; consider risk:benefit (ACOG, 2008).

Healthcare providers are encouraged to enroll women 18-45 years of age exposed to quetiapine during pregnancy in the Atypical Antipsychotics Pregnancy Registry (1-866-961-2388 or http://www.womensmentalhealth.org/pregnancyregistry).

Breast-Feeding Considerations Quetiapine is excreted into breast milk. Based on information from 8 mother-infant pairs, concentrations of quetiapine in breast milk have been reported from undetectable to 170 µg/L. The estimated exposure to the breast-feeding infant would be up to 0.1 mg/kg/day (relative infant dose up to 0.43% based on a weight adjusted maternal dose of 400 mg/day). Breast-feeding is not recommended by the manufacturer.

Medication Guide Available Yes

Contraindications Hypersensitivity to quetiapine or any component of the formulation

Warnings/Precautions [U.S. Boxed Warning]: Antidepressants increase the risk of suicidal thinking and behavior in children, adolescents, and young adults (18-24 years of age) with major depressive disorder (MDD) and other psychiatric disorders; consider risk prior to prescribing. Short-term studies did not show an increased risk in patients >24 years of age and showed a decreased risk in patients ≥65 years. Closely monitor all patients for clinical worsening, suicidality, or unusual changes in behavior; particularly during the initial 1-2 months of therapy or during periods of dosage adjustments (increased or decreases); the patient's family or caregiver should be instructed to closely observe the patient and communicate condition with healthcare provider. A medication guide concerning the use of antidepressants should be dispensed with each prescription. **Quetiapine is not approved in the U.S. for use in children <10 years of age.**

Leukopenia, neutropenia, and agranulocytosis (sometimes fatal) have been reported in clinical trials and postmarketing reports with antipsychotic use; presence of risk factors (eg, pre-existing low WBC or history of drug-induced leuko-/neutropenia) should prompt periodic blood count assessment. Discontinue therapy at first signs of blood dyscrasias or if absolute neutrophil count <1000/mm^3.

May worsen psychosis in some patients or precipitate a shift to mania or hypomania in patients with bipolar disorder; quetiapine is approved in the U.S. for the treatment of bipolar depression. May be sedating, use with caution in disorders where CNS depression is a feature. Use with caution in Parkinson's disease. May induce orthostatic hypotension associated with dizziness, tachycardia, and, in some cases, syncope, especially during the initial dose titration period. Should be used with particular caution in patients with known cardiovascular disease (history of MI or ischemic heart disease, heart failure, or conduction abnormalities), cerebrovascular disease, or conditions that predispose to hypotension. Use has been associated with QT prolongation; postmarketing reports have occurred in patients with concomitant illness, quetiapine overdose, or who were receiving concomitant therapy known to affect QT interval or cause electrolyte imbalance. Esophageal dysmotility and aspiration have been associated with antipsychotic use; use with caution in patients at risk of aspiration pneumonia (eg, Alzheimer's disease). May cause dose-related decreases in thyroid levels, including cases requiring thyroid replacement therapy. Measure both TSH and free T_4, along with clinical assessment, at baseline and follow-up to determine thyroid status; measurement of TSH alone may not be accurate (exact mechanism of quetiapine's effect on the thyroid axis is unknown). Development of cataracts has been observed in animal studies; lens changes have been observed in humans during long-term treatment. Lens examination on initiation of therapy and every 6 months thereafter is recommended. May cause hyperglycemia; in some cases may be extreme and associated with ketoacidosis, hyperosmolar coma, or death. Use with caution in patients with diabetes or other disorders of glucose regulation; monitor for worsening of glucose control. Significant weight gain has been observed with antipsychotic therapy; incidence varies with product. Monitor waist circumference and BMI.

Due to anticholinergic effects, use with caution in patients with decreased gastrointestinal motility, urinary retention, BPH, xerostomia, visual problems, and narrow-angle glaucoma. Relative to other antipsychotics, quetiapine has a moderate potency of cholinergic blockade. May cause extrapyramidal symptoms (EPS), pseudoparkinsonism, and/or tardive dyskinesia. Risk of dystonia (and probably other EPS) may be greater with increased doses, use of conventional antipsychotics, males, and younger patients. Impaired core body temperature regulation may occur; caution with strenuous exercise, heat exposure, dehydration, and concomitant medication possessing anticholinergic effects. Neuroleptic malignant syndrome (NMS) is a potentially fatal symptom complex that has been reported in association with administration of antipsychotic drugs. Clinical manifestations of NMS are hyperpyrexia, muscle rigidity, altered mental status, and evidence of autonomic instability (irregular pulse or blood pressure, tachycardia, diaphoresis, and cardiac dysrhythmia). Management of NMS should include immediate discontinuation of antipsychotic drugs and other drugs not essential to concurrent therapy, intensive symptomatic treatment and medication monitoring, and treatment of any concomitant medical problems for which specific treatment are available.

Use caution in patients with a history of seizures. May cause decreases in total free thyroxine, elevations of liver enzymes, cholesterol levels, and/or triglyceride increases. Rare cases of priapism have been reported. May increase prolactin levels; clinical significance of hyperprolactinemia in patients with breast cancer or other prolactin-dependent tumors is unknown.

[U.S. Boxed Warning]: Elderly patients with dementia-related psychosis treated with antipsychotics are at an increased risk of death compared to placebo. Most deaths appeared to be either cardiovascular (eg, heart failure, sudden death) or infectious (eg, pneumonia) in nature. Quetiapine is not approved for the treatment of dementia-related psychosis. An increased incidence of cerebrovascular effects (eg, transient ischemic attack, stroke), including fatalities, has also been reported in placebo-controlled trials of other atypical antipsychotic agents. Avoid antipsychotic use for behavioral problems associated with dementia unless alternative nonpharmacologic therapies have failed and patient may harm self or others. In addition, use may cause or exacerbate syndrome of inappropriate antidiuretic hormone secretion or hyponatremia; monitor sodium closely with initiation or dosage adjustments in older adults (Beers Criteria).

Pharmacologic treatment for pediatric bipolar I disorder or schizophrenia should be initiated only after thorough diagnostic evaluation and a careful consideration of potential risks vs benefits. If a pharmacologic agent is initiated, it should be a component of a total treatment program including psychological, educational and social interventions. Increased blood pressure (including hypertensive crisis) has been reported in children and adolescents; monitor blood pressure at baseline and periodically during use.

Potentially significant drug-drug interactions may exist, requiring dose or frequency adjustment, additional monitoring, and/or selection of alternative therapy. May cause withdrawal symptoms (rare) with abrupt cessation; gradually taper dose during discontinuation.

Adverse Reactions Actual frequency may be dependent upon dose and/or indication. Unless otherwise noted, frequency of adverse effects is reported for adult patients; spectrum and incidence of adverse effects similar in children (with significant exceptions noted).

>10%:

Cardiovascular: Hypertension (diastolic; children and adolescents 41%), systolic hypertension (children and adolescents 15%), tachycardia (1% to 11%)

Central nervous system: Drowsiness (18% to 57%), headache (7% to 21%), agitation (5% to 20%), dizziness (1% to 19%), fatigue (3% to 14%), extrapyramidal reaction (1% to 13%)

Endocrine & metabolic: Weight gain (dose related; 3% to 23%), increased serum triglycerides (≥200 mg/dL, 8% to 22%), decreased HDL cholesterol (≤40 mg/dL, 6% to 19%), total cholesterol increased (≥240 mg/dL, 7% to 18%), increased LDL cholesterol (≥160 mg/dL, 4% to 17%), hyperglycemia (≥200 mg/dL post glucose challenge or fasting glucose ≥126 mg/dL, 2% to 12%)

Gastrointestinal: Xerostomia (9% to 44%; children and adolescents 4% to 10%), increased appetite (2% to 12%), constipation (2% to 11%)

1% to 10%:

Cardiovascular: Orthostatic hypotension (2% to 7%; children and adolescents <1%), syncope (<5%), palpitations (4%), peripheral edema (4%), increased heart rate (2% to 4%), hypotension (3%), hypertension (1% to 2%)

Central nervous system: Insomnia (9%), akathisia (≤8%), pain (1% to 7%), dystonia (≤6%), dysarthria (1% to 5%), irritability (1% to 5%), lethargy (1% to 5%), drooling (<5%), tardive dyskinesia (<5%), hypertonia (4%), twitching (4%), anxiety (2% to 4%), ataxia (2% to 4%), drug-induced Parkinson's disease (≤4%), abnormal dreams (2% to 3%), aggressive behavior (children and adolescents 1% to 3%), depression (1% to 3%), hypersomnia (1% to 3%), paresthesia (≤3%), abnormality in thinking (2%), decreased mental acuity (2%), disorientation (2%), hypoesthesia (2%), lack of concentration (2%), migraine (2%), restless leg syndrome (2%), vertigo (2%), confusion (1% to 2%), restlessness (1% to 2%), falling (≤2%), chills (1%)

Dermatologic: Skin rash (4%), acne vulgaris (children and adolescents 2% to 3%), diaphoresis (2%), hyperhidrosis (2%), pallor (children and adolescents 1% to 2%)

Endocrine & metabolic: Hyperprolactinemia (4%), decreased libido (≤2%), hypothyroidism (≤2%), increased thirst (children and adolescents ≤2%), increased gamma-glutamyl transferase (1%)

Gastrointestinal: Nausea (5% to 10%), vomiting (1% to 8%), dyspepsia (dose related; 2% to 7%), abdominal pain (1% to 7%),gastroenteritis (2% to 4%), toothache (2% to 3%), periodontal abscess (adolescents 1% to 3%), decreased appetite (2%), dysphagia (2%), flatulence (2%), gastroesophageal reflux disease (2%), anorexia (≥1%), unpleasant taste (1%), abdominal distension (≤1%)

Genitourinary: Pollakiuria (2%), urinary tract infection (2%), impotence (1%), lactation (female 1%)

Hematologic & oncologic: Neutropenia (≤2%), leukopenia (≥1%), hemorrhage (1%), lymphadenopathy (1%)

Hepatic: Increased serum transaminases (1% to 6%)

Hypersensitivity: Seasonal allergy (2%)

Neuromuscular & skeletal: Weakness (1% to 10%), tremor (2% to 8%), back pain (1% to 5%), dyskinesia (≤4%), arthralgia (1% to 4%), muscle rigidity (≤3%), muscle spasm (1% to 3%), stiffness (children and adolescents 1% to 3%), limb pain (2%), myalgia (2%), neck pain (2%), neck stiffness (1%)

Ophthalmic: Blurred vision (1% to 4%), amblyopia (2% to 3%)

Otic: Otalgia (≤2%)

Respiratory: Pharyngitis (4% to 6%), nasal congestion (3% to 6%), rhinitis (3% to 4%), cough (3%), upper respiratory tract infection (2% to 3%), epistaxis (adolescents ≤3%), sinus congestion (≤3%), sinus headache (2%), sinusitis (2%), flu-like symptoms (1% to 2%), dyspnea (≥1%), dry throat (1%)

Miscellaneous: Fever (1% to 4%)

<1% (Limited to important or life-threatening): Abnormal T waves on ECG, acute renal failure, agranulocytosis, amnesia, anaphylaxis, anemia, angina pectoris, asthma, atrial arrhythmia, atrioventricular block, bradycardia, bundle branch block, cardiac failure, cardiomyopathy, cataract, cerebral ischemia, cerebrovascular accident, dehydration, diabetes mellitus, dysuria, eosinophilia, exfoliative dermatitis, galactorrhea, hallucination, hematemesis, hypersensitivity, hypoglycemia, hypokalemia, hyponatremia, increased creatinine, increased serum alkaline phosphatase, increased serum creatinine, increased ST segment on ECG, intestinal obstruction, inversion T wave on ECG, involuntary body movements, leukocytosis, myocarditis, neuroleptic malignant syndrome, nocturia, palpitations, pancreatitis, pneumonia, priapism, prolonged Q-T interval on ECG, rectal hemorrhage, retrograde amnesia, rhabdomyolysis, seizure, SIADH, Stevens-Johnson syndrome, suicidal ideation, suicidal tendencies, thrombocytopenia, toxic epidermal necrolysis, urinary retention, widened QRS complex on ECG

Drug Interactions

Metabolism/Transport Effects **Substrate** of CYP2D6 (minor), CYP3A4 (major); **Note:** Assignment of Major/Minor substrate status based on clinically relevant drug interaction potential

Avoid Concomitant Use

Avoid concomitant use of QUEtiapine with any of the following: Aclidinium; Amisulpride; Azelastine (Nasal); Fusidic Acid (Systemic); Highest Risk QTc-Prolonging Agents; Ipratropium (Oral Inhalation); Ivabradine; Metoclopramide; Mifepristone; Moderate Risk QTc-Prolonging Agents; Paraldehyde; Sulpiride; Tiotropium; Umeclidinium

Increased Effect/Toxicity

QUEtiapine may increase the levels/effects of: Alcohol (Ethyl); Amisulpride; Analgesics (Opioid); Anticholinergics; Azelastine (Nasal); Buprenorphine; CNS Depressants; Highest Risk QTc-Prolonging Agents; Hydrocodone; Hypotensive Agents; Methotrimeprazine; Methylphenidate; Paraldehyde; Serotonin Modulators; St Johns Wort; Sulpiride; Tiotropium; Zolpidem

The levels/effects of QUEtiapine may be increased by: Acetylcholinesterase Inhibitors (Central); Aclidinium; Brimonidine (Topical); CYP3A4 Inhibitors (Moderate); CYP3A4 Inhibitors (Strong); Dasatinib; Doxylamine; Fusidic Acid (Systemic); HydrOXYzine; Ipratropium (Oral Inhalation); Ivabradine; Ivacaftor; Lithium formulations; Luliconazole; Magnesium Sulfate; Methotrimeprazine; Methylphenidate; Metoclopramide; Metyrosine; Mifepristone; Moderate Risk QTc-Prolonging Agents; Perampanel; Pramlintide; QTc-Prolonging Agents (Indeterminate Risk and Risk Modifying); Serotonin Modulators; Simeprevir; Sodium Oxybate; Tetrabenazine; Umeclidinium

Decreased Effect

QUEtiapine may decrease the levels/effects of: Amphetamines; Anti-Parkinson's Agents (Dopamine Agonist); Quinagolide

The levels/effects of QUEtiapine may be decreased by: Bosentan; CYP3A4 Inducers (Strong); Dabrafenib; Deferasirox; Lithium formulations; Peginterferon Alfa-2b; St Johns Wort; Tocilizumab

Ethanol/Nutrition/Herb Interactions

Ethanol: May increase CNS depression; monitor for increased effects with coadministration. Caution patients about effects.

Food: In healthy volunteers, administration of quetiapine (immediate release) with food resulted in an increase in the peak serum concentration and AUC by 25% and 15%, respectively, compared to the fasting state. Administration of the extended release formulation with a high-fat meal (~800-1000 calories) resulted in an increase in peak serum concentration by 44% to 52% and AUC by 20% to 22% for the 50 mg and 300 mg tablets; administration with a light meal (≤300 calories) had no significant effect on the C_{max} or AUC.

Herb/Nutraceutical: St John's wort may decrease quetiapine levels. Avoid valerian, St John's wort, kava kava, gotu kola (may increase CNS depression).

Storage/Stability Store at controlled room temperature of 25°C (77°F); excursions permitted to 15°C to 30°C (59°F to 86°F).

Mechanism of Action Quetiapine is a dibenzothiazepine atypical antipsychotic. It has been proposed that this drug's antipsychotic activity is mediated through a combination of dopamine type 2 (D_2) and serotonin type 2 ($5\text{-}HT_2$) antagonism. It is an antagonist at multiple neurotransmitter receptors in the brain: Serotonin $5\text{-}HT_{1A}$ and

5-HT_2, dopamine D_1 and D_2, histamine H_1, and adrenergic alpha$_1$- and alpha$_2$-receptors; but appears to have no appreciable affinity at cholinergic muscarinic and benzodiazepine receptors. Norquetiapine, an active metabolite, differs from its parent molecule by exhibiting high affinity for muscarinic M1 receptors.

Antagonism at receptors other than dopamine and 5-HT_2 with similar receptor affinities may explain some of the other effects of quetiapine. The drug's antagonism of histamine H_1-receptors may explain the somnolence observed. The drug's antagonism of adrenergic alpha$_1$-receptors may explain the orthostatic hypotension observed.

Pharmacodynamics/Kinetics

Absorption: Rapidly absorbed following oral administration

Distribution: V_d: 6-14 L/kg

Protein binding, plasma: 83%

Metabolism: Primarily hepatic; via CYP3A4; forms the metabolite N-desalkyl quetiapine (active) and two inactive metabolites

Bioavailability: 100% (relative to oral solution)

Half-life elimination:

Mean: Terminal: Quetiapine: ~6 hours; Extended release: ~7 hours

Metabolite: N-desalkyl quetiapine: 9-12 hours

Time to peak, plasma: Immediate release: 1.5 hours; Extended release: 6 hours

Excretion: Urine (73% as metabolites, <1% of total dose as unchanged drug); feces (20%)

Dosage

Bipolar disorder:

Children ≥10 years and Adolescents ≤17 years: Oral:

Mania (monotherapy):

Immediate release: Initial: 25 mg twice daily on day 1; increase to 50 mg twice daily on day 2, then increase by 100 mg daily (administered twice daily) each day until 200 mg twice day is reached on day 5. May further increase up to 600 mg daily in increments of ≤100 mg daily. Usual dosage range: 400-600 mg daily; maximum: 600 mg daily. **Note:** Total daily doses may also be divided into 3 doses per day, based on response and tolerability.

Extended release: Initial: 50 mg once daily on day 1; increase to 100 mg once daily on day 2, further increase by 100 mg once daily until 400 mg once daily is reached on day 5. Usual dosage range: 400-600 mg once daily; maximum dose: 600 mg once daily.

Adults: Oral:

Depressive episodes:

Immediate release: Initial: 50 mg once daily at bedtime on day 1; increase to 100 mg once daily on day 2, further increase by 100 mg daily each day until 300 mg once daily is reached by day 4. Usual dose: 300 mg once daily; maximum dose: 300 mg once daily.

Extended release: Initial: 50 mg once daily on day 1; increase to 100 mg once daily on day 2, further increase by 100 mg once daily until 300 mg once daily is reached by day 4. Usual dose: 300 mg once daily; maximum dose: 300 mg once daily.

Mania (monotherapy or as an adjunct to lithium or divalproex):

Immediate release: Initial: 50 mg twice daily on day 1, further increase by 100 mg daily (administered twice daily) until 200 mg twice daily is reached by day 4; may further increase to 800 mg daily by day 6 in increments of ≤200 mg daily. Usual dosage range: 400-800 mg daily; maximum dose: 800 mg daily.

Extended release: Initial: 300 mg once daily on day 1; increase to 600 mg once daily on day 2 and increase dose to between 400-800 mg once daily on day 3; usual dosage range: 400-800 mg once daily; maximum dose: 800 mg once daily.

Maintenance therapy (adjunct to lithium or divalproex): Immediate release or extended release: Usual dosage range: 400-800 mg daily; maximum dose: 800 mg daily. **Note:** In the maintenance phase, patients generally continue on the same dose on which they were stabilized. Average time of stabilization was 15 weeks in clinical trials. During maintenance treatment, periodically reassess need for continued therapy and the appropriate dose. Patients who have discontinued therapy for >1 week should generally be retitrated following reinitiation of therapy; patients who have discontinued <1 week, can generally be reinitiated on their previous maintenance dose.

Elderly: Oral:

Immediate release: Initial: 50 mg daily; may increase in increments of 50 mg daily to an effective dose, based on individual clinical response and tolerability

Extended release: 50 mg once daily; may increase by 50 mg once daily to an effective dose, based on individual clinical response and tolerability

Major depressive disorder (adjunct to antidepressants): Adults: Oral: Extended release: Initial: 50 mg once daily on days 1 and 2; increase to 150 mg once daily on day 3. Usual dosage range: 150-300 mg daily; maximum dose: 300 mg once daily.

Schizophrenia:

Adolescents 13 to ≤17 years: Oral:

Immediate release: Initial: 25 mg twice daily on day 1; increase to 50 mg twice daily on day 2, further increase by 100 mg daily each day (divided twice daily) until 400 mg twice daily is reached on day 5. May further increase up to 800 mg daily in increments of ≤100 mg daily. Usual dosage range: 400-800 mg daily; maximum dose: 800 mg daily. **Note:** Total daily doses may also be divided into 3 doses per day, based on response and tolerability.

Extended release: Initial: 50 mg once daily on day 1; increase to 100 mg once daily on day 2, further increase by 100 mg once daily until 400 mg once daily is reached on day 5. Usual dosage range: 400-800 mg once daily; maximum dose: 800 mg once daily.

Adults: Oral:

Immediate release: Initial: 25 mg twice daily; increase in increments of 25-50 mg divided 2-3 times daily on days 2 and 3 to a range of 300-400 mg daily in 2-3 divided doses by day 4. Further adjustments as needed at intervals of at least 2 days in increments of 25-50 mg twice daily. Usual dosage range: 150-750 mg daily; maximum dose: 750 mg daily.

Extended release: Initial: 300 mg once daily; increase in increments of up to 300 mg once daily (in intervals of ≥1 day). Usual dosage range: 400-800 mg once daily; maximum dose: 800 mg once daily.

Maintenance therapy (monotherapy): Extended release: Usual dosage range: 400-800 mg once daily; maximum dose: 800 mg once daily. **Note:** During maintenance treatment, periodically reassess need for continued therapy and the appropriate dose. Patients who have discontinued therapy for >1 week should generally be retitrated following reinitiation of therapy; patients who have discontinued <1 week, can generally be reinitiated on their previous maintenance dose.

Elderly: Oral:

Immediate release: Initial: 50 mg daily; may increase in increments of 50 mg daily to an effective dose, based on individual clinical response and tolerability

Extended release: 50 mg once daily; may increase by 50 mg once daily to an effective dose, based on individual clinical response and tolerability

ICU delirium (unlabeled use): Adults: Oral: Immediate release: Initial: 50 mg twice daily; may increase as necessary on a daily basis in increments of 50 mg twice daily to a maximum dose of 400 mg daily (Devlin, 2010)

Psychosis/agitation related to Alzheimer's dementia (unlabeled use): Elderly: Oral: Initial: 12.5-50 mg daily; if necessary, gradually increase as tolerated not to exceed 200-300 mg daily (Rabins, 2007)

Switching from immediate release to extended release: Children ≥10 years, Adolescents, Adults, and Elderly: May convert patients from immediate release to extended release tablets at the equivalent total daily dose and administer once daily; individual dosage adjustments may be necessary.

Dosage adjustment for concomitant therapy: Children ≥10 years, Adolescents, Adults, and Elderly:

Concomitant use with a strong CYP3A4 inhibitor (eg, ketoconazole, itraconazole, indinavir, ritonavir, nefazodone): Immediate release or extended release: Decrease quetiapine to one-sixth of the original dose; when strong CYP3A4 inhibitor is discontinued, increase quetiapine by sixfold.

Concomitant use with a strong CYP3A4 inducer (eg, phenytoin, carbamazepine, rifampin, St John's wort): Immediate release or extended release: Increase quetiapine up to fivefold of the original dose when combined with chronic treatment (>7-14 days) of a strong CYP3A4 inducer; titrate based on clinical response and tolerance; when the strong CYP3A4 inducer is discontinued, decrease quetiapine to the original dose within 7-14 days.

Dosage adjustment in renal impairment: No dosage adjustment necessary.

Dosage adjustment in hepatic impairment:

Immediate release tablet: Initial: 25 mg daily, increase dose by 25-50 mg daily to effective dose, based on individual clinical response and tolerability

Extended release tablet: Initial: 50 mg once daily; increase dose by 50 mg once daily to effective dose, based on individual clinical response and tolerability

Dietary Considerations Immediate-release tablet may be taken without regard to meals. Extended release tablet should be taken without food or with a light meal (≤300 calories).

Administration

Oral:

Immediate release tablet: May be administered with or without food.

Extended release tablet: Administer without food or with a light meal (≤300 calories), preferably in the evening. Swallow tablet whole; do not break, crush, or chew.

Nasogastric/enteral tube (unlabeled route): Hold tube feeds for 30 minutes before administration; flush with 25 mL of sterile water. Crush dose using immediate-release formulation, mix in 10 mL water and administer via NG/enteral tube; follow with a 50 mL flush of sterile water (Devlin, 2010).

Monitoring Parameters Vital signs including baseline and periodic blood pressure monitoring during therapy, particularly in children and adolescents; fasting lipid profile and fasting blood glucose/Hgb A_{1c} (prior to treatment, at 3 months, then annually); CBC frequently during first few months of therapy in patients with pre-existing low WBC or a history of drug-induced leukopenia/neutropenia; TSH and free T_4 (baseline and follow-up); BMI, personal/family history of obesity, waist circumference; mental status, abnormal involuntary movement scale (AIMS). Weight should be assessed prior to treatment, at 4 weeks, 8 weeks, 12 weeks, and then at quarterly intervals. Consider titrating to a different antipsychotic agent for a weight gain ≥5% of the initial weight. Patients should have eyes checked for cataracts every 6 months while on this medication. Observe for new or worsening depression, anxiety, irritability, aggression, or other symptoms of unusual behavior, mood, or suicide ideation (especially at the beginning of therapy or when doses are increased or decreased).

Test Interactions May interfere with urine detection of methadone (false-positives); may cause false-positive serum TCA screen

Dosage Forms Excipient information presented when available (limited, particularly for generics); consult specific product labeling.

Tablet, Oral:

SEROquel: 25 mg, 50 mg, 100 mg, 200 mg, 300 mg, 400 mg

Generic: 25 mg, 50 mg, 100 mg, 200 mg, 300 mg, 400 mg

Tablet Extended Release 24 Hour, Oral:

SEROquel XR: 50 mg, 150 mg, 200 mg, 300 mg, 400 mg

Dosage Forms: Canada Excipient information presented when available (limited, particularly for generics); consult specific product labeling.

Tablet:

Seroquel: 25 mg, 50 mg, 100 mg, 200 mg, 300 mg, 400 mg

Tablet, extended release:

Seroquel XR: 50 mg, 150 mg, 200 mg, 300 mg, 400 mg

◆ **Quetiapine Fumarate** *see* QUEtiapine *on page 1757*

◆ **Quillivant XR** *see* Methylphenidate *on page 1336*

◆ **Quinalbarbitone Sodium** *see* Secobarbital *on page 1884*

Quinapril (KWIN a pril)

Brand Names: U.S. Accupril

Brand Names: Canada Accupril; Apo-Quinapril

Index Terms Quinapril Hydrochloride

Pharmacologic Category Angiotensin-Converting Enzyme (ACE) Inhibitor; Antihypertensive

Additional Appendix Information

Angiotensin Agents *on page 2280*

Use

Hypertension: Treatment of hypertension

Heart failure: Adjunctive treatment of heart failure

Unlabeled Use Treatment of left ventricular dysfunction after myocardial infarction; pediatric hypertension; to delay the progression of nephropathy and reduce risks of cardiovascular events in hypertensive patients with type 1 or 2 diabetes mellitus

Pregnancy Risk Factor D

Pregnancy Considerations [U.S. Boxed Warning]: Drugs that act on the renin-angiotensin system can cause injury and death to the developing fetus. Discontinue as soon as possible once pregnancy is detected. Quinapril crosses the placenta; teratogenic effects may occur following maternal use during pregnancy. Drugs that act on the renin-angiotensin system are associated with oligohydramnios. Oligohydramnios, due to decreased fetal renal function, may lead to fetal lung hypoplasia and skeletal malformations. Their use in pregnancy is also associated with anuria, hypotension, renal failure, skull hypoplasia, and death in the fetus/neonate. Chronic maternal hypertension itself is also associated with adverse events in the fetus/infant. ACE inhibitors are not recommended during pregnancy to treat maternal hypertension or heart failure. Use of an ACE inhibitor should also be avoided in any woman of reproductive age. Women who are planning a pregnancy should be considered for other medication options if an ACE inhibitor is currently prescribed or the ACE inhibitor should be discontinued as soon as possible once pregnancy is detected. The exposed fetus should be monitored for fetal growth, amniotic fluid volume, and organ formation. Infants exposed to an ACE inhibitor *in utero* should be monitored for hyperkalemia, hypotension, and oliguria.

Breast-Feeding Considerations Quinapril is excreted in breast milk. The manufacturer recommends that caution be exercised when administering quinapril to nursing women. The Canadian labeling contraindicates use in nursing women.

Contraindications

Hypersensitivity to quinapril or any component of the formulation; angioedema related to previous treatment with an ACE inhibitor; concomitant use with aliskiren in patients with diabetes mellitus.

Documentation of allergenic cross-reactivity for ACE inhibitors is limited. However, because of similarities in chemical structure and/or pharmacologic actions, the possibility of cross-sensitivity cannot be ruled out with certainty.

Canadian labeling: Additional contraindications (not in U.S. labeling): Women who are pregnant, intend to become pregnant, or of childbearing potential and not using adequate contraception; breast-feeding; concomitant use with aliskiren in patients with moderate-to-severe renal impairment (GFR <60 mL/minute/1.73 m^2)

Warnings/Precautions Anaphylactic reactions may occur rarely with ACE inhibitors. At any time during treatment (especially following first dose) angioedema may occur rarely with ACE inhibitors; it may involve the head and neck (potentially compromising airway) or the intestine (presenting with abdominal pain). African-Americans and patients with idiopathic or hereditary angioedema may be at an increased risk. Prolonged frequent monitoring may be required especially if tongue, glottis, or larynx are involved as they are associated with airway obstruction. Patients with a history of airway surgery may have a higher risk of airway obstruction. Aggressive early and appropriate management is critical. Use in patients with previous angioedema associated with ACE inhibitor therapy is contraindicated. Severe anaphylactoid reactions may be seen during hemodialysis (eg, CVVHD) with high-flux dialysis membranes (eg, AN69), and rarely, during low density lipoprotein apheresis with dextran sulfate cellulose. Rare cases of anaphylactoid reactions have been reported in patients undergoing sensitization treatment with hymenoptera (bee, wasp) venom while receiving ACE inhibitors. Formulation may contain lactose.

Symptomatic hypotension with or without syncope can occur with ACE inhibitors (usually with the first several doses); effects are most often observed in volume-depleted patients; close monitoring of patient is required especially with initial dosing and dosing increases; blood pressure must be lowered at a rate appropriate for the patient's clinical condition. Initiation of therapy in patients with ischemic heart disease or cerebrovascular disease warrants close observation due to the potential consequences posed by falling blood pressure (eg, MI, stroke). Use with caution in hypertrophic cardiomyopathy with outflow tract obstruction, severe aortic stenosis, or before, during, or immediately after major surgery. **[U.S. Boxed Warning]: Drugs that act on the renin-angiotensin system can cause injury and death to the developing fetus. Discontinue as soon as possible once pregnancy is detected.**

Hyperkalemia may occur with ACE inhibitors; risk factors include renal dysfunction, diabetes mellitus, concomitant use of potassium-sparing diuretics, potassium supplements, and/or potassium-containing salts. Use cautiously, if at all, with these agents and monitor potassium closely. Cough may occur with ACE inhibitors. Other causes of cough should be considered (eg, pulmonary congestion in patients with heart failure) and excluded prior to discontinuation.

May be associated with deterioration of renal function and/or increases in serum creatinine, particularly in patients with low renal blood flow (eg, renal artery stenosis, heart failure) whose glomerular filtration rate (GFR) is dependent on efferent arteriolar vasoconstriction by angiotensin II; deterioration may result in oliguria, acute renal failure, and progressive azotemia. Small increases in serum creatinine may occur following initiation; consider discontinuation only in patients with progressive and/or significant deterioration in renal function. Use with caution in patients with unstented unilateral/bilateral renal artery stenosis. When unstented bilateral renal artery stenosis is present, use is generally avoided due to the elevated risk of deterioration in renal function unless possible benefits outweigh risks. Potentially significant drug-drug interactions may exist, requiring dose or frequency adjustment, additional monitoring, and/or selection of alternative therapy.

Rare toxicities associated with ACE inhibitors include cholestatic jaundice (which may progress to fulminant hepatic necrosis), agranulocytosis, neutropenia, or leukopenia with myeloid hypoplasia. Patients with collagen vascular diseases (especially with concomitant renal impairment) or renal impairment alone may be at increased risk for hematologic toxicity; periodically monitor CBC with differential in these patients.

Adverse Reactions Note: Frequency ranges include data from hypertension and heart failure trials. Higher rates of adverse reactions have generally been noted in patients with CHF. However, the frequency of adverse effects associated with placebo is also increased in this population.

1% to 10%:

- Cardiovascular: Hypotension (3%), chest pain (2%), first-dose hypotension (up to 3%)
- Central nervous system: Dizziness (4% to 8%), headache (2% to 6%), fatigue (3%)
- Dermatologic: Rash (1%)
- Endocrine & metabolic: Hyperkalemia (2%)
- Gastrointestinal: Vomiting/nausea (1% to 2%), diarrhea (1.7%)
- Neuromuscular & skeletal: Myalgias (2% to 5%), back pain (1%)
- Renal: BUN/serum creatinine increased (2%, transient elevations may occur with a higher frequency), worsening of renal function (in patients with bilateral renal artery stenosis or hypovolemia)
- Respiratory: Upper respiratory symptoms, cough (2% to 4%; up to 13% in some studies), dyspnea (2%)

<1% (Limited to important or life-threatening): Acute renal failure, agranulocytosis, alopecia, amblyopia, anaphylactoid reaction, angina, angioedema, arrhythmia, cerebrovascular accident, depression, dermatopolymyositis, eosinophilic pneumonitis, exfoliative dermatitis, gastrointestinal hemorrhage, heart failure, hemolytic anemia, hepatitis, hyperkalemia, hypertensive crisis, impotence, insomnia, MI, orthostatic hypotension, pancreatitis, pemphigus, photosensitivity, shock, stroke, syncope, thrombocytopenia, viral infection, visual hallucinations (Doane, 2013)

A syndrome which may include fever, myalgia, arthralgia, interstitial nephritis, vasculitis, rash, eosinophilia and positive ANA, and elevated ESR has been reported with ACE inhibitors. In addition, pancreatitis, hepatic necrosis, neutropenia, and/or agranulocytosis (particularly in patients with collagen-vascular disease or renal impairment) have been associated with many ACE inhibitors.

Drug Interactions

Metabolism/Transport Effects None known.

Avoid Concomitant Use There are no known interactions where it is recommended to avoid concomitant use.

Increased Effect/Toxicity

Quinapril may increase the levels/effects of: Allopurinol; Amifostine; Antihypertensives; AzaTHIOprine; CycloSPORINE (Systemic); Ferric Gluconate; Gold Sodium Thiomalate; Hypotensive Agents; Iron Dextran Complex; Lithium; Nonsteroidal Anti-Inflammatory Agents; Obinutuzumab; RiTUXimab; Sodium Phosphates

The levels/effects of Quinapril may be increased by: Alfuzosin; Aliskiren; Angiotensin II Receptor Blockers; Brimonidine (Topical); Canagliflozin; Diazoxide; DPP-IV Inhibitors; Eplerenone; Everolimus; Heparin; Heparin (Low Molecular Weight); Herbs (Hypotensive Properties); Loop Diuretics; MAO Inhibitors; Pentoxifylline; Phosphodiesterase 5 Inhibitors; Potassium Salts; Potassium-Sparing Diuretics; Prostacyclin Analogues; Sirolimus; Temsirolimus; Thiazide Diuretics; TiZANidine; Tolvaptan; Trimethoprim

Decreased Effect

Quinapril may decrease the levels/effects of: Quinolone Antibiotics; Tetracycline Derivatives

The levels/effects of Quinapril may be decreased by: Antacids; Aprotinin; Herbs (Hypertensive Properties); Icatibant; Lanthanum; Methylphenidate; Nonsteroidal Anti-Inflammatory Agents; Salicylates; Yohimbine

Ethanol/Nutrition/Herb Interactions

Food: Potassium supplements and/or potassium-containing salts may cause or worsen hyperkalemia. Management: Consult prescriber before consuming a potassium-rich diet, potassium supplements, or salt substitutes.

Herb/Nutraceutical: Some herbal medications may worsen hypertension (eg, licorice); others may increase the antihypertensive effects of quinapril (eg, shepherd's purse). Management: Avoid bayberry, blue cohosh, cayenne, ephedra, ginger, ginseng (American), kola, licorice, and yohimbe. Avoid black cohosh, California poppy, coleus, golden seal, hawthorn, mistletoe, periwinkle, quinine, and shepherd's purse.

Storage/Stability Store at 15°C to 30°C (59°F to 86°F). Protect from light.

Mechanism of Action Competitive inhibitor of angiotensin-converting enzyme (ACE); prevents conversion of angiotensin I to angiotensin II, a potent vasoconstrictor; results in lower levels of angiotensin II which causes an increase in plasma renin activity and a reduction in aldosterone secretion; a CNS mechanism may also be involved in hypotensive effect as angiotensin II increases adrenergic outflow from CNS; vasoactive kallikreins may be decreased in conversion to active hormones by ACE inhibitors, thus reducing blood pressure

Pharmacodynamics/Kinetics

Onset of action: 1 hour

Duration: 24 hours

Absorption: Quinapril: ≥60%

Protein binding: Quinapril: 97%; Quinaprilat: 97%

Metabolism: Rapidly hydrolyzed to quinaprilat, the active metabolite

Half-life elimination: Quinapril: 0.8 hours; Quinaprilat: 3 hours; increases as Cl_{cr} decreases

Time to peak, serum: Quinapril: 1 hour; Quinaprilat: ~2 hours

Excretion: Urine (50% to 60% primarily as quinaprilat)

Dosage

Children and Adolescents (unlabeled use): Hypertension: Oral: Initial 5-10 mg once daily; maximum: 80 mg daily (National High Blood Pressure Education Program Working Group on High Blood Pressure in Children and Adolescents, 2004)

Adults:

Heart failure: Oral: Initial: 5 mg twice daily (monitor for hypotension/orthostasis for at least 2 hours after initial dose; if present, monitor until blood pressure stabilizes); as tolerated, titrate at weekly intervals to 20-40 mg daily in 2 divided doses; target dose (heart failure): 20 mg twice daily (Yancy, 2013)

Canadian labeling: Oral: Initial: 5 mg once daily; as tolerated, may double daily dose (eg, 10 mg once daily) at weekly intervals to a maximum of 40 mg daily given in 2 divided doses.

Hypertension: Oral: Initial: 10-20 mg once daily in patients not on diuretics, adjust according to blood pressure response at peak (2-6 hours post-dose) and trough blood levels; initial dose may be reduced to 5 mg in patients receiving diuretics if the diuretic is continued. Usual dose range: 10-80 mg once daily (Chobanian, 2003). **Note:** The Canadian labeling recommends a maximum dose of 40 mg daily.

Elderly:

Heart failure: Refer to adult dosing.

Hypertension: Oral: Initial: 10 mg once daily; titrate to optimal response.

Dosage adjustment in renal impairment: Lower initial doses should be used; after initial dose (if tolerated), administer initial dose twice daily; may be increased at weekly intervals to optimal response:

Heart failure: Initial:

Cl_{cr} >30 mL/minute: Administer 5 mg daily

Cl_{cr} 10-30 mL/minute: Administer 2.5 mg daily

Cl_{cr} <10 mL/minute: No dosage adjustment provided in manufacturer's labeling.

Hypertension: Initial:

Cl_{cr} >60 mL/minute: Administer 10 mg daily

Cl_{cr} 30-60 mL/minute: Administer 5 mg daily

Cl_{cr} 10-30 mL/minute: Administer 2.5 mg daily

Cl_{cr} <10 mL/minute: No dosage adjustment provided in manufacturer's labeling.

Dosage adjustment in hepatic impairment: No dosage adjustment provided in manufacturer's labeling (has not been studied).

Administration Administer without regard to meals.

Monitoring Parameters Blood pressure; serum creatinine and potassium; if patient has collagen vascular disease and/or renal impairment, periodically monitor CBC with differential

Dosage Forms Excipient information presented when available (limited, particularly for generics); consult specific product labeling.

Tablet, Oral:

Accupril: 5 mg [scored; contains magnesium carbonate]

Accupril: 10 mg, 20 mg, 40 mg [contains magnesium carbonate]

Generic: 5 mg, 10 mg, 20 mg, 40 mg

Extemporaneous Preparations A 1 mg/mL quinapril oral suspension may be made with tablets, K-Phos® Neutral (equivalent to 250 mg elemental phosphorus, 13 mEq sodium, and 1.1 mEq potassium per tablet), Bicitra®, and Ora-Sweet SF™. Place ten quinapril 20 mg tablets in an amber plastic prescription bottle (eg, 240 mL). In a separate container, prepare a buffer solution by crushing one K-Phos® Neutral tablet and dissolving it in 100 mL sterile water for irrigation. Add 30 mL of the prepared K-Phos® buffer solution to the quinapril tablets. Shake for at least 2 minutes, then remove cap and allow the concentrate to stand for 15 minutes, then shake the concentrate again for an additional minute. Add 30 mL of Bicitra® and shake for 2 minutes. Add quantity sufficient of Ora-Sweet SF® (~140 mL) to make 200 mL and shake the suspension. Store in amber plastic prescription bottles; label "shake well" and "refrigerate." Stable for 28 days refrigerated (Freed, 2005).

Freed A, Silbering SB, Kolodsick KJ, et al, "The Development and Stability Assessment of Extemporaneous Pediatric Formulations of Accupril," *Int J Pharm*, 2005, 304(1-2):135-44.

◆ **Quinapril Hydrochloride** *see* Quinapril *on page 1761*
◆ **Quinate® (Can)** *see* QuiNIDine *on page 1764*

QuiNIDine (KWIN i deen)

Brand Names: Canada Apo-Quinidine®; BioQuin® Durules™; Novo-Quinidin; Quinate®

Index Terms Quinidine Gluconate; Quinidine Polygalacturonate; Quinidine Sulfate

Pharmacologic Category Antiarrhythmic Agent, Class Ia; Antimalarial Agent

Additional Appendix Information

Beers Criteria – Potentially Inappropriate Medications for Geriatrics *on page 2368*

Use

Quinidine gluconate and sulfate salts: Conversion and prevention of relapse into atrial fibrillation and/or flutter; suppression of ventricular arrhythmias. **Note:** Due to proarrhythmic effects, use should be reserved for life-threatening arrhythmias. Moreover, the use of quinidine has largely been replaced by more effective/safer antiarrhythmic agents and/or nonpharmacologic therapies (eg, radiofrequency ablation).

Quinidine gluconate (I.V. formulation): Conversion of atrial fibrillation/flutter and ventricular tachycardia. **Note:** The use of I.V. quinidine gluconate for these indications has been replaced by more effective/safer antiarrhythmic agents (eg, amiodarone and procainamide).

Quinidine gluconate (I.V. formulation) and quinidine sulfate: Treatment of malaria (*Plasmodium falciparum*)

Unlabeled Use Paroxysmal supraventricular tachycardia, paroxysmal AV junctional rhythm, and symptomatic atrial or ventricular premature contractions; short QT syndrome; Brugada syndrome

Pregnancy Risk Factor C

Pregnancy Considerations Animal reproduction studies have not been conducted. Quinidine crosses the placenta and can be detected in the amniotic fluid, cord blood, and neonatal serum. Quinidine is indicated for use in the treatment of severe malaria infection in pregnant women (CDC, 2011; Smereck, 2011) and has also been used to treat arrhythmias in pregnancy when other agents are ineffective (European Society of Cardiology, 2003).

Breast-Feeding Considerations Quinidine can be detected in breast milk at concentrations slightly lower than those in the maternal serum. The manufacturer recommends avoiding use in nursing women.

Contraindications Hypersensitivity to quinidine or any component of the formulation; thrombocytopenia; thrombocytopenic purpura; myasthenia gravis; heart block greater than first degree; idioventricular conduction delays (except in patients with a functioning artificial pacemaker); those adversely affected by anticholinergic activity; concurrent use of quinolone antibiotics which prolong QT interval, cisapride, amprenavir, or ritonavir

Warnings/Precautions Watch for proarrhythmic effects; may cause QT prolongation and subsequent torsade de pointes. Monitor and adjust dose to prevent QT_c prolongation. Avoid use in patients with diagnosed or suspected congenital long QT syndrome. Correct hypokalemia before initiating therapy. Hypokalemia may worsen toxicity. **[U.S. Boxed Warning]: Antiarrhythmic drugs have not been shown to enhance survival in non-life-threatening ventricular arrhythmias and may increase mortality; the risk is greatest with structural heart disease. Quinidine may increase mortality in treatment of atrial fibrillation/flutter.** May precipitate or exacerbate HF. Reduce dosage in hepatic impairment. Use may cause digoxin-induced toxicity (adjust digoxin's dose). Use caution with concurrent use of other antiarrhythmics. Hypersensitivity reactions can occur. Can unmask sick sinus syndrome (causes bradycardia); use with caution in patients with heart block. In the treatment of atrial fibrillation in the elderly, avoid antiarrhythmics as first-line treatment. In older adults, data suggests rate control may provide more benefits than risks compared to rhythm control for most patients (Beers Criteria).

Has been associated with severe hepatotoxic reactions, including granulomatous hepatitis. Hemolysis may occur in patients with G6PD (glucose-6-phosphate dehydrogenase) deficiency. Different salt products are not interchangeable.

Adverse Reactions

Frequency not defined: Hypotension, syncope

>10%:

- Cardiovascular: QT_c prolongation (modest prolongation is common, however, excessive prolongation is rare and indicates toxicity)
- Central nervous system: Lightheadedness (15%)
- Gastrointestinal: Diarrhea (35%), upper GI distress, bitter taste, diarrhea, anorexia, nausea, vomiting, stomach cramping (22%)

1% to 10%:

- Cardiovascular: Angina (6%), palpitation (7%), new or worsened arrhythmia (proarrhythmic effect)
- Central nervous system: Syncope (1% to 8%), headache (7%), fatigue (7%), sleep disturbance (3%), tremor (2%), nervousness (2%), incoordination (1%)
- Dermatologic: Rash (5%)
- Neuromuscular & skeletal: Weakness (5%)
- Ocular: Blurred vision
- Otic: Tinnitus
- Respiratory: Wheezing

<1% (Limited to important or life-threatening): Abnormal pigmentation, acute psychotic reactions, agranulocytosis, angioedema, arthralgia, bronchospasm, cerebral hypoperfusion (possibly resulting in ataxia, apprehension, and seizure), cholestasis, confusion, delirium, depression, drug-induced lupus-like syndrome, eczematous dermatitis, esophagitis, exacerbated bradycardia (in sick sinus syndrome), exfoliative rash, fever, flushing, granulomatous hepatitis, hallucinations, heart block, hemolytic anemia, hepatotoxic reaction (rare), hearing impaired, CPK increased, lichen planus, livedo reticularis, lymphadenopathy, melanin pigmentation of the hard palate, myalgia, mydriasis, nephropathy, optic neuritis, pancytopenia, paradoxical increase in ventricular rate during atrial fibrillation/flutter, photosensitivity, pneumonitis, pruritus, psoriaform rash, QT_c prolongation (excessive), respiratory depression, sicca syndrome, tachycardia, thrombocytopenia, thrombocytopenic purpura, torsade de pointes, urticaria, uveitis, vascular collapse, vasculitis, ventricular fibrillation, ventricular tachycardia, vertigo, visual field loss

Note: Cinchonism, a syndrome which may include tinnitus, high-frequency hearing loss, deafness, vertigo, blurred vision, diplopia, photophobia, headache, confusion, and delirium has been associated with quinidine use. Usually associated with chronic toxicity, this syndrome has also been described after brief exposure to a moderate dose in sensitive patients. Vomiting and diarrhea may also occur as isolated reactions to therapeutic quinidine levels.

Drug Interactions

Metabolism/Transport Effects Substrate of CYP2C9 (minor), CYP2E1 (minor), CYP3A4 (major), P-glycoprotein; **Note:** Assignment of Major/Minor substrate status based on clinically relevant drug interaction potential; **Inhibits** CYP2C9 (weak), CYP2D6 (strong), CYP3A4 (weak), P-glycoprotein

Avoid Concomitant Use

Avoid concomitant use of QuiNIDine with any of the following: Amiodarone; Antifungal Agents (Azole Derivatives, Systemic); Bosutinib; Conivaptan; Crizotinib; Enzalutamide; Fingolimod; Fusidic Acid (Systemic); Haloperidol; Highest Risk QTc-Prolonging Agents; Ivabradine; Macrolide Antibiotics; Mefloquine; Mifepristone; Moderate Risk QTc-Prolonging Agents; Pimozide; Pomalidomide; Propafenone; Protease Inhibitors; Silodosin; Tamoxifen; Thioridazine; Topotecan; VinCRIStine (Liposomal)

Increased Effect/Toxicity

QuiNIDine may increase the levels/effects of: Afatinib; ARIPiprazole; AtoMOXetine; Bosutinib; Calcium Channel Blockers (Dihydropyridine); Cardiac Glycosides; Colchicine; CYP2D6 Substrates; Dabigatran Etexilate; Dalfampridine; Dextromethorphan; Everolimus; Fesoterodine; Haloperidol; Highest Risk QTc-Prolonging Agents; Iloperidone; Lomitapide; Mefloquine; Metoprolol; Nebivolol; Neuromuscular-Blocking Agents; P-glycoprotein/ABCB1 Substrates; Pimozide; Pomalidomide; Propafenone; Propranolol; Prucalopride; Rivaroxaban; Silodosin; Tetrabenazine; Thioridazine; Topotecan; Tricyclic Antidepressants; Verapamil; VinCRIStine (Liposomal); Vitamin K Antagonists; Vortioxetine

The levels/effects of QuiNIDine may be increased by: Amiodarone; Antacids; Antifungal Agents (Azole Derivatives, Systemic); Boceprevir; Calcium Channel Blockers (Dihydropyridine); Carbonic Anhydrase Inhibitors; Cimetidine; Conivaptan; Crizotinib; CYP3A4 Inhibitors (Moderate); CYP3A4 Inhibitors (Strong); Dasatinib; Diltiazem; Fingolimod; Fosphenytoin; Fusidic Acid (Systemic); Haloperidol; Ivabradine; Ivacaftor; Luliconazole; Lurasidone; Macrolide Antibiotics; Mifepristone; Moderate Risk QTc-Prolonging Agents; P-glycoprotein/ABCB1 Inhibitors; PHENobarbital; Protease Inhibitors; QTc-Prolonging Agents (Indeterminate Risk and Risk Modifying); Reserpine; Selective Serotonin Reuptake Inhibitors; Simeprevir; Telaprevir; Tricyclic Antidepressants; Verapamil

Decreased Effect

QuiNIDine may decrease the levels/effects of: Codeine; Dihydrocodeine; Hydrocodone; Iloperidone; Tamoxifen; TraMADol

The levels/effects of QuiNIDine may be decreased by: Bosentan; Calcium Channel Blockers (Dihydropyridine); CYP3A4 Inducers (Strong); Dabrafenib; Deferasirox; Enzalutamide; Etravirine; Fosphenytoin; Herbs (CYP3A4 Inducers); Kaolin; Mitotane; P-glycoprotein/ABCB1 Inducers; PHENobarbital; Phenytoin; Potassium-Sparing Diuretics; Primidone; Rifamycin Derivatives; Sucralfate; Tocilizumab

Ethanol/Nutrition/Herb Interactions

Food: Changes in dietary salt intake may alter the rate and extent of quinidine absorption. Quinidine serum levels may be increased if taken with food. Food has a variable effect on absorption of sustained release formulation. The rate of absorption of quinidine may be decreased following the ingestion of grapefruit juice. Excessive intake of fruit juice or vitamin C may decrease urine pH and result in increased clearance of quinidine with decreased serum concentration. Alkaline foods may result in increased quinidine serum concentrations. Management: Avoid changes in dietary salt intake. Grapefruit juice should be avoided. Take around-the-clock to avoid variation in serum levels and with food or milk to avoid GI irritation.

Herb/Nutraceutical: St John's wort may decrease quinidine levels. Ephedra may worsen arrhythmia. Management: Avoid St John's wort and ephedra.

Storage/Stability

Solution for injection: Store at room temperature of 25°C (77°F).

Tablets: Store at controlled room temperature of 20°C to 25°C (68°F to 77°F). Protect from light.

Mechanism of Action Class Ia antiarrhythmic agent; depresses phase O of the action potential; decreases myocardial excitability and conduction velocity, and myocardial contractility by decreasing sodium influx during depolarization and potassium efflux in repolarization; also reduces calcium transport across cell membrane

Pharmacodynamics/Kinetics

Distribution: V_d: Adults: 2-3 L/kg, decreased with congestive heart failure (0.5 L/kg), malaria; increased with cirrhosis

Protein binding: Newborns: 50% to 70%; Adults: 80% to 88%

Binds mainly to alpha$_1$-acid glycoprotein and to a lesser extent albumin; protein-binding changes may occur in periods of stress due to increased alpha$_1$-acid glycoprotein concentrations (eg, acute myocardial infarction) or in certain disease states due to decreased alpha$_1$-acid glycoprotein concentrations (eg, cirrhosis,hyperthyroidism, malnutrition)

Metabolism: Extensively hepatic (50% to 90%) to inactive compounds

Bioavailability: Sulfate: ~70% with wide variability between patients (45% to 100%); Gluconate: 70% to 80%

Half-life elimination, plasma: Children: 3-4 hours; Adults: 6-8 hours; prolonged with elderly, cirrhosis, and congestive heart failure

Time to peak, serum: Sulfate: 2 hours; Gluconate: 3-6 hours

Excretion: Urine (15% to 25% as unchanged drug)

Dosage Note: Dosage expressed in terms of the salt: 267 mg of quinidine gluconate = 200 mg of quinidine sulfate.

Antiarrhythmic: Adults: Oral:

Immediate release formulations: Quinidine sulfate: Initial: 200-400 mg/dose every 6 hours the dose may be increased cautiously to desired effect

Extended release formulations:

Quinidine sulfate: Initial: 300 mg every 8-12 hours; the dose may be increased cautiously to desired effect

Quinidine gluconate: Initial: 324 mg every 8-12 hours; the dose may be increased cautiously to desired effect

Severe malaria, treatment: Children and Adults: I.V. (quinidine gluconate): 10 mg/kg infused over 60-120 minutes followed by 0.02 mg/kg/minute continuous infusion for ≥24 hours; alternatively, may administer 24 mg/kg loading dose over 4 hours, followed by 12 mg/kg over 4 hours every 8 hours (beginning 8 hours after initiation of the loading dose); complete treatment with oral quinine once parasite density <1% and patient can receive oral medication; total duration of treatment (quinidine/quinine): 3 days (Africa or South America) or 7 days (Southeast Asia); use in combination with doxycycline, tetracycline or clindamycin (CDC malaria guidelines, 2009). **Note:** Close monitoring, including telemetry, required.

Dosing adjustment in renal impairment: No dosage adjustment provided in manufacturer's labeling. Use with caution. The following guidelines have been used by some clinicians (Aronoff, 2007): Oral:

Cl_{cr} ≥10 mL/minute: No dosage adjustment necessary.

Cl_{cr} <10 mL/minute: Administer 75% of normal dose.

Hemodialysis: Dose following hemodialysis

Peritoneal dialysis: Supplemental dose is not necessary

CRRT: No dosage adjustment required; monitor serum concentrations

Dosing adjustment/comments in hepatic impairment: No dosage adjustment provided in manufacturer's labeling. Use with caution due to reduced clearance.

Dietary Considerations Administer with food or milk to decrease gastrointestinal irritation. Avoid changes in dietary salt intake.

Usual Infusion Concentrations: Adult I.V. infusion: Quinidine gluconate: 800 mg in 50 mL (concentration: 16 mg/mL) of D_5W

Administration Administer around-the-clock to promote less variation in peak and trough serum levels

Oral: Do not crush, chew, or break sustained release dosage forms. Some preparations of quinidine gluconate extended release tablets may be split in half to facilitate dosage titration; tablets are not scored.

Parenteral: Minimize use of PVC tubing to enhance bioavailability; shorter tubing lengths are recommended by the manufacturer

Monitoring Parameters Cardiac monitor required during I.V. administration; CBC, liver and renal function tests, should be routinely performed during long-term administration

Consult individual institutional policies and procedures.

Reference Range Therapeutic: 2-5 mcg/mL (SI: 6.2-15.4 micromole/L). Patient-dependent therapeutic response occurs at levels of 3-6 mcg/mL (SI: 9.2-18.5 micromole/L). Optimal therapeutic level is method dependent; >6 mcg/mL (SI: >18 micromole/L).

Dosage Forms Excipient information presented when available (limited, particularly for generics); consult specific product labeling.

Solution, Injection, as gluconate:
Generic: 80 mg/mL (10 mL)

Tablet, Oral, as sulfate:
Generic: 200 mg, 300 mg

Tablet Extended Release, Oral, as gluconate:
Generic: 324 mg

Tablet Extended Release, Oral, as sulfate:
Generic: 300 mg

Extemporaneous Preparations A 10 mg/mL oral liquid preparation may be made with tablets and one of three different vehicles (cherry syrup, a 1:1 mixture of Ora-Sweet® and Ora-Plus®, or a 1:1 mixture of Ora-Sweet® SF and Ora-Plus®). Crush six 200 mg tablets in a mortar and reduce to a fine powder. Add 15 mL of the chosen vehicle and mix to a uniform paste; mix while adding vehicle in incremental proportions to **almost** 120 mL; transfer to a calibrated bottle, rinse mortar with vehicle, and add quantity of vehicle sufficient to make 120 mL. Label "shake well" and "protect from light". Stable for 60 days when stored in amber plastic prescription bottles in the dark at room temperature or refrigerated.

Allen LV and Erickson MA, "Stability of Bethanechol Chloride, Pyrazinamide, Quinidine Sulfate, Rifampin, and Tetracycline in Extemporaneously Compounded Oral Liquids," *Am J Health Syst Pharm*, 1998, 55(17):1804-9.

◆ **Quinidine and Dextromethorphan** *see* Dextromethorphan and Quinidine *on page 592*

◆ **Quinidine Gluconate** *see* QuiNIDine *on page 1764*

◆ **Quinidine Polygalacturonate** *see* QuiNIDine *on page 1764*

◆ **Quinidine Sulfate** *see* QuiNIDine *on page 1764*

QuiNINE (KWYE nine)

Brand Names: U.S. Qualaquin

Brand Names: Canada Apo-Quinine®; Novo-Quinine; Quinine-Odan

Index Terms Quinine Sulfate

Pharmacologic Category Antimalarial Agent

Use In conjunction with other antimalarial agents, treatment of uncomplicated chloroquine-resistant *P. falciparum* malaria

Unlabeled Use Treatment of *Babesia microti* infection in conjunction with clindamycin; treatment of uncomplicated chloroquine-resistant *P. vivax* malaria (in conjunction with other antimalarial agents)

Pregnancy Risk Factor C

Pregnancy Considerations Teratogenic effects have been reported in some animal studies. Quinine crosses the human placenta. Cord plasma to maternal plasma quinine ratios have been reported as 0.18-0.46 and should not be considered therapeutic to the infant. Teratogenic effects, optic nerve hypoplasia, and deafness have been reported in the infant following maternal use of very high doses; however, therapeutic doses used for malaria are generally considered safe. Quinine may also cause significant hypoglycemia when used during pregnancy. Malaria infection in pregnant women may be more severe than in nonpregnant women. Because *P. falciparum* malaria can cause maternal death and fetal loss, pregnant women traveling to malaria-endemic areas must use personal protection against mosquito bites. Quinine may be used for the treatment of malaria in pregnant women; consult current CDC guidelines. Pregnant women should be advised not to travel to areas of *P. falciparum* resistance to chloroquine.

Breast-Feeding Considerations Based on limited data, it is estimated that nursing infants would receive <0.4% of the maternal dose from breast-feeding.

Medication Guide Available Yes

Contraindications Hypersensitivity to quinine or any component of the formulation; hypersensitivity to mefloquine or quinidine (cross sensitivity reported); history of potential hypersensitivity reactions (including black water fever, thrombotic thrombocytopenia purpura [TTP], hemolytic uremic syndrome [HUS], or thrombocytopenia) associated with prior quinine use; prolonged QT interval; myasthenia gravis; optic neuritis; G6PD deficiency

Warnings/Precautions [U.S. Boxed Warning]: Quinine is not recommended for the prevention/treatment of nocturnal leg cramps due to the potential for severe and/or life-threatening side effects (eg, cardiac arrhythmias, thrombocytopenia, HUS/TTP, severe hypersensitivity reactions). These risks, as well as the absence of clinical effectiveness, do not justify its use in the unapproved/unlabeled prevention and/or treatment of leg cramps.

Quinine may cause QT-interval prolongation, with maximum increase corresponding to maximum plasma concentration. Fatal torsade de pointes and ventricular fibrillation has been reported. Use contraindicated in patients with QT prolongation. Concurrent use of Class IA (eg, quinidine, procainamide) or Class III (eg, amiodarone, dofetilide, sotalol) antiarrhythmic agents or with other drugs known to prolong the QT interval is not recommended. Quinine may also cause concentration-dependent prolongation of the PR and QRS intervals. Risk of prolonged PR and/or QRS intervals is higher in patients with underlying structural heart disease, myocardial ischemia, pre-existing conduction system abnormalities, elderly patients with sick sinus syndrome, patients with atrial fibrillation with slow ventricular response and concomitant use of drugs known to prolong the PR interval (eg, verapamil) or QRS interval (eg, flecainide or quinidine). Use caution with clinical conditions which may further prolong the QT interval or cause cardiac arrhythmias. Use caution with atrial fibrillation or flutter (paradoxical increase in heart rate may occur), or renal impairment. Use with caution with mild-to-moderate hepatic impairment; avoid use with severe hepatic impairment. Potentially significant drug-drug interactions may exist, requiring dose or frequency adjustment, additional monitoring, and/or selection of alternative therapy.

Severe hypersensitivity reactions (eg, Stevens-Johnson syndrome, anaphylactic shock) have occurred; discontinue following any signs of sensitivity. Other events (including acute interstitial nephritis, neutropenia, and granulomatous hepatitis) may also be attributed to hypersensitivity reactions. Immune-mediated thrombocytopenia, including life-threatening cases and hemolytic uremic syndrome/thrombotic thrombocytopenic purpura (HUS/TTP), has occurred with use. Chronic renal failure associated with TTP has also been reported. Thrombocytopenia generally resolves within a week upon discontinuation. Re-exposure may result in increased severity of thrombocytopenia and faster onset.

Use may cause significant hypoglycemia due to quinine-induced insulin release. Use with caution in patients with hepatic impairment. Use with caution in patients with renal impairment; dosage adjustment recommended. Quinine should not be used for the prevention of malaria or in the treatment of complicated or severe *P. falciparum* malaria (oral antimalarial agents are not appropriate for initial therapy of severe malaria).

Adverse Reactions

Frequency not defined.

Cardiovascular: Atrial fibrillation, atrioventricular block, bradycardia, cardiac arrest, chest pain, hypotension, irregular rhythm, nodal escape beats, orthostatic hypotension, palpitation, QT prolongation, syncope, tachycardia, torsade de pointes, unifocal premature ventricular contractions, U waves, vasodilation, ventricular fibrillation, ventricular tachycardia

Central nervous system: Aphasia, ataxia, chills, coma, confusion, disorientation, dizziness, dystonic reaction, fever, flushing, headache, mental status altered, restlessness, seizure, suicide, vertigo

Dermatologic: Acral necrosis, allergic contact dermatitis, bullous dermatitis, bruising, cutaneous rash (urticaria, papular, scarlatinal), cutaneous vasculitis, exfoliative dermatitis, erythema multiforme, petechiae, photosensitivity, pruritus, Stevens-Johnson syndrome, toxic epidermal necrolysis

Endocrine & metabolic: Hypoglycemia

Gastrointestinal: Abdominal pain, anorexia, diarrhea, esophagitis, gastric irritation, nausea, vomiting

Hematologic: Agranulocytosis, aplastic anemia, coagulopathy, disseminated intravascular coagulation, hemolytic anemia, hemolytic uremic syndrome, hemorrhage, hypoprothrombinemia, immune thrombocytopenia (ITP), leukopenia, neutropenia, pancytopenia, thrombocytopenia, thrombotic thrombocytopenic purpura

Hepatic: Granulomatous hepatitis, hepatitis, jaundice, liver function test abnormalities

Neuromuscular & skeletal: Myalgia, tremor, weakness

Ocular: Blindness, blurred vision (with or without scotomata), color vision disturbance, diminished visual fields, diplopia, night blindness, optic neuritis, photophobia, pupillary dilation, vision loss (sudden)

Otic: Deafness, hearing impaired, tinnitus

Renal: Acute interstitial nephritis, hemoglobinuria, renal failure, renal impairment

Respiratory: Asthma, dyspnea, pulmonary edema

Miscellaneous: Black water fever, diaphoresis, hypersensitivity reaction, lupus anticoagulant, lupus-like syndrome

Drug Interactions

Metabolism/Transport Effects **Substrate** of CYP1A2 (minor), CYP2C19 (minor), CYP3A4 (major), P-glycoprotein; **Note:** Assignment of Major/Minor substrate status based on clinically relevant drug interaction potential; **Inhibits** CYP2C8 (moderate), CYP2C9 (moderate), CYP2D6 (moderate), CYP3A4 (weak), P-glycoprotein

Avoid Concomitant Use

Avoid concomitant use of QuiNINE with any of the following: Antacids; Artemether; Bosutinib; Conivaptan; Fusidic Acid (Systemic); Halofantrine; Highest Risk QTc-Prolonging Agents; Ivabradine; Lopinavir; Lumefantrine; Macrolide Antibiotics; Mefloquine; Mifepristone; Moderate Risk QTc-Prolonging Agents; Neuromuscular-Blocking Agents; Pomalidomide; Rifampin; Ritonavir; Silodosin; Thioridazine; Topotecan; VinCRIStine (Liposomal)

Increased Effect/Toxicity

QuiNINE may increase the levels/effects of: Afatinib; Antihypertensives; Antipsychotic Agents (Phenothiazines); ARIPiprazole; Bosentan; Bosutinib; CarBAMazepine; Cardiac Glycosides; Carvedilol; Colchicine; CYP2C8 Substrates; CYP2C9 Substrates; CYP2D6 Substrates; Dabigatran Etexilate; Dapsone (Systemic); Dapsone (Topical); Everolimus; Fesoterodine; Halofantrine; Herbs (Hypotensive Properties); Highest Risk QTc-Prolonging Agents; HMG-CoA Reductase Inhibitors; Lomitapide; Lumefantrine; Mefloquine; Metoprolol; Nebivolol; Neuromuscular-Blocking Agents; P-glycoprotein/ABCB1 Substrates; PHENobarbital; Pomalidomide; Prilocaine; Prucalopride; Ritonavir; Rivaroxaban; Silodosin; Sodium Nitrite; Theophylline Derivatives; Thioridazine; Topotecan; VinCRIStine (Liposomal); Vitamin K Antagonists

The levels/effects of QuiNINE may be increased by: Alkalinizing Agents; Artemether; Cimetidine; Conivaptan; CYP3A4 Inhibitors (Moderate); CYP3A4 Inhibitors (Strong); Dapsone (Systemic); Dasatinib; Fusidic Acid (Systemic); Ivabradine; Ivacaftor; Luliconazole; Macrolide Antibiotics; Mefloquine; Mifepristone; Moderate Risk QTc-Prolonging Agents; Nitric Oxide; P-glycoprotein/ABCB1 Inhibitors; QTc-Prolonging Agents (Indeterminate Risk and Risk Modifying); Ritonavir; Simeprevir; Tetracycline

Decreased Effect

QuiNINE may decrease the levels/effects of: Codeine; Tamoxifen; TraMADol

The levels/effects of QuiNINE may be decreased by: Antacids; Bosentan; CarBAMazepine; CYP3A4 Inducers (Strong); Dabrafenib; Deferasirox; Fosphenytoin; Herbs (CYP3A4 Inducers); Lopinavir; Mitotane; P-glycoprotein/ABCB1 Inducers; PHENobarbital; Phenytoin; Rifampin; Ritonavir; Tocilizumab

Ethanol/Nutrition/Herb Interactions Herb/Nutraceutical: St John's wort may decrease quinine levels. Black cohosh, California poppy, coleus, golden seal, hawthorn, mistletoe, periwinkle, and shepherd's purse may cause excessive decreases in blood pressure.

Storage/Stability Store at 20°C to 25°C (68°F to 77°F).

Mechanism of Action Depresses oxygen uptake and carbohydrate metabolism; intercalates into DNA, disrupting the parasite's replication and transcription; cardiovascular effects similar to quinidine

Pharmacodynamics/Kinetics

Absorption: Readily, mainly from upper small intestine

Distribution: Children: ~0.9 L/kg (subjects with malaria); Adults: 2.5-7.1 L/kg (varies with severity of infection)

Intraerythrocytic levels are ~30% to 50% of the plasma concentration; distributes poorly to the CSF (~2% to 7% of plasma concentration)

Protein binding: 69% to 92% in healthy subjects; 78% to 95% with malaria (due to increase in alpha$_1$-acid glycoprotein)

Metabolism: Hepatic via CYP450 enzymes, primarily CYP3A4; forms metabolites; major metabolite, 3-hydroxyquinine, is less active than parent

Bioavailability: 76% to 88% in healthy subjects; increased with malaria

Half-life elimination:
Children: ~3 hours in healthy subjects; ~12 hours with malaria
Healthy adults: 10-13 hours
Healthy elderly subjects: 18 hours
Time to peak, serum:
Children: 2 hours in healthy subjects; 4 hours with malaria
Adults: 2-4 hours in healthy subjects; 1-11 hours with malaria
Excretion: Urine (~20% as unchanged drug)

Dosage Note: Actual duration of quinine treatment for malaria may be dependent upon the geographic region or pathogen. Dosage expressed in terms of the salt; 1 capsule Qualaquin® = 324 mg of quinine sulfate = 269 mg of base.
Children: Oral:
Treatment of uncomplicated chloroquine-resistant *P. falciparum* malaria (CDC guidelines): 30 mg/kg/day in divided doses every 8 hours for 3-7 days. Tetracycline, doxycycline, or clindamycin (consider risk versus benefit of using tetracycline or doxycycline in children <8 years) should also be given.
Treatment of uncomplicated chloroquine-resistant *P. vivax* malaria (unlabeled use; CDC guidelines): 30 mg/kg/day in divided doses every 8 hours for 3-7 days. Tetracycline or doxycycline (consider risk versus benefit of using tetracycline or doxycycline in children <8 years) plus primaquine should also be given.
Adults: Oral:
Treatment of uncomplicated chloroquine-resistant *P. falciparum* malaria (CDC guidelines): 648 mg every 8 hours for 3-7 days. Tetracycline, doxycycline, or clindamycin should also be given.
Treatment of uncomplicated chloroquine-resistant *P. vivax* malaria (unlabeled use; CDC guidelines): 648 mg every 8 hours for 3-7 days. Tetracycline or doxycycline plus primaquine should also be given.
Babesiosis (unlabeled use): 650 mg every 6-8 hours for 7-10 days with clindamycin (Wormser, 2006; Vannier, 2012). **Note:** Relapsing infection may require at least 6 weeks of therapy (Vannier, 2012).

Dosing interval/adjustment in renal impairment:
Cl_{cr} 10-50 mL/minute: Administer every 8-12 hours
Cl_{cr} <10 mL/minute: Administer every 24 hours
Severe chronic renal failure not on dialysis: Initial dose: 648 mg followed by 324 mg every 12 hours
Dialysis: Administer dose after dialysis. **Note:** Clearance of ~6.5% achieved with 1 hour of hemodialysis.
Peritoneal dialysis: Dose as for Cl_{cr} <10 mL/minute
Continuous arteriovenous or hemodialysis: Dose as for Cl_{cr} 10-50 mL/minute

Dosing adjustment in hepatic impairment:
Mild-to-moderate impairment (Child-Pugh classes A and B): No dosing adjustment required; monitor closely.
Severe impairment (Child-Pugh class C): Avoid use.

Dietary Considerations Take with food to decrease incidence of gastric upset.

Administration Avoid use of aluminum- or magnesium-containing antacids because of drug absorption problems. Swallow dose whole to avoid bitter taste. May be administered with food.

Monitoring Parameters Monitor CBC with platelet count, liver function tests, blood glucose; ECG; ophthalmologic examination

Test Interactions May interfere with urine detection of opioids (false-positive); positive Coombs' [direct]; false elevation of urinary steroids (when assayed by Zimmerman method) and catecholamines; qualitative and quantitative urine dipstick protein assays

Dosage Forms Excipient information presented when available (limited, particularly for generics); consult specific product labeling.
Capsule, Oral, as sulfate:
Qualaquin: 324 mg
Generic: 324 mg

◆ **Quinine-Odan (Can)** *see* QuiNINE *on page 1766*
◆ **Quinine Sulfate** *see* QuiNINE *on page 1766*
◆ **Quinol** *see* Hydroquinone *on page 1017*

Quinupristin and Dalfopristin

(kwi NYOO pris tin & dal FOE pris tin)

Brand Names: U.S. Synercid®
Brand Names: Canada Synercid®
Index Terms Dalfopristin and Quinupristin; RP-59500
Pharmacologic Category Antibiotic, Streptogramin
Additional Appendix Information
Antibiotic Treatment of Adults With Infective Endocarditis *on page 2355*
Dosing Considerations for the Critically-Ill Patient With Morbid Obesity *on page 2379*

Use Treatment of complicated skin and skin structure infections caused by methicillin-susceptible *Staphylococcus aureus* or *Streptococcus pyogenes*

Unlabeled Use Treatment of persistent MRSA bacteremia associated with vancomycin failure

Pregnancy Risk Factor B

Pregnancy Considerations Because adverse effects were not observed in animal reproduction studies, quinupristin/dalfopristin is classified pregnancy category B. There are no adequate and well-controlled studies of quinupristin/dalfopristin in pregnant women.

Breast-Feeding Considerations It is not known if quinupristin/dalfopristin is excreted in human milk. The manufacturer recommends caution if administering quinupristin/dalfopristin to a nursing woman. The increased molecular weight of quinupristin/dalfopristin may minimize excretion into human milk. Nondose-related effects could include modification of bowel flora.

Contraindications Hypersensitivity to quinupristin, dalfopristin, pristinamycin, or virginiamycin, or any component of the formulation

Warnings/Precautions Use with caution in patients with hepatic or renal dysfunction. May cause pain and phlebitis when infused through a peripheral line (not relieved by hydrocortisone or diphenhydramine). Prolonged use may result in fungal or bacterial superinfection, including *C. difficile*-associated diarrhea (CDAD) and pseudomembranous colitis; CDAD has been observed >2 months post-antibiotic treatment. May cause arthralgias, myalgias, and hyperbilirubinemia. May inhibit the metabolism of many drugs metabolized by CYP3A4. Concurrent therapy with cisapride (which may prolong QT_c interval and lead to arrhythmias) should be avoided.

Adverse Reactions
>10%:
Hepatic: Hyperbilirubinemia (3% to 35%)
Local: Local pain (40% to 44%), inflammation at infusion site (38% to 42%), local edema (17% to 18%), infusion site reaction (12% to 13%)
Neuromuscular & skeletal: Arthralgia (up to 47%), myalgia (up to 47%)
1% to 10%:
Central nervous system: Pain (2% to 3%), headache (2%)
Dermatologic: Rash (3%), pruritus (2%)
Endocrine & metabolic: Hyperglycemia (1%)
Gastrointestinal: Nausea (3% to 5%), vomiting (3% to 4%), diarrhea (3%)
Hematologic: Anemia (3%)

Hepatic: GGT increased (2%), LDH increased (3%)
Local: Thrombophlebitis (2%)
Neuromuscular & skeletal: CPK increased (2%)

<1% (Limited to important or life-threatening): Allergic reaction, anaphylactoid reaction, angina, apnea, arrhythmia, cardiac arrest, coagulation disorder, dysautonomia, dyspnea, encephalopathy, gout, hematuria, hemolytic anemia, hepatitis, hyperkalemia, hypotension, maculopapular rash, mesenteric artery occlusion, myasthenia, neuropathy, pancreatitis, pancytopenia, paraplegia, paresthesia, pericarditis, pleural effusion, pseudomembranous colitis, respiratory distress, seizure, shock, stomatitis, syncope, thrombocytopenia, urticaria

Drug Interactions

Metabolism/Transport Effects Refer to individual components.

Avoid Concomitant Use

Avoid concomitant use of Quinupristin and Dalfopristin with any of the following: Pimozide

Increased Effect/Toxicity

Quinupristin and Dalfopristin may increase the levels/effects of: ARIPiprazole; CycloSPORINE (Systemic); Dofetilide; Lomitapide; Pimozide

Decreased Effect There are no known significant interactions involving a decrease in effect.

Preparation for Administration Reconstitute single dose vial with 5 mL of 5% dextrose in water or sterile water for injection. Swirl gentle to dissolve; do not shake (to limit foam formation). The reconstituted solution should be diluted within 30 minutes. Stability of the diluted solution prior to the infusion is established as 5 hours at room temperature or 54 hours if refrigerated at 2°C to 8°C (36°F to 46°F). Reconstituted solution should be added to at least 250 mL of 5% dextrose in water for peripheral administration (increase to 500 mL or 750 mL if necessary to limit venous irritation). An infusion volume of 100 mL may be used for central line infusions. Do not freeze solution.

Storage/Stability Store unopened vials under refrigeration at 2°C to 8°C (36°F to 46°F). The following stability information has also been reported: May be stored at room temperature for up to 7 days (Cohen, 2007).

Mechanism of Action Quinupristin/dalfopristin inhibits bacterial protein synthesis by binding to different sites on the 50S bacterial ribosomal subunit thereby inhibiting protein synthesis

Pharmacodynamics/Kinetics

Distribution: Quinupristin: 0.45 L/kg; Dalfopristin: 0.24 L/kg

Metabolism: To active metabolites via nonenzymatic reactions

Half-life elimination: Quinupristin: 0.85 hour; Dalfopristin: 0.7 hour (mean elimination half-lives, including metabolites: 3 and 1 hours, respectively)

Excretion: Feces (75% to 77% as unchanged drug and metabolites); urine (15% to 19%)

Dosage I.V.: Children ≥12 years and Adults:

Complicated skin and skin structure infection: 7.5 mg/kg every 12 hours for at least 7 days

Bacteremia, MRSA (persistent, vancomycin failure) (unlabeled use): 7.5 mg/kg every 8 hours (Liu, 2011)

Dosage adjustment in renal impairment: No dosage adjustment necessary.

Dosage adjustment in hepatic impairment: No dosage adjustment provided in manufacturer's labeling. However, pharmacokinetic data suggest dosage adjustment may be necessary.

Administration Line should be flushed with 5% dextrose in water prior to and following administration. Infusion should be completed over 60 minutes (toxicity may be increased with shorter infusion). If severe venous irritation occurs following peripheral administration, quinupristin/dalfopristin may be further diluted (to 500 mL or 750 mL), infusion site changed, or infused by a peripherally-inserted central catheter (PICC) or a central venous catheter.

Monitoring Parameters Culture and sensitivity

Dosage Forms Excipient information presented when available (limited, particularly for generics); consult specific product labeling.

Injection, powder for reconstitution:

Synercid®: 500 mg: Quinupristin 150 mg and dalfopristin 350 mg

- ◆ **Qvar** *see* Beclomethasone (Systemic) *on page 227*
- ◆ **QVAR® (Can)** *see* Beclomethasone (Systemic) *on page 227*
- ◆ **R & C™ II (Can)** *see* Pyrethrins and Piperonyl Butoxide *on page 1752*
- ◆ **R & C™ Shampoo/Conditioner (Can)** *see* Pyrethrins and Piperonyl Butoxide *on page 1752*
- ◆ **R-1569** *see* Tocilizumab *on page 2080*
- ◆ **R7159** *see* Obinutuzumab *on page 1482*
- ◆ **R207910** *see* Bedaquiline *on page 229*
- ◆ **R05072759** *see* Obinutuzumab *on page 1482*
- ◆ **RabAvert** *see* Rabies Vaccine *on page 1772*

RABEprazole (ra BEP ra zole)

Brand Names: U.S. Aciphex; AcipHex Sprinkle

Brand Names: Canada Apo-Rabeprazole; Pariet; Pat-Rabeprazole; PMS-Rabeprazole EC; PRO-Rabeprazole; Rabeprazole EC; RAN-Rabeprazole; Riva-Rabeprazole EC; Sandoz-Rabeprazole; Teva-Rabeprazole EC

Index Terms Pariprazole

Pharmacologic Category Proton Pump Inhibitor; Substituted Benzimidazole

Use

Duodenal ulcers: Short-term (4 weeks or fewer) treatment in the healing and symptomatic relief of duodenal ulcers in adults.

Gastroesophageal reflux disease:

Erosive or ulcerative: Short-term (4 to 8 weeks) treatment in the healing and symptomatic relief of erosive or ulcerative gastroesophageal reflux disease (GERD) in adults; for maintaining healing and reduction in relapse rates of heartburn symptoms in adults with erosive or ulcerative GERD.

Symptomatic: Treatment of symptomatic GERD in adults and pediatric patients 1 year and older.

***Helicobacter pylori* eradication:** In combination with amoxicillin and clarithromycin as a 3-drug regimen for the treatment of adults with *H. pylori* infection and duodenal ulcer disease (active or history of within the past 5 years) to eradicate *H. pylori*.

Pathological hypersecretory conditions: Long-term treatment of pathological hypersecretory conditions, including Zollinger-Ellison syndrome in adults.

Canadian labeling: Additional uses (not in U.S. labeling): Treatment of nonerosive reflux disease (NERD); treatment of gastric ulcers

Unlabeled Use Maintenance of healing and prevention of relapse for duodenal ulcer; treatment and prevention of NSAID-induced ulcer

Pregnancy Risk Factor B

Pregnancy Considerations Adverse events were not observed in animal reproduction studies. Available studies have not shown an increased risk of major birth defects following maternal use of proton pump inhibitors during pregnancy; however, information specific to rabeprazole is limited (Pasternak, 2010); most information available for omeprazole. When treating GERD in pregnancy, PPIs may be used when clinically indicated (Katz, 2013).

Breast-Feeding Considerations It is not known if rabeprazole is excreted into breast milk. The manufacturer recommends that caution be exercised when administering rabeprazole to nursing women.

Medication Guide Available Yes

Contraindications Hypersensitivity to rabeprazole, substituted benzimidazoles, or any component of the formulation

Warnings/Precautions Use of proton pump inhibitors (PPIs) may increase the risk of gastrointestinal infections (eg, *Salmonella, Campylobacter*). Use caution in severe hepatic impairment. Relief of symptoms with rabeprazole does not preclude the presence of a gastric malignancy. Use of PPIs may increase risk of *Clostridium difficile*-associated diarrhea (CDAD), especially in hospitalized patients; consider CDAD diagnosis in patients with persistent diarrhea that does not improve. Use the lowest dose and shortest duration of PPI therapy appropriate for the condition being treated. Decreased *H. pylori* eradication rates have been observed with short-term (≤7 days) combination therapy. The American College of Gastroenterology recommends 10-14 days of therapy (triple or quadruple) for eradication of *H. pylori* (Chey, 2007).

PPIs may diminish the therapeutic effect of clopidogrel, thought to be due to reduced formation of the active metabolite of clopidogrel. The manufacturer of clopidogrel recommends either avoidance of both omeprazole (even when scheduled 12 hours apart) and esomeprazole or use of a PPI with comparatively less effect on the active metabolite of clopidogrel. Avoidance of rabeprazole appears prudent due to potent *in vitro* CYP2C19 inhibition (Li, 2004) and lack of sufficient comparative *in vivo* studies with other PPIs. In contrast to these warnings, others have recommended the continued use of PPIs, regardless of the degree of inhibition, in patients with a history of GI bleeding or multiple risk factors for GI bleeding who are also receiving clopidogrel since no evidence has established clinically meaningful differences in outcome; however, a clinically-significant interaction cannot be excluded in those who are poor metabolizers of clopidogrel (Abraham, 2010; Levine, 2011). Potentially significant drug-drug interactions may exist, requiring dose or frequency adjustment, additional monitoring, and/or selection of alternative therapy.

Increased incidence of osteoporosis-related bone fractures of the hip, spine, or wrist may occur with PPI therapy. Patients on high-dose (multiple daily doses) or long-term therapy (≥1 year) should be monitored. Use the lowest effective dose for the shortest duration of time, use vitamin D and calcium supplementation, and follow appropriate guidelines to reduce risk of fractures in patients at risk.

Hypomagnesemia, reported rarely, usually with prolonged PPI use of >3 months (most cases >1 year of therapy); may be symptomatic or asymptomatic; severe cases may cause tetany, seizures, and cardiac arrhythmias. Consider obtaining serum magnesium concentrations prior to beginning long-term therapy, especially if taking concomitant digoxin, diuretics, or other drugs known to cause hypomagnesemia; and periodically thereafter. Hypomagnesemia may be corrected by magnesium supplementation, although discontinuation of rabeprazole may be necessary; magnesium levels typically return to normal within 1 week of stopping.

Adverse Reactions Frequency not always defined.

1% to 10%:

Cardiovascular: Peripheral edema

Central nervous system: Headache (2% to 10%), pain (3%), dizziness

Gastrointestinal: Diarrhea (2% to 5%), nausea (2% to 5%), abdominal pain (4%), vomiting (4%), flatulence (3%), constipation (2%), xerostomia

Hepatic: Hepatic encephalopathy, hepatic enzymes increased, hepatitis

Neuromuscular & skeletal: Arthralgia, myalgia

Respiratory: Pharyngitis (3%)

Miscellaneous: Infection (2%)

<1% (Limited to important or life-threatening): Agitation, agranulocytosis, albuminuria, allergic reaction, alopecia, amblyopia, anaphylaxis, anemia, angioedema, bullous skin eruption, chest pain, cholecystitis, cholelithiasis, *Clostridium difficile*-associated diarrhea (CDAD), colitis, coma, delirium, disorientation, erythema multiforme, fever, fracture, gynecomastia, hematuria, hemolytic anemia, hyperammonemia, hypertension, hypokalemia, hypomagnesemia, hyponatremia, interstitial nephritis, jaundice, leukocytosis, leukopenia, melena, migraine, osteoporosis-related fracture, palpitation, pancreatitis, pancytopenia, pneumonia, pruritus, rhabdomyolysis, sinus bradycardia, somnolence, Stevens-Johnson syndrome, sudden death, taste abnormal, thrombocytopenia, toxic epidermal necrolysis, TSH increased, weakness

Drug Interactions

Metabolism/Transport Effects Substrate of CYP2C19 (major), CYP3A4 (major); **Note:** Assignment of Major/Minor substrate status based on clinically relevant drug interaction potential; **Inhibits** CYP2C19 (weak), CYP2C8 (moderate), CYP2D6 (weak), CYP3A4 (weak)

Avoid Concomitant Use

Avoid concomitant use of RABEprazole with any of the following: Dasatinib; Delavirdine; Erlotinib; Nelfinavir; Pimozide; PONATinib; Rilpivirine; Risedronate

Increased Effect/Toxicity

RABEprazole may increase the levels/effects of: Amphetamines; ARIPiprazole; CYP2C8 Substrates; Dexmethylphenidate; Dofetilide; Lomitapide; Methotrexate; Methylphenidate; Pimozide; Raltegravir; Risedronate; Saquinavir; Tacrolimus (Systemic); Voriconazole

The levels/effects of RABEprazole may be increased by: Fluconazole; Ketoconazole (Systemic); Voriconazole

Decreased Effect

RABEprazole may decrease the levels/effects of: Atazanavir; Bisphosphonate Derivatives; Bosutinib; Cefditoren; Clopidogrel; Dabigatran Etexilate; Dabrafenib; Dasatinib; Delavirdine; Erlotinib; Gefitinib; Indinavir; Iron Salts; Itraconazole; Ketoconazole (Systemic); Mesalamine; Multivitamins/Minerals (with ADEK, Folate, Iron); Mycophenolate; Nelfinavir; Nilotinib; PONATinib; Posaconazole; Rilpivirine; Riociguat; Risedronate; Vismodegib

The levels/effects of RABEprazole may be decreased by: Bosentan; CYP2C19 Inducers (Strong); CYP3A4 Inducers (Strong); Dabrafenib; Deferasirox; Herbs (CYP3A4 Inducers); Mitotane; Tipranavir; Tocilizumab

Ethanol/Nutrition/Herb Interactions

Ethanol: Ethanol may cause gastric mucosal irritation. Management: Avoid concomitant administration of ethanol.

Food: High-fat meals may delay absorption of tablets, but C_{max} and AUC are not altered. Administration of capsule granules (sprinkled on applesauce) with a high-fat meal resulted in a decrease in C_{max} and AUC by 55% and 35%, respectively. Management: Tablets may be administered with or without food; capsules should be administered before a meal.

Herb/Nutraceutical: St John's wort may increase the metabolism and thus decrease the levels/effects of rabeprazole. Management: Avoid concomitant administration of St. John's wort.

Storage/Stability Store at 25°C (77°F); excursions are permitted between 15° and 30°C (59° and 86°F). Protect from moisture.

Mechanism of Action Potent proton pump inhibitor; suppresses gastric acid secretion by inhibiting the parietal cell H+/K+ ATP pump

Pharmacodynamics/Kinetics

Onset of action: Within 1 hour

Duration: 24 hours

Absorption: Oral: Well absorbed within 1 hour

Protein binding, serum: ~96%

Metabolism: Hepatic via CYP3A and 2C19 to inactive metabolites

Bioavailability: Tablet: ~52%

Half-life elimination (dose dependent): 1-2 hours

Time to peak, plasma: Tablet: 2-5 hours; Capsule: 1-6.5 hours

Excretion: Urine (90% primarily as thioether carboxylic acid metabolites); remainder in feces

Dosage

Duodenal ulcer: Adults: Oral: 20 mg once daily for ≤4 weeks; additional therapy may be required for some patients

Gastric ulcers: *Canadian labeling:* Adults: Oral: 20 mg once daily up to 6 weeks; additional therapy may be required for some patients

Gastroesophageal reflux disease (GERD):

Children 1-11 years: Oral:

<15 kg: 5 mg once daily for ≤12 weeks; if inadequate response may increase to 10 mg once daily

≥15 kg: 10 mg once daily for ≤12 weeks

Children ≥12 years and Adolescents: Oral: 20 mg once daily for ≤8 weeks

Adults: Oral:

Erosive or ulcerative GERD: Treatment: 20 mg once daily for 4-8 weeks; if inadequate response, may repeat up to an additional 8 weeks; maintenance: 20 mg once daily

Canadian labeling: 20 mg once daily for 4 weeks; if inadequate response, may repeat for an additional 4 weeks (lack of symptom control after 4 weeks warrants further evaluation); maintenance: 10 mg once daily (maximum: 20 mg once daily).

Symptomatic GERD: Treatment: 20 mg once daily for 4 weeks; if inadequate response, may repeat for an additional 4 weeks.

Canadian labeling: 10 mg once daily (maximum: 20 mg once daily) for 4 weeks; lack of symptom control after 4 weeks warrants further evaluation

***Helicobacter pylori* eradication:** Adults: Oral:

Manufacturer labeling: 20 mg twice daily administered with amoxicillin 1000 mg *and* clarithromycin 500 mg twice daily for 7 days

American College of Gastroenterology guidelines (Chey, 2007):

Nonpenicillin allergy: 20 mg twice daily administered with amoxicillin 1000 mg *and* clarithromycin 500 mg twice daily for 10-14 days

Penicillin allergy: 20 mg twice daily administered with clarithromycin 500 mg *and* metronidazole 500 mg twice daily for 10-14 days **or** 20 mg once or twice daily administered with bismuth subsalicylate 525 mg *and* metronidazole 250 mg *plus* tetracycline 500 mg 4 times daily for 10-14 days

Hypersecretory conditions: Adults: Oral: 60 mg once daily; dose may need to be adjusted as necessary. Doses as high as 100 mg once daily and 60 mg twice daily have been used, and continued as long as necessary (up to 1 year in some patients).

Nonerosive reflux disease (NERD): *Canadian labeling:* Adults: Oral: Treatment: 10 mg (maximum: 20 mg once daily) for 4 weeks; lack of symptom control after 4 weeks warrants further evaluation

Dosage adjustment in renal impairment: No dosage adjustment necessary

Dosage adjustment in hepatic impairment:

Mild-to-moderate: No dosage adjustment necessary.

Severe: No dosage adjustment provided in manufacturer's labeling (has not been studied). Use with caution.

Dietary Considerations

Capsules: Take 30 minutes before a meal.

Tablets: May be taken with or without food. However, when used for the healing of duodenal ulcers, it is best if taken after breakfast. When used for the eradication of *Helicobacter pylori*, take with the morning and evening meals.

Administration May be administered with an antacid.

Capsules: Administer 30 minutes before a meal. Open capsule and sprinkle contents on a small amount of soft food (eg, applesauce, fruit or vegetable based baby food, yogurt) or empty contents into a small amount of liquid (eg, infant formula, apple juice, pediatric electrolyte solution); food or liquid should be at or below room temperature. Do not chew or crush granules; administer whole dose within 15 minutes of preparation (do not store for future use).

Tablets: May be administered with or without food. However, when used for the healing of duodenal ulcers, administration after breakfast is recommended. When used for the eradication of *H. pylori*, administration with the morning and evening meals is recommended. Swallow tablets whole; do not crush, split, or chew.

Monitoring Parameters Magnesium levels in patients on long-term treatment or those taking digoxin, diuretics, or other drugs that cause hypomagnesemia; susceptibility testing recommended in patients who fail *H. pylori* eradication regimen.

Dosage Forms Excipient information presented when available (limited, particularly for generics); consult specific product labeling.

Capsule Sprinkle, Oral, as sodium:

AcipHex Sprinkle: 5 mg [contains fd&c blue #2 aluminum lake]

AcipHex Sprinkle: 10 mg [contains fd&c yellow #6 (sunset yellow)]

Tablet Delayed Release, Oral, as sodium:

Aciphex: 20 mg

Generic: 20 mg

Dosage Forms: Canada Excipient information presented when available (limited, particularly for generics); consult specific product labeling.

Note: Sprinkle capsules are not available in Canada

Tablet, delayed release, enteric coated, as sodium:

Pariet®: 10 mg, 20 mg

◆ **Rabeprazole EC (Can)** *see* RABEprazole *on page 1769*

Rabies Immune Globulin (Human)

(RAY beez i MYUN GLOB yoo lin, HYU man)

Brand Names: U.S. HyperRAB S/D; Imogam Rabies-HT

Brand Names: Canada HyperRAB® S/D; Imogam® Rabies Pasteurized

Index Terms HRIG; RIG

Pharmacologic Category Blood Product Derivative; Immune Globulin

Additional Appendix Information

Immunization Administration Recommendations *on page 2334*

Immunization Recommendations *on page 2339*

Use Part of postexposure prophylaxis of persons with rabies exposure. Provides passive immunity until active immunity with rabies vaccine is established. Not for use in persons with a history of pre-exposure vaccination, history of postexposure prophylaxis, or previous vaccination with rabies vaccine and documentation of antibody response.

Pregnancy Risk Factor C

Pregnancy Considerations Reproduction studies have not been conducted. Pregnancy is not a contraindication to postexposure prophylaxis.

Contraindications There are no contraindications listed within the FDA-approved manufacturer's labeling.

Warnings/Precautions Hypersensitivity and anaphylactic reactions can occur; immediate treatment (including epinephrine 1:1000) should be available. Use with caution in patients with isolated immunoglobulin A deficiency or a history of systemic hypersensitivity to human immunoglobulins. Use with caution in patients with thrombocytopenia or coagulation disorders; I.M. injections may be contraindicated. Product of human plasma; may potentially contain infectious agents which could transmit disease. Screening of donors, as well as testing and/or inactivation or removal of certain viruses, reduces the risk. Infections thought to be transmitted by this product should be reported to the manufacturer. Not for intravenous administration.

Adverse Reactions Frequency not defined.

Central nervous system: Fever (mild), headache, malaise
Dermatologic: Angioneurotic edema, rash
Local: Injection site: Pain, stiffness, soreness, tenderness
Renal: Nephrotic syndrome
Miscellaneous: Anaphylaxis

Drug Interactions

Metabolism/Transport Effects None known.

Avoid Concomitant Use There are no known interactions where it is recommended to avoid concomitant use.

Increased Effect/Toxicity There are no known significant interactions involving an increase in effect.

Decreased Effect

Rabies Immune Globulin (Human) may decrease the levels/effects of: Vaccines (Live)

Storage/Stability Store between 2°C to 8°C (36°F to 46°F); do not freeze. Discard product exposed to freezing. The following stability information has also been reported for HyperRAB® S/D: May be exposed to room temperature for a cumulative 7 days (Cohen, 2007).

Mechanism of Action Rabies immune globulin is a solution of globulins dried from the plasma or serum of selected adult human donors who have been immunized with rabies vaccine and have developed high titers of rabies antibody. It generally contains 10% to 18% of protein of which not less than 80% is monomeric immunoglobulin G.

Dosage Children and Adults: Postexposure prophylaxis: Local wound infiltration: 20 units/kg in a single dose, RIG should always be administered as part of rabies vaccine regimen. If anatomically feasible, the full rabies immune globulin dose should be infiltrated around and into the wound(s); remaining volume should be administered I.M. at a site distant from the vaccine administration site. If rabies vaccine was initiated without rabies immune globulin, rabies immune globulin may be administered through the seventh day after the administration of the first dose of the vaccine. Administration of RIG is not recommended after the seventh day post vaccine since an antibody response to the vaccine is expected during this time period.

Note: Not for use in persons with a history of pre-exposure vaccination, history of postexposure prophylaxis, or previous vaccination with rabies vaccine and documentation of antibody response.

Dosage adjustment in renal impairment: No dosage adjustment provided in manufacturer's labeling.

Dosage adjustment in hepatic impairment: No dosage adjustment provided in manufacturer's labeling.

Administration Do not administer I.V.

Postexposure wound infiltration: If anatomically feasible, the full rabies immune globulin dose should be infiltrated around and into the wound(s); remaining volume should be administered I.M. in the deltoid muscle of the upper arm or lateral thigh muscle. The gluteal area should be avoided to reduce the risk of sciatic nerve damage. Do not administer rabies vaccine in the same syringe or at the same administration site as RIG.

Measles-containing vaccines should be given ≥4 months after rabies immune globulin.

Dosage Forms Excipient information presented when available (limited, particularly for generics); consult specific product labeling.

Injectable, Intramuscular:
Imogam Rabies-HT: 150 units/mL (2 mL, 10 mL)
Injectable, Intramuscular [preservative free]:
HyperRAB S/D: 150 units/mL (2 mL, 10 mL)

Rabies Vaccine (RAY beez vak SEEN)

Brand Names: U.S. Imovax Rabies; RabAvert

Brand Names: Canada Imovax Rabies; RabAvert

Index Terms HDCV; Human Diploid Cell Cultures Rabies Vaccine; PCEC; Purified Chick Embryo Cell

Pharmacologic Category Vaccine, Inactivated (Viral)

Additional Appendix Information

Immunization Administration Recommendations *on page 2334*

Immunization Recommendations *on page 2339*

Use Pre-exposure and postexposure vaccination against rabies

The Advisory Committee on Immunization Practices (ACIP) recommends a primary course of prophylactic immunization (pre-exposure vaccination) for the following:

- Persons with continuous risk of infection, including rabies research laboratory and biologics production workers
- Persons with frequent risk of infection in areas where rabies is enzootic, including rabies diagnostic laboratory workers, cavers, veterinarians and their staff, and animal control and wildlife workers; persons who frequently handle bats
- Persons with infrequent risk of infection, including veterinarians and animal control staff with terrestrial animals in areas where rabies infection is rare, veterinary students, and travelers visiting areas where rabies is enzootic and immediate access to medical care and biologicals is limited

The ACIP recommends the use of postexposure vaccination for a particular person be assessed by the severity and likelihood versus the actual risk of acquiring rabies. Consideration should include the type of exposure, epidemiology of rabies in the area, species of the animal, circumstances of the incident, and the availability of the exposing animal for observation or rabies testing. Postexposure vaccination is used in both previously vaccinated and previously unvaccinated individuals.

Pregnancy Risk Factor C

Pregnancy Considerations Animal reproduction studies have not been conducted. Pregnancy is not a contraindication to postexposure prophylaxis. Pre-exposure prophylaxis during pregnancy may also be considered if risk of rabies is great.

Breast-Feeding Considerations Breast-feeding mothers may be vaccinated. Inactivated virus vaccines do not affect the safety of breast-feeding for the mother or the infant. Breast-feeding infants should be vaccinated according to the recommended schedules (CDC, 2011)

Contraindications

Pre-exposure prophylaxis: Hypersensitivity to rabies vaccine or any component of the formulation

Postexposure prophylaxis: There are no contraindications listed within the FDA-approved manufacturer's labeling.

Warnings/Precautions Rabies vaccine should not be used in persons with a confirmed diagnosis of rabies; use after the onset of symptoms may be detrimental. Postexposure vaccination may begin regardless of the length of time from documented or likely exposure, as long as clinical signs of rabies are not present. Immediate treatment (including epinephrine 1:1000) for anaphylactoid and/or hypersensitivity reactions should be available during vaccine use. Once postexposure prophylaxis has begun, administration should generally not be interrupted or discontinued due to local or mild adverse events. Continuation of vaccination following severe systemic reactions should consider the persons risk of developing rabies. Report serious reactions to the State Health Department or the manufacturer/distributor. An immune complex reaction is possible 2-21 days following booster doses of HDCV. Symptoms may include arthralgia, arthritis, angioedema, fever, generalized urticaria, malaise, nausea, and vomiting. Syncope has been reported with use of injectable vaccines and may be accompanied by transient visual disturbances, weakness, or tonic-clonic movements. Procedures should be in place to avoid injuries from falling and to restore cerebral perfusion if syncope occurs. Vaccination may not result in effective immunity in all patients. Response depends upon multiple factors (eg, type of vaccine, age of patient) and may be improved by administering the vaccine at the recommended dose, route, and interval. Vaccines may not be effective if administered during periods of altered immune competence (CDC, 2011). Use with caution in severely immunocompromised patients (eg, patients receiving chemo/radiation therapy or other immunosuppressive therapy [including high-dose corticosteroids]); may have a reduced response to vaccination. Withhold nonessential immunosuppressive agents during postexposure prophylaxis; if possible postpone pre-exposure prophylaxis until the immunocompromising condition is resolved. Persons with altered immunocompetence should receive the five-dose postexposure vaccine regimen. In general, household and close contacts of persons with altered immunocompetence may receive all age appropriate vaccines. Products may contain albumin and therefore carry a remote risk of transmitting Creutzfeldt-Jakob or other viral diseases. Imovax® Rabies contains neomycin. RabAvert® contains amphotericin B, bovine gelatin, chicken protein, chlortetracycline, and neomycin. For I. M. administration only.

Adverse Reactions All serious adverse reactions must be reported to the U.S. Department of Health and Human Services (DHHS) Vaccine Adverse Event Reporting System (VAERS) 1-800-822-7967 or online at https://vaers.hhs.gov/esub/index. In Canada, adverse reactions may be reported to local provincial/territorial health agencies or to the Vaccine Safety Section at Public Health Agency of Canada (1-866-844-0018).

>10%:

Central nervous system: Dizziness, headache, malaise
Gastrointestinal: Abdominal pain, nausea
Local: Erythema, itching, pain, swelling
Neuromuscular & skeletal: Myalgia
Miscellaneous: Lymphadenopathy

Uncommon, frequency not defined, postmarketing, and/or case reports:

Cardiovascular: Circulatory reactions, edema, palpitation
Central nervous system: Chills, fatigue, fever >38°C (100°F), Guillain-Barré syndrome, encephalitis, meningitis, multiple sclerosis, myelitis, neuroparalysis, seizures, vertigo
Dermatologic: Pruritus, urticaria, urticaria pigmentosa
Endocrine & metabolic: Hot flashes
Gastrointestinal: Diarrhea, vomiting
Local: Hematoma, limb swelling (extensive)
Neuromuscular & skeletal: Arthralgia, limb pain, monoarthritis, neuropathy, paralysis (transient), paresthesias (transient), weakness
Ocular: Retrobulbar neuritis, visual disturbances
Respiratory: Bronchospasm, dyspnea, wheezing
Miscellaneous: Allergic reactions, anaphylaxis, hypersensitivity reactions, serum sickness, swollen lymph nodes

Drug Interactions

Metabolism/Transport Effects None known.

Avoid Concomitant Use There are no known interactions where it is recommended to avoid concomitant use.

Increased Effect/Toxicity There are no known significant interactions involving an increase in effect.

Decreased Effect

The levels/effects of Rabies Vaccine may be decreased by: Belimumab; Chloroquine; Fingolimod; Immunosuppressants

Preparation for Administration Reconstitute with provided diluent; gently swirl to dissolve. Use immediately after reconstitution.

Imovax®: Suspension will appear pink to red

RabAvert®: Suspension will appear clear to slightly opaque

Storage/Stability Prior to reconstitution, store under refrigeration at 2°C to 8°C (36°F to 46°F); do not freeze. Protect from light.

Mechanism of Action Rabies vaccine is an inactivated virus vaccine which promotes immunity by inducing an active immune response. The production of specific antibodies requires about 7-10 days to develop. Rabies immune globulin or antirabies serum, equine (ARS) is given in conjunction with rabies vaccine to provide immune protection until an antibody response can occur.

Pharmacodynamics/Kinetics

Onset of action: I.M.: Rabies antibody: ~7-10 days
Peak effect: ~30-60 days
Duration: ≥1 year

Dosage

Pre-exposure vaccination: I.M: A total of 3 doses, 1 mL each, on days 0, 7, and 21-28. **Note:** Prolonging the interval between doses does not interfere with immunity achieved after the concluding dose of the basic series.

Postexposure vaccination: All postexposure treatment should begin with immediate cleansing of the wound with soap and water

Persons not previously immunized as above: I.M.: 5 doses (1 mL each) on days 0, 3, 7, 14, 28. In addition, patients should also receive rabies immune globulin with the first dose (day 0). **Note:** A regimen of 4 doses (1 mL each) on days 0, 3, 7, 14 may be used in persons who are not immunosuppressed (ACIP recommendations, 2010).

Persons who have previously received postexposure prophylaxis with rabies vaccine, received a recommended I.M. pre-exposure series of rabies vaccine or have a previously documented rabies antibody titer considered adequate: I.M.: Two doses (1 mL each) on days 0 and 3; do not administer rabies immune globulin

Booster (for persons with continuous or frequent risk of infection): 1 mL I.M. based on antibody titers

Dosage adjustment in renal impairment: No dosage adjustment provided in manufacturer's labeling.

Dosage adjustment in hepatic impairment: No dosage adjustment provided in manufacturer's labeling.

Administration For I.M. administration only; this rabies vaccine product must not be administered intradermally; in adults and children, administer I.M. injections in the deltoid muscle, not the gluteal; for younger children, use the outer aspect of the thigh. Postexposure prophylaxis should begin with immediate cleansing of wounds with soap and water; if available, a virucidal agent (eg, povidone-iodine solution) should be used to irrigate the wounds.

For patients at risk of hemorrhage following intramuscular injection, the ACIP recommends "it should be administered intramuscularly if, in the opinion of the physician familiar with the patient's bleeding risk, the vaccine can be administered by this route with reasonable safety. If the patient receives antihemophilia or other similar therapy, intramuscular vaccination can be scheduled shortly after such therapy is administered. A fine needle (23 gauge or smaller) can be used for the vaccination and firm pressure applied to the site (without rubbing) for at least 2 minutes. The patient should be instructed concerning the risk of hematoma from the injection." Patients on anticoagulant therapy should be considered to have the same bleeding risks and treated as those with clotting factor disorders (CDC, 2011).

Simultaneous administration of vaccines helps ensure the patients will be fully vaccinated by the appropriate age. Simultaneous administration of vaccines is defined as administering >1 vaccine on the same day at different anatomic sites. The use of licensed combination vaccines is generally preferred over separate injections of the equivalent components. Separate vaccines should not be combined in the same syringe unless indicated by product specific labeling. Separate needles and syringes should be used for each injection. The ACIP prefers each dose of a specific vaccine in a series come from the same manufacturer when possible. Adolescents and adults should be vaccinated while seated or lying down. In general, preterm infants should be vaccinated at the same chronological age as full-term infants (CDC, 2011).

Antipyretics have not been shown to prevent febrile seizures. Antipyretics may be used to treat fever or discomfort following vaccination (CDC, 2011). One study reported that routine prophylactic administration of acetaminophen to prevent fever prior to vaccination decreased the immune response of some vaccines; the clinical significance of this reduction in immune response has not been established (Prymula, 2009).

Monitoring Parameters Monitor for syncope for 15 minutes following administration. If seizure-like activity associated with syncope occurs, maintain patient in supine or Trendelenburg position to reestablish adequate cerebral perfusion.

Antibody response to vaccination is not recommended for otherwise healthy persons who complete the pre-exposure or postexposure regimen. Serologic testing to determine if the antibody titer is at an acceptable level is required for the following persons (booster vaccination recommended if titer is below the acceptable level):

- Persons with continuous risk of infection: Serologic testing every 6 months
- Persons with frequent risk of infection: Serologic testing every 2 years
- Persons who are immunocompromised: Serologic testing after completion of pre-exposure or postexposure prophylaxis series

Monitoring of antibody response to vaccination is not recommended for otherwise healthy persons who complete the pre-exposure or postexposure regimen.

Reference Range Adequate adaptive immune response: antibody titers of 0.5 units/mL [WHO] or complete virus neutralization at a 1:5 serum dilution by the rapid fluorescent focus inhibition test (RFFIT) [ACIP]

Additional Information U.S. federal law requires that the name of medication, date of administration, the vaccine manufacturer, lot number of vaccine, and the administering person's name, title, and address be entered into the patient's permanent medical record.

Dosage Forms Excipient information presented when available (limited, particularly for generics); consult specific product labeling.

Injectable, Intramuscular [preservative free]:

Imovax Rabies: 2.5 units/mL (1 ea) [contains albumin human, neomycin sulfate]

Suspension Reconstituted, Intramuscular:

RabAvert: (1 ea) [contains albumin human, chicken protein, edetate disodium, gelatin (bovine), neomycin]

- **Racemic Epinephrine** *see* EPINEPHrine (Systemic, Oral Inhalation) *on page 714*
- **Racepinephrine** *see* EPINEPHrine (Systemic, Oral Inhalation) *on page 714*
- **RAD001** *see* Everolimus *on page 807*
- **Radiogardase®** *see* Ferric Hexacyanoferrate *on page 853*
- **rAHF** *see* Antihemophilic Factor (Recombinant) *on page 144*
- **RAL** *see* Raltegravir *on page 1776*
- **R-albuterol** *see* Levalbuterol *on page 1192*
- **Ralivia (Can)** *see* TraMADol *on page 2099*

Raloxifene (ral OKS i feen)

Brand Names: U.S. Evista

Brand Names: Canada Apo-Raloxifene®; Evista®; Novo-Raloxifene; Teva-Raloxifene

Index Terms Keoxifene Hydrochloride; Raloxifene Hydrochloride

Pharmacologic Category Selective Estrogen Receptor Modulator (SERM)

Use Prevention and treatment of osteoporosis in postmenopausal women; risk reduction for invasive breast cancer in postmenopausal women with osteoporosis and in postmenopausal women with high risk for invasive breast cancer

Pregnancy Risk Factor X

Pregnancy Considerations Adverse events were observed in in animal reproduction studies. Raloxifene is contraindicated for use in women who are or may become pregnant.

Breast-Feeding Considerations It is not known if raloxifene is excreted into breast milk. Breast-feeding is contraindicated by the manufacturer.

Medication Guide Available Yes

Contraindications History of or current venous thromboembolic disorders (including DVT, PE, and retinal vein thrombosis); pregnancy or women who could become pregnant; breast-feeding

Warnings/Precautions Hazardous agent - use appropriate precautions for handling and disposal (NIOSH, 2012). **[U.S. Boxed Warning]: May increase the risk for DVT or PE; use contraindicated in patients with history of or current venous thromboembolic disorders.** Use with caution in patients at high risk for venous thromboembolism; the risk for DVT and PE are higher in the first 4 months of treatment. Discontinue at least 72 hours prior to and during prolonged immobilization (postoperative recovery or prolonged bedrest). **[U.S. Boxed Warning]: The risk of death due to stroke may be increased in**

women with coronary heart disease or in women at risk for coronary events; use with caution in patients with cardiovascular disease. Not be used for the prevention of cardiovascular disease. Use caution with moderate-to-severe renal dysfunction, hepatic impairment, unexplained uterine bleeding, and in women with a history of elevated triglycerides in response to treatment with oral estrogens (or estrogen/progestin). Safety with concomitant estrogen therapy has not been established. Safety and efficacy in premenopausal women or men have not been established. Not indicated for treatment of invasive breast cancer, to reduce the risk of recurrence of invasive breast cancer or to reduce the risk of noninvasive breast cancer. The efficacy (for breast cancer risk reduction) in women with inherited BRCA1 and BRCA1 mutations has not been established.

Adverse Reactions Note: Raloxifene has been associated with increased risk of thromboembolism (DVT, PE) and superficial thrombophlebitis; risk is similar to reported risk of HRT

>10%:

- Cardiovascular: Peripheral edema (3% to 14%)
- Endocrine & metabolic: Hot flashes (8% to 29%)
- Neuromuscular & skeletal: Arthralgia (11% to 16%), leg cramps/muscle spasm (6% to 12%)
- Miscellaneous: Flu syndrome (14% to 15%), infection (11%)

1% to 10%:

- Cardiovascular: Chest pain (3%), venous thromboembolism (1% to 2%)
- Central nervous system: Insomnia (6%)
- Dermatologic: Rash (6%)
- Endocrine & metabolic: Breast pain (4%)
- Gastrointestinal: Weight gain (9%), abdominal pain (7%), vomiting (5%), flatulence (2% to 3%), cholelithiasis (≤3%), gastroenteritis (≤3%)
- Genitourinary: Vaginal bleeding (6%), leukorrhea (3%), urinary tract disorder (3%), uterine disorder (3%), vaginal hemorrhage (3%), endometrial disorder (≤3%)
- Neuromuscular & skeletal: Myalgia (8%), tendon disorder (4%)
- Respiratory: Bronchitis (10%), sinusitis (10%), pharyngitis (8%), pneumonia (3%), laryngitis (≤2%)
- Miscellaneous: Diaphoresis (3%)

<1% (Limited to important or life-threatening): Apolipoprotein A-1 increased, apolipoprotein B decreased, death related to VTE, fibrinogen decreased, hypertriglyceridemia (in women with a history of increased triglycerides in response to oral estrogens), intermittent claudication, LDL cholesterol decreased, lipoprotein decreased, retinal vein occlusion, stroke related to VTE, superficial thrombophlebitis, total serum cholesterol decreased

Drug Interactions

Metabolism/Transport Effects None known.

Avoid Concomitant Use

Avoid concomitant use of Raloxifene with any of the following: Ospemifene

Increased Effect/Toxicity

Raloxifene may increase the levels/effects of: Ospemifene

Decreased Effect

Raloxifene may decrease the levels/effects of: Levothyroxine; Ospemifene

The levels/effects of Raloxifene may be decreased by: Bile Acid Sequestrants

Ethanol/Nutrition/Herb Interactions Ethanol: Avoid ethanol (may increase risk of osteoporosis).

Storage/Stability Store at controlled room temperature of 20°C to 25°C (68°F to 77°F); excursions permitted to 15°C to 30°C (59°F to 86°F).

Mechanism of Action A selective estrogen receptor modulator (SERM), meaning that it affects some of the same receptors that estrogen does, but not all, and in some instances, it antagonizes or blocks estrogen; it acts like estrogen to prevent bone loss and has the potential to block some estrogen effects in the breast and uterine tissues. Raloxifene decreases bone resorption, increasing bone mineral density and decreasing fracture incidence.

Pharmacodynamics/Kinetics

Onset of action: 8 weeks

Absorption: Rapid; ~60%

Distribution: 2348 L/kg

Protein binding: >95% to albumin and α-glycoprotein; does not bind to sex-hormone-binding globulin

Metabolism: Hepatic, extensive first-pass effect; metabolized to glucuronide conjugates

Bioavailability: ~2%

Half-life elimination: 28-33 hours

Excretion: Primarily feces; urine (<0.2% as unchanged drug; <6% as glucuronide conjugates)

Dosage Adults: Females: Oral:

Osteoporosis: 60 mg once daily

Invasive breast cancer risk reduction: 60 mg once daily for 5 years per ASCO guidelines (Visvanathan, 2009)

Dosage adjustment in renal impairment: No dosage adjustment provided in manufacturer's labeling. Use caution in moderate-to-severe impairment.

Dosage adjustment in hepatic impairment: No dosage adjustment provided in manufacturer's labeling (has not been studied). Use with caution.

Dietary Considerations May be taken without regard to meals. Osteoporosis prevention or treatment: Ensure adequate calcium and vitamin D intake; if dietary intake is inadequate, dietary supplementation is recommended. Women and men should consume:

Calcium: 1000 mg/day (men: 50-70 years) **or** 1200 mg/day (women ≥51 years and men ≥71 years) (IOM, 2011; NOF, 2013)

Vitamin D: 800-1000 IU/day (men and women ≥50 years) (NOF, 2013). Recommended Dietary Allowance (RDA): 600 IU/day (men and women ≤70 years) **or** 800 IU/day (men and women ≥71 years) (IOM, 2011).

Administration May be administered without regard to meals.

Hazardous agent; use appropriate precautions for handling and disposal (NIOSH, 2012).

Monitoring Parameters Lipid profile; adequate diagnostic measures, including endometrial sampling, if indicated, should be performed to rule out malignancy in all cases of undiagnosed abnormal vaginal bleeding

Osteoporosis: Bone mineral density (BMD) should be re-evaluated every 2 years (or more frequently) after initiating therapy (NOF, 2013); annual measurements of height and weight; serum calcium and 25(OH)D; may consider monitoring biochemical markers of bone turnover

Reference Range

Calcium (total): Adults: 9.0-11.0 mg/dL (2.05-2.54 mmol/L), may slightly decrease with aging

Phosphorus: 2.5-4.5 mg/dL (0.81-1.45 mmol/L)

Vitamin D: There is no clear consensus on a reference range for total serum 25(OH)D concentrations or the validity of this level as it relates clinically to bone health. In addition, there is significant variability in the reporting of serum 25(OH)D levels as a result of different assay types in use; however, the following ranges have been suggested:

Adults (IOM, 2011): Sufficient levels in practically all persons: ≥20 ng/mL (50 nmol/L); concern for risk of toxicity: >50 ng/mL (125 nmol/L)

Osteoporosis patients (NOF, 2013): Recommended level to reach and maintain: ~30 ng/mL (75 nmol/L)

Additional Information The decrease in estrogen-related adverse effects with the selective estrogen-receptor modulators in general and raloxifene in particular should improve compliance and decrease the incidence of cardiovascular events and fractures while not increasing breast cancer.

Oncology Comment: The American Society of Clinical Oncology (ASCO) guidelines for breast cancer risk reduction (Visvanathan, 2009) recommend raloxifene (for 5 years) as an option to reduce the risk of ER-positive invasive breast cancer in postmenopausal women with a 5-year projected risk (based on NCI trial model) of ≥1.66%, or with lobular carcinoma *in situ*. Raloxifene should not be used in premenopausal women. Women with osteoporosis may use raloxifene beyond 5 years of treatment. According to the NCCN breast cancer risk reduction guidelines (v.2.2009), raloxifene is only recommended for postmenopausal women (≥35 years of age), and is equivalent to tamoxifen although, raloxifene has a better adverse event profile; however, tamoxifen is superior in reducing the risk on noninvasive breast cancer.

Dosage Forms Excipient information presented when available (limited, particularly for generics); consult specific product labeling.

Tablet, Oral, as hydrochloride:

Evista: 60 mg

◆ **Raloxifene Hydrochloride** *see* Raloxifene *on page 1774*

Raltegravir (ral TEG ra vir)

Brand Names: U.S. Isentress

Brand Names: Canada Isentress

Index Terms MK-0518; RAL

Pharmacologic Category Antiretroviral Agent, Integrase Inhibitor (Anti-HIV)

Use HIV-1 infection: Treatment of HIV-1 infection in combination with other antiretroviral agents

Unlabeled Use Postexposure prophylaxis for occupational exposure to HIV

Pregnancy Risk Factor C

Pregnancy Considerations Adverse events were observed in some animal reproduction studies. Raltegravir crosses the placenta and can be detected in neonatal serum after delivery. Standard doses appear to be appropriate in pregnant women. The DHHS Perinatal HIV Guidelines note that raltegravir may be used under special circumstances in pregnant women (eg, when preferred or alternative agents cannot be used).

Regardless of CD4 count or HIV RNA copy number, all HIV-infected pregnant women should receive a combination antepartum antiretroviral (ARV) drug regimen; this includes women who require therapy for their own health, as well as women who do not yet require therapy for their own health. ARV therapy should be started as soon as possible if required for the woman's health. Although earlier initiation may be more effective in reducing the perinatal transmission of HIV, also consider maternal conditions (eg, nausea and vomiting) and the potential risks of first trimester fetal exposure for specific agents. Plasma HIV RNA levels should be assessed at ~34-36 weeks gestation in order to help determine mode of delivery. If ARV therapy must be interrupted for <24 hours during the peripartum period, stop then restart all medications simultaneously in order to decrease the chance of developing resistance. Long-term follow-up is recommended for all infants exposed to ARV medications.

Healthcare providers are encouraged to enroll pregnant women exposed to antiretroviral medications in the Antiretroviral Pregnancy Registry (1-800-258-4263 or www.-APRegistry.com). Healthcare providers caring for HIV-infected women and their infants may contact the National Perinatal HIV Hotline (888-448-8765) for clinical consultation (DHHS [perinatal], 2012).

Breast-Feeding Considerations Maternal or infant antiretroviral therapy does not completely eliminate the risk of postnatal HIV transmission. In addition, multiclass-resistant virus has been detected in breast-feeding infants despite maternal therapy. Therefore, in the United States, where formula is accessible, affordable, safe, and sustainable, and the risk of infant mortality due to diarrhea and respiratory infections is low, complete avoidance of breast-feeding by HIV-infected women is recommended to decrease potential transmission of HIV (DHHS [perinatal], 2012).

Contraindications There are no contraindications listed in the manufacturer's labeling.

Canadian labeling: Hypersensitivity to raltegravir or any other component of the formulation

Warnings/Precautions Patients may develop immune reconstitution syndrome resulting in the occurrence of an inflammatory response to an indolent or residual opportunistic infection during initial HIV treatment or activation of autoimmune disorders (eg, Graves' disease, polymyositis, Guillain-Barré syndrome) later in therapy; further evaluation and treatment may be required. Severe, life-threatening or fatal cases of Stevens-Johnson syndrome and toxic epidermal necrolysis have been reported. Hypersensitivity reactions (rash [may occur with fever, fatigue, malaise, conjunctivitis, or other constitutional symptoms], organ dysfunction and/or hepatic failure) have also been reported. Discontinue immediately if a severe skin reaction or hypersensitivity symptoms develop. Monitor liver transaminases and start supportive therapy. Myopathy and rhabdomyolysis have been reported; use caution in patients with risk factors for CK elevations and/or skeletal muscle abnormalities. Potentially significant drug-drug interactions may exist, requiring dose or frequency adjustment, additional monitoring, and/or selection of alternative therapy. Avoid use as a boosted PI replacement in antiretroviral experienced patients with documented resistance to nucleoside reverse transcriptase inhibitors. Chewable tablet contains phenylalanine.

Adverse Reactions

>10%:

Hepatic: Increased serum ALT (1% to 11%; incidence higher with hepatitis B and/or C coinfection)

2% to 10%:

Central nervous system: Insomnia (4%), headache (2% to 4%), dizziness (2%), fatigue (2%)

Endocrine & metabolic: Increased serum glucose (126 to 250 mg/dL: 7% to 10%; 251 to 500 mg/dL: 2% to 3%)

Gastrointestinal: Increased serum lipase (2% to 5%), increased serum amylase (2% to 4%), nausea (3%)

Hematologic: Abnormal absolute neutrophil count (2% to 3%), thrombocytopenia (1% to 3%)

Hepatic: Increased serum AST (1% to 9%; incidence higher with hepatitis B and/or C coinfection), hyperbilirubinemia (<1% to 6%), increased serum alkaline phosphatase (<1% to 2%)

Neuromuscular & skeletal: Increased creatine phosphokinase (10 to 19.9 x ULN: 4%; ≥20 x ULN: 3%)

<2% (Limited to important or life-threatening): Anemia, cerebellar ataxia, depression (particularly in subjects with a pre-existing history of psychiatric illness), drug rash with eosinophilia and systemic symptoms (DRESS; Perry, 2013), gastritis, hepatic failure, hepatitis, hypersensitivity, myopathy, nephrolithiasis, psychomotor agitation (children; grade 3), renal failure, rhabdomyolysis,

Stevens-Johnson syndrome, suicidal tendencies, toxic epidermal necrolysis

Drug Interactions

Metabolism/Transport Effects None known.

Avoid Concomitant Use

Avoid concomitant use of Raltegravir with any of the following: Aluminum Hydroxide; Magnesium Salts

Increased Effect/Toxicity

Raltegravir may increase the levels/effects of: Fibric Acid Derivatives; HMG-CoA Reductase Inhibitors; Zidovudine

The levels/effects of Raltegravir may be increased by: Proton Pump Inhibitors

Decreased Effect

Raltegravir may decrease the levels/effects of: Fosamprenavir

The levels/effects of Raltegravir may be decreased by: Aluminum Hydroxide; Efavirenz; Fosamprenavir; Magnesium Salts; Rifabutin; Rifampin; Tipranavir

Ethanol/Nutrition/Herb Interactions

Food: Variable absorption depending upon meal type (low- vs high-fat meal) and dosage form; raltegravir was administered without regard to meals in clinical trials.

Herb/Nutraceutical: Avoid St John's wort (may decrease the levels/effects of raltegravir).

Storage/Stability

Chewable tablet: Store in the original package with the bottle tightly closed, at room temperature of 20°C to 25°C (68°F to 77°F); excursions permitted to 15°C to 30°C (59°F to 86°F). Keep the desiccant in the bottle to protect from moisture.

Film-coated tablet: Store at room temperature of 20°C to 25°C (68°F to 77°F); excursions permitted to 15°C to 30°C (59°F to 86°F).

Mechanism of Action Incorporation of viral DNA into the host cell's genome is required to produce a self-replicating provirus and propagation of infectious virion particles. The viral cDNA strand produced by reverse transcriptase is subsequently processed and inserted into the human genome by the enzyme HIV-1 integrase (encoded by the pol gene of HIV). Raltegravir inhibits the catalytic activity of integrase, thus preventing integration of the proviral gene into human DNA.

Pharmacodynamics/Kinetics

Absorption: Film-coated tablet: AUC increased twofold with high-fat meal; Chewable tablet: AUC decreased by ~6% with high-fat meal

Protein binding: ~83%

Metabolism: Primarily hepatic glucuronidation mediated by UGT1A1

Bioavailability: Film-coated tablet: Not established; however, chewable tablet has higher oral bioavailability compared to film-coated tablet

Half-life elimination: ~9 hours

Time to peak, plasma: Film-coated tablet: ~3 hours

Excretion: Feces (~51%, as unchanged drug); urine (~32%; 9% as unchanged drug)

Dosage

HIV treatment:

Children 2 to <12 years: Oral: Chewable tablet: Weight-based dosing based on ~6 mg/kg/dose twice daily.

7 to <10 kg: Canadian labeling (dosing for <10 kg is not found in U.S. labeling): 50 mg twice daily

10 to <14 kg: 75 mg twice daily

14 to <20 kg: 100 mg twice daily

20 to <28 kg: 150 mg twice daily (see **"Note"**)

28 to <40 kg: 200 mg twice daily (see **"Note"**)

≥40 kg: 300 mg twice daily (see **"Note"**)

Note: Children 6 to <12 years who are ≥25 kg may use either weight-based dosing (chewable tablet) **or** adult dosing (film-coated tablet).

Adolescents ≥12 years and Adults: Oral: Film-coated tablet: 400 mg twice daily. Recommended as a preferred therapy with emtricitabine/tenofovir in antiretroviral-naive naive patients (DHHS [adult], 2013; DHHS [adult, INSTI], 2013; Lennox, 2009).

Occupational HIV postexposure, prophylaxis (unlabeled use): Adults: Oral: Film-coated tablet: 400 mg twice daily for 4 weeks with concomitant emtricitabine/tenofovir. Recommended as preferred therapy (Kuhar, 2013).

Dosage adjustment for rifampin coadministration: 800 mg twice daily. There are no data to guide dose adjustment in patients <18 years of age.

Dosage adjustment in renal impairment: No dosage adjustment necessary.

Dosage adjustment in hepatic impairment:

Mild-to-moderate hepatic impairment: No dosage adjustment necessary.

Severe impairment: No dosage adjustment provided in manufacturer's labeling (has not been studied).

Dietary Considerations May be taken without regard to meals. Some products may contain phenylalanine.

Administration May be administered without regard to meals.

Monitoring Parameters Viral load, CD4 count, lipid profile

HIV occupational postexposure prophylaxis (PEP) (Kuhar, 2013): Documented HIV test (at baseline and 6 weeks, 12 weeks and 6 months after exposure); if confirmation that a fourth generation HIV p2 antigen-HIV antibody test is being used, monitor at baseline, 6 weeks and 4 months after exposure. CBC, renal and hepatic function assessments at baseline and 2 weeks after exposure (minimum recommendations, others dictated by clinical assessment)

Product Availability Isentress (100 mg single use packets for oral suspension): FDA approved December 2013; anticipated availability is the third quarter of 2014.

Dosage Forms Excipient information presented when available (limited, particularly for generics); consult specific product labeling.

Tablet, Oral:

Isentress: 400 mg [contains polyethylene glycol]

Tablet Chewable, Oral:

Isentress: 25 mg [contains aspartame, saccharin sodium; orange banana flavor]

Isentress: 100 mg [scored; contains aspartame, saccharin sodium; orange banana flavor]

Ramelteon (ra MEL tee on)

Brand Names: U.S. Rozerem

Index Terms TAK-375

Pharmacologic Category Hypnotic, Miscellaneous

Use Treatment of insomnia characterized by difficulty with sleep onset

Pregnancy Risk Factor C

Pregnancy Considerations Animal studies have demonstrated teratogenic effects. May cause disturbances of reproductive hormonal regulation (eg, disruption of menses or decreased libido). There are no adequate and well-controlled studies in pregnant women.

Breast-Feeding Considerations It is not known if ramelteon is excreted in breast milk. The manufacturer recommends that caution be exercised when administering ramelteon to nursing women.

Medication Guide Available Yes

Contraindications History of angioedema with previous ramelteon therapy (do not rechallenge); concurrent use with fluvoxamine

Warnings/Precautions Symptomatic treatment of insomnia should be initiated only after careful evaluation of potential causes of sleep disturbance. Failure of sleep disturbance to resolve after a reasonable period of treatment may indicate psychiatric and/or medical illness. Because of the rapid onset of action, administer immediately prior to bedtime or after the patient has gone to bed and is having difficulty falling asleep. Hypnotics/sedatives have been associated with abnormal thinking and behavior changes including decreased inhibition, aggression, bizarre behavior, agitation, hallucinations, and depersonalization. These changes may occur unpredictably and may indicate previously unrecognized psychiatric disorders; evaluate appropriately. Postmarketing studies have indicated that the use of hypnotic/sedative agents (including ramelteon) for sleep has been associated with hypersensitivity reactions including anaphylaxis as well as angioedema. Do not rechallenge patients who have developed angioedema with ramelteon therapy. An increased risk for hazardous sleep-related activities such as sleep-driving; cooking and eating food, and making phone calls while asleep have also been noted. Use caution with preexisting depression or other psychiatric conditions. Caution when using with other CNS depressants; avoid engaging in hazardous activities or activities requiring mental alertness. Not recommended for use in patients with severe sleep apnea or COPD. Use caution with moderate hepatic impairment; not recommended in patients with severe impairment. May cause disturbances of hormonal regulation. Use caution when administered concomitantly with strong CYP1A2 inhibitors.

Adverse Reactions 1% to 10%:

Central nervous system: Dizziness (4% to 5%), somnolence (3% to 5%), fatigue (3% to 4%), insomnia worsened (3%), depression (2%)

Endocrine & metabolic: Serum cortisol decreased (1%)

Gastrointestinal: Nausea (3%), taste perversion (2%)

Neuromuscular & skeletal: Myalgia (2%), arthralgia (2%)

Respiratory: Upper respiratory infection (3%)

Miscellaneous: Influenza (1%)

Postmarketing and/or case reports: Anaphylaxis, angioedema, complex sleep-related behavior (sleep-driving, cooking or eating food, making phone calls), prolactin levels increased, testosterone levels decreased

Drug Interactions

Metabolism/Transport Effects **Substrate** of CYP1A2 (major), CYP2C19 (minor), CYP3A4 (minor); **Note:** Assignment of Major/Minor substrate status based on clinically relevant drug interaction potential

Avoid Concomitant Use

Avoid concomitant use of Ramelteon with any of the following: Azelastine (Nasal); FluvoxaMINE; Paraldehyde; Sodium Oxybate

Increased Effect/Toxicity

Ramelteon may increase the levels/effects of: Alcohol (Ethyl); Azelastine (Nasal); Buprenorphine; CNS Depressants; Hydrocodone; Methotrimeprazine; Metyrosine; Mirtazapine; Paraldehyde; Pramipexole; ROPINIRole; Rotigotine; Selective Serotonin Reuptake Inhibitors; Sodium Oxybate; Zolpidem

The levels/effects of Ramelteon may be increased by: Abiraterone Acetate; Brimonidine (Topical); CYP1A2 Inhibitors (Moderate); CYP1A2 Inhibitors (Strong); Deferasirox; Doxylamine; Droperidol; Fluconazole; FluvoxaMINE; HydrOXYzine; Ketoconazole (Systemic); Magnesium Sulfate; Methotrimeprazine; Perampanel; Tapentadol; Vemurafenib

Decreased Effect

The levels/effects of Ramelteon may be decreased by: Rifamycin Derivatives

Ethanol/Nutrition/Herb Interactions

Ethanol: May increase CNS depression. Management: Avoid or limit ethanol.

Food: Taking with high-fat meal delays T_{max} and increases AUC (~31%). Management: Do not take with a high-fat meal.

Herb/Nutraceutical: Some herbal medications may increase CNS depression. Management: Avoid valerian, St John's wort, kava kava, and gotu kola.

Storage/Stability Store at 25°C (77°F); excursions permitted to 15°C to 30°C (59°F to 86°F). Protect from moisture.

Mechanism of Action Potent, selective agonist of melatonin receptors MT_1 and MT_2 (with little affinity for MT_3) within the suprachiasmic nucleus of the hypothalamus, an area responsible for determination of circadian rhythms and synchronization of the sleep-wake cycle. Agonism of MT_1 is thought to preferentially induce sleepiness, while MT_2 receptor activation preferentially influences regulation of circadian rhythms. Ramelteon is eightfold more selective for MT_1 than MT_2 and exhibits nearly sixfold higher affinity for MT_1 than melatonin, presumably allowing for enhanced effects on sleep induction.

Pharmacodynamics/Kinetics

Onset of action: 30 minutes

Absorption: Rapid; high-fat meal delays T_{max} and increases AUC (~31%)

Distribution: 74 L

Protein binding: ~82%

Metabolism: Extensive first-pass effect; oxidative metabolism primarily through CYP1A2 and to a lesser extent through CYP2C and CYP3A4; forms active metabolite (M-II)

Bioavailability: Absolute: 1.8%

Half-life elimination: Ramelteon: 1-2.6 hours; M-II: 2-5 hours

Time to peak, plasma: Median: 0.5-1.5 hours

Excretion: Primarily as metabolites: Urine (84%); feces (4%)

Dosage Oral: Adults: One 8 mg tablet within 30 minutes of bedtime

Dosage adjustment in renal impairment: No dosage adjustment necessary.

Dosage adjustment in hepatic impairment:

Mild-to-moderate impairment: No dosage adjustment necessary. Use with caution.

Severe impairment: Use is not recommended.

Dietary Considerations Do not take with high-fat meal.

Administration Do not administer with a high-fat meal. Swallow tablet whole; do not break.

Dosage Forms Excipient information presented when available (limited, particularly for generics); consult specific product labeling.

Tablet, Oral:

Rozerem: 8 mg

Ramipril (RA mi pril)

Brand Names: U.S. Altace

Brand Names: Canada Altace; Apo-Ramipril; Auro-Ramipri; Ava-Ramipril; CO Ramipril; Dom-Ramipril; JAMP-Ramipril; Mylan-Ramipril; PMS-Ramipril; Pro-Ramipril; RAN-Ramipril; ratio-Ramipril; Sandoz-Ramipril; Teva-Ramipril

Pharmacologic Category Angiotensin-Converting Enzyme (ACE) Inhibitor; Antihypertensive

Additional Appendix Information

Angiotensin Agents *on page 2280*

Use

Heart failure post-myocardial infarction: Treatment of heart failure after myocardial infarction (MI)

Hypertension: Treatment of hypertension, alone or in combination with thiazide diuretics

Reduction in risk of MI, stroke, and death from cardiovascular causes: To reduce the risk of MI, stroke, and death in patients ≥55 years of age at high risk of developing major cardiovascular events

Unlabeled Use Treatment of heart failure; to delay the progression of nephropathy and reduce risks of cardiovascular events in hypertensive patients with type 1 or 2 diabetes mellitus

Pregnancy Risk Factor D

Pregnancy Considerations [U.S. Boxed Warning]: Drugs that act on the renin-angiotensin system can cause injury and death to the developing fetus. Discontinue as soon as possible once pregnancy is detected. Ramipril crosses the placenta; teratogenic effects may occur following maternal use during pregnancy. Drugs that act on the renin-angiotensin system are associated with oligohydramnios. Oligohydramnios, due to decreased fetal renal function, may lead to fetal lung hypoplasia and skeletal malformations. Their use in pregnancy is also associated with anuria, hypotension, renal failure, skull hypoplasia, and death in the fetus/neonate. Chronic maternal hypertension itself is also associated with adverse events in the fetus/infant. ACE inhibitors are not recommended during pregnancy to treat maternal hypertension or heart failure. Use of an ACE inhibitor should also be avoided in any woman of reproductive age. Women who are planning a pregnancy should be considered for other medication options if an ACE inhibitor is currently prescribed or the ACE inhibitor should be discontinued as soon as possible once pregnancy is detected. The exposed fetus should be monitored for fetal growth, amniotic fluid volume, and organ formation. Infants exposed to an ACE inhibitor in utero should be monitored for hyperkalemia, hypotension, and oliguria.

Breast-Feeding Considerations Ramipril and its metabolites were not detected in breast milk following a single oral dose of 10 mg. It is not known if multiple doses will produce detectable levels. Breast-feeding is not recommended by the manufacturer.

Contraindications Hypersensitivity to ramipril or any component of the formulation; prior hypersensitivity (including angioedema) to ACE inhibitors; concomitant use with aliskiren in patients with diabetes mellitus

Warnings/Precautions Anaphylactic reactions may occur rarely with ACE inhibitors. At any time during treatment (especially following first dose) angioedema may occur rarely with ACE inhibitors; it may involve the head and neck (potentially compromising airway) or the intestine (presenting with abdominal pain). African-Americans and patients with idiopathic or hereditary angioedema may be at an increased risk. Prolonged frequent monitoring may be required especially if tongue, glottis, or larynx are involved as they are associated with airway obstruction. Patients with a history of airway surgery may have a higher risk of airway obstruction. Aggressive early and appropriate management is critical. Use in patients with previous angioedema associated with ACE inhibitor therapy is contraindicated. Severe anaphylactoid reactions may be seen during hemodialysis (eg, CVVHD) with high-flux dialysis membranes (eg, AN69), and rarely, during low density lipoprotein apheresis with dextran sulfate cellulose. Rare cases of anaphylactoid reactions have been reported in patients undergoing sensitization treatment with hymenoptera (bee, wasp) venom while receiving ACE inhibitors.

Symptomatic hypotension with or without syncope can occur with ACE inhibitors (usually with the first several doses); effects are most often observed in volume-depleted patients; close monitoring of patient is required especially with initial dosing and dosing increases; blood pressure must be lowered at a rate appropriate for the patient's clinical condition. Initiation of therapy in patients with ischemic heart disease or cerebrovascular disease warrants close observation due to the potential consequences posed by falling blood pressure (eg, MI, stroke). Use with caution in hypertrophic cardiomyopathy with outflow tract obstruction, severe aortic stenosis, or before, during, or immediately after major surgery. **[U.S. Boxed Warning]: Drugs that act on the renin-angiotensin system can cause injury and death to the developing fetus. Discontinue as soon as possible once pregnancy is detected.**

Hyperkalemia may occur with ACE inhibitors; risk factors include renal dysfunction, diabetes mellitus, concomitant use of potassium-sparing diuretics, potassium supplements, and/or potassium containing salts. Use cautiously, if at all, with these agents and monitor potassium closely. Cough may occur with ACE inhibitors. Other causes of cough should be considered (eg, pulmonary congestion in patients with heart failure) and excluded prior to discontinuation.

May be associated with deterioration of renal function and/or increases in serum creatinine, particularly in patients with low renal blood flow (eg, renal artery stenosis, heart failure) whose glomerular filtration rate (GFR) is dependent on efferent arteriolar vasoconstriction by angiotensin II; deterioration may result in oliguria, acute renal failure, and progressive azotemia. Small increases in serum creatinine may occur following initiation; consider discontinuation only in patients with progressive and/or significant deterioration in renal function. Use with caution in patients with unstented unilateral/bilateral renal artery stenosis. When unstented bilateral renal artery stenosis is present, use is generally avoided due to the elevated risk of deterioration in renal function unless possible benefits outweigh risks. Potentially significant drug-drug interactions may exist, requiring dose or frequency adjustment, additional monitoring, and/or selection of alternative therapy.

Rare toxicities associated with ACE inhibitors include cholestatic jaundice (which may progress to fulminant hepatic necrosis), agranulocytosis, neutropenia, or leukopenia with myeloid hypoplasia. Patients with collagen vascular diseases (especially with concomitant renal impairment) or renal impairment alone may be at increased risk for hematologic toxicity; periodically monitor CBC with differential in these patients.

Adverse Reactions Note: Frequency ranges include data from hypertension and heart failure trials. Higher rates of adverse reactions have generally been noted in patients with CHF. However, the frequency of adverse effects associated with placebo is also increased in this population.

>10%: Respiratory: Cough increased (7% to 12%)

1% to 10%:

- Cardiovascular: Hypotension (11%), angina (up to 3%), orthostatic hypotension (2%), syncope (up to 2%)
- Central nervous system: Headache (1% to 5%), dizziness (2% to 4%), fatigue (2%), vertigo (up to 2%)
- Endocrine & metabolic: Hyperkalemia (1% to 10%)
- Gastrointestinal: Nausea/vomiting (1% to 2%)
- Neuromuscular & skeletal: Chest pain (noncardiac) (1%)
- Renal: Renal dysfunction (1%), serum creatinine increased (1% to 2%), BUN increased (<1% to 3%); transient increases of creatinine and/or BUN may occur more frequently
- Respiratory: Cough (estimated 1% to 10%)

<1% (Limited to important or life-threatening): Agranulocytosis, amnesia, anaphylactoid reaction, angioedema, arrhythmia, bone marrow depression, convulsions, depression, dysphagia, eosinophilia, erythema multiforme, hearing loss, hemolytic anemia, hepatitis, hypersensitivity reactions (urticaria, rash, fever), impotence, insomnia, MI, neuropathy, onycholysis, pancreatitis,

pancytopenia, pemphigoid, pemphigus, photosensitivity, proteinuria, Stevens-Johnson syndrome, symptomatic hypotension, thrombocytopenia, toxic epidermal necrolysis, visual hallucinations (Doane, 2013)

Worsening of renal function may occur in patients with bilateral renal artery stenosis or in hypovolemia. In addition, a syndrome which may include fever, myalgia, arthralgia, interstitial nephritis, vasculitis, rash, eosinophilia and positive ANA, and elevated ESR has been reported with ACE inhibitors. Risk of pancreatitis and/or agranulocytosis may be increased in patients with collagen vascular disease or renal impairment.

Drug Interactions

Metabolism/Transport Effects None known.

Avoid Concomitant Use

Avoid concomitant use of Ramipril with any of the following: Telmisartan

Increased Effect/Toxicity

Ramipril may increase the levels/effects of: Allopurinol; Amifostine; Antihypertensives; AzaTHIOprine; CycloSPORINE (Systemic); Ferric Gluconate; Gold Sodium Thiomalate; Hypotensive Agents; Iron Dextran Complex; Lithium; Nonsteroidal Anti-Inflammatory Agents; Obinutuzumab; RiTUXimab; Sodium Phosphates

The levels/effects of Ramipril may be increased by: Alfuzosin; Aliskiren; Angiotensin II Receptor Blockers; Brimonidine (Topical); Canagliflozin; Diazoxide; DPP-IV Inhibitors; Eplerenone; Everolimus; Heparin; Heparin (Low Molecular Weight); Herbs (Hypotensive Properties); Loop Diuretics; MAO Inhibitors; Pentoxifylline; Phosphodiesterase 5 Inhibitors; Potassium Salts; Potassium-Sparing Diuretics; Prostacyclin Analogues; Sirolimus; Telmisartan; Temsirolimus; Thiazide Diuretics; TiZANidine; Tolvaptan; Trimethoprim

Decreased Effect

The levels/effects of Ramipril may be decreased by: Aprotinin; Herbs (Hypertensive Properties); Icatibant; Lanthanum; Methylphenidate; Nonsteroidal Anti-Inflammatory Agents; Salicylates; Yohimbine

Ethanol/Nutrition/Herb Interactions

Food: Potassium supplements and/or potassium-containing salts may cause or worsen hyperkalemia. Management: Advise patient to consult prescriber before consuming a potassium-rich diet, potassium supplements, or salt substitutes.

Herb/Nutraceutical: Bayberry, blue cohosh, cayenne, ephedra, ginger, ginseng (American), kola, licorice (may worsen hypertension). Black cohosh, California poppy, coleus, golden seal, hawthorn, mistletoe, periwinkle, quinine, shepherd's purse (may have increased antihypertensive effect). Management: Advise patients to consult prescriber before taking herbs with hyper/hypotensive properties during therapy.

Storage/Stability Store at 15°C to 30°C (59°F to 86°F). Ramipril mixed with applesauce, apple juice, or water may be stored at room temperature for up to 24 hours or for up to 48 hours under refrigeration.

Mechanism of Action Ramipril is an ACE inhibitor which prevents the formation of angiotensin II from angiotensin I and exhibits pharmacologic effects that are similar to captopril. Ramipril must undergo enzymatic saponification by esterases in the liver to its biologically active metabolite, ramiprilat. The pharmacodynamic effects of ramipril result from the high-affinity, competitive, reversible binding of ramiprilat to angiotensin-converting enzyme, thus preventing the formation of the potent vasoconstrictor angiotensin II. This isomerized enzyme-inhibitor complex has a slow rate of dissociation, which results in high potency and a long duration of action; a CNS mechanism may also be involved in the hypotensive effect as angiotensin II increases adrenergic outflow from CNS; vasoactive kallikreins may be decreased in conversion to active hormones by ACE inhibitors, thus reducing blood pressure

Pharmacodynamics/Kinetics

Onset of action: 1-2 hours

Duration: 24 hours

Absorption: Well absorbed (50% to 60%)

Distribution: Plasma levels decline in a triphasic fashion; rapid decline is a distribution phase to peripheral compartment, plasma protein and tissue ACE (half-life: 2-4 hours); second phase is an apparent elimination phase representing the clearance of free ramiprilat (half-life: 9-18 hours); and final phase is the terminal elimination phase representing the equilibrium phase between tissue binding and dissociation

Protein binding: Ramipril: 73%; Ramiprilat: 56%

Metabolism: Hepatic to the active form, ramiprilat

Bioavailability: Ramipril: 28%; Ramiprilat: 44%

Half-life elimination: Ramiprilat: Effective: 13-17 hours; Terminal: >50 hours

Time to peak, serum: Ramipril: ~1 hour; Ramiprilat: 2-4 hours

Excretion: Urine (60%) and feces (40%) as parent drug and metabolites

Dosage

Adults: Oral: **Note:** Consider discontinuation or dose reduction of concomitant diuretic when initiating ramipril. If diuretic cannot be discontinued or dose reduced, consider reduced initial ramipril dose. Monitor blood pressure closely until stabilized.

Heart failure post-myocardial infarction: Initial: 2.5 mg twice daily (patient should be monitored for at least 2 hours after initial dose and for at least an additional hour after blood pressure has stabilized); may reduce dose to 1.25 mg twice daily for hypotension. Reduce the dose of any concomitant diuretics, if possible. Continue initial dose for one week then titrate upward every 3 weeks as tolerated to target dose of 5 mg twice daily

Heart failure (unlabeled use): Initial: 1.25-2.5 mg once daily; target dose: 10 mg once daily (ACC/AHA 2009 Heart Failure Guidelines)

Hypertension: Initial dose in patients not receiving a diuretic is 2.5 mg once daily; titrate to effect. Usual maintenance: 2.5-20 mg daily in 1 or 2 divided doses (consider twice daily administration for patients unable to maintain adequate blood pressure control with once daily administration).

Reduction in risk of MI, stroke, and death from cardiovascular causes: Initial: 2.5 mg once daily for 1 week, then 5 mg once daily for the next 3 weeks, then increase as tolerated to 10 mg once daily (may be given as divided dose in hypertensive or recently post-MI patients)

Elderly: Oral: Adjust for renal function for elderly since glomerular filtration rates are decreased; may see exaggerated hypotensive effects if renal clearance is not considered. In the management of hypertension, consider lower initial doses and titrate to response (Aronow, 2011).

Dosage adjustment for patients with volume depletion: Initial: Administer 1.25 mg once daily; titrate as tolerated to effect.

Dosage adjustment in renal impairment:

Cl_{cr} >40 mL/minute: No dosage adjustment necessary.

Cl_{cr} <40 mL/minute: Administer 25% of normal dose.

Renal artery stenosis: Initial: 1.25 mg once daily; titrate as tolerated to effect

Renal failure and heart failure post-MI: Initial: 1.25 mg once daily, may increase to 1.25 mg twice daily and then up to 2.5 mg twice daily as tolerated

Renal failure and hypertension: Initial: 1.25 mg once daily, titrated as tolerated to effect; maximum: 5 mg daily

Dosage adjustment in hepatic impairment: No dosage adjustment provided in manufacturer's labeling; discontinue use for jaundice or marked elevation of hepatic enzymes.

Administration Swallow capsule whole; may open the capsule and the mix contents with 120 mL of water, apple juice, or applesauce.

Monitoring Parameters Blood pressure; serum creatinine and potassium; if patient has collagen vascular disease and/or renal impairment, periodically monitor CBC with differential

Test Interactions Positive Coombs' [direct]; may cause false-positive results in urine acetone determinations using sodium nitroprusside reagent

Dosage Forms Excipient information presented when available (limited, particularly for generics); consult specific product labeling.

Capsule, Oral:

Altace: 1.25 mg

Altace: 2.5 mg [contains fd&c red #40, fd&c yellow #10 (quinoline yellow)]

Altace: 5 mg [contains brilliant blue fcf (fd&c blue #1), fd&c red #40]

Altace: 10 mg [contains brilliant blue fcf (fd&c blue #1)]

Generic: 1.25 mg, 2.5 mg, 5 mg, 10 mg

Dosage Forms: Canada Note: Also refer to Dosage Forms. Excipient information presented when available (limited, particularly for generics); consult specific product labeling.

Capsule, Oral:

Altace: 15 mg

- **Ran-Alendronate (Can)** *see* Alendronate *on page 69*
- **RAN™-Amlodipine (Can)** *see* AmLODIPine *on page 109*
- **RAN™-Atenolol (Can)** *see* Atenolol *on page 186*
- **RAN-Atorvastatin (Can)** *see* AtorvaSTATin *on page 190*
- **Ran-Candesartan (Can)** *see* Candesartan *on page 327*
- **RAN™-Carvedilol (Can)** *see* Carvedilol *on page 355*
- **RAN™-Cefprozil (Can)** *see* Cefprozil *on page 377*
- **RAN-Ciproflox (Can)** *see* Ciprofloxacin (Systemic) *on page 430*
- **RAN™-Citalo (Can)** *see* Citalopram *on page 440*
- **RAN-Clarithromycin (Can)** *see* Clarithromycin *on page 446*
- **RAN-Clopidogrel (Can)** *see* Clopidogrel *on page 471*
- **RAN-Enalapril (Can)** *see* Enalapril *on page 701*
- **Ranexa** *see* Ranolazine *on page 1785*
- **RAN-Fentanyl Matrix Patch (Can)** *see* FentaNYL *on page 842*
- **RAN-Fentanyl Transdermal System (Can)** *see* FentaNYL *on page 842*
- **RAN-Fosinopril (Can)** *see* Fosinopril *on page 923*
- **RAN-Gabapentin (Can)** *see* Gabapentin *on page 933*

Ranibizumab (ra ni BIZ oo mab)

Brand Names: U.S. Lucentis

Brand Names: Canada Lucentis®

Index Terms rhuFabV2

Pharmacologic Category Angiogenesis Inhibitor; Monoclonal Antibody; Ophthalmic Agent; Vascular Endothelial Growth Factor (VEGF) Inhibitor

Use Treatment of neovascular (wet) age-related macular degeneration (AMD); treatment of macular edema following retinal vein occlusion (RVO); diabetic macular edema (DME)

Pregnancy Risk Factor C

Pregnancy Considerations Adverse fetal effects have been observed in some animal reproduction studies. Based on its mechanism of action, adverse effects on pregnancy would be expected. Canadian labeling recommends that women of childbearing potential use effective contraception during therapy and to wait 3 months after therapy before trying to conceive.

Breast-Feeding Considerations It is not known if ranibizumab is excreted in breast milk. The manufacturer recommends that caution be exercised when administering ranibizumab to nursing women.

Contraindications Hypersensitivity to ranibizumab or any component of the formulation; ocular or periocular infection

Canadian labeling: Additional contraindications (not in U.S. labeling): Active intraocular inflammation

Warnings/Precautions Intravitreous injections may be associated with endophthalmitis and retinal detachments. Proper aseptic injection techniques should be used. Patients should be monitored for potential infection following the injection and instructed to report any signs of infection immediately. Prior to and following intravitreal injection, Intraocular pressure may increase following injection. Onset postinjection is seen within 60 minutes. Monitor intraocular pressure before and after injection and manage accordingly. Intravitreal injections of ranibizumab may induce temporary visual disturbances that impair the ability to drive or operate machinery. Affected patients should be advised to abstain from driving or using machinery until resolution of disturbances. Risk of thromboembolic events, particularly stroke, may be increased following intravitreal administration of VEGF inhibitors. Use caution in patients with known risk factors (eg, history of stroke, TIA). Hypersensitivity may present as severe intraocular inflammation; instruct patients to report intraocular inflammation that increases with severity. Rare hypersensitivity reactions (including anaphylaxis) have been associated with another VEGF inhibitor, pegaptanib, occurring within several hours of use; monitor closely. Equipment and appropriate personnel should be available for monitoring and treatment of anaphylaxis.

Pooled analysis of trials involving diabetic macular edema (DME) patients revealed a higher incidence of fatal events in DME patients treated with ranibizumab compared to control (3% in patients treated with 0.3 mg in the first 2 years compared to 1% in the control). Overall, the incidence of fatalities was consistent with deaths normally observed in patients with advanced diabetic complications, however, a potential association between fatal events and intravitreal administration of VEGF inhibitors cannot be excluded.

Adverse Reactions Note: Rates of ocular adverse reactions reported for control group when percentages overlapped with treatment group.

As reported with AMD, RVO, and DME studies:

>10%:

Cardiovascular: Arterial thromboembolic events (AMD trials during first year: 2%; control: 1%; DME trials at 3 years: 11%; control rate not given)

Ocular: Conjunctival hemorrhage (48% to 74%; control: 32% to 60%), eye pain (17% to 35%; control 12% to 30%), vitreous floaters (7% to 27%), intraocular pressure increased (7% to 24%), blurred vision/visual disturbance (5% to 18%), intraocular inflammation (1% to 18%; control 3% to 8%), foreign body sensation (7% to 16%; control: 5% to 14%)

Note: Cataract, blepharitis, dry eye, eye irritation, lacrimation increased, maculopathy, ocular hyperemia, pruritus, and vitreous detachment occurred in >10% of patients, but also occurred either in similar percentages to the control or more often in the control in some studies.

1% to 10%:

Cardiovascular: Stroke (AMD trials during 2 years: 3%; control: 1%; DME trials at 3 years: 2%; control rate not given)

Ocular: Retinal degeneration (1% to 8%), injection site hemorrhage (≤5%)

Note: Conjunctival hyperemia, ocular discomfort, posterior capsule opacification, and retinal disorder occurred in 1% to 10% of patients, but also occurred in similar percentages to the control or more often in the control in some of the studies.

Miscellaneous: Ranibizumab antibodies (1% to 8%), influenza (3% to 7%; control: 2% to 5%)

All indications: <1% (Limited to important or life-threatening): Anterior chamber inflammation, anxiety, back pain, corneal edema, corneal epithelium defect, corneal erosion, coronary artery occlusion, dizziness, endophthalmitis, eyelid pain, hypoglycemia, iatrogenic traumatic cataracts, intestinal obstruction, lid margin discharge, photophobia, retinal pigment epithelium tear, rhegmatogenous retinal detachments, rhinorrhea, urticaria, visual acuity decreased

Drug Interactions

Metabolism/Transport Effects None known.

Avoid Concomitant Use There are no known interactions where it is recommended to avoid concomitant use.

Increased Effect/Toxicity There are no known significant interactions involving an increase in effect.

Decreased Effect There are no known significant interactions involving a decrease in effect.

Storage/Stability Store in original carton under refrigeration at 2°C to 8°C (36°F to 46°F). Protect from light. Do not freeze.

Mechanism of Action Ranibizumab is a recombinant humanized monoclonal antibody fragment which binds to and inhibits human vascular endothelial growth factor A (VEGF-A). Ranibizumab inhibits VEGF from binding to its receptors and thereby suppressing neovascularization and slowing vision loss.

Pharmacodynamics/Kinetics

Absorption: Low levels are detected in the serum following intravitreal injection

Half-life elimination: Vitreous: ~9 days

Dosage

Age-related macular degeneration (AMD): Adults: Intravitreal:

U.S. labeling: 0.5 mg once a month. Frequency may be reduced (eg, 4-5 injections over 9 months) after the first 3 injections or may be reduced after the first 4 injections to once every 3 months if monthly injections are not feasible.

Canadian labeling: 0.5 mg once a month. Frequency may be reduced after the first 3 injections to once every 3 months if monthly injections are not feasible.

Note: A regimen averaging 4-5 doses over 9 months is expected to maintain visual acuity and an every-3-month dosing regimen has reportedly resulted in a ~5 letter (1 line) loss of visual acuity over 9 months, as compared to monthly dosing which may result in an additional ~1-2 letter gain.

Diabetic macular edema (DME): Adults: Intravitreal:

U.S. labeling: 0.3 mg once a month

Canadian labeling: 0.5 mg once a month until achievement of stable visual acuity for 3 consecutive months. Upon discontinuation, may resume monthly therapy if monitoring identifies a loss of visual acuity.

Macular edema following retinal vein occlusion (RVO): Adults: Intravitreal: 0.5 mg once a month. **Note:** Canadian labeling recommends continuing therapy until achievement of stable visual acuity for 3 consecutive months; upon discontinuation, may resume monthly therapy if monitoring identifies a loss of visual acuity.

Dosage adjustment in renal impairment: No dosage adjustment necessary.

Dosage adjustment in hepatic impairment: No dosage adjustment provided in manufacturer's labeling. However, significant systemic exposure is not expected.

Administration For ophthalmic intravitreal injection only. Remove contents from vial using a 5 micron 19-gauge filter needle attached to a tuberculin syringe. Discard filter needle and replace with a sterile 30 gauge 1/2 inch needle for injection (do not use filter needle for intravitreal injection). Adequate anesthesia and a topical broad-spectrum antimicrobial agent should be administered prior to the procedure. Canadian labeling recommends administering ranibizumab at least 30 minutes after laser photocoagulation therapy when administered on the same day.

Monitoring Parameters Intraocular pressure (prior to and 30 minutes following injection via tonometry); consider checking for perfusion of the optic nerve head immediately following injection; signs of infection/inflammation (for first week following injection); retinal perfusion, endophthalmitis; visual acuity

Dosage Forms Excipient information presented when available (limited, particularly for generics); consult specific product labeling.

Solution, Intraocular [preservative free]:

Lucentis: 0.3 mg/0.05 mL (0.05 mL); 0.5 mg/0.05 mL (0.05 mL)

Dosage Forms: Canada Excipient information presented when available (limited, particularly for generics); consult specific product labeling.

Injection, solution [preservative free]:

Lucentis®: 10 mg/mL (0.3 mL)

◆ **RAN™-Imipenem-Cilastatin (Can)** *see* Imipenem and Cilastatin *on page 1052*

◆ **Ran-Irbesartan HCTZ (Can)** *see* Irbesartan and Hydrochlorothiazide *on page 1115*

Ranitidine (ra NI ti deen)

Brand Names: U.S. Acid Reducer Maximum Strength [OTC] [DSC]; Acid Reducer [OTC]; Ranitidine Acid Reducer [OTC]; Zantac; Zantac 150 Maximum Strength [OTC]; Zantac 75 [OTC]; Zantac EFFERdose [DSC]; Zantac in NaCl [DSC]

Brand Names: Canada Acid Reducer; Apo-Ranitidine®; CO Ranitidine; Dom-Ranitidine; Myl-Ranitidine; Mylan-Ranitidine; Nu-Ranit; PHL-Ranitidine; PMS-Ranitidine; Ranitidine Injection, USP; RAN™-Ranitidine; ratio-Ranitidine; Riva-Ranitidine; Sandoz-Ranitidine; ScheinPharm Ranitidine; Teva-Ranitidine; Zantac 75®; Zantac Maximum Strength Non-Prescription; Zantac®

Index Terms Ranitidine Hydrochloride

Pharmacologic Category Histamine H_2 Antagonist

Use

Zantac®: Short-term and maintenance therapy of duodenal ulcer, gastric ulcer, gastroesophageal reflux disease (GERD), active benign ulcer, erosive esophagitis, and pathological hypersecretory conditions; as part of a multidrug regimen for *H. pylori* eradication to reduce the risk of duodenal ulcer recurrence

Zantac 75® [OTC]: Relief of heartburn, acid indigestion, and sour stomach

Unlabeled Use Recurrent postoperative ulcer, upper GI bleeding, prevention of acid-aspiration pneumonitis during surgery, and prevention of stress-induced ulcers

Pregnancy Risk Factor B

Pregnancy Considerations Adverse events were not observed in animal studies; therefore, ranitidine is classified as pregnancy category B. Ranitidine crosses the placenta. An increased risk of congenital malformations or adverse events in the newborn has generally not been observed following maternal use of ranitidine during pregnancy. Histamine H_2 antagonists have been evaluated for the treatment of gastroesophageal reflux disease (GERD) as well as gastric and duodenal ulcers during pregnancy. If needed, ranitidine is the agent of choice. Histamine H_2 antagonists may be used for aspiration prophylaxis prior to cesarean delivery.

Breast-Feeding Considerations Ranitidine is excreted into breast milk. The manufacturer recommends that caution be exercised when administering ranitidine to nursing women. Peak milk concentrations of ranitidine occur ~5.5 hours after the dose (case report).

Contraindications Hypersensitivity to ranitidine or any component of the formulation

Warnings/Precautions Ranitidine has been associated with confusional states (rare). Use with caution in patients with hepatic impairment; use with caution in renal impairment, dosage modification required. Avoid use in patients with history of acute porphyria (may precipitate attacks); long-term therapy may be associated with vitamin B_{12} deficiency. Symptoms of GI distress may be associated with a variety of conditions; symptomatic response to H_2 antagonists does not rule out the potential for significant pathology (eg, malignancy). EFFERdose® formulation contains phenylalanine.

Adverse Reactions Frequency not defined.

Cardiovascular: Asystole, atrioventricular block, bradycardia (with rapid I.V. administration), premature ventricular beats, tachycardia, vasculitis

Central nervous system: Agitation, dizziness, depression, hallucinations, headache, insomnia, malaise, mental confusion, somnolence, vertigo

Dermatologic: Alopecia, erythema multiforme, rash

Endocrine & metabolic: Prolactin levels increased

Gastrointestinal: Abdominal discomfort/pain, constipation, diarrhea, nausea, necrotizing enterocolitis (VLBW neonates; Guillet, 2006), pancreatitis, vomiting

Hematologic: Acquired immune hemolytic anemia, acute porphyritic attack, agranulocytosis, aplastic anemia, granulocytopenia, leukopenia, pancytopenia, thrombocytopenia

Hepatic: Cholestatic hepatitis, hepatic failure, hepatitis, jaundice

Local: Transient pain, burning or itching at the injection site

Neuromuscular & skeletal: Arthralgia, involuntary motor disturbance, myalgia

Ocular: Blurred vision

Renal: Acute interstitial nephritis, serum creatinine increased

Respiratory: Pneumonia (causal relationship not established)

Miscellaneous: Anaphylaxis, angioneurotic edema, hypersensitivity reactions (eg, bronchospasm, fever, eosinophilia)

Drug Interactions

Metabolism/Transport Effects Substrate of CYP1A2 (minor), CYP2C19 (minor), CYP2D6 (minor), P-glycoprotein; **Note:** Assignment of Major/Minor substrate status based on clinically relevant drug interaction potential; **Inhibits** CYP1A2 (weak), CYP2D6 (weak)

Avoid Concomitant Use

Avoid concomitant use of Ranitidine with any of the following: Dasatinib; Delavirdine; PONATinib; Risedronate

Increased Effect/Toxicity

Ranitidine may increase the levels/effects of: ARIPiprazole; Dexmethylphenidate; Methylphenidate; Procainamide; Risedronate; Saquinavir; Sulfonylureas; Varenicline; Warfarin

The levels/effects of Ranitidine may be increased by: P-glycoprotein/ABCB1 Inhibitors

Decreased Effect

Ranitidine may decrease the levels/effects of: Atazanavir; Bosutinib; Cefditoren; Cefpodoxime; Cefuroxime; Dabrafenib; Dasatinib; Delavirdine; Erlotinib; Fosamprenavir; Gefitinib; Indinavir; Iron Salts; Itraconazole; Ketoconazole (Systemic); Mesalamine; Multivitamins/Minerals (with ADEK, Folate, Iron); Nelfinavir; Nilotinib; PONATinib; Posaconazole; Prasugrel; Rilpivirine; Vismodegib

The levels/effects of Ranitidine may be decreased by: Peginterferon Alfa-2b; P-glycoprotein/ABCB1 Inducers

Ethanol/Nutrition/Herb Interactions

Ethanol: Avoid ethanol (may cause gastric mucosal irritation).

Food: Does not interfere with absorption of ranitidine.

Preparation for Administration Vials can be mixed with NS or D_5W.

Intermittent bolus injection, continuous infusion: Dilute to maximum of 2.5 mg/mL.

Intermittent infusion: Dilute to maximum of 0.5 mg/mL.

Storage/Stability

Injection: Vials: Store between 4°C to 25°C (39°F to 77°F); excursion permitted to 30°C (86°F). Protect from light. Solution is a clear, colorless to yellow solution; slight darkening does not affect potency. Vials mixed with NS or D_5W are stable for 48 hours at room temperature.

Premixed bag: Store between 2°C to 25°C (36°F to 77°F). Protect from light.

EFFERdose® formulations: Store between 2°C to 30°C (36°F to 86°F).

Syrup: Store between 4°C to 25°C (39°F to 77°F). Protect from light.

Tablets: Store in dry place, between 15°C to 30°C (59°F to 86°F). Protect from light.

Mechanism of Action Competitive inhibition of histamine at H_2-receptors of the gastric parietal cells, which inhibits gastric acid secretion, gastric volume, and hydrogen ion concentration are reduced. Does not affect pepsin secretion, pentagastrin-stimulated intrinsic factor secretion, or serum gastrin.

Pharmacodynamics/Kinetics

Absorption: Oral: 50%

Distribution: Normal renal function: V_d: ~1.4 L/kg; Cl_{cr} 25-35 mL/minute: 1.76 L/kg minimally penetrates the blood-brain barrier

Protein binding: 15%

Metabolism: Hepatic to N-oxide, S-oxide, and N-desmethyl metabolites

Bioavailability: Oral: 48% to 50%; I.M.: 90% to 100%

Half-life elimination:

Oral: Normal renal function: 2.5-3 hours; Cl_{cr} 25-35 mL/minute: 4.8 hours

I.V.: Normal renal function: 2-2.5 hours

Time to peak, serum: Oral: 2-3 hours; I.M.: ≤15 minutes

Excretion: Urine: Oral: 30%, I.V.: 70% (as unchanged drug); feces (as metabolites)

Dosage

Children 1 month to 16 years:

Duodenal and gastric ulcer:

Oral:

Treatment: 4-8 mg/kg/day divided twice daily; maximum: 300 mg/day

Maintenance: 2-4 mg/kg/day once daily; maximum: 150 mg/day

I.V.: 2-4 mg/kg/day divided every 6-8 hours; maximum: 200 mg/day

GERD and erosive esophagitis:

Oral: 5-10 mg/kg/day divided twice daily; maximum: GERD: 300 mg/day, erosive esophagitis: 600 mg/day

I.V. (unlabeled): 2-4 mg/kg/day divided every 6-8 hours; maximum: 200 mg/day **or as an alternative**

Continuous infusion: Initial: 1 mg/kg/dose for one dose followed by infusion of 0.08-0.17 mg/kg/hour or 2-4 mg/kg/day

Children ≥12 years: Prevention of heartburn: Oral: Zantac 75® [OTC]: 75 mg 30-60 minutes before eating food or drinking beverages which cause heartburn; maximum: 150 mg/24 hours; do not use for more than 14 days

Adults:

Duodenal ulcer: Oral: Treatment: 150 mg twice daily, or 300 mg once daily after the evening meal or at bedtime; maintenance: 150 mg once daily at bedtime

Helicobacter pylori eradication: 150 mg twice daily; requires combination therapy

Pathological hypersecretory conditions:

Oral: 150 mg twice daily; adjust dose or frequency as clinically indicated; doses of up to 6 g/day have been used

I.V.: Continuous infusion for Zollinger-Ellison: Initial: 1 mg/kg/hour; measure gastric acid output at 4 hours, if >10 mEq or if patient is symptomatic, increase dose in increments of 0.5 mg/kg/hour; doses of up to 2.5 mg/kg/hour (or 220 mg/hour) have been used

Gastric ulcer, benign: Oral: 150 mg twice daily; maintenance: 150 mg once daily at bedtime

GERD: Oral: 150 mg twice daily

Erosive esophagitis: Oral: Treatment: 150 mg 4 times/day; maintenance: 150 mg twice daily

Prevention of heartburn: Oral: Zantac 75® [OTC]: 75 mg 30-60 minutes before eating food or drinking beverages which cause heartburn; maximum: 150 mg in 24 hours; do not use for more than 14 days

Stress ulcer prophylaxis, ICU patients (unlabeled use; ASHP, 1999): **Note:** Intended for patients with associated risk factors (eg, coagulopathy, mechanical ventilation for >48 hours, severe sepsis); discontinue use once risk factors have resolved. The Surviving Sepsis Campaign guidelines suggest the use of proton pump inhibitors rather than H_2 antagonist therapy (Dellinger, 2013).

Oral, nasogastric (NG) tube: 150 mg twice daily; may administer a 300 mg loading dose prior to maintenance dosing (Pemberton, 1993)

I.V.: Intermittent bolus: 50 mg every 6-8 hours (Cook, 1998; Geus 1993)

Patients not able to take oral medication:

I.M.: 50 mg every 6-8 hours

I.V.: Intermittent bolus or infusion: 50 mg every 6-8 hours

Continuous I.V. infusion: 6.25 mg/hour

Elderly: Ulcer healing rates and incidence of adverse effects are similar in the elderly, when compared to younger patients; dosing adjustments not necessary based on age alone

Dosage adjustment in renal impairment: Adults:

Cl_{cr} <50 mL/minute:

Oral: 150 mg every 24 hours; adjust dose cautiously if needed

I.V.: 50 mg every 18-24 hours; adjust dose cautiously if needed

Hemodialysis: Adjust dosing schedule so that dose coincides with the end of hemodialysis

Stress ulcer prophylaxis (ASHP, 1999): Cl_{cr} <50 mL/minute:

Oral, nasogastric (NG) tube: 150 mg 1-2 times daily

I.V.: Intermittent bolus: 50 mg every 12-24 hours

Dosage adjustment in hepatic disease: No dosage adjustment provided in manufacturer's labeling. However, no adjustment expected since undergoes minimal hepatic metabolism.

Dietary Considerations Some products may contain phenylalanine and/or sodium. Oral dosage forms may be taken with or without food.

Usual Infusion Concentrations: Pediatric Note: Premixed solutions available

I.V. infusion: 0.5 mg/mL

Usual Infusion Concentrations: Adult Note: Premixed solutions available

I.V. infusion: 50 mg in 50 mL (concentration: 1 mg/mL) **or** 500 mg in 250 mL (concentration: 2 mg/mL) of D_5W or NS

Administration

Ranitidine injection may be administered I.M. or I.V.:

I.M.: Injection is administered undiluted

I.V.: Must be diluted; may be administered I.V. push, intermittent I.V. infusion, or continuous I.V. infusion

I.V. push: Manufacturer recommends a maximum rate of administration of 10 mg/minute (or over 5 minutes); however, may also be administered at a maximum rate of 25 mg/minute (or over 2 minutes) if necessary (Coursin, 1988; Goelzer, 1988; Smith, 1987).

Intermittent I.V. infusion: Administer over 15-20 minutes

Continuous I.V. infusion: Titrate dosage based on gastric pH.

EFFERdose®: Should not be chewed, swallowed whole, or dissolved on tongue: 25 mg tablet: Dissolve in at least 5 mL of water; wait until completely dissolved before administering

Monitoring Parameters AST, ALT, serum creatinine; when used to prevent stress-related GI bleeding, measure the intragastric pH and try to maintain pH >4; signs and symptoms of peptic ulcer disease, occult blood with GI bleeding, monitor renal function to correct dose

Test Interactions False-positive urine protein using Multistix®; gastric acid secretion test; skin test allergen extracts. May also interfere with urine detection of amphetamine/methamphetamine (false-positive).

Dosage Forms Excipient information presented when available (limited, particularly for generics); consult specific product labeling. [DSC] = Discontinued product

Capsule, Oral:

Generic: 150 mg, 300 mg

Solution, Injection:

Zantac: 50 mg/2 mL (2 mL); 150 mg/6 mL (6 mL); 1000 mg/40 mL (40 mL) [contains phenol]

Generic: 50 mg/2 mL (2 mL); 150 mg/6 mL (6 mL); 1000 mg/40 mL (40 mL)

Solution, Intravenous [preservative free]:

Zantac in NaCl: 50 mg (50 mL [DSC])

Syrup, Oral:

Zantac: 15 mg/mL (480 mL [DSC]) [contains alcohol, usp, butylparaben, propylparaben, saccharin sodium; peppermint flavor]

Generic: 15 mg/mL (10 mL, 473 mL, 474 mL, 480 mL); 75 mg/5 mL (473 mL, 480 mL); 150 mg/10 mL (10 mL)

Tablet, Oral:

Acid Reducer: 75 mg

Acid Reducer: 75 mg [DSC] [sugar free]

Acid Reducer Maximum Strength: 150 mg [DSC] [sugar free; contains fd&c yellow #6 (sunset yellow)]

Ranitidine Acid Reducer: 75 mg

Zantac 75: 75 mg

Zantac: 150 mg, 300 mg

Zantac 150 Maximum Strength: 150 mg

Zantac 150 Maximum Strength: 150 mg [sodium free, sugar free; contains brilliant blue fcf (fd&c blue #1); mint flavor]

Generic: 75 mg, 150 mg, 300 mg

Tablet Effervescent, Oral:

Zantac EFFERdose: 25 mg [DSC] [contains aspartame, sodium benzoate]

◆ **Ranitidine Acid Reducer [OTC]** *see* Ranitidine *on page* 1782

◆ **Ranitidine Hydrochloride** *see* Ranitidine *on page* 1782

- ◆ **Ranitidine Injection, USP (Can)** *see* Ranitidine *on page 1782*
- ◆ **RAN-Letrozole (Can)** *see* Letrozole *on page 1185*
- ◆ **RAN-Levetiracetam (Can)** *see* LevETIRAcetam *on page 1194*
- ◆ **RAN-Lisinopril (Can)** *see* Lisinopril *on page 1226*
- ◆ **RAN-Losartan (Can)** *see* Losartan *on page 1247*
- ◆ **RAN™-Metformin (Can)** *see* MetFORMIN *on page 1310*

Ranolazine (ra NOE la zeen)

Brand Names: U.S. Ranexa

Pharmacologic Category Antianginal Agent; Cardiovascular Agent, Miscellaneous

Use Chronic angina: Treatment of chronic angina

Pregnancy Risk Factor C

Pregnancy Considerations Adverse events have been observed in animal reproduction studies.

Breast-Feeding Considerations It is not known if ranolazine is excreted into breast milk. Due to the potential for serious adverse reactions in the nursing infant, the manufacturer recommends a decision be made whether to discontinue nursing or to discontinue the drug, taking into account the importance of treatment to the mother.

Contraindications Hepatic cirrhosis; concurrent strong CYP3A inhibitors; concurrent CYP3A inducers

Warnings/Precautions Ranolazine has been shown to prolong QT interval in a dose/plasma concentration-related manner. Cirrhotic patients with mild to moderate hepatic impairment demonstrated a 3-fold increase in QT prolongation. The incidence of symptomatic arrhythmias was similar to placebo in one trial (Morrow, 2007). Risk versus benefit should be assessed in patient maintained on a higher dose (>2000 mg/day) or exposure, concurrent use of other QT-prolonging drugs, potassium-channel variants known to cause QT prolongation, family history of or congenital long QT syndrome, or known acquired QT interval prolongation. Use is contraindicated in patients with hepatic cirrhosis. Ranolazine plasma levels increase in patients with mild and moderate hepatic impairment. Acute renal failure has been observed in some patients with severe renal impairment (Cl_{cr} <30 mL/minute); if acute renal failure develops (marked increase in serum creatinine associated with increased BUN), discontinue ranolazine and manage appropriately. Monitor renal function periodically in patients with moderate to severe renal impairment; particularly for increases in serum creatinine accompanied but increased BUN. In a renal impairment study, patients with severe impairment exhibited an initial elevation in diastolic blood pressure (~12-17 mm Hg at day 3), however this diminished to ~4 mm Hg increase by day 5 (Jerling, 2005); consider monitoring blood pressure in patients with renal dysfunction. Ranolazine has not been evaluated in patients requiring dialysis.

Ranolazine will not relieve acute angina episode and has not demonstrated benefit in acute coronary syndrome. Although ranolazine produces small reductions in hemoglobin A_{1c}, it is not a treatment for diabetes. Potentially significant drug-drug interactions may exist, requiring dose or frequency adjustment, additional monitoring, and/or selection of alternative therapy. Use is contraindicated with inducers and strong inhibitors of CYP3A. Use with caution in patients ≥75 years of age; they may experience more adverse events (including serious adverse events) and drug discontinuations due to adverse events.

Adverse Reactions

>0.5% to 10%:

Cardiovascular: Bradycardia (≤4%), hypotension (≤4%), orthostatic hypotension (≤4%), palpitation (≤4%), peripheral edema (≤4%), QT_c prolongation (>500 msec: ≤1%)

Central nervous system: Headache (≤6%), dizziness (1% to 6%), confusion (≤4%), vasovagal attacks (≤4%), vertigo (≤4%)

Dermatologic: Hyperhidrosis (≤4%)

Gastrointestinal: Constipation (≤9%), abdominal pain (≤4%), anorexia (≤4%), dyspepsia (≤4%), nausea (≤4%; dose related), vomiting (≤4%), xerostomia (≤4%)

Neuromuscular: Weakness (≤4%)

Ocular: Blurred vision (≤4%)

Otic: Tinnitus (≤4%)

Renal: Hematuria (≤4%)

Respiratory: Dyspnea (≤4%)

≤0.5% (Limited to important or life-threatening): Angioedema, blood pressure increased, blood urea nitrogen increased, eosinophilia, hallucination, hemoglobin A_{1c} decreased, hypoesthesia, leukopenia, pancytopenia, paresthesia, pruritus, pulmonary fibrosis, rash, renal failure, serum creatinine increased, thrombocytopenia, T-wave amplitude decreased, T-wave changes (notched), torsade de pointes (case report [Morrow, 2007]), tremor

Drug Interactions

Metabolism/Transport Effects Substrate of CYP2D6 (minor), CYP3A4 (major), P-glycoprotein; **Note:** Assignment of Major/Minor substrate status based on clinically relevant drug interaction potential; **Inhibits** CYP2D6 (weak), CYP3A4 (weak), P-glycoprotein

Avoid Concomitant Use

Avoid concomitant use of Ranolazine with any of the following: Antifungal Agents (Azole Derivatives, Systemic); Bosutinib; CYP3A4 Inducers (Strong); CYP3A4 Inhibitors (Strong); Fusidic Acid (Systemic); Highest Risk QTc-Prolonging Agents; Ivabradine; Mifepristone; Pomalidomide; Rifampin; Silodosin; St Johns Wort; Topotecan; VinCRIStine (Liposomal)

Increased Effect/Toxicity

Ranolazine may increase the levels/effects of: Afatinib; ARIPiprazole; AtorvaSTATin; Bosutinib; Colchicine; Dabigatran Etexilate; Digoxin; Everolimus; Highest Risk QTc-Prolonging Agents; Lomitapide; Lovastatin; MetFORMIN; Moderate Risk QTc-Prolonging Agents; P-glycoprotein/ABCB1 Substrates; Pomalidomide; Prucalopride; Rivaroxaban; Silodosin; Simvastatin; Tacrolimus (Systemic); Topotecan; VinCRIStine (Liposomal)

The levels/effects of Ranolazine may be increased by: Antifungal Agents (Azole Derivatives, Systemic); Calcium Channel Blockers (Nondihydropyridine); CYP3A4 Inhibitors (Moderate); CYP3A4 Inhibitors (Strong); Dasatinib; Fusidic Acid (Systemic); Ivabradine; Ivacaftor; Luliconazole; Mifepristone; P-glycoprotein/ABCB1 Inhibitors; QTc-Prolonging Agents (Indeterminate Risk and Risk Modifying); Simeprevir

Decreased Effect

The levels/effects of Ranolazine may be decreased by: Bosentan; CYP3A4 Inducers (Strong); Dabrafenib; Deferasirox; Peginterferon Alfa-2b; P-glycoprotein/ABCB1 Inducers; Rifampin; St Johns Wort; Tocilizumab

Ethanol/Nutrition/Herb Interactions

Food: Grapefruit, grapefruit juice, or grapefruit-containing products may increase the serum concentration of ranolazine. Management: Avoid grapefruit-containing products or dose adjustment of ranolazine may be required.

Herb/Nutraceutical: St John's wort may decrease the serum concentration of ranolazine. Management: Avoid St John's wort.

Storage/Stability Store at 25°C (77°F); excursions permitted to 15°C to 30°C (59°F to 86°F).

Mechanism of Action Ranolazine exerts antianginal and anti-ischemic effects without changing hemodynamic parameters (heart rate or blood pressure). At therapeutic levels, ranolazine inhibits the late phase of the inward sodium channel (late I_{Na}) in ischemic cardiac myocytes during cardiac repolarization reducing intracellular sodium concentrations and thereby reducing calcium influx via Na^+-Ca^{2+} exchange. Decreased intracellular calcium reduces ventricular tension and myocardial oxygen consumption. It is thought that ranolazine produces myocardial relaxation and reduces anginal symptoms through this mechanism although this is uncertain. At higher concentrations, ranolazine inhibits the rapid delayed rectifier potassium current (I_{Kr}) thus prolonging the ventricular action potential duration and subsequent prolongation of the QT interval.

Pharmacodynamics/Kinetics

Absorption: Highly variable

Protein binding: ~62%

Metabolism: Extensive; Hepatic via CYP3A (major) and 2D6 (minor); intestines

Bioavailability: Tablet: 76% (compared to solution)

Half-life elimination: Ranolazine: Terminal: 7 hours; Metabolites (activity undefined): 6-22 hours

Time to peak, plasma: 2-5 hours

Excretion: Primarily urine (75% mostly as metabolites; <5% as unchanged drug); feces (25% mostly as metabolites; <5% as unchanged drug)

Dosage Note: May be used with beta-blockers, nitrates, calcium channel blockers, antiplatelet therapy, lipid-lowering therapy, angiotensin-converting enzyme (ACE) inhibitors, and angiotensin-receptor blockers.

Chronic angina: Oral:

Adults: Initial: 500 mg twice daily; may increase to 1000 mg twice daily as needed (based on symptoms); maximum recommended dose: 1000 mg twice daily

Elderly: Select dose cautiously, starting at the lower end of the dosing range

Missed doses: If a dose is missed, it should be taken at the next scheduled time; the next dose should not be doubled.

Dosage adjustment for ranolazine with concomitant medications:

Diltiazem, erythromycin, fluconazole, verapamil, and other moderate CYP3A inhibitors: Ranolazine dose should not exceed 500 mg twice daily

P-glycoprotein inhibitors (eg, cyclosporine): Titrate ranolazine based on clinical response

Dosage adjustment in renal impairment: No dosage adjustments provided in the manufacturer's labeling. However, plasma ranolazine levels increased ~40% to 50% in patients with varying degrees of renal dysfunction. Discontinue if acute renal failure develops. Ranolazine has not been evaluated in patients requiring dialysis.

Dosage adjustment in hepatic impairment: No dosage adjustment provided in the manufacturer's labeling. Use is contraindicated with hepatic cirrhosis.

Dietary Considerations Limit the use of grapefruit juice; the ranolazine dose should not exceed 500 mg twice daily when taken with grapefruit juice or grapefruit-containing products.

Administration Administer with or without meals. Swallow tablet whole; do not crush, break, or chew.

Monitoring Parameters Baseline and follow up ECG to evaluate QT interval; monitor renal function periodically in patients with moderate to severe renal impairment, particularly for increases in serum creatinine accompanied but increased BUN; consider monitoring blood pressure in patients with renal dysfunction; correct and maintain serum potassium in normal limits

Dosage Forms Excipient information presented when available (limited, particularly for generics); consult specific product labeling.

Tablet Extended Release 12 Hour, Oral:

Ranexa: 500 mg, 1000 mg

◆ **RAN™-Omeprazole (Can)** *see* Omeprazole *on page 1505*

◆ **RAN™-Ondansetron (Can)** *see* Ondansetron *on page 1510*

◆ **RAN™-Pantoprazole (Can)** *see* Pantoprazole *on page 1563*

◆ **RAN™-Pioglitazone (Can)** *see* Pioglitazone *on page 1649*

◆ **RAN-Pravastatin (Can)** *see* Pravastatin *on page 1700*

◆ **RAN™-Pregabalin (Can)** *see* Pregabalin *on page 1710*

◆ **RAN-Rabeprazole (Can)** *see* RABEprazole *on page 1769*

◆ **RAN-Ramipril (Can)** *see* Ramipril *on page 1778*

◆ **RAN™-Ranitidine (Can)** *see* Ranitidine *on page 1782*

◆ **RAN-Risperidone (Can)** *see* RisperiDONE *on page 1826*

◆ **RAN™-Ropinirole (Can)** *see* ROPINIRole *on page 1851*

◆ **RAN™-Rosuvastatin (Can)** *see* Rosuvastatin *on page 1858*

◆ **Ran-Sertraline (Can)** *see* Sertraline *on page 1889*

◆ **RAN-Simvastatin (Can)** *see* Simvastatin *on page 1899*

◆ **RAN™-Tamsulosin (Can)** *see* Tamsulosin *on page 1990*

◆ **Ran-Telmisartan (Can)** *see* Telmisartan *on page 2002*

◆ **RAN-Telmisartan HCTZ (Can)** *see* Telmisartan and Hydrochlorothiazide *on page 2004*

◆ **Ran-Valsartan (Can)** *see* Valsartan *on page 2154*

◆ **Ran-Venlafaxine XR (Can)** *see* Venlafaxine *on page 2178*

◆ **Rapaflo** *see* Silodosin *on page 1896*

◆ **Rapaflo® (Can)** *see* Silodosin *on page 1896*

◆ **Rapamune** *see* Sirolimus *on page 1902*

◆ **Rapamune® (Can)** *see* Sirolimus *on page 1902*

◆ **Rapamycin** *see* Sirolimus *on page 1902*

◆ **RapiMed Children's [OTC]** *see* Acetaminophen *on page 28*

◆ **RapiMed Junior [OTC]** *see* Acetaminophen *on page 28*

Rasagiline (ra SA ji leen)

Brand Names: U.S. Azilect

Brand Names: Canada Azilect®

Index Terms AGN 1135; Rasagiline Mesylate; TVP-1012

Pharmacologic Category Anti-Parkinson's Agent, MAO Type B Inhibitor

Additional Appendix Information

Antiparkinsonian Agents *on page 2289*

Tyramine Content of Foods *on page 2394*

Use Treatment of idiopathic Parkinson's disease (initial monotherapy or as adjunct to levodopa)

Pregnancy Risk Factor C

Pregnancy Considerations Animal studies have documented decreased offspring survival and birth weight. An increased incidence of teratogenic effects, embryo-fetal deaths, and cardiovascular abnormalities were also noted with rasagiline in combination with levodopa/carbidopa. There are no adequate and well-controlled studies in pregnant women.

Breast-Feeding Considerations Animal studies have shown rasagiline is capable of inhibiting prolactin secretion.

Contraindications Concomitant use of cyclobenzaprine, dextromethorphan, methadone, propoxyphene, St John's wort, or tramadol; concomitant use of meperidine or an MAO inhibitor (including selective MAO-B inhibitors) within 14 days of rasagiline

Warnings/Precautions Hazardous agent - use appropriate precautions for handling and disposal (NIOSH, 2012).

Cardiovascular system: May cause orthostatic hypotension, particularly in combination with levodopa; use with caution in patients with hypotension or patients who would not tolerate transient hypotensive episodes (cardiovascular or cerebrovascular disease); orthostasis is usually most problematic during first 2 months of therapy and tends to abate thereafter. Due to the potential for hemodynamic instability, patients should not undergo elective surgery requiring general anesthesia and should avoid local anesthesia containing sympathomimetic vasoconstrictors within 14 days of discontinuing rasagiline. If surgery is required, benzodiazepines, mivacurium, fentanyl, morphine or codeine may be used cautiously. In patients taking recommended doses of rasagiline, dietary restriction of most tyramine-containing products is not necessary; however, certain foods (eg, aged cheeses) may contain high amounts (>150 mg) of tyramine and could lead to hypertensive crisis. Avoid concomitant use with foods high in tyramine.

Central nervous system: Serotonin syndrome (SS)/neuroleptic malignant syndrome (NMS)-like reactions may occur rarely, particularly when used at doses exceeding recommendations or when used in combination with an antidepressant (eg, SSRI, SNRI, TCA). May cause hallucinations; signs of severe CNS toxicity (some fatal), including hyperpyrexia, hyperthermia, rigidity, altered mental status, seizure and coma have been reported with selective and nonselective MAO inhibitor use in combination with antidepressants. Do not use within 5 weeks of fluoxetine discontinuation; do not initiate tricyclic, SSRI, or SNRI therapy within 2 weeks of discontinuing rasagiline. Addition to levodopa therapy may result in exacerbation of dyskinesias, requiring a reduction in levodopa dosage.

Dermatologic: Risk of melanoma may be increased with rasagiline, although increased risk has been associated with Parkinson's disease itself; patients should have regular and frequent skin examinations.

Organ dysfunction: Use caution in mild hepatic impairment; dose reduction recommended. Do not use with moderate-to-severe hepatic impairment.

Adverse Reactions Unless otherwise noted, the following adverse reactions are as reported for monotherapy. Spectrum of adverse events was generally similar with adjunctive (levodopa) therapy, though the incidence tended to be higher.

>10%:

Cardiovascular: Orthostatic hypotension (6% to 13% adjunct therapy, dose dependent)

Central nervous system: Dyskinesia (18% adjunct therapy), headache (14%)

Gastrointestinal: Nausea (10% to 12% adjunct therapy)

1% to 10%:

Cardiovascular: Angina, bundle branch block, chest pain, syncope

Central nervous system: Depression (5%), hallucinations (4% to 5% adjunct therapy), fever (3%), malaise (2%), vertigo (2%), anxiety, dizziness

Dermatologic: Bruising (2%), alopecia, skin carcinoma, vesiculobullous rash

Endocrine & metabolic: Impotence, libido decreased

Gastrointestinal: Constipation (4% to 9% adjunct therapy), weight loss (2% to 9% adjunct therapy; dose dependent), dyspepsia (7%), xerostomia (2% to 6% adjunct therapy; dose dependent), gastroenteritis (3%), anorexia, diarrhea, gastrointestinal hemorrhage, vomiting

Genitourinary: Hematuria, urinary incontinence

Hematologic: Leukopenia

Hepatic: Liver function tests increased

Neuromuscular & skeletal: Arthralgia (7%), neck pain (2%), arthritis (2%), paresthesia (2%), abnormal gait, hyperkinesias, hypertonia, neuropathy, tremor, weakness

Ocular: Conjunctivitis (3%)

Renal: Albuminuria

Respiratory: Rhinitis (3%), asthma, cough increased

Miscellaneous: Fall (5%), flu-like syndrome (5%), allergic reaction

<1%, postmarketing, and/or case reports (limited to important or life-threatening): Acute kidney failure, aphasia, apnea, atrial arrhythmia, AV block, bigeminy, blepharitis, blindness, bone necrosis, cerebral hemorrhage, cerebral ischemia, circumoral paresthesia, deafness, deep thrombophlebitis, delirium, diplopia, dysautonomia, dysesthesia, emphysema, esophageal ulcer, exfoliative dermatitis, facial paralysis, glaucoma, gynecomastia, heart failure, hematemesis, hemiplegia, hemorrhage (various locations), hostility, hypersexuality, hypertension, hypocalcemia, impulse control symptoms, interstitial pneumonia, intestinal obstruction, intestinal perforation, intestinal stenosis, jaundice, keratitis, kidney calculus, large intestine perforation, laryngismus, larynx edema, leukoderma, leukorrhea, libido increased, lung fibrosis, macrocytic anemia, manic depressive reaction, mania, megacolon, menstrual abnormalities, MI, muscle atrophy, myelitis, neuralgia, neuritis, neurosis, nocturia, paranoid reaction, parosmia, pathological gambling, personality disorder, pleural effusion, pneumothorax, polyuria, psychosis, psychotic depression, ptosis, purpura, retinal degeneration, retinal detachment, seizure, stomach ulcer, strabismus, stupor, thrombocythemia, thrombosis, tongue edema, urinary disorders, vaginal moniliasis, ventricular fibrillation, ventricular tachycardia, vestibular disorder, visual field defect

Drug Interactions

Metabolism/Transport Effects Substrate of CYP1A2 (major); **Note:** Assignment of Major/Minor substrate status based on clinically relevant drug interaction potential; **Inhibits** Monoamine Oxidase

Avoid Concomitant Use

Avoid concomitant use of Rasagiline with any of the following: Alpha-/Beta-Agonists (Indirect-Acting); Alpha1-Agonists; Amphetamines; Anilidopiperidine Opioids; Antidepressants (Serotonin Reuptake Inhibitor/Antagonist); Apraclonidine; AtoMOXetine; Bezafibrate; Buprenorphine; BuPROPion; BusPIRone; CarBAMazepine; Cyclobenzaprine; Dexmethylphenidate; Dextromethorphan; Diethylpropion; Hydrocodone; HYDROmorphone; Isometheptene; Levonordefrin; Linezolid; Maprotiline; Meperidine; Methyldopa; Methylene Blue; Methylphenidate; Mirtazapine; Morphine (Liposomal); Morphine (Systemic); Oxymorphone; Pizotifen; Selective Serotonin Reuptake Inhibitors; Serotonin 5-HT1D Receptor Agonists; Serotonin/Norepinephrine Reuptake Inhibitors; Tapentadol; Tetrabenazine; Tetrahydrozoline (Nasal); Tricyclic Antidepressants; Tryptophan

Increased Effect/Toxicity

Rasagiline may increase the levels/effects of: Alpha-/Beta-Agonists (Indirect-Acting); Alpha1-Agonists; Amphetamines; Antidepressants (Serotonin Reuptake Inhibitor/Antagonist); Antihypertensives; Antipsychotics; Apraclonidine; AtoMOXetine; Beta2-Agonists; Betahistine; Bezafibrate; Brimonidine (Ophthalmic); Brimonidine

(Topical); BuPROPion; Dexmethylphenidate; Dextromethorphan; Diethylpropion; Domperidone; Doxapram; Doxylamine; EPINEPHrine (Nasal); Epinephrine (Racemic); EPINEPHrine (Systemic, Oral Inhalation); Hydrocodone; HYDROmorphone; Hypoglycemic Agents; Isometheptene; Levonordefrin; Linezolid; Lithium; Meperidine; Methadone; Methyldopa; Methylene Blue; Methylphenidate; Metoclopramide; Mirtazapine; Morphine (Liposomal); Morphine (Systemic); Norepinephrine; Orthostatic Hypotension Producing Agents; OxyCODONE; Pizotifen; Reserpine; Selective Serotonin Reuptake Inhibitors; Serotonin 5-HT1D Receptor Agonists; Serotonin Modulators; Serotonin/Norepinephrine Reuptake Inhibitors; Tetrahydrozoline (Nasal); Tricyclic Antidepressants

The levels/effects of Rasagiline may be increased by: Abiraterone Acetate; Altretamine; Anilidopiperidine Opioids; Antipsychotics; Buprenorphine; BusPIRone; CarBAMazepine; COMT Inhibitors; Cyclobenzaprine; CYP1A2 Inhibitors (Moderate); CYP1A2 Inhibitors (Strong); Deferasirox; Levodopa; MAO Inhibitors; Maprotiline; Oxymorphone; Tapentadol; Tetrabenazine; TraMADol; Tryptophan; Vemurafenib

Decreased Effect

Rasagiline may decrease the levels/effects of: Domperidone

The levels/effects of Rasagiline may be decreased by: CYP1A2 Inducers (Strong); Cyproterone; Domperidone

Ethanol/Nutrition/Herb Interactions

Ethanol: Management: Avoid ethanol.

Food: Concurrent ingestion of foods rich in tyramine may cause sudden and severe high blood pressure (hypertensive crisis). Management: Avoid foods containing high amounts (>150 mg) of tyramine (aged or matured cheese, air-dried or cured meats including sausages and salamis; fava or broad bean pods, tap/draft beers, Marmite concentrate, sauerkraut, soy sauce, and other soybean condiments). Food's freshness is also an important concern; improperly stored or spoiled food can create an environment in which tyramine concentrations may increase. Avoid these foods during and for 2 weeks after discontinuation of medication.

Herb/Nutraceutical: Some herbal medications may cause excessive sedation; others may increase the risk of serotonin syndrome or hypertensive reactions. Management: Avoid valerian, St John's wort, SAMe, and kava kava; avoid supplements containing caffeine, tyrosine, tryptophan, or phenylalanine.

Storage/Stability Store at 25°C (77°F); excursions permitted to 15°C to 30°C (59°F to 86°F).

Mechanism of Action Potent, irreversible and selective inhibitor of brain monoamine oxidase (MAO) type B, which plays a major role in the catabolism of dopamine. Inhibition of dopamine depletion in the striatal region of the brain reduces the symptomatic motor deficits of Parkinson's disease. There is also experimental evidence of rasagiline conferring neuroprotective effects (antioxidant, antiapoptotic), which may delay onset of symptoms and progression of neuronal deterioration.

Pharmacodynamics/Kinetics

Onset of action: Therapeutic: Within 1 hour

Duration: ~1 week (irreversible inhibition); may require ~14-40 days for complete restoration of (brain) MAO-B activity

Absorption: Rapid

Protein binding: 88% to 94%, primarily to albumin

Metabolism: Hepatic N-dealkylation and/or hydroxylation via CYP1A2 to multiple inactive metabolites (nonamphetamine derivatives)

Distribution: V_{dss}: 87 L

Bioavailability: ~36%

Half-life elimination: ~1.3-3 hours (no correlation with biologic effect due to irreversible inhibition)

Time to peak, plasma: ~1 hour

Excretion: Urine (62%, <1% of total dose as unchanged drug); feces (7%)

Dosage Oral: Adults: Parkinson's disease:

Monotherapy: 1 mg once daily

Adjunctive therapy with levodopa: Initial: 0.5 mg once daily; may increase to 1 mg once daily based on response and tolerability

Note: When added to existing levodopa therapy, a dose reduction of levodopa may be required to avoid exacerbation of dyskinesias; typical dose reductions of ~9% to 13% were employed in clinical trials

Dose reduction with concomitant ciprofloxacin or other CYP1A2 inhibitors: 0.5 mg once daily

Dosage adjustment in renal impairment:

Mild-to-moderate impairment: No dosage adjustment necessary.

Severe impairment: No dosage adjustment provided in manufacturer's labeling (has not been studied).

Dosage adjustment in hepatic impairment:

Mild impairment (Child-Pugh class A): Maximum dose: 0.5 mg once daily

Moderate-to-severe impairment: Use is not recommended.

Dietary Considerations May be taken without regard to meals. Avoid products containing high amounts of tyramine (>150 mg), such as aged cheeses (eg, Stilton cheese). Restriction of tyramine-containing products with lower amounts (<150 mg) of tyramine is not necessary in patients taking recommended doses. Some examples of tyramine-containing products include aged or matured cheese, air-dried or cured meats (including sausages and salamis), fava or broad bean pods, tap/draft beers, Marmite concentrate, sauerkraut, soy sauce and other soybean condiments. Food's freshness is also an important concern; improperly stored or spoiled food can create an environment where tyramine concentrations may increase.

Administration Administer without regard to meals.

Hazardous agent; use appropriate precautions for handling and disposal (NIOSH, 2012).

Monitoring Parameters Blood pressure; symptoms of parkinsonism; general mood and behavior (increased anxiety, or presence of mania or agitation); skin examination for presence of melanoma (higher incidence in Parkinson's patients- drug causation not established)

Additional Information When adding rasagiline to levodopa/carbidopa, the dose of the latter can usually be decreased. Studies are investigating the use of rasagiline in early Parkinson's disease to slow the progression of the disease.

Dosage Forms Excipient information presented when available (limited, particularly for generics); consult specific product labeling.

Tablet, Oral:

Azilect: 0.5 mg, 1 mg

◆ **Rasagiline Mesylate** *see* Rasagiline *on page 1786*

Rasburicase (ras BYOOR i kayse)

Brand Names: U.S. Elitek

Brand Names: Canada Fasturtec®

Index Terms Recombinant Urate Oxidase; Urate Oxidase

Pharmacologic Category Enzyme; Enzyme, Urate-Oxidase (Recombinant)

Additional Appendix Information

Dosing Considerations for the Critically-Ill Patient With Morbid Obesity *on page 2379*

Use Initial management of uric acid levels in patients with leukemia, lymphoma, and solid tumor malignancies receiving chemotherapy expected to result in tumor lysis and elevation of plasma uric acid

Pregnancy Risk Factor C

Pregnancy Considerations Adverse effects were observed in animal reproduction studies. There are no adequate and well-controlled studies in pregnant women. Use during pregnancy only if the benefit to the mother outweighs the potential risk to the fetus.

Breast-Feeding Considerations Due to the potential for serious adverse reactions in the nursing infant, the decision to discontinue breast-feeding or to discontinue rasburicase should take into account the benefits of treatment to the mother.

Contraindications History of anaphylaxis or severe hypersensitivity to rasburicase or any component of the formulation; history of hemolytic reaction or methemoglobinemia associated with rasburicase; glucose-6-phosphatase dehydrogenase (G6PD) deficiency

Warnings/Precautions [U.S. Boxed Warning]: Severe hypersensitivity reactions (including anaphylaxis) have been reported; immediately and permanently discontinue in patients developing serious hypersensitivity reaction; reactions may occur at any time during treatment, including the initial dose. Signs and symptoms of hypersensitivity may include bronchospasm, chest pain/tightness, dyspnea, hypotension, hypoxia, shock, or urticaria. The safety and efficacy of more than one course of administration has not been established. **[U.S. Boxed Warning]: Due to the risk for hemolysis (<1%), rasburicase is contraindicated in patients with G6PD deficiency; discontinue immediately and permanently in any patient developing hemolysis. Patients at higher risk for G6PD deficiency (eg, African, Mediterranean, or Southeast Asian descent) should be screened prior to therapy;** severe hemolytic reactions occurred within 2-4 days of rasburicase initiation. **[U.S. Boxed Warning]: Methemoglobinemia has been reported (<1%). Discontinue immediately and permanently in any patient developing methemoglobinemia;** initiate appropriate treatment (eg, transfusion, methylene blue) if methemoglobinemia occurs.

[U.S. Boxed Warning]: Enzymatic degradation of uric acid in blood samples will occur if left at room temperature, which may interfere with serum uric acid measurements; specific guidelines for the collection of plasma uric acid samples must be followed, including collection in prechilled tubes with heparin anticoagulant, immediate ice water bath immersion and assay within 4 hours. Patients at risk for tumor lysis syndrome should receive appropriate I.V. hydration as part of uric acid management; however, alkalinization (with sodium bicarbonate) concurrently with rasburicase is not recommended (Coiffier, 2008). Rasburicase is immunogenic and can elicit an antibody response; efficacy may be reduced with subsequent courses of therapy.

Adverse Reactions

>10%:

Cardiovascular: Peripheral edema (≤50%), fluid overload (≤12%)

Central nervous system: Fever (46%; serious: 5%), headache (26%), anxiety (≤24%)

Dermatologic: Rash (13%; serious: 1%)

Endocrine & metabolic: Hypophosphatemia (≤17%)

Gastrointestinal: Vomiting (50%), nausea (27%), abdominal pain (20%), constipation (20%), diarrhea (20%), mucositis (15%; serious: 2%)

Hepatic: Hyperbilirubinemia (≤16%), ALT increased (≤11%)

Respiratory: Pharyngolaryngeal pain (≤14%)

Miscellaneous: Antibody formation (healthy volunteers: 61% to 64%; patients with malignancies: 11%), sepsis (≤12%; serious: 3% to 5%)

1% to 10%:

Cardiovascular: Ischemic coronary disorder, supraventricular arrhythmia

Endocrine & metabolic: Hyperphosphatemia (≤10%)

Gastrointestinal: Abdominal/gastrointestinal infection

Hematologic: Neutropenic fever (serious: 4%), neutropenia (serious: 2%)

Respiratory: Respiratory distress (serious: 3%), pulmonary hemorrhage, respiratory failure

Miscellaneous: Hypersensitivity (≤4%)

<1% (Limited to important or life-threatening): Acute renal failure, anaphylaxis, arrhythmia, cardiac arrest, cardiac failure, cellulitis, cerebrovascular disorder, chest pain, cyanosis, dehydration, hemolysis, hemorrhage, hot flashes, ileus, infection, intestinal obstruction, liver enzymes increased, methemoglobinemia, MI, pancytopenia, paresthesia, pneumonia, pulmonary edema, pulmonary hypertension, retinal hemorrhage, rigors, seizure, thrombosis, thrombophlebitis

Drug Interactions

Metabolism/Transport Effects None known.

Avoid Concomitant Use There are no known interactions where it is recommended to avoid concomitant use.

Increased Effect/Toxicity There are no known significant interactions involving an increase in effect.

Decreased Effect There are no known significant interactions involving a decrease in effect.

Preparation for Administration Reconstitute with provided diluent (use 1 mL diluent for the 1.5 mg vial and 5 mL diluent for the 7.5 mg vial). Mix by gently swirling; do **not** shake or vortex. Discard if discolored or containing particulate matter. Total dose should be further diluted in NS to a final volume of 50 mL.

Storage/Stability Prior to reconstitution, store with diluent at 2°C to 8°C (36°F to 46°F); do not freeze. Protect from light. Reconstituted and final solution may be stored up to 24 hours at 2°C to 8°C (36°F to 46°F). Discard unused product.

Mechanism of Action Rasburicase is a recombinant urate-oxidase enzyme, which converts uric acid to allantoin (an inactive and soluble metabolite of uric acid); it does not inhibit the formation of uric acid.

Pharmacodynamics/Kinetics

Onset: Uric acid levels decrease within 4 hours of initial administration

Distribution: Children: 110-127 mL/kg; Adults: 76-138 mL/kg

Half-life elimination: ~16-23 hours

Dosage I.V.: Hyperuricemia associated with malignancy:

Children: 0.2 mg/kg once daily for up to 5 days (manufacturer-recommended dose) **or**

Alternate dosing (unlabeled; Coiffier, 2008): 0.05-0.2 mg/kg once daily for 1-7 days (average of 2-3 days) with the duration of treatment dependent on plasma uric acid levels and clinical judgment (patients with significant tumor burden may require an increase to twice daily); the following dose levels are recommended based on risk of tumor lysis syndrome (TLS):

High risk: 0.2 mg/kg once daily (duration is based on plasma uric acid levels)

Intermediate risk: 0.15 mg/kg once daily (duration is based on plasma uric acid levels); may consider managing initially with a single dose

Low risk: 0.1 mg/kg once daily (duration is based on clinical judgment); a dose of 0.05 mg/kg was used effectively in one trial

Single-dose rasburicase (unlabeled use; based on limited data): 0.15 mg/kg; additional doses may be needed based on serum uric acid levels (Liu, 2005)

Adults: 0.2 mg/kg once daily for up to 5 days (manufacturer-recommended dose) **or**

Alternate dosing (unlabeled; Coiffier, 2008): 0.05-0.2 mg/kg once daily for 1-7 days (average of 2-3 days) with the duration of treatment dependent on plasma uric acid levels and clinical judgment (patients with significant tumor burden may require an increase to twice daily); the following dose levels are recommended based on risk of tumor lysis syndrome (TLS):

High risk: 0.2 mg/kg once daily (duration is based on plasma uric acid levels)

Intermediate risk: 0.15 mg/kg once daily (duration is based on plasma uric acid levels)

Low risk: 0.1 mg/kg once daily (duration is based on clinical judgment); a dose of 0.05 mg/kg was used effectively in one trial

Single-dose rasburicase (unlabeled use; based on limited data): 0.15 mg/kg (Campara, 2009; Liu, 2005) **or** 3-7.5 mg as a single dose (Hutcherson, 2006; McDonnell, 2006; Reeves, 2008; Trifilio, 2006); repeat doses (1.5-6 mg) may be needed based on serum uric acid levels

Dosage adjustment in renal impairment: No dosage adjustment provided in manufacturer's labeling.

Dosage adjustment in hepatic impairment: No dosage adjustment provided in manufacturer's labeling.

Administration I.V. infusion over 30 minutes; do **not** administer as a bolus infusion. Do **not** filter during infusion. If not possible to administer through a separate line, I.V. line should be flushed with at least 15 mL saline prior to and following rasburicase infusion. The optimal timing of rasburicase administration (with respect to chemotherapy administration) is not specified in the manufacturer's labeling. In some studies, chemotherapy was administered 4-24 hours after the first rasburicase dose (Cortes, 2010; Kikuchi, 2009; Vadhan-Raj, 2012); however, rasburicase generally may be administered irrespective of chemotherapy timing.

Monitoring Parameters Plasma uric acid levels (4 hours after rasburicase administration, then every 6-8 hours until TLS resolution), CBC, G6PD deficiency screening (in patients at high risk for deficiency); monitor for hypersensitivity

Test Interactions Specific handling procedures must be followed to prevent the degradation of uric acid in plasma samples. Blood must be collected in prechilled tubes containing heparin anticoagulant. Samples must then be **immediately** immersed in an ice water bath. Prepare samples by centrifugation in a precooled centrifuge (4°C). Samples must be kept in ice water bath and analyzed within 4 hours of collection.

Dosage Forms Excipient information presented when available (limited, particularly for generics); consult specific product labeling.

Solution Reconstituted, Intravenous:

Elitek: 1.5 mg (1 ea); 7.5 mg (1 ea)

- ◆ **Rasilez (Can)** *see* Aliskiren *on page* 74
- ◆ **Rasilez HCT® (Can)** *see* Aliskiren and Hydrochlorothiazide *on page* 76
- ◆ **rATG** *see* Antithymocyte Globulin (Rabbit) *on page* 150
- ◆ **ratio-Aclavulanate (Can)** *see* Amoxicillin and Clavulanate *on page* 119
- ◆ **ratio-Acyclovir (Can)** *see* Acyclovir (Systemic) *on page* 42
- ◆ **ratio-Alendronate (Can)** *see* Alendronate *on page* 69
- ◆ **ratio-Amiodarone (Can)** *see* Amiodarone *on page* 101
- ◆ **ratio-Amlodipine (Can)** *see* AmLODIPine *on page* 109
- ◆ **ratio-Atenolol (Can)** *see* Atenolol *on page* 186
- ◆ **ratio-Atorvastatin (Can)** *see* AtorvaSTATin *on page* 190
- ◆ **ratio-Azithromycin (Can)** *see* Azithromycin (Systemic) *on page* 214
- ◆ **ratio-Baclofen (Can)** *see* Baclofen *on page* 221
- ◆ **ratio-Bicalutamide (Can)** *see* Bicalutamide *on page* 258
- ◆ **ratio-Bisacodyl [OTC] (Can)** *see* Bisacodyl *on page* 259
- ◆ **ratio-Brimonidine (Can)** *see* Brimonidine (Ophthalmic) *on page* 280
- ◆ **ratio-Bupropion SR (Can)** *see* BuPROPion *on page* 296
- ◆ **ratio-Carvedilol (Can)** *see* Carvedilol *on page* 355
- ◆ **ratio-Cefuroxime (Can)** *see* Cefuroxime *on page* 386
- ◆ **ratio-Ciprofloxacin (Can)** *see* Ciprofloxacin (Systemic) *on page* 430
- ◆ **ratio-Citalopram (Can)** *see* Citalopram *on page* 440
- ◆ **ratio-Clarithromycin (Can)** *see* Clarithromycin *on page* 446
- ◆ **ratio-Clobetasol (Can)** *see* Clobetasol *on page* 457
- ◆ **ratio-Clonazepam (Can)** *see* ClonazePAM *on page* 465
- ◆ **ratio-Codeine (Can)** *see* Codeine *on page* 482
- ◆ **ratio-Cyclobenzaprine (Can)** *see* Cyclobenzaprine *on page* 502
- ◆ **ratio-Dexamethasone (Can)** *see* Dexamethasone (Systemic) *on page* 580
- ◆ **ratio-Diltiazem CD (Can)** *see* Diltiazem *on page* 613
- ◆ **ratio-Ectosone (Can)** *see* Betamethasone *on page* 247
- ◆ **ratio-Emtec-30 (Can)** *see* Acetaminophen and Codeine *on page* 32
- ◆ **ratio-Enalapril (Can)** *see* Enalapril *on page* 701
- ◆ **ratio-Fenofibrate MC (Can)** *see* Fenofibrate and Derivatives *on page* 837
- ◆ **ratio-Fentanyl (Can)** *see* FentaNYL *on page* 842
- ◆ **ratio-Finasteride (Can)** *see* Finasteride *on page* 862
- ◆ **ratio-Fluoxetine (Can)** *see* FLUoxetine *on page* 885
- ◆ **ratio-Fluticasone (Can)** *see* Fluticasone (Nasal) *on page* 896
- ◆ **ratio-Fluvoxamine (Can)** *see* FluvoxaMINE *on page* 903
- ◆ **ratio-Gabapentin (Can)** *see* Gabapentin *on page* 933
- ◆ **ratio-Glimepiride (Can)** *see* Glimepiride *on page* 956
- ◆ **ratio-Glyburide (Can)** *see* GlyBURIDE *on page* 963
- ◆ **ratio-Indomethacin (Can)** *see* Indomethacin *on page* 1070
- ◆ **ratio-Ipra-Sal (Can)** *see* Albuterol *on page* 61
- ◆ **ratio-Ipra Sal UDV (Can)** *see* Ipratropium and Albuterol *on page* 1113
- ◆ **ratio-Ipratropium UDV (Can)** *see* Ipratropium (Systemic) *on page* 1111
- ◆ **ratio-Irbesartan (Can)** *see* Irbesartan *on page* 1113
- ◆ **ratio-Irbesartan HCTZ (Can)** *see* Irbesartan and Hydrochlorothiazide *on page* 1115
- ◆ **ratio-Ketorolac (Can)** *see* Ketorolac (Ophthalmic) *on page* 1155
- ◆ **ratio-Lamotrigine (Can)** *see* LamoTRIgine *on page* 1165
- ◆ **ratio-Lenoltec (Can)** *see* Acetaminophen and Codeine *on page* 32
- ◆ **Ratio-Levobunolol (Can)** *see* Levobunolol *on page* 1196
- ◆ **ratio-Lisinopril P (Can)** *see* Lisinopril *on page* 1226
- ◆ **ratio-Lisinopril Z (Can)** *see* Lisinopril *on page* 1226
- ◆ **ratio-Meloxicam (Can)** *see* Meloxicam *on page* 1284
- ◆ **ratio-Memantine (Can)** *see* Memantine *on page* 1289
- ◆ **ratio-Metformin (Can)** *see* MetFORMIN *on page* 1310

Raxibacumab (rax i BAK ue mab)

Index Terms ABthrax

Pharmacologic Category Antidote; Monoclonal Antibody

Use Treatment of inhalational anthrax following exposure to *Bacillus anthracis* in combination with appropriate antimicrobial therapy; prophylaxis of inhalational anthrax when alternative therapies are unavailable or not appropriate

Pregnancy Risk Factor B

Pregnancy Considerations Adverse events were not observed in animal reproduction studies. In general, medications used as antidotes should take into consideration the health and prognosis of the mother; antidotes should be administered to pregnant women if there is a clear indication for use and should not be withheld because of fears of teratogenicity (Bailey, 2003).

Breast-Feeding Considerations In general, an increase in maternal immunoglobulins is not observed in infants following nursing. The potential effects of raxibacumab on a nursing infant are not known.

Prescribing and Access Restrictions Raxibacumab is not available for general public use. All supplies are currently owned by the federal government for inclusion in the Strategic National Stockpile and for use by the U.S. military.

Contraindications There are no contraindications listed in the manufacturer's labeling.

Warnings/Precautions Raxibacumab is not an antimicrobial agent; use should always be in combination with appropriate antimicrobial therapy. Raxibacumab does not cross the blood brain barrier and is not appropriate for the prevention or treatment of meningitis due to anthrax infection. The efficacy of raxibacumab in humans is presumptive and based solely on efficacy studies in animals.

Infusion-related reactions (eg, rash, urticaria, pruritus) have been reported. Premedication with diphenhydramine is recommended to reduce the risk. The administration rate is slowed over the first 20 minutes to monitor for adverse reactions; slow or interrupt infusion if adverse reactions (including infusion-related reactions) occur.

Adverse Reactions

>10%: Local: Infusion-related rash (22% [without diphenhydramine premedication]; ~3% [with diphenhydramine premedication])

1.5% to 10%:

Central nervous system: Pain (3%)

Dermatologic: Pruritus (3%)

<1.5% (Limited to important or life-threatening): Amylase increased, anemia, back pain, creatinine phosphokinase increased, fatigue, flushing, hypertension, insomnia, leukopenia, lymphadenopathy, muscle spasm, pain (infusion site), palpitations, peripheral edema, prothrombin time increased, somnolence, syncope (vasovagal), vertigo

Drug Interactions

Metabolism/Transport Effects None known.

Avoid Concomitant Use There are no known interactions where it is recommended to avoid concomitant use.

Increased Effect/Toxicity There are no known significant interactions involving an increase in effect.

Decreased Effect There are no known significant interactions involving a decrease in effect.

Preparation for Administration Product requires dilution with 0.45% or 0.9% NS in patients <11 kg or with 0.9% NS in patients ≥11 kg prior to administration; may be prepared for administration in a syringe or infusion bag depending on volume required for administration. Gently mix solution; do not shake.

Body weight: ≤1 kg: Dilute to a final volume of 7 mL

Body weight 1.1 to 2 kg: Dilute to a final volume of 15 mL

Body weight 2.1 to 3 kg: Dilute to a final volume of 20 mL

Body weight 3.1 to 4.9 kg: Dilute to a final volume of 25 mL

Body weight 5 to 10 kg: Dilute to a final volume of 50 mL

Body weight 11 to 30 kg: Dilute to a final volume of 100 mL

Body weight ≥31 kg: Dilute to a final volume of 250 mL

Storage/Stability Unused vials should be stored at 2°C to 8°C (36°F to 46°F); do not freeze. Protect from light. Diluted solutions are stable for 8 hours at room temperature.

Mechanism of Action Raxibacumab is a recombinant human IgG1 lambda monoclonal antibody which binds and neutralizes free protective antigen (PA) component of *Bacillus anthracis* toxin; as a result, PA-mediated delivery of lethal toxin and edema toxin via the anthrax toxin receptor (ATR) into host cells of anthrax-infected individuals is inhibited.

Pharmacodynamics/Kinetics

Distribution: V_d: 0.07 L/kg (Migone, 2009)

Half-life elimination: Terminal: 20-22 days (Migone, 2009)

Excretion: Nonrenal (Migone, 2009)

Dosage Anthrax, prophylaxis or treatment: Note: Administer diphenhydramine (adult dose: 25-50 mg; in all patients, may administer oral or I.V. depending on the proximity to start of raxibacumab infusion) ≤1 hour prior to administration of raxibacumab to reduce the risk of infusion reactions. Must be administered in combination with antimicrobial therapy.

Children and Adolescents: I.V.:

- ≤15 kg: 80 mg/kg as a single dose
- >15 kg to 50 kg: 60 mg/kg as a single dose
- >50 kg: 40 mg/kg as a single dose

Adults: I.V.: 40 mg/kg as a single dose

Dosage adjustment in renal impairment: No dosage adjustment provided in manufacturer's labeling. However, dosage adjustment unlikely as clearance is nonrenal.

Dosage adjustment in hepatic impairment: No dosage adjustment provided in manufacturer's labeling (has not been studied).

Administration I.V.: Premedicate with diphenhydramine ≤1 hour prior to raxibacumab infusion. Administer over 2 hours and 15 minutes; administration rate should be slower over the first 20 minutes to monitor for adverse reactions; slow or interrupt infusion if adverse reactions (including infusion-related reactions) occur. Administer as follows:

- Body weight: ≤1 kg: Infuse at 0.5 mL/hour for 20 minutes; increase rate to 3.5 mL/hour for the remaining infusion
- Body weight 1.1 to 2 kg: Infuse at 1 mL/hour for 20 minutes; increase rate to 7 mL/hour for the remaining infusion
- Body weight 2.1 to 3 kg: Infuse at 1.2 mL/hour for 20 minutes; increase rate to 10 mL/hour for the remaining infusion
- Body weight 3.1 to 4.9 kg: Infuse at 1.5 mL/hour for 20 minutes; increase rate to 12 mL/hour for the remaining infusion
- Body weight 5 to 10 kg: Infuse at 3 mL/hour for 20 minutes; increase rate to 25 mL/hour for the remaining infusion
- Body weight 11 to 30 kg: Infuse at 6 mL/hour for 20 minutes; increase rate to 50 mL/hour for the remaining infusion
- Body weight ≥31 kg: Infuse at 15 mL/hour for 20 minutes; increase rate to 125 mL/hour for the remaining infusion

Dosage Forms Excipient information presented when available (limited, particularly for generics); consult specific product labeling.

Injection, solution: 50 mg/mL (34 mL) [contains polysorbate 80, sucrose 10 mg/mL]

- ◆ Rayos® *see* PredniSONE *on page 1707*
- ◆ Rayos *see* PredniSONE *on page 1707*
- ◆ Razadyne *see* Galantamine *on page 937*
- ◆ Razadyne ER *see* Galantamine *on page 937*
- ◆ 6R-BH4 *see* Sapropterin *on page 1875*
- ◆ Reactine [OTC] (Can) *see* Cetirizine *on page 396*
- ◆ Rea-Lo [OTC] *see* Urea *on page 2140*
- ◆ Rebetol *see* Ribavirin *on page 1804*
- ◆ Rebetron® *see* Interferon Alfa-2b and Ribavirin *on page 1102*
- ◆ Rebif® *see* Interferon Beta-1a *on page 1104*
- ◆ Rebif® Rebidose® *see* Interferon Beta-1a *on page 1104*
- ◆ Rebif® Rebidose® Titration Pack *see* Interferon Beta-1a *on page 1104*
- ◆ Rebif® Titration Pack *see* Interferon Beta-1a *on page 1104*
- ◆ Reclast *see* Zoledronic Acid *on page 2235*
- ◆ Reclipsen *see* Ethinyl Estradiol and Desogestrel *on page 784*
- ◆ Recombinant α-L-Iduronidase (Glycosaminoglycan α-L-Iduronohydrolase) *see* Laronidase *on page 1176*
- ◆ Recombinant Desulfatohirudin *see* Desirudin *on page 574*
- ◆ Recombinant Granulocyte-Macrophage Colony Stimulating Factor *see* Sargramostim *on page 1877*
- ◆ Recombinant Hirudin *see* Desirudin *on page 574*
- ◆ Recombinant Human Deoxyribonuclease *see* Dornase Alfa *on page 654*
- ◆ Recombinant Human Interleukin-2 *see* Aldesleukin *on page 63*
- ◆ Recombinant Human Interleukin-11 *see* Oprelvekin *on page 1514*
- ◆ Recombinant Human Luteinizing Hormone *see* Lutropin Alfa *on page 1258*
- ◆ Recombinant Human Parathyroid Hormone (1-34) *see* Teriparatide *on page 2023*
- ◆ Recombinant Human Platelet-Derived Growth Factor B *see* Becaplermin *on page 227*
- ◆ Recombinant Human Thyrotropin *see* Thyrotropin Alfa *on page 2053*
- ◆ Recombinant Interleukin-11 *see* Oprelvekin *on page 1514*
- ◆ Recombinant Plasminogen Activator *see* Reteplase *on page 1800*
- ◆ Recombinant Urate Oxidase *see* Rasburicase *on page 1788*
- ◆ Recombinant Urate Oxidase, Pegylated *see* Pegloticase *on page 1599*
- ◆ Recombinate *see* Antihemophilic Factor (Recombinant) *on page 144*
- ◆ Recombivax HB® *see* Hepatitis B Vaccine (Recombinant) *on page 995*
- ◆ Recort Plus [OTC] *see* Hydrocortisone (Topical) *on page 1011*
- ◆ Rectacort-HC *see* Hydrocortisone (Topical) *on page 1011*
- ◆ RectiCare [OTC] *see* Lidocaine (Topical) *on page 1212*
- ◆ Rectiv *see* Nitroglycerin *on page 1466*
- ◆ Rederm [OTC] *see* Hydrocortisone (Topical) *on page 1011*
- ◆ Reeses Pinworm Medicine [OTC] *see* Pyrantel Pamoate *on page 1750*
- ◆ Refenesen [OTC] *see* GuaiFENesin *on page 974*
- ◆ Refenesen 400 [OTC] *see* GuaiFENesin *on page 974*
- ◆ Refenesen DM [OTC] *see* Guaifenesin and Dextromethorphan *on page 976*
- ◆ Refenesen™ PE [OTC] *see* Guaifenesin and Phenylephrine *on page 978*
- ◆ Refenesen Plus [OTC] *see* Guaifenesin and Pseudoephedrine *on page 978*
- ◆ Refissa *see* Tretinoin (Topical) *on page 2120*

◆ **Refresh Eye Itch Relief [OTC] [DSC]** *see* Ketotifen (Ophthalmic) *on page 1156*

◆ **Regitine [DSC]** *see* Phentolamine *on page 1634*

◆ **Reglan** *see* Metoclopramide *on page 1345*

◆ **Regonol** *see* Pyridostigmine *on page 1752*

Regorafenib (re goe RAF e nib)

Brand Names: U.S. Stivarga
Brand Names: Canada Stivarga
Index Terms BAY 73-4506
Pharmacologic Category Antineoplastic Agent, Tyrosine Kinase Inhibitor; Vascular Endothelial Growth Factor (VEGF) Inhibitor

Use

Gastrointestinal stromal tumors: Treatment of locally-advanced, unresectable, or metastatic gastrointestinal stromal tumor (GIST) in patients previously treated with imatinib and sunitinib

Metastatic colorectal cancer: Treatment of metastatic colorectal cancer in patients previously treated with fluoropyrimidine-, oxaliplatin-, and irinotecan-based chemotherapy, anti-VEGF therapy, or anti-EGFR therapy (if *KRAS* wild type)

Pregnancy Risk Factor D

Pregnancy Considerations In animal reproduction studies, teratogenic effects were observed with doses less than the equivalent human dose. Patients (male and female) should use effective contraception during therapy and for at least 2 months following treatment.

Breast-Feeding Considerations It is not known if regorafenib is excreted into breast milk. According to the manufacturer, the decision to discontinue regorafenib or to discontinue breast-feeding during therapy should take into account the benefits of treatment to the mother.

Prescribing and Access Restrictions Regorafenib is available only through the REACH support program. Information regarding program enrollment may be found at http://www.stivarga-us.com/hcp/mcrc/support.html or by calling 1-866-639-2827.

Contraindications There are no contraindications listed in the manufacturer's U.S. product labeling.

Canadian labeling: Hypersensitivity to regorafenib, any component of the formulation, or sorafenib.

Warnings/Precautions Hazardous agent - use appropriate precautions for handling and disposal (meets NIOSH, 2012 criteria). Myocardial ischemia and infarction were observed at a higher incidence than placebo in a clinical trial. Interrupt therapy in patients who develop new or acute onset ischemia or infarction; resume only if the benefit of therapy outweighs the cardiovascular risk. Hand-foot skin reaction (HFSR), also known as palmar-plantar erythrodysesthesia (PPE), and rash were commonly seen in clinical trials; erythema multiforme and Stevens Johnson syndrome were also observed more frequently in regorafenib-treated patients. Toxic epidermal necrolysis occurred rarely. Onset of dermatologic toxicity typically occurs in the first cycle of treatment. Therapy interruptions, dosage reductions, and/or discontinuation may be necessary depending on the severity and persistence. Supportive treatment may be of benefit for symptomatic relief. Gastrointestinal perforation or fistula has occurred in a small number of patients treated with regorafenib; some cases were fatal. Monitor for signs/symptoms of perforation (fever, abdominal pain with constipation, and/or nausea/vomiting); permanently discontinue therapy if perforation or fistula develop. The incidence of hemorrhage was increased with regorafenib. Hemorrhage of the respiratory, gastrointestinal, or genitourinary tracts was observed in trials; some cases were fatal. Permanently discontinue in patients who experience severe or life-threatening bleeding. In patients receiving concomitant warfarin, monitor INR frequently.

[U.S. Boxed Warning]: Severe liver toxicity and hepatic failure (sometimes resulting in death) have been observed in clinical trials; hepatocyte necrosis with lymphocyte infiltration has been demonstrated with liver biopsy. Monitor hepatic function at baseline and during treatment. Interrupt therapy for hepatotoxicity; dose reductions or discontinuation are necessary depending on the severity and persistence.

Elevated blood pressure was observed in clinical trials (onset typically in the first cycle of therapy); ensure blood pressure is adequately controlled prior to initiation. Monitor blood pressure weekly for the first 6 weeks and monthly thereafter or as clinically indicated; if hypertension develops, interrupt therapy or permanently discontinue for severe or uncontrolled hypertension. Hypertensive crisis has occurred in some patients. Reversible posterior leukoencephalopathy syndrome (RPLS) occurred very rarely in regorafenib-treated patients; evaluate promptly if symptoms (eg, seizures, headache, visual disturbances, confusion, or altered mental function) occur. Discontinue if diagnosis is confirmed. Regorafenib inhibits vascular endothelial growth factor, which may lead to impaired wound healing. Stop therapy at least 2 weeks prior to scheduled surgery; resume regorafenib postsurgery based on clinical judgment of wound healing; discontinue therapy if wound dehiscence occurs.

Potentially significant drug-drug or drug-food interactions may exist, requiring dose or frequency adjustment, additional monitoring, and/or selection of alternative therapy.

Adverse Reactions

>10%:

Cardiovascular: Hypertension (30% to 59%; grade ≥3: 8% to 28%)

Central nervous system: Fatigue (52% to 64%), dysphonia (30% to 39%), pain (29%), fever (21% to 28%), headache (10% to 16%)

Dermatologic: Palmar-plantar erythrodysesthesia (45% to 67%; grade ≥3: 17% to 22%), rash (26% to 30%; grade ≥3: 6% to 7%), alopecia (8% to 24%)

Endocrine & metabolic: Hypocalcemia (17% to 59%), hypophosphatemia (55% to 57%), hyponatremia (30%), hypokalemia (21% to 26%), hypothyroidism (4% to 18%)

Gastrointestinal: Appetite decreased (31% to 47%), lipase increased (14% to 46%), diarrhea (43% to 47%), mucositis (33% to 40%), weight loss (14% to 32%), amylase increased (26%), nausea (20%), vomiting (17%)

Hematologic: Anemia (79%; grade 3: 5%; grade 4: 1%), lymphopenia (30% to 54%; grade 3: 8% to 9%), thrombocytopenia (13% to 41%; grade 3: 1% to 2%; grade 4: <1%), INR increased (24%), hemorrhage (11% to 21%; grade ≥3: 2% to 4%), neutropenia (3% to 16%; grade 3: 1% to 2%)

Hepatic: AST increased (58% to 65%; grade 3: 3% to 5%; grade 4: 1%), ALT increased (39% to 45%; grade 3: 4% to 5%; grade 4: 1%), hyperbilirubinemia (33% to 45%)

Neuromuscular & skeletal: Stiffness (14%)

Renal: Proteinuria (33% to 60%; grade 3: 3%)

Miscellaneous: Infection (31% to 32%; grade ≥3: 5% to 9%)

1% to 10%:

Cardiovascular: Myocardial ischemia and infarction (1%)

Gastrointestinal: Taste disturbance (8%), xerostomia (5%), gastroesophageal reflux (1%)

Neuromuscular & skeletal: Tremor (2%)

Respiratory: Dyspnea (2%)

<1% (Limited to important or life-threatening): Bradycardia, erythema multiforme, gastrointestinal fistula, hypertensive crisis, liver injury (severe), liver failure, reversible posterior encephalopathy syndrome (RPLS), skin cancer (keratoacanthoma, squamous cell carcinoma), Stevens-Johnson syndrome, toxic epidermal necrolysis

Drug Interactions

Metabolism/Transport Effects Substrate of CYP3A4 (major), UGT1A9; **Note:** Assignment of Major/Minor substrate status based on clinically relevant drug interaction potential; **Inhibits** BCRP, P-glycoprotein, UGT1A1, UGT1A9

Avoid Concomitant Use

Avoid concomitant use of Regorafenib with any of the following: CYP3A4 Inducers (Strong); CYP3A4 Inhibitors (Strong); Fusidic Acid (Systemic); Grapefruit Juice; St Johns Wort

Increased Effect/Toxicity

Regorafenib may increase the levels/effects of: Beta-Blockers; Bisphosphonate Derivatives; Calcium Channel Blockers (Nondihydropyridine); Digoxin; Irinotecan; Ivabradine; Vitamin K Antagonists

The levels/effects of Regorafenib may be increased by: CYP3A4 Inhibitors (Moderate); CYP3A4 Inhibitors (Strong); Dasatinib; Fusidic Acid (Systemic); Grapefruit Juice; Ivacaftor; Luliconazole; Mifepristone; Simeprevir; Warfarin

Decreased Effect

Regorafenib may decrease the levels/effects of: Vitamin K Antagonists

The levels/effects of Regorafenib may be decreased by: Bosentan; CYP3A4 Inducers (Strong); Dabrafenib; Deferasirox; St Johns Wort; Tocilizumab

Ethanol/Nutrition/Herb Interactions

Food: Regorafenib serum concentrations may be altered when taken with grapefruit or grapefruit juice. Management: Avoid concurrent use.

Herb/Nutraceutical: St John's wort may alter the levels/effects of regorafenib. Management: Avoid St John's wort.

Storage/Stability Store at 25°C (77°F); excursions permitted to 15°C to 30°C (59°F to 86°F). Store tablets in the original bottle and protect from moisture (do not remove the desiccant); keep container tightly closed. Any unused tablets remaining 28 days after opening the bottle should be discarded.

Mechanism of Action Regorafenib is a multikinase inhibitor; it targets kinases involved with tumor angiogenesis, oncogenesis, and maintenance of the tumor microenvironment which results in inhibition of tumor growth. Specifically, it inhibits VEGF receptors 1-3, KIT, PDGFR-alpha, PDGFR-beta, RET, FGFR1 and 2, TIE2, DDR2, TrkA, Eph2A, RAF-1. BRAF, BRAF^{V600E}, SAPK2, PTK5, and Abl.

Pharmacodynamics/Kinetics

Absorption: A high-fat meal increased the mean AUC of the parent drug by 48% compared to the fasted state and decreased the mean AUC of the M-2 (N-oxide) and M-5 (N-oxide and N-desmethyl) active metabolites by 20% and 51%, respectively. A low-fat meal increased the mean AUC of regorafenib, M-2, and M-5 by 36%, 40% and 23%, respectively (as compared to the fasted state).

Protein binding: 99.5% (active metabolites M-2 and M-5 are also highly protein bound)

Metabolism: Hepatic via CYP3A4 and UGT1A9, primarily to active metabolites M-2 (N-oxide) and M-5 (N-oxide and N-desmethyl)

Bioavailability: Tablets: 69%; Oral solution: 83%

Half-life elimination: Regorafenib: 28 hours (range: 14-58 hours); M-2 metabolite: 25 hours (range: 14-32 hours); M-5 metabolite: 51 hours (range: 32-70 hours)

Time to peak: 4 hours

Excretion: Feces (71%; 47% as parent compound; 24% as metabolites); Urine (19%)

Dosage

Colorectal cancer, metastatic: Adults: Oral: 160 mg once daily for the first 21 days of each 28-day cycle; continue until disease progression or unacceptable toxicity (Grothey, 2013)

Gastrointestinal stromal tumor (GIST), locally-advanced, unresectable, or metastatic: Adults: Oral: 160 mg once daily for the first 21 days of each 28-day cycle; continue until disease progression or unacceptable toxicity (Demetri, 2013)

Missed doses: Do not administer 2 doses on the same day to make up for a missed dose from the previous day.

Dosage adjustment for toxicity:

Dermatologic:

Grade 2 hand-foot skin reaction (HFSR; palmar-plantar erythrodysesthesia [PPE]) of any duration: Reduce dose to 120 mg once daily for first occurrence. If grade 2 HFSR recurs at this dose, further reduce the dose to 80 mg once daily. Interrupt therapy for grade 2 HFSR that is recurrent or fails to improve within 7 days in spite of dosage reduction.

Grade 3 HFSR: Interrupt therapy for a minimum of 7 days. Upon recovery, reduce dose to 120 mg once daily. If grade 2-3 toxicity recurs at this dose, further reduce dose to 80 mg once daily upon recovery. Interrupt therapy for grade 2-3 HFSR that is recurrent or fails to improve within 7 days in spite of dosage reduction.

Recurrent or persistent HFSR at 80 mg once daily: Discontinue treatment.

Hypertension: Grade 2 (symptomatic): Interrupt therapy.

Other toxicity: Any grade 3 or 4 adverse reaction (other than hepatotoxicity): Interrupt therapy; upon recovery, reduce dose to 120 mg once daily. If any grade 3 or 4 adverse reaction occurs while on this reduced dose, may further reduce dose to 80 mg once daily upon recovery. For any grade 4 adverse reaction, only resume therapy if the benefit outweighs the risk. Permanently discontinue therapy if unable to tolerate 80 mg once daily.

Gastrointestinal perforation/fistula: Discontinue permanently.

Hemorrhage (severe or life-threatening): Discontinue permanently.

Reversible posterior leukoencephalopathy syndrome (RPLS): Discontinue.

Wound dehiscence: Discontinue.

Dosage adjustment for renal impairment:

Pre-existing mild impairment (Cl_{cr} 60-89 mL/minute): No dosage adjustment necessary.

Pre-existing moderate impairment (Cl_{cr} 30-59 mL/minute): No dosage adjustment provided in manufacturer's labeling (limited pharmacokinetic data available).

Pre-existing severe impairment (Cl_{cr} <30 mL/minute): No dosage adjustment provided in manufacturer's labeling (has not been studied).

Dosage adjustment for hepatic impairment:

Pre-existing mild or moderate impairment (Child-Pugh Class A or B): No dosage adjustment necessary; closely monitor for adverse effects.

Pre-existing severe impairment (Child-Pugh Class C): Use is not recommended (has not been studied).

Hepatotoxicity during treatment:

Grade 3 AST and/or ALT elevation: Withhold dose until recovery. If benefit of treatment outweighs toxicity risk, resume therapy at a reduced dose of 120 mg once daily.

AST or ALT >20 times ULN: Discontinue permanently.

AST or ALT >3 times ULN **and** bilirubin >2 times ULN: Discontinue permanently.

Recurrence of AST or ALT >5 times ULN despite dose reduction to 120 mg: Discontinue permanently.

Dietary Considerations Take with a low-fat breakfast (<30% fat)

Administration Take at the same time each day with a low-fat (<30% fat) breakfast; swallow tablets whole.

Hazardous agent; use appropriate precautions for handling and disposal (meets NIOSH, 2012 criteria).

Monitoring Parameters Monitor for hand-foot skin reaction (HFSR)/palmar-plantar erythrodysesthesia (PPE); signs/symptoms of cardiac ischemia or infarction; bleeding; signs/symptoms of GI perforation or fistula; signs/symptoms of reversible posterior leukoencephalopathy syndrome (severe headaches, seizure, confusion, or change in vision). Monitor for impaired wound healing. Obtain liver function tests at baseline, every 2 weeks during the first 2 months of treatment, then monthly or more frequently if clinically necessary (weekly until improvement if liver function tests are elevated). Monitor blood pressure weekly for the first 6 weeks of therapy and with every subsequent cycle, or more frequently if indicated. CBC with differential and platelets and serum electrolytes (baseline and periodic). Monitor INR more frequently if receiving warfarin.

Dosage Forms Excipient information presented when available (limited, particularly for generics); consult specific product labeling.

Tablet, Oral:

Stivarga: 40 mg [contains soybean lecithin]

- ◆ **Regranex** *see* Becaplermin *on page 227*
- ◆ **Regular Insulin** *see* Insulin Regular *on page 1094*
- ◆ **Regulex® (Can)** *see* Docusate *on page 644*
- ◆ **Reguloid [OTC]** *see* Psyllium *on page 1748*
- ◆ **Rejuva-A® (Can)** *see* Tretinoin (Topical) *on page 2120*
- ◆ **Relafen** *see* Nabumetone *on page 1413*
- ◆ **Relafen® (Can)** *see* Nabumetone *on page 1413*
- ◆ **Relaxa (Can)** *see* Polyethylene Glycol 3350 *on page 1668*
- ◆ **Relenza® (Can)** *see* Zanamivir *on page 2222*
- ◆ **Relenza Diskhaler** *see* Zanamivir *on page 2222*
- ◆ **Relistor** *see* Methylnaltrexone *on page 1335*
- ◆ **Relpax** *see* Eletriptan *on page 692*
- ◆ **Relpax® (Can)** *see* Eletriptan *on page 692*
- ◆ **Remedy Antifungal [OTC]** *see* Miconazole (Topical) *on page 1358*
- ◆ **Remergent HQ** *see* Hydroquinone *on page 1017*
- ◆ **Remeron** *see* Mirtazapine *on page 1379*
- ◆ **Remeron® (Can)** *see* Mirtazapine *on page 1379*
- ◆ **Remeron® RD (Can)** *see* Mirtazapine *on page 1379*
- ◆ **Remeron SolTab** *see* Mirtazapine *on page 1379*
- ◆ **Remeven** *see* Urea *on page 2140*
- ◆ **Remicade** *see* InFLIXimab *on page 1073*
- ◆ **Remicade® (Can)** *see* InFLIXimab *on page 1073*

Remifentanil (rem i FEN ta nil)

Brand Names: U.S. Ultiva

Brand Names: Canada Ultiva®

Index Terms GI87084B

Pharmacologic Category Analgesic, Opioid; Anilidopiperidine Opioid

Additional Appendix Information

Dosing Considerations for the Critically-Ill Patient With Morbid Obesity *on page 2379*

Use Analgesic for use during the induction and maintenance of general anesthesia; for continued analgesia into the immediate postoperative period; analgesic component of monitored anesthesia

Unlabeled Use Management of pain in mechanically-ventilated patients

Pregnancy Risk Factor C

Pregnancy Considerations Adverse events were not observed in animal reproduction studies. Remifentanil has been shown to cross the placenta; fetal and maternal concentrations may be similar.

Breast-Feeding Considerations It is not known if remifentanil is excreted into breast milk. The manufacturer recommends that caution be used if administered to a nursing woman. Remifentanil has a limited duration of action; use may be appropriate for breast-feeding women undergoing short procedures (Montgomery, 2012).

Contraindications Not for intrathecal or epidural administration, due to the presence of glycine in the formulation; hypersensitivity to remifentanil, fentanyl, or fentanyl analogs, or any component of the formulation

Warnings/Precautions Remifentanil is not recommended as the sole agent for induction of anesthesia, because the loss of consciousness cannot be assured. Due to the high incidence of apnea, hypotension, respiratory depression, tachycardia and muscle rigidity remifentanil should only be administered by individuals specifically trained in the use of anesthetic agents and should not be used in diagnostic or therapeutic procedures outside the monitored anesthesia setting; resuscitative and intubation equipment should be readily available. May cause hypotension; use with caution in patients with hypovolemia, cardiovascular disease (including acute MI), or drugs which may exaggerate hypotensive effects (including phenothiazines or general anesthetics). Shares the toxic potentials of opioid agonists, and precautions of opioid agonist therapy should be observed. In patients <55 years of age, intraoperative awareness has been reported when used with propofol rates of ≤75 mcg/kg/minute.

Rapid I.V. infusion (single dose >1 mcg/kg over 30-60 seconds and infusion rates >0.1 mcg/kg/minute) should only be used during maintenance of general anesthesia; may result in skeletal muscle and chest wall rigidity, impaired ventilation, or respiratory distress/arrest; nondepolarizing skeletal muscle relaxant may be required. Chest wall rigidity may resolve by decreasing the infusion rate or temporarily stopping the infusion. Inadequate clearing of I.V. tubing following remifentanil administration could result in chest wall rigidity, respiratory depression, and apnea when another fluid is administered through the same line. Interruption of an infusion will result in offset of effects within 5-10 minutes; the discontinuation of remifentanil infusion should be preceded by the establishment of adequate postoperative analgesia orders, especially for patients in whom postoperative pain is anticipated. Use caution in the morbidly obese. Use with caution in patients with a history of drug abuse or acute alcoholism; potential for drug dependency exists. Tolerance, psychological and physical dependence may occur with prolonged use.

Adverse Reactions Frequency of adverse events may vary based on surgical procedures and rate of infusion.

>10%:

Cardiovascular: Hypotension (2% to 19%), bradycardia (1% to 7%; dose dependent)

Central nervous system: Headache (<2% to 18%)

Dermatologic: Pruritus (<2% to 18%)

Gastrointestinal: Nausea (<36% to 44%), vomiting (<16% to 22%)

Neuromuscular & skeletal: Muscle rigidity (<1% to 11%; includes chest wall rigidity)

1% to 10%:

Cardiovascular: Hypertension (1% to 2%; dose dependent), tachycardia (≤1%; dose dependent), flushing (1%)

Central nervous system: Fever (<5%), dizziness (<5%), postoperative pain (<2%), chills (1%), agitation (≤1%)

Local: Pain at injection site (1%)

Respiratory: Respiratory depression (<7%), apnea (<3%), hypoxia (≤1%)

Miscellaneous: Diaphoresis (6%), shivering (<5%), warm sensation (1%)

<1% (Limited to important or life-threatening): Abdominal discomfort, amnesia, anaphylaxis, anxiety, arrhythmias, awareness under anesthesia without pain, bronchitis, bronchospasm, chest pain, confusion, constipation, cough, CPK increased, diarrhea, disorientation, dysphagia, dysphoria, dyspnea, dysuria, ECG changes, electrolyte disorders, erythema, gastroesophageal reflux, hallucinations, heart block, heartburn, hiccups, hyperglycemia, ileus, incontinence, involuntary movement, laryngospasm, leukocytosis, liver dysfunction, lymphopenia, nasal congestion, nightmares, nystagmus, oliguria, paresthesia, pharyngitis, pleural effusion, prolonged emergence from anesthesia, pulmonary edema, rales, rapid awakening from anesthesia, rash, rhinorrhea, rhonchi, seizure, sleep disturbance, stridor, syncope, temperature regulation impaired, thrombocytopenia, tremors, twitching, urine retention, urticaria, xerostomia

Drug Interactions

Metabolism/Transport Effects None known.

Avoid Concomitant Use

Avoid concomitant use of Remifentanil with any of the following: Azelastine (Nasal); MAO Inhibitors; Paraldehyde

Increased Effect/Toxicity

Remifentanil may increase the levels/effects of: Alcohol (Ethyl); Alvimopan; Azelastine (Nasal); Beta-Blockers; Calcium Channel Blockers (Nondihydropyridine); CNS Depressants; Desmopressin; Diuretics; Hydrocodone; MAO Inhibitors; Metyrosine; Mirtazapine; Paraldehyde; Pramipexole; ROPINIRole; Rotigotine; Selective Serotonin Reuptake Inhibitors; Zolpidem

The levels/effects of Remifentanil may be increased by: Amphetamines; Anticholinergics; Antipsychotic Agents (Phenothiazines); Brimonidine (Topical); Cannabinoids; Doxylamine; Droperidol; HydrOXYzine; Magnesium Sulfate; Perampanel; Sodium Oxybate; Succinylcholine; Tapentadol

Decreased Effect

Remifentanil may decrease the levels/effects of: Pegvisomant

The levels/effects of Remifentanil may be decreased by: Ammonium Chloride; Mixed Agonist / Antagonist Opioids

Preparation for Administration Prepare solution by adding 1 mL of diluent per 1 mg of remifentanil. Shake well. Further dilute to a final concentration of 20, 25, 50, or 250 mcg/mL.

Storage/Stability Prior to reconstitution, store at 2°C to 25°C (36°F to 77°F). Stable for 24 hours at room temperature after reconstitution and further dilution to concentrations of 20-250 mcg/mL (4 hours if diluted with LR).

Mechanism of Action Binds with stereospecific mu-opioid receptors at many sites within the CNS, increases pain threshold, alters pain reception, inhibits ascending pain pathways

Pharmacodynamics/Kinetics

Onset of action: I.V.: 1-3 minutes

Distribution: V_d: 100 mL/kg; increased in children

Protein binding: ~70% (primarily $alpha_1$ acid glycoprotein)

Metabolism: Rapid via blood and tissue esterases

Half-life elimination (dose dependent): Terminal: 10-20 minutes; effective: 3-10 minutes

Excretion: Urine

Dosage I.V. continuous infusion:

Children Birth to 2 months: Maintenance of anesthesia with nitrous oxide (70%): 0.4 mcg/kg/minute (range: 0.4-1 mcg/kg/minute); supplemental bolus dose of 1 mcg/kg may be administered, smaller bolus dose may be required with potent inhalation agents, potent neuraxial anesthesia, significant comorbidities, significant fluid shifts, or without atropine pretreatment. Clearance in neonates is highly variable; dose should be carefully titrated.

Children 1-12 years: Maintenance of anesthesia with halothane, sevoflurane, or isoflurane: 0.25 mcg/kg/minute (range: 0.05-1.3 mcg/kg/minute); supplemental bolus dose of 1 mcg/kg may be administered every 2-5 minutes. Consider increasing concomitant anesthetics with infusion rate >1 mcg/kg/minute. Infusion rate can be titrated upward in increments up to 50% or titrated downward in decrements of 25% to 50%. May titrate every 2-5 minutes.

Adults:

Induction of anesthesia: 0.5-1 mcg/kg/minute; if endotracheal intubation is to occur in <8 minutes, an initial dose of 1 mcg/kg may be given over 30-60 seconds

Coronary bypass surgery: 1 mcg/kg/minute

Maintenance of anesthesia: **Note:** Supplemental bolus dose of 1 mcg/kg may be administered every 2-5 minutes. Consider increasing concomitant anesthetics with infusion rate >1 mcg/kg/minute. Infusion rate can be titrated upward in increments of 25% to 100% or downward in decrements of 25% to 50%. May titrate every 2-5 minutes.

With nitrous oxide (66%): 0.4 mcg/kg/minute (range: 0.1-2 mcg/kg/minute)

With isoflurane: 0.25 mcg/kg/minute (range: 0.05-2 mcg/kg/minute)

With propofol: 0.25 mcg/kg/minute (range: 0.05-2 mcg/kg/minute)

Coronary bypass surgery: 1 mcg/kg/minute (range: 0.125-4 mcg/kg/minute); supplemental dose: 0.5-1 mcg/kg

Continuation as an analgesic in immediate postoperative period: 0.1 mcg/kg/minute (range: 0.025-0.2 mcg/kg/minute). Infusion rate may be adjusted every 5 minutes in increments of 0.025 mcg/kg/minute. Bolus doses are not recommended. Infusion rates >0.2 mcg/kg/minute are associated with respiratory depression.

Coronary bypass surgery, continuation as an analgesic into the ICU: 1 mcg/kg/minute (range: 0.05-1 mcg/kg/minute)

Analgesic component of monitored anesthesia care: **Note:** Supplemental oxygen is recommended:

Single I.V. dose given 90 seconds prior to local anesthetic:

Remifentanil alone: 1 mcg/kg over 30-60 seconds

With midazolam: 0.5 mcg/kg over 30-60 seconds

Continuous infusion beginning 5 minutes prior to local anesthetic:

Remifentanil alone: 0.1 mcg/kg minute

With midazolam: 0.05 mcg/kg/minute

Continuous infusion given after local anesthetic:

Remifentanil alone: 0.05 mcg/kg/minute (range: 0.025-0.2 mcg/kg/minute)

With midazolam: 0.025 mcg/kg/minute (range: 0.025-0.2 mcg/kg/minute)

Note: Following local or anesthetic block, infusion rate should be decreased to 0.05 mcg/kg/minute; rate adjustments of 0.025 mcg/kg/minute may be done at 5-minute intervals

Critically-ill patients (unlabeled dose): Loading dose: 1.5 mcg/kg; followed by 0.008-0.25 mcg/kg/minute (**or** 0.5-15 mcg/kg/**hour**) (Barr, 2013)

Elderly: Elderly patients have an increased sensitivity to effect of remifentanil; doses should be decreased by 50% and titrated.

Dosage adjustment in renal impairment: No dosage adjustment necessary.

Dosage adjustment in hepatic impairment: No dosage adjustment necessary.

Dosing in obesity: Dose should be based on ideal body weight (IBW) in obese patients (>30% over IBW).

Administration An infusion device should be used to administer continuous infusions. During the maintenance of general anesthesia, I.V. boluses may be administered over 30-60 seconds. Injections should be given into I.V. tubing close to the venous cannula; tubing should be cleared after treatment to prevent residual effects when other fluids are administered through the same I.V. line.

Monitoring Parameters Respiratory and cardiovascular status, blood pressure, heart rate

Additional Information Ultra short-acting opioid that is unique compared to other short-acting opioids. This agent is not considered suitable as the sole agent for induction; remifentanil should be used in combination with other induction agents. Bolus doses are not recommended for sedation cases and in treatment of postoperative pain due to risk of respiratory depression and muscle rigidity. Due to remifentanil's short duration of action, when postoperative pain is anticipated, discontinuation of an infusion of remifentanil should be preceded by an adequate postoperative analgesic (ie, fentanyl, morphine).

Dosage Forms Excipient information presented when available (limited, particularly for generics); consult specific product labeling.

Solution Reconstituted, Intravenous [preservative free]:

Ultiva: 1 mg (1 ea); 2 mg (1 ea); 5 mg (1 ea)

Controlled Substance C-II

- **Reminyl® (Can)** *see* Galantamine *on page 937*
- **Reminyl® ER (Can)** *see* Galantamine *on page 937*
- **Remodulin** *see* Treprostinil *on page 2115*
- **Renagel** *see* Sevelamer *on page 1892*
- **Renal Replacement Solution** *see* Electrolyte Solution, Renal Replacement *on page 691*
- **Renedil® (Can)** *see* Felodipine *on page 836*
- **Renova** *see* Tretinoin (Topical) *on page 2120*
- **Renova® (Can)** *see* Tretinoin (Topical) *on page 2120*
- **Renova Pump** *see* Tretinoin (Topical) *on page 2120*
- **Renvela** *see* Sevelamer *on page 1892*
- **ReoPro** *see* Abciximab *on page 22*
- **ReoPro® (Can)** *see* Abciximab *on page 22*

Repaglinide (re PAG li nide)

Brand Names: U.S. Prandin

Brand Names: Canada CO-Repaglinide; GlucoNorm®; PMS-Repaglinide; Sandoz-Repaglinide

Pharmacologic Category Antidiabetic Agent, Meglitinide Derivative

Additional Appendix Information

Oral Antidiabetic Agents Comparison Table *on page 2312*

Use Management of type 2 diabetes mellitus (noninsulin dependent, NIDDM) as an adjunct to diet and exercise; may be used in combination with metformin or thiazolidinediones

Pregnancy Risk Factor C

Pregnancy Considerations Adverse events have been observed in some animal reproduction studies. Repaglinide was shown to have a low potential to cross the placenta using an *ex vivo* perfusion model (Tertti, 2011). Information describing the effects of repaglinide on pregnancy outcomes is limited.

For women with diabetes, maternal hyperglycemia can be associated with adverse effects in the fetus, neonate, and mother. To prevent adverse events, prior to conception and throughout pregnancy, the maternal Hb A_{1c} should be kept close to normal but without causing significant hypoglycemia. The use of meglitinide derivatives in pregnant women is not recommended; insulin is the drug of choice for the control of diabetes mellitus during pregnancy (ACOG, 2005; ADA, 2013; Kitzmiller, 2008; Metzger, 2007).

Breast-Feeding Considerations It is not known if repaglinide is excreted in breast milk. Breast-feeding is not recommended by the manufacturer.

Contraindications Hypersensitivity to repaglinide or any component of the formulation; diabetic ketoacidosis, with or without coma; type 1 diabetes (insulin dependent, IDDM); concurrent gemfibrozil therapy

Warnings/Precautions Use with caution in patients with hepatic impairment. Use caution in severe renal dysfunction, elderly, malnourished, or patients with adrenal/pituitary dysfunction; may be more susceptible to glucose-lowering effects. May cause hypoglycemia; appropriate patient selection, dosage, and patient education are important to avoid hypoglycemic episodes. It may be necessary to discontinue repaglinide and administer insulin if the patient is exposed to stress (fever, trauma, infection, surgery). Theoretically, repaglinide may increase cardiovascular events as observed in some studies using sulfonylureas, but there are no long-term studies assessing this concern. Not indicated for use in combination with NPH insulin as there have been case reports of myocardial ischemia; further evaluation required to assess the safety of this combination.

Adverse Reactions

>10%:

Central nervous system: Headache (9% to 11%)

Endocrine & metabolic: Hypoglycemia (16% to 31%)

Respiratory: Upper respiratory tract infection (10% to 16%)

1% to 10%:

Cardiovascular: Ischemia (4%), chest pain (2% to 3%)

Gastrointestinal: Diarrhea (4% to 5%), constipation (2% to 3%)

Genitourinary: Urinary tract infection (2% to 3%)

Neuromuscular & skeletal: Back pain (5% to 6%), arthralgia (3% to 6%)

Respiratory: Sinusitis (3% to 6%), bronchitis (2% to 6%)

Miscellaneous: Allergy (1% to 2%)

<1% (Limited to important or life-threatening): Anaphylactoid reaction, arrhythmia, hemolytic anemia, hepatic dysfunction (severe), hepatitis, hypertension, leukopenia, MI, pancreatitis, Stevens-Johnson syndrome, thrombocytopenia, visual disturbances (transient)

Drug Interactions

Metabolism/Transport Effects Substrate of CYP2C8 (major), CYP3A4 (major), SLCO1B1; **Note:** Assignment of Major/Minor substrate status based on clinically relevant drug interaction potential

Avoid Concomitant Use

Avoid concomitant use of Repaglinide with any of the following: Gemfibrozil

Increased Effect/Toxicity

Repaglinide may increase the levels/effects of: Hypoglycemic Agents

The levels/effects of Repaglinide may be increased by: CycloSPORINE (Systemic); CYP2C8 Inhibitors (Moderate); CYP2C8 Inhibitors (Strong); CYP3A4 Inhibitors (Strong); Deferasirox; Eltrombopag; Gemfibrozil; Herbs (Hypoglycemic Properties); Macrolide Antibiotics; MAO Inhibitors; Mifepristone; Pegvisomant; Salicylates; Selective Serotonin Reuptake Inhibitors; Telaprevir; Teriflunomide; Trimethoprim

Decreased Effect

The levels/effects of Repaglinide may be decreased by: Bosentan; Corticosteroids (Orally Inhaled); Corticosteroids (Systemic); CYP2C8 Inducers (Strong); CYP3A4 Inducers (Strong); Dabrafenib; Herbs (CYP3A4 Inducers); Loop Diuretics; Luteinizing Hormone-Releasing Hormone Analogs; Mitotane; Rifampin; Somatropin; Thiazide Diuretics; Tocilizumab

Ethanol/Nutrition/Herb Interactions

Ethanol: Ethanol may increase risk of hypoglycemia. Management: Avoid ethanol.

Food: When given with food, the AUC of repaglinide is decreased. Taking medication without eating may cause hypoglycemia. Management: Administer 15-30 minutes prior to a meal. If a meal is skipped, skip dose for that meal.

Herb/Nutraceutical: St John's wort may decrease the levels/effect of repaglinide. Other herbal medications may enhance the hypoglycemic effects of repaglinide. Management: Avoid St John's wort, alfalfa, aloe, bilberry, bitter melon, burdock, celery, damiana, fenugreek, garcinia, garlic, ginger, ginseng (American), gymnema, marshmallow, and stinging nettle.

Storage/Stability Do not store above 25°C (77°F). Protect from moisture.

Mechanism of Action Nonsulfonylurea hypoglycemic agent which blocks ATP-dependent potassium channels, depolarizing the membrane and facilitating calcium entry through calcium channels. Increased intracellular calcium stimulates insulin release from the pancreatic beta cells. Repaglinide-induced insulin release is glucose-dependent.

Pharmacodynamics/Kinetics

Onset of action: Single dose: Increased insulin levels: ~15-60 minutes

Duration: 4-6 hours

Absorption: Rapid and complete

Distribution: V_d: 31 L

Protein binding, plasma: >98% to albumin

Metabolism: Hepatic via CYP3A4 and CYP2C8 isoenzymes and glucuronidation to inactive metabolites

Bioavailability: ~56%

Half-life elimination: ~1 hour

Time to peak, plasma: ~1 hour

Excretion: Feces (~90%, <2% as unchanged drug); Urine (~8%, 0.1% as unchanged drug)

Dosage Oral: Adults:

Initial: For patients not previously treated or whose Hb A_{1c} is <8%, the starting dose is 0.5 mg before each meal. For patients previously treated with blood glucose-lowering agents whose Hb A_{1c} is ≥8%, the initial dose is 1 or 2 mg before each meal.

Dose adjustment: Determine dosing adjustments by blood glucose response, usually fasting blood glucose. Double the preprandial dose up to 4 mg until satisfactory blood glucose response is achieved. At least 1 week should elapse to assess response after each dose adjustment.

Dose range: 0.5-4 mg taken with meals. Repaglinide may be dosed preprandially 2, 3, or 4 times/day in response to changes in the patient's meal pattern. Maximum recommended daily dose: 16 mg.

Patients receiving other oral hypoglycemic agents: When repaglinide is used to replace therapy with other oral hypoglycemic agents, it may be started the day after the final dose is given. Observe patients carefully for hypoglycemia because of potential overlapping of drug effects. When transferred from longer half-life sulfonylureas (eg, chlorpropamide), close monitoring may be indicated for up to ≥1 week.

Combination therapy: If repaglinide monotherapy does not result in adequate glycemic control, metformin or a thiazolidinedione may be added. Or, if metformin or thiazolidinedione therapy does not provide adequate control, repaglinide may be added. The starting dose and dose adjustments for combination therapy are the same as repaglinide monotherapy. Carefully adjust the dose of each drug to determine the minimal dose required to achieve the desired pharmacologic effect. Failure to do so could result in an increase in the incidence of hypoglycemic episodes. Use appropriate monitoring of FPG and Hb A_{1c} measurements to ensure that the patient is not subjected to excessive drug exposure or increased probability of secondary drug failure. If glucose is not achieved after a suitable trial of combination therapy, consider discontinuing these drugs and using insulin.

Dosage adjustment in renal impairment:

Cl_{cr} 40-80 mL/minute (mild-to-moderate renal dysfunction): Initial: No dosage adjustment necessary.

Cl_{cr} 20-40 mL/minute (severe renal impairment): Initial: 0.5 mg with meals; titrate carefully.

Cl_{cr} <20 mL/minute: No dosage adjustment provided in manufacturer's labeling (has not been studied).

Hemodialysis: No dosage adjustment provided in manufacturer's labeling (has not been studied).

Dosage adjustment in hepatic impairment: No dosage adjustment provided in manufacturer's labeling. Use with caution; use conservative initial and maintenance doses. Use longer intervals between dosage adjustments.

Dietary Considerations Take repaglinide 15-30 minutes before meals. Individualized medical nutrition therapy (MNT) based on ADA recommendations is an integral part of therapy. May cause hypoglycemia. Must be able to recognize symptoms of hypoglycemia (palpitations, tachycardia, sweaty palms, diaphoresis, lightheadedness).

Administration Administer 15 minutes before meals; however, time may vary from immediately preceding a meal to as long as 30 minutes before a meal. If the patient misses a meal or is unable to take anything by mouth, repaglinide should not be administered to avoid hypoglycemia. Patients consuming extra meals should be instructed to add a dose for the extra meal.

Monitoring Parameters Monitor fasting blood glucose (periodically) and glycosylated hemoglobin (Hb A_{1c}) levels (every 3 months) with a goal of decreasing these levels towards the normal range. During dose adjustment, fasting glucose can be used to determine response.

Reference Range Recommendations for glycemic control in nonpregnant adults with diabetes (ADA, 2013):

Hb A_{1c}: <7% (a more aggressive [<6.5%] or less aggressive [<8%] Hb A_{1c} goal may be targeted based on patient-specific characteristics)

Preprandial capillary plasma glucose: 70-130 mg/dL

Peak postprandial capillary blood glucose: <180 mg/dL

Dosage Forms Excipient information presented when available (limited, particularly for generics); consult specific product labeling.

Tablet, Oral:

Prandin: 0.5 mg, 1 mg, 2 mg

Generic: 0.5 mg, 1 mg, 2 mg

Repaglinide and Metformin

(re PAG li nide & met FOR min)

Brand Names: U.S. PrandiMet®

Index Terms Metformin and Repaglinide; Repaglinide and Metformin Hydrochloride

Pharmacologic Category Antidiabetic Agent, Biguanide; Antidiabetic Agent, Meglitinide Derivative; Hypoglycemic Agent, Oral

Use Management of type 2 diabetes mellitus (noninsulin dependent, NIDDM), as an adjunct to diet and exercise, in patients currently receiving or not adequately controlled on metformin and/or a meglitinide

Pregnancy Risk Factor C

Dosage Oral: Adults: Type 2 diabetes mellitus: **Note:** Daily doses should be divided and given 2-3 times daily with meals (maximum single dose: 4 mg/dose [repaglinide], 1000 mg/dose [metformin]; maximum daily dose: 10 mg/day [repaglinide], 2500 mg/day [metformin])

Patients currently taking repaglinide and metformin: Initial doses should be based on (but not exceeding) the patient's current doses of repaglinide and metformin; titrate as needed to the maximum daily dose to achieve targeted glycemic control

Patients inadequately controlled on metformin alone: Initial dose: Repaglinide 1 mg/ metformin 500 mg twice daily with meals. Titrate slowly to reduce the risk of repaglinide-induced hypoglycemia.

Patients inadequately controlled on a meglitinide alone: Initial dose: Metformin 500 mg twice daily plus repaglinide at a dose similar to (but not exceeding) the patient's current dose. Titrate slowly to reduce the risk of metformin-induced gastrointestinal adverse effects.

Dosing adjustment in renal impairment: Do not use in renal impairment; metformin use is contraindicated in patients with renal impairment (serum creatinine ≥1.5 mg/dL in males or ≥1.4 mg/dL in females)

Dosing adjustment in hepatic impairment: Avoid use in patients with impaired liver function

Additional Information Complete prescribing information should be consulted for additional detail.

Dosage Forms Excipient information presented when available (limited, particularly for generics); consult specific product labeling.

Tablet:

PrandiMet®:

1/500: Repaglinide 1 mg and metformin hydrochloride 500 mg

2/500: Repaglinide 2 mg and metformin hydrochloride 500 mg

- **Repaglinide and Metformin Hydrochloride** *see* Repaglinide and Metformin *on page 1799*
- **Repan** *see* Butalbital, Acetaminophen, and Caffeine *on page 305*
- **Reprexain** *see* Hydrocodone and Ibuprofen *on page 1008*
- **Repronex®** *see* Menotropins *on page 1295*
- **Requip** *see* ROPINIRole *on page 1851*
- **Requip® (Can)** *see* ROPINIRole *on page 1851*
- **Requip XL** *see* ROPINIRole *on page 1851*
- **Rescon DM [OTC]** *see* Chlorpheniramine, Pseudoephedrine, and Dextromethorphan *on page 414*
- **Rescon GG [OTC]** *see* Guaifenesin and Phenylephrine *on page 978*
- **Rescriptor** *see* Delavirdine *on page 565*
- **Rescriptor® (Can)** *see* Delavirdine *on page 565*
- **Resectisol** *see* Mannitol *on page 1266*

Reserpine

(re SER peen)

Pharmacologic Category Central Monoamine-Depleting Agent; Rauwolfia Alkaloid

Additional Appendix Information

Beers Criteria – Potentially Inappropriate Medications for Geriatrics *on page 2368*

Use Management of mild-to-moderate hypertension; treatment of agitated psychotic states (schizophrenia)

Unlabeled Use Management of tardive dyskinesia

Pregnancy Risk Factor C

Dosage Note: When used for management of hypertension, full antihypertensive effects may take as long as 3 weeks.

Oral:

Children: Hypertension: 0.01-0.02 mg/kg/24 hours divided every 12 hours; maximum dose: 0.25 mg/day (not recommended in children)

Adults:

Hypertension:

Manufacturer's labeling: Initial: 0.5 mg/day for 1-2 weeks; maintenance: 0.1-0.25 mg/day

Note: Clinically, the need for a "loading" period (as recommended by the manufacturer) is not well supported, and alternative dosing is preferred.

Alternative dosing (unlabeled): Initial: 0.1 mg once daily; adjust as necessary based on response.

Usual dose range (JNC 7): 0.05-0.25 mg once daily; 0.1 mg every other day may be given to achieve 0.05 mg once daily

Schizophrenia (labeled use) or tardive dyskinesia (unlabeled use): Dosing recommendations vary; initial dose recommendations generally range from 0.05-0.25 mg (although manufacturer recommends 0.5 mg once daily initially in schizophrenia). May be increased in increments of 0.1-0.25 mg; maximum dose in tardive dyskinesia: 5 mg/day.

Elderly: Initial: 0.05 mg once daily, increasing by 0.05 mg every week as necessary (Beers Criteria: Avoid doses >0.25 mg daily)

Dosage adjustment in renal impairment: No dosage adjustment provided in manufacturer's labeling. The following dosing adjustments have been used by some clinicians (Aronoff, 2007):

Cl_{cr} <10 mL/minute: Avoid use.

Hemodialysis, peritoneal dialysis: Not removed by hemo- or peritoneal dialysis; supplemental dose is not necessary.

Dosage adjustment in renal impairment: No dosage adjustment provided in manufacturer's labeling.

Additional Information Complete prescribing information should be consulted for additional detail.

Dosage Forms Excipient information presented when available (limited, particularly for generics); consult specific product labeling.

Tablet, Oral:

Generic: 0.1 mg, 0.25 mg

- **Resistant Dextrin** *see* Wheat Dextrin *on page 2215*
- **Resistant Maltodextrin** *see* Wheat Dextrin *on page 2215*
- **Respa-BR** *see* Brompheniramine *on page 282*
- **Restasis** *see* CycloSPORINE (Ophthalmic) *on page 515*
- **Restasis® (Can)** *see* CycloSPORINE (Ophthalmic) *on page 515*
- **Restoril** *see* Temazepam *on page 2005*
- **Restylane** *see* Hyaluronate and Derivatives *on page 1000*
- **Restylane-L** *see* Hyaluronate and Derivatives *on page 1000*

Retapamulin (re te PAM ue lin)

Brand Names: U.S. Altabax

Pharmacologic Category Antibiotic, Pleuromutilin; Antibiotic, Topical

Use Treatment of impetigo caused by susceptible strains of *S. pyogenes* or methicillin-susceptible *S. aureus*

Pregnancy Risk Factor B

Dosage Topical: Impetigo:

Children ≥9 months: Apply to affected area twice daily for 5 days. Total treatment area should not exceed 2% of total body surface area.

Adults: Apply to affected area twice daily for 5 days. Total treatment area should not exceed 100 cm^2 total body surface area.

Additional Information Complete prescribing information should be consulted for additional detail.

Dosage Forms Excipient information presented when available (limited, particularly for generics); consult specific product labeling.

Ointment, External:

Altabax: 1% (15 g, 30 g)

◆ Retavase *see* Reteplase *on page 1800*

◆ Retavase® (Can) *see* Reteplase *on page 1800*

◆ Retavase Half-Kit *see* Reteplase *on page 1800*

Reteplase (RE ta plase)

Brand Names: U.S. Retavase; Retavase Half-Kit

Brand Names: Canada Retavase®

Index Terms r-PA; Recombinant Plasminogen Activator

Pharmacologic Category Thrombolytic Agent

Use Management of ST-elevation myocardial infarction (STEMI) for the improvement of ventricular function, the reduction of the incidence of CHF, and the reduction of mortality following STEMI

Recommended criteria for treatment of STEMI (ACCF/AHA; O'Gara, 2013): Ischemic symptoms within 12 hours of treatment or evidence of ongoing ischemia 12-24 hours after symptom onset with a large area of myocardium at risk or hemodynamic instability.

STEMI ECG definition: New ST-segment elevation at the J point in at least 2 contiguous leads of ≥2 mm (0.2 mV) in men or ≥1.5 mm (0.15 mV) in women in leads V_2-V_3 and/or of ≥1 mm (0.1 mV) in other contiguous precordial leads or limb leads on ECG. New or presumably new left bundle branch block (LBBB) may interfere with ST-elevation analysis and should not be considered diagnostic in isolation.

At non-PCI-capable hospitals, the ACCF/AHA recommends thrombolytic therapy administration when the anticipated first medical contact (FMC)-to-device time at a PCI-capable hospital is >120 minutes due to unavoidable delays.

Pregnancy Risk Factor C

Pregnancy Considerations Adverse events have been observed in some animal reproduction studies. The risk of bleeding may be increased in pregnant women.

Breast-Feeding Considerations It is not known if reteplase is excreted in breast milk. The manufacturer recommends that caution be exercised when administering reteplase to nursing women.

Contraindications Active internal bleeding; history of cerebrovascular accident; recent (ie, within 2 months) intracranial or intraspinal surgery or trauma; intracranial neoplasm, arteriovenous malformations, or aneurysm; known bleeding diathesis; severe uncontrolled hypertension

Additional contraindications (ACCF/AHA; O'Gara, 2013): Ischemic stroke within 3 months; prior intracranial hemorrhage; active bleeding (excluding menses); suspected aortic dissection; significant closed head or facial trauma within 3 months

Warnings/Precautions Use with caution in patients receiving oral anticoagulants; increased risk of bleeding. Adjunctive use of parenteral anticoagulants (eg, enoxaparin, heparin, or fondaparinux) is recommended to improve vessel patency and prevent reocclusion (ACCF/AHA; O'Gara, 2013); however, these may also contribute to bleeding; monitor for bleeding. I.M. injections and nonessential handling of the patient should be avoided. Venipunctures should be performed carefully and only when necessary. If arterial puncture is necessary, use an upper extremity vessel that can be manually compressed. If serious bleeding occurs then the infusion of reteplase and heparin should be stopped.

For the following conditions the risk of bleeding is higher with use of reteplase and should be weighed against the benefits of therapy: recent major surgery (eg, CABG, obstetrical delivery, organ biopsy), recent puncture of noncompressible vessels, cerebrovascular disease, recent gastrointestinal or genitourinary bleeding, recent trauma including CPR, hypertension (systolic BP >180 mm Hg and/or diastolic BP >110 mm Hg), high likelihood of left heart thrombus (eg, mitral stenosis with atrial fibrillation), acute pericarditis, subacute bacterial endocarditis, hemostatic defects including ones caused by severe renal or hepatic dysfunction, significant hepatic or renal dysfunction, diabetic hemorrhagic retinopathy or other hemorrhagic ophthalmic conditions, septic thrombophlebitis or occluded AV cannula at seriously infected site, advanced age (eg, >75 years), patients receiving oral anticoagulants, any other condition in which bleeding constitutes a significant hazard or would be particularly difficult to manage because of location.

Coronary thrombolysis may result in reperfusion arrhythmias. Follow standard MI management. Rare anaphylactic reactions can occur.

Adverse Reactions Bleeding is the most frequent adverse effect associated with reteplase. Heparin and aspirin have been administered concurrently with reteplase in clinical trials. The incidence of adverse events is a reflection of these combined therapies, and is comparable to comparison thrombolytics.

>10%: Local: Injection site bleeding (5% to 49%)

1% to 10%:

Gastrointestinal: Bleeding (2% to 9%)

Genitourinary: Bleeding (1% to 10%)

Hematologic: Anemia (1% to 3%)

<1% (Limited to important or life-threatening): Intracranial hemorrhage (0.8%), allergic/anaphylactoid reactions, cholesterol embolization

Other adverse effects noted are frequently associated with MI (and therefore may or may not be attributable to Retavase®) and include arrhythmia, AV block, cardiac arrest, cardiogenic shock, embolism, heart failure, hypotension, myocardial rupture, mitral regurgitation, pericardial effusion, pericarditis, pulmonary edema, recurrent ischemia, reinfarction, tamponade, thrombosis

Drug Interactions

Metabolism/Transport Effects None known.

Avoid Concomitant Use There are no known interactions where it is recommended to avoid concomitant use.

Increased Effect/Toxicity

Reteplase may increase the levels/effects of: Anticoagulants; Dabigatran Etexilate

The levels/effects of Reteplase may be increased by: Agents with Antiplatelet Properties; Herbs (Anticoagulant/Antiplatelet Properties); Nonsteroidal Anti-Inflammatory Agents; Salicylates

Decreased Effect

The levels/effects of Reteplase may be decreased by: Aprotinin

Preparation for Administration Reteplase should be reconstituted using the diluent, syringe, needle, and dispensing pin provided with each kit. Do not shake while reconstituting; swirl gently. Once reconstituted, use within 4 hours.

Storage/Stability Dosage kits should be stored at 2°C to 25°C (36°F to 77°F) and remain sealed until use in order to protect from light.

Mechanism of Action Reteplase is a nonglycosylated form of tPA produced by recombinant DNA technology using *E. coli*; it initiates local fibrinolysis by binding to fibrin in a thrombus (clot) and converts entrapped plasminogen to plasmin

Pharmacodynamics/Kinetics

Onset of action: Thrombolysis: 30-90 minutes

Half-life elimination: 13-16 minutes

Excretion: Feces and urine

Clearance: Plasma: 250-450 mL/minute

Dosage

Children: Not recommended

Adults: 10 units I.V. over 2 minutes, followed by a second dose 30 minutes later of 10 units I.V. over 2 minutes; withhold second dose if serious bleeding or anaphylaxis occurs

Note: Thrombolytic should be administered within 30 minutes of hospital arrival. Administer concurrent aspirin, clopidogrel, and anticoagulant therapy (ie, unfractionated heparin, enoxaparin, or fondaparinux) with reteplase (O'Gara, 2013).

Dosage adjustment in renal impairment: No dosage adjustment provided in manufacturer's labeling. However, risks of reteplase therapy may be increased.

Dosage adjustment in hepatic disease: No dosage adjustment provided in manufacturer's labeling. However, risks of reteplase therapy may be increased.

Administration Reconstituted dose should be administered I.V. over 2 minutes; no other medication should be added to the injection solution.

Monitoring Parameters Monitor for signs of bleeding (hematuria, GI bleeding, gingival bleeding); CBC, PTT; ECG monitoring

Test Interactions Altered results of coagulation and fibrinolytic activity tests

Dosage Forms Excipient information presented when available (limited, particularly for generics); consult specific product labeling.

Kit, Intravenous [preservative free]:

Retavase: 10.4 units

Retavase Half-Kit: 10.4 units

◆ **Retigabine** *see* Ezogabine *on page 819*
◆ **Retin-A** *see* Tretinoin (Topical) *on page 2120*
◆ **Retin-A® (Can)** *see* Tretinoin (Topical) *on page 2120*
◆ **Retin-A Micro** *see* Tretinoin (Topical) *on page 2120*
◆ **Retin-A Micro® (Can)** *see* Tretinoin (Topical) *on page 2120*
◆ **Retin-A Micro Pump** *see* Tretinoin (Topical) *on page 2120*
◆ **Retinoic Acid** *see* Tretinoin (Topical) *on page 2120*
◆ **Retinova® (Can)** *see* Tretinoin (Topical) *on page 2120*
◆ **Retrovir** *see* Zidovudine *on page 2226*
◆ **Retrovir® (Can)** *see* Zidovudine *on page 2226*
◆ **Retrovir® (AZT™) (Can)** *see* Zidovudine *on page 2226*
◆ **Revatio** *see* Sildenafil *on page 1894*
◆ **Revatio® (Can)** *see* Sildenafil *on page 1894*
◆ **ReVia** *see* Naltrexone *on page 1423*
◆ **Revitalose C-1000® (Can)** *see* Ascorbic Acid *on page 172*
◆ **Revlimid** *see* Lenalidomide *on page 1180*
◆ **Revlimid® (Can)** *see* Lenalidomide *on page 1180*
◆ **Revolade®** *see* Eltrombopag *on page 693*
◆ **Revolade™ (Can)** *see* Eltrombopag *on page 693*
◆ **Revonto** *see* Dantrolene *on page 537*
◆ **Reyataz** *see* Atazanavir *on page 182*
◆ **rFSH-alpha** *see* Follitropin Alfa *on page 908*
◆ **rFSH-beta** *see* Follitropin Beta *on page 909*
◆ **rFVIIa** *see* Factor VIIa (Recombinant) *on page 821*
◆ **RG7204** *see* Vemurafenib *on page 2176*
◆ **R-Gene 10** *see* Arginine *on page 163*
◆ **rhAT** *see* Antithrombin *on page 148*
◆ **rhATIII** *see* Antithrombin *on page 148*
◆ **r-hCG** *see* Chorionic Gonadotropin (Recombinant) *on page 420*
◆ **rhDNase** *see* Dornase Alfa *on page 654*
◆ **Rheumatrex** *see* Methotrexate *on page 1324*
◆ **rhFSH-alpha** *see* Follitropin Alfa *on page 908*
◆ **rhFSH-beta** *see* Follitropin Beta *on page 909*
◆ **rhGAA** *see* Alglucosidase Alfa *on page 74*
◆ **r-h α-GAL** *see* Agalsidase Beta *on page 57*
◆ **RhIG** *see* Rh_o(D) Immune Globulin *on page 1801*
◆ **rhIL-11** *see* Oprelvekin *on page 1514*
◆ **Rhinalar® (Can)** *see* Flunisolide (Nasal) *on page 878*
◆ **Rhinaris [OTC]** *see* Sodium Chloride *on page 1914*
◆ **Rhinaris-CS Anti-Allergic Nasal Mist (Can)** *see* Cromolyn (Nasal) *on page 500*
◆ **Rhinocort Aqua** *see* Budesonide (Nasal) *on page 286*
◆ **Rhinocort® Aqua® (Can)** *see* Budesonide (Nasal) *on page 286*
◆ **Rhinocort® Turbuhaler® (Can)** *see* Budesonide (Nasal) *on page 286*
◆ **r-Hirudin** *see* Desirudin *on page 574*
◆ **rhKGF** *see* Palifermin *on page 1548*
◆ **r-hLH** *see* Lutropin Alfa *on page 1258*
◆ **Rho(D) Immune Globulin (Human)** *see* Rh_o(D) Immune Globulin *on page 1801*

Rh_o(D) Immune Globulin

(ar aych oh (dee) i MYUN GLOB yoo lin)

Brand Names: U.S. HyperRHO S/D; MICRhoGAM Ultra-Filtered Plus; RhoGAM Ultra-Filtered Plus; Rhophylac; WinRho SDF

Brand Names: Canada WinRho® SDF

Index Terms Anti-D Immunoglobulin; RhIG; Rho(D) Immune Globulin (Human); RhoIGIV; RhoIVIM

Pharmacologic Category Blood Product Derivative; Immune Globulin

Use

Suppression of Rh isoimmunization: Use in the following situations when an Rh_o(D)-negative individual is exposed to Rh_o(D)-positive blood: During delivery of an Rh_o(D)-positive infant; abortion; amniocentesis; chorionic villus sampling; ruptured tubal pregnancy; abdominal trauma; hydatidiform mole; transplacental hemorrhage. Used when the mother is Rh_o(D)-negative, the father of the child is either Rh$_o$(D)-positive or Rh$_o$(D)-unknown, or the baby is either Rh$_o$(D)-positive or Rh$_o$(D)-unknown.

Transfusion: Suppression of Rh isoimmunization in Rh$_o$(D)-negative individuals transfused with Rh$_o$(D) antigen-positive RBCs or blood components containing Rh$_o$(D) antigen-positive RBCs

Treatment of immune thrombocytopenia (ITP): Used intravenously in the following nonsplenectomized Rh$_o$(D)-positive individuals: Children with acute or chronic ITP, adults with chronic ITP, and children and adults with ITP secondary to HIV infection

Pregnancy Risk Factor C

Pregnancy Considerations Animal studies have not been conducted. Available evidence suggests that Rh$_o$(D) immune globulin administration during pregnancy does not harm the fetus or affect future pregnancies.

Breast-Feeding Considerations Adverse events in the nursing infant have not been observed when administered to women for the suppression of Rh isoimmunization.

Contraindications Hypersensitivity to immune globulins or any component of the formulation; prior sensitization to Rh$_o$(D)

WinRho® SDF product labeling: Patients with autoimmune hemolytic anemia; patients with pre-existing hemolysis or at high risk for hemolysis; IgA-deficient patients with antibodies against IgA; suppression of isoimmunization in infants

WinRho® SDF Canadian labeling: Additional contraindications (not in U.S. labeling):

Rh immunization prophylaxis: Rh$_o$(D)-negative women who are not pregnant or have had a recent delivery or abortion and who are Rh sensitized

Treatment of ITP: Patients who are Rh$_o$(D)-negative or have had splenectomy, ITP secondary to conditions including leukemia, lymphoma, or active infections with Epstein-Barr virus (EBV) or hepatits C virus (HCV), elderly with comorbidities predisposing to acute hemolytic reaction (AHR), evidence of autoimmune hemolytic anemia (Evan's syndrome), systemic lupus erythematosus (SLE) or antiphospholipid antibody syndrome

Warnings/Precautions [U.S. Boxed Warning]: May cause IVH in patients treated for immune thrombocytopenia (ITP) (WinRho® SDF product labeling). Rare but serious signs and symptoms (eg, back pain, shaking, chills, fever, discolored urine; onset within 4 hours of infusion) of intravascular hemolysis (IVH) have been reported in postmarketing experience in patients treated for ITP and may result in clinically-compromising anemia and multiorgan system failure including acute respiratory distress syndrome. Acute renal insufficiency and disseminated intravascular coagulation (DIC) have also been reported. ITP patients should be advised of the signs and symptoms of IVH and instructed to report them immediately.

Product of human plasma; may potentially contain infectious agents which could transmit disease. Screening of donors, as well as testing and/or inactivation or removal of certain viruses, reduces the risk. Infections thought to be transmitted by this product should be reported to the manufacturer. Not for replacement therapy in immune globulin deficiency syndromes. Pulmonary edema may occur following IVIG treatment in patients being treated for ITP. Symptoms are usually present within 1-6 hours after administration; monitor patients for pulmonary reactions. Use caution with IgA deficiency, may contain trace amounts of IgA; patients who are IgA deficient may have the potential for developing IgA antibodies, anaphylactic reactions may occur. Administer I.M. injections with caution in patients with thrombocytopenia or coagulation disorders. Some products may contain maltose, which may result in falsely-elevated blood glucose readings. Use caution with renal dysfunction. Thrombotic events have been reported with administration of intravenous immune globulins (IVIG); use with caution in patients with a history of atherosclerosis or cardiovascular and/or thrombotic risk factors or patients with known/suspected hyperviscosity. Consider a baseline assessment of blood viscosity in patients at risk for hyperviscosity.

Administer at the minimum practical infusion rate in patients with renal impairment or in patients at risk for thrombotic events. Monitor for signs and symptoms of transfusion-related acute lung injury.

ITP: Do not administer I.M. or SubQ for the treatment of ITP; administer dose I.V. only. Safety and efficacy not established in Rh$_o$(D) negative, non-ITP thrombocytopenia, or splenectomized patients. When using WinRho® SDF, decrease dose with hemoglobin <10 g/dL; use with extreme caution if hemoglobin <8 g/dL. Safety and efficacy have not been established for Rhophylac® in patients with anemia.

Rh$_o$(D) suppression: For use in the mother; do not administer to the neonate.

Adverse Reactions Frequency not defined.

Cardiovascular: Hyper-/hypotension, pallor, vasodilation

Central nervous system: Chills, dizziness, fever, headache, malaise, somnolence

Dermatologic: Pruritus, rash

Gastrointestinal: Abdominal pain, diarrhea, nausea, vomiting

Hematologic: Haptoglobin decreased, hemoglobin decreased (patients with ITP), intravascular hemolysis (patients with ITP)

Hepatic: Bilirubin increased, LDH increased

Local: Injection site reaction: Discomfort, induration, mild pain, redness, swelling

Neuromuscular & skeletal: Arthralgia, back pain, hyperkinesia, myalgia, weakness

Renal: Acute renal insufficiency

Miscellaneous: Anaphylaxis, diaphoresis, infusion-related reactions, positive anti-C antibody test (transient), shivering

Postmarketing and/or case reports: Anemia (clinically-compromising), anuria, ARDS, cardiac arrest, cardiac failure, chest pain, chromaturia, DIC, edema, erythema, fatigue, hematuria, hemoglobinemia, hemoglobinuria (transient in patients with ITP), hyperhidrosis, hypersensitivity, injection site irritation, jaundice, myocardial infarction, muscle spasm, nausea, pain in extremities, renal failure, renal impairment, tachycardia, transfusion-related acute lung injury

Drug Interactions

Metabolism/Transport Effects None known.

Avoid Concomitant Use There are no known interactions where it is recommended to avoid concomitant use.

Increased Effect/Toxicity There are no known significant interactions involving an increase in effect.

Decreased Effect

Rho(D) Immune Globulin may decrease the levels/effects of: Vaccines (Live)

Storage/Stability Store at 2°C to 8°C (35°F to 46°F); do not freeze.

RhoGAM® UF Plus, MICRhoGAM® UF Plus: May be stored at 25°C (77°F) for up to 10 days (data on file [Ortho Clinical Diagnostics, 2011]). However, the manufacturer recommends storage under refrigeration. Room temperature stability information should only be utilized in situations where the drug has been inadvertently exposed to prolonged room temperature.

HyperRHO™ SD may be stored at 25°C (77°F) for ~2 weeks (data on file [Talecris Biotherapeutics, 2011]). However, the manufacturer recommends storage under refrigeration. Room temperature stability information should only be utilized in situations where the drug has been inadvertently exposed to prolonged room temperature.

Rhophylac®: Protect from light.

WinRho® SDF: After reconstitution, store at room temperature for no longer than 12 hours. Do not shake or freeze.

Mechanism of Action

Rh suppression: Prevents isoimmunization by suppressing the immune response and antibody formation by $Rh_o(D)$ negative individuals to $Rh_o(D)$ positive red blood cells.

ITP: Not completely characterized; $Rh_o(D)$ immune globulin is thought to form anti-D-coated red blood cell complexes which bind to macrophage Fc receptors within the spleen; blocking or saturating the spleens ability to clear antibody-coated cells, including platelets. In this manner, platelets are spared from destruction.

Pharmacodynamics/Kinetics

Onset of platelet increase: ITP: Platelets should rise within 1-2 days

Peak effect: In 7-14 days

Duration: Suppression of Rh isoimmunization: ~12 weeks; Treatment of ITP: 30 days (variable)

Distribution: V_d: I.M.: 8.59 L

Bioavailability: I.M.: Rhophylac®: 69%

Half-life elimination: ~24-30 days

Time to peak, plasma: I.M.: 5-10 days; I.V. (WinRho® SDF): ≤2 hours

Dosage

ITP: Children and Adults:

Rhophylac®: I.V.: 50 mcg/kg

WinRho® SDF: I.V.:

Initial: 50 mcg/kg as a single injection, or can be given as a divided dose on separate days. If hemoglobin is <10 g/dL: Dose should be reduced to 25-40 mcg/kg.

Subsequent dosing: 25-60 mcg/kg can be used if required to increase platelet count

Maintenance dosing if patient **did respond** to initial dosing: 25-60 mcg/kg based on platelet count and hemoglobin concentration

Maintenance dosing if patient **did not respond** to initial dosing:

Hemoglobin <8 g/dL: Alternative treatment should be used

Hemoglobin 8-10 g/dL: Redose between 25-40 mcg/kg

Hemoglobin >10 g/dL: Redose between 50-60 mcg/kg

$Rh_o(D)$ suppression: Adults: **Note:** One "full dose" (300 mcg) provides enough antibody to prevent Rh sensitization if the volume of RBC entering the circulation is ≤15 mL. When >15 mL is suspected, a fetal red cell count should be performed to determine the appropriate dose.

Pregnancy:

Antepartum prophylaxis: In general, dose is given at 28 weeks. If given early in pregnancy, administer every 12 weeks to ensure adequate levels of passively acquired anti-Rh

HyperRHO™ S/D Full Dose, RhoGAM®: I.M.: 300 mcg

Rhophylac®, WinRho® SDF: I.M., I.V.: 300 mcg

Postpartum prophylaxis: In general, dose is administered as soon as possible after delivery, preferably within 72 hours. Can be given up to 28 days following delivery

HyperRHO™ S/D Full Dose, RhoGAM®: I.M.: 300 mcg

Rhophylac®: I.M., I.V.: 300 mcg

WinRho® SDF: I.M., I.V.: 120 mcg

Threatened abortion, any time during pregnancy (with continuation of pregnancy):

HyperRHO™ S/D Full Dose, RhoGAM®: I.M.: 300 mcg; administer as soon as possible

Rhophylac®, WinRho® SDF: I.M., I.V.: 300 mcg; administer as soon as possible

Abortion, miscarriage, termination of ectopic pregnancy:

RhoGAM®: I.M.: ≥13 weeks gestation: 300 mcg.

HyperRHO™ S/D Mini Dose, MICRhoGAM®: <13 weeks gestation: I.M.: 50 mcg

Rhophylac®: I.M., I.V.: 300 mcg

WinRho® SDF: I.M., I.V.: After 34 weeks gestation: 120 mcg; administer immediately or within 72 hours

Amniocentesis, chorionic villus sampling:

HyperRHO™ S/D Full Dose, RhoGAM®: I.M.: At 15-18 weeks gestation or during the 3rd trimester: 300 mcg. If dose is given between 13-18 weeks, repeat at 26-28 weeks and within 72 hours of delivery.

Rhophylac®: I.M., I.V.: 300 mcg

WinRho® SDF: I.M., I.V.: Before 34 weeks gestation: 300 mcg; administer immediately, repeat dose every 12 weeks during pregnancy; After 34 weeks gestation: 120 mcg, administered immediately or within 72 hours

Excessive fetomaternal hemorrhage (>15 mL): Rhophylac®: I.M., I.V.: 300 mcg within 72 hours plus 20 mcg/mL fetal RBCs in excess of 15 mL if excess transplacental bleeding is quantified **or** 300 mcg/dose if bleeding cannot be quantified

Abdominal trauma, manipulation:

HyperRHO™ S/D Full Dose, RhoGAM®: I.M.: 2nd or 3rd trimester: 300 mcg. If dose is given between 13-18 weeks, repeat at 26-28 weeks and within 72 hours of delivery

Rhophylac®: I.M., I.V.: 300 mcg within 72 hours

WinRho® SDF: I.M./I.V.: After 34 weeks gestation: 120 mcg; administer immediately or within 72 hours

Transfusion:

Children and Adults: WinRho® SDF: Administer within 72 hours after exposure of incompatible blood transfusions or massive fetal hemorrhage.

I.V.: Calculate dose as follows; administer 600 mcg every 8 hours until the total dose is administered:

Exposure to $Rh_o(D)$ positive whole blood: 9 mcg/mL blood

Exposure to $Rh_o(D)$ positive red blood cells: 18 mcg/mL cells

I.M.: Calculate dose as follows; administer 1200 mcg every 12 hours until the total dose is administered:

Exposure to $Rh_o(D)$ positive whole blood: 12 mcg/mL blood

Exposure to $Rh_o(D)$ positive red blood cells: 24 mcg/mL cells

Adults:

HyperRHO™ S/D Full Dose, RhoGAM®: I.M.: Multiply the volume of Rh positive whole blood administered by the hematocrit of the donor unit to equal the volume of RBCs transfused. The volume of RBCs is then divided by 15 mL, providing the number of 300 mcg doses (vials/syringes) to administer. If the dose calculated results in a fraction, round up to the next higher whole 300 mcg dose (vial/syringe).

Rhophylac®: I.M., I.V.: 20 mcg/2 mL transfused blood or 20 mcg/mL erythrocyte concentrate

Elderly: Patients >65 years of age with a concurrent comorbid condition (eg, infection, malignancy, autoimmune disorders) may be at increased risk of developing acute hemolytic reactions. Fatal outcomes associated with IVH have occurred most frequently in those >65 years. Careful consideration should be used when selecting dosage for elderly patients due to a higher probability of decreased hepatic, renal, or cardiac function; consider starting at lower doses.

Dosage adjustment in renal impairment: No dosage adjustment provided in manufacturer's labeling.

Dosage adjustment in hepatic disease: No dosage adjustment provided in manufacturer's labeling.

Administration The total volume can be administered in divided doses at different sites at one time or may be divided and given at intervals, provided the total dosage is given within 72 hours of the fetomaternal hemorrhage or transfusion.

I.M.: Administer into the deltoid muscle of the upper arm or anterolateral aspect of the upper thigh; avoid gluteal region due to risk of sciatic nerve injury. If large doses (>5 mL) are needed, administration in divided doses at different sites is recommended. **Note:** Do not administer I.M. Rh_o(D) immune globulin for ITP.

I.V.:

Rhophylac®: ITP: Infuse at 2 mL per 15-60 seconds

WinRho® SDF: Infuse over at least 3-5 minutes; do not administer with other medications

Note: If preparing dose using liquid formulation, withdraw the entire contents of the vial to ensure accurate calculation of the dosage requirement.

Monitoring Parameters Signs and symptoms of intravascular hemolysis (IVH), anemia, renal insufficiency, back pain, shaking, chills, discolored urine, or hematuria; observe patient for side effects for 8 hours following administration

Patients with suspected IVH: CBC, haptoglobin, plasma hemoglobin, urine dipstick, BUN, serum creatinine, liver function tests, DIC-specific tests (D-dimer, fibrin degradation products [FDP] or fibrin split products [FSP]) for differential diagnosis. In patients at increased risk of developing acute renal failure, periodically monitor renal function and urine output. Clinical response may be determined by monitoring platelets, red blood cell (RBC) counts, hemoglobin, and reticulocyte levels.

ITP: Check blood type, CBC, reticulocyte count, DAT, urine dipstick before initiating treatment with WinRho® SDF, repeat urine dipstick at 2 and 4 hours after administration and prior to end of the 8-hour monitoring period.

Test Interactions Some infants born to women given Rh_o(D) antepartum have a weakly positive Coombs' test at birth. Fetal-maternal hemorrhage may cause false blood-typing result in the mother; when there is any doubt to the patients' Rh type, Rh_o(D) immune globulin should be administered. WinRho® SDF liquid contains maltose; may result in falsely elevated blood glucose levels with dehydrogenase pyrroloquinolinequinone or glucose-dye-oxidoreductase testing methods. WinRho® SDF contains trace amounts of anti-A, B, C and E; may alter Coombs' tests following administration.

Additional Information A "full dose" of Rh_o(D) immune globulin has previously been referred to as a 300 mcg dose. It is not the actual anti-D content. Although dosing has traditionally been expressed in mcg, potency is listed in units (1 mcg = 5 units). ITP patients requiring transfusions should be transfused with Rho-negative blood cells to avoid exacerbating hemolysis; platelet products may contain red blood cells; caution should be exercised if platelets are from Rh_o-positive donors.

Dosage Forms Excipient information presented when available (limited, particularly for generics); consult specific product labeling. [DSC] = Discontinued product

Injectable, Intramuscular:

HyperRHO S/D: 50 mcg (1 ea [DSC])

Injectable, Intramuscular [preservative free]:

HyperRHO S/D: 50 mcg (1 ea); 300 mcg (1 ea) [latex free]

MICRhoGAM Ultra-Filtered Plus: 50 mcg (1 ea) [latex free, thimerosal free; contains polysorbate 80]

RhoGAM Ultra-Filtered Plus: 300 mcg (1 ea) [latex free, thimerosal free; contains polysorbate 80]

Solution, Injection:

WinRho SDF: 2500 units/2.2 mL (2.2 mL); 5000 units/4.4 mL (4.4 mL); 1500 units/1.3 mL (1.3 mL); 15,000 units/13 mL (13 mL)

Solution, Injection [preservative free]:

Rhophylac: 1500 units/2 mL (2 mL)

WinRho SDF: 2500 units/2.2 mL (2.2 mL); 5000 units/4.4 mL (4.4 mL); 1500 units/1.3 mL (1.3 mL); 15,000 units/13 mL (13 mL) [contains polysorbate 80]

◆ RhoGAM Ultra-Filtered Plus *see* Rh_o(D) Immune Globulin *on page* *1801*

◆ RhoIGIV *see* Rh_o(D) Immune Globulin *on page* *1801*

◆ RhoIVIM *see* Rh_o(D) Immune Globulin *on page* *1801*

◆ Rho®-Loperamine (Can) *see* Loperamide *on page* *1235*

◆ Rho-Nitro Pump Spray (Can) *see* Nitroglycerin *on page* *1466*

◆ Rhophylac *see* Rh_o(D) Immune Globulin *on page* *1801*

◆ Rhotral (Can) *see* Acebutolol *on page* *28*

◆ Rhoxal-loperamide (Can) *see* Loperamide *on page* *1235*

◆ Rhoxal-nabumetone (Can) *see* Nabumetone *on page* *1413*

◆ Rhoxal-orphendrine (Can) *see* Orphenadrine *on page* *1517*

◆ Rhoxal-sotalol (Can) *see* Sotalol *on page* *1942*

◆ rhPTH(1-34) *see* Teriparatide *on page* *2023*

◆ Rh-TSH *see* Thyrotropin Alfa *on page* *2053*

◆ *r*HuEPO *see* Epoetin Alfa *on page* *723*

◆ rhuFabV2 *see* Ranibizumab *on page* *1781*

◆ rhuGM-CSF *see* Sargramostim *on page* *1877*

◆ rhu Keratinocyte Growth Factor *see* Palifermin *on page* *1548*

◆ rHu-KGF *see* Palifermin *on page* *1548*

◆ rhuMAb-2C4 *see* Pertuzumab *on page* *1625*

◆ rhuMAb-E25 *see* Omalizumab *on page* *1502*

◆ rHuMAb-EGFr *see* Panitumumab *on page* *1561*

◆ rhuMAb HER2 *see* Trastuzumab *on page* *2109*

◆ rhuMAb-VEGF *see* Bevacizumab *on page* *251*

◆ RiaSTAP® *see* Fibrinogen Concentrate (Human) *on page* *858*

◆ Ribasphere *see* Ribavirin *on page* *1804*

◆ Ribasphere RibaPak *see* Ribavirin *on page* *1804*

Ribavirin (rye ba VYE rin)

Brand Names: U.S. Copegus; Rebetol; Ribasphere; Ribasphere RibaPak; Virazole

Brand Names: Canada Virazole

Index Terms RTCA; Tribavirin

Pharmacologic Category Antiviral Agent

Use

Inhalation: Treatment of hospitalized infants and young children with respiratory syncytial virus (RSV) infections; specially indicated for treatment of severe lower respiratory tract RSV infections in patients with an underlying compromising condition (prematurity, cardiopulmonary disease, or immunosuppression)

Oral capsule: In combination with interferon alfa 2b (pegylated or nonpegylated) injection for the treatment of chronic hepatitis C in interferon alfa-naive or experienced-patients with compensated liver disease. Patients likely to fail retreatment after a prior failed course include previous nonresponders, those who received previous pegylated interferon treatment, patients who have significant bridging fibrosis or cirrhosis, or those with genotype 1 infection.

Oral solution: In combination with interferon alfa-2b (pegylated or nonpegylated) injection for the treatment of chronic hepatitis C in interferon alfa-naive or experienced patients ≥3 years of age with compensated liver disease. Patients likely to fail retreatment after a prior failed course include previous nonresponders, those who received previous pegylated interferon treatment, patients who have significant bridging fibrosis or cirrhosis, or those with genotype 1 infection.

Oral tablet: In combination with peginterferon alfa-2a (Pegasys®) injection for the treatment of chronic hepatitis C in patients with compensated liver disease who were previously untreated with alpha interferons, and in adult chronic hepatitis C patients coinfected with HIV.

Unlabeled Use

Inhalation: Treatment for RSV in adult hematopoietic stem cell or heart/lung transplant recipients

Used in other viral infections including influenza A and B and adenovirus

Pregnancy Risk Factor X

Pregnancy Considerations **[U.S. Boxed Warning]: Significant teratogenic effects have been observed in all animal studies** at ~0.01 times the maximum recommended daily human dose. Use is contraindicated in pregnancy. Negative pregnancy test is required before initiation and monthly thereafter. Avoid pregnancy in female patients and female partners of male patients during therapy by using two effective forms of contraception; continue contraceptive measures for at least 6 months after completion of therapy. If patient or female partner becomes pregnant during treatment, she should be counseled about potential risks of exposure. If pregnancy occurs during use or within 6 months after treatment, report to the ribavirin pregnancy registry (800-593-2214).

Breast-Feeding Considerations It is not known if ribavirin is excreted in breast milk. Due to the potential for serious adverse reactions in the nursing infant, a decision should be made whether to discontinue nursing or to discontinue the drug, taking into account the importance of treatment to the mother.

Medication Guide Available Yes

Contraindications

Inhalation: Hypersensitivity to ribavirin or any component of the formulation; women who are pregnant or may become pregnant

Oral formulations: Hypersensitivity to ribavirin or any component of the formulation; women who are pregnant or may become pregnant; males whose female partners are pregnant; patients with hemoglobinopathies (eg, thalassemia major, sickle cell anemia); patients with autoimmune hepatitis; concomitant use with didanosine

Ribasphere® capsules and Rebetol® capsules/solution: Additional contraindications: Patients with a Cl_{cr} <50 mL/minute

Oral combination therapy: Refer to individual monographs for Interferon Alfa-2b (Intron® A), Peginterferon Alfa-2b, and Peginterferon Alfa-2a (Pegasys®) for additional contraindication information.

Warnings/Precautions Hazardous agent - use appropriate precautions for handling and disposal (NIOSH, 2012).

Oral: **[U.S. Boxed Warning]: Significant teratogenic effects have been observed in all animal studies.** A negative pregnancy test is required before initiation and monthly thereafter. Avoid pregnancy in female patients and female partners of male patients, during therapy, and for at least 6 months after treatment; two forms of contraception should be used. Safety and efficacy have not been established in patients who have received organ transplants, or been coinfected with hepatitis B or HIV (ribavirin tablets [Copegus®, Ribasphere®] may be used in HIV coinfected patients unless CD4+ cell count is <100 cells/microliter and HIV-1 RNA <5000 cells/mm^3). Hemoglobin at initiation must be ≥12 g/dL (women) or ≥13 g/dL (men) in CHC monoinfected patients and ≥11 g/dL (women) or ≥12 g/dL (men) in CHC and HIV coinfected patients. Oral ribavirin should not be used for adenovirus, RSV, influenza or parainfluenza infections; ribavirin inhalation is approved for severe RSV infection in children.

[U.S. Boxed Warning]: Monotherapy not effective for chronic hepatitis C infection. Severe psychiatric events have occurred including depression and suicidal behavior during combination therapy. Avoid use in patients with a psychiatric history; discontinue if severe psychiatric symptoms occur. Acute hypersensitivity reactions (eg, anaphylaxis, angioedema, bronchoconstriction, and urticaria) have been observed (rarely) with ribavirin and alfa interferon combination therapy. Severe cutaneous reactions, including Stevens-Johnson syndrome and exfoliative dermatitis have been reported (rarely) with ribavirin and alfa interferon combination therapy; discontinue with signs or symptoms of severe skin reactions. Use with caution in patients with renal impairment; dosage adjustment or discontinuation may be required. Elderly patients are more susceptible to adverse effects; use caution.

[U.S. Boxed Warning]: Hemolytic anemia is the primary clinical toxicity of oral therapy; anemia associated with ribavirin may worsen underlying cardiac disease and lead to fatal and nonfatal myocardial infarctions. Avoid use in patients with significant/unstable cardiac disease. Anemia usually occurs within 1-2 weeks of therapy initiation; observed in ~10% to 13% of patients when alfa interferons were combined with ribavirin. Assess cardiac function before initiation of therapy. If patient has underlying cardiac disease, assess electrocardiogram prior to and periodically during treatment. If any deterioration in cardiovascular status occurs, discontinue therapy. Use caution in patients with baseline risk of severe anemia. Assess hemoglobin and hematocrit at baseline and, at minimum, weeks 2 and 4 of therapy since initial drop may be significant. Patients with renal dysfunction and/or those >50 years of age should be carefully assessed for development of anemia. Pancytopenia and bone marrow suppression have been reported with the combination of ribavirin, interferon, and azathioprine. Use caution in pulmonary disease; pulmonary symptoms have been associated with administration. Discontinue therapy if evidence of hepatic decompensation is observed. Use caution in patients with sarcoidosis (exacerbation reported). Dental and periodontal disorders have been reported with ribavirin and interferon therapy; patients should be instructed to brush teeth twice daily and have regular dental exams. Serious ophthalmologic disorders have occurred with combination therapy. All patients require an eye exam at baseline; those with pre-existing ophthalmologic disorders (eg, diabetic or hypertensive retinopathy) require periodic follow up. Delay in weight and height increases have been noted in children treated with combination therapy for CHC. In clinical studies, decreases were noted in weight and height for age z-scores and normative growth curve percentiles. Following treatment, rebound growth and weight gain occurred in most patients; however, a small percentage did not. Long-term data indicate that combination therapy may inhibit growth resulting in reduced adult height. Growth should be closely monitored in pediatric patients during therapy and post-treatment for growth catch-up.

Inhalation: **[U.S. Boxed Warning]: Use with caution in patients requiring assisted ventilation because precipitation of the drug in the respiratory equipment may interfere with safe and effective patient ventilation; sudden deterioration of respiratory function has been**

observed; monitor carefully in patients with COPD and asthma for deterioration of respiratory function. Ribavirin is potentially mutagenic, tumor-promoting, and gonadotoxic. Although anemia has not been reported with inhalation therapy, consider monitoring for anemia 1-2 weeks post-treatment. Pregnant healthcare workers may consider unnecessary occupational exposure; ribavirin has been detected in healthcare workers' urine. Healthcare professionals or family members who are pregnant (or may become pregnant) should be counseled about potential risks of exposure and counseled about risk reduction strategies. Hazardous agent - use appropriate precautions for handling and disposal.

Adverse Reactions

Inhalation:

1% to 10%:

Central nervous system: Fatigue, headache, insomnia

Gastrointestinal: Nausea, anorexia

Hematologic: Anemia

<1% (Limited to important or life-threatening): Hypotension, cardiac arrest, digitalis toxicity, conjunctivitis, mild bronchospasm, worsening of respiratory function, apnea

Note: Incidence of adverse effects (approximate) in healthcare workers: Headache (51%); conjunctivitis (32%); rhinitis, nausea, rash, dizziness, pharyngitis, and lacrimation (10% to 20%); bronchospasm and/or chest pain (case reports in individuals with underlying airway disease)

Oral (all adverse reactions are documented while receiving combination therapy with alfa interferons; percentages as reported in adults unless noted, most common pediatric adverse reactions were similar to adults); asterisked (*) percentages are those similar to interferon therapy alone:

>10%:

Central nervous system: Fatigue (60% to 70% [30% in pediatric patients])*, headache (43% to 66%)*, fever (32% to 55%)*, insomnia (26% to 41% [9% in pediatric patients]), depression (20% to 36%)*, irritability (23% to 33%), dizziness (14% to 26%), impaired concentration (10% to 21%)*, emotional lability (7% to 12%)*

Dermatologic: Alopecia (27% to 36% [17% in pediatric patients]), pruritus (13% to 29% [11% in pediatric patients]), rash (5% to 28%), dry skin (10% to 24%), dermatitis (≤16%)

Endocrine and metabolic: Growth suppression (pediatric) percentile decrease (≥15 percentiles: weight 43%; height 25%), hyperuricemia (33% to 38%)

Gastrointestinal: Nausea (25% to 47% [18% in pediatric patients]), anorexia (21% to 32%), weight decrease (10% to 29%), vomiting (9% to 25%)*, diarrhea (10% to 22%), dyspepsia (6% to 16%), abdominal pain (8% to 13%), xerostomia (≤12%), RUQ pain (≤12%)

Hematologic: Leukopenia (6% to 45%), neutropenia (8% to 42%; grade 4: 2% to 11%; 40% with HIV coinfection), hemoglobin decreased (11% to 35%), anemia (11% to 17%), thrombocytopenia (<1% to 15%), lymphopenia (12% to 14%), hemolytic anemia (10% to 13%)

Hepatic: Bilirubin increase (10% to 32%)

Neuromuscular & skeletal: Myalgia (40% to 64% [17% in pediatric patients])*, rigors (25% to 48%), arthralgia (22% to 34%)*, musculoskeletal pain (19% to 28% [35% in pediatric patients])

Respiratory: Upper respiratory tract infection (60% in pediatric patients), dyspnea (13% to 26%), cough (7% to 23%), pharyngitis (≤13%), sinusitis (≤12%)*

Miscellaneous: Flu-like syndrome (13% to 18% [up to 91% in pediatric patients])*, viral infection (≤12%), diaphoresis (≤11%)

1% to 10%:

Cardiovascular: Chest pain (5% to 9%)*, flushing (≤4%)

Central nervous system: Pain (≤10%), mood alteration (≤6%; 9% with HIV coinfection), agitation (5% to 8%), nervousness (6%)*, memory impairment (≤6%), malaise (≤6%), suicidal ideation (adolescents: 2%; adults: 1%)

Dermatologic: Eczema (4% to 5%)

Endocrine & metabolic: Menstrual disorder (≤7%), hypothyroidism (≤5%)

Gastrointestinal: Taste perversion (4% to 9%), constipation (5%)

Hepatic: Hepatomegaly (4%), transaminases increased (1% to 3%), hepatic decompensation (2% with HIV coinfection)

Neuromuscular & skeletal: Weakness (9% to 10%), back pain (5%)

Ocular: Blurred vision (≤6%), conjunctivitis (≤5%)

Respiratory: Rhinitis (≤8%), exertional dyspnea (≤7%)

Miscellaneous: Fungal infection (≤6%), bacterial infection (3% to 5%)

<1% (Limited to important or life-threatening): Aggression, angina, anxiety, aplastic anemia, arrhythmia; autoimmune disorders (systemic lupus erythematosus, rheumatoid arthritis, sarcoidosis); bone marrow suppression, cerebral hemorrhage, cholangitis, colitis, coma, corneal ulcer, dehydration, diabetes mellitus, drug abuse relapse/overdose, exfoliative dermatitis, fatty liver, hearing impairment/loss, gastrointestinal bleeding, gout, hallucination, hepatic dysfunction, hyper-/hypothyroidism, hypersensitivity (including anaphylaxis, angioedema, bronchoconstriction, and urticaria), macular edema, myositis, optic neuritis, papilledema, pancreatitis, peptic ulcer, peripheral neuropathy, pneumonitis, psychosis, psychotic disorder, pulmonary dysfunction, pulmonary embolism, pulmonary infiltrates, pure red cell aplasia, retinal artery/vein thrombosis, retinal detachment, retinal hemorrhage, retinopathy, sarcoidosis exacerbation; skin reactions (erythema multiforme, exfoliative dermatitis, urticaria, vesiculobullous eruptions); Stevens-Johnson syndrome, suicide, thrombotic thrombocytopenic purpura, thyroid function test abnormalities; transplant rejection (kidney, liver); vision loss

Note: Incidence of headache, fever, suicidal ideation, and vomiting are higher in children.

Drug Interactions

Metabolism/Transport Effects None known.

Avoid Concomitant Use

Avoid concomitant use of Ribavirin with any of the following: Didanosine

Increased Effect/Toxicity

Ribavirin may increase the levels/effects of: AzaTHIOprine; Didanosine; Reverse Transcriptase Inhibitors (Nucleoside)

The levels/effects of Ribavirin may be increased by: Interferons (Alfa); Zidovudine

Decreased Effect

Ribavirin may decrease the levels/effects of: Influenza Virus Vaccine (Live/Attenuated)

Ethanol/Nutrition/Herb Interactions Food: Oral: High-fat meal increases the AUC and C_{max}. Management: Capsule (in combination with peginterferon alfa-2b) and tablet should be administered with food. Other dosage forms and combinations should be taken consistently in regards to food.

Preparation for Administration Hazardous agent; use appropriate precautions for handling and disposal (NIOSH, 2012).

Inhalation: Do not use any water containing an antimicrobial agent to reconstitute drug. Reconstituted solution is stable for 24 hours at room temperature.

Storage/Stability

Inhalation: Store vials in a dry place at 15°C to 30°C (59°F to 86°F).

Oral: Store at controlled room temperature of 25°C (77°F); excursions permitted between 15°C and 30°C (59°F and 86°F). Keep bottle tightly closed. Solution may also be refrigerated at 2°C to 8°C (36°F to 46°F).

Mechanism of Action Inhibits replication of RNA and DNA viruses; inhibits influenza virus RNA polymerase activity and inhibits the initiation and elongation of RNA fragments resulting in inhibition of viral protein synthesis

Pharmacodynamics/Kinetics

Absorption: Inhalation: Systemic; dependent upon respiratory factors and method of drug delivery; maximal absorption occurs with the use of aerosol generator via endotracheal tube; highest concentrations in respiratory tract and erythrocytes

Distribution: Oral capsule: Single dose: V_d: 2825 L; distribution significantly prolonged in the erythrocyte (16-40 days), which can be used as a marker for intracellular metabolism

Protein binding: Oral: None

Metabolism: Hepatically and intracellularly (forms active metabolites); may be necessary for drug action

Bioavailability: Oral: 64%

Half-life elimination, plasma:

Children: Inhalation: 6.5-11 hours

Adults: Oral:

Capsule, single dose (Rebetol®, Ribasphere®): 24 hours in healthy adults, 44 hours with chronic hepatitis C infection (increases to ~298 hours at steady state)

Tablet, single dose (Copegus®): ~120-170 hours

Time to peak, serum: Inhalation: At end of inhalation period; Oral capsule: Multiple doses: 3 hours; Tablet: 2 hours

Excretion: Inhalation: Urine (40% as unchanged drug and metabolites); Oral capsule: Urine (61%), feces (12%)

Dosage

Infants and Children: Aerosol inhalation: RSV infection: Use with Viratek® small particle aerosol generator (SPAG-2) at a concentration of 20 mg/mL (6 **g** reconstituted with 300 mL of sterile water without preservatives). Continuous aerosol administration: 12-18 hours per day for 3 days, up to 7 days in length

Children ≥3 years: Oral capsule or solution (Rebetol®, Ribasphere®): Chronic hepatitis C monoinfection (in combination with pegylated or nonpegylated interferon alfa-2b): **Note:** Oral solution should be used in children <47 kg, or those unable to swallow capsules. Children who start treatment prior to age 18 years should continue on pediatric dosing regimen through therapy completion. Recommended therapy duration (manufacturer labeling): Genotypes 2,3: 24 weeks; all other genotypes: 48 weeks

Capsule, oral solution dosing recommendations:

<47 kg: 15 mg/kg/day in 2 divided doses (morning and evening) as oral solution

47-59 kg: 800 mg daily (400 mg in morning and evening)

60-73 kg: 1000 mg daily (400 mg in morning and 600 mg in the evening)

>73 kg: 1200 mg daily (600 mg in morning and evening)

Alternative recommendations: *American Association for the Study of Liver Diseases (AASLD) guidelines:* Children 2-17 years with chronic hepatitis C infection (Ghany, 2009): Treatment of choice: Ribavirin 15 mg/kg daily (in combination with SubQ peginterferon alfa-2b) once weekly for 48 weeks

Children ≥5 years: Oral tablet (Copegus®): Chronic hepatitis C monoinfection (in combination with peginterferon alfa-2a): **Note:** Assess child's ability to swallow tablet; children who start treatment prior to age 18 years should continue on pediatric dosing regimen through therapy completion. Recommended therapy duration (manufacturer labeling): Genotypes 2,3: 24 weeks; all other genotypes: 48 weeks

23-33 kg: 400 mg daily (200 mg in the morning and evening)

34-46 kg: 600 mg daily (200 mg in the morning and 400 mg in the evening)

47-59 kg: 800 mg daily (400 mg in the morning and evening)

60-74 kg: 1000 mg daily (400 mg in the morning and 600 mg in the evening)

≥75 kg: 1200 mg daily (600 mg in the morning and evening)

Adults: **Note:** Oral solution may be used those unable to swallow capsules.

Oral capsule, oral solution (Rebetol®, Ribasphere®):

Chronic hepatitis C monoinfection (in combination with peginterferon alfa-2b) (recommended therapy duration [manufacturer labeling]: Genotype 1: 48 weeks; genotypes 2,3: 24 weeks); recommended therapy duration for patients who previously failed therapy: 48 weeks [regardless of genotype])

<66 kg: 800 mg daily (400 mg in the morning and evening)

66-80 kg: 1000 mg daily (400 mg in the morning, 600 mg in the evening)

81-105 kg: 1200 mg daily (600 mg in the morning, 600 mg in the evening)

>105 kg: 1400 mg daily (600 mg in the morning, 800 mg in the evening)

Chronic hepatitis C monoinfection (in combination with interferon alfa-2b) (individualized therapy duration [manufacturer labeling] 24-48 weeks):

≤75 kg: 1000 mg daily (400 mg in the morning, 600 mg in the evening)

>75 kg: 1200 mg daily (600 mg in the morning, 600 mg in the evening)

Oral tablet (Copegus®, Ribasphere®):

Chronic hepatitis C monoinfection (in combination with peginterferon alfa-2a):

Genotype 1,4:

<75 kg: 1000 mg daily in 2 divided doses for 48 weeks

≥75 kg: 1200 mg daily in 2 divided doses for 48 weeks

Genotype 2,3: 800 mg daily in 2 divided doses for 24 weeks

Chronic hepatitis C coinfection with HIV (in combination with peginterferon alfa-2a): 800 mg daily in 2 divided doses for 48 weeks (regardless of genotype)

Alternative recommendations: *American Association for the Study of Liver Diseases (AASLD) guidelines:* Adults with chronic hepatitis C infection (Ghany, 2009): Treatment of choice: Ribavirin plus peginterferon; clinical condition and ability of patient to tolerate therapy should be evaluated to determine length and/or likely benefit of therapy. Recommended treatment duration (AASLD guidelines): Genotypes 1,4: 48 weeks; Genotypes 2,3: 24 weeks; Coinfection with HIV: 48 weeks.

Aerosol inhalation: RSV infection in hematopoietic cell or heart/lung transplant recipients (unlabeled use): 2000 mg (over 2 hours) every 8 hours (Boeckh, 2007; Liu, 2010)

Note: Heart/lung transplant recipients also received IVIG, methylprednisolone and palivizumab. Dosage and protocol may be institution specific. (Boeckh, 2007; Chemaly, 2006; Liu, 2010).

Dosage adjustment for toxicity:

Patient **without** cardiac history:

Hemoglobin 8.5 to <10 g/dL:

Children ≥3 years: Oral capsules, oral solution:

First reduction: Decrease to 12 mg/kg/day

Second reduction: Decrease to 8 mg/kg/day
Children ≥5 years: Oral tablets (Copegus®):
23-33 kg: Decrease dose to 200 mg daily (in the morning)
34-59 kg: Decrease dose to 400 mg daily (200 mg in the morning and evening)
≥60 kg: Decrease dose to 600 mg daily (200 mg in the morning and 400 mg in the evening)
Adults:
Oral capsules, oral solution:
First reduction: ≤105 kg: Decrease by 200 mg daily; >105 kg: Decrease by 400 mg daily
Second reduction: Decrease by an additional 200 mg daily (not weight-based)
Oral tablets: Decrease dose to 600 mg daily (200 mg in the morning, 400 mg in the evening)
Hemoglobin <8.5 g/dL: Children and Adults: Oral capsules, solution, tablets: Permanently discontinue treatment.
WBC <1000 mm^3, neutrophils <500 mm^3: Children and Adults: Oral capsules, solution: Permanently discontinue treatment.
Platelets <50 x 10^9/L: Children: Oral capsules, solution: Permanently discontinue treatment.
Platelets <25 x 10^9/L: Adults: Oral capsules, solution: Permanently discontinue treatment.
Patient **with** stable cardiac history:
Hemoglobin has decreased ≥2 g/dL during any 4-week period of treatment:
Children: Oral capsules, solution: Decrease ribavirin by 200 mg daily (regardless of the patient's initial dose); decrease peginterferon alfa-2b dose by 50%; monitor and evaluate weekly. If hemoglobin <8.5 g/dL any time after dose reduction or <12 g/dL after 4 weeks of dose reduction, permanently discontinue treatment.
Children ≥5 years: Oral tablets (Copegus®):
23-33 kg: Decrease dose to 200 mg daily (in the morning)
34-59 kg: Decrease dose to 400 mg daily (200 mg in the morning and evening)
≥60 kg: 600 mg daily (200 mg in the morning, 400 mg in the evening)
Hemoglobin has decreased >2 g/dL during any 4-week period of treatment: Adults:
Oral capsules, solution: Decrease dose by 200 mg daily; decrease peginterferon alfa-2b dose by 50%. If hemoglobin <8.5 g/dL any time after dose reduction or <12 g/dL after 4 weeks of dose reduction, permanently discontinue treatment.
Oral tablets: Decrease dose to 600 mg daily (200 mg in the morning, 400 mg in the evening). If hemoglobin <8.5 g/dL any time after dose reduction or <12 g/dL after 4 weeks of dose reduction, permanently discontinue treatment.
Hemoglobin <8.5 g/dL: Children and Adults: Oral capsules, solution, tablets: Permanently discontinue treatment.
WBC <1000 mm^3, neutrophils <500 mm^3: Children and Adults: Oral capsules, solution: Permanently discontinue treatment.
Platelets <50 x 10^9/L: Children: Oral capsules, solution: Permanently discontinue treatment.
Platelets <25 x 10^9/L: Adults: Oral capsules, solution: Permanently discontinue treatment.

Dosage adjustment in renal impairment: Chronic hepatitis C infection: Oral:
Rebetol capsules/solution, Ribasphere® capsules:
Children: Serum creatinine >2 mg/dL: Permanently discontinue treatment.
Adults:
Cl_{cr} ≥50 mL/minute: No dosage adjustment necessary.
Cl_{cr} <50 mL/minute: Use is contraindicated
Ribasphere® tablets: Adults:
Cl_{cr} ≥50 mL/minute: No dosage adjustment necessary.
Cl_{cr} <50 mL/minute: Use is not recommended
Copegus® tablets: Adults:
Cl_{cr} >50 mL/minute: No dosage adjustment necessary.
Cl_{cr} 30-50 mL/minute: Alternate 200 mg and 400 mg every other day
Cl_{cr} <30 mL/minute: 200 mg once daily
ESRD requiring hemodialysis: 200 mg once daily
Note: The dose of Copegus® should not be further modified in patients with renal impairment. If severe adverse reactions or laboratory abnormalities develop it should be discontinued, if appropriate, until the adverse reactions resolve or decrease in severity. If abnormalities persist after restarting, therapy should be discontinued.

Dosage adjustment in hepatic impairment: Chronic hepatitis C infection: Hepatic decompensation (Child-Pugh class B and C): Manufacturer's labeling: Oral tablets: Use contraindicated.

Dietary Considerations Capsules, solution, and tablets should be taken with food.

Administration

Inhalation: Ribavirin should be administered in well-ventilated rooms (at least 6 air changes/hour). In mechanically-ventilated patients, ribavirin can potentially be deposited in the ventilator delivery system depending on temperature, humidity, and electrostatic forces; this deposition can lead to malfunction or obstruction of the expiratory valve, resulting in inadvertently high positive end-expiratory pressures. The use of one-way valves in the inspiratory lines, a breathing circuit filter in the expiratory line, and frequent monitoring and filter replacement have been effective in preventing these problems. Solutions in SPAG-2 unit should be discarded at least every 24 hours and when the liquid level is low before adding newly reconstituted solution. Should not be mixed with other aerosolized medication.
Oral: Administer concurrently with interferon alfa injection. Capsule should not be opened, crushed, chewed, or broken. Use oral solution for children <47 kg, or those who cannot swallow capsules.
Capsule, solution, tablet: Administer with food.

Hazardous agent; use appropriate precautions for handling and disposal (NIOSH, 2012).

Monitoring Parameters

Inhalation: Respiratory function, hemoglobin, reticulocyte count, CBC with differential, I & O

Oral: For combination treatment: pretreatment hematological and biochemical tests are recommended for all patients; pregnancy screening (if woman of childbearing age) and ECG (if pre-existing cardiac abnormalities) are also recommended. In adults, hematologic tests should be at treatment weeks 2 and 4, biochemical tests at week 4, TSH at week 12, and pregnancy tests monthly during and for 6 months after treatment discontinuation.
In pediatric clinical studies, hematologic and biochemical assessments were made at weeks 1, 3, 5 and 8, then every 4 weeks thereafter. Growth velocity and weight should also be monitored during and periodically after treatment discontinuation.
Baseline values used in adult clinical trials:
Platelet count ≥90,000/mm^3 (75,000/mm^3 for cirrhosis or 70,000/mm^3 for coinfection with HIV)
ANC ≥1500/mm^3
Hemoglobin ≥12 g/dL for women and ≥13 g/dL for men (11 g/dL for HIV coinfected women and 12 g/dL for HIV coinfected men)
TSH and T_4 within normal limits or adequately controlled
$CD4^+$ cell count ≥200 cells/microL or $CD4^+$ cell count 100-200 cells/microL and HIV-1 RNA <5000 copies/mL for coinfection with HIV

Serum HCV RNA (pretreatment, week 12 and week 24, and 24 weeks after completion of therapy). **Note:** Discontinuation of therapy may be considered after 12 weeks in patients with HCV (genotypes 1,4) who fail to achieve an early virologic response (EVR) (defined as ≥2-log decrease in HCV RNA compared to pretreatment) or after 24 weeks with detectable HCV RNA. Treat patients with HCV (genotypes 2,3) for 24 weeks (if tolerated) and then evaluate HCV RNA levels (Ghany, 2009).

Pretreatment and monthly pregnancy test up to 6 months following discontinuation of therapy for women of childbearing age; pretreatment ECG in patients with preexisting cardiac disease; dental exams; ophthalmic exam pretreatment (all patients) and periodically for those with pre-existing ophthalmologic disorders. In pediatric patients, monitor growth closely during and after treatment.

Reference Range

Rapid virological response (RVR): Absence of detectable HCV RNA after 4 weeks of treatment

Early viral response (EVR): ≥2-log decrease in HCV RNA after 12 weeks of treatment

End of treatment response (ETR): Absence of detectable HCV RNA at end of the recommended treatment period

Sustained treatment response (STR) or sustained virologic response (SVR): Absence of HCV RNA in the serum 6 months following completion of full treatment course

Dosage Forms Excipient information presented when available (limited, particularly for generics); consult specific product labeling.

Capsule, oral: 200 mg
- Rebetol: 200 mg
- Ribasphere: 200 mg

Powder for solution, for nebulization:
- Virazole: 6 g [reconstituted product contains ribavirin 20 mg/mL]

Solution, oral:
- Rebetol: 40 mg/mL (100 mL) [contains propylene glycol, sodium benzoate; bubblegum flavor]

Tablet, oral: 200 mg
- Copegus: 200 mg
- Ribasphere: 200 mg, 400 mg, 600 mg

Tablet, oral [dose-pack]:
- Ribasphere RibaPak 600: 200 mg AM dose, 400 mg PM dose (14s, 56s)
- Ribasphere RibaPak 800: 400 mg AM dose, 400 mg PM dose (14s, 56s)
- Ribasphere RibaPak 1000: 600 mg AM dose, 400 mg PM dose (14s, 56s)
- Ribasphere RibaPak 1200: 600 mg AM dose, 600 mg PM dose (14s, 56s)

◆ **Ribavirin and Interferon Alfa-2b Combination Pack** *see* Interferon Alfa-2b and Ribavirin *on page 1102*

Riboflavin (RYE boe flay vin)

Brand Names: U.S. B-2-400 [OTC]

Index Terms Lactoflavin; Vitamin B_2; Vitamin G

Pharmacologic Category Vitamin, Water Soluble

Use Dietary supplement

Unlabeled Use Migraine prophylaxis

Dosage Oral:

Dietary supplement: Adults: 100 mg once or twice daily

Adequate intake:
- 1-6 months: 0.3 mg/day
- 7-12 months: 0.4 mg/day

Recommended daily intake:
- 1-3 years: 0.5 mg
- 4-8 years: 0.6 mg
- 9-13 years: 0.9 mg
- 14-18 years: Females: 1 mg; Males: 1.3 mg
- ≥19 years: Females: 1.1 mg; Males: 1.3 mg
- Pregnancy: 1.4 mg
- Lactation 1.6 mg

Additional Information Complete prescribing information should be consulted for additional detail.

Dosage Forms Excipient information presented when available (limited, particularly for generics); consult specific product labeling.

Capsule, Oral:
- B-2-400: 400 mg
- Generic: 50 mg

Tablet, Oral:
- Generic: 25 mg, 50 mg, 100 mg

Tablet, Oral [preservative free]:
- Generic: 100 mg

◆ **Ridaura** *see* Auranofin *on page 201*

◆ **Ridaura® (Can)** *see* Auranofin *on page 201*

◆ **RID® Maximum Strength [OTC]** *see* Pyrethrins and Piperonyl Butoxide *on page 1752*

◆ **RID® Mousse (Can)** *see* Pyrethrins and Piperonyl Butoxide *on page 1752*

Rifabutin (rif a BYOO tin)

Brand Names: U.S. Mycobutin

Brand Names: Canada Mycobutin®

Index Terms Ansamycin

Pharmacologic Category Antibiotic, Miscellaneous; Antitubercular Agent

Use Prevention of disseminated *Mycobacterium avium* complex (MAC) in patients with advanced HIV infection

Unlabeled Use Utilized in multidrug regimens for treatment of MAC; alternative to rifampin as prophylaxis for latent tuberculosis infection (LTBI) or part of multidrug regimen for treatment active tuberculosis infection

Pregnancy Risk Factor B

Pregnancy Considerations Adverse events were seen in some animal reproduction studies.

Breast-Feeding Considerations In the United States, where formula is accessible, affordable, safe, and sustainable, and the risk of infant mortality due to diarrhea and respiratory infections is low, complete avoidance of breastfeeding by HIV-infected women is recommended to decrease potential transmission of HIV (DHHS [perinatal], 2011).

Contraindications Hypersensitivity to rifabutin, any other rifamycins, or any component of the formulation

Warnings/Precautions Rifabutin must not be administered for MAC prophylaxis to patients with active tuberculosis since its use may lead to the development of tuberculosis that is resistant to both rifabutin and rifampin. May be associated with neutropenia and/or thrombocytopenia (rarely). Dosage reduction recommended in severe impairment (Cl_{cr} <30 mL/minute). Prolonged use may result in fungal or bacterial superinfection, including *C. difficile*-associated diarrhea (CDAD) and pseudomembranous colitis; CDAD has been observed >2 months postantibiotic treatment. May cause brown/orange discoloration of urine, feces, saliva, sweat, tears, and skin. Remove soft contact lenses during therapy since permanent staining may occur.

Adverse Reactions

>10%:
- Dermatologic: Rash (11%)
- Genitourinary: Discoloration of urine (30%)
- Hematologic: Neutropenia (25%), leukopenia (17%)

1% to 10%:
- Central nervous system: Headache (3%), fever (2%)

Gastrointestinal: Nausea (3% to 6%), abdominal pain (4%), dyspepsia (3%), eructation (3%), taste perversion (3%), vomiting (3%), flatulence (2%)
Hematologic: Thrombocytopenia (5%)
Hepatic: ALT increased (7% to 9%; incidence less than placebo), AST increased (7% to 9%; incidence less than placebo)
Neuromuscular & skeletal: Myalgia (2%)
<1% (Limited to important or life-threatening): Aphasia, arthralgia, chest pain, confusion, dyspnea, flu-like syndrome, hepatitis, hemolysis, myositis, parasthesia, seizures, skin discoloration, T-wave abnormalities, uveitis

Drug Interactions

Metabolism/Transport Effects **Substrate** of CYP1A2 (minor), CYP3A4 (major); **Note:** Assignment of Major/Minor substrate status based on clinically relevant drug interaction potential; **Induces** CYP3A4 (strong)

Avoid Concomitant Use

Avoid concomitant use of Rifabutin with any of the following: Abiraterone Acetate; Apixaban; Artemether; Atovaquone; Axitinib; BCG; Bedaquiline; Boceprevir; Bortezomib; Bosutinib; Cabozantinib; CloZAPine; Cobicistat; Crizotinib; Dienogest; Dronedarone; Elvitegravir; Enzalutamide; Everolimus; Ibrutinib; Itraconazole; Ivacaftor; Lapatinib; Lumefantrine; Lurasidone; Macitentan; Mifepristone; Mycophenolate; NIFEdipine; Nilotinib; Nisoldipine; PAZOPanib; Perampanel; Pomalidomide; PONATinib; Praziquantel; Ranolazine; Regorafenib; Rilpivirine; Rivaroxaban; Roflumilast; RomiDEPsin; Simeprevir; Sofosbuvir; SORAfenib; Telaprevir; Ticagrelor; Tofacitinib; Tolvaptan; Toremifene; Ulipristal; Vandetanib; Vemurafenib; VinCRIStine (Liposomal); Voriconazole

Increased Effect/Toxicity

Rifabutin may increase the levels/effects of: Clarithromycin; Clopidogrel; Darunavir; Fosamprenavir; Ifosfamide; Isoniazid; Lopinavir; Pitavastatin

The levels/effects of Rifabutin may be increased by: Antifungal Agents (Azole Derivatives, Systemic); Atazanavir; Boceprevir; Clarithromycin; Darunavir; Delavirdine; Fosamprenavir; Indinavir; Lopinavir; Macrolide Antibiotics; Nelfinavir; Nevirapine; Ritonavir; Saquinavir; Telaprevir; Tipranavir; Voriconazole

Decreased Effect

Rifabutin may decrease the levels/effects of: Abiraterone Acetate; Alfentanil; Angiotensin II Receptor Blockers; Antiemetics (5HT3 Antagonists); Antifungal Agents (Azole Derivatives, Systemic); Apixaban; ARIPiprazole; Artemether; Atovaquone; Axitinib; Barbiturates; BCG; Bedaquiline; Benzodiazepines (metabolized by oxidation); Boceprevir; Bortezomib; Bosutinib; Brentuximab Vedotin; BusPIRone; Cabozantinib; Calcium Channel Blockers; Clarithromycin; CloZAPine; Cobicistat; Contraceptives (Estrogens); Contraceptives (Progestins); Corticosteroids (Systemic); Crizotinib; CycloSPORINE (Systemic); CYP3A4 Substrates; Dapsone (Systemic); Dasatinib; Delavirdine; Dienogest; Dronedarone; Efavirenz; Elvitegravir; Enzalutamide; Etravirine; Everolimus; Exemestane; FentaNYL; Gefitinib; GuanFACINE; HMG-CoA Reductase Inhibitors; Ibrutinib; Imatinib; Indinavir; Itraconazole; Ivacaftor; Ixabepilone; Lapatinib; Linagliptin; Lumefantrine; Lurasidone; Macitentan; Maraviroc; Mifepristone; Morphine (Systemic); Mycophenolate; Nelfinavir; Nevirapine; NIFEdipine; Nilotinib; Nisoldipine; PAZOPanib; Perampanel; Pomalidomide; PONATinib; Praziquantel; Propafenone; QUEtiapine; QuiNIDine; Raltegravir; Ramelteon; Ranolazine; Regorafenib; Rilpivirine; Rivaroxaban; Roflumilast; RomiDEPsin; Saxagliptin; Simeprevir; Sodium Picosulfate; Sofosbuvir; SORAfenib; SUNItinib; Tacrolimus (Systemic); Tadalafil; Tamoxifen; Telaprevir; Temsirolimus; Ticagrelor; Tofacitinib; Tolvaptan; Toremifene; Typhoid Vaccine; Ulipristal; Vandetanib; Vemurafenib; VinCRIStine (Liposomal); Vitamin K Antagonists; Voriconazole; Vortioxetine; Zaleplon; Zolpidem; Zuclopenthixol

The levels/effects of Rifabutin may be decreased by: Bosentan; CYP3A4 Inducers (Strong); Dabrafenib; Deferasirox; Efavirenz; Herbs (CYP3A4 Inducers); Mitotane; Nevirapine; Tocilizumab

Ethanol/Nutrition/Herb Interactions Food: High-fat meal may decrease the rate but not the extent of absorption.

Storage/Stability Store at 25°C (77°F); excursions permitted to 15°C to 30°C (59°F to 86°F).

Mechanism of Action Inhibits DNA-dependent RNA polymerase at the beta subunit which prevents chain initiation

Pharmacodynamics/Kinetics

Absorption: Readily, 53%
Distribution: V_d: 9.32 L/kg; distributes to body tissues including the lungs, liver, spleen, eyes, and kidneys
Protein binding: 85%
Metabolism: To 5 metabolites; predominantly 25-O-desacetyl-rifabutin (antimicrobial activity equivalent to parent drug; serum AUC 10% of parent drug) and 31-hydroxy-rifabutin (serum AUC 7% of parent drug)
Bioavailability: Absolute: HIV: 20%
Half-life elimination: Terminal: 45 hours (range: 16-69 hours)
Time to peak, serum: 2-4 hours
Excretion: Urine (53% as metabolites); feces (30%)

Dosage Oral:

Infants and Children:
Prophylaxis for recurrence of *Mycobacterium avium* complex (MAC) in HIV-exposed/-infected patients (unlabeled use; CDC, 2009): 5 mg/kg (maximum dose: 300 mg) once daily as an optional add-on to primary therapy of clarithromycin and ethambutol
Treatment of active TB (as alternative to rifampin) in HIV-exposed/-infected patients (unlabeled use; CDC, 2009): 10-20 mg/kg (maximum dose: 300 mg) once daily or intermittently 2-3 times weekly
Treatment of severe MAC in HIV-exposed/-infected patients (unlabeled use; CDC, 2009): 10-20 mg/kg (maximum dose: 300 mg) once daily, in addition to primary therapy of clarithromycin and ethambutol
Children ≥6 years: Prophylaxis for first episode of MAC in HIV-exposed/-infected patients (unlabeled use; CDC, 2009): 300 mg once daily
Adolescents and Adults:
Disseminated MAC in advanced HIV infection:
Prophylaxis: 300 mg once daily or 150 mg twice daily to reduce gastrointestinal upset
Treatment (unlabeled use; AIDS*info* guidelines): 300 mg once daily as an optional add-on to primary therapy of clarithromycin and ethambutol
Tuberculosis (unlabeled use as alternative to rifampin; AIDS*info* guidelines):
Prophylaxis of LTBI: 300 mg once daily for 4 months
Treatment of active TB: 300 mg once daily or intermittently 2-3 times weekly as part of multidrug regimen

Dosage adjustment for concurrent nelfinavir, amprenavir, indinavir: Reduce rifabutin dose to 150 mg/day; no change in dose if administered twice weekly

Dosage adjustment for concurrent efavirenz (no concomitant protease inhibitor): Increase rifabutin dose to 450-600 mg daily, or 600 mg 3 times/week

Dosage adjustment in renal impairment:
Cl_{cr} ≥30 mL/minute: No dosage adjustment necessary.
Cl_{cr} <30 mL/minute: Reduce dose by 50%

Dosage adjustment in hepatic impairment:
Mild impairment: No dosage adjustment necessary.
Moderate impairment: No dosage adjustment provided in manufacturer's labeling.

Severe impairment: No dosage adjustment provided in manufacturer's labeling; consider dosage reduction.

Dietary Considerations May be taken with meals.

Administration May be taken with meals to minimize nausea or vomiting.

Monitoring Parameters Periodic liver function tests, CBC with differential, platelet count

Dosage Forms Excipient information presented when available (limited, particularly for generics); consult specific product labeling.

Capsule, Oral:

Mycobutin: 150 mg

Extemporaneous Preparations A 20 mg/mL rifabutin oral suspension may be made with capsules and a 1:1 mixture of Ora-Sweet® and Ora-Plus®. Empty the the powder from eight 150 mg rifabutin capsules into a glass mortar; add 20 mL of vehicle and mix to a uniform paste. Mix while adding vehicle in incremental proportions to **almost** 60 mL; transfer to a calibrated bottle, rinse mortar with vehicle, and add quantity of vehicle sufficient to make 60 mL. Label "shake well". Stable for 12 weeks at 4°C, 25°C, 30°C, and 40°C.

Haslam JL, Egodage KL, Chen Y, et al, "Stability of Rifabutin in Two Extemporaneously Compounded Oral Liquids," *Am J Health Syst Pharm*, 1999, 56(4):333-6.

◆ **Rifadin** *see* Rifampin *on page 1811*

◆ **Rifadin® (Can)** *see* Rifampin *on page 1811*

◆ **Rifampicin** *see* Rifampin *on page 1811*

Rifampin (rif AM pin)

Brand Names: U.S. Rifadin

Brand Names: Canada Rifadin®; Rofact™

Index Terms Rifampicin

Pharmacologic Category Antibiotic, Miscellaneous; Antitubercular Agent

Additional Appendix Information

Antibiotic Treatment of Adults With Infective Endocarditis *on page 2355*

Desensitization Protocols *on page 2325*

Use Management of active tuberculosis in combination with other agents; elimination of meningococci from the nasopharynx in asymptomatic carriers

Unlabeled Use Prophylaxis of *Haemophilus influenzae* type b infection; *Legionella* pneumonia; used in combination with other anti-infectives in the treatment of staphylococcal infections; treatment of *M. leprae* infections; used in combination with penicillin for the treatment of chronic carriers of pharyngeal group A streptococci

Pregnancy Risk Factor C

Pregnancy Considerations Teratogenic effects have been reported in animal studies. Rifampin crosses the human placenta. Due to the risk of tuberculosis to the fetus, treatment is recommended when the probability of maternal disease is moderate to high. Postnatal hemorrhages have been reported in the infant and mother with isoniazid administration during the last few weeks of pregnancy.

Breast-Feeding Considerations The manufacturer does not recommend breast-feeding due to tumorigenicity observed in animal studies; however, the CDC does not consider rifampin a contraindication to breast-feeding.

Contraindications Hypersensitivity to rifampin, any rifamycins, or any component of the formulation; concurrent use of amprenavir, saquinavir/ritonavir (possibly other protease inhibitors)

Warnings/Precautions Use with caution and modify dosage in patients with liver impairment; observe for hyperbilirubinemia; discontinue therapy if this in conjunction with clinical symptoms or any signs of significant hepatocellular damage develop. Use with caution in patients receiving concurrent medications associated with hepatotoxicity. Use with caution in patients with a history of alcoholism (even if ethanol consumption is discontinued during therapy). Since rifampin since rifampin has enzyme-inducing properties, porphyria exacerbation is possible; use with caution in patients with porphyria; do not use for meningococcal disease, only for short-term treatment of asymptomatic carrier states

Regimens of >600 mg once or twice weekly have been associated with a high incidence of adverse reactions including a flu-like syndrome, hypersensitivity, thrombocytopenia, leukopenia, and anemia. Urine, feces, saliva, sweat, tears, and CSF may be discolored to red/orange; remove soft contact lenses during therapy since permanent staining may occur. Do not administer I.V. form via I.M. or SubQ routes; restart infusion at another site if extravasation occurs. Prolonged use may result in fungal or bacterial superinfection, including *C. difficile*-associated diarrhea (CDAD) and pseudomembranous colitis; CDAD has been observed >2 months postantibiotic treatment. Monitor for compliance in patients on intermittent therapy.

Adverse Reactions

1% to 10%:

Dermatologic: Rash (1% to 5%)

Gastrointestinal (1% to 2%): Anorexia, cramps, diarrhea, epigastric distress, flatulence, heartburn, nausea, pseudomembranous colitis, pancreatitis, vomiting

Hepatic: LFTs increased (up to 14%)

Frequency not defined:

Cardiovascular: Edema, flushing

Central nervous system: Ataxia, behavioral changes, concentration impaired, confusion, dizziness, drowsiness, fatigue, fever, headache, numbness, psychosis

Dermatologic: Pemphigoid reaction, pruritus, urticaria

Endocrine & metabolic: Adrenal insufficiency, menstrual disorders

Hematologic: Agranulocytosis (rare), DIC, eosinophilia, hemoglobin decreased, hemolysis, hemolytic anemia, leukopenia, thrombocytopenia (especially with high-dose therapy)

Hepatic: Hepatitis (rare), jaundice

Neuromuscular & skeletal: Myalgia, osteomalacia, weakness

Ocular: Exudative conjunctivitis, visual changes

Renal: Acute renal failure, BUN increased, hemoglobinuria, hematuria, interstitial nephritis, uric acid increased

Miscellaneous: Flu-like syndrome

Drug Interactions

Metabolism/Transport Effects Substrate of P-glycoprotein, SLCO1B1; **Induces** CYP1A2 (strong), CYP2A6 (strong), CYP2B6 (strong), CYP2C19 (strong), CYP2C8 (strong), CYP2C9 (strong), CYP3A4 (strong), P-glycoprotein

Avoid Concomitant Use

Avoid concomitant use of Rifampin with any of the following: Abiraterone Acetate; Apixaban; Artemether; Atazanavir; Atovaquone; Axitinib; BCG; Bedaquiline; Boceprevir; Bortezomib; Bosutinib; Cabozantinib; CloZAPine; Cobicistat; Crizotinib; Dabigatran Etexilate; Darunavir; Dienogest; Dronedarone; Elvitegravir; Enzalutamide; Esomeprazole; Etravirine; Everolimus; Fosamprenavir; Ibrutinib; Indinavir; Itraconazole; Ivacaftor; Lapatinib; Lopinavir; Lumefantrine; Lurasidone; Macitentan; Mifepristone; Mycophenolate; Nelfinavir; NIFEdipine; Nilotinib; Nisoldipine; Omeprazole; PAZOPanib; Perampanel; Pirfenidone; Pomalidomide; PONATinib; Praziquantel; QuiNINE; Ranolazine; Regorafenib; Rilpivirine; Ritonavir; Rivaroxaban; Roflumilast; RomiDEPsin; Saquinavir; Simeprevir; Sofosbuvir; SORAfenib; Telaprevir; Ticagrelor; Tipranavir; Tofacitinib; Tolvaptan; Toremifene; Ulipristal; Vandetanib; Vemurafenib; VinCRIStine (Liposomal); Voriconazole

Increased Effect/Toxicity

Rifampin may increase the levels/effects of: Bosentan; Clarithromycin; Clopidogrel; Fexofenadine; Ifosfamide; Isoniazid; Leflunomide; Lopinavir; Pitavastatin; Propofol; RomiDEPsin; Saquinavir

The levels/effects of Rifampin may be increased by: Antifungal Agents (Azole Derivatives, Systemic); Clarithromycin; Delavirdine; Eltrombopag; Macrolide Antibiotics; P-glycoprotein/ABCB1 Inhibitors; Pyrazinamide; Voriconazole

Decreased Effect

Rifampin may decrease the levels/effects of: Abiraterone Acetate; Afatinib; Alfentanil; Amiodarone; Angiotensin II Receptor Blockers; Antidiabetic Agents (Thiazolidinedione); Antiemetics (5HT3 Antagonists); Antifungal Agents (Azole Derivatives, Systemic); Apixaban; Aprepitant; ARIPiprazole; Artemether; Atazanavir; Atovaquone; Axitinib; Barbiturates; Bazedoxifene; BCG; Bedaquiline; Bendamustine; Benzodiazepines (metabolized by oxidation); Beta-Blockers; Boceprevir; Bortezomib; Bosentan; Bosutinib; Brentuximab Vedotin; BusPIRone; Cabozantinib; Calcium Channel Blockers; Canagliflozin; Caspofungin; Chloramphenicol; Citalopram; Clarithromycin; CloZAPine; Cobicistat; Contraceptives (Estrogens); Contraceptives (Progestins); Corticosteroids (Systemic); Crizotinib; CycloSPORINE (Systemic); CYP1A2 Substrates; CYP2A6 Substrates; CYP2B6 Substrates; CYP2C19 Substrates; CYP2C8 Substrates; CYP2C9 Substrates; CYP3A4 Substrates; Dabigatran Etexilate; Dapsone (Systemic); Darunavir; Dasatinib; Deferasirox; Delavirdine; Diclofenac (Systemic); Dienogest; Disopyramide; Dolutegravir; Doxycycline; Dronedarone; Efavirenz; Elvitegravir; Enzalutamide; Erlotinib; Esomeprazole; Etravirine; Everolimus; Exemestane; FentaNYL; Fexofenadine; Fosamprenavir; Fosaprepitant; Fosphenytoin; Gefitinib; GuanFACINE; HMG-CoA Reductase Inhibitors; Ibrutinib; Imatinib; Indinavir; Itraconazole; Ivacaftor; Ixabepilone; LamoTRIgine; Lapatinib; Linagliptin; Lopinavir; Lumefantrine; Lurasidone; Macitentan; Maraviroc; Methadone; Mifepristone; Mirabegron; Morphine (Systemic); Mycophenolate; Nelfinavir; Nevirapine; NIFEdipine; Nilotinib; Nisoldipine; Omeprazole; OxyCODONE; PAZOPanib; Perampanel; P-glycoprotein/ABCB1 Substrates; Phenytoin; Pirfenidone; Pomalidomide; PONATinib; Prasugrel; Praziquantel; Propafenone; QUEtiapine; QuiNIDine; QuiNINE; Raltegravir; Ramelteon; Ranolazine; Regorafenib; Repaglinide; Rilpivirine; Ritonavir; Rivaroxaban; Roflumilast; Saquinavir; Saxagliptin; Simeprevir; Sirolimus; Sodium Picosulfate; Sofosbuvir; SORAfenib; Sulfonylureas; SUNItinib; Tacrolimus (Systemic); Tadalafil; Tamoxifen; Telaprevir; Temsirolimus; Terbinafine (Systemic); Thyroid Products; Ticagrelor; Tipranavir; Tofacitinib; Tolvaptan; Toremifene; Treprostinil; Typhoid Vaccine; Ulipristal; Valproic Acid and Derivatives; Vandetanib; Vemurafenib; VinCRIStine (Liposomal); Vitamin K Antagonists; Voriconazole; Vortioxetine; Zaleplon; Zidovudine; Zolpidem; Zuclopenthixol

The levels/effects of Rifampin may be decreased by: P-glycoprotein/ABCB1 Inducers

Ethanol/Nutrition/Herb Interactions

Ethanol: Avoid ethanol (may increase risk of hepatotoxicity).

Food: Food decreases the extent of absorption; rifampin concentrations may be decreased if taken with food.

Herb/Nutraceutical: St John's wort may decrease rifampin levels.

Preparation for Administration Reconstitute vial with 10 mL SWFI. Prior to injection, dilute in appropriate volume of a compatible solution (eg, 100 mL D_5W).

Storage/Stability Store capsules and intact vials at 25°C (77°F); excursions permitted to 15°C to 30°C (59°F to 86°F); avoid excessive heat (>40°C [104°F]). Protect the intact vials from light. Reconstituted vials are stable for 24 hours at room temperature.

Stability of parenteral admixture at room temperature (25°C [77°F]) is 4 hours for D_5W and 24 hours for NS.

Mechanism of Action Inhibits bacterial RNA synthesis by binding to the beta subunit of DNA-dependent RNA polymerase, blocking RNA transcription

Pharmacodynamics/Kinetics

Duration: ≤24 hours

Absorption: Oral: Well absorbed; food may delay or slightly reduce peak

Distribution: Highly lipophilic; crosses blood-brain barrier well

Relative diffusion from blood into CSF: Adequate with or without inflammation (exceeds usual MICs)

CSF:blood level ratio: Inflamed meninges: 25%

Protein binding: 80%

Metabolism: Hepatic; undergoes enterohepatic recirculation

Half-life elimination: 3-4 hours; prolonged with hepatic impairment; End-stage renal disease: 1.8-11 hours

Time to peak, serum: Oral: 2-4 hours

Excretion: Feces (60% to 65%) and urine (~30%) as unchanged drug

Dosage

Usual dosage ranges: *Oral, I.V.:*

Infants and Children: 10-20 mg/kg/day as a single dose or in 2 divided doses; maximum: 600 mg/day

Adults: 600 mg once or twice daily

Indication-specific dosing: *Oral:*

Pharyngeal chronic carriers of group A streptococci, treatment (unlabeled use; IDSA guidelines): Children, Adolescents, and Adults: 20 mg/kg/day once daily (maximum: 600 mg daily) for the last 4 days of treatment when combined with oral penicillin V **or** 20 mg/kg/day in 2 divided doses (maximum: 600 mg daily) for 4 days when combined with intramuscular benzathine penicillin G (Shulman, 2012)

Indication-specific dosing: *Oral, I.V.:*

Endocarditis, prosthetic valve due to MRSA (unlabeled use): Adults: 300 mg every 8 hours for at least 6 weeks (combine with vancomycin for the entire duration of therapy and gentamicin for the first 2 weeks) (Liu, 2011)

***H. influenzae* prophylaxis (unlabeled use):**

Infants and Children: 20 mg/kg/day every 24 hours for 4 days, not to exceed 600 mg/dose

Adults: 600 mg every 24 hours for 4 days

Leprosy (unlabeled use): Adults:

Multibacillary: 600 mg once monthly for 24 months in combination with ofloxacin and minocycline

Paucibacillary: 600 mg once monthly for 6 months in combination with dapsone

Single lesion: 600 mg as a single dose in combination with ofloxacin 400 mg and minocycline 100 mg

Meningitis *(Pneumococcus* or *Staphylococcus)* (unlabeled use): Adults: 600 mg once daily

Note: Recommended only for organisms known to be rifampin-susceptible and highly penicillin- or cephalosporin-resistant. May be used in place of or in addition to vancomycin when dexamethasone therapy employed.

Meningococcal meningitis prophylaxis (unlabeled use):

Infants <1 month: 10 mg/kg/day in divided doses every 12 hours for 2 days

Infants ≥1 month and Children: 20 mg/kg/day in divided doses every 12 hours for 2 days (maximum: 600 mg/dose)

Adults: 600 mg every 12 hours for 2 days

Nasal carriers of *Staphylococcus aureus* (unlabeled use): Note: Must use in combination with at least one other systemic antistaphylococcal antibiotic. Not recommended as first-line drug for decolonization; evidence is weak for use in patients with recurrent infections (Liu, 2011).

Children: 15 mg/kg/day divided every 12 hours for 5-10 days in combination with other antibiotics

Adults: 600 mg/day for 5-10 days in combination with other antibiotics

Nontuberculous mycobacterium *(M. kansasii)* (unlabeled use): Adults: 10 mg/kg/day (maximum: 600 mg/day) for duration to include 12 months of culture-negative sputum; typically used in combination with ethambutol and isoniazid

Prosthetic joint infection (unlabeled use): *Staphylococci (oxacillin-susceptible or -resistant):* Oral: Adults:

Debridement and prosthesis retention or following 1-stage exchange, acute treatment: 300-450 mg every 12 hours in combination with an I.V. antistaphylococcal antibiotic for 2-6 weeks (Osmon, 2013)

Debridement and prosthesis retention or following 1-stage exchange, chronic treatment:

Total ankle, elbow, hip, or shoulder arthroplasty: 300-450 mg every 12 hours in combination with an oral antistaphylococcal antibiotic for 3 months (Osmon, 2013)

Total knee arthroplasty: 300-450 mg every 12 hours in combination with an oral antistaphylococcal antibiotic for 6 months (Osmon, 2013)

Following resection arthroplasty with or without planned staged reimplantation: 300-450 mg every 12 hours in combination with an I.V. antistaphylococcal antibiotics for 4-6 weeks (Osmon, 2013)

***Staphylococcus aureus* infections, adjunctive therapy (unlabeled use):** Adults: 600 mg once daily or 300-450 mg every 12 hours with other antibiotics. **Note:** Must be used in combination with another antistaphylococcal antibiotic to avoid rapid development of resistance (Liu, 2011).

Tuberculosis, active: Note: A four-drug regimen (isoniazid, rifampin, pyrazinamide, and ethambutol) is preferred for the initial, empiric treatment of TB. When the drug susceptibility results are available, the regimen should be altered as appropriate.

Infants and Children <12 years:

Daily therapy: 10-20 mg/kg/day usually as a single dose (maximum: 600 mg/day)

Twice weekly directly observed therapy (DOT): 10-20 mg/kg (maximum: 600 mg)

Adults:

Daily therapy: 10 mg/kg/day (maximum: 600 mg/day)

Directly observed therapy (DOT): 10 mg/kg (maximum: 600 mg) administered 2 or 3 times/week (*MMWR*, 2003)

Tuberculosis, latent infection (LTBI): As an alternative to isoniazid:

Children: 10-20 mg/kg/day (maximum: 600 mg/day) for 6 months

Adults: 10 mg/kg/day (maximum: 600 mg/day) for 4 months. **Note:** Combination with pyrazinamide should not generally be offered (*MMWR*, Aug 8, 2003).

Dosage adjustment in renal impairment: No dosage adjustment necessary.

Poorly dialyzed; no supplemental dose or dosage adjustment necessary, including patients on intermittent hemodialysis, peritoneal dialysis, or continuous renal replacement therapy (eg, CVVHD).

Dosage adjustment in hepatic impairment: No dosage adjustment provided in manufacturer's labeling.

Dietary Considerations Rifampin should be taken on an empty stomach.

Administration

I.V.: Administer I.V. preparation by slow I.V. infusion over 30 minutes to 3 hours at a final concentration not to exceed 6 mg/mL.

Oral: Administer on an empty stomach (ie, 1 hour prior to, or 2 hours after meals or antacids) to increase total absorption. The compounded oral suspension must be shaken well before using. May mix contents of capsule with applesauce or jelly.

Monitoring Parameters Periodic (baseline and every 2-4 weeks during therapy) monitoring of liver function (AST, ALT, bilirubin), CBC, mental status, sputum culture, chest x-ray 2-3 months into treatment

Test Interactions May interfere with urine detection of opioids (false-positive); positive Coombs' reaction [direct], rifampin inhibits standard assay's ability to measure serum folate and B_{12}; transient increase in LFTs and decreased biliary excretion of contrast media

Dosage Forms Excipient information presented when available (limited, particularly for generics); consult specific product labeling.

Capsule, Oral:

Rifadin: 150 mg, 300 mg

Generic: 150 mg, 300 mg

Solution Reconstituted, Intravenous:

Rifadin: 600 mg (1 ea)

Generic: 600 mg (1 ea)

Extemporaneous Preparations A rifampin 1% w/v suspension (10 mg/mL) may be made with capsules and one of four syrups (Syrup NF, simple syrup, Syrpalta® syrup, or raspberry syrup). Empty the contents of four 300 mg capsules or eight 150 mg capsules onto a piece of weighing paper. If necessary, crush contents to produce a fine powder. Transfer powder to a 4-ounce amber glass or plastic prescription bottle. Rinse paper and spatula with 20 mL of chosen syrup and add the rinse to bottle; shake vigorously. Add 100 mL syrup to the bottle and shake vigorously. Label "shake well". Stable for 4 weeks at room temperature or refrigerated.

A 25 mg/mL oral suspension may be made with capsules and cherry syrup concentrate diluted 1:4 with simple syrup, NF. Empty the contents of ten 300 mg capsules into a mortar and reduce to a fine powder. Add 20 mL of the vehicle and mix to a uniform paste; mix while adding the vehicle in incremental proportions to **almost** 120 mL; transfer to a calibrated bottle, rinse mortar with vehicle, and add quantity of vehicle sufficient to make 120 mL. Label "shake well" and "refrigerate". Stable for 28 days refrigerated (preferred) or at room temperature.

Nahata MC, Pai VB, and Hipple TF, *Pediatric Drug Formulations*, 5th ed, Cincinnati, OH: Harvey Whitney Books Co, 2004.

Rifapentine (rif a PEN teen)

Brand Names: U.S. Priftin

Brand Names: Canada Priftin®

Pharmacologic Category Antitubercular Agent

Use Treatment of pulmonary tuberculosis; rifapentine must always be used in conjunction with at least one other antituberculosis drug to which the isolate is susceptible; it may also be necessary to add additional agents (eg, streptomycin, ethambutol) until susceptibility is known.

Unlabeled Use Treatment of latent tuberculosis infection (LTBI) in combination with isoniazid

Pregnancy Risk Factor C

Pregnancy Considerations Teratogenic effects have been observed in animal reproduction studies. Postnatal hemorrhages have been reported in the infant and mother with rifampin (another rifamycin) administration during the last few weeks of pregnancy. Due to the risk of tuberculosis to the fetus, treatment is recommended when the probability of maternal disease is moderate to high. The

CDC does not currently recommend rifapentine as part of the treatment regimen due to insufficient data in pregnant women (CDC, 2003).

Breast-Feeding Considerations May discolor breast milk

Contraindications Hypersensitivity to rifapentine, rifampin, rifabutin, any rifamycin analog, or any component of the formulation

Warnings/Precautions Patients with abnormal liver tests and/or liver disease should only be given rifapentine when absolutely necessary and under strict medical supervision. Monitoring of liver function tests (eg, serum transaminases) should be carried out prior to therapy and then every 2-4 weeks during therapy. Combination therapy should be discontinued if ALT is ≥5 times the upper limit of normal (ULN) even in the absence of liver dysfunction symptoms or ≥3 times ULN in the presence of symptoms (CDC, 2012). Use is not recommended in patients with porphyria; exacerbation is possible due to enzyme-inducing properties.

Use of rifapentine during the **initial phase** of treatment in HIV–seropositive patients has not been evaluated. Rifapentine should not be used during the **continuation phase** of treatment in HIV-seropositive patients; rifampin relapse and resistance have been reported. Use with caution in patients with cavitary pulmonary lesions and/or positive sputum cultures after initial treatment phase and patients with bilateral pulmonary disease; higher relapse rates may occur in these patients. Rifapentine may produce a red-orange discoloration of body tissues/fluids including skin, teeth, tongue, urine, feces, saliva, sputum, tears, sweat, and cerebral spinal fluid. Contact lenses may become permanently stained; remove soft contact lenses during therapy. Prolonged use may result in fungal or bacterial superinfection, including *C. difficile*-associated diarrhea (CDAD) and pseudomembranous colitis; CDAD has been observed >2 months postantibiotic treatment. Compliance with dosing regimen is absolutely necessary for successful drug therapy.

Adverse Reactions Frequency may vary based on treatment phase; adverse reaction data is based on rifapentine combination therapy.

>10%:

- Endocrine & metabolic: Hyperuricemia (≤32%; most likely due to pyrazinamide from initiation phase)
- Genitourinary: Hematuria (10% to 18%), pyuria (11% to 22%), urinary tract infection (7% to 13%)
- Hematologic: Neutropenia (6% to 13%), lymphopenia (3% to 13%)

1% to 10%:

- Cardiovascular: Chest pain (3% to 6%), edema (1%)
- Central nervous system: Fatigue (≤1%), fever (≤1%)
- Dermatologic: Acne (≤3%), maculopapular rash (2%), pruritus (1%)
- Endocrine & metabolic: Hypoglycemia (5% to 10%), hyperglycemia (1% to 4%)
- Gastrointestinal: Anorexia (3%), nausea (1% to 3%), abdominal pain (1% to 2%), constipation (1% to 2%), diarrhea (1% to 2%), hemorrhoids (1%), hyperphosphatemia (1%)
- Genitourinary: Urinary casts (4% to 8%), cystitis (1%)
- Hematologic: Thrombocytosis (≤6%), leukopenia (4% to 6%), leukocytosis (2% to 3%), neutrophilia (1% to 3%), thrombocytopenia (1% to 3%), polycythemia (≤2%), lymphadenopathy (≤1%)
- Hepatic: ALT increased (2% to 7%), AST increased (2% to 6%)
- Neuromuscular & skeletal: Back pain (4% to 7%), pain (3% to 6%), arthrosis (1%), gout (1%), tremor (1%)
- Ocular: Conjunctivitis (2% to 3%)
- Respiratory: Hemoptysis (8%), cough (6% to 8%), bronchitis (3%), pharyngitis (1% to 2%), epistaxis (1%) pleuritis (1%)
- Miscellaneous: Influenza (3% to 8%), injury (1% to 5%), infection (1% to 3%), diaphoresis (2%), herpes zoster (1%)

<1% (Limited to important or life-threatening): Alopecia, anxiety, bilirubinemia, bronchospasm, BUN increased, diabetes mellitus, dyspnea, dysuria, erythematous rash, hepatomegaly, hypercalcemia, jaundice, loss of taste, muscle weakness, orthostatic hypotension, palpitation, pancreatitis, pyelonephritis, seizure, somnolence, syncope, tachycardia, urinary incontinence, weight gain/loss, xerostomia

Drug Interactions

Metabolism/Transport Effects Induces CYP2C8 (strong), CYP2C9 (strong), CYP3A4 (strong)

Avoid Concomitant Use

Avoid concomitant use of Rifapentine with any of the following: Abiraterone Acetate; Apixaban; Artemether; Atovaquone; Axitinib; Bedaquiline; Boceprevir; Bortezomib; Bosutinib; Cabozantinib; CloZAPine; Cobicistat; Crizotinib; Dienogest; Dronedarone; Elvitegravir; Enzalutamide; Etravirine; Everolimus; Ibrutinib; Itraconazole; Ivacaftor; Lapatinib; Lumefantrine; Lurasidone; Macitentan; Mifepristone; Mycophenolate; NIFEdipine; Nilotinib; Nisoldipine; PAZOPanib; Perampanel; Pomalidomide; PONATinib; Praziquantel; Ranolazine; Regorafenib; Rilpivirine; Rivaroxaban; Roflumilast; RomiDEPsin; Simeprevir; Sofosbuvir; SORAfenib; Telaprevir; Ticagrelor; Tofacitinib; Tolvaptan; Toremifene; Ulipristal; Vandetanib; Vemurafenib; VinCRIStine (Liposomal); Voriconazole

Increased Effect/Toxicity

Rifapentine may increase the levels/effects of: Clarithromycin; Clopidogrel; Ifosfamide; Isoniazid; Pitavastatin

The levels/effects of Rifapentine may be increased by: Antifungal Agents (Azole Derivatives, Systemic); Clarithromycin; Delavirdine; Voriconazole

Decreased Effect

Rifapentine may decrease the levels/effects of: Abiraterone Acetate; Alfentanil; Angiotensin II Receptor Blockers; Antiemetics (5HT3 Antagonists); Antifungal Agents (Azole Derivatives, Systemic); Apixaban; ARIPiprazole; Artemether; Atovaquone; Axitinib; Barbiturates; Bedaquiline; Benzodiazepines (metabolized by oxidation); Beta-Blockers; Boceprevir; Bortezomib; Bosutinib; Brentuximab Vedotin; BusPIRone; Cabozantinib; Calcium Channel Blockers; Clarithromycin; CloZAPine; Cobicistat; Contraceptives (Estrogens); Contraceptives (Progestins); Corticosteroids (Systemic); Crizotinib; CycloSPORINE (Systemic); CYP2C8 Substrates; CYP2C9 Substrates; CYP3A4 Substrates; Dapsone (Systemic); Dasatinib; Delavirdine; Diclofenac (Systemic); Dienogest; Dronedarone; Elvitegravir; Enzalutamide; Etravirine; Everolimus; Exemestane; FentaNYL; Gefitinib; GuanFACINE; HMG-CoA Reductase Inhibitors; Ibrutinib; Imatinib; Itraconazole; Ivacaftor; Ixabepilone; Lapatinib; Linagliptin; Lumefantrine; Lurasidone; Macitentan; Maraviroc; Methadone; Mifepristone; Morphine (Systemic); Mycophenolate; NIFEdipine; Nilotinib; Nisoldipine; PAZOPanib; Perampanel; Pomalidomide; PONATinib; Praziquantel; Propafenone; QUEtiapine; QuiNIDine; Ramelteon; Ranolazine; Regorafenib; Rilpivirine; Rivaroxaban; Roflumilast; RomiDEPsin; Saxagliptin; Simeprevir; Sofosbuvir; SORAfenib; SUNItinib; Tacrolimus (Systemic); Tadalafil; Tamoxifen; Telaprevir; Temsirolimus; Ticagrelor; Tofacitinib; Tolvaptan; Toremifene; Treprostinil; Ulipristal; Vandetanib; Vemurafenib; VinCRIStine (Liposomal); Vitamin K Antagonists; Voriconazole; Vortioxetine; Zaleplon; Zidovudine; Zolpidem; Zuclopenthixol

Ethanol/Nutrition/Herb Interactions Food: High-fat meals increase AUC and maximum serum concentration by 43% and 44% respectively as compared to fasting conditions.

Storage/Stability Store at 25°C (77°F); excursions permitted to 15°C to 30°C (59°F to 86°F). Protect from excessive heat and humidity.

Mechanism of Action Inhibits DNA-dependent RNA polymerase in susceptible strains of *Mycobacterium tuberculosis* (MTB) (but not in mammalian cells). Rifapentine is bactericidal against both intracellular and extracellular MTB organisms.

Pharmacodynamics/Kinetics

Absorption: High-fat meals increase AUC and C_{max} by 43% and 44% respectively.

Distribution: V_d: ~70 L; rifapentine and metabolite accumulate in human monocyte-derived macrophages with intracellular/extracellular ratios of 24:1 and 7:1 respectively

Protein binding: Rifapentine: ~98%, primarily to albumin; 25-desacetyl rifapentine: ~93%

Metabolism: Hepatic; hydrolyzed by an esterase enzyme to form the active metabolite 25-desacetyl rifapentine

Bioavailability: 70%

Half-life elimination: Rifapentine: 12-15 hours; 25-desacetyl rifapentine: 11-16 hours

Time to peak, serum: 5-6 hours

Excretion: Feces (70%); urine (17%, primarily as metabolites)

Dosage Oral:

Tuberculosis: Adults: **Rifapentine should not be used alone**; initial phase should include a 3- to 4-drug regimen

Initial phase of short-term therapy: 600 mg twice weekly (with an interval ≥72 hours between doses) by direct observation therapy for 2 months

Continuation phase of short-term therapy: 600 mg once weekly by direct observation therapy for 4 months

Latent tuberculosis infection (unlabeled use):

Children ≥12 years and Adolescents (CDC, 2011): Use once weekly for 3 months; **Note:** Must be administered under direct observation therapy and given in combination with isoniazid (maximum dose: 900 mg):

10-14 kg: 300 mg
14.1-25 kg: 450 mg
25.1-32 kg: 600 mg
32.1-49.9 kg: 750 mg
≥50 kg: 900 mg

Adults: 900 mg once weekly for 3 months; **Note:** Must be administered under direct observation therapy and given in combination with isoniazid (Sterling, 2011; CDC, 2011).

Alternative regimen based on weight (CDC, 2011): Refer to Children ≥12 years and Adolescents dosing.

Dosing adjustment in renal impairment: No dosage adjustment provided in manufacturer's labeling (has not been studied).

Dosing adjustment in hepatic impairment: No dosage adjustment provided in manufacturer's labeling. However, dosage adjustment unlikely since pharmacokinetics in varying degrees of hepatic impairment were similar to those in healthy volunteers.

Administration Administer with meals.

Monitoring Parameters Patients with pre-existing hepatic problems should have liver function tests monitored (eg, serum transaminases) prior to therapy and then every 2-4 weeks during therapy. In treatment of latent infection with rifapentine and isoniazid combination therapy, patients with HIV infection, liver disorders, immediate postpartum (≤3 months after delivery) or regular ethanol use should have liver function (at least alanine aminotransferase [ALT]) monitored prior to therapy and then at subsequent clinical visits whose baseline testing is abnormal or for others at risk for liver disease disease (CDC, 2012).

Test Interactions Rifampin has been shown to inhibit standard microbiological assays for serum folate and vitamin B_{12}; this should be considered for rifapentine; therefore, alternative assay methods should be considered.

Additional Information Rifapentine has been studied in patients with tuberculosis receiving a 6-month short-course intensive regimen approval. Outcomes were based on 6-month follow-up treatment observed in clinical trial 008 as a surrogate for the 2-year follow-up generally accepted as evidence for efficacy in the treatment of pulmonary tuberculosis. In a study of rifapentine and isoniazid given weekly by direct observation therapy for 12 weeks in latent tuberculosis, the regimen was as effective as 36 weeks of daily isoniazid alone and had higher treatment completion rates (Sterling, 2011). CDC recommends the combination of rifapentine and isoniazid once weekly for 12 weeks as an equal alternative to daily isoniazid for 9 months (CDC, 2011).

Dosage Forms Excipient information presented when available (limited, particularly for generics); consult specific product labeling.

Tablet, Oral:

Priftin: 150 mg

Rifaximin (rif AX i min)

Brand Names: U.S. Xifaxan

Pharmacologic Category Antibiotic, Miscellaneous

Use Treatment of travelers' diarrhea caused by noninvasive strains of *E. coli*; reduction in the risk of overt hepatic encephalopathy (HE) recurrence

Unlabeled Use Treatment of hepatic encephalopathy; alternative treatment for *Clostridium difficile*-associated diarrhea (CDAD)

Pregnancy Risk Factor C

Pregnancy Considerations Adverse events have been observed in animal reproduction studies; therefore, the manufacturer classifies rifaximin as pregnancy category C. Due to the limited oral absorption of rifaximin in patients with normal hepatic function, exposure to the fetus is expected to be extremely low.

Breast-Feeding Considerations It is not known if rifaximin is excreted in human milk. Due to the limited oral absorption of rifaximin in patients with normal hepatic function, exposure to the nursing infant is expected to be extremely low. Use of rifaximin during breast-feeding is not recommended by the manufacturer.

Contraindications Hypersensitivity to rifaximin, other rifamycin antibiotics, or any component of the formulation

Warnings/Precautions Efficacy has not been established for the treatment of diarrhea due to pathogens other than *E. coli*, including *C. jejuni*, *Shigella* and *Salmonella*. Consider alternative therapy if symptoms persist or worsen after 24-48 hours of treatment. Not for treatment of systemic infections; <1% is absorbed orally. Prolonged use may result in fungal or bacterial superinfection, including *C. difficile*-associated diarrhea (CDAD) and pseudomembranous colitis; CDAD has been observed >2 months postantibiotic treatment. Use caution in severe hepatic impairment (Child-Pugh class C); efficacy for prevention of encephalopathy has not been established in patients with a Model for End-Stage Liver Disease (MELD) score >25.

Adverse Reactions Note: Frequency of adverse events generally higher following treatment for hepatic encephalopathy (HE). Percentages are presented for HE unless otherwise stated.

>10%:
Cardiovascular: Peripheral edema (15%)
Central nervous system: Dizziness (13%), fatigue (12%)
Hepatic: Ascites (11%)
Gastrointestinal: Nausea (14%)
2% to 10%:
Cardiovascular: Chest pain (>2% to 5%), edema (>2% to 5%), hypotension (>2% to 5%)
Central nervous system: Headache (travelers' diarrhea 10%), depression (7%), fever (6%), amnesia (>2% to 5%), attention disturbance (>2% to 5%), confusion (>2% to 5%), hypoesthesia (>2% to 5%), pain (>2% to 5%), tremor (>2% to 5%), vertigo (>2% to 5%)
Dermatological: Pruritus (9%), rash (5%), cellulitis (>2% to 5%)
Endocrine and metabolism: Hyper-/hypoglycemia (>2% to 5%), hyperkalemia (>2% to 5%), hyponatremia (>2% to 5%)
Gastrointestinal: Abdominal pain (>2% to 9%), abdominal tenderness (>2% to 5%), anorexia (>2% to 5%), dehydration (>2% to 5%), esophageal varices (>2% to 5%), weight gain (>2% to 5%), xerostomia (>2% to 5%)
Hematologic: Anemia (8%)
Neuromuscular & skeletal: Muscle spasms (9%), arthralgia (6%), myalgia (>2% to 5%)
Respiratory: Nasopharyngitis (7%), dyspnea (6%), epistaxis(>2% to 5%), pneumonia (>2% to 5%), rhinitis (>2% to 5%), upper respiratory tract infection (>2% to 5%)
Miscellaneous: Influenza-like illness (>2% to 5%)

All indications: <2% (Limited to important or life-threatening): Abnormal dreams, allergic dermatitis, anaphylaxis, angioneurotic edema, AST increased, choluria, CDAD, dry lips, dysuria, ear pain, exfoliative dermatitis, flushing, gingival disorder, hematuria, hot flashes, hypersensitivity reactions, lymphocytosis, migraine, monocytosis, motion sickness, nasal irritation, nasopharyngitis, neck pain, neutropenia, pharyngitis, pharyngolaryngeal pain, polyuria, proteinuria, sunburn, syncope, taste loss, tinnitus, urticaria, weakness, weight loss

Drug Interactions

Metabolism/Transport Effects None known.

Avoid Concomitant Use

Avoid concomitant use of Rifaximin with any of the following: BCG

Increased Effect/Toxicity There are no known significant interactions involving an increase in effect.

Decreased Effect

Rifaximin may decrease the levels/effects of: BCG; Sodium Picosulfate

Storage/Stability Store at controlled room temperature of 20°C to 25°C (68°F to 77°F).

Mechanism of Action Rifaximin inhibits bacterial RNA synthesis by binding to bacterial DNA-dependent RNA polymerase.

Pharmacodynamics/Kinetics

Absorption: Oral: Travelers' diarrhea: Low; Increased in prevention of hepatic encephalopathy with Child-Pugh class C having a greater exposure than A
Protein binding: Healthy subjects: ~68%; Hepatic impairment: 62%
Half-life elimination: ~2-5 hours
Time to peak: Hepatic encephalopathy prevention: ~1 hour
Excretion: Feces (~97% as unchanged drug); urine (<1%)

Dosage Oral:
Children ≥12 years and Adults: Travelers' diarrhea: 200 mg 3 times/day for 3 days
Adults:
Hepatic encephalopathy:
Reduction of overt hepatic encephalopathy recurrence: 550 mg 2 times/day. **Note:** Supporting clinical trial evaluated efficacy over 6-month treatment period.
Treatment of hepatic encephalopathy (unlabeled use): 400 mg every 8 hours for 5-10 days (Mas, 2003)
Clostridium difficile-associated diarrhea (unlabeled use): 200-400 mg 2-3 times/day for 14 days (Johnson, 2007)

Dosage adjustment in renal impairment: No dosage adjustment provided in manufacturer's labeling (has not been studied).

Dosage adjustment in hepatic impairment: No dosage adjustment necessary. Use with caution in severe impairment (Child-Pugh class C) as systemic absorption does occur and pharmacokinetic parameters are highly variable

Dietary Considerations May be taken with or without food.

Administration May be administered with or without food.

Monitoring Parameters Temperature, blood in stool, change in symptoms; monitor changes in mental status in hepatic encephalopathy

Dosage Forms Excipient information presented when available (limited, particularly for generics); consult specific product labeling.
Tablet, Oral:
Xifaxan: 200 mg, 550 mg [contains edetate disodium]

Extemporaneous Preparations A 20 mg/mL oral suspension may be made using tablets. Crush six 200 mg tablets and reduce to a fine powder. Add 30 mL of a 1:1 mixture of Ora-Sweet® and Ora-Plus® or a 1:1 mixture of Ora-Sweet® SF and Ora-Plus®; mix well while adding the vehicle in geometric proportions to **almost** 60 mL; transfer to a calibrated bottle, rinse mortar with vehicle, and add quantity of vehicle sufficient to make 60 mL. Label "shake well". Stable 60 days at room temperature.

Cober MP, Johnson CE, Lee J, et al, "Stability of Extemporaneously Prepared Rifaximin Oral Suspensions," *Am J Health Syst Pharm*, 2010, 67(4):287-89.

◆ rIFN beta-1a *see* Interferon Beta-1a *on page 1104*
◆ rIFN beta-1b *see* Interferon Beta-1b *on page 1106*
◆ RIG *see* Rabies Immune Globulin (Human) *on page 1771*

Rilonacept (ri LON a sept)

Brand Names: U.S. Arcalyst

Pharmacologic Category Interleukin-1 Inhibitor

Use Treatment of cryopyrin-associated periodic syndromes (CAPS) including familial cold autoinflammatory syndrome (FCAS) and Muckle-Wells syndrome (MWS)

Pregnancy Risk Factor C

Pregnancy Considerations Adverse events have been observed in animal reproduction studies.

Breast-Feeding Considerations It is not known if rilonacept is excreted in breast milk. The manufacturer recommends that caution be exercised when administering rilonacept to nursing women.

Contraindications There are no contraindications listed in the manufacturer's labeling.

Warnings/Precautions May cause rare hypersensitivity reactions; discontinue use and initiate appropriate therapy if reaction occurs. Caution should be exercised when considering use in patients with a history of new/recurrent infections, with conditions that predispose them to infections, or with latent or localized infections. Therapy should not be initiated in patients with active or chronic infections. May increase risk of reactivation of latent tuberculosis; follow current guidelines for evaluation and treatment of latent tuberculosis prior to initiating rilonacept therapy. Use may impair defenses against malignancies; impact on the development and course of malignancies is not fully defined. Use may increase total cholesterol, HDL, LDL, and triglycerides; periodic assessment of lipid profile should occur. Tumor necrosis factor (TNF)-blocking agents should not be used in combination with rilonacept; risk of serious infection is increased. Immunizations should be up to date including pneumococcal and influenza vaccines before initiating therapy. Live vaccines should not be given concurrently. Administration of inactivated (killed) vaccines while on therapy may not be effective.

Adverse Reactions

>10%:

Immunologic: Antibody development (35%)

Infection: Increased susceptibility to infection (34% to 48%; incidence higher during winter months)

Local: Injection site reaction (48%; majority mild-moderate; typically lasting 1-2 days; characterized by bleeding, bruising, erythema, induration, inflammation, itching, pain, swelling, urticaria; other local reactions include dermatitis, vesicles)

Respiratory: Upper respiratory tract infection (26%)

1% to 10%:

Central nervous system: Hypoesthesia (9%)

Respiratory: Cough (9%), sinusitis (9%)

<1%, postmarketing, and/or case reports: Bacterial meningitis (*Streptococcus pneumoniae*), bronchitis, colitis, gastrointestinal hemorrhage, hypercholesterolemia, hypersensitivity reaction, increased HDL cholesterol, increased LDL cholesterol, increased serum triglycerides, mycobacterium infection (*Mycobacterium intracellulare*), neutropenia (transient)

Drug Interactions

Metabolism/Transport Effects None known.

Avoid Concomitant Use

Avoid concomitant use of Rilonacept with any of the following: Anti-TNF Agents; BCG; Canakinumab; Natalizumab; Pimecrolimus; Tacrolimus (Topical); Tofacitinib; Vaccines (Live)

Increased Effect/Toxicity

Rilonacept may increase the levels/effects of: Canakinumab; Leflunomide; Natalizumab; Tofacitinib; Vaccines (Live)

The levels/effects of Rilonacept may be increased by: Anti-TNF Agents; Denosumab; Pimecrolimus; Roflumilast; Tacrolimus (Topical); Trastuzumab

Decreased Effect

Rilonacept may decrease the levels/effects of: BCG; Coccidioidin Skin Test; Sipuleucel-T; Vaccines (Inactivated); Vaccines (Live)

The levels/effects of Rilonacept may be decreased by: Echinacea

Preparation for Administration Reconstitute rilonacept 220 mg powder for injection with preservative free SWFI 2.3 mL. After reconstituting with preservative free SWFI, gently shake the vial for 1 minute, then allow solution to sit for 1 minute. If the powder is not completely dissolved, gently shake the vial for an additional 30 seconds, then allow solution to sit for 1 minute; repeat if necessary. Each reconstituted vial allows for withdrawal of 2 mL (160 mg) for SubQ administration.

Storage/Stability Store intact vials in refrigerator at 2°C to 8°C (36°F to 46°F); do not freeze. Do not shake. Protect from light. After reconstitution, may be stored at controlled room temperature. Protect from light. Use within 3 hours of reconstitution.

Mechanism of Action Cryopyrin-associated periodic syndromes (CAPS) refers to rare genetic syndromes caused by mutations in the nucleotide-binding domain, leucine rich family (NLR), pyrin domain containing 3 (NLRP-3) gene or the cold-induced autoinflammatory syndrome-1 (*CIAS1*) gene. Cryopyrin, a protein encoded by this gene, regulates interleukin-1 beta (IL-1β) activation. Deficiency of cryopyrin results in excessive inflammation. Rilonacept reduces inflammation by binding to IL-1β (some binding of IL-1α and IL-1 receptor antagonist) and preventing interaction with cell surface receptors.

Pharmacodynamics/Kinetics

Onset of action: Steady state reached by 6 weeks

Half-life elimination: 8.6 days

Dosage Cryopyrin-associated periodic syndromes: SubQ:

Children ≥12 years: Loading dose 4.4 mg/kg (maximum dose: 320 mg) given as 1-2 separate injections (maximum: 2 mL/injection; administer at 2 different sites if multiple injections are necessary) on the same day, followed by a once-weekly dose of 2.2 mg/kg (maximum dose: 160 mg). **Note:** Do not administer more frequently than once weekly.

Adults: Loading dose 320 mg given as 2 separate injections (160 mg each) on the same day at 2 different sites, followed by a once-weekly dose of 160 mg. **Note:** Do not administer more frequently than once weekly.

Dosage adjustment in renal impairment: No dosage adjustment provided in manufacturer's labeling (has not been studied).

Dosage adjustment in hepatic impairment: No dosage adjustment provided in manufacturer's labeling (has not been studied).

Administration SubQ: Rotate injection sites (thigh, abdomen, upper arm); injections should never be made at sites that are bruised, red, tender, or hard. If 2 injections are necessary to complete a dose, administer at different injection sites. Discard any unused portion.

Monitoring Parameters CBC with differential, lipid profile, C-reactive protein (CRP), serum amyloid A; signs of infection

Dosage Forms Excipient information presented when available (limited, particularly for generics); consult specific product labeling.

Solution Reconstituted, Subcutaneous [preservative free]:

Arcalyst: 220 mg (1 ea) [contains polyethylene glycol]

Rilpivirine (ril pi VIR een)

Brand Names: U.S. Edurant

Brand Names: Canada Edurant®

Index Terms TMC278

Pharmacologic Category Antiretroviral, Reverse Transcriptase Inhibitor, Non-nucleoside (Anti-HIV)

Use Treatment of HIV-1 infections in treatment-naive patients with HIV-1 RNA ≤100,000 copies/mL in combination with at least 2 other antiretroviral agents

Pregnancy Risk Factor B

Pregnancy Considerations No evidence of fetal toxicity has been noted in animal reproduction studies. Available data in pregnant women are insufficient and the DHHS Perinatal HIV Guidelines do not recommend use unless other alternatives are not available. Hypersensitivity reactions (including hepatic toxicity and rash) are more common in women on NNRTI therapy; it is not known if pregnancy increases this risk.

Regardless of CD4 count or HIV RNA copy number, all HIV-infected pregnant women should receive a combination antepartum antiretroviral (ARV) drug regimen; this includes women who require therapy for their own health, as well as women who do not yet require therapy for their own health. ARV therapy should be started as soon as possible if required for the woman's health. Although earlier initiation may be more effective in reducing the perinatal transmission of HIV), also consider maternal conditions (eg, nausea and vomiting) and the potential risks of first trimester fetal exposure for specific agents. Plasma HIV RNA levels should be assessed at ~34-36 weeks gestation in order to help determine mode of delivery. If ARV therapy must be interrupted for <24 hours during the peripartum period, stop then restart all medications simultaneously in order to decrease the chance of developing resistance. Long-term follow-up is recommended for all infants exposed to ARV medications.

Healthcare providers are encouraged to enroll pregnant women exposed to antiretroviral medications in the Antiretroviral Pregnancy Registry (1-800-258-4263 or www.-APRegistry.com). Healthcare providers caring for HIV-infected women and their infants may contact the National Perinatal HIV Hotline (888-448-8765) for clinical consultation (DHHS [perinatal], 2012).

Breast-Feeding Considerations Maternal or infant antiretroviral therapy does not completely eliminate the risk of postnatal HIV transmission. In addition, multiclass-resistant virus has been detected in breast-feeding infants despite maternal therapy. Therefore, in the United States, where formula is accessible, affordable, safe, and sustainable, and the risk of infant mortality due to diarrhea and respiratory infections is low, complete avoidance of breast-feeding by HIV-infected women is recommended to decrease potential transmission of HIV (DHHS [perinatal], 2012).

Contraindications Concurrent use of carbamazepine, dexamethasone (>1 dose), oxcarbazepine, phenobarbital, phenytoin, proton pump inhibitors (PPIs), rifabutin, rifampin, rifapentine, or St John's wort

Warnings/Precautions Use in treatment-naive patients with HIV-1 RNA ≤100,000 copies/mL; not for use in treatment-experienced patients. May cause depressive disorders (depression, depressed mood, dysphoria, mood changes, negative thoughts, suicide attempts, or suicidal ideation); monitor for changes and need for intervention. Causes hepatotoxicity; patients with significant transaminase elevations or hepatitis B or C prior to treatment may be at greater risk; has occurred in a few patients with no prior hepatic disease or risk factors. Baseline and periodic laboratory LFT evaluation during therapy is recommended. May cause redistribution of fat (eg, buffalo hump, peripheral wasting with increased abdominal girth, cushingoid appearance). Patients may develop immune reconstitution syndrome resulting in the occurrence of an inflammatory response to an indolent or residual opportunistic infection during initial HIV treatment or activation of autoimmune disorders (eg, Graves' disease, polymyositis, Guillain-Barré syndrome) later in therapy; further evaluation and treatment may be required.

Potentially significant interactions may exist, requiring dose or frequency adjustment, additional monitoring, and/or selection of alternative therapy. Doses >25 mg daily (ie, 75 mg daily, 300 mg daily) have been associated with QT_c prolongation; use caution when coadministering with a drug with a known risk of torsade de pointes (DHHS, 2013).

Adverse Reactions

>10%:

Endocrine & metabolic: Cholesterol increased (7% to 17%; grade 3: <1%), LDL increased (5% to 14%; grade 3: 1%)

Hepatic: ALT increased (5% to 18%; grade 3/4: 1%), AST increased (4% to 16%; grade 3/4: 1% to 2%)

2% to 10%:

Central nervous system: Depressive disorders (depression, depressed mood, dysphoria, mood changes, negative thoughts, suicide attempts, suicidal ideation) (4% to 9%; grades 3/4: 1%), headache (3%), insomnia (3%), abnormal dreams (2%), fatigue (2%)

Dermatologic: Rash (3%)

Endocrine & metabolic: Triglycerides increased (2%; grade 3/4: ≤1%)

Gastrointestinal: Abdominal pain (2%)

Hepatic: Total bilirubin increased (3% to 5%; grade 3/4: ≤1%)

Renal: Creatinine increased (1% to 6%; grade 3/4: ≤1%)

<2% (Limited to important or life-threatening): Abdominal discomfort, anxiety, appetite decreased, cholecystitis, cholelithiasis, diarrhea, dizziness, glomerulonephritis (membranous and mesangioproliferative), nausea, nephrolithiasis, nephrotic syndrome, sleep disorders, somnolence, vomiting

Drug Interactions

Metabolism/Transport Effects Substrate of CYP3A4 (major); **Note:** Assignment of Major/Minor substrate status based on clinically relevant drug interaction potential

Avoid Concomitant Use

Avoid concomitant use of Rilpivirine with any of the following: CarBAMazepine; Dexamethasone (Systemic); Etravirine; Fosphenytoin; OXcarbazepine; PHENobarbital; Phenytoin; Primidone; Proton Pump Inhibitors; Reverse Transcriptase Inhibitors (Non-Nucleoside); Rifamycin Derivatives; St Johns Wort

Increased Effect/Toxicity

Rilpivirine may increase the levels/effects of: Etravirine; Highest Risk QTc-Prolonging Agents; Moderate Risk QTc-Prolonging Agents

The levels/effects of Rilpivirine may be increased by: Boceprevir; CYP3A4 Inhibitors (Strong); Darunavir; Ketoconazole (Systemic); Lopinavir; Macrolide Antibiotics; Mifepristone; Reverse Transcriptase Inhibitors (Non-Nucleoside); Simeprevir

Decreased Effect

Rilpivirine may decrease the levels/effects of: CarBAMazepine; Didanosine; Etravirine; Ketoconazole (Systemic); Methadone

The levels/effects of Rilpivirine may be decreased by: Antacids; Bosentan; CarBAMazepine; CYP3A4 Inducers (Strong); Dabrafenib; Deferasirox; Dexamethasone (Systemic); Didanosine; Fosphenytoin; H2-Antagonists; Mitotane; OXcarbazepine; PHENobarbital; Phenytoin; Primidone; Proton Pump Inhibitors; Reverse Transcriptase Inhibitors (Non-Nucleoside); Rifamycin Derivatives; St Johns Wort; Tocilizumab

Ethanol/Nutrition/Herb Interactions

Food: Absorption increased by ~40% when taken with a normal- to high-calorie meal. Management: Administer with a normal- to high-calorie meal. Administration with a protein supplement drink alone does not increase absorption.

Herb/Nutraceutical: St John's wort may decrease the levels/effects of rilpivirine. Management: Avoid St John's wort; concurrent use is contraindicated.

Storage/Stability Store at 25°C (77°F); excursions permitted to 15°C to 30°C (59°F to 86°F). Keep in original container; protect from light.

Mechanism of Action As a non-nucleoside reverse transcriptase inhibitor, rilpivirine has activity against HIV-1 by binding to reverse transcriptase. It consequently blocks the RNA-dependent and DNA-dependent DNA polymerase activities, including HIV-1 replication. It does not require intracellular phosphorylation for antiviral activity.

Pharmacodynamics/Kinetics

Absorption: Increased 40% with a meal (normal-to-high calorie)

Protein binding: 99.7% (primarily albumin)

Metabolism: Hepatic, primarily by CYP3A4

Half-life elimination: ~50 hours

Time to peak, plasma: 4-5 hours

Excretion: Feces (85%, ~25% as unchanged drug); urine (~6%; <1% as unchanged drug)

Dosage Oral: Adults: 25 mg once daily. **Note:** Recommended only in antiretroviral treatment-naive patients with HIV-1 RNA ≤100,000 copies/mL at the start of therapy (DHHS, 2013).

Dosage adjustment in renal impairment:

Mild-to-moderate renal impairment: No dosage adjustment necessary

Severe or end-stage renal impairment: Use with caution; no dosage adjustment necessary (DHHS, 2012)

Hemodialysis/peritoneal dialysis: Due to extensive protein binding, significant removal by hemodialysis or peritoneal dialysis is unlikely.

Dosage adjustment in hepatic impairment:

Mild-to-moderate impairment (Child-Pugh class A or B): No dosage adjustment necessary

Severe impairment (Child-Pugh class C): No dosage adjustment provided in the manufacturer's labeling (has not been studied); DHHS HIV guidelines also have no dosage recommendation (DHHS, 2012).

Dietary Considerations Take with a normal- to high-calorie meal. Taking with a protein supplement drink alone does not increase absorption.

Administration Administer with a normal- to high-calorie meal. Taking with a protein supplement drink alone does not increase absorption.

Monitoring Parameters Cholesterol, triglycerides, hepatic transaminases; signs of skin rash, signs and symptoms of infection

Additional Information Rilpivirine has been shown in several studies to be noninferior to efavirenz in treatment-naive HIV-1 patients. Efficacy data in clinical studies exist for up to 96 weeks. Patients with CD4+ counts <200 cells/mm^3 (regardless of HIV-1 RNA at the start of therapy) are more likely to experience virologic failure (defined as HIV-1 RNA ≥50 copies/mL) than patients with CD4+ counts ≥200 cells/mm^3. Additionally, patients with increased HIV-1 viral loads at treatment initiation (HIV-1 RNA >100,000 copies/mL) are more likely to develop virologic failure. Increased viral load patients also are more likely to develop rilpivirine-resistance, tenofovir and emtricitabine/lamivudine resistance and NNRTI class cross-resistance. Rilpivirine resistance patterns are very similar to those of etravirine (including cross resistance with single substitutions at K101P, Y181I, and Y181V) (Azijn, 2010). In rilpivirine-treated patients who experience virologic failure, rilpivirine-resistant mutations are very common (DHHS, 2013).

Dosage Forms Excipient information presented when available (limited, particularly for generics); consult specific product labeling.

Tablet, Oral:

Edurant: 25 mg

◆ **Rilpivirine, Emtricitabine, and Tenofovir** *see* Emtricitabine, Rilpivirine, and Tenofovir *on page 700*

◆ **Rilutek** *see* Riluzole *on page 1819*

◆ **Rilutek® (Can)** *see* Riluzole *on page 1819*

Riluzole (RIL yoo zole)

Brand Names: U.S. Rilutek

Brand Names: Canada Apo-Riluzole®; Mylan-Riluzole; Rilutek®

Index Terms 2-Amino-6-Trifluoromethoxy-benzothiazole; RP-54274

Pharmacologic Category Glutamate Inhibitor

Use Treatment of amyotrophic lateral sclerosis (ALS); riluzole can extend survival or time to tracheostomy

Pregnancy Risk Factor C

Pregnancy Considerations Impaired fertility, decreased implantation, increased intrauterine death, and adverse effects on offspring growth and viability were observed in animal studies. There are no adequate or well-controlled studies in pregnant women.

Breast-Feeding Considerations It is not known if riluzole is excreted in breast milk. Breast-feeding is not recommended by the manufacturer.

Contraindications Severe hypersensitivity reactions to riluzole or any component of the formulation

Warnings/Precautions Among 4000 patients given riluzole for ALS, there were 3 cases of marked neutropenia (ANC <500/mm^3), all seen within the first 2 months of treatment. Interstitial lung disease (primarily hypersensitivity pneumonitis) has occurred, requires prompt evaluation and possible discontinuation. Use with caution in patients with concomitant renal insufficiency. Use with caution in patients with current evidence or history of abnormal liver function; do not administer if baseline liver function tests are elevated. May cause elevations in transaminases (usually transient). May cause elevations in transaminases (usually transient) within first 3 months of therapy; discontinue if ALT levels are ≥5 times upper limit of normal or if jaundice develops. The elderly or female patients may have decreased clearance of riluzole; use with caution. May cause dizziness or somnolence; caution should be used performing tasks which require alertness (operating machinery or driving).

Adverse Reactions

>10%:

Gastrointestinal: Nausea (16%)

Neuromuscular & skeletal: Weakness (19%)

1% to 10%:

Cardiovascular: Hypertension (5%), peripheral edema (3%), tachycardia (3%)

Central nervous system: Dizziness (4%), somnolence (2%), vertigo (2%), malaise (1%)

Dermatologic: Pruritus (4%), eczema (2%), exfoliative dermatitis (1%)

Gastrointestinal: Abdominal pain (5%), vomiting (4%), flatulence (3%), oral moniliasis (1%), stomatitis (1%), tooth caries (1%)

Genitourinary: Urinary tract infection (3%), dysuria (1%)

Hepatic: Liver function tests increased (8% >3 x ULN; 2% >5 x ULN)

Neuromuscular & skeletal: Arthralgia (4%), paresthesia (circumoral; 2%), tremor (1%)

Respiratory: Lung function decreased (10%), cough increased (3%)

<1% (Limited to important or life-threatening): Alkaline phosphatase increased, amblyopia, anaphylactoid reaction, anaphylaxis, angioedema, aplastic anemia, arthrosis, asthma, ataxia, bone necrosis, bradycardia, bundle branch block, cataract, cerebral hemorrhage, deafness, dementia, diabetes mellitus, diabetes insipidus, edema, erythema multiforme, extrapyramidal syndrome, facial paralysis, gastrointestinal hemorrhage, gastrointestinal ulcer, GGT increased, glaucoma, hallucination, heart failure, hematemesis, hematuria, hemoptysis, hepatitis, hypercalcemia, hypokalemia, hypokinesia, hyponatremia, hypotension, hypersensitivity pneumonitis, interstitial lung disease, jaundice, LDH increased, leukocytosis, leukopenia, lymphadenopathy, mania, myoclonus, neutropenia, osteoporosis, pancreatitis, peripheral neuritis, pleural effusion, pseudomembranous colitis, purpura, respiratory acidosis, seizure, subarachnoid hemorrhage, thrombosis, urinary retention, urticaria, uterine hemorrhage, ventricular fibrillation, ventricular tachycardia

Drug Interactions

Metabolism/Transport Effects Substrate of CYP1A2 (major); **Note:** Assignment of Major/Minor substrate status based on clinically relevant drug interaction potential

Avoid Concomitant Use There are no known interactions where it is recommended to avoid concomitant use.

Increased Effect/Toxicity There are no known significant interactions involving an increase in effect.

Decreased Effect

The levels/effects of Riluzole may be decreased by: CYP1A2 Inducers (Strong); Cyproterone

Ethanol/Nutrition/Herb Interactions

Ethanol: Avoid ethanol (due to CNS depression and possible risk of liver toxicity).

Food: A high-fat meal decreases absorption of riluzole (decreasing AUC by 20% and peak blood levels by 45%). Charbroiled food may increase riluzole elimination.

Storage/Stability Store at 20°C to 25°C (68°F to 77°F). Protect from bright light.

Mechanism of Action Mechanism of action is not known. Pharmacologic properties include inhibitory effect on glutamate release, inactivation of voltage-dependent sodium channels; and ability to interfere with intracellular events that follow transmitter binding at excitatory amino acid receptors

Pharmacodynamics/Kinetics

Absorption: ~90%; high-fat meal decreases AUC by 20% and peak blood levels by 45%

Protein binding, plasma: 96%, primarily to albumin and lipoproteins

Metabolism: Extensively hepatic to six major and a number of minor metabolites via CYP1A2 dependent hydroxylation and glucuronidation

Bioavailability: Oral: Absolute: ~60%

Half-life elimination: 12 hours

Excretion: Urine (90%; 85% as metabolites, 2% as unchanged drug) and feces (5%) within 7 days

Dosage Adults: Oral: 50 mg every 12 hours; no increased benefit can be expected from higher daily doses, but adverse events are increased

Dosage adjustment in smoking: Cigarette smoking is known to induce CYP1A2; patients who smoke cigarettes would be expected to eliminate riluzole faster. There is no information, however, on the effect of, or need for, dosage adjustment in these patients.

Dosage adjustment in renal impairment: No dosage adjustment provided in manufacturer's labeling. Use with caution.

Dosage adjustment in hepatic impairment: No dosage adjustment provided in manufacturer's labeling. Use with caution.

Dietary Considerations Take at least 1 hour before or 2 hours after a meal.

Administration Administer at the same time each day, at least 1 hour before or 2 hours after a meal.

Monitoring Parameters Monitor serum aminotransferases including ALT levels before and during therapy. Evaluate serum ALT levels every month during the first 3 months of therapy, every 3 months during the remainder of the first year and periodically thereafter. Evaluate ALT levels more frequently in patients who develop elevations. Maximum increases in serum ALT usually occurred within 3 months after the start of therapy and were usually transient when <5 times ULN (upper limits of normal). Discontinue therapy if ALT levels are ≥5 times upper limit of normal or if jaundice develops.

In trials, if ALT levels were <5 times ULN, treatment continued and ALT levels usually returned to below 2 times ULN within 2-6 months. There is no experience with continued treatment of ALS patients once ALT values exceed 5 times ULN.

Dosage Forms Excipient information presented when available (limited, particularly for generics); consult specific product labeling.

Tablet, Oral:

Rilutek: 50 mg

Generic: 50 mg

RimabotulinumtoxinB

(rime uh BOT yoo lin num TOKS in bee)

Brand Names: U.S. Myobloc

Index Terms Botulinum Toxin Type B

Pharmacologic Category Neuromuscular Blocker Agent, Toxin

Use Treatment of cervical dystonia (spasmodic torticollis)

Unlabeled Use Treatment of cervical dystonia in patients who have developed resistance to onabotulinumtoxinA or abobotulinumtoxinA

Pregnancy Risk Factor C (manufacturer)

Medication Guide Available Yes

Dosage

Children: Not established in pediatric patients

Adults: Cervical dystonia: I.M.: Initial: 2500-5000 units divided among the affected muscles in patients **previously treated** with botulinum toxin; initial dose in **previously untreated** patients should be lower. Subsequent dosing should be optimized according to patient's response.

Elderly: No dosage adjustments required, but limited experience in patients ≥75 years old

Dosage adjustment in renal impairment: No dosage adjustment provided in manufacturer's labeling.

Dosage adjustment in hepatic impairment: No dosage adjustment provided in manufacturer's labeling.

Additional Information Complete prescribing information should be consulted for additional detail.

Dosage Forms Excipient information presented when available (limited, particularly for generics); consult specific product labeling.

Solution, Intramuscular [preservative free]:

Myobloc: 2500 units/0.5 mL (0.5 mL); 5000 units/mL (1 mL); 10,000 units/2 mL (2 mL) [contains albumin human]

Rimantadine (ri MAN ta deen)

Brand Names: U.S. Flumadine

Brand Names: Canada Flumadine®

Index Terms Rimantadine Hydrochloride

Pharmacologic Category Antiviral Agent; Antiviral Agent, Adamantane

Use Prophylaxis (adults and children >1 year of age) and treatment (adults) of influenza A viral infection (per manufacturer labeling; also refer to current ACIP guidelines for recommendations during current flu season)

Note: In certain circumstances, the ACIP recommends use of rimantadine in combination with oseltamivir for the treatment or prophylaxis of influenza A infection when resistance to oseltamivir is suspected.

Pregnancy Risk Factor C

Pregnancy Considerations Animal data suggest embryotoxicity, maternal toxicity, and offspring mortality at doses 7-11 times the recommended human dose. There are no adequate and well-controlled studies in pregnant women.

Influenza infection may be more severe in pregnant women. Untreated influenza infection is associated with an increased risk of adverse events to the fetus and an increased risk of complications or death to the mother. Oseltamivir and zanamivir are currently recommended for the treatment or prophylaxis influenza in pregnant women and women up to 2 weeks postpartum. Appropriate antiviral agents are currently recommended as an adjunct to vaccination and should not be used as a substitute for vaccination in pregnant women (consult current CDC guidelines).

Healthcare providers are encouraged to refer women exposed to influenza vaccine, or who have taken an antiviral medication during pregnancy to the Vaccines and Medications in Pregnancy Surveillance System (VAMPSS) by contacting The Organization of Teratology Information Specialists (OTIS) at (877) 311-8972.

Breast-Feeding Considerations Do not use in nursing mothers due to potential adverse effect in infants. The CDC recommends that women infected with the influenza virus follow general precautions (eg, frequent hand washing) to decrease viral transmission to the child. Mothers with influenza-like illnesses at delivery should consider avoiding close contact with the infant until they have received 48 hours of antiviral medication, fever has resolved, and cough and secretions can be controlled. These measures may help decrease (but not eliminate) the risk of transmitting influenza to the newborn during breast-feeding. During this time, breast milk can be expressed and bottle-fed to the infant by another person who is not infected. Protective measures, such as wearing a face mask, changing into a clean gown or clothing, and strict hand hygiene should be continued by the mother for ≥7 days after the onset of symptoms or until symptom-free for 24 hours. Infant care should be performed by a non-infected person when possible (consult current CDC guidelines).

Contraindications Hypersensitivity to drugs of the adamantine class, including rimantadine and amantadine, or any component of the formulation

Warnings/Precautions Use with caution in patients with renal and hepatic dysfunction; avoid use, if possible, in patients with uncontrolled psychosis or severe psychoneurosis. An increase in seizure incidence may occur in patients with seizure disorders; discontinue drug if seizures occur; resistance may develop during treatment; viruses exhibit cross-resistance between amantadine and rimantadine. Due to increased resistance, the ACIP has recommended that rimantadine and amantadine no longer be used for the treatment or prophylaxis of influenza A in the United States until susceptibility has been re-established; consult current guidelines. Rimantadine is not effective in the prevention or treatment of influenza B virus infections. The elderly are at higher risk for CNS (eg, dizziness, headache, weakness) and gastrointestinal (eg, nausea/vomiting, abdominal pain) adverse events; dosage adjustment is recommended in elderly patients >65 years of age.

Adverse Reactions

1% to 10%:

Central nervous system: Insomnia (2% to 3%), concentration impaired (≤2%), dizziness (1% to 2%), nervousness (1% to 2%), fatigue (1%), headache (1%)

Gastrointestinal: Nausea (3%), anorexia (2%), vomiting (2%), xerostomia (2%), abdominal pain (1%)

Neuromuscular & skeletal: Weakness (1%)

<1% (Limited to important or life-threatening): Agitation, ataxia, bronchospasm, cardiac failure, confusion, convulsions, depression, diarrhea, dyspnea, euphoria, gait abnormality, hallucinations, heart block, hyperkinesias, hypertension, lactation, palpitation, parosmia, pedal edema, rash, syncope, tachycardia, taste alteration, tremor

Drug Interactions

Metabolism/Transport Effects None known.

Avoid Concomitant Use There are no known interactions where it is recommended to avoid concomitant use.

Increased Effect/Toxicity

The levels/effects of Rimantadine may be increased by: MAO Inhibitors

Decreased Effect

Rimantadine may decrease the levels/effects of: Influenza Virus Vaccine (Live/Attenuated)

Ethanol/Nutrition/Herb Interactions Food: Food does not affect rate or extent of absorption

Storage/Stability Store at 25°C (77°F); excursions permitted to 15°C to 30°C (59°F to 86°F).

Mechanism of Action Exerts its inhibitory effect on three antigenic subtypes of influenza A virus (H1N1, H2N2, H3N2) early in the viral replicative cycle, possibly inhibiting the uncoating process; it has no activity against influenza B virus and is two- to eightfold more active than amantadine

Pharmacodynamics/Kinetics

Onset of action: Antiviral activity: No data exist establishing a correlation between plasma concentration and antiviral effect

Protein Binding: ~40%, primarily to albumin

Metabolism: Extensively hepatic

Half-life elimination: 25.4 hours; prolonged in elderly, severe liver and severe renal impairment

Time to peak: 6 hours

Excretion: Urine (<25% as unchanged drug)

Clearance: Hemodialysis does not contribute to clearance

Dosage Oral:

Prophylaxis:

Children

1-9 years: 5 mg/kg/day in 1-2 divided doses; maximum: 150 mg/day

≥10 years and <40 kg: 5 mg/kg/day in 2 divided doses (CDC, 2011)

Children ≥10 years (and ≥40 kg) and Adults: 100 mg twice daily

Elderly: 100 mg daily in the elderly (≥65 years), including elderly nursing home patients

Note: Prophylaxis (institutional outbreak): In order to control outbreaks in institutions, if influenza A virus subtyping is unavailable and oseltamivir resistant viruses are circulating, rimantadine may be used in combination with oseltamivir if zanamivir cannot be used. Treatment should continue for ≥2 weeks and until ~10 days after illness onset in the last patient (CDC, 2011; Harper, 2009).

Treatment:

Children ≥17 years and Adults: 100 mg twice daily

Elderly: 100 mg daily in the elderly (≥65 years) or nursing home patients

Dosage adjustment in renal impairment:

Cl_{cr} ≥30 mL/minute: No dosage adjustment necessary.

Cl_{cr} <30 mL/minute: Maximum: 100 mg daily

Dosage adjustment in hepatic impairment: Severe dysfunction: Maximum: 100 mg daily

Administration Initiation of rimantadine within 48 hours of the onset of influenza A illness halves the duration of illness and significantly reduces the duration of viral shedding and increased peripheral airways resistance; continue therapy for 5-7 days after symptoms begin; discontinue as soon as clinically warranted to reduce the emergence of antiviral drug resistant viruses

Monitoring Parameters Monitor for CNS or GI effects in elderly or patients with renal or hepatic impairment

Dosage Forms Excipient information presented when available (limited, particularly for generics); consult specific product labeling.

Tablet, Oral, as hydrochloride:

Flumadine: 100 mg [contains fd&c yellow #6 (sunset yellow), fd&c yellow #6 aluminum lake]

Generic: 100 mg

Extemporaneous Preparations Rimantadine 10 mg/mL Suspension:

To prepare suspension, 10 mL of Ora-Sweet® will be required for every 100 mg tablet of rimantadine. (Do not prepare more than a 14-day supply).

- Calculate the total dose needed (daily dose x number of days = mg of rimantadine needed) and round the final mg of rimantadine needed up to the next 100 mg (eg, 750 mg would be 800 mg, or eight 100 mg tablets).
- Calculate the total volume of Ora-Sweet® by taking the rounded mg of rimantadine and dividing by 10 mg/mL (eg, 800 mg divided by 10 mg/mL = 80 mL).
- Grind required number of tablets in mortar and triturate to a fine powder. Slowly add 1/3 of the total volume of Ora-Sweet® to the mortar and triturate until a uniform suspension is achieved.
- Transfer to an amber glass or PET plastic bottle. Slowly add another 1/3 of the total volume of Ora-Sweet® to the mortar, rinsing the mortar, then transferring the contents into the bottle. Repeat using the final 1/3 of Ora-Sweet®. Add additional vehicle to bottle, if needed, to achieve the total calculated volume.
- Shake well to ensure homogeneous suspension. Some inert ingredients in the tablet may be insoluble.
- Label: Shake gently prior to each use.
- Suspension is stable for 14 days when stored at room temperature (25°C/77°F).

◆ **Rimantadine Hydrochloride** *see* Rimantadine *on page 1820*

Rimexolone (ri MEKS oh lone)

Brand Names: U.S. Vexol

Brand Names: Canada Vexol®

Pharmacologic Category Corticosteroid, Ophthalmic

Use Treatment of inflammation after ocular surgery and the treatment of anterior uveitis

Pregnancy Risk Factor C

Dosage Ophthalmic: Adults:

Anti-inflammatory: Instill 1-2 drops in conjunctival sac of affected eye 4 times/day beginning 24 hours after surgery and continuing through the first 2 weeks of the postoperative period

Anterior uveitis: Instill 1-2 drops in conjunctival sac of affected eye every hour during waking hours for the first week, then 1 drop every 2 hours during waking hours of the second week, and then taper until uveitis is resolved

Dosage adjustment in renal impairment: No dosage adjustment provided in manufacturer's labeling.

Dosage adjustment in hepatic impairment: No dosage adjustment provided in manufacturer's labeling.

Additional Information Complete prescribing information should be consulted for additional detail.

Dosage Forms Excipient information presented when available (limited, particularly for generics); consult specific product labeling.

Suspension, Ophthalmic:

Vexol: 1% (5 mL, 10 mL)

Riociguat (rye oh SIG ue at)

Brand Names: U.S. Adempas

Index Terms Adempas; BAY 63-2521

Pharmacologic Category Soluble Guanylate Cyclase (sGC) Stimulator

Use

Chronic thromboembolic pulmonary hypertension: Treatment of adults with persistent/recurrent chronic thromboembolic pulmonary hypertension (CTEPH) (WHO group 4) after surgical treatment or inoperable CTEPH to improve exercise capacity and WHO functional class

Pulmonary arterial hypertension: Treatment of adults with pulmonary artery hypertension (PAH) (WHO group 1) to improve exercise capacity, improve WHO functional class and to delay clinical worsening

Pregnancy Risk Factor X

Pregnancy Considerations Reproduction studies in animals have shown evidence of fetal abnormalities and use is contraindicated in women who are or may become pregnant. **[U.S. Boxed Warnings]: Riociguat may cause fetal harm if given to pregnant women. Riociguat is available to females only through the restricted Adempas Risk Evaluation and Mitigation Strategy (REMS) Program. All females of reproductive potential should have a negative pregnancy test prior to beginning therapy and testing should continue monthly during treatment and one month after discontinuing therapy. Females of childbearing potential should not become pregnant during therapy or for 1 month following discontinuation riociguat.** All females regardless of their reproductive potential must be enrolled in the REMS program; prescribers and pharmacies must also be enrolled in the program. Females of reproductive potential must be able to comply with pregnancy testing and contraception requirements of the program. Women may use one highly effective form of contraception (intrauterine device, contraceptive implant, or tubal sterilization) or a combination of methods (hormonal contraceptive with a barrier method or two barrier methods). A hormonal contraceptive or barrier method must be used in addition to a partner's vasectomy, if that method is chosen. Females should be counseled on pregnancy prevention and planning and instructed to notify their prescriber immediately if a pregnancy should occur. Women with pulmonary arterial hypotension (PAH) are encouraged to avoid pregnancy (Badesch, 2007; McLaughlin, 2009).

Breast-Feeding Considerations It is not known if riociguat is excreted into breast milk. Due to the potential for adverse reactions in the nursing infant, the manufacturer recommends a decision be made whether to discontinue nursing or to discontinue the drug, taking into account the importance of treatment to the mother.

Prescribing and Access Restrictions As a requirement of the REMS program, access to this medication is restricted. Female patients, prescribers, and pharmacies must register and be active in the Adempas REMS Program. Additional information, including certified pharmacies, is provided at www.adempasREMS.com or by calling 1-855-423-3672.

Contraindications Pregnancy; coadministration with nitrates or nitric oxide donors (eg, amyl nitrite) in any form; concomitant administration with phosphodiesterase (PDE) inhibitors, including specific PDE-5 inhibitors (eg, sildenafil, tadalafil, vardenafil) or nonspecific PDE inhibitors (eg, dipyridamole, theophylline)

Warnings/Precautions Reduces blood pressure. Use with caution in patients at increased risk for symptomatic hypotension or ischemia (eg, patients with hypovolemia, severe left ventricular outflow obstruction, resting hypotension, autonomic dysfunction) or concurrent use of antihypertensives or strong CYP and P-gp/BCRP inhibitors. Consider initiating at a lower dose for patients at risk of hypotension and/or dose reduction if hypotension develops. Patients must be cautioned about performing tasks which require mental alertness (eg, operating machinery or driving). Serious bleeding has been observed.

Use is not recommended in patients with pulmonary veno-occlusive disease (PVOD). Discontinue in any patient with pulmonary edema suggestive of PVOD. Use with caution in patients with renal and hepatic impairment. Use in patients with severe hepatic impairment and patients with Cl_{cr} <15 mL/minute or receiving dialysis have not been evaluated.

[U.S. Boxed Warning] May cause fetal harm if given to pregnant women. All females of reproductive potential should have a negative pregnancy test prior to beginning therapy and testing should continue monthly during treatment and one month after discontinuing therapy. Females of childbearing potential should not become pregnant during therapy or for 1 month following discontinuation of riociguat. Women may use one highly effective form of contraception (intrauterine device, contraceptive implant, or tubal sterilization) or a combination of methods (hormonal contraceptive with a barrier method or two barrier methods). A hormonal contraceptive or barrier method must be used in addition to a partner's vasectomy, if that method is chosen. Females should be counseled on pregnancy prevention and planning and instructed to notify their prescriber immediately if a pregnancy should occur. **[U.S. Boxed Warning]: Riociguat is available to females only through the restricted Adempas Risk Evaluation and Mitigation Strategy (REMS) Program.** All females, regardless of their reproductive potential, must be enrolled in the REMS program; prescribers and pharmacies must also be enrolled in the program. Females of reproductive potential must be able to comply with pregnancy testing and contraception requirements of the program. Call 855-4-ADEMPAS or visit www.AdempasREMS.com for more information.

Riociguat concentrations are 50% to 60% lower in patients who smoke compared to nonsmokers; consider titrating dose to >2.5 mg 3 times daily, if tolerated. A decreased dose may be necessary in patients who stop smoking during therapy. Potentially significant drug-drug interactions may exist, requiring dose or frequency adjustment, additional monitoring, and/or selection of alternative therapy.

Adverse Reactions Frequency not always defined.

Cardiovascular: Hypotension (3% to 10%; Ghofrani, 2013), palpitations, peripheral edema

Central nervous system: Headache (27%), dizziness (20%)

Gastrointestinal: Dyspepsia (13% to 19%; Ghofrani, 2013), nausea (14%), diarrhea (12%), vomiting (10%), gastritis (2% to 6%; Ghofrani, 2013), constipation (5%), gastroesophageal reflux disease (5%), abdominal distention, dysphagia

Hematologic & oncologic: Anemia (7%), major hemorrhage (2%; including vaginal hemorrhage, catheter site hemorrhage, subdural hematoma, hematemesis, and intra-abdominal hemorrhage)

Respiratory: Hemoptysis (1%), epistaxis, nasal congestion

Drug Interactions

Metabolism/Transport Effects Substrate of BCRP, CYP2C8 (major), CYP3A4 (major), P-glycoprotein; **Note:** Assignment of Major/Minor substrate status based on clinically relevant drug interaction potential

Avoid Concomitant Use

Avoid concomitant use of Riociguat with any of the following: Amyl Nitrite; Anagrelide; Cilostazol; Dipyridamole; Milrinone; Phosphodiesterase 5 Inhibitors; Theophylline Derivatives; Vasodilators (Organic Nitrates)

Increased Effect/Toxicity

Riociguat may increase the levels/effects of: Hypotensive Agents

The levels/effects of Riociguat may be increased by: Amyl Nitrite; Anagrelide; Cilostazol; Cobicistat; Dipyridamole; Itraconazole; Ketoconazole (Systemic); Milrinone; P-glycoprotein/ABCB1 Inhibitors; Phosphodiesterase 5 Inhibitors; Protease Inhibitors; Theophylline Derivatives; Vasodilators (Organic Nitrates)

Decreased Effect

The levels/effects of Riociguat may be decreased by: Antacids; Bosentan; CYP2C8 Inducers (Strong); CYP3A4 Inducers (Strong); Dabrafenib; Deferasirox; Herbs (CYP3A4 Inducers); Mitotane; P-glycoprotein/ABCB1 Inducers; Proton Pump Inhibitors; Tocilizumab

Storage/Stability Store at 25°C (77°F); excursions are permitted from 15°C to 30°C (59°F to 86°F).

Mechanism of Action Riociguat has a dual mode of action. It sensitizes soluble guanylate cyclase (sGC) to endogenous nitric oxide (NO) by stabilizing the NO-sGC binding. Riociguat also directly stimulates sGC independent of NO. Riociguat stimulates the NO-sGC-cGMP pathway and leads to increased generation of cGMP with subsequent vasodilation.

Pharmacodynamics/Kinetics

Distribution: ~30 L

Protein binding: Plasma: ~95%

Metabolism: Mainly cleared by metabolism by CYP1A1, CYP3A, CYP2C8 and CYP2J2. Formation of the major active metabolite, M1, is catalyzed by CYP1A1, which is inducible by polycyclic aromatic hydrocarbons such as those present in cigarette smoke. M1 is only 1/3 to 1/10 as potent as the parent drug and is further metabolized to the inactive N-glucuronide. Plasma concentrations of M1 in patients with pulmonary arterial hypertension are about half those for riociguat.

Bioavailability: ~94%

Half-life elimination: Patients: 12 hours; Healthy subjects: 7 hours

Time to peak, plasma: 1.5 hours

Excretion: Feces (~53%); urine (~40%)

Dosage Chronic thromboembolic pulmonary hypertension, pulmonary arterial hypertension: Adults: Oral: Initial: 1 mg 3 times daily; may initiate dose at 0.5 mg 3 times daily in patients who may not tolerate the hypotensive effects. If tolerated, may increase the dose by 0.5 mg 3 times daily if systolic blood pressure remains >95 mm Hg and the patient has no signs or symptoms of hypotension; increase dose at intervals of ≥2 weeks. Maximum dose: 2.5 mg 3 times daily.

Missed doses: If a dose is missed, continue with the next regularly scheduled dose. If therapy is interrupted for ≥3 days, retitration is required.

Dosage adjustment for concurrent use in patients receiving strong CYP and P-gp/BCRP inhibitors (eg, azole antifungals [ketoconazole, itraconazole] or protease inhibitors [ritonavir]): Consider a starting dose of 0.5 mg 3 times daily.

Dosage adjustment for patients who smoke: Dose may be titrated to >2.5 mg 3 times daily, if tolerated. A decreased dose may be necessary in patients who stop smoking during therapy.

Dosage adjustment for toxicity:

Hypotension: Decrease dose by 0.5 mg 3 times daily if hypotensive effects are not tolerated.

Pulmonary edema: Consider the possibility of pulmonary veno-occlusive disease (PVOD); if confirmed discontinue treatment with riociguat.

Dosage adjustment in renal impairment:

Cl_{cr} ≥15 mL/minute: No dosage adjustment provided in manufacturer's labeling.

Cl_{cr} <15 mL/minute: No dosage adjustment provided in manufacturer's labeling (has not been studied).

Dialysis: No dosage adjustment provided in manufacturer's labeling (has not been studied).

Dosage adjustment in hepatic impairment:

Mild to moderate hepatic impairment (Child Pugh class A and B): No dosage adjustment provided in manufacturer's labeling.

Severe hepatic impairment (Child Pugh class C): No dosage adjustment provided in manufacturer's labeling (has not been studied).

Administration Oral: Administer with or without food.

Monitoring Parameters Monitor blood pressure and signs and symptoms of hypotension. Monitor for significant peripheral edema and improvements in pulmonary function and exercise tolerance. Women of childbearing potential must have a negative pregnancy test prior to the initiation of therapy, monthly during treatment, and 1 month after discontinuation of therapy.

Product Availability Adempas: FDA approved October 2013; anticipated availability is October 2013.

Dosage Forms Excipient information presented when available (limited, particularly for generics); consult specific product labeling.

Tablet, Oral:

Adempas: 0.5 mg, 1 mg, 1.5 mg, 2 mg, 2.5 mg

◆ **Riomet** *see* MetFORMIN *on page 1310*

◆ **Riopan Plus** *see* Magaldrate and Simethicone *on page 1259*

Risedronate (ris ED roe nate)

Brand Names: U.S. Actonel; Atelvia

Brand Names: Canada Actonel®; Actonel® DR; Apo-Risedronate®; Dom-Risedronate; Novo-Risedronate; PMS-Risedronate; ratio-Risedronate; Riva-Risedronate; Sandoz-Risedronate; Teva-Risedronate

Index Terms Risedronate Sodium

Pharmacologic Category Bisphosphonate Derivative

Use

Actonel®: Treatment of Paget's disease of the bone; treatment and prevention of glucocorticoid-induced osteoporosis; treatment and prevention of osteoporosis in postmenopausal women; treatment of osteoporosis in men

Atelvia™: Treatment of osteoporosis in postmenopausal women

Pregnancy Risk Factor C

Pregnancy Considerations Adverse events were observed in some animal reproduction studies. It is not known if bisphosphonates cross the placenta, but fetal exposure is expected (Djokanovic, 2008; Stathopoulos, 2011). Bisphosphonates are incorporated into the bone matrix and gradually released over time. The amount available in the systemic circulation varies by dose and duration of therapy. Theoretically, there may be a risk of fetal harm when pregnancy follows the completion of therapy; however, available data have not shown that exposure to bisphosphonates during pregnancy significantly increases the risk of adverse fetal events (Djokanovic, 2008; Levy, 2009; Stathopoulos, 2011). Until additional data is available, most sources recommend discontinuing bisphosphonate therapy in women of reproductive potential as early as possible prior to a planned pregnancy; use in premenopausal women should be reserved for special circumstances when rapid bone loss is occurring (Bhalla, 2010; Pereira, 2012; Stathopoulos, 2011). Because hypocalcemia has been described following *in utero* bisphosphonate exposure, exposed infants should be monitored for hypocalcemia after birth (Djokanovic, 2008; Stathopoulos, 2011).

Breast-Feeding Considerations It is not known if risedronate is excreted into breast milk. Due to the potential for serious adverse reactions in the nursing infant, the manufacturer recommends a decision be made whether to discontinue nursing or to discontinue the drug, taking into account the importance of treatment to the mother.

Medication Guide Available Yes

Contraindications Hypersensitivity to risedronate, bisphosphonates, or any component of the formulation; hypocalcemia; inability to stand or sit upright for at least 30 minutes; abnormalities of the esophagus (eg, stricture, achalasia) which delay esophageal emptying

Warnings/Precautions Bisphosphonates may cause upper gastrointestinal disorders such as dysphagia, esophagitis, esophageal ulcer, and gastric ulcer; risk increases in patients unable to comply with dosing instructions. Use with caution in patients with dysphagia, esophageal disease, gastritis, duodenitis, or ulcers (may worsen underlying condition). Discontinue if new or worsening symptoms occur. Use caution in patients with renal impairment (not recommended in patients with a Cl_{cr} <30 mL/minute). Hypocalcemia must be corrected before therapy initiation with risedronate. Ensure adequate calcium and vitamin D intake, especially for patients with Paget's disease in whom the pretreatment rate of bone turnover may be greatly elevated.

Bisphosphonate therapy has been associated with osteonecrosis, primarily of the jaw. Risk factors for osteonecrosis of the jaw (ONJ) include invasive dental procedures (eg, tooth extraction, dental implants, boney surgery); a diagnosis of cancer, with concomitant chemotherapy or corticosteroids; poor oral hygiene, ill-fitting dentures; and comorbid disorders (anemia, coagulopathy, infection, preexisting dental disease); risk may increase with duration of bisphosphonate use. Most reported cases occurred after I.V. bisphosphonate therapy; however, cases have been reported following oral therapy. A dental exam and preventative dentistry should be performed prior to placing patients with risk factors on chronic bisphosphonate therapy. The manufacturer's labeling states that discontinuing bisphosphonates in patients requiring invasive dental procedures may reduce the risk of ONJ. However, other experts suggest that there is no evidence that discontinuing therapy reduces the risk of developing ONJ (Assael, 2009). The benefit/risk must be assessed by the treating physician and/or dentist/surgeon prior to any invasive dental procedure. Patients developing ONJ while on bisphosphonates should receive care by an oral surgeon.

Atypical femur fractures have been reported in patients receiving bisphosphonates for treatment/prevention of osteoporosis. The fractures include subtrochanteric femur (bone just below the hip joint) and diaphyseal femur (long segment of the thigh bone). Some patients experience prodromal pain weeks or months before the fracture occurs. It is unclear if bisphosphonate therapy is the cause for these fractures, although the majority of cases have been reported in patients taking bisphosphonates. Patients receiving long-term (>3-5 years) therapy may be at an increased risk. Discontinue bisphosphonate therapy in patients who develop a femoral shaft fracture.

Infrequently, severe (and occasionally debilitating) bone, joint, and/or muscle pain have been reported during bisphosphonate treatment. The onset of pain ranged from a single day to several months. Consider discontinuing therapy in patients who experience severe symptoms; symptoms usually resolve upon discontinuation. Some patients experienced recurrence when rechallenged with same drug or another bisphosphonate; avoid use in patients with a history of these symptoms in association with bisphosphonate therapy.

In the management of osteoporosis, re-evaluate the need for continued therapy periodically; the optimal duration of treatment has not yet been determined. Consider discontinuing after 3-5 years of use in patients at low-risk for fracture; following discontinuation, re-evaluate fracture risk periodically. When using for glucocorticoid-induced osteoporosis, evaluate sex steroid hormonal status prior to treatment initiation; consider appropriate hormone replacement if necessary. Not approved for use in pediatric patients with osteogenesis imperfecta due to lack of efficacy in reducing the risk of fracture. Potentially significant drug-drug interactions may exist, requiring dose or frequency adjustment, additional monitoring, and/or selection of alternative therapy.

Adverse Reactions Frequency may vary with product, dose, and indication.

>10%:

Cardiovascular: Hypertension (11%)

Central nervous system: Headache (3% to 18%)

Dermatologic: Skin rash (8% to 12%)

Endocrine & metabolic: Increased parathyroid hormone (transient; <30%)

Gastrointestinal: Diarrhea (5% to 20%), nausea (4% to 13%), constipation (3% to 13%), abdominal pain (2% to 12%), dyspepsia (4% to 11%)

Genitourinary: Urinary tract infection (11%)

Infection: Increased susceptibility to infection (≤31%)

Neuromuscular & skeletal: Arthralgia (7% to 33%), back pain (6% to 28%)

1% to 10%:

Cardiovascular: Peripheral edema (8%), chest pain (5% to 7%), cardiac arrhythmia (2%)

Central nervous system: Depression (7%), dizziness (3% to 7%)

Endocrine & metabolic: Hypocalcemia (≤5%), hypophosphatemia (<3%)

Gastrointestinal: Vomiting (2% to 5%), gastritis (3%), duodenitis (≤1%), glossitis (≤1%)

Genitourinary: Benign prostatic hyperplasia (5%), nephrolithiasis (3%)

Immunologic: Acute phase reaction (≤8%; includes fever, influenza-like illness)

Neuromuscular & skeletal: Myalgia (2% to 7%), neck pain (5%), muscle spasm (1% to 2%)

Ophthalmic: Cataract (7%)

Respiratory: Flu-like symptoms (10%), bronchitis (3% to 10%), pharyngitis (6%), rhinitis (6%), dyspnea (4%)

<1% (Limited to important or life-threatening): Dysphagia, esophageal ulcer, esophagitis, exacerbation of asthma, femur fracture (diaphyseal, subtrochanteric), gastric ulcer, hypersensitivity reaction, malignant neoplasm of esophagus, musculoskeletal pain (rarely severe or incapacitating), osteonecrosis (primarily of the jaw)

Drug Interactions

Metabolism/Transport Effects None known.

Avoid Concomitant Use

Avoid concomitant use of Risedronate with any of the following: H2-Antagonists; Proton Pump Inhibitors

Increased Effect/Toxicity

Risedronate may increase the levels/effects of: Deferasirox; Phosphate Supplements

The levels/effects of Risedronate may be increased by: Aminoglycosides; H2-Antagonists; Nonsteroidal Anti-Inflammatory Agents; Proton Pump Inhibitors; Systemic Angiogenesis Inhibitors

Decreased Effect

The levels/effects of Risedronate may be decreased by: Antacids; Calcium Salts; Iron Salts; Magnesium Salts; Multivitamins/Minerals (with ADEK, Folate, Iron); Multivitamins/Minerals (with AE, No Iron); Proton Pump Inhibitors; Sucroferric Oxyhydroxide

Ethanol/Nutrition/Herb Interactions

Ethanol: Avoid ethanol (may increase risk of osteoporosis).

Food: Food reduces absorption (similar to other bisphosphonates); mean oral bioavailability is decreased when given with food.

Storage/Stability Store at room temperature of 20°C to 25°C (68°F to 77°F).

Mechanism of Action A bisphosphonate which inhibits bone resorption via actions on osteoclasts or on osteoclast precursors; decreases the rate of bone resorption, leading to an indirect increase in bone mineral density. In Paget's disease, characterized by disordered resorption and formation of bone, inhibition of resorption leads to an indirect decrease in bone formation; but the newly-formed bone has a more normal architecture.

Pharmacodynamics/Kinetics

Onset of action: May require weeks

Absorption: Rapid

Distribution: V_d: 13.8 L/kg

Protein binding: ~24%

Metabolism: None

Bioavailability: Poor, ~0.54% to 0.75%

Half-life elimination: Initial: 1.5 hours; Terminal: 480-561 hours

Time to peak, serum: 1-3 hours

Excretion: Urine (up to 85%); feces (as unabsorbed drug)

Dosage Note: Patients should receive supplemental calcium and vitamin D if dietary intake is inadequate. Consider discontinuing after 3-5 years of use for osteoporosis in patients at low-risk for fracture.

Paget's disease of bone: Adults: Oral: *Immediate release tablet:* 30 mg once daily for 2 months

Note: Retreatment may be considered (following post-treatment observation of at least 2 months) if relapse occurs, or if treatment fails to normalize serum alkaline phosphatase. For retreatment, the dose and duration of therapy are the same as for initial treatment. No data are available on more than one course of retreatment.

Osteoporosis (postmenopausal): Adults: Oral:

Immediate release tablet: Prevention and treatment: 5 mg once daily **or** 35 mg once weekly **or** 150 mg once a month

Delayed release tablet: Treatment: 35 mg once weekly

Osteoporosis (males) treatment: Adults: Oral: *Immediate release tablet:* 35 mg once weekly

Osteoporosis (glucocorticoid-induced) prevention and treatment: Adults: Oral: *Immediate release tablet:* 5 mg once daily

Missed doses: Immediate release tablet:

Once-weekly: If a once-weekly dose is missed, it should be given the next morning after remembered; may then return to the original once-weekly schedule (original scheduled day of the week), however, do not give 2 doses on the same day.

Monthly (150 mg once monthly): If 150 mg once-monthly dose is missed, it should be given the next morning after remembered if the next month's scheduled dose is >7 days away. If the next month's scheduled dose is within 7 days, wait until the next month's scheduled dose. For either scenario, may then return to the original monthly schedule (original scheduled day of the month). Do not give >150 mg within 7 days.

Dosage adjustment in renal impairment:

Cl_{cr} ≥30 mL/minute: No dosage adjustment necessary.

Cl_{cr} <30 mL/minute: Use is not recommended.

Dosage adjustment in hepatic impairment: No dosage adjustment provided in manufacturer's labeling (has not been studied). However, dosage adjustment unlikely because risendronate is not metabolized by the liver.

Dietary Considerations Ensure adequate calcium and vitamin D intake; if dietary intake is inadequate, dietary supplementation is recommended. Women and men should consume:

Calcium: 1000 mg/day (men: 50-70 years) **or** 1200 mg/day (women ≥51 years and men ≥71 years) (IOM, 2011; NOF, 2013)

Vitamin D: 800-1000 IU/day (men and women ≥50 years) (NOF, 2013). Recommended Dietary Allowance (RDA): 600 IU/day (men and women ≤70 years) **or** 800 IU/day (men and women ≥71 years) (IOM, 2011).

Take immediate release tablet with at least 6 oz of **plain water** (not mineral water) ≥30 minutes before the first food or drink of the day other than water. Take delayed release tablet with at least 4 ounces of **plain water** immediately **after** breakfast.

Administration Note: Avoid administration of oral calcium supplements, antacids, magnesium supplements/laxatives, and iron preparations within 30 minutes of risedronate administration.

Immediate release tablet: Risedronate immediate release tablets must be taken on an empty stomach with a full glass (6-8 oz) of **plain water** (not mineral water) at least 30 minutes before any food, drink, or other medications orally to avoid interference with absorption. Patient must remain sitting upright or standing for at least 30 minutes after taking (to reduce esophageal irritation). Tablet should be swallowed whole; do not crush or chew.

Delayed release tablet: Risedronate delayed release tablets must be taken with at least 4 oz of **plain water** (not mineral water) immediately after breakfast. Patient must remain sitting upright or standing for at least 30 minutes after taking (to reduce esophageal irritation). Tablet should be swallowed whole; do not cut, split, crush, or chew.

Monitoring Parameters

Osteoporosis: Bone mineral density (BMD) should be reevaluated every 2 years (or more frequently) after initiating therapy (NOF, 2013); in patients with combined risedronate and glucocorticoid treatment, BMD should be made at initiation and repeated after 6-12 months; annual measurements of height and weight, assessment of chronic back pain; serum calcium and 25(OH)D; consider measuring biochemical markers of bone turnover

Paget's disease: Alkaline phosphatase; pain; serum calcium and 25(OH)D

Reference Range

Calcium (total): Adults: 9.0-11.0 mg/dL (2.05-2.54 mmol/L), may slightly decrease with aging

Phosphorus: 2.5-4.5 mg/dL (0.81-1.45 mmol/L)

Vitamin D: There is no clear consensus on a reference range for total serum 25(OH)D concentrations or the validity of this level as it relates clinically to bone health. In addition, there is significant variability in the reporting of serum 25(OH)D levels as a result of different assay types in use; however, the following ranges have been suggested:

Adults (IOM, 2011): Sufficient levels in practically all persons: ≥20 ng/mL (50 nmol/L); concern for risk of toxicity: >50 ng/mL (125 nmol/L)

Osteoporosis patients (NOF, 2013): Recommended level to reach and maintain: ~30 ng/mL (75 nmol/L)

Test Interactions Bisphosphonates may interfere with diagnostic imaging agents such as technetium-99m-diphosphonate in bone scans.

Dosage Forms Excipient information presented when available (limited, particularly for generics); consult specific product labeling.

Tablet, Oral, as sodium:

Actonel: 5 mg, 30 mg, 35 mg

Actonel: 150 mg [contains fd&c blue #2 aluminum lake]

Tablet Delayed Release, Oral, as sodium:

Atelvia: 35 mg [contains edetate disodium]

◆ **Risedronate Sodium** *see* Risedronate *on page 1824*

◆ **RisperDAL** *see* RisperiDONE *on page 1826*

◆ **Risperdal (Can)** *see* RisperiDONE *on page 1826*

◆ **Risperdal M-Tab** *see* RisperiDONE *on page 1826*

◆ **RisperDAL M-TAB** *see* RisperiDONE *on page 1826*

◆ **RisperDAL Consta** *see* RisperiDONE *on page 1826*

◆ **Risperdal Consta (Can)** *see* RisperiDONE *on page 1826*

RisperiDONE (ris PER i done)

Brand Names: U.S. RisperDAL; RisperDAL Consta; RisperDAL M-TAB; RisperiDONE M-TAB

Brand Names: Canada Apo-Risperidone; Ava-Risperidone; CO Risperidone; Dom-Risperidone; JAMP-Risperidone; Mar-Risperidone; Mint-Risperidon; Mylan-Risperidone; PHL-Risperidone; PMS-Risperidone; PMS-Risperidone ODT; PRO-Risperidone; RAN-Risperidone; ratio-Risperidone; Risperdal; Risperdal Consta; Risperdal M-Tab; Riva-Risperidone; Sandoz-Risperidone; Teva-Risperidone

Index Terms Risperdal M-Tab

Pharmacologic Category Antimanic Agent; Antipsychotic Agent, Atypical

Additional Appendix Information

Antipsychotic Agents *on page 2290*

Beers Criteria – Potentially Inappropriate Medications for Geriatrics *on page 2368*

Use

Oral: Treatment of schizophrenia; treatment of acute mania or mixed episodes associated with bipolar I disorder (as monotherapy in children or adults, or in combination with lithium or valproate in adults); treatment of irritability/aggression associated with autistic disorder

Injection: Treatment of schizophrenia; maintenance treatment of bipolar I disorder in adults as monotherapy or in combination with lithium or valproate

Unlabeled Use Treatment of Tourette's syndrome; psychosis/agitation related to Alzheimer's dementia; post-traumatic stress disorder (PTSD)

Pregnancy Risk Factor C

Pregnancy Considerations Adverse events were observed in animal reproduction studies. In human studies, risperidone and its metabolite cross the placenta (Newport, 2007). An increased risk of teratogenic effects has not been observed following maternal use of risperidone (limited data) (Coppola, 2007). Agenesis of the corpus callosum has been noted in one case report of an infant exposed *in utero*; relationship to risperidone exposure is not known. Antipsychotic use during the third trimester of pregnancy has a risk for extrapyramidal symptoms (EPS) and/or withdrawal symptoms in newborns following delivery. Symptoms in the newborn may include agitation, feeding disorder, hypertonia, hypotonia, respiratory distress, somnolence, and tremor. These effects may be self-limiting and allow recovery within hours or days with no specific treatment, or they may be severe requiring prolonged hospitalization. When using Risperdal® Consta®, patients should notify healthcare provider if they become or intend to become pregnant during therapy or within 12 weeks of last injection. Risperidone may cause hyperprolactinemia, which may decrease reproductive function in both males and females.

The ACOG recommends that therapy during pregnancy be individualized; treatment with psychiatric medications during pregnancy should incorporate the clinical expertise of the mental health clinician, obstetrician, primary healthcare provider, and pediatrician. Safety data related to atypical antipsychotics during pregnancy is limited and routine use is not recommended. However, if a woman is inadvertently exposed to an atypical antipsychotic while pregnant, continuing therapy may be preferable to switching to a typical antipsychotic that the fetus has not yet been exposed to; consider risk:benefit (ACOG, 2008).

Healthcare providers are encouraged to enroll women 18-45 years of age exposed to risperidone during pregnancy in the Atypical Antipsychotics Pregnancy Registry (1-866-961-2388 or http://www.womensmentalhealth.org/pregnancyregistry).

Breast-Feeding Considerations Risperidone and its metabolite are excreted in breast milk. Due to the potential for serious adverse reactions in the nursing infant, the manufacturer recommends a decision be made whether to discontinue nursing or to discontinue the drug, taking into account the importance of treatment to the mother. It is also recommended that women using Risperdal Consta not breast-feed during therapy or for 12 weeks after the last injection.

Contraindications Hypersensitivity to risperidone or any component of the formulation

Warnings/Precautions Hazardous agent - use appropriate precautions for handling and disposal (NIOSH, 2012). **[U.S. Boxed Warning]: Elderly patients with dementia-related psychosis treated with antipsychotics are at an increased risk of death compared to placebo.** Most deaths appeared to be either cardiovascular (eg, heart failure, sudden death) or infectious (eg, pneumonia) in nature. In addition, an increased incidence of cerebrovascular effects (eg, transient ischemic attack, cerebrovascular accidents) has been reported in studies of placebo-controlled trials of risperidone in elderly patients with dementia-related psychosis. Risperidone is not approved for the treatment of dementia-related psychosis.

Leukopenia, neutropenia, and agranulocytosis (sometimes fatal) have been reported in clinical trials and postmarketing reports with antipsychotic use; presence of risk factors (eg, pre-existing low WBC or history of drug-induced leuko-/neutropenia) should prompt periodic blood count assessment. Discontinue therapy at first signs of blood dyscrasias or if absolute neutrophil count <1000/mm^3.

Low to moderately sedating, use with caution in disorders where CNS depression is a feature. Use with caution in Parkinson's disease. Caution in patients with predisposition to seizures. Use with caution in renal or hepatic dysfunction; dose reduction recommended. Esophageal dysmotility and aspiration have been associated with antipsychotic use; use with caution in patients at risk of aspiration pneumonia (ie, Alzheimer's disease). Risperidone is associated with greater increases in prolactin levels as compared to other antipsychotic agents; clinical significance of hyperprolactinemia in patients with breast cancer or other prolactin-dependent tumors is unknown. May alter temperature regulation. May mask toxicity of other drugs or conditions (eg, intestinal obstruction, Reyes syndrome, brain tumor) due to antiemetic effects. Neutropenia has been reported with antipsychotic use, including fatal cases of agranulocytosis. Pre-existing myelosuppression (disease or drug-induced) increases risk and these patients should have frequent CBC monitoring; decreased blood counts in absence of other causative factors should prompt discontinuation of therapy.

Use with caution in patients with cardiovascular diseases (eg, heart failure, history of myocardial infarction or ischemia, cerebrovascular disease, conduction abnormalities). May cause orthostatic hypotension; use with caution in patients at risk of this effect (eg, concurrent medication use which may predispose to hypotension/bradycardia or presence of hypovolemia) or in those who would not tolerate transient hypotensive episodes. May alter cardiac conduction (low risk relative to other neuroleptics); life-threatening arrhythmias have occurred with therapeutic doses of neuroleptics.

May cause anticholinergic effects (confusion, agitation, constipation, xerostomia, blurred vision, urinary retention); therefore, they should be used with caution in patients with decreased gastrointestinal motility, urinary retention, BPH, xerostomia, or visual problems (including narrow-angle glaucoma). Relative to other neuroleptics, risperidone has a low potency of cholinergic blockade. Few case reports describe intraoperative floppy iris syndrome (IFIS) in patients receiving risperidone and undergoing cataract surgery (Ford, 2011). Prior to cataract surgery, evaluate for prior or current risperidone use. The benefits or risks of interrupting risperidone prior to surgery have not been established; clinicians are advised to proceed with surgery cautiously.

May cause extrapyramidal symptoms (EPS), including pseudoparkinsonism, acute dystonic reactions, akathisia, and tardive dyskinesia (risk of these reactions is low relative to other neuroleptics, and is dose dependent). Risk of dystonia (and probably other EPS) may be greater with increased doses, use of conventional antipsychotics, males, and younger patients. Risk of neuroleptic malignant syndrome (NMS) may be increased in patients with Parkinson's disease or Lewy body dementia; monitor for symptoms of confusion, obtundation, postural instability and extrapyramidal symptoms. May cause hyperglycemia; in some cases may be extreme and associated with ketoacidosis, hyperosmolar coma, or death. Use with caution in patients with diabetes or other disorders of glucose regulation; monitor for worsening of glucose control. Dyslipidemia has been reported with atypical antipsychotics; risk profile may differ between agents. Discrepant results have been reported in clinical trials, regarding lipid changes associated with risperidone (American Diabetes Association, 2004). Significant weight gain has been observed with antipsychotic therapy; incidence varies with product. Monitor waist circumference and BMI. Rare cases of priapism have been reported.

Use in elderly patients with dementia is associated with an increased risk of mortality and cerebrovascular accidents; avoid antipsychotic use for behavioral problems associated with dementia unless alternative nonpharmacologic therapies have failed and patient may harm self or others. In addition, use may cause or exacerbate syndrome of inappropriate antidiuretic hormone secretion or hyponatremia; monitor sodium closely with initiation or dosage adjustments in older adults (Beers Criteria).

The possibility of a suicide attempt is inherent in psychotic illness or bipolar disorder; use caution in high-risk patients during initiation of therapy. Prescriptions should be written for the smallest quantity consistent with good patient care. Long-term effects on growth or sexual maturation have not been evaluated. Vehicle used in injectable (polylactide-co-glycolide microspheres) has rarely been associated with retinal artery occlusion in patients with abnormal arteriovenous anastomosis.

Adverse Reactions

>10%:

Central nervous system: Sedation (children 12% to 63%; adults 5% to 11%), parkinsonism (children: 28% to 62%; adults 8% to 25%), somnolence (adults 5% to 41%; children 4% to 11%), insomnia (≤32%), fatigue (children 18% to 31%; adults 1% to 9%), headache (12% to 21%), anxiety (≤8% to 16%), dizziness (3% to 16%), fever (children 16%; adults 1% to 2%), akathisia (5% to 11%)

Gastrointestinal: Appetite increased (children 4% to 44%; adults 4%), weight gain (≥7% kg increase from baseline: children 8% to 33%; adults 4% to 21%), vomiting (children 10% to 20%; adults <4%), constipation (5% to 17%), nausea (5% to 16%), abdominal pain (children 6% to 16%; adults <4%), drooling (children 12%; adults <4%)

Genitourinary: Urinary incontinence (children 5% to 22%; adults <4%), enuresis (children 16%; adults <1%)
Neuromuscular & skeletal: Tremor (adults ≤24%; children ≤11%)
Respiratory: Nasopharyngitis (children 19%; adults ≤4%), cough (children ≤17%; adults ≤4%), rhinorrhea (children 12%; adults <4%)

1% to 10%:
Cardiovascular: Atrioventricular block first degree (<4%), bradycardia (<4%), bundle branch block (<4%), chest pain (<4%), ECG changes (<4%), facial edema (<4%), hypotension (<4%), orthostatic hypotension (<4%), palpitation (<4%), QT prolongation (<4%), tachycardia (adults <4%; children <1%), hypertension (≤3%), peripheral edema (≤3%), syncope (1% to 2%)
Central nervous system: Gait disturbance (4%), pain (1% to 4%), attention span decreased (≤4%), agitation (<4%), akinesia (<4%), coordination impaired (<4%), depression (<4%), malaise (<4%), nervousness (<4%), postural dizziness (<4%), seizure (<4%), sleep disturbances (<4%), sluggishness (<4%), vertigo (<4%), lethargy (2%), hypoesthesia (≤2%)
Dermatologic: Rash (<4% to 8%), eczema (<4%), pruritus (<4%), dry skin (≤3%), acne (<1% to 2%)
Endocrine & metabolic: Menorrhea (≤4%), breast discomfort (<4%), ejaculation disorder/delayed (<4%), erectile dysfunction (<4%), galactorrhea (<4%), gynecomastia (<4%), hyperglycemia (<4%), hyperprolactinemia (<4%), libido decreased (<4%), menstrual irregularities (<4%), sexual dysfunction (<4%)
Gastrointestinal: Dyspepsia (3% to 10%), xerostomia (≤7% to 10%), salivation increased (1% to 10%), diarrhea (<4% to 8%), appetite decreased (≤6%), anorexia (<1% to <4%), weight loss (≤4%), gastritis (<4%), gastroenteritis (<4%), toothache (≤3%)
Genitourinary: Cystitis (<4%), glucosuria (<4%), urinary tract infection (<4%)
Hematologic: Anemia (<4%), neutropenia (<4%)
Hepatic: ALT increased (<4%), AST increased (<4%), GGT increased (<4%)
Local: Abscess (<4%); injection site induration, pain, reaction, swelling (<4%)
Neuromuscular & skeletal: Dystonia (2% to 6%), limb pain (2% to 6%), dyskinesia (adults ≤6%; children <1%), arthralgia (2% to 4%), back pain (≤4%), buttock pain (<4%), dysarthria (<4%), hypokinesia (<4%), musculoskeletal chest pain (<4%), myalgia (<4%), neck pain (<4%), paresthesia (<4%), posture abnormal (<4%), tardive dyskinesia (<4%), weakness (<4%), creatine phosphokinase increased (≤2%)
Ocular: Blurred vision (2% to 7%), conjunctivitis (<4%), visual acuity reduced (<4%)
Otic: Earache (≤4%), otitis media (<4%)
Respiratory: Nasal congestion (≤6% to 10%), pharyngolaryngeal pain (3% to 10%), rhinitis (<4% to 9%), respiratory infection (≤6% to 8%), bronchitis (<4%), dyspnea (<4%), pharyngitis (<4%), pneumonia (<4%), sinusitis (<4%), epistaxis (≤2%)
Miscellaneous: Thirst (children ≤7%; adults <1%), flu-like syndrome (<4%), hypersensitivity (<4%), infection (<4%), viral infection (<4%)

<1% (Limited to important or life-threatening): Acarodermatitis, agranulocytosis, allergic reaction, alopecia, anaphylactic reaction, angioedema, antidiuretic hormone disorder, apnea, aspiration, atrial fibrillation, cerebral ischemia, cerebrovascular accident, cholestatic hepatitis, cholesterol increased, cholinergic syndrome, coma, cyst formation, delirium, diabetes mellitus, diabetic coma, diabetic ketoacidosis, diverticulitis, esophageal dysmotility, eye infection, eye swelling, fecal incontinence, fecaloma, glaucoma, granulocytopenia, hematoma, hemorrhage, hepatic failure, hepatocellular damage, hyperkeratosis, hypertonia, hypertriglyceridemia, hyperuricemia, hypoglycemia, hypokalemia, hyponatremia, hypothermia, intestinal obstruction, intraoperative floppy iris syndrome, leukocytosis, leukopenia, leukorrhea, lower respiratory tract infection, lymphadenopathy, mania, migraine, myocardial infarction, myocarditis, necrosis, neuroleptic malignant syndrome (NMS), nystagmus, ocular hyperemia, pancreatitis, Pelger-Huët anomaly, pituitary adenomas, precocious puberty, premature atrial contractions, priapism, pulmonary embolism, RBC disorders, renal insufficiency, retinal artery occlusion, retrograde ejaculation, rhabdomyolysis, skin ulceration, ST depression, stroke, superficial phlebitis, synostosis, temperature regulation impairment, thrombocytopenia, thrombophlebitis, thrombotic thrombocytopenic purpura, tongue paralysis, torticollis, transient ischemic attack, urinary retention, ventricular extrasystoles, ventricular tachycardia, water intoxication, withdrawal syndrome

Drug Interactions

Metabolism/Transport Effects Substrate of CYP2D6 (major), CYP3A4 (minor), P-glycoprotein; **Note:** Assignment of Major/Minor substrate status based on clinically relevant drug interaction potential; **Inhibits** CYP2D6 (weak), CYP3A4 (weak)

Avoid Concomitant Use

Avoid concomitant use of RisperiDONE with any of the following: Aclidinium; Amisulpride; Azelastine (Nasal); Ipratropium (Oral Inhalation); Metoclopramide; Paraldehyde; Pimozide; Sulpiride; Tiotropium; Umeclidinium

Increased Effect/Toxicity

RisperiDONE may increase the levels/effects of: Alcohol (Ethyl); Amisulpride; Analgesics (Opioid); Anticholinergics; ARIPiprazole; Azelastine (Nasal); Buprenorphine; CNS Depressants; Dofetilide; Highest Risk QTc-Prolonging Agents; Hydrocodone; Lomitapide; Methotrimeprazine; Methylphenidate; Moderate Risk QTc-Prolonging Agents; Paliperidone; Paraldehyde; Pimozide; Serotonin Modulators; Sulpiride; Tiotropium; Zolpidem

The levels/effects of RisperiDONE may be increased by: Abiraterone Acetate; Acetylcholinesterase Inhibitors (Central); Aclidinium; Brimonidine (Topical); CYP2D6 Inhibitors (Moderate); CYP2D6 Inhibitors (Strong); Darunavir; Doxylamine; Droperidol; HydrOXYzine; Ipratropium (Oral Inhalation); Lithium formulations; Loop Diuretics; Magnesium Sulfate; Methotrimeprazine; Methylphenidate; Metoclopramide; Metyrosine; Mifepristone; Perampanel; P-glycoprotein/ABCB1 Inhibitors; Pramlintide; Selective Serotonin Reuptake Inhibitors; Serotonin Modulators; Sodium Oxybate; Tetrabenazine; Umeclidinium; Valproic Acid and Derivatives; Verapamil

Decreased Effect

RisperiDONE may decrease the levels/effects of: Amphetamines; Anti-Parkinson's Agents (Dopamine Agonist); Quinagolide

The levels/effects of RisperiDONE may be decreased by: CarBAMazepine; Lithium formulations; Peginterferon Alfa-2b; P-glycoprotein/ABCB1 Inducers

Ethanol/Nutrition/Herb Interactions

Ethanol: Ethanol may increase CNS depression. Management: Limit or avoid ethanol.
Food: Oral solution is not compatible with beverages containing tannin or pectinate (cola or tea). Management: Administer oral solution with water, coffee, orange juice, or low-fat milk.
Herb/Nutraceutical: Some herbal medications may increase CNS depression. Management: Avoid kava kava, gotu kola, valerian, and St John's wort.

Preparation for Administration Hazardous agent; use appropriate precautions for handling and disposal (NIOSH, 2012). Risperdal® Consta®: Bring to room temperature prior to reconstitution. Reconstitute with provided diluent only. Shake vigorously to mix; will form thick, milky suspension. Following reconstitution, store at room temperature and use within 6 hours. Suspension settles in ~2 minutes; shake vigorously to resuspend prior to administration.

Storage/Stability

Injection: Risperdal® Consta®: Store in refrigerator at 2°C to 8°C (36°F to 46°F) and protect from light. May be stored at room temperature of 25°C (77°F) for up to 7 days prior to administration. Following reconstitution, store at room temperature and use within 6 hours. Suspension settles in ~2 minutes; shake vigorously to resuspend prior to administration.

Oral solution, tablet: Store at 15°C to 25°C (59°F to 77°F). Protect from light and moisture. Keep orally-disintegrating tablets sealed in foil pouch until ready to use. Do not freeze solution.

Mechanism of Action Risperidone is a benzisoxazole atypical antipsychotic with mixed serotonin-dopamine antagonist activity that binds to 5-HT_2-receptors in the CNS and in the periphery with a very high affinity; binds to dopamine-D_2 receptors with less affinity. The binding affinity to the dopamine-D_2 receptor is 20 times lower than the 5-HT_2 affinity. The addition of serotonin antagonism to dopamine antagonism (classic neuroleptic mechanism) is thought to improve negative symptoms of psychoses and reduce the incidence of extrapyramidal side effects. $Alpha_1$, $alpha_2$ adrenergic, and histaminergic receptors are also antagonized with high affinity. Risperidone has low to moderate affinity for 5-HT_{1C}, 5-HT_{1D}, and 5-HT_{1A} receptors, weak affinity for D_1 and no affinity for muscarinics or $beta_1$ and $beta_2$ receptors

Pharmacodynamics/Kinetics

Absorption:

Oral: Rapid and well absorbed; food does not affect rate or extent

Injection: <1% absorbed initially; main release occurs at ~3 weeks and is maintained from 4-6 weeks

Distribution: V_d: 1-2 L/kg

Protein binding, plasma: Risperidone 90%; 9-hydroxyrisperidone: 77%

Metabolism: Extensively hepatic via CYP2D6 to 9-hydroxyrisperidone (similar pharmacological activity as risperidone); *N*-dealkylation is a second minor pathway

Bioavailability: Oral: 70%; Tablet (relative to solution): 94%; orally-disintegrating tablets and oral solution are bioequivalent to tablets

Half-life elimination: Active moiety (risperidone and its active metabolite 9-hydroxyrisperidone)

Oral: 20 hours (mean)

Extensive metabolizers: Risperidone: 3 hours; 9-hydroxyrisperidone: 21 hours

Poor metabolizers: Risperidone: 20 hours; 9-hydroxyrisperidone: 30 hours

Injection: 3-6 days; related to microsphere erosion and subsequent absorption of risperidone

Time to peak, plasma: Oral: Risperidone: Within 1 hour; 9-hydroxyrisperidone: Extensive metabolizers: 3 hours; Poor metabolizers: 17 hours

Excretion: Urine (70%); feces (14%)

Dosage Note: When reinitiating treatment after discontinuation, the initial titration schedule should be followed.

Oral:

Children ≥5 years and Adolescents: Autism:

<15 kg: Use with caution; specific dosing recommendations not available

15 to <20 kg: Initial: 0.25 mg daily; may increase dose to 0.5 mg daily after ≥4 days, maintain dose for ≥14 days. In patients not achieving sufficient clinical response, may increase dose by 0.25 mg daily in ≥2-week intervals. Doses ranging from 0.5-3 mg daily have been evaluated; however, therapeutic effect reached plateau at 1 mg daily in clinical trials. Following clinical response, consider gradually lowering dose. May be administered once daily or in divided doses twice daily.

≥20 kg: Initial: 0.5 mg daily; may increase dose to 1 mg daily after ≥4 days, maintain dose for ≥14 days. In patients not achieving sufficient clinical response, may increase dose by 0.5 mg daily in ≥2-week intervals. Doses ranging from 0.5-3 mg daily have been evaluated; however, therapeutic effect reached plateau at 2.5 mg daily (3 mg daily in children >45 kg) in clinical trials. Following clinical response, consider gradually lowering dose. May be administered once daily or in divided doses twice daily.

Children and Adolescents:

Schizophrenia: Adolescents 13-17 years: Initial: 0.5 mg once daily; dose may be adjusted in increments of 0.5-1 mg daily at intervals ≥24 hours to a dose of 3 mg daily. Doses ranging from 1-6 mg daily have been evaluated, however, doses >3 mg daily do not confer additional benefit and are associated with increased adverse events.

Bipolar mania: Children and Adolescents 10-17 years: Initial: 0.5 mg once daily; dose may be adjusted in increments of 0.5-1 mg daily at intervals ≥24 hours to a dose of 1-2.5 mg daily. Doses ranging from 0.5-6 mg daily have been evaluated; however doses >2.5 mg daily do not confer additional benefit and are associated with increased adverse events.

Maintenance: No dosing recommendation available for treatment >3 weeks duration

Adolescents and Adults: Tourette's syndrome (unlabeled use): Initial: 0.25 mg once daily for 2 days, then 0.25 mg twice daily for 3 days, then 0.5 mg twice daily for 2 days; titrate slowly thereafter in increments/decrements ≤0.5 mg twice daily and at intervals ≥3 days; maximum dose: 6 mg daily (Dion, 2002)

Adults:

Schizophrenia:

Initial: 2 mg daily in 1-2 divided doses; may be increased by 1-2 mg daily at intervals ≥24 hours to a recommended dosage range of 4-8 mg daily; may be given as a single daily dose once maintenance dose is achieved; daily dosages >6 mg do not appear to confer any additional benefit, and the incidence of extrapyramidal symptoms is higher than with lower doses. Further dose adjustments should be made in increments/decrements of 1-2 mg daily on a weekly basis. Dose range studied in clinical trials: 4-16 mg daily.

Maintenance: Recommended dosage range: 2-8 mg daily

Bipolar mania:

Initial: 2-3 mg once daily; if needed, adjust dose by 1 mg daily in intervals ≥24 hours; dosing range: 1-6 mg daily

Maintenance: No dosing recommendation available for treatment >3 weeks duration.

Post-traumatic stress disorder (PTSD) (unlabeled use): 0.5-8 mg daily (Bandelow, 2008; Benedek, 2009)

Elderly:

Initial: 0.5 mg twice daily; titration should progress slowly in increments of no more than 0.5 mg twice daily; increases to dosages >1.5 mg twice daily should occur at intervals of ≥1 week.

Note: Additional monitoring of renal function and orthostatic blood pressure may be warranted. If once-a-day dosing in the elderly or debilitated patient is considered, a twice daily regimen should be used to titrate to the target dose, and this dose should be maintained for 2-3 days prior to attempts to switch to a once-daily regimen.

Psychosis/agitation related to Alzheimer's dementia (unlabeled use): Initial: 0.25-1 mg daily; if necessary, gradually increase as tolerated not to exceed 1.5-2 mg daily; doses >1 mg daily are associated with higher rates of extrapyramidal symptoms (Rabins, 2007)

I.M.: **Note:** Oral risperidone (or other antipsychotic) should be administered with the initial injection of Risperdal® Consta® and continued for 3 weeks (then discontinued) to maintain adequate therapeutic plasma concentrations prior to main release phase of risperidone from injection site. When switching from depot administration to a short-acting formulation, administer short-acting agent in place of the next regularly-scheduled depot injection.

Adults: Schizophrenia, bipolar I maintenance (Risperdal® Consta®): Initial: 25 mg every 2 weeks; if unresponsive, some may benefit from larger doses (37.5-50 mg); maximum dose: 50 mg every 2 weeks. Dosage adjustments should not be made more frequently than every 4 weeks. A lower initial dose of 12.5 mg may be appropriate in some patients (eg, demonstrated poor tolerability to other psychotropic medications).

Elderly (Risperdal® Consta®): 25 mg every 2 weeks; a lower initial dose of 12.5 mg may be appropriate in some patients

Dosing adjustment in renal impairment: Adults:

Oral: Cl_{cr} <30 mL/minute: Starting dose of 0.5 mg twice daily; titration should progress slowly in increments of no more than 0.5 mg twice daily; increases to dosages >1.5 mg twice daily should occur at intervals of ≥1 week. Clearance of the active moiety is decreased by 60% in patients with moderate-to-severe renal disease (Cl_{cr} <60 mL/minute) compared to healthy subjects.

I.M.: Initiate with **oral** dosing (0.5 mg twice daily for 1 week then 2 mg daily for 1 week); if tolerated, begin 25 mg **I.M.** every 2 weeks; continue oral dosing for 3 weeks after the first I.M. injection. An initial I.M. dose of 12.5 mg may also be considered.

Dosing adjustment in hepatic impairment: Adults:

Oral: Child-Pugh class C: Starting dose of 0.5 mg twice daily; titration should progress slowly in increments of no more than 0.5 mg twice daily; increases to dosages >1.5 mg twice daily should occur at intervals of ≥1 week. The mean free fraction of risperidone in plasma was increased by 35% in patients with hepatic impairment compared to healthy subjects.

I.M.: Initiate with **oral** dosing (0.5 mg twice daily for 1 week then 2 mg daily for 1 week); if tolerated, begin 25 mg **I.M.** every 2 weeks; continue oral dosing for 3 weeks after the first I.M. injection. An initial I.M. dose of 12.5 mg may also be considered.

Dietary Considerations May be taken without regard to meals. Some products may contain phenylalanine.

Administration

Oral: May be administered without regard to meals.

Oral solution can be administered directly from the provided pipette or may be mixed with water, coffee, orange juice, or low-fat milk, but is **not compatible** with cola or tea.

In children or adolescents experiencing somnolence, half the daily dose may be administered twice daily **or** the once-daily dose may be administered at bedtime.

Risperdal® M-Tab® should not be removed from blister pack until administered. Do not push tablet through foil (tablet may become damaged); peel back foil to expose tablet. Using dry hands, place immediately on tongue. Tablet will dissolve within seconds, and may be swallowed with or without liquid. Do not split or chew.

I.M.: Risperdal® Consta® should be administered into either the deltoid muscle or the upper outer quadrant of the gluteal area. Avoid inadvertent injection into vasculature. Injection should alternate between the two arms or buttocks. Do not combine two different dosage strengths into one single administration. Do not substitute any components of the dose-pack; administer with needle provided (1-inch needle for deltoid administration or 2-inch needle for gluteal administration).

Hazardous agent; use appropriate precautions for handling and disposal (NIOSH, 2012).

Monitoring Parameters Vital signs; fasting lipid profile and fasting blood glucose/Hgb A_{1c} (prior to treatment, at 3 months, then annually); CBC; BMI, personal/family history of obesity, waist circumference; blood pressure; mental status, abnormal involuntary movement scale (AIMS), extrapyramidal symptoms; orthostatic blood pressure changes for 3-5 days after starting or increasing dose. Weight should be assessed prior to treatment, at 4 weeks, 8 weeks, 12 weeks, and then at quarterly intervals. Consider titrating to a different antipsychotic agent for a weight gain ≥5% of the initial weight.

Additional Information Risperdal® Consta® is an injectable formulation of risperidone using the extended release Medisorb® drug-delivery system; small polymeric microspheres degrade slowly, releasing the medication at a controlled rate.

Dosage Forms Excipient information presented when available (limited, particularly for generics); consult specific product labeling.

Solution, Oral:
- RisperDAL: 1 mg/mL (30 mL) [contains benzoic acid]
- Generic: 1 mg/mL (30 mL)

Suspension Reconstituted, Intramuscular:
- RisperDAL Consta: 12.5 mg (1 ea); 25 mg (1 ea); 37.5 mg (1 ea); 50 mg (1 ea)

Tablet, Oral:
- RisperDAL: 0.25 mg, 0.5 mg, 1 mg
- RisperDAL: 2 mg [contains fd&c yellow #6 aluminum lake]
- RisperDAL: 3 mg [contains fd&c yellow #10 (quinoline yellow)]
- RisperDAL: 4 mg [contains fd&c blue #2 aluminum lake, fd&c yellow #10 (quinoline yellow)]
- Generic: 0.25 mg, 0.5 mg, 1 mg, 2 mg, 3 mg, 4 mg

Tablet Dispersible, Oral:
- RisperDAL M-TAB: 0.5 mg, 1 mg, 2 mg, 3 mg, 4 mg [contains aspartame, peppermint oil (mentha piperita oil)]
- RisperiDONE M-TAB: 0.5 mg, 1 mg, 2 mg, 3 mg, 4 mg [contains aspartame]
- Generic: 0.25 mg, 0.5 mg, 1 mg, 2 mg, 3 mg, 4 mg

◆ **RisperiDONE M-TAB** *see* RisperiDONE *on page* 1826
◆ **Ritalin** *see* Methylphenidate *on page* 1336
◆ **Ritalin LA** *see* Methylphenidate *on page* 1336
◆ **Ritalin SR** *see* Methylphenidate *on page* 1336

Ritonavir (ri TOE na veer)

Brand Names: U.S. Norvir

Brand Names: Canada Norvir®; Norvir® SEC

Pharmacologic Category Antiretroviral, Protease Inhibitor (Anti-HIV)

Use Treatment of HIV infection; should always be used as part of a multidrug regimen

Unlabeled Use Used as a pharmacokinetic "booster" for other protease inhibitors

Pregnancy Risk Factor B

Pregnancy Considerations Adverse events were observed in animal reproduction studies only with doses which were also maternally toxic. Ritonavir crosses the placenta in minimal amounts; no increased risk of overall birth defects has been observed following first trimester exposure according to data collected by the antiretroviral pregnancy registry. Early studies have shown lower plasma levels during pregnancy compared to postpartum. The DHHS Perinatal HIV Guidelines consider ritonavir to be a preferred protease inhibitor (PI) for use during pregnancy when used as a booster for other PIs. The oral solution contains alcohol and therefore may not be the best formulation for use in pregnancy. A small increased risk of preterm birth has been associated with maternal use of protease inhibitor-based combination antiretroviral (ARV) therapy during pregnancy; however, the benefits of use generally outweigh this risk and PIs should not be withheld if otherwise recommended. Hyperglycemia, new onset of diabetes mellitus, or diabetic ketoacidosis have been reported with protease inhibitors; it is not clear if pregnancy increases this risk.

Regardless of CD4 count or HIV RNA copy number, all HIV-infected pregnant women should receive a combination antepartum ARV drug regimen; this includes women who require therapy for their own health, as well as women who do not yet require therapy for their own health. ARV therapy should be started as soon as possible if required for the woman's health. Although earlier initiation may be more effective in reducing the perinatal transmission of HIV, also consider maternal conditions (eg, nausea and vomiting) and the potential risks of first trimester fetal exposure for specific agents. Plasma HIV RNA levels should be assessed at ~34-36 weeks gestation in order to help determine mode of delivery. If ARV therapy must be interrupted for <24 hours during the peripartum period, stop then restart all medications simultaneously in order to decrease the chance of developing resistance. Long-term follow-up is recommended for all infants exposed to ARV medications.

Healthcare providers are encouraged to enroll pregnant women exposed to antiretroviral medications in the Antiretroviral Pregnancy Registry (1-800-258-4263 or www.-APRegistry.com). Healthcare providers caring for HIV-infected women and their infants may contact the National Perinatal HIV Hotline (888-448-8765) for clinical consultation (DHHS [perinatal], 2012).

Breast-Feeding Considerations Maternal or infant antiretroviral therapy does not completely eliminate the risk of postnatal HIV transmission. In addition, multiclass-resistant virus has been detected in breast-feeding infants despite maternal therapy. Therefore, in the United States, where formula is accessible, affordable, safe, and sustainable, and the risk of infant mortality due to diarrhea and respiratory infections is low, complete avoidance of breast-feeding by HIV-infected women is recommended to decrease potential transmission of HIV (DHHS [perinatal], 2012).

Contraindications Hypersensitivity to ritonavir or any component of the formulation; concurrent alfuzosin, amiodarone, cisapride, dihydroergotamine, ergonovine, ergotamine, flecainide, lovastatin, methylergonovine, midazolam (oral), pimozide, propafenone, quinidine, sildenafil (when used for the treatment of pulmonary arterial hypertension [eg, Revatio®]), simvastatin, St John's wort, triazolam, and voriconazole (when ritonavir ≥800 mg/day)

Canadian labeling: Additional contraindications (not in U.S. labeling): Concurrent use with rivaroxaban, voriconazole (regardless of ritonavir dose), salmeterol, vardenafil, bepridil, astemizole, or terfenadine

Warnings/Precautions **[U.S. Boxed Warning]: Ritonavir may interact with many medications, including antiarrhythmics, ergot alkaloids, and sedatives/hypnotics, resulting in potentially serious and/or life-threatening adverse events.** Some interactions may require dose or frequency adjustment, additional monitoring, and/or selection of alternative therapy. Pancreatitis has been observed (including fatalities); use with caution in patients with increased triglycerides; monitor serum lipase and amylase and for gastrointestinal symptoms. Increases in total cholesterol and triglycerides have been reported; screening should be done prior to therapy and periodically throughout treatment. Temporary or permanent discontinuation may be clinically indicated.

Protease inhibitors have been associated with a variety of hypersensitivity events (some severe), including rash, anaphylaxis (rare), angioedema, bronchospasm, erythema multiforme, toxic epidermal necrolysis, and/or Stevens-Johnson syndrome (rare). It is generally recommended to discontinue treatment if severe rash or moderate symptoms accompanied by other systemic symptoms occur. Use with caution in patients with cardiomyopathy, ischemic heart disease, pre-existing conduction abnormalities, or structural heart disease; may be at increased risk of conduction abnormalities (eg, second- or third-degree AV block). Ritonavir has been associated with AV block due to prolongation of PR interval; use caution with drugs that prolong the PR interval. Use with caution in patients with hemophilia A or B; increased bleeding during protease inhibitor therapy has been reported and additional Factor VIII may be needed. Changes in glucose tolerance, hyperglycemia, exacerbation of diabetes, DKA, and new-onset diabetes mellitus have been reported in patients receiving protease inhibitors. May be associated with fat redistribution (buffalo hump, increased abdominal girth, breast engorgement, facial atrophy, and dyslipidemia). Immune reconstitution syndrome may develop resulting in the occurrence of an inflammatory response to an indolent or residual opportunistic infection during initial HIV treatment or activation of autoimmune disorders (eg, Graves' disease, polymyositis, Guillain-Barré syndrome) later in therapy; further evaluation and treatment may be required. May cause hepatitis or exacerbate pre-existing hepatic dysfunction (including fatalities); use with caution in patients with hepatitis B or C, cirrhosis, or those with high baseline transaminases; consider increased monitoring of transaminases in these patients. Norvir® tablets are **not** bioequivalent to Norvir® capsules. Gastrointestinal side effects (eg, nausea, vomiting, abdominal pain, diarrhea) or paresthesias may be more common when patients are switching from the capsule to the tablet formulation due to a higher C_{max} (26% increase) observed with the tablet formulation compared to the capsule. These side effects should decrease as therapy is continued.

Oral solution contains ethanol and propylene glycol; healthcare providers should pay special attention to accurate calculation, measurement, and administration of dose; ethanol competitively inhibits propylene glycol metabolism; preterm infants may be at increased risk of toxicity due to decreased ability to metabolize propylene glycol. Postmarketing adverse reactions (cardiac toxicity, lactic acidosis, renal failure, CNS depression, respiratory complications, acute renal failure including fatalities) have been reported in preterm neonates receiving ritonavir-containing solutions. Do not use in neonates with a postmenstrual age (first day of mother's last menstrual period to birth plus elapsed time after birth) <44 weeks, unless benefit outweighs risk and neonate is closely monitored (serum creatinine and osmolality, CNS depression, renal toxicity, lactic acidosis, cardiac conduction abnormalities, hemolysis).

Adverse Reactions Percentages as reported for combined experiences in both treatment-naive and experienced adults:

>10%:

Endocrine & metabolic: Hypercholesterolemia (>240 mg/dL: 37% to 45%), increased serum triglycerides (>800 mg/dL: 17% to 34%; >1500 mg/dL: 1% to 13%)

Gastrointestinal: Nausea (26% to 30%), diarrhea (15% to 23%), vomiting (14% to 17%), dysgeusia (7% to 11%)
Hepatic: Increased gamma-glutamyl transferase (5% to 20%)
Neuromuscular & skeletal: Weakness (10% to 15%), increased creatine phosphokinase (9% to 12%)

2% to 10%:
Cardiovascular: Vasodilatation (2%), syncope (1% to 2%)
Central nervous system: Headache (6% to 7%), paresthesia (3% to 7%), dizziness (3% to 4%), insomnia (2% to 3%), drowsiness (2% to 3%), depression (2%), anxiety (≤2%), malaise (1% to 2%)
Dermatologic: Skin rash (≤4%), diaphoresis (2% to 3%)
Genitourinary: Uricosuria (≤4%)
Gastrointestinal: Abdominal pain (6% to 8%), anorexia (2% to 8%), dyspepsia (≤6%), throat irritation (local, 2% to 3%), flatulence (1% to 2%)
Hepatic: Increased serum transaminases (6% to 10%)
Neuromuscular & skeletal: Arthralgia (≤2%), myalgia (2%)
Respiratory: Pharyngitis (≤1% to 3%)
Miscellaneous: Fever (1% to 5%)

<2% (Limited to important or life-threatening): Adrenal suppression, adrenocortical cortex insufficiency, adrenal suppression, amnesia, anaphylaxis, anemia, angioedema, aphasia, asthma, atrioventricular block (first, second, or third degree), cachexia, cerebral ischemia, chest pain, cholestatic jaundice, coma, Cushing's syndrome, dementia, depersonalization, diabetes mellitus, diabetic ketoacidosis, edema, esophageal ulcer, gastroenteritis, gastrointestinal hemorrhage, hallucination, hematologic disease (myeloproliferative), hemorrhage (in patients with hemophilia A or B), hepatic coma, hepatitis, hepatomegaly, hepatosplenomegaly, hyperglycemia, hypersensitivity reaction, hypertension, hypotension, hypothermia, hypoventilation, immune reconstitution syndrome, intestinal obstruction, leukemia (acute myeloblastic), leukopenia, lymphadenopathy, lymphocytosis, malignant melanoma, manic behavior, myocardial infarction, neuropathy, orthostatic hypotension, palpitations, pancreatitis, paralysis, pneumonia, prolongation P-R interval on ECG, prolonged Q-T interval on ECG, pseudomembranous colitis, rectal hemorrhage, redistribution of body fat, renal failure, right bundle branch block, seizure, Stevens-Johnson syndrome, subdural hematoma, syncope, tachycardia, thrombocytopenia, torsades de pointes, toxic epidermal necrolysis, ulcerative colitis, vasospasm, venous thrombosis (cerebral)

Drug Interactions

Metabolism/Transport Effects Substrate of CYP1A2 (minor), CYP2B6 (minor), CYP2D6 (minor), CYP3A4 (major), P-glycoprotein; **Note:** Assignment of Major/Minor substrate status based on clinically relevant drug interaction potential; **Inhibits** CYP2C19 (weak), CYP2C8 (strong), CYP2C9 (weak), CYP2D6 (strong), CYP2E1 (weak), CYP3A4 (strong), P-glycoprotein; **Induces** CYP1A2 (weak/moderate), CYP2C9 (weak/moderate), CYP3A4 (weak/moderate)

Avoid Concomitant Use

Avoid concomitant use of Ritonavir with any of the following: Ado-Trastuzumab Emtansine; Alfuzosin; Amiodarone; Apixaban; Atovaquone; Avanafil; Axitinib; Bosutinib; Cabozantinib; Cisapride; Conivaptan; Crizotinib; Disulfiram; Dronedarone; Eplerenone; Ergot Derivatives; Etravirine; Everolimus; Flecainide; Fluticasone (Nasal); Fusidic Acid (Systemic); Halofantrine; Ibrutinib; Imatinib; Ivabradine; Lapatinib; Lomitapide; Lovastatin; Lurasidone; Macitentan; Midazolam; Nilotinib; Nisoldipine; Pimozide; Pomalidomide; Propafenone; QuiNIDine; QuiNINE; Ranolazine; Red Yeast Rice; Regorafenib; Rifampin; Rivaroxaban; Salmeterol; Silodosin; Simeprevir; Simvastatin; St Johns Wort; Tamoxifen; Tamsulosin; Thioridazine; Ticagrelor; Tolvaptan; Topotecan; Toremifene; Triazolam; Ulipristal; Vemurafenib; VinCRIStine (Liposomal); Voriconazole

Increased Effect/Toxicity

Ritonavir may increase the levels/effects of: Ado-Trastuzumab Emtansine; Afatinib; Alfuzosin; Almotriptan; Alosetron; ALPRAZolam; Amiodarone; Apixaban; ARIPiprazole; AtoMOXetine; AtorvaSTATin; Avanafil; Axitinib; Bedaquiline; Bortezomib; Bosentan; Bosutinib; Brentuximab Vedotin; Brinzolamide; Budesonide (Nasal); Budesonide (Systemic, Oral Inhalation); Cabozantinib; Calcium Channel Blockers (Dihydropyridine); Calcium Channel Blockers (Nondihydropyridine); CarBAMazepine; Cisapride; Clarithromycin; Clorazepate; Colchicine; Conivaptan; Corticosteroids (Orally Inhaled); Crizotinib; CycloSPORINE (Systemic); CYP2C8 Substrates; CYP2D6 Substrates; CYP3A4 Substrates; Dabigatran Etexilate; Diazepam; Dienogest; Digoxin; Dofetilide; Dronabinol; Dronedarone; Dutasteride; Efavirenz; Enfuvirtide; Enzalutamide; Eplerenone; Ergot Derivatives; Estazolam; Everolimus; FentaNYL; Fesoterodine; Flecainide; Flurazepam; Fluticasone (Nasal); Fluticasone (Oral Inhalation); Fusidic Acid (Systemic); GuanFACINE; Halofantrine; Highest Risk QTc-Prolonging Agents; Ibrutinib; Iloperidone; Imatinib; Itraconazole; Ivabradine; Ivacaftor; Ixabepilone; Ketoconazole (Systemic); Lacosamide; Lapatinib; Levomilnacipran; Linagliptin; Lomitapide; Lovastatin; Lumefantrine; Lurasidone; Macitentan; Maraviroc; Meperidine; MethylPREDNISolone; Metoprolol; Midazolam; Mifepristone; Moderate Risk QTc-Prolonging Agents; Nebivolol; Nefazodone; Nilotinib; Nisoldipine; Ospemifene; OxyCODONE; Paricalcitol; PAZOPanib; P-glycoprotein/ABCB1 Substrates; Pimecrolimus; Pimozide; Pioglitazone; Pomalidomide; PONATinib; PrednisoLONE (Systemic); PredniSONE; Propafenone; Protease Inhibitors; Prucalopride; QUEtiapine; QuiNIDine; QuiNINE; Ranolazine; Red Yeast Rice; Regorafenib; Repaglinide; Rifabutin; Rilpivirine; Riociguat; Rivaroxaban; RomiDEPsin; Rosuvastatin; Ruxolitinib; Salmeterol; Saxagliptin; Sildenafil; Silodosin; Simeprevir; Simvastatin; SORAfenib; Tacrolimus (Systemic); Tacrolimus (Topical); Tadalafil; Tamsulosin; Telaprevir; Temsirolimus; Tetrabenazine; Thioridazine; Ticagrelor; Tofacitinib; Tolterodine; Tolvaptan; Topotecan; Toremifene; Treprostinil; Triamcinolone (Systemic); Triazolam; Tricyclic Antidepressants; Ulipristal; Vardenafil; Vemurafenib; Vilazodone; VinBLAStine; VinCRIStine; VinCRIStine (Liposomal); Vortioxetine; Zuclopenthixol

The levels/effects of Ritonavir may be increased by: ARIPiprazole; Clarithromycin; CycloSPORINE (Systemic); Delavirdine; Disulfiram; Efavirenz; Enfuvirtide; Fusidic Acid (Systemic); MetroNIDAZOLE (Topical); P-glycoprotein/ABCB1 Inhibitors; Posaconazole; QuiNINE; Simeprevir

Decreased Effect

Ritonavir may decrease the levels/effects of: Abacavir; Atovaquone; Boceprevir; BuPROPion; Canagliflozin; Clarithromycin; Codeine; Contraceptives (Estrogens); Deferasirox; Delavirdine; Etravirine; Fosphenytoin; Ifosfamide; Iloperidone; LamoTRIgine; Meperidine; Methadone; Phenytoin; Prasugrel; Proguanil; QuiNINE; Tamoxifen; Telaprevir; Theophylline Derivatives; Ticagrelor; TraMADol; Valproic Acid and Derivatives; Voriconazole; Warfarin; Zidovudine

The levels/effects of Ritonavir may be decreased by: Antacids; Boceprevir; CarBAMazepine; CYP3A4 Inducers (Strong); Dabrafenib; Fosphenytoin; Garlic; Mitotane; Peginterferon Alfa-2b; P-glycoprotein/ABCB1 Inducers; Phenytoin; Rifampin; St Johns Wort; Tocilizumab

Ethanol/Nutrition/Herb Interactions

Food: Food enhances absorption. Management: Manufacturer recommends taking with food. Maintain adequate hydration, unless instructed to restrict fluid intake.

Herb/Nutraceutical: St John's wort may decrease ritonavir serum levels. Garlic may decrease the serum concentration of ritonavir. Management: Avoid St John's wort; concurrent use is contraindicated. Garlic supplementation is not recommended.

Storage/Stability

Capsule: Store under refrigeration at 2°C to 8°C (36°F to 46°F); may be left out at room temperature of <25°C (<77°F) if used within 30 days. Protect from light. Avoid exposure to excessive heat.

Solution: Store at room temperature at 20°C to 25°C (68°F to 77°F); do not refrigerate. Avoid exposure to excessive heat. Keep cap tightly closed.

Tablet: Store at ≤30 (86°F); exposure to temperatures ≤50°C (122°F) permitted for ≤7 days. Exposure to high humidity outside of the original container (or a USP equivalent container) for >2 weeks is not recommended.

Mechanism of Action Binds to the site of HIV-1 protease activity and inhibits cleavage of viral Gag-Pol polyprotein precursors into individual functional proteins required for infectious HIV. This results in the formation of immature, noninfectious viral particles.

Pharmacodynamics/Kinetics

Absorption: Variable; increased with food; In the fed state, mean C_{max} of the tablet formulation increased by 26% compared to the capsule.

Distribution: High concentrations in serum and lymph nodes; V_d: 0.16-0.66 L/kg

Protein binding: 98% to 99%

Metabolism: Hepatic via CYP3A4 and 2D6; five metabolites, low concentration of an active metabolite (M-2) achieved in plasma (oxidative)

Half-life elimination: 3-5 hours

Time to peak, plasma: Oral solution: 2 hours (fasted); 4 hours (nonfasted)

Excretion: Urine (~11%, ~4% as unchanged drug); feces (~86%, ~34% as unchanged drug)

Dosage Note: Must be given in combination with other antiretroviral agents. Norvir® tablets are **not** bioequivalent to Norvir® capsules. Gastrointestinal side effects or paresthesias may be more common initially when patients are switching from the capsule to the tablet formulation.

Treatment of HIV infection: Oral: Manufacturer's labeling:

Infants >1 month and Children: Initiate dose at 250 mg/m²/dose twice daily; titrate dose upward every 2-3 days by 50 mg/m² twice daily to recommended dosage of 350-400 mg/m²/dose twice daily (maximum dose: 600 mg twice daily). If 400 mg/m²/dose twice daily is not tolerated, the highest tolerated dose may be used for maintenance therapy. **Note:** Oral solution should not be administered to neonates before a postmenstrual age (first day of mother's last period to birth plus the time elapsed after birth) <44 weeks.

Adolescents and Adults (**Note:** Not recommended as the primary protease inhibitor in any regimen [DHHS, 2013]): Initiate dose at 300 mg twice daily, then increase by 100 mg twice daily every 2-3 days to recommended dosage of 600 mg twice daily (maximum: 600 mg twice daily)

Pharmacokinetic "booster" in combination with other protease inhibitors (unlabeled use): Adults: 100-400 mg daily in 1-2 divided doses (DHHS, 2013)

Note: Recommended as the "booster" component in the following preferred regimens in treatment-naive patients: Atazanavir and tenofovir/emtricitabine, or darunavir and tenofovir/emtricitabine (DHHS, 2013). In patients without evidence of PI resistance, once-daily booster-dosing of 100 mg ritonavir may be preferred to 200 mg daily due to less gastrointestinal and metabolic adverse events. Refer to individual protease inhibitor monographs; specific dosage recommendations often require adjustment of both agents.

Dosage adjustment in renal impairment: No dosage adjustment necessary.

Dosage adjustment in hepatic impairment:

Mild-to-moderate impairment (Child-Pugh class A or B): No dosage adjustment necessary; however, ritonavir levels may be decreased in moderate impairment and patient response should be monitored.

Severe impairment (Child-Pugh class C): Not recommended (has not been studied).

Dietary Considerations The manufacturer recommends taking with food. Oral solution contains 43% ethanol by volume.

Administration Administer all formulations with food, per the manufacturer. DHHS guidelines recommend administering the tablets with food and administering capsules or oral solution with food, if possible, to improve tolerability (DHHS, 2013). Liquid formulations usually have an unpleasant taste. Consider mixing it with chocolate milk or a liquid nutritional supplement and taking within 60 minutes. Whenever possible, administer oral solution with calibrated dosing syringe. Shake solution well before use. Tablets should be swallowed whole; do not chew, break, or crush.

Monitoring Parameters Triglycerides, cholesterol, CBC, LFTs, CPK, uric acid, basic HIV monitoring, viral load, CD4 count, glucose, serum amylase and lipase

Additional Information Potential compliance problems, frequency of administration and adverse effects should be discussed with patients before initiating therapy to help prevent the emergence of resistance.

Dosage Forms Excipient information presented when available (limited, particularly for generics); consult specific product labeling.

Capsule, Oral:

Norvir: 100 mg [contains alcohol, usp]

Solution, Oral:

Norvir: 80 mg/mL (240 mL) [contains alcohol, usp, fd&c yellow #6 (sunset yellow), propylene glycol, saccharin sodium; peppermint-caramel flavor]

Tablet, Oral:

Norvir: 100 mg

◆ **Ritonavir and Lopinavir** *see* Lopinavir and Ritonavir *on page 1237*

◆ **Rituxan** *see* RiTUXimab *on page 1833*

RiTUXimab (ri TUK si mab)

Brand Names: U.S. Rituxan

Brand Names: Canada Rituxan

Index Terms Anti-CD20 Monoclonal Antibody; C2B8 Monoclonal Antibody; IDEC-C2B8

Pharmacologic Category Antineoplastic Agent, Monoclonal Antibody; Antirheumatic Miscellaneous; Immunosuppressant Agent; Monoclonal Antibody

Additional Appendix Information

Desensitization Protocols *on page 2325*

Use

Treatment of CD20-positive non-Hodgkin lymphomas (NHL):

Relapsed or refractory, low-grade or follicular B-cell NHL (as a single agent)

Follicular B-cell NHL, previously untreated (in combination with first-line chemotherapy, and as single-agent maintenance therapy if response to first-line rituximab with chemotherapy)

Nonprogressing, low-grade B-cell NHL (as a single agent after first-line CVP treatment)

Diffuse large B-cell NHL, previously untreated (in combination with CHOP chemotherapy [or other anthracycline-based regimen])

Treatment of CD20-positive chronic lymphocytic leukemia (CLL) (in combination with fludarabine and cyclophosphamide)

Treatment of moderately- to severely-active rheumatoid arthritis (in combination with methotrexate) in adult patients with inadequate response to one or more TNF antagonists

Treatment of granulomatosis with polyangiitis (GPA; Wegener's granulomatosis) (in combination with glucocorticoids)

Treatment of microscopic polyangiitis (MPA) (in combination with glucocorticoids)

Unlabeled Use Treatment of Burkitt's lymphoma, central nervous system lymphoma, Hodgkin's lymphoma (lymphocyte predominant); mucosal associated lymphoid tissue (MALT) lymphoma (gastric and nongastric), splenic marginal zone lymphoma; Waldenström's macroglobulinemia (WM); post-transplant lymphoproliferative disorder (PTLD); autoimmune hemolytic anemia (AIHA) in children; chronic immune thrombocytopenia (ITP); refractory pemphigus vulgaris; treatment of steroid-refractory chronic graft-versus-host disease (GVHD); refractory lupus nephritis; relapsed/refractory thrombotic thrombocytopenic purpura-hemolytic uremic syndrome (TTP-HUS), resistant idiopathic membranous nephropathy (IMN), refractory nephrotic syndrome (children)

Pregnancy Risk Factor C

Pregnancy Considerations Animal reproduction studies have demonstrated adverse effects including decreased (reversible) B-cells and immunosuppression. Rituximab crosses the placenta and can be detected in the newborn. In one infant born at 41 weeks gestation, *in utero* exposure occurred from week 16-37; rituximab concentrations were higher in the neonate at birth (32,095 ng/mL) than the mother (9750 ng/mL) and still measurable at 18 weeks of age (700 ng/mL infant; 500 ng/mL mother) (Friedrichs, 2006).

B-cell lymphocytopenia lasting <6 months may occur in exposed infants. Limited information is available following maternal use of rituximab for the treatment of lymphomas and hematologic disorders (Ton, 2011). Retrospective case reports of inadvertent pregnancy during rituximab treatment collected by the manufacturer (often combined with concomitant teratogenic therapies) describe premature births and infant hematologic abnormalities and infections; no specific pattern of birth defects has been observed (limited data) (Chakravarty, 2010). Use is not recommended to treat non-life-threatening maternal conditions (eg, rheumatoid arthritis) during pregnancy (Makol, 2011; Østensen, 2008) and other agents are preferred for treating lupus nephritis in pregnant women (Hahn, 2012).

Effective contraception should be used during and for 12 months following treatment. Healthcare providers are encouraged to enroll women with rheumatoid arthritis exposed to rituximab during pregnancy in the Mother-ToBabyAutoImmune Diseases Study by contacting the Organization of Teratology Information Specialists (OTIS) (877-311-8972).

Breast-Feeding Considerations It is not known if rituximab is excreted in human milk. However, human IgG is excreted in breast milk, and therefore, rituximab may also be excreted in milk. Although rituximab would not be expected to enter the circulation of a nursing infant in significant amounts, the decision to discontinue rituximab or discontinue breast-feeding should take into account the benefits of treatment to the mother.

Medication Guide Available Yes

Contraindications There are no contraindications listed in the FDA-approved manufacturer's labeling.

Canadian labeling (not in U.S. labeling): Type 1 hypersensitivity or anaphylactic reaction to murine proteins, Chinese Hamster Ovary (CHO) cell proteins, or any component of the formulation; patients who have or have had progressive multifocal leukoencephalopathy (PML)

Warnings/Precautions [U.S. Boxed Warning]: Severe (occasionally fatal) infusion-related reactions have been reported, usually with the first infusion; fatalities have been reported within 24 hours of infusion; monitor closely during infusion; discontinue for severe reactions and provide medical intervention for grades 3 or 4 infusion reactions. Reactions usually occur within 30-120 minutes and may include hypotension, angioedema, bronchospasm, hypoxia, urticaria, and in more severe cases pulmonary infiltrates, acute respiratory distress syndrome, myocardial infarction, ventricular fibrillation, cardiogenic shock and/or anaphylaxis. Risk factors associated with fatal outcomes include chronic lymphocytic leukemia, female gender, mantle cell lymphoma, or pulmonary infiltrates. Closely monitor patients with a history of prior cardiopulmonary reactions or with pre-existing cardiac or pulmonary conditions and patients with high numbers of circulating malignant cells (>25,000/mm^3). Prior to infusion, premedicate patients with acetaminophen and an antihistamine (and methylprednisolone for patients with RA). Discontinue infusion for severe reactions; treatment is symptomatic. Medications for the treatment of hypersensitivity reactions (eg, bronchodilators, epinephrine, antihistamines, corticosteroids) should be available for immediate use. Discontinue infusion for serious or life-threatening cardiac arrhythmias. Perform cardiac monitoring during and after the infusion in patients who develop clinically significant arrhythmias or who have a history of arrhythmia or angina. Mild-to-moderate infusion-related reactions (eg, chills, fever, rigors) occur frequently and are typically managed through slowing or interrupting the infusion. Infusion may be resumed at a 50% infusion rate reduction upon resolution of symptoms. Due to the potential for hypotension, consider withholding antihypertensives 12 hours prior to treatment.

[U.S. Boxed Warning]: Hepatitis B virus (HBV) reactivation may occur with use and may result in fulminant hepatitis, hepatic failure, and death. Screen all patients for HBV infection by measuring hepatitis B surface antigen (HBsAG) and hepatitis B core antibody (anti-HBc) prior to therapy initiation; monitor patients for clinical and laboratory signs of hepatitis or HBV during and for several months after treatment. Discontinue rituximab (and concomitant medications) if viral hepatitis develops and initiate appropriate antiviral therapy. Reactivation has occurred in patients who are HBsAg positive as well as in those who are HBsAg negative but are anti-HBc positive; HBV reactivation has also been observed in patients who had previously resolved HBV infection. HBV reactivation has been reported up to 24 months after therapy discontinuation. Use cautiously in patients who show evidence of prior HBV infection (eg, HBsAg positive [regardless of antibody status] or HBsAG negative but anti-HBc positive); consult with appropriate clinicians regarding monitoring and consideration of antiviral therapy before and/or during rituximab treatment. The safety of resuming rituximab treatment following HBV reactivation is not known; discuss reinitiation of therapy in patients with resolved HBV reactivation with physicians experienced in HBV management.

[U.S. Boxed Warning]: Progressive multifocal leukoencephalopathy (PML) due to JC virus infection has been reported with rituximab use; may be fatal. Cases were reported in patients with hematologic malignancies receiving rituximab either with combination chemotherapy, or with hematopoietic stem cell transplant. Cases were also reported in patients receiving rituximab for autoimmune diseases who had received prior or concurrent immunosuppressant therapy. Onset may be delayed, although most cases were diagnosed within 12 months of the last rituximab dose. A retrospective analysis of patients (n=57) diagnosed with PML following rituximab therapy, found a median of 16 months (following rituximab initiation), 5.5 months (following last rituximab dose), and 6 rituximab doses preceded PML diagnosis. Clinical findings included confusion/disorientation, motor weakness/hemiparesis, altered vision/speech, and poor motor coordination with symptoms progressing over weeks to months (Carson, 2009). Promptly evaluate any patient presenting with neurological changes; consider neurology consultation, brain MRI and lumbar puncture for suspected PML. Discontinue rituximab in patients who develop PML; consider reduction/discontinuation of concurrent chemotherapy or immunosuppressants. Avoid use if severe active infection is present. Serious and potentially fatal bacterial, fungal, and either new or reactivated viral infections may occur during treatment and after completing rituximab. Infections have been observed in patients with prolonged hypogammaglobulinemia, defined as hypogammaglobulinemia >11 months after rituximab exposure; monitor immunoglobulin levels as necessary. Associated new or reactivated viral infections have included cytomegalovirus, herpes simplex virus, parvovirus B19, varicella zoster virus, West Nile virus, and hepatitis B and C. Discontinue rituximab in patients who develop other serious infections and initiate appropriate anti-infective treatment.

Tumor lysis syndrome leading to acute renal failure requiring dialysis (some fatal) may occur 12-24 hours following the first dose when used as a single agent in the treatment of NHL. Hyperkalemia, hypocalcemia, hyperuricemia, and/or hyperphosphatemia may occur. Administer prophylaxis (antihyperuricemic therapy, hydration) in patients at high risk (high numbers of circulating malignant cells ≥25,000/mm^3 or high tumor burden). May cause fatal renal toxicity in patients with hematologic malignancies. Patients who received combination therapy with cisplatin and rituximab for NHL experienced renal toxicity during clinical trials; this combination is not an approved treatment regimen. Monitor for signs of renal failure; discontinue rituximab with increasing serum creatinine or oliguria. Correct electrolyte abnormalities; monitor hydration status.

[U.S. Boxed Warning]: Severe and sometimes fatal mucocutaneous reactions (lichenoid dermatitis, paraneoplastic pemphigus, Stevens-Johnson syndrome, toxic epidermal necrolysis and vesiculobullous dermatitis) have been reported; onset has been variable but has occurred as early as the first day of exposure. Discontinue in patients experiencing severe mucocutaneous skin reactions; the safety of re-exposure following mucocutaneous reactions has not been evaluated. Use caution with pre-existing cardiac or pulmonary disease, or prior cardiopulmonary events. Rheumatoid arthritis patients are at increased risk for cardiovascular events; monitor closely during and after each infusion. Elderly patients are at higher risk for cardiac (supraventricular arrhythmia) and pulmonary adverse events (pneumonia, pneumonitis). Abdominal pain, bowel obstruction, and perforation (rarely fatal) have been reported with an average onset of symptoms of ~6 days (range: 1-77 days); complaints of abdominal pain or repeated vomiting should be evaluated, especially if early in the treatment course. Live vaccines should not be given concurrently with rituximab; there is no data available concerning secondary transmission of live vaccines with or following rituximab treatment. RA patients should be brought up to date with nonlive immunizations (following current guidelines) at least 4 weeks before initiating therapy; evaluate risks of therapy delay versus benefit (of nonlive vaccines) for NHL patients. Safety and efficacy of rituximab in combination with biologic agents or disease-modifying antirheumatic drugs (DMARDs) other than methotrexate have not been established. Rituximab is not recommended for use in RA patients who have not had prior inadequate response to TNF antagonists. Safety and efficacy of retreatment for RA have not been established. The safety of concomitant immunosuppressants other than corticosteroids has not been evaluated in patients with granulomatosis with polyangiitis (GPA; Wegener's granulomatosis) or microscopic polyangiitis (MPA) after rituximab-induced B-cell depletion. There are only limited data on subsequent courses of rituximab for GPA or MPA; safety and efficacy of retreatment have not been established.

Adverse Reactions Note: Patients treated with rituximab for rheumatoid arthritis (RA) may experience fewer adverse reactions.

>10%:

- Cardiovascular: Peripheral edema (8% to 16%), hypertension (6% to 12%)
- Central nervous system: Fever (5% to 53%), fatigue (13% to 39%), chills (3% to 33%), headache (17% to 19%), insomnia (≤14%), pain (12%)
- Dermatologic: Rash (10% to 17%; grades 3/4: 1%), pruritus (5% to 17%), angioedema (11%; grades 3/4: 1%)
- Gastrointestinal: Nausea (8% to 23%), diarrhea (10% to 17%), abdominal pain (2% to 14%), weight gain (11%)
- Hematologic: Cytopenias (grades 3/4: ≤48%; may be prolonged), lymphopenia (48%; grades 3/4: 40%; median duration 14 days), anemia (8% to 35%; grades 3/4: 3%), leukopenia (NHL: 14%; grades 3/4: 4%; CLL: grades 3/4: 23%; GPA/MPA: 10%), neutropenia (NHL: 14%; grades 3/4: 4% to 6%; median duration 13 days; CLL: grades 3/4: 30% to 49%), neutropenic fever (CLL: grades 3/4: 9% to 15%), thrombocytopenia (12%; grades 3/4: 2% to 11%)
- Hepatic: ALT increased (≤13%)
- Neuromuscular & skeletal: Neuropathy (≤30%), weakness (2% to 26%), muscle spasm (≤17%), arthralgia (6% to 13%)
- Respiratory: Cough (13%), rhinitis (3% to 12%), epistaxis (≤11%)
- Miscellaneous: Infusion-related reactions (lymphoma: first dose 77%; decreases with subsequent infusions; may include angioedema, bronchospasm, chills, dizziness, fever, headache, hyper-/hypotension, myalgia, nausea, pruritus, rash, rigors, urticaria, and vomiting; reactions reported are lower [first infusion: 32%] in RA; CLL: 59%; grades 3/4: 7% to 9%; GPA/MPA: 12%); infection (19% to 62%; grades 3/4: 4%; bacterial: 19%; viral 10%; fungal: 1%), human antichimeric antibody (HACA) positive (1% to 23%), night sweats (15%)

1% to 10%:

- Cardiovascular: Hypotension (10%; grades 3/4: 2%), flushing (5%)
- Central nervous system: Dizziness (10%), anxiety (2% to 5%), migraine (RA: 2%)
- Dermatologic: Urticaria (2% to 8%)
- Endocrine & metabolic: Hyperglycemia (9%)
- Gastrointestinal: Vomiting (10%), dyspepsia (RA: 3%)
- Neuromuscular & skeletal: Back pain (10%), myalgia (10%), paresthesia (2%)
- Respiratory: Dyspnea (≤10%), throat irritation (2% to 9%), bronchospasm (8%), dyspnea (7%), upper respiratory tract infection (RA: 7%), sinusitis (6%)
- Miscellaneous: LDH increased (7%)

Postmarketing and/or case reports: Acute renal failure, anaphylactoid reaction/anaphylaxis, angina, aplastic anemia, ARDS, arrhythmia, bowel obstruction/perforation, bronchiolitis obliterans, cardiac failure, cardiogenic shock, encephalomyelitis, fatal infusion-related reactions, fulminant hepatitis, gastrointestinal perforation, hemolytic anemia, hepatic failure, hepatitis, hepatitis B reactivation, hyperviscosity syndrome (in Waldenström's macroglobulinemia), hypogammaglobulinemia (prolonged), hypoxia, interstitial pneumonitis, laryngeal edema, lichenoid dermatitis, lupus-like syndrome, marrow hypoplasia, MI, mucositis, mucocutaneous reaction, neutropenia (late-onset occurring >40 days after last dose), optic neuritis, pancytopenia (prolonged), paraneoplastic pemphigus (uncommon), pleuritis, pneumonia, pneumonitis, polyarticular arthritis, polymyositis, posterior reversible encephalopathy syndrome (PRES), progressive multifocal leukoencephalopathy (PML), pure red cell aplasia, renal toxicity, reversible posterior leukoencephalopathy syndrome (RPLS), serum sickness, Stevens-Johnson syndrome, supraventricular arrhythmia, systemic vasculitis, toxic epidermal necrolysis, tuberculosis reactivation, tumor lysis syndrome, uveitis, vasculitis with rash, ventricular fibrillation, ventricular tachycardia, vesiculobullous dermatitis, viral reactivation (includes JC virus, cytomegalovirus, herpes simplex virus, parvovirus B19, varicella zoster virus, West Nile virus, and hepatitis C), wheezing

Drug Interactions

Metabolism/Transport Effects None known.

Avoid Concomitant Use

Avoid concomitant use of RiTUXimab with any of the following: Abatacept; BCG; Belimumab; Certolizumab Pegol; CloZAPine; Natalizumab; Pimecrolimus; Tacrolimus (Topical); Tofacitinib; Vaccines (Live)

Increased Effect/Toxicity

RiTUXimab may increase the levels/effects of: Abatacept; Belimumab; Certolizumab Pegol; CloZAPine; Leflunomide; Natalizumab; Tofacitinib; Vaccines (Live)

The levels/effects of RiTUXimab may be increased by: Abciximab; Antihypertensives; Denosumab; Pimecrolimus; Roflumilast; Tacrolimus (Topical); Trastuzumab

Decreased Effect

RiTUXimab may decrease the levels/effects of: BCG; Coccidioidin Skin Test; Sipuleucel-T; Vaccines (Inactivated); Vaccines (Live)

The levels/effects of RiTUXimab may be decreased by: Echinacea

Ethanol/Nutrition/Herb Interactions Herb/Nutraceutical: Avoid echinacea (may diminish the therapeutic effect of immunosuppressants). Avoid hypoglycemic herbs, including alfalfa, aloe, bilberry, bitter melon, burdock, celery, damiana, fenugreek, garcinia, garlic, ginger, ginseng (American), gymnema, marshmallow, and stinging nettle (may enhance the hypoglycemic effect of rituximab).

Preparation for Administration Withdraw necessary amount of rituximab and dilute to a final concentration of 1-4 mg/mL with 0.9% sodium chloride or 5% dextrose in water. Gently invert the bag to mix the solution. Do not shake.

Storage/Stability Store intact vials refrigerated at 2°C to 8°C (36°F to 46°F); do not freeze. Do not shake. Protect vials from direct sunlight. Solutions for infusion are stable at 2°C to 8°C (36°F to 46°F) for 24 hours and at room temperature for an additional 24 hours.

Mechanism of Action Rituximab is a monoclonal antibody directed against the CD20 antigen on B-lymphocytes. CD20 regulates cell cycle initiation; and, possibly, functions as a calcium channel. Rituximab binds to the antigen on the cell surface, activating complement-dependent B-cell cytotoxicity; and to human Fc receptors, mediating cell killing through an antibody-dependent cellular toxicity. B-cells are believed to play a role in the development and progression of rheumatoid arthritis. Signs and symptoms of RA are reduced by targeting B-cells and the progression of structural damage is delayed.

Pharmacodynamics/Kinetics

Duration: Detectable in serum 3-6 months after completion of treatment; B-cell recovery begins ~6 months following completion of treatment; median B-cell levels return to normal by 12 months following completion of treatment

Absorption: I.V.: Immediate and results in a rapid and sustained depletion of circulating and tissue-based B cells

Distribution: RA: 3.1 L; GPA/MPA: 4.5 L

Half-life elimination:

CLL: Median terminal half-life: 32 days (range: 14-62 days)

NHL: Median terminal half-life: 22 days (range: 6-52 days)

RA: Mean terminal half-life: 18 days (range: 5-78 days)

GPA/MPA: 23 days (range: 9-49 days)

Excretion: Uncertain; may undergo phagocytosis and catabolism in the reticuloendothelial system (RES)

Dosage Note: Details concerning dosing in combination regimens should also be consulted. Pretreatment with acetaminophen and an antihistamine is recommended for all indications. For oncology uses, antihyperuricemic therapy and aggressive hydration are recommended for patients at risk for tumor lysis syndrome (high tumor burden or lymphocytes >25,000/mm^3). In patients with CLL, *Pneumocystis jirovecii* pneumonia (PCP) and anti-herpetic viral prophylaxis is recommended during treatment (and for up to 12 months following treatment). In patients with granulomatosis with polyangiitis (GPA) and microscopic polyangiitis (MPA), PCP prophylaxis is recommended during and for 6 months after rituximab treatment. For patients with RA, premedication with methylprednisolone 100 mg I.V. (or equivalent) is recommended 30 minutes prior to each dose.

Children: I.V. infusion:

AIHA (unlabeled use): 375 mg/m^2 once weekly for 2-4 doses (Zecca, 2003)

Chronic ITP (unlabeled use): 375 mg/m^2 once weekly for 4 doses (Parodi, 2009; Wang, 2005)

Nephrotic syndrome, severe, refractory (unlabeled use): 375 mg/m^2 once weekly for 1-4 doses has been used in small case series, case reports, and retrospective analyses, including reports of successful remission induction of severe or refractory nephrotic syndromes that are poorly responsive to standard therapies (Dello Strologo, 2009; Fujinaga, 2010; Guigonis, 2008; Prytula, 2010)

Adults: I.V. infusion:

CLL: 375 mg/m^2 on the day prior to fludarabine/cyclophosphamide in cycle 1, then 500 mg/m^2 on day 1 (every 28 days) of cycles 2-6

Granulomatosis with polyangiitis (GPA; Wegener's granulomatosis): 375 mg/m^2 once weekly for 4 doses (in combination with methylprednisolone I.V. for 1-3 days followed by daily prednisone)

NHL (relapsed/refractory, low-grade or follicular CD20-positive, B-cell): 375 mg/m^2 once weekly for 4 or 8 doses

Retreatment following disease progression: 375 mg/m^2 once weekly for 4 doses

NHL (diffuse large B-cell): 375 mg/m^2 given on day 1 of each chemotherapy cycle for up to 8 doses

NHL (follicular, CD20-positive, B-cell, previously untreated): 375 mg/m^2 given on day 1 of each chemotherapy cycle for up to 8 doses

Maintenance therapy (as a single agent, in patients with partial or complete response to rituximab plus chemotherapy; begin 8 weeks after completion of combination chemotherapy): 375 mg/m^2 every 8 weeks for 12 doses

NHL (nonprogressing, low-grade, CD20-positive, B-cell, after 6-8 cycles of first-line CVP are completed): 375 mg/m^2 once weekly for 4 doses every 6 months for a maximum of 16 doses

NHL: Combination therapy with ibritumomab: 250 mg/m^2 I.V. day 1; repeat in 7-9 days with ibritumomab

Canadian labeling: NHL, low grade or follicular:

Initial: 375 mg/m^2 once weekly for 4 doses (as a single agent) or 375 mg/m^2 on day 1 of each 21-day cycle for 8 cycles (in combination with CVP chemotherapy)

Maintenance (responding to induction therapy): 375 mg/m^2 every 3 months until disease progression or up to a maximum of 2 years

Rheumatoid arthritis: 1000 mg on days 1 and 15 in combination with methotrexate; subsequent courses may be administered every 24 weeks (based on clinical evaluation), if necessary may be repeated no sooner than every 16 weeks

Microscopic polyangiitis (MPA): 375 mg/m^2 once weekly for 4 doses (in combination with methylprednisolone I.V. for 1-3 days followed by daily prednisone)

Chronic GVHD, refractory (unlabeled use): 375 mg/m^2 once weekly for 4 doses (Cutler, 2006)

Chronic ITP (unlabeled use): 375 mg/m^2 once weekly for 4 doses (Arnold, 2007; Godeau, 2008)

Hodgkin's lymphoma (unlabeled use): 375 mg/m^2 once weekly for 4 weeks (Ekstrand, 2003; Schulz, 2008)

Idiopathic membranous nephropathy (IMN), resistant (unlabeled use): 375 mg/m^2 once weekly for 4 doses with retreatment at 6 months (Fervenza, 2010) **or** 1000 mg on days 1 and 15 (Fervenza, 2008) **or** 375 mg/m^2 single doses titrated to B cell response (Cravedi, 2007)

Lupus nephritis, refractory (unlabeled use): 375 mg/m^2 once weekly for 4 doses (Melander, 2009) **or** 500-1000 mg on days 1 and 15 (Vigna-Perez, 2006)

Pemphigus vulgaris, refractory (unlabeled use): 375 mg/m^2 once weekly of weeks 1, 2, and 3 of a 4-week cycle, repeat for 1 additional cycle, then 1 dose per month for 4 months (total of 10 doses in 6 months) (Ahmed, 2006)

Post-transplant lymphoproliferative disorder (unlabeled use): 375 mg/m^2 once weekly for 4 doses (Choquet, 2006)

Thrombotic thrombocytopenic purpura (TTP), relapsed/refractory (unlabeled use): 375 mg/m^2 once weekly for 4 doses (Scully, 2007; Scully, 2011)

Waldenström's macroglobulinemia (unlabeled use): 375 mg/m^2 once weekly for 4 doses (Dimopoulos, 2002)

Dosage adjustment in renal impairment: No dosage adjustment provided in manufacturer's labeling (has not been studied).

Dosage adjustment in hepatic impairment: No dosage adjustment provided in manufacturer's labeling (has not been studied)

Administration Do **not** administer I.V. push or bolus. If a reaction occurs, slow or stop the infusion. If the reaction abates, restart infusion at 50% of the previous rate. Discontinue infusion in the event of serious or life-threatening cardiac arrhythmias.

I.V.: Initial infusion: Start rate of 50 mg/hour; if there is no reaction, increase the rate by 50 mg/hour increments every 30 minutes, to a maximum rate of 400 mg/hour.

Subsequent infusions:

Standard infusion rate: If patient tolerated initial infusion, start at 100 mg/hour; if there is no reaction, increase the rate by 100 mg/hour increments every 30 minutes, to a maximum rate of 400 mg/hour.

Accelerated infusion rate (90 minutes): For patients with previously untreated follicular NHL and diffuse large B-cell NHL who are receiving a corticosteroid as part of their combination chemotherapy regimen, have a circulating lymphocyte count <5000/mm^3, or have no significant cardiovascular disease. After tolerance has been established (no grade 3 or 4 infusion-related event) at the recommended infusion rate in cycle 1, a rapid infusion rate may be used beginning with cycle 2. The daily corticosteroid, acetaminophen, and diphenhydramine are administered prior to treatment, then the rituximab dose is administered over 90 minutes, with 20% of the dose administered over the first 30 minutes and the remaining 80% is given over 60 minutes (Sehn, 2007). If the 90-minute infusion in cycle 2 is tolerated, the same rate may be used for the remainder of the treatment regimen (through cycles 6 or 8).

Monitoring Parameters CBC with differential and platelets (obtain at weekly to monthly intervals and more frequently in patients with cytopenias, or at 2-4 month intervals in rheumatoid arthritis patients, GPA and MPA), peripheral CD20$^+$ cells; HAMA/HACA titers (high levels may increase the risk of allergic reactions); renal function, fluid balance; vital signs; monitor for infusion reactions, cardiac monitoring during and after infusion in rheumatoid arthritis patients and in patients with pre-existing cardiac disease or if arrhythmias develop during or after subsequent infusions.

Screen all patients for HBV infection prior to therapy initiation (eg, HBsAG and anti-HBc measurements). In addition, carriers and patients with evidence of current infection or recovery from prior hepatitis B infection should be monitored closely for clinical and laboratory signs of HBV reactivation and/or infection during therapy and for up to 2 years following completion of treatment. High-risk patients should be screened for hepatitis C (per NCCN NHL guidelines v.2.2013).

Complaints of abdominal pain, especially early in the course of treatment, should prompt a thorough diagnostic evaluation and appropriate treatment. Signs or symptoms of progressive multifocal leukoencephalopathy (focal neurologic deficits, which may present as hemiparesis, visual field deficits, cognitive impairment, aphasia, ataxia, and/or cranial nerve deficits). If PML is suspected, obtain brain MRI scan and lumbar puncture.

Dosage Forms Excipient information presented when available (limited, particularly for generics); consult specific product labeling.

Concentrate, Intravenous [preservative free]:

Rituxan: 10 mg/mL (10 mL, 50 mL) [contains polysorbate 80]

◆ **Riva-Alendronate (Can)** *see* Alendronate *on page* 69

◆ **Riva-Amiodarone (Can)** *see* Amiodarone *on page* 101

◆ **Riva-Amlodipine (Can)** *see* AmLODIPine *on page* 109

◆ **Riva-Anastrozole (Can)** *see* Anastrozole *on page* 137

◆ **Riva-Atenolol (Can)** *see* Atenolol *on page* 186

◆ **RIVA-Atomoxetine (Can)** *see* AtoMOXetine *on page* 187

◆ **Riva-Azithromycin (Can)** *see* Azithromycin (Systemic) *on page* 214

◆ **Riva-Baclofen (Can)** *see* Baclofen *on page* 221

◆ **Riva-Buspirone (Can)** *see* BusPIRone *on page* 300

◆ **Riva-Ciprofloxacin (Can)** *see* Ciprofloxacin (Systemic) *on page* 430

◆ **Riva-Citalopram (Can)** *see* Citalopram *on page* 440

◆ **Riva-Clarithromycin (Can)** *see* Clarithromycin *on page* 446

◆ **Riva-Clindamycin (Can)** *see* Clindamycin (Systemic) *on page* 451

◆ **Riva-Clonazepam (Can)** *see* ClonazePAM *on page* 465

- ◆ Riva-Cycloprine (Can) *see* Cyclobenzaprine *on page 502*
- ◆ Riva-Dicyclomine (Can) *see* Dicyclomine *on page 601*
- ◆ Riva-Enalapril (Can) *see* Enalapril *on page 701*
- ◆ Riva-Fenofibrate Micro (Can) *see* Fenofibrate and Derivatives *on page 837*
- ◆ Riva-Fluconazole (Can) *see* Fluconazole *on page 868*
- ◆ Riva-Fluoxetine (Can) *see* FLUoxetine *on page 885*
- ◆ Riva-Fluvox (Can) *see* FluvoxaMINE *on page 903*
- ◆ Riva-Fosinopril (Can) *see* Fosinopril *on page 923*
- ◆ Riva-Gabapentin (Can) *see* Gabapentin *on page 933*
- ◆ Riva-Glyburide (Can) *see* GlyBURIDE *on page 963*
- ◆ Riva-Hydroxyzine (Can) *see* HydrOXYzine *on page 1025*
- ◆ Riva-Indapamide (Can) *see* Indapamide *on page 1066*
- ◆ Riva-Lisinopril (Can) *see* Lisinopril *on page 1226*
- ◆ Riva-Loperamide (Can) *see* Loperamide *on page 1235*
- ◆ Riva-Lovastatin (Can) *see* Lovastatin *on page 1250*
- ◆ Riva-Memantine (Can) *see* Memantine *on page 1289*
- ◆ Riva-Metformin (Can) *see* MetFORMIN *on page 1310*
- ◆ Riva-Metoprolol-L (Can) *see* Metoprolol *on page 1348*
- ◆ Riva-Minocycline (Can) *see* Minocycline *on page 1373*
- ◆ Riva-Mirtazapine (Can) *see* Mirtazapine *on page 1379*
- ◆ Rivanase AQ (Can) *see* Beclomethasone (Nasal) *on page 229*
- ◆ Riva-Norfloxacin (Can) *see* Norfloxacin *on page 1475*
- ◆ Riva-Olanzapine (Can) *see* OLANZapine *on page 1493*
- ◆ Riva-Olanzapine ODT (Can) *see* OLANZapine *on page 1493*
- ◆ Riva-Oxazepam (Can) *see* Oxazepam *on page 1529*
- ◆ Riva-Oxybutynin (Can) *see* Oxybutynin *on page 1533*
- ◆ Riva-Pantoprazole (Can) *see* Pantoprazole *on page 1563*
- ◆ Riva-Paroxetine (Can) *see* PARoxetine *on page 1575*
- ◆ Riva-Pravastatin (Can) *see* Pravastatin *on page 1700*
- ◆ Riva-Pregabalin (Can) *see* Pregabalin *on page 1710*
- ◆ Riva-Quetiapine (Can) *see* QUEtiapine *on page 1757*
- ◆ Riva-Rabeprazole EC (Can) *see* RABEprazole *on page 1769*
- ◆ Riva-Ranitidine (Can) *see* Ranitidine *on page 1782*
- ◆ Riva-Risedronate (Can) *see* Risedronate *on page 1824*
- ◆ Riva-Risperidone (Can) *see* RisperiDONE *on page 1826*

Rivaroxaban (riv a ROX a ban)

Brand Names: U.S. Xarelto

Brand Names: Canada Xarelto®

Index Terms BAY 59-7939

Pharmacologic Category Factor Xa Inhibitor

Additional Appendix Information

Antithrombotic Therapy in Patients With Atrial Fibrillation *on page 2366*

Oral Anticoagulant Comparison Chart *on page 2307*

Reversal of Oral Anticoagulants *on page 2308*

Use Postoperative thromboprophylaxis in patients who have undergone hip or knee replacement surgery; prevention of stroke and systemic embolism in patients with nonvalvular atrial fibrillation; treatment of deep vein thrombosis (DVT) and pulmonary embolism (PE); to reduce the risk of recurrent DVT and/or PE

Pregnancy Risk Factor C

Pregnancy Considerations Adverse events were observed in animal reproduction studies. Data are insufficient to evaluate the safety of oral factor Xa inhibitors during pregnancy; use during pregnancy should be avoided (Guyatt, 2012). Use may increase the risk of pregnancy related hemorrhage. Clinicians should note that the anticoagulant effect cannot be easily monitored or readily reversed. Prompt clinical evaluation is warranted with any unexplained decrease in hemoglobin, hematocrit or blood pressure, or fetal distress. Pregnancy planning should be discussed if use is needed in women of reproductive potential. Use during pregnancy is contraindicated in the Canadian labeling.

Breast-Feeding Considerations It is not known if rivaroxaban is excreted into breast milk. Due to the potential for serious adverse reactions in the nursing infant, the decision to continue or discontinue breast-feeding during therapy should take into account the risk of exposure to the infant and the benefits of treatment to the mother; use of alternative anticoagulants is preferred (Guyatt, 2012). Use in breast-feeding mothers is contraindicated in the Canadian labeling.

Medication Guide Available Yes

Contraindications Severe hypersensitivity to rivaroxaban or any component of the formulation; active pathological bleeding

Canadian labeling: Additional contraindications (not in U.S. labeling): Hepatic disease (including Child-Pugh classes B and C) associated with coagulopathy and clinically relevant bleeding risk; clinically significant active bleeding, including hemorrhagic manifestations and bleeding diathesis; lesions at increased risk of clinically significant bleeding (eg, hemorrhagic or ischemic cerebral infarction) within previous 6 months; spontaneous hemostasis impairment; concomitant systemic treatment with strong CYP3A4 and P-glycoprotein (P-gp) inhibitors; pregnancy; lactation

Warnings/Precautions Most common complication is bleeding; major hemorrhages (eg, intracranial, GI, retinal, epidural hematoma, adrenal bleeding) have been reported. Certain patients are at increased risk of bleeding; risk factors include bacterial endocarditis, congenital or acquired bleeding disorders, thrombocytopenia, recent puncture of large vessels or organ biopsy, stroke, intracerebral surgery, or other neuraxial procedure, severe uncontrolled hypertension, renal impairment, recent major surgery, recent major bleeding (intracranial, GI, intraocular, or pulmonary), concomitant use of drugs that affect hemostasis, and advanced age. Monitor for signs and symptoms of bleeding. Prompt clinical evaluation is warranted with any unexplained decrease in hemoglobin or blood pressure. Avoid use with direct thrombin inhibitors (eg, bivalirudin), unfractionated heparin or heparin derivatives, low molecular weight heparins (eg, enoxaparin), aspirin, coumarin derivatives, and sulfinpyrazone. NSAIDs and other platelet aggregation inhibitors (eg, clopidogrel) should be used cautiously.

[U.S. Boxed Warning]: Spinal or epidural hematomas, including subsequent paralysis, may occur with neuraxial anesthesia (epidural or spinal anesthesia) or spinal puncture in patients who are anticoagulated; the risk is increased with concomitant administration of other drugs that affect hemostasis (eg, NSAIDS, platelet inhibitors, other anticoagulants), in patients with a history of traumatic or repeated epidural or spinal punctures, or a history of spinal deformity or surgery. In patients who receive both rivaroxaban and neuraxial anesthesia, avoid removal of epidural catheter for at least 18 hours following last rivaroxaban dose; avoid rivaroxaban administration for at least 6 hours following epidural catheter removal; if traumatic puncture occurs, avoid rivaroxaban administration for at least 24 hours. Monitor for signs of neurologic impairment (eg, numbness/weakness of legs, bowel/bladder dysfunction); prompt diagnosis and treatment are necessary.

[U.S. Boxed Warning]: As with any oral anticoagulant in the absence of adequate alternative anticoagulation, an increased risk of thrombotic events (including stroke) may occur with premature discontinuation of rivaroxaban. Consider the addition of alternative anticoagulant therapy when discontinuing rivaroxaban for reasons other than pathological bleeding or completion of a course of therapy. An increased rate of stroke was observed during the transition from rivaroxaban to warfarin in clinical trials in atrial fibrillation patients. In a post-hoc analysis of the ROCKET AF trial, patients who temporarily (>3 days) or permanently discontinued anticoagulation, the risk of stroke or non-CNS embolism was similar with rivaroxaban as compared to warfarin (Patel, 2013).

Avoid use in patients with moderate-to-severe hepatic impairment (Child-Pugh classes B and C) or in patients with any hepatic disease associated with coagulopathy; use in this patient population is contraindicated in the Canadian labeling. Use with caution in patients with moderate renal impairment (Cl_{cr} 30-49 mL/minute) when used for postoperative thromboprophylaxis including patients receiving concomitant drug therapy that may increase rivaroxaban systemic exposure and those with deteriorating renal function. Monitor for any signs or symptoms of blood loss. Avoid use in severe renal impairment (DVT/PE, postoperative thromboprophylaxis: Cl_{cr} <30 mL/minute; nonvalvular atrial fibrillation: Cl_{cr} <15 mL/minute) since rivaroxaban exposure is expected to increase; discontinue use in patients who develop acute renal failure. Use with caution in the elderly. Elderly patients exhibit higher rivaroxaban concentrations compared to younger patients due primarily to reduced clearance. Overall, efficacy of rivaroxaban in the elderly (age ≥65 years) was similar to that of patients <65 years of age. Both thrombotic and bleeding events were higher in the elderly; however, the risk to benefit profile was favorable among all age groups.

Potentially significant interactions may exist, requiring dose or frequency adjustment, additional monitoring, and/or selection of alternative therapy. In patients with renal impairment, concomitant use of rivaroxaban with combined P-gp and weak or moderate CYP3A4 inhibitors should only occur if the potential benefit outweighs the risk of bleeding. Formulation contains lactose; use is not recommended in patients with lactose or galactose intolerance (eg, Lapp lactase deficiency, glucose-galactose malabsorption).

Discontinue rivaroxaban at least 24 hours prior to surgery/invasive procedures; reinitiate when adequate hemostasis has been achieved unless oral therapy cannot be administered then consider administration of a parenteral anticoagulant. Safety and efficacy have not been established in patients with prosthetic heart valves or significant rheumatic heart disease (eg, mitral stenosis); use is not recommended. Non-valvular atrial fibrillation is defined as atrial fibrillation that occurs in the absence of rheumatic mitral valve disease, mitral valve repair, or prosthetic heart valve (Fuster, 2011).

Adverse Reactions

1% to 10%:

- Cardiovascular: Peripheral edema (≤6%)
- Central nervous system: Dizziness (≤6%), headache (3% to 5%), pyrexia (1% to 3%), fatigue (≤3%), syncope (≤2%)
- Dermatologic: Bruising (3%), pruritus (≤2%), rash (2%), blister (1%)
- Gastrointestinal: Diarrhea (≤5%), constipation (≤3%), abdominal pain (≤2%), nausea (1% to 3%), dyspepsia (≤2%), vomiting (≤2%), oropharyngeal pain (≤1%), toothache (≤1%)
- Genitourinary: Hematuria (≤4%), urinary tract infection (≤1%)
- Hematologic: Bleeding (atrial fibrillation: 21% [major: 6%]; DVT prophylaxis: 5% to 6% [major: <1%]; DVT treatment: 6% to 10% [major: 1%]), hematoma (≤3%), anemia (1% to 3%)
- Local: Wound secretion (≤3%)
- Neuromuscular & skeletal: Extremity pain (≤5%), back pain (≤4%), osteoarthritis (≤2%), muscle spasm (1%)
- Respiratory: Epistaxis (4% to 10%), hemoptysis (≤1%), sinusitis (≤1%)

<1% (Limited to important or life-threatening): Agranulocytosis, alkaline phosphatase increased, allergic dermatitis, amylase increased, anaphylactic reaction, anaphylactic shock, anaphylaxis, angioedema, BUN increased, cholestasis, cytolytic hepatitis, creatinine increased, dysuria, ecchymosis, fatal bleeding, GI hemorrhage, hematoma (epidural/subdural), hemiparesis, hemoglobin decrease (≥2 g/dL), hemorrhage (cerebral/retroperitoneal), hypersensitivity, hypotension, intracranial bleeding, intraocular bleeding, jaundice, LDH increased, lipase increased, menorrhagia, pain, pulmonary hemorrhage (with and without bronchiectasis), retroperitoneal bleeding, Stevens-Johnson syndrome, tachycardia, thrombocythemia, thrombocytopenia (<100,000/mm^3 or <50% baseline), urticaria, xerostomia

Drug Interactions

Metabolism/Transport Effects Substrate of CYP3A4 (major), P-glycoprotein; **Note:** Assignment of Major/Minor substrate status based on clinically relevant drug interaction potential

Avoid Concomitant Use

Avoid concomitant use of Rivaroxaban with any of the following: Anticoagulants; Apixaban; CYP3A4 Inducers (Strong); CYP3A4 Inhibitors (Strong); Dabigatran Etexilate; Omacetaxine; St Johns Wort

Increased Effect/Toxicity

Rivaroxaban may increase the levels/effects of: Collagenase (Systemic); Deferasirox; Ibritumomab; Omacetaxine; Tositumomab and Iodine I 131 Tositumomab

The levels/effects of Rivaroxaban may be increased by: Agents with Antiplatelet Properties; Anticoagulants; Apixaban; Azithromycin (Systemic); Clarithromycin; CYP3A4 Inhibitors (Moderate); CYP3A4 Inhibitors (Strong); Dabigatran Etexilate; Dasatinib; Diltiazem; Erythromycin (Systemic); Fusidic Acid (Systemic); Herbs (Anticoagulant/Antiplatelet Properties); Ibrutinib; Ivacaftor; Luliconazole; Mifepristone; Nonsteroidal Anti-Inflammatory Agents; Omega-3 Fatty Acids; Pentosan Polysulfate Sodium; P-glycoprotein/ABCB1 Inhibitors; Prostacyclin Analogues; Salicylates; Simeprevir; Sugammadex; Thrombolytic Agents; Tibolone; Tipranavir; Verapamil; Vitamin E

Decreased Effect

The levels/effects of Rivaroxaban may be decreased by: Bosentan; CYP3A4 Inducers (Strong); Dabrafenib; Deferasirox; Estrogen Derivatives; P-glycoprotein/ABCB1 Inducers; Progestins; St Johns Wort; Tocilizumab

Ethanol/Nutrition/Herb Interactions

Food: Grapefruit juice may increase levels/effects of rivaroxaban; use caution.

Herb/Nutraceutical: Avoid concomitant use of St John's wort if possible (may decrease levels/effects of rivaroxaban; use with caution and consider dosage adjustment of rivaroxaban if concomitant use cannot be avoided).

Storage/Stability Store at 25°C (77°F); excursions permitted to 15°C to 30°C (59°F to 86°F).

Mechanism of Action Inhibits platelet activation and fibrin clot formation via direct, selective and reversible inhibition of factor Xa (FXa) in both the intrinsic and extrinsic coagulation pathways. FXa, as part of the prothrombinase complex consisting also of factor Va, calcium ions, factor II and phospholipid, catalyzes the conversion of prothrombin to thrombin. Thrombin both activates platelets and catalyzes the conversion of fibrinogen to fibrin.

Pharmacodynamics/Kinetics

Absorption: Rapid

Distribution: V_{dss}: ~50 L

Protein binding: ~92% to 95% (primarily to albumin)

Metabolism: Hepatic via CYP3A4/5 and CYP2J2

Bioavailability: Absolute bioavailability: 10 mg dose: ~80% to 100%; 20 mg dose: ~66% (fasting; increased with food)

Half-life elimination: Terminal: 5-9 hours; Elderly: 11-13 hours

Time to peak, plasma: 2-4 hours

Excretion: Urine (66% primarily via active tubular secretion [36% as unchanged drug; 30% as inactive metabolites]); feces (28% [7% as unchanged drug; 21% as inactive metabolites])

Dosage

Adults: Oral: **Note:** Extremes of body weight (<50 kg or >120 kg) did not significantly influence rivaroxaban exposure (Kubitza, 2007).

Deep vein thrombosis (DVT), pulmonary embolism (PE): Initial: 15 mg twice daily with food for 3 weeks followed by 20 mg once daily with food. **Note:** The American College of Chest Physicians (ACCP) recommends anticoagulant treatment for 3 months in patients with provoked DVT or ≥3 months with unprovoked DVT (duration depends on bleeding risk) (Guyatt, 2012). Canadian labeling recommends continuation of treatment for at least 3 months if first episode of DVT is secondary to transient risk factors (eg, recent trauma, surgery, immobilization) and an extended duration of treatment if patient has permanent risk factors or idiopathic DVT/PE.

Reduction in the risk of recurrent DVT/PE (in select patients): 20 mg once daily with food; duration of treatment in the EINSTEIN-Extension Study was 6-12 months in addition to the initial treatment duration of 6-12 months (EINSTEIN Investigators, 2010).

Nonvalvular atrial fibrillation (to prevent stroke and systemic embolism): 20 mg once daily with the evening meal. **Note:** The American Heart Association/American Stroke Association recommends rivaroxaban as a reasonable alternative to warfarin in patients who are at moderate-to-high risk of stroke (prior history of TIA, stroke, or systemic embolism or ≥2 additional risk factors for stroke) (Furie, 2012).

Conversion from warfarin: Discontinue warfarin and initiate rivaroxaban as soon as INR falls to <3.0 (U.S. labeling) or ≤2.5 (Canadian labeling)

Conversion to warfarin: **Note:** Rivaroxaban affects INR; therefore, initial INR measurements after initiating warfarin may be unreliable.

U.S. labeling: Initiate warfarin and a parenteral anticoagulant 24 hours after discontinuation of rivaroxaban (other approaches to conversion may be acceptable).

Canadian labeling: Continue rivaroxaban concomitantly with warfarin until INR ≥2.0 and then discontinue rivaroxaban. **Note:** Caution must be employed with this strategy given the lack of an antidote for rivaroxaban reversal. During concomitant therapy, measure INR daily at least 24 hours after previous rivaroxaban dose and just prior to the next scheduled rivaroxaban dose.

Conversion from continuous infusion unfractionated heparin: Initiate rivaroxaban at the time of heparin discontinuation

Conversion to continuous infusion unfractionated heparin: Initiate continuous infusion unfractionated heparin 24 hours after discontinuation of rivaroxaban

Conversion from anticoagulants (other than warfarin and continuous infusion unfractionated heparin):

U.S. labeling: Discontinue current anticoagulant and initiate rivaroxaban ≤2 hours prior to the next regularly scheduled evening dose of the discontinued anticoagulant.

Canadian labeling: Discontinue current anticoagulant and initiate rivaroxaban ≤2 hours prior to the next regularly scheduled evening dose of the discontinued anticoagulant; patients previously receiving prophylactic doses of anticoagulant may initiate rivaroxaban ≥6 hours after last prophylactic dose.

Conversion to other anticoagulants (other than warfarin): Initiate the anticoagulant 24 hours after discontinuation of rivaroxaban

Postoperative thromboprophylaxis: **Note:** Initiate therapy after hemostasis has been established, 6-10 hours postoperatively.

Knee replacement: 10 mg once daily; recommended total duration of therapy: 12-14 days; ACCP recommendation: Minimum of 10-14 days; extended duration of up to 35 days suggested (Guyatt, 2012).

Hip replacement: 10 mg once daily; total duration of therapy: 35 days; ACCP recommendation: Minimum of 10-14 days; extended duration of up to 35 days suggested (Guyatt, 2012).

Elderly: Refer to adult dosing.

Dosing adjustment in renal impairment: Note: Clinical trials evaluating safety and efficacy utilized the Cockcroft-Gault formula with the use of actual body weight (weight range of patients enrolled in clinical trials: 33-209 kg) (data on file; Janssen Pharmaceuticals Inc, 2012).

DVT, PE, reduction of the risk of recurrent DVT/PE:

U.S. labeling:

Cl_{cr} ≥30 mL/minute: No dosage adjustment provided in manufacturer's labeling.

Cl_{cr} <30 mL/minute: Avoid use.

Canadian labeling:

Cl_{cr} ≥30 mL/minute: No dosage adjustment necessary.

Cl_{cr} <30 mL/minute: Avoid use.

Nonvalvular atrial fibrillation:

U.S. labeling:

Cl_{cr} >50 mL/minute: No dosage adjustment necessary.

Cl_{cr} 15-50 mL/minute: 15 mg once daily with the evening meal.

Cl_{cr} <15 mL/minute: Avoid use.

ESRD requiring hemodialysis: Avoid use

Canadian labeling:

Cl_{cr} ≥50 mL/minute: No dosage adjustment necessary.

Cl_{cr} 30-49 mL/minute: 15 mg once daily

Cl_{cr} <30 mL/minute: Avoid use.

Postoperative thromboprophylaxis:

Cl_{cr} >50 mL/minute: No dosage adjustment necessary.

Cl_{cr} 30-50 mL/minute: No dosage adjustment necessary; use with caution.

Cl_{cr} <30 mL/minute: Avoid use.

ESRD requiring hemodialysis: Avoid use.

Dosing adjustment in hepatic impairment:

Mild hepatic impairment: No dosage adjustment provided in manufacturer's labeling. Limited data indicates pharmacokinetics and pharmacodynamic response were similar to healthy subjects.

Moderate-to-severe hepatic impairment (Child-Pugh class B or C) and patients with any hepatic disease associated with coagulopathy: Avoid use. **Note:** The Canadian labeling contraindicates use in these patient populations.

Dosing in obesity: Body weight >120 kg did not significantly influence rivaroxaban exposure (Kubitza, 2007). Clinical outcomes in postoperative thromboprophylaxis trials were also not affected by weight (up to 190 kg) (Turpie, 2011). Therefore, dosage adjustment is not required.

Administration Administer doses ≥15 mg/day with food; dose of 10 mg/day may be administered without regard to meals. For nonvalvular atrial fibrillation, administer with the evening meal. For patients who cannot swallow whole tablets, the manufacturer's labeling states the 15 mg and 20 mg tablets may be crushed and mixed with applesauce immediately prior to use (**Note:** The manufacturer's labeling does not specify the 10 mg tablets can be crushed although the 10 mg, 15 mg, and 20 mg tablets are all biconvex film-coated tablets); immediately follow administration with food.

For nasogastric/gastric feeding tube administration, the manufacturer's labeling states the 15 mg and 20 mg tablets may be crushed and mixed in 50 mL of water (**Note:** The manufacturer's labeling does not specify the 10 mg tablets can be crushed although the 10 mg, 15 mg, and 20 mg tablets are all biconvex film-coated tablets); administer the suspension within 4 hours of preparation and follow administration immediately with enteral feeding. Avoid administration distal to the stomach; a decrease in the AUC and C_{max} (29% and 56%, respectively) was observed when rivaroxaban was delivered to the proximal small intestine; further decreases may be seen with delivery to the distal small intestine or ascending colon.

Missed doses: Patients receiving 15 mg twice daily dosing who miss a dose should take a dose immediately to ensure 30 mg of rivaroxaban is administered per day (two 15 mg tablets may be taken together); resume therapy the following day as previously taken. Patients receiving once-daily dosing who miss a dose should take a dose as soon as possible on the same day; resume therapy the following day as previously taken.

Monitoring Parameters Routine monitoring of coagulation tests not required; in major clinical trials, monitoring of coagulation tests (eg, aPTT, PT/INR, or antifactor Xa activity) did not occur. Prothrombin time (PT) or antifactor Xa activity may be used to detect presence of rivaroxaban (neither is intended to be used for dosage adjustment). However, variability exists among PT assays and even more so when converted to INR. Therefore, antifactor Xa activity measurement is the preferred test (Asmis, 2012; Barrett, 2010; Kubitza, 2005). A therapeutic range has not been defined, and dosage adjustment based on results has not been established.

CBC with differential, renal function, hepatic function

Test Interactions Prolongs activated partial thromboplastin time (aPTT), HepTest®, and Russell viper venom time

Dosage Forms Excipient information presented when available (limited, particularly for generics); consult specific product labeling.

Tablet, Oral:

Xarelto: 10 mg, 15 mg, 20 mg

- ◆ **Riva-Sertraline (Can)** *see* Sertraline *on page* 1889
- ◆ **Riva-Simvastatin (Can)** *see* Simvastatin *on page* 1899
- ◆ **Rivasol (Can)** *see* Zinc Sulfate *on page* 2230
- ◆ **Rivasone (Can)** *see* Betamethasone *on page* 247
- ◆ **Riva-Sotalol (Can)** *see* Sotalol *on page* 1942

Rivastigmine (ri va STIG meen)

Brand Names: U.S. Exelon

Brand Names: Canada Apo-Rivastigmine; Exelon; Mylan-Rivastigmine; Novo-Rivastigmine; PMS-Rivastigmine; ratio-Rivastigmine; Sandoz-Rivastigmine

Index Terms ENA 713; Rivastigmine Tartrate; SDZ ENA 713

Pharmacologic Category Acetylcholinesterase Inhibitor (Central)

Use Dementia associated with Alzheimer's or Parkinson's disease:

U.S. labeling: Treatment of mild, moderate, or severe dementia associated with Alzheimer's disease; treatment of mild-to-moderate dementia associated with Parkinson's disease

Canadian labeling: Treatment of mild-to-moderate dementia associated with Alzheimer's disease; treatment of mild-to-moderate dementia associated with Parkinson's disease

Unlabeled Use Treatment of dementia with Lewy bodies

Pregnancy Risk Factor B

Pregnancy Considerations Adverse events were observed in some animal reproduction studies. Use in women of reproductive age is not recommended.

Breast-Feeding Considerations It is not known if rivastigmine is excreted in breast milk. Rivastigmine is not indicated in nursing mothers.

Contraindications Hypersensitivity to rivastigmine, other carbamate derivatives (eg, neostigmine, pyridostigmine, physostigmine), or any component of the formulation; history of application site reactions with rivastigmine patch

Canadian labeling: Additional contraindications (not in U.S. labeling): Severe hepatic impairment

Warnings/Precautions Significant nausea/vomiting/diarrhea or anorexia/weight loss/decreased appetite are associated with use; occurs more frequently in women and during the titration phase. The incidence and severity of these reactions are dose-related. Monitor weight during therapy. Therapy should be initiated at lowest dose and titrated; if treatment is interrupted for >3 days, reinstate at the lowest daily dose. May have vagotonic effects which may cause bradycardia and/or heart block with or without a history of cardiac disease. Alzheimer's treatment guidelines consider bradycardia to be a relative contraindication for use of centrally-active cholinesterase inhibitors. Postmarketing cases of overdose (including fatalities) have been reported in association with medication errors/improper use of rivastigmine transdermal patches. No more than 1 patch should be applied daily and existing patch must be removed prior to applying new patch.

Use of patch may result in allergic contact dermatitis; discontinue therapy if an intense local reaction occurs (eg, increasing erythema, edema, papules, vesicles) and if symptoms do not improve after 48 hours of patch removal. If therapy is still required, oral rivastigmine may be used following negative allergy testing; some patients may not be able to take rivastigmine in any form. Postmarketing reports of disseminated hypersensitivity skin reactions have occurred with use of oral or transdermal products; discontinue use of all rivastigmine therapy in these cases.

Use caution in patients with a history of peptic ulcer disease or concurrent NSAID use; may increase gastric acid secretion. Monitor for active or occult bleeding. Use caution in patients with sick-sinus syndrome, bradycardia or supraventricular conduction conditions, urinary obstruction, seizure disorders, or pulmonary conditions such as asthma or COPD. May exacerbate or induce extrapyramidal symptoms; worsening of symptoms (eg, tremor) in patients with Parkinson's disease has been observed. May cause CNS depression, which may impair physical or mental abilities; patients must be cautioned about performing tasks which require mental alertness (eg, operating machinery or driving). Systemic exposure may be increased in patients <50 kg and decreased in patients >100 kg. Consider dose reduction if toxicities develop in patients <50 kg (oral and transdermal). Consider a dose increase in patients >100 kg (transdermal). Potentially significant drug-drug interactions may exist, requiring dose or frequency adjustment, additional monitoring, and/or selection of alternative therapy.

Adverse Reactions Note: Many concentration-related effects are reported at a lower frequency by transdermal route.

>10%:

Central nervous system: Dizziness (1% to 21%), headache (3% to 17%)

Gastrointestinal: Nausea (5% to 47%), vomiting (5% to 31%), diarrhea (<1% to 19%), anorexia (3% to 17%), abdominal pain (1% to 13%)

1% to 10%:

Cardiovascular: Syncope (3%), hypertension (3%)

Central nervous system: Fatigue (1% to 9%), insomnia (1% to 9%), confusion (8%), falling (6% to 8%), depression (4% to 6%), agitation (5%), anxiety (2% to 5%), malaise (5%), somnolence (4% to 5%), hallucinations (4%), aggressiveness (2% to 3%), parkinsonism symptoms worsening (2% to 3%), psychomotor hyperactivity (3%), vertigo (≤2%), paranoia (>1%)

Dermatologic: Application site reactions (including erythema <1% to 6%)

Gastrointestinal: Dyspepsia (9%), appetite decreased (3% to 9%), weight loss (3% to 8%), constipation (5%), flatulence (4%), dehydration (2%), eructation (2%)

Genitourinary: Urinary tract infection (1% to 7%), urinary incontinence (2% to 3%)

Neuromuscular & skeletal: Weakness (2% to 6%), tremor (1%; up to 10% in Parkinson's patients), back pain (>1%)

Respiratory: Rhinitis (4%)

Miscellaneous: Accidental trauma (10%), diaphoresis (4%), flu-like syndrome (3%)

<1% (Limited to important or life-threatening): Allergy, anemia, angina, apraxia, atrial fibrillation, AV block, bradycardia, bundle branch block, cardiac arrest, cardiac failure, cholecystitis, diplopia, diverticulitis, gastritis, gastroesophageal reflux, glaucoma, hyper-/hypoglycemia, hypercholesterolemia, hypersensitivity reactions, hypotension, hypothyroidism, ileus, intracranial hemorrhage, mastitis, MI, migraine, neuralgia, pancreatitis, peripheral ischemia, peripheral neuropathy, pneumonia, psychiatric disorders (eg, delirium, depersonalization, psychosis, emotional lability, suicidal ideation or tendencies), renal failure, respiratory depression, retinopathy, seizure, sick-sinus syndrome, Stevens-Johnson syndrome, sudden cardiac death, supraventricular tachycardia, thrombocytopenia, thrombophlebitis, thrombosis, transient ischemic attack, ulcerative stomatitis, vasovagal syncope

Drug Interactions

Metabolism/Transport Effects None known.

Avoid Concomitant Use There are no known interactions where it is recommended to avoid concomitant use.

Increased Effect/Toxicity

Rivastigmine may increase the levels/effects of: Antipsychotics; Beta-Blockers; Cholinergic Agonists; Succinylcholine

The levels/effects of Rivastigmine may be increased by: Corticosteroids (Systemic)

Decreased Effect

Rivastigmine may decrease the levels/effects of: Anticholinergics; Neuromuscular-Blocking Agents (Nondepolarizing)

The levels/effects of Rivastigmine may be decreased by: Anticholinergics; Dipyridamole

Ethanol/Nutrition/Herb Interactions

Smoking: Nicotine increases the clearance of rivastigmine by 23%.

Ethanol: Avoid ethanol (due to risk of sedation; may increase GI irritation).

Food: Food delays absorption by 90 minutes, lowers C_{max} by 30% and increases AUC by 30%.

Herb/Nutraceutical: Avoid ginkgo biloba (may increase cholinergic effects).

Storage/Stability

Oral: Store at 25°C (77°F); excursions permitted between 15°C and 30°C (59°F to 86°F); do not freeze. Store solution in an upright position. Stable at room temperature for up to 4 hours when solution is mixed with cold fruit juice or soda.

Transdermal patch: Store at 25°C (77°F); excursions permitted between 15°C and 30°C (59°F to 86°F). Patches should be kept in sealed pouch until use.

Mechanism of Action A deficiency of cortical acetylcholine is thought to account for some of the symptoms of Alzheimer's disease and the dementia of Parkinson's disease; rivastigmine increases acetylcholine in the central nervous system through reversible inhibition of its hydrolysis by cholinesterase

Pharmacodynamics/Kinetics

Duration: Anticholinesterase activity (CSF): ~10 hours (6 mg oral dose)

Absorption: Oral: Fasting: Rapid and complete within 1 hour; Transdermal patch: Within 30-60 minutes

Distribution: V_d: 1.8-2.7 L/kg; penetrates blood-brain barrier (CSF levels are ~40% of plasma levels following oral administration)

Protein binding: 40%

Metabolism: Extensively via cholinesterase-mediated hydrolysis in the brain; metabolite undergoes N-demethylation and/or sulfate conjugation hepatically; CYP minimally involved; linear kinetics at 3 mg twice daily, but nonlinear at higher doses

Bioavailability: Oral: 36%

Half-life elimination: Oral: 1.5 hours; Transdermal patch: ~3 hours (after removal)

Time to peak: Oral: 1 hour; Transdermal patch: 8-16 hours following first dose

Excretion: Urine (97% as metabolites); feces (0.4%)

Dosage Note: Exelon oral solution and capsules are bioequivalent.

Alzheimer's dementia, mild-to-moderate: Adults:

Oral: Initial: 1.5 mg twice daily; may increase by 3 mg daily (1.5 mg/dose) every 2 weeks based on tolerability (maximum recommended dose: 6 mg twice daily)

Low body weight: Careful titration and monitoring should be performed in patients with low body weight. In patients <50 kg, monitor closely for toxicities (eg, excessive nausea, vomiting) and consider reducing the dose if such toxicities develop.

Note: If GI adverse events occur, discontinue treatment for several doses then restart at the same or next lower dosage level; antiemetics have been used to control GI symptoms. If dosing is interrupted for ≤3 days, restart the treatment at the lowest dose and titrate as previously described.

Transdermal patch:

U.S. labeling: Initial: Apply 4.6 mg/24 hours patch once daily; if well tolerated, may titrate (no sooner than every 4 weeks) to 9.5 mg/24 hours (continue as long as therapeutically beneficial), and then to 13.3 mg/24 hours (maximum dose); doses >13.3 mg/24 hours have not been shown to be more effective and are associated with significant increases in adverse events. Remove old patch and replace with a new patch every 24 hours. Recommended effective dose: Apply 9.5 mg/24 hours or 13.3 mg/24 hours patch once daily; remove old patch and replace with a new patch every 24 hours

Canadian labeling: Initial: Apply 4.6 mg/24 hours patch once daily; if well tolerated, may titrate (no sooner than after 4 weeks) to 9.5 mg/24 hours (maximum recommended dose); continue as long as therapeutically beneficial.

Low body weight: Careful titration and monitoring should be performed in patients with low body weight. In patients <50 kg, monitor closely for toxicities (eg, excessive nausea, vomiting) and consider reducing the maintenance dose to 4.6 mg/24 hour if such toxicities develop. Consider doses >9.5 mg/24 hours in patients >100 kg.

Note: If dosing is interrupted for ≤3 days, restart treatment with the same or a lower strength patch. If interrupted for >3 days, reinitiate at 4.6 mg/24 hours and titrate (no sooner than every 4 weeks) to lowest effective maintenance dose.

Conversion from oral therapy: If oral daily dose <6 mg, switch to 4.6 mg/24 hours patch; if oral daily dose 6-12 mg, switch to 9.5 mg/24 hours patch. Apply patch on the next day following last oral dose.

Alzheimer's dementia, severe: Adults: Transdermal patch: Initial: Apply 4.6 mg/24 hours patch once daily. Titrate dose as recommended for transdermal dosing for mild-to-moderate Alzheimer's dementia. Recommended effective dose: Apply 13.3 mg/24 hours patch once daily; remove old patch and replace with a new patch every 24 hours

Low body weight: Careful titration and monitoring should be performed in patients with low body weight. In patients <50 kg, monitor closely for toxicities (eg, excessive nausea, vomiting) and consider reducing the maintenance dose to 4.6 mg/24 hour if such toxicities develop. Consider doses >9.5 mg/24 hours in patients >100 kg.

Note: If dosing is interrupted for ≤3 days, restart treatment with the same or a lower strength patch. If interrupted for >3 days, reinitiate at 4.6 mg/24 hours and titrate (no sooner than every 4 weeks) to lowest effective maintenance dose.

Parkinson's-related dementia, mild-to-moderate: Adults:

Oral: Initial: 1.5 mg twice daily; may increase by 3 mg daily (1.5 mg per dose) every 4 weeks based on tolerability (maximum recommended dose: 6 mg twice daily)

Low body weight: Careful titration and monitoring should be performed in patients with low body weight. In patients <50 kg, monitor closely for toxicities (eg, excessive nausea, vomiting) and consider reducing the dose if such toxicities develop.

Note: If GI adverse events occur, discontinue treatment for several doses then restart at the same or next lower dosage level; antiemetics have been used to control GI symptoms. If dosing is interrupted for ≤3 days, restart the treatment at the lowest dose and titrate as previously described.

Transdermal patch: Initial: Apply 4.6 mg/24 hours patch once daily. If well tolerated, may titrate (no sooner than every 4 weeks) to 9.5 mg/24 hours (continue as long as therapeutically beneficial), and then to 13.3 mg/24 hours (maximum dose); doses >13.3 mg/24 hours have not been shown to be more effective and are associated with significant increases in adverse events. Recommended effective dose: Apply 9.5 mg/24 hours or 13.3 mg/24 hours patch once daily; remove old patch and replace with a new patch every 24 hours

Low body weight: Careful titration and monitoring should be performed in patients with low body weight. In patients <50 kg, monitor closely for toxicities (eg, excessive nausea, vomiting) and consider reducing the maintenance dose to 4.6 mg/24 hour if such toxicities develop. Consider doses >9.5 mg/24 hours in patients >100 kg.

Note: If dosing is interrupted for ≤3 days, restart treatment with the same or a lower strength patch. If interrupted for >3 days, reinitiate at 4.6 mg/24 hours and titrate (no sooner than every 4 weeks) to lowest effective maintenance dose.

Dementia with Lewy bodies (unlabeled use): Adults: Oral: Initial: 1.5 mg twice daily; may increase by 3 mg daily (1.5 mg per dose) every 2 weeks based on tolerability up to a maximum of 6 mg twice daily (titration lasted up to 8 weeks); study duration was 23 weeks (McKeith, 2000). An extension study was conducted in a limited number of patients (at the same dose) for up to 96 weeks (Grace, 2001).

Elderly: Following oral administration, clearance is significantly lower in patients >60 years of age, but dosage adjustments are not recommended. Age was not associated with exposure in patients treated transdermally. Titrate dose to individual's tolerance. **Note:** Canadian labeling recommends an initial oral dose of 1.5 mg once daily in patients >85 years of age with low body weight (<50 kg) or serious comorbidities, with a slower titration rate than used for adults.

Dosage adjustment in renal impairment:

U.S. labeling:

Oral: Moderate-to-severe impairment (Cl_{cr} ≤50 mL/minute): No dosage adjustment provided in manufacturer's labeling; clearance is reduced and patients may require lower doses.

Transdermal: No dosage adjustment necessary.

Canadian labeling:

Oral: Initial dose: 1.5 mg once daily; titrate dose at a rate slower than recommended for healthy adults

Transdermal: No dosage adjustment provided in manufacturer's labeling (has not been studied); titrate dose cautiously

Dosage adjustment in hepatic impairment:

U.S. labeling:

Oral:

Mild-to-moderate impairment (Child-Pugh class A and B): No dosage adjustment provided in manufacturer's labeling; clearance is reduced and patients may require lower doses.

Severe impairment (Child-Pugh class C): No dosage adjustment provided in manufacturer's labeling (has not been studied).

Transdermal:

Mild-to-moderate impairment (Child-Pugh class A and B): Initial and maximum dose: 4.6 mg/24 hours

Severe impairment (Child-Pugh class C): No dosage adjustment provided in manufacturer's labeling (has not been studied).

Canadian labeling:
Oral:
Mild-to-moderate impairment (Child-Pugh class A and B): Initial dose: 1.5 mg once daily; titrate dose at a rate slower than recommended for healthy adults
Severe impairment (Child-Pugh class C): Use is contraindicated.
Transdermal:
Mild-to-moderate impairment (Child-Pugh class A and B): No dosage adjustment provided in manufacturer's labeling; titrate dose cautiously
Severe impairment (Child-Pugh class C): Use is contraindicated.

Administration
Oral: Administer with meals (breakfast and dinner). Capsule should be swallowed whole. Liquid form, which is available for patients who cannot swallow capsules, can be swallowed directly from syringe or mixed with water, soda, or cold fruit juice. Stir well and drink within 4 hours of mixing.
Topical: Apply transdermal patch to upper or lower back (alternatively, may apply to upper arm or chest). Do not use patch if the pouch seal is broken or if the patch is cut, altered, or damaged. Avoid reapplication to same spot of skin for 14 days (eg, may rotate sections of back). Apply to clean, dry, and hairless skin. Patch should be pressed down firmly by applying pressure with the hand over the entire patch for at least 30 seconds, making sure edges stick well. Do not apply to red, irritated, or broken skin. Avoid areas of recent application of lotion or powder. After removal, fold patch to press adhesive surfaces together, place in previously saved pouch, and discard. Avoid eye contact; wash hands after handling patch. Remove old patch and replace with a new patch every 24 hours (at the same time each day). If a dose is missed or if the patch falls off, apply a new patch immediately and replace the following day at the usual application time. Avoid exposing the patch to external sources of heat (eg, sauna, excessive light) for prolonged periods of time. No more than 1 patch should be applied daily and existing patch must be removed prior to applying new patch.

Monitoring Parameters Cognitive function at periodic intervals, symptoms of GI intolerance, weight

Dosage Forms Excipient information presented when available (limited, particularly for generics); consult specific product labeling.
Capsule, Oral:
Exelon: 1.5 mg, 3 mg, 4.5 mg, 6 mg
Generic: 1.5 mg, 3 mg, 4.5 mg, 6 mg
Patch 24 Hour, Transdermal:
Exelon: 4.6 mg/24 hr (1 ea, 30 ea); 9.5 mg/24 hr (1 ea, 30 ea); 13.3 mg/24 hr (1 ea, 30 ea)
Solution, Oral:
Exelon: 2 mg/mL (120 mL)

Dosage Forms: Canada Refer to Dosage Forms. **Note:** Exelon 13.3 mg/24 hour transdermal patch is not available in Canada.

- **Rivastigmine Tartrate** *see* Rivastigmine *on page 1841*
- **Riva-Terbinafine (Can)** *see* Terbinafine (Systemic) *on page 2017*
- **Riva-Valacyclovir (Can)** *see* ValACYclovir *on page 2145*
- **Riva-Venlafaxine XR (Can)** *see* Venlafaxine *on page 2178*
- **Riva-Verapamil SR (Can)** *see* Verapamil *on page 2182*
- **Riva-Zolmitriptan (Can)** *see* ZOLMitriptan *on page 2240*
- **Rivotril (Can)** *see* ClonazePAM *on page 465*
- **Rixubis** *see* Factor IX (Recombinant) *on page 827*

Rizatriptan (rye za TRIP tan)

Brand Names: U.S. Maxalt; Maxalt-MLT

Brand Names: Canada Apo-Rizatriptan®; CO Rizatriptan; CO Rizatriptan ODT; JAMP-Rizatriptan; Mar-Rizatriptan; Maxalt RPD™; Maxalt™; Mylan-Rizatriptan ODT; Sandoz-Rizatriptan ODT

Index Terms MK462

Pharmacologic Category Antimigraine Agent; Serotonin 5-$HT_{1B,\ 1D}$ Receptor Agonist

Additional Appendix Information
Antimigraine Drugs: 5-HT_1 Receptor Agonists *on page 2288*

Use Acute treatment of migraine with or without aura

Pregnancy Risk Factor C

Pregnancy Considerations Adverse events were observed in animal reproduction studies. Information related to rizatriptan use in pregnancy is limited (Källén, 2011; Nezvalová-Henriksen, 2010; Nezvalová-Henriksen, 2012).

A pregnancy registry has been established to monitor outcomes of women exposed to rizatriptan during pregnancy (800-986-8999). Preliminary data from the pregnancy registry (prospectively collected from 65 live births 1998-2004) does not show an increased risk of congenital malformations (Fiore, 2005). Until additional information is available, other agents are preferred for the initial treatment of migraine in pregnancy (Da Silva, 2012; MacGregor, 2012; Williams, 2012).

Breast-Feeding Considerations It is not known if rizatriptan is excreted in breast milk. The manufacturer recommends that caution be exercised when administering rizatriptan to nursing women.

Contraindications Hypersensitivity to rizatriptan or any component of the formulation; documented ischemic heart disease or other significant cardiovascular disease; coronary artery vasospasm (including Prinzmetal's angina); history of stroke or transient ischemic attack; peripheral vascular disease; ischemic bowel disease; uncontrolled hypertension; basilar or hemiplegic migraine; during or within 2 weeks of MAO inhibitors; during or within 24 hours of treatment with another 5-HT_1 agonist, or an ergot-containing or ergot-type medication (eg, methysergide, dihydroergotamine)

Warnings/Precautions Only indicated for treatment of acute migraine; not for the prevention of migraines or the treatment of cluster headache. If a patient does not respond to the first dose, the diagnosis of migraine should be reconsidered. Coronary artery vasospasm, transient ischemia, myocardial infarction, ventricular tachycardia/fibrillation, cardiac arrest, and death have been reported with 5-HT_1 agonist administration. Patients who experience sensations of chest pain/pressure/tightness or symptoms suggestive of angina following dosing should be evaluated for coronary artery disease or Prinzmetal's angina before receiving additional doses; if dosing is resumed and similar symptoms recur, monitor with ECG. Should not be given to patients who have risk factors for CAD (eg, hypertension, hypercholesterolemia, smoker, obesity, diabetes, strong family history of CAD, menopause, male >40 years of age) without adequate cardiac evaluation. Patients with suspected CAD should have cardiovascular evaluation to rule out CAD before considering use; if cardiovascular evaluation is "satisfactory," first dose should be given in the healthcare provider's office (consider ECG monitoring). Periodic evaluation of cardiovascular status should be done in all patients. Significant elevation in blood pressure, including hypertensive crisis, has also been reported on rare occasions in patients with and without a history of hypertension. Cerebral/subarachnoid hemorrhage, stroke, peripheral vascular ischemia, gastrointestinal ischemia/infarction, splenic infarction and Raynaud's syndrome have been reported with 5-HT_1 agonist administration. Use is contraindicated in patients with a history of stroke or transient ischemic attack. Rarely, partial vision loss and blindness (transient and permanent) have been reported with 5-HT_1 agonists.

Use with caution in elderly or patients with hepatic or renal impairment (including dialysis patients). Symptoms of agitation, confusion, hallucinations, hyper-reflexia, myoclonus, shivering, and tachycardia may occur with concomitant proserotonergic drugs (eg, SSRIs/SNRIs or triptans) or agents which reduce rizatriptan's metabolism. Concurrent use of serotonin precursors (eg, tryptophan) is not recommended. If concomitant administration with SSRIs is warranted, monitor closely, especially at initiation and with dose increases. Overuse of medications for acute migraine, including 5-HT_1 agonists, may lead to headache exacerbation. Maxalt-MLT® tablets contain phenylalanine.

Adverse Reactions

1% to 10%:

Cardiovascular: Chest pain (<2% to 3%), flushing (>1%), palpitation (>1%)

Central nervous system: Dizziness (4% to 9%), somnolence (4% to 8%), fatigue (adults 4% to 7%; children >1%), pain (3%), headache (≤2%), euphoria (>1%), hypoesthesia (>1%)

Dermatologic: Skin flushing

Gastrointestinal: Nausea (4% to 6%), xerostomia (3%), abdominal discomfort (children >1%), diarrhea (>1%), vomiting (>1%)

Neuromuscular & skeletal: Weakness (4% to 7%), paresthesia (3% to 4%); neck, throat, and jaw pain/tightness/pressure (≤2%), tremor (>1%)

Respiratory: Dyspnea (>1%)

Miscellaneous: Feeling of heaviness (<1% to 2%)

<1% (Limited to important or life-threatening): Anaphylaxis/anaphylactoid reactions, angina, angioedema, blurred vision, bradycardia, confusion, edema, hallucination (children), hearing impairment, hypertensive crisis, memory impairment, MI, myocardial ischemia, pruritus, seizure, syncope, tachycardia, tinnitus, tongue edema, toxic epidermal necrolysis, vasospasm, vertigo, wheezing

Drug Interactions

Metabolism/Transport Effects None known.

Avoid Concomitant Use

Avoid concomitant use of Rizatriptan with any of the following: Ergot Derivatives; MAO Inhibitors

Increased Effect/Toxicity

Rizatriptan may increase the levels/effects of: Antipsychotics; Ergot Derivatives; Metoclopramide; Serotonin Modulators

The levels/effects of Rizatriptan may be increased by: Antipsychotics; Ergot Derivatives; MAO Inhibitors; Propranolol

Decreased Effect There are no known significant interactions involving a decrease in effect.

Ethanol/Nutrition/Herb Interactions Food: Food delays absorption.

Storage/Stability Store at room temperature of 15°C to 30°C (59°F to 86°F); orally disintegrating tablets should be stored in blister pack until administration.

Mechanism of Action Selective agonist for serotonin (5-HT_{1B} and 5-HT_{1D} receptors) in cranial arteries; causes vasoconstriction and reduces sterile inflammation associated with antidromic neuronal transmission correlating with relief of migraine

Pharmacodynamics/Kinetics

Onset of action: Most patients have response to treatment within 2 hours

Distribution: V_d: Females: 110 L; Males 140 L

Protein binding: 14%

Metabolism: Via monoamine oxidase-A; forms metabolites; significant first-pass metabolism

Bioavailability: ~45%

Half-life elimination: 2-3 hours

Time to peak: Maxalt®: 1-1.5 hours (delayed up to 0.7 hour with Maxalt-MLT®)

Excretion: Urine (82%, 14% as unchanged drug); feces (12%)

Dosage Note: In patients with risk factors for coronary artery disease, following adequate evaluation to establish the absence of coronary artery disease, the initial dose should be administered in a setting where response may be evaluated (physician's office or similarly staffed setting). ECG monitoring may be considered.

Children 6-17 years: Oral: **Note:** Safety and efficacy of multiple rizatriptan doses in a 24-hour period have not been established for pediatric patients.

<40 kg: 5 mg as a single dose

≥40 kg: 10 mg as a single dose

Dose adjustment with concomitant propranolol therapy:

<40 kg: Use not recommended

≥40 kg: 5 mg as a single dose (maximum: 5 mg/24 hours)

Adults: Oral: 5-10 mg, repeat after 2 hours if significant relief is not attained; maximum: 30 mg/24 hours

Dose adjustment with concomitant propranolol therapy: 5 mg/dose (maximum: 15 mg/24 hours)

Dosage adjustment in renal impairment: No dosage adjustment provided in manufacturer's labeling; however, the AUC was 44% greater in patients on hemodialysis.

Dosage adjustment in hepatic impairment: No dosage adjustment provided in manufacturer's labeling; however, plasma concentrations are increased by 30% in patients with moderate hepatic dysfunction.

Dietary Considerations Some products may contain phenylalanine.

Administration May be administered with or without food. For orally-disintegrating tablets (Maxalt-MLT®), patient should be instructed to place tablet on tongue and allow to dissolve. Dissolved tablet will be swallowed with saliva.

Monitoring Parameters Headache severity, signs/symptoms suggestive of angina; consider monitoring blood pressure, heart rate, and/or ECG with first dose in patients with likelihood of unrecognized coronary disease, such as patients with significant hypertension, hypercholesterolemia, obese patients, patients with diabetes, smokers with other risk factors or strong family history of coronary artery disease

Dosage Forms Excipient information presented when available (limited, particularly for generics); consult specific product labeling.

Tablet, Oral:

Maxalt: 5 mg, 10 mg

Generic: 5 mg, 10 mg

Tablet Dispersible, Oral:

Maxalt-MLT: 5 mg, 10 mg [contains aspartame; peppermint flavor]

Generic: 5 mg, 10 mg

◆ **rLFN-α2** *see* Interferon Alfa-2b *on page 1099*

◆ **R-modafinil** *see* Armodafinil *on page 167*

◆ **Ro 5488** *see* Tretinoin (Systemic) *on page 2117*

◆ **RO5185426** *see* Vemurafenib *on page 2176*

◆ **RoActemra** *see* Tocilizumab *on page 2080*

◆ **Robafen [OTC]** *see* GuaiFENesin *on page 974*

◆ **Robafen AC** *see* Guaifenesin and Codeine *on page 976*

◆ **Robafen DM [OTC]** *see* Guaifenesin and Dextromethorphan *on page 976*

◆ **Robaxin** *see* Methocarbamol *on page 1322*

◆ **Robaxin® (Can)** *see* Methocarbamol *on page 1322*

Rocuronium (roe kyoor OH nee um)

Brand Names: U.S. Zemuron

Brand Names: Canada Rocuronium Bromide Injection; Zemuron®

Index Terms ORG 9426; Rocuronium Bromide

Pharmacologic Category Neuromuscular Blocker Agent, Nondepolarizing

Additional Appendix Information

Dosing Considerations for the Critically-Ill Patient With Morbid Obesity *on page 2379*

Use Facilitate both rapid sequence and routine endotracheal intubation and to relax skeletal muscles during surgery; to facilitate mechanical ventilation in ICU patients

Pregnancy Risk Factor C

Pregnancy Considerations Teratogenic effects were not observed in animal reproduction studies. Rocuronium crosses the placenta; umbilical venous plasma levels are ~18% of the maternal concentration following a maternal dose of 0.6 mg/kg (Abouleish, 1994). The manufacturer does not recommend use for rapid sequence induction during cesarean section.

Breast-Feeding Considerations Information related to rocuronium use and breast-feeding has not been located. If present in breast milk, oral absorption by a nursing infant would be expected to be minimal (Lee, 1993).

Contraindications Hypersensitivity (eg, anaphylaxis) to rocuronium, other neuromuscular-blocking agents, or any component of the formulation

Warnings/Precautions Use with caution in patients with cardiovascular disease and pulmonary disease; ventilation must be supported during neuromuscular blockade; certain clinical conditions may result in potentiation or antagonism of neuromuscular blockade:

Potentiation: Electrolyte abnormalities, severe hyponatremia, severe hypocalcemia, severe hypokalemia, hypermagnesemia, cachexia, neuromuscular diseases, metabolic acidosis, metabolic alkalosis, Eaton-Lambert syndrome, and myasthenia gravis

Antagonism: Respiratory alkalosis, hypercalcemia, demyelinating lesions, peripheral neuropathies, denervation, infection, and muscle trauma

Use with caution in patients with hepatic impairment; clinical duration may be prolonged. Resistance may occur in burn patients (>30% of body) for period of 5-70 days postinjury or in immobilized patients. Cross-sensitivity with other neuromuscular-blocking agents may occur; use is contraindicated in patients with previous anaphylactic reactions to other neuromuscular blockers. Use with caution in patients with pulmonary hypertension or valvular heart disease. Use caution in the elderly. Should be administered by adequately trained individuals familiar with its use. Use appropriate anesthesia, pain control, and sedation. In patients requiring long-term administration in the ICU, use of a peripheral nerve stimulator to monitor drug effects is strongly recommended. Additional doses of rocuronium or any other neuromuscular-blocking agent should be avoided unless definite excessive response to nerve stimulation is present.

Some patients may experience prolonged recovery of neuromuscular function after administration (especially after prolonged use). Patients should be adequately recovered prior to extubation. Other factors associated with prolonged recovery should be considered (eg, corticosteroid use, patient condition). In addition to prolonging recovery from neuromuscular blockade, concomitant use with corticosteroids has been associated with development of acute quadriplegic myopathy syndrome (AQMS). Current guidelines recommend neuromuscular blockers be discontinued as soon as possible in patients receiving corticosteroids or interrupted daily until necessary to restart them based on clinical condition (Murray, 2002). Numerous drugs either *antagonize* (eg, acetylcholinesterase inhibitors) or *potentiate* (eg, calcium channel blockers, certain antimicrobials, inhalation anesthetics, lithium, magnesium salts, procainamide, and quinidine) the effects of neuromuscular blockade; use with caution in patients receiving these agents. Immediate treatment (including epinephrine 1:1000) for anaphylactoid and/or hypersensitivity reactions should be available during use. Not recommended by the manufacturer for rapid sequence intubation in pediatric patients; however, it has been used successfully in clinical trials for this indication. If extravasation occurs, local irritation may ensue; discontinue administration immediately and restart in another vein.

Adverse Reactions

>1%: Cardiovascular: Hypertension (≤2%), hypotension (transient; ≤2%)

<1% (Limited to important or life-threatening): Abnormal ECG, anaphylactoid reaction, anaphylaxis, arrhythmia, bronchospasm, injection site edema, hiccups, pruritus, nausea, pulmonary vascular resistance (increased), rash, rhonchi, shock, tachycardia, vomiting, wheezing

Drug Interactions

Metabolism/Transport Effects None known.

Avoid Concomitant Use

Avoid concomitant use of Rocuronium with any of the following: QuiNINE

Increased Effect/Toxicity

Rocuronium may increase the levels/effects of: Cardiac Glycosides; Corticosteroids (Systemic); OnabotulinumtoxinA; RimabotulinumtoxinB

The levels/effects of Rocuronium may be increased by: AbobotulinumtoxinA; Aminoglycosides; Calcium Channel Blockers; Capreomycin; Colistimethate; CycloSPORINE (Systemic); Fosphenytoin-Phenytoin; Inhalational Anesthetics; Ketorolac (Nasal); Ketorolac (Systemic); Lincosamide Antibiotics; Lithium; Loop Diuretics; Magnesium Salts; Polymyxin B; Procainamide; QuiNIDine; QuiNINE; Spironolactone; Tetracycline Derivatives; Vancomycin

Decreased Effect

The levels/effects of Rocuronium may be decreased by: Acetylcholinesterase Inhibitors; Fosphenytoin-Phenytoin; Loop Diuretics

Storage/Stability Store unopened/undiluted vials under refrigeration at 2°C to 8°C (36°F to 46°F); do not freeze. When stored at room temperature, it is stable for 60 days; once opened, use within 30 days. Dilutions up to 5 mg/mL in 0.9% sodium chloride, dextrose 5% in water, 5% dextrose in sodium chloride 0.9%, or lactated Ringer's are stable for up to 24 hours at room temperature.

Mechanism of Action Blocks acetylcholine from binding to receptors on motor endplate inhibiting depolarization

Pharmacodynamics/Kinetics

Onset of action: Good intubation conditions within 1-2 minutes (depending on dose administered); maximum neuromuscular blockade within 4 minutes

Duration: ~30 minutes (with standard doses, increases with higher doses and inhalational anesthetic agents; patient age dependent)

Distribution: V_d: ~0.25 L/kg

Protein binding: ~30%

Metabolism: Minimally hepatic; 17-desacetylrocuronium (5% to 10% activity of parent drug)

Half-life elimination: 60-144 minutes

Excretion: Feces (50%); urine (30%)

Dosage Dose to effect; doses will vary due to interpatient variability. Dosing also dependent on anesthetic technique and age of patient.

Infants 28 days to 3 months and Children ≥3 months:

Note: In general, onset is shortened and duration is prolonged as dose increases. Duration is shortest in children >2 to ≤11 years and longest in neonates and infants.

Rapid sequence intubation (unlabeled use): I.V.: 0.9 mg/kg or 1.2 mg/kg. Not recommended, per the manufacturer, for rapid sequence intubation in pediatric patients; however, it has been used successfully in clinical trials for this indication in children >1 year of age (Cheng, 2002; Fuchs-Buder, 1996; Mazurek, 1998; Naguib, 1997).

Tracheal intubation: I.V.: 0.45 mg/kg or 0.6 mg/kg

Maintenance for continued surgical relaxation: I.V.: 0.075-0.15 mg/kg; redosing interval is guided by monitoring with a peripheral nerve stimulator **or** 7-12 **mcg**/kg/**minute** (0.42-0.72 **mg**/kg/**hour**) as a continuous infusion; use lower end of the continuous infusion dosing range for neonates and infants up to age 28 days and the upper end for children >2 to ≤11 years of age

Adults:

Rapid sequence intubation: I.V.: 0.6-1.2 mg/kg

Obesity: In adult patients with morbid obesity (BMI >40 kg/m^2), the use of 1.2 mg/kg using ideal body weight (IBW) provided a short onset of action and excellent or good intubating conditions at 60 seconds in one study (Gaszynski, 2011).

Tracheal intubation: I.V.:

Initial: 0.45-0.6 mg/kg; administration of 0.3 mg/kg may also provide optimal conditions for tracheal intubation (Barclay, 1997)

Obesity: May use ideal body weight (IBW) for morbidly obese (BMI >40 kg/m^2) adult patients (Leykin, 2004); onset time may be slightly delayed using IBW. The manufacturer recommends dosing based on actual body weight in all obese patients.

Maintenance for continued surgical relaxation: 0.1-0.2 mg/kg; repeat as needed **or** a continuous infusion of 10-12 **mcg**/kg/**minute** (0.6-0.72 **mg**/kg/**hour**) only after recovery of neuromuscular function is evident; infusion rates have ranged from 4-16 **mcg**/kg/**minute** (0.24-0.96 **mg**/kg/**hour**)

Note: Inhaled anesthetic agents prolong the duration of action of rocuronium. Use lower end of the dosing range; redosing interval guided by monitoring with a peripheral nerve stimulator.

Preinduction defasciculating dose: I.V.: 0.03-0.06 mg/kg given 1.5-3 minutes before administration of succinylcholine (Harvey, 1998; Martin, 1998)

ICU paralysis (eg, facilitate mechanical ventilation) in selected adequately sedated patients (Greenberg, 2013; Murray, 2002; Rudis, 1996; Sparr, 1997; Warr, 2011): Initial bolus dose: 0.6-1 mg/kg, then a continuous I.V. infusion of 8-12 **mcg**/kg/**minute** (0.48-0.72 **mg**/kg/**hour**); monitor depth of blockade every 2-3 hours initially until stable dose, then every 8-12 hours; adjust rate of administration by 10% increments according to peripheral nerve stimulation response or desired clinical response

Note: When possible, minimize depth and duration of paralysis. Stopping the infusion for some time until forced to restart based on patient condition is recommended to reduce post-paralytic complications (eg, acute quadriplegic myopathy syndrome [AQMS]) (Murray, 2002).

Intermittent dosing has also been described with an initial loading dose of 50 mg followed by 25 mg given when peripheral nerve stimulation returns (Sparr, 1997).

Dosage adjustment in renal impairment: No dosage adjustment necessary. Duration of neuromuscular blockade may vary in patients with renal impairment.

Dosage adjustment in hepatic impairment: No dosage adjustment provided in manufacturer's labeling. However, dosage reductions may be necessary in patients with liver disease; duration of neuromuscular blockade may be prolonged due to increased volume of distribution. When rapid sequence intubation is required in adult patients with ascites, a dose on the higher end of the dosage range may be necessary to achieve adequate neuromuscular blockade.

Administration Administer I.V. only; may be administered undiluted as a bolus injection or via a continuous infusion using an infusion pump

Monitoring Parameters Peripheral nerve stimulator measuring twitch response, heart rate, blood pressure, assisted ventilation status

Additional Information Rocuronium is classified as an intermediate-duration neuromuscular-blocking agent. Do not mix in the same syringe with barbiturates. Rocuronium does not relieve pain or produce sedation.

Dosage Forms Excipient information presented when available (limited, particularly for generics); consult specific product labeling.

Solution, Intravenous, as bromide:

Zemuron: 50 mg/5 mL (5 mL); 100 mg/10 mL (10 mL)

Generic: 50 mg/5 mL (5 mL); 100 mg/10 mL (10 mL)

Solution, Intravenous, as bromide [preservative free]:

Generic: 50 mg/5 mL (5 mL); 100 mg/10 mL (10 mL)

◆ **Rocuronium Bromide** *see* Rocuronium *on page 1846*

◆ **Rocuronium Bromide Injection (Can)** *see* Rocuronium *on page 1846*

◆ **Rofact™ (Can)** *see* Rifampin *on page 1811*

Roflumilast (roe FLUE mi last)

Brand Names: U.S. Daliresp

Brand Names: Canada Daxas™

Pharmacologic Category Phosphodiesterase-4 Enzyme Inhibitor

Use Adjunct to bronchodilator therapy in the maintenance treatment of severe chronic obstructive pulmonary disease (COPD) associated with chronic bronchitis

Pregnancy Risk Factor C

Pregnancy Considerations Animal studies have demonstrated reproductive toxicity (incomplete ossification, postimplantive losses) at doses greater than the human recommended dose. There are no adequate and well controlled studies in pregnant women. Avoid use during pregnancy.

Breast-Feeding Considerations Roflumilast and/or its metabolites are excreted into the breast milk of lactating rats. Excretion into human breast milk is likely. Avoid use while breast-feeding.

Medication Guide Available Yes

Contraindications Moderate or severe hepatic impairment (Child-Pugh class B or C)

Canadian labeling: Additional contraindication (not in U.S. labeling): Hypersensitivity to roflumilast or any component of the formulation

Warnings/Precautions Not indicated for relieving acute bronchospasms or for use as monotherapy of COPD; use only as adjunctive therapy to bronchodilator therapy. Neuropsychiatric effects (eg, anxiety, depression) have been reported with use; rarely, suicidal behavior/ ideation and completed suicide were reported. Avoid use in patients with a history of depression with suicidal behavior/ideations; instruct patients/caregivers to report psychiatric symptoms and consider discontinuation of therapy in such patients. Systemic exposure may be increased in patients with mild hepatic impairment; use in moderate-to-severe impairment is contraindicated.

May cause weight loss and/or diarrhea (sometimes severe); weight loss usually observed within 6 months of initiating therapy and diarrhea within 4 weeks. Instruct patients to monitor weight regularly. Avoid initiation of therapy or discontinue therapy with unexplained/pronounced weight loss.

Adverse Reactions

2% to 10%:

Central nervous system: Headache (4%), dizziness (2%), insomnia (2%)

Endocrine & metabolic: Weight loss (5% to 10% of body weight: 8% to 20%; >10% loss: 7%)

Gastrointestinal: Diarrhea (10%), nausea (5%), decreased appetite (2%)

Infection: Influenza (3%)

Neuromuscular & skeletal: Back pain (3%)

<2% (Limited to important or life-threatening): Abdominal pain, anemia, arthritis, atrial fibrillation, depression, dysgeusia, epistaxis, gastritis, gastroesophageal reflux disease, gynecomastia, hematochezia, hypersensitivity, increased gamma-glutamyl transferase, increased lactate dehydrogenase, increased serum AST, lung carcinoma, muscle spasm, myalgia, myasthenia, pancreatitis, paresthesia, prostate carcinoma, renal failure, respiratory tract infection, rhinitis, sinusitis, suicidal ideation, suicidal tendencies, suicide completed, supraventricular cardiac arrhythmia, urinary tract infection

Drug Interactions

Metabolism/Transport Effects Substrate of CYP1A2 (minor), CYP3A4 (major); **Note:** Assignment of Major/ Minor substrate status based on clinically relevant drug interaction potential

Avoid Concomitant Use

Avoid concomitant use of Roflumilast with any of the following: CYP3A4 Inducers (Strong); Rifampin

Increased Effect/Toxicity

Roflumilast may increase the levels/effects of: Immunosuppressants

The levels/effects of Roflumilast may be increased by: Cimetidine; Ciprofloxacin (Systemic); FluvoxaMINE

Decreased Effect

The levels/effects of Roflumilast may be decreased by: Bosentan; CYP3A4 Inducers (Strong); Dabrafenib; Deferasirox; Herbs (CYP3A4 Inducers); Rifampin

Storage/Stability Store at 20°C to 25°C (68°F to 77°F), excursions permitted from 15°C to 30°C (59°F to 86°F).

Mechanism of Action Roflumilast and its active N-oxide metabolite selectively inhibit phosphodiesterase-4 (PDE4) leading to an accumulation of cyclic AMP (cAMP) within inflammatory and structural cells important in the pathogenesis of COPD. Anti-inflammatory effects include suppression of cytokine release and inhibition of lung infiltration by neutrophils and other leukocytes. Pulmonary remodeling and mucociliary malfunction are also attenuated.

Pharmacodynamics/Kinetics

Distribution: V_d: 2.9 L/kg

Protein binding: 99%; N-oxide metabolite: 97%

Metabolism: Hepatic via CYP3A4 and CYP1A2 to active N-oxide metabolite; also undergoes conjugation

Bioavailability: ~80%

Half-life elimination: 17 hours; N-oxide metabolite: 30 hours

Time to peak: ~1 hour (delayed by food); N-oxide metabolite: ~8 hours

Excretion: Urine (~70% as metabolites)

Dosage Oral: Adults: COPD: 500 mcg once daily

Dosage adjustment in renal impairment: No dosage adjustment necessary.

Dosage adjustment in hepatic impairment:

Mild impairment (Child-Pugh class A): No dosage adjustment necessary. Use with caution; 500 mcg once daily dose has not been evaluated in mild impairment.

Moderate-to-severe impairment (Child-Pugh class B or C): Use is contraindicated.

Dietary Considerations May be given with or without food.

Administration Administer without regard to meals.

Monitoring Parameters Liver function tests. Measure weight regularly during therapy

Dosage Forms Excipient information presented when available (limited, particularly for generics); consult specific product labeling.

Tablet, Oral:

Daliresp: 500 mcg

Dosage Forms: Canada Excipient information presented when available (limited, particularly for generics); consult specific product labeling.

Tablet, oral:

Daxas™: 500 mcg

◆ **Rogaine® (Can)** *see* Minoxidil (Topical) *on page 1375*

◆ **Rogaine Mens Extra Strength [OTC]** *see* Minoxidil (Topical) *on page 1375*

◆ **Rogitine® (Can)** *see* Phentolamine *on page 1634*

◆ **Rolene (Can)** *see* Betamethasone *on page 247*

◆ **Romazicon (Can)** *see* Flumazenil *on page 877*

RomiDEPsin (roe mi DEP sin)

Brand Names: U.S. Istodax

Index Terms Depsipeptide; FK228; FR901228

Pharmacologic Category Antineoplastic Agent, Histone Deacetylase Inhibitor

Use Treatment of refractory cutaneous T-cell lymphoma (CTCL) and refractory peripheral T-cell lymphoma (PTCL)

Pregnancy Risk Factor D

Pregnancy Considerations Adverse events were observed in animal reproduction studies. Based on the mechanism of action, romidepsin may cause fetal harm if administered during pregnancy.

Breast-Feeding Considerations According to the manufacturer, the decision to continue or discontinue breast-feeding during therapy should take into account the risk of exposure to the infant and the benefits of treatment to the mother.

Contraindications There are no contraindications listed within the manufacturer's labeling.

Warnings/Precautions Hazardous agent - use appropriate precautions for handling and disposal (NIOSH, 2012). Anemia, leukopenia, neutropenia, lymphopenia and thrombocytopenia may occur; may require dosage modification; monitor blood counts during treatment. Serious infections (occasionally fatal), including pneumonia and sepsis have occurred during or within 30 days of treatment; the risk of life-threatening infection is increased in patients who have received prior intensive or extensive chemotherapy. QT_c prolongation has been observed; use caution in patients with a history of QT_c prolongation, congenital long QT syndrome, with medications known to prolong the QT interval, or with pre-existing cardiac disease. Obtain baseline and periodic ECG (12-lead); monitor and correct electrolyte (potassium, magnesium, and calcium) abnormalities prior to and during treatment. T-wave and ST-segment changes have also been reported. Use with caution in patients with moderate-to-severe hepatic impairment or end-stage renal disease. Avoid use with strong CYP3A4 inhibitors or inducers. Use with caution with moderate CYP3A4 inhibitors and P-glycoprotein inhibitors. Tumor lysis syndrome (TLS) has been observed; closely monitor patients with advanced disease and/or with a high tumor burden; if TLS occurs, initiate appropriate treatment.

Adverse Reactions

>10%:

Cardiovascular: ST-T wave changes (2% to 63%), hypotension (7% to 23%)

Central nervous system: Fatigue (53% to 77%), fever (20% to 47%), headache (15% to 34%), chills (11% to 17%)

Dermatologic: Pruritus (7% to 31%), dermatitis/exfoliative dermatitis (4% to 27%)

Endocrine & metabolic: Hypocalcemia (4% to 52%), hyperglycemia (2% to 51%), hypoalbuminemia (3% to 48%), hyperuricemia (≤33%), hypomagnesemia (22% to 28%), hypermagnesemia (≤27%), hypophosphatemia (≤27%), hypokalemia (6% to 20%), hyponatremia (≤20%)

Gastrointestinal: Nausea (56% to 86%; grades 3/4: 2% to 6%), anorexia (23% to 54%), vomiting (34% to 52%; grades 3/4: ≤10%), taste alteration (15% to 40%), constipation (12% to 40%), diarrhea (20% to 36%), weight loss (10% to 15%), abdominal pain (13% to 14%)

Hematologic: Anemia (19% to 72%; grades 3/4: 3% to 28%), thrombocytopenia (17% to 72%; grades 3/4: ≤36%), neutropenia (11% to 66%; grades 3/4: 4% to 47%), lymphopenia (4% to 57%; grades 3/4: ≤37%), leukopenia (4% to 55%; grades 3/4: ≤45%)

Hepatic: AST increased (3% to 28%), ALT increased (3% to 22%)

Neuromuscular & skeletal: Weakness (53% to 77%)

Respiratory: Cough (18% to 21%), dyspnea (13% to 21%)

Miscellaneous: Infection (46% to 54%; grades 3/4: 11% to 33%)

1% to 10%:

Cardiovascular: Peripheral edema (6% to 10%), tachycardia (≤10%), chest pain, DVT, edema, QT prolongation, supraventricular arrhythmia, syncope, ventricular arrhythmia

Dermatologic: Cellulitis

Endocrine & metabolic: Dehydration

Gastrointestinal: Stomatitis (6% to 10%)

Hematologic: Neutropenic fever

Hepatic: Hyperbilirubinemia

Respiratory: Hypoxia, pneumonia, pneumonitis, pulmonary embolism

Miscellaneous: Central line infection, hypersensitivity, sepsis, tumor lysis syndrome (1% to 2%)

<1% (Limited to important or life-threatening): Acute renal failure, acute respiratory distress syndrome, atrial fibrillation, bacteremia, candida infection, cardiopulmonary failure, cardiogenic shock, Epstein-Barr virus reactivation, multiorgan failure, septic shock

Drug Interactions

Metabolism/Transport Effects Substrate of CYP3A4 (major), P-glycoprotein; **Note:** Assignment of Major/Minor substrate status based on clinically relevant drug interaction potential

Avoid Concomitant Use

Avoid concomitant use of RomiDEPsin with any of the following: CYP3A4 Inducers (Strong); Highest Risk QTc-Prolonging Agents; Ivabradine; Mifepristone; Rifampin

Increased Effect/Toxicity

RomiDEPsin may increase the levels/effects of: Highest Risk QTc-Prolonging Agents; Moderate Risk QTc-Prolonging Agents; Warfarin

The levels/effects of RomiDEPsin may be increased by: CYP3A4 Inhibitors (Strong); Ivabradine; Mifepristone; P-glycoprotein/ABCB1 Inhibitors; QTc-Prolonging Agents (Indeterminate Risk and Risk Modifying); Rifampin

Decreased Effect

The levels/effects of RomiDEPsin may be decreased by: Bosentan; CYP3A4 Inducers (Strong); Dabrafenib; Deferasirox; Herbs (CYP3A4 Inducers); P-glycoprotein/ABCB1 Inducers; Tocilizumab

Ethanol/Nutrition/Herb Interactions

Food: Avoid grapefruit juice (may increase the levels/effects of romidepsin).

Herb/Nutraceutical: Avoid St John's wort (may increase metabolism and decrease romidepsin concentrations).

Preparation for Administration Hazardous agent; use appropriate precautions for handling and disposal (NIOSH, 2012). Reconstitute each 10 mg vial with 2 mL of supplied diluent to a reconstituted concentration of 5 mg/mL; swirl until dissolved. (**Note:** Although the reconstituted vial contains a final volume of 2 mL, due to the viscosity of the reconstituted solution, a total volume <2 mL [usually ~1.6-1.8 mL] can be withdrawn from each vial.) Further dilute in 500 mL normal saline; compatible with polyvinyl chloride (PVC), ethylene vinyl acetate (EVA), polyethylene (PE) and glass infusion containers.

Storage/Stability Store intact vials at room temperature of 20°C to 25°C (68°F to 77°F); excursions permitted between 15°C and 30°C (59°F and 86°F). The reconstituted solution is stable for 8 hours at room temperature. Solutions diluted for infusion are stable for 24 hours at room temperature; however, the manufacturer recommends use as soon as possible after dilution.

Mechanism of Action Histone deacetylase inhibitor; catalyzes acetyl group removal from protein lysine residues (including histone and transcription factors). Inhibition of histone deacetylase results in accumulation of acetyl groups, leading to alterations in chromatin structure and transcription factor activation causing termination of cell growth (induces arrest in cell cycle at G_1 and G_2/M phases) leading to cell death.

Pharmacodynamics/Kinetics

Protein binding: 92% to 94%; primarily to α_1-acid glycoprotein

Metabolism: Hepatic, primarily via CYP3A4, minor metabolism from CYP3A5, 1A1, 2B6, and 2C19

Half-life elimination: ~3 hours

Dosage I.V.: Adults:

Cutaneous T-cell lymphoma: 14 mg/m² days 1, 8, and 15 of a 28-day treatment cycle; repeat cycle as long as benefit continues and treatment is tolerated

Peripheral T-cell lymphoma: 14 mg/m² days 1, 8, and 15 of a 28-day treatment cycle; repeat cycle as long as benefit continues and treatment is tolerated

Dosage adjustment for toxicity:

Nonhematologic toxicity (excluding alopecia):

Grade 2 or 3: Delay treatment until toxicity returns to ≤grade 1 or baseline, may restart at 14 mg/m²

Grade 4 or recurrent grade 3 toxicity: Delay treatment until toxicity returns to ≤grade 1 or baseline, permanently reduce dose to 10 mg/m²

Recurrent grade 3 or 4 toxicity despite dosage reduction: Discontinue treatment

Hematologic toxicity:

Grade 3 or 4 neutropenia or thrombocytopenia: Delay treatment until ANC ≥1500/mm³ and/or platelets ≥75,000/mm³ or baseline, may restart at 14 mg/m²

Grade 4 febrile neutropenia or thrombocytopenia requiring platelet transfusion: Delay treatment until toxicity returns to ≤grade 1 or baseline, permanently reduce dose to 10 mg/m²

Dosage adjustment in renal impairment: No dosage adjustment provided in manufacturer's labeling (has not been studied). However, dosage adjustment unlikely since pharmacokinetics are unaffected by renal impairment. Use with caution in patients with end-stage renal disease (has not been studied).

Dosage adjustment in hepatic impairment:

Mild impairment: No dosage adjustment provided in manufacturer's labeling. However, Mild hepatic impairment does not significantly influence the pharmacokinetics of romidepsin.

Moderate or severe impairment: No dosage adjustment provided in manufacturer's labeling.. Use with caution.

Dosing in obesity: *ASCO Guidelines for appropriate chemotherapy dosing in obese adults with cancer:* Utilize patient's actual body weight (full weight) for calculation of body surface area- or weight-based dosing, particularly when the intent of therapy is curative; manage regimen-related toxicities in the same manner as for nonobese patients; if a dose reduction is utilized due to toxicity, consider resumption of full weight-based dosing with subsequent cycles, especially if cause of toxicity (eg, hepatic or renal impairment) is resolved (Griggs, 2012).

Dietary Considerations Avoid grapefruit juice.

Administration Infuse over 4 hours. Antiemetics to prevent nausea and vomiting were used in clinical trials (Piekarz, 2009; Piekarz, 2011).

Hazardous agent; use appropriate precautions for handling and disposal (NIOSH, 2012).

Monitoring Parameters Serum electrolytes (baseline and periodic; especially potassium and magnesium); CBC with differential and platelets, ECG (baseline and periodic; in patients with significant cardiovascular disease, congenital long QT syndrome, and in patients taking QT-prolonging medications); signs/symptoms of infection or tumor lysis syndrome

Dosage Forms Excipient information presented when available (limited, particularly for generics); consult specific product labeling.

Solution Reconstituted, Intravenous:

Istodax: 10 mg (1 ea) [contains alcohol, usp, propylene glycol]

RomiPLOStim (roe mi PLOE stim)

Brand Names: U.S. Nplate

Brand Names: Canada Nplate®

Index Terms AMG 531

Pharmacologic Category Colony Stimulating Factor; Thrombopoietic Agent

Use Treatment of thrombocytopenia in patients with chronic immune thrombocytopenia (ITP) who have had insufficient response to corticosteroids, immune globulin, or splenectomy

Note: Should be used only when the degree of thrombocytopenia and clinical condition increase the risk for bleeding; should not be used in attempt to normalize platelet counts; **not** indicated for the treatment of thrombocytopenia due to myelodysplastic syndrome or any cause of thrombocytopenia other than chronic ITP.

Pregnancy Risk Factor C

Pregnancy Considerations Adverse effects were observed in animal reproduction studies. Use during pregnancy only if the potential benefit to the mother outweighs the potential risk to the fetus. The Nplate® pregnancy registry has been established to monitor outcomes of women exposed to romiplostim during pregnancy (1-800-772-6436).

Breast-Feeding Considerations It is not known if romiplostim is excreted in breast milk. According to the manufacturer, the decision to discontinue romiplostim or discontinue breast-feeding during therapy should take into account the benefits of treatment to the mother.

Medication Guide Available Yes

Contraindications There are no contraindications listed within the manufacturer's labeling.

Warnings/Precautions May increase the risk for bone marrow reticulin formation or progression. In patients where reticulin formation occurred, doses were ≥5 mcg/kg. A baseline peripheral blood smear is recommended prior to treatment to establish baseline level of cellular morphologic abnormalities, then monthly (after stable dose achieved) for new or worsening abnormalities (teardrop or nucleated RBC, immature WBCs) or cytopenias. Progression to marrow fibrosis with cytopenias was not observed in clinical trials, although the risk has not been excluded. Onset of new or worsening cellular abnormalities or cytopenias may warrant therapy discontinuation and subsequent bone marrow biopsy. Thromboembolism or thrombotic complications may occur with increased platelets; maintain appropriate platelet levels with dosage adjustments; portal vein thrombosis has been reported in patients with chronic liver disease; use with caution in patients with a history of cerebrovascular disease and in ITP patients with chronic liver disease. Progression of underlying myelodysplastic syndrome (MDS) to acute myeloid leukemia (AML) has been observed in MDS clinical trials (not indicated for the treatment of thrombocytopenia due to MDS). An increase in the percentage of circulating myeloblasts in peripheral blood smears was also noted (both in patients who progressed to AML and in those who did not); blast cells decreased to baseline after discontinuation in some patients.

Inadequate platelet response may be due to neutralizing antibodies (to romiplostim or TPO) or bone marrow fibrosis. Indicated only when the degree of thrombocytopenia and clinical conditions increase the risk for bleeding; use the lowest dose necessary to achieve and maintain platelet count ≥50,000/mm³. Do not use to normalize platelet counts. Discontinue if platelet count does not respond to a level to avoid clinically important bleeding after 4 weeks at the maximum recommended dose. May be used in combination with other therapies for ITP, including corticosteroids, danazol, azathioprine, immune globulin, or Rho(D) immune globulin; not indicated for the treatment of thrombocytopenia due to any cause other than chronic ITP. Reduce dose or discontinue ITP medications when platelet count ≥50,000/mm^3. Lack of response or failure to maintain platelet response should trigger investigation in to causative factors, including neutralizing antibodies to romiplostim.

Overdose may result in thrombotic/thromboembolic complications due to excessive platelet levels; underdose may result in lack of platelet response and potential for bleeding. Use caution when calculating dose and appropriate volume for administration (volume may be very small; administer with syringe that allows for 0.01 mL graduations).

Upon discontinuation of therapy, thrombocytopenia may worsen. Severity may be greater than pretreatment level. Risk of bleeding is increased, particularly in patients receiving anticoagulants or antiplatelet agents; monitor CBCs and platelet counts weekly for at least 2 weeks after discontinuation. Rebound thrombocytopenia generally resolves within 14 days.

Use with caution in patients with hepatic and renal impairment (has not been studied).

Adverse Reactions

>10%:

Central nervous system: Headache (35%), dizziness (17%), insomnia (16%)

Gastrointestinal: Abdominal pain (11%)

Hematologic: Circulating myeloblasts increased (MDS patients: 17%)

Neuromuscular & skeletal: Arthralgia (26%), myalgia (14%), limb pain (13%)

1% to 10%:

Gastrointestinal: Dyspepsia (7%)

Hematologic: Rebound thrombocytopenia (7%), AML (MDS patients: 4% to 6%), bone marrow reticulin formation/deposition (4%)

Neuromuscular & skeletal: Shoulder pain (8%), paresthesia (6%)

Miscellaneous: Antibody formation (romiplostim 6%; TPO 4%)

<1% (Limited to important or life-threatening): Angioedema, erythromelalgia, hypersensitivity, marrow fibrosis with collagen, thromboembolism, thrombotic complications

Drug Interactions

Metabolism/Transport Effects None known.

Avoid Concomitant Use There are no known interactions where it is recommended to avoid concomitant use.

Increased Effect/Toxicity There are no known significant interactions involving an increase in effect.

Decreased Effect There are no known significant interactions involving a decrease in effect.

Preparation for Administration Reconstitute with preservative free SWFI (add 0.72 mL to 250 mcg vial or 1.2 mL to 500 mcg vial) to a final concentration of 500 mcg/mL. Gently invert vial and swirl; do not shake. Usually dissolves within 2 minutes.

Storage/Stability Store intact vials refrigerated at 2°C to 8°C (36°F to 46°F); do not freeze. Protect from light. Store in original carton until use. Reconstituted solution may be stored at room temperature of 25°C (77°F) or refrigerated at 2°C to 8°C (36°F to 46°F) for up to 24 hours prior to administration. Protect reconstituted solution from light; discard any unused portion.

Mechanism of Action Thrombopoietin (TPO) peptide mimetic which increases platelet counts in ITP by binding to and activating the human TPO receptor.

Pharmacodynamics/Kinetics

Onset of action: Platelet count increase: SubQ: 4-9 days; Peak platelet count increase: Days 12-16

Duration: Platelet counts return to baseline by day 28

Absorption: SubQ: Slow

Half-life elimination: Median: 3.5 days (range: 1-34 days)

Time to peak, plasma: SubQ: Median: 14 hours (range: 7-50 hours)

Dosage Note: Initial dose is based on actual body weight. Use the lowest dose sufficient to maintain platelet count ≥50,000/mm^3 as necessary to reduce the risk of bleeding. Adjust dose based on platelet count response; discontinue if platelet count does not respond to a level that avoids clinically important bleeding after 4 weeks at the maximum recommended dose.

SubQ: Adults: Chronic ITP: Initial: 1 mcg/kg once weekly; adjust dose by 1 mcg/kg/week increments to achieve platelet count ≥50,000/mm^3 and to reduce the risk of bleeding; Maximum dose: 10 mcg/kg/week (median dose needed to achieve response in clinical trials: 2 mcg/kg)

Dosage adjustment recommendations:

Platelet count <50,000/mm^3: Increase weekly dose by 1 mcg/kg

Platelet count >200,000/mm^3 for 2 consecutive weeks: Reduce weekly dose by 1 mcg/kg

Platelet count >400,000/mm^3: Withhold dose; assess platelet count weekly; when platelet count <200,000/mm^3, resume with the weekly dose reduced by 1 mcg/kg

Dosage adjustment in renal impairment: No dosage adjustment provided in manufacturer's labeling (has not been studied)

Dosage adjustment in hepatic impairment: No dosage adjustment provided in manufacturer's labeling (has not been studied)

Dietary Considerations Some products may contain sucrose.

Administration Administer SubQ. Administration volume may be small; use appropriate syringe (with graduations to 0.01 mL) for administration. Verify calculations, final concentration, and volume drawn up for administration.

Monitoring Parameters CBC with differential and platelets (baseline, during treatment [weekly until platelet response stable for at least 4 weeks then monthly] and weekly for at least 2 weeks following completion of treatment)

Evaluate for neutralizing antibodies in patients with inadequate response (blood samples may be submitted to Amgen for assay [1-800-772-6436]).

Reference Range Target platelet count of 50,000-200,000/mm^3; platelet life span: 8-11 days

Additional Information Restricted access to Nplate® was previously a REMS requirement via the Nplate® NEXUS (Network of Experts Understanding and Supporting Nplate® and Patients) program. Patients, prescribers, and pharmacies were required to be enrolled in this program. However, the FDA eliminated this REMS requirement in December 2011. There is currently no restricted access to obtaining Nplate®.

Dosage Forms Excipient information presented when available (limited, particularly for generics); consult specific product labeling.

Solution Reconstituted, Subcutaneous [preservative free]: Nplate: 250 mcg (1 ea); 500 mcg (1 ea)

◆ **Romycin** *see* Erythromycin (Ophthalmic) *on page* 744

ROPINIRole (roe PIN i role)

Brand Names: U.S. Requip; Requip XL

Brand Names: Canada CO Ropinirole; JAMP-Ropinirole; PMS-Ropinirole; RAN™-Ropinirole; Requip®

Index Terms Ropinirole Hydrochloride

Pharmacologic Category Anti-Parkinson's Agent, Dopamine Agonist

Additional Appendix Information

Antiparkinsonian Agents *on page 2289*

Use Treatment of idiopathic Parkinson's disease; in patients with early Parkinson's disease who were not receiving concomitant levodopa therapy as well as in patients with advanced disease on concomitant levodopa; treatment of moderate-to-severe primary Restless Legs Syndrome (RLS)

Pregnancy Risk Factor C

Pregnancy Considerations Adverse events were observed in animal reproduction studies. Information related to the use of ropinirole for the treatment of restless legs syndrome (RLS) in pregnant women is limited. Current guidelines note that the available information is insufficient to make a recommendation for use in pregnant women (Aurora, 2012; Dostal, 2013).

Breast-Feeding Considerations It is not known if ropinirole is excreted into breast milk. Ropinirole inhibits prolactin secretion in humans and may potentially inhibit lactation. Due to the potential for serious adverse reactions, the manufacturer recommends that a decision be made whether to discontinue nursing or discontinue the drug, taking into account the importance of the drug to the mother.

Contraindications Hypersensitivity to ropinirole or any component of the formulation

Warnings/Precautions Syncope, sometimes associated with bradycardia, was observed in association with ropinirole in both early Parkinson's disease (without levodopa) patients and advanced Parkinson's disease (with levodopa) patients. Dopamine agonists appear to impair the systemic regulation of blood pressure resulting in postural hypotension, especially during dose escalation. Parkinson's disease patients appear to have an impaired capacity to respond to a postural challenge; use with caution in patients at risk of hypotension (ie, those receiving antihypertensive or antiarrhythmic drugs) or where transient hypotensive episodes would be poorly tolerated (cardiovascular disease or cerebrovascular disease). Parkinson's patients being treated with dopaminergic agonists ordinarily require careful monitoring for signs and symptoms of postural hypotension, especially during dose escalation, and should be informed of this risk.

May cause hallucinations (dose dependent); risk may be increased in the elderly. Use with caution in patients with pre-existing dyskinesia, hepatic or severe renal dysfunction (use in patients with severe renal impairment and who are not undergoing regular hemodialysis is not recommended in the Canadian labeling). Avoid use in patients with a major psychotic disorder; may exacerbate psychosis.

Patients treated with ropinirole have reported falling asleep while engaging in activities of daily living; this has been reported to occur without significant warning signs. Monitor for daytime somnolence or pre-existing sleep disorder; caution with concomitant sedating medication; discontinue if significant daytime sleepiness or episodes of falling asleep occur. Patients must be cautioned about performing tasks which require mental alertness (eg, operating machinery or driving). Use with caution in patients receiving other CNS depressants or psychoactive agents. Effects with other sedative drugs or ethanol may be potentiated.

Dopamine agonists have been associated with compulsive behaviors and/or loss of impulse control, which has manifested as pathological gambling, libido increases (hypersexuality), and/or binge eating. Causality has not been established, and controversy exists as to whether this phenomenon is related to the underlying disease, prior behaviors/addictions and/or drug therapy. Dose reduction or discontinuation of therapy has been reported to reverse these behaviors in some, but not all cases. Risk for melanoma development is increased in Parkinson's disease patients; drug causation or factors contributing to risk have not been established. Patients should be monitored closely and periodic skin examinations should be performed.

Some patients treated for RLS may experience worsening of symptoms in the early morning hours (rebound) or an increase and/or spread of daytime symptoms (augmentation); clinical management of these phenomena has not been evaluated in controlled clinical trials. Pathologic degenerative changes were observed in the retinas of albino rats during studies with this agent, but were not observed in the retinas of albino mice or in other species. The significance of these data for humans remains uncertain.

Other dopaminergic agents have been associated with a syndrome resembling neuroleptic malignant syndrome on withdrawal or significant dosage reduction after long-term use. Risk of fibrotic complications (eg, pleural effusion/fibrosis, interstitial lung disease) and melanoma has been reported in patients receiving ropinirole; drug causation has not been established.

Adverse Reactions

Data inclusive of trials in early Parkinson's disease (without levodopa) and Restless Legs Syndrome:

>10%:

- Cardiovascular: Syncope (1% to 12%)
- Central nervous system: Somnolence (11% to 40%), dizziness (6% to 40%), fatigue (8% to 11%)
- Gastrointestinal: Nausea (immediate release: 40% to 60%; extended release: 19%), vomiting (11% to 12%)
- Miscellaneous: Viral infection (11%)

1% to 10%:

- Cardiovascular: Dependent/leg edema (2% to 7%), orthostasis (1% to 6%), hypertension (5%), chest pain (4%), flushing (3%), palpitation (3%), peripheral ischemia (2% to 3%), atrial fibrillation (2%), extrasystoles (2%), hypotension (2%), tachycardia (2%)
- Central nervous system: Pain (3% to 8%), headache (extended release: 6%), confusion (5%), hallucinations (up to 5%; dose related), hypoesthesia (4%), amnesia (3%), malaise (3%), yawning (3%), concentration impaired (2%), vertigo (2%)
- Dermatologic: Hyperhidrosis (3%)
- Gastrointestinal: Dyspepsia (4% to 10%), abdominal pain (3% to 7%), constipation (≥5%), xerostomia (3% to 5%), diarrhea (5%), anorexia (4%), flatulence (3%)
- Genitourinary: Urinary tract infection (5%), impotence (3%)
- Hepatic: Alkaline phosphatase increased (3%)
- Neuromuscular & skeletal: Weakness (6%), arthralgia (4%), muscle cramps (3%), paresthesia (3%), hyperkinesia (2%)
- Ocular: Abnormal vision (6%), xerophthalmia (2%)
- Respiratory: Pharyngitis (6% to 9%), rhinitis (4%), sinusitis (4%), bronchitis (3%), dyspnea (3%), influenza (3%), cough (3%), nasal congestion (2%)
- Miscellaneous: Diaphoresis increased (3% to 6%)

Advanced Parkinson's disease (with levodopa):

>10%:

- Central nervous system: Dizziness (immediate release: 26%; extended-release: 8%), somnolence (immediate release: 20%, extended release: 7%), headache (17%)
- Gastrointestinal: Nausea (immediate release: 30%; extended-release: 11%)
- Neuromuscular & skeletal: Dyskinesias (immediate release: 34%; extended-release: 13%; dose related)

1% to 10%:

- Cardiovascular: Hypotension (2% to 5%; including orthostatic), peripheral edema (4%), syncope (3%), hypertension (3%; dose related)

Central nervous system: Hallucinations (7% to 10%; dose related), confusion (9%), anxiety (2% to 6%), amnesia (5%), nervousness (5%), pain (5%), vertigo (4%), abnormal dreaming (3%), paresis (3%), aggravated parkinsonism, insomnia

Gastrointestinal: Abdominal pain (6% to 9%), vomiting (7%), constipation (4% to 6%), diarrhea (3% to 5%), xerostomia (2% to 5%), dysphagia (2%), flatulence (2%), salivation increased (2%), weight loss (2%)

Genitourinary: Urinary tract infection (6%), pyuria (2%), urinary incontinence (2%)

Hematologic: Anemia (2%)

Neuromuscular & skeletal: Falls (2% to 10%; dose related), arthralgia (7%), tremor (6%), hypokinesia (5%), paresthesia (5%), arthritis (3%), back pain (3%)

Ocular: Diplopia (2%)

Respiratory: Upper respiratory tract infection (9%), dyspnea (3%)

Miscellaneous: Injury, diaphoresis increased (7%), viral infection, increased drug level (7%)

Other adverse effects (all phase 2/3 trials for Parkinson's disease and Restless Leg Syndrome):

≥1%: Asthma, BUN increased, depression, gastroenteritis, gastrointestinal reflux, irritability, migraine, muscle spasm, myalgia, neck pain, neuralgia, osteoarthritis, pharyngolaryngeal pain, rash, rigors, sleep disorder, tendonitis

<1% (Limited to important or life-threatening): Abnormal coordination, acidosis, agitation, aneurysm, angina, aphasia, behavioral disorders, bradycardia, bundle branch block, cardiac arrest, cardiac failure, cardiac valvulopathy, cardiomegaly, cellulitis, cholecystitis, cholelithiasis, choreoathetosis, colitis, coma, conjunctival hemorrhage, dehydration, delusion, delirium, diabetes mellitus, diverticulitis, Dupuytren's contracture, dysphonia, electrolyte disturbances, eosinophilia, extrapyramidal symptoms, gangrene, gastrointestinal hemorrhage, gastrointestinal ulceration, glaucoma, goiter, gynecomastia, hematuria, hemiparesis, hemiplegia, hepatitis (ischemic), hyperbilirubinemia, hypercholesterolemia, hyper-/hypothyroidism, hyper-/hypotonia, hypoglycemia, hyponatremia, hyperphosphatemia, hypersensitivity reactions (angioedema, pruritus), hyperuricemia, impulsive/compulsive behaviors (eg, pathological gambling, hypersexuality, binge eating), infections (bacterial, viral, or fungal); interstitial lung disease, intestinal obstruction, leukocytosis, leukopenia, limb embolism, liver enzymes increased, lymphadenopathy, lymphedema, lymphocytosis, lymphopenia, menstrual abnormalities, mitral insufficiency, MI, neoplasms (various), pancreatitis, paralysis, paranoia, peripheral neuropathy, photosensitivity, pleural effusion, pleural fibrosis, proteinuria, psychiatric disorders, pulmonary edema, pulmonary embolism, renal calculus, renal failure (acute), seizure, sepsis, SIADH, skin disorders, stomatitis, stupor, subarachnoid hemorrhage, suicide attempt, SVT, thrombocytopenia, thrombosis, tinnitus, tongue edema, torticollis, urticaria, vagina/uterine hemorrhage, ventricular tachycardia, visual disturbances

Drug Interactions

Metabolism/Transport Effects Substrate of CYP1A2 (major), CYP3A4 (minor); **Note:** Assignment of Major/Minor substrate status based on clinically relevant drug interaction potential; **Inhibits** CYP1A2 (weak), CYP2D6 (weak)

Avoid Concomitant Use

Avoid concomitant use of ROPINIRole with any of the following: Amisulpride; Sulpiride

Increased Effect/Toxicity

The levels/effects of ROPINIRole may be increased by: Abiraterone Acetate; Alcohol (Ethyl); Ciprofloxacin (Systemic); CNS Depressants; CYP1A2 Inhibitors (Moderate); CYP1A2 Inhibitors (Strong); Deferasirox; Estrogen Derivatives; MAO Inhibitors; Methylphenidate; Vemurafenib

Decreased Effect

ROPINIRole may decrease the levels/effects of: Amisulpride; Antipsychotics (Typical); Sulpiride

The levels/effects of ROPINIRole may be decreased by: Amisulpride; Antipsychotics (Atypical); Antipsychotics (Typical); CYP1A2 Inducers (Strong); Cyproterone; Metoclopramide; Sulpiride

Ethanol/Nutrition/Herb Interactions

Ethanol: Avoid ethanol (may increase CNS depression).

Herb/Nutraceutical: Avoid kava kava, gotu kola, valerian, St John's wort (may increase CNS depression).

Storage/Stability Store at controlled room temperature of 20°C to 25°C (68°F to 77°F). Protect from light.

Mechanism of Action Ropinirole has a high relative *in vitro* specificity and full intrinsic activity at the D_2 and D_3 dopamine receptor subtypes, binding with higher affinity to D_3 than to D_2 or D_4 receptor subtypes; relevance of D_3 receptor binding in Parkinson's disease is unknown. Ropinirole has moderate *in vitro* affinity for opioid receptors. Ropinirole and its metabolites have negligible *in vitro* affinity for dopamine D_1, 5-HT_1, 5-HT_2, benzodiazepine, GABA, muscarinic, $alpha_1$-, $alpha_2$-, and beta-adrenoreceptors. Although precise mechanism of action of ropinirole is unknown, it is believed to be due to stimulation of postsynaptic dopamine D_2-type receptors within the caudate putamen in the brain. Ropinirole caused decreases in systolic and diastolic blood pressure at doses >0.25 mg. The mechanism of ropinirole-induced postural hypotension is believed to be due to D_2-mediated blunting of the noradrenergic response to standing and subsequent decrease in peripheral vascular resistance.

Pharmacodynamics/Kinetics

Absorption: Not affected by food

Distribution: V_d: 525 L

Protein binding: 40%

Metabolism: Extensively hepatic via CYP1A2 to inactive metabolites; first-pass effect

Bioavailability: Absolute: 45% to 55%

Half-life elimination: ~6 hours

Time to peak: Immediate release: ~1-2 hours; Extended release: 6-10 hours; T_{max} increased by 2.5-3 hours when drug taken with food

Excretion: Urine (<10% as unchanged drug, 60% as metabolites)

Clearance: Reduced by 15% to 30% in patients >65 years of age

Dosage Oral: Adults:

Parkinson's disease:

Immediate release tablet: The dosage should be increased to achieve a maximum therapeutic effect, balanced against the principal side effects of nausea, dizziness, somnolence and dyskinesia. Recommended starting dose is 0.25 mg 3 times/day; based on individual patient response, the dosage should be titrated with weekly increments as described below:

- Week 1: 0.25 mg 3 times/day; total daily dose: 0.75 mg
- Week 2: 0.5 mg 3 times/day; total daily dose: 1.5 mg
- Week 3: 0.75 mg 3 times/day; total daily dose: 2.25 mg
- Week 4: 1 mg 3 times/day; total daily dose: 3 mg

Note: After week 4, if necessary, daily dosage may be increased by 1.5 mg/day on a weekly basis up to a dose of 9 mg/day, and then by up to 3 mg/day weekly to a total of 24 mg/day

Parkinson's disease discontinuation taper: Ropinirole should be gradually tapered over 7 days as follows: reduce frequency of administration from 3 times daily to twice daily for 4 days, then reduce to once daily for remaining 3 days.

Extended release tablet: Initial: 2 mg once daily for 1-2 weeks, followed by increases of 2 mg/day at weekly or longer intervals based on therapeutic response and tolerability (maximum: 24 mg/day); **Note:** When discontinuing gradually taper over 7 days.

Restless legs syndrome: Immediate release tablets: Initial: 0.25 mg once daily 1-3 hours before bedtime. Dose may be increased after 2 days to 0.5 mg daily, and after 7 days to 1 mg daily. Dose may be further titrated upward in 0.5 mg increments every week until reaching a daily dose of 3 mg during week 6. If symptoms persist or reappear, the daily dose may be increased to a maximum of 4 mg beginning week 7.

Note: Doses up to 4 mg per day may be discontinued without tapering.

Converting from ropinirole immediate release tablets to ropinirole extended-release tablets: Choose a once daily extended-release dose that most closely matches current immediate-release daily dose.

Elderly: Clearance is reduced; however, no dosage adjustment necessary. Titrate dose to clinical response. Refer to adult dosing.

Dosage adjustment in renal impairment:

Moderate renal impairment (Cl_{cr} 30-50 mL/minute): No dosage adjustment necessary.

Severe renal impairment (Cl_{cr} <30 mL/minute): No dosage adjustment provided in manufacturer's labeling (has not been studied). Use with caution. **Note:** The Canadian labeling recommends to avoid use in patients with severe renal impairment and who are not undergoing regular hemodialysis.

Hemodialysis: Canadian labeling (not in U.S. labeling): Initial: 0.25 mg 3 times daily; may titrate dose upward based on tolerability and efficacy (maximum dose: 18 mg daily); postdialysis supplemental doses are not required

Dosage adjustment in hepatic impairment: No dosage adjustment provided in manufacturer's labeling (has not been studied). Titrate with caution.

Dietary Considerations May be taken without regard to meals; taking with food may reduce nausea.

Administration May be administered without regard to meals; taking with food may reduce nausea. Swallow extended-release tablet whole; do not crush, split, or chew.

Monitoring Parameters Blood pressure (orthostatic); daytime alertness

Additional Information If therapy with a drug known to be a potent inhibitor of CYP1A2 is stopped or started during treatment with ropinirole, adjustment of ropinirole dose may be required. Ropinirole binds to melanin-containing tissues (ie, eyes, skin) in pigmented rats. After a single dose, long-term retention of drug was demonstrated, with a half-life in the eye of 20 days; not known if ropinirole accumulates in these tissues over time.

Dosage Forms Excipient information presented when available (limited, particularly for generics); consult specific product labeling.

Tablet, Oral:

Requip: 0.25 mg, 0.5 mg, 1 mg, 2 mg, 3 mg, 4 mg, 5 mg [contains fd&c blue #2 aluminum lake, fd&c yellow #6 aluminum lake, polysorbate 80]

Generic: 0.25 mg, 0.5 mg, 1 mg, 2 mg, 3 mg, 4 mg, 5 mg

Tablet Extended Release 24 Hour, Oral:

Requip XL: 2 mg, 4 mg, 6 mg, 8 mg, 12 mg [contains fd&c blue #2 aluminum lake, fd&c yellow #6 aluminum lake]

Generic: 2 mg, 4 mg, 6 mg, 8 mg, 12 mg

◆ Ropinirole Hydrochloride *see* ROPINIRole *on page 1851*

Ropivacaine (roe PIV a kane)

Brand Names: U.S. Naropin

Brand Names: Canada Naropin®; Ropivacaine Hydrochloride Injection, USP

Index Terms Ropivacaine Hydrochloride

Pharmacologic Category Local Anesthetic

Use Local anesthetic for use in surgery, postoperative pain management, and obstetrical procedures when local or regional anesthesia is needed

Pregnancy Risk Factor B

Pregnancy Considerations Teratogenic events were not observed in animal studies. When used for epidural block during labor and delivery, systemically absorbed ropivacaine may cross the placenta, resulting in varying degrees of fetal or neonatal effects (eg, CNS or cardiovascular depression). Fetal or neonatal adverse events include fetal bradycardia (12%), neonatal jaundice (8%), low Apgar scores (3%), fetal distress (2%), neonatal respiratory disorder (3%). Maternal hypotension may also result from systemic absorption. In cases of hypotension, position pregnant woman in left lateral decubitus position to prevent aortocaval compression by the gravid uterus. Epidural anesthesia may prolong the second stage of labor.

Breast-Feeding Considerations It is not known if ropivacaine is excreted into breast milk; however, exposure to a nursing infant is expected to be low. The manufacturer recommends that caution be exercised when administering ropivacaine to nursing women.

Contraindications Hypersensitivity to ropivacaine, amide-type local anesthetics (eg, bupivacaine, mepivacaine, lidocaine), or any component of the formulation

Warnings/Precautions Careful and constant monitoring of the patient's state of consciousness should be done following each local anesthetic injection; at such times, restlessness, anxiety, tinnitus, dizziness, blurred vision, tremors, depression, or drowsiness may be early warning signs of CNS toxicity. Treatment is primarily symptomatic and supportive. Intravascular injections should be avoided. Continuous intra-articular infusion of local anesthetics after arthroscopic or other surgical procedures is **not** an approved use; chondrolysis (primarily in the shoulder joint) has occurred following infusion, with some cases requiring arthroplasty or shoulder replacement. Local anesthetics have been associated with rare occurrences of sudden respiratory arrest, seizures, and cardiac arrest. When administering this agent, have ready access to drugs and equipment for resuscitation. Use with caution in patients with liver disease, cardiovascular disease, neurological or psychiatric disorders, and in the elderly or debilitated; these patients may be at greater risk for toxicity. Cardiovascular adverse events (bradycardia, hypotension) may be age-related (more common in patients >61 years of age). Use caution in patients on type III antiarrhythmics (eg, amiodarone); consider ECG monitoring since cardiac effects may be additive. Use cautiously in hypotension, hypovolemia, or heart block. Ropivacaine is not recommended for use in emergency situations where rapid administration is necessary. Safety and efficacy have not been established in pediatric patients.

Adverse Reactions

>10%:

Cardiovascular: Hypotension (dose-related and age-related: 32% to 69%), bradycardia (6% to 20%)

Gastrointestinal: Nausea (11% to 29%), vomiting (7% to 14%)

Neuromuscular & skeletal: Back pain (7% to 16%)

1% to 10%:
- Cardiovascular: Hypertension, tachycardia, chest pain (1% to 5%)
- Central nervous system: Fever (3% to 9%), headache (5% to 8%), dizziness (3%), chills (2% to 3%), anxiety (1%), lightheadedness
- Dermatologic: Pruritus (1% to 5%)
- Endocrine & metabolic: Hypokalemia
- Genitourinary: Urinary retention (1% to 5%), urinary tract infection (1% to 5%)
- Hematologic: Anemia (6%)
- Neuromuscular & skeletal: Paresthesia (2% to 6%), hypoesthesia, rigors, circumoral paresthesia
- Renal: Oliguria
- Respiratory: Dyspnea
- Miscellaneous: Shivering

<1% (Limited to important or life-threatening): Accidental I.V. injection (0.2%), angioedema, allergic reaction, apnea (usually associated with epidural block in head/neck region), bronchospasm, cardiac arrest, cardiovascular collapse, chondrolysis (continuous intra-articular administration), dyskinesia, hallucination, hyperthermia, laryngeal edema, myocardial depression, MI, rash, seizure, syncope, tinnitus, urticaria, ventricular arrhythmia

Drug Interactions

Metabolism/Transport Effects Substrate of CYP1A2 (major), CYP2B6 (minor), CYP2D6 (minor), CYP3A4 (minor); **Note:** Assignment of Major/Minor substrate status based on clinically relevant drug interaction potential

Avoid Concomitant Use There are no known interactions where it is recommended to avoid concomitant use.

Increased Effect/Toxicity

The levels/effects of Ropivacaine may be increased by: Abiraterone Acetate; Ciprofloxacin (Systemic); CYP1A2 Inhibitors (Moderate); CYP1A2 Inhibitors (Strong); Deferasirox; FluvoxaMINE; Hyaluronidase; Propofol; Vemurafenib

Decreased Effect

Ropivacaine may decrease the levels/effects of: Technetium Tc 99m Tilmanocept

The levels/effects of Ropivacaine may be decreased by: Peginterferon Alfa-2b

Storage/Stability Store at 20°C to 25°C (68°F to 77°F). Infusions should be discarded after 24 hours.

Mechanism of Action Blocks both the initiation and conduction of nerve impulses by decreasing the neuronal membrane's permeability to sodium ions, which results in inhibition of depolarization with resultant blockade of conduction

Pharmacodynamics/Kinetics

Onset of action: Anesthesia (route dependent): 3-15 minutes

Duration (dose and route dependent): 3-15 hours

Metabolism: Hepatic, via CYP1A2 to metabolites

Half-life elimination: Epidural: 5-7 hours; I.V.: Terminal: 111 ± 62 minutes (Lee, 1989)

Excretion: Urine (86% as metabolites)

Dosage Dose varies with procedure, onset and depth of anesthesia desired, vascularity of tissues, duration of anesthesia, and condition of patient: Adults:

Surgical anesthesia:
- Lumbar epidural: 15-30 mL of 0.5% to 1% solution
- Lumbar epidural block for cesarean section:
  - 20-30 mL dose of 0.5% solution
  - 15-20 mL dose of 0.75% solution
- Thoracic epidural block: 5-15 mL dose of 0.5% or 0.75% solution
- Major nerve block:
  - 35-50 mL dose of 0.5% solution (175-250 mg)
  - 10-40 mL dose of 0.75% solution (75-300 mg)
- Field block: 1-40 mL dose of 0.5% solution (5-200 mg)

Labor pain management: Lumbar epidural: Initial: 10-20 mL 0.2% solution; continuous infusion dose: 6-14 mL/hour of 0.2% solution with incremental injections of 10-15 mL/hour of 0.2% solution

Postoperative pain management:
- Peripheral nerve block: Continuous infusion dose: 5-10 mL/hour of 0.2% solution (Bagry, 2008; Klein, 2000)
- Lumbar or thoracic epidural: Continuous infusion dose: 6-14 mL/hour of 0.2% solution
- Infiltration/minor nerve block:
  - 1-100 mL dose of 0.2% solution
  - 1-40 mL dose of 0.5% solution

Dosage adjustment in renal impairment: No dosage adjustment provided in manufacturer's labeling. However, ropivacaine and its metabolites are renally excreted, and the risk of toxic reactions may be greater.

Dosage comment in hepatic impairment: No dosage adjustment provided in manufacturer's labeling. Use with caution since patients may be at a greater risk for developing toxic drug levels.

Administration Administered via local infiltration, epidural block and epidural infusion, or intermittent bolus

Monitoring Parameters Heart rate, blood pressure, ECG monitoring (if used with antiarrhythmics)

Dosage Forms Excipient information presented when available (limited, particularly for generics); consult specific product labeling.

Solution, Injection [preservative free]:
- Naropin: 5 mg/mL (30 mL)

Solution, Injection, as hydrochloride [preservative free]:
- Naropin: 2 mg/mL (10 mL, 20 mL, 100 mL, 200 mL); 5 mg/mL (20 mL, 30 mL, 100 mL, 200 mL); 7.5 mg/mL (20 mL); 10 mg/mL (10 mL, 20 mL)

◆ **Ropivacaine Hydrochloride** *see* Ropivacaine *on page 1854*

◆ **Ropivacaine Hydrochloride Injection, USP (Can)** *see* Ropivacaine *on page 1854*

◆ **Rosadan** *see* MetroNIDAZOLE (Topical) *on page 1354*

◆ **Rosanil** *see* Sulfur and Sulfacetamide *on page 1966*

◆ **Rosasol® (Can)** *see* MetroNIDAZOLE (Topical) *on page 1354*

Rosiglitazone (roh si GLI ta zone)

Brand Names: U.S. Avandia

Brand Names: Canada Avandia

Pharmacologic Category Antidiabetic Agent, Thiazolidinedione

Additional Appendix Information

Oral Antidiabetic Agents Comparison Table *on page 2312*

Use Type 2 diabetes: Adjunct to diet and exercise to improve glycemic control in adults with type 2 diabetes mellitus (noninsulin dependent, NIDDM); may be used as monotherapy or in combination with metformin or a sulfonylurea.

Pregnancy Risk Factor C

Pregnancy Considerations Adverse effects were observed in initial animal reproduction studies. Rosiglitazone has been found to cross the placenta during the first trimester of pregnancy. Inadvertent use early in pregnancy has not been shown to increase the risk of adverse fetal effects, although in the majority of cases, the medication was stopped as soon as pregnancy was detected (Chan, 2005; Kalyoncu, 2005; Yaris, 2004). For women with diabetes, maternal hyperglycemia itself can be associated with adverse effects in the fetus, neonate, and mother. To prevent adverse events, prior to conception and throughout pregnancy the maternal Hb A_{1c} should be kept close to normal but without causing significant hypoglycemia. Maternal hyperglycemia can be associated with adverse effects in the mother. The use of thiazolidinediones in pregnant women is not recommended; insulin is the drug of choice for the control of diabetes mellitus during pregnancy (ACOG, 2005; ADA, 2013; Kitzmiller, 2008; Metzger, 2007).

Thiazolidinediones may cause ovulation in anovulatory premenopausal women, increasing the risk of pregnancy; adequate contraception in premenopausal women is recommended. Insulin-sensitizing agents, including rosiglitazone, have been evaluated for the treatment of polycystic ovary syndrome (POS) (ASRM, 2008). However, due to long-term safety concerns associated with their use, thiazolidinediones should be avoided in women of reproductive age (Fauser, 2012).

Breast-Feeding Considerations It is not known if rosiglitazone is excreted in breast milk. Although breast-feeding is encouraged for all women, including those with diabetes, the safety of rosiglitazone during breast-feeding has not yet been established (Metzger, 2007). Breast-feeding is not recommended by the manufacturer.

Prescribing and Access Restrictions As a requirement of the REMS program, the prescribing and dispensing of any rosiglitazone-containing medication in the U.S. requires physician and patient enrollment in the Avandia-Rosiglitazone Medicines Access Program™. Complete program details are available at www.avandia.com or by calling the program Coordinating Center at 800-282-6342.

Health Canada requires written informed consent for new and current patients receiving rosiglitazone.

Medication Guide Available Yes

Contraindications

U.S. labeling: NYHA Class III/IV heart failure (initiation of therapy)

Canadian labeling: Hypersensitivity to rosiglitazone or any component of the formulation; any stage of heart failure (eg, NYHA Class I, II, III, IV); serious hepatic impairment; pregnancy

Warnings/Precautions [U.S. Boxed Warning]: Thiazolidinediones, including rosiglitazone, may cause or exacerbate congestive heart failure; closely monitor for signs/symptoms of congestive heart failure (eg, rapid weight gain, dyspnea, edema), particularly after initiation or dose increases. If heart failure develops, treat accordingly and consider dose reduction or discontinuation. Not recommended for use in any patient with symptomatic heart failure. In the U.S., initiation of therapy is contraindicated in patients with NYHA class III or IV heart failure; in Canada use is contraindicated in patients with any stage of heart failure (NYHA class I, II, III, IV). Use with caution in patients with edema; may increase plasma volume and/or cause fluid retention, leading to heart failure. Monitor for signs/symptoms of heart failure. Dose-related weight gain observed with use; mechanism unknown but likely associated with fluid retention and fat accumulation. Use may also be associated with an increased risk of angina and MI. Use caution in patients at risk for cardiovascular events and monitor closely. Discontinue if any deterioration in cardiac status occurs.

[U.S. Boxed Warning]: Due to cardiovascular risks, rosiglitazone-containing medications are only available through the Avandia-Rosiglitazone Medicines Access Program™. Patients and prescribers must be registered with and meet conditions of the program. Call 1-800-282-6342 or visit www.avandia.com for more information.

Should not be used in diabetic ketoacidosis. Mechanism requires the presence of insulin; therefore, use in type 1 diabetes (insulin dependent, IDDM) is not recommended. It may be necessary to discontinue therapy and administer insulin if the patient is exposed to stress (fever, trauma, infection, surgery). Do not initiate in patients with stable ischemic heart disease due to an increased risk of cardiovascular complications (Fihn, 2012).

Potentially significant drug-drug interactions may exist, requiring dose or frequency adjustment, additional monitoring, and/or selection of alternative therapy.

Use with caution in patients with elevated transaminases (AST or ALT); do not initiate in patients with active liver disease or ALT >2.5 times ULN at baseline; evaluate patients with ALT ≤2.5 times ULN at baseline or during therapy for cause of enzyme elevation; during therapy, if ALT >3 times ULN, reevaluate levels promptly and discontinue if elevation persists or if jaundice occurs at any time during use. Idiosyncratic hepatotoxicity has been reported with another thiazolidinedione agent (troglitazone); avoid use in patients who previously experienced jaundice during troglitazone therapy. Monitoring should include periodic determinations of liver function. Increased incidence of bone fractures in females treated with rosiglitazone observed during analysis of long-term trial; majority of fractures occurred in the upper arm, hand, and foot (differing from the hip or spine fractures usually associated with postmenopausal osteoporosis). May decrease hemoglobin/hematocrit and/or WBC count (slight); effects may be related to increased plasma volume and/or dose related; use with caution in patients with anemia; may reduce hemoglobin and hematocrit.

Rosiglitazone has been associated with new onset and/or worsening of macular edema in patients with diabetes. Rosiglitazone should be used with caution in patients with a pre-existing macular edema or diabetic retinopathy. Discontinuation of rosiglitazone should be considered in any patient who reports visual deterioration. In addition, ophthalmological consultation should be initiated in these patients. Use with caution in premenopausal, anovulatory women; may result in resumption of ovulation, increasing the risk of pregnancy.

Additional Canadian warnings (not included in U.S. labeling): If glycemic control is inadequate, rosiglitazone may be added to metformin or a sulfonylurea (if metformin use is contraindicated or not tolerated); use of triple therapy (rosiglitazone in combination with both metformin and a sulfonylurea) is not indicated due to increased risks of heart failure and fluid retention.

Adverse Reactions Note: The rate of certain adverse reactions (eg, anemia, edema, hypoglycemia) may be higher with some combination therapies.

>10%: Endocrine & metabolic: HDL-cholesterol increased, LDL-cholesterol increased, total cholesterol increased, weight gain

1% to 10%:

Cardiovascular: Edema (5%), hypertension (4%); heart failure/CHF (up to 2% to 3% in patients receiving insulin; incidence likely higher in patients with pre-existing HF; myocardial ischemia (3%; incidence likely higher in patients with pre-existing CAD)

Central nervous system: Headache (6%)

Endocrine & metabolic: Hypoglycemia (1% to 3%; combination therapy with insulin: 12% to 14%)

Gastrointestinal: Diarrhea (3%)

Hematologic: Anemia (2%)

Neuromuscular & skeletal: Fractures (up to 9%; incidence greater in females; usually upper arm, hand, or foot), arthralgia (5%), back pain (4% to 5%)

Respiratory: Upper respiratory tract infection (4% to 10%), nasopharyngitis (6%)

Miscellaneous: Injury (8%)

<1% (Limited to important or life-threatening): Anaphylaxis, angina, angioedema, bilirubin increased, blurred vision, cardiac arrest, dyspnea, coronary artery disease, coronary thrombosis, hematocrit decreased, hemoglobin decreased, hepatic failure, hepatitis, HDL-cholesterol decreased, jaundice (reversible), macular edema, MI, pleural effusion, pruritus, pulmonary edema, rash, Stevens-Johnson syndrome, thrombocytopenia, transaminases increased, urticaria, visual acuity decreased, weight gain (rapid, excessive; usually due to fluid accumulation), WBC count decreased

Note: Rare cases of hepatocellular injury have been reported in men in their 60s within 2-3 weeks after initiation of rosiglitazone therapy. LFTs in these patients revealed severe hepatocellular injury which responded with rapid improvement of liver function and resolution of symptoms upon discontinuation of rosiglitazone. Patients were also receiving other potentially hepatotoxic medications (Al-Salman, 2000; Freid, 2000).

Drug Interactions

Metabolism/Transport Effects Substrate of CYP2C8 (major), CYP2C9 (minor); **Note:** Assignment of Major/Minor substrate status based on clinically relevant drug interaction potential; **Inhibits** CYP2C19 (weak), CYP2C8 (moderate), CYP2C9 (weak)

Avoid Concomitant Use There are no known interactions where it is recommended to avoid concomitant use.

Increased Effect/Toxicity

Rosiglitazone may increase the levels/effects of: CYP2C8 Substrates; Hypoglycemic Agents

The levels/effects of Rosiglitazone may be increased by: CYP2C8 Inhibitors (Moderate); CYP2C8 Inhibitors (Strong); Deferasirox; Gemfibrozil; Herbs (Hypoglycemic Properties); Insulin; MAO Inhibitors; Mifepristone; Pegvisomant; Pregabalin; Salicylates; Selective Serotonin Reuptake Inhibitors; Trimethoprim; Vasodilators (Organic Nitrates)

Decreased Effect

The levels/effects of Rosiglitazone may be decreased by: Bile Acid Sequestrants; Corticosteroids (Orally Inhaled); Corticosteroids (Systemic); CYP2C8 Inducers (Strong); Dabrafenib; Loop Diuretics; Luteinizing Hormone-Releasing Hormone Analogs; Rifampin; Somatropin; Thiazide Diuretics

Ethanol/Nutrition/Herb Interactions

Ethanol: Ethanol may cause hypoglycemia. Management: Avoid ethanol during therapy.

Herb/Nutraceutical: Concurrent use of some herbal products may enhance hypoglycemic effects. Management: Avoid alfalfa, aloe, bilberry, bitter melon, burdock, celery, damiana, fenugreek, garcinia, garlic, ginger, ginseng (American), gymnema, marshmallow, stinging nettle.

Storage/Stability Store at 25°C (77°F); excursions are permitted between 15°C and 30°C (59°F and 86°F). Protect from light.

Mechanism of Action Thiazolidinedione antidiabetic agent that lowers blood glucose by improving target cell response to insulin, without increasing pancreatic insulin secretion. It has a mechanism of action that is dependent on the presence of insulin for activity. Rosiglitazone is an agonist for peroxisome proliferator-activated receptor-gamma (PPARgamma). Activation of nuclear PPAR-gamma receptors influences the production of a number of gene products involved in glucose and lipid metabolism. PPARgamma is abundant in the cells within the renal collecting tubules; fluid retention results from stimulation by thiazolidinediones which increases sodium reabsorption.

Pharmacodynamics/Kinetics

Onset of action: Delayed; Maximum effect: Up to 12 weeks

Distribution: V_{dss} (apparent): 17.6 L

Protein binding: 99.8%; primarily albumin

Metabolism: Hepatic (99%) via CYP2C8; minor metabolism via CYP2C9

Bioavailability: 99%

Half-life elimination: 3-4 hours

Time to peak, plasma: 1 hour; delayed with food

Excretion: Urine (~64%) and feces (~23%) as metabolites

Dosage Type 2 diabetes: Oral: **Note:** All patients should be initiated at the lowest recommended dose.

Adults: Initial: 4 mg daily as a single daily dose or in divided doses twice daily. If response is inadequate after 8-12 weeks of treatment, the dosage may be increased to 8 mg daily (maximum dose) as a single daily dose or in divided doses twice daily. In clinical trials, the 4 mg twice-daily regimen resulted in the greatest reduction in fasting plasma glucose and Hb A_{1c}. **Note:** When used in combination therapy with other hypoglycemic agents, a dose reduction of the concurrent agent may be necessary if hypoglycemia occurs. The Canadian labeling recommends a maximum rosiglitazone dose of 4 mg daily when used in combination with a sulfonylurea.

Elderly: Refer to adult dosing. No dosage adjustment is recommended.

Dosage adjustment in renal impairment: No dosage adjustment is necessary.

Dosage adjustment in hepatic impairment: No dosage adjustment provided in manufacturer's labeling. Clearance is significantly lower in hepatic impairment; therapy should not be initiated if the patient exhibits active liver disease or increased transaminases (ALT >2.5 times the upper limit of normal) at baseline.

Dietary Considerations Management of type 2 diabetes mellitus (noninsulin dependent, NIDDM) should include diet control.

Administration May be administered without regard to meals.

Monitoring Parameters

Hemoglobin A_{1c}, fasting serum glucose; signs and symptoms of fluid retention or heart failure; ophthalmic exams.

Liver enzymes (prior to initiation of therapy, then periodically thereafter); evaluate patients with ALT ≤2.5 times ULN at baseline or during therapy for cause of enzyme elevation. Patients with an elevation in ALT >3 times ULN during therapy should be rechecked as soon as possible. If the ALT levels remain >3 times ULN, therapy with rosiglitazone should be discontinued.

Reference Range Recommendations for glycemic control in nonpregnant adults with diabetes (ADA, 2013):

Hb A_{1c}: <7% (a more aggressive [<6.5%] or less aggressive [<8%] Hb A_{1c} goal may be targeted based on patient-specific characteristics)

Preprandial capillary plasma glucose: 70-130 mg/dL

Peak postprandial capillary blood glucose: <180 mg/dL

Dosage Forms Excipient information presented when available (limited, particularly for generics); consult specific product labeling.

Tablet, Oral:

Avandia: 2 mg, 4 mg, 8 mg

Rosiglitazone and Glimepiride

(roh si GLI ta zone & GLYE me pye ride)

Brand Names: U.S. Avandaryl

Index Terms Glimepiride and Rosiglitazone Maleate

Pharmacologic Category Antidiabetic Agent, Sulfonylurea; Antidiabetic Agent, Thiazolidinedione

Use Type 2 diabetes: Adjunct to diet and exercise to improve glycemic control in adults with type 2 diabetes mellitus (noninsulin dependent, NIDDM) and in whom dual rosiglitazone/glimepiride therapy is appropriate

Pregnancy Risk Factor C

Prescribing and Access Restrictions As a requirement of the REMS program, the prescribing and dispensing of any rosiglitazone-containing medication in the U.S. requires physician and patient enrollment in the Avandia-Rosiglitazone Medicines Access Program™. Complete program details are available at www.avandia.com or by calling the program Coordinating Center at 800-282-6342.

Medication Guide Available Yes

Dosage Type 2 diabetes mellitus: Adults: Oral:

Initial: Rosiglitazone 4 mg and glimepiride 1 mg once daily **or** rosiglitazone 4 mg and glimepiride 2 mg once daily (for patients previously treated with sulfonylurea or thiazolidinedione monotherapy)

Patients switching from combination rosiglitazone and glimepiride as separate tablets: Use current dose

Titration:

Dose adjustment in patients previously on sulfonylurea monotherapy: May take 2 weeks to observe decreased blood glucose and 2-3 months to see full effects of rosiglitazone component. If not adequately controlled after 8-12 weeks, increase daily dose of rosiglitazone component.

Dose adjustment in patients previously on thiazolidinedione monotherapy: If not adequately controlled after 1-2 weeks, increase daily dose of glimepiride component in ≤2 mg increments in 1-2 week intervals.

Maximum dose: Rosiglitazone 8 mg and glimepiride 4 mg once daily

Elderly: Rosiglitazone 4 mg and glimepiride 1 mg once daily; carefully titrate dose.

Dosage adjustment in renal impairment: Dose conservatively to avoid hypoglycemia.

Dosage adjustment in hepatic impairment: No dosage adjustment provided in manufacturer's labeling. Therapy should not be initiated if the patient exhibits symptoms of active liver disease or increased transaminases (ALT >2.5 times the upper limit of normal) at baseline since clearance is significantly lower in hepatic impairment. Discontinue if ALT >3 times ULN or jaundice occurs.

Additional Information Complete prescribing information should be consulted for additional detail.

Dosage Forms Excipient information presented when available (limited, particularly for generics); consult specific product labeling.

Tablet:

Avandaryl® 4 mg/1 mg: Rosiglitazone maleate 4 mg and glimepiride 1 mg

Avandaryl® 4 mg/2 mg: Rosiglitazone maleate 4 mg and glimepiride 2 mg

Avandaryl® 4 mg/4 mg: Rosiglitazone maleate 4 mg and glimepiride 4 mg

Avandaryl® 8 mg/2 mg: Rosiglitazone maleate 8 mg and glimepiride 2 mg

Avandaryl® 8 mg/4 mg: Rosiglitazone maleate 8 mg and glimepiride 4 mg

Rosiglitazone and Metformin

(roh si GLI ta zone & met FOR min)

Brand Names: U.S. Avandamet

Brand Names: Canada Avandamet

Index Terms Metformin and Rosiglitazone; Metformin Hydrochloride and Rosiglitazone Maleate; Rosiglitazone Maleate and Metformin Hydrochloride

Pharmacologic Category Antidiabetic Agent, Biguanide; Antidiabetic Agent, Thiazolidinedione

Use Type 2 diabetes: As an adjunct to diet and exercise to improve glycemic control in adults with type 2 diabetes mellitus (noninsulin dependent, NIDDM) when treatment with both rosiglitazone and metformin is appropriate.

Pregnancy Risk Factor C

Prescribing and Access Restrictions As a requirement of the REMS program, the prescribing and dispensing of any rosiglitazone-containing medication in the U.S. requires physician and patient enrollment in the Avandia-Rosiglitazone Medicines Access Program™. Complete program details are available at www.avandia.com or by calling the program Coordinating Center at 800-282-6342.

Health Canada requires written informed consent for new and current patients receiving rosiglitazone.

Medication Guide Available Yes

Dosage Type 2 diabetes mellitus: Adults: Oral: **Note:** Daily dose should be divided.

Patients inadequately controlled on **metformin alone**: Initial dose: Rosiglitazone 4 mg daily plus current dose of metformin

Patients inadequately controlled on **rosiglitazone alone**: Initial dose: Metformin 1000 mg daily plus current dose of rosiglitazone

Note: When switching from combination rosiglitazone and metformin as separate tablets: Use current dose

Dose adjustment: Titrate daily dose gradually in increments of rosiglitazone 4 mg/metformin 500 mg up to a maximum of rosiglitazone 8 mg/metformin 2000 mg.

Elderly: The initial and maintenance dosing should be conservative, due to the potential for decreased renal function (monitor). Generally, elderly patients should not be titrated to the maximum; do not use in patients ≥80 years unless normal renal function has been established.

Dosage adjustment in renal impairment: Contraindicated in the presence of renal disease or renal dysfunction (serum creatinine ≥1.5 mg/dL [males], ≥1.4 mg/dL [females] or abnormal clearance)

Dosage adjustment in hepatic impairment: Do not initiate therapy with active liver disease or ALT >2.5 times the upper limit of normal

Additional Information Complete prescribing information should be consulted for additional detail.

Dosage Forms Excipient information presented when available (limited, particularly for generics); consult specific product labeling.

Tablet, Oral:

Avandamet: 2/500: Rosiglitazone 2 mg and metformin hydrochloride 500 mg

Avandamet: 4/500: Rosiglitazone 4 mg and metformin hydrochloride 500 mg

Avandamet: 2/1000: Rosiglitazone 2 mg and metformin hydrochloride 1000 mg

Avandamet: 4/1000: Rosiglitazone 4 mg and metformin hydrochloride 1000 mg

Dosage Forms: Canada Note: Refer also to dosage forms.

Excipient information presented when available (limited, particularly for generics); consult specific product labeling.

Tablet, Oral:

Avandamet: 1/500: Rosiglitazone 1 mg and metformin hydrochloride 500 mg

◆ **Rosiglitazone Maleate and Metformin Hydrochloride** *see* Rosiglitazone and Metformin *on page 1858*

◆ **Rosone (Can)** *see* Betamethasone *on page 247*

Rosuvastatin (roe soo va STAT in)

Brand Names: U.S. Crestor

Brand Names: Canada Apo-Rosuvastatin; CO Rosuvastatin; Crestor; Jamp-Rosuvastatin; Mylan-Rosuvastatin; PMS-Rosuvastatin; RAN™-Rosuvastatin; Sandoz-Rosuvastatin; Teva-Rosuvastatin

Index Terms Rosuvastatin Calcium

Pharmacologic Category Antilipemic Agent, HMG-CoA Reductase Inhibitor

Use

Heterozygous familial hypercholesterolemia in children: Adjunct to diet to reduce total cholesterol, low-density lipoprotein cholesterol (LDL-C), and apolipoprotein B (apo B) levels in adolescent males and females who are at least 1 year postmenarche and are 10-17 years of age with heterozygous familial hypercholesteremia if after an adequate trial of diet therapy the following findings are present: LDL-C more than 190 mg/dL or more than 160 mg/dL and there is a positive family history of premature cardiovascular (CV) disease or 2 or more other CV disease risk factors.

Homozygous familial hypercholesterolemia: To reduce LDL-C, total cholesterol, and apo B in adults with homozygous familial hypercholesterolemia as an adjunct to other lipid-lowering treatments (eg, LDL apheresis) or alone if such treatments are unavailable.

Hyperlipidemia and mixed dyslipidemia: Adjunctive therapy to diet to reduce elevated total cholesterol, LDL-C, apo B, non–high-density lipoprotein cholesterol (non-HDL-C), and triglyceride levels, and to increase HDL-C in patients with primary hyperlipidemia or mixed dyslipidemia.

Hypertriglyceridemia: Adjunct to diet for the treatment of adults with hypertriglyceridemia.

Primary dysbetalipoproteinemia (type III hyperlipoproteinemia): Adjunct to diet for the treatment of patients with primary dysbetalipoproteinemia (type III hyperlipoproteinemia).

Prevention of cardiovascular disease:

Primary prevention: To reduce the risk of stroke, myocardial infarction, or arterial revascularization procedures in patients without clinically evident coronary heart disease or lipid abnormalities but with all of the following: 1) an increased risk of cardiovascular disease based on age ≥50 years old in men and ≥60 years old in women, 2) hsCRP ≥2 mg/L, and 3) the presence of at least one additional cardiovascular disease risk factor such as hypertension, low HDL-C, smoking, or a family history of premature coronary heart disease.

Secondary prevention: Adjunctive therapy to diet to slow the progression of atherosclerosis in adults as part of a treatment strategy to lower total cholesterol and LDL-C to target levels.

Primary and secondary prevention of atherosclerotic cardiovascular disease (ASCVD) according to the American College of Cardiology/American Heart Association: To reduce the risk of ASCVD in patients with clinical ASCVD (eg, coronary heart disease, stroke/TIA, or peripheral arterial disease presumed to be of atherosclerotic origin) who are less than 75 years of age; in patients without clinical ASCVD if LDL-C is 190 mg/dL or greater; in patients without clinical ASCVD who have type 1 or type 2 diabetes and are between 40 and 75 years of age with an estimated 10-year ASCVD risk 7.5% or greater; in patients with an estimated 10-year ASCVD risk 7.5% or greater and who are between 40 and 75 years of age. (Stone, 2013).

Pregnancy Risk Factor X

Pregnancy Considerations Adverse events were observed in some animal reproduction studies. There are reports of congenital anomalies following maternal use of HMG-CoA reductase inhibitors in pregnancy; however, maternal disease, differences in specific agents used, and the low rates of exposure limit the interpretation of the available data (Godfrey, 2012; Lecarpentier, 2012). Cholesterol biosynthesis may be important in fetal development; serum cholesterol and triglycerides increase normally during pregnancy. The discontinuation of lipid lowering medications temporarily during pregnancy is not expected to have significant impact on the long term outcomes of primary hypercholesterolemia treatment.

Use of rosuvastatin is contraindicated in pregnancy. HMG-CoA reductase inhibitors should be discontinued prior to pregnancy (ADA, 2013). If treatment of dyslipidemias is needed in pregnant women or in women of reproductive age, other agents are preferred (Berglund, 2012; Stone, 2013). The manufacturer recommends administration to women of childbearing potential only when conception is highly unlikely and patients have been informed of potential hazards.

Breast-Feeding Considerations It is not known if rosuvastatin is excreted into breast milk. Due to the potential for serious adverse reactions in a nursing infant, use while breast-feeding is contraindicated by the manufacturer.

Contraindications

Known hypersensitivity to any component of the formulation; active liver disease or unexplained persistent elevations of serum transaminases; pregnancy; breast-feeding.

Canadian labeling: Additional contraindications (not in U.S. labeling): Concomitant administration of cyclosporine; use of 40 mg dose in Asian patients, patients with predisposing risk factors for myopathy/rhabdomyolysis (eg, hereditary muscle disorders, history of myotoxicity with other HMG-CoA reductase inhibitors, concomitant use with fibrates or niacin, severe hepatic impairment, severe renal impairment [Cl_{cr} <30 mL/minute/1.73 m^2], hypothyroidism, alcohol abuse)

Warnings/Precautions Secondary causes of hyperlipidemia should be ruled out prior to therapy. Rosuvastatin has not been studied when the primary lipid abnormality is chylomicron elevation (Fredrickson types I and V). Postmarketing reports of fatal and nonfatal hepatic failure are rare. If serious hepatotoxicity with clinical symptoms and/or hyperbilirubinemia or jaundice occurs during treatment, interrupt therapy. If an alternate etiology is not identified, do not restart rosuvastatin. Liver enzyme tests should be obtained at baseline and as clinically indicated; routine periodic monitoring of liver enzymes is not necessary. Use with caution in patients who consume large amounts of ethanol or have a history of liver disease; use is contraindicated with active liver disease or unexplained transaminase elevations. Hematuria (microscopic) and proteinuria have been observed; more commonly reported in patients receiving rosuvastatin 40 mg daily, but typically transient and not associated with a decrease in renal function. Consider dosage reduction if unexplained hematuria and proteinuria persists. HMG-CoA reductase inhibitors may cause rhabdomyolysis with acute renal failure and/or myopathy. Discontinue in any patient in which CPK levels are markedly elevated (>10 times ULN) or if myopathy is suspected/diagnosed. This risk is dose-related and is increased with concurrent use of other lipid-lowering medications (fibric acid derivatives or niacin doses ≥1 g/day), other interacting drugs, drugs associated with myopathy (eg, colchicine), age ≥65 years, female gender, certain subgroups of Asian ancestry, uncontrolled hypothyroidism, and renal dysfunction. Dose reductions may be necessary. Immune-mediated necrotizing myopathy (IMNM), an autoimmune-mediated myopathy, has been reported (rarely) with HMG-CoA reductase inhibitor therapy. IMNM presents as proximal muscle weakness with elevated CPK levels, which persists despite discontinuation of HMG-CoA reductase inhibitor therapy; additionally, muscle biopsy may show necrotizing myopathy with limited inflammation; immunosuppressive therapy (eg, corticosteroids, azathioprine) may be used for treatment.

The manufacturer recommends temporary discontinuation for elective major surgery, acute medical or surgical conditions, or in any patient experiencing an acute or serious condition predisposing to renal failure (eg, sepsis, dehydration, electrolyte disorders, hypotension, trauma, uncontrolled seizures). However, based upon current evidence,

HMG-CoA reductase inhibitor therapy should be continued in the perioperative period unless risk outweighs cardioprotective benefit. Patients should be instructed to report unexplained muscle pain, tenderness, weakness, or dark urine; in Canada, concomitant use with cyclosporine or niacin is contraindicated, and rosuvastatin at a dose of 40 mg/day in Asian patients is contraindicated. Small increases in Hb A_{1c} (mean: ~0.1%) and fasting blood glucose have been reported with rosuvastatin; however, the benefits of statin therapy far outweigh the risk of dysglycemia.

Potentially significant interactions may exist, requiring dose or frequency adjustment, additional monitoring, and/or selection of alternative therapy. Consult drug interactions database for more detailed information. Dosage adjustment required in patients with a Cl_{cr} <30 mL/minute/1.73 m^2 and not receiving hemodialysis (contraindicated in the Canadian labeling. Use with caution in elderly patients as they are more predisposed to myopathy.

Adverse Reactions

>10%: Neuromuscular & skeletal: Myalgia (3% to 13%)

2% to 10%:

Central nervous system: Headache (6%), dizziness (4%)

Endocrine & metabolic: Diabetes mellitus (3%)

Gastrointestinal: Nausea (3%), abdominal pain (2%), constipation (2%)

Hepatic: Increased serum ALT (2%; >3 times ULN)

Neuromuscular & skeletal: Arthralgia (4% to 10%), increased creatine phosphokinase (3%; >10 x ULN: Children 3%), weakness (3%)

<2% (Limited to important or life-threatening): Abnormal thyroid function test, amnesia (reversible), cataract, cognitive dysfunction (reversible), confusion (reversible), depression, elevated glycosylated hemoglobin (Hb A_{1c}), gynecomastia, hematuria (microscopic), hepatic failure, hepatitis, hyperglycemia, hypersensitivity reaction (including angioedema, pruritus, rash, urticaria), immune-mediated necrotizing myopathy, increased gamma-glutamyl transferase, increased serum alkaline phosphatase, increased serum AST, increased serum bilirubin, increased serum glucose, insomnia, jaundice, memory impairment (reversible), myoglobinuria, myositis, myopathy, nightmares, pancreatitis, proteinuria (dose related), renal failure, rhabdomyolysis, thrombocytopenia

Drug Interactions

Metabolism/Transport Effects Substrate of CYP2C9 (minor), CYP3A4 (minor), SLCO1B1; **Note:** Assignment of Major/Minor substrate status based on clinically relevant drug interaction potential

Avoid Concomitant Use

Avoid concomitant use of Rosuvastatin with any of the following: Fusidic Acid (Systemic); Gemfibrozil; Red Yeast Rice

Increased Effect/Toxicity

Rosuvastatin may increase the levels/effects of: DAPTOmycin; PAZOPanib; Trabectedin; Vitamin K Antagonists

The levels/effects of Rosuvastatin may be increased by: Amiodarone; Bezafibrate; Boceprevir; Colchicine; CycloSPORINE (Systemic); Dronedarone; Eltrombopag; Fenofibrate and Derivatives; Fusidic Acid (Systemic); Gemfibrozil; Itraconazole; Niacin; Niacinamide; Protease Inhibitors; Raltegravir; Red Yeast Rice; Simeprevir; Telaprevir

Decreased Effect

Rosuvastatin may decrease the levels/effects of: Lanthanum

The levels/effects of Rosuvastatin may be decreased by: Antacids; Eslicarbazepine

Ethanol/Nutrition/Herb Interactions

Ethanol: Avoid excessive ethanol consumption (due to potential hepatic effects).

Food: Red yeast rice contains an estimated 2.4 mg lovastatin per 600 mg rice.

Storage/Stability Store between 20°C and 25°C (68°F to 77°F). Protect from moisture.

Mechanism of Action Inhibitor of 3-hydroxy-3-methylglutaryl coenzyme A (HMG-CoA) reductase, the rate-limiting enzyme in cholesterol synthesis (reduces the production of mevalonic acid from HMG-CoA); this then results in a compensatory increase in the expression of LDL receptors on hepatocyte membranes and a stimulation of LDL catabolism

Pharmacodynamics/Kinetics

Onset of action: Within 1 week; maximal at 4 weeks

Distribution: V_d: 134 L

Protein binding: 88%

Metabolism: Hepatic (10%), via CYP2C9 (1 active metabolite identified: N-desmethyl rosuvastatin, one-sixth to one-half the HMG-CoA reductase activity of the parent compound)

Bioavailability: 20% (high first-pass extraction by liver)

Asian patients have been noted to have increased bioavailability.

Half-life elimination: 19 hours

Time to peak, plasma: 3-5 hours

Excretion: Feces (90%), primarily as unchanged drug

Dosage Oral: **Note:** Doses should be individualized according to the baseline LDL-cholesterol levels, the recommended goal of therapy, and patient response; adjustments should be made at intervals of 4 weeks or more

Children and Adolescents 10-17 years (females >1 year postmenarche): Heterozygous familial hypercholesterolemia (HeFH):

U.S. labeling: 5-20 mg once daily; maximum: 20 mg daily

Dosage adjustment for rosuvastatin with concomitant cyclosporine, gemfibrozil, atazanavir/ritonavir, or lopinavir/ritonavir: Refer to adult dosing.

Canadian labeling: 5-10 mg once daily; maximum: 10 mg daily

Adults:

Hyperlipidemia, mixed dyslipidemia, hypertriglyceridemia, primary dysbetalipoproteinemia, slowing progression of atherosclerosis, primary prevention of cardiovascular disease:

Initial dose:

General dosing: 10-20 mg once daily; 20 mg once daily may be used in patients with severe hyperlipidemia (LDL >190 mg/dL) and aggressive lipid targets (McKenney, 2009)

Conservative dosing: Patients requiring less aggressive treatment or predisposed to myopathy (including patients of Asian descent): 5 mg once daily

Titration: After initiation or upon titration, analyze lipid levels within 2-4 weeks (peak, steady-state lowering effects usually seen between 4-6 weeks [McKenney, 2009]) and adjust dose accordingly; dosing range: 5-40 mg daily (maximum dose: 40 mg once daily).

Note: The 40 mg dose should be reserved for patients who have not achieved goal cholesterol levels on a dose of 20 mg daily, including patients switched from another HMG-CoA reductase inhibitor.

Homozygous familial hypercholesterolemia (FH): Initial: 20 mg once daily (maximum dose: 40 mg daily)

ACC/AHA Blood Cholesterol Guideline recommendations to reduce the risk of atherosclerotic cardiovascular disease (ASCVD) (Stone, 2013): Adults ≥21 years:

Primary prevention:

LDL-C ≥190 mg/dL: High-intensity therapy: 20-40 mg once daily.

Type 1 or 2 diabetes and age 40-75 years: Moderate-intensity therapy: 5-10 mg once daily.

Type 1 or 2 diabetes, age 40-75 years, and an estimated 10-year ASCVD risk ≥7.5%: High intensity therapy: 20-40 mg once daily

Age 40-75 years and an estimated 10-year ASCVD risk ≥7.5%: Moderate to high intensity therapy: 5-40 mg once daily

Secondary prevention:

Patient has clinical ASCVD (eg, coronary heart disease, stroke/TIA, or peripheral arterial disease presumed to be of atherosclerotic origin) **and**:

Age ≤75 years: High-intensity therapy: 20-40 mg once daily.

Age >75 years or not a candidate for high-intensity therapy: Moderate-intensity therapy: 5-10 mg once daily.

Dosage adjustment for rosuvastatin with concomitant medications:

U.S. labeling:

Cyclosporine: Rosuvastatin dose should not exceed 5 mg once daily

Gemfibrozil: Avoid concurrent use; if unable to avoid concurrent use, initiate rosuvastatin at 5 mg once daily; dose should not exceed 10 mg once daily

Atazanavir/ritonavir or lopinavir/ritonavir: Initiate rosuvastatin at 5 mg once daily; dose should not exceed 10 mg once daily

Canadian labeling:

Cyclosporine: Concomitant use is contraindicated

Gemfibrozil: Rosuvastatin dose should not exceed 20 mg daily

Dosage adjustment for toxicity:

Severe muscle symptoms or fatigue: Promptly discontinue use; evaluate CPK, creatinine, and urinalysis for myoglobinuria (Stone, 2013).

Mild to moderate muscle symptoms: Discontinue use until symptoms can be evaluated; evaluate patient for conditions that may increase the risk for muscle symptoms (eg, hypothyroidism, reduced renal or hepatic function, rheumatologic disorders such as polymyalgia rheumatica, steroid myopathy, vitamin D deficiency, or primary muscle diseases). Upon resolution, resume the original or lower dose of rosuvastatin. If muscle symptoms recur, discontinue rosuvastatin use. After muscle symptom resolution, may then use a low dose of a different statin; gradually increase if tolerated. In the absence of continued statin use, if muscle symptoms or elevated CPK continues after 2 months, consider other causes of muscle symptoms. If determined to be due to another condition aside from statin use, may resume statin therapy at the original dose (Stone, 2013).

Dosage adjustment for hematuria and/or persistent, unexplained proteinuria while on 40 mg daily: Reduce dose and evaluate causes

Dosage adjustment in renal impairment:

Cl_{cr} ≥30 mL/minute/1.73 m^2: No dosage adjustment necessary.

Cl_{cr} <30 mL/minute/1.73 m^2: Initial: 5 mg once daily; maximum: 10 mg once daily

Dosage adjustment in hepatic impairment:

U.S. labeling: Manufacturer labeling does not provide specific dosing recommendations; however, systemic exposure may be increased in patients with liver disease (increased AUC and C_{max}); use is contraindicated in active liver disease or unexplained transaminase elevations.

Canadian labeling:

Active hepatic disease or unexplained persistent transaminase >3 x ULN: Use is contraindicated

Mild-to-moderate impairment: No dosage adjustment necessary.

Severe impairment: Initial: 5 mg daily. Maximum: 20 mg once daily

Dietary Considerations Red yeast rice contains an estimated 2.4 mg lovastatin per 600 mg rice.

Administration May be administered with or without food. May be taken at any time of the day.

Monitoring Parameters

2013 ACC/AHA Blood Cholesterol Guideline recommendations (Stone, 2013):

Lipid panel (total cholesterol, HDL, LDL, triglycerides): Baseline lipid panel; fasting lipid profile within 4-12 weeks after initiation or dose adjustment and every 3-12 months (as clinically indicated) thereafter. If 2 consecutive LDL levels are <40 mg/dL, consider decreasing the dose.

Hepatic transaminase levels: Baseline measurement of hepatic transaminase levels (ie, ALT); measure hepatic function if symptoms suggest hepatotoxicity (eg, unusual fatigue or weakness, loss of appetite, abdominal pain, dark-colored urine or yellowing of skin or sclera) during therapy.

CPK: CPK should not be routinely measured. Baseline CPK measurement is reasonable for some individuals (eg, family history of statin intolerance or muscle disease, clinical presentation, concomitant drug therapy that may increase risk of myopathy). May measure CPK in any patient with symptoms suggestive of myopathy (pain, tenderness, stiffness, cramping, weakness, or generalized fatigue).

Evaluate for new-onset diabetes mellitus during therapy; if diabetes develops, continue statin therapy and encourage adherence to a heart-healthy diet, physical activity, a healthy body weight, and tobacco cessation.

If patient develops a confusional state or memory impairment, may evaluate patient for nonstatin causes (eg, exposure to other drugs), systemic and neuropsychiatric causes, and the possibility of adverse effects associated with statin therapy.

Manufacturer recommendations: Liver enzyme tests at baseline and repeated when clinically indicated. Upon initiation or titration, lipid panel should be analyzed within 2-4 weeks.

Dosage Forms Excipient information presented when available (limited, particularly for generics); consult specific product labeling.

Tablet, Oral:

Crestor: 5 mg, 10 mg, 20 mg, 40 mg

◆ **Rosuvastatin Calcium** *see* Rosuvastatin *on page 1858*

◆ **Rotarix** *see* Rotavirus Vaccine *on page 1861*

◆ **RotaTeq** *see* Rotavirus Vaccine *on page 1861*

Rotavirus Vaccine (ROE ta vye rus vak SEEN)

Brand Names: U.S. Rotarix; RotaTeq

Brand Names: Canada Rotarix; RotaTeq

Index Terms Human Rotavirus Vaccine, Attenuated (HRV); Pentavalent Human-Bovine Reassortant Rotavirus Vaccine (PRV); Rotavirus Vaccine, Pentavalent; RV1 (Rotarix); RV5 (RotaTeq)

Pharmacologic Category Vaccine, Live (Viral)

Additional Appendix Information

Immunization Administration Recommendations *on page 2334*

Immunization Recommendations *on page 2339*

Use Prevention of rotavirus gastroenteritis in infants and children

The Advisory Committee on Immunization Practices (ACIP) recommends routine vaccination of all infants (CDC, 2009).

Pregnancy Risk Factor C

Pregnancy Considerations Reproduction studies have not been conducted. Not indicated for use in women of reproductive age. Infants living in households with pregnant women may be vaccinated (CDC, 2009).

Breast-Feeding Considerations Infants receiving vaccine may be breast fed (CDC, 2009).

Contraindications Hypersensitivity to rotavirus vaccine or any component of the formulation; use in infants with severe combined immunodeficiency disease (SCID); infants with a history of intussusception

Rotarix: Additional contraindication: Contraindicated with a history of an uncorrected congenital malformation of the GI tract

Warnings/Precautions Information is not available for use in postexposure prophylaxis. May consider deferring administration in patients with moderate or severe acute illness (with or without fever); may administer to patients with mild acute illness (with or without fever). Vaccination may not result in effective immunity in all patients. Response depends upon multiple factors (eg, type of vaccine, age of patient) and may be improved by administering the vaccine at the recommended dose, route, and interval. Vaccines may not be effective if administered during periods of altered immune competence (CDC, 2011). Use caution with history of GI disorders, acute GI illness, chronic diarrhea, failure to thrive, congenital abdominal disorders, and abdominal surgery. Vaccine may be used with controlled gastroesophageal reflux disease. Consider delaying administration to infants with acute diarrhea or vomiting. An increased risk of intussusception was observed with a previously licensed rotavirus vaccine. Cases have been noted in postmarketing reports and a temporal association has been observed in postmarketing observational studies with current vaccines. Cases were noted within 21-31 days of the first dose, with a clustering of cases within the first 7 days following administration. Use of RotaTeq and Rotarix is contraindicated with a history of intussusception.

Virus from live virus vaccines may be transmitted to nonvaccinated contacts; use caution in presence immunocompromised family members. Viral shedding occurs within the first weeks of administration; peak viral shedding generally occurs ~7 days after the first dose. The ACIP recommends vaccination of infants living in households with persons who are immunocompromised (CDC, 2009). Safety and efficacy have not been established for use in immunocompromised infants (including blood dyscrasias, leukemia, lymphoma, malignant neoplasms affecting bone marrow or lymphatic system), infants on immunosuppressants (including high-dose corticosteroids; may be administered with topical corticosteroids or inhaled steroids), or infants with primary and acquired immunodeficiencies (including HIV/AIDS, cellular immune deficiencies, hypogammaglobulinemic and dysgammaglobulinemic states). The ACIP recommendations support vaccination of HIV-exposed or infected infants, since the diagnosis of infection may not be made prior to the first dose of the vaccine and also because strains of rotavirus vaccine are considerably attenuated (CDC, 2009).

Immediate treatment (including epinephrine 1:1000) for anaphylactoid and/or hypersensitivity reactions should be available during vaccine use. Some packaging may contain natural latex/natural rubber. Not intended for use in adults. In order to maximize vaccination rates, the ACIP recommends simultaneous administration of all age-appropriate vaccines (live or inactivated) for which a person is eligible at a single clinic visit, unless contraindications exist (CDC, 2011).

Adverse Reactions All serious adverse reactions must be reported to the U.S. Department of Health and Human Services (DHHS) Vaccine Adverse Event Reporting System (VAERS) 1-800-822-7967 or online at https://vaers.hhs.gov/esub/index.

Note: Ranges reported; actual percentage may vary between products.

>10%:

Central nervous system: Fever ≥38.1°C (17% to 43%; equal to or less than placebo), fussiness/irritability (3% to 52%)

Gastrointestinal: Diarrhea (4% to 24%), vomiting (3% to 15%)

Otic: Otitis media (15%)

1% to 10%:

Gastrointestinal: Flatulence (2%)

Respiratory: Nasopharyngitis (7%), bronchospasm (1%)

<1% (Limited to important or life-threatening): Anaphylaxis, angioedema, gastroenteritis with severe diarrhea and prolonged vaccine viral shedding in infants with SCID, hematochezia, immune thrombocytopenia (ITP), intussusception, Kawasaki disease, seizure, transmission of vaccine virus from recipient to nonvaccinated contacts, urticaria

Drug Interactions

Metabolism/Transport Effects None known.

Avoid Concomitant Use

Avoid concomitant use of Rotavirus Vaccine with any of the following: Belimumab; Fingolimod; Immunosuppressants

Increased Effect/Toxicity

The levels/effects of Rotavirus Vaccine may be increased by: AzaTHIOprine; Belimumab; Corticosteroids (Systemic); Dimethyl Fumarate; Fingolimod; Hydroxychloroquine; Immunosuppressants; Leflunomide; Mercaptopurine; Methotrexate

Decreased Effect

Rotavirus Vaccine may decrease the levels/effects of: Tuberculin Tests

The levels/effects of Rotavirus Vaccine may be decreased by: Dimethyl Fumarate; Fingolimod; Immune Globulins; Immunosuppressants

Preparation for Administration Rotarix: Reconstitute only with provided diluent and transfer adapter. Shake to form suspension.

Storage/Stability

Rotarix: Prior to reconstitution, store powder under refrigeration at 2°C to 8°C (36°F to 46°F); diluent may be stored at room temperature 20°C to 25°C (68°F to 77°F). Protect from light; discard if frozen. Following reconstitution, may be refrigerated or stored at room temperature for up to 24 hours. Discard if frozen. **Note:** In Canada, Rotarix is available as an oral suspension ready for use and does not need reconstituted. The oral suspension may be stored at 2°C to 8°C (36°F to 46°F); do not freeze. Protect from light.

RotaTeq: Store and transport under refrigeration at 2°C to 8°C (36°F to 46°F). Use as soon as possible once removed from refrigerator. Protect from light. Canadian labeling suggests that once the vaccine is removed from refrigeration, it may be stored at temperatures up to 25°C (77°F) for up to 4 hours; do not freeze. Protect from light.

Mechanism of Action A live vaccine; replicates in the small intestine and promotes active immunity to rotavirus gastroenteritis. Rotarix is specifically indicated for prevention of rotavirus gastroenteritis caused by serotypes G1, G3, G4, and G9 and RotaTeq is specifically indicated for prevention of rotavirus gastroenteritis caused by serotypes G1, G2, G3, and G4. However, vaccines may provide immunity to other serotypes.

Pharmacodynamics/Kinetics Note: There is no established relationship between antibody response and protection against gastroenteritis.

Seroconversion:

Rotarix: Antirotavirus IgA antibodies were noted 1-2 months following completion of the 2-dose series in 77% to 87% of infants.

RotaTeq: A threefold increase in antirotavirus IgA was noted following completion of the 3-dose regimen in 93% to 100% of infants.

Duration: Following administration of rotavirus vaccine, efficacy of protecting against any grade of rotavirus gastroenteritis through two seasons was 70% to 79%

Dosage Oral:

Manufacturer's labeling:

Infants 6-24 weeks of age: Rotarix: A total of two 1 mL doses, the first dose given at 6 weeks of age. The first and second dose should be separated by ≥4 weeks. The 2-dose series should be completed by 24 weeks of age.

Infants 6-32 weeks: RotaTeq: A total of three 2 mL doses, the first dose given at 6-12 weeks of age, followed by subsequent doses at 4- to 10-week intervals. Administer all doses by 32 weeks of age.

ACIP recommendations (CDC, 2009): The first dose can be given at 6-14 weeks of age. The series should not be started in infants ≥15 weeks. The final dose in the series should be administered by 8 months 0 days of age. The minimum interval between doses is 4 weeks. RotaTeq should be given in 3 doses administered at 2-, 4-, and 6 months of age. Rotarix should be given in 2 doses administered at 2- and 4 months of age. For infants inadvertently administered rotavirus vaccine at ≥15 weeks of age, the vaccine series may be completed according to schedule. The ACIP recommendations for vaccination recommend completing the vaccine series with the same product whenever possible. If continuing with same product will cause vaccination to be deferred, or if product used previously is unknown, vaccination should be completed with the product available. If RotaTeq was used in any previous doses, or if the specific product used was unknown, a total of 3 doses should be given. Infants who have had rotavirus gastroenteritis before getting the full course of vaccine should still initiate or complete the recommended schedule; initial infection provides only partial immunity.

Dosage adjustment in renal impairment: No dosage adjustment provided in manufacturer's labeling.

Dosage adjustment in hepatic impairment: No dosage adjustment provided in manufacturer's labeling.

Dietary Considerations Do not mix or dilute vaccine. May be administered before or after food, milk, or breast milk.

Administration

Rotarix: Using oral applicator, administer contents into infant's inner cheek. Dispose of applicator and vaccine vial in biologic waste container.

RotaTeq: Gently squeeze dose from ready-to-use dosing tube into infant's inner cheek. After use, dispose of the empty tube and cap in a biologic waste container.

Note: A single dose of the rotavirus vaccine should not be readministered to an infant who regurgitates, spits out, or vomits the vaccine during administration. Any remaining dose(s) should be administered on schedule (CDC, 2009).

Simultaneous administration of vaccines helps ensure the patients will be fully vaccinated by the appropriate age. Simultaneous administration of vaccines is defined as administering >1 vaccine on the same day at different anatomic sites. Separate vaccines should not be combined in the same syringe unless indicated by product specific labeling. The ACIP prefers each dose of a specific vaccine in a series come from the same manufacturer when possible. In general, preterm infants should be vaccinated at the same chronological age as full-term infants (CDC, 2011).

Antipyretics have not been shown to prevent febrile seizures. Antipyretics may be used to treat fever or discomfort following vaccination (CDC, 2011). One study reported that routine prophylactic administration of acetaminophen to prevent fever prior to vaccination decreased the immune response of some vaccines; the clinical significance of this reduction in immune response has not been established (Prymula, 2009).

Test Interactions Tuberculin tests: Rotavirus vaccine may diminish the diagnostic effect of tuberculin tests.

Additional Information U.S. federal law requires that the name of medication, date of administration, the vaccine manufacturer, lot number of vaccine, and the administering person's name, title and address be entered into the patient's permanent medical record.

Dosage Forms Excipient information presented when available (limited, particularly for generics); consult specific product labeling.

Powder, for suspension, oral [preservative free; human derived]:

Rotarix: G1P[8] ≥10^6 $CCID_{50}$ per 1 mL [contains sorbitol, sucrose; supplied with diluent which may contain natural rubber/natural latex in packaging]

Solution, oral [preservative free; bovine and human derived]:

RotaTeq: G1 ≥2.2 x 10^6 infectious units, G2 ≥2.8 x 10^6 infectious units, G3 ≥2.2 x 10^6 infectious units, G4 ≥2 x 10^6 infectious units, and P1A [8] ≥2.3 x 10^6 infectious units per 2 mL (2 mL)

Dosage Forms: Canada Excipient information presented when available (limited, particularly for generics); consult specific product labeling.

Suspension, oral [human derived]:

Rotarix: ≥10^6 $CCID_{50}$ per 1.5 mL (1.5 mL)

◆ **Rotavirus Vaccine, Pentavalent** *see* Rotavirus Vaccine *on page 1861*

Rotigotine (roe TIG oh teen)

Brand Names: U.S. Neupro

Index Terms N-0923

Pharmacologic Category Anti-Parkinson's Agent, Dopamine Agonist

Additional Appendix Information

Antiparkinsonian Agents *on page 2289*

Use Treatment of the signs and symptoms of idiopathic Parkinson's disease (early-stage to advanced-stage disease); treatment of moderate-to-severe primary restless legs syndrome (RLS)

Pregnancy Risk Factor C

Pregnancy Considerations Adverse events were observed in animal reproduction studies.

Breast-Feeding Considerations Prolactin secretion is decreased and lactation may be inhibited.

Contraindications Hypersensitivity to rotigotine or any component of the formulation

Warnings/Precautions Use is commonly associated with somnolence. In addition, falling asleep during activities of daily living, including while driving, has also been reported and may occur without significant warning signs. Monitor for daytime somnolence or pre-existing sleep disorder. Patients must be cautioned about performing tasks which require mental alertness (eg, operating machinery or driving). Use with caution in patients receiving other CNS depressants or psychoactive agents; discontinue if significant daytime sleepiness or episodes of falling asleep ▶

occur. Effects with other sedative drugs or ethanol may be potentiated.

Dopamine agonists may cause orthostatic hypotension and syncope; Parkinson's disease patients appear to have an impaired capacity to respond to a postural challenge. Use with caution in patients at risk of hypotension (such as those receiving antihypertensive drugs) or where transient hypotensive episodes would be poorly tolerated (cardiovascular disease or cerebrovascular disease). Parkinson's and restless legs syndrome (RLS) patients being treated with dopaminergic agonists ordinarily require careful monitoring for signs and symptoms of postural hypotension, especially during dose escalation, and should be informed of this risk. Weight gain and fluid retention have been reported, primarily associated with development of peripheral edema in Parkinson's disease patients; use caution in patients with heart failure or renal insufficiency. Therapy has also been associated with increases in blood pressure (may be significant), and increased heart rate; use caution in pre-existing cardiovascular disease.

Dopamine agonists have been associated with compulsive behaviors and/or loss of impulse control, which has manifested as pathological gambling, libido increases (hypersexuality), and/or binge eating. Causality has not been established, and controversy exists as to whether this phenomenon is related to the underlying disease, prior behaviors/addictions and/or drug therapy. Dose reduction or discontinuation of therapy has been reported to reverse these behaviors in some, but not all cases.

In RLS patents, augmentation (earlier onset of symptoms each day and/or an overall increase in symptom severity) or rebound (considered to be an end of dose effect) may occur.

Use with caution in patients with pre-existing dyskinesia; therapy may exacerbate. Therapy may also cause hallucinations (dose-related) and other psychotic like behaviors (eg, agitation, delirium, delusions, aggression); in general, avoid use in patients with pre-existing major psychotic disorders. Risk for melanoma development is increased in Parkinson's disease patients; drug causation or factors contributing to risk have not been established. Patients receiving therapy for any indication should be monitored closely and periodic skin examinations should be performed. Other dopaminergic agents have been associated with a syndrome resembling neuroleptic malignant syndrome on withdrawal and/or significant dosage reduction. Taper treatment when discontinuing therapy; do not stop abruptly. Rare cases of pleural effusion, pleural thickening, pulmonary infiltrates, retroperitoneal fibrosis, pericarditis and/or cardiac valvulopathy have been reported in patients treated with ergot-derived dopamine agonists, generally with prolonged use. The potential of rotigotine, a non-ergot-derived dopamine agonist, to cause similar fibrotic complications is unknown.

Patch contains aluminum; remove patch prior to magnetic resonance imaging or cardioversion to avoid skin burns. Patch also contains sodium metabisulfite which may cause allergic reaction in susceptible individuals. Dose-dependent application site reactions, potentially severe, have been observed; daily rotation of application sites has been shown to decrease incidence of reactions. If a generalized (nonapplication site) skin reaction occurs; discontinue therapy. Avoid exposure of application site to any direct external heat sources (eg, hair dryers, heating pads, electric blankets, saunas, hot tubs, direct sunlight); heat exposure has not been studied with the rotigotine patch, but an increase in the rate and extent of absorption has been observed with other transdermal products.

Adverse Reactions

>10%:

- Cardiovascular: Peripheral edema (dose related; 2% to 14%)
- Central nervous system: Somnolence (dose related; 5% to 32%), dizziness (5% to 23%), headache (8% to 18%), fatigue (6% to 18%), orthostatic hypotension (1% to 18%), sleep disorder (disturbance in initiating/maintaining sleep; dose related; 2% to 14%), hallucinations (dose related; 7% to 14%), insomnia (5% to 11%)
- Dermatologic: Application site reactions (dose related; 27% to 46%), hyperhidrosis (dose related; 1% to 11%)
- Gastrointestinal: Nausea (dose related; 15% to 48%), vomiting (dose related; 2% to 20%)
- Neuromuscular & skeletal: Dyskinesia (dose related; 14% to 17%), arthralgia (8% to 11%)

1% to 10%:

- Cardiovascular: Hypertension (dose related; 1% to 5%), T-wave abnormalities on ECG (≤3%), syncope
- Central nervous system: Abnormal dreams (dose related; 1% to 7%), nightmare (dose related; 3% to 5%), depression (≤5%), vertigo (1% to 4%), early morning awakening (dose related; ≤3%), balance disorder (2% to 3%), lethargy (1% to 2%), postural dizziness (1% to 2%), sleep attacks (dose related; ≤2%)
- Dermatologic: Pruritus (3% to 7%), erythema (dose related; ≤6%), pruritic rash (dose related; ≤3%)
- Endocrine & metabolic: Hot flash (≤3%), serum ferritin decreased (dose related; 1% to 2%); serum glucose decreased
- Gastrointestinal: Constipation (2% to 9%), weight gain (2% to 9%), diarrhea (5% to 7%), anorexia (≤8%), xerostomia (dose related; 3% to 7%), appetite decreased (≤3%), dyspepsia (dose related; ≤3%), weight loss (dose related; ≤3%)
- Genitourinary: Erectile dysfunction (dose related; ≤3%), urinary WBC positive (≤3%)
- Hematologic: Contusion (dose related; ≤4%), hemoglobin decreased, hematocrit decreased
- Neuromuscular & skeletal: Paresthesia (dose related 5% to 6%), tremor (3% to 4%), weakness (3% to 4%), muscle spasms (dose related; 1% to 4%), musculoskeletal pain (2%)
- Ocular: Vision changes
- Otic: Tinnitus (≤3%)
- Renal: BUN increased
- Respiratory: Nasopharyngitis (7% to 10%), upper respiratory tract infection (≤5%), cough (3%), nasal congestion (3%), sinus congestion (2% to 3%), sinusitis (dose related; ≤3%), pharyngolaryngeal pain (≤2%)
- Miscellaneous: Hiccups (dose related; 2% to 3%)

<1% (Limited to important or life-threatening): Agitation, aggression, confusion, delirium, delusions, disorientation, generalized skin reaction, impulsive/compulsive behaviors (eg, binge eating, hypersexuality, pathological gambling, shopping), paranoid ideation, psychotic-like behavior

Drug Interactions

Metabolism/Transport Effects None known.

Avoid Concomitant Use

Avoid concomitant use of Rotigotine with any of the following: Amisulpride

Increased Effect/Toxicity

The levels/effects of Rotigotine may be increased by: Alcohol (Ethyl); CNS Depressants; MAO Inhibitors; Methylphenidate

Decreased Effect

Rotigotine may decrease the levels/effects of: Amisulpride; Antipsychotics (Typical)

The levels/effects of Rotigotine may be decreased by: Amisulpride; Antipsychotics (Atypical); Antipsychotics (Typical); Metoclopramide

Ethanol/Nutrition/Herb Interactions Ethanol: Avoid ethanol (may increase CNS depression).

Storage/Stability Store at 20°C to 25°C (68°F to 77°F). Store in original pouch until application.

Mechanism of Action Rotigotine is a nonergot dopamine agonist with specificity for D_3-, D_2-, and D_1-dopamine receptors. Although the precise mechanism of action of rotigotine is unknown, it is believed to be due to stimulation of postsynaptic dopamine D_2-type auto receptors within the substantia nigra in the brain, leading to improved dopaminergic transmission in the motor areas of the basal ganglia, notably the caudate nucleus/putamen regions.

Pharmacodynamics/Kinetics

Distribution: V_d: 84 L/kg

Protein binding: ~90%

Metabolism: Extensive via conjugation and N-dealkylation; multiple CYP isoenzymes, sulfotransferases, and two UDP-glucuronosyltransferases involved in catalyzing the metabolism

Half-life elimination: After removal of patch: ~5-7 hours

Time to peak, plasma: 15-18 hours; can occur 4-27 hours post application

Excretion: Urine (~71% as inactive conjugates and metabolites, <1% as unchanged drug); feces (~23%)

Dosage Topical: Transdermal: Adults:

Parkinson's disease:

Early-stage: Initial: Apply 2 mg/24 hours patch once daily; may increase by 2 mg/24 hours weekly, based on clinical response and tolerability; lowest effective dose: 4 mg/24 hours (maximum dose: 6 mg/24 hours)

Advanced-stage: Initial: Apply 4 mg/24 hours patch once daily; may increase by 2 mg/24 hours weekly, based on clinical response and tolerability (maximum dose: 8 mg/24 hours)

Discontinuation of treatment in Parkinson's disease: Decrease by ≤2 mg/24 hours preferably every other day until withdrawal complete

Restless legs syndrome (RLS): Initial: Apply 1 mg/24 hours patch once daily; may increase by 1 mg/24 hours weekly, based on clinical response and tolerability; lowest effective dose: 1 mg/24 hours (maximum dose: 3 mg/24 hours)

Discontinuation of treatment for RLS: Decrease by 1 mg/24 hours preferably every other day until withdrawal complete

Dosage adjustment in renal impairment: Mild-to-severe impairment (Cl_{cr} ≥15 mL/minute): No dosage adjustment necessary.

Dosage adjustment in hepatic impairment:

Mild-to-moderate hepatic impairment (Child-Pugh class A or B): No dosage adjustment necessary.

Severe hepatic impairment: No dosage adjustment provided in manufacturer's labeling (has not been studied).

Administration Transdermal patch: Apply patch to clean, dry, hairless area of intact healthy skin on the front of the abdomen, thigh, hip, flank, shoulder, or upper arm at approximately the same time daily. Remove from pouch immediately before use and press patch firmly in place on skin for 30 seconds. Application sites should be rotated on a daily basis. Do not apply to same application site more than once every 14 days or apply patch to oily, irritated or damaged skin. Avoid exposing patch to external heat sources (eg, heating pad, electric blanket, heat lamp, hot tub, direct sunlight). If applied to hairy area, shave ≥3 days prior to applying patch. If patch falls off, immediately apply a new one to a new site.

Monitoring Parameters Blood pressure (including orthostatic); daytime alertness; periodic skin evaluations (melanoma development)

Additional Information In April 2008, Neupro® was removed from the market following a recall due to the formation of rotigotine crystals (resembling snowflakes) on the patch. The crystallization resulted in decreased drug available for absorption and altered efficacy. Reintroduction of a reformulated Neupro® into the U.S. market was announced in 2012.

Dosage Forms Excipient information presented when available (limited, particularly for generics); consult specific product labeling.

Patch 24 Hour, Transdermal:

Neupro: 1 mg/24 hr (30 ea); 2 mg/24 hr (30 ea); 3 mg/24 hr (30 ea); 4 mg/24 hr (30 ea); 6 mg/24 hr (30 ea); 8 mg/24 hr (30 ea) [contains sodium metabisulfite]

- ◆ **Rowasa** *see* Mesalamine *on page* 1305
- ◆ **Roxanol** *see* Morphine (Systemic) *on page* 1398
- ◆ **Roxicet** *see* Oxycodone and Acetaminophen *on page* 1538
- ◆ **Roxicet 5/500** *see* Oxycodone and Acetaminophen *on page* 1538
- ◆ **Roxicodone** *see* OxyCODONE *on page* 1535
- ◆ **Roychlor (Can)** *see* Potassium Chloride *on page* 1684
- ◆ **Rozerem** *see* Ramelteon *on page* 1777
- ◆ **RP-6976** *see* DOCEtaxel *on page* 638
- ◆ **RP-54274** *see* Riluzole *on page* 1819
- ◆ **RP-59500** *see* Quinupristin and Dalfopristin *on page* 1768
- ◆ **r-PA** *see* Reteplase *on page* 1800
- ◆ **rPDGF-BB** *see* Becaplermin *on page* 227
- ◆ **RPR-116258A** *see* Cabazitaxel *on page* 307
- ◆ **(R,R)-Formoterol L-Tartrate** *see* Arformoterol *on page* 160
- ◆ **RS-25259** *see* Palonosetron *on page* 1554
- ◆ **RS-25259-197** *see* Palonosetron *on page* 1554
- ◆ **RTCA** *see* Ribavirin *on page* 1804
- ◆ **RTG** *see* Ezogabine *on page* 819
- ◆ **RU 0211** *see* Lubiprostone *on page* 1254
- ◆ **RU-486** *see* Mifepristone *on page* 1364
- ◆ **RU-23908** *see* Nilutamide *on page* 1459
- ◆ **RU-38486** *see* Mifepristone *on page* 1364
- ◆ **Rubella, Measles and Mumps Vaccines** *see* Measles, Mumps, and Rubella Virus Vaccine *on page* 1272
- ◆ **Rubella, Varicella, Measles, and Mumps Vaccine** *see* Measles, Mumps, Rubella, and Varicella Virus Vaccine *on page* 1273
- ◆ **Rubidomycin Hydrochloride** *see* DAUNOrubicin (Conventional) *on page* 553
- ◆ **RUF 331** *see* Rufinamide *on page* 1865

Rufinamide (roo FIN a mide)

Brand Names: U.S. Banzel

Brand Names: Canada Banzel™

Index Terms CGP 33101; E 2080; RUF 331; Xilep

Pharmacologic Category Anticonvulsant, Triazole Derivative

Use Adjunctive therapy in the treatment of generalized seizures of Lennox-Gastaut syndrome

Pregnancy Risk Factor C

Pregnancy Considerations Adverse effects were seen in animal studies. There are no adequate and well-controlled studies in pregnant women; use during pregnancy only if clearly needed. Hormonal contraceptives may be less effective with concurrent rufinamide use; additional forms of nonhormonal contraceptives should be used.

Patients exposed to rufinamide during pregnancy are encouraged to enroll themselves into the AED Pregnancy Registry by calling 1-888-233-2334. Additional information is available at www.aedpregnancyregistry.org.

Breast-Feeding Considerations Excretion into breast milk is unknown, but may be expected. Breast-feeding is not recommended by the manufacturer due to the potential for adverse effects in the nursing infant.

Medication Guide Available Yes

Contraindications Patients with familial short QT syndrome

Canadian labeling: Additional contraindications (not in U.S. labeling): Family history of short QT syndrome; presence or history of short QT interval; hypersensitivity to rufinamide, triazole derivatives, or any component of the formulation

Warnings/Precautions Has been associated with shortening of the QT interval. Use caution in patients receiving concurrent medications that shorten the QT interval. Contraindicated in patients with familial short-QT syndrome (Canadian labeling also contraindicates use in patients with a family history of short QT syndrome or presence or history of short QT interval). Use has been associated with CNS-related adverse events, most significant of these were cognitive symptoms (including somnolence or fatigue) and coordination abnormalities (including ataxia, dizziness, and gait disturbances). Caution patients about performing tasks which require mental alertness (eg, operating machinery or driving). Effects with other sedative drugs or ethanol may be potentiated. Potentially serious, sometimes fatal, multiorgan hypersensitivity reactions have been reported with some antiepileptic drugs, including rufinamide; monitor for signs and symptoms of possible disparate manifestations associated with lymphatic, hepatic, renal, and/or hematologic organ systems; gradual discontinuation and conversion to alternate therapy may be required. Closely monitor any patient who develops a rash; instruct patients to report any rash associated with fever.

Antiepileptics are associated with an increased risk of suicidal behavior/thoughts with use (regardless of indication); patients should be monitored for signs/symptoms of depression, suicidal tendencies, and other unusual behavior changes during therapy and instructed to inform their healthcare provider immediately if symptoms occur. Use with caution in patients with mild-to-moderate hepatic impairment; use in not recommended in patients with severe hepatic impairment. Concurrent use with hormonal contraceptives may lead to contraceptive failure. Anticonvulsants should not be discontinued abruptly because of the possibility of increasing seizure frequency; therapy should be withdrawn gradually to minimize the potential of increased seizure frequency, unless safety concerns require a more rapid withdrawal. Reducing dose by ~25% every two days was effective in trials.

Adverse Reactions

>10%:

Cardiovascular: QT shortening (46% to 65%; dose related)

Central nervous system: Headache (16% to 27%), somnolence (11% to 24%), dizziness (3% to 19%), fatigue (9% to 16%)

Gastrointestinal: Vomiting (5% to 17%), nausea (7% to 12%)

1% to 10%:

Central nervous system: Ataxia (4% to 5%), seizure (children 5%), status epilepticus (≤4%), aggression (children 3%), anxiety (adults 3%), attention disturbance (children 3%), hyperactivity (children 3%), vertigo (adults 3%)

Dermatologic: Rash (children 4%), pruritus (children 3%)

Gastrointestinal: Appetite decreased (≥1% to 5%), abdominal pain (3%), constipation (adults 3%), dyspepsia (adults 3%), appetite increased (≥1%)

Hematologic: Leukopenia (≤4%), anemia (≥1%)

Neuromuscular & skeletal: Tremor (adults 6%), back pain (adults 3%), gait disturbance (1% to 3%)

Ocular: Diplopia (4% to 9%), blurred vision (adults 6%), nystagmus (adults 6%)

Otic: Otitis media (children 3%)

Renal: Pollakiuria (≥1%)

Respiratory: Nasopharyngitis (children 5%), bronchitis (children 3%), sinusitis (children 3%)

Miscellaneous: Influenza (children 5%)

<1% (Limited to important or life-threatening): Atrioventricular block (first degree), bundle branch block (right), dysuria, enuresis, hematuria; hypersensitivity (multiorgan; includes eosinophilia, facial edema, fever, hepatitis [severe], LFTs increased, rash, stupor, urticaria); incontinence, iron-deficiency anemia, lymphadenopathy, nephrolithiasis, neutropenia, nocturia, polyuria, thrombocytopenia, urinary incontinence

Drug Interactions

Metabolism/Transport Effects Inhibits CYP2E1 (weak); **Induces** CYP3A4 (weak/moderate)

Avoid Concomitant Use

Avoid concomitant use of Rufinamide with any of the following: Axitinib; Simeprevir

Increased Effect/Toxicity

Rufinamide may increase the levels/effects of: Fosphenytoin; PHENobarbital; Phenytoin

The levels/effects of Rufinamide may be increased by: Valproic Acid and Derivatives

Decreased Effect

Rufinamide may decrease the levels/effects of: ARIPiprazole; Axitinib; CarBAMazepine; Ethinyl Estradiol; Ibrutinib; Norethindrone; Saxagliptin; Simeprevir

The levels/effects of Rufinamide may be decreased by: CarBAMazepine; Fosphenytoin; PHENobarbital; Phenytoin; Primidone

Ethanol/Nutrition/Herb Interactions

Ethanol: Ethanol may increase CNS depression. Management: Avoid ethanol.

Food: Food increases the absorption of rufinamide. Management: Take with food.

Herb/Nutraceutical: Evening primrose may decrease seizure threshold. Management: Avoid evening primrose.

Storage/Stability Store at 25°C (77°F); excursions permitted to 15°C to 30°C (59°F to 86°F). Protect tablets from moisture. The cap to the oral suspension bottle fits over the adapter.

Mechanism of Action A triazole-derivative antiepileptic whose exact mechanism is unknown. *In vitro*, it prolongs the inactive state of the sodium channels, thereby limiting repetitive firing of sodium-dependent action potentials mediating anticonvulsant effects.

Pharmacodynamics/Kinetics

Absorption: Slow; extensive ≥85%; increased with food

Distribution: V_d: ~50 L

Protein binding: 34%, primarily to albumin

Metabolism: Extensively via carboxylesterase-mediated hydrolysis of the carboxylamide group to CGP 47292 (inactive metabolite); weak inhibitor of CYP2E1 and weak inducer of CYP3A4

Bioavailability: Extent decreased with increased dose; oral tablets and oral suspension are bioequivalent

Half-life elimination: ~6-10 hours

Time to peak, plasma: 4-6 hours

Excretion: Urine (85%, ~66% as CGP 47292, <2% as unchanged drug)

Dosage Oral: Lennox-Gastaut (adjunctive):

U.S. labeling:

Children ≥4 years: Initial: 10 mg/kg/day in 2 equally divided doses; increase dose by ~10 mg/kg every other day to a target dose of 45 mg/kg/day **or** 3200 mg/day (whichever is lower) in 2 equally divided doses

Adults: Initial: 400-800 mg/day in 2 equally divided doses; increase dose by 400-800 mg/day every other day to a maximum dose of 3200 mg/day in 2 equally divided doses

Canadian labeling: Children ≥4 years and Adults:

<30 kg: Initial: 100 mg twice daily; increase dose by 5 mg/kg/day every 2 weeks until satisfactory control (maximum dose: 1300 mg/day)

≥30 kg: Initial: 200 mg twice daily; increase dose by 5 mg/kg/day every 2 weeks until satisfactory control (maximum dose: 30-50 kg: 1800 mg/day; 50.1-70 kg: 2400 mg/day; ≥70.1 kg: 3200 mg/day). **Note:** Dose was increased as frequently as every other day in clinical trials.

Dosage adjustment for concomitant medications: Valproate:

U.S. labeling: Initial rufinamide dose should be <10 mg/kg/day (children) or 400 mg/day (adults)

Canadian labeling: Initial rufinamide dose should be less than the initial daily recommended dosage; however, a specific dosage recommendation is not included in the manufacturer's labeling.

Dosage adjustment in renal impairment: Cl_{cr} <30 mL/minute: No dosage adjustment necessary.

Hemodialysis: No dosage adjustment provided in manufacturer's labeling. However, consider dosage adjustment for loss of drug.

Dosage adjustment in hepatic impairment:

Mild-to-moderate impairment: Use with caution

Severe impairment: No dosage adjustment provided in manufacturer's labeling (has not been studied). Use with caution. Use in severe impairment is not recommended.

Dietary Considerations Take with food.

Administration Administer with food. Tablets may be swallowed whole, split in half, or crushed. Oral suspension should be administered using the provided adapter and oral syringe; shake well before every administration.

Monitoring Parameters Seizure (frequency and duration); serum levels of concurrent anticonvulsants; suicidality (eg, suicidal thoughts, depression, behavioral changes)

Dosage Forms Excipient information presented when available (limited, particularly for generics); consult specific product labeling.

Suspension, Oral:

Banzel: 40 mg/mL (460 mL) [contains methylparaben, propylene glycol, propylparaben; orange flavor]

Tablet, Oral:

Banzel: 200 mg, 400 mg [scored]

Dosage Forms: Canada Excipient information presented when available (limited, particularly for generics); consult specific product labeling.

Tablet, oral:

Banzel™: 100 mg [scored]

Extemporaneous Preparations A 40 mg/mL oral suspension may be made using tablets. Crush twelve 400 mg tablets (or twenty-four 200 mg tablets) and reduce to a fine powder. Add 60 mL of Ora-Plus® in incremental proportions until a smooth suspension is obtained; then mix well while adding 60 mL of Ora-Sweet® or Ora-Sweet® SF; transfer to a calibrated bottle. Label "shake well". Stable 90 days at room temperature.

Hutchinson DJ, Liou Y, Best R, et al, "Stability of Extemporaneously Prepared Rufinamide Oral Suspensions," *Ann Pharmacother*, 2010, 44(3):462-5.

◆ **Rulox [OTC]** *see* Aluminum Hydroxide, Magnesium Hydroxide, and Simethicone *on page 90*

Ruxolitinib (rux oh LI ti nib)

Brand Names: U.S. Jakafi

Brand Names: Canada Jakavi™

Index Terms INCB 18424; INCB018424; INCB424; Ruxolitinib Phosphate

Pharmacologic Category Antineoplastic Agent, Janus Associated Kinase Inhibitor; Antineoplastic Agent, Tyrosine Kinase Inhibitor; Janus Associated Kinase Inhibitor

Use Treatment of intermediate or high-risk myelofibrosis, including primary myelofibrosis, post-polycythemia vera (post-PV) myelofibrosis and post-essential thrombocythemia (post-ET) myelofibrosis

Pregnancy Risk Factor C

Pregnancy Considerations Increased resorptions (late) and reduced fetal weights were observed in animal reproduction studies. Use during human pregnancy only if the potential treatment benefits outweigh risks.

Breast-Feeding Considerations It is not known if ruxolitinib is excreted in breast milk. According to the manufacturer, the decision to continue or discontinue breast-feeding during therapy should take into account the risk of exposure to the infant and the benefits of treatment to the mother.

Prescribing and Access Restrictions Available through specialty/network pharmacies. Further information may be obtained from the manufacturer, Incyte, at 1-855-452-5234 or at www.Jakafi.com.

Contraindications There are no contraindications listed within the manufacturer's U.S. labeling.

Canadian labeling: Hypersensitivity to ruxolitinib or any component of the formulation or container

Warnings/Precautions Hazardous agent - use appropriate precautions for handling and disposal (meets NIOSH, 2012 criteria). Hematologic toxicity, including thrombocytopenia, anemia and neutropenia may occur; may require dosage modification; monitor complete blood counts at baseline, every 2-4 weeks during dose stabilization, and then as clinically necessary. Thrombocytopenia is generally reversible with treatment interruption or dose reduction; platelet transfusions may be administered during treatment if clinically indicated. Anemia may require blood transfusion; may consider dose modification. Neutropenia (ANC <500/mm^3) is generally reversible and managed by treatment interruption.

Serious bacterial, mycobacterial (including tuberculosis), fungal, or viral infections may occur; monitor for infections during treatment. Active serious infections should be resolved prior to treatment initiation. Prompt treatment is recommended if symptoms of herpes zoster infection develop. Progressive multifocal leukoencephalopathy (PML) has been reported; discontinue and evaluate if suspected. May require initial dosage reduction for hepatic impairment; avoid use if platelets <100,000/mm^3 and with hepatic impairment (any degree). May require initial dosage reduction for renal impairment; avoid use if platelets <100,000/mm^3 and with moderate-to-severe renal impairment or in patients with ESRD not requiring dialysis. Ruxolitinib is not removed by dialysis, however, some active metabolites may be removed. On dialysis days, patients are advised to take their dose following dialysis sessions. Potentially significant drug-drug interactions may exist, requiring dose or frequency adjustment, additional monitoring, and/or selection of alternative therapy. Reduced initial doses are recommended with concomitant use of strong CYP3A4 inhibitors (eg, clarithromycin, conivaptin, itraconazole, ketoconazole, nefazodone, posaconazole, protease inhibitors, telithromycin, voriconazole, grapefruit juice); if platelets <100,000/mm^3, avoid concomitant use with strong CYP3A4 inhibitors. No adjustment is recommended with concomitant use of mild or moderate CYP3A4 inhibitors or with CYP3A4 inducers (monitor closely for efficacy and titrate dose appropriately). Discontinue treatment after 6 months if no reduction in spleen size or no improvement in symptoms. Consider gradually tapering off if discontinuing for reasons other than thrombocytopenia. Within ~1 week after discontinuation, symptoms of myelofibrosis generally return to pretreatment levels. Acute relapse of myelofibrosis symptoms, splenomegaly, worsening cytopenias, hemodynamic compensation, and septic shock-like syndrome have been reported with treatment discontinuation (Tefferi, 2011); consider gradually tapering off if discontinuing for reasons other than thrombocytopenia.

Use with caution in patients with a history of bradycardia, conduction disturbances, ischemic heart disease, heart failure and/or receiving other drugs that also affect heart rate/conduction; decreased heart rate (mean change 6-8 bpm) and prolongation of the PR interval (mean change 6-9 msec) and of the QT interval (mean 4-5 msec) were observed during some clinical trials. Canadian labeling recommends obtaining an ECG at baseline and periodically; monitor heart rate and blood pressure during treatment.

Adverse Reactions

>10%:

Cardiovascular: Peripheral edema (22%)

Central nervous system: Dizziness (15% to 18%), headache (10% to 15%), insomnia (12%)

Dermatologic: Ecchymoses (19% to 23%)

Endocrine & metabolic: Increased serum cholesterol (17%; grade 2: <1%)

Gastrointestinal: Diarrhea (23%), constipation (13%), nausea (13%), vomiting (12%)

Hematologic & oncologic: Anemia (96%; grade 3: 34%; grade 4: 11%), thrombocytopenia (70%; grade 3: 9%; grade 4: 4%), neutropenia (19%; grade 3: 5%; grade 4: 2%)

Hepatic: Increased serum ALT (25%; grades 2/3: 1% to 2%), increased serum AST (17%; grade 2: <1%)

Respiratory: Dyspnea (16%), nasopharyngitis (16%)

1% to 10%:

Endocrine & metabolic: Weight gain (7%)

Gastrointestinal: Flatulence (5%)

Genitourinary: Urinary tract infection (9%)

Infection: Herpes zoster (2%)

<1% (Limited to important or life-threatening): Edema, heart murmur, peripheral neuropathy, withdrawal syndrome (acute relapse of myelofibrosis symptoms, splenomegaly, severe cytopenia, and septic shock

Drug Interactions

Metabolism/Transport Effects Substrate of CYP3A4 (major); **Note:** Assignment of Major/Minor substrate status based on clinically relevant drug interaction potential

Avoid Concomitant Use

Avoid concomitant use of Ruxolitinib with any of the following: BCG; CloZAPine; Fusidic Acid (Systemic); Natalizumab; Pimecrolimus; Tacrolimus (Topical); Tofacitinib; Vaccines (Live)

Increased Effect/Toxicity

Ruxolitinib may increase the levels/effects of: CloZAPine; Leflunomide; Natalizumab; Tofacitinib; Vaccines (Live)

The levels/effects of Ruxolitinib may be increased by: CYP3A4 Inhibitors (Moderate); CYP3A4 Inhibitors (Strong); Dasatinib; Denosumab; Fusidic Acid (Systemic); Grapefruit Juice; Ivacaftor; Luliconazole; Mifepristone; Pimecrolimus; Roflumilast; Simeprevir; Tacrolimus (Topical); Trastuzumab

Decreased Effect

Ruxolitinib may decrease the levels/effects of: BCG; Coccidioidin Skin Test; Sipuleucel-T; Vaccines (Inactivated); Vaccines (Live)

The levels/effects of Ruxolitinib may be decreased by: Bosentan; CYP3A4 Inducers (Strong); Dabrafenib; Deferasirox; Echinacea; Herbs (CYP3A4 Inducers); Mitotane; Tocilizumab

Ethanol/Nutrition/Herb Interactions Food: Avoid grapefruit juice (may increase the effects of ruxolitinib).

Storage/Stability Store at room temperature of 20°C to 25°C (68°F to 77°F); excursions permitted to 15°C to 30°C (59°F to 86°F).

Mechanism of Action Kinase inhibitor which selectively inhibits Janus Associated Kinases (JAKs), JAK1 and JAK2. JAK1 and JAK2 mediate signaling of cytokine and growth factors responsible for hematopoiesis and immune function; JAK mediated signaling involves recruitment of STATs (signal transducers and activators of transcription) to cytokine receptors which leads to modulation of gene expression. In myelofibrosis, JAK1/2 activity is dysregulated; ruxolitinib modulates the affected JAK1/2 activity.

Pharmacodynamics/Kinetics

Absorption: Rapid

Distribution: V_d: 53-65 L

Protein binding: ~97%; primarily to albumin

Metabolism: Hepatic, primarily via CYP3A4; forms active metabolites responsible for 20% to 50% of activity

Half-life elimination: Ruxolitinib: 2.8-3 hours (hepatic impairment: 5 hours); Ruxolitinib + metabolites: ~6 hours

Time to peak: Within 1-2 hours

Excretion: Urine (74%, <1% as unchanged drug); feces (22%, <1% as unchanged drug)

Dosage Oral: Adults: Myelofibrosis: Initial dose (based on platelet count, titrate dose thereafter based on efficacy and safety):

U.S. labeling:

Platelets >200,000/mm^3: 20 mg twice daily

Platelets 100,000-200,000/mm^3: 15 mg twice daily

Platelets 50,000 to <100,000/mm^3: 5 mg twice daily

Canadian labeling:

Platelets >200,000/mm^3: 20 mg twice daily

Platelets 100,000-200,000/mm^3: 15 mg twice daily

Platelets 50,000-100,000/ mm^3: Initial dose should not exceed 5 mg twice daily; titrate dose cautiously

Dosage modification based on response in patients with baseline platelet count ≥100,000/mm^3 prior to initial treatment with ruxolitinib: For insufficient response (with adequate platelet and neutrophil counts), may increase the dose in 5 mg twice daily increments to a maximum dose of 25 mg twice daily. Do not increase during initial 4 weeks and no more frequently than every 2 weeks. Discontinue treatment after 6 months if no reduction in spleen size or no improvement in symptoms. When discontinuing for reasons other than thrombocytopenia, consider gradually tapering by ~5 mg twice daily per week.

Dose increases may be considered if meet all of the following situations:

- Failure to achieve either a 50% reduction (from baseline) in palpable spleen length or a 35% reduction (from baseline) in spleen volume (measured by CT or MRI)
- Platelet count >125,000/mm^3 at 4 weeks (and never <100,000/mm^3)
- Absolute neutrophil count (ANC) >750/mm^3

Dosage modification based on response in patients with baseline platelet 50,000 to <100,000/mm^3 prior to initial treatment with ruxolitinib: For insufficient response (with adequate platelet and neutrophil counts), may increase the dose in 5 mg daily increments to a maximum dose of 10 mg twice daily. Do not increase during initial 4 weeks and no more frequently than every 2 weeks. Discontinue treatment after 6 months if no reduction in spleen size or no improvement in symptoms.

Dose increases may be considered if meet all of the following situations:

- Platelet count remains ≥40,000/mm^3 and did not decrease more than 20% in prior 4 weeks
- Absolute neutrophil count (ANC) >1000/mm^3
- No adverse event or hematological toxicity resulting in dose reduction or interruption occurred in prior 4 weeks

Dosage modification for bleeding requiring intervention (regardless of platelet count): Interrupt treatment until bleeding resolved; may consider resuming at the prior dose if the underlying cause of bleeding has resolved or at a reduced dose if the underlying cause of bleeding persists.

Dosage modification for treatment interruption:

U.S. labeling:

If baseline platelet count ≥100,000/mm^3 prior to initial treatment with ruxolitinib and:

Platelets <50,000/mm^3 and ANC <500/mm^3: Interrupt treatment; upon platelet recovery (to ≥50,000/mm^3) or ANC recovery (to ≥750/mm^3), dosing may be restarted or increased based on the following platelet or ANC levels

Platelets ≥125,000/mm^3: Dose should be at least 5 mg twice daily below the dose at treatment interruption, up to a maximum of 20 mg twice daily

Platelets 100,000 to <125,000/mm^3: Dose should be at least 5 mg twice daily below the dose at treatment interruption, up to a maximum of 15 mg twice daily

Platelets 75,000 to <100,000/mm^3: Dose should be at least 5 mg twice daily below the dose at treatment interruption, up to a maximum of 10 mg twice daily for at least 2 weeks; may increase to 15 mg twice daily if stable

Platelets 50,000 to <75,000/mm^3: 5 mg twice daily for at least 2 weeks; may increase to 10 mg twice daily if stable

Platelets <50,000/mm^3: Continue to withhold treatment

ANC ≥750/mm^3: Resume at 5 mg once daily or 5 mg twice daily below the largest dose in the week prior to treatment interruption, whichever is greater

Note: Long-term maintenance at 5 mg twice daily has not demonstrated responses; limit use of the dose level to patients where the benefits outweigh risks

If baseline platelet count 50,000 to <100,000/mm^3 prior to initial treatment with ruxolitinib and:

Platelets <25,000/mm^3 and ANC <500/mm^3: Interrupt treatment; upon platelet recovery (to ≥35,000/mm^3) or ANC recovery (to ≥750/mm^3), resume at 5 mg once daily or 5 mg twice daily below the largest dose in the week prior to treatment interruption, whichever is greater

Note: Long-term maintenance at 5 mg twice daily has not demonstrated responses; limit use of the dose level to patients where the benefits outweigh risks

Canadian labeling: Platelets <50,000/mm^3 or ANC <500 mm^3: Interrupt treatment; upon recovery of platelets to ≥50,000/mm^3 or ANC to ≥500/mm^3, dosing may be restarted at 5 mg twice daily and then gradually titrated based on blood cell counts.

Dosage reduction for thrombocytopenia in patients with baseline platelet count ≥100,000/mm^3 prior to initial treatment with ruxolitinib:

Platelet Count	Dose at Time of Thrombocytopenia				
	25 mg twice/day	20 mg twice/day	15 mg twice/day	10 mg twice/day	5 mg twice/day
	New Dose	New Dose	New Dose	New Dose	New Dose
100,000 to <125,000/mm^3	20 mg twice/day	15 mg twice/day	No change	No change	No change
75,000 to <100,000/mm^3	10 mg twice/day	10 mg twice/day	10 mg twice/day	No change	No change
50,000 to <75,000/mm^3	5 mg twice/day	5 mg twice/day	5 mg twice/day	5 mg twice/day	No change
<50,000/mm^3	Hold dose	Hold dose	Hold dose	Hold dose	Hold dose

Note: Long-term maintenance at 5 mg twice daily has not demonstrated responses; limit use of the dose level to patients where the benefits outweigh risks

Dosage reduction for thrombocytopenia in patients with baseline platelet 50,000 to <100,000/mm^3 prior to initial treatment with ruxolitinib:

Platelets 25,000 to <35,000/mm^3 **and** platelet count decreased <20% during prior 4 weeks:

If current daily dose >5 mg: Reduce dose by 5 mg once daily

If current dose 5 mg once daily: Continue 5 mg once daily

Platelets 25,000 to <35,000/mm^3 **and** platelet count decreased ≥20% during prior four weeks:

If current daily dose >10 mg: Reduce dose by 5 mg twice daily

If current dose 5 mg twice daily: Reduce dose to 5 mg once daily

If current dose 5 mg once daily: Continue 5 mg once daily

Platelets <25,000 mm^3: Continue to withhold treatment

Note: Long-term maintenance at 5 mg twice daily has not demonstrated responses; limit use of the dose level to patients where the benefits outweigh risks

Dosage adjustment with concomitant strong CYP3A4 inhibitors: Initial dose: 10 mg twice daily (if platelet count ≥100,000/mm^3); additional dose adjustments should be made with careful monitoring. Avoid concomitant use if platelet count <100,000/mm^3.

Dosage adjustment in renal impairment:

U.S. labeling:

Cl_{cr} 15-59 mL/minute and platelets >150,000/mm^3: No dosage adjustment provided in manufacturer's labeling.

Cl_{cr} 15-59 mL/minute and platelets 100,000-150,000/mm^3: Initial dose: 10 mg twice daily; additional dose adjustments should be made with careful monitoring.

Cl_{cr} 15-59 mL/minute and platelets <100,000/mm^3: Avoid use.

End-stage renal disease (ESRD) on dialysis and platelets 100,000-200,000/mm^3: Initial dose: 15 mg; administer subsequent doses after dialysis on dialysis days. Additional dose adjustments should be made with careful monitoring.

ESRD on dialysis and platelets >200,000/mm^3: Initial dose: 20 mg; administer subsequent doses after dialysis on dialysis days. Additional dose adjustments should be made with careful monitoring.

ESRD not requiring dialysis: Avoid use.

Canadian labeling:

Cl_{cr} <50 mL/minute and platelets ≥100,000/mm^3: Initial dose: 10 mg twice daily; additional dose adjustments should be made with careful monitoring

Cl_{cr} <50 mL/minute and platelets <100,000/mm^3: Avoid use

ESRD on dialysis and platelets 100,000-200,000/mm^3: Initial dose: 15 mg; administer subsequent doses after dialysis on dialysis days. Additional dose adjustments should be made with careful monitoring.

ESRD on dialysis and platelets >200,000/mm^3: Initial dose: 20 mg; administer subsequent doses after dialysis on dialysis days. Additional dose adjustments should be made with careful monitoring.

Dosage adjustment in hepatic impairment:

U.S. labeling:

Mild-to-severe impairment and platelets >150,000/mm^3: No dosage adjustment provided in manufacturer's labeling.

Mild-to-severe impairment and platelets 100,000-150,000/mm^3: Initial dose: 10 mg twice daily; additional dose adjustments should be made with careful monitoring.

Mild-to-severe impairment and platelets <100,000/mm^3: Avoid use.

Canadian labeling:

Hepatic impairment and platelets >100,000/mm^3: Initial dose: 10 mg twice daily; additional dose adjustments should be made with careful monitoring.

Hepatic impairment and platelets <100,000/mm^3: Avoid use.

Dietary Considerations May be taken with or without food. Avoid grapefruit juice (may increase the effects of ruxolitinib).

Administration May be administered orally with or without food. If a dose is missed, return to the usual dosing schedule and do **not** administer an additional dose.

If unable to ingest tablets, may administer through a nasogastric (NG) tube (≥8 Fr): Suspend 1 tablet in ~40 mL water and stir for ~10 minutes and administer (within 6 hours after dispersion) with appropriate syringe; rinse NG tube with ~75 mL water (effect of enteral tube feeding on ruxolitinib exposure has not been evaluated)

Hazardous agent; use appropriate precautions for handling and disposal (meets NIOSH, 2012 criteria).

Monitoring Parameters CBC (baseline, every 2-4 weeks until dose stabilized, then as clinically indicated), renal function, hepatic function. Canadian labeling recommends obtaining an ECG at baseline and then periodically during therapy; monitor heart rate and blood pressure during therapy.

Dosage Forms Excipient information presented when available (limited, particularly for generics); consult specific product labeling.

Tablet, Oral:

Jakafi: 5 mg, 10 mg, 15 mg, 20 mg, 25 mg

Extemporaneous Preparations Hazardous agent; use appropriate precautions for handling and disposal.

A suspension for nasogastric administration may be prepared with tablets. Place one tablet into ~40 mL water; stir for approximately 10 minutes. Administer within 6 hour after preparation.

Jakafi™ prescribing information November, 2011. Incyte Corporation, Wilmington, DE.

- **Ruxolitinib Phosphate** *see* Ruxolitinib *on page 1867*
- **RV1 (Rotarix)** *see* Rotavirus Vaccine *on page 1861*
- **RV5 (RotaTeq)** *see* Rotavirus Vaccine *on page 1861*
- **Rybix ODT [DSC]** *see* TraMADol *on page 2099*
- **Rylosol (Can)** *see* Sotalol *on page 1942*
- **Rythmodan® (Can)** *see* Disopyramide *on page 636*
- **Rythmodan®-LA (Can)** *see* Disopyramide *on page 636*
- **Rythmol** *see* Propafenone *on page 1731*
- **Rythmol® Gen-Propafenone (Can)** *see* Propafenone *on page 1731*
- **Rythmol SR** *see* Propafenone *on page 1731*
- **S2 [OTC]** *see* EPINEPHrine (Systemic, Oral Inhalation) *on page 714*
- **S-(+)-3-isobutylgaba** *see* Pregabalin *on page 1710*
- **S-4661** *see* Doripenem *on page 653*
- **Sabril** *see* Vigabatrin *on page 2186*

Sacrosidase (sak ROE si dase)

Brand Names: U.S. Sucraid

Brand Names: Canada Sucraid®

Pharmacologic Category Enzyme, Gastrointestinal

Use Oral replacement therapy in sucrase deficiency, as seen in congenital sucrase-isomaltase deficiency (CSID)

Pregnancy Risk Factor C

Prescribing and Access Restrictions Sucraid® is not available in retail pharmacies or via mail-order pharmacies. To obtain the product, please refer to http://www.sucraid.net/how-to-order-sucraid or call 1-866-740-2743.

Dosage Oral:

Infants ≥5 months and Children ≤15 kg: 8500 units (1 mL) per meal or snack

Children >15 kg, Adolescents, and Adults: 17,000 units (2 mL) per meal or snack

Doses should be diluted with 2-4 oz of cold or room temperature water, milk, or formula. Approximately one-half of the dose should be taken before and the remainder of a dose taken during each meal or snack.

Dosage adjustment in renal impairment: No dosage adjustment provided in manufacturer's labeling.

Dosage adjustment in hepatic impairment: No dosage adjustment provided in manufacturer's labeling.

Additional Information Complete prescribing information should be consulted for additional detail.

Dosage Forms Excipient information presented when available (limited, particularly for generics); consult specific product labeling.

Solution, Oral:

Sucraid: 8500 units/mL (118 mL) [contains papain]

- **Safetussin® CD [OTC]** *see* Dextromethorphan and Phenylephrine *on page 591*
- **Safe Tussin DM [OTC]** *see* Guaifenesin and Dextromethorphan *on page 976*
- **Safe Wash [OTC]** *see* Sodium Chloride *on page 1914*
- **Safyral** *see* Ethinyl Estradiol, Drospirenone, and Levomefolate *on page 797*
- **SAHA** *see* Vorinostat *on page 2207*
- **Saizen** *see* Somatropin *on page 1934*
- **Saizen Click.Easy** *see* Somatropin *on page 1934*
- **Salagen** *see* Pilocarpine (Systemic) *on page 1646*
- **Salagen® (Can)** *see* Pilocarpine (Systemic) *on page 1646*
- **Salazopyrin (Can)** *see* SulfaSALAzine *on page 1964*
- **Salazopyrin En-Tabs (Can)** *see* SulfaSALAzine *on page 1964*
- **Salbutamol** *see* Albuterol *on page 61*
- **Salbutamol and Ipratropium** *see* Ipratropium and Albuterol *on page 1113*
- **Salbutamol Sulphate** *see* Albuterol *on page 61*
- **Salflex® (Can)** *see* Salsalate *on page 1873*
- **Salicylazosulfapyridine** *see* SulfaSALAzine *on page 1964*
- **Salicylsalicylic Acid** *see* Salsalate *on page 1873*

- ◆ **Saline** *see* Sodium Chloride *on page 1914*
- ◆ **Saline Flush ZR** *see* Sodium Chloride *on page 1914*
- ◆ **Saline Mist Spray [OTC]** *see* Sodium Chloride *on page 1914*
- ◆ **Saljet [OTC]** *see* Sodium Chloride *on page 1914*
- ◆ **Saljet Rinse [OTC]** *see* Sodium Chloride *on page 1914*
- ◆ **Salk Vaccine** *see* Poliovirus Vaccine (Inactivated) *on page 1666*

Salmeterol (sal ME te role)

Brand Names: U.S. Serevent Diskus

Brand Names: Canada Serevent® Diskhaler® Disk; Serevent® Diskus®

Index Terms Salmeterol Xinafoate

Pharmacologic Category $Beta_2$ Agonist; $Beta_2$-Adrenergic Agonist, Long-Acting

Use Maintenance treatment of asthma and prevention of bronchospasm (as concomitant therapy) in patients with reversible obstructive airway disease, including patients with symptoms of nocturnal asthma; prevention of exercise-induced bronchospasm (monotherapy may be indicated in patients without persistent asthma); maintenance treatment of bronchospasm associated with COPD

Pregnancy Risk Factor C

Pregnancy Considerations Adverse events were observed in some animal reproduction studies. Salmeterol has the potential to affect uterine contractility if administered during labor.

Uncontrolled asthma is associated with adverse events on pregnancy (increased risk of perinatal mortality, pre-eclampsia, preterm birth, low birth weight infants). Although data related to its use in pregnancy is limited, salmeterol may be used when a long-acting beta agonist is needed to treat moderate persistent or severe persistent asthma in pregnant women (NAEPP, 2005).

Breast-Feeding Considerations It is not known if salmeterol is excreted into breast milk. According to the manufacturer, the decision to continue or discontinue breast-feeding during therapy should take into account the risk of exposure to the infant and the benefits of treatment to the mother. The use of $beta_2$-receptor agonists are not considered a contraindication to breast-feeding (NAEPP, 2005).

Medication Guide Available Yes

Contraindications Hypersensitivity to salmeterol or any component of the formulation (milk proteins); monotherapy in the treatment of asthma (ie, use without a concomitant long-term asthma control medication, such as an inhaled corticosteroid); status asthmaticus or other acute episodes of asthma or COPD

Warnings/Precautions Asthma treatment: [U.S. Boxed Warning]: Long-acting $beta_2$-agonists (LABAs) increase the risk of asthma-related deaths. Salmeterol should only be used in asthma patients as adjuvant therapy in patients who are currently receiving but are not adequately controlled on a long-term asthma control medication (ie, an inhaled corticosteroid). Monotherapy with an LABA is contraindicated in the treatment of asthma. In a large, randomized, placebo-controlled U.S. clinical trial (SMART, 2006), salmeterol was associated with an increase in asthma-related deaths (when added to usual asthma therapy); risk is considered a class effect among all LABAs. Data are not available to determine if the addition of an inhaled corticosteroid lessens this increased risk of death associated with LABA use. Assess patients at regular intervals once asthma control is maintained on combination therapy to determine if step-down therapy is appropriate and the LABA can be discontinued (without loss of asthma control), and the patient can be maintained on an inhaled corticosteroid. LABAs are not appropriate in patients whose asthma is adequately controlled on low- or medium-dose inhaled corticosteroids. Do **not** use for acute bronchospasm. Short-acting $beta_2$-agonist (eg, albuterol) should be used for acute symptoms and symptoms occurring between treatments. Do **not** initiate in patients with significantly worsening or acutely deteriorating asthma; reports of severe (sometimes fatal) respiratory events have been reported when salmeterol has been initiated in this situation. Corticosteroids should not be stopped or reduced when salmeterol is initiated. During initiation, watch for signs of worsening asthma. Patients must be instructed to use short-acting $beta_2$-agonists (eg, albuterol) for acute asthmatic or COPD symptoms and to seek medical attention in cases where acute symptoms are not relieved or a previous level of response is diminished. The need to increase frequency of use of short-acting $beta_2$-agonist may indicate deterioration of asthma, and treatment must not be delayed. Because LABAs may disguise poorly controlled persistent asthma, frequent or chronic use of LABAs for exercise-induced bronchospasm is discouraged by the NIH Asthma Guidelines (NIH, 2007). Salmeterol should not be used more than twice daily; do not use with other long-acting $beta_2$-agonists. **[U.S. Boxed Warning]: LABAs may increase the risk of asthma-related hospitalization in pediatric and adolescent patients.** In general, a combination product containing a LABA and an inhaled corticosteroid is preferred in patients <18 years of age to ensure compliance.

COPD treatment: Appropriate use: Do **not** use for acute episodes of COPD. Do **not** initiate in patients with significantly worsening or acutely deteriorating COPD. Data are not available to determine if LABA use increases the risk of death in patients with COPD.

Concurrent diseases: Use caution in patients with cardiovascular disease (eg, arrhythmia, hypertension, or HF), seizure disorders, diabetes, hyperthyroidism, hepatic impairment, or hypokalemia. Beta-agonists may cause elevation in blood pressure, heart rate, CNS stimulation/ excitation, increased risk of arrhythmia, increase serum glucose, or decrease serum potassium.

Adverse events: Immediate hypersensitivity reactions (urticaria, angioedema, rash, bronchospasm) have been reported. There have been reports of laryngeal spasm, irritation, swelling (stridor, choking) with use. Salmeterol should not be used more than twice daily; do not exceed recommended dose; do not use with other long-acting $beta_2$-agonists; serious adverse events have been associated with excessive use of inhaled sympathomimetics. Rarely, paradoxical bronchospasm may occur with use of inhaled bronchodilating agents; this should be distinguished from inadequate response. Use with strong CYP3A4 inhibitors (see Drug Interactions) is not recommended due to potential for an increased risk of cardiovascular events. Powder for oral inhalation contains lactose; very rare anaphylactic reactions have been reported in patients with severe milk protein allergy.

Adverse Reactions

>10%:

Central nervous system: Headache (13% to 17%)

Neuromuscular & skeletal: Pain (1% to 12%)

1% to 10%:

Cardiovascular: Hypertension (4%), edema (1% to 3%), pallor

Central nervous system: Dizziness (4%), sleep disturbance (1% to 3%), fever (1% to 3%), anxiety (1% to 3%), migraine (1% to 3%)

Dermatologic: Rash (1% to 4%), contact dermatitis (1% to 3%), eczema (1% to 3%), urticaria (3%), photodermatitis (1% to 2%)

Endocrine & metabolic: Hyperglycemia (1% to 3%)
Gastrointestinal: Throat irritation (7%), nausea (1% to 3%), dyspepsia (1% to 3%), dental pain (1% to 3%), gastrointestinal infection (1% to 3%), oropharyngeal candidiasis (1% to 3%), xerostomia (1% to 3%)
Hepatic: Liver enzymes increased
Neuromuscular & skeletal: Muscular cramps/spasm (3%), articular rheumatism (1% to 3%), arthralgia (1% to 3%), joint pain (1% to 3%), muscular stiffness (1% to 3%), paresthesia (1% to 3%), rigidity (1% to 3%)
Ocular: Keratitis/conjunctivitis (1% to 3%)
Respiratory: Nasal congestion (4% to 9%), tracheitis/bronchitis (7%), pharyngitis (≤6%), cough (5%), influenza (5%), viral respiratory tract infection (5%), sinusitis (4% to 5%), rhinitis (4% to 5%), asthma (3% to 4%)

<1% (Limited to important or life-threatening): Abdominal pain, agitation, aggression, anaphylactic reaction (some in patients with severe milk allergy [Diskus®]), angioedema, aphonia, arrhythmia, atrial fibrillation, cataracts, chest congestion, chest tightness, choking, contusions, Cushing syndrome, Cushingoid features, depression, dysmenorrhea, dyspnea, earache, ecchymoses, edema (facial, oropharyngeal), eosinophilic conditions, glaucoma, growth velocity reduction in children/adolescents, hypercorticism, hypersensitivity reaction (immediate and delayed), hypokalemia, hypothyroidism, intraocular pressure increased, laryngeal spasm/irritation, irregular menstruation, myositis, oropharyngeal irritation, osteoporosis, pallor, paradoxical bronchospasm, paradoxical tracheitis, paranasal sinus pain, PID, QTc prolongation, restlessness, stridor, supraventricular tachycardia, syncope, tremor, vaginal candidiasis, vaginitis, vulvovaginitis, rare cases of vasculitis (Churg-Strauss syndrome), ventricular tachycardia, weight gain

Drug Interactions

Metabolism/Transport Effects **Substrate** of CYP3A4 (major); **Note:** Assignment of Major/Minor substrate status based on clinically relevant drug interaction potential

Avoid Concomitant Use

Avoid concomitant use of Salmeterol with any of the following: Beta-Blockers (Nonselective); Cobicistat; CYP3A4 Inhibitors (Strong); Fusidic Acid (Systemic); Iobenguane I 123; Long-Acting Beta2-Agonists; Telaprevir

Increased Effect/Toxicity

Salmeterol may increase the levels/effects of: Atosiban; Highest Risk QTc-Prolonging Agents; Long-Acting Beta2-Agonists; Loop Diuretics; Moderate Risk QTc-Prolonging Agents; Sympathomimetics; Thiazide Diuretics

The levels/effects of Salmeterol may be increased by: AtoMOXetine; Cannabinoids; Cobicistat; CYP3A4 Inhibitors (Moderate); CYP3A4 Inhibitors (Strong); Dasatinib; Fusidic Acid (Systemic); Ivacaftor; Luliconazole; MAO Inhibitors; Mifepristone; Simeprevir; Telaprevir; Tricyclic Antidepressants

Decreased Effect

Salmeterol may decrease the levels/effects of: Iobenguane I 123

The levels/effects of Salmeterol may be decreased by: Beta-Blockers (Beta1 Selective); Beta-Blockers (Nonselective); Betahistine

Storage/Stability Inhalation powder (Serevent® Diskus®): Store at controlled room temperature 20°C to 25°C (68°F to 77°F) in a dry place away from direct heat or sunlight. Stable for 6 weeks after removal from foil pouch.

Mechanism of Action Relaxes bronchial smooth muscle by selective action on beta$_2$-receptors with little effect on heart rate; salmeterol acts locally in the lung.

Pharmacodynamics/Kinetics

Onset of action: Asthma: 30-48 minutes, COPD: 2 hours
Peak effect: Asthma: 3 hours, COPD: 2-5 hours
Duration: 12 hours
Absorption: Systemic: Inhalation: Undetectable to poor
Protein binding: 96%
Metabolism: Hepatic; hydroxylated via CYP3A4
Half-life elimination: 5.5 hours
Time to peak, serum: ~20 minutes
Excretion: Feces (60%); urine (25%)

Dosage Inhalation, powder (50 mcg/inhalation):

Asthma, maintenance and prevention: Children ≥4 years and Adults: One inhalation twice daily (~12 hours apart); maximum: 1 inhalation twice daily. **Note:** For asthma control, long acting beta$_2$-agonists (LABAs) should be used in combination with inhaled corticosteroids and not as monotherapy.

Exercise-induced asthma, prevention: Children ≥4 years and Adults: One inhalation at least 30 minutes prior to exercise; additional doses should not be used for 12 hours; should not be used in individuals already receiving salmeterol twice daily. **Note:** Because LABAs may disguise poorly controlled persistent asthma, frequent or chronic use of LABAs for exercise-induced bronchospasm is discouraged by the NIH Asthma Guidelines (NIH, 2007).

COPD maintenance: Adults: One inhalation twice daily (~12 hours apart); maximum: 1 inhalation twice daily

Dosage adjustment in renal impairment: No dosage adjustment provided in manufacturer's labeling.

Dosage adjustment in hepatic impairment: No dosage adjustment provided in manufacturer's labeling (has not been studied). Use with caution.

Dietary Considerations Some products may contain lactose; very rare anaphylactic reactions have been reported in patients with severe milk protein allergy.

Administration Inhalation: **Not** to be used for the relief of acute attacks. Not for use with a spacer device. Administer with Diskus® in a level, horizontal position. Do not wash mouthpiece; Diskus® should be kept dry. Discard device 6 weeks after removal from foil pouch or when the dose counter reads "0" (whichever comes first).

Monitoring Parameters FEV$_1$, peak flow, and/or other pulmonary function tests; blood pressure, heart rate; CNS stimulation. Monitor for increased use of short-acting beta$_2$-agonist inhalers; may be marker of a deteriorating asthma condition.

Dosage Forms Excipient information presented when available (limited, particularly for generics); consult specific product labeling.

Aerosol Powder Breath Activated, Inhalation:
Serevent Diskus: 50 mcg/dose (28 ea, 60 ea) [contains lactose]

Dosage Forms: Canada Excipient information presented when available (limited, particularly for generics); consult specific product labeling.

Powder for oral inhalation:
Serevent® Diskhaler® Disk: Salmeterol xinafoate 50 mcg (60s) [delivers 50 mcg/inhalation; contains lactose]

◆ **Salmeterol and Fluticasone** *see* Fluticasone and Salmeterol *on page* 897

◆ **Salmeterol Xinafoate** *see* Salmeterol *on page* 1871

◆ **Salofalk (Can)** *see* Mesalamine *on page* 1305

◆ **Salofalk 5-ASA (Can)** *see* Mesalamine *on page* 1305

◆ **Salonpas® Arthritis Pain® [OTC]** *see* Methyl Salicylate and Menthol *on page* 1344

◆ **Salonpas® Jet Spray [OTC]** *see* Methyl Salicylate and Menthol *on page* 1344

◆ **Salonpas® Massage Foam [OTC]** *see* Methyl Salicylate and Menthol *on page* 1344

◆ **Salonpas® Pain Relief Patch® [OTC]** *see* Methyl Salicylate and Menthol *on page* 1344

Salsalate (SAL sa late)

Brand Names: Canada Amigesic®; Salflex®

Index Terms Disalicylic Acid; Salicylsalicylic Acid

Pharmacologic Category Salicylate

Use Treatment of rheumatoid arthritis, osteoarthritis, and related rheumatic disorders

Pregnancy Risk Factor C

Dosage Oral:

Adults: 3 g/day in 2-3 divided dose

Elderly: May require lower dosage

Dosage adjustment in renal impairment: No dosage adjustment provided in manufacturer's labeling. Use is not recommended in patients with advanced renal disease.

Dosage adjustment in hepatic impairment: No dosage adjustment provided in manufacturer's labeling.

Additional Information Complete prescribing information should be consulted for additional detail.

Dosage Forms Excipient information presented when available (limited, particularly for generics); consult specific product labeling.

Tablet, Oral:

Generic: 500 mg, 750 mg

- ◆ **Salt** *see* Sodium Chloride *on page 1914*
- ◆ **Salt Poor Albumin** *see* Albumin *on page 59*
- ◆ **Samsca** *see* Tolvaptan *on page 2089*
- ◆ **Samsca™ (Can)** *see* Tolvaptan *on page 2089*
- ◆ **Sanctura** *see* Trospium *on page 2132*
- ◆ **Sanctura XR** *see* Trospium *on page 2132*
- ◆ **Sanctura® XR (Can)** *see* Trospium *on page 2132*
- ◆ **Sancuso** *see* Granisetron *on page 972*
- ◆ **SandIMMUNE** *see* CycloSPORINE (Systemic) *on page 508*
- ◆ **Sandimmune I.V. (Can)** *see* CycloSPORINE (Systemic) *on page 508*
- ◆ **SandoSTATIN** *see* Octreotide *on page 1485*
- ◆ **Sandostatin® (Can)** *see* Octreotide *on page 1485*
- ◆ **Sandostatin LAR (Can)** *see* Octreotide *on page 1485*
- ◆ **SandoSTATIN LAR Depot** *see* Octreotide *on page 1485*
- ◆ **Sandoz-Acebutolol (Can)** *see* Acebutolol *on page 28*
- ◆ **Sandoz-Alendronate (Can)** *see* Alendronate *on page 69*
- ◆ **Sandoz-Alfuzosin (Can)** *see* Alfuzosin *on page 73*
- ◆ **Sandoz-Almotriptan (Can)** *see* Almotriptan *on page 79*
- ◆ **Sandoz-Amiodarone (Can)** *see* Amiodarone *on page 101*
- ◆ **Sandoz Amlodipine (Can)** *see* AmLODIPine *on page 109*
- ◆ **Sandoz-Anagrelide (Can)** *see* Anagrelide *on page 136*
- ◆ **Sandoz-Anastrozole (Can)** *see* Anastrozole *on page 137*
- ◆ **Sandoz-Atenolol (Can)** *see* Atenolol *on page 186*
- ◆ **Sandoz-Atomoxetine (Can)** *see* AtoMOXetine *on page 187*
- ◆ **Sandoz-Atorvastatin (Can)** *see* AtorvaSTATin *on page 190*
- ◆ **Sandoz-Azithromycin (Can)** *see* Azithromycin (Systemic) *on page 214*
- ◆ **Sandoz-Betaxolol (Can)** *see* Betaxolol (Ophthalmic) *on page 250*
- ◆ **Sandoz-Bicalutamide (Can)** *see* Bicalutamide *on page 258*
- ◆ **Sandoz-Bisoprolol (Can)** *see* Bisoprolol *on page 261*
- ◆ **Sandoz-Bosentan (Can)** *see* Bosentan *on page 273*
- ◆ **Sandoz-Brimonidine (Can)** *see* Brimonidine (Ophthalmic) *on page 280*
- ◆ **Sandoz-Bupropion SR (Can)** *see* BuPROPion *on page 296*
- ◆ **Sandoz-Calcitonin (Can)** *see* Calcitonin *on page 312*
- ◆ **Sandoz-Candesartan (Can)** *see* Candesartan *on page 327*
- ◆ **Sandoz-Candesartan Plus (Can)** *see* Candesartan and Hydrochlorothiazide *on page 329*
- ◆ **Sandoz-Carbamazepine (Can)** *see* CarBAMazepine *on page 336*
- ◆ **Sandoz-Cefprozil (Can)** *see* Cefprozil *on page 377*
- ◆ **Sandoz-Ciprofloxacin (Can)** *see* Ciprofloxacin (Systemic) *on page 430*
- ◆ **Sandoz-Citalopram (Can)** *see* Citalopram *on page 440*
- ◆ **Sandoz-Clarithromycin (Can)** *see* Clarithromycin *on page 446*
- ◆ **Sandoz-Clonazepam (Can)** *see* ClonazePAM *on page 465*
- ◆ **Sandoz-Clopidogrel (Can)** *see* Clopidogrel *on page 471*
- ◆ **Sandoz-Cyclosporine (Can)** *see* CycloSPORINE (Systemic) *on page 508*
- ◆ **Sandoz-Diclofenac (Can)** *see* Diclofenac (Systemic) *on page 597*
- ◆ **Sandoz-Diclofenac Rapide (Can)** *see* Diclofenac (Systemic) *on page 597*
- ◆ **Sandoz-Diclofenac SR (Can)** *see* Diclofenac (Systemic) *on page 597*
- ◆ **Sandoz-Diltiazem CD (Can)** *see* Diltiazem *on page 613*
- ◆ **Sandoz-Diltiazem T (Can)** *see* Diltiazem *on page 613*
- ◆ **Sandoz-Dimenhydrinate [OTC] (Can)** *see* DimenhyDRINATE *on page 616*
- ◆ **Sandoz-Dorzolamide (Can)** *see* Dorzolamide *on page 655*
- ◆ **Sandoz-Dorzolamide/Timolol (Can)** *see* Dorzolamide and Timolol *on page 655*
- ◆ **Sandoz-Enalapril (Can)** *see* Enalapril *on page 701*
- ◆ **Sandoz-Entacapone (Can)** *see* Entacapone *on page 710*
- ◆ **Sandoz-Estradiol Derm 50 (Can)** *see* Estradiol (Systemic) *on page 754*
- ◆ **Sandoz-Estradiol Derm 75 (Can)** *see* Estradiol (Systemic) *on page 754*
- ◆ **Sandoz-Estradiol Derm 100 (Can)** *see* Estradiol (Systemic) *on page 754*
- ◆ **Sandoz-Famciclovir (Can)** *see* Famciclovir *on page 830*
- ◆ **Sandoz-Felodipine (Can)** *see* Felodipine *on page 836*
- ◆ **Sandoz-Fenofibrate E (Can)** *see* Fenofibrate and Derivatives *on page 837*
- ◆ **Sandoz-Fenofibrate S (Can)** *see* Fenofibrate and Derivatives *on page 837*
- ◆ **Sandoz Fentanyl Patch (Can)** *see* FentaNYL *on page 842*
- ◆ **Sandoz-Finasteride (Can)** *see* Finasteride *on page 862*
- ◆ **Sandoz-Fluoxetine (Can)** *see* FLUoxetine *on page 885*
- ◆ **Sandoz-Fluvoxamine (Can)** *see* FluvoxaMINE *on page 903*
- ◆ **Sandoz-Glimepiride (Can)** *see* Glimepiride *on page 956*
- ◆ **Sandoz-Glyburide (Can)** *see* GlyBURIDE *on page 963*
- ◆ **Sandoz-Indomethacin (Can)** *see* Indomethacin *on page 1070*
- ◆ **Sandoz-Irbesartan (Can)** *see* Irbesartan *on page 1113*

◆ **Santyl® (Can)** *see* Collagenase (Topical) *on page 490*
◆ **Saphris** *see* Asenapine *on page 173*
◆ **Saphris® (Can)** *see* Asenapine *on page 173*

Sapropterin (sap roe TER in)

Brand Names: U.S. Kuvan

Index Terms 6R-BH4; Phenoptin; Sapropterin Dihydrochloride

Pharmacologic Category Enzyme Cofactor

Use Adjunct to dietary management in the treatment of tetrahydrobiopterin (BH4) responsive phenylketonuria (PKU)

Pregnancy Risk Factor C

Dosage Oral: PKU: Children ≥4 years and Adults: Initial: 10 mg/kg once daily; adjust after 1 month based on blood phenylalanine levels (if phenylalanine levels do not decrease from baseline, increase dose to 20 mg/kg once daily); discontinue if phenylalanine levels do not decrease after 1 month of treatment at 20 mg/kg/day (nonresponder). Maintenance range: 5-20 mg/kg once daily

Dosage adjustment in renal impairment: No dosage adjustment provided in manufacturer's labeling (has not been studied). Use with caution.

Dosage adjustment in hepatic impairment: No dosage adjustment provided in manufacturer's labeling (has not been studied). Use with caution.

Additional Information Complete prescribing information should be consulted for additional detail.

Product Availability Kuvan powder for oral solution: FDA approved December 2013; availability anticipated in the first quarter of 2014.

Dosage Forms Excipient information presented when available (limited, particularly for generics); consult specific product labeling.

Tablet Soluble, Oral, as dihydrochloride:
Kuvan: 100 mg

◆ **Sapropterin Dihydrochloride** *see* Sapropterin *on page 1875*

Saquinavir (sa KWIN a veer)

Brand Names: U.S. Invirase

Brand Names: Canada Invirase®

Index Terms Saquinavir Mesylate; SQV

Pharmacologic Category Antiretroviral, Protease Inhibitor (Anti-HIV)

Use Treatment of HIV infection; used in combination with ritonavir and other antiretroviral agents

Pregnancy Risk Factor B

Pregnancy Considerations Adverse events were not observed in animal reproduction studies. Saquinavir crosses the human placenta in minimal amounts. Based on limited data, saquinavir administered twice daily with ritonavir 100 mg twice daily provide adequate levels in pregnant women. The DHHS Perinatal HIV Guidelines consider saquinavir and ritonavir to be an alternative combination for use during pregnancy; use without ritonavir is **not** recommended. A small increased risk of preterm birth has been associated with maternal use of protease inhibitor-based combination antiretroviral (ARV) therapy during pregnancy; however, the benefits of use generally outweigh this risk and protease inhibitors (PIs) should not be withheld if otherwise recommended. Hyperglycemia, new onset of diabetes mellitus, or diabetic ketoacidosis have been reported with PIs; it is not clear if pregnancy increases this risk.

Regardless of CD4 count or HIV RNA copy number, all HIV-infected pregnant women should receive a combination antepartum ARV drug regimen; this includes women who require therapy for their own health, as well as women who do not yet require therapy for their own health. ARV therapy should be started as soon as possible if required for the woman's health. Although earlier initiation may be more effective in reducing the perinatal transmission of HIV, also consider maternal conditions (eg, nausea and vomiting) and the potential risks of first trimester fetal exposure for specific agents. Plasma HIV RNA levels should be assessed at ~34-36 weeks gestation in order to help determine mode of delivery. If ARV therapy must be interrupted for <24 hours during the peripartum period, stop then restart all medications simultaneously in order to decrease the chance of developing resistance. Long-term follow-up is recommended for all infants exposed to ARV medications.

Healthcare providers are encouraged to enroll pregnant women exposed to antiretroviral medications in the Antiretroviral Pregnancy Registry (1-800-258-4263 or www.APRegistry.com). Healthcare providers caring for HIV-infected women and their infants may contact the National Perinatal HIV Hotline (888-448-8765) for clinical consultation (DHHS [perinatal], 2012).

Breast-Feeding Considerations Maternal or infant antiretroviral therapy does not completely eliminate the risk of postnatal HIV transmission. In addition, multiclass-resistant virus has been detected in breast-feeding infants despite maternal therapy. Therefore, in the United States, where formula is accessible, affordable, safe, and sustainable, and the risk of infant mortality due to diarrhea and respiratory infections is low, complete avoidance of breast-feeding by HIV-infected women is recommended to decrease potential transmission of HIV (DHHS [perinatal], 2012).

Medication Guide Available Yes

Contraindications Hypersensitivity to saquinavir or any component of the formulation; congenital or acquired QT prolongation, refractory hypokalemia or hypomagnesemia, concomitant use of other medications that both increase saquinavir plasma concentrations and prolong the QT interval; complete AV block (without implanted ventricular pacemaker) or patients at high risk of complete AV block; severe hepatic impairment; coadministration of saquinavir/ritonavir with alfuzosin, amiodarone, bepridil, cisapride, dofetilide, ergot derivatives, flecainide, lidocaine (systemic), lovastatin, midazolam (oral), pimozide, propafenone, quinidine, rifampin, sildenafil (when used for pulmonary artery hypertension [eg, Revatio®]), simvastatin, trazodone, or triazolam

Canadian labeling: Additional contraindications (not in U.S. labeling): Concurrent use with procainamide, sotalol, astemizole, or terfenadine

Warnings/Precautions Use caution in patients with hepatic insufficiency. May exacerbate pre-existing hepatic dysfunction; use with caution in patients with hepatitis B or C and in cirrhosis. May be associated with fat redistribution (buffalo hump, increased abdominal girth, breast engorgement, facial atrophy). Use caution in hemophilia. May increase cholesterol and/or triglycerides. Changes in glucose tolerance, hyperglycemia, exacerbation of diabetes, DKA, and new-onset diabetes mellitus have been reported in patients receiving protease inhibitors.

Altered cardiac conduction: Saquinavir/ritonavir prolongs the QT interval, potentially leading to torsade de pointes, and prolongs the PR interval, potentially leading to heart block. Second- or third-degree AV block has been reported (rare). An ECG should be performed for all patients prior to starting saquinavir/ritonavir therapy; do not initiate therapy in patients with a baseline QT interval >450 msec or diagnosed with long QT syndrome. If baseline QT interval <450 msec, may initiate therapy but a subsequent ECG is recommended after ~3-4 days of therapy. If subsequent QT interval is >480 msec or is prolonged over baseline by >20 msec, therapy should be discontinued. Patients who may be at increased risk for QT- or PR-interval prolongation include those with heart failure, bradyarrhythmias, hepatic impairment, electrolyte abnormalities, ischemic heart disease, cardiomyopathy, structural heart disease, or those with pre-existing cardiac conduction abnormalities; ECG monitoring is recommended for these patients.

Must be used in combination with ritonavir. Continued administration after loss of viral suppression efficacy may increase the likelihood of cross-resistance to other protease inhibitors. Promptly discontinue therapy if viral suppression response is lost. High potential for drug interactions; concomitant use of saquinavir with some drugs may require cautious use, may not be recommended, may require dosage adjustments, or may be contraindicated. Consult drug interactions database for more detailed information. Patients may develop immune reconstitution syndrome resulting in the occurrence of an inflammatory response to an indolent or residual opportunistic infection during initial HIV treatment or activation of autoimmune disorders (eg, Graves' disease, polymyositis, Guillain-Barré syndrome) later in therapy; further evaluation and treatment may be required. Formulation contains lactose; Canadian product labeling recommends against use in patients with galactose intolerance, Lapp lactase deficiency or glucose-galactose malabsorption.

Adverse Reactions

Incidence data shown for saquinavir soft gel capsule formulation (no longer available) in combination with ritonavir.

10%: Gastrointestinal: Nausea (11%)

1% to 10%:

Cardiovascular: Chest pain

Central nervous system: Fatigue (6%), fever (3%), anxiety, depression, headache, insomnia, pain

Dermatologic: Pruritus (3%), rash (3%), dry lips/skin (2%), eczema (2%), verruca

Endocrine & metabolic: Lipodystrophy (5%), hyperglycemia (3%), hypoglycemia, hyperkalemia, libido disorder, serum amylase increased

Gastrointestinal: Diarrhea (8%), vomiting (7%), abdominal pain (6%), constipation (2%), abdominal discomfort, appetite decreased, buccal mucosa ulceration, dyspepsia, flatulence, taste alteration

Hepatic: AST increased, ALT increased, bilirubin increased

Neuromuscular & skeletal: Back pain (2%), CPK increased, paresthesia, weakness

Renal: Creatinine kinase increased

Respiratory: Pneumonia (5%), bronchitis (3%), sinusitis (3%)

Miscellaneous: Influenza (3%)

Incidence not currently defined (limited to significant reactions; reported for hard or soft gel capsule with/without ritonavir)

Cardiovascular: Cyanosis, heart valve disorder (including murmur), hyper-/hypotension, peripheral vasoconstriction, prolonged QT interval, prolonged PR interval, syncope, thrombophlebitis

Central nervous system: Agitation, amnesia, ataxia, confusion, hallucination, hyper-/hyporeflexia, myelopolyradiculoneuritis, neuropathies, poliomyelitis, progressive multifocal encephalopathy, psychosis, seizures, somnolence, speech disorder, suicide attempt

Dermatologic: Alopecia, bullous eruption, dermatitis, erythema, maculopapular rash, photosensitivity, Stevens-Johnson syndrome, skin ulceration, urticaria

Endocrine & metabolic: Dehydration, diabetes, electrolyte changes, TSH increased

Gastrointestinal: Ascites, colic, dysphagia, esophagitis, bloody stools, gastritis, intestinal obstruction, hemorrhage (rectal), pancreatitis, stomatitis

Genitourinary: impotence, prostate enlarged, hematuria, UTI

Hematologic; Acute myeloblastic leukemia, anemia (including hemolytic), leukopenia, neutropenia, pancytopenia, splenomegaly, thrombocytopenia

Hepatic: Alkaline phosphatase increased, GGT increased, hepatitis, hepatomegaly, hepatosplenomegaly, jaundice, liver disease exacerbation

Neuromuscular & skeletal: Arthritis, LDH increased

Ocular: Blepharitis, visual disturbance

Otic: Otitis, hearing decreased, tinnitus

Renal: Nephrolithiasis, renal calculus

Respiratory: Dyspnea, hemoptysis, pharyngitis, upper respiratory tract infection

Miscellaneous: Immune reconstitution syndrome, infections (bacterial, fungal, viral)

Postmarketing and/or case reports: AV block (second or third degree), torsade de pointes

Drug Interactions

Metabolism/Transport Effects Substrate of CYP2D6 (minor), CYP3A4 (major), P-glycoprotein; **Note:** Assignment of Major/Minor substrate status based on clinically relevant drug interaction potential; **Inhibits** CYP2C19 (weak), CYP2C9 (weak), CYP2D6 (weak), CYP3A4 (strong), P-glycoprotein

Avoid Concomitant Use

Avoid concomitant use of Saquinavir with any of the following: Ado-Trastuzumab Emtansine; Alfuzosin; Amiodarone; Apixaban; Avanafil; Axitinib; Bepridil [Off Market]; Bosutinib; Cabozantinib; Cisapride; Conivaptan; Crizotinib; Darunavir; Dofetilide; Dronedarone; Eplerenone; Ergot Derivatives; Everolimus; Flecainide; Fusidic Acid (Systemic); Halofantrine; Highest Risk QTc-Prolonging Agents; Ibrutinib; Imatinib; Ivabradine; Lapatinib; Lidocaine (Systemic); Lomitapide; Lovastatin; Lurasidone; Macitentan; Midazolam; Mifepristone; Nilotinib; Nisoldipine; Pimozide; Pomalidomide; Propafenone; QuiNIDine; Ranolazine; Red Yeast Rice; Regorafenib; Rifampin; Rivaroxaban; Salmeterol; Silodosin; Simeprevir; Simvastatin; St Johns Wort; Tamsulosin; Ticagrelor; Tolvaptan; Topotecan; Toremifene; TraZODone; Triazolam; Ulipristal; Vemurafenib; VinCRIStine (Liposomal)

Increased Effect/Toxicity

Saquinavir may increase the levels/effects of: Ado-Trastuzumab Emtansine; Afatinib; Alfuzosin; Almotriptan; Alosetron; ALPRAZolam; Amiodarone; Apixaban; ARIPiprazole; AtorvaSTATin; Avanafil; Axitinib; Bedaquiline; Bepridil [Off Market]; Bortezomib; Bosentan; Bosutinib; Brentuximab Vedotin; Brinzolamide; Budesonide (Nasal); Budesonide (Systemic, Oral Inhalation); Cabozantinib; Calcium Channel Blockers (Dihydropyridine); Calcium Channel Blockers (Nondihydropyridine); CarBAMazepine; Cisapride; Clarithromycin; Clorazepate; Colchicine; Conivaptan; Corticosteroids (Orally Inhaled); Crizotinib; CycloSPORINE (Systemic); CYP3A4 Substrates; Dabigatran Etexilate; Diazepam; Dienogest; Digoxin; Dofetilide; Dronedarone; Dutasteride; Efavirenz; Enfuvirtide; Enzalutamide; Eplerenone; Ergot Derivatives; Everolimus; FentaNYL; Fesoterodine; Flecainide; Flurazepam; Fluticasone (Nasal); Fluticasone (Oral Inhalation); Fusidic Acid (Systemic); GuanFACINE; Halofantrine; Highest Risk QTc-Prolonging Agents; Ibrutinib; Iloperidone; Imatinib; Itraconazole; Ivabradine; Ivacaftor; Ixabepilone; Ketoconazole (Systemic); Lacosamide; Lapatinib; Levomilnacipran; Lidocaine (Systemic); Lomitapide; Lovastatin; Lumefantrine; Lurasidone; Macitentan; Maraviroc; Meperidine; MethylPREDNISolone;

Midazolam; Mifepristone; Moderate Risk QTc-Prolonging Agents; Nefazodone; Nilotinib; Nisoldipine; Ospemifene; OxyCODONE; Paricalcitol; PAZOPanib; P-glycoprotein/ABCB1 Substrates; Pimecrolimus; Pimozide; Pomalidomide; PONATinib; Propafenone; Protease Inhibitors; Prucalopride; QUEtiapine; QuiNIDine; Ranolazine; Red Yeast Rice; Regorafenib; Repaglinide; Rifabutin; Rilpivirine; Riociguat; Rivaroxaban; RomiDEPsin; Rosuvastatin; Ruxolitinib; Salmeterol; Saxagliptin; Sildenafil; Silodosin; Simeprevir; Simvastatin; SORAfenib; Tacrolimus (Systemic); Tacrolimus (Topical); Tadalafil; Tamsulosin; Temsirolimus; Ticagrelor; Tofacitinib; Tolterodine; Tolvaptan; Topotecan; Toremifene; TraZODone; Triazolam; Tricyclic Antidepressants; Ulipristal; Vardenafil; Vemurafenib; Vilazodone; VinCRIStine (Liposomal); Warfarin; Zuclopenthixol

The levels/effects of Saquinavir may be increased by: Bepridil [Off Market]; Clarithromycin; CycloSPORINE (Systemic); Delavirdine; Enfuvirtide; Etravirine; Fusidic Acid (Systemic); H2-Antagonists; Itraconazole; Ivabradine; Ketoconazole (Systemic); Methadone; Mifepristone; P-glycoprotein/ABCB1 Inhibitors; Proton Pump Inhibitors; QTc-Prolonging Agents (Indeterminate Risk and Risk Modifying); Rifampin; Simeprevir

Decreased Effect

Saquinavir may decrease the levels/effects of: Abacavir; Boceprevir; Clarithromycin; Contraceptives (Estrogens); Darunavir; Delavirdine; Etravirine; Ifosfamide; Meperidine; Methadone; Prasugrel; Pravastatin; Theophylline Derivatives; Ticagrelor; Valproic Acid and Derivatives; Zidovudine

The levels/effects of Saquinavir may be decreased by: Antacids; Boceprevir; Bosentan; CarBAMazepine; CYP3A4 Inducers (Strong); Dabrafenib; Deferasirox; Efavirenz; Garlic; Mitotane; Nevirapine; Peginterferon Alfa-2b; P-glycoprotein/ABCB1 Inducers; Rifampin; St Johns Wort; Tocilizumab

Ethanol/Nutrition/Herb Interactions

Food: A high-fat meal maximizes bioavailability. Saquinavir levels may increase if taken with grapefruit juice. Management: Administer within 2 hours of a full meal.

Herb/Nutraceutical: Saquinavir serum concentrations may be decreased by St John's wort and garlic capsules. Management: Avoid St John's wort. Avoid garlic supplementation.

Storage/Stability Invirase®: Store at 25°C (77°F); excursions permitted to 15°C to 30°C (59°F to 86°F).

Mechanism of Action Binds to the site of HIV-1 protease activity and inhibits cleavage of viral Gag-Pol polyprotein precursors into individual functional proteins required for infectious HIV. This results in the formation of immature, noninfectious viral particles.

Pharmacodynamics/Kinetics

Absorption: Poor; increased with high-fat meal

Distribution: V_d: 700 L; does not distribute into CSF

Protein binding, plasma: ~98%

Metabolism: Extensively hepatic via CYP3A4; extensive first-pass effect

Bioavailability: Invirase®: ~4%

Excretion: Feces (81% to 88%), urine (1% to 3%) within 5 days

Dosage Note: ECG should be done prior to starting therapy; do not initiate therapy if pretreatment QT interval >450 msec. Saquinavir should always be used with concomitant ritonavir.

Oral: Children >16 years and Adults: 1000 mg twice daily given in combination with ritonavir 100 mg twice daily. This combination should be given together and within 2 hours after a full meal in combination with a nucleoside analog.

Dosage adjustments when administered in combination therapy: Saquinavir: 1000 mg twice daily administered with lopinavir 400 mg/ritonavir 100 mg (Kaletra™) twice daily; no additional ritonavir is necessary

Elderly: Clinical studies did not include sufficient numbers of patients ≥65 years of age; use caution due to increased frequency of organ dysfunction

Dosage adjustment in renal impairment: No dosage adjustment necessary. However, has not been studied in severe renal impairment or ESRD.

Dosage adjustment in hepatic impairment:

Mild to moderate impairment (Child-Pugh classes A and B): No dosage adjustment necessary.

Severe impairment (Child-Pugh class C): Use is contraindicated when coadministered with ritonavir.

Dietary Considerations Take within 2 hours of a meal. Invirase® capsules and tablets contain lactose (not expected to induce symptoms of intolerance).

Administration Administer saquinavir and ritonavir at the same time and within 2 hours after a full meal. Patients unable to swallow capsules may open capsules and mix contents with 15 mL of syrup (or sorbitol if diabetic or glucose intolerant) or with 3 teaspoons of jam. Mixture should be stirred for 30-60 seconds and then administered entirely. Suspension should be at room temperature prior to administration.

Monitoring Parameters Monitor ECG (prior to therapy and after 3-4 days of therapy); serum potassium and magnesium levels, triglycerides and cholesterol (prior to initiation and periodically during therapy); viral load, CD4 count; glucose

Dosage Forms Excipient information presented when available (limited, particularly for generics); consult specific product labeling.

Capsule, Oral:

Invirase: 200 mg

Tablet, Oral:

Invirase: 500 mg

◆ **Saquinavir Mesylate** *see* Saquinavir *on page 1875*

◆ **Sarafem** *see* FLUoxetine *on page 885*

Sargramostim (sar GRAM oh stim)

Brand Names: U.S. Leukine

Brand Names: Canada Leukine

Index Terms GM-CSF; GMCSF; Granulocyte-Macrophage Colony Stimulating Factor; Prokine; Recombinant Granulocyte-Macrophage Colony Stimulating Factor; rhuGM-CSF

Pharmacologic Category Colony Stimulating Factor

Use

Acute myelogenous leukemia (AML): To shorten time to neutrophil recovery and to reduce the incidence of severe and life-threatening infections and infections resulting in death following induction chemotherapy in older adults (≥55 years of age)

Bone marrow transplant (allogeneic or autologous): For graft failure or engraftment delay

Myeloid reconstitution after allogeneic bone marrow transplantation: To accelerate myeloid recovery

Myeloid reconstitution after autologous bone marrow transplantation: To accelerate myeloid recovery following transplantation in non-Hodgkin lymphoma (NHL), acute lymphoblastic leukemia (ALL), Hodgkin lymphoma

Peripheral stem cell transplantation: Mobilization of hematopoietic progenitor cells for leukapheresis and myeloid reconstitution following autologous peripheral stem cell transplantation

Unlabeled Use

Primary prophylaxis of neutropenia in patients receiving chemotherapy (outside transplant and AML) or who are at high risk for neutropenic fever

Treatment of radiation-induced myelosuppression of the bone marrow

Pregnancy Risk Factor C

Pregnancy Considerations Animal reproduction studies have not been conducted.

Breast-Feeding Considerations It is not known if sargramostim is excreted in breast milk. Breast-feeding is not recommended by the manufacturer.

Contraindications Hypersensitivity to sargramostim, yeast-derived products, or any component of the formulation; concurrent (24 hours preceding/following) use with myelosuppressive chemotherapy or radiation therapy; patients with excessive (≥10%) leukemic myeloid blasts in bone marrow or peripheral blood

Warnings/Precautions Simultaneous administration or administration 24 hours preceding/following cytotoxic chemotherapy or radiotherapy is contraindicated due to the sensitivity of rapidly dividing hematopoietic progenitor cells. If there is a rapid increase in blood counts (ANC >20,000/mm^3, WBC >50,000/mm^3, or platelets >500,000/mm^3), decrease the dose by 50% or discontinue therapy. Excessive blood counts should fall to normal within 3-7 days after the discontinuation of therapy. Monitor CBC with differential twice weekly during treatment. Limited response to sargramostim may be seen in patients who have received bone marrow purged by chemical agents which do not preserve an adequate number of responsive hematopoietic progenitors (eg, <1.2 x 10^4/kg progenitors). In patients receiving autologous bone marrow transplant, response to sargramostim may be limited if extensive radiotherapy to the abdomen or chest or multiple myelotoxic agents were administered prior to transplantation. May potentially act as a growth factor for any tumor type, particularly myeloid malignancies; caution should be exercised when using in any malignancy with myeloid characteristics. Tumors of nonhematopoietic origin may have surface receptors for sargramostim. Discontinue use if disease progression occurs during treatment.

Anaphylaxis or other serious allergic reactions have been reported; discontinue immediately and initiate appropriate therapy if a serious allergic or anaphylactic reaction occurs. A "first-dose effect", characterized by respiratory distress, hypoxia, flushing, hypotension, syncope, and/or tachycardia, may occur (rarely) with the first dose of a cycle and resolve with appropriate symptomatic treatment; symptoms do not usually occur with subsequent doses within that cycle. Dyspnea may occur; monitor respiratory symptoms during and following I.V. infusion. Decrease infusion rate by 50% if dyspnea occurs; discontinue the infusion if dyspnea persists despite reduction in the rate of administration. Subsequent doses may be administered at the standard rate with careful monitoring. Use with caution in patients with hypoxia or pre-existing pulmonary disease. Edema, capillary leak syndrome, pleural and/or pericardial effusion have been reported; fluid retention has been shown to be reversible with dosage reduction or discontinuation of sargramostim with or without concomitant use of diuretics. Use with caution in patients with pre-existing fluid retention, pulmonary infiltrates, or congestive heart failure; may exacerbate fluid retention.

Use with caution in patients with pre-existing cardiac disease. Reversible transient supraventricular arrhythmias have been reported, especially in patients with a history of arrhythmias. Use with caution in patients with hepatic impairment (hyperbilirubinemia and elevated transaminases have been observed) or renal impairment (serum creatinine elevations have been observed). Monitor hepatic and renal function at least every other week in patients with history of impairment. Solution contains benzyl alcohol; do not use in premature infants or neonates.

Adverse Reactions

>10%:

Cardiovascular: Hypertension (34%), edema (13% to 25%), pericardial effusion (4% to 25%), thrombosis (19%), chest pain (15%), peripheral edema (11%), tachycardia (11%)

Central nervous system: Malaise (57%), headache (26%), chills (25%), anxiety (11%), insomnia (11%)

Dermatologic: Skin rash (44% to 77%), pruritus (23%)

Endocrine & metabolic: Weight loss (37%), hyperglycemia (25%), hypercholesterolemia (17%), hypomagnesemia (15%)

Gastrointestinal: Diarrhea (81% to 89%), nausea (58% to 70%), vomiting (46% to 70%), gastric ulcer (50%), abdominal pain (38%), anorexia (13%), hematemesis (13%), dysphagia (11%), gastrointestinal hemorrhage (11%)

Hepatic: Hyperbilirubinemia (30%)

Neuromuscular & skeletal: Weakness (66%), ostealgia (21%), arthralgia (11% to 21%), myalgia (18%)

Ophthalmic: Retinal hemorrhage (11%)

Renal: Increased blood urea nitrogen (23%), increased serum creatinine (15%)

Respiratory: Pharyngitis (23%), epistaxis (17%), dyspnea (15%)

Miscellaneous: Fever (81%)

1% to 10%:

Immunologic: Antibody development (2%)

Respiratory: Pleural effusion (1%)

<1% (Limited to important or life-threatening): Anaphylaxis, capillary leak syndrome, cardiac arrhythmia, eosinophilia, hypoxia, leukocytosis, liver function impairment (transient), pericarditis, prolonged prothrombin time, respiratory distress, rigors, sore throat, supraventricular cardiac arrhythmia, syncope, thrombocythemia, thrombophlebitis

Drug Interactions

Metabolism/Transport Effects None known.

Avoid Concomitant Use There are no known interactions where it is recommended to avoid concomitant use.

Increased Effect/Toxicity

Sargramostim may increase the levels/effects of: Bleomycin

Decreased Effect There are no known significant interactions involving a decrease in effect.

Preparation for Administration

Powder for injection: May be reconstituted with 1 mL of preservative free SWFI or bacteriostatic water for injection. Direct the diluent toward the side of the vial and gently swirl to reconstitute; do not shake. Do not mix the contents of vials which have been reconstituted with different diluents.

SubQ: May be administered without further dilution.

I.V.: Further dilution with NS is required. If the final sargramostim concentration is <10 mcg/mL, 1 mg of human albumin per 1 mL of NS should be added (eg, add 1 mL of 5% human albumin per 50 mL of NS).

Storage/Stability Store intact vials at 2°C to 8°C (36°F to 46°F); do not freeze. Do not shake.

Solution for injection: May be stored for up to 20 days at 2°C to 8°C (36°F to 46°F) once the vial has been entered. Discard remaining solution after 20 days.

Powder for injection: Preparations made with SWFI should be administered as soon as possible, and discarded within 6 hours of reconstitution. Solutions reconstituted with bacteriostatic water may be stored for up to 20 days at 2°C to 8°C (36°F to 46°F); do not freeze.

Mechanism of Action Stimulates proliferation, differentiation and functional activity of neutrophils, eosinophils, monocytes, and macrophages.

Pharmacodynamics/Kinetics
Onset of action: Increase in WBC: 7-14 days
Duration: WBCs return to baseline within 1 week of discontinuing drug
Half-life elimination: I.V.: 60 minutes; SubQ: 2.7 hours
Time to peak, serum: SubQ: 1-3 hours

Dosage Note: May round the dose to the nearest vial size (Ozer, 2000).

Acute myeloid leukemia (AML), neutrophil recovery following chemotherapy: Adults ≥55 years: I.V.: 250 mcg/m²/day (infused over 4 hours) starting approximately on day 11 or 4 days following the completion of induction chemotherapy (if day 10 bone marrow is hypoplastic with <5% blasts), continue until ANC >1500/mm³ for 3 consecutive days or a maximum of 42 days. If WBC >50,000/mm³ and/or ANC >20,000/mm³, interrupt treatment or reduce the dose by 50%.

If a second cycle of chemotherapy is necessary, administer ~4 days after the completion of chemotherapy if the bone marrow is hypoplastic with <5% blasts

Discontinue sargramostim immediately if leukemic regrowth occurs. If a severe adverse reaction occurs, reduce the dose by 50% or temporarily discontinue the dose until the reaction abates.

Bone marrow transplant (BMT), failure or engraftment delay: Adults: I.V.: 250 mcg/m²/day (infused over 2 hours) for 14 days; If engraftment has not occurred after 7 days off sargramostim, may repeat. If engraftment still has not occurred after 7 days off sargramostim, a third course of 500 mcg/m²/day for 14 days may be attempted. If there is still no improvement, it is unlikely that further dose escalation will be of benefit.

If a severe adverse reaction occurs, reduce the dose by 50% or temporarily discontinue the dose until the reaction abates

If blast cells appear or disease progression occurs, discontinue treatment

If WBC >50,000/mm³ and/or ANC >20,000 cells/mm³, interrupt treatment or reduce the dose by 50%.

Myeloid reconstitution after allogeneic or autologous bone marrow transplant: Adults: I.V.: 250 mcg/m²/day (infused over 2 hours), begin 2-4 hours after the marrow infusion and ≥24 hours after chemotherapy or radiotherapy, when the post marrow infusion ANC is <500 /mm³, and continue until ANC >1500 /mm³ for 3 consecutive days. If WBC >50,000/mm³ and/or ANC >20,000/mm³, interrupt treatment or reduce the dose by 50%.

If a severe adverse reaction occurs, reduce dose by 50% or temporarily discontinue the dose until the reaction abates

If blast cells appear or progression of the underlying disease occurs, discontinue treatment

Peripheral stem cell transplant, mobilization of peripheral blood progenitor cells (PBPC): Adults: I.V., SubQ: 250 mcg/m²/day I.V. (infused over 24 hours) or SubQ once daily; continue the same dose throughout PBPC collection. If WBC >50,000/mm³, reduce the dose by 50%.

Note: The optimal schedule for PBPC collection has not been established (usually begun by day 5 and performed daily until protocol specified targets are achieved). If adequate numbers of progenitor cells are not collected, consider other mobilization therapy.

Postperipheral blood progenitor cell transplantation: Adults: I.V., SubQ: 250 mcg/m²/day I.V. (infused over 24 hours) or SubQ once daily beginning immediately following infusion of progenitor cells; continue until ANC is >1500/mm³ for 3 consecutive days.

Primary prophylaxis of neutropenia in patients receiving chemotherapy (outside transplant and AML) or who are at high risk for neutropenic fever (unlabeled use): Adults: SubQ: 250 mcg/m²/day (may round to the nearest vial size) beginning at least 24 hours after chemotherapy administration; continue until ANC >1500/mm³ for 3 consecutive days (Ozer, 2000; Smith, 2006).

Treatment of radiation-induced myelosuppression of the bone marrow (unlabeled use): Adults: SubQ: 250 mcg/m²/day; continue until ANC >1000/mm³ (Smith, 2006; Waselenko, 2004).

Dosage adjustment in renal impairment: No dosage adjustment provided in manufacturer's labeling.

Dosage adjustment in hepatic impairment: No dosage adjustment provided in manufacturer's labeling.

Administration Sargramostim is administered as a subcutaneous injection or intravenous infusion.

I.V.: Infuse over 2 hours, 4 hours or 24 hours (indication specific). An in-line membrane filter should **NOT** be used for intravenous administration. When administering GM-CSF subcutaneously, rotate injection sites.

SubQ: Administer undiluted; rotate injection sites, avoiding navel/waistline.

Monitoring Parameters CBC with differential (twice weekly during treatment), renal/liver function tests (at least every 2 weeks in patients displaying renal or hepatic dysfunction prior to treatment initiation); pulmonary function; vital signs; hydration status; weight

Test Interactions May interfere with bone imaging studies; increased hematopoietic activity of the bone marrow may appear as transient positive bone imaging changes

Dosage Forms Excipient information presented when available (limited, particularly for generics); consult specific product labeling. [DSC] = Discontinued product

Solution, Injection:
Leukine: 500 mcg/mL (1 mL) [contains benzyl alcohol]

Solution Reconstituted, Intravenous:
Leukine: 250 mcg (1 ea [DSC])

Solution Reconstituted, Intravenous [preservative free]:
Leukine: 250 mcg (1 ea)

◆ **Sarna® HC (Can)** *see* Hydrocortisone (Topical) *on page 1011*

◆ **Sarnol-HC [OTC]** *see* Hydrocortisone (Topical) *on page 1011*

◆ **Saturated Potassium Iodide Solution** *see* Potassium Iodide *on page 1687*

◆ **Saturated Solution of Potassium Iodide** *see* Potassium Iodide *on page 1687*

◆ **Savella** *see* Milnacipran *on page 1369*

◆ **Savella Titration Pack** *see* Milnacipran *on page 1369*

Saxagliptin (sax a GLIP tin)

Brand Names: U.S. Onglyza

Brand Names: Canada Onglyza™

Index Terms BMS-477118

Pharmacologic Category Antidiabetic Agent, Dipeptidyl Peptidase IV (DPP-IV) Inhibitor

Additional Appendix Information
Oral Antidiabetic Agents Comparison Table *on page 2312*

Use Treatment of type 2 diabetes mellitus (noninsulin dependent, NIDDM) as an adjunct to diet and exercise as monotherapy or in combination therapy with other antidiabetic agents to improve glycemic control

Pregnancy Risk Factor B

Pregnancy Considerations Teratogenic effects were not observed in animal reproduction studies. For women with diabetes, maternal hyperglycemia can be associated with adverse effects in the fetus, neonate, and mother. To prevent adverse events, prior to conception and throughout pregnancy, the maternal Hb A_{1c} should be kept close to normal but without causing significant hypoglycemia. The use of dipeptidyl peptidase IV (DPP-IV) inhibitors in pregnant women is not currently recommended; insulin is the drug of choice for the control of diabetes mellitus during pregnancy (ACOG, 2005; ADA, 2013; Kitzmiller, 2008; Metzger, 2007).

Breast-Feeding Considerations It is not known if saxagliptin is excreted in breast milk. The manufacturer recommends that caution be exercised when administering saxagliptin to nursing women.

Medication Guide Available Yes

Contraindications Hypersensitivity to saxagliptin or any component of the formulation

Canadian labeling: Additional contraindications (not in U.S. labeling): Diabetic ketoacidosis, diabetic coma/precoma, type 1 diabetes mellitus

Warnings/Precautions Use with caution in patients with moderate-to-severe renal dysfunction, end-stage renal disease (ESRD) requiring hemodialysis, and in patients taking strong CYP3A4/5 inhibitors (eg, atazanavir, clarithromycin, indinavir, itraconazole, nefazodone, nelfinavir, ritonavir, saquinavir, telithromycin [also see Drug Interactions]); dosing adjustment required. Clinical trials included only a limited number of patients with heart failure (HF). No specific recommendations regarding this population are provided in the U.S. manufacturer labeling (Canadian labeling recommends against use in this population). Use caution when used in conjunction with insulin or insulin secretagogues (eg, sulfonylureas); risk of hypoglycemia is increased. Monitor blood glucose closely; dosage adjustments of insulin or the insulin secretagogue may be necessary. Rare hypersensitivity reactions, including anaphylaxis, angioedema, and/or exfoliative dermatologic reactions have been reported; discontinue if signs/symptoms of severe hypersensitivity reactions occur. Cases of acute pancreatitis have been reported; discontinue immediately if suspected. Contains lactose; Canadian labeling recommends avoiding use in patients with galactose intolerance, Lapp lactase deficiency, or glucose-galactose malabsorption syndromes.

Adverse Reactions Note: Frequencies and adverse reactions reported with monotherapy unless otherwise noted.

1% to 10%:

- Cardiovascular: Peripheral edema (≤4%; incidence increased in conjunction with thiazolidinediones: ≤8%)
- Central nervous system: Headache (7%)
- Endocrine & metabolic: Hypoglycemia (≤6%; incidence increased in conjunction with insulin secretagogues: ≤15%)
- Gastrointestinal: Abdominal pain (2%), gastroenteritis (2%), vomiting (2%)
- Genitourinary: Urinary tract infection (7%)
- Hematologic: Lymphopenia (≤2%; dose related)
- Respiratory: Sinusitis (3%)
- Miscellaneous: Hypersensitivity reactions (2%; including urticaria and facial edema)

<1% (Limited to important or life-threatening): Angioedema, anaphylaxis, creatinine increased, creatine phosphokinase increased, exfoliative skin reactions, immune thrombocytopenia (ITP), pancreatitis (acute), rash

Drug Interactions

Metabolism/Transport Effects Substrate of CYP3A4 (major), P-glycoprotein; **Note:** Assignment of Major/Minor substrate status based on clinically relevant drug interaction potential

Avoid Concomitant Use

Avoid concomitant use of Saxagliptin with any of the following: Fusidic Acid (Systemic)

Increased Effect/Toxicity

Saxagliptin may increase the levels/effects of: ACE Inhibitors; Hypoglycemic Agents

The levels/effects of Saxagliptin may be increased by: CYP3A4 Inhibitors (Moderate); CYP3A4 Inhibitors (Strong); Dasatinib; Fusidic Acid (Systemic); Herbs (Hypoglycemic Properties); Ivacaftor; Luliconazole; MAO Inhibitors; Mifepristone; Pegvisomant; P-glycoprotein/ABCB1 Inhibitors; Salicylates; Selective Serotonin Reuptake Inhibitors; Simeprevir

Decreased Effect

The levels/effects of Saxagliptin may be decreased by: Corticosteroids (Orally Inhaled); Corticosteroids (Systemic); CYP3A4 Inducers; Loop Diuretics; Luteinizing Hormone-Releasing Hormone Analogs; P-glycoprotein/ABCB1 Inducers; Somatropin; Thiazide Diuretics

Storage/Stability Store at 20°C to 25°C (68°F to 77°F); excursions permitted between 15°C to 30°C (59°F to 86°F).

Mechanism of Action Saxagliptin inhibits dipeptidyl peptidase IV (DPP-IV) enzyme resulting in prolonged active incretin levels. Incretin hormones (eg, glucagon-like peptide-1 [GLP-1] and glucose-dependent insulinotropic polypeptide [GIP]) regulate glucose homeostasis by increasing insulin synthesis and release from pancreatic beta cells and decreasing glucagon secretion from pancreatic alpha cells. Decreased glucagon secretion results in decreased hepatic glucose production. Under normal physiologic circumstances, incretin hormones are released by the intestine throughout the day and levels are increased in response to a meal; incretin hormones are rapidly inactivated by the DPP-IV enzyme.

Pharmacodynamics/Kinetics

Duration: 24 hours

Protein binding: Negligible

Metabolism: Hepatic via CYP3A4/5 to 5-hydroxy saxagliptin (active; ~50% potency of the parent compound)

Half-life elimination: Saxagliptin: 2.5 hours; 5-hydroxy saxagliptin: 3.1 hours

Time to peak, plasma: Saxagliptin: 2 hours; 5-hydroxy saxagliptin: 4 hours

Excretion: Urine (75%, 24% of the total dose as saxagliptin, 36% of the total dose as 5-hydroxy saxagliptin); feces (22%)

Dosage Oral: Adults: Type 2 diabetes: 2.5-5 mg once daily

Concomitant use with strong CYP3A4/5 inhibitors: 2.5 mg once daily

Concomitant use with insulin or insulin secretagogues: Reduced dose of insulin or insulin secretagogues (eg, sulfonylureas) may be needed

Dosage adjustment in renal impairment:

Note: Renal function may be estimated using the Cockcroft-Gault formula or the MDRD formula for dosage adjustment purposes.

Cl_{cr} >50 mL/minute: No dosage adjustment necessary

Cl_{cr} ≤50 mL/minute: 2.5 mg once daily

ESRD requiring hemodialysis:

U.S. labeling: 2.5 mg once daily; administer postdialysis

Canadian labeling: Use is not recommended.

Peritoneal dialysis: Not studied

Dosage adjustment in hepatic impairment:

U.S. labeling: Mild-to-severe impairment: No dosage adjustment necessary.

Canadian labeling:

Mild impairment: No dosage adjustment provided in manufacturer's labeling.

Moderate-to-severe impairment: Use is not recommended.

Dietary Considerations May be taken without regard to meals. Individualized medical nutrition therapy (MNT) is an integral part of therapy (ADA, 2013).

Administration May be administered without regard to meals. Swallow whole; do not split or cut tablets.

Monitoring Parameters Plasma glucose, Hb A_{1c}, renal function

Reference Range Recommendations for glycemic control in nonpregnant adults with diabetes (ADA, 2013):

Hb A_{1c}: <7% (a more aggressive [<6.5%] or less aggressive [<8%] Hb A_{1c} goal may be targeted based on patient-specific characteristics)

Preprandial capillary plasma glucose: 70-130 mg/dL

Peak postprandial capillary blood glucose: <180 mg/dL

Dosage Forms Excipient information presented when available (limited, particularly for generics); consult specific product labeling.

Tablet, Oral:

Onglyza: 2.5 mg, 5 mg

Saxagliptin and Metformin

(sax a GLIP tin & met FOR min)

Brand Names: U.S. Kombiglyze™ XR

Brand Names: Canada Komboglyze™

Index Terms Metformin and Saxagliptin; Metformin Hydrochloride and Saxagliptin; Saxagliptin and Metformin Hydrochloride

Pharmacologic Category Antidiabetic Agent, Biguanide; Antidiabetic Agent, Dipeptidyl Peptidase IV (DPP-IV) Inhibitor

Use Management of type 2 diabetes mellitus (noninsulin dependent, NIDDM) as an adjunct to diet and exercise when treatment with both saxagliptin and metformin is appropriate

Pregnancy Risk Factor B

Medication Guide Available Yes

Dosage Oral: Type 2 diabetes mellitus:

Adults:

U.S. labeling: Initial doses should be based on current dose of saxagliptin and metformin; daily doses should be given once daily with the evening meal. Maximum: Saxagliptin 5 mg/metformin 2000 mg daily

Patients inadequately controlled on metformin alone: Initial dose: Saxagliptin 2.5-5 mg daily plus current dose of metformin. **Note:** Patients who require saxagliptin 2.5 mg (eg, dose adjusted for concomitant use of strong CYP3A4/5 inhibitors) and metformin >1000 mg should not be switched to the combination product.

Patients inadequately controlled on saxagliptin alone: Initial dose: Metformin 500 mg daily plus saxagliptin 5 mg daily. **Note:** Metformin-naive patients currently receiving saxagliptin 2.5 mg daily (eg, dose adjusted for concomitant use of strong CYP3A4/5 inhibitors) should not be switched to the combination product.

Concomitant use with strong CYP3A4/5 inhibitors: Maximum: Saxagliptin 2.5 mg/metformin 1000 mg daily

Concomitant use with insulin or insulin secretagogues: Reduced dose of insulin or insulin secretagogues (eg, sulfonylureas) may be needed.

Canadian labeling: Initial doses should be based on current dose of saxagliptin and metformin; daily dose should be divided into 2 equal doses given with meals. Maximum: Saxagliptin 5 mg/metformin 2000 mg daily

Patients inadequately controlled on metformin alone: Initial dose: Saxagliptin 2.5 mg twice daily plus current dose of metformin.

Concomitant use with insulin: Reduced dose of insulin may be needed.

Elderly: The initial and maintenance dosing should be conservative, due to the potential for decreased renal function (monitor). Do not use in patients ≥80 years of age unless normal renal function has been established.

Dosage adjustment in renal impairment:

U.S. labeling: Do not use in patients with renal disease or renal dysfunction (serum creatinine ≥1.5 mg/dL [≥136 micromole/L] in males or ≥1.4 mg/dL [≥124 micromole/L] in females or abnormal clearance).

Canadian labeling: Use is contraindicated.

Dosage adjustment in hepatic impairment:

U.S. labeling: Avoid metformin; liver disease is a risk factor for the development of lactic acidosis during metformin therapy.

Canadian labeling: Use is not recommended with clinical or laboratory evidence of disease and contraindicated in the presence of moderate-to-severe impairment.

Additional Information Complete prescribing information should be consulted for additional detail.

Dosage Forms Excipient information presented when available (limited, particularly for generics); consult specific product labeling.

Tablet, variable release, oral:

Kombiglyze™ XR 2.5/1000: Saxagliptin 2.5 mg [immediate release] and metformin hydrochloride 1000 mg [extended release]

Kombiglyze™ XR 5/500: Saxagliptin 5 mg [immediate release] and metformin hydrochloride 500 mg [extended release]

Kombiglyze™ XR 5/1000: Saxagliptin 5 mg [immediate release] and metformin hydrochloride 1000 mg [extended release]

Dosage Forms: Canada Excipient information presented when available (limited, particularly for generics); consult specific product labeling.

Tablet, oral:

Komboglyze™ 2.5/500: Saxagliptin 2.5 mg [immediate release] and metformin hydrochloride 500 mg [immediate release]

Komboglyze™ 2.5/850: Saxagliptin 2.5 mg [immediate release] and metformin hydrochloride 850 mg [immediate release]

Komboglyze™ 2.5/1000: Saxagliptin 2.5 mg [immediate release] and metformin hydrochloride 1000 mg [immediate release]

◆ Saxagliptin and Metformin Hydrochloride *see* Saxagliptin and Metformin *on page* 1881

◆ SB-265805 *see* Gemifloxacin *on page* 948

◆ SB-497115 *see* Eltrombopag *on page* 693

◆ SB-497115-GR *see* Eltrombopag *on page* 693

◆ SB659746-A *see* Vilazodone *on page* 2186

◆ SC 33428 *see* IDArubicin *on page* 1039

◆ Scalacort *see* Hydrocortisone (Topical) *on page* 1011

◆ Scalacort DK *see* Hydrocortisone (Topical) *on page* 1011

◆ Scalpicin Maximum Strength [OTC] *see* Hydrocortisone (Topical) *on page* 1011

◆ SCH 13521 *see* Flutamide *on page* 892

◆ SCH 52365 *see* Temozolomide *on page* 2005

◆ SCH 56592 *see* Posaconazole *on page* 1679

◆ SCH503034 *see* Boceprevir *on page* 267

◆ ScheinPharm Ranitidine (Can) *see* Ranitidine *on page* 1782

◆ SCIG *see* Immune Globulin *on page* 1059

◆ S-Citalopram *see* Escitalopram *on page* 745

◆ Scleromate *see* Morrhuate Sodium *on page* 1403

◆ Sclerosol Intrapleural *see* Talc (Sterile) *on page* 1986

Scopolamine (Systemic) (skoe POL a meen)

Brand Names: U.S. Transderm-Scop

Brand Names: Canada Buscopan®; Scopolamine Hydrobromide Injection; Transderm-V®

Index Terms Hyoscine Butylbromide; Scopolamine Base; Scopolamine Butylbromide; Scopolamine Hydrobromide

Pharmacologic Category Anticholinergic Agent

Additional Appendix Information

Beers Criteria – Potentially Inappropriate Medications for Geriatrics *on page 2368*

Use

Scopolamine base: Transdermal: Prevention of nausea/vomiting associated with motion sickness and recovery from anesthesia and surgery

Scopolamine hydrobromide: Injection: Preoperative medication to produce amnesia, sedation, tranquilization, antiemetic effects, and decrease salivary and respiratory secretions

Scopolamine butylbromide [not available in the U.S.]: Oral/injection: Treatment of smooth muscle spasm of the genitourinary or gastrointestinal tract; injection may also be used prior to radiological/diagnostic procedures to prevent spasm

Unlabeled Use Scopolamine base: Transdermal: Breakthrough treatment of nausea and vomiting associated with chemotherapy

Pregnancy Risk Factor C

Pregnancy Considerations Adverse events were observed in some animal reproduction studies. Scopolamine crosses the placenta; may cause respiratory depression and/or neonatal hemorrhage when used during pregnancy. Transdermal scopolamine has been used as an adjunct to epidural anesthesia for cesarean delivery without adverse CNS effects on the newborn. Parenteral administration does not increase the duration of labor or affect uterine contractions. Except when used prior to cesarean section, use during pregnancy only if the benefit to the mother outweighs the potential risk to the fetus.

Breast-Feeding Considerations Scopolamine is excreted into breast milk. The manufacturer recommends caution be used if scopolamine is administered to a nursing woman.

Contraindications

Transdermal, oral: Hypersensitivity to scopolamine, other belladonna alkaloids, or any component of the formulation; narrow-angle glaucoma

Injection: Hypersensitivity to scopolamine, other belladonna alkaloids, or any component of the formulation; narrow-angle glaucoma; chronic lung disease (repeated administration)

Canadian labeling: Additional contraindications (not in U.S. labeling):

Oral: Glaucoma, megacolon, myasthenia gravis, obstructive prostatic hypertrophy

Injection:

Hyoscine butylbromide: Untreated narrow-angle glaucoma; megacolon, prostatic hypertrophy with urinary retention; stenotic lesions of the GI tract; myasthenia gravis; tachycardia, angina, or heart failure; I.M. administration in patients receiving anticoagulant therapy

Scopolamine hydrobromide: Glaucoma or predisposition to narrow-angle glaucoma; paralytic ileus; prostatic hypertrophy; pyloric obstruction; tachycardia secondary to cardiac insufficiency or thyrotoxicosis

Warnings/Precautions Use with caution in patients with coronary artery disease, tachyarrhythmias, heart failure, hypertension, or hyperthyroidism; evaluate tachycardia prior to administration. Use caution in hepatic or renal impairment; adverse CNS effects occur more often in these patients. Use injectable and transdermal products with caution in patients with prostatic hyperplasia or urinary retention. Discontinue if patient reports unusual visual disturbances or pain within the eye. Use caution in GI obstruction, hiatal hernia, reflux esophagitis, and ulcerative colitis. Use with caution in patients with a history of seizure or psychosis; may exacerbate these conditions.

Anaphylaxis including episodes of shock has been reported following parenteral administration; observe for signs/symptoms of hypersensitivity following parenteral administration. Patients with a history of allergies or asthma may be at increased risk of hypersensitivity reactions. Adverse events (including dizziness, headache, nausea, vomiting) may occur following abrupt discontinuation of large doses or in patients with Parkinson's disease; adverse events may also occur following removal of the transdermal patch although symptoms may not appear until ≥24 hours after removal.

Idiosyncratic reactions may rarely occur; patients may experience acute toxic psychosis, agitation, confusion, delusions, hallucinations, paranoid behavior, and rambling speech. May cause CNS depression, which may impair physical or mental abilities; patients must be cautioned about performing tasks which require mental alertness (eg, operating machinery or driving).

Transdermal patch may contain conducting metal (eg, aluminum); remove patch prior to MRI. Use of the transdermal product in patients with open-angle glaucoma may necessitate adjustments in glaucoma therapy.

Scopolamine (hyoscine) hydrobromide should not be interchanged with scopolamine butylbromide formulations; dosages are not equivalent.

Avoid use in the elderly due to potent anticholinergic adverse effects and uncertain effectiveness (Beers Criteria). Use with caution in infants and children since they may be more susceptible to adverse effects of scopolamine. Safety and efficacy have not been established for the use of transdermal and oral scopolamine in children. Tablets may contain sucrose; avoid use of tablets in patients who are fructose intolerant.

Adverse Reactions Frequency not defined.

Cardiovascular: Bradycardia, flushing, orthostatic hypotension, tachycardia

Central nervous system: Acute toxic psychosis (rare), agitation (rare), ataxia, confusion, delusion (rare), disorientation, dizziness, drowsiness, fatigue, hallucination (rare), headache, irritability, loss of memory, paranoid behavior (rare), restlessness, sedation

Dermatologic: Drug eruptions, dry skin, dyshidrosis, erythema, pruritus, rash, urticaria

Endocrine & metabolic: Thirst

Gastrointestinal: Constipation, diarrhea, dry throat, dysphagia, nausea, vomiting, xerostomia

Genitourinary: Dysuria, urinary retention

Neuromuscular & skeletal: Tremor, weakness

Ocular: Accommodation impaired, blurred vision, conjunctival infection, cycloplegia, dryness, glaucoma (narrow-angle), increased intraocular pain, itching, photophobia, pupil dilation, retinal pigmentation

Respiratory: Dry nose, dyspnea

Miscellaneous: Anaphylaxis (rare), anaphylactic shock (rare), angioedema, diaphoresis decreased, heat intolerance, hypersensitivity reactions

Drug Interactions

Metabolism/Transport Effects None known.

Avoid Concomitant Use

Avoid concomitant use of Scopolamine (Systemic) with any of the following: Aclidinium; Azelastine (Nasal); Ipratropium (Oral Inhalation); Paraldehyde; Potassium Chloride; Tiotropium; Umeclidinium

Increased Effect/Toxicity

Scopolamine (Systemic) may increase the levels/effects of: AbobotulinumtoxinA; Alcohol (Ethyl); Analgesics (Opioid); Anticholinergics; Azelastine (Nasal); Buprenorphine; Cannabinoids; CNS Depressants; Hydrocodone; Methotrimeprazine; Metyrosine; Mirabegron; Mirtazapine; OnabotulinumtoxinA; Paraldehyde; Potassium Chloride; Pramipexole; RimabotulinumtoxinB;

ROPINIRole; Rotigotine; Selective Serotonin Reuptake Inhibitors; Thiazide Diuretics; Tiotropium; Topiramate; Zolpidem

The levels/effects of Scopolamine (Systemic) may be increased by: Aclidinium; Brimonidine (Topical); Doxylamine; Droperidol; HydrOXYzine; Ipratropium (Oral Inhalation); Magnesium Sulfate; Methotrimeprazine; Perampanel; Pramlintide; Sodium Oxybate; Tapentadol; Umeclidinium

Decreased Effect

Scopolamine (Systemic) may decrease the levels/effects of: Acetylcholinesterase Inhibitors (Central); Secretin

The levels/effects of Scopolamine (Systemic) may be decreased by: Acetylcholinesterase Inhibitors (Central)

Ethanol/Nutrition/Herb Interactions Ethanol: May increase CNS depression; monitor for increased effects with coadministration. Caution patients about effects.

Preparation for Administration Solution for injection:

I.M.: Butylbromide: No dilution required.

I.V.:

Butylbromide: No dilution is necessary prior to injection.

Hydrobromide: Dilute with an equal volume of sterile water.

Storage/Stability

Solution for injection:

Butylbromide (Canadian availability): Store at room temperature. Do not freeze. Protect from light and heat. Stable in D_5W, $D_{10}W$, NS, Ringer's solution, and LR for up to 8 hours.

Hydrobromide: Store at room temperature of 20°C to 25°C (68°F to 77°F). Protect from light. Avoid acid solutions; hydrolysis occurs at pH <3.

Tablet (Canadian availability): Store at room temperature. Protect from light and heat.

Transdermal system: Store at 20°C to 25°C (68°F to 77°F).

Mechanism of Action Blocks the action of acetylcholine at parasympathetic sites in smooth muscle, secretory glands and the CNS; increases cardiac output, dries secretions, antagonizes histamine and serotonin

Pharmacodynamics/Kinetics

Onset of action: Oral, I.M.: 0.5-1 hour; I.V.: 10 minutes; Transdermal: 6-8 hours

Duration: I.M., I.V., SubQ: 4 hours

Absorption: I.M., SubQ: Rapid; Oral: Quaternary salts (butylbromide) are poorly absorbed (local concentrations in the GI tract following oral dosing may be high)

Distribution: V_d: Butylbromide: 128 L

Protein binding: Butylbromide: ~4% (albumin)

Metabolism: Hepatic

Bioavailability: Oral: 8%

Half-life elimination: Butylbromide: ~5-11 hours; Hydrobromide: ~1-4 hours; Scopolamine base: 9.5 hours

Time to peak: Hydrobromide: I.M.: ~20 minutes, SubQ: ~15 minutes; Butylbromide: Oral: ~2 hours; Scopolamine base: Transdermal: 24 hours

Excretion: Urine (<10%, as parent drug and metabolites); I.V.: Butylbromide: Urine (42% to 61% [half as parent drug]), feces (28% to 37%)

Dosage Note: Scopolamine (hyoscine) hydrobromide should not be interchanged with scopolamine butylbromide formulations. Dosages are not equivalent.

Scopolamine base: Transdermal patch: Adults:

Preoperative: Apply 1 patch to hairless area behind ear the night before surgery or 1 hour prior to cesarean section (apply no sooner than 1 hour before surgery to minimize newborn exposure); remove 24 hours after surgery

Motion sickness: Apply 1 patch to hairless area behind the ear at least 4 hours prior to exposure and every 3 days as needed; effective if applied as soon as 2-3 hours before anticipated need, best if 12 hours before

Chemotherapy-induced nausea and vomiting, breakthrough (unlabeled use): Apply 1 patch every 72 hours (NCCN Antiemesis guidelines v.1.2012)

Scopolamine hydrobromide:

Antiemetic: SubQ:

Children: 0.006 mg/kg

Adults: 0.6-1 mg

Preoperative: I.M., I.V., SubQ:

Children 6 months to 3 years: 0.1-0.15 mg

Children 3-6 years: 0.2-0.3 mg

Adults: 0.3-0.65 mg

Sedation, tranquilization: I.M., I.V., SubQ: Adults:

U.S. labeling: 0.6 mg 3-4 times/day

Canadian labeling: 0.3-0.6 mg 3-4 times/day

Scopolamine butylbromide: Gastrointestinal/genitourinary spasm (Buscopan® [CAN]; not available in the U.S.): Adults:

Oral: Acute therapy: 10-20 mg daily (1-2 tablets); prolonged therapy: 10 mg (1 tablet) 3-5 times/day; maximum: 60 mg/day

I.M., I.V., SubQ: 10-20 mg; maximum: 100 mg/day

Elderly: Lower dosages may be required. Refer to adult dosing.

Dosage adjustment in renal impairment: No dosage adjustment provided in manufacturer's labeling. However, caution is recommended due to increased risks of adverse effects.

Dosage adjustment in hepatic impairment: No dosage adjustment provided in manufacturer's labeling. However, caution is recommended due to increased risks of adverse effects.

Administration Note: Butylbromide or hydrobromide may be administered by I.M., I.V., or SubQ injection.

I.M.: **Butylbromide:** Intramuscular injections should be administered 10-15 minutes prior to radiological/diagnostic procedures.

I.V.:

Butylbromide: No dilution is necessary prior to injection; inject at a rate of 1 mL/minute

Hydrobromide: Dilute with an equal volume of sterile water and administer by direct I.V.; inject over 2-3 minutes

Oral: Tablet should be swallowed whole and taken with a full glass of water.

Transdermal: Apply to hairless area of skin behind the ear. Wash hands before and after applying the disc to avoid drug contact with eyes. Do not use any patch that has been damaged, cut, or manipulated in any way. Topical patch is programmed to deliver 1 mg over 3 days. Once applied, do not remove the patch for 3 full days (motion sickness). When used postoperatively for nausea/vomiting, the patch should be removed 24 hours after surgery. If patch becomes displaced, discard and apply a new patch.

Monitoring Parameters Body temperature, heart rate, urinary output, intraocular pressure

Test Interactions Interferes with gastric secretion test

Dosage Forms Excipient information presented when available (limited, particularly for generics); consult specific product labeling.

Patch 72 Hour, Transdermal:

Transderm-Scop: 1.5 mg (1 ea, 4 ea, 10 ea, 24 ea)

Solution, Injection, as hydrobromide:

Generic: 0.4 mg/mL (1 mL)

Dosage Forms: Canada Excipient information presented when available (limited, particularly for generics); consult specific product labeling.

Tablet, oral, as butylbromide:

Buscopan®: 10 mg

◆ **Scopolamine Base** *see* Scopolamine (Systemic) *on page 1881*

◆ **Scopolamine Butylbromide** *see* Scopolamine (Systemic) *on page 1881*

◆ **Scopolamine Hydrobromide** *see* Scopolamine (Systemic) *on page 1881*

◆ **Scopolamine Hydrobromide Injection (Can)** *see* Scopolamine (Systemic) *on page 1881*

◆ **Scopolamine, Hyoscyamine, Atropine, and Phenobarbital** *see* Hyoscyamine, Atropine, Scopolamine, and Phenobarbital *on page 1028*

◆ **Scorpion Antivenin** *see Centruroides* Immune $F(ab')_2$ (Equine) *on page 390*

◆ **Scorpion Antivenom** *see Centruroides* Immune $F(ab')_2$ (Equine) *on page 390*

◆ **Scot-Tussin Allergy Relief [OTC]** *see* DiphenhydrAMINE (Systemic) *on page 622*

◆ **Scot-Tussin® DM Maximum Strength [OTC]** *see* Dextromethorphan and Chlorpheniramine *on page 591*

◆ **Scot-Tussin Expectorant [OTC]** *see* GuaiFENesin *on page 974*

◆ **Scot-Tussin Senior [OTC]** *see* Guaifenesin and Dextromethorphan *on page 976*

◆ **Sculptra®** *see* Poly-L-Lactic Acid *on page 1671*

◆ **Sculptra® Aesthetic** *see* Poly-L-Lactic Acid *on page 1671*

◆ **SD/01** *see* Pegfilgrastim *on page 1588*

◆ **SDX-105** *see* Bendamustine *on page 237*

◆ **SDZ ENA 713** *see* Rivastigmine *on page 1841*

◆ **Se-100 [OTC]** *see* Selenium *on page 1888*

◆ **Sea-Clens Wound Cleanser [OTC]** *see* Sodium Chloride *on page 1914*

◆ **Sea Soft Nasal Mist [OTC]** *see* Sodium Chloride *on page 1914*

◆ **Seasonale (Can)** *see* Ethinyl Estradiol and Levonorgestrel *on page 787*

◆ **Seasonique** *see* Ethinyl Estradiol and Levonorgestrel *on page 787*

◆ **Se Aspartate [OTC]** *see* Selenium *on page 1888*

◆ **Seb-Prev** *see* Sulfacetamide (Topical) *on page 1957*

◆ **Seb-Prev Wash** *see* Sulfacetamide (Topical) *on page 1957*

Secobarbital (see koe BAR bi tal)

Brand Names: U.S. Seconal

Index Terms Quinalbarbitone Sodium; Secobarbital Sodium

Pharmacologic Category Barbiturate

Additional Appendix Information

Beers Criteria – Potentially Inappropriate Medications for Geriatrics *on page 2368*

Use Preanesthetic agent; short-term treatment of insomnia

Pregnancy Risk Factor D

Dosage Oral: Adults:

Insomnia (hypnotic): Usual: 100 mg at bedtime. **Note:** Limit to short-term use only; efficacy for sleep induction and maintenance is lost after 14 days.

Preoperative sedation: 200-300 mg 1-2 hours before procedure

Elderly: Manufacturer's labeling recommends a dose reduction, but does not provide specific dosing recommendations.

Dosage adjustment in renal impairment: No specific dosage adjustment provided in manufacturer's labeling. However, a dosage reduction is recommended. Slightly dialyzable (5% to 20%).

Dosage adjustment in hepatic impairment: No dosage adjustment provided in manufacturer's labeling. However, dosage reduction is recommended.

Additional Information Complete prescribing information should be consulted for additional detail.

Dosage Forms Excipient information presented when available (limited, particularly for generics); consult specific product labeling.

Capsule, Oral, as sodium:

Seconal: 100 mg [contains fd&c yellow #10 (quinoline yellow)]

Controlled Substance C-II

◆ **Secobarbital Sodium** *see* Secobarbital *on page 1884*

◆ **Seconal** *see* Secobarbital *on page 1884*

◆ **Sectral** *see* Acebutolol *on page 28*

◆ **Sectral® (Can)** *see* Acebutolol *on page 28*

◆ **Secura Antifungal [OTC]** *see* Miconazole (Topical) *on page 1358*

◆ **Secura Antifungal Extra Thick [OTC]** *see* Miconazole (Topical) *on page 1358*

◆ **Seebri® Breezhaler® (Can)** *see* Glycopyrrolate *on page 965*

◆ **Selax® (Can)** *see* Docusate *on page 644*

◆ **Select 1/35 (Can)** *see* Ethinyl Estradiol and Norethindrone *on page 793*

Selegiline (se LE ji leen)

Brand Names: U.S. Eldepryl; Emsam; Zelapar

Brand Names: Canada Apo-Selegiline; Gen-Selegiline; Mylan-Selegiline; Novo-Selegiline; Nu-Selegiline

Index Terms Deprenyl; L-Deprenyl; Selegiline Hydrochloride

Pharmacologic Category Anti-Parkinson's Agent, MAO Type B Inhibitor; Antidepressant, Monoamine Oxidase Inhibitor

Additional Appendix Information

Antidepressant Agents *on page 2284*

Antiparkinsonian Agents *on page 2289*

Tyramine Content of Foods *on page 2394*

Use Adjunct in the management of parkinsonian patients in which levodopa/carbidopa therapy is deteriorating (oral products); treatment of major depressive disorder (transdermal product)

Unlabeled Use Early Parkinson's disease; attention-deficit/hyperactivity disorder (ADHD)

Pregnancy Risk Factor C

Pregnancy Considerations Adverse events were observed in some animal reproduction studies.

Breast-Feeding Considerations It is not known if selegiline is excreted in breast milk. The manufacturer recommends discontinuing all unessential drugs in nursing women.

Medication Guide Available Yes

Contraindications Hypersensitivity to selegiline or any component of the formulation; concomitant use of meperidine

Orally disintegrating tablet: Additional contraindications: Concomitant use of dextromethorphan, methadone, propoxyphene, tramadol, oral selegiline, other MAO inhibitors

Transdermal: Additional contraindications: Pheochromocytoma; concomitant use of bupropion, selective or dual serotonin reuptake inhibitors (including SSRIs and SNRIs), tricyclic antidepressants, tramadol, propoxyphene, methadone, dextromethorphan, St. John's wort, mirtazapine, cyclobenzaprine, oral selegiline and other MAO inhibitors; carbamazepine, and oxcarbazepine; elective surgery requiring general anesthesia (selegiline should be discontinued at least 10 days prior to elective surgery), local anesthesia containing sympathomimetic vasoconstrictors; sympathomimetics (and related compounds); foods high in tyramine content; supplements containing tyrosine, phenylalanine, tryptophan, or caffeine

Warnings/Precautions

Oral: MAO-B selective inhibition should not pose a problem with tyramine-containing products as long as the typical oral doses are employed, however, rare reactions have been reported. Increased risk of nonselective MAO inhibition occurs with oral capsule/tablet doses >10 mg/day or orally disintegrating tablet doses >2.5 mg/day. Use of oral selegiline with tricyclic antidepressants and SSRIs has also been associated with rare reactions and should generally be avoided. Addition to levodopa therapy may result in exacerbation of levodopa adverse effects, requiring a reduction in levodopa dosage. Dopaminergic agents used for Parkinson's disease or restless legs syndrome have been associated with compulsive behaviors and/or loss of impulse control, which has manifested as pathological gambling, libido increases (hypersexuality), and/or binge eating. Causality has not been established, and controversy exists as to whether this phenomenon is related to the underlying disease, prior behaviors/addictions and/or drug therapy. Dose reduction or discontinuation of therapy has been reported to reverse these behaviors in some, but not all cases. Use caution in patients with hepatic or renal impairment. Incidence of orthostatic hypotension may be increased in older adults and when titrating to the 2.5 mg dosage in patients taking the orally disintegrating tablet. Risk for melanoma development is increased in Parkinson's disease patients; drug causation or factors contributing to risk have not been established. Patients should be monitored closely and periodic skin examinations should be performed. Orally disintegrating tablet may cause oral mucosa edema, irritation, pain, ulceration and/or swallowing pain. Do not use orally disintegrating tablet concurrently with other selegiline products; wait at least 14 days from discontinuation before initiating treatment with another selegiline dosage form. Some products may contain phenylalanine.

Transdermal: Nonselective MAO inhibition occurs with transdermal delivery and is necessary for antidepressant efficacy. Hypertensive crisis as a result of ingesting tyramine-rich foods is always a concern with nonselective MAO inhibition. Although transdermal delivery minimizes inhibition of MAO-A in the gut, there is limited data with higher transdermal doses; dietary modifications are recommended with doses >6 mg/24 hours.

Transdermal patch: May cause orthostatic hypotension; use with caution in patients at risk of this effect or in those who would not tolerate transient hypotensive episodes (cerebrovascular disease, cardiovascular disease, hypovolemia, or concurrent medication use which may predispose to hypotension/bradycardia). May contain conducting metal (eg, aluminum); remove patch prior to MRI. Avoid exposure of application site and surrounding area to direct external heat sources.

Transdermal: **[U.S. Boxed Warning]: Antidepressants increase the risk of suicidal thinking and behavior in children, adolescents, and young adults (18-24 years of age) with major depressive disorder (MDD) and other psychiatric disorders;** consider risk prior to prescribing. Short-term studies did not show an increased risk in patients >24 years of age and showed a decreased risk in patients ≥65 years. Closely monitor patients for worsening of depression, suicidality and/or associated behaviors, particularly during the initial 1-2 months of therapy or during periods of dosage adjustments (increases or decreases); the patient's family or caregiver should be instructed to closely observe the patient and communicate condition with healthcare provider. A medication guide concerning the use of antidepressants should be dispensed with each prescription. **Transdermal selegiline is not FDA approved for use in children <12 years of age.**

Transdermal: The possibility of a suicide attempt is inherit in major depression and may persist until remission occurs. Patients treated with antidepressants (for any indication) should be observed for clinical worsening and suicidality, especially during the initial few months of a course of drug therapy, or at times of dose changes, either increases or decreases. Use caution in high-risk patients. Worsening depression and severe abrupt suicidality that are not part of the presenting symptoms may require discontinuation or modification of drug therapy. Use caution in high-risk patients during initiation of therapy. The patient's family or caregiver should be alerted to monitor patients for the emergence of suicidality and associated behaviors (such as agitation, irritability, hostility, and hypomania) and call healthcare provider.

Transdermal selegiline may worsen psychosis in some patients or precipitate a shift to mania or hypomania in patients with bipolar disorder. Monotherapy in patients with bipolar disorder should be avoided. Patients presenting with depressive symptoms should be screened for bipolar disorder. **Selegiline is not FDA approved for the treatment of bipolar depression.**

Abrupt discontinuation or interruption of antidepressant therapy has been associated with a discontinuation syndrome. Symptoms arising may vary with antidepressant however commonly include nausea, vomiting, diarrhea, headaches, lightheadedness, dizziness, diminished appetite, sweating, chills, tremors, paresthesias, fatigue, somnolence, and sleep disturbances (eg, vivid dreams, insomnia). Greater risks for developing a discontinuation syndrome have been associated with antidepressants with shorter half-lives, longer durations of treatment, and abrupt discontinuation. More severe symptoms have also been associated with MAO inhibitors. For antidepressants of short or intermediate half-lives, symptoms may emerge within 2-5 days after treatment discontinuation and last 7-14 days (APA, 2010; Fava, 2006; Haddad, 2001; Shelton, 2001; Warner, 2006).

Adverse Reactions Unless otherwise noted, the percentage of adverse events is reported for the transdermal patch (**Note:** ODT = orally disintegrating tablet, Oral = capsule/tablet)

>10%:

- Central nervous system: Headache (18%; ODT 7%; oral 4%), insomnia (12%; ODT 7%), dizziness (oral 14%; ODT 11%)
- Gastrointestinal: Nausea (oral 20%; ODT 11%)
- Local: Application site reaction (24%)

1% to 10%:

- Cardiovascular: Hypotension (including postural 3% to 10%), palpitation (oral 2%), chest pain (≥1%; ODT 2%), hypertension (≥1%; ODT 3%), peripheral edema (≥1%)
- Central nervous system: Pain (ODT 8%; oral 2%), hallucinations (oral 6%; ODT 4%), confusion (oral 6%; ODT 4%), vivid dreams (oral 4%), ataxia (ODT 3%), somnolence (ODT 3%), lethargy (oral 2%), agitation (≥1%), amnesia (≥1%), paresthesia (≥1%), thinking abnormal (≥1%), depression (<1%; ODT 2%)
- Dermatologic: Rash (4%), bruising (≥1%; ODT 2%), pruritus (≥1%), acne (≥1%)
- Endocrine & metabolic: Weight loss (5%; oral 2%), hypokalemia (ODT 2%), sexual side effects (≤1%)

Gastrointestinal: Diarrhea (9%; ODT 2%; oral 2%), xerostomia (8%; oral 6%; ODT 4%), stomatitis (ODT 5%), abdominal pain (oral 8%), dyspepsia (4%; ODT 5%), dysphagia (ODT 2%), dental caries (ODT 2%), constipation (≥1%; ODT 4%), flatulence (≥1%; ODT 2%), anorexia (≥1%), gastroenteritis (≥1%), taste perversion (≥1%; ODT 2%), vomiting (≥1%; ODT 3%)

Genitourinary: Urinary retention (oral 2%), dysmenorrhea (≥1%), metrorrhagia (≥1%), UTI (≥1%), urinary frequency (≥1%)

Neuromuscular & skeletal: Dyskinesia (ODT 6%), back pain (ODT 5%; oral 2%), ataxia (<1%; ODT 3%), leg cramps (ODT 3%; oral 2%), myalgia (≥1%; ODT 3%), neck pain (≥1%), tremor (<1%; ODT 3%)

Otic: Tinnitus (≥1%)

Respiratory: Rhinitis (ODT 7%), pharyngitis (3%; ODT 4%), sinusitis (3%), cough (≥1%), bronchitis (≥1%), dyspnea (<1%; ODT 3%)

Miscellaneous: Diaphoresis (≥1%)

Oral and/or transdermal patch: <1% or frequency not defined (limited to important or life-threatening): Abnormal liver function tests, alkaline phosphatase increased, appetite increased, arrhythmia, asthma, ataxia, atrial fibrillation, bacterial infection, behavior/mood changes, bilirubinemia, bradycardia, bradykinesia, breast neoplasm (female), breast pain, chorea, circumoral paresthesia, colitis, dehydration, delusions, depersonalization, depression, emotional lability, epistaxis, eructation, euphoria, face edema, fever, fungal infection, gastritis, generalized spasm, glossitis, heat stroke, hematuria (female), hernia, hostility, hypercholesterolemia, hyperesthesia, hyperglycemia, hyperkinesias, hypertonia, hypoglycemic reaction, hyponatremia, impulsive/compulsive behaviors (eg, pathological gambling, hypersexuality, binge eating), kidney calculus (female), lactate dehydrogenase increased, laryngismus, leukocytosis, leukopenia, libido increased, loss of balance, lymphadenopathy, maculopapular rash, manic reaction, melena, MI, migraine, moniliasis, myasthenia, myoclonus, neoplasia, neurosis, osteoporosis, otitis external, palpitation, paranoid reaction, parasitic infection, parosmia, pelvic pain, periodontal abscess, peripheral vascular disorder, pneumonia, polyuria (female), prostatic hyperplasia, rectal hemorrhage, salivation increased, skin hypertrophy, skin benign neoplasm, suicide attempt, syncope, tachycardia, tenosynovitis, tongue edema, twitching, urinary retention, urinary urgency (male and female), urination impaired (male), urticaria, vaginal hemorrhage, vaginal moniliasis, vaginitis, vasodilatation, vertigo, vesiculobullous rash, viral infection, visual field defect

Drug Interactions

Metabolism/Transport Effects

Substrate of CYP1A2 (minor), CYP2A6 (minor), CYP2B6 (major), CYP2C8 (minor), CYP2D6 (minor), CYP3A4 (minor); **Note:** Assignment of Major/Minor substrate status based on clinically relevant drug interaction potential; **Inhibits** CYP1A2 (weak), CYP2A6 (weak), CYP2C19 (weak), CYP2D6 (weak), CYP2E1 (weak), CYP3A4 (weak), Monoamine Oxidase

Avoid Concomitant Use

Avoid concomitant use of Selegiline with any of the following: Alpha-/Beta-Agonists (Indirect-Acting); Alpha1-Agonists; Amphetamines; Anilidopiperidine Opioids; Antidepressants (Serotonin Reuptake Inhibitor/Antagonist); Apraclonidine; AtoMOXetine; Bezafibrate; Buprenorphine; BuPROPion; BusPIRone; CarBAMazepine; Cyclobenzaprine; Dexmethylphenidate; Dextromethorphan; Diethylpropion; Hydrocodone; HYDROmorphone; Isometheptene; Levonordefrin; Linezolid; Maprotiline; Meperidine; Methyldopa; Methylene Blue; Methylphenidate; Mirtazapine; Morphine (Liposomal); Morphine (Systemic); OXcarbazepine; Oxymorphone; Pizotifen; Selective Serotonin Reuptake Inhibitors; Serotonin 5-HT1D Receptor Agonists; Serotonin/Norepinephrine Reuptake Inhibitors; Tapentadol; Tetrabenazine; Tetrahydrozoline (Nasal); Tricyclic Antidepressants; Tryptophan

Increased Effect/Toxicity

Selegiline may increase the levels/effects of: Alpha-/Beta-Agonists (Indirect-Acting); Alpha1-Agonists; Amphetamines; Antidepressants (Serotonin Reuptake Inhibitor/Antagonist); Antihypertensives; Antipsychotics; Apraclonidine; AtoMOXetine; Beta2-Agonists; Betahistine; Bezafibrate; Brimonidine (Ophthalmic); Brimonidine (Topical); BuPROPion; Dexmethylphenidate; Dextromethorphan; Diethylpropion; Dofetilide; Domperidone; Doxapram; Doxylamine; EPINEPHrine (Nasal); Epinephrine (Racemic); EPINEPHrine (Systemic, Oral Inhalation); Hydrocodone; HYDROmorphone; Hypoglycemic Agents; Isometheptene; Levonordefrin; Linezolid; Lithium; Lomitapide; Meperidine; Methadone; Methyldopa; Methylene Blue; Methylphenidate; Metoclopramide; Mirtazapine; Morphine (Liposomal); Morphine (Systemic); Norepinephrine; Orthostatic Hypotension Producing Agents; OxyCODONE; Pizotifen; Reserpine; Selective Serotonin Reuptake Inhibitors; Serotonin 5-HT1D Receptor Agonists; Serotonin Modulators; Serotonin/Norepinephrine Reuptake Inhibitors; Tetrahydrozoline (Nasal); Tricyclic Antidepressants

The levels/effects of Selegiline may be increased by: Altretamine; Anilidopiperidine Opioids; Antipsychotics; Buprenorphine; BusPIRone; CarBAMazepine; COMT Inhibitors; Contraceptives (Estrogens); Contraceptives (Progestins); Cyclobenzaprine; CYP2B6 Inhibitors (Moderate); CYP2B6 Inhibitors (Strong); Levodopa; MAO Inhibitors; Maprotiline; OXcarbazepine; Oxymorphone; Quazepam; Tapentadol; Tetrabenazine; TraMADol; Tryptophan

Decreased Effect

Selegiline may decrease the levels/effects of: Domperidone; Ioflupane I 123

The levels/effects of Selegiline may be decreased by: CYP2B6 Inducers (Strong); Dabrafenib; Domperidone; Peginterferon Alfa-2b

Ethanol/Nutrition/Herb Interactions

Ethanol: Ethanol may enhance the adverse/toxic effects of selegiline. Beverages containing tyramine (eg, hearty red wine and beer) may increase toxic effects. Management: Avoid ethanol and beverages containing tyramine.

Food: Concurrent ingestion of foods rich in tyramine, dopamine, tyrosine, phenylalanine, tryptophan, or caffeine may cause sudden and severe high blood pressure (hypertensive crisis or serotonin syndrome). Management: Avoid tyramine-containing foods (aged or matured cheese, air-dried or cured meats including sausages and salamis; fava or broad bean pods, tap/draft beers, Marmite concentrate, sauerkraut, soy sauce, and other soybean condiments). Food's freshness is also an important concern; improperly stored or spoiled food can create an environment in which tyramine concentrations may increase. Avoid foods containing dopamine, tyrosine, phenylalanine, tryptophan, or caffeine.

Herb/Nutraceutical: Kava kava, valerian, St John's wort, and SAMe may increase risk of serotonin syndrome and/or excessive sedation. Supplements containing caffeine, tyrosine, tryptophan, or phenylalanine may increase the risk of severe side effects like hypertensive reactions or serotonin syndrome. Management: Avoid kava kava, valerian, St John's wort, SAMe, and supplements containing caffeine, tyrosine, tryptophan, or phenylalanine.

Storage/Stability

Capsule, tablet, transdermal: Store at 20°C to 25°C (68°F to 77°F). Store patch in sealed pouch and apply immediately after removal.

Orally disintegrating tablet: Store at controlled room temperature 25°C (77°F); excursions permitted to 15°C to 30°C (59°F to 86°F). Use within 3 months of opening pouch and immediately after opening individual blister.

Mechanism of Action Potent, irreversible inhibitor of monoamine oxidase (MAO). Plasma concentrations achieved via administration of oral dosage forms in recommended doses confer selective inhibition of MAO type B, which plays a major role in the metabolism of dopamine; selegiline may also increase dopaminergic activity by interfering with dopamine reuptake at the synapse. When administered transdermally in recommended doses, selegiline achieves higher blood levels and effectively inhibits both MAO-A and MAO-B, which blocks catabolism of other centrally-active biogenic amine neurotransmitters.

Pharmacodynamics/Kinetics

Onset of action: Therapeutic: Oral: Within 1 hour

Duration: Oral: 24-72 hours

Absorption:

Orally disintegrating tablet: Rapid; greater bioavailability than capsule/tablet

Transdermal: 25% to 30% (of total selegiline content) over 24 hours

Protein binding: ~90%

Metabolism: Hepatic, primarily via CYP2B6 to active (N-desmethylselegiline, amphetamine, methamphetamine) and inactive metabolites

Half-life elimination: Oral: 10 hours; Transdermal: 18-25 hours

Excretion: Urine (primarily metabolites); feces

Dosage

Capsule/tablet:

Children and Adolescents: ADHD (unlabeled use): Oral: 5-15 mg/day (Jankovic, 1993)

Adults: Parkinson's disease: 5 mg twice daily with breakfast and lunch

Elderly: Parkinson's disease: ≤5 mg/day (when combined with levodopa) is recommended by some clinicians to decrease the enhanced dopaminergic side effects (Olanow, 2001)

Orally disintegrating tablet (Zelapar®): Adults: Parkinson's disease: Initial 1.25 mg daily for at least 6 weeks; may increase to 2.5 mg daily based on clinical response (maximum: 2.5 mg daily)

Transdermal (Emsam®): Depression:

Adults: Initial: 6 mg/24 hours once daily; may titrate based on clinical response in increments of 3 mg/day every 2 weeks up to a maximum of 12 mg/24 hours

Elderly: 6 mg/24 hours

Discontinuation of therapy: Upon discontinuation of antidepressant therapy, gradually taper the dose to minimize the incidence of withdrawal symptoms and allow for the detection of re-emerging symptoms. Evidence supporting ideal taper rates is limited. APA and NICE guidelines suggest tapering therapy over at least several weeks with consideration to the half-life of the antidepressant; antidepressants with a shorter half-life and MAO inhibitors may need to be tapered more conservatively. In addition for long-term treated patients, WFSBP guidelines recommend tapering over 4-6 months. If intolerable withdrawal symptoms occur following a dose reduction, consider resuming the previously prescribed dose and/or decrease dose at a more gradual rate (APA, 2010; Bauer, 2002; Haddad, 2001; NCCMH, 2010; Schatzberg, 2006; Shelton, 2001; Warner, 2006).

MAO inhibitor recommendations:

Switching to or from an MAO inhibitor intended to treat psychiatric disorders:

Allow 14 days to elapse between discontinuing an alternative antidepressant without long half-life metabolites (eg, TCAs, paroxetine, fluvoxamine, venlafaxine) or MAO inhibitor intended to treat psychiatric disorders and initiation of selegiline.

Allow 5 weeks to elapse between discontinuing fluoxetine (with long half-life metabolites) intended to treat psychiatric disorders and initiation of selegiline.

Allow 14 days to elapse between discontinuing selegiline and initiation of an alternative antidepressant or MAO inhibitor intended to treat psychiatric disorders.

Use with other MAO inhibitors (such as linezolid or I.V. methylene blue):

Do not initiate selegiline in patients receiving linezolid or I.V. methylene blue; consider other interventions for psychiatric condition.

If urgent treatment with linezolid or I.V. methylene blue is required in a patient already receiving selegiline and potential benefits outweigh potential risks, discontinue selegiline promptly and administer linezolid or I.V. methylene blue. Monitor for serotonin syndrome for 2 weeks or until 24 hours after the last dose of linezolid or I.V. methylene blue, whichever comes first. May resume selegiline 24 hours after the last dose of linezolid or I.V. methylene blue.

Dosage adjustment in renal impairment:

Oral: No dosage adjustment provided in manufacturer's labeling (has not been studied). Use with caution.

Transdermal: No dosage adjustment necessary.

Dosage adjustment in hepatic impairment:

Oral: No dosage adjustment provided in manufacturer's labeling (has not been studied). Use with caution.

Transdermal:

Mild to moderate impairment: No dosage adjustment necessary.

Severe impairment: No dosage adjustment provided in manufacturer's labeling.

Dietary Considerations Avoid or limit tyramine-containing foods/beverages (product and/or dose-dependent). Some examples include aged or matured cheese, air-dried or cured meats (including sausages and salamis), fava or broad bean pods, tap/draft beers, Marmite concentrate, sauerkraut, soy sauce and other soybean condiments. Food's freshness is also an important concern; improperly stored or spoiled food can create an environment where tyramine concentrations may increase.

Emsam®: 9 mg/24 hours or 12 mg/24 hours: Avoid tyramine-rich foods or beverages beginning the first day of treatment or for 2 weeks after discontinuation or dose reduction to 6 mg/24 hours.

Zelapar®: Do not take with food or liquid.

Some products may contain phenylalanine.

Administration

Oral: Orally disintegrating tablet (Zelapar®): Take in morning before breakfast; place on top of tongue and allow to dissolve. Avoid food or liquid 5 minutes before and after administration.

Topical: Transdermal (Emsam®): Apply to clean, dry, intact skin to the upper torso (below the neck and above the waist), upper thigh, or outer surface of the upper arm. Avoid exposure of application site to external heat source, which may increase the amount of drug absorbed. Apply at the same time each day and rotate application sites. Wash hands with soap and water after handling. Avoid touching the sticky side of the patch.

Monitoring Parameters Blood pressure; symptoms of parkinsonism; general mood and behavior (increased anxiety, presence of mania or agitation); suicidal ideation (especially at the beginning of therapy or when doses are increased or decreased)

Test Interactions May interfere with urine detection of amphetamine/methamphetamine (false-positive).

Additional Information When adding selegiline to levodopa/carbidopa, the dose of the latter can usually be decreased.

Dosage Forms Excipient information presented when available (limited, particularly for generics); consult specific product labeling.

Capsule, Oral, as hydrochloride:
- Eldepryl: 5 mg
- Generic: 5 mg

Patch 24 Hour, Transdermal:
- Emsam: 6 mg/24 hr (30 ea); 9 mg/24 hr (30 ea); 12 mg/24 hr (30 ea)

Tablet, Oral, as hydrochloride:
- Generic: 5 mg

Tablet Dispersible, Oral, as hydrochloride:
- Zelapar: 1.25 mg [contains aspartame; grapefruit flavor]

◆ **Selegiline Hydrochloride** *see* Selegiline *on page* 1884
◆ **Selenicaps-200 [OTC]** *see* Selenium *on page* 1888
◆ **Selenimin [OTC]** *see* Selenium *on page* 1888
◆ **Selenimin-200 [OTC]** *see* Selenium *on page* 1888

Selenium (se LEE nee um)

Brand Names: U.S. Aqueous Selenium [OTC]; Oceanic Selenium [OTC]; Se Aspartate [OTC]; Se-100 [OTC]; Se-Plus Protein [OTC]; Selenicaps-200 [OTC]; Selenimin [OTC]; Selenimin-200 [OTC]

Pharmacologic Category Trace Element, Parenteral

Use Trace metal supplement

Pregnancy Risk Factor C

Dosage Nutritional supplement:

Oral:

Adequate intake (AI):
- 1-6 months: 15 mcg/day
- 7-12 months: 20 mcg/day

Recommended daily allowance (RDA):
- 1-3 years: 20 mcg/day
- 4-8 years: 30 mcg/day
- 9-13 years 40 mcg/day
- ≥14 years and Adults: 55 mcg/day
- Pregnancy: 60 mcg/day
- Lactation: 70 mcg/day

I.V. in TPN solutions:
- Children: 3 mcg/kg/day
- Adults:
  - Metabolically stable: 20-40 mcg/day
  - Deficiency from prolonged TPN support: 100 mcg/day

Additional Information Complete prescribing information should be consulted for additional detail.

Dosage Forms Excipient information presented when available (limited, particularly for generics); consult specific product labeling.

Capsule, Oral:
- Selenicaps-200: 200 mcg [corn free, no artificial color(s), rye free, sugar free, wheat free, yeast free]

Capsule, Oral [preservative free]:
- Se-100: 100 mcg [dye free, yeast free]

Liquid, Oral:
- Aqueous Selenium: 95 mcg/drop (15 mL) [contains sodium benzoate]

Solution, Intravenous:
- Generic: 40 mcg/mL (10 mL)

Tablet, Oral:
- Oceanic Selenium: 50 mcg, 200 mcg [animal products free, gelatin free, gluten free, kosher certified, lactose free, no artificial color(s), no artificial flavor(s), starch free, sugar free, yeast free]
- Se Aspartate: 50 mcg
- Se-Plus Protein: 200 mcg
- Selenimin: 125 mcg [corn free, rye free, starch free, sugar free, wheat free]
- Selenimin-200: 200 mcg [corn free, rye free, starch free, sugar free, wheat free, yeast free]
- Generic: 50 mcg, 200 mcg

Tablet, Oral [preservative free]:
- Generic: 50 mcg, 200 mcg

Tablet Extended Release, Oral [preservative free]:
- Generic: 200 mcg

Selenium Sulfide (se LEE nee um SUL fide)

Brand Names: U.S. Anti-Dandruff [OTC]; Dandrex [OTC]; Selsun [DSC]; Tersi

Brand Names: Canada Versel®

Pharmacologic Category Topical Skin Product

Use Treatment of itching and flaking of the scalp associated with dandruff, to control scalp seborrheic dermatitis; treatment of tinea versicolor

Pregnancy Risk Factor C

Dosage Topical: Adults:

Dandruff, seborrhea: Massage 5-10 mL of shampoo into wet scalp, leave on scalp 2-3 minutes, rinse thoroughly. Usually 2 applications each week for 2 weeks will provide control. After this, may repeat at less frequent intervals (eg, once weekly, every 2-4 weeks). Rub foam into affected skin twice daily.

Tinea versicolor: Apply the 2.5% lotion to affected area and lather with small amounts of water; leave on skin for 10 minutes, then rinse thoroughly; apply every day for 7 days; rub foam into affected skin twice daily

Additional Information Complete prescribing information should be consulted for additional detail.

Dosage Forms Excipient information presented when available (limited, particularly for generics); consult specific product labeling. [DSC] = Discontinued product

Foam, External:
- Tersi: 2.25% (70 g) [contains trolamine (triethanolamine)]

Lotion, External:
- Selsun: 2.5% (120 mL [DSC])
- Generic: 2.5% (118 mL, 120 mL)

Shampoo, External:
- Anti-Dandruff: 1% (207 mL) [contains brilliant blue fcf (fd&c blue #1), menthol]
- Dandrex: 1% (240 mL)

◆ **Selsun [DSC]** *see* Selenium Sulfide *on page* 1888
◆ **Selzentry** *see* Maraviroc *on page* 1269
◆ **Semprex®-D** *see* Acrivastine and Pseudoephedrine *on page* 41
◆ **Senexon®-S [OTC]** *see* Docusate and Senna *on page* 645
◆ **Senna and Docusate** *see* Docusate and Senna *on page* 645
◆ **SennaLax-S [OTC]** *see* Docusate and Senna *on page* 645
◆ **Senna Plus [OTC]** *see* Docusate and Senna *on page* 645
◆ **Senna-S** *see* Docusate and Senna *on page* 645
◆ **Senokot-S® [OTC]** *see* Docusate and Senna *on page* 645
◆ **SenoSol™-SS [OTC]** *see* Docusate and Senna *on page* 645
◆ **Sensipar** *see* Cinacalcet *on page* 428
◆ **Sensorcaine** *see* Bupivacaine *on page* 289
◆ **Sensorcaine® (Can)** *see* Bupivacaine *on page* 289
◆ **Sensorcaine-MPF** *see* Bupivacaine *on page* 289
◆ **Sensorcaine-MPF Spinal** *see* Bupivacaine *on page* 289
◆ **Se-Plus Protein [OTC]** *see* Selenium *on page* 1888
◆ **Septa-Amlodipine (Can)** *see* AmLODIPine *on page* 109
◆ **Septa-Atenolol (Can)** *see* Atenolol *on page* 186
◆ **Septa-Citalopram (Can)** *see* Citalopram *on page* 440

◆ **Septa-Metformin (Can)** *see* MetFORMIN *on page 1310*

◆ **Septra** *see* Sulfamethoxazole and Trimethoprim *on page 1959*

◆ **Septra DS** *see* Sulfamethoxazole and Trimethoprim *on page 1959*

◆ **Septra Injection (Can)** *see* Sulfamethoxazole and Trimethoprim *on page 1959*

◆ **Serax** *see* Oxazepam *on page 1529*

◆ **Serevent® Diskhaler® Disk (Can)** *see* Salmeterol *on page 1871*

◆ **Serevent Diskus** *see* Salmeterol *on page 1871*

◆ **Serevent® Diskus® (Can)** *see* Salmeterol *on page 1871*

◆ **Serophene** *see* ClomiPHENE *on page 461*

◆ **Serophene® (Can)** *see* ClomiPHENE *on page 461*

◆ **SEROquel** *see* QUEtiapine *on page 1757*

◆ **Seroquel (Can)** *see* QUEtiapine *on page 1757*

◆ **SEROquel XR** *see* QUEtiapine *on page 1757*

◆ **Seroquel XR (Can)** *see* QUEtiapine *on page 1757*

◆ **Serostim** *see* Somatropin *on page 1934*

Sertaconazole (ser ta KOE na zole)

Brand Names: U.S. Ertaczo

Index Terms Sertaconazole Nitrate

Pharmacologic Category Antifungal Agent, Topical

Use Topical treatment of tinea pedis (athlete's foot)

Pregnancy Risk Factor C

Dosage Topical: Children ≥12 years and Adults: Apply between toes and to surrounding healthy skin twice daily for 4 weeks

Additional Information Complete prescribing information should be consulted for additional detail.

Dosage Forms Excipient information presented when available (limited, particularly for generics); consult specific product labeling.

Cream, External, as nitrate:

Ertaczo: 2% (60 g) [contains methylparaben]

◆ **Sertaconazole Nitrate** *see* Sertaconazole *on page 1889*

Sertraline (SER tra leen)

Brand Names: U.S. Zoloft

Brand Names: Canada Apo-Sertraline; Auro-Sertraline; CO Sertraline; Dom-Sertraline; GD-Sertraline; JAMP-Sertraline; MINT-Sertraline; Mylan-Sertraline; PHL-Sertraline; PMS-Sertraline; Q-Sertraline; Ran-Sertraline; ratio-Sertraline; Riva-Sertraline; Sandoz-Sertraline; Teva-Sertraline; Zoloft

Index Terms Sertraline Hydrochloride

Pharmacologic Category Antidepressant, Selective Serotonin Reuptake Inhibitor

Additional Appendix Information

Antidepressant Agents *on page 2284*

Selective Serotonin Reuptake Inhibitors (SSRIs) Pharmacokinetics *on page 2314*

Use

Major depressive disorder: Treatment of major depressive disorder (MDD) in adults.

Obsessive-compulsive disorder: Treatment of obsessions and compulsions in patients with obsessive-compulsive disorder (OCD).

Panic disorder: Treatment of panic disorder in adults with or without agoraphobia.

Post-traumatic stress disorder: Treatment of post-traumatic stress disorder (PTSD) in adults.

Premenstrual dysphoric disorder: Treatment of premenstrual dysphoric disorder (PMDD) in adults.

Social anxiety disorder: Treatment of social anxiety disorder (social phobia) in adults.

Unlabeled Use Binge-eating disorder; bulimia nervosa; generalized anxiety disorder (GAD)

Pregnancy Risk Factor C

Pregnancy Considerations Adverse events have been observed in animal reproduction studies. Sertraline crosses the human placenta. An increased risk of teratogenic effects, including cardiovascular defects, may be associated with maternal use of sertraline or other SSRIs; however, available information is conflicting. Nonteratogenic effects in the newborn following SSRI/SNRI exposure late in the third trimester include respiratory distress, cyanosis, apnea, seizures, temperature instability, feeding difficulty, vomiting, hypoglycemia, hypo- or hypertonia, hyper-reflexia, jitteriness, irritability, constant crying, and tremor. Symptoms may be due to the toxicity of the SSRIs/SNRIs or a discontinuation syndrome and may be consistent with serotonin syndrome associated with SSRI treatment. Persistent pulmonary hypertension of the newborn (PPHN) has also been reported with SSRI exposure. The long-term effects of *in utero* SSRI exposure on infant development and behavior are not known.

Due to pregnancy-induced physiologic changes, women who are pregnant may require adjusted doses of sertraline to achieve euthymia. The ACOG recommends that therapy with SSRIs or SNRIs during pregnancy be individualized; treatment of depression during pregnancy should incorporate the clinical expertise of the mental health clinician, obstetrician, primary healthcare provider, and pediatrician. According to the American Psychiatric Association (APA), the risks of medication treatment should be weighed against other treatment options and untreated depression. For women who discontinue antidepressant medications during pregnancy and who may be at high risk for postpartum depression, the medications can be restarted following delivery. Treatment algorithms have been developed by the ACOG and the APA for the management of depression in women prior to conception and during pregnancy.

Breast-Feeding Considerations Sertraline and desmethylsertraline are excreted in breast milk. Adverse events have been reported in nursing infants exposed to some SSRIs. The American Academy of Breast-feeding Medicine suggests that sertraline may be considered for the treatment of postpartum depression in appropriately selected women who are nursing. Infants exposed to sertraline while breast-feeding generally receive a low relative dose and serum concentrations are not detectable in most infants. Sertraline concentrations in the hindmilk are higher than in foremilk. If the benefits of the mother receiving the sertraline and breast-feeding outweigh the risks, the mother may consider pumping and discarding breast milk with the feeding 7-9 hours after the daily dose to decrease sertraline exposure to the infant. The long-term effects on development and behavior have not been studied. The manufacturer recommends that caution be exercised when administering sertraline to nursing women. Maternal use of an SSRI during pregnancy may cause delayed milk secretion.

Medication Guide Available Yes

Contraindications

Use of MAOIs intended to treat psychiatric disorders (concurrently or within 14 days of stopping an MAOI or sertraline); concurrent use with pimozide; initiation in patients treated with linezolid or methylene blue IV; hypersensitivity to sertraline or any component of the formulation; concurrent use with disulfiram (oral concentrate only).

Documentation of allergenic cross-reactivity for SSRIs is limited. However, because of similarities in chemical structure and/or pharmacologic actions, the possibility of cross-sensitivity cannot be ruled out with certainty.

Warnings/Precautions [U.S. Boxed Warning]: Antidepressants increase the risk of suicidal thinking and behavior in children, adolescents, and young adults (18-24 years of age) with major depressive disorder (MDD) and other psychiatric disorders; consider risk prior to prescribing. Short-term studies did not show an increased risk in patients >24 years of age and showed a decreased risk in patients ≥65 years. Closely monitor patients for clinical worsening, suicidality, or unusual changes in behavior, particularly during the initial 1-2 months of therapy or during periods of dosage adjustments (increases or decreases); the patient's family or caregiver should be instructed to closely observe the patient and communicate condition with healthcare provider. A medication guide concerning the use of antidepressants should be dispensed with each prescription. **Sertraline is not FDA approved for use in children with major depressive disorder (MDD). However, it is approved for the treatment of obsessive-compulsive disorder (OCD) in children ≥6 years of age.**

The possibility of a suicide attempt is inherent in major depression and may persist until remission occurs. Use caution in high-risk patients. Worsening depression and severe abrupt suicidality that are not part of the presenting symptoms may require discontinuation or modification of drug therapy. The patient's family or caregiver should be alerted to monitor patients for the emergence of suicidality and associated behaviors (such as agitation, irritability, hostility, impulsivity, and hypomania) and call healthcare provider.

May precipitate a mixed/manic episode in patients at risk for bipolar disorder. Use with caution in patients with a family history of bipolar disorder, mania, or hypomania. Patients presenting with depressive symptoms should be screened for bipolar disorder. **Sertraline is not FDA approved for the treatment of bipolar depression.**

Potentially life-threatening serotonin syndrome (SS) has occurred with serotonergic agents (eg, SSRIs, SNRIs), particularly when used in combination with other serotonergic agents (eg, triptans, TCAs, fentanyl, lithium, tramadol, buspirone, St John's wort, tryptophan) or agents that impair metabolism of serotonin (eg, MAO inhibitors intended to treat psychiatric disorders, other MAO inhibitors [ie, linezolid and intravenous methylene blue]). Discontinue treatment (and any concomitant serotonergic agent) immediately if signs/symptoms arise. Has a very low potential to impair cognitive or motor performance. However, caution patients regarding activities requiring alertness until response to sertraline is known. Does not appear to potentiate the effects of alcohol, however, ethanol use is not advised.

Use with caution in patients with risk factors for QTc prolongation; cases of QTc prolongation and torsade de pointes have been reported. Use caution in patients with a previous seizure disorder or condition predisposing to seizures such as brain damage, alcoholism, or concurrent therapy with other drugs which lower the seizure threshold. May increase the risks associated with electroconvulsive therapy. Use with caution in patients with narrow-angle glaucoma or a history of glaucoma; may cause mydriasis, which can exacerbate symptoms. Use with caution in patients with hepatic dysfunction and in elderly patients. May cause hyponatremia/SIADH (elderly at increased risk); volume depletion (diuretics may increase risk). Use caution in elderly patients; may cause or exacerbate syndrome of inappropriate antidiuretic hormone secretion or hyponatremia; monitor sodium closely with initiation or dosage adjustments in older adults (Beers Criteria). Sertraline acts as a mild uricosuric; use with caution in patients at risk of uric acid nephropathy. Use with caution in patients where weight loss is undesirable. May cause or exacerbate sexual dysfunction. Potentially significant drug-drug interactions may exist, requiring dose or frequency adjustment, additional monitoring, and/or selection of alternative therapy.

Use oral concentrate formulation with caution in patients with latex sensitivity; dropper dispenser contains dry natural rubber. Monitor growth in pediatric patients. Given their lower body weight, lower doses are advisable in pediatric patients in order to avoid excessive plasma levels, despite slightly greater metabolism efficiency than adults.

Abrupt discontinuation or interruption of antidepressant therapy has been associated with a discontinuation syndrome. Symptoms arising may vary with antidepressant however commonly include nausea, vomiting, diarrhea, headaches, lightheadedness, dizziness, diminished appetite, sweating, chills, tremors, paresthesias, fatigue, somnolence, and sleep disturbances (eg, vivid dreams, insomnia). Greater risks for developing a discontinuation syndrome have been associated with antidepressants with shorter half-lives, longer durations of treatment, and abrupt discontinuation. For antidepressants of short or intermediate half-lives, symptoms may emerge within 2-5 days after treatment discontinuation and last 7-14 days (APA, 2010; Fava, 2006; Haddad, 2001; Shelton, 2001; Warner, 2006).

Adverse Reactions

>10%:

Central nervous system: Dizziness, fatigue, headache, insomnia, somnolence

Endocrine & metabolic: Libido decreased

Gastrointestinal: Anorexia, diarrhea, nausea, xerostomia

Genitourinary: Ejaculatory disturbances

Neuromuscular & skeletal: Tremors

Miscellaneous: Diaphoresis

1% to 10%:

Cardiovascular: Chest pain, palpitation

Central nervous system: Agitation, anxiety, hypoesthesia, malaise, nervousness, pain

Dermatologic: Rash

Endocrine & metabolic: Impotence

Gastrointestinal: Appetite increased, constipation, dyspepsia, flatulence, vomiting, weight gain

Neuromuscular & skeletal: Back pain, hypertonia, myalgia, paresthesia, weakness

Ocular: Visual difficulty, abnormal vision

Otic: Tinnitus

Respiratory: Rhinitis

Miscellaneous: Yawning

<1% (Limited to important or life-threatening): Abdominal pain, acute renal failure, agranulocytosis, allergic reaction, anaphylactoid reaction, angioedema, aplastic anemia, atrial arrhythmia, AV block, bilirubin increased, blindness, bradycardia, Call-Fleming syndrome, cataract, cerebral vasoconstriction syndrome (reversible), cerebrovascular spasm, diabetes mellitus, dystonia, extrapyramidal symptoms, galactorrhea, gum hyperplasia, gynecomastia, hallucinations, hepatic failure, hepatitis, hepatomegaly, hyperglycemia, hyperprolactinemia, hypothyroidism, jaundice, leukopenia, lupus-like syndrome, micturition disorders, neuroleptic malignant syndrome, oculogyric crisis, serotonin syndrome, SIADH, Stevens-Johnson syndrome (and other severe dermatologic reactions), optic neuritis, pancreatitis (rare), photosensitivity, priapism, psychosis, PT/INR increased, pulmonary hypertension, QT_c prolongation, serum sickness, thrombocytopenia, torsade de pointes, transaminases increased, vasculitis, ventricular tachycardia

Pediatric patients: Additional adverse reactions reported in pediatric patients (frequency >2%): Aggressiveness, epistaxis, hyperkinesia, purpura, sinusitis, urinary incontinence

Drug Interactions

Metabolism/Transport Effects Substrate of CYP2B6 (minor), CYP2C19 (minor), CYP2C9 (minor), CYP2D6 (minor), CYP3A4 (minor); **Note:** Assignment of Major/Minor substrate status based on clinically relevant drug interaction potential; **Inhibits** CYP1A2 (weak), CYP2B6 (moderate), CYP2C19 (moderate), CYP2C8 (weak), CYP2C9 (weak), CYP2D6 (moderate), CYP3A4 (weak)

Avoid Concomitant Use

Avoid concomitant use of Sertraline with any of the following: Disulfiram; Dosulepin; Iobenguane I 123; Linezolid; MAO Inhibitors; Methylene Blue; Pimozide; Thioridazine; Tryptophan

Increased Effect/Toxicity

Sertraline may increase the levels/effects of: Agents with Antiplatelet Properties; Anticoagulants; Antidepressants (Serotonin Reuptake Inhibitor/Antagonist); Antipsychotics; ARIPiprazole; Aspirin; Beta-Blockers; BusPIRone; CarBAMazepine; CloZAPine; Collagenase (Systemic); CYP2B6 Substrates; CYP2C19 Substrates; CYP2D6 Substrates; Dabigatran Etexilate; Desmopressin; Dextromethorphan; Dofetilide; Dosulepin; Fesoterodine; Fosphenytoin; Galantamine; Highest Risk QTc-Prolonging Agents; Hypoglycemic Agents; Ibritumomab; Lomitapide; Methadone; Methylene Blue; Metoclopramide; Metoprolol; Moderate Risk QTc-Prolonging Agents; NSAID (COX-2 Inhibitor); NSAID (Nonselective); Phenytoin; Pimozide; Propafenone; RisperiDONE; Rivaroxaban; Salicylates; Serotonin Modulators; Thiazide Diuretics; Thioridazine; Thrombolytic Agents; Tositumomab and Iodine I 131 Tositumomab; TraMADol; Tricyclic Antidepressants; Vitamin K Antagonists

The levels/effects of Sertraline may be increased by: Alcohol (Ethyl); Analgesics (Opioid); Antipsychotics; BusPIRone; Cimetidine; CNS Depressants; Cobicistat; Dasatinib; Disulfiram; Glucosamine; Grapefruit Juice; Herbs (Anticoagulant/Antiplatelet Properties); Ibrutinib; Linezolid; Lithium; Macrolide Antibiotics; MAO Inhibitors; Metoclopramide; Metyrosine; Mifepristone; Multivitamins/Fluoride (with ADE); Multivitamins/Minerals (with ADEK, Folate, Iron); Multivitamins/Minerals (with AE, No Iron); Omega-3 Fatty Acids; Pentosan Polysulfate Sodium; Pentoxifylline; Prostacyclin Analogues; Tipranavir; TraMADol; Tryptophan; Vitamin E

Decreased Effect

Sertraline may decrease the levels/effects of: Clopidogrel; Iobenguane I 123; Ioflupane I 123; Tamoxifen; Thyroid Products

The levels/effects of Sertraline may be decreased by: CarBAMazepine; Cyproheptadine; Darunavir; Efavirenz; Fosphenytoin; NSAID (COX-2 Inhibitor); NSAID (Nonselective); Peginterferon Alfa-2b; Phenytoin

Ethanol/Nutrition/Herb Interactions

Ethanol: Concurrent use with ethanol may increase CNS depression. Management: Monitor for increased effects with coadministration. Caution patients about effects.

Food: Sertraline average peak serum levels may be increased if taken with food.

Herb/Nutraceutical: Concurrent use with some herbal medications may increase the risk of serotonin syndrome and/or CNS depression. Management: Avoid valerian, St John's wort, tryptophan, kava kava, gotu kola.

Preparation for Administration Oral concentrate: Must be diluted before use. **Immediately before administration**, use the dropper provided to measure the required amount of concentrate; mix with 4 ounces (1/2 cup) of water, ginger ale, lemon/lime soda, lemonade, or orange juice only. Do not mix with any other liquids than these. The dose should be taken immediately after mixing; do not mix in advance. A slight haze may appear after mixing; this is normal.

Storage/Stability Store at 25°C (77°F); excursions are permitted between 15°C and 30°C (59°F and 86°F).

Mechanism of Action Antidepressant with selective inhibitory effects on presynaptic serotonin (5-HT) reuptake and only very weak effects on norepinephrine and dopamine neuronal uptake. *In vitro* studies demonstrate no significant affinity for adrenergic, cholinergic, GABA, dopaminergic, histaminergic, serotonergic, or benzodiazepine receptors.

Pharmacodynamics/Kinetics

Onset of action: Depression: The onset of action is within a week, however, individual response varies greatly and full response may not be seen until 8-12 weeks after initiation of treatment.

Absorption: Area under the plasma concentration time curve (AUC) slightly increased and mean peak plasma concentrations (C_{max}) 25% greater when administered with food.

Protein binding: 98%

Metabolism: Hepatic; may involve CYP2C19 and CYP2D6; extensive first pass metabolism; forms metabolite N-desmethylsertraline (APA, 2010)

Bioavailability: Bioavailability of tablets and solution are equivalent

Half-life elimination: Sertraline: 26 hours; N-desmethylsertraline: 66 hours (range: 62-104 hours)

Time to peak, plasma: Sertraline: 4.5-8.4 hours

Excretion: Urine and feces

Dosage

Children 6-12 years: Oral:

Obsessive-compulsive disorder (OCD): Initial: 25 mg once daily. **Note:** May increase daily dose, at intervals of not less than 1 week, to a maximum of 200 mg daily.

Depression (unlabeled use): Initial: 12.5-25 mg once daily; titrate dose upwards if clinically needed; may increase by 25-50 mg daily increments at intervals of at least 1 week; mean final dose in 21 children (8-18 years of age) was 100 ± 53 mg or 1.6 mg/kg/day (n=11); range: 25-200 mg daily; maximum dose: 200 mg daily (Dopheide, 2006; Tierney, 1995); avoid excessive dosing

Adolescents 13-17 years: Oral:

Obsessive-compulsive disorder (OCD): Initial: 50 mg once daily. **Note:** May increase daily dose, at intervals of not less than 1 week, to a maximum of 200 mg daily.

Depression (unlabeled use): Initial 25-50 mg once daily; titrate dose upwards if clinically needed; may increase by 50 mg daily increments at intervals of at least 1 week; mean final dose in 13 adolescents was 110 ± 50 mg or about 2 mg/kg/day (McConville, 1996); in another study using a slower titration, the mean dose at week 6 was 93 mg (n=41) and at week 10 was 127 mg (n=34) (Ambrosini, 1999); range: 25-200 mg daily; maximum dose: 200 mg daily (Dopheide, 2006).

Adults: Oral:

Depression/obsessive-compulsive disorder: Initial: 50 mg daily. **Note:** May increase daily dose, at intervals of not less than 1 week, to a maximum of 200 mg daily.

Panic disorder, post-traumatic stress disorder (PTSD), social anxiety disorder: Initial: 25 mg once daily; increase to 50 mg once daily after 1 week; maximum dose: 200 mg daily

Premenstrual dysphoric disorder (PMDD): 50 mg daily either daily throughout menstrual cycle **or** limited to the luteal phase of menstrual cycle. Patients not responding to 50 mg daily may benefit from dose increases (50 mg increments per menstrual cycle) up to 150 mg daily when dosing throughout menstrual cycle **or** up to 100 mg day when dosing during luteal phase only. If a 100 mg daily dose has been established with luteal phase dosing, a 50 mg daily titration step for 3 days should be utilized at the beginning of each luteal phase dosing period.

Binge-eating disorder (unlabeled use): Initial: 25 mg daily after lunch for 3 days; increase at 25 mg increments every 3 days based on response and tolerability. Usual dose range: 100-200 mg daily. Maximum dose: 200 mg daily (Leombruni P, 2008).

Bulimia nervosa (unlabeled use): Initial: 50 mg daily; increase at 50 mg increments each week based on response and tolerability. Maximum dose: 200 mg daily (Milano, 2004; Sloan, 2003).

Generalized anxiety disorder (GAD) (unlabeled use): Initial dose: 25 mg once daily for 1week; increase based on response and tolerability. Maximum dose: 200 mg daily (Ball, 2005; Brawman, 2006; Dahl, 2005).

Discontinuation of therapy: Upon discontinuation of antidepressant therapy, gradually taper the dose to minimize the incidence of withdrawal symptoms and allow for the detection of re-emerging symptoms. Evidence supporting ideal taper rates is limited. APA and NICE guidelines suggest tapering therapy over at least several weeks with consideration to the half-life of the antidepressant; antidepressants with a shorter half-life may need to be tapered more conservatively. In addition for long-term treated patients, WFSBP guidelines recommend tapering over 4-6 months. If intolerable withdrawal symptoms occur following a dose reduction, consider resuming the previously prescribed dose and/or decrease dose at a more gradual rate (APA, 2010; Bauer, 2002; Haddad, 2001; NCCMH, 2010; Schatzberg, 2006; Shelton, 2001; Warner, 2006).

MAO inhibitor recommendations:

Switching to or from an MAO inhibitor intended to treat psychiatric disorders:

Allow 14 days to elapse between discontinuing an MAO inhibitor intended to treat psychiatric disorders and initiation of sertraline.

Allow 14 days to elapse between discontinuing sertraline and initiation of an MAO inhibitor intended to treat psychiatric disorders.

Use with other MAO inhibitors (linezolid or I.V. methylene blue):

Do not initiate sertraline in patients receiving linezolid or I.V. methylene blue; consider other interventions for psychiatric condition.

If urgent treatment with linezolid or I.V. methylene blue is required in a patient already receiving sertraline and potential benefits outweigh potential risks, discontinue sertraline promptly and administer linezolid or I.V. methylene blue. Monitor for serotonin syndrome for 2 weeks or until 24 hours after the last dose of linezolid or I.V. methylene blue, whichever comes first. May resume sertraline 24 hours after the last dose of linezolid or I.V. methylene blue.

Dosage adjustment/comment in renal impairment: No dosage adjustment is provided in manufacturer's labeling; however, sertraline pharmacokinetics does not appear to be affected by renal impairment.

Dosage adjustment/comment in hepatic impairment: No specific dosage adjustment provided in manufacturer's labeling (has not been studied). Use with caution due to extensive hepatic metabolism and risk of increased exposure. A lower dose or less frequent dosing is recommended.

Administration Administer once daily either in the morning or evening; if somnolence is noted, administer at bedtime.

Oral concentrate: Must be diluted immediately before use. **Note:** Use with caution in patients with latex sensitivity; dropper dispenser contains dry natural rubber.

Monitoring Parameters Weight, height, BMI (longitudinal monitoring); mental status for depression, suicide ideation (especially at the beginning of therapy or when doses are increased or decreased), anxiety, social functioning, mania, panic attacks, or other unusual changes in behavior; signs/symptoms of serotonin syndrome.

Test Interactions May interfere with urine detection of benzodiazepines (false-positive)

Dosage Forms Excipient information presented when available (limited, particularly for generics); consult specific product labeling.

Concentrate, Oral:

Zoloft: 20 mg/mL (60 mL) [contains alcohol, usp, menthol]

Generic: 20 mg/mL (60 mL)

Tablet, Oral:

Zoloft: 25 mg [scored; contains fd&c blue #1 aluminum lake, fd&c red #40 aluminum lake, fd&c yellow #10 aluminum lake, polysorbate 80]

Zoloft: 50 mg [scored; contains fd&c blue #2 aluminum lake]

Zoloft: 100 mg [scored; contains polysorbate 80]

Generic: 25 mg, 50 mg, 100 mg

◆ **Sertraline Hydrochloride** *see* Sertraline *on page 1889*

◆ **Serzone** *see* Nefazodone *on page 1434*

Sevelamer (se VEL a mer)

Brand Names: U.S. Renagel; Renvela

Brand Names: Canada Renagel; Renvela

Index Terms Sevelamer Carbonate; Sevelamer Hydrochloride

Pharmacologic Category Phosphate Binder

Use Reduction or control of serum phosphorous in patients with chronic kidney disease on hemodialysis

Pregnancy Risk Factor C

Pregnancy Considerations Adverse events were observed in animal reproduction studies. Sevelamer is not absorbed systemically; however, it may cause a reduction in the absorption of some vitamins.

Breast-Feeding Considerations Sevelamer is not absorbed systemically; however, it may cause a reduction in the absorption of some vitamins.

Contraindications Bowel obstruction

Warnings/Precautions Use with caution in patients with gastrointestinal disorders including dysphagia, swallowing disorders, severe gastrointestinal motility disorders (including constipation), or major gastrointestinal surgery. May cause reductions in vitamin D, E, K, or folic acid absorption. May bind to some drugs in the gastrointestinal tract and decrease their absorption; when changes in absorption of oral medications may have significant clinical consequences (such as antiarrhythmic and antiseizure medications), these medications should be taken at least 1 hour before or 3 hours after a dose of sevelamer. Tablets should not be taken apart or chewed; broken or crushed tablets will rapidly expand in water/saliva and may be a choking hazard.

Adverse Reactions

>10%:

Endocrine & metabolic: Metabolic acidosis (children: 34% [Pieper, 2006]); adults: Frequency not defined)

Gastrointestinal: Vomiting (22%), nausea (20%), diarrhea (19%), dyspepsia (16%)

1% to 10%:

Endocrine & metabolic: Hypercalcemia (5% to 7%)

Gastrointestinal: Abdominal pain (9%), constipation (8%), flatulence (8%), peritonitis (peritoneal dialysis: 8%)

Postmarketing and/or case reports: Fecal impaction, intestinal obstruction (rare), intestinal perforation (rare)

Drug Interactions

Metabolism/Transport Effects None known.

Avoid Concomitant Use There are no known interactions where it is recommended to avoid concomitant use.

Increased Effect/Toxicity There are no known significant interactions involving an increase in effect.

Decreased Effect

Sevelamer may decrease the levels/effects of: Calcitriol; Levothyroxine; Mycophenolate; Quinolone Antibiotics

Ethanol/Nutrition/Herb Interactions Food: May cause reductions in vitamin D, E, K, or folic acid absorption. Management: Must be administered with meals. Consider vitamin supplementation.

Preparation for Administration Powder for oral suspension: Mix powder with water prior to administration. The 0.8 g packet should be mixed with 30 mL of water and the 2.4 g packet should be mixed with 60 mL of water (multiple packets may be mixed together using the appropriate amount of water).

Storage/Stability Store at controlled room temperature of 25°C (77°F); excursions permitted to 15°C to 30°C (59°F to 86°F). Protect from moisture.

Mechanism of Action Sevelamer (a polymeric compound) binds phosphate within the intestinal lumen, limiting absorption and decreasing serum phosphate concentrations without altering calcium, aluminum, or bicarbonate concentrations.

Pharmacodynamics/Kinetics

Onset of action: Reduction in serum phosphorus has been demonstrated after 1-2 weeks (Burke, 1997; Chertow, 1997).

Absorption: Not systemically absorbed

Excretion: Feces

Dosage Oral: **Note:** The dosing of sevelamer carbonate and sevelamer hydrochloride are similar; when switching from one product to another, the same dose (on a mg per mg basis) should be utilized.

Children (unlabeled use): In a pilot study of 17 pediatric patients aged 11.8 ± 3.7 years on hemodialysis (n=3) or peritoneal dialysis (n=14), initial doses of 121 ± 50 mg/kg/day (4.5 ± 5 g/day) were used. Doses were adjusted based on the serum phosphorus with final doses of 163 ± 46 mg/kg (6.7 ± 2.4 g/day) without any adverse effects (Mahdavi, 2003). In a study of 18 patients aged 0.9-18 years with chronic kidney disease, a mean dose of 140 ± 86 mg/kg/day (5.38 ± 3.24 g/day) resulted in good phosphorus control with minimal adverse effects. Initial doses were based on prior phosphate-binder dose and were adjusted based on the serum phosphorus (Pieper, 2006).

Adults: Patients not taking a phosphate binder: 800-1600 mg 3 times/day with meals; the initial dose may be based on serum phosphorous levels:

>5.5 mg/dL to <7.5 mg/dL: 800 mg 3 times/day

≥7.5 mg/dL to <9.0 mg/dL: 1200-1600 mg 3 times/day

≥9.0 mg/dL: 1600 mg 3 times/day

Maintenance dose adjustment based on serum phosphorous concentration (goal range of 3.5-5.5 mg/dL; maximum dose studied was equivalent to 13 g/day [sevelamer hydrochloride] or 14 g/day [sevelamer carbonate]):

>5.5 mg/dL: Increase by 400-800 mg per meal at 2-week intervals

3.5-5.5 mg/dL: Maintain current dose

<3.5 mg/dL: Decrease by 400-800 mg per meal

Dosage adjustment when switching between phosphate-binder products: 667 mg of calcium acetate is equivalent to ~800 mg sevelamer (carbonate or hydrochloride)

Conversion based on dose per meal:

Calcium acetate 667 mg: Convert to 800 mg Renagel/Renvela

Calcium acetate 1334 mg: Convert to 1600 mg as Renagel/Renvela (800 mg tablets x 2) **or** 1200 mg as Renagel (400 mg tablets x 3)

Calcium acetate 2001 mg: Convert to 2400 mg as Renagel/Renvela (800 mg tablets x 3) **or** 2000 mg as Renagel (400 mg tablets x 5)

Dosage adjustment in renal impairment: No dosage adjustment provided in manufacturer's labeling (has not been studied).

Dosage adjustment in hepatic impairment: No dosage adjustment provided in manufacturer's labeling.

Dietary Considerations Take with meals. Reduced levels of folic acid, and vitamins D, E, and K may occur; most hemodialysis patients in clinical trials received vitamin supplementation.

Administration Must be administered with meals.

Powder for oral suspension: Stir vigorously to suspend mixture just prior to drinking; powder does not dissolve. Drink within 30 minutes of preparing and resuspend just prior to drinking.

Tablets: Swallow whole; do not crush, chew, or break.

Monitoring Parameters

Serum chemistries, including bicarbonate and chloride

Serum calcium and phosphorus: Frequency of measurement may be dependent upon the presence and magnitude of abnormalities, the rate of progression of CKD, and the use of treatments for CKD-mineral and bone disorders (KDIGO, 2009):

CKD stage 3: Every 6-12 months

CKD stage 4: Every 3-6 months

CKD stage 5 and 5D: Every 1-3 months

Periodic 24-hour urinary calcium and phosphorus; magnesium; alkaline phosphatase every 12 months or more frequently in the presence of elevated PTH; creatinine, BUN, albumin; intact parathyroid hormone (iPTH) every 3-12 months depending on CKD severity

Reference Range

Corrected total serum calcium (K/DOQI, 2003): CKD stages 3 and 4: 8.4-10.2 mg/dL (2.1-2.6 mmol/L); CKD stage 5: 8.4-9.5 mg/dL (2.1-2.37 mmol/L); KDIGO guidelines recommend maintaining normal ranges for all stages of CKD (3-5D) (KDIGO, 2009)

Phosphorus (K/DOQI, 2003):

CKD stages 3 and 4: 2.7-4.6 mg/dL (0.87-1.48 mmol/L) (adults); maintain within age-appropriate limits (children)

CKD stage 5 (including those treated with dialysis): 3.5-5.5 mg/dL (1.13-1.78 mmol/L) (children >12 years and adults); 4-6 mg/dL (1.29-1.94 mmol/L) (children 1-12 years)

KDIGO guidelines recommend maintaining normal ranges for CKD stages 3-5 and lowering elevated phosphorus levels toward the normal range for CKD stage 5D (KDIGO, 2009)

Serum calcium-phosphorus product (K/DOQI, 2003): CKD stage 3-5: <55 mg^2/dL^2 (children >12 years and adults); <65 mg2/dL2 (children ≤12 years)

PTH: Whole molecule, immunochemiluminometric assay (ICMA): 1.0-5.2 pmol/L; whole molecule, radioimmunoassay (RIA): 10.0-65.0 pg/mL; whole molecule, immunoradiometric, double antibody (IRMA): 1.0-6.0 pmol/L

Target ranges by stage of chronic kidney disease (KDIGO, 2009): CKD stage 3-5: Optimal iPTH is unknown; maintain normal range (assay-dependent); CKD stage 5D: Maintain iPTH within 2-9 times the upper limit of normal for the assay used

Dosage Forms Excipient information presented when available (limited, particularly for generics); consult specific product labeling.

Packet, Oral, as carbonate:
Renvela: 0.8 g (1 ea, 90 ea); 2.4 g (1 ea, 90 ea) [citrus flavor]

Tablet, Oral, as carbonate:
Renvela: 800 mg

Tablet, Oral, as hydrochloride:
Renagel: 400 mg, 800 mg

- **Sevelamer Carbonate** *see* Sevelamer *on page 1892*
- **Sevelamer Hydrochloride** *see* Sevelamer *on page 1892*
- **SfRowasa** *see* Mesalamine *on page 1305*
- **SGN-35** *see* Brentuximab Vedotin *on page 278*
- **Shingles Vaccine** *see* Zoster Vaccine *on page 2247*
- **Shohl's Solution (Modified)** *see* Sodium Citrate and Citric Acid *on page 1917*
- **Shur-Seal Contraceptive [OTC]** *see* Nonoxynol 9 *on page 1471*
- **Sig-Enalapril (Can)** *see* Enalapril *on page 701*
- **Signifor** *see* Pasireotide *on page 1579*
- **Silace [OTC]** *see* Docusate *on page 644*
- **Siladryl Allergy [OTC]** *see* DiphenhydrAMINE (Systemic) *on page 622*
- **Silapap Children's [OTC]** *see* Acetaminophen *on page 28*
- **Silapap Infant's [OTC]** *see* Acetaminophen *on page 28*

Sildenafil (sil DEN a fil)

Brand Names: U.S. Revatio; Viagra

Brand Names: Canada Apo-Sildenafil®; CO Sildenafil; GD-Sildenafil; PMS-Sildenafil; ratio-Sildenafil R; Revatio®; Teva-Sildenafil; Viagra®

Index Terms Sildenafil Citrate; UK92480

Pharmacologic Category Phosphodiesterase-5 Enzyme Inhibitor

Use

Revatio®: Treatment of pulmonary arterial hypertension (PAH) (WHO Group I) to improve exercise ability and delay clinical worsening. Efficacy established based upon short-term studies (12-16 weeks).

Viagra®: Treatment of erectile dysfunction (ED)

Unlabeled Use Pulmonary hypertension (WHO Group II, III, and IV); persistent pulmonary hypertension after recent left ventricular assist device placement

Pregnancy Risk Factor B

Pregnancy Considerations Adverse events were not observed in animal reproduction studies. Information related to the use of sildenafil for the treatment of pulmonary arterial hypertension (PAH) in pregnant women is limited (Hsu, 2012). Current guidelines recommend that women with PAH use effective contraception and avoid pregnancy (Badesch, 2007; McLaughlin, 2009). Less than 0.001% appears in the semen.

Breast-Feeding Considerations It is not known if sildenafil is excreted in breast milk. The manufacturer recommends that caution be exercised when administering sildenafil to nursing women.

Contraindications Hypersensitivity to sildenafil or any component of the formulation; concurrent use (regularly/intermittently) of organic nitrates in any form (eg, nitroglycerin, isosorbide dinitrate); concurrent use with a protease inhibitor regimen when sildenafil used for pulmonary artery hypertension (eg, Revatio®)

Warnings/Precautions Decreases in blood pressure may occur due to vasodilator effects; use with caution in patients with left ventricular outflow obstruction (aortic stenosis or hypertrophic obstructive cardiomyopathy), those on antihypertensive therapy, with resting hypotension (BP <90/50 mm Hg), fluid depletion, or autonomic dysfunction; may be more sensitive to hypotensive actions. Patients should be hemodynamically stable prior to initiating therapy at the lowest possible dose. Avoid or limit concurrent substantial alcohol consumption as this may increase the risk of symptomatic hypotension. Use with caution in patients with uncontrolled hypertension (>170/110 mm Hg); life-threatening arrhythmias, stroke or MI within the last 6 months; cardiac failure or coronary artery disease causing unstable angina; safety and efficacy have not been studied in these patients. There is a degree of cardiac risk associated with sexual activity; therefore, physicians should consider the cardiovascular status of their patients prior to initiating any treatment for erectile dysfunction. If pulmonary edema occurs when treating pulmonary arterial hypertension (PAH), consider the possibility of pulmonary veno-occlusive disease (PVOD); continued use is not recommended in patient with PVOD.

Sildenafil should be used with caution in patients with anatomical deformation of the penis (angulation, cavernosal fibrosis, or Peyronie's disease) and in patients who have conditions which may predispose them to priapism (sickle cell anemia, multiple myeloma, leukemia). All patients should be instructed to seek medical attention if erection persists >4 hours.

Vision loss may occur rarely and be a sign of nonarteritic anterior ischemic optic neuropathy (NAION). Risk may be increased with history of vision loss. Other risk factors for NAION include low cup-to-disc ratio ("crowded disc"), coronary artery disease, diabetes, hypertension, hyperlipidemia, smoking, and age >50 years. May cause dose-related impairment of color discrimination. Use caution in patients with retinitis pigmentosa; a minority have genetic disorders of retinal phosphodiesterases (no safety information available). Sudden decrease or loss of hearing has been reported rarely; hearing changes may be accompanied by tinnitus and dizziness. A direct relationship between therapy and vision or hearing loss has not been determined.

The potential underlying causes of erectile dysfunction should be evaluated prior to treatment. The safety and efficacy of sildenafil with other treatments for erectile dysfunction have not been established; use is not recommended. Efficacy with concurrent bosentan therapy has not been evaluated; use with caution. Use with caution in patients taking strong CYP3A4 inhibitors or alpha-blockers. Concomitant use with all forms of nitrates is contraindicated. If nitrate administration is medically necessary, it is not known when nitrates can be safely administered following the use of sildenafil (per manufacturer); the ACC/AHA 2007 guidelines supports administration of nitrates only if 24 hours have elapsed.

Avoid abrupt discontinuation, especially if used as monotherapy in PAH as exacerbation may occur. Use caution in patients with bleeding disorders or with active peptic ulcer disease; safety and efficacy have not been established. Efficacy has not be established for treatment of pulmonary hypertension associated with sickle cell disease. Use with caution in the elderly, or patients with renal or hepatic dysfunction; dose adjustment may be needed. Use of Revatio®, especially chronic use, is not recommended in children. After 2 years of treatment, increased mortality seen in long-term (median treatment exposure: 3.8 years) study at higher doses (20-80 mg [depending upon weight] 3 times/day) (Barst, 2012a; Barst, 2012b).

Adverse Reactions Based upon normal doses for either indication or route. (Adverse effects such as flushing, diarrhea, myalgia, and visual disturbances may be increased with adult doses >100 mg/24 hours.)

>10%:

Central nervous system: Headache (16% to 46%)

Gastrointestinal: Dyspepsia (7% to 17%; dose related)

2% to 10%:

Cardiovascular: Flushing (10%)

Central nervous system: Insomnia (≤7%), pyrexia (6%), dizziness (2%)

Dermatologic: Erythema (6%), rash (2%)

Gastrointestinal: Diarrhea (3% to 9%), gastritis (≤3%)

Genitourinary: Urinary tract infection (3%)

Hepatic: LFTs increased

Neuromuscular & skeletal: Myalgia (≤7%), paresthesia (≤3%)

Ocular: Abnormal vision (color changes, blurred vision, or increased sensitivity to light 3% to 11%; dose related)

Respiratory: Epistaxis (9% to 13%), dyspnea exacerbated (≤7%), nasal congestion (4%), rhinitis (4%), sinusitis (3%)

<2% (Limited to important or life-threatening): Allergic reaction, amnesia (transient global), anemia, angina pectoris, anorgasmia, asthma, AV block, cardiac arrest, cardiomyopathy, cataract, cerebral thrombosis, cerebrovascular hemorrhage, colitis, cystitis, depression, dysphagia, edema, exfoliative dermatitis, eye hemorrhage, gout, hearing decreased, hearing loss, heart failure, hematuria, hemorrhage, hyper-/hypoglycemia, hypernatremia, hyper-/hypotension, hyperuricemia, intracerebral hemorrhage, intraocular pressure increased, leukopenia, migraine, myocardial ischemia, MI, myasthenia, mydriasis, neuralgia, nonarteritic ischemic optic neuropathy (NAION), orthostatic hypotension, palpitation, priapism, pulmonary hemorrhage, rectal hemorrhage, retinal vascular disease or bleeding, seizure, shock, sickle cell crisis (vaso-occlusive crisis in patients with pulmonary hypertension associated with sickle cell disease), stomatitis, subarachnoid hemorrhage, syncope, tachycardia, tendon rupture, TIA, urinary incontinence, ventricular arrhythmia, vertigo, visual field loss, vitreous detachment/traction, vomiting

Drug Interactions

Metabolism/Transport Effects **Substrate** of CYP1A2 (minor), CYP2C19 (minor), CYP2C9 (minor), CYP2D6 (minor), CYP2E1 (minor), CYP3A4 (major); **Note:** Assignment of Major/Minor substrate status based on clinically relevant drug interaction potential; **Inhibits** CYP2C9 (weak), CYP3A4 (weak)

Avoid Concomitant Use

Avoid concomitant use of Sildenafil with any of the following: Alprostadil; Amyl Nitrite; Boceprevir; Cobicistat; Fusidic Acid (Systemic); Phosphodiesterase 5 Inhibitors; Pimozide; Riociguat; Telaprevir; Vasodilators (Organic Nitrates)

Increased Effect/Toxicity

Sildenafil may increase the levels/effects of: Alpha1-Blockers; Alprostadil; Amyl Nitrite; Antihypertensives; ARIPiprazole; Bosentan; Dofetilide; HMG-CoA Reductase Inhibitors; Lomitapide; Phosphodiesterase 5 Inhibitors; Pimozide; Riociguat; Vasodilators (Organic Nitrates)

The levels/effects of Sildenafil may be increased by: Alcohol (Ethyl); Boceprevir; Cobicistat; CYP3A4 Inhibitors (Moderate); CYP3A4 Inhibitors (Strong); Dasatinib; Erythromycin (Systemic); Fluconazole; Fusidic Acid (Systemic); Itraconazole; Ivacaftor; Ketoconazole (Systemic); Lorcaserin; Luliconazole; Mifepristone; Posaconazole; Protease Inhibitors; Sapropterin; Simeprevir; Telaprevir; Voriconazole

Decreased Effect

The levels/effects of Sildenafil may be decreased by: Bosentan; CYP3A4 Inducers (Strong); Dabrafenib; Deferasirox; Etravirine; Herbs (CYP3A4 Inducers); Mitotane; Peginterferon Alfa-2b; Tocilizumab

Ethanol/Nutrition/Herb Interactions Ethanol: Substantial consumption of ethanol may increase the risk of hypotension and orthostasis. Lower ethanol consumption has not been associated with significant changes in blood pressure or increase in orthostatic symptoms. Management: Avoid or limit ethanol consumption.

Food: Avoid grapefruit juice.

Herb/Nutraceutical: St John's wort may decrease sildenafil levels. Management: Avoid St John's wort.

Storage/Stability Store at controlled room temperature of 25°C (77°F); excursions permitted to 15°C to 30°C (59°F to 86°F).

Mechanism of Action

Erectile dysfunction: Does not directly cause penile erections, but affects the response to sexual stimulation. The physiologic mechanism of erection of the penis involves release of nitric oxide (NO) in the corpus cavernosum during sexual stimulation. NO then activates the enzyme guanylate cyclase, which results in increased levels of cyclic guanosine monophosphate (cGMP), producing smooth muscle relaxation and inflow of blood to the corpus cavernosum. Sildenafil enhances the effect of NO by inhibiting phosphodiesterase type 5 (PDE-5), which is responsible for degradation of cGMP in the corpus cavernosum; when sexual stimulation causes local release of NO, inhibition of PDE-5 by sildenafil causes increased levels of cGMP in the corpus cavernosum, resulting in smooth muscle relaxation and inflow of blood to the corpus cavernosum; at recommended doses, it has no effect in the absence of sexual stimulation.

Pulmonary arterial hypertension (PAH): Inhibits phosphodiesterase type 5 (PDE-5) in smooth muscle of pulmonary vasculature where PDE-5 is responsible for the degradation of cyclic guanosine monophosphate (cGMP). Increased cGMP concentration results in pulmonary vasculature relaxation; vasodilation in the pulmonary bed and the systemic circulation (to a lesser degree) may occur.

Pharmacodynamics/Kinetics

Onset of action: ~60 minutes

Duration: 2-4 hours

Absorption: Rapid; slower with a high-fat meal

Distribution: V_{dss}: 105 L

Protein binding, plasma: ~96%

Metabolism: Hepatic via CYP3A4 (major) and CYP2C9 (minor route); forms N-desmethyl metabolite (active)

Bioavailability: 40% (25% to 63%)

Half-life elimination: ~4 hours; the elderly and those with severe renal impairment have reduced clearance of sildenafil and its active N-desmethyl metabolite

Time to peak: 30-120 minutes; delayed by 60 minutes with a high-fat meal

Excretion: Feces (~80%); urine (~13%)

Dosage

I.V.: Adults: Pulmonary arterial hypertension (PAH) (Revatio): 10 mg 3 times/day

Oral:

Adults:

Erectile dysfunction (Viagra): Usual dose: 50 mg once daily 1 hour (range: 30 minutes to 4 hours) before sexual activity; dosing range: 25-100 mg once daily

PAH (Revatio): 20 mg 3 times/day, taken 4-6 hours apart; maximum recommended dose: 20 mg 3 times/day

Elderly >65 years: Use with caution.

Revatio: Refer to adult dosing.

Viagra: Starting dose of 25 mg should be considered.

Dosage considerations for patients stable on alpha-blockers: Viagra: Initial 25 mg

Dosage adjustment for concomitant use of potent CYP34A inhibitors:

Revatio:

Erythromycin: No dosage adjustment

Itraconazole, ketoconazole: Not recommended

Protease inhibitors: Contraindicated

Viagra:

Erythromycin, itraconazole, ketoconazole: Starting dose of 25 mg should be considered

Protease inhibitors: Maximum sildenafil dose: 25 mg every 48 hours

Dosage adjustment in renal impairment:

Cl_{cr} ≥30 mL/minute:

Revatio: No dosage adjustment necessary.

Viagra: No dosage adjustment recommended.

Cl_{cr} <30 mL/minute:

Revatio: No dosage adjustment necessary.

Viagra: Starting dose of 25 mg should be considered.

Dosage adjustment in hepatic impairment:

Mild to moderate impairment (Child-Pugh classes A and B):

Revatio: No dosage adjustment necessary.

Viagra: Starting dose of 25 mg should be considered.

Severe impairment (Child-Pugh class C): Revatio, Viagra: No dosage adjustment provided in manufacturer's labeling (has not been studied).

Dietary Considerations Avoid grapefruit juice.

Administration

Revatio®: Administer tablets without regard to meals at least 4-6 hours apart. Administer injection as an I.V. bolus.

Viagra®: Administer orally 30 minutes to 4 hours before sexual activity

Monitoring Parameters PAH: Monitor blood pressure and pulse when used concurrently with medications that lower blood pressure

Additional Information Sildenafil is ~10 times more selective for PDE-5 as compared to PDE6. This enzyme is found in the retina and is involved in phototransduction. At higher plasma levels, interference with PDE6 is believed to be the basis for changes in color vision noted in some patients.

Product Availability Revatio oral suspension is not currently available in the U.S. Launch date for U.S. availability is unknown.

Dosage Forms Excipient information presented when available (limited, particularly for generics); consult specific product labeling.

Solution, Intravenous:

Revatio: 10 mg/12.5 mL (12.5 mL)

Tablet, Oral:

Revatio: 20 mg

Viagra: 25 mg, 50 mg, 100 mg [contains fd&c blue #2 aluminum lake]

Generic: 20 mg

Extemporaneous Preparations A 2.5 mg/mL sildenafil citrate oral suspension may be made with tablets and either a 1:1 mixture of methylcellulose 1% and simple syrup NF or a 1:1 mixture of Ora-Sweet® and Ora-Plus®. Crush thirty sildenafil 25 mg tablets (Viagra®) in a mortar and reduce to a fine powder. Add small portions of chosen vehicle and mix to a uniform paste; mix while adding vehicle in incremental proportions to **almost** 300 mL; transfer to a graduated cylinder, rinse mortar with vehicle, and add quantity of vehicle sufficient to make 300 mL. Store in amber plastic bottles and label "shake well". Stable for 90 days at room temperature or refrigerated.

Nahata MC, Morosco RS, and Brady MT, "Extemporaneous Sildenafil Citrate Oral Suspensions for the Treatment of Pulmonary Hypertension in Children," *Am J Health-Syst Pharm*, 2006, 63(3):254-7.

◆ **Sildenafil Citrate** *see* Sildenafil *on page* *1894*

◆ **Silenor** *see* Doxepin (Systemic) *on page* *658*

◆ **Silenor® (Can)** *see* Doxepin (Systemic) *on page* *658*

◆ **Silexin [OTC]** *see* Guaifenesin and Dextromethorphan *on page* *976*

◆ **Silkis™ (Can)** *see* Calcitriol *on page* *314*

Silodosin (SI lo doe sin)

Brand Names: U.S. Rapaflo

Brand Names: Canada Rapaflo®

Index Terms KMD 3213

Pharmacologic Category $Alpha_1$ Blocker

Use Treatment of signs and symptoms of benign prostatic hyperplasia (BPH)

Pregnancy Risk Factor B

Dosage Oral: Adults: BPH: 8 mg once daily with a meal

Dosage adjustment in renal impairment:

Cl_{cr} >50 mL/minute: No dosage adjustment necessary.

Cl_{cr} 30-50 mL/minute: 4 mg once daily

Cl_{cr} <30 mL/minute: Use is contraindicated.

Dosage adjustment in hepatic impairment:

Mild-to-moderate impairment (Child-Pugh class A or B): No dosage adjustment necessary.

Severe impairment (Child-Pugh class C): Use is contraindicated (has not been studied).

Additional Information Complete prescribing information should be consulted for additional detail.

Dosage Forms Excipient information presented when available (limited, particularly for generics); consult specific product labeling.

Capsule, Oral:

Rapaflo: 4 mg, 8 mg

◆ **Silphen Cough [OTC]** *see* DiphenhydrAMINE (Systemic) *on page* *622*

◆ **Siltussin DAS [OTC]** *see* GuaiFENesin *on page* *974*

◆ **Siltussin DM [OTC]** *see* Guaifenesin and Dextromethorphan *on page* *976*

◆ **Siltussin DM DAS [OTC]** *see* Guaifenesin and Dextromethorphan *on page* *976*

◆ **Siltussin SA [OTC]** *see* GuaiFENesin *on page* *974*

◆ **Silvadene** *see* Silver Sulfadiazine *on page* *1897*

◆ **Silver Bullet Suppository [OTC] (Can)** *see* Bisacodyl *on page* *259*

Silver Nitrate (SIL ver NYE trate)

Index Terms $AgNO_3$

Pharmacologic Category Antibiotic, Topical; Cauterizing Agent, Topical; Topical Skin Product, Antibacterial

Use Astringent, cauterization of wounds, germicidal, removal of granulation tissue, corns and warts

Dosage Children and Adults:

Sticks: Apply to mucous membranes and other moist skin surfaces only on area to be treated

Topical solution: Usual: Apply a cotton applicator dipped in solution on the affected area 2-3 times/week for 2-3 weeks

Additional Information Complete prescribing information should be consulted for additional detail.

Dosage Forms Excipient information presented when available (limited, particularly for generics); consult specific product labeling.

Applicator sticks, topical: Silver nitrate 75% and potassium nitrate 25%

Solution, topical: 0.5% (960 mL); 10% (30 mL); 25% (30 mL); 50% (30 mL)

Silver Sulfadiazine (SIL ver sul fa DYE a zeen)

Brand Names: U.S. Silvadene; SSD; Thermazene

Brand Names: Canada Flamazine®

Pharmacologic Category Antibiotic, Topical

Use Prevention and treatment of infection in second and third degree burns

Pregnancy Risk Factor B

Dosage Children and Adults: Topical: Apply once or twice daily with a sterile-gloved hand; apply to a thickness of 1/16"; burned area should be covered with cream at all times

Additional Information Complete prescribing information should be consulted for additional detail.

Dosage Forms Excipient information presented when available (limited, particularly for generics); consult specific product labeling.

Cream, External:

Silvadene: 1% (20 g, 50 g, 85 g, 400 g, 1000 g) [contains methylparaben, propylene glycol]

SSD: 1% (25 g, 50 g, 85 g, 400 g) [contains cetyl alcohol, methylparaben, propylene glycol]

Thermazene: 1% (20 g, 50 g, 85 g, 400 g, 1000 g) [contains methylparaben, propylene glycol]

Generic: 1% (20 g, 25 g, 50 g, 85 g, 400 g)

Simeprevir (sim E pre vir)

Brand Names: U.S. Olysio

Brand Names: Canada Galexos

Index Terms TMC435

Pharmacologic Category Antihepaciviral, Protease Inhibitor (Anti-HCV)

Use Chronic hepatitis C: Treatment of genotype 1 chronic hepatitis C (in combination with peginterferon alfa and ribavirin) in patients with compensated liver disease (including cirrhosis)

Pregnancy Risk Factor X

Pregnancy Considerations Adverse events were observed in animal reproduction studies. Because simeprevir is used in combination with ribavirin, use is contraindicated in pregnant women and males with female partners who are pregnant. A negative pregnancy test is required before initiation and monthly thereafter. Female patients (and their male partners) as well as male patients (and their female partners) should use two forms of effective contraception during therapy and for 6 months after therapy is discontinued. Pregnancy testing should be done monthly during this time.

Health care providers are encouraged to enroll women exposed to ribavirin during pregnancy or within 6 months after treatment in the ribavirin pregnancy registry (800-593-2214); patients may also enroll themselves.

Breast-Feeding Considerations It is not known if simeprevir is excreted into breast milk. Due to the potential for serious adverse reactions in the nursing infant, the manufacturer recommends a decision be made whether to discontinue nursing or to discontinue the drug, taking into account the importance of treatment to the mother.

Contraindications Combination treatment with peginterferon alfa and ribavirin: Pregnancy; male partners of pregnant women

Warnings/Precautions Higher simeprevir exposures have been associated with an increased risk of adverse effects (including rash and photosensitivity) in people of East Asian ancestry. An appropriate dose in these patients has not been determined. Use with caution. Rash has been typically observed within first 4 weeks of therapy initiation but may occur at any time. Severe rashes and rash requiring discontinuation have occurred. If a patient experiences a mild to moderate rash, follow for progression and/or development of mucosal signs (eg, oral lesions, conjunctivitis) or systemic symptoms. If rash becomes severe, discontinue simeprevir and monitor for rash resolution. Avoid excessive sunlight, tanning devices, and take precautions to limit exposure (eg, loose fitting clothing, sunscreen); may cause moderate to severe phototoxicity reactions. Most reactions have occurred within the first 4 weeks of therapy. Discontinue use if photosensitivity occurs and monitor until the reaction resolves. If therapy is to be continued in a patient who has experienced photosensitivity, expert consultation is advised. Contains a sulfonamide moiety. In patients with a history of sulfa allergy, no increased incidence of rash or photosensitivity has been reported, although the risk of reaction (or potential severity) cannot be excluded. Discontinue if signs of hypersensitivity are noted.

Not recommended in moderate or severe hepatic impairment (Child-Pugh class B or C). Combination therapy with ribavirin may cause birth defects; avoid pregnancy in females and female partners of male patients. Combination therapy with ribavirin is contraindicated in pregnancy. Use 2 effective forms of contraception during treatment and for 6 months after completion of treatment. Routine monthly pregnancy tests must be performed during this time period as well. Should only be used in combination with peginterferon alfa and ribavirin (do not use as monotherapy). Safety and efficacy have not been established in patients who have received liver transplants, who have HCV genotypes other than genotype 1, or who have failed to respond to other HCV direct-acting inhibitors or on repeated courses of simeprevir. Potentially significant drug-drug interactions may exist, requiring dose or frequency adjustments, additional monitoring, and/or selection of alternative therapy.

Adverse Reactions Percentages reported for combination therapy.

>10%:

Dermatologic: Skin rash (28%; including erythema, eczema, rash maculopapular, urticaria, toxic skin eruption, dermatitis exfoliative, cutaneous vasculitis, photosensitivity reaction), pruritus (22%)

Gastrointestinal: Nausea (22%)

Hepatic: Increased serum bilirubin (<50%)

Neuromuscular & skeletal: Myalgia (16%)

Respiratory: Dyspnea (12%)

1% to 10%:

Dermatologic: Skin photosensitivity (5%; grade 3: 1%)

Hepatic: Increased serum alkaline phosphatase (<4%)

Drug Interactions

Metabolism/Transport Effects Substrate of CYP3A4 (major), P-glycoprotein, SLCO1B1; **Note:** Assignment of Major/Minor substrate status based on clinically relevant drug interaction potential; **Inhibits** CYP1A2 (weak), P-glycoprotein, SLCO1B1

Avoid Concomitant Use

Avoid concomitant use of Simeprevir with any of the following: Bosutinib; Cisapride; CYP3A4 Inducers (Strong); CYP3A4 Inducers (Weakly to Moderately Effective); CYP3A4 Inhibitors (Moderate); CYP3A4 Inhibitors (Strong); Erythromycin (Systemic); Fusidic Acid (Systemic); Milk Thistle; PAZOPanib; Pomalidomide; Protease Inhibitors; Silodosin; St Johns Wort; Topotecan; VinCRIStine (Liposomal)

Increased Effect/Toxicity

Simeprevir may increase the levels/effects of: Afatinib; AtorvaSTATin; Bosutinib; Cisapride; Colchicine; CYP3A4 Substrates; Dabigatran Etexilate; Digoxin; Everolimus; Lovastatin; Midazolam; PAZOPanib; P-glycoprotein/ABCB1 Substrates; Phosphodiesterase 5 Inhibitors; Pitavastatin; Pomalidomide; Porfimer; Pravastatin; Protease Inhibitors; Prucalopride; Rilpivirine; Rivaroxaban;

Rosuvastatin; Silodosin; Simvastatin; Tenofovir; Topotecan; Triazolam; VinCRIStine (Liposomal)

The levels/effects of Simeprevir may be increased by: CYP3A4 Inhibitors (Moderate); CYP3A4 Inhibitors (Strong); Dasatinib; Eltrombopag; Erythromycin (Systemic); Fusidic Acid (Systemic); Ivacaftor; Luliconazole; Mifepristone; Milk Thistle; Protease Inhibitors

Decreased Effect

The levels/effects of Simeprevir may be decreased by: Bosentan; CYP3A4 Inducers (Strong); CYP3A4 Inducers (Weakly to Moderately Effective); Dabrafenib; Deferasirox; Escitalopram; St Johns Wort; Tenofovir; Tocilizumab

Storage/Stability Store at room temperature below 30°C (86°F). Store in the original bottle. Protect from light.

Mechanism of Action Considered a direct-acting antiviral treatment for HCV, also called a specifically targeted antiviral therapy for HCV (STAT-C).

Pharmacodynamics/Kinetics

Absorption: Food enhances absorption.

Protein binding: >99% (albumin and alpha 1-acid glycoprotein)

Metabolism: Primarily oxidative metabolism by CYP3A4 (and possibly CYP2C8 and CYP2C19) to unchanged drug and metabolites (minor).

Half-life elimination: Plasma: 10-13 hours (healthy volunteers); 41 hours (hepatitis C–infected patients)

Time to peak, serum: 4-6 hours

Excretion: Feces (~91%); urine (<1%)

Dosage Note: If peginterferon alfa or ribavirin is discontinued for any reason, simeprevir must also be discontinued.

Treatment of chronic hepatitis C (CHC): Adults: Oral: 150 mg once daily (in combination with peginterferon alfa and ribavirin). Treatment duration is indication and response-specific.

Missed dose: If a dose is missed within 12 hours of the time it is usually taken, take as soon as possible. If more than 12 hours have passed since the dose is usually taken, do not take the missed dose and the patient should resume the usual schedule.

Treatment-naive or prior relapse patients (including those with cirrhosis): **Note:** Prior relapsers include patients with an undetectable HCV-RNA upon completion of treatment (prior interferon-based regimen) but with detectable HCV-RNA during the follow up period.

Weeks 1-12: Triple therapy: Simeprevir 150 mg once daily in combination with peginterferon alfa and ribavirin

HCV-RNA **detectable** (level ≥25 units/mL) at week 4: Discontinue simeprevir, peginterferon alfa, and ribavirin at week 4

Weeks 13-23 (based on HCV-RNA results at weeks 4 and 12):

HCV-RNA **undetectable** (level <25 units/mL) at week 12: Discontinue simeprevir (treatment completed). Dual therapy: Peginterferon alfa and ribavirin only (through week 24)

HCV-RNA **detectable** (level ≥25 units/mL) at week 12: Discontinue simeprevir (treatment completed), peginterferon alfa, and ribavirin

Week 24 (based on HCV-RNA results at week 24):

HCV-RNA **undetectable** (level <25 units/mL) at week 24: Dual therapy: Peginterferon alfa and ribavirin only through week 24

HCV-RNA **detectable** (level ≥25 units/mL) at week 24: Discontinue peginterferon alfa and ribavirin

Previously treated patients (partial response or null responders) including those with cirrhosis: **Note:** Partial response includes patients with a ≥2-$\log_{10}$ HCV-RNA decrease at week 12 but detectable HCV-RNA at the end of prior interferon-based therapy. Prior null responders include patients with a <2-$\log_{10}$ HCV-RNA decrease at week 12 during interferon-based therapy.

Weeks 1-12: Triple therapy: Simeprevir 150 mg daily in combination with peginterferon alfa and ribavirin

HCV-RNA **undetectable** (level <25 units/mL) at week 12: Dual therapy: Peginterferon alfa and ribavirin only (through week 48)

HCV-RNA **detectable** (level ≥25 units/mL) at week 4: Discontinue simeprevir, peginterferon alfa, and ribavirin at week 4

Weeks 13-48 (based on HCV-RNA results at weeks 4, 12, and 24):

HCV-RNA **undetectable** (level <25 units/mL) at week 24: Discontinued simeprevir (treatment was completed after week 12). Dual therapy: Peginterferon alfa and ribavirin through week 48

HCV-RNA **detectable** (level ≥25 units/mL) at week 12: Discontinue simeprevir (treatment completed), peginterferon alfa, and ribavirin

Dosage adjustment in renal impairment:

Simeprevir: No dosage adjustment necessary. Not studied in patients with Cl_{cr} ≤30 mL/minute or with end stage renal disease, including those requiring hemodialysis.

Dosage adjustment in hepatic impairment:

Simeprevir:

Mild impairment (Child-Pugh class A): No dosage adjustment necessary.

Moderate or severe impairment (Child-Pugh class B or C): Use is not recommended in patients with decompensated liver disease or with moderate or severe hepatic impairment (has not been studied).

Administration Administer orally with food. Administer concurrently with peginterferon alfa and ribavirin. Maintain adequate fluid intake/hydration. Swallow capsules whole; do not chew, crush, break, cut, or dissolve the capsule.

Monitoring Parameters

Bilirubin, liver enzymes, and uric acid at baseline and periodically when clinically indicated

Serum HCV-RNA at baseline, weeks 4, 12, and 24, at end of treatment, during treatment follow-up, and when clinically indicated

Pretreatment and monthly pregnancy tests up to 6 months following discontinuation of therapy for women of childbearing age

Dosage Forms

Capsule, Oral:

Olysio: 150 mg

- **Simethicone, Aluminum Hydroxide, and Magnesium Hydroxide** *see* Aluminum Hydroxide, Magnesium Hydroxide, and Simethicone *on page* 90
- **Simethicone and Loperamide Hydrochloride** *see* Loperamide and Simethicone *on page* 1237
- **Simethicone and Magaldrate** *see* Magaldrate and Simethicone *on page* 1259
- **Simply Allergy [OTC]** *see* DiphenhydrAMINE (Systemic) *on page* 622
- **Simply Sleep [OTC]** *see* DiphenhydrAMINE (Systemic) *on page* 622
- **Simply Sleep® (Can)** *see* DiphenhydrAMINE (Systemic) *on page* 622
- **Simply Stuffy [OTC]** *see* Pseudoephedrine *on page* 1746
- **Simponi** *see* Golimumab *on page* 968
- **Simponi Aria** *see* Golimumab *on page* 968
- **Simponi I.V. (Can)** *see* Golimumab *on page* 968
- **Simulect** *see* Basiliximab *on page* 224
- **Simulect® (Can)** *see* Basiliximab *on page* 224

Simvastatin (sim va STAT in)

Brand Names: U.S. Zocor

Brand Names: Canada Apo-Simvastatin; Ava-Simvastatin; CO Simvastatin; Dom-Simvastatin; JAMP-Simvastatin; Mint-Simvastatin; Mylan-Simvastatin; Nu-Simvastatin; PHL-Simvastatin; PMS-Simvastatin; Q-Simvastatin; RAN-Simvastatin; ratio-Simvastatin; Riva-Simvastatin; Sandoz-Simvastatin; Simvastatin-Odan; Taro-Simvastatin; Teva-Simvastatin; Zocor; ZYM-Simvastatin

Pharmacologic Category Antilipemic Agent, HMG-CoA Reductase Inhibitor

Use Used with dietary therapy for the following:

Secondary prevention of cardiovascular events in hypercholesterolemic patients with established coronary heart disease (CHD) or at high risk for CHD: To reduce cardiovascular morbidity (myocardial infarction, coronary/noncoronary revascularization procedures) and mortality; to reduce the risk of stroke

Hyperlipidemias: To reduce elevations in total cholesterol (total-C), LDL-C, apolipoprotein B, triglycerides, and VLDL-C, and to increase HDL-C in patients with primary hypercholesterolemia (elevations of 1 or more components are present in Fredrickson type IIa, IIb, III, and IV hyperlipidemias); treatment of homozygous familial hypercholesterolemia

Heterozygous familial hypercholesterolemia (HeFH): In adolescent patients (10-17 years of age, females >1 year postmenarche) with HeFH having LDL-C ≥190 mg/dL **or** LDL-C ≥160 mg/dL with positive family history of premature cardiovascular disease (CVD), or 2 or more CVD risk factors in the adolescent patient

Primary and secondary prevention of atherosclerotic cardiovascular disease (ASCVD) according to the American College of Cardiology/American Heart Association: To reduce the risk of ASCVD in patients with clinical ASCVD (eg, coronary heart disease, stroke/TIA, or peripheral arterial disease presumed to be of atherosclerotic origin) who are greater than 75 years of age or not a candidate for high-intensity statin therapy; in patients without clinical ASCVD if LDL-C is 190 mg/dL or greater and not a candidate for high-intensity statin therapy; in patients without clinical ASCVD who have type 1 or type 2 diabetes and are between 40 and 75 years of age; in patients with an estimated 10-year ASCVD risk 7.5% or greater and who are between 40 and 75 years of age (Stone, 2013).

Pregnancy Risk Factor X

Pregnancy Considerations Adverse events were not observed in animal reproduction studies. There are reports of congenital anomalies following maternal use of HMG-CoA reductase inhibitors in pregnancy; however, maternal disease, differences in specific agents used, and the low rates of exposure limit the interpretation of the available data (Godfrey, 2012; Lecarpentier, 2012). Cholesterol biosynthesis may be important in fetal development; serum cholesterol and triglycerides increase normally during pregnancy. The discontinuation of lipid lowering medications temporarily during pregnancy is not expected to have significant impact on the long term outcomes of primary hypercholesterolemia treatment.

Use of simvastatin is contraindicated in pregnancy. HMG-CoA reductase inhibitors should be discontinued prior to pregnancy (ADA, 2013). If treatment of dyslipidemias is needed in pregnant women or in women of reproductive age, other agents are preferred (Berglund, 2012; Stone, 2013). The manufacturer recommends administration to women of childbearing potential only when conception is highly unlikely and patients have been informed of potential hazards.

Breast-Feeding Considerations It is not known if simvastatin is excreted into breast milk. Due to the potential for serious adverse reactions in a nursing infant, breast-feeding is contraindicated by the manufacturer.

Contraindications Hypersensitivity to simvastatin or any component of the formulation; active liver disease; unexplained persistent elevations of serum transaminases; concomitant use of strong CYP3A4 inhibitors (eg, clarithromycin, erythromycin, itraconazole, ketoconazole, nefazodone, posaconazole, voriconazole, protease inhibitors [including boceprevir and telaprevir], telithromycin), cyclosporine, danazol, and gemfibrozil; pregnancy; breast-feeding

Warnings/Precautions Secondary causes of hyperlipidemia should be ruled out prior to therapy. Liver enzyme tests should be obtained at baseline and as clinically indicated; routine periodic monitoring of liver enzymes is not necessary. Use with caution in patients who consume large amounts of ethanol or have a history of liver disease; use is contraindicated with active liver disease and with unexplained transaminase elevations. Rhabdomyolysis with acute renal failure has occurred. Risk of rhabdomyolysis is dose-related and increased with high doses (80 mg), concurrent use of lipid-lowering agents which may also cause rhabdomyolysis (other fibrates or niacin doses ≥1 g/day), or moderate-to-strong CYP3A4 inhibitors (eg, amiodarone, grapefruit juice in large quantities, or verapamil), age ≥65 years, female gender, uncontrolled hypothyroidism, and renal dysfunction. In Chinese patients, do not use high-dose simvastatin (80 mg) if concurrently taking niacin ≥1 g/day; may increase risk of myopathy. Immune-mediated necrotizing myopathy (IMNM), an autoimmune-mediated myopathy, has been reported (rarely) with HMG-CoA reductase inhibitor therapy. IMNM presents as proximal muscle weakness with elevated CPK levels, which persists despite discontinuation of HMG-CoA reductase inhibitor therapy; additionally, muscle biopsy may show necrotizing myopathy with limited inflammation; immunosuppressive therapy (eg, corticosteroids, azathioprine) may be used for treatment. Concomitant use of simvastatin with some drugs may require cautious use, may not be recommended, may require dosage adjustments, or may be contraindicated. If concurrent use of a contraindicated interacting medication is unavoidable, treatment with simvastatin should be suspended during use or consider the use of an alternative HMG-CoA reductase inhibitor void of CYP3A4 metabolism. Monitor closely if used with other drugs associated with myopathy (eg, colchicine). Increases in Hb A_{1c} and fasting blood glucose have been reported with HMG-CoA reductase inhibitors; however, the benefits of statin therapy far outweigh the risk of dysglycemia. The manufacturer recommends temporary discontinuation for elective major surgery, acute medical or surgical conditions, or in any patient experiencing an acute or serious condition predisposing to renal failure (eg, sepsis, hypotension, trauma, uncontrolled seizures). However, based upon current evidence, HMG-CoA reductase inhibitor therapy should be continued in the perioperative period unless risk outweighs cardioprotective benefit. Use with caution in patients with severe renal impairment; initial dosage adjustment is necessary; monitor closely.

Adverse Reactions

1% to 10%:

Cardiovascular: Atrial fibrillation (6%; placebo 5%), edema (3%; placebo 2%)

Central nervous system: Headache (3% to 7%), vertigo (5%)

Dermatologic: Eczema (5%)

Gastrointestinal: Abdominal pain (7%), constipation (2% to 7%), gastritis (5%), nausea (5%)

Hepatic: Transaminases increased (>3 x ULN; 1%)

Neuromuscular & skeletal: CPK increased (>3 x normal; 5%), myalgia (4%)

Respiratory: Upper respiratory infections (9%), bronchitis (7%)

<1% (Limited to important or life-threatening): Alkaline phosphatase increased, alopecia, amnesia (reversible), anaphylaxis, anemia, angioedema, arthralgia, arthritis, blood glucose increased, chills, cognitive impairment (reversible), confusion (reversible), depression, dermatomyositis, diabetes mellitus (new onset), diarrhea, dizziness, dryness of skin/mucous membranes, dyspepsia, dyspnea, eosinophilia, erythema multiforme, ESR increased, fever, flatulence, flushing, glycosylated hemoglobin (Hb A_{1c}) increased, GGT increased, hemolytic anemia, hepatic failure, hepatitis, hypersensitivity reaction, jaundice, leukopenia, malaise, memory disturbance (reversible), memory impairment (reversible), muscle cramps, nail changes, nodules, pancreatitis, paresthesia, peripheral neuropathy, photosensitivity, polymyalgia rheumatica, positive ANA, pruritus, purpura, rash, rhabdomyolysis, skin discoloration, Stevens-Johnson syndrome, systemic lupus erythematosus-like syndrome, thrombocytopenia, toxic epidermal necrolysis, urticaria, vasculitis, vomiting, weakness

Additional class-related events or case reports (not necessarily reported with simvastatin therapy): Alteration in taste, anorexia, anxiety, bilirubin increased, cataracts, cholestatic jaundice, cirrhosis, decreased libido, depression, erectile dysfunction/impotence, facial paresis, fatty liver, fulminant hepatic necrosis, gynecomastia, hepatoma, hyperbilirubinemia, immune-mediated necrotizing myopathy (IMNM), impaired extraocular muscle movement, increased CPK (>10 x normal), interstitial lung disease, ophthalmoplegia, peripheral nerve palsy, psychic disturbance, renal failure (secondary to rhabdomyolysis), thyroid dysfunction, tremor, vertigo

Drug Interactions

Metabolism/Transport Effects **Substrate** of CYP3A4 (major), SLCO1B1; **Note:** Assignment of Major/Minor substrate status based on clinically relevant drug interaction potential; **Inhibits** CYP2C8 (weak), CYP2C9 (weak), CYP2D6 (weak)

Avoid Concomitant Use

Avoid concomitant use of Simvastatin with any of the following: Boceprevir; Clarithromycin; CycloSPORINE (Systemic); CYP3A4 Inhibitors (Strong); Erythromycin (Systemic); Fusidic Acid (Systemic); Gemfibrozil; Mifepristone; Protease Inhibitors; Red Yeast Rice; Telaprevir; Telithromycin

Increased Effect/Toxicity

Simvastatin may increase the levels/effects of: ARIPiprazole; DAPTOmycin; Diltiazem; PAZOPanib; Trabectedin; Vitamin K Antagonists

The levels/effects of Simvastatin may be increased by: Amiodarone; AmLODIPine; Azithromycin (Systemic); Bezafibrate; Boceprevir; Clarithromycin; Colchicine; CycloSPORINE (Systemic); CYP3A4 Inhibitors (Moderate); CYP3A4 Inhibitors (Strong); Cyproterone; Danazol; Dasatinib; Diltiazem; Dronedarone; Eltrombopag; Erythromycin (Systemic); Fenofibrate and Derivatives; Fluconazole; Fusidic Acid (Systemic); Gemfibrozil; Grapefruit Juice; Green Tea; Imatinib; Ivacaftor; Lomitapide; Luliconazole; Mifepristone; Niacin; Niacinamide; Protease Inhibitors; QuiNINE; Raltegravir; Ranolazine; Red Yeast Rice; Sildenafil; Simeprevir; Telaprevir; Telithromycin; Ticagrelor; Verapamil

Decreased Effect

Simvastatin may decrease the levels/effects of: Lanthanum

The levels/effects of Simvastatin may be decreased by: Antacids; Bosentan; CYP3A4 Inducers (Strong); Dabrafenib; Deferasirox; Efavirenz; Eslicarbazepine; Etravirine; Fosphenytoin; Mitotane; Phenytoin; Rifamycin Derivatives; St Johns Wort; Tocilizumab

Ethanol/Nutrition/Herb Interactions

Ethanol: Excessive ethanol consumption has the potential to cause hepatic effects. Management: Avoid or limit ethanol consumption.

Food: Simvastatin serum concentration may be increased when taken with grapefruit juice. Red yeast rice contains an estimated 2.4 mg lovastatin per 600 mg rice. Management: Avoid concurrent intake of large quantities of grapefruit juice (>1 quart/day).

Herb/Nutraceutical: St John's wort may decrease simvastatin levels. Management: Avoid St John's wort.

Storage/Stability Tablets should be stored in tightly-closed containers at temperatures between 5°C to 30°C (41°F to 86°F).

Mechanism of Action Simvastatin is a methylated derivative of lovastatin that acts by competitively inhibiting 3-hydroxy-3-methylglutaryl-coenzyme A (HMG-CoA) reductase, the enzyme that catalyzes the rate-limiting step in cholesterol biosynthesis

Pharmacodynamics/Kinetics

Onset of action: >3 days

Peak effect: 2 weeks

Absorption: 85%

Protein binding: ~95%

Metabolism: Hepatic via CYP3A4; extensive first-pass effect

Bioavailability: <5%

Half-life elimination: Unknown

Time to peak: 1.3-2.4 hours

Excretion: Feces (60%); urine (13%)

Dosage Oral: **Note:** Doses should be individualized according to the baseline LDL-cholesterol levels, the recommended goal of therapy, and the patient's response; adjustments should be made at intervals of 4 weeks or more; doses may need adjusted based on concomitant medications

Children 10-17 years (females >1 year postmenarche):

HeFH: 10 mg once daily in the evening; range: 10-40 mg/day (maximum: 40 mg/day)

Dosage adjustment for simvastatin with concomitant amiodarone, amlodipine, diltiazem, dronedarone, lomitapide, ranolazine, or verapamil: Refer to drug-specific dosing in adult dosing section

Adults:

Note: Dosing limitation: Simvastatin 80 mg is limited to patients that have been taking this dose for >12 consecutive months without evidence of myopathy and are not currently taking or beginning to take a simvastatin dose-limiting or contraindicated interacting medication. If patient is unable to achieve low-density lipoprotein cholesterol (LDL-C) goal using the 40 mg dose of simvastatin, increasing to 80 mg dose is not recommended. Instead, switch patient to an alternative LDL-C-lowering treatment providing greater LDL-C reduction.

Homozygous familial hypercholesterolemia: 40 mg once daily in the evening

Prevention of cardiovascular events (also see ACC/AHA Blood Cholesterol Guideline recommendations), hyperlipidemias: 10-20 mg once daily in the evening; range: 5-40 mg/day

Patients requiring only moderate reduction of LDL-C may be started at 5-10 mg once daily in the evening; adjust to achieve recommended LDL-C goal

Patients requiring reduction of >40% of LDL-C may be started at 40 mg once daily in the evening; adjust to achieve recommended LDL-C goal

Patients with CHD or at high risk for cardiovascular events (patients with diabetes, PVD, history of stroke or other cerebrovascular disease): Dosing should be started at 40 mg once daily in the evening; start simultaneously with diet therapy.

ACC/AHA Blood Cholesterol Guideline recommendations to reduce the risk of atherosclerotic cardiovascular disease (ASCVD) (Stone, 2013): Adults ≥21 years:

Primary prevention:

LDL-C ≥190 mg/dL: High intensity therapy necessary; use alternate statin therapy (eg, atorvastatin or rosuvastatin)

Type 1 or 2 diabetes and age 40-75 years: Moderate intensity therapy: 20-40 mg once daily

Type 1 or 2 diabetes, age 40-75 years, and an estimated 10-year ASCVD risk ≥7.5%: High intensity therapy necessary; use alternate statin therapy (eg, atorvastatin or rosuvastatin)

Age 40-75 years and an estimated 10-year ASCVD risk ≥7.5%: Moderate to high intensity therapy: 20-40 mg once daily or consider using high intensity statin therapy (eg, atorvastatin or rosuvastatin)

Secondary prevention:

Patient has clinical ASCVD (eg, coronary heart disease, stroke/TIA, or peripheral arterial disease presumed to be of atherosclerotic origin) **and**:

Age ≤75 years: High intensity therapy necessary; use alternate statin therapy (eg, atorvastatin or rosuvastatin)

Age >75 years or not a candidate for high intensity therapy: Moderate intensity therapy: 20-40 mg once daily

Dosage adjustment with concomitant medications: Note: Patients currently tolerating and requiring a dose of simvastatin 80 mg who require initiation of an interacting drug with a dose cap for simvastatin should be switched to an alternative statin with less potential for drug-drug interaction.

Amiodarone, amlodipine, or ranolazine: Simvastatin dose should **not** exceed 20 mg/day

Diltiazem, dronedarone, or verapamil: Simvastatin dose should **not** exceed 10 mg/day

Lomitapide: Reduce simvastatin dose by 50% when initiating lomitapide. Simvastatin dose should not exceed 20 mg/day (or 40 mg daily for those who previously tolerated simvastatin 80 mg daily for ≥1 year without evidence of muscle toxicity)

Dosage adjustment in Chinese patients on niacin doses ≥1 g/day: Use caution with simvastatin doses exceeding 20 mg/day; because of an increased risk of myopathy, do not administer simvastatin 80 mg concurrently.

Dosing adjustment for toxicity:

Severe muscle symptoms or fatigue: Promptly discontinue use; evaluate CPK, creatinine, and urinalysis for myoglobinuria (Stone, 2013).

Mild to moderate muscle symptoms: Discontinue use until symptoms can be evaluated; evaluate patient for conditions that may increase the risk for muscle symptoms (eg, hypothyroidism, reduced renal or hepatic function, rheumatologic disorders such as polymyalgia rheumatica, steroid myopathy, vitamin D deficiency, or primary muscle diseases). Upon resolution, resume the original or lower dose of simvastatin. If muscle symptoms recur, discontinue simvastatin use. After muscle symptom resolution, may then use a low dose of a different statin; gradually increase if tolerated. In the absence of continued statin use, if muscle symptoms or elevated CPK continues after 2 months, consider other causes of muscle symptoms. If determined to be due to another condition aside from statin use, may resume statin therapy at the original dose (Stone, 2013).

Dosage adjustment in renal impairment: Manufacturer's recommendations:

Mild to moderate impairment: No dosage adjustment necessary; simvastatin does not undergo significant renal excretion

Severe impairment: Cl_{cr} <30 mL/minute: Initial: 5 mg/day with close monitoring.

Dosage adjustment in hepatic impairment: Use is contraindicated in the setting of active liver disease.

Dietary Considerations May be taken without regard to meals. Red yeast rice contains an estimated 2.4 mg lovastatin per 600 mg rice.

Administration May be administered without regard to meals. Administer in the evening for maximal efficacy.

Monitoring Parameters ***2013 ACC/AHA Blood Cholesterol Guideline recommendations (Stone, 2013):***

Lipid panel (total cholesterol, HDL, LDL, triglycerides): Baseline lipid panel; fasting lipid profile within 4-12 weeks after initiation or dose adjustment and every 3-12 months (as clinically indicated) thereafter. If 2 consecutive LDL levels are <40 mg/dL, consider decreasing the dose.v

Hepatic transaminase levels: Baseline measurement of hepatic transaminase levels (ie, ALT); measure hepatic function if symptoms suggest hepatotoxicity (eg, unusual fatigue or weakness, loss of appetite, abdominal pain, dark-colored urine or yellowing of skin or sclera) during therapy.

CPK: CPK should not be routinely measured. Baseline CPK measurement is reasonable for some individuals (eg, family history of statin intolerance or muscle disease, clinical presentation, concomitant drug therapy that may increase risk of myopathy). May measure CPK in any patient with symptoms suggestive of myopathy (pain, tenderness, stiffness, cramping, weakness, or generalized fatigue).

Evaluate for new-onset diabetes mellitus during therapy; if diabetes develops, continue statin therapy and encourage adherence to a heart-healthy diet, physical activity, a healthy body weight, and tobacco cessation.

If patient develops a confusional state or memory impairment, may evaluate patient for nonstatin causes (eg, exposure to other drugs), systemic and neuropsychiatric causes, and the possibility of adverse effects associated with statin therapy.

Manufacturer recommendations: Liver enzyme tests at baseline and repeated when clinically indicated. Measure CPK when myopathy is being considered or may measure CPK periodically in high risk patients (eg, drug-drug interaction). Lipid panel should be analyzed after 4 weeks of therapy and periodically thereafter.

Dosage Forms Excipient information presented when available (limited, particularly for generics); consult specific product labeling.

Tablet, Oral:

Zocor: 5 mg, 10 mg, 20 mg, 40 mg, 80 mg

Generic: 5 mg, 10 mg, 20 mg, 40 mg, 80 mg

◆ **Simvastatin and Ezetimibe** *see* Ezetimibe and Simvastatin *on page 818*

◆ **Simvastatin and Sitagliptin** *see* Sitagliptin and Simvastatin *on page 1908*

◆ **Simvastatin-Odan (Can)** *see* Simvastatin *on page 1899*

◆ **Sinemet®** *see* Carbidopa and Levodopa *on page 340*

◆ **Sinemet® CR** *see* Carbidopa and Levodopa *on page 340*

◆ **Sinequan® (Can)** *see* Doxepin (Systemic) *on page 658*

◆ **Singulair** *see* Montelukast *on page 1396*

◆ **Singulair® (Can)** *see* Montelukast *on page 1396*

◆ **Sinutab® Non Drowsy (Can)** *see* Acetaminophen and Pseudoephedrine *on page 33*

Sipuleucel-T (si pu LOO sel tee)

Brand Names: U.S. Provenge

Index Terms APC8015; Prostate Cancer Vaccine, Cell-Based

Pharmacologic Category Cellular Immunotherapy, Autologous

Use Treatment of metastatic hormone-refractory prostate cancer in patients who are asymptomatic or minimally symptomatic

Prescribing and Access Restrictions Patients may receive Sipuleucel-T at a participating site. Physicians must go through an inservice and register to prescribe the treatment; patients must also complete an enrollment form. Information on registration and enrollment is available at 1-877-336-3736.

Dosage Note: Premedicate with oral acetaminophen 650 mg and an antihistamine (eg, diphenhydramine 50 mg) ~30 minutes prior to infusion. For autologous use only. Do not infuse until confirmation of product release has been received from the company.

I.V.: Adults: Prostate cancer, metastatic: Each dose contains ≥50 million autologous CD54+ cells (obtained through leukapheresis) activated with PAP-GM-CSF; administer doses at ~2 week intervals for a total of 3 doses (Kantoff, 2010)

Dosage adjustment for toxicity: Acute infusion reaction: Interrupt or slow infusion rate (depending on the severity of infusion reaction); may require acetaminophen, I.V. H_1 and/or H_2 antagonists, or low-dose meperidine to manage acute symptoms.

Dosage adjustment in renal impairment: No dosage adjustment provided in manufacturer's labeling.

Dosage adjustment in hepatic impairment: No dosage adjustment provided in manufacturer's labeling.

Additional Information Complete prescribing information should be consulted for additional detail.

Dosage Forms Excipient information presented when available (limited, particularly for generics); consult specific product labeling.

Suspension, Intravenous [preservative free]:
Provenge: (250 mL)

◆ **Sirdalud** *see* TiZANidine *on page 2074*

Sirolimus (sir OH li mus)

Brand Names: U.S. Rapamune

Brand Names: Canada Rapamune®

Index Terms Rapamycin

Pharmacologic Category Immunosuppressant Agent; mTOR Kinase Inhibitor

Use Prophylaxis of organ rejection in patients receiving renal transplants

Unlabeled Use Prophylaxis of organ rejection and allograft vasculopathy in heart transplant recipients; prevention acute graft-versus-host disease (GVHD) in allogeneic stem cell transplantation; treatment of refractory acute or chronic GVHD; treatment of chordoma, renal angiomyolipoma, or lymphangioleiomyomatosis

Pregnancy Risk Factor C

Pregnancy Considerations Adverse events have been observed in animal reproduction studies. Effective contraception must be initiated before therapy with sirolimus and continued for 12 weeks after discontinuation.

The National Transplantation Pregnancy Registry (NTPR, Temple University) is a registry for pregnant women taking immunosuppressants following any solid organ transplant. The NTPR encourages reporting of all immunosuppressant exposures during pregnancy in transplant recipients at 877-955-6877.

Breast-Feeding Considerations It is not known if sirolimus is excreted in breast milk. Due to the potential for adverse reactions in the breast-fed infant, including possible immunosuppression, breast-feeding is not recommended.

Medication Guide Available Yes

Contraindications Hypersensitivity to sirolimus or any component of the formulation

Warnings/Precautions Hazardous agent - use appropriate precautions for handling and disposal (NIOSH, 2012). **[U.S. Boxed Warning]: Immunosuppressive agents, including sirolimus, increase the risk of infection and may be associated with the development of lymphoma.** Immune suppression may also increase the risk of opportunistic infections (including activation of latent viral infections including BK virus-associated nephropathy), fatal infections, and sepsis. Prophylactic treatment for *Pneumocystis jirovecii* pneumonia (PCP) should be administered for 1 year post-transplant; prophylaxis for cytomegalovirus (CMV) should be taken for 3 months post-transplant in patients at risk for CMV. Progressive multifocal leukoencephalopathy (PML), an opportunistic CNS infection caused by reactivation of the JC virus, has been reported in patients receiving immunosuppressive therapy, including sirolimus. Clinical findings of PML include apathy, ataxia, cognitive deficiency, confusion, and hemiparesis; promptly evaluate any patient presenting with neurological changes; consider decreasing the degree of immunosuppression with consideration to the risk of organ rejection in transplant patients.

[U.S. Boxed Warning]: Sirolimus is not recommended for use in liver or lung transplantation. Bronchial anastomotic dehiscence cases have been reported in lung transplant patients when sirolimus was used as part of an immunosuppressive regimen; most of these reactions were fatal. Studies indicate an association with an increased risk of hepatic artery thrombosis (HAT), graft failure, and increased mortality (with evidence of infection) in liver transplant patients when sirolimus is used in combination with cyclosporine and/or tacrolimus. Most cases of HAT occurred within 30 days of transplant.

In renal transplant patients, *de novo* use without cyclosporine has been associated with higher rates of acute rejection. Sirolimus should be used in combination with cyclosporine (and corticosteroids) initially. Cyclosporine may be withdrawn in low-to-moderate immunologic risk patients after 2-4 months, in conjunction with an increase in sirolimus dosage. In high immunologic risk patients, use in combination with cyclosporine and corticosteroids is recommended for the first year. Safety and efficacy of combination therapy with cyclosporine in high immunologic risk patients has not been studied beyond 12 months of treatment; adjustment of immunosuppressive therapy beyond 12 months should be considered based on clinical judgement. Monitor renal function closely when combined with cyclosporine; consider dosage adjustment or discontinue in patients with increasing serum creatinine.

May increase serum creatinine and decrease GFR. Use caution when used concurrently with medications which may alter renal function. May delay recovery of renal function in patients with delayed allograft function. Increased urinary protein excretion has been observed when converting renal transplant patients from calcineurin inhibitors to sirolimus during maintenance therapy. A higher level of proteinuria prior to sirolimus conversion correlates with a higher degree of proteinuria after conversion. In some patients, proteinuria may reach nephrotic levels; nephrotic syndrome (new onset) has been reported. Increased risk of BK viral-associated nephropathy which may impair renal function and cause graft loss; consider decreasing immunosuppressive burden if evidence of deteriorating renal function.

Use caution with hepatic impairment; a reduction in the maintenance dose is recommended. Has been associated with an increased risk of fluid accumulation and lymphocele; peripheral edema, lymphedema, ascites, and pleural and pericardial effusions (including significant effusions and tamponade) were reported; use with caution in patients in whom fluid accumulation may be poorly tolerated, such as in cardiovascular disease (heart failure or hypertension) and pulmonary disease. Cases of interstitial lung disease (eg, pneumonitis, bronchiolitis obliterans organizing pneumonia [BOOP], pulmonary fibrosis) have been observed; risk may be increased with higher trough levels. Potentially significant drug-drug interactions may exist, requiring dose or frequency adjustment, additional monitoring, and/or selection of alternative therapy. Concurrent use with a calcineurin inhibitor (cyclosporine, tacrolimus) may increase the risk of calcineurin inhibitor-induced hemolytic uremic syndrome/thrombotic thrombocytopenic purpura/thrombotic microangiopathy (HUS/TTP/TMA).

Hypersensitivity reactions, including anaphylactic/anaphylactoid reactions, angioedema, exfoliative dermatitis, and hypersensitivity vasculitis have been reported. Concurrent use with other drugs known to cause angioedema (eg, ACE inhibitors) may increase risk. Immunosuppressant therapy is associated with an increased risk of skin cancer; limit sun and ultraviolet light exposure; use appropriate sun protection. May increase serum lipids (cholesterol and triglycerides); use with caution in patients with hyperlipidemia; monitor cholesterol/lipids; if hyperlipidemia occurs, follow current guidelines for management (diet, exercise, lipid lowering agents); antihyperlipidemic therapy may not be effective in normalizing levels. May be associated with wound dehiscence and impaired healing; use caution in the perioperative period. Patients with a body mass index (BMI) >30 kg/m^2 are at increased risk for abnormal wound healing.

Sirolimus tablets and oral solution are not bioequivalent, due to differences in absorption. Clinical equivalence was seen using 2 mg tablet and 2 mg solution. It is not known if higher doses are also clinically equivalent. Monitor sirolimus levels if changes in dosage forms are made. **[U.S. Boxed Warning]: Should only be used by physicians experienced in immunosuppressive therapy and management of transplant patients. Adequate laboratory and supportive medical resources must be readily available.** Sirolimus concentrations are dependent on the assay method (eg, chromatographic and immunoassay) used; assay methods are not interchangeable. Variations in methods to determine sirolimus whole blood concentrations, as well as interlaboratory variations, may result in improper dosage adjustments, which may lead to subtherapeutic or toxic levels. Determine the assay method used to assure consistency (or accommodations if changes occur), and for monitoring purposes, be aware of alterations to assay method or reference range. The manufacturer recommends high performance liquid chromatography (HPLC) as the reference standard to determine sirolimus trough concentrations.

Adverse Reactions Incidence of many adverse effects is dose related.

>20%:

Cardiovascular: Peripheral edema (54% to 58%), hypertension (45% to 49%), edema (18% to 20%)

Central nervous system: Headache (34%), pain (29% to 33%), insomnia (13% to 22%)

Dermatologic: Acne (22%)

Endocrine & metabolic: Hypertriglyceridemia (45% to 57%), hypercholesterolemia (43% to 46%)

Gastrointestinal: Constipation (36% to 38%), abdominal pain (29% to 36%), diarrhea (25% to 36%), nausea (25% to 31%)

Genitourinary: Urinary tract infection (26% to 33%)

Hematologic: Anemia (23% to 33%), thrombocytopenia (14% to 30%)

Neuromuscular & skeletal: Arthralgia (25% to 31%)

Renal: Serum creatinine increased (39% to 40%)

3% to 20%:

Cardiovascular: Atrial fibrillation, CHF, DVT, facial edema, hypervolemia, hypotension, orthostatic hypotension, palpitation, peripheral vascular disorder, syncope, tachycardia, thrombosis, vasodilation

Central nervous system: Anxiety, chills, confusion, depression, dizziness, emotional lability, hypoesthesia, malaise, neuropathy, somnolence

Dermatologic: Rash (10% to 20%), skin carcinoma (up to 3%; includes basal cell carcinoma, squamous cell carcinoma, melanoma), cellulitis, dermal ulcer, dermatitis (fungal), ecchymosis, hirsutism, pruritus, skin hypertrophy, wound healing abnormal

Endocrine & metabolic: Acidosis, Cushing's syndrome, dehydration, diabetes mellitus, glycosuria, hypercalcemia, hyperglycemia, hyperphosphatemia, hypocalcemia, hypoglycemia, hypomagnesemia, hyponatremia

Gastrointestinal: Abdomen enlarged, anorexia, dysphagia, eructation, esophagitis, flatulence, gastritis, gastroenteritis, gingival hyperplasia, gingivitis, ileus, mouth ulceration, oral moniliasis, stomatitis, weight loss

Genitourinary: Amenorrhea, hypermenorrhea, impotence, menstrual disease, ovarian cyst, pelvic pain, scrotal edema, testis disorder

Hematologic: Hemolytic-uremic syndrome, hemorrhage, leukopenia, leukocytosis, polycythemia, TTP

Hepatic: Abnormal liver function tests, alkaline phosphatase increased, LDH increased

Local: Thrombophlebitis

Neuromuscular & skeletal: Arthrosis, bone necrosis, CPK increased, hyper-/hypotonia, leg cramps, myalgia, osteoporosis, paresthesia, tetany

Ocular: Abnormal vision, cataract, conjunctivitis

Otic: Ear pain, otitis media, tinnitus

Renal: Albuminuria, bladder pain, BUN increased, dysuria, hematuria, hydronephrosis, kidney pain, nephropathy (toxic), nocturia, oliguria, pyelonephritis, pyuria, tubular necrosis, urinary frequency, urinary incontinence, urinary retention

Respiratory: Asthma, atelectasis, bronchitis, cough, epistaxis, hypoxia, lung edema, pleural effusion, pneumonia, pulmonary embolism, rhinitis, sinusitis

Miscellaneous: Lymphoproliferative disease/lymphoma (1% to 3%), abscess, diaphoresis, flu-like syndrome, hernia, herpesvirus infection, infection (including opportunistic), lymphadenopathy, lymphocele, peritonitis, sepsis

<3% (Limited to important or life-threatening): ALT increased, alveolar proteinosis, anaphylactoid reaction, anaphylaxis, anastomotic disruption, angioedema, ascites, AST increased, azoospermia, *Clostridium difficile* colitis, cytomegalovirus, Epstein-Barr virus, exfoliative

dermatitis, fascial dehiscence, focal segmental glomerulosclerosis, hepatic necrosis, hepatotoxicity, hypersensitivity reaction, hypersensitivity vasculitis, hypophosphatemia, incisional hernia; interstitial lung disease (dose-related; includes pneumonitis, pulmonary fibrosis, and bronchiolitis obliterans organizing pneumonia [BOOP] with no identified infectious etiology); joint disorders, lymphedema, myocardial infarction, mycobacterial infection, nephropathy (BK virus-associated), nephrotic syndrome, neutropenia, pancreatitis, pancytopenia, pericardial effusion, *Pneumocystis* pneumonia, progressive multifocal leukoencephalopathy (PML), proteinuria, pulmonary hemorrhage, reversible posterior leukoencephalopathy syndrome (RPLS), tamponade, tuberculosis, wound dehiscence

Note: Hepatic artery thrombosis (HAT) and graft failure have been reported in liver transplant patients (not an approved use); bronchial anastomotic dehiscence has been reported in lung transplant patients (not an approved use)

Drug Interactions

Metabolism/Transport Effects Substrate of CYP3A4 (major), P-glycoprotein; **Note:** Assignment of Major/Minor substrate status based on clinically relevant drug interaction potential; **Inhibits** CYP3A4 (weak)

Avoid Concomitant Use

Avoid concomitant use of Sirolimus with any of the following: BCG; CloZAPine; Conivaptan; Crizotinib; Enzalutamide; Fusidic Acid (Systemic); Mifepristone; Natalizumab; Pimecrolimus; Pimozide; Posaconazole; Tacrolimus (Systemic); Tacrolimus (Topical); Tofacitinib; Vaccines (Live); Voriconazole

Increased Effect/Toxicity

Sirolimus may increase the levels/effects of: ACE Inhibitors; ARIPiprazole; CloZAPine; CycloSPORINE (Systemic); Dofetilide; Leflunomide; Lomitapide; Natalizumab; Pimozide; Tacrolimus (Systemic); Tacrolimus (Topical); Tofacitinib; Vaccines (Live)

The levels/effects of Sirolimus may be increased by: Boceprevir; Conivaptan; Crizotinib; CycloSPORINE (Systemic); CYP3A4 Inhibitors (Moderate); CYP3A4 Inhibitors (Strong); Dasatinib; Denosumab; Fluconazole; Fusidic Acid (Systemic); Itraconazole; Ivacaftor; Ketoconazole (Systemic); Luliconazole; Macrolide Antibiotics; Mifepristone; Nelfinavir; P-glycoprotein/ABCB1 Inhibitors; Pimecrolimus; Posaconazole; Roflumilast; Tacrolimus (Systemic); Tacrolimus (Topical); Telaprevir; Trastuzumab; Voriconazole

Decreased Effect

Sirolimus may decrease the levels/effects of: BCG; Coccidioidin Skin Test; Sipuleucel-T; Tacrolimus (Systemic); Vaccines (Inactivated); Vaccines (Live)

The levels/effects of Sirolimus may be decreased by: Bosentan; CYP3A4 Inducers (Strong); Dabrafenib; Deferasirox; Echinacea; Efavirenz; Enzalutamide; Fosphenytoin; Herbs (CYP3A4 Inducers); Mitotane; P-glycoprotein/ABCB1 Inducers; Phenytoin; Rifampin; Tocilizumab

Ethanol/Nutrition/Herb Interactions

Food: Grapefruit juice may decrease clearance of sirolimus. Ingestion with high-fat meals decreases peak concentrations but increases AUC by 23% to 35%. Management: Avoid grapefruit juice. Take consistently (either with or without food) to minimize variability.

Herb/Nutraceutical: St John's wort may decrease sirolimus levels. Some herbal medications have immunostimulant properties (eg, echinacea). Herbs with hypoglycemic properties may increase the risk of sirolimus-induced hypoglycemia (eg, alfalfa). Management: Avoid St John's wort, cat's claw, and echinacea. Avoid alfalfa, aloe, bilberry, bitter melon, burdock, celery, damiana, fenugreek, garcinia, garlic, ginger, ginseng (American), gymnema, marshmallow, and stinging nettle.

Storage/Stability

Oral solution: Store under refrigeration, 2°C to 8°C (36°F to 46°F). Protect from light. A slight haze may develop in refrigerated solutions, but the quality of the product is not affected. After opening, solution should be used in 1 month. If necessary, may be stored at temperatures up to 25°C (77°F) for ≤15 days after opening. Product may be stored in amber syringe for a maximum of 24 hours (at room temperature or refrigerated). Discard syringe after single use. Solution should be used immediately following dilution.

Tablet: Store at room temperature of 20°C to 25°C (68°F to 77°F). Protect from light.

Mechanism of Action Sirolimus inhibits T-lymphocyte activation and proliferation in response to antigenic and cytokine stimulation and inhibits antibody production. Its mechanism differs from other immunosuppressants. Sirolimus binds to FKBP-12, an intracellular protein, to form an immunosuppressive complex which inhibits the regulatory kinase, mTOR (mammalian target of rapamycin). This inhibition suppresses cytokine mediated T-cell proliferation, halting progression from the G1 to the S phase of the cell cycle. It inhibits acute rejection of allografts and prolongs graft survival.

Pharmacodynamics/Kinetics

Absorption: Rapid

Distribution: 12 L/kg (range: 4-20 L/kg)

Protein binding: ~92%, primarily to albumin

Metabolism: Extensive; in intestinal wall via P-glycoprotein and hepatic via CYP3A4; to 7 major metabolites

Bioavailability: Oral solution: 14%; Oral tablet: 18%

Half-life elimination: Mean: 62 hours (range: 46-78 hours); extended in hepatic impairment (Child-Pugh class A or B) to 113 hours

Time to peak: Oral solution: 1-3 hours; Tablet: 1-6 hours

Excretion: Feces (91% due to P-glycoprotein-mediated efflux into gut lumen); urine (2%)

Dosage

Low-to-moderate immunologic risk renal transplant patients: Adolescents ≥13 years and Adults: Dosing by body weight: Oral:

<40 kg: Loading dose: 3 mg/m^2 on day 1, followed by maintenance dosing of 1 mg/m^2 once daily

≥40 kg: Loading dose: 6 mg on day 1; maintenance: 2 mg once daily

High immunologic risk renal transplant patients: Adults: Oral: Loading dose: Up to 15 mg on day 1; maintenance: 5 mg/day; obtain trough concentration between days 5-7 and adjust accordingly. Continue concurrent cyclosporine/sirolimus therapy for 1 year following transplantation. Further adjustment of the regimen must be based on clinical status.

Dosage adjustment: Sirolimus dosages should be adjusted to maintain trough concentrations within desired range based on risk and concomitant therapy. Maximum daily dose: 40 mg. Dosage should be adjusted at intervals of 7-14 days to account for the long half-life of sirolimus. In general, dose proportionality may be assumed. New sirolimus dose **equals** current dose **multiplied by** (target concentration **divided by** current concentration). **Note:** If large dose increase is required, consider loading dose calculated as:

Loading dose **equals** (new maintenance dose **minus** current maintenance dose) **multiplied by** 3

Maximum dose in 1 day: 40 mg; if required dose is >40 mg (due to loading dose), divide loading dose over 2 days. Whole blood concentrations should not be used as the sole basis for dosage adjustment (monitor clinical signs/symptoms, tissue biopsy, and laboratory parameters).

Maintenance therapy after withdrawal of cyclosporine: Cyclosporine withdrawal is not recommended in high immunological risk patients. Following 2-4 months of combined therapy, withdrawal of cyclosporine may be considered in low-to-moderate immunologic risk patients. Cyclosporine should be discontinued over 4-8 weeks, and a necessary increase in the dosage of sirolimus (up to fourfold) should be anticipated due to removal of metabolic inhibition by cyclosporine and to maintain adequate immunosuppressive effects. Dose-adjusted trough target concentrations are typically 16-24 ng/mL for the first year post-transplant and 12-20 ng/mL thereafter (measured by chromatographic methodology).

Graft-versus-host disease (GVHD): Adults: Oral:

GVHD prophylaxis (unlabeled use): 12 mg loading dose on day -3, followed by 4 mg daily (target trough level: 3-12 ng/mL); taper off after 6-9 months (Armand, 2008; Cutler, 2007)

Treatment of refractory acute GVHD (unlabeled use): 4-5 mg/m^2 for 14 days (no loading dose) (Benito, 2001)

Treatment of chronic GVHD (unlabeled use): 6 mg loading dose, followed by 2 mg daily (target trough level: 7-12 ng/mL) for 6-9 months (Couriel, 2005)

Heart transplantation (unlabeled use): Adults: Oral: **Note:** The use of sirolimus in the immediate post-cardiac transplant period (ie, *de novo* heart transplant) as a primary immunosuppressant has fallen out of favor due to adverse effects (eg, impaired wound healing and infection); however, patients may be converted to sirolimus from a calcineurin inhibitor (after at least 6 months from time of transplant [Costanzo, 2010]) or may have sirolimus added to a calcineurin inhibitor to prevent or minimize further transplant related vasculopathy or renal toxicity due to calcineurin inhibitor use.

Conversion from a calcineurin inhibitor (CNI) (ie, cyclosporine, tacrolimus): Reduce cyclosporine by 25 mg twice daily or tacrolimus by 1 mg twice daily followed by initiation of sirolimus 1 mg once daily; adjust sirolimus dose to target trough level of 8-14 ng/mL, withdraw CNI, repeat biopsy 2 weeks after CNI withdrawal (Topilsky, 2012). Alternatively, maintain CNI concentrations and initiate sirolimus 1 mg once daily for 1 week; adjust sirolimus to target trough levels of 10-15 ng/mL over 2 weeks, then reduce CNI to target 50% of therapeutic concentrations and after 2 weeks evaluate for rejection. If no rejection, continue same regimen for an additional month, then reduce CNI to 25% of therapeutic concentrations with repeat biopsy 2 weeks later; if no rejection, may discontinue CNI after 2 weeks and continue to maintain sirolimus trough levels of 10-15 ng/mL (usual doses required to maintain target levels: 1-8 mg daily) (Kushwaha, 2005).

Conversion from antiproliferative drug (ie, azathioprine or mycophenolate) while maintaining calcineurin inhibitor: Upon discontinuation of antiproliferative, administer sirolimus 6 mg loading dose followed by 2 mg once daily titrated to a target trough level of 4-15 ng/mL (Mancini, 2003) or 4-12 ng/mL per ISHLT recommendations (Costanzo, 2010).

Renal angiomyolipoma or lymphangioleiomyomatosis (unlabeled use): Adults: Oral: Initial: 0.5 mg/m^2 once daily titrated to a target trough level of 3-6 ng/mL (may increase to target trough level of 6-10 ng/mL if <10% reduction in lesion diameters at 2 months) for 2 years (Davies, 2011) **or** Initial: 2 mg once daily titrated to a target trough level of 5-15 ng/mL for 1 year (McCormack, 2011)

Dosage adjustment in renal impairment: No dosage adjustment necessary. However, adjustment of regimen (including discontinuation of therapy) should be considered when used concurrently with cyclosporine and elevated or increasing serum creatinine is noted.

Dosage adjustment in hepatic impairment:

Loading dose: No dosage adjustment necessary.

Maintenance dose:

Mild to moderate impairment (Child-Pugh classes A and B): Reduce maintenance dose by ~33%.

Severe impairment (Child-Pugh class C): Reduce maintenance dose by ~50%.

Dietary Considerations Take consistently (either with or without food) to minimize variability of absorption.

Administration Initial dose should be administered as soon as possible after transplant. Sirolimus should be taken 4 hours after oral cyclosporine (Neoral® or Gengraf®). Should be administered consistently (either with or without food).

Solution: Mix (by stirring vigorously) with at least 2 ounces of water or orange juice. No other liquids should be used for dilution. Patient should drink diluted solution immediately. The cup should then be refilled with an additional 4 ounces of water or orange juice, stirred vigorously, and the patient should drink the contents at once.

Tablet: Do not crush, split, or chew.

Hazardous agent; use appropriate precautions for handling and disposal (NIOSH, 2012).

Monitoring Parameters Monitor LFTs and CBC during treatment. Monitor sirolimus levels in all patients (especially in pediatric patients, patients ≥13 years of age weighing <40 kg, patients with hepatic impairment, or on concurrent potent inhibitors or inducers of CYP3A4 or P-gp, and/or if cyclosporine dosing is markedly reduced or discontinued), and when changing dosage forms of sirolimus. Also monitor serum cholesterol and triglycerides, blood pressure, serum creatinine, and urinary protein. Serum drug concentrations should be determined 3-4 days after loading doses and 7-14 days after dosage adjustments; however, these concentrations should not be used as the sole basis for dosage adjustment, especially during withdrawal of cyclosporine (monitor clinical signs/symptoms, tissue biopsy, and laboratory parameters). **Note:** Concentrations and ranges are dependent on and will vary with assay methodology (chromatographic or immunoassay); assay methods are not interchangeable.

Reference Range Note: Sirolimus concentrations are dependent on the assay method (eg, chromatographic and immunoassay) used; assay methods are not interchangeable. Determine the assay method used to assure consistency (or accommodations if changes occur) and for monitoring purposes, be aware of alterations to assay method or reference range.

Serum trough concentration goals for renal transplantation (based on HPLC methods):

Concomitant cyclosporine: 4-12 ng/mL

Low-to-moderate immunologic risk (after cyclosporine withdrawal): 16-24 ng/mL for the first year after transplant; after 1 year: 12-20 ng/mL

High immunologic risk (with cyclosporine): 10-15 ng/mL

Note: Trough concentrations vary based on clinical context and use of additional immunosuppressants. The following represents typical ranges.

When combined with tacrolimus and mycophenolate mofetil (MMF) without steroids: 6-8 ng/mL

As a substitute for tacrolimus (starting 4-8 weeks post-transplant), in combination with MMF and steroids: 8-12 ng/mL

Following conversion from tacrolimus to sirolimus >6 months post-transplant due to chronic allograft nephropathy: 4-6 ng/mL

Serum trough concentrations for heart transplantation (unlabeled use):

With calcineurin inhibitor (eg, cyclosporine): 4-12 ng/mL (Costanzo, 2010)

Without calcineurin inhibitor: 10-15 ng/mL (Raichlin, 2007a; Raichlin, 2007b)

Following conversion from cyclosporine or tacrolimus to sirolimus: Initial (maintained until completion of conversion [~2 weeks]): 8-14 ng/mL (Topilsky, 2012) **or** 9-15 ng/mL (Zuckermann, 2012); Maintenance: 10-15 ng/mL (Kushwaha, 2005) **or** 7-15 ng/mL (Zuckermann, 2012)

Serum trough concentrations for GVHD prophylaxis in allogeneic stem cell transplant (unlabeled use): 3-12 ng/mL (Armand, 2008; Cutler, 2007)

Serum trough concentrations for advanced chordoma (unlabeled use): 15-20 ng/mL (Stacchiotti, 2009)

Serum trough concentrations for renal angiomyolipoma or lymphangioleiomyomatosis (unlabeled use): 3-6 ng/mL; may increase to 6-10 ng/mL if <10% reduction in lesion diameters at 2 months (Davies, 2011) **or** 5-15 ng/mL (McCormack, 2011)

Additional Information Sirolimus tablets and oral solution are not bioequivalent, due to differences in absorption. Clinical equivalence was seen using 2 mg tablet and 2 mg solution. It is not known if higher doses are also clinically equivalent. Monitor sirolimus levels if changes in dosage forms are made.

Sirolimus solution may cause irritation if administered undiluted.

High-risk renal transplant patients are defined (per the manufacturer's labeling) as African-American transplant recipients and/or repeat renal transplant recipients who lost a previous allograft based on an immunologic process and/or patients with high PRA (panel-reactive antibodies; peak PRA level >80%). Individual transplant centers may have differences in their definitions. For example, some centers would consider a PRA >50% to be at higher risk of rejection.

Dosage Forms Excipient information presented when available (limited, particularly for generics); consult specific product labeling.

Solution, Oral:
- Rapamune: 1 mg/mL (60 mL) [contains alcohol, usp]

Tablet, Oral:
- Rapamune: 0.5 mg, 1 mg, 2 mg
- Generic: 0.5 mg

◆ **Sirturo** *see* Bedaquiline *on page 229*

SitaGLIPtin (sit a GLIP tin)

Brand Names: U.S. Januvia

Brand Names: Canada Januvia®

Index Terms MK-0431; Sitagliptin Phosphate

Pharmacologic Category Antidiabetic Agent, Dipeptidyl Peptidase IV (DPP-IV) Inhibitor

Additional Appendix Information

Oral Antidiabetic Agents Comparison Table *on page 2312*

Use Management of type 2 diabetes mellitus (noninsulin dependent, NIDDM) as an adjunct to diet and exercise as monotherapy or in combination therapy with other antidiabetic agents

Pregnancy Risk Factor B

Pregnancy Considerations Adverse events have not been observed in animal reproduction studies. For women with diabetes, maternal hyperglycemia can be associated with adverse effects in the fetus, neonate, and mother. To prevent adverse events, prior to conception and throughout pregnancy, the maternal Hb A_{1c} should be kept close to normal but without causing significant hypoglycemia. The use of dipeptidyl peptidase IV (DPP-IV) inhibitors in pregnant women is not currently recommended; insulin is the drug of choice for the control of diabetes mellitus during pregnancy (ACOG, 2005; ADA, 2013; Kitzmiller, 2008; Metzger, 2007).

Breast-Feeding Considerations It is not known if sitagliptin is excreted in breast milk. The manufacturer recommends that caution be used if administered to breast-feeding women.

Medication Guide Available Yes

Contraindications Serious hypersensitivity (eg, anaphylaxis, angioedema) to sitagliptin or any component of the formulation

Warnings/Precautions Avoid use in type 1 diabetes mellitus (insulin dependent, IDDM) and diabetic ketoacidosis (DKA) due to lack of efficacy in these populations. Use caution when used in conjunction with insulin or insulin secretagogues; risk of hypoglycemia is increased. Monitor blood glucose closely; dosage adjustments of insulin or insulin secretagogues may be necessary. Use with caution in patients with moderate-to-severe renal dysfunction and end-stage renal disease (ESRD) requiring hemodialysis or peritoneal dialysis; dosing adjustment required. Safety and efficacy have not been established in severe hepatic dysfunction.

Rare hypersensitivity reactions, including anaphylaxis, angioedema, and/or severe dermatologic reactions (such as Stevens-Johnson syndrome), have been reported in postmarketing surveillance; discontinue if signs/symptoms of hypersensitivity reactions occur. Use with caution if patient has experienced angioedema with other DPP-IV inhibitor use. Cases of acute pancreatitis (including hemorrhagic and necrotizing with some fatalities) have been reported with use; monitor for signs/symptoms of pancreatitis. Discontinue use immediately if pancreatitis is suspected and initiate appropriate management. Use with caution in patients with a history of pancreatitis (not known if this population is at greater risk).

Clinical trials included only a limited number of patients with heart failure (HF). No specific recommendations regarding this population are provided in the approved U.S. labeling (Canadian labeling recommends against use in this population). Diabetes self-management education (DSME) is essential to maximize the effectiveness of therapy.

Adverse Reactions As reported with monotherapy:

1% to 10%:
- Cardiovascular: Peripheral edema (2%)
- Endocrine & metabolic: Hypoglycemia (1%)
- Gastrointestinal: Diarrhea (4%), constipation (3%), nausea (2%)
- Neuromuscular & skeletal: Osteoarthritis (1%)
- Respiratory: Nasopharyngitis (5%), pharyngitis (1%), upper respiratory tract infection (viral; 1%)

<1% (Limited to important or life-threatening): Acute renal failure (possibly requiring dialysis), anaphylaxis, anemia, angioedema, bundle branch block, depression, erectile dysfunction, exfoliative dermatitis, gastritis (*Helicobacter*), GERD, hepatic steatosis, hyper-/hypotension, hypersensitivity, liver enzymes increased, migraine, orthostasis, pancreatitis (acute cases including hemorrhagic or necrotizing forms with some fatalities), peripheral neuropathy, renal function decreased, rosacea, Stevens-Johnson syndrome

Drug Interactions

Metabolism/Transport Effects **Substrate** of P-glycoprotein

Avoid Concomitant Use There are no known interactions where it is recommended to avoid concomitant use.

Increased Effect/Toxicity

SitaGLIPtin may increase the levels/effects of: ACE Inhibitors; Digoxin; Hypoglycemic Agents

The levels/effects of SitaGLIPtin may be increased by: Herbs (Hypoglycemic Properties); MAO Inhibitors; Pegvisomant; P-glycoprotein/ABCB1 Inhibitors; Salicylates; Selective Serotonin Reuptake Inhibitors

Decreased Effect

The levels/effects of SitaGLIPtin may be decreased by: Corticosteroids (Orally Inhaled); Corticosteroids (Systemic); Loop Diuretics; Luteinizing Hormone-Releasing Hormone Analogs; P-glycoprotein/ABCB1 Inducers; Somatropin; Thiazide Diuretics

Storage/Stability Store at 20°C to 25°C (68°F to 77°F); excursions permitted to 15°C to 30°C (59°F to 86°F).

Mechanism of Action Sitagliptin inhibits dipeptidyl peptidase IV (DPP-IV) enzyme resulting in prolonged active incretin levels. Incretin hormones (eg, glucagon-like peptide-1 [GLP-1] and glucose-dependent insulinotropic polypeptide [GIP]) regulate glucose homeostasis by increasing insulin synthesis and release from pancreatic beta cells and decreasing glucagon secretion from pancreatic alpha cells. Decreased glucagon secretion results in decreased hepatic glucose production. Under normal physiologic circumstances, incretin hormones are released by the intestine throughout the day and levels are increased in response to a meal; incretin hormones are rapidly inactivated by the DPP-IV enzyme.

Pharmacodynamics/Kinetics

Absorption: Rapid

Distribution: ~198 L

Protein binding: 38%

Metabolism: Not extensively metabolized; minor metabolism via CYP3A4 and 2C8 to metabolites (inactive) suggested by *in vitro* studies

Bioavailability: ~87%

Half-life elimination: 12 hours

Time to peak, plasma: 1-4 hours

Excretion: Urine 87% (79% as unchanged drug, 16% as metabolites); feces 13%

Dosage Oral: Adults: Type 2 diabetes: 100 mg once daily

Concomitant use with insulin and/or insulin secretagogues (eg, sulfonylureas): Reduced dose of insulin and/or insulin secretagogues may be needed.

Dosage adjustment in renal impairment: Note: Renal function may be estimated using the Cockcroft-Gault formula for dosage adjustment purposes.

Cl_{cr} ≥50 mL/minute: No dosage adjustment necessary.

Cl_{cr} ≥30 to <50 mL/minute (approximate S_{cr} of >1.7 to ≤3.0 mg/dL [males] or >1.5 to ≤2.5 mg/dL [females]): 50 mg once daily

Cl_{cr} <30 mL/minute (approximate S_{cr} of >3.0 mg/dL [males] or >2.5 mg/dL [females]): 25 mg once daily

ESRD requiring hemodialysis or peritoneal dialysis: 25 mg once daily; administered without regard to timing of hemodialysis

Dosage adjustment in hepatic impairment:

Mild to moderate impairment (Child-Pugh classes A and B): No dosage adjustment necessary.

Severe impairment (Child-Pugh class C): No dosage adjustment provided in manufacturer's labeling (has not been studied).

Dietary Considerations May be taken with or without food. Individualized medical nutrition therapy (MNT) based on ADA recommendations is an integral part of therapy.

Administration May be administered with or without food.

Monitoring Parameters Hb A_{1c}, serum glucose; renal function prior to initiation and periodically during treatment

Reference Range Recommendations for glycemic control in nonpregnant adults with diabetes (ADA, 2013):

Hb A_{1c}: <7% (a more aggressive [<6.5%] or less aggressive [<8%] Hb A_{1c} goal may be targeted based on patient-specific characteristics)

Preprandial capillary plasma glucose: 70-130 mg/dL

Peak postprandial capillary blood glucose: <180 mg/dL

Dosage Forms Excipient information presented when available (limited, particularly for generics); consult specific product labeling.

Tablet, Oral:

Januvia: 25 mg, 50 mg, 100 mg

Sitagliptin and Metformin

(sit a GLIP tin & met FOR min)

Brand Names: U.S. Janumet; Janumet XR

Brand Names: Canada Janumet

Index Terms Metformin and Sitagliptin; Sitagliptin Phosphate and Metformin Hydrochloride

Pharmacologic Category Antidiabetic Agent, Biguanide; Antidiabetic Agent, Dipeptidyl Peptidase IV (DPP-IV) Inhibitor; Hypoglycemic Agent, Oral

Use Type 2 diabetes mellitus: As an adjunct to diet and exercise to improve glycemic control in adults with type 2 diabetes mellitus when treatment with both sitagliptin and metformin is appropriate

Pregnancy Risk Factor B

Medication Guide Available Yes

Dosage Oral: Type 2 diabetes mellitus: **Note:** Patients receiving concomitant insulin and/or insulin secretagogues (eg, sulfonylureas) may require dosage adjustments of these agents.

Adults: Initial doses should be based on current dose of sitagliptin and metformin.

Patients inadequately controlled on metformin alone: Initial dose:

Immediate release: Sitagliptin 100 mg daily plus current daily dose of metformin given in 2 equally divided doses; maximum: sitagliptin 100 mg/metformin 2000 mg daily. **Note:** The U.S. labeling recommends patients currently receiving metformin 850 mg twice daily receive an initial dose of sitagliptin 50 mg and metformin 1000 mg twice daily.

Extended release: Sitagliptin 100 mg daily plus current daily dose of metformin given once daily; maximum: sitagliptin 100 mg/metformin 2000 mg daily. **Note:** The U.S. labeling recommends patients currently receiving immediate release metformin 850-1000 mg twice daily receive an initial dose of sitagliptin 100 mg and metformin 2000 mg once daily.

Patients inadequately controlled on sitagliptin alone: Initial dose: **Note:** Patients currently receiving a renally-adjusted dose of sitagliptin should not be switched to a combination product.

Immediate release: Metformin 1000 mg daily plus sitagliptin 100 mg daily given in 2 equally divided doses

Extended release: Metformin 1000 mg and sitagliptin 100 mg once daily

Conversion from immediate release to extended release: Convert using same total daily dose (up to the maximum recommended dose), but adjust frequency as indicated for immediate (twice daily) or extended (once daily) release products.

Patients inadequately controlled on combination metformin and either pioglitazone, a sulfonylurea, or insulin: Canadian labeling (not in U.S. labeling): Sitagliptin 100 mg daily plus current daily dose of metformin given in 2 equally divided doses. If taking insulin or a sulfonylurea concomitantly with sitagliptin/metformin, the dosage of insulin or sulfonylurea may need adjusted.

Patients inadequately controlled on combination therapy with sitagliptin and insulin: Canadian labeling (not in U.S. labeling): Sitagliptin 100 mg daily plus metformin (dose based on glycemic control) given in 2 equally divided doses. Insulin dose may need adjusted.

Dosing adjustment: Metformin component may be gradually increased up to the maximum dose. Maximum dose: Sitagliptin 100 mg/metformin 2000 mg daily

Elderly: The initial and maintenance dosing should be conservative, due to the potential for decreased renal function (monitor). Do not use in patients ≥80 years of age unless normal renal function has been established.

Dosage adjustment in renal impairment:

U.S. labeling: Use is contraindicated in patients with renal impairment (eg, serum creatinine ≥1.5 mg/dL in males or ≥1.4 mg/dL in females or abnormal clearance).

Canadian labeling: Use is contraindicated.

Dosage adjustment in hepatic impairment:

U.S. labeling: Avoid metformin; liver disease is a risk factor for the development of lactic acidosis during metformin therapy.

Canadian labeling: Use is not recommended with clinical or laboratory evidence of disease and contraindicated in the presence of severe impairment.

Additional Information Complete prescribing information should be consulted for additional detail.

Dosage Forms Excipient information presented when available (limited, particularly for generics); consult specific product labeling.

Tablet, oral:

Janumet 50/500: Sitagliptin 50 mg and metformin hydrochloride 500 mg

Janumet 50/1000: Sitagliptin 50 mg and metformin hydrochloride 1000 mg

Tablet, extended release, oral:

Janumet XR: 50/500: Sitagliptin 50 mg and metformin hydrochloride 500 mg

Janumet XR: 50/1000: Sitagliptin 50 mg and metformin hydrochloride 1000 mg

Janumet XR: 100/1000: Sitagliptin 100 mg and metformin hydrochloride 1000 mg

Dosage Forms: Canada Excipient information presented when available (limited, particularly for generics); consult specific product labeling.

Tablet, oral:

Janumet 50/500: Sitagliptin 50 mg and metformin hydrochloride 500 mg

Janumet 50/850: Sitagliptin 50 mg and metformin hydrochloride 850 mg

Janumet 50/1000: Sitagliptin 50 mg and metformin hydrochloride 1000 mg

Sitagliptin and Simvastatin

(sit a GLIP tin & sim va STAT in)

Brand Names: U.S. Juvisync™ [DSC]

Index Terms Simvastatin and Sitagliptin; Sitagliptin Phosphate and Simvastatin

Pharmacologic Category Antidiabetic Agent, Dipeptidyl Peptidase IV (DPP-IV) Inhibitor; Antilipemic Agent, HMG-CoA Reductase Inhibitor

Use For use when treatment with both sitagliptin and simvastatin is appropriate:

Sitagliptin: Management of type 2 diabetes mellitus (noninsulin dependent, NIDDM) as an adjunct to diet and exercise as monotherapy or in combination therapy with other antidiabetic agents

Simvastatin: Used with dietary therapy for the following:

Secondary prevention of cardiovascular events in hypercholesterolemic patients with established coronary heart disease (CHD) or at high risk for CHD: To reduce cardiovascular morbidity (myocardial infarction, coronary/noncoronary revascularization procedures) and mortality; to reduce the risk of stroke

Hyperlipidemias: To reduce elevations in total cholesterol (total-C), LDL-C, apolipoprotein B, triglycerides, and VLDL-C, and to increase HDL-C in patients with primary hypercholesterolemia (elevations of 1 or more components are present in Fredrickson type IIa, IIb, III, and IV hyperlipidemias); treatment of homozygous familial hypercholesterolemia

Pregnancy Risk Factor X

Medication Guide Available Yes

Dosage Hyperlipidemia and type 2 diabetes: Adults: Oral: Initial dose: Sitagliptin 100 mg and simvastatin 40 mg once daily. **Note:** Patients already taking simvastatin <40 mg daily (with or without sitagliptin 100 mg daily) can be converted to the comparable equivalent of the combination product. Dose adjustments should be made at intervals of ≥4 weeks.

Concomitant use with insulin and/or insulin secretagogues (eg, sulfonylureas): Reduced dose of insulin and/or insulin secretagogues may be needed.

Dosage adjustment for simvastatin with concomitant medications:

Amiodarone, amlodipine, or ranolazine: Simvastatin dose should **not** exceed 20 mg daily

Diltiazem, dronedarone, or verapamil: Simvastatin dose should **not** exceed 10 mg daily

Lomitapide: Reduce simvastatin dose by 50% when initiating lomitapide. Simvastatin dose should not exceed 20 mg daily (or 40 mg daily for those who previously tolerated simvastatin 80 mg daily for ≥1 year without evidence of muscle toxicity)

Dosage adjustment for simvastatin in Chinese patients on niacin doses ≥1 g daily: Use caution with simvastatin doses of 40 mg daily because of an increased risk of myopathy

Dosage adjustment in renal impairment: Note: Renal function may be estimated using Cockcroft-Gault formula for dosage adjustment purposes.

Cl_{cr} ≥50 mL/minute: No dosage adjustment necessary.

Cl_{cr} ≥30 to <50 mL/minute (approximate S_{cr} of >1.7 to ≤3.0 mg/dL [males] or >1.5 to ≤2.5 mg/dL [females]): Initial: Sitagliptin 50 mg and simvastatin 40 mg once daily. **Note:** Patients already taking simvastatin <40 mg daily (with or without sitagliptin 50 mg daily) can be converted to the comparable equivalent of the combination product.

Cl_{cr} <30 mL/minute (approximate S_{cr} of >3.0 mg/dL [males] or >2.5 mg/dL [females]): Use is not recommended.

End-stage renal disease (ESRD): Use is not recommended

Dosage adjustment in hepatic impairment: Use is contraindicated

Additional Information Complete prescribing information should be consulted for additional detail.

Dosage Forms Excipient information presented when available (limited, particularly for generics); consult specific product labeling.

Tablet, oral:

Juvisync 50/10: Sitagliptin 50 mg and simvastatin 10 mg [DSC]

Juvisync 50/20: Sitagliptin 50 mg and simvastatin 20 mg [DSC]

Juvisync 50/40: Sitagliptin 50 mg and simvastatin 40 mg [DSC]

Juvisync 100/10: Sitagliptin 100 mg and simvastatin 10 mg [DSC]

Juvisync 100/20: Sitagliptin 100 mg and simvastatin 20 mg [DSC]

Juvisync 100/40: Sitagliptin 100 mg and simvastatin 40 mg [DSC]

◆ **Sitagliptin Phosphate** *see* SitaGLIPtin *on page* 1906

◆ **Sitagliptin Phosphate and Metformin Hydrochloride** *see* Sitagliptin and Metformin *on page* 1907

◆ **Sitagliptin Phosphate and Simvastatin** *see* Sitagliptin and Simvastatin *on page 1908*

◆ **Sitavig®** *see* Acyclovir (Topical) *on page 44*

◆ **Skelaxin** *see* Metaxalone *on page 1309*

◆ **Skelaxin® (Can)** *see* Metaxalone *on page 1309*

◆ **Skelid** *see* Tiludronate *on page 2063*

◆ **SKF 104864** *see* Topotecan *on page 2093*

◆ **SKF 104864-A** *see* Topotecan *on page 2093*

◆ **SKI-606** *see* Bosutinib *on page 275*

◆ **Skin Bleaching** *see* Hydroquinone *on page 1017*

◆ **Skin Bleaching-Sunscreen** *see* Hydroquinone *on page 1017*

◆ **Sklice** *see* Ivermectin (Topical) *on page 1139*

◆ **Skyla** *see* Levonorgestrel *on page 1202*

◆ **Sleep Tabs [OTC]** *see* DiphenhydrAMINE (Systemic) *on page 622*

◆ **S-leucovorin** *see* LEVOleucovorin *on page 1201*

◆ **6S-leucovorin** *see* LEVOleucovorin *on page 1201*

◆ **Slo-Niacin [OTC]** *see* Niacin *on page 1447*

◆ **Slo-Pot (Can)** *see* Potassium Chloride *on page 1684*

◆ **Slow Fe [OTC]** *see* Ferrous Sulfate *on page 854*

◆ **Slow Iron [OTC]** *see* Ferrous Sulfate *on page 854*

◆ **Slow-K (Can)** *see* Potassium Chloride *on page 1684*

◆ **Slow-Mag [OTC]** *see* Magnesium Chloride *on page 1259*

◆ **Slow Magnesium/Calcium [OTC]** *see* Magnesium Chloride *on page 1259*

◆ **Slow Release Iron [OTC] [DSC]** *see* Ferrous Sulfate *on page 854*

◆ **SM-13496** *see* Lurasidone *on page 1255*

Smallpox Vaccine (SMAL poks vak SEEN)

Brand Names: U.S. ACAM2000®

Index Terms Live Smallpox Vaccine; Vaccinia Vaccine

Pharmacologic Category Vaccine, Live (Viral)

Additional Appendix Information

Immunization Administration Recommendations *on page 2334*

Immunization Recommendations *on page 2339*

Use Active immunization against smallpox disease in persons determined to be at high risk for smallpox infection.

The Advisory Committee on Immunization Practices (ACIP) recommends routine vaccination for the following:

- Laboratory workers at risk of exposure from cultures or contaminated animals which may be a source of vaccinia or related Orthopoxviruses capable of causing infections in humans (eg, monkeypox, cowpox, variola, vaccinia).
- Consideration may also be given for vaccination of healthcare workers having contact with clinical specimens, contaminated material, or patients receiving vaccinia or recombinant vaccinia viruses.

In a Pre-Event Vaccination Program, the ACIP recommends vaccination for the following:

- Persons designated by authorities to investigate smallpox cases with the likelihood of direct patient contact
- Persons responsible for administering smallpox vaccine

In the event of an intentional release of smallpox virus, the ACIP recommends vaccination for the following:

- Persons exposed to the initial release of the virus
- Persons who had close contact with a confirmed or suspected smallpox patient at any time from the onset of the patient's fever until all scabs have separated
- Healthcare providers involved in evaluation, care, or transport of confirmed or suspected smallpox patients
- Laboratory personnel involved in processing specimens of confirmed or suspected smallpox patients
- Persons likely to have increased contact with infectious materials from smallpox patients

Pregnancy Risk Factor D

Pregnancy Considerations [U.S. Boxed Warning]: Pregnant women are at increased risk for severe adverse reactions. Animal reproduction studies have not been conducted with this vaccine. Vaccinia vaccine has not been associated with the development of congenital malformations. On rare occasions, vaccination has been reported to cause fetal infection. Fetal vaccinia infection is associated with stillbirth or neonatal mortality. Vaccination of pregnant women is not recommended in a pre-event setting. Pregnancy should be avoided for at least 4 weeks following vaccination. Healthcare providers may enroll pregnant women who were inadvertently vaccinated during pregnancy (or who were a close contact of a vaccinee within 4 weeks of vaccination) in the CDC pregnancy registry by calling 404-639-8253 or 877-554-4625. Military cases should be reported to the Department of Defense.

Breast-Feeding Considerations Not recommended for use in a breast-feeding woman in a nonemergency situation. Breast-feeding should be interrupted if the vaccine is administered in an emergency situation. Breast-feeding women should take precautions to avoid inadvertent contact with a vaccinee. One case of tertiary transfer to an infant has been reported following secondary transfer to a breast-feeding woman.

Prescribing and Access Restrictions ACAM2000® is deemed to have an approved REMS program. The smallpox vaccine is not available for general public use. All supplies are currently owned by the federal government for inclusion in the Strategic National Stockpile. In October 2002, the FDA approved the licensing of the stockpile of smallpox vaccine. This approval allows the vaccine to be distributed and administered in the event of a smallpox attack. The bulk of current supplies have been designated for use by the U.S. military. Additionally, laboratory workers who may be at risk of exposure may require vaccination. Bioterrorism experts have proposed immunization of first responders (including police, fire, and emergency workers), but these plans may not be implemented until additional stocks of vaccine are licensed.

Medication Guide Available Yes

Contraindications Manufacturer labeling: Severe immune deficiency (eg, persons undergoing bone marrow transplant, individuals with primary or acquired immunodeficiency requiring isolation). There are very few absolute contraindications regarding vaccination of individuals at high-risk for exposure to smallpox. The decision to vaccinate must be based on a careful analysis of potential benefits and possible risks.

ACIP contraindications in a pre-event vaccination program: Hypersensitivity to the vaccine or any component of the formulation; history or presence of atopic dermatitis, eczema or other acute, chronic or exfoliative skin conditions (or persons with household contacts with these conditions); immunosuppression (or persons with household contacts who are immunosuppressed); pregnant or breast-feeding women (or household contacts of pregnant women); children <1 year of age

According to ACIP, persons exposed to smallpox virus in an emergency situation have no contraindications to vaccination.

Warnings/Precautions [U.S. Boxed Warning]: Acute myocarditis and/or pericarditis, encephalitis, encephalomyelitis, and encephalopathy have been observed following vaccination. [U.S. Boxed Warning]: Progressive vaccinia, general vaccinia, and severe vaccinial skin infections have been observed following

vaccination. [U.S. Boxed Warning]: Severe skin and systemic reactions, including Stevens-Johnson syndrome, have also occurred. [U.S. Boxed Warning]: Patients with congenital or acquired immune deficiency disorders (including those on immunosuppressive medications), patients with or with a history of cardiovascular disease, patients with eye diseases treated with topical steroids, infants <12 months of age, and pregnant women may be at an increased risk for severe adverse reactions and should not be vaccinated in nonemergency situations. **[U.S. Boxed Warning]: Following vaccination, eczema vaccinatum has been reported. Patients with eczema, a history of eczema, or other acute or chronic exfoliative skin conditions may be at an increased risk for severe skin infections;** these patients should not be vaccinated in nonemergency situations. **[U.S. Boxed Warning]: The risk of vaccination complications must be weighed against the risk of experiencing a potentially fatal smallpox infection.** Patients at greatest risk for adverse reactions from the vaccine are also at increased risk for death from smallpox infection. **[U.S. Boxed Warning]: Live vaccinia virus may be transmitted to close contacts of the vaccinee; risks for the close contact are the same as those receiving the vaccine.**

For percutaneous administration only. Vaccination is given by scarification (multiple punctures into superficial layers of the skin) only. **Not for I.M., I.V., or SubQ injection.** Some dosage forms may contain neomycin, polymyxin B, and/or human albumin. Virus may be cultured from vaccination sites until scab separates from lesion. Individuals should be instructed to avoid contact with patients at high risk of transmission/adverse effects, including pregnant or breast-feeding women and patients with eczema or immunodeficiency during this time. Patients should be advised not to donate blood or organs for 21-30 days; contacts who have inadvertently contracted vaccinia should avoid donating blood for 14 days. Use appropriate precautions for handling and disposal. Personnel responsible for preparation and administration should observe appropriate contact precautions to avoid inadvertent inoculation (eg, wear surgical or protective gloves and avoid contact of vaccine with skin, eyes, or mucous membranes). Dispose of all materials for preparation and administration in a biohazard waste container. All materials must be burned, boiled, or autoclaved. Vaccinees should change bandages away from others and launder their own linens separately to prevent transmission. Per the ACIP, vaccine is contraindicated for use in infants <12 months of age (nonemergency situation) and use is not recommended in pediatric patients <18 years of age (nonemergency situations). In order to maximize vaccination rates, the ACIP recommends simultaneous administration of all age-appropriate vaccines (live or inactivated) for which a person is eligible at a single clinic visit, unless contraindications exist.

Vaccination may not result in effective immunity in all patients. Response depends upon multiple factors (eg, type of vaccine, age of patient) and may be improved by administering the vaccine at the recommended dose, route, and interval. Vaccines may not be effective if administered during periods of altered immune competence (CDC, 2011).

Adverse Reactions All serious adverse reactions must be reported to the U.S. Department of Health and Human Services (DHHS) Vaccine Adverse Event Reporting System (VAERS) 1-800-822-7967 or online at https://vaers.hhs.gov/esub/index. In addition, clinicians may enroll patients with adverse reactions in the CDC Registry at 877-554-4625. Serious adverse reactions to ACAM2000® may also be reported to the manufacturer, Acambis Inc, at 866-440-9440.

>10%:

Central nervous system: Headache (32% to 51%), fatigue (34% to 48%), malaise (28% to 37%)

Dermatologic: Erythema (18% to 24%); rash (6% to 11% erythematous, folliculitis, papulovesicular, urticarial, nonspecific)

Gastrointestinal: Nausea (10% to 19%), diarrhea (12% to 16%)

Local: Injection site: Pruritus (82% to 92%), erythema (61% to 74%), pain (37% to 67%), edema (28% to 48%)

Neuromuscular & skeletal: Myalgia (27% to 46%), rigors (12% to 21%)

Miscellaneous: Lymph node pain (19% to 57%), feeling hot (20% to 32%), exercise tolerance decreased (8% to 11%)

1% to 10%:

Gastrointestinal: Constipation (6%), vomiting (3% to 5%)

Neuromuscular & skeletal: Arthralgia, back pain

Respiratory: Dyspnea (3% to 4%)

Miscellaneous: Lymphadenopathy (6% to 8%)

Frequency not defined: Abdominal pain, Bell's palsy, blindness, cardiomyopathy (nonischemic/dilated), contact dermatitis, corneal scarring, death, dizziness, eczema vaccinatum, encephalitis, encephalomyelitis, encephalopathy, erythema multiforme, fever, generalized vaccinia, Guillain-Barré syndrome, hypersensitivity reactions; inadvertent inoculation at other sites (including autoinoculation to eyelid, face, genitalia, lips, mouth, nose, rectum); ischemic heart disease, keratitis, meningitis, myelitis, myocarditis, myopericarditis (asymptomatic or symptomatic), ocular vaccinia, paresthesia, pericarditis, photophobia, progressive vaccinia, secondary pyogenic infection, seizure, Stevens-Johnson syndrome, toothache, vaccinial skin infection, vertigo

Drug Interactions

Metabolism/Transport Effects None known.

Avoid Concomitant Use

Avoid concomitant use of Smallpox Vaccine with any of the following: Belimumab; Fingolimod; Immunosuppressants

Increased Effect/Toxicity

Smallpox Vaccine may increase the levels/effects of: Varicella Virus Vaccine

The levels/effects of Smallpox Vaccine may be increased by: AzaTHIOprine; Belimumab; Corticosteroids (Systemic); Dimethyl Fumarate; Fingolimod; Hydroxychloroquine; Immunosuppressants; Leflunomide; Mercaptopurine; Methotrexate

Decreased Effect

Smallpox Vaccine may decrease the levels/effects of: Tuberculin Tests

The levels/effects of Smallpox Vaccine may be decreased by: Dimethyl Fumarate; Fingolimod; Immune Globulins; Immunosuppressants

Preparation for Administration Bring to room temperature prior to reconstitution. Using the syringe provided, inject 0.3 mL of provided diluent into the vaccine vial. Swirl gently until the solution becomes a slightly hazy, colorless to straw-colored liquid free from particulate matter; avoid contact between the solution and the rubber stopper.

Storage/Stability Prior to reconstitution, store frozen at -15°C to -25°C (5°F to -13°F); may also be stored at 2°C to 8°C (36°F to 46°F) for up to 18 months. Following reconstitution, stable for 6 to 8 hours at room temperature of 20°C to 25°C (68°F to 77°F) or for up to 30 days when refrigerated at 2°C to 8°C (36°F to 46°F). The provided diluent should be stored at room temperature of 15°C to 30°C (59°F to 86°F).

Mechanism of Action Vaccinia virus is similar to the variola (smallpox) virus. By inducing a localized infection with vaccinia virus, immunity to both vaccinia and variola is achieved. Vaccination results in viral replication, production of neutralizing antibodies, immunity, and cellular hypersensitivity; revaccination is recommended every 3-10 years (depending on type of anticipated exposure) to maintain immunity in patients eligible for pre-event vaccination.

Pharmacodynamics/Kinetics Onset of action: Neutralizing antibodies appear 15-20 days after vaccination; time to appearance of neutralizing antibodies may be shorter (~7 days) following revaccination (CDC, 2001).

Dosage Percutaneous: Not for I.M., I.V., or SubQ injection: Vaccination by scarification (multiple-puncture technique) only: **Note:** A trace of blood should appear at vaccination site after 15-20 seconds; if no trace of blood is visible, an additional 3 insertions should be made using the same needle, without reinserting the needle into the vaccine bottle.

Children ≥12 months (in emergency conditions only) and Adults:

Primary vaccination and revaccination: Use a single drop of vaccine suspension and 15 needle punctures (using the same bifurcated needle) into the superficial skin

Note: According to the manufacturer, revaccination is recommended every 3 years for patients at a continued high risk for smallpox infection. The ACIP recommends routine nonemergency revaccination every 3-10 years, depending on type of exposure. Additional information can be obtained from the Department of Defense and the CDC.

Dosage adjustment in renal impairment: No dosage adjustment provided in manufacturer's labeling.

Dosage adjustment in hepatic impairment: No dosage adjustment provided in manufacturer's labeling.

Administration Vaccination should only be performed by healthcare providers trained in the safe and efficacious administration of the smallpox vaccine via the percutaneous route.

A single-use bifurcated needle should be dipped carefully into the reconstituted vaccine (following removal of rubber stopper). Visually confirm that the needle picks up a drop of vaccine solution. Using a bifurcated needle, 1 drop of vaccine is introduced into the superficial layers of the skin using a multiple-puncture technique. The skin over the insertion of the deltoid muscle is the preferred site for vaccination. Deposit the drop of vaccine onto clean, dry skin at the vaccination site. If alcohol is used to clean the skin, allow site to dry completely prior to administration to prevent the inactivation of the vaccine by the alcohol. Holding the bifurcated needle perpendicular to the skin, punctures are to be made rapidly within a diameter of about 5 mm into the superficial skin of the vaccination site. The puncture strokes should be vigorous enough to allow a trace of blood to appear after approximately 15-20 seconds. Wipe off any remaining vaccine with dry sterile gauze. Dispose of all materials in a biohazard waste container; do not reuse the bifurcated needle. All materials must be burned, boiled, or autoclaved. If no evidence of vaccine "take" (major cutaneous reaction characterized by a pustule at the site of inoculation) is apparent after 6-8 days in patients vaccinated for the first time, the individual may be vaccinated again. Previously vaccinated patients may not experience a cutaneous response following revaccination.

To prevent transmission of the virus, avoid scratching the vaccination site and cover with gauze (using first aid adhesive tape to keep gauze in place); cover gauze with a semipermeable barrier (eg, semiocclusive dressing) or clothing. Ointment or salves should not be applied to the vaccination site. Good handwashing prevents inadvertent inoculation. Vaccinees should change bandages away from others and launder their own linens separately to prevent transmission.

Simultaneous administration of vaccines helps ensure the patients will be fully vaccinated by the appropriate age. Simultaneous administration of vaccines is defined as administering >1 vaccine on the same day at different anatomic sites. Separate vaccines should not be combined in the same syringe unless indicated by product specific labeling. Separate needles and syringes should be used for each injection. The ACIP prefers each dose of a specific vaccine in a series come from the same manufacturer when possible. Adolescents and adults should be vaccinated while seated or lying down. In general, preterm infants should be vaccinated at the same chronological age as full-term infants (CDC, 2011).

Antipyretics have not been shown to prevent febrile seizures. Antipyretics may be used to treat fever or discomfort following vaccination (CDC, 2011). One study reported that routine prophylactic administration of acetaminophen to prevent fever prior to vaccination decreased the immune response of some vaccines; the clinical significance of this reduction in immune response has not been established (Prymula, 2009).

Monitoring Parameters

Primary vaccines: Monitor vaccination site; inspect after 6-8 days. Evidence of a major reaction (vesicular or pustular lesion or an area of palpable induration surrounding a central lesion) confirms success of vaccination. An equivocal reaction (all responses other than a major reaction) requires revaccination in patients undergoing primary vaccination only (preferably with another vial or vaccine lot, if available). Consult CDC or state or local health department if response to a second vaccination from a different vial or lot is equivocal.

Revaccination: Successful vaccination is confirmed when a major cutaneous reaction is observed 6-8 days post-vaccination. Prior vaccinations may reduce the cutaneous response and does not necessarily indicate a vaccination failure. A revaccinated individual without a cutaneous response does not require revaccination.

Test Interactions Rapid plasma regain (RPR) test: Smallpox vaccine may induce false-positive RPR test for syphilis; confirm positive RPR test using a more specific test (eg, FTA assay).

Tuberculin skin (PPD) and blood tests: Smallpox vaccine may diminish the diagnostic utility of tuberculin skin (PPD) and blood tests; avoid skin test for ≥1 month after vaccine to prevent false-negative results.

Additional Information Initial reaction of the vaccine includes formation of a papule (2-5 days following vaccination). The papule forms a vesicle on day 5 or day 6, which becomes pustular, with surrounding erythema and induration. The maximal area of erythema usually occurs between day 8 and day 10, and crusting of the lesion normally occurs between day 14 and day 21. Formation of a major cutaneous reaction in patients undergoing primary vaccination by day 6-8 is indicative of successful acquisition of protective immunity. In patients previously vaccinated, the major cutaneous reaction typically seen by day 6-8 may be modified and/or reduced; a lack of cutaneous response does not indicate vaccination failure and revaccination is not required in these patients. At the peak of the reaction, systemic symptoms (fever, malaise) and lymphadenopathy may occur. All materials used in vaccination must be burned, boiled, or autoclaved. Vaccination can decrease the rate of severe or fatal smallpox if administered during the first 4 days of exposure. If vaccination failure occurs, revaccination should be attempted using a different vial or vaccine lot. If the second vaccination (from a different vial or lot) also fails, contact the Centers for Disease Control and Prevention (CDC) at 404-639-3670 and/or the state or local health department prior to administering any additional vaccine. Vaccinia immune globulin (VIG) is available from the CDC for the treatment of severe adverse reactions.

If vaccination failure occurs, revaccination should be attempted using a different vial or vaccine lot. If the second vaccination (from a different vial or lot) also fails, contact the Centers for Disease Control and Prevention (CDC) at 404-639-3670 and/or the state or local health department prior to administering any additional vaccine.

Vaccinia immune globulin (VIG) is available from the CDC for the treatment of severe adverse reactions; administration of VIG does not blunt response to vaccination.

U.S. federal law requires that the name of medication, date of administration, the vaccine manufacturer, lot number of vaccine, and the administering person's name, title and address be entered into the patient's permanent medical record.

Dosage Forms Excipient information presented when available (limited, particularly for generics); consult specific product labeling. [DSC] = Discontinued product

Injection, powder for reconstitution [purified monkey cell source]:

ACAM2000®: 1-5 x 10^8 plaque-forming units per mL [contains polymyxin B, neomycin (trace amounts) and human albumin; packed with diluent, tuberculin syringes for reconstitution, and 100 bifurcated needles for administration]

◆ **SMX-TMP** *see* Sulfamethoxazole and Trimethoprim *on page 1959*

◆ **SMZ-TMP** *see* Sulfamethoxazole and Trimethoprim *on page 1959*

◆ **(+)-(*S*)-*N*-Methyl-γ-(1-naphthyloxy)-2-thiophenepropylamine Hydrochloride** *see* DULoxetine *on page 677*

◆ **Sochlor [OTC]** *see* Sodium Chloride *on page 1914*

◆ **Sodium 2-Mercaptoethane Sulfonate** *see* Mesna *on page 1307*

◆ **Sodium 4-Hydroxybutyrate** *see* Sodium Oxybate *on page 1922*

◆ **Sodium *L*-Triiodothyronine** *see* Liothyronine *on page 1222*

Sodium Acetate (SOW dee um AS e tate)

Pharmacologic Category Electrolyte Supplement, Parenteral

Use Sodium source in large volume I.V. fluids to prevent or correct hyponatremia in patients with restricted intake; used to counter acidosis through conversion to bicarbonate

Pregnancy Risk Factor C

Pregnancy Considerations Animal reproduction studies have not been conducted. Sodium requirements do not change during pregnancy (IOM, 2004).

Breast-Feeding Considerations Sodium is found in breast milk. Sodium requirements do not change during lactation (IOM, 2004).

Contraindications Hypernatremia and fluid retention

Warnings/Precautions Avoid extravasation, use with caution in patients with edema, heart failure, severe hepatic failure, or renal impairment. Use with caution in patients with acid/base alterations; contains acetate, monitor closely during acid/base correction. Close monitoring of serum sodium concentrations is needed to avoid hypernatremia. Solution for injection contains aluminum; use with caution in patients with impaired renal function and in premature infants.

Adverse Reactions 1% to 10%:

Cardiovascular: Thrombosis, hypervolemia

Dermatologic: Chemical cellulitis at injection site (extravasation)

Endocrine & metabolic: Hypernatremia, dilution of serum electrolytes, overhydration, hypokalemia, metabolic alkalosis, hypocalcemia

Gastrointestinal: Gastric distension, flatulence

Local: Phlebitis

Respiratory: Pulmonary edema

Miscellaneous: Congestive conditions

Drug Interactions

Metabolism/Transport Effects None known.

Avoid Concomitant Use There are no known interactions where it is recommended to avoid concomitant use.

Increased Effect/Toxicity There are no known significant interactions involving an increase in effect.

Decreased Effect There are no known significant interactions involving a decrease in effect.

Storage/Stability Store at room temperature of 20°C to 25°C (68°F to 77°F).

Dosage Sodium acetate is metabolized to bicarbonate on an equimolar basis outside the liver; administer in large volume I.V. fluids as a sodium source. Refer to Sodium Bicarbonate monograph.

Maintenance electrolyte requirements of sodium in parenteral nutrition solutions:

Daily requirements: 3-4 mEq/kg/24 hours or 25-40 mEq/1000 kcal/24 hours

Maximum: 100-150 mEq/24 hours

Dosage adjustment in renal impairment: No dosage adjustment provided in manufacturer's labeling. Use with caution.

Dosage adjustment in hepatic impairment: No dosage adjustment provided in manufacturer's labeling. Use with caution.

Dietary Considerations Sodium acetate anhydrous (2 mEq/mL): 1 mL = 164 mg sodium acetate anhydrous = 2 mEq of sodium (46 mg) and acetate (118 mg)

Administration Must be diluted prior to I.V. administration; infuse hypertonic solutions (>154 mEq/L) via a central line; maximum rate of administration: 1 mEq/kg/hour

Dosage Forms Excipient information presented when available (limited, particularly for generics); consult specific product labeling.

Solution, Intravenous, as anhydrous:

Generic: 2 mEq/mL (20 mL, 50 mL, 100 mL); 4 mEq/mL (50 mL, 100 mL)

◆ **Sodium Acid Carbonate** *see* Sodium Bicarbonate *on page 1912*

◆ **Sodium Acid Phosphate and Methenamine** *see* Methenamine and Sodium Acid Phosphate *on page 1319*

◆ **Sodium Artesunate** *see* Artesunate *on page 171*

◆ **Sodium Benzoate and Caffeine** *see* Caffeine *on page 309*

◆ **Sodium Benzoate and Sodium Phenylacetate** *see* Sodium Phenylacetate and Sodium Benzoate *on page 1922*

Sodium Bicarbonate (SOW dee um bye KAR bun ate)

Brand Names: U.S. Neut

Index Terms Baking Soda; $NaHCO_3$; Sodium Acid Carbonate; Sodium Hydrogen Carbonate

Pharmacologic Category Alkalinizing Agent; Antacid; Electrolyte Supplement, Oral; Electrolyte Supplement, Parenteral

Additional Appendix Information

Contrast Media Reactions, Premedication for Prophylaxis *on page 2373*

Use

Management of metabolic acidosis; gastric hyperacidity; as an alkalinization agent for the urine; treatment of hyperkalemia; management of overdose of certain drugs, including tricyclic antidepressants and aspirin

Neutralizing additive (dental use): Improves onset of analgesia and reduces injection site pain by adjusting lidocaine with epinephrine solution to a more physiologic pH.

Unlabeled Use Prevention of contrast-induced nephropathy (CIN)

Pregnancy Risk Factor C

Pregnancy Considerations Animal reproduction studies have not been conducted. The use of sodium bicarbonate in pregnant women for the management of cardiac arrest and metabolic acidosis is the same as in nonpregnant women (Campbell, 2009; Vanden Hoek, 2010). Antacids containing sodium bicarbonate should not be used during pregnancy due to their potential to cause metabolic alkalosis and fluid overload (Mahadevan, 2007).

Breast-Feeding Considerations Sodium is found in breast milk (IOM, 2004).

Contraindications

Alkalosis, hypernatremia, severe pulmonary edema, hypocalcemia, unknown abdominal pain

Neutralizing additive (dental use): Not for use as a systemic alkalizer

Warnings/Precautions Rapid administration in neonates and children <2 years of age has led to hypernatremia, decreased CSF pressure and intracranial hemorrhage. **Use of I.V. $NaHCO_3$ should be reserved for documented metabolic acidosis and for hyperkalemia-induced cardiac arrest.** Routine use in cardiac arrest is not recommended. Avoid extravasation, tissue necrosis can occur due to the hypertonicity of $NaHCO_3$. May cause sodium retention especially if renal function is impaired; not to be used in treatment of peptic ulcer; use with caution in patients with HF, edema, cirrhosis, or renal failure. Not the antacid of choice for the elderly because of sodium content and potential for systemic alkalosis.

Adverse Reactions Frequency not defined.

Cardiovascular: Cerebral hemorrhage, CHF (aggravated), edema

Central nervous system: Tetany

Gastrointestinal: Belching, flatulence (with oral), gastric distension

Endocrine & metabolic: Hypernatremia, hyperosmolality, hypocalcemia, hypokalemia, increased affinity of hemoglobin for oxygen-reduced pH in myocardial tissue necrosis when extravasated, intracranial acidosis, metabolic alkalosis, milk-alkali syndrome (especially with renal dysfunction)

Respiratory: Pulmonary edema

Drug Interactions

Metabolism/Transport Effects None known.

Avoid Concomitant Use

Avoid concomitant use of Sodium Bicarbonate with any of the following: PONATinib

Increased Effect/Toxicity

Sodium Bicarbonate may increase the levels/effects of: Alpha-/Beta-Agonists; Amphetamines; Calcium Polystyrene Sulfonate; Dexmethylphenidate; Flecainide; Memantine; Methylphenidate; QuiNIDine; QuiNINE

The levels/effects of Sodium Bicarbonate may be increased by: AcetaZOLAMIDE

Decreased Effect

Sodium Bicarbonate may decrease the levels/effects of: ACE Inhibitors; Anticonvulsants (Hydantoin); Antipsychotic Agents (Phenothiazines); Atazanavir; Bisacodyl; Bosutinib; Cefditoren; Cefpodoxime; Cefuroxime; Chloroquine; Corticosteroids (Oral); Dabigatran Etexilate; Dabrafenib; Dasatinib; Delavirdine; Elvitegravir; Erlotinib; Flecainide; Gabapentin; HMG-CoA Reductase Inhibitors; Hyoscyamine; Iron Salts; Isoniazid; Itraconazole; Ketoconazole (Systemic); Lithium; Mesalamine; Methenamine; Multivitamins/Minerals (with ADEK, Folate, Iron); Nilotinib; PenicillAMINE; Phosphate Supplements; PONATinib; Potassium Acid Phosphate; Protease Inhibitors; Rilpivirine; Riociguat; Sulpiride; Tetracycline Derivatives; Trientine; Vismodegib

Ethanol/Nutrition/Herb Interactions Herb/Nutraceutical: Concurrent doses with iron may decrease iron absorption.

Preparation for Administration

Prevention of contrast-induced nephropathy (unlabeled use): Remove 154 mL from 1000 mL bag of D_5W; replace with 154 mL of 8.4% sodium bicarbonate; resultant concentration is 154 mEq/L (Merten, 2004); more practically, institutions may remove 150 mL from 1000 mL bag of D_5W and replace with 150 mL of 8.4% sodium bicarbonate; resultant concentration is 150 mEq/L

Neutralizing additive (dental use): Add specified volume of 8.4% sodium bicarbonate directly with lidocaine and epinephrine injection and mix; use immediately after mixing.

Storage/Stability

Store injection at room temperature. Protect from heat and from freezing. Use only clear solutions.

Neutralizing additive (dental use): Store at 20°C to 25°C (68°F to 77°F).

Mechanism of Action

Dissociates to provide bicarbonate ion which neutralizes hydrogen ion concentration and raises blood and urinary pH

Neutralizing additive (dental use): Increases pH of lidocaine and epinephrine solution to improve tolerability and increase tissue uptake

Pharmacodynamics/Kinetics

Onset of action: Oral: Rapid; I.V.: 15 minutes

Duration: Oral: 8-10 minutes; I.V.: 1-2 hours

Absorption: Oral: Well absorbed

Excretion: Urine (<1%)

Dosage

Cardiac arrest (ACLS, 2010; PALS, 2010): **Routine use of $NaHCO_3$ is not recommended.** May be considered in the setting of prolonged cardiac arrest only after adequate alveolar ventilation has been established and effective cardiac compressions. **Note:** In some cardiac arrest situations (eg, metabolic acidosis, hyperkalemia, or tricyclic antidepressant overdose), sodium bicarbonate may be beneficial.

Infants and Children: I.V., I.O.: 1 mEq/kg/dose; repeat doses should be guided by arterial blood gases; children <2 years of age should receive 4.2% (0.5 mEq/mL) solution. **Note:** If I.O. route is used for administration and is subsequently used to obtain blood samples for acid-base analysis, results will be inaccurate.

Adults: I.V.: Initial: 1 mEq/kg/dose; repeat doses should be guided by arterial blood gases

Metabolic acidosis: Infants, Children, and Adults: Dosage should be based on the following formula if blood gases and pH measurements are available:

HCO_3^-(mEq) = 0.5 x weight (kg) x [24 - serum HCO_3^- (mEq/L)] **or** HCO_3^-(mEq) = 0.5 x weight (kg) x [desired increase in serum HCO_3^-(mEq/L)]

Administer $1/2$ dose initially, then remaining $1/2$ dose over the next 24 hours; monitor pH, serum HCO_3^-, and clinical status. **Note:** These equations provide an estimated replacement dose. The underlying cause and degree of acidosis may result in the need for larger or smaller replacement doses. In most cases, the initial goal of therapy is to target a pH of ~7.2 and a plasma bicarbonate level of ~10 mEq/L to prevent overalkalinization.

Note: If acid-base status is not available: Dose for older Children and Adults: 2-5 mEq/kg I.V. infusion over 4-8 hours; subsequent doses should be based on patient's acid-base status

Chronic renal failure: Oral: Initiate when plasma HCO_3^- <15 mEq/L

Children: 1-3 mEq/kg/day

Adults: Start with 20-36 mEq/day in divided doses, titrate to bicarbonate level of 18-20 mEq/L

Hyperkalemia (ACLS, 2010): Adults: I.V.: 50 mEq over 5 minutes (as appropriate, consider methods of enhancing potassium removal/excretion)

Renal tubular acidosis: Oral:

Distal:

Children: 2-3 mEq/kg/day

Adults: 0.5-2 mEq/kg/day in 4-5 divided doses

Proximal: Children and Adults: Initial: 5-10 mEq/kg/day; maintenance: Increase as required to maintain serum bicarbonate in the normal range

Urine alkalinization: Oral:

Children: 1-10 mEq (84-840 mg)/kg/day in divided doses every 4-6 hours; dose should be titrated to desired urinary pH

Adults: Initial: 48 mEq (4 g), then 12-24 mEq (1-2 g) every 4 hours; dose should be titrated to desired urinary pH; doses up to 16 g/day (200 mEq) in patients <60 years and 8 g (100 mEq) in patients >60 years

Antacid: Adults: Oral: 325 mg to 2 g 1-4 times/day

Neutralize lidocaine with epinephrine dental anesthetic: Children, Adolescents, and Adults: Neutralizing additive: Mix 10 parts anesthetic (lidocaine with epinephrine) to 1 part 8.4% sodium bicarbonate:

Add 0.18 mL sodium bicarbonate to 1.8 mL cartridge of lidocaine 2% with epinephrine 1:50,000 or 1:100,000

Add 2 mL sodium bicarbonate to 20 mL vial of lidocaine 2% with epinephrine 1:100,000

Add 3 mL sodium bicarbonate to 30 mL vial of lidocaine 2% with epinephrine 1:100,000

Add 5 mL sodium bicarbonate to 50 mL vial of lidocaine 2% with epinephrine 1:100,000

Prevention of contrast-induced nephropathy (unlabeled use): Adults: I.V. infusion: 154 mEq/L sodium bicarbonate in D_5W solution: 3 mL/kg/hour for 1 hour immediately before contrast injection, then 1mL/kg/hour during contrast exposure and for 6 hours after procedure

To prepare solution, remove 154 mL from 1000 mL bag of D_5W; replace with 154 mL of 8.4% sodium bicarbonate; resultant concentration is 154 mEq/L (Merten, 2004); more practically, institutions may remove 150 mL from 1000 mL bag of D_5W and replace with 150 mL of 8.4% sodium bicarbonate; resultant concentration is 150 mEq/L

Dietary Considerations Some products may contain sodium. Oral product should be taken 1-3 hours after meals.

Administration For I.V. administration to infants, use the 0.5 mEq/mL solution or dilute the 1 mEq/mL solution 1:1 with **sterile water**; for direct I.V. infusion in emergencies, administer slowly (maximum rate in infants: 10 mEq/minute); for infusion, dilute to a maximum concentration of 0.5 mEq/mL in dextrose solution and infuse over 2 hours (maximum rate of administration: 1 mEq/kg/hour)

Oral product should be administered 1-3 hours after meals.

Infiltration (dental use; Onpharma): Add specified volume of 8.4% sodium bicarbonate directly with lidocaine and epinephrine injection and mix; use immediately after mixing.

Dosage Forms Considerations

Sodium bicarbonate solution 4.2% [42 mg/mL] provides 0.5 mEq/mL each of sodium and bicarbonate

Sodium bicarbonate solution 7.5% [75 mg/mL] provides 0.9 mEq/mL each of sodium and bicarbonate

Sodium bicarbonate solution 8.4% [84 mg/mL] provides 1 mEq/mL each of sodium and bicarbonate

Dosage Forms Excipient information presented when available (limited, particularly for generics); consult specific product labeling.

Powder, Oral:

Generic: (1 g, 120 g, 454 g, 500 g, 1000 g, 2270 g, 2500 g, 12000 g, 45000 g)

Solution, Intravenous:

Neut: 4% (5 mL)

Generic: 4.2% (5 mL, 10 mL); 7.5% (50 mL); 8.4% (10 mL, 50 mL)

Tablet, Oral:

Generic: 325 mg, 650 mg

- **Sodium Bicarbonate and Omeprazole** *see* Omeprazole and Sodium Bicarbonate *on page 1508*
- **Sodium Biphosphate, Methenamine, Methylene Blue, Phenyl Salicylate, and Hyoscyamine** *see* Methenamine, Sodium Biphosphate, Phenyl Salicylate, Methylene Blue, and Hyoscyamine *on page 1320*

Sodium Chloride (SOW dee um KLOR ide)

Brand Names: U.S. 4-Way Saline [OTC]; Afrin Saline Nasal Mist [OTC]; Altachlore [OTC]; Altamist Spray [OTC]; Ayr Nasal Mist Allergy/Sinus [OTC]; Ayr Saline Nasal Drops [OTC]; Ayr Saline Nasal Gel [OTC]; Ayr Saline Nasal No-Drip [OTC]; AYR Saline Nasal Rinse [OTC]; Ayr Saline Nasal [OTC]; Ayr [OTC]; Baby Ayr Saline [OTC]; Broncho Saline [OTC]; Deep Sea Nasal Spray [OTC]; Entsol Nasal Wash [OTC]; Entsol Nasal [OTC]; Entsol [OTC]; Humist [OTC]; HyperSal; Little Noses Decongestant [OTC]; Muro 128 [OTC]; Na-Zone [OTC]; Nasal Moist [OTC]; Nebusal; Ocean Complete Sinus Rinse [OTC]; Ocean for Kids [OTC]; Ocean Nasal Spray [OTC]; Ocean Ultra Saline Mist [OTC]; Optics Eye Wash [OTC]; Pretz Irrigation [OTC]; Pretz [OTC]; Rhinaris [OTC]; Safe Wash [OTC]; Saline Flush ZR; Saline Mist Spray [OTC]; Saljet Rinse [OTC]; Saljet [OTC]; Sea Soft Nasal Mist [OTC]; Sea-Clens Wound Cleanser [OTC]; Sochlor [OTC]; Sodium Chloride Thermoject Sys; SwabFlush Saline Flush; Wound Wash Saline [OTC]

Index Terms Hypertonic Saline; NaCl; Normal Saline; Saline; Salt

Pharmacologic Category Electrolyte Supplement, Parenteral; Genitourinary Irrigant; Irrigant; Lubricant, Ocular; Sodium Salt

Additional Appendix Information

Contrast Media Reactions, Premedication for Prophylaxis *on page 2373*

Use

Parenteral: Restores sodium ion in patients with restricted oral intake (especially hyponatremia states or low salt syndrome).

Concentrated sodium chloride: Additive for parenteral fluid therapy

Hypertonic sodium chloride: For severe hyponatremia and hypochloremia

Hypotonic sodium chloride: Hydrating solution

Normal saline: Restores water/sodium losses

Ophthalmic: Reduces corneal edema

Inhalation: Restores moisture to pulmonary system; loosens and thins congestion caused by colds or allergies; diluent for bronchodilator solutions that require dilution before inhalation

Intranasal: Restores moisture to nasal membranes

Irrigation: Wound cleansing, irrigation, and flushing

Unlabeled Use Parenteral:

Hypertonic saline: Refractory elevated intracranial pressure (ICP) due to various etiologies (eg, subarachnoid hemorrhage, neoplasm); transtentorial herniation syndrome; traumatic brain injury with elevated ICP. **Note:** May be used in patients in whom mannitol may not be recommended (eg, renal failure).

Normal saline: Fluid resuscitation

Pregnancy Risk Factor C

Pregnancy Considerations Animal reproduction studies have not been conducted. Sodium requirements do not change during pregnancy (IOM, 2004). Nasal saline rinses may be used for the treatment of pregnancy rhinitis (Wallace, 2008)

Breast-Feeding Considerations Sodium is found in breast milk. Sodium requirements do not change during lactation (IOM, 2004).

Contraindications Hypersensitivity to sodium chloride or any component of the formulation; hypertonic uterus, hypernatremia, fluid retention

Warnings/Precautions The use of hypotonic saline solutions (eg, 0.225% sodium chloride) may result in hemolysis if administered rapidly and for prolonged periods. If hypotonic saline solutions become necessary, administration as D_5W/0.2% NaCl or 0.45% NaCl is recommended for most patients (eg, those without hyperglycemia). Use with caution in patients with HF, renal insufficiency, liver cirrhosis, hypertension, edema.

Administration of low sodium or sodium-free I.V. solutions may result in significant hyponatremia or water intoxication; monitor serum sodium concentration closely. In the treatment of acute hypernatremia (ie, development over a couple of hours), serum sodium concentration should be corrected no faster than 1-2 mEq/L per hour. If patient has been chronically hypernatremic, correct serum sodium no faster than 0.5 mEq/L per hour and by no more than 10-12 mEq/L in a given 24-hour period; use extreme caution since rapid correction may result in cerebral edema, herniation, coma, and death (Adrogue, 2000; Kraft, 2005).

When treating hyponatremia, rate of correction is dependent upon whether or not it is acute or chronic. Sodium toxicity (eg, osmotic demyelination syndrome) is almost exclusively related to how fast a sodium deficit is corrected; both rate and magnitude are extremely important. For patients with acute (<24 hours) or chronic (>48 hours), severe (<120 mEq/L) hyponatremia, a serum sodium concentration increase of 4-6 mEq/L within a 24-hour period is sufficient for most patients. In chronic severe hyponatremia, overcorrection risks iatrogenic osmotic demyelination syndrome. For patients with severe symptoms or other need for urgent correction, may increase by 4-6 mEq/L within the first 6 hours and postpone any further correction until the next day at a correction rate of 4-6 mEq/L per day. Choice of infusate sodium concentration is dependent upon the severity of the hyponatremia with more concentrated solutions (eg, 3% NaCl) for more severe cases; monitor serum sodium closely during administration (Sterns, 2013).

Do not use bacteriostatic sodium chloride in newborns since benzyl alcohol preservatives have been associated with toxicity. Wound Wash Saline is for single-patient use only.

Irrigants: For external use only; not for parenteral use. Do not use during electrosurgical procedures. Irrigating fluids may be absorbed into systemic circulation; monitor for fluid or solute overload.

Adverse Reactions Frequency not defined.

Cardiovascular: Congestive heart failure, transient hypotension (especially with adult administration of 23.4% NaCl)

Central nervous system: Central pontine myelinolysis (due to rapid correction of hyponatremia)

Endocrine & metabolic: Dilution of serum electrolytes, extravasation, hypernatremia, hypervolemia, hypokalemia, overhydration

Gastrointestinal: Nausea, vomiting (oral use)

Local: Thrombosis, phlebitis, extravasation

Respiratory: Bronchospasm (inhalation with hypertonic solutions), pulmonary edema

Drug Interactions

Metabolism/Transport Effects None known.

Avoid Concomitant Use

Avoid concomitant use of Sodium Chloride with any of the following: Tolvaptan

Increased Effect/Toxicity

Sodium Chloride may increase the levels/effects of: Tolvaptan

Decreased Effect

Sodium Chloride may decrease the levels/effects of: Lithium

Storage/Stability Store injection at room temperature; do not freeze. Protect from heat. Use only clear solutions.

Mechanism of Action Principal extracellular cation; functions in fluid and electrolyte balance, osmotic pressure control, and water distribution

Pharmacodynamics/Kinetics

Absorption: Oral: Rapid

Distribution: Widely distributed

Excretion: Primarily urine; also sweat, tears, saliva

Dosage

Children: I.V.: Hypertonic solutions (>0.9%) should only be used for the initial treatment of acute serious symptomatic hyponatremia or increased intracranial pressure in the setting of traumatic brain injury.

Maintenance: 3-4 mEq/kg/day; maximum: 100-150 mEq/day; dosage varies widely depending on clinical condition

Replacement: Determined by laboratory determinations mEq

Sodium deficiency (mEq/kg) = [% dehydration (L/kg)/100 x 70 (mEq/L)] + [0.6 (L/kg) x (140 - serum sodium) (mEq/L)]

Hypovolemic septic shock, initial fluid resuscitation (unlabeled use): I.V.: Normal saline (0.9% NaCl): Up to 20 mL/kg/dose over 5-10 minutes; titrate to hypotension reversal, increasing urine output, and attainment of normal capillary refill, peripheral pulses, and level of consciousness (Dellinger, 2013)

Increased intracranial pressure (unlabeled use): Hypertonic saline (3%): 0.1-1 mL/kg/hour continuous infusion titrated to maintain ICP <20 mm Hg (Addleson, 2003)

Children ≥2 years and Adults:

Intranasal: 2-3 sprays in each nostril as needed

Irrigation: Spray affected area

Children and Adults: Inhalation: Bronchodilator diluent: 1-3 sprays (1-3 mL) to dilute bronchodilator solution in nebulizer prior to administration

Adults:

Refractory elevated ICP due to various etiologies (eg, subarachnoid hemorrhage, trauma, neoplasm), transtentorial herniation syndromes (unlabeled use): I.V.: Hypertonic saline: 23.4% (30-60 mL) given over 2-20 minutes administered via central venous access only (Koenig, 2008; Suarez, 1998; Ware, 2005)

Severe sepsis, initial fluid resuscitation (unlabeled use): I.V.: Normal saline (0.9% NaCl): Minimum of 30 mL/kg. **Note:** Administer within 3 hours of sepsis recognition for hypotension or lactate ≥4 mmol/L (≥36 mg/dL). Some patients may require more rapid administration and/or greater amount of fluid for complete resuscitation (Dellinger, 2013).

Subarachnoid hemorrhage with hyponatremia (ie, ≤135 mEq/L) to enhance cerebral perfusion (unlabeled use): I.V.: Hypertonic saline: 3% sodium chloride/acetate (50:50 mixture) 100-200 mL/hour administered via central venous catheter; titrate to clinical response up to a maximum serum sodium between 150-160 mEq/L (achieved at a rate of 0.5-1 mEq/L/hour) (Suarez, 1999)

Traumatic brain injury with elevated ICP (unlabeled use): I.V.: Hypertonic saline: **Note:** Optimal dose has not been established; due to insufficient evidence, the Brain Trauma Foundation guidelines (Bratton, 2007) do not make specific recommendations on the use of hypertonic saline for the treatment of traumatic intracranial hypertension. Clinical trials are small; few are prospective. **Some concentrations may not be commercially available; administer via central venous catheter;** protocols include:

3%: 300 mL administered over 20 minutes when ICP values exceed 20 mm Hg (Huang, 2006)

7.2%: 1.5 mL/kg administered over 15 minutes when ICP values exceed 15 mm Hg (Munar, 2000)

7.5%: 2 mL/kg administered over 20 minutes when ICP values exceed 25 mm Hg (Vialet, 2003)

23.4%: 30 mL administered over 2 minutes (Ware, 2005) **or** over >30 minutes when ICP values exceed 20 mm Hg (Kerwin, 2009)

GU irrigant: 1-3 L/day by intermittent irrigation

Replacement I.V.: Determined by laboratory determinations mEq

Hyponatremia: I.V.: To correct acute (<24 hours) or chronic (>48 hours), severe (<120 mEq/L) hyponatremia: In general, a serum sodium concentration increase of 4-6 mEq/L within a 24-hour period is sufficient to improve most symptoms of hyponatremia. In chronic severe hyponatremia, overcorrection risks iatrogenic osmotic demyelination syndrome. For patients with severe symptoms or other need for urgent correction, one approach is to increase serum sodium concentration by 4-6 mEq/L within the first 6 hours and postpone any further correction until the next day at a correction rate of 4-6 mEq/L per day. Choice of sodium correction fluid concentration is dependent upon the severity of the hyponatremia with more concentrated solutions (eg, 3% NaCl) for more severe cases; monitor serum sodium closely during administration (Sterns, 2013).

Chloride maintenance electrolyte requirement in parenteral nutrition: I.V.: As needed to maintain acid-base balance with parenteral nutrition; use equal amounts of chloride and acetate to maintain balance and adjust ratio based on individual patient needs (Mirtallo, 2004).

Sodium maintenance electrolyte requirement in parenteral nutrition: I.V.: 1-2 mEq/kg/24 hours; customize amounts based on individual patient needs (Mirtallo, 2004).

Ophthalmic:

Ointment: Apply once daily or more often

Solution: Instill 1-2 drops into affected eye(s) every 3-4 hours

Administration

Irrigation solution: Do not warm >66°C (150°F); not for I.V. use. Wound Wash Saline: Before use, expel a short stream into air to clear nozzle.

I.V.: ≥3% solutions: Administration through a central line is recommended due to high osmolarity and tonicity

Monitoring Parameters Serum sodium, potassium, chloride, and bicarbonate concentrations; I & O, weight

Reference Range Serum/plasma sodium concentration:

Neonates:

Full-term: 133-142 mEq/L

Premature: 132-140 mEq/L

Children ≥2 months to Adults: 135-145 mEq/L

Additional Information

Normal saline (0.9%) = 154 mEq/L; 3% NaCl = 513 mEq/L; 5% NaCl = 856 mEq/L

Tablet 1g = 17.1 mEq

Dosage Forms Considerations

1 g sodium chloride = elemental sodium 393.3 mg = 17.1 mEq sodium = sodium 17.1 mmol

Dosage Forms Excipient information presented when available (limited, particularly for generics); consult specific product labeling.

Aerosol Solution, Inhalation:

Broncho Saline: 0.9% (90 mL, 240 mL)

Aerosol Solution, Nasal [preservative free]:

Ocean Complete Sinus Rinse: (177 mL) [drug free]

Gel, Nasal:

Ayr Saline Nasal: (14.1 g) [contains aloe barbadensis, brilliant blue fcf (fd&c blue #1), methylparaben, propylparaben, soybean oil]

Ayr Saline Nasal No-Drip: (22 mL) [contains aloe barbadensis, benzalkonium chloride, benzyl alcohol, soybean oil]

Entsol Nasal: (20 g)

Rhinaris: 0.2% (28.4 g) [contains benzalkonium chloride, propylene glycol]

Liquid, External:

Sea-Clens Wound Cleanser: (355 mL)

Nebulization Solution, Inhalation:

Generic: 0.9% (3 mL)

Nebulization Solution, Inhalation [preservative free]:

HyperSal: 3.5% (4 mL) [latex free]

HyperSal: 7% (4 mL)

Nebusal: 3% (4 mL); 6% (4 mL)

Generic: 0.9% (3 mL, 5 mL, 15 mL); 3% (4 mL, 15 mL); 7% (4 mL); 10% (4 mL, 15 mL)

Ointment, Ophthalmic:

Altachlore: 5% (3.5 g)

Muro 128: 5% (3.5 g)

Generic: 5% (3.5 g)

Packet, Nasal [preservative free]:

AYR Saline Nasal Rinse: 1.57 g (50 ea, 100 ea) [iodine free]

Solution, External:

Saljet: 0.9% (30 mL)

Wound Wash Saline: 0.9% (210 mL)

Solution, External [preservative free]:

Safe Wash: 0.9% (210 mL) [drug free, latex free]

Saljet Rinse: 0.9% (30 mL)

Solution, Injection:

Sodium Chloride Thermoject Sys: 0.9% (10 mL)

Generic: 0.9% (2 mL, 2.5 mL, 3 mL, 5 mL, 10 mL, 20 mL, 30 mL, 100 mL); 23.4% (20 mL, 40 mL, 250 mL)

Solution, Injection [preservative free]:

Generic: 0.9% (1 mL, 2 mL, 2.5 mL, 3 mL, 5 mL, 10 mL, 20 mL, 30 mL, 50 mL)

Solution, Intravenous:

SwabFlush Saline Flush: 0.9% (10 mL)

Generic: 0.45% (25 mL, 50 mL, 100 mL, 250 mL, 500 mL, 1000 mL); 0.9% (2.5 mL, 3 mL, 10 mL, 25 mL, 50 mL, 100 mL, 150 mL, 250 mL, 500 mL, 1000 mL); 3% (500 mL); 5% (500 mL); 14.6% (30 mL, 100 mL, 200 mL, 250 mL)

Solution, Intravenous [preservative free]:

Saline Flush ZR: 0.9% (2.5 mL, 5 mL, 10 mL) [latex free]

Generic: 0.9% (1 mL, 2 mL, 2.5 mL, 3 mL, 5 mL, 10 mL)

Solution, Irrigation:

Generic: 0.9% (250 mL, 500 mL, 1000 mL, 1500 mL, 2000 mL, 3000 mL, 4000 mL, 5000 mL)

Solution, Nasal:
4-Way Saline: (29.6 mL)
Afrin Saline Nasal Mist: 0.65% (30 mL, 45 mL)
Altamist Spray: 0.65% (45 mL, 60 mL)
Ayr: 0.65% (50 mL)
Ayr Nasal Mist Allergy/Sinus: 2.65% (50 mL) [contains benzalkonium chloride]
Ayr Saline Nasal Drops: 0.65% (50 mL)
Baby Ayr Saline: 0.65% (30 mL)
Deep Sea Nasal Spray: 0.65% (44 mL) [contains benzalkonium chloride]
Entsol: (30 mL)
Humist: 0.65% (45 mL)
Little Noses Decongestant: 0.125% (15 mL) [alcohol free; contains benzalkonium chloride, polyethylene glycol]
Na-Zone: 0.65% (59 mL)
Nasal Moist: 0.65% (15 mL, 45 mL)
Ocean for Kids: 0.65% (37.5 mL) [alcohol free, drug free; contains benzalkonium chloride]
Ocean Nasal Spray: 0.65% (45 mL, 104 mL, 480 mL) [contains benzalkonium chloride]
Pretz: (50 mL, 946 mL)
Pretz Irrigation: (237 mL)
Rhinaris: 0.2% (30 mL) [contains benzalkonium chloride, propylene glycol]
Saline Mist Spray: 0.65% (45 mL) [contains benzalkonium chloride]
Sea Soft Nasal Mist: 0.65% (45 mL)
Generic: 0.65% (44 mL, 45 mL)
Solution, Nasal [preservative free]:
Entsol Nasal: 3% (100 mL) [drug free]
Entsol Nasal Wash: (237 mL)
Ocean Ultra Saline Mist: (90 mL) [drug free]
Solution, Ophthalmic:
Altachlore: 5% (15 mL, 30 mL)
Muro 128: 2% (15 mL); 5% (15 mL, 30 mL)
Sochlor: 5% (15 mL)
Generic: 5% (15 mL)
Solution, Ophthalmic [preservative free]:
Optics Eye Wash: 0.9% (20 mL)
Swab, Nasal:
Ayr Saline Nasal Gel: (20 ea) [contains methylparaben, propylparaben, soybean oil, trolamine (triethanolamine)]
Tablet, Oral:
Generic: 1 g

◆ **Sodium Chloride Thermoject Sys** *see* Sodium Chloride *on page 1914*

Sodium Chondroitin Sulfate and Sodium Hyaluronate

(SOW de um kon DROY tin SUL fate & SOW de um hye al yoor ON ate)

Brand Names: U.S. DisCoVisc®; Viscoat®

Index Terms Chondroitin Sulfate and Sodium Hyaluronate; Sodium Hyaluronate and Chondroitin Sulfate

Pharmacologic Category Ophthalmic Agent, Viscoelastic

Use Ophthalmic surgical aid in the anterior segment during cataract extraction and intraocular lens implantation

Dosage Ophthalmic: Adults: Carefully introduce (using a 27-gauge cannula) into anterior chamber during surgery

Dosage adjustment in renal impairment: No dosage adjustment provided in manufacturer's labeling.

Dosage adjustment in hepatic impairment: No dosage adjustment provided in manufacturer's labeling.

Additional Information Complete prescribing information should be consulted for additional detail.

Dosage Forms Excipient information presented when available (limited, particularly for generics); consult specific product labeling.

Injection, solution, intraocular:
DisCoVisc®: Sodium chondroitin sulfate ≤4% and sodium hyaluronate ≤1.7% (1 mL) [provided in a kit which also contains 27-gauge cannula and cannula locking ring]
Viscoat®: Sodium chondroitin sulfate ≤4% and sodium hyaluronate ≤3% (0.5 mL, 0.75 mL) [packaged with 27-gauge cannula and cannula locking ring]

Sodium Citrate and Citric Acid

(SOW dee um SIT rate & SI trik AS id)

Brand Names: U.S. Cytra-2; Oracit®; Shohl's Solution (Modified)

Brand Names: Canada PMS-Dicitrate

Index Terms Bicitra; Citric Acid and Sodium Citrate; Modified Shohl's Solution

Pharmacologic Category Alkalinizing Agent, Oral

Use Treatment of metabolic acidosis; alkalinizing agent in conditions where long-term maintenance of an alkaline urine is desirable

Pregnancy Risk Factor Not established

Dosage Oral: Systemic alkalization:
Infants and Children: 2-3 mEq/kg/day in divided doses 3-4 times/day **or** 5-15 mL with water after meals and at bedtime
Adults: 10-30 mL with water after meals and at bedtime

Dosage adjustment in renal impairment: Use is contraindicated.

Dosage adjustment in hepatic impairment: No dosage adjustment provided in manufacturer's labeling.

Additional Information Complete prescribing information should be consulted for additional detail.

Dosage Forms Considerations
Each mL provides 1 mEq sodium, and is equivalent to 1 mEq bicarbonate

Dosage Forms Excipient information presented when available (limited, particularly for generics); consult specific product labeling.

Solution, oral:
Generic: Sodium citrate 500 mg and citric acid 334 mg per 5 mL (480 mL)
Cytra-2: Sodium citrate 500 mg and citric acid 334 mg per 5 mL (480 mL) [alcohol free, dye free, sugar free; contains propylene glycol and sodium benzoate; grape flavor]
Oracit®: Sodium citrate 490 mg and citric acid 640 mg per 5 mL (15 mL, 30 mL, 500 mL, 3840 mL)
Shohl's Solution (Modified): Sodium citrate 500 mg and citric acid 300 mg per 5 mL (480 mL) [contains alcohol]

◆ **Sodium Citrate, Citric Acid, and Potassium Citrate** *see* Citric Acid, Sodium Citrate, and Potassium Citrate *on page 443*
◆ **Sodium Diuril** *see* Chlorothiazide *on page 411*
◆ **Sodium Edecrin** *see* Ethacrynic Acid *on page 782*
◆ **Sodium Edecrin® (Can)** *see* Ethacrynic Acid *on page 782*
◆ **Sodium Etidronate** *see* Etidronate *on page 798*
◆ **Sodium Ferric Gluconate** *see* Ferric Gluconate *on page 853*
◆ **Sodium Ferric Gluconate Complex** *see* Ferric Gluconate *on page 853*
◆ **Sodium Fluorescein** *see* Fluorescein *on page 880*
◆ **Sodium Fluoride** *see* Fluoride *on page 880*

Sodium Glycerophosphate Pentahydrate

(SOE dee um glis er oh FOS fate pen ta HYE drate)

Index Terms Glycophos

Pharmacologic Category Electrolyte Supplement, Parenteral

Use Supplement in intravenous nutrition to meet the requirements of phosphate

Unlabeled Use General phosphate repletion during sodium phosphate and potassium phosphate shortages

Dosage Note: When converting from inorganic phosphate products (ie, sodium phosphate and potassium phosphate), maintain the same mmol amount of phosphate. Doses are listed as mmol of phosphate. Sodium glycerophosphate pentahydrate 306.1 mg = sodium glycerophosphate 216 mg = phosphate 1 **mmol**. Sodium glycerophosphate pentahydrate will provide 2 mEq of sodium for every 1 mmol of phosphate delivered.

Phosphate replacement, parenteral nutrition: Manufacturer's labeling: I.V.:

Infants: 1-1.5 mmol/kg per day admixed within parenteral nutrition solution. Dosage should be individualized.

Adults: 10-20 mmol per day admixed within parenteral nutrition solution. Dosage should be individualized.

Phosphate repletion, general (unlabeled use):

Caution: With orders for I.V. phosphate, there is considerable confusion associated with the use of millimoles (mmol) versus milliequivalents (mEq) to express the phosphate requirement. The most reliable method of ordering I.V. phosphate is by millimoles.

Acute treatment of hypophosphatemia: I.V.: It is difficult to provide concrete guidelines for the treatment of severe hypophosphatemia because the extent of total body deficits and response to therapy are difficult to predict. Aggressive doses of phosphate may result in a transient serum elevation followed by redistribution into intracellular compartments or bone tissue. It is recommended that repletion of severe hypophosphatemia be done I.V. because large doses of oral phosphate may cause diarrhea and intestinal absorption may be unreliable. Intermittent I.V. infusion should be reserved for severe depletion situations; requires continuous cardiac monitoring. Guidelines differ based on degree of illness, need/use of TPN, and severity of hypophosphatemia. Obese patients and/or severe renal impairment were excluded from phosphate supplement trials. **Note:** 1 mmol phosphate = 31 mg phosphorus; 1 mg phosphorus = 0.032 mmol phosphate.

There are no prospective studies of parenteral phosphate replacement in children. **The following weight-based guidelines for adult dosing may be cautiously employed in pediatric patients.** Guidelines differ based on degree of illness, use of TPN, and severity of hypophosphatemia.

General replacement guidelines (Lentz, 1978):

Low dose, serum phosphorus losses are recent and uncomplicated: 0.08 mmol/kg over 6 hours

Intermediate dose, serum phosphorus level 0.5-1 mg/dL (0.16-0.32 mmol/L): 0.16-0.24 mmol/kg over 6 hours

Note: The initial dose may be increased by 25% to 50% if the patient is symptomatic secondary to hypophosphatemia, and lowered by 25% to 50% if the patient is hypercalcemic.

Critically-ill adult patients receiving concurrent enteral/parenteral nutrition (Brown, 2006; Clark, 1995): **Note:** Round doses to the nearest 7.5 mmol for ease of preparation. If administering with phosphate-containing parenteral nutrition, do not exceed 15 mmol/L within parenteral nutrition. May use adjusted body weight for patients weighing >130% of ideal body weight (and BMI <40 kg/m^2) by using [IBW + 0.25 (ABW-IBW)]:

Low dose, serum phosphorus level 2.3-3 mg/dL (0.74-0.96 mmol/L): 0.16-0.32 mmol/kg over 4-6 hours

Intermediate dose, serum phosphorus level 1.6-2.2 mg/dL (0.51-0.71 mmol/L): 0.32-0.64 mmol/kg over 4-6 hours

High dose, serum phosphorus <1.5 mg/dL (<0.5 mmol/L): 0.64-1 mmol/kg over 8-12 hours

Parenteral nutrition: I.V.:

Infants and Children: 0.5-2 mmol/kg/24 hours (Mirtallo, 2004 [ASPEN guidelines])

Children >50 kg and Adolescents: 10-40 mmol/24 hours (Mirtallo, 2004 [ASPEN guidelines])

Adults: 10-15 mmol/1000 kcal (Hicks, 2001) **or** 20-40 mmol/24 hours (Mirtallo, 2004 [ASPEN guidelines])

Dosage adjustment in renal impairment: No dosage adjustment provided in manufacturer's labeling (has not been studied); use with caution since phosphate excretion is primarily renal.

Dosage adjustment in hepatic impairment: No dosage adjustment provided in manufacturer's labeling (has not been studied); however, phosphate excretion is primarily renal

Additional Information Complete prescribing information should be consulted for additional detail.

◆ **Sodium Hyaluronate** *see* Hyaluronate and Derivatives *on page 1000*

◆ **Sodium Hyaluronate and Chondroitin Sulfate** *see* Sodium Chondroitin Sulfate and Sodium Hyaluronate *on page 1917*

◆ **Sodium Hydrogen Carbonate** *see* Sodium Bicarbonate *on page 1912*

Sodium Hypochlorite Solution

(SOW dee um hye poe KLOR ite soe LOO shun)

Brand Names: U.S. Di-Dak-Sol [OTC]; H-Chlor 12 [OTC]; HySept [OTC]

Index Terms Modified Dakin's Solution

Pharmacologic Category Disinfectant, Antibacterial (Topical)

Use

Atrapro™ Dermal (0.004%): Management (via debridement) of wounds such as stage I-IV pressure ulcers; partial and full thickness wounds; diabetic foot ulcers; post surgical and donor sites; first- and second-degree burns

Dakin's Solution (0.125%, 0.25%, 0.5%); Di-Dak-Sol (0.0125%): Prevention/treatment of skin and tissue infections, cuts, abrasions, skin ulcers; pre- and postsurgery

Dosage Children and Adults:

Atrapro™ Dermal spray: Apply to affected area 3 times daily.

Dakin's solution, Di-Dak-Sol: Topical via irrigation:

Lightly-to-moderately exudative wounds: Apply once daily.

Highly exudative or contaminated wounds: Apply twice daily.

Additional Information Complete prescribing information should be consulted for additional detail.

Dosage Forms Excipient information presented when available (limited, particularly for generics); consult specific product labeling.

Solution, External:

Di-Dak-Sol: 0.0125% (473 mL)

H-Chlor 12: 0.125% (473 mL)

HySept: 0.25% (473 mL); 0.5% (473 mL)

Generic: 0.125% (473 mL); 0.25% (473 mL); 0.5% (473 mL)

◆ **Sodium Hyposulfate** *see* Sodium Thiosulfate *on page 1931*

◆ **Sodium Nafcillin** *see* Nafcillin *on page 1417*

Sodium Nitrite (SOW dee um NYE trite)

Pharmacologic Category Antidote

Use **Cyanide poisoning:** Treatment of acute, life-threatening cyanide poisoning in combination with sodium thiosulfate. Consider consultation with a poison control center at 1-800-222-1222.

Unlabeled Use Treatment of hydrogen sulfide exposure

Pregnancy Risk Factor C

Pregnancy Considerations Teratogenic effects have been observed following maternal exposure to high concentrations of sodium nitrite in drinking water. Teratogenic effects were not observed in animal reproduction studies of sodium nitrite. Embryotoxic and nonteratogenic effects were observed in animal reproduction studies of sodium nitrite. Methemoglobin reductase is lower in the fetus compared to adults and may result in adverse effects due to nitrite-induced prenatal hypoxia. In general, medications used as antidotes should take into consideration the health and prognosis of the mother; antidotes should be administered to pregnant women if there is a clear indication for use and should not be withheld because of fears of teratogenicity (Bailey, 2003).

Breast-Feeding Considerations It is not known if sodium nitrite is excreted in breast milk. The manufacturer recommends that caution be exercised when administering sodium nitrite to nursing women.

Contraindications There are no contraindications listed within the manufacturer's labeling.

Warnings/Precautions [U.S. Boxed Warning]: Sodium nitrite may cause methemoglobin formation and severe hypotension resulting in diminished oxygen-carrying capacity; serious adverse effects may occur at doses less than twice the recommended therapeutic dose. Monitor for adequate perfusion and oxygenation; ensure patient is euvolemic. Use with caution in patients where the diagnosis of cyanide poisoning is uncertain, patients with pre-existing diminished oxygen or cardiovascular reserve (eg, smoke inhalation victims, anemia, substantial blood loss, and cardiac or respiratory compromise), in patients at greater risk for developing methemoglobinemia (eg, congenital methemoglobin reductase deficiency), and in patients who may be susceptible to injury from vasodilation; the use of hydroxocobalamin is recommended in these patients. Sodium nitrite is generally discontinued for methemoglobin levels >30%. Use with caution with concomitant medications known to cause methemoglobinemia (eg, nitroglycerin, phenazopyridine). Due to the risk for serious adverse effects, use with caution in patients where the diagnosis of cyanide poisoning is uncertain. However, if clinical suspicion of cyanide poisoning is high, treatment should not be delayed. Signs of cyanide poisoning may include altered mental status, cardiovascular collapse, chest tightness, mydriasis, nausea/vomiting, dyspnea, hyper-/hypotension, plasma lactate ≥8 mmol/L. Treatment of cyanide poisoning should include external decontamination and supportive therapy. Collection of pretreatment blood cyanide concentrations does not preclude administration and should not delay administration in the emergency management of highly suspected or confirmed cyanide toxicity. Pretreatment levels may be useful as postinfusion levels may be inaccurate. Monitor patients for return of symptoms for 24-48 hours; repeat treatment (one-half the original dose) should be administered if symptoms return. Fire victims and patients with cyanide poisoning related to smoke inhalation may present with both cyanide and carbon monoxide poisoning. In these patients, the induction of methemoglobinemia (due to sodium nitrite) is contraindicated until carbon monoxide levels return to normal due to the risk of tissue hypoxia. Methemoglobinemia decreases the oxygen-carrying capacity of hemoglobin and the presence of carbon monoxide prevents hemoglobin from releasing oxygen to the tissues. In this scenario, sodium thiosulfate may be used alone to promote the clearance of cyanide. Hydroxocobalamin, however, should be considered to avoid the nitrite-related problems and because sodium thiosulfate has a slow onset of action. Consider consultation with a poison control center at 1-800-222-1222.

Potentially significant drug-drug interactions may exist, requiring dose or frequency adjustment, additional monitoring, and/or selection of alternative therapy. Patients with anemia will form more methemoglobin; dosage reduction in proportion to oxygen-carrying capacity is recommended. Patients with G6PD deficiency are at an increased risk for hemolytic crisis following sodium nitrite administration; consider alternative treatment options if possible. Monitor for an acute drop in hematocrit; exchange transfusion may be necessary. Use with caution in renal impairment and in the elderly.

Methemoglobin reductase, which is responsible for converting methemoglobin back to hemoglobin, has reduced activity in pediatric patients. In addition, infants and young children have some proportion of fetal hemoglobin which forms methemoglobin more readily than adult hemoglobin. Therefore, pediatric patients (eg, neonates and infants <6 months of age) are more susceptible to excessive nitrite-induced methemoglobinemia. Hydroxocobalamin will circumvent this problem and may be a more effective and rapid alternative. Nitrites should be avoided in pregnant patients due to fetal hemoglobin's susceptibility to oxidative stress.

Adverse Reactions

Cardiovascular: Arrhythmias, cyanosis, flushing, hypotension, palpitations, syncope, tachycardia

Central nervous system: Anxiety, coma, confusion, dizziness, fatigue, headache, lightheadedness, seizure

Dermatologic: Urticaria

Endocrine & metabolic: Acidosis

Gastrointestinal: Abdominal pain, nausea, vomiting

Hematologic: Methemoglobinemia

Local: Injection site tingling

Neuromuscular & skeletal: Numbness, paresthesia, weakness

Ocular: Blurred vision

Respiratory: Dyspnea, tachypnea

Miscellaneous: Diaphoresis

Drug Interactions

Metabolism/Transport Effects None known.

Avoid Concomitant Use There are no known interactions where it is recommended to avoid concomitant use.

Increased Effect/Toxicity

Sodium Nitrite may increase the levels/effects of: Prilocaine

The levels/effects of Sodium Nitrite may be increased by: Methemoglobinemia Associated Agents; Nitric Oxide

Decreased Effect There are no known significant interactions involving a decrease in effect.

Storage/Stability Store at 20°C to 25°C (68°F to 77°F); excursions permitted to 15°C to 30°C (59°F to 86°F); do not freeze. Protect from direct light.

Mechanism of Action Sodium nitrite promotes the formation of methemoglobin which competes with cytochrome oxidase for the cyanide ion. Cyanide combines with methemoglobin to form cyanomethemoglobin, thereby freeing the cytochrome oxidase and allowing aerobic metabolism to continue.

Pharmacodynamics/Kinetics

Onset: Peak effect: Methemoglobinemia: 30-60 minutes

Duration of action: Methemoglobinemia: ~55 minutes

Metabolism: To ammonia and other metabolites

Excretion: Urine (~40% as unchanged drug)

Dosage Cyanide poisoning: I.V.: **Note:** Given in conjunction with sodium thiosulfate. Administer sodium nitrite first, followed immediately by the administration of sodium thiosulfate. Sodium nitrite is generally discontinued for methemoglobin levels >30%.

Children: 6 mg/kg (0.2 mL/kg or 6-8 mL/m^2 of a 3% solution); maximum dose: 300 mg (10 mL of a 3% solution); may repeat at one-half the original dose if symptoms of cyanide toxicity return

Adults: 300 mg (10 mL of a 3% solution); may repeat at one-half the original dose if symptoms of cyanide toxicity return

Alternatively, in patients who are unable to tolerate significant methemoglobinemia (eg, patients with comorbidities that compromise oxygen delivery, such as heart disease, lung disease), dosing may be based on hemoglobin levels (when rapid bedside testing is available) to prevent fatal methemoglobinemia; see table (Berlin, 1970):

Hemoglobin Level (g/dL)	Dose of 3% Sodium Nitrite Solution (maximum dose: 10 mL)
7	0.19 mL/kg
8	0.22 mL/kg
9	0.25 mL/kg
10	0.27 mL/kg
11	0.3 mL/kg
12	0.33 mL/kg
13	0.36 mL/kg
14	0.39 mL/kg

Note: Monitor the patient for 24-48 hours; if symptoms return, repeat sodium nitrite and sodium thiosulfate at one-half the original dose.

Elderly: Refer to adult dosing; use with caution due to the likelihood of decreased renal function

Dosage adjustment in renal impairment: No dosage adjustment provided in the manufacturer's labeling; however, renal elimination of sodium nitrite is significant and risk of adverse effects may be increased in patients with renal impairment.

Dosage adjustment in hepatic impairment: No dosage adjustment provided in manufacturer's labeling (has not been studied).

Administration Administer via slow I.V. injection (2.5-5 mL/minute) as soon as possible after diagnosis of acute, life-threatening cyanide poisoning; follow immediately with the administration of sodium thiosulfate. Decrease rate of infusion in the event of significant hypotension.

Monitoring Parameters Monitor for at least 24-48 hours after administration; blood pressure and heart rate during and after infusion; hemoglobin/hematocrit; co-oximetry; serum lactate levels; venous-arterial PO_2 gradient; serum methemoglobin and oxyhemoglobin. Pretreatment cyanide levels may be useful diagnostically.

Dosage Forms Excipient information presented when available (limited, particularly for generics); consult specific product labeling.

Solution, Intravenous:

Generic: 30 mg/mL (10 mL)

Sodium Nitrite and Sodium Thiosulfate

(SOW dee um NYE trite & SOW dee um thye oh SUL fate)

Brand Names: U.S. Nithiodote

Index Terms Sodium Thiosulfate and Sodium Nitrite

Pharmacologic Category Antidote

Use Acute, life-threatening cyanide poisoning

Pregnancy Risk Factor C

Pregnancy Considerations Teratogenic effects have been observed following maternal exposure to high concentrations of sodium nitrite in drinking water. Teratogenic effects were not observed in animal reproduction studies of sodium nitrite or sodium thiosulfate. Embryotoxic and nonteratogenic effects were observed in animal reproduction studies of sodium nitrite. Methemoglobin reductase is lower in the fetus compared to adults and may result in adverse effects due to nitrite-induced prenatal hypoxia. There are no adequate and well-controlled studies of Nithiodote™ in pregnant women. In general, medications used as antidotes should take into consideration the health and prognosis of the mother; antidotes should be administered to pregnant women if there is a clear indication for use and should not be withheld because of fears of teratogenicity (Bailey, 2003).

Contraindications There are no contraindications listed within the manufacturer's labeling.

Warnings/Precautions [U.S. Boxed Warning]: Sodium nitrite may cause methemoglobin formation and severe hypotension resulting in diminished oxygen-carrying capacity; serious adverse effects may occur at doses less than twice the recommended therapeutic dose. Monitor for adequate perfusion and oxygenation; ensure patient is euvolemic. Use with caution in patients where the diagnosis of cyanide poisoning is uncertain, patients with pre-existing diminished oxygen or cardiovascular reserve (eg, smoke inhalation victims, anemia, substantial blood loss, and cardiac or respiratory compromise), in patients at greater risk for developing methemoglobinemia (eg, congenital methemoglobin reductase deficiency), and in patients who may be susceptible to injury from vasodilation; the use of hydroxocobalamin is recommended in these patients. Use with caution with concomitant medications known to cause methemoglobinemia (eg, nitroglycerin, phenazopyridine). Collection of pretreatment blood cyanide concentrations does not preclude administration and should not delay administration in the emergency management of highly suspected or confirmed cyanide toxicity. Pretreatment levels may be useful as postinfusion levels may be inaccurate. Treatment of cyanide poisoning should include external decontamination and supportive therapy. Monitor patients for return of symptoms for 24-48 hours; repeat treatment should be administered if symptoms return. Fire victims and patients with cyanide poisoning related to smoke inhalation may present with both cyanide and carbon monoxide poisoning. In these patients, the induction of methemoglobinemia (due to amyl nitrite, sodium nitrite) is contraindicated until carbon monoxide levels return to normal due to the risk of tissue hypoxia. Methemoglobinemia decreases the oxygen-carrying capacity of hemoglobin and the presence of carbon monoxide prevents hemoglobin from releasing oxygen to the tissues. In this scenario, sodium thiosulfate may be used alone to promote the clearance of cyanide. Hydroxocobalamin, however, should be considered to avoid the nitrite-related problems and because sodium thiosulfate has a slow onset of action. Consider consultation with a poison control center at 1-800-222-1222.

Concurrent use of antihypertensives, diuretics, and phosphodiesterase-5 enzyme (PDE5) inhibitors should be done with caution. Patients with anemia will form more methemoglobin; dosage reduction in proportion to oxygen-carrying capacity is recommended. Patients with G6PD deficiency are at an increased risk for hemolytic crisis following sodium nitrite administration; monitor for an acute drop in hematocrit. The presence of sulfite hypersensitivity should not preclude the use of this medication.

Methemoglobin reductase, which is responsible for converting methemoglobin back to hemoglobin, has reduced activity in pediatric patients. In addition, infants and young children have some proportion of fetal hemoglobin which forms methemoglobin more readily than adult hemoglobin. Therefore, pediatric patients (eg, neonates and infants <6 months of age) are more susceptible to excessive nitrite-induced methemoglobinemia. Hydroxocobalamin may be a more effective and rapid alternative. Nitrites should be avoided in pregnant patients due to fetal hemoglobin's susceptibility to oxidative stress. Hydroxocobalamin will circumvent this problem and may be a more effective and rapid alternative.

Adverse Reactions Frequency not defined.

Sodium nitrite:

Cardiovascular: Arrhythmias, cyanosis, flushing, hypotension, palpitations, syncope, tachycardia

Central nervous system: Anxiety, coma, confusion, dizziness, fatigue, headache, lightheadedness, seizure

Dermatologic: Urticaria

Endocrine & metabolic: Acidosis

Gastrointestinal: Abdominal pain, nausea, vomiting

Hematologic: Methemoglobinemia

Local: Injection site tingling

Neuromuscular & skeletal: Numbness, paresthesia, weakness

Ocular: Blurred vision

Respiratory: Dyspnea, tachypnea

Miscellaneous: Diaphoresis

Sodium thiosulfate:

Cardiovascular: Hypotension

Central nervous system: Disorientation, headache

Gastrointestinal: Nausea, salty taste, vomiting

Hematologic: Bleeding time prolonged

Miscellaneous: Warmth

Drug Interactions

Metabolism/Transport Effects None known.

Avoid Concomitant Use There are no known interactions where it is recommended to avoid concomitant use.

Increased Effect/Toxicity

Sodium Nitrite and Sodium Thiosulfate may increase the levels/effects of: Prilocaine

The levels/effects of Sodium Nitrite and Sodium Thiosulfate may be increased by: Methemoglobinemia Associated Agents; Nitric Oxide

Decreased Effect There are no known significant interactions involving a decrease in effect.

Storage/Stability Store at 20°C to 25°C (68°F to 77°F); excursions permitted to 15°C to 30°C (59°F to 86°F); do not freeze. Protect from direct light.

Mechanism of Action

Sodium nitrite: Promotes the formation of methemoglobin which competes with cytochrome oxidase for the cyanide ion. Cyanide combines with methemoglobin to form cyanomethemoglobin, thereby freeing the cytochrome oxidase and allowing aerobic metabolism to continue.

Sodium thiosulfate: Serves as a sulfur donor in rhodanese-catalyzed formation of thiocyanate (much less toxic than cyanide).

Pharmacodynamics/Kinetics

Sodium nitrite:

Onset: Peak effect: Methemoglobinemia: 30-60 minutes

Duration: Methemoglobinemia: ~55 minutes

Metabolism: To ammonia and other metabolites

Excretion: Urine (~40% as unchanged drug)

Sodium thiosulfate:

Half-life elimination: Thiosulfate: ~3 hours; Thiocyanate: ~3 days; Renal impairment: ≤9 days

Excretion: Urine (~20% to 50% as unchanged drug)

Dosage I.V.: **Note:** Administer sodium nitrite first, followed immediately by the administration of sodium thiosulfate.

Sodium nitrite:

Children: 6 mg/kg (0.2 mL/kg or 6-8 mL/m^2 of a 3% solution); maximum dose: 300 mg (10 mL of a 3% solution); may repeat at one-half the original dose if symptoms of cyanide toxicity return

Adults: 300 mg (10 mL of a 3% solution); may repeat at one-half the original dose if symptoms of cyanide toxicity return

Alternatively, in patients who are unable to tolerate significant methemoglobinemia (eg, patients with comorbidities that compromise oxygen delivery, such as heart disease, lung disease), dosing may be based on hemoglobin levels (when rapid bedside testing is available) to prevent fatal methemoglobinemia; see table (Berlin, 1970):

Hemoglobin Level (g/dL)	Dose of 3% Sodium Nitrite Solution (maximum dose: 10 mL)
7	0.19 mL/kg
8	0.22 mL/kg
9	0.25 mL/kg
10	0.27 mL/kg
11	0.3 mL/kg
12	0.33 mL/kg
13	0.36 mL/kg
14	0.39 mL/kg

Sodium thiosulfate:

Children: 7 g/m^2 or 250 mg/kg (1 mL/kg or 28-40 mL/m^2 of a 25% solution); maximum dose: 12.5 g (50 mL of a 25% solution); may repeat at one-half the original dose if symptoms of cyanide toxicity return

Adults: 12.5 g (50 mL of a 25% solution); may repeat at one-half the original dose if symptoms of cyanide toxicity return

Note: Monitor the patient for 24-48 hours; if symptoms return, repeat both sodium nitrite and sodium thiosulfate at one-half the original doses.

Dosage adjustment in renal impairment: No dosage adjustment provided in manufacturer's labeling. However, the risk of toxic reactions may be greater in patients with impaired renal function due to decreased excretion.

Dosage adjustment in hepatic impairment: No dosage adjustment provided in manufacturer's labeling.

Administration Administer via slow I.V. injection as soon as possible after diagnosis of acute, life-threatening cyanide poisoning. Administer sodium nitrite first at a rate of 2.5-5 mL/minute, followed immediately by the administration of sodium thiosulfate over 10-20 minutes. Decrease rate of infusion in the event of significant hypotension, nausea, or vomiting.

Monitoring Parameters Monitor for at least 24-48 hours after administration; blood pressure and heart rate during and after infusion; hemoglobin/hematocrit; co-oximetry; serum lactate levels; venous-arterial PO_2 gradient; serum methemoglobin and oxyhemoglobin. Pretreatment cyanide levels may be useful diagnostically.

Dosage Forms Excipient information presented when available (limited, particularly for generics); consult specific product labeling.

Injection, solution [combination package]:

Nithiodote: Sodium nitrite 300 mg/10 mL (10 mL) and sodium thiosulfate 12.5 g/50 mL (50 mL)

- ◆ **Sodium Nitroferricyanide** *see* Nitroprusside *on page 1469*
- ◆ **Sodium Nitroprusside** *see* Nitroprusside *on page 1469*

Sodium Oxybate (SOW dee um ox i BATE)

Brand Names: U.S. Xyrem

Brand Names: Canada Xyrem®

Index Terms 4-Hydroxybutyrate; Gamma Hydroxybutyric Acid; GHB; Oxybate; Sodium 4-Hydroxybutyrate

Pharmacologic Category Central Nervous System Depressant

Additional Appendix Information

Patient Information for Disposal of Unused Medications *on page 2393*

Use Treatment of cataplexy and excessive daytime sleepiness in patients with narcolepsy

Pregnancy Risk Factor C

Prescribing and Access Restrictions Sodium oxybate is deemed to have an approved REMS program. As a requirement of the REMS program, access to this medication is restricted. Sodium oxybate oral solution will be available only to prescribers and patients enrolled in the Xyrem® Patient Success Program® and dispensed to the patient through the designated centralized pharmacy (1-866-997-3688). Prior to dispensing the first prescription, prescribers will be sent educational materials to be reviewed with the patient and enrollment forms for the postmarketing surveillance program. Patients must be seen at least every 3 months; prescriptions can be written for a maximum of 3 months (the first prescription may only be written for a 1-month supply).

Medication Guide Available Yes

Dosage Oral:

Adults: Narcolepsy: Initial: 2.25 g at bedtime after the patient is in bed, and 2.25 g 2.5-4 hours later (4.5 g per night). Titrate to effect; usual effective dosage range: 6-9 g per night

Dose titration:

U.S. labeling: Increase dose by 1.5 g per night (0.75 g per dose) in weekly intervals (maximum dose: 9 g per night)

Canadian labeling: Increase dose by 1.5 g per night (0.75 g per dose) at 2-week intervals (maximum dose: 9 g per night). Dosage may be decreased using the same titration schedule.

Elderly: Use with caution; initiate at lower dosage range. Limited studies available in patients >65 years. Refer to adult dosing.

Dosage adjustment in renal impairment: No dosage adjustment provided in manufacturer's labeling (has not been studied).

Dosage adjustment in hepatic impairment: Initial: ~1.13 g at bedtime after the patient is in bed and ~1.13 g 2.5-4 hours later (2.25 g per night)

Additional Information Complete prescribing information should be consulted for additional detail.

Dosage Forms Excipient information presented when available (limited, particularly for generics); consult specific product labeling.

Solution, Oral:

Xyrem: 500 mg/mL (180 mL)

Controlled Substance C-I (illicit use); C-III (medical use)

Sodium Phenylacetate and Sodium Benzoate

(SOW dee um fen il AS e tate & SOW dee um BENZ oh ate)

Brand Names: U.S. Ammonul®

Index Terms NAPA and NABZ; Sodium Benzoate and Sodium Phenylacetate

Pharmacologic Category Antidote; Urea Cycle Disorder (UCD) Treatment Agent

Use Adjunct to treatment of acute hyperammonemia and encephalopathy in patients with urea cycle disorders involving partial or complete deficiencies of carbamyl-phosphate synthetase (CPS), ornithine transcarbamoylase (OTC), argininosuccinate lysase (ASL), or argininosuccinate synthetase (ASS); for use with hemodialysis in acute neonatal hyperammonemic coma, moderate-to-severe hyperammonemic encephalopathy and hyperammonemia which fails to respond to initial therapy

Pregnancy Risk Factor C

Dosage Administer as a loading dose over 90-120 minutes, followed by an equivalent maintenance infusion given over 24 hours. Dosage based on weight and specific enzyme deficiency; therapy should continue until ammonia levels are in normal range. Repeat loading doses are not recommended due to the prolonged plasma levels.

Children ≤20 kg:

CPS and OTC deficiency: Ammonul® 2.5 mL/kg and arginine 10% 2 mL/kg (provides sodium phenylacetate 250 mg/kg, sodium benzoate 250 mg/kg, and arginine hydrochloride 200 mg/kg).

ASS and ASL deficiency: Ammonul® 2.5 mL/kg and arginine 10% 6 mL/kg (provides sodium phenylacetate 250 mg/kg, sodium benzoate 250 mg/kg, and arginine hydrochloride 600 mg/kg)

Note: Pending a specific diagnosis in infants, the bolus and maintenance dose of arginine should be 6 mL/kg. If ASS or ASL are excluded as diagnostic possibilities, reduce dose of arginine to 2 mL/kg/day.

Children >20 kg and Adults:

CPS and OTC deficiency: Ammonul® 55 mL/m^2 and arginine 10% 2 mL/kg (provides sodium phenylacetate 5.5 g/m^2, sodium benzoate 5.5 g/m^2, and arginine hydrochloride 200 mg/kg)

ASS and ASL deficiency: Ammonul® 55 mL/m^2 and arginine 10% 6 mL/kg (provides sodium phenylacetate 5.5 g/m^2, sodium benzoate 5.5 g/m^2, and arginine hydrochloride 600 mg/kg)

Dosage adjustment in renal impairment: No dosage adjustment provided in manufacturer's labeling. However, renal impairment increases systemic exposure to sodium phenylacetate and sodium benzoate..Use with caution; monitor closely.

Dialysis: Ammonia clearance is ~10 times greater with hemodialysis than by peritoneal dialysis or hemofiltration. Exchange transfusion is ineffective.

Dosage adjustment in hepatic impairment: No dosage adjustment provided in manufacturer's labeling. Use with caution.

Additional Information Complete prescribing information should be consulted for additional detail.

Dosage Forms Excipient information presented when available (limited, particularly for generics); consult specific product labeling.

Injection, solution [concentrate]:

Ammonul®: Sodium phenylacetate 100 mg and sodium benzoate 100 mg per 1 mL (50 mL)

Sodium Phenylbutyrate

(SOW dee um fen il BYOO ti rate)

Brand Names: U.S. Buphenyl

Index Terms Ammonapse

Pharmacologic Category Urea Cycle Disorder (UCD) Treatment Agent

Use Adjunctive therapy in the chronic management of patients with urea cycle disorder involving deficiencies of carbamoylphosphate synthetase, ornithine transcarbamylase, or argininosuccinic acid synthetase

Pregnancy Risk Factor C

Dosage Oral: Management of urea cycle disorders:

Children <20 kg: Powder: 450-600 mg/kg/day, administered in equally divided amounts with each meal or feeding, 3-6 times daily (maximum dose: 20 g/day)

Children ≥20 kg and Adults: Powder or tablet: 9.9-13 g/m^2/day, administered in equally divided amounts with each meal or feeding, 3-6 times daily (maximum dose: 20 g/day)

Dosage adjustment in renal impairment: No dosage adjustment provided in manufacturer's labeling. Use with caution.

Dosage adjustment in hepatic impairment: No dosage adjustment provided in manufacturer's labeling. Use with caution.

Additional Information Complete prescribing information should be consulted for additional detail.

Dosage Forms Considerations

Powder products: 1 level teaspoon provides 3 g sodium phenylbutyrate, 1 level tablespoon provides 8.6 g sodium phenylbutyrate. Measurers provided with the product.

Dosage Forms Excipient information presented when available (limited, particularly for generics); consult specific product labeling.

Powder, Oral:

Buphenyl: (250 g) [contains sodium 125 mg/g]

Generic: (250 g)

Tablet, Oral:

Buphenyl: 500 mg [contains sodium 62 mg/tablet]

◆ **Sodium Phosphate and Potassium Phosphate** *see* Potassium Phosphate and Sodium Phosphate *on page 1691*

Sodium Phosphates (SOW dee um FOS fates)

Brand Names: U.S. Fleet Enema Extra [OTC]; Fleet Enema [OTC]; Fleet Pedia-Lax Enema [OTC]; LaCrosse Complete [OTC]; OsmoPrep

Brand Names: Canada Fleet Enema

Index Terms Phosphates, Sodium

Pharmacologic Category Cathartic; Electrolyte Supplement, Parenteral; Laxative, Bowel Evacuant

Additional Appendix Information

Laxatives, Classification and Properties *on page 2304*

Use

Oral solution, rectal: Short-term treatment of constipation

Oral tablets: Bowel cleansing prior to colonoscopy

I.V.: Source of phosphate in large volume I.V. fluids and parenteral nutrition; treatment and prevention of hypophosphatemia

Pregnancy Risk Factor C

Pregnancy Considerations Reproduction studies have not been conducted with these products. Use with caution in pregnant women.

Breast-Feeding Considerations Phosphorus, sodium, and potassium are normal constituents of human milk.

Medication Guide Available Yes

Contraindications Hypersensitivity to sodium phosphate salts or any component of the formulation; additional contraindications vary by product:

Enema: Ascites, clinically significant renal impairment, heart failure, imperforate anus, known or suspected GI obstruction, megacolon (congenital or acquired)

Intravenous preparation: Diseases with hyperphosphatemia, hypocalcemia, or hypernatremia

Oral preparation: Acute phosphate nephropathy (biopsy proven), bowel obstruction, bowel perforation, gastric bypass or stapling surgery, toxic colitis, toxic megacolon

Warnings/Precautions [U.S. Boxed Warning]: Acute phosphate nephropathy has been reported (rarely) with use of oral products as a colon cleanser prior to colonoscopy. Some cases have resulted in permanent renal impairment (some requiring dialysis). Risk factors for acute phosphate nephropathy may include increased age (>55 years of age), pre-existing renal dysfunction, bowel obstruction, active colitis, or dehydration, and the use of medicines that affect renal perfusion or function (eg, ACE inhibitors, angiotensin receptor blockers, diuretics, and possibly NSAIDs), although some cases have been reported in patients without apparent risk factors. Other preventive measures may include avoid exceeding maximum recommended doses and concurrent use of other laxatives containing sodium phosphate; encourage patients to adequately hydrate before, during, and after use; obtain baseline and postprocedure labs in patients at risk; consider hospitalization and intravenous hydration during bowel cleansing for patients unable to hydrate themselves (eg, frail patients). Use is contraindicated in patients with acute phosphate nephropathy (biopsy proven).

Use with caution in patients with impaired renal dysfunction, pre-existing electrolyte imbalances, risk of electrolyte disturbance (hypocalcemia, hyperphosphatemia, hypernatremia), or dehydration. If using as a bowel evacuant, correct electrolyte abnormalities before administration. Use caution in patients with unstable angina, history of myocardial infarction arrhythmia, cardiomyopathy; use caution in patients with or at risk for arrhythmias (eg, cardiomyopathy, prolonged QT interval, history of uncontrolled arrhythmias, recent MI) or with concurrent use of other QT-prolonging medications; pre-/postdose ECGs should be considered in high-risk patients.

Use caution in inflammatory bowel disease or severe active ulcerative colitis; may induce colonic aphthous ulceration and ischemic colitis (some requiring hospitalization). Use caution in patients with any of the following: Gastric retention or hypomotility, ileus, severe, chronic constipation, colitis. Use is contraindicated in patients with bowel obstruction (including pseudo) or perforation, congenital megacolon, gastric bypass or bariatric surgery, toxic colitis, or toxic megacolon. Use with caution in patients with impaired gag reflex and those prone to regurgitation or aspiration.

Use with caution in patients with a history of seizures and those at higher risk of seizures. Ensure adequate clear liquid intake prior to and during bowel evacuation regimens; inadequate fluid intake may lead to dehydration. Other oral medications may not be well absorbed when given during bowel evacuation because of rapid intestinal peristalsis. Use with caution in debilitated patients; consider each patient's ability to hydrate properly. Use with caution in geriatric patients. Laxatives and purgatives have the potential for abuse by bulimia nervosa patients. Solutions for injection may contain aluminum; toxic levels may occur following prolonged administration in premature neonates or patients with renal impairment. Enemas and oral solution are available in pediatric and adult sizes; prescribe by "volume" not by "bottle."

Adverse Reactions Frequency not always defined.

Central nervous system: Dizziness, headache

Gastrointestinal: Bloating (31% to 47%), nausea (26% to 35%), abdominal pain (23% to 30%), vomiting (4% to 7%), mucosal bleeding, superficial mucosal ulcerations

Endocrine & metabolic: Hyperphosphatemia (≤96%), hypocalcemia (on colonoscopy day; 47%), hypophosphatemia (2-3 days postcolonoscopy; 34%), hypokalemia (on colonoscopy day; 28%), hypernatremia

Postmarketing and/or case reports (Limited to important or life-threatening): Acute phosphate nephropathy, anaphylaxis, bronchospasm, calcium nephrolithiasis, cardiac arrhythmia, dehydration, dysphagia, dyspnea, facial edema, increased blood urea nitrogen, increased serum creatinine, ischemic colitis, lip edema, paresthesia, pharyngeal edema, pruritus, rectal bleeding, renal failure, renal insufficiency, renal tubular necrosis, seizure, skin rash, tightness in throat, tongue edema, urticaria

Drug Interactions

Metabolism/Transport Effects None known.

Avoid Concomitant Use There are no known interactions where it is recommended to avoid concomitant use.

Increased Effect/Toxicity

Sodium Phosphates may increase the levels/effects of: Nonsteroidal Anti-Inflammatory Agents

The levels/effects of Sodium Phosphates may be increased by: ACE Inhibitors; Angiotensin II Receptor Blockers; Bisphosphonate Derivatives; Diuretics; Tricyclic Antidepressants

Decreased Effect

The levels/effects of Sodium Phosphates may be decreased by: Antacids; Calcium Salts; Iron Salts; Magnesium Salts; Multivitamins/Minerals (with ADEK, Folate, Iron); Sucralfate

Preparation for Administration Solution for injection: In general, the dose, concentration of infusion, and rate of administration may be dependent on patient condition and specific institution policy. Intermittent infusion doses are typically prepared in 100-250 mL of NS or D_5W (usual concentration range: 0.15-0.6 mmol/mL). Observe the vial for the presence of crystals. Do not use vial if crystals are present. **Note:** Due to the potential for solution crystallization, American Regent, Inc recommends the use of a 5 micron filter when preparing I.V. sodium phosphate containing solutions (Important Drug Safety Information, American Regent, 2013); a similar recommendation has not been noted by other manufacturers.

Storage/Stability

Enema: Store at room temperature.

Oral solution: Store at room temperature.

Solution for injection: Store intact vials at 20°C to 25°C (68°F to 77°F); excursions permitted between 15°C and 30°C (59°F and 86°F).

Tablet: Store at 25°C (77°F); excursions permitted between 15°C and 30°C (59°F and 86°F).

Mechanism of Action As a laxative, exerts osmotic effect in the small intestine by drawing water into the lumen of the gut, producing distention and promoting peristalsis and evacuation of the bowel; phosphorous participates in bone deposition, calcium metabolism, utilization of B complex vitamins, and as a buffer in acid-base equilibrium

Pharmacodynamics/Kinetics

Onset of action: Cathartic: 3-6 hours; Rectal: 2-5 minutes

Absorption: Oral: ~1% to 20%

Excretion: Urine

Dosage

Note: If phosphate repletion is required and a phosphate product is not available at your institution, consider the use of sodium glycerophosphate pentahydrate (Glycophos) as a suitable substitute. Concentration and dosing are different from FDA-approved products; use caution when switching between products. Refer to Sodium Glycerophosphate Pentahydrate monograph.

Caution: With orders for I.V. phosphate, there is considerable confusion associated with the use of millimoles (mmol) versus milliequivalents (mEq) to express the phosphate requirement. The most reliable method of ordering I.V. phosphate is by millimoles, then specifying the potassium or sodium salt. Intravenous doses listed as mmol of phosphate.

Acute treatment of hypophosphatemia: I.V.: It is difficult to provide concrete guidelines for the treatment of severe hypophosphatemia because the extent of total body deficits and response to therapy are difficult to predict. Aggressive doses of phosphate may result in a transient serum elevation followed by redistribution into intracellular compartments or bone tissue. It is recommended that repletion of severe hypophosphatemia be done I.V. because large doses of oral phosphate may cause diarrhea and intestinal absorption may be unreliable. Intermittent I.V. infusion should be reserved for severe depletion situations; requires continuous cardiac monitoring. Guidelines differ based on degree of illness, need/use of TPN, and severity of hypophosphatemia. If hypokalemia exists (some clinicians recommend threshold of <4 mmol/L), consider phosphate replacement strategy with potassium (eg, potassium phosphates). Obese patients and/or severe renal impairment were excluded from phosphate supplement trials.

Children and Adults: There are no prospective studies of parenteral phosphate replacement in children. The following weight-based guidelines for adult dosing may be cautiously employed in pediatric patients. **Note:** 1 mmol phosphate = 31 mg phosphorus; 1 mg phosphorus = 0.032 mmol phosphate

General replacement guidelines (Lentz, 1978):

Low dose, serum phosphorus losses are recent and uncomplicated: 0.08 mmol/kg over 6 hours

Intermediate dose, serum phosphorus level 0.5-1 mg/dL (0.16-0.32 mmol/L): 0.16-0.24 mmol/kg over 6 hours

Note: The initial dose may be increased by 25% to 50% if the patient is symptomatic secondary to hypophosphatemia and lowered by 25% to 50% if the patient is hypercalcemic.

Critically-ill adult patients receiving concurrent enteral/parenteral nutrition (Brown, 2006; Clark, 1995): **Note:** Round doses to the nearest 7.5 mmol for ease of preparation. If administering with phosphate-containing parenteral nutrition, do not exceed 15 mmol/L within parenteral nutrition. May use adjusted body weight for patients weighing >130% of ideal body weight (and BMI <40 kg/m^2) by using [IBW + 0.25 (ABW-IBW)]:

Low dose, serum phosphorus level 2.3-3 mg/dL (0.74-0.96 mmol/L): 0.16-0.32 mmol/kg over 4-6 hours

Intermediate dose, serum phosphorus level 1.6-2.2 mg/dL (0.51-0.71 mmol/L): 0.32-0.64 mmol/kg over 4-6 hours

High dose, serum phosphorus <1.5 mg/dL (<0.5 mmol/L): 0.64-1 mmol/kg over 8-12 hours

Parenteral nutrition: I.V.:

Infants and Children: 0.5-2 mmol/kg/24 hours (Mirtallo, 2004 [ASPEN guidelines])

Children >50 kg and Adolescents: 10-40 mmol/24 hours (Mirtallo, 2004 [ASPEN guidelines])

Adults: 10-15 mmol/1000 kcal (Hicks, 2001) **or** 20-40 mmol/24 hours (Mirtallo, 2004 [ASPEN guidelines])

Laxative (Fleet): Rectal:

Children 2-4 years: One-half contents of one 2.25 oz pediatric enema

Children 5-11 years: Contents of one 2.25 oz pediatric enema

Children ≥12 years and Adults: Contents of one 4.5 oz enema as a single dose

Laxative: Oral solution:

Children 5-9 years: 7.5 mL as a single dose; maximum single daily dose: 7.5 mL

Children 10-11 years: 15 mL as a single dose; maximum single daily dose: 15 mL

Children ≥12 years and Adults: 15 mL as a single dose; maximum single daily dose: 45 mL

Bowel cleansing prior to colonoscopy: Oral tablets:

Adults: **Note:** Do not use additional agents, especially other sodium phosphate products.

OsmoPrep: A total of 32 tablets and 2 quarts of clear liquids (8 ounces of clear liquids with each dose) divided as follows:

Evening before colonoscopy: 4 tablets every 15 minutes for 5 doses (total of 20 tablets)

3-5 hours prior to colonoscopy: 4 tablets every 15 minutes for 3 doses (total of 12 tablets)

Elderly: Use with caution due to increased risk of renal impairment in the elderly.

Dosage adjustment in renal impairment: No dosage adjustment provided in manufacturer's labeling. Use with caution; ionized inorganic phosphate is excreted by the kidneys. Oral solution is contraindicated in patients with kidney disease.

Dosage adjustment in hepatic impairment: No dosage adjustment provided in manufacturer's labeling.

Dietary Considerations Bowel cleansing: Should be taken on an empty stomach with clear liquids; a clear liquid diet should be used for 12 hours prior to and during tablet administration. Clear liquids may include water, flavored water, pulp-free lemonade, ginger ale, or apple juice; purple or red colored liquids should be avoided. Some products may contain phenylalanine and/or sodium.

Administration

Intermittent I.V. infusion; do **not** administer I.V. push. Must be diluted prior to parenteral administration. In general, the dose, concentration of infusion, and rate of administration may be dependent on patient condition and specific institution policy. For adult patients with severe symptomatic hypophosphatemia (ie, <1.5 mg/dL), may administer at rates up to 15 mmol/hour (Charron, 2003; Rosen, 1995). In patients with renal dysfunction and/or less severe hypophosphatemia, slower administration rates (eg, over 4-6 hours) or oral repletion is recommended. **Note:** Due to the potential for solution crystallization, American Regent, Inc recommends the use of a 0.22 micron in-line filter for I.V. administration (1.2 micron filter if admixture contains lipids) (Important Drug Safety Information, American Regent, 2013); a similar recommendation has not been noted by other manufacturers.

Bowel cleansing (oral tablets): Have patient drink 8 ounces of clear liquids with each dose of sodium phosphate; have patient rehydrate before and after colonoscopy. Clear liquids may include water, flavored water, pulp-free lemonade, ginger ale, or apple juice; purple or red colored liquids should be avoided.

Constipation (oral solution): Take on an empty stomach; dilute dose with 8 ounces cool water, then follow dose with 8 ounces water; **do not repeat dose within 24 hours**

Monitoring Parameters

I.V.: Serum calcium, sodium and phosphorus levels; renal function; after I.V. phosphate repletion, repeat serum phosphorus level should be checked 2-4 hours later

Oral: Bowel cleansing: Baseline and postprocedure labs (electrolytes, calcium, phosphorus, BUN, creatinine) in patients at risk for acute renal nephropathy, seizure, or who have a history of electrolyte abnormality; ECG in patients with risks for prolonged QT or arrhythmias. Ensure euvolemia before initiating bowel preparation.

Reference Range Note: Reference ranges may vary depending on the laboratory

Serum calcium: 8.4-10.2 mg/dL

Serum phosphorus: Both low and high ends of the normal range are higher in children than in adults.

Infants: 4.5-7.5 mg/dL (1.45-2.42 mmol/L)

Children: ~4.0-6.0 mg/dL (1.29-1.94 mmol/L)

Adults: 2.5-4.5 mg/dL (0.81-1.45 mmol/L)

Additional Information Phosphate salts may precipitate when mixed with calcium salts; solubility is improved in amino acid parenteral nutrition solutions; check with a pharmacist to determine compatibility.

Dosage Forms Considerations

Sodium 4 mEq is equivalent to sodium 92 mg

Phosphorous 3 mmol is equivalent to phosphorus 93 mg

Dosage Forms Excipient information presented when available (limited, particularly for generics); consult specific product labeling.

Injection, solution [concentrate; preservative free]: Phosphorus 3 mmol and sodium 4 mEq per 1 mL (5 mL, 15 mL, 50 mL) [equivalent to phosphorus 93 mg and sodium 92 mg per 1 mL; source of electrolytes: monobasic and dibasic sodium phosphate]

Solution, oral: Monobasic sodium phosphate monohydrate 2.4 g and dibasic sodium phosphate heptahydrate 0.9 g per 5 mL (45 mL) [sugar free; contains sodium 556 mg/5 mL, sodium benzoate; ginger-lemon flavor]

Solution, rectal [enema]: Monobasic sodium phosphate monohydrate 19 g and dibasic sodium phosphate heptahydrate 7 g per 118 mL delivered dose (133 mL)

Fleet Enema: Monobasic sodium phosphate monohydrate 19 g and dibasic sodium phosphate heptahydrate 7 g per 118 mL delivered dose (133 mL) [contains sodium 4.4 g/118 mL]

Fleet Enema Extra: Monobasic sodium phosphate monohydrate 19 g and dibasic sodium phosphate heptahydrate 7 g per 197 mL delivered dose (230 mL) [contains sodium 4.4 g/197 mL]

Fleet Pedia-Lax™ Enema: Monobasic sodium phosphate monohydrate 9.5 g and dibasic sodium phosphate heptahydrate 3.5 g per 59 mL delivered dose (66 mL) [contains sodium 2.2 g/59 mL]

LaCrosse Complete: Monobasic sodium phosphate monohydrate 19 g and dibasic sodium phosphate heptahydrate 7 g per 118 mL delivered dose (133 mL) [contains sodium 4.4 g/118 mL]

Tablet, oral [scored]:

OsmoPrep: Monobasic sodium phosphate monohydrate 1.102 g and dibasic sodium phosphate anhydrous 0.398 g [sodium phosphate 1.5 g per tablet; gluten free]

Sodium Picosulfate, Magnesium Oxide, and Citric Acid

(SOW dee um pye ko SUL fate mag NEE zhum OKS ide & SI trik AS id)

Brand Names: U.S. Prepopik™

Brand Names: Canada Oral Purgative; Pico-Salax®; Picodan; Picoflo; Purg-Odan™

Index Terms Citric Acid, Sodium Picosulfate, and Magnesium Oxide; DA-1773; Magnesium Oxide, Sodium Picosulfate, and Citric Acid; Prepopik™; Sodium Picosulphate, Magnesium Oxide, and Citric Acid

Pharmacologic Category Laxative, Osmotic; Laxative, Stimulant

Additional Appendix Information

Laxatives, Classification and Properties *on page 2304*

Use Bowel cleansing prior to colonoscopy

Canadian labeling: Additional uses (not in U.S. labeling): Bowel cleansing prior to x-ray examination, endoscopy, or surgery

Pregnancy Risk Factor B

Pregnancy Considerations Adverse events were not observed in animal reproduction studies using doses similar to a human dose.

Breast-Feeding Considerations Lactating women (n=8) were administered sodium picosulfate 10 mg as an oral solution once daily for 8 days. The active metabolite, BPHM, was detected in plasma and urine, but below the limit of detection in breast milk (<1 ng/mL) (Friedrich, 2011). Also refer to individual monographs.

Medication Guide Available Yes

Contraindications Hypersensitivity to sodium picosulfate, magnesium oxide, anhydrous citric acid, or any component of the formulation; GI obstruction or ileus; bowel perforation; gastric retention; toxic colitis; toxic megacolon; severe renal impairment (Cl_{cr} <30 mL/minute).

Canadian labeling: Additional contraindications (not in U.S. labeling): Congestive heart failure; GI ulceration; nausea; vomiting; acute surgical abdominal conditions (eg, acute appendicitis)

Warnings/Precautions Serious arrhythmias have occurred rarely with the use of ionic osmotic laxative products; use caution in patients at increased risk for arrhythmias (eg, recent MI, unstable angina, cardiomyopathy, history of prolonged QT, HF, uncontrolled arrhythmias); consider baseline and post-colonoscopy ECGs in patients at increased risk for arrhythmias. Administration may cause fluid and electrolyte disturbances, particularly in patients at increased risk (eg, renal impairment, concomitant mediations that alter electrolyte balance). Any pre-existing electrolyte abnormalities should be corrected prior to use and patients should be adequately hydrated before, during, and after use. Consider evaluating for and treating post-colonoscopy electrolyte abnormalities in patients who develop significant vomiting, dehydration, or orthostatic hypotension. Seizures associated with electrolyte abnormalities (eg, hyponatremia, hypokalemia) and low serum osmolality have occurred; use with caution in patients with underlying electrolyte disturbances and in patients at increased risk for seizures (eg, concomitant medications that lower seizure threshold, withdrawal from alcohol or benzodiazepines). Osmotic laxatives may produce colonic mucosal aphthous ulcerations, including cases of ischemic colitis. Use caution when interpreting colonoscopy results in patients with inflammatory bowel disease.

Use with caution in patients with renal impairment and/or in patients taking medications that may adversely affect renal function (eg, diuretics, NSAIDs, ACE inhibitors); adequate hydration is particularly important in these patients. Patients with impaired renal function who develop severe vomiting should be closely monitored including measurement of electrolytes. Use with caution in patients with severe ulcerative colitis. Observe unconscious or semiconscious patients with impaired gag reflex or those who are otherwise prone to regurgitation or aspiration during administration of this product.

Patients with symptoms of bowel obstruction/perforation (nausea, vomiting, abdominal pain or distension) should be evaluated prior to use of this product. Each packet must be diluted with water prior to use, because inadvertent administration of undiluted solution may increase the risk of nausea, vomiting, and fluid/electrolyte abnormalities.

Oral medications administered ≤1 hour prior to the start of the bowel preparation regimen may not be absorbed. Chlorpromazine, digoxin, fluoroquinolones, iron, penicillamine, and tetracycline should be administered at least 2 hours before and 6 hours after administration of magnesium oxide to avoid chelation with magnesium. Sodium picosulfate requires the presence of colonic bacteria for the conversion to an active metabolite; prior or concomitant administration of antibiotics may reduce the efficacy of sodium picosulfate.

Adverse Reactions

>10%:

Endocrine & metabolic: Hypermagnesemia (9% to 12%)

Renal: GFR decreased (≤48 hours after colonoscopy: 10% to 29%)

1% to 10%:

Central nervous system: Headache (2% to 3%)

Endocrine & metabolic: Hypokalemia (5% to 7%), hypochloremia (1% to 4%), hyponatremia (1% to 4%)

Gastrointestinal: Nausea (3%), vomiting (1%)

Renal: Serum creatinine increased (<1% to 5%)

<1% (Limited to important or life-threatening): Aphthoid ileal ulcers, hypersensitivity, ischemic colitis, seizure

Drug Interactions

Metabolism/Transport Effects None known.

Avoid Concomitant Use

Avoid concomitant use of Sodium Picosulfate, Magnesium Oxide, and Citric Acid with any of the following: Calcium Polystyrene Sulfonate; Raltegravir; Sodium Polystyrene Sulfonate

Increased Effect/Toxicity

Sodium Picosulfate, Magnesium Oxide, and Citric Acid may increase the levels/effects of: Aluminum Hydroxide; Calcium Channel Blockers; Calcium Polystyrene Sulfonate; Neuromuscular-Blocking Agents; Sodium Polystyrene Sulfonate

The levels/effects of Sodium Picosulfate, Magnesium Oxide, and Citric Acid may be increased by: Alfacalcidol; Calcitriol; Calcium Channel Blockers

Decreased Effect

Sodium Picosulfate, Magnesium Oxide, and Citric Acid may decrease the levels/effects of: Bisphosphonate Derivatives; Deferiprone; Dolutegravir; Eltrombopag; Gabapentin; Multivitamins/Fluoride (with ADE); Mycophenolate; Phosphate Supplements; Quinolone Antibiotics; Raltegravir; Tetracycline Derivatives; Trientine

The levels/effects of Sodium Picosulfate, Magnesium Oxide, and Citric Acid may be decreased by: Antibiotics; Trientine

Preparation for Administration Reconstitute immediately prior to each administration; do not prepare the solution in advance. To reconstitute, fill the supplied dosing cup with 5 ounces of cold water (up to the lower line) and add the contents of one packet to the cup; stir for 2-3 minutes.

Storage/Stability Store at 25°C (77°F); excursions permitted to15°C to 30°C (59°F to 86°F). Use the reconstituted solution immediately.

Mechanism of Action

Sodium picosulfate, a prodrug, is hydrolyzed by colonic bacteria to an active metabolite which stimulates colonic peristalsis.

Magnesium oxide and citric acid react to create magnesium citrate which induces catharsis by the osmotic effects of the unabsorbed ions in the GI tract.

Pharmacodynamics/Kinetics

Absorption: Magnesium cation: ≥20%

Metabolism: Sodium picosulfate: Hydrolyzed by colonic bacteria to the active compound bis-(*p*-hydroxy-phenyl)-pyridyl-2-methane (BHPM)

Half-life elimination: Sodium picosulfate: ~7.5 hours

Time to peak: Sodium picosulfate: ~7 hours; Magnesium: 10 hours

Excretion: Urine

Dosage Bowel cleansing:

Prepopik™: Adults: Oral:

Split-dose regimen (preferred): 150 mL (5 oz) the evening before the colonoscopy (5 PM-9 PM), followed by a second 150 mL (5 oz) dose ~5 hours before the colonoscopy.

Day-before regimen (alternative): 150 mL (5 oz) in the early evening before the colonoscopy (4 PM-6 PM), followed by a second 150 mL (5 oz) dose 6 hours later (10 PM-12 AM) the night before the colonoscopy.

Purg-Odan™ (Canadian availability): Oral:

Children 1-5 years: One-fourth (1/4) of one sachet (mixed and dissolved in water) in the morning (8 AM) the day prior to the procedure, followed by a second dose of one-fourth (1/4) of one sachet in the afternoon (2 PM-4 PM) on the day prior to the procedure.

Children 6-12 years: One-half (1/2) of one sachet (mixed and dissolved in water) in the morning (8 AM) the day prior to the procedure, followed by a second dose of one-half (1/2) of one sachet in the afternoon (2 PM-4 PM) on the day prior to the procedure.

Adults: One sachet (mixed and dissolved in water) in the morning (8 AM) the day prior to the procedure followed by a second dose of one sachet in the afternoon (2 PM-4 PM) on the day prior to the procedure.

Pico-Salax® (Canadian availability): Oral:

Children 1-5 years: One-fourth (1/4) of one sachet (mixed and dissolved in water) in the evening (6 PM) the day prior to the procedure, followed by a second dose of one-fourth (1/4) of one sachet in the morning (8 AM) on the day of the procedure

Children 6-12 years: One-half (1/2) of one sachet (mixed and dissolved in water) in the evening (6 PM) the day prior to the procedure, followed by a second dose of one-half (1/2) of one sachet in the morning (8 AM) on the day of the procedure

Adults:

Early colonoscopy (before 12 PM): One sachet (mixed and dissolved in water) in the evening (5 PM) the day prior to the procedure, followed by a second dose of one sachet 5 hours later (10 PM) the night before the procedure

Late colonoscopy (after 12 PM): One sachet (mixed and dissolved in water) in the late evening (7 PM) the day prior to the procedure, followed by a second dose of one sachet in the morning (6 AM) on the day of the procedure

Administration Oral:

Prepopik™: Following the first dose, administer five 8-ounce clear liquid drinks (eg, water, clear broth, apple juice, white cranberry juice, white grape juice, ginger ale, plain gelatin [not purple or red], frozen juice bars [not purple or red]) within 5 hours. Following the second dose, administer three 8-ounce clear liquid drinks within 5 hours of administration. Clear liquids may be consumed up until 2 hours prior to the colonoscopy. In patients who develop bloating, distension, or abdominal pain, temporarily discontinue administration or increase the dosing interval until symptoms improve.

Purg-Odan™ (Canadian availability): Drink ~250 mL (8 oz) of clear liquids every hour while the effects of the bowel preparation regimen are apparent. Clear liquids may be consumed up until 2 hours prior to the procedure.

Pico-Salax® (Canadian availability):

At least 3 days prior to the procedure: Avoid eating seeds, nuts, fresh fruits and vegetables, and multigrain bread.

Day prior to the procedure: Consume clear liquids only (eg, water, clear power drinks, apple juice, white [not red] cranberry juice, white [not purple] grape juice, ginger ale, broth, tea [without milk, cream, or soy]), and no solid food. Patients with diabetes may drink a fiber-free supplement.

Following each dose: Adults should drink 1.5-2 L of clear fluids up until 2 hours prior to the procedure; children should drink one 8-ounce drink every hour while awake and up until 2 hours prior to the procedure.

Monitoring Parameters Serum electrolytes and renal function tests (baseline and post-colonoscopy) in patients with or at risk for renal impairment or seizure, and in patients who have a history of electrolyte abnormality; consider ECG (baseline and post-colonoscopy) in patients at risk for prolonged QT or arrhythmias.

Dosage Forms Excipient information presented when available (limited, particularly for generics); consult specific product labeling.

Powder for solution, oral [kit]:

Prepopik™: Sodium picosulfate 10 mg, magnesium oxide 3.5 g, and citric acid 12 g per packet (2s) [orange flavor]

Dosage Forms: Canada Excipient information presented when available (limited, particularly for generics); consult specific product labeling.

Powder for solution, oral [kit]:

Pico-Salax®: Sodium picosulphate 10 mg, magnesium oxide 3.5 g, and citric acid 12 g per sachet (1s, 2s) [orange or cranberry flavor]

Purg-Odan™: Sodium picosulphate 10 mg, magnesium oxide 3.5 g, and citric acid 12 g per sachet (1s, 2s) [orange flavor]

◆ **Sodium Picosulphate, Magnesium Oxide, and Citric Acid** *see* Sodium Picosulfate, Magnesium Oxide, and Citric Acid *on page 1925*

Sodium Polystyrene Sulfonate

(SOW dee um pol ee STYE reen SUL fon ate)

Brand Names: U.S. Kalexate; Kayexalate; Kionex; SPS

Brand Names: Canada Kayexalate®; PMS-Sodium Polystyrene Sulfonate

Pharmacologic Category Antidote

Use Treatment of hyperkalemia

Pregnancy Risk Factor C

Pregnancy Considerations Animal reproduction studies have not been conducted. There are no adequate and well-controlled studies in pregnant women. Use during pregnancy only if benefits outweigh the risks.

Breast-Feeding Considerations It is not known if sodium polystyrene sulfonate is excreted in breast milk. The manufacturer recommends that caution be exercised when administering sodium polystyrene sulfonate to nursing women.

Contraindications Hypersensitivity to sodium polystyrene sulfonate or any component of the formulation; hypokalemia; obstructive bowel disease; neonates with reduced gut motility (postoperatively or drug-induced); oral administration in neonates

Additional contraindications: Sodium polystyrene sulfonate suspension (**with** sorbitol): Rectal administration in neonates (particularly in premature infants); any postoperative patient until normal bowel function resumes

Warnings/Precautions Intestinal necrosis (including fatalities) and other serious gastrointestinal events (eg, bleeding, ischemic colitis, perforation) have been reported, especially when administered with sorbitol. Increased risk may be associated with a history of intestinal disease or surgery, hypovolemia, prematurity, and renal insufficiency or failure; use with sorbitol is not recommended. Avoid use in any postoperative patient until normal bowel function resumes or in patients at risk for constipation or impaction; discontinue use if constipation occurs. Oral or rectal administration of sorbitol-containing sodium polystyrene sulfonate suspensions is contraindicated in neonates (particularly with prematurity). Use with caution in patients with severe HF, hypertension, or edema; sodium load may exacerbate condition. Effective lowering of serum potassium from sodium polystyrene sulfonate may take hours to days after administration; consider alternative measures (eg, dialysis) or concomitant therapy (eg, I.V. sodium bicarbonate) in situations where rapid correction of severe hyperkalemia is required. Severe hypokalemia may occur; frequent monitoring of serum potassium is recommended within each 24-hour period; ECG monitoring may be appropriate in select patients. In addition to serum potassium-lowering effects, cation-exchange resins may also affect other cation concentrations possibly resulting in decreased serum magnesium and calcium. Large oral doses may cause fecal impaction (especially in elderly).

Concomitant administration of oral sodium polystyrene sulfonate with nonabsorbable cation-donating antacids or laxatives (eg, magnesium hydroxide) may result in systemic alkalosis and may diminish ability to reduce serum potassium concentrations; use with such agents is not recommended. In addition, intestinal obstruction has been reported with concomitant administration of aluminum hydroxide due to concretion formation. Enema will reduce the serum potassium faster than oral administration, but the oral route will result in a greater reduction over several hours. Oral administration in neonates and use in neonates with reduced gut motility (postoperatively or drug-induced) is contraindicated. Oral or rectal administration of sorbitol-containing sodium polystyrene sulfonate suspensions in neonates (particularly with prematurity) is also contraindicated due to propylene glycol content and risk of intestinal necrosis and digestive hemorrhage. Use sodium polystyrene sulfonate (**without** sorbitol) with caution in premature or low-birth-weight infants. Use with caution in children when administering rectally; excessive dosage or inadequate dilution may result in fecal impaction.

Adverse Reactions

Frequency not defined:

Endocrine & metabolic: Hypernatremia, hypocalcemia, hypokalemia, hypomagnesemia, sodium retention

Gastrointestinal: Anorexia, constipation, diarrhea, fecal impaction, intestinal necrosis (rare), intestinal obstruction (due to concretions in association with aluminum hydroxide), nausea, vomiting

<1% (Limited to important or life-threatening): Acute bronchitis (rare; associated with inhalation of particles), concretions, gastrointestinal bleeding, gastrointestinal ulceration, intestinal perforation, ischemic colitis

Drug Interactions

Metabolism/Transport Effects None known.

Avoid Concomitant Use

Avoid concomitant use of Sodium Polystyrene Sulfonate with any of the following: Laxatives; Meloxicam; Sorbitol

Increased Effect/Toxicity

Sodium Polystyrene Sulfonate may increase the levels/effects of: Aluminum Hydroxide; Digoxin

The levels/effects of Sodium Polystyrene Sulfonate may be increased by: Antacids; Laxatives; Meloxicam; Sorbitol

Decreased Effect

Sodium Polystyrene Sulfonate may decrease the levels/effects of: Lithium; Thyroid Products

Ethanol/Nutrition/Herb Interactions Food: Some liquids may contain potassium: Management: Do not mix in orange juice or in any fruit juice known to contain potassium.

Storage/Stability Store at 25°C (77°F); excursions permitted to 15°C to 30°C (59°F to 86°F). Store repackaged product in refrigerator and use within 14 days. Freshly prepared suspensions should be used within 24 hours. Do not heat resin suspension.

Mechanism of Action Removes potassium by exchanging sodium ions for potassium ions in the intestine (especially the large intestine) before the resin is passed from the body; exchange capacity is 1 mEq/g *in vivo*, and *in vitro* capacity is 3.1 mEq/g, therefore, a wide range of exchange capacity exists such that close monitoring of serum electrolytes is necessary

Pharmacodynamics/Kinetics

Onset of action: 2-24 hours

Absorption: None

Excretion: Completely feces (primarily as potassium polystyrene sulfonate)

Dosage

Children: Hyperkalemia:

Oral: 1 g/kg/dose every 6 hours

Rectal: 1 g/kg/dose every 2-6 hours (In small children and infants, employ lower doses by using the practical exchange ratio of 1 mEq K^+/g of resin as the basis for calculation)

Adults: Hyperkalemia:

Oral: 15 g 1-4 times/day

Rectal: 30-50 g every 6 hours

Dosage adjustment in renal impairment: No dosage adjustment provided in manufacturer's labeling. Use with caution; risks of gastrointestinal adverse effects are greater in patients with renal insufficiency or failure.

Dosage adjustment in hepatic impairment: No dosage adjustment provided in manufacturer's labeling.

Dietary Considerations Do **not** mix in orange juice or in any fruit juice known to contain potassium. Some products may contain sodium.

Administration

Oral: Shake suspension well prior to administration. Administer orally (or via NG tube) as a suspension. **Do not mix in orange juice.** Chilling the oral mixture will increase palatability.

Powder for suspension: For each 1 g of the powdered resin, add 3-4 mL of water or syrup (amount of fluid usually ranges from 20-100 mL)

Rectal: Enema route is less effective than oral administration. Administer cleansing enema first. Each dose of the powder for suspension should be suspended in 100 mL of aqueous vehicle and administered as a warm emulsion (body temperature). The commercially available suspension should also be warmed to body temperature. During administration, the solution should be agitated gently. Retain enema in colon for at least 30-60 minutes and for several hours, if possible. Once retention time is complete, irrigate colon with a non-sodium-containing solution to remove resin.

Monitoring Parameters Serum electrolytes (potassium, sodium, calcium, magnesium); ECG in select patients

Reference Range Serum potassium: Adults: 3.5-5.2 mEq/L

Additional Information 1 g of resin binds approximately 1 mEq of potassium

Historically, sorbitol was often recommended as a cathartic agent to be administered with sodium polystyrene sulfonate (SPS) to prevent SPS-induced fecal impaction.

However, SPS, particularly when used with sorbitol, has been associated with cases of intestinal necrosis and other serious GI adverse events. Due to the concern that sorbitol may increase the risk of intestinal necrosis, concomitant use of sorbitol is no longer recommended.

Sodium polystyrene sulfonate is commercially available in a liquid suspension containing 33% sorbitol (~20 g sorbitol per 60 mL suspension).

Dosage Forms Excipient information presented when available (limited, particularly for generics); consult specific product labeling.

Powder, Oral:

Kalexate: (454 g) [sorbitol free; contains sodium 100 mg (4.1 mEq)/g]

Kayexalate: (453.6 g) [contains sodium 100 mg (4.1 mEq)/g]

Kionex: (454 g) [contains sodium 100 mg (4.1 mEq)/g]

Generic: (453.6 g, 454 g)

Suspension, Oral:

Kionex: 15 g/60 mL (60 mL, 473 mL) [contains alcohol, usp, methylparaben, propylene glycol, propylparaben, saccharin sodium, sodium 1500 mg (65 mEq)/60 mL, sorbitol; raspberry flavor]

SPS: 15 g/60 mL (60 mL, 120 mL, 473 mL) [contains alcohol, usp, methylparaben, propylene glycol, propylparaben, saccharin sodium, sodium 1500 mg (65 mEq)/ 60 mL, sorbitol; cherry flavor]

Generic: 15 g/60 mL (60 mL, 480 mL, 500 mL)

Suspension, Rectal:

Generic: 30 g/120 mL (120 mL); 50 g/200 mL (200 mL)

◆ **Sodium Sulamyd (Can)** *see* Sulfacetamide (Ophthalmic) *on page 1956*

◆ **Sodium Sulfacetamide** *see* Sulfacetamide (Ophthalmic) *on page 1956*

◆ **Sodium Sulfacetamide** *see* Sulfacetamide (Topical) *on page 1957*

◆ **Sodium Sulfacetamide and Sulfur** *see* Sulfur and Sulfacetamide *on page 1966*

◆ **Sodium Sulfate, Magnesium Sulfate, and Potassium Sulfate** *see* Sodium Sulfate, Potassium Sulfate, and Magnesium Sulfate *on page 1929*

Sodium Sulfate, Potassium Sulfate, and Magnesium Sulfate

(SOW dee um SUL fate, poe TASS ee um SUL fate, & mag NEE zhum SUL fate)

Brand Names: U.S. Suprep® Bowel Prep Kit

Index Terms Magnesium Sulfate, Potassium Sulfate, and Sodium Sulfate; Magnesium Sulfate, Sodium Sulfate, and Potassium Sulfate; Potassium Sulfate, Magnesium Sulfate, and Sodium Sulfate; Potassium Sulfate, Sodium Sulfate, and Magnesium Sulfate; Sodium Sulfate, Magnesium Sulfate, and Potassium Sulfate

Pharmacologic Category Laxative, Osmotic

Use Bowel cleansing prior to GI examination

Pregnancy Risk Factor C

Medication Guide Available Yes

Dosage Oral: Adults: Bowel cleansing prior to GI exam:

Split-dose regimen: Total volume of liquid consumed over the course of treatment: 2880 mL (96 oz)

Evening before colonoscopy: Drink the entire contents of 1 bottle, diluted to a final volume of 480 mL (16 oz). Then drink 2 additional containers of water each (filled to the 16-ounce line) over the next hour, for an additional volume of 960 mL (32 oz).

Morning of the colonoscopy (10-12 hours after the evening dose): Repeat entire process with the second bottle: Drink entire contents of second bottle diluted to a final volume of 480 mL (16 oz); then drink 2 additional containers of water (each filled to the 16-ounce line) over the next hour, for an additional volume of 960 mL (32 oz). Complete at least 2 hours before the procedure.

Dosage adjustment in renal impairment: No adjustments provided in manufacturer's labeling. Use with caution, ensure adequate hydration, and consider baseline and post-colonoscopy renal function assessment.

Dosage adjustment in hepatic impairment: No dosage adjustment provided in manufacturer's labeling. However, no adjustment expected due to similar disposition to healthy patients in pharmacokinetic studies.

Additional Information Complete prescribing information should be consulted for additional detail.

Dosage Forms Excipient information presented when available (limited, particularly for generics); consult specific product labeling. [DSC] = Discontinued product

Solution, oral:

Suprep® Bowel Prep Kit: Sodium sulfate 17.5 g, potassium sulfate 3.13 g, and magnesuim sulfate 1.6 g per 180 mL (180 mL) [contains sodium benzoate]

◆ **Sodium Sulfate, Potassium Sulfate, Magnesium Sulfate and PEG-Electrolyte Solution** *see* Sodium Sulfate, Potassium Sulfate, Magnesium Sulfate, and Polyethylene Glycol-Electrolyte Solution *on page 1929*

◆ **Sodium Sulfate, Potassium Sulfate, Magnesium Sulfate and PEG Solution** *see* Sodium Sulfate, Potassium Sulfate, Magnesium Sulfate, and Polyethylene Glycol-Electrolyte Solution *on page 1929*

Sodium Sulfate, Potassium Sulfate, Magnesium Sulfate, and Polyethylene Glycol-Electrolyte Solution

(SOW dee um SUL fate, poe TASS ee um SUL fate, mag NEE zhum SUL fate, & pol i ETH i leen GLY kol ee LEK troe lite soe LOO shun)

Brand Names: U.S. Suclear™

Index Terms Sodium Sulfate, Potassium Sulfate, Magnesium Sulfate and PEG Solution; Sodium Sulfate, Potassium Sulfate, Magnesium Sulfate and PEG-Electrolyte Solution

Pharmacologic Category Laxative, Osmotic

Use Bowel cleansing prior to colonoscopy

Pregnancy Risk Factor C

Pregnancy Considerations Animal reproduction studies have not been conducted.

Breast-Feeding Considerations It is not known if the components from this preparation are excreted into breast milk. The manufacturer recommends that caution be used if administered to breast-feeding women.

Medication Guide Available Yes

Contraindications Hypersensitivity to sodium sulfate, potassium sulfate, magnesium sulfate, polyethylene glycol or any component of the formulation; GI obstruction, bowel perforation, gastric retention, ileus, toxic colitis, toxic megacolon

Warnings/Precautions Fluid and electrolyte disturbances can lead to arrhythmias, seizures, and renal impairment. Advise patients to maintain adequate hydration before, during, and after treatment. Use caution in patients at increased risk for cardiac arrhythmias (eg, recent MI, uncontrolled arrhythmias, unstable angina, cardiomyopathy, history of prolonged QT, HF); consider pre-dose and post-colonoscopy ECGs in these patients. Use with caution in patients with underlying electrolyte disturbances and in patients at increased risk for seizures (eg, concomitant medications that lower seizure threshold, withdrawal from alcohol or benzodiazepines). Use caution in patients with renal impairment; adequate hydration is particularly important in these patients or in patients receiving concomitant medications that may affect renal function (eg, diuretics, angiotensin converting enzyme inhibitors, angiotensin receptor blockers, NSAIDs). Consider baseline and post-colonoscopy electrolytes, creatinine, and BUN levels in patients at increased risk for renal impairment. If patient becomes dehydrated or experiences significant vomiting after treatment, consider post-colonoscopy lab tests (electrolytes, creatinine, and BUN).

Osmotic laxatives may produce colonic mucosal aphthous ulcerations, including cases of ischemic colitis requiring hospitalization. Concomitant use of stimulant laxatives and this preparation may increase the risk and should be avoided. Use caution when interpreting colonoscopy results in patients with known or suspected inflammatory bowel disease. Use with caution in patients with severe, active ulcerative colitis; increased risk of exacerbation of ulcerative colitis with use. Evaluate patients with symptoms of GI obstruction/perforation (nausea, vomiting, abdominal pain or distension) to rule out these conditions prior to use.

Use may cause an increase in uric acid; use caution in patients with gout. Observe patients with impaired gag reflex or those who are otherwise prone to regurgitation or aspiration during administration; use with caution in these patients. Each bottle must be diluted with water prior to use; inadvertent administration of the undiluted oral solution may increase the risk of nausea, vomiting, and fluid/electrolyte abnormalities.

Adverse Reactions

>10%:

Central nervous system: Malaise (62% to 69%)

Gastrointestinal: Abdominal distension (52%), nausea (42% to 46%), abdominal pain (38% to 40%), vomiting (11% to 14%)

Hepatic: Increased serum bilirubin (8% to 11%)

Renal: Renal insufficiency (9% to 25%)

1% to 10%:

Central nervous system: Headache (1% to 2%)

Endocrine & metabolic: Acidosis (3% to 10%), hypercalcemia (4% to 9%), increased serum glucose (2% to 7%), hyperuricemia (4% to 6%), hypokalemia (4%), decreased serum bicarbonate (3% to 4%), increased urine osmolality (2% to 4%), hypophosphatemia (≤3%), hypochloremia (1%), hyponatremia (≤1%), decreased serum magnesium (≤1%)

Neuromuscular & skeletal: Increased creatine phosphokinase (7%)

Renal: Increased serum creatinine (1% to 2%)

Ethanol/Nutrition/Herb Interactions Ethanol: Avoid alcohol beginning the day before colonoscopy and until after the completion of the colonoscopy; alcohol consumption may increase risk of dehydration.

Preparation for Administration Prior to administration, each component of the dosing regimen (oral solution and powder for oral solution) must be diluted with water as follows:

Oral solution: Further dilute the 6 ounce oral solution by pouring the entire contents of the bottle into the provided 16 ounce mixing container and filling that container with cool water to the fill line for a final volume of 16 ounces (480 mL). Following dilution, the oral solution should be consumed within 20 minutes.

Powder for oral solution: Dissolve the powder in the provided 2 L bottle by adding water to the fill line for a final volume of 2 L (2000 mL). Close tightly and shake the container until all powder is dissolved; solution should be clear and colorless. Flavor packs (provided with the product) may also be added if desired. Following reconstitution of the powder for oral solution, the solution may be refrigerated and should be used within 48 hours.

Storage/Stability Store unused kits at 20°C to 25°C (68°F to 77°F); excursions permitted between 15°C to 30°C (59°F to 86°F). Keep out of reach of children. Following dilution, the oral solution should be consumed within 20 minutes. Following reconstitution of the powder for oral solution, the solution may be refrigerated and should be used within 48 hours.

Mechanism of Action Induces catharsis by the osmotic effects of the unabsorbed sulfate salts and polyethylene glycol (PEG) in the GI tract. Specifically, sulfate salts provide sulfate anions, which are poorly absorbed, and PEG, which is primarily unabsorbed, causes water to be retained in the GI tract resulting in watery diarrhea.

Pharmacodynamics/Kinetics Note: Moderate renal impairment (Cl_{cr} 30-49 mL/minute) resulted in a 43% higher C_{max} and a 16% lower urinary clearance of serum sulfates compared to healthy patients

Absorption: PEG 3350: Minimal; Sulfates: Poor; ~20% absorbed systemically

Half-life elimination: Serum sulfate: 8.5 hours

Time to peak: Serum sulfate: ~5.5 hours

Excretion: Feces/rectal effluent (primary route of excretion for unabsorbed sulfates and PEG); urine (predominant route for absorbed sulfates and PEG)

Dosage Bowel cleansing prior to colonoscopy: Adults:

Oral: May be administered as the *split-dose (2-day) regimen* (preferred method) or the *day-before (1-day) regimen* (alternative method).

Split-dose (2-day) regimen: Total volume of liquid consumed over the course of treatment: 3440 mL (~115 oz)

Dose 1: Evening before colonoscopy (10-12 hours prior to Dose 2): Dilute the contents of the 6-ounce oral solution bottle to a final volume of 480 mL (16 oz), and drink the contents within 20 minutes. Refill container with 16 ounces of water and drink over the next 2 hours. Refill the container with the second refill of 16 oz of water, and finish drinking before bedtime (2 refills totaling 960 mL [32 oz]). Total volume of liquid consumed with Dose 1: 1440 mL (48 oz).

Dose 2: Morning of the colonoscopy (beginning at least 3.5 hours prior to colonoscopy): Drink the entire contents of the reconstituted powder which has been diluted to a final volume of 2000 mL (2 L [~67 oz]) as follows: Using the 16-ounce container provided, drink at a rate of 480 mL (16 oz) every 20 minutes (four 16-ounce containers over ~1.5 hours). Complete at least 2 hours prior to colonoscopy. Total volume of liquid consumed with Dose 2: 2000 mL (~67 oz)

Day-before (1-day) regimen: Total volume of liquid consumed over the course of treatment: 3440 mL (~115 oz)

Dose 1: Evening before colonoscopy (beginning at least 3.5 hours prior to bedtime): Drink the diluted contents of the 6-ounce oral solution bottle, which has been further diluted to a final volume of 480 mL (16 oz), preferably within 20 minutes. Refill container with 480 mL (16 oz) of water, and drink over the next 2 hours. Total volume of liquid consumed with Dose 1: 960 mL (32 oz).

Dose 2: Evening before colonoscopy (~2 hours after starting Dose 1): Drink the entire contents of the reconstituted powder which has been diluted to a final volume of 2000 mL (2 L [~67 oz]) as follows: Using the 16-ounce container provided, drink at a rate of 480 mL (16 oz) every 20 minutes (four 16-ounce containers over ~1.5 hours). Refill the container with 480 mL (16 oz) of water and finish drinking before bedtime. Total volume of liquid consumed with Dose 2: 2480 mL (~83 oz).

Dosage adjustment in renal impairment: No dosage adjustment provided in manufacturer's labeling (safety has not been adequately studied); however, use caution and ensure adequate hydration in patients with renal impairment or at risk for impairment. Moderate renal impairment (Cl_{cr} 30-49 mL/minute) resulted in a 43% higher C_{max} and a 16% lower urinary clearance of serum sulfates compared to healthy patients.

Dosage adjustment in hepatic impairment: No dosage adjustment provided in manufacturer's labeling.

Dietary Considerations Patient should not eat solid food from start of solution administration until after colonoscopy. Patient may have clear liquids (no solid food or milk) until 2 hours prior to colonoscopy.

Administration Oral: Each bottle must be diluted prior to use. The entire contents should be consumed followed by each postdose hydration amount, as directed depending on the regimen. Only clear liquids should be consumed from the start of the dosing regimen until 2 hours prior to colonoscopy; thereafter, nothing should be consumed until after colonoscopy. Patients should avoid solid foods, red and purple liquids, milk, and alcoholic beverages on the day prior and the day of the colonoscopy. Oral medications should not be administered within 1 hour of start of therapy.

Monitoring Parameters Consider baseline and postprocedure labwork (eg, electrolytes, BUN, creatinine) in patients at risk for renal impairment, seizure, or who have a history of electrolyte abnormality; post-colonoscopy labwork (electrolytes, creatinine, and BUN) is recommended in any patient experiencing significant vomiting or signs of dehydration following use. ECG (prior to therapy and post-colonoscopy) in patients with risks for prolonged QT or arrhythmias.

Dosage Forms Excipient information presented when available (limited, particularly for generics); consult specific product labeling.

Kit, oral [each kit contains]:

Suclear™: Powder for solution, oral: PEG 3350 210 g, sodium bicarbonate 2.86 g, sodium chloride 5.6 g, potassium chloride 0.74 g (2000 mL) [contains cherry, lemon-lime, orange, and pineapple flavor packs] and Solution, oral: Sodium sulfate 17.5 g, potassium sulfate 3.13 g, and magnesium sulfate 1.6 g (177 mL) [contains sodium benzoate]

Sodium Tetradecyl Sulfate

(SOW dee um tetra DEK il SUL fate)

Brand Names: U.S. Sotradecol

Brand Names: Canada Trombovar

Pharmacologic Category Sclerosing Agent

Use Treatment of small, uncomplicated varicose veins of the lower extremities

Pregnancy Risk Factor C

Dosage I.V.: Test dose: 0.5 mL given several hours prior to administration of larger dose; 0.5-2 mL (preferred maximum: 1 mL) in each vein, maximum: 10 mL per treatment session; 3% solution reserved for large varices

Dosage adjustment in renal impairment: No dosage adjustment provided in manufacturer's labeling.

Dosage adjustment in hepatic impairment: No dosage adjustment provided in manufacturer's labeling.

Additional Information Complete prescribing information should be consulted for additional detail.

Dosage Forms Excipient information presented when available (limited, particularly for generics); consult specific product labeling.

Solution, Intravenous, as sulfate:

Sotradecol: 1% (2 mL); 3% (2 mL) [contains benzyl alcohol]

Sodium Thiosulfate (SOW dee um thye oh SUL fate)

Index Terms Disodium Thiosulfate Pentahydrate; Pentahydrate; Sodium Hyposulfate; Sodium Thiosulphate; Thiosulfuric Acid Disodium Salt

Pharmacologic Category Antidote; Antidote, Extravasation

Use Treatment of cyanide poisoning

Unlabeled Use Management of mechlorethamine extravasation; management of concentrated cisplatin (≥0.4 mg/mL) extravasation; management of bendamustine extravasation

Pregnancy Risk Factor C

Pregnancy Considerations Teratogenic effects were not observed in animal reproduction studies of sodium thiosulfate. In general, medications used as antidotes should take into consideration the health and prognosis of the mother; antidotes should be administered to pregnant women if there is a clear indication for use and should not be withheld because of fears of teratogenicity (Bailey, 2003).

Breast-Feeding Considerations It is not known if sodium thiosulfate is excreted in breast milk. Because sodium thiosulfate may be used as an antidote in life-threatening situations, breast-feeding is not a contraindication to use. It is not known when breast-feeding may safely be restarted following administration; the manufacturer recommends caution be used following administration to nursing women.

Contraindications There are no contraindications listed within the manufacturer's labeling.

Warnings/Precautions Due to the risk for serious adverse effects, use with caution in patients where the diagnosis of cyanide poisoning is uncertain. However, if clinical suspicion of cyanide poisoning is high, treatment should not be delayed. Treatment of cyanide poisoning should include external decontamination and supportive therapy. Collection of pretreatment blood cyanide concentrations does not preclude administration and should not delay administration in the emergency management of highly suspected or confirmed cyanide toxicity. Pretreatment levels may be useful as postinfusion levels may be inaccurate. Monitor patients for return of symptoms for 24-48 hours; repeat treatment should be administered if symptoms return. Fire victims may present with both cyanide and carbon monoxide poisoning. In these patients, the induction of methemoglobinemia with amyl nitrite or sodium nitrite is contraindicated until carbon monoxide levels return to normal due to the risk of tissue hypoxia. Methemoglobinemia decreases the oxygen-carrying capacity of hemoglobin and the presence of carbon monoxide prevents hemoglobin from releasing oxygen to the tissues. In this scenario, sodium thiosulfate may be used alone to promote the clearance of cyanide. Hydroxocobalamin, however, should be considered to avoid the nitrite-related problems and because sodium thiosulfate has a slow onset of action. Hydroxocobalamin, however, should be considered to avoid the nitrite-related problems and because sodium thiosulfate has a slow onset of action. Consider consultation with a poison control center at 1-800-222-1222.

The presence of sulfite hypersensitivity should not preclude the use of this medication.

Adverse Reactions Frequency not defined

Cardiovascular: Hypotension

Central nervous system: Disorientation, headache

Gastrointestinal: Nausea, salty taste, vomiting

Hematologic: Bleeding time prolonged

Miscellaneous: Warmth

Drug Interactions

Metabolism/Transport Effects None known.

Avoid Concomitant Use There are no known interactions where it is recommended to avoid concomitant use.

Increased Effect/Toxicity There are no known significant interactions involving an increase in effect.

Decreased Effect There are no known significant interactions involving a decrease in effect.

Preparation for Administration Extravasation management (unlabeled use/route): To prepare a 1/6 M solution for SubQ administration (unlabeled route), add 4 mL of a 10% sodium thiosulfate solution to 6 mL SWFI or 1.6 mL of a 25% sodium thiosulfate solution to 8.4 mL SWFI.

Storage/Stability Store at 20°C to 25°C (68°F to 77°F); excursions permitted to 15°C to 30°C (59°F to 86°F). Protect from light. Do not freeze.

Extravasation management (unlabeled use/route): Store the 1/6 M solution for SubQ administration at 15°C to 30°C (59°F to 86°F) (Polovich, 2009).

Mechanism of Action

Cyanide toxicity: Serves as a sulfur donor in rhodanese-catalyzed formation of thiocyanate (much less toxic than cyanide)

Extravasation management: Neutralizes the reactive species of mechlorethamine; reduces the formation of hydroxyl radicals which cause tissue injury

Pharmacodynamics/Kinetics

Half-life elimination: Thiosulfate: ~3 hours; Thiocyanate: ~3 days; Renal impairment: ≤9 days

Excretion: Urine (~20% to 50% as unchanged drug)

Dosage

Cyanide poisoning: I.V.: **Note:** Usually given in conjunction with sodium nitrite. Administer sodium nitrite first, followed immediately by the administration of sodium thiosulfate.

Children: 7 g/m^2 or 250 mg/kg (1 mL/kg or 28-40 mL/m^2 of a 25% solution); maximum dose: 12.5 g (50 mL of a 25% solution); may repeat at one-half the original dose if symptoms of cyanide toxicity return

Adults: 12.5 g (50 mL of a 25% solution); may repeat at one-half the original dose if symptoms of cyanide toxicity return

Note: Monitor the patient for 24-48 hours; if symptoms return, repeat both sodium nitrite and sodium thiosulfate at one-half the original doses.

Extravasation management (unlabeled use): Adults:

Mechlorethamine: SubQ (unlabeled route): Inject 2 mL of a 1/6 M (~4%) sodium thiosulfate solution (into the extravasation site) for each mg of mechlorethamine suspected to have extravasated (Pérez Fidalgo, 2012; Polovich, 2009)

Cisplatin, concentrated: Inject 2 mL of a 1/6 M (~4%) sodium thiosulfate solution into existing I.V. line for each 100 mg of cisplatin extravasated; consider also injecting 1 mL of a 1/6 M (~4%) sodium thiosulfate solution as 0.1 mL subcutaneous injections (clockwise) into the area around the extravasation, may repeat subcutaneous injections several times over the next 3-4 hours (Ener, 2004)

Bendamustine: SubQ: Bendamustine extravasation may be managed with 1/6 M (~4%) sodium thiosulfate solution in the same manner as mechlorethamine extravasation (Schulmeister, 2011)

Dosage adjustment in renal impairment: No dosage adjustment provided in manufacturer's labeling. However, use with caution since the risk of toxic reactions may be greater in those with renal impairment.

Dosage adjustment in hepatic impairment: No dosage adjustment provided in the manufacturer's labeling.

Administration

I.V.: Administer over 10-20 minutes.

Extravasation management (unlabeled use): Stop vesicant infusion immediately and disconnect I.V. line (leave needle/cannula in place); gently aspirate extravasated solution from the I.V. line (do **NOT** flush the line); remove needle/cannula (temporarily keep in place for cisplatin extravasation to allow for sodium thiosulfate administration through the needle/cannula); elevate extremity.

Mechlorethamine: Inject subcutaneously (unlabeled route) into the extravasation site using ≤25-gauge needle; change needle with each injection (Pérez Fidalgo, 2012; Polovich, 2009).

Cisplatin, concentrated: Inject into the existing I.V. line; consider also injecting 1 mL as 0.1 mL subcutaneous injections (clockwise) into the area around the extravasation using a new 25- or 27-gauge needle for each injection (Ener, 2004).

Bendamustine: SubQ: Bendamustine extravasation may be managed with sodium thiosulfate in the same manner as mechlorethamine extravasation (Schulmeister, 2011).

Monitoring Parameters

Cyanide poisoning: Monitor for at least 24-48 hours after administration; blood pressure and heart rate during and after infusion; hemoglobin/hematocrit; co-oximetry; serum lactate levels; venous-arterial PO_2 gradient; serum methemoglobin and oxyhemoglobin. Pretreatment cyanide levels may be useful diagnostically.

Extravasation management: Monitor and document extravasation site for pain, blister formation, skin sloughing, arm/hand swelling/stiffness; monitor for fever, chills, or worsening pain

Dosage Forms Excipient information presented when available (limited, particularly for generics); consult specific product labeling.

Injection, solution [preservative free]: 100 mg/mL (10 mL); 250 mg/mL (50 mL)

Injection, solution: 250 mg/mL (50 mL)

◆ **Sodium Thiosulfate and Sodium Nitrite** *see* Sodium Nitrite and Sodium Thiosulfate *on page* 1920

◆ **Sodium Thiosulphate** *see* Sodium Thiosulfate *on page* 1931

◆ **Sof-Lax [OTC]** *see* Docusate *on page* 644

◆ **Soflax [OTC] (Can)** *see* Bisacodyl *on page* 259

◆ **Soflax™ (Can)** *see* Docusate *on page* 644

◆ **Solaquin® (Can)** *see* Hydroquinone *on page* 1017

◆ **Solaquin Forte® (Can)** *see* Hydroquinone *on page* 1017

Solifenacin (sol i FEN a sin)

Brand Names: U.S. VESIcare

Index Terms Solifenacin Succinate; YM905

Pharmacologic Category Anticholinergic Agent

Additional Appendix Information

Beers Criteria – Potentially Inappropriate Medications for Geriatrics *on page* 2368

Use Treatment of overactive bladder with symptoms of urinary frequency, urgency, or urge incontinence

Pregnancy Risk Factor C

Pregnancy Considerations Adverse events were observed in some animal reproduction studies.

Breast-Feeding Considerations It is not known if solifenacin is excreted in breast milk. The manufacturer recommends a decision be made whether to discontinue nursing or to discontinue the drug.

Contraindications Hypersensitivity to solifenacin or any component of the formulation; urinary retention; gastric retention; uncontrolled narrow-angle glaucoma.

Warnings/Precautions Cases of angioedema involving the face, lips, tongue, and/or larynx have been reported during treatment; some cases have occurred after the first dose. Immediately discontinue if tongue, hypopharynx, or larynx is involved. Anaphylactic reactions have been reported rarely with solifenacin; immediately discontinue therapy if anaphylactic reaction develops. Do not use in patients with a known or suspected hypersensitivity. Central nervous system effects have been reported (eg, headache, confusion, hallucinations, somnolence); monitor, particularly at treatment initiation or dose increase, reduce dose or discontinue if necessary. May cause drowsiness and/or blurred vision, which may impair physical or mental abilities; patients must be cautioned about performing tasks which require mental alertness (eg, operating machinery or driving). Heat prostration may occur in the presence of increased environmental temperature; use caution in hot weather and/or exercise. Use with caution in patients with bladder outflow obstruction, gastrointestinal obstructive disorders, and decreased gastrointestinal motility. Use with caution in patients with a known history of QT prolongation or other risk factors for QT prolongation (eg, concomitant use of medications known to prolong QT interval and/or electrolyte abnormalities); the risk for QT prolongation is dose-related. Use with caution in patients with controlled (treated) narrow-angle glaucoma; use is contraindicated with uncontrolled narrow-angle glaucoma. Dosage adjustment is required for patients with severe renal impairment (Cl_{cr} <30 mL/minute) or moderate (Child-Pugh class B) hepatic impairment; use is not recommended with severe hepatic impairment (Child-Pugh class C). Patients on potent CYP3A4 inhibitors require the lower dose of solifenacin. This medication is associated with potent anticholinergic properties which may be inappropriate in older adults depending on comorbidities (eg, dementia, delirium) (Beers Criteria).

Adverse Reactions

>10%: Gastrointestinal: Xerostomia (11% to 28%; dose-related), constipation (5% to 13%; dose-related)

1% to 10%:

Cardiovascular: Edema (≤1%), hypertension (≤1%)

Central nervous system: Fatigue (1% to 2%), depression (≤1%)

Gastrointestinal: Dyspepsia (1% to 4%), nausea (2% to 3%), upper abdominal pain (1% to 2%)

Genitourinary: Urinary tract infection (3% to 5%), urinary retention (≤1%)

Ocular: Blurred vision (4% to 5%), dry eye syndrome (≤2%)

Respiratory: Cough (≤1%)

Miscellaneous: Influenza (≤2%)

<1% (Limited to important or life-threatening): Abnormal hepatic function tests, anaphylaxis, angioedema, confusion, delirium, erythema multiforme, exfoliative dermatitis, fecal impaction, gastroesophageal reflux disease, gastrointestinal obstruction, glaucoma, hallucination, hyperkalemia, hypersensitivity reactions, intestinal obstruction, prolonged Q-T interval on ECG, renal insufficiency, torsades de pointes, voice disorder

Drug Interactions

Metabolism/Transport Effects Substrate of CYP3A4 (major); **Note:** Assignment of Major/Minor substrate status based on clinically relevant drug interaction potential

Avoid Concomitant Use

Avoid concomitant use of Solifenacin with any of the following: Aclidinium; Conivaptan; Fusidic Acid (Systemic); Ipratropium (Oral Inhalation); Potassium Chloride; Tiotropium; Umeclidinium

Increased Effect/Toxicity

Solifenacin may increase the levels/effects of: AbobotulinumtoxinA; Analgesics (Opioid); Anticholinergics; Cannabinoids; Highest Risk QTc-Prolonging Agents; Moderate Risk QTc-Prolonging Agents; OnabotulinumtoxinA; Potassium Chloride; RimabotulinumtoxinB; Thiazide Diuretics; Tiotropium; Topiramate

The levels/effects of Solifenacin may be increased by: Aclidinium; Antifungal Agents (Azole Derivatives, Systemic); Conivaptan; CYP3A4 Inhibitors (Moderate); CYP3A4 Inhibitors (Strong); Dasatinib; Fusidic Acid (Systemic); Ipratropium (Oral Inhalation); Ivacaftor; Luliconazole; Mifepristone; Mirabegron; Pramlintide; Simeprevir; Umeclidinium

Decreased Effect

Solifenacin may decrease the levels/effects of: Acetylcholinesterase Inhibitors (Central); Secretin

The levels/effects of Solifenacin may be decreased by: Acetylcholinesterase Inhibitors (Central); Bosentan; CYP3A4 Inducers (Strong); Dabrafenib; Deferasirox; Herbs (CYP3A4 Inducers); Mitotane; Tocilizumab

Ethanol/Nutrition/Herb Interactions

Food: Grapefruit juice may increase the serum level effects of solifenacin.

Herb/Nutraceutical: St John's wort (*Hypericum*) may decrease the levels/effects of solifenacin.

Storage/Stability Store at controlled room temperature of 25°C (77°F); excursions permitted to 15°C to 30°C (59°F to 86°F).

Mechanism of Action Inhibits muscarinic receptors resulting in decreased urinary bladder contraction, increased residual urine volume, and decreased detrusor muscle pressure.

Pharmacodynamics/Kinetics

Distribution: V_d: ~600 L

Protein binding: ~98% bound primarily to alpha$_1$-acid glycoprotein

Metabolism: Extensively hepatic; via N-oxidation and 4 R-hydroxylation, forms 1 active and 3 inactive metabolites; primary pathway for elimination is via CYP3A4

Bioavailability: ~90%

Half-life elimination: 45-68 hours following chronic dosing; prolonged in severe renal (Cl_{cr} <30 mL/minute) or moderate hepatic (Child-Pugh class B) impairment

Time to peak, plasma: 3-8 hours

Excretion: Urine (69%; <15% as unchanged drug); feces (23%)

Dosage Oral: Adults: 5 mg once daily; if tolerated, may increase to 10 mg once daily

Dosage adjustment with concomitant CYP3A4 inhibitors: Maximum solifenacin dose: 5 mg/day

Dosage adjustment in renal impairment: Use with caution in reduced renal function

Cl_{cr} <30 mL/minute: Maximum dose: 5 mg/day

Dosage adjustment in hepatic impairment: Use with caution in reduced hepatic function

Moderate (Child-Pugh class B): Maximum dose: 5 mg/day

Severe (Child-Pugh class C): Use is not recommended

Dietary Considerations May be taken without regard to meals.

Administration Swallow tablet whole; administer with liquids; may be administered without regard to meals.

Monitoring Parameters Anticholinergic effects (eg, fixed and dilated pupils, blurred vision, tremors, or dry skin); creatinine clearance (prior to treatment for dosing adjustment); liver function

Dosage Forms Excipient information presented when available (limited, particularly for generics); consult specific product labeling.

Tablet, Oral, as succinate:

VESIcare: 5 mg, 10 mg

◆ **Solifenacin Succinate** *see* Solifenacin *on page 1932*

◆ **Soliris** *see* Eculizumab *on page 683*

◆ **Soliris® (Can)** *see* Eculizumab *on page 683*

◆ **Solodyn** *see* Minocycline *on page 1373*

◆ **Soltamox** *see* Tamoxifen *on page 1987*

◆ **Soluble Fluorescein** *see* Fluorescein *on page 880*

◆ **Solu-CORTEF** *see* Hydrocortisone (Systemic) *on page 1008*

◆ **Solu-Cortef® (Can)** *see* Hydrocortisone (Systemic) *on page 1008*

◆ **Solumedrol** *see* MethylPREDNISolone *on page 1340*
◆ **Solu-MEDROL** *see* MethylPREDNISolone *on page 1340*
◆ **Solu-Medrol® (Can)** *see* MethylPREDNISolone *on page 1340*
◆ **Solzira** *see* Gabapentin Enacarbil *on page 936*
◆ **SOM230** *see* Pasireotide *on page 1579*
◆ **Soma** *see* Carisoprodol *on page 351*
◆ **Soma Compound** *see* Carisoprodol and Aspirin *on page 352*
◆ **Soma Compound w/Codeine** *see* Carisoprodol, Aspirin, and Codeine *on page 352*

Somatropin (soe ma TROE pin)

Brand Names: U.S. Genotropin; Genotropin MiniQuick; Humatrope; Norditropin FlexPro; Norditropin NordiFlex Pen; Nutropin AQ NuSpin 10; Nutropin AQ NuSpin 20; Nutropin AQ NuSpin 5; Nutropin AQ Pen; Nutropin [DSC]; Omnitrope; Saizen; Saizen Click.Easy; Serostim; Tev-Tropin; Zorbtive

Brand Names: Canada Humatrope; Norditropin Simplexx; Nutropin; Nutropin AQ; Nutropin AQ NuSpin™; Nutropin AQ Pen; Omnitrope; Saizen; Serostim

Index Terms Growth Hormone, Human; hGH; Human Growth Hormone

Pharmacologic Category Growth Hormone

Additional Appendix Information

Beers Criteria – Potentially Inappropriate Medications for Geriatrics *on page 2368*

Use

Children:

Treatment of growth failure due to inadequate endogenous growth hormone secretion (Genotropin®, Humatrope®, Norditropin®, Nutropin®, Nutropin AQ®, Omnitrope®, Saizen®, Tev-Tropin®)

Treatment of short stature associated with Turner syndrome (Genotropin®, Humatrope®, Norditropin®, Nutropin®, Nutropin AQ®, Omnitrope®)

Treatment of Prader-Willi syndrome (Genotropin®, Omnitrope®)

Treatment of growth failure associated with chronic renal insufficiency (CRI) up until the time of renal transplantation (Nutropin®, Nutropin AQ®)

Treatment of growth failure in children born small for gestational age who fail to manifest catch-up growth by 2 years of age (Genotropin®, Omnitrope®) or by 2-4 years of age (Humatrope®, Norditropin®)

Treatment of idiopathic short stature (nongrowth hormone-deficient short stature) defined by height standard deviation score (SDS) ≤-2.25 and growth rate not likely to attain normal adult height (Genotropin®, Humatrope®, Nutropin®, Nutropin AQ®, Omnitrope®)

Treatment of short stature or growth failure associated with short stature homeobox gene (SHOX) deficiency (Humatrope®)

Treatment of short stature associated with Noonan syndrome (Norditropin®)

Adults:

HIV patients with wasting or cachexia with concomitant antiviral therapy (Serostim®)

Replacement of endogenous growth hormone in patients with adult growth hormone deficiency who meet both of the following criteria (Genotropin®, Humatrope®, Norditropin®, Nutropin®, Nutropin AQ®, Omnitrope®, Saizen®):

Biochemical diagnosis of adult growth hormone deficiency by means of a subnormal response to a standard growth hormone stimulation test (peak growth hormone ≤5 mcg/L). Confirmatory testing may not be required in patients with congenital/genetic growth hormone deficiency or multiple pituitary hormone deficiencies due to organic diseases.

and

Adult-onset: Patients who have adult growth hormone deficiency whether alone or with multiple hormone deficiencies (hypopituitarism) as a result of pituitary disease, hypothalamic disease, surgery, radiation therapy, or trauma

or

Childhood-onset: Patients who were growth hormone deficient during childhood, confirmed as an adult before replacement therapy is initiated

Treatment of short-bowel syndrome (Zorbtive®)

Unlabeled Use Pediatric HIV patients with wasting/cachexia (Serostim®); HIV-associated adipose redistribution syndrome (HARS) (Serostim®)

Pregnancy Risk Factor B/C (depending upon manufacturer)

Pregnancy Considerations Teratogenic effects were not observed in animal studies. Reproduction studies have not been conducted with all agents. During normal pregnancy, maternal production of endogenous growth hormone decreases as placental growth hormone production increases. Data with somatropin use during pregnancy is limited.

Breast-Feeding Considerations It is not known if somatropin is excreted in breast milk. The manufacturer recommends that caution be exercised when administering somatropin to nursing women.

Contraindications Hypersensitivity to growth hormone or any component of the formulation; growth promotion in pediatric patients with closed epiphyses; progression or recurrence of any underlying intracranial lesion or actively growing intracranial tumor; acute critical illness due to complications following open heart or abdominal surgery; multiple accidental trauma or acute respiratory failure; evidence of active malignancy; active proliferative or severe nonproliferative diabetic retinopathy; use in patients with Prader-Willi syndrome **without** growth hormone deficiency (except Genotropin®) or in patients with Prader-Willi syndrome **with** growth hormone deficiency who are severely obese, have a history of upper airway obstruction or sleep apnea, or have severe respiratory impairment

Warnings/Precautions Initiation of somatropin is contraindicated with acute critical illness due to complications following open heart or abdominal surgery, multiple accidental trauma, or acute respiratory failure; mortality may be increased. The safety of continuing somatropin in patients who develop these illnesses during therapy has not been established; use with caution. Use in contraindicated with active malignancy; monitor patients with pre-existing tumors or growth failure secondary to an intracranial lesion for recurrence or progression of underlying disease; discontinue therapy with evidence of recurrence. An increased risk of second neoplasm has been reported in childhood cancer survivors treated with somatropin; the most common second neoplasms were meningiomas in patients treated with radiation to the head for their first neoplasm. Monitor patients for any malignant transformation of skin lesions.

Somatropin may decrease insulin sensitivity; use with caution in patients with diabetes or with risk factors for impaired glucose tolerance. Adjustment of antidiabetic medications may be necessary. Pancreatitis has been rarely reported; incidence in children (especially girls) with Turner syndrome may be greater than adults. Monitor for hypersensitivity reactions. Patients with hypoadrenalism may require increased dosages of glucocorticoids (especially cortisone acetate and prednisone) due to somatropin-mediated inhibition of 11 beta-hydroxysteroid dehydrogenase type 1; undiagnosed central hypoadrenalism may be unmasked. Excessive glucocorticoid therapy may inhibit the growth promoting effects of somatropin in children; monitor and adjust glucocorticoids carefully. Untreated/undiagnosed hypothyroidism may decrease response to therapy; monitor thyroid function test periodically and initiate/adjust thyroid replacement therapy as needed. Closely monitor other hormonal replacement treatments in patients with hypopituitarism. Obese patients may experience an increased incidence of adverse events when using a weight-based dosing regimen. Intracranial hypertension (IH) with headache, nausea, papilledema, visual changes, and/or vomiting has been reported with somatropin; funduscopic examination prior to initiation of therapy and periodically thereafter is recommended. Treatment should be discontinued in patients who develop papilledema; resuming treatment at a lower dose may be considered once IH-associated signs and symptoms have resolved. Patients with Turner syndrome, chronic renal failure and Prader-Willi syndrome may be at increased risk for IH. Progression of scoliosis may occur in children experiencing rapid growth. Patients with growth hormone deficiency may develop slipped capital epiphyses more frequently, evaluate any child with new onset of a limp or with complaints of hip or knee pain. Patients with Turner syndrome are at increased risk for otitis media and other ear/hearing disorders, cardiovascular disorders (including stroke, aortic aneurysm, hypertension), and thyroid disease, monitor carefully. Fluid retention may occur frequently in adults during use; manifestations of fluid retention (eg, edema, arthralgia, myalgia, nerve compression syndromes/paresthesias) are generally transient and dose dependent. Products may contain benzyl alcohol or m-cresol. When administering to newborns, reconstitute with sterile water or saline for injection. Not for I.V. injection. According to the Centers for Disease Control and Prevention (CDC), pen-shaped injection devices should never be used for more than one person (even when the needle is changed) because of the risk of infection. The injection device should be clearly labeled with individual patient information to ensure that the correct pen is used (CDC, 2012).

Fatalities have been reported in pediatric patients with Prader-Willi syndrome following the use of growth hormone. The reported fatalities occurred in patients with one or more risk factors, including severe obesity, sleep apnea, respiratory impairment, or unidentified respiratory infection; male patients with one or more of these factors may be at greater risk. Treatment interruption is recommended in patients who show signs of upper airway obstruction, including the onset of, or increased, snoring. In addition, evaluation of and/or monitoring for sleep apnea and respiratory infections are recommended.

Patients with HIV infection should be maintained on antiretroviral therapy to prevent the potential increase in viral replication.

Avoid use in the elderly, except as hormone replacement following pituitary gland removal; use results in minimal effect on body composition and is associated with edema, arthralgia, carpal tunnel syndrome, gynecomastia, and impaired fasting glucose (Beers Criteria). Elderly may be more sensitive to the actions of somatropin; consider lower starting doses.

Safety and efficacy have not been established for the treatment of Noonan syndrome in children with significant cardiac disease. Children with epiphyseal closure who are treated for adult GHD need reassessment of therapy and dose. Administration site rotation is necessary to prevent tissue atrophy.

Adverse Reactions

Growth hormone deficiency: Adverse reactions reported with growth hormone deficiency vary greatly by age. Generally, percentages are less in pediatric patients than adults, and many of the reactions reported in adults are dose related. Percentages reported also vary by product. Below is a listing by age group; events reported more commonly overall are noted with an asterisk (*).

Children: Antibodies development, arthralgia, benign intracranial hypertension, edema, eosinophilia, glycosuria, Hb A_{1c} increased, headache, hematoma, hematuria, hyperglycemia (mild), hypertriglyceridemia, hypoglycemia, hypothyroidism, injection site reaction, intracranial tumor, leg pain, lipoatrophy, leukemia, meningioma, muscle pain, papilledema, pseudotumor cerebri, psoriasis exacerbation, rash, scoliosis progression, seizure, slipped capital femoral epiphysis, weakness

Adults: Acne, ALT increased, AST increased, arthralgia*, back pain, bronchitis, carpal tunnel syndrome, chest pain, cough, depression, diabetes mellitus (type 2), diaphoresis, dizziness, edema*, fatigue, flu-like syndrome*, gastritis, glucose intolerance, glucosuria, headache*, hyperglycemia (mild), hypertension, hypoesthesia, hypothyroidism, infection, insomnia, insulin resistance, joint disorder, leg edema, muscle pain, myalgia*, nausea, pain in extremities, paresthesia*, peripheral edema*, pharyngitis, retinopathy, rhinitis, skeletal pain*, stiffness in extremities, surgical procedure, upper respiratory tract infection, weakness

Additional/postmarketing reactions observed with growth hormone deficiency: Gynecomastia, increased growth of pre-existing nevi, pancreatitis

HARS: Serostim®: Limited to >10%: Edema (peripheral) (19% to 45%), arthralgia (28% to 37%), pain (extremity) (5% to 19%), hypoesthesia (9% to 15%), headache (4% to 14%), blood glucose increased (4% to 14%), paresthesia (11% to 13%), myalgia (3% to 13%)

Idiopathic short stature: Percentages reported using Humatrope® versus placebo: Myalgia (24%), scoliosis (19%), otitis media (16%), arthralgia (11%), arthrosis (11%), hyperlipidemia (8%), gynecomastia (5%), hip pain (3%), hypertension (3%). Additional adverse reactions listed as reported using other products from ISS NCGS Cohort (frequencies <1%): Aggressiveness, benign intracranial hypertension, diabetes, edema, hair loss, headache, injection site reaction

Prader-Willi syndrome: Genotropin® (frequency not defined): Aggressiveness, arthralgia, edema, hair loss, headache, benign intracranial hypertension, myalgia; fatalities associated with use in this population have been reported

Turner syndrome: Percentages reported using Humatrope® compared to untreated patients. Additional adverse reactions reported from other products, frequency not specified: Surgical procedures (45%), otitis media (43%), ear disorders (18%), joint pain, respiratory illness, urinary tract infection

HIV patients with wasting or cachexia: Serostim® (limited to ≥5%): Musculoskeletal disorders (arthralgia, arthrosis, myalgia: 78%), peripheral edema (26%), headache (13%), nausea (9%), paresthesia (8%), edema (6%), gynecomastia (6%), hypoesthesia (5%)

Short-bowel syndrome: Zorbtive® (limited to >10%): Peripheral edema (69% to 81%), facial edema (44% to 50%), arthralgia (31% to 44%), nausea (13% to 31%), injection site pain (up to 31%), flatulence (25%), injection site reaction (19% to 25%), abdominal pain (13% to 25%), vomiting (19%), pain (6% to 19%), chest pain (up to 19%), dehydration (up to 19%), infection (up to 19%), rhinitis (up to 19%), hearing symptoms (13%), dizziness (6% to 13%), rash (6% to 13%), diaphoresis (up to 13%), generalized edema (up to 13%), malaise (up to 13%), moniliasis (up to 13%), myalgia (up to 13%)

SHOX deficiency: Humatrope®: Arthralgia (11%), gynecomastia (8%), excessive cutaneous nevi (7%), scoliosis (4%)

Small for gestational age: Genotropin®, Humatrope® (frequency not defined): Mild, transient hyperglycemia; benign intracranial hypertension (rare); central precocious puberty; jaw prominence (rare); aggravation of pre-existing scoliosis (rare); injection site reactions; progression of pigmented nevi; carpal tunnel syndrome (rare) diabetes mellitus (rare); otitis media; headache; slipped capital femoral epiphysis

Drug Interactions

Metabolism/Transport Effects None known.

Avoid Concomitant Use There are no known interactions where it is recommended to avoid concomitant use.

Increased Effect/Toxicity There are no known significant interactions involving an increase in effect.

Decreased Effect

Somatropin may decrease the levels/effects of: Antidiabetic Agents; Cortisone; PredniSONE

The levels/effects of Somatropin may be decreased by: Estrogen Derivatives

Preparation for Administration

Genotropin®: Reconstitute with diluent provided.

Genotropin MiniQuick®: Reconstitute with diluent provided. Consult the instructions provided with the reconstitution device.

Humatrope®:

Cartridge: Consult HumatroPen™ User Guide for complete instructions for reconstitution. **Dilute with solution provided with cartridges ONLY; do not use diluent provided with vials.**

Vial: 5 mg: Reconstitute with 1.5-5 mL diluent provided. Swirl gently; do not shake.

Nutropin®: Vial:

5 mg: Reconstitute with 1-5 mL bacteriostatic water for injection. Swirl gently, do not shake.

10 mg: Reconstitute with 1-10 mL bacteriostatic water for injection. Swirl gently, do not shake.

Omnitrope® powder: Reconstitute with provided diluent. Swirl gently; do not shake.

Saizen®: Vial:

5 mg: Reconstitute with 1-3 mL bacteriostatic water for injection or sterile water for injection. Gently swirl; do not shake.

8.8 mg: Reconstitute with 2-3 mL bacteriostatic water for injection or sterile water for injection. Gently swirl; do not shake.

Serostim®: Vial: Reconstitute with 0.5-1 mL sterile water for injection.

Tev-Tropin®: Reconstitute with 1-5 mL of diluent provided. Gently swirl; do not shake. May use preservative-free NS for use in newborns.

Zorbtive®: 8.8 mg vial: Reconstitute with 1-2 mL bacteriostatic water for injection. Swirl gently.

Storage/Stability

Genotropin®: Store at 2°C to 8°C (36°F to 46°F); do not freeze. Protect from light. Following reconstitution of 5.8 mg and 13.8 mg cartridge, store under refrigeration and use within 28 days.

Genotropin® Miniquick®: Store in refrigerator prior to dispensing, but may be stored ≤25°C (77°F) for up to 3 months after dispensing. Once reconstituted, solution must be refrigerated and used within 24 hours. Discard unused portion.

Humatrope®:

Vial: Before and after reconstitution, store at 2°C to 8°C (36°F to 46°F); do not freeze. When reconstituted with provided diluent or bacteriostatic water for injection, use within 14 days. When reconstituted with sterile water for injection, use within 24 hours and discard unused portion.

Cartridge: Before and after reconstitution, store at 2°C to 8°C (36°F to 46°F); do not freeze. Following reconstitution with provided diluent, stable for 28 days under refrigeration.

Norditropin®: Store at 2°C to 8°C (36°F to 46°F); do not freeze. Avoid direct light.

Cartridge: When refrigerated, must be used within 4 weeks once inserted into pen. Orange cartridges (5 mg/1.5 mL) may also be stored up to 3 weeks at ≤25°C (77°F).

Prefilled pen: When refrigerated, must be used within 4 weeks after initial injection. Orange and blue prefilled pens may also be stored up to 3 weeks at ≤25°C (77°F).

Nutropin®: Before and after reconstitution, store at 2°C to 8°C (36°F to 46°F); do not freeze.

Nutropin® vial: Use reconstituted vials within 14 days. When reconstituted with sterile water for injection, use immediately and discard unused portion.

Nutropin® AQ formulations: Use within 28 days following initial use.

Omnitrope®:

Powder for injection: Prior to reconstitution, store under refrigeration at 2°C to 8°C (36°F to 46°F); do not freeze. Protect from light. Reconstitute with provided diluent. Swirl gently; do not shake. Following reconstitution with the provided diluents, the 5.8 mg vial may be stored under refrigeration for up to 3 weeks. Store vial in carton to protect from light.

Solution: Prior to use, store under refrigeration at 2°C to 8°C (36°F to 46°F). Once the cartridge is loaded into the pen delivery system, store under refrigeration for up to 21 days after first use.

Saizen®: Prior to reconstitution, store at room temperature 15°C to 30°C (59°F to 86°F). Following reconstitution with bacteriostatic water for injection, reconstituted solution should be refrigerated and used within 14 days. When reconstituted with sterile water for injection, use immediately and discard unused portion. The Saizen® easy click cartridge, when reconstituted with the provided bacteriostatic water, should be stored under refrigeration and used within 21 days.

Serostim®: Prior to reconstitution, store at room temperature 15°C to 30°C (59°F to 86°F). When reconstituted with sterile water for injection, use immediately and discard unused portion.

Tev-Tropin®: Prior to reconstitution, store at 2°C to 8°C (36°F to 46°F). Following reconstitution with bacteriostatic NS, solution should be refrigerated and used within 14 days. Some cloudiness may occur; do not use if cloudiness persists after warming to room temperature.

Zorbtive®: Store unopened vials and diluent at room temperature of 15°C to 30°C (59°F to 86°F). Store reconstituted vial under refrigeration at 2°C to 8°C (36°F to 46°F) for up to 14 days; do not freeze.

Mechanism of Action Somatropin is a purified polypeptide hormones of recombinant DNA origin; somatropin contains the identical sequence of amino acids found in human growth hormone; human growth hormone assists growth of linear bone, skeletal muscle, and organs by stimulating chondrocyte proliferation and differentiation, lipolysis, protein synthesis, and hepatic glucose output; stimulates erythropoietin which increases red blood cell mass; exerts both insulin-like and diabetogenic effects; enhances the transmucosal transport of water, electrolytes, and nutrients across the gut

Pharmacodynamics/Kinetics

Duration: Maintains supraphysiologic levels for 18-20 hours

Absorption: I.M., SubQ: Well absorbed

Distribution: ~1 L/kg

Metabolism: Hepatic and renal (~90%)

Bioavailability: SubQ: ~70% to 90%; **Note:** Variable; product-dependent

Half-life elimination: Preparation and route of administration dependent; SubQ: ~2-4 hours
Excretion: Urine (small amount)

Dosage

Children (individualize dose):

Chronic renal insufficiency (CRI): Nutropin®, Nutropin® AQ: SubQ: Weekly dosage: 0.35 mg/kg divided into daily injections; continue until the time of renal transplantation

Dosage recommendations in patients treated for CRI who require dialysis:

Hemodialysis: Administer dose at night prior to bedtime or at least 3-4 hours after hemodialysis to prevent hematoma formation from heparin

CCPD: Administer dose in the morning following dialysis

CAPD: Administer dose in the evening at the time of overnight exchange

Growth hormone deficiency:

Genotropin®, Omnitrope®: SubQ: Weekly dosage: 0.16-0.24 mg/kg divided into equal doses 6-7 days per week

Humatrope®: SubQ: Weekly dosage: 0.18-0.3 mg/kg divided into equal doses 6-7 days per week

Norditropin®: SubQ: 0.024-0.034 mg/kg/day, 6-7 days per week

Nutropin®, Nutropin® AQ: SubQ: Weekly dosage: 0.3 mg/kg divided into equal daily doses; pubertal patients: ≤0.7 mg/kg divided into equal daily doses

Tev-Tropin®: SubQ: Up to 0.1 mg/kg/dose administered 3 days per week

Saizen®: I.M., SubQ: Weekly dosage: 0.18 mg/kg divided into equal daily doses **or** as 0.06 mg/kg/dose administered 3 days per week **or** as 0.03 mg/kg/dose administered 6 days per week

Note: Therapy should be discontinued when patient has reached satisfactory adult height, when epiphyses have fused, or when the patient ceases to respond. Growth of 5 cm/year or more is expected, if growth rate does not exceed 2.5 cm in a 6-month period, double the dose for the next 6 months; if there is still no satisfactory response, discontinue therapy

HIV patients with wasting or cachexia (unlabeled use): Serostim®: SubQ: Limited data; doses of 0.04 mg/kg/day were reported in five children, 6-17 years of age; doses of 0.07 mg/kg/day were reported in six children, 8-14 years of age

Idiopathic short stature:

Genotropin®, Omnitrope®: SubQ: Weekly dosage: 0.47 mg/kg divided into equal doses 6-7 days per week

Humatrope®: SubQ: Weekly dosage: 0.37 mg/kg divided into equal doses 6-7 days per week

Nutropin®, Nutropin AQ®: SubQ: Weekly dosage: Up to 0.3 mg/kg divided into equal daily doses

Noonan syndrome: Norditropin®: SubQ: Up to 0.066 mg/kg/day

Prader-Willi syndrome: Genotropin®, Omnitrope®: SubQ: Weekly dosage: 0.24 mg/kg divided into equal doses 6-7 days per week

SHOX deficiency: Humatrope®: SubQ: Weekly dosage: 0.35 mg/kg divided into equal doses 6-7 days per week

Small for gestational age:

Genotropin®, Omnitrope®: SubQ: Weekly dosage: 0.48 mg/kg divided into equal doses 6-7 days per week

Humatrope®: SubQ: Weekly dosage: 0.47 mg/kg divided into equal doses 6-7 days per week

Norditropin®: SubQ: Up to 0.067 mg/kg/day

Alternate dosing (small for gestational age): In older/early pubertal children or children with very short stature, consider initiating therapy at higher doses (0.067 mg/kg/day) and then consider reducing the dose (0.033 mg/kg/day) if substantial catch-up growth observed. In younger children (<4 years) with less severe short stature, consider initiating therapy with lower doses (0.033 mg/kg/day) and then titrating the dose upwards as needed.

Turner syndrome:

Genotropin®, Omnitrope®: SubQ: Weekly dosage: 0.33 mg/kg divided into equal doses 6-7 days per week

Humatrope®: SubQ: Weekly dosage: 0.375 mg/kg divided into equal doses 6-7 days per week

Norditropin®: SubQ: Up to 0.067 mg/kg/day

Nutropin®, Nutropin® AQ: SubQ: Weekly dosage: ≤0.375 mg/kg divided into equal doses 3-7 days per week

Adults:

Growth hormone deficiency: Adjust dose based on individual requirements: To minimize adverse events in older or overweight patients, reduced dosages may be necessary. During therapy, dosage should be decreased if required by the occurrence of side effects or excessive IGF-I levels.

Weight-based dosing:

Norditropin®: SubQ: Initial dose ≤0.004 mg/kg/day; after 6 weeks of therapy, may increase dose up to 0.016 mg/kg/day

Nutropin®, Nutropin® AQ: SubQ: ≤0.006 mg/kg/day; dose may be increased up to a maximum of 0.025 mg/kg/day in patients <35 years of age, or up to a maximum of 0.0125 mg/kg/day in patients ≥35 years of age

Humatrope®: SubQ: ≤0.006 mg/kg/day; dose may be increased up to a maximum of 0.0125 mg/kg/day

Genotropin®, Omnitrope®: SubQ: Weekly dosage: ≤0.04 mg/kg divided into equal doses 6-7 days per week; dose may be increased at 4- to 8-week intervals to a maximum of 0.08 mg/kg/week

Saizen®: SubQ: ≤0.005 mg/kg/day; dose may be increased to not more than 0.01 mg/kg/day after 4 weeks

Nonweight-based dosing: SubQ: Initial: 0.2 mg/day (range: 0.15-0.3 mg/day); may increase every 1-2 months by 0.1-0.2 mg/day based on response and/or serum IGF-I levels

Dosage adjustment with estrogen supplementation (growth hormone deficiency): Larger doses of somatropin may be needed for women taking oral estrogen replacement products; dosing not affected by topical products

HIV-associated adipose redistribution syndrome (HARS) (unlabeled use): Serostim®: SubQ: Induction: 4 mg once daily at bedtime for 12 weeks; Maintenance: 2 mg or 4 mg every other day at bedtime for 12-24 weeks. **Note:** Every-other-day dosing during induction has also been studied. Although a greater response was seen with daily dosing, it was associated with an increased incidence of adverse events.

HIV patients with wasting or cachexia: Serostim®: SubQ: 0.1 mg/kg once daily at bedtime (maximum: 6 mg/day). Alternately, patients at risk for side effects may be started at 0.1 mg/kg every other day. Patients who continue to lose weight after 12 weeks should be re-evaluated for opportunistic infections or other clinical events; rotate injection sites to avoid lipodystrophy Adjust dose if needed to manage side effects.

Daily dose based on body weight:

<35 kg: 0.1 mg/kg

35-45 kg: 4 mg

45-55 kg: 5 mg

>55 kg: 6 mg

Short-bowel syndrome (Zorbtive®): SubQ: 0.1 mg/kg once daily for 4 weeks (maximum: 8 mg/day)

Fluid retention (moderate) or arthralgias: Treat symptomatically or reduce dose by 50%
Severe toxicity: Discontinue therapy for up to 5 days; when symptoms resolve, restart at 50% of dose. If severe toxicity recurs or does not disappear within 5 days after discontinuation, permanently discontinue treatment.

Elderly: Patients ≥65 years of age may be more sensitive to the action of growth hormone and more prone to adverse effects; in general, dosing should be cautious, beginning at low end of dosing range

Dosage adjustment in renal impairment No dosage adjustment provided in manufacturer's labeling (has not been studied).

Dosage adjustment in hepatic impairment: No dosage adjustment provided in manufacturer's labeling (has not been studied).

Dietary Considerations

Prader-Willi syndrome: All patients should have effective weight control (use is contraindicated in severely-obese patients).

Short-bowel syndrome: Intravenous parenteral nutrition requirements may need reassessment as gastrointestinal absorption improves.

Administration Do not shake; administer SubQ or I.M. (not all products are approved for I.M. administration). Rotate administration sites to avoid tissue atrophy. When administering to newborns, do not reconstitute with a diluent that contains benzyl alcohol; sterile water for injection may be used as an alternative.

Norditropin® cartridge must be administered using the corresponding color-coded NordiPen® injection pen.

Omnitrope®: Solution in the cartridges must be administered using the Omnitrope® pen; when installing a new cartridge, prime pen prior to first use.

Humatrope®: When administering for growth hormone deficiency, SubQ route is preferred

Tev-Tropin®: SubQ injections of solutions >1 mL not recommended.

Monitoring Parameters Growth curve, Tanner staging (children), periodic thyroid function tests, bone age (annually), periodical urine testing for glucose, somatomedin C (IGF-I) levels; funduscopic examinations at initiation of therapy and periodically during treatment; serum phosphorus, alkaline phosphatase and parathyroid hormone. If growth deceleration is observed in children treated for growth hormone deficiency, and not due to other causes, evaluate for presence of antibody formation. Periodic blood glucose monitoring; strict blood glucose monitoring in patients with diabetes. Progression or recurrence of preexisting tumors or malignant transformation of skin lesions.

Note: Practice guidelines recommend monitoring for efficacy and adverse effects every 1-2 months during dose titration and semiannually, thereafter (TES, 2006).

CRI: Progression of renal osteodystrophy

Prader-Willi syndrome: Monitor for sleep apnea, respiratory infections, snoring (onset of or increased)

Turner syndrome: Ear disorders including otitis media; cardiovascular disorders

Noonan syndrome: Prior to use, verify short stature syndrome.

Dosage Forms Excipient information presented when available (limited, particularly for generics); consult specific product labeling. [DSC] = Discontinued product

Solution, Subcutaneous:

Norditropin FlexPro: 5 mg/1.5 mL (1.5 mL); 10 mg/1.5 mL (1.5 mL); 15 mg/1.5 mL (1.5 mL) [contains phenol]

Norditropin NordiFlex Pen: 30 mg/3 mL (3 mL) [contains phenol]

Nutropin AQ NuSpin 5: 5 mg/2 mL (2 mL) [contains phenol]

Nutropin AQ NuSpin 10: 10 mg/2 mL (2 mL) [contains phenol]

Nutropin AQ NuSpin 20: 20 mg/2 mL (2 mL) [contains phenol]

Nutropin AQ Pen: 10 mg/2 mL (2 mL)

Nutropin AQ Pen: 20 mg/2 mL (2 mL) [contains phenol]

Omnitrope: 5 mg/1.5 mL (1.5 mL) [contains benzyl alcohol]

Omnitrope: 10 mg/1.5 mL (1.5 mL) [contains phenol]

Solution Reconstituted, Injection:

Humatrope: 5 mg (1 ea)

Humatrope: 6 mg (1 ea); 12 mg (1 ea); 24 mg (1 ea) [contains glycerin, metacresol]

Saizen: 5 mg (1 ea); 8.8 mg (1 ea)

Saizen Click.Easy: 8.8 mg (1 ea)

Solution Reconstituted, Subcutaneous:

Genotropin: 5 mg (1 ea); 12 mg (1 ea) [contains metacresol]

Nutropin: 10 mg (1 ea [DSC]) [contains benzyl alcohol]

Omnitrope: 5.8 mg (1 ea)

Serostim: 4 mg (1 ea); 5 mg (1 ea); 6 mg (1 ea)

Tev-Tropin: 5 mg (1 ea)

Zorbtive: 8.8 mg (1 ea) [contains benzyl alcohol]

Solution Reconstituted, Subcutaneous [preservative free]:

Genotropin MiniQuick: 0.2 mg (1 ea); 0.4 mg (1 ea); 0.6 mg (1 ea); 0.8 mg (1 ea); 1 mg (1 ea); 1.2 mg (1 ea); 1.4 mg (1 ea); 1.6 mg (1 ea); 1.8 mg (1 ea); 2 mg (1 ea)

◆ **Somatuline® Autogel® (Can)** *see* Lanreotide *on page 1170*

◆ **Somatuline Depot** *see* Lanreotide *on page 1170*

◆ **Somavert** *see* Pegvisomant *on page 1600*

◆ **Somavert® (Can)** *see* Pegvisomant *on page 1600*

◆ **Sominex [OTC]** *see* DiphenhydrAMINE (Systemic) *on page 622*

◆ **Sominex® (Can)** *see* DiphenhydrAMINE (Systemic) *on page 622*

◆ **Sominex Maximum Strength [OTC]** *see* DiphenhydrAMINE (Systemic) *on page 622*

◆ **Som Pam (Can)** *see* Flurazepam *on page 892*

◆ **Sonata** *see* Zaleplon *on page 2220*

◆ **Soothe & Cool INZO Antifungal [OTC]** *see* Miconazole (Topical) *on page 1358*

SORAfenib (sor AF e nib)

Brand Names: U.S. NexAVAR

Brand Names: Canada Nexavar

Index Terms BAY 43-9006; Sorafenib Tosylate

Pharmacologic Category Antineoplastic Agent, Tyrosine Kinase Inhibitor; Vascular Endothelial Growth Factor (VEGF) Inhibitor

Use

Hepatocellular cancer: Treatment of unresectable hepatocellular cancer (HCC)

Renal cell cancer, advanced: Treatment of advanced renal cell cancer (RCC)

Thyroid cancer, differentiated: Treatment of locally recurrent or metastatic, progressive, differentiated thyroid cancer (refractory to radioactive iodine treatment)

Unlabeled Use Treatment of recurrent or metastatic angiosarcoma, resistant gastrointestinal stromal tumor (GIST)

Pregnancy Risk Factor D

Pregnancy Considerations Animal reproduction studies have demonstrated teratogenicity and fetal loss. Based on its mechanism of action and because sorafenib inhibits angiogenesis, a critical component of fetal development, adverse effects on pregnancy would be expected. Women of childbearing potential should be advised to avoid pregnancy. Men and women of reproductive potential should use effective birth control during treatment and for at least 2 weeks after treatment is discontinued.

Breast-Feeding Considerations It is not known if sorafenib is excreted in human milk. Due to the potential for serious adverse reactions in the nursing infant, the decision to discontinue sorafenib or to discontinue breast-feeding during therapy should take into account the benefits of treatment to the mother.

Prescribing and Access Restrictions Available from specialty pharmacies. Further information may be obtained at 1-866-639-2827 or www.nexavar-us.com.

Contraindications Known severe hypersensitivity to sorafenib or any component of the formulation; use in combination with carboplatin and paclitaxel in patients with squamous cell lung cancer

Warnings/Precautions Hazardous agent - use appropriate precautions for handling and disposal (NIOSH, 2012). May cause hypertension (generally mild-to-moderate), especially in the first 6 weeks of treatment; monitor; use caution in patients with underlying or poorly-controlled hypertension; consider discontinuing (temporary or permanent) in patients who develop severe or persistent hypertension while on appropriate antihypertensive therapy. May cause cardiac ischemia or infarction; consider discontinuing (temporarily or permanently) in patients who develop these conditions; use in patients with unstable coronary artery disease or recent myocardial infarction has not been studied. QT prolongation has been observed; may increase the risk for ventricular arrhythmia. Avoid use in patients with congenital long QT syndrome; monitor electrolytes and ECG in patients with heart failure, bradyarrhythmias, and concurrent medications known to prolong the QT interval; correct electrolyte (calcium, magnesium, potassium) imbalances; interrupt treatment for QTc interval >500 msec or for ≥60 msec increase from baseline.

Serious bleeding events may occur (consider permanently discontinuing if serious); monitor PT/INR in patients on warfarin therapy. Thyroid cancer patients with tracheal, bronchial, and esophageal infiltration should be treated with local therapy prior to administering sorafenib due to the potential bleeding risk. May complicate wound healing; temporarily withhold treatment for patients undergoing major surgical procedures (the appropriate timing for reinitiation after surgical procedures has not been determined). Gastrointestinal perforation has been reported (rare); monitor patients for signs/symptoms (abdominal pain, constipation, or vomiting); discontinue treatment if gastrointestinal perforation occurs. Potentially significant drug-drug interactions may exist, requiring dose or frequency adjustment, additional monitoring, and/or selection of alternative therapy. Avoid concurrent use with strong CYP3A4 inducers (eg, carbamazepine, dexamethasone, phenobarbital, phenytoin, rifampin, St John's wort); may decrease sorafenib levels/effects. Use caution when administering sorafenib with compounds that are metabolized predominantly via UGT1A1 (eg, irinotecan). Use in combination with carboplatin and paclitaxel in patients with squamous cell lung cancer is contraindicated.

Hand-foot skin reaction and rash (generally grades 1 or 2) are the most common drug-related adverse events, and typically appear within the first 6 weeks of treatment; usually managed with topical treatment, treatment delays, and/or dose reductions. Consider permanently discontinuing with severe or persistent dermatological toxicities. The risk for hand-foot syndrome increased with cumulative doses of sorafenib (Azad, 2009). The incidence of hand-foot syndrome is also increased in patients treated with sorafenib plus bevacizumab in comparison to those treated with sorafenib monotherapy (Azad, 2009). Severe dermatologic toxicities, including Stevens-Johnson syndrome (SJS) and toxic epidermal necrolysis (TEN) have been reported; may be life-threatening; discontinue sorafenib for suspected SJS or TEN.

Sorafenib impairs exogenous thyroid suppression; TSH level elevations were commonly observed in the thyroid cancer study; monitor TSH levels monthly and as clinically necessary, and adjust thyroid replacement as needed. Sorafenib levels in patients with mild-to-moderate hepatic impairment (Child-Pugh classes A and B) were similar to levels observed in patients without hepatic impairment; has not been studied in patients with severe hepatic impairment. In a small study of Asian patients with advanced HCC, sorafenib demonstrated efficacy with adequate tolerability in a hepatitis B-endemic area (Yau, 2009). There have been reports of sorafenib-induced hepatitis (including hepatic failure and death) which is characterized by hepatocellular liver damage and transaminase increases (significant); increased bilirubin and INR may also occur. Monitor hepatic function regularly; discontinue sorafenib for unexplained significant transaminase increases.

Adverse Reactions

>10%:

Cardiovascular: Hypertension (9% to 17%; grade 3: 3% to 4%; grade 4: <1%; onset: ~3 weeks)
Central nervous system: Fatigue (37% to 46%), sensory neuropathy (≤13%), pain (11%)
Dermatologic: Rash/desquamation (19% to 40%; grade 3: ≤1%), hand-foot syndrome (21% to 30%; grade 3: 6% to 8%), alopecia (14% to 27%), pruritus (14% to 19%), dry skin (10% to 11%), erythema
Endocrine & metabolic: Hypoalbuminemia (≤59%), hypophosphatemia (35% to 45%; grade 3: 11% to 13%; grade 4: <1%), hypocalcemia (12% to 27%)
Gastrointestinal: Diarrhea (43% to 55%; grade 3: 2% to 10%; grade 4: <1%), lipase increased (40% to 41% [usually transient]), amylase increased (30% to 34% [usually transient]), abdominal pain (11% to 31%), weight loss (10% to 30%), anorexia (16% to 29%), nausea (23% to 24%), vomiting (15% to 16%), constipation (14% to 15%)
Hematologic: Lymphopenia (23% to 47%; grades 3/4: ≤13%), thrombocytopenia (12% to 46%; grades 3/4: 1% to 4%), INR increased (≤42%), neutropenia (≤18%; grades 3/4: ≤5%), hemorrhage (15% to 18%; grade 3: 2% to 3%; grade 4: ≤2%), leukopenia
Hepatic: Liver dysfunction (≤11%; grade 3: 2%; grade 4: 1%)
Neuromuscular & skeletal: Muscle pain, weakness
Respiratory: Dyspnea (≤14%), cough (≤13%)

1% to 10%:

Cardiovascular: Cardiac ischemia/infarction (≤3%), heart failure (2%, congestive), flushing
Central nervous system: Headache (≤10%), depression, fever
Dermatologic: Acne, exfoliative dermatitis
Endocrine & Metabolic: Hypokalemia (5% to 9%)
Gastrointestinal: Appetite decreased, dyspepsia, dysphagia, esophageal varices bleeding (2%), glossodynia, mucositis, stomatitis, xerostomia
Genitourinary: Erectile dysfunction
Hematologic: Anemia
Hepatic: Transaminases increased (transient)
Neuromuscular & skeletal: Joint pain (≤10%), arthralgia, myalgia
Renal: Proteinuria, renal failure
Respiratory: Hoarseness
Miscellaneous: Flu-like syndrome

<1% (Limited to important or life-threatening): Acute renal failure, alkaline phosphatase increased, anaphylactic reaction, angioedema, aortic dissection, arrhythmia, bilirubin increased, bone pain, cardiac failure, cerebral hemorrhage, cholangitis, cholecystitis, dehydration, eczema,

epistaxis, erythema multiforme, folliculitis, gastritis, gastrointestinal hemorrhage, gastrointestinal perforation, gastrointestinal reflux, gynecomastia, hepatic failure, hepatitis, hypersensitivity (skin reaction, urticaria), hypertensive crisis, hyper-/hypothyroidism, hyponatremia, infection, interstitial lung disease (acute respiratory distress, interstitial pneumonia, lung inflammation, pneumonitis, pulmonitis, radiation pneumonitis), jaundice, MI, mouth pain, muscle wasting, myocardial ischemia, nephrotic syndrome, osteonecrosis of the jaw, pancreatitis, pleural effusion, preeclampsia-like syndrome (reversible hypertension and proteinuria), QT prolongation, respiratory hemorrhage, reversible posterior leukoencephalopathy syndrome (RPLS), rhabdomyolysis, rhinorrhea, skin cancer (squamous cell/keratoacanthomas), Stevens-Johnson syndrome, thromboembolism, tinnitus, toxic epidermal necrolysis (TEN), transient ischemic attack, tumor lysis syndrome, tumor pain, voice alteration

Drug Interactions

Metabolism/Transport Effects Substrate of CYP3A4 (minor), UGT1A9; **Note:** Assignment of Major/Minor substrate status based on clinically relevant drug interaction potential; **Inhibits** CYP2B6 (moderate), CYP2C8 (weak), CYP2C9 (moderate), UGT1A1, UGT1A9

Avoid Concomitant Use

Avoid concomitant use of SORAfenib with any of the following: BCG; CARBOplatin; CloZAPine; CYP3A4 Inducers (Strong); Highest Risk QTc-Prolonging Agents; Ivabradine; Mifepristone; Natalizumab; PACLitaxel; Pimecrolimus; St Johns Wort; Tacrolimus (Topical); Tofacitinib; Vaccines (Live)

Increased Effect/Toxicity

SORAfenib may increase the levels/effects of: Acetaminophen; Bisphosphonate Derivatives; Bosentan; CARBOplatin; Carvedilol; CloZAPine; CYP2B6 Substrates; CYP2C9 Substrates; DOCEtaxel; DOXOrubicin; Fluorouracil (Systemic); Fluorouracil (Topical); Highest Risk QTc-Prolonging Agents; Irinotecan; Leflunomide; Moderate Risk QTc-Prolonging Agents; Natalizumab; PACLitaxel; Tofacitinib; Vaccines (Live); Vitamin K Antagonists; Warfarin

The levels/effects of SORAfenib may be increased by: Acetaminophen; Bevacizumab; CYP3A4 Inhibitors (Strong); Denosumab; Ivabradine; Mifepristone; Pimecrolimus; QTc-Prolonging Agents (Indeterminate Risk and Risk Modifying); Roflumilast; Tacrolimus (Topical); Trastuzumab

Decreased Effect

SORAfenib may decrease the levels/effects of: BCG; Cardiac Glycosides; Coccidioidin Skin Test; Dacarbazine; Fluorouracil (Systemic); Fluorouracil (Topical); Sipuleucel-T; Vaccines (Inactivated); Vaccines (Live); Vitamin K Antagonists

The levels/effects of SORAfenib may be decreased by: CYP3A4 Inducers (Strong); Echinacea; Neomycin; St Johns Wort

Ethanol/Nutrition/Herb Interactions

Food: Bioavailability is decreased 29% with a high-fat meal (bioavailability is similar to fasting state when administered with a moderate-fat meal). Management: Administer on an empty stomach 1 hour before or 2 hours after eating.

Herb/Nutraceutical: St John's wort may decrease the levels/effects of sorafenib. Management: Avoid St John's wort.

Storage/Stability Store at 25°C (77°F); excursions are permitted between 15°C and 30°C (59°F and 86°F). Protect from moisture.

Mechanism of Action Multikinase inhibitor; inhibits tumor growth and angiogenesis by inhibiting intracellular Raf kinases (CRAF, BRAF, and mutant BRAF), and cell surface kinase receptors (VEGFR-1, VEGFR-2, VEGFR-3, PDGFR-beta, cKIT, FLT-3, RET, and RET/PTC)

Pharmacodynamics/Kinetics

Protein binding: 99.5%

Metabolism: Hepatic, via CYP3A4 (primarily oxidated to the pyridine N-oxide; active, minor) and UGT1A9 (glucuronidation)

Bioavailability: 38% to 49%; reduced by 29% when administered with a high-fat meal

Half-life elimination: 25-48 hours

Time to peak, plasma: ~3 hours

Excretion: Feces (77%, 51% of dose as unchanged drug); urine (19%, as metabolites)

Dosage Note: Interrupt treatment (temporarily) in patients undergoing major surgical procedures.

Hepatocellular cancer (HCC): Adults: Oral: 400 mg twice daily; continue until no longer clinically benefiting or until unacceptable toxicity occurs (Llovet, 2008)

Renal cell cancer (RCC), advanced: Adults: Oral: 400 mg twice daily; continue until no longer clinically benefiting or until unacceptable toxicity occurs (Escudier, 2007; Escudier, 2009)

Thyroid cancer, differentiated: Adults: Oral: 400 mg twice daily; continue until no longer clinically benefiting or until unacceptable toxicity occurs (Brose, 2013)

Angiosarcoma (unlabeled use): 400 mg twice daily (Maki, 2009)

GIST (unlabeled use): 400 mg twice daily (Wiebe, 2008)

Dosage adjustment for toxicity: Temporary interruption and/or dosage reduction may be necessary for management of adverse drug reactions.

Cardiovascular toxicity:

Cardiac ischemia or infarction: Consider temporary interruption or permanent discontinuation.

Hypertension, severe or persistent (despite antihypertensive therapy): Consider temporary interruption or permanent discontinuation.

QT prolongation (QTc interval >500 msec or ≥60 msec increase from baseline): Interrupt treatment.

Gastrointestinal perforation: Permanently discontinue.

Hemorrhage requiring medical intervention: Consider permanent discontinuation.

Dermatologic toxicity:

Suspected Stevens-Johnson syndrome or toxic epidermal necrolysis: Discontinue.

RCC and HCC: If dosage reductions are necessary, decrease dose to 400 mg once daily. If further reductions are needed, decrease dose to 400 mg every other day.

Grade 1 (numbness, dysesthesia, paresthesia, tingling, painless swelling, erythema, or discomfort of the hands or feet which do not disrupt normal activities): Continue sorafenib and consider symptomatic treatment with topical therapy.

Grade 2 (painful erythema and swelling of the hands or feet and/or discomfort affecting normal activities):

First occurrence: Continue sorafenib and consider symptomatic treatment with topical therapy. **Note:** If no improvement within 7 days, see dosing for second or third occurrence.

Second or third occurrence (or no improvement after 7 days of 1st occurrence): Hold treatment until resolves to grade 0-1; resume treatment with dose reduced by one dose level (400 mg daily or 400 mg every other day).

Fourth occurrence: Discontinue treatment.

Grade 3 (moist desquamation, ulceration, blistering, or severe pain of the hands or feet or severe discomfort that prevents working or performing daily activities):

First or second occurrence: Hold treatment until resolves to grade 0-1; resume treatment with dose reduced by one dose level (400 mg daily or 400 mg every other day).

Third occurrence: Discontinue treatment.

Thyroid cancer:

First dose level reduction: Reduce to 600 mg daily (in 2 divided doses, as 400 mg and 200 mg, separated by 12 hours).

Second dose level reduction: Reduce dose to 200 mg twice daily.

Third dose level reduction: Reduce dose to 200 mg once daily.

Grade 1 (numbness, dysesthesia, paresthesia, tingling, painless swelling, erythema, or discomfort of the hands or feet which do not disrupt normal activities): Continue sorafenib treatment.

Grade 2 (painful erythema and swelling of the hands or feet and/or discomfort affecting normal activities):

First occurrence: Decrease dose to 600 mg daily (in divided doses). **Note:** If no improvement within 7 days, see dosing for 2nd occurrence.

Second occurrence (or no improvement after 7 days of the reduced dose after 1st occurrence): Hold treatment until resolved or improved to grade 1; if resumed, decrease the dose by 1 dose level.

Third occurrence: Hold treatment until resolved or improved to grade 1; if resumed, decrease the dose by 1 dose level.

Fourth occurrence: Permanently discontinue.

Grade 3 (moist desquamation, ulceration, blistering, or severe pain of the hands or feet or severe discomfort that prevents working or performing daily activities):

First occurrence: Hold treatment until resolved or improved to grade 1; if resumed, decrease by 1 dose level.

Second occurrence: Hold treatment until resolved or improved to grade 1; if resumed, decrease by 2 dose levels.

Third occurrence: Permanently discontinue.

Following improvement of grade 2 or 3 dermatologic toxicity to grade 0 or 1 after at least 28 days of a reduced dose, the sorafenib dose may be increased 1 dose level from the reduced dose (~50% of patients requiring dose reduction for dermatologic toxicity may meet the criteria for increased dosing; and half of those patients may tolerate the increased dose without recurrent grade 2 or higher dermatologic toxicity).

Dosage adjustment in renal impairment:

Manufacturer's labeling: No dosage adjustment necessary for mild, moderate, or severe impairment (not dependent on dialysis); has not been studied in dialysis patients.

The following adjustments have also been reported: Safety and pharmacokinetics were studied in varying degrees of renal dysfunction with the following empiric dose levels recommended based on patient tolerance (Miller, 2009):

Mild renal dysfunction (Cl_{cr} 40-59 mL/minute): 400 mg twice daily

Moderate renal dysfunction (Cl_{cr} 20-39 mL/minute): 200 mg twice daily

Severe renal dysfunction (Cl_{cr} <20 mL/minute): Data inadequate to define dose

Hemodialysis (any Cl_{cr}): 200 mg once daily

Dosage adjustment in hepatic impairment:

Hepatic impairment at baseline:

Manufacturer's labeling:

Mild to moderate (Child-Pugh class A and B) impairment: No dosage adjustment is necessary.

Severe impairment (Child-Pugh class C): No dosage adjustment provided (has not been studied).

The following adjustments have also been reported: Safety and pharmacokinetics were studied in varying degrees of hepatic dysfunction with the following empiric dose levels recommended based on patient tolerance (Miller, 2009):

Mild hepatic dysfunction (bilirubin >1 to ≤1.5 times ULN and/or AST >ULN): 400 mg twice daily

Moderate hepatic dysfunction (bilirubin >1.5 to ≤3 times ULN; any AST): 200 mg twice daily

Severe hepatic dysfunction:

Bilirubin >3-10 x ULN (any AST): 200 mg every 3 days was **not** tolerated

Albumin <2.5 g/dL (any bilirubin and any AST): 200 mg once daily

Drug-induced liver injury during treatment: Unexplained (eg, not due to viral hepatitis or progressive underlying malignancy) significantly increased transaminases: Discontinue treatment.

Dietary Considerations Take without food (1 hour before or 2 hours after eating).

Administration Administer on an empty stomach (1 hour before or 2 hours after eating).

Hazardous agent; use appropriate precautions for handling and disposal (NIOSH, 2012).

Monitoring Parameters

CBC with differential, electrolytes (magnesium, potassium, calcium), phosphorus, lipase and amylase levels; liver function tests; blood pressure (baseline, weekly for the first 6 weeks, then periodic); monitor for hand-foot syndrome and other dermatologic toxicities; monitor ECG in patients at risk for prolonged QT interval; signs/symptoms of bleeding

Thyroid function testing:

Patients with differentiated thyroid cancer: Monitor TSH monthly.

Patients with RCC and HCC (Hamnvik, 2011):

Pre-existing levothyroxine therapy: Obtain baseline TSH levels, then monitor every 4 weeks until levels and levothyroxine dose are stable, then monitor every 2 months

Without pre-existing thyroid hormone replacement: TSH at baseline, then every 4 weeks for 4 months, then every 2-3 months

Additional Information Hand-foot skin reaction (HFSR) management (Lacouture, 2008): The following treatments may be used in addition to the recommended dosage modifications. Prior to treatment initiation, a pedicure is recommended to remove hyperkeratotic areas/calluses, which may predispose to HFSR; avoid vigorous exercise/activities which may stress hands or feet. During therapy, patients should reduce exposure to hot water (may exacerbate hand-foot symptoms); avoid constrictive footwear and excessive skin friction. Patients may also wear thick cotton gloves or socks and should wear shoes with padded insoles. Grade 1 HFSR may be relieved with moisturizing creams, cotton gloves and socks (at night) and/or keratolytic creams such as urea (20% to 40%) or salicylic acid (6%). Apply topical steroid (eg, clobetasol ointment) twice daily to erythematous areas of Grade 2 HFSR; topical anesthetics (eg, lidocaine 2%) and then systemic analgesics (if appropriate) may be used for pain control. Resolution of acute erythema may result in keratotic areas which may be softened with keratolytic agents.

Dosage Forms Excipient information presented when available (limited, particularly for generics); consult specific product labeling.

Tablet, Oral:

NexAVAR: 200 mg

Extemporaneous Preparations Hazardous agent: Use appropriate precautions for handling and disposal.

An oral suspension may be prepared with tablets. Place two 200 mg tablets into a glass containing 60 mL (2 oz) water; let stand 5 minutes before stirring. Stir until tablets are completely disintegrated, forming a uniform suspension. Administer within 1 hour after preparation. Stir suspension again immediately before administration. To ensure the full dose is administered, rinse glass several times with a total of 180 mL (6 oz) water and administer residue. **Note:** Brown tablet coating may initially form a thin film but has no effect on the dosing accuracy.

Nexavar® data on file, Bayer Healthcare Pharmaceuticals.

◆ **Sorafenib Tosylate** *see* SORAfenib *on page 1938*

Sorbitol (SOR bi tole)

Brand Names: U.S. Ora-Sweet SF [OTC]

Pharmacologic Category Genitourinary Irrigant; Laxative, Osmotic

Additional Appendix Information

Laxatives, Classification and Properties *on page 2304*

Use Genitourinary irrigant in transurethral prostatic resection or other transurethral resection or other transurethral surgical procedures; diuretic; humectant; sweetening agent; hyperosmotic laxative; facilitate the passage of sodium polystyrene sulfonate through the intestinal tract

Pregnancy Risk Factor C

Dosage

Hyperosmotic laxative (as single dose, at infrequent intervals):

Children 2-11 years:

Oral: 2 mL/kg (as 70% solution)

Rectal enema: 30-60 mL as 25% to 30% solution

Children >12 years and Adults:

Oral: 30-150 mL (as 70% solution)

Rectal enema: 120 mL as 25% to 30% solution

Adjunct to sodium polystyrene sulfonate: Adults: 15 mL as 70% solution orally until diarrhea occurs (10-20 mL/2 hours) or 20-100 mL as an oral vehicle for the sodium polystyrene sulfonate resin

Transurethral surgical procedures: Adults: Irrigation: Topical: 3% to 3.3% as transurethral surgical procedure irrigation

Additional Information Complete prescribing information should be consulted for additional detail.

Dosage Forms Excipient information presented when available (limited, particularly for generics); consult specific product labeling.

Solution, Irrigation:

Generic: 3% (3000 mL, 5000 mL); 3.3% (2000 mL, 4000 mL)

Solution, Oral:

Generic: 70% (30 mL, 473 mL, 474 mL, 480 mL, 3840 mL)

Syrup, Oral:

Ora-Sweet SF: (473 mL) [alcohol free, sugar free; contains saccharin sodium; fruit flavor]

◆ **Sorbulax [OTC]** *see* Psyllium *on page 1748*

◆ **Sore Throat Relief [OTC]** *see* Benzocaine *on page 240*

◆ **Soriatane** *see* Acitretin *on page 39*

◆ **Soriatane® (Can)** *see* Acitretin *on page 39*

◆ **Sorilux** *see* Calcipotriene *on page 311*

◆ **Sorine** *see* Sotalol *on page 1942*

Sotalol (SOE ta lole)

Brand Names: U.S. Betapace; Betapace AF; Sorine

Brand Names: Canada Apo-Sotalol®; CO Sotalol; Dom-Sotalol; Med-Sotalol; Mylan-Sotalol; Novo-Sotalol; Nu-Sotalol; PHL-Sotalol; PMS-Sotalol; PRO-Sotalol; ratio-Sotalol; Rhoxal-sotalol; Riva-Sotalol; Rylosol; Sandoz-Sotalol; ZYM-Sotalol

Index Terms Sotalol Hydrochloride

Pharmacologic Category Antiarrhythmic Agent, Class II; Antiarrhythmic Agent, Class III; Beta-Adrenergic Blocker, Nonselective

Additional Appendix Information

Adult ACLS Algorithms *on page 2363*

Beers Criteria – Potentially Inappropriate Medications for Geriatrics *on page 2368*

Beta-Blockers *on page 2294*

Use Treatment of documented ventricular arrhythmias (ie, sustained ventricular tachycardia), that in the judgment of the physician are life-threatening; maintenance of normal sinus rhythm in patients with symptomatic atrial fibrillation and atrial flutter who are currently in sinus rhythm. Manufacturer states substitutions should not be made for Betapace AF® since Betapace AF® is distributed with a patient package insert specific for atrial fibrillation/flutter.

Injection: Substitution for oral sotalol in those who are unable to take sotalol orally

Unlabeled Use Fetal tachycardia; alternative antiarrhythmic for the treatment of atrial fibrillation in patients with hypertrophic cardiomyopathy (HCM)

Pregnancy Risk Factor B

Pregnancy Considerations Adverse events were not observed in the initial animal reproduction studies; therefore, the manufacturer classifies sotalol as pregnancy category B. Sotalol crosses the placenta and is found in amniotic fluid. In a cohort study, an increased risk of cardiovascular defects was observed following maternal use of beta-blockers during pregnancy. Intrauterine growth restriction (IUGR), small placentas, as well as fetal/neonatal bradycardia, hypoglycemia, and/or respiratory depression have been observed following *in utero* exposure to beta-blockers as a class. Adequate facilities for monitoring infants at birth should be available. Untreated chronic maternal hypertension and pre-eclampsia are also associated with adverse events in the fetus, infant, and mother; however, sotalol is currently not recommended for the initial treatment of hypertension in pregnancy. Because sotalol crosses the placenta in concentrations similar to the maternal serum, it has been used for the treatment of fetal atrial flutter or fetal supraventricular tachycardia without hydrops. The clearance of sotalol is increased during the third trimester of pregnancy, but other pharmacokinetic parameters do not significantly differ from nonpregnant values.

Breast-Feeding Considerations Sotalol is excreted into breast milk in concentrations higher than those found in the maternal serum. Although adverse events in nursing infants have not been observed in case reports, close monitoring for bradycardia, hypotension, respiratory distress, and hypoglycemia is advised. According to the manufacturer, the decision to continue or discontinue breast-feeding during therapy should take into account the risk of exposure to the infant and the benefits of treatment to the mother.

Contraindications Hypersensitivity to sotalol or any component of the formulation; bronchial asthma; sinus bradycardia; second- or third-degree AV block (unless a functioning pacemaker is present); congenital or acquired long QT syndromes; cardiogenic shock; uncontrolled heart failure

Additional contraindications: Betapace AF® and the injectable formulation: Baseline QT_c interval >450 msec; bronchospastic conditions; Cl_{cr} <40 mL/minute; serum potassium <4 mEq/L; sick sinus syndrome

Warnings/Precautions [U.S. Boxed Warning] Manufacturer recommends initiation (or reinitiation) and doses increased in a hospital setting with continuous monitoring and staff familiar with the recognition and treatment of life-threatening arrhythmias. Some experts will initiate therapy on an outpatient basis in a patient without heart disease or bradycardia, who has a baseline uncorrected QT interval <450 msec, and normal serum potassium and magnesium levels; close ECG monitoring during this time is necessary. ACC/AHA guidelines for management of atrial fibrillation also recommend that for outpatient initiation the patient not have risk factors predisposing to drug-induced ventricular proarrhythmia (Fuster, 2006). Dosage should be adjusted gradually with 3 days between dosing increments to achieve steady-state concentrations, and to allow time to monitor QT intervals. **[U.S. Boxed Warning]: Adjust dosing interval based on creatinine clearance to decrease risk of proarrhythmia; QT interval prolongation is directly related to sotalol concentration.** Creatinine clearance must be calculated with dose initiation and dose increases. Use cautiously in the renally-impaired (dosage adjustment required). Betapace AF® and the injectable formulation are contraindicated in patients with Cl_{cr} <40 mL/minute.

[U.S. Boxed Warning]: Sotalol injection: Sotalol can cause life-threatening ventricular tachycardia associated with QT-interval prolongation (ie, torsade de pointes). Do not initiate if baseline QTc interval is >450 msec. If QT_c exceeds 500 msec during therapy, reduce the dose, prolong the infusion duration, or discontinue use. If while on oral sotalol therapy baseline QT_c interval is >500 msec, use I.V. sotalol with particular caution; serious consideration should be given to reducing the dose or discontinuing I.V. sotalol when QT_c exceeds 520 msec. QT_c prolongation is directly related to the concentration of sotalol; reduced creatinine clearance, female gender, and large doses increase the risk of QT_c prolongation and subsequent torsade de pointes. Monitor and adjust dose to prevent QT_c prolongation. Concurrent use with other QT_c-prolonging drugs (including Class I and Class III antiarrhythmics) and use within 3 months of discontinuing amiodarone is generally not recommended. To reduce the chance of excessive QT_c-prolongation, withhold QT_c-prolonging drugs for at least 3 half-lives (or 3 months for amiodarone) before initiating sotalol.

Correct electrolyte imbalances before initiating (especially hypokalemia and hypomagnesemia). Consider pre-existing conditions such as sick sinus syndrome before initiating. Conduction abnormalities can occur particularly sinus bradycardia. Use cautiously within the first 2 weeks post-MI especially in patients with markedly impaired ventricular function (experience limited). Administer cautiously in compensated heart failure and monitor for a worsening of the condition. May precipitate or aggravate symptoms of arterial insufficiency in patients with PVD and Raynaud's disease; use with caution and monitor for progression of arterial obstruction. Bradycardia may be observed more frequently in elderly patients (>65 years of age); dosage reductions may be necessary. In the treatment of atrial fibrillation, avoid antiarrhythmics as first-line treatment. In older adults, data suggests rate control may provide more benefits than risks compared to rhythm control for most patients (Beers Criteria). Beta-blocker therapy should not be withdrawn abruptly (particularly in patients with CAD), but gradually tapered to avoid acute tachycardia, hypertension, and/or ischemia. Chronic beta-blocker therapy should not be routinely withdrawn prior to major surgery. Use caution with concurrent use of digoxin, verapamil, or diltiazem; bradycardia or heart block can occur. Use with caution in patients receiving inhaled anesthetic agents known to depress myocardial contractility. Use cautiously in diabetics because it can mask prominent hypoglycemic symptoms. Use with caution in patients with bronchospastic disease, myasthenia gravis or psychiatric disease. Adequate alpha-blockade is required prior to use of any beta-blocker for patients with untreated pheochromocytoma. May mask signs of hyperthyroidism (eg, tachycardia); if hyperthyroidism is suspected, carefully manage and monitor; abrupt withdrawal may exacerbate symptoms of hyperthyroidism or precipitate thyroid storm. Use caution with history of severe anaphylaxis to allergens; patients taking beta-blockers may become more sensitive to repeated challenges. Treatment of anaphylaxis (eg, epinephrine) in patients taking beta-blockers may be ineffective or promote undesirable effects.

[U.S. Boxed Warning]: Betapace® should not be substituted for Betapace® AF; Betapace® AF is distributed with an educational insert specifically for patients with atrial fibrillation/flutter.

Adverse Reactions Note: No clinical experience with I.V. sotalol; however, since exposure is similar between I.V. and oral sotalol, adverse reactions are expected to be similar.

>10%:

Cardiovascular: Bradycardia (13% to 16%), chest pain (3% to 16%), palpitation (14%)

Central nervous system: Fatigue (20%), dizziness (20%), lightheadedness (12%)

Neuromuscular & skeletal: Weakness (13%)

Respiratory: Dyspnea (21%)

1% to 10%:

Cardiovascular: Edema (8%), abnormal ECG (7%), hypotension (6%), proarrhythmia (5%), syncope (5%), CHF (5%), torsade de pointes (dose related; 1% to 4%), peripheral vascular disorders (3%), ventricular tachycardia worsened (1%), QT_c interval prolongation (dose related)

Central nervous system: Headache (8%), sleep problems (8%), mental confusion (6%), anxiety (4%), depression (4%)

Dermatologic: Itching/rash (5%)

Endocrine & metabolic: Sexual ability decreased (3%)

Gastrointestinal: Nausea/vomiting (10%), diarrhea (7%), stomach discomfort (3% to 6%), flatulence (2%)

Genitourinary: Impotence (2%)

Hematologic: Bleeding (2%)

Neuromuscular & skeletal: Extremity pain (7%), paresthesia (4%), back pain (3%)

Ocular: Visual problems (5%)

Respiratory: Upper respiratory problems (5% to 8%), asthma (2%)

<1% (Limited to important or life-threatening): Alopecia, bronchiolitis obliterans with organized pneumonia (BOOP), cold extremities, diaphoresis, eosinophilia, leukocytoclastic vasculitis, leukopenia, paralysis, phlebitis, photosensitivity reaction, pruritus, pulmonary edema, Raynaud's phenomenon, red crusted skin, retroperitoneal fibrosis, serum transaminases increased, skin necrosis after extravasation, thrombocytopenia, vertigo

Drug Interactions

Metabolism/Transport Effects None known.

Avoid Concomitant Use

Avoid concomitant use of Sotalol with any of the following: Beta2-Agonists; Fingolimod; Floctafenine; Highest Risk QTc-Prolonging Agents; Ivabradine; Methacholine; Mifepristone; Moderate Risk QTc-Prolonging Agents; Propafenone

Increased Effect/Toxicity

Sotalol may increase the levels/effects of: Alpha-/Beta-Agonists (Direct-Acting); Alpha1-Blockers; Alpha2-Agonists; Amifostine; Antihypertensives; Antipsychotic Agents (Phenothiazines); Bupivacaine; Cardiac Glycosides; Cholinergic Agonists; Ergot Derivatives; Fingolimod; Highest Risk QTc-Prolonging Agents; Hypotensive Agents; Insulin; Lidocaine (Systemic); Lidocaine (Topical); Mepivacaine; Methacholine; Midodrine; Obinutuzumab; RiTUXimab; Sulfonylureas

The levels/effects of Sotalol may be increased by: Acetylcholinesterase Inhibitors; Alpha2-Agonists; Aminoquinolines (Antimalarial); Amiodarone; Anilidopiperidine Opioids; Antipsychotic Agents (Phenothiazines); Brimonidine (Topical); Calcium Channel Blockers (Dihydropyridine); Calcium Channel Blockers (Nondihydropyridine); Diazoxide; Dipyridamole; Disopyramide; Dronedarone; Fingolimod; Floctafenine; Herbs (Hypotensive Properties); Ivabradine; Lidocaine (Topical); MAO Inhibitors; Mifepristone; Moderate Risk QTc-Prolonging Agents; Pentoxifylline; Phosphodiesterase 5 Inhibitors; Propafenone; Prostacyclin Analogues; QTc-Prolonging Agents (Indeterminate Risk and Risk Modifying); Regorafenib; Reserpine

Decreased Effect

Sotalol may decrease the levels/effects of: Beta2-Agonists; Theophylline Derivatives

The levels/effects of Sotalol may be decreased by: Barbiturates; Herbs (Hypertensive Properties); Methylphenidate; Nonsteroidal Anti-Inflammatory Agents; Rifamycin Derivatives; Yohimbine

Ethanol/Nutrition/Herb Interactions

Food: Sotalol peak serum concentrations may be decreased if taken with food.

Herb/Nutraceutical: Avoid ephedra (may worsen arrhythmia).

Storage/Stability Store at 25°C (77°F); excursions permitted to 15°C to 30°C (59°F to 86°F). To prepare sotalol infusion, see manufacturer's prescribing information.

Mechanism of Action

Beta-blocker which contains both beta-adrenoreceptor-blocking (Vaughan Williams Class II) and cardiac action potential duration prolongation (Vaughan Williams Class III) properties

Class II effects: Increased sinus cycle length, slowed heart rate, decreased AV nodal conduction, and increased AV nodal refractoriness Sotalol has both $beta_1$- and $beta_2$-receptor blocking activity. The beta-blocking effect of sotalol is a noncardioselective (half maximal at about 80 mg/day and maximal at doses of 320-640 mg/day). Significant beta-blockade occurs at oral doses as low as 25 mg/day.

Class III effects: Prolongation of the atrial and ventricular monophasic action potentials, and effective refractory prolongation of atrial muscle, ventricular muscle, and atrioventricular accessory pathways in both the antegrade and retrograde directions. Sotalol is a racemic mixture of *d*- and *l*-sotalol; both isomers have similar Class III antiarrhythmic effects while the *l*-isomer is responsible for virtually all of the beta-blocking activity. The Class III effects are seen only at oral doses ≥160 mg/day

Pharmacodynamics/Kinetics

Onset of action: Oral: Rapid, 1-2 hours; when administered I.V. for ongoing VT over 5 minutes, onset of action is ~5-10 minutes (Ho, 1994)

Duration: 8-16 hours

Absorption: Oral: Decreased 20% to 30% by meals compared to fasting

Distribution: V_d: 1.2-2.4 L/kg

Protein binding: None

Metabolism: None

Bioavailability: Oral: 90% to 100%

Half-life elimination: 12 hours; Children: 9.5 hours; terminal half-life decreases with age <2 years (time to steady state may be ≥1 week in neonates); increases with renal dysfunction

Time to peak, serum: Oral: 2.5-4 hours

Excretion: Urine (as unchanged drug)

Dosage Baseline QT_c interval and creatinine clearance must be determined prior to initiation. Sotalol should be initiated and doses increased in a hospital with facilities for cardiac rhythm monitoring and assessment. Proarrhythmic events can occur after initiation of therapy and with each upward dosage adjustment.

Children: Oral: The safety and efficacy of sotalol in children have not been established

Note: Dosing per manufacturer, based on pediatric pharmacokinetic data; wait at least 36 hours between dosage adjustments to allow monitoring of QT intervals

≤2 years: Dosage should be adjusted (decreased) by plotting of the child's age on a logarithmic scale; see graph or refer to manufacturer's package labeling.

Sotalol Age Factor Nomogram for Patients ≤2 Years of Age

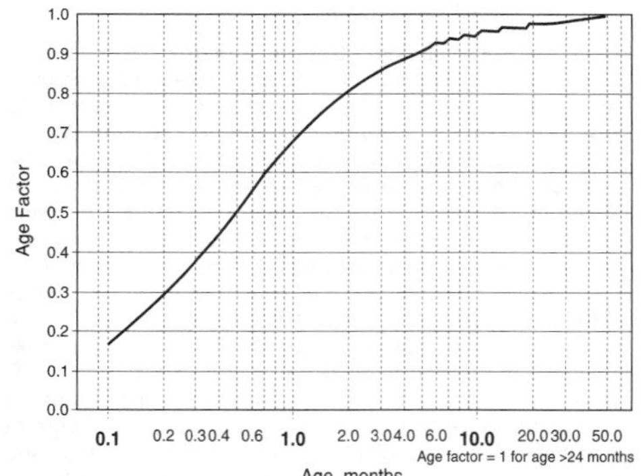

Adapted from U.S. Food and Drug Administration.
http://www.fda.gov/cder/foi/label/2001/2115s3lbl.PDF

>2 years: Initial: 90 mg/m²/day in 3 divided doses; may be incrementally increased to a maximum of 180 mg/m²/day

Adults:

I.V.: **Note:** The effects of the initial I.V. dose must be monitored and the dose titrated either upward or downward, if needed, based on clinical effect, QT_c interval, or adverse reactions.

Symptomatic atrial fibrillation/flutter, ventricular arrhythmias: Substitution for oral sotalol: *Initial dose:* 75 mg infused over 5 hours twice daily

Dose adjustment: If the frequency of relapse does not reduce and excessive QT_c prolongation does not occur, may increase to 112.5 mg twice daily. For ventricular arrhythmias, may increase dose every 3 days in increments of 75 mg/day.

Dose range for symptomatic atrial fibrillation/flutter: Usual therapeutic dose: 112.5 mg twice daily; maximum dose: 150 mg twice daily

Dose range for ventricular arrhythmias: Usual therapeutic dose: 75-150 mg twice daily; maximum dose: 300 mg twice daily.

Hemodynamically stable monomorphic VT, ongoing (unlabeled use): 1.5 mg/kg over 5 minutes (ACLS, 2010); **Note:** Clinical trial employed standard dose of 100 mg (Ho, 1994).

Conversion from oral sotalol to I.V. sotalol:

80 mg oral equivalent to 75 mg I.V.

120 mg oral equivalent to 112.5 mg I.V.

160 mg oral equivalent to 150 mg I.V.

Oral:

Ventricular arrhythmias (Betapace®, Sorine®):

Initial: 80 mg twice daily

Dose may be increased gradually to 240-320 mg/day; allow 3 days between dosing increments in order to attain steady-state plasma concentrations and to allow monitoring of QT intervals

Most patients respond to a total daily dose of 160-320 mg/day in 2-3 divided doses.

Some patients, with life-threatening refractory ventricular arrhythmias, may require doses as high as 480-640 mg/day; however, these doses should only be prescribed when the potential benefit outweighs the increased of adverse events.

Atrial fibrillation or atrial flutter (Betapace AF®): Initial: 80 mg twice daily. If the frequency of relapse does not reduce and excessive QT_c prolongation does not occur after 3 days, the dose may be increased to 120 mg twice daily; may further increase to 160 mg twice daily if response is inadequate and QT_c prolongation is not excessive.

Elderly: Age does not significantly alter the pharmacokinetics of sotalol, but impaired renal function in elderly patients can increase the terminal half-life, resulting in increased drug accumulation

Dosage adjustment for toxicity:

QT_c ≥500 msec during initiation period:

Betapace AF®: Reduce dose or discontinue sotalol

Injectable formulation: Reduce dose, decrease infusion rate, or discontinue sotalol

QT_c ≥520 msec (or JT interval ≥430 msec if the QRS >100 msec) during maintenance therapy (Betapace AF®, injectable formulation): Reduce dose and carefully monitor QT_c until <520 msec. If QT_c interval ≥520 msec on the lowest maintenance dose, discontinue sotalol.

QT_c ≥550 msec (Betapace®, Sorine®): Reduce dose or discontinue sotalol.

Dosage adjustment in renal impairment: Adults: Impaired renal function can increase the terminal half-life, resulting in increased drug accumulation. Sotalol (Betapace AF®, injectable formulation) is contraindicated per the manufacturers for treatment of atrial fibrillation/flutter in patients with a Cl_{cr} <40 mL/minute.

Ventricular arrhythmias (Betapace®, Sorine®):

Cl_{cr} >60 mL/minute: Administer every 12 hours

Cl_{cr} 30-60 mL/minute: Administer every 24 hours

Cl_{cr} 10-29 mL/minute: Administer every 36-48 hours

Cl_{cr} <10 mL/minute: Individualize dose

Atrial fibrillation/flutter (Betapace AF®):

Cl_{cr} >60 mL/minute: Administer every 12 hours

Cl_{cr} 40-60 mL/minute: Administer every 24 hours

Cl_{cr} <40 mL/minute: Use is contraindicated

Note: The manufacturer of the injectable formulation recommends adjustment similar to that used for Betapace AF®. However, the injectable formulation may be used for either indication.

Hemodialysis: Hemodialysis would be expected to reduce sotalol plasma concentrations because sotalol is not bound to plasma proteins and does not undergo extensive metabolism; administer dose postdialysis or administer supplemental 80 mg dose.

Peritoneal dialysis: Peritoneal dialysis does not remove sotalol; supplemental dose is not necessary.

Dosage adjustment in hepatic impairment: No dosage adjustment provided in manufacturer's labeling. However, dosage adjustment unlikely because sotalol is not metabolized by the liver.

Dietary Considerations May be taken without regard to meals.

Administration

Oral: Administer without regard to meals.

I.V.:

Substitution for oral: Administer over 5 hours.

Hemodynamically stable monomorphic VT: Administer I.V. push over 5 minutes; use with caution due to increased risk of adverse events (eg, bradycardia, hypotension, torsade de pointes) (ACLS, 2010)

Monitoring Parameters Serum creatinine, magnesium, potassium; heart rate, blood pressure; ECG (eg, QT_c interval, PR interval). If baseline QT_c >450 msec (or JT interval >330 msec if QRS over 100 msec), sotalol is contraindicated.

For oral use (Betapace AF®) during initiation period, monitor QT_c interval 2-4 hours after each dose. If QT_c interval ≥500 msec, discontinue use; if QT_c interval <500 msec after 3 days (after fifth or sixth dose if patient receiving once-daily dosing), patient may be discharged on current regimen. Monitor QT_c interval periodically thereafter.

For I.V. use, measure QT_c interval after completion of each infusion.

Consult individual institutional policies and procedures.

Test Interactions May falsely increase urinary metanephrine values when fluorimetric or photometric methods are used; does not interact with HPLC assay with solid phase extraction for determination of urinary catecholamines

Additional Information Pharmacokinetics in children are more relevant for BSA than age.

Dosage Forms Excipient information presented when available (limited, particularly for generics); consult specific product labeling. [DSC] = Discontinued product

Solution, Intravenous, as hydrochloride:

Generic: 150 mg/10 mL (10 mL [DSC])

Tablet, Oral, as hydrochloride:

Betapace: 80 mg, 120 mg, 160 mg [scored]

Betapace AF: 80 mg, 120 mg, 160 mg [scored]

Sorine: 80 mg, 120 mg, 160 mg, 240 mg [scored]

Generic: 80 mg, 120 mg, 160 mg, 240 mg

Extemporaneous Preparations A 5 mg/mL sotalol hydrochloride syrup may be made with Betapace® or Betapace AF® tablets and Simple Syrup containing sodium benzoate 0.1% (Syrup, NF). Place 120 mL Syrup, NF in a 6-ounce amber plastic (polyethylene terephthalate) prescription bottle; add five Betapace® or Betapace AF® 120 mg tablets and shake the bottle to wet the tablets. Allow tablets to hydrate for at least 2 hours, then shake intermittently over ≥2 hours until the tablets are completely disintegrated; a dispersion of fine particles (water-insoluble inactive ingredients) in syrup should be obtained. **Note:** To simplify the disintegration process, tablets can hydrate overnight; tablets may also be crushed, carefully transferred into the bottle and shaken well until a dispersion of fine particles in syrup is obtained. Label "shake well". Stable for 3 months at controlled room temperature (15°C to 30°C [59°F to 86°F]) and ambient humidity.

Betapace® prescribing information, Bayer HealthCare Pharmaceuticals Inc, Wayne, NJ, 2007.

Betapace AF® prescribing information, Bayer HealthCare Pharmaceuticals Inc, Wayne, NJ, 2009.

◆ **Sotalol Hydrochloride** *see* Sotalol *on page* 1942

◆ **Sotradecol** *see* Sodium Tetradecyl Sulfate *on page* 1931

◆ **SP-303** *see* Crofelemer *on page* 500

◆ **SPA** *see* Albumin *on page* 59

◆ **SPD417** *see* CarBAMazepine *on page* 336

◆ **Spectracef** *see* Cefditoren *on page 366*

◆ **SPI 0211** *see* Lubiprostone *on page 1254*

Spinosad (SPIN oh sad)

Brand Names: U.S. Natroba

Index Terms NatrOVA

Pharmacologic Category Antiparasitic Agent, Topical; Pediculocide

Use Topical treatment of head lice (*Pediculosis capitis*) infestation in adults and children ≥4 years of age

Unlabeled Use Topical treatment of head lice (*Pediculosis capitis*) infestation in children ≥6 months and <4 years of age

Pregnancy Risk Factor B

Pregnancy Considerations Teratogenic effects were not observed in animal reproduction studies. Human studies did not assess the absorption of benzyl alcohol, an ingredient in the product.

Breast-Feeding Considerations Spinosad used topically is not systemically absorbed and will not be present in human milk. The suspension formulation does include benzyl alcohol, which may be systemically absorbed and may be excreted in human milk. Lactating women may choose to pump and discard breast milk for five benzyl alcohol half-lives (8 hours) after use to avoid ingestion of benzyl alcohol by an infant.

Contraindications There are no contraindications listed in the manufacturer's labeling

Warnings/Precautions For topical use on scalp and scalp hair only; avoid contact with eyes. Wash hands after application. The suspension contains benzyl alcohol and is not recommended for use in children <6 months of age.

Adverse Reactions

1% to 10%:

Dermatologic: Application site erythema (3%), application site irritation (1%), skin irritation

Ocular: Erythema (2%), hyperemia (2%), irritation

<1% (Limited to important or life-threatening): Alopecia, application site reactions (dryness, exfoliation), dry skin

Drug Interactions

Metabolism/Transport Effects None known.

Avoid Concomitant Use There are no known interactions where it is recommended to avoid concomitant use.

Increased Effect/Toxicity There are no known significant interactions involving an increase in effect.

Decreased Effect There are no known significant interactions involving a decrease in effect.

Storage/Stability Store at 25°C (77°F); excursions permitted between 15°C to 30°C (59°F to 86°F).

Mechanism of Action Insect paralysis and death is caused by central nervous system excitation and involuntary muscle contractions. Spinosad is thought to be both pediculocidal and ovicidal (Stough, 2009).

Pharmacodynamics/Kinetics Absorption: Not absorbed topically (not detectable in a pediatric patient plasma sampling study); absorption of the benzyl alcohol was not analyzed in this study.

Dosage Topical:

Children ≥6 months to <4 years (unlabeled use): Head lice: Apply to dry scalp; may repeat in 7 days if needed (Stough, 2009)

Children ≥4 years and Adults: Head lice: Apply sufficient amount to cover dry scalp and completely cover dry hair; 120 mL may be necessary depending on the length of hair. If live lice are seen 7 days after first treatment, repeat with second application.

Administration Topical suspension. For external use only. Shake bottle well. Apply to dry scalp and rub gently until the scalp is thoroughly moistened, then apply to dry hair; completely covering scalp and hair. Leave on for 10 minutes (start timing treatment after the scalp and hair have been completely covered). The hair should then be rinsed thoroughly with warm water. Shampoo may be used immediately after the product is completely rinsed off. If live lice are seen 7 days after the first treatment, repeat with second application. Avoid contact with the eyes. Nit combing is not required, although a fine-tooth comb may be used to remove treated lice and nits.

Spinosad should be a portion of a whole lice removal program, which should include washing or dry cleaning all clothing, hats, bedding and towels recently worn or used by the patient and washing combs, brushes, and hair accessories in hot water.

Monitoring Parameters Monitor scalp for lice

Dosage Forms Excipient information presented when available (limited, particularly for generics); consult specific product labeling.

Suspension, External:

Natroba: 0.9% (120 mL) [contains benzyl alcohol, cetearyl alcohol, fd&c yellow #6 (sunset yellow), isopropyl alcohol, propylene glycol]

Generic: 0.9% (120 mL)

◆ **Spiriva® (Can)** *see* Tiotropium *on page 2069*

◆ **Spiriva HandiHaler** *see* Tiotropium *on page 2069*

Spironolactone (speer on oh LAK tone)

Brand Names: U.S. Aldactone

Brand Names: Canada Aldactone; Teva-Spironolactone

Pharmacologic Category Antihypertensive; Diuretic, Potassium-Sparing; Selective Aldosterone Blocker

Additional Appendix Information

Beers Criteria – Potentially Inappropriate Medications for Geriatrics *on page 2368*

Use Management of edema associated with excessive aldosterone excretion or with congestive heart failure (HF) unresponsive to other therapies; hypertension; primary hyperaldosteronism (establishing diagnosis, short-term preoperative treatment, and long-term maintenance therapy in selected patients); hypokalemia; cirrhosis of liver accompanied by edema or ascites; nephrotic syndrome; severe HF (NYHA class III-IV) to increase survival and reduce hospitalization when added to standard therapy

Unlabeled Use Female acne (adjunctive therapy); hirsutism; hypertension (pediatric); diuretic (pediatric); HF (NYHA class II) with LVEF ≤35% in patients who have a history of prior cardiovascular hospitalization or elevated plasma natriuretic peptide levels to reduce morbidity and mortality; to reduce morbidity and mortality following acute MI with LVEF ≤40% in patients who develop HF symptoms or have a history of diabetes mellitus

Pregnancy Risk Factor C

Pregnancy Considerations Adverse events were observed in some animal reproduction studies. The antiandrogen effects of spironolactone have been shown to cause feminization of the male fetus in animal studies. Spironolactone crosses the placenta (Regitz-Zagrosek, 2011).

The treatment of heart failure is generally the same in pregnant and nonpregnant women; however, spironolactone should be avoided in the first trimester due to its antiandrogenic effects (Regitz-Zagrosek, 2011). When treatment for hypertension in pregnancy is needed, other agents are preferred (Chobanian, 2003). Use of diuretics to treat edema during normal pregnancies is not appropriate; use may be considered when edema is due to pathologic causes (as in the nonpregnant patient); monitor.

Breast-Feeding Considerations The active metabolite of spironolactone (canrenone) has been found in breast milk. Information is available from a case report following maternal use of spironolactone 25 mg twice daily throughout pregnancy, then 4 times daily after delivery. Milk and maternal serum samples were obtained 17 days after birth. Two hours after the maternal dose, canrenone concentrations were ~144 ng/mL (serum) and ~104 ng/mL (milk). When measured 14.5 hours after the dose, canrenone concentrations were ~92 ng/mL (serum) and ~47 ng/mL (milk). The authors calculated the estimated maximum amount of canrenone to the nursing infant to be ~0.2% of the maternal dose (Phelps, 1977). Effects to humans are not known; however, this metabolite was found to be carcinogenic in rats. Diuretics have the potential to decrease milk volume and suppress lactation. Breast-fed infants of mothers taking medications for hypertension should be monitored for adverse effects (Chobanian, 2003). According to the manufacturer, the decision to continue or discontinue breast-feeding during therapy should take into account the risk of exposure to the infant and the benefits of treatment to the mother; if use of spironolactone is essential, an alternative method of feeding should be used.

Contraindications Anuria; acute renal insufficiency; significant impairment of renal excretory function; hyperkalemia; Addison's disease or other conditions associated with hyperkalemia; concomitant use with eplerenone

Canadian labeling: Additional contraindications (not in U.S. labeling): Hypersensitivity to spironolactone or any component of the formulation; concomitant use with heparin or low molecular weight heparin

Warnings/Precautions [U.S. Boxed Warning]: Shown to be a tumorigen in chronic toxicity animal studies. Avoid unnecessary use.

Monitor serum potassium closely in patients being treated for heart failure. Avoid potassium supplements, potassium-containing salt substitutes, a diet rich in potassium, or other drugs that can cause hyperkalemia. Potentially significant interactions may exist, requiring dose or frequency adjustment, additional monitoring, and/or selection of alternative therapy. Somnolence and dizziness have been reported with use; advise patients to use caution when driving or operating machinery until response to initial treatment has been determined. Excess amounts can lead to profound diuresis with fluid and electrolyte loss; close medical supervision and dose evaluation are required. Watch for and correct electrolyte disturbances; adjust dose to avoid dehydration. In cirrhosis, avoid electrolyte and acid/base imbalances that might lead to hepatic encephalopathy. Gynecomastia is related to dose and duration of therapy; typically is reversible following discontinuation of therapy but may persist (rare). Discontinue use prior to adrenal vein catheterization. When evaluating a heart failure patient for spironolactone treatment, creatinine should be <2.5 mg/dL or eGFR >30 mL/minute/1.73 m^2) with no recent worsening and potassium <5 mEq/L with no history of severe hyperkalemia (Yancy, 2013). Serum potassium levels require close monitoring and management if elevated. Discontinue or interrupt therapy if serum potassium >5 mEq/L or serum creatinine >4 mg/dL. The ACCF/AHA recommends considering discontinuation upon the development of worsening renal function with careful evaluation of the entire medical regimen. Avoid routine triple therapy with the combined use of an ACE inhibitor, ARB, and spironolactone. Instruct patients with heart failure to discontinue use during an episode of diarrhea or dehydration or when loop diuretic therapy is interrupted (Yancy, 2013). In the elderly, avoid use of doses >25 mg/day in patients with heart failure or in patients with reduced renal function (Cl_{cr} <30 mL/minute or eGFR ≤30 mL/minute/1.73 m^2 [Yancy, 2013]); risk of hyperkalemia is increased for heart failure patients receiving >25 mg/day, particularly if taking concomitant medications such as NSAIDS, ACE inhibitor, angiotensin receptor blocker, or potassium supplements (Beers Criteria).

Adverse Reactions Frequency not defined.

Cardiovascular: Vasculitis

Central nervous system: Ataxia, confusion, drowsiness, headache, lethargy

Dermatologic: Erythematous maculopapular rash, Stevens-Johnson syndrome, toxic epidermal necrolysis, urticaria

Endocrine & metabolic: Amenorrhea, gynecomastia, hyperkalemia

Gastrointestinal: Abdominal cramps, diarrhea, gastritis, gastrointestinal hemorrhage, gastrointestinal ulcer, nausea, vomiting

Genitourinary: Impotence, irregular menses, postmenopausal bleeding

Hematologic & oncologic: Agranulocytosis, malignant neoplasm of breast

Hepatic: Hepatotoxicity

Hypersensitivity: Anaphylaxis

Immunologic: DRESS syndrome

Renal: Increased blood urea nitrogen, renal failure, renal insufficiency

Miscellaneous: Fever

Drug Interactions

Metabolism/Transport Effects None known.

Avoid Concomitant Use

Avoid concomitant use of Spironolactone with any of the following: AMILoride; CycloSPORINE (Systemic); Tacrolimus (Systemic); Triamterene

Increased Effect/Toxicity

Spironolactone may increase the levels/effects of: ACE Inhibitors; Amifostine; Ammonium Chloride; Antihypertensives; Cardiac Glycosides; CycloSPORINE (Systemic); Digoxin; Hypotensive Agents; Neuromuscular-Blocking Agents (Nondepolarizing); Obinutuzumab; RiTUXimab; Sodium Phosphates; Tacrolimus (Systemic)

The levels/effects of Spironolactone may be increased by: Alfuzosin; AMILoride; Analgesics (Opioid); Angiotensin II Receptor Blockers; AtorvaSTATin; Brimonidine (Topical); Canagliflozin; Cholestyramine Resin; Diazoxide; Drospirenone; Eplerenone; Heparin; Heparin (Low Molecular Weight); Herbs (Hypotensive Properties); MAO Inhibitors; Nitrofurantoin; Nonsteroidal Anti-Inflammatory Agents; Pentoxifylline; Phosphodiesterase 5 Inhibitors; Potassium Salts; Prostacyclin Analogues; Tolvaptan; Triamterene; Trimethoprim

Decreased Effect

Spironolactone may decrease the levels/effects of: Abiraterone Acetate; Alpha-/Beta-Agonists; Cardiac Glycosides; Mitotane; QuiNIDine

The levels/effects of Spironolactone may be decreased by: Herbs (Hypertensive Properties); Methylphenidate; Nonsteroidal Anti-Inflammatory Agents; Yohimbine

Ethanol/Nutrition/Herb Interactions

Ethanol: Increases risk of orthostasis.

Food: Food increases absorption.

Herb/Nutraceutical: Avoid natural licorice (due to mineralocorticoid activity)

Storage/Stability Store below 25°C (77°F).

Mechanism of Action Competes with aldosterone for receptor sites in the distal renal tubules, increasing sodium chloride and water excretion while conserving potassium and hydrogen ions; may block the effect of aldosterone on arteriolar smooth muscle as well

Pharmacodynamics/Kinetics

Duration: 2-3 days

Protein binding: >90%

Metabolism: Hepatic to multiple metabolites, including active metabolites canrenone and 7-alpha-spirolactone

Half-life elimination: Spironolactone: ~1.4 hours; Canrenone: 12-20 hours (Skluth, 1990); 7-alpha-spirolactone: ~13.8 hours

Time to peak, serum: 3-4 hours (primarily as the active metabolite)

Excretion: Urine and feces

Dosage Oral:

Children: Diuretic, hypertension (unlabeled use): Children 1-17 years: Initial: 1 mg/kg/day divided every 12-24 hours (maximum dose: 3.3 mg/kg/day, up to 100 mg daily) (NHBPEP, 2004)

Adults:

Edema: 25-200 mg daily in 1-2 divided doses

Hypokalemia: 25-100 mg once daily

Hypertension (JNC 7): 25-50 mg daily in 1-2 divided doses

Diagnosis of primary aldosteronism: Long test: 400 mg once daily for 3-4 weeks; short test: 400 mg once daily for 4 days; maintenance until surgical correction: 100-400 mg once daily

Heart failure (HF), severe (NYHA class III-IV; with ACE inhibitor and a loop diuretic with or without digoxin): 12.5-25 mg once daily; maximum daily dose: 50 mg. If 25 mg once daily not tolerated, may reduce to 25 mg every other day. The ACCF/AHA 2013 HF guidelines also recommend the use of aldosterone receptor antagonists (eg, spironolactone) in patients with NYHA class II HF and LVEF ≤35% who have a history of prior cardiovascular hospitalization or elevated plasma natriuretic peptide levels and postmyocardial infarction patients with LVEF ≤40% who develop HF symptoms or have a history of diabetes mellitus (Yancy, 2013).

Note: If potassium >5 mEq/L or serum creatinine >4 mg/dL (or worsening renal function [Yancy, 2013]), discontinue or interrupt therapy.

Acne in women (unlabeled use): 50-200 mg once daily (Goodfellow, 1984; Muhlemann, 1986)

Hirsutism in women (unlabeled use): 50-200 mg daily in 1-2 divided doses (Koulouri, 2008; Martin, 2008)

Elderly:

Hypertension: No initial dosage adjustment necessary (Aronow, 2011).

Heart failure: Avoid using doses >25 mg daily (Beers Criteria); monitor potassium closely/use with caution.

Dosage adjustment in renal impairment: Heart failure (Yancy, 2013):

eGFR ≥50 mL/minute/1.73 m^2: Initial dose: 12.5-25 mg once daily; Maintenance dose (after 4 weeks of treatment with potassium ≤5 mEq/L): 25 mg once or twice daily

eGFR 30-49 mL/minute/1.73 m^2: Initial dose: 12.5 mg once daily or every other day; Maintenance dose (after 4 weeks of treatment with potassium ≤5 mEq/L): 12.5-25 mg once daily

eGFR <30 mL/minute/1.73 m^2: Not recommended.

Note: Contraindicated in patients with anuria, acute renal insufficiency, or significant impairment of renal excretory function.

Dosage adjustment in hepatic impairment: No dosage adjustment provided in manufacturer's labeling.

Dietary Considerations Should be taken with food to decrease gastrointestinal irritation and to increase absorption. Excessive potassium intake (eg, salt substitutes, low-salt foods, bananas, nuts) should be avoided.

Monitoring Parameters Blood pressure, serum electrolytes (potassium, sodium), renal function, I & O ratios and daily weight throughout therapy

HF: Potassium levels and renal function should be checked in 3 days and 1 week after initiation or increase in dose, then every 2-4 weeks for 3 months, then quarterly for a year, then every 6 months thereafter. Discontinue or interrupt spironolactone if serum potassium is >5 mEq/L or serum creatinine is >4 mg/dL (or renal function worsens [Yancy, 2013]).

Test Interactions May interfere with the radioimmunoassay for digoxin.

Additional Information Maximum diuretic effect may be delayed 2-3 days and maximum antihypertensive effects may be delayed 2-3 weeks.

Dosage Forms Excipient information presented when available (limited, particularly for generics); consult specific product labeling.

Tablet, Oral:

Aldactone: 25 mg

Aldactone: 50 mg, 100 mg [scored]

Generic: 25 mg, 50 mg, 100 mg

Dosage Forms: Canada Refer to Dosage Forms. **Note:** Aldactone 50 mg tablets are not available in Canada.

Extemporaneous Preparations A 1 mg/mL oral suspension may be made with tablets. Crush ten 25 mg tablets in a mortar and reduce to a fine powder. Add a small amount of purified water and soak for 5 minutes; add 50 mL 1.5% carboxymethylcellulose, 100 mL syrup NF, and mix to a uniform paste; mix while adding purified water in incremental proportions to **almost** 250 mL; transfer to a calibrated bottle, rinse mortar with purified water, and add quantity of purified water sufficient to make 250 mL. Label "shake well". Stable for 3 months at room temperature or refrigerated (Nahata, 1993).

A 2.5 mg/mL oral suspension may be made with tablets. Crush twelve 25 mg tablets in a mortar and reduce to a fine powder. Add small portions of distilled water or glycerin and mix to a uniform paste; mix while adding cherry syrup to **almost** 120 mL; transfer to a calibrated bottle, rinse mortar with cherry syrup, and add quantity of cherry syrup sufficient to make 120 mL. Label "shake well" and "refrigerate". This method may also be used with twenty-four 25 mg tablets for a 5 mg/mL oral suspension. Both concentrations are stable for 28 days refrigerated (Mathur, 1989).

A 25 mg/mL oral suspension may be made with tablets and either a 1:1 mixture of Ora-Sweet and Ora-Plus or a 1:1 mixture of Ora-Sweet SF and Ora-Plus. Crush one-hundred-twenty 25 mg tablets in a mortar and reduce to a fine powder. Add small portions of chosen vehicle and mix to a uniform paste; mix while adding vehicle in incremental proportions to **almost** 120 mL; transfer to a calibrated bottle, rinse mortar with vehicle, and add quantity of vehicle sufficient to make 120 mL. Store in amber bottles; label "shake well" and "refrigerate". Stable for 60 days refrigerated (Allen, 1996).

Allen LV Jr and Erickson MA 3rd, "Stability of Ketoconazole, Metolazone, Metronidazole, Procainamide Hydrochloride, and Spironolactone in Extemporaneously Compounded Oral Liquids," *Am J Health Syst Pharm*, 1996, 53(17):2073-8.

Mathur LK and Wickman A, "Stability of Extemporaneously Compounded Spironolactone Suspensions," *Am J Hosp Pharm*, 1989, 46(10):2040-2.

Nahata MC, Morosco RS, and Hipple TF, "Stability of Spironolactone in an Extemporaneously Prepared Suspension at Two Temperatures," *Ann Pharmacother*, 1993, 27(10):1198-9.

◆ **SPM 927** *see* Lacosamide *on page* 1159

◆ **Sporanox** *see* Itraconazole *on page* 1132

◆ **Sporanox Pulsepak** *see* Itraconazole *on page* 1132

◆ **SPP100** *see* Aliskiren *on page* 74

◆ **Sprintec** *see* Ethinyl Estradiol and Norgestimate *on page* 795

◆ **Sprix** *see* Ketorolac (Nasal) *on page* 1155

◆ **Sprycel** *see* Dasatinib *on page 550*
◆ **Sprycel® (Can)** *see* Dasatinib *on page 550*
◆ **SPS** *see* Sodium Polystyrene Sulfonate *on page 1927*
◆ **SQV** *see* Saquinavir *on page 1875*
◆ **SR33589** *see* Dronedarone *on page 675*
◆ **Sronyx** *see* Ethinyl Estradiol and Levonorgestrel *on page 787*
◆ **SS734** *see* Besifloxacin *on page 246*
◆ **SSD** *see* Silver Sulfadiazine *on page 1897*
◆ **SSKI** *see* Potassium Iodide *on page 1687*
◆ **SSS 10-4** *see* Sulfur and Sulfacetamide *on page 1966*
◆ **SSS 10-5** *see* Sulfur and Sulfacetamide *on page 1966*
◆ **Stadol** *see* Butorphanol *on page 306*
◆ **Stagesic™** *see* Hydrocodone and Acetaminophen *on page 1006*
◆ **Stalevo®** *see* Levodopa, Carbidopa, and Entacapone *on page 1197*
◆ **StanGard® Perio** *see* Fluoride *on page 880*
◆ **Stannous Fluoride** *see* Fluoride *on page 880*
◆ **Starlix** *see* Nateglinide *on page 1431*
◆ **Statex® (Can)** *see* Morphine (Systemic) *on page 1398*

Stavudine (STAV yoo deen)

Brand Names: U.S. Zerit

Brand Names: Canada Zerit®

Index Terms d4T

Pharmacologic Category Antiretroviral, Reverse Transcriptase Inhibitor, Nucleoside (Anti-HIV)

Use Treatment of HIV infection in combination with other antiretroviral agents

Pregnancy Risk Factor C

Pregnancy Considerations Adverse events were observed in some animal reproduction studies. Stavudine crosses the placenta. No increased risk of overall birth defects has been observed following first trimester exposure according to data collected by the antiretroviral pregnancy registry. Pharmacokinetics of stavudine are not significantly altered during pregnancy; dose adjustments are not needed. Cases of lactic acidosis/hepatic steatosis syndrome related to mitochondrial toxicity have been reported in pregnant women with prolonged use of nucleoside analogues. It is not known if pregnancy itself potentiates this known side effect; however, women may be at increased risk of lactic acidosis and liver damage. In addition, these adverse events are similar to other rare but life-threatening syndromes which occur during pregnancy (eg, HELLP syndrome). Combination treatment with didanosine may also contribute to the risk of lactic acidosis, and should be considered only if benefit outweighs risk. Hepatic enzymes and electrolytes should be monitored in women receiving nucleoside analogues and clinicians should watch for early signs of the syndrome. In addition, mitochondrial dysfunction may develop in infants following *in utero* exposure. The DHHS Perinatal HIV Guidelines recommend stavudine to be used only in special circumstances during pregnancy; do not use with didanosine or zidovudine.

Regardless of CD4 count or HIV RNA copy number, all HIV-infected pregnant women should receive a combination antepartum antiretroviral (ARV) drug regimen; this includes women who require therapy for their own health, as well as women who do not yet require therapy for their own health. ARV therapy should be started as soon as possible if required for the woman's health. Although earlier initiation may be more effective in reducing the perinatal transmission of HIV), also consider maternal conditions (eg, nausea and vomiting) and the potential risks of first trimester fetal exposure for specific agents. Plasma HIV RNA levels should be assessed at ~34-36 weeks gestation in order to help determine mode of delivery. If ARV therapy must be interrupted for <24 hours during the peripartum period, stop then restart all medications simultaneously in order to decrease the chance of developing resistance. Long-term follow-up is recommended for all infants exposed to ARV medications.

Healthcare providers are encouraged to enroll pregnant women exposed to antiretroviral medications in the Antiretroviral Pregnancy Registry (1-800-258-4263 or www.-APRegistry.com). Healthcare providers caring for HIV-infected women and their infants may contact the National Perinatal HIV Hotline (888-448-8765) for clinical consultation (DHHS [perinatal], 2012).

Breast-Feeding Considerations Maternal or infant antiretroviral therapy does not completely eliminate the risk of postnatal HIV transmission. In addition, multiclass-resistant virus has been detected in breast-feeding infants despite maternal therapy. Therefore, in the United States, where formula is accessible, affordable, safe, and sustainable, and the risk of infant mortality due to diarrhea and respiratory infections is low, complete avoidance of breast-feeding by HIV-infected women is recommended to decrease potential transmission of HIV (DHHS [perinatal], 2012).

Medication Guide Available Yes

Contraindications Hypersensitivity to stavudine or any component of the formulation

Warnings/Precautions Use with caution in patients who demonstrate previous hypersensitivity to zidovudine, didanosine, zalcitabine, pre-existing bone marrow suppression, renal insufficiency (dosage adjustment recommended), hepatic impairment, or peripheral neuropathy. Peripheral neuropathy may be a treatment-limiting side effect; consider permanent discontinuation. Zidovudine should not be used in combination with stavudine. **[U.S. Boxed Warning]: Lactic acidosis and severe hepatomegaly with steatosis have been reported with stavudine use, including fatal cases;** combination therapy with didanosine may increase risk; use with caution in patients with risk factors for liver disease (although acidosis has occurred in patients without known risk factors, risk may be increased with female gender, obesity, pregnancy, or prolonged exposure). Suspend treatment in any patient who develops clinical or laboratory findings suggestive of lactic acidosis or hepatotoxicity. Mortality of 50% associated in some case series, notably with serum lactate >10 mmol/L (DHHS, 2012). Severe motor weakness (resembling Guillain-Barré syndrome) has been reported (including fatal cases, usually in association with lactic acidosis); manufacturer recommends discontinuation if motor weakness develops (with or without lactic acidosis). May cause redistribution of fat (eg, buffalo hump, peripheral wasting with increased abdominal girth, cushingoid appearance). Patients may develop immune reconstitution syndrome resulting in the occurrence of an inflammatory response to an indolent or residual opportunistic infection during initial HIV treatment or activation of autoimmune disorders (eg, Graves' disease, polymyositis, Guillain-Barré syndrome) later in therapy; further evaluation and treatment may be required. **[U.S. Boxed Warning]: Pancreatitis (including some fatal cases) has occurred during combination therapy with didanosine.** Suspend stavudine and didanosine combination therapy, and any other agents toxic to the pancreas, in patients with suspected pancreatitis. If pancreatitis diagnosis confirmed, use extreme caution if reinitiating stavudine; monitor closely and do not use didanosine in regimen. Use with caution in combination with interferon alfa with or without ribavirin in HIV/HBV coinfected patients; monitor closely for hepatic decompensation, anemia, or neutropenia; dose reduction or discontinuation of interferon and/or ribavirin may be required if toxicity evident. Combination therapy with didanosine or hydroxyurea may increase risk of hepatotoxicity, pancreatitis, or severe peripheral neuropathy; avoid stavudine or hydroxyurea combination.

Adverse Reactions Adverse reactions reported below represent experience with combination therapy with other nucleoside analogues and protease inhibitors.

>10%:

Central nervous system: Headache (25% to 46%)
Dermatologic: Rash (18% to 30%)
Gastrointestinal: Nausea (43% to 53%; less than comparator group), vomiting (18% to 30%; less than comparator group), diarrhea (34% to 45%)
Hepatic: Hyperbilirubinemia (65% to 68%; grade 3/4: 7% to 16%), AST increased (42% to 53%; grade 3/4: 5% to 7%), ALT increased (40% to 50%; grade 3/4: 6% to 8%), GGT increased (15% to 28%; grade 3/4: 2% to 5%)
Neuromuscular & skeletal: Peripheral neuropathy (8% to 21%)
Miscellaneous: Amylase increased (21% to 31%; grade 3/4: 4% to 8%), lipase increased (~27%; grade 3/4: 5% to 6%)

Postmarketing and/or case reports: Abdominal pain, allergic reaction, anemia, anorexia, chills, diabetes mellitus, fever, hepatic failure, hepatitis, hepatomegaly (with steatosis; some fatal), hyperglycemia, hyperlactatemia (symptomatic), hyperlipidemia, immune reconstitution syndrome, insomnia, insulin resistance, lactic acidosis (some fatal), leukopenia, macrocytosis, myalgia, neuromuscular weakness (severe-resembling Guillain-Barré), neutropenia, pancreatitis (some fatal), redistribution/accumulation/atrophy of body fat, thrombocytopenia

Drug Interactions

Metabolism/Transport Effects None known.

Avoid Concomitant Use

Avoid concomitant use of Stavudine with any of the following: Hydroxyurea; Zidovudine

Increased Effect/Toxicity

Stavudine may increase the levels/effects of: Didanosine; Hydroxyurea

The levels/effects of Stavudine may be increased by: Hydroxyurea; Ribavirin

Decreased Effect

The levels/effects of Stavudine may be decreased by: DOXOrubicin; DOXOrubicin (Liposomal); Zidovudine

Preparation for Administration Reconstitute powder for oral suspension with 202 mL of purified water as specified on the bottle. Shake vigorously until suspended. Final suspension will be 1 mg/mL (200 mL).

Storage/Stability Capsules and powder for reconstitution may be stored at controlled room temperature of 25°C (77°F). Reconstituted oral solution should be stored in refrigerator at 2°C to 8°C (36°F to 46°F) and is stable for 30 days.

Mechanism of Action Stavudine is a thymidine analog which interferes with HIV viral DNA dependent DNA polymerase resulting in inhibition of viral replication; nucleoside reverse transcriptase inhibitor

Pharmacodynamics/Kinetics

Distribution: V_d: 46 L
Metabolism: Undergoes intracellular phosphorylation to an active metabolite (stavudine triphosphate)
Bioavailability: Children: 76.9%; Adults: 86.4%
Half-life elimination: HIV-infected Children: 0.96 hours, HIV-infected Adults: 1.6 hours
Time to peak, serum: 1 hour
Excretion: Urine 95% (74% as unchanged drug); feces 3% (62% as unchanged drug)

Dosage Oral:

Newborns (Birth to 13 days): 0.5 mg/kg every 12 hours
Children:
≥14 days and <30 kg: 1 mg/kg every 12 hours
≥30 kg: Refer to adult dosing
Adults:
<60 kg: 30 mg every 12 hours
≥60 kg: 40 mg every 12 hours
Note: The World Health Organization recommends 30 mg every 12 hours in all adult and adolescent patients regardless of body weight (DHHS, 2012).
Elderly: Older patients should be closely monitored for signs and symptoms of peripheral neuropathy; dosage should be carefully adjusted to renal function

Dosage adjustment in renal impairment:

Children: Specific recommendations not available. Reduction in dose or increase in dosing interval should be considered.
Adults:
Cl_{cr} >50 mL/minute:
<60 kg: 30 mg every 12 hours
≥60 kg: 40 mg every 12 hours
Cl_{cr} 26-50 mL/minute:
<60 kg: 15 mg every 12 hours
≥60 kg: 20 mg every 12 hours
Cl_{cr} 10-25 mL/minute, hemodialysis (administer dose after hemodialysis on day of dialysis):
<60 kg: 15 mg every 24 hours
≥60 kg: 20 mg every 24 hours

Dosage adjustment in hepatic impairment: No dosage adjustment provided in manufacturer's labeling. Use with caution.

Dietary Considerations May be taken without regard to meals. Some products may contain sucrose.

Administration May be administered without regard to meals. Oral solution should be shaken vigorously prior to use.

Monitoring Parameters Monitor liver function tests and renal function tests; signs and symptoms of peripheral neuropathy; monitor viral load and CD4 count

Additional Information Potential compliance problems, frequency of administration and adverse effects should be discussed with patients before initiating therapy to help prevent the emergence of resistance. Concomitant use of stavudine and lamivudine is discouraged; additive toxicities include life-threatening lactic acidosis and pancreatitis; concomitant stavudine with zidovudine, or stavudine with didanosine use should be avoided (DHHS, 2012).

Dosage Forms Excipient information presented when available (limited, particularly for generics); consult specific product labeling.

Capsule, Oral:
Zerit: 15 mg, 20 mg, 30 mg, 40 mg
Generic: 15 mg, 20 mg, 30 mg, 40 mg
Solution Reconstituted, Oral:
Zerit: 1 mg/mL (200 mL) [dye free; fruit flavor]
Generic: 1 mg/mL (200 mL)

◆ **Stavzor** *see* Valproic Acid and Derivatives *on page 2149*
◆ **Staxyn** *see* Vardenafil *on page 2164*
◆ **Stelara** *see* Ustekinumab *on page 2142*
◆ **Stelazine** *see* Trifluoperazine *on page 2125*
◆ **Stendra** *see* Avanafil *on page 202*
◆ **Sterile Talc** *see* Talc (Sterile) *on page 1986*
◆ **Sterile Talc Powder** *see* Talc (Sterile) *on page 1986*
◆ **Sterile Vancomycin Hydrochloride, USP (Can)** *see* Vancomycin *on page 2157*
◆ **STI-571** *see* Imatinib *on page 1048*
◆ **Stieprox (Can)** *see* Ciclopirox *on page 423*

Streptomycin (strep toe MYE sin)

Brand Names: Canada Streptomycin for Injection

Index Terms Streptomycin Sulfate

Pharmacologic Category Antibiotic, Aminoglycoside; Antitubercular Agent

Use Part of combination therapy of active tuberculosis; used in combination with other agents for treatment of bacteremia caused by susceptible gram-negative bacilli, brucellosis, chancroid granuloma inguinale, *H. influenzae* (respiratory, endocardial, meningeal infections), *K. pneumoniae*, plague, streptococcal or enterococcal endocarditis, tularemia, urinary tract infections (caused by *A. aerogenes, E. coli, E. faecalis, K. pneumoniae, Proteus* spp)

Unlabeled Use Buruli ulcer (*Mycobacterium ulcerans*), Ménière's disease, *Mycobacterium kansasii* infection; *Mycobacterium avium* complex (MAC)

Pregnancy Risk Factor D

Pregnancy Considerations Streptomycin crosses the placenta. Many case reports of hearing impairment in children exposed *in utero* have been published. Impairment has ranged from mild hearing loss to bilateral deafness. Because of several reports of total irreversible bilateral congenital deafness in children whose mothers received streptomycin during pregnancy, the manufacturer classifies streptomycin as pregnancy risk factor D.

Breast-Feeding Considerations Streptomycin is excreted into breast milk; however, it is not well absorbed when taken orally. This limited oral absorption may minimize exposure to the nursing infant. Nondose-related effects could include modification of bowel flora. Breast-feeding is not recommended by the manufacturer.

Contraindications Hypersensitivity to streptomycin, other aminoglycosides, or any component of the formulation

Warnings/Precautions [U.S. Boxed Warnings]: May cause neurotoxicity, nephrotoxicity, and/or neuromuscular blockade and respiratory paralysis; usual risk factors include pre-existing renal impairment, concomitant neuro-/nephrotoxic medications, advanced age and dehydration. The drug's neurotoxicity can result in respiratory paralysis from neuromuscular blockade, especially when the drug is given soon after anesthesia or muscle relaxants. Use with caution in patients with pre-existing vertigo, tinnitus, hearing loss, neuromuscular disorders, or renal impairment; modify dosage in patients with renal impairment; ototoxicity is directly proportional to the amount of drug given and the duration of treatment; tinnitus or vertigo are indications of vestibular injury and impending bilateral irreversible damage; renal damage is usually reversible. Monitor renal function closely; peak serum concentrations should not surpass 20-25 mcg/mL in patients with renal impairment. Formulation contains metabisulfite; may cause allergic reactions in patients with sulfite sensitivity. **[U.S. Boxed Warning]: Parenteral form should be used only where appropriate audiometric and laboratory testing facilities are available.** Prolonged use may result in fungal or bacterial superinfection, including *C. difficile*-associated diarrhea (CDAD) and pseudomembranous colitis; CDAD has been observed >2 months postantibiotic treatment. I.M. injections should be administered in a large muscle well within the body to avoid peripheral nerve damage and local skin reactions.

Adverse Reactions Frequency not defined.

Cardiovascular: Hypotension

Central nervous system: Drug fever, headache, neurotoxicity, paresthesia of face

Dermatologic: Angioedema, exfoliative dermatitis, skin rash, urticaria

Gastrointestinal: Nausea, vomiting

Hematologic: Eosinophilia, hemolytic anemia, leukopenia, pancytopenia, thrombocytopenia

Neuromuscular & skeletal: Arthralgia, tremor, weakness

Ocular: Amblyopia

Otic: Ototoxicity (auditory), ototoxicity (vestibular)

Renal: Azotemia, nephrotoxicity

Respiratory: Difficulty in breathing

Miscellaneous: Anaphylaxis

Postmarketing and/or case reports: Drug reaction with eosinophilia and systemic symptoms (DRESS), toxic epidermal necrolysis

Drug Interactions

Metabolism/Transport Effects None known.

Avoid Concomitant Use

Avoid concomitant use of Streptomycin with any of the following: BCG; Gallium Nitrate

Increased Effect/Toxicity

Streptomycin may increase the levels/effects of: AbobotulinumtoxinA; Bisphosphonate Derivatives; CARBOplatin; Colistimethate; CycloSPORINE (Systemic); Gallium Nitrate; Neuromuscular-Blocking Agents; OnabotulinumtoxinA; RimabotulinumtoxinB; Tenofovir

The levels/effects of Streptomycin may be increased by: Amphotericin B; Capreomycin; Cephalosporins (2nd Generation); Cephalosporins (3rd Generation); Cephalosporins (4th Generation); CISplatin; Loop Diuretics; Nonsteroidal Anti-Inflammatory Agents; Tenofovir; Vancomycin

Decreased Effect

Streptomycin may decrease the levels/effects of: BCG; Sodium Picosulfate; Typhoid Vaccine

The levels/effects of Streptomycin may be decreased by: Penicillins

Storage/Stability

Lyophilized powder: Store dry powder at controlled room temperature 20°C to 25°C (68°F to 77°F). Protect from light.

Solution: Store in refrigerator at 2°C to 8°C (36°F to 46°F).

Depending upon manufacturer, reconstituted solution remains stable for 24 hours at room temperature. Exposure to light causes darkening of solution without apparent loss of potency.

Mechanism of Action Inhibits bacterial protein synthesis by binding directly to the 30S ribosomal subunits causing faulty peptide sequence to form in the protein chain

Pharmacodynamics/Kinetics

Absorption: Oral: Poorly absorbed; I.M.: Well absorbed

Distribution: To extracellular fluid including serum, abscesses, ascitic, pericardial, pleural, synovial, lymphatic, and peritoneal fluids; poorly distributed into CSF

Half-life elimination: Adults: ~5 hours

Time to peak: I.M.: Within 1 hour

Excretion: Urine (29% to 89% as unchanged drug); feces, saliva, sweat, and tears (minimal)

Dosage Note: For I.M. administration; I.V. use is not recommended.

Usual dosage range: I.M.:
Children: 20-40 mg/kg/day (maximum: 1 g)
Adults: 15-30 mg/kg/day or 1-2 g/day

Indication-specific dosing:
Children: I.M.:
***Mycobacterium ulcerans* (Buruli ulcers):** 15 mg/kg once daily (maximum: 1 g) for 8 weeks (WHO, 2004)
Plague: 30 mg/kg/day divided every 12 hours for 10 days (WHO, 2010)
Tularemia: 15 mg/kg twice daily (maximum: 2 g) for 10 days (WHO, 2007)
Tuberculosis:
Daily therapy: 20-40 mg/kg/day (maximum: 1 g daily)
Directly observed therapy (DOT), twice weekly: 25-30 mg/kg (maximum: 1.5 g)
Directly observed therapy (DOT), 3 times weekly: 25-30 mg/kg (maximum: 1.5 g)
Adults: I.M.:
Brucellosis: 1 g daily in 2-4 divided doses for 14-21 days (with doxycycline) (Skalsky, 2008)
Endocarditis:
Enterococcal: 1 g every 12 hours for 2 weeks, 500 mg every 12 hours for 4 weeks in combination with penicillin
Streptococcal: 1 g every 12 hours for 1 week, 500 mg every 12 hours for 1 week in combination with penicillin. **Note:** For patients >60 years, 500 mg every 12 hours for 2 weeks is recommended.
***Mycobacterium avium* complex:** Adjunct therapy (with macrolide, rifamycin, and ethambutol): 8-25 mg/kg 2-3 times weekly for first 2-3 months for severe disease (maximum single dose for age >50 years: 500 mg) (Griffith, 2007)
***Mycobacterium kansasii* disease (rifampin-resistant):** 750 mg to 1 g daily (as part of a three-drug regimen based on susceptibilities) (Campbell, 2000; Griffith, 2007)
***Mycobacterium ulcerans* (Buruli ulcers):** 15 mg/kg once daily for 8 weeks (WHO, 2004)
Plague: 30 mg/kg/day (or 2 g) divided every 12 hours until the patient is afebrile for at least 3 days. **Note:** Full course is considered 10 days (WHO, 2010).
Tuberculosis:
Daily therapy: 15 mg/kg/day (maximum: 1 g)
Directly observed therapy (DOT), twice weekly: 25-30 mg/kg (maximum: 1.5 g)
Directly observed therapy (DOT), 3 times weekly: 25-30 mg/kg (maximum: 1.5 g)
Tularemia:
Manufacturer's labeling: 1-2 g daily in divided doses every 12 hours (maximum: 2 g daily) for 7-14 days until the patients is afebrile for 5-7 days
Alternative regimen: 2 g daily in 2 divided doses (maximum: 2 g daily) for 10 days (WHO, 2007)

Elderly: I.M.: Manufacturer states dose reductions are necessary in patients >60 years.

Dosage adjustment in renal impairment: The following adjustments have been recommended (Aronoff, 2007):
Cl_{cr} 10-50 mL/minute: Administer every 24-72 hours.
Cl_{cr} <10 mL/minute: Administer every 72-96 hours.
Intermittent hemodialysis (IHD): One-half the dose administered after hemodialysis on dialysis days. **Note:** Dosing dependent on the assumption of 3 times weekly complete IHD sessions.
Peritoneal dialysis (PD): Administration via PD fluid: 20-40 mg/L (20-40 mcg/mL) of PD fluid
Continuous renal replacement therapy (CRRT): Administer every 24-72 hours; monitor levels. **Note:** Drug clearance is highly dependent on the method of renal replacement, filter type, and flow rate. Appropriate dosing requires close monitoring of pharmacologic response, signs of adverse reactions due to drug accumulation, as well as drug concentrations in relation to target trough (if appropriate).

Dosage adjustment in hepatic impairment: No dosage adjustment provided in manufacturer's labeling.

Administration Inject deep I.M. into large muscle mass; midlateral thigh muscle (preferred site for children); midlateral thigh muscle or upper buttocks (adults); alternate injection site areas. I.V. administration is not recommended; has been administered intravenously over 30-60 minutes.

Monitoring Parameters Hearing (audiogram), BUN, creatinine; serum concentration of the drug should be monitored in all patients; eighth cranial nerve damage is usually preceded by high-pitched tinnitus, roaring noises, sense of fullness in ears, or impaired hearing and may persist for weeks after drug is discontinued

Reference Range Therapeutic: Peak: 20-30 mcg/mL; Trough: <5 mcg/mL; Toxic: Peak: >50 mcg/mL; Trough: >10 mcg/mL

Dosage Forms Excipient information presented when available (limited, particularly for generics); consult specific product labeling.
Solution Reconstituted, Intramuscular:
Generic: 1 g (1 ea)

- **Streptomycin for Injection (Can)** *see* Streptomycin *on page 1951*
- **Streptomycin Sulfate** *see* Streptomycin *on page 1951*
- **Striant** *see* Testosterone *on page 2026*
- **Stribild** *see* Elvitegravir, Cobicistat, Emtricitabine, and Tenofovir *on page 696*
- **Stromectol** *see* Ivermectin (Systemic) *on page 1137*
- **Strong Iodine Solution** *see* Potassium Iodide and Iodine *on page 1689*
- **SU011248** *see* SUNItinib *on page 1973*
- **Suberoylanilide Hydroxamic Acid** *see* Vorinostat *on page 2207*
- **Sublinox (Can)** *see* Zolpidem *on page 2242*
- **Suboxone** *see* Buprenorphine and Naloxone *on page 295*
- **Subsys** *see* FentaNYL *on page 842*

Succimer (SUKS si mer)

Brand Names: U.S. Chemet
Brand Names: Canada Chemet
Index Terms DMSA
Pharmacologic Category Antidote
Use Treatment of lead poisoning in children with serum lead levels >45 mcg/dL
Unlabeled Use Treatment of lead poisoning in symptomatic adults
Pregnancy Risk Factor C
Pregnancy Considerations Adverse events were observed in animal reproduction studies.

Lead poisoning: Lead is known to cross the placenta in amounts related to maternal plasma levels. Prenatal lead exposure may be associated with adverse events such as spontaneous abortion, preterm delivery, decreased birth weight, and impaired neurodevelopment. Some adverse outcomes may occur with maternal blood lead levels <10 mcg/dL. In addition, pregnant women exposed to lead may have an increased risk of gestational hypertension. Consider chelation therapy in pregnant women with confirmed blood lead levels ≥45 mcg/dL (pregnant women with blood lead levels ≥70 mcg/dL should be considered for chelation regardless of trimester); consultation with experts in lead poisoning and high-risk pregnancy is recommended. Encephalopathic pregnant women should be chelated regardless of trimester (CDC, 2010).

Breast-Feeding Considerations It is not known if succimer is excreted in breast milk. When used for the treatment of lead poisoning, the amount of lead in breast milk may range from 0.6% to 3% of the maternal serum concentration. Women with confirmed blood lead levels ≥40 mcg/dL should not initiate breast-feeding; pumping and discarding breast milk is recommended until blood lead levels are <40 mcg/dL, at which point breast-feeding may resume (CDC, 2010). Calcium supplementation may reduce the amount of lead in breast milk.

Contraindications Hypersensitivity to succimer or any component of the formulation

Warnings/Precautions Investigate, identify, and remove sources of lead exposure prior to treatment; do not permit patients to re-enter the contaminated environment until lead abatement has been completed. Primary care providers should consult experts in chemotherapy of heavy metal toxicity before using chelation drug therapy. Succimer is not used to prevent lead poisoning. A rebound rise in serum lead levels may occur after treatment as lead is released from storage sites into blood. The severity of rebound may guide the frequency of future monitoring and the need for additional chelation therapy. Succimer does not cross blood-brain barrier and should not be used to treat encephalopathy associated with lead toxicity. Adequate hydration should be maintained during therapy.

Transient elevations in serum transaminases have been reported. Evaluate serum transaminases at baseline and weekly during treatment; more frequent monitoring may be required in patients with a history of liver disease. Use with caution in patients with renal impairment. Succimer is dialyzable; however, the lead chelates are not. Mild-to-moderate neutropenia has been reported; evaluate CBC with differential at baseline, weekly during treatment, and immediately upon the development of any sign of infection. The manufacturer recommends withholding treatment for ANC <1200/mm^3; treatment may be cautiously resumed when ANC returns to baseline or >1500/mm^3. Consultation with a medical toxicologist to determine the risk versus benefit of withholding treatment is recommended. Monitor for the development of allergic or other mucocutaneous reactions. A reversible mucocutaneous vesicular eruption of the oral mucosa, external urethral meatus, or perianal area has been reported (rarely).

Adverse Reactions

>10%: Gastrointestinal: Appetite decreased, diarrhea, hemorrhoid symptoms, metallic taste, loose stools, nausea, vomiting

1% to 10%:

Cardiovascular: Arrhythmia (adults 2%)

Central nervous system: Chills, dizziness, drowsiness, fatigue, fever, headache, sleepiness

Dermatologic: Rash (including papular rash, herpetic rash and mucocutaneous eruptions); pruritus

Endocrine & metabolic: Cholesterol increased

Gastrointestinal: Abdominal cramps, mucosal irritation, sore throat

Genitourinary: Proteinuria (adults), urine output decreased (adults), voiding difficulty (adults)

Hematologic & oncologic: Eosinophilia, increased platelet count

Hepatic: Alkaline phosphatase increased, ALT increased, AST increased

Infection: Common cold

Neuromuscular & skeletal: Back pain, flank pain, knee pain (adults), leg pain (adults), neuropathy, paresthesia, rib pain

Ocular: Cloudy film in eye, watery eyes

Otic: Otitis media, plugged ears

Respiratory: Cough, nasal congestion, rhinorrhea

Miscellaneous: Flu-like syndrome, moniliasis

<1% (Limited to important or life-threatening): Allergic reactions (especially with retreatment), neutropenia (causal relationship not established)

Drug Interactions

Metabolism/Transport Effects None known.

Avoid Concomitant Use There are no known interactions where it is recommended to avoid concomitant use.

Increased Effect/Toxicity There are no known significant interactions involving an increase in effect.

Decreased Effect There are no known significant interactions involving a decrease in effect.

Storage/Stability Store between 15°C to 25°C (59°F to 77°F); avoid excessive heat.

Mechanism of Action Succimer is an analog of dimercaprol. It forms water soluble chelates with heavy metals which are subsequently excreted renally. Succimer binds heavy metals; however, the chemical form of these chelates is not known.

Pharmacodynamics/Kinetics

Absorption: Rapid but incomplete

Distribution: Primarily extracellular (Aposhian, 1992)

Protein binding: >95% primarily to albumin (Aposhian, 1992)

Metabolism: Rapidly and extensively to mixed succimer cysteine disulfides

Half-life elimination: ~3 hours (Aposhian, 1992)

Time to peak, serum: ~1-2 hours

Excretion: Urine (~25%) with peak urinary excretion between 2-4 hours (90% as mixed succimer-cysteine disulfide conjugates, 10% as unchanged drug); feces (as unabsorbed drug)

Dosage Lead poisoning: **Note:** For the treatment of high blood lead levels in children, the CDC recommends chelation treatment when blood lead levels are >45 mcg/dL (CDC, 2002). Children with blood lead levels >70 mcg/dL or symptomatic lead poisoning should be treated with parenteral agents (AAP, 2005). In adults, available guidelines recommend chelation therapy with blood lead levels >50 mcg/dL and significant symptoms; chelation therapy may also be indicated with blood lead levels ≥100 mcg/dL and/or symptoms. (Kosnett, 2007).

Children: Oral: 10 mg/kg/dose (or 350 mg/m^2/dose) every 8 hours for 5 days followed by 10 mg/kg/dose (or 350 mg/m^2/dose) every 12 hours for 14 days. Maximum: 500 mg/dose.

Adults (unlabeled use; Kosnett, 2007): Oral: Consider using labeled dose for children: 10 mg/kg/dose (or 350 mg/m^2/dose) every 8 hours for 5 days, followed by 10 mg/kg/dose (or 350 mg/m^2/dose) every 12 hours for 14 days; Maximum: 500 mg/dose

Note: Treatment courses may be repeated, but 2-week intervals between courses is generally recommended.

Dosage adjustment for toxicity: ANC <1200 mm^3: The manufacturer recommends withholding treatment; treatment may be cautiously resumed when ANC returns to baseline or >1500/mm^3. Consultation with a medical toxicologist to determine the risk versus benefit of withholding treatment is recommended.

Dosage adjustment in renal impairment: No dosage adjustment provided in the manufacturer's labeling; use with caution. Succimer is dialyzable; however, the lead chelates are not.

Dosage adjustment in hepatic impairment: No dosage adjustment provided in the manufacturer's labeling; has not been studied. More frequent monitoring of serum transaminases may be required in patients with a history of liver disease due to the risk of transient increases.

Administration If unable to swallow whole, capsule may be separated and contents sprinkled on a small amount of soft food, or the contents placed on a spoon and administered followed by fruit drink.

Monitoring Parameters Blood lead levels (baseline and 7-21 days after completing chelation therapy); serum aminotransferase (baseline and weekly during treatment; may require more frequent monitoring in patients with a history of liver disease), CBC with differential and platelets (baseline, and weekly during treatment); hemoglobin or hematocrit, iron status, free erythrocyte protoporphyrin or zinc protoporphyrin; neurodevelopmental changes

Test Interactions False-positive ketones (U) using nitroprusside methods, falsely decreased serum CPK; falsely decreased uric acid measurement

Dosage Forms Excipient information presented when available (limited, particularly for generics); consult specific product labeling.

Capsule, Oral:

Chemet: 100 mg

Succinylcholine (suks in il KOE leen)

Brand Names: U.S. Anectine; Quelicin; Quelicin-1000

Brand Names: Canada Quelicin®

Index Terms Succinylcholine Chloride; Suxamethonium Chloride

Pharmacologic Category Neuromuscular Blocker Agent, Depolarizing

Additional Appendix Information

Dosing Considerations for the Critically-Ill Patient With Morbid Obesity *on page 2379*

Use To facilitate both rapid sequence and routine endotracheal intubation and to relax skeletal muscles during surgery

Note: Does not relieve pain or produce sedation

Unlabeled Use To reduce the intensity of muscle contractions of electroconvulsive therapy (ECT)

Pregnancy Risk Factor C

Pregnancy Considerations Reproduction studies have not been conducted. Small amounts cross the placenta. Sensitivity to succinylcholine may be increased due to a ~24% decrease in plasma cholinesterase activity during pregnancy and several days postpartum.

Breast-Feeding Considerations It is not known if succinylcholine is excreted in breast milk. The manufacturer recommends that caution be exercised when administering succinylcholine to nursing women.

Contraindications Hypersensitivity to succinylcholine or any component of the formulation; personal or familial history of malignant hyperthermia; myopathies associated with elevated serum creatine phosphokinase (CPK) values; acute phase of injury following major burns, multiple trauma, extensive denervation of skeletal muscle or upper motor neuron injury

Warnings/Precautions [U.S. Boxed Warning]: Use caution in children and adolescents. Acute rhabdomyolysis with hyperkalemia, ventricular arrhythmias and cardiac arrest have been reported (rarely) in children with undiagnosed skeletal muscle myopathy. Use in children should be reserved for emergency intubation or where immediate airway control is necessary. Use with caution in patients with pre-existing hyperkalemia, extensive or severe burns; severe hyperkalemia may develop in patients with chronic abdominal infections, burn injuries, children with skeletal muscle myopathy, subarachnoid hemorrhage, or conditions which cause degeneration of the nervous system. Alkalosis, hypercalcemia, demyelinating lesions, peripheral neuropathies, denervation, infection, muscle trauma, and diabetes mellitus may result in antagonism of neuromuscular blockade. Electrolyte abnormalities, severe hyponatremia, severe hypocalcemia, severe hypokalemia, hypermagnesemia, neuromuscular diseases, acidosis, acute intermittent porphyria, Eaton-Lambert syndrome, myasthenia gravis, renal failure, and hepatic failure may result in potentiation of neuromuscular blockade. May increase vagal tone.

Succinylcholine is metabolized by plasma cholinesterase; use with caution (if at all) in patients suspected of being homozygous for the atypical plasma cholinesterase gene.

Use with caution in patients with extensive or severe burns; risk of hyperkalemia is increased following injury. May increase intraocular pressure; use caution with narrow angle glaucoma or penetrating eye injuries. Risk of bradycardia may be increased with second dose and may occur more in children. Use may be associated with acute onset of malignant hyperthermia; risk may be increased with concomitant administration of volatile anesthetics. Use with caution in the elderly; effects and duration are more variable.

Maintenance of an adequate airway and respiratory support is critical. Should be administered by adequately trained individuals familiar with its use.

Adverse Reactions

Frequency not defined.

Cardiovascular: Arrhythmias, bradycardia (higher with second dose, more frequent in children), cardiac arrest, hyper-/hypotension, tachycardia

Dermatologic: Rash

Endocrine & metabolic: Hyperkalemia

Gastrointestinal: Salivation (excessive)

Neuromuscular & skeletal: Jaw rigidity, muscle fasciculation, postoperative muscle pain, rhabdomyolysis (with possible myoglobinuric acute renal failure)

Ocular: Intraocular pressure increased

Renal: Acute renal failure (secondary to rhabdomyolysis)

Respiratory: Apnea, respiratory depression (prolonged)

Miscellaneous: Anaphylaxis, malignant hyperthermia

Postmarketing and/or case reports: Acute quadriplegic myopathy syndrome (prolonged use), myositis ossificans (prolonged use)

Drug Interactions

Metabolism/Transport Effects None known.

Avoid Concomitant Use

Avoid concomitant use of Succinylcholine with any of the following: QuiNINE

Increased Effect/Toxicity

Succinylcholine may increase the levels/effects of: Analgesics (Opioid); Cardiac Glycosides; OnabotulinumtoxinA; RimabotulinumtoxinB

The levels/effects of Succinylcholine may be increased by: AbobotulinumtoxinA; Acetylcholinesterase Inhibitors; Aminoglycosides; Capreomycin; Colistimethate; Cyclophosphamide; CycloSPORINE (Systemic); Echothiophate Iodide; Lincosamide Antibiotics; Lithium; Loop Diuretics; Magnesium Salts; Phenelzine; Polymyxin B; Procainamide; QuiNIDine; QuiNINE; Tetracycline Derivatives; Vancomycin

Decreased Effect

The levels/effects of Succinylcholine may be decreased by: Loop Diuretics

Preparation for Administration May dilute to a final concentration of 1-2 mg/mL. Do not mix with alkaline solutions (pH >8.5).

Storage/Stability Manufacturer recommends refrigeration at 2°C to 8°C (36°F to 46°F) and may be stored at room temperature for 14 days; however, additional testing has demonstrated stability for ≤6 months unrefrigerated (25°C) (Ross, 1988; Roy, 2008). Stability in polypropylene syringes (20 mg/mL) at room temperature (25°C) is 45 days (Storms, 2003). Stability of parenteral admixture

(1-2 mg/mL) at refrigeration temperature (4°C) is 24 hours in D_5W or NS.

Mechanism of Action Acts similar to acetylcholine, produces depolarization of the motor endplate at the myoneural junction which causes sustained flaccid skeletal muscle paralysis produced by state of accommodation that develops in adjacent excitable muscle membranes

Pharmacodynamics/Kinetics

Onset of action: I.M.: 2-3 minutes; I.V.: Complete muscular relaxation: 30-60 seconds

Duration: I.M.: 10-30 minutes; I.V.: 4-6 minutes with single administration

Metabolism: Rapidly hydrolyzed by plasma pseudocholinesterase

Excretion: Urine

Dosage I.M., I.V.: Dose to effect; doses will vary due to interpatient variability. Use carefully and/or consider dose reduction in patients with reduced plasma cholinesterase activity due to genetic abnormalities of plasma cholinesterase or when associated with other conditions (eg, pregnancy, severe liver disease, renal disease); prolonged neuromuscular blockade may occur.

I.M.: Children and Adults: Up to 3-4 mg/kg, total dose should not exceed 150 mg

I.V.:

Smaller Children: Intermittent: Initial: 2 mg/kg/dose; maintenance: 0.3-0.6 mg/kg/dose every 5-10 minutes as needed

Older Children and Adolescents: Intermittent: Initial: 1 mg/kg/dose; maintenance: 0.3-0.6 mg/kg every 5-10 minutes as needed

Adults:

Intubation: 0.6 mg/kg (range: 0.3-1.1 mg/kg)

Rapid sequence intubation: 1-1.5 mg/kg (Sluga, 2005; Weiss, 1997)

Note: Initial dose of succinylcholine must be increased when nondepolarizing agent pretreatment used because of the antagonism between succinylcholine and nondepolarizing neuromuscular-blocking agents.

Dosing adjustment in renal impairment: No dosage adjustment provided in manufacturer's labeling.

Dosing adjustment in hepatic impairment: No dosage adjustment provided in manufacturer's labeling.

Dosing in obesity: Use total body weight for obese patients (Bentley, 1982; Brunette, 2004; Rose, 2000).

Administration May be administered by rapid I.V. injection without further dilution. I.M. injections should be made deeply, preferably high into deltoid muscle; use only when I.V. access is not available.

Monitoring Parameters Monitor cardiac, blood pressure, and oxygenation during administration; temperature, serum potassium and calcium, assisted ventilator status; neuromuscular function with a peripheral nerve stimulator

Dosage Forms Excipient information presented when available (limited, particularly for generics); consult specific product labeling.

Solution, Injection, as chloride:

Anectine: 20 mg/mL (10 mL) [contains methylparaben]

Quelicin: 20 mg/mL (10 mL) [contains methylparaben, propylparaben]

Quelicin-1000: 100 mg/mL (10 mL)

- **Succinylcholine Chloride** *see* Succinylcholine *on page 1954*
- **Suclear™** *see* Sodium Sulfate, Potassium Sulfate, Magnesium Sulfate, and Polyethylene Glycol-Electrolyte Solution *on page 1929*
- **Sucraid** *see* Sacrosidase *on page 1870*
- **Sucraid® (Can)** *see* Sacrosidase *on page 1870*

Sucralfate (soo KRAL fate)

Brand Names: U.S. Carafate

Brand Names: Canada Apo-Sucralfate; Dom-Sucralfate; Novo-Sucralate; Nu-Sucralate; PMS-Sucralate; Sucralfate-1; Sulcrate®; Sulcrate® Suspension Plus; Teva-Sucralfate

Index Terms Aluminum Sucrose Sulfate, Basic

Pharmacologic Category Gastrointestinal Agent, Miscellaneous

Use Short-term (≤8 weeks) management of duodenal ulcers; maintenance therapy for duodenal ulcers

Pregnancy Risk Factor B

Dosage Oral:

Children (unlabeled use): Doses of 40-80 mg/kg/day divided every 6 hours have been used

Adults: Duodenal ulcer:

Treatment: 1 g 4 times daily on an empty stomach for 4-8 weeks

Maintenance: Prophylaxis: 1 g twice daily

Dosage adjustment in renal impairment: No dosage adjustment provided in manufacturer's labeling. Aluminum salt is minimally absorbed; however, may accumulate in renal impairment; use with caution in patients with chronic renal failure.

Dosage adjustment in hepatic impairment: No dosage adjustment provided in manufacturer's labeling.

Additional Information Complete prescribing information should be consulted for additional detail.

Dosage Forms Excipient information presented when available (limited, particularly for generics); consult specific product labeling.

Suspension, Oral:

Carafate: 1 g/10 mL (420 mL) [contains fd&c red #40, methylparaben; cherry flavor]

Tablet, Oral:

Carafate: 1 g [scored; contains fd&c blue #1 aluminum lake]

Generic: 1 g

- **Sucralfate-1 (Can)** *see* Sucralfate *on page 1955*
- **Sucrets® Children's [OTC]** *see* Dyclonine *on page 681*
- **Sucrets® Maximum Strength [OTC]** *see* Dyclonine *on page 681*
- **Sucrets® Regular Strength [OTC]** *see* Dyclonine *on page 681*
- **Sudafed** *see* Pseudoephedrine *on page 1746*
- **Sudafed [OTC]** *see* Pseudoephedrine *on page 1746*
- **Sudafed 12 Hour [OTC]** *see* Pseudoephedrine *on page 1746*
- **Sudafed 24 Hour [OTC]** *see* Pseudoephedrine *on page 1746*
- **Sudafed Childrens [OTC]** *see* Pseudoephedrine *on page 1746*
- **Sudafed® Children's Cold & Cough [OTC]** *see* Pseudoephedrine and Dextromethorphan *on page 1748*
- **Sudafed® Decongestant (Can)** *see* Pseudoephedrine *on page 1746*
- **Sudafed® Head Cold and Sinus Extra Strength (Can)** *see* Acetaminophen and Pseudoephedrine *on page 33*
- **Sudafed PE Childrens [OTC]** *see* Phenylephrine (Systemic) *on page 1636*
- **Sudafed PE® Children's Cold & Cough [OTC]** *see* Dextromethorphan and Phenylephrine *on page 591*
- **Sudafed PE Maximum Strength [OTC]** *see* Phenylephrine (Systemic) *on page 1636*
- **Sudafed PE® Non-Drying Sinus [OTC]** *see* Guaifenesin and Phenylephrine *on page 978*

◆ **Sudafed PE® Sinus + Allergy [OTC]** *see* Chlorpheniramine and Phenylephrine *on page 412*

◆ **Sudafed® Sinus Advance (Can)** *see* Pseudoephedrine and Ibuprofen *on page 1748*

◆ **Sudanyl [OTC]** *see* Pseudoephedrine *on page 1746*

◆ **SudoGest [OTC]** *see* Pseudoephedrine *on page 1746*

◆ **SudoGest 12 Hour [OTC]** *see* Pseudoephedrine *on page 1746*

◆ **Sudogest PE [OTC]** *see* Phenylephrine (Systemic) *on page 1636*

◆ **SudoGest™ Sinus & Allergy [OTC]** *see* Chlorpheniramine and Pseudoephedrine *on page 412*

◆ **Sufenta** *see* SUFentanil *on page 1956*

◆ **Sufenta® (Can)** *see* SUFentanil *on page 1956*

SUFentanil (soo FEN ta nil)

Brand Names: U.S. Sufenta

Brand Names: Canada Sufentanil Citrate Injection, USP; Sufenta®

Index Terms Sufentanil Citrate

Pharmacologic Category Analgesic, Opioid; Anilidopiperidine Opioid; General Anesthetic

Additional Appendix Information

Dosing Considerations for the Critically-Ill Patient With Morbid Obesity *on page 2379*

Use Analgesic supplement in maintenance of general anesthesia; epidural analgesic in conjunction with a local anesthetic

Pregnancy Risk Factor C

Dosage

I.V.:

Children 2-12 years: Induction: 10-25 mcg/kg (10-15 mcg/kg most common dose) with 100% O_2; Maintenance: Up to 1-2 mcg/kg total dose

Adults: Surgical analgesia (surgery 1-2 hours long): Total dose: 1-2 mcg/kg; ≥75% of dose administered prior to intubation; administered with N_2O/O_2; Maintenance: 5-20 mcg as needed. Total dose should not exceed 1 mcg/kg/hour of expected surgical time.

Epidural: Adults: Analgesia: Labor and delivery: 10-15 mcg with 10 mL bupivacaine 0.125% with/without epinephrine. May repeat at ≥1-hour interval for 2 additional doses.

Dosage adjustment in renal impairment: No dosage adjustment provided in manufacturer's labeling. Use with caution.

Dosage adjustment in hepatic impairment: No dosage adjustment provided in manufacturer's labeling. Use with caution.

Dosing in obesity: I.V.: In adult obese patients (eg, >20% above ideal body weight), use lean body weight to determine dosage.

Additional Information Complete prescribing information should be consulted for additional detail.

Dosage Forms Excipient information presented when available (limited, particularly for generics); consult specific product labeling.

Solution, Intravenous [preservative free]:

Sufenta: 50 mcg/mL (1 mL); 100 mcg/2 mL (2 mL); 250 mcg/5 mL (5 mL)

Generic: 50 mcg/mL (1 mL); 100 mcg/2 mL (2 mL); 250 mcg/5 mL (5 mL)

Controlled Substance C-II

◆ **Sufentanil Citrate** *see* SUFentanil *on page 1956*

◆ **Sufentanil Citrate Injection, USP (Can)** *see* SUFentanil *on page 1956*

◆ **Sulamyd** *see* Sulfacetamide (Ophthalmic) *on page 1956*

◆ **Sulamyd** *see* Sulfacetamide (Topical) *on page 1957*

◆ **Sular** *see* Nisoldipine *on page 1461*

◆ **Sulbactam and Ampicillin** *see* Ampicillin and Sulbactam *on page 133*

Sulconazole (sul KON a zole)

Brand Names: U.S. Exelderm

Brand Names: Canada Exelderm®

Index Terms Sulconazole Nitrate

Pharmacologic Category Antifungal Agent, Topical

Use Treatment of superficial fungal infections of the skin, including tinea cruris (jock itch), tinea corporis (ringworm), tinea versicolor, and tinea pedis (athlete's foot, cream only)

Pregnancy Risk Factor C

Dosage Adults: Topical: Apply a small amount to the affected area and gently massage once or twice daily (tinea pedis apply twice daily) for 3 weeks (tinea cruris, tinea corporis, tinea versicolor) to 4 weeks (tinea pedis).

Additional Information Complete prescribing information should be consulted for additional detail.

Dosage Forms Excipient information presented when available (limited, particularly for generics); consult specific product labeling.

Cream, External, as nitrate:

Exelderm: 1% (15 g, 30 g, 60 g) [contains cetyl alcohol, propylene glycol]

Solution, External, as nitrate:

Exelderm: 1% (30 mL) [contains propylene glycol]

◆ **Sulconazole Nitrate** *see* Sulconazole *on page 1956*

◆ **Sulcrate® (Can)** *see* Sucralfate *on page 1955*

◆ **Sulcrate® Suspension Plus (Can)** *see* Sucralfate *on page 1955*

Sulfacetamide (Ophthalmic) (sul fa SEE ta mide)

Brand Names: U.S. Bleph-10

Brand Names: Canada AK Sulf Liq; Bleph 10 DPS; Diosulf™; PMS-Sulfacetamide; Sodium Sulamyd

Index Terms Sodium Sulfacetamide; Sulamyd; Sulfacetamide Sodium

Pharmacologic Category Antibiotic, Ophthalmic

Use Treatment and prophylaxis of conjunctivitis and other superficial ocular infections due to susceptible organisms; adjunctive treatment with systemic sulfonamides for therapy of trachoma

Pregnancy Risk Factor C

Dosage Children >2 months and Adults: Ophthalmic:

Conjunctivitis:

Ointment: Instill 1/2" (1.25 cm) ribbon into the conjunctival sac of affected eye(s) every 3-4 hours and at bedtime; increase dosing interval as condition responds. Usual duration of treatment: 7-10 days.

Solution: Instill 1-2 drops several times daily up to every 2-3 hours in lower conjunctival sac during waking hours and less frequently at night; increase dosing interval as condition responds. Usual duration of treatment: 7-10 days

Trachoma: Solution: Instill 2 drops into the conjunctival sac every 2 hours; must be used in conjunction with systemic therapy

Additional Information Complete prescribing information should be consulted for additional detail.

Dosage Forms Excipient information presented when available (limited, particularly for generics); consult specific product labeling.

Ointment, Ophthalmic, as sodium:

Generic: 10% (3.5 g)

Solution, Ophthalmic, as sodium:

Bleph-10: 10% (5 mL)

Generic: 10% (15 mL)

Sulfacetamide (Topical) (sul fa SEE ta mide)

Brand Names: U.S. Klaron; Mexar Wash; Ovace Plus; Ovace Plus Wash; Ovace Wash; Seb-Prev; Seb-Prev Wash

Brand Names: Canada Sulfacet-R

Index Terms Sodium Sulfacetamide; Sulamyd; Sulfacetamide Sodium

Pharmacologic Category Acne Products; Antibiotic, Sulfonamide Derivative; Topical Skin Product, Acne

Use

Cleansing gel, wash: Scaling dermatoses (seborrheic dermatitis and seborrhea sicca [dandruff]); bacterial infections of the skin

Lotion: Acne vulgaris

Shampoo: Scaling dermatoses (seborrheic dermatitis and seborrhea sicca [dandruff])

Pregnancy Risk Factor C

Dosage Topical: Children ≥12 years and Adults:

Acne: Lotion: Apply thin film to affected area twice daily

Seborrheic dermatitis:

Cleansing gel, wash: Wash affected areas twice daily; repeat application for 8-10 days. Dosing interval may be increased as eruption subsides. Applications once or twice weekly, or every other week may be used for prevention. If treatment needs to be reinitiated, start therapy as a twice daily regimen.

Shampoo: Wash hair at least twice weekly

Secondary cutaneous bacterial infections: Cleansing gel, wash: Apply to affected areas daily; duration of therapy is usually for 8-10 days

Additional Information Complete prescribing information should be consulted for additional detail.

Dosage Forms Excipient information presented when available (limited, particularly for generics); consult specific product labeling.

Cream, External, as sodium:

Ovace Plus: 10% (57 g) [contains benzyl alcohol, butylparaben, cetyl alcohol, disodium edta, ethylparaben, methylparaben, propylparaben]

Gel, External, as sodium:

Ovace Plus Wash: 10% (355 mL) [contains cetearyl alcohol, edetate disodium dihydrate, methylparaben]

Generic: 10% (355 mL)

Liquid, External, as sodium:

Mexar Wash: 10% (170 mL) [contains methylparaben]

Ovace Plus Wash: 10% (180 mL, 473 mL) [contains cetearyl alcohol, edetate disodium, methylparaben]

Ovace Wash: 10% (180 mL, 355 mL) [contains edetate disodium, methylparaben]

Seb-Prev Wash: 10% (340 mL) [contains edetate disodium, methylparaben]

Generic: 10% (177 mL, 354.8 mL, 355 mL, 480 mL)

Lotion, External, as sodium:

Klaron: 10% (118 mL)

Klaron: 10% (118 mL) [contains disodium edta, methylparaben, propylene glycol, sodium metabisulfite]

Seb-Prev: 10% (118 mL) [contains methylparaben, sodium metabisulfite]

Generic: 10% (118 mL)

Pad, External, as sodium:

Generic: 10% (30 ea)

Shampoo, External, as sodium:

Ovace Plus: 10% (237 mL) [contains cetearyl alcohol, methylparaben, propylparaben]

Generic: 10% (237 mL)

Suspension, External, as sodium:

Generic: 10% (118 mL)

Sulfacetamide and Prednisolone

(sul fa SEE ta mide & pred NIS oh lone)

Brand Names: U.S. Blephamide®

Brand Names: Canada AK Cide Oph; Blephamide®; Dioptimyd®

Index Terms Prednisolone and Sulfacetamide

Pharmacologic Category Antibiotic/Corticosteroid, Ophthalmic

Use Steroid-responsive inflammatory ocular conditions in which a corticosteroid is indicated and where infection is present or there is a risk of infection

Pregnancy Risk Factor C

Dosage Ophthalmic:

Children ≥6 years and Adults:

Ointment: Apply ~1/2 inch ribbon to lower conjunctival sac 3-4 times/day and 1-2 times at night

Solution: Instill 2 drops every 4 hours

Suspension: Instill 2 drops every 4 hours during the day and at bedtime

Additional Information Complete prescribing information should be consulted for additional detail.

Dosage Forms Excipient information presented when available (limited, particularly for generics); consult specific product labeling.

Ointment, ophthalmic:

Blephamide®: Sulfacetamide sodium 10% and prednisolone acetate 0.2% (3.5 g)

Solution, ophthalmic [drops]: Sulfacetamide sodium 10% and prednisolone sodium phosphate 0.25% (5 mL, 10 mL)

Suspension, ophthalmic [drops]:

Blephamide®: Sulfacetamide sodium 10% and prednisolone acetate 0.2% (5 mL, 10 mL) [contains benzalkonium chloride]

◆ **Sulfacetamide and Sulfur** *see* Sulfur and Sulfacetamide *on page 1966*

◆ **Sulfacetamide Sodium** *see* Sulfacetamide (Ophthalmic) *on page 1956*

◆ **Sulfacetamide Sodium** *see* Sulfacetamide (Topical) *on page 1957*

◆ **Sulfacet-R (Can)** *see* Sulfacetamide (Topical) *on page 1957*

◆ **Sulfacet-R (Can)** *see* Sulfur and Sulfacetamide *on page 1966*

◆ **SulfaCleanse 8/4** *see* Sulfur and Sulfacetamide *on page 1966*

SulfADIAZINE (sul fa DYE a zeen)

Pharmacologic Category Antibiotic, Sulfonamide Derivative

Use Treatment of the following conditions (per product labeling): Chancroid, trachoma, inclusion conjunctivitis, nocardiosis, urinary tract infections, toxoplasmosis encephalitis, malaria, meningococcal meningitis, acute otitis media, rheumatic fever (prophylaxis), meningitis (adjunctive)

Refer to current guidelines for appropriate use.

Pregnancy Risk Factor C

Pregnancy Considerations Adverse events have been observed in animal reproduction studies. Sulfadiazine crosses the placenta (Speert, 1943). Available studies and case reports have failed to show an increased risk for congenital malformations after sulfadiazine use (Heinonen, 1977); however, studies with sulfonamides as a class have shown mixed results (ACOG, 2011).

Sulfadiazine is recommended for use in pregnant women to prevent *T. gondii* infection of the fetus, for the maternal treatment of *Toxoplasmic gondii* encephalitis, and as an alternative agent for the secondary prevention of rheumatic fever (CDC, 2009; DHHS, 2013; Gerber, 2009). Sulfonamides may be used to treat other infections in pregnant women when clinically appropriate for confirmed infections caused by susceptible organisms; use during the first trimester should be limited to situations where no alternative therapies are available (ACOG, 2011). Because safer options are available for the treatment of urinary tract infections in pregnant women, use of sulfonamide-containing products >32 weeks gestation should be avoided (Lee, 2008). Due to the theoretical increased risk for hyperbilirubinemia and kernicterus, sulfadiazine is contraindicated by the manufacturer for use near term. Neonatal healthcare providers should be informed if maternal sulfonamide therapy is used near the time of delivery (DHHS, 2013).

Breast-Feeding Considerations Sulfadiazine distributes into human milk. Sulfonamides should not be used while nursing an infant with G6PD deficiency or hyperbilirubinemia (Della-Giustina, 2003). Per the manufacturer, sulfadiazine is contraindicated in nursing mothers since sulfonamides cross into the milk and may cause kernicterus in the newborn. Nondose-related effects could include modification of bowel flora.

Contraindications Hypersensitivity to any sulfa drug or any component of the formulation; children <2 months of age unless indicated for the treatment of congenital toxoplasmosis; pregnancy (at term); breast-feeding

Warnings/Precautions Fatalities associated with severe reactions including agranulocytosis, aplastic anemia and other blood dyscrasias, hepatic necrosis, Stevens-Johnson syndrome, and toxic epidermal necrolysis have occurred; discontinue use at first sign of rash or signs of serious adverse reactions. Use with caution in patients with allergies or asthma.

Chemical similarities are present among sulfonamides, sulfonylureas, carbonic anhydrase inhibitors, thiazides, and loop diuretics (except ethacrynic acid). Use in patients with sulfonamide allergy is specifically contraindicated in product labeling; however, a risk of cross-reaction exists in patients with allergy to any of these compounds; avoid use when previous reaction has been severe.

Prolonged use may result in fungal or bacterial superinfection, including *C. difficile*-associated diarrhea (CDAD) and pseudomembranous colitis; CDAD has been observed >2 months postantibiotic treatment. Use with caution in patients with G6PD deficiency; hemolysis may occur. Use with caution in patients with hepatic impairment. Use with caution in patients with renal impairment; dosage modification required. Maintain adequate hydration to prevent crystalluria. Not for the treatment of group A beta-hemolytic streptococcal infections.

Adverse Reactions Frequency not defined.

Cardiovascular: Allergic myocarditis, periarteritis nodosa

Central nervous system: Ataxia, chills, convulsions, depression, fever, hallucinations, headache, insomnia, vertigo

Dermatologic: Epidermal necrolysis, erythema multiforme, exfoliative dermatitis, photosensitivity, pruritus, purpura, rash, skin eruptions, Stevens-Johnson syndrome, urticaria

Endocrine & metabolic: Hypoglycemia, thyroid function disturbance

Gastrointestinal: Abdominal pain, anorexia, diarrhea, nausea, pancreatitis, stomatitis, vomiting

Genitourinary: Crystalluria, stone formation, toxic nephrosis with oliguria and anuria

Hematologic: Agranulocytopenia, aplastic anemia, hemolytic anemia, hypoprothrombinemia, leukopenia, methemoglobinemia, thrombocytopenia

Hepatic: Hepatitis

Neuromuscular & skeletal: Arthralgia, peripheral neuritis

Ocular: Conjunctival/scleral injection, periorbital edema

Otic: Tinnitus

Renal: Diuresis

Miscellaneous: Anaphylactoid reactions, lupus erythematosus, serum sickness-like reactions

Drug Interactions

Metabolism/Transport Effects **Substrate** of CYP2C9 (major), CYP2E1 (minor), CYP3A4 (minor); **Note:** Assignment of Major/Minor substrate status based on clinically relevant drug interaction potential; **Inhibits** CYP2C9 (strong)

Avoid Concomitant Use

Avoid concomitant use of SulfADIAZINE with any of the following: BCG; Methenamine; Potassium P-Aminobenzoate; Procaine

Increased Effect/Toxicity

SulfADIAZINE may increase the levels/effects of: Bosentan; Carvedilol; CycloSPORINE (Systemic); CYP2C9 Substrates; Diclofenac (Systemic); Lacosamide; Methotrexate; Ospemifene; Porfimer; Prilocaine; Sodium Nitrite; Sulfonylureas; Vitamin K Antagonists

The levels/effects of SulfADIAZINE may be increased by: CYP2C9 Inhibitors (Moderate); CYP2C9 Inhibitors (Strong); Methenamine; Mifepristone; Nitric Oxide

Decreased Effect

SulfADIAZINE may decrease the levels/effects of: BCG; CycloSPORINE (Systemic); Sodium Picosulfate; Typhoid Vaccine

The levels/effects of SulfADIAZINE may be decreased by: CYP2C9 Inducers (Strong); Dabrafenib; Peginterferon Alfa-2b; Potassium P-Aminobenzoate; Procaine

Ethanol/Nutrition/Herb Interactions

Food: Avoid large quantities of vitamin C or acidifying agents (cranberry juice) to prevent crystalluria.

Herb/Nutraceutical: Avoid dong quai, St John's wort (may also cause photosensitization).

Storage/Stability Store at controlled room temperature of 20°C to 25°C (68°F to 77°F). Protect from light.

Mechanism of Action Interferes with bacterial growth by inhibiting bacterial folic acid synthesis through competitive antagonism of PABA

Pharmacodynamics/Kinetics

Absorption: Well absorbed

Distribution: Throughout body tissues and fluids including pleural, peritoneal, synovial, and ocular fluids; throughout total body water; readily diffused into CSF

Protein binding: 38% to 48%

Metabolism: Via N-acetylation

Half-life elimination: 10 hours

Time to peak: Within 3-6 hours

Excretion: Urine (43% to 60% as unchanged drug, 15% to 40% as metabolites)

Dosage Oral:

General dosing guidelines:

Children >2 months of age: Initial: 75 mg/kg; Maintenance: 150 mg/kg/day in 4-6 divided doses (maximum: 6 g/24 hours)

Adults: 2-4 g/day in 3-6 divided doses

Rheumatic fever prophylaxis: Children and Adults:

<30 kg: 0.5 g/day

≥30 kg: 1 g/day

Toxoplasmosis (HIV-exposed/-positive patients) (CDC, 2009):

Congenital toxoplasmosis: Infants: 100 mg/kg/day in divided doses every 12 hours for 12 months in combination with pyrimethamine plus leucovorin calcium

Acquired toxoplasmosis: Infants and Children:

Acute induction therapy: 25-50 mg/kg/dose given 4 times/day (maximum: 1-1.5 g/dose) in combination with pyrimethamine and leucovorin calcium. Continue acute induction therapy for ≥6 weeks, then follow with chronic suppressive therapy.

Prophylaxis to prevent recurrence (prior to encephalitis): 85-120 mg/kg/day divided every 6-12 hours (maximum: 2-4 g/day) in combination with pyrimethamine plus leucovorin calcium

Toxoplasma gondii encephalitis: Adolescents and Adults:

Acute therapy (duration of therapy: ≥6 weeks): 1000 mg (<60 kg) or 1500 mg (≥60 kg) every 6 hours in combination with pyrimethamine plus leucovorin calcium (preferred) **or** alternatively, may give 1000-1500 mg every 6 hours in combination with atovaquone

Prophylaxis to prevent recurrence: 2000-4000 mg/day in 2-4 divided doses in combination with pyrimethamine and leucovorin calcium (preferred) **or** alternatively, may give 2000-4000 mg/day in 2-4 divided doses in combination with atovaquone

Dietary Considerations Supplemental leucovorin calcium should be administered to reverse symptoms or prevent problems due to folic acid deficiency.

Administration Administer with at least 8 ounces of water and around-the-clock to promote less variation in peak and trough serum levels. Oral sodium bicarbonate may be used to alkalinize the urine of patients unable to maintain adequate fluid intake (in order to prevent crystalluria, azotemia, oliguria) (Lerner, 1996).

Monitoring Parameters Perform culture and sensitivity testing prior to initiating therapy; frequent CBC and urinalysis during therapy; signs of serious blood disorders (sore throat, fever, pallor, purpura, jaundice); CD4+ count in HIV-exposed/-positive patients treated for toxoplasmosis; sulfonamide blood concentrations may be monitored for severe infections (target: 12-15 mg/100 mL)

Dosage Forms Excipient information presented when available (limited, particularly for generics); consult specific product labeling.

Tablet, Oral:

Generic: 500 mg

Extemporaneous Preparations A 200 mg/mL oral suspension may be made with sulfadiazine powder and sterile water. Place 50 g sulfadiazine powder in a glass mortar. Add small portions of sterile water and mix to a uniform paste; mix while incrementally adding sterile water to **almost** 250 mL; transfer to a calibrated bottle, rinse mortar with sterile water, and add sufficient quantity of sterile water to make 250 mL. Label "shake well" and "refrigerate". Stable for 3 days refrigerated. **Note:** Suspension may also be prepared by crushing one-hundred 500 mg tablets; however, it is stable for only 2 days.

Pathmanathan U, Halgrain D, Chiadmi F, et al, "Stability of Sulfadiazine Oral Liquids Prepared From Tablets and Powder," *J Pharm Pharm Sci*, 2004, 7(1):84-7.

Sulfadoxine and Pyrimethamine

(sul fa DOKS een & peer i METH a meen)

Brand Names: U.S. Fansidar® [DSC]

Index Terms Pyrimethamine and Sulfadoxine

Pharmacologic Category Antimalarial Agent

Use Treatment of *Plasmodium falciparum* malaria in patients in whom chloroquine resistance is suspected; malaria prophylaxis for travelers to areas where chloroquine-resistant malaria is endemic

Pregnancy Risk Factor C

Dosage Children and Adults: Oral:

Treatment of acute attack of malaria: A single dose of the following number of Fansidar® tablets is used in sequence with quinine or alone:

- 2-11 months: 1/4 tablet
- 1-3 years: 1/2 tablet
- 4-8 years: 1 tablet
- 9-14 years: 2 tablets
- >14 years: 3 tablets

Malaria prophylaxis: A single dose should be carried for self-treatment in the event of febrile illness when medical attention is not immediately available:

- 2-11 months: 1/4 tablet
- 1-3 years: 1/2 tablet
- 4-8 years: 1 tablet
- 9-14 years: 2 tablets
- >14 years and Adults: 3 tablets

Additional Information Complete prescribing information should be consulted for additional detail.

Dosage Forms Excipient information presented when available (limited, particularly for generics); consult specific product labeling. [DSC] = Discontinued product

Tablet:

Fansidar®: Sulfadoxine 500 mg and pyrimethamine 25 mg [DSC]

Sulfamethoxazole and Trimethoprim

(sul fa meth OKS a zole & trye METH oh prim)

Brand Names: U.S. Bactrim; Bactrim DS; Septra DS; Sulfatrim

Brand Names: Canada Apo-Sulfatrim; Apo-Sulfatrim DS; Apo-Sulfatrim Pediatric; Novo-Trimel; Novo-Trimel D.S.; Nu-Cotrimox; Septra Injection

Index Terms Co-Trimoxazole; Septra; SMX-TMP; SMZ-TMP; Sulfatrim; TMP-SMX; TMP-SMZ; Trimethoprim and Sulfamethoxazole

Pharmacologic Category Antibiotic, Miscellaneous; Antibiotic, Sulfonamide Derivative

Additional Appendix Information

Desensitization Protocols *on page 2325*

Use

Oral: Treatment of urinary tract infections due to *E. coli, Klebsiella* and *Enterobacter* sp, *M. morganii, P. mirabilis* and *P. vulgaris*; acute otitis media; acute exacerbations of chronic bronchitis due to susceptible strains of *H. influenzae* or *S. pneumoniae*; treatment and prophylaxis of *Pneumocystis jirovecii* pneumonia (PCP); traveler's diarrhea due to enterotoxigenic *E. coli*; treatment of enteritis caused by *Shigella flexneri* or *Shigella sonnei*

I.V.: Treatment of *Pneumocystis jirovecii* pneumonia (PCP); treatment of enteritis caused by *Shigella flexneri* or *Shigella sonnei*; treatment of severe or complicated urinary tract infections due to *E. coli, Klebsiella* and *Enterobacter* spp, *M. morganii, P. mirabilis,* and *P. vulgaris*

Unlabeled Use Cholera and *Salmonella*-type infections and nocardiosis; chronic prostatitis; as prophylaxis in neutropenic patients with *P. jirovecii* infections, in leukemia patients, and in patients following renal transplantation, to decrease incidence of PCP; treatment of *Cyclospora* infection, typhoid fever, *Nocardia asteroides* infection; prophylaxis against urinary tract infection; alternative treatment for MRSA infections; oral phase treatment of prosthetic joint infection; chronic antimicrobial suppression of prosthetic joint infection, treatment of Q fever (*Coxiella burnetii*)

Pregnancy Risk Factor D

Pregnancy Considerations Adverse events have been observed in animal reproduction studies. Trimethoprim-sulfamethoxazole (TMP-SMX) crosses the placenta and distributes to amniotic fluid (Ylikorkala, 1973). An increased risk of congenital malformations (neural tube defects, cardiovascular malformations, urinary tract defects, oral clefts, club foot) following maternal use of TMP-SMX during pregnancy has been observed in some studies. Folic acid supplementation may decrease this risk (Crider, 2009; Czeizel, 2001; Hernandez-Diaz, 2000; Hernandez-Diaz, 2001; Matok, 2009). Due to theoretical concerns that sulfonamides pass the placenta and may cause kernicterus in the newborn, neonatal healthcare providers should be informed if maternal sulfonamide therapy is used near the time of delivery (DHHS, 2013).

The pharmacokinetics of TMP-SMX are similar to nonpregnant values in early pregnancy (Ylikorkala, 1973). TMP-SMX is recommended for the prophylaxis or treatment of *Pneumocystis jirovecii* pneumonia (PCP), prophylaxis of *Toxoplasmic gondii* encephalitis (TE), and for the acute and chronic treatment of Q fever in pregnancy (CDC, 2013; DHHS, 2013). Sulfonamides may also be used to treat other infections in pregnant women when clinically appropriate; use during the first trimester should be limited to situations where no alternative therapies are available (ACOG, 2011). Because safer options are available for the treatment of urinary tract infections in pregnant women, use of TMP-containing products in the first trimester and sulfonamide-containing products >32 weeks gestation should be avoided (Lee, 2008).

Breast-Feeding Considerations Small amounts of TMP and SMX are transferred into breast milk. The manufacturer recommends that caution be used if administered to nursing women, especially if breast-feeding ill, jaundiced, premature, or stressed infants due to the potential risk of bilirubin displacement and kernicterus. Sulfonamides should not be used while nursing an infant with G6PD deficiency or hyperbilirubinemia (Della-Giustina, 2003). Maternal indications for TMP-SMX must also be considered prior to nursing. Nondose-related effects could include modification of bowel flora.

Contraindications Hypersensitivity to any sulfa drug, trimethoprim, or any component of the formulation; history of drug induced-immune thrombocytopenia with use of sulfonamides or trimethoprim; megaloblastic anemia due to folate deficiency; infants <2 months of age; marked hepatic damage or severe renal disease (if patient not monitored)

Warnings/Precautions Use with caution in patients with G6PD deficiency, impaired renal or hepatic function or potential folate deficiency (malnourished, chronic anticonvulsant therapy, or elderly); maintain adequate hydration to prevent crystalluria; adjust dosage in patients with renal impairment. Injection vehicle may contain benzyl alcohol and sodium metabisulfite.

Chemical similarities are present among sulfonamides, sulfonylureas, carbonic anhydrase inhibitors, thiazides, and loop diuretics (except ethacrynic acid). Use in patients with sulfonamide allergy is specifically contraindicated in product labeling, however, a risk of cross-reaction exists in patients with allergy to any of these compounds; avoid use when previous reaction has been severe.

Fatalities associated with severe reactions including Stevens-Johnson syndrome, toxic epidermal necrolysis, hepatic necrosis, agranulocytosis, aplastic anemia, thrombocytopenia and other blood dyscrasias have been reported; discontinue use at first sign of rash or serious adverse reactions. Elderly patients appear at greater risk for more severe adverse reactions. May cause hypoglycemia, particularly in malnourished, or patients with renal or hepatic impairment. Use with caution in patients with porphyria or thyroid dysfunction. Potentially significant interactions may exist, requiring dose or frequency adjustment, additional monitoring, and/or selection of alternative therapy. Slow acetylators may be more prone to adverse reactions. Caution in patients with allergies or asthma. May cause hyperkalemia (associated with high doses of trimethoprim) or hyponatremia. Incidence of adverse effects appears to be increased in patients with AIDS. Prolonged use may result in fungal or bacterial superinfection, including *C. difficile*-associated diarrhea (CDAD) and pseudomembranous colitis; CDAD has been observed >2 months postantibiotic treatment. Avoid concomitant use with leucovorin when treating *Pneumocystis jirovecii* pneumonia (PCP) in HIV patients; may increase risk of treatment failure and death.

When used for uncomplicated urinary tract infections, this combination should not be used if a single agent is effective. Additionally, sulfonamides should not be used to treat group A beta-hemolytic streptococcal infections.

Adverse Reactions Frequency not defined:

Cardiovascular: Allergic myocarditis, periarteritis nodosa (rare)

Central nervous system: Apathy, aseptic meningitis, ataxia, chills, depression, fatigue, hallucination, headache, insomnia, nervousness, peripheral neuritis, seizure, vertigo

Dermatologic: Erythema multiforme (rare), exfoliative dermatitis (rare), pruritus, skin photosensitivity, skin rash, Stevens-Johnson syndrome (rare), toxic epidermal necrolysis (rare), urticaria

Endocrine & metabolic: Hyperkalemia (generally at high dosages), hypoglycemia (rare), hyponatremia

Gastrointestinal: Abdominal pain, anorexia, diarrhea, glottis edema, kernicterus (in neonates), nausea, pancreatitis, pseudomembranous colitis, stomatitis, vomiting

Genitourinary: Crystalluria, diuresis (rare), nephrotoxicity (in association with cyclosporine), toxic nephrosis (with anuria and oliguria)

Hematologic & oncologic: Agranulocytosis, anaphylactoid purpura (IgA vasculitis; rare), aplastic anemia, eosinophilia, hemolysis (with G6PD deficiency), hemolytic anemia, hypoprothrombinemia, leukopenia, megaloblastic anemia, methemoglobinemia, neutropenia, thrombocytopenia

Hepatic: Cholestatic jaundice, hepatotoxicity (including hepatitis, cholestasis, and hepatic necrosis), hyperbilirubinemia, increased transaminases

Hypersensitivity: Anaphylaxis, angioedema, hypersensitivity reaction, serum sickness

Neuromuscular & skeletal: Arthralgia, myalgia, rhabdomyolysis (mainly in AIDS patients), systemic lupus erythematosus (rare), weakness

Ophthalmic: Conjunctival injection, injected sclera

Otic: Tinnitus

Renal: Increased blood urea nitrogen, increased serum creatinine, interstitial nephritis, renal failure

Respiratory: Cough, dyspnea, pulmonary infiltrates

Miscellaneous: Fever

<1% (Limited to important or life-threatening): Idiopathic thrombocytopenic purpura, prolonged Q-T interval on ECG, thrombotic thrombocytopenic purpura

Drug Interactions

Metabolism/Transport Effects Refer to individual components.

Avoid Concomitant Use

Avoid concomitant use of Sulfamethoxazole and Trimethoprim with any of the following: BCG; Dofetilide; Leucovorin Calcium-Levoleucovorin; Methenamine; Potassium P-Aminobenzoate; Procaine

Increased Effect/Toxicity

Sulfamethoxazole and Trimethoprim may increase the levels/effects of: ACE Inhibitors; Amantadine; Angiotensin II Receptor Blockers; Antidiabetic Agents (Thiazolidinedione); AzaTHIOprine; Bosentan; Carvedilol; CycloSPORINE (Systemic); CYP2C8 Substrates; CYP2C9 Substrates; Dapsone (Systemic); Dapsone (Topical); Digoxin; Dofetilide; Eplerenone; Fosphenytoin;

Highest Risk QTc-Prolonging Agents; LamiVUDine; Memantine; Mercaptopurine; MetFORMIN; Methotrexate; Moderate Risk QTc-Prolonging Agents; Phenytoin; Porfimer; PRALAtrexate; Prilocaine; Procainamide; Repaglinide; Sodium Nitrite; Spironolactone; Sulfonylureas; Varenicline; Vitamin K Antagonists

The levels/effects of Sulfamethoxazole and Trimethoprim may be increased by: Amantadine; CYP2C9 Inhibitors (Moderate); CYP2C9 Inhibitors (Strong); Dapsone (Systemic); Memantine; Methenamine; Mifepristone; Nitric Oxide

Decreased Effect

Sulfamethoxazole and Trimethoprim may decrease the levels/effects of: BCG; CycloSPORINE (Systemic); Sodium Picosulfate; Typhoid Vaccine

The levels/effects of Sulfamethoxazole and Trimethoprim may be decreased by: Bosentan; CYP2C9 Inducers (Strong); CYP3A4 Inducers (Strong); Dabrafenib; Deferasirox; Fosphenytoin; Herbs (CYP3A4 Inducers); Leucovorin Calcium-Levoleucovorin; Mitotane; Peginterferon Alfa-2b; Phenytoin; Potassium P-Aminobenzoate; Procaine; Tocilizumab

Ethanol/Nutrition/Herb Interactions Herb/Nutraceutical: Avoid dong quai; St John's wort (may diminish effects and also cause photosensitization).

Preparation for Administration I.V.: Must dilute well prior to administration (ie, 1:15 to 1:25, which equates to 5 mL of drug solution diluted in 75-125 mL base solution)

Storage/Stability

Injection: Store at room temperature; do not refrigerate. Less soluble in more alkaline pH. Protect from light. Solution must be diluted prior to administration. Following dilution, store at room temperature; do not refrigerate. Manufacturer recommended dilutions and stability of parenteral admixture at room temperature (25°C):

5 mL/125 mL D_5W; stable for 6 hours.

5 mL/100 mL D_5W; stable for 4 hours.

5 mL/75 mL D_5W; stable for 2 hours.

Studies have also confirmed limited stability in NS; detailed references should be consulted.

Suspension, tablet: Store at controlled room temperature of 15°C to 25°C (59°F to 77°F). Protect from light.

Mechanism of Action Sulfamethoxazole interferes with bacterial folic acid synthesis and growth via inhibition of dihydrofolic acid formation from para-aminobenzoic acid; trimethoprim inhibits dihydrofolic acid reduction to tetrahydrofolate resulting in sequential inhibition of enzymes of the folic acid pathway

Pharmacodynamics/Kinetics

Absorption: Oral: Rapid

Distribution: Both SMX and TMP distribute to middle ear fluid, sputum, vaginal fluid; TMP also distributes into bronchial secretions

Protein binding: SMX: ~70%, TMP: ~44%

Metabolism: Hepatic, both to multiple metabolites; SMX to hydroxy (via CYP2C9) and acetyl derivatives, and also conjugated with glucuronide; TMP to oxide and hydroxy derivatives; the free forms of both SMX and TMP are therapeutically active

Half-life elimination: Oral (mean): SMX: 10 hours, TMP: 8-10 hours; both are prolonged in renal failure

Time to peak, serum: Oral: 1-4 hours

Excretion: Both are excreted in urine as metabolites and unchanged drug

Dosage Dosage recommendations are based on the trimethoprim component. Double-strength tablets are equivalent to sulfamethoxazole 800 mg and trimethoprim 160 mg.

Usual dosage ranges:

Children >2 months: Manufacturer's labeling:

Mild-to-moderate infections: Oral: 8 mg TMP/kg/day in divided doses every 12 hours

Serious infection:

Oral: 15-20 mg TMP/kg/day in divided doses every 6 hours

I.V.: 8-12 mg TMP/kg/day in divided doses every 6-12 hours

Adults:

Oral: 1-2 double-strength tablets (sulfamethoxazole 800 mg; trimethoprim 160 mg) every 12-24 hours

I.V.: 8-20 mg TMP/kg/day divided every 6-12 hours

Indication-specific dosing:

Children >2 months:

Acute otitis media: Oral: 8 mg TMP/kg/day in divided doses every 12 hours for 10 days. **Note:** Recommended by the American Academy of Pediatrics as an alternative agent in penicillin-allergic patients at a dose of 6-10 mg TMP/kg/day (AOM guidelines, 2004).

Cyclosporiasis (unlabeled use): Oral, I.V.: 5 mg TMP/kg twice daily for 7-10 days (*Red Book*, 2009)

Pneumocystis jirovecii:

Treatment: Oral, I.V.: 15-20 mg TMP/kg/day in divided doses every 6-8 hours for 21 days

Prophylaxis: Oral, 150 mg TMP/m^2/day in divided doses every 12 hours and administered for 3 days/week on consecutive or alternate days; an alternative dosing regimen allows for same dose to be administered in 2 divided doses daily (maximum: trimethoprim 320 mg and sulfamethoxazole 1600 mg daily) (CDC, 2009)

Q fever (unlabeled use): Oral:

Acute: Infants ≥2 months and Children <8 years with mild or uncomplicated illness (if patient remains febrile past 5 days of doxycycline treatment): 4-20 mg TMP/kg/day in divided doses every 12 hours (maximum: trimethoprim 320 mg daily) (CDC, 2013). **Note:** Some clinicians may recommend initial treatment with sulfamethoxazole and trimethoprim for children <8 years with mild or uncomplicated illness (CDC, 2013; Hartzell, 2008).

Chronic: Infectious Disease consult recommended for treatment of chronic Q fever (CDC, 2013)

Shigellosis: Note: Due to reported widespread resistance, empiric therapy with sulfamethoxazole and trimethoprim is not recommended (CDC-NARMS, 2010; WHO, 2005).

Oral:

Manufacturer's recommendation: 8 mg TMP/kg/day in divided doses every 12 hours for 5 days

Alternate recommendations (unlabeled dose): 10 mg TMP/kg/day in divided doses every 12 hours for 5 days (Ashkenazi, 1993)

I.V.: 8-10 mg TMP/kg/day in divided doses every 6, 8, or 12 hours for up to 5 days

Skin/soft tissue infection due to community-acquired MRSA (unlabeled use): Oral: 4-6 mg TMP/kg/dose every 12 hours for 5-10 days (Liu, 2011); **Note:** If beta-hemolytic *Streptococcus* spp are also suspected, a beta-lactam antibiotic should be added to the regimen (Liu, 2011)

Toxoplasmosis primary prophylaxis in HIV-exposed/infected patients (unlabeled use; CDC, 2009): Oral: 150 mg TMP/m^2/day in 2 divided doses (preferred) or 150 mg TMP/m^2/day in a single dose 3 times/week on consecutive days; or 150 mg TMP/m^2/day in 2 divided doses 3 times/week on alternate days

Urinary tract infection:

Treatment:

Oral: Manufacturer's labeling: 8 mg TMP/kg/day in divided doses every 12 hours for 10 days

I.V.: Manufacturer's labeling: 8-10 mg TMP/kg/day in divided doses every 6, 8, or 12 hours for up to 14 days with serious infections

Prophylaxis: Oral: 2 mg TMP/kg/dose daily or 5 mg TMP/kg/dose twice weekly

Adults:

Chronic bronchitis (acute): Oral: One double-strength tablet every 12 hours for 10-14 days

Cyclosporiasis (unlabeled use): Oral, I.V.: 160 mg TMP twice daily for 7-10 days. **Note:** AIDS patients: Oral: One double-strength tablet 2-4 times/day for 10 days, then 1 double-strength tablet 3 times/week for 10 weeks (Pape, 1994; Verdier, 2000)

Granuloma inguinale (donovanosis) (unlabeled use): Oral: One double-strength tablet every 12 hours for at least 3 weeks and until lesions have healed (CDC, 2010)

Isosporiasis (*Isospora belli* infection) in HIV-positive patients (unlabeled use; CDC, 2009):

Treatment: Oral, I.V.: 160 mg TMP 4 times/day for 10 days **or** 160 mg TMP 2 times/day for 7-10 days. May increase dose and/or duration up to 3-4 weeks if symptoms worsen or persist

Secondary prophylaxis (in patients with CD4+ count <200 /microL): Oral: 160 mg TMP 3 times/week (preferred) **or** alternatively, 160 mg TMP daily **or** 320 mg TMP 3 times/week

Meningitis (bacterial): I.V.: 10-20 mg TMP/kg/day in divided doses every 6-12 hours

Nocardia (unlabeled use): Oral, I.V.:

Cutaneous infections: 5-10 mg TMP/kg/day in 2-4 divided doses

Severe infections (pulmonary/cerebral): 15 mg TMP/kg/day in 2-4 divided doses for 3-4 weeks, then 10 mg TMP/kg/day in 2-4 divided doses. Treatment duration is controversial; an average of 7 months has been reported.

Note: Therapy for severe infection may be initiated I.V. and converted to oral therapy (frequently converted to approximate dosages of oral solid dosage forms: 2 DS tablets every 8-12 hours). Although not widely available, sulfonamide levels should be considered in patients with questionable absorption, at risk for dose-related toxicity, or those with poor therapeutic response.

Osteomyelitis due to MRSA (unlabeled use): Oral, I.V.: 3.5-4 mg TMP/kg/dose every 8-12 hours for a minimum of 8 weeks with rifampin 600 mg once daily (Liu, 2011)

***Pneumocystis jirovecii* pneumonia (PCP):** Oral: Manufacturer's labeling:

Prophylaxis: 160 mg TMP daily

Treatment: 15-20 mg TMP/kg/day divided every 6 hours for 14-21 days

***Pneumocystis jirovecii* pneumonia (PCP) prophylaxis and treatment in HIV-positive patients (CDC, 2009):** **Note:** Sulfamethoxazole and trimethoprim is the preferred regimen for this indication.

Prophylaxis: Oral: 80-160 mg TMP daily **or** alternatively, 160 mg TMP 3 times/week

Treatment:

Mild-to-moderate: Oral: 15-20 mg TMP/kg/day in 3 divided doses for 21 days **or** alternatively, 320 mg TMP 3 times/day for 21 days

Moderate-to-severe: Oral, I.V.: 15-20 mg TMP/kg/day in 3-4 divided doses for 21 days

Prosthetic joint infection (unlabeled use): Oral phase treatment (after completion of pathogen-specific I.V. therapy) following debridement and prosthesis retention or 1-stage exchange:

Total ankle, elbow, hip, or shoulder arthroplasty: 160 mg TMP 2 times daily for 3 months. **Note:** Must be used in combination with rifampin (Cordero-Ampuero, 2007; Osmon, 2013).

Total knee arthroplasty: Adults: 160 mg TMP 2 times daily for 6 months. **Note:** Must be used in combination with rifampin (Cordero-Ampuero, 2007; Osmon, 2013).

Q fever (unlabeled use): Oral:

Acute (in pregnant women) (CDC, 2013): 160 mg TMP twice daily throughout pregnancy but not beyond 32 weeks gestation. **Note:** Discontinue therapy for the final 8 weeks of pregnancy due to hyperbilirubinemia risk

Chronic: Infectious Disease consult recommended for treatment of chronic Q fever

Sepsis: I.V.: 20 mg TMP/kg/day divided every 6 hours

Septic arthritis due to MRSA (unlabeled use): Oral, I.V.: 3.5-4 mg TMP/kg/dose every 8-12 hours for 3-4 weeks (some experts combine with rifampin) (Liu, 2011)

Shigellosis: **Note:** Due to reported widespread resistance, empiric therapy with sulfamethoxazole and trimethoprim is not recommended (CDC-NARMS, 2010; WHO, 2005).

Oral: One double-strength tablet every 12 hours for 5 days

I.V.: 8-10 mg TMP/kg/day in divided doses every 6, 8, or 12 hours for up to 5 days

Skin/soft tissue infection due to community-acquired MRSA (unlabeled use): Oral: 1-2 double-strength tablets every 12 hours for 5-10 days (Liu, 2011); **Note:** If beta-hemolytic *Streptococcus* spp are also suspected, a beta-lactam antibiotic should be added to the regimen (Liu, 2011)

***Stenotrophomonas maltophilia* (ventilator-associated pneumonia):** I.V.: Most clinicians have utilized 12-15 mg TMP/kg/day for the treatment of VAP caused by *Stenotrophomonas maltophilia*. Higher doses (up to 20 mg TMP/kg/day) have been mentioned for treatment of severe infection in patients with normal renal function (Looney, 2009; Vartivarian, 1989; Wood, 2010)

***Toxoplasma gondii* encephalitis (unlabeled use; CDC, 2009):** Oral:

Primary prophylaxis: Oral: 160 mg TMP daily (preferred) **or** 160 mg TMP 3 times/week **or** 80 mg TMP daily

Treatment (alternative to sulfadiazine, pyrimethamine and leucovorin calcium): Oral, I.V.: 5 mg/kg TMP twice daily

Travelers' diarrhea: Oral: One double-strength tablet every 12 hours for 5 days

Urinary tract infection:

Oral: One double-strength tablet every 12 hours

Duration of therapy: Uncomplicated: 3-5 days; Complicated: 7-10 days

Pyelonephritis: 14 days

Prostatitis: Acute: 2 weeks; Chronic: 2-3 months

I.V.: 8-10 mg TMP/kg/day in divided doses every 6, 8, or 12 hours for up to 14 days with severe infections

Dosage adjustment in renal impairment: Oral, I.V.:

Manufacturer's recommendation: Children and Adults:

Cl_{cr} >30 mL/minute: No dosage adjustment required

Cl_{cr} 15-30 mL/minute: Administer 50% of recommended dose

Cl_{cr} <15 mL/minute: Use is not recommended

Alternate recommendations:

Cl_{cr} 15-30 mL/minute:

Treatment: Administer full daily dose (divided every 12 hours) for 24-48 hours, then decrease daily dose by 50% and administer every 24 hours (**Note:** For serious infections including *Pneumocystis jirovecii* pneumonia (PCP), full daily dose is given in divided doses every 6-8 hours for 2 days, followed by reduction to 50% daily dose divided every 12 hours) (Nahata, 1995).

PCP prophylaxis: One-half single-strength tablet (40 mg trimethoprim) daily **or** 1 single-strength tablet (80 mg trimethoprim) daily or 3 times weekly (Masur, 2002).

Cl_{cr} <15 mL/minute:

Treatment: Administer full daily dose every 48 hours (Nahata, 1995)

PCP prophylaxis: One-half single-strength tablet (40 mg trimethoprim) daily **or** 1 single-strength tablet (80 mg trimethoprim) 3 times weekly (Masur, 2002). While the guidelines do acknowledge the alternative of giving 1 single-strength tablet daily, this may be inadvisable in the uremic/ESRD patient.

GFR <10 mL/minute/1.73 m^2: Children: Use is not recommended, but if required, administer 5-10 mg trimethoprim/kg every 24 hours (Aronoff, 2007).

Intermittent Hemodialysis (IHD) (administer after hemodialysis on dialysis days):

Children: Use is not recommended, but if required, administer 5-10 mg trimethoprim/kg every 24 hours (Aronoff, 2007).

Adults: 2.5-10 mg/kg trimethoprim every 24 hours or 5-20 mg/kg trimethoprim 3 times weekly after IHD. **Note:** Dosing is highly dependent upon indication for use (eg, treatment of cystitis versus treatment of PCP pneumonia (Heinz, 2009).

PCP prophylaxis: One single-strength tablet (80 mg trimethoprim) after each dialysis session (Masur, 2002)

Note: Dosing dependent on the assumption of 3 times/week, complete IHD sessions.

Peritoneal dialysis (PD):

Use Cl_{cr} <15 mL/minute dosing recommendations. Not significantly removed by PD; supplemental dosing is not required (Aronoff, 2007):

GFR <10 mL/minute/1.73 m^2: Children: Use is not recommended, but if required 5-10 mg TMP/kg every 24 hours.

Exit-site and tunnel infections: Oral: One single-strength tablet daily (Li, 2010)

Intraperitoneal: Loading dose: TMP-SMX 320/1600 mg/L; Maintenance: TMP-SMX 80/400 mg/L (Aronoff, 2007; Warady, 2000)

Peritonitis: Oral: One double-strength tablet twice daily (Li, 2010)

Continuous renal replacement therapy (CRRT) (Heintz, 2009; Trotman, 2005): Drug clearance is highly dependent on the method of renal replacement, filter type, and flow rate. Appropriate dosing requires close monitoring of pharmacologic response, signs of adverse reactions due to drug accumulation, as well as drug concentrations in relation to target trough (if appropriate). The following are general recommendations only (based on dialysate flow/ultrafiltration rates of 1-2 L/hour and minimal residual renal function) and should not supersede clinical judgment:

CVVH/CVVHD/CVVHDF: 2.5-7.5 mg/kg of TMP every 12 hours. **Note:** Dosing regimen dependent on clinical indication. Critically-ill patients with *P. jirovecii* pneumonia receiving CVVHDF may require up to 10 mg/kg every 12 hours (Heintz, 2009).

Dosage adjustment in renal impairment: No dosage adjustment provided in manufacturer's labeling. Use with caution; use is contraindicated in cases of marked hepatic damage.

Dietary Considerations Should be taken with 8 oz of water. May be taken without regard to meals.

Administration

I.V.: Infuse diluted solution over 60-90 minutes; not for I.M. injection

Oral: Administer without regard to meals. Administer with at least 8 ounces of water.

Monitoring Parameters Perform culture and sensitivity testing prior to initiating therapy; CBC, serum potassium, creatinine, BUN

Test Interactions Increased creatinine (Jaffé alkaline picrate reaction); increased serum methotrexate by dihydrofolate reductase method

Dosage Forms Excipient information presented when available (limited, particularly for generics); consult specific product labeling. **Note:** The 5:1 ratio (SMX:TMP) remains constant in all dosage forms.

Injection, solution: Sulfamethoxazole 80 mg and trimethoprim 16 mg per mL (5 mL, 10 mL, 30 mL)

Suspension, oral: Sulfamethoxazole 200 mg and trimethoprim 40 mg per 5 mL (20 mL, 480 mL)

Sulfatrim: Sulfamethoxazole 200 mg and trimethoprim 40 mg per 5 mL (480 mL) [contains alcohol <0.5%, propylene glycol; cherry flavor]

Tablet, oral: Sulfamethoxazole 400 mg and trimethoprim 80 mg

Bactrim: Sulfamethoxazole 400 mg and trimethoprim 80 mg

Tablet, double-strength, oral: Sulfamethoxazole 800 mg and trimethoprim 160 mg

Bactrim DS: Sulfamethoxazole 800 mg and trimethoprim 160 mg

Septra DS: Sulfamethoxazole 800 mg and trimethoprim 160 mg

◆ **Sulfamylon** *see* Mafenide *on page 1259*

Sulfanilamide (sul fa NIL a mide)

Brand Names: U.S. AVC Vaginal

Index Terms p-amino-benzenesulfonamide

Pharmacologic Category Antifungal Agent, Vaginal

Use Treatment of vulvovaginitis caused by *Candida albicans*

Pregnancy Risk Factor C

Pregnancy Considerations Adverse events have been observed in animal reproduction studies with sulfonamides, including sulfanilamide. Sulfonamides cross the placenta and distribute to amniotic fluid. The fetal concentration is 50% to 90% of that measured in the maternal blood. Use of vaginal products (eg, applicators and inserts) should be used with caution after the seventh month of pregnancy. Because of the theoretical increased risk for hyperbilirubinemia and kernicterus, neonatal healthcare providers should be informed if maternal sulfonamide therapy is used near the time of delivery.

Breast-Feeding Considerations Sulfanilamide is excreted into breast milk. Absorbed sulfonamides are transferred to breast milk and have caused kernicterus in the newborn. Due to the potential for serious adverse reactions in the nursing infant, breast-feeding is not recommended.

Contraindications Hypersensitivity to sulfanilamide or any component of the formulation

Warnings/Precautions Severe reactions, including agranulocytosis, aplastic anemia, and other blood dyscrasias, have occurred with sulfonamides (regardless of route). Severe dermatologic reactions, including Stevens-Johnson syndrome and toxic epidermal necrolysis, have occurred with sulfonamides (regardless of route). Fatalities associated with fulminant hepatic necrosis have occurred with sulfonamides (regardless of route). Chemical similarities are present among sulfonamides, sulfonylureas, carbonic anhydrase inhibitors, thiazides, and loop diuretics (except ethacrynic acid). Use in patients with sulfonamide allergy is specifically contraindicated in product labeling; however, a risk of cross-reaction exists in patients with allergy to any of these compounds; avoid use when previous reaction has been severe.

Topical antifungal agents or oral fluconazole are generally considered to be the preferred treatment for uncomplicated vulvovaginal candidiasis (Pappas, 2009; Reef, 1993; Sobel, 2007). Sulfanilamide is not recognized as a preferred or as an alternative agent for the treatment of uncomplicated vulvovaginitis candidiasis in the available literature.

Adverse Reactions <1% (Limited to important or life-threatening): Local: Sensitivity reactions (burning, discomfort)

Drug Interactions

Metabolism/Transport Effects None known.

Avoid Concomitant Use There are no known interactions where it is recommended to avoid concomitant use.

Increased Effect/Toxicity There are no known significant interactions involving an increase in effect.

Decreased Effect There are no known significant interactions involving a decrease in effect.

Mechanism of Action Interferes with microbial folic acid synthesis and growth via inhibition of para-aminiobenzoic acid metabolism; exerts a bacteriostatic action

Dosage Intravaginal: Adults: Females: Insert one applicatorful intravaginally once or twice daily; treatment should continue for a period of 30 days

Dosage Forms Excipient information presented when available (limited, particularly for generics); consult specific product labeling.

Cream, Vaginal:

AVC Vaginal: 15% (120 g) [contains methylparaben, propylparaben, trolamine (triethanolamine)]

SulfaSALAzine (sul fa SAL a zeen)

Brand Names: U.S. Azulfidine; Azulfidine EN-tabs; Sulfazine; Sulfazine EC

Brand Names: Canada Apo-Sulfasalazine; PMS-Sulfasalazine; Salazopyrin; Salazopyrin En-Tabs

Index Terms Salicylazosulfapyridine

Pharmacologic Category 5-Aminosalicylic Acid Derivative

Use

U.S. labeling: Treatment of mild-to-moderate ulcerative colitis or as adjunctive therapy in severe ulcerative colitis; enteric coated tablets are also used for rheumatoid arthritis (including juvenile idiopathic arthritis [JIA]) in patients who inadequately respond to analgesics and NSAIDs

Canadian labeling: Adjunctive therapy in severe ulcerative colitis, distal ulcerative colitis or proctitis, and Crohn's disease; enteric coated tablets are also used for rheumatoid arthritis unsuccessfully treated with first-line therapy

Unlabeled Use Ankylosing spondylitis, Crohn's disease, psoriasis, psoriatic arthritis

Pregnancy Risk Factor B

Pregnancy Considerations Adverse events have not been observed in animal reproduction studies. Sulfasalazine and sulfapyridine cross the placenta; a potential for kernicterus in the newborn exists. Agranulocytosis was noted in an infant following maternal use of sulfasalazine during pregnancy. Additionally, cases of neural tube defects have been reported (causation undetermined); sulfasalazine is known to inhibit the absorption and metabolism of folic acid and may diminish the effects of folic acid supplementation. Based on available data, an increase in fetal malformations has not been observed following maternal use of sulfasalazine for the treatment of inflammatory bowel disease or ulcerative colitis. When treatment for inflammatory bowel disease is needed during pregnancy, sulfasalazine may be used, although supplementation with folic acid is recommended (Habal, 2012; Mahadevan, 2009; Mottet, 2009).

Breast-Feeding Considerations Sulfasalazine is excreted in breast milk; sulfapyridine concentrations are ~30% to 60% of the maternal serum. Bloody stools or diarrhea have been reported in nursing infants. Although sulfapyridine has poor bilirubin-displacing ability, exposure may cause kernicterus in the newborn. The manufacturer recommends that caution be used in women who are breast-feeding. Other sources consider use of sulfasalazine to be safe while breast-feeding; monitoring of the infant is recommended (Habal, 2012; Mahadevan, 2009; Mottet, 2009).

Contraindications Hypersensitivity to sulfasalazine, sulfa drugs, salicylates, or any component of the formulation; porphyria; GI or GU obstruction

Canadian labeling: Additional contraindications (not in U.S. labeling): Use in pediatric patients <2 years of age; patients in whom acute asthmatic attacks, urticaria, rhinitis or other allergic manifestations are precipitated by acetyl salicylic acid (ASA) or other NSAIDs

Warnings/Precautions Use with extreme caution in patients with renal impairment, impaired hepatic function or blood dyscrasias. Use caution in patients with severe allergies or asthma, or G6PD deficiency. May decrease folic acid absorption. Deaths from irreversible neuromuscular or central nervous system changes, fibrosing alveolitis, agranulocytosis, aplastic anemia, and other blood dyscrasias have been reported. In males, oligospermia (rare) and infertility has been reported. Chemical similarities are present among sulfonamides, sulfonylureas, carbonic anhydrase inhibitors, thiazides, and loop diuretics (except ethacrynic acid). Nausea, vomiting, and abdominal discomfort commonly occur; titration of dose and/or using the enteric coated formulation may decrease GI adverse effects. Use in patients with sulfonamide allergy is specifically contraindicated in product labeling, however, a risk of cross-reaction exists in patients with allergy to any of these compounds; avoid use when previous reaction has been severe. Slow acetylators may be more prone to adverse reactions. Discontinue enteric coated tablets if noted to pass without disintegrating. Severe skin reactions (some fatal), including Stevens-Johnson syndrome (SJS), exfoliative dermatitis, and toxic epidermal necrolysis (TEN) have occurred with sulfonamides, most commonly during the first month of treatment; discontinue use at first sign of rash. Severe hypersensitivity reactions, including drug rash with eosinophilia and systemic symptoms (DRESS) syndrome have been reported; discontinue treatment for severe reactions.

Adverse Reactions

>10%:

Central nervous system: Headache (RA 9%)

Dermatologic: Skin rash (RA 13%)

Gastrointestinal: Nausea (RA 19%), dyspepsia (RA 13%), anorexia, gastric distress, vomiting

Genitourinary: Oligospermia (reversible)

1% to 10%:

Central nervous system: Dizziness

Dermatologic: Pruritus (RA 4%), urticaria

Gastrointestinal: Abdominal pain (RA 8%), stomatitis (RA 4%)

Hematologic & oncologic: Leukopenia (RA 3%), thrombocytopenia (RA 1%), Heinz body anemia, hemolytic anemia

Hepatic: Abnormal hepatic function tests (RA 4%)

Respiratory: Cyanosis

Miscellaneous: Fever

<1% (limited to important or life-threatening; includes reactions reported with mesalamine or other sulfonamides): Agranulocytosis, alopecia, anaphylaxis, angioedema, aplastic anemia, arthralgia, ataxia, cauda equina syndrome, cholestatic jaundice, conjunctival injection, crystalluria, depression, diarrhea, DRESS syndrome, drowsiness, eosinophilia, exfoliative dermatitis, fulminant

hepatitis, Guillain-Barré syndrome, hallucination, hearing loss, hematuria, hemolytic-uremic syndrome, hepatic cirrhosis, hepatic failure, hepatic necrosis, hepatitis, hypoglycemia, hypoprothrombinemia, injected sclera, insomnia, interstitial nephritis, interstitial pulmonary disease, jaundice, Kawasaki syndrome (single case report), lupus-like syndrome, megaloblastic anemia, meningitis, methemoglobinemia, myelitis, myelodysplastic syndrome, myocarditis (allergic), nephropathy (acute), nephrotic syndrome, neutropenia (congenital), neutropenic enterocolitis, pancreatitis, parapsoriasis varioliformis acuta, periarteritis nodosa, pericarditis, periorbital edema, peripheral neuropathy, pleurisy, pneumonitis, proteinuria, pulmonary alveolitis, purpura, rhabdomyolysis, seizure, serum sickness-like reaction (children with JRA have frequent and severe reaction), skin discoloration, skin photosensitivity, Stevens-Johnson syndrome, thyroid function impairment, toxic epidermal necrolysis, toxic nephrosis, urine discoloration, vasculitis

Drug Interactions

Metabolism/Transport Effects None known.

Avoid Concomitant Use There are no known interactions where it is recommended to avoid concomitant use.

Increased Effect/Toxicity

SulfaSALAzine may increase the levels/effects of: Heparin; Heparin (Low Molecular Weight); Methotrexate; Prilocaine; Sodium Nitrite; Thiopurine Analogs; Varicella Virus-Containing Vaccines

The levels/effects of SulfaSALAzine may be increased by: Nitric Oxide; Nonsteroidal Anti-Inflammatory Agents

Decreased Effect

SulfaSALAzine may decrease the levels/effects of: Cardiac Glycosides; Folic Acid; Methylfolate

Ethanol/Nutrition/Herb Interactions

Food: May decrease folic acid absorption.

Herb/Nutraceutical: Avoid dong quai, St John's wort (may also cause photosensitization)

Storage/Stability Store at 25°C (77°F); excursions permitted to 15°C to 30°C (59°F to 86°F).

Mechanism of Action 5-aminosalicylic acid (5-ASA) is the active component of sulfasalazine; the specific mechanism of action of 5-ASA is unknown; however, it is thought that it modulates local chemical mediators of the inflammatory response, especially leukotrienes, and is also postulated to be a free radical scavenger or an inhibitor of tumor necrosis factor (TNF); action appears topical rather than systemic

Pharmacodynamics/Kinetics

Absorption: ≤15% as unchanged drug from small intestine

Protein binding: Sulfasalazine: >99% to albumin; Sulfapyridine: ~70% to albumin; Acetylsulfapyridine (AcSP): ~90% to plasma proteins

Distribution: V_d: Sulfasalazine ~7.5 L

Metabolism: Via colonic intestinal flora to sulfapyridine and 5-aminosalicylic acid (5-ASA). Following absorption, sulfapyridine undergoes acetylation to form AcSP and ring hydroxylation while 5-ASA undergoes N-acetylation (non-acetylation phenotype dependent process); rate of metabolism via acetylation dependent on acetylation phenotype

Bioavailability: Sulfasalazine: <15%; Sulfapyridine: ~60%; 5-aminosalicylic acid: ~10% to 30%

Half-life elimination: Sulfasalazine: 5.7-10 hours (prolonged in elderly); Sulfapyridine: 14.8 hours (slow acetylators) and 10.4 hours (fast acetylators)

Time to peak: Sulfasalazine: 3-12 hours (mean: 6 hours); Metabolites: ~10 hours

Excretion: Primarily urine (as unchanged drug, conjugates, and acetylated metabolites); feces (small amounts)

Dosage Oral:

U.S. labeling:

Children ≥6 years:

Juvenile idiopathic arthritis (JIA): Enteric coated tablet: 30-50 mg/kg/day in 2 divided doses; Initial: Begin with 1/4 to 1/3 of expected maintenance dose; increase weekly; maximum: 2 g daily typically

Ulcerative colitis: Initial: 40-60 mg/kg/day in 3-6 divided doses; maintenance dose: 30 mg/kg/day in 4 divided doses

Adults:

Rheumatoid arthritis: Enteric coated tablet: Initial: 0.5-1 g daily; increase weekly to maintenance dose of 2 g daily in 2 divided doses; maximum: 3 g daily (if response to 2 g daily is inadequate after 12 weeks of treatment)

Ulcerative colitis:

Initial: 3-4 g daily in evenly divided doses at ≤8-hour intervals; may initiate therapy with 1-2 g daily to reduce GI intolerance. **Note:** American College of Gastroenterology guideline recommendations: Titrate to 4-6 g daily in 4 divided doses (Kornbluth, 2010).

Maintenance dose: 2 g daily in evenly divided doses at ≤8-hour intervals; if GI intolerance occurs reduce dosage by 50% and gradually increase to target dose after several days. If GI intolerance persists, stop drug for 5-7 days and reintroduce at a lower daily dose.

Crohn's disease, active mild/moderate, ileocolonic or colonic disease (unlabeled use): 3-6 g daily in divided doses (Lichtenstein, 2009)

Desensitization regimen: For patients who may be sensitive to treatment, it is suggested to start with a total dose of 50-250 mg daily and double it every 4-7 days until the desired dose is achieved. Discontinue if symptoms of sensitivity occur. Do not attempt in patients with a history of agranulocytosis or those who have had a previous anaphylactoid reaction on sulfasalazine therapy

Canadian labeling:

Children: Ulcerative colitis, inflammatory bowel disease, Crohn's disease: **Note:** Consider dose reduction or use of enteric coated tablet in patients experiencing adverse gastrointestinal effects with uncoated tablet.

Acute attacks:

Body weight 25 to <35 kg: 500 mg 3 times daily

Body weight 35-50 kg: 1 g 2-3 times daily

Maintenance of remission:

Body weight 25 to <35 kg: 500 mg 2 times daily

Body weight 35-50 kg: 500 mg 2-3 times daily

Adults:

Rheumatoid arthritis: Enteric coated tablet: Initial: 500 mg daily; increase dose weekly by 500 mg (total daily dose given in 2 divided doses) to maintenance dose of 1 g twice daily; if inadequate response to 1 g twice daily after 2 months, may increase dose to 3 g daily. Clinical improvement usually observed 1-2 months after initiating therapy. Concurrent use of analgesics and/or anti-inflammatory agents is recommended until therapeutic effect of sulfasalazine is observed.

Ulcerative colitis, inflammatory bowel disease, Crohn's disease: **Note:** Consider dose reduction or use of enteric coated tablet in patients experiencing adverse gastrointestinal effects with uncoated tablet.

Acute attacks: Severe: 1-2 g 3-4 times daily; mild-to-moderate: 1 g 3-4 times daily

Maintenance of remission: 1 g 2-3 times daily; continue dose indefinitely unless patient experiences adverse effects. In the event patient condition worsens, increase dose to 1-2 g 3-4 times daily.

Dosage adjustment in renal impairment: No dosage adjustment provided in manufacturer's labeling; use with extreme caution.

Dosage adjustment in hepatic impairment: No dosage adjustment provided in manufacturer's labeling; use with extreme caution.

Dietary Considerations Sulfasalazine impairs folate absorption. Adequate fluid intake is required to prevent crystalluria and stone formation.

Administration Tablets should be administered in evenly divided doses, preferably after meals. Enteric coated tablets should be swallowed whole.

Monitoring Parameters CBC with differential and liver function tests (prior to therapy, then every other week for first 3 months of therapy, followed by every month for the second 3 months, then once every 3 months thereafter); periodic urinalysis and renal function tests; stool frequency; signs of infection

Reference Range Sulfapyridine concentrations >50 mcg/mL are associated with increased adverse events.

Dosage Forms Excipient information presented when available (limited, particularly for generics); consult specific product labeling.

Tablet, Oral:
- Azulfidine: 500 mg [scored]
- Sulfazine: 500 mg [scored]
- Generic: 500 mg

Tablet Delayed Release, Oral:
- Azulfidine EN-tabs: 500 mg
- Sulfazine EC: 500 mg
- Generic: 500 mg

Extemporaneous Preparations A 100 mg/mL oral suspension may be made with tablets. Place twenty 500 mg tablets in a mortar and add a small amount of a 1:1 mixture of Ora-Sweet® and Ora-Plus® to cover the tablets. Let soak for 20-30 minutes. Crush the tablets and mix to a uniform paste; mix while adding the vehicle in equal proportions to **almost** 100 mL; transfer to a calibrated bottle, rinse mortar with vehicle, and add sufficient quantity of vehicle to make 100 mL. Label "shake well". Stable 91 days under refrigeration or at room temperature.

Lingertat-Walsh K, Walker SE, Law S, et al, "Stability of Sulfasalazine Oral Suspension," *Can J Hosp Pharm*, 2006, 59(4):194-200.

◆ **Sulfatrim** *see* Sulfamethoxazole and Trimethoprim *on page 1959*

◆ **Sulfazine** *see* SulfaSALAzine *on page 1964*

◆ **Sulfazine EC** *see* SulfaSALAzine *on page 1964*

◆ **Sulfisoxazole and Erythromycin** *see* Erythromycin and Sulfisoxazole *on page 744*

Sulfur and Sulfacetamide

(SUL fur & sul fa SEE ta mide)

Brand Names: U.S. AVAR; AVAR LS; AVAR-e; AVAR-e Green; AVAR-e LS; BP 10-1; BP Cleansing Wash; Clarifoam EF; Claris; Clenia [DSC]; Prascion; Prascion FC; Prascion RA; Rosanil; SSS 10-4; SSS 10-5; SulfaCleanse 8/4; Sumadan; Sumadan XLT; Sumaxin; Sumaxin TS; Verti-sulf; Zencia

Brand Names: Canada Sulfacet-R

Index Terms Sodium Sulfacetamide and Sulfur; Sulfacetamide and Sulfur; Sulfur and Sulfacetamide Sodium

Pharmacologic Category Acne Products; Antibiotic, Sulfonamide Derivative; Antiseborrheic Agent, Topical; Topical Skin Product, Acne

Use Aid in the treatment of acne vulgaris, acne rosacea, and seborrheic dermatitis

Pregnancy Risk Factor C

Dosage Topical: Children ≥12 years and Adults: Apply in a thin film 1-3 times/day. Cleansing products should be used 1-2 times/day.

Dosage adjustment in renal impairment: Use is contraindicated.

Dosage adjustment in hepatic impairment: No dosage adjustment provided in manufacturer's labeling.

Additional Information Complete prescribing information should be consulted for additional detail.

Dosage Forms Excipient information presented when available (limited, particularly for generics); consult specific product labeling. [DSC] = Discontinued product

Aerosol, foam, topical: Sulfur 5% and sulfacetamide sodium 10% (60 g)
- Clarifoam EF: Sulfur 5% and sulfacetamide sodium 10% (60 g, 100 g)
- SSS 10-4: Sulfur 4% and sulfacetamide sodium 10% (100 g)
- SSS 10-5: Sulfur 5% and sulfacetamide sodium 10% (60 g, 100 g)

Cleanser, topical: Sulfur 5% and sulfacetamide sodium 10% (170 g, 340 g)
- AVAR: Sulfur 5% and sulfacetamide sodium 10% (227 g) [contains benzyl alcohol]
- AVAR LS: Sulfur 2% and sulfacetamide sodium 10% (227 g) [contains benzyl alcohol]
- Prascion: Sulfur 5% and sulfacetamide sodium 10% (170 g, 340 g)
- Rosanil: Sulfur 5% and sulfacetamide sodium 10% (170 g)

Cream, topical: Sulfur 5% and sulfacetamide sodium 10% (28 g)
- AVAR-e: Sulfur 5% and sulfacetamide sodium 10% (45 g [DSC], 57 g) [contains benzyl alcohol]
- AVAR-e Green: Sulfur 5% and sulfacetamide sodium 10% (45 g [DSC], 57 g) [contains benzyl alcohol; color corrective cream]
- AVAR-e LS: Sulfur 2% and sulfacetamide sodium 10% (45 g [DSC], 57 g) [contains benzyl alcohol]
- Clenia: Sulfur 5% and sulfacetamide sodium 10% (28 g) [DSC]
- Prascion RA: Sulfur 5% and sulfacetamide sodium 10% (45 g) [contains benzyl alcohol and sunscreen]
- SSS 10-5: Sulfur 5% and sulfacetamide sodium 10% (28 g)
- Virti-sulf: Sulfur 5% and sulfacetamide sodium 10% (28 g)

Gel, topical: Sulfur 5% and sulfacetamide sodium 10% (45 g)

Pad, topical [cleansing cloth]: Sulfur 4% and sulfacetamide sodium 10% (60s)
- Avar: Sulfur 5% and sulfacetamide sodium 9.5% (30s, 60s)
- Avar LS: Sulfur 2% and sulfacetamide sodium 10% (30s, 60s)
- Prascion FC: Sulfur 5% and sulfacetamide sodium 10% (30s, 60s)
- Sumaxin: Sulfur 4% and sulfacetamide sodium 10% (60s) [contains aloe]

Suspension, topical: Sulfur 4% and sulfacetamide sodium 8% (473 mL)
- SulfaCleanse 8/4: Sulfur 4% and sulfacetamide sodium 8% (473 mL) [contains aloe]
- Sumaxin TS: Sulfur 4% and sulfacetamide sodium 8% (473 mL) [contains aloe]

Wash, topical: Sulfur 4% and sulfacetamide sodium 9% (480 mL); Sulfur 4.5% and sulfacetamide sodium 9% (454 g)
- BP 10-1: Sulfur 1% and sulfacetamide sodium 10% (170 g)
- BP Cleansing Wash: Sulfur 5% and sulfacetamide sodium 10% (480 mL) [contains urea]

Clenia: Sulfur 5% and sulfacetamide sodium 10% (170 g, 340 g) [DSC]
Sumaxin: Sulfur 4% and sulfacetamide sodium 9% (473 mL) [contains aloe]
Zencia: Sulfur 4% and sulfacetamide sodium 9% (480 mL) [contains aloe]
Wash, topical [emulsion-based]:
BP Cleansing Wash: Sulfur 4% and sulfacetamide sodium 10% (473 mL) [contains urea]
Claris: Sulfur 4% and sulfacetamide sodium 10% (473 mL) [contains urea 10%]
Sumadan: Sulfur 4.5% and sulfacetamide sodium 9% (454 g)
Sumadan XLT: Sulfur 4.5% and sulfacetamide sodium 9% (454 g) [packaged in a kit with Niseko sunscreen SPF 25]

◆ **Sulfur and Sulfacetamide Sodium** *see* Sulfur and Sulfacetamide *on page 1966*

Sulindac (SUL in dak)

Brand Names: Canada Apo-Sulin®; Novo-Sundac; Nu-Sulindac; Nu-Sundac; Teva-Sulindac

Pharmacologic Category Nonsteroidal Anti-inflammatory Drug (NSAID), Oral

Additional Appendix Information

Beers Criteria – Potentially Inappropriate Medications for Geriatrics *on page 2368*

Use Management of inflammatory diseases including osteoarthritis, rheumatoid arthritis, acute gouty arthritis, ankylosing spondylitis, acute painful shoulder (bursitis/tendonitis)

Unlabeled Use Management of preterm labor

Pregnancy Risk Factor C

Pregnancy Considerations Adverse events were not observed in the initial animal reproduction studies; therefore, the manufacturer classifies sulindac as pregnancy category C. Sulindac and the sulfide metabolite have been found to cross the placenta. NSAID exposure during the first trimester is not strongly associated with congenital malformations; however, cardiovascular anomalies and cleft palate have been observed following NSAID exposure in some studies. The use of an NSAID in the first trimester may be associated with an increased risk of miscarriage. Nonteratogenic effects have been observed following NSAID administration during the third trimester including myocardial degenerative changes, prenatal constriction of the ductus arteriosus, failure of the ductus arteriosus to close postnatally, and fetal tricuspid regurgitation; renal dysfunction or failure, oligohydramnios; gastrointestinal bleeding or perforation, increased risk of necrotizing enterocolitis; intracranial bleeding, platelet dysfunction with resultant bleeding; or pulmonary hypertension. Because they may cause premature closure of the ductus arteriosus, use of NSAIDs late in pregnancy should be avoided (use after 31-32 weeks gestation is not recommended by some clinicians). Sulindac has been used in the management of preterm labor. The chronic use of NSAIDs in women of reproductive age may be associated with infertility that is reversible upon discontinuation of the medication. A registry is available for pregnant women exposed to autoimmune medications including sulindac. For additional information contact the Organization of Teratology Information Specialists, OTIS Autoimmune Diseases Study, at (877) 311-8972.

Breast-Feeding Considerations It is not known if sulindac is excreted into breast milk. Breast-feeding is not recommended by the manufacturer.

Medication Guide Available Yes

Contraindications Hypersensitivity or allergic-type reactions to sulindac, aspirin, other NSAIDs, or any component of the formulation; perioperative pain in the setting of coronary artery bypass graft (CABG) surgery

Warnings/Precautions [U.S. Boxed Warning]: NSAIDs are associated with an increased risk of adverse cardiovascular thrombotic events, including MI and stroke. Use caution with fluid retention. Avoid use in heart failure. Concurrent administration of ibuprofen, and potentially other nonselective NSAIDs, may interfere with aspirin's cardioprotective effect. May cause new-onset hypertension or worsening of existing hypertension. NSAID use may compromise existing renal function; dose-dependent decreases in prostaglandin synthesis may result from NSAID use, reducing renal blood flow which may cause renal decompensation. NSAID use may increase the risk for hyperkalemia. Patients with impaired renal function, dehydration, heart failure, liver dysfunction, those taking diuretics, and ACE inhibitors, and the elderly are at greater risk of renal toxicity and hyperkalemia. Rehydrate patient before starting therapy; monitor renal function closely. Not recommended for use in patients with advanced renal disease. Long-term NSAID use may result in renal papillary necrosis. Use caution in patients with renal lithiasis; sulindac metabolites have been reported as components of renal stones. Maintain adequate hydration in patients with a history of renal stones. Use with caution in patients with decreased hepatic function. May require dosage adjustment in hepatic dysfunction; sulfide and sulfone metabolites may accumulate. The elderly are at increased risk for adverse effects. **[U.S. Boxed Warning]: Use is contraindicated for treatment of perioperative pain in the setting of coronary artery bypass graft (CABG) surgery.** Risk of MI and stroke may be increased with use following CABG surgery.

[U.S. Boxed Warning]: NSAIDs may increase risk of gastrointestinal irritation, inflammation, ulceration, bleeding, and perforation. Use the lowest effective dose for the shortest duration of time, consistent with individual patient goals, to reduce risk of cardiovascular or GI adverse events. When used concomitantly with ≤325 mg of aspirin, a substantial increase in the risk of gastrointestinal complications (eg, ulcer) occurs; concomitant gastroprotective therapy (eg, proton pump inhibitors) is recommended (Bhatt, 2008). Pancreatitis has been reported; discontinue with suspected pancreatitis.

Avoid chronic use in the elderly (unless alternative agents ineffective and patient can receive concomitant gastroprotective agent); nonselective oral NSAID use is associated with an increased risk of GI bleeding and peptic ulcer disease in older adults in high risk category (eg, >75 years or age or receiving concomitant oral/parenteral corticosteroids, anticoagulants, or antiplatelet agents) (Beers Criteria).

NSAIDS may cause drowsiness, dizziness, blurred vision and other neurologic effects which may impair physical or mental abilities; patients must be cautioned about performing tasks which require mental alertness (eg, operating machinery or driving). Discontinue use with blurred or diminished vision and perform ophthalmologic exam. Monitor vision with long-term therapy.

Platelet adhesion and aggregation may be decreased, may prolong bleeding time; patients with coagulation disorders or who are receiving anticoagulants should be monitored closely. Anemia may occur; patients on long-term NSAID therapy should be monitored for anemia. Rarely, NSAID use may cause severe blood dyscrasias (eg, agranulocytosis, aplastic anemia, thrombocytopenia). NSAIDs may cause serious skin adverse events including exfoliative dermatitis, Stevens-Johnson syndrome (SJS) and toxic epidermal necrolysis (TEN); discontinue use at first sign of skin rash or hypersensitivity. Anaphylactoid reactions may occur. Do not use in patients who experience bronchospasm, asthma, rhinitis, or urticaria with NSAID or aspirin therapy. Use caution in other forms of asthma. May increase the risk of aseptic meningitis, especially in patients with systemic lupus erythematosus (SLE) and mixed connective tissue disorders.

Withhold for at least 4-6 half-lives prior to surgical or dental procedures.

Adverse Reactions

1% to 10%:

Cardiovascular: Edema (1% to 3%)

Central nervous system: Dizziness (3% to 9%), headache (3% to 9%), nervousness (1% to 3%)

Dermatologic: Rash (3% to 9%), pruritus (1% to 3%)

Gastrointestinal: GI pain (10%), constipation (3% to 9%), diarrhea (3% to 9%), dyspepsia (3% to 9%), nausea (3% to 9%), abdominal cramps (1% to 3%), anorexia (1% to 3%), flatulence (1% to 3%), vomiting (1% to 3%)

Otic: Tinnitus (1% to 3%)

<1% (Limited to important or life-threatening): Agranulocytosis, ageusia, alopecia, anaphylaxis, angioneurotic edema, aplastic anemia, arrhythmia, aseptic meningitis, bitter taste, blurred vision, bone marrow depression, bronchial spasm, bruising, CHF, cholestasis, colitis, conjunctivitis, crystalluria, depression, dry mucous membranes, dyspnea, dysuria, epistaxis, erythema multiforme, exfoliative dermatitis, fever, gastritis, GI bleeding, GI perforation, glossitis, gynecomastia, hearing decreased, hematuria, hemolytic anemia, hepatitis, hepatic failure, hyperglycemia, hyperkalemia, hypersensitivity reaction, hypersensitivity syndrome (includes chills, diaphoresis, fever, flushing), hypersensitivity vasculitis, hypertension, insomnia, intestinal stricture, interstitial nephritis, jaundice, leukopenia, liver function abnormal, metallic taste, necrotizing fascitis, nephrotic syndrome, neuritis, neutropenia, palpitation, pancreatitis, paresthesia, peptic ulcer, photosensitivity, proteinuria, psychosis, purpura, renal calculi, renal failure, renal impairment, retinal disturbances, seizure, somnolence, Stevens-Johnson syndrome, stomatitis, syncope, thrombocytopenia, toxic epidermal necrolysis, urine discoloration, urticaria, vaginal bleeding, vertigo, visual disturbance, weakness

Drug Interactions

Metabolism/Transport Effects None known.

Avoid Concomitant Use

Avoid concomitant use of Sulindac with any of the following: Floctafenine; Ketorolac (Nasal); Ketorolac (Systemic); NSAID (COX-2 Inhibitor); Omacetaxine

Increased Effect/Toxicity

Sulindac may increase the levels/effects of: 5-ASA Derivatives; Agents with Antiplatelet Properties; Aliskiren; Aminoglycosides; Anticoagulants; Bisphosphonate Derivatives; Collagenase (Systemic); CycloSPORINE (Systemic); Dabigatran Etexilate; Deferasirox; Desmopressin; Digoxin; Eplerenone; Haloperidol; Ibritumomab; Methotrexate; Nonsteroidal Anti-Inflammatory Agents; NSAID (COX-2 Inhibitor); Omacetaxine; PEMEtrexed; Porfimer; Potassium-Sparing Diuretics; PRALAtrexate; Quinolone Antibiotics; Rivaroxaban; Salicylates; Tenofovir; Thrombolytic Agents; Tositumomab and Iodine I 131 Tositumomab; Vancomycin; Vitamin K Antagonists

The levels/effects of Sulindac may be increased by: ACE Inhibitors; Angiotensin II Receptor Blockers; Antidepressants (Tricyclic, Tertiary Amine); Corticosteroids (Systemic); CycloSPORINE (Systemic); Dasatinib; Dimethyl Sulfoxide; Floctafenine; Glucosamine; Herbs (Anticoagulant/Antiplatelet Properties); Ibrutinib; Ketorolac (Nasal); Ketorolac (Systemic); Multivitamins/Fluoride (with ADE); Multivitamins/Minerals (with ADEK, Folate, Iron); Multivitamins/Minerals (with AE, No Iron); Nonsteroidal Anti-Inflammatory Agents; Omega-3 Fatty Acids; Pentosan Polysulfate Sodium; Pentoxifylline; Probenecid; Prostacyclin Analogues; Selective Serotonin Reuptake Inhibitors; Serotonin/Norepinephrine Reuptake Inhibitors; Sodium Phosphates; Tipranavir; Treprostinil; Vitamin E

Decreased Effect

Sulindac may decrease the levels/effects of: ACE Inhibitors; Agents with Antiplatelet Properties; Aliskiren; Angiotensin II Receptor Blockers; Beta-Blockers; Eplerenone; HydrALAZINE; Loop Diuretics; Potassium-Sparing Diuretics; Prostaglandins (Ophthalmic); Salicylates; Selective Serotonin Reuptake Inhibitors; Thiazide Diuretics

The levels/effects of Sulindac may be decreased by: Bile Acid Sequestrants; Nonsteroidal Anti-Inflammatory Agents; Salicylates

Ethanol/Nutrition/Herb Interactions

Ethanol: Avoid ethanol (may enhance gastric mucosal irritation).

Herb/Nutraceutical: Avoid alfalfa, anise, bilberry, bladderwrack, bromelain, cat's claw, celery, chamomile, coleus, cordyceps, dong quai, evening primrose, fenugreek, feverfew, garlic, ginger, ginkgo biloba, ginseng (American, Panax, Siberian), grapeseed, green tea, guggul, horse chestnut seed, horseradish, licorice, prickly ash, red clover, reishi, SAMe (S-adenosylmethionine), sweet clover, turmeric, white willow (all have additional antiplatelet activity).

Storage/Stability Store at room temperature of 15°C to 30°C (59°F to 86°F).

Mechanism of Action Reversibly inhibits cyclooxygenase-1 and 2 (COX-1 and 2) enzymes, which results in decreased formation of prostaglandin precursors; has antipyretic, analgesic, and anti-inflammatory properties

Other proposed mechanisms not fully elucidated (and possibly contributing to the anti-inflammatory effect to varying degrees), include inhibiting chemotaxis, altering lymphocyte activity, inhibiting neutrophil aggregation/activation, and decreasing proinflammatory cytokine levels.

Pharmacodynamics/Kinetics

Absorption: 90%

Distribution: Crosses blood-brain barrier (brain concentrations <4% of plasma concentrations)

Protein binding: Sulindac: 93%, sulfone metabolite: 95%, sulfide metabolite: 98%; primarily to albumin

Metabolism: Hepatic; prodrug metabolized to sulfide metabolite (active) for therapeutic effects and to sulfone metabolites (inactive); parent and inactive sulfone metabolite undergo extensive enterohepatic recirculation

Half-life elimination: Sulindac: ~8 hours; Sulfide metabolite: ~16 hours

Time to peak: Sulindac: 3-4 hours; Sulfide and sulfone metabolites: 5-6 hours

Excretion: Urine (~50%, primarily as inactive metabolites, <1% as active metabolite); feces (~25%, primarily as metabolites)

Dosage Oral:

Children: Dose not established

Adults: **Note:** Maximum daily dose: 400 mg

Osteoarthritis, rheumatoid arthritis, ankylosing spondylitis: 150 mg twice daily

Acute painful shoulder (bursitis/tendonitis): 200 mg twice daily; usual treatment: 7-14 days

Acute gouty arthritis: 200 mg twice daily; usual treatment: 7 days

Dosing adjustment in renal impairment: No dosage adjustment provided in manufacturer's labeling. However, sulindac is not recommended with advanced renal impairment; if required, decrease dose and monitor closely.

Dosing adjustment in hepatic impairment: No dosage adjustment provided in manufacturer's labeling. However, dosage reduction may be necessary; discontinue if abnormal liver function tests occur.

Dietary Considerations Drug may cause GI upset, bleeding, ulceration, perforation; take with food or milk to minimize GI upset.

Administration Should be administered with food or milk.

Monitoring Parameters Liver enzymes, BUN, serum creatinine, CBC, blood pressure; signs and symptoms of GI bleeding; ophthalmic exam (if ocular complaints develop during treatment)

Test Interactions Increased chloride (S), increased sodium (S), increased bleeding time

Dosage Forms Excipient information presented when available (limited, particularly for generics); consult specific product labeling.

Tablet, Oral:

Generic: 150 mg, 200 mg

◆ **Sumadan** *see* Sulfur and Sulfacetamide *on page 1966*

◆ **Sumadan XLT** *see* Sulfur and Sulfacetamide *on page 1966*

SUMAtriptan (soo ma TRIP tan)

Brand Names: U.S. Alsuma; Imitrex; Imitrex STATdose Refill; Imitrex STATdose System; Sumavel DosePro

Brand Names: Canada Apo-Sumatriptan; Ava-Sumatriptan; CO Sumatriptan; Dom-Sumatriptan; Imitrex; Imitrex DF; Imitrex Injection; Imitrex Nasal Spray; Mylan-Sumatriptan; PHL-Sumatriptan; PMS-Sumatriptan; Sandoz-Sumatriptan; Sumatriptan DF; Taro-Sumatriptan; Teva-Sumatriptan; Teva-Sumatriptan DF

Index Terms Sumatriptan Succinate

Pharmacologic Category Antimigraine Agent; Serotonin 5-$HT_{1B, 1D}$ Receptor Agonist

Additional Appendix Information

Antimigraine Drugs: 5-HT_1 Receptor Agonists *on page 2288*

Use

Intranasal, Oral, SubQ, Transdermal: Acute treatment of migraine with or without aura

SubQ: Acute treatment of cluster headache episodes

Pregnancy Risk Factor C

Pregnancy Considerations Adverse events were observed in animal reproduction studies. In a study using full term healthy human placentas, limited amounts of sumatriptan were found to cross the placenta (Schenker, 1995).

An overall increased risk of major congenital malformations has not been observed following first trimester exposure to sumatriptan in several studies. Pregnancy outcome information for sumatriptan is available from a pregnancy registry sponsored by GlaxoSmithKline. As of October 2008, data was available for 558 infants/fetuses exposed to sumatriptan, and seven exposed to both sumatriptan and naratriptan. The risk of major birth defects following sumatriptan exposure was 4.6% (95% CI: 2.9-7.2) (Cunnington, 2009). The pregnancy registry was closed in January, 2012 and additional information may be obtained from the manufacturer (800-336-2176). An analysis of data collected between 1995-2008 using the Swedish Medical Birth Register reported pregnancy outcomes following 5-$HT_{1B/1D}$ agonist exposure. An increased risk of major congenital malformations was not observed following sumatriptan exposure (2229 exposed during the first trimester) (Källén, 2011). An increased risk of major congenital malformations was not observed in the prospective Norwegian Mother and Child Cohort Study. The study included women with 5-$HT_{1B/1D}$ agonist exposure between 1999-2006 (n=455); of these, 217 were exposed to sumatriptan (Nezvalová-Henriksen, 2010; Nezvalová-Henriksen, 2012).

If treatment for cluster headaches is needed during pregnancy, sumatriptan may be used (Jürgens, 2009). Other agents are preferred for the initial treatment of migraine in pregnancy (Da Silva, 2012; MacGregor, 2012; Williams, 2012); however, sumatriptan may be considered if first-line agents fail (MacGregor, 2012).

Breast-Feeding Considerations The excretion of sumatriptan into breast milk was studied in five lactating women, 10-28 weeks postpartum (mean: 22.2 weeks). Sumatriptan 6 mg SubQ was administered and maternal milk and blood samples were collected over 8 hours after the dose. Sumatriptan was detected in breast milk. Maximum concentrations in the maternal blood (mean: 80.2 mcg/L; 0.25 hours after the dose) and milk (mean: 87.2 mcg/L; 2.5 hours after the dose) were similar. However, the amount of sumatriptan an infant would be exposed to following breast-feeding is considered to be small (although the mean milk-to-plasma ratio is ~4.9, weight-adjusted doses estimates suggest breast-fed infants receive 3.5% of a maternal dose). Expressing and discarding the milk for 8-12 hours after a single dose is suggested to reduce the amount present even further (Wojnar-Horton, 1996). Breast-feeding is not recommended by some manufacturers; however, according to other sources if treatment is needed, breast-feeding does not need to be discontinued (Jürgens, 2009; MacGregor, 2012).

Contraindications Hypersensitivity to sumatriptan or any component of the formulation, including allergic contact dermatitis to the transdermal patch; patients with ischemic heart disease or signs or symptoms of ischemic heart disease (including Prinzmetal's angina, angina pectoris, myocardial infarction, silent myocardial ischemia); cerebrovascular syndromes (including strokes, transient ischemic attacks); peripheral vascular disease (including ischemic bowel disease); uncontrolled hypertension; use within 24 hours of ergotamine derivatives; use within 24 hours of another 5-HT_1 agonist; concurrent administration or within 2 weeks of discontinuing an MAO type A inhibitors (oral, transdermal, and nasal sumatriptan only; see Warnings/Precautions); management of hemiplegic or basilar migraine; Wolff-Parkinson-White syndrome or arrhythmias associated with other cardiac accessory conduction pathway disorders (injectable Imitrex and transdermal only); severe hepatic impairment (oral, transdermal, and nasal sumatriptan, and injectable Imitrex only); not for I.V. administration

Warnings/Precautions Sumatriptan is only indicated for the acute treatment of migraine or cluster headache (product dependent); not indicated for migraine prophylaxis, or for the treatment of hemiplegic or basilar migraine. Acute migraine agents (eg, triptans, opioids, ergotamine, or a combination of the agents) used for 10 or more days per month may lead to worsening of headaches (medication overuse headache); withdrawal treatment may be necessary in the setting of overuse. May cause CNS depression, such as dizziness, weakness, or drowsiness, which may impair physical or mental abilities; patients must be cautioned about performing tasks which require mental alertness (eg, operating machinery or driving). If a patient does not respond to the first dose, the diagnosis of migraine or cluster headache should be reconsidered; rule out underlying neurologic disease in patients with atypical headache and in patients with no prior history of migraine or cluster headache. Cardiac events (coronary artery vasospasm, transient ischemia, myocardial infarction, ventricular tachycardia/fibrillation, cardiac arrest and death), cerebral/subarachnoid hemorrhage, and stroke have been reported with 5-HT_1 agonist administration. Patients who experience sensations of chest pain/pressure/tightness or symptoms suggestive of angina following dosing should be evaluated for coronary artery disease or Prinzmetal's angina before receiving additional doses; if dosing is resumed and similar symptoms recur, monitor with ECG. Do not give to patients with risk factors for CAD until a cardiovascular evaluation has been performed; if evaluation is satisfactory, the healthcare provider should administer the first dose (consider ECG monitoring) and cardiovascular status should be periodically evaluated.

Significant elevation in blood pressure, including hypertensive crisis, has also been reported on rare occasions in patients with and without a history of hypertension; use is contraindicated in patients with uncontrolled hypertension. Vasospasm-related reactions have been reported other than coronary artery vasospasm. Peripheral vascular ischemia, colonic ischemia with abdominal pain and bloody diarrhea, splenic infarction, and Raynaud syndrome have occurred. Transient and permanent blindness and significant partial vision loss have been very rarely reported. Use with caution in patients with a history of seizure disorder or in patients with a lowered seizure threshold. Use the oral formulation with caution (and with dosage limitations) in patients with hepatic impairment where treatment is necessary and advisable. Presystemic clearance of orally administered sumatriptan is reduced in hepatic impairment, leading to increased plasma concentrations; dosage reduction of the oral product is recommended. Non-oral routes of administration (nasal, subcutaneous formulations) do not undergo similar hepatic first-pass metabolism and are not expected to result in significantly altered pharmacokinetics in patients with hepatic impairment. Use of the oral, nasal, transdermal, or Imitrex injectable is contraindicated in severe hepatic impairment. Allergic contact dermatitis may occur with use of transdermal patch; erythematous plaque and/or erythemato-vesicular or erythemato-bullous eruptions may develop. Erythema alone is common and not by itself an indication of sensitization. Discontinue use if allergic contact dermatitis is suspected. Patients sensitized from use of transdermal system may develop systemic sensitization or other systemic reactions if sumatriptan-containing products are taken by other routes (oral, subcutaneous); if treatment with sumatriptan by other routes is required, first dose should be taken under close medical supervision. Do not apply transdermal patch in areas near or over electrically-active implantable or body-worn medical devices (eg, implantable cardiac pacemaker, body-worn insulin pump, implantable deep brain stimulator);patch contains metal parts and must be removed before magnetic resonance imaging (MRI) procedures.

Potentially significant drug-drug interactions may exist, requiring dose or frequency adjustment, additional monitoring, and/or selection of alternative therapy. Serotonin syndrome may occur with triptans, particularly when used concomitantly with other serotonergic drugs; symptoms (eg, mental status changes, tachycardia, hyperthermia, nausea, vomiting, diarrhea, hyperreflexia, incoordination) typically occur minutes to hours after initiation/dose increase of a serotonergic drug. Discontinue use if serotonin syndrome is suspected. Not recommended for use in elderly patients; older adults are at a higher risk for coronary artery disease and may be more likely to have reduced hepatic function.

Adverse Reactions

Injection:

>10%:

Central nervous system: Paresthesia (5% to 14%), dizziness (12%), localized warm feeling (11%)

Local: Injection site reaction (≤86%; includes bleeding, bruising, swelling, and erythema)

1% to 10%:

Cardiovascular: Flushing (7%), chest discomfort (2% to 5%)

Central nervous system: Burning sensation (7%), feeling of heaviness (7%), pressure sensation (7%), feeling of tightness (5%), drowsiness (3%), feeling strange (2%), headache (2%), tight feeling in head (2%), anxiety (1%), cold sensation (1%), malaise (1%)

Dermatologic: Diaphoresis (2%)

Gastrointestinal: Nausea and vomiting (4%), sore throat (3%), abdominal distress (1%), dysphagia (1%)

Neuromuscular & skeletal: Neck pain (5%), numbness (5%), weakness (5%), jaw pain (2%), myalgia (2%), muscle cramps (1%)

Ophthalmic: Visual disturbance (1%)

Respiratory: Nasal signs and symptoms (2%), bronchospasm (1%)

Nasal spray:

>10%: Gastrointestinal: Unpleasant taste (13% to 24%), nausea (11% to 13%), vomiting (11% to 13%)

1% to 10%:

Central nervous system: Dizziness (1% to 2%)

Gastrointestinal: Sore throat (1% to 2%)

Respiratory: Nasal signs and symptoms (2% to 4%)

Tablet:

1% to 10%:

Cardiovascular: Hot and cold flashes (2% to 3%, placebo 2%), chest pain (1% to 2%), palpitations (1%), syncope (1%)

Central nervous system: Paresthesia (3% to 5%), sensation of pressure (neck/throat/jaw: 2% to 3%; nonspecified: 1% to 3%, placebo 2%), burning sensation (1%), dizziness (>1%), drowsiness (>1%), malaise (2% to 3%), headache (>1%), pain (nonspecified; 1% to 2%, placebo 1%), vertigo (<1% to 2%), migraine (>1%), sleepiness (>1%), hyperacusis (1%), numbness (1%)

Gastrointestinal: Diarrhea (1%), nausea (>1%), vomiting (>1%), reduced salivation (>1%)

Genitourinary: Hematuria (1%)

Hematologic & oncologic: Hemolytic anemia (1%), hemorrhage (ear: 1%; nose/throat: 1%)

Hypersensitivity: Hypersensitivity reaction (1%)

Neuromuscular & skeletal: Myalgia (1%)

Otic: Hearing loss (1%), tinnitus (1%)

Respiratory: Allergic rhinitis (1%), dyspnea (1%), rhinitis (1%), sinusitis (1%), upper respiratory tract inflammation (1%)

Transdermal system:

>10%: Local: Localized pain (26%)

1% to 10%:

Central nervous system: Localized warm feeling (6%), feeling abnormal (paresthesia, warm/cold sensation: 2%), sensation of pressure (chest/neck/throat/jaw: 2%)

Dermatologic: Skin discoloration (application site: 3% to 5%), allergic contact dermatitis (4%), skin vesicle (application site: 3%)

Hematologic & oncologic: Bruise (application site: 1% to 2%)

Local: Localized pruritus (8%), localized irritation (4%)

<1%: Skin erosion (application site)

Route unspecified: <1%: (Limited to important or life-threatening): Abdominal aortic aneurysm, abnormal hepatic function tests, accommodation disturbance, acute renal failure, anaphylactoid reaction, anaphylaxis, anemia, angioedema, atrial fibrillation, cardiac arrhythmia, cardiomyopathy, cerebral ischemia, cerebrovascular accident, colonic ischemia, coronary artery vasospasm, cyanosis, deafness, dystonic reaction, ECG changes, fluid retention, hallucination, heart block, hemorrhage (nose/throat), hematuria, hemolytic anemia, hypersensitivity reaction, hypertensive crisis, hypertension, hypotension, increased intracranial pressure, increased serum transaminases, increased thyroid stimulating hormone level, intestinal obstruction, ischemic colitis, muscle rigidity, myocardial infarction, myocardial ischemia (transient), optic neuropathy (ischemic), pancytopenia, phlebitis, Prinzmetal angina, psychomotor disturbance, pulmonary embolism, Raynaud's phenomenon, retinal blood vessel occlusion (artery), retinal thrombosis, seizure, serotonin syndrome, shock, skin photosensitivity, subarachnoid hemorrhage, syncope, giant-cell arteritis, thrombocytopenia, thrombophlebitis, thrombosis, vasculitis, ventricular fibrillation, ventricular tachycardia, vision loss

Drug Interactions

Metabolism/Transport Effects None known.

Avoid Concomitant Use

Avoid concomitant use of SUMAtriptan with any of the following: Ergot Derivatives; MAO Inhibitors

Increased Effect/Toxicity

SUMAtriptan may increase the levels/effects of: Antipsychotics; Ergot Derivatives; Metoclopramide; Serotonin Modulators

The levels/effects of SUMAtriptan may be increased by: Antipsychotics; Ergot Derivatives; MAO Inhibitors

Decreased Effect There are no known significant interactions involving a decrease in effect.

Storage/Stability

Alsuma: Store at 25°C (77°F); excursions permitted between 15°C and 30°C (59°F and 86°F); do not refrigerate. Protect from light.

Imitrex injectable, tablet, nasal spray: Store at 2°C to 30°C (36°F to 86°F). Protect from light.

Sumavel DosePro: Store at 20°C to 25°C (68°F to 77°F); excursions permitted between 15°C and 30°C (59°F and 86°F); do not freeze.

Zecuity: Store at 20°C to 25°C (68°F to 77°F); excursions permitted between 15°C and 30°C (59°F and 86°F); do not refrigerate or freeze.

Mechanism of Action Selective agonist for serotonin (5-HT_{1B} and 5-HT_{1D} receptors) in cranial arteries; causes vasoconstriction and reduces neurogenic inflammation associated with antidromic neuronal transmission correlating with relief of migraine

Pharmacodynamics/Kinetics

Onset of action: Oral: ~30 minutes; Nasal: ~15-30 minutes; SubQ: ~10 minutes

Distribution: V_d: 2.4 L/kg

Protein binding: 14% to 21%

Metabolism: Hepatic, primarily via MAO-A isoenzyme; extensive first-pass metabolism following oral administration

Bioavailability: Nasal: 17% (compared to SubQ); Oral: 15%; SubQ: 97% ± 16%

Half-life elimination: ~2-3 hours

Time to peak, serum: Oral: 2-2.5 hours; SubQ: 12 minutes (range: 4-20 minutes); Transdermal patch: ~1 hour

Excretion:

Nasal spray: Urine (42% of total dose as indole acetic acid metabolite; 3% of total dose as unchanged drug)

Oral: Urine (~60% of total dose, mostly as indole acetic acid metabolite; 3% of total dose as unchanged drug); feces (~40%)

SubQ: Urine (38% of total dose as indole acetic acid metabolite; 22% of total dose as unchanged drug)

Transdermal patch: Urine (69% of total dose as indole acetic acid metabolite; 11% of total dose as unchanged drug)

Dosage

Adults:

Oral: A single dose of 25 mg, 50 mg, or 100 mg (taken with fluids). If a satisfactory response has not been obtained at 2 hours, a second dose may be administered. Results from clinical trials show that initial doses of 50 mg and 100 mg are more effective than doses of 25 mg, and that 100 mg doses do not provide a greater effect than 50 mg and may have increased incidence of side effects. Although doses of up to 300 mg/day have been studied, the total daily dose should not exceed 200 mg. The safety of treating an average of >4 headaches in a 30-day period have not been established.

Intranasal: A single dose of 5 mg, 10 mg, or 20 mg administered in one nostril. A 10 mg dose may be achieved by administering a single 5 mg dose in each nostril. If headache returns, the dose may be repeated once after 2 hours, not to exceed a total daily dose of 40 mg. In clinical trials, a greater number of patients responded to initial doses of 20 mg versus 5 or 10 mg. The safety of treating an average of >4 headaches in a 30-day period has not been established.

SubQ: Initial: Up to 6 mg; may repeat if needed ≥1 hour after initial dose (maximum: Two 6 mg injections per 24-hour period). However, controlled clinical trials have failed to document a benefit with administration of a second 6 mg dose in nonresponders.

Transdermal patch: Initial: Apply one patch (provides 6.5 mg per 4 hour); if necessary, may apply a second patch no sooner than 2 hours after activation of the first patch (maximum: 2 patches per 24-hour period). The safety of using >4 transdermal systems in 1 month has not been established.

Elderly: Use is not recommended (due to increased potential for adverse effects).

Dosage adjustment in renal impairment: No dosage adjustment provided in manufacturer's labeling (has not been studied). However, dosage adjustment not expected due to extensive metabolism to inactive agents.

Dosage adjustment in hepatic impairment:

Mild-to-moderate hepatic impairment:

Oral: Bioavailability of oral sumatriptan is increased with liver disease. If treatment is needed, do not exceed single doses of 50 mg.

Nasal spray: No dosage adjustment provided in manufacturer's labeling (has not been studied). However, because the spray does not undergo first-pass metabolism, levels would not be expected to be altered.

Subcutaneous: No dosage adjustment necessary.

Transdermal patch: No dosage adjustment provided in the manufacturer's labeling (has not been studied).

Severe hepatic impairment: Oral, nasal, subcutaneous (limited to Imitrex injection, per prescribing information), and transdermal formulations are contraindicated with severe hepatic impairment.

Administration Should be administered as soon as symptoms appear.

Intranasal: Each nasal spray unit is preloaded with 1 dose; **do not** test the spray unit before use; remove unit from plastic pack when ready to use; while sitting down, gently blow nose to clear nasal passages; keep head upright and close one nostril gently with index finger; hold container with other hand, with thumb supporting bottom and index and middle fingers on either side of nozzle;

insert nozzle into nostril about 1/2 inch; close mouth; take a breath through nose while releasing spray into nostril by pressing firmly on blue plunger; remove nozzle from nostril; keep head level for 10-20 seconds and gently breathe in through nose and out through mouth; **do not breathe deeply**

SubQ: Not for I.M. or I.V. use. Needle penetrates 1/4 inch of skin; use in areas of the body with adequate skin and subcutaneous thickness. Alsuma™ is a prefilled single-use autoinjector device.

Needleless administration (Sumavel® DosePro®): Administer to the abdomen (>2 inches from the navel) or thigh; not for I.M. or I.V. administration. Do not administer to other areas of the body (eg, arm). Device is for single use only, discard after use; do not use if the tip of the device is tilted or broken.

Transdermal: Apply transdermal system to dry intact, non-irritated skin on the upper arm or thigh on a site that is relatively hair free and without scars, tattoos, abrasions, or other skin conditions (ie, generalized skin irritation, eczema, psoriasis, melanoma, contact dermatitis); secure with medical tape if needed. Do not apply to a previous application site until the site remains erythema free for at least 3 days. After application, the activation button must be pushed, and the red light emitting diode (LED) will turn on; the system will stop operating when dosing is completed and the LED will turn off, signaling that the system can be removed; if the LED turns off before 4 hours, dosing has stopped and the system can be removed. If headache relief is incomplete, a second system can be applied to a different site, if >2 hours have elapsed since the first system was applied. Patient should not swim, bathe, or shower while wearing patch. After use, fold the system so the adhesive side sticks to itself and discard away from children and pets. The system contains lithium-manganese dioxide batteries; dispose in accordance with state and local regulations.

Monitoring Parameters Headache severity, blood pressure, signs/symptoms suggestive of angina; perform a cardiovascular evaluation in triptan-naïve patients who have multiple cardiovascular risk factors (eg, increased age, diabetes, hypertension, smoking, obesity, strong family history of CAD), monitor ECG with first dose in patients with multiple cardiovascular risk factors who have a negative cardiovascular evaluation and consider periodic cardiovascular evaluation in such patients if they are intermittent long-term users.

Product Availability Zecuity (transdermal system): FDA approved January 2013; availability anticipated in fourth quarter of 2013. Refer to prescribing information for additional information.

Dosage Forms Excipient information presented when available (limited, particularly for generics); consult specific product labeling.

Device, Subcutaneous, as succinate [strength expressed as base]:
- Sumavel DosePro: 6 mg/0.5 mL (0.5 mL)

Solution, Nasal:
- Imitrex: 5 mg/actuation (1 ea); 20 mg/actuation (1 ea)
- Generic: 5 mg/actuation (1 ea); 20 mg/actuation (1 ea)

Solution, Subcutaneous, as succinate:
- Generic: 6 mg/0.5 mL (0.5 mL)

Solution, Subcutaneous, as succinate [strength expressed as base]:
- Alsuma: 6 mg/0.5 mL (0.5 mL)
- Imitrex: 6 mg/0.5 mL (0.5 mL)
- Imitrex STATdose Refill: 4 mg/0.5 mL (0.5 mL); 6 mg/0.5 mL (0.5 mL)
- Imitrex STATdose System: 4 mg/0.5 mL (0.5 mL); 6 mg/0.5 mL (0.5 mL)
- Generic: 4 mg/0.5 mL (0.5 mL); 6 mg/0.5 mL (0.5 mL)

Solution, Subcutaneous, as succinate [strength expressed as base, preservative free]:
- Generic: 6 mg/0.5 mL (0.5 mL)

Tablet, Oral, as succinate [strength expressed as base]:
- Imitrex: 25 mg, 50 mg, 100 mg
- Generic: 25 mg, 50 mg, 100 mg

Extemporaneous Preparations A 5 mg/mL oral liquid preparation made from tablets and one of three different vehicles (Ora-Sweet®, Ora-Sweet® SF, or Syrpalta® syrups). **Note:** Ora-Plus® Suspending Vehicle is used with Ora-Sweet® or Ora-Sweet® SF to facilitate dispersion of the tablets (Ora-Plus® is not necessary if Syrpalta® is the vehicle). Crush nine 100 mg tablets in a mortar and reduce to a fine powder. Add 40 mL of Ora-Plus® in 5 mL increments and mix thoroughly between each addition; rinse mortar and pestle 5 times with 10 mL of Ora-Plus®, pouring into bottle each time, and add quantity of appropriate syrup (Ora-Sweet® or Ora-Sweet® SF) sufficient to make 180 mL. Store in amber glass bottles in the dark; label "shake well", "refrigerate", and "protect from light". Stable for 21 days refrigerated.

Fish DN, Beall HD, Goodwin SD, et al, "Stability of Sumatriptan Succinate in Extemporaneously Prepared Oral Liquids," *Am J Health Syst Pharm*, 1997, 54(14):1619-22.

Sumatriptan and Naproxen

(soo ma TRIP tan & na PROKS en)

Brand Names: U.S. Treximet®

Index Terms Naproxen and Sumatriptan; Naproxen Sodium and Sumatriptan; Naproxen Sodium and Sumatriptan Succinate; Sumatriptan Succinate and Naproxen; Sumatriptan Succinate and Naproxen Sodium

Pharmacologic Category Antimigraine Agent; Nonsteroidal Anti-inflammatory Drug (NSAID), Oral; Serotonin 5-$HT_{1B,\ 1D}$ Receptor Agonist

Use Acute treatment of migraine with or without aura

Pregnancy Risk Factor C

Medication Guide Available Yes

Dosage Oral: Adults: 1 tablet (sumatriptan 85 mg and naproxen 500 mg). If a satisfactory response has not been obtained at 2 hours, a second dose may be administered (maximum: 2 tablets/24 hours). **Note:** The safety of treating an average of >5 migraine headaches in a 30-day period has not been established.

Dosage adjustment in renal impairment:

Cl_{cr} ≥30 mL/minute: No dosage adjustmentprovided in manufacturer's labeling(has not been studied). Use with caution.

Cl_{cr} <30 mL/minute: Use not recommended.

Dosage adjustment in hepatic impairment: Use is contraindicated.

Additional Information Complete prescribing information should be consulted for additional detail.

Dosage Forms Excipient information presented when available (limited, particularly for generics); consult specific product labeling.

Tablet, oral:
- Treximet® 85/500: Sumatriptan 85 mg and naproxen sodium 500 mg [contains sodium 61.2 mg/tablet (~2.7 mEq/tablet)]

- ◆ **Sumatriptan DF (Can)** *see* SUMAtriptan *on page* 1969
- ◆ **Sumatriptan Succinate** *see* SUMAtriptan *on page* 1969
- ◆ **Sumatriptan Succinate and Naproxen** *see* Sumatriptan and Naproxen *on page* 1972
- ◆ **Sumatriptan Succinate and Naproxen Sodium** *see* Sumatriptan and Naproxen *on page* 1972
- ◆ **Sumavel DosePro** *see* SUMAtriptan *on page* 1969
- ◆ **Sumaxin** *see* Sulfur and Sulfacetamide *on page* 1966
- ◆ **Sumaxin TS** *see* Sulfur and Sulfacetamide *on page* 1966

SUNItinib (su NIT e nib)

Brand Names: U.S. Sutent

Brand Names: Canada Sutent

Index Terms SU011248; SU11248; Sunitinib Malate

Pharmacologic Category Antineoplastic Agent, Tyrosine Kinase Inhibitor; Vascular Endothelial Growth Factor (VEGF) Inhibitor

Use

Pancreatic neuroendocrine tumors, advanced: Treatment of progressive, well-differentiated pancreatic neuroendocrine tumors in patients with unresectable locally advanced or metastatic disease

Renal cell carcinoma, advanced: Treatment of advanced renal cell carcinoma

Gastrointestinal stromal tumor: Treatment of Gastrointestinal stromal tumor (GIST) after disease progression on or intolerance to imatinib

Unlabeled Use Treatment of advanced thyroid cancer; treatment of non-GIST soft tissue sarcomas

Pregnancy Risk Factor D

Pregnancy Considerations Animal reproduction studies have demonstrated teratogenicity, embryotoxicity, and fetal loss. Because sunitinib inhibits angiogenesis, a critical component of fetal development, adverse effects on pregnancy would be expected. Women of childbearing potential should be advised to avoid pregnancy if receiving sunitinib.

Breast-Feeding Considerations It is not known if sunitinib is excreted in human milk. Due to the potential for serious adverse reactions in the nursing infant, the decision to discontinue breast-feeding or discontinue sunitinib should take into account the benefits of treatment to the mother.

Medication Guide Available Yes

Contraindications There are no contraindications listed in the manufacturer's labeling.

Canadian labeling: Hypersensitivity to sunitinib or any component of the formulation; pregnancy

Warnings/Precautions Hazardous agent - use appropriate precautions for handling and disposal (NIOSH, 2012). **[U.S. Boxed Warning]: Hepatotoxicity, which may be severe and/or result in fatal liver failure, has been observed in clinical trials and in postmarketing surveillance.** Signs of liver failure include jaundice, elevated transaminases, and/or hyperbilirubinemia, in conjunction with encephalopathy, coagulopathy and/or renal failure. Monitor liver function tests at baseline, with each treatment cycle and if clinically indicated. Withhold treatment for grade 3 or 4 hepatotoxicity; discontinue if hepatotoxicity does not resolve. Do not reinitiate in patients with severe changes in liver function tests or other signs/symptoms of liver failure. Sunitinib has not been studied in patients with ALT or AST >2.5 times ULN (or >5 times ULN if due to liver metastases).

May cause a decrease in left ventricular ejection fraction (LVEF), including grade 3 reductions; consider obtaining LVEF evaluation prior to treatment. Mean onset of symptomatic heart failure (HF) is 22 days from treatment initiation. Interrupt therapy or decrease dose with LVEF <50% or >20% reduction from baseline. Discontinue with clinical signs and symptoms of HF. Cardiovascular events (some fatal), including symptomatic HF, myocardial disorders and cardiomyopathy have been reported with use. QT_c prolongation and torsade de pointes have been observed (dose dependent); a baseline and periodic ECG should be obtained; correct electrolyte abnormalities prior to treatment and monitor and correct potassium, calcium and magnesium levels during therapy; use caution in patients with a history of QT_c prolongation, with medications known to prolong the QT_c interval, or patients with pre-existing (relevant) cardiac disease, bradycardia, or electrolyte imbalance. Use with caution in patients with cardiac dysfunction; monitor for clinical signs/symptoms of HF, obtain baseline and periodic LVEF evaluation patients with MI, bypass grafts, symptomatic HF, vascular diseases (including CVA and TIA), and PE were excluded from clinical trials. May cause hypertension; monitor and control with antihypertensives if needed; interrupt therapy until hypertension is controlled for severe hypertension. Use caution and closely monitor in patients with underlying or poorly-controlled hypertension. Potentially significant drug-drug interactions may exist, requiring dose or frequency adjustment, additional monitoring, and/or selection of alternative therapy.

Hemorrhagic events have been reported including epistaxis, rectal, gingival, upper GI, urinary tract, genital, brain, wound bleeding, tumor-related, and hemoptysis/pulmonary hemorrhage; may be serious and/or fatal. Proteinuria and (rare) cases of nephrotic syndrome have been reported; discontinue treatment in patients with nephrotic syndrome. Renal impairment and/or failure resulting in death haves been reported in postmarketing experience. Microangiopathic hemolytic anemia (MAHA) and dose-limiting hypertension have been reported when sunitinib has been used in combination with bevacizumab. Impaired wound healing has been reported with sunitinib; temporarily withhold treatment for patients undergoing major surgical procedures; the optimal time to resume treatment after a procedure has not been determined. Serious and fatal gastrointestinal complications, including gastrointestinal perforation, have occurred (rarely). Pancreatitis has been observed in RCC patients; discontinue sunitinib if symptoms are present. Thyroid dysfunction (eg, hypothyroidism, hyperthyroidism, and thyroiditis) may occur; the risk for hypothyroidism appears to increase with therapy duration; hyperthyroidism, sometimes followed by hypothyroidism has also been reported; monitor thyroid function at baseline and if symptomatic. Adrenal function abnormalities have been reported; monitor for adrenal insufficiency in patients with stress such as trauma, severe infection, or who are undergoing surgery. May cause skin and/or hair depigmentation or discoloration. Reversible posterior leukoencephalopathy syndrome (RPLS) has been reported (rarely, some fatal); symptoms include confusion, headache, hypertension, lethargy, seizure, blindness and/or other vision, or neurologic disturbances; interrupt treatment and begin hypertension management. Tumor lysis syndrome (TLS), including fatalities, has been reported, predominantly in patients with RCC or GIST; risk for TLS is higher in patients with a high tumor burden prior to treatment; monitor closely; correct clinically significant dehydration and treat high uric acid levels prior to initiation of treatment. An increased incidence of fatigue, thyroid dysfunction and treatment-induced hypertension was reported in patients with renal insufficiency (Cl_{cr} ≤60 mL/minute) who received sunitinib for the treatment of renal cell cancer (Gupta, 2011). Osteonecrosis of the jaw (ONJ) has been observed with sunitinib; concurrent bisphosphonate use or dental disease may increase the risk for ONJ. If possible, avoid invasive dental procedures in patients with current or prior bisphosphonate use. Consider a dental exam and appropriate prophylactic dentistry prior to treatment initiation Dosing schedules vary by indication; some treatment regimens are continuous daily dosing; other treatment schedules are daily dosing for 4 weeks of a 6-week cycle (4 weeks on, 2 weeks off).

Adverse Reactions

>10%:

Cardiovascular: Hypertension (15% to 34%; grade 3: 4% to 13%), peripheral edema (24%), decreased left ventricular ejection fraction (11% to 16%; grades 3/4: 1% to 3%), heart failure (≤15%), chest pain (13%)

Central nervous system: Fatigue (33% to 62%), headache (≤23%), insomnia (15% to 18%), chills (14%), mouth pain (6% to 14%), depression (11%), dizziness (11%), glossalgia (11%)

Dermatologic: Skin discoloration (25% to 30%), skin rash (14% to 29%), palmar-plantar erythrodysesthesia (14% to 29%; grades 3/4: 4% to 8%), hair discoloration (7% to 29%), xeroderma (≤23%), alopecia (5% to 14%), erythema (12%), pruritus (12%)

Endocrine & metabolic: Hyperglycemia (23% to 71%), hyperuricemia (≤46%), hypocalcemia (34% to 42%), hypoalbuminemia (28% to 41%), hypophosphatemia (≤36%), hyponatremia (≤29%), hypoglycemia (17% to 22%), hypokalemia (12% to 21%), hypomagnesemia (≤19%), hyperkalemia (≤18%), hypothyroidism (4% to 16%; grades 3/4: ≤2%), hypercalcemia (13%), hypernatremia (10% to 13%)

Gastrointestinal: Diarrhea (40% to 66%), nausea (45% to 58%), increased serum lipase (17% to 56%), anorexia (33% to 48%), mucositis (29% to 48%), dysgeusia (21% to 47%), abdominal pain (39%), vomiting (34% to 39%), increased serum amylase (17% to 35%), dyspepsia (15% to 34%), constipation (20% to 23%), weight loss (16%), flatulence (14%), xerostomia (13%), gastroesophageal reflux disease (12%)

Hematologic & oncologic: Anemia (26% to 79%; grades 3/4: ≤8%), leukopenia (78%; grades 3/4: 8%), neutropenia (53% to 77%; grades 3/4: 10% to 17%), lymphocytopenia (38% to 68%; grades 3/4: ≤18%), thrombocytopenia (38% to 68%; grades 3/4: 5% to 9%), hemorrhage (18% to 37%)

Hepatic: Increased serum AST (39% to 72%; grades 3/4: 2% to 5%), increased serum alkaline phosphatase (24% to 63%; grades 3/4: 2% to 10%), increased serum ALT (39% to 61%; grades 3/4: 2% to 4%), hyperbilirubinemia (10% to 37%; grades 3/4 ≤1%)

Neuromuscular & skeletal: Increased creatine kinase (49%), limb pain (14% to 40%), weakness (22% to 34%), arthralgia (15% to 30%), back pain (≤28%), myalgia (14%)

Renal: Increased serum creatinine (12% to 70%)

Respiratory: Cough (27%), dyspnea (26%), epistaxis (21%), nasopharyngitis (14%), upper respiratory tract infection (11%)

Miscellaneous: Fever (≤22%)

1% to 10%:

Cardiovascular: Venous thrombosis (1% to 3%), deep vein thrombosis (2% to 3%), pulmonary embolism (2%)

Gastrointestinal: Hemorrhoids (10%), pancreatitis (1%)

Respiratory: Flu-like symptoms (5%)

<1% (Limited to important or life-threatening): Acute renal failure, adrenocortical insufficiency, angioedema, arterial thrombosis, atrial flutter, cardiomyopathy, cerebral hemorrhage, cerebral infarction, cerebrovascular accident, cholecystitis (particularly acalculous), coma, coronary artery dissection (aortic), erythema multiforme, esophagitis, febrile neutropenia, fistula (sometimes associated with tumor necrosis and/or regression), gastrointestinal perforation, glomerulonephritis (segmental glomerular sclerosis), hemorrhage (tumor), hepatic failure, hepatotoxicity, hypersensitivity, hyperthyroidism, hypotension, hypothyroidism (myxedema coma), infection, macrocytosis, hemolytic anemia (microangiopathic; when used in combination with bevacizumab), myocardial infarction, myopathy, necrotizing fasciitis (including of the perineum), nephrotic syndrome, neutropenic infection, osteonecrosis (jaw), pneumonitis (recall), pre-eclampsia, prolonged Q-T interval on ECG, proteinuria, pulmonary hemorrhage, pyoderma gangrenosum (including positive dechallenges), renal impairment, reversible posterior leukoencephalopathy syndrome, rhabdomyolysis, seizure, septic shock, sepsis, skin infection, Stevens-Johnson syndrome, thrombotic microangiopathy, thyroiditis, tissue necrosis (tumor), torsades de pointes, toxic epidermal necrolysis, transient ischemic attacks, tumor lysis syndrome, urinary tract infection, ventricular arrhythmia, wound healing impairment

Drug Interactions

Metabolism/Transport Effects Substrate of CYP3A4 (major); **Note:** Assignment of Major/Minor substrate status based on clinically relevant drug interaction potential; **Inhibits** BCRP, P-glycoprotein

Avoid Concomitant Use

Avoid concomitant use of SUNItinib with any of the following: BCG; Bevacizumab; Bosutinib; Conivaptan; Fusidic Acid (Systemic); Highest Risk QTc-Prolonging Agents; Ivabradine; Mifepristone; Natalizumab; PAZOPanib; Pimecrolimus; Pomalidomide; Silodosin; St Johns Wort; Tacrolimus (Topical); Temsirolimus; Tofacitinib; Vaccines (Live); VinCRIStine (Liposomal)

Increased Effect/Toxicity

SUNItinib may increase the levels/effects of: Afatinib; Bevacizumab; Bisphosphonate Derivatives; Bosutinib; Colchicine; Dabigatran Etexilate; Everolimus; Highest Risk QTc-Prolonging Agents; Leflunomide; Moderate Risk QTc-Prolonging Agents; Natalizumab; PAZOPanib; P-glycoprotein/ABCB1 Substrates; Pomalidomide; Prucalopride; Rivaroxaban; Silodosin; Tofacitinib; Topotecan; Vaccines (Live); VinCRIStine (Liposomal); Vitamin K Antagonists

The levels/effects of SUNItinib may be increased by: Antifungal Agents (Azole Derivatives, Systemic); Bevacizumab; Conivaptan; CYP3A4 Inhibitors (Moderate); CYP3A4 Inhibitors (Strong); Dasatinib; Denosumab; Fusidic Acid (Systemic); Ivabradine; Ivacaftor; Luliconazole; Mifepristone; Pimecrolimus; QTc-Prolonging Agents (Indeterminate Risk and Risk Modifying); Roflumilast; Simeprevir; Tacrolimus (Topical); Temsirolimus; Trastuzumab

Decreased Effect

SUNItinib may decrease the levels/effects of: BCG; Cardiac Glycosides; Coccidioidin Skin Test; Sipuleucel-T; Vaccines (Inactivated); Vaccines (Live); Vitamin K Antagonists

The levels/effects of SUNItinib may be decreased by: Bosentan; CYP3A4 Inducers (Strong); Dabrafenib; Deferasirox; Echinacea; St Johns Wort; Tocilizumab

Ethanol/Nutrition/Herb Interactions

Food: Grapefruit juice may increase the levels/effects of sunitinib. Food has no effect on the bioavailability of sunitinib. Management: Avoid grapefruit juice.

Herb/Nutraceutical: St John's wort may increase metabolism and decrease sunitinib concentrations. Management: Avoid St John's wort.

Storage/Stability Store at 25°C (77°F); excursions are permitted between 15°C to 30°C (59°F to 86°F).

Mechanism of Action Exhibits antitumor and antiangiogenic properties by inhibiting multiple receptor tyrosine kinases, including platelet-derived growth factors (PDGFRα and PDGFRβ), vascular endothelial growth factors (VEGFR1, VEGFR2, and VEGFR3), FMS-like tyrosine kinase-3 (FLT3), colony-stimulating factor type 1 (CSF-1R), and glial cell-line-derived neurotrophic factor receptor (RET).

Pharmacodynamics/Kinetics

Distribution: V_d/F: 2230 L

Protein binding: Sunitinib: 95%; SU12662: 90%

Metabolism: Hepatic; primarily metabolized by CYP3A4 to the N-desethyl metabolite SU12662 (active)

Half-life elimination: Terminal: Sunitinib: 40-60 hours; SU12662: 80-110 hours

Time to peak, plasma: 6-12 hours

Excretion: Feces (61%); urine (16%)

Dosage Note: Dosage modifications should be done in increments or decrements of 12.5 mg; individualize based on safety and tolerability.

Gastrointestinal stromal tumor (GIST): Adults: Oral: 50 mg once daily for 4 weeks of a 6-week treatment cycle (4 weeks on, 2 weeks off)

GIST unlabeled dosing: Adults: Oral: 37.5 mg once daily, continuous daily dosing (George, 2009, *EJC*)

Pancreatic neuroendocrine tumors, advanced (PNET): Adults: Oral: 37.5 mg once daily, continuous daily dosing (maximum daily dose used in clinical trials: 50 mg)

Renal cell cancer, advanced (RCC): Adults: Oral: 50 mg once daily for 4 weeks of a 6-week treatment cycle (4 weeks on, 2 weeks off)

Soft tissue sarcoma, non-GIST (unlabeled use): Adults: Oral: 37.5 mg once daily, continuous daily dosing (George, 2009, *JCO*)

Thyroid cancer, refractory (unlabeled use): Adults: Oral: 50 mg once daily for 4 weeks of a 6-week treatment cycle (4 weeks on, 2 weeks off) (Cohen, 2008; Ravaud, 2008)

Dosage adjustment with concurrent CYP3A4 inhibitor: Avoid concomitant administration with strong CYP3A4 inhibitors (eg, clarithromycin, erythromycin, itraconazole, ketoconazole, nefazodone, protease inhibitors, telithromycin, voriconazole); if concomitant administration with a strong CYP3A4 inhibitor cannot be avoided, consider a dose reduction to a minimum of 37.5 mg/day (GIST, RCC) or 25 mg/day (PNET).

Dosage adjustment with concurrent CYP3A4 inducer: Avoid concomitant administration with strong CYP3A4 inducers (eg, carbamazepine, dexamethasone, phenobarbital, phenytoin, rifampin, St John's wort); if concomitant administration with a strong CYP3A4 inducer cannot be avoided, consider a dosage increase (with careful monitoring for toxicity) to a maximum of 87.5 mg/day (GIST, RCC) or 62.5 mg/day (PNET).

Dosage adjustment for toxicity: Dosage modifications should be done in increments or decrements of 12.5 mg; individualize based on safety and tolerability.

Cardiac toxicity:

Ejection fraction <50% and >20% below baseline without evidence of CHF: Interrupt treatment and/or reduce dose

LV dysfunction with CHF clinical manifestations: Discontinue treatment

Severe hypertension: Temporarily interrupt treatment until hypertension is controlled

Nephrotic syndrome or pancreatitis: Discontinue treatment

Reversible posterior leukoencephalopathy (RPLS) or thrombotic microangiopathy: Temporarily withhold treatment; after resolution, may resume with discretion.

Dosage adjustment in renal impairment:

Mild, moderate, or severe impairment: No initial dosage adjustment necessary; subsequent adjustments may be needed based on safety and tolerance.

ESRD on hemodialysis: No initial dosage adjustment necessary; subsequent dosage increases (up to 2 fold) may be required due to reduced (47%) exposure.

Dosage adjustment in hepatic impairment:

Pre-existing hepatic impairment: No adjustment is necessary with mild-to-moderate (Child-Pugh class A or B) hepatic impairment; not studied in patients with severe (Child-Pugh class C) hepatic impairment. Studies excluded patients with ALT or AST >2.5 x ULN, or if due to liver metastases, ALT or AST >5 x ULN.

Hepatotoxicity during treatment: Hepatic adverse events ≥ grade 3 or 4: Withhold treatment; discontinue if hepatotoxicity does not resolve. Do not reinitiate in patients with severe changes in liver function tests or other signs/symptoms of liver failure.

Dietary Considerations Avoid grapefruit juice.

Administration May be administered with or without food.

Hazardous agent; use appropriate precautions for handling and disposal (NIOSH, 2012).

Monitoring Parameters LVEF, baseline (and periodic with cardiac risk factors), ECG (12-lead; baseline and periodic), blood pressure; adrenal function CBC with differential and platelets (prior to each treatment cycle), liver function tests (baseline, with each cycle and if clinically indicated), serum chemistries including magnesium, phosphate, and potassium (prior to each treatment cycle), urinalysis (for proteinuria development or worsening); consider dental exam prior to treatment initiation; symptoms of hypothyroidism, hyperthyroidism, or thyroiditis

Thyroid function testing (Hamnvik, 2011):

Pre-existing levothyroxine therapy: Obtain baseline TSH levels, then monitor every 4 weeks until levels and levothyroxine dose are stable, then monitor every 2 months

Without pre-existing thyroid hormone replacement: TSH at baseline, then every 4 weeks for 4 months, then every 2-3 months

Additional Information Hand-foot skin reaction (HFSR) observed with tyrosine kinase inhibitors (TKIs) is distinct from hand-foot syndrome (palmar-plantar erythrodysesthesia) associated with traditional chemotherapy agents; HFSR due to TKIs is localized with defined hyperkeratotic lesions; symptoms include burning, dysesthesia, paresthesia, or tingling on the palms/soles, and generally occur within the first 2-4 weeks of treatment; pressure and flexor areas may develop blisters (callus-like), dry/cracked skin, edema, erythema, desquamation, or hyperkeratosis (Appleby, 2011).

HFSR management (Lacouture, 2008): The following treatments may be used in addition to the recommended dosage modifications. Prior to treatment initiation, a pedicure is recommended to remove hyperkeratotic areas/calluses, which may predispose to HFSR; avoid vigorous exercise/activities which may stress hands or feet. During therapy, patients should reduce exposure to hot water (may exacerbate hand-foot symptoms); avoid constrictive footwear and excessive skin friction. Patients may also wear thick cotton gloves or socks and should wear shoes with padded insoles. Grade 1 HFSR may be relieved with moisturizing creams, cotton gloves and socks (at night) and/or keratolytic creams such as urea (20% to 40%) or salicylic acid (6%). Apply topical steroid (eg, clobetasol ointment) twice daily to erythematous areas of Grade 2 HFSR; topical anesthetics (eg, lidocaine 2%) and then systemic analgesics (if appropriate) may be used for pain control. Resolution of acute erythema may result in keratotic areas which may be softened with keratolytic agents.

Dosage Forms Excipient information presented when available (limited, particularly for generics); consult specific product labeling.

Capsule, Oral:

Sutent: 12.5 mg, 25 mg, 50 mg

Extemporaneous Preparations Hazardous agent: Use appropriate precautions for handling and disposal.

A 10 mg/mL sunitinib oral suspension may be made with capsules and a 1:1 mixture of Ora-Sweet and Ora-Plus. Empty the contents of three 50 mg sunitinib capsules into a mortar; add small portions of vehicle and mix to a uniform paste. Mix while adding vehicle in incremental proportions to 15 mL. Transfer to amber plastic bottle and label "shake well". This suspension maintains an average concentration of 96% to 106% (of the original concentration) at room temperature or refrigerated for up to 60 days in plastic amber prescription bottles.

Navid F, Christensen R, Minkin P, et al, "Stability of Sunitinib in Oral Suspension," *Ann Pharmacother*, 2008, 42(7):962-6.

- ◆ **Sunitinib Malate** *see* SUNItinib *on page 1973*
- ◆ **Supartz** *see* Hyaluronate and Derivatives *on page 1000*
- ◆ **Supeudol (Can)** *see* OxyCODONE *on page 1535*
- ◆ **Suphedrine [OTC]** *see* Pseudoephedrine *on page 1746*
- ◆ **Suplasyn (Can)** *see* Hyaluronate and Derivatives *on page 1000*
- ◆ **Supprelin LA** *see* Histrelin *on page 998*
- ◆ **Suprax** *see* Cefixime *on page 369*
- ◆ **Suprax® (Can)** *see* Cefixime *on page 369*
- ◆ **Suprenza** *see* Phentermine *on page 1632*
- ◆ **Suprep® Bowel Prep Kit** *see* Sodium Sulfate, Potassium Sulfate, and Magnesium Sulfate *on page 1929*
- ◆ **Surfaxin** *see* Lucinactant *on page 1254*
- ◆ **Sur-Q-Lax [OTC]** *see* Docusate *on page 644*
- ◆ **Survanta** *see* Beractant *on page 245*
- ◆ **Survanta® (Can)** *see* Beractant *on page 245*
- ◆ **Sustiva** *see* Efavirenz *on page 688*
- ◆ **Sutent** *see* SUNItinib *on page 1973*
- ◆ **Suxamethonium Chloride** *see* Succinylcholine *on page 1954*
- ◆ **SwabFlush Saline Flush** *see* Sodium Chloride *on page 1914*
- ◆ **Sween Cream® [OTC]** *see* Vitamin A and Vitamin D (Topical) *on page 2202*
- ◆ **Syeda™** *see* Ethinyl Estradiol and Drospirenone *on page 785*
- ◆ **Sylatron** *see* Peginterferon Alfa-2b *on page 1594*
- ◆ **Symax Duotab** *see* Hyoscyamine *on page 1026*
- ◆ **Symax FasTabs** *see* Hyoscyamine *on page 1026*
- ◆ **Symax-SL** *see* Hyoscyamine *on page 1026*
- ◆ **Symax-SR** *see* Hyoscyamine *on page 1026*
- ◆ **Symbicort®** *see* Budesonide and Formoterol *on page 287*
- ◆ **SymlinPen 60** *see* Pramlintide *on page 1697*
- ◆ **SymlinPen 120** *see* Pramlintide *on page 1697*
- ◆ **Symmetrel** *see* Amantadine *on page 92*
- ◆ **Sympt-X [OTC]** *see* Glutamine *on page 962*
- ◆ **Sympt-X G.I. [OTC]** *see* Glutamine *on page 962*
- ◆ **Synacthen** *see* Cosyntropin *on page 495*
- ◆ **Synacthen® Depot (Can)** *see* Cosyntropin *on page 495*
- ◆ **Synagis** *see* Palivizumab *on page 1553*
- ◆ **Synagis® (Can)** *see* Palivizumab *on page 1553*
- ◆ **Synalar** *see* Fluocinolone (Topical) *on page 878*
- ◆ **Synalar® (Can)** *see* Fluocinolone (Topical) *on page 878*
- ◆ **Synalar (Cream)** *see* Fluocinolone (Topical) *on page 878*
- ◆ **Synalar (Ointment)** *see* Fluocinolone (Topical) *on page 878*
- ◆ **Synalar TS** *see* Fluocinolone (Topical) *on page 878*
- ◆ **Synalgos®-DC** *see* Dihydrocodeine, Aspirin, and Caffeine *on page 611*
- ◆ **Synarel** *see* Nafarelin *on page 1417*
- ◆ **Synarel® (Can)** *see* Nafarelin *on page 1417*
- ◆ **Synera®** *see* Lidocaine and Tetracaine *on page 1215*
- ◆ **Synercid®** *see* Quinupristin and Dalfopristin *on page 1768*
- ◆ **Synphasic (Can)** *see* Ethinyl Estradiol and Norethindrone *on page 793*
- ◆ **Synribo** *see* Omacetaxine *on page 1501*
- ◆ **Synthroid** *see* Levothyroxine *on page 1206*
- ◆ **Synthroid® (Can)** *see* Levothyroxine *on page 1206*
- ◆ **Synvisc** *see* Hyaluronate and Derivatives *on page 1000*
- ◆ **Synvisc-One** *see* Hyaluronate and Derivatives *on page 1000*
- ◆ **Syprine** *see* Trientine *on page 2125*
- ◆ **Syprine® (Can)** *see* Trientine *on page 2125*
- ◆ **T_3 Sodium (error-prone abbreviation)** *see* Liothyronine *on page 1222*
- ◆ **T_3/T_4 Liotrix** *see* Liotrix *on page 1222*
- ◆ **T_4** *see* Levothyroxine *on page 1206*
- ◆ **T-20** *see* Enfuvirtide *on page 704*
- ◆ **T-91825** *see* Ceftaroline Fosamil *on page 378*
- ◆ **Tabloid** *see* Thioguanine *on page 2045*
- ◆ **Taclonex®** *see* Calcipotriene and Betamethasone *on page 312*

Tacrolimus (Systemic) (ta KROE li mus)

Brand Names: U.S. Astagraf XL; Hecoria; Prograf

Brand Names: Canada Advagraf; Prograf

Index Terms FK506

Pharmacologic Category Calcineurin Inhibitor; Immunosuppressant Agent

Use Organ rejection prophylaxis:

U.S. labeling:

Astagraf XL: Prevention of organ rejection in kidney transplant recipients

Hecoria: Prevention of organ rejection in heart, kidney, and liver transplant recipients

Prograf: Prevention of organ rejection in heart, kidney, and liver transplant recipients

Canadian labeling:

Advagraf: Prevention of organ rejection in kidney transplant recipients

Prograf: Prevention of organ rejection in heart, kidney, or liver transplant recipients; treatment of refractory rejection in kidney or liver transplant recipients; treatment of active rheumatoid arthritis in adult patients nonresponsive to disease-modifying antirheumatic drug (DMARD) therapy or when DMARD therapy is inappropriate

Unlabeled Use Prevention of organ rejection in lung, small bowel transplant recipients; prevention and treatment of graft-versus-host disease (GVHD) in allogeneic hematopoietic stem cell transplantation

Pregnancy Risk Factor C

Pregnancy Considerations Adverse events were observed in animal reproduction studies. Tacrolimus crosses the human placenta and is measurable in the cord blood, amniotic fluid, and newborn serum. Tacrolimus concentrations in the placenta may be higher than the maternal serum (Jain, 1997). Infants with lower birth weights have been found to have higher tacrolimus concentrations (Bramham, 2013). Transient neonatal hyperkalemia and renal dysfunction have been reported.

Tacrolimus pharmacokinetics are altered during pregnancy. Whole blood concentrations decrease as pregnancy progresses; however, unbound concentrations increase. Measuring unbound concentrations may be preferred, especially in women with anemia or hypoalbuminemia. If unbound concentration measurement is not available, interpretation of whole blood concentrations should account for RBC count and serum albumin concentration (Hebert, 2013; Zheng, 2012).

In general, women who have had a kidney transplant should be instructed that fertility will be restored following the transplant but that pregnancy should be avoided for ~2 years. Tacrolimus may be used as an immunosuppressant during pregnancy. The risk of infection, hypertension, and pre-eclampsia may be increased in pregnant women who have had a kidney transplant (EPBG, 2002).

The National Transplantation Pregnancy Registry (NTPR) is a registry which follows pregnancies which occur in maternal transplant recipients or those fathered by male transplant recipients. The NTPR encourages reporting of pregnancies following solid organ transplant by contacting them at 877-955-6877.

Breast-Feeding Considerations Tacrolimus is excreted into breast milk; concentrations are variable and lower than that of the maternal serum. The low bioavailability of tacrolimus following oral absorption may also decrease the amount of exposure to a nursing infant (Bramham, 2013; French, 2003; Gardiner, 2006). In one study, tacrolimus serum concentrations in the infants did not differ between those who were bottle fed or breast-fed (all infants were exposed to tacrolimus throughout pregnancy) (Bramham, 2013). Available information suggests that tacrolimus exposure to the nursing infant is ≤0.5% of the weight-adjusted maternal dose (Bramham, 2013; French, 2003; Gardiner, 2006). The manufacturer recommends that nursing be discontinued, taking into consideration the importance of the drug to the mother.

Medication Guide Available Yes

Contraindications Hypersensitivity to tacrolimus or any component of the formulation

Warnings/Precautions Hazardous agent: Use appropriate precautions for handling and disposal (NIOSH, 2012). **[U.S. Boxed Warning]: Risk of developing infections (including bacterial, viral [including CMV], fungal, and protozoal infections [including opportunistic infections]) is increased.** Latent viral infections may be activated, including BK virus (associated with polyoma virus-associated nephropathy [PVAN]) and JC virus (associated with progressive multifocal leukoencephalopathy [PML]); may result in serious adverse effects. Immunosuppression increases the risk for CMV viremia and/or CMV disease; the risk of CMV disease is increased for patients who are CMV-seronegative prior to transplant and receive a graft from a CMV-seropositive donor. Consider reduction in immunosuppression if PVAN, PML, CMV viremia and/or CMV disease occurs. **[U.S. Boxed Warning]: Immunosuppressive therapy may result in the development of lymphoma and other malignancies (predominantly skin malignancies).** The risk for new-onset diabetes and insulin-dependent post-transplant diabetes mellitus (PTDM) is increased with tacrolimus use after transplantation, including in patients without pretransplant history of diabetes mellitus; insulin dependence may be reversible; monitor blood glucose frequently; risk is increased in African-American and Hispanic kidney transplant patients. Nephrotoxicity (acute or chronic) has been reported, especially with higher doses; to avoid excess nephrotoxicity do not administer simultaneously with other nephrotoxic drugs (eg, sirolimus, cyclosporine). Neurotoxicity may occur especially when used in high doses; tremor headache, coma and delirium have been reported and are associated with serum concentrations. Seizures may also occur. Posterior reversible encephalopathy syndrome (PRES) has been reported; symptoms (altered mental status, headache, hypertension, seizures, and visual disturbances) are reversible with dose reduction or discontinuation of therapy; stabilize blood pressure and reduce dose with suspected or confirmed PRES diagnosis.

Pure red cell aplasia (PRCA) has been reported in patients receiving tacrolimus. Use with caution in patients with risk factors for PRCA including parvovirus B19 infection, underlying disease, or use of concomitant medications associated with PRCA (eg, mycophenolate). Discontinuation of therapy should be considered with diagnosis of PRCA. Monitoring of serum concentrations (trough for oral therapy) is essential to prevent organ rejection and reduce drug-related toxicity. Use caution in renal or hepatic dysfunction, dosing adjustments may be required. Delay initiation of therapy in kidney transplant patients if postoperative oliguria occurs; begin therapy no sooner than 6 hours and within 24 hours post-transplant, but may be delayed until renal function has recovered. Mild-to-severe hyperkalemia may occur; monitor serum potassium levels. Hypertension may commonly occur; antihypertensive treatment may be necessary; avoid use of potassium-sparing diuretics due to risk of hyperkalemia; concurrent use of calcium channel blockers may require tacrolimus dosage adjustment. Gastrointestinal perforation may occur; all reported cases were considered to be a complication of transplant surgery or accompanied by infection, diverticulum, or malignant neoplasm. Myocardial hypertrophy has been reported (rare). Prolongation of the QT/QTc and torsade de pointes may occur; avoid use in patients with congenital long QT syndrome. Consider obtaining electrocardiograms and monitoring electrolytes (magnesium, potassium, calcium) periodically during treatment in patients with congestive heart failure, bradyarrhythmias, those taking certain antiarrhythmic medications or other medicinal products that lead to QT prolongation, and those with electrolyte disturbances such as hypokalemia, hypocalcemia, or hypomagnesemia. Potentially significant drug-drug/drug-food interactions may exist, requiring dose or frequency adjustment, additional monitoring, and/or selection of alternative therapy. In liver transplantation, the tacrolimus dose and target range should be reduced to minimize the risk of nephrotoxicity when used in combination with everolimus. Extended release tacrolimus in combination with sirolimus is not recommended in renal transplant patients; the safety and efficacy of immediate release tacrolimus in combination with sirolimus has not been established in this patient population. Concomitant use was associated with increased mortality, graft loss, and hepatic artery thrombosis in liver transplant patients, as well as increased risk of renal impairment, wound healing complications, and PTDM in heart transplant recipients.

Immediate release and extended release capsules are NOT interchangeable or substitutable. The extended release formulation is a once daily preparation; and immediate release is intended for twice daily administration. Serious adverse events, including organ rejection may occur if inadvertently substituted. **[U.S. Boxed Warning]: Extended release tacrolimus was associated with increased mortality in female liver transplant recipients; the use of extended release tacrolimus is not recommended in liver transplantation.** Mortality at 12 months was 18% in females who received extended release tacrolimus compared to 8% for females who received regular release tacrolimus. Each mL of injection contains polyoxyl 60 hydrogenated castor oil (HCO-60) (200 mg) and dehydrated alcohol USP 80% v/v. Anaphylaxis has been reported with the injection, use should be reserved for those patients not able to take oral medications. Patients should not be immunized with live vaccines during or shortly after treatment and should avoid close contact with recently vaccinated (live vaccine) individuals. Oral formulations contain lactose; the Canadian labeling does not recommend use of these products in patients who may be lactose intolerant (eg, Lapp lactase deficiency, glucose-galactose malabsorption, galactose intolerance). **[U.S. Boxed Warning]: Should be administered under the supervision of a physician experienced in immunosuppressive therapy and organ transplantation in a facility appropriate for monitoring and managing therapy.**

Adverse Reactions As reported for kidney, liver, and heart transplantation:

≥15%:

Cardiovascular: Hypertension (13% to 89%), peripheral edema (11% to 36%), chest pain (19%), edema (<15% to 18%), pericardial effusion (heart transplant 15%; Astagraf XL <15%)

Central nervous system: Headache (10% to 64%), insomnia (9% to 64%), pain (24% to 63%), paresthesia (<15% to 40%), dizziness (<15% to 19%), fatigue (2% to 16%)

Dermatologic: Pruritus (<15% to 36%), skin rash (10% to 24%)

Endocrine & metabolic: Diabetes mellitus (post-transplant; kidney transplant 20% to 75%; heart transplant 13% to 22%; liver transplant 11% to 18%), hyperglycemia (16% to 70%), hypertriglyceridemia (65%), hypoglycemia (<15% to 61%), hypercholesterolemia (<15% to 57%), hypophosphatemia (5% to 49%), hypomagnesemia (3% to 48%), hyperkalemia (13% to 45%), hyperlipidemia (7% to 34%), hypokalemia (13% to 29%)

Gastrointestinal: Diarrhea (25% to 72%), abdominal pain (29% to 59%; Astagraf XL <15%), nausea (13% to 46%), constipation (14% to 40%), anorexia (7% to 34%), vomiting (13% to 29%), dyspepsia (18% to 28%; Astagraf XL <15%)

Genitourinary: Urinary tract infection (1% to 34%), oliguria (<15% to 19%)

Hematologic & oncologic: Anemia (5% to 50%; hemoglobin <10 g/dL 65%), leukopenia (11% to 48%), leukocytosis (8% to 32%), thrombocytopenia (14% to 24%)

Hepatic: Abnormal hepatic function tests (6% to 36%), ascites (7% to 27%)

Infection: Infection (15% to 45%), bacterial infection (8% to 41%), cytomegalovirus disease (heart transplant 32%; kidney transplant 6% to 12%), serious infection (19% to 24%)

Local: Postoperative wound complication (kidney transplant 28%)

Neuromuscular & skeletal: Tremor (15% to 56%; heart transplant 15%), weakness (11% to 52%), back pain (17% to 30%), arthralgia (25%; Astagraf XL <15%)

Renal: Renal function abnormality (36% to 56%), increased serum creatinine (16% to 45%), increased blood urea nitrogen (12% to 30%)

Respiratory: Pleural effusion (30% to 36%), respiratory tract infection (22% to 34%), dyspnea (5% to 29%), atelectasis (5% to 28%), cough (<15% to 18%), bronchitis (17%)

Miscellaneous: Fever (19% to 48%), postoperative pain (kidney transplant 29%), graft complications (kidney transplant 14% to 24%)

<15%:

Cardiovascular: Angina pectoris, atrial fibrillation, atrial flutter, bradycardia, cardiac arrest, cardiac arrhythmia, cardiac failure, cardiorespiratory arrest, cerebral infarction, cerebral ischemia, decreased heart rate, deep vein thrombophlebitis, deep vein thrombosis, ECG abnormality (QRS or ST segment or T wave), flushing, hemorrhagic stroke, hypertrophic cardiomyopathy, hypotension, ischemic heart disease, myocardial infarction, orthostatic hypotension, peripheral vascular disease, phlebitis, syncope, tachycardia, thrombosis, vasodilatation, ventricular premature contractions

Central nervous system: Abnormal dreams, abnormality in thinking, agitation, amnesia, anxiety, aphasia, ataxia, brain disease, carpal tunnel syndrome, chills, confusion, convulsions, depression, drowsiness, emotional lability, excessive crying, falling, flaccid paralysis, hallucination, hypertonia, hypoesthesia, mental status changes, mood elevation, myasthenia, myoclonus, nervousness, neurotoxicity, nightmares, paresis, peripheral neuropathy, psychosis, seizure, vertigo, voice disorder, writing difficulty

Dermatologic: Acne vulgaris, alopecia, bruise, cellulitis, condyloma acuminatum, dermal ulcer, dermatitis (including fungal), dermatological reaction, diaphoresis, exfoliative dermatitis, hypotrichosis, skin discoloration, skin photosensitivity

Endocrine & metabolic: Acidosis, albuminuria, alkalosis, anasarca, Cushing's syndrome, decreased serum bicarbonate, decreased serum iron, dehydration, gout, hirsutism, hypercalcemia, hyperphosphatemia, hyperuricemia, hypervolemia, hypocalcemia, hyponatremia, increased gamma-glutamyl transferase, increased lactate dehydrogenase, weight changes

Gastrointestinal: Gastroenteritis (2% to 7%), aphthous stomatitis, cholangitis, colitis, delayed gastric emptying, duodenitis, dysphagia, enlargement of abdomen, esophagitis (including ulcerative), flatulence, gastric ulcer, gastritis, gastroesophageal reflux disease, gastrointestinal hemorrhage, gastrointestinal perforation, hernia, hiccups, increased appetite, intestinal obstruction, oral candidiasis, pancreatic disease (pseudocyst), pancreatitis (including hemorrhagic and necrotizing), peritonitis, rectal disease, stomach cramps, stomatitis

Genitourinary: Anuria, bladder spasm, cystitis, dysuria, hematuria, nocturia, proteinuria, toxic nephrosis, urinary frequency, urinary incontinence, urinary retention, urinary urgency, vaginitis

Hematologic & oncologic: Blood coagulation disorder, decreased prothrombin time, hemolytic anemia, hemorrhage, hypochromic anemia, hypoproteinemia, increased hematocrit, increased INR, Kaposi's sarcoma, malignant neoplasm of bladder, malignant neoplasm of thyroid (papillary), neutropenia, pancytopenia, polycythemia, skin neoplasm

Hepatic: Cholestatic jaundice, hepatic injury, hepatitis (including acute, chronic, and granulomatous), hyperbilirubinemia, increased liver enzymes, increased serum alkaline phosphatase, jaundice

Hypersensitivity: Hypersensitivity reaction

Infection: Polyoma virus infection (≤5%), abscess, Epstein Barr virus infection, herpes simplex infection, sepsis, tinea versicolor

Local: Localized phlebitis

Neuromuscular & skeletal: Arthropathy, leg cramps, muscle spasm, muscle weakness of the extremities, myalgia, neuropathy (including compression), osteopenia, osteoporosis

Ophthalmic: Amblyopia, blurred vision, conjunctivitis, visual disturbance

Otic: Hearing loss, otalgia, otitis externa, otitis media, tinnitus

Renal: Acute renal failure, hydronephrosis, renal disease (BK nephropathy), renal tubular necrosis

Respiratory: Allergic rhinitis, asthma, emphysema, flu-like symptoms, pharyngitis, pneumonia, pneumothorax, pulmonary disease, pulmonary edema, pulmonary infiltrates, respiratory depression, respiratory failure, rhinitis, sinusitis

Miscellaneous: Wound healing impairment

Postmarketing and/or case reports (limited to important or life-threatening): Adult respiratory distress syndrome, agranulocytosis, anaphylactoid reaction, anaphylaxis, angioedema, basal cell carcinoma, biliary tract disease (stenosis), blindness, cerebrovascular accident, coma, deafness, decreased serum fibrinogen, delirium, disseminated intravascular coagulation, dysarthria, graft versus host disease (acute and chronic), hemiparesis, hemolytic-uremic syndrome, hemorrhagic cystitis, hepatic cirrhosis, hepatic failure, hepatic necrosis, hepatic veno-occlusive disease, hepatosplenic T-cell lymphomas, hepatotoxicity, hyperpigmentation, interstitial pulmonary disease, leukemia, leukoencephalopathy, liver steatosis, lymphoproliferative disorder (post-transplant or related to EBV), malignant melanoma, multi-organ failure, mutism, optic atrophy, osteomyelitis, photophobia, polyarthritis, progressive multifocal leukoencephalopathy (PML), prolonged partial thromboplastin time, prolonged Q-T interval on ECG, pulmonary hypertension, pure red cell aplasia, quadriplegia, reversible posterior leukoencephalopathy syndrome, rhabdomyolysis, septicemia, squamous cell carcinoma, status epilepticus, Stevens-Johnson syndrome, supraventricular extrasystole, supraventricular tachycardia, thrombocytopenic purpura, thrombotic thrombocytopenic purpura, torsades de pointes, toxic epidermal necrolysis, venous thrombosis, ventricular fibrillation

Note: Calcineurin inhibitor-induced hemolytic uremic syndrome/thrombotic thrombocytopenic purpura/thrombotic microangiopathy (HUS/TTP/TMA) have been reported (with concurrent sirolimus).

Drug Interactions

Metabolism/Transport Effects Substrate of CYP3A4 (major), P-glycoprotein; **Note:** Assignment of Major/Minor substrate status based on clinically relevant drug interaction potential; **Inhibits** CYP3A4 (weak), P-glycoprotein

Avoid Concomitant Use

Avoid concomitant use of Tacrolimus (Systemic) with any of the following: BCG; Bosutinib; CloZAPine; Conivaptan; Crizotinib; CycloSPORINE (Systemic); Enzalutamide; Eplerenone; Fusidic Acid (Systemic); Grapefruit Juice; Mifepristone; Natalizumab; PAZOPanib; Pimecrolimus; Pimozide; Pomalidomide; Potassium-Sparing Diuretics; Silodosin; Sirolimus; Tacrolimus (Topical); Temsirolimus; Tofacitinib; Topotecan; Vaccines (Live); VinCRIStine (Liposomal)

Increased Effect/Toxicity

Tacrolimus (Systemic) may increase the levels/effects of: Afatinib; ARIPiprazole; Bosutinib; CloZAPine; Colchicine; CycloSPORINE (Systemic); Dabigatran Etexilate; Dofetilide; Everolimus; Fenofibrate and Derivatives; Fosphenytoin; Highest Risk QTc-Prolonging Agents; Leflunomide; Lomitapide; Moderate Risk QTc-Prolonging Agents; Natalizumab; PAZOPanib; P-glycoprotein/ABCB1 Substrates; Phenytoin; Pimozide; Pomalidomide; Prucalopride; Rivaroxaban; Silodosin; Sirolimus; Temsirolimus; Tofacitinib; Topotecan; Vaccines (Live); VinCRIStine (Liposomal)

The levels/effects of Tacrolimus (Systemic) may be increased by: Antidepressants (Serotonin Reuptake Inhibitor/Antagonist); Boceprevir; Calcium Channel Blockers (Dihydropyridine); Calcium Channel Blockers (Nondihydropyridine); Chloramphenicol; Clotrimazole (Oral); Conivaptan; Crizotinib; CycloSPORINE (Systemic); CYP3A4 Inhibitors (Moderate); CYP3A4 Inhibitors (Strong); Danazol; Dasatinib; Denosumab; Eplerenone; Ertapenem; Fluconazole; Fusidic Acid (Systemic); Grapefruit Juice; Itraconazole; Ivacaftor; Ketoconazole (Systemic); Levofloxacin (Systemic); Luliconazole; Macrolide Antibiotics; MetroNIDAZOLE (Systemic); Mifepristone; P-glycoprotein/ABCB1 Inhibitors; Pimecrolimus; Posaconazole; Potassium-Sparing Diuretics; Protease Inhibitors; Proton Pump Inhibitors; Ranolazine; Roflumilast; Sirolimus; Tacrolimus (Topical); Telaprevir; Temsirolimus; Trastuzumab; Voriconazole

Decreased Effect

Tacrolimus (Systemic) may decrease the levels/effects of: BCG; Coccidioidin Skin Test; Sipuleucel-T; Vaccines (Inactivated); Vaccines (Live)

The levels/effects of Tacrolimus (Systemic) may be decreased by: Bosentan; Caspofungin; Cinacalcet; CYP3A4 Inducers (Strong); Dabrafenib; Deferasirox; Echinacea; Efavirenz; Enzalutamide; Fosphenytoin; Mitotane; P-glycoprotein/ABCB1 Inducers; Phenytoin; Rifamycin Derivatives; Sirolimus; St Johns Wort; Temsirolimus; Tocilizumab

Ethanol/Nutrition/Herb Interactions

Ethanol: Alcohol may increase the rate of release of extended-release tacrolimus and adversely affect tacrolimus safety and/or efficacy. Management: Avoid alcohol.

Food: Food decreases rate and extent of absorption. High-fat meals have most pronounced effect (37% and 25% decrease in AUC, respectively, and 77% and 25% decrease in C_{max}, respectively, for immediately release and extended release formulations). Grapefruit juice, a CYP3A4 inhibitor, may increase serum level and/or toxicity of tacrolimus. Management: Administer with or without food (immediate release), but be consistent. Administer extended release on an empty stomach. Avoid concurrent use of grapefruit juice.

Herb/Nutraceutical: St John's wort may reduce tacrolimus serum concentrations. Management: Avoid St John's wort.

Preparation for Administration Hazardous agent - use appropriate precautions for handling and disposal (NIOSH, 2012).

Injection: Dilute with 5% dextrose injection or 0.9% sodium chloride injection to a final concentration between 0.004 mg/mL and 0.02 mg/mL.

Storage/Stability

Injection: Prior to dilution, store at 5°C to 25°C (41°F to 77°F). Following dilution, stable for 24 hours in D_5W or NS in glass or polyethylene containers.

Capsules:

Astagraf XL, Prograf: Store at 25°C (77°F); excursions permitted between 15°C and 30°C (59°F and 86°F).

Hecoria: Store at 20°C to 25°C (68°F to 77°F).

Mechanism of Action Suppresses cellular immunity (inhibits T-lymphocyte activation), by binding to an intracellular protein, FKBP-12 and complexes with calcineurin dependent proteins to inhibit calcineurin phosphatase activity

Pharmacodynamics/Kinetics

Absorption: Better in resected patients with a closed stoma; unlike cyclosporine, clamping of the T-tube in liver transplant patients does not alter trough concentrations or AUC; Oral: Incomplete and variable; the rate and extent of absorption is affected by food and may be most pronounced with a high-fat meal. Oral absorption may be variable in stem cell transplant patients with mucositis due to the conditioning regimen.

Distribution: V_d: Children: 0.5-4.7 L/kg; Adults: 0.55-2.47 L/kg

Protein binding: ~99% primarily to albumin and alpha$_1$-acid glycoprotein glycoprotein

Metabolism: Extensively hepatic via CYP3A4 to eight possible metabolites (major metabolite, 31-demethyl tacrolimus, shows same activity as tacrolimus *in vitro*)

Bioavailability: Oral: Children: 7% to 55%, Adults: 7% to 32%; Absolute: Unknown

Half-life elimination:

Immediate release: Variable, 23-46 hours in healthy volunteers; 2.1-36 hours in transplant patients

Extended release: 34.5-41 hours

Time to peak: 0.5-6 hours

Excretion: Feces (~93%); urine (<1% as unchanged drug)

Dosage

Children:

Liver transplant:

Oral: Immediate release: Initial: 0.15-0.20 mg/kg/day in 2 divided doses, given every 12 hours (titrate to target trough concentrations)

I.V.: Initial: 0.03-0.05 mg/kg/day as a continuous infusion

Note: The initial postoperative dose of tacrolimus should begin no sooner than 6 hours after liver and heart transplant and within 24 hours of kidney transplant (but may be delayed until renal function has recovered). Adjunctive therapy with corticosteroids is recommended early post-transplant. I.V. route should only be used in patients not able to take oral medications and continued only until oral medication can be tolerated; anaphylaxis has been reported with I.V. administration. If switching from I.V. to oral, the oral dose should be started 8-12 hours after stopping the infusion. Patients without pre-existing renal or hepatic dysfunction have required (and tolerated) higher doses than adults to achieve similar blood concentrations. It is recommended that therapy be initiated at the **high end** of the recommended adult I.V. and oral dosing ranges; dosage adjustments may be required.

Prevention of graft-vs-host disease (GVHD) (unlabeled use): Oral, I.V.: Refer to adult dosing.

Adults:

Prevention of organ rejection in transplant recipients: **Note:** The initial postoperative dose of tacrolimus (immediate release) should begin no sooner than 6 hours after liver and heart transplant and within 24 hours of kidney transplant (but may be delayed until renal function has recovered); titrate to target trough concentrations. Adjunctive therapy with corticosteroids is recommended early post-transplant. I.V. route should only be used in patients not able to take oral medications and continued only until oral medication can be tolerated; anaphylaxis has been reported with I.V. administration. If switching from I.V. to oral, the oral dose should be started 8-12 hours after stopping the infusion.

Liver transplant:

Oral: Immediate release: Initial: 0.1-0.15 mg/kg/day in 2 divided doses, given every 12 hours (titrate to target trough concentrations)

I.V.: Initial: 0.03-0.05 mg/kg/day as a continuous infusion

Heart transplant: Use in combination with azathioprine or mycophenolate mofetil is recommended.

Oral: Immediate release: Initial: 0.075 mg/kg/day in 2 divided doses, given every 12 hours (titrate to target trough concentrations)

I.V.: Initial: 0.01 mg/kg/day as a continuous infusion

Kidney transplant: Use in combination with azathioprine or mycophenolate mofetil is recommended. **Note:** African-American patients may require larger doses to attain trough concentration.

Oral:

U.S. labeling:

Immediate release (Hecoria, Prograf): Initial: 0.2 mg/kg/day in combination with azathioprine or 0.1 mg/kg/day in combination with mycophenolate mofetil; titrate to target trough concentrations. Administer in 2 divided doses, given every 12 hours.

Extended release (Astagraf XL):

With basiliximab induction (prior to or within 48 hours of transplant completion): 0.15 mg/kg once daily (in combination with corticosteroids and mycophenolate); titrate to target trough concentrations

Without basiliximab induction: Preoperative dose (administer within 12 hours prior to reperfusion): 0.1 mg/kg

Without basiliximab induction: Postoperative dosing (administer at least 4 hours after preoperative dose and within 12 hours of reperfusion): 0.2 mg/kg once daily (in combination with corticosteroids and mycophenolate); titrate to target trough concentrations

Conversion from I.V. to extended release: Administer the first oral extended release dose 8-12 hours after discontinuation of I.V. tacrolimus

Canadian labeling:

Immediate release (Prograf): Initial: 0.2-0.3 mg/kg/day in 2 divided doses, given every 12 hours in combination with corticosteroids and other immunosuppressive agents; titrate to target trough concentrations

Extended release (Advagraf): Initial: 0.15-0.2 mg/kg once daily; titrate to target trough concentrations. Administer in combination with corticosteroids and mycophenolate mofetil (MMF) in *de novo* kidney transplant recipients. Antibody induction therapy should also be used.

Conversion from immediate release to extended release: Initiate extended release treatment using previously established total daily dose of immediate release. Administer once daily.

I.V.: Initial: 0.03-0.05 mg/kg/day as a continuous infusion

Graft-versus-host disease (GVHD) (unlabeled use):

Adults:

Prevention:

Oral: Convert from I.V. to immediate release oral dose (1:4 ratio): Multiply total daily I.V. dose times 4 and administer in 2 divided oral doses per day, every 12 hours (Uberti, 1999; Yanik, 2000).

I.V.: Initial: 0.03 mg/kg/day (based on lean body weight) as continuous infusion. Treatment should begin at least 24 hours prior to stem cell infusion and continued only until oral medication can be tolerated (Przepiorka, 1999; Yanik, 2000).

Treatment:

Oral: Immediate release: 0.06 mg/kg twice daily (Furlong, 2000; Przepiorka, 1999)

I.V.: Initial: 0.03 mg/kg/day (based on lean body weight) as continuous infusion (Furlong, 2000; Przepiorka, 1999)

Rheumatoid arthritis: Canadian labeling (not in U.S. labeling): Oral: Immediate release: 3 mg once daily; carefully monitor serum creatinine during therapy

Dosing adjustment in renal impairment: Systemic therapy: Evidence suggests that lower doses should be used; patients should receive doses at the lowest value of the recommended I.V. and oral dosing ranges; further reductions in dose below these ranges may be required. May also require dose reductions due to nephrotoxicity.

Kidney transplant: Tacrolimus therapy in patients with postoperative oliguria should begin no sooner than 6 hours and within 24 hours (immediate release) or 48 hours (extended release) post-transplant, but may be delayed until renal function displays evidence of recovery.

Hemodialysis: Not removed by hemodialysis; supplemental dose is not necessary.

Peritoneal dialysis: Significant drug removal is unlikely based on physiochemical characteristics.

Dosing adjustment in hepatic impairment: Systemic therapy: Use of tacrolimus in liver transplant recipients experiencing post-transplant hepatic impairment may be associated with increased risk of developing renal insufficiency related to high whole blood levels of tacrolimus. The presence of moderate-to-severe hepatic dysfunction (serum bilirubin >2 mg/dL; Child-Pugh score ≥10) appears to affect the metabolism of tacrolimus. The half-life of the drug was prolonged and the clearance reduced after I.V. administration. The bioavailability of tacrolimus was also increased after oral administration. The higher plasma concentrations as determined by ELISA, in patients with severe hepatic dysfunction are probably due to the accumulation of metabolites of lower activity. These patients should be monitored closely and dosage adjustments should be considered. Some evidence indicates that lower doses could be used in these patients.

Dietary Considerations Capsule: Administer immediate release with or without food; be consistent with timing and composition of meals, food decreases bioavailability. Administer extended release on an empty stomach 1 hour before or 2 hours after a meal. Avoid grapefruit juice. Avoid alcohol.

Administration

I.V.: If I.V. administration is necessary, administer by continuous infusion only. Do not use PVC tubing when administering diluted solutions. Tacrolimus is usually intended to be administered as a continuous infusion over 24 hours. Do not mix with solutions with a pH ≥9 (eg, acyclovir or ganciclovir) due to chemical degradation of tacrolimus (use different ports in multilumen lines). Do not alter dose with concurrent T-tube clamping. Adsorption of the drug to PVC tubing may become clinically significant with low concentrations.

Oral:

Immediate release: Administer with or without food; be consistent with timing and composition of meals if GI intolerance occurs and administration with food becomes necessary (per manufacturer). If dosed once daily, administer in the morning. If dosed twice daily, doses should be 12 hours apart. If the morning and evening doses differ, the larger dose (differences are never >0.5-1 mg) should be given in the morning. If dosed 3 times daily, separate doses by 8 hours.

Combination therapy with everolimus for liver transplantation: Administer tacrolimus at the same time as everolimus.

Extended release: Administer on an empty stomach at least 1 hour before or 2 hours after a meal. Swallow whole, do not chew, crush, or divide. Take once daily in the morning at a consistent time each day. Missed doses may be taken up to 14 hours after scheduled time; if >14 hours, resume at next regularly scheduled time; do not double a dose to make up for a missed dose.

Hazardous agent - use appropriate precautions for handling and disposal (NIOSH, 2012).

Monitoring Parameters Renal function, hepatic function, serum electrolytes (calcium, magnesium, potassium), glucose and blood pressure, measure 3 times/week for first few weeks, then gradually decrease frequency as patient stabilizes. Whole blood concentrations should be used for monitoring (trough for oral therapy). Signs/symptoms of anaphylactic reactions during I.V. infusion should also be monitored. Patients should be monitored during the first 30 minutes of the infusion, and frequently thereafter. Monitor for QT prolongation; consider echocardiographic evaluation in patients who develop renal failure, electrolyte abnormalities, or clinical manifestations of ventricular dysfunction.

Tacrolimus serum levels may be falsely elevated in infected liver transplant patients due to interference from β-galactosidase antibodies.

Reference Range

Heart transplant: Typical whole blood trough concentrations:
- Months 1-3: 10-20 ng/mL
- Months ≥4: 5-15 ng/mL

Kidney transplant: Whole blood trough concentrations:

Immediate release:

In combination with azathioprine:
- Months 1-3: 7-20 ng/mL
- Months 4-12: 5-15 ng/mL

In combination with mycophenolate mofetil/IL-2 receptor antagonist (eg, daclizumab): Months 1-12: 4-11 ng/mL

Extended release:

With basiliximab induction:
- Days 1-60: 5-17 ng/mL
- Month 3-12: 4-12 ng/mL

Without induction:
- Days 1-60: 6-20 ng/mL
- Month 3-12: 6-14 ng/mL

Liver transplant: Whole blood trough concentrations:

Months 1-12: 5-20 ng/mL

Recommended therapeutic ranges when administered in combination with everolimus for liver transplant (Zortress product labeling, 2013): By 3 weeks after first everolimus dose and through month 12 post-transplant: 3-5 ng/mL

Prevention of graft-versus-host disease (unlabeled use): 10-20 ng/mL (Uberti, 1999) although some institutions use a lower limit of 5 ng/mL and an upper limit of 15 ng/mL (Przepiorka, 1999; Yanik, 2000)

Dosage Forms Excipient information presented when available (limited, particularly for generics); consult specific product labeling.

Capsule, Oral:
- Hecoria: 0.5 mg, 1 mg, 5 mg
- Prograf: 0.5 mg, 1 mg, 5 mg
- Generic: 0.5 mg, 1 mg, 5 mg

Capsule Extended Release 24 Hour, Oral:
- Astagraf XL: 0.5 mg, 1 mg, 5 mg

Solution, Intravenous:
- Prograf: 5 mg/mL (1 mL) [contains alcohol, usp, cremophor el]

Dosage Forms: Canada Excipient information presented when available (limited, particularly for generics); consult specific product labeling.

Capsule, oral:
- Advagraf®: 0.5 mg, 1 mg, 3 mg, 5 mg

Extemporaneous Preparations Hazardous agent: Use appropriate precautions for handling and disposal.

A 0.5 mg/mL tacrolimus oral suspension may be made with immediate release capsules and a 1:1 mixture of Ora-Plus® and Simple Syrup, N.F. Mix the contents of six 5 mg tacrolimus capsules with quantity of vehicle sufficient to make 60 mL. Store in glass or plastic amber prescription bottles; label "shake well". Stable for 56 days at room temperature (Esquivel, 1996; Foster, 1996).

A 1 mg/mL tacrolimus oral suspension may be made with immediate release capsules, sterile water, Ora-Plus®, and Ora-Sweet®. Pour the contents of six 5 mg capsules into a plastic amber prescription bottle. Add ~5 mL of sterile water and agitate bottle until drug disperses into a slurry. Add equal parts Ora-Plus® and Ora-Sweet® in sufficient quantity to make 30 mL. Store in plastic amber prescription bottles; label "shake well". Stable for 4 months at room temperature (Elefante, 2006).

Elefante A, Muindi J, West K, et al, "Long-Term Stability of a Patient-Convenient 1 mg/mL Suspension of Tacrolimus for Accurate Maintenance of Stable Therapeutic Levels," *Bone Marrow Transplant*, 2006, 37(8):781-4.

Esquivel C, So S, McDiarmid S, Andrews W, and Colombani PM, "Suggested Guidelines for the Use of Tacrolimus in Pediatric Liver Transplant Patients," *Transplantation*, 1996, 61(5):847-8.

Foster JA, Jacobson PA, Johnson CE, et al, "Stability of Tacrolimus in an Extemporaneously Compounded Oral Liquid (Abstract of Meeting Presentation)," *American Society of Health-System Pharmacists Annual Meeting*, 1996, 53:P-52(E).

Tacrolimus (Topical) (ta KROE li mus)

Brand Names: U.S. Protopic

Brand Names: Canada Protopic®

Pharmacologic Category Calcineurin Inhibitor; Immunosuppressant Agent; Topical Skin Product

Use Moderate-to-severe atopic dermatitis in immunocompetent patients not responsive to conventional therapy or when conventional therapy is not appropriate

Canadian labeling: Additional use (not in U.S. labeling): Maintenance therapy to prevent flares and extend flare-free intervals in patients with moderate-to-severe atopic dermatitis who are responsive to initial therapy and experiencing ≥5 flares per year

Pregnancy Risk Factor C

Pregnancy Considerations Adverse events were observed in animal reproduction studies. Tacrolimus crosses the human placenta and is measurable in the cord blood, amniotic fluid, and newborn serum following systemic use. Refer to the Tacrolimus (Systemic) monograph for additional information.

Breast-Feeding Considerations Tacrolimus is excreted into breast milk following systemic administration. Refer to the Tacrolimus (Systemic) monograph for additional information.

Medication Guide Available Yes

Contraindications Hypersensitivity to tacrolimus or any component of the formulation

Warnings/Precautions Hazardous agent - use appropriate precautions for handling and disposal (NIOSH, 2012). **[U.S. Boxed Warning]: Topical calcineurin inhibitors have been associated with rare cases of malignancy (including skin and lymphoma); therefore, it should be limited to short-term and intermittent treatment using the minimum amount necessary for the control of symptoms and only on involved areas. Use in children <2 years of age is not recommended, children ages 2-15 should only use the 0.03% ointment.** Avoid use on malignant or premalignant skin conditions (eg, cutaneous T-cell lymphoma). Should not be used in immunocompromised patients. Do not apply to areas of active bacterial or viral infection; infections at the treatment site should be cleared prior to therapy. Topical calcineurin agents are considered second-line therapies in the treatment of atopic dermatitis/eczema, and should be limited to use in patients who have failed treatment with other therapies. Patients with atopic dermatitis are predisposed to skin infections, and tacrolimus therapy has been associated with risk of developing eczema herpeticum, varicella zoster, and herpes simplex. If atopic dermatitis is not improved in <6 weeks, re-evaluate to confirm diagnosis. May be associated with development of lymphadenopathy; possible infectious causes should be investigated. Discontinue use in patients with unknown cause of lymphadenopathy or acute infectious mononucleosis. Acute renal failure has been observed (rarely) with topical use. Not recommended for use in patients with skin disease which may increase systemic absorption (eg, Netherton's syndrome). Minimize sunlight exposure during treatment. Safety not established in patients with generalized erythroderma. Safety of intermittent use for >1 year has not been established, particularly since the effect on immune system development is unknown. Should not be used in immunocompromised patients; safety and efficacy have not been evaluated.

Adverse Reactions As reported in children and adults, unless otherwise noted:

>10%:

Central nervous system: Headache (5% to 20%), fever (1% to 21%)

Dermatologic: Skin burning (43% to 58%; tends to improve as lesions resolve), pruritus (41% to 46%), erythema (12% to 28%)

Respiratory: Increased cough (children 18%)

Miscellaneous: Flu-like syndrome (23% to 31%), allergic reaction (4% to 12%)

1% to 10%:

Cardiovascular: Peripheral edema (adults 3% to 4%)

Central nervous system: Hyperesthesia (adults 3% to 7%), pain (1% to 2%)

Dermatologic: Skin tingling (2% to 8%), acne (adults 4% to 7%), localized flushing (following ethanol consumption; adults 3% to 7%), folliculitis (2% to 6%), urticaria (1% to 6%), rash (2% to 5%), pustular rash (2% to 4%), vesiculobullous rash (children 4%), contact dermatitis (3% to 4%), cyst (adults 1% to 3%), eczema herpeticum (1% to 2%), fungal dermatitis (adults 1% to 2%), sunburn (adults 1% to 2%), alopecia (adults 1%), dry skin (children 1%)

Endocrine & metabolic: Dysmenorrhea (adult females 4%)

Gastrointestinal: Diarrhea (3% to 5%), dyspepsia (adults 1% to 4%), abdominal pain (children 3%), vomiting (adults 1%), gastroenteritis (adults 2%), nausea (children 1%)

Neuromuscular & skeletal: Paresthesia (adults 3%), myalgia (adults 2% to 3%), weakness (adults 2% to 3%), arthralgia (adults 1% to 3%), back pain (adults 2%)

Ocular: Conjunctivitis (2% adults)

Otic: Otitis media (12% children)

Respiratory: Rhinitis (6% children), sinusitis (2% to 4% adults), bronchitis (2% adults), pneumonia (1% adults)

Miscellaneous: Varicella/herpes zoster (1% to 5%), lymphadenopathy (3% children)

<1% (Limited to important or life-threatening): Acute renal failure, anaphylaxis, anaphylactoid reaction, anemia, basal cell carcinoma, chest pain, hypercholesterolemia, malignant melanoma, osteomyelitis, photosensitivity reaction, seizure, septicemia, skin discoloration, squamous cell carcinoma

Drug Interactions

Metabolism/Transport Effects Substrate of CYP3A4 (minor), P-glycoprotein; **Note:** Assignment of Major/Minor substrate status based on clinically relevant drug interaction potential

Avoid Concomitant Use

Avoid concomitant use of Tacrolimus (Topical) with any of the following: CycloSPORINE (Systemic); Immunosuppressants; Sirolimus; Temsirolimus

Increased Effect/Toxicity

Tacrolimus (Topical) may increase the levels/effects of: Alcohol (Ethyl); CycloSPORINE (Systemic); Immunosuppressants; Sirolimus; Temsirolimus

The levels/effects of Tacrolimus (Topical) may be increased by: Antidepressants (Serotonin Reuptake Inhibitor/Antagonist); Antifungal Agents (Azole Derivatives, Systemic); Calcium Channel Blockers (Nondihydropyridine); CycloSPORINE (Systemic); Danazol; Fluconazole; Grapefruit Juice; Macrolide Antibiotics; Protease Inhibitors; Sirolimus; Temsirolimus

Decreased Effect There are no known significant interactions involving a decrease in effect.

Ethanol/Nutrition/Herb Interactions Ethanol: Localized flushing (redness, warm sensation) may occur at application site of topical tacrolimus following ethanol consumption.

Storage/Stability Store at room temperature of 25°C (77°F); excursions permitted to 15°C to 30°C (59°F to 86°F).

Mechanism of Action Suppresses cellular immunity (inhibits T-lymphocyte activation), by binding to an intracellular protein, FKBP-12 and complexes with calcineurin dependent proteins to inhibit calcineurin phosphatase activity

Pharmacodynamics/Kinetics

Absorption: Minimally absorbed; serum concentrations range from undetectable to 20 ng/mL (~2 ng/mL in majority of adult patients studied)

Bioavailability: ~0.5%

Dosage Topical: Atopic dermatitis (moderate-to-severe):

Treatment:

Children ≥2-15 years: Apply thin layer of 0.03% ointment to affected area twice daily; rub in gently and completely. Discontinue use when symptoms have cleared. If no improvement within 6 weeks, patients should be re-examined to confirm diagnosis.

Children >15 years and Adults: Apply thin layer of 0.03% or 0.1% ointment to affected area twice daily; rub in gently and completely. Discontinue use when symptoms have cleared. If no improvement within 6 weeks, patients should be re-examined to confirm diagnosis.

Maintenance therapy (Canadian labeling; not in U.S. labeling):

Children ≥2-15 years: Apply one application (thin layer of 0.03% ointment) to areas usually affected twice a week, allowing 2-3 days between applications (eg, one application on Monday and Thursday). Reevaluate after 12 months. Safety of maintenance therapy >12 months has not been established.

Children >15 years and Adults: Apply one application (thin layer of 0.03% or 0.1% ointment) to areas usually affected twice a week, allowing 2-3 days between applications (eg, one application on Monday and Thursday). Re-evaluate after 12 months. Safety of maintenance therapy >12 months has not been established.

Note: Patients experiencing flares should resume twice daily treatment.

Administration Do not use with occlusive dressings. Burning at the application site is most common in first few days; improves as atopic dermatitis improves. Limit application to involved areas. Continue as long as signs and symptoms persist; discontinue if resolution occurs; re-evaluate if symptoms persist >6 weeks.

Hazardous agent; use appropriate precautions for handling and disposal (NIOSH, 2012).

Dosage Forms Excipient information presented when available (limited, particularly for generics); consult specific product labeling.

Ointment, External:

Protopic: 0.03% (30 g, 60 g, 100 g); 0.1% (30 g, 60 g, 100 g)

◆ **Tactuo™ (Can)** *see* Adapalene and Benzoyl Peroxide *on page 48*

Tadalafil (tah DA la fil)

Brand Names: U.S. Adcirca; Cialis

Brand Names: Canada Adcirca; Cialis

Index Terms GF196960

Pharmacologic Category Phosphodiesterase-5 Enzyme Inhibitor

Use

Benign prostatic hyperplasia (Cialis only): For the treatment of the signs and symptoms of benign prostatic hyperplasia (BPH).

Erectile dysfunction (Cialis only): For the treatment of erectile dysfunction.

Erectile dysfunction and benign prostatic hyperplasia (Cialis only): For the treatment of erectile dysfunction and the signs and symptoms of BPH.

Pulmonary arterial hypertension (Adcirca only): Pulmonary arterial hypertension (Adcirca only):

Studies establishing effectiveness included predominately patients with New York Heart Association (NYHA) functional class II to III symptoms and etiologies of idiopathic or heritable pulmonary arterial hypertension (61%) or pulmonary arterial hypertension associated with connective tissue diseases (23%).

Pregnancy Risk Factor B

Pregnancy Considerations Teratogenic events were not reported in animal reproduction studies. Postnatal development and pup survival was decreased at some doses. There are no adequate and well-controlled studies in pregnant women. Less than 0.0005% is found in the semen of healthy males.

Breast-Feeding Considerations It is not known if tadalafil is excreted in breast milk. The manufacturer recommends that caution be exercised when administering tadalafil to nursing women.

Contraindications Known serious hypersensitivity to tadalafil or any component of the formulation; concurrent use (regularly/intermittently) of organic nitrates in any form (eg, nitroglycerin, isosorbide dinitrate)

Warnings/Precautions There is a degree of cardiac risk associated with sexual activity; therefore, physicians should consider the cardiovascular status of their patients prior to initiation. Use is not recommended in patients with hypotension (<90/50 mm Hg), uncontrolled hypertension (>170/100 mm Hg), NYHA class II-IV heart failure within the last 6 months, uncontrolled arrhythmias, stroke within the last 6 months, MI within the last 3 months, unstable angina or angina during sexual intercourse; safety and efficacy have not been evaluated in these patients. Safety and efficacy in PAH have not been evaluated in patients with clinically significant aortic and/or mitral valve disease, life-threatening arrhythmias, hypotension (<90/50 mm Hg), uncontrolled hypertension, significant left ventricular dysfunction, pericardial constriction, restrictive or congestive cardiomyopathy, symptomatic coronary artery disease. Use caution in patients with left ventricular outflow obstruction (eg, aortic stenosis, hypertrophic obstructive cardiomyopathy); may be more sensitive to vasodilator effects.

Patients experiencing anginal chest pain after tadalafil administration should seek immediate medical attention. Concomitant use (regularly/intermittently) with all forms of nitrates is contraindicated. When used for BPH, erectile dysfunction, or PAH and nitrate administration is medically necessary following use, at least 48 hours should elapse after the tadalafil dose and nitrate administration. When used for PAH, per the manufacturer, nitrate may be administered within 48 hours of tadalafil. For both situations, administration of nitrates should only be done under close medical supervision with hemodynamic monitoring.

Concurrent use with alpha-adrenergic antagonist therapy may cause symptomatic hypotension; patients should be hemodynamically stable prior to initiating tadalafil therapy at the lowest possible dose. Avoid or limit concurrent substantial alcohol consumption as this may increase the risk of symptomatic hypotension. When used for BPH or erectile dysfunction, use caution in patients receiving strong CYP3A4 inhibitors. When used for PAH, avoid use in patients taking strong CYP3A4 inducers/inhibitors. Use in patients receiving or about to receive ritonavir requires dosage adjustment or interruption of therapy, respectively. Canadian labeling does not recommend use of tadalafil in patients with PAH who are also receiving protease inhibitors.

Pulmonary vasodilators may exacerbate the cardiovascular status in patients with pulmonary veno-occlusive disease (PVOD); use is not recommended. In patients with unrecognized PVOD, signs of pulmonary edema should prompt investigation into this diagnosis. Use with caution in patients with mild-to-moderate hepatic impairment; dosage adjustment/limitation is needed. Use is not recommended in patients with severe hepatic impairment or cirrhosis. Use with caution in patients with renal impairment; dosage adjustment/limitation is needed. Safety and efficacy with other tadalafil brands or other PDE-5 inhibitors (ie, sildenafil and vardenafil) have not been established. Patients should be informed not to take with other tadalafil brands or other PDE-5 inhibitors. Use caution in patients with bleeding disorders or peptic ulcer disease due to effect on platelets (bleeding).

When used to treat BPH or erectile dysfunction, potential underlying causes of BPH or erectile dysfunction should be evaluated prior to treatment. Use with caution in patients with anatomical deformation of the penis (angulation, cavernosal fibrosis, or Peyronie's disease), or who have conditions which may predispose them to priapism (sickle cell anemia, multiple myeloma, leukemia). Instruct patients to seek immediate medical attention if erection persists >4 hours. Safety and efficacy with other tadalafil brands or other PDE-5 inhibitors (ie, sildenafil and vardenafil) have not been established. Patients should be informed not to take with other tadalafil brands or other PDE-5 inhibitors. The safety and efficacy of tadalafil with other treatments for erectile dysfunction have not been studied and are, therefore, not recommended as combination therapy.

Rare cases of nonarteritic anterior ischemic optic neuropathy (NAION) have been reported; risk may be increased with history of vision loss or NAION in one eye. Other risk factors for NAION include heart disease, diabetes, hypertension, smoking, age >50 years, or history of certain eye problems. Sudden decrease or loss of hearing has been reported rarely; hearing changes may be accompanied by tinnitus and dizziness. A direct relationship between therapy and vision or hearing loss has not been determined. Instruct patients to seek medical assistance for sudden loss of vision in one or both eyes, sudden decrease in hearing, or sudden loss of hearing.

Patients with genetic retinal disorders (eg, retinitis pigmentosa) were not evaluated in clinical trials; use is not recommended. Use with caution in the elderly.

Adverse Reactions Based upon usual doses for either indication. For erectile dysfunction, similar adverse events are reported with once-daily versus intermittent dosing, but are generally lower than with doses used intermittently.

>10%:

- Cardiovascular: Flushing (1% to 13%; dose related)
- Central nervous system: Headache (3% to 42%; dose related)
- Gastrointestinal: Dyspepsia (1% to 13%), nausea (10% to 11%)
- Neuromuscular & skeletal: Myalgia (1% to 14%; dose related), back pain (2% to 12%), extremity pain (1% to 11%)
- Respiratory: Respiratory tract infection (3% to 13%), nasopharyngitis (2% to 13%)

2% to 10%:

- Cardiovascular: Hypertension (1% to 3%)
- Gastrointestinal: Gastroenteritis (viral; 3% to 5%), GERD (1% to 3%), abdominal pain (1% to 2%), diarrhea (1% to 2%)
- Genitourinary: Urinary tract infection (≤2%)
- Respiratory: Nasal congestion (≤9%), cough (2% to 4%), bronchitis (≤2%)
- Miscellaneous: Flu-like syndrome (2% to 5%)

<2% (Limited to important or life-threatening): Amnesia (transient global), angina pectoris, arthralgia, blurred vision, chest pain, color vision decreased, conjunctival hyperemia, conjunctivitis, diaphoresis, dizziness, dysphagia, dyspnea, epistaxis, esophagitis, exfoliative dermatitis, eye pain, eyelid swelling, facial edema, fatigue, gastritis, GGTP increased, hearing decreased, hearing loss, hepatic enzymes increased, hypoesthesia, hypotension, insomnia, lacrimation, migraine, MI, neck pain, nonarteritic ischemic optic neuropathy (NAION), orthostatic hypotension, pain, palpitation, paresthesia, pharyngitis, priapism, pruritus, rash, retinal artery occlusion, retinal vein occlusion, seizure, somnolence, spontaneous penile erection, Stevens-Johnson syndrome, stroke, sudden cardiac death, syncope, tachycardia, tinnitus, urticaria, vertigo, visual field loss, vomiting, weakness, xerostomia

Drug Interactions

Metabolism/Transport Effects Substrate of CYP3A4 (major); **Note:** Assignment of Major/Minor substrate status based on clinically relevant drug interaction potential

Avoid Concomitant Use

Avoid concomitant use of Tadalafil with any of the following: Alprostadil; Amyl Nitrite; Fusidic Acid (Systemic); Phosphodiesterase 5 Inhibitors; Riociguat; Vasodilators (Organic Nitrates)

Increased Effect/Toxicity

Tadalafil may increase the levels/effects of: Alpha1-Blockers; Alprostadil; Amyl Nitrite; Antihypertensives; Bosentan; Phosphodiesterase 5 Inhibitors; Riociguat; Vasodilators (Organic Nitrates)

The levels/effects of Tadalafil may be increased by: Alcohol (Ethyl); Boceprevir; Cobicistat; CYP3A4 Inhibitors (Moderate); CYP3A4 Inhibitors (Strong); Dasatinib; Fluconazole; Fusidic Acid (Systemic); Itraconazole; Ivacaftor; Ketoconazole (Systemic); Lorcaserin; Luliconazole; Mifepristone; Posaconazole; Ritonavir; Sapropterin; Simeprevir; Telaprevir; Voriconazole

Decreased Effect

The levels/effects of Tadalafil may be decreased by: Bosentan; CYP3A4 Inducers (Strong); Etravirine

Ethanol/Nutrition/Herb Interactions

Ethanol: Substantial consumption of ethanol may increase the risk of hypotension and orthostasis. Lower ethanol consumption has not been associated with significant changes in blood pressure or increase in orthostatic symptoms. Management: Avoid or limit ethanol consumption.

Food: Rate and extent of absorption are not affected by food. Grapefruit juice may increase serum levels/toxicity of tadalafil. Management: Use of grapefruit juice should be limited or avoided.

Herb/Nutraceutical: St John's wort may decrease the levels/effectiveness of tadalafil. Management: Avoid or use caution with concomitant use.

Storage/Stability Store at 25°C (77°F); excursions permitted to 15°C to 30°C (59°F to 86°F).

Mechanism of Action

BPH: Exact mechanism unknown; effects likely due to PDE-5 mediated reduction in smooth muscle and endothelial cell proliferation, decreased nerve activity, and increased smooth muscle relaxation and tissue perfusion of the prostate and bladder

Erectile dysfunction: Does not directly cause penile erections, but affects the response to sexual stimulation. The physiologic mechanism of erection of the penis involves release of nitric oxide (NO) in the corpus cavernosum during sexual stimulation. NO then activates the enzyme guanylate cyclase, which results in increased levels of cyclic guanosine monophosphate (cGMP), producing smooth muscle relaxation and inflow of blood to the corpus cavernosum. Tadalafil enhances the effect of NO by inhibiting phosphodiesterase type 5 (PDE-5), which is responsible for degradation of cGMP in the corpus cavernosum; when sexual stimulation causes local release of NO, inhibition of PDE-5 by tadalafil causes increased levels of cGMP in the corpus cavernosum, resulting in smooth muscle relaxation and inflow of blood to the corpus cavernosum. At recommended doses, it has no effect in the absence of sexual stimulation.

PAH: Inhibits phosphodiesterase type 5 (PDE-5) in smooth muscle of pulmonary vasculature where PDE-5 is responsible for the degradation of cyclic guanosine monophosphate (cGMP). Increased cGMP concentration results in pulmonary vasculature relaxation; vasodilation in the pulmonary bed and the systemic circulation (to a lesser degree) may occur.

Pharmacodynamics/Kinetics

Onset of action: Within 1 hour

Peak effect (pulmonary artery vasodilation): 75-90 minutes (Ghofrani, 2004)

Duration: Erectile dysfunction: Up to 36 hours

Distribution: V_d: 63-77 L

Protein binding: 94%

Metabolism: Hepatic, via CYP3A4 to metabolites (inactive)

Half-life elimination: 15-17.5 hours; Pulmonary hypertension (not receiving bosentan): 35 hours

Time to peak, plasma: ~2-4 hours (range: 30 minutes to 8 hours)

Excretion: Feces (~61%, predominantly as metabolites); urine (~36%, predominantly as metabolites)

Dosage Oral: Adults:

Benign prostatic hyperplasia (with or without concomitant erectile dysfunction) (Cialis): 5 mg once daily. **Note:** When tadalafil is used with finasteride to initiate BPH therapy, the recommended duration of therapy is ≤26 weeks.

Dosing adjustment with concomitant medications: CYP3A4 inhibitors (strong): 2.5 mg once daily; maximum: 2.5 mg once daily

Erectile dysfunction (Cialis):

As-needed dosing: 10 mg (U.S. labeling) or 20 mg (Canadian labeling) at least 30 minutes prior to anticipated sexual activity (dosing range: 5-20 mg); to be given as one single dose and not given more than once daily. **Note:** Erectile function may be improved for up to 36 hours following a single dose; adjust dose.

Once-daily dosing: 2.5 mg once daily (U.S. labeling) or 5 mg once daily (Canadian labeling) to be given at approximately the same time daily without regard to timing of sexual activity. Dose may be adjusted based on tolerability (dosage range: 2.5-5 mg/day).

Dosing adjustment with concomitant medications:

U.S. labeling: $Alpha_1$-blockers: If stabilized on either alpha-blockers or tadalafil therapy, initiate new therapy with the other agent at the lowest possible dose.

Canadian labeling: Nonselective alpha-blockers (eg, doxazosin): *As-needed dosing:* 10 mg at least 30 minutes prior to anticipated sexual activity

CYP3A4 inhibitors (strong):

As-needed dosing:

U.S. labeling: Maximum: 10 mg, not to be given more frequently than every 72 hours

Canadian labeling: 10 mg, not to be given more frequently than every 48 hours (maximum 3 doses/week); may increase to 20 mg if lower dose is tolerated but ineffective. Discontinue use if 10 mg dose is not tolerated.

Once-daily dosing:

U.S. labeling: 2.5 mg once daily; maximum: 2.5 mg once daily

Canadian labeling: 2.5-5 mg once daily

Pulmonary arterial hypertension (Adcirca®): 40 mg once daily

Dosing adjustment with concomitant medications:

Coadministration with protease inhibitor regimen:

Concurrent use with atazanavir/ritonavir, darunavir/ritonavir, fosamprenavir, ritonavir, saquinavir/ritonavir, tipranavir/ritonavir:

Coadministration of tadalafil in patients currently receiving one of these protease inhibitor regimens for at least 1 week: Initiate tadalafil at 20 mg once daily; increase to 40 mg once daily based on individual tolerability.

Coadministration of one of these protease inhibitor regimens in patients currently receiving tadalafil: Discontinue tadalafil at least 24 hours prior to the initiation of the protease inhibitor regimen. After at least 1 week of the protease inhibitor regimen, resume tadalafil at 20 mg once daily; increase to 40 mg once daily based on individual tolerability.

Concurrent use with indinavir or nelfinavir:

Patient receiving indinavir/nelfinavir when initiating tadalafil: Initiate tadalafil at 20 mg once daily; increase to 40 mg once daily based on individual tolerability

Patient receiving tadalafil when initiating indinavir/nelfinavir: Adjust tadalafil to 20 mg once daily; increase to 40 mg once daily based on individual tolerability

Elderly: No dose adjustment for patients >65 years of age in the absence of renal or hepatic impairment

Dosage adjustment in renal impairment:

Benign prostatic hyperplasia (with or without concomitant erectile dysfunction) (Cialis®):

Cl_{cr} ≥51 mL/minute: No dosage adjustment necessary

Cl_{cr} 30-50 mL/minute: Initial: 2.5 mg once daily; maximum: 5 mg once daily

Cl_{cr} <30 mL/minute: Use not recommended

ESRD requiring hemodialysis: Use not recommended

Erectile dysfunction (Cialis®):

As-needed use:

U.S. labeling:

Cl_{cr} ≥51 mL/minute: No dosage adjustment necessary

Cl_{cr} 30-50 mL/minute: Initial: 5 mg once daily; maximum: 10 mg (not to be given more frequently than every 48 hours)

Cl_{cr} <30 mL/minute: Maximum: 5 mg (not to be given more frequently than every 72 hours)

ESRD requiring hemodialysis: Maximum: 5 mg (not to be given more frequently than every 72 hours)

Canadian labeling:

Cl_{cr} >80 mL/minute: No dosage adjustment necessary

Cl_{cr} ≥31-80 mL/minute: 10 mg, not to be given more frequently than every 48 hours (maximum: 3 doses/week); may increase to 20 mg if lower dose is tolerated but ineffective. Discontinue use if 10 mg dose is not tolerated.

Cl_{cr} <30 mL/minute: Use with extreme caution; has not been adequately studied

ESRD requiring hemodialysis: Use with extreme caution; has not been adequately studied

Once-daily use:

Cl_{cr} ≥31 mL/minute: No dosage adjustment necessary

Cl_{cr} <30 mL/minute: Use not recommended

ESRD requiring hemodialysis: Use not recommended

Pulmonary arterial hypertension (Adcirca®):

Cl_{cr} >80 mL/minute: No dosage adjustment necessary

Cl_{cr} 31-80 mL/minute: Initial: 20 mg once daily; increase to 40 mg once daily based on individual tolerability

Cl_{cr} ≤30 mL/minute: Avoid use due to increased tadalafil exposure, limited clinical experience, and lack of ability to influence clearance by dialysis.

Dosage adjustment in hepatic impairment:

Benign prostatic hyperplasia (with or without concomitant erectile dysfunction) (Cialis®):

Mild-to-moderate impairment (Child-Pugh class A or B): Use with caution

Severe impairment (Child-Pugh class C): Use is not recommended

Erectile dysfunction (Cialis®):
As-needed use:
U.S. labeling:
Mild-to-moderate impairment (Child-Pugh class A or B): Use with caution; dose should not exceed 10 mg once daily
Severe impairment (Child-Pugh class C): Use is not recommended
Canadian labeling:
Mild-to-moderate impairment (Child-Pugh class A or B): 10 mg, not to be given more frequently than every 48 hours (maximum 3 doses/week); may increase to 20 mg if lower dose is tolerated but ineffective. Discontinue use if 10 mg dose is not tolerated.
Severe impairment (Child-Pugh class C): Use with extreme caution; has not been adequately studied
Once-daily use:
U.S. labeling:
Mild-to-moderate impairment (Child-Pugh class A or B): Use with caution
Severe impairment (Child-Pugh class C): Use is not recommended
Canadian labeling:
Mild-to-moderate impairment (Child-Pugh class A or B): No dosage adjustment necessary
Severe impairment (Child-Pugh class C): Use with extreme caution; has not been adequately studied
Pulmonary arterial hypertension (Adcirca®):
Mild-to-moderate impairment (Child-Pugh class A or B): Use with caution; consider initial dose of 20 mg once daily
Severe impairment (Child-Pugh class C): Avoid use; has not been studied in patients with severe hepatic cirrhosis.

Dietary Considerations May be taken with or without food.

Administration May be administered with or without food.
Adcirca®: Administer daily dose all at once; dividing doses throughout the day is not advised.
Cialis®: When used on an as-needed basis, should be taken at least 30 minutes prior to sexual activity. When used on a once-daily basis, should be taken at the same time each day, without regard to timing of sexual activity.

Monitoring Parameters Blood pressure, response and adverse effects; urine flow, PSA

Dosage Forms Excipient information presented when available (limited, particularly for generics); consult specific product labeling.
Tablet, Oral:
Adcirca: 20 mg
Cialis: 2.5 mg, 5 mg, 10 mg, 20 mg

Extemporaneous Preparations A 5 mg/mL tadalafil oral suspension may be made with tablets in a 1:1 mixture of Ora-Plus® and Ora-Sweet®. Crush fifteen 20 mg tadalafil tablets in a glass mortar and reduce to a fine powder. Prepare the vehicle by mixing 30 mL of Ora-Plus® and 30 mL of Ora-Sweet®; stir vigorously. Add 30 mL of the vehicle in geometric proportions to the powder and mix to form a smooth suspension. Transfer the mixture to a 2 ounce amber plastic prescription bottle. Rinse mortar with a quantity of the vehicle sufficient to make a final volume of 60 mL. Label "shake well." Stable for 91 days when stored in amber plastic prescription bottles at room temperature.

Pettit RS, Johnson CE, and Caruthers RL, "Stability of an Extemporaneously Prepared Tadalafil Suspension," *Am J Health Syst Pharm*, 2012, 69(7):592-4.

◆ **Tafinlar** *see* Dabrafenib *on page* 528
◆ **Tagamet HB [OTC]** *see* Cimetidine *on page* 427
◆ **TAK-375** *see* Ramelteon *on page* 1777
◆ **TAK-390MR** *see* Dexlansoprazole *on page* 584
◆ **TAK-599** *see* Ceftaroline Fosamil *on page* 378
◆ **Talc** *see* Talc (Sterile) *on page* 1986
◆ **Talc for Pleurodesis** *see* Talc (Sterile) *on page* 1986

Talc (Sterile) (talk STARE il)

Brand Names: U.S. Sclerosol Intrapleural; Sterile Talc Powder

Index Terms Intrapleural Talc; Sterile Talc; Talc; Talc for Pleurodesis

Pharmacologic Category Sclerosing Agent

Use Prevention of recurrence of malignant pleural effusion in symptomatic patients

Pregnancy Risk Factor B

Dosage Adults: Pleural effusion:
Intrapleural aerosol: 4-8 g (1-2 cans) as a single dose
Intrapleural instillation: 5 g

Additional Information Complete prescribing information should be consulted for additional detail.

Dosage Forms Excipient information presented when available (limited, particularly for generics); consult specific product labeling.
Aerosol Powder, Intrapleural:
Sclerosol Intrapleural: 4 g (30 g) [contains dichlorodifluoromethane]
Suspension Reconstituted, Intrapleural:
Sterile Talc Powder: 5 g (1 ea)

Taliglucerase Alfa (tal i GLOO ser ase AL fa)

Brand Names: U.S. Elelyso

Pharmacologic Category Enzyme

Use Long-term enzyme replacement therapy for patients with type 1 Gaucher's disease

Pregnancy Risk Factor B

Pregnancy Considerations Adverse events were not observed in animal reproduction studies.

Breast-Feeding Considerations It is not known if taliglucerase alfa is excreted in breast milk. Enzyme ingested by a nursing infant would likely degrade in their digestive system. The benefits of nursing to the infant should be weighed against the potential for additional bone loss in the mother (Zimran, 2009). The manufacturer recommends that caution be exercised when administering taliglucerase alfa to nursing women.

Prescribing and Access Restrictions Product access is restricted to the Gaucher Personal Support (GPS) program. Healthcare providers and patients may obtain additional information by contacting the GPS program at 855-353-5976.

Contraindications There are no contraindications listed in the manufacturer's labeling.

Warnings/Precautions Use with caution in patients who have exhibited hypersensitivity reactions to taliglucerase alfa or other enzyme replacement therapies; anaphylaxis has occurred; appropriate medical support should be readily available in the event of a serious reaction. Infusion-related reactions (eg, headache, chest pain, fatigue, urticaria, arthralgia), including allergic reactions, may occur; management strategies include symptomatic treatment, pretreatment with antihistamines, antipyretics, and/or corticosteroids, and slowing of the infusion rate. The development of IgG anti-drug antibodies (ADA) has been reported; the clinical significance is unknown. Patients who develop immune or infusion reactions to taliglucerase alfa or who have had an immune response to other enzyme replacement therapies and who are switching to taliglucerase alfa should be monitored for antibody development.

Adverse Reactions
≥10%:
Central nervous system: Headache (11% to 19%)

Genitourinary: Urinary tract infection/pyelonephritis (9% to 11%)
Neuromuscular & skeletal: Arthralgia (11% to 13%), back pain (3% to 11%), limb pain (≤11%)
Respiratory: Upper respiratory tract infection/nasopharyngitis (18% to 22%), pharyngitis (4% to 19%)
Miscellaneous: IgG antibody formation (14% to 53%), infusion reactions (44% to 46%, including headache [16%], chest discomfort/pain [6%], asthenia [7%], back pain/arthralgia [7%], urticaria [7%], flushing [6%], erythema [5%], fatigue [5%], blood pressure increased [5%]), flu-like syndrome (4% to 13%)

>2% to <10%:
Cardiovascular: Chest discomfort, flushing, peripheral edema
Central nervous system: Dizziness, fatigue, insomnia, pain
Dermatologic: Erythema, pruritus, rash, skin irritation
Gastrointestinal: Abdominal pain, diarrhea, nausea, throat irritation
Hepatic: ALT increased
Local: Infusion site pain
Neuromuscular & skeletal: Bone pain, muscle spasm, musculoskeletal discomfort/pain, paresthesia, weakness
Respiratory: Dyspnea, pharyngolaryngeal pain

≤2% (Limited to important or life-threatening): Anaphylaxis, infusion/allergic reactions (including angioedema, wheezing, cough, cyanosis, hypotension)

Drug Interactions

Metabolism/Transport Effects None known.

Avoid Concomitant Use There are no known interactions where it is recommended to avoid concomitant use.

Increased Effect/Toxicity There are no known significant interactions involving an increase in effect.

Decreased Effect There are no known significant interactions involving a decrease in effect.

Preparation for Administration Reconstitute each vial with 5.1 mL of SWFI; mix gently; do not shake. Solution should be clear and colorless. Withdraw 5 mL of reconstituted solution from each vial (reconstituted vials contain 5.3 mL) and further dilute in NS to a final volume of 100-200 mL in a low protein binding container; slight flocculation may occur following dilution.

Storage/Stability Store unused vials at 2°C to 8°C (36°F to 46°F); may be stored at room temperature for ≤24 hours; protect from light. If not used immediately, diluted solutions for infusion may be stored at 2°C to 8°C (36°F to 46°F) for ≤24 hours; protect from light; do not freeze.

Mechanism of Action Taliglucerase alfa is an analogue of glucocerebrosidase; it is produced by recombinant DNA technology using plant (carrot) cell culture. Glucocerebrosidase is an enzyme deficient in Gaucher's disease. It is needed to catalyze the hydrolysis of glucocerebroside to glucose and ceramide, thereby reducing liver and spleen size and improving anemia and thrombocytopenia.

Pharmacodynamics/Kinetics

Distribution: V_{ss}: 7.3-11.7 L (dose-dependent; increased with higher doses)

Half-life elimination: 19-29 minutes (dose-dependent; increased with higher doses)

Dosage Note: Pretreatment with antihistamines and/or corticosteroids can be considered for prevention of subsequent infusion reactions in patients with an infusion reaction requiring symptomatic treatment; during clinical studies, patients were not routinely premedicated prior to infusion. Round up to the next whole vial when determining the number of vials needed.

I.V.: Adults: Initial: 60 units/kg every 2 weeks; dosing is individualized based on disease severity. Dosing range: 11-73 units/kg every 2 weeks.

Conversion from imiglucerase: Initiate taliglucerase alfa using the patient's same previous imiglucerase dose and administer every 2 weeks. **Note:** Conversion to taliglucerase alfa is based on a single study of patients stabilized on a biweekly imiglucerase dose for ≥6 months.

Dosage adjustment in renal impairment: No dosage adjustment necessary.

Dosage adjustment in hepatic impairment: No dosage adjustment necessary.

Administration Initiate infusion at a rate of 1.3 mL/minute; rate may be increased to 2.3 mL/minute based on patient tolerance and/or a minimal infusion time of 60 minutes (usual infusion time: 60-120 minutes). Administer using a low protein-binding infusion set with a 0.2 micron in-line filter.

Monitoring Parameters Hemoglobin, platelet count, angiotensin converting enzyme, tartrate-resistant acid phosphatase, chitotriosidase, IgG anti-drug antibody formation (in patients who experience, or previously experienced, immune or infusion reactions to enzyme replacement therapy); liver volume, spleen volume; bone density; ECG, echocardiogram, chest x-ray

Additional Information Gaucher Disease Registry: https://www.registrynxt.com/Gaucher/Pages/Home.aspx

Dosage Forms Excipient information presented when available (limited, particularly for generics); consult specific product labeling.

Solution Reconstituted, Intravenous [preservative free]:
Elelyso: 200 units (1 ea) [contains polysorbate 80]

- **Talwin** *see* Pentazocine *on page 1615*
- **Talwin® (Can)** *see* Pentazocine *on page 1615*
- **Tambocor [DSC]** *see* Flecainide *on page 866*
- **Tambocor™ (Can)** *see* Flecainide *on page 866*
- **Tamiflu** *see* Oseltamivir *on page 1518*

Tamoxifen (ta MOKS i fen)

Brand Names: U.S. Soltamox

Brand Names: Canada Apo-Tamox®; Mylan-Tamoxifen; Nolvadex®-D; PMS-Tamoxifen; Teva-Tamoxifen

Index Terms ICI-46474; Nolvadex; Tamoxifen Citras; Tamoxifen Citrate

Pharmacologic Category Antineoplastic Agent, Estrogen Receptor Antagonist; Selective Estrogen Receptor Modulator (SERM)

Use Treatment of metastatic (female and male) breast cancer; adjuvant treatment of breast cancer after primary treatment with surgery and radiation; reduce risk of invasive breast cancer in women with ductal carcinoma *in situ* (DCIS) after surgery and radiation; reduce the incidence of breast cancer in women at high risk

Unlabeled Use Treatment of mastalgia, gynecomastia, ovarian cancer, endometrial cancer, and desmoid tumors; risk reduction in women with Paget's disease of the breast (with ER-positive DCIS or without associated cancer); induction of ovulation; treatment of precocious puberty in females, secondary to McCune-Albright syndrome

Pregnancy Risk Factor D

Pregnancy Considerations Animal reproduction studies have demonstrated fetal adverse effects and fetal loss. There have been reports of vaginal bleeding, birth defects and fetal loss in pregnant women. Tamoxifen use during pregnancy may have a potential long term risk to the fetus of a DES-like syndrome. For sexually-active women of childbearing age, initiate during menstruation (negative β-hCG immediately prior to initiation in women with irregular cycles). Tamoxifen may induce ovulation. Barrier or nonhormonal contraceptives are recommended. Pregnancy should be avoided during treatment and for 2 months after treatment has been discontinued.

Breast-Feeding Considerations It is not known if tamoxifen is excreted in breast milk, however, it has been shown to inhibit lactation. Due to the potential for adverse reactions, women taking tamoxifen should not breast-feed.

Medication Guide Available Yes

Contraindications Hypersensitivity to tamoxifen or any component of the formulation; concurrent warfarin therapy or history of deep vein thrombosis or pulmonary embolism (when tamoxifen is used for breast cancer risk reduction in women at high risk for breast cancer or with ductal carcinoma *in situ* [DCIS])

Warnings/Precautions Hazardous agent - use appropriate precautions for handling and disposal (NIOSH, 2012). **[U.S. Boxed Warning]: Serious and life-threatening events (some fatal), including stroke, pulmonary emboli, and uterine or endometrial malignancies, have occurred at an incidence greater than placebo during use for breast cancer risk reduction in women at high-risk for breast cancer and in women with ductal carcinoma *in situ* (DCIS). In women already diagnosed with breast cancer, the benefits of tamoxifen treatment outweigh risks; evaluate risks versus benefits (and discuss with patients) when used for breast cancer risk reduction.** An increased incidence of thromboembolic events, including DVT and pulmonary embolism, has been associated with use for breast cancer; risk is increased with concomitant chemotherapy; use with caution in individuals with a history of thromboembolic events. Thrombocytopenia and/or leukopenia may occur; neutropenia and pancytopenia have been reported rarely. Although the relationship to tamoxifen therapy is uncertain, rare hemorrhagic episodes have occurred in patients with significant thrombocytopenia. Use with caution in patients with hyperlipidemias; infrequent postmarketing cases of hyperlipidemias have been reported. Decreased visual acuity, retinal vein thrombosis, retinopathy, corneal changes, color perception changes, and increased incidence of cataracts (and the need for cataract surgery), have been reported. Hypercalcemia has occurred in some patients with bone metastasis, usually within a few weeks of therapy initiation; institute appropriate hypercalcemia management; discontinue if severe. Local disease flare and increased bone and tumor pain may occur in patients with metastatic breast cancer; may be associated with (good) tumor response.

Potentially significant drug-drug interactions may exist, requiring dose or frequency adjustment, additional monitoring, and/or selection of alternative therapy. Decreased efficacy and an increased risk of breast cancer recurrence has been reported with concurrent moderate or strong CYP2D6 inhibitors (Aubert, 2009; Dezentje, 2009). Concomitant use with select SSRIs may result in decreased tamoxifen efficacy. Strong CYP2D6 inhibitors (eg, fluoxetine, paroxetine) and moderate CYP2D6 inhibitors (eg, sertraline) are reported to interfere with transformation to the active metabolite endoxifen; when possible, select alternative medications with minimal or no impact on endoxifen levels (NCCN Breast Cancer Risk Reduction Guidelines v.1.2013; Sideras, 2010). Weak CYP2D6 inhibitors (eg, venlafaxine, citalopram) have minimal effect on the conversion to endoxifen (Jin, 2005; NCCN Breast Cancer Risk Reduction Guidelines v.1.2013); escitalopram is also a weak CYP2D6 inhibitor. In a retrospective analysis of breast cancer patients taking tamoxifen and SSRIs, concomitant use of paroxetine and tamoxifen was associated with an increased risk of death due to breast cancer (Kelly, 2010). Lower plasma concentrations of endoxifen have been observed in patients associated with reduced CYP2D6 activity (Jin, 2005; Schroth, 2009) and may be associated with reduced efficacy, although data is conflicting. Routine CYP2D6 testing is not recommended at this time in order to determine optimal endocrine therapy (NCCN Breast Cancer Guidelines v.2.2013; Visvanathan, 2009).

Tamoxifen use may be associated with changes in bone mineral density (BMD) and the effects may be dependent upon menstrual status. In postmenopausal women, tamoxifen use is associated with a protective effect on bone mineral density (BMD), preventing loss of BMD which lasts over the 5-year treatment period. In premenopausal women, a decline (from baseline) in BMD mineral density has been observed in women who continued to menstruate; may be associated with an increased risk of fractures. Liver abnormalities such as cholestasis, fatty liver, hepatitis, and hepatic necrosis have occurred. Hepatocellular carcinomas have been reported in some studies; relationship to treatment is unclear. Tamoxifen is associated with an increased incidence of uterine or endometrial cancers. Endometrial hyperplasia, polyps, endometriosis, uterine fibroids, and ovarian cysts have occurred. Monitor and promptly evaluate any report of abnormal vaginal bleeding. Amenorrhea and menstrual irregularities have been reported with tamoxifen use.

Adverse Reactions

>10%:

- Cardiovascular: Vasodilation (41%), flushing (33%), hypertension (11%), peripheral edema (11%)
- Central nervous system: Mood changes (12% to 18%), pain (3% to 16%), depression (2% to 12%)
- Dermatologic: Skin changes (6% to 19%), rash (13%)
- Endocrine & metabolic: Hot flashes (3% to 80%), fluid retention (32%), altered menses (13% to 25%), amenorrhea (16%)
- Gastrointestinal: Nausea (5% to 26%), weight loss (23%), vomiting (12%)
- Genitourinary: Vaginal discharge (13% to 55%), vaginal bleeding (2% to 23%)
- Neuromuscular & skeletal: Weakness (18%), arthritis (14%), arthralgia (11%)
- Respiratory: Pharyngitis (14%)
- Miscellaneous: Lymphedema (11%)

1% to 10%:

- Cardiovascular: Chest pain (5%), venous thrombotic events (5%), edema (4%), cardiovascular ischemia (3%), angina (2%), deep venous thrombus (≤2%), MI (1%)
- Central nervous system: Insomnia (9%), dizziness (8%), headache (8%), anxiety (6%), fatigue (4%)
- Dermatologic: Alopecia (≤5%)
- Endocrine & metabolic: Oligomenorrhea (9%), breast pain (6%), menstrual disorder (6%), breast neoplasm (5%), hypercholesterolemia (4%)
- Gastrointestinal: Abdominal pain (9%), weight gain (9%), constipation (4% to 8%), diarrhea (7%), dyspepsia (6%), throat irritation (oral solution 5%), abdominal cramps (1%), anorexia (1%)
- Genitourinary: Urinary tract infection (10%), leukorrhea (9%), vaginal hemorrhage (6%), vaginitis (5%), vulvovaginitis (5%), ovarian cyst (3%)
- Hematologic: Thrombocytopenia (≤10%), anemia (5%)
- Hepatic: AST increased (5%), serum bilirubin increased (2%)
- Neuromuscular & skeletal: Back pain (10%), bone pain (6% to 10%), osteoporosis (7%), fracture (7%), arthrosis (5%), joint disorder (5%), myalgia (5%), paresthesia (5%), musculoskeletal pain (3%)
- Ocular: Cataract (7%)
- Renal: Serum creatinine increased (≤2%)
- Respiratory: Cough (4% to 9%), dyspnea (8%), bronchitis (5%), sinusitis (5%)
- Miscellaneous: Infection/sepsis (≤9%), diaphoresis (6%), flu-like syndrome (6%), cyst (5%), neoplasm (5%), allergic reaction (3%)

<1 or frequency not defined (limited to important or life-threatening): Angioedema, bullous pemphigoid, cholestasis, corneal changes, endometrial cancer, endometrial hyperplasia, endometrial polyps, endometriosis, erythema multiforme, fatty liver, hepatic necrosis, hepatitis, hypercalcemia, hyperlipidemia, hypersensitivity reactions, hypertriglyceridemia, impotence (males), interstitial pneumonitis, loss of libido (males), pancreatitis, phlebitis, pruritus vulvae, pulmonary embolism, retinal vein thrombosis, retinopathy, second primary tumors, Stevens-Johnson syndrome, stroke; tumor pain and local disease flare (including increase in lesion size and erythema) during treatment of metastatic breast cancer (generally resolves with continuation); uterine fibroids, vaginal dryness, visual color perception changes

Drug Interactions

Metabolism/Transport Effects Substrate of CYP2A6 (minor), CYP2B6 (minor), CYP2C9 (major), CYP2D6 (major), CYP2E1 (minor), CYP3A4 (major); **Note:** Assignment of Major/Minor substrate status based on clinically relevant drug interaction potential; **Inhibits** CYP2B6 (weak), CYP2C8 (moderate), CYP2C9 (weak), CYP3A4 (weak), P-glycoprotein

Avoid Concomitant Use

Avoid concomitant use of Tamoxifen with any of the following: Bosutinib; Conivaptan; CYP2D6 Inhibitors (Strong); Fusidic Acid (Systemic); Ospemifene; PAZOPanib; Pimozide; Pomalidomide; Silodosin; Topotecan; VinCRIStine (Liposomal); Vitamin K Antagonists

Increased Effect/Toxicity

Tamoxifen may increase the levels/effects of: Afatinib; ARIPiprazole; Bosutinib; Colchicine; CYP2C8 Substrates; Dabigatran Etexilate; Dofetilide; Everolimus; Highest Risk QTc-Prolonging Agents; Lomitapide; Mipomersen; Moderate Risk QTc-Prolonging Agents; Ospemifene; PAZOPanib; P-glycoprotein/ABCB1 Substrates; Pimozide; Pomalidomide; Prucalopride; Rivaroxaban; Silodosin; Topotecan; VinCRIStine (Liposomal); Vitamin K Antagonists

The levels/effects of Tamoxifen may be increased by: Abiraterone Acetate; Conivaptan; CYP2C9 Inhibitors (Moderate); CYP2C9 Inhibitors (Strong); CYP3A4 Inhibitors (Moderate); CYP3A4 Inhibitors (Strong); Darunavir; Dasatinib; Fusidic Acid (Systemic); Ivacaftor; Luliconazole; Mifepristone; Simeprevir

Decreased Effect

Tamoxifen may decrease the levels/effects of: Anastrozole; Letrozole; Ospemifene

The levels/effects of Tamoxifen may be decreased by: Aminoglutethimide; Bexarotene (Systemic); Bosentan; CYP2C9 Inducers (Strong); CYP2D6 Inhibitors (Moderate); CYP2D6 Inhibitors (Strong); CYP3A4 Inducers (Strong); Dabrafenib; Deferasirox; Herbs (CYP3A4 Inducers); Mitotane; Peginterferon Alfa-2b; Rifamycin Derivatives; Tocilizumab

Ethanol/Nutrition/Herb Interactions

Food: Grapefruit juice may decrease the metabolism of tamoxifen. Management: Avoid grapefruit juice.

Herb/Nutraceutical: Black cohosh and dong quai have estrogenic properties. St John's wort may decrease levels/effects of tamoxifen. Management: Avoid black cohosh and dong quai in estrogen-dependent tumors. Avoid St John's wort.

Storage/Stability

Oral solution: Store at ≤25°C (77°F); do not freeze or refrigerate. Protect from light. Discard opened bottle after 3 months.

Tablets: Store at 20°C to 25°C (68°F to 77°F). Protect from light.

Mechanism of Action Competitively binds to estrogen receptors on tumors and other tissue targets, producing a nuclear complex that decreases DNA synthesis and inhibits estrogen effects; nonsteroidal agent with potent antiestrogenic properties which compete with estrogen for binding sites in breast and other tissues; cells accumulate in the G_0 and G_1 phases; therefore, tamoxifen is cytostatic rather than cytocidal.

Pharmacodynamics/Kinetics

Absorption: Well absorbed

Distribution: High concentrations found in uterus, endometrial and breast tissue

Protein binding: 99%

Metabolism: Hepatic; via CYP2D6 to 4-hydroxytamoxifen and via CYP3A4/5 to N-desmethyl-tamoxifen. Each is then further metabolized into endoxifen (4-hydroxy-tamoxifen via CYP3A4/5 and N-desmethyl-tamoxifen via CYP2D6); both 4-hydroxy-tamoxifen and endoxifen are 30- to 100-fold more potent than tamoxifen

Half-life elimination: Tamoxifen: ~5-7 days; N-desmethyl tamoxifen: ~14 days

Time to peak, serum: ~5 hours

Excretion: Feces (26% to 51%); urine (9% to 13%)

Dosage Oral: **Note:** For the treatment of breast cancer, patients receiving both tamoxifen and chemotherapy should receive treatment sequentially, with tamoxifen following completion of chemotherapy.

Children: Females: Precocious puberty secondary to McCune-Albright syndrome (unlabeled use): A dose of 20 mg daily has been reported in patients 2-10 years of age; safety and efficacy have not been established for treatment of longer than 1 year duration (Eugster, 2003)

Adults:

Breast cancer treatment:

Adjuvant therapy (females): 20 mg once daily for 5 years

Premenopausal women: Duration of treatment is 5 years (Burstein, 2010; NCCN Breast Cancer guidelines v.2.2013)

Postmenopausal women: Duration of tamoxifen treatment is 2-3 years followed by an aromatase inhibitor (AI) to complete 5 years; may take tamoxifen for the full 5 years (if contraindications or intolerance to AI) or extended therapy: 4.5-6 years of tamoxifen followed by 5 years of an AI (Burstein, 2010; NCCN Breast Cancer guidelines v.2.2013)

ER-positive early breast cancer: Extended duration: Duration of treatment of 10 years demonstrated a reduced risk of recurrence and mortality (Davies, 2012)

Metastatic (males and females): 20-40 mg daily (doses >20 mg should be given in 2 divided doses). **Note:** Although the FDA-approved labeling recommends dosing up to 40 mg daily, clinical benefit has not been demonstrated with doses above 20 mg daily (Bratherton, 1984).

Ductal carcinoma *in situ* (DCIS) (females), to reduce the risk for invasive breast cancer: 20 mg once daily for 5 years

Breast cancer risk reduction (pre- and postmenopausal high-risk females): 20 mg once daily for 5 years

Endometrial carcinoma, recurrent, metastatic, or high-risk (endometrioid histologies only) (unlabeled use):

Monotherapy: 20 mg twice daily until disease progression or unacceptable toxicity (Thigpen, 2001)

Combination therapy: 20 mg twice daily for 3 weeks (alternating with megestrol acetate every 3 weeks); continue alternating until disease progression or unacceptable toxicity) (Fiorica, 2004)

Induction of ovulation (unlabeled use): 20 mg once daily (range: 20-80 mg once daily) for 5 days (Steiner, 2005)

Ovarian cancer, advanced and/or recurrent (unlabeled use): 20 mg twice daily (Hatch, 1991; Markman, 1996)

Paget's disease of the breast (risk reduction; with DCIS or without associated cancer): 20 mg once daily for 5 years (NCCN Breast Cancer Guidelines, v.2.2013)

Dosage adjustment for DVT, pulmonary embolism, cerebrovascular accident, or prolonged immobilization: Discontinue tamoxifen (NCCN Breast Cancer Risk Reduction Guidelines, v.1.2013)

Dosage adjustment in renal impairment: No dosage adjustment provided in manufacturer's labeling.

Chronic dialysis: No dosage adjustment necessary (Janus, 2013).

Dosage adjustment in hepatic impairment: No dosage adjustment provided in manufacturer's labeling (has not been studied).

Dietary Considerations Tablets and oral solution may be taken with or without food. Avoid grapefruit and grapefruit juice.

Administration Administer tablets or oral solution orally with or without food. Use supplied dosing cup for oral solution.

Hazardous agent; use appropriate precautions for handling and disposal (NIOSH, 2012).

Monitoring Parameters CBC with platelets, serum calcium, LFTs; triglycerides and cholesterol (in patients with pre-existing hyperlipidemias); INR and PT (in patients on vitamin K antagonists); abnormal vaginal bleeding; breast and gynecologic exams (baseline and routine), mammogram (baseline and routine); signs/symptoms of DVT (leg swelling, tenderness) or PE (shortness of breath); ophthalmic exam (if vision problem or cataracts); bone mineral density (premenopausal women)

Test Interactions T_4 elevations (which may be explained by increases in thyroid-binding globulin) have been reported; not accompanied by clinical hyperthyroidism

Additional Information Estrogen receptor status may predict if adjuvant treatment with tamoxifen is of benefit. In metastatic breast cancer, patients with estrogen receptor positive tumors are more likely to benefit from tamoxifen treatment. With tamoxifen use to reduce the incidence of breast cancer in high risk-women, high risk is defined as women ≥35 years of age with a 5 year NCI Gail model predicted risk of breast cancer ≥1.67%.

Oncology Comment: The American Society of Clinical Oncology (ASCO) guidelines for adjuvant endocrine therapy in postmenopausal women with HR-positive breast cancer (Burstein, 2010) recommend considering aromatase inhibitor (AI) therapy at some point in the treatment course (primary, sequentially, or extended). Optimal duration at this time is not known; however, treatment with an AI should not exceed 5 years in primary and extended therapies, and 2-3 years if followed by tamoxifen in sequential therapy (total of 5 years). If initial therapy with AI has been discontinued before the 5 years, consideration should be taken to receive tamoxifen for a total of 5 years. The optimal time to switch to an AI is also not known; but data supports switching after 2-3 years of tamoxifen (sequential) or after 5 years of tamoxifen (extended). If patient becomes intolerant or has poor adherence, consideration should be made to switch to another AI or initiate tamoxifen.

Recent data suggest that continuing tamoxifen for 10 years (rather than stopping after 5 years of therapy) may provide a further reduction in breast cancer recurrence and mortality in women with early stage disease (Davies, 2012). The Adjuvant Tamoxifen: Longer Against Shorter (ATLAS) trial randomized 6846 patients with estrogen receptor positive disease to continue tamoxifen for a total of 10 years of treatment or to stop after 5 years. Breast cancer recurrence was observed in 617 patients in the 10-year arm versus 711 recurrences in the 5-year arm (p=0.002). Breast cancer mortality was significantly reduced with 10 years of tamoxifen therapy versus 5 years (331 deaths vs 397 deaths, respectively; p=0.01) (Davies, 2012).

The adjuvant endocrine therapy of choice is tamoxifen for men with breast cancer and for pre- or perimenopausal women at diagnosis. CYP2D6 genotyping is not recommended, however, due to the potential for drug-drug interactions use caution and consider avoiding concomitant therapy with tamoxifen and known CYP2D6 inhibitors.

Dosage Forms Excipient information presented when available (limited, particularly for generics); consult specific product labeling.

Solution, Oral:

Soltamox: 10 mg/5 mL (150 mL) [sugar free; contains alcohol, usp, propylene glycol; licorice-aniseed flavor]

Tablet, Oral:

Generic: 10 mg, 20 mg

Extemporaneous Preparations Hazardous agent: Use appropriate precautions for handling and disposal.

A 0.5 mg/mL oral suspension may be prepared with tablets. Place two 10 mg tablets into 40 mL purified water and let stand ~2-5 minutes. Stir until tablets are completely disintegrated (dispersion time for each 10 mg tablet is ~2-5 minutes). Administer immediately after preparation. To ensure the full dose is administered, rinse glass several times with water and administer residue.

Lam MS, "Extemporaneous Compounding of Oral Liquid Dosage Formulations and Alternative Drug Delivery Methods for Anticancer Drugs," *Pharmacotherapy*, 2011, 31(2):164-92.

◆ **Tamoxifen Citras** *see* Tamoxifen *on page 1987*

◆ **Tamoxifen Citrate** *see* Tamoxifen *on page 1987*

Tamsulosin (tam SOO loe sin)

Brand Names: U.S. Flomax

Brand Names: Canada Ava-Tamsulosin CR; Flomax® CR; JAMP-Tamsulosin; Mylan-Tamsulosin; RAN™-Tamsulosin; ratio-Tamsulosin; Sandoz-Tamsulosin; Sandoz-Tamsulosin CR; Teva-Tamsulosin

Index Terms Tamsulosin Hydrochloride

Pharmacologic Category Alpha$_1$ Blocker

Use Treatment of signs and symptoms of benign prostatic hyperplasia (BPH)

Unlabeled Use Symptomatic treatment of bladder outlet obstruction or dysfunction; facilitation of expulsion of ureteral stones

Pregnancy Risk Factor B

Pregnancy Considerations Adverse events were not observed in animal reproduction studies. For pregnant women with kidney stones, other treatments such as stents or ureteroscopy, are recommended if stone removal is needed (Preminger, 2007; Tan, 2013).

Contraindications Hypersensitivity to tamsulosin or any component of the formulation

Warnings/Precautions Not intended for use as an antihypertensive drug. May cause significant orthostatic hypotension and syncope, especially with first dose; anticipate a similar effect if therapy is interrupted for a few days, if dosage is rapidly increased, or if another antihypertensive drug (particularly vasodilators) or a PDE-5 inhibitor (eg, sildenafil, tadalafil, vardenafil) is introduced. "First-dose" orthostatic hypotension may occur 4-8 hours after dosing; may be dose related. Patients should be cautioned about performing hazardous tasks when starting new therapy or adjusting dosage upward. Discontinue if symptoms of angina occur or worsen. Rule out prostatic carcinoma before beginning therapy with tamsulosin. Intraoperative floppy iris syndrome (IFIS) has been observed in cataract surgery patients who were on or were previously treated with alpha$_1$-blockers, particularly with tamsulosin use (Abdel-Aziz, 2009); in some cases, patients had discontinued the alpha1-blocker 5 weeks to 9 months prior to the surgery. The benefit of discontinuing alpha-blocker therapy prior to cataract surgery has not been established. IFIS may increase the risk of ocular complications during and after surgery. May require modifications to surgical technique; instruct patients to inform ophthalmologist of current or previous alpha$_1$-blocker use when considering eye surgery. Initiation of tamsulosin therapy in patients with planned cataract surgery is not recommended. Priapism has been associated with use (rarely). Rarely, patients with a sulfa allergy have also developed an allergic reaction to tamsulosin; avoid use when previous reaction has been severe.

Adverse Reactions

>10%:

Cardiovascular: Orthostatic hypotension (6% to 19%)

Central nervous system: Headache (19% to 21%), dizziness (15% to 17%)

Genitourinary: Abnormal ejaculation (8% to 18%)

Respiratory: Rhinitis (13% to 18%)

Miscellaneous: Infection (9% to 11%)

1% to 10%:

Cardiovascular: Chest pain (4%)

Central nervous system: Somnolence (3% to 4%), insomnia (1% to 2%), vertigo (≤1%)

Endocrine & metabolic: Libido decreased (1% to 2%)

Gastrointestinal: Diarrhea (4% to 6%), nausea (3% to 4%), gum pain, toothache

Neuromuscular & skeletal: Weakness (8% to 9%), back pain (7% to 8%)

Ocular: Blurred vision (≤2%)

Respiratory: Pharyngitis (5% to 6%), cough (3% to 5%), sinusitis (2% to 4%)

<1% (Limited to important or life-threatening): Allergic reactions (angioedema, pruritus, rash, urticaria, respiratory symptoms); constipation, hypotension, intraoperative floppy iris syndrome, lightheadedness, orthostasis (symptomatic), palpitation, priapism, skin desquamation, syncope, vomiting

Drug Interactions

Metabolism/Transport Effects Substrate of CYP2D6 (minor), CYP3A4 (major); **Note:** Assignment of Major/Minor substrate status based on clinically relevant drug interaction potential

Avoid Concomitant Use

Avoid concomitant use of Tamsulosin with any of the following: Alpha1-Blockers; CYP3A4 Inhibitors (Strong); Fusidic Acid (Systemic)

Increased Effect/Toxicity

Tamsulosin may increase the levels/effects of: Alpha1-Blockers; Calcium Channel Blockers

The levels/effects of Tamsulosin may be increased by: Beta-Blockers; CYP3A4 Inhibitors (Moderate); CYP3A4 Inhibitors (Strong); Dasatinib; Fusidic Acid (Systemic); Ivacaftor; Luliconazole; MAO Inhibitors; Mifepristone; Phosphodiesterase 5 Inhibitors; Simeprevir

Decreased Effect

Tamsulosin may decrease the levels/effects of: Alpha-/Beta-Agonists; Alpha1-Agonists

The levels/effects of Tamsulosin may be decreased by: Bosentan; CYP3A4 Inducers (Strong); Dabrafenib; Deferasirox; Herbs (CYP3A4 Inducers); Mitotane; Peginterferon Alfa-2b; Tocilizumab

Ethanol/Nutrition/Herb Interactions

Food: Fasting increases bioavailability by 30% and peak concentration 40% to 70%. Management: Administer 30 minutes after the same meal each day.

Herb/Nutraceutical: St John's wort may decrease the levels/effects of tamsulosin. Some herbal medications have hypotensive properties or may increase the hypotensive effect of tamsulosin. Limited information is available regarding combination with saw palmetto. Management: Avoid St John's wort, black cohosh, California poppy, coleus, golden seal, hawthorn, mistletoe, periwinkle, quinine, and shepherd's purse. Avoid saw palmetto.

Storage/Stability Store at room temperature of 25°C (77°F); excursions permitted to 15°C to 30°C (59°F to 86°F).

Mechanism of Action Tamsulosin is an antagonist of alpha$_{1A}$-adrenoreceptors in the prostate. Smooth muscle tone in the prostate is mediated by alpha$_{1A}$-adrenoreceptors; blocking them leads to relaxation of smooth muscle in the bladder neck and prostate causing an improvement of urine flow and decreased symptoms of BPH. Approximately 75% of the alpha$_1$-receptors in the prostate are of the alpha$_{1A}$ subtype.

Pharmacodynamics/Kinetics

Absorption: >90%

Distribution: V_d: 16 L

Protein binding: 94% to 99%, primarily to alpha$_1$ acid glycoprotein (AAG)

Metabolism: Hepatic (extensive) via CYP3A4 and 2D6; metabolites undergo extensive conjugation to glucuronide or sulfate

Bioavailability: Fasting: 30% increase

Steady-state: By the fifth day of once-daily dosing

Half-life elimination: Healthy volunteers: 9-13 hours; Target population: 14-15 hours

Time to peak: Fasting: 4-5 hours; With food: 6-7 hours

Excretion: Urine (76%, <10% as unchanged drug); feces (21%)

Dosage Oral: Adults:

Benign prostatic hyperplasia (BPH): 0.4 mg once daily ~30 minutes after the same meal each day; dose may be increased after 2-4 weeks to 0.8 mg once daily in patients who fail to respond. If therapy is interrupted for several days, restart with 0.4 mg once daily.

Bladder outlet obstruction symptoms (unlabeled use): 0.4 mg once daily (Rossi, 2001)

Ureteral stones, expulsion (unlabeled use): 0.4 mg once daily, discontinue after successful expulsion (average time to expulsion was 1-2 weeks) (Agrawal, 2009; Ahmed, 2010). **Note:** Patients with stones >10 mm were excluded from studies.

Dosage adjustment in renal impairment:

Cl_{cr} ≥10 mL/minute: No dosage adjustment necessary.

Cl_{cr} <10 mL/minute: No dosage adjustment provided in manufacturer's labeling (has not been studied).

Dosage adjustment in hepatic impairment:

Mild-to-moderate impairment: No adjustment needed

Severe impairment: Not studied

Dietary Considerations Take once daily, 30 minutes after the same meal each day.

Administration Administer 30 minutes after the same meal each day. Capsules should be swallowed whole; do not crush, chew, or open.

Dosage Forms Excipient information presented when available (limited, particularly for generics); consult specific product labeling.

Capsule, Oral, as hydrochloride:

Flomax: 0.4 mg [contains fd&c blue #2 (indigotine)]

Generic: 0.4 mg

◆ **Tamsulosin and Dutasteride** *see* Dutasteride and Tamsulosin *on page* 681

◆ **Tamsulosin Hydrochloride** *see* Tamsulosin *on page* 1990

◆ **Tamsulosin Hydrochloride and Dutasteride** *see* Dutasteride and Tamsulosin *on page* 681

◆ **Tanta-Orciprenaline® (Can)** *see* Metaproterenol *on page* 1309

◆ **TAP-144** *see* Leuprolide *on page* 1189

◆ **Tapazole** *see* Methimazole *on page* 1321

◆ **Tapazole® (Can)** *see* Methimazole *on page* 1321

Tapentadol (ta PEN ta dol)

Brand Names: U.S. Nucynta; Nucynta ER

Brand Names: Canada Nucynta CR; Nucynta IR

Index Terms CG5503; Tapentadol Hydrochloride

Pharmacologic Category Analgesic, Opioid

Use

Immediate release formulation: Relief of moderate-to-severe acute pain

Long acting formulation: Relief of moderate-to-severe chronic pain or neuropathic pain associated with diabetic peripheral neuropathy (DPN) when continuous, around-the-clock analgesia is necessary for an extended period of time

Pregnancy Risk Factor C

Pregnancy Considerations Adverse events were observed in animal reproduction studies. Opioids cross the placenta. Tapentadol is not recommended for use during labor and delivery and if exposure occurs the neonate should be monitored for respiratory depression. Use in pregnant women is contraindicated in the Canadian labeling.

If chronic opioid exposure occurs in pregnancy, adverse events in the newborn (including withdrawal) may occur; monitoring of the neonate is recommended. The minimum effective dose should be used if opioids are needed (Chou, 2009). Neonatal abstinence syndrome following opioid exposure may present with autonomic (eg, fever, temperature instability), gastrointestinal (eg, diarrhea, vomiting, poor feeding/weight gain), or neurologic (eg, high-pitched crying, increased muscle tone, irritability, seizure, tremor) symptoms (Dow, 2012; Hudak, 2012).

Breast-Feeding Considerations Limited information is available on the excretion of tapentadol in human milk; however, data suggests it may be excreted in human milk. The possibility of sedation or respiratory depression in the nursing infant should be considered; withdrawal may occur when maternal therapy is stopped. Due to the potential for serious adverse reactions in the nursing infant, the U.S. manufacturer recommends a decision be made whether to discontinue nursing or to discontinue the drug, taking into account the importance of treatment to the mother. Use while breast-feeding is contraindicated in the Canadian labeling.

Medication Guide Available Yes

Contraindications Hypersensitivity to tapentadol or any component of the formulation; significant respiratory depression; acute or severe asthma or hypercapnia in unmonitored settings or in absence of resuscitative equipment or ventilatory support; known or suspected paralytic ileus; use with or within 14 days of MAO inhibitors

Canadian labeling: Additional contraindications (not in U.S. labeling): Hypersensitivity to opioids; acute respiratory depression, cor pulmonale; gastrointestinal obstruction or any disease/condition that affects bowel transit (eg, ileus of any type, strictures); severe renal impairment (Cl_{cr} <30 mL/minute); severe hepatic impairment (Child-Pugh class C); mild, intermittent, or short-duration pain that can be managed with alternative pain medication; management of perioperative pain (controlled release tablets); acute alcoholism, delirium tremens, and seizure disorders; severe CNS depression, increased cerebrospinal or intracranial pressure or head injury; pregnancy; breast-feeding; use during labor/delivery

Warnings/Precautions Use with caution in patients with respiratory disease or respiratory compromise (eg, asthma, chronic obstructive pulmonary disease [COPD], cor pulmonale, sleep apnea, severe obesity, kyphoscoliosis, hypoxia, hypercapnia); critical respiratory depression may occur, even at therapeutic dosages. Use with caution in debilitated or cachectic patients; there is a greater potential for critical respiratory depression, even at therapeutic dosages. Use with extreme caution in patients with head injury, intracranial lesions, or elevated intracranial pressure (ICP); exaggerated elevation of ICP may occur. Use caution in patients with a history of seizures or conditions predisposing patients to seizures; patients with a history of seizures were excluded in clinical trials of tapentadol. Tramadol, an analgesic with similar pharmacologic properties to tapentadol, has been associated with seizures, particularly in patients with predisposing factors. May cause severe hypotension; use with caution in patients with risk factors (eg, hypovolemia, concomitant use of other hypotensive agents). Avoid use in patients with circulatory shock.

Opioids may obscure diagnosis or clinical course of patients with acute abdominal conditions. May cause CNS depression, which may impair physical or mental abilities; patients must be cautioned about performing tasks which require mental alertness (eg, operating machinery or driving). Effects may be potentiated when used with other sedative drugs or ethanol. Potentially significant drug-drug interactions may exist, requiring dose or frequency adjustment, additional monitoring, and/or selection of alternative therapy.

Use with caution in patients with adrenal insufficiency (including Addison's disease), patients with biliary tract dysfunction or acute pancreatitis (opioids may cause spasm of the sphincter of Oddi), patients with CNS depression (avoid use in patients with impaired consciousness or coma as these patients are susceptible to intracranial effects of CO_2 retention), patients with hypothyroidism, prostatic hyperplasia and/or urinary stricture. Use opioids with caution in the elderly; consider decreasing initial dose. May have a greater potential for critical respiratory depression. Serum concentrations are increased in hepatic impairment; use with caution in patients with moderate hepatic impairment (dosage adjustment required). Not recommended for use in severe hepatic impairment (not studied). Use with caution in patients with mild-to-moderate renal impairment; no dosage adjustments recommended. Not recommended for use in severe renal impairment (not studied).

Prolonged use increases risk of abuse, addiction, and withdrawal symptoms. An opioid-containing regimen should be tailored to each patient's needs with respect to degree of tolerance for opioids (naïve versus chronic user), age, weight, and medical condition. Abrupt discontinuation may lead to withdrawal symptoms. Symptoms may be decreased by tapering prior to discontinuation. Mixed agonist/antagonist opioids may diminish the analgesic effect of tapentadol or precipitate withdrawal symptoms. Abuse of products by crushing, chewing, snorting, or injecting may result in severe overdose, adverse effects, or death.

After chronic maternal exposure to opioids, neonatal withdrawal syndrome may occur in the newborn; monitor neonate closely. Signs and symptoms include irritability, hyperactivity and abnormal sleep pattern, high pitched cry, tremor, vomiting, diarrhea and failure to gain weight. Onset, duration and severity depend on the drug used, duration of use, maternal dose, and rate of drug elimination by the newborn. Opioid withdrawal syndrome in the neonate, unlike in adults, may be life-threatening and should be treated according to protocols developed by neonatology experts.

Extended release tablets:

[U.S. Boxed Warning]: Respiratory depression, possibly fatal, may occur. Proper dosing, titration, and monitoring are essential. Extended release tablets must be swallowed whole and should NOT be split,

crushed, broken, chewed, or dissolved in order to avoid rapid release and potential for fatal dose. Risk for respiratory depression is greatest during the initiation of therapy or with dose increases. Use is contraindicated in patients with significant respiratory depression or conditions that may increase that risk.

[U.S. Boxed Warning]: Accidental exposure, especially in children, may lead to fatal overdose. Not intended for use as an as-needed analgesic; **not** intended for the management of acute or postoperative pain; approved for the treatment of chronic pain only (not an as-needed basis).

[U.S. Boxed Warning]: Use of alcohol may increase tapentadol systemic exposure which may lead to possible fatal overdose. Avoid alcohol or alcohol containing medications during therapy.

[U.S. Boxed Warning]: Healthcare provider should be alert to problems of abuse, misuse, and diversion. Potential for abuse may be increased in patients with a history of or family history of substance abuse or mental illness. Use with caution in patients with a history of drug abuse or acute alcoholism. Tolerance, psychological and physical dependence may occur with prolonged use.

Adverse Reactions

Immediate release:

>10%:

Central nervous system: Dizziness (24%), somnolence (15%)

Gastrointestinal: Nausea (30%), vomiting (18%)

1% to 10%:

Central nervous system: Fatigue (3%), insomnia (2%), anxiety (1%), confusion (1%), dreams abnormal (1%), lethargy (1%)

Dermatologic: Pruritus (3% to 5%), hyperhidrosis (3%), rash (1%)

Endocrine & metabolic: Hot flushes (1%)

Gastrointestinal: Constipation (8%), xerostomia (4%), appetite decreased (2%), dyspepsia (2%)

Genitourinary: Urinary tract infection (1%)

Neuromuscular & skeletal: Arthralgia (1%), tremor (1%)

Respiratory: Nasopharyngitis (1%), upper respiratory tract infection (1%)

Extended release:

>10%:

Central nervous system: Dizziness (17% to 18%), headache (10% to 15%), somnolence (12% to 14%)

Gastrointestinal: Nausea (21% to 27%), constipation (13% to 17%), vomiting (8% to 12%)

1% to 10%:

Cardiovascular: Hypotension (1%)

Central nervous system: Fatigue (9%), anxiety (2% to 5%), insomnia (4%), irritability (2%), lethargy (2%), abnormal dreams (1% to 2%), vertigo (1% to 2%), attention disturbances (1%), chills (1%), depression/depressed mood (1%), hypoesthesia (1%), nervousness (1%), sedation (1%), withdrawal syndrome (1%)

Dermatologic: Pruritus (1% to 8%), hyperhidrosis (3% to 5%), rash (1%)

Endocrine & metabolic: Hot flushes (2% to 3%)

Gastrointestinal: Diarrhea (7%), xerostomia (7%), appetite decreased (2% to 6%), dyspepsia (1% to 3%), abdominal discomfort (1%)

Genitourinary: Erectile dysfunction (1%)

Neuromuscular & skeletal: Tremor (1% to 3%), weakness (2%)

Ocular: Vision blurred (1%)

Respiratory: Dyspnea (1%)

Immediate and/or extended release: <1% (Limited to important or life-threatening): Anaphylaxis, abnormal thinking, agitation, angioedema, ataxia, blood pressure decreased, consciousness depressed, coordination abnormal, disorientation, drug withdrawal, drunk feeling, dysarthria, euphoria, gastric emptying impaired, hallucination, hypersensitivity, memory impaired, paresthesia, pollakiuria, presyncope, respiratory depression, seizure, syncope, urinary hesitation, urticaria, visual disturbance

Drug Interactions

Metabolism/Transport Effects Substrate of CYP2C9 (minor), CYP2D6 (minor); **Note:** Assignment of Major/Minor substrate status based on clinically relevant drug interaction potential

Avoid Concomitant Use

Avoid concomitant use of Tapentadol with any of the following: Alcohol (Ethyl); Azelastine (Nasal); MAO Inhibitors; Paraldehyde

Increased Effect/Toxicity

Tapentadol may increase the levels/effects of: Alvimopan; Antipsychotics; Azelastine (Nasal); CNS Depressants; Desmopressin; Diuretics; Hydrocodone; MAO Inhibitors; Metoclopramide; Metyrosine; Paraldehyde; Pramipexole; ROPINIRole; Rotigotine; Selective Serotonin Reuptake Inhibitors; Serotonin Modulators; Zolpidem

The levels/effects of Tapentadol may be increased by: Alcohol (Ethyl); Amphetamines; Anticholinergics; Antipsychotic Agents (Phenothiazines); Antipsychotics; Brimonidine (Topical); Cannabinoids; Doxylamine; HydrOXYzine; Magnesium Sulfate; Perampanel; Sodium Oxybate; Succinylcholine

Decreased Effect

Tapentadol may decrease the levels/effects of: Pegvisomant

The levels/effects of Tapentadol may be decreased by: Ammonium Chloride; Antiemetics (5HT3 Antagonists); Mixed Agonist / Antagonist Opioids; Peginterferon Alfa-2b

Ethanol/Nutrition/Herb Interactions

Ethanol: Concomitant use with alcohol may increase CNS depression and can increase the bioavailability of extended release tablets. Management: Avoid use of alcohol during therapy.

Food: When administered after a high fat/calorie meal, the AUC and C_{max} increased by 25% and 16%, respectively; may administer without regard to meals.

Herb/Nutraceutical: Avoid St John's wort (may increase CNS depression and risk of serotonin syndrome).

Storage/Stability Store at room temperature up to 25°C (77°F); excursions permitted to 15°C to 30°C (59°F to 86°F). Protect from moisture.

Mechanism of Action Binds to µ-opiate receptors in the CNS causing inhibition of ascending pain pathways, altering the perception of and response to pain; also inhibits the reuptake of norepinephrine, which also modifies the ascending pain pathway

Pharmacodynamics/Kinetics

Absorption: Rapid and complete

Distribution: V_d: I.V.: 442-638 L

Protein binding: ~20%

Metabolism: Extensive metabolism, including first pass metabolism; metabolized primarily via phase 2 glucuronidation to glucuronides (major metabolite: tapentadol-O-glucuronide); minimal phase 1 oxidative metabolism; also metabolized to a lesser degree by CYP2C9, CYP2C19, and CYP2D6; all metabolites pharmacologically inactive

Bioavailability: ~32%

Half-life elimination: Immediate release: ~4 hours; Long acting formulations: ~5-6 hours

Time to peak, plasma: Immediate release: 1.25 hours; Long acting formulations: 3-6 hours

Excretion: Urine (99%: 70% conjugated metabolites; 3% unchanged drug)

Dosage Adults: **Note:** Dose and dosage intervals should be individualized according to pain severity with respect to patient's previous experience with similar opioid analgesics. In patients receiving extended release tapentadol, immediate-release opioid or nonopioid medication may be used for rescue relief of breakthrough pain and during dosage adjustments. The Canadian labeling does not recommend use of fentanyl as rescue medication. To reduce the risk of withdrawal symptoms, it is recommended to taper the dose when discontinuing therapy.

Acute moderate-severe pain: Oral: *Immediate release:* Day 1: 50-100 mg every 4-6 hours as needed; may administer a second dose ≥1 hour after the initial dose (maximum dose on first day: 700 mg daily); Day 2 and subsequent dosing: 50-100 mg every 4-6 hours as needed (maximum: 600 mg daily)

Chronic moderate-severe pain (U.S. and Canadian labeling), neuropathic pain associated with diabetic peripheral neuropathy (U.S. labeling): Oral: *Extended release:*

Opioid naive: Initial: 50 mg twice daily (recommended interval: every 12 hours)

Opioid experienced: No adequate data on converting patients from other opioids to tapentadol extended release. In general, begin with a dose that is 50% of the estimated daily tapentadol requirement and use immediate release rescue medications to supplement dose. Per the Canadian product labeling, comparable pain relief was observed between tapentadol CR and oxycodone CR at a dose ratio of 5:1 in clinical studies.

Conversion from Nucynta immediate release to extended release: Convert using same total daily dose but divide into 2 equal doses and administer twice daily (recommended interval: ~12 hours) (maximum dose: 500 mg daily).

Dose titration: Titrate in increments of 50 mg no more frequently than twice daily every 3 days to effective dose (therapeutic range: 100-250 mg twice daily) (maximum dose: 500 mg daily)

Elderly: Initial: Consider initiating at lower range of dosing. Refer to adult dosing.

Dosage adjustment in renal impairment:

Cl_{cr} ≥30 mL/minute: No dosage adjustment necessary.

Cl_{cr} <30 mL/minute: Use not recommended (not studied); use is contraindicated in the Canadian labeling.

Dosage adjustment in hepatic impairment:

Mild impairment: No dosage adjustment necessary.

Moderate impairment:

Immediate release: Initial: 50 mg every 8 hours or longer (maximum: 3 doses/24 hours). Further treatment for maintenance of analgesia may be achieved by either shortening or lengthening the dosing interval.

Extended release: Initial: 50 mg every 24 hours or longer; maximum: 100 mg once daily

Severe impairment: Use not recommended (not studied); use is contraindicated in the Canadian labeling.

Dietary Considerations May be taken without regard to meals.

Administration Administer orally with or without food. Long acting formulations must be swallowed whole and should **not** be split, crushed, broken, chewed, or dissolved; patients should be instructed to swallow 1 tablet at a time, immediately after placing in mouth. The Canadian product labeling recommends that immediate release tablets be swallowed whole.

Monitoring Parameters Respiratory and cardiovascular status, blood pressure, heart rate; signs of misuse, abuse, or addiction

Extended release tablets: Monitor for respiratory depression for 72 hours of initiating dose.

Product Availability Nucynta Oral Solution: FDA approved October 2012; anticipated availability currently unknown. Refer to prescribing information for additional information.

Dosage Forms Excipient information presented when available (limited, particularly for generics); consult specific product labeling.

Tablet, Oral:

Nucynta: 50 mg, 75 mg, 100 mg

Tablet Extended Release 12 Hour, Oral:

Nucynta ER: 50 mg

Nucynta ER: 100 mg, 150 mg [contains fd&c blue #2 aluminum lake]

Nucynta ER: 200 mg, 250 mg [scored; contains fd&c blue #2 aluminum lake]

Dosage Forms: Canada Excipient information presented when available (limited, particularly for generics); consult specific product labeling.

Tablet, Oral:

Nucynta: 50 mg, 75 mg, 100 mg

Tablet, Controlled Release, Oral, as hydrochloride:

Nucynta CR: 50 mg, 100 mg, 150 mg, 200 mg, 250 mg

Controlled Substance C-II

- Tapentadol Hydrochloride *see* Tapentadol *on page 1992*
- Tarceva *see* Erlotinib *on page 735*
- Tarceva® (Can) *see* Erlotinib *on page 735*
- Targretin *see* Bexarotene (Systemic) *on page 255*
- Targretin *see* Bexarotene (Topical) *on page 257*
- Tarka® *see* Trandolapril and Verapamil *on page 2104*
- Taro-Anastrozole (Can) *see* Anastrozole *on page 137*
- Taro-Carbamazepine Chewable (Can) *see* CarBAMazepine *on page 336*
- Taro-Ciclopirox (Can) *see* Ciclopirox *on page 423*
- Taro-Ciprofloxacin (Can) *see* Ciprofloxacin (Systemic) *on page 430*
- Taro-Clindamycin (Can) *see* Clindamycin (Topical) *on page 454*
- Taro-Clobetasol (Can) *see* Clobetasol *on page 457*
- Taro-Enalapril (Can) *see* Enalapril *on page 701*
- Taro-Fluconazole (Can) *see* Fluconazole *on page 868*
- Taro-Mometasone (Can) *see* Mometasone (Topical) *on page 1395*
- Taro-Phenytoin (Can) *see* Phenytoin *on page 1638*
- Taro-Simvastatin (Can) *see* Simvastatin *on page 1899*
- Taro-Sone (Can) *see* Betamethasone *on page 247*
- Taro-Sumatriptan (Can) *see* SUMAtriptan *on page 1969*
- Taro-Terconazole (Can) *see* Terconazole *on page 2021*
- Taro-Warfarin (Can) *see* Warfarin *on page 2211*
- Tasigna *see* Nilotinib *on page 1458*
- Tasmar *see* Tolcapone *on page 2085*
- Tavist Allergy [OTC] *see* Clemastine *on page 449*
- Tavist ND *see* Loratadine *on page 1240*
- Taxol *see* PACLitaxel *on page 1543*
- Taxotere *see* DOCEtaxel *on page 638*

Tazarotene (taz AR oh teen)

Brand Names: U.S. Avage; Fabior; Tazorac

Brand Names: Canada Tazorac

Pharmacologic Category Acne Products; Keratolytic Agent; Topical Skin Product, Acne

Use Topical treatment of facial acne vulgaris; topical treatment of stable plaque psoriasis; mitigation (palliation) of facial skin wrinkling, facial mottled hyper-/hypopigmentation, and benign facial lentigines

Pregnancy Risk Factor X

Dosage Topical: **Note:** In patients experiencing excessive pruritus, burning, skin redness, or peeling, discontinue until integrity of the skin is restored, or reduce dosing to an interval the patient is able to tolerate.

Children ≥12 years, Adolescents, and Adults:

Acne:

Fabior foam 0.1%: Apply once daily.

Tazorac cream/gel 0.1%: Apply a thin film (2 mg/cm^2) to affected area once daily.

Psoriasis: Tazorac gel: Initial: 0.05%: Apply once daily to psoriatic lesions using enough (2 mg/cm^2) to cover only the lesion with a thin film to no more than 20% of body surface area. May increase strength to 0.1% if tolerated and necessary.

Children ≥17 years and Adults: Palliation of fine facial wrinkles, facial mottled hyper-/hypopigmentation, benign facial lentigines: Avage: Apply a pea-sized amount once daily.

Adults: Psoriasis: Tazorac cream: Initial: 0.05%: Apply once daily to psoriatic lesions using enough (2 mg/cm^2) to cover only the lesion with a thin film. May increase strength to 0.1% if tolerated and necessary.

Additional Information Complete prescribing information should be consulted for additional detail.

Dosage Forms Excipient information presented when available (limited, particularly for generics); consult specific product labeling.

Cream, External:

Avage: 0.1% (30 g) [contains benzyl alcohol]

Tazorac: 0.05% (30 g, 60 g); 0.1% (30 g, 60 g) [contains benzyl alcohol]

Foam, External:

Fabior: 0.1% (50 g, 100 g)

Gel, External:

Tazorac: 0.05% (30 g, 100 g); 0.1% (30 g, 100 g) [contains benzyl alcohol]

◆ **Tazicef** *see* CefTAZidime *on page 379*

◆ **Tazobactam and Piperacillin** *see* Piperacillin and Tazobactam *on page 1653*

◆ **Tazocin (Can)** *see* Piperacillin and Tazobactam *on page 1653*

◆ **Tazorac** *see* Tazarotene *on page 1994*

◆ **Taztia XT** *see* Diltiazem *on page 613*

◆ **TBC** *see* Trypsin, Balsam Peru, and Castor Oil *on page 2133*

◆ **Tbo-Filgrastim** *see* Filgrastim *on page 859*

◆ **TB Skin Test** *see* Tuberculin Tests *on page 2134*

◆ **3TC** *see* LamiVUDine *on page 1162*

◆ **3TC® (Can)** *see* LamiVUDine *on page 1162*

◆ **3TC, Abacavir, and Zidovudine** *see* Abacavir, Lamivudine, and Zidovudine *on page 20*

◆ **T-Cell Growth Factor** *see* Aldesleukin *on page 63*

◆ **TCGF** *see* Aldesleukin *on page 63*

◆ **TCN** *see* Tetracycline *on page 2034*

◆ **Td** *see* Diphtheria and Tetanus Toxoid *on page 626*

◆ **TD-6424** *see* Telavancin *on page 1999*

◆ **Td Adsorbed (Can)** *see* Diphtheria and Tetanus Toxoid *on page 626*

◆ **Tdap** *see* Diphtheria and Tetanus Toxoids, and Acellular Pertussis Vaccine *on page 630*

◆ **TDF** *see* Tenofovir *on page 2012*

◆ **T-DM1** *see* Ado-Trastuzumab Emtansine *on page 52*

◆ **Tebrazid™ (Can)** *see* Pyrazinamide *on page 1751*

◆ **Tecfidera** *see* Dimethyl Fumarate *on page 618*

◆ **Tecnu First Aid [OTC]** *see* Lidocaine (Topical) *on page 1212*

◆ **Tecta® (Can)** *see* Pantoprazole *on page 1563*

Teduglutide (te due GLOO tide)

Brand Names: U.S. Gattex

Index Terms ALX-0600; Teduglutide Recombinant; Teduglutide [rDNA origin]

Pharmacologic Category Glucagon-Like Peptide-2 (GLP-2) Analog

Use Treatment of short bowel syndrome (SBS) in patients requiring parenteral nutrition support

Pregnancy Risk Factor B

Pregnancy Considerations Adverse events were not observed in animal reproduction studies.

Breast-Feeding Considerations It is not known if teduglutide is excreted into breast milk. Due to the potential for serious adverse reactions in the nursing infant, a decision should be made whether to discontinue nursing or to discontinue the drug, taking into account the importance of treatment to the mother.

Medication Guide Available Yes

Contraindications There are no contraindications listed in the manufacturer's labeling.

Warnings/Precautions Teduglutide may increase the risk of hyperplastic changes, including neoplasia. In patients at increased risk for malignancy, consider treatment only if benefits outweigh the risks. Discontinue treatment in patients with active gastrointestinal malignancy (GI tract, hepatobiliary, pancreatic); evaluate risk versus benefit in patients with active non-GI malignancy. Monitor for small bowel neoplasia; remove any benign neoplasm. Development of colorectal polyps has been described in patients receiving teduglutide. A baseline colonoscopy of the entire colon with polyp removal is recommended ≤6 months prior to initiation of therapy. Follow-up colonoscopy (or alternative imaging) should be performed at 1 year and at least every 5 years, thereafter. Discontinue teduglutide in patients who develop colorectal cancer.

Intestinal and stomal obstructions have been reported (onset usually 1 day to 7 months); temporarily discontinue treatment in patients that develop obstruction. Teduglutide may be resumed (if clinically indicated) once the obstruction is resolved. Increased fluid absorption and subsequent fluid overload/congestive heart failure has been reported; consider modification of parenteral support in patients who develop fluid overload, especially in patients with underlying cardiovascular disease; if significant cardiac deterioration develops, reassess the need for continued teduglutide treatment. Cholecystitis, cholangitis, cholelithiasis, and pancreatitis have been reported; monitor serum bilirubin, alkaline phosphatase, lipase, and amylase at least every 6 months for duration of therapy; if clinically meaningful changes are detected, perform gallbladder/biliary tract/pancreatic imaging and reassess the need for continued teduglutide treatment.

Teduglutide may increase absorption of oral medications; monitor therapy of medications with a narrow therapeutic index. Treatment discontinuation may result in fluid and electrolyte imbalance; carefully monitor fluid/electrolyte status.

Adverse Reactions

>10%:

Central nervous system: Headache (16%)

Endocrine & metabolic: Fluid overload (12%)

Gastrointestinal: Stoma complications (42%), abdominal pain (30% to 38%), nausea (18% to 25%), abdominal distension (14% to 20%), vomiting (12%)
Local: Injection site reaction (12% to 22%)
Respiratory: Upper respiratory tract infection (12% to 26%)

1% to 10%:
Central nervous system: Sleep disturbances (5%)
Dermatologic: Cutaneous hemorrhage (5%)
Gastrointestinal: Flatulence (9%), appetite disorders (7%), intestinal obstruction/stenosis (4%), colorectal polyps (2%)
Respiratory: Cough (5%)
Miscellaneous: Hypersensitivity reactions (8%)

<1% (Limited to important or life-threatening): Cholecystitis, cholelithiasis, cholestasis, congestive heart failure, gallbladder perforation, malignancy, pancreatic pseudocyst, pancreatitis

Drug Interactions

Metabolism/Transport Effects None known.

Avoid Concomitant Use There are no known interactions where it is recommended to avoid concomitant use.

Increased Effect/Toxicity There are no known significant interactions involving an increase in effect.

Decreased Effect There are no known significant interactions involving a decrease in effect.

Preparation for Administration Reconstitute each vial with 0.5 mL of SWFI (provided in syringe); let stand for 30 seconds and then roll vial between palms for 15 seconds. Do not shake. Allow vial to stand for an additional ~2 minutes; if undissolved material remains, roll between palms again. If particles are not dissolved after second attempt, discard vial. Once reconstituted, each vial provides 3.8 mg/0.38 mL (concentration is 10 mg/mL).

Storage/Stability Prior to dispensing, store intact vials refrigerated at 2°C to 8°C (36°F to 46°F); do not freeze. The carton of ancillary supplies should be stored at 25°C (77°F). After dispensing, store vials at 25°C (77°F); once dispensed, vials must be used within 90 days. Once reconstituted, use within 3 hours. Discard any unused portion.

Mechanism of Action Teduglutide is an analog of glucagon-like peptide-2 (GLP-2), which is secreted in the distal intestine. Endogenous GLP-2 increases intestinal and portal blood flow while inhibiting gastric acid secretion and reducing gastric motility, thereby reducing intestinal losses and improving intestinal absorption. Teduglutide binds and activates GLP-2 receptors, resulting in release of mediators including insulin-like growth factor (IGF)-1, nitric oxide and keratinocyte growth factor (KGF).

Pharmacodynamics/Kinetics

Distribution: 0.1 L/kg
Metabolism: Similar to endogenous catabolism of GLP-2 but slower due to a single amino acid substitution (Ferrone, 2006)
Bioavailability: SubQ: 88%
Half-life elimination: 1.3 hours
Time to peak, plasma: 3-5 hours
Excretion: Urine

Dosage Short bowel syndrome: Adults: SubQ: 0.05 mg/kg once daily

Missed doses: If a dose is missed, take as soon as possible on that day; do **NOT** take 2 doses on the same day.

Dosage adjustment in renal impairment:
Cl_{cr} ≥50 mL/minute: No dosage adjustment necessary.
Cl_{cr} <50 mL/minute: Administer 50% of the usual dose.
ESRD: Administer 50% of the usual dose.

Dosage adjustment in hepatic impairment:
Mild-to-moderate impairment (Child-Pugh class B): No dosage adjustment necessary.
Severe impairment: No dosage adjustment provided in manufacturer's labeling (has not been studied).

Administration SubQ: Rotate injection site between thighs, upper arms, and quadrants of the abdomen. Do not administer I.M. or I.V.

Monitoring Parameters Serum bilirubin, alkaline phosphatase, lipase and amylase (baseline [within 6 months prior to initiation] and every 6 months thereafter); colonoscopy of entire colon and removal of polyps (baseline [within 6 months prior to initiation], 1 year, and ≤5 years thereafter); monitor fluid status in patients with cardiovascular disease; signs/symptoms of intestinal obstruction; signs/symptoms suggestive of gall bladder disease or pancreatitis; monitor fluid and electrolyte balance following therapy discontinuation

Dosage Forms Excipient information presented when available (limited, particularly for generics); consult specific product labeling.

Kit, Subcutaneous [preservative free]:
Gattex: 5 mg

- ◆ Teduglutide [rDNA origin] *see* Teduglutide *on page 1995*
- ◆ Teduglutide Recombinant *see* Teduglutide *on page 1995*
- ◆ Teflaro *see* Ceftaroline Fosamil *on page 378*
- ◆ Tegaderm CHG Dressing [OTC] *see* Chlorhexidine Gluconate *on page 408*
- ◆ TEGretol *see* CarBAMazepine *on page 336*
- ◆ Tegretol® (Can) *see* CarBAMazepine *on page 336*
- ◆ TEGretol-XR *see* CarBAMazepine *on page 336*
- ◆ TEI-6720 *see* Febuxostat *on page 834*
- ◆ Tekturna *see* Aliskiren *on page 74*
- ◆ Tekturna HCT *see* Aliskiren and Hydrochlorothiazide *on page 76*

Telaprevir (tel A pre vir)

Brand Names: U.S. Incivek

Brand Names: Canada Incivek™

Index Terms LY570310; MP-424; MP424; VRT111950; VX-950; VX950

Pharmacologic Category Antihepaciviral, Protease Inhibitor (Anti-HCV)

Use Chronic hepatitis C: Treatment of genotype 1 chronic hepatitis C (in combination with peginterferon alfa and ribavirin) in adult patients with compensated liver disease (including cirrhosis) who are treatment naive or who have received previous interferon-based treatment, including null or partial responders, and treatment relapsers.

Pregnancy Risk Factor B / X (in combination with ribavirin)

Pregnancy Considerations Adverse events were not observed in telaprevir animal developmental studies; however, telaprevir must not be used as monotherapy (must be used in combination with peginterferon alfa and ribavirin). Significant ribavirin teratogenic effects have been observed in all animal studies at ~0.01 times the maximum recommended daily human dose. Use of ribavirin is contraindicated in pregnancy. In addition, animal studies with interferons have demonstrated abortifacient effects. Negative pregnancy test is required before initiation and monthly thereafter. Hormonal contraceptive measures may not be effective in patients taking telaprevir or for 2 weeks after discontinuing therapy. Avoid pregnancy in female patients and female partners of male patients during therapy by using two effective nonhormonal forms of contraception; continue contraceptive measures for at least 6 months after completion of therapy. If patient or female partner becomes pregnant during treatment, she should be counseled about potential risks of exposure. If pregnancy occurs during use or within 6 months after treatment, report to the ribavirin pregnancy registry (800-593-2214).

Breast-Feeding Considerations It is not known if telaprevir or ribavirin are excreted into breast milk. The manufacturer recommends that breast-feeding be discontinued prior to the initiation of treatment.

Medication Guide Available Yes

Contraindications

Combination treatment with ribavirin: Pregnancy; male partners of pregnant women

Coadministration with alfuzosin, cisapride, ergot derivatives (eg, dihydroergotamine, ergonovine, ergotamine, methylergonovine), lovastatin, midazolam [oral], pimozide, sildenafil/tadalafil [when used for treatment of pulmonary arterial hypertension], simvastatin, triazolam), rifampin, St John's wort, carbamazepine, phenobarbital, phenytoin

Canadian labeling: Additional contraindications (not in U.S. labeling): Hypersensitivity to telaprevir or any component of the formulation; coadministration with amiodarone, atorvastatin, eletriptan, flecainide, propafenone, quinidine, terfenadine, vardenafil

Warnings/Precautions [U.S. Boxed Warning] Serious skin reactions (some fatal) including Stevens-Johnson syndrome (SJS), drug reaction with eosinophilia and systemic symptoms (DRESS), and toxic epidermal necrolysis (TEN), have been reported with telaprevir combination therapy. Fatal cases have been reported in patients with progressive rash and systemic symptoms who received ongoing therapy after diagnoses of serious skin reactions. Discontinue telaprevir, peginterferon alfa, and ribavirin immediately for serious skin reactions (including rash with systemic symptoms or a progressive severe rash) and refer for immediate medical care. Rash has been typically observed within first 4 weeks of therapy initiation but may occur at any time. Severe rashes (other than DRESS, SJS) are generalized, bullous, vesicular or ulcerative; may also have an eczematous appearance. Discontinue telaprevir (may continue peginterferon alfa and ribavirin) for severe rash or for mild-to-moderate rash that progresses; if no improvement in rash within 1 week of stopping telaprevir, interruption or discontinuation of peginterferon alfa and/or ribavirin should be considered (or sooner if clinically indicated). May use oral antihistamines/topical corticosteroids for rash treatment; do not use systemic corticosteroids. Do not restart telaprevir if discontinued due to any skin reaction.

Prerenal azotemia (with or without acute renal failure) and uric acid nephropathy have been reported. Assess serum electrolytes, creatinine, and uric acid pretreatment, at weeks 2, 4, 8, and 12, and when clinically indicated. Maintain adequate hydration. Anemia has been reported with peginterferon alfa and ribavirin; addition of telaprevir is associated with further hemoglobin decreases. Low hemoglobin levels were measured during the first 4 weeks of treatment, and the lowest at the end of telaprevir treatment (week 12). Dose modifications of ribavirin were needed more often in patients also taking telaprevir. Assess hematologic parameters (CBC with differential and platelet count) pretreatment, at weeks 2, 4, 8, and 12, and when clinically indicated. May require ribavirin dose reduction, interruption or discontinuation of treatment; if ribavirin dose reductions are inadequate, may consider discontinuing telaprevir. Do not reduce telaprevir dose. If ribavirin is discontinued, telaprevir must also be discontinued. Do not restart telaprevir if ribavirin therapy is reinitiated.

Avoid pregnancy in female patients and female partners of male patients, during therapy, and for at least 6 months after treatment; two forms of nonhormonal contraception should be used. Hormonal contraceptives may not be effective in patients taking telaprevir or for two weeks after discontinuing therapy. Safety and efficacy have not been established in patients who have uncompensated cirrhosis, received liver transplants, or who have failed to respond to other NS3/4A inhibitors (including repeated courses of telaprevir). Monotherapy is not effective for chronic hepatitis C infection. Not recommended in moderate or severe hepatic impairment (Child-Pugh class B or C) or decompensated hepatic disease. Potentially significant drug-drug interactions may exist, requiring dose or frequency adjustments, additional monitoring, and/or selection of alternative therapy.

Adverse Reactions

>10%:

Central nervous system: Fatigue (56%)

Dermatologic: Rash (56%), pruritus (47%)

Endocrine and Metabolic: Hyperuricemia (<12.1 mg/dL: 66%; ≥12.1 mg/dL: 7%)

Gastrointestinal: Nausea (39%), diarrhea (26%), vomiting (13%), hemorrhoids (12%), anorectal discomfort (11%)

Hematologic: Anemia (36%), lymphopenia (15%)

Hepatic: Hyperbilirubinemia (<2.6 x ULN: 37%; ≥2.6 x ULN: 4%)

1% to 10%:

Gastrointestinal: Abnormal taste (10%), anal pruritus (6%)

Hematologic: Thrombocytopenia (3%)

<1% (Limited to important or life-threatening): Drug reaction with eosinophilia and systemic symptoms (DRESS), erythema multiforme, prerenal azotemia (with or without acute renal failure/insufficiency), Stevens-Johnson syndrome, toxic epidermal necrolysis, uric acid nephropathy

Drug Interactions

Metabolism/Transport Effects Substrate of CYP3A4 (major), P-glycoprotein; **Note:** Assignment of Major/Minor substrate status based on clinically relevant drug interaction potential; **Inhibits** CYP3A4 (strong), P-glycoprotein, SLCO1B1

Avoid Concomitant Use

Avoid concomitant use of Telaprevir with any of the following: Ado-Trastuzumab Emtansine; Alfuzosin; Apixaban; AtorvaSTATin; Avanafil; Axitinib; Bosutinib; Cabozantinib; CarBAMazepine; Cisapride; Conivaptan; Crizotinib; CYP3A4 Inducers (Strong); Darunavir; Dihydroergotamine; Dronedarone; Eplerenone; Ergoloid Mesylates; Ergonovine; Ergotamine; Everolimus; Fosamprenavir; Fosphenytoin; Fusidic Acid (Systemic); Halofantrine; Ibrutinib; Imatinib; Ivabradine; Lapatinib; Lomitapide; Lopinavir; Lovastatin; Lurasidone; Macitentan; Methylergonovine; Midazolam; Nilotinib; Nisoldipine; PHENobarbital; Phenytoin; Pimozide; Pomalidomide; Ranolazine; Red Yeast Rice; Regorafenib; Rifabutin; Rifampin; Rivaroxaban; Salmeterol; Sildenafil; Silodosin; Simeprevir; Simvastatin; St Johns Wort; Tamsulosin; Ticagrelor; Tolvaptan; Topotecan; Toremifene; Triazolam; Ulipristal; Vemurafenib; VinCRIStine (Liposomal)

Increased Effect/Toxicity

Telaprevir may increase the levels/effects of: Ado-Trastuzumab Emtansine; Afatinib; Alfuzosin; Almotriptan; Alosetron; ALPRAZolam; Amiodarone; Apixaban; ARIPiprazole; Atazanavir; AtorvaSTATin; Avanafil; Axitinib; Bedaquiline; Bepridil [Off Market]; Bortezomib; Bosentan; Bosutinib; Brentuximab Vedotin; Brinzolamide; Budesonide (Nasal); Budesonide (Systemic, Oral Inhalation); Cabozantinib; CarBAMazepine; Cisapride; Clarithromycin; Colchicine; Conivaptan; Corticosteroids; Corticosteroids (Orally Inhaled); Corticosteroids (Systemic); Crizotinib; CycloSPORINE (Systemic); CYP3A4 Substrates; Dabigatran Etexilate; Dienogest; Digoxin; Dihydroergotamine; Dofetilide; Dronedarone; Dutasteride; Enzalutamide; Eplerenone; Ergoloid Mesylates; Ergonovine; Ergotamine; Erythromycin (Systemic); Everolimus; FentaNYL; Fesoterodine; Flecainide; Fluticasone

(Nasal); Fluticasone (Oral Inhalation); Fluvastatin; Fosphenytoin; GuanFACINE; Halofantrine; Ibrutinib; Iloperidone; Imatinib; Itraconazole; Ivabradine; Ivacaftor; Ixabepilone; Ketoconazole (Systemic); Lacosamide; Lapatinib; Levomilnacipran; Lidocaine (Systemic); Lomitapide; Lovastatin; Lumefantrine; Lurasidone; Macitentan; Maraviroc; Methylergonovine; MethylPREDNISolone; Midazolam; Mifepristone; Nilotinib; Nisoldipine; Ospemifene; OxyCODONE; Paricalcitol; PAZOPanib; P-glycoprotein/ABCB1 Substrates; Phenytoin; Pimecrolimus; Pimozide; Pitavastatin; Pomalidomide; PONATinib; Posaconazole; Pravastatin; Propafenone; Prucalopride; QUEtiapine; QuiNIDine; Ranolazine; Red Yeast Rice; Regorafenib; Repaglinide; Rifabutin; Rilpivirine; Rivaroxaban; RomiDEPsin; Rosuvastatin; Ruxolitinib; Salmeterol; Saxagliptin; Sildenafil; Silodosin; Simeprevir; Simvastatin; Sirolimus; SORAfenib; Tacrolimus (Systemic); Tadalafil; Tamsulosin; Telithromycin; Tenofovir; Ticagrelor; Tofacitinib; Tolterodine; Tolvaptan; Topotecan; Toremifene; TraZODone; Triazolam; Ulipristal; Vardenafil; Vemurafenib; Vilazodone; VinCRIStine (Liposomal); Voriconazole; Warfarin; Zuclopenthixol

The levels/effects of Telaprevir may be increased by: Clarithromycin; CYP3A4 Inhibitors (Moderate); CYP3A4 Inhibitors (Strong); Dasatinib; Erythromycin (Systemic); Fusidic Acid (Systemic); Itraconazole; Ketoconazole (Systemic); Luliconazole; P-glycoprotein/ABCB1 Inhibitors; Posaconazole; Ritonavir; Telithromycin; Voriconazole

Decreased Effect

Telaprevir may decrease the levels/effects of: Contraceptives (Estrogens); Contraceptives (Progestins); Darunavir; Efavirenz; Escitalopram; Fosamprenavir; Ifosfamide; Methadone; Prasugrel; Ticagrelor; Voriconazole; Warfarin; Zolpidem

The levels/effects of Telaprevir may be decreased by: Atazanavir; Bosentan; CarBAMazepine; Corticosteroids; Corticosteroids (Systemic); CYP3A4 Inducers (Strong); Dabrafenib; Darunavir; Deferasirox; Efavirenz; Etravirine; Fosamprenavir; Fosphenytoin; Lopinavir; P-glycoprotein/ABCB1 Inducers; PHENobarbital; Phenytoin; Rifabutin; Rifampin; Ritonavir; St Johns Wort; Tocilizumab

Storage/Stability Store at 25°C (77°F); excursions permitted to 15°C to 30°C (59°F to 86°F).

Mechanism of Action Binds reversibly to nonstructural protein 3 (NS 3) serine protease and inhibits replication of the hepatitis C virus. Considered a direct-acting antiviral treatment for HCV, also called a specifically targeted antiviral therapy for HCV (STAT-C).

Pharmacodynamics/Kinetics Note: Telaprevir total exposure ($AUC_{24h,ss}$) was similar regardless of whether the total daily dose of 2250 mg was administered as 750 mg every 8 hours or 1125 mg twice daily.

Absorption: Food (not low fat) enhances absorption
Distribution: V_d: ~252 L
Protein binding: 59% to 76%
Metabolism: Primarily hepatic to less active (30x) and inactive metabolites. Some oxidative CYP3A4 metabolism.
Half-life elimination: Plasma: Adults: ~4-5 hours (single dose); steady state: ~9-11 hours
Time to peak, serum: 4-5 hours
Excretion: Feces (82%); urine (1%)

Dosage Oral: Adults: 1125 mg twice daily (in combination with peginterferon alfa and ribavirin)

Treatment-naive or prior relapse patients: **Note:** Relapse includes patients with an undetectable HCV-RNA upon completion of treatment (non-telaprevir based regimen) but with detectable HCV-RNA during the follow up period.

Weeks 1-12: Triple therapy: Telaprevir 1125 mg twice daily in combination with peginterferon alfa and ribavirin

Weeks 13-23 (based on HCV-RNA results at weeks 4 and 12):

HCV-RNA **undetectable** (level less than ~10-15 units/mL) at both weeks 4 and 12 (eRVR): Dual therapy: Peginterferon alfa and ribavirin only (through week 24)

HCV-RNA **detectable** (level greater than ~10-15 units/mL but ≤1000 units/mL) at week 4 and/or week 12: Dual therapy: Peginterferon alfa and ribavirin only (through week 48 discussed below)

HCV-RNA **detectable** (level >1000 units/mL) at week 4 or week 12 (treatment futility): Discontinue telaprevir, peginterferon alfa and ribavirin at week 12

Weeks ≥24 (based on HCV-RNA results at week 24):

HCV-RNA **detectable** (level greater than ~10-15 units/mL but ≤1000 units/mL) at week 4 and/or week 12: Peginterferon alfa with concomitant ribavirin only (through week 48)

HCV-RNA **detectable** (level greater than ~10-15 units/mL) at week 24 (treatment futility): Discontinue peginterferon alfa and concomitant ribavirin

Treatment naïve patients with cirrhosis, compensated:

Weeks 1-12: Triple therapy: Telaprevir 1125 mg twice daily in combination with peginterferon alfa and ribavirin

Weeks 13-24 (based on HCV-RNA results at weeks 4 and 12):

HCV-RNA **undetectable** at both weeks 4 and 12 (eRVR): Dual therapy: Peginterferon alfa and ribavirin only (through week 48 discussed below)

HCV-RNA **detectable** (level greater than ~10-15 units/mL but ≤1000 units/mL) at week 4 and/or week 12: Dual therapy: Peginterferon alfa and ribavirin only (through week 48 discussed below)

HCV-RNA **detectable** (level >1000 units/mL) at week 4 or week 12 (treatment futility): Discontinue telaprevir, peginterferon alfa and ribavirin at week 12

Weeks ≥24 (based on HCV-RNA results at week 24):

HCV-RNA **undetectable** at week 24: Peginterferon alfa with concomitant ribavirin only (through week 48)

HCV-RNA **detectable** (level greater than ~10-15 units/mL) at week 24 (treatment futility): Discontinue peginterferon alfa and ribavirin

Previously-treated patients (partial response or null responders): **Note:** Previously treated does not include prior treatment with telaprevir. Partial response includes patients with a >2-$\log_{10}$ HCV-RNA decrease by week 12 but a nonsustained virologic response thereafter. Null response includes patients with a <2-$\log_{10}$ HCV-RNA decrease at week 12.

Weeks 1-12: Triple therapy: Telaprevir 1125 mg twice daily with peginterferon alfa and ribavirin

Weeks 13-48 (based on HCV-RNA results at weeks 4 and 12):

HCV-RNA **undetectable** (level less than ~10-15 units/mL) or detectable (level ≤1000 units/mL) at both weeks 4 and 12: Dual therapy: Peginterferon alfa and ribavirin only (through week 48)

HCV-RNA **detectable** (level >1000 units/mL) at week 4 or week 12: Discontinue telaprevir, peginterferon alfa, and ribavirin at week 12

HCV-RNA **detectable** (level greater than ~10-15 units/mL) at week 24: Discontinue peginterferon alfa and concomitant ribavirin

Missed dose: If a dose is missed within 6 hours of the time it is usually taken, take as soon as possible. If more than 6 hours have passed since the dose is usually taken, do not take the missed dose and the patient should resume the usual schedule.

Dosage adjustment in renal impairment:

Telaprevir: No dosage adjustment necessary. Not studied in patients with Cl_{cr} ≤50 mL/minute or in hemodialysis.

Dosage adjustment in hepatic impairment: Telaprevir:

Mild impairment (Child-Pugh class A): No dosage adjustment necessary.

Moderate or severe impairment (Child-Pugh class B or C): Use is not recommended in patients with decompensated liver disease or with moderate or severe hepatic impairment (has not been studied).

Dietary Considerations Take with a meal (not low fat).

Administration Administer with a meal (not low fat) within 30 minutes prior to each dose. Doses should be taken approximately every 10-14 hours. Administer concurrently with peginterferon alfa and ribavirin. Maintain adequate fluid intake/hydration. Swallow tablets whole; do not chew, crush, break, cut, or dissolve the tablets. If a dose is missed within 6 hours of the time it is usually taken, take as soon as possible. If more than 6 hours have passed since the dose is usually taken, the missed dose should not be taken and the patient should resume the usual schedule.

Monitoring Parameters

CBC with differential and platelet count, serum electrolytes, serum creatinine, TSH, bilirubin, liver enzymes, and uric acid at baseline and weeks 2, 4, 8 and 12, then periodically (and when clinically indicated)

Serum HCV-RNA at baseline, weeks 4, 8, 12 and 24, end of treatment, during treatment follow up, and when clinically indicated

Pretreatment and monthly pregnancy test up to 6 months following discontinuation of therapy for women of childbearing age

Hydration status, including fluid intake/output, urine output, signs/symptoms of dehydration

Reference Range

Treatment futility: HCV-RNA ≥1000 units/mL at treatment week 4 or 12 or confirmed, detectable HCV-RNA at treatment week 24

Rapid virologic response (RVR): Absence of detectable HCV-RNA after 4 weeks of treatment

Extended rapid virologic response (eRVR): Absence of detectable HCV-RNA after 4 and 12 weeks of treatment

Early virologic response (EVR): Absence of detectable HCV-RNA after 12 weeks of treatment

Sustained virologic response (SVR): Absence of HCV-RNA in the serum 32-78 weeks after completion of a 24 week treatment course or 56-78 weeks after a 48 week treatment course.

Additional Information In clinical studies of treatment-naive patients, a sustained virologic response (SVR) of ~75% (~65% in African-Americans) was observed with peginterferon alfa, ribavirin, and telaprevir versus 46% with peginterferon and ribavirin alone. Adherence to 3 times/day dosing is needed; resistance is increased and efficacy is affected when dosed every 12 hours.

Dosage Forms Excipient information presented when available (limited, particularly for generics); consult specific product labeling.

Tablet, Oral:

Incivek: 375 mg [contains fd&c blue #2 (indigotine), fd&c red #40]

Telavancin (tel a VAN sin)

Brand Names: U.S. Vibativ

Index Terms TD-6424; Telavancin Hydrochloride

Pharmacologic Category Glycopeptide

Use

Complicated skin and skin structure infections: Treatment of complicated skin and skin structure infections caused by susceptible gram-positive organisms including methicillin-susceptible or -resistant *Staphylococcus aureus*, vancomycin-susceptible *Enterococcus faecalis*, and *Streptococcus pyogenes*, *Streptococcus agalactiae*, or *Streptococcus anginosus* group

Hospital-acquired and ventilator-associated bacterial pneumonia (HABP/VABP): Treatment of HABP/VABP caused by susceptible isolates of *Staphylococcus aureus* when alternative treatments are not appropriate

Pregnancy Risk Factor C

Pregnancy Considerations [U.S. Boxed Warning]: Based on animal data, adverse developmental outcomes have been observed. Prior to use, women of childbearing potential should have a serum pregnancy test. Use of telavancin is not recommended during pregnancy unless the potential benefit to the mother outweighs the possible risk to the fetus. Telavancin crosses the placenta (Nanovskaya, 2012). In women of childbearing potential, effective contraception should be used during therapy.

Healthcare providers are encouraged to enroll women exposed to telavancin during pregnancy in the Vibativ Pregnancy Registry 855-633-8479).

Breast-Feeding Considerations It is not known if telavancin is excreted in breast milk. The manufacturer recommends that caution be exercised when administering telavancin to nursing women.

Medication Guide Available Yes

Contraindications Hypersensitivity to telavancin or any component of the formulation

Warnings/Precautions Hazardous agent - use appropriate precautions for handling and disposal (NIOSH, 2012). **[U.S. Boxed Warning]: Based on animal data, adverse developmental outcomes have been observed. Prior to use, women of childbearing potential should have a serum pregnancy test. Use of telavancin is not recommended during pregnancy unless the potential benefit outweighs the risk to the fetus. [U.S. Boxed Warning]: New-onset or worsening renal impairment has occurred. Monitor renal function prior to, during (at least every 48-72 hours; more frequently if indicated), and following therapy in all patients.** May cause nephrotoxicity; usual risk factors include concomitant nephrotoxic medications or baseline comorbidities associated with decreased renal function (eg, baseline renal dysfunction, diabetes, hypertension, or heart failure). **[U.S. Boxed Warning]: In clinical studies, patients with pre-existing moderate-to-severe renal impairment (Cl_{cr} ≤50 mL/minute) treated for hospital-acquired/ventilator-associated bacterial pneumonia (HABP/VABP) had increased (all cause) mortality versus vancomycin. Use in HABP/VABP only when benefit outweighs risk.** Serious hypersensitivity reactions, including anaphylaxis, have been reported after first or subsequent doses; some have been fatal. Discontinue if hypersensitivity or rash occurs. Telavancin is a semisynthetic derivative of vancomycin; cross-reactivity rates are unknown. Use with caution in patients with known vancomycin hypersensitivity.

May prolong QT_c interval; avoid use in patients with a history of QT_c prolongation, uncompensated heart failure, severe left ventricular hypertrophy, or concurrent administration of other medications known to prolong the QT interval. Clinical studies indicate mean maximal QT_c prolongation of 12-15 msec at the end of 10 mg/kg infusion. Contains solubilizer cyclodextrin (hydroxypropyl-beta-cyclodextrin) which may accumulate in patients with renal dysfunction. Prolonged use may result in fungal or bacterial superinfection, including *C. difficile*-associated diarrhea (CDAD) and pseudomembranous colitis; CDAD has been observed >2 months postantibiotic treatment. Potentially significant drug-drug interactions may exist, requiring dose or frequency adjustment, additional monitoring, and/or selection of alternative therapy.

May interfere with tests used to monitor coagulation (eg, prothrombin time, INR, activated partial thromboplastin time, activated clotting time, coagulation based factor Xa tests) when samples drawn ≤18 hours after drug administration. Blood samples should be collected as close to the next dose of telavancin as possible. Rapid I.V. administration may result in flushing, rash, urticaria, and/or pruritus; slowing or stopping the infusion may alleviate these symptoms. In the elderly, lower doses are often required secondary to age-related decreases in renal function.

Adverse Reactions

>10%:

Central nervous system: Insomnia (13%), psychiatric disturbance (12%), headache (11%)

Gastrointestinal: Metallic taste (33%), nausea (5% to 27%), vomiting (5% to 14%)

Genitourinary: Proteinuria (13%)

Renal: Increased serum creatinine (8% to 16%)

1% to 10%:

Central nervous system: Dizziness (6%), paresthesia (5%), local pain (4%), rigors (4%)

Dermatologic: Pruritus (3% to 6%), skin rash (4%), localized erythema (3%)

Endocrine & metabolic: Albuminuria (micro) (7%), hypokalemia (7%)

Gastrointestinal: Diarrhea (7%), decreased appetite (3%), abdominal pain (2%)

Genitourinary: Acute renal failure (5%)

Hematologic & oncologic: Thrombocytopenia (7%)

Renal: Renal insufficiency (3%)

Respiratory: Dyspnea (8%)

<1% (Limited to important or life-threatening): *Clostridium difficile* associated diarrhea, hearing loss (transient), hypersensitivity reaction, nephrotoxicity, prolonged Q-T interval on ECG, urticaria

Drug Interactions

Metabolism/Transport Effects None known.

Avoid Concomitant Use

Avoid concomitant use of Telavancin with any of the following: BCG; Highest Risk QTc-Prolonging Agents; Ivabradine; Mifepristone

Increased Effect/Toxicity

Telavancin may increase the levels/effects of: Highest Risk QTc-Prolonging Agents; Moderate Risk QTc-Prolonging Agents

The levels/effects of Telavancin may be increased by: Ivabradine; Mifepristone; QTc-Prolonging Agents (Indeterminate Risk and Risk Modifying)

Decreased Effect

Telavancin may decrease the levels/effects of: BCG; Sodium Picosulfate; Typhoid Vaccine

Preparation for Administration Hazardous agent; use appropriate precautions for handling and disposal (NIOSH, 2012). Reconstitute 250 mg vial with 15 mL of D_5W, NS, or SWFI to yield 15 mg/mL (total volume of ~17 mL). Reconstitute 750 mg vial with 45 mL of of D_5W, NS, or SWFI to yield 15 mg/mL (total volume of ~50 mL). Allow vacuum to pull the diluent into the vial; discard vial if this did not occur. Reconstitution generally takes <2 minutes, although may take up to 20 minutes. Do not shake the vial or final solution for infusion. Prior to administration, dilute dose in 100-250 mL D_5W, LR, or NS to a final concentration of 0.6-8 mg/mL.

Storage/Stability Store intact vials at 2°C to 8°C (35°F to 46°F); excursions permitted up to 25°C (77°F); avoid excess heat. **Note:** Vials contain no bacteriostatic agent. Reconstituted solution in the vial should be used within 4 hours at room temperature or 72 hours refrigerated; solutions admixed for infusion are stable at room temperature for 4 hours or under refrigeration for 72 hours. Total time in vial **plus** time in infusion bag should not exceed 4 hours at room temperature or 72 hours if refrigerated at 2°C to 8°C (35°F to 46°F).

Mechanism of Action Exerts concentration-dependent bactericidal activity; inhibits bacterial cell wall synthesis by blocking polymerization and cross-linking of peptidoglycan by binding to D-Ala-D-Ala portion of cell wall. Unlike vancomycin, additional mechanism involves disruption of membrane potential and changes cell permeability due to presence of lipophilic side chain moiety.

Pharmacodynamics/Kinetics

Distribution: V_{ss}: 0.13 L/kg

Protein binding: ~90%; primarily to albumin

Half-life elimination: 6.6-9.6 hours

Excretion: Urine (~76%); feces (<1%)

Dosage

Complicated skin and skin structure infection: Adults: I.V.: 10 mg/kg every 24 hours for 1-2 weeks

Hospital-acquired and ventilator-associated bacterial pneumonia (HABP/VABP): Adults: I.V.: 10 mg/kg every 24 hours for 1-3 weeks

Dosage adjustment in renal impairment: Note: Renal function may be estimated using the Cockcroft-Gault formula for dosage adjustment purposes.

Cl_{cr} >50 mL/minute: No dosage adjustment necessary

Cl_{cr} 30-50 mL/minute: 7.5 mg/kg every 24 hours

Cl_{cr} 10 to <30 mL/minute: 10 mg/kg every 48 hours

Cl_{cr} <10 mL/minute: No dosage adjustment provided in manufacturer's labeling (has not been studied).

ESRD and hemodialysis patients: No dosage adjustment provided in manufacturer's labeling (has not been studied).

Dosage adjustment in hepatic impairment:

Mild-to-moderate hepatic impairment (Child-Pugh class A or B): No dosage adjustment necessary.

Severe hepatic impairment (Child-Pugh class C): No dosage adjustment provided in manufacturer's labeling (has not been studied).

Administration Administer I.V. over 60 minutes. Other medications should not be infused simultaneously through the same I.V. line. When the same intravenous line is used for sequential infusion of other medications, flush line with D_5W, LR, or NS before and after infusing telavancin.

Red-man syndrome may occur if the infusion is too rapid. It is not an allergic reaction, but may be characterized by hypotension and/or a maculopapular rash appearing on the face, neck, trunk, and/or upper extremities. If this should occur, discontinuing or slowing the infusion rate may eliminate these reactions.

Hazardous agent; use appropriate precautions for handling and disposal (NIOSH, 2012).

Monitoring Parameters Renal function (prior to start, every 48-72 hours; more frequently if indicated, and following therapy), pregnancy test

Test Interactions Interferes with the following coagulation assessments (causes artificially increased clotting times): PT, INR, aPTT, ACT, Xa; interferes with urine protein via qualitative dipstick and quantitative dye methods

Dosage Forms Excipient information presented when available (limited, particularly for generics); consult specific product labeling.

Solution Reconstituted, Intravenous [preservative free]:

Vibativ: 750 mg (1 ea)

◆ **Telavancin Hydrochloride** *see* Telavancin *on page 1999*

Telithromycin (tel ith roe MYE sin)

Brand Names: U.S. Ketek

Brand Names: Canada Ketek®

Index Terms HMR 3647

Pharmacologic Category Antibiotic, Ketolide

Use Treatment of community-acquired pneumonia (mild-to-moderate) caused by susceptible strains of *Streptococcus pneumoniae* (including multidrug-resistant isolates), *Haemophilus influenzae, Chlamydophila pneumoniae, Moraxella catarrhalis*, and *Mycoplasma pneumoniae*

Pregnancy Risk Factor C

Pregnancy Considerations Because adverse effects were observed in some animal studies, telithromycin is classified pregnancy category C. There are no adequate and well-controlled studies of telithromycin in pregnant women.

Breast-Feeding Considerations It is not known if telithromycin is excreted in breast milk. The manufacturer recommends caution if using telithromycin in a breast-feeding woman.

Medication Guide Available Yes

Contraindications Hypersensitivity to telithromycin, macrolide antibiotics, or any component of the formulation; myasthenia gravis; history of hepatitis and/or jaundice associated with telithromycin or other macrolide antibiotic use; concurrent use of colchicine (if patient has concomitant renal or hepatic impairment), cisapride, pimozide, lovastatin, or simvastatin

Warnings/Precautions Acute hepatic failure and severe liver injury, including hepatitis and hepatic necrosis (leading to some fatalities) have been reported, in some cases after only a few doses; if signs/symptoms of hepatitis or liver damage occur, discontinue therapy and initiate liver function tests. **[U.S. Boxed Warning]: Life-threatening (including fatal) respiratory failure has occurred in patients with myasthenia gravis;** use in these patients is contraindicated. May prolong QT_c interval, leading to a risk of ventricular arrhythmias; closely-related antibiotics have been associated with malignant ventricular arrhythmias and torsade de pointes. Avoid in patients with prolongation of QT_c interval due to congenital causes, history of long QT syndrome, uncorrected electrolyte disturbances (hypokalemia or hypomagnesemia), significant bradycardia (<50 bpm), or concurrent therapy with QT_c-prolonging drugs (eg, class Ia and class III antiarrhythmics). Avoid use in patients with a prior history of confirmed cardiogenic syncope or ventricular arrhythmias while receiving macrolide antibiotics or other QT_c-prolonging drugs. May cause severe visual disturbances (eg, changes in accommodation ability, diplopia, blurred vision). May cause loss of consciousness (possibly vagal-related); caution patients that these events may interfere with ability to operate machinery or drive, and to use caution until effects are known. Use caution in renal impairment; severe impairment (Cl_{cr} <30 mL/minute) requires dosage adjustment. Pseudomembranous colitis has been reported. Safety and efficacy not established in pediatric patients <13 years of age per Canadian approved labeling and <18 years of age per U.S. approved labeling.

Adverse Reactions

>10%: Gastrointestinal: Diarrhea (10% to 11%)

2% to 10%:

Central nervous system: Headache (2% to 6%), dizziness (3% to 4%)

Gastrointestinal: Nausea (7% to 8%), vomiting (2% to 3%), loose stools (2%), dysgeusia (2%)

≥0.2% to <2%:

Central nervous system: Fatigue, insomnia, somnolence, vertigo

Dermatologic: Rash

Gastrointestinal: Abdominal distension, abdominal pain, anorexia, constipation, dyspepsia, flatulence, gastritis, gastroenteritis, GI upset, glossitis, stomatitis, watery stools, xerostomia

Genitourinary: Vaginal candidiasis, vaginitis

Hematologic: Platelets increased

Hepatic: Transaminases increased

Ocular: Blurred vision, accommodation delayed, diplopia

Miscellaneous: Candidiasis, diaphoresis increased

<0.2% (Limited to important or life-threatening): Acute repiratory failure, alkaline phosphatase increased, allergic reaction, anaphylaxis, angioedema, anxiety, arrhythmia, bilirubin increased, bradycardia, edema (facial), eosinophilia, erythema multiforme, flushing, hepatitis, hepatitis, hepatocellular injury (including necrosis), hypotension, jaundice, liver failure, loss of consciousness (may be vagal-related), muscle cramps, myasthenia gravis exacerbation (rare), palpitation, pancreatitis, paresthesia, pruritus, pseudomembranous colitis, QT_c prolongation, syncope, torsade de pointes

Drug Interactions

Metabolism/Transport Effects Substrate of CYP1A2 (minor), CYP3A4 (major); **Note:** Assignment of Major/Minor substrate status based on clinically relevant drug interaction potential; **Inhibits** CYP2D6 (weak), CYP3A4 (strong)

Avoid Concomitant Use

Avoid concomitant use of Telithromycin with any of the following: Ado-Trastuzumab Emtansine; Alfuzosin; Apixaban; Avanafil; Axitinib; BCG; Bosutinib; Cabozantinib; Cisapride; Conivaptan; Crizotinib; Disopyramide; Dronedarone; Eplerenone; Everolimus; Fusidic Acid (Systemic); Halofantrine; Highest Risk QTc-Prolonging Agents; Ibrutinib; Imatinib; Ivabradine; Lapatinib; Lomitapide; Lovastatin; Lurasidone; Macitentan; Mifepristone; Nilotinib; Nisoldipine; Pimozide; Pomalidomide; QuiNIDine; QuiNINE; Ranolazine; Red Yeast Rice; Regorafenib; Rivaroxaban; Salmeterol; Silodosin; Simeprevir; Simvastatin; Tamsulosin; Terfenadine; Ticagrelor; Tolvaptan; Toremifene; Ulipristal; Vemurafenib; VinCRIStine (Liposomal)

Increased Effect/Toxicity

Telithromycin may increase the levels/effects of: Ado-Trastuzumab Emtansine; Alfentanil; Alfuzosin; Almotriptan; Alosetron; ALPRAZolam; Antifungal Agents (Azole Derivatives, Systemic); Antineoplastic Agents (Vinca Alkaloids); Apixaban; ARIPiprazole; AtorvaSTATin; Avanafil; Axitinib; Bedaquiline; Bortezomib; Bosentan; Bosutinib; Brentuximab Vedotin; Brinzolamide; Budesonide (Nasal); Budesonide (Systemic, Oral Inhalation); BusPIRone; Cabozantinib; Calcium Channel Blockers; CarBAMazepine; Cardiac Glycosides; Cilostazol; Cisapride; CloZAPine; Cobicistat; Colchicine; Conivaptan; Corticosteroids (Orally Inhaled); Corticosteroids (Systemic); Crizotinib; CycloSPORINE (Systemic); CYP3A4 Substrates; Dienogest; Disopyramide; Dofetilide; Dronedarone; Dutasteride; Eletriptan; Enzalutamide; Eplerenone; Ergot Derivatives; Estazolam; Everolimus; FentaNYL; Fesoterodine; Fluticasone (Nasal); Fluticasone (Oral Inhalation); GuanFACINE; Halofantrine; Highest Risk QTc-Prolonging Agents; Ibrutinib; Iloperidone; Imatinib; Ivabradine; Ivacaftor; Ixabepilone; Lacosamide; Lapatinib; Levomilnacipran; Lomitapide; Lovastatin; Lumefantrine; Lurasidone; Macitentan; Maraviroc; MethylPREDNISolone; Midazolam; Mifepristone; Moderate Risk QTc-Prolonging Agents; Nilotinib; Nisoldipine; Ospemifene; OxyCODONE; Paricalcitol; PAZOPanib; Pimecrolimus; Pimozide; Pitavastatin; Pomalidomide; PONATinib; Pravastatin; Propafenone; QUEtiapine; QuiNIDine; QuiNINE; Ranolazine; Red Yeast Rice; Regorafenib; Repaglinide; Rifamycin Derivatives; Rilpivirine; Rivaroxaban; RomiDEPsin; Ruxolitinib; Salmeterol; Saxagliptin; Selective Serotonin Reuptake Inhibitors; Sildenafil; Silodosin; Simeprevir; Simvastatin; Sirolimus; SORAfenib; Tacrolimus (Systemic); Tacrolimus (Topical); Tadalafil; Tamsulosin; Telaprevir; Temsirolimus; Terfenadine; Ticagrelor; Tofacitinib; Tolterodine; Tolvaptan; Toremifene; Triazolam; Ulipristal; Vardenafil; Vemurafenib; Verapamil; Vilazodone; VinCRIStine (Liposomal); Vitamin K Antagonists; Zopiclone; Zuclopenthixol

The levels/effects of Telithromycin may be increased by: Antifungal Agents (Azole Derivatives, Systemic); Cobicistat; CYP3A4 Inhibitors (Moderate); CYP3A4 Inhibitors (Strong); Dasatinib; Fusidic Acid (Systemic); Ivabradine; Luliconazole; Mifepristone; QTc-Prolonging Agents (Indeterminate Risk and Risk Modifying); Telaprevir

Decreased Effect

Telithromycin may decrease the levels/effects of: BCG; Clopidogrel; Ifosfamide; Prasugrel; Sodium Picosulfate; Ticagrelor; Typhoid Vaccine

The levels/effects of Telithromycin may be decreased by: CYP3A4 Inducers (Strong); Dabrafenib; Deferasirox; Etravirine; Herbs (CYP3A4 Inducers); Mitotane; Tocilizumab

Ethanol/Nutrition/Herb Interactions Herb/Nutraceutical: St John's wort: May decrease the levels/effects of telithromycin.

Storage/Stability Store at 15°C to 30°C (59°F to 86°F).

Mechanism of Action Inhibits bacterial protein synthesis by binding to two sites on the 50S ribosomal subunit. Telithromycin has also been demonstrated to alter secretion of IL-1alpha and TNF-alpha; the clinical significance of this immunomodulatory effect has not been evaluated.

Pharmacodynamics/Kinetics

Absorption: Rapid

Distribution: 2.9 L/kg

Protein binding: 60% to 70%; primarily to albumin

Metabolism: Hepatic, via CYP3A4 (50%) and non-CYP-mediated pathways

Bioavailability: 57% (significant first-pass metabolism)

Half-life elimination: 10 hours

Time to peak, plasma: 1 hour

Excretion: Urine (13% unchanged drug, remainder as metabolites); feces (7%)

Dosage Oral:

Children ≥13 years and Adults: Tonsillitis/pharyngitis (unlabeled use; Canadian indication): 800 mg once daily for 5 days

Adults: Community-acquired pneumonia: 800 mg once daily for 7-10 days

Dosage adjustment in renal impairment:

U.S. product labeling: Cl_{cr} <30 mL/minute, including dialysis: 600 mg once daily; when renal impairment is accompanied by hepatic impairment, reduce dosage to 400 mg once daily

Canadian product labeling: Cl_{cr} <30 mL/minute: Reduce dose to 400 mg once daily

Hemodialysis: Administer following dialysis

Dosage adjustment in hepatic impairment: No dosage adjustment necessary, unless concurrent severe renal impairment is present

Dietary Considerations May be taken with or without food.

Administration May be administered with or without food.

Monitoring Parameters Liver function tests; signs/symptoms of liver failure (eg, jaundice, fatigue, malaise, anorexia, nausea, bilirubinemia, acholic stools, liver tenderness, hepatomegaly); visual acuity

Dosage Forms Excipient information presented when available (limited, particularly for generics); consult specific product labeling.

Tablet, Oral:

Ketek: 300 mg, 400 mg

Dosage Forms: Canada Excipient information presented when available (limited, particularly for generics); consult specific product labeling.

Tablet:

Ketek®: 400 mg

Telmisartan (tel mi SAR tan)

Brand Names: U.S. Micardis

Brand Names: Canada CO Telmisartan; Micardis; Mylan-Telmisartan; PMS-Telmisartan; Ran-Telmisartan; Sandoz-Telmisartan; Teva-Telmisartan

Pharmacologic Category Angiotensin II Receptor Blocker; Antihypertensive

Additional Appendix Information

Angiotensin Agents *on page 2280*

Use

Cardiovascular risk reduction: Cardiovascular risk reduction in patients ≥55 years of age unable to take ACE inhibitors and who are at high risk of major cardiovascular events (eg, MI, stroke, death)

Hypertension: For the treatment of hypertension, alone or in combination with other antihypertensive agents

Pregnancy Risk Factor D

Pregnancy Considerations [U.S. Boxed Warning]: Drugs that act on the renin-angiotensin system can cause injury and death to the developing fetus. Discontinue as soon as possible once pregnancy is detected. The use of drugs which act on the renin-angiotensin system are associated with oligohydramnios. Oligohydramnios, due to decreased fetal renal function, may lead to fetal lung hypoplasia and skeletal malformations. Use is also associated with anuria, hypotension, renal failure, skull hypoplasia, and death in the fetus/neonate. The exposed fetus should be monitored for fetal growth, amniotic fluid volume, and organ formation. Infants exposed *in utero* should be monitored for hyperkalemia, hypotension, and oliguria.

Untreated chronic maternal hypertension is also associated with adverse events in the fetus, infant, and mother. If treatment for hypertension during pregnancy is needed, other agents are preferred (ACOG, 2012; Chobanian, 2003). In women of reproductive potential, angiotensin II receptor blockers should be discontinued prior to conception or as soon as pregnancy is confirmed (Chobanian, 2003). The Canadian labeling contraindicates use during pregnancy.

Breast-Feeding Considerations It is not known if telmisartan is excreted in breast milk. Due to the potential for serious adverse reactions in the nursing infant, a decision should be made whether to discontinue nursing or to discontinue the drug, taking into account the importance of treatment to the mother. The Canadian labeling contraindicates use in nursing women. Breast-fed infants of mothers taking medications for hypertension should be monitored for adverse effects (Chobanian, 2003).

Contraindications Known hypersensitivity (eg, anaphylaxis, angioedema) to telmisartan or any component of the formulation; concurrent use of aliskiren in patients with diabetes

Canadian labeling: Additional contraindications: Concomitant use with aliskiren in patients with moderate-to-severe renal impairment (GFR <60 mL/min/1.73m^2); pregnancy; breast-feeding; fructose intolerance

Warnings/Precautions [U.S. Boxed Warning]: Drugs that act on the renin-angiotensin system can cause injury and death to the developing fetus. Discontinue as soon as possible once pregnancy is detected. May cause hyperkalemia; avoid potassium supplementation unless specifically required by healthcare provider. Avoid use or use a smaller dose in patients who are volume depleted; correct depletion first. May be associated with deterioration of renal function and/or increases in serum creatinine, particularly in patients with low renal blood flow (eg, renal artery stenosis, heart failure) whose glomerular filtration rate (GFR) is dependent on efferent arteriolar vasoconstriction by angiotensin II. Use with caution in unstented unilateral/bilateral renal artery stenosis. When unstented bilateral renal artery stenosis is present, use is generally avoided due to the elevated risk of deterioration in renal function unless possible benefits outweigh risks. Use with caution with pre-existing renal insufficiency; significant aortic/mitral stenosis. Potentially significant drug-drug interactions may exist, requiring dose or frequency adjustment, additional monitoring, and/or selection of alternative therapy. Use with caution in patients who have biliary obstructive disorders or hepatic dysfunction. Product contains sorbitol. The Canadian labeling contraindicates use in fructose intolerant patients.

Angioedema has been reported rarely with some angiotensin II receptor antagonists (ARBs) and may occur at any time during treatment (especially following first dose). It may involve the head and neck (potentially compromising airway) or the intestine (presenting with abdominal pain). Patients with idiopathic or hereditary angioedema or previous angioedema associated with ACE-inhibitor therapy may be at an increased risk. Prolonged frequent monitoring may be required, especially if tongue, glottis, or larynx are involved, as they are associated with airway obstruction. Patients with a history of airway surgery may have a higher risk of airway obstruction. Discontinue therapy immediately if angioedema occurs. Aggressive early management is critical. Intramuscular (I.M.) administration of epinephrine may be necessary. Do not readminister to patients who have had angioedema with ARBs.

Adverse Reactions May be associated with worsening of renal function in patients dependent on renin-angiotensin-aldosterone system.

1% to 10%:

Cardiovascular: Intermittent claudication (7%; placebo 6%), chest pain (≥1%), hypertension (≥1%), peripheral edema (≥1%)

Central nervous system: Dizziness (≥1%), fatigue (≥1%), headache (≥1%), pain (≥1%)

Dermatologic: Skin ulcer (3%; placebo 2%)

Gastrointestinal: Diarrhea (3%), abdominal pain (≥1%), dyspepsia (≥1%), nausea (≥1%)

Genitourinary: Urinary tract infection (≥1%)

Neuromuscular & skeletal: Back pain (3%), myalgia (≥1%)

Respiratory: Upper respiratory infection (7%), sinusitis (3%), cough (≥1%), pharyngitis (1%)

<1% (Limited to important or life-threatening): Abnormal ECG, abscess, allergic reaction, anaphylaxis, anemia, angina, angioedema, arthritis, asthma, atrial fibrillation, bradycardia, cerebrovascular disorder, CHF, conjunctivitis, creatinine kinase increased, depression, diabetes mellitus, eczema, edema, epistaxis, erectile dysfunction, fixed drug eruption, fungal infection, gastroenteritis, gout, hepatic dysfunction, hypercholesterolemia, hyperkalemia, hypersensitivity, hypoglycemia (diabetic patients), hypotension, impotence, insomnia, MI, migraine, neoplasm, orthostatic hypotension (more frequent in dialysis patients), otitis media, renal failure, rhabdomyolysis, reflux, serum creatinine increased, syncope, tachycardia, tendon pain, thrombocytopenia, uric acid increased

Drug Interactions

Metabolism/Transport Effects **Inhibits** CYP2C19 (weak)

Avoid Concomitant Use

Avoid concomitant use of Telmisartan with any of the following: Ramipril

Increased Effect/Toxicity

Telmisartan may increase the levels/effects of: ACE Inhibitors; Amifostine; Antihypertensives; Cardiac Glycosides; CycloSPORINE (Systemic); Hypotensive Agents; Lithium; Nonsteroidal Anti-Inflammatory Agents; Obinutuzumab; Potassium-Sparing Diuretics; Ramipril; RiTUXimab; Sodium Phosphates

The levels/effects of Telmisartan may be increased by: Alfuzosin; Aliskiren; Brimonidine (Topical); Canagliflozin; Diazoxide; Eplerenone; Heparin; Heparin (Low Molecular Weight); Herbs (Hypotensive Properties); MAO Inhibitors; Pentoxifylline; Phosphodiesterase 5 Inhibitors; Potassium Salts; Prostacyclin Analogues; Tolvaptan; Trimethoprim

Decreased Effect

The levels/effects of Telmisartan may be decreased by: Herbs (Hypertensive Properties); Methylphenidate; Nonsteroidal Anti-Inflammatory Agents; Yohimbine

Ethanol/Nutrition/Herb Interactions Herb/Nutraceutical: Some herbal medications may have hypertensive or hypotensive properties; others may increase or decrease the antihypertensive effect of telmisartan. Management: Avoid bayberry, blue cohosh, cayenne, ephedra, ginger, ginseng (American), kola, licorice, and yohimbe. Avoid black cohosh, California poppy, coleus, golden seal, hawthorn, mistletoe, periwinkle, quinine, and shepherd's purse.

Storage/Stability Store at 25°C (77°F); excursions are permitted between 15°C and 30°C (59°F and 86°F). Tablets should not be removed from blisters until immediately before administration.

Mechanism of Action Angiotensin II acts as a vasoconstrictor. In addition to causing direct vasoconstriction, angiotensin II also stimulates the release of aldosterone. Once aldosterone is released, sodium as well as water is reabsorbed. The end result is an elevation in blood pressure. Telmisartan is a nonpeptide AT1 angiotensin II receptor antagonist. This binding prevents angiotensin II from binding to the receptor thereby blocking the vasoconstriction and the aldosterone secreting effects of angiotensin II.

Pharmacodynamics/Kinetics Orally active, not a prodrug

Onset of action: 1-2 hours

Duration: Up to 24 hours

Distribution: V_d: 500 L

Protein binding: >99.5%; primarily to albumin and alpha$_1$-acid glycoprotein

Metabolism: Hepatic via conjugation to inactive metabolites; not metabolized via CYP

Bioavailability (dose dependent): 42% to 58%; Hepatic impairment: Approaches 100%

Half-life elimination: Terminal: 24 hours

Time to peak, plasma: 0.5-1 hours

Excretion: Feces (97%)

Clearance: Total body: 800 mL/minute

Dosage

Adults: Oral:

Hypertension: Initial: 40 mg once daily; usual maintenance dose range: 20-80 mg daily. Patients with volume depletion should be initiated on the lower dosage with close supervision.

Cardiovascular risk reduction: Oral: 80 mg once daily. **Note:** It is unknown whether doses <80 mg daily are associated with a reduction in risk of cardiovascular morbidity or mortality.

Elderly: Refer to adult dosing.

Dosage adjustment in renal impairment: No dosage adjustment necessary; hemodialysis patients are more susceptible to orthostatic hypotension

Dosage adjustment in hepatic impairment: Initiate therapy with low dose; titrate slowly and monitor closely.

Canadian labeling: Recommended initial dose: 40 mg daily

Dietary Considerations May be taken without regard to meals. Product contains sorbitol.

Administration May be administered without regard to meals.

Monitoring Parameters Blood pressure; electrolytes, serum creatinine, BUN

Dosage Forms Excipient information presented when available (limited, particularly for generics); consult specific product labeling.

Tablet, Oral:

Micardis: 20 mg, 40 mg, 80 mg

Generic: 20 mg, 40 mg, 80 mg

Dosage Forms: Canada Refer to Dosage Forms. **Note:** Telmisartan 20 mg tablet is not available in Canada.

Telmisartan and Amlodipine

(tel mi SAR tan & am LOE di peen)

Brand Names: U.S. Twynsta

Brand Names: Canada Twynsta

Index Terms Amlodipine and Telmisartan; Amlodipine Besylate and Telmisartan

Pharmacologic Category Angiotensin II Receptor Blocker; Antianginal Agent; Antihypertensive; Calcium Channel Blocker; Calcium Channel Blocker, Dihydropyridine

Use Hypertension:

U.S. labeling: Treatment of hypertension, including initial treatment in patients who will require multiple antihypertensives for adequate control

Canadian labeling: Treatment of mild-to-moderate hypertension in patients whom combination therapy is appropriate; not indicated for initial therapy

Pregnancy Risk Factor D

Dosage Oral: Adults: Dose is individualized; combination product may be substituted for individual components in patients currently maintained on both agents separately or in patients not adequately controlled with monotherapy (using one of the agents or an agent within the same antihypertensive class). May also be used as initial therapy in patients who are likely to need >1 antihypertensive to control blood pressure. **Note:** Use as initial therapy is not an approved indication in the Canadian labeling.

Hypertension:

Initial therapy (antihypertensive naive): Telmisartan 40 mg/amlodipine 5 mg once daily; dose may be increased after 2 weeks of therapy. Patients requiring larger blood pressure reductions may be started on telmisartan 80 mg/amlodipine 5 mg once daily. Maximum recommended dose: Telmisartan 80 mg/day, amlodipine 10 mg/day

Add-on/replacement therapy: Telmisartan 40-80 mg and amlodipine 5-10 mg once daily depending upon previous doses, current control, and goals of therapy; dose may be titrated after 2 weeks of therapy. Maximum recommended dose: Telmisartan 80 mg/day; amlodipine 10 mg/day

Elderly: Not recommended for initial therapy in patients ≥75 years of age. For add-on/replacement therapy, initiate amlodipine therapy at 2.5 mg once daily and titrate slowly. **Note:** Use of individual agents may be necessary if the appropriate combination dose is not available.

Dosage adjustment in renal impairment: No dosage adjustment necessary; titrate slowly in severe impairment.

Dosage adjustment in hepatic impairment: Not recommended for initial therapy. For add-on/replacement therapy, initiate amlodipine at 2.5 mg once daily with low-dose telmisartan and titrate slowly; **Note:** Use of individual agents is necessary as the appropriate combination dose is not available. Upon titration to therapeutic dose, may initiate combination dose if available. Canadian labeling contraindicates use in severe hepatic impairment or with biliary obstructive disorders.

Additional Information Complete prescribing information should be consulted for additional detail.

Dosage Forms Excipient information presented when available (limited, particularly for generics); consult specific product labeling.

Tablet, oral:

Twynsta® 40/5: Telmisartan 40 mg and amlodipine 5 mg

Twynsta® 40/10: Telmisartan 40 mg and amlodipine 10 mg

Twynsta® 80/5: Telmisartan 80 mg and amlodipine 5 mg

Twynsta® 80/10: Telmisartan 80 mg and amlodipine 10 mg

Generic: Telmisartan 40 mg and amlodipine 5 mg; telmisartan 40 mg and amlodipine 10 mg; telmisartan 80 mg and amlodipine 5 mg; telmisartan 80 mg and amlodipine 10 mg

Telmisartan and Hydrochlorothiazide

(tel mi SAR tan & hye droe klor oh THYE a zide)

Brand Names: U.S. Micardis HCT

Brand Names: Canada CO Telmisartan HCT; Micardis Plus; Mylan-Telmisartan HCTZ; PMS-Telmisartan HCTZ; RAN-Telmisartan HCTZ; Sandoz-Telmisartan HCT; Telmisartan HCTZ; Teva-Telmisartan HCTZ

Index Terms Hydrochlorothiazide and Telmisartan

Pharmacologic Category Angiotensin II Receptor Blocker; Antihypertensive; Diuretic, Thiazide

Use Hypertension: Treatment of hypertension; **Note:** A fixed-dose combination product should not be used for initial therapy

Pregnancy Risk Factor D

Dosage

Hypertension: Adults: Oral:

Replacement therapy: Combination product can be substituted for individual titrated agents.

Initiation of combination therapy when monotherapy has failed to achieve desired effects:

Patients currently on telmisartan:

U.S. labeling: Initial dose if blood pressure is not currently controlled on monotherapy of 80 mg telmisartan: Telmisartan 80 mg/hydrochlorothiazide 12.5 mg once daily; manufacturer labeling suggests that dose may be titrated up to telmisartan 160 mg/hydrochlorothiazide 25 mg if needed; however, in mild to moderate hypertension, doses of telmisartan >80 mg were not associated with a greater reduction in blood pressure (Smith, 2000).

Canadian labeling: If blood pressure is not currently controlled on monotherapy of telmisartan 80 mg: Telmisartan 80 mg/hydrochlorothiazide 12.5 mg once daily; may titrate up to telmisartan 80 mg/hydrochlorothiazide 25 mg if needed.

Patients currently on hydrochlorothiazide:

U.S. labeling: Initial dose if blood pressure is not currently controlled on monotherapy of 25 mg once daily: Telmisartan 80 mg/hydrochlorothiazide 12.5 mg once daily or telmisartan 80 mg/hydrochlorothiazide 25 mg once daily; manufacturer labeling suggests that dose may be titrated up to telmisartan 160 mg/hydrochlorothiazide 25 mg if blood pressure remains uncontrolled after 2-4 weeks of therapy. In mild to moderate hypertension, doses of telmisartan >80 mg were not associated with a greater reduction in blood pressure (Smith, 2000). Patients who develop hypokalemia while on hydrochlorothiazide 25 mg may be switched to telmisartan 80 mg/hydrochlorothiazide 12.5 mg.

Canadian labeling: Specific dosing recommendations for the combination product are not provided by the manufacturer. When possible, discontinue the diuretic 2-3 days prior to initiation of telmisartan monotherapy. If diuretic therapy is necessary, use of individual agents may be necessary to allow for dose titration.

Dosage adjustment in renal impairment:
Cl_{cr} >30 mL/minute: No dosage adjustment necessary
Cl_{cr} ≤30 mL/minute: Not recommended

Dosage adjustment in hepatic impairment:
Mild to moderate hepatic impairment or biliary obstructive disorders: Initial: Telmisartan 40 mg/hydrochlorothiazide 12.5 mg
Severe hepatic impairment: Not recommended

Additional Information Complete prescribing information should be consulted for additional detail.

Dosage Forms Excipient information presented when available (limited, particularly for generics); consult specific product labeling.
Tablet, oral:
Micardis® HCT:
40/12.5: Telmisartan 40 mg and hydrochlorothiazide 12.5 mg
80/12.5: Telmisartan 80 mg and hydrochlorothiazide 12.5 mg
80/25: Telmisartan 80 mg and hydrochlorothiazide 25 mg

Dosage Forms: Canada Excipient information presented when available (limited, particularly for generics); consult specific product labeling.
Tablet, oral:
Micardis Plus:
80/12.5: Telmisartan 80 mg and hydrochlorothiazide 12.5 mg
80/25: Telmisartan 80 mg and hydrochlorothiazide 25 mg

◆ **Telmisartan HCTZ (Can)** *see* Telmisartan and Hydrochlorothiazide *on page 2004*

◆ **Telzir® (Can)** *see* Fosamprenavir *on page 916*

Temazepam (te MAZ e pam)

Brand Names: U.S. Restoril

Brand Names: Canada Apo-Temazepam; CO Temazepam; Dom-Temazepam; Novo-Temazepam; PHL-Temazepam; PMS-Temazepam; ratio-Temazepam; Restoril; Temazepam-15; Temazepam-30

Pharmacologic Category Benzodiazepine

Additional Appendix Information
Beers Criteria – Potentially Inappropriate Medications for Geriatrics *on page 2368*
Benzodiazepine Comparison Table *on page 2292*

Use Insomnia: Short-term treatment of insomnia

Pregnancy Risk Factor X

Medication Guide Available Yes

Dosage Oral:
Adults: Usual dose: 15-30 mg at bedtime; some patients may respond to 7.5 mg in transient insomnia
Elderly or debilitated patients:
U.S. labeling: Initial: 7.5 mg at bedtime.
Canadian labeling: Initial: 15 mg at bedtime.
Dosage adjustment in renal impairment: No dosage adjustment provided in manufacturer's labeling.
Dosage adjustment in hepatic impairment: No dosage adjustment provided in manufacturer's labeling.

Additional Information Complete prescribing information should be consulted for additional detail.

Dosage Forms Excipient information presented when available (limited, particularly for generics); consult specific product labeling.
Capsule, Oral:
Restoril: 7.5 mg, 15 mg, 22.5 mg, 30 mg [contains brilliant blue fcf (fd&c blue #1)]
Generic: 7.5 mg, 15 mg, 22.5 mg, 30 mg

Dosage Forms: Canada Excipient information presented when available (limited, particularly for generics); consult specific product labeling.
Capsule, Oral:
Restoril: 15 mg, 30 mg

Controlled Substance C-IV

◆ **Temazepam-15 (Can)** *see* Temazepam *on page 2005*

◆ **Temazepam-30 (Can)** *see* Temazepam *on page 2005*

◆ **Temodal (Can)** *see* Temozolomide *on page 2005*

◆ **Temodar** *see* Temozolomide *on page 2005*

◆ **Temovate** *see* Clobetasol *on page 457*

◆ **Temovate E** *see* Clobetasol *on page 457*

Temozolomide (te moe ZOE loe mide)

Brand Names: U.S. Temodar

Brand Names: Canada Ahi-Temozolomide Capsules; Co-Temozolomide; Temodal

Index Terms SCH 52365; TMZ

Pharmacologic Category Antineoplastic Agent, Alkylating Agent (Triazene)

Use
Anaplastic astrocytoma: Treatment of refractory anaplastic astrocytoma (refractory to a regimen containing a nitrosourea and procarbazine)
Glioblastoma multiforme: Treatment of newly-diagnosed glioblastoma multiforme (initially in combination with radiotherapy, then as maintenance treatment)
Canadian labeling: Treatment of newly-diagnosed glioblastoma multiforme (initially in combination with radiotherapy, then as maintenance treatment), treatment of recurrent or progressive glioblastoma multiforme or anaplastic astrocytoma

Unlabeled Use Treatment of recurrent glioblastoma multiforme, low-grade astrocytoma, low-grade oligodendroglioma, anaplastic oligodendroglioma, metastatic CNS lesions, refractory primary CNS lymphoma, advanced or metastatic melanoma, advanced cutaneous T-cell lymphomas (mycosis fungoides [MF] and Sézary syndrome [SS]), advanced neuroendocrine tumors (carcinoid or islet cell), Ewing's sarcoma (recurrent or progressive), soft tissue sarcomas (extremity/retroperitoneal/intra-abdominal or hemangiopericytoma/solitary fibrous tumor), treatment of pediatric neuroblastoma

Pregnancy Risk Factor D

Pregnancy Considerations Adverse events were observed in animal reproduction studies. May cause fetal harm when administered to pregnant women. Male and female patients should avoid pregnancy while receiving temozolomide.

Breast-Feeding Considerations It is not known if temozolomide is excreted in breast milk. Due to the potential for serious adverse reactions in the nursing infant, a decision should be made to discontinue nursing or to discontinue temozolomide, taking into account the importance of treatment to the mother.

Contraindications Hypersensitivity (eg, allergic reaction, anaphylaxis, urticaria, Stevens-Johnson syndrome, toxic epidermal necrolysis) to temozolomide or any component of the formulation; hypersensitivity to dacarbazine (both drugs are metabolized to MTIC)

Canadian labeling: Additional contraindications (not in U.S. labeling): Not recommended in patients with severe myelosuppression

Warnings/Precautions Hazardous agent - use appropriate precautions for handling and disposal (NIOSH, 2012). *Pneumocystis jirovecii* pneumonia (PCP) may occur; risk is increased in those receiving steroids or longer dosing regimens; monitor all patients for development of PCP (particularly if also receiving corticosteroids); PCP prophylaxis is required in patients receiving radiotherapy in combination with the 42-day temozolomide regimen. Myelosuppression may occur; may require treatment interruption, dose reduction, and/or discontinuation; monitor blood counts; an increased incidence has been reported in geriatric and female patients. Prolonged pancytopenia resulting in aplastic anemia has been reported (may be fatal); concurrent use of temozolomide with medications associated with aplastic anemia (eg, carbamazepine, co-trimoxazole, phenytoin) may obscure assessment for development of aplastic anemia. Rare cases of myelodysplastic syndrome and secondary malignancies, including acute myeloid leukemia have been reported. Use caution in patients with severe hepatic or renal impairment; has not been studied in dialysis patients.

Temozolomide is associated with a moderate emetic potential (Dupuis, 2011; Roila, 2010); antiemetics are recommended to prevent nausea and vomiting. Increased MGMT (O-6-methylguanine-DNA methyltransferase) activity/levels within tumor tissue is associated with temozolomide resistance. Glioblastoma patients with decreased levels (due to methylated MGMT promoter) may be more likely to benefit from the combination of radiation therapy and temozolomide (Hegi, 2008; Stupp, 2009). Determination of MGMT status may be predictive for response to alkylating agents. Potentially significant drug-drug interactions may exist, requiring dose or frequency adjustment, additional monitoring, and/or selection of alternative therapy. Bioequivalence has only been established when I.V. temozolomide is administered over 90 minutes; shorter or longer infusion times may result in suboptimal dosing.

Adverse Reactions Note: With CNS malignancies, it may be difficult to distinguish between CNS adverse events caused by temozolomide versus the effects of progressive disease.

>10%:

Cardiovascular: Peripheral edema (11%)

Central nervous system: Fatigue (34% to 61%), headache (23% to 41%), seizure (6% to 23%), hemiparesis (18%), fever (13%), dizziness (5% to 12%), coordination abnormality (11%)

Dermatologic: Alopecia (55%), rash (8% to 13%)

Gastrointestinal: Nausea (49% to 53%; grades 3/4: 1% to 10%), vomiting (29% to 42%; grades 3/4: 2% to 6%), constipation (22% to 33%), anorexia (9% to 27%), diarrhea (10% to 16%)

Hematologic: Lymphopenia (grades 3/4: 55%), thrombocytopenia (grades 3/4: adults: 4% to 19%; children: 25%), neutropenia (grades 3/4: adults: 8% to 14%; children: 20%), leukopenia (grades 3/4: 11%)

Neuromuscular & skeletal: Weakness (7% to 13%)

Miscellaneous: Viral infection (11%)

1% to 10%:

Central nervous system: Amnesia (10%), insomnia (4% to 10%), somnolence (9%), ataxia (8%), paresis (8%), anxiety (7%), memory impairment (7%), depression (6%), confusion (5%)

Dermatologic: Pruritus (5% to 8%), dry skin (5%), radiation injury (2% maintenance phase after radiotherapy), erythema (1%)

Endocrine & metabolic: Hypercorticism (8%), breast pain (females 6%)

Gastrointestinal: Stomatitis (9%), abdominal pain (5% to 9%), dysphagia (7%), taste perversion (5%), weight gain (5%)

Genitourinary: Incontinence (8%), urinary tract infection (8%), urinary frequency (6%)

Hematologic: Anemia (grades 3/4: 4%)

Neuromuscular & skeletal: Paresthesia (9%), back pain (8%), abnormal gait (6%), arthralgia (6%), myalgia (5%)

Ocular: Blurred vision (5% to 8%), diplopia (5%), vision abnormality (visual deficit/vision changes 5%)

Respiratory: Pharyngitis (8%), upper respiratory tract infection (8%), cough (5% to 8%), sinusitis (6%), dyspnea (5%)

Miscellaneous: Allergic reaction (≤3%)

<1% (Limited to important or life-threatening): Alkaline phosphatase increased, alveolitis, anaphylaxis, aplastic anemia, cholestasis, emotional lability, erythema multiforme, febrile neutropenia, flu-like syndrome, hallucination, hematoma, hemorrhage, hepatitis, hepatotoxicity, herpes simplex, herpes zoster, hyperbilirubinemia, hyperglycemia, hypokalemia, injection site reactions (erythema, irritation, pain, pruritus, swelling, warmth), interstitial pneumonia/pneumonitis, myelodysplastic syndrome, opportunistic infection (eg, PCP), oral candidiasis, pancytopenia (may be prolonged), peripheral neuropathy, petechiae, pneumonitis, pulmonary fibrosis, secondary malignancies (including myeloid leukemia), Stevens-Johnson syndrome, toxic epidermal necrolysis, transaminases increased

Drug Interactions

Metabolism/Transport Effects None known.

Avoid Concomitant Use

Avoid concomitant use of Temozolomide with any of the following: BCG; CloZAPine; Natalizumab; Pimecrolimus; Tacrolimus (Topical); Tofacitinib; Vaccines (Live)

Increased Effect/Toxicity

Temozolomide may increase the levels/effects of: CloZAPine; Leflunomide; Natalizumab; Tofacitinib; Vaccines (Live)

The levels/effects of Temozolomide may be increased by: Denosumab; Pimecrolimus; Roflumilast; Tacrolimus (Topical); Trastuzumab; Valproic Acid and Derivatives

Decreased Effect

Temozolomide may decrease the levels/effects of: BCG; Coccidioidin Skin Test; Sipuleucel-T; Vaccines (Inactivated); Vaccines (Live)

The levels/effects of Temozolomide may be decreased by: Echinacea

Ethanol/Nutrition/Herb Interactions Food: Food reduces rate and extent of absorption. Management: Administer consistently either with food or without food (was administered in studies under fasting and nonfasting conditions).

Preparation for Administration Hazardous agent; use appropriate precautions for handling and disposal (NIOSH, 2012). Bring to room temperature prior to reconstitution. Reconstitute each 100 mg vial with 41 mL sterile water for injection to a final concentration of 2.5 mg/mL. Swirl gently; do not shake. Place dose without further dilution into a 250 mL empty sterile infusion bag. Infusion must be completed within 14 hours of reconstitution.

Storage/Stability

Capsule: Store at room temperature of 25°C (77°F); excursions permitted to 15°C to 30°C (59°F to 86°F).

Injection: Store intact vials refrigerated at 2°C to 8°C (36°F to 46°F). Reconstituted vials may be stored for up to 14 hours at room temperature of 25°C (77°F); infusion must be completed within 14 hours of reconstitution.

Mechanism of Action Temozolomide is a prodrug which is rapidly and nonenzymatically converted to the active alkylating metabolite MTIC [(methyl-triazene-1-yl)-imidazole-4-carboxamide]; this conversion is spontaneous, nonenzymatic, and occurs under physiologic conditions in all tissues to which it distributes. The cytotoxic effects of MTIC are manifested through alkylation (methylation) of DNA at the O^6, N^7 guanine positions which lead to DNA double strand breaks and apoptosis. Non-cell cycle specific.

Pharmacodynamics/Kinetics

Absorption: Oral: Rapid and complete

Distribution: V_d: Parent drug: 0.4 L/kg; penetrates blood-brain barrier; CSF levels are ~35% to 39% of plasma levels (Yung, 1999)

Protein binding: 15%

Metabolism: Prodrug, hydrolyzed to the active form, MTIC; MTIC is eventually eliminated as CO_2 and 5-aminoimidazole-4-carboxamide (AIC), a natural constituent in urine; CYP isoenzymes play only a minor role in metabolism (of temozolomide and MTIC)

Bioavailability: Oral: 100% (on a mg-per-mg basis, I.V. temozolomide, infused over 90 minutes, is bioequivalent to an oral dose)

Half-life elimination: Mean: Parent drug: 1.8 hours

Time to peak: Oral: Empty stomach: 1 hour; with food (high-fat meal): 2.25 hours

Excretion: Urine (~38%; parent drug 6%); feces <1%

Dosage Note: Temozolomide is associated with a moderate emetic potential; antiemetics are recommended to prevent nausea and vomiting. Prior to dosing, ANC should be ≥1500/mm^3 and platelets ≥100,000/mm^3.

Anaplastic astrocytoma (refractory): Adults: Oral, I.V.: Initial dose: 150 mg/m^2 once daily for 5 consecutive days of a 28-day treatment cycle. If ANC ≥1500/mm^3 and platelets ≥100,000/mm^3, on day 1 of subsequent cycles, may increase to 200 mg/m^2 once daily for 5 consecutive days of a 28-day treatment cycle. May continue until disease progression.

Dosage modification for toxicity:

ANC <1000/mm^3 or platelets <50,000/mm^3 on day 22 or day 29 (day 1 of next cycle): Postpone therapy until ANC >1500/mm^3 and platelets >100,000/mm^3; reduce dose by 50 mg/m^2/day (but not below 100 mg/m^2) for subsequent cycle

ANC 1000-1500/mm^3 or platelets 50,000-100,000/mm^3 on day 22 or day 29 (day 1 of next cycle): Postpone therapy until ANC >1500/mm^3 and platelets >100,000/mm^3; maintain initial dose

Glioblastoma multiforme (newly diagnosed, high-grade glioma): Adults: Oral, I.V.:

Concomitant phase: 75 mg/m^2/day for 42 days with focal radiotherapy (60 Gy administered in 30 fractions). **Note:** PCP prophylaxis is required during concomitant phase and should continue in patients who develop lymphocytopenia until lymphocyte recovery to ≤grade 1. Obtain weekly CBC.

Continue at 75 mg/m^2/day throughout the 42-day concomitant phase (up to 49 days) as long as ANC ≥1500/mm^3, platelet count ≥100,000/mm^3, and nonhematologic toxicity ≤grade 1 (excludes alopecia, nausea/vomiting)

Dosage modification for toxicity:

ANC ≥500/mm^3 but <1500/mm^3 **or** platelet count ≥10,000/mm^3 but <100,000/mm^3 **or** grade 2 nonhematologic toxicity (excludes alopecia, nausea/vomiting): Interrupt therapy

ANC <500/mm^3 **or** platelet count <10,000/mm^3 **or** grade 3/4 nonhematologic toxicity (excludes alopecia, nausea/vomiting): Discontinue therapy

Maintenance phase (consists of 6 treatment cycles): Begin 4 weeks after concomitant phase completion. **Note:** Each subsequent cycle is 28 days (consisting of 5 days of drug treatment followed by 23 days without treatment). Draw CBC within 48 hours of day 22; hold next cycle and do weekly CBC until ANC >1500/mm^3 and platelet count >100,000/mm^3; dosing modification should be based on lowest blood counts and worst nonhematologic toxicity during the previous cycle.

Cycle 1: 150 mg/m^2 once daily for 5 days of a 28-day treatment cycle

Cycles 2-6: May increase to 200 mg/m^2 once daily for 5 days; repeat every 28 days (if ANC ≥1500/mm^3, platelets ≥100,000/mm^3 and nonhematologic toxicities for cycle 1 are ≤grade 2 [excludes alopecia, nausea/vomiting]); **Note:** If dose was not escalated at the onset of cycle 2, do not increase for cycles 3-6)

Dosage modification (during maintenance phase) for toxicity:

ANC <1000/mm^3, platelet count <50,000/mm^3, or grade 3 nonhematologic toxicity (excludes alopecia, nausea/vomiting) during previous cycle: Decrease dose by 1 dose level (by 50 mg/m^2/day for 5 days), unless dose has already been lowered to 100 mg/m^2/day, then discontinue therapy.

If dose reduction <100 mg/m^2/day is required or grade 4 nonhematologic toxicity (excludes alopecia, nausea/vomiting), or if the same grade 3 nonhematologic toxicity occurs after dose reduction: Discontinue therapy

Glioblastoma multiforme (recurrent glioma): *Canadian labeling (unlabeled use in the U.S.):* Adults: Oral: 200 mg/m^2/day for 5 days every 28 days; if previously treated with chemotherapy, initiate at 150 mg/m^2/day for 5 days every 28 days and increase to 200 mg/m^2/day for 5 days every 28 days with cycle 2 if no hematologic toxicity (Brada, 2001; Yung, 2000)

Cutaneous T-cell lymphoma, advanced (mycosis fungoides [MF] and Sézary syndrome [SS]; unlabeled use): Adults: Oral: 200 mg/m^2 once daily for 5 days every 28 days for up to 1 year (Querfeld, 2011)

Ewing's sarcoma, recurrent or progressive (unlabeled use): Children, Adolescents, and Adults: Oral: 100 mg/m^2/dose days 1-5 every 21 days (in combination with irinotecan) (Casey, 2009)

Melanoma, advanced or metastatic (unlabeled use): Adults: Oral: 200 mg/m^2/day for 5 days every 28 days (for up to 12 cycles). For subsequent cycles, reduce dose to 75% of the original dose for grade 3/4 hematologic toxicity and reduce the dose to 50% of the original dose for grade 3/4 nonhematologic toxicity (Middleton, 2000).

Neuroblastoma, relapsed or refractory (unlabeled use): Children and Adolescents: Oral: 100 mg/m^2/dose days 1-5 every 21 days (in combination with irinotecan) for up to 6 cycles (Bagatell, 2011)

Neuroendocrine tumors, advanced (unlabeled use): Adults: Oral: 150 mg/m^2/day for 7 days every 14 days (in combination with thalidomide) until disease progression (Kulke, 2006) **or** 200 mg/m^2 once daily (at bedtime) days 10 to 14 of a 28-day treatment cycle (in combination with capecitabine) (Strosberg, 2011)

Primary CNS lymphoma, refractory (unlabeled use): Adults: Oral: 150 mg/m^2/day for 5 days every 28 days, initially in combination with rituximab, followed by temozolomide monotherapy: 150 mg/m^2/day for 5 days every 28 days (Wong, 2004) **or** 150 mg/m^2/day for 7 days every 14 days, initially in combination with rituximab, followed by temozolomide monotherapy: 150 mg/m^2/day for 5 days every 28 days (Enting, 2004)

Soft tissue sarcoma (unlabeled use): Adults: Oral:

Soft tissue sarcoma, metastatic or unresectable: 75 mg/m^2/day for 6 weeks (Garcia del Muro, 2005)

Hemangiopericytoma/solitary fibrous tumor: 150 mg/m^2 once daily days 1 to 7 and days 15 to 21 of a 28-day treatment cycle (in combination with bevacizumab) (Park, 2011)

Elderly: Refer to adult dosing. **Note:** Patients ≥70 years of age in the anaplastic astrocytoma study had a higher incidence of grade 4 neutropenia and thrombocytopenia in the first cycle of therapy than patients <70 years of age.

Dosage adjustment in renal impairment: Oral:

Cl_{cr} ≥36 mL/minute/m^2: No dosage adjustment provided in the manufacturer's labeling, however, dosage adjustment is not likely needed as no effect on temozolomide clearance was demonstrated.

Severe renal impairment (Cl_{cr} <36 mL/minute/m^2): No dosage adjustment provided in manufacturer's labeling; use with caution (has not been studied).

Dialysis patients: No dosage adjustment provided in manufacturer's labeling (has not been studied).

Dosage adjustment in hepatic impairment:

Mild-to-moderate impairment: No dosage adjustment provided in manufacturer's labeling; however, pharmacokinetics are similar to patients with normal hepatic function.

Severe hepatic impairment: No dosage adjustment provided in manufacturer's labeling; use with caution (has not been studied).

Dosing in obesity: *ASCO Guidelines for appropriate chemotherapy dosing in obese adults with cancer:* Utilize patient's actual body weight (full weight) for calculation of body surface area- or weight-based dosing, particularly when the intent of therapy is curative; manage regimen-related toxicities in the same manner as for nonobese patients; if a dose reduction is utilized due to toxicity, consider resumption of full weight-based dosing with subsequent cycles, especially if cause of toxicity (eg, hepatic or renal impairment) is resolved (Griggs, 2012).

Dietary Considerations The incidence of nausea/vomiting is decreased when taken on an empty stomach. Take capsules consistently either with food or without food (absorption is affected by food).

Administration

Oral: Swallow capsules whole with a glass of water. Absorption is affected by food; therefore, administer consistently either with food or without food (was administered in studies under fasting and nonfasting conditions). May administer on an empty stomach or at bedtime to reduce nausea and vomiting. Do not repeat if vomiting occurs after dose is administered; wait until the next scheduled dose. Do not open or chew capsules; avoid contact with skin or mucous membranes if capsules are accidentally opened or damaged.

I.V.: Infuse over 90 minutes. Flush line before and after administration. May be administered through the same I.V. line as sodium chloride 0.9%; do not administer other medications through the same I.V. line.

Note: Temozolomide is associated with a moderate emetic potential; antiemetics are recommended to prevent nausea and vomiting.

Hazardous agent; use appropriate precautions for handling and disposal (NIOSH, 2012).

Monitoring Parameters CBC with differential and platelets (prior to each cycle; weekly during glioma concomitant phase treatment; at or within 48 hours of day 22 and weekly until ANC >1500/mm^3 and platelets >100,000/mm^3 for glioma maintenance and astrocytoma treatment)

Dosage Forms Excipient information presented when available (limited, particularly for generics); consult specific product labeling.

Capsule, Oral:

Temodar: 5 mg [contains fd&c blue #2 (indigotine)]

Temodar: 20 mg, 100 mg

Temodar: 140 mg [contains fd&c blue #2 (indigotine)]

Temodar: 180 mg, 250 mg

Generic: 5 mg, 20 mg, 100 mg, 140 mg, 180 mg, 250 mg

Solution Reconstituted, Intravenous:

Temodar: 100 mg (1 ea) [pyrogen free; contains polysorbate 80]

Extemporaneous Preparations Hazardous agent: Use appropriate precautions for handling and disposal.

A 10 mg/mL temozolomide oral suspension may be compounded in a vertical flow hood. Mix the contents of ten 100 mg capsules and 500 mg of povidone K-30 powder in a glass mortar; add 25 mg anhydrous citric acid dissolved in 1.5 mL purified water and mix to a uniform paste; mix while adding 50 mL Ora-Plus® in incremental proportions. Transfer to an amber plastic bottle, rinse mortar 4 times with small portions of either Ora-Sweet® or Ora-Sweet® SF, and add quantity of Ora-Sweet® or Ora-Sweet® SF sufficient to make 100 mL. Store in plastic amber prescription bottles; label "shake well" and "refrigerate"; include the beyond-use date. Stable for 7 days at room temperature or 60 days refrigerated (preferred).

Trissel LA, Yanping Z, and Koontz SE, "Temozolomide Stability in Extemporaneously Compounded Oral Suspension," *Int J Pharm Compound*, 2006, 10(5):396-9.

◆ Tempra (Can) *see* Acetaminophen *on page 28*

Temsirolimus (tem sir OH li mus)

Brand Names: U.S. Torisel

Brand Names: Canada Torisel®

Index Terms CCI-779

Pharmacologic Category Antineoplastic Agent, mTOR Kinase Inhibitor

Use Treatment of advanced renal cell cancer (RCC)

Pregnancy Risk Factor D

Pregnancy Considerations Embryotoxicity and fetotoxicity (as evidenced by increased mortality, reduced fetal weights, and delayed ossification) occurred in animal reproduction studies at oral doses lower than the usual human dose. Women of childbearing potential should be advised to avoid pregnancy. Men and women should use effective birth control during temsirolimus treatment, and continue for 3 months after temsirolimus discontinuation.

Breast-Feeding Considerations Due to the potential for serious adverse reactions in the nursing infant, the decision to discontinue breast-feeding or discontinue temsirolimus should take into account the benefits of treatment to the mother.

Contraindications Bilirubin >1.5 times the upper limit of normal (ULN)

Canadian labeling: Additional contraindications (not in U.S. labeling): History of anaphylaxis after exposure to temsirolimus, sirolimus, or any component of the formulation

Warnings/Precautions Hazardous agent - use appropriate precautions for handling and disposal (NIOSH, 2012).

Hypersensitivity/infusion reactions (eg, anaphylaxis, apnea, dyspnea, flushing, loss of consciousness, hypotension, and/or chest pain) have been reported. Infusion reaction may occur during the initial infusion (early in infusion) or with subsequent infusions. Premedicate with an antihistamine (H_1 antagonist) prior to infusion; monitor throughout infusion (appropriate supportive care should be available); interrupt infusion for hypersensitivity reaction and observe patient for 30-60 minutes. With discretion, treatment may be resumed at a slower infusion rate; administer an H_1 antagonist (if not given as premedication) and/or an I.V. H_2 antagonist ~30 minutes prior to resuming infusion. For severe infusion reactions, asses risk versus benefit of continued treatment. Use with caution in patients with hypersensitivity temsirolimus, sirolimus (a metabolite), or polysorbate 80. Angioneurotic edema has been reported; concurrent use with other drugs known to cause angioedema (eg, ACE inhibitors) may increase risk.

Temsirolimus is predominantly cleared by the liver; use with caution and reduce dose in patients with mild hepatic impairment (bilirubin >1-1.5 x ULN or AST >ULN with bilirubin ≤ULN). Toxicities were increased in patients with baseline bilirubin >1.5 x ULN. Use is contraindicated in patients with moderate-to-severe hepatic impairment (bilirubin >1.5 x ULN).

Avoid concomitant use with strong CYP3A4 inhibitors and strong CYP3A4 inducers (see Drug Interactions); consider alternative agents that avoid or lessen the potential for CYP-mediated interactions. Patients should not be immunized with live, viral vaccines during or shortly after treatment and should avoid close contact with recently vaccinated (live vaccine) individuals. Patients who are receiving anticoagulant therapy or those with CNS tumors/metastases may be at increased risk for developing intracerebral bleeding. Combination therapy with temsirolimus and sunitinib has resulted in dose-limiting toxicities, including grade 3 or 4 rash, gout, and/or cellulitis.

Increases in serum glucose commonly occur during treatment; initiation or alteration of insulin and/or oral hypoglycemic therapy may be required; monitor serum glucose before and during treatment; use with caution in patients with diabetes. Use with caution in patients with hyperlipidemia; may increase serum lipids (cholesterol and triglycerides); initiation or dosage adjustment of of antihyperlipidemic agents may be required; monitor cholesterol/triglyceride panel. Treatment may result in immunosuppression, may increase risk of opportunistic infections and/or sepsis. Interstitial lung disease (ILD), sometimes fatal, has been reported; symptoms include dyspnea, cough, hypoxia, and/or fever, although asymptomatic or mild cases may present; promptly evaluate worsening respiratory symptoms; may require corticosteroids, antibiotic therapy, and/or treatment discontinuation; baseline chest radiographic assessment (CT scan or xray) is recommended. Cases of bowel perforation (fatal) have occurred (usually presenting with abdominal pain, bloody stools, diarrhea, fever, or metabolic acidosis); promptly evaluate any new or worsening abdominal pain or bloody stools. Temsirolimus may be associated with impaired wound healing; use caution in the perioperative period. Cases of acute renal failure with rapid progression have been reported (unrelated to disease progression), including cases unresponsive to dialysis. An increased incidence of rash, infection and dose interruptions have been reported in patients with renal insufficiency (Cl_{cr} ≤60 mL/minute) who received mTOR inhibitors for the treatment of renal cell cancer (Gupta, 2011).

Adverse Reactions

>10%:

Cardiovascular: Edema (35%), peripheral edema (27%), chest pain (16%)

Central nervous system: Pain (28%), fever (24%), headache (15%), insomnia (12%)

Dermatologic: Rash (47%), pruritus (19%), nail disorder/thinning (14%), dry skin (11%)

Endocrine & metabolic: Hyperglycemia (26% to 89%; grades 3/4: 16%), hypercholesterolemia (24% to 87%; grades 3/4: 2%), hypertriglyceridemia (83%; grades 3/4: 44%), hypophosphatemia (49%; grades 3/4: 18%), hyperlipidemia (27%), hypokalemia (21%; grades 3/4: 5%)

Gastrointestinal: Mucositis (41%), nausea (37%), anorexia (32%), diarrhea (27%), abdominal pain (21%), constipation (20%), stomatitis (20%), taste disturbance (20%), vomiting (19%), weight loss (19%)

Genitourinary: Urinary tract infection (15%)

Hematologic: Anemia (45% to 94%; grades 3/4: 20%), lymphopenia (53%; grades 3/4: 16%), thrombocytopenia (14% to 40%; grades 3/4: 1%; dose-limiting toxicity), leukopenia (6% to 32%; grades 3/4: 1%), neutropenia (7% to 19%; grades 3/4: 3% to 5%)

Hepatic: Alkaline phosphatase increased (68%; grades 3/4: 3%), AST increased (8% to 38%; grades 3/4: 1% to 2%)

Neuromuscular & skeletal: Weakness (51%), back pain (20%), arthralgia (18%)

Renal: Creatinine increased (14% to 57%; grades 3/4: 3%)

Respiratory: Dyspnea (28%), cough (26%), epistaxis (12%), pharyngitis (12%)

Miscellaneous: Infection (20% to 27%; includes abscess, bronchitis, cellulitis, herpes simplex, herpes zoster)

1% to 10%:

Cardiovascular: Hypertension, thrombophlebitis, venous thromboembolism (includes DVT and PE)

Central nervous system: Chills, depression

Dermatologic: Acne, wound healing impaired

Gastrointestinal: Bowel perforation

Hepatic: Hyperbilirubinemia

Neuromuscular & skeletal: Myalgia

Ocular: Conjunctivitis

Respiratory: Interstitial lung disease (ILD), pneumonia, rhinitis, upper respiratory tract infection

Miscellaneous: Allergic/hypersensitivity/infusion reaction (includes anaphylaxis, apnea, chest pain, dyspnea, flushing, hypotension, loss of consciousness)

<1% (Limited to important or life-threatening): Acute renal failure, angioneurotic edema, glucose intolerance, infusion site extravasation (with pain, swelling, warmth, erythema), pericardial effusion, pleural effusion, pneumonitis, reflex sympathetic dystrophy, rhabdomyolysis, seizure, Stevens-Johnson syndrome

Drug Interactions

Metabolism/Transport Effects Substrate of CYP3A4 (major), P-glycoprotein; **Note:** Assignment of Major/Minor substrate status based on clinically relevant drug interaction potential; **Inhibits** CYP2D6 (weak), CYP3A4 (weak)

Avoid Concomitant Use

Avoid concomitant use of Temsirolimus with any of the following: BCG; CloZAPine; Conivaptan; Fusidic Acid (Systemic); Natalizumab; Pimecrolimus; Pimozide; SUNItinib; Tacrolimus (Systemic); Tacrolimus (Topical); Tofacitinib; Vaccines (Live)

Increased Effect/Toxicity

Temsirolimus may increase the levels/effects of: ACE Inhibitors; ARIPiprazole; CloZAPine; CycloSPORINE (Systemic); Dofetilide; Leflunomide; Lomitapide; Natalizumab; Pimozide; SUNItinib; Tacrolimus (Systemic); Tacrolimus (Topical); Tofacitinib; Vaccines (Live)

The levels/effects of Temsirolimus may be increased by: Conivaptan; CYP3A4 Inhibitors (Moderate); CYP3A4 Inhibitors (Strong); Dasatinib; Denosumab; Fluconazole; Fusidic Acid (Systemic); Itraconazole; Ivacaftor; Ketoconazole (Systemic); Luliconazole; Macrolide Antibiotics; Mifepristone; P-glycoprotein/ABCB1 Inhibitors; Pimecrolimus; Posaconazole; Protease Inhibitors; Roflumilast; Simeprevir; Tacrolimus (Systemic); Tacrolimus (Topical); Trastuzumab

Decreased Effect

Temsirolimus may decrease the levels/effects of: BCG; Coccidioidin Skin Test; Sipuleucel-T; Tacrolimus (Systemic); Vaccines (Inactivated); Vaccines (Live)

The levels/effects of Temsirolimus may be decreased by: Bosentan; CarBAMazepine; CYP3A4 Inducers (Strong); Dabrafenib; Deferasirox; Echinacea; Fosphenytoin; Herbs (CYP3A4 Inducers); Mitotane; P-glycoprotein/ABCB1 Inducers; Phenytoin; Rifamycin Derivatives; Tocilizumab

Ethanol/Nutrition/Herb Interactions

Food: Grapefruit and grapefruit juice may increase the levels/effects of sirolimus. Management: Avoid grapefruit and grapefruit juice.

Herb/Nutraceutical: Herbs with hypoglycemic properties may increase the risk of temsirolimus-induced hypoglycemia. St John's wort may decrease sirolimus (the active metabolite of temsirolimus) levels. Management: Avoid concurrent use of St John's wort. Avoid alfalfa, aloe, bilberry, bitter melon, burdock, celery, damiana, fenugreek, garcinia, garlic, ginger, ginseng (American), gymnema, marshmallow, and stinging nettle.

Preparation for Administration Hazardous agent; use appropriate precautions for handling and disposal (NIOSH, 2012). Preparation requires a two-step dilution process (do not add undiluted temsirolimus to aqueous solution; addition to aqueous solution prior to step 1 will result in precipitation). *Step 1:* Total amount in undiluted vial is 30 mg/1.2 mL (25 mg/mL concentration); contains overfill. Vials should initially be diluted with 1.8 mL of provided diluent to a concentration of 10 mg/mL. Once diluted with provided diluent, mix by inverting vial. *Step 2:* After allowing air bubbles to subside, the intended dose should be withdrawn from the 10 mg/mL diluted vial (ie, 2.5 mL for a 25 mg dose) and further diluted in 250 mL of NS in a non-DEHP/non-PVC container (glass, polyolefin, or polypropylene). Mix by inverting bottle or bag; avoid excessive shaking (may result in foaming).

Storage/Stability Store intact vials refrigerated at 2°C to 8°C (36°F to 46°F). Diluted solution in the vial (10 mg/mL) is stable for 24 hours at room temperature. Solutions diluted for infusion (in NS) must be infused within 6 hours of preparation. Protect from light during storage, preparation, and handling.

Mechanism of Action Temsirolimus and its active metabolite, sirolimus, are targeted inhibitors of mTOR (mammalian target of rapamycin) kinase activity. Temsirolimus (and sirolimus) bind to FKBP-12, an intracellular protein, to form a complex which inhibits mTOR signaling, halting the cell cycle at the G1 phase in tumor cells. In renal cell carcinoma, mTOR inhibition also exhibits anti-angiogenesis activity by reducing levels of HIF-1 and HIF-2 alpha (hypoxia inducible factors) and vascular endothelial growth factor (VEGF).

Pharmacodynamics/Kinetics

Distribution: V_{dss}: 172 L

Metabolism: Hepatic; via CYP3A4 to sirolimus (primary active metabolite) and 4 minor metabolites

Half-life elimination: Temsirolimus: ~17 hours; Sirolimus: ~55 hours

Time to peak, plasma: Temsirolimus: At end of infusion; Sirolimus: 0.5-2 hours after temsirolimus infusion

Excretion: Feces (78%); urine (<5%)

Dosage Note: For infusion reaction prophylaxis, premedicate with an H_1 antagonist (eg, diphenhydramine 25-50 mg I.V.) 30 minutes prior to infusion.

I.V.: Adults: Renal cell cancer (RCC), advanced: 25 mg once weekly; continue until disease progression or unacceptable toxicity

Dosage adjustment for concomitant CYP3A4 inhibitors/inducers:

CYP3A4 inhibitors: Avoid concomitant administration with strong CYP3A4 inhibitors (eg, clarithromycin, itraconazole, ketoconazole, nefazodone, protease inhibitors, telithromycin, voriconazole); if concomitant administration with a strong CYP3A4 inhibitor cannot be avoided, consider a dose reduction to 12.5 mg/week. When a strong CYP3A4 inhibitor is discontinued; allow ~1 week to elapse prior to adjusting the temsirolimus upward to the dose used prior to initiation of the CYP3A4 inhibitor.

CYP3A4 inducers: Avoid concomitant administration with strong CYP3A4 inducers (eg, carbamazepine, dexamethasone, phenobarbital, phenytoin, rifampin, St John's wort); if concomitant administration with a strong CYP3A4 inducer cannot be avoided, consider adjusting temsirolimus dose up to 50 mg/week. If the strong CYP3A4 enzyme inducer is discontinued, reduce the temsirolimus to the dose used prior to initiation of the CYP3A4 inducer.

Dosage adjustment for toxicity:

Hematologic toxicity: ANC <1000/mm^3 or platelets <75,000/mm^3: Withhold treatment until resolves and reinitiate treatment with the dose reduced by 5 mg/week; minimum dose: 15 mg/week if adjustment for toxicity is needed.

Nonhematologic toxicity: Any toxicity ≥grade 3: Withhold treatment until resolves to ≤grade 2; reinitiate treatment with the dose reduced by 5 mg/week; minimum dose: 15 mg/week if adjustment for toxicity is needed.

Infusion/hypersensitivity reaction: Interrupt infusion and observe for 30-60 minutes; treatment may be resumed with discretion at a slower infusion rate (up to 60 minutes); administer an H_1 antagonist (if not given as premedication) and/or an I.V. H_2 antagonist 30 minutes prior to resuming infusion.

Interstitial lung disease: Consider withholding treatment for clinically significant respiratory symptoms until after recovery of symptoms or radiographic improvement.

Dosage adjustment in renal impairment: No dosage adjustment necessary.

Hemodialysis: No dosage adjustment provided in manufacturer's labeling (has not been studied).

Dosage adjustment in hepatic impairment:

Mild hepatic impairment (bilirubin >1-1.5 x ULN or AST >ULN with bilirubin ≤ULN): Reduce dose to 15 mg once weekly

Moderate-to-severe hepatic impairment (bilirubin >1.5 x ULN): Use is contraindicated

Dietary Considerations Avoid grapefruit juice (may increase the levels of the major metabolite, sirolimus).

Administration Infuse over 30-60 minutes via an infusion pump (preferred). Use polyethylene-lined non-DEHP administration tubing. Administer through an inline polyethersulfone filter ≤5 micron; if set does not contain an inline filter, a polyethersulfone end filter (0.2-5 micron) should be added (do not use both an inline and an end filter). Premedicate with an H_1 antagonist (eg, diphenhydramine 25-50 mg I.V.) ~30 minutes prior to infusion. Monitor during infusion; interrupt infusion for hypersensitivity/infusion reaction; monitor for 30-60 minutes; may reinitiate at a reduced infusion rate (over 60 minutes) with discretion, 30 minutes after administration of a histamine H_1 antagonist and/or a histamine H_2 antagonist (eg, famotidine or ranitidine). Administration should be completed within 6 hours of admixture.

Hazardous agent; use appropriate precautions for handling and disposal (NIOSH, 2012).

Monitoring Parameters CBC with differential and platelets (weekly), serum chemistries including glucose (baseline and every other week), serum cholesterol and triglycerides (baseline and periodic), liver function (baseline and periodic), renal function tests (baseline and periodic)

Monitor for infusion reactions; infection; symptoms of ILD (or radiographic changes), symptoms of hyperglycemia (excessive thirst, polyuria)

Dosage Forms Excipient information presented when available (limited, particularly for generics); consult specific product labeling.

Solution, Intravenous:

Torisel: 25 mg/mL (1 mL) [contains alcohol, usp, polyethylene glycol, polysorbate 80, propylene glycol]

Tenecteplase (ten EK te plase)

Brand Names: U.S. TNKase

Brand Names: Canada TNKase®

Pharmacologic Category Thrombolytic Agent

Use Management of ST-elevation myocardial infarction (STEMI) for the lysis of thrombi in the coronary vasculature to restore perfusion and reduce mortality.

Recommended criteria for treatment of STEMI (ACCF/AHA; O'Gara, 2013): Ischemic symptoms within 12 hours of treatment or evidence of ongoing ischemia 12-24 hours after symptom onset with a large area of myocardium at risk or hemodynamic instability.

STEMI ECG definition: New ST-segment elevation at the J point in at least 2 contiguous leads of ≥2 mm (0.2 mV) in men or ≥1.5 mm (0.15 mV) in women in leads V_2-V_3 and/or of ≥1 mm (0.1 mV) in other contiguous precordial leads or limb leads on ECG. New or presumably new left bundle branch block (LBBB) may interfere with ST-elevation analysis and should not be considered diagnostic in isolation.

At non-PCI-capable hospitals, the ACCF/AHA recommends thrombolytic therapy administration when the anticipated first medical contact (FMC)-to-device time at a PCI-capable hospital is >120 minutes due to unavoidable delays.

Pregnancy Risk Factor C

Pregnancy Considerations Adverse events have been observed in some animal reproduction studies. The risk of bleeding may be increased in pregnant women. Administer to pregnant women only if the potential benefits justify the risk to the fetus.

Breast-Feeding Considerations It is not known if tenecteplase is excreted in breast milk. The manufacturer recommends that caution be exercised when administering tenecteplase to nursing women.

Contraindications Active internal bleeding; history of cerebrovascular accident; recent (ie, within 2 months) intracranial/intraspinal surgery or trauma; intracranial neoplasm; arteriovenous malformation or aneurysm; bleeding diathesis; severe uncontrolled hypertension

Additional contraindications (ACCF/AHA; O'Gara, 2013): Ischemic stroke within 3 months; prior intracranial hemorrhage; active bleeding (excluding menses); suspected aortic dissection; significant closed head or facial trauma within 3 months

Warnings/Precautions Use with caution in patients receiving oral anticoagulants; increased risk of bleeding. Adjunctive use of parenteral anticoagulants (eg, enoxaparin, heparin, or fondaparinux) is recommended to improve vessel patency and prevent reocclusion and may also contribute to bleeding; monitor for bleeding (ACCF/AHA; O'Gara, 2013). Stop antiplatelet agents and heparin if serious bleeding occurs. Avoid I.M. injections and nonessential handling of the patient for a few hours after administration. Monitor for bleeding complications. Venipunctures should be performed carefully and only when necessary. If arterial puncture is necessary, then use an upper extremity that can be easily compressed manually. For the following conditions, the risk of bleeding is higher with use of tenecteplase and the use of tenecteplase should be weighed against the benefits: Recent major surgery, cerebrovascular disease, recent GI or GU bleed, recent trauma, uncontrolled hypertension (systolic BP >180 mm Hg and/or diastolic BP >110 mm Hg), suspected left heart thrombus, acute pericarditis, subacute bacterial endocarditis, hemostatic defects, severe hepatic dysfunction, hemorrhagic diabetic retinopathy or other hemorrhagic ophthalmic conditions, pregnancy, septic thrombophlebitis or occluded arteriovenous cannula at seriously infected site, advanced age, anticoagulants, recent administration of GP IIb/IIIa inhibitors. Use with caution in patients with advanced age; increased risk of bleeding. Mortality and rate of intracranial hemorrhage increases with increasing age >65 years of age; the risks and benefits of use should be weighed carefully in the elderly. Coronary thrombolysis may result in reperfusion arrhythmias. Caution with readministration of tenecteplase.

Adverse Reactions As with all drugs which may affect hemostasis, bleeding is the major adverse effect associated with tenecteplase. Hemorrhage may occur at virtually any site. Risk is dependent on multiple variables, including the dosage administered, concurrent use of multiple agents which alter hemostasis, and patient predisposition. Rapid lysis of coronary artery thrombi by thrombolytic agents may be associated with reperfusion-related arterial and/or ventricular arrhythmia.

>10%:

Local: Hematoma (12% minor)

Hematologic: Bleeding (22% minor: ASSENT-2 trial)

1% to 10%:

Central nervous system: Stroke (2%)

Gastrointestinal: Epistaxis (2% minor), GI hemorrhage (1% major, 2% minor)

Genitourinary: GU bleeding (4% minor)

Hematologic: Bleeding (5% major; ASSENT-2 trial)

Local: Bleeding at catheter puncture site (4% minor), hematoma (2% major)

Respiratory: Pharyngeal (3% minor)

The incidence of stroke and bleeding increase with age above 65 years.

<1% (Limited to important or life-threatening): Anaphylaxis, angioedema, bleeding at catheter puncture site (<1% major), cholesterol embolism (clinical features may include livedo reticularis, "purple toe" syndrome, acute renal failure, gangrenous digits, hypertension, pancreatitis, MI, cerebral infarction, spinal cord infarction, retinal artery occlusion, bowel infarction, rhabdomyolysis), GU bleeding (<1% major), intracranial hemorrhage (0.9%), laryngeal edema, rash, respiratory tract bleeding, retroperitoneal bleeding, urticaria

Additional cardiovascular events associated with use in MI: Arrhythmia, AV block, cardiac arrest, cardiac tamponade, cardiogenic shock, embolism, electromechanical dissociation, fever, heart failure, hypotension, mitral regurgitation, myocardial reinfarction, myocardial rupture, nausea, pericardial effusion, pericarditis, pulmonary edema, recurrent myocardial ischemia, thrombosis, vomiting

Drug Interactions

Metabolism/Transport Effects None known.

Avoid Concomitant Use There are no known interactions where it is recommended to avoid concomitant use.

Increased Effect/Toxicity

Tenecteplase may increase the levels/effects of: Anticoagulants; Dabigatran Etexilate

The levels/effects of Tenecteplase may be increased by: Agents with Antiplatelet Properties; Herbs (Anticoagulant/Antiplatelet Properties); Nonsteroidal Anti-Inflammatory Agents; Salicylates

Decreased Effect

The levels/effects of Tenecteplase may be decreased by: Aprotinin

Preparation for Administration Tenecteplase should be reconstituted using the supplied 10 mL syringe with Twin-Pak™ Dual Cannula Device and 10 mL sterile water for injection. Do not shake when reconstituting. Slight foaming is normal and will dissipate if left standing for several minutes. The reconstituted solution is 5 mg/mL. Any unused solution should be discarded. If reconstituted and not used immediately, store in refrigerator and use within 8 hours.

Storage/Stability Store under refrigeration of 2°C to 8°C (36°F to 46°F) or at room temperature; do not exceed 30°C (86°F). If reconstituted and not used immediately, store in refrigerator and use within 8 hours.

Mechanism of Action Promotes initiation of fibrinolysis by binding to fibrin and converting plasminogen to plasmin. Tenecteplase is essentially alteplase with the exception of 3 point mutations and is more fibrin specific, more resistant to plasminogen activator inhibitor -1 (PAI-1), with a longer duration of action compared to alteplase. Produced by recombinant DNA technology using a mammalian cell line (Chinese hamster ovary cells).

Pharmacodynamics/Kinetics

Distribution: V_d is weight related and approximates plasma volume

Metabolism: Primarily hepatic

Half-life elimination: Biphasic: Initial: 20-24 minutes; Terminal: 90-130 minutes

Excretion: Clearance: Plasma: 99-119 mL/minute

Dosage I.V.:

Adult: Recommended total dose should not exceed 50 mg and is based on patient's weight; administer as a single bolus over 5 seconds

If patient's weight:

<60 kg: 30 mg

≥60 to <70 kg: 35 mg

≥70 to <80 kg: 40 mg

≥80 to <90 kg: 45 mg

≥90 kg: 50 mg

Note: Thrombolytic should be administered within 30 minutes of hospital arrival. Administer concurrent aspirin, clopidogrel, and anticoagulant therapy (ie, unfractionated heparin, enoxaparin, or fondaparinux) with tenecteplase (O'Gara, 2013).

Elderly: Refer to adult dosing. Although dosage adjustments are not recommended, the elderly have a higher incidence of morbidity and mortality with the use of tenecteplase.

Dosage adjustment in renal impairment: No dosage adjustment necessary.

Dosage adjustment in hepatic impairment:

Mild to moderate impairment: No dosage adjustment provided in manufacturer's labeling.

Severe impairment: No dosage adjustment provided in manufacturer's labeling; weigh the risk of bleeding against the benefits with tenecteplase especially in those with a coagulopathy.

Administration Tenecteplase is **incompatible** with dextrose solutions. Dextrose-containing lines must be flushed with a saline solution before and after administration. Administer as a single I.V. bolus over 5 seconds. Avoid I.M. injections and nonessential handling of patient.

Monitoring Parameters CBC, aPTT, signs and symptoms of bleeding, ECG monitoring

Test Interactions Altered results of coagulation and fibrinolytic activity tests

Dosage Forms Excipient information presented when available (limited, particularly for generics); consult specific product labeling.

Kit, Intravenous:

TNKase: 50 mg

◆ **Tenex** *see* GuanFACINE *on page* 979

Teniposide (ten i POE side)

Brand Names: U.S. Vumon

Brand Names: Canada Vumon®

Index Terms EPT; PTG; VM-26

Pharmacologic Category Antineoplastic Agent, Podophyllotoxin Derivative

Use Treatment of refractory childhood acute lymphoblastic leukemia (ALL) in combination with other chemotherapy

Unlabeled Use Treatment of refractory acute lymphoblastic leukemia (ALL) in adults

Pregnancy Risk Factor D

Dosage I.V.: **Note:** Patients with Down syndrome and leukemia may be more sensitive to the myelosuppressive effects; administer the first course at half the usual dose and adjust dose in subsequent cycles upward based on degree of toxicities (myelosuppression and mucositis) in the previous course(s).

Children: Acute lymphoblastic leukemia (ALL; combination chemotherapy): 165 mg/m^2 twice weekly for 8-9 doses **or** 250 mg/m^2 weekly for 4-8 weeks **or** (unlabeled dosing) 165 mg/m^2/dose days 1 and 2 of weeks 3, 13, and 23 (Lauer, 2001)

Adults: ALL consolidation treatment (unlabeled use; combination chemotherapy): 165 mg/m^2/dose days 1, 4, 8, and 11 of alternating consolidation cycles (Linker, 1991)

Dosage adjustment in renal impairment: No dosage adjustment provided in manufacturer's labeling (has not been studied). However, dosage adjustment may be necessary in patient with significant renal impairment.

Dosage adjustment in hepatic impairment: No dosage adjustment provided in manufacturer's labeling (has not been studied). However, dosage adjustment may be necessary in patient with significant hepatic impairment.

Dosing in obesity: *ASCO Guidelines for appropriate chemotherapy dosing in obese adults with cancer:* Utilize patient's actual body weight (full weight) for calculation of body surface area- or weight-based dosing, particularly when the intent of therapy is curative; manage regimen-related toxicities in the same manner as for nonobese patients; if a dose reduction is utilized due to toxicity, consider resumption of full weight-based dosing with subsequent cycles, especially if cause of toxicity (eg, hepatic or renal impairment) is resolved (Griggs, 2012).

Additional Information Complete prescribing information should be consulted for additional detail.

Dosage Forms Excipient information presented when available (limited, particularly for generics); consult specific product labeling.

Solution, Intravenous:

Vumon: 10 mg/mL (5 mL) [contains alcohol, usp, benzyl alcohol, cremophor el, dimethylacetamide]

Generic: 10 mg/mL (5 mL)

◆ **Tenivac** *see* Diphtheria and Tetanus Toxoid *on page* 626

Tenofovir (ten OF oh vir)

Brand Names: U.S. Viread

Brand Names: Canada Viread

Index Terms PMPA; TDF; Tenofovir Disoproxil Fumarate

Pharmacologic Category Antiretroviral, Reverse Transcriptase Inhibitor, Nucleotide (Anti-HIV)

Use

U.S. labeling:

Chronic hepatitis B: Treatment of chronic hepatitis B virus (HBV) in patients ≥12 years of age

HIV infection: In combination with other antiretroviral agents for the treatment of HIV-1 infection in adults and pediatric patients ≥2 years of age

Canadian labeling: Management of HIV infections in combination with at least two other antiretroviral agents in patients ≥12 years of age; treatment of chronic hepatitis B virus (HBV) in patients with compensated or decompensated liver disease in patients ≥18 years of age

Pregnancy Risk Factor B

Pregnancy Considerations Adverse events were not observed in rat and rabbit reproduction studies. Decreased fetal growth and reduced fetal bone porosity were observed in monkeys. Clinical studies in children have shown bone demineralization with chronic use. Tenofovir crosses the human placenta. No increased risk of overall birth defects has been observed following first trimester exposure according to data collected by the antiretroviral pregnancy registry. Limited data indicate decreased maternal bioavailability during the third trimester. Cases of lactic acidosis/hepatic steatosis syndrome related to mitochondrial toxicity have been reported in pregnant women with prolonged use of nucleoside analogues. It is not known if pregnancy itself potentiates this known side effect; however, women may be at increased risk of lactic acidosis and liver damage. In addition, these adverse events are similar to other rare but life-threatening syndromes which occur during pregnancy (eg, HELLP syndrome). Hepatic enzymes and electrolytes should be monitored in women receiving nucleoside analogues and clinicians should watch for early signs of the syndrome. In addition, mitochondrial dysfunction may develop in infants following *in utero* exposure. Renal function should also be monitored. The DHHS Perinatal HIV Guidelines consider tenofovir to be an alternative NRTI in dual nucleoside combination regimens. The DHHS Perinatal HIV Guidelines consider emtricitabine plus tenofovir, or lamivudine plus tenofovir as recommended dual NRTI/NtRTI backbones for HIV/HBV coinfected pregnant women. Hepatitis B flare may occur if tenofovir is discontinued postpartum.

Regardless of CD4 count or HIV RNA copy number, all HIV-infected pregnant women should receive a combination antepartum antiretroviral (ARV) drug regimen; this includes women who require therapy for their own health, as well as women who do not yet require therapy for their own health. ARV therapy should be started as soon as possible if required for the woman's health. Although earlier initiation may be more effective in reducing the perinatal transmission of HIV), also consider maternal conditions (eg, nausea and vomiting) and the potential risks of first trimester fetal exposure for specific agents. Plasma HIV RNA levels should be assessed at ~34-36 weeks gestation in order to help determine mode of delivery. If ARV therapy must be interrupted for <24 hours during the peripartum period, stop then restart all medications simultaneously in order to decrease the chance of developing resistance. Long-term follow-up is recommended for all infants exposed to ARV medications.

Healthcare providers are encouraged to enroll pregnant women exposed to antiretroviral medications in the Antiretroviral Pregnancy Registry (1-800-258-4263 or www.APRegistry.com). Healthcare providers caring for HIV-infected women and their infants may contact the National Perinatal HIV Hotline (888-448-8765) for clinical consultation (DHHS [perinatal], 2012).

Breast-Feeding Considerations Maternal or infant antiretroviral therapy does not completely eliminate the risk of postnatal HIV transmission. In addition, multiclass-resistant virus has been detected in breast-feeding infants despite maternal therapy. Therefore, in the United States, where formula is accessible, affordable, safe, and sustainable, and the risk of infant mortality due to diarrhea and respiratory infections is low, complete avoidance of breast-feeding by HIV-infected women is recommended to decrease potential transmission of HIV (DHHS [perinatal], 2012).

Contraindications

U.S. labeling: There are no contraindications listed in the manufacturer's labeling.

Canadian labeling: Hypersensitivity to tenofovir or any component of the formulation; concurrent use with fixed-dose combination products that contain tenofovir (Truvada, Atripla, Complera, or Stribild); concurrent use with adefovir (Hepsera)

Warnings/Precautions [U.S Boxed Warning]: Lactic acidosis and severe hepatomegaly with steatosis have been reported with tenofovir and other nucleoside analogues, including fatal cases; use with caution in patients with risk factors for liver disease (risk may be increased in obese patients or prolonged exposure) and suspend treatment in any patient who develops clinical or laboratory findings suggestive of lactic acidosis (transaminase elevation may/may not accompany hepatomegaly and steatosis). May cause redistribution of fat (eg, buffalo hump, peripheral wasting with increased abdominal girth, cushingoid appearance). Immune reconstitution syndrome may develop resulting in the occurrence of an inflammatory response to an indolent or residual opportunistic infection during initial HIV treatment or activation of autoimmune disorders (eg, Graves' disease, polymyositis, Guillain-Barré syndrome) later in therapy; further evaluation and treatment may be required. Use caution in hepatic impairment; limited data supporting treatment of chronic hepatitis B in patients with decompensated liver disease; observe for increased adverse reactions, including renal dysfunction.

In clinical trials, use has been associated with decreases in bone mineral density in HIV-1 infected adults and increases in bone metabolism markers. Serum parathyroid hormone and 1,25 vitamin D levels were also higher. Decreases in bone mineral density have also been observed in clinical trials of HIV-1 infected pediatric patients. Observations in chronic hepatitis B infected pediatric patients (aged 12-18 years) were similar. Consider monitoring of bone density in adult and pediatric patients with a history of pathologic fractures or with other risk factors for bone loss or osteoporosis. Consider calcium and vitamin D supplementation for all patients; effect of supplementation has not been studied but may be beneficial. Long-term bone health and fracture risk unknown. Skeletal growth (height) appears to be unaffected in tenofovir-treated children and adolescents.

May cause osteomalacia with proximal renal tubulopathy. Bone pain, extremity pain, fractures, arthralgias, weakness and muscle pain have been reported. In patients at risk for renal dysfunction, persistent or worsening bone or muscle symptoms should be evaluated for hypophosphatemia and osteomalacia.

Do not use as monotherapy in treatment of HIV. Clinical trials in HIV-infected patients whose regimens contained only three nucleoside reverse transcriptase inhibitors (NRTI) show less efficacy, early virologic failure and high rates of resistance substitutions. Use three NRTI regimens with caution and monitor response carefully. Triple drug regimens with two NRTIs in combination with a non-nucleoside reverse transcriptase inhibitor or a HIV-1 protease inhibitor are usually more effective. Treatment of HIV in patients with unrecognized/untreated hepatitis B virus (HBV) may lead to rapid HBV resistance. Patients should be tested for presence of chronic hepatitis B infection prior to initiation of therapy. In patients coinfected with HIV and HBV, an appropriate antiretroviral combination should be selected due to HIV resistance potential; these patients should receive tenofovir dosed for HIV therapy.

Tenofovir is predominately eliminated renally; use caution in renal impairment. May cause acute renal failure or Fanconi syndrome; use caution with other nephrotoxic agents (including high dose or multiple NSAID use or those which compete for active tubular secretion). Acute renal failure has occurred in HIV-infected patients with risk factors for renal impairment who were on a stable tenofovir regimen to which a high dose or multiple NSAID therapy was added. Consider alternatives to NSAIDS in patients taking tenofovir and at risk for renal impairment. Calculate creatinine clearance prior to initiation of therapy and monitor renal function (including recalculation of creatinine clearance and serum phosphorus) during therapy. Dosage adjustment required in patients with Cl_{cr} <50 mL/minute. Use caution in patients with low body weight, or concurrent medications which increase tenofovir levels. Use caution in the elderly; dosage adjustment based on renal function may be required.

[U.S. Boxed Warning]: If treating HBV, acute exacerbation of hepatitis B may occur upon discontinuation. Monitor liver function closely for several months after discontinuing treatment; reinitiation of antihepatitis B therapy may be required. Treatment of HBV in patients with unrecognized/untreated HIV may lead to HIV resistance; patients should be tested for presence of HIV infection prior to initiating therapy. Do not use as monotherapy in treatment of HIV. Treatment of HIV in patients with unrecognized/untreated HBV may lead to rapid HBV resistance. Patients should be tested for presence of chronic hepatitis B prior to initiation of therapy. Potentially significant drug-drug interactions may exist, requiring dose or frequency adjustment, additional monitoring, and/or selection of alternative therapy. Do not use concurrently with adefovir or tenofovir combination products.

Adverse Reactions Frequencies listed are treatment-emergent adverse effects noted at higher frequency than in the placebo group or comparator group. Only adverse events from treatment-naive studies which varied significantly were noted (eg, rash event). Patients treated for chronic hepatitis B had similar reactions and frequencies.

>10%:

- Central nervous system: Insomnia (3% to 4%; decompensated liver disease 18%), pain (7% to 13%), dizziness (3%; treatment naïve 8%; decompensated liver disease 13%), depression (4% to 8%; treatment naïve 9% to 11%), fever (2% to 4%; treatment naïve 8%; decompensated liver disease 11%)
- Dermatologic: Rash event (includes maculopapular, pustular, or vesiculobullous rash, pruritus or urticaria 5% to 7%; treatment naïve 18%)
- Endocrine & metabolic: Triglycerides increased (grades 3/4: 11%; treatment naïve 4%)
- Gastrointestinal: Abdominal pain (4% to 7%; decompensated liver disease 22%), nausea (8% to 11%; decompensated liver disease 20%), diarrhea (11% to 16%), vomiting (4% to 7%; decompensated liver disease 13%)
- Neuromuscular & skeletal: Creatine kinase increased (9% to 12%), weakness (7% to 11%)

1% to 10%:

- Cardiovascular: Chest pain (3%)
- Central nervous system: Fatigue (9%), headache (5% to 8%), anxiety (6%)
- Endocrine & metabolic: Hyperglycemia (grades 3/4: 3%)
- Gastrointestinal: Serum amylase increased (grades 3/4: 4% to 7%; treatment naïve 8% to 9%), anorexia (3% to 4%), dyspepsia (3% to 4%), flatulence (3% to 4%), weight loss (2% to 4%)
- Genitourinary: Hematuria (grades 3/4: 3% to 7%)
- Hematologic: Neutropenia (1% to 3%)
- Hepatic: Transaminases increased (2% to 5%), alkaline phosphatase increased (1%)
- Neuromuscular & skeletal: Back pain (3% to 4%; treatment naive 9%), peripheral neuropathy (3% to 5%), myalgia (3% to 4%)
- Renal: Serum creatinine increased (decompensated liver disease 9%), renal failure (decompensated liver disease 7%), glycosuria (grades 3/4: 3%)
- Respiratory: Upper respiratory tract infection (8%), sinusitis (8%), nasopharyngitis (5%), pneumonia (2% to 3%; treatment naive 5%)
- Miscellaneous: Diaphoresis (3%)

Postmarketing and/or case reports: Acute tubular necrosis, allergic reaction, angioedema, bone mineral density decreased, dyspnea, Fanconi syndrome, hepatic steatosis, hepatitis, hypokalemia, hypophosphatemia, immune reconstitution syndrome, interstitial nephritis, lactic acidosis, muscle weakness, myopathy, nephrogenic diabetes insipidus, nephrotoxicity, osteomalacia, pancreatitis, polyuria, proteinuria, proximal renal tubulopathy, renal insufficiency, renal myopathy, rhabdomyolysis

Drug Interactions

Metabolism/Transport Effects **Inhibits** CYP1A2 (weak); **Induces** P-glycoprotein

Avoid Concomitant Use

Avoid concomitant use of Tenofovir with any of the following: Adefovir; Dabigatran Etexilate; Didanosine; Pomalidomide; VinCRIStine (Liposomal)

Increased Effect/Toxicity

Tenofovir may increase the levels/effects of: Adefovir; Aminoglycosides; Darunavir; Didanosine; Ganciclovir-Valganciclovir

The levels/effects of Tenofovir may be increased by: Acyclovir-Valacyclovir; Adefovir; Aminoglycosides; Atazanavir; Cidofovir; Darunavir; Diclofenac (Systemic); Ganciclovir-Valganciclovir; Lopinavir; Nonsteroidal Anti-Inflammatory Agents; Simeprevir; Telaprevir

Decreased Effect

Tenofovir may decrease the levels/effects of: Afatinib; Atazanavir; Dabigatran Etexilate; Didanosine; Linagliptin; P-glycoprotein/ABCB1 Substrates; Pomalidomide; Simeprevir; Tipranavir; VinCRIStine (Liposomal)

The levels/effects of Tenofovir may be decreased by: Adefovir; Tipranavir

Ethanol/Nutrition/Herb Interactions Food: Fatty meals may increase the bioavailability of tenofovir. Tenofovir may be taken with or without food.

Storage/Stability Store at 25°C (77°F); excursions are permitted between 15°C and 30°C (59°F and 86°F). Dispense only in original container.

Mechanism of Action Tenofovir disoproxil fumarate (TDF), a nucleotide reverse transcriptase inhibitor, is an analog of adenosine 5'-monophosphate; it interferes with the HIV viral RNA dependent DNA polymerase resulting in inhibition of viral replication. TDF is first converted intracellularly by hydrolysis to tenofovir and subsequently phosphorylated to the active tenofovir diphosphate. Tenofovir inhibits replication of HBV by inhibiting HBV polymerase.

Pharmacodynamics/Kinetics

- Distribution: V_d: 1.2-1.3 L/kg
- Protein binding: <7% to serum proteins
- Metabolism: Tenofovir disoproxil fumarate (TDF) is converted intracellularly by hydrolysis (by non-CYP enzymes) to tenofovir, then phosphorylated to the active tenofovir diphosphate
- Bioavailability: ~25% (fasting); increases ~40% with high-fat meal
- Half-life elimination: ~17 hours
- Time to peak, serum: Fasting: 36-84 minutes; With high-fat meal: 96-144 minutes
- Excretion: Urine (70% to 80%) via filtration and active secretion, primarily as unchanged tenofovir

Dosage Oral: **Note:** Concurrent use with adefovir and/or tenofovir combination products should be avoided.

Children 2 to <12 years: HIV infection: 8 mg/kg once daily (maximum: 300 mg once daily) (in combination with other antiretrovirals)

Dosing recommendations based on body weight if using the **oral powder**: **Note:** One level scoop of powder = 40 mg tenofovir

10 to <12 kg: 80 mg once daily
12 to <14 kg: 100 mg once daily
14 to <17 kg: 120 mg once daily
17 to <19 kg: 140 mg once daily
19 to <22 kg: 160 mg once daily
22 to <24 kg: 180 mg once daily
24 to <27 kg: 200 mg once daily
27 to <29 kg: 220 mg once daily
29 to <32 kg: 240 mg once daily
32 to <34 kg: 260 mg once daily
34 to <35 kg: 280 mg once daily
≥35 kg: 300 mg once daily

Dosing recommendations based on body weight if using the **oral tablets**:

17 to <22 kg: 150 mg once daily
22 to <28 kg: 200 mg once daily
28 to <35 kg: 250 mg once daily
≥35 kg: 300 mg once daily

Children ≥12 years (and ≥35 kg), Adolescents, and Adults:

Hepatitis B infection: 300 mg once daily; **Note:** Tenofovir is recommended for first-line treatment of HBV (Lok, 2009)

Treatment duration (AASLD practice guidelines, 2009):

Note: Patients not achieving <2 log decrease in serum HBV DNA after at least 6 months of therapy should either receive additional treatment or be switched to an alternative therapy (Lok, 2009).

Hepatitis Be antigen (HBeAg) positive chronic hepatitis: Treat ≥1 year until HBeAg seroconversion and undetectable serum HBV DNA; continue therapy for ≥6 months after HBeAg seroconversion

HBeAg negative chronic hepatitis: Treat >1 year until hepatitis B surface antigen (HBsAg) clearance

Decompensated liver disease: Lifelong treatment is recommended

HIV infection: 300 mg once daily (in combination with other antiretrovirals)

Dosage adjustment in renal impairment:

Children: No dosage adjustment provided in manufacturer's labeling (has not been studied).

Adults: **Note:** Use of powder formulation has not been evaluated in renal impairment.

Cl_{cr} ≥50 mL/minute: No dosage adjustment necessary
Cl_{cr} 30-49 mL/minute: 300 mg every 48 hours
Cl_{cr} 10-29 mL/minute: 300 mg every 72-96 hours
Cl_{cr} <10 mL/minute without hemodialysis: No dosage adjustment provided in manufacturer's labeling; has not been studied.

Hemodialysis: 300 mg following dialysis every 7 days or after a total of ~12 hours of dialysis (usually once weekly assuming 3 dialysis sessions lasting about 4 hours each)

Dosage adjustment in hepatic impairment: No dosage adjustment necessary.

Dietary Considerations Consider calcium and vitamin D supplementation.

Administration Tablets may be administered without regard to meals. Powder should be mixed with 2-4 ounces of soft food (applesauce, baby food, yogurt) and swallowed immediately (avoids bitter taste); do not mix in liquid (powder may float on top of the liquid even after stirring). Measure powder using only the supplied dosing scoop.

Monitoring Parameters

Patients with HIV: CBC with differential, reticulocyte count, creatine kinase, CD4 count, HIV RNA plasma levels, serum phosphorus; serum creatinine (prior to initiation and as clinically indicated during therapy), urine glucose and urine protein (in patients at risk for renal impairment or who experienced renal impairment while taking adefovir), hepatic function tests, bone density (patients with a history of bone fracture or have risk factors for bone loss); testing for HBV is recommended prior to the initiation of antiretroviral therapy; weight (children)

Patients with HBV: HIV status (prior to initiation of therapy); serum phosphorus; serum creatinine (prior to initiation and as clinically indicated during therapy), urine glucose and urine protein (in patients at risk for renal impairment or who experienced renal impairment while taking adefovir); bone density (patients with a history of bone fracture or have risk factors for bone loss); HBV DNA (every 3-6 months during therapy); HBeAg and anti-HBe; LFTs every 3 months during therapy and for several months following discontinuation of tenofovir; signs/symptoms of HBV relapse/exacerbation following discontinuation of therapy

Patients with HIV and HBV coinfection should be monitored for several months following tenofovir discontinuation.

Dosage Forms Excipient information presented when available (limited, particularly for generics); consult specific product labeling.

Powder, Oral, as disoproxil fumarate:
Viread: 40 mg/g (60 g)

Tablet, Oral, as disoproxil fumarate:
Viread: 150 mg, 200 mg, 250 mg
Viread: 300 mg [contains fd&c blue #2 aluminum lake]

◆ **Tenofovir and Emtricitabine** *see* Emtricitabine and Tenofovir *on page 700*

◆ **Tenofovir Disoproxil Fumarate** *see* Tenofovir *on page 2012*

◆ **Tenofovir Disoproxil Fumarate, Efavirenz, and Emtricitabine** *see* Efavirenz, Emtricitabine, and Tenofovir *on page 690*

◆ **Tenofovir Disoproxil Fumarate, Rilpivirine, and Emtricitabine** *see* Emtricitabine, Rilpivirine, and Tenofovir *on page 700*

◆ **Tenofovir, Elvitegravir, Cobicistat, and Emtricitabine** *see* Elvitegravir, Cobicistat, Emtricitabine, and Tenofovir *on page 696*

◆ **Tenofovir, Emtricitabine, and Rilpivirine** *see* Emtricitabine, Rilpivirine, and Tenofovir *on page 700*

◆ **Tenormin** *see* Atenolol *on page 186*

◆ **Tenormin® (Can)** *see* Atenolol *on page 186*

◆ **Tensilon® (Can)** *see* Edrophonium *on page 686*

◆ **Tenuate** *see* Diethylpropion *on page 604*

◆ **Tenuate Dospan** *see* Diethylpropion *on page 604*

◆ **Terazol (Can)** *see* Terconazole *on page 2021*

◆ **Terazol 3** *see* Terconazole *on page 2021*

◆ **Terazol 7** *see* Terconazole *on page 2021*

Terazosin (ter AY zoe sin)

Brand Names: Canada Apo-Terazosin®; Dom-Terazosin; Hytrin®; Nu-Terazosin; PHL-Terazosin; PMS-Terazosin; ratio-Terazosin; Teva-Terazosin

Index Terms Hytrin

Pharmacologic Category $Alpha_1$ Blocker; Antihypertensive

Additional Appendix Information

Beers Criteria – Potentially Inappropriate Medications for Geriatrics *on page 2368*

Use Management of mild-to-moderate hypertension; alone or in combination with other agents such as diuretics or beta-blockers; benign prostate hyperplasia (BPH)

Unlabeled Use Pediatric hypertension

Pregnancy Risk Factor C

Pregnancy Considerations Teratogenic effects have not been observed in animal studies. Decreased fetal weight and increased risk of fetal mortality were noted in some animal reproduction studies. There are no adequate and well-controlled studies in pregnant women. Use only if benefit outweighs risk.

Breast-Feeding Considerations It is not known if terazosin is excreted in breast milk. The manufacturer recommends that caution be exercised when administering terazosin to nursing women.

Contraindications Hypersensitivity to terazosin or any component of the formulation

Warnings/Precautions Can cause significant orthostatic hypotension and syncope, especially with first dose; anticipate a similar effect if therapy is interrupted for a few days, if dosage is rapidly increased, or if another antihypertensive drug (particularly vasodilators) or a PDE-5 inhibitor is introduced. Discontinue if symptoms of angina occur or worsen. Patients should be cautioned about performing hazardous tasks when starting new therapy or adjusting dosage upward. Prostate cancer should be ruled out before starting for BPH. Intraoperative floppy iris syndrome has been observed in cataract surgery patients who were on or were previously treated with alpha$_1$-blockers. Causality has not been established and there appears to be no benefit in discontinuing alpha-blocker therapy prior to surgery. Priapism has been associated with use (rarely). In the elderly, avoid use as an antihypertensive due to high risk of orthostatic hypotension; alternative agents preferred due to a more favorable risk/benefit profile (Beers Criteria).

Adverse Reactions

>10%:

- Central nervous system: Dizziness (9% to 19%)
- Neuromuscular & skeletal: Muscle weakness (7% to 11%)

1% to 10%:

- Cardiovascular: Peripheral edema (1% to 6%), orthostatic hypotension (1% to 4%), palpitation (≤4%), tachycardia (≤2%), syncope (≤1%
- Central nervous system: Somnolence (4% to 5%), vertigo (1%)
- Gastrointestinal: Nausea (2% to 4%), weight gain (≤1%)
- Genitourinary: Impotence (≤2%), libido decreased (≤1%)
- Neuromuscular & skeletal: Extremity pain (≤4%), paresthesia (≤3%), back pain (≤2%)
- Ocular: Blurred vision (≤2%)
- Respiratory: Nasal congestion (2% to 6%), dyspnea (2% to 3%), sinusitis (≤3%)

<1% (Limited to important or life-threatening): Abdominal pain, abnormal vision, allergic reactions, anaphylaxis, anxiety, arrhythmia, arthralgia, arthritis, atrial fibrillation, bronchitis, chest pain, conjunctivitis, constipation, cough, diaphoresis, diarrhea, dyspepsia, epistaxis, facial edema, fever, flatulence, flu-like syndrome, gout, insomnia, intraoperative floppy iris syndrome (IFIS), joint disorder, myalgia, neck pain, pharyngitis, polyuria, priapism, pruritus, rash, rhinitis, shoulder pain, thrombocytopenia, tinnitus, urinary incontinence, urinary tract infection, vasodilation, vomiting, xerostomia

Drug Interactions

Metabolism/Transport Effects None known.

Avoid Concomitant Use

Avoid concomitant use of Terazosin with any of the following: Alpha1-Blockers

Increased Effect/Toxicity

Terazosin may increase the levels/effects of: Alpha1-Blockers; Amifostine; Antihypertensives; Calcium Channel Blockers; Hypotensive Agents; Obinutuzumab; RiTUXimab

The levels/effects of Terazosin may be increased by: Beta-Blockers; Brimonidine (Topical); Diazoxide; Herbs (Hypotensive Properties); MAO Inhibitors; Pentoxifylline; Phosphodiesterase 5 Inhibitors; Prostacyclin Analogues

Decreased Effect

Terazosin may decrease the levels/effects of: Alpha-/Beta-Agonists; Alpha1-Agonists

The levels/effects of Terazosin may be decreased by: Herbs (Hypertensive Properties); Methylphenidate; Yohimbine

Ethanol/Nutrition/Herb Interactions Herb/Nutraceutical: Avoid dong quai if using for hypertension (has estrogenic activity). Avoid ephedra, yohimbe, ginseng (may worsen hypertension). Avoid saw palmetto. Avoid garlic (may have increased antihypertensive effect).

Storage/Stability Store below 30°C (86°F).

Mechanism of Action Alpha$_1$-specific blocking agent with minimal alpha$_2$ effects; this allows peripheral postsynaptic blockade, with the resultant decrease in arterial tone, while preserving the negative feedback loop which is mediated by the peripheral presynaptic alpha$_2$-receptors; terazosin relaxes the smooth muscle of the bladder neck, thus reducing bladder outlet obstruction

Pharmacodynamics/Kinetics

Onset of action: 1-2 hours

Absorption: Rapid and complete

Protein binding: 90% to 95%

Metabolism: Hepatic; minimal first-pass

Half-life elimination: ~12 hours

Time to peak, serum: ~1 hour

Excretion: Feces (~60%, ~20% as unchanged drug); urine (~40%, ~10% as unchanged drug)

Dosage Oral: **Note:** If drug is discontinued for greater than several days, consider beginning with initial dose and retitrate as needed.

Hypertension:

- Children (unlabeled use): Initial: 1 mg once daily; gradually increase dose as necessary, up to maximum of 20 mg/day
- Adults: Initial: 1 mg at bedtime; slowly increase dose to achieve desired blood pressure, up to 20 mg/day; usual dose range (JNC 7): 1-20 mg once daily. **Note:** Dosage may be given on a twice daily regimen if response is diminished at 24 hours and hypotension is observed at 2-4 hours following a dose.
- Elderly: Consider lower initial doses (eg, immediate release: 0.5 mg once daily) and titrate to response (Aronow, 2011)

Benign prostatic hyperplasia: Adults: Initial: 1 mg at bedtime; thereafter, titrate upwards, if needed, over several weeks, balancing therapeutic benefit with terazosin-induced postural hypotension; most patients require 10 mg day; if no response after 4-6 weeks of 10 mg/day, may increase to 20 mg/day

Dosage adjustment with concurrent medication:

Concurrent use with a diuretic or other antihypertensive agent (especially verapamil): Dosage reduction may be needed when adding

Concurrent use with PDE-5 inhibitors: Initiate PDE-5 inhibitor therapy at the lowest dose due to additive orthostatic and blood pressure lowering effects

Dosage adjustment in renal impairment: No dosage adjustment necessary.

Hemodialysis: No supplemental dose necessary.

Dosage adjustment in hepatic impairment: No dosage adjustment provided in manufacturer's labeling.

Dietary Considerations May be taken without regard to meals at the same time each day.

Administration Administer without regard to meals at the same time each day.

Monitoring Parameters Standing and sitting/supine blood pressure, especially following the initial dose at 2-4 hours following the dose and thereafter at the trough point to ensure adequate control throughout the dosing interval; urinary symptoms

Dosage Forms Excipient information presented when available (limited, particularly for generics); consult specific product labeling.

Capsule, Oral:

Generic: 1 mg, 2 mg, 5 mg, 10 mg

Dosage Forms: Canada Excipient information presented when available (limited, particularly for generics); consult specific product labeling.

Tablet, Oral: 1 mg, 2 mg, 5 mg, 10 mg

Terbinafine (Systemic) (TER bin a feen)

Brand Names: U.S. LamISIL; Terbinex

Brand Names: Canada Apo-Terbinafine; Auro-Terbinafine; CO Terbinafine; Dom-Terbinafine; GD-Terbinafine; JAMP-Terbinafine; Lamisil; Mylan-Terbinafine; PHL-Terbinafine; PMS-Terbinafine; Q-Terbinafine; Riva-Terbinafine; Sandoz-Terbinafine; Teva-Terbinafine

Index Terms Terbinafine Hydrochloride

Pharmacologic Category Antifungal Agent, Oral

Additional Appendix Information

Antifungal Agents *on page 2286*

Use

Onychomycosis (tablets only): Treatment of onychomycosis of the toenail or fingernail caused by dermatophytes (tinea unguium).

Tinea capitis (granules only): Treatment of tinea capitis in patients 4 years and older.

Canadian labeling: Additional use (not in U.S. labeling): Severe tineal skin infections (tinea cruris and tinea pedis) unresponsive to topical therapy

Unlabeled Use Sporotrichosis: Treatment of sporotrichosis (lymphocutaneous and cutaneous)

Pregnancy Risk Factor B

Pregnancy Considerations Adverse events were not observed in animal reproduction studies. Avoid use in pregnancy since treatment of onychomycosis is postponable.

Breast-Feeding Considerations Terbinafine is excreted in breast milk; the milk/plasma ratio is 7:1. Breast-feeding is not recommended by the manufacturer.

Contraindications Hypersensitivity to terbinafine or any component of the formulation

Warnings/Precautions Due to potential toxicity, confirmation of diagnostic testing of nail or skin specimens prior to treatment of onychomycosis or dermatomycosis is recommended. Use caution in patients sensitive to allylamine antifungals (eg, naftifine, butenafine); cross sensitivity to terbinafine may exist. Transient decreases in absolute lymphocyte counts were observed in clinical trials; severe neutropenia (reversible upon discontinuation) has also been reported. Monitor CBC in patients with pre-existing immunosuppression if therapy is to continue >6 weeks and discontinue therapy if ANC ≤1000/mm^3.

Serious skin and hypersensitivity reactions (eg, Stevens-Johnson syndrome, toxic epidermal necrolysis, erythema multiforme, exfoliative dermatitis, bullous dermatitis, drug reaction with eosinophilia and systemic symptoms [DRESS] syndrome) have occurred. If progressive skin rash or signs and symptoms of a hypersensitivity reaction occur, discontinue treatment. Cases of hepatic failure, some leading to liver transplant or death, have been reported; not recommended for use in patients with active or chronic liver disease. If clinical evidence of liver injury develops (eg, nausea, anorexia, fatigue, vomiting, right upper abdominal pain, jaundice, dark urine, pale stools), assess hepatic function immediately; discontinue therapy in cases of elevated liver function tests. Use with caution in patients with renal dysfunction (Cl_{cr} ≤50 mL/minute) (per Canadian labeling, not recommended for use); clearance is reduced by ~50%.

Disturbances of taste and/or smell may occur; resolution may be delayed (eg, >1 year) following discontinuation of therapy or in some cases, disturbance may be permanent. Discontinue therapy in patients with symptoms of taste or smell disturbance.

Adverse Reactions Adverse events listed for tablets unless otherwise specified. Granules were studied in patients 4-12 years of age.

>10%: Central nervous system: Headache (13%; granules 7%)

1% to 10%:

Dermatologic: Skin rash (6%; granules 2%), pruritus (3%; granules 1%), urticaria (1%)

Gastrointestinal: Diarrhea (6%; granules 3%), vomiting (<1%; granules 5%), dyspepsia (4%), dysgeusia (may be severe and result in weight loss and depression; 3%), nausea (3%; granules 2%), abdominal pain (2%; granules 2% to 4%), flatulence (2%), sore throat (granules 2%), toothache (granules 1%)

Hepatic: Liver enzyme disorder (3%)

Infection: Influenza (granules 2%)

Ophthalmic: Visual disturbance (1%)

Respiratory: Nasopharyngitis (granules 10%), cough (granules 6%), upper respiratory tract infection (granules 5%), nasal congestion (granules 2%), rhinorrhea (granules 2%)

Miscellaneous: Fever (granules 7%)

<1% (Limited to important or life-threatening): Acute generalized exanthematous pustulosis, acute pancreatitis, agranulocytosis, alopecia, altered sense of smell, anaphylaxis, angioedema, depression, DRESS syndrome, exacerbation of psoriasis, exacerbation of systemic lupus erythematosus, hepatic disease, hepatic failure, hypersensitivity reaction, pancytopenia, rhabdomyolysis, severe neutropenia, Stevens-Johnson syndrome, thrombocytopenia, toxic epidermal necrolysis, vasculitis, visual field loss

Drug Interactions

Metabolism/Transport Effects Substrate of CYP1A2 (minor), CYP2C19 (minor), CYP2C9 (minor), CYP3A4 (minor); **Note:** Assignment of Major/Minor substrate status based on clinically relevant drug interaction potential; **Inhibits** CYP2D6 (strong); **Induces** CYP3A4 (weak/moderate)

Avoid Concomitant Use

Avoid concomitant use of Terbinafine (Systemic) with any of the following: Axitinib; Pimozide; Simeprevir; Tamoxifen; Thioridazine

Increased Effect/Toxicity

Terbinafine (Systemic) may increase the levels/effects of: ARIPiprazole; AtoMOXetine; CYP2D6 Substrates; Fesoterodine; Iloperidone; Metoprolol; Nebivolol; Pimozide; Propafenone; Tetrabenazine; Thioridazine; Tricyclic Antidepressants; Vortioxetine

Decreased Effect

Terbinafine (Systemic) may decrease the levels/effects of: Axitinib; Codeine; Ibrutinib; Iloperidone; Saccharomyces boulardii; Saxagliptin; Simeprevir; Tamoxifen; TraMADol

The levels/effects of Terbinafine (Systemic) may be decreased by: Rifampin

Storage/Stability

Granules: Store at 25°C (77°F); excursions permitted between 15°C to 30°C (59°F to 86°F).

Tablet: Store below 25°C (77°F). Protect from light.

Mechanism of Action Synthetic allylamine derivative which inhibits squalene epoxidase, a key enzyme in sterol biosynthesis in fungi. This results in a deficiency in ergosterol within the fungal cell wall and results in fungal cell death.

Pharmacodynamics/Kinetics

Absorption: >70%

Distribution: Distributed to sebum and skin predominantly

Protein binding: Plasma: >99%

Metabolism: Hepatic predominantly via CYP1A2, 3A4, 2C8, 2C9, and 2C19 to inactive metabolites

Bioavailability: ~40%; Children 36% to 64%

Half-life elimination: Terminal half-life: 200-400 hours; very slow release of drug from skin and adipose tissues occurs; effective half-life: ~36 hours; Children: 27-31 hours

Time to peak, plasma: Within 2 hours

Excretion: Urine (~70%)

Dosage Oral:

Children ≥4 years, Adolescents, and Adults: Granules: Tinea capitis:

<25 kg: 125 mg once daily for 6 weeks

25-35 kg: 187.5 mg once daily for 6 weeks

>35 kg: 250 mg once daily for 6 weeks

Children and Adolescents: Tablet: Onychomycosis (unlabeled use; Gupta, 1997):

10-20 kg: 62.5 mg once daily for 6 weeks (fingernails) **or** 12 weeks (toenails)

20-40 kg: 125 mg once daily for 6 weeks (fingernails) **or** 12 weeks (toenails)

>40 kg: 250 mg once daily for 6 weeks (fingernails) **or** 12 weeks (toenails)

Adults:

Tablet:

U.S. labeling: Onychomycosis: Fingernail: 250 mg once daily for 6 weeks; Toenail: 250 mg once daily for 12 weeks

Missed doses: If a dose is missed, take as soon as remembered, unless it is less than 4 hours before the next dose is due.

Canadian labeling: **Note:** Mycologic cure may precede complete resolution of symptoms by several weeks (skin infections) or by several months (onychomycosis).

Onychomycosis (finger or toenail): 250 mg/day in 1-2 divided doses for 6 weeks to 3 months (≥6 months may be necessary in some patients with infections of the big toenail)

Tinea corporis, tinea cruris: 250 mg/day in 1-2 divided doses for 2-4 weeks

Tinea pedis (interdigital and plantar/moccasin type): 250 mg/day in 1-2 divided doses for 2-6 weeks

Sporotrichosis, lymphocutaneous and cutaneous (unlabeled use): 500 mg twice daily as alternative therapy; treat for 2-4 weeks after resolution of all lesions (usual duration: 3-6 months) (Kauffman, 2007)

Elderly: Use with caution; refer to adult dosing.

Dosing adjustment in renal impairment:

U.S. labeling: No dosage adjustment provided in manufacturer's labeling (has not been studied); however, clearance is decreased 50% in patients with Cl_{cr} ≤50 mL/minute.

Canadian labeling: Use is not recommended in patients with Cl_{cr} ≤50 mL/minute.

Dosing adjustment in hepatic impairment: Use is not recommended in chronic or active hepatic disease.

Administration Administer tablets without regard to meals. Administer granules with food; sprinkle granules on a spoonful of pudding or other soft, nonacidic food (eg, mashed potatoes); swallow entire spoonful without chewing; do not mix granules with applesauce or other fruit-based foods.

Monitoring Parameters AST/ALT prior to initiation, repeat if used >6 weeks; CBC; taste and/or smell disturbances

Dosage Forms Excipient information presented when available (limited, particularly for generics); consult specific product labeling.

Cream, External, as hydrochloride:

LamISIL AT: 1% (12 g) [contains benzyl alcohol, cetyl alcohol]

Kit, Combination:

Terbinex: 250 MG & 1%

Packet, Oral:

LamISIL: 125 mg (1 ea, 14 ea); 187.5 mg (1 ea, 14 ea) [contains polyethylene glycol]

Tablet, Oral:

LamISIL: 250 mg

Generic: 250 mg

Dosage Forms: Canada Excipient information presented when available (limited, particularly for generics); consult specific product labeling.

Tablet, oral:

LamISIL: 125 mg [contains lactose]

Extemporaneous Preparations A 25 mg/mL oral suspension may be made using tablets. Crush twenty 250 mg tablets and reduce to a fine powder. Add small amount of a 1:1 mixture of Ora-Sweet® and Ora-Plus® and mix to a uniform paste; mix while adding the vehicle in geometric proportions to **almost** 200 mL; transfer to a calibrated bottle, rinse mortar with vehicle, and add quantity of vehicle sufficient to make 200 mL. Label "shake well" and "refrigerate". Stable 42 days.

Nahata MC, Pai VB, and Hipple TF, *Pediatric Drug Formulations*, 5th ed, Cincinnati, OH: Harvey Whitney Books Co, 2004.

Terbinafine (Topical) (TER bin a feen)

Brand Names: U.S. LamISIL Advanced [OTC]; LamISIL AT Jock Itch [OTC]; LamISIL AT Spray [OTC]; LamISIL AT [OTC]

Brand Names: Canada Lamisil®

Index Terms Terbinafine Hydrochloride

Pharmacologic Category Antifungal Agent, Topical

Use Antifungal for the treatment of tinea pedis (athlete's foot), tinea cruris (jock itch), and tinea corporis (ringworm) [OTC/Canadian prescription formulations]; cutaneous candidiasis and tinea versicolor [Canadian prescription formulations]

Dosage Topical:

Children ≥12 years and Adolescents:

Tinea pedis:

Cream: Apply between the toes to affected area twice daily for at least 1 week [OTC formulations]; apply on the bottom or sides of feet twice daily for 2 weeks [OTC formulations]

Gel: Apply to affected area once daily for at least 1 week [OTC formulations]

Solution: Apply to affected area once daily for at least 1 week [OTC formulations]

Tinea corporis, Tinea cruris:

Cream: Apply to affected area once daily for 1 week [OTC formulations]

Gel: Apply to affected area once daily for 1 week [OTC formulations]

Solution: Apply to affected area once daily for 1 week [OTC formulations]

Adults:

Tinea pedis:

Cream: Apply between the toes to affected area once or twice daily for at least 1 week [OTC/Canadian prescription formulations]; apply on the bottom or sides of feet twice daily for 2 weeks [OTC formulations]

Gel: Apply to affected area once daily for at least 1 week [OTC formulations]

Solution: Apply to affected area once daily for at least 1 week [OTC/Canadian prescription formulations]

Tinea corporis, Tinea cruris:

Cream: Apply to affected area once daily for 1 week [OTC/Canadian prescription formulations]

Gel: Apply to affected area once daily for 1 week [OTC formulations]

Solution: Apply to affected area once daily for 1 week [OTC/Canadian prescription formulations]

Cutaneous candidiasis: Apply to affected area once or twice daily for 1-2 weeks [Canadian prescription formulation]

Tinea versicolor:

Cream: Apply to affected area once or twice daily for 1-2 weeks [Canadian prescription formulation]

Solution: Apply to affected area twice daily for 1 week [Canadian prescription formulation]

Additional Information Complete prescribing information should be consulted for additional detail.

Dosage Forms Excipient information presented when available (limited, particularly for generics); consult specific product labeling.

Cream, External, as hydrochloride:

LamISIL AT: 1% (12 g, 24 g, 30 g, 36 g, 42 g) [contains benzyl alcohol, cetyl alcohol]

LamISIL AT Jock Itch: 1% (12 g) [contains benzyl alcohol, cetyl alcohol]

Generic: 1% (12 g, 15 g, 24 g, 30 g)

Gel, External:

LamISIL Advanced: 1% (12 g) [contains alcohol, usp]

Solution, External, as hydrochloride:

LamISIL AT Spray: 1% (30 mL, 125 mL) [contains alcohol, usp, propylene glycol]

LamISIL Spray: 1% (30 mL) [contains alcohol, usp]

Dosage Forms: Canada Excipient information presented when available (limited, particularly for generics); consult specific product labeling.

Cream, topical, as hydrochloride: 1% (12 g, 24 g)

Lamisil®: 1% (15 g, 30 g)

Solution, topical, as hydrochloride [spray]:

Lamisil®: 1% (30 mL)

◆ **Terbinafine Hydrochloride** *see* Terbinafine (Systemic) *on page 2017*

◆ **Terbinafine Hydrochloride** *see* Terbinafine (Topical) *on page 2018*

◆ **Terbinex** *see* Terbinafine (Systemic) *on page 2017*

Terbutaline (ter BYOO ta leen)

Brand Names: Canada Bricanyl® Turbuhaler®

Index Terms Brethaire; Brethine; Bricanyl; Terbutaline Sulfate

Pharmacologic Category Antidote, Extravasation; Beta$_2$ Agonist

Use Bronchodilator in reversible airway obstruction and bronchial asthma

Unlabeled Use Injection: Tocolytic agent (short-term [≤72 hours]) prevention or management of preterm labor; management of extravasation of sympathomimetic vasoconstrictors (based on limited case reports)

Pregnancy Risk Factor C

Pregnancy Considerations Adverse events have been observed in animal reproduction studies. Terbutaline crosses the placenta; umbilical cord concentrations are ~11% to 48% of maternal blood levels.

Uncontrolled asthma is associated with adverse events on pregnancy (increased risk of perinatal mortality, preeclampsia, preterm birth, low birth weight infants). Terbutaline is not recommended for the treatment of asthma during pregnancy; inhaled beta$_2$-receptor agonists are preferred (NAEPP, 2005).

[U.S. Boxed Warning]: Terbutaline is not FDA approved for and should not be used for prolonged tocolysis (>48-72 hours). Use for maintenance tocolysis should not be done in the outpatient setting. Adverse events observed in pregnant women include arrhythmias, increased heart rate, hyperglycemia (transient), hypokalemia, myocardial ischemia, and pulmonary edema. Heart rate may be increased in the fetus and hypoglycemia may occur in the neonate. Terbutaline has been used in the management of preterm labor. Tocolytics may be used for the short-term (48 hour) prolongation of pregnancy to allow for the administration of antenatal steroids and should not be used prior to fetal viability or when the risks of use to the fetus or mother are greater than the risk of preterm birth (ACOG, 2012).

Breast-Feeding Considerations Terbutaline is excreted in breast milk; concentrations are similar to or higher than those in the maternal plasma. Based on information from four cases, exposure to the breast-fed infant would be <1% of the weight-adjusted maternal dose. Adverse events were not observed in nursing infants (Boréus, 1982; Lönnerholm, 1982). The manufacturer recommends that terbutaline be used in breast-feeding women only if the potential benefit to the mother outweighs the possible risk to the infant. The use of beta$_2$-receptor agonists are not considered a contraindication to breast-feeding (NAEPP, 2005).

Contraindications

Hypersensitivity to terbutaline, sympathomimetic amines, or any component of the formulation

Injection: Additional contraindications: Prolonged (>72 hours) prevention or management of preterm labor

Oral: Additional contraindications: Prevention or treatment of preterm labor

Warnings/Precautions [U.S. Boxed Warning]: Terbutaline is not FDA approved for and should not be used for prolonged tocolysis (>48-72 hours). Use for maintenance tocolysis should not be done in the outpatient setting. Adverse events observed in pregnant women include arrhythmias, increased heart rate, hyperglycemia (transient), hypokalemia, myocardial ischemia, and pulmonary edema. Heart rate may be increased in the fetus and hypoglycemia may occur in the neonate. Oral terbutaline is contraindicated for acute or chronic use in the management of preterm labor.

Use caution in patients with cardiovascular disease (arrhythmia or hypertension or HF), convulsive disorders, diabetes, glaucoma, hyperthyroidism, or hypokalemia. Beta-agonists may cause elevation in blood pressure, heart rate, and result in CNS stimulation/excitation. Beta$_2$-agonists may increase risk of arrhythmia, increase serum glucose, or decrease serum potassium.

When used as a bronchodilator, optimize anti-inflammatory treatment before initiating maintenance treatment with terbutaline. Do not use as a component of chronic therapy without an anti-inflammatory agent. Only the mildest form of asthma (Step 1 and/or exercise-induced) would not require concurrent use based upon asthma guidelines. Patient must be instructed to seek medical attention in cases where acute symptoms are not relieved or a previous level of response is diminished. The need to increase frequency of use may indicate deterioration of asthma, and treatment must not be delayed.

Immediate hypersensitivity reactions (urticaria, angioedema, rash, bronchospasm) have been reported. Do not exceed recommended dose; serious adverse events including fatalities, have been associated with excessive use of inhaled sympathomimetics. Rarely, paradoxical bronchospasm may occur with use of inhaled bronchodilating agents; this should be distinguished from inadequate response.

Adverse Reactions

>10%:

Central nervous system: Nervousness, restlessness

Endocrine & metabolic: Serum glucose increased, serum potassium decreased

Neuromuscular & skeletal: Trembling

1% to 10%:

Cardiovascular: Tachycardia, hypertension, pounding heartbeat

Central nervous system: Dizziness, lightheadedness, drowsiness, headache, insomnia

Gastrointestinal: Dry mouth, nausea, vomiting, bad taste in mouth

Neuromuscular & skeletal: Muscle cramps, weakness

Miscellaneous: Diaphoresis

<1% (Limited to important or life-threatening): Arrhythmia, cardiac arrest (preterm labor), chest pain, hyperglycemia (preterm labor), hypokalemia (preterm labor), hypotension (preterm labor), paradoxical bronchospasm, myocardial infarction (preterm labor), myocardial ischemia (preterm labor), pulmonary edema (preterm labor)

Drug Interactions

Metabolism/Transport Effects None known.

Avoid Concomitant Use

Avoid concomitant use of Terbutaline with any of the following: Beta-Blockers (Nonselective); Iobenguane I 123

Increased Effect/Toxicity

Terbutaline may increase the levels/effects of: Atosiban; Loop Diuretics; Sympathomimetics; Thiazide Diuretics

The levels/effects of Terbutaline may be increased by: AtoMOXetine; Cannabinoids; MAO Inhibitors; Tricyclic Antidepressants

Decreased Effect

Terbutaline may decrease the levels/effects of: Iobenguane I 123

The levels/effects of Terbutaline may be decreased by: Beta-Blockers (Beta1 Selective); Beta-Blockers (Nonselective); Betahistine

Ethanol/Nutrition/Herb Interactions Herb/Nutraceutical: Avoid ephedra, yohimbe (may cause CNS stimulation).

Preparation for Administration For extravasation management (unlabeled use): Using vial for injection, dilute 1 mg with 9 mL (total volume: 10 mL) (large extravasation site) **or** 1 mg with 1 mL (total volume: 2 mL) (small/distal extravasation site) of 0.9% sodium chloride (Stier, 1999).

Storage/Stability Store injection at room temperature; do not freeze. Protect from heat and light. Use only clear solutions. Store powder for inhalation (Bricanyl® Turbuhaler [Canadian availability]) at room temperature between 15°C and 30°C (58°F and 86°F).

Mechanism of Action Relaxes bronchial and uterine smooth muscle by action on beta$_2$-receptors with less effect on heart rate

Pharmacodynamics/Kinetics

Onset of action: Oral: 30-45 minutes; SubQ: 6-15 minute; Inhalation: 5 minutes (maximum effect: 15-60 minutes)

Duration: Inhalation: 4-7 hours

Protein binding: 25%

Metabolism: Hepatic to inactive sulfate conjugates

Bioavailability: SubQ doses are more bioavailable than oral

Half-life elimination: 11-16 hours

Excretion: Urine

Dosage

Children <12 years: Bronchoconstriction:

Oral: Initial: 0.05 mg/kg/dose 3 times/day, increased gradually as required; maximum: 0.15 mg/kg/dose 3-4 times/day or a total of 5 mg/24 hours

SubQ: 0.005-0.01 mg/kg/dose to a maximum of 0.4 mg/dose every 15-20 minutes for 3 doses; may repeat every 2-6 hours as needed

Children ≥6 years and Adults: Bronchospasm (acute): Inhalation: Bricanyl® Turbuhaler®: (Canadian labeling; not available in U.S.): One puff as needed; may repeat with 1 inhalation (after 5 minutes); more than 6 inhalations should not be necessary in any 24-hour period. **Note:** If adequate relief is not obtained with previously effective dose, or if effects of inhalation last <3 hours, patient should be reassessed; may indicate worsening asthma.

Children >12 years and Adults: Bronchoconstriction:

Oral:

12-15 years: 2.5 mg every 6 hours 3 times/day; not to exceed 7.5 mg in 24 hours

>15 years: 5 mg/dose every 6 hours 3 times/day; if side effects occur, reduce dose to 2.5 mg every 6 hours; not to exceed 15 mg in 24 hours

SubQ:

Manufacturer's labeling: 0.25 mg/dose; may repeat in 15-30 minutes (maximum: 0.5 mg/4-hour period)

Unlabeled dose: 0.25 mg/dose; may repeat every 20 minutes for 3 doses (maximum: 0.75 mg/1-hour period) (NIH Guidelines, 2007)

Adults: Premature labor (acute; short-term [≤72 hours] tocolysis; unlabeled use):

I.V.: 2.5-5 mcg/minute; increased gradually every 20-30 minutes by 2.5-5 mcg/minute; effective maximum dosages from 17.5-30 mcg/minute have been used with caution. Duration of infusion is at least 12 hours (Travis, 1993).

SubQ: 0.25 mg every 20 minutes to 3 hours; hold for pulse >120 beats per minute. Terbutaline has not been approved for and should not be used for prolonged tocolysis (beyond 48-72 hours) (ACOG, 2012; Hearne, 2000).

Adults: Extravasation management, sympathomimetic vasoconstrictors (unlabeled use; based on limited case reports): SubQ:

Large extravasations: Infiltrate extravasation area using a solution of 1 mg diluted in 9 mL (total volume: 10 mL) of 0.9% sodium chloride; volume of terbutaline solution administered varied from 3-10 mL (Stier, 1999).

Small/distal extravasations: Infiltrate extravasation area using a solution of 1 mg diluted in 1 mL (total volume: 2 mL) of 0.9% sodium chloride; volume of terbutaline solution administered varied from 0.5-1 mL (Stier, 1999).

Dosage adjustment in renal impairment: No dosage adjustment provided in manufacturer's labeling.

Dosage adjustment in hepatic impairment: No dosage adjustment provided in manufacturer's labeling.

Administration

I.V.: Use infusion pump.

Oral: Administer around-the-clock to promote less variation in peak and trough serum levels

Inhalation: Bricanyl® Turbuhaler® (Canadian availability): After removing lid, patient should hold inhaler upright and turn blue grip as far as it will go in one direction then turn it back to original position. Clicking sound indicates that inhaler is ready for use. Patient should exhale fully but not into the inhaler and then place mouthpiece gently between teeth, close lips around inhaler and inhale deeply. Inhaler should be removed from mouth prior to exhaling. Instruct patients to rinse mouth with water after each inhalation as some medication may stick to the inside of the mouth and throat. If inhaler is dropped or shaken, or if patient exhales into the inhaler after a dose is loaded, the dose will be lost and a new dose should be loaded and inhaled. Outside of mouthpiece should be cleaned once weekly with a dry tissue. Instruct patient to keep inhaler dry. First appearance of red mark in dose indicator (window underneath mouthpiece) indicates that 20 doses remain. When red mark reaches bottom of dose indicator no doses remain and Turbuhaler should be discarded.

SubQ: Extravasation management, sympathomimetic vasopressors (unlabeled use): Stop vesicant infusion immediately and disconnect I.V. line (leave needle/cannula in place); gently aspirate extravasated solution from the I.V. line (do **NOT** flush the line); remove needle/cannula; elevate extremity. Infiltrate extravasation area with terbutaline solution 1 mg diluted with 9 mL (large extravasation site) **or** 1 mg diluted with 1 mL (small/distal extravasation site) of 0.9% sodium chloride into extravasation site (Stier, 1999).

Monitoring Parameters Serum potassium, glucose; intake/output; heart rate, blood pressure, respiratory rate; chest pain, shortness of breath; monitor for signs and symptoms of pulmonary edema (when used as a tocolytic); monitor FEV_1, peak flow, and/or other pulmonary function tests (when used as bronchodilator). If used for extravasation management, monitor and document extravasation site.

Dosage Forms Excipient information presented when available (limited, particularly for generics); consult specific product labeling.

Solution, Injection, as sulfate:
Generic: 1 mg/mL (1 mL)

Tablet, Oral, as sulfate:
Generic: 2.5 mg, 5 mg

Dosage Forms: Canada Excipient information presented when available (limited, particularly for generics); consult specific product labeling.

Powder for oral inhalation:
Bricanyl® Turbuhaler®: 500 mcg/actuation [100 or 200 metered actuations]

Extemporaneous Preparations A 1 mg/mL oral suspension may be made with tablets. Crush twenty-four 5 mg tablets in a mortar and reduce to a fine powder. Add 5 mL purified water USP and mix to a uniform paste; mix while adding simple syrup, NF in incremental proportions to **almost** 120 mL; transfer to a calibrated bottle, rinse mortar with vehicle, and add quantity of simple syrup, NF sufficient to make 120 mL. Label "shake well" and "refrigerate". Stable for 30 days.

Nahata MC, Pai VB, and Hipple TF, *Pediatric Drug Formulations*, 5th ed, Cincinnati, OH: Harvey Whitney Books Co, 2004.

◆ Terbutaline Sulfate *see* Terbutaline *on page 2019*

Terconazole (ter KONE a zole)

Brand Names: U.S. Terazol 3; Terazol 7; Zazole

Brand Names: Canada Taro-Terconazole; Terazol

Index Terms Triaconazole

Pharmacologic Category Antifungal Agent, Vaginal

Use Candidiasis: For the local treatment of vulvovaginal candidiasis (moniliasis). As terconazole is effective only for vulvovaginitis caused by the genus *Candida*, the diagnosis should be confirmed by KOH smears or cultures.

Pregnancy Risk Factor C

Dosage Intravaginal: Adults: Females:

Vaginal cream 0.4%: Insert 1 applicatorful intravaginally at bedtime for 7 consecutive days

Vaginal cream 0.8%: Insert 1 applicatorful intravaginally at bedtime for 3 consecutive days

Vaginal suppository: Insert 1 suppository intravaginally at bedtime for 3 consecutive days

Additional Information Complete prescribing information should be consulted for additional detail.

Dosage Forms Excipient information presented when available (limited, particularly for generics); consult specific product labeling.

Cream, Vaginal:
Terazol 7: 0.4% (45 g)
Terazol 3: 0.8% (20 g)
Zazole: 0.4% (45 g); 0.8% (20 g)
Generic: 0.4% (45 g); 0.8% (20 g)

Suppository, Vaginal:
Terazol 3: 80 mg (3 ea)
Zazole: 80 mg (3 ea)
Generic: 80 mg (3 ea)

◆ Terfluzine (Can) *see* Trifluoperazine *on page 2125*

Teriflunomide (ter i FLOO noh mide)

Brand Names: U.S. Aubagio

Brand Names: Canada Aubagio

Index Terms A771726; HMR1726

Pharmacologic Category Pyrimidine Synthesis Inhibitor

Use Multiple sclerosis: Treatment of relapsing forms of multiple sclerosis

Pregnancy Risk Factor X

Pregnancy Considerations Adverse events have been observed in animal reproduction studies conducted using doses lower than the expected human exposure. **[U.S. Boxed Warning]: Based on animal data, teriflunomide may cause major birth defects if used in pregnant women. Teriflunomide is contraindicated in pregnant women or women of childbearing potential who are not using reliable contraception. Pregnancy must be avoided during therapy or prior to completing the accelerated elimination treatment protocol.** Pregnancy must be excluded prior to initiating treatment. Women of childbearing potential should not receive therapy until pregnancy has been excluded, they have been counseled concerning fetal risk, and reliable contraceptive measures have been confirmed. Following treatment, pregnancy should be avoided until undetectable serum concentrations (<0.02 mg/L) are verified. This may be accomplished by the use of an enhanced drug elimination procedure using cholestyramine or activated charcoal powder. If pregnancy occurs during treatment, discontinue therapy and initiate the accelerated elimination procedure. Pregnant women exposed to teriflunomide should be registered with the pregnancy registry (800-745-4447, option 2). Teriflunomide is also found in semen. Males and their female partners should use reliable contraception during therapy. Males taking teriflunomide who wish to father a child should consider discontinuing therapy and using the accelerated elimination procedure to decrease the potential risk of fetal exposure. (**Note:** Without use of the accelerated elimination procedure, teriflunomide may remain in the serum for up to 2 years)

Breast-Feeding Considerations It is not known whether teriflunomide is secreted in human milk. Because the potential for serious adverse reactions exists in the nursing infant, a decision should be made whether to discontinue nursing or discontinue the drug, taking into account the importance of the drug to the mother.

Medication Guide Available Yes

Contraindications

Severe hepatic impairment; concomitant use with leflunomide; women of childbearing age who will not use contraception reliably; pregnancy

Canadian labeling: Additional contraindications (not in U.S. labeling): Hypersensitivity to teriflunomide, leflunomide or any component of the formulation; immunodeficiency states (eg, AIDS); impaired bone marrow function or significant anemias, leucopenia, neutropenia, or thrombocytopenia; serious active infections

Warnings/Precautions Hazardous agent; use appropriate precautions for handling and disposal (meets NIOSH, 2012 criteria). **[U.S. Boxed Warning]: Use of leflunomide has been associated with rare reports of hepatotoxicity, hepatic failure, and death, therefore, a similar risk is expected with teriflunomide. Treatment should not be initiated in patients with pre-existing acute or chronic liver disease or ALT >2 x ULN; use is contraindicated in patients with severe impairment. Use caution in patients with concurrent exposure to potentially hepatotoxic drugs. Monitor ALT levels at least monthly for first 6 months during therapy; discontinue if ALT >3 x ULN occurs and, if hepatotoxicity is likely teriflunomide-induced, start drug elimination procedures** (eg, cholestyramine, activated charcoal) and monitor liver function tests weekly until normalized.

Use of leflunomide has been associated (rarely) with interstitial lung disease; discontinue in patients who develop new onset or worsening of pulmonary symptoms. Drug elimination procedures should be considered (eg, cholestyramine, activated charcoal) if evidence of interstitial lung disease; fatal outcomes have been reported. May increase susceptibility to infection, including opportunistic pathogens. Severe infections, sepsis, and fatalities have been reported with leflunomide. One case of fatal sepsis has been reported with teriflunomide. Not recommended in patients with severe immunodeficiency, bone marrow dysplasia, or severe, uncontrolled infections. Caution should be exercised when considering the use in patients with a history of new/recurrent infections, with conditions that predispose them to infections, or with chronic, latent, or localized infections. Patients who develop a new infection while undergoing treatment should be monitored closely; consider discontinuation of therapy and drug elimination procedures if infection is serious.

Use may affect defenses against malignancies; impact on the development and course of malignancies is not fully defined. As compared to the general population, an increased risk of lymphoma has been noted in clinical trials with use of some immunosuppressive medications. Use with caution in patients with a prior history of significant hematologic abnormalities; avoid use with bone marrow dysplasia. Neutropenia, leukopenia, and thrombocytopenia have been reported in clinical trials. Use of leflunomide has been associated with rare pancytopenia, agranulocytosis, and thrombocytopenia, therefore, a similar risk may be expected with teriflunomide. Monitoring of hematologic function is required; discontinue if evidence of bone marrow suppression and begin drug elimination procedures (eg, cholestyramine, activated charcoal). If coadministered with other potential immunosuppressive agents or switching from teriflunomide to another known immunosuppressant, increased monitoring for hematological adverse effects is necessary. Rare cases of dermatologic reactions (including Stevens-Johnson syndrome and toxic epidermal necrolysis) have been reported with leflunomide, therefore patients taking teriflunomide may also be at risk; discontinue if evidence of severe dermatologic reaction occurs, and begin drug elimination procedures (eg, cholestyramine or activated charcoal). Cases of peripheral neuropathy have been reported; use with caution in patients >60 years of age, receiving concomitant neurotoxic medications, or patients with diabetes; discontinue if evidence of peripheral neuropathy occurs and begin drug elimination procedures (eg, cholestyramine, activated charcoal).

Transient acute renal failure, most likely due to acute uric acid nephropathy has been reported. Increased serum creatinine typically occurred 12 weeks to 2 years after the first dose; serum creatinine usually normalized with continued use. Severe hyperkalemia (>7.0 mmol/L) has been reported. Monitor levels in patients with symptoms or acute renal failure. Increases in blood pressure have been reported; monitor at initiation of therapy and periodically thereafter.

Safety has not been established in patients with latent tuberculosis infection. Patients should be screened for tuberculosis and if necessary, treated prior to initiating therapy. Potentially significant drug-drug interactions may exist, requiring dose or frequency adjustment, additional monitoring, and/or selection of alternative therapy. Patients should be brought up to date with all immunizations before initiating therapy. Live vaccines should not be given concurrently; there is no data available concerning secondary transmission of live vaccines in patients receiving therapy. Due to variations in clearance, it may take up to 2 years to reach low levels of teriflunomide metabolite serum concentrations. A drug elimination procedure using cholestyramine or activated charcoal is recommended when a more rapid elimination is needed. If a response to teriflunomide had already been observed, the use of a rapid elimination procedure may result in the return of disease activity. **[U.S. Boxed Warning]: Based on animal data, teriflunomide may cause major birth defects if used in pregnant women. Teriflunomide is contraindicated in pregnant women or women of childbearing potential who are not using reliable contraception. Pregnancy must be avoided during therapy or prior to completing the accelerated elimination treatment protocol.**

Adverse Reactions

>10%:

- Central nervous system: Headache (19% to 22%)
- Dermatologic: Alopecia (10% to 13%)
- Endocrine & metabolic: Hypophosphatemia (5% to 18%)
- Gastrointestinal: Diarrhea (15% to 18%), nausea (9% to 14%)
- Hematologic: Neutropenia (2% to 15%)
- Hepatic: ALT increased (12% to 14%)
- Miscellaneous: Influenza (12%)

1% to 10%:

- Cardiovascular: Hypertension (4%), palpitation (2% to 3%)
- Central nervous system: Anxiety (3% to 4%)
- Dermatologic: Pruritus (3% to 4%), acne (3%), burning sensation (2% to 3%)
- Endocrine & metabolic: Hyperkalemia (1%)
- Gastrointestinal: Abdominal pain (5% to 6%), toothache (4%), viral gastroenteritis (2% to 4%), weight loss (2% to 3%), abdominal distension (1% to 2%)
- Genitourinary: Cystitis (2% to 4%)
- Hematologic: Thrombocytopenia (10%), lymphocytopenia (7% to 10%), leukopenia (1% to 2%)
- Hepatic: GGT increased (3% to 5%), AST increased (2% to 3%)
- Neuromuscular & skeletal: Paresthesia (9% to 10%), musculoskeletal pain (4% to 5%), myalgia (3% to 4%), sciatica (3%), carpal tunnel syndrome (1% to 3%), peripheral neuropathy (1% to 2%)
- Ocular: Blurred vision (3%), conjunctivitis (3%)
- Renal: Renal failure (transient, 1%)
- Respiratory: Upper respiratory tract infection (9%), bronchitis (8%), sinusitis (6%)
- Miscellaneous: Herpes simplex (4%), seasonal allergy (2% to 3%)

<1% (Limited to important or life-threatening): Cytomegalovirus hepatitis reactivation, jaundice, infection, MI

Drug Interactions

Metabolism/Transport Effects Substrate of BCRP; **Inhibits** BCRP, CYP2C8 (moderate), SLCO1B1; **Induces** CYP1A2 (weak/moderate)

Avoid Concomitant Use

Avoid concomitant use of Teriflunomide with any of the following: BCG; Leflunomide; Natalizumab; Pimecrolimus; Tacrolimus (Topical); Tofacitinib; Vaccines (Live)

Increased Effect/Toxicity

Teriflunomide may increase the levels/effects of: CYP2C8 Substrates; Natalizumab; Repaglinide; Tofacitinib; Vaccines (Live)

The levels/effects of Teriflunomide may be increased by: Denosumab; Leflunomide; Pimecrolimus; Roflumilast; Tacrolimus (Topical); Trastuzumab

Decreased Effect

Teriflunomide may decrease the levels/effects of: BCG; Caffeine; Coccidioidin Skin Test; Sipuleucel-T; Vaccines (Inactivated); Vaccines (Live); Warfarin

The levels/effects of Teriflunomide may be decreased by: Bile Acid Sequestrants; Charcoal, Activated; Echinacea

Storage/Stability Store at 20°C to 25°C (68°F to 77°F); excursions permitted to 15°C to 30°C (59°F to 86°F).

Mechanism of Action Teriflunomide is an immunomodulatory agent that inhibits pyrimidine synthesis, resulting in antiproliferative and anti-inflammatory effects. It may reduce the number of activated lymphocytes in the CNS.

Pharmacodynamics/Kinetics

Distribution: V_d: I.V.: 11 L

Protein binding: >99%

Metabolism: Primarily by hydrolysis to minor metabolites; secondary pathways include oxidation, conjugation, and N-acetylation

Half-life elimination: Median: 18-19 days; enterohepatic recycling appears to contribute to the long half-life of this agent, since activated charcoal and cholestyramine substantially reduce plasma half-life

Time to peak, plasma: 1-4 hours

Excretion: Feces (~38%); urine (~23%)

Dosage

Multiple sclerosis: Adults: Oral:

U.S. labeling: 7 mg or 14 mg once daily

Canadian labeling: 14 mg once daily

Dosage adjustment in renal impairment:

Mild, moderate, or severe impairment: No dosage adjustment necessary.

Severe impairment requiring dialysis: Data from a small pharmacokinetic study (n=5) suggest that hemodialysis removes a negligible amount of teriflunomide (Bergner, 2013); the Canadian labeling recommends avoiding use in this patient population.

Dosage adjustment in hepatic impairment:

Mild to moderate impairment: No dosage adjustment necessary.

Severe impairment: Use is contraindicated (has not been studied).

Dosage adjustment in hepatic toxicity: ALT elevations >3 times ULN: Discontinue teriflunomide and initiate cholestyramine or activated charcoal to enhance elimination

Drug elimination procedure: To achieve nondetectable serum concentrations (<0.02 mg/L) of teriflunomide administer either of the following:

Cholestyramine: 8 g every 8 hours for 11 days. If not tolerated, may decrease to 4 g every 8 hours for 11 days. The 11 days do not need to be consecutive unless plasma concentrations need to be lowered rapidly.

or

Activated charcoal: 50 g every 12 hours for 11 days

Note: Both treatments have successfully lead to >98% decrease in teriflunomide concentrations.

Dietary Considerations May be taken with or without food.

Administration Administer without regard to meals.

Hazardous agent; use appropriate precautions for handling and disposal (meets NIOSH, 2012 criteria).

Monitoring Parameters CBC within 6 months of initiation and periodically thereafter based on signs/symptoms of infection; serum potassium, serum creatinine, serum transaminase and bilirubin within 6 months of initiation of therapy and monthly during the initial 6 months of treatment. In addition, monitor for signs/symptoms of severe infection, abnormalities in hepatic function tests, symptoms of hepatotoxicity, and blood pressure (baseline and periodically thereafter). Screen for tuberculosis and pregnancy prior to therapy.

Dosage Forms Excipient information presented when available (limited, particularly for generics); consult specific product labeling.

Tablet, Oral:

Aubagio: 7 mg

Aubagio: 14 mg [contains fd&c blue #2 aluminum lake]

Dosage Forms: Canada Excipient information presented when available (limited, particularly for generics); consult specific product labeling.

Tablet, Oral:

Aubagio: 14 mg

Teriparatide (ter i PAR a tide)

Brand Names: U.S. Forteo

Brand Names: Canada Forteo®

Index Terms Parathyroid Hormone (1-34); Recombinant Human Parathyroid Hormone (1-34); rhPTH(1-34)

Pharmacologic Category Parathyroid Hormone Analog

Use Treatment of osteoporosis in postmenopausal women at high risk of fracture; treatment of primary or hypogonadal osteoporosis in men at high risk of fracture; treatment of glucocorticoid-induced osteoporosis in men and women at high risk for fracture

Pregnancy Risk Factor C

Pregnancy Considerations Adverse events were observed in animal studies; the effect on human fetal development has not been studied. Teriparatide is not indicated for use in pregnant or premenopausal women.

Breast-Feeding Considerations Indicated for use in postmenopausal women. Studies have not been conducted to determine excretion in breast milk. Not recommended for use in breast-feeding women.

Medication Guide Available Yes

Contraindications Hypersensitivity to teriparatide or any component of the formulation

Canadian labeling: Additional contraindications (not in U.S. labeling): Pre-existing hypercalcemia; severe renal impairment; metabolic bone diseases other than primary osteoporosis (including hyperparathyroidism and Paget's disease of the bone); unexplained elevations of alkaline phosphatase; prior external beam or implant radiation therapy involving the skeleton; bone metastases or history of skeletal malignancies; pregnancy; breast-feeding mothers; pediatric patients or young adults with open epiphysis

Warnings/Precautions [U.S. Boxed Warning]: In animal studies, teriparatide has been associated with an increase in osteosarcoma; risk was dependent on both dose and duration. Avoid use in patients with an increased risk of osteosarcoma (including Paget's disease, prior radiation, unexplained elevation of alkaline phosphatase, or in patients with open epiphyses). Do not use in patients with a history of skeletal metastases, hyperparathyroidism, or pre-existing hypercalcemia. Not for use in patients with metabolic bone disease other than osteoporosis. Use caution in patients with active or recent urolithiasis. Use caution in patients at risk of orthostasis (including concurrent antihypertensive therapy), or in patients who may not tolerate transient hypotension (cardiovascular or cerebrovascular disease). Use caution in patients with cardiac, renal or hepatic impairment (limited data available concerning safety and efficacy). Use in severe renal impairment is contraindicated in the Canadian labeling. Use of teriparatide for longer than 2 years is not recommended. Not approved for use in pediatric patients.

Adverse Reactions

>10%: Endocrine & metabolic: Hypercalcemia (transient increases noted 4-6 hours postdose [women 11%; men 6%])

1% to 10%:

Cardiovascular: Orthostatic hypotension (5%; transient), chest pain (3%), syncope (3%)

Central nervous system: Dizziness (8%), insomnia (4% to 5%), anxiety (≤4%), depression (4%), vertigo (4%)

Dermatologic: Rash (5%)

Endocrine & metabolic: Hyperuricemia (3%)

Gastrointestinal: Nausea (9% to 14%), gastritis (≤7%), dyspepsia (5%), vomiting (3%)

Neuromuscular & skeletal: Arthralgia (10%), weakness (9%), leg cramps (3%)

Respiratory: Rhinitis (10%), pharyngitis (6%), dyspnea (4% to 6%), pneumonia (4% to 6%)

Miscellaneous: Antibodies to teriparatide (3% of women in long-term treatment; hypersensitivity reactions or decreased efficacy were not associated in preclinical trials), herpes zoster (≤3%)

Postmarketing and/or case reports: Acute dyspnea, allergic reactions, edema (facial/oral), hypercalcemia >13 mg/dL, injection site reactions (bruising, pain, swelling), muscle spasm, osteosarcoma, urticaria

Drug Interactions

Metabolism/Transport Effects None known.

Avoid Concomitant Use There are no known interactions where it is recommended to avoid concomitant use.

Increased Effect/Toxicity There are no known significant interactions involving an increase in effect.

Decreased Effect There are no known significant interactions involving a decrease in effect.

Ethanol/Nutrition/Herb Interactions

Ethanol: Excessive intake may increase risk of osteoporosis.

Herb/Nutraceutical: Ensure adequate calcium and vitamin D intake.

Storage/Stability Store at 2°C to 8°C (36°F to 46°F); do not freeze. Protect from light. Discard pen 28 days after first injection. Do not use if solution is cloudy, colored, or contains solid particles.

Mechanism of Action Teriparatide is a recombinant formulation of endogenous parathyroid hormone (PTH), containing a 34-amino-acid sequence which is identical to the N-terminal portion of this hormone. The pharmacologic activity of teriparatide, which is similar to the physiologic activity of PTH, includes stimulating osteoblast function, increasing gastrointestinal calcium absorption, and increasing renal tubular reabsorption of calcium. Treatment with teriparatide results in increased bone mineral density, bone mass, and strength. In postmenopausal women, teriparatide has been shown to decrease osteoporosis-related fractures.

Pharmacodynamics/Kinetics

Distribution: V_d: ~0.12 L/kg

Metabolism: Hepatic (nonspecific proteolysis)

Bioavailability: 95%

Half-life elimination: I.V.: 5 minutes; SubQ: ~1 hour

Time to peak, serum: ~30 minutes

Excretion: Urine (as metabolites)

Dosage SubQ: Adults: 20 mcg once daily; **Note:** Initial administration should occur under circumstances in which the patient may sit or lie down, in the event of orthostasis.

Dosage adjustment in renal impairment: No dosage adjustment necessary. Bioavailability and half-life increase with Cl_{cr} <30 mL/minute. Use in severe renal impairment is contraindicated in the Canadian labeling.

Dosage adjustment in hepatic impairment: No dosage adjustment provided in manufacturer's labeling (has not been studied).

Dietary Considerations Ensure adequate calcium and vitamin D intake; if dietary intake is inadequate, dietary supplementation is recommended. Women and men should consume:

Calcium: 1000 mg/day (men: 50-70 years) **or** 1200 mg/day (women ≥51 years and men ≥71 years) (IOM, 2011; NOF, 2013)

Vitamin D: 800-1000 IU/day (men and women ≥50 years) (NOF, 2013). Recommended Dietary Allowance (RDA): 600 IU/day (men and women ≤70 years) **or** 800 IU/day (men and women ≥71 years) (IOM, 2011).

Administration Administer by subcutaneous injection into the thigh or abdominal wall. Initial administration should occur under circumstances in which the patient may sit or lie down, in the event of orthostasis. **Note:** The 3 mL prefilled pen (Canadian availability; not available in U.S.) must be primed prior to each dose.

Monitoring Parameters

Osteoporosis: Bone mineral density (BMD) should be reevaluated every 2 years (or more frequently) after initiating therapy (NOF, 2013); annual measurements of height and weight, assessment of chronic back pain; serum calcium and 25(OH)D; consider measuring biochemical markers of bone turnover

Paget's disease: Alkaline phosphatase; pain; serum calcium and 25(OH)D

Reference Range

Calcium (total): Adults: 9.0-11.0 mg/dL (2.05-2.54 mmol/L), may slightly decrease with aging

Phosphorus: 2.5-4.5 mg/dL (0.81-1.45 mmol/L)

Vitamin D: There is no clear consensus on a reference range for total serum 25(OH)D concentrations or the validity of this level as it relates clinically to bone health. In addition, there is significant variability in the reporting of serum 25(OH)D levels as a result of different assay types in use; however, the following ranges have been suggested:

Adults (IOM, 2011): Sufficient levels in practically all persons: ≥20 ng/mL (50 nmol/L); concern for risk of toxicity: >50 ng/mL (125 nmol/L)

Osteoporosis patients (NOF, 2013): Recommended level to reach and maintain: ~30 ng/mL (75 nmol/L)

Test Interactions Transiently increases serum calcium; maximal effect 4-6 hours postdose; generally returns to baseline ~16 hours postdose

Additional Information Teriparatide was formerly marketed as a diagnostic agent (Perithar™); that agent was withdrawn from the market in 1997. Teriparatide (Forteo®) is manufactured through recombinant DNA technology using a strain of *E. coli*.

Patients are encouraged to enroll in the Forteo® Patient Registry which is designed to monitor the potential risk of osteosarcoma and teriparatide treatment. Enrollment information may be found at www.forteoregistry.rti.org or by calling 1-866-382-6813.

Dosage Forms Excipient information presented when available (limited, particularly for generics); consult specific product labeling.

Solution, Subcutaneous:

Forteo: 600 mcg/2.4 mL (2.4 mL) [contains metacresol]

Dosage Forms: Canada Excipient information presented when available (limited, particularly for generics); consult specific product labeling.

Injection, solution:

Forteo®: 250 mcg/mL (3 mL) [delivers teriparatide 20 mcg/dose]

◆ **Tersi** *see* Selenium Sulfide *on page 1888*

Tesamorelin (tes a moe REL in)

Brand Names: U.S. Egrifta

Index Terms Tesamorelin Acetate; TH9507

Pharmacologic Category Growth Hormone Releasing Factor

Use Lipodystrophy in HIV-infected patients: For the reduction of excess abdominal fat in HIV-infected patients with lipodystrophy

Pregnancy Risk Factor X

Pregnancy Considerations Adverse effects were noted in animal reproduction studies. During pregnancy, there is an increased deposition of visceral adipose tissue due to metabolic and hormonal changes. Tesamorelin decreases the deposition of visceral fat and could potentially cause harm to the unborn fetus. Therefore, use during pregnancy is contraindicated; if pregnancy occurs during treatment, discontinue tesamorelin.

Breast-Feeding Considerations It is not known if tesamorelin is excreted into breast milk. Maternal or infant antiretroviral therapy does not completely eliminate the risk of postnatal HIV transmission. Therefore, in the United States, where formula is accessible, affordable, safe, and sustainable, and the risk of infant mortality due to diarrhea and respiratory infections is low, complete avoidance of breast-feeding by HIV-infected women is recommended to decrease potential transmission of HIV (DHHS [perinatal], 2012).

Prescribing and Access Restrictions In order to prescribe Egrifta, healthcare providers must call the Axis Center at 1-877-714-2947. Egrifta is only available through specialty pharmacy distribution.

Contraindications Hypersensitivity to tesamorelin, mannitol, or any component of the formulation; disruption of hypothalamic-pituitary-axis due to hypophysectomy, hypopituitarism, pituitary tumor/surgery, head irradiation or head trauma; active malignancy (newly diagnosed or recurrent); pregnancy

Warnings/Precautions Hypersensitivity reactions (eg, pruritus, erythema, flushing, urticaria, rash) may occur. If hypersensitivity is suspected, discontinue and instruct patient to seek immediate medical attention. Tesamorelin use may result in peripheral edema manifested by increased skin turgor and musculoskeletal discomfort; edema may be transient or resolve upon treatment discontinuation. Injection site reactions (including erythema, pruritus, pain, irritation, and bruising) may occur; incidence decreases with treatment continued beyond 26 weeks; rotating the site of injection to different areas of the abdomen may reduce incidence of reactions. Tesamorelin may increase risk of development of diabetes due to glucose intolerance; evaluate glucose status prior to treatment initiation; monitor periodically for glucose metabolism changes. Patients with diabetes should be monitored for the development or worsening of retinopathy due to increased IGF-1 levels.

Release of endogenous growth hormone and increased serum IGF-1 may increase the risk for development or reactivation of malignancies. Use is contraindicated in patients with active malignancies; treatment for prior malignancy should be completed prior to initiation of tesamorelin. IGF-1 levels should be monitored during treatment; consider discontinuing with persistent IGF-1 elevations (eg, >3 standard deviation scores). Growth hormone is associated with an increased risk of mortality in patients with acute critical illness due to complications following open heart surgery, abdominal surgery, trauma, or acute respiratory failure; consider discontinuing in critically ill patients. Should not be used in children due to risk of excess growth (gigantism) when epiphyses are open and is not indicated for weight loss management. Due to a lack of long-term cardiovascular safety/benefit data, carefully consider whether continuation of treatment is warranted in patients who do not demonstrate efficacy (based on degree of reduction of visceral adipose tissue). There is no data supporting improved compliance of antiretroviral therapy with concomitant tesamorelin.

Adverse Reactions

10%:

Immunologic: Development of IgG antibodies (48% to 50%)

Local: Injection site reactions (6% to 25%; includes erythema [1% to 9%], pruritus [2% to 8%], pain [4%], irritation [3%], hemorrhage [2%], swelling [2%], urticaria [2%], rash [1%])

Neuromuscular & skeletal: Arthralgia (13%)

1% to 10%:

Cardiovascular: Peripheral edema (2% to 6%), hypertension (1% to 2%), chest pain (1%), palpitation (1%)

Central nervous system: Hypoesthesia (2% to 4%), depression (2%), pain (2%), insomnia (1%)

Dermatologic: Rash (4%), pruritus (1% to 2%), urticaria (1%)

Endocrine & metabolic: Diabetes mellitus (5%), Hb A_{1c} increased (5%), hot flush (1%), hyperglycemia

Gastrointestinal: Nausea (4%), vomiting (2% to 3%), dyspepsia (2%), abdominal pain (1%)

Immunologic: Antibody development (neutralizing; tesamorelin: 10%; hGHRH: 5%)

Neuromuscular & skeletal: Pain in extremity (3% to 6%), myalgia (1% to 6%), paresthesia (2% to 5%), carpal tunnel syndrome (2%), creatine phosphokinase increased (2%), muscle stiffness (2%), musculoskeletal pain (2%), joint stiffness (2%), peripheral neuropathy (2%), joint swelling (1%), muscle spasm (1%), muscle strain (1%)

Miscellaneous: Hypersensitivity reactions (1% to 4%), night sweats (1%)

<1% (Limited to important or life-threatening): Anemia, abdominal abscess, basal cell carcinoma, bipolar II disorder, cellulitis, cerebellar syndrome, chorioretinopathy, coronary artery arteriosclerosis, dehydration, diarrhea, fracture, heart failure (congestive), impaired glucose tolerance, mental status changes, pneumonia, rectal cancer, sepsis, small intestinal obstruction, spontaneous abortion, trigeminal neuralgia, upper respiratory tract infection, viral bronchitis

Drug Interactions

Metabolism/Transport Effects None known.

Avoid Concomitant Use There are no known interactions where it is recommended to avoid concomitant use.

Increased Effect/Toxicity There are no known significant interactions involving an increase in effect.

Decreased Effect

Tesamorelin may decrease the levels/effects of: Cortisone; PredniSONE

Preparation for Administration Reconstitute each 2 mg vial with 2.1 mL diluent, use provided diluent only. Gently roll vial for 30 seconds to mix; do not shake. Use reconstituted solution immediately after prepared.

Storage/Stability Store refrigerated at 2°C to 8°C (36°F to 46°F). Protect from light and store in original container until time of use. Store diluent, (sterile water for injection), syringes, and needles at 20°C to 25°C (68°F to 77°F). Upon dispensing, patient may store unreconstituted vials ≤25°C (77°F) for 3 months or until the expiration date, whichever comes first. Use reconstituted solution immediately after prepared; do not refrigerate or freeze. Discard if not used immediately.

Mechanism of Action Tesamorelin binds to pituitary growth hormone-releasing factor (GRF) receptors and stimulates the secretion of endogenous growth hormone which has anabolic and lipolytic properties. Growth hormone exerts its effects by interacting with receptors on target cells such as osteoblasts, myocytes, hepatocytes, and adipocytes to promote the reduction of total fat mass. These effects are primarily mediated by IGF-1 produced in the liver and in peripheral tissues.

Pharmacodynamics/Kinetics

Distribution: V_d: Healthy adults: 9.4 ± 3.1 L/kg; HIV-infected patients: 10.5 ± 6.1 L/kg

Bioavailability: SubQ: Healthy adults: <4%

Half-life elimination: Healthy adults: 26 minutes; HIV-infected patients: 38 minutes

Time to peak: 9 minutes

Dosage SubQ: Adults: HIV-associated lipodystrophy: 2 mg once daily

Dosing adjustment for toxicity: Consider discontinuing with persistent elevations of IGF-1 (eg, >3 standard deviation scores). Discontinue if symptoms of hypersensitivity occur.

Dosage adjustment in renal impairment: No dosage adjustment provided in the manufacturer's labeling (has not been studied).

Dosage adjustment in hepatic impairment: No dosage adjustment provided in the manufacturer's labeling (has not been studied).

Administration SubQ: The abdomen is the preferred site of administration; rotate site within the abdomen. Avoid injection into scar tissue, bruises, or the navel.

Monitoring Parameters Serum IGF-1 levels should be monitored at baseline and during therapy due to the potential increased risk of malignancy from sustained elevation of IGF-1 levels. Serum glucose (prior to treatment initiation); monitor periodically for glucose metabolism changes. Monitor for retinopathy in patients with diabetes. Visceral adipose tissue (by waist circumference or CT scan). Monitor for fluid retention.

Dosage Forms Excipient information presented when available (limited, particularly for generics); consult specific product labeling. [DSC] = Discontinued product

Solution Reconstituted, Subcutaneous [preservative free]:
Egrifta: 1 mg (1 ea [DSC]); 2 mg (1 ea)

- ◆ **Tesamorelin Acetate** *see* Tesamorelin *on page 2025*
- ◆ **TESPA** *see* Thiotepa *on page 2049*
- ◆ **Tessalon Perles** *see* Benzonatate *on page 243*
- ◆ **Testim** *see* Testosterone *on page 2026*
- ◆ **Testim® (Can)** *see* Testosterone *on page 2026*
- ◆ **Testopel** *see* Testosterone *on page 2026*

Testosterone (tes TOS ter one)

Brand Names: U.S. Androderm; AndroGel; AndroGel Pump; Axiron; Delatestryl; Depo-Testosterone; First-Testosterone; First-Testosterone MC; Fortesta; Striant; Testim; Testopel

Brand Names: Canada Andriol®; Androderm®; AndroGel®; Andropository; Delatestryl®; Depotest® 100; Everone® 200; PMS-Testosterone; Testim®

Index Terms Axiron®; Testosterone Cypionate; Testosterone Enanthate; Testosterone Undecanoate

Pharmacologic Category Androgen

Additional Appendix Information

Beers Criteria – Potentially Inappropriate Medications for Geriatrics *on page 2368*

Use

Injection: Androgen replacement therapy in the treatment of delayed male puberty; male hypogonadism (primary or hypogonadotropic); inoperable metastatic female breast cancer (enanthate only)

Pellet: Androgen replacement therapy in the treatment of delayed male puberty; male hypogonadism (primary or hypogonadotropic)

Buccal system, topical gel, topical solution, transdermal system: Male hypogonadism (primary or hypogonadotropic)

Capsule (not available in U.S.): Conditions associated with a deficiency or absence of endogenous testosterone

Pregnancy Risk Factor X

Pregnancy Considerations Testosterone may cause adverse effects, including masculinization of the female fetus, if used during pregnancy. Females who are or may become pregnant should also avoid skin-to-skin contact to areas where testosterone has been applied topically on another person.

Breast-Feeding Considerations High levels of endogenous maternal testosterone, such as those caused by certain ovarian cysts, suppress milk production. Maternal serum testosterone levels generally fall following pregnancy and return to normal once breast-feeding is stopped. The amount of testosterone present in breast milk or the effect to the nursing infant following maternal supplementation is not known. Some products are contraindicated while breast-feeding. Females who are nursing should avoid skin-to-skin contact to areas where testosterone has been applied topically on another person.

Medication Guide Available Yes

Contraindications Hypersensitivity to testosterone or any component of the formulation; males with known or suspected carcinoma of the breast or prostate; women who are breast-feeding, pregnant, or who may become pregnant (**Note:** Striant® is contraindicated in all women.)

Depo-Testosterone: Also contraindicated in serious hepatic, renal, or cardiac disease

Warnings/Precautions Hazardous agent; use appropriate precautions for handling and disposal (NIOSH, 2012).

When used to treat delayed male puberty, perform radiographic examination of the hand and wrist every 6 months to determine the rate of bone maturation. May cause hypercalcemia in patients with prolonged immobilization or cancer. May accelerate bone maturation without producing compensating gain in linear growth. Has both androgenic and anabolic activity, the anabolic action may enhance hypoglycemia. May alter serum lipid profile; use caution with history of MI or coronary artery disease. Use caution in elderly patients or patients with other demographic factors which may increase the risk of prostatic carcinoma; careful monitoring is required. Discontinue therapy if urethral obstruction develops in patients with BPH (use lower dose if restarted). Withhold therapy pending urological evaluation in patients with palpable prostate nodule or induration, PSA >4 ng/mL, or PSA >3 ng/mL in men at high risk of prostate cancer (Bhasin, 2010). Use with caution in patients with conditions influenced by edema (eg, cardiovascular disease, migraine, seizure disorder, renal or hepatic impairment) or medications that enhance edema formation (eg, corticosteroids); testosterone may cause fluid retention. May cause gynecomastia. Large doses may suppress spermatogenesis. During treatment for metastatic breast cancer, women should be monitored for signs of virilization; discontinue if mild virilization is present to prevent irreversible symptoms.

May be inappropriate in the elderly due to potential risk of cardiac problems and contraindication for use in men with prostate cancer; in general, avoid use in older adults except in the setting of moderate-to-severe hypogonadism (Beers Criteria). In addition, elderly patients may be at greater risk for prostatic hyperplasia, prostate cancer, fluid retention, and transaminase elevations.

Prolonged use of high doses of oral androgens has been associated with serious hepatic effects (peliosis hepatis, hepatic neoplasms, cholestatic hepatitis, jaundice). Prolonged use of intramuscular testosterone enanthate has been associated with multiple hepatic adenomas. May potentiate sleep apnea in some male patients (obesity or chronic lung disease). May increase hematocrit requiring dose adjustment or discontinuation; discontinue therapy if hematocrit exceeds 54%; may reinitiate at lower dose (Bhasin, 2010).

[U.S. Boxed Warning]: Virilization in children has been reported following contact with unwashed or unclothed application sites of men using topical testosterone. Patients should strictly adhere to instructions for use in order to prevent secondary exposure. Virilization of female sexual partners has also been reported with male use of topical testosterone. Symptoms of virilization generally regress following removal of exposure; however, in some children, enlarged genitalia and bone age did not fully return to age appropriate normal. Signs of inappropriate virilization in women or children following secondary exposure to topical testosterone should be brought to the attention of a healthcare provider. Topical testosterone products (gels and solution) may have different doses, strengths, or application instructions that may result in different systemic exposure; these products are not interchangeable. Transdermal patch may contain conducting metal (eg, aluminum); remove patch prior to MRI. Gels, solution, transdermal, and buccal system have not been evaluated in males <18 years of age; safety and efficacy of injection have not been established in males <12 years of age. Some testosterone products may be chemically synthesized from soy. Some products may contain benzyl alcohol. Use of Axiron® in males with BMI >35 kg/m^2 has not been established.

Adverse Reactions Frequency not always defined.

Cardiovascular: Deep venous thrombosis, edema, hypertension, vasodilation

Central nervous system: Abnormal dreams, aggressive behavior, anger, amnesia, anxiety, blood pressure increased/decreased, chills, depression, dizziness, emotional lability, excitation, fatigue, headache, hostility, insomnia, malaise, memory loss, mood swings, nervousness, seizure, sleep apnea, sleeplessness

Dermatologic: Acne, alopecia, contact dermatitis, dry skin, erythema, folliculitis, hair discoloration, hirsutism (increase in pubic hair growth), pruritus, rash, seborrhea

Endocrine & metabolic: Breast pain/soreness, gonadotropin secretion decreased, growth acceleration, gynecomastia, hot flashes, hypercalcemia, hyperchloremia, hypercholesterolemia, hyper-/hypoglycemia, hyper-/hypokalemia, hyperlipidemia, hypernatremia, inorganic phosphate retention, libido changes, menstrual problems (including amenorrhea), virilism, water retention

Gastrointestinal: Appetite increased, diarrhea, gastroesophageal reflux, GI bleeding, GI irritation, nausea, taste disorder, vomiting, weight gain

Following buccal administration (most common): Bitter taste, gum edema, gum or mouth irritation, gum pain, gum tenderness, taste perversion

Genitourinary: Bladder irritability, impotence, oligospermia, penile erections (spontaneous), priapism, prostatic carcinoma, prostatic hyperplasia, prostatitis, PSA increased, testicular atrophy, urination impaired

Hepatic: Bilirubin increased, cholestatic hepatitis, cholestatic jaundice, hepatic dysfunction, hepatic necrosis, hepatocellular neoplasms, liver function test changes, peliosis hepatis

Hematologic: Anemia, bleeding, hematocrit/hemoglobin increased, leukopenia, polycythemia, suppression of clotting factors

Local: Application site reaction (gel, solution), injection site inflammation/pain

Transdermal system: Pruritus at application site (17% to 37%), burn-like blisters under system (12%), erythema at application site (≤7%), vesicles at application site (6%), allergic contact dermatitis to system (4%), burning at application site (3%), induration at application site (3%), exfoliation at application site (<3%)

Neuromuscular & skeletal: Back pain, hemarthrosis, hyperkinesias, paresthesia, weakness

Ocular: Lacrimation increased

Renal: Creatinine increased, hematuria, polyuria

Respiratory: Dyspnea, nasopharyngitis

Miscellaneous: Anaphylactoid reactions, diaphoresis, hypersensitivity reactions, smell disorder

Postmarketing and/or case reports: Injection: Cough, coughing fits, respiratory distress; migraine; virilization of children following secondary exposure to topical gel (advanced bone age, aggressive behavior, enlargement of clitoris requiring surgery, enlargement of penis, erections increased, libido increased, pubic hair development); vitreous detachment

Drug Interactions

Metabolism/Transport Effects Substrate of CYP2B6 (minor), CYP2C19 (minor), CYP2C9 (minor), CYP3A4 (minor); **Note:** Assignment of Major/Minor substrate status based on clinically relevant drug interaction potential

Avoid Concomitant Use

Avoid concomitant use of Testosterone with any of the following: Dehydroepiandrosterone

Increased Effect/Toxicity

Testosterone may increase the levels/effects of: CycloSPORINE (Systemic); Vitamin K Antagonists

The levels/effects of Testosterone may be increased by: Dehydroepiandrosterone

Decreased Effect There are no known significant interactions involving a decrease in effect.

Ethanol/Nutrition/Herb Interactions Herb/Nutraceutical: St John's wort may decrease testosterone levels.

Storage/Stability

Androderm: Store at room temperature. Do not store outside of pouch. Excessive heat may cause system to burst.

AndroGel 1%, AndroGel 1.62%, Axiron, Delatestryl, Striant, Testim: Store at room temperature.

Depo-Testosterone: Store at room temperature. Protect from light.

Fortesta: Store at room temperature; do not freeze

Testopel: Store in a cool location.

Mechanism of Action Principal endogenous androgen responsible for promoting the growth and development of the male sex organs and maintaining secondary sex characteristics in androgen-deficient males

Pharmacodynamics/Kinetics

Duration (route and ester dependent): I.M.: Cypionate and enanthate esters have longest duration, ≤2-4 weeks; gel: 24-48 hours

Absorption: Transdermal gel: ~10% of applied dose

Protein binding: 98%; bound to sex hormone-binding globulin (40%) and albumin

Metabolism: Hepatic; forms metabolites, including dihydrotestosterone (DHT) and estradiol (both active)

Half-life elimination: Variable: 10-100 minutes

Excretion: Urine (90%); feces (6%)

Dosage

Adolescents and Adults: Males:

I.M.:

Primary hypogonadism or hypogonadotropic hypogonadism: Testosterone enanthate or testosterone cypionate: 50-400 mg every 2-4 weeks (FDA-approved dosing range); 75-100 mg/week or 150-200 mg every 2 weeks (Bhasin, 2010)

Delayed puberty: Testosterone enanthate: 50-200 mg every 2-4 weeks for a limited duration

Pellet (for subcutaneous implantation): Delayed puberty, primary hypogonadism or hypogonadotropic hypogonadism: 150-450 mg every 3-6 months

Adults:

I.M.: Females: Inoperable metastatic breast cancer: Testosterone enanthate: 200-400 mg every 2-4 weeks

Oral: Males: Conditions associated with a deficiency or absence of endogenous testosterone: Capsule (Andriol®; not available in U.S.): Initial: 120-160 mg daily in 2 divided doses for 2-3 weeks; adjust according to individual response; usual maintenance dose: 40-120 mg daily (in divided doses)

Topical: Primary male hypogonadism **or** hypogonadotropic hypogonadism:

Buccal: 30 mg twice daily (every 12 hours) applied to the gum region above the incisor tooth

Gel: Apply to clean, dry, intact skin. **Do not apply testosterone gel to the genitals.**

AndroGel® 1%: 50 mg applied once daily in the morning to the shoulder and upper arms, or abdomen. Dosage may be increased to a maximum of 100 mg daily.

Dose adjustment based on testosterone levels:

Less than normal range: Increase dose from 50 mg to 75 mg or from 75 mg to 100 mg once daily

Greater than normal range: Decrease dose. Discontinue if consistently above normal at 50 mg daily

AndroGel® 1.62%: 40.5 mg applied once daily in the morning to the shoulder and upper arms. Dosage may be increased to a maximum of 81 mg daily.

Dose adjustment based on testosterone levels:

>750 ng/dL: Decrease dose by 20.25 mg daily

≥350 ng/dL to ≤750 ng/dL: Maintain current dose

<350 ng/dL: Increase dose by 20.25 mg daily

Fortesta™: 40 mg once daily in the morning. Apply to the thighs. Dosing range: 10-70 mg daily

Dose adjustment based on serum testosterone levels:

≥2500 ng/dL: Decrease dose by 20 mg daily

≥1250 to <2500 ng/dL: Decrease dose by 10 mg daily

≥500 and <1250 ng/dL: Maintain current dose

<500 ng/dL: Increase dose by 10 mg daily

Testim®: 50 mg applied once daily (preferably in the morning) to the shoulder and upper arms. Dosage may be increased to a maximum of 100 mg daily.

Dose adjustment based on testosterone levels:

Less than normal range: Increase dose from 50 mg to 100 mg once daily

Greater than normal range: Decrease dose

Solution: Axiron®: 60 mg once daily (dosage range: 30-120 mg daily). Apply to the axilla at the same time each morning; do not apply to other parts of the body. Apply to clean, dry, intact skin. **Do not apply testosterone solution to the genitals.**

Dose adjustment based on serum testosterone levels:

>1050 ng/dL: Decrease 60 mg daily dose to 30 mg daily; if levels >1050 ng/dL persist after dose reduction discontinue therapy

<300 ng/dL: Increase 60 mg daily dose to 90 mg daily, or increase 90 mg daily dose to 120 mg daily

Transdermal system (Androderm®): **Note:** Initial dose is either 4 mg daily or 5 mg and dose adjustment varies as follows:

Initial: 4 mg daily (as one 4 mg/day patch; do **not** use two 2 mg/day patches)

Dose adjustment based on testosterone levels:

>930 ng/dL: Decrease dose to 2 mg daily

400-930 ng/dL: Continue 4 mg daily

<400 ng/dL: Increase dose to 6 mg daily (as one 4 mg/day and one 2 mg/day patch)

Initial: 5 mg daily (as one 5 mg/day or two 2.5 mg/day patches)

Dose adjustment based on testosterone levels:

>1030 ng/dL: Decrease dose to 2.5 mg daily

300-1030 ng/dL: Continue 5 mg daily

<300 ng/dL: Increase dose to 7.5 mg daily (as one 5 mg/day and one 2.5 mg/day patch)

Dosing conversion: The 2.5 mg/day and the 5 mg/day patches have been discontinued in the U.S.; patients may be switched from the 2.5 mg/day patch, 5 mg/day patch, or the combination (ie, 7.5 mg/day) as follows:

From 2.5 mg/day patch to 2 mg/day patch

From 5 mg/day patch to 4 mg/day patch

From 7.5 mg daily (one 2.5 mg/day and one 5 mg/day patch) to 6 mg daily (one 2 mg/day and one 4 mg/day patch)

Note: Patch change should occur at the next scheduled dosing. Measure early morning testosterone concentrations ~2 weeks after switching therapy.

Dosing adjustment in renal impairment: No dosage adjustment provided in manufacturer's labeling (has not been studied). Use with caution; may enhance edema formation.

Dosing adjustment in hepatic impairment: No dosage adjustment provided in manufacturer's labeling (has not been studied). Use with caution; may enhance edema formation.

Dietary Considerations Testosterone USP may be synthesized from soy. Food and beverages have not been found to interfere with buccal system; ensure system is in place following eating, drinking, or brushing teeth.

Administration

I.M.: Warm to room temperature; shaking vial will help redissolve crystals that have formed after storage. Administer by deep I.M. injection into the gluteal muscle.

Oral, buccal application (Striant®): One mucoadhesive for buccal application (buccal system) should be applied to a comfortable area above the incisor tooth. Place the flat side of the system on your fingertip. Gently push the curved side against your upper gum. Rotate to alternate sides of mouth with each application. Hold buccal system firmly in place for 30 seconds to ensure adhesion. The buccal system should adhere to gum for 12 hours. If the buccal system falls out, replace with a new system. If the system falls out within 4 hours of next dose, the new buccal system should remain in place until the time of the following scheduled dose. System will soften and mold to shape of gum as it absorbs moisture from mouth. Do not chew or swallow the buccal system. The buccal system will not dissolve; gently remove by sliding downwards from gum; avoid scratching gum.

Oral, capsule (Andriol®; not available in the U.S.): Should be administered with meals. Should be swallowed whole; do not crush or chew.

Subcutaneous implant (Testopel®): Using strict sterile technique, must be surgically implanted.

Transdermal patch (Androderm®): Apply patch to clean, dry area of skin on the back, abdomen, upper arms, or thigh. Do not apply to bony areas or parts of the body that are subject to prolonged pressure while sleeping or sitting. **Do not apply to the scrotum.** Avoid showering, washing the site, or swimming for 3 hours after application. Following patch removal, mild skin irritation may be treated with OTC hydrocortisone cream. A small amount of triamcinolone acetonide 0.1% cream may be applied under the system to decrease irritation; do not use ointment. Patch should be applied nightly. Rotate administration sites, allowing 7 days between applying to the same site.

Topical gel and solution: Apply to clean, dry, intact skin. Application sites should be allowed to dry for a few minutes prior to dressing. Hands should be washed with soap and water after application. **Do not apply testosterone gel or solution to the genitals.** Alcohol-based gels and solutions are flammable; avoid fire, flames, or smoking until dry. Testosterone may be transferred to another person following skin-to-skin contact with the application site. Strict adherence to application instructions is needed in order to decrease secondary exposure. Thoroughly wash hands after application and cover application site with clothing (ie, shirt) once gel or solution has dried, or clean application site thoroughly with soap and water prior to contact in order to minimize transfer. In addition to skin-to-skin contact, secondary exposure has also been reported following exposure to secondary items (eg, towel, shirt, sheets). If secondary exposure occurs, the other person should thoroughly wash the skin with soap and water as soon as possible.

AndroGel® 1%, AndroGel® 1.62%, Testim®: Apply (preferably in the morning) to the shoulder and upper arms. AndroGel® 1% may also be applied to the abdomen; do not apply AndroGel® 1.62% or Testim® to the abdomen. Area of application should be limited to what will be covered by a short sleeve t-shirt. Apply at the same time each day. Upon opening the packet(s), the entire contents should be squeezed into the palm of the hand and immediately applied to the application site(s). Alternatively, a portion may be squeezed onto palm of hand and applied, repeating the process at the same or other site until entire packet has been applied. Application site(s) should not be washed for ≥2 hours following application of AndroGel® 1.62% or Testim®, or >5 hours for AndroGel® 1%.

AndroGel® 1% multidose pump: Prime pump 3 times (and discard this portion of product) prior to initial use. Each actuation delivers 12.5 mg of testosterone (4 actuations = 50 mg; 6 actuations = 75 mg; 8 actuations = 100 mg); each actuation may be applied individually or all at the same time. Application site should not be washed for >5 hours following application.

AndroGel® 1.62% multidose pump: Prime pump 3 times (and discard this portion of product) prior to initial use. Each actuation delivers 20.25 mg of testosterone (2 actuations = 40.5 mg; 3 actuations = 60.75 mg; 4 actuations = 81 mg); each actuation may be applied individually or all at the same time. Avoid washing the site or swimming for ≥2 hours following application.

Axiron®: Apply using the applicator to the axilla at the same time each morning. Do not apply to other parts of the body (eg, abdomen, genitals, shoulders, upper arms). Avoid washing the site or swimming for 2 hours after application. Prior to first use, prime the applicator pump by depressing it 3 times (discard this portion of the product). After priming, position the nozzle over the applicator cup and depress pump fully one time; ensure liquid enters cup. Each pump actuation delivers testosterone 30 mg. No more than 30 mg (one pump) should be added to the cup at one time. The total dose should be divided between axilla (example, 30 mg/day: apply to one axilla only; 60 mg/day: apply 30 mg to each axilla; 90 mg/day: apply 30 mg to each axilla, allow to dry, then apply an additional 30 mg to one axilla; etc). To apply dose, keep applicator upright and wipe into the axilla; if solution runs or drips, use cup to wipe. Do not rub into skin with fingers or hand. If more than one 30 mg dose is needed, repeat process. Apply roll-on or stick antiperspirants or deodorants prior to testosterone. Once application site is dry, cover with clothing. After use, rinse applicator under running water and pat dry with a tissue. The application site and dose of this product are not interchangeable with other topical testosterone products.

Fortesta™: Apply to skin of front and inner thighs. Do not apply to other parts of the body. Use one finger to rub gel evenly onto skin of each thigh. Avoid showering, washing the site, or swimming for 2 hours after application. Prior to first dose, prime the pump by holding canister upright and fully depressing the pump 8 times (discard this portion of the product). Each pump actuation delivers testosterone 10 mg. The total dose should be divided between thighs (example, 10 mg/day: apply 10 mg to one thigh only; 20 mg/day: apply 10 mg to each thigh; 30 mg/day: apply 20 mg to one thigh and 10 mg to the other thigh; etc). Once application site is dry, cover with clothing. The application site and dose of this product are not interchangeable with other topical testosterone products.

Hazardous agent; use appropriate precautions for handling and disposal (NIOSH, 2012).

Monitoring Parameters Periodic liver function tests, lipid panel, hemoglobin and hematocrit (prior to therapy, at 3-6 months, then annually); radiologic examination of wrist and hand every 6 months (when using in prepubertal children). Withhold initial treatment with hematocrit >50% (discontinue therapy if hematocrit exceeds 54% [Bhasin, 2010]), hyperviscosity, untreated obstructive sleep apnea, or uncontrolled severe heart failure. Monitor urine and serum calcium and signs of virilization in women treated for breast cancer. Serum glucose (may be decreased by testosterone, monitor patients with diabetes). Evaluate males for response to treatment and adverse events 3-6 months after initiation and then annually.

Bone mineral density: Monitor after 1-2 years of therapy in hypogonadal men with osteoporosis or low trauma fracture (Bhasin, 2010)

PSA: In men >40 years of age with baseline PSA >0.6 ng/mL, PSA and prostate exam (prior to therapy, at 3-6 months, then as based on current guidelines). Withhold treatment pending urological evaluation in patients with palpable prostate nodule or induration or PSA >4 ng/mL or if PSA >3 ng/mL in men at high risk of prostate cancer (Bhasin, 2010).

Do not treat with severe untreated BPH with IPSS symptom score >19.

Serum testosterone: After initial dose titration (if applicable), monitor 3-6 months after initiating treatment, then annually.

Injection: Measure midway between injections. Adjust dose or frequency if testosterone concentration is <400 ng/dL or >700 ng/dL (Bhasin, 2010).

AndroGel® 1%, Testim®: Morning serum testosterone levels ~14 days after start of therapy or dose adjustments

AndroGel® 1.62%: Morning serum testosterone levels after 14 and 28 days of starting therapy or dose adjustments and periodically thereafter

Androderm®: Morning serum testosterone levels (following application the previous evening) ~14 days after start of therapy or dose adjustments

Axiron®: Serum testosterone levels can be measured 2-8 hours after application and after 14 days of starting therapy or dose adjustments

Fortesta™: Serum testosterone levels can be measured 2 hours after application and after 14 and 35 days of starting therapy or dose adjustments

Striant®: Application area of gums; total serum testosterone 4-12 weeks after initiating treatment, prior to morning dose

Testopel®: Measure at the end of the dosing interval (Bhasin, 2010)

Reference Range

Total testosterone, males:

12-13 years: <800 ng/dL

14 years: <1200 ng/dL

15-16 years: 100-1200ng/dL

17-18 years: 300-1200 ng/dL

19-40 years: 300-950 ng/dL

>40 years: 240-950 ng/dL

Free testosterone, males: 9-30 ng/dL

Test Interactions Testosterone may decrease thyroxine-binding globulin, resulting in decreased total T_4; free thyroid hormone levels are not changed.

Dosage Forms Excipient information presented when available (limited, particularly for generics); consult specific product labeling.

Cream, Transdermal:

First-Testosterone MC: 2% (60 g) [contains benzyl alcohol, sesame oil]

Gel, Transdermal:

AndroGel: 25 mg/2.5 g (2.5 g); 50 mg/5 g (5 g); 40.5 MG/2.5GM (1.62%) (2.5 g); 20.25 MG/1.25GM (1.62%) (1.25 g) [contains alcohol, usp]

AndroGel Pump: 12.5 MG/ACT (1%) (75 g); 20.25 MG/ACT (1.62%) (75 g) [contains alcohol, usp]

Fortesta: 10 MG/ACT (2%) (60 g) [odorless; contains propylene glycol, trolamine (triethanolamine)]

Testim: 50 mg/5 g (5 g) [contains alcohol, usp, tromethamine]

Miscellaneous, Buccal:

Striant: 30 mg (60 ea)

Oil, Intramuscular, as cypionate:

Depo-Testosterone: 100 mg/mL (10 mL); 200 mg/mL (1 mL, 10 mL) [contains benzyl alcohol, benzyl benzoate]

Generic: 100 mg/mL (10 mL); 200 mg/mL (1 mL, 10 mL)

Oil, Intramuscular, as enanthate:

Delatestryl: 200 mg/mL (5 mL)

Generic: 200 mg/mL (5 mL)

Ointment, Transdermal:

First-Testosterone: 2% (60 g) [contains benzyl alcohol, butylated hydroxytoluene (bht), petrolatum, sesame oil]

Patch 24 Hour, Transdermal:

Androderm: 2 mg/24 hr (1 ea, 60 ea); 4 mg/24 hr (1 ea, 30 ea)

Pellet, Implant:

Testopel: 75 mg (10 ea, 100 ea)

Solution, Transdermal:

Axiron: 30 mg/actuation (90 mL)

Dosage Forms: Canada Excipient information presented when available (limited, particularly for generics); consult specific product labeling.

Capsule, gelatin, as undecanoate:

Andriol™: 40 mg (10s)

Controlled Substance C-III

◆ **Testosterone Cypionate** *see* Testosterone *on page 2026*

◆ **Testosterone Enanthate** *see* Testosterone *on page 2026*

◆ **Testosterone Undecanoate** *see* Testosterone *on page 2026*

◆ **Testred** *see* MethylTESTOSTERone *on page 1344*

◆ **Tetanus and Diphtheria Toxoid** *see* Diphtheria and Tetanus Toxoid *on page 626*

Tetanus Immune Globulin (Human)

(TET a nus i MYUN GLOB yoo lin HYU man)

Brand Names: U.S. HyperTET S/D

Brand Names: Canada HyperTET™ S/D

Index Terms TIG

Pharmacologic Category Immune Globulin

Additional Appendix Information

Immunization Administration Recommendations *on page 2334*

Immunization Recommendations *on page 2339*

Use Prophylaxis against tetanus following injury in patients where immunization status is not known or uncertain

The Advisory Committee on Immunization Practices (ACIP) recommends passive immunization with TIG for the following:

- Persons with a wound that is not clean or minor and in whom contraindications to a tetanus-toxoid containing vaccine exist and they have not completed a primary series of tetanus toxoid immunization.
- Persons who are wounded in bombings or similar mass casualty events who have penetrating injuries or non-intact skin exposure and who cannot confirm receipt of a tetanus booster within the previous 5 years. In case of shortage, use should be reserved for persons ≥60 years of age.

Pregnancy Risk Factor C

Pregnancy Considerations Animal reproduction studies have not been conducted. Tetanus immune globulin and a tetanus toxoid containing vaccine are recommended by the ACIP as part of the standard wound management to prevent tetanus in pregnant women.

Warnings/Precautions Hypersensitivity and anaphylactic reactions can occur; immediate treatment (including epinephrine 1:1000) should be available. Use caution in patients with isolated immunoglobulin A deficiency or a history of systemic hypersensitivity to human immunoglobulins. Use with caution in patients with thrombocytopenia or coagulation disorders; I.M. injections may be contraindicated. Product of human plasma; may potentially contain infectious agents which could transmit disease. Screening of donors, as well as testing and/or inactivation or removal of certain viruses, reduces the risk. Infections thought to be transmitted by this product should be reported to the manufacturer. Skin testing should not be performed as local irritation can occur and be misinterpreted as a positive reaction. Not for intravenous administration.

Adverse Reactions Frequency not defined.

Central nervous system: Temperature increased

Dermatologic: Angioneurotic edema (rare)

Local: Injection site: Pain, soreness, tenderness

Renal: Nephritic syndrome (rare)

Miscellaneous: Anaphylactic shock (rare)

Drug Interactions

Metabolism/Transport Effects None known.

Avoid Concomitant Use There are no known interactions where it is recommended to avoid concomitant use.

Increased Effect/Toxicity There are no known significant interactions involving an increase in effect.

Decreased Effect

Tetanus Immune Globulin (Human) may decrease the levels/effects of: Vaccines (Live)

Storage/Stability Store at 2°C to 8°C (26°F to 46°F). Do not use if frozen. The following stability information has also been reported for HyperTET™ S/D: May be exposed to room temperature for a cumulative 7 days (Cohen, 2007).

Mechanism of Action Passive immunity toward tetanus

Pharmacodynamics/Kinetics Absorption: Well absorbed

Dosage I.M.:

Prophylaxis of tetanus:

Children <7 years: 4 units/kg; some recommend administering 250 units to small children

Children ≥7 years and Adults: 250 units

Tetanus prophylaxis in wound management: Children and Adults: Tetanus prophylaxis in patients with wounds should consider if the wound is clean or contaminated, the immunization status of the patient, proper use of tetanus toxoid and/or tetanus immune globulin (TIG), wound cleaning, and (if required) surgical debridement and the proper use of antibiotics. Patients with an uncertain or incomplete tetanus immunization status should have additional follow up to ensure a series is completed. Patients with a history of Arthus reaction following a previous dose of a tetanus toxoid-containing vaccine should not receive a tetanus toxoid-containing vaccine until >10 years after the most recent dose even if they have a wound that is neither clean nor minor. See table.

Tetanus Prophylaxis in Wound Management

History of Tetanus Immunization Doses	Clean, Minor Wounds		All Other Wounds[1]	
	Tetanus Toxoid[2]	TIG	Tetanus Toxoid[2]	TIG
Uncertain or <3 doses	Yes	No	Yes	Yes
3 or more doses	No[3]	No	No[4]	No

[1]Such as, but not limited to, wounds contaminated with dirt, feces, soil, and saliva; puncture wounds; wounds from crushing, tears, burns, and frostbite.

[2]Tetanus toxoid in this chart refers to a tetanus toxoid-containing vaccine. For children <7 years of age, DTaP (DT, if pertussis vaccine contraindicated) is preferred to tetanus toxoid alone. For children ≥7 years and Adults, Td preferred to tetanus toxoid alone; Tdap may be preferred if the patient has not previously been vaccinated with Tdap.

[3]Yes, if ≥10 years since last dose.

[4]Yes, if ≥5 years since last dose.

Adapted from CDC "Yellow Book" (*Health Information for International Travel 2010*), "Routine Vaccine-Preventable Diseases, Tetanus" (available at http://www.cdc.gov/yellowbook) and *MMWR* 2006, 55 (RR-17).

Abbreviations: **DT** = Diphtheria and Tetanus Toxoids (formulation for age ≤6 years); **DTaP** = Diphtheria and Tetanus Toxoids, and Acellular Pertussis (formulation for age ≤6 years; Daptacel®, Infanrix®); **Td** = Diphtheria and Tetanus Toxoids (formulation for age ≥7 years; Decavac®, Tenivac™); **TT**= Tetanus toxoid (adsorbed [formulation for age ≥7 years]); **Tdap** = Diphtheria and Tetanus Toxoids, and Acellular Pertussis (Adacel® or Boostrix® [formulations for age ≥7 years]); **TIG** = Tetanus Immune Globulin

Treatment of tetanus: Children and Adults: 500-6000 units. Infiltration of part of the dose around the wound is recommended.

Dosage adjustment in renal impairment: No dosage adjustment provided in the manufacturer's labeling.

Dosage adjustment in hepatic impairment: No dosage adjustment provided in the manufacturer's labeling.

Administration Do not administer I.V.; I.M. use only. Administer in the anterolateral aspects of the upper thigh or the deltoid muscle of the upper arm. Avoid gluteal region due to risk of injury to sciatic nerve; if gluteal region is used, administer only in the upper outer quadrant. If tetanus vaccine and tetanus immune globulin are administered simultaneously, separate sites should be used for each injection. When used for the treatment of tetanus, infiltration of part of the dose around the wound is recommended.

Additional Information Tetanus immune globulin (TIG) must not contain <50 units/mL. Protein makes up 10% to 18% of TIG preparations. The great majority of this (≥90%) is IgG. TIG has almost no color or odor and it is a sterile, nonpyrogenic, concentrated preparation of immunoglobulins that has been derived from the plasma of adults hyperimmunized with tetanus toxoid. The pooled material from which the immunoglobulin is derived may be from fewer than 1000 donors. This plasma has been shown to be free of hepatitis B surface antigen.

Dosage Forms Excipient information presented when available (limited, particularly for generics); consult specific product labeling.

Injectable, Intramuscular:

HyperTET S/D: 250 units/mL (1 ea)

◆ **Tetanus Toxoid** *see* Diphtheria and Tetanus Toxoids, Acellular Pertussis, Poliovirus and *Haemophilus* b Conjugate Vaccine *on page 629*

Tetanus Toxoid (Adsorbed)

(TET a nus TOKS oyd, ad SORBED)

Index Terms TT

Pharmacologic Category Vaccine, Inactivated (Bacterial)

Additional Appendix Information

Immunization Administration Recommendations *on page 2334*

Immunization Recommendations *on page 2339*

Use Active immunization against tetanus when combination antigen preparations are not indicated; tetanus prophylaxis in wound management. **Note:** Tetanus and diphtheria toxoids for adult use (Td) is the preferred immunizing agent for most adults and for children after their seventh birthday. Young children should receive trivalent DTaP (diphtheria/tetanus/acellular pertussis) as part of their childhood immunization program, unless pertussis is contraindicated, then DT is warranted.

Pregnancy Risk Factor C

Pregnancy Considerations Animal studies have not been conducted. Inactivated bacterial vaccines have not been shown to cause increased risks to the fetus (CDC, 2011). The ACIP recommends vaccination in previously unvaccinated women or in women with an incomplete vaccination series, whose child may be born in unhygienic conditions. Tetanus immune globulin and a tetanus toxoid-containing vaccine are recommended by the ACIP as part of the standard wound management to prevent tetanus in pregnant women. Vaccination using Td is preferred.

Breast-Feeding Considerations Inactivated vaccines do not affect the safety of breast-feeding for the mother or the infant. Breast-feeding infants should be vaccinated according to the recommended schedules (CDC, 2011).

Contraindications Hypersensitivity to tetanus toxoid or any component of the formulation

Warnings/Precautions Avoid injection into a blood vessel; allergic reactions may occur; epinephrine 1:1000 must be available. Patients who are immunocompromised may have reduced response; may be used in patients with HIV infection. In general, household and close contacts of persons with altered immunocompetence may receive all age appropriate vaccines. May defer elective immunization during febrile illness or acute infection. In patients with a history of severe local reaction (Arthus-type) following previous dose, do not give further routine or emergency doses of tetanus and diphtheria toxoids for 10 years. Use caution in patients on anticoagulants, with thrombocytopenia, or bleeding disorders (bleeding may occur following intramuscular injection). Use with caution if Guillain-Barré syndrome occurred within 6 weeks of prior tetanus toxoid. Syncope has been reported with use of injectable vaccines and may be accompanied by transient visual disturbances, weakness, or tonic-clonic movements. Procedures should be in place to avoid injuries from falling and to restore cerebral perfusion if syncope occurs. Contains thimerosal. This product is not indicated for use in children <7 years of age. In order to maximize vaccination rates, the ACIP recommends simultaneous administration of all age-appropriate vaccines (live or inactivated) for which a person is eligible at a single clinic visit, unless contraindications exist. The use of combination vaccines is generally preferred over separate injections, taking into consideration provider assessment, patient preference, and adverse events. When using combination vaccines, the minimum age for administration is the oldest minimum age for any individual component; the minimum interval between dosing is the greatest minimum interval between any individual component.

Vaccination may not result in effective immunity in all patients. Response depends upon multiple factors (eg, type of vaccine, age of patient) and may be improved by administering the vaccine at the recommended dose, route, and interval. Vaccines may not be effective if administered during periods of altered immune competence (CDC, 2011).

Adverse Reactions All serious adverse reactions must be reported to the U.S. Department of Health and Human Services (DHHS) Vaccine Adverse Event Reporting System (VAERS) 1-800-822-7967 or online at https://vaers.hhs.gov/esub/index.

Frequency not defined.

Cardiovascular: Hypotension

Central nervous system: Brachial neuritis, fever, malaise, pain

Gastrointestinal: Nausea

Local: Edema, induration (with or without tenderness), rash, redness, urticaria, warmth

Neuromuscular: Arthralgia, Guillain-Barré syndrome

Miscellaneous: Anaphylactic reaction, Arthus-type hypersensitivity reaction

Drug Interactions

Metabolism/Transport Effects None known.

Avoid Concomitant Use There are no known interactions where it is recommended to avoid concomitant use.

Increased Effect/Toxicity There are no known significant interactions involving an increase in effect.

Decreased Effect

The levels/effects of Tetanus Toxoid (Adsorbed) may be decreased by: Belimumab; Fingolimod; Immunosuppressants

Storage/Stability Store at 2°C to 8°C (26°F to 46°F); do not freeze.

Mechanism of Action Tetanus toxoid preparations contain the toxin produced by virulent tetanus bacilli (detoxified growth products of *Clostridium tetani*). The toxin has been modified by treatment with formaldehyde so that it has lost toxicity but still retains ability to act as antigen and produce active immunity; the aluminum salt, a mineral adjuvant, delays the rate of absorption and prolongs and enhances its properties; duration ~10 years.

Pharmacodynamics/Kinetics Duration: Primary immunization: ~10 years

Dosage Note: In most patients, Td is the recommended product for primary immunization, booster doses, and tetanus immunization in wound management (refer to Diphtheria and Tetanus Toxoid monograph).

Children ≥7 years and Adults: I.M.:

Primary immunization: 0.5 mL; repeat 0.5 mL at 4-8 weeks after first dose and at 6-12 months after second dose

Routine booster dose: Recommended every 10 years

Tetanus prophylaxis in wound management: Tetanus prophylaxis in patients with wounds should consider if the wound is clean or contaminated, the immunization status of the patient, proper use of tetanus toxoid and/or tetanus immune globulin (TIG), wound cleaning, and (if required) surgical debridement and the proper use of antibiotics. Patients with an uncertain or incomplete tetanus immunization status should have additional follow up to ensure a series is completed. Patients with a history of Arthus reaction following a previous dose of a tetanus toxoid-containing vaccine should not receive a tetanus toxoid-containing vaccine until >10 years after the most recent dose even if they have a wound that is neither clean nor minor. See table.

Tetanus Prophylaxis in Wound Management

History of Tetanus Immunization Doses	Clean, Minor Wounds		All Other Wounds[1]	
	Tetanus Toxoid[2]	TIG	Tetanus Toxoid[2]	TIG
Uncertain or <3 doses	Yes	No	Yes	Yes
3 or more doses	No[3]	No	No[4]	No

[1]Such as, but not limited to, wounds contaminated with dirt, feces, soil, and saliva; puncture wounds; wounds from crushing, tears, burns, and frostbite.

[2]Tetanus toxoid in this chart refers to a tetanus toxoid-containing vaccine. For children <7 years of age, DTaP (DT, if pertussis vaccine contraindicated) is preferred to tetanus toxoid alone. For children ≥7 years and Adults, Td preferred to tetanus toxoid alone; Tdap may be preferred if the patient has not previously been vaccinated with Tdap.

[3]Yes, if ≥10 years since last dose.

[4]Yes, if ≥5 years since last dose.

Adapted from CDC "Yellow Book" (*Health Information for International Travel 2010*), "Routine Vaccine-Preventable Diseases, Tetanus" (available at http://www.cdc.gov/yellowbook) and *MMWR* 2006, 55 (RR-17).

Abbreviations: **DT** = Diphtheria and Tetanus Toxoids (formulation for age ≤6 years); **DTaP** = Diphtheria and Tetanus Toxoids, and Acellular Pertussis (formulation for age ≤6 years; Daptacel®, Infanrix®); **Td** = Diphtheria and Tetanus Toxoids (formulation for age ≥7 years; Decavac®,Tenivac™); **TT**= Tetanus toxoid (adsorbed [formulation for age ≥7 years]); **Tdap** = Diphtheria and Tetanus Toxoids, and Acellular Pertussis (Adacel® or Boostrix® [formulations for age ≥7 years]); **TIG** = Tetanus Immune Globulin

Administration Inject intramuscularly in the area of the vastus lateralis (midthigh laterally) or deltoid. Do not inject into gluteal area. Shake well prior to withdrawing dose; do not use if product does not form a suspension.

For patients at risk of hemorrhage following intramuscular injection, the ACIP recommends "it should be administered intramuscularly if, in the opinion of the physician familiar with the patient's bleeding risk, the vaccine can be administered by this route with reasonable safety. If the patient receives antihemophilia or other similar therapy, intramuscular vaccination can be scheduled shortly after such therapy is administered. A fine needle (23 gauge or smaller) can be used for the vaccination and firm pressure applied to the site (without rubbing) for at least 2 minutes. The patient should be instructed concerning the risk of hematoma from the injection." Patients on anticoagulant therapy should be considered to have the same bleeding risks and treated as those with clotting factor disorders (CDC, 2011).

Simultaneous administration of vaccines helps ensure the patients will be fully vaccinated by the appropriate age. Simultaneous administration of vaccines is defined as administering >1 vaccine on the same day at different anatomic sites. The use of licensed combination vaccines is generally preferred over separate injections of the equivalent components. Separate vaccines should not be combined in the same syringe unless indicated by product specific labeling. Separate needles and syringes should be used for each injection. The ACIP prefers each dose of a specific vaccine in a series come from the same manufacturer when possible. Adolescents and adults should be vaccinated while seated or lying down. In general, preterm infants should be vaccinated at the same chronological age as full-term infants (CDC, 2011).

Antipyretics have not been shown to prevent febrile seizures. Antipyretics may be used to treat fever or discomfort following vaccination (CDC, 2011). One study reported that routine prophylactic administration of acetaminophen to prevent fever prior to vaccination decreased the immune response of some vaccines; the clinical significance of this reduction in immune response has not been established (Prymula, 2009).

Monitoring Parameters Monitor for syncope for 15 minutes following administration. If seizure-like activity associated with syncope occurs, maintain patient in supine or Trendelenburg position to reestablish adequate cerebral perfusion.

Additional Information U.S. federal law requires that the name of medication, date of administration, the vaccine manufacturer, lot number of vaccine, and the administering person's name, title and address be entered into the patient's permanent medical record.

Dosage Forms Excipient information presented when available (limited, particularly for generics); consult specific product labeling.

Solution, Intramuscular:

Generic: 5 units (0.5 mL)

◆ **Tetanus Toxoid, Reduced Diphtheria Toxoid, and Acellular Pertussis, Adsorbed** *see* Diphtheria and Tetanus Toxoids, and Acellular Pertussis Vaccine *on page 630*

◆ **Tetcaine** *see* Tetracaine (Ophthalmic) *on page 2034*

Tetrabenazine (tet ra BEN a zeen)

Brand Names: U.S. Xenazine

Brand Names: Canada Nitoman; PMS-Tetrabenazine

Pharmacologic Category Central Monoamine-Depleting Agent

Use Treatment of chorea associated with Huntington's disease

Canadian labeling: Treatment of hyperkinetic movement disorders, including Huntington's chorea, hemiballismus, senile chorea, Tourette syndrome, and tardive dyskinesia

Pregnancy Risk Factor C

Prescribing and Access Restrictions Xenazine® is available only through specialty pharmacies. For more information regarding the procurement of Xenazine®, healthcare providers, patients, and caregivers may contact the Xenazine® Information Center (XIC) at 1-888-882-6013 or at:

Healthcare providers: http://www.xenazineusa.com/HCP/PrescribingXenazine/Default.aspx

Patients and caregivers: http://www.xenazineusa.com/AboutXenazine/Getting-Your-Prescription.aspx

Medication Guide Available Yes

Dosage Oral: Dose should be individualized; titrate slowly

Chorea associated with Huntington's disease: Adults:

Initial: 12.5 mg once daily, may increase to 12.5 mg twice daily after 1 week

Maintenance: May be increased by 12.5 mg/day at weekly intervals; doses >37.5 mg/day should be divided into 3 doses (maximum single dose: 25 mg)

Patients requiring doses >50 mg/day: Genotype for CYP2D6:

Extensive/intermediate metabolizers: Maximum: 100 mg/day; 37.5 mg/dose

Poor metabolizers: Maximum: 50 mg/day; 25 mg/dose

Concomitant use with strong CYP2D6 inhibitors (eg, fluoxetine, paroxetine, quinidine): Dose of tetrabenazine should be reduced by 50% in patients receiving strong CYP2D6 inhibitors, follow dosing for poor CYP2D6 metabolizers. Use caution when adding a CYP2D6 inhibitor to patients already taking tetrabenazine.

Note: If treatment is interrupted for >5 days, retitration is recommended. If treatment is interrupted for <5 days resume at previous maintenance dose.

Canadian labeling: Hyperkinetic movement disorders:

Adults: Initial: 12.5 mg twice daily (may be given 3 times/day); may be increased by 12.5 mg/day every 3-5 days; should be titrated slowly to maximal tolerated and effective dose (dose is individualized)

Usual maximum tolerated dosage: 25 mg 3 times/day; maximum recommended dose: 200 mg/day

Note: If there is no improvement at the maximum tolerated dose after 7 days, improvement is unlikely; discontinuation should be considered.

Elderly and/or debilitated patients: Consider initiation at lower doses; must be titrated slowly to individualize dosage

Dosage adjustment for toxicity: For toxicity/adverse reaction, including akathisia, restlessness, parkinsonism, insomnia, depression, suicidality, anxiety, sedation (intolerable): Suspend upward dosage titration and reduce dose; consider discontinuing if adverse reaction does not resolve (may be discontinued without tapering).

Dosage adjustment in renal impairment: No dosage adjustment provided in manufacturer's labeling (has not been studied).

Dosage adjustment in hepatic impairment: Use is contraindicated

Additional Information Complete prescribing information should be consulted for additional detail.

Dosage Forms Excipient information presented when available (limited, particularly for generics); consult specific product labeling.

Tablet, Oral:

Xenazine: 12.5 mg

Xenazine: 25 mg [scored]

Dosage Forms: Canada Excipient information presented when available (limited, particularly for generics); consult specific product labeling.

Tablet:

Nitoman™: 25 mg

Tetracaine (Systemic) (TET ra kane)

Brand Names: U.S. Pontocaine

Brand Names: Canada Pontocaine®

Index Terms Amethocaine Hydrochloride; Tetracaine Hydrochloride

Pharmacologic Category Local Anesthetic

Use Spinal anesthesia

Pregnancy Risk Factor C

Dosage Injection: Adults: Spinal anesthesia: **Note:** Dosage varies with the anesthetic procedure, the degree of anesthesia required, and the individual patient response; it is administered by subarachnoid injection for spinal anesthesia.

Perineal anesthesia: 5 mg

Perineal and lower extremities: 10 mg

Anesthesia extending up to costal margin: 15 mg; doses up to 20 mg may be given, but are reserved for exceptional cases

Low spinal anesthesia (saddle block): 2-5 mg

Dosage adjustment in renal impairment: No dosage adjustment provided in manufacturer's labeling.

Dosage adjustment in hepatic impairment: No dosage adjustment provided in manufacturer's labeling.

Additional Information Complete prescribing information should be consulted for additional detail.

Dosage Forms Excipient information presented when available (limited, particularly for generics); consult specific product labeling.

Solution, Injection, as hydrochloride [preservative free]:

Pontocaine: 1% (2 mL)

Generic: 1% (2 mL)

Solution Reconstituted, Injection, as hydrochloride:

Pontocaine: 20 mg (1 ea)

Tetracaine (Ophthalmic) (TET ra kane)

Brand Names: U.S. Altacaine; Tetcaine; TetraVisc; TetraVisc Forte

Brand Names: Canada Pontocaine®

Index Terms Amethocaine Hydrochloride; Tetracaine Hydrochloride

Pharmacologic Category Local Anesthetic

Use Local anesthesia for various ophthalmic procedures of short duration (eg, tonometry, gonioscopy); minor ophthalmic surgical procedures (eg, removal of corneal foreign bodies, suture removal); and for various diagnostic purposes (eg, conjunctival scrapings)

Pregnancy Risk Factor C

Dosage Ophthalmic: Adults:

Short-term (nonsurgical procedures) anesthesia: Instill 1-2 drops into affected eye just prior to evaluation

Minor surgical procedures: Instill 1-2 drops into affected eye every 5-10 minutes for up to 3 doses

Prolonged surgical procedures: Instill 1-2 drops into affected eye every 5-10 minutes for up to 5 doses

Dosage adjustment in renal impairment: No dosage adjustment provided in manufacturer's labeling.

Dosage adjustment in hepatic impairment: No dosage adjustment provided in manufacturer's labeling.

Additional Information Complete prescribing information should be consulted for additional detail.

Dosage Forms Excipient information presented when available (limited, particularly for generics); consult specific product labeling.

Solution, Ophthalmic, as hydrochloride:

Altacaine: 0.5% (1 ea, 15 mL, 30 mL)

Tetcaine: 0.5% (15 mL) [contains chlorobutanol (chlorobutol), edetate disodium]

TetraVisc: 0.5% (1 ea, 5 mL) [contains benzalkonium chloride]

TetraVisc Forte: 0.5% (1 ea, 5 mL) [contains benzalkonium chloride, edetate disodium]

Generic: 0.5% (1 mL, 2 mL, 15 mL)

Tetracaine (Topical) (TET ra kane)

Brand Names: U.S. Pontocaine

Brand Names: Canada Ametop™; Pontocaine®

Index Terms Amethocaine Hydrochloride; Tetracaine Hydrochloride

Pharmacologic Category Local Anesthetic

Use Applied to nose and throat for diagnostic procedures

Pregnancy Risk Factor C

Dosage Adults: Topical mucous membranes (rhinolaryngology): Used as a 0.25% or 0.5% solution by direct application or nebulization; total dose should not exceed 20 mg

Additional Information Complete prescribing information should be consulted for additional detail.

Dosage Forms Excipient information presented when available (limited, particularly for generics); consult specific product labeling.

Solution, Mouth/Throat, as hydrochloride:

Pontocaine: 2% (30 mL)

◆ **Tetracaine and Lidocaine** *see* Lidocaine and Tetracaine *on page 1215*

◆ **Tetracaine, Benzocaine, and Butamben** *see* Benzocaine, Butamben, and Tetracaine *on page 242*

◆ **Tetracaine Hydrochloride** *see* Tetracaine (Ophthalmic) *on page 2034*

◆ **Tetracaine Hydrochloride** *see* Tetracaine (Systemic) *on page 2033*

◆ **Tetracaine Hydrochloride** *see* Tetracaine (Topical) *on page 2034*

◆ **Tetracosactide** *see* Cosyntropin *on page 495*

Tetracycline (tet ra SYE kleen)

Brand Names: Canada Apo-Tetra; Nu-Tetra

Index Terms Achromycin; TCN; Tetracycline Hydrochloride

Pharmacologic Category Antibiotic, Tetracycline Derivative

Use Treatment of susceptible bacterial infections of both gram-positive and gram-negative organisms; also infections due to *Mycoplasma*, *Chlamydia*, and *Rickettsia*; indicated for acne, exacerbations of chronic bronchitis, and treatment of gonorrhea and syphilis in patients who are allergic to penicillin; as part of a multidrug regimen for *H. pylori* eradication to reduce the risk of duodenal ulcer recurrence

Unlabeled Use Treatment of periodontitis associated with presence of *Actinobacillus actinomycetemcomitans* (AA)

Pregnancy Risk Factor D

Pregnancy Considerations Tetracyclines cross the placenta and accumulate in developing teeth and long tubular bones. Tetracyclines may discolor fetal teeth following maternal use during pregnancy; the specific teeth involved and the portion of the tooth affected depends on the timing and duration of exposure relative to tooth calcification. The pharmacokinetics of tetracycline are not altered in pregnant patients with normal renal function. Hepatic toxicity during pregnancy, potentially associated with tetracycline use, has been widely reported in the literature. As a class, tetracyclines are generally considered second-line antibiotics in pregnant women and their use should be avoided (Mylonas, 2011; Whalley, 1966; Whalley, 1970).

Breast-Feeding Considerations Tetracycline is excreted into breast milk (Matsuda, 1984). According to the manufacturer, the decision to continue or discontinue breast-feeding during therapy should take into account the risk of exposure to the infant and the benefits of treatment to the mother. Tetracycline binds to calcium. The calcium in the maternal milk will decrease the amount of tetracycline absorbed by the breast-feeding infant (Mitrano, 2009). Nondose-related effects could include modification of bowel flora.

Contraindications Hypersensitivity to tetracycline or any component of the formulation

Warnings/Precautions Hazardous agent - use appropriate precautions for handling and disposal (NIOSH, 2012). Use with caution in patients with renal or hepatic impairment (eg, elderly); dosage modification required in patients with renal impairment since it may increase BUN as an antianabolic agent. Hepatotoxicity has been reported rarely; risk may be increased in patients with pre-existing hepatic or renal impairment. Pseudotumor cerebri has been reported with tetracycline use (usually resolves with discontinuation); outdated drug can cause nephropathy; use protective measure to avoid photosensitivity. Prolonged use may result in fungal or bacterial superinfection, including *C. difficile*-associated diarrhea (CDAD) and pseudomembranous colitis; CDAD has been observed >2 months postantibiotic treatment. May cause tissue hyperpigmentation, enamel hypoplasia, or permanent tooth discoloration; use of tetracyclines should be avoided during tooth development (children <8 years of age) unless other drugs are not likely to be effective or are contraindicated. Do not use during pregnancy. In addition to affecting tooth development, tetracycline use has been associated with retardation of skeletal development and reduced bone growth.

Adverse Reactions Frequency not defined.

Cardiovascular: Pericarditis

Central nervous system: Bulging fontanels in infants, increased intracranial pressure, paresthesia, pseudotumor cerebri

Dermatologic: Exfoliative dermatitis, photosensitivity, pigmentation of nails, pruritus

Gastrointestinal: Abdominal cramps, anorexia, antibiotic-associated pseudomembranous colitis, diarrhea, discoloration of teeth and enamel hypoplasia (young children), esophagitis, nausea, pancreatitis, staphylococcal enterocolitis, vomiting

Hematologic: Thrombophlebitis

Hepatic: Hepatotoxicity

Renal: Acute renal failure, azotemia, renal damage

Miscellaneous: Anaphylaxis, candidal superinfection, hypersensitivity reactions, superinfection

Drug Interactions

Metabolism/Transport Effects **Substrate** of CYP3A4 (major); **Note:** Assignment of Major/Minor substrate status based on clinically relevant drug interaction potential; **Inhibits** CYP3A4 (moderate)

Avoid Concomitant Use

Avoid concomitant use of Tetracycline with any of the following: BCG; Bosutinib; Ibrutinib; Ivabradine; Lomitapide; Pimozide; Retinoic Acid Derivatives; Simeprevir; Strontium Ranelate; Tolvaptan; Ulipristal

Increased Effect/Toxicity

Tetracycline may increase the levels/effects of: ARIPiprazole; Avanafil; Bosentan; Bosutinib; Budesonide (Systemic, Oral Inhalation); Colchicine; CYP3A4 Substrates; Dofetilide; Eplerenone; Everolimus; FentaNYL; Halofantrine; Ibrutinib; Imatinib; Ivabradine; Ivacaftor; Lomitapide; Lurasidone; Mipomersen; Neuromuscular-Blocking Agents; OxyCODONE; Pimecrolimus; Pimozide; Porfimer; Propafenone; QuiNINE; Ranolazine; Retinoic Acid Derivatives; Salmeterol; Saxagliptin; Simeprevir; Tolvaptan; Ulipristal; Vilazodone; Vitamin K Antagonists; Zuclopenthixol

Decreased Effect

Tetracycline may decrease the levels/effects of: Atovaquone; BCG; Ifosfamide; Penicillins; Sodium Picosulfate; Typhoid Vaccine

The levels/effects of Tetracycline may be decreased by: Antacids; Bile Acid Sequestrants; Bismuth; Bismuth Subsalicylate; Bosentan; Calcium Salts; CYP3A4 Inducers (Strong); Dabrafenib; Deferasirox; Herbs (CYP3A4 Inducers); Iron Salts; Lanthanum; Magnesium Salts; Mitotane; Multivitamins/Minerals (with ADEK, Folate, Iron); Multivitamins/Minerals (with AE, No Iron); Quinapril; Strontium Ranelate; Sucralfate; Sucroferric Oxyhydroxide; Tocilizumab; Zinc Salts

Ethanol/Nutrition/Herb Interactions

Food: Serum concentrations may be decreased if taken with dairy products. Take on an empty stomach 1 hour before or 2 hours after meals to increase total absorption. Administer around-the-clock to promote less variation in peak and trough serum levels.

Herb/Nutraceutical: Dong quai and St John's wort may also cause photosensitization. Management: Avoid dong quai and St John's wort.

Storage/Stability Outdated tetracyclines have caused a Fanconi-like syndrome (nausea, vomiting, acidosis, proteinuria, glycosuria, aminoaciduria, polydipsia, polyuria, hypokalemia). Protect oral dosage forms from light.

Mechanism of Action Inhibits bacterial protein synthesis by binding with the 30S and possibly the 50S ribosomal subunit(s) of susceptible bacteria; may also cause alterations in the cytoplasmic membrane

Pharmacodynamics/Kinetics

Absorption: Oral: 75%

Distribution: Small amount appears in bile

Relative diffusion from blood into CSF: Good only with inflammation (exceeds usual MICs)

CSF:blood level ratio: Inflamed meninges: 25%

Protein binding: ~65%

Half-life elimination: Normal renal function: 8-11 hours; End-stage renal disease: 57-108 hours

Time to peak, serum: Oral: 2-4 hours

Excretion: Urine (60% as unchanged drug); feces (as active form)

Dosage

Usual dosage range:

Children >8 years: Oral: 25-50 mg/kg/day in divided doses every 6 hours

Adults: Oral: 250-500 mg/dose every 6 hours

Indication-specific dosing:

Children ≥8 years: Oral:

Malaria, severe, treatment (unlabeled use): 25 mg/kg/day in divided doses every 6 hours (maximum dose: 250 mg every 6 hours) for 7 days with quinidine gluconate. **Note:** Quinidine gluconate duration is region specific; consult CDC for current recommendations (CDC, 2009).

Malaria, uncomplicated, treatment (unlabeled use): 25 mg/kg/day in divided doses every 6 hours (maximum dose: 250 mg every 6 hours) for 7 days with quinine sulfate. **Note:** Quinine sulfate duration is region specific; consult CDC for current recommendations (CDC, 2009).

Adults: Oral:

Acne: 250-500 twice daily

Chronic bronchitis, acute exacerbation: 500 mg 4 times daily

Erlichiosis: 500 mg 4 times daily for 7-14 days

Malaria, severe, treatment (unlabeled use): 250 mg 4 times daily for 7 days with quinidine gluconate. **Note:** Quinidine gluconate duration is region specific; consult CDC for current recommendations (CDC, 2009).

Malaria, uncomplicated, treatment (unlabeled use): 250 mg 4 times daily for 7 days with quinine sulfate. **Note:** Quinine sulfate duration is region specific; consult CDC for current recommendations (CDC, 2009).

Peptic ulcer disease: Eradication of *Helicobacter pylori*: 500 mg 2-4 times daily depending on regimen; requires combination therapy with at least one other antibiotic and an acid-suppressing agent (proton pump inhibitor or H_2 blocker)

Periodontitis (unlabeled use): 250 mg every 6 hours until improvement (usually 10 days)

Syphilis:

Early syphilis (primary or secondary infection): 500 mg 4 times daily for 14 days. **Note:** Alternative treatment for non-pregnant, penicillin-allergic patients (CDC, 2010).

Latent syphilis (late or of unknown duration): 500 mg 4 times daily for 28 days. **Note:** Alternative treatment for non-pregnant, penicillin-allergic patients. Effectiveness not well documented; close clinical and serologic follow-up recommended (CDC, 2010).

Vibrio cholerae: 500 mg 4 times/day for 3 days

Dosage adjustment in renal impairment:

Cl_{cr} 50-80 mL/minute: Administer every 8-12 hours

Cl_{cr} 10-50 mL/minute: Administer every 12-24 hours

Cl_{cr} <10 mL/minute: Administer every 24 hours

Dialysis: Slightly dialyzable (5% to 20%) via hemo- and peritoneal dialysis or via continuous arteriovenous or venovenous hemofiltration; no supplemental dosage necessary

Dosage adjustment in hepatic impairment: No dosage adjustment necessary. Use with caution.

Dietary Considerations Take on an empty stomach (ie, 1 hour prior to, or 2 hours after meals). Take at least 1-2 hours prior to, or 4 hours after antacid.

Administration Should be administered on an empty stomach (ie, 1 hour prior to, or 2 hours after meals) to increase total absorption. Administer at least 1-2 hours prior to, or 4 hours after antacid because aluminum and magnesium cations may chelate with tetracycline and reduce its total absorption.

Hazardous agent; use appropriate precautions for handling and disposal (NIOSH, 2012).

Monitoring Parameters Renal, hepatic, and hematologic function test, temperature, WBC, cultures and sensitivity, appetite, mental status

Dosage Forms Excipient information presented when available (limited, particularly for generics); consult specific product labeling.

Capsule, Oral, as hydrochloride:

Generic: 250 mg, 500 mg

Extemporaneous Preparations Hazardous agent: Use appropriate precautions for handling and disposal.

A 25 mg/mL oral suspension may be made using capsules. Empty the contents of six 500 mg capsules into mortar. Add a small amount (~20 mL) of a 1:1 mixture of Ora-Sweet® and Ora-Plus® and mix to a uniform paste; mix while adding the vehicle in geometric proportions to **almost** 120 mL; transfer to a calibrated bottle, rinse mortar with vehicle, and add quantity of vehicle sufficient to make 120 mL. Label "shake well" and "refrigerate". Stable 28 days refrigerated.

Nahata MC, Pai VB, and Hipple TF, *Pediatric Drug Formulations*, 5th ed, Cincinnati, OH: Harvey Whitney Books Co, 2004.

- ◆ **Tetracycline Hydrochloride** *see* Tetracycline *on page 2034*
- ◆ **Tetra-Formula Nighttime Sleep [OTC]** *see* DiphenhydrAMINE (Systemic) *on page 622*
- ◆ **Tetrahydrocannabinol** *see* Dronabinol *on page 674*
- ◆ **Tetraiodothyronine and Triiodothyronine** *see* Thyroid, Desiccated *on page 2052*
- ◆ **2,2,2-tetramine** *see* Trientine *on page 2125*

Tetrastarch (TET ra starch)

Brand Names: U.S. Voluven

Brand Names: Canada Volulyte; Voluven

Index Terms Etherified Starch; HES; HES 130/0.4; Hydroxyethyl Starch

Pharmacologic Category Plasma Volume Expander, Colloid

Use Blood volume expander used in treatment and prevention of hypovolemia

Pregnancy Risk Factor C

Dosage I.V. infusion: Plasma volume expansion: **Note:** With severe dehydration, administer crystalloid first. Daily dose and rate of infusion dependent on amount of blood lost, on maintenance or restoration of hemodynamics, and on amount of hemodilution. Titrate to individual colloid needs, hemodynamics, and hydration status. Do not use in the critically ill including patients with sepsis, those with pre-existing renal dysfunction or receiving dialysis, those with pre-existing bleeding disorders or those with intracranial bleeding.

Children ≤12 years and Adolescents: May administer up to 50 mL/kg/day (or up to 3500 mL per day in a 70 kg patient); may administer repetitively over several days.

Mean daily dose ± SD in pediatric clinical trials:

Children <2 years: 16 ± 9 mL/kg

Children 2-12 years: 36 ± 11 mL/kg

Adults: May administer up to 50 mL/kg/day (or up to 3500 mL per day in a 70 kg patient); may administer repetitively over several days

Dosage adjustment in renal impairment: Avoid use in patients with pre-existing renal dysfunction. Use is contraindicated in oliguric/anuric renal failure unrelated to hypovolemia or patients receiving dialysis. Discontinue use at the first sign of renal injury.

Dosage adjustment in hepatic impairment: No dosage adjustment provided in manufacturer's labeling; use is contraindicated in severe liver disease.

Additional Information Complete prescribing information should be consulted for additional detail.

Dosage Forms Excipient information presented when available (limited, particularly for generics); consult specific product labeling.

Solution, Intravenous:

Voluven: 6% (500 mL) [dehp free, latex free, pvc free]

Dosage Forms: Canada

Excipient information presented when available (limited, particularly for generics); consult specific product labeling.

Infusion, premixed in isotonic electrolyte solution:

Volulyte: 6% (250 mL, 500 mL)

- ◆ **TetraVisc** *see* Tetracaine (Ophthalmic) *on page 2034*
- ◆ **TetraVisc Forte** *see* Tetracaine (Ophthalmic) *on page 2034*
- ◆ **Teva-Acebutolol (Can)** *see* Acebutolol *on page 28*
- ◆ **Teva-Acyclovir (Can)** *see* Acyclovir (Systemic) *on page 42*
- ◆ **Teva-Alendronate (Can)** *see* Alendronate *on page 69*
- ◆ **Teva-Alfuzosin PR (Can)** *see* Alfuzosin *on page 73*
- ◆ **Teva-Alprazolam (Can)** *see* ALPRAZolam *on page 81*
- ◆ **Teva-Amiodarone (Can)** *see* Amiodarone *on page 101*
- ◆ **Teva-Amlodipine (Can)** *see* AmLODIPine *on page 109*
- ◆ **Teva-Anastrozole (Can)** *see* Anastrozole *on page 137*
- ◆ **Teva-Atenolol (Can)** *see* Atenolol *on page 186*
- ◆ **Teva-Atomoxetine (Can)** *see* AtoMOXetine *on page 187*
- ◆ **Teva-Azathioprine (Can)** *see* AzaTHIOprine *on page 208*
- ◆ **Teva-Candesartan (Can)** *see* Candesartan *on page 327*
- ◆ **Teva-Candesartan/HCTZ (Can)** *see* Candesartan and Hydrochlorothiazide *on page 329*
- ◆ **Teva-Capecitabine (Can)** *see* Capecitabine *on page 329*
- ◆ **Teva-Captopril (Can)** *see* Captopril *on page 333*
- ◆ **Teva-Carbamazepine (Can)** *see* CarBAMazepine *on page 336*
- ◆ **Teva-Cefadroxil (Can)** *see* Cefadroxil *on page 361*
- ◆ **Teva-Chlorpromazine (Can)** *see* ChlorproMAZINE *on page 415*
- ◆ **Teva-Citalopram (Can)** *see* Citalopram *on page 440*
- ◆ **Teva-Clarithromycin (Can)** *see* Clarithromycin *on page 446*
- ◆ **Teva-Clindamycin (Can)** *see* Clindamycin (Systemic) *on page 451*
- ◆ **Teva-Clonazepam (Can)** *see* ClonazePAM *on page 465*
- ◆ **Teva-Clopidogrel (Can)** *see* Clopidogrel *on page 471*
- ◆ **Teva-Combo Sterinebs (Can)** *see* Ipratropium and Albuterol *on page 1113*

- ◆ **Teva-Tamsulosin (Can)** *see* Tamsulosin *on page 1990*
- ◆ **Teva-Telmisartan (Can)** *see* Telmisartan *on page 2002*
- ◆ **Teva-Telmisartan HCTZ (Can)** *see* Telmisartan and Hydrochlorothiazide *on page 2004*
- ◆ **Teva-Terazosin (Can)** *see* Terazosin *on page 2015*
- ◆ **Teva-Terbinafine (Can)** *see* Terbinafine (Systemic) *on page 2017*
- ◆ **Teva-Theophylline SR (Can)** *see* Theophylline *on page 2042*
- ◆ **Teva-Ticlopidine (Can)** *see* Ticlopidine *on page 2059*
- ◆ **Teva-Timolol (Can)** *see* Timolol (Systemic) *on page 2064*
- ◆ **TEVA-Tramadol/Acetaminophen (Can)** *see* Acetaminophen and Tramadol *on page 33*
- ◆ **Teva-Trazodone (Can)** *see* TraZODone *on page 2112*
- ◆ **Teva-Triamterene HCTZ (Can)** *see* Hydrochlorothiazide and Triamterene *on page 1006*
- ◆ **Teva-Valsartan (Can)** *see* Valsartan *on page 2154*
- ◆ **Teva-Valsartan HCTZ (Can)** *see* Valsartan and Hydrochlorothiazide *on page 2156*
- ◆ **Teva-Venlafaxine XR (Can)** *see* Venlafaxine *on page 2178*
- ◆ **Teva-Zolmitriptan (Can)** *see* ZOLMitriptan *on page 2240*
- ◆ **Teva-Zolmitriptan OD (Can)** *see* ZOLMitriptan *on page 2240*
- ◆ **Teveten** *see* Eprosartan *on page 729*
- ◆ **Teveten® (Can)** *see* Eprosartan *on page 729*
- ◆ **Teveten® HCT** *see* Eprosartan and Hydrochlorothiazide *on page 731*
- ◆ **Teveten® Plus (Can)** *see* Eprosartan and Hydrochlorothiazide *on page 731*
- ◆ **Tev-Tropin** *see* Somatropin *on page 1934*
- ◆ **Texacort** *see* Hydrocortisone (Topical) *on page 1011*
- ◆ **TG** *see* Thioguanine *on page 2045*
- ◆ **6-TG (error-prone abbreviation)** *see* Thioguanine *on page 2045*
- ◆ **TH9507** *see* Tesamorelin *on page 2025*

Thalidomide (tha LI doe mide)

Brand Names: U.S. Thalomid

Brand Names: Canada Thalomid

Pharmacologic Category Angiogenesis Inhibitor; Antineoplastic Agent; Immunomodulator, Systemic

Use Treatment of newly-diagnosed multiple myeloma; treatment and maintenance of cutaneous manifestations of erythema nodosum leprosum (ENL)

Unlabeled Use Treatment of refractory Crohn's disease; treatment of chronic graft-versus-host disease (GVHD) in hematopoietic stem cell transplantation; AIDS-related aphthous stomatitis; Waldenström's macroglobulinemia; maintenance therapy of multiple myeloma (following autologous stem cell transplant); systemic light chain amyloidosis

Pregnancy Risk Factor X

Pregnancy Considerations **[U.S. Boxed Warning]: Thalidomide may cause severe birth defects or embryo-fetal death if taken during pregnancy. Thalidomide cannot be used in women who are pregnant or may become pregnant during therapy as even a single dose may cause birth defects. In order to decrease the risk of fetal exposure, thalidomide is available only through a special restricted distribution program (Thalomid REMS™).** Reproduction studies in animals and data from pregnant women have shown evidence of fetal abnormalities; use is contraindicated in women who are or may become pregnant. Anomalies observed in humans include amelia, phocomelia, bone defects, ear and eye abnormalities, facial palsy, congenital heart defects, urinary and genital tract malformations; mortality in ~40% of infants at or shortly after birth has also been reported.

Women of reproductive potential must avoid pregnancy 4 weeks prior to therapy, during therapy, during therapy interruptions, and for ≥4 weeks after therapy is discontinued. Two forms of effective contraception or total abstinence from heterosexual intercourse must be used by females who are not infertile or who have not had a hysterectomy. A negative pregnancy test (sensitivity of at least 50 mIU/mL) 10-14 days prior to therapy, within 24 hours prior to beginning therapy, weekly during the first 4 weeks, and every 4 weeks (every 2 weeks for women with irregular menstrual cycles) thereafter is required for women of childbearing potential. Thalidomide must be immediately discontinued for a missed period, abnormal pregnancy test or abnormal menstrual bleeding; refer patient to a reproductive toxicity specialist if pregnancy occurs during treatment.

Females of reproductive potential must also avoid contact with thalidomide capsules.

Thalidomide is also present in the semen of males. Males (even those vasectomized) must use a latex or synthetic condom during any sexual contact with women of childbearing potential and for up to 28 days following discontinuation of therapy. Males taking thalidomide must not donate sperm.

The parent or legal guardian for patients between 12-18 years of age must agree to ensure compliance with the required guidelines.

If pregnancy occurs during treatment, thalidomide must be immediately discontinued and the patient referred to a reproductive toxicity specialist. Any suspected fetal exposure to thalidomide must be reported to the FDA via the MedWatch program (1-800-FDA-1088) and to Celgene Corporation (1-888-423-5436). In Canada, thalidomide is available only through a restricted-distribution program called RevAid® (1-888-738-2431).

Breast-Feeding Considerations It is not known if thalidomide is excreted in breast milk. Due to the potential for serious adverse reactions in the infant, a decision should be made to discontinue nursing or discontinue treatment with thalidomide, taking into account the importance of treatment to the mother. Use in breast-feeding women is contraindicated in the Canadian labeling.

Prescribing and Access Restrictions U.S.: As a requirement of the REMS program, access to this medication is restricted. Thalidomide is approved for marketing only under a special distribution program, the Thalomid REMS™ (www.celgeneriskmanagment.com or 1-888-423-5436), which has been approved by the FDA. Prescribers, patients, and pharmacies must be certified with the program to prescribe or dispense thalidomide. No more than a 4-week supply should be dispensed. Blister packs should be dispensed intact (do not repackage capsules). Prescriptions must be filled within 7 days (for females of reproductive potential) or within 30 days (for all other patients) after authorization number obtained. Subsequent prescriptions may be filled only if fewer than 7 days of therapy remain on the previous prescription. A new prescription is required for further dispensing (a telephone prescription may not be accepted.) Pregnancy testing is required for females of childbearing potential.

Canada: Access to thalidomide is restricted through a controlled distribution program called RevAid®. Only physicians and pharmacists enrolled in this program are authorized to prescribe or dispense thalidomide. Patients must be enrolled in the program by their physicians.

Further information is available at www.RevAid.ca or by calling 1-888-738-2431.

Medication Guide Available Yes

Contraindications Hypersensitivity to thalidomide or any component of the formulation; pregnancy

Canadian labeling: Additional contraindications (not in U.S. labeling): Hypersensitivity to lenalidomide; breast-feeding

Warnings/Precautions Hazardous agent - use appropriate precautions for handling and disposal (NIOSH, 2012).

[U.S. Boxed Warning]: Associated with an increased risk for venous thromboembolism, including deep vein thrombosis (DVT) and pulmonary embolism (PE) in multiple myeloma patients; the risk is increased when used in combination with dexamethasone. Monitor for signs and symptoms of thromboembolism (shortness of breath, chest pain, or arm or leg swelling) and instruct patients to seek prompt medical attention with development of these symptoms. Patients at risk may benefit from prophylactic anticoagulation. Arterial thromboembolic events (ATEE) including fatal myocardial infarction, cerebrovascular accident, and transient ischemic attack have also been reported; risk appears greatest within first 5 months of therapy. The NCCN multiple myeloma guidelines (v.1.2013) recommend anticoagulant prophylaxis with thalidomide-based therapy. Anticoagulant prophylaxis should be individualized and selected based on the venous thromboembolism risk of the combination treatment regimen, using the safest and easiest to administer (Palumbo, 2008). The Canadian labeling recommends anticoagulant prophylaxis for at least the first 5 months of thalidomide-based therapy. Patients with a high tumor burden may be at risk for tumor lysis syndrome; monitor closely; institute appropriate management for hyperuricemia.

May cause neutropenia; avoid initiating therapy if ANC <750/mm^3; monitor blood counts. Persistent neutropenia may require treatment interruption. Anemia and thrombocytopenia have also been observed. May cause bradycardia; use with caution in patients with cardiovascular disease. May require dose reduction or discontinuation. Use caution when administering with concomitant medications which may decrease heart rate. Stevens-Johnson syndrome (SJS) and toxic epidermal necrolysis (TEN) have been reported (may be fatal); withhold therapy and evaluate with skin rashes; permanently discontinue if rash is exfoliative, purpuric, bullous or if SJS or TEN is suspected. Hypersensitivity, including erythematous macular rash, possibly associated with fever, tachycardia and hypotension has been reported. May require treatment interruption for severe reactions; discontinue if recurs with rechallenge.

Increased incidence of second primary malignancies (SPMs), including acute myeloid leukemia (AML) and myelodysplastic syndrome (MDS), has been observed in previously untreated multiple myeloma patients receiving thalidomide in combination with melphalan, and prednisone. In addition to AML and MDS, solid tumors have been reported with thalidomide maintenance treatment for multiple myeloma (Usmani, 2012). Carefully evaluate patients for SPMs prior to and during treatment and manage as clinically indicated.

Associated with the development of peripheral neuropathy, which may be irreversible; generally occurs following chronic use (over months), but may occur with short-term use; onset may be delayed. Use caution with other medications which may also cause peripheral neuropathy. Monitor for signs/symptoms of neuropathy monthly for the first 3 months of therapy and regularly thereafter. Electrophysiological testing may be considered at baseline and every 6 months to detect asymptomatic neuropathy. Consider immediate discontinuation (if clinically appropriate) in patients who develop neuropathy. Reinitiate therapy only if neuropathy returns to baseline; may require dosage reduction or permanent discontinuation. Seizures have been reported in postmarketing data; use caution in patients with a history of seizures, concurrent therapy with drugs which alter seizure threshold, or conditions which predispose to seizures. May cause dizziness, drowsiness, and/or somnolence; caution patients about performing tasks which require mental alertness (eg, operating machinery or driving). Avoid concomitant medications which may exacerbate these symptoms; dose reductions may be necessary for excessive drowsiness or somnolence. May cause orthostatic hypotension; use with caution in patients who would not tolerate transient hypotensive episodes. When arising from a recumbent position, advise patients to sit upright for a few minutes prior to standing. Constipation may commonly occur. May require treatment interruption or dosage reduction. Certain adverse reactions (constipation, fatigue, weakness, nausea, hypokalemia, hyperglycemia, DVT, pulmonary embolism, atrial fibrillation) are more likely in elderly patients. In studies conducted prior to the use of highly active antiretroviral therapy, use was associated with increased viral loads in HIV infected patients. Monitor viral load after the 1st and 3rd months of therapy and every 3 months thereafter.

Potentially significant drug-drug interactions may exist, requiring dose or frequency adjustment, additional monitoring, and/or selection of alternative therapy. Patients should not donate blood during thalidomide treatment and for 1 month after therapy discontinuation

[U.S. Boxed Warning]: Thalidomide may cause severe birth defects or embryo-fetal death if taken during pregnancy. Thalidomide cannot be used in women who are pregnant or may become pregnant during therapy as even a single dose may cause birth defects. In order to decrease the risk of fetal exposure, thalidomide is available only through a special restricted distribution program (Thalomid REMS™). Use is contraindicated in women who are or may become pregnant. Pregnancy must be excluded prior to therapy initiation with 2 negative pregnancy tests. Women of reproductive potential must avoid pregnancy 4 weeks prior to therapy, during therapy, during therapy interruptions, and for ≥4 weeks after therapy is discontinued; two reliable methods of birth control, or abstinence from heterosexual intercourse, must be used. Males taking thalidomide (even those vasectomized) must use a latex or synthetic condom during any sexual contact with women of childbearing potential and for up to 28 days following discontinuation of therapy. Males taking thalidomide must not donate sperm. Some forms of contraception may not be appropriate in certain patients. An intrauterine device (IUD) or implantable contraceptive may increase the risk of infection or bleeding; estrogen containing products may increase the risk of thromboembolism.

[U.S. Boxed Warning]: Thalidomide should only be prescribed to patients who can understand and comply with the conditions of the Thalomid REMS™ program. Prescribers, patients, and pharmacies must be certified with the program to prescribe or dispense thalidomide.

Adverse Reactions

>10%:

Cardiovascular: Edema (57%), thrombosis/embolism (23%; grade 3: 13%, grade 4: 9%), hypotension (16%)

Central nervous system: Fatigue (79%; grade 3: 14%, grade 4: 3%), somnolence (36% to 38%), dizziness (4% to 20%), sensory neuropathy (54%), confusion (28%), anxiety/agitation (9% to 26%), fever (19% to 23%), motor neuropathy (22%), headache (13% to 19%)

Dermatologic: Rash/desquamation (21% to 30%; grade 3: 4%), dry skin (21%), maculopapular rash (4% to 19%), acne (3% to 11%)
Endocrine & metabolic: Hypocalcemia (72%)
Gastrointestinal: Constipation (3% to 55%), nausea (4% to 28%), anorexia (3% to 28%), weight loss (23%), weight gain (22%), diarrhea (4% to 19%), oral moniliasis (4% to 11%)
Hematologic: Leukopenia (17% to 35%), neutropenia (31%), anemia (6% to 13%), lymphadenopathy (6% to 13%)
Hepatic: AST increased (3% to 25%), bilirubin increased (14%)
Neuromuscular & skeletal: Muscle weakness (40%), tremor (4% to 26%), weakness (6% to 22%), myalgia (17%), paresthesia (6% to 16%), arthralgia (13%)
Renal: Hematuria (11%)
Respiratory: Dyspnea (42%)
Miscellaneous: Diaphoresis (13%)

1% to 10%:
Cardiovascular: Peripheral edema (3% to 8%), facial edema (4%)
Central nervous system: Insomnia (9%), nervousness (3% to 9%), malaise (8%), vertigo (8%), pain (3% to 8%)
Dermatologic: Dermatitis (fungal 4% to 9%), pruritus (3% to 8%), nail disorder (3% to 4%)
Endocrine & metabolic: Hyperlipemia (6% to 9%)
Gastrointestinal: Xerostomia (8% to 9%), flatulence (8%), tooth pain (4%)
Genitourinary: Impotence (3% to 8%)
Hepatic: LFTs abnormal (9%)
Neuromuscular & skeletal: Neuropathy (8%), back pain (4% to 6%), neck pain (4%), neck rigidity (4%)
Renal: Albuminuria (3% to 8%)
Respiratory: Pharyngitis (4% to 8%), rhinitis (4%), sinusitis (3% to 8%)
Miscellaneous: Infection (6% to 8%)

Postmarketing and/or case reports (limited to important or life-threatening): Acute renal failure, alkaline phosphatase increased, ALT increased, amenorrhea, angioedema, aphthous stomatitis, arrhythmia, atrial fibrillation, bile duct obstruction, bradycardia, BUN increased, carpal tunnel, cerebral vascular accident, CML, creatinine clearance decreased, creatinine increased, deafness, depression, diplopia, dysesthesia, ECG abnormalities, enuresis, eosinophilia, epistaxis, erythema multiforme, erythema nodosum, erythroleukemia, exfoliative dermatitis, febrile neutropenia, foot drop, galactorrhea, granulocytopenia, gynecomastia, hearing loss, hepatomegaly, Hodgkin's disease, hypercalcemia, hyper-/hypokalemia, hypersensitivity, hypertension, hyper-/hypothyroidism, hypersensitivity, hyperuricemia, hypomagnesemia, hyponatremia, hypoproteinemia, intestinal obstruction, intestinal perforation, interstitial pneumonitis, LDH increased, lethargy, leukocytosis, loss of consciousness, lymphedema, lymphopenia, mental status changes, metrorrhagia, MI, myxedema, nystagmus, oliguria, orthostatic hypotension, pancytopenia, paresthesia, petechiae, peripheral neuritis, photosensitivity, pleural effusion, prothrombin time changes, psychosis, pulmonary embolus, pulmonary hypertension, purpura, Raynaud's syndrome, renal failure, secondary malignancy (AML, MDS, solid tumors), seizure, sepsis, septic shock, sexual dysfunction, sick sinus syndrome, status epilepticus, Stevens-Johnson syndrome, stomach ulcer, stupor, suicide attempt, syncope, tachycardia, thrombocytopenia, toxic epidermal necrolysis, transient ischemic attack, tumor lysis syndrome, urticaria

Drug Interactions

Metabolism/Transport Effects None known.

Avoid Concomitant Use

Avoid concomitant use of Thalidomide with any of the following: Abatacept; Anakinra; Azelastine (Nasal); BCG; Canakinumab; Certolizumab Pegol; CloZAPine; Natalizumab; Paraldehyde; Pimecrolimus; Rilonacept; Tacrolimus (Topical); Tocilizumab; Tofacitinib; Vaccines (Live)

Increased Effect/Toxicity

Thalidomide may increase the levels/effects of: Abatacept; Alcohol (Ethyl); Anakinra; Azelastine (Nasal); Bisphosphonate Derivatives; Buprenorphine; Canakinumab; Certolizumab Pegol; CloZAPine; CNS Depressants; Hydrocodone; Leflunomide; Methotrimeprazine; Metyrosine; Mirtazapine; Natalizumab; Pamidronate; Paraldehyde; Pramipexole; Rilonacept; ROPINIRole; Rotigotine; Selective Serotonin Reuptake Inhibitors; Tofacitinib; Vaccines (Live); Zoledronic Acid; Zolpidem

The levels/effects of Thalidomide may be increased by: Brimonidine (Topical); Denosumab; Dexamethasone (Systemic); Doxylamine; Droperidol; HydrOXYzine; Magnesium Sulfate; Methotrimeprazine; Perampanel; Pimecrolimus; Roflumilast; Sodium Oxybate; Tacrolimus (Topical); Tapentadol; Tocilizumab; Trastuzumab

Decreased Effect

Thalidomide may decrease the levels/effects of: BCG; Coccidioidin Skin Test; Sipuleucel-T; Vaccines (Inactivated); Vaccines (Live)

The levels/effects of Thalidomide may be decreased by: Echinacea

Ethanol/Nutrition/Herb Interactions

Ethanol: May increase CNS depression; monitor for increased effects with coadministration. Caution patients about effects.

Herb/Nutraceutical: Avoid cat's claw and echinacea (have immunostimulant properties; consider therapy modifications).

Storage/Stability Store at 20°C to 25°C (68°F to 77°F); excursions permitted to 15°C to 30°C (59°F to 86°F). Protect from light. Keep in original package.

Mechanism of Action Immunomodulatory and antiangiogenic characteristics; immunologic effects may vary based on conditions; may suppress excessive tumor necrosis factor-alpha production in patients with ENL, yet may increase plasma tumor necrosis factor-alpha levels in HIV-positive patients. In multiple myeloma, thalidomide is associated with an increase in natural killer cells and increased levels of interleukin-2 and interferon gamma. Other proposed mechanisms of action include suppression of angiogenesis, prevention of free-radical-mediated DNA damage, increased cell mediated cytotoxic effects, and altered expression of cellular adhesion molecules.

Pharmacodynamics/Kinetics

Absorption: Slow, good
Protein binding: 55% to 66%
Metabolism: Nonenzymatic hydrolysis in plasma; forms multiple metabolites
Bioavailability: Capsule: 90%
Half-life elimination: 5.5-7.3 hours
Time to peak, plasma: 2-5 hours
Excretion: Urine (92%; <41% as unchanged drug); feces (<2%)

Dosage

Children ≥3 years: Oral: Chronic graft-versus-host disease (refractory), treatment (unlabeled second-line use; limited data): 3 mg/kg 4 times daily (dose adjusted to goal thalidomide concentration of ≥5 mcg/mL 2 hours post-dose) (Vogelsang, 1992) **or** Initial: 3-6 mg/kg/day in 2-4 divided doses; target dose 12 mg/kg/day; Maximum daily dose: 800 mg (Rovelli, 1998)

Children ≥12 years and Adults: Oral: Cutaneous erythema nodosum leprosum (ENL): Initial: 100-300 mg once daily at bedtime

Adjustments to initial dose:

Patients weighing <50 kg: Initiate at lower end of the dosing range

Severe cutaneous reaction or patients previously requiring high dose may be initiated at 400 mg daily; doses may be divided

Duration and tapering/maintenance:

Maintenance: Dosing should continue until active reaction subsides (usually at least 2 weeks), then tapered in 50 mg decrements every 2-4 weeks

Patients who flare during tapering or with a history of requiring prolonged maintenance should be maintained on the minimum dosage necessary to control the reaction. Efforts to taper should be repeated every 3-6 months, in decrements of 50 mg every 2-4 weeks.

Adults: Oral:

Multiple myeloma: **Note:** Details concerning dosing for multiple myeloma with combination regimens should also be consulted.

200 mg once daily at bedtime (in combination with dexamethasone 40 mg daily on days 1-4, 9-12, and 17-20 of a 28-day treatment cycle)

In combination with bortezomib and dexamethasone (unlabeled combination): Induction therapy: 100 mg once daily for the first 14 days, then 200 mg once daily for 3 (21-day) cycles (Cavo, 2010) **or** 100 mg once daily for up to 8 (21-day) cycles (Kaufman, 2010)

In combination with melphalan and prednisone (unlabeled combination in U.S.): 200-400 mg once daily (Facon, 2007) **or** 100 mg once daily (Palumbo, 2008)

Canadian labeling: Adults ≥65 years: 200 mg once daily; maximum: 12 six-week cycles (in combination with melphalan and prednisone)

Multiple myeloma, maintenance (following autologous stem cell transplant; unlabeled use): 200 mg once daily starting 3-6 months after transplant; continue until disease progression or unacceptable toxicity (Brinker, 2006) or 100 mg once daily starting 42-60 days following transplant; increase to 200 mg once daily after 2 weeks if tolerated; continue for up to 12 months (in combination with prednisolone) (Spencer, 2009)

AIDS-related aphthous stomatitis (unlabeled use): 200 mg once daily at bedtime for up to 8 weeks, if no response, then 200 mg twice daily for 4 weeks (Jacobson, 1997)

Chronic graft-versus-host disease (refractory), treatment (unlabeled second-line use; optimum dose not determined): Initial: 100 mg once daily at bedtime, with dose escalation up to 400 mg daily in 3-4 divided doses (Wolff, 2010) **or** Initial: 50-100 mg 3 times daily; maximum dose: 600-1200 mg daily (Kulkarni, 2003) **or** 200 mg 4 times daily (dose adjusted to goal thalidomide concentration of ≥5 mcg/mL 2 hours postdose) (Vogelsang, 1992) **or** 100-300 mg 4 times daily (Parker, 1995)

Crohn's disease, refractory (unlabeled use): 50-100 mg once daily at bedtime (Vasiliauskas, 1999) **or** 200-300 mg once daily at bedtime (Ehrenpreis, 1999)

Systemic light chain amyloidosis (unlabeled use): 200 mg once daily (starting dose 50-100 mg once daily; titrate at 4-week intervals) in combination with cyclophosphamide and dexamethasone (Wechalekar, 2007)

Waldenström's macroglobulinemia (unlabeled use): 200 mg once daily for up to 52 weeks (in combination with rituximab) (Treon, 2008)

Dosing adjustment for toxicity:

ANC ≤750/mm^3: Withhold treatment if clinically appropriate

Multiple myeloma:

U.S. labeling: Constipation, oversedation, peripheral neuropathy: Temporarily withhold or continue with a reduced dose

Canadian labeling:

ANC <1500/mm^3: Withhold melphalan and prednisone for 1 week; resume melphalan and prednisone after 1 week if ANC >1500/mm^3 **or** if ANC 1000-1500/mm^3 reduce melphalan dose by 50% **or** if ANC <1000/mm^3 adjust chemotherapy dose based on clinical status of patient.

Constipation, oversedation: Temporarily withhold thalidomide treatment or continue with a reduced dose

Peripheral neuropathy, Grade 1 (paresthesia, weakness and/or loss of reflexes) without loss of function): Evaluate patient and consider dose reduction with worsening of symptoms; symptom improvement may not follow dose reduction, however.

Peripheral neuropathy, Grade 2 (interferes with function but not with daily activities), Grade 3 (interferes with daily activities), or Grade 4 (disabling neuropathy): Discontinue thalidomide treatment

Thromboembolic events: Withhold therapy and initiate standard anticoagulant treatment; may resume thalidomide therapy at original dose following stabilization of patient and resolution of thromboembolic event; maintain anticoagulant treatment for duration of thalidomide therapy

Unlabeled recommendation (Richardson, 2012): Peripheral neuropathy:

Grade 1: Reduce dose by 50%

Grade 2: Temporarily interrupt therapy; once resolved to ≤ grade 1, resume therapy with a 50% dosage reduction (if clinically appropriate)

Grade 3 or higher: Discontinue therapy

Dosage adjustment in renal impairment: No dosage adjustment necessary for patients with renal impairment and on dialysis (per manufacturer). In a study of 6 patients with end-stage renal disease on dialysis, although clearance was increased by dialysis, a supplemental dose was not needed (Eriksson, 2003).

Multiple myeloma: An evaluation of 29 newly-diagnosed myeloma patients with renal failure (serum creatinine ≥2 mg/dL) treated with thalidomide and dexamethasone (some also received cyclophosphamide) found that toxicities and efficacy were similar to patients with normal renal function (Seol, 2010). A study evaluating induction therapy with thalidomide and dexamethasone in 31 newly-diagnosed myeloma patients with renal failure (Cl_{cr} <50 mL/minute), including 16 patients with severe renal impairment (Cl_{cr} <30 mL/minute) and 7 patients on chronic hemodialysis found that toxicities were similar to patients without renal impairment and that thalidomide and dexamethasone could be administered safely (Tosi, 2009).

Dosage adjustment in hepatic impairment: No dosage adjustment provided in manufacturer's labeling (has not been studied). However, thalidomide does not appear to undergo significant hepatic metabolism.

Dietary Considerations Should be taken at least 1 hour after the evening meal.

Administration Avoid extensive handling of capsules; capsules should remain in blister pack until ingestion. If exposed to the powder content from broken capsules or body fluids from patients receiving thalidomide, the exposed area should be washed with soap and water.

U.S. labeling: Administer orally with water, preferably at bedtime once daily on an empty stomach, at least 1 hour after the evening meal. Doses >400 mg/day may be given in 2-3 divided doses at least 1 hour after meals. For missed doses, if <12 hours patient may receive dose; if >12 hours wait till next dose due.

Canadian labeling: Administer orally as a single dose at the same time each day; may be taken without regard to meals. May be administered at bedtime to decrease somnolence. Capsules should be swallowed whole, preferably with water.

Hazardous agent; use appropriate precautions for handling and disposal (NIOSH, 2012).

Monitoring Parameters CBC with differential, platelets; thyroid function tests (TSH at baseline then every 2-3 months during thalidomide treatment [Hamnvik, 2011]). In HIV-seropositive patients: viral load after 1 and 3 months, then every 3 months. Pregnancy testing (sensitivity of at least 50 mIU/mL) is required within 24 hours prior to initiation of therapy, weekly during the first 4 weeks, then every 4 weeks in women with regular menstrual cycles or every 2 weeks in women with irregular menstrual cycles. Signs of neuropathy monthly for the first 3 months, then periodically during treatment; consider monitoring of sensory nerve application potential amplitudes (at baseline and every 6 months) to detect asymptomatic neuropathy. Monitor for signs and symptoms of thromboembolism (shortness of breath, chest pain, arm/leg swelling).

Reference Range Graft-vs-host disease: Therapeutic plasma thalidomide levels are 5-8 mcg/mL, although it has been suggested that lower plasma levels (0.5-1.5 mcg/mL) may be therapeutic; peak serum thalidomide level after a 200 mg dose: 1.8 mcg/mL

Dosage Forms Excipient information presented when available (limited, particularly for generics); consult specific product labeling.

Capsule, Oral:

Thalomid: 50 mg, 100 mg

Thalomid: 150 mg, 200 mg [contains fd&c blue #2 (indigotine)]

Extemporaneous Preparations Hazardous agent: Use appropriate precautions for handling and disposal.

A 20 mg/mL oral suspension may be prepared with capsules and a 1:1 mixture of Ora-Sweet® and Ora-Plus®. Empty the contents of twelve 100 mg capsules into a glass mortar. Add small portions of the vehicle and mix to a uniform paste; mix while adding the vehicle in incremental proportions to almost 60 mL; transfer to an amber calibrated bottle, rinse mortar with vehicle, and add quantity of vehicle sufficient to make 60 mL. Label "shake well," "protect from light," and "refrigerate". Stable for 35 days refrigerated.

Kraft S, Johnson CE, and Tyler RP, "Stability of an Extemporaneously Prepared Thalidomide Suspension," *Am J Health Syst Pharm*, 2011, 69(1):56-8.

- ◆ **Thalomid** *see* Thalidomide *on page 2038*
- ◆ **Tham** *see* Tromethamine *on page 2132*
- ◆ **THC** *see* Dronabinol *on page 674*
- ◆ **The Magic Bullett [OTC] (Can)** *see* Bisacodyl *on page 259*
- ◆ **Theo-24** *see* Theophylline *on page 2042*
- ◆ **Theochron** *see* Theophylline *on page 2042*
- ◆ **Theo ER (Can)** *see* Theophylline *on page 2042*
- ◆ **Theolair (Can)** *see* Theophylline *on page 2042*

Theophylline (thee OFF i lin)

Brand Names: U.S. Elixophyllin; Theo-24; Theochron

Brand Names: Canada Apo-Theo LA®; Novo-Theophyl SR; PMS-Theophylline; Pulmophylline; ratio-Theo-Bronc; Teva-Theophylline SR; Theo ER; Theolair; Uniphyl

Index Terms Theophylline Anhydrous

Pharmacologic Category Phosphodiesterase Enzyme Inhibitor, Nonselective

Use Treatment of symptoms and reversible airway obstruction due to chronic asthma, or other chronic lung diseases

Note: The Global Initiative for Asthma Guidelines (2009) and the National Heart, Lung and Blood Institute Guidelines (2007) do not recommend oral theophylline as a long-term control medication for asthma in children ≤5 years of age; use has been shown to be effective as an add-on (but not preferred) agent in older children and adults with severe asthma treated with inhaled or oral glucocorticoids. The guidelines do not recommend theophylline for the treatment of exacerbations of asthma.

The Global Initiative for Chronic Obstructive Lung Disease Guidelines (2013) suggest that while higher doses of slow release formulations of theophylline have been proven to be effective for use in COPD, it is not a preferred agent due to its potential for toxicity.

Pregnancy Risk Factor C

Pregnancy Considerations Teratogenic effects were observed in animal reproduction studies. Theophylline crosses the placenta; adverse effects may be seen in the newborn. Use is generally safe when used at the recommended doses (serum concentrations 5-12 mcg/mL) however maternal adverse events may be increased and efficacy may be decreased in pregnant women. Theophylline metabolism may change during pregnancy; the half-life is similar to that observed in otherwise healthy, nonsmoking adults with asthma during the first and second trimesters (~8.7 hours), but may increase to 13 hours (range: 8-18 hours) during the third trimester. The volume of distribution is also increased during the third trimester. Monitor serum levels. The recommendations for the use of theophylline in pregnant women with asthma are similar to those used in nonpregnant adults (National Heart, Lung, and Blood Institute Guidelines, 2004).

Breast-Feeding Considerations The concentration of theophylline in breast milk is similar to the maternal serum concentration. Irritability may be observed in the nursing infant. Serious adverse events in the infant are unlikely unless toxic serum levels are present in the mother.

Contraindications Hypersensitivity to theophylline or any component of the formulation; premixed injection may contain corn-derived dextrose and its use is contraindicated in patients with allergy to corn-related products

Warnings/Precautions If a patient develops signs and symptoms of theophylline toxicity (eg, persistent, repetitive vomiting), a serum theophylline level should be measured and subsequent doses held. Serum theophylline monitoring may be lessened as lower therapeutic ranges are established. More intense monitoring may be required during acute illness or when interacting drugs are introduced into the regimen. Use with caution in patients with peptic ulcer, hyperthyroidism, seizure disorders, and patients with tachyarrhythmias (eg, sinus tachycardia, atrial fibrillation); use may exacerbate these conditions. Theophylline-induced nonconvulsive status epilepticus has been reported (rarely) and should be considered in patients who develop CNS abnormalities. Theophylline clearance may be decreased in patients with acute pulmonary edema, congestive heart failure, cor-pulmonale, fever, hepatic disease, acute hepatitis, cirrhosis, hypothyroidism, sepsis with multiorgan failure, and shock; clearance may also be decreased in neonates, infants <3 months of age with decreased renal function, children <1 year of age, the elderly >60 years, and patients following cessation of smoking.

Adverse Reactions Frequency not defined. Adverse events observed at therapeutic serum levels:

Cardiovascular: Flutter, tachycardia

Central nervous system: Headache, hyperactivity (children), insomnia, restlessness, seizures, status epilepticus (nonconvulsive)

Endocrine & metabolic: Hypercalcemia (with concomitant hyperthyroid disease)
Gastrointestinal: Nausea, reflux or ulcer aggravation, vomiting
Genitourinary: Difficulty urinating (elderly males with prostatism)
Neuromuscular & skeletal: Tremor
Renal: Diuresis (transient)

Drug Interactions

Metabolism/Transport Effects Substrate of CYP1A2 (major), CYP2C9 (minor), CYP2D6 (minor), CYP2E1 (major), CYP3A4 (major); **Note:** Assignment of Major/Minor substrate status based on clinically relevant drug interaction potential; **Inhibits** CYP1A2 (weak)

Avoid Concomitant Use

Avoid concomitant use of Theophylline with any of the following: Conivaptan; Deferasirox; Fusidic Acid (Systemic); Iobenguane I 123; Riociguat

Increased Effect/Toxicity

Theophylline may increase the levels/effects of: Formoterol; Indacaterol; Pancuronium; Riociguat; Sympathomimetics

The levels/effects of Theophylline may be increased by: Abiraterone Acetate; Allopurinol; Antithyroid Agents; AtoMOXetine; Cannabinoids; Cimetidine; Conivaptan; CYP1A2 Inhibitors (Moderate); CYP1A2 Inhibitors (Strong); CYP3A4 Inhibitors (Moderate); CYP3A4 Inhibitors (Strong); Dasatinib; Deferasirox; Disulfiram; Estrogen Derivatives; Febuxostat; FluvoxaMINE; Fusidic Acid (Systemic); Interferons; Isoniazid; Ivacaftor; Linezolid; Luliconazole; Macrolide Antibiotics; Methotrexate; Mexiletine; Mifepristone; Pentoxifylline; Propafenone; QuiNINE; Quinolone Antibiotics; Simeprevir; Thiabendazole; Ticlopidine; Vemurafenib; Zafirlukast; Zileuton

Decreased Effect

Theophylline may decrease the levels/effects of: Adenosine; Benzodiazepines; CarBAMazepine; Fosphenytoin; Iobenguane I 123; Lithium; Pancuronium; Phenytoin; Regadenoson; Zafirlukast

The levels/effects of Theophylline may be decreased by: Adalimumab; Aminoglutethimide; Barbiturates; Beta-Blockers (Beta1 Selective); Beta-Blockers (Nonselective); Bosentan; CarBAMazepine; CYP1A2 Inducers (Strong); CYP3A4 Inducers (Strong); Cyproterone; Dabrafenib; Fosphenytoin; Herbs (CYP3A4 Inducers); Isoproterenol; Mitotane; Phenytoin; Protease Inhibitors; Thyroid Products; Tocilizumab

Ethanol/Nutrition/Herb Interactions Food: Food does not appreciably affect the absorption of liquid, fast-release products, and most sustained release products; however, food may induce a sudden release (dose-dumping) of once-daily sustained release products resulting in an increase in serum drug levels and potential toxicity. Changes in diet may affect the elimination of theophylline; charbroiled foods may increase elimination, reducing half-life by 50%. Management: Should be taken with water 1 hour before or 2 hours after meals. Avoid excessive amounts of caffeine. Avoid extremes of dietary protein and carbohydrate intake.

Storage/Stability Tablet, premixed infusion, solution: Store at controlled room temperature of 25°C (77°F).

Mechanism of Action Causes bronchodilatation, diuresis, CNS and cardiac stimulation, and gastric acid secretion by blocking phosphodiesterase which increases tissue concentrations of cyclic adenine monophosphate (cAMP) which in turn promotes catecholamine stimulation of lipolysis, glycogenolysis, and gluconeogenesis and induces release of epinephrine from adrenal medulla cells

Pharmacodynamics/Kinetics

Absorption: Oral: Dosage form dependent

Distribution: 0.45 L/kg (range: 0.3-0.7 L/kg) based on ideal body weight; distributes poorly into body fat; V_d may increase in premature neonates, patients with hepatic cirrhosis, acidemia (uncorrected), the elderly

Metabolism: Children >1 year and Adults: Hepatic; involves CYP1A2, 2E1 and 3A4; forms active metabolites (caffeine and 3-methylxanthine)

Protein binding: 40%, primarily to albumin

Half-life elimination: Highly variable and dependent upon age, liver function, cardiac function, lung disease, and smoking history
- Premature infants, postnatal age 3-15 days: 30 hours (range: 17-43 hours)
- Premature infants, postnatal age 25-57 days: 20 hours (range: 9.4-30.6 hours)
- Children 6-17 years: 3.7 hours (range: 1.5-5.9 hours)
- Adults 16-60 years with asthma, nonsmoking, otherwise healthy: 8.7 hours (range: 6.1-12.8 hours)

Time to peak, serum:
- Oral: Liquid: 1 hour
- I.V.: Within 30 minutes

Excretion: Urine
- Neonates: 50% as unchanged theophylline
- Children >3 months and Adults: ~10% as unchanged theophylline

Dosage Doses should be individualized based on steady-state serum concentrations and ideal body weight.

Acute symptoms: Loading dose: Children and Adults: Oral, I.V.:

Asthma exacerbations: While theophylline may be considered for relief of asthma symptoms, the role of treating exacerbations is not supported by current practice.

COPD treatment: Theophylline is currently considered second-line intravenous therapy in the emergency department or hospital setting when there is inadequate or insufficient response to short acting bronchodilators (Global Initiative for COPD Guidelines, 2013).

If no theophylline received within the previous 24 hours: 4.6 mg/kg loading dose (~5.8 mg/kg hydrous aminophylline) I.V. or 5 mg/kg orally. Loading dose intended to achieve a serum level of approximately 10 mcg/mL; loading doses should be given intravenously (preferred) or with a rapidly absorbed oral product (not an extended-release product). **Note:** On the average, for every 1 mg/kg theophylline given, blood levels will rise 2 mcg/mL.

If theophylline has been administered in the previous 24 hours: A loading dose is not recommended without obtaining a serum theophylline concentration. The loading dose should be calculated as follows:

Dose = (desired serum theophylline concentration - measured serum theophylline concentration) (V_d)

Acute symptoms: Maintenance dose: Children and Adults: I.V.: **Note:** To achieve a target concentration of 10 mcg/mL unless otherwise noted. Lower initial doses may be required in patients with reduced theophylline clearance. Dosage should be adjusted according to serum level measurements during the first 12- to 24-hour period.
- Infants 6-52 weeks: mg/kg/hour = (0.008) (age in weeks) + 0.21
- Children 1-9 years: 0.8 mg/kg/hour
- Children 9-12 years: 0.7 mg/kg/hour
- Adolescents 12-16 years (cigarette or marijuana smokers): 0.7 mg/kg/hour
- Adolescents 12-16 years (nonsmokers): 0.5 mg/kg/hour; maximum: 900 mg/day unless serum levels indicate need for larger dose
- Adults 16-60 years (otherwise healthy, nonsmokers): 0.4 mg/kg/hour; maximum: 900 mg/day unless serum levels indicate need for larger dose

Adults >60 years: 0.3 mg/kg/hour; maximum: 400 mg/day unless serum levels indicate need for larger dose

Treatment of chronic conditions: With newer guidelines suggesting lower therapeutic theophylline ranges, it is unlikely that doses larger than >10 mg/kg/day will be required in children ≥1 year or adults.

Oral solution:

Infants <1 year: **Note:** Doses should be adjusted to maintain the peak steady state serum concentrations. The time to reach steady state will vary based on age and the presence of risk factors which may affect theophylline clearance.

Full-term Infants and Infants <26 weeks: Total daily dose (mg)= [(0.2 x age in weeks) +5] x (weight in kg); divide dose into 3 equal amounts and administer at 8-hour intervals

Full-term Infants and Infants ≥26 weeks and <52 weeks: Total daily dose (mg) = [(0.2 x age in weeks) +5] x (weight in kg); divide dose into 4 equal amounts and administer at 6-hour intervals

Children ≥1 year and <45 kg: Initial dose: 10-14 mg/kg/day (maximum: 300 mg/day) administered in divided doses every 4-6 hours; Maintenance: Up to 20 mg/kg/day (maximum: 600 mg/day)

Children >45 kg and Adults: Initial dose: 300 mg/day administered in divided doses every 6-8 hours; Maintenance: 400-600 mg/day (maximum: 600 mg/day)

Oral extended release formulations:

Children ≥1 year and <45 kg: Initial: 10-14 mg/kg once daily (maximum: 300 mg/day); Maintenance up to 20 mg/kg/day (maximum: 600 mg/day)

Children >45 kg and Adults: Initial dose: 300-400 mg once daily; Maintenance: 400-600 mg once daily (maximum: 600 mg/day)

Dosage adjustment in renal impairment: Oral, I.V.:

Infants 1-3 months: Consider dose reduction and frequent monitoring of serum theophylline concentrations.

Infants >3 months, Children, Adolescents, and Adults: No dosage adjustment necessary.

Dosage adjustment in hepatic impairment:

Oral: Infants, Children, Adolescents, and Adults: No dosage adjustment provided in manufacturer's labeling. However, dose reduction and frequent monitoring of serum theophylline concentration are required in patients with decreased hepatic function (eg, cirrhosis, acute hepatitis, cholestasis).

I.V.: Infants, Children, Adolescents, and Adults: Initial: 0.25 mg/kg/hour; maximum daily dose: 400 mg daily unless serum concentrations indicate need for larger dose. Use with caution and monitor serum theophylline concentrations frequently.

Dosing in obesity: Use ideal body weight for obese patients.

Dosage adjustment after serum theophylline measurement: Asthma: Within normal limits: Children: 5-10 mcg/mL; Adults: 5-15 mcg/mL: Maintain dosage if tolerated. Recheck serum theophylline concentration at 24-hour intervals (for acute I.V. dosing) or at 6- to 12-month intervals (for oral dosing). Finer adjustments in dosage may be needed for some patients. If levels ≥15 mcg/mL, consider 10% dose reduction to improve safety margin.

Note: Recheck serum theophylline levels after 3 days when using oral dosing, or after 12 hours (children) or 24 hours (adults) when dosing intravenously. Patients maintained with oral therapy may be reassessed at 6- to 12-month intervals.

Dietary Considerations Should be taken with water 1 hour before or 2 hours after meals. Premixed injection may contain corn-derived dextrose and its use is contraindicated in patients with allergy to corn-related products.

Administration

I.V.: Administer loading dose over 30 minutes; follow with a continuous infusion as appropriate

Oral: Long-acting preparations should be taken with a full glass of water, swallowed whole, or cut in half if scored. Do **not** crush. Extended release capsule forms may be opened and the contents sprinkled on soft foods; do **not** chew beads.

Monitoring Parameters Monitor heart rate, CNS effects (insomnia, irritability); respiratory rate (COPD patients often have resting controlled respiratory rates in low 20s); arterial or capillary blood gases (if applicable)

Theophylline levels: Serum theophylline levels should be monitored prior to making dose increases; in the presence of signs or symptoms of toxicity; or when a new illness, worsening of a present illness, or medication changes occur that may change theophylline clearance

I.V. loading dose: Measure serum concentrations 30 minutes after the end of an I.V. loading dose

I.V. infusion: Measure serum concentrations one half-life after starting a continuous infusion, then every 12-24 hours

Reference Range Therapeutic levels: Asthma:

Children: 5-10 mcg/mL

Adults: 5-15 mcg/mL

Test Interactions Plasma glucose, uric acid, free fatty acids, total cholesterol, HDL, HDL/LDL ratio, and urinary free cortisol excretion may be increased by theophylline. Theophylline may decrease triiodothyronine.

Dosage Forms Excipient information presented when available (limited, particularly for generics); consult specific product labeling.

Capsule Extended Release 24 Hour, Oral:

Theo-24: 100 mg, 200 mg, 300 mg, 400 mg

Elixir, Oral:

Elixophyllin: 80 mg/15 mL (473 mL) [contains fd&c red #40, saccharin sodium; mixed fruit flavor]

Solution, Intravenous:

Generic: 400 mg (250 mL, 500 mL); 800 mg (500 mL)

Solution, Oral:

Generic: 80 mg/15 mL (473 mL)

Tablet Extended Release 12 Hour, Oral:

Theochron: 100 mg, 200 mg, 300 mg [scored]

Generic: 100 mg, 200 mg, 300 mg, 450 mg

Tablet Extended Release 24 Hour, Oral:

Generic: 400 mg, 600 mg

Extemporaneous Preparations Note: An alcohol-containing commercial oral solution is available (80 mg/15mL).

A 5 mg/mL oral suspension may be made with tablets. Crush one 300 mg extended release tablet in a mortar and reduce to a fine powder. Add small portions of a 1:1 mixture of Ora-Sweet® and Ora-Plus® and mix to a uniform paste; mix while adding the vehicle in equal proportions to **almost** 60 mL; transfer to a calibrated bottle, rinse mortar with vehicle, and add sufficient quantity of vehicle to make 60 mL. Label "shake well". Stable for 90 days at room temperature.

Johnson CE, VanDeKoppel S, and Myers E, "Stability of Anhydrous Theophylline in Extemporaneously Prepared Alcohol-Free Oral Suspensions," *Am J Health-Syst Pharm*, 2005, 62(23):2518-20.

◆ Theophylline Anhydrous *see* Theophylline *on page 2042*

◆ TheraCort [OTC] *see* Hydrocortisone (Topical) *on page 1011*

◆ TheraCys *see* BCG *on page 226*

◆ Thera-Ear [OTC] *see* Carbamide Peroxide *on page 340*

◆ Thera-Gesic® [OTC] *see* Methyl Salicylate and Menthol *on page 1344*

◆ Thera-Gesic® Plus [OTC] *see* Methyl Salicylate and Menthol *on page 1344*

◆ **Thermazene** *see* Silver Sulfadiazine *on page 1897*
◆ **Thiamazole** *see* Methimazole *on page 1321*
◆ **Thiamin** *see* Thiamine *on page 2045*

Thiamine (THYE a min)

Brand Names: Canada Betaxin®
Index Terms Aneurine Hydrochloride; Thiamin; Thiamine Hydrochloride; Thiaminium Chloride Hydrochloride; Vitamin B_1
Pharmacologic Category Vitamin, Water Soluble
Use Treatment of thiamine deficiency including beriberi, Wernicke's encephalopathy, Korsakoff's syndrome, neuritis associated with pregnancy, or in alcoholic patients; dietary supplement
Pregnancy Risk Factor A
Dosage
Adequate Intake:
0-6 months: 0.2 mg/day
7-12 months: 0.3 mg/day
Recommended daily intake:
1-3 years: 0.5 mg
4-8 years: 0.6 mg
9-13 years: 0.9 mg
14-18 years: Females: 1 mg; Males: 1.2 mg
≥19 years: Females: 1.1 mg; Males: 1.2 mg
Pregnancy, lactation: 1.4 mg
Parenteral nutrition supplementation:
Infants: 1.2 mg/day
Adults: 6 mg/day; may be increased to 25-50 mg/day with history of alcohol abuse
Thiamine deficiency (beriberi):
Children: 10-25 mg/dose I.M. or I.V. daily (if critically ill), or 10-50 mg/dose orally every day for 2 weeks, then 5-10 mg/dose orally daily for 1 month
Adults: 5-30 mg/dose I.M. or I.V. 3 times/day (if critically ill); then orally 5-30 mg/day in single or divided doses 3 times/day for 1 month
Alcohol withdrawal syndrome: Adults: 100 mg/day I.M. or I.V. for several days, followed by 50-100 mg/day orally
Wernicke's encephalopathy: Adults: Treatment (manufacturer labeling): Initial: 100 mg I.V., then 50-100 mg/day I.M. or I.V. until consuming a regular, balanced diet. However, larger doses may be required based on failure of lower doses to produce clinical improvement in some patients.
Alternate dosage: The Royal College of Physicians (U.K.) has recommended the use of higher doses of thiamine (in combination with other B vitamins, ascorbic acid, potassium, phosphate, and magnesium) for the management of Wernicke's encephalopathy (Thomson, 2002):
Prophylaxis: 250 mg I.V. once daily for 3-5 days
Treatment: Initial: 500 mg I.V. 3 times/day for 3 days. If response to thiamine after 3 days, continue with 250 mg I.M. or I.V. once daily for an additional 5 days or until clinical improvement.

Dosage adjustment in renal impairment: No dosage adjustment provided in manufacturer's labeling.
Dosage adjustment in hepatic impairment: No dosage adjustment provided in manufacturer's labeling.
Additional Information Complete prescribing information should be consulted for additional detail.
Dosage Forms Excipient information presented when available (limited, particularly for generics); consult specific product labeling.
Capsule, Oral, as hydrochloride:
Generic: 50 mg
Solution, Injection, as hydrochloride:
Generic: 100 mg/mL (2 mL)
Tablet, Oral, as hydrochloride:
Generic: 50 mg, 100 mg, 250 mg
Tablet, Oral, as hydrochloride [preservative free]:
Generic: 100 mg

◆ **Thiamine Hydrochloride** *see* Thiamine *on page 2045*
◆ **Thiaminium Chloride Hydrochloride** *see* Thiamine *on page 2045*

Thioguanine (thye oh GWAH neen)

Brand Names: U.S. Tabloid
Brand Names: Canada Lanvis®
Index Terms 2-Amino-6-Mercaptopurine; 6-TG (error-prone abbreviation); 6-Thioguanine (error-prone abbreviation); TG; Tioguanine
Pharmacologic Category Antineoplastic Agent, Antimetabolite (Purine Analog)
Use Treatment of acute myelogenous (nonlymphocytic) leukemia (AML)
Unlabeled Use Treatment of pediatric acute lymphoblastic leukemia (ALL)
Pregnancy Risk Factor D
Pregnancy Considerations Animal studies have demonstrated adverse effects. There are no adequate and well-controlled studies in pregnant women. May cause fetal harm if administered during pregnancy. Women of child-bearing potential should avoid becoming pregnant during treatment.
Breast-Feeding Considerations Due to the potential for serious adverse reactions in the nursing infant, the manufacturer recommends to discontinue breast-feeding during therapy.
Contraindications Prior resistance to thioguanine (or mercaptopurine)

Canadian labeling: Additional contraindications (not in US labeling): Hypersensitivity to thioguanine or any component of the formulation
Warnings/Precautions Hazardous agent - use appropriate precautions for handling and disposal (NIOSH, 2012).

Not recommended for maintenance therapy or long-term continuous treatment; long-term continuous therapy or maintenance treatment is associated with a high risk for hepatotoxicity, hepatic sinusoidal obstruction syndrome (SOS; formerly called veno-occlusive disease), or portal hypertension; monitor liver function carefully for liver toxicity and discontinue in patients with evidence of hepatic SOS (eg, hyperbilirubinemia, hepatomegaly [tender], and weight gain due to ascites and fluid retention) or portal hypertension (eg, splenomegaly, thrombocytopenia, esophageal varices); hepatotoxicity with or without transaminase elevations may occur; pathologic findings of hepatotoxicity include hepatoportal sclerosis, nodular regenerative hyperplasia, peliosis hepatitis, and periportal fibrosis.

Myelosuppression (anemia, leukopenia, and/or thrombocytopenia) is a common dose-related toxicity (may be delayed); monitor for infection (due to leukopenia) or bleeding(due to thrombocytopenia); withhold treatment with abnormally significant drop in blood counts. Patients with genetic enzyme deficiency of thiopurine methyltransferase (TPMT) or who are receiving drugs which inhibit this enzyme (mesalazine, olsalazine, sulfasalazine) may be highly sensitive to myelosuppressive effects and may require substantial dose reductions.

Hyperuricemia occurs commonly with treatment; institute adequate hydration and prophylactic allopurinol. Thioguanine is potentially carcinogenic. Cross resistance with mercaptopurine generally occurs. Avoid vaccination with live vaccines during treatment.

Adverse Reactions Frequency not defined.

Endocrine & metabolic: Fluid retention, hyperuricemia (common)

Gastrointestinal: Anorexia, intestinal necrosis, intestinal perforation, nausea, splenomegaly, stomatitis, vomiting, weight gain

Hematologic: Anemia (may be delayed), bleeding, granulocytopenia, leukopenia (common; may be delayed), marrow hypoplasia, pancytopenia, thrombocytopenia (common; may be delayed)

Hepatic: Ascites, esophageal varices, hepatic necrosis (centrilobular), hepatic sinusoidal obstruction syndrome (SOS; veno-occlusive disease), hepatitis, hepatomegaly [tender], hepatoportal sclerosis, hepatotoxicity, hyperbilirubinemia, jaundice, LFTs increased, nodular regenerative hyperplasia, peliosis hepatitis, periportal fibrosis, portal hypertension

Miscellaneous: Infection

Drug Interactions

Metabolism/Transport Effects None known.

Avoid Concomitant Use

Avoid concomitant use of Thioguanine with any of the following: BCG; CloZAPine; Natalizumab; Pimecrolimus; Tacrolimus (Topical); Tofacitinib; Vaccines (Live)

Increased Effect/Toxicity

Thioguanine may increase the levels/effects of: CloZAPine; Leflunomide; Natalizumab; Tofacitinib; Vaccines (Live)

The levels/effects of Thioguanine may be increased by: 5-ASA Derivatives; Denosumab; Pimecrolimus; Roflumilast; Tacrolimus (Topical); Trastuzumab

Decreased Effect

Thioguanine may decrease the levels/effects of: BCG; Coccidioidin Skin Test; Sipuleucel-T; Vaccines (Inactivated); Vaccines (Live)

The levels/effects of Thioguanine may be decreased by: Echinacea

Ethanol/Nutrition/Herb Interactions Ethanol: Avoid; may increase the risk for hepatotoxicity.

Storage/Stability Store tablet at room temperature at 15°C to 25°C (59°F to 77°F). Protect from moisture.

Mechanism of Action Purine analog that is incorporated into DNA and RNA resulting in the blockage of synthesis and metabolism of purine nucleotides

Pharmacodynamics/Kinetics

Absorption: ~30% (range: 14% to 46%; highly variable)

Distribution: Does not reach therapeutic concentrations in the CSF

Metabolism: Hepatic; rapidly and extensively via thiopurine methyltransferase (TPMT) to 2-amino-6-methylthioguanine (MTG; active) and inactive compounds

Half-life elimination: Terminal: 5-9 hours

Time to peak, serum: Within 8 hours; predominantly metabolite(s)

Dosage

Oral: Children: Pediatric ALL (unlabeled use; combination therapy): Delayed intensification treatment phase: 60 mg/m^2/day for 14 days (Lange, 2002; Nachman, 1998)

Dosing comments in renal impairment: Children: No adjustment required (Aronoff, 2007).

Dosing comments in hepatic impairment: Deterioration in transaminases, alkaline phosphatase or bilirubin, toxic hepatitis, biliary stasis, clinical jaundice, evidence of hepatic sinusoidal obstruction syndrome (veno-occlusive disease), or evidence of portal hypertension: Discontinue treatment.

Administration Administer orally; total daily dose can be given at one time.

Hazardous agent; use appropriate precautions for handling and disposal (NIOSH, 2012).

Monitoring Parameters CBC with differential and platelet count; liver function tests (weekly when beginning therapy then monthly, more frequently in patients with liver disease or concurrent hepatotoxic drugs); serum uric acid; some laboratories offer testing for TPMT deficiency

Hepatotoxicity may present with signs of portal hypertension (splenomegaly, esophageal varices, thrombocytopenia) or sinusoidal obstruction syndrome (veno-occlusive disease; fluid retention, ascites, hepatomegaly with tenderness, or hyperbilirubinemia)

Dosage Forms Excipient information presented when available (limited, particularly for generics); consult specific product labeling. [DSC] = Discontinued product

Tablet, Oral:

Tabloid: 40 mg

Tabloid: 40 mg [DSC] [scored]

Extemporaneous Preparations Hazardous agent: Use appropriate precautions for handling and disposal.

A 20 mg/mL oral suspension may be made with tablets, methylcellulose 1%, and simple syrup NF. Crush fifteen 40 mg tablets in a mortar and reduce to a fine powder. Add 10 mL methylcellulose 1% in incremental proportions and mix to a uniform paste. Transfer to a graduated cylinder, rinse mortar with simple syrup, and add quantity of simple syrup sufficient to make 30 mL. Label "shake well" and "refrigerate". Stable for 84 days refrigerated (preferred) or at room temperature.

Dressman JB and Poust RI, "Stability of Allopurinol and Five Antineoplastics in Suspension," *Am J Hosp Pharm*, 1983, 40(4):616-8.

Nahata MC, Pai VB, and Hipple TF, *Pediatric Drug Formulations*, 5th ed, Cincinnati, OH: Harvey Whitney Books Co, 2004.

◆ **6-Thioguanine (error-prone abbreviation)** *see* Thioguanine *on page 2045*

Thiopental (thye oh PEN tal)

Index Terms Thiopental Sodium; Thiopentone

Pharmacologic Category Anticonvulsant, Barbiturate; Barbiturate; General Anesthetic

Additional Appendix Information

Dosing Considerations for the Critically-Ill Patient With Morbid Obesity *on page 2379*

Use Induction of anesthesia; control of convulsive states; treatment of elevated intracranial pressure

Pregnancy Risk Factor C

Contraindications Hypersensitivity to thiopental, barbiturates, or any component of the formulation; status asthmaticus; severe cardiovascular disease; porphyria (variegate or acute intermittent); should not be administered by intra-arterial injection

Warnings/Precautions Laryngospasm or bronchospasms may occur; use with extreme caution in patients with reactive airway diseases (asthma or COPD). Use with caution when the hypnotic may be prolonged or potentiated (excessive premedication, Addison's disease, hepatic or renal dysfunction, myxedema, increased blood urea, severe anemia, or myasthenia gravis). Potential for drug dependency exists, abrupt cessation may precipitate withdrawal, including status epilepticus in epileptic patients. Do not administer to patients in acute pain. Use caution in patients with unstable aneurysms, cardiovascular disease, renal impairment, or hepatic disease. Use caution in elderly, debilitated, or pediatric patients. May cause paradoxical responses, including agitation and hyperactivity, particularly in acute pain and pediatric patients. Effects with other sedative drugs or ethanol may be potentiated. May cause respiratory depression or hypotension. Use with caution in hemodynamically unstable patients (hypotension or shock) or patients with respiratory disease. Repeated dosing or continuous infusions may cause cumulative effects. Administer only by I.V. route.

Adverse Reactions Frequency not defined.

Cardiovascular: Bradycardia, hypotension, syncope

Central nervous system: Drowsiness, lethargy, CNS excitation or depression, impaired judgment, "hangover" effect, confusion, somnolence, agitation, hyperkinesia, ataxia, nervousness, headache, insomnia, nightmares, hallucinations, anxiety, dizziness, shivering

Dermatologic: Rash, exfoliative dermatitis, Stevens-Johnson syndrome

Gastrointestinal: Nausea, vomiting, constipation

Hematologic: Agranulocytosis, thrombocytopenia, megaloblastic anemia, immune hemolytic anemia (rare)

Local: Pain at injection site, thrombophlebitis with I.V. use

Renal: Oliguria

Respiratory: Laryngospasm, respiratory depression, apnea (especially with rapid I.V. use), hypoventilation, sneezing, cough, bronchospasm

Miscellaneous: Gangrene with inadvertent intra-arterial injection, anaphylaxis, anaphylactic reactions

Drug Interactions

Metabolism/Transport Effects None known.

Avoid Concomitant Use

Avoid concomitant use of Thiopental with any of the following: Azelastine (Nasal); Paraldehyde

Increased Effect/Toxicity

Thiopental may increase the levels/effects of: Alcohol (Ethyl); Azelastine (Nasal); Buprenorphine; CNS Depressants; Hydrocodone; Meperidine; Methotrimeprazine; Metyrosine; Mirtazapine; Paraldehyde; Pramipexole; ROPINIRole; Rotigotine; Selective Serotonin Reuptake Inhibitors; Thiazide Diuretics; Zolpidem

The levels/effects of Thiopental may be increased by: Brimonidine (Topical); Carbonic Anhydrase Inhibitors; Chloramphenicol; Doxylamine; Droperidol; Felbamate; HydrOXYzine; Magnesium Sulfate; Methotrimeprazine; Perampanel; Primidone; Sodium Oxybate; Tapentadol; Valproic Acid and Derivatives

Decreased Effect

Thiopental may decrease the levels/effects of: Acetaminophen; Beta-Blockers; Calcium Channel Blockers; Chloramphenicol; Contraceptives (Estrogens); Contraceptives (Progestins); Corticosteroids (Systemic); CycloSPORINE (Systemic); Doxycycline; Etoposide; Etoposide Phosphate; Felbamate; LamoTRIgine; Propafenone; Teniposide; Theophylline Derivatives; Tricyclic Antidepressants; Valproic Acid and Derivatives; Vitamin K Antagonists

The levels/effects of Thiopental may be decreased by: Ketorolac (Nasal); Ketorolac (Systemic); Mefloquine; Multivitamins/Minerals (with ADEK, Folate, Iron); Orlistat; Pyridoxine; Rifamycin Derivatives

Storage/Stability Reconstituted solutions remain stable for 3 days at room temperature and 7 days when refrigerated.

Mechanism of Action Short-acting barbiturate with sedative, hypnotic, and anticonvulsant properties. Barbiturates depress the sensory cortex, decrease motor activity, alter cerebellar function, and produce drowsiness, sedation, and hypnosis. In high doses, barbiturates exhibit anticonvulsant activity; barbiturates produce dose-dependent respiratory depression.

Pharmacodynamics/Kinetics

Onset of action: Anesthetic: I.V.: 30-60 seconds

Duration: 5-30 minutes

Distribution: V_d: ~1.6 L/kg

Protein binding: 72% to 86%

Metabolism: Hepatic, primarily to inactive metabolites but pentobarbital is also formed

Half-life elimination: 3-11.5 hours; decreased in children

Dosage I.V.:

Induction anesthesia:

Infants: 5-8 mg/kg

Children 1-12 years: 5-6 mg/kg

Adults: 3-5 mg/kg

Maintenance anesthesia:

Children: 1 mg/kg as needed

Adults: 25-100 mg as needed

Increased intracranial pressure: Children and Adults: 1.5-5 mg/kg/dose; repeat as needed to control intracranial pressure

Seizures:

Children: 2-3 mg/kg/dose; repeat as needed

Adults: 75-250 mg/dose; repeat as needed

Dosage adjustment in renal impairment: Cl_{cr} <10 mL/minute: Administer at 75% of normal dose. **Note:** Accumulation may occur with chronic dosing due to lipid solubility; prolonged recovery may result from redistribution of thiopental from fat stores.

Dosage adjustment in hepatic impairment: No dosage adjustment provided in manufacturer's labeling.

Dietary Considerations Some products may contain sodium.

Administration Administer slowly over 20-30 seconds. Rapid I.V. injection may cause hypotension or decreased cardiac output; avoid extravasation, necrosis may occur. Check I.V. catheter placement prior to administration. If inadvertent intra-arterial administration occurs, treat with a local anesthetic (eg, lidocaine 1%, 5 mL) and/or papaverine (20-40 mg), preferably through the catheter used for the thiopental injection.

Monitoring Parameters Respiratory rate, heart rate, blood pressure

Reference Range Therapeutic: Hypnotic: 1-5 mcg/mL (SI: 4.1-20.7 micromole/L); Coma: 30-100 mcg/mL (SI: 124-413 micromole/L); Anesthesia: 7-130 mcg/mL (SI: 29-536 micromole/L); Toxic: >10 mcg/mL (SI: >41 micromole/L)

Additional Information Thiopental switches from linear to nonlinear pharmacokinetics following prolonged continuous infusions.

Product Availability Pentothal® (thiopental injection): Hospira Pharmaceuticals, the sole manufacturer, has discontinued all Pentothal® products. Product is currently unavailable in the U.S. and in Canada.

Controlled Substance C-III

◆ **Thiopental Sodium** *see* Thiopental *on page 2046*

◆ **Thiopentone** *see* Thiopental *on page 2046*

◆ **Thiophosphoramide** *see* Thiotepa *on page 2049*

◆ **Thioplex** *see* Thiotepa *on page 2049*

Thioridazine (thye oh RID a zeen)

Index Terms Mellaril; Thioridazine Hydrochloride

Pharmacologic Category Antipsychotic Agent, Typical, Phenothiazine

Additional Appendix Information

Antipsychotic Agents *on page 2290*

Beers Criteria – Potentially Inappropriate Medications for Geriatrics *on page 2368*

Use Management of schizophrenic patients who fail to respond adequately to treatment with other antipsychotic drugs, either because of insufficient effectiveness or the inability to achieve an effective dose due to intolerable adverse effects from those medications

Unlabeled Use Behavior problems (children); severe psychoses (children); schizophrenia/psychoses (children); depressive disorders/dementia (children and adults); behavioral symptoms associated with dementia (elderly); psychosis/agitation related to Alzheimer's dementia

Pregnancy Risk Factor C

Pregnancy Considerations Jaundice or hyper-/hyporeflexia have been reported in newborn infants following maternal use of phenothiazines. Antipsychotic use during the third trimester of pregnancy has a risk for abnormal muscle movements (extrapyramidal symptoms [EPS]) and withdrawal symptoms in newborns following delivery. Symptoms in the newborn may include agitation, feeding disorder, hypertonia, hypotonia, respiratory distress, somnolence, and tremor; these effects may be self-limiting or require hospitalization.

Breast-Feeding Considerations Other phenothiazines are excreted in human milk; excretion of thioridazine is not known.

Contraindications Severe CNS depression; severe hyper-/hypotensive heart disease; coma; in combination with other drugs that are known to prolong the QT_c interval and/or CYP2D6 inhibitors; in patients with congenital long QT syndrome or a history of cardiac arrhythmias; concurrent use with medications that inhibit the metabolism of thioridazine (fluoxetine, paroxetine, fluvoxamine, propranolol, pindolol); patients known to have genetic defect leading to reduced levels of activity of CYP2D6

Warnings/Precautions [U.S. Boxed Warning]: Thioridazine has dose-related effects on ventricular repolarization leading to QT_c prolongation, a potentially life-threatening effect. Therefore, it should be reserved for patients with schizophrenia who have failed to respond to adequate levels of other antipsychotic drugs. Due to potential for QT_c prolongation; use contraindicated with concomitant CYP2D6 inhibitors and/or concomitant use with other agents that prolong the QT_c interval. May cause orthostatic hypotension; use with caution in patients at risk of this effect or those who would tolerate transient hypotensive episodes (cerebrovascular disease, cardiovascular disease, or other medications which may predispose). **[U.S. Boxed Warning]: Elderly patients with dementia-related psychosis treated with antipsychotics are at an increased risk of death compared to placebo.** Most deaths appeared to be either cardiovascular (eg, heart failure, sudden death) or infectious (eg, pneumonia) in nature. Thioridazine is not approved for the treatment of dementia-related psychosis.

Leukopenia, neutropenia, and agranulocytosis (sometimes fatal) have been reported in clinical trials and postmarketing reports with antipsychotic use; presence of risk factors (eg, pre-existing low WBC or history of drug-induced leuko-/neutropenia) should prompt periodic blood count assessment. Discontinue therapy at first signs of blood dyscrasias or if absolute neutrophil count <1000/mm^3.

Highly sedating, use with caution in disorders where CNS depression is a feature. Use with caution in Parkinson's disease. Use caution in patients with hemodynamic instability; predisposition to seizures; subcortical brain damage; severe cardiac, hepatic, or renal disease. Esophageal dysmotility and aspiration have been associated with antipsychotic use; use with caution in patients at risk of pneumonia (ie, Alzheimer's disease). Use associated with increased prolactin levels; clinical significance of hyperprolactinemia in patients with breast cancer or other prolactin-dependent tumors is unknown. May alter temperature regulation or mask toxicity of other drugs due to antiemetic effects.

Phenothiazines may cause anticholinergic effects (confusion, agitation, constipation, xerostomia, blurred vision, urinary retention); therefore, they should be used with caution in patients with decreased gastrointestinal motility, urinary retention, BPH, xerostomia, visual problems, or narrow-angle glaucoma (screening is recommended). Relative to other neuroleptics, thioridazine has a high potency of cholinergic blockade.

May cause extrapyramidal symptoms (EPS), including pseudoparkinsonism, acute dystonic reactions, akathisia, and tardive dyskinesia. Risk of dystonia (and possibly other EPS) may be greater with increased doses, use of conventional antipsychotics, males, and younger patients. In the elderly, avoid use; potent anticholinergic agent with potential to cause QT-interval prolongation. Use in elderly patients with dementia is associated with an increased risk of mortality and cerebrovascular accidents; avoid antipsychotic use for behavioral problems associated with dementia unless alternative nonpharmacologic therapies have failed and patient may harm self or others. In addition, use may cause or exacerbate syndrome of inappropriate antidiuretic hormone secretion or hyponatremia; monitor sodium closely with initiation or dosage adjustments in older adults (Beers Criteria). May be associated with neuroleptic malignant syndrome (NMS). May cause pigmentary retinopathy, and lenticular and corneal deposits, particularly with prolonged therapy.

Adverse Reactions Frequency not defined.

Cardiovascular: Hypotension, orthostatic hypotension, peripheral edema, ECG changes

Central nervous system: EPS (pseudoparkinsonism, akathisia, dystonias, tardive dyskinesia), dizziness, drowsiness, neuroleptic malignant syndrome (NMS), impairment of temperature regulation, lowering of seizure threshold

Dermatologic: Increased sensitivity to sun, rash, discoloration of skin (blue-gray)

Endocrine & metabolic: Changes in menstrual cycle, libido (changes in), breast pain, galactorrhea, amenorrhea

Gastrointestinal: Constipation, weight gain, nausea, vomiting, stomach pain, xerostomia, diarrhea

Genitourinary: Difficulty in urination, ejaculatory disturbances, urinary retention, priapism

Hematologic: Agranulocytosis, leukopenia

Hepatic: Cholestatic jaundice, hepatotoxicity

Neuromuscular & skeletal: Tremor, seizure

Ocular: Pigmentary retinopathy, blurred vision, cornea and lens changes

Respiratory: Nasal congestion

Drug Interactions

Metabolism/Transport Effects Substrate of CYP2C19 (minor), CYP2D6 (major); **Note:** Assignment of Major/Minor substrate status based on clinically relevant drug interaction potential; **Inhibits** CYP1A2 (weak), CYP2C9 (weak), CYP2D6 (strong), CYP2E1 (weak)

Avoid Concomitant Use

Avoid concomitant use of Thioridazine with any of the following: Aclidinium; Amisulpride; Azelastine (Nasal); CYP2D6 Inhibitors; FLUoxetine; FluvoxaMINE; Highest Risk QTc-Prolonging Agents; Ipratropium (Oral Inhalation); Ivabradine; Metoclopramide; Mifepristone; Moclobemide; Moderate Risk QTc-Prolonging Agents; Paraldehyde; Pimozide; Sulpiride; Tamoxifen; Tiotropium; Umeclidinium

Increased Effect/Toxicity

Thioridazine may increase the levels/effects of: Alcohol (Ethyl); Amisulpride; Analgesics (Opioid); Anticholinergics; Antidepressants (Serotonin Reuptake Inhibitor/Antagonist); ARIPiprazole; AtoMOXetine; Azelastine (Nasal); Beta-Blockers; Chlorpheniramine; CNS Depressants; CYP2D6 Substrates; Fesoterodine; Highest Risk QTc-Prolonging Agents; Iloperidone; Methylphenidate; Metoprolol; Nebivolol; Paraldehyde; Pimozide; Porfimer; Propafenone; Serotonin Modulators; Sulpiride; Tetrabenazine; Tiotropium; Vortioxetine; Zolpidem

The levels/effects of Thioridazine may be increased by: Acetylcholinesterase Inhibitors (Central); Aclidinium; Antidepressants (Serotonin Reuptake Inhibitor/Antagonist); Antimalarial Agents; Beta-Blockers; Brimonidine (Topical); Chlorpheniramine; CYP2D6 Inhibitors;

Darunavir; Doxylamine; FLUoxetine; FluvoxaMINE; HydrOXYzine; Ipratropium (Oral Inhalation); Ivabradine; Lithium formulations; Magnesium Sulfate; Methylphenidate; Metoclopramide; Metyrosine; Mifepristone; Moclobemide; Moderate Risk QTc-Prolonging Agents; Perampanel; Pramlintide; QTc-Prolonging Agents (Indeterminate Risk and Risk Modifying); Serotonin Modulators; Sodium Oxybate; Tetrabenazine; Umeclidinium

Decreased Effect

Thioridazine may decrease the levels/effects of: Amphetamines; Anti-Parkinson's Agents (Dopamine Agonist); Codeine; Iloperidone; Quinagolide; Tamoxifen; TraMADol

The levels/effects of Thioridazine may be decreased by: Antacids; Anti-Parkinson's Agents (Dopamine Agonist); Lithium formulations; Peginterferon Alfa-2b

Ethanol/Nutrition/Herb Interactions

Ethanol: May increase CNS depression; monitor for increased effects with coadministration. Caution patients about effects.

Herb/Nutraceutical: Avoid kava kava, valerian, St John's wort, gotu kola (may increase CNS depression). Avoid dong quai, St John's wort (may also cause photosensitization).

Storage/Stability Protect from light.

Mechanism of Action Thioridazine is a piperidine phenothiazine which blocks postsynaptic mesolimbic dopaminergic receptors in the brain; exhibits a strong alpha-adrenergic blocking effect and depresses the release of hypothalamic and hypophyseal hormones

Pharmacodynamics/Kinetics

Duration: 4-5 days

Half-life elimination: 21-25 hours

Time to peak, serum: ~1 hour

Dosage Oral:

Children >2-12 years (unlabeled use): Range: 0.5-3 mg/kg/day in 2-3 divided doses; usual: 1 mg/kg/day; maximum: 3 mg/kg/day

Behavior problems (unlabeled use): Initial: 10 mg 2-3 times/day, increase gradually

Severe psychoses (unlabeled use): Initial: 25 mg 2-3 times/day, increase gradually

Children >12 years (unlabeled use) and Adults:

Schizophrenia/psychoses: Initial: 50-100 mg 3 times/day with gradual increments as needed and tolerated; maximum: 800 mg/day in 2-4 divided doses

Depressive disorders/dementia (unlabeled use): Initial: 25 mg 3 times/day; maintenance dose: 20-200 mg/day

Elderly: Behavioral symptoms associated with dementia (unlabeled use): Oral: Initial: 10-25 mg 1-2 times/day; increase at 4- to 7-day intervals by 10-25 mg/day; increase dose intervals (once daily, twice daily, etc) as necessary to control response or side effects. Maximum daily dose: 400 mg; gradual increases (titration) may prevent some side effects or decrease their severity.

Dosage adjustment in renal impairment: No dosage adjustment provided in manufacturer's labeling

Hemodialysis: Not dialyzable (0% to 5%)

Dosage adjustment in hepatic impairment: No dosage adjustment provided in manufacturer's labeling

Administration Do not take antacid within 2 hours of taking drug.

Monitoring Parameters Baseline and periodic ECG; vital signs; serum potassium, lipid profile, fasting blood glucose and Hgb A_{1c}; BMI; mental status, abnormal involuntary movement scale (AIMS); periodic eye exam; do not initiate if QT_c >450 msec

Reference Range Toxic: >1 mg/mL; lethal: 2-8 mg/dL

Test Interactions False-positives for phenylketonuria, urinary amylase, uroporphyrins, urobilinogen; may interfere with urine detection of methadone and PCP (false-positives)

Dosage Forms Excipient information presented when available (limited, particularly for generics); consult specific product labeling.

Tablet, Oral, as hydrochloride:

Generic: 10 mg, 25 mg, 50 mg, 100 mg

◆ **Thioridazine Hydrochloride** *see* Thioridazine *on page 2047*

◆ **Thiosulfuric Acid Disodium Salt** *see* Sodium Thiosulfate *on page 1931*

Thiotepa (thye oh TEP a)

Index Terms TESPA; Thiophosphoramide; Thioplex; Triethylenethiophosphoramide; TSPA

Pharmacologic Category Antineoplastic Agent, Alkylating Agent

Use Treatment of superficial papillary bladder cancer; palliative treatment of adenocarcinoma of breast or ovary; controlling intracavitary effusions caused by metastatic tumors

Unlabeled Use Intrathecal treatment of leptomeningeal metastases

Pregnancy Risk Factor D

Pregnancy Considerations Animal reproduction studies have demonstrated teratogenicity and fetal loss. There are no adequate and well-controlled studies in pregnant women. May cause harm if administered during pregnancy. Effective contraception is recommended for men and women of childbearing potential.

Breast-Feeding Considerations Due to the potential for serious adverse reactions in the nursing infant, breastfeeding is not recommended.

Contraindications Hypersensitivity to thiotepa or any component of the formulation

Note: May be contraindicated in certain circumstances of hepatic, renal, and/or bone marrow failure; evaluate on an individual basis as lower dose treatment (with close monitoring) may still be appropriate if the potential benefit outweighs the risks

Warnings/Precautions Hazardous agent - use appropriate precautions for handling and disposal (NIOSH, 2012). Myelosuppression is common; monitor for infection or bleeding. Myelosuppression has also been reported with intravesicular administration (due to systemic absorption). Potentially teratogenic, mutagenic, and carcinogenic; myelodysplastic syndrome and acute myeloid leukemia (AML) have been reported. Reduce dosage and use extreme caution in patients with hepatic, renal, or bone marrow damage. Use may be contraindicated with impairment/damage and should be limited to cases where benefit outweighs risk.

When used for intrathecal administration, should not be prepared during the preparation of any other agents; after preparation, keep intrathecal medications in an isolated location or container clearly marked with a label identifying as "intrathecal" use only; delivery of intrathecal medications to the patient should only be with other medications intended for administration into the central nervous system (Jacobson, 2009).

Adverse Reactions

Frequency not defined:

Central nervous system: Chills, dizziness, fatigue, fever, headache

Dermatologic: Alopecia, contact dermatitis, depigmentation (with topical treatment), dermatitis, rash, urticaria

Endocrine & metabolic: Amenorrhea, spermatogenesis inhibition

Gastrointestinal: Abdominal pain, anorexia, nausea, vomiting

Genitourinary: Dysuria, urinary retention

Hematologic: Anemia, bleeding, leukopenia, thrombocytopenia
Local: Injection site pain
Neuromuscular & skeletal: Weakness
Ocular: Blurred vision, conjunctivitis
Renal: Hematuria
Respiratory: Asthma, epistaxis, laryngeal edema, wheezing
Miscellaneous: Allergic reaction, anaphylactic shock, infection

Infrequent, postmarketing, and/or case reports: Acute myeloid leukemia (AML), chemical cystitis (bladder instillation), hemorrhagic cystitis (bladder instillation), myelodysplastic syndrome

Drug Interactions

Metabolism/Transport Effects Inhibits CYP2B6 (strong)

Avoid Concomitant Use

Avoid concomitant use of Thiotepa with any of the following: BCG; CloZAPine; Natalizumab; Pimecrolimus; Tacrolimus (Topical); Tofacitinib; Vaccines (Live)

Increased Effect/Toxicity

Thiotepa may increase the levels/effects of: CloZAPine; CYP2B6 Substrates; Leflunomide; Natalizumab; Tofacitinib; Vaccines (Live)

The levels/effects of Thiotepa may be increased by: Denosumab; Pimecrolimus; Roflumilast; Tacrolimus (Topical); Trastuzumab

Decreased Effect

Thiotepa may decrease the levels/effects of: BCG; Coccidioidin Skin Test; Sipuleucel-T; Vaccines (Inactivated); Vaccines (Live)

The levels/effects of Thiotepa may be decreased by: Echinacea

Ethanol/Nutrition/Herb Interactions

Ethanol: Avoid ethanol (due to GI irritation).
Herb/Nutraceutical: Avoid black cohosh, dong quai in estrogen-dependent tumors.

Preparation for Administration Hazardous agent; use appropriate precautions for handling and disposal (NIOSH, 2012). Reconstitute each 15 mg vial with 1.5 mL SWFI to a concentration of 10 mg/mL. Solutions for I.V. use should be further diluted in 0.9% sodium chloride injection prior to infusion. Filter through a 0.22 micron filter (polysulfone membrane [eg, Sterile Aerodisc®] or triton-free cellulose mixed ester [eg, Millex®-GS]) prior to administration; do not use solutions which precipitate or remain opaque after filtering. Solutions for intravesicular administration should be diluted in 30-60 mL NS. Solutions for intrathecal administration should be diluted to a concentration of 1-5 mg/mL in preservative-free NS. Intrathecal medications should not be prepared during the preparation of any other agents.

Storage/Stability Store intact vials under refrigeration (2°C to 8°C). Protect from light. Reconstituted solutions (10 mg/mL) are stable for up to 28 days under refrigeration (4°C to 8°C) or 7 days at room temperature (25°C), although the manufacturer recommends use within 8 hours when reconstituted solutions are stored under refrigeration. Solutions further diluted (for I.V. use) in NS to 1 mg/mL are stable for 24 hours and to 3 mg/mL are stable for 48 hours at room temperature, although the manufacturer recommends immediate use. After preparation, keep intrathecal medications in an isolated location or container clearly marked with a label identifying as "intrathecal" use only.

Mechanism of Action Alkylating agent that reacts with DNA phosphate groups to produce cross-linking of DNA strands leading to inhibition of DNA, RNA, and protein synthesis; mechanism of action has not been explored as thoroughly as the other alkylating agents, it is presumed that the aziridine rings open and react as nitrogen mustard; reactivity is enhanced at a lower pH

Pharmacodynamics/Kinetics

Absorption: Intracavitary instillation: Unreliable (10% to 100%) through bladder mucosa
Metabolism: Extensively hepatic; major metabolite (active): TEPA
Half-life elimination: Terminal (dose-dependent clearance): ~2 hours
Excretion: Urine (as metabolites and unchanged drug)

Dosage

Children: HSCT for CNS malignancy (unlabeled use; combination chemotherapy): I.V.: 300 mg/m^2/day for 3 days beginning 8 days prior to transplant (Gilheeney, 2010) **or** 300 mg/m^2/day for 3 days beginning 5 days prior to transplant (Dunkel, 2010; Grodman, 2009)

Adults:

Bladder cancer: Intravesical: 60 mg in 30-60 mL NS retained for 2 hours once weekly for 4 weeks
Ovarian, breast cancer: I.V.: 0.3-0.4 mg/kg by rapid I.V. administration every 1-4 weeks
Effusions: Intracavitary: 0.6-0.8 mg/kg
Leptomeningeal metastases (unlabeled use): Intrathecal: 10 mg twice a week for 4 weeks, then (if CSF cytology is negative) weekly for 4 weeks, then monthly for 4 doses (NCCN CNS cancer guidelines v.1.2010)
Hematopoietic stem cell transplant (HSCT) for CNS malignancy (unlabeled use; combination chemotherapy): I.V.: 250 mg/m^2/day for 3 days beginning 9 days prior to transplant (Soussain, 2008) **or** 150 mg/m^2/dose every 12 hours for 6 doses, followed by stem cell reinfusion 96 hours after completion of thiotepa (Abrey, 2006)

Dosage adjustment for hematologic toxicity: I.V.:
WBC ≤3000/mm^3: Discontinue treatment
Platelets ≤150,000/mm^3: Discontinue treatment
Note: Use may be contraindicated with pre-existing marrow damage and should be limited to cases where benefit outweighs risk.

Dosage adjustment in renal impairment: No dosage adjustment provided in manufacturer's labeling. Use with caution; reduced dose may be warranted. Use may be contraindicated with existing renal impairment and should be limited to cases where benefit outweighs risk.

Dosage adjustment in hepatic impairment: No dosage adjustment provided in manufacturer's labeling. Use with caution; reduced dose may be warranted. Use may be contraindicated with existing hepatic impairment and should be limited to cases where benefit outweighs risk.

Dosing in obesity: *ASCO Guidelines for appropriate chemotherapy dosing in obese adults with cancer (**Note:** Excludes HSCT dosing):* Utilize patient's actual body weight (full weight) for calculation of body surface area- or weight-based dosing, particularly when the intent of therapy is curative; manage regimen-related toxicities in the same manner as for nonobese patients; if a dose reduction is utilized due to toxicity, consider resumption of full weight-based dosing with subsequent cycles, especially if cause of toxicity (eg, hepatic or renal impairment) is resolved (Griggs, 2012).

Administration

I.V.: Administer as a rapid injection. Infusion times may be longer for high-dose (unlabeled use) treatment; refer to specific protocols
Intravesical instillation: Instill directly into the bladder and retain for 2 hours; patient should be repositioned every 15-30 minutes for maximal exposure

Hazardous agent; use appropriate precautions for handling and disposal (NIOSH, 2012).

Monitoring Parameters CBC with differential and platelet count (monitor weekly during treatment and for at least 3 weeks after treatment); renal and liver function tests; uric acid, urinalysis

Dosage Forms Excipient information presented when available (limited, particularly for generics); consult specific product labeling.

Solution Reconstituted, Injection:

Generic: 15 mg (1 ea)

Thiothixene (thye oh THIKS een)

Brand Names: Canada Navane

Index Terms Navane; Tiotixene

Pharmacologic Category Antipsychotic Agent, Typical

Additional Appendix Information

Antipsychotic Agents *on page 2290*

Beers Criteria – Potentially Inappropriate Medications for Geriatrics *on page 2368*

Use Schizophrenia: For the management of schizophrenia

Unlabeled Use Schizophrenia (children); psychosis/agitation related to Alzheimer dementia

Pregnancy Considerations Adverse events were observed in some animal reproduction studies. Antipsychotic use during the third trimester of pregnancy has a risk for abnormal muscle movements (extrapyramidal symptoms [EPS]) and withdrawal symptoms in newborns following delivery. Symptoms in the newborn may include agitation, feeding disorder, hypertonia, hypotonia, respiratory distress, somnolence, and tremor; these effects may be self-limiting or require hospitalization. The ACOG recommends that therapy during pregnancy be individualized; treatment with psychiatric medications during pregnancy should incorporate the clinical expertise of the mental health clinician, obstetrician, primary healthcare provider, and pediatrician. When treating schizophrenia during pregnancy, atypical antipsychotics may be better tolerated by the mother however more information related to fetal effects may be available for agents considered typical (or first generation) antipsychotics (ACOG, 2008). Information related to the use of thiothixene in pregnancy is limited and other agents may be preferred.

Breast-Feeding Considerations It is not known if thiothixene is excreted into breast milk; other agents are preferred for use in nursing women (Klinger, 2013).

Contraindications Hypersensitivity to thiothixene or any component of the formulation; severe CNS depression; circulatory collapse; blood dyscrasias; coma

Warnings/Precautions [U.S. Boxed Warning]: Elderly patients with dementia-related psychosis treated with antipsychotics are at an increased risk of death compared to placebo. Most deaths appeared to be either cardiovascular (eg, heart failure, sudden death) or infectious (eg, pneumonia) in nature. Thiothixene is not approved for the treatment of dementia-related psychosis.

May alter cardiac conduction; life-threatening arrhythmias have occurred with therapeutic doses of antipsychotics. Avoid use in patients with underlying QT prolongation, in those taking medicines that prolong the QT interval, or cause polymorphic ventricular tachycardia; monitor ECG closely for dose-related QT effects (Haddad, 2002; Stollberger, 2005).

Leukopenia, neutropenia, and agranulocytosis (sometimes fatal) have been reported in clinical trials and postmarketing reports with antipsychotic use; presence of risk factors (eg, pre-existing low WBC or history of drug-induced leuko-/neutropenia) should prompt periodic blood count assessment. Discontinue therapy at first signs of blood dyscrasias or if absolute neutrophil count <1000/mm^3.

Antipsychotic use has been associated with esophageal dysmotility and aspiration; use with caution in patients at risk of aspiration pneumonia (ie, Alzheimer disease) (Maddalena, 2004). May cause extrapyramidal symptoms (EPS), including pseudoparkinsonism, acute dystonic reactions, akathisia, and tardive dyskinesia. Risk of dystonia (and possibly other EPS) may be greater with increased doses, use of conventional antipsychotics, males, and younger patients. Use may be associated with NMS; monitor for mental status changes, fever, muscle rigidity, and/or autonomic instability. May cause orthostatic hypotension; use with caution in patients at risk of this effect or in those who would not tolerate transient hypotensive episodes (cerebrovascular disease, cardiovascular disease, hypovolemia, or concurrent medication use which may predispose to hypotension/bradycardia). May rarely cause pigmentary retinopathy and lenticular pigmentation. Impaired core body temperature regulation may occur; caution with strenuous exercise, heat exposure, dehydration, and concomitant medication possessing anticholinergic effects.

Photosensitivity has been reported with thiothixene; avoid undue exposure to sunlight. May be sedating, use with caution in disorders where CNS depression is a feature; patients must be cautioned about performing tasks which require mental alertness (eg, operating machinery or driving). Effects may be potentiated when used with other sedative drugs or ethanol. May cause anticholinergic effects (constipation, xerostomia, blurred vision, urinary retention); use with caution in patients with decreased gastrointestinal motility, paralytic ileus, urinary retention, BPH, xerostomia, or visual problems. Relative to other neuroleptics, thiothixene has a low potency of cholinergic blockade. May mask toxicity of other drugs or conditions (eg, intestinal obstruction, Reye's syndrome, brain tumor) due to antiemetic effects. Use is associated with increased prolactin levels; clinical significance of hyperprolactinemia in patients with breast cancer or other prolactin-dependent tumors is unknown.

Use with caution in patients with severe cardiovascular disease, narrow-angle glaucoma, hepatic impairment, Parkinson disease, renal impairment, or seizure disorder. Potentially significant drug-drug interactions may exist, requiring dose or frequency adjustment, additional monitoring, and/or selection of alternative therapy.

Use in elderly patients with dementia is associated with an increased risk of mortality and cerebrovascular accidents; avoid antipsychotic use for behavioral problems associated with dementia unless alternative nonpharmacologic therapies have failed and patient may harm self or others. In addition, use may cause or exacerbate syndrome of inappropriate antidiuretic hormone secretion or hyponatremia; monitor sodium closely with initiation or dosage adjustments in older adults May also be inappropriate in older adults depending on comorbidities (eg, dementia, delirium) due to its potent anticholinergic effects (Beers Criteria). Increased risk for developing tardive dyskinesia, particularly elderly women.

Adverse Reactions Frequency not defined.

Cardiovascular: Cardiac arrest, ECG changes, hypotension, peripheral edema, syncope, tachycardia

Central nervous system: Abnormal cerebrospinal fluid, agitation, cerebral edema, dizziness, drowsiness, extrapyramidal reaction (akathisia, dystonias, pseudoparkinsonism, tardive dyskinesia), fatigue, hyperreflexia (infants), hypertonia (neonates), hypotonia (neonates), insomnia, Neuroleptic Malignant Syndrome, restlessness, seizure

Dermatologic: Contact dermatitis, diaphoresis, exfoliative dermatitis, pruritus, skin discoloration (blue-gray), skin photosensitivity, skin rash, urticaria

Endocrine & metabolic: Amenorrhea, change in libido, galactorrhea, glycosuria, gynecomastia, hyperglycemia, hyperprolactinemia, hypoglycemia, menstrual disease, polydipsia, weight gain

Gastrointestinal: Anorexia, constipation, diarrhea, increased appetite, nausea, paralytic ileus, sialorrhea, stomach pain, vomiting, xerostomia

Genitourinary: Breast hypertrophy, difficulty in micturition, ejaculatory disorder, impotence, lactation, mastalgia

Hematologic & oncologic: Leukocytosis, leukopenia

Hepatic: Increased serum alkaline phosphatase, increased serum transaminase

Hypersensitivity: Anaphylaxis (rare)

Neuromuscular & skeletal: Lupus-like syndrome, tremor, weakness

Ophthalmic: Blurred vision, miosis, mydriasis, retinitis pigmentosa

Respiratory: Asphyxia, nasal congestion, respiratory distress (neonates)

Miscellaneous: Fever, paradoxical reaction (excerbation of psychotic symptoms)

Drug Interactions

Metabolism/Transport Effects Substrate of CYP1A2 (major); **Note:** Assignment of Major/Minor substrate status based on clinically relevant drug interaction potential; **Inhibits** CYP2D6 (weak)

Avoid Concomitant Use

Avoid concomitant use of Thiothixene with any of the following: Aclidinium; Amisulpride; Azelastine (Nasal); Ipratropium (Oral Inhalation); Metoclopramide; Paraldehyde; Sulpiride; Tiotropium; Umeclidinium

Increased Effect/Toxicity

Thiothixene may increase the levels/effects of: Alcohol (Ethyl); Amisulpride; Analgesics (Opioid); Anticholinergics; ARIPiprazole; Azelastine (Nasal); Buprenorphine; CNS Depressants; Highest Risk QTc-Prolonging Agents; Hydrocodone; Methotrimeprazine; Methylphenidate; Moderate Risk QTc-Prolonging Agents; Paraldehyde; Serotonin Modulators; Sulpiride; Tiotropium; Zolpidem

The levels/effects of Thiothixene may be increased by: Abiraterone Acetate; Acetylcholinesterase Inhibitors (Central); Aclidinium; Brimonidine (Topical); CYP1A2 Inhibitors (Moderate); CYP1A2 Inhibitors (Strong); Deferasirox; Doxylamine; Droperidol; HydrOXYzine; Ipratropium (Oral Inhalation); Lithium formulations; Magnesium Sulfate; Methotrimeprazine; Methylphenidate; Metoclopramide; Metyrosine; Mifepristone; Perampanel; Pramlintide; Serotonin Modulators; Sodium Oxybate; Tetrabenazine; Umeclidinium; Vemurafenib

Decreased Effect

Thiothixene may decrease the levels/effects of: Amphetamines; Anti-Parkinson's Agents (Dopamine Agonist); Quinagolide

The levels/effects of Thiothixene may be decreased by: Anti-Parkinson's Agents (Dopamine Agonist); CYP1A2 Inducers (Strong); Cyproterone; Lithium formulations

Ethanol/Nutrition/Herb Interactions

Ethanol: Concomitant use with ethanol may increase CNS depression. Management: Advise patient that ethanol may enhance CNS depression; monitor for increased effects.

Herb/Nutraceutical: Some herbal medications should be avoided due to the risk of CNS depression with concomitant use. Management: Avoid kava kava, valerian, St John's wort, gotu kola.

Storage/Stability Store at 20°C to 25°C (68°F to 77°F). Protect from moisture. Dispense in a tight, light-resistant container.

Mechanism of Action Thiothixene is a thioxanthene antipsychotic which elicits antipsychotic activity by postsynaptic blockade of CNS dopamine receptors resulting in inhibition of dopamine-mediated effects; also has alpha-adrenergic blocking activity

Pharmacodynamics/Kinetics

Absorption: Erratic; high lipophilicity (Wilson, 2011)

Protein binding: 90% (Wilson, 2011)

Metabolism: Hepatic; substrate of CYP1A2 (Wilson, 2011)

Half-life elimination: 34 hours (Lehman, 2004)

Dosage Schizophrenia: Children >12 years (unlabeled use), Adolescents (unlabeled use), and Adults: Oral: Initial: Mild-to-moderate symptoms: 2 mg 3 times daily; usual dose 15 mg daily; severe symptoms: 5 mg 2 times daily; usual dose 20-30 mg daily. Increase dose gradually. Maximum 60 mg daily.

Dosage adjustment in renal impairment: No dosage adjustment provided in manufacturer's labeling.

Dosage adjustment in hepatic impairment: No dosage adjustment provided in manufacturer's labeling.

Monitoring Parameters Mental status; vital signs (as clinically indicated); weight, height, BMI, waist circumference (baseline; at every visit for the first 6 months; quarterly with stable antipsychotic dose); CBC (as clinically indicated); electrolytes and liver function (annually and as clinically indicated); fasting plasma glucose level/HGA1C (baseline, then yearly; in patients with diabetes risk factors or if gaining weight repeat 4 months after starting antipsychotic, then yearly); lipid panel (baseline; repeat every 2 years if LDL level is normal; repeat every 6 months if LDL level is >130 mg/dL); changes in menstruation, libido, development of galactorrhea, erectile and ejaculatory function (at each visit for the first 12 weeks after the antipsychotic is initiated or until the dose is stable, then yearly); abnormal involuntary movements or parkinsonian signs (baseline; repeat weekly until dose stabilized for at least 2 weeks after introduction and for 2 weeks after any significant dose increase); tardive dyskinesia (every 6 months; high-risk patients every 3 months); visual changes (inquire yearly); ocular examination (yearly in patients >40 years; every 2 years in younger patients) (Lehman, 2004; Marder, 2004; ADA, 2004)

Test Interactions May cause false-positive pregnancy test

Dosage Forms Excipient information presented when available (limited, particularly for generics); consult specific product labeling.

Capsule, Oral:

Generic: 1 mg, 2 mg, 5 mg, 10 mg

- **Thonzonium, Neomycin, Colistin, and Hydrocortisone** *see* Neomycin, Colistin, Hydrocortisone, and Thonzonium *on page 1439*
- **Thorazine** *see* ChlorproMAZINE *on page 415*
- **Three-Factor PCC** *see* Factor IX Complex (Human) [(Factors II, IX, X)] *on page 822*
- **Thrive [OTC]** *see* Nicotine *on page 1453*
- **Thrombate III** *see* Antithrombin *on page 148*
- **Thrombate III® (Can)** *see* Antithrombin *on page 148*
- **Thymocyte Stimulating Factor** *see* Aldesleukin *on page 63*
- **Thymoglobulin** *see* Antithymocyte Globulin (Rabbit) *on page 150*
- **Thyrogen** *see* Thyrotropin Alfa *on page 2053*

Thyroid, Desiccated (THYE roid DES i kay tid)

Brand Names: U.S. Armour Thyroid; Nature-Throid; NP Thyroid; Westhroid; Westhroid-P [DSC]; WP Thyroid

Index Terms Desiccated Thyroid; Levothyroxine and Liothyronine; Tetraiodothyronine and Triiodothyronine; Thyroid Extract; Thyroid USP

Pharmacologic Category Thyroid Product

Additional Appendix Information

Beers Criteria – Potentially Inappropriate Medications for Geriatrics *on page 2368*

Use Replacement or supplemental therapy in hypothyroidism; pituitary TSH suppressants (thyroid nodules, thyroiditis, multinodular goiter, thyroid cancer)

Pregnancy Risk Factor A

Dosage Oral: **Note:** The American Association of Clinical Endocrinologists does not recommend the use of desiccated thyroid for thyroid replacement therapy for hypothyroidism (Baskin, 2002). Tablet strengths may vary by manufacturer in terms of grains or mg; dosing recommendations are based on general clinical equivalencies that 1 grain = 60 mg or 65 mg; 1/2 grain = 30 mg or 32.5 mg; and 1/4 grain = 15 mg or 16.25 mg.

Children: See table.

Recommended Pediatric Dosage for Congenital Hypothyroidism

Age	Daily Dose (mg)	Daily Dose/kg (mg)
0-6 mo	15-30	4.8-6
6-12 mo	30-45	3.6-4.8
1-5 y	45-60	3-3.6
6-12 y	60-90	2.4-3
>12 y	>90	1.2-1.8

Adults: Initial: 15-30 mg; increase with 15 mg increments every 2-3 weeks; use 15 mg in patients with cardiovascular disease or long-standing myxedema. Maintenance dose: Usually 60-120 mg/day; monitor TSH and clinical symptoms.

Dosage adjustment in renal impairment: No dosage adjustment provided in manufacturer's labeling.

Dosage adjustment in hepatic impairment: No dosage adjustment provided in manufacturer's labeling.

Additional Information Complete prescribing information should be consulted for additional detail.

Dosage Forms Excipient information presented when available (limited, particularly for generics); consult specific product labeling. [DSC] = Discontinued product

Tablet, Oral:

Armour Thyroid: 15 mg, 30 mg, 60 mg, 90 mg, 120 mg
Armour Thyroid: 180 mg [scored]
Armour Thyroid: 240 mg
Armour Thyroid: 300 mg [scored]
Nature-Throid: 16.25 mg, 32.5 mg, 48.75 mg
Nature-Throid: 65 mg, 81.25 mg, 97.5 mg, 113.75 mg, 130 mg, 146.25 mg, 162.5 mg, 195 mg, 260 mg, 325 mg [scored]
NP Thyroid: 30 mg, 60 mg, 90 mg
Westhroid: 16.25 mg, 32.5 mg
Westhroid: 48.75 mg, 65 mg [scored]
Westhroid: 81.25 mg
Westhroid: 97.5 mg, 113.75 mg, 130 mg, 146.25 mg, 162.5 mg, 195 mg, 260 mg, 325 mg [scored]
Westhroid-P: 16.25 mg [DSC], 32.5 mg [DSC]
Westhroid-P: 48.75 mg [DSC], 65 mg [DSC], 97.5 mg [DSC], 130 mg [DSC] [scored]
WP Thyroid: 16.25 mg, 32.5 mg
WP Thyroid: 48.75 mg, 65 mg, 97.5 mg, 130 mg [scored]

◆ **Thyroid Extract** *see* Thyroid, Desiccated *on page* 2052

◆ **Thyroid USP** *see* Thyroid, Desiccated *on page* 2052

◆ **Thyrolar®** *see* Liotrix *on page* 1222

◆ **ThyroShield [OTC]** *see* Potassium Iodide *on page* 1687

Thyrotropin Alfa (thye roe TROH pin AL fa)

Brand Names: U.S. Thyrogen

Brand Names: Canada Thyrogen

Index Terms Human Thyroid Stimulating Hormone; Recombinant Human Thyrotropin; Rh-TSH; Thyrotropin Alpha; TSH

Pharmacologic Category Diagnostic Agent

Use

Diagnostic imaging: Adjunctive diagnostic tool for serum thyroglobulin (Tg) testing (with or without radioiodine imaging) in follow up of patients with well-differentiated thyroid cancer.

Thyroid tissue remnant ablation: Adjunctive treatment for radioiodine ablation of thyroid tissue remnants after total or near-total thyroidectomy in patients with well-differentiated thyroid cancer without evidence of metastatic disease

Potential clinical uses: Patients with an undetectable Tg on thyroid hormone suppressive therapy to exclude the diagnosis of residual or recurrent thyroid cancer, patients requiring serum Tg testing and radioiodine imaging who are unwilling to undergo thyroid hormone withdrawal testing and a less sensitive test is justified; patients who are either unable to mount an adequate endogenous TSH response to thyroid hormone withdrawal or in whom withdrawal is medically contraindicated, and patients without evidence of metastatic disease to ablate thyroid remnants (in combination with radioiodine [I^{131}]) following near-total thyroidectomy.

Pregnancy Risk Factor C

Dosage Note: Consider pretreatment with glucocorticoids for patients in whom local tumor expansion may compromise vital anatomic structures (such as trachea, CNS, or extensive macroscopic lung metastases).

Diagnostic imaging: I.M.:

U.S. labeling: Adolescents ≥16 years and Adults: 0.9 mg, followed 24 hours later by a second 0.9 mg dose; obtain serum Tg sample 72 hours after the second thyrotropin alfa injection

Canadian labeling: Adults: 0.9 mg, followed 24 hours later by a second 0.9 mg dose; obtain serum Tg sample 72 hours after the second thyrotropin alfa injection

Thyroid tissue remnant ablation: I.M.:

U.S. labeling: Adolescents ≥16 years and Adults: 0.9 mg, followed 24 hours later by a second 0.9 mg dose

Canadian labeling: Adults: 0.9 mg, followed 24 hours later by a second 0.9 mg dose

Radioiodine administration should be given 24 hours following the second thyrotropin alfa injection. Perform diagnostic scanning 48 hours after radioiodine administration (72 hours after the second thyrotropin alfa injection). Post-therapy scanning may be delayed (additional days) to allow decline of background activity.

Dosage adjustment in renal impairment: No dosage adjustment provided in the manufacturer's labeling; however, elimination is significantly slower in dialysis-dependent end-stage renal impairment and TSH level elevation may be prolonged.

Dosage adjustment in hepatic impairment: No dosage adjustment provided in the manufacturer's labeling (has not been studied).

Additional Information Complete prescribing information should be consulted for additional detail.

Dosage Forms Excipient information presented when available (limited, particularly for generics); consult specific product labeling.

Solution Reconstituted, Intramuscular:

Thyrogen: 1.1 mg (1 ea)

◆ **Thyrotropin Alpha** *see* Thyrotropin Alfa *on page* 2053

◆ **Tiacumicin B** *see* Fidaxomicin *on page* 859

TiaGABine (tye AG a been)

Brand Names: U.S. Gabitril

Index Terms Tiagabine Hydrochloride

Pharmacologic Category Anticonvulsant, Miscellaneous

Use Adjunctive therapy in adults and children ≥12 years of age in the treatment of partial seizures

Pregnancy Risk Factor C

Pregnancy Considerations Adverse events were observed in animal reproduction studies. Patients exposed to tiagabine during pregnancy are encouraged to enroll themselves into the AED Pregnancy Registry by calling 1-888-233-2334. Additional information is available at www.aedpregnancyregistry.org.

Breast-Feeding Considerations Levels of excretion of tiagabine and/or its metabolites in human milk have not been determined and effects on the nursing infant are unknown. According to the manufacturer, the decision to continue or discontinue breast-feeding during therapy should take into account the risk of exposure to the infant and the benefits of treatment to the mother.

Medication Guide Available Yes

Contraindications Hypersensitivity to tiagabine or any component of the formulation

Warnings/Precautions Antiepileptics are associated with an increased risk of suicidal behavior/thoughts with use (regardless of indication); patients should be monitored for signs/symptoms of depression, suicidal tendencies, and other unusual behavior changes during therapy and instructed to inform their healthcare provider immediately if symptoms occur. New-onset seizures and status epilepticus have been associated with tiagabine use when taken for unlabeled indications. Often these seizures have occurred shortly after the initiation of treatment or shortly after a dosage increase. Seizures have also occurred with very low doses or after several months of therapy. In most cases, patients were using concomitant medications (eg, antidepressants, antipsychotics, stimulants, opioids). In these instances, the discontinuation of tiagabine, followed by an evaluation for an underlying seizure disorder, is suggested. Use for unapproved indications, however, has not been proven to be safe or effective and is not recommended. When tiagabine is used as an adjunct in partial seizures (an FDA-approved indication), it should not be abruptly discontinued because of the possibility of increasing seizure frequency, unless safety concerns require a more rapid withdrawal. Rarely, nonconvulsive status epilepticus has been reported following abrupt discontinuation or dosage reduction.

Use with caution in patients with hepatic impairment. Experience in patients not receiving enzyme-inducing drugs has been limited; caution should be used in treating any patient who is not receiving one of these medications (decreased dose and slower titration may be required). Weakness, sedation, and confusion may occur with tiagabine use. Patients must be cautioned about performing tasks which require mental alertness (eg, operating machinery or driving). Effects with other sedative drugs or ethanol may be potentiated. May cause serious rash, including Stevens-Johnson syndrome.

Adverse Reactions

>10%:

Central nervous system: Concentration decreased, dizziness, nervousness, somnolence

Gastrointestinal: Nausea

Neuromuscular & skeletal: Weakness, tremor

1% to 10%:

Cardiovascular: Chest pain, edema, hypertension, palpitation, peripheral edema, syncope, tachycardia, vasodilation

Central nervous system: Agitation, ataxia, chills, confusion, difficulty with memory, confusion, depersonalization, depression, euphoria, hallucination, hostility, insomnia, malaise, migraine, paranoid reaction, personality disorder, speech disorder

Dermatologic: Alopecia, bruising, dry skin, pruritus, rash

Gastrointestinal: Abdominal pain, diarrhea, gingivitis, increased appetite, mouth ulceration, stomatitis, vomiting, weight gain/loss

Neuromuscular & skeletal: Abnormal gait, arthralgia, dysarthria, hyper-/hypokinesia, hyper-/hypotonia, myasthenia, myalgia, myoclonus, neck pain, paresthesia, reflexes decreased, stupor, twitching, vertigo

Ocular: Abnormal vision, amblyopia, nystagmus

Otic: Ear pain, hearing impairment, otitis media, tinnitus

Respiratory: Bronchitis, cough, dyspnea, epistaxis, pneumonia

Miscellaneous: Allergic reaction, cyst, diaphoresis, flu-like syndrome, lymphadenopathy

<1% (Limited to important or life-threatening): Abortion, abscess, anemia, angina, apnea, asthma, blepharitis, blindness, cellulitis, cerebral ischemia, cholelithiasis, CNS neoplasm, coma, deafness, dehydration, dysphagia, dystonia, electrocardiogram abnormal, encephalopathy, hemorrhage, erythrocytes abnormal, leukopenia, fecal incontinence, herpes simplex/zoster, glossitis, goiter, hematuria, hemoptysis, hepatomegaly, hypercholesteremia, hyper-/hypoglycemia, hyperlipemia, hypokalemia, hyponatremia, hypotension, hypothyroidism, impotence, kidney failure, liver function tests abnormal, MI, neoplasm, peripheral vascular disorder, paralysis, photophobia, psychosis, petechia, photosensitivity, seizure (when used for unlabeled uses), sepsis, spasm, suicide attempt, thrombocytopenia, thrombophlebitis, urinary retention, urinary urgency, urticaria, visual field defect

Drug Interactions

Metabolism/Transport Effects Substrate of CYP3A4 (major); **Note:** Assignment of Major/Minor substrate status based on clinically relevant drug interaction potential

Avoid Concomitant Use

Avoid concomitant use of TiaGABine with any of the following: Azelastine (Nasal); Conivaptan; Fusidic Acid (Systemic); Paraldehyde

Increased Effect/Toxicity

TiaGABine may increase the levels/effects of: Alcohol (Ethyl); Azelastine (Nasal); Buprenorphine; CNS Depressants; Hydrocodone; Methotrimeprazine; Metyrosine; Mirtazapine; Paraldehyde; Pramipexole; ROPINIRole; Rotigotine; Selective Serotonin Reuptake Inhibitors; Zolpidem

The levels/effects of TiaGABine may be increased by: Brimonidine (Topical); Conivaptan; CYP3A4 Inhibitors (Moderate); CYP3A4 Inhibitors (Strong); Dasatinib; Doxylamine; Droperidol; Fusidic Acid (Systemic); HydrOXYzine; Ivacaftor; Luliconazole; Magnesium Sulfate; Methotrimeprazine; Mifepristone; Perampanel; Simeprevir; Sodium Oxybate; Tapentadol

Decreased Effect

The levels/effects of TiaGABine may be decreased by: Bosentan; CYP3A4 Inducers (Strong); Dabrafenib; Deferasirox; Herbs (CYP3A4 Inducers); Ketorolac (Nasal); Ketorolac (Systemic); Mefloquine; Mitotane; Orlistat; Tocilizumab

Ethanol/Nutrition/Herb Interactions

Ethanol: May increase CNS depression; monitor for increased effects with coadministration. Caution patients about effects.

Food: Food reduces the rate but not the extent of absorption.

Herb/Nutraceutical: St John's wort may decrease tiagabine levels. Avoid valerian, St John's wort, kava kava, gotu kola (may increase CNS depression).

Mechanism of Action The exact mechanism by which tiagabine exerts antiseizure activity is not definitively known; however, *in vitro* experiments demonstrate that it enhances the activity of gamma aminobutyric acid (GABA), the major neuroinhibitory transmitter in the nervous system; it is thought that binding to the GABA uptake carrier inhibits the uptake of GABA into presynaptic neurons, allowing an increased amount of GABA to be available to postsynaptic neurons; based on *in vitro* studies, tiagabine does not inhibit the uptake of dopamine, norepinephrine, serotonin, glutamate, or choline

Pharmacodynamics/Kinetics

Absorption: Rapid (45 minutes); prolonged with food

Protein binding: 96%, primarily to albumin and α_1-acid glycoprotein

Metabolism: Hepatic via CYP (primarily 3A4)

Bioavailability: Oral: Absolute: 90%

Half-life elimination: 2-5 hours when administered with enzyme inducers; 7-9 hours when administered without enzyme inducers

Time to peak, plasma: 45 minutes

Excretion: Feces (63%); urine (25%); 2% as unchanged drug; primarily as metabolites

Dosage Oral (administer with food):

Patients receiving enzyme-inducing AED regimens:

Children 12-18 years: 4 mg once daily for 1 week; may increase to 8 mg daily in 2 divided doses for 1 week; then may increase by 4-8 mg weekly to response or up to 32 mg daily in 2-4 divided doses

Adults: 4 mg once daily for 1 week; may increase by 4-8 mg weekly to response or up to 56 mg daily in 2-4 divided doses; usual maintenance: 32-56 mg/day

Patients **not** receiving enzyme-inducing AED regimens: The estimated plasma concentrations of tiagabine in patients not taking enzyme-inducing medications is twice that of patients receiving enzyme-inducing AEDs. Lower doses are required; slower titration may be necessary.

Dosage adjustment in renal impairment: No dosage adjustment necessary.

Dosage adjustment in hepatic impairment: No specific dosage adjustment provided in manufacturer's labeling. However, dosage reduction may be necessary since clearance is reduced in the setting of hepatic impairment.

Dietary Considerations Take with food.

Monitoring Parameters A reduction in seizure frequency is indicative of therapeutic response to tiagabine in patients with partial seizures; complete blood counts, renal function tests, liver function tests, and routine blood chemistry should be monitored periodically during therapy; suicidality (eg, suicidal thoughts, depression, behavioral changes)

Reference Range Maximal plasma level after a 24 mg/dose: 552 ng/mL

Additional Information Animal studies suggest that tiagabine may bind to retina and uvea; however, no treatment-related ophthalmoscopic changes were seen long-term; periodic monitoring may be considered.

Dosage Forms Excipient information presented when available (limited, particularly for generics); consult specific product labeling.

Tablet, Oral, as hydrochloride:

Gabitril: 2 mg [contains fd&c yellow #6 (sunset yellow)]

Gabitril: 4 mg [contains fd&c yellow #10 (quinoline yellow)]

Gabitril: 12 mg [contains brilliant blue fcf (fd&c blue #1), fd&c yellow #10 (quinoline yellow)]

Gabitril: 16 mg [contains fd&c blue #2 (indigotine)]

Generic: 2 mg, 4 mg

Extemporaneous Preparations A 1 mg/mL tiagabine hydrochloride oral suspension may be made with tablets and a 1:1 mixture of Ora-Sweet® and Ora-Plus®. Crush ten 12 mg tablets in a mortar and reduce to a fine powder. Add small portions of the vehicle and mix to a uniform paste; mix while adding the vehicle in incremental proportions to **almost** 120 mL; transfer to a graduated cylinder; rinse mortar with vehicle, and add quantity of vehicle sufficient to make 120 mL. Label "shake well" and "refrigerate". Store in amber plastic prescription bottles; stable for 70 days at room temperature or 91 days refrigerated (preferred).

A 1 mg/mL oral suspension may be made with tablets and a 6:1 mixture of simple syrup, NF and methylcellulose 1%. Crush ten 12 mg tablets in a mortar and reduce to a fine powder. Add 17 mL of methylcellulose 1% gel and mix to a uniform paste; mix while adding simple syrup, NF in incremental proportions to **almost** 120 mL; transfer to a graduated cylinder, rinse mortar with syrup, and add quantity of syrup sufficient to make 120 mL. Label "shake well" and "refrigerate". Store in amber plastic prescription bottles; stable for 42 days at room temperature or 91 days refrigerated (preferred).

Nahata MC, Pai VB, and Hipple TF, *Pediatric Drug Formulations*, 5th ed, Cincinnati, OH: Harvey Whitney Books Co, 2004.

- **Tiagabine Hydrochloride** *see* TiaGABine *on page 2053*
- **Tiamol® (Can)** *see* Fluocinonide *on page 879*
- **Tiazac** *see* Diltiazem *on page 613*
- **Tiazac® (Can)** *see* Diltiazem *on page 613*
- **Tiazac® XC (Can)** *see* Diltiazem *on page 613*

Ticagrelor (tye KA grel or)

Brand Names: U.S. Brilinta

Brand Names: Canada Brilinta™

Index Terms AZD6140

Pharmacologic Category Antiplatelet Agent; Antiplatelet Agent, Cyclopentyltriazolopyrimidine

Additional Appendix Information

Oral Antiplatelet Comparison Chart *on page 2313*

Use Used in conjunction with aspirin for secondary prevention of thrombotic events in patients with unstable angina (UA), non-ST-elevation myocardial infarction (NSTEMI), or ST-elevation myocardial infarction (STEMI) managed medically or with percutaneous coronary intervention (PCI) and/or coronary artery bypass graft (CABG)

Unlabeled Use In patients with allergy or major gastrointestinal intolerance to aspirin, initial treatment of UA/NSTEMI; **Note:** Dual antiplatelet therapy with another $P2Y_{12}$ receptor inhibitor is not recommended in this situation (Jneid, 2012).

Pregnancy Risk Factor C

Pregnancy Considerations Fetal mortality and/or abnormalities were observed in animal studies at doses greater than maximum recommended human doses. There are no adequate and well-controlled studies in pregnant women. Use only if potential benefits outweigh potential risk to fetus. The Canadian labeling recommends women of childbearing potential use appropriate contraceptive measures.

Breast-Feeding Considerations Excretion into breast milk is unknown; use is not recommended.

Medication Guide Available Yes

Contraindications Hypersensitivity (eg, angioedema) to ticagrelor or any component of the formulation; active pathological bleeding (eg, peptic ulcer or intracranial hemorrhage); history of intracranial hemorrhage; severe hepatic impairment

Canadian labeling: Additional contraindications (not in U.S. labeling): Moderate hepatic impairment; concomitant use of strong CYP3A4 inhibitors (eg, ketoconazole, clarithromycin, ritonavir, atazanavir, nefazodone)

Warnings/Precautions [U.S. Boxed Warning]: Ticagrelor increases the risk of bleeding including significant and sometimes fatal bleeding. Use is contraindicated in patients with active pathological bleeding and presence or history of intracranial hemorrhage. Additional risk factors for bleeding include propensity to bleed (eg, recent trauma or surgery, recent or recurrent GI bleeding, active PUD, moderate-to-severe hepatic impairment), CABG or other surgical procedure, concomitant use of medications that increase risk of bleeding (eg, warfarin, NSAIDs), and advanced age. Bleeding should be suspected if patient becomes hypotensive after undergoing recent coronary angiography, PCI, CABG, or other surgical procedure even if overt signs of bleeding do not exist. **Where possible, manage bleeding without discontinuing ticagrelor as the risk of cardiovascular events is increased upon discontinuation.** If discontinuation of ticagrelor is necessary, resume as soon as possible after the bleeding source is identified and controlled. Hemostatic benefits of platelet transfusions are not known; may inhibit transfused platelets. Premature discontinuation of therapy may increase the risk of cardiac events (eg, stent thrombosis with subsequent fatal or nonfatal MI). Duration of therapy, in general, is determined by the type of stent placed (bare metal or drug eluting) and whether an ACS event was ongoing at the time of placement. Use with caution in patients who are at an increased risk of bradycardia (eg, second- or third-degree AV block, sick sinus syndrome) or taking other bradycardic-inducing agents (eg, beta blockers, nondihydropyridine calcium channel blockers). Ventricular pauses ≥3 seconds were noted more frequently with ticagrelor than with clopidogrel in a substudy of the Platelet Inhibition and Patient Outcomes (PLATO) trial. Dyspnea (often mild-to-moderate and transient) was observed more frequently in patients receiving ticagrelor than clopidogrel during clinical trials. Ticagrelor-related dyspnea does not require specific treatment nor does it warrant therapy interruption; however, therapy should be discontinued in patients unable to tolerate ticagrelor-related dyspnea.

[U.S. Boxed Warning]: Maintenance doses of aspirin greater than 100 mg/day reduce the efficacy of ticagrelor and should be avoided. Use of higher maintenance doses of aspirin (ie, >100 mg/day) was associated with relatively unfavorable outcomes for ticagrelor versus clopidogrel in the PLATO trial (Gaglia, 2011; Wallentin, 2009). Canadian labeling recommends a maximum maintenance aspirin dose of 150 mg/day.

[U.S. Boxed Warning]: Avoid initiation of ticagrelor when urgent CABG surgery is planned; when possible discontinue use at least 5 days before any surgery. Discontinue 5 days before elective surgery (except in patients with cardiac stents that have not completed their full course of dual antiplatelet therapy; patient-specific situations need to be discussed with cardiologist). When urgent CABG is necessary, the ACCF/AHA CABG guidelines recommend discontinuation for at least 24 hours prior to surgery (Hillis, 2011).

Use is contraindicated in patients with severe hepatic impairment (Canadian labeling also contraindicates use in moderate-to-severe hepatic impairment). Use with caution in patients with renal impairment, a history of hyperuricemia or gouty arthritis. Canadian labeling does not recommend use in patients with uric acid nephropathy. Avoid concomitant use with strong CYP3A4 inhibitors (eg, ketoconazole, ritonavir, nefazodone) or strong CYP3A4 inducers (eg, rifampin, carbamazepine, dexamethasone, phenobarbital, phenytoin). Canadian labeling contraindicates use with strong CYP3A4 inhibitors.

Adverse Reactions Note: As with all drugs which may affect hemostasis, bleeding is associated with ticagrelor. Hemorrhage may occur at virtually any site. Risk is dependent on multiple variables, including the concurrent use of multiple agents which alter hemostasis and patient susceptibility.

Frequencies as reported in PLATO trial versus clopidogrel:

>10%: Respiratory: Dyspnea (≤14%)

1% to 10%:

- Cardiovascular: Ventricular pauses (6%; 2% after 1 month of therapy), atrial fibrillation (4%), hypertension (4%), angina (3%), hypotension (3%), bradycardia (1% to 3%), cardiac failure (2%), peripheral edema (2%), ventricular tachycardia (2%), palpitation (1%), syncope (1%), ventricular extrasystoles (1%), ventricular fibrillation (1%)
- Central nervous system: Headache (7%), dizziness (5%), fatigue (3%), fever (3%), anxiety (2%), insomnia (2%), vertigo (2%), depression (1%)
- Dermatologic: Bruising (2% to 4%), rash (2%), pruritus (1%), subcutaneous or dermal bleeding
- Endocrine & metabolic: Hypokalemia (2%), diabetes mellitus (1%), dyslipidemia (1%), hypercholesterolemia (1%)
- Gastrointestinal: Diarrhea (4%), nausea (4%), vomiting (3%), abdominal pain (2%), constipation (2%), dyspepsia (2%), GI hemorrhage
- Genitourinary: Urinary tract infection (2%), urinary tract bleeding
- Hematologic: Major bleeding (12%; composite of major fatal/life threatening and other major bleeding events), minor bleeding (~5%), anemia (2%), hematoma (2%), postprocedural hemorrhage (2%)
- Local: Puncture site hematoma (2%)
- Neuromuscular & skeletal: Back pain (4%), noncardiac chest pain (4%), extremity pain (2%), arthralgia (2%), musculoskeletal pain (2%), weakness (2%), myalgia (1%)
- Renal: Creatinine increased (7%; mechanism undetermined), hematuria (2%), renal failure (1%)
- Respiratory: Epistaxis (6%), cough (5%), nasopharyngitis (2%), bronchitis (1%), pneumonia (1%)

<1% (Limited to important or life-threatening): Angioedema, confusion, conjunctival hemorrhage, gastritis, gout, gynecomastia, hemarthrosis, hemoptysis, hypersensitivity, intracranial hemorrhage (including fatalities), intraocular hemorrhage, paresthesia, retinal hemorrhage, retroperitoneal hemorrhage

Drug Interactions

Metabolism/Transport Effects Substrate of CYP3A4 (major); **Note:** Assignment of Major/Minor substrate status based on clinically relevant drug interaction potential; **Inhibits** CYP2B6 (weak), CYP2C9 (moderate), CYP2D6 (weak)

Avoid Concomitant Use

Avoid concomitant use of Ticagrelor with any of the following: CYP3A4 Inducers (Strong); CYP3A4 Inhibitors (Strong)

Increased Effect/Toxicity

Ticagrelor may increase the levels/effects of: Agents with Antiplatelet Properties; Anticoagulants; ARIPiprazole; Bosentan; Carvedilol; Collagenase (Systemic); CycloSPORINE (Systemic); CYP2C9 Substrates; Dabigatran Etexilate; Digoxin; Ibritumomab; Lovastatin; Rivaroxaban; Salicylates; Simvastatin; Thrombolytic Agents; Tositumomab and Iodine I 131 Tositumomab

The levels/effects of Ticagrelor may be increased by: Aspirin; CycloSPORINE (Systemic); CYP3A4 Inhibitors (Strong); Dasatinib; Glucosamine; Grapefruit Juice; Herbs (Anticoagulant/Antiplatelet Properties); Ibrutinib; Multivitamins/Fluoride (with ADE); Multivitamins/Minerals (with ADEK, Folate, Iron); Multivitamins/Minerals (with AE, No Iron); Nonsteroidal Anti-Inflammatory Agents; Omega-3 Fatty Acids; Pentosan Polysulfate Sodium; Pentoxifylline; Prostacyclin Analogues; Tipranavir; Vitamin E

Decreased Effect

The levels/effects of Ticagrelor may be decreased by: Aspirin; Bosentan; CYP3A4 Inducers (Strong); CYP3A4 Inhibitors (Strong); Dabrafenib; Deferasirox; Herbs (CYP3A4 Inducers); Nonsteroidal Anti-Inflammatory Agents; Tocilizumab

Storage/Stability Store at 25°C (77°F); excursions permitted to 15°C to 30°C (59°F to 86°F).

Mechanism of Action Reversibly and noncompetitively binds the adenosine diphosphate (ADP) $P2Y_{12}$ receptor on the platelet surface which prevents ADP-mediated activation of the GPIIb/IIIa receptor complex thereby reducing platelet aggregation. Due to the reversible antagonism of the $P2Y_{12}$ receptor, recovery of platelet function is likely to depend on serum concentrations of ticagrelor and its active metabolite.

Pharmacodynamics/Kinetics

Onset of inhibition of platelet aggregation (IPA): 180 mg loading dose: ~41% within 30 minutes (similar to clopidogrel 600 mg at 8 hours)

Peak effect: Time to maximal IPA: 180 mg loading dose: IPA ~88% at 2 hours post administration

Duration of IPA: 180 mg loading dose: 87% to 89% maintained from 2-8 hours; 24 hours after the last maintenance dose, IPA is 58% (similar to maintenance clopidogrel)

Time after discontinuation when IPA is 30%: ~56 hours; IPA 10%: ~110 hours (Gurbel, 2009). Mean IPA observed with ticagrelor at 3 days post-discontinuation was comparable to that observed with clopidogrel at 5 days post discontinuation.

Absorption: Rapid

Distribution: 88 L

Protein binding: >99% (parent drug and active metabolite)

Metabolism: Hepatic via CYP3A4/5 to active metabolite (AR-C124910XX)

Bioavailability: ~36% (range: 30% to 42%)

Half-life elimination: Parent drug: ~7 hours; active metabolite: ~9 hours

Time to peak: Parent drug: ~1.5 hours; active metabolite (AR-C124910XX): ~2.5 hours

Excretion: Feces (58%); urine (26%); actual amount of parent drug and active metabolite excreted in urine was <1% of total dose administered

Dosage Oral: Adults:

Acute coronary syndrome: Unstable angina, non-ST-segment elevation myocardial infarction (NSTEMI), ST-segment elevation myocardial infarction (STEMI): Initial: 180 mg loading dose (with a loading dose of aspirin [eg, 325 mg] if not already receiving); Maintenance: 90 mg twice daily; initiated 12 hours after initial loading dose (with low-dose aspirin 75-100 mg/day or 81 mg/day in patients with UA/NSTEMI as recommended by the ACC/AHA [Jneid, 2012]). For UA/NSTEMI patients managed medically, continue ticagrelor for up to 12 months (Jneid, 2012). **Note:** Canadian labeling recommends a maintenance aspirin dose of 75-150 mg/day. Safety and efficacy of therapy beyond 12 months has not been established.

Duration of ticagrelor (in combination with aspirin) after stent placement: **Premature interruption of therapy may result in stent thrombosis with subsequent fatal and nonfatal MI.** Those with ACS receiving either stent type (bare metal [BMS] or drug-eluting stent [DES]) or those receiving a DES for a non-ACS indication, ticagrelor for at least 12 months is recommended. Those receiving a BMS for a non-ACS indication should be given at least 1 month and ideally up to 12 months; if patient is at increased risk of bleeding, give for a minimum of 2 weeks (Levine, 2011). A duration >12 months, regardless of indication, may be considered in patients with DES placement (Jneid, 2012; Levine, 2011).

Conversion from clopidogrel to ticagrelor: May initiate ticagrelor 90 mg twice daily beginning 24 hours after last clopidogrel dose (loading or maintenance); patients who are in the acute phase of an acute coronary syndrome, especially if determined to be clopidogrel nonresponsive, may be considered for administration of ticagrelor 180 mg loading dose followed by 90 mg twice daily regardless of previous clopidogrel exposure, taking into consideration the administration of other antiplatelet agents (eg, GP IIb/IIIa inhibitors) (Gurbel, 2010; Wallentin, 2009). **Note:** In general, conversion to ticagrelor results in an absolute inhibition of platelet aggregation (IPA) increase of 26.4%.

Dosage adjustment in renal impairment: No dosage adjustment necessary.

Hemodialysis: Use caution; drug is thought to be non-dialyzable

Dosage adjustment in hepatic impairment:

Mild impairment: No dosage adjustment necessary.

Moderate impairment: No dosage adjustment provided in manufacturer's labeling (has not been studied); however, undergoes hepatic metabolism; use caution. Use is contraindicated in the Canadian labeling.

Severe impairment: Use is contraindicated.

Dietary Considerations May be taken without regard to meals.

Administration May be administered without regard to meals. Missed doses should be taken at their next regularly scheduled time. For patients unable to swallow whole, tablets may be crushed to create a suspension for oral or NG use (data on file, AstraZeneca).

Monitoring Parameters Signs of bleeding; hemoglobin and hematocrit periodically; renal function; uric acid levels (patients with gout or at risk of hyperuricemia); signs/symptoms of dyspnea; may consider platelet function testing to determine platelet inhibitory response if results of testing may alter management (Jneid, 2012).

Additional Information Unlike thienopyridines (eg, clopidogrel, prasugrel) which are prodrugs and require metabolic transformation to their active metabolites for their activity, ticagrelor and its active metabolite both exhibit antiplatelet activity by reversibly and noncompetitively binding to the adenosine diphosphate (ADP) $P2Y_{12}$ receptor on the platelet surface. Due to the reversible antagonism of the $P2Y_{12}$ receptor, recovery of platelet function is faster than with use of irreversible $P2Y_{12}$ receptor antagonists such as clopidogrel or prasugrel.

Dosage Forms Excipient information presented when available (limited, particularly for generics); consult specific product labeling.

Tablet, Oral:

Brilinta: 90 mg

Dosage Forms: Canada Excipient information presented when available (limited, particularly for generics); consult specific product labeling.

Tablet, oral:

Brilinta®: 90 mg

Extemporaneous Preparations A suspension for oral administration may be prepared by crushing 1 or 2 tablets and placing in a dosing cup. To ensure the full dose is received, rinse mortar with 100 mL purified water, transfer to dosing cup, and repeat rinse (data on file, AstraZeneca).

A suspension for NG tube administration may be prepared by crushing one 90 mg tablet and diluting with 50 mL purified water; transfer to an oral enteral syringe and administer via NG tube. To ensure the full dose is received, flush mortar, syringe, and NG tube with 50 mL purified water, and repeat rinse (data on file, AstraZeneca).

When stored in a PVC oral syringe for up to 2 hours, there was no degradation of the suspension detected (data on file, AstraZeneca).

Ticarcillin and Clavulanate Potassium

(tye kar SIL in & klav yoo LAN ate poe TASS ee um)

Brand Names: U.S. Timentin

Brand Names: Canada Timentin

Index Terms Ticarcillin and Clavulanic Acid

Pharmacologic Category Antibiotic, Penicillin

Use

Bone and joint infections: Treatment of bone and joint infections caused by beta-lactamase-producing isolates of *Staphylococcus aureus*.

Endometritis: Treatment of endometritis caused by beta-lactamase-producing isolates of *Prevotella melaninogenicus*, *Enterobacter* species (including *E. cloacae*), *Klebsiella pneumoniae*, *Escherichia coli*, *S. aureus*, or *Staphylococcus epidermidis*.

Lower respiratory tract infections: Treatment of lower respiratory tract infections caused by beta-lactamase-producing isolates of *S. aureus*, *Haemophilus influenzae*, or *Klebsiella* species.

Peritonitis: Treatment of peritonitis caused by beta-lactamase-producing isolates of *E. coli*, *K. pneumonia*, or *Bacteroides fragilis* group.

Septicemia: Treatment of septicemia (including bacteremia) caused by beta-lactamase-producing isolates of *Klebsiella* species, *E. coli*, *S. aureus*, or *Pseudomonas aeruginosa* (or other *Pseudomonas* species).

Skin and skin structure infections: Treatment of skin and skin structure infections caused by beta-lactamase-producing isolates of *S. aureus*, *Klebsiella* species, or *E. coli*.

Urinary tract infections: Treatment of complicated and uncomplicated urinary tract infections caused by beta-lactamase-producing isolates of *E. coli*, *Klebsiella* species, *P. aeruginosa* (and other *Pseudomonas* species), *Citrobacter* species, *Enterobacter cloacae*, *Serratia marcescens*, or *S. aureus*.

Unlabeled Use Treatment of complicated intra-abdominal infections (Solomkin 2010), cystic fibrosis exacerbations (Zobell, 2013)

Pregnancy Risk Factor B

Pregnancy Considerations Adverse events were not observed in animal reproduction studies. Ticarcillin and clavulanate cross the placenta (Maberry, 1992). Maternal use of penicillins has generally not resulted in an increased risk of adverse fetal effects (Crider, 2009; Santos, 2011). Ticarcillin/clavulanate is approved for the treatment of postpartum gynecologic infections, including endometritis, caused by susceptible organisms.

Breast-Feeding Considerations Small amounts of ticarcillin are found in breast milk (Matsuda, 1984; von Kobyletzki, 1983); however, it is not orally absorbed (Brogden, 1980). The manufacturer recommends that caution be exercised when administering ticarcillin/clavulanate to nursing women.

Contraindications Hypersensitivity (history of a serious reaction [eg, anaphylaxis, Stevens-Johnson syndrome]) to ticarcillin, clavulanate, or to other beta-lactams (eg, penicillins, cephalosporins)

Warnings/Precautions Use with caution and modify dosage in patients with renal impairment; serious and occasionally severe or fatal hypersensitivity (anaphylactoid) reactions have been reported in patients on penicillin therapy (especially with a history of beta-lactam hypersensitivity and/or a history of sensitivity to multiple allergens); use with caution in patients with seizures and in patients with HF due to high sodium load. Particularly in patients with renal impairment, bleeding disorders have been observed; discontinue if thrombocytopenia or bleeding occurs. Prolonged use may result in fungal or bacterial superinfection, including *C. difficile*-associated diarrhea (CDAD) and pseudomembranous colitis; CDAD has been observed >2 months postantibiotic treatment.

Adverse Reactions Frequency not defined.

Central nervous system: Confusion, drowsiness, fever, headache, Jarisch-Herxheimer reaction, seizure

Dermatologic: Erythema multiforme, pruritus, rash, Stevens-Johnson syndrome, toxic epidermal necrolysis, urticaria

Endocrine & metabolic: Electrolyte imbalance

Gastrointestinal: *Clostridium difficile* colitis, diarrhea, nausea, vomiting

Hematologic: Bleeding, eosinophilia, hemolytic anemia, leukopenia, neutropenia, positive Coombs' reaction, prothrombin time prolonged, thrombocytopenia

Hepatic: Hepatotoxicity, jaundice

Local: Injection site reaction (pain, burning, induration); thrombophlebitis

Neuromuscular & skeletal: Myoclonus

Renal: BUN increased, interstitial nephritis (acute), serum creatinine increased

Miscellaneous: Anaphylaxis, hypersensitivity reactions

Drug Interactions

Metabolism/Transport Effects None known.

Avoid Concomitant Use

Avoid concomitant use of Ticarcillin and Clavulanate Potassium with any of the following: BCG

Increased Effect/Toxicity

Ticarcillin and Clavulanate Potassium may increase the levels/effects of: Methotrexate; Vitamin K Antagonists

The levels/effects of Ticarcillin and Clavulanate Potassium may be increased by: Probenecid

Decreased Effect

Ticarcillin and Clavulanate Potassium may decrease the levels/effects of: Aminoglycosides; BCG; Mycophenolate; Sodium Picosulfate; Typhoid Vaccine

The levels/effects of Ticarcillin and Clavulanate Potassium may be decreased by: Tetracycline Derivatives

Preparation for Administration

Reconstitute 3.1 g vials with 13 mL sterile water for injection or NS; shake well; resulting concentration is ticarcillin 200 mg/mL and clavulanic acid 6.7 mg/mL. Reconstitute 31 g bulk vials with 76 mL sterile water for injection or NS; shake well; resulting concentration is ticarcillin 300 mg/mL and clavulanic acid 10 mg/mL. Further dilute to a final concentration of 10-100 mg/mL in D_5W, LR, or NS.

Storage/Stability

Vials: Store intact vials at ≤24°C (≤75°F). Reconstituted solution is stable for 6 hours at room temperature and 72 hours when refrigerated. I.V. infusion in NS or LR is stable for 24 hours at room temperature (21°C to 24°C [70°F to 75°F]), 7 days when refrigerated (4°C [39°F]), or 30 days when frozen (-18°C [0°F]). I.V. infusion in D_5W solution is stable for 24 hours at room temperature (21°C to 24°C [70°F to 75°F]), 3 days when refrigerated (4°C [39°F]), or 7 days when frozen (-18°C [0°F]. After freezing, thawed solution is stable for 8 hours at room temperature. Do not refreeze. Darkening of drug indicates loss of potency of clavulanate potassium.

Premixed solution: Store frozen at ≤-20°C (-4°F). Thawed solution is stable for 24 hours at room temperature (22°C [72°F]) or 7 days under refrigeration at (4°C [39°F]); do not refreeze.

Mechanism of Action Inhibits bacterial cell wall synthesis by binding to one or more of the penicillin-binding proteins (PBPs), which in turn inhibits the final transpeptidation step of peptidoglycan synthesis in bacterial cell walls, thus inhibiting cell wall biosynthesis. Bacteria eventually lyse due to ongoing activity of cell wall autolytic enzymes (autolysins and murein hydrolases) while cell wall assembly is arrested.

Pharmacodynamics/Kinetics

Protein binding: Ticarcillin: ~45%; Clavulanic acid: ~25%

Half-life elimination: Ticarcillin: 1.1 hours; Clavulanic acid: 1.1 hours

Time to peak, plasma: Immediately following completion of 30-minute infusion

Excretion: Ticarcillin: Urine (60% to 70%); Clavulanic acid: Urine (35% to 45% as unchanged drug)

Dosage Note: Timentin (ticarcillin/clavulanate) is a combination product; each 3.1 g dosage form contains 3 g ticarcillin disodium and 0.1 g clavulanic acid.

Usual dosage range: Note: Dosage adjustment recommended in patients with renal impairment.

Infants ≥3 months, Children, Adolescents, and Adults: I.V.:

<60 kg: 200-300 mg ticarcillin/kg/day in divided doses every 4-6 hours (maximum: 18 g daily)

≥60 kg: 3.1 g every 4-6 hours

Indication-specific dosing:

Infants ≥3 months, Children, and Adolescents:

Mild to moderate infections: I.V.:

<60 kg: 200 mg ticarcillin/kg/day in divided doses every 6 hours (maximum: 12 g daily)

≥60 kg: 3.1 g every 6 hours

Severe infections: I.V.:

<60 kg: 300 mg ticarcillin/kg/day in divided doses every 4 hours. (maximum: 18 g daily)

≥60 kg: 3.1 g every 4 hours

Cystic fibrosis (unlabeled use): I.V.: 400 mg ticarcillin/kg/day in divided doses every 6 hours; higher doses have been used: 400-750 mg ticarcillin/kg/day in divided doses every 6 hours (maximum, 24-30 g ticarcillin daily) (Zobell, 2013)

Intra-abdominal infection, complicated (unlabeled use): I.V.: 200-300 mg ticarcillin/kg/day in divided every 4-6 hours (Solomkin, 2010)

Adults:

Gynecologic infections (eg, endometritis): I.V.:

Moderate infections: 200 mg ticarcillin/kg/day in divided doses every 6 hours (maximum: 12 g daily)

Severe infections: 300 mg ticarcillin/kg/day in divided doses every 4 hours (maximum: 18 g daily)

Systemic infections, urinary tract infections: I.V.:

<60 kg: 200-300 mg ticarcillin/kg/day in divided doses every 4-6 hours (maximum: 18 g daily)

≥60 kg: 3.1 g every 4-6 hours

Intra-abdominal infection, complicated, community-acquired, mild-to-moderate (unlabeled use): 3.1 g every 6 hours for 4-7 days (provided source controlled) (Solomkin, 2010)

Dosing adjustment in renal impairment: Loading dose: I.V.: 3.1 g one dose, followed by maintenance dose based on creatinine clearance:

Cl_{cr} 30-60 mL/minute: Administer 2 g of ticarcillin component every 4 hours

Cl_{cr} 10-30 mL/minute: Administer 2 g of ticarcillin component every 8 hours

Cl_{cr} <10 mL/minute: Administer 2 g of ticarcillin component every 12 hours

Cl_{cr} <10 mL/minute with concomitant hepatic dysfunction: 2 g of ticarcillin component every 24 hours

Intermittent hemodialysis (IHD) (administer after hemodialysis on dialysis days): Dialyzable (20% to 50%): 2 g of ticarcillin component every 12 hours; supplemented with 3.1 g (ticarcillin/clavulanate) after each dialysis session. Alternatively, administer 2 g every 8 hours without a supplemental dose for deep-seated infections (Heintz, 2009). **Note:** Dosing dependent on the assumption of 3 times/week, complete IHD sessions.

Peritoneal dialysis (PD): 3.1 g every 12 hours

Continuous renal replacement therapy (CRRT) (Heintz, 2009; Trotman, 2005): Drug clearance is highly dependent on the method of renal replacement, filter type, and flow rate. Appropriate dosing requires close monitoring of pharmacologic response, signs of adverse reactions due to drug accumulation, as well as drug concentrations in relation to target trough (if appropriate). The following are general recommendations only (based on dialysate flow/ultrafiltration rates of 1-2 L/hour and minimal residual renal function) and should not supersede clinical judgment:

CVVH: Loading dose of 3.1g followed by 2 g every 6-8 hours

CVVHD: Loading dose of 3.1 g followed by 3.1 g every 6-8 hours

CVVHDF: Loading dose of 3.1 g followed by 3.1 g every 6 hours

Note: Do not administer in intervals exceeding every 8 hours. Clavulanate component is hepatically eliminated; extending the dosing interval beyond 8 hours may result in loss of beta-lactamase inhibition.

Dosing adjustment in hepatic dysfunction: With concomitant renal dysfunction (Cl_{cr} <10 mL/minute): 2 g of ticarcillin component every 24 hours

Dietary Considerations Some products may contain potassium and/or sodium.

Administration Infuse over 30 minutes.

Some penicillins (eg, carbenicillin, ticarcillin, and piperacillin) have been shown to inactivate aminoglycosides *in vitro*. This has been observed to a greater extent with tobramycin and gentamicin, while amikacin has shown greater stability against inactivation. Concurrent use of these agents may pose a risk of reduced antibacterial efficacy *in vivo*, particularly in the setting of profound renal impairment. However, definitive clinical evidence is lacking. If combination penicillin/aminoglycoside therapy is desired in a patient with renal dysfunction, separation of doses (if feasible), and routine monitoring of aminoglycoside levels, CBC, and clinical response should be considered.

Monitoring Parameters Observe for signs and symptoms of anaphylaxis during first dose; serum electrolytes, bleeding time, and periodic tests of renal, hepatic, and hematologic function

Test Interactions Positive Coombs' test, false-positive urinary proteins

Some penicillin derivatives may accelerate the degradation of aminoglycosides *in vitro*, leading to a potential underestimation of aminoglycoside serum concentration.

Dosage Forms Excipient information presented when available (limited, particularly for generics); consult specific product labeling.

Infusion [premixed, frozen]: Ticarcillin 3 g and clavulanic acid 0.1 g (100 mL) [contains sodium 4.51 mEq and potassium 0.15 mEq per g]

Injection, powder for reconstitution: Ticarcillin 3 g and clavulanic acid 0.1 g (3.1 g, 31 g) [contains sodium 4.51 mEq and potassium 0.15 mEq per g]

◆ **Ticarcillin and Clavulanic Acid** *see* Ticarcillin and Clavulanate Potassium *on page* 2058

◆ **Tice BCG** *see* BCG *on page* 226

Ticlopidine (tye KLOE pi deen)

Brand Names: Canada Apo-Ticlopidine®; Dom-Ticlopidine; Gen-Ticlopidine; Mylan-Ticlopidine; Novo-Ticlopidine; Nu-Ticlopidine; PMS-Ticlopidine; Sandoz-Ticlopidine; Teva-Ticlopidine

Index Terms Ticlopidine Hydrochloride

Pharmacologic Category Antiplatelet Agent; Antiplatelet Agent, Thienopyridine

Additional Appendix Information

Beers Criteria – Potentially Inappropriate Medications for Geriatrics *on page 2368*

Oral Antiplatelet Comparison Chart *on page 2313*

Use Platelet aggregation inhibitor that reduces the risk of thrombotic stroke in patients who have had a stroke or stroke precursors (**Note:** Due to its association with life-threatening hematologic disorders, ticlopidine should be reserved for patients who are intolerant to aspirin, or who have failed aspirin therapy); adjunctive therapy (with aspirin) following successful coronary stent implantation to reduce the incidence of subacute stent thrombosis.

Unlabeled Use Protection of aortocoronary bypass grafts, diabetic microangiopathy, ischemic heart disease, prevention of postoperative DVT, reduction of graft loss following renal transplant

Pregnancy Risk Factor B

Pregnancy Considerations Teratogenic effects have not been observed in animal reproduction studies; a case report has demonstrated the safe use of ticlopidine in pregnant women (Ueno, 2001).

Breast-Feeding Considerations It is not known if ticlopidine is excreted in breast milk. Due to the potential for serious adverse reactions in the nursing infant, a decision should be made whether to discontinue nursing or to discontinue the drug, taking into account the importance of treatment to the mother.

Contraindications Hypersensitivity to ticlopidine or any component of the formulation; active pathological bleeding such as peptic ulcer bleeding or intracranial hemorrhage; severe liver impairment; hematopoietic disorders (neutropenia, thrombocytopenia, or a past history of TTP or aplastic anemia)

Warnings/Precautions Use with caution in patients who may be at risk of increased bleeding (eg, PUD, trauma, or surgery). Consider discontinuing 10-14 days before elective surgery (except in patients with cardiac stents that have not completed their full course of dual antiplatelet therapy; patient-specific situations need to be discussed with cardiologist; AHA/ACC/SCAI/ACS/ADA Science Advisory provides recommendations). In patients who have received bare-metal or drug-eluting stents (sirolimus or paclitaxel), premature interruption of antiplatelet therapy may result in stent thrombosis with subsequent fatal and nonfatal myocardial infarction. If ticlopidine is used, duration of therapy, in general, is determined by the type of stent placed (bare metal or drug eluting) and whether an ACS event was ongoing at the time of placement (Levine, 2011). Use caution in concurrent treatment with anticoagulants (eg, heparin, warfarin) or other antiplatelet drugs; bleeding risk is increased.

Because of structural similarities, cross-reactivity is possible among the thienopyridines (clopidogrel, prasugrel, and ticlopidine); use with caution or avoid in patients with previous thienopyridine hypersensitivity. Use of ticlopidine is contraindicated in patients with hypersensitivity to ticlopidine.

Use with caution in patients with mild-to-moderate hepatic impairment; use is contraindicated with severe hepatic impairment. Use with caution in patients with moderate-to-severe renal impairment (experience is limited); bleeding times may be significantly prolonged and the risk of hematologic adverse effects (eg, neutropenia) may be increased. **[U.S. Boxed Warning]: May cause life-threatening hematologic reactions, including neutropenia, agranulocytosis, thrombotic thrombocytopenia purpura (TTP), and aplastic anemia.** Routine monitoring is required (see Monitoring Parameters). Monitor for signs and symptoms of neutropenia including WBC count. Discontinue if the absolute neutrophil count falls to $<1200/mm^3$ or if the platelet count falls to $<80,000/mm^3$. Avoid use in the elderly due to availability of safer alternative agents (Beers Criteria).

Adverse Reactions As with all drugs which may affect hemostasis, bleeding is associated with ticlopidine. Hemorrhage may occur at virtually any site. Risk is dependent on multiple variables, including the use of multiple agents which alter hemostasis and patient susceptibility.

>10%:

Endocrine & metabolic: Total cholesterol increased (increases of ~8% to 10% within 1 month of therapy), triglycerides increased

Gastrointestinal: Diarrhea (13%)

1% to 10%:

Central nervous system: Dizziness (1%)

Dermatologic: Rash (5%), purpura (2%), pruritus (1%)

Gastrointestinal: Nausea (7%), dyspepsia (7%), gastrointestinal pain (4%), vomiting (2%), flatulence (2%), anorexia (1%)

Hematologic: Neutropenia (2%)

Hepatic: Alkaline phosphatase increased (>2 x upper limit of normal; 8%), abnormal liver function test (1%)

<1% (Limited to important or life-threatening): Agranulocytosis, anaphylaxis, angioedema, aplastic anemia, arthropathy, bilirubin increased, bone marrow suppression, bronchiolitis obliterans-organized pneumonia, chronic diarrhea, conjunctival bleeding, eosinophilia, erythema multiforme, erythema nodosum, exfoliative dermatitis, gastrointestinal bleeding, hematuria, hemolytic anemia, hepatic necrosis, hepatitis, hyponatremia, intracranial bleeding (rare), jaundice, maculopapular rash, menorrhagia, myositis, nephrotic syndrome, pancytopenia, peptic ulcer, peripheral neuropathy, pneumonitis (allergic), positive ANA, renal failure, sepsis, serum creatinine increased, serum sickness, Stevens-Johnson syndrome, systemic lupus erythematosus, thrombocytopenia (immune), thrombocytosis, thrombotic thrombocytopenic purpura, urticaria, vasculitis

Drug Interactions

Metabolism/Transport Effects Substrate of CYP3A4 (major); **Note:** Assignment of Major/Minor substrate status based on clinically relevant drug interaction potential; **Inhibits** CYP1A2 (weak), CYP2B6 (moderate), CYP2C19 (strong), CYP2C9 (weak), CYP2D6 (moderate), CYP2E1 (weak), CYP3A4 (weak)

Avoid Concomitant Use

Avoid concomitant use of Ticlopidine with any of the following: Pimozide; Thioridazine

Increased Effect/Toxicity

Ticlopidine may increase the levels/effects of: Agents with Antiplatelet Properties; Anticoagulants; ARIPiprazole; Citalopram; Collagenase (Systemic); CYP2B6 Substrates; CYP2C19 Substrates; CYP2D6 Substrates; Dabigatran Etexilate; Dofetilide; Fesoterodine; Fosphenytoin; Ibritumomab; Lomitapide; Metoprolol; Nebivolol; Phenytoin; Pimozide; Rivaroxaban; Salicylates; Theophylline Derivatives; Thioridazine; Thrombolytic Agents; Tositumomab and Iodine I 131 Tositumomab

The levels/effects of Ticlopidine may be increased by: Dasatinib; Glucosamine; Herbs (Anticoagulant/Antiplatelet Properties); Ibrutinib; Multivitamins/Fluoride (with ADE); Multivitamins/Minerals (with ADEK, Folate, Iron); Multivitamins/Minerals (with AE, No Iron); Nonsteroidal Anti-Inflammatory Agents; Omega-3 Fatty Acids; Pentosan Polysulfate Sodium; Pentoxifylline; Propafenone; Prostacyclin Analogues; Tipranavir; Vitamin E

Decreased Effect

Ticlopidine may decrease the levels/effects of: Clopidogrel; Codeine; Tamoxifen; TraMADol

The levels/effects of Ticlopidine may be decreased by: Bosentan; CYP3A4 Inducers (Strong); Dabrafenib; Deferasirox; Herbs (CYP3A4 Inducers); Mitotane; Nonsteroidal Anti-Inflammatory Agents; Tocilizumab

Ethanol/Nutrition/Herb Interactions

Food: Ticlopidine bioavailability may be increased (20%) if taken with food. High-fat meals increase absorption, antacids decrease absorption. May cause upset stomach. Management: Take with food to reduce stomach upset.

Herb/Nutraceutical: Some herbal medications have additional antiplatelet activity. Management: Avoid alfalfa, anise, bilberry, bladderwrack, bromelain, cat's claw, chamomile, coleus, cordyceps, dong quai, evening primrose oil, fenugreek, feverfew, garlic, ginger, ginkgo biloba, ginseng (American), ginseng (Panax), ginseng (Siberian), grapeseed, green tea, guggul, horse chestnut seed, horseradish, licorice, prickly ash, red clover, reishi, SAMe (S-adenosylmethionine), sweet clover, turmeric, and white willow.

Mechanism of Action Ticlopidine requires *in vivo* biotransformation to an unidentified active metabolite. This active metabolite irreversibly blocks the P2Y12 component of ADP receptors, which prevents activation of the GPIIb/IIIa receptor complex, thereby reducing platelet aggregation. Platelets blocked by ticlopidine are affected for the remainder of their lifespan.

Pharmacodynamics/Kinetics

Onset of action: ~6 hours

Peak effect: 3-5 days; serum levels do not correlate with clinical antiplatelet activity

Absorption: Well absorbed

Protein binding: Parent drug: 98%; <15% bound to alpha$_1$-acid glycoprotein

Metabolism: Extensively hepatic; has at least 1 active metabolite

Half-life elimination: 13 hours

Time to peak, serum: ~2 hours

Excretion: Urine (60%); feces (23%)

Dosage Oral: Adults:

Stroke prevention: 250 mg twice daily

Coronary artery stenting (initiate after successful implantation): 250 mg twice daily (in combination with antiplatelet doses of aspirin). If initiated prior to percutaneous coronary intervention, a loading dose of 500 mg may be administered (Berger, 1999). May continue treatment for up to 30 days per the manufacturer; however, in general, duration of therapy may extend up to 12 months in patients with drug-eluting stents or those with stent implantation (bare metal or drug eluting) for acute coronary syndrome (Levine, 2011).

Note: Overall, the use of ticlopidine has largely been replaced by newer P2Y$_{12}$ inhibitors (ie, clopidogrel, prasugrel, ticagrelor).

Dosage adjustment in renal impairment: No dosage adjustment provided in manufacturer's labeling. While there were no statistically significant differences in ADP-induced platelet aggregation, AUC increases and clearance decreases were seen in patients with mild to moderate renal impairment. However, bleeding time may be prolonged in patients with moderate renal impairment

Dosage adjustment in hepatic impairment: No dosage adjustment provided in manufacturer's labeling. Use with caution. Use is contraindicated in severe hepatic diseaseimpairment.

Dietary Considerations Should be taken with food to reduce stomach upset.

Administration Administer with food.

Monitoring Parameters Signs of bleeding; CBC with differential every 2 weeks starting the second week through the third month of treatment; more frequent monitoring is recommended for patients whose absolute neutrophil counts have been consistently declining or are 30% less than baseline values. The peak incidence of TTP occurs between 3-4 weeks, the peak incidence of neutropenia occurs at approximately 4-6 weeks, and the incidence of aplastic anemia peaks after 4-8 weeks of therapy. Few cases have been reported after 3 months of treatment. Liver function tests (alkaline phosphatase and transaminases) should be performed in the first 4 months of therapy if liver dysfunction is suspected.

Dosage Forms Excipient information presented when available (limited, particularly for generics); consult specific product labeling.

Tablet, Oral, as hydrochloride:

Generic: 250 mg

◆ **Ticlopidine Hydrochloride** *see* Ticlopidine *on page 2059*

◆ **TIG** *see* Tetanus Immune Globulin (Human) *on page 2030*

◆ **Tigan** *see* Trimethobenzamide *on page 2128*

◆ **Tigan® (Can)** *see* Trimethobenzamide *on page 2128*

Tigecycline (tye ge SYE kleen)

Brand Names: U.S. Tygacil

Brand Names: Canada Tygacil

Index Terms GAR-936

Pharmacologic Category Antibiotic, Glycylcycline

Use

Community-acquired bacterial pneumonia: Treatment of community-acquired pneumonia in patients 18 years and older caused by *Streptococcus pneumoniae* (penicillin-susceptible isolates), including cases with concurrent bacteremia, *Haemophilus influenzae* (beta-lactamase negative isolates), and *Legionella pneumophila*.

Complicated intra-abdominal infections: Treatment of complicated intra-abdominal infections in patients 18 years and older caused by *Citrobacter freundii*, *Enterobacter cloacae*, *Escherichia coli*, *Klebsiella oxytoca*, *Klebsiella pneumoniae*, *Enterococcus faecalis* (vancomycin-susceptible isolates), *Staphylococcus aureus* (methicillin-susceptible and methicillin-resistant isolates), *Streptococcus anginosus* group (includes *S. anginosus*, *Streptococcus intermedius*, and *Streptococcus constellatus*), *Bacteroides fragilis*, *Bacteroides thetaiotaomicron*, *Bacteroides uniformis*, *Bacteroides vulgatus*, *Clostridium perfringens*, and *Peptostreptococcus micros*.

Complicated skin and skin structure infections: Treatment of skin and skin structure infections in patients 18 years and older caused by *E. coli*, *E. faecalis* (vancomycin-susceptible isolates), *S. aureus* (methicillin-susceptible and methicillin-resistant isolates), *Streptococcus agalactiae*, *S. anginosus* group (includes *S. anginosus*, *S. intermedius*, and *S. constellatus*), *Streptococcus pyogenes*, *E. cloacae*, *K. pneumoniae*, and *B. fragilis*.

Pregnancy Risk Factor D

Pregnancy Considerations Because adverse effects were observed in animals and because of the potential for permanent tooth discoloration, tigecycline is classified pregnancy category D. Tigecycline frequently causes nausea and vomiting and, therefore, may not be ideal for use in a patient with pregnancy-related nausea.

Breast-Feeding Considerations It is not known if tigecycline is found in breast milk. The manufacturer recommends caution if giving tigecycline to a nursing woman. Nondose-related effects could include modification of bowel flora.

Contraindications

Hypersensitivity to tigecycline or any component of the formulation

Documentation of allergenic cross-reactivity for tetracyclines is limited. However, because of similarities in chemical structure and/or pharmacologic actions, the possibility of cross-sensitivity cannot be ruled out with certainty.

Canadian labeling: Additional contraindications (not in U.S. labeling): Hypersensitivity to tetracycline class of antibiotics

Warnings/Precautions [U.S. Boxed Warning]: In Phase 3 and 4 clinical trials, an increase in all-cause mortality was observed in patients treated with tigecycline compared to those treated with comparator antibiotics; cause has not been established. Use should be reserved for situations in which alternative treatments are not appropriate. In general, deaths were the result of worsening infection, complications of infection, or underlying comorbidity. May cause life-threatening anaphylaxis/anaphylactoid reactions. Due to structural similarity with tetracyclines, use caution in patients with prior hypersensitivity and/or severe adverse reactions associated with tetracycline use (Canadian labeling contraindicates use in patients with hypersensitivity to tetracyclines). Due to structural similarities with tetracyclines, may be associated with photosensitivity, pseudotumor cerebri, pancreatitis, and antianabolic effects (including increased BUN, azotemia, acidosis, and hyperphosphatemia) observed with this class. Acute pancreatitis (including fatalities) has been reported, including patients without known risk factors; discontinue use when suspected. May cause fetal harm if used during pregnancy; patients should be advised of potential risks associated with use. Permanent discoloration of the teeth may occur if used during tooth development (fetal stage through children up to 8 years of age).

Safety and efficacy in children <18 years of age have not been established due to increased mortality observed in trials of adult patients. Use only if no alternative antibiotics are available. Because of effects on tooth development (yellow-gray-brown discoloration), use in patients <8 years is not recommended.

Use caution in hepatic impairment; dosage adjustment recommended in severe hepatic impairment. Abnormal liver function tests (increased total bilirubin, prothrombin time, transaminases) have been reported. Isolated cases of significant hepatic dysfunction and hepatic failure have occurred. Closely monitor for worsening hepatic function in patients that develop abnormal liver function tests during therapy. Adverse hepatic effects may occur after drug discontinuation.

Prolonged use may result in fungal or bacterial superinfection, including *C. difficile*-associated diarrhea (CDAD) and pseudomembranous colitis; CDAD has been observed >2 months postantibiotic treatment. Use with caution if using as monotherapy for patients with intestinal perforation (in the small sample of available cases, septic shock occurred more frequently than patients treated with imipenem/cilastatin comparator). Do not use for diabetic foot infections; on-inferiority was not demonstrated in studies. Do not use for healthcare-acquired pneumonia (HAP) or ventilator-associated pneumonia (VAP); increased mortality and decreased efficacy have been reported in HAP and VAP trials.

Adverse Reactions Note: Frequencies relative to placebo are not available; some frequencies are lower than those experienced with comparator drugs.

>10%: Gastrointestinal: Nausea (26%; severe: 1%), vomiting (18%; severe: 1%), diarrhea (12%)

2% to 10%:

Cardiovascular: Localized phlebitis (3%)

Central nervous system: Headache (6%), dizziness (3%)

Dermatologic: Skin rash (3%)

Endocrine & metabolic: Hyponatremia (2%), increased amylase (3%)

Gastrointestinal: Abdominal pain (6%), dyspepsia (2%)

Hematologic & oncologic: Anemia (5%), hypoproteinemia (5%)

Hepatic: Increased serum ALT (5%), increased serum AST (4%), increased serum alkaline phosphatase (3%), hyperbilirubinemia (2%)

Infection: Infection (7%), abscess (2%)

Neuromuscular & skeletal: Weakness (3%)

Renal: Increased blood urea nitrogen (3%)

Respiratory: Pneumonia (2%)

Miscellaneous: Abnormal healing (3%)

<2% (Limited to important or life-threatening): Acute pancreatitis, allergic skin reaction, anaphylactoid reaction, anaphylaxis, anorexia, *Clostridium difficile* associated diarrhea, dysgeusia, eosinophilia, hepatic insufficiency, hepatic failure, hypocalcemia, hypoglycemia, increased INR, increased serum creatinine, increased serum transaminases, increased INR, increased serum creatinine, increased serum transaminases, prolonged partial thromboplastin time, prolonged prothrombin time, pruritus, septic shock, Stevens-Johnson syndrome, swelling at injection site, thrombocytopenia, thrombophlebitis, vaginal moniliasis, vaginitis

Drug Interactions

Metabolism/Transport Effects None known.

Avoid Concomitant Use There are no known interactions where it is recommended to avoid concomitant use.

Increased Effect/Toxicity

Tigecycline may increase the levels/effects of: Warfarin

Decreased Effect There are no known significant interactions involving a decrease in effect.

Preparation for Administration Add 5.3 mL NS, D_5W, or LR to each 50 mg vial. Swirl gently to dissolve. Resulting solution is 10 mg/mL. Reconstituted solution must be further diluted to allow I.V. administration. Transfer to 100 mL I.V. bag for infusion (final concentration should not exceed 1 mg/mL). Reconstituted solution should be yellow-orange; discard if not this color.

Storage/Stability Prior to reconstitution, store at 20°C to 25°C (68°F to 77°F); excursions are permitted between 15°C and 30°C (59°F and 86°F). Reconstituted solution may be stored at room temperature (not to exceed 25°C [77°F]) for up to 6 hours in the vial or up to 24 hours if further diluted in a compatible I.V. solution. Alternatively, may be stored refrigerated at 2°C to 8°C (36°F to 46°F) for up to 48 hours following immediate transfer of the reconstituted solution into NS or D_5W.

Mechanism of Action A glycylcycline antibiotic that binds to the 30S ribosomal subunit of susceptible bacteria, thereby, inhibiting protein synthesis. Generally considered bacteriostatic; however, bactericidal activity has been demonstrated against isolates of *S. pneumoniae* and *L. pneumophila*. Tigecycline is a derivative of minocycline (9-t-butylglycylamido minocycline), and while not classified as a tetracycline, it may share some class-associated adverse effects. Tigecycline has demonstrated activity against a variety of gram-positive and -negative bacterial pathogens including methicillin-resistant staphylococci.

Pharmacodynamics/Kinetics

Distribution: V_d: 7-9 L/kg; extensive tissue distribution

Protein binding: 71% to 89%

Metabolism: Hepatic, via glucuronidation, N-acetylation, and epimerization to several metabolites, each <10% of the dose

Half-life elimination: Single dose: 27 hours; following multiple doses: 42 hours

Excretion: Feces (59%, primarily as unchanged drug); urine (33%, with 22% of the total dose as unchanged drug)

Dosage

Children ≥8 years and Adolescents: Limited data available:

Note: Use should be reserved for situations when no effective alternative therapy is available

General dosing, susceptible infection: I.V.: Dosing based on data from pharmacokinetic trials.

Children 8-11 years: 1.2 mg/kg/dose every 12 hours; maximum dose: 50 mg

Children ≥12 years and Adolescents: 50 mg every 12 hours

Adults: **Note:** Duration of therapy dependent on severity/site of infection and clinical status and response to therapy.

Intra-abdominal infections, complicated (cIAI): I.V.: Initial: 100 mg as a single dose; Maintenance dose: 50 mg every 12 hours for 5-14 days; **Note:** 2010 IDSA guidelines recommend a treatment duration of 4-7 days (provided source controlled) for community-acquired, mild-to-moderate IAI

Pneumonia, community-acquired: I.V.: Initial: 100 mg as a single dose; Maintenance dose: 50 mg every 12 hours for 7-14 days

Skin/skin structure infections, complicated: I.V.: Initial: 100 mg as a single dose; Maintenance dose: 50 mg every 12 hours for 5-14 days

Dosage adjustment in renal impairment: No dosage adjustment necessary.

Poorly dialyzed; no supplemental dose or dosage adjustment necessary, including patients on intermittent hemodialysis, peritoneal dialysis, or continuous renal replacement therapy (eg, CVVHD).

Dosage adjustment in hepatic impairment:

Mild to moderate hepatic impairment (Child-Pugh class A or B): No dosage adjustment necessary.

Severe hepatic impairment (Child-Pugh class C): Initial: 100 mg single dose; Maintenance: 25 mg every 12 hours

Administration Infuse over 30-60 minutes through dedicated line or via Y-site

Dosage Forms Excipient information presented when available (limited, particularly for generics); consult specific product labeling.

Solution Reconstituted, Intravenous:

Tygacil: 50 mg (1 ea)

◆ **Tikosyn** *see* Dofetilide *on page* 645

◆ **Tikosyn® (Can)** *see* Dofetilide *on page* 645

◆ **Tilia Fe** *see* Ethinyl Estradiol and Norethindrone *on page* 793

Tiludronate (tye LOO droe nate)

Brand Names: U.S. Skelid

Index Terms Tiludronate Disodium

Pharmacologic Category Bisphosphonate Derivative

Use Treatment of Paget's disease of the bone (osteitis deformans) in patients who have a level of serum alkaline phosphatase (SAP) at least twice the upper limit of normal, or who are symptomatic, or who are at risk for future complications of their disease

Pregnancy Risk Factor C

Pregnancy Considerations Adverse events were observed in some animal reproduction studies. It is not known if bisphosphonates cross the placenta, but fetal exposure is expected (Djokanovic, 2008; Stathopoulos, 2011). Bisphosphonates are incorporated into the bone matrix and gradually released over time. The amount available in the systemic circulation varies by dose and duration of therapy. Theoretically, there may be a risk of fetal harm when pregnancy follows the completion of therapy; however, available data have not shown that exposure to bisphosphonates during pregnancy significantly increases the risk of adverse fetal events (Djokanovic, 2008; Levy, 2009; Stathopoulos, 2011). Until additional data is available, most sources recommend discontinuing bisphosphonate therapy in women of reproductive potential as early as possible prior to a planned pregnancy; use in premenopausal women should be reserved for special circumstances when rapid bone loss is occurring (Bhalla, 2010; Pereira, 2012; Stathopoulos, 2011). Because hypocalcemia has been described following *in utero* bisphosphonate exposure, exposed infants should be monitored for hypocalcemia after birth (Djokanovic, 2008; Stathopoulos, 2011).

Breast-Feeding Considerations It is now known if tiludronate is excreted into breast milk. The manufacturer recommends caution be exercised when administering tiludronate to nursing women.

Contraindications Hypersensitivity to tiludronate, bisphosphonates, or any component of the formulation; inability to stand or sit upright for at least 30 minutes

Warnings/Precautions Not recommended in patients with severe renal impairment (Cl_{cr} <30 mL/minute). Use with caution in patients with active upper GI problems (eg, dysphagia, symptomatic esophageal diseases, gastritis, duodenitis, ulcers); discontinue use if new or worsening symptoms develop.

Osteonecrosis of the jaw (ONJ) has been reported in patients receiving bisphosphonates. Risk factors include invasive dental procedures (eg, tooth extraction, dental implants, boney surgery); a diagnosis of cancer, with concomitant chemotherapy or corticosteroids; poor oral hygiene, ill-fitting dentures; and comorbid disorders (anemia, coagulopathy, infection, pre-existing dental disease). Most reported cases occurred after I.V. bisphosphonate therapy; however, cases have been reported following oral therapy. A dental exam and preventative dentistry should be performed prior to placing patients with risk factors on chronic bisphosphonate therapy. The manufacturer's labeling states that discontinuing bisphosphonates in patients requiring invasive dental procedures may reduce the risk of ONJ. However, other experts suggest that there is no evidence that discontinuing therapy reduces the risk of developing ONJ (Assael, 2009). The benefit/risk must be assessed by the treating physician and/or dentist/surgeon prior to any invasive dental procedure. Patients developing ONJ while on bisphosphonates should receive care by an oral surgeon.

Infrequently, severe (and occasionally debilitating) bone, joint, and/or muscle pain have been reported during bisphosphonate treatment. The onset of pain ranged from a single day to several months. Consider discontinuing therapy in patients who experience severe symptoms; symptoms usually resolve upon discontinuation. Some patients experienced recurrence when rechallenged with same drug or another bisphosphonate; avoid use in patients with a history of these symptoms in association with bisphosphonate therapy.

Adverse Reactions

1% to 10%:

Cardiovascular: Chest pain (3%), edema (3%), peripheral edema (3%), flushing, hypertension, syncope

Central nervous system: Anxiety, fatigue, insomnia, nervousness, somnolence, vertigo

Dermatologic: Rash (3%), skin disorder (3%), pruritus

Endocrine & metabolic: Hyperparathyroidism (3%)

Gastrointestinal: Nausea (9%), diarrhea (9%), dyspepsia (5%), vomiting (4%), flatulence (3%), abdominal pain, anorexia, constipation, gastritis, xerostomia

Genitourinary: Urinary tract infection

Neuromuscular & skeletal: Paresthesia (4%), arthrosis (3%), fractures, muscle spasm, weakness

Ocular: Cataract (3%), conjunctivitis (3%), glaucoma (3%)

Respiratory: Rhinitis (5%), sinusitis (5%), pharyngitis (3%), bronchitis

Miscellaneous: Accidental injury (4%), infection (3%), diaphoresis

<1% (Limited to important or life-threatening): Musculoskeletal pain (sometimes severe and/or incapacitating), osteonecrosis (primarily of the jaw), Stevens-Johnson syndrome

Drug Interactions

Metabolism/Transport Effects None known.

Avoid Concomitant Use There are no known interactions where it is recommended to avoid concomitant use.

Increased Effect/Toxicity

Tiludronate may increase the levels/effects of: Deferasirox; Phosphate Supplements

The levels/effects of Tiludronate may be increased by: Aminoglycosides; Indomethacin; Nonsteroidal Anti-Inflammatory Agents; Systemic Angiogenesis Inhibitors

Decreased Effect

The levels/effects of Tiludronate may be decreased by: Antacids; Aspirin; Calcium Salts; Iron Salts; Magnesium Salts; Multivitamins/Minerals (with ADEK, Folate, Iron); Multivitamins/Minerals (with AE, No Iron); Proton Pump Inhibitors; Sucroferric Oxyhydroxide

Ethanol/Nutrition/Herb Interactions Food: In single-dose studies, the bioavailability of tiludronate was reduced by 90% when an oral dose was administered with, or 2 hours after, a standard breakfast compared to the same dose administered after an overnight fast and 4 hours before a standard breakfast. Management: Administer as a single oral dose with 6-8 oz of plain water. Should not be taken with beverages containing minerals (eg, mineral water), food, or with other medications. Do not take within 2 hours of food. Take calcium or mineral supplements at least 2 hours before or after tiludronate.

Storage/Stability Store at 25°C (77°F); excursions permitted to 15°C to 30°C (59°F to 86°F). Do not remove tablets from foil strips until they are to be used.

Mechanism of Action Inhibition of normal and abnormal bone resorption. Inhibits osteoclasts through at least two mechanisms: disruption of the cytoskeletal ring structure, possibly by inhibition of protein-tyrosine-phosphatase, thus leading to the detachment of osteoclasts from the bone surface area and the inhibition of the osteoclast proton pump.

Pharmacodynamics/Kinetics

Onset of action: Delayed, may require several weeks

Absorption: Rapid

Distribution: Widely to bone and soft tissue

Protein binding: ~90%, primarily to albumin

Metabolism: Little, if any

Bioavailability: ~6% (range: 2% to 11%); reduced by 90% when given with food

Half-life elimination: Healthy volunteers: Single dose: 50 hours; Cl_{cr} 11-18 mL/minute: 205 hours; Pagetic patients: Repeated dosing: 150 hours

Time to peak, plasma: Within 2 hours

Excretion: Urine (~60%, as tiludronic acid within 13 days)

Dosage Oral: Adults: 400 mg (2 tablets of tiludronic acid) daily for a period of 3 months; allow an interval of 3 months to assess response

Dosage adjustment in renal impairment: No dosage adjustment provided in manufacturer's labeling. However, tiludronate is excreted renally. It is not recommended for use in patients with severe renal impairment (Cl_{cr} <30 mL/minute) and is not removed by dialysis.

Dosage adjustment in hepatic impairment: No dosage adjustment necessary.

Dietary Considerations Do not take within 2 hours of food. Ensure adequate intake of vitamin D and calcium supplements during treatment.

Administration Administer as a single oral dose, take with 6-8 oz of plain water. Should not be taken with beverages containing minerals (eg, mineral water), food, or with other medications (may reduce absorption). Do not take within 2 hours of food. Take calcium or mineral supplements at least 2 hours before or after tiludronate. Take aluminum- or magnesium-containing antacids at least 2 hours after taking tiludronate. Patients should be instructed to stay upright (not to lie down) for at least 30 minutes and until after first food of the day (to reduce esophageal irritation).

Monitoring Parameters Alkaline phosphatase; pain; serum calcium and 25(OH)D

Test Interactions Bisphosphonates may interfere with diagnostic imaging agents such as technetium-99m-diphosphonate in bone scans.

Dosage Forms Excipient information presented when available (limited, particularly for generics); consult specific product labeling.

Tablet, Oral, as tiludronic acid:

Skelid: 200 mg

- Tiludronate Disodium *see* Tiludronate *on page 2063*
- Tim-AK (Can) *see* Timolol (Ophthalmic) *on page 2064*
- Timentin *see* Ticarcillin and Clavulanate Potassium *on page 2058*

Timolol (Systemic) (TIM oh lol)

Brand Names: Canada Apo-Timol®; Nu-Timolol; Teva-Timolol

Index Terms Timolol Maleate

Pharmacologic Category Antihypertensive; Beta-Blocker, Nonselective

Additional Appendix Information

Beta-Blockers *on page 2294*

Use Treatment of hypertension and angina; to reduce mortality following myocardial infarction; prophylaxis of migraine

Pregnancy Risk Factor C

Dosage Oral: Adults:

Hypertension: Initial: 10 mg twice daily, increase gradually every 7 days, usual dosage: 20-40 mg/day in 2 divided doses; maximum: 60 mg/day

Prevention of myocardial infarction: 10 mg twice daily initiated within 1-4 weeks after infarction

Migraine headache: Initial: 10 mg twice daily, increase to maximum of 30 mg/day

Dosage adjustment in renal impairment: No specific dosage adjustment provided in manufacturer's labeling. However, timolol is primarily eliminated renally; dosage reduction may be necessary. Significant hypotension has been seen in patients with severe impairment and undergoing dialysis. Use with caution.

Dosage adjustment in hepatic impairment: No specific dosage adjustment provided in manufacturer's labeling. However, timolol is partially metabolized by the liver; dosage reduction may be necessary.

Additional Information Complete prescribing information should be consulted for additional detail.

Dosage Forms Excipient information presented when available (limited, particularly for generics); consult specific product labeling.

Tablet, Oral, as maleate:

Generic: 5 mg, 10 mg, 20 mg

Timolol (Ophthalmic) (TIM oh lol)

Brand Names: U.S. Betimol; Istalol; Timoptic; Timoptic Ocudose; Timoptic-XE

Brand Names: Canada Apo-Timop®; Dom-Timolol; Mylan-Timolol; Novo-Timol; PMS-Timolol; Sandoz-Timolol; Tim-AK; Timolol Maleate-EX; Timoptic-XE®; Timoptic®

Index Terms Timolol Hemihydrate; Timolol Maleate

Pharmacologic Category Beta-Blocker, Nonselective; Ophthalmic Agent, Antiglaucoma

Use Treatment of elevated intraocular pressure such as glaucoma or ocular hypertension

Pregnancy Risk Factor C

Pregnancy Considerations Adverse events were not observed in animal reproduction studies; therefore, the manufacturer classifies timolol ophthalmic as pregnancy category C. Timolol crosses the placenta. Decreased fetal heart rate has been observed following maternal use of oral and ophthalmic timolol during pregnancy. In a cohort study, an increased risk of cardiovascular defects was observed following maternal use of beta-blockers during pregnancy. Intrauterine growth restriction (IUGR), small placentas, as well as fetal/neonatal bradycardia, hypoglycemia, and/or respiratory depression have been observed following *in utero* exposure to beta-blockers as a class. Adequate facilities for monitoring infants at birth should be available. Untreated chronic maternal hypertension and pre-eclampsia are also associated with adverse events in the fetus, infant, and mother. If timolol is required for the treatment of glaucoma during pregnancy, the minimum effective dose should be used in combination with punctual occlusion to decrease exposure to the fetus. Also refer to the Timolol (Systemic) monograph for additional information.

Breast-Feeding Considerations Timolol is excreted into breast milk following ophthalmic administration. According to the manufacturer, the decision to continue or discontinue breast-feeding during therapy should take into account the risk of exposure to the infant and the benefits of treatment to the mother. Due to the potential for adverse events, nursing infants (especially those with cardiorespiratory problems) should be monitored. Also refer to the Timolol (Systemic) monograph for additional information.

Contraindications Hypersensitivity to timolol or any component of the formulation; sinus bradycardia; sinus node dysfunction; heart block greater than first degree (except in patients with a functioning artificial pacemaker); cardiogenic shock; uncompensated cardiac failure; bronchospastic disease

Warnings/Precautions Consider pre-existing conditions such as sick sinus syndrome before initiating. Use with caution in patients with compensated heart failure and monitor for a worsening of the condition. Use with caution in patients on concurrent digoxin, verapamil, or diltiazem; bradycardia or heart block can occur. Concomitant use with other topical beta-blockers should be avoided; monitor for increased effects (systemic or intraocular) with concomitant use of a systemic beta-blocker. Use with caution in patients receiving inhaled anesthetic agents known to depress myocardial contractility. In general, patients with bronchospastic disease should not receive beta-blockers; if used at all, should be used cautiously with close monitoring. Use with caution in patients with diabetes mellitus; may potentiate hypoglycemia and/or mask signs and symptoms. Can precipitate or aggravate symptoms of arterial insufficiency in patients with PVD and Raynaud's disease. Use with caution and monitor for progression of arterial obstruction. May mask signs of hyperthyroidism (eg, tachycardia); if hyperthyroidism is suspected, carefully manage and monitor; abrupt withdrawal may exacerbate symptoms of hyperthyroidism or precipitate thyroid storm. Use caution with history of severe anaphylaxis to allergens; patients taking beta-blockers may become more sensitive to repeated challenges. Treatment of anaphylaxis (eg, epinephrine) in patients taking beta-blockers may be ineffective or promote undesirable effects. Should not be used alone in angle-closure glaucoma (has no effect on pupillary constriction). Multidose vials have been associated with development of bacterial keratitis; avoid contamination. Beta-blockade and/or other suppressive therapy have been associated with choroidal detachment following filtration procedures. Some products contain benzalkonium chloride which may be absorbed by soft contact lenses; remove lens prior to administration and wait 15 minutes before reinserting.

Adverse Reactions

>10%: Ocular: Burning, stinging

Frequency not defined:

Cardiovascular: Angina pectoris, arrhythmia, bradycardia, cardiac arrest, cardiac failure, cerebral ischemia, cerebral vascular accident, edema, heart block, hypertension, hypotension, palpitation, Raynaud's phenomenon

Central nervous system: Anxiety, confusion, depression, disorientation, dizziness, hallucinations, headache, insomnia, memory loss, nervousness, nightmares, somnolence

Dermatologic: Alopecia, angioedema, pseudopemphigoid, psoriasiform rash, psoriasis exacerbation, rash, urticaria

Endocrine & metabolic: Hypoglycemia masked, libido decreased

Gastrointestinal: Anorexia, diarrhea, dyspepsia, nausea, xerostomia

Genitourinary: Impotence, retoperitoneal fibrosis

Hematologic: Claudication

Neuromuscular & skeletal: Myasthenia gravis exacerbation, paresthesia

Ocular: Blepharitis, blurred vision, cataract, choroidal detachment (following filtration surgery), conjunctival injection, conjunctivitis, corneal sensitivity decreased, cystoid macular edema, diplopia, dry eyes, foreign body sensation, hyperemia, itching, keratitis, ocular discharge, ocular pain, ptosis, tearing, visual acuity decreased refractive changes, visual disturbances

Otic: Tinnitus

Respiratory: Bronchospasm, cough, dyspnea, nasal congestion, pulmonary edema, respiratory failure

Miscellaneous: Allergic reactions, cold hands/feet, Peyronie's disease, systemic lupus erythematosus

Drug Interactions

Metabolism/Transport Effects Substrate of CYP2D6 (major); **Note:** Assignment of Major/Minor substrate status based on clinically relevant drug interaction potential; **Inhibits** CYP2D6 (weak)

Avoid Concomitant Use

Avoid concomitant use of Timolol (Ophthalmic) with any of the following: Beta2-Agonists; Floctafenine; Methacholine

Increased Effect/Toxicity

Timolol (Ophthalmic) may increase the levels/effects of: Alpha-/Beta-Agonists (Direct-Acting); Alpha1-Blockers; Alpha2-Agonists; Amifostine; Antihypertensives; Antipsychotic Agents (Phenothiazines); ARIPiprazole; Bupivacaine; Cardiac Glycosides; Cholinergic Agonists; Ergot Derivatives; Fingolimod; Hypotensive Agents; Insulin; Lidocaine (Systemic); Lidocaine (Topical); Mepivacaine; Methacholine; Midodrine; Obinutuzumab; RiTUXimab; Sulfonylureas

The levels/effects of Timolol (Ophthalmic) may be increased by: Abiraterone Acetate; Acetylcholinesterase Inhibitors; Alpha2-Agonists; Aminoquinolines (Antimalarial); Amiodarone; Anilidopiperidine Opioids; Antipsychotic Agents (Phenothiazines); Brimonidine (Topical); Calcium Channel Blockers (Dihydropyridine); Calcium Channel Blockers (Nondihydropyridine); CYP2D6 Inhibitors (Moderate); CYP2D6 Inhibitors (Strong); Darunavir; Diazoxide; Dipyridamole; Disopyramide; Dronedarone; Floctafenine;

Herbs (Hypotensive Properties); MAO Inhibitors; Pentoxifylline; Phosphodiesterase 5 Inhibitors; Propafenone; Prostacyclin Analogues; Regorafenib; Reserpine; Selective Serotonin Reuptake Inhibitors

Decreased Effect

Timolol (Ophthalmic) may decrease the levels/effects of: Beta2-Agonists; Theophylline Derivatives

The levels/effects of Timolol (Ophthalmic) may be decreased by: Barbiturates; Herbs (Hypertensive Properties); Methylphenidate; Nonsteroidal Anti-Inflammatory Agents; Rifamycin Derivatives; Yohimbine

Storage/Stability Drops: Store at room temperature of 15°C to 25°C (59°F to 77°F); do not freeze. Protect from light.

Timolol GFS: Store at 2°C to 25°C (36°F to 77°F). Protect from light.

Timoptic® in OcuDose®: Store in the protective foil wrap and use within 1 month after opening foil package.

Mechanism of Action Blocks both $beta_1$- and $beta_2$-adrenergic receptors, reduces intraocular pressure by reducing aqueous humor production or possibly outflow; reduces blood pressure by blocking adrenergic receptors and decreasing sympathetic outflow, produces a negative chronotropic and inotropic activity through an unknown mechanism

Pharmacodynamics/Kinetics

Onset of action: Intraocular pressure reduction: 30 minutes

Peak effect: 1-2 hours

Duration: 24 hours

Absorption: Timolol is measurable in the serum following ophthalmic use

Dosage Ophthalmic:

Children and Adults:

Solution: Initial: Instill 1 drop (0.25% solution) into affected eye(s) twice daily; increase to 0.5% solution if response not adequate; decrease to 1 drop/day if controlled; do not exceed 1 drop twice daily of 0.5% solution

Gel-forming solution (Timolol GFS, Timoptic-XE®): Instill 1 drop (either 0.25% or 0.5% solution) once daily

Adults: Solution (Istalol®): Instill 1 drop (0.5% solution) once daily in the morning

Dosage adjustment in renal impairment: No dosage adjustment provided in manufacturer's labeling.

Dosage adjustment in hepatic impairment: No dosage adjustment provided in manufacturer's labeling.

Administration Administer other topically-applied ophthalmic medications at least 10 minutes before Timoptic-XE®; wash hands before use; invert closed bottle and shake once before use; remove cap carefully so that tip does not touch anything; hold bottle between thumb and index finger; use index finger of other hand to pull down the lower eyelid to form a pocket for the eye drop and tilt head back; place the dispenser tip close to the eye and gently squeeze the bottle to administer 1 drop; remove pressure after a single drop has been released; **do not allow the dispenser tip to touch the eye**; replace cap and store bottle in an upright position in a clean area; do **not** enlarge hole of dispenser; do **not** wash tip with water, soap, or any other cleaner. Some solutions contain benzalkonium chloride; wait at least 10 minutes after instilling solution before inserting soft contact lenses.

Dosage Forms Excipient information presented when available (limited, particularly for generics); consult specific product labeling.

Gel Forming Solution, Ophthalmic, as maleate [strength expressed as base]:

Timoptic-XE: 0.25% (5 mL); 0.5% (5 mL)

Generic: 0.25% (5 mL); 0.5% (5 mL)

Solution, Ophthalmic, as hemihydrate [strength expressed as base]:

Betimol: 0.25% (5 mL)

Betimol: 0.5% (5 mL, 10 mL, 15 mL) [contains benzalkonium chloride]

Solution, Ophthalmic, as maleate [strength expressed as base]:

Istalol: 0.5% (2.5 mL, 5 mL) [contains benzalkonium chloride]

Timoptic: 0.25% (5 mL); 0.5% (5 mL, 10 mL) [contains benzalkonium chloride]

Generic: 0.25% (5 mL, 10 mL, 15 mL); 0.5% (5 mL, 10 mL, 15 mL)

Solution, Ophthalmic, as maleate [strength expressed as base, preservative free]:

Timoptic Ocudose: 0.25% (60 ea); 0.5% (60 ea)

- **Timolol and Brimonidine** *see* Brimonidine and Timolol *on page 281*
- **Timolol and Dorzolamide** *see* Dorzolamide and Timolol *on page 655*
- **Timolol Hemihydrate** *see* Timolol (Ophthalmic) *on page 2064*
- **Timolol Maleate** *see* Timolol (Ophthalmic) *on page 2064*
- **Timolol Maleate** *see* Timolol (Systemic) *on page 2064*
- **Timolol Maleate-EX (Can)** *see* Timolol (Ophthalmic) *on page 2064*
- **Timoptic** *see* Timolol (Ophthalmic) *on page 2064*
- **Timoptic® (Can)** *see* Timolol (Ophthalmic) *on page 2064*
- **Timoptic Ocudose** *see* Timolol (Ophthalmic) *on page 2064*
- **Timoptic-XE** *see* Timolol (Ophthalmic) *on page 2064*
- **Timoptic-XE® (Can)** *see* Timolol (Ophthalmic) *on page 2064*
- **Tinactin [OTC]** *see* Tolnaftate *on page 2087*
- **Tinactin Deodorant [OTC]** *see* Tolnaftate *on page 2087*
- **Tinactin Jock Itch [OTC]** *see* Tolnaftate *on page 2087*
- **Tinamar [OTC]** *see* Tolnaftate *on page 2087*
- **Tinaspore [OTC]** *see* Tolnaftate *on page 2087*
- **Tincture of Opium** *see* Opium Tincture *on page 1513*

Tinzaparin (tin ZA pa rin)

Brand Names: Canada Innohep®

Index Terms Tinzaparin Sodium

Pharmacologic Category Low Molecular Weight Heparin

Use Treatment of deep vein thrombosis (DVT) and/or pulmonary embolism (PE) (except in patients with severe hemodynamic instability); prevention of venous thromboembolism (VTE) following orthopedic surgery or following general surgery in patients at high risk of VTE; prevention of clotting in indwelling intravenous lines and extracorporeal circuit during hemodialysis (in patients without high bleeding risk)

Pregnancy Considerations Teratogenic events were not observed in animal reproduction studies. Tinzaparin does not cross the human placenta. A pharmacokinetic study in pregnant women found no dose adjustment was needed during pregnancy. Vaginal bleeding was reported in ~10% of pregnant patients during tinzaparin therapy. LMWH is recommended over unfractionated heparin for the treatment of acute venous thromboembolism (VTE) in pregnant women. LMWH is also recommended over unfractionated heparin for VTE prophylaxis in pregnant women with certain risk factors. LMWH should be discontinued prior to induction of labor or a planned cesarean delivery. When choosing therapy, fetal outcomes (ie, pregnancy loss, malformations), maternal outcomes (ie, VTE, hemorrhage), burden of therapy, and maternal preference should be considered (Guyatt, 2012). Contains benzyl alcohol; use with caution in pregnant women due to association with gasping syndrome in premature infants.

Breast-Feeding Considerations Small amounts of LMWH have been detected in breast milk; however, because it has a low oral bioavailability, it is unlikely to cause adverse events in a nursing infant. Use of LMWH may be continued in breast-feeding women (Guyatt, 2012).

Contraindications Hypersensitivity to tinzaparin sodium, heparin or other low molecular weight heparins (LMWH), or any component of the formulation; active bleeding; history of confirmed or suspected immunologically mediated heparin-induced thrombocytopenia (HIT) or positive *in vitro* platelet-aggregation test in the presence of tinzaparin; acute or subacute endocarditis; generalized hemorrhage tendency and other conditions involving increased risks of hemorrhage (eg, severe hepatic insufficiency, imminent abortion); hemophilia or major blood clotting disorders; acute cerebral insult or hemorrhagic cerebrovascular accidents without systemic emboli; uncontrolled severe hypertension; diabetic or hemorrhagic retinopathy; injury or surgery involving the brain, spinal cord, eyes or ears; spinal/epidural anesthesia in patients requiring treatment dosages of tinzaparin; use of multidose vials containing benzyl alcohol in children <2 years of age, premature infants, and neonates

Note: Use of tinzaparin in patients with current HIT or HIT with thrombosis is **not** recommended and considered contraindicated due to high cross-reactivity to heparin-platelet factor-4 antibody (Guyatt [ACCP], 2012; Warkentin, 1999).

Warnings/Precautions Spinal or epidural hematomas, including subsequent paralysis, may occur with recent or anticipated neuraxial anesthesia (epidural or spinal) or spinal puncture in patients anticoagulated with low molecular weight heparin (LMWH) or heparinoids. Consider risk versus benefit prior to spinal procedures; risk is increased by the use of concomitant agents which may alter hemostasis, the use of indwelling epidural catheters for analgesia, a history of spinal deformity or spinal surgery, as well as traumatic or repeated epidural or spinal punctures. Avoid invasive spinal procedures for 12 hours following tinzaparin administration and withhold the next tinzaparin dose for at least 2 hours after the spinal procedure. Patient should be observed closely for signs and symptoms of neurological impairment. Not to be used interchangeably (unit for unit) with heparin or any other LMWHs.

Monitor patient closely for signs or symptoms of bleeding. Certain patients are at increased risk of bleeding. Risk factors include bacterial endocarditis; congenital or acquired bleeding disorders; active ulcerative or angiodysplastic GI diseases; severe uncontrolled hypertension; history of hemorrhagic stroke; use shortly after brain, spinal, or ophthalmologic surgery; those concomitantly treated with drugs that increase bleeding risk (eg, antiplatelet agents, anticoagulants); recent GI bleeding; thrombocytopenia or platelet defects; severe liver disease; hypertensive or diabetic retinopathy; or in patients undergoing invasive procedures. Withhold or discontinue for minor bleeding. Protamine infusion may be necessary for serious bleeding. Cases of thrombocytopenia including thrombocytopenia with thrombosis have occurred. Use with caution in patients with history of thrombocytopenia (drug-induced or congenital) or platelet defects; monitor platelet count closely. Use is contraindicated in patients with history of confirmed or suspected heparin-induced thrombocytopenia (HIT) or positive *in vitro* test for antiplatelet antibodies in the presence of tinzaparin. Discontinue therapy and consider alternative treatment if platelets are <100,000/mm^3 and/or thrombosis develops. Asymptomatic thrombocytosis has been observed with use, particularly in patients undergoing orthopedic surgery or with concurrent inflammatory process; discontinue use with increased platelet counts and evaluate the risks/necessity of further therapy. Prosthetic valve thrombosis has been reported in patients receiving thromboprophylaxis therapy with LMWHs. Pregnant women may be at increased risk.

Use with caution in hepatic impairment; associated with transient, dose-dependent increases in AST/ALT which typically resolve within 2-4 weeks of therapy discontinuation. Use with caution in patients with renal insufficiency. Reduced tinzaparin clearance has been observed in patients with moderate-to-severe renal impairment; Consider dosage reduction in patients with Cl_{cr} <30 mL/minute. Use with caution in the elderly (delayed elimination may occur). Use is not recommended in patients >70 years of age with renal impairment. An increase in all-cause mortality has been observed in patients ≥70 years (mean age: >82 years) with Cl_{cr} ≤60 mL/minute treated with tinzaparin compared to unfractionated heparin for acute DVT (Leizorovicz, 2011).

Heparin can cause hyperkalemia by suppressing aldosterone production; similar reactions could occur with LMWHs. Monitor for hyperkalemia which most commonly occurs in patients with risk factors for the development of hyperkalemia (eg, renal dysfunction, concomitant use of potassium-sparing diuretics or potassium supplements, hematoma in body tissues). For subcutaneous use only; do not administer intramuscularly or intravenously. Use with caution in patients <45 kg or >120 kg; limited experience in these patients. Individualized clinical and laboratory monitoring are recommended. Derived from porcine intestinal mucosa. Some dosage forms may contain benzyl alcohol or sodium metabisulfite.

Adverse Reactions As with all anticoagulants, bleeding is the major adverse effect of tinzaparin. Hemorrhage may occur at virtually any site. Risk is dependent on multiple variables. **Note:** Incidence not always reported.

>10%:

- Hepatic: ALT increased (≤13%)
- Local: Injection site hematoma

1% to 10%:

- Cardiovascular: Chest pain (2%), angina pectoris (≥1%), arrhythmia (≥1%), coronary thrombosis/MI (≥1%), dependent edema (≥1%), thromboembolism (≥1%)
- Central nervous system: Fever (2%), headache (2%), pain (2%)
- Dermatologic: Bullous eruption (≥1%), erythematous rash (≥1%), maculopapular rash (≥1%), skin necrosis (≥1%)
- Gastrointestinal: Nausea (2%), abdominal pain (1%), constipation (1%), diarrhea (1%), vomiting (1%)
- Genitourinary: Urinary tract infection (4%)
- Hematologic: Bleeding events (major events including intracranial, retroperitoneal, or bleeding into a major prosthetic joint: ≤3%; hemorrhage site not specified (2%); other bleeding events reported at an incidence of ≥1% include anorectal bleeding, GI hemorrhage, hemarthrosis, hematemesis, hematuria, hemopericardium, injection site bleeding, melena, purpura, intra-abdominal bleeding, vaginal bleeding, wound hemorrhage), granulocytopenia (≥1%), thrombocytopenia (≥1%)
- Hepatic: AST increased (9%)
- Local: Injection site cellulitis (≥1%)
- Neuromuscular & skeletal: Back pain (2%)
- Respiratory: Epistaxis (2%), dyspnea (1%)
- Miscellaneous: Allergic reaction (≥1%), neoplasm (≥1%)

<1% (Limited to important or life-threatening): Agranulocytosis, angioedema, anaphylactoid reaction, GGT increased, hemoptysis, hypoaldosteronism, hyperkalemia, LDH increased, lipase increased, metabolic acidosis, ocular hemorrhage, osteopenia, osteoporosis, priapism, pruritus, rash, spinal epidural hematoma, Stevens-Johnson syndrome, thrombocytosis, toxic epidermal necrolysis, urticaria

Drug Interactions

Metabolism/Transport Effects None known.

Avoid Concomitant Use

Avoid concomitant use of Tinzaparin with any of the following: Apixaban; Dabigatran Etexilate; Omacetaxine; Rivaroxaban

Increased Effect/Toxicity

Tinzaparin may increase the levels/effects of: ACE Inhibitors; Aliskiren; Angiotensin II Receptor Blockers; Anticoagulants; Canagliflozin; Collagenase (Systemic); Deferasirox; Eplerenone; Ibritumomab; Omacetaxine; Palifermin; Potassium Salts; Potassium-Sparing Diuretics; Rivaroxaban; Tositumomab and Iodine I 131 Tositumomab

The levels/effects of Tinzaparin may be increased by: 5-ASA Derivatives; Agents with Antiplatelet Properties; Apixaban; Dabigatran Etexilate; Dasatinib; Herbs (Anticoagulant/Antiplatelet Properties); Ibrutinib; Nonsteroidal Anti-Inflammatory Agents; Omega-3 Fatty Acids; Pentosan Polysulfate Sodium; Pentoxifylline; Prostacyclin Analogues; Salicylates; Sugammadex; Thrombolytic Agents; Tibolone; Tipranavir; Vitamin E

Decreased Effect

The levels/effects of Tinzaparin may be decreased by: Estrogen Derivatives; Progestins

Storage/Stability Store at 15°C to 25°C (59°F to 77°F).

Mechanism of Action Tinzaparin is a low molecular weight heparin (average molecular weight ranges between 5500 and 7500 daltons, distributed as <2000 daltons [<10%], 2000-8000 daltons [60% to 72%], and >8000 daltons [22% to 36%]) that binds antithrombin III, enhancing the inhibition of several clotting factors, particularly factor Xa. Tinzaparin anti-Xa activity (70-120 units/mg) is greater than anti-IIa activity (~55 units/mg) and it has a higher ratio of antifactor Xa to antifactor IIa activity compared to unfractionated heparin. Low molecular weight heparins have a small effect on the activated partial thromboplastin time.

Pharmacodynamics/Kinetics Note: Values reflective of anti-Xa activity.

Onset of action: 2-3 hours

Duration: Detectable anti-Xa activity persists for 24 hours

Absorption: Slow; absorption half-life ~3 hours after subcutaneous administration

Distribution: 4 L

Metabolism: Does not undergo hepatic metabolism

Bioavailability: SubQ: ~90%

Half-life elimination: 82 minutes; prolonged in renal impairment

Time to peak: 4-6 hours

Excretion: Urine

Dosage Note: 1 mg of tinzaparin equals 70-120 units of anti-Xa activity

SubQ:

Infants, Children, and Adolescents: VTE treatment (unlabeled use; Monagle, 2012): **Note:** May initiate a vitamin K antagonist on day 1 of tinzaparin therapy; discontinue tinzaparin on day 6 or later if INR is not >2.

Birth to 2 months: 275 anti-Xa units/kg once daily

2-12 months: 250 anti-Xa units/kg once daily

1-5 years: 240 anti-Xa units/kg once daily

5-10 years: 200 anti-Xa units/kg once daily

10-16 years: 175 anti-Xa units/kg once daily

Adults:

DVT and/or PE treatment: 175 anti-Xa units/kg once daily (maximum: 18,000 anti-Xa units/day). The 2012 *Chest* guidelines recommend starting warfarin on the first or second treatment day and continuing tinzaparin until INR is ≥2 for at least 24 hours (usually 5-7 days) (Guyatt, 2012). Body weight dosing using prefilled syringes may also be considered. Refer to manufacturer labeling for detailed dosing recommendations.

DVT prophylaxis:

Hip replacement surgery: **Note:** The American College of Chest Physicians recommends initiation of LMWH ≥12 hours preoperatively **or** ≥12 hours postoperatively; extended duration up to 35 days suggested (Guyatt, 2012).

Preoperative regimen: 50 anti-Xa units/kg given 2 hours preoperatively followed by 50 anti-Xa units/kg once daily for 7-10 days

Postoperative regimen: 75 anti-Xa units/kg once daily, with initial dose given postoperatively and continued for 7-10 days

Knee replacement surgery: 75 anti-Xa units/kg once daily, with initial dose given postoperatively and continued for 7-10 days. **Note:** The American College of Chest Physicians recommends initiation of LMWH ≥12 hours preoperatively **or** ≥12 hours postoperatively; extended duration of up to 35 days suggested (Guyatt, 2012). Body weight dosing using prefilled syringes may also be considered. Refer to manufacturer labeling for detailed dosing recommendations.

General surgery: 3500 anti-Xa units once daily, with initial dose given 2 hours prior to surgery and then continued postoperatively for 7-10 days

I.V.: Adults: Anticoagulant in extracorporeal circuit during hemodialysis (recommendations apply to stable patients with chronic renal failure):

Dialysis session ≤4 hours (no hemorrhage risk): Initial bolus (via arterial side of circuit or I.V.): 4500 anti-Xa units at beginning of dialysis; typically achieves plasma concentrations of 0.5-1 anti-Xa units/mL; may give larger bolus for dialysis sessions >4 hours. For subsequent dialysis sessions, may adjust dose as necessary in increments of 500 anti-Xa units based on previous outcome.

Dialysis session ≤4 hours (hemorrhage risk): Initial bolus (I.V. only): 2250 anti-Xa units at beginning of dialysis (do not add to dialysis circuit). A smaller second I.V. dose may be administered during dialysis sessions >4 hours. For subsequent dialysis sessions, adjust dose as necessary to achieve plasma concentrations of 0.2-0.4 anti-Xa units/mL.

Elderly: No significant differences in safety or response were seen when used in patients ≥65 years of age. However, increased sensitivity to tinzaparin in elderly patients may be possible due to a decline in renal function. Use is not recommended in patients >70 years of age with renal impairment.

Dosage adjustment in renal impairment:

Cl_{cr} ≥30 mL/minute: No dosage adjustment provided in manufacturer's labeling; however, primarily undergoes renal elimination. Clearance is decreased in renal impairment; use with caution.

Cl_{cr} <30 mL/minute: Manufacturer's labeling suggests that a reduction in dose be considered but does not provide specific dose recommendations. Use with caution.

Dosage adjustment in hepatic impairment: No dosage adjustment provided in manufacturer's labeling. Does not undergo hepatic metabolism; however, has been associated with transient increases in transaminase levels; use with caution.

Dosing in obesity: A pharmacokinetic study confirmed that weight-based dosing (single doses of 75 or 175 units/kg) using actual body weight in heavy/obese patients between 100 and 165 kg led to achievement of similar anti-Xa activity levels compared to normal-weight patients (Hainer, 2002). However, there is limited clinical experience in patients with a BMI >40 kg/m^2.

Administration Patient should be lying down or sitting. Administer by deep SubQ injection into the lower abdomen, outer thigh, lower back, or upper arm. Injection site should be varied daily. To minimize bruising, do not rub the injection site. In hemodialysis patients, may be administered I.V. (patients with high or low hemorrhage risk) or added to the dialyzer circuit (patients with low hemorrhage risk).

Monitoring Parameters CBC (at baseline then twice weekly throughout therapy); renal function (use Cockcroft-Gault formula); hepatic function; potassium (baseline in patients at risk for hyperkalemia, monitor regularly if duration >7 days); stool for occult blood. Routine monitoring of anti-Xa levels is generally not recommended; however, anti-Xa levels may be beneficial in certain patients (eg, children, obese patients, patients with severe renal insufficiency receiving therapeutic doses, and possibly pregnant women receiving therapeutic doses) (Guyatt, 2012). Peak anti-Xa levels are measured 4-6 hours after administration. Monitoring of PT and/or aPTT is not of clinical benefit.

Reference Range Anti-Xa level (measured 4 hours after administration): Fixed-dose (3500 units): 0.15 anti-Xa units/mL; weight-based (75-175 units/kg): 0.34-0.70 anti-Xa units/mL; in treatment of venous thromboembolism, a target of 0.85 anti-Xa units/mL has been recommended (Garcia, 2012)

Children: Target anti-Xa level: 0.5-1 anti-Xa units/mL 4-6 hours after administration or 0.5-0.8 anti-Xa units/mL 2-6 hours after administration (Monagle, 2012)

Additional Information Neutralization of tinzaparin (in overdose) with protamine 1% solution: Manufacturer's recommendations: 1 mg protamine for each 100 anti-Xa units of tinzaparin; if PTT prolonged 2-4 hours after first dose (or if bleeding continues), consider additional dose of 0.5 mg for each 100 anti-Xa units of tinzaparin.

Dosage Forms: Canada Excipient information presented when available (limited, particularly for generics); consult specific product labeling. [DSC] = Discontinued product

Injection, solution, as sodium:
- Innohep®: 10,000 anti-Xa units/mL (2 mL) [contains benzyl alcohol, sodium metabisulfite]
- Innohep®: 20,000 anti-Xa units/mL (0.5 mL, 0.7 mL, 0.9 mL) [contains sodium metabisulfite]
- Innohep®: 20,000 anti-Xa units/mL (2 mL) [contains benzyl alcohol, sodium metabisulfite]

Injection, solution, as sodium [preservative free]:
- Innohep®: 10,000 anti-Xa units/mL (0.25 mL, 0.35 mL, 0.45 mL)

◆ **Tinzaparin Sodium** *see* Tinzaparin *on page 2066*

◆ **Tioguanine** *see* Thioguanine *on page 2045*

◆ **Tiotixene** *see* Thiothixene *on page 2051*

Tiotropium (ty oh TRO pee um)

Brand Names: U.S. Spiriva HandiHaler
Brand Names: Canada Spiriva®
Index Terms Tiotropium Bromide Monohydrate
Pharmacologic Category Anticholinergic Agent; Anticholinergic Agent, Long-Acting
Use Maintenance treatment of bronchospasm associated with COPD (including bronchitis and emphysema); reduction of COPD exacerbations

Pregnancy Risk Factor C

Pregnancy Considerations Adverse events (fetal loss, decreased birth weights, delayed sexual maturation) were observed in some animal studies. There are no adequate and well-controlled studies in pregnant women. Use only when expected benefit to mother outweighs potential risk to the fetus.

Breast-Feeding Considerations It is not known if tiotropium is excreted in breast milk. The manufacturer recommends that caution be exercised when administering tiotropium to nursing women.

Contraindications Hypersensitivity to tiotropium or ipratropium, or any component of the formulation (contains lactose)

Warnings/Precautions Rarely, paradoxical bronchospasm may occur with use of inhaled bronchodilating agents; discontinue use and consider other therapy if bronchospasm occurs.

Not indicated for the initial (rescue) treatment of acute episodes of bronchospasm. Use with caution in patients with myasthenia gravis, narrow-angle glaucoma, prostatic hyperplasia, moderate-severe renal impairment (Cl_{cr} ≤50 mL/minute), or bladder neck obstruction; avoid inadvertent instillation of powder into the eyes. Immediate hypersensitivity reactions may occur; discontinue immediately if signs/symptoms occur. Use with caution in patients with a history of hypersensitivity to atropine.

The contents of Spiriva® capsules are for inhalation only via the HandiHaler® device. There have been reports of incorrect administration (swallowing of the capsules). Capsule for oral inhalation contains lactose; use with caution in patients with severe milk protein allergy.

Adverse Reactions

>10%:
- Gastrointestinal: Xerostomia (5% to 16%)
- Respiratory: Upper respiratory tract infection (41%), pharyngitis (9% to 13%), sinusitis (7% to 11%)

1% to 10%:
- Cardiovascular: Chest pain (1% to 7%), edema (dependent, 5%)
- Central nervous system: Headache (6%), insomnia (4%), depression (1% to 4%), dysphonia (1% to 3%)
- Dermatologic: Rash (4%)
- Endocrine & metabolic: Hypercholesterolemia (1% to 3%), hyperglycemia (1% to 3%)
- Gastrointestinal: Dyspepsia (6%), abdominal pain (5%), constipation (4% to 5%), vomiting (4%), gastroesophageal reflux (1% to 3%), stomatitis (including ulcerative; 1% to 3%)
- Genitourinary: Urinary tract infection (7%)
- Neuromuscular & skeletal: Arthralgia (4%), myalgia (4%), arthritis (≥3%), leg pain (1% to 3%), paresthesia (1% to 3%), skeletal pain (1% to 3%)
- Ocular: Cataract (1% to 3%)
- Respiratory: Rhinitis (6%), epistaxis (4%), cough (≥3%), laryngitis (1% to 3%)
- Miscellaneous: Infection (4%), moniliasis (4%), flu-like syndrome (≥3%), allergic reaction (1% to 3%), herpes zoster (1% to 3%)

<1% (Limited to important or life-threatening): Angioedema; application site irritation (glossitis, mouth ulceration, pharyngolaryngeal pain); atrial fibrillation, blurred vision, candidiasis (oral), dizziness, dehydration, dry skin, dysphagia, gingivitis, glaucoma, hoarseness, hypersensitivity reactions, ileus (paralytic), intestinal obstruction, intraocular pressure increased, joint swelling, palpitation, paradoxical bronchospasm, pruritus, pupil dilation (if powder comes in contact with eyes), skin infection, skin ulcer, supraventricular tachycardia, tachycardia, throat irritation, urinary difficulty, urinary retention, urticaria

Drug Interactions

Metabolism/Transport Effects Substrate of CYP2D6 (minor), CYP3A4 (minor); **Note:** Assignment of Major/ Minor substrate status based on clinically relevant drug interaction potential

Avoid Concomitant Use

Avoid concomitant use of Tiotropium with any of the following: Aclidinium; Anticholinergics; Ipratropium (Oral Inhalation); Potassium Chloride; Umeclidinium

Increased Effect/Toxicity

Tiotropium may increase the levels/effects of: AbobotulinumtoxinA; Analgesics (Opioid); Anticholinergics; Cannabinoids; Mirabegron; OnabotulinumtoxinA; Potassium Chloride; RimabotulinumtoxinB; Thiazide Diuretics; Topiramate

The levels/effects of Tiotropium may be increased by: Aclidinium; Anticholinergics; Ipratropium (Oral Inhalation); Pramlintide; Umeclidinium

Decreased Effect

Tiotropium may decrease the levels/effects of: Acetylcholinesterase Inhibitors (Central); Secretin

The levels/effects of Tiotropium may be decreased by: Acetylcholinesterase Inhibitors (Central); Peginterferon Alfa-2b

Storage/Stability Store at 25°C (77°F); excursions permitted to 15°C to 30°C (59°F to 86°F). Avoid excessive temperatures and moisture. Do not store capsules in HandiHaler® device. Capsules should be stored in the blister pack and only removed immediately before use. Once protective foil is peeled back and/or removed the capsule should be used immediately; if capsule is not used immediately it should be discarded.

Mechanism of Action Competitively and reversibly inhibits the action of acetylcholine at type 3 muscarinic (M_3) receptors in bronchial smooth muscle causing bronchodilation

Pharmacodynamics/Kinetics

Absorption: Poorly absorbed from GI tract, systemic absorption may occur from lung

Distribution: V_d: 32 L/kg

Protein binding: 72%

Metabolism: Hepatic (minimal), via CYP2D6 and CYP3A4

Bioavailability: Following inhalation, 19.5%; oral solution: 2% to 3%

Half-life elimination: 5-6 days

Time to peak, plasma: 5 minutes (following inhalation)

Excretion: Urine (14% of an inhaled dose); feces (primarily nonabsorbed drug)

Dosage Oral inhalation: Adults: Contents of 1 capsule (18 mcg) inhaled once daily using HandiHaler® device. **Note:** To ensure drug delivery the contents of each capsule should be inhaled twice.

Dosage adjustment in renal impairment: No dosage adjustment necessary. However, plasma concentrations may increase in renal impairment. Use caution in moderate-to-severe impairment (Cl_{cr} ≤50 mL/minute); although no dosage adjustment is required, monitor closely.

Dosage adjustment in hepatic impairment: No dosage adjustment necessary.

Administration Administer once daily at the same time each day. Remove capsule from foil blister immediately before use. Capsule should not be swallowed. Place capsule in the capsule-chamber in the base of the HandiHaler® Inhaler. Must only use the HandiHaler® Inhaler. Close mouthpiece until a click is heard, leaving dustcap open. Exhale fully. Do not exhale into inhaler. Tilt head slightly back and inhale (rapidly, steadily and deeply); the capsule vibration may be heard within the device. Hold breath as long as possible. If any powder remains in capsule, exhale and inhale again. Repeat until capsule is empty. Throw away empty capsule; do not leave in inhaler. Do not use a spacer with the HandiHaler® Inhaler. Do not use HandiHaler® device for other medications. Always keep capsules and inhaler dry.

Delivery of dose: Instruct patient to place mouthpiece gently between teeth, closing lips around inhaler. Instruct patient to inhale deeply and hold breath for 5-10 seconds. The amount of drug delivered is small, and the individual will not sense the medication as it is inhaled. Remove mouthpiece prior to exhalation. Patient should not breathe out through the mouthpiece.

Monitoring Parameters FEV_1, peak flow (or other pulmonary function studies)

Dosage Forms Excipient information presented when available (limited, particularly for generics); consult specific product labeling.

Capsule, Inhalation:

Spiriva HandiHaler: 18 mcg [contains milk protein]

Dosage Forms: Canada Excipient information presented when available (limited, particularly for generics); consult specific product labeling.

Powder, for oral inhalation:

Spiriva®: 18 mcg/capsule (10s) [contains lactose]

◆ **Tiotropium Bromide Monohydrate** *see* Tiotropium *on page 2069*

Tipranavir (tip RA na veer)

Brand Names: U.S. Aptivus

Brand Names: Canada Aptivus®

Index Terms PNU-140690E; TPV

Pharmacologic Category Antiretroviral, Protease Inhibitor (Anti-HIV)

Use Treatment of HIV-1 infections in combination with ritonavir and other antiretroviral agents; limited to highly treatment-experienced or multiprotease inhibitor-resistant patients.

Pregnancy Risk Factor C

Pregnancy Considerations Teratogenic effects were not observed in animal reproduction studies; fetotoxity was observed with some doses. Tipranavir crosses the human placenta. The DHHS Perinatal HIV Guidelines note there are insufficient data to recommend use during pregnancy; however, if used, tipranavir must be given with low-dose ritonavir boosting. A small increased risk of preterm birth has been associated with maternal use of protease inhibitor-based combination antiretroviral (ARV) therapy during pregnancy; however, the benefits of use generally outweigh this risk and protease inhibitors (PIs) should not be withheld if otherwise recommended. Hyperglycemia, new onset of diabetes mellitus, or diabetic ketoacidosis have been reported with PIs; it is not clear if pregnancy increases this risk.

Regardless of CD4 count or HIV RNA copy number, all HIV-infected pregnant women should receive a combination antepartum ARV drug regimen; this includes women who require therapy for their own health, as well as women who do not yet require therapy for their own health. ARV therapy should be started as soon as possible if required for the woman's health. Although earlier initiation may be more effective in reducing the perinatal transmission of HIV, also consider maternal conditions (eg, nausea and vomiting) and the potential risks of first trimester fetal exposure for specific agents. Plasma HIV RNA levels should be assessed at ~34-36 weeks gestation in order to help determine mode of delivery. If ARV therapy must be interrupted for <24 hours during the peripartum period, stop then restart all medications simultaneously in order to decrease the chance of developing resistance. Long-term follow-up is recommended for all infants exposed to ARV medications.

Healthcare providers are encouraged to enroll pregnant women exposed to antiretroviral medications in the Antiretroviral Pregnancy Registry (1-800-258-4263 or www.-APRegistry.com). Healthcare providers caring for HIV-infected women and their infants may contact the National Perinatal HIV Hotline (888-448-8765) for clinical consultation (DHHS [perinatal], 2012).

Women receiving estrogen (as hormonal contraception or replacement therapy) may have an increased incidence of rash.

Breast-Feeding Considerations Maternal or infant antiretroviral therapy does not completely eliminate the risk of postnatal HIV transmission. In addition, multiclass-resistant virus has been detected in breast-feeding infants despite maternal therapy. Therefore, in the United States, where formula is accessible, affordable, safe, and sustainable, and the risk of infant mortality due to diarrhea and respiratory infections is low, complete avoidance of breast-feeding by HIV-infected women is recommended to decrease potential transmission of HIV (DHHS [perinatal], 2012).

Contraindications Concurrent therapy of tipranavir/ritonavir with alfuzosin, amiodarone, bepridil, cisapride, ergot derivatives (eg, dihydroergotamine, ergonovine, ergotamine, methylergonovine), flecainide, lovastatin, midazolam (oral), pimozide, propafenone, quinidine, rifampin, sildenafil (for pulmonary arterial hypertension [eg, Revatio®]), simvastatin, St John's wort, and triazolam; moderate-to-severe hepatic impairment (Child-Pugh class B or C)

Warnings/Precautions [U.S. Boxed Warning]: In combination with ritonavir, may cause hepatitis (including fatalities) and/or exacerbate pre-existing hepatic dysfunction (causal relationship not established); patients with chronic hepatitis B or C are at increased risk. Monitor patients closely; discontinue use if signs or symptoms of toxicity occur or if asymptomatic AST/ALT elevations >10 times upper limit of normal or AST/ALT elevations >5-10 times upper limit of normal concurrently with total bilirubin >2.5 times the upper limit of normal occur. Use with caution in patients with mild hepatic impairment; contraindicated in moderate-to-severe impairment. May be associated with fat redistribution (buffalo hump, increased abdominal girth, breast engorgement, facial atrophy). Use caution in hemophilia. May increase cholesterol and/or triglycerides; hypertriglyceridemia may increase risk of pancreatitis. May cause hyperglycemia. Use with caution in patients with sulfonamide allergy. Protease inhibitors have been associated with a variety of hypersensitivity events (some severe), including rash, anaphylaxis (rare), angioedema, bronchospasm, erythema multiforme, and/or Stevens-Johnson syndrome (rare). It is generally recommended to discontinue treatment if severe rash or moderate symptoms accompanied by other systemic symptoms occur. Patients may develop immune reconstitution syndrome resulting in the occurrence of an inflammatory response to an indolent or residual opportunistic infection during initial HIV treatment or activation of autoimmune disorders (eg, Graves' disease, polymyositis, Guillain-Barré syndrome) later in therapy; further evaluation and treatment may be required.

[U.S. Boxed Warning]: Tipranavir in combination with ritonavir has been associated with rare reports of fatal and nonfatal intracranial hemorrhage; causal relationship not established. Events often occurred in patients with medical conditions (eg, CNS lesions, head trauma, recent neurosurgery, coagulopathy, alcohol abuse) or concurrent therapy which may have influenced these events. Tipranavir may inhibit platelet aggregation. Use with caution in patients who may be at risk for increased bleeding (trauma, surgery or other medical conditions) or in patients receiving concurrent medications which may increase the risk of bleeding, including antiplatelet agents and anticoagulants.

High potential for drug interactions; concomitant use of tipranavir with some drugs may require cautious use, may not be recommended, may require dosage adjustments, or may be contraindicated.

Adverse Reactions

>10%:

Dermatologic: Rash (children 21%; adults 3% to 10%)

Endocrine & metabolic: Hypertriglyceridemia (>400 mg/dL: 61%), hypercholesterolemia (>300 mg/dL: 22%)

Gastrointestinal: Diarrhea (15%)

Hepatic: Transaminases increased (>2.5 x ULN: 26% to 32%; grade 3/4: 10% to 20%)

Neuromuscular & skeletal: CPK increased (grade 3/4: children 11%)

2% to 10%:

Central nervous system: Fever (6% to 8%), fatigue (6%), headache (5%)

Endocrine & metabolic: Dehydration (2%)

Gastrointestinal: Nausea (5% to 9%), amylase increased (grade 3: 6% to 8%), vomiting (6%), abdominal pain (4%), diarrhea (children 4%), weight loss (3%)

Hematologic: Bleeding (children 8%), WBC decreased (grades 3: 5%), anemia (3%), neutropenia (2%)

Hepatic: ALT increased (2%, grades 3/4: 10%), AST increased (grades 3/4: 6%), GGT increased (2%)

Neuromuscular & skeletal: Myalgia (2%)

Respiratory: Cough (children 6%), dyspnea (2%), epistaxis (children 4%)

<2% (Limited to important or life-threatening): Abdominal distension, anorexia, appetite decreased, diabetes mellitus, dizziness, dyspepsia, exanthem, facial wasting, flatulence, flu-like syndrome, gastroesophageal reflux, hepatic failure, hepatic steatosis, hepatitis, hyperbilirubinemia, hyperglycemia, hypersensitivity, immune reconstitution syndrome, insomnia, intracranial hemorrhage, lipase increased, lipoatrophy, lipodystrophy (acquired), lipohypertrophy, malaise, mitochondrial toxicity, muscle cramp, neuropathy (peripheral), pancreatitis, pruritus, renal insufficiency, sleep disorder, somnolence, thrombocytopenia

Drug Interactions

Metabolism/Transport Effects Substrate of CYP3A4 (major); **Note:** Assignment of Major/Minor substrate status based on clinically relevant drug interaction potential; **Inhibits** CYP2D6 (strong); **Induces** P-glycoprotein

Avoid Concomitant Use

Avoid concomitant use of Tipranavir with any of the following: Alfuzosin; Amiodarone; AtorvaSTATin; Bepridil [Off Market]; Cisapride; Dabigatran Etexilate; Ergot Derivatives; Etravirine; Flecainide; Ketoconazole (Systemic); Lovastatin; Midazolam; Pimozide; Pomalidomide; Propafenone; QuiNIDine; Rifampin; Simeprevir; Simvastatin; Sofosbuvir; St Johns Wort; Tamoxifen; Thioridazine; Triazolam; VinCRIStine (Liposomal)

Increased Effect/Toxicity

Tipranavir may increase the levels/effects of: Agents with Antiplatelet Properties; Alfuzosin; ALPRAZolam; Amiodarone; Anticoagulants; ARIPiprazole; AtoMOXetine; AtorvaSTATin; Bepridil [Off Market]; Bosentan; Calcium Channel Blockers (Dihydropyridine); Calcium Channel Blockers (Nondihydropyridine); CarBAMazepine; Cisapride; Clarithromycin; CycloSPORINE (Systemic); CYP2D6 Substrates; Digoxin; Enfuvirtide; Ergot Derivatives; Fesoterodine; Flecainide; Iloperidone; Itraconazole; Ketoconazole (Systemic); Lovastatin; Meperidine; Metoprolol; Midazolam; Nebivolol; Nefazodone; Pimozide; Propafenone; Protease Inhibitors; QuiNIDine; Rifabutin; Riociguat; Rosuvastatin; Sildenafil; Simeprevir; Simvastatin; Tacrolimus (Systemic); Tacrolimus (Topical);

Temsirolimus; Tetrabenazine; Thioridazine; TraZODone; Triazolam; Tricyclic Antidepressants; Vardenafil; Vitamin E; Vortioxetine

The levels/effects of Tipranavir may be increased by: Clarithromycin; CycloSPORINE (Systemic); Delavirdine; Disulfiram; Enfuvirtide; Estrogen Derivatives; Fluconazole; MetroNIDAZOLE (Systemic); MetroNIDAZOLE (Topical); Simeprevir

Decreased Effect

Tipranavir may decrease the levels/effects of: Abacavir; Afatinib; Boceprevir; Clarithromycin; Codeine; Contraceptives (Estrogens); Dabigatran Etexilate; Delavirdine; Didanosine; Dolutegravir; Estrogen Derivatives; Etravirine; Fosphenytoin; Iloperidone; Linagliptin; Meperidine; Methadone; P-glycoprotein/ABCB1 Substrates; PHENObarbital; Phenytoin; Pomalidomide; Proton Pump Inhibitors; Raltegravir; Sofosbuvir; Tamoxifen; Tenofovir; Theophylline Derivatives; TraMADol; Valproic Acid and Derivatives; VinCRIStine (Liposomal); Zidovudine

The levels/effects of Tipranavir may be decreased by: Antacids; Boceprevir; Bosentan; CarBAMazepine; CYP3A4 Inducers (Strong); Dabrafenib; Deferasirox; Fosphenytoin; Garlic; Mitotane; PHENobarbital; Phenytoin; Rifampin; St Johns Wort; Tenofovir; Tocilizumab

Ethanol/Nutrition/Herb Interactions

Ethanol: Capsules contain dehydrated alcohol 7% w/w (0.1 g per capsule)

Herb/Nutraceutical: St John's wort may decrease the levels/effects of tipranavir/ritonavir. Vitamin E (high dose) may increase the risk of bleeding. Garlic may decrease the serum concentration of tipranavir. Management: Avoid St John's wort; concurrent use is contraindicated. Avoid vitamin E supplementation. Garlic supplementation is not recommended.

Storage/Stability

Capsule: Prior to opening bottle, store under refrigeration at 2°C to 8°C (36°F to 46°F). After bottle is opened, may be stored at controlled room temperature of 25°C (77°F) for up to 60 days.

Oral solution: Store at 15°C to 30°C (59°F to 86°F). After bottle is open, use within 60 days. Do not refrigerate or freeze oral solution.

Mechanism of Action Binds to the site of HIV-1 protease activity and inhibits cleavage of viral Gag-Pol polyprotein precursors into individual functional proteins required for infectious HIV. This results in the formation of immature, noninfectious viral particles.

Pharmacodynamics/Kinetics

Absorption: Incomplete (percentage not established)

Distribution: V_d: 7.7-10 L

Protein binding: >99% (albumin, alpha$_1$-acid glycoprotein)

Metabolism: Hepatic, via CYP3A4 (minimal when coadministered with ritonavir)

Bioavailability: Not established

Half-life elimination: Children 2-<6 years of age: ~8 hours, 6-<12 years of age: ~7 hours, 12-18 years: ~5 hours; Adults: 6 hours

Time to peak, plasma: 3 hours

Excretion: Feces (82%); urine (4%); primarily as unchanged drug (when coadministered with ritonavir)

Dosage Oral:

Children ≥2 years: 14 mg/kg or 375 mg/m^2 (maximum: 500 mg/dose) twice daily. **Note:** Coadministration with ritonavir (6 mg/kg or 150 mg/m^2 [maximum: 200 mg/dose] twice daily) is required.

If intolerance or toxicity develops and virus is not resistant to multiple protease inhibitors: May decrease dose to 12 mg/kg or 290 mg/m^2 twice daily. **Note:** Coadministration with ritonavir (5 mg/kg or 115 mg/m^2 twice daily) is required.

Adults: 500 mg twice daily; **Note:** Coadministration with ritonavir (200 mg twice daily) is required.

Dosage adjustment in renal impairment: No dosage adjustment provided in manufacturer's labeling (has not been studied). However, dosage adjustment not expected since renal clearance is negligible.

Dosage adjustment in hepatic impairment:

Mild impairment (Child-Pugh class A): No dosage adjustment necessary.

Moderate-to-severe impairment (Child-Pugh class B or C): Concurrent use is contraindicated

Dietary Considerations Capsule contains dehydrated ethanol. Oral solution formulation contains vitamin E; additional vitamin E supplements should be avoided.

Administration Coadministration with ritonavir is required. Administer with ritonavir capsules or solution without regard to meals; administer with ritonavir tablets with meals.

Monitoring Parameters Viral load, CD4, serum glucose, liver function tests, bilirubin

Dosage Forms Excipient information presented when available (limited, particularly for generics); consult specific product labeling.

Capsule, Oral:

Aptivus: 250 mg

Solution, Oral:

Aptivus: 100 mg/mL (95 mL) [contains polyethylene glycol, propylene glycol, tocophersolan; buttermint-butter toffee flavor]

Tirofiban (tye roe FYE ban)

Brand Names: U.S. Aggrastat

Brand Names: Canada Aggrastat

Index Terms MK383; Tirofiban Hydrochloride

Pharmacologic Category Antiplatelet Agent, Glycoprotein IIb/IIIa Inhibitor

Use Unstable angina/non-ST-elevation myocardial infarction: To decrease the rate of thrombotic cardiovascular events (combined end point of death, MI, or refractory ischemia/repeat cardiac procedure) in patients with non-ST-elevation acute coronary syndrome (unstable angina/non-ST-elevation myocardial infarction [UA/NSTEMI]).

Unlabeled Use To support PCI (administered at the time of PCI) for ST-elevation myocardial infarction (STEMI), UA/NSTEMI, and stable ischemic heart disease (ie, elective PCI)

Pregnancy Risk Factor B

Pregnancy Considerations Adverse events have not been observed in animal reproduction studies. Information related to use in pregnancy is limited; successful use during pregnancy has been described in a case report (Boztosun, 2008).

Breast-Feeding Considerations It is not known if tirofiban is excreted in breast milk. Due to the potential for serious adverse reactions in the nursing infant, a decision should be made whether to discontinue nursing or to discontinue the drug, taking into account the importance of treatment to the mother.

Contraindications Severe hypersensitivity reaction (ie, anaphylactic reaction) to tirofiban or any component of the formulation; history of thrombocytopenia following prior exposure to tirofiban; active internal bleeding or a history of bleeding diathesis, major surgical procedure, or severe physical trauma within the previous month

Warnings/Precautions Bleeding is the most common complication encountered during this therapy; most major bleeding occurs at the arterial access site for cardiac catheterization. Caution in patients with platelets <150,000/mm^3; patients with hemorrhagic retinopathy; chronic dialysis patients; when used in combination with other drugs impacting on coagulation. Percutaneous coronary intervention (unlabeled use): Prior to pulling the sheath, ACT should be <180 seconds or aPTT <50 seconds (Levine, 2011). Use standard compression techniques after sheath removal. Watch the site closely afterwards for further bleeding. Sheath hemostasis should be achieved at least 4 hours before hospital discharge. Other trauma and vascular punctures should be minimized. Avoid obtaining vascular access through a noncompressible site (eg, subclavian or jugular vein).

Profound thrombocytopenia has been reported with use of tirofiban. If during therapy platelet count decreases to <90,000/mm^3, monitor platelet counts to exclude pseudothrombocytopenia. If thrombocytopenia is confirmed, discontinue tirofiban and heparin if administered concurrently. Previous exposure to a glycoprotein IIb/IIIa inhibitor may increase the risk of thrombocytopenia. Use is contraindicated in patients with a history of thrombocytopenia following exposure to tirofiban.

Discontinue at least 2-4 hours prior to coronary artery bypass graft surgery (Anderson, 2013; Hillis, 2011). Dosage reduction of the maintenance infusion rate is necessary in patients with Cl_{cr} ≤60 mL/minute.

Adverse Reactions Bleeding is the major drug-related adverse effect. Patients received background treatment with aspirin and heparin. Major bleeding was reported in 1.4% to 2.2%; minor bleeding in 10.5% to 12%; transfusion was required in 4% to 4.3%.

>1% (nonbleeding adverse events):
- Cardiovascular: Coronary artery dissection (5%), bradycardia (4%), edema (2%)
- Central nervous system: Dizziness (3%), vasovagal reaction (2%), fever (>1%), headache (>1%)
- Gastrointestinal: Nausea (>1%)
- Genitourinary: Pelvic pain (6%)
- Hematologic: Thrombocytopenia: <90,000/mm^3 (1.5%), <50,000/mm^3 (0.3%)
- Neuromuscular & skeletal: Leg pain (3%)
- Miscellaneous: Diaphoresis (2%)

<1% (Limited to important or life-threatening): Acutely decreased platelets in association with fever, anaphylaxis, GI bleeding (0.1% to 0.2%), GU bleeding (up to 0.1%), hemopericardium, intracranial bleeding (up to 0.1%), pulmonary alveolar hemorrhage, rash, retroperitoneal bleeding (up to 0.6%), severe (<10,000/mm^3) thrombocytopenia (rare), spinal-epidural hematoma

Drug Interactions

Metabolism/Transport Effects None known.

Avoid Concomitant Use There are no known interactions where it is recommended to avoid concomitant use.

Increased Effect/Toxicity

Tirofiban may increase the levels/effects of: Agents with Antiplatelet Properties; Anticoagulants; Collagenase (Systemic); Dabigatran Etexilate; Ibritumomab; Rivaroxaban; Salicylates; Thrombolytic Agents; Tositumomab and Iodine I 131 Tositumomab

The levels/effects of Tirofiban may be increased by: Dasatinib; Glucosamine; Herbs (Anticoagulant/Antiplatelet Properties); Ibrutinib; Multivitamins/Fluoride (with ADE); Multivitamins/Minerals (with ADEK, Folate, Iron); Multivitamins/Minerals (with AE, No Iron); Nonsteroidal Anti-Inflammatory Agents; Omega-3 Fatty Acids; Pentosan Polysulfate Sodium; Pentoxifylline; Prostacyclin Analogues; Tipranavir; Vitamin E

Decreased Effect

The levels/effects of Tirofiban may be decreased by: Nonsteroidal Anti-Inflammatory Agents

Storage/Stability Store at 25°C (77°F); excursions are permitted between 15°C and 30°C (59°F and 86°F); do not freeze. Protect from light during storage.

Mechanism of Action A reversible antagonist of fibrinogen binding to the glycoprotein (GP) IIb/IIIa receptor, the major platelet surface receptor involved in platelet aggregation. When administered intravenously, it inhibits *ex vivo* platelet aggregation in a dose- and concentration-dependent manner. When given according to the recommended regimen, >90% inhibition is attained within 10 minutes after initiation. Platelet aggregation inhibition is reversible following cessation of the infusion.

Pharmacodynamics/Kinetics

Onset: >90% inhibition of platelet aggregation (reversible after discontinuation) seen within 10 minutes

Distribution: V_{dss}: 22-42 L

Protein Binding: 65% (concentration dependent)

Metabolism: Negligible

Half-life elimination: 2 hours; **Note:** In ~90% of patients, *ex vivo* platelet aggregation returns to near baseline in 4-8 hours after discontinuation.

Excretion: Urine (65%) and feces (25%) primarily as unchanged drug

Dosage Adults: I.V.:

Unstable angina/non-ST-elevation myocardial infarction (UA/NSTEMI): Loading dose: 25 mcg/kg over 3 minutes; Maintenance infusion: 0.15 mcg/kg/minute continued for up to 18 hours.

Percutaneous coronary intervention (PCI) (unlabeled use): Loading dose: 25 mcg/kg over 3 minutes at the time of PCI; Maintenance infusion: 0.15 mcg/kg/minute continued for up to 18 hours (Anderson, 2013; Levine, 2011).

Stable ischemic heart disease (high-risk features) undergoing elective PCI (unlabeled use): Loading dose: 25 mcg/kg over 3 minutes at the time of PCI; Maintenance infusion: 0.15 mcg/kg/minute continued for up to 48 hours (Levine, 2011; Valgimigli, 2004). **Note:** Reserve for patients who were not pretreated with clopidogrel or who are undergoing elective PCI with stent implantation with adequate clopidogrel pretreatment (Levine, 2011).

ST-elevation myocardial infarction (STEMI) undergoing primary PCI (unlabeled use): Loading dose: 25 mcg/kg over 3 minutes at the time of PCI; Maintenance infusion: 0.15 mcg/kg/minute continued for up to 18-24 hours in combination with heparin or bivalirudin in selected patients (O'Gara, 2013; Levine, 2011; Valgimigli, 2008; Van't Hof, 2008).

Dosage adjustment in renal impairment:

Cl_{cr} >60 mL/minute: No dosage reduction necessary

Cl_{cr} ≤60 mL/minute: Loading dose: 25 mcg/kg over 3 minutes; Maintenance infusion: 0.075 mcg/kg/minute continued for up to 18 hours. **Note:** When used to support PCI in STEMI or UA/NSTEMI, current ACCF/AHA guidelines recommend reducing the maintenance infusion by 50% for patients with Cl_{cr} <30 mL/minute (Anderson, 2013; O'Gara, 2013).

Administration I.V.: Infuse loading dose over 3 minutes, followed by continuous infusion. May be administered through the same catheter as heparin.

Monitoring Parameters Platelet count (baseline; 6 hours after initiation and daily thereafter during therapy). Monitor platelet counts more closely in patients who have had previous exposure to glycoprotein IIb/IIa antagonists. Persistent reductions of platelet counts <90,000/mm^3 may require interruption or discontinuation of infusion; hemoglobin and hematocrit; signs of bleeding.

Standard post-PCI assessment if patient undergoes PCI (eg, monitoring vascular access site, monitoring for chest pain and signs of bleeding)

Dosage Forms Excipient information presented when available (limited, particularly for generics); consult specific product labeling.

Solution, Intravenous:

Aggrastat: 50 mcg/mL (100 mL, 250 mL)

◆ **Tirofiban Hydrochloride** *see* Tirofiban *on page 2072*

◆ **Tirosint** *see* Levothyroxine *on page 1206*

◆ **Titralac [OTC]** *see* Calcium Carbonate *on page 318*

◆ **Ti-U-Lac® H (Can)** *see* Urea and Hydrocortisone *on page 2141*

◆ **TIV (Trivalent Inactivated Influenza Vaccine)** *see* Influenza Virus Vaccine (Inactivated) *on page 1078*

TiZANidine (tye ZAN i deen)

Brand Names: U.S. Zanaflex

Brand Names: Canada Apo-Tizanidine; Gen-Tizanidine; Mylan-Tizanidine; Pal-Tizanidine; Zanaflex

Index Terms Sirdalud

Pharmacologic Category Alpha$_2$-Adrenergic Agonist

Additional Appendix Information

Beers Criteria – Potentially Inappropriate Medications for Geriatrics *on page 2368*

Use Muscle spasticity: Management of spasticity; reserve treatment with tizanidine for daily activities and times when relief of spasticity is most important.

Unlabeled Use Tension headaches, acute low back pain

Pregnancy Risk Factor C

Pregnancy Considerations Adverse events were observed in some animal reproduction studies.

Breast-Feeding Considerations Excretion in breast milk is unknown, but expected due to lipid solubility.

Contraindications Concomitant therapy with ciprofloxacin or fluvoxamine (potent CYP1A2 inhibitors)

Warnings/Precautions Significant hypotension, syncope, and sedation may occur; use caution in patients at risk for severe hypotensive effects (eg, patients taking concurrent medications which may predispose to hypotension) or sedative effects (patients must be cautioned about performing tasks which require mental alertness [eg, operating machinery or driving]). Potentially significant drug-drug interactions may exist, requiring dose or frequency adjustment, additional monitoring, and/or selection of alternative therapy. Use caution in any patient with renal impairment. Clearance decreased significantly in patients with severe impairment (Cl_{cr} <25 mL/minute); dose reductions recommended. Use not recommended in patients with hepatic impairment; potential for hepatotoxicity likely due to extensive hepatic metabolism. Monitor aminotransferases prior to and during use or if hepatic injury is suspected.

May be inappropriate in older adults depending on comorbidities (eg, dementia, delirium) due to its potent anticholinergic effects (Beers Criteria). Use with caution; clearance decreased fourfold in the elderly; may increase risk of adverse effects and/or duration of effects. Elderly with severe renal impairment (Cl_{cr} <25 mL/minute) may have clearance reduced by >50% compared to healthy elderly subjects.

Use has been associated with visual hallucinations or delusions; use caution in patients with psychiatric disorders. Consider discontinuation of therapy if hallucinations occur. Withdrawal resulting in rebound hypertension, tachycardia, and hypertonia may occur upon discontinuation; doses should be decreased slowly, particularly in patients taking concomitant narcotics or receiving high doses (20-28 mg daily) for prolonged periods (≥9 weeks). Food alters absorption profile relative to administration under fasting conditions. In addition, bioequivalence between capsules and tablets is altered by food; capsules and tablets are bioequivalent under fasting conditions, but not under nonfasting conditions.

Adverse Reactions Frequency percentages below reported during multiple-dose studies, unless specified otherwise.

>10%:

Cardiovascular: Hypotension (16% to 33%)

Central nervous system: Somnolence (48%), dizziness (16%)

Gastrointestinal: Xerostomia (49%)

Neuromuscular & skeletal: Weakness (41%)

1% to 10%:

Cardiovascular: Bradycardia (12% to 10%)

Central nervous system: Nervousness (3%), speech disorder (3%), visual hallucinations/delusions (3%), anxiety (1%), depression (1%), fever (1%)

Dermatologic: Rash (1%), skin ulcer (1%)

Gastrointestinal: Constipation (4%), vomiting (3%), abdominal pain (1%), diarrhea (1%), dyspepsia (1%)

Genitourinary: UTI (10%), urinary frequency (3%)

Hepatic: Liver enzymes increased (3% to 5%)

Neuromuscular & skeletal: Dyskinesia (3%), back pain (1%), myasthenia (1%), paresthesia (1%)

Ocular: Blurred vision (3%)

Respiratory: Pharyngitis (3%), rhinitis (3%)

Miscellaneous: Infection (6%), flu-like syndrome (3%), diaphoresis (1%)

<1%, frequency not defined, and postmarketing experience (limited to important or life-threatening): Abnormal dreams, abnormal thinking, abscess, adrenal insufficiency, allergic reaction, anemia, angina pectoris, arrhythmia, carcinoma (including skin), cholelithiasis, deafness, dementia, depersonalization, dyslipidemia, gastrointestinal hemorrhage, glaucoma, heart failure, hepatomegaly, hemiplegia, hepatic failure, hepatitis, hepatoma, herpes infections, hypercholesterolemia, hyperglycemia, hypokalemia, hyponatremia, hypoproteinemia, hypothyroidism, intestinal obstruction, jaundice, leukopenia, leukocytosis, MI, migraine, neuralgia, optic neuritis, orthostatic hypotension, palpitation, paralysis, psychotic-like symptoms, pulmonary embolus, purpura, respiratory acidosis, retinal hemorrhage, seizure, sepsis, suicide attempt, syncope, thrombocythemia, thrombocytopenia, ventricular extrasystoles, ventricular tachycardia, vertigo

Drug Interactions

Metabolism/Transport Effects Substrate of CYP1A2 (major); **Note:** Assignment of Major/Minor substrate status based on clinically relevant drug interaction potential

Avoid Concomitant Use

Avoid concomitant use of TiZANidine with any of the following: Azelastine (Nasal); Ciprofloxacin (Systemic); FluvoxaMINE; Iobenguane I 123; Paraldehyde

Increased Effect/Toxicity

TiZANidine may increase the levels/effects of: ACE Inhibitors; Alcohol (Ethyl); Azelastine (Nasal); Beta-Blockers; Buprenorphine; CNS Depressants; Highest Risk QTc-Prolonging Agents; Hydrocodone; Hypotensive Agents; Lisinopril; Methotrimeprazine; Metyrosine; Moderate Risk QTc-Prolonging Agents; Paraldehyde; Pramipexole; ROPINIRole; Rotigotine; Selective Serotonin Reuptake Inhibitors; Zolpidem

The levels/effects of TiZANidine may be increased by: Abiraterone Acetate; Beta-Blockers; Brimonidine (Topical); Ciprofloxacin (Systemic); Contraceptives (Estrogens); CYP1A2 Inhibitors (Moderate); CYP1A2 Inhibitors (Strong); Deferasirox; Doxylamine; Droperidol; FluvoxaMINE; HydrOXYzine; Magnesium Sulfate; MAO Inhibitors; Methotrimeprazine; Mifepristone; Perampanel; Sodium Oxybate; Tapentadol; Vemurafenib

Decreased Effect

TiZANidine may decrease the levels/effects of: Iobenguane I 123

The levels/effects of TiZANidine may be decreased by: Antidepressants (Alpha2-Antagonist); Serotonin/Norepinephrine Reuptake Inhibitors; Tricyclic Antidepressants

Ethanol/Nutrition/Herb Interactions

Ethanol: May increase CNS depression; monitor for increased effects with coadministration. Caution patients about effects.

Food: The tablet and capsule dosage forms are not bioequivalent when administered with food. Food increases both the time to peak concentration and the extent of absorption for both the tablet and capsule. However, maximal concentrations of tizanidine achieved when administered with food were increased by 30% for the tablet, but decreased by 20% for the capsule. Under fed conditions, the capsule is approximately 80% bioavailable relative to the tablet.

Herb/Nutraceutical: Avoid valerian, St John's wort, kava kava, gotu kola (may increase CNS depression). Avoid black cohosh, California poppy, coleus, golden seal, hawthorn, mistletoe, periwinkle, quinine, shepherd's purse (may increase hypotensive effects).

Storage/Stability Store at 25°C (77°F); excursions are permitted between 15°C and 30°C (59°F and 86°F).

Mechanism of Action An alpha$_2$-adrenergic agonist agent which decreases spasticity by increasing presynaptic inhibition; effects are greatest on polysynaptic pathways; overall effect is to reduce facilitation of spinal motor neurons.

Pharmacodynamics/Kinetics

Onset: Single dose (8 mg): Peak effect: 1-2 hours

Duration: Single dose (8 mg): 3-6 hours

Absorption: Tablets and capsules are bioequivalent under fasting conditions, but not under nonfasting conditions.

Tablets administered with food: Peak plasma concentration is increased by ~30%; time to peak increased by 25 minutes; extent of absorption increased by ~30%.

Capsules administered with food: Peak plasma concentration decreased by 20%; time to peak increased by 2-3 hours; extent of absorption increased by ~10%.

Capsules opened and sprinkled on applesauce are not bioequivalent to administration of intact capsules under fasting conditions. Peak plasma concentration and AUC are increased by 15% to 20%; time to peak decreased by 15 minutes.

Distribution: IV: 2.4 L/kg

Protein binding: ~30%

Metabolism: Extensively hepatic via CYP1A2 to inactive metabolites

Bioavailability: ~40% (extensive first-pass metabolism)

Half-life elimination: ~2.5 hours

Time to peak, serum:

Fasting state: Capsule, tablet: 1 hour

Fed state: Capsule: 3-4 hours, Tablet: 1.5 hours

Excretion: Urine (60%); feces (20%)

Dosage Spasticity: Oral:

Adults: Initial: 2 mg up to 3 times daily (at 6- to 8-hour intervals) as needed; may titrate to optimal effect in 2-4 mg increments per dose (with a minimum of 1-4 days between dose increases); maximum: 36 mg daily. **Note:** Single doses >16 mg have not been studied.

Discontinuation of therapy: Gradually taper dose by 2-4 mg daily.

Elderly: Refer to adult dosing. Use with caution; clearance is decreased.

Dosage adjustment in renal impairment:

Cl_{cr} ≥25 mL/minute: No dosage adjustment provided in manufacturer's labeling; however, caution may be needed as creatinine clearance decreases.

Cl_{cr} <25 mL/minute: Use with caution; clearance reduced >50%. During initial dose titration, use reduced doses. If higher doses are necessary, increase dose instead of increasing dosing frequency.

Dosage adjustment in hepatic impairment: Avoid use in hepatic impairment; if used, reduce dose during initial dose titration. If higher doses are necessary, increase dose instead of increasing dosing frequency. Monitor aminotransferases.

Dietary Considerations Administration with food compared to administration in the fasting state results in clinically-significant differences in absorption and other pharmacokinetic parameters. Patients should be consistent and should not switch administration of the tablets or the capsules between the fasting and nonfasting state. In addition, switching between the capsules and the tablets in the fed state will also result in significant differences. Opening capsule contents to sprinkle on applesauce compared to swallowing intact capsules whole will also result in significant absorption differences. Patients should be consistent with regards to administration.

Administration Capsules may be opened and contents sprinkled on food; however, extent of absorption is increased up to 20% relative to administration of the capsule under fasted conditions.

Monitoring Parameters Monitor liver function (aminotransferases) at baseline and 1 month after maximum dose achieved or if hepatic injury suspected; blood pressure; renal function

Dosage Forms Excipient information presented when available (limited, particularly for generics); consult specific product labeling.

Capsule, Oral:

Zanaflex: 2 mg, 4 mg, 6 mg

Generic: 2 mg, 4 mg, 6 mg

Tablet, Oral:

Zanaflex: 4 mg [scored]

Generic: 2 mg, 4 mg

- ◆ **TL Hydroquinone** *see* Hydroquinone *on page 1017*
- ◆ **TL Urea [DSC]** *see* Urea *on page 2140*
- ◆ **TMC-114** *see* Darunavir *on page 547*
- ◆ **TMC125** *see* Etravirine *on page 807*
- ◆ **TMC207** *see* Bedaquiline *on page 229*
- ◆ **TMC278** *see* Rilpivirine *on page 1817*
- ◆ **TMC435** *see* Simeprevir *on page 1897*
- ◆ **TMP** *see* Trimethoprim *on page 2129*
- ◆ **TMP-SMX** *see* Sulfamethoxazole and Trimethoprim *on page 1959*
- ◆ **TMP-SMZ** *see* Sulfamethoxazole and Trimethoprim *on page 1959*
- ◆ **TMX-67** *see* Febuxostat *on page 834*
- ◆ **TMZ** *see* Temozolomide *on page 2005*
- ◆ **TNKase** *see* Tenecteplase *on page 2011*
- ◆ **TNKase® (Can)** *see* Tenecteplase *on page 2011*
- ◆ **Tobi** *see* Tobramycin (Systemic, Oral Inhalation) *on page 2076*
- ◆ **TOBI (Can)** *see* Tobramycin (Systemic, Oral Inhalation) *on page 2076*
- ◆ **Tobi Podhaler** *see* Tobramycin (Systemic, Oral Inhalation) *on page 2076*
- ◆ **TOBI Podhaler (Can)** *see* Tobramycin (Systemic, Oral Inhalation) *on page 2076*
- ◆ **TobraDex®** *see* Tobramycin and Dexamethasone *on page 2079*
- ◆ **Tobradex® (Can)** *see* Tobramycin and Dexamethasone *on page 2079*
- ◆ **TobraDex® ST** *see* Tobramycin and Dexamethasone *on page 2079*

Tobramycin (Systemic, Oral Inhalation)

(toe bra MYE sin)

Brand Names: U.S. Bethkis; Tobi; Tobi Podhaler

Brand Names: Canada TOBI; TOBI Podhaler; Tobramycin Injection, USP

Index Terms Tobramycin Sulfate

Pharmacologic Category Antibiotic, Aminoglycoside

Use Treatment of documented or suspected infections caused by susceptible gram-negative bacilli, including *Pseudomonas aeruginosa*. Tobramycin solution for inhalation and powder for inhalation are indicated for the management of cystic fibrosis patients with *Pseudomonas aeruginosa*.

Pregnancy Risk Factor D

Pregnancy Considerations [U.S. Boxed Warning]: Aminoglycosides may cause fetal harm if administered to a pregnant woman. There are several reports of total irreversible bilateral congenital deafness in children whose mothers received another aminoglycoside (streptomycin) during pregnancy; therefore, tobramycin is classified as pregnancy category D. Tobramycin crosses the placenta and produces detectable serum levels in the fetus. Although serious side effects to the fetus have not been reported following maternal use of tobramycin, a potential for harm exists.

Due to pregnancy-induced physiologic changes, some pharmacokinetic parameters of tobramycin may be altered. Pregnant women have an average-to-larger volume of distribution which may result in lower serum peak levels than for the same dose in nonpregnant women. Serum half-life is also shorter.

Breast-Feeding Considerations Tobramycin is excreted into breast milk and breast-feeding is not recommended by the manufacturer; however, tobramycin is not well absorbed when taken orally. This limited oral absorption may minimize exposure to the nursing infant. Nondose-related effects could include modification of bowel flora.

Contraindications Hypersensitivity to tobramycin, other aminoglycosides, or any component of the formulation

Warnings/Precautions [U.S. Boxed Warning]: Aminoglycosides may cause neurotoxicity and/or nephrotoxicity; usual risk factors include pre-existing renal impairment, concomitant neuro-/nephrotoxic medications, advanced age, and dehydration. Ototoxicity may be directly proportional to the amount of drug given and the duration of treatment; tinnitus or vertigo are indications of vestibular injury and impending hearing loss; renal damage is usually reversible. Tinnitus and/or hearing loss have also been reported with powder for oral inhalation use. May cause neuromuscular blockade and respiratory paralysis, especially when given soon after anesthesia or muscle relaxants. **[U.S. Boxed Warnings]: Aminoglycosides may cause fetal harm if administered to a pregnant woman.**

Not intended for long-term therapy due to toxic hazards associated with extended administration; use caution in pre-existing renal insufficiency, vestibular or cochlear impairment, myasthenia gravis, Parkinson's disease, hypocalcemia, and conditions which depress neuromuscular transmission. Dosage modification required in patients with impaired renal function during systemic therapy. Prolonged use may result in fungal or bacterial superinfection, including *C. difficile*-associated diarrhea (CDAD) and pseudomembranous colitis; CDAD has been observed >2 months postantibiotic treatment. Solution may contain sodium metabisulfate; use caution in patients with sulfite allergy. Solution for injection may contain sodium metabisulfate; use caution in patients with sulfite allergy. Bronchospasm may occur with tobramycin solution for inhalation; bronchospasm or wheezing should be treated appropriately if either arise. Safety and efficacy of the solution for inhalation have not been demonstrated in patients with FEV_1 <40% or >80% predicted (Bethkis, TOBI), or FEV_1 <25% or >80% predicted (TOBI Podhaler), in patients colonized with *Burkholderia cepacia*, or in patients ≤6 years of age. With powder for inhalation, consider baseline audiogram in patients at increased risk of auditory dysfunction. If any patient experiences tinnitus or hearing loss during treatment, audiological assessment should be performed. Serum tobramycin concentrations do not need to be monitored; one hour after powder inhalation, serum concentrations of 1-2 mcg/mL have been observed. If ototoxicity or nephrotoxicity occur, discontinue therapy until serum concentrations fall below 2 mcg/mL.

Potentially significant drug-drug interactions may exist, requiring dose or frequency adjustment, additional monitoring, and/or selection of alternative therapy.

Adverse Reactions

Injection: Frequency not defined:

Central nervous system: Confusion, disorientation, dizziness, headache, lethargy, vertigo

Dermatologic: Exfoliative dermatitis, pruritus, skin rash, urticaria

Endocrine & metabolic: Decreased serum calcium, decreased serum magnesium, decreased serum potassium and/or decreased serum sodium, increased lactate dehydrogenase

Gastrointestinal: Diarrhea, nausea, vomiting

Genitourinary: Casts in urine, oliguria, proteinuria

Hematologic & oncologic: Anemia, eosinophilia, granulocytopenia, leukocytosis, leukopenia, thrombocytopenia

Hepatic: Increased serum ALT, increased serum AST, increased serum bilirubin

Local: Pain at injection site

Miscellaneous: Fever

Otic: Auditory ototoxicity, hearing loss, tinnitus, vestibular ototoxicity

Renal: Increased blood urea nitrogen, increased serum creatinine

Inhalation

>10%:

Central nervous system: Voice disorder (powder 14%, solution 4%), headache (11% to 12%)

Miscellaneous: Fever (12% to 16%)

Respiratory: Cough (powder 10% to 48%, solution 31%), pulmonary disease (30% to 34%), reduced forced expiratory volume (solution 1% to 31%, powder 4%), discoloration of sputum (solution 21%), productive cough (18% to 20%), rales (solution 6% to 19%, powder 7%), dyspnea (12% to 16%), respiratory depression (2% to 16%), oropharyngeal pain (11% to 14%), hemoptysis (12% to 13%), pharyngolaryngeal pain (powder 11%, solution 3%)

1% to 10%:

Cardiovascular: Chest discomfort (3% to 7%)

Central nervous system: Malaise (6%)

Dermatologic: Skin rash (2%)

Endocrine: Increased serum glucose (powder 3%, solution <1%)

Gastrointestinal: Nausea (8% to 10%), dysgeusia (powder 4% to 7%, solution <1%), vomiting (6%), diarrhea (2% to 4%), xerostomia (powder 2%)

Hematologic & oncologic: Increased erythrocyte sedimentation rate (solution 8%), eosinophilia (solution 2%), increased serum immunoglobulins (solution 2%)

Neuromuscular and Skeletal: Musculoskeletal chest pain (<1% to 5%)

Otic: Hypoacusis (powder 10%), tinnitus (2% to 3%)

Respiratory: Upper respiratory tract infection (7% to 9%), nasal congestion (1% to 8%), wheezing (5% to 7%), throat irritation (2% to 5%), bronchospasm (≤1% to 5%), bronchitis (solution 3%), epistaxis (2% to 3%), rhinitis (solution 2%), tonsillitis (solution 2%)

<1% (Limited to important or life-threatening): Abnormal breath sounds, deafness (including unilateral deafness, reported as mild to moderate hearing loss or increased hearing loss), decreased exercise tolerance, decrease in forced vital capacity, hypersensitivity reaction, increased bronchial secretions, lower respiratory tract infection, obstructive pulmonary disease, oral candidiasis, pneumonitis, pruritus, pulmonary congestion, urticaria

Drug Interactions

Metabolism/Transport Effects None known.

Avoid Concomitant Use

Avoid concomitant use of Tobramycin (Systemic, Oral Inhalation) with any of the following: BCG; Gallium Nitrate

Increased Effect/Toxicity

Tobramycin (Systemic, Oral Inhalation) may increase the levels/effects of: AbobotulinumtoxinA; Bisphosphonate Derivatives; CARBOplatin; Colistimethate; CycloSPORINE (Systemic); Gallium Nitrate; Neuromuscular-Blocking Agents; OnabotulinumtoxinA; RimabotulinumtoxinB; Tenofovir

The levels/effects of Tobramycin (Systemic, Oral Inhalation) may be increased by: Amphotericin B; Capreomycin; Cephalosporins (2nd Generation); Cephalosporins (3rd Generation); Cephalosporins (4th Generation); CISplatin; Loop Diuretics; Nonsteroidal Anti-Inflammatory Agents; Tenofovir; Vancomycin

Decreased Effect

Tobramycin (Systemic, Oral Inhalation) may decrease the levels/effects of: BCG; Sodium Picosulfate; Typhoid Vaccine

The levels/effects of Tobramycin (Systemic, Oral Inhalation) may be decreased by: Penicillins

Preparation for Administration Solution for injection: Dilute in 50-100 mL NS or D_5W for I.V. infusion.

Storage/Stability

Injection: Stable at room temperature both as the clear, colorless solution and as the dry powder. Reconstituted solutions remain stable for 24 hours at room temperature and 96 hours when refrigerated.

Powder, for inhalation (TOBI Podhaler): Store in original package at 25°C (77°F); excursions permitted to 15°C to 30°C (59°F to 86°F). Protect from moisture.

Solution, for inhalation (Bethkis, TOBI): Store under refrigeration at 2°C to 8°C (36°F to 46°F). May be stored in foil pouch (opened or unopened) at room temperature of 25°C (77°F) for up to 28 days. The colorless to pale yellow solution may darken over time if not stored under refrigeration; however, the color change does not affect product quality. Do not use if solution is cloudy, contains particles, or has been stored at room temperature for >28 days.

Mechanism of Action Interferes with bacterial protein synthesis by binding to 30S and 50S ribosomal subunits, resulting in a defective bacterial cell membrane

Pharmacodynamics/Kinetics

Absorption:

Oral: Poorly absorbed

I.M.: Rapid and complete

Inhalation: Peak serum concentrations:

Solution for inhalation: ~1 mcg/mL following a 300 mg dose

Powder for inhalation: ~1 mcg/mL (range: 0.49-1.55 mcg/mL) following a 112 mg dose

Distribution: V_d: 0.2-0.3 L/kg; Pediatrics: 0.2-0.7 L/kg; to extracellular fluid, including serum, abscesses, ascitic, pericardial, pleural, synovial, lymphatic, and peritoneal fluids; poor penetration into CSF, eye, bone, prostate

Inhalation: Tobramycin remains concentrated primarily in the airways

Powder for inhalation: V_d (central compartment) for a typical cystic fibrosis patient: 85.1 L

Protein binding: <30%

Half-life elimination:

Neonates: ≤1200 g: 11 hours; >1200 g: 2-9 hours

Adults: I.V.: 2-3 hours; directly dependent upon glomerular filtration rate; Inhalation: ~4 hours

Adults with impaired renal function: 5-70 hours

Inhalation: Powder for inhalation: Serum clearance: 14.5 L/hour; Half-life: ~3 hours after 112 mg single dose

Time to peak, serum: I.M.: 30-60 minutes; I.V.: ~30 minutes

Excretion: Normal renal function: Urine (~90% to 95%) within 24 hours

Dosage Note: Dosage individualization is **critical** because of the low therapeutic index.

In underweight and nonobese patients, use of total body weight (TBW) instead of ideal body weight for determining the initial mg/kg/dose is widely accepted (Nicolau, 1995). Ideal body weight (IBW) also may be used to determine doses for patients who are neither underweight nor obese (Gilbert, 2009).

Initial and periodic plasma drug levels (eg, peak and trough with conventional dosing, post dose level at a prespecified time with extended-interval dosing) should be determined, particularly in critically-ill patients with serious infections or in disease states known to significantly alter aminoglycoside pharmacokinetics (eg, cystic fibrosis, burns, or major surgery).

Usual dosage range:

Infants and Children <5 years: I.M., I.V.: 2.5 mg/kg/dose every 8 hours

Children ≥5 years: I.M., I.V.: 2-2.5 mg/kg/dose every 8 hours

Note: Higher individual doses and/or more frequent intervals (eg, every 6 hours) may be required in selected clinical situations (cystic fibrosis) or serum levels document the need.

Children ≥6 years and Adults: Inhalation:

Bethkis, TOBI: 300 mg every 12 hours (do not administer doses <6 hours apart); administer in repeated cycles of 28 days on drug followed by 28 days off drug.

TOBI Podhaler: 112 mg (4 x 28 mg capsules) every 12 hours (do not administer doses <6 hours apart); administer in repeated cycles of 28 days on drug followed by 28 days off drug.

Adults: I.M., I.V.:

Conventional: 1-2.5 mg/kg/dose every 8-12 hours; to ensure adequate peak concentrations early in therapy, higher initial dosage may be considered in selected patients when extracellular water is increased (edema, septic shock, postsurgical, and/or trauma)

Once-daily: 4-7 mg/kg/dose once daily; some clinicians recommend this approach for all patients with normal renal function; this dose is at least as efficacious with similar, if not less, toxicity than conventional dosing.

Indication-specific dosing:

Children:

CNS shunt infection: Intrathecal (unlabeled route): Refer to adult dosing

Cystic fibrosis:

I.M., I.V.: 2.5-3.3 mg/kg every 6-8 hours; **Note:** Some patients may require larger or more frequent doses if serum levels document the need (eg, cystic fibrosis or febrile granulocytopenic patients).

Inhalation: Children ≥6 years: Refer to adult dosing.

Adults:

I.M., I.V.:

Brucellosis: 240 mg (I.M.) daily or 5 mg/kg (I.V.) daily for 7 days; either regimen recommended in combination with doxycycline

Cholangitis: 4-6 mg/kg once daily with ampicillin

Diverticulitis, complicated: 1.5-2 mg/kg every 8 hours (with ampicillin and metronidazole)

Infective endocarditis or synergy (for gram-positive infections): I.M., I.V.: 1 mg/kg every 8 hours (with ampicillin)

Meningitis *(Enterococcus or Pseudomonas aeruginosa)*: I.V.: Loading dose: 2 mg/kg, then 1.7 mg/kg/dose every 8 hours (administered with another bactericidal drug)

Pelvic inflammatory disease: Loading dose: 2 mg/kg, then 1.5 mg/kg every 8 hours **or** 4.5 mg/kg once daily

Plague *(Yersinia pestis)*: Treatment: 5 mg/kg/day, followed by postexposure prophylaxis with doxycycline

Pneumonia, hospital- or ventilator-associated: 7 mg/kg/day (with antipseudomonal beta-lactam or carbapenem)

Prophylaxis against endocarditis (dental, oral, upper respiratory procedures, GI/GU procedures): 1.5 mg/kg with ampicillin (50 mg/kg) 30 minutes prior to procedure. **Note:** AHA guidelines now recommend prophylaxis only in patients undergoing invasive procedures and in whom underlying cardiac conditions may predispose to a higher risk of adverse outcomes should infection occur. As of April 2007, routine prophylaxis no longer recommended by the AHA.

Tularemia: 5 mg/kg/day divided every 8 hours for 1-2 weeks

Urinary tract infection: 1.5 mg/kg/dose every 8 hours

Inhalation: **Cystic fibrosis:**

Bethkis, TOBI: 300 mg every 12 hours (do not administer doses <6 hours apart); administer in repeated cycles of 28 days on drug followed by 28 days off drug.

TOBI Podhaler: 112 mg (4 x 28 mg capsules) every 12 hours (do not administer doses <6 hours apart); administer in repeated cycles of 28 days on drug followed by 28 days off drug.

Intrathecal (unlabeled route): **CNS shunt infection:** 5-20 mg/day (Tunkel, 2004)

Dosing in obesity: I.M., I.V.: In moderate obesity (TBW/IBW ≥1.25) or greater, (eg, morbid obesity [TBW/IBW >2]), initial dosage requirement may be estimated using a dosing weight of IBW + 0.4 (TBW - IBW) (Traynor, 1995).

Dosage adjustment in renal impairment:

I.M., I.V.

Conventional dosing:

Cl_{cr} ≥60 mL/minute: Administer every 8 hours

Cl_{cr} 40-60 mL/minute: Administer every 12 hours

Cl_{cr} 20-40 mL/minute: Administer every 24 hours

Cl_{cr} 10-20 mL/minute: Administer every 48 hours

Cl_{cr} <10 mL/minute: Administer every 72 hours

High-dose therapy: Interval may be extended (eg, every 48 hours) in patients with moderate renal impairment (Cl_{cr} 30-59 mL/minute) and/or adjusted based on serum level determinations.

Intermittent hemodialysis (IHD) (administer after hemodialysis on dialysis days) (Heintz, 2009): Dialyzable (25% to 70%; variable; dependent on filter, duration, and type of HD): I.V.:

Loading dose of 2-3 mg/kg, followed by:

Mild UTI or synergy: I.V.: 1 mg/kg every 48-72 hours; consider redosing for pre-HD or post-HD concentrations <1mg/L

Moderate-to-severe UTI: I.V. 1-1.5 mg/kg every 48-72 hours; consider redosing for pre-HD concentrations <1.5-2 mg/L or post-HD concentrations <1 mg/L

Systemic gram-negative infection: I.V.: 1.5-2 mg/kg every 48-72 hours; consider redosing for pre-HD concentrations <3-5 mg/L or post-HD concentrations <2 mg/L

Note: Dosing dependent on the assumption of 3 times/week, complete IHD sessions.

Peritoneal dialysis (PD):

Administration via peritoneal dialysis (PD) fluid:

Gram-negative infection: 4-8 mg/L (4-8 mcg/mL) of PD fluid

Gram-positive infection (ie, synergy): 3-4 mg/L (3-4 mcg/mL) of PD fluid

Administration IVPB/I.M.: Dose as for Cl_{cr} <10 mL/minute and follow levels

Continuous renal replacement therapy (CRRT) (Heintz, 2009; Trotman, 2005): Drug clearance is highly dependent on the method of renal replacement, filter type, and flow rate. Appropriate dosing requires close monitoring of pharmacologic response, signs of adverse reactions due to drug accumulation, as well as drug concentrations in relation to target trough (if appropriate). The following are general recommendations only (based on dialysate flow/ultrafiltration rates of 1-2 L/hour and minimal residual renal function) and should not supersede clinical judgment:

CVVH/CVVHD/CVVHDF: I.V.: Loading dose of 2-3 mg/kg, followed by:

Mild UTI or synergy: I.V. 1 mg/kg every 24-36 hours (redose when concentration <1 mg/L)

Moderate-severe UTI: I.V.: 1-1.5 mg/kg every 24-36 hours (redose when concentration <1.5-2 mg/L)

Systemic gram-negative infection: I.V.: 1.5-2.5 mg/kg every 24-48 hours (redose when concentration <3-5 mg/L)

Inhalation: No dosage adjustment provided in manufacturer's labeling (has not been studied).

Dosing adjustment in hepatic impairment: No dosage adjustment necessary; does not undergo hepatic metabolism.

Dietary Considerations May require supplementation of calcium, magnesium, potassium.

Administration

I.V.: Infuse over 30-60 minutes. Flush with saline before and after administration.

Inhalation:

Bethkis, TOBI: To be inhaled over ~15 minutes using a handheld reusable nebulizer (PARI-LC PLUS) with a PARI Vios air compressor (Bethkis) or a DeVilbiss Pulmo-Aide air compressor (TOBI). If multiple different nebulizer treatments are required, administer bronchodilator first, followed by chest physiotherapy, any other nebulized medications, and then TOBI or Bethkis last. Do not mix with other nebulizer medications.

TOBI Podhaler: Capsules should be administered by oral inhalation via Podhaler device following manufacturer recommendations for use and handling. Capsules should be removed from the blister packaging immediately prior to use and should not be swallowed. Patients requiring bronchodilator therapy should administer the bronchodilator 15-90 minutes prior to TOBI Podhaler. The sequence of chest physiotherapy and additional inhaled therapies is at the discretion of the healthcare provider; however, TOBI Podhaler should always be administered last. The Canadian labeling recommends that patients requiring bronchodilator therapy should administer the bronchodilator 15-90 minutes prior to administering TOBI Podhaler.

Some penicillins (eg, carbenicillin, ticarcillin, and piperacillin) have been shown to inactivate aminoglycosides *in vitro*. This has been observed to a greater extent with tobramycin and gentamicin, while amikacin has shown greater stability against inactivation. Concurrent use of these agents may pose a risk of reduced antibacterial efficacy *in vivo*, particularly in the setting of profound renal impairment. However, definitive clinical evidence is lacking. If combination penicillin/aminoglycoside therapy is desired in a patient with renal dysfunction, separation of doses (if feasible), and routine monitoring of aminoglycoside levels, CBC, and clinical response should be considered.

Monitoring Parameters Urinalysis, urine output, BUN, serum creatinine, peak and trough plasma tobramycin levels. Levels are typically obtained after the third dose in conventional dosing. Be alert to ototoxicity; hearing should be tested before and during treatment

Some penicillin derivatives may accelerate the degradation of aminoglycosides *in vitro*. This may be clinically-significant for certain penicillin (ticarcillin, piperacillin, carbenicillin) and aminoglycoside (gentamicin, tobramycin) combination therapy in patients with significant renal impairment. Close monitoring of aminoglycoside levels is warranted.

Inhalation: The utility of monitoring serum concentrations in patients with renal impairment should be per physician discretion; serum concentrations achieved following inhalation are significantly less than those achieved following parenteral therapy in patients with normal renal function. Serum tobramycin concentrations (patients with known or history of auditory dysfunction, renal dysfunction, or concomitant use of nephrotoxic drugs). One hour after oral powder inhalation, serum concentrations of 1-2 mcg/mL have been observed.

Reference Range

Timing of serum samples: Draw peak 30 minutes after 30-minute infusion has been completed or 1 hour following I.M. injection or beginning of infusion; draw trough immediately before next dose

Therapeutic levels:

Peak:

Serious infections: 6-8 mcg/mL (SI: 12-17 micromole/L)

Life-threatening infections: 8-10 mcg/mL (SI: 17-21 micromole/L)

Urinary tract infections: 4-6 mcg/mL (SI: 7-12 micromole/L)

Synergy against gram-positive organisms: 3-5 mcg/mL

Trough:

Serious infections: 0.5-1 mcg/mL

Life-threatening infections: 1-2 mcg/mL

The American Thoracic Society (ATS) recommends trough levels of <1 mcg/mL for patients with hospital-acquired pneumonia.

Monitor serum creatinine and urine output; obtain drug levels after the third dose unless otherwise directed

Inhalation: Serum levels are ~1 mcg/mL one hour following a 300 mg dose in patients with normal renal function.

Test Interactions Some penicillin derivatives may accelerate the degradation of aminoglycosides *in vitro*, leading to a potential underestimation of aminoglycoside serum concentration.

Additional Information Once-daily dosing: Higher peak serum drug concentration to MIC ratios, demonstrated aminoglycoside postantibiotic effect, decreased renal cortex drug uptake, and improved cost-time efficiency are supportive reasons for the use of once daily dosing regimens for aminoglycosides. Current research indicates these regimens to be as effective for non-life-threatening infections, with no higher incidence of nephrotoxicity, than those requiring multiple daily doses. Doses are determined by calculating the entire day's dose via usual multiple dose calculation techniques and administering this quantity as a single dose. Doses are then adjusted to maintain mean serum concentrations above the MIC(s) of the causative organism(s). (Example: 2.5-5 mg/kg as a single dose; expected Cp_{max}: 10-20 mcg/mL and Cp_{min}: <1 mcg/mL). Further research is needed for universal recommendation in all patient populations and gram-negative disease; exceptions may include those with known high clearance (eg, children, patients with cystic fibrosis, or burns who may require shorter dosage intervals) and patients with renal function impairment for whom longer than conventional dosage intervals are usually required.

Dosage Forms Excipient information presented when available (limited, particularly for generics); consult specific product labeling.

Capsule, Inhalation:

Tobi Podhaler: 28 mg

Nebulization Solution, Inhalation [preservative free]:

Bethkis: 300 mg/4 mL (4 mL)

Tobi: 300 mg/5 mL (5 mL) [contains sodium chloride, sodium hydroxide, sulfuric acid]

Generic: 300 mg/5 mL (5 mL)

Solution, Injection:

Generic: 10 mg/mL (2 mL); 80 mg/2 mL (2 mL); 1.2 g/30 mL (30 mL); 2 g/50 mL (50 mL)

Solution, Intravenous:

Generic: 60 mg (50 mL); 80 mg (100 mL)

Solution Reconstituted, Injection:

Generic: 1.2 g (1 ea)

Solution Reconstituted, Injection [preservative free]:

Generic: 1.2 g (1 ea)

Dosage Forms: Canada Also refer to Dosage Forms. Excipient information presented when available (limited, particularly for generics); consult specific product labeling.

Powder, for oral inhalation [capsule]:

TOBI Podhaler: 28 mg/capsule (224s)

Tobramycin (Ophthalmic) (toe bra MYE sin)

Brand Names: U.S. Tobrex

Brand Names: Canada PMS-Tobramycin; Sandoz-Tobramycin; Tobrex®

Index Terms Tobramycin Sulfate

Pharmacologic Category Antibiotic, Aminoglycoside; Antibiotic, Ophthalmic

Use Treatment of superficial ophthalmic infections caused by susceptible bacteria

Pregnancy Risk Factor B

Dosage Ophthalmic: Children ≥2 months and Adults:

Ointment: Instill 1/2" (1.25 cm) 2-3 times/day; for severe infections, apply every 3-4 hours

Solution: Instill 1-2 drops every 2-4 hours; for severe infections, instill up to 2 drops every hour until improved, then reduce to less frequent intervals

Additional Information Complete prescribing information should be consulted for additional detail.

Dosage Forms Excipient information presented when available (limited, particularly for generics); consult specific product labeling.

Ointment, Ophthalmic:

Tobrex: 0.3% (3.5 g)

Solution, Ophthalmic:

Tobrex: 0.3% (5 mL)

Generic: 0.3% (5 mL)

Tobramycin and Dexamethasone

(toe bra MYE sin & deks a METH a sone)

Brand Names: U.S. TobraDex®; TobraDex® ST

Brand Names: Canada Tobradex®

Index Terms Dexamethasone and Tobramycin

Pharmacologic Category Antibiotic/Corticosteroid, Ophthalmic

Use Treatment of external ocular infection caused by susceptible gram-negative bacteria and steroid responsive inflammatory conditions of the palpebral and bulbar conjunctiva, cornea, and anterior segment of the globe

Pregnancy Risk Factor C

Dosage Ophthalmic: Children ≥2 years and Adults: Ocular infection/inflammation:

Ointment: Apply a small amount (~1/2-inch ribbon of ointment) up to 3-4 times/day

Suspension: Instill 1-2 drops every 4-6 hours; may be increased to 1-2 drops every 2 hours for the first 24-48 hours, then reduce to less frequent intervals

Additional Information Complete prescribing information should be consulted for additional detail.

Dosage Forms Excipient information presented when available (limited, particularly for generics); consult specific product labeling.

Ointment, ophthalmic:

TobraDex®: Tobramycin 0.3% and dexamethasone 0.1% (3.5 g) [contains chlorobutanol]

Suspension, ophthalmic: Tobramycin 0.3% and dexamethasone 0.1% (2.5 mL, 5 mL, 10 mL)

TobraDex®: Tobramycin 0.3% and dexamethasone 0.1% (2.5 mL, 5 mL, 10 mL) [contains benzalkonium chloride]

TobraDex® ST: Tobramycin 0.3% and dexamethasone 0.05% (5 mL) [contains benzalkonium chloride]

◆ **Tobramycin and Loteprednol Etabonate** *see* Loteprednol and Tobramycin *on page 1250*

◆ **Tobramycin Injection, USP (Can)** *see* Tobramycin (Systemic, Oral Inhalation) *on page 2076*

◆ **Tobramycin Sulfate** *see* Tobramycin (Ophthalmic) *on page 2079*

◆ **Tobramycin Sulfate** *see* Tobramycin (Systemic, Oral Inhalation) *on page 2076*

◆ **Tobrex** *see* Tobramycin (Ophthalmic) *on page 2079*

◆ **Tobrex® (Can)** *see* Tobramycin (Ophthalmic) *on page 2079*

Tocilizumab (toe si LIZ oo mab)

Brand Names: U.S. Actemra

Brand Names: Canada Actemra

Index Terms Atlizumab; MRA; R-1569; RoActemra

Pharmacologic Category Antirheumatic, Disease Modifying; Interleukin-6 Receptor Antagonist

Use

Polyarticular juvenile idiopathic arthritis: Treatment of active polyarticular juvenile idiopathic arthritis in patients 2 years and older.

Rheumatoid arthritis: Treatment of adults with moderately to severely active rheumatoid arthritis (RA) who have had an inadequate response to one or more disease-modifying antirheumatic drugs (DMARDs).

Systemic juvenile idiopathic arthritis: Treatment of active systemic juvenile idiopathic arthritis in patients 2 years and older.

Pregnancy Risk Factor C

Pregnancy Considerations Adverse events have been observed in some animal reproduction studies. Monoclonal antibodies cross the placenta, with the largest amount transferred during the third trimester. A pregnancy registry has been established to monitor outcomes of women exposed to tocilizumab during pregnancy (877-311-8972).

Breast-Feeding Considerations It is not known if tocilizumab is excreted in human milk. Because many immunoglobulins are excreted in human milk and the potential for serious adverse reactions exists, a decision should be made whether to discontinue nursing or to discontinue the drug, taking into account the importance of the drug to the mother.

Medication Guide Available Yes

Contraindications Hypersensitivity to tocilizumab or any component of the formulation

Warnings/Precautions [U.S. Boxed Warning]: Serious and potentially fatal infections (including active tuberculosis, invasive fungal, bacterial, viral, protozoal, and other opportunistic infections) have been reported in patients receiving tocilizumab; infection may lead to hospitalization or death. Most of the serious infections have occurred in patients on concomitant immunosuppressive therapy. Patients should be closely monitored for signs and symptoms of infection during and after treatment. If serious infection occurs during treatment, withhold tocilizumab until infection is controlled. Prior to treatment initiation, carefully consider risk versus benefit in patients with chronic or recurrent infections, tuberculosis exposure, history of or current opportunistic infection, underlying conditions predisposing to infection, or patients residing in or with travel to areas of endemic tuberculosis or endemic mycosis, The most common serious infections occurring have included pneumonia, UTI, cellulitis, herpes zoster, gastroenteritis, diverticulitis, sepsis, and bacterial arthritis. Do not administer tocilizumab to a patient with an active infection, including localized infection. Interrupt treatment for opportunistic infection or sepsis. **[U.S. Boxed Warning]: Tuberculosis (pulmonary or extrapulmonary) has been reported in patients receiving tocilizumab; both reactivation of latent infection and new infections have been reported. Patients should be tested for latent tuberculosis infection before and during therapy; consider treatment of latent tuberculosis prior to tocilizumab treatment. Some patients who test negative prior to therapy may develop active infection; monitor for signs and symptoms of tuberculosis during and after treatment in all patients.** Patients should be evaluated for tuberculosis risk factors with a tuberculin skin test prior to starting therapy. Consider antituberculosis treatment in patients with a history of latent or active tuberculosis if adequate treatment course cannot be confirmed, and for patients with risk factors for tuberculosis despite a negative test. Rare reactivation of herpes zoster has been reported. Patients should be brought up to date with all immunizations before initiating therapy. Live vaccines should not be given concurrently; there is no data available concerning secondary transmission of infection from live vaccines in patients receiving therapy.

Use of tocilizumab may affect defenses against malignancies; impact on the development and course of malignancies is not fully defined, however, malignancies were observed in clinical trials. Use with caution in patients with pre-existing or recent onset CNS demyelinating disorders; rare cases of CNS demyelinating disorders (eg, multiple sclerosis) have occurred. All patients should be monitored for signs and symptoms of demyelinating disorders. May cause hypersensitivity or anaphylaxis; anaphylactic events including fatalities have been reported with I.V. administration; hypersensitivity reactions have occurred in patients who were premedicated, in patients with and without a prior history of hypersensitivity, and as early as the first infusion. Medications for the treatment of hypersensitivity reactions should be available for immediate use. Patients should seek medical attention if symptoms of hypersensitivity reaction occur with subcutaneous use. Stop infusion and permanently discontinue treatment in patients who develop a hypersensitivity reaction to tocilizumab. In clinical studies, reactions requiring treatment discontinuation included generalized erythema, rash, and urticaria. Use is not recommended in patients with active hepatic disease or hepatic impairment. Monitor ALT and AST. Do not initiate treatment if ALT or AST is >1.5 times ULN. Use with caution in patients at increased risk for gastrointestinal perforation; perforation has been reported, typically secondary to diverticulitis. Monitor for new-onset abdominal symptoms; promptly evaluate if new symptoms occur.

Use may cause increases in total cholesterol, triglycerides, LDL and HDL cholesterol; monitor ~4-8 weeks after initiation, then approximately every 6 months; hyperlipidemia should be managed according to current guidelines. Neutropenia and thrombocytopenia may occur; may require treatment interruption, dose or interval modification, or discontinuation. Monitor neutrophils and platelets. Do not initiate treatment in patients with an ANC <2000/mm^3 or platelet count <100,000/mm^3; discontinue treatment for ANC <500/mm^3 or platelet count <50,000/mm^3. Monitor transaminases; treatment should be discontinued in patients who develop elevated ALT or AST >5 x ULN. Patients receiving concomitant hepatotoxic drugs (eg, methotrexate) are at an increased risk of developing elevated transaminases; elevations are typically reversible and do not result in clinically evident hepatic injury.

Potentially significant drug/drug interactions may exist, requiring dose or frequency adjustment, additional monitoring, and/or selection of alternative therapy. Concomitant use with other biological DMARDs (eg, TNF blockers, IL-1 receptor blockers, anti-CD20 monoclonal antibodies, selective costimulation modulators) has not been studied and should should be avoided. Cautious use is recommended in elderly patients due to an increased incidence of serious infections. Subcutaneous administration is only indicated for adult patients with rheumatoid arthritis. Do not use subcutaneous injection for I.V. infusion. Product may contain polysorbate 80.

Adverse Reactions Incidence as reported for monotherapy, except where noted. Combination therapy refers to use in rheumatoid arthritis with nonbiological DMARDs or use in SJIA or PJIA in trials where most patients (~70% to 80%) were taking methotrexate at baseline.

>10%:

Endocrine & metabolic: Increased serum cholesterol (>240 mg/dL; 19% to 20%; >1.5-2 x ULN; combination therapy; children and adolescents <1% to 2%)

Hepatic: Increased serum ALT (≤36%; grades 3/4: <1%), increased serum AST (≤22%; grades 3/4: <1%)

Miscellaneous: Infusion-related reaction (combination therapy; 4% to 16%)

1% to 10%:

Cardiovascular: Hypertension (1% to 6%), peripheral edema (<2%)

Central nervous system: Headache (1% to 7%), dizziness (3%)

Dermatologic: Skin rash (2%), dermatological reaction (combination therapy; 1% [includes pruritus, urticaria])

Endocrine & metabolic: Increased LDL cholesterol (9% to 10%; >1.5-2 x ULN; combination therapy; children and adolescents <1% to 2%), hypothyroidism (<2%)

Gastrointestinal: Diarrhea (children and adolescents ≤5%), abdominal pain (2%), oral mucosa ulcer (2%), gastric ulcer (<2%), stomatitis (<2%), weight gain (<2%), gastritis (1%)

Hematologic & oncologic: Neutropenia (combination therapy; grade 3: 2% to 7%; grade 4: <1%), thrombocytopenia (combination therapy; 1% to 2%), leukopenia (<2%)

Hepatic: Increased serum bilirubin (<2%)

Immunologic: Antibody development (<2%)

Infection: Herpes simplex infection (<2%)

Local: Injection site reaction (SubQ: Including erythema, pruritus, pain, and hematoma; 4% to 10%)

Ophthalmic: Conjunctivitis (<2%)

Renal: Nephrolithiasis (<2%)

Respiratory: Upper respiratory tract infection (7%), nasopharyngitis (7%), bronchitis (3%), cough (<2%), dyspnea (<2%)

<1% (Limited to important or life-threatening): Anaphylaxis, anaphylactoid reaction, angioedema, aspergillosis, candidiasis, cellulitis, chronic inflammatory demyelinating polyneuropathy, cryptococcosis, diverticulitis, gastroenteritis, gastrointestinal perforation, herpes zoster, hypersensitivity, hypersensitivity pneumonitis, hypertriglyceridemia, hypotension, increased HDL cholesterol, malignant neoplasm (including breast and colon cancer), multiple sclerosis, otitis media, pneumonia, pneumocystosis, reactivation of latent Epstein-Barr virus, septic arthritis, sepsis, tuberculosis, urinary tract infection, varicella

Drug Interactions

Metabolism/Transport Effects None known.

Avoid Concomitant Use

Avoid concomitant use of Tocilizumab with any of the following: Abatacept; Anti-TNF Agents; BCG; Belimumab; Natalizumab; Pimecrolimus; Tacrolimus (Topical); Tofacitinib; Vaccines (Live)

Increased Effect/Toxicity

Tocilizumab may increase the levels/effects of: Abatacept; Anti-TNF Agents; Belimumab; Leflunomide; Natalizumab; Tofacitinib; Vaccines (Live)

The levels/effects of Tocilizumab may be increased by: Abciximab; Denosumab; Pimecrolimus; Roflumilast; Tacrolimus (Topical); Trastuzumab

Decreased Effect

Tocilizumab may decrease the levels/effects of: BCG; Coccidioidin Skin Test; CYP3A4 Substrates; Sipuleucel-T; Vaccines (Inactivated); Vaccines (Live)

The levels/effects of Tocilizumab may be decreased by: Echinacea

Preparation for Administration I.V.: Prior to administration, dilute to 50 mL (children <30 kg) or 100 mL (children ≥30 kg and adults) by slowly adding to 0.9% sodium chloride. Use vials for I.V. to prepare infusion solutions; do **not** use prefilled SubQ syringes to prepare I.V. solutions. Withdraw equal volume of 0.9% sodium chloride to the volume of tocilizumab required for dose; slowly add tocilizumab dose into infusion bag or bottle. Gently invert to mix (avoid foaming). Diluted solutions may be stored under refrigeration or at room temperature for up to 24 hours (protected from light) and are compatible with polypropylene, polyethylene (PE), polyvinyl chloride (PVC), and glass infusion containers. Allow diluted solution to reach room temperature prior to infusion.

Storage/Stability Store intact vials/syringes at 2°C to 8°C (36°F to 46°F). Do not freeze. Protect vials and syringes from light (store in the original package until time of use); keep syringes dry. Solutions diluted for I.V. infusion may be stored at 2°C to 8°C (36°F to 46°F) or room temperature for up to 24 hours and should be protected from light. Discard unused product remaining in the vials.

Mechanism of Action Antagonist of the interleukin-6 (IL-6) receptor. Endogenous IL-6 is induced by inflammatory stimuli and mediates a variety of immunological responses. Inhibition of IL-6 receptors by tocilizumab leads to a reduction in cytokine and acute phase reactant production.

Pharmacodynamics/Kinetics

Distribution: V_{dss}: Children: 2.54-4.08 L; Adults: 6.4 L

Bioavailability: SubQ: 80%

Half life elimination:

I.V.: Terminal, single dose: 6.3 days (concentration-dependent; may be increased up to 16-23 days [children] or 11-13 days [adults] at steady state)

SubQ: Concentration dependent: Adults: Up to 5 days (every other week dosing) or 13 days (every week dosing)

Dosage Note: Do not initiate if ANC is <2000/mm^3, platelets are <100,000/mm^3 or if ALT or AST are >1.5 times ULN.

Polyarticular juvenile idiopathic arthritis (PJIA): Children ≥2 years: I.V.: **Note:** Dose adjustment should not be made based solely on a single-visit body weight measurement due to fluctuations in body weight. May be used as monotherapy or in combination with methotrexate.

<30 kg: 10 mg/kg every 4 weeks

≥30 kg: 8 mg/kg every 4 weeks

Systemic juvenile idiopathic arthritis (SJIA): Children ≥2 years: I.V.: **Note:** Dose adjustment should not be made based solely on a single-visit body weight measurement due to fluctuations in body weight. May be used as monotherapy or in combination with methotrexate.

<30 kg: 12 mg/kg every 2 weeks

≥30 kg: 8 mg/kg every 2 weeks

Rheumatoid arthritis: Adults: **Note:** Methotrexate or other *nonbiologic* disease-modifying antirheumatic drugs (DMARDs) may be continued for the treatment of rheumatoid arthritis. Tocilizumab should not be used in combination with *biologic* DMARDs.

I.V.: Initial: 4 mg/kg every 4 weeks; increase to 8 mg/kg based on clinical response (maximum dose: 800 mg)

SubQ:

<100 kg: 162 mg every other week; increase to every week based on clinical response

≥100 kg: 162 mg every week

Transitioning from I.V. therapy to SubQ therapy: Administer the first SubQ dose instead of the next scheduled I.V. dose.

Dosage adjustment for toxicity:

Hypersensitivity (anaphylaxis or other clinically-significant hypersensitivity reaction): Stop immediately and discontinue permanently.

Infection (serious infection, opportunistic infection or sepsis): Interrupt treatment until the infection is controlled.

Polyarticular and systemic juvenile idiopathic arthritis: Dose reductions have not been studied; however, dose interruptions are recommended for liver enzyme abnormalities, low neutrophil counts, and low platelets similar to recommendations provided for rheumatoid arthritis. In addition, consider interrupting or discontinuing concomitant methotrexate and/or other medications and hold tocilizumab dosing until the clinical situation has been assessed.

Rheumatoid arthritis (RA):

Liver enzyme abnormalities:

>1 to 3 x ULN: Adjust concomitant DMARDs as appropriate. For patients receiving I.V. therapy with persistent increases >1 to 3 x ULN, reduce dose to 4 mg/kg or interrupt until ALT/AST have normalized. For patients receiving SubQ therapy with persistent increases >1 to 3 x ULN, reduce injection frequency to every other week or interrupt until ALT/AST have normalized; increase frequency to every week as clinically appropriate.

>3 to 5 x ULN (confirmed with repeat testing): Interrupt until ALT/AST <3 x ULN and follow dosage adjustments recommended for liver enzyme abnormalities >1 to 3 x ULN. For persistent increases >3 x ULN, discontinue.

>5 x ULN: Discontinue.

Low absolute neutrophil counts (ANC):

ANC >1000 cells/mm^3: Maintain dose.

ANC 500-1000 cells/mm^3: Interrupt therapy; when ANC >1000 cells/mm^3, resume I.V. tocilizumab at 4 mg/kg (may increase to 8 mg/kg as clinically appropriate) or resume SubQ tocilizumab at every other week dosing (increase frequency to every week as clinically appropriate).

ANC <500 cells/mm^3: Discontinue.

Low platelet counts:

Platelets 50,000-100,000 cells/mm^3: Interrupt therapy; when platelet count is >100,000 cells/mm^3, resume I.V. tocilizumab at 4 mg/kg (may increase to 8 mg/kg as clinically appropriate) or resume SubQ tocilizumab at every other week dosing (increase frequency to every week as clinically appropriate).

Platelets <50,000 cells/mm^3: Discontinue.

Dosage adjustment for renal impairment:

Mild renal impairment: No dosage adjustment necessary.

Moderate-to-severe renal impairment: No dosage adjustment provided in the manufacturer's labeling (has not been studied).

Dosage adjustment for hepatic impairment: No dosage adjustment provided in the manufacturer's labeling (has not been studied). Not recommended for use in patients with active hepatic disease or hepatic impairment

Administration

I.V.: Allow diluted solution for infusion to reach room temperature prior to administration; infuse over 60 minutes using a dedicated I.V. line. Do not infuse other agents through same I.V. line. Do not administer I.V. push or I.V. bolus. Do not use if opaque particles or discoloration is visible.

SubQ: Rheumatoid arthritis: When transitioning from I.V. administration to SubQ administration, give the first SubQ dose instead of the next scheduled I.V. dose. Administer the full amount in the prefilled syringe. Allow to reach room temperature prior to use. Do not use if particulate matter or discoloration is visible; solution should be clear and colorless to pale yellow. Rotate injection sites; avoid injecting into moles, scars, or tender, bruised, red, or hard skin. Prefilled syringe is available for use by patients (self-administration).

Monitoring Parameters Latent TB screening prior to therapy initiation; neutrophils, platelets, ALT/AST (prior to therapy, 4-8 weeks after start of therapy, and every 3 months thereafter [RA]); neutrophils, platelets, ALT/AST (prior to therapy, at 2nd infusion, and every 2-4 weeks [SJIA] or 4-8 weeks [PJIA] thereafter); additional liver function tests (eg, bilirubin) as clinically indicated; lipid panel (prior to, at 4-8 weeks following initiation, and every ~6 months during therapy); signs and symptoms of infection (prior to, during, and after therapy); signs and symptoms of CNS demyelinating disorders

Dosage Forms Excipient information presented when available (limited, particularly for generics); consult specific product labeling.

Solution, Intravenous [preservative free]:

Actemra: 80 mg/4 mL (4 mL); 200 mg/10 mL (10 mL); 400 mg/20 mL (20 mL) [contains polysorbate 80]

Solution Prefilled Syringe, Subcutaneous [preservative free]:

Actemra: 162 mg/0.9 mL (0.9 mL) [contains polysorbate 80]

Tofacitinib (toe fa SYE ti nib)

Brand Names: U.S. Xeljanz

Index Terms CP-690, 550; Tofacitinib Citrate

Pharmacologic Category Antirheumatic Miscellaneous; Antirheumatic, Disease Modifying; Janus Associated Kinase Inhibitor

Use Treatment of moderately- to severely-active rheumatoid arthritis (as monotherapy or in combination with methotrexate or other nonbiologic disease-modifying antirheumatic drugs [DMARDs]) in patients who have had an inadequate response to, or are intolerant of, methotrexate

Pregnancy Risk Factor C

Pregnancy Considerations Adverse events have been observed in animal reproduction studies. Healthcare providers are encouraged to enroll women exposed to tofacitinib during pregnancy in the Xeljanz® Pregnancy Registry (877-311-8972); patients may also enroll themselves.

Breast-Feeding Considerations It is not known if tofacitinib is excreted into breast milk. Due to the potential for adverse reactions in a nursing infant, the decision to continue or discontinue breast-feeding during therapy should take into account the risk of exposure to the infant and the benefits of treatment to the mother.

Prescribing and Access Restrictions Available through specialty/network pharmacies. Further information may be obtained from the manufacturer, Pfizer Inc, at 1-855-493-5526 or at http://www.xeljanz.com/.

Medication Guide Available Yes

Contraindications There are no contraindications listed in the manufacturer's labeling.

Warnings/Precautions [U.S. Boxed Warning]: Patients receiving tofacitinib are at increased risk for serious infections, which may result in hospitalization and/or fatality; infections often developed in patients receiving concomitant immunosuppressive agents (eg, methotrexate or corticosteroids) and may present as disseminated disease. Active tuberculosis (disseminated or extrapulmonary), invasive fungal (including cryptococcosis and pneumocystosis) and bacterial, viral or other opportunistic infections (including esophageal candidiasis, multidermatomal herpes zoster, cytomegalovirus, and BK virus) have been reported in patients receiving tofacitinib. Reactivation of viral infections (eg, herpes zoster) was observed in clinical trials; the incidence of chronic viral hepatitis reactivation is unknown. Use with caution in patients that have been exposed to tuberculosis, with a history of serious or opportunistic infection, taking concomitant immunosuppressants, with comorbid conditions that predispose them to infections (eg, diabetes), or in patients who live in or travel to/from areas of endemic mycoses (ie, blastomycosis, coccidioidomycosis, histoplasmosis). Consider risks versus benefits prior to use in patients with a history of chronic or recurrent infection; do not initiate tofacitinib in patients with active infections, including localized infections. Monitor closely for signs/symptoms of infection during therapy; interrupt therapy if serious infections or sepsis develop. Use with caution in elderly patients; general incidence of infection is higher in elderly.

[U.S. Boxed Warning]: Tuberculosis (disseminated or extrapulmonary) has been reported in patients receiving tofacitinib. Patients should be evaluated for tuberculosis risk factors and active or latent infection (with a tuberculin skin test) before and during therapy. Treatment of latent tuberculosis should be initiated before use. Patients with initial negative tuberculin skin tests should receive continued monitoring for tuberculosis throughout treatment; active tuberculosis has developed in this population during treatment with tofacitinib. Use with caution in patients who have resided in regions where tuberculosis is endemic. Consider antituberculosis therapy if an adequate course of treatment cannot be confirmed in patients with a history of latent or active tuberculosis or for patients with risk factors despite negative skin test.

[U.S. Boxed Warning]: Lymphoma and other malignancies have been reported in patients receiving tofacitinib; Epstein Barr Virus-associated post-transplant lymphoproliferative disorder has been observed at an increased rate in renal transplant patients receiving tofacitinib and concomitant immunosuppressive medications. The most common types of malignancy observed were lung, breast, gastric, colorectal, renal cell, prostate, lymphoma, and malignant melanoma. Consider risks versus benefits prior to use in patients with a known malignancy (other than successfully treated nonmelanoma skin cancers [NMSC]) or when continuing tofacitinib in patients who develop a new malignancy.

Lymphocytopenia (after an initial lymphocytosis), neutropenia (<2000 cells/mm^3), and anemia have been observed with tofacitinib therapy. Lymphocyte counts <500 cells/mm^3 were associated with increased incidence of treated and serious infections; avoid tofacitinib initiation in patients with lymphocytes <500 cells/mm^3 at baseline. Avoid use in patients with ANC <1000 cells/mm^3 at baseline; interrupt therapy if ANC is persistently between 500-1000 cells/mm^3 or if ANC <500 cells/mm^3 during treatment. Consider resuming tofacitinib when ANC ≥1000 cells/mm^3. Avoid use in patients with hemoglobin <9 g/dL; interrupt therapy if hemoglobin decreases >2 g/dL or if hemoglobin <8 g/dL. Monitor lymphocyte counts at baseline and every 3 months thereafter; ANC, platelet counts, and hemoglobin should be assessed at baseline, after 4-8 weeks of therapy, and every 3 months thereafter.

Use with caution in patients at increased risk for gastrointestinal perforation (eg, history of diverticulitis); perforations have been reported in clinical trials. Promptly evaluate new-onset abdominal symptoms in patients taking tofacitinib. Increases in lipid parameters (eg, total cholesterol, LDL, and HDL cholesterol) were observed in patients receiving tofacitinib; maximum lipid increases were typically seen within 6 weeks of initiation. Assess lipids 4-8 weeks after tofacitinib initiation and manage lipid abnormalities accordingly. Increased incidence of liver enzyme elevation was observed in patients taking tofacitinib compared to placebo. Routine liver function test monitoring is recommended; interrupt therapy if drug-induced liver injury is suspected.

Immunization status should be current before initiating therapy. Live vaccines should not be given concomitantly with tofacitinib; no data are available concerning vaccination response or secondary transmission of infection by live vaccines in patients receiving therapy.

Tofacitinib should not be administered in combination with strong immunosuppressive medications (eg, azathioprine, tacrolimus, cyclosporine) due to the risk of additive immunosuppression; such combinations have not been studied in rheumatoid arthritis. Tofacitinib should not be administered in combination with biologic DMARDs.

Use is not recommended in patients with severe hepatic impairment; dosage reduction required in patients with moderate hepatic impairment. Dosage reduction required in patients with moderate or severe renal impairment.

Adverse Reactions

Percentages noted include the highest frequency regardless of dosage. Frequencies may vary for specific doses; consult prescribing information.

>10%: Miscellaneous: Infections (20%)

1% to 10%:

- Cardiovascular: Hypertension (2%)
- Central nervous system: Headache (4%)
- Gastrointestinal: Diarrhea (4%)
- Genitourinary: Urinary tract infection (2%)
- Hepatic: ALT increased (>3 x upper limit of normal; 1%)
- Renal: Serum creatinine increased (<2%)
- Respiratory: Upper respiratory tract infections (5%), nasopharyngitis (4%)
- Miscellaneous: Serious infections (2%)

<1% (Limited to important or life-threatening): Abdominal pain, anemia, dehydration, drug-induced liver injury, dyspepsia, dyspnea, erythema, gastritis, hepatic steatosis, lymphocytopenia, malignancies, musculoskeletal pain, neutropenia, paresthesia, peripheral edema, pruritus, pyrexia, rash, sinus congestion, tendonitis, tuberculosis, vomiting

Drug Interactions

Metabolism/Transport Effects Substrate of CYP2C19 (minor), CYP3A4 (major); **Note:** Assignment of Major/Minor substrate status based on clinically relevant drug interaction potential

Avoid Concomitant Use

Avoid concomitant use of Tofacitinib with any of the following: Abatacept; Anakinra; Anti-TNF Agents; BCG; CloZAPine; CYP3A4 Inducers (Strong); Fusidic Acid (Systemic); Immunosuppressants; Natalizumab; Pimecrolimus; RiTUXimab; Tacrolimus (Topical); Tocilizumab; Vaccines (Live)

Increased Effect/Toxicity

Tofacitinib may increase the levels/effects of: CloZAPine; Leflunomide; Natalizumab; Vaccines (Live)

The levels/effects of Tofacitinib may be increased by: Abatacept; Anakinra; Anti-TNF Agents; CYP3A4 Inhibitors (Moderate); CYP3A4 Inhibitors (Strong); Denosumab; Fluconazole; Fusidic Acid (Systemic); Immunosuppressants; Ivacaftor; Luliconazole; Mifepristone; Pimecrolimus; RiTUXimab; Roflumilast; Simeprevir; Sitaxentan; Tacrolimus (Topical); Tocilizumab; Trastuzumab

Decreased Effect

Tofacitinib may decrease the levels/effects of: BCG; Coccidioidin Skin Test; Sipuleucel-T; Vaccines (Inactivated); Vaccines (Live)

The levels/effects of Tofacitinib may be decreased by: Bosentan; CYP3A4 Inducers (Strong); Dabrafenib; Deferasirox; Echinacea; Herbs (CYP3A4 Inducers)

Storage/Stability Store between 20°C and 25°C (68°F to 77°F).

Mechanism of Action Tofacitinib inhibits Janus kinase (JAK) enzymes, which are intracellular enzymes involved in stimulating hematopoiesis and immune cell function through a signaling pathway. In response to extracellular cytokine or growth factor signaling, JAKs activate signal transducers and activators of transcription (STATs), which regulate gene expression and intracellular activity. Inhibition of JAKs prevents cytokine- or growth factor-mediated gene expression and intracellular activity of immune cells, reduces circulating CD16/56+ natural killer cells, serum IgG, IgM, IgA, and C-reactive protein, and increases B cells.

Pharmacodynamics/Kinetics

Absorption: Oral: Rapid (74%); C_{max} is reduced by 32% when administered with high-fat meal, but AUC remains unchanged.

Distribution: V_d: 87 L

Protein binding: ~40% (predominantly to albumin)

Metabolism: Hepatic (70%): CYP3A4 and CYP2C19 to inactive metabolites

Half-life elimination: ~3 hours

Time to peak: 0.5-1 hour

Excretion: Primarily urine (30%) as unchanged drug

Dosage Rheumatoid arthritis (monotherapy or in combination with nonbiologic disease-modifying antirheumatic drugs (DMARDs): Adults: Oral: 5 mg twice daily

Note: Tofacitinib should not be used in combination with biologic DMARDs or with strong immunosuppressants, such as azathioprine, tacrolimus, or cyclosporine.

Dosage adjustment for toxicity:

Lymphopenia (lymphocytes ≥500 cells/mm^3): Maintain dose.

Lymphopenia (lymphocytes <500 cells/mm^3): Discontinue therapy.

Neutropenia (ANC >1000 cells/mm^3): Maintain dose.

Neutropenia (ANC persistently between 500-1000 cells/mm^3): Interrupt therapy; resume when ANC >1000 cells/mm^3.

Neutropenia (ANC <500 cells/mm^3): Discontinue therapy.

Anemia (hemoglobin ≥9 g/dL **and** decrease ≤2 g/dL): Maintain dose.

Anemia (hemoglobin <8 g/dL **or** decrease >2 g/dL): Interrupt therapy until hemoglobin values have normalized.

Dosage adjustment for strong CYP3A4 inhibitors (eg, ketoconazole): Reduce dose to 5 mg daily

Dosage adjustment for concomitant moderate CYP3A4 inhibitors and potent CYP2C19 inhibitors (eg, fluconazole): Reduce dose to 5 mg daily

Dosage adjustment in renal impairment:

Mild impairment: No dosage adjustment necessary.

Moderate-to-severe impairment: Reduce dose to 5 mg once daily. **Note:** Tofacitinib has not been studied in patients with baseline Cl_{cr} <40 mL/minute.

Dosage adjustment in hepatic impairment:

Mild impairment: No dosage adjustment necessary.

Moderate impairment: Reduce dose to 5 mg once daily.

Severe impairment: Use is not recommended (has not been studied in patients with severe hepatic impairment or in patients with hepatitis B or hepatitis C viruses).

Administration May be taken without regard to food.

Monitoring Parameters Lymphocyte count (baseline and every 3 months thereafter); neutrophil/platelet counts (baseline, after 4-8 weeks, and every 3 months thereafter); lipids (4-8 weeks after therapy initiation and periodically); hemoglobin (baseline, after 4-8 weeks, and every 3 months thereafter); LFTs; signs/symptoms of infections (including tuberculosis) during and after therapy; abdominal symptoms

Dosage Forms Excipient information presented when available (limited, particularly for generics); consult specific product labeling.

Tablet, Oral:

Xeljanz: 5 mg

- ◆ **Tofacitinib Citrate** *see* Tofacitinib *on page 2082*
- ◆ **Tofranil** *see* Imipramine *on page 1055*
- ◆ **Tofranil® (Can)** *see* Imipramine *on page 1055*
- ◆ **Tofranil-PM** *see* Imipramine *on page 1055*

TOLAZamide (tole AZ a mide)

Pharmacologic Category Antidiabetic Agent, Sulfonylurea

Additional Appendix Information

Oral Antidiabetic Agents Comparison Table *on page 2312*

Use Adjunct to diet for the management of mild-to-moderately severe, stable, type 2 diabetes mellitus (noninsulin dependent, NIDDM)

Pregnancy Risk Factor C

Dosage Oral: Adults: Doses >500 mg/day should be given in 2 divided doses:

Initial: 100-250 mg/day with breakfast or the first main meal of the day

Fasting blood sugar <200 mg/dL: 100 mg/day

Fasting blood sugar >200 mg/dL: 250 mg/day

Patient is malnourished, underweight, elderly, or not eating properly: 100 mg/day

Adjust dose in increments of 100-250 mg/day at weekly intervals to response; maximum daily dose: 1 g (doses >1 g/day are not likely to improve control)

Conversion from insulin to tolazamide:

<20 units day = 100 mg/day

21-<40 units/day = 250 mg/day

≥40 units/day = 250 mg/day and 50% of insulin dose

Dosing adjustment in renal impairment: No dosage adjustment provided in manufacturer's labeling. However, conservative initial and maintenance doses are recommended because tolazamide is metabolized to active metabolites, which are eliminated in the urine

Dosing comments in hepatic impairment: No dosage adjustment provided in manufacturer's labeling. However, conservative initial and maintenance doses and careful monitoring of blood glucose are recommended

Additional Information Complete prescribing information should be consulted for additional detail.

Dosage Forms Excipient information presented when available (limited, particularly for generics); consult specific product labeling.

Tablet, Oral:

Generic: 250 mg, 500 mg

TOLBUTamide (tole BYOO ta mide)

Brand Names: Canada Apo-Tolbutamide®

Index Terms Orinase; Tolbutamide Sodium

Pharmacologic Category Antidiabetic Agent, Sulfonylurea

Additional Appendix Information

Oral Antidiabetic Agents Comparison Table *on page 2312*

Use Adjunct to diet for the management of type 2 diabetes mellitus (noninsulin dependent, NIDDM)

Pregnancy Risk Factor C

Dosage Oral: **Note:** Divided doses may improve gastrointestinal tolerance.

Adults: Initial: 1-2 g/day as a single dose in the morning or in divided doses throughout the day. Maintenance dose: 0.25-3 g/day; however, a maintenance dose >2 g/day is seldom required.

Elderly: Initial: 250 mg 1-3 times/day; usual: 500-2000 mg; maximum: 3 g/day

Dosage adjustment in renal impairment: No dosage adjustment provided in manufacturer's labeling. However, conservative initial and maintenance doses are recommended.

Hemodialysis: Not dialyzable (0% to 5%)

Dosage adjustment in hepatic impairment: No dosage adjustment provided in manufacturer's labeling. However, conservative initial and maintenance doses and careful monitoring of blood glucose are recommended.

Additional Information Complete prescribing information should be consulted for additional detail.

Dosage Forms Excipient information presented when available (limited, particularly for generics); consult specific product labeling.

Tablet, Oral:

Generic: 500 mg

◆ **Tolbutamide Sodium** *see* TOLBUTamide *on page 2085*

Tolcapone (TOLE ka pone)

Brand Names: U.S. Tasmar

Pharmacologic Category Anti-Parkinson's Agent, COMT Inhibitor

Additional Appendix Information

Antiparkinsonian Agents *on page 2289*

Use Adjunct to levodopa and carbidopa for the treatment of signs and symptoms of idiopathic Parkinson's disease in patients with motor fluctuations not responsive to other therapies

Pregnancy Risk Factor C

Pregnancy Considerations Adverse events were observed in animal reproduction studies.

Breast-Feeding Considerations It is not known if tolcapone is excreted in breast milk. The manufacturer recommends that caution be exercised when administering tolcapone to nursing women.

Prescribing and Access Restrictions A patient signed consent form acknowledging the risks of hepatic injury should be obtained by the treating physician.

Contraindications Hypersensitivity to tolcapone or any component of the formulation; patients with liver disease or a history of tolcapone-induced hepatocellular injury; history of nontraumatic rhabdomyolysis or hyperpyrexia and confusion potentially related to medication

Warnings/Precautions [U.S. Boxed Warning]: Due to reports of fatal liver injury associated with use of this drug, the manufacturer is advising that tolcapone be reserved for patients who are experiencing inadequate symptom control or who are not appropriate candidates for other available treatments. Patients must provide written consent acknowledging the risks of hepatic injury. Close monitoring for potential hepatotoxicity is required during use. Do not initiate in patients with clinical evidence of liver disease or with two transaminases values greater than the upper limit of normal. Discontinue if signs and/or symptoms of hepatic injury are noted (eg, anorexia, jaundice, lethargy, transaminases >2 times upper limit of normal) or if clinical improvement is not evident after 3 weeks of therapy. Tolcapone should not be reinitiated in patients who discontinued therapy due to evidence of liver injury; may be at increased risk for liver injury. Use with caution in patients with pre-existing dyskinesias; exacerbation of pre-existing dyskinesia has been reported. Levodopa dosage reduction may be required, particularly in patients with levodopa dosages >600 mg daily or with moderate-to-severe dyskinesia prior to initiation.

May cause orthostatic hypotension and syncope; Parkinson's disease patients appear to have an impaired capacity to respond to a postural challenge; use with caution in patients at risk of hypotension (such as those receiving antihypertensive drugs) or where transient hypotensive episodes would be poorly tolerated (cardiovascular disease or cerebrovascular disease). Parkinson's patients being treated with dopaminergic agonists ordinarily require careful monitoring for signs and symptoms of postural hypotension, especially during dose escalation, and should be informed of this risk. Patients have reported falling asleep while engaging in activities of daily living; this has been reported to occur without significant warning signs. Monitor for daytime somnolence or pre-existing sleep disorder. Use caution with other CNS depressants, sedating agents, psychoactive drugs or ethanol. Patients must be cautioned about performing tasks which require mental alertness (eg, operating machinery or driving). Discontinuation of treatment may be required in patients experiencing significant drowsiness. May cause hallucinations (onset within 2 weeks), which may improve with reduction in levodopa therapy; incidence may be increased in patients >75 years of age. Abnormal thinking and behavior changes have been reported and may include paranoid ideation, delusions, confusion, psychotic-like behavior, disorientation, aggressive behavior, agitation, and delirium. Avoid use in patients with a major psychotic disorder; may exacerbate psychosis. Use with caution in patients with lower gastrointestinal disease or an increased risk of dehydration; tolcapone has been associated with delayed development of diarrhea (onset after 2-12 weeks).

Potentially significant interactions may exist, requiring dose or frequency adjustment, additional monitoring, and/or selection of alternative therapy. Concomitant use of tolcapone and nonselective MAO inhibitors should be avoided. Selegiline is a selective MAO type B inhibitor (when given orally at ≤10 mg/day) and can be taken with tolcapone. Dopaminergic agents used for Parkinson's disease or restless legs syndrome have been associated with compulsive behaviors and/or loss of impulse control, which has manifested as pathological gambling, libido increases (hypersexuality), and/or binge eating. Causality has not been established, and controversy exists as to whether this phenomenon is related to the underlying disease, prior behaviors/addictions and/or drug therapy. Dose reduction or discontinuation of therapy has been reported to reverse these behaviors in some, but not all cases. Severe rhabdomyolysis has been reported with use. Risk for melanoma development is increased in Parkinson's disease patients; drug causation or factors contributing to risk have not been established. Patients should be monitored closely and periodic skin examinations should be performed. Dopaminergic agents from the ergot class have also been associated with fibrotic complications, such as retroperitoneal fibrosis, pulmonary infiltrates or effusion and pleural thickening. It is unknown whether nonergot, pro-dopaminergic agents like tolcapone confer this risk. Use caution in patients with severe renal impairment. Dopaminergic agents have been associated with a syndrome resembling neuroleptic malignant syndrome upon withdrawal or abrupt dosage reduction; patients should be monitored closely if therapy is discontinued.

Adverse Reactions

>10%:

Cardiovascular: Orthostatic hypotension (17%)

Central nervous system: Somnolence (14% to 32%), sleep disorder (24% to 25%), hallucinations (8% to 24%), excessive dreaming (16% to 21%), dizziness (6% to 13%), headache (10% to 11%), confusion (10% to 11%)

Gastrointestinal: Nausea (28% to 50%), diarrhea (16% to 34%; approximately 3% to 4% severe), anorexia (19% to 23%)

Neuromuscular & skeletal: Dyskinesia (42% to 51%), dystonia (19% to 22%), muscle cramps (17% to 18%)

1% to 10%:

Cardiovascular: Syncope (4% to 5%), chest pain (1% to 3%), hypotension (2%), palpitation

Central nervous system: Fatigue (3% to 7%), loss of balance (2% to 3%), agitation (1%), euphoria (1%), hyperactivity (1%), malaise (1%), panic reaction (1%), irritability (1%), mental deficiency (1%), fever (1%), depression, hypoesthesia, tremor, speech disorder, vertigo, emotional lability, hyperkinesia

Dermatologic: Alopecia (1%), bleeding (1%), tumor (1%), rash

Gastrointestinal: Vomiting (8% to 10%), constipation (6% to 8%), xerostomia (5% to 6%), abdominal pain (5% to 6%), dyspepsia (3% to 4%), flatulence (2% to 4%)

Genitourinary: UTI (5%), hematuria (4% to 5%), urine discoloration (2% to 3%), urination disorder (1% to 2%), uterine tumor (1%), incontinence, impotence

Hepatic: Transaminases increased (1% to 3%; 3 times ULN, usually with first 6 months of therapy)

Neuromuscular & skeletal: Paresthesia (1% to 3%), hyper-/hypokinesia (1% to 3%), arthritis (1% to 2%), neck pain (2%), stiffness (2%), myalgia, rhabdomyolysis

Ocular: Cataract (1%), eye inflammation (1%)

Otic: Tinnitus

Respiratory: Upper respiratory infection (5% to 7%), dyspnea (3%), sinus congestion (1% to 2%), bronchitis, pharyngitis

Miscellaneous: Diaphoresis (4% to 7%), influenza (3% to 4%), burning (1% to 2%), flank pain, injury, infection

<1% (Limited to important or life-threatening): Abnormal stools, abscess, allergic reaction, amnesia, anemia, antisocial reaction, apathy, apnea, arteriosclerosis, arthrosis, asthma, bladder calculus, breast neoplasm, carcinoma, cardiovascular disorder, cellulitis, cerebral ischemia, cerebrovascular accident, chills, cholecystitis, cholelithiasis, choreoathetosis, colitis, cough increased, death, dehydration, delirium, delusions, diabetes mellitus, diplopia, duodenal ulcer, dysphagia, dysuria, ear pain, eczema, edema, encephalopathy, epistaxis, erythema multiforme, esophagitis, extrapyramidal syndrome, eye hemorrhage, eye pain, facial edema, furunculosis, gastroenteritis, gastrointestinal carcinoma, gastrointestinal hemorrhage, glaucoma, hemiplegia, hernia, herpes simplex, herpes zoster, hiccup, hostility, hypercholesteremia, hyperventilation, hypoxia, infection (bacterial), infection (fungal), joint disorder, kidney calculus, lacrimation disorder, laryngitis, leukemia, libido changes, lung edema, manic reaction, meningitis, mouth ulceration, myoclonus, neoplasm, nervousness, neuralgia, neuropathy, nocturia, oliguria, otitis media, ovarian carcinoma, pain, paranoid reaction, parosmia, pericardial effusion, polyuria, prostatic carcinoma, prostatic disorder, pruritus, psychosis, rectal disorder, rhinitis, salivation increased, seborrhea, skin discoloration, skin disorder, stomach atony, surgical procedure, tenosynovitis, thinking abnormal, thirst, thrombocytopenia, thrombosis, tongue disorder, twitching, urinary retention, urinary tract disorder, urticaria, uterine atony, uterine disorder, uterine hemorrhage, vaginitis, viral infection

Drug Interactions

Metabolism/Transport Effects **Inhibits** COMT, CYP2C9 (weak)

Avoid Concomitant Use

Avoid concomitant use of Tolcapone with any of the following: Azelastine (Nasal); Paraldehyde

Increased Effect/Toxicity

Tolcapone may increase the levels/effects of: Alcohol (Ethyl); Azelastine (Nasal); Buprenorphine; CNS Depressants; COMT Substrates; Hydrocodone; MAO Inhibitors; Methotrimeprazine; Metyrosine; Mirtazapine; Paraldehyde; Pramipexole; ROPINIRole; Rotigotine; Selective Serotonin Reuptake Inhibitors; Zolpidem

The levels/effects of Tolcapone may be increased by: Brimonidine (Topical); Doxylamine; Droperidol; HydrOXYzine; Magnesium Sulfate; MAO Inhibitors; Methotrimeprazine; Perampanel; Sodium Oxybate; Tapentadol

Decreased Effect There are no known significant interactions involving a decrease in effect.

Ethanol/Nutrition/Herb Interactions

Ethanol: May increase CNS depression; monitor for increased effects with coadministration. Caution patients about effects.

Food: Tolcapone, taken with food within 1 hour before or 2 hours after the dose, decreases bioavailability by 10% to 20%.

Avoid valerian, St John's wort, kava kava, gotu kola (may increase CNS depression).

Storage/Stability Store at 20°C to 25°C (68°F to 77°F).

Mechanism of Action Tolcapone is a selective and reversible inhibitor of catechol-o-methyltransferase (COMT). In the presence of a decarboxylase inhibitor (eg, carbidopa), COMT is the major degradation pathway for levodopa. Inhibition of COMT leads to more sustained plasma levels of levodopa and enhanced central dopaminergic activity.

Pharmacodynamics/Kinetics

Absorption: Rapid

Distribution: 9 L

Protein binding: >99.9%

Metabolism: Hepatic, via glucuronidation, to inactive metabolite (>99%)
Bioavailability: ~65%
Half-life elimination: 2-3 hours
Time to peak: ~2 hours
Excretion: Urine (60% as metabolites, 0.5% as unchanged drug); feces (40%)

Dosage Note: Tolcapone is only appropriate in patients receiving concomitant carbidopa and levodopa. If clinical improvement is not observed after 3 weeks of therapy (regardless of dose), tolcapone treatment should be discontinued.

Parkinson's disease: Adults: Oral: Initial: 100 mg 3 times daily; may increase as tolerated to 200 mg 3 times daily only if clinical benefit is justified (dosage associated with an increased incidence of ALT elevations). **Note:** Levodopa dose may need to be decreased upon initiation of tolcapone (average reduction in clinical trials was 30%). As many as 70% of patients receiving levodopa doses >600 mg daily required levodopa dosage reduction in clinical trials. Patients with moderate-to-severe dyskinesia prior to initiation are also more likely to require dosage reduction.

Dosage adjustment in renal impairment:
Mild-to-moderate impairment (Cl_{cr} ≥25 mL/minute): No dosage adjustment necessary.
Severe impairment (Cl_{cr} <25 mL/minute): No dosage adjustment provided in manufacturer's labeling (has not been studied). Use with caution.

Dosage adjustment in hepatic impairment: Use is contraindicated in patients with liver disease. Discontinue immediately if signs/symptoms of hepatic impairment develop.

Dietary Considerations May be taken without regard to meals.

Administration May be administered without regard to meals. In clinical studies, the first dose of the day was administered with carbidopa/levodopa, and the subsequent doses were administered 6 hours and 12 hours later.

Monitoring Parameters Blood pressure; symptoms of Parkinson's disease; mental status; liver enzymes at baseline and then every 2-4 weeks for the first 6 months of therapy; thereafter, periodic monitoring should be conducted as deemed clinically relevant. If the dose is increased to 200 mg 3 times/day, reinitiate LFT monitoring prior to dose increase and then every 2-4 weeks for 6 months, and then resume periodic monitoring. Discontinue therapy if the ALT or AST exceeds 2 times ULN or if the clinical signs and symptoms suggest the onset of liver failure.

Dosage Forms Excipient information presented when available (limited, particularly for generics); consult specific product labeling.
Tablet, Oral:
Tasmar: 100 mg

◆ Tolectin *see* Tolmetin *on page 2087*

Tolmetin (TOLE met in)

Index Terms Tolectin; Tolmetin Sodium

Pharmacologic Category Nonsteroidal Anti-inflammatory Drug (NSAID), Oral

Additional Appendix Information
Beers Criteria – Potentially Inappropriate Medications for Geriatrics *on page 2368*

Use Treatment of rheumatoid arthritis and osteoarthritis, juvenile idiopathic arthritis (JIA)

Pregnancy Risk Factor C

Medication Guide Available Yes

Dosage Oral:
Children ≥2 years:
Juvenile idiopathic arthritis (JIA): Initial: 20 mg/kg/day in 3-4 divided doses, then 15-30 mg/kg/day in 3-4 divided doses (maximum dose: 30 mg/kg/day)
Analgesic (unlabeled use): 5-7 mg/kg/dose every 6-8 hours
Adults: RA, osteoarthritis: 400 mg 3 times/day; usual dose: 600 mg to 1.8 g/day; maximum: 1.8 g/day

Dosage adjustment in renal impairment: No dosage adjustment provided in manufacturer's labeling. However, use may precipitate or worsen renal injury. Use is not recommended in patients with advanced renal disease.

Dosage adjustment in hepatic impairment: No dosage adjustment provided in manufacturer's labeling.

Additional Information Complete prescribing information should be consulted for additional detail.

Dosage Forms Excipient information presented when available (limited, particularly for generics); consult specific product labeling.
Capsule, Oral:
Generic: 400 mg
Tablet, Oral:
Generic: 200 mg, 600 mg

◆ Tolmetin Sodium *see* Tolmetin *on page 2087*

Tolnaftate (tole NAF tate)

Brand Names: U.S. Anti-Fungal [OTC]; Antifungal [OTC]; Athletes Foot Spray [OTC]; Dr Gs Clear Nail [OTC]; Fungi-Guard [OTC]; Fungoid-D [OTC]; Jock Itch Spray [OTC]; LamISIL AF Defense [OTC]; Medi-First Anti-Fungal [OTC]; Mycocide Clinical NS [OTC]; Podactin [OTC]; Tinactin Deodorant [OTC]; Tinactin Jock Itch [OTC]; Tinactin [OTC]; Tinamar [OTC]; Tinaspore [OTC]; Tolnaftate Antifungal [OTC]

Brand Names: Canada Pitrex

Pharmacologic Category Antifungal Agent, Topical

Use Treatment of tinea pedis, tinea cruris, tinea corporis

Dosage Children ≥2 years and Adults: Topical: Wash and dry affected area; spray aerosol or apply 1-3 drops of solution or a small amount of cream, or powder and rub into the affected areas 2 times/day
Note: May use for up to 4 weeks for tinea pedis or tinea corporis, and up to 2 weeks for tinea cruris

Additional Information Complete prescribing information should be consulted for additional detail.

Dosage Forms Excipient information presented when available (limited, particularly for generics); consult specific product labeling.
Aerosol, External:
Athletes Foot Spray: 1% (150 g) [contains sd alcohol 40]
Aerosol Powder, External:
Jock Itch Spray: 1% (130 g) [contains sd alcohol 40b]
LamISIL AF Defense: 1% (133 g)
Tinactin: 1% (133 g)
Tinactin Deodorant: 1% (133 g)
Cream, External:
Antifungal: 1% (15 g) [odorless]
Fungi-Guard: 1% (15 g)
Fungoid-D: 1% (113 g) [contains cetyl alcohol, methylparaben, propylene glycol, propylparaben, trolamine (triethanolamine)]
Medi-First Anti-Fungal: 1% (1 ea)
Tinactin: 1% (15 g, 30 g)
Tinactin Jock Itch: 1% (15 g)
Tinamar: 1% (15 g)
Tolnaftate Antifungal: 1% (114 g) [contains cetyl alcohol, methylparaben, polysorbate 80, propylene glycol, propylparaben]

Generic: 1% (15 g, 20 g, 28.3 g, 30 g)
Powder, External:
Anti-Fungal: 1% (45 g)
LamISIL AF Defense: 1% (113 g)
Podactin: 1% (45 g)
Tinactin: 1% (108 g)
Tinamar: 1% (45 g, 90 g)
Generic: 1% (45 g)
Solution, External:
Dr Gs Clear Nail: 1% (18 mL) [contains propylene glycol]
Mycocide Clinical NS: 1% (30 mL) [contains propylene glycol]
Tinamar: 1% (10 mL)
Tinaspore: 1% (10 mL)
Generic: 1% (10 mL)

◆ **Tolnaftate Antifungal [OTC]** *see* Tolnaftate *on page 2087*

◆ **Toloxin (Can)** *see* Digoxin *on page 605*

Tolterodine (tole TER oh deen)

Brand Names: U.S. Detrol; Detrol LA

Brand Names: Canada Detrol®; Detrol® LA; Unidet®

Index Terms Tolterodine Tartrate

Pharmacologic Category Anticholinergic Agent

Additional Appendix Information

Beers Criteria – Potentially Inappropriate Medications for Geriatrics *on page 2368*

Use Treatment of patients with an overactive bladder with symptoms of urinary frequency, urgency, or urge incontinence

Pregnancy Risk Factor C

Pregnancy Considerations Teratogenic effects were observed in some animal reproduction studies.

Breast-Feeding Considerations It is not known if tolterodine is excreted in breast milk. Due to the potential for serious adverse reactions in the nursing infant, a decision should be made whether to discontinue nursing or to discontinue the drug, taking into account the importance of treatment to the mother.

Contraindications Hypersensitivity to tolterodine or fesoterodine (both are metabolized to 5-hydroxymethyl tolterodine) or any component of the formulation; urinary retention; gastric retention; uncontrolled narrow-angle glaucoma

Warnings/Precautions Cases of angioedema have been reported; some cases have occurred after a single dose. Discontinue immediately if angioedema and associated difficulty breathing, airway obstruction, or hypotension develop. May cause drowsiness, dizziness, and/or blurred vision, which may impair physical or mental abilities; patients must be cautioned about performing tasks which require mental alertness (eg, operating machinery or driving). Consider dose reduction or discontinuation if CNS effects occur. Use with caution in patients with bladder flow obstruction, may increase the risk of urinary retention. Use with caution in patients with gastrointestinal obstructive disorders (ie, pyloric stenosis), may increase the risk of gastric retention. Use with caution in patients with myasthenia gravis and controlled (treated) narrow-angle glaucoma; metabolized in the liver and excreted in the urine and feces, dosage adjustment is required for patients with renal or hepatic impairment. Tolterodine has been associated with QT_c prolongation at high (supratherapeutic) doses. The manufacturer recommends caution in patients with congenital prolonged QT or in patients receiving concurrent therapy with QT_c-prolonging drugs (class Ia or III antiarrhythmics). However, the mean change in QT_c even at supratherapeutic dosages was less than 15 msec. Individuals who are CYP2D6 poor metabolizers or in the presence of inhibitors of CYP2D6 and CYP3A4 may be more likely to exhibit prolongation. Dosage adjustment is recommended in patients receiving CYP3A4 inhibitors (a lower dose of tolterodine is recommended). This medication is associated with potent anticholinergic properties which may be inappropriate in older adults depending on comorbidities (eg, dementia, delirium) (Beers Criteria).

Adverse Reactions As reported with immediate release tablet, unless otherwise specified

>10%: Gastrointestinal: Dry mouth (35%; extended release capsules 23%)

1% to 10%:

Cardiovascular: Chest pain (2%)

Central nervous system: Headache (7%; extended release capsules 6%), dizziness (5%; extended release capsules 2%), fatigue (4%; extended release capsules 2%), somnolence (3%; extended release capsules 3%), anxiety (extended release capsules 1%)

Dermatologic: Dry skin (1%)

Gastrointestinal: Constipation (7%; extended release capsules 6%), abdominal pain (5%; extended release capsules 4%), diarrhea (4%), dyspepsia (4%; extended release capsules 3%), weight gain (1%)

Genitourinary: Dysuria (2%; extended release capsules 1%)

Neuromuscular & skeletal: Arthralgia (2%)

Ocular: Dry eyes (3%; extended release capsules 3%), abnormal vision (2%; extended release capsules 1%)

Respiratory: Bronchitis (2%), sinusitis (extended release capsules 2%)

Miscellaneous: Flu-like syndrome (3%), infection (1%)

<1% (Limited to important or life-threatening): Anaphylaxis, angioedema, confusion, dementia aggravated, disorientation, hallucinations, memory impairment, palpitation, peripheral edema, QT_c prolongation, tachycardia

Drug Interactions

Metabolism/Transport Effects Substrate of CYP2C19 (minor), CYP2C9 (minor), CYP2D6 (major), CYP3A4 (major); **Note:** Assignment of Major/Minor substrate status based on clinically relevant drug interaction potential

Avoid Concomitant Use

Avoid concomitant use of Tolterodine with any of the following: Aclidinium; Fusidic Acid (Systemic); Ipratropium (Oral Inhalation); Potassium Chloride; Tiotropium; Umeclidinium

Increased Effect/Toxicity

Tolterodine may increase the levels/effects of: AbobotulinumtoxinA; Analgesics (Opioid); Anticholinergics; Cannabinoids; Highest Risk QTc-Prolonging Agents; Mirabegron; Moderate Risk QTc-Prolonging Agents; OnabotulinumtoxinA; Potassium Chloride; RimabotulinumtoxinB; Thiazide Diuretics; Tiotropium; Topiramate; Warfarin

The levels/effects of Tolterodine may be increased by: Abiraterone Acetate; Aclidinium; Antifungal Agents (Azole Derivatives, Systemic); CYP2D6 Inhibitors (Moderate); CYP2D6 Inhibitors (Strong); CYP3A4 Inhibitors (Moderate); CYP3A4 Inhibitors (Strong); Dasatinib; Fluconazole; Fusidic Acid (Systemic); Ipratropium (Oral Inhalation); Ivacaftor; Luliconazole; Mifepristone; Pramlintide; Simeprevir; Umeclidinium; VinBLAStine

Decreased Effect

Tolterodine may decrease the levels/effects of: Acetylcholinesterase Inhibitors (Central); Secretin

The levels/effects of Tolterodine may be decreased by: Acetylcholinesterase Inhibitors (Central); Bosentan; CYP3A4 Inducers (Strong); Dabrafenib; Deferasirox; Herbs (CYP3A4 Inducers); Mitotane; Peginterferon Alfa-2b; Tocilizumab

Ethanol/Nutrition/Herb Interactions

Food: Increases bioavailability (~53% increase) of tolterodine tablets (dose adjustment not necessary); does not affect the pharmacokinetics of tolterodine extended release capsules. As a CYP3A4 inhibitor, grapefruit juice may increase the serum level and/or toxicity of tolterodine, but unlikely secondary to high oral bioavailability.

Herb/Nutraceutical: St John's wort (*Hypericum*) appears to induce CYP3A enzymes.

Storage/Stability Store at 25°C (77°F); excursions permitted to 15°C to 30°C (59°F to 86°F). Protect from light.

Mechanism of Action Tolterodine is a competitive antagonist of muscarinic receptors. In animal models, tolterodine demonstrates selectivity for urinary bladder receptors over salivary receptors. Urinary bladder contraction is mediated by muscarinic receptors. Tolterodine increases residual urine volume and decreases detrusor muscle pressure.

Pharmacodynamics/Kinetics

Absorption: Immediate release tablet: Rapid; ≥77%

Distribution: I.V.: V_d: 113 ± 27 L

Protein binding: >96% (primarily to alpha$_1$-acid glycoprotein)

Metabolism: Extensively hepatic, primarily via CYP2D6 to 5-hydroxymethyltolterodine (active) and 3A4 usually (minor pathway). In patients with a genetic deficiency of CYP2D6, metabolism via 3A4 predominates.

Bioavailability: Immediate release tablet: Increased 53% with food

Half-life elimination:

Immediate release tablet: Extensive metabolizers: ~2 hours; Poor metabolizers: ~10 hours

Extended release capsule: Extensive metabolizers: ~7 hours; Poor metabolizers: ~18 hours

Time to peak: Immediate release tablet: 1-2 hours; Extended release capsule: 2-6 hours

Excretion: Urine (77%); feces (17%); primarily as metabolites (<1% unchanged drug) of which the active 5-hydroxymethyl metabolite accounts for 5% to 14% (<1% in poor metabolizers); as unchanged drug (<1%; <2.5% in poor metabolizers)

Dosage

Oral: Adults: Treatment of overactive bladder:

Immediate release tablet: 2 mg twice daily; the dose may be lowered to 1 mg twice daily based on individual response and tolerability

Dosing adjustment in patients concurrently taking strong CYP3A4 inhibitors (eg, ketoconazole, clarithromycin, ritonavir): 1 mg twice daily

Extended release capsule: 4 mg once daily; dose may be lowered to 2 mg once daily based on individual response and tolerability

Dosing adjustment in patients concurrently taking strong CYP3A4 inhibitors (eg, ketoconazole, clarithromycin, ritonavir): 2 mg once daily

Elderly: Safety and efficacy in patients >64 years was found to be similar to that in younger patients; no dosage adjustment is needed based on age

Dosing adjustment in renal impairment:

Immediate release tablet: Significantly reduced renal function (studies conducted in patients with Cl_{cr} 10-30 mL/minute): 1 mg twice daily; use with caution

Extended release capsule:

Cl_{cr} 10-30 mL/minute: 2 mg once daily

Cl_{cr} <10 mL/minute: Use is not recommended; has not been studied.

Dosing adjustment in hepatic impairment:

Immediate release tablet: Significantly reduced hepatic function: 1 mg twice daily; use with caution

Extended release capsule:

Mild-to-moderate impairment (Child-Pugh class A or B): 2 mg once daily

Severe impairment (Child-Pugh class C): Use is not recommended; has not been studied.

Administration Extended release capsule: Swallow whole; do not crush, chew, or open

Monitoring Parameters Renal function (BUN, creatinine); hepatic function

Dosage Forms Excipient information presented when available (limited, particularly for generics); consult specific product labeling.

Capsule Extended Release 24 Hour, Oral, as tartrate:

Detrol LA: 2 mg, 4 mg

Generic: 2 mg, 4 mg

Tablet, Oral, as tartrate:

Detrol: 1 mg, 2 mg

Generic: 1 mg, 2 mg

◆ **Tolterodine Tartrate** *see* Tolterodine *on page 2088*

Tolvaptan (tol VAP tan)

Brand Names: U.S. Samsca

Brand Names: Canada Samsca™

Index Terms OPC-41061

Pharmacologic Category Vasopressin Antagonist

Use Treatment of clinically significant hypervolemic or euvolemic hyponatremia associated with heart failure or SIADH with either a serum sodium <125 mEq/L or less marked hyponatremia that is symptomatic and resistant to fluid restriction

Pregnancy Risk Factor C

Medication Guide Available Yes

Dosage Oral: Adults: Hyponatremia: Initial: 15 mg once daily; after at least 24 hours, may increase to 30 mg once daily to a maximum of 60 mg once daily titrating at 24-hour intervals to desired serum sodium concentration. Avoid fluid restriction during the first 24 hours of therapy. Do not use for more than 30 days due to the risk of hepatotoxicity.

Dosage adjustment in renal impairment:

Cl_{cr} ≥10 mL/minute: No dosage adjustment necessary

Cl_{cr} <10 mL/minute: Use not recommended (not studied); contraindicated in anuria (no benefit expected)

Dosage adjustment in hepatic impairment: Avoid use in patients with underlying liver disease, including cirrhosis.

Additional Information Complete prescribing information should be consulted for additional detail.

Dosage Forms Excipient information presented when available (limited, particularly for generics); consult specific product labeling.

Tablet, Oral:

Samsca: 15 mg, 30 mg [contains fd&c blue #2 aluminum lake]

Dosage Forms: Canada Excipient information presented when available (limited, particularly for generics); consult specific product labeling.

Tablet, oral:

Samsca™: 15 mg, 30 mg, 60 mg

◆ **Tomoxetine** *see* AtoMOXetine *on page 187*

◆ **Topactin (Can)** *see* Fluocinonide *on page 879*

◆ **Topamax** *see* Topiramate *on page 2090*

◆ **Topamax Sprinkle** *see* Topiramate *on page 2090*

◆ **TopCare® Pain Relief PM [OTC]** *see* Acetaminophen and Diphenhydramine *on page 32*

◆ **Topex Topical Anesthetic** *see* Benzocaine *on page 240*

◆ **Topicaine [OTC]** *see* Lidocaine (Topical) *on page 1212*

◆ **Topicaine 5 [OTC]** *see* Lidocaine (Topical) *on page 1212*

◆ **Topicort** *see* Desoximetasone *on page 579*

◆ **Topicort® (Can)** *see* Desoximetasone *on page 579*

◆ **Topicort® Gel (Can)** *see* Desoximetasone *on page 579*

◆ **Topicort® Mild (Can)** *see* Desoximetasone *on page 579*

◆ **Topicort® Ointment (Can)** *see* Desoximetasone *on page 579*

◆ **Topicort Spray** *see* Desoximetasone *on page 579*

◆ **Topiragen** *see* Topiramate *on page 2090*

Topiramate (toe PYRE a mate)

Brand Names: U.S. Topamax; Topamax Sprinkle; Topiragen; Trokendi XR

Brand Names: Canada Apo-Topiramate; CO Topiramate; Dom-Topiramate; Mint-Topiramate; Mylan-Topiramate; Novo-Topiramate; PHL-Topiramate; PMS-Topiramate; PRO-Topiramate; ratio-Topiramate; Sandoz-Topiramate; Topamax; ZYM-Topiramate

Pharmacologic Category Anticonvulsant, Miscellaneous

Use

Epilepsy:

Monotherapy: As initial monotherapy in patients 2 years and older (immediate release) or 10 years and older (extended release [ER]) with partial-onset or primary generalized tonic-clonic seizures

Adjunctive therapy: As adjunctive therapy in patients 2 years and older (immediate release) or 6 years and older (ER) with partial-onset seizures, primary generalized tonic-clonic seizures, or seizures associated with Lennox-Gastaut syndrome

Migraine (immediate release only): For the prophylaxis of migraine headache in adults

Unlabeled Use Diabetic neuropathy, infantile spasms, neuropathic pain; prophylaxis of cluster headache

Pregnancy Risk Factor D

Pregnancy Considerations Adverse events have been observed in animal reproduction studies. Based on limited data (n=5), topiramate was found to cross the placenta and could be detected in neonatal serum (Ohman, 2002). Topiramate may cause fetal harm if administered to a pregnant woman. An increased risk of oral clefts (cleft lip and/or palate) has been observed following first trimester exposure. Data from the North American Antiepileptic Drug (NAAED) Pregnancy Registry reported that the prevalence of oral clefts was 1.2% for infants exposed to topiramate during the first trimester of pregnancy, versus 0.39% to 0.46% for infants exposed to other antiepileptic drugs and 0.12% with no exposure. Although not evaluated during pregnancy, metabolic acidosis may be induced by topiramate. In general, metabolic acidosis during pregnancy may result in adverse effects and fetal death. Pregnant women and their newborns should be monitored for metabolic acidosis. Maternal serum concentrations may decrease during the second and third trimesters of pregnancy therefore therapeutic drug monitoring should be considered in pregnant women who require therapy (Ohman, 2009; Westin, 2009).

Use for migraine prophylaxis is contraindicated per the Canadian labeling in pregnant women or women of childbearing potential who are not using effective contraception.

Patients exposed to topiramate during pregnancy are encouraged to enroll themselves into the AED Pregnancy Registry by calling 1-888-233-2334. Additional information is available at www.aedpregnancyregistry.org.

Breast-Feeding Considerations Topiramate is excreted into breast milk. Based on information from five nursing infants, infant plasma concentrations of topiramate have been reported as 10% to 20% of the maternal plasma concentration. The manufacturer recommends that caution be used if administered to a nursing woman.

Medication Guide Available Yes

Contraindications

Extended release: Recent alcohol use (ie, within 6 hours prior to and 6 hours after administration); patients with metabolic acidosis who are taking concomitant metformin

Immediate release: There are no contraindications listed in the manufacturer's labeling.

Canadian labeling (not in U.S. labeling): Hypersensitivity to topiramate or any component of the formulation or container; pregnancy and women in childbearing years not using effective contraception (migraine prophylaxis only)

Warnings/Precautions Antiepileptics are associated with an increased risk of suicidal behavior/thoughts with use (regardless of indication); patients should be monitored for signs/symptoms of depression, suicidal tendencies, and other unusual behavior changes during therapy and instructed to inform their healthcare provider immediately if symptoms occur. Use with caution in patients with hepatic, respiratory, or renal impairment. Topiramate may decrease serum bicarbonate concentrations (up to 67% of patients); treatment-emergent metabolic acidosis is less common. Risk may be increased in patients with a predisposing condition (organ dysfunction, diarrhea, ketogenic diet, status epilepticus, or concurrent treatment with other drugs which may cause acidosis). Metabolic acidosis may occur at dosages as low as 50 mg/day. Monitor serum bicarbonate as well as potential complications of chronic acidosis (nephrolithiasis, osteomalacia, and reduced growth rates and/or weight in children). Kidney stones have been reported in both children and adults; the risk of kidney stones is about 2-4 times that of the untreated population; the risk of this event may be reduced by increasing fluid intake.

Cognitive dysfunction, psychiatric disturbances (depression or mood disorders), and sedation (somnolence or fatigue) may occur with topiramate use; incidence may be related to rapid titration and higher doses. Patients must be cautioned about performing tasks which require mental alertness (eg, operating machinery or driving). Topiramate may also cause paresthesia, dizziness, and ataxia. Topiramate has been associated with acute myopia and secondary angle-closure glaucoma in adults and children, typically within 1 month of initiation; discontinue in patients with acute onset of decreased visual acuity or ocular pain. Hyperammonemia with or without encephalopathy may occur with or without concomitant valproate administration; valproic acid dose-dependency was observed in limited pediatric studies; use with caution in patients with inborn errors of metabolism or decreased hepatic mitochondrial activity. Hypothermia (core body temperature <35°C [95°F]) has been reported with concomitant use of topiramate and valproic acid; may occur with or without associated hyperammonemia and may develop after topiramate initiation or dosage increase; discontinuation of topiramate or valproic acid may be necessary. Topiramate may be associated (rarely) with severe oligohydrosis and hyperthermia, most frequently in children; use caution and monitor closely during strenuous exercise, during exposure to high environmental temperature, or in patients receiving receiving other carbonic anhydrase inhibitors and drugs with anticholinergic activity. Potentially significant interactions may exist, requiring dose or frequency adjustment, additional monitoring, and/or selection of alternative therapy. Consult drug interactions database for more detailed information.

Avoid abrupt withdrawal of topiramate therapy; it should be withdrawn/tapered slowly to minimize the potential of increased seizure frequency. Doses were also gradually withdrawn in migraine prophylaxis studies.

Adverse Reactions Adverse events are reported for placebo-controlled trials of adjunctive therapy in adult and pediatric patients. Unless otherwise noted, the percentages refer to incidence in epilepsy trials. **Note:** A wide range of dosages were studied; incidence of adverse events was frequently lower in the pediatric population studied.

>10%:

Central nervous system: Somnolence (15% to 29%), dizziness (4% to 25%; dose dependent), fatigue (9% to 16%; dose-dependent), nervousness (9% to 18%), ataxia (6% to 16%), psychomotor slowing (3% to 13%; dose dependent), speech problems (2% to 13%), memory difficulties (2% to 12%), behavior problems (children 11%), confusion (4% to 11%)

Endocrine & metabolic: Serum bicarbonate decreased (dose related: 7% to 67%; marked reductions [to <17 mEq/L] 1% to 11%)

Gastrointestinal: Anorexia (4% to 24%; dose dependent), nausea (6% to 10%; migraine trial: 9% to 14%)

Neuromuscular & skeletal: Paresthesia (1% to 11%; migraine trial: 35% to 51%)

Ocular: Abnormal vision (2% to 13%)

Respiratory: Upper respiratory infection (migraine trial: 12% to 14%)

Miscellaneous: Injury (14%)

1% to 10%:

Cardiovascular: Chest pain (2% to 4%), edema (2%), hypertension (1% to 2%), bradycardia (1%), pallor (1%), syncope (1%)

Central nervous system: Difficulty concentrating (5% to 10%), aggressive reactions (2% to 9%), depression (5% to 9%; dose dependent, insomnia (4% to 8%), mood problems (≤6%), abnormal coordination (4%), agitation (3%), cognitive problems (3%), emotional lability (3%), anxiety (2% to 3%; dose dependent), hypoesthesia (2%; migraine trial: 6% to 8%), stupor (2%), vertigo (2%), fever (migraine trial: 1% to 2%), apathy (1%), hallucination (1%), neurosis (1%), psychosis (1%), seizure (1%), suicide attempt (1%)

Dermatologic: Pruritus (migraine trial: 2% to 4%), skin disorder (2% to 3%), alopecia (2%), dermatitis (2%), hypertrichosis (2%), rash erythematous (1% to 2%), eczema (1%), seborrhea (1%), skin discoloration (1%)

Endocrine & metabolic: Breast pain (4%), hot flashes (1% to 2%), libido decreased (<1% to 2%), menstrual irregularities (1% to 2%), hypoglycemia (1%), metabolic acidosis (hyperchloremia, nonanion gap)

Gastrointestinal: Weight loss (4% to 9%), dyspepsia (2% to 7%), abdominal pain (5% to 6%), salivation increased (6%), constipation (4% to 5%), gastroenteritis (2% to 3%), vomiting (migraine trial: 1% to 3%), diarrhea (2%; migraine trial: 9% to 11%), dysgeusia (2%; migraine trial: 8% to 15%), xerostomia (2%), loss of taste (migraine trial: ≤2%), appetite increased (1%), dysphagia (1%), fecal incontinence (1%), flatulence (1%), GERD (1%), gingivitis (1%), glossitis (1%), gum hyperplasia (1%), weight gain (1%)

Genitourinary: Incontinence (2% to 4%), UTI (2%), premature ejaculation (migraine trial: ≤3%), cystitis (2%), leukorrhea (2%), impotence (1%), nocturia (1%)

Hematologic: Purpura (8%), leukopenia (2%), anemia (1%), hematoma (1%), prothrombin time increased (1%), thrombocytopenia (1%)

Neuromuscular & skeletal: Tremor (3% to 9%), gait abnormal (3% to 8%), arthralgia (migraine trial: 1% to 7%), weakness (6%), hyperkinesia (5%), back pain (1% to 5%), involuntary muscle contractions (2%; migraine trial: 2% to 4%), leg cramps (2%), leg pain (2%), myalgia (2%), hyporeflexia (2%), rigors (1%), skeletal pain (1%)

Ocular: Diplopia (1% to 10%), nystagmus (10%), conjunctivitis (1%), lacrimation abnormal (1%), myopia (1%)

Otic: Hearing decreased (2%), tinnitus (2%), otitis media (migraine trial: 1% to 2%)

Renal: Hematuria (2%), renal calculus (migraine trial ≤2%)

Respiratory: Rhinitis (4% to 7%), pharyngitis (6%), sinusitis (5%; migraine trial: 6% to 10%), pneumonia (5%), epistaxis (2% to 4%), cough (migraine trial: 2% to 4%), bronchitis (migraine trial: 3%), dyspnea (migraine trial: 1% to 3%)

Miscellaneous: Viral infection (2% to 7%: migraine trial: 3% to 4%), flu-like syndrome (3%), allergy (2%), infection (2%), thirst (2%), body odor (1%), diaphoresis (1%), moniliasis (1%)

<1% (Limited to important or life-threatening): Angina, apraxia, AV block, bone marrow depression, deep vein thrombosis, dehydration, delirium, delusion, diabetes mellitus, dyskinesia, eosinophilia, erythema multiforme, euphoria, granulocytopenia, hepatic failure, hepatitis, hyperammonemia/encephalopathy (with or without valproate therapy), hyperesthesia, hyperthermia (severe), hypokalemia, hypotension, lymphadenopathy, lymphopenia, maculopathy, manic reaction, neuropathy, oligohydrosis, pancreatitis, pancytopenia, paranoid reaction, pemphigus, photosensitivity, pulmonary embolism, renal tubular acidosis, Stevens-Johnson syndrome, suicidal behavior, suicide, suicidal ideation, syndrome of acute myopia/secondary angle-closure glaucoma, tongue edema, toxic epidermal necrolysis

Drug Interactions

Metabolism/Transport Effects Inhibits CYP2C19 (weak); **Induces** CYP3A4 (weak/moderate)

Avoid Concomitant Use

Avoid concomitant use of Topiramate with any of the following: Alcohol (Ethyl); Axitinib; Azelastine (Nasal); Carbonic Anhydrase Inhibitors; Paraldehyde; Simeprevir

Increased Effect/Toxicity

Topiramate may increase the levels/effects of: Alpha-/Beta-Agonists; Amphetamines; Anticonvulsants (Barbiturate); Anticonvulsants (Hydantoin); Azelastine (Nasal); Buprenorphine; Carbonic Anhydrase Inhibitors; CNS Depressants; Flecainide; Fosphenytoin; Hydrocodone; Lithium; Memantine; MetFORMIN; Methotrimeprazine; Metyrosine; Mirtazapine; Paraldehyde; Phenytoin; Pramipexole; Primidone; QuiNIDine; ROPINIRole; Rotigotine; Selective Serotonin Reuptake Inhibitors; Valproic Acid and Derivatives; Zolpidem

The levels/effects of Topiramate may be increased by: Alcohol (Ethyl); Anticholinergic Agents; Brimonidine (Topical); Doxylamine; Droperidol; HydrOXYzine; Loop Diuretics; Magnesium Sulfate; Methotrimeprazine; Perampanel; Salicylates; Sodium Oxybate; Tapentadol; Thiazide Diuretics

Decreased Effect

Topiramate may decrease the levels/effects of: ARIPiprazole; Axitinib; Contraceptives (Estrogens); Contraceptives (Progestins); Ibrutinib; Methenamine; Primidone; Saxagliptin; Simeprevir

The levels/effects of Topiramate may be decreased by: CarBAMazepine; Fosphenytoin; Ketorolac (Nasal); Ketorolac (Systemic); Mefloquine; Orlistat; Phenytoin

Ethanol/Nutrition/Herb Interactions

Ethanol: May increase CNS depression; monitor for increased effects with coadministration. Caution patients about effects.

Food: Ketogenic diet may increase the possibility of acidosis and/or kidney stones.

Herb/Nutraceutical: Avoid evening primrose (seizure threshold decreased).

Storage/Stability

Extended release capsules: Store at 25°C (77°F); excursions permitted at 15°C to 30°C (59°F to 86°F). Protect from moisture. Protect from light.

Sprinkle capsules: Store at or below 25°C (77°F). Protect from moisture.

Tablets: Store at 15°C to 30°C (59°F to 86°F). Protect from moisture.

Mechanism of Action Anticonvulsant activity may be due to a combination of potential mechanisms: Blocks neuronal voltage-dependent sodium channels, enhances GABA(A) activity, antagonizes AMPA/kainate glutamate receptors, and weakly inhibits carbonic anhydrase.

Pharmacodynamics/Kinetics

Absorption: Good, rapid; immediate release formulation is unaffected by food. A single extended release (ER) capsule with a high-fat meal increased the C_{max} by 37% and shortened the T_{max} to approximately 8 hours; this effect is significantly reduced following repeat administrations.

Protein binding: 15% to 41% (inversely related to plasma concentrations)

Metabolism: Minor amounts metabolized in liver via hydroxylation, hydrolysis, and glucuronidation; there is evidence of renal tubular reabsorption; percentage of dose metabolized in liver and clearance are increased in patients receiving enzyme inducers (eg, carbamazepine, phenytoin)

Bioavailability: ~80% (immediate release)

Half-life elimination: 21 hours (immediate release); ~31 hours (ER)

Time to peak, serum: ~1-4 hours (immediate release); ~24 hours (ER)

Excretion: Urine (~70% as unchanged drug)

Dialyzable: Significantly hemodialyzed; dialysis clearance: 120 mL/minute (4-6 times higher than in adults with normal renal function)

Dosage Note: Do not abruptly discontinue therapy; taper dosage gradually to prevent rebound effects. (In clinical trials, adult doses were withdrawn by decreasing in weekly intervals of 50-100 mg daily gradually over 2-8 weeks for seizure treatment, and by decreasing in weekly intervals by 25-50 mg daily for migraine prophylaxis.)

Epilepsy, monotherapy: Partial-onset seizure and primary generalized tonic-clonic seizure:

Children 2-9 years: Oral:

Immediate release: Initial: 25 mg once daily (in evening); may increase to 25 mg twice daily in week 2; thereafter, may increase by 25-50 mg daily at weekly intervals over 5-7 weeks up to the following minimum recommended maintenance dose:

≤11 kg: 150 mg daily in 2 divided doses
12-22 kg: 200 mg daily in 2 divided doses
23-31 kg: 200 mg daily in 2 divided doses
32-38 kg: 250 mg daily in 2 divided doses
≥39 kg: 250 mg daily in 2 divided doses

Maximum maintenance dose: If additional seizure control is needed and therapy is tolerated, may further increase by 25-50 mg daily at weekly intervals up to the following maximum recommended maintenance dose:

≤11 kg: 250 mg daily in 2 divided doses
12-22 kg: 300 mg daily in 2 divided doses
23-31 kg: 350 mg daily in 2 divided doses
32-38 kg: 350 mg daily in 2 divided doses
≥39 kg: 400 mg daily in 2 divided doses

Children ≥10 years and Adults: Oral:

Immediate release: Initial: 25 mg twice daily; may increase weekly by 50 mg daily up to 100 mg twice daily (week 4 dose); thereafter, may further increase weekly by 100 mg daily up to the recommended dose of 200 mg twice daily.

Extended release: Initial: 50 mg daily for 1 week; may increase weekly by 50 mg daily up to 200 mg once daily (week 4 dose); thereafter, may further increase weekly by 100 mg daily up to the recommended dose of 400 mg once daily.

Canadian labeling: Children ≥6 years and Adults: Oral: Immediate release: Initial: 25 mg once daily (in evening); may increase to 25 mg twice daily in weeks 2 or 3, and up to 50 mg twice daily by weeks 3 or 4; may further increase weekly in increments of 50 mg daily up to recommended maximum of 200 mg twice daily.

Epilepsy, adjunctive therapy: Partial-onset seizure, primary generalized tonic-clonic seizure, or Lennox-Gastaut syndrome:

Children 2-16 years: Oral: Immediate release: Initial: 25 mg (1-3 mg/kg/day) once daily (in evening) for 1 week; may increase every 1-2 weeks in increments of 1-3 mg/kg/day up to the recommended dose of 5-9 mg/kg/day in 2 divided doses.

Children 6-16 years: Oral: Extended release: Initial: 25 mg (1-3 mg/kg/day) once daily (in evening) for 1 week; may increase every 1-2 weeks in increments of 1-3 mg/kg/day up to the recommended dose of 5-9 mg/kg once daily.

Adolescents ≥17 years and Adults: Oral: **Note:** Doses >1600 mg have not been studied.

Immediate release: Initial: 25 mg once or twice daily for 1 week; may increase weekly by 25-50 mg daily until response; usual maintenance dose: 100-200 mg twice daily (partial-onset seizures) or 200 mg twice daily (primary generalized tonic-clonic seizures). Doses >400 mg daily have not shown additional benefit for treatment of partial-onset seizures.

Extended release: Initial: 25-50 mg once daily for 1 week; may increase weekly by 25-50 mg daily until response; usual maintenance dose: 200-400 mg once daily (partial-onset seizures, Lennox-Gastaut syndrome) or 400 mg once daily (primary generalized tonic-clonic seizures). Doses >400 mg daily have not shown additional benefit for treatment of partial-onset seizures.

Canadian labeling: Oral: Immediate release: Initial: 25 mg once or twice daily; may increase weekly by 50 mg daily up to the recommended dose of 100-200 mg twice daily (maximum recommended dose: 800 mg daily; doses >400 mg daily have shown no additional benefit).

Migraine prophylaxis: Adults: Oral: Immediate release: Initial: 25 mg once daily (in evening); may increase weekly by 25 mg daily up to the recommended dose of 100 mg daily given in 2 divided doses. Doses >100 mg daily have shown no additional benefit.

Cluster headache prophylaxis (unlabeled use): Adults: Initial: 25 mg daily, titrated at weekly intervals in 25 mg increments, up to 200 mg daily (Pascual, 2007)

Diabetic neuropathy (unlabeled use): Adults: Initial: 25 mg daily, titrated at weekly intervals in 25-50 mg increments to target dose of 400 mg daily in 2 divided doses (Raskin, 2004; Thienel, 2004)

Dosage adjustment in renal impairment: Cl_{cr} <70 mL/minute/1.73 m²: Administer 50% dose and titrate more slowly

Hemodialysis: Supplemental dose may be needed during hemodialysis

Dosage adjustment in hepatic impairment: No specific dosage adjustment provided in manufacturer's labeling. However, topiramate clearance in hepatic impairment may be reduced. Use with caution.

Administration Oral: Administer without regard to meals. Administer the immediate release formulation in divided doses; do not break the tablets. Swallow the extended release (ER) capsules whole; do not sprinkle on food, chew, or crush. Avoid alcohol use with topiramate ER within 6 hours prior to and 6 hours after administration.

Sprinkle capsules may be swallowed whole or opened to sprinkle the entire contents on a small amount (~1 teaspoon) of soft food; swallow immediately and do not chew. Do not store mixture for future use.

Monitoring Parameters Seizure frequency, hydration status; electrolytes (recommended monitoring includes serum bicarbonate at baseline and periodically during treatment), serum creatinine; monitor for symptoms of acute acidosis and complications of long-term acidosis (nephrolithiasis, osteomalacia, and reduced growth rates and/or weight in children); ammonia level in patients with unexplained lethargy, vomiting, or mental status changes; intraocular pressure, symptoms of secondary angle closure glaucoma; suicidality (eg, suicidal thoughts, depression, behavioral changes)

Additional Information May be associated with weight loss in some patients

Product Availability

Trokendi XR: FDA approved August 2013; availability anticipated in August 2013.

Trokendi XR is an extended release capsule formulation indicated for the treatment of partial-onset and primary generalized tonic-clonic seizures and Lennox-Gastaut syndrome.

Dosage Forms Excipient information presented when available (limited, particularly for generics); consult specific product labeling.

Capsule Extended Release 24 Hour, Oral:
- Trokendi XR: 25 mg [contains brilliant blue fcf (fd&c blue #1), sodium benzoate]
- Trokendi XR: 50 mg, 100 mg, 200 mg [contains brilliant blue fcf (fd&c blue #1), fd&c yellow #6 (sunset yellow), sodium benzoate]

Capsule Sprinkle, Oral:
- Topamax Sprinkle: 15 mg, 25 mg
- Generic: 15 mg, 25 mg

Tablet, Oral:
- Topamax: 25 mg, 50 mg, 100 mg, 200 mg
- Topiragen: 25 mg, 50 mg, 100 mg, 200 mg
- Generic: 25 mg, 50 mg, 100 mg, 200 mg

Dosage Forms: Canada Refer to Dosage Forms. **Note:** Extended release capsules not available in Canada.

Extemporaneous Preparations A 6 mg/mL topiramate oral suspension may be made with tablets and one of two different vehicles (a 1:1 mixture of Ora-Sweet® and Ora-Plus®, or a mixture of Simple Syrup, NF and methylcellulose 1% with parabens). Crush six 100 mg tablets in a mortar and reduce to a fine powder. Add a small amount of methylcellulose gel and mix to a uniform paste (**Note:** Use a small amount of methylcellulose gel when using the 1:1 Ora-Sweet® and Ora-Plus® mixture as the vehicle; use 10 mL methylcellulose 1% with parabens when using Simple Syrup, NF as the vehicle); mix while adding the chosen vehicle in incremental proportions to **almost** 100 mL; transfer to a graduated cylinder; rinse mortar with vehicle, and add quantity of vehicle sufficient to make 100 mL. Store in plastic prescription bottles; label "shake well" and "refrigerate". Stable for 90 days refrigerated (preferred) or at room temperature.

Nahata MC, Pai VB, and Hipple TF, *Pediatric Drug Formulations*, 5th ed, Cincinnati, OH: Harvey Whitney Books Co, 2004.

◆ **Toposar** *see* Etoposide *on page* 802

Topotecan (toe poe TEE kan)

Brand Names: U.S. Hycamtin

Brand Names: Canada Hycamtin; Topotecan For Injection; Topotecan Hydrochloride For Injection

Index Terms Hycamptamine; SKF 104864; SKF 104864-A; Topotecan Hydrochloride

Pharmacologic Category Antineoplastic Agent, Camptothecin; Antineoplastic Agent, Topoisomerase I Inhibitor

Use

Cervical cancer: Treatment of recurrent or resistant (stage IVB) cervical cancer (in combination with cisplatin)

Ovarian cancer: Treatment of metastatic ovarian cancer

Small cell lung cancer (SCLC): Treatment of relapsed or refractory SCLC

Unlabeled Use Treatment of acute myeloid leukemia (induction in older adults), central nervous system lesions (metastatic from lung cancer), central nervous system lymphoma (primary), Ewing's sarcoma, merkel cell cancer, osteosarcoma, rhabdomyosarcoma (pediatrics), neuroblastoma (pediatrics)

Pregnancy Risk Factor D

Pregnancy Considerations Adverse effects were observed in animal reproduction studies. May cause fetal harm in pregnant women. Women of childbearing potential should use effective contraception to prevent pregnancy during treatment.

Breast-Feeding Considerations It is not known if topotecan is excreted in breast milk. Due to then potential for serious adverse reactions in the nursing infant, the manufacturer recommends to discontinue breast-feeding in women who are receiving topotecan.

Contraindications Hypersensitivity to topotecan or any component of the formulation; severe bone marrow depression

Canadian labeling: Additional contraindications (not in U.S. labeling): Severe renal impairment (Cl_{cr} <20 mL/minute); pregnancy; breast-feeding

Warnings/Precautions Hazardous agent - use appropriate precautions for handling and disposal (NIOSH, 2012). **[U.S. Boxed Warning]: May cause neutropenia, which may be severe or lead to infection or fatalities. Monitor blood counts frequently. Do NOT administer to patients with baseline neutrophils <1500/mm^3 and platelets <100,000/mm^3.** The dose-limiting toxicity is bone marrow suppression (primarily neutropenia); may also cause thrombocytopenia and anemia. Neutropenia is not cumulative overtime. In a clinical study comparing I.V. to oral topotecan, G-CSF support was administered in a higher percentage of patients receiving oral topotecan (Eckerd, 2007). Topotecan-induced neutropenia may lead to neutropenic colitis (including fatalities); should be considered in patients presenting with neutropenia, fever and abdominal pain.

Diarrhea has been reported with oral topotecan; may be severe (requiring hospitalization); incidence may be higher in the elderly; educate patients on early recognition and proper management, including diet changes, increase in fluid intake, antidiarrheals, and antibiotics. Interstitial lung disease (ILD) (with fatalities) has been reported; discontinue use in patients with confirmed ILD diagnosis; risk factors for ILD include a history of ILD, pulmonary fibrosis, lung cancer, thoracic radiation, and the use of colony-stimulating factors or medication with pulmonary toxicity; monitor pulmonary symptoms (cough, fever, dyspnea, and/or hypoxia). Use caution in renal impairment; may require dose adjustment (use in severe renal impairment is contraindicated in the Canadian labeling). Potentially significant drug-drug interactions may exist, requiring dose or frequency adjustment, additional monitoring, and/or selection of alternative therapy. Topotecan exposure is increased when oral topotecan is used concurrently with P-glycoprotein inhibitors; avoid concurrent use.

Adverse Reactions

>10%:

Central nervous system: Fatigue (6% to 29%), fever (5% to 28%), pain (5% to 23%), headache (18%)

Dermatologic: Alopecia (10% to 49%), rash (16%)

Gastrointestinal: Nausea (8% to 64%), vomiting (10% to 45%), diarrhea (6% to 32%; Oral: grade 3: 4%; grade 4: ≤1%; onset: 9 days), constipation (5% to 29%), abdominal pain (5% to 22%), anorexia (7% to 19%), stomatitis (18%)

Hematologic: Anemia (89% to 98%; grade 4: 7% to 37%; nadir: 15 days), neutropenia (83% to 97%; grade 4: 32% to 80%; nadir 12-15 days; duration: 7 days), leukopenia (86% to 97%; grade 4: 15% to 32%), thrombocytopenia (69% to 81%; grade 4: 6% to 27%; nadir: 15 days; duration: 3-5 days), neutropenic fever/sepsis (2% to 43%)

Neuromuscular & skeletal: Weakness (3% to 25%)

Respiratory: Dyspnea (6% to 22%), cough (15%)

Miscellaneous: Infection (≤17%)

1% to 10%:

Gastrointestinal: Obstruction (5%)

Hepatic: Liver enzymes increased (transient; 8%; grades 3/4: 4%), bilirubin increased (grades 3/4: <2%)

Neuromuscular & skeletal: Paresthesia (7%)

Respiratory: Pneumonia (8%)

Miscellaneous: Sepsis (grades 3/4: 5%)

<1% (Limited to important or life-threatening): Allergic reactions, anaphylactoid reactions, angioedema, bleeding (severe, associated with thrombocytopenia), dermatitis (severe), extravasation (inadvertent), interstitial lung disease (ILD), neutropenic colitis, pancytopenia, pruritus (severe)

Drug Interactions

Metabolism/Transport Effects None known.

Avoid Concomitant Use

Avoid concomitant use of Topotecan with any of the following: BCG; CloZAPine; Natalizumab; P-glycoprotein/ABCB1 Inhibitors; Pimecrolimus; Tacrolimus (Topical); Tofacitinib; Vaccines (Live)

Increased Effect/Toxicity

Topotecan may increase the levels/effects of: CloZAPine; Leflunomide; Natalizumab; Tofacitinib; Vaccines (Live)

The levels/effects of Topotecan may be increased by: BCRP/ABCG2 Inhibitors; Denosumab; Filgrastim; P-glycoprotein/ABCB1 Inhibitors; Pimecrolimus; Platinum Derivatives; Roflumilast; Tacrolimus (Topical); Trastuzumab

Decreased Effect

Topotecan may decrease the levels/effects of: BCG; Coccidioidin Skin Test; Sipuleucel-T; Vaccines (Inactivated); Vaccines (Live)

The levels/effects of Topotecan may be decreased by: Echinacea; Fosphenytoin-Phenytoin

Ethanol/Nutrition/Herb Interactions Ethanol: Avoid ethanol (due to GI irritation).

Preparation for Administration Hazardous agent; use appropriate precautions for handling and disposal (NIOSH, 2012). Reconstitute lyophilized powder with 4 mL SWFI. Further dilute in 50-100 mL D_5W or NS for infusion.

Storage/Stability

I.V.:

Solution for injection: Store intact vials at 2°C to 8°C (36°F to 45°F). Protect from light. Single-use vials should be discarded after initial vial entry; solutions for infusion are stable for 24 hours at room temperature after diluted.

Lyophilized powder: Store intact vials at room temperature of 20°C to 25°C (68°F to 77°F). Protect from light. Reconstituted solution is stable for up to 28 days at room temperature of 20°C to 25°C (68°F to 77°F), although the manufacturer recommends use immediately after reconstitution. Further dilute in 50-100 mL D_5W or NS. This solution is stable for 24 hours at room temperature (manufacturer recommendation) or up to 7 days under refrigeration (Craig, 1997).

Oral: Store at 2°C to 8°C (36°F to 46°F). Protect from light.

Mechanism of Action Binds to topoisomerase I and stabilizes the cleavable complex so that religation of the cleaved DNA strand cannot occur. This results in the accumulation of cleavable complexes and single-strand DNA breaks. Topotecan acts in S phase of the cell cycle.

Pharmacodynamics/Kinetics

Absorption: Oral: Rapid

Distribution: V_d: 25-75 L/m^2 (Hartmann, 2006)

Protein binding: ~35%

Metabolism: Undergoes a rapid, pH-dependent hydrolysis of the lactone ring to yield a relatively inactive hydroxy acid in plasma; metabolized in the liver to N-demethylated metabolite

Bioavailability: Oral: ~40%

Half-life elimination: I.V.: 2-3 hours; renal impairment: ~5 hours; Oral: 3-6 hours

Time to peak, plasma: Oral: 1-2 hours; delayed with high-fat meal (3-4 hours)

Excretion:

I.V.: Urine (51%; 3% as N-desmethyl topotecan); feces (18%; 2% as N-desmethyl topotecan)

Oral: Urine (20%; 2% as N-desmethyl topotecan); feces (33%; <2% as N-desmethyl topotecan)

Dosage Note: Baseline neutrophil count should be ≥1500/mm^3 and platelets should be ≥100,000/mm^3 prior to treatment; for retreatment, neutrophil count should be >1000/mm^3; platelets >100,000/mm^3 and hemoglobin ≥9 g/dL:

Cervical cancer, recurrent or resistant: Adults: IVPB: 0.75 mg/m^2/day for 3 days (followed by cisplatin on day 1 only, [with hydration]) every 21 days

Ovarian cancer, metastatic: Adults: IVPB: 1.5 mg/m^2/day for 5 consecutive days every 21 days, minimum of 4 cycles recommended in the absence of tumor progression **or** (weekly administration; unlabeled dosing) 4 mg/m^2 on days 1, 8, and 15 every 28 days until disease progression or unacceptable toxicity or a maximum of 12 months (Sehouli, 2011)

Small cell lung cancer (SCLC), relapsed or refractory: Adults:

IVPB: 1.5 mg/m^2/day for 5 consecutive days every 21 days, minimum of 4 cycles recommended in the absence of tumor progression

Oral: 2.3 mg/m^2/day for 5 consecutive days every 21 days (round dose to the nearest 0.25 mg); if patient vomits after dose is administered, do not give a replacement dose.

Dosage adjustment for toxicity:

Cervical cancer (cisplatin may also require dosage adjustment): I.V.: Severe febrile neutropenia (<1000/mm^3 with temperature of 38°C) or platelet count <25,000/mm^3: Reduce topotecan to 0.6 mg/m^2/day for subsequent cycles (may consider G-CSF support [beginning on day 4] prior to instituting dose reduction for neutropenic fever.

For neutropenic fever despite G-CSF use, reduce dose to 0.45 mg/m^2/day for subsequent cycles.

Ovarian cancer: I.V.: Dosage adjustment for hematological effects: Severe neutropenia (<500/mm^3) or platelet count <25,000/mm^3: Reduce dose to 1.25 mg/m^2/day for subsequent cycles (may consider G-CSF support [beginning on day 6] prior to instituting dose reduction for severe neutropenia). **Note:** The Canadian labeling states that the dose may be further reduced to 1 mg/m^2/day if necessary.

Small cell lung cancer (SCLC):

I.V.: Dosage adjustment for hematological effects: Severe neutropenia (<500/mm^3) or platelet count <25,000/mm^3: Reduce dose to 1.25 mg/m^2/day for subsequent cycles (may consider G-CSF support [beginning on day 6] prior to instituting dose reduction for severe neutropenia). **Note:** The Canadian labeling states that the dose may be further reduced to 1 mg/m^2/day if necessary.

Oral: Severe neutropenia (neutrophils <500/mm^3 associated with fever or infection or lasting ≥7 days) or prolonged neutropenia (neutrophils ≥500/mm^3 to ≤1000/mm^3 lasting beyond day 21) or platelets <25,000/mm^3 or grades 3/4 diarrhea: Reduce dose by 0.4 mg/m^2/day for subsequent cycles (may consider same dosage reduction for grade 2 diarrhea if clinically indicated).

Dosing adjustment in renal impairment:
Manufacturer's recommendations:

I.V.:
- Cl_{cr} ≥40 mL/minute: No dosage adjustment necessary.
- Cl_{cr} 20-39 mL/minute: Reduce dose to 0.75 mg/m^2/dose
- Cl_{cr} <20 mL/minute: No dosage adjustment provided in manufacturer's U.S. labeling (insufficient data available for dosing recommendation); use is contraindicated in the Canadian labeling.

Note: For topotecan in combination with cisplatin for cervical cancer, do not initiate treatment in patients with serum creatinine >1.5 mg/dL; consider discontinuing treatment in patients with serum creatinine >1.5 mg/dL in subsequent cycles.

Oral:
- Cl_{cr} ≥50 mL/minute: No dosage adjustment necessary.
- Cl_{cr} 30-49 mL/minute: Reduce dose to 1.8 mg/m^2/day
- Cl_{cr} <30 mL/minute: No dosage adjustment provided in manufacturer's U.S. labeling (insufficient data available for dosing recommendation).

Alternate recommendations:

Aronoff, 2007: I.V.:

Children:
- Cl_{cr} 30-50 mL/minute: Administer 75% of dose
- Cl_{cr} 10-29 mL/minute: Administer 50% of dose or reduce by 0.75 mg/m^2/dose
- Cl_{cr} <10 mL/minute: Administer 25% of dose
- Hemodialysis: 0.75 mg/m^2
- Continuous renal replacement therapy (CRRT): Administer 50% of dose or reduce by 0.75 mg/m^2/dose

Adults:
- Cl_{cr} >50 mL/minute: Administer 75% of dose
- Cl_{cr} 10-50 mL/minute: Administer 50% of dose
- Cl_{cr} <10 mL/minute: Administer 25% of dose
- Hemodialysis: Avoid use
- Continuous ambulatory peritoneal dialysis (CAPD): Avoid use
- Continuous renal replacement therapy (CRRT): 0.75 mg/m^2

Kintzel, 1995: I.V.:
- Cl_{cr} 46-60 mL/minute: Administer 80% of dose
- Cl_{cr} 31-45 mL/minute: Administer 75% of dose
- Cl_{cr} ≤30 mL/minute: Administer 70% of dose

Dosing adjustment in hepatic impairment: *Manufacturer's labeling:*

I.V.: Bilirubin 1.7-15 mg/dL (U.S. labeling) or >1.5 - <10 mg/dL (Canadian labeling): No dosage adjustment necessary (the half-life is increased slightly; usual doses are generally tolerated).

Oral: Bilirubin >1.5 mg/dL: No dosage adjustment necessary.

Dosing in obesity: *ASCO Guidelines for appropriate chemotherapy dosing in obese adults with cancer:* Utilize patient's actual body weight (full weight) for calculation of body surface area- or weight-based dosing, particularly when the intent of therapy is curative; manage regimen-related toxicities in the same manner as for nonobese patients; if a dose reduction is utilized due to toxicity, consider resumption of full weight-based dosing with subsequent cycles, especially if cause of toxicity (eg, hepatic or renal impairment) is resolved (Griggs, 2012).

Dietary Considerations May be taken without regard to meals.

Administration

I.V.: Administer IVPB over 30 minutes. For combination chemotherapy with cisplatin, administer pretreatment hydration.

Oral: Administer without regard to meals. Swallow whole; do not crush, chew, or divide capsule. If vomiting occurs after dose, do not take replacement dose.

Hazardous agent; use appropriate precautions for handling and disposal (NIOSH, 2012).

Monitoring Parameters CBC with differential and platelet count, renal function tests, bilirubin; monitor for symptoms of interstitial lung disease; diarrhea symptoms/hydration status

Dosage Forms Excipient information presented when available (limited, particularly for generics); consult specific product labeling.

Capsule, Oral:
- Hycamtin: 0.25 mg, 1 mg

Solution, Intravenous:
- Generic: 4 mg/4 mL (4 mL)

Solution Reconstituted, Intravenous:
- Hycamtin: 4 mg (1 ea)
- Generic: 4 mg (1 ea)

Solution Reconstituted, Intravenous [preservative free]:
- Generic: 4 mg (1 ea)

◆ **Topotecan For Injection (Can)** *see* Topotecan *on page 2093*

◆ **Topotecan Hydrochloride** *see* Topotecan *on page 2093*

◆ **Topotecan Hydrochloride For Injection (Can)** *see* Topotecan *on page 2093*

◆ **Toprol XL** *see* Metoprolol *on page 1348*

◆ **Topsyn® (Can)** *see* Fluocinonide *on page 879*

◆ **Toradol** *see* Ketorolac (Systemic) *on page 1152*

◆ **Toradol® (Can)** *see* Ketorolac (Systemic) *on page 1152*

◆ **Toradol® IM (Can)** *see* Ketorolac (Systemic) *on page 1152*

Toremifene (tore EM i feen)

Brand Names: U.S. Fareston

Brand Names: Canada Fareston®

Index Terms FC1157a; Toremifene Citrate

Pharmacologic Category Antineoplastic Agent, Estrogen Receptor Antagonist; Selective Estrogen Receptor Modulator (SERM)

Use Treatment of metastatic breast cancer in postmenopausal women with estrogen receptor positive or estrogen receptor status unknown

Unlabeled Use Treatment of soft tissue sarcoma (desmoid tumors)

Pregnancy Risk Factor D

Pregnancy Considerations Animal studies have demonstrated embryotoxicity and fetal adverse effects. There are no adequate and well-controlled studies in pregnant women. Only approved for use in postmenopausal women. May cause fetal harm if administered during pregnancy.

Breast-Feeding Considerations It is not known if toremifene is excreted in breast milk. Due to the potential for serious adverse reactions in the nursing infant, the manufacturer recommends a decision be made whether to discontinue nursing or to discontinue the drug, taking into account the importance of treatment to the mother.

Contraindications Hypersensitivity to toremifene or any component of the formulation; long QT syndrome (congenital or acquired QT prolongation), uncorrected hypokalemia, uncorrected hypomagnesemia

Warnings/Precautions Hazardous agent - use appropriate precautions for handling and disposal (NIOSH, 2012).

[U.S. Boxed Warning]: May prolong the QT interval; QT_c prolongation is dose-dependent and concentration dependent. Torsade de pointes, syncope, seizure and/or sudden death may occur. Use is contraindicated in patients with congenital or acquired long QT syndrome, uncorrected hypokalemia, or uncorrected hypomagnesemia. Avoid use with other medications known to prolong the QT interval and with strong CYP3A4 inhibitors. Use with caution in patients with heart failure, hepatic impairment, or electrolyte abnormalities. Monitor electrolytes; correct hypokalemia and hypomagnesemia prior to treatment. Obtain ECG at baseline and as clinically indicated in patients at risk for QT prolongation

Hypercalcemia and tumor flare have been reported during the first weeks of treatment in some breast cancer patients with bone metastases; monitor closely for hypocalcemia. Institute appropriate measures if hypercalcemia occurs, and if severe, discontinue treatment. Tumor flare consists of diffuse musculoskeletal pain and erythema with initial increased size of tumor lesions that later regress; is often accompanied by hypercalcemia. Tumor flare does not imply treatment failure or represent tumor progression. Drugs that decrease renal calcium excretion (eg, thiazide diuretics) may increase the risk of hypercalcemia in patients receiving toremifene. Leukopenia and thrombocytopenia have been reported rarely; monitor leukocyte and platelet counts. Endometrial hyperplasia has been reported; some patients have developed endometrial cancer, although a role of toremifene in endometrial cancer development has not been established. Avoid long-term use in patients with pre-existing endometrial hyperplasia. Use with caution in patients with hepatic failure. Avoid use in patients with a history of thromboembolic disease.

Adverse Reactions

>10%:

Endocrine & metabolic: Hot flashes (35%)
Gastrointestinal: Nausea (14%)
Genitourinary: Vaginal discharge (13%)
Hepatic: Alkaline phosphatase increased (8% to 19%), AST increased (5% to 19%)
Miscellaneous: Diaphoresis (20%)

1% to 10%:

Cardiovascular: Edema (5%), arrhythmia (≤2%), CVA/TIA (≤2%), thrombosis (≤2%), cardiac failure (≤1%), MI (≤1%)
Central nervous system: Dizziness (9%)
Endocrine & metabolic: Hypercalcemia (≤3%)
Gastrointestinal: Vomiting (4%)
Genitourinary: Vaginal bleeding (2%)
Hepatic: Bilirubin increased (1% to 2%)
Local: Thrombophlebitis (≤2%)
Ocular: Cataracts (≤10%), xerophthalmia (≤9%), visual field abnormal (≤4%), corneal keratopathy (≤2%), glaucoma (≤2%), vision abnormal/diplopia (≤2%)
Respiratory: Pulmonary embolism (≤2%)

<1% (Limited to important or life-threatening): Alopecia, angina, ataxia, blurred vision, corneal opacity (reversible), corneal verticulata, depression, dermatitis, dyspnea, endometrial cancer, endometrial hyperplasia, hepatitis (toxic), incoordination, ischemic attack, jaundice, lethargy, leukopenia, paresis, pruritus, QT prolongation, rigors, skin discoloration, thrombocytopenia, tremor, tumor flare, vertigo, weakness

Drug Interactions

Metabolism/Transport Effects Substrate of CYP1A2 (minor), CYP3A4 (major); **Note:** Assignment of Major/Minor substrate status based on clinically relevant drug interaction potential

Avoid Concomitant Use

Avoid concomitant use of Toremifene with any of the following: CYP3A4 Inducers (Strong); CYP3A4 Inhibitors (Strong); Grapefruit Juice; Highest Risk QTc-Prolonging Agents; Ivabradine; Mifepristone; Moderate Risk QTc-Prolonging Agents; Ospemifene

Increased Effect/Toxicity

Toremifene may increase the levels/effects of: Highest Risk QTc-Prolonging Agents; Ospemifene; Vitamin K Antagonists

The levels/effects of Toremifene may be increased by: CYP3A4 Inhibitors (Strong); Grapefruit Juice; Ivabradine; Mifepristone; Moderate Risk QTc-Prolonging Agents; QTc-Prolonging Agents (Indeterminate Risk and Risk Modifying); Thiazide Diuretics

Decreased Effect

Toremifene may decrease the levels/effects of: Ospemifene; Sugammadex

The levels/effects of Toremifene may be decreased by: Bosentan; CYP3A4 Inducers (Strong); Dabrafenib; Deferasirox; Herbs (CYP3A4 Inducers); Tocilizumab

Ethanol/Nutrition/Herb Interactions

Food: Grapefruit juice may increase toremifene levels. Management: Avoid grapefruit juice.

Herb/Nutraceutical: St John's wort may decrease toremifene levels. Management: Avoid St John's wort.

Storage/Stability Store at 25°C (77°F); excursions permitted to 15°C to 30°C (59°F to 86°F); protect from heat. Protect from light.

Mechanism of Action Nonsteroidal, triphenylethylene derivative with potent antiestrogenic properties (also has estrogenic effects). Competitively binds to estrogen receptors on tumors and other tissue targets, producing a nuclear complex that decreases DNA synthesis and inhibits estrogen effects. Competes with estrogen for binding sites in breast and other tissues; cells accumulate in the G_0 and G_1 phases; therefore, toremifene is cytostatic rather than cytocidal.

Pharmacodynamics/Kinetics

Absorption: Well absorbed
Distribution: V_d: 580 L (range: 457-958 L)
Protein binding, plasma: >99.5%, primarily to albumin
Metabolism: Extensively hepatic, principally by CYP3A4 to N-demethyltoremifene (a weak antiestrogen)
Bioavailability: Not affected by food
Half-life elimination: Toremifene: ~5 days; N-demethyltoremifene: 6 days
Time to peak, serum: ≤3 hours
Excretion: Primarily feces; urine (10%) during a 1-week period

Dosage Oral: Adults: Metastatic breast cancer (postmenopausal): 60 mg once daily, continue until disease progression

Dosage adjustment in renal impairment: No dosage adjustment necessary.

Dosage adjustment in hepatic impairment: No dosage adjustment provided in manufacturer's labeling. However, hepatic impairment increases systemic exposure to toremifene. Use with caution.

Dietary Considerations May be taken with or without food. Avoid grapefruit juice.

Administration Administer orally, as a single daily dose, with or without food.

Hazardous agent; use appropriate precautions for handling and disposal (NIOSH, 2012).

Monitoring Parameters CBC with differential, electrolytes (calcium, magnesium, and potassium), hepatic function. Obtain ECG in patients at risk for QT prolongation. In patients with bone metastases, monitor closely for hypercalcemia during the first few weeks of treatment.

Dosage Forms Excipient information presented when available (limited, particularly for generics); consult specific product labeling.

Tablet, Oral:

Fareston: 60 mg

◆ **Toremifene Citrate** *see* Toremifene *on page 2095*

◆ **Torisel** *see* Temsirolimus *on page 2008*

◆ **Torisel® (Can)** *see* Temsirolimus *on page 2008*

Torsemide (TORE se mide)

Brand Names: U.S. Demadex

Pharmacologic Category Antihypertensive; Diuretic, Loop

Use Management of edema associated with heart failure and hepatic or renal disease (including chronic renal failure); treatment of hypertension

Pregnancy Risk Factor B

Pregnancy Considerations A decrease in fetal weight, an increase in fetal resorption, and delayed fetal ossification has occurred in animal studies.

Breast-Feeding Considerations It is not known if torsemide is excreted in breast milk. The manufacturer recommends that caution be exercised when administering torsemide to nursing women.

Contraindications Hypersensitivity to torsemide, any component of the formulation, or any sulfonylurea; anuria

Warnings/Precautions Loop diuretics are potent diuretics; excess amounts can lead to profound diuresis with fluid and electrolyte loss; close medical supervision and dose evaluation are required. Potassium supplementation and/or use of potassium-sparing diuretics may be necessary to prevent hypokalemia. Use with caution in patients with cirrhosis; avoid sudden changes in fluid and electrolyte balance and acid/base status which may lead to hepatic encephalopathy. Administration with an aldosterone antagonist or potassium-sparing diuretic may provide additional diuretic efficacy and maintain normokalemia. Coadministration of antihypertensives may increase the risk of hypotension.

Monitor fluid status and renal function in an attempt to prevent oliguria, azotemia, and reversible increases in BUN and creatinine; close medical supervision of aggressive diuresis required. Ototoxicity has been demonstrated following oral administration of torsemide and following rapid I.V. administration of other loop diuretics. Other possible risk factors may include use in renal impairment, excessive doses, and concurrent use of other ototoxins (eg, aminoglycosides).

Chemical similarities are present among sulfonamides, sulfonylureas, carbonic anhydrase inhibitors, thiazides, and loop diuretics (except ethacrynic acid). Use in patients with sulfonylurea allergy is specifically contraindicated in product labeling; a risk of cross-reaction exists in patients with allergy to any of these compounds; avoid use when previous reaction has been severe. Discontinue if signs of hypersensitivity are noted.

Adverse Reactions

1% to 10%:

Cardiovascular: ECG abnormality (2%), chest pain (1%)

Central nervous system: Nervousness (1%)

Gastrointestinal: Constipation (2%), diarrhea (2%), dyspepsia (2%), nausea (2%), sore throat (2%)

Genitourinary: Excessive urination (7%)

Neuromuscular & skeletal: Arthralgia (2%), myalgia (2%), weakness (2%)

Respiratory: Rhinitis (3%), cough (2%)

<1% (Limited to important or life-threatening): Angioedema, arthritis, atrial fibrillation, esophageal hemorrhage, GI hemorrhage, hyperglycemia, hyperuricemia, hypokalemia, hyponatremia, hypotension, hypovolemia, impotence, leukopenia, pancreatitis, rash, rectal bleeding, shunt thrombosis, Stevens-Johnson syndrome, syncope, thirst, thrombocytopenia, toxic epidermal necrolysis, ventricular tachycardia, vomiting

Drug Interactions

Metabolism/Transport Effects **Substrate** of CYP2C8 (minor), CYP2C9 (major), SLCO1B1; **Note:** Assignment of Major/Minor substrate status based on clinically relevant drug interaction potential; **Inhibits** CYP2C19 (weak)

Avoid Concomitant Use There are no known interactions where it is recommended to avoid concomitant use.

Increased Effect/Toxicity

Torsemide may increase the levels/effects of: ACE Inhibitors; Allopurinol; Amifostine; Aminoglycosides; Antihypertensives; Cardiac Glycosides; CISplatin; Dofetilide; Hypotensive Agents; Ivabradine; Lithium; Methotrexate; Neuromuscular-Blocking Agents; Obinutuzumab; RisperiDONE; RiTUXimab; Salicylates; Sodium Phosphates; Topiramate; Warfarin

The levels/effects of Torsemide may be increased by: Alfuzosin; Analgesics (Opioid); Beta2-Agonists; Brimonidine (Topical); Corticosteroids (Orally Inhaled); Corticosteroids (Systemic); CycloSPORINE (Systemic); CYP2C9 Inhibitors (Moderate); CYP2C9 Inhibitors (Strong); Diazoxide; Eltrombopag; Herbs (Hypotensive Properties); Licorice; MAO Inhibitors; Methotrexate; Mifepristone; Pentoxifylline; Phosphodiesterase 5 Inhibitors; Probenecid; Prostacyclin Analogues

Decreased Effect

Torsemide may decrease the levels/effects of: Hypoglycemic Agents; Lithium; Neuromuscular-Blocking Agents

The levels/effects of Torsemide may be decreased by: Bile Acid Sequestrants; CYP2C9 Inducers (Strong); Dabrafenib; Fosphenytoin; Herbs (Hypertensive Properties); Methotrexate; Methylphenidate; Nonsteroidal Anti-Inflammatory Agents; Peginterferon Alfa-2b; Phenytoin; Probenecid; Salicylates; Yohimbine

Ethanol/Nutrition/Herb Interactions Herb/Nutraceutical: Avoid herbs with *hypertensive* properties (bayberry, blue cohosh, cayenne, ephedra, ginger, ginseng [American], kola, licorice); may diminish the antihypertensive effect of torsemide. Avoid herbs with *hypotensive* properties (black cohosh, California poppy, coleus, golden seal, hawthorn, mistletoe, periwinkle, quinine, shepherd's purse); may enhance the hypotensive effect of torsemide.

Storage/Stability

I.V.: Store at 15°C to 30°C (59°F to 86°F). If torsemide is to be administered via continuous infusion, stability has been demonstrated through 24 hours at room temperature in plastic containers for the following fluids and concentrations:

200 mg torsemide (10 mg/mL) added to 250 mL D_5W, 250 mL NS or 500 mL 0.45% sodium chloride

50 mg torsemide (10 mg/mL) added to 500 mL D_5W, 500 mL NS, or 500 mL 0.45% sodium chloride

Tablets: Store at 15°C to 30°C (59°F to 86°F).

Mechanism of Action Inhibits reabsorption of sodium and chloride in the ascending loop of Henle and distal renal tubule, interfering with the chloride-binding cotransport system, thus causing increased excretion of water, sodium, chloride, magnesium, and calcium; does not alter GFR, renal plasma flow, or acid-base balance

Pharmacodynamics/Kinetics

Onset of action: Diuresis: Oral: Within 1hour

Peak effect: Diuresis: Oral: 1-2 hours; Antihypertensive: Oral: 4-6 weeks (up to 12 weeks)
Duration: Diuresis: Oral: ~6-8 hours
Absorption: Oral: Rapid
Distribution: V_d: 12-15 L; Cirrhosis: Approximately doubled
Protein binding: >99%
Metabolism: Hepatic (~80%) via CYP
Bioavailability: ~80%
Half-life elimination: ~3.5 hours; Cirrhosis: 7-8 hours
Time to peak, plasma: Oral: 1 hour; delayed ~30 minutes when administered with food
Excretion: Urine (~20% as unchanged drug)

Dosage Adults: **Note:** I.V. and oral dosing are equivalent.

Edema:

Chronic renal failure: Oral, I.V.: Initial: 20 mg once daily; may increase gradually by doubling dose until the desired diuretic response is obtained (maximum recommended daily dose: 200 mg)

Heart failure:

Oral: Initial: 10-20 mg once daily; may increase gradually by doubling dose until the desired diuretic response is obtained. **Note:** ACC/AHA 2009 guidelines for heart failure maximum daily dose: 200 mg (Hunt, 2009)

I.V.: Initial: 10-20 mg; may repeat every 2 hours with double the dose as needed. **Note:** ACC/AHA 2009 guidelines for heart failure recommend maximum single dose: 100-200 mg (Hunt, 2009)

Continuous I.V. infusion (unlabeled dose): Initial: 20 mg I.V. load, then 5-20 mg/hour (Hunt, 2009)

Hepatic cirrhosis: Oral: Initial: 5-10 mg once daily; may increase gradually by doubling dose until the desired diuretic response is obtained (maximum recommended single dose: 40 mg). **Note:** Administer with an aldosterone antagonist or a potassium-sparing diuretic.

Hypertension: Oral: Initial: 5 mg once daily; may increase to 10 mg once daily after 4-6 weeks if adequate antihypertensive response is not apparent; if still not effective, an additional antihypertensive agent may be added. Usual dosage range (JNC 7): 2.5-10 mg once daily. **Note:** Thiazide-type diuretics are preferred in the treatment of hypertension (Chobanian, 2003)

Dosage adjustment in renal impairment: No dosage adjustment necessary. However, higher doses may be required to achieve diuretic response.

Dosage adjustment in hepatic impairment: No dosage adjustment provided in manufacturer's labeling; use with caution.

Dietary Considerations May be taken without regard to meals; however, food slows the rate and reduces the extent of absorption and may reduce diuretic efficacy (Bard, 2004). May require increased intake of potassium-rich foods.

Administration

I.V.: Administer over ≥2 minutes; reserve I.V. administration for situations which require rapid onset of action

Oral: Administer without regard to meals; patients may be switched from the I.V. form to the oral (and vice-versa) with no change in dose

Monitoring Parameters Renal function, electrolytes, and fluid status (weight and I & O), blood pressure

Additional Information 10-20 mg torsemide is approximately equivalent to furosemide 40 mg or bumetanide 1 mg.

Dosage Forms Excipient information presented when available (limited, particularly for generics); consult specific product labeling.

Solution, Intravenous:
Generic: 20 mg/2 mL (2 mL); 50 mg/5 mL (5 mL)

Tablet, Oral:
Demadex: 5 mg, 10 mg, 20 mg, 100 mg [scored]
Generic: 5 mg, 10 mg, 20 mg, 100 mg

◆ **Total Allergy [OTC]** *see* DiphenhydrAMINE (Systemic) *on page 622*

◆ **Total Allergy Medicine [OTC]** *see* DiphenhydrAMINE (Systemic) *on page 622*

Total Parenteral Nutrition

(TOE tal par EN ter al noo TRISH un)

Index Terms Hyperal; Hyperalimentation; Parenteral Nutrition; PN; TPN

Pharmacologic Category Caloric Agent; Intravenous Nutritional Therapy

Use Infusion of nutrient solutions into the bloodstream to support nutritional needs during a time when patient is unable to absorb nutrients via the gastrointestinal tract, cannot take adequate nutrition orally or enterally, or have had (or are expected to have) inadequate oral intake for 7-14 days.

Dosage PN is a highly-individualized therapy. The following general guidelines may be used in the estimation of needs. Electrolytes, vitamins, and trace minerals should be added to TPN mixtures based on patients individualized needs.

Children: I.V.: **Note:** Give within 5-7 days if unable to meet needs orally or with enteral nutrition:

Total calories:
<6 months: 85-105 kcal/kg/day
6-12 months: 80-100 kcal/kg/day
1-7 years: 75-90 kcal/kg/day
7-12 years: 50-75 kcal/kg/day
12-18 years: 30-50 kcal/kg/day

Fluid:
2-10 kg: 100 mL/kg
>10-20 kg: 1000 mL for 10 kg plus 50 mL/kg for each kg >10
>20 kg: 1500 mL for 10 kg plus 20 mL/kg for each kg >20

Carbohydrate (dextrose): 40% to 50% of caloric intake
<1 year: Initial: 6-8 mg/kg/minute; goal: 10-14 mg/kg/minute
1-10 years: Initial: 10% to 12.5%; daily increase: 5% increments (maximum: 15 mg/kg/minute)
>10 years: Initial: 10% to 15%; daily increase: 5% increments (maximum: 8.5 mg/kg/minute)

Protein (amino acids):
1-12 months: Initial: 2-3 g/kg/day; daily increase: 1 g/kg/day (maximum: 3 g/kg/day)
1-10 years: Initial: 1-2 g/kg/day; daily increase: 1 g/kg/day (maximum: 2-2.5 g/kg/day)
>10 years: Initial: 0.8-1.5 g/kg/day; daily increase: 1 g/kg/day (maximum: 1.5-2 g/kg/day)

Fat: Initial: 1 g/kg/day; daily increase: 1 g/kg/day (maximum: 3 g/kg/day); **Note:** Monitor triglycerides while receiving intralipids.

Adults: I.V.:

Total calories: Calculate using Harris-Benedict equation or based on stress level as indicated below:

Harris-Benedict Equation (BEE):
Females: 655.1 + [(9.56 x W) + (1.85 x H) - (4.68 x A)]
Males: 66.47 + [(13.75 x W) + (5 x H) - (6.76 x A)]
Then multiply BEE x (activity factor) x (stress factor)
W = weight in kg; H = height in cm; A = age in years
Activity factor = 1.2 sedentary, 1.3 normal activity, 1.4 active, 1.5 very active
Stress factor = 1.5 for trauma, stressed, or surgical patients and underweight (to promote weight gain); 2.0 for severe burn patients

Stress level:
Normal/mild stress level: 20-25 kcal/kg/day
Moderate stress level: 25-30 kcal/kg/day
Severe stress level: 30-40 kcal/kg/day
Pregnant women in second or third trimester: Add an additional 300 kcal/day

Fluid: mL/day = 30-40 mL/kg

Carbohydrate (dextrose):
5 g/kg/day or 3.5 mg/kg/minute (maximum rate: 4-7 mg/kg/minute)
Minimum recommended amount: 400 calories/day or 100 g/day

Protein (amino acids):
Maintenance: 0.8-1 g/kg/day
Normal/mild stress level: 1-1.2 g/kg/day
Moderate stress level: 1.2-1.5 g/kg/day
Severe stress level: 1.5-2 g/kg/day
Burn patients (severe): Increase protein until significant wound healing achieved
Solid organ transplant: Perioperative: 1.5-2 g/kg/day
Renal failure:
Acute (severely malnourished or hypercatabolic): 1.5-1.8 g/kg/day
Chronic, with dialysis: 1.2-1.3 g/kg/day
Chronic, without dialysis: 0.6-0.8 g/kg/day
Continuous hemofiltration: ≥1 g/kg/day
Hepatic failure:
Acute management when other treatments have failed:
With encephalopathy: 0.6-1 g/kg/day
Without encephalopathy: 1-1.5 g/kg/day
Chronic encephalopathy: Use branch chain amino acid enriched diets only if unresponsive to pharmacotherapy
Pregnant women in second or third trimester: Add an additional 10-14 g/day

Fat:
Initial: 20% to 40% of total calories (maximum: 60% of total calories or 2.5 g/kg/day); **Note:** Monitor triglycerides while receiving intralipids.
Safe for use in pregnancy
I.V. lipids are safe in adults with pancreatitis if triglyceride levels <400 mg/dL

Additional Information Complete prescribing information should be consulted for additional detail.

Dosage Forms Excipient information presented when available (limited, particularly for generics); consult specific product labeling. TPN is usually compounded from optimal combinations of macronutrients (water, protein, dextrose, and lipids) and micronutrients (electrolytes, trace elements, and vitamins) to meet the specific nutritional requirements of a patient. Individual hospitals may have designated standard TPN formulas. There are a few commercially-available amino acids with electrolytes solutions; however, these products may not meet an individual's specific nutrition requirements.

- **Totect** *see* Dexrazoxane *on page 587*
- **Toviaz** *see* Fesoterodine *on page 855*
- **tPA** *see* Alteplase *on page 85*
- **TPN** *see* Total Parenteral Nutrition *on page 2098*
- **TPV** *see* Tipranavir *on page 2070*
- **tRA** *see* Tretinoin (Systemic) *on page 2117*
- **Tracleer** *see* Bosentan *on page 273*
- **Tracleer® (Can)** *see* Bosentan *on page 273*
- **Tradjenta** *see* Linagliptin *on page 1216*
- **Trajenta** *see* Linagliptin *on page 1216*
- **Tramacet (Can)** *see* Acetaminophen and Tramadol *on page 33*

TraMADol (TRA ma dole)

Brand Names: U.S. ConZip; Rybix ODT [DSC]; Ultram; Ultram ER

Brand Names: Canada Durela; Ralivia; Tridural; Ultram; Zytram XL

Index Terms Tramadol Hydrochloride

Pharmacologic Category Analgesic, Opioid

Use Relief of moderate to moderately-severe pain
Extended release formulations are indicated for patients requiring around-the-clock management of moderate to moderately-severe pain for an extended period of time

Pregnancy Risk Factor C

Pregnancy Considerations Adverse events were observed in animal reproduction studies. Tramadol has been shown to cross the human placenta when administered during labor. Postmarketing reports following tramadol use during pregnancy include neonatal seizures, withdrawal syndrome, fetal death, and stillbirth. Tramadol is not recommended for use during labor and delivery. Some Canadian products are contraindicated for use in pregnant women.

If chronic opioid exposure occurs in pregnancy, adverse events in the newborn (including withdrawal) may occur; monitoring of the neonate is recommended (Chou, 2009). Neonatal abstinence syndrome following opioid exposure may present with autonomic (eg, fever, temperature instability), gastrointestinal (eg, diarrhea, vomiting, poor feeding/weight gain), or neurologic (eg, high-pitched crying, increased muscle tone, irritability, seizure, tremor) symptoms (Dow, 2012; Hudak, 2012).

Breast-Feeding Considerations Tramadol is excreted into breast milk. Sixteen hours following a single 100 mg I.V. dose, the amount of tramadol found in breast milk was 0.1% of the maternal dose. Use is not recommended by the manufacturer for postdelivery analgesia in nursing mothers. Some Canadian products are contraindicated for use in nursing women. Nursing infants exposed to large doses of opioids should be monitored for apnea and sedation (Montgomery, 2012).

Contraindications Hypersensitivity to tramadol, opioids, or any component of the formulation
Additional contraindications for Ultram®, Rybix™ ODT, and Ultram® ER: Any situation where opioids are contraindicated, including acute intoxication with alcohol, hypnotics, centrally-acting analgesics, opioids, or psychotropic drugs
Additional contraindications for ConZip: Severe/acute bronchial asthma, hypercapnia, or significant respiratory depression in the absence of appropriately monitored setting and/or resuscitative equipment

Canadian product labeling:
Tramadol is contraindicated during or within 14 days following MAO inhibitor therapy
Extended release formulations: Additional contraindications:
Ralivia™, Tridural™: Severe (Cl_{cr} <30 mL/minute) renal dysfunction, severe (Child-Pugh class C) hepatic dysfunction
Durela™ and Zytram® XL: Severe (Cl_{cr} <30 mL/minute) renal dysfunction, severe (Child-Pugh class C) hepatic dysfunction; known or suspected mechanical GI obstruction or any disease/condition that affects bowel transit; mild, intermittent or short-duration pain that can be managed with other pain medication; management of peri-operative pain; obstructive airway, acute respiratory depression, cor pulmonale, delirium tremens, seizure disorder, severe CNS depression, increased cerebrospinal or intracranial pressure, head injury, breast-feeding, pregnancy; use during labor and delivery

Warnings/Precautions Rare but serious anaphylactoid reactions (including fatalities) often following initial dosing have been reported. Pruritus, hives, bronchospasm, angioedema, toxic epidermal necrolysis (TEN) and Stevens-Johnson syndrome also have been reported with use. Previous anaphylactoid reactions to opioids may increase risks for similar reactions to tramadol. Caution patients to swallow extended release tablets whole. Rapid release and absorption of tramadol from extended release tablets that are broken, crushed, or chewed may lead to a potentially lethal overdose. May cause CNS depression, which may impair physical or mental abilities; patients must be cautioned about performing tasks which require mental alertness (eg, operating machinery or driving). May cause CNS depression and/or respiratory depression, particularly when combined with other CNS depressants. Use with caution and reduce dosage when administered to patients receiving other CNS depressants. An increased risk of seizures may occur in patients receiving serotonin reuptake inhibitors (SSRIs or anorectics), tricyclic antidepressants or other cyclic compounds (including cyclobenzaprine, promethazine), neuroleptics, drugs which may lower seizure threshold, or drugs which impair metabolism of tramadol (ie, CYP2D6 and 3A4 inhibitors). Patients with a history of seizures, or with a risk of seizures (head trauma, metabolic disorders, CNS infection, or malignancy, or during ethanol/drug withdrawal) are also at increased risk. Potentially significant drug interactions may exist, requiring dose or frequency adjustment, additional monitoring, and/or selection of alternative therapy.

Elderly (particularly >75 years of age), debilitated patients and patients with chronic respiratory disorders may be at greater risk of adverse events. Use with caution in patients with increased intracranial pressure or head injury. Avoid use in patients who are suicidal or addiction prone; use with caution in patients taking tranquilizers and/or antidepressants, or those with an emotional disturbance including depression. Healthcare provider should be alert to problems of abuse, misuse, and diversion. Use caution in heavy alcohol users. Use caution in treatment of acute abdominal conditions; may mask pain. Use tramadol with caution and reduce dosage in patients with liver disease or renal dysfunction. Avoid using extended release tablets in severe hepatic impairment. Tolerance or drug dependence may result from extended use (withdrawal symptoms have been reported); abrupt discontinuation should be avoided. Tapering of dose at the time of discontinuation limits the risk of withdrawal symptoms. Some products may contain phenylalanine.

After chronic maternal exposure to opioids, neonatal withdrawal syndrome may occur in the newborn; monitor neonate closely. Signs and symptoms include irritability, hyperactivity and abnormal sleep pattern, high pitched cry, tremor, vomiting, diarrhea and failure to gain weight. Onset, duration and severity depend on the drug used, duration of use, maternal dose, and rate of drug elimination by the newborn. Opioid withdrawal syndrome in the neonate, unlike in adults, may be life-threatening and should be treated according to protocols developed by neonatology experts.

Adverse Reactions

>10%:

Cardiovascular: Flushing (8% to 16%)

Central nervous system: Dizziness (10% to 33%), headache (4% to 32%), somnolence (7% to 25%), insomnia (2% to 11%)

Dermatologic: Pruritus (3% to 12%)

Gastrointestinal: Constipation (9% to 46%), nausea (15% to 40%), vomiting (5% to 17%), dyspepsia (1% to 13%)

Neuromuscular & skeletal: Weakness (4% to 12%)

1% to 10%:

Cardiovascular: Orthostatic hypotension (2% to 5%), chest pain (1% to <5%), hypertension (1% to <5%), peripheral edema (1% to <5%), vasodilation (1% to <5%)

Central nervous system: Agitation (1% to <5%), anxiety (1% to <5%), apathy (1% to <5%), chills (1% to <5%), confusion (1% to <5%), coordination impaired (1% to <5%), depersonalization (1% to <5%), depression (1% to <5%), euphoria (1% to <5%), fever (1% to <5%), hypoesthesia (1% to <5%), lethargy (1% to <5%), nervousness (1% to <5%), pain (1% to <5%), pyrexia (1% to <5%), restlessness (1% to <5%), malaise (<1% to <5%), fatigue (2%), vertigo (2%)

Dermatologic: Dermatitis (1% to <5%), rash (1% to <5%)

Endocrine & metabolic: Hot flashes (2% to 9%), hyperglycemia (1% to <5%), menopausal symptoms (1% to <5%)

Gastrointestinal: Diarrhea (5% to 10%), xerostomia (3% to 13%), anorexia (1% to 6%), abdominal pain (1% to <5%), appetite decreased (1% to <5%), weight loss (1% to <5%), flatulence (<1% to <5%)

Genitourinary: Pelvic pain (1% to <5%), prostatic disorder (1% to <5%), urine abnormalities (1% to <5%), urinary tract infection (1% to <5%), urinary frequency (<1% to <5%), urinary retention (<1% to <5%)

Neuromuscular & skeletal: Arthralgia (1% to 5%), back pain (1% to <5%), creatine phosphokinase increased (1% to <5%), myalgia (1% to <5%), hypertonia (1% to <5%), neck pain (1% to <5%), rigors (1% to <5%), paresthesia (1% to <5%), tremor (1% to <5%)

Ocular: Blurred vision (1% to <5%), miosis (1% to <5%)

Respiratory: Bronchitis (1% to <5%), congestion (nasal/sinus) (1% to <5%), cough (1% to <5%), dyspnea (1% to <5%), nasopharyngitis (1% to <5%), pharyngitis (1% to <5%), rhinitis (1% to <5%), rhinorrhea (1% to <5%), sinusitis (1% to <5%), sneezing (1% to <5%), sore throat (1% to <5%), upper respiratory infection (1% to <5%)

Miscellaneous: Diaphoresis (2% to 9%), flu-like syndrome (1% to <5%), withdrawal syndrome (1% to <5%), shivering (<1% to <5%)

<1% (Limited to important or life-threatening): Abnormal gait, allergic reaction, amnesia, anaphylactoid reactions, anaphylaxis, anemia, angioedema, appendicitis, ALT increased/decreased, AST increased/decreased, bradycardia, bronchospasm, BUN increased, cataracts, cellulitis, cholecystitis, cholelithiasis, clamminess, cognitive dysfunction, concentration difficulty, creatinine increased, deafness, disorientation, diverticulitis, dreams abnormal, dysphagia, dysuria, ear infection, ECG abnormalities, edema, fecal impaction, gastroenteritis, gastrointestinal bleeding, GGT increased, gout, hallucination, hematuria, hemoglobin decreased, hepatitis, hypotension, hypersensitivity, irritability, joint stiffness, libido decreased, liver enzymes increased, liver failure, menstrual disorder, MI, migraine, muscle cramps, muscle spasms, muscle twitching, myocardial ischemia, night sweats, palpitation, pancreatitis, peripheral edema, peripheral ischemia, pneumonia, proteinuria, pulmonary edema, pulmonary embolism, sedation, seizure, serotonin syndrome, sleep disorder, speech disorder, Stevens-Johnson syndrome, stomatitis, suicidal tendency, syncope, taste perversion, tachycardia, thrombocytopenia, tinnitus, toxic epidermal necrolysis, urticaria, vesicles, visual disturbance

A withdrawal syndrome may include anxiety, diarrhea, hallucinations (rare), nausea, pain, piloerection, rigors, sweating, and tremor. Uncommon discontinuation symptoms may include severe anxiety, panic attacks, or paresthesia.

Drug Interactions

Metabolism/Transport Effects Substrate of CYP2B6 (minor), CYP2D6 (major), CYP3A4 (major); **Note:** Assignment of Major/Minor substrate status based on clinically relevant drug interaction potential

Avoid Concomitant Use

Avoid concomitant use of TraMADol with any of the following: Azelastine (Nasal); CarBAMazepine; Conivaptan; Fusidic Acid (Systemic); Paraldehyde

Increased Effect/Toxicity

TraMADol may increase the levels/effects of: Alcohol (Ethyl); Alvimopan; Antipsychotics; Azelastine (Nasal); CarBAMazepine; CNS Depressants; Desmopressin; Diuretics; Hydrocodone; MAO Inhibitors; Metoclopramide; Metyrosine; Paraldehyde; Pramipexole; ROPINIRole; Rotigotine; Selective Serotonin Reuptake Inhibitors; Serotonin Modulators; Tricyclic Antidepressants; Vitamin K Antagonists; Zolpidem

The levels/effects of TraMADol may be increased by: Amphetamines; Anticholinergics; Antipsychotic Agents (Phenothiazines); Antipsychotics; Brimonidine (Topical); Cannabinoids; Conivaptan; Cyclobenzaprine; CYP3A4 Inhibitors (Moderate); CYP3A4 Inhibitors (Strong); Dasatinib; Doxylamine; Fusidic Acid (Systemic); HydrOXYzine; Ivacaftor; Luliconazole; Magnesium Sulfate; Mifepristone; Perampanel; Selective Serotonin Reuptake Inhibitors; Simeprevir; Sodium Oxybate; Succinylcholine; Tricyclic Antidepressants

Decreased Effect

TraMADol may decrease the levels/effects of: CarBAMazepine; Pegvisomant

The levels/effects of TraMADol may be decreased by: Ammonium Chloride; Antiemetics (5HT3 Antagonists); Bosentan; CarBAMazepine; CYP2D6 Inhibitors (Moderate); CYP2D6 Inhibitors (Strong); CYP3A4 Inducers (Strong); Dabrafenib; Deferasirox; Mitotane; Mixed Agonist / Antagonist Opioids; Tocilizumab

Ethanol/Nutrition/Herb Interactions

Ethanol: May increase CNS depression; monitor for increased effects with coadministration. Caution patients about effects.

Food:

Immediate release tablet: Rate and extent of absorption were not significantly affected.

Extended release:

ConZip™: Rate and extent of absorption were unaffected.

Ultram® ER: High-fat meal reduced C_{max} and AUC, and increased T_{max} by 3 hours.

Orally disintegrating tablet: Food delays the time to peak serum concentration by 30 minutes; extent of absorption was not significantly affected.

Herb/Nutraceutical: Avoid valerian, St John's wort, kava kava, gotu kola (may increase CNS depression).

Storage/Stability Store at 25°C (77°F); excursions permitted to 15°C to 30°C (59°F to 86°F).

Mechanism of Action Tramadol and its active metabolite (M1) binds to μ-opiate receptors in the CNS causing inhibition of ascending pain pathways, altering the perception of and response to pain; also inhibits the reuptake of norepinephrine and serotonin, which are neurotransmitters involved in the descending inhibitory pain pathway responsible for pain relief (Grond, 2004)

Pharmacodynamics/Kinetics

Onset of action: Immediate release: ~1 hour

Duration: 9 hours

Absorption: Immediate release formulation: Rapid and complete; Extended release formulation: Delayed

Distribution: V_d: 2.5-3 L/kg

Protein binding, plasma: ~20%

Metabolism: Extensively hepatic via demethylation (mediated by CYP3A4 and CYP2B6), glucuronidation, and sulfation; has pharmacologically active metabolite formed by CYP2D6 (M1; O-desmethyl tramadol)

Bioavailability: Immediate release: 75%; Extended release: Ultram® ER: 85% to 90% (as compared to immediate release), Zytram® XL, Tridural™: 70%

Half-life elimination: Tramadol: ~6-8 hours; Active metabolite: 7-9 hours; prolonged in elderly, hepatic or renal impairment; Zytram® XL: Apparent half-life: ~16 hours; Durela™, Ralivia™, Tridural™: ~5-9 hours

Time to peak: Immediate release: ~2 hours; Extended release: ConZip™: ~10-12 hours, Tridural™: ~4 hours; Durela™, Ultram® ER: ~12 hours

Excretion: Urine (30% as unchanged drug; 60% as metabolites)

Dosage Oral: Moderate-to-severe pain:

Children ≥17 years and Adults:

Immediate release: 50-100 mg every 4-6 hours (not to exceed 400 mg/day).For patients not requiring rapid onset of effect, tolerability may be improved by starting dose at 25 mg/day and titrating dose by 25 mg every 3 days, until reaching 25 mg 4 times/day. The total daily dose may then be increased by 50 mg every 3 days as tolerated, to reach dose of 50 mg 4 times/day. After titration, 50-100 mg may be given every 4-6 hours as needed up to a maximum 400 mg/day.

Orally-disintegrating tablet (Rybix™ ODT): 50-100 mg every 4-6 hours (not to exceed 400 mg/day); for patients not requiring rapid onset of effect, tolerability may be improved by starting dose at 50 mg/day and titrating dose by 50 mg every 3 days, until reaching 50 mg 4 times/day. After titration, 50-100 mg may be given every 4-6 hours as needed up to a maximum 400 mg/day.

Adults: Extended release:

U.S. labeling: ConZip™, Ultram® ER:

Patients not currently on immediate-release tramadol: 100 mg once daily; titrate every 5 days (ConZip™, Ultram® ER); maximum dose: 300 mg daily

Patients currently on immediate-release tramadol: Calculate 24-hour immediate release total dose and initiate total extended release daily dose (round dose to the next lowest 100 mg increment); titrate as tolerated to desired effect (maximum: 300 mg daily)

Canadian labeling: **Note:** Patients currently on immediate-release tramadol: When switching to extended release, initiate at the same or lowest nearest total daily tramadol dose. Not to exceed recommended maximum daily dosing.

Durela™, Ralivia™, Tridural™: Patients not currently on immediate-release tramadol or opioids: Initial: 100 mg once daily; titrate every 5 days (Durela™, Ralivia™) or every 2 days (Tridural™) as needed based on clinical response and severity of pain (maximum: 300 mg daily)

Zytram® XL: Patients not currently on immediate-release tramadol or opioids: 150 mg once daily; if pain relief is not achieved may titrate by increasing dosage incrementally, with sufficient time to evaluate effect of increased dosage; generally not more often than every 7 days (maximum: 400 mg daily)

Elderly >65 years: Use caution and initiate at the lower end of the dosing range

Elderly >75 years:

Immediate release: Do not exceed 300 mg/day; see dosing adjustments for renal and hepatic impairment.

Extended release: Use with great caution. See adult, renal, and hepatic dosing.

Dosage adjustment in renal impairment:

Immediate release: Cl_{cr} <30 mL/minute: Administer 50-100 mg dose every 12 hours (maximum: 200 mg daily)

Extended release: Should not be used in patients with Cl_{cr} <30 mL/minute

Dosage adjustment in hepatic impairment:

Immediate release: Cirrhosis: Recommended dose: 50 mg every 12 hours

Extended release: Should not be used in patients with severe (Child-Pugh class C) hepatic dysfunction.

Dietary Considerations Some products may contain phenylalanine.

Administration

Immediate release: Administer without regard to meals.

Extended release: Swallow whole; do not crush, chew, or split. **Note:** Durela™, Ralivia™, and Tridural™: Canadian availability; products not available in U.S.:

ConZip™, Zytram® XL, Durela™: May administer without regard to meals.

Ultram® ER, Ralivia™, Tridural™: May administer without regard to meals, but administer in a consistent manner of either with or without meals.

Orally-disintegrating tablet: Remove from foil blister by peeling back (do not push tablet through the foil). Place tablet on tongue and allow to dissolve (may take ~1 minute); water is not needed, but may be administered with water. Do not chew, break, or split tablet.

Monitoring Parameters Pain relief, respiratory rate, blood pressure, and pulse; signs of tolerance, abuse, or suicidal ideation

Reference Range 100-300 ng/mL; however, serum level monitoring is not required

Test Interactions May interfere with urine detection of PCP (false-positive).

Dosage Forms Excipient information presented when available (limited, particularly for generics); consult specific product labeling.

Capsule, variable release, oral, as hydrochloride: 150 mg [37.5 mg (immediate release) and 112.5 mg (extended release)]

ConZip™: 100 mg [25 mg (immediate release) and 75 mg (extended release)]

ConZip™: 200 mg [50 mg (immediate release) and 150 mg (extended release)]

ConZip™: 300 mg [50 mg (immediate release) and 250 mg (extended release)]

Tablet, oral, as hydrochloride: 50 mg

Ultram®: 50 mg [scored]

Tablet, extended release, oral, as hydrochloride: 100 mg, 200 mg, 300 mg

Ultram® ER: 100 mg, 200 mg, 300 mg

Tablet, orally disintegrating, oral, as hydrochloride:

Rybix™ ODT: 50 mg [contains aspartame; mint flavor] [DSC]

Dosage Forms: Canada Excipient information presented when available (limited, particularly for generics); consult specific product labeling.

Tablet, extended release, as hydrochloride

Durela™: 100 mg, 200 mg, 300 mg

Ralivia™: 100 mg, 200 mg, 300 mg

Tridural™: 100 mg, 200 mg, 300 mg

Zytram® XL: 75 mg, 150 mg, 200 mg, 300 mg, 400 mg

Extemporaneous Preparations A 5 mg/mL oral suspension may be made with tablets and either Ora-Sweet® SF or a mixture of 30 mL Ora-Plus® and 30 mL strawberry syrup. Crush six 50 mg tramadol tablets in a mortar and reduce to a fine powder. Add small portions of the chosen vehicle and mix to a uniform paste; mix while adding vehicle in incremental proportions to **almost** 60 mL; transfer to a calibrated bottle, rinse mortar with vehicle, and add quantity of vehicle sufficient to make 60 mL. Label "shake well before use". Stable for 90 days refrigerated or at room temperature.

Wagner DS, Johnson CE, Cichon-Hensley BK, et al, "Stability of Oral Liquid Preparations of Tramadol in Strawberry Syrup and a Sugar-Free Vehicle," *Am J Health Syst Pharm*, 2003, 60(12):1268-70.

◆ **Tramadol Hydrochloride** *see* TraMADol *on page 2099*

◆ **Tramadol Hydrochloride and Acetaminophen** *see* Acetaminophen and Tramadol *on page 33*

◆ **Tramaphen-Odan (Can)** *see* Acetaminophen and Tramadol *on page 33*

Trametinib (tra ME ti nib)

Brand Names: U.S. Mekinist

Brand Names: Canada Mekinist

Index Terms GSK1120212

Pharmacologic Category Antineoplastic Agent, MEK Inhibitor

Use Melanoma, metastatic: Treatment of unresectable or metastatic melanoma in patients with a BRAF V600E or BRAF V600K mutation (as detected by an approved test). **Note:** Not recommended in patients who have received prior BRAF-inhibitor therapy.

Pregnancy Risk Factor D

Pregnancy Considerations Adverse effects were observed in animal reproduction studies. Based on its mechanism of action, trametinib would be expected to cause fetal harm if administered to a pregnant woman. Females of reproductive potential should use a highly effective contraceptive during therapy and for 4 months after treatment is complete. Fertility may also be impaired in females.

Breast-Feeding Considerations It is not known if trametinib is excreted into breast milk. Due to the potential for serious adverse reactions in the nursing infant, the manufacturer recommends a decision be made whether to discontinue nursing or to discontinue the drug, taking into account the importance of treatment to the mother.

Contraindications There are no contraindications listed in the manufacturer's U.S. labeling.

Canadian labeling: Hypersensitivity to trametinib or any component of the formulation.

Warnings/Precautions Hazardous agent - use appropriate precautions for handling and disposal (meets NIOSH, 2012 criteria). Cardiac events such as heart failure, left ventricular dysfunction, or decreased left ventricular ejection fraction (LVEF) were observed in clinical trials; the median time to onset of cardiomyopathy was ~2 months (range: 16-156 days). Assess LVEF (by echocardiogram or MUGA scan) prior to therapy initiation, at one month, and then at 2- to 3-month intervals while on therapy. Cardiac dysfunction may require treatment interruption, dosage reduction, or discontinuation; such measures resulted in resolution of cardiomyopathy in some patients. Interstitial lung disease and pneumonitis were observed in clinical trials; median time to initial presentation was 160 days (range: 60-172 days). Monitor for new or progressive pulmonary symptoms (eg, cough, dyspnea, hypoxia, pleural effusion, infiltrates); may require therapy interruption or permanent discontinuation.

Dermatologic toxicity (eg, rash, dermatitis, acneiform rash, palmar-plantar erythrodysesthesia syndrome, and erythema) was commonly observed in trametinib-treated patients; some patients required hospitalization for severe toxicity or for secondary skin infections. The median time to onset and resolution of skin toxicity was 15 days (range: 1-221 days) and 48 days (range: 1-282 days), respectively. Monitor for dermatologic toxicity and signs/symptoms of secondary infections. Treatment interruption, dose reductions, and/or therapy discontinuation may be necessary. Retinal pigment epithelial detachments (RPED) and retinal vein occlusion were seen in clinical trials (rare). Detachments were typically bilateral and multifocal and occurred in the macular area of the retina. RPED resolution occurred after a median of 11.5 days (range: 3-71 days) following therapy interruption, although some visual disturbances persisted beyond 1 month. Retinal vein occlusion may lead to macular edema, degeneration, decreased visual function, neovascularization, and glaucoma. Promptly refer patients for ophthalmological evaluations if visual disturbances occur; therapy interruption and/or discontinuation may be required. Prior to initiating therapy, confirm BRAF mutation status with an approved test; approved for use in patients with BRAF V600K and BRAF V600E mutations. Current data regarding use in patients with BRAF V600K mutation is limited; compared to BRAF V600E mutation, lower response rates have been observed with BRAF V600K mutation. Data regarding other less common BRAF V600 mutations is lacking.

Adverse Reactions

>10%:

Cardiovascular: Hypertension (15%), cardiomyopathy (5% to 11%)

Dermatologic: Skin rash (57%; grades 3/4: 8%), acneiform eruption (19%; grades 3/4: <1%), xeroderma (11%)

Endocrine & metabolic: Hypoalbuminemia (42%)

Gastrointestinal: Diarrhea (43%), stomatitis (15%), abdominal pain (13%)

Hematologic & oncologic: Anemia (38%; grades 3/4: 2%), lymphedema (32%), hemorrhage (epistaxis, gingival bleeding, hematochezia, rectal hemorrhage, melena, vaginal hemorrhage, hemorrhoidal hemorrhage, hematuria, conjunctival hemorrhage; 13%)

Hepatic: Increased serum AST (60%), increased serum ALT (39%), increased serum alkaline phosphatase (24%)

1% to 10%:

Cardiovascular: Bradycardia (≤10%)

Central nervous system: Dizziness (≤10%)

Dermatologic: Paronychia (10%), pruritus (10%), cellulitis (≤10%), folliculitis (≤10%), pustular rash (≤10%)

Gastrointestinal: Dysgeusia (≤10%), xerostomia (≤10%)

Ophthalmic: Blurred vision (≤10%), dry eye syndrome (≤10%)

Respiratory: Interstitial lung disease or pneumonitis (2%)

<1% (Limited to important or life-threatening): Dermatitis, erythema, palmar-plantar erythrodysesthesia, retinal pigment epithelial detachment, retinal vein occlusion, rhabdomyolysis

Drug Interactions

Metabolism/Transport Effects Inhibits CYP2C8 (weak); **Induces** CYP3A4 (weak/moderate)

Avoid Concomitant Use

Avoid concomitant use of Trametinib with any of the following: Axitinib; Simeprevir

Increased Effect/Toxicity There are no known significant interactions involving an increase in effect.

Decreased Effect

Trametinib may decrease the levels/effects of: ARIPiprazole; Axitinib; Ibrutinib; Saxagliptin; Simeprevir

Ethanol/Nutrition/Herb Interactions Food: Administration with a high-fat, high-calorie meal decreased AUC by 24%, C_{max} by 70%, and delayed T_{max} by ~4 hours. Management: Administer 1 hour before or 2 hours after a meal.

Storage/Stability Store refrigerated at 2°C to 8°C (36°F to 46°F); do not freeze. Dispense in original bottle; do not remove dessicant. Protect from light and moisture. Do not transfer to pill boxes.

Mechanism of Action Reversibly and selectively inhibits mitogen-activated extracellular kinase (MEK) 1 and 2 activation and kinase activity. MEK is a downstream effector of the protein kinase B-raf (BRAF); BRAFvV600 mutations result in constitutive activation of the BRAF pathway (including MEK1 and MEK2). Through inhibition of MEK 1 and 2 kinase activity, trametinib causes decreased cellular proliferation, cell cycle arrest, and increased apoptosis (Kim, 2013).

Pharmacodynamics/Kinetics

Absorption: Rapid; decreased with a high-fat, high-calorie meal

Distribution: 214 L

Protein binding: ~97% to plasma proteins

Metabolism: Predominantly deacetylation (via hydrolytic enzymes) alone or with mono-oxygenation or in combination with glucuronidation

Bioavailability: 72%

Half-life elimination: 4-5 days

Time to peak: 1.5 hours; delayed with a high-fat, high-calorie meal

Excretion: Feces (>80%); urine (<20% with <0.1% as unchanged drug)

Dosage

Melanoma, metastatic or unresectable (with BRAFvV600E or BRAF V600K mutations): Adults: Oral: 2 mg once daily until disease progression or unacceptable toxicity

Missed doses: Do not take a missed dose within 12 hours of the next dose.

Dosage adjustment for toxicity:

Cardiac:

Asymptomatic, 10% or greater absolute decrease in LVEF from baseline and LVEF is below institutional lower limits of normal (LLN): Interrupt therapy for up to 4 weeks. If LVEF improves to normal within 4 weeks following therapy interruption, resume at a reduced dose (decrease previous dose by 0.5 mg); if previous dose was 1 mg daily, discontinue therapy. If LVEF does not improve to normal within 4 weeks following therapy interruption, permanently discontinue.

>20% absolute decrease in LVEF from baseline and LVEF is below institutional LLN: Permanently discontinue.

Symptomatic heart failure: Permanently discontinue.

Dermatologic:

Grade 2 rash: Reduce dose by 0.5 mg; if taking 1 mg daily, discontinue therapy.

Intolerable Grade 2 rash that does not improve within 3 weeks of dosage reduction or Grade 3 or 4 rash: Interrupt therapy for up to 3 weeks. If rash improves within 3 weeks, resume at a reduced dose (decrease previous dose by 0.5 mg); if previous dose was 1 mg daily, discontinue therapy.

Intolerable Grade 2-4 rash that does not improve within 3 weeks despite therapy interruption: Permanently discontinue.

Ocular:

Grade 2 or 3 retinal pigment epithelial detachments (RPED): Interrupt therapy for up to 3 weeks (or discontinue use if dose is 1 mg daily).

Grade 2 or 3 RPED that improves to ≤ Grade 1 within 3 weeks: Resume at a reduced dose (decrease previous dose by 0.5 mg); if previous dose was 1 mg daily, discontinue therapy.

Grade 2 or 3 RPED that does not improve to ≤ Grade 1 within 3 weeks: Permanently discontinue.

Recurrence of RPED (any grade) after dose reduction/therapy interruption: *Canadian labeling (not in U.S. labeling):* Permanently discontinue.

Retinal vein occlusion: Permanently discontinue.

Pulmonary: Interstitial lung disease or pneumonitis: Permanently discontinue.

Other toxicity:

Grade 3 adverse reaction: Interrupt therapy for up to 3 weeks. If toxicity improves to ≤ Grade 1 within 3 weeks following therapy interruption, resume at a reduced dose (decrease previous dose by 0.5 mg); if previous dose was 1 mg daily, discontinue therapy.

Grade 3 adverse reaction that does not improve to ≤ Grade 1 within 3 weeks following therapy interruption: Permanently discontinue.

Grade 4 adverse reaction: Permanently discontinue.

Dosage adjustment for renal impairment:

Mild-to-moderate impairment (GFR 30-89 mL/minute/1.73 m^2): No dosage adjustment necessary.

Severe impairment (GFR <30 mL/minute/1.73 m^2): No dosage adjustment provided in manufacturer's labeling (has not been studied); however, renal excretion is low and is unlikely to affect drug exposure.

Dosage adjustment for hepatic impairment:

Mild impairment (total bilirubin ≤ ULN and AST > ULN **or** total bilirubin >1-1.5 times ULN with any AST): No dosage adjustment necessary.

Moderate-to-severe impairment: No dosage adjustment provided in manufacturer's labeling (has not been studied).

Dietary Considerations Take at least 1 hour before or 2 hours after a meal.

Administration Administer orally at least 1 hour before or 2 hours after a meal. Do not take a missed dose within 12 hours of the next dose.

Hazardous agent; use appropriate precautions for handling and disposal (meets NIOSH, 2012 criteria).

Monitoring Parameters CBC and liver function tests at baseline and periodically; assess LVEF (by echocardiogram or MUGA scan) at baseline, 1 month after therapy initiation, and then at 2- to 3-month intervals; ophthalmological evaluation as necessary (if reports of visual disturbance); monitor for signs/symptoms of pulmonary toxicity (eg, cough dyspnea, hypoxia, pleural effusion, or infiltrates); monitor for dermatologic toxicity and secondary skin infections; blood pressure; diarrhea

Dosage Forms Excipient information presented when available (limited, particularly for generics); consult specific product labeling.

Tablet, Oral:

Mekinist: 0.5 mg, 2 mg

◆ Trandate *see* Labetalol *on page 1156*

◆ Trandate® (Can) *see* Labetalol *on page 1156*

Trandolapril (tran DOE la pril)

Brand Names: U.S. Mavik

Brand Names: Canada Mavik

Pharmacologic Category Angiotensin-Converting Enzyme (ACE) Inhibitor; Antihypertensive

Additional Appendix Information

Angiotensin Agents *on page 2280*

Use Treatment of hypertension alone or in combination with other antihypertensive agents; treatment of heart failure (HF) or left ventricular (LV) dysfunction after myocardial infarction (MI)

Unlabeled Use To delay the progression of nephropathy and reduce risks of cardiovascular events in hypertensive patients with type 1 or 2 diabetes mellitus

Pregnancy Risk Factor D

Dosage Adults: Oral:

Hypertension: Initial dose in patients not receiving a diuretic: 1 mg once daily (2 mg/day in black patients). Adjust dosage at intervals of ≥1 week according to blood pressure response; most patients require 2-4 mg/day. There is little experience with doses >8 mg/day. Patients inadequately treated with once daily dosing at 4 mg may be treated with twice daily dosing. If blood pressure is not adequately controlled with trandolapril monotherapy, a diuretic may be added.

Usual dose range (JNC 7): 1-4 mg once daily

Post-MI heart failure or LV dysfunction: Initial: 1 mg once daily; titrate (as tolerated) towards target dose of 4 mg/day. If 4 mg dose is not tolerated, patients may continue therapy with the greatest tolerated dose.

Dosing adjustment in renal impairment: Cl_{cr} <30 mL/minute: Recommended starting dose: 0.5 mg once daily

Dosing adjustment in hepatic impairment: Cirrhosis: Recommended starting dose: 0.5 mg once daily

Additional Information Complete prescribing information should be consulted for additional detail.

Dosage Forms Excipient information presented when available (limited, particularly for generics); consult specific product labeling.

Tablet, Oral:

Mavik: 1 mg [scored]

Mavik: 2 mg, 4 mg

Generic: 1 mg, 2 mg, 4 mg

Dosage Forms: Canada Excipient information presented when available (limited, particularly for generics); consult specific product labeling.

Capsule, Oral:

Mavik: 0.5 mg, 1 mg, 2 mg, 4 mg

Trandolapril and Verapamil

(tran DOE la pril & ver AP a mil)

Brand Names: U.S. Tarka®

Brand Names: Canada Tarka®

Index Terms Verapamil and Trandolapril

Pharmacologic Category Angiotensin-Converting Enzyme (ACE) Inhibitor; Antihypertensive; Calcium Channel Blocker

Use Treatment of hypertension; however, not indicated for initial treatment of hypertension

Pregnancy Risk Factor D

Dosage Dose is individualized

Dosage adjustment in renal impairment: Usual regimen need not be adjusted unless patient's creatinine clearance is <30 mL/minute. Titration of individual components must be done prior to switching to combination product

Dosage adjustment in hepatic impairment: No dosage adjustment provided in manufacturer's labeling (has not been studied). However, verapamil is hepatically metabolized; adjustment of dosage in hepatic impairment is recommended.

Additional Information Complete prescribing information should be consulted for additional detail.

Dosage Forms Excipient information presented when available (limited, particularly for generics); consult specific product labeling.

Tablet, variable release: Trandolapril 2 mg [immediate release] and verapamil hydrochloride 180 mg [sustained release]; Trandolapril 2 mg [immediate release] and verapamil hydrochloride 240 mg [sustained release]; Trandolapril 4 mg [immediate release] and verapamil hydrochloride 240 mg [sustained release]

Tarka®:

1/240: Trandolapril 1 mg [immediate release] and verapamil hydrochloride 240 mg [sustained release]

2/180: Trandolapril 2 mg [immediate release] and verapamil hydrochloride 180 mg [sustained release]

2/240: Trandolapril 2 mg [immediate release] and verapamil hydrochloride 240 mg [sustained release]

4/240: Trandolapril 4 mg [immediate release] and verapamil hydrochloride 240 mg [sustained release]

Tranexamic Acid (tran eks AM ik AS id)

Brand Names: U.S. Cyklokapron; Lysteda

Brand Names: Canada Cyklokapron; Tranexamic Acid Injection BP

Pharmacologic Category Antifibrinolytic Agent; Antihemophilic Agent; Hemostatic Agent; Lysine Analog

Use

Injection: Short-term use (2-8 days) in hemophilia patients to reduce or prevent hemorrhage and reduce need for replacement therapy during and following tooth extraction

Oral: Treatment of cyclic heavy menstrual bleeding

Unlabeled Use Trauma-associated hemorrhage; treatment of traumatic hyphema; topical treatment (mouth rinse) of bleeding associated with dental procedures in patients on oral anticoagulant therapy; prevention of perioperative bleeding associated with cardiac surgery; prevention of bleeding associated with craniosynostosis surgery, extracorporeal membrane oxygenation (ECMO), orthognathic surgery, spinal surgery (eg, spinal fusion), total knee replacement surgery, or transurethral prostatectomy; reduction of blood loss associated with cesarean delivery; hereditary angioedema (long-term prophylaxis)

Pregnancy Risk Factor B

Dosage

Oral:

Children ≥12 years, Adolescents, and Adults: Menorrhagia: 1300 mg 3 times daily (3900 mg daily) for up to 5 days during monthly menstruation

Children:

Hereditary angioedema (HAE) (unlabeled use):

Long-term prophylaxis: 20-40 mg/kg/day in 2-3 divided doses (maximum dose: 3000 mg daily) (Farkas, 2007) **or** 50 mg/kg/day (or 1000-2000 mg daily; depending on age and size of patient); may consider alternate-day regimen or twice-weekly regimen when frequency of attacks reduces; diarrhea may be a dose-limiting side effect (Gompels, 2005)

Short-term prophylaxis: 20-40 mg/kg/day in 2-3 divided doses (maximum dose: 3000 mg daily) (Farkas, 2007) **or** 500 mg 4 times daily (Gompels, 2005). **Note:** For short-term prophylaxis (eg, dental work), initiate 2-5 days before and continue for 2 days after the procedure (Bowen, 2004; Gompels, 2005).

Children and Adults: Traumatic hyphema (unlabeled use): 25 mg/kg administered 3 times daily for 5-7 days (Rahmani, 1999; Vangsted, 1983; Varnek, 1980). **Note:** This same regimen may also be used for secondary hemorrhage after an initial traumatic hyphema event.

Adults:

Hereditary angioedema (HAE) (unlabeled use):

Long-term prophylaxis: 1000-1500 mg 2-3 times daily; reduce to 500 mg/dose once or twice daily when frequency of attacks reduces (Gompels, 2005; Levy, 2010) **or** 25 mg/kg/dose administered 2-3 times daily (Bowen, 2004)

Short-term prophylaxis (eg, for dental work): 75 mg/kg/day divided 2-3 times daily for 5 days before and 2 days after the event (Bowen, 2004) **or** 1000 mg 4 times daily for 48 hours before and after procedure (Gompels, 2005)

Treatment of acute HAE attack: 25 mg/kg/dose (maximum single dose: 1000 mg) every 3-4 hours (maximum: 75 mg/kg/day) (Bowen, 2004) **or** 1000 mg 4 times daily for 48 hours (Gompels, 2005)

Prevention of dental procedure bleeding in patients on oral anticoagulant therapy (unlabeled use): Oral rinse: 4.8% solution: Hold 10 mL in mouth and rinse for 2 minutes then spit out. Repeat 4 times daily for 2 days after procedure. **Note:** Patient should not eat or drink for 1 hour after using oral rinse (Carter, 2003).

Transurethral prostatectomy, blood loss reduction (unlabeled use): 2000 mg 3 times daily on the operative and first postoperative day (Rannikko, 2004)

I.V.:

Children:

Prevention of perioperative bleeding associated with cardiac surgery (unlabeled use): 10 mg/kg given over 30 minutes prior to incision, 10 mg/kg while on cardiopulmonary bypass, and 10 mg/kg administered after protamine reversal (Chauhan, 2004; Chauhan, 2004)

or

Loading dose of 100 mg/kg over 15 minutes prior to incision, followed by 10 mg/kg/hour infusion (continued until ICU transport); add 100 mg/kg to pump reservoir when cardiopulmonary bypass initiated (Reid, 1997)

Prevention of perioperative bleeding associated with craniosynostosis surgery (unlabeled use): Loading dose of 50 mg/kg over 15 minutes prior to incision, followed by 5 mg/kg/hour (Goobie, 2011) **or** 15 mg/kg over 15 minutes prior to incision, followed by 10 mg/kg/hour until skin closure (Dadure, 2011)

Children and Adolescents:

Prevention of perioperative bleeding associated with spinal surgery (eg, spinal fusion) (unlabeled use): 10 mg/kg given over 15 minutes prior to incision followed by 1 mg/kg/hour for the remainder of the surgery; discontinue at time of wound closure (Neilipovitz, 2001; Verma, 2010)

or

100 mg/kg over 15 minutes prior to incision followed by 10 mg/kg/hour until skin closure (Sethna, 2005)

or

30 mg/kg over 20 minutes prior to incision followed by 1 mg/kg/hour during surgery and for 5 hours postoperatively (Elwatidy, 2008)

Children and Adults: Tooth extraction in patients with hemophilia (in combination with appropriate factor replacement therapy): 10 mg/kg immediately before surgery, then 10 mg/kg/dose 3-4 times daily; may be used for 2-8 days

Adults:

Elective cesarean section, blood loss reduction (unlabeled use): 1000 mg over 5 minutes at least 10 minutes prior to skin incision (Gungorduk, 2011)

Hereditary angioedema (HAE), treatment of acute attack (unlabeled use): 25 mg/kg/dose (maximum single dose: 1000 mg) every 3-4 hours (maximum: 75 mg/kg/day) (Bowen, 2004) **or** 1000 mg 4 times daily for 48 hours (Gompels, 2005)

Orthognathic surgery, blood loss reduction (unlabeled use): 20 mg/kg over 15 minutes prior to incision (Choi, 2009)

Prevention of perioperative bleeding associated with cardiac surgery (unlabeled use): Loading dose of 30 mg/kg over 30 minutes (total loading dose includes a test dose administered over the first 10 minutes followed by the remainder of dose) prior to incision, followed by 16 mg/kg/hour until sternal closure; add an additional 2 mg/kg to cardiopulmonary bypass circuit (Fergusson, 2008)

or

Loading dose of 10 mg/kg over 20 minutes prior to incision followed by 2 mg/kg/hour continued for 2 hours after transfer to ICU; add a prime dose of 50 mg for a 2.5 L cardiopulmonary bypass circuit; maintenance infusion adjusted for renal insufficiency (Nuttall, 2008)

or

Loading dose of 10-15 mg/kg over 10-15 minutes, followed by 1-1.5 mg/kg/hour. The authors suggest adding 2–2.5 mg/kg to cardiopulmonary bypass circuit; however, amounts have varied widely in clinical trials (Gravlee, 2008).

Prevention of perioperative bleeding associated with spinal surgery (eg, spinal fusion) (unlabeled use): 2000 mg over 20 minutes prior to incision followed by 100 mg/hour during surgery and for 5 hours postoperatively (Elwatidy, 2008) **or** 10 mg/kg prior to incision followed by 1 mg/kg/hour for the remainder of the surgery; discontinue at time of wound closure (Wong, 2008)

Total knee replacement surgery, blood loss reduction (unlabeled use): 10 mg/kg over 30 minutes before inflation of tourniquet and 3 hours after first dose (Camarasa, 2006)

or

10 mg/kg over 10 minutes before inflation of tourniquet with a second dose (10 mg/kg) administered immediately after tourniquet release (Lozano, 2008)

or

10 mg/kg administered 30 minutes before deflation of tourniquet followed by 1 mg/kg/hour beginning at the end of the operation and continuing for 6 hours postoperatively (Alvarez, 2008)

Trauma-associated hemorrhage (unlabeled use): Loading dose: 1000 mg over 10 minutes, followed by 1000 mg over the next 8 hours. **Note:** Clinical trial included patients with significant hemorrhage (SBP <90 mm Hg, heart rate >110 bpm, or both) or those at risk of significant hemorrhage. Treatment began within 8 hours of injury (CRASH-2 Trial Collaborators, 2010).

Dosing adjustment/interval in renal impairment:

I.V. formulation:

Tooth extraction in patients with hemophilia:

Serum creatinine 1.36-2.83 mg/dL: Maintenance dose of 10 mg/kg/dose twice daily

Serum creatinine 2.83-5.66 mg/dL: Maintenance dose of 10 mg/kg/dose once daily

Serum creatinine >5.66 mg/dL: Maintenance dose of 10 mg/kg/dose every 48 hours **or** 5 mg/kg/dose once daily

Cardiac surgery (the following dose adjustments have been recommended [Nuttall, 2008]):

Serum creatinine 1.6-3.3 mg/dL: Reduce maintenance infusion to 1.5 mg/kg/hour (based on a 25% reduction from 2 mg/kg/hour)

Serum creatinine 3.3-6.6 mg/dL: Reduce maintenance infusion to 1 mg/kg/hour (based on a 50% reduction from 2 mg/kg/hour)

Serum creatinine >6.6 mg/dL: Reduce maintenance infusion to 0.5 mg/kg/hour (based on a 75% reduction from 2 mg/kg/hour)

Oral formulation: *Cyclic heavy menstrual bleeding:*

Serum creatinine >1.4-2.8 mg/dL: 1300 mg twice daily (2600 mg daily) for up to 5 days

Serum creatinine 2.9-5.7 mg/dL: 1300 mg once daily for up to 5 days

Serum creatinine >5.7 mg/dL: 650 mg once daily for up to 5 days

Dosing adjustment in hepatic impairment: No dosage adjustment is necessary.

Additional Information Complete prescribing information should be consulted for additional detail.

Dosage Forms Excipient information presented when available (limited, particularly for generics); consult specific product labeling.

Solution, Intravenous:

Cyklokapron: 100 mg/mL (10 mL)

Generic: 100 mg/mL (10 mL)

Tablet, Oral:

Lysteda: 650 mg

Generic: 650 mg

- ◆ **Tranexamic Acid Injection BP (Can)** *see* Tranexamic Acid *on page 2104*
- ◆ **Transamine Sulphate** *see* Tranylcypromine *on page 2106*
- ◆ **Transderm-V® (Can)** *see* Scopolamine (Systemic) *on page 1881*
- ◆ **Transderm-Nitro (Can)** *see* Nitroglycerin *on page 1466*
- ◆ **Transderm-Scop** *see* Scopolamine (Systemic) *on page 1881*
- ◆ ***trans*-Retinoic Acid** *see* Tretinoin (Systemic) *on page 2117*
- ◆ ***trans*-Retinoic Acid** *see* Tretinoin (Topical) *on page 2120*
- ◆ ***trans* Vitamin A Acid** *see* Tretinoin (Systemic) *on page 2117*
- ◆ **Tranxene-T** *see* Clorazepate *on page 475*
- ◆ **Tranxene T-Tab** *see* Clorazepate *on page 475*

Tranylcypromine (tran il SIP roe meen)

Brand Names: U.S. Parnate

Brand Names: Canada Parnate®

Index Terms Transamine Sulphate; Tranylcypromine Sulfate

Pharmacologic Category Antidepressant, Monoamine Oxidase Inhibitor

Additional Appendix Information

Antidepressant Agents *on page 2284*

Tyramine Content of Foods *on page 2394*

Use Treatment of major depressive episode without melancholia

Pregnancy Considerations Adverse events were observed in animal reproduction studies.

Breast-Feeding Considerations Tranylcypromine is excreted in breast milk.

Medication Guide Available Yes

Contraindications

Cardiovascular disease (including hypertension); cerebrovascular defect; history of headache; history of hepatic disease or abnormal liver function tests; pheochromocytoma

Concurrent use of antihistamines, antihypertensives, antiparkinson drugs, bupropion, buspirone, caffeine (excessive use), CNS depressants (including ethanol and opioids), dextromethorphan, diuretics, elective surgery requiring general anesthesia (discontinue tranylcypromine ≥10 days prior to elective surgery), local vasoconstrictors, meperidine, MAO inhibitors or dibenzazepine derivatives (eg, amitriptyline, clomipramine, desipramine, imipramine, nortriptyline, protriptyline, doxepin, carbamazepine, cyclobenzaprine, amoxapine, maprotiline, trimipramine), SSRIs or SNRIs, spinal anesthesia (hypotension may be exaggerated), sympathomimetics (including amphetamines, cocaine, phenylephrine, pseudoephedrine) or related compounds (methyldopa, reserpine, levodopa, tryptophan), or foods high in tyramine content

Bupropion: At least 14 days should elapse between MAO inhibitor discontinuation and bupropion initiation.

Buspirone: At least 10 days should elapse between tranylcypromine discontinuation and buspirone initiation.

MAO inhibitors or dibenzazepine derivatives: At least 1-2 weeks should elapse between the use of another MAO inhibitor or dibenzazepine derivative and tranylcypromine use.

Meperidine: At least 2-3 weeks should elapse between MAO inhibitor discontinuation and meperidine use.

SSRIs or SNRIs: At least 2 weeks should elapse between the discontinuation of sertraline or paroxetine and the initiation of tranylcypromine. At least 5 weeks should elapse between the discontinuation of fluoxetine and the initiation of tranylcypromine. At least 1 week should elapse between discontinuation of a SNRI and the initiation of tranylcypromine. At least 2 weeks should elapse between the discontinuation of tranylcypromine and the initiation of SNRIs and SSRIs.

Warnings/Precautions **Risk of suicide: [U.S. Boxed Warning]: Antidepressants increase the risk of suicidal thinking and behavior in children, adolescents, and young adults (18-24 years of age) with major depressive disorder (MDD) and other psychiatric disorders;** consider risk prior to prescribing. Short-term studies did not show an increased risk in patients >24 years of age and showed a decreased risk inpatients >65 years. Closely monitor for clinical worsening, suicidality, or unusual changes in behavior such as anxiety, agitation, panic attacks, insomnia, irritability, hostility, impulsivity, akathisia, hypomania, and mania. The patient's family or caregiver should be instructed to closely observe the patient and communicate condition with healthcare provider. Such observation would generally include at least weekly face-to-face contact with patients or their family members or caregivers during the first 4 weeks of treatment, then every other week visits for the next 4 weeks, then at 12 weeks, and as clinically indicated beyond 12 weeks. Additional contact by telephone may be appropriate between face-to-face visits. A medication guide should be dispensed with each prescription. **Tranylcypromine is not FDA approved for treatment of children and adolescents.**

All patients treated with antidepressants should be observed similarly for clinical worsening and suicidality, especially during the initial few months of a course of drug therapy, or at times of dose changes, either increases or decreases. The possibility of a suicide attempt is inherent in major depression and may persist until remission occurs. Worsening depression and severe abrupt suicidality that are not part of the presenting symptoms may require discontinuation or modification of drug therapy. Use caution in high-risk patients during initiation of therapy. Prescriptions should be written for the smallest quantity consistent with good patient care.

Hypertensive crisis may occur with foods/supplements high in tyramine, tryptophan, phenylalanine, or tyrosine content; treatment with phentolamine is recommended for hypertensive crisis. Use with caution in patients who have glaucoma, hyperthyroidism, diabetes or hypotension. May cause orthostatic hypotension (especially at dosages >30 mg/day). Use with caution in patients at risk of seizures, or in patients receiving other drugs which may lower seizure threshold. Use with caution in patients with a history of drug abuse or acute alcoholism; potential for drug dependency exists especially in patients using excessive doses. Discontinue at least 48 hours prior to myelography. May increase the risks associated with electroconvulsive therapy. Use with caution in patients with renal impairment. Do not use with other MAO inhibitors or antidepressants. Avoid products containing sympathomimetic stimulants or dextromethorphan. Concurrent use with antihypertensive agents may lead to exaggeration of hypotensive effects. Tranylcypromine is not generally considered a first-line agent for the treatment of depression; tranylcypromine is typically used in patients who have failed to respond to other treatments. May worsen psychosis in some patients or precipitate a shift to mania or hypomania in patients with bipolar disorder. **Tranylcypromine is not FDA approved for the treatment of bipolar depression.**

Abrupt discontinuation or interruption of antidepressant therapy has been associated with a discontinuation syndrome. Symptoms arising may vary with antidepressant however commonly include nausea, vomiting, diarrhea, headaches, lightheadedness, dizziness, diminished appetite, sweating, chills, tremors, paresthesias, fatigue, somnolence, and sleep disturbances (eg, vivid dreams, insomnia). Greater risks for developing a discontinuation syndrome have been associated with antidepressants with shorter half-lives, longer durations of treatment, and abrupt discontinuation. More severe symptoms have also been associated with MAO inhibitors. For antidepressants of short or intermediate half-lives, symptoms may emerge within 2-5 days after treatment discontinuation and last 7-14 days (APA, 2010; Fava, 2006; Haddad, 2001; Shelton, 2001; Warner, 2006).

Adverse Reactions

Frequency not defined:

Cardiovascular: Edema, orthostatic hypotension, palpitation, tachycardia

Central nervous system: Agitation, anxiety, chills, dizziness, drowsiness, headache, insomnia, mania, restlessness

Dermatologic: Alopecia (rare), rash (rare), urticaria

Endocrine & metabolic: Sexual dysfunction (anorgasmia, ejaculatory disturbances, impotence); SIADH

Gastrointestinal: Abdominal pain, anorexia, constipation, diarrhea, nausea, xerostomia

Genitourinary: Urinary retention

Hematologic: Agranulocytosis, anemia, leukopenia, thrombocytopenia

Hepatic: Hepatitis (rare)

Neuromuscular & skeletal: Muscle spasm, myoclonus, numbness, paresthesia, tremor, weakness

Ocular: Blurred vision

Otic: Tinnitus

Miscellaneous: Diaphoresis

Postmarketing and/or case reports: Akinesia, ataxia, confusion, cystic acne, disorientation, memory loss, mouth fissures, polyuria, scleroderma (localized), urinary incontinence, urticaria, withdrawal symptoms

Drug Interactions

Metabolism/Transport Effects **Inhibits** CYP1A2 (moderate), CYP2A6 (strong), CYP2C19 (moderate), CYP2C8 (weak), CYP2C9 (weak), CYP2D6 (moderate), CYP2E1 (weak), CYP3A4 (weak), Monoamine Oxidase

Avoid Concomitant Use

Avoid concomitant use of Tranylcypromine with any of the following: Aclidinium; Alpha-/Beta-Agonists (Indirect-Acting); Alpha1-Agonists; Amphetamines; Anilidopiperidine Opioids; Antidepressants (Serotonin Reuptake Inhibitor/Antagonist); Apraclonidine; AtoMOXetine; Bezafibrate; Buprenorphine; BuPROPion; BusPIRone; CarBAMazepine; Cyclobenzaprine; Dexmethylphenidate; Dextromethorphan; Diethylpropion; Hydrocodone; HYDROmorphone; Ipratropium (Oral Inhalation); Isometheptene; Levonordefrin; Linezolid; Maprotiline; Meperidine; Methyldopa; Methylene Blue; Methylphenidate; Mirtazapine; Morphine (Liposomal); Morphine (Systemic); Oxymorphone; Pirfenidone; Pizotifen; Selective Serotonin Reuptake Inhibitors; Serotonin 5-HT1D Receptor Agonists; Serotonin/Norepinephrine Reuptake Inhibitors; Tapentadol; Tegafur; Tetrabenazine; Tetrahydrozoline (Nasal); Thioridazine; Tiotropium; Tricyclic Antidepressants; Tryptophan; Umeclidinium

Increased Effect/Toxicity

Tranylcypromine may increase the levels/effects of: Agomelatine; Alpha-/Beta-Agonists (Indirect-Acting); Alpha1-Agonists; Amphetamines; Analgesics (Opioid); Anticholinergics; Antidepressants (Serotonin Reuptake Inhibitor/Antagonist); Antihypertensives; Antipsychotics; Apraclonidine; AtoMOXetine; Beta2-Agonists; Betahistine; Bezafibrate; Brimonidine (Ophthalmic); Brimonidine (Topical);

BuPROPion; CYP1A2 Substrates; CYP2A6 Substrates; CYP2C19 Substrates; CYP2D6 Substrates; Dexmethylphenidate; Dextromethorphan; Diethylpropion; Dofetilide; Domperidone; Doxapram; Doxylamine; EPINEPHrine (Nasal); Epinephrine (Racemic); EPINEPHrine (Systemic, Oral Inhalation); Fesoterodine; Hydrocodone; HYDROmorphone; Hypoglycemic Agents; Isometheptene; Levonordefrin; Linezolid; Lithium; Lomitapide; Meperidine; Methadone; Methyldopa; Methylene Blue; Methylphenidate; Metoclopramide; Metoprolol; Mirtazapine; Morphine (Liposomal); Morphine (Systemic); Norepinephrine; Orthostatic Hypotension Producing Agents; OxyCODONE; Pirfenidone; Pizotifen; Reserpine; Selective Serotonin Reuptake Inhibitors; Serotonin 5-HT1D Receptor Agonists; Serotonin Modulators; Serotonin/Norepinephrine Reuptake Inhibitors; Tetrahydrozoline (Nasal); Thioridazine; Tiotropium; Tricyclic Antidepressants

The levels/effects of Tranylcypromine may be increased by: Aclidinium; Altretamine; Anilidopiperidine Opioids; Antipsychotics; Buprenorphine; BusPIRone; CarBAMazepine; COMT Inhibitors; Cyclobenzaprine; Ipratropium (Oral Inhalation); Levodopa; MAO Inhibitors; Maprotiline; Oxymorphone; Pramlintide; Propafenone; Tapentadol; Tetrabenazine; TraMADol; Tryptophan; Umeclidinium

Decreased Effect

Tranylcypromine may decrease the levels/effects of: Acetylcholinesterase Inhibitors (Central); Clopidogrel; Codeine; Domperidone; Tamoxifen; Tegafur

The levels/effects of Tranylcypromine may be decreased by: Acetylcholinesterase Inhibitors (Central); Domperidone

Ethanol/Nutrition/Herb Interactions

Ethanol: Ethanol may increase CNS depression. Beverages containing tyramine (eg, hearty red wine and beer) may increase toxic effects. Management: Avoid ethanol and beverages containing tyramine.

Food: Concurrent ingestion of foods rich in tyramine, dopamine, tyrosine, phenylalanine, tryptophan, or caffeine may cause sudden and severe high blood pressure (hypertensive crisis or serotonin syndrome). Management: Avoid tyramine-containing foods (aged or matured cheese, air-dried or cured meats including sausages and salamis; fava or broad bean pods, tap/draft beers, Marmite concentrate, sauerkraut, soy sauce, and other soybean condiments). Food's freshness is also an important concern; improperly stored or spoiled food can create an environment in which tyramine concentrations may increase. Avoid foods containing dopamine, tyrosine, phenylalanine, tryptophan, or caffeine.

Herb/Nutraceutical: Kava kava, valerian, St John's wort, and SAMe may increase risk of serotonin syndrome and/or excessive sedation. Supplements containing caffeine, tyrosine, tryptophan, or phenylalanine may increase the risk of severe side effects like hypertensive reactions or serotonin syndrome. Management: Avoid kava kava, valerian, St John's wort, SAMe, and supplements containing caffeine, tyrosine, tryptophan, or phenylalanine.

Storage/Stability Store at room temperature of 15°C to 30°C (59°F to 86°F).

Mechanism of Action Tranylcypromine is a nonhydrazine monoamine oxidase inhibitor. It increases endogenous concentrations of epinephrine, norepinephrine, dopamine, and serotonin through inhibition of the enzyme (monoamine oxidase) responsible for the breakdown of these neurotransmitters.

Pharmacodynamics/Kinetics

Onset of action: Therapeutic: 2 days to 3 weeks continued dosing

Duration: MAO inhibition may persist for up to 10 days following discontinuation

Half-life elimination: 90-190 minutes

Time to peak, serum: ~2 hours

Excretion: Urine

Dosage Adults: Oral: Usual effective dose: 30 mg/day in divided doses; if symptoms don't improve after 2 weeks, increase by 10 mg increments at 1- to 3-week intervals; maximum: 60 mg/day

Discontinuation of therapy: Upon discontinuation of antidepressant therapy, gradually taper the dose to minimize the incidence of withdrawal symptoms and allow for the detection of re-emerging symptoms. Evidence supporting ideal taper rates is limited. APA and NICE guidelines suggest tapering therapy over at least several weeks with consideration to the half-life of the antidepressant; antidepressants with a shorter half-life and MAO inhibitors may need to be tapered more conservatively. In addition for long-term treated patients, WFSBP guidelines recommend tapering over 4-6 months. If intolerable withdrawal symptoms occur following a dose reduction, consider resuming the previously prescribed dose and/or decrease dose at a more gradual rate (APA, 2010; Bauer, 2002; Haddad, 2001; NCCMH, 2010; Schatzberg, 2006; Shelton, 2001; Warner, 2006).

MAO inhibitor recommendations:

Switching to or from an MAO inhibitor intended to treat psychiatric disorders:

Allow 14 days to elapse between discontinuing an alternative antidepressant without long half-life metabolites (eg, TCAs, paroxetine, fluvoxamine, venlafaxine) or MAO inhibitor intended to treat psychiatric disorders and initiation of tranylcypromine.

Allow 5 weeks to elapse between discontinuing fluoxetine (with long half-life metabolites) intended to treat psychiatric disorders and initiation of tranylcypromine.

Allow at least 7-14 days days to elapse between discontinuing tranylcypromine and initiation of an alternative antidepressant or MAO inhibitor intended to treat psychiatric disorders.

Use with other MAO inhibitors (such as linezolid or I.V. methylene blue):

Do not initiate tranylcypromine in patients receiving linezolid or I.V. methylene blue; consider other interventions for psychiatric condition.

If urgent treatment with linezolid or I.V. methylene blue is required in a patient already receiving tranylcypromine and potential benefits outweigh potential risks, discontinue tranylcypromine promptly and administer linezolid or I.V. methylene blue. Monitor for serotonin syndrome for 2 weeks or until 24 hours after the last dose of linezolid or I.V. methylene blue, whichever comes first. May resume tranylcypromine 24 hours after the last dose of linezolid or I.V. methylene blue.

Dosage adjustment in renal impairment: No dosage adjustment provided in manufacturer's labeling.

Dosage adjustment in hepatic impairment: No dosage adjustment provided in manufacturer's labeling. Use is contraindicated in patients with a history of liver disease or abnormal liver function tests.

Dietary Considerations Avoid tyramine-containing foods/beverages. Some examples include aged or matured cheese, air-dried or cured meats (including sausages and salamis), fava or broad bean pods, tap/draft beers, Marmite concentrate, sauerkraut, soy sauce and other soybean condiments. Food's freshness is also an important concern; improperly stored or spoiled food can create an environment where tyramine concentrations may increase.

Monitoring Parameters Blood glucose; blood pressure, mental status, suicide ideation (especially at the beginning of therapy or when doses are increased or decreased)

Additional Information Tranylcypromine has a more rapid onset of therapeutic effect than other MAO inhibitors, but causes more severe hypertensive reactions.

Dosage Forms Excipient information presented when available (limited, particularly for generics); consult specific product labeling.

Tablet, Oral:

Parnate: 10 mg [contains fd&c blue #2 (indigotine), fd&c red #40, fd&c yellow #6 (sunset yellow)]

Generic: 10 mg

◆ **Tranylcypromine Sulfate** *see* Tranylcypromine *on page 2106*

Trastuzumab (tras TU zoo mab)

Brand Names: U.S. Herceptin

Brand Names: Canada Herceptin®

Index Terms anti-c-erB-2; anti-ERB-2; Conventional Trastuzumab; MOAB HER2; rhuMAb HER2; Trastuzumab (Conventional)

Pharmacologic Category Antineoplastic Agent, Anti-HER2; Antineoplastic Agent, Monoclonal Antibody; Monoclonal Antibody

Use Treatment (adjuvant) of HER2 overexpressing breast cancer as part of a combination regimen with doxorubicin, cyclophosphamide, and either paclitaxel or docetaxel; in combination with docetaxel and carboplatin; as a single agent following anthracycline-based combination treatment; treatment of HER2 overexpressing metastatic breast cancer in combination with paclitaxel as first-line treatment or as a single agent in patients who have received prior chemotherapy regimens for treatment of metastatic disease; treatment of HER2 overexpressing metastatic gastric or gastroesophageal junction adenocarcinoma in combination with cisplatin and either capecitabine or fluorouracil in patients who have not received prior treatment for metastatic disease

Unlabeled Use Treatment of HER2-positive metastatic breast cancer (in combination with pertuzumab and docetaxel) in patients who have not received prior anti-HER2 therapy or chemotherapy to treat metastatic disease; treatment of HER2 overexpressing metastatic breast cancer (in combination with lapatinib) which had progressed on prior trastuzumab containing therapy

Pregnancy Risk Factor D

Pregnancy Considerations Reproductive studies in cynomolgus monkeys showed no evidence of impaired fertility or fetal harm. However, trastuzumab inhibits HER2 protein, which has a role in embryonic development. **[U.S. Boxed Warning]: Trastuzumab exposure during pregnancy may result in oligohydramnios and oligohydramnios sequence (pulmonary hypoplasia, skeletal malformations and neonatal death).** Oligohydramnios (reversible in some cases) has been reported with trastuzumab use alone or with combination chemotherapy. If trastuzumab exposure occurs during pregnancy, monitor for oligohydramnios. Effective contraception is recommended during and for 6 months after treatment for women of childbearing potential. Women exposed to trastuzumab during pregnancy are encouraged to enroll in MotHER (the Herceptin Pregnancy Registry; 1-800-690-6720).

The National Comprehensive Cancer Network (NCCN) breast cancer guidelines (v.1.2013) consider pregnancy a contraindication to trastuzumab treatment and recommend (if indicated) administering trastuzumab in the postpartum period.

Breast-Feeding Considerations It is not known whether trastuzumab is secreted in human milk. Because many immunoglobulins are secreted in milk, and the potential for serious adverse reactions in the nursing infant exists, the decision to discontinue trastuzumab or discontinue breast-feeding during treatment should take in account the benefits of treatment to the mother. The extended half-life should also be considered for decisions regarding breast-feeding after therapy completion.

Contraindications There are no contraindications listed within the manufacturer's labeling.

Canadian labeling: Hypersensitivity to trastuzumab, Chinese hamster ovary (CHO) cell proteins, or any component of the formulation

Warnings/Precautions Hazardous agent - use appropriate precautions for handling and disposal (meets NIOSH, 2012 criteria). **[U.S. Boxed Warning]: Trastuzumab is associated with symptomatic and asymptomatic reductions in left ventricular ejection fraction (LVEF) and heart failure (HF); the incidence is highest in patients receiving trastuzumab with an anthracycline-containing chemotherapy regimen. Evaluate LVEF in all patients prior to and during treatment; discontinue for cardiomyopathy.** Extreme caution should be used in patients with pre-existing cardiac disease or dysfunction. Prior or concurrent exposure to anthracyclines or radiation therapy significantly increases the risk of cardiomyopathy; other potential risk factors include advanced age, high or low body mass index, smoking, diabetes, hypertension, and hyper-/hypothyroidism. Discontinuation should be strongly considered in patients who develop a clinically significant reduction in LVEF during therapy; treatment with HF medications (eg, ACE inhibitors, beta-blockers) should be initiated. Withhold treatment for ≥16% decrease from pretreatment levels or LVEF below normal limits and ≥10% decrease from baseline (see dosage adjustment for cardiotoxicity in Dosage). Cardiomyopathy due to trastuzumab is generally reversible over a period of 1-3 months after discontinuation. Trastuzumab is also associated with arrhythmias, hypertension, mural thrombus formation, stroke, and even cardiac death.

[U.S. Boxed Warning]: Serious adverse events, including hypersensitivity reaction (anaphylaxis), infusion reactions (including fatalities), and pulmonary events (including acute respiratory distress syndrome [ARDS]) have been associated with trastuzumab. Discontinue for anaphylaxis, angioedema, ARDS or interstitial pneumonitis. Most of these events occur with the first infusion; pulmonary events may occur during or within 24 hours of the first infusion; delayed reactions have occurred. Interrupt infusion for dyspnea or significant hypotension; monitor until symptoms resolve. Infusion reactions may consist of fever and chills, and may also include nausea, vomiting, pain, headache dizziness, dyspnea, hypotension, rash and weakness. Retreatment of patients who experienced severe hypersensitivity reactions has been attempted (with premedication). Some patients tolerated retreatment, while others experienced a second severe reaction. When used in combination with myelosuppressive chemotherapy, trastuzumab may increase the incidence of neutropenia (moderate-to-severe) and febrile neutropenia; the incidence of anemia may be higher when trastuzumab is added to chemotherapy. Rare cases of nephrotic syndrome with evidence of glomerulopathy have been reported, with an onset of 4-18 months from trastuzumab initiation; complications may include volume overload and HF. The incidence of renal impairment was increased in metastatic gastric cancer patients when trastuzumab is added to chemotherapy.

May cause serious pulmonary toxicity (dyspnea, hypoxia, interstitial pneumonitis, pulmonary infiltrates, pleural effusion, noncardiogenic pulmonary edema, pulmonary insufficiency, acute respiratory distress syndrome, and/or pulmonary fibrosis); use caution in patients with pre-existing pulmonary disease or patients with extensive pulmonary tumor involvement. Establish HER2 status prior to treatment; has only been studied in patients with evidence of HER2 protein overexpression, either by validated immunohistochemistry (IHC) assay or fluorescence in situ hybridization (FISH) assay. Tests appropriate for the specific tumor type (breast or gastric) should be used to assess HER2 status. **[U.S. Boxed Warning]: Trastuzumab exposure during pregnancy may result in oligohydramnios and oligohydramnios sequence (pulmonary hypoplasia, skeletal malformations and neonatal death).** Effective contraception is recommended during and for 6 months after treatment for women of childbearing potential. Conventional trastuzumab and ado-trastuzumab emtansine are **not** interchangeable; verify product label prior to reconstitution and administration to prevent medication errors.

Adverse Reactions Note: Percentages reported with single-agent therapy.

>10%:

Cardiovascular: LVEF decreased (4% to 22%)

Central nervous system: Pain (47%), fever (6% to 36%), chills (5% to 32%), headache (10% to 26%), insomnia (14%), dizziness (4% to 13%)

Dermatologic: Rash (4% to 18%)

Gastrointestinal: Nausea (6% to 33%), diarrhea (7% to 25%), vomiting (4% to 23%), abdominal pain (2% to 22%), anorexia (14%)

Neuromuscular & skeletal: Weakness (4% to 42%), back pain (5% to 22%)

Respiratory: Cough (5% to 26%), dyspnea (3% to 22%), rhinitis (2% to 14%), pharyngitis (12%)

Miscellaneous: Infusion reaction (21% to 40%, chills and fever most common; severe: 1%), infection (20%)

1% to 10%:

Cardiovascular: Peripheral edema (5% to 10%), edema (8%), HF (2% to 7%; severe: <1%), tachycardia (5%), hypertension (4%), arrhythmia (3%), palpitation (3%)

Central nervous system: Depression (6%)

Dermatologic: Acne (2%), nail disorder (2%), pruritus (2%)

Gastrointestinal: Constipation (2%), dyspepsia (2%)

Genitourinary: Urinary tract infection (3% to 5%)

Hematologic: Anemia (4%), leukopenia (3%)

Neuromuscular & skeletal: Paresthesia (2% to 9%), bone pain (3% to 7%), arthralgia (6% to 8%), myalgia (4%), muscle spasm (3%), peripheral neuritis (2%), neuropathy (1%)

Respiratory: Sinusitis (2% to 9%), nasopharyngitis (8%), upper respiratory infection (3%), epistaxis (2%), pharyngolaryngeal pain (2%)

Miscellaneous: Flu-like syndrome (2% to 10%), accidental injury (6%), influenza (4%), allergic reaction (3%), herpes simplex (2%)

<1% (Limited to important or life-threatening; as a single-agent or with combination chemotherapy): Acute respiratory distress syndrome (ARDS), amblyopia, anaphylaxis, anaphylactoid reaction, angioedema, apnea, ascites, asthma, ataxia, bone necrosis, bronchospasm, cardiac arrest, cardiomyopathy, cellulitis, coagulopathy, colitis, confusion, deafness, esophageal ulcer, gastroenteritis, glomerulonephritis (membraneous, focal and fibrillary), glomerulopathy, glomerulosclerosis, hematemesis, hemorrhage, hemorrhagic cystitis, hepatic failure, hepatitis, herpes zoster, hydrocephalus, hydronephrosis, hypercalcemia, hypersensitivity, hypotension, hypothyroidism, hypoxia, ileus, intestinal obstruction, interstitial pneumonitis, laryngitis, leukemia (acute), lymphangitis, mania, mural thrombosis, myopathy, nephrotic syndrome, neutropenia, oligohydramnios, pancreatitis, pancytopenia, paroxysmal nocturnal dyspnea, pathological fracture, pericardial effusion, pleural effusion, pneumonitis, pneumothorax, pulmonary edema (noncardiogenic), pulmonary fibrosis, pulmonary hypertension, pulmonary infiltrate, pyelonephritis, radiation injury, renal failure, respiratory distress, respiratory failure, seizure, sepsis, shock, skin ulcers, stroke, syncope, stomatitis, thyroiditis (autoimmune), vascular thrombosis, ventricular dysfunction, volume overload

Drug Interactions

Metabolism/Transport Effects None known.

Avoid Concomitant Use

Avoid concomitant use of Trastuzumab with any of the following: Belimumab

Increased Effect/Toxicity

Trastuzumab may increase the levels/effects of: Antineoplastic Agents (Anthracycline, Systemic); Belimumab; Immunosuppressants

The levels/effects of Trastuzumab may be increased by: Abciximab; PACLitaxel

Decreased Effect

Trastuzumab may decrease the levels/effects of: PACLitaxel

Preparation for Administration Hazardous agent; use appropriate precautions for handling and disposal (meets NIOSH, 2012 criteria). Check vial labels to assure appropriate product is being reconstituted (conventional trastuzumab and ado-trastuzumab emtansine are different products and are **NOT** interchangeable).

Reconstitute each vial with 20 mL of bacteriostatic sterile water for injection to a concentration of 21 mg/mL. Swirl gently; do not shake. Allow vial to rest for ~5 minutes. If the patient has a known hypersensitivity to benzyl alcohol, trastuzumab may be reconstituted with sterile water for injection without preservatives, which must be used immediately. Further dilute the appropriate volume for the trastuzumab dose in 250 mL NS prior to administration. Gently invert bag to mix.

Storage/Stability Prior to reconstitution, store intact vials under refrigeration at 2°C to 8°C (36°F to 46°F). Following reconstitution with bacteriostatic SWFI, the solution in the vial is stable refrigerated for 28 days from the date of reconstitution; do not freeze. Solutions reconstituted with sterile water for injection without preservatives must be used immediately. The solution diluted in 250 mL NS for infusion is stable for 24 hours refrigerated; do not freeze.

Mechanism of Action Trastuzumab is a monoclonal antibody which binds to the extracellular domain of the human epidermal growth factor receptor 2 protein (HER-2); it mediates antibody-dependent cellular cytotoxicity by inhibiting proliferation of cells which overexpress HER-2 protein.

Pharmacodynamics/Kinetics

Distribution: V_d: 44 mL/kg; not likely to cross the (intact) blood-brain barrier (due to the large molecule size)

Half-life elimination: Weekly dosing: Mean: 6 days (range: 1-32 days); every 3 week regimen: Mean: 16 days (range: 11-23 days)

Dosage Note: Do **NOT** substitute conventional trastuzumab for or with ado-trastuzumab emtansine; products are different and are **NOT** interchangeable. Adults: I.V. infusion: Details concerning dosing in combination regimens should also be consulted.

Breast cancer, adjuvant treatment, HER2+:

With concurrent paclitaxel or docetaxel:

Initial loading dose: 4 mg/kg infused over 90 minutes, followed by

Maintenance dose: 2 mg/kg infused over 30 minutes weekly for total of 12 weeks, followed 1 week later (when concurrent chemotherapy completed) by 6 mg/kg infused over 30-90 minutes every 3 weeks for total therapy duration of 52 weeks

With concurrent docetaxel/carboplatin:
Initial loading dose: 4 mg/kg infused over 90 minutes, followed by
Maintenance dose: 2 mg/kg infused over 30 minutes weekly for total of 18 weeks, followed 1 week later (when concurrent chemotherapy completed) by 6 mg/kg infused over 30-90 minutes every 3 weeks for total therapy duration of 52 weeks

Following completion of anthracycline-based chemotherapy:
Initial loading dose: 8 mg/kg infused over 90 minutes, followed by
Maintenance dose: 6 mg/kg infused over 30-90 minutes every 3 weeks for total therapy duration of 52 weeks

Breast cancer, metastatic, HER2+ (either as a single agent or in combination with paclitaxel):
Initial loading dose: 4 mg/kg infused over 90 minutes, followed by
Maintenance dose: 2 mg/kg infused over 30 minutes weekly until disease progression

Gastric cancer, metastatic, HER2+ (in combination with cisplatin and either capecitabine or fluorouracil for 6 cycles followed by trastuzumab monotherapy; Bang, 2010; Van Cutsem, 2009):
Initial loading dose: 8 mg/kg infused over 90 minutes, followed by
Maintenance dose: 6 mg/kg infused over 30-90 minutes every 3 weeks until disease progression

Missed doses *(Canadian labeling, 2012):* If a dose is missed by ≤1 week, the usual maintenance dose (based on patient's schedule) should be administered as soon as possible (do not wait until the next planned cycle); if a dose is missed by >1 week, then a loading dose (4 mg/kg if patient receives trastuzumab weekly; 8 mg/kg if on an every-3-week schedule) should be administered, followed by the usual maintenance dose and schedule.

Breast cancer, metastatic, HER2+ (unlabeled combinations):
Trastuzumab, pertuzumab, and docetaxel (in patients with no prior anti-HER2 therapy or chemotherapy to treat metastatic disease): Initial: 8 mg/kg followed by a maintenance dose of 6 mg/kg every 3 weeks until disease progression or unacceptable toxicity (Baselga, 2012)
Trastuzumab and lapatinib (in patients with progression on prior trastuzumab containing therapy): Initial: 4 mg/kg followed by a maintenance dose of 2 mg/kg every week (Blackwell, 2010; Blackwell, 2012)

Dosage adjustment for toxicity:
Cardiotoxicity: LVEF ≥16% decrease from baseline or LVEF below normal limits and ≥10% decrease from baseline: Withhold treatment for at least 4 weeks and repeat LVEF every 4 weeks. May resume trastuzumab treatment if LVEF returns to normal limits within 4-8 weeks and remains at ≤15% decrease from baseline value. Discontinue permanently for persistent (>8 weeks) LVEF decline or for >3 incidents of treatment interruptions for cardiomyopathy.
Infusion-related events:
Mild-moderate infusion reactions: Decrease infusion rate
Dyspnea, clinically significant hypotension: Interrupt infusion
Severe or life-threatening infusion reactions: Discontinue

Dosing adjustment in renal impairment: No dosage adjustment provided in manufacturer's labeling, although data suggest that the disposition of trastuzumab is not altered based on serum creatinine (up to 2 mg/dL).

Dosing adjustment in hepatic impairment: No dosage adjustment provided in manufacturer's labeling.

Administration Check label to ensure appropriate product is being administered (conventional trastuzumab and ado-trastuzumab are different products and are **NOT** interchangeable).

Administered by I.V. infusion; loading doses are infused over 90 minutes; maintenance doses may be infused over 30 minutes if tolerated. Do not administer with D_5W. **Do not administer I.V. push or by rapid bolus.**

Observe patients closely during the infusion for fever, chills, or other infusion-related symptoms. Treatment with acetaminophen, diphenhydramine, and/or meperidine is usually effective for managing infusion-related events.

Hazardous agent; use appropriate precautions for handling and disposal (meets NIOSH, 2012 criteria).

Monitoring Parameters Assessment for HER2 overexpression and HER2 gene amplification by validated immunohistochemistry (IHC) or fluorescence *in situ* hybridization (FISH) methodology (pretherapy); test should be specific for cancer type (breast vs gastric cancer). Pregnancy test (prior to treatment). Monitor vital signs during infusion; signs and symptoms of cardiac dysfunction; LVEF (baseline, every 3 months during treatment, upon therapy completion and if component of adjuvant therapy, every 6 months for at least 2 years; if treatment is withheld for significant LVEF dysfunction, monitor LVEF at 4-week intervals); signs and symptoms of infusion reaction; if pregnancy inadvertently occurs during treatment, monitor amniotic fluid volume

Dosage Forms Excipient information presented when available (limited, particularly for generics); consult specific product labeling.
Solution Reconstituted, Intravenous:
Herceptin: 440 mg (1 ea) [contains benzyl alcohol]

◆ **Trastuzumab-MCC-DM1** *see* Ado-Trastuzumab Emtansine *on page 52*
◆ **Trastuzumab (Conventional)** *see* Trastuzumab *on page 2109*
◆ **Trastuzumab-DM1** *see* Ado-Trastuzumab Emtansine *on page 52*
◆ **Trastuzumab Emtansine** *see* Ado-Trastuzumab Emtansine *on page 52*
◆ **Trasylol** *see* Aprotinin *on page 159*
◆ **Trasylol® (Can)** *see* Aprotinin *on page 159*
◆ **Travatan Z** *see* Travoprost *on page 2111*
◆ **Travatan Z® (Can)** *see* Travoprost *on page 2111*
◆ **Travel Sickness [OTC]** *see* Meclizine *on page 1277*
◆ **Travel Tabs [OTC] (Can)** *see* DimenhyDRINATE *on page 616*

Travoprost (TRA voe prost)

Brand Names: U.S. Travatan Z
Brand Names: Canada Travatan Z®
Pharmacologic Category Ophthalmic Agent, Antiglaucoma; Prostaglandin, Ophthalmic
Use Reduction of elevated intraocular pressure in patients with open-angle glaucoma or ocular hypertension
Pregnancy Risk Factor C
Dosage
U.S. labeling: Glaucoma (open angle) or ocular hypertension: Adolescents ≥16 years and Adults: Ophthalmic: Instill 1 drop into affected eye(s) once daily in the evening; do not exceed once-daily dosing (may decrease IOP-lowering effect).

Canadian labeling: Glaucoma (open angle) or ocular hypertension: Adults: Ophthalmic: Instill 1 drop into affected eye(s) once daily in the evening; do not exceed once-daily dosing (may decrease IOP-lowering effect).

Dosage adjustment in renal impairment: No dosage adjustment necessary.

Dosage adjustment in hepatic impairment: No dosage adjustment necessary.

Additional Information Complete prescribing information should be consulted for additional detail.

Dosage Forms Excipient information presented when available (limited, particularly for generics); consult specific product labeling.

Solution, Ophthalmic:

Travatan Z: 0.004% (2.5 mL, 5 mL) [benzalkonium free]

Generic: 0.004% (2.5 mL, 5 mL)

TraZODone (TRAZ oh done)

Brand Names: U.S. Oleptro [DSC]

Brand Names: Canada Apo-Trazodone D®; Apo-Trazodone®; Dom-Trazodone; Mylan-Trazodone; Novo-Trazodone; Nu-Trazodone; Nu-Trazodone D; Oleptro™; PHL-Trazodone; PMS-Trazodone; ratio-Trazodone; Teva-Trazodone; Trazorel®; ZYM-Trazodone

Index Terms Desyrel; Trazodone Hydrochloride

Pharmacologic Category Antidepressant, Serotonin Reuptake Inhibitor/Antagonist

Additional Appendix Information

Antidepressant Agents *on page 2284*

Use Treatment of major depressive disorder

Unlabeled Use Potential augmenting agent for antidepressants, hypnotic

Pregnancy Risk Factor C

Pregnancy Considerations Adverse effects were observed in some animal reproduction studies. When trazodone is taken during pregnancy, an increased risk of major malformations has not been observed in the limited number of pregnancies studied (Einarson, 2003; Einarson, 2009). The long-term effects of *in utero* trazodone exposure on infant development and behavior are not known.

The ACOG recommends that therapy with antidepressants during pregnancy be individualized; treatment of depression during pregnancy should incorporate the clinical expertise of the mental health clinician, obstetrician, primary healthcare provider, and pediatrician. According to the American Psychiatric Association (APA), the risks of medication treatment should be weighed against other treatment options and untreated depression. Consideration should be given to using agents with safety data in pregnancy. For women who discontinue antidepressant medications during pregnancy and who may be at high risk for postpartum depression, the medications can be restarted following delivery. Treatment algorithms have been developed by the ACOG and the APA for the management of depression in women prior to conception and during pregnancy (ACOG, 2008; APA, 2010; Yonkers, 2009).

Breast-Feeding Considerations Trazodone is excreted into breast milk; breast milk concentrations peak ~2 hours following administration. It is not known if the trazodone metabolite is found in breast milk (Verbeeck, 1986). The long-term effects on neurobehavior have not been studied. The manufacturer recommends that caution be exercised when administering trazodone to nursing women.

Medication Guide Available Yes

Contraindications Hypersensitivity to trazodone or any component of the formulation; use of MAO inhibitors intended to treat psychiatric disorders (concurrently or within 14 days of discontinuing either trazodone or the MAO inhibitor); initiation of trazodone in a patient receiving linezolid or intravenous methylene blue

Warnings/Precautions [U.S. Boxed Warning]: Antidepressants increase the risk of suicidal thinking and behavior in children, adolescents, and young adults (18-24 years of age) with major depressive disorder (MDD) and other psychiatric disorders; consider risk prior to prescribing. Short-term studies did not show an increased risk in patients >24 years of age and showed a decreased risk in patients ≥65 years of age. Closely monitor for clinical worsening, suicidality, or unusual changes in behavior; the patient's family or caregiver should be instructed to closely observe the patient and communicate condition with healthcare provider. A medication guide should be dispensed with each prescription. **Trazodone is not FDA approved for use in children.**

The possibility of a suicide attempt is inherent in major depression and may persist until remission occurs. Monitor for worsening of depression or suicidality, especially during initiation of therapy (generally first 1-2 months) or with dose increases or decreases. Use caution in high-risk patients. Worsening depression and severe abrupt suicidality that are not part of the presenting symptoms may require discontinuation or modification of drug therapy. The patient's family or caregiver should be alerted to monitor patients for the emergence of suicidality and associated behaviors (such as agitation, irritability, hostility, impulsivity, and hypomania) and call healthcare provider.

May worsen psychosis in some patients or precipitate a shift to mania or hypomania in patients with bipolar disorder. Patients presenting with depressive symptoms should be screened for bipolar disorder. Monotherapy in patients with bipolar disorder should be avoided. **Trazodone is not FDA approved for the treatment of bipolar depression.**

Priapism, including cases resulting in permanent dysfunction, has occurred with the use of trazodone. Instruct patient to seek medical assistance for erection lasting >4 hours; use with caution in patients who have conditions which may predispose them to priapism (eg, sickle cell anemia, multiple myeloma, leukemia). Not recommended for use in a patient during the acute recovery phase of MI. The risks of sedation, postural hypotension, and/or syncope are high relative to other antidepressants. Trazodone frequently causes sedation, which may result in impaired performance of tasks requiring alertness (eg, operating machinery or driving).

Use with caution in patients with a history of cardiovascular disease (including previous MI, stroke, tachycardia, or conduction abnormalities). Although the risk of conduction abnormalities with this agent is low relative to other antidepressants, QT prolongation (with or without torsade de pointes), ventricular tachycardia, and other arrhythmias have been observed with the use of trazodone (reports limited to immediate-release formulation); use with caution in patients with pre-existing cardiac disease. May impair platelet aggregation resulting in increased risk of bleeding events (eg, epistaxis, life threatening bleeding).

Potentially life-threatening serotonin syndrome (SS) has occurred with serotonergic agents (eg, SSRIs, SNRIs), particularly when used in combination with other serotonergic agents (eg, triptans, TCAs, fentanyl, lithium, tramadol, buspirone, St John's wort, tryptophan) or agents that impair metabolism of serotonin (eg, MAO inhibitors intended to treat psychiatric disorders, other MAO inhibitors [ie, linezolid and intravenous methylene blue]).

Discontinue treatment (and any concomitant serotonergic agent) immediately if signs/symptoms arise.

Serotonin syndrome (SS)/neuroleptic malignant syndrome (NMS)-like reactions may occur with trazodone when used alone, particularly if used with other serotonergic agents (eg, serotonin/norepinephrine reuptake inhibitors [SNRIs], selective serotonin reuptake inhibitors [SSRIs], or triptans), drugs that impair serotonin metabolism (eg, MAO inhibitors), or antidopaminergic agents (eg, antipsychotics). If concurrent use is clinically warranted, carefully observe patient during treatment initiation and dose increases. Do not use concurrently with serotonin precursors (eg, tryptophan).

Use caution in patients with a previous seizure disorder or condition predisposing to seizures such as brain damage, or alcoholism. Bone fractures have been associated with antidepressant treatment. Consider the possibility of a fragility fracture if an antidepressant-treated patient presents with unexplained bone pain, point tenderness, swelling, or bruising (Rabenda, 2013; Rizzoli, 2012). Use with caution in patients with hepatic or renal dysfunction and in elderly patients. May cause SIADH and hyponatremia, predominantly in the elderly; volume depletion and/or concurrent use of diuretics likely increases risk. Potentially significant drug-drug interactions may exist, requiring dose or frequency adjustment, additional monitoring, and/or selection of alternative therapy.

Abrupt discontinuation or interruption of antidepressant therapy has been associated with a discontinuation syndrome. Symptoms arising may vary with antidepressant however commonly include nausea, vomiting, diarrhea, headaches, lightheadedness, dizziness, diminished appetite, sweating, chills, tremors, paresthesias, fatigue, somnolence, and sleep disturbances (eg, vivid dreams, insomnia). Greater risks for developing a discontinuation syndrome have been associated with antidepressants with shorter half-lives, longer durations of treatment, and abrupt discontinuation. For antidepressants of short or intermediate half-lives, symptoms may emerge within 2-5 days after treatment discontinuation and last 7-14 days (APA, 2010; Fava, 2006; Haddad, 2001; Shelton, 2001; Warner, 2006).

Adverse Reactions

>10%:

- Central nervous system: Sedation (≤46%), headache (10% to 33%), dizziness (20% to 28%), fatigue (6% to 15%)
- Gastrointestinal: Xerostomia (15% to 34%), nausea (10% to 21%)
- Ocular: Blurred vision (5% to 15%)

1% to 10%:

- Cardiovascular: Edema (3% to 7%), hypotension (≤7%), syncope (≤5%), hypertension (1% to 2%)
- Central nervous system: Confusion (5% to 6%), incoordination (2% to 5%), concentration decreased (1% to 3%), disorientation (≤2%), memory impairment (≤1%), agitation, migraine
- Endocrine & metabolic: Libido decreased (1% to 2%)
- Gastrointestinal: Diarrhea (5% to 9%), constipation (7% to 8%), abdominal pain, abnormal taste, flatulence, vomiting, weight gain/loss
- Genitourinary: Ejaculation disorder (2%), urinary urgency
- Neuromuscular & skeletal: Back pain (≤5%), tremor (1% to 5%), paresthesia (≤1%), myalgia
- Ocular: Visual disturbance
- Respiratory: Nasal congestion (3% to 6%), dyspnea
- Miscellaneous: Night sweats

<1% (Limited to important or life-threatening): Abnormal dreams, abnormal orgasm, acne, akathisia, allergic reactions, alopecia, amylase increased, anemia, anxiety, aphasia, apnea, appetite increased, arrhythmia, ataxia, atrial fibrillation, bladder pain, bradycardia, breast enlargement/engorgement, cardiac arrest, cardiospasm, cerebrovascular accident, chest pain, CHF, chills, cholestasis, clitorism, conduction block, diplopia, early menses, erectile dysfunction, extrapyramidal symptoms, eye pain, flushing, gait disturbance, hallucination, hearing loss (partial), hematuria, hemolytic anemia, hepatitis, hirsutism, hyperbilirubinemia, hyperhidrosis, hypersalivation, hypersensitivity, hypoesthesia, hypomania, impaired speech, impotence, insomnia, jaundice, lactation, leukocytosis, leukonychia, libido increased, liver enzyme alteration, methemoglobinemia, MI, muscle twitching, orthostatic hypotension, palpitation, paranoia, photophobia, photosensitivity reaction, priapism, pruritus, psoriasis, psychosis, QT prolongation, rash, reflux esophagitis, retrograde ejaculation, salivation increased, seizure, SIADH, speech impairment, stupor, tachycardia, tardive dyskinesia, tinnitus, torsade de pointes, urinary frequency increased, urinary retention, urinary incontinence, urticaria, vasodilation, ventricular ectopy, ventricular tachycardia, vertigo, dry eyes, weakness

Drug Interactions

Metabolism/Transport Effects Substrate of CYP2D6 (minor), CYP3A4 (major); **Note:** Assignment of Major/Minor substrate status based on clinically relevant drug interaction potential; **Inhibits** CYP3A4 (weak); **Induces** P-glycoprotein

Avoid Concomitant Use

Avoid concomitant use of TraZODone with any of the following: Conivaptan; Fusidic Acid (Systemic); Highest Risk QTc-Prolonging Agents; Ivabradine; Linezolid; MAO Inhibitors; Methylene Blue; Mifepristone; Saquinavir

Increased Effect/Toxicity

TraZODone may increase the levels/effects of: Antipsychotic Agents (Phenothiazines); Antipsychotics; Fosphenytoin; Highest Risk QTc-Prolonging Agents; Lomitapide; Methylene Blue; Metoclopramide; Moderate Risk QTc-Prolonging Agents; Phenytoin; Serotonin Modulators

The levels/effects of TraZODone may be increased by: Antipsychotic Agents (Phenothiazines); Antipsychotics; Atazanavir; Boceprevir; BusPIRone; Cobicistat; Conivaptan; CYP3A4 Inhibitors (Moderate); CYP3A4 Inhibitors (Strong); Darunavir; Dasatinib; Fosamprenavir; Fusidic Acid (Systemic); Indinavir; Ivabradine; Ivacaftor; Linezolid; Lopinavir; Luliconazole; MAO Inhibitors; Mifepristone; Nelfinavir; QTc-Prolonging Agents (Indeterminate Risk and Risk Modifying); Saquinavir; Selective Serotonin Reuptake Inhibitors; Simeprevir; Telaprevir; Tipranavir; Venlafaxine

Decreased Effect

TraZODone may decrease the levels/effects of: Warfarin

The levels/effects of TraZODone may be decreased by: Bosentan; CYP3A4 Inducers (Strong); Dabrafenib; Deferasirox; Fosphenytoin; Mitotane; Peginterferon Alfa-2b; Phenytoin; Tocilizumab

Ethanol/Nutrition/Herb Interactions

Ethanol: May increase CNS depression; monitor for increased effects with coadministration. Caution patients about effects.

Food: Time to peak serum levels may be increased if immediate release trazodone is taken with food.

Herb/Nutraceutical: Avoid valerian, St John's wort, tryptophan, SAMe, kava kava (may increase risk of serotonin syndrome and/or excessive sedation).

Storage/Stability

Immediate release tablet: Store at room temperature; avoid temperatures >40°C (>104°F). Protect from light.

Extended release tablet: Store at room temperature of 15°C to 30°C (59°F to 86°F). Protect from light.

Mechanism of Action Inhibits reuptake of serotonin, causes adrenoreceptor subsensitivity, and induces significant changes in 5-HT presynaptic receptor adrenoreceptors. Trazodone also significantly blocks histamine (H_1) and alpha$_1$-adrenergic receptors.

Pharmacodynamics/Kinetics

Onset of action: Therapeutic (antidepressant): Up to 6 weeks; sleep aid: 1-3 hours

Absorption: Well absorbed; Extended release: C_{max} increases ~86% when taken shortly after ingestion of a high-fat meal compared to fasting conditions

Protein binding: 85% to 95%

Metabolism: Hepatic via CYP3A4 (extensive) to an active metabolite (mCPP)

Half-life elimination: 7-10 hours

Time to peak, serum:

Immediate release: 30-100 minutes; delayed with food (up to 2.5 hours)

Extended release: 9 hours; not significantly affected by food

Excretion: Primarily urine (<1% excreted unchanged); secondarily feces

Dosage Oral: Therapeutic effects may take up to 6 weeks to occur; therapy is normally maintained for 6-12 months after optimum response is reached to prevent recurrence of depression

Children 6-12 years: Depression (unlabeled use): Initial: 1.5-2 mg/kg/day in divided doses; increase gradually every 3-4 days as needed; maximum: 6 mg/kg/day in 3 divided doses

Adolescents: Depression (unlabeled use): Initial: 25-50 mg/day; increase to 100-150 mg/day in divided doses

Adults:

Depression: Initial: 150 mg/day in 3 divided doses (may increase by 50 mg/day every 3-7 days); maximum dose: 600 mg/day

Extended release formulation: Initial: 150 mg once daily at bedtime (may increase by 75 mg/day every 3 days); maximum dose: 375 mg/day; once adequate response obtained, gradually reduce with adjustment based on therapeutic response

Note: Therapeutic effects may take up to 6 weeks. Therapy is normally maintained for 6-12 months after optimum response is reached to prevent recurrence of depression.

Sedation/hypnotic (unlabeled use): 25-50 mg at bedtime (often in combination with daytime SSRIs); may increase up to 200 mg at bedtime

Elderly: 25-50 mg at bedtime with 25-50 mg/day dose increase every 3 days for inpatients and weekly for outpatients, if tolerated; usual dose: 75-150 mg/day

Discontinuation of therapy: Upon discontinuation of antidepressant therapy, gradually taper the dose to minimize the incidence of withdrawal symptoms and allow for the detection of re-emerging symptoms. Evidence supporting ideal taper rates is limited. APA and NICE guidelines suggest tapering therapy over at least several weeks with consideration to the half-life of the antidepressant; antidepressants with a shorter half-life may need to be tapered more conservatively. In addition for long-term treated patients, WFSBP guidelines recommend tapering over 4-6 months. If intolerable withdrawal symptoms occur following a dose reduction, consider resuming the previously prescribed dose and/or decrease dose at a more gradual rate (APA, 2010; Bauer, 2002; Haddad, 2001; NCCMH, 2010; Schatzberg, 2006; Shelton, 2001; Warner, 2006)

MAO inhibitor recommendations:

Switching to or from an MAO inhibitor intended to treat psychiatric disorders:

Allow 14 days to elapse between discontinuing an MAO inhibitor intended to treat psychiatric disorders and initiation of trazodone.

Allow 14 days to elapse between discontinuing trazodone and initiation of an MAO inhibitor intended to treat psychiatric disorders.

Use with other MAO inhibitors (linezolid or I.V. methylene blue):

Do not initiate trazodone in patients receiving linezolid or I.V. methylene blue; consider other interventions for psychiatric condition.

If urgent treatment with linezolid or I.V. methylene blue is required in a patient already receiving trazodone and potential benefits outweigh potential risks, discontinue trazodone promptly and administer linezolid or I.V. methylene blue. Monitor for serotonin syndrome for 2 weeks or until 24 hours after the last dose of linezolid or I.V. methylene blue, whichever comes first. May resume trazodone 24 hours after the last dose of linezolid or I.V. methylene blue.

Dosage adjustment in renal impairment: No dosage adjustment provided in manufacturer's labeling (has not been studied). Use with caution.

Dosage adjustment in hepatic impairment: No dosage adjustment provided in manufacturer's labeling (has not been studied). Use with caution.

Administration

Immediate release tablet: Dosing after meals may decrease lightheadedness and postural hypotension

Extended release tablet: Take on an empty stomach; swallow whole or as a half tablet without food. Tablet may be broken along the score line, but do not crush or chew.

Monitoring Parameters Baseline liver function prior to and periodically during therapy; suicide ideation (especially at the beginning of therapy or when doses are increased or decreased); suicide ideation (especially at the beginning of therapy or when doses are increased or decreased); signs/symptoms of serotonin syndrome

Reference Range

Plasma levels do not always correlate with clinical effectiveness

Therapeutic: 0.5-2.5 mcg/mL

Potentially toxic: >2.5 mcg/mL

Toxic: >4 mcg/mL

Test Interactions May interfere with urine detection of amphetamine/methamphetamine (false-positive).

Dosage Forms Excipient information presented when available (limited, particularly for generics); consult specific product labeling. [DSC] = Discontinued product

Tablet, Oral:

Generic: 50 mg, 100 mg, 150 mg, 300 mg

Tablet, Oral, as hydrochloride:

Generic: 50 mg, 100 mg, 150 mg, 300 mg

Tablet Extended Release 24 Hour, Oral, as hydrochloride:

Oleptro: 150 mg [DSC], 300 mg [DSC] [scored]

◆ **Trazodone Hydrochloride** *see* TraZODone *on page 2112*

◆ **Trazorel® (Can)** *see* TraZODone *on page 2112*

◆ **Treanda** *see* Bendamustine *on page 237*

◆ **Trelstar® (Can)** *see* Triptorelin *on page 2131*

◆ **Trelstar Depot** *see* Triptorelin *on page 2131*

◆ **Trelstar Depot Mixject** *see* Triptorelin *on page 2131*

◆ **Trelstar LA** *see* Triptorelin *on page 2131*

◆ **Trelstar LA Mixject** *see* Triptorelin *on page 2131*

◆ **Trelstar Mixject** *see* Triptorelin *on page 2131*

◆ Tremytoine Inj (Can) *see* Phenytoin *on page 1638*

◆ TRENtal [DSC] *see* Pentoxifylline *on page 1619*

Treprostinil (tre PROST in il)

Brand Names: U.S. Remodulin; Tyvaso; Tyvaso Refill; Tyvaso Starter

Brand Names: Canada Remodulin

Index Terms Orenitram; Treprostinil Sodium

Pharmacologic Category Prostacyclin; Prostaglandin; Vasodilator

Use

Injection: Treatment of pulmonary arterial hypertension (PAH) (WHO Group I) in patients with NYHA Class II-IV symptoms to decrease exercise-associated symptoms; to diminish clinical deterioration when transitioning from epoprostenol (I.V.)

Inhalation: Treatment of pulmonary arterial hypertension (PAH) (WHO Group I) in patients with NYHA Class III symptoms to improve exercise ability. **Note:** Nearly all controlled clinical trial experience has been with concomitant bosentan or sildenafil.

Pregnancy Risk Factor B

Pregnancy Considerations Some skeletal malformations and maternal toxicity noted in animal studies. There are no adequate and well-controlled studies in pregnant women. Use with caution and only if clearly needed.

Breast-Feeding Considerations It is not known if treprostinil is excreted in breast milk. The manufacturer recommends that caution be exercised when administering treprostinil to nursing women

Contraindications There are no contraindications listed in the FDA-approved labeling.

Warnings/Precautions May produce symptomatic hypotension; use with caution in patients with low systemic arterial blood pressure. Abrupt withdrawal/large dosage reductions may worsen symptoms of PAH. If a SubQ or I.V. infusion is restarted within a few hours of discontinuation, the same dose rate may be used. Interruptions for longer periods may require retitration. Regardless of administration route (inhalation, I.V., or SubQ), treatment interruptions should be avoided. Immediate access to medication, back-up inhalation device, or pump and infusion sets is essential to prevent treatment interruptions. Chronic continuous I.V. infusion of treprostinil via a chronic indwelling central venous catheter has been associated with serious blood stream infections. This method of administration should be reserved for patients who are intolerant of the SubQ route or in whom the benefit outweighs the potential risks. Treprostinil should only be used by clinicians experienced in the treatment of PAH. Prior to initiation, patients should be carefully evaluated for ability to administer treprostinil, either as an I.V./SubQ infusion or inhalation, and care for the infusion system/inhalation device. Initiation of infusion must occur in a setting where adequate personnel and equipment necessary for hemodynamic monitoring and emergency treatment is available. Use with caution in patients with hepatic impairment; dose reduction is recommended for the initial dose (I.V./SubQ) in patients with mild-to-moderate hepatic insufficiency; titrate dose slowly in patients with hepatic insufficiency; has not been studied in severe hepatic impairment. Has not been studied in renal impairment; use with caution in renal impairment; titrate dose slowly in patients with renal insufficiency. Use with caution in patients ≥65 years of age. Inhalation: Safety and efficacy have not been established in patients with underlying pulmonary disease (eg, asthma, COPD). Patients with acute pulmonary infections should be monitored closely for exacerbation or reduced efficacy. Treprostinil inhibits platelet aggregation, increasing the risk of bleeding; use with caution in patients receiving concurrent anticoagulant/antiplatelet therapy.

Adverse Reactions

>10%:

- Cardiovascular: Flushing (11%; inhalation: 15%)
- Central nervous system: Headache (27% to 41%)
- Dermatologic: Rash (14%)
- Gastrointestinal: Diarrhea (25%), nausea (19% to 22%)
- Local: Infusion site pain (SubQ: 85%; may improve after several months of therapy), infusion site reaction (SubQ: 83%)
- Neuromuscular & skeletal: Jaw pain (13%)
- Respiratory: Cough (inhalation: 54%), throat irritation/pharyngolaryngeal pain (inhalation: 25%)

1% to 10%:

- Cardiovascular: Edema (9%), syncope (inhalation: 6%), hypotension (4%)
- Central nervous system: Dizziness (9%)
- Dermatologic: Pruritus (8%)
- Respiratory: Epistaxis (inhalation), hemoptysis, pneumonia, wheezing (inhalation)

<1% (Limited to important or life-threatening): Angioedema, anxiety, arm swelling, bone pain, cellulitis, central venous catheter-related line infections, central venous catheter-related sepsis, hematoma, pain, paresthesia, restlessness, thrombocytopenia, thrombophlebitis

Drug Interactions

Metabolism/Transport Effects Substrate of CYP2C8 (minor), CYP2C9 (minor); **Note:** Assignment of Major/Minor substrate status based on clinically relevant drug interaction potential

Avoid Concomitant Use There are no known interactions where it is recommended to avoid concomitant use.

Increased Effect/Toxicity

Treprostinil may increase the levels/effects of: Agents with Antiplatelet Properties; Anticoagulants; Antihypertensives; Highest Risk QTc-Prolonging Agents; Moderate Risk QTc-Prolonging Agents; Nonsteroidal Anti-Inflammatory Agents; Salicylates

The levels/effects of Treprostinil may be increased by: Alcohol (Ethyl); CYP2C8 Inhibitors (Strong); Mifepristone

Decreased Effect

The levels/effects of Treprostinil may be decreased by: CYP2C8 Inducers (Strong)

Preparation for Administration Injection solution: For SubQ infusion, **product should not be diluted prior to use**. For I.V. infusion, dilute in SWFI, NS, or Flolan® sterile diluent to a final volume of either 50 mL or 100 mL (dependent on system reservoir and calculated dose).

Storage/Stability

Injection solution: Store vials at 25°C (77°F); excursions permitted to 15°C to 30°C (59°F to 86°F). Contents of a vial should not be used past 30 days after initial needle access into the vial. Stability for up to 48 hours at 37°C has been shown for I.V. infusion concentrations as low as 4000 ng/mL.

Solution for inhalation: Store ampules in foil packs at 25°C (77°F); excursions permitted to 15°C to 30°C (59°F to 89°F). Protect from light. Once foil pack is opened, ampules should be used within 7 days. Following transfer of solution to inhalation device, solution should remain in device for no more than 24 hours; discard unused portion.

Mechanism of Action Treprostinil is a direct vasodilator of both pulmonary and systemic arterial vascular beds; also inhibits platelet aggregation.

Pharmacodynamics/Kinetics

Absorption: SubQ: Rapidly and completely

Distribution: 14 L/70 kg ideal body weight

Protein binding: 91%

Metabolism: Hepatic (primarily by CYP2C8); forms 5 inactive metabolites (HU1-HU5)

Bioavailability: Inhalation: 64% to 72% (dose-dependent); SubQ: 100%

Half-life elimination: Terminal: ~4 hours

Excretion: Urine (79%; 4% as unchanged drug, 64% as metabolites); feces (13%)

Dosage Pulmonary arterial hypertension (PAH):

Children: SubQ; I.V. infusion: Limited experience in patients ≤16 years of age.

Adults:

Inhalation: **Note:** Prior to initiation, patients should be carefully evaluated for ability to administer treprostinil and care for the inhalation system and accessories required for administration. Immediate access to a back-up inhalation device, accessories, and medication is essential to prevent treatment interruptions.

Initial: 18 mcg (or 3 inhalations) every 4 hours 4 times/day; if 3 inhalations are not tolerated, reduce to 1-2 inhalations, then increase to 3 inhalations as tolerated

Maintenance: If tolerated, increase dose by an additional 3 inhalations at approximately 1- to 2-week intervals; target dose and maximum dose: 54 mcg (or 9 inhalations) 4 times/day

SubQ (preferred) or I.V. infusion: **Note:** Prior to initiation, patients should be carefully evaluated for ability to administer treprostinil and care for the infusion system outside of inpatient setting. Immediate access to a back-up pump, infusion sets, and medication is essential to prevent treatment interruptions.

New to prostacyclin therapy: Initial: 1.25 ng/kg/minute; if dose cannot be tolerated due to systemic effects, reduce to 0.625 ng/kg/minute. Increase dose in increments of 1.25 ng/kg/minute per week for first 4 weeks, followed by increments of 2.5 ng/kg/minute per week for remainder of therapy. Limited experience with doses >40 ng/kg/minute. **Note:** Dose must be carefully and individually titrated (symptom improvement with minimal adverse effects). Avoid abrupt withdrawal. If infusion is restarted within a few hours of discontinuation, the same dose rate may be used. Interruptions for longer periods may require retitration.

Transitioning from epoprostenol (see table): **Note:** Transition should occur in a hospital setting to follow response (eg, walking distance, sign/symptoms of disease progression). May take 24-48 hours to transition. Transition is accomplished by initiating the infusion of treprostinil, and increasing it while simultaneously reducing the dose of intravenous epoprostenol. During transition, increases in PAH symptoms should be first treated with an increase in treprostinil dose. Occurrence of prostacyclin associated side effects should be treated by decreasing the dose of epoprostenol.

Transitioning From I.V. Epoprostenol to SubQ (Preferred) or I.V. Treprostinil

Step	Epoprostenol Dose	Treprostinil Dose
1	Maintain current dose	Initiate at 10% initial epoprostenol dose
2	Decrease to 80% initial dose	Increase to 30% initial epoprostenol dose
3	Decrease to 60% initial dose	Increase to 50% initial epoprostenol dose
4	Decrease to 40% initial dose	Increase to 70% initial epoprostenol dose
5	Decrease to 20% initial dose	Increase to 90% initial epoprostenol dose
6	Decrease to 5% initial dose	Increase to 110% initial epoprostenol dose
7	Discontinue epoprostenol	Maintain current dose plus additional 5% to 10% as needed

Elderly: Refer to adult dosing. Limited experience in patients ≥65 years; use caution.

Dosage adjustment in renal impairment: Inhalation, SubQ infusion, I.V. infusion: No dosage adjustment provided in manufacturer's labeling (has not been studied). Use with caution and titrate slowly.

Dosage adjustment in hepatic impairment:

Inhalation: No specific dosage adjustment provided in manufacturer's labeling. However, hepatic impairment increases systemic exposure to treprostinil. Use with caution and titrate slowly.

SubQ infusion, I.V. infusion:

Mild to moderate impairment: Initial: 0.625 ng/kg/minute (ideal body weight). Use with caution and titrate slowly.

Severe impairment: No dosage adjustment provided in manufacturer's labeling (has not been studied). Use with caution and titrate slowly.

Administration Regardless of administration route (inhalation, I.V., or SubQ), treatment interruptions or rapid large dosage reductions should be avoided. Immediate access to medication, a back-up inhalation device, or pump and infusion sets is essential to prevent treatment interruptions.

Inhalation: Do not mix with other medications. For inhalation only via the Tyvaso™ Inhalation System. Prior to the first treatment session of each day, transfer the entire contents of one ampule into the medicine chamber; one ampule contains sufficient volume of medication for all 4 treatment sessions in a single day. Between each session, the device should be capped and stored upright with the remaining medication inside. At the end of each day, the medicine chamber and any remaining medication must be discarded. Avoid contact of solution with eyes or skin; wash hands after handling.

I.V. infusion: I.V. use is recommended when SubQ infusion is not tolerated or when the benefit outweighs the potential risks of an indwelling central venous catheter. Solution must be diluted in SWFI, NS, or Flolan® sterile diluent prior to use and administered by continuous infusion using a central indwelling catheter and infusion pump. The ambulatory infusion pump should be small and lightweight; have occlusion/no delivery, low battery, programming error, and motor malfunction alarms; have ± 6% accuracy of the programmed rate; and be positive pressure driven. The reservoir should be made of polyvinyl chloride, polypropylene, or glass. Peripheral infusion may be used temporarily until central line is established. Infusion sets with an in-line 0.22 or 0.2 micron filter should be used for central and peripheral administration.

SubQ infusion (preferred): Administer undiluted via continuous SubQ infusion using an appropriately-designed infusion pump. The ambulatory infusion pump should be small and lightweight; be able to adjust infusion rates in ~0.002 mL/hour increments; have occlusion/no delivery, low battery, programming error, and motor malfunction alarms; have ± 6% accuracy of the programmed rate; and be positive pressure driven. The reservoir should be made of polyvinyl chloride, polypropylene, or glass. Infusion site reactions may be helped by moving the infusion site every 3 days, local application of topical hot and cold packs, topical or oral analgesics. Injection site pain and erythema may improve after several months of treprostinil therapy.

Monitoring Parameters BP, dyspnea, fatigue, activity tolerance, symptoms of excessive dose (eg, headache, nausea, vomiting)

Product Availability

Orenitram extended release tablets: FDA approved December 2013; anticipated availability is June 2014.

Orenitram is indicated for the treatment of pulmonary arterial hypertension (WHO Group 1) to improve exercise capacity.

Dosage Forms Excipient information presented when available (limited, particularly for generics); consult specific product labeling.

Solution, Inhalation:

Tyvaso: 0.6 mg/mL (2.9 mL)

Tyvaso Refill: 0.6 mg/mL (2.9 mL)

Tyvaso Starter: 0.6 mg/mL (2.9 mL)

Solution, Injection:

Remodulin: 1 mg/mL (20 mL); 2.5 mg/mL (20 mL); 5 mg/mL (20 mL); 10 mg/mL (20 mL) [contains metacresol, sodium chloride, sodium citrate]

◆ **Treprostinil Sodium** *see* Treprostinil *on page 2115*

◆ **Tretin-X** *see* Tretinoin (Topical) *on page 2120*

◆ **Tretinoin and Clindamycin** *see* Clindamycin and Tretinoin *on page 455*

◆ **Tretinoin, Fluocinolone Acetonide, and Hydroquinone** *see* Fluocinolone, Hydroquinone, and Tretinoin *on page 879*

Tretinoin (Systemic) (TRET i noyn)

Brand Names: Canada Vesanoid®

Index Terms *trans* Vitamin A Acid; *trans*-Retinoic Acid; All-*trans* Retinoic Acid; All-*trans* Vitamin A Acid; ATRA; Ro 5488; tRA; Tretinoinum; Vesanoid

Pharmacologic Category Antineoplastic Agent, Miscellaneous; Retinoic Acid Derivative

Use Induction of remission in patients with acute promyelocytic leukemia (APL), French American British (FAB) classification M3 (including the M3 variant) characterized by t(15;17) translocation and/or PML/RARα gene presence

Unlabeled Use Post consolidation and maintenance therapy in APL; combination therapy (with arsenic trioxide) for remission induction in APL

Pregnancy Risk Factor D

Pregnancy Considerations Adverse events were observed in animal reproduction studies. **[U.S. Boxed Warning]: High risk of teratogenicity; if treatment with tretinoin is required in women of childbearing potential, two reliable forms of contraception should be used simultaneously during and for 1 month after treatment, unless abstinence is the chosen method. Within 1 week prior to starting therapy, serum or urine pregnancy test (sensitivity at least 50 mIU/mL) should be collected. If possible, delay therapy until results are available. Repeat pregnancy testing and contraception counseling monthly throughout the period of treatment.** Contraception must be used even when there is a history of infertility or menopause, unless a hysterectomy has been preformed. Tretinoin was detected in the serum of a neonate at birth following maternal use of standard doses during pregnancy (Takitani, 2005). Use in humans for the treatment of acute promyelocytic leukemia (APL) is limited and exposure occurred after the first trimester in most cases (Valappil, 2007). However, major fetal abnormalities and spontaneous abortions have been reported with other retinoids; some of these abnormalities were fatal. If the clinical condition of a patient presenting with APL during pregnancy warrants immediate treatment, tretinoin use should be avoided in the first trimester; treatment with tretinoin may be considered in the second and third trimester with careful fetal monitoring, including cardiac monitoring (Sanz, 2009).

Breast-Feeding Considerations It is not known if tretinoin is excreted in breast milk. Due to the potential for serious adverse reactions in the nursing infant, breast-feeding should be discontinued prior to treatment initiation.

Contraindications Hypersensitivity to tretinoin, other retinoids, parabens, or any component of the formulation

Warnings/Precautions Hazardous agent: Use appropriate precautions for handling and disposal (NIOSH, 2012).

[U.S. Boxed Warning]: About 25% of patients with APL treated with tretinoin have experienced APL differentiation syndrome (DS) (formerly called retinoic-acid-APL [RA-APL] syndrome), which is characterized by fever, dyspnea, acute respiratory distress, weight gain, radiographic pulmonary infiltrates and pleural or pericardial effusions, edema, and hepatic, renal, and/or multiorgan failure. DS usually occurs during the first month of treatment, with some cases reported following the first dose. DS has been observed with or without concomitant leukocytosis and has occasionally been accompanied by impaired myocardial contractility and episodic hypotension; endotracheal intubation and mechanical ventilation have been required in some cases due to progressive hypoxemia, and several patients have expired with multiorgan failure. About one-half of DS cases are severe, which is associated with increased mortality. Management has not been defined, although high-dose steroids given at the first suspicion appear to reduce morbidity and mortality. Regardless of the leukocyte count, at the first signs suggestive of DS, immediately initiate steroid therapy with dexamethasone 10 mg I.V. every 12 hours for 3-5 days; taper off over 2 weeks. Most patients do not require termination of tretinoin therapy during treatment of DS.

[U.S. Boxed Warning]: During treatment, ~40% of patients will develop rapidly evolving leukocytosis. A high WBC at diagnosis increases the risk for further leukocytosis and may be associated with a higher risk of life-threatening complications. If signs and symptoms of the APL-DS syndrome are present together with leukocytosis, initiate treatment with high-dose steroids immediately. Consider adding full-dose chemotherapy (including an anthracycline, if not contraindicated) to the tretinoin therapy on day 1 or 2 for patients presenting with a WBC count of >5 x 10^9/L. Consider adding chemotherapy immediately in patients who presented with a WBC count of <5 x 10^9/L, yet the WBC count reaches ≥6 x 10^9/L by day 5, or ≥10 x 10^9/L by day 10, or ≥15 x 10^9/L by day 28.

[U.S. Boxed Warning]: High risk of teratogenicity; if treatment with tretinoin is required in women of childbearing potential, two reliable forms of contraception should be used during and for 1 month after treatment. Microdosed progesterone products ("minipill") may provide inadequate pregnancy protection. Repeat pregnancy testing and contraception counseling monthly throughout the period of treatment. If possible, initiation of treatment with tretinoin should be delayed until negative pregnancy test result is confirmed.

Retinoids have been associated with pseudotumor cerebri (benign intracranial hypertension), especially in children. Concurrent use of other drugs associated with this effect (eg, tetracyclines) may increase risk. Early signs and symptoms include papilledema, headache, nausea, vomiting, visual disturbances, intracranial noises, or pulsate tinnitus.

Up to 60% of patients experienced hypercholesterolemia or hypertriglyceridemia, which were reversible upon completion of treatment. Venous thrombosis and MI have been reported in patient without risk factors for thrombosis or MI; the risk for thrombosis (arterial and venous) is increased during the first month of treatment. Use with caution with antifibrinolytic agents; thrombotic complications have been reported (rarely) with concomitant use. Elevated liver function test results occur in 50% to 60% of patients during treatment. Carefully monitor liver function test results during treatment and give consideration to a temporary withdrawal of tretinoin if test results reach >5 times the upper ▶

limit of normal. Most liver function test abnormalities will resolve without interruption of treatment or after therapy completion. May cause headache, malaise, and/or dizziness; caution patients about performing tasks which require mental alertness (eg, operating machinery or driving). Patients with APL are at high risk and can have severe adverse reactions to tretinoin. **[U.S. Boxed Warning]: Should be administered under the supervision of an experienced cancer chemotherapy physician.** Tretinoin treatment for APL should be initiated early, discontinue if pending cytogenetic analysis does not confirm APL by t(15;17) translocation or the presence of the PML/RARα fusion protein (caused by translocation of the promyelocytic [PML] gene on chromosome 15 and retinoic acid receptor [RAR] alpha gene on chromosome 17).

Tretinoin (which is also known as all-*trans* retinoic acid, or ATRA) and isotretinoin may be confused, while both products may be used in cancer treatment, they are **not** interchangeable; verify product prior to dispensing and administration to prevent medication errors.

Adverse Reactions Most patients will experience drug-related toxicity, especially headache, fever, weakness and fatigue. These are seldom permanent or irreversible and do not typically require therapy interruption.

>10%:

- Cardiovascular: Peripheral edema (52%), chest discomfort (32%), edema (29%), arrhythmias (23%), flushing (23%), hypotension (14%), hypertension (11%)
- Central nervous system: Headache (86%), fever (83%), malaise (66%), pain (37%), dizziness (20%), anxiety (17%), depression (14%), insomnia (14%), confusion (11%)
- Dermatologic: Skin/mucous membrane dryness (77%), rash (54%), pruritus (20%), alopecia (14%), skin changes (14%)
- Endocrine & metabolic: Hypercholesterolemia and/or hypertriglyceridemia (≤60%)
- Gastrointestinal: Nausea/vomiting (57%), GI hemorrhage (34%), abdominal pain (31%), mucositis (26%), diarrhea (23%), weight gain (23%), anorexia (17%), constipation (17%), weight loss (17%), dyspepsia (14%), abdominal distention (11%)
- Hematologic: Hemorrhage (60%), leukocytosis (40%), disseminated intravascular coagulation (DIC) (26%)
- Hepatic: Liver function tests increased (50% to 60%)
- Local: Phlebitis (11%)
- Neuromuscular & skeletal: Bone pain (77%), paresthesia (17%), myalgia (14%)
- Ocular: Ocular disorder (17%), visual disturbances (17%)
- Otic: Earache/ear fullness (23%)
- Renal: Renal insufficiency (11%)
- Respiratory: Upper respiratory tract disorders (63%), dyspnea (60%), respiratory insufficiency (26%), pleural effusion (20%), expiratory wheezing (14%), pneumonia (14%), rales (14%)
- Miscellaneous: Shivering (63%), infections (58%), retinoic acid-acute promyelocytic leukemia syndrome differentiation syndrome (≤25%), diaphoresis (20%)

1% to 10%:

- Cardiovascular: Cerebral hemorrhage (9%), cardiac failure (6%), facial edema (6%), pallor (6%), cardiac arrest (3%), cardiomyopathy (3%), heart enlarged (3%), heart murmur (3%), ischemia (3%), MI (3%), myocarditis (3%), pericarditis (3%), stroke (3%)
- Central nervous system: Agitation (9%), intracranial hypertension (9%), hallucination (6%), aphasia (3%), cerebellar edema (3%), CNS depression (3%), coma (3%), dementia (3%), encephalopathy (3%), facial paralysis (3%), forgetfulness (3%), hypotaxia (3%), hypothermia (3%), light reflex absent (3%), seizure (3%), slow speech (3%), somnolence (3%), spinal cord disorder (3%), unconsciousness (3%)
- Dermatologic: Cellulitis (8%)
- Endocrine & metabolic: Fluid imbalance (6%), acidosis (3%)
- Gastrointestinal: Hepatosplenomegaly (9%), ulcer (3%)
- Genitourinary: Dysuria (9%), micturition frequency (3%), prostate enlarged (3%)
- Hepatic: Ascites (3%), hepatitis (3%)
- Neuromuscular & skeletal: Flank pain (9%), abnormal gait (3%), asterixis (3%), bone inflammation (3%), dysarthria (3%), hemiplegia (3%), hyporeflexia (3%), leg weakness (3%), tremor (3%)
- Ocular: Visual acuity change (6%), agnosia (3%), visual field deficit (3%)
- Otic: Hearing loss (6%)
- Renal: Acute renal failure (3%), renal tubular necrosis (3%)
- Respiratory: Lower respiratory tract disorders (9%), pulmonary infiltration (6%), bronchial asthma (3%), larynx edema (3%), pulmonary hypertension (3%)
- Miscellaneous: Lymph disorder (6%)

<1% (Limited to important or life-threatening): Arterial thrombosis, basophilia, erythema nodosum, genital ulceration, hypercalcemia, hyperhistaminemia, irreversible hearing loss, myositis, organomegaly, pancreatitis, pseudotumor cerebri, renal infarct, Sweet's syndrome, thrombocytosis, vasculitis (skin), venous thrombosis

Drug Interactions

Metabolism/Transport Effects Substrate of CYP2A6 (minor), CYP2B6 (minor), CYP2C8 (major), CYP2C9 (minor); **Note:** Assignment of Major/Minor substrate status based on clinically relevant drug interaction potential; **Inhibits** CYP2C9 (weak); **Induces** CYP2E1 (weak/moderate)

Avoid Concomitant Use

Avoid concomitant use of Tretinoin (Systemic) with any of the following: BCG; Multivitamins/Fluoride (with ADE); Multivitamins/Minerals (with ADEK, Folate, Iron); Multivitamins/Minerals (with AE, No Iron); Natalizumab; Pimecrolimus; Tacrolimus (Topical); Tetracycline Derivatives; Tofacitinib; Vaccines (Live); Vitamin A

Increased Effect/Toxicity

Tretinoin (Systemic) may increase the levels/effects of: Antifibrinolytic Agents; Leflunomide; Natalizumab; Porfimer; Tofacitinib; Vaccines (Live); Vitamin A

The levels/effects of Tretinoin (Systemic) may be increased by: CYP2C8 Inhibitors (Moderate); CYP2C8 Inhibitors (Strong); Deferasirox; Denosumab; Mifepristone; Multivitamins/Fluoride (with ADE); Multivitamins/Minerals (with ADEK, Folate, Iron); Multivitamins/Minerals (with AE, No Iron); Pimecrolimus; Roflumilast; Tacrolimus (Topical); Tetracycline Derivatives; Trastuzumab

Decreased Effect

Tretinoin (Systemic) may decrease the levels/effects of: BCG; Coccidioidin Skin Test; Contraceptives (Estrogens); Contraceptives (Progestins); Sipuleucel-T; Vaccines (Inactivated); Vaccines (Live)

The levels/effects of Tretinoin (Systemic) may be decreased by: CYP2C8 Inducers (Strong); Dabrafenib; Echinacea

Ethanol/Nutrition/Herb Interactions

Ethanol: Avoid ethanol (may increase CNS depression).

Food: Absorption of retinoids has been shown to be enhanced when taken with food.

Herb/Nutraceutical: St John's wort may decrease tretinoin levels. Avoid dong quai, St John's wort (may also cause photosensitization). Avoid additional vitamin A supplementation; may lead to vitamin A toxicity.

Storage/Stability Store capsule at 20°C to 25°C (68°F to 77°F). Protect from light.

Mechanism of Action Tretinoin appears to bind one or more nuclear receptors and decreases proliferation and induces differentiation of APL cells; initially produces maturation of primitive promyelocytes and repopulates the marrow and peripheral blood with normal hematopoietic cells to achieve complete remission

Pharmacodynamics/Kinetics

Absorption: Well absorbed

Protein binding: >95%, predominantly to albumin

Metabolism: Hepatic via CYP; primary metabolite: 4-oxo-all-*trans*-retinoic acid; displays autometabolism

Half-life elimination: Terminal: Parent drug: 0.5-2 hours

Time to peak, serum: 1-2 hours

Excretion: Urine (63%); feces (30%)

Dosage Details concerning dosing in combination regimens should also be consulted. **Note:** Induction treatment of APL with tretinoin should be initiated early; discontinue if pending cytogenetic analysis does not confirm t(15;17) translocation or the presence of the PML/RARα fusion protein.

Acute promyelocytic leukemia (APL): Oral:

Remission induction: Children and Adults: 45 mg/m^2/day in 2 equally divided doses until documentation of complete remission (CR); discontinue 30 days after CR or after 90 days of treatment, whichever occurs first

Remission induction (in combination with an anthracycline ± cytarabine; unlabeled use):

Children: 25 mg/m^2/day in 2 equally divided doses until complete remission or 90 days (Ortega, 2005)

Adults: 45 mg/m^2/day in 2 equally divided doses until complete remission or 90 days (Powell, 2010) or until complete hematologic remission (Ades, 2008; Sanz, 2008; Sanz, 2010)

Remission induction (in combination with arsenic trioxide; unlabeled use): Adults: 45 mg/m^2/day in 2 equally divided doses until <5% blasts in marrow and no abnormal promyelocytes or up to 85 days (Estey, 2006; Ravandi, 2009)

Consolidation therapy (unlabeled use):

Children: 25 mg/m^2/day in 2 equally divided doses for 15 days each month for 3 months (Ortega, 2005)

Adults: 45 mg/m^2/day in 2 equally divided doses for 15 days each month for 3 months (in combination with chemotherapy) (Lo-Coco, 2010; Sanz 2010) **or** 45 mg/m^2/day for 14 days every 4 weeks for 7 cycles (in combination with arsenic trioxide) (Ravandi, 2009)

Maintenance therapy, intermediate- and high-risk patients (unlabeled use):

Children: 25 mg/m^2/day in 2 equally divided doses for 15 days every 3 months for 2 years (Ortega, 2005)

Adults: 45 mg/m^2/day in 2 equally divided doses for 15 days every 3 months for 2 years (Sanz, 2004)

Dosage adjustment for toxicity:

APL differentiation syndrome: Initiate dexamethasone 10 mg I.V. every 12 hours for 3-5 days; consider interrupting tretinoin until resolution of hypoxia

Liver function tests >5 times the upper limit of normal: Consider temporarily withholding treatment.

Dosage adjustment in renal impairment: No dosage adjustment provided in the manufacturer's labeling (has not been studied).

Dosage adjustment in hepatic impairment: No dosage adjustment provided in the manufacturer's labeling (has not been studied).

Dosing in obesity: *ASCO Guidelines for appropriate chemotherapy dosing in obese adults with cancer:* Utilize patient's actual body weight (full weight) for calculation of body surface area- or weight-based dosing, particularly when the intent of therapy is curative; manage regimen-related toxicities in the same manner as for nonobese patients; if a dose reduction is utilized due to toxicity, consider resumption of full weight-based dosing with subsequent cycles, especially if cause of toxicity (eg, hepatic or renal impairment) is resolved (Griggs, 2012).

Dietary Considerations The absorption of retinoids (as a class) is enhanced when taken with food. Capsule contains soybean oil.

Administration Administer orally with a meal; do not crush capsules.

Although the manufacturer does not recommend the use of the capsule contents to extemporaneously prepare tretinoin suspension, there are limited case reports of use in patients who are unable to swallow the capsules whole. In a patient with a nasogastric (NG) tube, tretinoin capsules were cut open, with partial aspiration of the contents into a glass syringe, the residual capsule contents were mixed with soy bean oil and aspirated into the same syringe and administered (Shaw, 1995). Tretinoin capsules have also been mixed with sterile water (~20 mL) and heated in a water bath (37°C) to melt the capsules and create an oily suspension for NG tube administration (Bargetzi, 1996). Tretinoin has also been administered sublingually by squeezing the capsule contents beneath the tongue (Kueh, 1999). Low plasma concentrations have been reported when tretinoin has been administered through a feeding tube, although patient-specific impaired absorption or a lack of excipient (eg, soybean oil) may have been a contributing factor (Takitani, 2004).

Hazardous agent - use appropriate precautions for handling and disposal (NIOSH, 2012).

Monitoring Parameters Bone marrow cytology to confirm t(15;17) translocation or the presence of the PML/RARα fusion protein (do not withhold treatment initiation for results); monitor CBC with differential, coagulation profile, liver function test results, and triglyceride and cholesterol levels frequently; monitor closely for signs of APL differentiation syndrome (eg, monitor volume status, pulmonary status, temperature, respiration)

Dosage Forms Excipient information presented when available (limited, particularly for generics); consult specific product labeling.

Capsule, Oral:

Generic: 10 mg

Extemporaneous Preparations Hazardous agent: Use appropriate precautions for handling and disposal.

Although the manufacturer does not recommend the use of the capsule contents to extemporaneously prepare a suspension of tretinoin (due to reports of low plasma levels) (Vesanoid® data on file), there are limited case reports of use in patients who are unable to swallow the capsules whole. In a patient with a nasogastric (NG) tube, tretinoin capsules were cut open, with partial aspiration of the contents aspirated into a glass syringe. The residual capsule contents were mixed with soybean oil, aspirated into the syringe, and administered (Shaw, 1995). Tretinoin capsules have also been mixed with sterile water (~20 mL) and heated in a water bath to melt the capsules and create an oily suspension for NG tube administration (Bargetzi, 1996). Tretinoin has also been administered sublingually by squeezing the capsule contents beneath the tongue (Kueh, 1999).

Bargetzi MJ, Tichelli A, Gratwohl A, et al, "Oral All-Transretinoic Acid Administration in Intubated Patients With Acute Promyelocytic Leukemia," *Schweiz Med Wochenschr*, 1996, 126(45):1944-5.

Kueh YK, Liew PP, Ho PC, et al, "Sublingual Administration of All-*Trans*-Retinoic Acid to a Comatose Patient With Acute Promyelocytic Leukemia," *Ann Pharmacother*, 1999, 33(4):503-5.

Shaw PJ, Atkins MC, Nath CE, et al, "ATRA Administration in the Critically Ill Patient," *Leukemia*, 1995, 9(7):1288.

Vesanoid® data on file, Roche Pharmaceuticals

Tretinoin (Topical) (TRET i noyn)

Brand Names: U.S. Atralin; Avita; Refissa; Renova; Renova Pump; Retin-A; Retin-A Micro; Retin-A Micro Pump; Tretin-X

Brand Names: Canada Rejuva-A®; Renova®; Retin-A Micro®; Retin-A®; Retinova®; Stieva-A; Vitamin A Acid

Index Terms *trans*-Retinoic Acid; Retinoic Acid; Vitamin A Acid

Pharmacologic Category Acne Products; Retinoic Acid Derivative; Topical Skin Product, Acne

Use Treatment of acne vulgaris; photodamaged skin; palliation of fine wrinkles, mottled hyperpigmentation, and tactile roughness of facial skin as part of a comprehensive skin care and sun avoidance program

Unlabeled Use Some skin cancers

Pregnancy Risk Factor C

Pregnancy Considerations Oral tretinoin is teratogenic and fetotoxic in rats at doses 1000 and 500 times the topical human dose, respectively. Tretinoin does not appear to be teratogenic when used topically since it is rapidly metabolized by the skin; however, there are rare reports of fetal defects. Use for acne only if benefit to mother outweighs potential risk to fetus. During pregnancy, do not use for palliation of fine wrinkles, mottled hyperpigmentation, and tactile roughness of facial skin.

Breast-Feeding Considerations It is not known if tretinoin (topical) is excreted in breast milk. The manufacturer recommends that caution be exercised when administering tretinoin (topical) to nursing women.

Contraindications Hypersensitivity to tretinoin or any component of the formulation; sunburn

Warnings/Precautions Hazardous agent - use appropriate precautions for handling and disposal (NIOSH, 2012). Use with caution in patients with eczema; avoid excessive exposure to sunlight and sunlamps; avoid contact with abraded skin, sunburned skin, mucous membranes, eyes, mouth, angles of the nose. Treatment can increase skin sensitivity to weather extremes of wind or cold. Also, concomitant topical medications (eg, medicated or abrasive soaps, cleansers, or cosmetics with a strong drying effect) should be used with caution due to increased skin irritation. Palliation of fine wrinkles, mottled hyperpigmentation, and tactile roughness of facial skin: Do not use the 0.05% cream for longer than 48 weeks or the 0.02% cream for longer than 52 weeks. Not for use on moderate- to heavily-pigmented skin. Gel is flammable; do not expose to high temperatures or flame. Safety and efficacy have not been established in children <12 years of age.

Adverse Reactions

>10%: Dermatologic: Excessive dryness, erythema, scaling of the skin, pruritus

1% to 10%:

Dermatologic: Hyperpigmentation or hypopigmentation, photosensitivity, initial acne flare-up

Local: Edema, blistering, stinging

Drug Interactions

Metabolism/Transport Effects None known.

Avoid Concomitant Use

Avoid concomitant use of Tretinoin (Topical) with any of the following: Multivitamins/Fluoride (with ADE); Multivitamins/Minerals (with ADEK, Folate, Iron); Multivitamins/Minerals (with AE, No Iron)

Increased Effect/Toxicity

Tretinoin (Topical) may increase the levels/effects of: Porfimer

The levels/effects of Tretinoin (Topical) may be increased by: Multivitamins/Fluoride (with ADE); Multivitamins/Minerals (with ADEK, Folate, Iron); Multivitamins/Minerals (with AE, No Iron)

Decreased Effect

Tretinoin (Topical) may decrease the levels/effects of: Contraceptives (Progestins)

Ethanol/Nutrition/Herb Interactions

Food: Avoid excessive intake of vitamin A (cod liver oil, halibut fish oil).

Herb/Nutraceutical: Avoid dong quai, St John's wort (may also cause photosensitization). Avoid excessive amounts of vitamin A supplements.

Storage/Stability Store at 25°C (77°F). Gel is flammable; keep away from heat and flame.

Mechanism of Action Keratinocytes in the sebaceous follicle become less adherent which allows for easy removal; inhibits microcomedone formation and eliminates lesions already present

Pharmacodynamics/Kinetics

Absorption: Minimal

Metabolism: Hepatic for the small amount absorbed

Excretion: Urine and feces

Dosage Topical:

Children >12 years and Adults: Acne vulgaris: Begin therapy with a weaker formulation of tretinoin (0.025% cream, 0.04% microsphere gel, or 0.01% gel) and increase the concentration as tolerated; apply once daily to acne lesions before retiring or on alternate days; if stinging or irritation develop, decrease frequency of application

Adults ≥18: Palliation of fine wrinkles, mottled hyperpigmentation, and tactile roughness of facial skin: Pea-sized amount of the 0.02% or 0.05% cream applied to entire face once daily in the evening

Elderly: Use of the 0.02% cream in patients 65-71 years of age showed similar improvement in fine wrinkles as seen in patients <65 years. Safety and efficacy of the 0.02% cream have not been established in patients >71 years of age. Safety and efficacy of the 0.05% cream have not been established in patients >50 years of age.

Administration Palliation of fine wrinkles, mottled hyperpigmentation, and tactile roughness of facial skin: Cream: Prior to application, gently wash face with a mild soap. Pat dry. Wait 20-30 minutes to apply cream. Avoid eyes, ears, nostrils, and mouth.

Hazardous agent; use appropriate precautions for handling and disposal (NIOSH, 2012).

Dosage Forms Excipient information presented when available (limited, particularly for generics); consult specific product labeling. [DSC] = Discontinued product

Cream, External:

- Avita: 0.025% (20 g, 45 g)
- Refissa: 0.05% (20 g, 40 g) [contains edetate disodium, methylparaben, propylparaben]
- Renova: 0.02% (40 g, 60 g) [contains benzyl alcohol, cetyl alcohol, edetate disodium, methylparaben, propylparaben]
- Renova Pump: 0.02% (44 g) [contains benzyl alcohol, cetyl alcohol, edetate disodium, methylparaben, propylparaben]
- Retin-A: 0.025% (20 g, 45 g); 0.05% (20 g, 45 g); 0.1% (20 g, 45 g)
- Tretin-X: 0.0375% (35 g); 0.075% (35 g)
- Generic: 0.025% (20 g, 45 g); 0.05% (20 g, 40 g, 45 g, 60 g); 0.1% (20 g, 45 g)

Gel, External:

- Atralin: 0.05% (45 g) [contains alcohol, usp, butylparaben, ethylparaben, isobutylparaben, methylparaben, propylparaben, trolamine (triethanolamine)]
- Avita: 0.025% (20 g, 45 g)
- Retin-A: 0.01% (15 g, 45 g); 0.025% (15 g, 45 g) [contains alcohol, usp]
- Retin-A Micro: 0.04% (20 g, 45 g); 0.1% (20 g, 45 g) [contains benzyl alcohol, disodium edta, propylene glycol, trolamine (triethanolamine)]

Retin-A Micro Pump: 0.04% (50 g); 0.1% (50 g) [contains benzyl alcohol, disodium edta, propylene glycol, trolamine (triethanolamine)]
Generic: 0.01% (15 g, 45 g); 0.025% (15 g, 45 g); 0.04% (20 g, 45 g, 50 g); 0.1% (20 g, 45 g, 50 g)
Kit, External:
Tretin-X: 0.01% [DSC], 0.025%, 0.05%, 0.1% [contains benzyl alcohol, cetearyl alcohol, disodium edta, fd&c red #40, methylparaben, propylparaben, tartrazine (fd&c yellow #5), trolamine (triethanolamine)]

◆ **Tretinoinum** *see* Tretinoin (Systemic) *on page 2117*
◆ **Trexall** *see* Methotrexate *on page 1324*
◆ **Treximet®** *see* Sumatriptan and Naproxen *on page 1972*
◆ **Triacetyluridine** *see* Uridine Triacetate *on page 2141*
◆ **Triaconazole** *see* Terconazole *on page 2021*
◆ **Triaderm (Can)** *see* Triamcinolone (Topical) *on page 2123*

Triamcinolone (Systemic) (trye am SIN oh lone)

Brand Names: U.S. Aristospan Intra-Articular; Aristospan Intralesional; Kenalog
Brand Names: Canada Aristospan®
Index Terms Triamcinolone Acetonide, Parenteral; Triamcinolone Hexacetonide
Pharmacologic Category Corticosteroid, Systemic
Additional Appendix Information
Corticosteroids Systemic Equivalencies *on page 2297*
Use
Intra-articular (soft tissue): Acute gouty arthritis, acute/subacute bursitis, acute tenosynovitis, epicondylitis, rheumatoid arthritis, synovitis of osteoarthritis
Intralesional: Alopecia areata, discoid lupus erythematosus, keloids, granuloma annulare lesions (localized hypertrophic, infiltrated, or inflammatory), lichen planus plaques, lichen simplex chronicus plaques, psoriatic plaques, necrobiosis lipoidica diabeticorum, cystic tumors of aponeurosis or tendon (ganglia)
Systemic: Adrenocortical insufficiency, dermatologic diseases, endocrine disorders, gastrointestinal diseases, hematologic and neoplastic disorders, nervous system disorders, nephrotic syndrome, rheumatic disorders, allergic states, respiratory diseases, systemic lupus erythematosus (SLE), and other diseases requiring anti-inflammatory or immunosuppressive effects
Pregnancy Risk Factor C
Pregnancy Considerations Adverse events have been observed with corticosteroids in animal reproduction studies. Some studies have shown an association between first trimester systemic corticosteroid use and oral clefts (Park-Wyllie, 2000; Pradat, 2003). Systemic corticosteroids may also influence fetal growth (decreased birth weight); however, information is conflicting (Lunghi, 2010). Hypoadrenalism may occur in newborns following maternal use of corticosteroids in pregnancy; monitor.
Breast-Feeding Considerations Corticosteroids are excreted in human milk; information specific to triamcinolone has not been located. The manufacturer notes that when used systemically, maternal use of corticosteroids have the potential to cause adverse events in a nursing infant (eg, growth suppression, interfere with endogenous corticosteroid production); therefore, caution should be used if administered to a nursing woman. A case report notes a decrease in milk production following a high-dose triamcinolone injection in a nursing mother with a previously abundant milk supply (McGuire, 2012).
Contraindications Hypersensitivity to triamcinolone or any component of the formulation; systemic fungal infections; cerebral malaria; immune thrombocytopenia (ITP) (I.M. injection)
Warnings/Precautions May cause hypercorticism or suppression of hypothalamic-pituitary-adrenal (HPA) axis, particularly in younger children or in patients receiving high doses for prolonged periods. HPA axis suppression may lead to adrenal crisis. Withdrawal and discontinuation of a corticosteroid should be done slowly and carefully.

Acute myopathy has been reported with high-dose corticosteroids, usually in patients with neuromuscular transmission disorders; may involve ocular and/or respiratory muscles; monitor creatine kinase; recovery may be delayed. Corticosteroid use may cause psychiatric disturbances, including depression, euphoria, insomnia, mood swings, and personality changes. Pre-existing psychiatric conditions may be exacerbated by corticosteroid use. Prolonged use of corticosteroids may also increase the incidence of secondary infection, mask acute infection (including fungal infections), prolong or exacerbate viral infections, or limit response to vaccines. Exposure to chickenpox should be avoided; corticosteroids should not be used to treat ocular herpes simplex. Corticosteroids should not be used for cerebral malaria or viral hepatitis. Close observation is required in patients with latent tuberculosis and/or TB reactivity; restrict use in active TB (only in conjunction with antituberculosis treatment). Use with caution in patients with threadworm infection; may cause serious hyperinfection. Prolonged treatment with corticosteroids has been associated with the development of Kaposi's sarcoma (case reports); if noted, discontinuation of therapy should be considered. Avoid use in head injury patients.

Use with caution in patients with thyroid disease, hepatic impairment, renal impairment, cardiovascular disease, diabetes, myasthenia gravis, patients at risk for osteoporosis, patients at risk for seizures, or GI diseases (diverticulitis, peptic ulcer, ulcerative colitis) due to perforation risk. Avoid use in head injury patients. Use caution following acute MI (corticosteroids have been associated with myocardial rupture). Because of the risk of adverse effects, systemic corticosteroids should be used cautiously in the elderly in the smallest possible effective dose for the shortest duration. Patients should not be immunized with live, viral vaccines while receiving immunosuppressive doses of corticosteroids. The ability to respond to dead viral vaccines is unknown.

Withdraw therapy with gradual tapering of dose. There have been reports of systemic corticosteroid withdrawal symptoms (eg, joint/muscle pain, lassitude, depression) when withdrawing oral inhalation therapy. Injection suspension contains benzyl alcohol; benzyl alcohol has been associated with the "gasping syndrome" in neonates and low-birth-weight infants. Administer products only via recommended route (depending on product used). Do **not** administer any triamcinolone product via the epidural or intrathecal route; serious adverse events, including fatalities, have been reported.
Adverse Reactions Frequency not defined; reactions reported with corticosteroid therapy in general:
Cardiovascular: Arrhythmia, bradycardia, cardiac arrest, cardiac enlargement, CHF, circulatory collapse, edema, hypertension, hypertrophic cardiomyopathy (premature infants), myocardial rupture (following recent MI), syncope, tachycardia, thromboembolism, vasculitis
Central nervous system: Arachnoiditis (I.T.), depression, emotional instability, euphoria, headache, insomnia, intracranial pressure increased, malaise, meningitis (I.T.), mood changes, neuritis, neuropathy, personality change, pseudotumor cerebri (with discontinuation), seizure, spinal cord infarction, stroke, vertigo

Dermatologic: Abscess (sterile), acne, allergic dermatitis, angioedema, atrophy (cutaneous/subcutaneous), bruising, dry skin, erythema, hair thinning, hirsutism, hyper-/hypopigmentation, hypertrichosis, impaired wound healing, lupus erythematosus-like lesions, petechiae, purpura, rash, skin test suppression, striae, thin skin
Endocrine & metabolic: Carbohydrate intolerance, Cushingoid state, diabetes mellitus, fluid retention, glucose intolerance, growth suppression (children), hypokalemia, hypokalemic alkalosis, menstrual irregularities, negative nitrogen balance, sodium retention, sperm motility altered
Gastrointestinal: Abdominal distention, appetite increased, GI hemorrhage, GI perforation, nausea, pancreatitis, peptic ulcer, ulcerative esophagitis, weight gain
Hepatic: Hepatomegaly, liver function tests increased
Local: Thrombophlebitis
Neuromuscular & skeletal: Aseptic necrosis of femoral and humeral heads, calcinosis, Charcot-like arthropathy, fractures, joint tissue damage, muscle mass loss, myopathy, osteoporosis, parasthesia, paraplegia, quadriplegia, tendon rupture, vertebral compression fractures, weakness
Ocular: Cataracts, cortical blindness, exophthalmos, glaucoma, ocular pressure increased, papilledema
Renal: Glycosuria
Respiratory: Pulmonary edema
Miscellaneous: Abnormal fat deposits, anaphylactoid reaction, anaphylaxis, diaphoresis, hiccups, infection, moon face

Drug Interactions

Metabolism/Transport Effects Substrate of CYP3A4 (minor); **Note:** Assignment of Major/Minor substrate status based on clinically relevant drug interaction potential

Avoid Concomitant Use

Avoid concomitant use of Triamcinolone (Systemic) with any of the following: Aldesleukin; BCG; Mifepristone; Natalizumab; Pimecrolimus; Tacrolimus (Topical); Tofacitinib

Increased Effect/Toxicity

Triamcinolone (Systemic) may increase the levels/effects of: Acetylcholinesterase Inhibitors; Amphotericin B; Deferasirox; Leflunomide; Loop Diuretics; Natalizumab; NSAID (COX-2 Inhibitor); NSAID (Nonselective); Thiazide Diuretics; Tofacitinib; Vaccines (Live); Warfarin

The levels/effects of Triamcinolone (Systemic) may be increased by: Antifungal Agents (Azole Derivatives, Systemic); Aprepitant; Calcium Channel Blockers (Nondihydropyridine); Denosumab; Estrogen Derivatives; Fluconazole; Fosaprepitant; Indacaterol; Macrolide Antibiotics; Mifepristone; Neuromuscular-Blocking Agents (Nondepolarizing); Pimecrolimus; Quinolone Antibiotics; Ritonavir; Roflumilast; Salicylates; Tacrolimus (Topical); Telaprevir; Trastuzumab

Decreased Effect

Triamcinolone (Systemic) may decrease the levels/effects of: Aldesleukin; Antidiabetic Agents; BCG; Calcitriol; Coccidioidin Skin Test; Corticorelin; Hyaluronidase; Isoniazid; Salicylates; Sipuleucel-T; Telaprevir; Urea Cycle Disorder Agents; Vaccines (Inactivated)

The levels/effects of Triamcinolone (Systemic) may be decreased by: Aminoglutethimide; Barbiturates; Echinacea; Mifepristone; Mitotane; Primidone; Rifamycin Derivatives

Preparation for Administration Hexacetonide injectable suspension: Avoid diluents containing parabens, phenol, or other preservatives (may cause flocculation). Suspension for intralesional use may be diluted with D_5NS, $D_{10}NS$, NS, or SWFI to a 1:1, 1:2, or 1:4 concentration. Solutions for intra-articular use, may be diluted with lidocaine 1% or 2%.

Storage/Stability Injection, suspension:
Acetonide injectable suspension: Kenalog®: Store at 20°C to 25°C (68°F to 77°F); avoid freezing. Protect from light.
Hexacetonide injectable suspension: Store at 20°C to 25°C (68°F to 77°F); avoid freezing. Protect from light. Diluted suspension stable up to 1 week.

Mechanism of Action Decreases inflammation by suppression of migration of polymorphonuclear leukocytes and reversal of increased capillary permeability; suppresses the immune system by reducing activity and volume of the lymphatic system; suppresses adrenal function at high doses

Pharmacodynamics/Kinetics

Distribution: V_d: 99.5 L
Protein binding: ~68%
Half-life elimination: Biologic: 18-36 hours
Time to peak: I.M.: 8-10 hours
Excretion: Urine (~40%); feces (~60%)

Dosage The lowest possible dose should be used to control the condition; when dose reduction is possible, the dose should be reduced gradually.

Injection:
Acetonide:
Intra-articular, intrabursal, tendon sheaths: Adults: Initial: Smaller joints: 2.5-5 mg, larger joints: 5-15 mg; may require up to 10 mg for small joints and up to 40 mg for large joints; maximum dose/treatment (several joints at one time): 20-80 mg
Intradermal: Adults: Initial: 1 mg
I.M.: Range: 2.5-100 mg/day
Children: Initial: 0.11-1.6 mg/kg/day in 3-4 divided doses
Children 6-12 years: Initial: 40 mg
Children >12 years and Adults: Initial: 60 mg
Hay fever/pollen asthma: 40-100 mg as a single injection/season
Multiple sclerosis (acute exacerbation): 160 mg daily for 1 week, followed by 64 mg every other day for 1 month
Hexacetonide: Adults:
Intralesional, sublesional: Up to 0.5 mg/square inch of affected skin; range: 2-48 mg/day
Intra-articular: Average dose: 2-20 mg; smaller joints: 2-6 mg; larger joints: 10-20 mg. Frequency of injection into a single joint is every 3-4 weeks as necessary; to avoid possible joint destruction use as infrequently as possible.

Triamcinolone Dosing

	Acetonide	Hexacetonide
Intrasynovial	5-40 mg	
Intralesional	1-30 mg (usually 1 mg per injection site); 10 mg/mL suspension usually used	Up to 0.5 mg/sq inch affected area
Sublesional	1-30 mg	
Systemic I.M.	2.5-60 mg/dose (usual adult dose: 60 mg; may repeat with 20-100 mg dose when symptoms recur)	
Intra-articular	2.5-40 mg	2-20 mg average
large joints	5-15 mg	10-20 mg
small joints	2.5-5 mg	2-6 mg
Tendon sheaths	2.5-10 mg	
Intradermal	1 mg/site	

Dosage adjustment in renal impairment: No dosage adjustment provided in the manufacturer's labeling; use with caution.

Dosage adjustment in hepatic impairment: No dosage adjustment provided in the manufacturer's labeling.

Dietary Considerations Ensure adequate intake of calcium and vitamins (or consider supplementation) in patients on medium-to-high doses of systemic corticosteroids.

Administration Shake well before use to ensure suspension is uniform. Inspect visually to ensure no clumping; administer immediately after withdrawal so settling does not occur in the syringe. Do **not** administer any product I.V. or via the epidural or intrathecal route.

Aristospan® (20 mg/mL concentration): For intra-articular and soft tissue administration only; a ≥23-gauge needle is preferred.

Aristospan® (5 mg/mL concentration): For intralesional or sublesional administration only; a ≥23-gauge needle is preferred.

Kenalog®-10 injection: For intra-articular or intralesional administration only. When administered intralesionally, inject directly into the lesion (ie, intradermally or subcutaneously). Tuberculin syringes with a 23- to 25-gauge needle are preferable for intralesional injections.

Kenalog®-40 injection: For intra-articular, soft tissue or I.M. administration. When administered I.M., inject deep into the gluteal muscle using a minimum needle length of 1½ inches for adults. Obese patients may require a longer needle. Alternate sites for subsequent injections.

Dosage Forms Excipient information presented when available (limited, particularly for generics); consult specific product labeling.

Suspension, Injection, as acetonide:

Kenalog: 10 mg/mL (5 mL); 40 mg/mL (1 mL, 5 mL, 10 mL) [contains benzyl alcohol, polysorbate 80]

Suspension, Injection, as hexacetonide:

Aristospan Intra-Articular: 20 mg/mL (1 mL, 5 mL) [contains benzyl alcohol]

Aristospan Intralesional: 5 mg/mL (5 mL) [contains benzyl alcohol]

Triamcinolone (Nasal) (trye am SIN oh lone)

Brand Names: U.S. Nasacort AQ

Brand Names: Canada Nasacort AQ; Trinasal

Index Terms Nasacort Allergy 24HR [OTC]; Triamcinolone Acetonide

Pharmacologic Category Corticosteroid, Nasal

Use Management of seasonal and perennial allergic rhinitis

Unlabeled Use Adjunct to antibiotics in empiric treatment of acute bacterial rhinosinusitis (ABRS) (Chow, 2012)

Pregnancy Risk Factor C

Dosage Perennial allergic rhinitis, seasonal allergic rhinitis:

Intranasal: Nasal spray:

Children 2 to <6 years: One spray (55 mcg) in each nostril once daily (maximum: 1 spray [55 mcg] in each nostril once daily)

Children 6 to <12 years: Initial: One spray (55 mcg) in each nostril once daily; may increase to 2 sprays (110 mcg) in each nostril once daily if response not adequate; once symptoms controlled may reduce to 1 spray (55 mcg) in each nostril once daily (maximum: 2 sprays [110 mcg] in each nostril once daily)

Children ≥12 years, Adolescents, and Adults: Two sprays (110 mcg) in each nostril once daily; once symptoms controlled reduce to 1 spray (55 mcg) in each nostril once daily (maximum: 2 sprays [110 mcg] in each nostril once daily)

Dosage adjustment in renal impairment: No dosage adjustment provided in the manufacturer's labeling (has not been studied).

Dosage adjustment in hepatic impairment: No dosage adjustment provided in the manufacturer's labeling (has not been studied).

Additional Information Complete prescribing information should be consulted for additional detail.

Product Availability Nasacort Allergy 24HR OTC: FDA approved October 2013; availability anticipated in the Spring of 2014.

Dosage Forms Considerations

Nasacort AQ 16.5 g bottles contain 120 sprays.

Dosage Forms Excipient information presented when available (limited, particularly for generics); consult specific product labeling.

Aerosol Solution, Nasal, as acetonide:

Nasacort AQ: 55 mcg/actuation (16.5 g)

Inhaler, Nasal, as acetonide:

Generic: 55 mcg/actuation (16.5 g)

Triamcinolone (Ophthalmic)

(trye am SIN oh lone)

Brand Names: U.S. Triesence

Index Terms Triamcinolone acetonide

Pharmacologic Category Corticosteroid, Ophthalmic

Use

Intavitreal: Treatment of sympathetic ophthalmia, temporal arteritis, uveitis, ocular inflammatory conditions unresponsive to topical corticosteroids

Triesence™: Visualization during vitrectomy

Pregnancy Risk Factor D

Dosage Ophthalmic injection: Intravitreal: Children and Adults:

Ocular disease: Initial: 4 mg as a single dose; additional doses may be given as needed over the course of treatment

Visualization during vitrectomy (Triesence™): 1-4 mg

Dosage adjustment in renal impairment: No dosage adjustment provided in the manufacturer's labeling.

Dosage adjustment in hepatic impairment: No dosage adjustment provided in the manufacturer's labeling.

Additional Information Complete prescribing information should be consulted for additional detail.

Dosage Forms Excipient information presented when available (limited, particularly for generics); consult specific product labeling.

Suspension, Intraocular, as acetonide:

Triesence: 40 mg/mL (1 mL) [contains polysorbate 80]

Triamcinolone (Topical) (trye am SIN oh lone)

Brand Names: U.S. Dermasorb TA; Kenalog; Oralone; Pediaderm TA; Trianex; Triderm

Brand Names: Canada Kenalog®; Oracort; Triaderm

Pharmacologic Category Corticosteroid, Topical

Additional Appendix Information

Topical Corticosteroids *on page 2299*

Use

Oral topical: Adjunctive treatment and temporary relief of symptoms associated with oral inflammatory lesions and ulcerative lesions resulting from trauma

Topical: Inflammatory dermatoses responsive to steroids

Pregnancy Risk Factor C

Dosage

Oral topical: Oral inflammatory lesions/ulcers: Press a small dab (about ¼ inch) to the lesion until a thin film develops. A larger quantity may be required for coverage of some lesions. For optimal results use only enough to coat the lesion with a thin film; do not rub in.

Topical:

Cream, Ointment:

0.025% or 0.05%: Apply thin film to affected areas 2-4 times/day

0.1% or 0.5%: Apply thin film to affected areas 2-3 times/day

Spray: Apply to affected area 3-4 times/day

Additional Information Complete prescribing information should be consulted for additional detail.

Dosage Forms Excipient information presented when available (limited, particularly for generics); consult specific product labeling.

Aerosol Solution, External, as acetonide:
 Kenalog: (63 g, 100 g)
Cream, External, as acetonide:
 Triderm: 0.1% (28.4 g, 85.2 g) [contains propylene glycol]
 Generic: 0.025% (15 g, 80 g, 454 g); 0.1% (15 g, 30 g, 80 g, 453.6 g, 454 g); 0.5% (15 g)
Kit, External, as acetonide:
 Dermasorb TA: 0.1% [contains cetyl alcohol, milk protein, propylene glycol]
 Pediaderm TA: 0.1% [contains cetyl alcohol, methylparaben, polysorbate 80, propylene glycol, propylparaben]
Lotion, External, as acetonide:
 Generic: 0.025% (60 mL); 0.1% (60 mL)
Ointment, External, as acetonide:
 Trianex: 0.05% (17 g, 85 g)
 Generic: 0.025% (15 g, 80 g, 454 g); 0.1% (15 g, 80 g, 453.6 g, 454 g); 0.5% (15 g)
Paste, Mouth/Throat, as acetonide:
 Oralone: 0.1% (5 g)
 Generic: 0.1% (5 g)

- ◆ **Triamcinolone Acetonide** *see* Triamcinolone (Nasal) *on page 2123*
- ◆ **Triamcinolone acetonide** *see* Triamcinolone (Ophthalmic) *on page 2123*
- ◆ **Triamcinolone Acetonide, Parenteral** *see* Triamcinolone (Systemic) *on page 2121*
- ◆ **Triamcinolone and Nystatin** *see* Nystatin and Triamcinolone *on page 1482*
- ◆ **Triamcinolone Hexacetonide** *see* Triamcinolone (Systemic) *on page 2121*
- ◆ **Triaminic Allerchews [OTC]** *see* Loratadine *on page 1240*
- ◆ **Triaminic® Children's Chest & Nasal Congestion [OTC]** *see* Guaifenesin and Phenylephrine *on page 978*
- ◆ **Triaminic® Children's Cold & Allergy [OTC]** *see* Chlorpheniramine and Phenylephrine *on page 412*
- ◆ **Triaminic Children's Fever Reducer Pain Reliever [OTC]** *see* Acetaminophen *on page 28*
- ◆ **Triaminic® Children's Night Time Cold & Cough [OTC]** *see* Diphenhydramine and Phenylephrine *on page 625*
- ◆ **Triaminic® Children's Softchews® Cough & Runny Nose [OTC]** *see* Dextromethorphan and Chlorpheniramine *on page 591*
- ◆ **Triaminic® Cold & Allergy (Can)** *see* Chlorpheniramine and Pseudoephedrine *on page 412*
- ◆ **Triaminic Cough/Runny Nose [OTC]** *see* DiphenhydrAMINE (Systemic) *on page 622*
- ◆ **Triaminic® Day Time Cold & Cough [OTC]** *see* Dextromethorphan and Phenylephrine *on page 591*

Triamterene (trye AM ter een)

Brand Names: U.S. Dyrenium

Pharmacologic Category Antihypertensive; Diuretic, Potassium-Sparing

Use Edema: For the treatment of edema associated with congestive heart failure, cirrhosis of the liver and the nephrotic syndrome; also in steroid-induced edema, idiopathic edema and edema due to secondary hyperaldosteronism.

Unlabeled Use Hypertension: For the treatment of hypertension in children >1 year, adolescents, and adults.

Pregnancy Risk Factor C

Dosage

Edema: Adults: Oral: 100-300 mg daily in 1-2 divided doses; maximum dose: 300 mg daily
Hypertension (unlabeled use):
 Children ≥1 year and Adolescents: Oral: Initial: 1-2 mg/kg/day in 2 divided doses; maximum: 3-4 mg/kg/day, up to 300 mg daily (NHLBI, 2004)
 Adults: Oral: Usual dosage range: 50-100 mg daily (JNC7)
 Elderly: Consider lower initial doses and titrate to response (Aronow, 2011)

Dosage adjustment in renal impairment:
 Mild-to-moderate impairment: No dosage adjustment provided in manufacturer's labeling.
 Severe impairment or progressive kidney disease: Use is contraindicated.
 The following adjustments have also been recommended (Aronoff, 2007); **Note:** Renal function may be estimated using the Cockcroft-Gault formula for dosage adjustment purposes: Adults:
  Cl_{cr} >50 mL/minute: No dosage adjustment necessary.
  Cl_{cr} ≤50 mL/minute: Use not recommended.

Dosage adjustment in hepatic impairment:
 Mild-to-moderate impairment: No dosage adjustment provided in manufacturer's labeling (has not been studied).
 Severe hepatic disease: Use is contraindicated.

Additional Information Complete prescribing information should be consulted for additional detail.

Dosage Forms Excipient information presented when available (limited, particularly for generics); consult specific product labeling.

Capsule, Oral:
 Dyrenium: 50 mg, 100 mg

- ◆ **Triamterene and Hydrochlorothiazide** *see* Hydrochlorothiazide and Triamterene *on page 1006*
- ◆ **Trianex** *see* Triamcinolone (Topical) *on page 2123*
- ◆ **Triatec-8 (Can)** *see* Acetaminophen and Codeine *on page 32*
- ◆ **Triatec-8 Strong (Can)** *see* Acetaminophen and Codeine *on page 32*
- ◆ **Triatec-30 (Can)** *see* Acetaminophen and Codeine *on page 32*

Triazolam (trye AY zoe lam)

Brand Names: U.S. Halcion

Brand Names: Canada Apo-Triazo®; Gen-Triazolam; Halcion®; Mylan-Triazolam

Pharmacologic Category Benzodiazepine

Additional Appendix Information

 Beers Criteria – Potentially Inappropriate Medications for Geriatrics *on page 2368*
 Benzodiazepine Comparison Table *on page 2292*

Use Short-term (generally 7-10 days) treatment of insomnia

Unlabeled Use Oral sedation prior to outpatient dental procedures

Pregnancy Risk Factor X

Medication Guide Available Yes

Dosage

Insomnia (short-term use): Oral:
 Adults: Usual dose: 0.25 mg at bedtime; 0.125 mg at bedtime may be sufficient in some patients, such as those with low body weight; maximum dose: 0.5 mg daily
 Elderly and/or debilitated patients: Initial: 0.125 mg at bedtime; maximum dose: 0.25 mg daily
Dental preprocedure oral sedation (unlabeled use): Adults: 0.25 mg 1 hour before procedure; 0.125 mg used for elderly patients or patients sensitive to sedative effects (Dionne, 2006)

Dosage adjustment in renal impairment: No dosage adjustment provided in manufacturer's labeling; use with caution.

Dosage adjustment in hepatic impairment: No dosage adjustment provided in manufacturer's labeling; use with caution.

Additional Information Complete prescribing information should be consulted for additional detail.

Dosage Forms Excipient information presented when available (limited, particularly for generics); consult specific product labeling.

Tablet, Oral:
- Halcion: 0.25 mg [scored]
- Generic: 0.125 mg, 0.25 mg

Controlled Substance C-IV

- **Tri-B® [OTC]** *see* Folic Acid, Cyanocobalamin, and Pyridoxine *on page 908*
- **Tribavirin** *see* Ribavirin *on page 1804*
- **Tribenzor™** *see* Olmesartan, Amlodipine, and Hydrochlorothiazide *on page 1498*
- **Tri-Buffered Aspirin [OTC]** *see* Aspirin *on page 177*
- **Tricardio B** *see* Folic Acid, Cyanocobalamin, and Pyridoxine *on page 908*
- **Trichloroacetaldehyde Monohydrate** *see* Chloral Hydrate *on page 403*
- **Tricitrates** *see* Citric Acid, Sodium Citrate, and Potassium Citrate *on page 443*
- **Tricode® GF** *see* Guaifenesin, Pseudoephedrine, and Codeine *on page 979*
- **Tricor** *see* Fenofibrate and Derivatives *on page 837*
- **Tricosal** *see* Choline Magnesium Trisalicylate *on page 418*
- **Tri-Cyclen (Can)** *see* Ethinyl Estradiol and Norgestimate *on page 795*
- **Tri-Cyclen Lo (Can)** *see* Ethinyl Estradiol and Norgestimate *on page 795*
- **Triderm** *see* Triamcinolone (Topical) *on page 2123*
- **Tridesilon (Can)** *see* Desonide *on page 578*
- **Tridil** *see* Nitroglycerin *on page 1466*
- **Tridural (Can)** *see* TraMADol *on page 2099*
- **Trien** *see* Trientine *on page 2125*

Trientine (TRYE en teen)

Brand Names: U.S. Syprine

Brand Names: Canada Syprine®

Index Terms 2,2,2-tetramine; Trien; Trientine Hydrochloride; Triethylene Tetramine Dihydrochloride

Pharmacologic Category Chelating Agent

Use Treatment of Wilson's disease in patients intolerant to penicillamine

Pregnancy Risk Factor C

Dosage Oral:

Children <12 years: 500-750 mg/day in divided doses 2-4 times/day; maximum: 1.5 g/day. AASLD practice guidelines suggest 20 mg/kg/day rounded off to the nearest 250 mg, given in 2-3 divided doses (Roberts, 2008).

Children ≥12 years and Adults: 750-1250 mg/day in divided doses 2-4 times/day; maximum dose: 2 g/day. AASLD practice guidelines suggest typical doses of 750-1500 mg/day in 2-3 divided doses with maintenance therapy of 750-1000 mg/day (Roberts, 2008).

Dosage adjustment in renal impairment: No dosage adjustment provided in manufacturer's labeling.

Dosage adjustment in hepatic impairment: No dosage adjustment provided in manufacturer's labeling.

Additional Information Complete prescribing information should be consulted for additional detail.

Dosage Forms Excipient information presented when available (limited, particularly for generics); consult specific product labeling.

Capsule, Oral, as hydrochloride:
- Syprine: 250 mg

- **Trientine Hydrochloride** *see* Trientine *on page 2125*
- **Triesence** *see* Triamcinolone (Ophthalmic) *on page 2123*
- **Tri-Estarylla** *see* Ethinyl Estradiol and Norgestimate *on page 795*
- **Triethylene Tetramine Dihydrochloride** *see* Trientine *on page 2125*
- **Triethylenethiophosphoramide** *see* Thiotepa *on page 2049*

Trifluoperazine (trye floo oh PER a zeen)

Brand Names: Canada Apo-Trifluoperazine®; Novo-Trifluzine; PMS-Trifluoperazine; Terfluzine

Index Terms Stelazine; Trifluoperazine Hydrochloride

Pharmacologic Category Antipsychotic Agent, Typical, Phenothiazine

Additional Appendix Information

Antipsychotic Agents *on page 2290*

Beers Criteria – Potentially Inappropriate Medications for Geriatrics *on page 2368*

Use Treatment of schizophrenia; short-term treatment of generalized nonpsychotic anxiety

Unlabeled Use Management of psychotic disorders; behavioral symptoms associated with dementia behavior (elderly); psychosis/agitation related to Alzheimer's dementia

Pregnancy Considerations Adverse events were not observed in animal reproduction studies, except when using doses that were also maternally toxic. Jaundice or hyper-/hyporeflexia have been reported in newborn infants following maternal use of phenothiazines. Antipsychotic use during the third trimester of pregnancy has a risk for abnormal muscle movements (extrapyramidal symptoms [EPS]) and withdrawal symptoms in newborns following delivery. Symptoms in the newborn may include agitation, feeding disorder, hypertonia, hypotonia, respiratory distress, somnolence, and tremor; these effects may be self-limiting or require hospitalization.

Breast-Feeding Considerations Trifluoperazine is excreted into breast milk and was measurable in the serum of three nursing infants (adverse events were not reported). Milk concentrations may be higher than those found in the maternal serum. Infants should be monitored for signs of adverse events.

Contraindications Hypersensitivity to trifluoperazine or any component of the formulation (cross-reactivity between phenothiazines may occur); severe CNS depression; bone marrow suppression; blood dyscrasias; severe hepatic disease; coma

Warnings/Precautions [U.S. Boxed Warning]: Elderly patients with dementia-related psychosis treated with antipsychotics are at an increased risk of death compared to placebo. Most deaths appeared to be either cardiovascular (eg, heart failure, sudden death) or infectious (eg, pneumonia) in nature. Trifluoperazine is not approved for the treatment of dementia-related psychosis.

Leukopenia, neutropenia, and agranulocytosis (sometimes fatal) have been reported in clinical trials and postmarketing reports with antipsychotic use; presence of risk factors (eg, pre-existing low WBC or history of drug-induced leuko-/neutropenia) should prompt periodic blood count assessment. Discontinue therapy at first signs of blood dyscrasias or if absolute neutrophil count <1000/mm^3.

May be sedating, use with caution in disorders where CNS depression is a feature. Use with caution in Parkinson's disease. Caution in patients with hemodynamic instability; predisposition to seizures; subcortical brain damage; severe cardiac or renal disease. Liver damage and jaundice of the cholestatic type of hepatitis have been reported with use; use is contraindicated in patients with pre-existing hepatic disease. Esophageal dysmotility and aspiration have been associated with antipsychotic use - use with caution in patients at risk of pneumonia (ie, Alzheimer's disease). Use associated with increased prolactin levels; clinical significance of hyperprolactinemia in patients with breast cancer or other prolactin-dependent tumors is unknown. May alter temperature regulation or mask toxicity of other drugs due to antiemetic effects. May alter cardiac conduction - life-threatening arrhythmias have occurred with therapeutic doses of phenothiazines. May cause orthostatic hypotension - use with caution in patients at risk of this effect or those who would tolerate transient hypotensive episodes (cerebrovascular disease, cardiovascular disease or other medications which may predispose).

Due to anticholinergic effects, should be used with caution in patients with decreased gastrointestinal motility, urinary retention, BPH, xerostomia, visual problems, or narrow-angle glaucoma. Relative to other antipsychotics, trifluoperazine has a low potency of cholinergic blockade.

Use in elderly patients with dementia is associated with an increased risk of mortality and cerebrovascular accidents; avoid antipsychotic use for behavioral problems associated with dementia unless alternative nonpharmacologic therapies have failed and patient may harm self or others. In addition, use may cause or exacerbate syndrome of inappropriate antidiuretic hormone secretion or hyponatremia; monitor sodium closely with initiation or dosage adjustments in older adults. May also be inappropriate in older adults depending on comorbidities (eg, dementia, delirium) due to its potent anticholinergic effects (Beers Criteria). Increased risk for developing tardive dyskinesia, particularly elderly women.

May cause extrapyramidal symptoms (EPS), including pseudoparkinsonism, acute dystonic reactions, akathisia, and tardive dyskinesia. Risk of dystonia (and possibly other EPS) may be greater with increased doses, use of conventional antipsychotics, males, and younger patients. Use caution in the elderly. May be associated with neuroleptic malignant syndrome (NMS) or pigmentary retinopathy.

Adverse Reactions Frequency not defined.

Cardiovascular: Cardiac arrest, hypotension, orthostatic hypotension

Central nervous system: Dizziness; extrapyramidal symptoms (akathisia, dystonias, pseudoparkinsonism, tardive dyskinesia); headache, impairment of temperature regulation, lowering of seizure threshold, neuroleptic malignant syndrome (NMS)

Dermatologic: Discoloration of skin (blue-gray), increased sensitivity to sun, photosensitivity, rash

Endocrine & metabolic: Breast pain, galactorrhea, gynecomastia, hyperglycemia, hypoglycemia, lactation, libido (changes in), menstrual cycle (changes in)

Gastrointestinal: Constipation, nausea, stomach pain, vomiting, weight gain, xerostomia

Genitourinary: Difficulty in urination, ejaculatory disturbances, priapism, urinary retention

Hematologic: Agranulocytosis, aplastic anemia, eosinophilia, hemolytic anemia, leukopenia, pancytopenia, thrombocytopenic purpura

Hepatic: Cholestatic jaundice, hepatotoxicity

Neuromuscular & skeletal: Tremor

Ocular: Cornea and lens changes, pigmentary retinopathy

Respiratory: Nasal congestion

Drug Interactions

Metabolism/Transport Effects Substrate of CYP1A2 (major); **Note:** Assignment of Major/Minor substrate status based on clinically relevant drug interaction potential

Avoid Concomitant Use

Avoid concomitant use of Trifluoperazine with any of the following: Aclidinium; Amisulpride; Azelastine (Nasal); Ipratropium (Oral Inhalation); Metoclopramide; Paraldehyde; Sulpiride; Tiotropium; Umeclidinium

Increased Effect/Toxicity

Trifluoperazine may increase the levels/effects of: Alcohol (Ethyl); Amisulpride; Analgesics (Opioid); Anticholinergics; Antidepressants (Serotonin Reuptake Inhibitor/Antagonist); Azelastine (Nasal); Beta-Blockers; CNS Depressants; Methotrimeprazine; Methylphenidate; Paraldehyde; Porfimer; Serotonin Modulators; Sulpiride; Tiotropium; Zolpidem

The levels/effects of Trifluoperazine may be increased by: Abiraterone Acetate; Acetylcholinesterase Inhibitors (Central); Aclidinium; Antidepressants (Serotonin Reuptake Inhibitor/Antagonist); Antimalarial Agents; Beta-Blockers; Brimonidine (Topical); CYP1A2 Inhibitors (Moderate); CYP1A2 Inhibitors (Strong); Deferasirox; Doxylamine; Droperidol; HydrOXYzine; Ipratropium (Oral Inhalation); Lithium formulations; Magnesium Sulfate; Methotrimeprazine; Methylphenidate; Metoclopramide; Metyrosine; Perampanel; Pramlintide; Serotonin Modulators; Sodium Oxybate; Tetrabenazine; Umeclidinium; Vemurafenib

Decreased Effect

Trifluoperazine may decrease the levels/effects of: Amphetamines; Anti-Parkinson's Agents (Dopamine Agonist); Quinagolide

The levels/effects of Trifluoperazine may be decreased by: Antacids; Anti-Parkinson's Agents (Dopamine Agonist); CYP1A2 Inducers (Strong); Cyproterone; Lithium formulations

Ethanol/Nutrition/Herb Interactions

Ethanol: May increase CNS depression; monitor for increased effects with coadministration. Caution patients about effects.

Herb/Nutraceutical: Avoid kava kava, gotu kola, valerian, St John's wort (may increase CNS depression). Avoid dong quai, St John's wort (may also cause photosensitization).

Mechanism of Action Trifluoperazine is a piperazine phenothiazine antipsychotic which blocks postsynaptic mesolimbic dopaminergic receptors in the brain; exhibits alpha-adrenergic blocking effect and depresses the release of hypothalamic and hypophyseal hormones

Pharmacodynamics/Kinetics

Metabolism: Extensively hepatic

Half-life elimination: >24 hours with chronic use

Dosage Oral:

Children 6-12 years: Schizophrenia/psychoses: Hospitalized or well-supervised patients: Initial: 1 mg 1-2 times/day, gradually increase until symptoms are controlled or adverse effects become troublesome; maximum: 15 mg/day

Adults:

Schizophrenia/psychoses:

Outpatients: 1-2 mg twice daily

Hospitalized or well-supervised patients: Initial: 2-5 mg twice daily with optimum response in the 15-20 mg/day range; do not exceed 40 mg/day

Nonpsychotic anxiety: 1-2 mg twice daily; maximum: 6 mg/day; therapy for anxiety should not exceed 12 weeks; do not exceed 6 mg/day for longer than 12 weeks when treating anxiety; agitation, jitteriness, or insomnia may be confused with original neurotic or psychotic symptoms

Elderly:

Schizophrenia/psychoses: Refer to adult dosing. Dose selection should start at the low end of the dosage range and titration must be gradual.

Behavioral symptoms associated with dementia behavior (unlabeled use): Initial: 0.5-1 mg 1-2 times/day; increase dose at 4- to 7-day intervals by 0.5-1 mg/day; increase dosing intervals (bid, tid, etc) as necessary to control response or side effects. Maximum daily dose: 40 mg. Gradual increases (titration) may prevent some side effects or decrease their severity.

Dosage adjustment in renal impairment: No dosage adjustment provided in manufacturer's labeling.

Hemodialysis: Not dialyzable (0% to 5%)

Dosage adjustment in hepatic impairment: Use is contraindicated in pre-existing liver injury.

Dietary Considerations May be taken with food to decrease GI distress.

Monitoring Parameters Vital signs; lipid profile, fasting blood glucose/Hgb A_{1c}; BMI; mental status, abnormal involuntary movement scale (AIMS)

Reference Range Therapeutic response and blood levels have not been established

Test Interactions False-positive for phenylketonuria

Additional Information Do not exceed 6 mg/day for longer than 12 weeks when treating anxiety. Agitation, jitteriness, or insomnia may be confused with original neurotic or psychotic symptoms.

Dosage Forms Excipient information presented when available (limited, particularly for generics); consult specific product labeling.

Tablet, Oral:

Generic: 1 mg, 2 mg, 5 mg, 10 mg

◆ **Trifluoperazine Hydrochloride** *see* Trifluoperazine *on page 2125*

◆ **Trifluorothymidine** *see* Trifluridine *on page 2127*

Trifluridine (trye FLURE i deen)

Brand Names: U.S. Viroptic

Brand Names: Canada Sandoz-Trifluridine; Viroptic®

Index Terms F_3T; Trifluorothymidine

Pharmacologic Category Antiviral Agent, Ophthalmic

Use Treatment of primary keratoconjunctivitis and recurrent epithelial keratitis caused by herpes simplex virus types I and II

Pregnancy Risk Factor C

Dosage Children ≥6 years, Adolescents, and Adults: Instill 1 drop into affected eye every 2 hours while awake, to a maximum of 9 drops daily, until re-epithelialization of corneal ulcer occurs; then use 1 drop every 4 hours while awake for another 7 days (minimum daily dosage of 5 drops is recommended); do **not** exceed 21 days of treatment; if improvement has not taken place in 7-14 days, consider another form of therapy

Dosage adjustment in renal impairment: No dosage adjustment provided in manufacturer's labeling.

Dosage adjustment in hepatic impairment: No dosage adjustment provided in manufacturer's labeling.

Additional Information Complete prescribing information should be consulted for additional detail.

Dosage Forms Excipient information presented when available (limited, particularly for generics); consult specific product labeling.

Solution, Ophthalmic:

Viroptic: 1% (7.5 mL) [contains thimerosal]

Generic: 1% (7.5 mL)

◆ **Triglide** *see* Fenofibrate and Derivatives *on page 837*

◆ **Trihexyphen (Can)** *see* Trihexyphenidyl *on page 2127*

Trihexyphenidyl (trye heks ee FEN i dil)

Brand Names: Canada PMS-Trihexyphenidyl; Trihexyphen; Trihexyphenidyl

Index Terms Artane; Benzhexol Hydrochloride; Trihexyphenidyl Hydrochloride

Pharmacologic Category Anti-Parkinson's Agent, Anticholinergic; Anticholinergic Agent

Additional Appendix Information

Antiparkinsonian Agents *on page 2289*

Beers Criteria – Potentially Inappropriate Medications for Geriatrics *on page 2368*

Use Adjunctive treatment of Parkinson's disease; treatment of drug-induced extrapyramidal symptoms

Pregnancy Risk Factor C

Pregnancy Considerations Animal reproduction studies have not been conducted. One case report did not show evidence of adverse events after trihexyphenidyl administration during pregnancy (Robottom, 2011).

Breast-Feeding Considerations Anticholinergic agents may suppress lactation.

Contraindications There are no contraindications listed within the manufacturer's labeling.

Warnings/Precautions Use with caution in hot weather or during exercise, especially when administered concomitantly with other atropine-like drugs to chronically-ill patients, alcoholics, patients with CNS disease, or persons doing manual labor in a hot environment. Use with caution in patients with cardiovascular disease (including hypertension), glaucoma, prostatic hyperplasia or any tendency toward urinary retention, liver or kidney disorders, and obstructive disease of the GI tract. May exacerbate mental symptoms when used to treat extrapyramidal symptoms. When given in large doses or to susceptible patients, may cause weakness. May impair physical or mental abilities; patients must be cautioned about performing tasks which require mental alertness (eg, operating machinery or driving). Does not improve symptoms of tardive dyskinesias. Avoid use in older adults; not recommended for prevention of extrapyramidal symptoms with antipsychotics; alternative agents preferred in the treatment of Parkinson disease. May be inappropriate in older adults depending on comorbidities(eg, dementia, delirium) due to its potent anticholinergic effects (Beers Criteria).

Adverse Reactions Frequency not defined.

Cardiovascular: Tachycardia

Central nervous system: Agitation, confusion, delusions, dizziness, drowsiness, euphoria, hallucination, headache, nervousness, paranoia, psychiatric disturbance

Dermatologic: Skin rash

Gastrointestinal: Constipation, intestinal obstruction, nausea, parotitis, toxic megacolon, vomiting, xerostomia

Genitourinary: Urinary retention

Neuromuscular & skeletal: Weakness

Ophthalmic: Blurred vision, glaucoma, increased intraocular pressure, mydriasis

Drug Interactions

Metabolism/Transport Effects None known.

Avoid Concomitant Use

Avoid concomitant use of Trihexyphenidyl with any of the following: Aclidinium; Ipratropium (Oral Inhalation); Potassium Chloride; Tiotropium; Umeclidinium

Increased Effect/Toxicity

Trihexyphenidyl may increase the levels/effects of: AbobotulinumtoxinA; Analgesics (Opioid); Anticholinergics; Cannabinoids; Mirabegron; OnabotulinumtoxinA; Potassium Chloride; RimabotulinumtoxinB; Thiazide Diuretics; Tiotropium; Topiramate

The levels/effects of Trihexyphenidyl may be increased by: Aclidinium; Ipratropium (Oral Inhalation); Pramlintide; Umeclidinium

Decreased Effect

Trihexyphenidyl may decrease the levels/effects of: Acetylcholinesterase Inhibitors (Central); Secretin

The levels/effects of Trihexyphenidyl may be decreased by: Acetylcholinesterase Inhibitors (Central)

Ethanol/Nutrition/Herb Interactions Ethanol: Avoid ethanol (may increase CNS depression).

Storage/Stability Store at 20°C to 25°C (68°F to 77°F).

Mechanism of Action Exerts a direct inhibitory effect on the parasympathetic nervous system. It also has a relaxing effect on smooth musculature; exerted both directly on the muscle itself and indirectly through parasympathetic nervous system (inhibitory effect)

Pharmacodynamics/Kinetics

Metabolism: Hydroxylation of the alicyclic groups
Half-life elimination: 33 hours
Time to peak, serum: 1.3 hours
Excretion: Urine and bile

Dosage Oral:

Adults:

Parkinson's disease: Initial: 1 mg/day, increase by 2 mg increments at intervals of 3-5 days; usual dose: 6-10 mg/day in 3-4 divided doses; doses of 12-15 mg/day may be required

Drug-induced EPS: Initial: 1 mg/day; increase as necessary to usual range: 5-15 mg/day in 3-4 divided doses

Use in combination with levodopa: Usual range: 3-6 mg/day in divided doses

Elderly: Parkinson's disease: Refer to adult dosing. **Note:** Conservative initial doses and gradual titration is especially important in patients >60 years of age.

Dosage adjustment in renal impairment: No dosage adjustment provided in manufacturer's labeling; use with caution.

Dosage adjustment in hepatic impairment: No dosage adjustment provided in manufacturer's labeling; use with caution.

Dietary Considerations May be taken before or after meals; tolerated best if given with food.

Administration May be administered before or after meals; tolerated best if given in 3 daily doses and with food. High doses (>10 mg/day) may be divided into 4 doses, at meal times and at bedtime.

Monitoring Parameters IOP monitoring and gonioscopic evaluations should be performed periodically

Additional Information Incidence and severity of side effects are dose related. Patients may be switched to sustained-action capsules when stabilized on conventional dosage forms.

Dosage Forms Excipient information presented when available (limited, particularly for generics); consult specific product labeling.

Elixir, Oral, as hydrochloride:
Generic: 0.4 mg/mL (473 mL)

Tablet, Oral, as hydrochloride:
Generic: 2 mg, 5 mg

- **Trihexyphenidyl Hydrochloride** *see* Trihexyphenidyl *on page 2127*
- **Trilafon** *see* Perphenazine *on page 1624*
- **Tri-Legest Fe** *see* Ethinyl Estradiol and Norethindrone *on page 793*
- **Trileptal** *see* OXcarbazepine *on page 1530*
- **Trileptal® (Can)** *see* OXcarbazepine *on page 1530*
- **Trilipix** *see* Fenofibrate and Derivatives *on page 837*
- **Trilisate** *see* Choline Magnesium Trisalicylate *on page 418*
- **Tri-Luma®** *see* Fluocinolone, Hydroquinone, and Tretinoin *on page 879*
- **TriLyte** *see* Polyethylene Glycol-Electrolyte Solution *on page 1669*

Trimethobenzamide (trye meth oh BEN za mide)

Brand Names: U.S. Tigan

Brand Names: Canada Tigan®

Index Terms Trimethobenzamide Hydrochloride

Pharmacologic Category Antiemetic

Additional Appendix Information

Beers Criteria – Potentially Inappropriate Medications for Geriatrics *on page 2368*

Use Treatment of postoperative nausea and vomiting; treatment of nausea associated with gastroenteritis

Pregnancy Considerations Teratogenic effects were not observed in animal studies. Safety and efficacy have not been established in pregnant patients. Trimethobenzamide has been used to treat nausea and vomiting of pregnancy.

Breast-Feeding Considerations It is not known if trimethobenzamide is excreted in breast milk.

Contraindications Hypersensitivity to trimethobenzamide or any component of the formulation; injection contraindicated in children

Warnings/Precautions May mask emesis due to Reye's syndrome or mimic CNS effects of Reye's syndrome in patients with emesis of other etiologies. Antiemetic effects may mask toxicity of other drugs or conditions (eg, intestinal obstruction). May cause drowsiness; patient should avoid tasks requiring alertness (eg, driving, operating machinery). May cause extrapyramidal symptoms (EPS) which may be confused with CNS symptoms of primary disease responsible for emesis. Avoid use in the elderly due to the risk of EPS adverse effects combined with lower efficacy, as compared to other antiemetics (Beers Criteria). Risk of CNS adverse effects (eg, coma, EPS, seizure) may be increased in patients with acute febrile illness, dehydration, electrolyte imbalance, encephalitis, or gastroenteritis; use caution. Allergic-type skin reactions have been reported with use; discontinue with signs of sensitization. Trimethobenzamide clearance is predominantly renal; dosage reductions may be recommended in patient with renal impairment. Use capsule formulation with caution in children; antiemetics are not recommended for uncomplicated vomiting in children, limit antiemetic use to prolonged vomiting of known etiology. Use of injection is contraindicated in children.

Adverse Reactions Frequency not defined.

Cardiovascular: Hypotension (I.V. administration)
Central nervous system: Coma, depression, disorientation, dizziness, drowsiness, EPS, headache, Parkinson-like symptoms, seizure
Dermatologic: Allergic-type skin reactions
Gastrointestinal: Diarrhea
Hematologic: Blood dyscrasias
Hepatic: Jaundice
Local: Injection site burning, pain, redness, stinging, or swelling
Neuromuscular & skeletal: Muscle cramps, opisthotonos
Ocular: Blurred vision
Miscellaneous: Hypersensitivity reactions

Drug Interactions

Metabolism/Transport Effects None known.

Avoid Concomitant Use

Avoid concomitant use of Trimethobenzamide with any of the following: Aclidinium; Ipratropium (Oral Inhalation); Potassium Chloride; Tiotropium; Umeclidinium

Increased Effect/Toxicity

Trimethobenzamide may increase the levels/effects of: AbobotulinumtoxinA; Analgesics (Opioid); Anticholinergics; Cannabinoids; Mirabegron; OnabotulinumtoxinA; Potassium Chloride; RimabotulinumtoxinB; Thiazide Diuretics; Tiotropium; Topiramate

The levels/effects of Trimethobenzamide may be increased by: Aclidinium; Ipratropium (Oral Inhalation); Pramlintide; Umeclidinium

Decreased Effect

Trimethobenzamide may decrease the levels/effects of: Acetylcholinesterase Inhibitors (Central); Secretin

The levels/effects of Trimethobenzamide may be decreased by: Acetylcholinesterase Inhibitors (Central)

Ethanol/Nutrition/Herb Interactions Ethanol: Concomitant use should be avoided (sedative effects may be additive).

Storage/Stability Store capsules and injection solution at room temperature of 25°C (77°F); excursions permitted to 15°C to 30°C (59°F to 86°F).

Mechanism of Action Acts centrally to inhibit the medullary chemoreceptor trigger zone by blocking emetic impulses to the vomiting center

Pharmacodynamics/Kinetics

Onset of action: Antiemetic: Oral: 10-40 minutes; I.M.: 15-35 minutes

Duration: 3-4 hours

Metabolism: Via oxidation, forms metabolite trimethobenzamide N-oxide

Bioavailability: Oral: 60% to 100%

Half-life elimination: 7-9 hours

Time to peak: Oral: ~45 minutes; I.M.: ~30 minutes

Excretion: Urine (30% to 50%, as unchanged drug)

Dosage

Children >40 kg: Oral: 300 mg 3-4 times/day

Adults:

Oral: 300 mg 3-4 times/day

I.M.: 200 mg 3-4 times/day

Postoperative nausea and vomiting (PONV): I.M.: 200 mg, followed 1 hour later by a second 200 mg dose

Elderly: Refer to adult dosing. Consider dosage reduction or increasing dosing interval in elderly patients with renal impairment (specific adjustment guidelines are not provided in the manufacturer's labeling).

Dosage adjustment in renal impairment: Cl_{cr} ≤70 mL/minute: No specific dosage adjustment provided in manufacturer's labeling. However, dosage reduction or increased dosing interval should be considered.

Dosage adjustment in hepatic impairment: No dosage adjustment provided in manufacturer's labeling.

Administration

Injection: Administer I.M. only; not for I.V. administration. Inject deep into upper outer quadrant of gluteal muscle.

Capsule: Administer capsule orally without regard to meals.

Monitoring Parameters Renal function (at baseline)

Dosage Forms Excipient information presented when available (limited, particularly for generics); consult specific product labeling.

Capsule, Oral, as hydrochloride:

Tigan: 300 mg

Generic: 300 mg

Solution, Intramuscular, as hydrochloride:

Tigan: 100 mg/mL (2 mL)

Tigan: 100 mg/mL (20 mL) [contains phenol]

Generic: 100 mg/mL (2 mL, 20 mL)

◆ **Trimethobenzamide Hydrochloride** *see* Trimethobenzamide *on page 2128*

Trimethoprim (trye METH oh prim)

Brand Names: U.S. Primsol

Brand Names: Canada Apo-Trimethoprim®

Index Terms TMP

Pharmacologic Category Antibiotic, Miscellaneous

Use Treatment of urinary tract infections due to susceptible strains of *E. coli*, *P. mirabilis*, *K. pneumoniae*, *Enterobacter* spp and coagulase-negative *Staphylococcus* including *S. saprophyticus*; acute otitis media due to susceptible strains of *S. pneumoniae* and *H. influenzae* in children

Unlabeled Use Alternative agent for *Pneumocystis jirovecii* pneumonia (in combination with dapsone)

Pregnancy Risk Factor C

Pregnancy Considerations Adverse effects have been observed in animal reproduction studies. Trimethoprim crosses the placenta and can be detected in the fetal serum and amniotic fluid (Reid, 1975). Adverse events may be associated with trimethoprim use during pregnancy (Andersen, 2012; Andersen, 2013; Mølgaard-Nielsen, 2012). Untreated urinary tract infections may cause adverse pregnancy outcomes (Nicolle, 2005); because safer options are available for the treatment of UTIs in pregnant women, use of TMP containing products in the first trimester should be avoided (Lee, 2008). Studies evaluating the effects of trimethoprim administration in pregnancy have also been conducted with sulfamethoxazole/trimethoprim (see the Sulfamethoxazole and Trimethoprim monograph for details).

Breast-Feeding Considerations Trimethoprim is excreted in breast milk. The manufacturer recommends caution while using trimethoprim in a breast-feeding woman because trimethoprim may interfere with folic acid metabolism. Nondose-related effects could include modification of bowel flora. Also see the Sulfamethoxazole and Trimethoprim monograph for additional information.

Contraindications Hypersensitivity to trimethoprim or any component of the formulation; megaloblastic anemia due to folate deficiency

Warnings/Precautions Use with caution in patients with impaired renal or hepatic function or with possible folate deficiency. Prolonged use may result in fungal or bacterial superinfection, including *C. difficile*-associated diarrhea (CDAD) and pseudomembranous colitis; CDAD has been observed >2 months postantibiotic treatment.

Adverse Reactions Frequency not defined.

Central nervous system: Aseptic meningitis (rare), fever

Dermatologic: Maculopapular rash (3% to 7% at 200 mg/day; incidence higher with larger daily doses), erythema multiforme (rare), exfoliative dermatitis (rare), pruritus (common), phototoxic skin eruptions, Stevens-Johnson syndrome (rare), toxic epidermal necrolysis (rare)

Endocrine & metabolic: Hyperkalemia, hyponatremia

Gastrointestinal: Epigastric distress, glossitis, nausea, vomiting

Hematologic: Leukopenia, megaloblastic anemia, methemoglobinemia, neutropenia, thrombocytopenia

Hepatic: Cholestatic jaundice (rare), liver enzymes increased

Renal: BUN and creatinine increased

Miscellaneous: Anaphylaxis, hypersensitivity reactions

Drug Interactions

Metabolism/Transport Effects Substrate of CYP2C9 (major), CYP3A4 (major); **Note:** Assignment of Major/Minor substrate status based on clinically relevant drug interaction potential; **Inhibits** CYP2C8 (moderate), CYP2C9 (moderate)

Avoid Concomitant Use

Avoid concomitant use of Trimethoprim with any of the following: BCG; Dofetilide; Leucovorin Calcium-Levoleucovorin

Increased Effect/Toxicity

Trimethoprim may increase the levels/effects of: ACE Inhibitors; Amantadine; Angiotensin II Receptor Blockers; Antidiabetic Agents (Thiazolidinedione); AzaTHIOprine; Bosentan; Carvedilol; CYP2C8 Substrates; CYP2C9 Substrates; Dapsone (Systemic); Dapsone (Topical);

Digoxin; Dofetilide; Eplerenone; Fosphenytoin; Highest Risk QTc-Prolonging Agents; LamiVUDine; Memantine; Mercaptopurine; MetFORMIN; Methotrexate; Moderate Risk QTc-Prolonging Agents; Phenytoin; PRALAtrexate; Procainamide; Repaglinide; Spironolactone; Varenicline

The levels/effects of Trimethoprim may be increased by: Amantadine; CYP2C9 Inhibitors (Moderate); CYP2C9 Inhibitors (Strong); Dapsone (Systemic); Memantine; Mifepristone

Decreased Effect

Trimethoprim may decrease the levels/effects of: BCG; Sodium Picosulfate; Typhoid Vaccine

The levels/effects of Trimethoprim may be decreased by: Bosentan; CYP2C9 Inducers (Strong); CYP3A4 Inducers (Strong); Dabrafenib; Deferasirox; Fosphenytoin; Herbs (CYP3A4 Inducers); Leucovorin Calcium-Levoleucovorin; Mitotane; Peginterferon Alfa-2b; Phenytoin; Tocilizumab

Storage/Stability

Solution: Store between 15°C to 25°C (59°F to 77°F). Protect from light.

Tablets: Store at 20°C to 25°C (68°F to 77°F). Protect from light.

Mechanism of Action Inhibits folic acid reduction to tetrahydrofolate, and thereby inhibits microbial growth

Pharmacodynamics/Kinetics

Absorption: Readily and extensive

Distribution: Widely into body tissues and fluids (middle ear, prostate, bile, aqueous humor, CSF)

Protein binding: 42% to 46%

Metabolism: Partially hepatic

Half-life elimination: 8-14 hours; prolonged with renal impairment

Time to peak, serum: 1-4 hours

Excretion: Urine (60% to 80%) as unchanged drug

Dosage Oral:

Children:

Susceptible infections: Children ≥2 months: 4-6 mg/kg/day in divided doses every 12 hours (dosing for UTI in Schleiss, 2007); **Note:** AAP guidelines on treatment of UTI recommend 6-12 mg trimethoprim/kg/day (in combination with sulfamethoxazole) in 2 divided doses (AAP, 1999)

Acute otitis media: Children ≥6 months: 10 mg/kg/day in divided doses every 12 hours for 10 days

Adults:

***Pneumocystis jirovecii* pneumonia, mild-to-moderate (unlabeled use) (CDC, 2009):** 15 mg/kg/day in 3 divided doses in combination with dapsone

Susceptible infections: 100 mg every 12 hours or 200 mg every 24 hours for 10 days

Urinary tract infection, uncomplicated (unlabeled duration):

Treatment: 100 mg every 12 hours for 3 days (Gupta, 2011)

Prophylaxis: 100 mg once daily (Kodner, 2010)

Dosage adjustment in renal impairment:

Cl_{cr} 15-30 mL/minute: Administer 50 mg every 12 hours

Cl_{cr} <15 mL/minute: Not recommended

Hemodialysis: Moderately dialyzable (20% to 50%)

Dosage adjustment in hepatic impairment: No dosage adjustment provided in manufacturer's labeling; use with caution.

Dietary Considerations May cause folic acid deficiency, supplements may be needed. Should be taken with milk or food.

Administration Administer with milk or food.

Monitoring Parameters Periodic CBC and serum potassium during long-term therapy

Reference Range Therapeutic: Peak: 5-15 mg/L; Trough: 2-8 mg/L

Test Interactions May falsely increase creatinine determination measured by the Jaffé alkaline picrate assay; may interfere with determination of serum methotrexate when measured by methods that use a bacterial dihydrofolate reductase as the binding protein (eg, the competitive binding protein technique); does **not** interfere with RIA for methotrexate

Dosage Forms Excipient information presented when available (limited, particularly for generics); consult specific product labeling.

Solution, Oral [strength expressed as base]:

Primsol: 50 mg/5 mL (473 mL) [alcohol free, dye free]

Tablet, Oral:

Generic: 100 mg

Extemporaneous Preparations Note: Commercial oral solution is available (10 mg/mL [dye free, ethanol free; contains propylene glycol, sodium benzoate; bubblegum flavor])

A 10 mg/mL oral suspension may be made with tablets. Crush ten 100 mg tablets in a mortar and reduce to a fine powder. Add 20 mL of a 1:1 mixture of Simple Syrup, NF, and Methylcellulose 1% and mix to a uniform paste; mix while adding the vehicle in incremental proportions to **almost** 100 mL; transfer to a calibrated bottle, rinse mortar with vehicle, and add quantity of vehicle sufficient to make 100 mL. Label "shake well" and "refrigerate". Stable for 91 days.

Nahata MC, Pai VB, and Hipple TF, *Pediatric Drug Formulations*, 5th ed, Cincinnati, OH: Harvey Whitney Books Co, 2004.

Trimethoprim and Polymyxin B

(trye METH oh prim & pol i MIKS in bee)

Brand Names: U.S. Polytrim®

Brand Names: Canada PMS-Polytrimethoprim; Polytrim™

Index Terms Polymyxin B and Trimethoprim

Pharmacologic Category Antibiotic, Ophthalmic

Use Treatment of surface ocular bacterial conjunctivitis and blepharoconjunctivitis

Pregnancy Risk Factor C

Dosage Ophthalmic:

Children ≥2 months and Adults: Instill 1 drop in affected eye(s) every 3 hours (maximum: 6 doses per day) for 7-10 days; has also been used 4 times daily for 5-7 days (Williams, 2013; *The Wills Eye Manual*, 2004)

Elderly: No overall differences observed between elderly and other adults

Dosage adjustment in renal impairment: No dosage adjustment provided in manufacturer's labeling.

Dosage adjustment in hepatic impairment: No dosage adjustment provided in manufacturer's labeling.

Additional Information Complete prescribing information should be consulted for additional detail.

Dosage Forms Excipient information presented when available (limited, particularly for generics); consult specific product labeling.

Solution, ophthalmic: Trimethoprim 1 mg and polymyxin B sulfate 10,000 units per 1 mL (10 mL)

Polytrim®: Trimethoprim 1 mg and polymyxin B sulfate 10,000 units per 1 mL (10 mL) [contains benzalkonium chloride]

◆ **Trimethoprim and Sulfamethoxazole** *see* Sulfamethoxazole and Trimethoprim *on page* 1959

◆ **Trinasal (Can)** *see* Triamcinolone (Nasal) *on page* 2123

◆ **TriNessa** *see* Ethinyl Estradiol and Norgestimate *on page* 795

◆ **Trinipatch (Can)** *see* Nitroglycerin *on page* 1466

◆ **Tri-Norinyl** *see* Ethinyl Estradiol and Norethindrone *on page* 793

- **Triostat** *see* Liothyronine *on page 1222*
- **Tripedia** *see* Diphtheria and Tetanus Toxoids, and Acellular Pertussis Vaccine *on page 630*
- **Triphasil (Can)** *see* Ethinyl Estradiol and Levonorgestrel *on page 787*
- **Triple Antibiotic** *see* Bacitracin, Neomycin, and Polymyxin B *on page 221*
- **Triple Paste AF [OTC]** *see* Miconazole (Topical) *on page 1358*
- **Tri-Previfem** *see* Ethinyl Estradiol and Norgestimate *on page 795*

Triprolidine and Pseudoephedrine

(trye PROE li deen & soo doe e FED rin)

Brand Names: U.S. Aprodine [OTC]; Pediatex® TD

Brand Names: Canada Actifed®

Index Terms Pseudoephedrine and Triprolidine

Pharmacologic Category Alkylamine Derivative; Alpha/Beta Agonist; Decongestant; Histamine H_1 Antagonist; Histamine H_1 Antagonist, First Generation

Use Temporary relief of nasal congestion, decongest sinus openings, running nose, sneezing, itching of nose or throat and itchy, watery eyes due to common cold, hay fever, or other upper respiratory allergies

Dosage Oral:

Liquid (Pediatex® TD):

Children 6-12 years: 1.33 mL every 6 hours (maximum: 4 doses/24 hours)

Children ≥12 years and Adults: 2.67 mL every 6 hours (maximum: 4 doses/24 hours)

Syrup (Aprodine):

Children 6-12 years: 5 mL every 4-6 hours; do not exceed 4 doses in 24 hours

Children >12 years and Adults: 10 mL every 4-6 hours; do not exceed 4 doses in 24 hours

Tablet (Aprodine):

Children 6-12 years: 1/2 tablet every 4-6 hours; do not exceed 4 doses in 24 hours

Children >12 years and Adults: One tablet every 4-6 hours; do not exceed 4 doses in 24 hours

Additional Information Complete prescribing information should be consulted for additional detail.

Dosage Forms Excipient information presented when available (limited, particularly for generics); consult specific product labeling. [DSC] = Discontinued product

Liquid, oral:

Pediatex® TD: Triprolidine hydrochloride 0.938 mg and pseudoephedrine hydrochloride 10 mg per 1 mL (30 mL) [cotton candy flavor]

Syrup, oral: Triprolidine hydrochloride 1.25 mg and pseudoephedrine hydrochloride 30 mg per 5 mL (120 mL) [DSC]

Aprodine: Triprolidine hydrochloride 1.25 mg and pseudoephedrine hydrochloride 30 mg per 5 mL (120 mL)

Tablet, oral:

Aprodine: Triprolidine hydrochloride 2.5 mg and pseudoephedrine hydrochloride 60 mg

Triptorelin (trip toe REL in)

Brand Names: U.S. Trelstar Depot; Trelstar Depot Mixject; Trelstar LA; Trelstar LA Mixject; Trelstar Mixject

Brand Names: Canada Decapeptyl®; Trelstar®

Index Terms AY-25650; CL-118,532; D-Trp(6)-LHRH; Detryptoreline; Triptorelin Pamoate; Tryptoreline

Pharmacologic Category Gonadotropin Releasing Hormone Agonist

Use Palliative treatment of advanced prostate cancer

Decapeptyl® (Canadian labeling; not available in U.S.): Adjunctive therapy in women undergoing controlled ovarian hyperstimulation for assisted reproductive technologies (ART)

Unlabeled Use Treatment of endometriosis, *in vitro* fertilization, precocious puberty, uterine sarcoma; treatment of paraphilia/hypersexuality

Pregnancy Risk Factor X

Dosage

Prostate cancer, advanced: Adults: I.M.:

3.75 mg once every 4 weeks **or**

11.25 mg once every 12 weeks **or**

22.5 mg once every 24 weeks

Controlled ovarian hyperstimulation for assisted reproductive technologies (ART) (adjunctive therapy): Canadian labeling (Decapeptyl®; not available in U.S.): Adults: Females: SubQ: Usual dose: 0.1 mg once daily initiated on day 2 or 3 or days 21-23 of cycle (or 5-7 days prior to expected onset of menses). Dose may be adjusted according to ovarian response as measured by ovarian ultrasound with or without serum estradiol levels. Treatment is continued until follicles achieve suitable size (typically 4-7 weeks).

Treatment of paraphilia/hypersexuality (unlabeled use; Guay, 2009; Thibaut, 1993): Adults: Males:

Note: May cause an initial increase in androgen concentrations which may be treated with an antiandrogen (eg, flutamide, cyproterone) for 1-2 months (Guay, 2009). Avoid use in patients with osteoporosis or active pituitary pathology.

SubQ: Test dose: 1 mg (observe for hypersensitivity)

I.M.: 3.75 mg monthly

Dosage adjustment in renal impairment: No dosage adjustment provided in manufacturer's labeling. However, renal impairment increases systemic exposure to triptorelin.

Dosage adjustment in hepatic impairment: No dosage adjustment provided in manufacturer's labeling. However, hepatic impairment increases systemic exposure to triptorelin.

Additional Information Complete prescribing information should be consulted for additional detail.

Dosage Forms Excipient information presented when available (limited, particularly for generics); consult specific product labeling.

Suspension Reconstituted, Intramuscular:

Trelstar Depot: 3.75 mg (1 ea) [contains carboxymethylcellulose sodium]

Trelstar Depot Mixject: 3.75 mg (1 ea) [contains polysorbate 80]

Trelstar LA: 11.25 mg (1 ea) [contains carboxymethylcellulose sodium]

Trelstar LA Mixject: 11.25 mg (1 ea) [contains polysorbate 80]

Trelstar Mixject: 22.5 mg (1 ea) [contains polysorbate 80]

Dosage Forms: Canada Excipient information presented when available (limited, particularly for generics); consult specific product labeling.

Injection, solution, as acetate [preservative free]:

Decapeptyl®: 100 mcg/mL (equivalent to 95.6 mcg triptorelin free base) (1 mL) [prefilled syringe]

- **Triptorelin Pamoate** *see* Triptorelin *on page 2131*
- **Triquilar (Can)** *see* Ethinyl Estradiol and Levonorgestrel *on page 787*
- **Tris Buffer** *see* Tromethamine *on page 2132*
- **Trisenox** *see* Arsenic Trioxide *on page 169*
- **Tris(hydroxymethyl)aminomethane** *see* Tromethamine *on page 2132*
- **Tri-Sprintec** *see* Ethinyl Estradiol and Norgestimate *on page 795*

◆ **Trivagizole-3® (Can)** *see* Clotrimazole (Topical) *on page 476*

◆ **Trivora** *see* Ethinyl Estradiol and Levonorgestrel *on page 787*

◆ **Trizivir®** *see* Abacavir, Lamivudine, and Zidovudine *on page 20*

◆ **Trocaine Throat [OTC]** *see* Benzocaine *on page 240*

◆ **Trokendi XR** *see* Topiramate *on page 2090*

◆ **Trombovar (Can)** *see* Sodium Tetradecyl Sulfate *on page 1931*

Tromethamine (troe METH a meen)

Brand Names: U.S. Tham

Index Terms Tris Buffer; Tris(hydroxymethyl)aminomethane

Pharmacologic Category Alkalinizing Agent, Parenteral

Use Correction of metabolic acidosis associated with cardiac bypass surgery or cardiac arrest; to correct excess acidity of stored blood that is preserved with acid citrate dextrose (ACD); indicated in infants needing alkalinization after receiving maximum sodium bicarbonate (8-10 mEq/kg/24 hours)

Pregnancy Risk Factor C

Dosage Dose depends on buffer base deficit; when deficit is known: tromethamine (mL of 0.3 M solution) = body weight (kg) x base deficit (mEq/L) x 1.1

Metabolic acidosis with cardiac arrest: Adults:

I.V.: 3.6-10.8 g (111-333 mL); additional amounts may be required to control acidosis after arrest reversed

Open chest: Intraventricular: 2-6 g (62-185 mL). **Note:** Do not inject into cardiac muscle

Acidosis associated with cardiac bypass surgery: Adults:

I.V.: Average dose: 9 mL/kg (2.7 mEq/kg); 500 mL is adequate for most adults; maximum dose: 500 mg/kg over at least 1 hour

Excess acidity of acid citrate dextrose (ACD) blood in cardiac bypass surgery: Adults: 15-77 mL of 0.3 molar solution added to each 500 mL of ACD blood

Dosage adjustment in renal impairment: No dosage adjustment provided in manufacturer's labeling. Tromethamine is substantially excreted by the kidneys; use with caution; monitor ECG and potassium levels.

Dosage adjustment in hepatic impairment: No dosage adjustment provided in manufacturer's labeling.

Additional Information Complete prescribing information should be consulted for additional detail.

Dosage Forms Excipient information presented when available (limited, particularly for generics); consult specific product labeling.

Solution, Intravenous:

Tham: 30 mEq/100 mL (500 mL)

Tropicamide (troe PIK a mide)

Brand Names: U.S. Mydral; Mydriacyl

Brand Names: Canada Diotrope®; Mydriacyl®

Index Terms Bistropamide

Pharmacologic Category Ophthalmic Agent, Mydriatic

Use Short-acting mydriatic used in diagnostic procedures; as well as preoperatively and postoperatively; treatment of some cases of acute iritis, iridocyclitis, and keratitis

Pregnancy Risk Factor C

Dosage Ophthalmic: Children and Adults (individuals with heavily pigmented eyes may require larger doses):

Cycloplegia: Instill 1-2 drops (1%); may repeat in 5 minutes

Exam must be performed within 30 minutes after the repeat dose; if the patient is not examined within 20-30 minutes, instill an additional drop

Mydriasis: Instill 1-2 drops (0.5%) 15-20 minutes before exam; may repeat every 30 minutes as needed

Dosage adjustment in renal impairment: No dosage adjustment provided in manufacturer's labeling.

Dosage adjustment in hepatic impairment: No dosage adjustment provided in manufacturer's labeling.

Additional Information Complete prescribing information should be consulted for additional detail.

Dosage Forms Excipient information presented when available (limited, particularly for generics); consult specific product labeling.

Solution, Ophthalmic:

Mydral: 0.5% (15 mL); 1% (15 mL)

Mydriacyl: 1% (3 mL, 15 mL)

Generic: 0.5% (15 mL); 1% (2 mL, 3 mL, 15 mL)

◆ **Trosec (Can)** *see* Trospium *on page 2132*

Trospium (TROSE pee um)

Brand Names: U.S. Sanctura; Sanctura XR

Brand Names: Canada Sanctura® XR; Trosec

Index Terms Trospium Chloride

Pharmacologic Category Anticholinergic Agent

Additional Appendix Information

Beers Criteria – Potentially Inappropriate Medications for Geriatrics *on page 2368*

Use Treatment of overactive bladder with symptoms of urgency, incontinence, and urinary frequency

Pregnancy Risk Factor C

Pregnancy Considerations Adverse events were observed in animal studies. There are no adequate or well-controlled studies in pregnant women; use only if clearly needed.

Breast-Feeding Considerations It is not known if trospium is excreted in breast milk. According to the manufacturer, the decision to continue or discontinue breast-feeding during therapy should take into account the risk of exposure to the infant and the benefits of treatment to the mother.

Contraindications Hypersensitivity to trospium or any component of the formulation; urinary retention; gastric retention; uncontrolled narrow-angle glaucoma

Warnings/Precautions Cases of angioedema involving the face, lips, tongue, and/or larynx have been reported. Immediately discontinue if tongue, hypopharynx, or larynx are involved. May cause drowsiness, confusion, dizziness, hallucinations, and/or blurred vision, which may impair physical or mental abilities; patients must be cautioned about performing tasks which require mental alertness (eg, operating machinery or driving). May occur in the presence of increased environmental temperature; use caution in hot weather and/or exercise. Use with caution in patients with bladder flow obstruction, may increase the risk of urinary retention. Use with caution in patients with gastrointestinal obstructive disorders (eg, pyloric stenosis); may increase the risk of gastric retention. Use caution in patients with decreased GI motility (eg, myasthenia gravis, ulcerative colitis). Use immediate release formulation with caution in renal dysfunction; dosage adjustment is required. Use of the extended release formulation is contraindicated in patients with severe renal impairment (Cl_{cr} <30 mL/minute). Ethanol should not be ingested within 2 hours of the administration of the extended release formulation. Concurrent ethanol use may increase the incidence of drowsiness. Active tubular secretion (ATS) is a route of elimination; use caution with other medications that are eliminated by ATS (eg, procainamide, pancuronium, vancomycin, morphine, metformin, and tenofovir). Use with extreme caution in patients with controlled (treated) narrow-angle glaucoma. Use caution in patients with moderate or severe hepatic dysfunction. Use caution in Alzheimer's patients. Use caution in the elderly (≥65 years of age); increased anticholinergic side effects are seen. This medication is associated with potent anticholinergic properties which may be inappropriate in older adults depending on comorbidities (eg, dementia, delirium) (Beers Criteria).

Adverse Reactions

>10%: Gastrointestinal: Xerostomia (9% to 22%)

1% to 10%:

Cardiovascular: Tachycardia (<2%)

Central nervous system: Headache (4% to 7%), fatigue (2%)

Dermatologic: Skin rash (<2%), xeroderma

Gastrointestinal: Constipation (9% to 10%), abdominal pain (1% to 3%), dyspepsia (1% to 2%), flatulence (1% to 2%), abdominal distention (<2%), nausea (1%), dysgeusia, vomiting

Genitourinary: Urinary tract infection (1% to 7%), urinary retention (≤1%)

Infection: Influenza (2%)

Ophthalmic: Dry eye syndrome (1% to 2%), blurred vision (1%)

Respiratory: Nasopharyngitis (3%), dry nose (1%)

<1% (Limited to important or life-threatening): Anaphylaxis, angioedema, confusion, delirium, drowsiness, fecal impaction, gastritis, hallucination, heat intolerance, hypertensive crisis, inversion T wave on ECG, palpitations, rhabdomyolysis, Stevens-Johnson syndrome, supraventricular tachycardia, syncope, visual disturbance

Drug Interactions

Metabolism/Transport Effects None known.

Avoid Concomitant Use

Avoid concomitant use of Trospium with any of the following: Aclidinium; Ipratropium (Oral Inhalation); Potassium Chloride; Tiotropium; Umeclidinium

Increased Effect/Toxicity

Trospium may increase the levels/effects of: AbobotulinumtoxinA; Analgesics (Opioid); Anticholinergics; Cannabinoids; Mirabegron; OnabotulinumtoxinA; Potassium Chloride; RimabotulinumtoxinB; Thiazide Diuretics; Tiotropium; Topiramate

The levels/effects of Trospium may be increased by: Aclidinium; Alcohol (Ethyl); Ipratropium (Oral Inhalation); Pramlintide; Umeclidinium

Decreased Effect

Trospium may decrease the levels/effects of: Acetylcholinesterase Inhibitors (Central); Secretin

The levels/effects of Trospium may be decreased by: Acetylcholinesterase Inhibitors (Central); MetFORMIN

Ethanol/Nutrition/Herb Interactions

Ethanol: Ethanol may enhance the sedative effects of trospium. Ethanol may increase the peak (maximum) serum concentration of trospium when consumed within 2 hours of taking extended release trospium. Management: Avoid use of ethanol. Avoid consuming any alcohol within 2 hours of taking a dose of extended release trospium.

Food: Administration with a fatty meal reduces the absorption and bioavailability of trospium. Management: Administer 1 hour prior to meals or an empty stomach. Administer extended release capsules in the morning with a full glass of water.

Storage/Stability Store at 20°C to 25°C (68°F to 77°F); excursions permitted between 15°C to 30°C (59°F to 86°F).

Mechanism of Action Trospium antagonizes the effects of acetylcholine on muscarinic receptors in cholinergically innervated organs. It reduces the smooth muscle tone of the bladder.

Pharmacodynamics/Kinetics

Absorption: <10%; decreased with a high-fat meal

Distribution: V_d: 395 - >600 L, primarily in plasma

Protein binding: 48% to 85% *in vitro*

Metabolism: Hypothesized to be via esterase hydrolysis and conjugation; forms metabolites

Bioavailability: Immediate release formulation: ~10% (range: 4% to 16%)

Half-life elimination: Immediate release formulation: 20 hours

Severe renal insufficiency (Cl_{cr} <30 mL/minute): ~33 hours; extended release formulation: ~35 hours

Time to peak, plasma: 5-6 hours

Excretion: Feces (85%); urine (~6%; mostly as unchanged drug) primarily via active tubular secretion

Dosage Oral:

Adults:

Immediate release: 20 mg twice daily

Extended release: 60 mg once daily

Elderly ≥75 years: Immediate release: Consider initial dose of 20 mg once daily (based on tolerability); Extended release: Refer to adult dosing.

Dosage adjustment in renal impairment:

Cl_{cr} ≥30 mL/minute: No dosage adjustment provided in manufacturer's labeling. However, renal impairment increases systemic exposure to trospium. Monitor for increased adverse effects.

Cl_{cr} <30 mL/minute:

Immediate release: 20 mg once daily at bedtime

Extended release: Use not recommended

Dosage adjustment in hepatic impairment:

Mild impairment: No dosage adjustment provided in manufacturer's labeling.

Moderate to severe impairment: No dosage adjustment provided in manufacturer's labeling; use with caution.

Dietary Considerations Take1 hour prior to meals or on an empty stomach.

Administration Administer 1 hour prior to meals or on an empty stomach. Administer extended release capsules in the morning with a full glass of water.

Dosage Forms Excipient information presented when available (limited, particularly for generics); consult specific product labeling.

Capsule Extended Release 24 Hour, Oral, as chloride:

Sanctura XR: 60 mg

Generic: 60 mg

Tablet, Oral, as chloride:

Sanctura: 20 mg

Generic: 20 mg

◆ **Trospium Chloride** *see* Trospium *on page* 2132

◆ **Trusopt** *see* Dorzolamide *on page* 655

◆ **Trusopt® (Can)** *see* Dorzolamide *on page* 655

◆ **Truvada** *see* Emtricitabine and Tenofovir *on page* 700

Trypsin, Balsam Peru, and Castor Oil

(TRIP sin, BAL sam pe RUE, & KAS tor oyl)

Brand Names: U.S. Granulex®; TBC; Vasolex™; Xenaderm®

Index Terms Balsam Peru, Castor Oil, and Trypsin; Castor Oil, Trypsin, and Balsam Peru

Pharmacologic Category Protectant, Topical

Use

Granulex®: Treatment of decubitus ulcers, varicose ulcers, debridement of eschar, dehiscent wounds and sunburn; promote wound healing; reduce odor from necrotic wounds

Vasolex™, Xenaderm ®: Treatment of decubitus ulcers, varicose ulcers, and dehiscent wounds; promote wound healing; reduce odor from necrotic wounds

Dosage Topical: Apply a minimum of twice daily or as often as necessary

Additional Information Complete prescribing information should be consulted for additional detail.

Dosage Forms Excipient information presented when available (limited, particularly for generics); consult specific product labeling.

Aerosol, spray, topical:
- Granulex®: Trypsin 0.12 mg, balsam Peru 87 mg, and castor oil 788 mg per gram (60 g, 120 g)
- TBC: Trypsin 0.1 mg, balsam Peru 72.5 mg, and castor oil 650 mg per 0.82 mL (60 g, 120 g)

Ointment, topical:
- Vasolex™: Trypsin 90 USP units, balsam Peru 87 mg, and castor oil 788 mg per gram (5 g, 30 g, 60 g)
- Xenaderm®: Trypsin 90 USP units, balsam Peru 87 mg, and castor oil 788 mg per gram (30 g, 60 g)

◆ **Tryptoreline** *see* Triptorelin *on page* 2131
◆ **TSH** *see* Thyrotropin Alfa *on page* 2053
◆ **TSPA** *see* Thiotepa *on page* 2049
◆ **TST** *see* Tuberculin Tests *on page* 2134
◆ **TT** *see* Tetanus Toxoid (Adsorbed) *on page* 2031
◆ **Tuberculin Purified Protein Derivative** *see* Tuberculin Tests *on page* 2134
◆ **Tuberculin Skin Test** *see* Tuberculin Tests *on page* 2134

Tuberculin Tests (too BER kyoo lin tests)

Brand Names: U.S. Aplisol; Tubersol

Index Terms Mantoux; PPD; TB Skin Test; TST; Tuberculin Purified Protein Derivative; Tuberculin Skin Test

Pharmacologic Category Diagnostic Agent

Use Skin test in diagnosis of tuberculosis

Pregnancy Risk Factor C

Pregnancy Considerations Reproduction studies have not been conducted. Pregnancy is not a contraindication to testing.

Breast-Feeding Considerations Breast-feeding is not a contraindication to testing.

Contraindications Hypersensitivity to tuberculin purified protein derivative (PPD) or any component of the formulation; previous severe reaction to tuberculin PPD skin test (TST)

Warnings/Precautions Patients with a previous severe reaction to TST (vesiculation, ulceration, necrosis) at the injection site should not receive tuberculin PPD again. Do not administer to persons with documented tuberculosis or a clear history of treatment for tuberculosis; persons with extensive burns or eczema. Skin testing may be deferred with major viral infections or live-virus vaccination within 1 month. Tuberculous or other bacterial infections, viral infection, live virus vaccination, malignancy, immunosuppressive agents, and conditions which impair immune response may cause a decreased response to test. Very young children (<6 weeks of age) may also have an absent or delayed response. For intradermal administration only; do not administer I.V., I.M., or SubQ. Epinephrine (1:1000) should be available to treat possible allergic reactions.

Adverse Reactions Suspected adverse reactions should be reported to the Food and Drug Administration (FDA) MedWatch Program at 1-800-332-1088

Frequency not defined:
- Dermatologic: Rash
- Local: Injection site reactions: Bleeding, bruising, discomfort, erythematous reaction, hematoma, necrosis, pain, pruritus, redness, scarring, ulceration, vesiculation
- Miscellaneous: Anaphylaxis

Drug Interactions

Metabolism/Transport Effects None known.

Avoid Concomitant Use There are no known interactions where it is recommended to avoid concomitant use.

Increased Effect/Toxicity There are no known significant interactions involving an increase in effect.

Decreased Effect

The levels/effects of Tuberculin Tests may be decreased by: Vaccines (Live)

Storage/Stability Aplisol®, Tubersol®: Store under refrigeration at 2°C to 8°C (36°F to 46°F); do not freeze. Protect from light. Opened vials should be discarded after 30 days.

Mechanism of Action Tuberculosis results in individuals becoming sensitized to certain antigenic components of the *M. tuberculosis* organism. Culture extracts called tuberculins are contained in tuberculin skin test preparations. Upon intracutaneous injection of these culture extracts, a classic delayed (cellular) hypersensitivity reaction occurs. This reaction is characteristic of a delayed course (peak occurs >24 hours after injection, induration of the skin secondary to cell infiltration, and occasional vesiculation and necrosis). Delayed hypersensitivity reactions to tuberculin may indicate infection with a variety of nontuberculosis mycobacteria, or vaccination with the live attenuated mycobacterial strain of *M. bovis* vaccine, BCG, in addition to previous natural infection with *M. tuberculosis*.

Pharmacodynamics/Kinetics

Onset of action: Delayed hypersensitivity reactions: 5-6 hours
- Peak effect: 48-72 hours

Duration: Reactions subside over a few days

Dosage Children and Adults: Intradermal: 0.1 mL

TST interpretation: Criteria for positive TST read at 48-72 hours (see "Note" below for healthcare workers):

Induration ≥5 mm: Persons with HIV infection (or risk factors for HIV infection, but unknown status), recent close contact to person with known active TB, persons with chest x-ray consistent with healed TB, persons who are immunosuppressed

Induration ≥10 mm: Persons with clinical conditions which increase risk of TB infection, recent immigrants, I.V. drug users, residents and employees of high-risk settings, children <4 years of age

Induration ≥15 mm: Persons who do not meet any of the above criteria (no risk factors for TB)

Note: A two-step test is recommended when testing will be performed at regular intervals (eg, for healthcare workers). If the first test is negative, a second TST should be administered 1-3 weeks after the first test was read.

TST interpretation (CDC guidelines) in a healthcare setting:

Baseline test: ≥10 mm is positive (either first or second step)

Serial testing without known exposure: Increase of ≥10 mm is positive

Known exposure:
- ≥5 mm is positive in patients with baseline of 0 mm
- ≥10 mm is positive in patients with negative baseline or previous screening result of ≥0 mm

Read test at 48-72 hours following placement. Test results with 0 mm induration or measured induration less than the defined cutoff point are considered to signify absence of infection with *M. tuberculosis*. Test results should be documented in millimeters even if classified as negative. Erythema and redness of skin are not indicative of a positive test result.

Administration For intradermal administration only. Administer to upper third of forearm (palm up) ≥2 inches from elbow, wrist, or other injection site. If neither arm can be used, may administer to back of shoulder. Administer using inch 1/4 to 1/2 inch 27-gauge needle or finer tuberculin syringe. Should form wheal (6-10 mm in diameter) as liquid is injected which will remain ~10 minutes. Avoid pressure or bandage at injection site. Document date and time of injection, person placing TST, location of injection site, and lot number of solution.

Monitoring Parameters Monitor for immediate hypersensitivity reactions for ~15 minutes following injection.

Test Interactions False-positive reactions may occur with BCG vaccination or previous mycobacteria (nonTB) infection (previous BCG vaccination is not a contraindication to testing). False-negative reactions may occur with impaired cell mediated immunity.

Additional Information Situations where risk of tuberculosis infection may be increased are with contacts of recently-diagnosed persons with active disease, contact with immigrants from countries where tuberculosis is still common, or reactivation with impaired immunity (HIV infection, diabetes, renal failure, immunosuppressant use, pulmonary silicosis). Healthcare workers, staff of correctional facilities, and travelers at high risk of exposure should have routine testing. Patients with HIV infection should be tested as soon as possible following diagnosis.

The date of administration, the product manufacturer, and lot number of product must be entered into the patient's permanent medical record. Results should be recorded in millimeters (even if 0), not "negative" or "positive".

Dosage Forms Excipient information presented when available (limited, particularly for generics); consult specific product labeling.

Solution, Intradermal:

Aplisol: 5 units/0.1 mL (1 mL, 5 mL) [latex free; contains phenol, polysorbate 80]

Tubersol: 5 units/0.1 mL (1 mL, 5 mL) [contains phenol]

◆ **Tubersol** *see* Tuberculin Tests *on page 2134*
◆ **Tums [OTC]** *see* Calcium Carbonate *on page 318*
◆ **Tums® Chews Extra Strength (Can)** *see* Calcium Carbonate *on page 318*
◆ **Tums E-X 750 [OTC]** *see* Calcium Carbonate *on page 318*
◆ **Tums Extra Strength (Can)** *see* Calcium Carbonate *on page 318*
◆ **Tums Freshers [OTC]** *see* Calcium Carbonate *on page 318*
◆ **Tums Kids [OTC]** *see* Calcium Carbonate *on page 318*
◆ **Tums Lasting Effects [OTC]** *see* Calcium Carbonate *on page 318*
◆ **Tums® Regular Strength (Can)** *see* Calcium Carbonate *on page 318*
◆ **Tums Smoothies [OTC]** *see* Calcium Carbonate *on page 318*
◆ **Tums Smoothies (Can)** *see* Calcium Carbonate *on page 318*
◆ **Tums Ultra 1000 [OTC]** *see* Calcium Carbonate *on page 318*
◆ **Tums® Ultra Strength (Can)** *see* Calcium Carbonate *on page 318*
◆ **Tusscough DHC™** *see* Dihydrocodeine, Chlorpheniramine, and Phenylephrine *on page 611*
◆ **TussiCaps** *see* Hydrocodone and Chlorpheniramine *on page 1007*
◆ **Tussigon®** *see* Hydrocodone and Homatropine *on page 1008*
◆ **Tussin [OTC]** *see* GuaiFENesin *on page 974*
◆ **Tussionex** *see* Hydrocodone and Chlorpheniramine *on page 1007*
◆ **Tussionex Pennkinetic** *see* Hydrocodone and Chlorpheniramine *on page 1007*
◆ **TVP-1012** *see* Rasagiline *on page 1786*
◆ **Twinject (Can)** *see* EPINEPHrine (Systemic, Oral Inhalation) *on page 714*
◆ **Twinrix®** *see* Hepatitis A and Hepatitis B Recombinant Vaccine *on page 990*
◆ **Twinrix® Junior (Can)** *see* Hepatitis A and Hepatitis B Recombinant Vaccine *on page 990*
◆ **Twynsta** *see* Telmisartan and Amlodipine *on page 2004*
◆ **Ty21a Vaccine** *see* Typhoid Vaccine *on page 2135*
◆ **Tygacil** *see* Tigecycline *on page 2061*
◆ **Tykerb** *see* Lapatinib *on page 1174*
◆ **Tykerb® (Can)** *see* Lapatinib *on page 1174*
◆ **Tylenol [OTC]** *see* Acetaminophen *on page 28*
◆ **Tylenol (Can)** *see* Acetaminophen *on page 28*
◆ **Tylenol #2** *see* Acetaminophen and Codeine *on page 32*
◆ **Tylenol #3** *see* Acetaminophen and Codeine *on page 32*
◆ **Tylenol 8 Hour [OTC]** *see* Acetaminophen *on page 28*
◆ **Tylenol Arthritis Pain Extended Relief [OTC]** *see* Acetaminophen *on page 28*
◆ **Tylenol Children's [OTC]** *see* Acetaminophen *on page 28*
◆ **Tylenol Children's Meltaways [OTC]** *see* Acetaminophen *on page 28*
◆ **Tylenol Codeine** *see* Acetaminophen and Codeine *on page 32*
◆ **Tylenol® Decongestant (Can)** *see* Acetaminophen and Pseudoephedrine *on page 33*
◆ **Tylenol Elixir with Codeine (Can)** *see* Acetaminophen and Codeine *on page 32*
◆ **Tylenol Extra Strength [OTC]** *see* Acetaminophen *on page 28*
◆ **Tylenol Infant's Concentrated [OTC] [DSC]** *see* Acetaminophen *on page 28*
◆ **Tylenol Jr. Meltaways [OTC]** *see* Acetaminophen *on page 28*
◆ **Tylenol No. 1 (Can)** *see* Acetaminophen and Codeine *on page 32*
◆ **Tylenol No. 1 Forte (Can)** *see* Acetaminophen and Codeine *on page 32*
◆ **Tylenol No. 2 with Codeine (Can)** *see* Acetaminophen and Codeine *on page 32*
◆ **Tylenol No. 3 with Codeine (Can)** *see* Acetaminophen and Codeine *on page 32*
◆ **Tylenol No. 4 with Codeine (Can)** *see* Acetaminophen and Codeine *on page 32*
◆ **Tylenol® PM [OTC]** *see* Acetaminophen and Diphenhydramine *on page 32*
◆ **Tylenol® Severe Allergy [OTC]** *see* Acetaminophen and Diphenhydramine *on page 32*
◆ **Tylenol® Sinus (Can)** *see* Acetaminophen and Pseudoephedrine *on page 33*
◆ **Tylenol® with Codeine No. 3** *see* Acetaminophen and Codeine *on page 32*
◆ **Tylenol® with Codeine No. 4** *see* Acetaminophen and Codeine *on page 32*
◆ **Tylox** *see* Oxycodone and Acetaminophen *on page 1538*
◆ **Typherix® (Can)** *see* Typhoid Vaccine *on page 2135*
◆ **Typhim Vi®** *see* Typhoid Vaccine *on page 2135*

Typhoid Vaccine (TYE foid vak SEEN)

Brand Names: U.S. Typhim Vi®; Vivotif®

Brand Names: Canada Typherix®; Typhim Vi®; Vivotif®

Index Terms Ty21a Vaccine; Typhoid Vaccine Live Oral Ty21a; Vi Vaccine

Pharmacologic Category Vaccine, Inactivated (Bacterial); Vaccine, Live (Bacterial)

Additional Appendix Information

Immunization Administration Recommendations *on page 2334*

Immunization Recommendations *on page 2339*

Use Active immunization against typhoid fever caused by *Salmonella typhi*

Not for routine vaccination. In the United States and Canada, use should be limited to:

- Travelers to areas with a prolonged risk of exposure to *S. typhi*
- Persons with intimate exposure to a *S. typhi* carrier
- Laboratory technicians with exposure to *S. typhi*
- Travelers with achlorhydria or hypochlorhydria (Canadian recommendation)

Pregnancy Risk Factor C

Pregnancy Considerations Reproduction studies have not been conducted. The manufacturer of the Typhim Vi® injection suggests delaying vaccination until the 2nd or 3rd trimester if possible. Untreated typhoid fever may lead to miscarriage or vertical intrauterine transmission causing neonatal typhoid (rare).

Breast-Feeding Considerations It is not known if typhoid vaccine is excreted in breast milk.

Contraindications Hypersensitivity to any component of the vaccine. In addition, the oral vaccine is contraindicated with congenital or acquired immunodeficient state, acute febrile illness

Warnings/Precautions Not all recipients of typhoid vaccine will be fully protected against typhoid fever. Travelers should take all necessary precautions to avoid contact or ingestion of potentially contaminated food or water sources. Should not be used to treat typhoid fever.

Injection: Administer at least 2 weeks prior to expected exposure. Vaccination may be deferred during acute infection or febrile illness. Immune response may be decreased in those receiving immunosuppressive therapy or are otherwise immunocompromised. In general, household and close contacts of persons with altered immunocompetence may receive all age appropriate vaccines. Use caution with coagulation disorders (including thrombocytopenia) where intramuscular injections should not be used. Epinephrine 1:1000 should be readily available. Syncope has been reported with use of injectable vaccines and may be accompanied by transient visual disturbances, weakness, or tonic-clonic movements. Procedures should be in place to avoid injuries from falling and to restore cerebral perfusion if syncope occurs.

Oral: Full immunization schedule should be completed at least 1 week prior to expected exposure. The complete immunization schedule must be followed to achieve optimum immune response. Do not administer during acute GI illness; vaccination may be deferred with persistent diarrhea or vomiting.

In order to maximize vaccination rates, the ACIP recommends simultaneous administration of all age-appropriate vaccines (live or inactivated) for which a person is eligible at a single clinic visit, unless contraindications exist. Vaccination may not result in effective immunity in all patients. Response depends upon multiple factors (eg, type of vaccine, age of patient) and may be improved by administering the vaccine at the recommended dose, route, and interval. Vaccines may not be effective if administered during periods of altered immune competence (CDC, 2011).

Adverse Reactions In the U.S., all serious adverse reactions must be reported to the Department of Health and Human Services (DHHS) Vaccine Adverse Event Reporting System (VAERS) 1-800-822-7967 or online at https://vaers.hhs.gov/esub/index. In Canada, adverse reactions may be reported to local provincial/territorial health agencies or to the Vaccine Safety Section at Public Health Agency of Canada (1-866-844-0018).

Injection (incidence may vary based on age and/or product used):

>10%:

Central nervous system: Fever (undefined; 2% to 32%), malaise (4% to 24%), headache (16% to 20%)

Local: Injection site: Tenderness (97% to 98%), pain (27% to 41%), soreness (up to 16%), induration (5% to 15%)

Neuromuscular & skeletal: General aches (1% to 13%)

1% to 10%:

Central nervous system: Fever ≥100°F (2%), >102°F (2%)

Dermatologic: Pruritus (up to 8%)

Gastrointestinal: Nausea (up to 8%), vomiting (2%)

Local: Injection site: Erythema (up to 5%), swelling (up to 4%)

Neuromuscular & skeletal: Myalgia (3% to 7%)

Postmarketing and/or case reports: Abdominal pain, allergic reactions, anaphylaxis, arthralgia, cervical pain, diarrhea, dizziness, flu-like syndrome, Guillain-Barré syndrome, hypotension, injection site inflammation (including angioedema and urticaria), loss of consciousness, lymphadenopathy, malaise, perforated jejunum, rash, serum sickness, tremor, urticaria, vasodilation, weakness

Oral:

1% to 10%:

Central nervous system: Headache (5%), fever (3%)

Dermatologic: Rash (1%)

Gastrointestinal: Abdominal pain (6%), nausea (6%), diarrhea (3%), vomiting (2%)

Postmarketing and/or case reports: Anaphylactic reaction, demyelinating disease, myalgia, pain, RA, urticaria, sepsis, weakness

Drug Interactions

Metabolism/Transport Effects None known.

Avoid Concomitant Use

Avoid concomitant use of Typhoid Vaccine with any of the following: Belimumab; Fingolimod; Immunosuppressants

Increased Effect/Toxicity

The levels/effects of Typhoid Vaccine may be increased by: AzaTHIOprine; Belimumab; Corticosteroids (Systemic); Dimethyl Fumarate; Fingolimod; Hydroxychloroquine; Immunosuppressants; Leflunomide; Mercaptopurine; Methotrexate

Decreased Effect

Typhoid Vaccine may decrease the levels/effects of: Tuberculin Tests

The levels/effects of Typhoid Vaccine may be decreased by: Antibiotics; Dimethyl Fumarate; Fingolimod; Immune Globulins; Immunosuppressants

Ethanol/Nutrition/Herb Interactions Ethanol: Avoid alcohol within 2 hours of taking the capsule; may disrupt the enteric coating

Storage/Stability

Typherix®: Store between 2°C to 8°C (35°F to 46°F); do not freeze. Discard if vaccine has been frozen. Protect from light.

Typhim Vi®: Store between 2°C to 8°C (35°F to 46°F); do not freeze.

Vivotif®: Store between 2°C to 8°C (35°F to 46°F).

Mechanism of Action Virulent strains of *Salmonella typhi* cause disease by penetrating the intestinal mucosa and entering the systemic circulation via the lymphatic vasculature. One possible mechanism of conferring immunity may be the provocation of a local immune response in the intestinal tract induced by oral ingesting of a live strain with subsequent aborted infection. The ability of *Salmonella typhi* to produce clinical disease (and to elicit an immune response) is dependent on the bacteria having a complete lipopolysaccharide. The live attenuate Ty21a strain lacks the enzyme UDP-4-galactose epimerase so that lipopolysaccharide is only synthesized under conditions that induce bacterial autolysis. Thus, the strain remains avirulent despite the production of sufficient lipopolysaccharide to evoke a protective immune response. Despite low levels of lipopolysaccharide synthesis, cells lyse before gaining a virulent phenotype due to the intracellular accumulation of metabolic intermediates.

Pharmacodynamics/Kinetics

Onset of action: Immunity to *Salmonella typhi*: Oral: ~1 week

Duration: Immunity: Oral: ~4-7 years; Parenteral: Typhim Vi®: >17-21 months, Typherix®: ~3 years

Dosage Immunization:

Oral: Children ≥6 years and Adults:

Primary immunization: One capsule on alternate days (day 1, 3, 5, and 7) for a total of 4 doses; all doses should be complete at least 1 week prior to potential exposure

Booster immunization (with repeated or continued exposure to typhoid fever):

U.S. labeling: Repeat full course of primary immunization every 5 years

Canadian labeling: Repeat full course of primary immunization every 7 years

I.M.: Children ≥2 years and Adults: 0.5 mL given at least 2 weeks prior to expected exposure

Reimmunization:

Typhim Vi®: 0.5 mL; optimal schedule has not been established; a single dose every 2 years is currently recommended for repeated or continued exposure

Typherix® (Canadian labeling; not available in U.S.): 0.5 mL every 3 years

Dosage adjustment in renal impairment: No dosage adjustment provided in manufacturer's labeling.

Dosage adjustment in hepatic impairment: No dosage adjustment provided in manufacturer's labeling.

Administration

Injection: Typhim Vi® and Typherix® may be given I.M. and are indicated for children ≥2 years of age; administer as a single 0.5 mL (25 mcg) injection in deltoid muscle. **Do not administer Typhim Vi® or Typherix® intravascularly. Note:** For patients at risk of hemorrhage following intramuscular injection, the ACIP recommends "it should be administered intramuscularly if, in the opinion of the physician familiar with the patient's bleeding risk, the vaccine can be administered by this route with reasonable safety. If the patient receives antihemophilia or other similar therapy, intramuscular vaccination can be scheduled shortly after such therapy is administered. A fine needle (23 gauge or smaller) can be used for the vaccination and firm pressure applied to the site (without rubbing) for at least 2 minutes. The patient should be instructed concerning the risk of hematoma from the injection." Patients on anticoagulant therapy should be considered to have the same bleeding risks and treated as those with clotting factor disorders (CDC, 2011).

Oral: Swallow capsule whole soon after placing into mouth; do not chew or open capsule. Capsule should be taken with a cold or lukewarm beverage (≤37°C/98.6°F). Take 1 hour prior to a meal. Avoid alcohol 1 hour before or 2 hours after administration.

Simultaneous administration of vaccines helps ensure patients will be fully vaccinated by the appropriate age. Simultaneous administration of vaccines is defined as administering >1 vaccine on the same day at different anatomic sites. The ACIP prefers each dose of a specific vaccine in a series come from the same manufacturer when possible. Adolescents and adults should be vaccinated while seated or lying down. In general, preterm infants should be vaccinated at the same chronological age as full-term infants (CDC, 2011).

Antipyretics have not been shown to prevent febrile seizures. Antipyretics may be used to treat fever or discomfort following vaccination (CDC, 2011). One study reported that routine prophylactic administration of acetaminophen to prevent fever prior to vaccination decreased the immune response of some vaccines; the clinical significance of this reduction in immune response has not been established (Prymula, 2009).

Monitoring Parameters Monitor for syncope for 15 minutes following administration. If seizure-like activity associated with syncope occurs, maintain patient in supine or Trendelenburg position to reestablish adequate cerebral perfusion.

Additional Information U.S. federal law requires that the name of medication, date of administration, the vaccine manufacturer, lot number of vaccine, and the administering person's name, title, and address be entered into the patient's permanent medical record.

Dosage Forms Excipient information presented when available (limited, particularly for generics); consult specific product labeling.

Capsule, enteric coated [live]:

Vivotif®: Viable *S. typhi* Ty21a 2-6.8 x 10^9 colony-forming units and nonviable *S. typhi* Ty21a 5-50 x 10^9 bacterial cells [contains lactose 100-180 mg/capsule and sucrose 26-130 mg/capsule]

Injection, solution [inactivated]:

Typhim Vi®: Purified Vi capsular polysaccharide 25 mcg/ 0.5 mL (0.5 mL, 10 mL) [derived from *S. typhi* Ty2 strain]

Dosage Forms: Canada Excipient information presented when available (limited, particularly for generics); consult specific product labeling.

Injection, solution:

Typherix®: Vi capsular polysaccharide 25 mcg/0.5 mL (0.5 mL) [derived from *S. typhi* Ty2 strain]

- ◆ **Typhoid Vaccine Live Oral Ty21a** *see* Typhoid Vaccine *on page 2135*
- ◆ **Tysabri** *see* Natalizumab *on page 1431*
- ◆ **Tysabri® (Can)** *see* Natalizumab *on page 1431*
- ◆ **Tyvaso** *see* Treprostinil *on page 2115*
- ◆ **Tyvaso Refill** *see* Treprostinil *on page 2115*
- ◆ **Tyvaso Starter** *see* Treprostinil *on page 2115*
- ◆ **506U78** *see* Nelarabine *on page 1434*
- ◆ **U-90152S** *see* Delavirdine *on page 565*
- ◆ **UCB-P071** *see* Cetirizine *on page 396*
- ◆ **Uceris™** *see* Budesonide (Systemic) *on page 282*
- ◆ **Uceris** *see* Budesonide (Systemic) *on page 282*
- ◆ **U-Cort** *see* Hydrocortisone (Topical) *on page 1011*
- ◆ **UK-88,525** *see* Darifenacin *on page 546*
- ◆ **UK-427,857** *see* Maraviroc *on page 1269*
- ◆ **UK92480** *see* Sildenafil *on page 1894*
- ◆ **UK109496** *see* Voriconazole *on page 2203*
- ◆ **U-Kera E** *see* Urea *on page 2140*
- ◆ **Ulcidine (Can)** *see* Famotidine *on page 832*
- ◆ **Ulesfia** *see* Benzyl Alcohol *on page 245*

Ulipristal (ue li PRIS tal)

Brand Names: U.S. Ella

Brand Names: Canada Fibristal

Index Terms CDB-2914; Ulipristal Acetate

Pharmacologic Category Contraceptive; Progestin Receptor Modulator

Use Ella: Emergency contraception following unprotected intercourse or possible contraceptive failure

Fibristal [Canadian product]: Treatment of moderate-to-severe signs/symptoms of uterine fibroids in premenopausal adult women eligible for surgery. **Note:** Treatment is limited to 3 months.

Pregnancy Risk Factor X

Pregnancy Considerations Embryofetal loss was observed following administration of ulipristal to pregnant rats and rabbits during the period of organogenesis at doses that were 1/3 and 1/2 the human dose (based on BSA), respectively. Teratogenic effects were not observed in surviving fetuses. Pregnancy terminations were also observed in pregnant monkeys following administration of ulipristal during the first trimester in doses ~3 times the human dose (based on BSA). Exclude pregnancy prior to therapy; not indicated for terminating an existing pregnancy. A rapid return of fertility is expected following use for emergency contraception; routine contraceptive measures should be initiated or continued following use to ensure ongoing prevention of pregnancy. Barrier contraception is recommended immediately following emergency contraception and throughout the same menstrual cycle; efficacy of hormonal contraceptives may be decreased. When ulipristal is used for treatment of uterine fibroids (Canadian labeling; not in U.S. labeling) a nonhormonal method of contraception is recommended.

Breast-Feeding Considerations It is not known if ulipristal is excreted in breast milk. Breast-feeding is not recommended by the U.S. manufacturer.

Fibristal [Canadian product] is contraindicated in women who are breast-feeding.

Contraindications

Ella: Known or suspected pregnancy

Fibristal [Canadian product]: Hypersensitivity to ulipristal acetate or any component of the formulation; pregnancy; breast-feeding; genital bleeding of unknown etiology or for reasons other than uterine fibroids; cancer of the breast, cervix, uterus, or ovaries; continuous use longer than 3 months

Warnings/Precautions Hazardous agent - use appropriate precautions for handling and disposal (NIOSH, 2012). Use is contraindicated in patients known or suspected to be pregnant. Exclude pregnancy prior to therapy via history, physical exam or pregnancy testing; not indicated for terminating an existing pregnancy. Not intended for routine contraception. Barrier contraception is recommended immediately following emergency contraception and throughout the same menstrual cycle; efficacy of hormonal contraception may be decreased. Repeated use within the same menstrual cycle is not recommended. Menstrual bleeding patterns may be altered (cycle length may be delayed or shortened by a few days) but returns to normal in subsequent cycles. Intermenstrual bleeding (spotting) has also been observed. The possibility of pregnancy should be considered if menstruation is delayed for >7 days of the expected menstrual period. A history of ectopic pregnancy is not a contraindication to use in emergency contraception. The possibility of ectopic pregnancy should be considered in patients with abdominal pain after administration of ulipristal.

In Canada, ulipristal is approved for the treatment of uterine fibroids. A nonhormonal method of contraception is recommended during treatment of uterine fibroids. Following initiation of therapy, a significant reduction in menstrual blood loss or amenorrhea is usually observed within 10 days of initiation; menses generally returns within 4 weeks after discontinuation. Endometrial thickening has been observed in the treatment of uterine fibroids; effects are reversible following discontinuation of therapy. Persistent endometrial thickening (>3 months after discontinuation of therapy and return of menses) should be further evaluated. Changes in endometrial tissue observed with use are referred to as progesterone receptor modulator-associated endometrial changes (PAEC); may be mistaken for endometrial hyperplasia. Pathologists should be informed of ulipristal therapy when submitting endometrial tissue for histologic evaluation.

Safety and efficacy have not been established for use in hepatic or renal impairment. In the treatment of uterine fibroids (Canadian labeling; not an approved indication in U.S. labeling), use is not recommended in hepatic impairment or moderate-to-severe renal impairment unless patient is closely monitored, and is not recommended with uncontrolled severe asthma. Not for use prior to menarche or in postmenopausal women. Does not protect against HIV infection or other sexually-transmitted diseases. Potentially significant drug-drug interactions may exist, requiring dose or frequency adjustment, additional monitoring, and/or selection of alternative therapy.

Adverse Reactions

Emergency contraception (Ella):

>10%:

Central nervous system: Headache (18% to 19%)

Endocrine & metabolic: Suppressed menstruation (≥7 days later than expected: 19%)

Gastrointestinal: Abdominal pain (8% to 15%), nausea (12% to 13%)

Genitourinary: Dysmenorrhea (7% to 13%)

1% to 10%:

Central nervous system: Fatigue (6%), dizziness (5%)

Endocrine & metabolic: Intermenstrual bleeding (9%)

Genitourinary: Early menses (≥7 days earlier than expected: 7%)

Postmarketing and/or case reports: Acne vulgaris

Treatment of moderate-to-severe signs/symptoms of uterine fibroids (Fibristal [Canadian product]):

>10%:

Central nervous system: Headache (1% to 16%)

Endocrine & metabolic: Hot flash (1% to 25%)

1% to 10%:

Cardiovascular: Edema (≤1%), hypotension (≤1%), sinus bradycardia (≤1%)

Central nervous system: Fatigue (≤4%), vertigo (≤4%), insomnia (≤2%), dizziness (1%), aggressive behavior (≤1%), drowsiness (≤1%), emotional lability (≤1%), migraine (≤1%), sleep disorder (≤1%)

Dermatologic: Night sweats (≤2%), acne vulgaris (≤1%), alopecia (≤1%), seborrhea (≤1%), xeroderma (≤1%)

Endocrine & metabolic: Hypercholesterolemia (3%), hypertriglyceridemia (≤3%), hypothyroidism (≤2%), obesity (1%), amenorrhea (≤1%), increased gamma-glutamyl transferase (≤1%), ovarian cyst (≤1%), ovarian hyperstimulation (≤1%), thyroid disease (≤1%)

Gastrointestinal: Nausea (3%), constipation (1%), dyspepsia (≤1%), upper abdominal pain (≤1%)

Genitourinary: Mastalgia (2%), pelvic pain (1% to 2%), endometrial hyperplasia (≤2%), genital bleeding (≤2%), breast swelling (≤1%), breast tenderness (≤1%), genital discharge (≤1%), uterine disease (≤1%), uterine hemorrhage (≤1%), vaginal dryness (≤1%), vulvovaginal candidiasis (≤1%)

Infection: Herpes virus infection (≤1%)

Neuromuscular & skeletal: Arthralgia (2%), muscle spasm (≤2%), back pain (≤1%), limb pain (≤1%)

Respiratory: Dyspnea (≤1%), epistaxis (≤1%), pharyngitis (≤1%)
Miscellaneous: Fever (≤1%)

Drug Interactions

Metabolism/Transport Effects Substrate of CYP3A4 (major); **Note:** Assignment of Major/Minor substrate status based on clinically relevant drug interaction potential; **Inhibits** P-glycoprotein

Avoid Concomitant Use

Avoid concomitant use of Ulipristal with any of the following: Bosutinib; CYP3A4 Inducers (Strong); CYP3A4 Inhibitors (Moderate); CYP3A4 Inhibitors (Strong); PAZOPanib; Pomalidomide; Progestins; Silodosin; Topotecan; VinCRIStine (Liposomal)

Increased Effect/Toxicity

Ulipristal may increase the levels/effects of: Afatinib; Bosutinib; Colchicine; Dabigatran Etexilate; Everolimus; PAZOPanib; P-glycoprotein/ABCB1 Substrates; Pomalidomide; Prucalopride; Rivaroxaban; Silodosin; Topotecan; VinCRIStine (Liposomal)

The levels/effects of Ulipristal may be increased by: CYP3A4 Inhibitors (Moderate); CYP3A4 Inhibitors (Strong)

Decreased Effect

Ulipristal may decrease the levels/effects of: Progestins

The levels/effects of Ulipristal may be decreased by: Bosentan; CYP3A4 Inducers (Strong); Dabrafenib; Deferasirox; Herbs (CYP3A4 Inducers); Tocilizumab

Ethanol/Nutrition/Herb Interactions Herb/Nutraceutical: St John's wort (an enzyme inducer) may decrease serum levels of ulipristal. Management: Avoid concomitant use; monitor for decreased ulipristal effects if used concomitantly.

Storage/Stability

Ella: Store at 20°C to 25°C (68°F to 77°F). Protect from light.

Fibristal [Canadian product]: Store at 15°C to 30°C (59°F to 86°F). Protect from light.

Mechanism of Action Prevents progestin from binding to the progesterone receptor. Ulipristal postpones follicular rupture when administered prior to ovulation, thereby inhibiting or delaying ovulation. May also alter the normal endometrium, impairing implantation. When used for the treatment of signs and symptoms of uterine fibroids, ulipristal reduces the size of uterine fibroids by inhibiting cellular proliferation and inducing apoptosis.

Pharmacodynamics/Kinetics

Absorption: Rapid

Protein binding: Ulipristal: >98% to plasma proteins including albumin, alpha$_1$-acid glycoprotein, high-density lipoprotein, and low-density lipoprotein

Metabolism: Hepatic via CYP3A4; forms monodemethylated metabolite (active) and inactive metabolites

Half-life elimination: Ulipristal: ~32-38 hours; Monodemethylated metabolite: ~27 hours

Time to peak, serum: 1 hour (ulipristal and monodemethylated metabolite)

Excretion: Feces (primary route of elimination); urine (<10%)

Dosage

Emergency contraception (Ella): Oral:

Children and Adolescents (prepubertal): Not indicated for use prior to menarche

Adolescents (postpubertal) and Adults: 30 mg as soon as possible, but within 120 hours (5 days) of unprotected intercourse or contraceptive failure

Treatment of moderate-to-severe signs/symptoms of uterine fibroids (Fibristal [Canadian product]): Oral:

Adults: Females (premenopausal): 5 mg daily for 3 consecutive months. **Note:** Treatment is limited to 3 months.

Note: Not indicated for use in postmenopausal women.

Dosage adjustment in renal impairment: No dosage adjustment provided in manufacturer's labeling (has not been studied).

Dosage adjustment in hepatic impairment: No dosage adjustment provided in manufacturer's labeling (has not been studied).

Dietary Considerations May be taken with or without food.

Administration

Ella: Administer orally with or without food at anytime during menstrual cycle. If vomiting occurs within 3 hours of administration, consider repeating dose.

Fibristal [Canadian product]: Administer orally with or without food; initiate during the first 7 days of menstrual cycle.

Hazardous agent; use appropriate precautions for handling and disposal (NIOSH, 2012).

Monitoring Parameters Evaluate for pregnancy or ectopic pregnancy if menses is delayed for ≥1 week following emergency contraception, or if lower abdominal pain (3-5 weeks after administration) or persistent irregular bleeding develops.

Dosage Forms Excipient information presented when available (limited, particularly for generics); consult specific product labeling.

Tablet, Oral, as acetate:

Ella: 30 mg

Dosage Forms: Canada Excipient information presented when available (limited, particularly for generics); consult specific product labeling.

Tablet, Oral, as acetate:

Fibristal: 5 mg

- **Ulipristal Acetate** *see* Ulipristal *on page* 2138
- **Uloric** *see* Febuxostat *on page* 834
- **Uloric® (Can)** *see* Febuxostat *on page* 834
- **Ultiva** *see* Remifentanil *on page* 1795
- **Ultiva® (Can)** *see* Remifentanil *on page* 1795
- **Ultracet®** *see* Acetaminophen and Tramadol *on page* 33
- **Ultram** *see* TraMADol *on page* 2099
- **Ultram ER** *see* TraMADol *on page* 2099
- **Ultra Mide 25 [OTC]** *see* Urea *on page* 2140
- **UltraMide 25™ (Can)** *see* Urea *on page* 2140
- **Ultramop (Can)** *see* Methoxsalen (Systemic) *on page* 1331
- **Ultraquin™ (Can)** *see* Hydroquinone *on page* 1017
- **Ultrase (Can)** *see* Pancrelipase *on page* 1558
- **Ultrase MT (Can)** *see* Pancrelipase *on page* 1558
- **Ultravate** *see* Halobetasol *on page* 983
- **Ultravate® (Can)** *see* Halobetasol *on page* 983
- **Ultresa** *see* Pancrelipase *on page* 1558
- **Umecta** *see* Urea *on page* 2140
- **Umecta Mousse** *see* Urea *on page* 2140
- **Umecta Nail Film** *see* Urea *on page* 2140
- **Umecta PD** *see* Urea *on page* 2140
- **Unasyn®** *see* Ampicillin and Sulbactam *on page* 133
- **Unidet® (Can)** *see* Tolterodine *on page* 2088
- **Unifed [OTC]** *see* Pseudoephedrine *on page* 1746
- **Uniphyl (Can)** *see* Theophylline *on page* 2042
- **Uniretic®** *see* Moexipril and Hydrochlorothiazide *on page* 1392
- **Unithroid** *see* Levothyroxine *on page* 1206
- **Unithroid Direct** *see* Levothyroxine *on page* 1206
- **Univasc** *see* Moexipril *on page* 1392
- **UniVert** *see* Meclizine *on page* 1277

- Unna's Boot *see* Zinc Gelatin *on page 2229*
- Unna's Paste *see* Zinc Gelatin *on page 2229*
- Uramaxin *see* Urea *on page 2140*
- Uramaxin GT *see* Urea *on page 2140*
- Urasal® (Can) *see* Methenamine *on page 1319*
- Urate Oxidase *see* Rasburicase *on page 1788*
- Urate Oxidase, Pegylated *see* Pegloticase *on page 1599*

Urea (yoor EE a)

Brand Names: U.S. Aluvea; Aquaphilic/Carbamide [OTC]; Atrac-Tain [OTC]; Beta Care Betamide [OTC]; Carb-O-Lac HP [OTC]; Carb-O-Lac5 [OTC]; Carmol 10 [OTC]; Carmol 20 [OTC]; Carmol [OTC]; CEM-Urea; Cerovel; Dermal Therapy Finger Care [OTC]; Dermasorb XM; DPM [OTC]; Gordons Urea; Gordons Urea [OTC]; Gormel 10 [OTC]; Gormel [OTC]; Hydro 35; Hydro 40; Kerafoam; Kerafoam 42; Lanaphilic/Urea [OTC]; Latrix XM; Mycocide CX Callus Exfoliator [OTC]; Nutraplus [OTC]; Rea-Lo [OTC]; Remeven; TL Urea [DSC]; U-Kera E; Ultra Mide 25 [OTC]; Umecta; Umecta Mousse; Umecta Nail Film; Umecta PD; Uramaxin; Uramaxin GT; Urea Hydrating; Urea Nail; Urea-C40; Ureacin-10 [OTC]; Ureacin-20 [OTC]; Utopic; X-Viate

Brand Names: Canada UltraMide 25™; Uremol®; Urisec®

Index Terms Carbamide

Pharmacologic Category Diuretic, Osmotic; Keratolytic Agent; Topical Skin Product

Use Keratolytic agent to soften nails or skin; OTC: Moisturizer for dry, rough skin

Pregnancy Risk Factor B/C (manufacturer specific)

Dosage Topical: Adults: Hyperkeratotic conditions, dry skin: Apply 1-3 times/day

Additional Information Complete prescribing information should be consulted for additional detail.

Dosage Forms Excipient information presented when available (limited, particularly for generics); consult specific product labeling. [DSC] = Discontinued product

Cream, External:
- Aluvea: 39% (227 g)
- Atrac-Tain: 10% (2 g, 57 g, 142 g)
- Carb-O-Lac5: Urea 20% and Ammonium Lactate 10% (236 g) [contains propylene glycol]
- Carb-O-Lac HP: Urea 20% and Ammonium Lactate 10% (277 g) [contains propylene glycol]
- Carmol 20: 20% (85 g)
- DPM: (170 g) [lanolin free, mineral oil free, paraben free; contains brilliant blue fcf (fd&c blue #1), propylene glycol, tartrazine (fd&c yellow #5), trolamine (triethanolamine)]
- Gormel: 20% (75 g, 120 g, 480 g, 2400 g) [contains cetyl alcohol, methylparaben, propylene glycol, propylparaben, trolamine (triethanolamine)]
- Mycocide CX Callus Exfoliator: 12% (100 mL) [contains methylparaben, propylene glycol, propylparaben]
- Nutraplus: 10% (453 g) [odorless; contains cetearyl alcohol, methylparaben, propylene glycol, propylparaben]
- Nutraplus: 10% (85 g) [odorless; contains cetyl alcohol, methylparaben, propylene glycol, propylparaben]
- Rea-Lo: 30% (227 g, 59 mL)
- Remeven: 50% (142 g, 255 g) [contains disodium edta]
- U-Kera E: 40% (28.35 g, 85.05 g, 198.45 g) [contains trolamine (triethanolamine)]
- Uramaxin: 45% (255 g) [contains alcohol, usp, edetate disodium, menthol]
- Ureacin-20: 20% (113.4 g)
- Utopic: 41% (227 g) [contains cetyl alcohol, propylene glycol]
- X-Viate: 40% (28.3 g, 85 g, 199 g)
- Generic: 10% (85 g); 20% (85 g); 39% (226.8 g, 227 g); 40% (28.35 g, 85 g, 85.05 g, 198.6 g); 45% (255 g); 50% (142 g, 255 g); 39% (227 g)

Emulsion, External:
- Latrix XM: 45% (240 mL) [contains cetyl alcohol, disodium edta, propylene glycol, trolamine (triethanolamine)]
- Umecta: 40% (120 g, 227 g) [contains trolamine (triethanolamine)]
- Umecta PD: 40% (198.5 g) [contains disodium edta, glycine soja (soybean) sterol]
- Generic: 50% (284 g, 300 g)

Foam, External:
- Hydro 35: 35% (150 g) [contains ethylparaben, methylparaben, propylene glycol, propylparaben, trolamine (triethanolamine)]
- Hydro 40: 40% (150 g) [contains ethylparaben, methylparaben, propylene glycol, propylparaben, trolamine (triethanolamine)]
- Kerafoam: 30% (60 g, 100 g) [contains cetyl alcohol, methylparaben, propylene glycol, propylparaben]
- Kerafoam 42: 42% (60 g, 100 g) [contains cetearyl alcohol, edetate disodium, methylparaben, propylene glycol, propylparaben]
- Umecta Mousse: 40% (113.4 g) [contains soya sterol, trolamine (triethanolamine)]
- Uramaxin: 20% (100 g) [contains cetyl alcohol, propylene glycol]
- Urea Hydrating: 35% (150 g) [contains ethylparaben, methylparaben, propylene glycol, propylparaben, trolamine (triethanolamine)]

Gel, External:
- Cerovel: 40% (25 mL)
- Uramaxin: 45% (28 mL) [contains edetate disodium, menthol, propylene glycol]
- Uramaxin GT: 45% (20 mL) [contains edetate disodium, menthol, propylene glycol]
- Urea Nail: 45% (28 mL) [contains edetate disodium, menthol, propylene glycol]
- X-Viate: 40% (15 mL) [contains methylparaben]
- Generic: 40% (15 mL)

Kit, External:
- Dermasorb XM: 39% [contains ceteareth-20, cetyl alcohol, chlorocresol (chloro-m-cresol)]
- Uramaxin GT: 45% [contains edetate disodium, menthol, propylene glycol]
- Urea Nail: 40 & 0.2% [contains disodium edta, methylparaben, propylparaben, trolamine (triethanolamine)]

Lotion, External:
- Atrac-Tain: 5% (118 mL, 237 mL)
- Beta Care Betamide: 25% (120 mL, 480 mL)
- Carmol 10: 10% (177 mL)
- Cerovel: 40% (325 mL) [contains alcohol, usp, trolamine (triethanolamine)]
- Dermal Therapy Finger Care: 20% (18 mL)
- Gormel 10: 10% (240 mL)
- Nutraplus: 10% (236 mL, 473 mL) [odorless; contains methylparaben, propylparaben]
- Rea-Lo: 15% (120 mL)
- TL Urea: 45% (480 g [DSC]) [contains alcohol, usp, edetate disodium, menthol]
- Ultra Mide 25: 25% (236 mL) [paraben free; contains cetyl alcohol, edetate sodium (tetrasodium)]
- Uramaxin: 45% (480 g) [contains alcohol, usp, edetate disodium, menthol]
- Urea-C40: 40% (236.6 mL)
- Ureacin-10: 10% (236.56 mL)
- X-Viate: 40% (237 mL) [contains cetyl alcohol, methylparaben, propylene glycol, propylparaben, trolamine (triethanolamine)]
- Generic: 10% (180 mL, 240 mL, 480 mL); 40% (236.6 mL); 45% (480 g)

Ointment, External:
Aquaphilic/Carbamide: 10% (180 g, 454 g); 20% (454 g)
Gordons Urea: 22% (30 g); 40% (30 g)
Lanaphilic/Urea: 10% (454 g); 20% (454 g)
Shampoo, External:
Carmol: 10% (240 mL)
Solution, External:
CEM-Urea: 45% (20 mL) [contains edetate disodium, menthol, methylparaben, propylene glycol]
Stick, External:
Urea Nail: 50% (2.4 mL) [contains cetyl alcohol, disodium edta]
Suspension, External:
Umecta: 40% (283.4 g) [contains trolamine (triethanolamine)]
Umecta Nail Film: 40% (3 g, 18 mL) [contains disodium edta]
Umecta PD: 40% (255.1 g) [contains disodium edta, glycine soja (soybean) sterol]
Generic: 40% (283.4 g, 18 mL); 50% (284 g)

Urea and Hydrocortisone

(yoor EE a & hye droe KOR ti sone)

Brand Names: U.S. Carmol-HC®
Brand Names: Canada Ti-U-Lac® H; Uremol® HC
Index Terms Hydrocortisone and Urea
Pharmacologic Category Corticosteroid, Topical
Use Inflammation of corticosteroid-responsive dermatoses
Pregnancy Risk Factor C
Dosage Topical: Children and Adults: Steroid-responsive dermatoses: Apply thin film and rub in well 2-4 times/day. Therapy should be discontinued when control is achieved; if no improvement is seen, reassessment of diagnosis may be necessary.
Additional Information Complete prescribing information should be consulted for additional detail.
Dosage Forms Excipient information presented when available (limited, particularly for generics); consult specific product labeling.
Cream, topical:
Carmol-HC®: Urea 10% and hydrocortisone acetate 1% (28 g) [in water soluble vanishing cream base]

◆ **Urea-C40** *see* Urea *on page 2140*
◆ **Ureacin-10 [OTC]** *see* Urea *on page 2140*
◆ **Ureacin-20 [OTC]** *see* Urea *on page 2140*
◆ **Urea Hydrating** *see* Urea *on page 2140*
◆ **Urea Nail** *see* Urea *on page 2140*
◆ **Urea Peroxide** *see* Carbamide Peroxide *on page 340*
◆ **Urecholine** *see* Bethanechol *on page 250*
◆ **Urelle®** *see* Methenamine, Sodium Biphosphate, Phenyl Salicylate, Methylene Blue, and Hyoscyamine *on page 1320*
◆ **Uremol® (Can)** *see* Urea *on page 2140*
◆ **Uremol® HC (Can)** *see* Urea and Hydrocortisone *on page 2141*
◆ **Urex** *see* Methenamine *on page 1319*
◆ **Uribel™** *see* Methenamine, Sodium Biphosphate, Phenyl Salicylate, Methylene Blue, and Hyoscyamine *on page 1320*

Uridine Triacetate

(URE i deen trye AS e tate)

Index Terms PN401; Triacetyluridine; Vistonuridine
Pharmacologic Category Antidote
Unlabeled Use Antidote for fluorouracil overdose or overexposure
Prescribing and Access Restrictions Uridine triacetate (formerly called vistonuridine) is supplied for emergency use under a single-patient Investigational New Drug (IND) provision. Procurement information is available from Wellstat Therapeutics at 1-443-831-5626.
Dosage Oral: Adults: Fluorouracil overdose (unlabeled use): 10 g every 6 hours for 20 doses beginning as soon as possible (8 hours to 4 days) after fluorouracil overdose (von Borstel, 2009)
Additional Information Complete prescribing information should be consulted for additional detail.

◆ **Urimar-T** *see* Methenamine, Sodium Biphosphate, Phenyl Salicylate, Methylene Blue, and Hyoscyamine *on page 1320*
◆ **Urinary Pain Relief [OTC]** *see* Phenazopyridine *on page 1627*
◆ **Urisec® (Can)** *see* Urea *on page 2140*
◆ **Urispas** *see* FlavoxATE *on page 865*
◆ **Urispas® (Can)** *see* FlavoxATE *on page 865*

Urofollitropin

(yoor oh fol li TROE pin)

Brand Names: U.S. Bravelle
Brand Names: Canada Bravelle®; Fertinorm® H.P.
Index Terms Follicle-Stimulating Hormone, Human; FSH; hFSH
Pharmacologic Category Gonadotropin; Ovulation Stimulator
Use Ovulation induction in patients who previously received pituitary suppression; development of multiple follicles with Assisted Reproductive Technologies (ART)
Pregnancy Risk Factor X
Dosage Note: Dose should be individualized. Use the lowest dose consistent with the expectation of good results. Over the course of treatment, doses may vary depending on individual patient response.
Adults: Females:
Ovulation induction: I.M., SubQ: Initial: 150 units daily for the first 5 days of treatment. Dose adjustments ≤75-150 units can be made every ≥2 days; maximum daily dose: 450 units; treatment >12 days is not recommended. If response to follitropin is appropriate, hCG is given 1 day following the last dose. Withhold hCG if serum estradiol is >2000 pg/mL, if the ovaries are abnormally enlarged, or if abdominal pain occurs.
ART: SubQ: 225 units daily for the first 5 days; dose may be adjusted based on patient response, but adjustments should not be made more frequently than once every 2 days; maximum adjustment: 75-150 units; maximum daily dose: 450 units; maximum duration of treatment: 12 days. When a sufficient number of follicles of adequate size are present, the final maturation of the follicles is induced by administering hCG. Withhold hCG in cases where the ovaries are abnormally enlarged on the last day of therapy.

Dosage adjustment in renal impairment: No dosage adjustment provided in manufacturer's labeling (has not been studied).
Dosage adjustment in hepatic impairment: No dosage adjustment provided in manufacturer's labeling (has not been studied).
Additional Information Complete prescribing information should be consulted for additional detail.
Dosage Forms Excipient information presented when available (limited, particularly for generics); consult specific product labeling.
Solution Reconstituted, Injection:
Bravelle: 75 units (1 ea)

◆ **Uro-Mag [OTC]** *see* Magnesium Oxide *on page 1262*

◆ Uromax (Can) *see* Oxybutynin *on page 1533*
◆ Uromitexan (Can) *see* Mesna *on page 1307*
◆ Uroqid-Acid® No. 2 *see* Methenamine and Sodium Acid Phosphate *on page 1319*
◆ Uroxatral *see* Alfuzosin *on page 73*
◆ Urso (Can) *see* Ursodiol *on page 2142*
◆ Urso 250 *see* Ursodiol *on page 2142*
◆ Ursodeoxycholic Acid *see* Ursodiol *on page 2142*

Ursodiol (ur soe DYE ol)

Brand Names: U.S. Actigall; Urso 250; Urso Forte
Brand Names: Canada Dom-Ursodiol C; PHL-Ursodiol C; PMS-Ursodiol C; Urso; Urso DS
Index Terms Ursodeoxycholic Acid
Pharmacologic Category Gallstone Dissolution Agent
Use
Actigall: Gallbladder stone dissolution; prevention of gallstones in obese patients experiencing rapid weight loss
Urso, Urso Forte: Primary biliary cirrhosis
Pregnancy Risk Factor B
Dosage Oral: Adults:
Gallstone dissolution (Actigall): 8-10 mg/kg/day in 2-3 divided doses; use beyond 24 months is not established
Gallstone prevention (Actigall): 300 mg twice daily
Primary biliary cirrhosis (Urso, Urso Forte): 13-15 mg/kg/day in 2-4 divided doses (with food)

Dosage adjustment in renal impairment: No dosage adjustment provided in manufacturer's labeling.
Dosage adjustment in hepatic impairment: No dosage adjustment provided in manufacturer's labeling.
Additional Information Complete prescribing information should be consulted for additional detail.
Dosage Forms Excipient information presented when available (limited, particularly for generics); consult specific product labeling.
Capsule, Oral:
Actigall: 300 mg
Generic: 300 mg
Tablet, Oral:
Urso 250: 250 mg
Urso Forte: 500 mg [scored]
Generic: 250 mg, 500 mg

◆ Urso DS (Can) *see* Ursodiol *on page 2142*
◆ Urso Forte *see* Ursodiol *on page 2142*

Ustekinumab (yoo stek in YOO mab)

Brand Names: U.S. Stelara
Brand Names: Canada Stelara
Index Terms CNTO 1275
Pharmacologic Category Antipsoriatic Agent; Interleukin-12 Inhibitor; Interleukin-23 Inhibitor; Monoclonal Antibody
Use
Plaque psoriasis: Treatment of adults with moderate-to-severe plaque psoriasis who are candidates for phototherapy or systemic therapy
Psoriatic arthritis: Treatment of adults with active psoriatic arthritis (as monotherapy or in combination with methotrexate)
Pregnancy Risk Factor B
Pregnancy Considerations Adverse events were not observed in animal reproduction studies. There is limited information related to the use of ustekinumab in pregnancy (Andrulonis, 2012). In general, other agents are preferred for the treatment of plaque psoriasis in pregnant women (Hsu, 2012).
Breast-Feeding Considerations It is not known whether ustekinumab is secreted in human milk. Because many immunoglobulins are secreted in milk it is expected that ustekinumab will be present in breast milk. The manufacturer recommends caution be used in nursing women.
Medication Guide Available Yes
Contraindications Clinically significant hypersensitivity to ustekinumab or any component of the formulation

Canadian labeling: Additional contraindications (not in U.S. labeling): Severe infections such as sepsis, tuberculosis, and opportunistic infections
Warnings/Precautions May increase the risk for malignancy although the impact on the development and course of malignancies is not fully defined. Rapidly appearing cutaneous squamous cell carcinomas (multiple) have been reported in patients receiving ustekinumab who were at risk for developing nonmelanoma skin cancer. Monitor all patients closely for the development of nonmelanoma skin cancer; closely follow patients >60 years of age, with a history of prolonged immunosuppression, and in patients with a history of PUVA treatment. Use with caution in patients with prior malignancy (use not studied in this population).

May increase the risk for infections or reactivation of latent infections. Serious bacterial, fungal, and viral infections have been observed with use. Avoid use in patients with clinically important active infection. Caution should be exercised when considering use in patients with a history of new/recurrent infections, with conditions that predispose them to infections (eg, diabetes or residence/travel from areas of endemic mycoses), or with chronic, latent, or localized infections, or who are genetically deficient in IL-12/IL-23 (IL-12/IL-23 genetic deficiency may predispose patients to disseminated infection). Patients who develop a new infection while undergoing treatment should be monitored closely. If a patient develops a serious infection, therapy should be discontinued or withheld until successful resolution of infection.

Do not use in patients with active tuberculosis (TB). Patients should be evaluated for latent tuberculosis infection with a tuberculin skin test prior to starting therapy. Treatment of latent TB should be initiated before ustekinumab therapy is used. Consider antituberculosis treatment in patients with a history of latent or active tuberculosis if an adequate prior treatment course cannot be confirmed. During and following treatment, monitor for signs/symptoms of active TB.

Antibody formation to ustekinumab has been observed with therapy and has been associated with decreased serum levels and therapeutic response in some patients. Hypersensitivity, including anaphylaxis and angioedema, has been reported. Discontinue immediately with signs/symptoms of hypersensitivity reaction and treat appropriately as indicated. Reversible posterior leukoencephalopathy syndrome (RPLS) has been observed (rare). RPLS symptoms include headache, seizures, confusion, and visual disturbances; may be fatal. Monitor; discontinue ustekinumab if symptoms occur and administer appropriate therapy. Use in combination with other immunosuppressive drugs or phototherapy has not been studied. Patients should be brought up to date with all immunizations before initiating therapy. **Live vaccines should not be given concurrently;** inactivated or nonlive vaccines may be given concurrently, but may not elicit a proper immune response. BCG vaccines should not be given 1 year prior to, during, or 1 year following treatment. Patients >100 kg may require higher dose to achieve adequate serum levels. Use in hepatic or renal impairment has not been studied.

The packaging may contain latex. Product may contain polysorbate 80. Potentially significant interactions may exist, requiring dose or frequency adjustment, additional monitoring, and/or selection of alternative therapy.

Adverse Reactions

>10%: Infection: Increased susceptibility to infection (27% to 70%; severe infection: ≤2%)

1% to 10%:

Central nervous system: Headache (5%), fatigue (3%), dizziness (2%), depression (1%)

Dermatologic: Pruritus (2%)

Local: Erythema at injection site (1% to 2%)

Neuromuscular & skeletal: Back pain (2%)

Respiratory: Pharyngolaryngeal pain (2%)

Immunologic: Antibody development (3% to 5%)

<1%, postmarketing, and/or case reports: Anaphylaxis, angina pectoris, angioedema, bacterial infection, bleeding at injection site, bruising at injection site, cellulitis, cerebrovascular accident, dactylitis, diverticulitis, erythrodermic psoriasis, fungal infection, gastroenteritis, herpes zoster, hypersensitivity reaction, hypertension, induration at injection site, irritation at injection site, itching at injection site, malignant neoplasm (breast, colon, head and neck, kidney, prostate, thyroid); malignant melanoma (*in situ*), myocardial infarction, nephrolithiasis, osteomyelitis, pain at injection site, pneumonia, pustular psoriasis, reversible posterior leukoencephalopathy syndrome, skin rash, squamous cell carcinoma of skin, swelling at injection site, urinary tract infection, urticaria, viral infection

Drug Interactions

Metabolism/Transport Effects None known.

Avoid Concomitant Use

Avoid concomitant use of Ustekinumab with any of the following: BCG; Belimumab; InFLIXimab; Natalizumab; Pimecrolimus; Tacrolimus (Topical); Tofacitinib; Vaccines (Live)

Increased Effect/Toxicity

Ustekinumab may increase the levels/effects of: Belimumab; InFLIXimab; Leflunomide; Natalizumab; Tofacitinib; Vaccines (Live)

The levels/effects of Ustekinumab may be increased by: Abciximab; Denosumab; Pimecrolimus; Roflumilast; Tacrolimus (Topical); Trastuzumab

Decreased Effect

Ustekinumab may decrease the levels/effects of: BCG; Coccidioidin Skin Test; Sipuleucel-T; Vaccines (Inactivated); Vaccines (Live)

The levels/effects of Ustekinumab may be decreased by: Echinacea

Storage/Stability Refrigerate at 2° to 8°C (36° to 46°F); do not freeze. Store vials upright. Keep the product in the original carton to protect from light until the time of use. Do not shake. Discard any unused portion.

Mechanism of Action Ustekinumab is a human monoclonal antibody that binds to and interferes with the proinflammatory cytokines, interleukin (IL)-12 and IL-23. Biological effects of IL-12 and IL-23 include natural killer (NK) cell activation, CD4+ T-cell differentiation and activation. Ustekinumab also interferes with the expression of monocyte chemotactic protein-1 (MCP-1), tumor necrosis factor-alpha (TNF-α), interferon-inducible protein-10 (IP-10), and interleukin-8 (IL-8). Significant clinical improvement in psoriasis and psoriatic arthritis patients is seen in association with reduction of these proinflammatory signalers.

Pharmacodynamics/Kinetics

Distribution: V_d (terminal elimination phase): 45 mg: 0.161 ± 0.065 L/kg; 90 mg: 0.179 ± 0.085 L/kg

Bioavailability: Absolute bioavailability: SubQ: ~57%

Half-life elimination: 10-126 days

Time to peak, plasma: 45 mg: 13.5 days; 90 mg: 7 days

Dosage

Plaque psoriasis: Adults: SubQ:

Initial and maintenance: **Note:** Following an interruption in therapy, retreatment may be initiated at the initial dosing interval. Consider therapy discontinuation in any patient failing to demonstrate a response after 12 weeks of therapy.

≤100 kg: 45 mg at 0- and 4 weeks, and then every 12 weeks thereafter

>100 kg: 90 mg at 0- and 4 weeks, and then every 12 weeks thereafter. **Note:** Doses of 45 mg given to patients >100 kg were also efficacious; however, 90 mg is the recommended dose in these patients due to greater efficacy.

Canadian labeling: If response inadequate on every-12-week therapy, consider increasing frequency to every 8 weeks.

Psoriatic arthritis: Adults: SubQ: **Note:** When used for psoriatic arthritis, may be administered alone or in combination with methotrexate.

Initial and maintenance: 45 mg at 0- and 4 weeks, and then every 12 weeks thereafter.

Coexistent psoriatic arthritis and moderate-to-severe plaque psoriasis in patients >100 kg: Initial and maintenance: 90 mg at 0- and 4 weeks, and then every 12 weeks thereafter.

Dosage adjustment in renal impairment: No dosage adjustment provided in manufacturer's labeling (has not been studied).

Dosage adjustment in hepatic impairment: No dosage adjustment provided in manufacturer's labeling (has not been studied).

Administration Do not use if cloudy or discolored. Administer by subcutaneous injection into the top of the thigh, abdomen, upper arms, or buttocks. Rotate sites. Do not inject into tender, bruised, erythematous, or indurated skin. Avoid areas of skin where psoriasis is present. Discard any unused portion.

Monitoring Parameters Tuberculosis screening (prior to initiating and periodically during therapy); CBC; ustekinumab-antibody formation; monitor for signs/symptoms of infection, reversible posterior leukoencephalopathy syndrome (RPLS), and squamous cell skin carcinoma

Dosage Forms Excipient information presented when available (limited, particularly for generics); consult specific product labeling.

Solution, Subcutaneous [preservative free]:

Stelara: 45 mg/0.5 mL (0.5 mL); 90 mg/mL (1 mL) [contains polysorbate 80]

◆ **Uta®** *see* Methenamine, Sodium Biphosphate, Phenyl Salicylate, Methylene Blue, and Hyoscyamine *on page 1320*

◆ **Utopic** *see* Urea *on page 2140*

◆ **Utradol™ (Can)** *see* Etodolac *on page 799*

◆ **Uvadex** *see* Methoxsalen (Systemic) *on page 1331*

Vaccinia Immune Globulin (Intravenous)

(vax IN ee a i MYUN GLOB yoo lin IN tra VEE nus)

Brand Names: U.S. CNJ-016®

Index Terms VIGIV

Pharmacologic Category Blood Product Derivative; Immune Globulin

Use Treatment of infectious complications of smallpox (vaccinia virus) vaccination, such as eczema vaccinatum, progressive vaccinia, and severe generalized vaccinia; treatment of vaccinia infections in individuals with concurrent skin conditions or accidental virus exposure to eyes (except vaccinia keratitis), mouth, or other areas where viral infection would pose significant risk

CDC guidelines for use:

Use is recommended for:

- Inadvertent inoculation (considering severity, toxicity of affected person, and pain)
- Eczema vaccinatum
- Generalized vaccinia (severe form or if underlying illness is present)
- Progressive vaccinia

Use may be considered for:

- Severe ocular complications except isolated keratitis

Use is not recommended for:

- Inadvertent inoculation that is not severe
- Mild or limited generalized vaccinia
- Nonspecific rashes, erythema multiforme, or Stevens-Johnson syndrome
- Postvaccinial encephalitis or encephalomyelitis

Pregnancy Risk Factor C

Pregnancy Considerations Animal reproduction studies have not been conducted. Immune globulins cross the placenta in increased amounts after 30 weeks gestation. There are no adequate and well-controlled studies in pregnant women. Vaccinia immune globulin is currently not recommended for use in persons with contraindications to smallpox vaccine; inadvertent exposure to smallpox vaccine in high risk populations (eg, pregnant women) should be reported to the CDC so that standardized treatment may be provided.

Prescribing and Access Restrictions Vaccinia immune globulin is not available for general public use. All supplies are currently owned by the federal government for inclusion in the Strategic National Stockpile. The CDC Smallpox Adverse Events Clinical Consultation team will coordinate shipment. The State Health Department should be contacted first concerning severe or unexpected adverse events from smallpox vaccination.

Contraindications Hypersensitivity to immune globulin or any component of the formulation; isolated vaccinia keratitis; selective IgA deficiency

Warnings/Precautions Vaccinia immune globulin is currently not recommended for use in persons with contraindications to smallpox vaccine; inadvertent exposure to smallpox vaccine in high risk populations should be reported to the CDC so that standardized treatment may be provided.

Hypersensitivity and anaphylactic reactions can occur; immediate treatment (including epinephrine 1:1000) should be available. Contains trace amounts of IgA; use caution in IgA-deficient patients. Aseptic meningitis syndrome (AMS) has been reported with intravenous immune globulin administration (rare); may occur with high doses (≥2 g/kg). Intravenous immune globulin has been associated with antiglobulin hemolysis; monitor for signs of hemolytic anemia. Monitor for transfusion-related acute lung injury (TRALI); noncardiogenic pulmonary edema has been reported with intravenous immune globulin use. TRALI is characterized by severe respiratory distress, pulmonary edema, hypoxemia, and fever in the presence of normal left ventricular function. Usually occurs within 1-6 hours after infusion.

Acute renal dysfunction (increased serum creatinine, oliguria, acute renal failure) can rarely occur; usually within 7 days of use (more likely with products stabilized with sucrose). Use with caution in the elderly, patients with renal disease, diabetes mellitus, volume depletion, sepsis, paraproteinemia, and nephrotoxic medications due to risk of renal dysfunction. In patients at risk of renal dysfunction, the rate of infusion and concentration of solution should be minimized. discontinue if renal function deteriorates. Patients should not be volume depleted prior to therapy. Thrombotic events have been reported with administration of intravenous immune globulin; use with caution in patients with cardiovascular risk factors. Product of human plasma; may potentially contain infectious agents which could transmit disease. Screening of donors, as well as testing and/or inactivation or removal of certain viruses, reduces the risk. Infections thought to be transmitted by this product should be reported to the manufacturer. Product may contain maltose. **[U.S. Boxed Warning]: Maltose in vaccinia immune globulin can interact with glucose monitoring systems and test strips.** Falsely-elevated blood glucose readings may result in unnecessary insulin use and life-threatening hypoglycemia. Glucose specific monitoring systems and test strips are recommended. For intravenous administration only.

Adverse Reactions Note: Actual frequency varies by dose and rate of infusion

Cardiovascular: Peripheral edema

Central nervous system: Cold or hot feeling, dizziness, fatigue, headache, pain, pallor, pyrexia

Dermatologic: Erythema

Gastrointestinal: Appetite decreased, nausea, vomiting

Local: Injection site reaction

Neuromuscular & skeletal: Back pain, paraesthesia, muscle spasm, rigors, tremor, weakness

Miscellaneous: Diaphoresis

Postmarketing and/or case reports: Abdominal pain, anaphylaxis, apnea, acute respiratory distress syndrome, arthralgia, aseptic meningitis, blood pressure changes, bronchospasm, bullous dermatitis, cardiac arrest, chills, coma, Coombs' test positive, cyanosis, diarrhea, dyspnea, epidermolysis, erythema multiforme, flushing, hemolysis, hepatic dysfunction, hypersensitivity reactions, hypoxemia, hypotension, intravascular hemolysis, leukopenia, loss of consciousness, lung injury (transfusion associated), malaise, myalgia, osmotic nephropathy, pancytopenia, proximal tubular nephropathy, pulmonary edema, renal dysfunction/failure (acute), seizure, Stevens-Johnson syndrome, syncope, tachycardia, thrombocytopenia, thromboembolism, transfusion-related acute lung injury (TRALI), urticaria, vascular collapse, wheezing

Drug Interactions

Metabolism/Transport Effects None known.

Avoid Concomitant Use There are no known interactions where it is recommended to avoid concomitant use.

Increased Effect/Toxicity There are no known significant interactions involving an increase in effect.

Decreased Effect

Vaccinia Immune Globulin (Intravenous) may decrease the levels/effects of: Vaccines (Live)

Storage/Stability Store between 2°C and 8°C (36°F to 46°F); may also be frozen. If frozen, use within 60 days of thawing at 2°C and 8°C. Infusion should begin within 4 hours after entering vial.

Mechanism of Action Antibodies obtained from pooled human plasma of individuals immunized with the smallpox vaccine provide passive immunity

Pharmacodynamics/Kinetics

Distribution: V_d: 6630 L

Half-life elimination: 30 days (range: 13-67 days)

Time to peak, plasma: ≤2 hours

Dosage I.V.: **Note:** Vaccinia immune globulin is currently not recommended for use in persons with contraindications to smallpox vaccine; inadvertent exposure to smallpox vaccine in high-risk populations should be reported to the CDC so that standardized treatment may be provided.

Adults: 6000 units/kg; may repeat dose based on severity of symptoms and response to treatment (specific data are lacking); 9000 units/kg may be considered if patient does not respond to initial dose. Doses up to 24,000 unit/kg were tolerated in healthy volunteers.

Dosage adjustment in renal impairment: Use caution. In patients at risk of renal dysfunction, the rate of infusion and concentration of solution should be minimized; discontinue if renal function deteriorates.

Dosage adjustment in hepatic impairment: No dosage adjustment provided in manufacturer's labeling.

Administration Do not shake; avoid foaming. For intravenous use only. Predilution is not recommended. If dedicated line is not available, flush with NS prior to administration of VIGIV. Do not exceed recommended rates of infusion.

Patients ≥50 kg: Infuse at ≤2 mL/minute; Patients <50 kg: Infuse at ≤0.04 mL/kg/minute. Maximum assessed rate of infusion: 4 mL/minute. Decrease rate of infusion in patients who develop minor adverse reactions (eg, flushing) and in patients with risk factors for thrombosis/ thromboembolism and/or renal insufficiency.

Monitoring Parameters Renal function and urine output (at baseline and at appropriate intervals). Baseline assessment of blood viscosity in patients at risk for hyperviscosity. During infusion, monitor patient for signs of infusion-related reactions, including (but not limited to) flushing, fever, chills, respiratory distress, blood pressure or heart rate changes. Transfusion-related lung injury (typically 1-6 hours after infusion) and hemolysis have been reported with infusion.

Test Interactions [U.S. Boxed Warning]: Maltose in vaccinia immune globulin can interact with glucose monitoring systems and test strips. CNJ-016® contains maltose. Falsely-elevated blood glucose levels may occur when glucose monitoring devices and test strips utilizing the glucose dehydrogenase pyrroloquinolinequinone (GDH-PQQ) based methods are used. Glucose monitoring devices and test strips which utilize the glucose-specific method are recommended.

Positive direct Coombs' test due to transitory increase of antibodies.

Dosage Forms Excipient information presented when available (limited, particularly for generics); consult specific product labeling.

Injection, solution [preservative free; solvent-detergent treated]:

CNJ-016®: ≥50,000 units/15 mL (15 mL) [contains maltose 10% and polysorbate 80 0.03%]

- **Vaccinia Vaccine** *see* Smallpox Vaccine *on page 1909*
- **Vacuant Mini-Enema [OTC] [DSC]** *see* Docusate *on page 644*
- **Vagifem** *see* Estradiol (Topical) *on page 759*
- **Vagifem® (Can)** *see* Estradiol (Topical) *on page 759*
- **Vagifem® 10 (Can)** *see* Estradiol (Topical) *on page 759*
- **Vagistat-3 [OTC]** *see* Miconazole (Topical) *on page 1358*

ValACYclovir (val ay SYE kloe veer)

Brand Names: U.S. Valtrex

Brand Names: Canada Apo-Valacyclovir®; CO Valacyclovir; DOM-Valacyclovir; Mylan-Valacyclovir; PHL-Valacyclovir; PMS-Valacyclovir; PRO-Valacyclovir; Riva-Valacyclovir; Valtrex®

Index Terms Valacyclovir Hydrochloride

Pharmacologic Category Antiviral Agent; Antiviral Agent, Oral

Use Treatment of herpes zoster (shingles) in immunocompetent patients; treatment of first-episode and recurrent genital herpes; suppression of recurrent genital herpes and reduction of transmission of genital herpes in immunocompetent patients; suppression of genital herpes in HIV-infected individuals; treatment of herpes labialis (cold sores); chickenpox in immunocompetent children

Unlabeled Use Prophylaxis of cancer-related HSV, VZV, and CMV infections; treatment of cancer-related HSV, VZV infection

Pregnancy Risk Factor B

Pregnancy Considerations Adverse events were not observed in animal reproduction studies. Valacyclovir is metabolized to acyclovir. In a pharmacokinetic study, maternal acyclovir serum concentrations were higher in pregnant women receiving valacyclovir than those given acyclovir for the suppression of recurrent herpes simplex virus (HSV) infection late in pregnancy. Amniotic fluid concentrations were also higher; however, there was no evidence that fetal exposure differed between the groups (Kimberlin, 1998). Data from an acyclovir pregnancy registry has shown no increased rate of birth defects than that of the general population; however, the registry is small and the manufacturer notes that use during pregnancy is only warranted if the potential benefit to the mother justifies the risk of the fetus. Because more data is available for acyclovir, that agent is preferred for the treatment of genital herpes in pregnant women (ACOG, 2000; CDC, 2010); however, valacyclovir may be considered for use due to its simplified dosing schedule (DHHS, 2013). Pregnant women who have a history of genital herpes recurrence, suppressive therapy is recommended starting at 36 weeks gestation (ACOG, 2000; DHHS, 2013).

Breast-Feeding Considerations Valacyclovir is metabolized to acyclovir; acyclovir (but not unchanged valacyclovir) can be detected in breast milk. Peak concentrations in breast milk range from 0.5-2.3 times the corresponding maternal acyclovir serum concentration. This is expected to provide a nursing infant with a dose of acyclovir equivalent to ~0.6 mg/kg/day following ingestion of valacyclovir 500 mg twice daily by the mother. The manufacturer recommends that caution be used if administered to a nursing woman. Other sources note that women with HSV infection taking valacyclovir may breast-feed as long as there are not lesions on the breast, body lesions are covered, and strict hand hygiene is practiced (ACOG, 2000; Jaiyeoba, 2012). Women with HSV who also have HIV infection should not breast-feed; complete avoidance of breast-feeding by HIV-infected women is recommended to decrease potential transmission of HIV (DHHS [perinatal], 2012).

Contraindications Hypersensitivity to valacyclovir, acyclovir, or any component of the formulation

Warnings/Precautions Thrombotic thrombocytopenic purpura/hemolytic uremic syndrome has occurred in immunocompromised patients (at doses of 8 g/day). Safety and efficacy have not been established for treatment/suppression of recurrent genital herpes or disseminated herpes in patients with profound immunosuppression (eg, advanced HIV with CD4 <100 cells/mm^3). CNS adverse effects (including agitation, hallucinations, confusion, delirium, seizures, and encephalopathy) have been reported. Use caution in patients with renal impairment, the elderly, and/ or those receiving nephrotoxic agents. Acute renal failure has been observed in patients with renal dysfunction; dose adjustment may be required. Decreased precipitation in renal tubules may occur leading to urinary precipitation; adequately hydrate patient. For cold sores, treatment should begin at with earliest symptom (tingling, itching, burning). For genital herpes, treatment should begin as soon as possible after the first signs and symptoms (within 72 hours of onset of first diagnosis or within 24 hours of onset of recurrent episodes). For herpes zoster, treatment should begin within 72 hours of onset of rash. For chickenpox, treatment should begin with earliest sign or symptom. Use with caution in the elderly; CNS effects have been reported. Safety and efficacy have not been established in patients <2 years of age.

Adverse Reactions

>10%:

Central nervous system: Headache (13% to 38%)
Gastrointestinal: Nausea (5% to 15%), abdominal pain (1% to 11%)
Hepatic: ALT increased (≤14%), AST increased (2% to 16%)
Respiratory: Nasopharyngitis (≤16%)

1% to 10%:

Central nervous system: Fatigue (≤8%), depression (≤7%), fever (children 4%), dizziness (2% to 4%)
Dermatologic: Rash (≤8%)
Endocrine: Dysmenorrhea (≤1% to 8%), dehydration (children 2%)
Gastrointestinal: Vomiting (<1% to 6%), diarrhea (children 5%; adults <1%)
Hematologic: Thrombocytopenia (≤3%), mild leukopenia (≤1%)
Hepatic: Alkaline phosphatase increased (≤4%)
Neuromuscular & skeletal: Arthralgia (<1 to 6%)
Respiratory: Rhinorrhea (children 2%)
Miscellaneous: Herpes simplex (children 2%)

<1% (Limited to important or life-threatening): Acute hypersensitivity reactions (angioedema, anaphylaxis, dyspnea, pruritus, rash, urticaria); aggression, agitation, alopecia, anemia, aplastic anemia, ataxia, creatinine increased, coma, confusion, consciousness decreased, delirium, dysarthria, encephalopathy, erythema multiforme, facial edema, hallucinations (auditory and visual), hemolytic uremic syndrome (HUS), hepatitis, hypertension, leukocytoclastic vasculitis, mania, photosensitivity reaction, psychosis, renal failure, renal pain, seizure, tachycardia, thrombotic thrombocytopenic purpura (TTP), tremor, urinary precipitation, visual disturbances

Drug Interactions

Metabolism/Transport Effects None known.

Avoid Concomitant Use

Avoid concomitant use of ValACYclovir with any of the following: Zoster Vaccine

Increased Effect/Toxicity

ValACYclovir may increase the levels/effects of: Mycophenolate; Tenofovir; Zidovudine

The levels/effects of ValACYclovir may be increased by: Mycophenolate

Decreased Effect

ValACYclovir may decrease the levels/effects of: Zoster Vaccine

Storage/Stability Store at 15°C to 25°C (59°F to 77°F).

Mechanism of Action Valacyclovir is rapidly and nearly completely converted to acyclovir by intestinal and hepatic metabolism. Acyclovir is converted to acyclovir monophosphate by virus-specific thymidine kinase then further converted to acyclovir triphosphate by other cellular enzymes. Acyclovir triphosphate inhibits DNA synthesis and viral replication by competing with deoxyguanosine triphosphate for viral DNA polymerase and being incorporated into viral DNA.

Pharmacodynamics/Kinetics

Absorption: Rapid
Distribution: Acyclovir is widely distributed throughout the body including brain, kidney, lungs, liver, spleen, muscle, uterus, vagina, and CSF
Protein binding: ~14% to 18%
Metabolism: Hepatic; valacyclovir is rapidly and nearly completely converted to acyclovir and L-valine by first-pass effect; acyclovir is hepatically metabolized to a very small extent by aldehyde oxidase and by alcohol and aldehyde dehydrogenase (inactive metabolites)
Bioavailability: ~55% once converted to acyclovir
Half-life elimination: Normal renal function: Adults: Acyclovir: 2.5-3.3 hours, Valacyclovir: ~30 minutes; End-stage renal disease: Acyclovir: 14-20 hours; During hemodialysis: 4 hours
Excretion: Urine, primarily as acyclovir (89%); **Note:** Following oral administration of radiolabeled valacyclovir, 46% of the label is eliminated in the feces (corresponding to nonabsorbed drug), while 47% of the radiolabel is eliminated in the urine.

Dosage Oral:

Children 2 to <18 years: Chickenpox: 20 mg/kg/dose 3 times/day for 5 days (maximum: 1 g 3 times/day)
Children ≥12 and Adults: Herpes labialis (cold sores): 2 g twice daily for 1 day (separate doses by ~12 hours)
Adults:
CMV prophylaxis in allogeneic HSCT recipients (unlabeled use): 2 g 4 times/day
Herpes zoster (shingles): 1 g 3 times/day for 7 days
HSV, VZV in cancer patients (unlabeled use): Prophylaxis: 500 mg 2-3 times/day; Treatment: 1 g 3 times/day
Genital herpes:
Initial episode: 1 g twice daily for 10 days
Recurrent episode: 500 mg twice daily for 3 days
Reduction of transmission: 500 mg once daily (source partner)
Suppressive therapy:
Immunocompetent patients: 1 g once daily (500 mg once daily in patients with <9 recurrences per year)
HIV-infected patients (CD4 ≥100 cells/mm^3): 500 mg twice daily

Dosage adjustment in renal impairment:

Herpes zoster: Adults:
U.S. labeling:
Cl_{cr} 30-49 mL/minute: 1 g every 12 hours
Cl_{cr} 10-29 mL/minute: 1 g every 24 hours
Cl_{cr} <10 mL/minute: 500 mg every 24 hours
Canadian labeling:
Cl_{cr} >30 mL/minute: No dosage adjustment required
Cl_{cr} 15-30 mL/minute: 1 g every 12 hours
Cl_{cr} <15 mL/minute: 1 g every 24 hours

Genital herpes: Adults:
U.S. labeling:
Initial episode:
Cl_{cr} 10-29 mL/minute: 1 g every 24 hours
Cl_{cr} <10 mL/minute: 500 mg every 24 hours
Recurrent episode: Cl_{cr} <29 mL/minute: 500 mg every 24 hours
Suppressive therapy: Cl_{cr} <29 mL/minute:
For usual dose of 1 g every 24 hours, decrease dose to 500 mg every 24 hours
For usual dose of 500 mg every 24 hours, decrease dose to 500 mg every 48 hours
HIV-infected patients: 500 mg every 24 hours
Canadian labeling:
Initial episode:
Cl_{cr} 15-30 mL/minute: 1 g every 24 hours
Cl_{cr} <15 mL/minute: 500 mg every 24 hours
Recurrent episode:
Cl_{cr} 15-30 mL/minute: 500 mg every 12 hours
Cl_{cr} <15 mL/minute: 500 mg every 24 hours
Suppressive therapy:
Cl_{cr} 15-30 mL/minute: 500 mg every 24 hours
Cl_{cr} <15 mL/minute:
Immunocompetent or HIV-infected patients: 500 mg every 24 hours
Immunocompetent patients and ≤9 recurrences/year: 500 mg every 48 hours

Herpes labialis: Adolescents and Adults *(U.S. labeling)* or Adults *(Canadian labeling)*:
Cl_{cr} 30-49 mL/minute: 1 g every 12 hours for 2 doses
Cl_{cr} 10-29 mL/minute: 500 mg every 12 hours for 2 doses
Cl_{cr} <10 mL/minute: 500 mg as a single dose

Hemodialysis: Dialyzable (~33% removed during 4-hour session); administer dose postdialysis

Chronic ambulatory peritoneal dialysis/continuous arteriovenous hemofiltration dialysis: Pharmacokinetic parameters are similar to those in patients with ESRD; supplemental dose not needed following dialysis

Dosage adjustment in hepatic impairment: No dosage adjustment necessary.

Dietary Considerations May be taken with or without food.

Administration If GI upset occurs, administer with meals.

Monitoring Parameters Urinalysis, BUN, serum creatinine, liver enzymes, and CBC

Dosage Forms Excipient information presented when available (limited, particularly for generics); consult specific product labeling.

Tablet, Oral:

Valtrex: 500 mg [contains fd&c blue #2 aluminum lake]

Valtrex: 1 g [scored; contains fd&c blue #2 aluminum lake]

Generic: 500 mg, 1 g

Extemporaneous Preparations A 50 mg/mL oral suspension may be made with caplets and either Ora-Sweet® or Ora-Sweet SF®. Crush eighteen 500 mg caplets in a mortar and reduce to a fine powder. Add 5 mL portions of chosen vehicle (40 mL total) and mix to a uniform paste; transfer to a 180 mL calibrated amber glass bottle, rinse mortar with 10 mL of vehicle 5 times, and add quantity of vehicle sufficient to make 180 mL. Label "shake well" and "refrigerate". Stable for 21 days refrigerated.

Fish DN, Vidaurri VA, and Deeter RG, "Stability of Valacyclovir Hydrochloride in Extemporaneously Prepared Oral Liquids," *Am J Health Syst Pharm*, 1999, 56(19):1957-60.

◆ **Valacyclovir Hydrochloride** *see* ValACYclovir *on page 2145*

◆ **Valchlor** *see* Mechlorethamine (Topical) *on page 1275*

◆ **Valcyte** *see* ValGANciclovir *on page 2147*

◆ **23-Valent Pneumococcal Polysaccharide Vaccine** *see* Pneumococcal Polysaccharide Vaccine (Polyvalent) *on page 1664*

ValGANciclovir (val gan SYE kloh veer)

Brand Names: U.S. Valcyte

Brand Names: Canada Apo-Valganciclovir; Valcyte

Index Terms Valganciclovir Hydrochloride

Pharmacologic Category Antiviral Agent

Use Treatment of cytomegalovirus (CMV) retinitis in patients with acquired immunodeficiency syndrome (AIDS); prevention of CMV disease in high-risk patients (donor CMV positive/recipient CMV negative) undergoing kidney, heart, or kidney/pancreas transplantation

Pregnancy Risk Factor C

Pregnancy Considerations Valganciclovir is converted to ganciclovir and shares its reproductive toxicity. **[U.S. Boxed Warning]: Ganciclovir may be teratogenic and cause aspermatogenesis.** Based on animal data, temporary or permanent impairment of fertility may occur in males and females. Ganciclovir is also teratogenic in animals. Females should use effective contraception during treatment and for 30 days after; males should use barrier contraception during treatment and for 90 days after.

Breast-Feeding Considerations HIV-infected mothers are discouraged from breast-feeding to decrease the potential transmission of HIV.

Contraindications Hypersensitivity to valganciclovir, ganciclovir, or any component of the formulation

Warnings/Precautions Hazardous agent - use appropriate precautions for handling and disposal (NIOSH, 2012). **[U.S. Boxed Warning]: May cause dose- or therapy-limiting granulocytopenia, anemia, and/or thrombocytopenia;** do not use in patients with an absolute neutrophil count <500/mm³, platelet count <25,000/mm³, or hemoglobin <8 g/dL. Use with caution in patients with impaired renal function (dose adjustment required). Acute renal failure (ARF) may occur; ensure adequate hydration and use with caution in patients receiving concomitant nephrotoxic agents. Elderly patients with or without pre-existing renal impairment may develop ARF; use with caution and adjust dose as needed. **[U.S. Boxed Warning]: Ganciclovir may be teratogenic, carcinogenic, and cause aspermatogenesis.** Due to its teratogenic potential, contraceptive precautions for female and male patients need to be followed during and for at least 90 days after therapy with the drug. Fertility may be temporarily or permanently impaired in males and females. Due to differences in bioavailability, valganciclovir tablets cannot be substituted for ganciclovir capsules on a one-to-one basis. The preferred dosage form for pediatric patients is the oral solution; however, valganciclovir tablets may used so long as the calculated dose is within 10% of the available tablet strength (450 mg). Not indicated for use in liver transplant patients (higher incidence of tissue-invasive CMV relative to oral ganciclovir was observed in trials). Use of valganciclovir for the treatment of congenital CMV disease has not been evaluated.

Adverse Reactions

>10%:

Cardiovascular: Hypertension (12% to 18%)

Central nervous system: Fever (9% to 31%), headache (6% to 22%), insomnia (6% to 20%)

Gastrointestinal: Diarrhea (16% to 41%), nausea (8% to 30%), vomiting (3% to 21%), abdominal pain (15%), constipation

Hematologic: Anemia (≤31%), thrombocytopenia (≤22%), neutropenia (3% to 19%)

Neuromuscular & skeletal: Tremor (12% to 28%)

Ocular: Retinal detachment (15%)

Renal: Serum creatinine increased (S_{cr} >1.5-2.5 mg/dL: 12% to 50%; S_{cr} >2.5: 3% to 17%)

Respiratory: Cough, upper respiratory tract infection

5% to 10%: Central nervous system: Peripheral neuropathy (9%), paresthesia (8%)

<5%:

Cardiovascular: Edema, hypotension, peripheral edema

Central nervous system: Agitation, confusion, depression, dizziness, fatigue, hallucination, pain, psychosis, seizure

Dermatologic: Acne, dermatitis, pruritus

Endocrine & metabolic: Dehydration, hyperglycemia, hyper-/hypokalemia, hypocalcemia, hypomagnesemia, hypophosphatemia

Gastrointestinal: Abdominal distention/pain, appetite (decreased), dyspepsia

Genitourinary: Urinary tract infection

Hematologic: Aplastic anemia, bleeding (potentially life-threatening due to thrombocytopenia), bone marrow depression, pancytopenia

Hepatic: Ascites

Neuromuscular & skeletal: Arthralgia, back pain, limb pain, muscle cramps, weakness

Renal: Creatinine clearance (decreased), dysuria, renal impairment

Respiratory: Dyspnea, nasopharyngitis, pharyngitis, pleural effusion, rhinorrhea

Miscellaneous: Allergic reaction, local and systemic infection (including sepsis)

<1% (Limited to important or life-threatening): Valganciclovir is expected to share the toxicities which may occur at a low incidence or due to idiosyncratic reactions which have been associated with ganciclovir

Drug Interactions

Metabolism/Transport Effects None known.

Avoid Concomitant Use

Avoid concomitant use of ValGANciclovir with any of the following: Imipenem

Increased Effect/Toxicity

ValGANciclovir may increase the levels/effects of: Imipenem; Mycophenolate; Reverse Transcriptase Inhibitors (Nucleoside); Tenofovir

The levels/effects of ValGANciclovir may be increased by: Mycophenolate; Probenecid; Tenofovir

Decreased Effect There are no known significant interactions involving a decrease in effect.

Ethanol/Nutrition/Herb Interactions Food: Coadministration with a high-fat meal increased AUC by 30%. Management: Valganciclovir should be taken with meals.

Preparation for Administration Hazardous agent; use appropriate precautions for handling and disposal (NIOSH, 2012).

Oral solution: Prior to dispensing, prepare the oral solution by adding 91 mL of purified water to the bottle; shake well. Discard any unused medication after 49 days. A reconstituted 100 mL bottle will only provide 88 mL of solution for administration.

Storage/Stability

Oral solution: Store dry powder at 25°C (77°F); excursions permitted to 15°C to 30°C (59°F to 86°F). Store oral solution under refrigeration at 2°C to 8°C (36°F to 46°F); do not freeze. Discard any unused medication after 49 days.

Tablet: Store at 25°C (77°F); excursions permitted to 15°C to 30°C (59°F to 86°F).

Mechanism of Action Valganciclovir is rapidly converted to ganciclovir in the body. The bioavailability of ganciclovir from valganciclovir is increased 10-fold compared to oral ganciclovir. A dose of 900 mg achieved systemic exposure of ganciclovir comparable to that achieved with the recommended doses of intravenous ganciclovir of 5 mg/kg. Ganciclovir is phosphorylated to a substrate which competitively inhibits the binding of deoxyguanosine triphosphate to DNA polymerase resulting in inhibition of viral DNA synthesis.

Pharmacodynamics/Kinetics

Absorption: Well absorbed; high-fat meal increases AUC by 30%

Distribution: V_{dss}: Ganciclovir: 0.7 L/kg; widely to all tissue including CSF and ocular tissue

Protein binding: Ganciclovir: 1% to 2%

Metabolism: Converted to ganciclovir by intestinal mucosal cells and hepatocytes

Bioavailability: With food: 60%

Half-life elimination: Ganciclovir: 4.08 hours; prolonged with renal impairment; Severe renal impairment: Up to 68 hours

Time to peak: Ganciclovir: 1-3 hours

Excretion: Urine (primarily as ganciclovir)

Dosage Oral:

Children 4 months to 16 years: Prevention of CMV disease following kidney or heart transplantation: Dose (mg) = 7 x body surface area x creatinine clearance* once daily beginning within 10 days of transplantation; continue therapy until 100 days post-transplantation. Doses should be rounded to the nearest 25 mg increment; maximum dose: 900 mg/day.

*Cl_{cr} (mL/minute/1.73 m^2) = [k x Height (cm)] divided by serum creatinine (mg/dL)

Note: If the calculated Cl_{cr} is >150 mL/minute/1.73 m^2, then a maximum value of 150 mL/minute/1.73 m^2 should be used to calculate the dose.

Note: Calculated using *modified* Schwartz formula where k is as follows:

Patients <2 years: k = 0.45

Girls 2-16 years: k = 0.55

Boys 2 to <13 years: k = 0.55

Boys 13-16 years: k = 0.7

Children >16 years and Adults:

CMV retinitis:

Induction: 900 mg twice daily for 21 days

Maintenance: Following induction treatment, or for patients with inactive CMV retinitis who require maintenance therapy: 900 mg once daily

Prevention of CMV disease following transplantation: 900 mg once daily beginning within 10 days of transplantation; continue therapy until 100 days (heart or kidney-pancreas transplant) or 200 days (kidney transplant) post-transplantation

Dosage adjustment in renal impairment:

Children 4 months to 16 years: No dosage adjustment necessary; calculation for all patients adjusts for renal function.

Children >16 years and Adults:

Induction dose:

Cl_{cr} 40-59 mL/minute: 450 mg twice daily

Cl_{cr} 25-39 mL/minute: 450 mg once daily

Cl_{cr} 10-24 mL/minute: 450 mg every 2 days

Maintenance dose:

Cl_{cr} 40-59 mL/minute: 450 mg once daily

Cl_{cr} 25-39 mL/minute: 450 mg every 2 days

Cl_{cr} 10-24 mL/minute: 450 mg twice weekly

Note: Valganciclovir is not recommended in patients receiving hemodialysis. For patients on hemodialysis (Cl_{cr} <10 mL/minute), it is recommended that ganciclovir be used (dose adjusted as specified for ganciclovir).

Dosage adjustment in hepatic impairment: No dosage adjustment provided in manufacturer's labeling (has not been studied).

Dietary Considerations Should be taken with meals.

Administration Valganciclovir should be taken with meals. The preferred dosage form for pediatric patients is the oral solution; however, valganciclovir tablets may used so long as the calculated dose is within 10% of the available tablet strength (450 mg).

Due to the carcinogenic and mutagenic potential, avoid direct contact with broken or crushed tablets, powder for oral solution, and oral solution. Consideration should be given to handling and disposal according to guidelines issued for antineoplastic drugs. However, there is no consensus on the need for these precautions.

Hazardous agent; use appropriate precautions for handling and disposal (NIOSH, 2012).

Monitoring Parameters Retinal exam (at least every 4-6 weeks), CBC, platelet counts, serum creatinine

Dosage Forms Excipient information presented when available (limited, particularly for generics); consult specific product labeling.

Solution Reconstituted, Oral:

Valcyte: 50 mg/mL (88 mL) [contains saccharin sodium, sodium benzoate; tutti-frutti flavor]

Tablet, Oral:

Valcyte: 450 mg

Extemporaneous Preparations Hazardous agent: Use appropriate precautions for handling and disposal.

Note: Commercial preparation is available (50 mg/mL)

A 60 mg/mL oral suspension may be with tablets and a 1:1 mixture of Ora-Sweet® and Ora-Plus®. Crush sixteen 450 mg tablets and reduce to a fine powder. Add 1 mL portions of chosen vehicle (10 mL total) and mix to a uniform paste; mix while adding the vehicle in incremental proportions to **almost** 120 mL; transfer to a calibrated amber glass bottle, rinse mortar with vehicle, and add quantity of vehicle sufficient to make 120 mL. Label "shake well" and "refrigerate". Stable for 35 days refrigerated.

Henkin CC, Griener JC, and Ten Eick AP, "Stability of Valganciclovir in Extemporaneously Compounded Liquid Formulations," *Am J Health Syst Pharm*, 2003, 60(7):687-90.

◆ **Valganciclovir Hydrochloride** *see* ValGANciclovir *on page* 2147

◆ **Valisone® Scalp Lotion (Can)** *see* Betamethasone *on page* 247

◆ **Valium** *see* Diazepam *on page* 594

◆ **Valium® (Can)** *see* Diazepam *on page* 594

◆ **Valorin [OTC]** *see* Acetaminophen *on page* 28

◆ **Valorin Extra [OTC]** *see* Acetaminophen *on page* 28

◆ **Valproate Semisodium** *see* Valproic Acid and Derivatives *on page* 2149

◆ **Valproate Sodium** *see* Valproic Acid and Derivatives *on page* 2149

◆ **Valproic Acid** *see* Valproic Acid and Derivatives *on page* 2149

◆ **Valproic Acid Derivative** *see* Valproic Acid and Derivatives *on page* 2149

Valproic Acid and Derivatives

(val PROE ik AS id & dah RIV ah tives)

Brand Names: U.S. Depacon; Depakene; Depakote; Depakote ER; Depakote Sprinkles; Stavzor

Brand Names: Canada Apo-Divalproex; Apo-Valproic; Depakene; Dom-Divalproex; Dom-Valproic Acid; Dom-Valproic Acid E.C.; Epival; Mylan-Divalproex; Mylan-Valproic; Novo-Divalproex; PHL-Divalproex; PHL-Valproic Acid; PHL-Valproic Acid E.C.; PMS-Divalproex; PMS-Valproic Acid; PMS-Valproic Acid E.C.; ratio-Valproic; Sandoz-Valproic

Index Terms 2-Propylpentanoic Acid; 2-Propylvaleric Acid; Dipropylacetic Acid; Divalproex Sodium; DPA; Valproate Semisodium; Valproate Sodium; Valproic Acid; Valproic Acid Derivative

Pharmacologic Category Anticonvulsant, Miscellaneous; Antimanic Agent; Histone Deacetylase Inhibitor

Additional Appendix Information

Status Epilepticus *on page* 2375

Use

Oral, I.V.: Monotherapy and adjunctive therapy in the treatment of patients with complex partial seizures; monotherapy and adjunctive therapy of simple and complex absence seizures; adjunctive therapy in patients with multiple seizure types that include absence seizures

Additional indications: Depakote, Depakote ER, Stavzor: Mania associated with bipolar disorder; migraine prophylaxis

Unlabeled Use Refractory status epilepticus, diabetic neuropathy

Pregnancy Risk Factor X (migraine prophylaxis)/D (all other indications)

Pregnancy Considerations [U.S. Boxed Warning]: May cause teratogenic effects such as neural tube defects (eg, spina bifida) and decreased IQ scores following *in utero* exposure. Teratogenic effects have been reported in animals and humans. Valproic acid crosses the placenta (Harden, 2009b). Neural tube, cardiac, facial (characteristic pattern of dysmorphic facial features), skeletal, multiple other defects reported. Information from the North American Antiepileptic Drug Pregnancy Registry notes a fourfold increase in congenital malformations with exposure to valproic acid monotherapy during the 1st trimester of pregnancy when compared to monotherapy with other antiepileptic drugs (AED). The risk of spinal bifida is ~1% to 2% (general population risk estimated to be 0.06% to 0.07%). The effect of folic acid supplementation to decrease this risk is unknown, however, folic acid supplementation is recommended for all women contemplating pregnancy.

Nonteratogenic adverse effects have also been reported. Afibrinogenemia leading to fatal hemorrhage and hepatotoxicity have been noted in case reports of infants following *in utero* exposure to valproic acid. Developmental delay, decreased IQ scores, autism and/or autism spectrum disorder have also been reported.

Use is contraindicated in pregnant women for the prevention of migraine. Current guidelines recommend complete avoidance of valproic acid and derivatives for the treatment of epilepsy in pregnant women whenever possible (Harden, 2009a). **Use is not recommended in women of childbearing potential for any condition unless alternative therapies are not appropriate,** especially when used for conditions not associated with permanent injury or risk of death. Effective contraception should be used during treatment. When pregnancy is being planned, consider tapering off of therapy prior to conception if appropriate and supplementing with folic acid.

A pregnancy registry is available for women who have been exposed to valproic acid. Patients may enroll themselves in the North American Antiepileptic Drug (NAAED) Pregnancy Registry by calling (888) 233-2334. Additional information is available at www.aedpregnancyregistry.org.

Breast-Feeding Considerations Valproate is excreted into breast milk. Breast milk concentrations of valproic acid have been reported as 1% to 10% of maternal concentration. The weight-adjusted dose to the infant has been calculated to be ~4% (Hagg, 2000). The manufacturer recommends that caution be used if administered to nursing women.

Medication Guide Available Yes

Contraindications Hypersensitivity to valproic acid, divalproex, derivatives, or any component of the formulation; hepatic disease or significant impairment; urea cycle disorders; pregnant women for the prevention of migraine; known mitochondrial disorders caused by mutations in mitochondrial DNA polymerase gamma (POLG; eg, Alpers-Huttenlocher syndrome [AHS]) or children <2 years of age suspected of having a POLG-related disorder

Warnings/Precautions Hazardous agent; use appropriate precautions for handling and disposal (NIOSH, 2012). **[U.S. Boxed Warning]: Hepatic failure resulting in fatalities has occurred in patients, usually in the initial 6 months of therapy; children <2 years of age are at considerable risk. Risk is also increased in patients with hereditary neurometabolic syndromes caused by DNA mutations of the mitochondrial DNA polymerase gamma (POLG) gene (eg, Alpers-Huttenlocher syndrome [AHS]).** Other risk factors include organic brain disease, mental retardation with severe seizure disorders, congenital metabolic disorders, and patients on multiple anticonvulsants. Monitor patients closely for appearance of malaise, weakness, facial edema, anorexia, jaundice, and vomiting; discontinue immediately with signs/symptom of significant or suspected impairment. Liver function tests should be performed at baseline and at regular intervals after initiation of therapy, especially within the first 6 months. Hepatic dysfunction may progress despite discontinuing treatment. Should only be used as monotherapy and with extreme caution in children <2 years of age and/or patients at high risk for hepatotoxicity. Contraindicated with significant hepatic impairment.

[U.S. Boxed Warning]: Risk of valproate-induced acute liver failure and death is increased in patients with hereditary neurometabolic syndromes caused by DNA mutations of the mitochondrial polymerase gamma (POLG) gene (eg, Alpers-Huttenlocher syndrome [AHS]). Use is contraindicated in patients with known mitochondrial disorders caused by POLG mutations and children <2 years of age suspected of having a POLG-related disorder. Use in children ≥2 years of age suspected of having a POLG-related disorder only after other anticonvulsants have failed and with close monitoring for the development of acute liver injury. POLG mutation testing should be performed in accordance with current clinical practice.

[U.S. Boxed Warning]: Cases of life-threatening pancreatitis, occurring at the start of therapy or following years of use, have been reported in adults and children. Some cases have been hemorrhagic with rapid progression of initial symptoms to death. Promptly evaluate symptoms of abdominal pain, nausea, vomiting, and/or anorexia; should generally be discontinued if pancreatitis is diagnosed.

[U.S. Boxed Warning]: May cause teratogenic effects such as neural tube defects (eg, spina bifida) and decreased IQ scores following *in utero* exposure. Use is contraindicated in pregnant women for the prevention of migraine. **Use is not recommended in women of childbearing potential for any indication unless alternative therapies are not appropriate**, especially when used for conditions not associated with permanent injury or risk of death (eg, migraine).

May cause severe thrombocytopenia, inhibition of platelet aggregation, and bleeding. Hypersensitivity reactions affecting multiple organs have been reported in association with valproate use; may include dermatologic and/or hematologic changes (eosinophilia, neutropenia, thrombocytopenia) or symptoms of organ dysfunction.

Hyperammonemia and/or encephalopathy, sometimes fatal, have been reported following the initiation of valproate therapy and may be present with normal transaminase levels. Ammonia levels should be measured in patients who develop unexplained lethargy and vomiting, changes in mental status, or in patients who present with hypothermia (unintentional drop in core body temperature to <35°C/95°F). Discontinue therapy if ammonia levels are increased and evaluate for possible urea cycle disorder (UCD); contraindicated in patients with UCD. Evaluation of UCD should be considered for the following patients prior to the start of therapy: History of unexplained encephalopathy or coma; encephalopathy associated with protein load; pregnancy or postpartum encephalopathy; unexplained mental retardation; history of elevated plasma ammonia or glutamine; history of cyclical vomiting and lethargy; episodic extreme irritability, ataxia; low BUN or protein avoidance; family history of UCD or unexplained infant deaths (particularly male); or signs or symptoms of UCD (hyperammonemia, encephalopathy, respiratory alkalosis). Hypothermia has been reported with valproate therapy; hypothermia may or may not be associated with hyperammonemia; may also occur with concomitant topiramate therapy following topiramate initiation or dosage increase.

In vitro studies have suggested valproate stimulates the replication of HIV and CMV viruses under experimental conditions. The clinical consequence of this is unknown, but should be considered when monitoring affected patients.

Antiepileptics are associated with an increased risk of suicidal behavior/thoughts with use (regardless of indication); patients should be monitored for signs/symptoms of depression, suicidal tendencies, and other unusual behavior changes during therapy and instructed to inform their healthcare provider immediately if symptoms occur.

Intravenous valproate is not recommended for post-traumatic seizure prophylaxis in patients with acute head trauma; study results for this indication suggested increased mortality with I.V. valproate use compared to I.V. phenytoin. Anticonvulsants should not be discontinued abruptly because of the possibility of increasing seizure frequency; valproate should be withdrawn gradually to minimize the potential of increased seizure frequency, unless safety concerns require a more rapid withdrawal. Patients treated for bipolar disorder should be monitored closely for clinical worsening or suicidality; prescriptions should be written for the smallest quantity consistent with good patient care.

Reversible and irreversible cerebral and cerebellar atrophy have been reported; motor and cognitive function should be routinely monitored to assess for signs and symptoms of brain atrophy. CNS depression may occur with valproate use. Patients must be cautioned about performing tasks which require mental alertness (operating machinery or driving). Effects with other sedative drugs or ethanol may be potentiated. Use with caution in the elderly as the elderly may be more sensitive to sedating effects and dehydration; in some elderly patients with somnolence, concomitant decreases in nutritional intake and weight loss were observed. Reduce initial dosages in elderly and closely monitor fluid status, nutritional intake, somnolence, and other adverse events. Potentially significant drug-drug interactions may exist, requiring dose or frequency adjustment, additional monitoring, and/or selection of alternative therapy.

Medication residue in stool has been reported (rarely) with oral Depakote (divalproex sodium) formulations; some reports have occurred in patients with shortened GI transit times (eg, diarrhea) or anatomic GI disorders (eg, ileostomy, colostomy). In patients reporting medication residue in stool, it is recommended to monitor valproate level and clinical condition.

Adverse Reactions

>10%:

- Central nervous system: Headache (≤31%), somnolence (≤30%), dizziness (12% to 25%), insomnia (>1% to 15%), nervousness (>1% to 11%), pain (1% to 11%)
- Dermatologic: Alopecia (>1% to 24%)
- Gastrointestinal: Nausea (15% to 48%), vomiting (7% to 27%), diarrhea (7% to 23%), abdominal pain (7% to 23%), dyspepsia (7% to 23%), anorexia (>1% to 12%)
- Hematologic: Thrombocytopenia (1% to 24%; dose related)
- Neuromuscular & skeletal: Tremor (≤57%), weakness (6% to 27%)
- Ocular: Diplopia (>1% to 16%), amblyopia/blurred vision (≤12%)
- Miscellaneous: Infection (≤20%), flu-like syndrome (12%)

1% to 10%:

- Cardiovascular: Peripheral edema (>1% to 8%), chest pain (>1% to <5%), edema (>1% to <5%), facial edema (>1% to <5%), hypertension (>1% to <5%), hypotension (>1% to <5%), orthostatic hypotension (>1% to <5%), palpitation (>1% to <5%), tachycardia (>1% to <5%), vasodilation (>1% to <5%), arrhythmia
- Central nervous system: Ataxia (>1% to 8%), amnesia (>1% to 7%), emotional lability (>1% to 6%), fever (>1% to 6%), abnormal thinking (≤6%), depression (>1% to 5%), abnormal dreams (>1% to <5%), agitation (>1% to <5%), anxiety (>1% to <5%), catatonia (>1% to <5%),

chills (>1% to <5%), confusion (>1% to <5%), coordination abnormal (>1% to <5%), hallucination (>1% to <5%), malaise (>1% to <5%), personality disorder (>1% to <5%), speech disorder (>1% to <5%), tardive dyskinesia (>1% to <5%), vertigo (>1% to <5%), euphoria (1%), hypoesthesia (1%)

Dermatologic: Rash (>1% to 6%), bruising (>1% to 5%), discoid lupus erythematosus (>1% to <5%), dry skin (>1% to <5%), furunculosis (>1% to <5%), petechia (>1% to <5%), pruritus (>1% to <5), seborrhea (>1% to <5%)

Endocrine & metabolic: Amenorrhea (>1% to <5%), dysmenorrhea (>1% to <5%), metrorrhagia (>1% to <5%), hypoproteinemia

Gastrointestinal: Weight gain (4% to 9%), weight loss (6%), appetite increased (≤6%), constipation (>1% to 5%), xerostomia (>1% to 5%), eructation (>1% to <5%), fecal incontinence (>1% to <5%), flatulence (>1% to <5%), gastroenteritis (>1% to <5%), glossitis (>1% to <5%), hematemesis (>1% to <5%), pancreatitis (>1% to <5%), periodontal abscess (>1% to <5%), stomatitis (>1% to <5%), taste perversion (>1% to <5%), dysphagia, gum hemorrhage, mouth ulceration

Genitourinary: Cystitis (>1% to 5%), dysuria (>1% to 5%), urinary frequency (>1% to <5%), urinary incontinence (>1% to <5%), vaginal hemorrhage (>1% to 5%), vaginitis (>1% to <5%)

Hepatic: ALT increased (>1% to <5%), AST increased (>1% to <5%)

Local: Injection site pain (3%), injection site reaction (2%), injection site inflammation (1%)

Neuromuscular & skeletal: Back pain (≤8%), abnormal gait (>1% to <5%), arthralgia (>1% to <5%), arthrosis (>1% to <5%), dysarthria (>1% to <5%), hypertonia (>1% to <5%), hypokinesia (>1% to <5%), leg cramps (>1% to <5%), myalgia (>1% to <5%), myasthenia (>1% to <5%), neck pain (>1% to <5%), neck rigidity (>1% to <5%), paresthesia (>1% to <5%), reflex increased (>1% to <5%), twitching (>1% to <5%)

Ocular: Nystagmus (1% to 8%), dry eyes (>1% to 5%), eye pain (>1% to 5%), abnormal vision (>1% to <5%), conjunctivitis (>1% to <5%)

Otic: Tinnitus (1% to 7%), ear pain (>1% to 5%), deafness (>1% to <5%), otitis media (>1% to <5%)

Respiratory: Pharyngitis (2% to 8%), bronchitis (5%), rhinitis (>1% to 5%), dyspnea (1% to 5%), cough (>1% to <5%), epistaxis (>1% to <5%), pneumonia (>1% to <5%), sinusitis (>1% to <5%)

Miscellaneous: Diaphoresis (1%), hiccups

<1% (Limited to important and/or life-threatening): Aggression, agranulocytosis, allergic reaction, anaphylaxis, anemia, aplastic anemia, asterixis, behavioral deterioration, bilirubin increased, bleeding time altered, bone marrow suppression, bone pain, bradycardia, breast enlargement, cutaneous vasculitis, carnitine decreased, cerebral atrophy (reversible), coma (rare), dementia, encephalopathy (rare), enuresis, eosinophilia, erythema multiforme, Fanconi-like syndrome (rare, in children), galactorrhea, hematoma formation, hemorrhage, hepatic failure, hepatotoxicity, hostility, hyperactivity, hyperammonemia, hyperammonemic encephalopathy (in patients with UCD), hyperglycinemia, hypersensitivity reactions (severe, with multiorgan dysfunction), hypofibrinogenemia, hyponatremia, hypothermia, inappropriate ADH secretion, intermittent porphyria, LDH increased, leukopenia, lupus, lymphocytosis, macrocytosis, menstrual irregularities, pancytopenia parkinsonism, parotid gland swelling, photosensitivity, platelet aggregation inhibited, polycystic ovary disease (rare), psychosis, seeing "spots before the eyes," Stevens-Johnson syndrome, suicidal behavior/ideation, thyroid function tests abnormal, toxic epidermal necrolysis (rare), urinary tract infection

Drug Interactions

Metabolism/Transport Effects **Substrate** of CYP2A6 (minor), CYP2B6 (minor), CYP2C19 (minor), CYP2C9 (minor), CYP2E1 (minor); **Note:** Assignment of Major/Minor substrate status based on clinically relevant drug interaction potential; **Inhibits** CYP2C9 (weak); **Induces** CYP2A6 (weak/moderate)

Avoid Concomitant Use

Avoid concomitant use of Valproic Acid and Derivatives with any of the following: Cosyntropin

Increased Effect/Toxicity

Valproic Acid and Derivatives may increase the levels/effects of: Barbiturates; Ethosuximide; LamoTRIgine; LORazepam; Paliperidone; Primidone; RisperiDONE; Rufinamide; Temozolomide; Tricyclic Antidepressants; Vorinostat; Zidovudine

The levels/effects of Valproic Acid and Derivatives may be increased by: ChlorproMAZINE; Cosyntropin; Felbamate; GuanFACINE; Primidone; Salicylates; Topiramate

Decreased Effect

Valproic Acid and Derivatives may decrease the levels/effects of: CarBAMazepine; Fosphenytoin-Phenytoin; OLANZapine; OXcarbazepine; Urea Cycle Disorder Agents

The levels/effects of Valproic Acid and Derivatives may be decreased by: Barbiturates; CarBAMazepine; Carbapenems; Ethosuximide; Fosphenytoin-Phenytoin; Methylfolate; Protease Inhibitors; Rifampin

Ethanol/Nutrition/Herb Interactions

Ethanol: Avoid ethanol (may increase CNS depression).

Food: Food may delay but does not affect the extent of absorption.

Preparation for Administration Hazardous agent; use appropriate precautions for handling and disposal (NIOSH, 2012).

I.V.: Prior to administration of the injectable solution, dilute in 50 mL of a compatible diluent.

Storage/Stability

Oral: Store at controlled room temperature.

I.V.: Store at controlled room temperature. Stable in D_5W, NS, and LR for at least 24 hours when stored in glass or PVC.

Mechanism of Action Causes increased availability of gamma-aminobutyric acid (GABA), an inhibitory neurotransmitter, to brain neurons or may enhance the action of GABA or mimic its action at postsynaptic receptor sites

Pharmacodynamics/Kinetics

Distribution: Total valproate: 11 L/1.73 m^2; free valproate 92 L/1.73 m^2

Protein binding (concentration dependent): 80% to 90%; free fraction: ~10% at 40 mcg/mL and ~18.5% at 130 mcg/mL; protein binding decreased in the elderly and with hepatic or renal dysfunction

Metabolism: Extensively hepatic via glucuronide conjugation (30% to 50% of administered dose) and 40% via mitochondrial beta-oxidation; other oxidative metabolic pathways occur to a lesser extent. The relationship between dose and total valproate concentration is nonlinear; concentration does not increase proportionally with the dose, but increases to a lesser extent due to saturable plasma protein binding. The kinetics of unbound drug are linear.

Bioavailability: Depakote ER: ~90% relative to I.V. dose and ~89% relative to delayed release formulation

Half-life elimination (increased in neonates, elderly and those with liver disease): Children >2 months: 7-13 hours; Adults: 9-19 hours

Time to peak, serum:

Oral: Depakote tablet: ~4 hours; Depakote ER: 4-17 hours; Stavzor: 2 hours

Rectal (unlabeled route): 1-3 hours (Graves, 1987)

Excretion: Urine (30% to 50% as glucuronide conjugate, <3% as unchanged drug)

Dosage

Seizure disorders: **Note:** Administer doses >250 mg daily in divided doses.

Oral:

Simple and complex absence seizures: Children and Adults: Initial: 15 mg/kg/day; increase by 5-10 mg/kg/day at weekly intervals until therapeutic levels are achieved; maximum: 60 mg/kg/day. Larger maintenance doses may be required in younger children.

Complex partial seizures: Children ≥10 years and Adults: Initial: 10-15 mg/kg/day; increase by 5-10 mg/kg/day at weekly intervals until therapeutic levels are achieved; maximum: 60 mg/kg/day. Larger maintenance doses may be required in younger children.

Note: Regular release and delayed release formulations are usually given in 2-4 divided doses per day; extended release formulation (Depakote ER) is usually given once daily. Depakote ER is not recommended for use in children <10 years of age. In patients previously maintained on regular release valproic acid therapy (Depakene) who convert to delayed release valproate tablets or capsules (Depakote, Stavzor), the same daily dose and frequency as the regular release should be used; once therapy is stabilized, the frequency of Depakote or Stavzor may be adjusted to 2-3 times daily.

Conversion to Depakote ER from a stable dose of Depakote: Children ≥10 years and Adults: May require an increase in the total daily dose between 8% and 20% to maintain similar serum concentrations.

Conversion to monotherapy from adjunctive therapy: The concomitant antiepileptic drug (AED) can be decreased by ~25% every 2 weeks; dosage reduction of the concomitant AED may begin when valproate therapy is initiated or 1-2 weeks following valproate initiation.

I.V.: Total daily I.V. dose should be equivalent to the total daily dose of the oral valproate product; administer dose as a 60-minute infusion (≤20 mg/minute) with the same frequency as oral products; switch patient to oral products as soon as possible. Alternatively, rapid infusions of 1.5-6 mg/kg/minute have been used in clinical trials to quickly achieve therapeutic concentrations, and were generally well tolerated (Ramsay, 2003; Wheless, 2004; Venkataraman, 1999). One study reported undiluted valproic acid administered at ≤10 mg/kg/minute (dose of ≤30 mg/kg) was well tolerated (Limdi, 2007).

Rectal (unlabeled route): Children: Dilute syrup 1:1 with water for use as a retention enema; acute and maintenance dose: 6-15 mg/kg/dose (Graves, 1987)

Status epilepticus, refractory (unlabeled use): Adults: I.V.: Loading dose: 15-20 mg/kg administered at 20 mg/minute; maintenance dose: I.V. infusion: 1-5 mg/kg/hour (Gaitanis, 2003). Alternatively, median loading doses of 25-30 mg/kg (maximum dose: 45 mg/kg) administered at ≤6 mg/kg/minute have also been reported (Limdi, 2005; Misra, 2006; Sinha, 2000).

Mania: Adults: Oral:

Depakote tablet, Stavzor: Initial: 750 mg/day in divided doses; dose should be adjusted as rapidly as possible to desired clinical effect; maximum recommended dosage: 60 mg/kg/day

Depakote ER: Initial: 25 mg/kg/day given once daily; dose should be adjusted as rapidly as possible to desired clinical effect; maximum recommended dose: 60 mg/kg/day.

Migraine prophylaxis: Oral:

Children ≥12 years (Stavzor): 250 mg twice daily; adjust dose based on patient response, up to 1000 mg/day

Children ≥16 years and Adults (Depakote tablet): 250 mg twice daily; adjust dose based on patient response, up to 1000 mg/day

Adults (Depakote ER): 500 mg once daily for 7 days, then increase to 1000 mg once daily; adjust dose based on patient response; usual dosage range 500-1000 mg/day

Diabetic neuropathy (unlabeled use): Adults: Oral: 500-1200 mg/day (Bril, 2011)

Elderly: Oral, I.V.: Lower initial doses are recommended due to decreased elimination and increased incidences of somnolence in the elderly; no specific dosage recommendations are provided by the manufacturer. Upward titration should be done slowly and with close monitoring for adverse events (eg, sedation, dehydration, decreased nutritional intake). Safety and efficacy for use in patients >65 years have not been studied for migraine prophylaxis.

Dosage adjustment in renal impairment: Mild-to-severe impairment: No dosage adjustment necessary; however, due to decreased protein binding in renal impairment, monitoring only total valproate concentrations may be misleading.

Dosage adjustment in hepatic impairment:

Mild-to-moderate impairment: Not recommended for use in hepatic disease; clearance is decreased with liver impairment. Hepatic disease is also associated with decreased albumin concentrations and 2- to 2.6-fold increase in the unbound fraction. Free concentrations of valproate may be elevated while total concentrations appear normal, therefore, monitoring only total valproate concentrations may be misleading.

Severe impairment: Use is contraindicated.

Administration

Oral: Oral valproate products may cause GI upset; taking with food or slowly increasing the dose may decrease GI upset should it occur.

Depakote ER: Swallow whole; do not crush or chew.

Depakote Sprinkle capsules may be swallowed whole or capsule opened and sprinkled on small amount (1 teaspoonful) of soft food (eg, pudding, applesauce) to be used immediately (do not store or chew).

Depakene capsule, Stavzor: Swallow whole; do not chew.

I.V.: Following dilution to final concentration, manufacturer's labeling recommends administering over 60 minutes at a rate ≤20 mg/minute. Alternatively, more rapid infusion rates of 1.5-6 mg/kg/minute have been used in clinical trials to quickly achieve therapeutic concentrations, and were generally well tolerated (Ramsay, 2003; Wheless, 2004). One study reported undiluted valproic acid administered at ≤10 mg/kg/minute (dose of ≤30 mg/kg) was well tolerated (Limdi, 2007).

Hazardous agent; use appropriate precautions for handling and disposal (NIOSH, 2012).

Monitoring Parameters Liver enzymes (at baseline and frequently during therapy especially during the first 6 months), CBC with platelets (baseline and periodic intervals), PT/PTT (especially prior to surgery), serum ammonia (with symptoms of lethargy, mental status change), serum valproate levels; suicidality (eg, suicidal thoughts, depression, behavioral changes); motor and cognitive function (for signs or symptoms of brain atrophy)

Reference Range Note: In general, trough concentrations should be used to assess adequacy of therapy; peak concentrations may also be drawn if clinically necessary (eg, concentration-related toxicity). Within 2-4 days of initiation or dose adjustment, trough concentrations should be drawn just before the next dose (extended-release preparations) or before the morning dose (for immediate-release preparations). Patients with epilepsy should not delay taking their dose for >2-3 hours. Additional patient-specific factors must be taken into consideration when interpreting drug levels, including indication, age, clinical response, pregnancy status, adherence, comorbidities, adverse effects, and concomitant medications (Patsalos, 2008; Reed, 2006).

Therapeutic:

Epilepsy: 50-100 mcg/mL (SI: 350-700 micromole/L); although seizure control may improve at levels >100 mcg/mL (SI: 700 micromole/L), toxicity may occur at levels of 100-150 mcg/mL (SI: 700-1040 micromole/L)

Mania: 50-125 mcg/mL (SI: 350-875 micromole/L)

Toxic: Some laboratories may report >200 mcg/mL (SI: >1390 micromole/L) as a toxic threshold, although clinical toxicity can occur at lower concentrations. Probability of thrombocytopenia increases with total valproate levels ≥110 mcg/mL in females or ≥135 mcg/mL in males.

Epilepsy: Although seizure control may improve at levels >100 mcg/mL (SI: 700 micromole/L), toxicity may occur at levels of 100-150 mcg/mL (SI: 700-1050 micromole/L)

Mania: Clinical response seen with trough levels between 50-125 mcg/mL (SI: 350-875 micromole/L); risk of toxicity increases at levels >125 mcg/mL (SI: 875 micromole/L)

Test Interactions May cause a false-positive result for urine ketones (valproate partially eliminated as a keto-metabolite in the urine); may alter thyroid function tests

Additional Information

Divalproex sodium is a compound of sodium valproate and valproic acid; divalproex dissociates to valproate in the GI tract.

Extended release tablets have 10% to 20% less fluctuation in serum concentration than delayed release tablets. Extended release tablets are not bioequivalent to delayed release tablets.

Dosage Forms Considerations

Strengths of divalproex sodium and valproate sodium products are expressed in terms of valproic acid

Dosage Forms Excipient information presented when available (limited, particularly for generics); consult specific product labeling.

Capsule, Oral, as valproic acid:
- Depakene: 250 mg
- Generic: 250 mg

Capsule Delayed Release, Oral, as valproic acid:
- Stavzor: 125 mg, 250 mg, 500 mg [contains fd&c yellow #6 (sunset yellow)]

Capsule Sprinkle, Oral, as divalproex sodium:
- Depakote Sprinkles: 125 mg [contains brilliant blue fcf (fd&c blue #1)]
- Generic: 125 mg

Solution, Intravenous, as valproate sodium:
- Depacon: 100 mg/mL (5 mL)
- Generic: 100 mg/mL (5 mL)

Solution, Intravenous, as valproate sodium [preservative free]:
- Generic: 100 mg/mL (5 mL); 500 mg/5 mL (5 mL); 100 mg/mL (5 mL)

Solution, Oral, as valproate sodium:
- Generic: 250 mg/5 mL (473 mL)

Syrup, Oral, as valproate sodium:
- Depakene: 250 mg/5 mL (480 mL)
- Generic: 250 mg/5 mL (5 mL, 10 mL, 473 mL)

Tablet Delayed Release, Oral, as divalproex sodium:
- Depakote: 125 mg [contains brilliant blue fcf (fd&c blue #1), fd&c red #40]
- Depakote: 250 mg [contains fd&c yellow #6 (sunset yellow)]
- Depakote: 500 mg [contains fd&c blue #2 (indigotine)]
- Generic: 125 mg, 250 mg, 500 mg

Tablet Extended Release 24 Hour, Oral, as divalproex sodium:
- Depakote ER: 250 mg, 500 mg
- Generic: 250 mg, 500 mg

Valrubicin (val ROO bi sin)

Brand Names: U.S. Valstar

Brand Names: Canada Valtaxin®

Index Terms *N*-trifluoroacetyladriamycin-14-valerate; AD32

Pharmacologic Category Antineoplastic Agent, Anthracycline

Use Intravesical treatment of BCG-refractory bladder carcinoma *in situ*

Pregnancy Risk Factor C

Pregnancy Considerations Embryotoxicity and teratogenic effects were observed in animal reproduction studies. Systemic exposure (eg, with bladder perforation) during human pregnancy may result in fetal harm. Women of childbearing potential should avoid becoming pregnant during treatment. All patients of reproductive age should use an effective method of contraception during the treatment period.

Breast-Feeding Considerations Due to the potential for serious adverse reactions in the nursing infant, breast-feeding should be discontinued prior to initiation of therapy.

Contraindications Hypersensitivity to anthracyclines, polyoxyl castor oil (Cremophor® EL), or any component of the formulation; concurrent urinary tract infection; small bladder capacity (unable to tolerate a 75 mL instillation)

Warnings/Precautions Hazardous agent - use appropriate precautions for handling and disposal (NIOSH, 2012). Delay valrubicin therapy for at least 2 weeks after transurethral resection and/or fulguration. Evaluate bladder status prior to instillation; do not administer if mucosal integrity of bladder has been compromised or bladder perforation is present (delay treatment until restoration of bladder integrity). Use aseptic technique to prevent urinary tract infection or traumatizing urinary mucosa. Although clamping of the urinary catheter after administration is not recommended, use caution and appropriate medical supervision if performed. Irritable bladder symptoms may occur during instillation and retention, and for a brief time after voiding. Use caution in patients with severe irritable bladder symptoms. Red-tinged urine is typical for the first 24 hours after instillation. Prolonged symptoms or discoloration should prompt contact with the physician.

Contains polyoxyl castor oil (Cremophor® EL) which is associated with hypersensitivity reactions; use is contraindicated in patients with hypersensitivity to polyoxyl castor oil. Delaying cystectomy during treatment may lead to metastatic bladder cancer; reconsider cystectomy if complete response to treatment does not occur within 3 months.

Adverse Reactions Note: In general, local adverse reactions occur during or shortly after instillation and resolve within 1-7 days.

>10%: Genitourinary: Bladder irritation (88%), urinary frequency (61%), urinary urgency (57%), dysuria (56%), bladder spasm (31%), hematuria (29%; gross: 1%), bladder pain (28%), urinary incontinence (22%), cystitis (15%), urinary tract infection (15%), urine red-tinged

1% to 10%:
Cardiovascular: Chest pain (3%), vasodilation (2%), peripheral edema (1%)
Central nervous system: Headache (4%), malaise (4%), dizziness (3%), fever (2%)
Dermatologic: Rash (3%)
Endocrine & metabolic: Hyperglycemia (1%)
Gastrointestinal: Abdominal pain (5%), nausea (5%), diarrhea (3%), vomiting (2%), flatulence (1%)
Genitourinary: Nocturia (7%), burning symptoms (5%), urinary retention (4%), urethral pain (3%), pelvic pain (1%), hematuria (microscopic) (3%)
Hematologic: Anemia (2%)
Neuromuscular & skeletal: Weakness (4%), back pain (3%), myalgia (1%)
Respiratory: Pneumonia (1%)
<1% (Limited to important or life-threatening): Hematologic toxicity (following instillation into perforated bladder), nonprotein nitrogen increased, pruritus, skin irritation (local), taste loss, tenesmus, urine flow decreased, urethritis

Drug Interactions

Metabolism/Transport Effects None known.

Avoid Concomitant Use There are no known interactions where it is recommended to avoid concomitant use.

Increased Effect/Toxicity There are no known significant interactions involving an increase in effect.

Decreased Effect There are no known significant interactions involving a decrease in effect.

Preparation for Administration Hazardous agent; use appropriate precautions for handling and disposal (NIOSH, 2012). Allow vials to slowly warm to room temperature (without heating) prior to use. A waxy precipitate (due to polyoxyl castor oil) may form at temperatures <4°C, warm vial in the hand until solution is clear (do not use vial if particulate still present). Dilute 800 mg (20 mL) with 55 mL NS (total volume of 75 mL). Use non-PVC containers (glass, polyolefin, or polypropylene) and administration sets to avoid leaching of DEHP plasticizers. Stable for 12 hours at room temperature when diluted in 0.9% sodium chloride. Do not mix with other drugs.

Storage/Stability Store unopened vials refrigerated at 2°C to 8°C (36°F to 48°F). Stable for 12 hours at room temperature when diluted in 0.9% sodium chloride.

Mechanism of Action Blocks function of DNA topoisomerase II; inhibits DNA synthesis, causes extensive chromosomal damage, and arrests cell development (G_2 phase); unlike other anthracyclines, does not appear to intercalate DNA; readily penetrates cells.

Pharmacodynamics/Kinetics

Absorption: Intravesical: Penetrates into bladder wall; negligible systemic absorption (dependent on bladder wall condition; trauma to mucosa may increase absorption, bladder wall perforation may significantly increase absorption and systemic myelotoxicity).

Metabolism: Negligible after intravesical instillation and 2-hour retention

Excretion: Urine (post 2-hour retention): 98.6% as intact drug; 0.4% as *N*-trifluoroacetyladriamycin)

Dosage Adults: Intravesical: Bladder cancer: 800 mg once weekly (retain for 2 hours) for 6 weeks

Dosage adjustment for toxicity: In clinical trials (Steinberg, 2000), treatment was delayed for 1 week for the following adverse events: Grade 3 dysuria (not controlled with phenazopyridine), frequency/urgency lasting >24 hours, grade 2 gross hematuria (without clots) lasting >48 hours, grade 3 hematuria (with clots) lasting >48 hours. For local toxicities <grade 4 (eg, dysuria [not controlled with phenazopyridine] or severe bladder spasm), anticholinergic therapy (systemic or topical) or topical anesthesia was administered prior to subsequent instillations.

Dosage adjustment in renal impairment: No dosage adjustment provided in manufacturer's labeling. However, dosage adjustment unlikely due to low systemic absorption.

Dosage adjustment in hepatic impairment: No dosage adjustment provided in manufacturer's labeling. However, dosage adjustment unlikely due to low systemic absorption.

Administration Intravesicular bladder instillation: Insert urinary catheter, empty bladder prior to instillation, slowly by gravity flow, instill 800 mg/75 mL (in 0.9% sodium chloride injection), remove catheter. Retain in the bladder for 2 hours, then void. Administer through non-PVC tubing due to the polyoxyl castor oil (Cremophor® EL) diluent. Maintain adequate hydration following treatment. Use appropriate protective gown, goggles, and gloves during administration.

Hazardous agent; use appropriate precautions for handling and disposal (NIOSH, 2012).

Monitoring Parameters Cystoscopy, biopsy, and urine cytology every 3 months for recurrence or progression

Dosage Forms Excipient information presented when available (limited, particularly for generics); consult specific product labeling.

Solution, Intravesical [preservative free]:
Valstar: 40 mg/mL (5 mL) [contains alcohol, usp, cremophor el]

Valsartan (val SAR tan)

Brand Names: U.S. Diovan

Brand Names: Canada Apo-Valsartan; Ava-Valsartan; CO Valsartan; Diovan; Mylan-Valsartan; PMS-Valsartan; Ran-Valsartan; Sandoz-Valsartan; Teva-Valsartan

Pharmacologic Category Angiotensin II Receptor Blocker; Antihypertensive

Additional Appendix Information

Angiotensin Agents *on page* 2280

Use Alone or in combination with other antihypertensive agents in the treatment of primary hypertension; reduction of cardiovascular mortality in patients with left ventricular dysfunction postmyocardial infarction; treatment of heart failure (NYHA Class II-IV)

Pregnancy Risk Factor D

Pregnancy Considerations [U.S. Boxed Warning]: Drugs that act on the renin-angiotensin system can cause injury and death to the developing fetus. Discontinue as soon as possible once pregnancy is detected. The use of drugs which act on the renin-angiotensin system are associated with oligohydramnios. Oligohydramnios, due to decreased fetal renal function, may lead to fetal lung hypoplasia and skeletal malformations. Use is also associated with anuria, hypotension, renal failure, skull hypoplasia, and death in the fetus/neonate. The exposed fetus should be monitored for fetal growth, amniotic fluid volume, and organ formation. Infants exposed *in utero* should be monitored for hyperkalemia, hypotension, and oliguria.

Untreated chronic maternal hypertension is also associated with adverse events in the fetus, infant, and mother. If treatment for hypertension during pregnancy is needed, other agents are preferred (ACOG, 2012; Chobanian, 2003). In women of reproductive potential, angiotensin II receptor blockers should be discontinued prior to conception or as soon as pregnancy is confirmed (Chobanian, 2003). The Canadian labeling contraindicates use in pregnancy.

Breast-Feeding Considerations It is not known if valsartan is found in breast milk. Due to the potential for serious adverse reactions in the nursing infant, the manufacturer recommends a decision be made whether to discontinue nursing or to discontinue the drug, taking into account the importance of treatment to the mother. The Canadian labeling contraindicates use in nursing women. Breast-fed infants of mothers taking medications for hypertension should be monitored for adverse effects (Chobanian, 2003).

Contraindications Hypersensitivity to valsartan or any component of the formulation; concomitant use with aliskiren in patients with diabetes mellitus

Canadian labeling: Additional contraindications (not in U.S. labeling): Concomitant use with aliskiren in patients with moderate-to-severe renal impairment (GFR <60 mL/minute/1.73m^2); pregnancy; breast-feeding

Warnings/Precautions [U.S. Boxed Warning]: Drugs that act on the renin-angiotensin system can cause injury and death to the developing fetus. Discontinue as soon as possible once pregnancy is detected. May cause hyperkalemia; avoid potassium supplementation unless specifically required by healthcare provider. During the initiation of therapy, hypotension may occur, particularly in patients with heart failure or post-MI patients. Use extreme caution with concurrent administration of potassium-sparing diuretics or potassium supplements, in patients with mild-to-moderate hepatic dysfunction (adjust dose), in those who may be sodium/water depleted (eg, on high-dose diuretics), and in the elderly; correct depletion first.

Use caution with unstented unilateral/bilateral renal artery stenosis. When unstented bilateral renal artery stenosis is present, use is generally avoided due to the elevated risk of deterioration in renal function unless possible benefits outweigh risks. Use with caution with pre-existing renal insufficiency; significant aortic/mitral stenosis. May be associated with deterioration of renal function and/or increases in serum creatinine, particularly in patients with low renal blood flow (eg, renal artery stenosis, heart failure) whose glomerular filtration rate (GFR) is dependent on efferent arteriolar vasoconstriction by angiotensin II. Use caution in patients with severe renal impairment or significant hepatic dysfunction. Monitor renal function closely in patients with severe heart failure; changes in renal function should be anticipated and dosage adjustments of valsartan or concomitant medications may be needed. Concomitant use of an angiotensin-converting enzyme (ACE) inhibitor or renin inhibitor (eg, aliskiren) is associated with an increased risk of hypotension, hyperkalemia, and renal dysfunction; concomitant use with aliskiren should be avoided in patients with GFR <60 mL/minute and is contraindicated in patients with diabetes mellitus (regardless of GFR). The Canadian labeling contraindicates concomitant use of aliskiren in both of these patient populations. In Canada, use is not approved in patients <18 years of age.

Angioedema has been reported rarely with some angiotensin II receptor antagonists (ARBs) and may occur at any time during treatment (especially following first dose). It may involve the head and neck (potentially compromising airway) or the intestine (presenting with abdominal pain). Patients with idiopathic or hereditary angioedema or previous angioedema associated with ACE-inhibitor therapy may be at an increased risk. Prolonged frequent monitoring may be required, especially if tongue, glottis, or larynx are involved, as they are associated with airway obstruction. Patients with a history of airway surgery may have a higher risk of airway obstruction. Discontinue therapy immediately if angioedema occurs. Aggressive early management is critical. Intramuscular (I.M.) administration of epinephrine may be necessary. Do not readminister to patients who have had angioedema with ARBs.

Adverse Reactions

>10%:

Central nervous system: Dizziness (heart failure trials 17%)

Renal: BUN increased >50% (heart failure trials 17%)

1% to 10%:

Cardiovascular: Hypotension (heart failure trials 7%; MI trial 1%), orthostatic hypotension (heart failure trials 2%), syncope (up to >1%)

Central nervous system: Dizziness (hypertension trial 2% to 8%), fatigue (heart failure trials 3%; hypertension trial 2%), postural dizziness (heart failure trials 2%), headache (heart failure trials >1%), vertigo (up to >1%)

Endocrine & metabolic: Serum potassium increased by >20% (4% to 10%), hyperkalemia (heart failure trials 2%)

Gastrointestinal: Diarrhea (heart failure trials 5%), abdominal pain (2%), nausea (heart failure trials >1%), upper abdominal pain (heart failure trials >1%)

Hematologic: Neutropenia (2%)

Neuromuscular & skeletal: Arthralgia (heart failure trials 3%), back pain (up to 3%)

Ocular: Blurred vision (heart failure trials >1%)

Renal: Creatinine doubled (MI trial 4%), creatinine increased >50% (heart failure trials 4%), renal dysfunction (up to >1%)

Respiratory: Cough (1% to 3%)

Miscellaneous: Viral infection (3%)

All indications: <1% (Limited to important or life-threatening): Allergic reactions, alopecia, anaphylaxis, anemia, angioedema, anorexia, anxiety, chest pain, constipation, dyspepsia, dyspnea, flatulence, hematocrit/hemoglobin decreased, hepatitis (rare), impotence, insomnia, liver function tests increased, microcytic anemia, muscle cramps, myalgia, palpitation, paresthesia, photosensitivity, pruritus, rash, renal failure, rhabdomyolysis, somnolence, taste disorder, thrombocytopenia (very rare), vasculitis, vomiting, weakness, xerostomia

Drug Interactions

Metabolism/Transport Effects Substrate of SLCO1B1; **Inhibits** CYP2C9 (weak)

Avoid Concomitant Use There are no known interactions where it is recommended to avoid concomitant use.

Increased Effect/Toxicity

Valsartan may increase the levels/effects of: ACE Inhibitors; Amifostine; Antihypertensives; CycloSPORINE (Systemic); Hydrochlorothiazide; Hypotensive Agents; Lithium; Nonsteroidal Anti-Inflammatory Agents; Obinutuzumab; Potassium-Sparing Diuretics; RiTUXimab; Sodium Phosphates

The levels/effects of Valsartan may be increased by: Alfuzosin; Aliskiren; Brimonidine (Topical); Canagliflozin; Diazoxide; Eltrombopag; Eplerenone; Heparin; Heparin (Low Molecular Weight); Herbs (Hypotensive Properties); Hydrochlorothiazide; MAO Inhibitors; Pentoxifylline; Phosphodiesterase 5 Inhibitors; Potassium Salts; Prostacyclin Analogues; Tolvaptan; Trimethoprim

Decreased Effect

The levels/effects of Valsartan may be decreased by: Herbs (Hypertensive Properties); Methylphenidate; Nonsteroidal Anti-Inflammatory Agents; Yohimbine

Ethanol/Nutrition/Herb Interactions

Food: Decreases the peak plasma concentration and extent of absorption by 50% and 40%, respectively. Potassium supplements and/or potassium-containing salts may cause or worsen hyperkalemia. Management: Take consistently with regard to food. Consult prescriber before consuming a potassium-rich diet, potassium supplements, or salt substitutes.

Herb/Nutraceutical: Some herbal medications may worsen hypertension (eg, licorice); others may increase the antihypertensive effect of valsartan (eg, shepherd's purse).

Management: Avoid bayberry, blue cohosh, cayenne, ephedra, ginger, ginseng (American), kola, licorice, and yohimbe. Avoid black cohosh, California poppy, coleus, golden seal, hawthorn, mistletoe, periwinkle, quinine, and shepherd's purse.

Storage/Stability Store at 25°C (77°F); excursions permitted to 15°C to 30°C (59°F to 86°F). Protect from moisture.

Mechanism of Action Valsartan produces direct antagonism of the angiotensin II (AT2) receptors, unlike the ACE inhibitors. It displaces angiotensin II from the AT1 receptor and produces its blood pressure-lowering effects by antagonizing AT1-induced vasoconstriction, aldosterone release, catecholamine release, arginine vasopressin release, water intake, and hypertrophic responses. This action results in more efficient blockade of the cardiovascular effects of angiotensin II and fewer side effects than the ACE inhibitors.

Pharmacodynamics/Kinetics

Onset of action: ~2 hours

Duration: 24 hours

Distribution: V_d: 17 L (adults)

Protein binding: 95%, primarily albumin

Metabolism: To inactive metabolite

Bioavailability: Tablet: 25% (range: 10% to 35%); suspension: ~40% (~1.6 times more than tablet)

Half-life elimination: ~6 hours

Time to peak, serum: 2-4 hours

Excretion: Feces (83%) and urine (13%) as unchanged drug

Dosage Oral:

Hypertension:

Children 6-16 years: Initial: 1.3 mg/kg once daily (maximum: 40 mg/day); dose may be increased to achieve desired effect; doses >2.7 mg/kg (maximum: 160 mg) have not been studied.

Adults: Initial: 80 mg or 160 mg once daily (in patients who are not volume depleted); dose may be increased to achieve desired effect; maximum recommended dose: 320 mg daily

Heart failure: Adults: Initial: 40 mg twice daily; titrate dose to 80-160 mg twice daily, as tolerated; maximum daily dose: 320 mg

Left ventricular dysfunction after MI: Adults: Initial: 20 mg twice daily; titrate dose to target of 160 mg twice daily as tolerated; may initiate ≥12 hours following MI

Dosing adjustment in renal impairment:

Cl_{cr} ≥30 mL/minute: No dosage adjustment necessary.

Cl_{cr} <30 mL/minute: No dosage adjustment provided in manufacturer's labeling; safety and efficacy have not been established.

Dialysis: Not significantly removed

Dosing adjustment in hepatic impairment:

Mild-to-moderate impairment: No dosage adjustment necessary; use caution in patients with liver disease. Patients with mild-to-moderate chronic disease have twice the exposure as healthy volunteers.

Severe impairment: No dosage adjustment provided in manufacturer's labeling; has not been studied

Dietary Considerations Avoid salt substitutes which contain potassium. May be taken with or without food.

Administration Administer with or without food.

Monitoring Parameters Baseline and periodic electrolyte panels, renal function, BP; in HF, serum potassium during dose escalation and periodically thereafter

Additional Information Valsartan may have an advantage over losartan due to minimal metabolism requirements and consequent use in mild-to-moderate hepatic impairment.

Dosage Forms Excipient information presented when available (limited, particularly for generics); consult specific product labeling.

Tablet, Oral:

Diovan: 40 mg [scored]

Diovan: 80 mg, 160 mg, 320 mg

Extemporaneous Preparations A 4 mg/mL oral suspension may be made from tablets, Ora-Plus®, and Ora-Sweet® SF. Add 80 mL of Ora-Plus® to an 8-ounce amber glass bottle containing eight valsartan 80 mg tablets. Shake well for ≥2 minutes. Allow the suspension to stand for a minimum of 1 hour, then shake for ≥1 minute. Add 80 mL of Ora-Sweet SF® to the bottle and shake for ≥10 seconds. Store in amber glass prescription bottles; label "shake well". Stable for 30 days at room temperature or 75 days refrigerated.

Diovan® prescribing information, Novartis Pharmaceuticals Corp, East Hanover, NJ, 2012.

◆ **Valsartan and Amlodipine** *see* Amlodipine and Valsartan *on page 112*

Valsartan and Hydrochlorothiazide

(val SAR tan & hye droe klor oh THYE a zide)

Brand Names: U.S. Diovan HCT

Brand Names: Canada Apo-Valsartan/HCTZ; Ava-Valsartan/HCT; Diovan HCT; Mylan-Valsartan HCTZ; Sandoz Valsartan HCT; Teva-Valsartan HCTZ; Valsartan-HCT; Valsartan-HCTZ

Index Terms Hydrochlorothiazide and Valsartan

Pharmacologic Category Angiotensin II Receptor Blocker; Antihypertensive; Diuretic, Thiazide

Use

U.S. labeling: Treatment of hypertension (initial, add-on, or as substitute for titrated components)

Canadian labeling: Treatment of mild-to-moderate hypertension where combination therapy is appropriate. Not indicated for initial treatment.

Pregnancy Risk Factor D

Dosage

Hypertension: Adults: Oral:

U.S. labeling: Dose is individualized; combination product may be used as initial therapy or substituted for individual components in patients currently maintained on both agents separately or in patients not adequately controlled with monotherapy (using one of the agents or an agent within same antihypertensive class).

Initial therapy: Valsartan 160 mg and hydrochlorothiazide 12.5 mg once daily; dose may be titrated after 1-2 weeks of therapy. Maximum recommended daily doses: Valsartan 320 mg; hydrochlorothiazide 25 mg.

Add-on/replacement therapy: Valsartan 80-320 mg and hydrochlorothiazide 12.5-25 mg once daily; dose may be titrated after 3-4 weeks of therapy. Maximum recommended daily dose: Valsartan 320 mg; hydrochlorothiazide 25 mg.

Canadian labeling: Dose is individualized; combination product may be used as substitute for individual components following successful titration of each component. Maximum recommended daily dose: Valsartan 320 mg; hydrochlorothiazide 25 mg. Not approved for initial therapy.

Dosage adjustment in renal impairment:

Cl_{cr} ≥30 mL/minute: No dosage adjustment necessary.

Cl_{cr} <30 mL/minute: No dosage adjustment provided in manufacturer's labeling (has not been studied). Use is contraindicated in patients with anuria (U.S. and Canadian labeling) and not recommended in severe impairment (Canadian labeling).

Dosage adjustment in hepatic impairment:

Mild-to-moderate impairment: No dosage adjustment necessary; use with caution. Patients with mild-to-moderate chronic disease have twice the exposure of valsartan as healthy volunteers.

Severe impairment: No dosage adjustment provided in manufacturer's labeling (has not been studied). The Canadian labeling does not recommend use in severe impairment.

Additional Information Complete prescribing information should be consulted for additional detail.

Dosage Forms Excipient information presented when available (limited, particularly for generics); consult specific product labeling.

Tablet, oral: 80 mg/12.5 mg: Valsartan 80 mg and hydrochlorothiazide 12.5 mg; 160 mg/12.5 mg: Valsartan 160 mg and hydrochlorothiazide 12.5 mg; 160 mg/25 mg: Valsartan 160 mg and hydrochlorothiazide 25 mg; 320 mg/12.5 mg: Valsartan 320 mg and hydrochlorothiazide 12.5 mg; 320 mg/25 mg: Valsartan 320 mg and hydrochlorothiazide 25 mg

Diovan HCT® 80 mg/12.5 mg: Valsartan 80 mg and hydrochlorothiazide 12.5 mg

Diovan HCT® 160 mg/12.5 mg: Valsartan 160 mg and hydrochlorothiazide 12.5 mg

Diovan HCT® 160 mg/25 mg: Valsartan 160 mg and hydrochlorothiazide 25 mg

Diovan HCT® 320 mg/12.5 mg: Valsartan 320 mg and hydrochlorothiazide 12.5 mg

Diovan HCT® 320 mg/25 mg: Valsartan 320 mg and hydrochlorothiazide 25 mg

◆ **Valsartan-HCT (Can)** *see* Valsartan and Hydrochlorothiazide *on page 2156*

◆ **Valsartan-HCTZ (Can)** *see* Valsartan and Hydrochlorothiazide *on page 2156*

◆ **Valsartan, Hydrochlorothiazide, and Amlodipine** *see* Amlodipine, Valsartan, and Hydrochlorothiazide *on page 113*

◆ **Valstar** *see* Valrubicin *on page 2153*

◆ **Valtaxin® (Can)** *see* Valrubicin *on page 2153*

◆ **Valtrex** *see* ValACYclovir *on page 2145*

◆ **Valtrex® (Can)** *see* ValACYclovir *on page 2145*

◆ **Val-Vancomycin (Can)** *see* Vancomycin *on page 2157*

◆ **Vanceril** *see* Beclomethasone (Systemic) *on page 227*

◆ **Vancocin (Can)** *see* Vancomycin *on page 2157*

◆ **Vancocin HCl** *see* Vancomycin *on page 2157*

Vancomycin (van koe MYE sin)

Brand Names: U.S. Vancocin HCl

Brand Names: Canada PMS-Vancomycin; Sterile Vancomycin Hydrochloride, USP; Val-Vancomycin; Vancocin; Vancomycin Hydrochloride for Injection; Vancomycin Hydrochloride for Injection, USP

Index Terms Vancomycin Hydrochloride

Pharmacologic Category Glycopeptide

Additional Appendix Information

Antibiotic Treatment of Adults With Infective Endocarditis *on page 2355*

Desensitization Protocols *on page 2325*

Dosing Considerations for the Critically-Ill Patient With Morbid Obesity *on page 2379*

Prevention of Infective Endocarditis *on page 2353*

Use

I.V.: Treatment of patients with infections caused by staphylococcal species and streptococcal species

Oral: Treatment of *C. difficile*-associated diarrhea and treatment of enterocolitis caused by *Staphylococcus aureus* (including methicillin-resistant strains)

Unlabeled Use Bacterial endophthalmitis; treatment of infections caused by gram-positive organisms in patients who have serious allergies to beta-lactam agents; treatment of beta-lactam resistant gram-positive infections; surgical (perioperative) prophylaxis; treatment of prosthetic joint infection; group B streptococcus maternal use for neonatal prophylaxis; rectal administration for treatment of *Clostridium difficile* infection

Pregnancy Risk Factor B (oral); C (injection)

Pregnancy Considerations Adverse events have not been observed in animal reproduction studies. Vancomycin crosses the placenta and can be detected in fetal serum, amniotic fluid, and cord blood (Bourget, 1991; Reyes, 1989). Adverse fetal effects, including sensorineural hearing loss or nephrotoxicity, have not been reported following maternal use during the second or third trimesters of pregnancy.

The pharmacokinetics of vancomycin may be altered during pregnancy and pregnant patients may need a higher dose of vancomycin. Maternal half-life is unchanged, but the volume of distribution and the total plasma clearance may be increased (Bourget, 1991). Individualization of therapy through serum concentration monitoring may be warranted. Vancomycin is recommended for the treatment of mild, moderate, or severe *Clostridium difficile* infections in pregnant women (Surawicz, 2013). Vancomycin is recommended as an alternative agent to prevent the transmission of group B streptococcal (GBS) disease from mothers to newborns (ACOG, 2011; CDC, 2010).

Breast-Feeding Considerations Vancomycin is excreted in human milk following I.V. administration. If given orally to the mother, the minimal systemic absorption of the dose would limit the amount available to pass into the milk. Vancomycin is recommended for the treatment of mild, moderate, or severe *Clostridium difficile* infections in breast-feeding women (Surawicz, 2013). Due to the potential for serious adverse reactions in the nursing infant, the manufacturer recommends a decision be made whether to discontinue nursing or to discontinue the drug, taking into account the importance of treatment to the mother. Nondose-related effects could include modification of bowel flora.

Contraindications Hypersensitivity to vancomycin or any component of the formulation

Warnings/Precautions May cause nephrotoxicity although limited data suggest direct causal relationship; usual risk factors include pre-existing renal impairment, concomitant nephrotoxic medications, advanced age, and dehydration (nephrotoxicity has also been reported following treatment with oral vancomycin, typically in patients >65 years of age). If multiple sequential (≥2) serum creatinine concentrations demonstrate an increase of 0.5 mg/dL or ≥50% increase from baseline (whichever is greater) in the absence of an alternative explanation, the patient should be identified as having vancomycin-induced nephrotoxicity (Rybak, 2009). Discontinue treatment if signs of nephrotoxicity occur; renal damage is usually reversible.

May cause neurotoxicity; usual risk factors include preexisting renal impairment, concomitant neuro-/nephrotoxic medications, advanced age, and dehydration. Ototoxicity, although rarely associated with monotherapy, is proportional to the amount of drug given and the duration of treatment. Tinnitus or vertigo may be indications of vestibular injury and impending bilateral irreversible damage. Discontinue treatment if signs of ototoxicity occur. Prolonged therapy (>1 week) or total doses exceeding 25 g may increase the risk of neutropenia; prompt reversal of neutropenia is expected after discontinuation of therapy. Prolonged use may result in fungal or bacterial superinfection, including *C. difficile*-associated diarrhea (CDAD) and pseudomembranous colitis; CDAD has been observed >2 months postantibiotic treatment. Use with caution in patients with renal impairment or those receiving other nephrotoxic or ototoxic drugs; dosage modification required in patients with impaired renal function (especially elderly). Accumulation may occur after multiple oral doses of vancomycin in patients with renal impairment; consider monitoring trough concentrations in this circumstance.

Rapid I.V. administration may result in hypotension, flushing, erythema, urticaria, and/or pruritus. Oral vancomycin is only indicated for the treatment of pseudomembranous colitis due to *C. difficile* and enterocolitis due to *S. aureus* and is not effective for systemic infections; parenteral vancomycin is not effective for the treatment of colitis due to *C. difficile* and enterocolitis due to *S. aureus*. Clinically significant serum concentrations have been reported in patients with inflammatory disorders of the intestinal mucosa who have taken oral vancomycin (multiple doses) for the treatment of *C. difficile*-associated diarrhea. Although use may be warranted, the risk for adverse reactions may be higher in this situation; consider monitoring serum trough concentrations, especially with renal insufficiency, severe colitis, concurrent rectal vancomycin administration, and/or concomitant I.V. aminoglycosides. The IDSA suggests that it is appropriate to obtain trough concentrations when a patient is receiving long courses of ≥2 g/day (Cohen, 2010). **Note:** The Infectious Disease Society of America (IDSA) and American College of Gastroenterology (ACG) recommend the use of oral metronidazole for initial treatment of mild-to-moderate *C. difficile* infection and the use of oral vancomycin for initial treatment of severe *C. difficile* infection (Cohen, 2010; Surawicz, 2013).

Adverse Reactions

Injection:

>10%:

- Cardiovascular: Hypotension accompanied by flushing
- Dermatologic: Erythematous rash on face and upper body (red neck or red man syndrome)

1% to 10%:

- Central nervous system: Chills, drug fever
- Hematologic: Eosinophilia, reversible neutropenia
- Local: Phlebitis

<1% (Limited to important or life-threatening): Drug rash with eosinophilia and systemic symptoms (DRESS), ototoxicity (rare; use of other ototoxic agents may increase risk), renal failure (limited data suggesting direct relationship), Stevens-Johnson syndrome, thrombocytopenia, vasculitis

Oral:

>10%: Gastrointestinal: Abdominal pain, bad taste (with oral solution), nausea

1% to 10%:

- Cardiovascular: Peripheral edema
- Central nervous system: Fatigue, fever, headache
- Gastrointestinal: Diarrhea, flatulence, vomiting
- Genitourinary: Urinary tract infection
- Neuromuscular & skeletal: Back pain

<1% (Limited to important or life-threatening): Creatinine increased, interstitial nephritis, ototoxicity, renal failure, renal impairment, thrombocytopenia, vasculitis

Drug Interactions

Metabolism/Transport Effects None known.

Avoid Concomitant Use

Avoid concomitant use of Vancomycin with any of the following: BCG; Gallium Nitrate

Increased Effect/Toxicity

Vancomycin may increase the levels/effects of: Aminoglycosides; Colistimethate; Gallium Nitrate; Neuromuscular-Blocking Agents

The levels/effects of Vancomycin may be increased by: Nonsteroidal Anti-Inflammatory Agents

Decreased Effect

Vancomycin may decrease the levels/effects of: BCG; Sodium Picosulfate; Typhoid Vaccine

The levels/effects of Vancomycin may be decreased by: Bile Acid Sequestrants

Preparation for Administration Injection: Reconstitute vials with 20 mL of SWFI for each 1 g of vancomycin (10 mL/500 mg vial; 20 mL/1 g vial; 100 mL/5 g vial; 200 mL/10 g vial). The reconstituted solution must be further diluted with at least 100 mL of a compatible diluent per 500 mg of vancomycin prior to parenteral administration.

Intrathecal (unlabeled route): Vancomycin is available as a powder for injection and may be diluted to 1-5 mg/mL concentration in preservative free 0.9% sodium chloride for administration into the CSF.

Storage/Stability

Capsules: Store at controlled room temperature of 15°C to 30°C (59°F to 86°F).

Injection: Reconstituted 500 mg and 1 g vials are stable for at either room temperature or under refrigeration for 14 days. **Note:** Vials contain no bacteriostatic agent. Solutions diluted for administration in either D_5W or NS are stable under refrigeration for 14 days or at room temperature for 7 days.

Mechanism of Action Inhibits bacterial cell wall synthesis by blocking glycopeptide polymerization through binding tightly to D-alanyl-D-alanine portion of cell wall precursor

Pharmacodynamics/Kinetics

Absorption: Oral: Poor; may be enhanced with bowel inflammation; I.M.: Erratic; Intraperitoneal: ~38%

Distribution: V_d: 0.4-1 L/kg; Distributes widely in body tissue and fluids, except for CSF

- Relative diffusion from blood into CSF: Good only with inflammation (exceeds usual MICs)
  - Uninflamed meninges: 0-4 mcg/mL; serum concentration dependent
  - Inflamed meninges: 6-11 mcg/mL; serum concentration dependent
- CSF:blood level ratio: Normal meninges: Nil; Inflamed meninges: 20% to 30%

Protein binding: ~50%

Half-life elimination: Biphasic: Terminal:

- Newborns: 6-10 hours
- Infants and Children 3 months to 4 years: 4 hours
- Children >3 years: 2.2-3 hours
- Adults: 5-11 hours; significantly prolonged with renal impairment
- End-stage renal disease: 200-250 hours

Time to peak, serum: I.V.: Immediately after completion of infusion

Excretion: I.V.: Urine (80% to 90% as unchanged drug); Oral: Primarily feces

Dosage

Usual dosage range:

Infants >1 month and Children: I.V.: 10-15 mg/kg every 6 hours

Adults: Initial intravenous dosing should be based on actual body weight; subsequent dosing adjusted based on serum trough vancomycin concentrations.

- I.V.: 2000-3000 mg/day (or 30-60 mg/kg/day) in divided doses every 8-12 hours (Rybak, 2009); **Note:** Dose requires adjustment in renal impairment
- Oral: 500-2000 mg daily in divided doses every 6 hours

Indication-specific dosing:

Catheter-related infections: Adults: Antibiotic lock technique (Mermel, 2009): 2 mg/mL ± 10 units heparin/mL **or** 2.5 mg/mL ± 2500 **or** 5000 units heparin/mL **or** 5 mg/mL ± 5000 units heparin/mL (preferred regimen); instill into catheter port with a volume sufficient to fill the catheter (2-5 mL). **Note:** May use SWFI/NS or D_5W as diluents. Do not mix with any other solutions. Dwell times generally should not exceed 48 hours before renewal of lock solution. Remove lock solution prior to catheter use, then replace.

***C. difficile*-associated diarrhea (CDAD):**

Infants >1 month and Children: Oral: 40 mg/kg/day in 3-4 divided doses for 7-10 days (maximum: 2000 mg daily)

Adults:

Oral:

Manufacturer recommendations: 125 mg 4 times daily for 10 days

Mild to moderate disease unresponsive to metronidazole: 125 mg 4 times daily for 10 days (Surawica, 2013)

Severe disease (defined as serum albumin <3 g/dL and either WBC ≥15,000 or abdominal tenderness): 125 mg times daily for 10 days (Surawica, 2013)

Severe, complicated infection: 500 mg every 6 hours for 10-14 days with or without concurrent I.V. metronidazole. May consider vancomycin retention enema (in patients with complete ileus) (Cohen, 2010)

Severe and complicated disease, without abdominal distention: 125 mg 4 times daily with I.V. metronidazole (Surawica, 2013)

Severe and complicated disease with significant abdominal distention, ileus, and/or toxic colon: 500 mg 4 times daily plus rectal vancomycin in combination with I.V. metronidazole (Surawica, 2013)

Recurrent, severe infection (if initial regimen did not include vancomycin): 125 mg 4 times daily for 10 days

Rectal (unlabeled route): Retention enema:

Severe, complicated infection in patients with ileus: 500 mg every 6 hours (in 100 mL 0.9% sodium chloride) with oral vancomycin with or without concurrent I.V. metronidazole (Cohen, 2010)

Severe and complicated disease with abdominal distention, ileus, and/or toxic colon: 500 mg 4 times daily (in 500 mL NS) in combination with oral vancomycin and I.V. metronidazole (Surawicz, 2013)

Complicated infections in seriously-ill patients: Adults: I.V.: Loading dose: 25-30 mg/kg (based on actual body weight) may be used to rapidly achieve target concentration; then 15-20 mg/kg/dose every 8-12 hours (Rybak, 2009)

Enterocolitis *(S. aureus)*:

Infants >1 months and Children: Oral: 40 mg/kg/day in 3-4 divided doses for 7-10 days (maximum: 2000 mg/day)

Adults: Oral: 500-2000 mg/day in 3-4 divided doses for 7-10 days (usual dose: 125-500 mg every 6 hours)

Group B streptococcus (neonatal prophylaxis): Adults: I.V.: 1000 mg every 12 hours until delivery. **Note:** reserved for penicillin allergic patients at high risk for anaphylaxis if organism is resistant to clindamycin or where no susceptibility data are available (CDC, 2010).

Meningitis:

Infants >1 month and Children:

I.V.: 15 mg/kg every 6 hours (Tunkel, 2004)

Intrathecal, intraventricular (unlabeled route): 5-20 mg/day (Tunkel, 2004)

Children: Alternate regimen: *S. aureus* (methicillin-resistant) (unlabeled use; Liu, 2011): I.V.: 15 mg/kg/dose every 6 hours for 2 weeks (some experts combine with rifampin)

Adults:

I.V.: 30-60 mg/kg/day in divided doses every 8-12 hours (Rybak, 2009) **or** 500-750 mg every 6 hours. **Note:** For PCN-resistant *Streptococcus pneumoniae* (MIC ≥2 mcg/mL), combine with a third-generation cephalosporin.

Alternate regimen: *S. aureus* (methicillin-resistant) (unlabeled use; Liu, 2011): 15-20 mg/kg/dose every 8-12 hours for 2 weeks (some experts combine with rifampin)

Intrathecal, intraventricular (unlabeled route): 5-20 mg/day

Pneumonia:

Community-acquired pneumonia (CAP):

Infants >3 months and Children (IDSA/PIDS, 2011): I.V.: **Note:** In children ≥5 years, a macrolide antibiotic should be added if atypical pneumonia cannot be ruled out.

Group A *Streptococcus* (alternative to ampicillin or penicillin in beta-lactam allergic patients): 40-60 mg/kg/day divided every 6-8 hours

Presumed bacterial (in addition to recommended antibiotic therapy), *S. pneumoniae*, moderate-to-severe infection (MICs to penicillin ≤2.0 mcg/mL) (alternative to ampicillin or penicillin): 40-60 mg/kg/day divided every 6-8 hours

S. aureus (methicillin-susceptible) (alternative to cefazolin/oxacillin): 40-60 mg/kg/day divided every 6-8 hours

S. aureus, moderate-to-severe infection (methicillin-resistant +/- clindamycin susceptible) (preferred): 40-60 mg/kg/day divided every 6-8 hours **or** dosing to achieve AUC/MIC >400

Alternate regimen: 60 mg/kg/day divided every 6 hours for 7-21 days, depending on severity (Liu, 2011)

S. pneumoniae, moderate-to-severe infection (MICs to penicillin ≥4.0 mcg/mL) (alternative to ceftriaxone in beta-lactam allergic patients): 40-60 mg/kg/day divided every 6-8 hours

Adults: *S. aureus* (methicillin-resistant): I.V.: 45-60 mg/kg/day divided every 8-12 hours (maximum: 2000 mg/dose) for 7-21 days depending on severity (Liu, 2011)

Healthcare-associated pneumonia (HAP): *S. aureus* (methicillin-resistant): I.V.:

Infants and Children: 60 mg/kg/day divided every 6 hours for 7-21 days depending on severity (Liu, 2011)

Adults: 45-60 mg/kg/day divided every 8-12 hours (maximum: 2000 mg/dose) for 7-21 days depending on severity (American Thoracic Society [ATS], 2005; Liu, 2011; Rybak 2009)

Prophylaxis against infective endocarditis: I.V.:

Children:

Dental, oral, or upper respiratory tract surgery: 20 mg/kg/dose administered 1 hour prior to the procedure. **Note:** American Heart Association (AHA) guidelines recommend prophylaxis only in patients undergoing invasive procedures and in whom underlying cardiac conditions may predispose to a higher risk of adverse outcomes should infection occur.

GI/GU procedure: 20 mg/kg (plus gentamicin 1.5 mg/kg) administered 1 hour prior to surgery. **Note:** Routine prophylaxis no longer recommended by the AHA.

Adults:

Dental, oral, or upper respiratory tract surgery: 1000 mg 1 hour before surgery. **Note:** AHA guidelines now recommend prophylaxis only in patients undergoing invasive procedures and in whom underlying cardiac conditions may predispose to a higher risk of adverse outcomes should infection occur.

GI/GU procedure: 1000 mg plus 1.5 mg/kg gentamicin 1 hour prior to surgery. **Note:** As of April 2007, routine prophylaxis no longer recommended by the AHA.

Susceptible gram-positive infections (MIC ≤1 mcg/mL; Rybak, 2009): I.V.:

Infants >1 month and Children: 10 mg/kg/dose every 6 hours (manufacturer recommendations) **or** 15 mg/kg/dose (maximum: 2000 mg/dose) every 6 hours (Liu, 2011)

Adults: 15-20 mg/kg/dose (usual: 750-1500 mg) every 8-12 hours

Note: If MIC ≥2 mcg/mL, alternative therapies are recommended.

Bacteremia (*S. aureus* [methicillin-resistant]) (unlabeled use; Liu, 2011): I.V.:

Children: 15 mg/kg/dose every 6 hours for 2-6 weeks depending on severity

Adults: 15-20 mg/kg/dose every 8-12 hours for 2-6 weeks depending on severity

Brain abscess, subdural empyema, spinal epidural abscess (*S. aureus* [methicillin-resistant]) (unlabeled use; Liu, 2011): I.V.:

Children: 15 mg/kg/dose every 6 hours for 4-6 weeks (some experts combine with rifampin)

Adults: 15-20 mg/kg/dose every 8-12 hours for 4-6 weeks (some experts combine with rifampin)

Endocarditis:

Native valve (*Enterococcus*, vancomycin MIC ≤4 mg/L) (unlabeled use; Gould, 2012): I.V.: Adults: 1000 mg every 12 hours for 4-6 weeks (combine with gentamicin for 4-6 weeks)

Native valve (*S. aureus* [methicillin-resistant]) (unlabeled use; Liu, 2011): I.V.:

Children: 15 mg/kg/dose every 6 hours for 6 weeks

Adults: 15-20 mg/kg/dose every 8-12 hours for 6 weeks (European guidelines support the entire duration of therapy to be 4 weeks and in combination with rifampin [Gould, 2012])

Native or prosthetic valve (streptococcal [penicillin MIC >0.5 mg/L or patient intolerant to penicillin]) (unlabeled use; Gould, 2012): I.V.: Adults: 1000 mg every 12 hours for 4-6 weeks (combine with gentamicin for at least the first 2 weeks); **Note:** The longer duration of treatment (ie, 6 weeks) should be used for patients with prosthetic valve endocarditis.

Prosthetic valve (*Enterococcus*, vancomycin MIC ≤4 mg/L) (unlabeled use; Gould, 2012): I.V.: Adults: 1000 mg every 12 hours for 6 weeks (combine with gentamicin for 4-6 weeks)

Prosthetic valve (*S. aureus* [methicillin-resistant]) (unlabeled use; Liu, 2011): I.V.:

Children: 15 mg/kg/dose every 6 hours for at least 6 weeks

Adults: 15-20 mg/kg/dose every 8-12 hours for at least 6 weeks (combine with rifampin for the entire duration of therapy and gentamicin for the first 2 weeks)

Endophthalmitis (unlabeled use): Adults: Intravitreal: Usual dose: 1 mg/0.1 mL NS instilled into vitreum; may repeat administration, if necessary, in 2-3 days, usually in combination with ceftazidime or an aminoglycoside (Kelsey, 1995). **Note:** Based on concerns for retinotoxicity, some clinicians have recommended using a lower dose of 0.2 mg/0.1mL; may repeat in 3-4 days, if necessary (Gan, 2001).

Osteomyelitis (*S. aureus* [methicillin-resistant]) (unlabeled use; Liu, 2011): I.V.:

Children: 15 mg/kg/dose every 6 hours for 4-6 weeks

Adults: 15-20 mg/kg/dose every 8-12 hours for a minimum of 8 weeks (some experts combine with rifampin)

Prosthetic joint infection (unlabeled use; Osman, 2013): I.V.: Adults:

Enterococcus spp (penicillin-susceptible or –resistant), *Propionibacterium acnes,* streptococci (beta-hemolytic): 15 mg/kg every 12 hours for 4-6 weeks, followed by an oral antibiotic suppressive regimen

Note: For penicillin-susceptible or -resistant *Enterococcus* spp, consider addition of an aminoglycoside; in penicillin-susceptible *Enterococcus*, beta-hemolytic streptococcus or *Propionibacterium acnes* infections, only use vancomycin if patient has penicillin allergy.

Staphylococci (oxacillin-susceptible or –resistant): 15 mg/kg every 12 hours for 2-6 weeks in combination with rifampin followed by oral antibiotic treatment and suppressive regimens

Septic arthritis (*S. aureus* [methicillin-resistant]) (unlabeled use; Liu, 2011): I.V.:

Children: 15 mg/kg/dose every 6 hours for minimum of 3-4 weeks

Adults: 15-20 mg/kg/dose every 8-12 hours for 3-4 weeks

Septic thrombosis of cavernous or dural venous sinus (*S. aureus* [methicillin-resistant]) (unlabeled use; Liu, 2011): I.V.:

Children: 15 mg/kg/dose every 6 hours for 4-6 weeks (some experts combine with rifampin)

Adults: 15-20 mg/kg/dose every 8-12 hours for 4-6 weeks (some experts combine with rifampin)

Skin and skin structure infections, complicated (*S. aureus* [methicillin-resistant]) (unlabeled use; Liu, 2011): I.V.:

Children: 15 mg/kg/dose every 6 hours for 7-14 days

Adults: 15-20 mg/kg/dose every 8-12 hours for 7-14 days

Surgical (perioperative) prophylaxis (unlabeled use): I.V.:

Children: 15 mg/kg/dose within 120 minutes prior to surgical incision. May be administered in combination with other antibiotics depending upon the surgical procedure (Bratzler, 2013).

Adults: 15 mg/kg within 120 minutes prior to surgical incision. May be administered in combination with other antibiotics depending upon the surgical procedure (Bratzler, 2013).

Note: For patients known to be colonized with methicillin-resistant *S. aureus*, a single 15 mg/kg preoperative dose may be added to other recommended agents for the specific procedure (Bratzler, 2013)

The Society of Thoracic Surgeons recommends 1000-1500 mg or 15 mg/kg over 60 minutes with completion within 1 hour of skin incision. Although not well established, a second dose of 7.5 mg/kg may be considered during cardiopulmonary bypass (Engelman, 2007).

Dosage adjustment in renal impairment:

Oral: No dosage adjustment provided in manufacturer's labeling, However, dosage adjustment unlikely due to low systemic absorption.

I.V.: Vancomycin levels should be monitored in patients with any renal impairment:

Cl_{cr} >50 mL/minute: Start with 15-20 mg/kg/dose (usual: 750-1500 mg) every 8-12 hours

Cl_{cr} 20-49 mL/minute: Start with 15-20 mg/kg/dose (usual: 750-1500 mg) every 24 hours

Cl_{cr} <20 mL/minute: Will need longer intervals; determine by serum concentration monitoring

Note: In the critically-ill patient with renal insufficiency, the initial loading dose (25-30 mg/kg) should not be reduced. However, subsequent dosage adjustments should be made based on renal function and trough serum concentrations.

Poorly dialyzable by intermittent hemodialysis (0% to 5%); however, use of high-flux membranes and continuous renal replacement therapy (CRRT) increases vancomycin clearance, and generally requires replacement dosing.

Intermittent hemodialysis (IHD) (administer after hemodialysis on dialysis days): Following loading dose of 15-25 mg/kg, give either 500-1000 mg **or** 5-10 mg/kg after each dialysis session. (Heintz, 2009). **Note:** Dosing dependent on the assumption of 3 times/week, complete IHD sessions.

Redosing based on pre-HD concentrations:

<10 mg/L: Administer 1000 mg after HD

10-25 mg/L: Administer 500-750 mg after HD

>25 mg/L: Hold vancomycin

Redosing based on post-HD concentrations: <10-15 mg/L: Administer 500-1000 mg

Peritoneal dialysis (PD):

Administration via PD fluid: 15-30 mg/L (15-30 mcg/mL) of PD fluid

Systemic: Loading dose of 1000 mg, followed by 500-1000 mg every 48-72 hours with close monitoring of levels

Continuous renal replacement therapy (CRRT) (Heintz, 2009; Trotman, 2005): Drug clearance is highly dependent on the method of renal replacement, filter type, and flow rate. Appropriate dosing requires close monitoring of pharmacologic response, signs of adverse reactions due to drug accumulation, as well as drug concentrations in relation to target trough (if appropriate). The following are general recommendations only (based on dialysate flow/ultrafiltration rates of 1-2 L/hour and minimal residual renal function) and should not supersede clinical judgment:

CVVH: Loading dose of 15-25 mg/kg, followed by either 1000 mg every 48 hours **or** 10-15 mg/kg every 24-48 hours

CVVHD: Loading dose of 15-25 mg/kg, followed by either 1000 mg every 24 hours **or** 10-15 mg/kg every 24 hours

CVVHDF: Loading dose of 15-25 mg/kg, followed by either 1000 mg every 24 hours **or** 7.5-10 mg/kg every 12 hours

Note: Consider redosing patients receiving CRRT for vancomycin concentrations <10-15 mg/L.

Dosage adjustment in hepatic impairment:

Oral: No dosage adjustment provided in the manufacturer's labeling. However, dosage adjustment unlikely due to low systemic absorption.

I.V.: No dosage adjustment provided in manufacturer's labeling. However, degrees of hepatic dysfunction do not affect the pharmacokinetics of vancomycin (Marti, 1996).

Dietary Considerations May be taken with food.

Administration

Intravenous: Administer vancomycin with a final concentration not to exceed 5 mg/mL by I.V. intermittent infusion over at least 60 minutes (recommended infusion period of ≥30 minutes for every 500 mg administered).

If a maculopapular rash appears on the face, neck, trunk, and/or upper extremities (red man syndrome), slow the infusion rate to over 1½ to 2 hours and increase the dilution volume. Hypotension, shock, and cardiac arrest (rare) have also been reported with too rapid of infusion. Reactions are often treated with antihistamines and steroids.

Intrathecal (unlabeled route): Vancomycin is available as a powder for injection and may be diluted to 1-5 mg/mL concentration in preservative free 0.9% sodium chloride for intrathecal administration.

Intravitreal: (unlabeled use): Administer vancomycin intravitreally with a final concentration of 1.0 mg/0.1 mL NS (Kelsey, 1995). **Note:** Due to retinotoxicity, some clinicians recommend using a lower dose of 0.2 mg/0.1 mL NS (Gan, 2001).

Oral: Vancomycin powder for injection may be reconstituted and used for oral administration (Cohen, 2010). Reconstituted powder for injection (not premixed solution) may be administered orally by diluting the reconstituted solution in 30 mL of water; common flavoring syrups may be added to improve taste. The unflavored, diluted solution may also be administered via nasogastric tube. Also see Extemporaneous Preparations section.

Rectal (unlabeled route): May be administered as a retention enema per rectum (Cohen, 2010); 500 mg in 100-500 mL of NS, volume may depend on length of segment being treated. If sodium chloride causes hyperchloremia could use solution with lower chloride concentration (eg, LR) (Surawicz, 2013).

Not for I.M. administration.

Extravasation treatment: Monitor I.V. site closely; extravasation will cause serious injury with possible necrosis and tissue sloughing. Rotate infusion site frequently.

Monitoring Parameters Intravenous: Periodic renal function tests, urinalysis, WBC; serum trough vancomycin concentrations in select patients (eg, aggressive dosing, unstable renal function, concurrent nephrotoxins, prolonged courses)

Suggested frequency of trough vancomycin concentration monitoring (Rybak, 2009):

Hemodynamically stable patients: Draw trough concentrations at least once-weekly.

Hemodynamically unstable patients: Draw trough concentrations more frequently or in some instances daily.

Prolonged courses (>3-5 days): Draw at least one steady-state trough concentration; repeat as clinically appropriate.

Note: Drawing >1 trough concentration prior to the fourth dose for short course (<3 days) or lower intensity dosing (target trough concentrations <15 mcg/mL) is not recommended.

Oral/rectal therapy: Serum sample monitoring is not typically required; consider monitoring serum trough concentrations, especially with renal insufficiency, severe colitis, concurrent rectal vancomycin administration, and/or concomitant I.V. aminoglycosides.

Reference Range

Timing of serum samples: Draw trough just before the administration of a dose at steady-state conditions. Steady state conditions generally occur approximately after the fourth dose. Drawing peak concentrations is no longer recommended.

Therapeutic levels: Trough: ≥10 mcg/mL. For pathogens with an MIC ≤1 mcg/mL, the minimum trough concentration should be 15 mcg/mL to meet target AUC/MIC of ≥400 (see **"Note"** below). For complicated infections (eg, bacteremia, endocarditis, osteomyelitis, meningitis, and hospital-acquired pneumonia caused by *S. aureus*), trough concentrations of 15-20 mcg/mL are recommended to improve penetration and improve clinical outcomes (Liu, 2011; Rybak, 2009). The American Thoracic Society (ATS) guidelines for hospital-acquired pneumonia and the Infectious Disease Society of America (IDSA) meningitis guidelines also recommend trough concentrations of 15-20 mcg/mL.

Note: Although AUC/MIC is the preferred pharmacokinetic-pharmacodynamic parameter used to determine clinical effectiveness, trough serum concentrations may be used as a surrogate marker for AUC and are recommended as the most accurate and practical method of vancomycin monitoring (Liu, 2011; Rybak, 2009).

Toxic: >80 mcg/mL (SI: >54 micromole/L)

Additional Information Because of its long half-life, vancomycin should be dosed on an every 8- to 12-hour basis. Monitoring of trough serum concentrations is advisable in certain situations. "Red man syndrome", characterized by skin rash and hypotension, is not an allergic reaction but rather is associated with too rapid infusion of the drug. To alleviate or prevent the reaction, infuse vancomycin at a rate of ≥30 minutes for each 500 mg of drug being administered (eg, 1 g over ≥60 minutes); 1.5 g over ≥90 minutes.

Dosage Forms Excipient information presented when available (limited, particularly for generics); consult specific product labeling.

Capsule, Oral:
- Vancocin HCl: 125 mg, 250 mg
- Generic: 125 mg, 250 mg

Solution, Intravenous:
- Generic: 500 mg/100 mL (100 mL); 750 mg/150 mL (150 mL); 1 g/200 mL (200 mL)

Solution Reconstituted, Intravenous:
- Generic: 500 mg (1 ea); 750 mg (1 ea); 1000 mg (1 ea); 5000 mg (1 ea); 10 g (1 ea)

Solution Reconstituted, Intravenous [preservative free]:
- Generic: 1000 mg (1 ea); 5000 mg (1 ea); 10 g (1 ea)

Extemporaneous Preparations Using a vial of vancomycin powder for injection (reconstituted to 50 mg/mL), add the appropriate volume for the dose to 30 mL of water and administer orally or via NG tube. For oral administration, common flavoring syrups may be added to improve taste.

Vancomycin Hydrochloride for Injection, USP (prescribing information), Schaumburg, Il, APP Pharmaceuticals, LLC, 2011.

A vancomycin 25 mg/mL solution in Ora-Sweet® and water (1:1) may be prepared by reconstituting vancomycin for injection with sterile water, then dilute with a 1:1 mixture of Ora-Sweet® and distilled water to a final concentration of 25 mg/mL; transfer to amber prescription bottle. Stable for 75 days refrigerated or for 26 days at room temperature.

Ensom MH, Decarie D, and Lakhani A, "Stability of Vancomycin 25 mg/mL in Ora-Sweet and Water in Unit-Dose Cups and Plastic Bottles at 4°C and 25°C," *Can J Hosp Pharm*, 2010, 63(5):366-72.

◆ **Vancomycin Hydrochloride** *see* Vancomycin *on page 2157*

◆ **Vancomycin Hydrochloride for Injection (Can)** *see* Vancomycin *on page 2157*

◆ **Vancomycin Hydrochloride for Injection, USP (Can)** *see* Vancomycin *on page 2157*

◆ **Vandazole** *see* MetroNIDAZOLE (Topical) *on page 1354*

Vandetanib (van DET a nib)

Brand Names: U.S. Caprelsa

Brand Names: Canada Caprelsa

Index Terms AZD6474; Zactima; ZD6474; Zictifa

Pharmacologic Category Antineoplastic Agent, Tyrosine Kinase Inhibitor; Epidermal Growth Factor Receptor (EGFR) Inhibitor; Vascular Endothelial Growth Factor (VEGF) Inhibitor

Use Thyroid cancer: Treatment of metastatic or unresectable locally-advanced medullary thyroid cancer (symptomatic or progressive)

Pregnancy Risk Factor D

Pregnancy Considerations Animal reproduction studies have demonstrated teratogenic effects and fetal loss. Because vandetanib inhibits angiogenesis, a critical component of fetal development, adverse effects on pregnancy would be expected. Women of childbearing potential should be advised to avoid pregnancy and use effective contraception during and for 4 months following treatment with vandetanib. Canadian labeling recommends that nonsterile males employ reliable contraceptive methods (barrier method in conjunction with spermicide) during and for 2 months after vandetanib treatment.

Breast-Feeding Considerations It is not known if vandetanib is excreted in human breast milk. Due to the potential for serious adverse reactions in the nursing infant, a decision should be made to discontinue vandetanib or to discontinue breast-feeding, taking into account the importance of treatment to the mother.

Prescribing and Access Restrictions As a requirement of the REMS program, access to vandetanib is restricted. Vandetanib is approved for marketing under a Food and Drug Administration (FDA) approved, risk management program, and through a restricted distribution program, the Vandetanib REMS Program (1-800-236-9933). Prescribers and pharmacies must be certified with the program to prescribe or dispense vandetanib.

In Canada, vandetanib is available only through the CAPRELSA Restricted Distribution Program. Prescribers and pharmacies must be certified with the program to prescribe or dispense vandetanib. Further information may be obtained at 1-800-668-6000.

Medication Guide Available Yes

Contraindications Congenital long QT syndrome

Canadian labeling: Additional contraindications (not in U.S. labeling): Hypersensitivity to vandetanib or any component of the formulation; persistent Fridericia-corrected QT interval (QTcF) ≥500 ms; uncorrected hypokalemia, hypomagnesemia, or hypocalcemia; uncontrolled hypertension

Warnings/Precautions Hazardous agent - use appropriate precautions for handling and disposal (meets NIOSH, 2012 criteria). **[U.S. Boxed Warning]: May prolong the QT interval; torsade de pointes and sudden death have been reported. Do not use in patients with hypocalcemia, hypokalemia, hypomagnesemia, or long QT syndrome. Correct electrolyte imbalance prior to initiating therapy. Monitor electrolytes and ECG (to monitor QT interval) at baseline, at 2-4 weeks, at 8-12 weeks, and every 3 months thereafter; monitoring (at the same frequency) is required following dose reductions for QT prolongation or with dose interruptions >2 weeks. Avoid the use of QT-prolonging agents; if concomitant use with QT prolonging agents cannot be avoided, monitor ECG more frequently. Vandetanib has a long half-life (19 days), therefore, adverse reactions (including QT prolongation) may resolve slowly; monitor appropriately.** Ventricular tachycardia has also been reported. The potential for QT prolongation is dose-dependent. Do not initiate treatment unless QT interval, Fridericia-corrected QT interval (QTcF) is <450 msec. During treatment, if QTcF >500 msec, withhold vandetanib and resume at a reduced dose when QTcF is <450 msec. Do not use in patients with a history of torsade de pointes, congenital long QT syndrome, bradyarrhythmias or uncompensated heart failure. Patients with ventricular arrhythmias or recent MI were excluded from clinical trials. To reduce the risk of QT prolongation, maintain serum calcium and magnesium within normal limits and maintain serum potassium ≥4 mEq/L. Heart failure (HF) has been reported; monitor for signs and symptoms of HF; may require discontinuation (HF may not be reversible upon discontinuation). Hypertension and hypertensive crisis have been observed with vandetanib; monitor blood pressure and initiate or adjust antihypertensive therapy as needed; may require vandetanib dosage adjustment or treatment interruption; discontinue vandetanib (permanently) if blood pressure cannot be adequately controlled. Canadian labeling contraindicates use in uncontrolled hypertension.

Diarrhea has been reported with use; may cause electrolyte imbalance (closely monitor electrolytes and ECGs to detect QT prolongation resulting from dehydration); routine antidiarrheals are recommended; withhold vandetanib treatment until resolution for severe diarrhea; dose reduction is recommended when treatment is resumed. Stevens-Johnson syndrome and other serious skin reactions (including fatal) have been reported. Mild-to-moderate skin reactions, including acne, dermatitis, dry skin, palmar-plantar erythrodysesthesia syndrome, pruritus, and rash have also been reported. Withhold treatment for dermatologic toxicity of grade 3 or higher; consider a reduced dose or permanent discontinuation upon improvement in symptoms. Consider discontinuation for severe dermatologic toxicity. Mild-to-moderate toxicity has responded to corticosteroids (systemic or topical), oral antihistamines, and antibiotics (topical or systemic). Increased risk of photosensitivity is associated with use; effective sunscreen and protective clothing are recommended during and for at least 4 months after treatment discontinuation.

Reversible posterior leukoencephalopathy syndrome (RPLS) been observed with vandetanib; symptoms of RPLS include altered mental function, confusion, headache, seizure, or visual disturbances; generally associated with hypertension; consider discontinuing treatment if RPLS occurs. Serious and sometimes fatal hemorrhagic events have been reported with use; discontinue in patients with severe hemorrhage; do not administer in patients with a recent history of hemoptysis with ≥2.5 mL of red blood. Ischemic cerebrovascular events (some fatal) have been observed with vandetanib; discontinue treatment in patients with severe ischemic events (the safety of resuming treatment after an ischemic event has not been studied). Interstitial lung disease (ILD) or pneumonitis (including fatalities) has been reported with vandetanib. Patients should be advised to report any new or worsening respiratory symptoms; ILD should be suspected with nonspecific respiratory symptoms such as hypoxia, pleural effusion, cough or dyspnea. Interrupt therapy for acute or worsening pulmonary symptoms; discontinue if ILD diagnosis is confirmed.

Increased doses of thyroid replacement therapy have been required in patients with prior thyroidectomy; obtain TSH at baseline, at 2-4 weeks, 8-12 weeks, and every 3 months after vandetanib initiation; if signs and symptoms of hypothyroidism occur during treatment, evaluate thyroid hormone levels and adjust replacement therapy if needed. Dosage reduction is recommended in patients with moderate-to-severe renal impairment. Exposure is increased in patients with impaired renal function; closely monitor QT interval; has not been studied in patients with end stage renal disease requiring dialysis. Not recommended for use in patients with moderate-to-severe hepatic impairment. Potentially significant drug-drug interactions may exist, requiring dose or frequency adjustment, additional monitoring, and/or selection of alternative therapy. Due to the risk for serious treatment-related adverse events, use in patients whose disease is not progressive or symptomatic should be only be undertaken after careful consideration. **[U.S. Boxed Warning]: Vandetanib is only available through a restricted access program; prescribers and pharmacies must be certified with the restricted distribution program to prescribe and dispense vandetanib.**

Adverse Reactions

>10%:

Cardiovascular: Hypertension (33%; grades 3/4: 9%), prolonged Q-T interval on ECG (14%; grades 3/4: 8%)

Central nervous system: Headache (26%; grades 3/4: 1%), fatigue (24%; grades 3/4: 6%), insomnia (13%)

Dermatologic: Skin rash (53%; grades 3/4: 5%), acne vulgaris (35%; grades 3/4: 1%), xeroderma (15%), skin photosensitivity (13%; grades 3/4: 2%), pruritus (11%; grades 3/4: 1%)

Endocrine & metabolic: Hypocalcemia (11% to 57%; grades 3/4: 2%), hypoglycemia (24%)

Gastrointestinal: Pseudomembranous colitis (57%; grades 3/4: 11%), nausea (33%; grades 3/4: 1%), abdominal pain (21%; grades 3/4: 3%), decreased appetite (21%; grades 3/4: 1% to 4%), vomiting (15%; grades 3/4: 1%), dyspepsia (11%)

Hematologic & oncologic: Leukopenia (19%), hemorrhage (13% to 14%), anemia (13%; grades 3/4: <1%)

Hepatic: Increased serum ALT (51%), increased serum bilirubin (13%)

Neuromuscular & skeletal: Weakness (15%)

Ophthalmic: Corneal changes (13%; corneal edema, corneal opacity, corneal dystrophy, iris hyperpigmentation, keratopathy, arcus lipoides, corneal deposits, acquired corneal dystrophy)

Renal: Increased serum creatinine (16%)

Respiratory: Upper respiratory tract infection (23%), cough (11%), nasopharyngitis (11%)

1% to 10%:

Cardiovascular: Cardiac failure (2%), cerebral ischemia (1%)

Central nervous system: Depression (10%; grades 3/4: 2%)

Dermatologic: Nail disease (9%; inflammation, tenderness, paronychia), alopecia (8%)

Endocrine & metabolic: Weight loss (10%), hypercalcemia (7%), hypomagnesemia (7%), hyperkalemia (6%), hypokalemia (6%), hypothyroidism (6%), hyperglycemia (5%), hypermagnesemia (3%)

Gastrointestinal: Xerostomia (9%), dysgeusia (8%)

Genitourinary: Proteinuria (10%)

Hematologic & oncologic: Neutropenia (10%; grades 3/4: <1%), thrombocytopenia (9%)

Infection: Sepsis (2%)

Neuromuscular & skeletal: Muscle spasm (6%)

Ophthalmic: Blurred vision (9%)

Respiratory: Aspiration pneumonia (2%), respiratory arrest (2%), respiratory failure (2%)

<1% (Limited to important or life-threatening): Cardiorespiratory arrest, interstitial pulmonary disease, palmar-plantar erythrodysesthesia, pancreatitis, pneumonitis, reversible posterior leukoencephalopathy syndrome, Stevens-Johnson syndrome, torsades de pointes, ventricular tachycardia

Drug Interactions

Metabolism/Transport Effects Substrate of CYP3A4 (major); **Note:** Assignment of Major/Minor substrate status based on clinically relevant drug interaction potential; **Inhibits** BCRP, P-glycoprotein

Avoid Concomitant Use

Avoid concomitant use of Vandetanib with any of the following: Bosutinib; CYP3A4 Inducers (Strong); Highest Risk QTc-Prolonging Agents; Ivabradine; Mifepristone; Moderate Risk QTc-Prolonging Agents; PAZOPanib; Pomalidomide; Silodosin; St Johns Wort; VinCRIStine (Liposomal)

Increased Effect/Toxicity

Vandetanib may increase the levels/effects of: Afatinib; Bisphosphonate Derivatives; Bosutinib; Colchicine; Dabigatran Etexilate; Everolimus; Highest Risk QTc-Prolonging Agents; PAZOPanib; P-glycoprotein/ABCB1 Substrates; Pomalidomide; Prucalopride; Rivaroxaban; Silodosin; Topotecan; VinCRIStine (Liposomal); Vitamin K Antagonists

The levels/effects of Vandetanib may be increased by: Ivabradine; Mifepristone; Moderate Risk QTc-Prolonging Agents; QTc-Prolonging Agents (Indeterminate Risk and Risk Modifying)

Decreased Effect

Vandetanib may decrease the levels/effects of: Cardiac Glycosides; Vitamin K Antagonists

The levels/effects of Vandetanib may be decreased by: Bosentan; CYP3A4 Inducers (Strong); Dabrafenib; Deferasirox; St Johns Wort; Tocilizumab

Ethanol/Nutrition/Herb Interactions Herb/Nutraceutical: St John's wort may decrease vandetanib exposure. Management: Avoid St John's wort.

Storage/Stability Store at 25°C (77°F); excursions permitted to 15°C to 30°C (59°F to 86°F).

Mechanism of Action Multikinase inhibitor; inhibits tyrosine kinases including epidermal growth factor reception (EGFR), vascular endothelial growth factor (VEGF), rearranged during transfection (RET), protein tyrosine kinase 6 (BRK), TIE2, EPH kinase receptors and SRC kinase receptors, selectively blocking intracellular signaling, angiogenesis and cellular proliferation

Pharmacodynamics/Kinetics

Absorption: Slow

Protein binding: ~90%; to albumin and alpha 1-acid-glycoprotein

Distribution: V_d: ~7450 L

Metabolism: Hepatic, via CYP3A4 to N-desmethyl vandetanib and via flavin-containing monooxygenase enzymes to vandetanib-N-oxide

Bioavailability: Not affected by food

Half life, elimination: 19 days

Time to peak: 6 hours (range: 4-10 hours)

Excretion: Feces (~44%); urine (~25%)

Dosage Note: Do not initiate treatment unless QTcF <450 msec. Avoid concomitant use of QT-prolonging agents and strong CYP3A4 inducers. To reduce the risk of QT prolongation, maintain serum calcium and magnesium within normal limits and maintain serum potassium ≥4 mEq/L.

Medullary thyroid cancer, locally-advanced or metastatic: Adults: Oral: 300 mg once daily, continue treatment until no longer clinically benefiting or until unacceptable toxicity

Dosage adjustment for toxicity:

Toxicity ≥ grade 3: Interrupt dose until resolves or improves to grade 1, then resume at a reduced dose

Dosage reduction: Reduce from 300 mg once daily to 200 mg once daily, further reduce if needed to 100 mg once daily. For recurrent toxicities, reduce dose to 100 mg once daily after symptom improvement to ≤ grade 1 toxicity, if continued treatment is warranted.

Management of specific toxicities:

Cardiac: QTcF >500 msec: Withhold dose until QTcF returns to <450 msec, then resume at a reduced dose

Diarrhea (severe): Withhold treatment until resolution. Dose reduction is recommended when treatment is resumed. Routine antidiarrheals are recommended. Closely monitor electrolytes and ECGs to detect QT prolongation resulting from dehydration.

Heart failure: May require discontinuation.

Hemorrhage (severe): Discontinue.

Hypertension: Initiate or adjust antihypertensive therapy as needed; may require vandetanib dosage adjustment or treatment interruption; discontinue permanently if blood pressure cannot be adequately controlled.

Interstitial lung disease (ILD)/pneumonitis: Interrupt therapy for acute or worsening pulmonary symptoms. Discontinue if ILD diagnosis is confirmed.

Ischemic cerebrovascular events (severe): Discontinue treatment (safety of resuming treatment after an ischemic event has not been studied).

Reversible posterior leukoencephalopathy syndrome (RPLS): Discontinue treatment.

Skin reactions: Withhold treatment for dermatologic toxicity of grade 3 or higher. Consider a reduced dose or permanent discontinuation upon improvement in symptoms. Consider permanent discontinuation for severe dermatologic toxicity. Mild-to-moderate toxicity has responded to corticosteroids (systemic or topical), oral antihistamines, and antibiotics (topical or systemic).

Dosage adjustment in renal impairment:

Cl_{cr} ≥50 mL/minute: No dosage adjustment necessary

Cl_{cr} <50 mL/minute: Reduce initial dose to 200 mg once daily; closely monitor QT interval

Dosage adjustment in hepatic impairment:

Mild impairment (Child-Pugh class A): No dosage adjustment provided in manufacturer's labeling.

Moderate and severe impairment (Child-Pugh class B or C): Use is not recommended.

Dietary Considerations May be taken with or without food.

Administration May be administered with or without food. Missed doses should be omitted if within 12 hours of the next scheduled dose. Do not crush tablet. If unable to swallow tablet whole or if nasogastric or gastrostomy tube administration is necessary, disperse one tablet in 2 ounces of water (noncarbonated only) and stir for 10 minutes to disperse (will not dissolve completely) and administer immediately. Rinse residue in glass with additional 4 ounces of water (noncarbonated only) and administer.

Hazardous agent; use appropriate precautions for handling and disposal (meets NIOSH, 2012 criteria).

Monitoring Parameters Monitor electrolytes (calcium, magnesium, potassium), TSH, and ECG (QT interval) at baseline, at 2-4 weeks, at 8-12 weeks, and every 3 months thereafter; also monitor QT interval at same frequency for dose reduction due to QT interval or treatment delays >2 weeks (monitor electrolytes and ECG more frequently if diarrhea). Monitor renal function, hepatic function, blood pressure; monitor for signs and symptoms of heart failure, reversible posterior leukoencephalopathy syndrome (RPLS), pulmonary and skin toxicities

Dosage Forms Excipient information presented when available (limited, particularly for generics); consult specific product labeling.

Tablet, Oral:

Caprelsa: 100 mg, 300 mg

Extemporaneous Preparations Hazardous agent: Use appropriate precautions for handling and disposal.

An oral solution may be prepared using the tablet. Disperse one tablet in 2 ounces of water (noncarbonated only) and stir for 10 minutes to disperse (will not dissolve completely) and administer immediately. Rinse residue in glass with additional 4 ounces of water (noncarbonated only) and administer.

- Vaniqa *see* Eflornithine *on page* 691
- Vaniqa® (Can) *see* Eflornithine *on page* 691
- Vanos *see* Fluocinonide *on page* 879
- Vanoxide-HC® *see* Benzoyl Peroxide and Hydrocortisone *on page* 243
- Vanquish® Extra Strength Pain Reliever [OTC] *see* Acetaminophen, Aspirin, and Caffeine *on page* 33
- Vantas *see* Histrelin *on page* 998
- Vantin *see* Cefpodoxime *on page* 376
- Vaprisol *see* Conivaptan *on page* 491
- VAQTA *see* Hepatitis A Vaccine *on page* 990
- VAR *see* Varicella Virus Vaccine *on page* 2168

Vardenafil (var DEN a fil)

Brand Names: U.S. Levitra; Staxyn

Brand Names: Canada Levitra; Staxyn

Index Terms Vardenafil Hydrochloride

Pharmacologic Category Phosphodiesterase-5 Enzyme Inhibitor

Use Erectile dysfunction: Treatment of erectile dysfunction (ED)

Pregnancy Risk Factor B

Pregnancy Considerations Teratogenic effects were not observed in animal studies; however, vardenafil is not indicated for use in women. No effects on sperm motility or morphology were observed in healthy males.

Breast-Feeding Considerations It is not known if vardenafil is excreted in breast milk. Vardenafil is not indicated for use in women.

Contraindications Hypersensitivity to vardenafil or any component of the formulation; concurrent (regular or intermittent) use of organic nitrates in any form (eg, nitroglycerin, isosorbide dinitrate)

Warnings/Precautions There is a degree of cardiac risk associated with sexual activity; therefore, physicians may wish to consider the patient's cardiovascular status prior to initiating any treatment for erectile dysfunction. Use caution in patients with anatomical deformation of the penis (angulation, cavernosal fibrosis, or Peyronie's disease) and in patients who have conditions which may predispose them to priapism (sickle cell anemia, multiple myeloma, leukemia). Instruct patients to seek immediate medical attention if erection persists >4 hours.

Use is not recommended in patients with hypotension (<90/50 mm Hg); uncontrolled hypertension (>170/100 mm Hg); unstable angina or angina during intercourse; life-threatening arrhythmias, stroke, or MI within the last 6 months; cardiac failure or coronary artery disease causing unstable angina. Safety and efficacy have not been studied in these patients. Use caution in patients with left ventricular outflow obstruction (eg, aortic stenosis or hypertrophic cardiomyopathy [HCM] with outflow tract obstruction). Use caution with alpha-blockers, effective CYP3A4 inhibitors, the elderly, or those with hepatic impairment (Child-Pugh class B); dosage adjustment is needed. Concurrent use with alpha-adrenergic antagonist therapy may cause symptomatic hypotension; patients should be hemodynamically stable prior to initiating tadalafil therapy at the lowest possible dose. Avoid or limit concurrent substantial alcohol consumption as this may increase the risk of symptomatic hypotension.

Rare cases of nonarteritic ischemic optic neuropathy (NAION) have been reported; risk may be increased with history of vision loss. Other risk factors for NAION include heart disease, diabetes, hypertension, smoking, age >50 years, or history of certain eye problems. Sudden decrease or loss of hearing has been reported rarely; hearing changes may be accompanied by tinnitus and dizziness.

Safety and efficacy have not been studied in patients with the following conditions, therefore, use in these patients is not recommended at this time: Congenital QT prolongation, patients taking medications known to prolong the QT interval (avoid use in patients taking Class Ia or III antiarrhythmics); severe hepatic impairment (Child-Pugh class C); end-stage renal disease requiring dialysis; retinitis pigmentosa or other degenerative retinal disorders. The safety and efficacy of vardenafil with other treatments for erectile dysfunction have not been studied and are not recommended as combination therapy. Concomitant use with all forms of nitrates is contraindicated. If nitrate administration is medically necessary, it is not known when nitrates can be safely administered following the use of vardenafil; however, when a 20 mg (film-coated tablet) was administered 24 hours prior to a 0.4 mg sublingual dose of nitroglycerin, no changes in blood pressure or heart rate were detected. Potential underlying causes of erectile dysfunction should be evaluated prior to treatment. Some products may contain phylalanine. Some products may contain sorbitol; do not use in patients with fructose intolerance.

Adverse Reactions

>10%:
- Cardiovascular: Flushing (8% to 11%)
- Central nervous system: Headache (14% to 15%)

2% to 10%:
- Central nervous system: Dizziness (2%)
- Gastrointestinal: Dyspepsia (3% to 4%), nausea (2%)
- Neuromuscular & skeletal: Back pain (2%), CPK increased (2%)
- Respiratory: Rhinitis (9%), nasal congestion (3%), sinusitis (3%)
- Miscellaneous: Flu-like syndrome (3%)

<2% (Limited to important or life-threatening): Abnormal ejaculation, amnesia (transient global), anaphylactic reaction, angina, angioedema, arthralgia, dyspnea, hearing decreased, hearing loss, hyper-/hypotension, insomnia, liver function tests abnormal, MI, myalgia, nonarteritic ischemic optic neuropathy (NAION), orthostatic hypotension, pain, photophobia, photosensitivity, priapism, pruritus, rash, somnolence, syncope, tachycardia, tinnitus, ventricular tachyarrhythmia, vertigo, vision abnormal, visual acuity reduced, visual field defects, vision loss (temporary or permanent)

Drug Interactions

Metabolism/Transport Effects Substrate of CYP3A4 (major); **Note:** Assignment of Major/Minor substrate status based on clinically relevant drug interaction potential

Avoid Concomitant Use

Avoid concomitant use of Vardenafil with any of the following: Alprostadil; Amyl Nitrite; Cobicistat; Fusidic Acid (Systemic); Phosphodiesterase 5 Inhibitors; Riociguat; Vasodilators (Organic Nitrates)

Increased Effect/Toxicity

Vardenafil may increase the levels/effects of: Alpha1-Blockers; Alprostadil; Amyl Nitrite; Antihypertensives; Bosentan; Highest Risk QTc-Prolonging Agents; Moderate Risk QTc-Prolonging Agents; Phosphodiesterase 5 Inhibitors; Riociguat; Vasodilators (Organic Nitrates)

The levels/effects of Vardenafil may be increased by: Alcohol (Ethyl); Boceprevir; Clarithromycin; Cobicistat; CYP3A4 Inhibitors (Moderate); CYP3A4 Inhibitors (Strong); Dasatinib; Erythromycin (Systemic); Fluconazole; Fusidic Acid (Systemic); Itraconazole; Ivacaftor; Ketoconazole (Systemic); Lorcaserin; Luliconazole; Mifepristone; Posaconazole; Protease Inhibitors; Sapropterin; Simeprevir; Telaprevir; Voriconazole

Decreased Effect

The levels/effects of Vardenafil may be decreased by: Bosentan; Etravirine

Ethanol/Nutrition/Herb Interactions

Ethanol: Substantial consumption of ethanol may increase the risk of hypotension and orthostasis. Lower ethanol consumption has not been associated with significant changes in blood pressure or increase in orthostatic symptoms. Management: Avoid or limit ethanol consumption.

Food: High-fat meals decrease maximum serum concentration 18% to 50%. Serum concentrations/toxicity may be increased with grapefruit juice. Management: Do not take with a high-fat meal. Avoid grapefruit juice.

Storage/Stability Store at 25°C (77°F); excursions permitted to 15°C to 25°C (59°F to 86°F). Keep oral disintegrating tablets sealed in blisterpack until ready to use.

Mechanism of Action Does not directly cause penile erections, but affects the response to sexual stimulation. The physiologic mechanism of erection of the penis involves release of nitric oxide (NO) in the corpus cavernosum during sexual stimulation. NO then activates the enzyme guanylate cyclase, which results in increased levels of cyclic guanosine monophosphate (cGMP), producing smooth muscle relaxation and inflow of blood to the corpus cavernosum. Vardenafil enhances the effect of NO by inhibiting phosphodiesterase type 5 (PDE-5), which is responsible for degradation of cGMP in the corpus cavernosum; when sexual stimulation causes local release of NO, inhibition of PDE-5 by vardenafil causes increased levels of cGMP in the corpus cavernosum, resulting in smooth muscle relaxation and inflow of blood to the corpus cavernosum; at recommended doses, it has no effect in the absence of sexual stimulation.

Pharmacodynamics/Kinetics

Onset of action: ~60 minutes

Absorption: Rapid

Distribution: V_d: 208 L

Protein binding: ~95% (parent drug and metabolite)

Metabolism: Hepatic via CYP3A4 (major), CYP2C and 3A5 (minor); forms metabolite (active)

Bioavailability: ~15%

Film-coated tablet: Elderly (≥65 years): AUC increased by 52%; Hepatic impairment (moderate, Child-Pugh class B): AUC increased by 160%

Oral disintegrating tablet: Elderly (≥65 years): AUC increased by 21% more compared to film-coated tablet. When administered with water, AUC decreases by 29%.

Half-life elimination: Terminal: Vardenafil and metabolite: 3-6 hours

Time to peak, plasma: 0.5-2 hours

Excretion: Feces (~91% to 95% as metabolites); urine (~2% to 6%)

Dosage Note: Oral disintegrating tablets should not be used interchangeably with film-coated tablets; patients requiring a dose other than 10 mg should use the film-coated tablets.

Oral: Erectile dysfunction:

Adults:

Film-coated tablet (Levitra): 10 mg administered ~60 minutes prior to sexual activity; dosing range: 5-20 mg; to be given as one single dose and not given more than once daily

Oral disintegrating tablet (Staxyn): 10 mg administered ~60 minutes prior to sexual activity; maximum: 10 mg per day

Elderly ≥65 years: Film-coated tablet (Levitra): Consider a starting dose of 5 mg administered ~60 minutes prior to sexual activity; to be given as one single dose and not given more than once daily

Dosing adjustment with concomitant medications:

Alpha-blocker (dose should be stable at time of vardenafil initiation):

Film-coated tablet (Levitra): Initial vardenafil dose: 5 mg per day; if an alpha-blocker is added to vardenafil therapy, it should be initiated at the smallest possible dose and titrated carefully.

Oral disintegrating tablet (Staxyn): Do not use to initiate therapy. Initial therapy should be with film-coated tablets at lower doses. Patients who have previously used film-coated tablets may be switched to oral disintegrating tablets as recommended by healthcare provider. With coadministration, consider a time interval between dosing (eg, 6-hour interval).

Film-coated tablet (Levitra):

Atazanavir: Maximum vardenafil dose: 2.5 mg/24 hours

Clarithromycin: Maximum vardenafil dose: 2.5 mg/24 hours

Darunavir: Maximum vardenafil dose: 2.5 mg/72 hours

Erythromycin: Maximum vardenafil dose: 5 mg/24 hours

Fosamprenavir: Maximum vardenafil dose: 2.5 mg/24 hours

Fosamprenavir/ritonavir: Maximum vardenafil dose: 2.5 mg/72 hours

Indinavir: Maximum vardenafil dose: 2.5 mg/24 hours

Itraconazole:

200 mg/day: Maximum vardenafil dose: 5 mg/24 hours

400 mg/day: Maximum vardenafil dose: 2.5 mg/24 hours

Ketoconazole:

200 mg/day: Maximum vardenafil dose: 5 mg/24 hours

400 mg/day: Maximum vardenafil dose: 2.5 mg/24 hours

Lopinavir/ritonavir: Maximum vardenafil dose: 2.5 mg/72 hours

Nelfinavir: Maximum vardenafil dose: 2.5 mg/24 hours

Ritonavir: Maximum vardenafil dose: 2.5 mg/72 hours

Saquinavir: Maximum vardenafil dose: 2.5 mg/24 hours

Tipranavir: Maximum vardenafil dose: 2.5 mg/72 hours

Oral disintegrating tablet (Staxyn): Concurrent use not recommended with potent or moderate CYP3A4 inhibitors (atazanavir, clarithromycin, erythromycin, indinavir, itraconazole, ketoconazole, ritonavir, saquinavir)

Dosage adjustment in renal impairment:

Mild, moderate, or severe impairment: No dosage adjustment necessary.

Hemodialysis: Use not recommended.

Dosage adjustment in hepatic impairment:

Child-Pugh class A: No dosage adjustment necessary.

Child-Pugh class B:

Film-coated tablet (Levitra): Initial: 5 mg adminsitered ~60 minutes prior to sexual activity (maximum dose: 10 mg); to be given as one single dose and not given more than once daily

Oral disintegrating tablet (Staxyn): Use not recommended.

Child-Pugh class C: Has not been studied; use is not recommended by the manufacturer.

Dietary Considerations Avoid grapefruit juice. Some products may contain phenylalanine. Some products may contain sorbitol; do not use in patients with fructose intolerance.

Administration May be administered with or without food, 60 minutes prior to sexual activity.

Oral disintegrating tablet should not be removed from blister pack until administered. Using dry hands, place immediately on tongue. Tablet will dissolve within seconds; do not take with liquid. Do not crush, split, or chew.

Monitoring Parameters Monitor for response, adverse reactions, blood pressure, and heart rate.

Dosage Forms Excipient information presented when available (limited, particularly for generics); consult specific product labeling.

Tablet, Oral:

Levitra: 2.5 mg, 5 mg, 10 mg, 20 mg

Tablet Dispersible, Oral:

Staxyn: 10 mg [contains aspartame; peppermint flavor]

◆ **Vardenafil Hydrochloride** *see* Vardenafil *on page 2164*

Varenicline (var e NI kleen)

Brand Names: U.S. Chantix; Chantix Continuing Month Pak; Chantix Starting Month Pak

Brand Names: Canada Champix®

Index Terms Varenicline Tartrate

Pharmacologic Category Partial Nicotine Agonist; Smoking Cessation Aid

Use Smoking cessation: Aid to smoking cessation treatment

Pregnancy Risk Factor C

Pregnancy Considerations Teratogenic effects were not observed in animal studies; however, decreased fertility, decreased fetal weight, and increased auditory startle response were observed in the offspring. There are no adequate or well-controlled studies in pregnant women. Use only if benefit outweighs the potential risk to fetus.

Breast-Feeding Considerations It is not known if varenicline is excreted in breast milk. Due to the potential for serious adverse reactions in the nursing infant, breast-feeding is not recommended.

Medication Guide Available Yes

Contraindications Serious hypersensitivity or skin reactions to varenicline or any component of the formulation

Warnings/Precautions **[U.S. Boxed Warning]: Serious neuropsychiatric events (including depression, suicidal thoughts, and suicide) have been reported with use;** some cases may have been complicated by symptoms of nicotine withdrawal following smoking cessation. Smoking cessation (with or without treatment) is associated with nicotine withdrawal symptoms and the exacerbation of underlying psychiatric illness; however, some of the behavioral disturbances were reported in treated patients who continued to smoke. Neuropsychiatric symptoms (eg, mood disturbances, psychosis, hostility) have occurred in patients with and without pre-existing psychiatric disease; many cases resolved following therapy discontinuation although in some cases, symptoms persisted. Ethanol consumption may increase the risk of psychiatric adverse events. Monitor all patients for behavioral changes and psychiatric symptoms (eg, agitation, depression, suicidal behavior, suicidal ideation); inform patients to discontinue treatment and contact their healthcare provider immediately if they experience any behavioral and/or mood changes. **[U.S. Boxed Warning]: Before prescribing, the risks of serious neuropsychiatric events must be weighed against the immediate and long term benefits of smoking abstinence for each patient.**

Hypersensitivity reactions (including angioedema) and rare cases of serious skin reactions (including Stevens-Johnson syndrome and erythema multiforme) have been reported. Patients should be instructed to discontinue use and contact healthcare provider if signs/symptoms occur. Treatment may increase risk of cardiovascular events. A meta-analysis of 15 clinical trials, including a placebo-controlled trial in patients with stable cardiovascular disease, showed an increased incidence of major cardiovascular events (combined outcome of cardiovascular-related death, nonfatal MI, nonfatal stroke) in patients using varenicline compared with placebo. Cardiovascular events were uncommon in both the varenicline and placebo groups. These findings did not reach statistical significance, although data was consistent. Events occurred primarily in patients with known cardiovascular disease. The meta-analysis also showed a lower incidence of all-cause and cardiovascular mortality in varenicline-treated patients, although this was not statistically significant either. Dose-dependent nausea may occur; both transient and persistent nausea has been reported. Dosage reduction may be considered for intolerable nausea. May cause CNS depression, which may impair physical or mental abilities; patients must be cautioned about performing tasks which require mental alertness (eg, operating machinery or driving). There have been postmarketing reports of traffic accidents, near-miss incidents in traffic, or other accidental injuries in patients taking varenicline.

Use caution in renal dysfunction; dosage adjustment required. Safety and efficacy of varenicline with other smoking cessation therapies have not been established; increased adverse events when used concurrently with nicotine replacement therapy.

Adverse Reactions

>10%:

Central nervous system: Headache (15% to 19%), insomnia (10% to 19%), abnormal dreams (9% to 13%), suicidal ideation (11%)

Gastrointestinal: Nausea (16% to 40%), vomiting (≤5% to 11%)

1% to 10%:

Cardiovascular: Angina pectoris (4%), peripheral edema (2%), myocardial infarction (1%)

Central nervous system: Malaise (≤7%), sleep disorder (≤5%), drowsiness (3%), lethargy (1% to 2%), nightmares (1% to 2%)

Dermatologic: Skin rash (≤3%)

Gastrointestinal: Flatulence (6% to 9%), constipation (5% to 8%), dysgeusia (5% to 8%), abdominal pain (≤7%), xerostomia (≤6%), dyspepsia (5%), increased appetite (3% to 4%), anorexia (≤2%), gastroesophageal reflux disease (1%)

Respiratory: Upper respiratory tract infection (5% to 7%), dyspnea (≤2%), rhinorrhea (≤1%)

<1% (Limited to important or life-threatening): Acute coronary syndrome, acute renal failure, amnesia, anemia, angioedema, asthma, atrial fibrillation, Bell's palsy, bradycardia, cardiac arrhythmia, cardiac flutter, cataract, cerebrovascular accident, conjunctivitis, cor pulmonale, coronary artery disease, deafness, delusions, depression, diabetes mellitus, dissociative disorder, dysarthria, dysphagia, ECG abnormality, eczema, enterocolitis, equilibrium disturbance, erectile dysfunction, erythema multiforme, gallbladder disease, gastric ulcer, gastrointestinal hemorrhage, hallucination, homicidal ideation, hostility, hyperhidrosis, hyperlipidemia, hypersensitivity, hypoglycemia, hypokalemia, intestinal obstruction, leukocytosis, loss of consciousness, lymphadenopathy, mania, Meniere's disease, migraine, multiple sclerosis, myositis, nephrolithiasis, nocturia, nocturnal amblyopia, nystagmus, ophthalmic vascular disease, oral mucosa ulcer, osteoporosis, pancreatitis, panic, photophobia, pleurisy, polyuria, psoriasis, psychomotor retardation, psychosis, psychotic reaction, pulmonary embolism, restless leg syndrome, seizure, skin photosensitivity, splenomegaly, Stevens-Johnson syndrome, syncope, tachycardia, thrombocytopenia, thrombosis, thyroid disease, transient blindness, transient ischemic attacks, urinary retention, ventricular premature contractions

Drug Interactions

Metabolism/Transport Effects None known.

Avoid Concomitant Use There are no known interactions where it is recommended to avoid concomitant use.

Increased Effect/Toxicity

The levels/effects of Varenicline may be increased by: Alcohol (Ethyl); H2-Antagonists; Quinolone Antibiotics; Trimethoprim

Decreased Effect There are no known significant interactions involving a decrease in effect.

Ethanol/Nutrition/Herb Interactions Ethanol: May increase the risk of psychiatric adverse events. Caution patients about the potential effects of ethanol consumption during therapy.

Storage/Stability Store at 25°C (77°F); excursions permitted to 15°C to 30°C (59°F to 86°F).

Mechanism of Action Partial neuronal α_4 β_2 nicotinic receptor agonist; prevents nicotine stimulation of mesolimbic dopamine system associated with nicotine addiction. Also binds to 5-HT_3 receptor (significance not determined) with moderate affinity. Varenicline stimulates dopamine activity but to a much smaller degree than nicotine does, resulting in decreased craving and withdrawal symptoms.

Pharmacodynamics/Kinetics

Absorption: Well absorbed; unaffected by food

Protein binding: ≤20%

Metabolism: Minimal (<10% of clearance is through metabolism)
Half-life elimination: ~24 hours
Time to peak, plasma: ~3-4 hours
Excretion: Urine (92% as unchanged drug)

Dosage Oral: Adults:
Initial:
Days 1-3: 0.5 mg once daily
Days 4-7: 0.5 mg twice daily
Maintenance (≥ Day 8):
U.S. labeling: 1 mg twice daily for 11 weeks
Canadian labeling: 0.5-1 mg twice daily for 11 weeks

Note: Start 1 week before target quit date. Alternatively, patients may consider setting a quit date up to 35 days after initiation of varenicline and then quit smoking between 8-35 days of treatment (some data suggest that an extended pretreatment regimen may result in higher abstinence rates [Hajek, 2011]). If patient successfully quits smoking at the end of the 12 weeks, may continue for another 12 weeks to help maintain success. If not successful in first 12 weeks, then stop medication and reassess factors contributing to failure.

Dosage adjustment for toxicity: Patients who cannot tolerate adverse events may require temporary (or permanent) reduction in dose. Lower dose for a period of time, then may increase dose again or remain on lower dose.

Dosage adjustment in renal impairment:
Cl_{cr} ≥30 mL/minute: No dosage adjustment necessary.
Cl_{cr} <30 mL/minute: Initial: 0.5 mg once daily; maximum dose: 0.5 mg twice daily
End-stage renal disease (ESRD) (receiving hemodialysis): Maximum dose: 0.5 mg once daily

Dosage adjustment in hepatic impairment: No dosage adjustment necessary.

Dietary Considerations Should be given with food and a full glass of water to decrease gastric upset.

Administration Administer after eating and with a full glass of water.

Monitoring Parameters Monitor for behavioral changes and psychiatric symptoms (eg, agitation, depression, suicidal behavior, suicidal ideation).

Additional Information In all studies, patients received an educational booklet on smoking cessation and received up to 10 minutes of counseling at each weekly visit. Dosing started 1 week before target quit date. Successful cessation of smoking may alter pharmacokinetic properties of other medications (eg, theophylline, warfarin, insulin).

Dosage Forms Excipient information presented when available (limited, particularly for generics); consult specific product labeling.
Tablet, Oral:
Chantix: 0.5 mg, 1 mg
Chantix Continuing Month Pak: 1 mg
Chantix Starting Month Pak: 0.5 MG X 11 & 1 MG X 42

◆ **Varenicline Tartrate** *see* Varenicline *on page 2166*

◆ **Varicella, Measles, Mumps, and Rubella Vaccine** *see* Measles, Mumps, Rubella, and Varicella Virus Vaccine *on page 1273*

Varicella Virus Vaccine

(var i SEL a VYE rus vak SEEN)

Brand Names: U.S. Varivax
Brand Names: Canada Varilrix; Varivax III
Index Terms Chickenpox Vaccine; VAR; Varicella-Zoster Virus (VZV) Vaccine (Varicella); VZV Vaccine (Varicella)
Pharmacologic Category Vaccine, Live (Viral)

Additional Appendix Information
Immunization Administration Recommendations *on page 2334*
Immunization Recommendations *on page 2339*

Use
Varicella prevention: For the prevention of varicella in persons 12 months and older
The Advisory Committee on Immunization Practices (ACIP) recommends vaccination for all children, adolescents, and adults who do not have evidence of immunity (CDC, 2007). Vaccination is especially important for:
- Healthcare personnel
- Household contacts of immunocompromised persons
- Persons living or working in environments where transmission is likely (teachers, child-care workers, residents and staff of institutional settings)
- Persons in environments where transmission has been reported
- Nonpregnant women of childbearing age
- Adolescents and adults in households with children
- International travelers

Postexposure prophylaxis: Vaccination within 3 days (possibly 5 days) after exposure to rash is effective in preventing illness or modifying severity of disease in persons without other evidence of immunity (CDC, 2007).

Pregnancy Considerations Varicella virus vaccine is contraindicated for use in pregnant females and pregnancy should be avoided for 3 months (per manufacturer labeling; 1 month per ACIP) following vaccination. Varicella disease during the 1st or 2nd trimesters may result in congenital varicella syndrome. The onset of maternal varicella infection from 5 days prior to 2 days after delivery may cause varicella infection in the newborn. All women should be assessed for immunity during a prenatal visit; those without evidence of immunity should be vaccinated upon completion or termination of pregnancy (CDC, 2007). Based on information collected from 1995-2013 using the manufacturer's pregnancy registry, of 820 women who received a varicella containing vaccine, there were no infants born with abnormalities consistent with congenital varicella syndrome. Any exposures to the vaccine during pregnancy or within 3 months prior to pregnancy should be reported to the manufacturer (Merck & Co, 877-888-4231) or to VAERS (800-822-7967) as suspected adverse reactions.

Breast-Feeding Considerations Following immunization, varicella virus was not detected in the milk samples of 12 breast-feeding women and none of the breast-fed infants seroconverted. Immunization should not be delayed due to breast-feeding (CDC, 2007). The manufacturer recommends that caution be exercised when administering varicella virus vaccine to nursing women. Breast-feeding infants should be vaccinated according to the recommended schedules (CDC, 2011).

Contraindications
U.S. labeling: Severe allergic or anaphylactic reaction to the vaccine, neomycin, gelatin, or any component of the formulation; immunosuppressed or immunodeficient individuals including individuals with leukemia, lymphomas, or other malignant neoplasms affecting the bone marrow or lymphatic systems; persons with AIDs or other clinical manifestations of HIV; those receiving immunosuppressive therapy (including immunosuppressive doses of corticosteroids); history of primary and acquired immunodeficiency states; active, untreated tuberculosis; current febrile illness (per manufacturer labeling); pregnancy
Canadian labeling: Additional contraindications (not in U.S. labeling): Varivax III: Family history of congenital or hereditary immunodeficiency (unless immune competence of vaccine recipient is demonstrated); Varilrix: Primary or acquired immunodeficiency with a total lymphocyte count <1200/mm^3

Warnings/Precautions Immediate treatment for anaphylactoid reaction should be available during vaccine use. Varicella vaccine and antibody-containing products (eg, immune globulin, blood products) should **not** be administered simultaneously. Guidelines with suggested administration intervals are available (CDC, 2011). Vaccination may not result in effective immunity in all patients. Response depends upon multiple factors (eg, type of vaccine, age of patient) and may be improved by administering the vaccine at the recommended dose, route, and interval. Vaccines may not be effective if administered during periods of altered immune competence (CDC, 2011). The manufacturer notes that vaccinated individuals should not have close association with susceptible high-risk individuals for 6 weeks following vaccination. High-risk individuals include immunocompromised persons, pregnant women without evidence of immunity, newborns of mothers without evidence of immunity, and all infants born <28 weeks' gestation (regardless of maternal immunity). However, the CDC notes that transmission of the virus is rare and recommends that vaccine recipients who develop a vaccine-related rash avoid contact with susceptible individuals at high risk for complications until the lesions are resolved (crusted over or fade away) or until no new lesions appear for 24 hours. According to the CDC guidelines, having a pregnant household member is not a contraindication to vaccination (CDC, 2007). May administer to patients with mild acute illness with or without low grade fever (CDC, 2007). Syncope has been reported with use of injectable vaccines and may be accompanied by transient visual disturbances, weakness, or tonic-clonic movements. Procedures should be in place to avoid injuries from falling and to restore cerebral perfusion if syncope occurs (CDC, 2008). Although the manufacturer contraindicates administration to persons with HIV, guidelines for use are available. Children with HIV infection with age-specific CD4+ T-lymphocyte percentages ≥15% may receive live attenuated varicella vaccine. Vaccination may be considered for children >8 years, adolescents, and adults with CD4+ T-lymphocyte counts ≥200 cells/microliter (CDC, 2007). Defer use in patients with a family history of congenital or hereditary immunodeficiency until immune competence in the vaccine recipient is demonstrated (CDC, 2007). Products may contain gelatin, neomycin, or albumin; patients with history of anaphylaxis should not receive vaccine (CDC, 2007). Contact dermatitis to neomycin is not a contraindication to the vaccine. In order to maximize vaccination rates, the ACIP recommends simultaneous administration of all age-appropriate vaccines (live or inactivated) for which a person is eligible at a single clinic visit, unless contraindications exist. The use of combination vaccines is generally preferred over separate injections, taking into consideration provider assessment, patient preference, and adverse events (CDC, 2011). Use of this vaccine for specific medical and/or other indications (eg, immunocompromising conditions, hepatic or kidney disease, diabetes) is also addressed in the ACIP Recommended Immunization Schedule (CDC, 2013a; CDC, 2013b).

Varilrix (Canadian availability; not available in U.S.): Approved for use in high-risk patients (eg, acute leukemia, chronic disease, organ transplantation) if complete remission ≥12 months (acute leukemia), lymphocyte count ≥1200/mm^3 and evidence of immune competence can be demonstrated prior to vaccination. Canadian National Advisory Committee on Immunization (NACI) suggests that Varivax® III may also be used for select groups (NACI, 2012). Consult product labeling and/or NACI for specific recommendations regarding appropriate use in high risk patients.

Adverse Reactions All serious adverse reactions must be reported to the U.S. Department of Health and Human Services (DHHS) Vaccine Adverse Event Reporting System (VAERS) 1-800-822-7967 or online at https://vaers.hhs.gov/esub/index. In Canada, adverse reactions may be reported to local provincial/territorial health agencies or to the Vaccine Safety Section at Public Health Agency of Canada (1-866-844-0018).

>10%:
- Central nervous system: Fever (10% to 15%)
- Local: Injection site reaction (19% to 33%)

1% to 10%:
- Central nervous system: Chills, fatigue, headache, irritability, malaise, nervousness, sleep disturbance
- Dermatologic: Generalized varicella-like rash (1% to 6%), contact rash, dermatitis, diaper rash, dry skin, eczema, heat rash, itching, urticaria
- Gastrointestinal: Abdominal pain, appetite decreased, cold/canker sore, constipation, diarrhea, nausea, vomiting
- Hematologic: Lymphadenopathy
- Local: Varicella-like rash at the injection site (1% to 3%)
- Neuromuscular & skeletal: Arthralgia, myalgia, stiff neck
- Otic: Otitis
- Respiratory: Cough, lower/upper respiratory illness
- Miscellaneous: Allergic reactions, teething

<1% (Limited to important or life-threatening): Anaphylaxis, anaphylactic shock, angioneurotic edema, aplastic anemia, aseptic meningitis, ataxia, Bell's palsy, cerebellar ataxia (acute), cerebrovascular accident, disseminated varicella infection, encephalitis, erythema multiforme, febrile seizure, Guillain-Barré syndrome, hemiparesis (acute), Henoch-Schönlein purpura (IgA vasculitis), hepatitis, herpes zoster, nonfebrile seizure, pneumonitis, Stevens-Johnson syndrome, thrombocytopenia (including immune thrombocytopenia [ITP]), transverse myelitis, varicella (vaccine strain)

Drug Interactions

Metabolism/Transport Effects None known.

Avoid Concomitant Use

Avoid concomitant use of Varicella Virus Vaccine with any of the following: Belimumab; Fingolimod; Immunosuppressants

Increased Effect/Toxicity

The levels/effects of Varicella Virus Vaccine may be increased by: 5-ASA Derivatives; AzaTHIOprine; Belimumab; Corticosteroids (Systemic); Dimethyl Fumarate; Fingolimod; Hydroxychloroquine; Immunosuppressants; Leflunomide; Mercaptopurine; Methotrexate; Salicylates; Smallpox Vaccine

Decreased Effect

Varicella Virus Vaccine may decrease the levels/effects of: Tuberculin Tests

The levels/effects of Varicella Virus Vaccine may be decreased by: Dimethyl Fumarate; Fingolimod; Immune Globulins; Immunosuppressants

Preparation for Administration Use the total volume of the provided diluent to reconstitute vaccine. Gently agitate to mix thoroughly. (Total volume of reconstituted vaccine will be ~0.5 mL.) Administer vaccine within 30 minutes of preparation.

Storage/Stability Prior to reconstitution and during shipping, store vaccine in freezer at -50°C to -15°C (-58°F to 5°F). Use of dry ice may subject vaccine to temperatures colder than -58°F (-50°C). Vaccine may be stored under refrigeration at 2°C to 8°C (36°F to 46°F) for up to 72 hours. Protect from light. Store diluent at room temperature of 20°C to 25°C (68°F to 77°F) or in refrigerator. Gently agitate to mix thoroughly. (Total volume of reconstituted vaccine will be ~0.5 mL.) Administer immediately following reconstitution, discard reconstituted vaccine if not used within 30 minutes.

Canadian formulations:

Varilrix: Prior to reconstitution, store vaccine under refrigeration at 2°C to 8°C (36°F to 46°F). Vaccine not affected by freezing. Store diluent at 25°C (77°F) or under refrigeration. Following reconstitution, vaccine may be stored for 90 minutes at 25°C (77°F) or up to 8 hours under refrigeration. Discard if not used within recommended times.

Varivax III: Maintain vaccine at -50°C to 8°C (-58°F to 46°F) during transport. Prior to reconstitution, vaccine may be stored in a freezer at temperatures above -50°C (-58°F) or under refrigeration at 2°C to 8°C (36°F to 46°F). Vials transferred from freezer to a refrigerator may be placed back in freezer as long as they have not been reconstituted. Store diluent at room temperature 20°C to 25°C (68°F to77°F) or under refrigeration. Administer immediately following reconstitution; discard reconstituted vaccine if not administered within 90 minutes.

Mechanism of Action As a live, attenuated vaccine, varicella virus vaccine offers active immunity to disease caused by the varicella-zoster virus by inducing cell mediated and humoral immune responses

Pharmacodynamics/Kinetics

Onset of action: Seroconversion occurred in 97% of healthy children ~4-6 weeks following a one dose regimen; using a two dose regimen, the seroconversion rate was 99.9% 6 weeks after the second dose. In adolescents ≥13 years of age and adults, the seroconversion rate was ~75% 4 weeks after the first dose and 99% 4 weeks after the second dose

Duration: Antibody titers detectable at 10 years postvaccination. Actual antibody titers vary by year and age group, but are ~99% to 100% for children at 10 years and 100% for adolescents and adults at 6 years postvaccination. Exposure to wild-type varicella may boost antibody levels.

Dosage SubQ:

U.S. labeling:

Children ≥12 months: 0.5 mL; a second dose may be administered ≥3 months later

Note: The ACIP recommends the routine childhood vaccination be 2 doses, with the first dose administered at 12-15 months of age. The second dose should be administered at 4-6 years of age before school entry, but it may be administered earlier provided ≥3 months have elapsed after the first dose. All children and adolescents who received only 1 dose of vaccine should receive a second dose (CDC, 2007). If the second dose was administered ≥4 weeks after the first dose, it may be considered as valid (CDC, 2013).

Adolescents ≥13 years and Adults: Two doses of 0.5 mL separated by ≥4 weeks (4-8 weeks apart per ACIP). **Note:** The ACIP recommends that all children and adults without evidence of immunity receive 2 doses of the vaccine; those who received only 1 dose of vaccine receive a second dose (CDC, 2007).

Canadian labeling:

Children ≥12 months:

Varilrix: Two doses of 0.5 mL separated by ≥6 weeks

Varivax III: 0.5 mL as a single dose

Alternative recommendations (NACI, 2012): Two doses of 0.5 mL with first dose administered at 12-15 months of age. Separate doses by ≥3 months; however, if rapid protection is necessary, may administer second dose after ≥6 weeks.

Adolescents ≥13 years and Adults: Two single doses 0.5 mL separated by 4-8 weeks (Varivax III) or ≥6 weeks (Varilrix); **Note:** The NACI recommends that adolescents (≥13 years of age) and adults (<50 years of age) who received only 1 dose of vaccine receive a second dose (NACI, 2012).

Dosage adjustment in renal impairment: No dosage adjustment provided in manufacturer's labeling.

Dosage adjustment in hepatic impairment: No dosage adjustment provided in manufacturer's labeling.

Administration For SubQ injection only; inject in the outer aspect of upper arm or the anterolateral thigh. Administer immediately following reconstitution.

Simultaneous administration of vaccines helps ensure the patient will be fully vaccinated by the appropriate age. Simultaneous administration of vaccines is defined as administering >1 vaccine on the same day at different anatomic sites. The use of licensed combination vaccines is generally preferred over separate injections of the equivalent components. Separate vaccines should not be combined in the same syringe unless indicated by product specific labeling. Separate needles and syringes should be used for each injection. The ACIP prefers each dose of a specific vaccine in a series come from the same manufacturer when possible. Adolescents and adults should be vaccinated while seated or lying down. In general, preterm infants should be vaccinated at the same chronological age as full-term infants (CDC, 2011).

Antipyretics have not been shown to prevent febrile seizures. Antipyretics may be used to treat fever or discomfort following vaccination (CDC, 2011). One study reported that routine prophylactic administration of acetaminophen to prevent fever prior to vaccination decreased the immune response of some vaccines; the clinical significance of this reduction in immune response has not been established (Prymula, 2009).

Monitoring Parameters Rash, fever; monitor for syncope for 15 minutes following administration. If seizure-like activity associated with syncope occurs, maintain patient in supine or Trendelenburg position to reestablish adequate cerebral perfusion (CDC, 2011).

Additional Information U.S. federal law requires that the name of medication, date of administration, the vaccine manufacturer, lot number of vaccine, and the administering person's name, title, and address be entered into the patient's permanent medical record.

Evidence of immunity to varicella includes any of the following (CDC, 2007):

Documentation of age appropriate vaccination with varicella vaccine.

Laboratory evidence of immunity or laboratory confirmation of disease.

Birth in the United States prior to 1980 (except for health care personnel, pregnant women and the immunocompromised).

Diagnosis or verification of varicella disease by healthcare provider.

Diagnosis or verification of herpes zoster by healthcare provider.

Persons who lack evidence of immunity should be vaccinated.

Dosage Forms Excipient information presented when available (limited, particularly for generics); consult specific product labeling.

Injectable, Subcutaneous [preservative free]:

Varivax: 1350 PFU/0.5 mL (1 ea)

Dosage Forms: Canada Excipient information presented when available (limited, particularly for generics); consult specific product labeling.

Injection, powder for reconstitution [preservative free]:

Varivax III: 1350 plaque-forming units (PFU) [contains gelatin and trace amounts of neomycin; packaged with diluent]

Injection, powder for reconstitution:

Valrilix: $10^{3.3}$ plaque-forming units (PFU) [contains albumin and gelatin; packaged with diluent]

Varicella-Zoster Immune Globulin (Human)

(var i SEL a- ZOS ter i MYUN GLOB yoo lin HYU man)

Brand Names: U.S. VariZIG
Brand Names: Canada VariZIG
Index Terms VZIG
Pharmacologic Category Blood Product Derivative; Immune Globulin
Additional Appendix Information

Immunization Administration Recommendations *on page 2334*

Immunization Recommendations *on page 2339*

Use

U.S. labeling: Postexposure prophylaxis of varicella in high-risk individuals. High-risk groups include:

- Immunocompromised children and adults
- Newborns of mothers with varicella shortly before or after delivery
- Premature infants
- Neonates and infants <1 year of age
- Adults without evidence of immunity
- Pregnant women

Canadian labeling: In pregnant women, for the prevention or reduction in severity of maternal infection within 4 days of exposure to the varicella zoster virus.

The Advisory Committee on Immunization Practices (ACIP) recommends varicella-zoster immune globulin (VZIG) to patients who are at high risk for severe varicella infection and complications; and who were exposed to varicella or herpes zoster; and for whom varicella vaccine is contraindicated. The decision to use VZIG should take into consideration if the patient lacks evidence of immunity; if exposure is likely to result in an infection; and if the patient is at greater risk for varicella complications than the general population. The following are patient groups for whom VZIG is recommended (CDC, 2013):

- Immunocompromised patients without evidence of immunity, including those with neoplastic disease (eg, leukemia or lymphoma); primary or acquired immunodeficiency; immunosuppressive therapy (including steroid therapy equivalent to prednisone ≥2 mg/kg or 20 mg/day)
- Newborn of mother who had onset of varicella (chickenpox) within 5 days before delivery or within 48 hours after delivery
- Hospitalized premature infants (≥28 weeks gestation) who were exposed during the neonatal period and whose mother has no evidence of immunity
- Hospitalized premature infants (<28 weeks gestation or ≤1000 g) regardless of maternal history and who were exposed during the neonatal period
- Pregnant women without evidence of immunity who have been exposed

Pregnancy Risk Factor C

Pregnancy Considerations Animal reproduction studies have not been conducted. Endogenous immune globulins cross the placenta. Clinical use of other immunoglobulins suggest that there are no adverse effects on the fetus. Women who do not have evidence of immunity to varicella may be at increased risk of complications if infected during pregnancy. Varicella infection in the mother can also lead to intrauterine infection in the fetus. VZIG is primarily used to prevent maternal complications, not fetal infection (CDC, 2007).

Breast-Feeding Considerations It is not known if this preparation is excreted into breast milk; endogenous immune globulins can be found in breast milk (Agarwal, 2011). The manufacturer recommends that caution be used if administered to breast-feeding women.

Contraindications *U.S. labeling:* History of anaphylaxis or other severe reaction associated with past human immune globulin administration; IgA deficiency

Canadian labeling: Additional contraindications (not in US labeling): Hypersensitivity to any component of the formulation; patients with evidence of immunity to varicella zoster virus (ie, with previous varicella infection or vaccination)

Warnings/Precautions [Canadian Boxed Warning]: Hypersensitivity and anaphylactic reactions can occur; immediate treatment (including epinephrine 1:1000) should be available. Reactions can occur in patients with IgA deficiency or hypersensitivity reactions to human globulin.

Noncardiogenic pulmonary edema has been reported with intravenous administration of immune globulin. Monitor for symptoms of transfusion-related acute lung injury (TRALI) including severe respiratory distress, hypoxemia, fever, and pulmonary edema which typically occur within 1-6 hours after administration. Use caution with pre-existing respiratory conditions. Per Canadian labeling, I.M. administration may be preferred in this patient population. Acute renal dysfunction (increased serum creatinine, oliguria, acute renal failure) can rarely occur; usually within 7 days of use (more likely with products stabilized with sucrose). Use with caution in patients with renal disease, diabetes mellitus, volume depletion, sepsis, paraproteinemia, nephrotoxic medications, and in the elderly due to risk of renal dysfunction. Thrombotic events have been reported with administration of intravenous immune globulin; use with caution in patients with cardiovascular risk factors, history of atherosclerosis, advanced age, impaired cardiac output, coagulation disorders, prolonged periods of immobilization, and/or known hyperviscosity disorders. Per Canadian labeling, I.M. administration may be preferred in this patient population. Use with caution in patients with a history of bleeding disorders (including thrombocytopenia) and/or patients on anticoagulant therapy; bleeding/hematoma may occur from I.M. administration.

[Canadian Boxed Warnings]: Product of human plasma; may potentially contain infectious agents which could transmit disease. Screening of donors, as well as testing and/or inactivation or removal of certain viruses, reduces the risk. Infections thought to be transmitted by this product should be reported to the manufacturer (Cangene Corporation 800-768-2304).

Varicella zoster immune globulin should be administered as soon as possible following exposure (within 96 hours, preferred) to reduce the severity of varicella. There is no evidence which shows therapy will reduce the incidence of chickenpox infection after exposure to varicella zoster virus, or that it will effect established varicella zoster virus infections. According to the U.S. CDC guidelines, healthy and immunocompromised patients (except bone marrow transplant recipients [BMT]) with positive history of varicella infection are considered immune. BMT patients who had varicella infection *prior* to transplant are **not** considered immune. BMT patients who develop varicella infection *after* transplant **are** considered immune. Patients who are fully vaccinated, but later became immunocompromised should be monitored closely; treatment with VZIG is not indicated, but other therapy may be needed if disease occurs (CDC, 2007).

Adverse Reactions

U.S. labeling:

1% to 10%:

Central nervous system: Headache (4%), chills (2%), fatigue (2%)

Local: Injection site pain (9%)

Postmarketing and/or case reports: DVT, serum sickness

Canadian labeling:

>10%:

Central nervous system: Headache (7% to 11%)

Local: Injection site pain (17% to 47%)

1% to 10%:

Cardiovascular: Flushing (≤2%)

Central nervous system: Dizziness (≤5%), fever (≤5%), pain (≤5%), chills (≤2%), fatigue (≤2%), insomnia (≤2%)

Dermatologic: Rash (≤5%), dermatitis (≤2%), erythematous rash (≤2%)

Gastrointestinal: Nausea (2% to 5%), dysgeusia (≤2%)

Local: Injection site bruising, itching, or tenderness (≤2%)

Neuromuscular & skeletal: Neck pain (≤5%), myalgia (≤2%)

Drug Interactions

Metabolism/Transport Effects None known.

Avoid Concomitant Use There are no known interactions where it is recommended to avoid concomitant use.

Increased Effect/Toxicity There are no known significant interactions involving an increase in effect.

Decreased Effect

Varicella-Zoster Immune Globulin (Human) may decrease the levels/effects of: Vaccines (Live)

Preparation for Administration Reconstitute only with provided diluent. Inject diluent slowly and at an angle onto the inside glass wall of the vial. Gently invert vial and swirl to dissolve; do not shake. For I.V. administration (Canadian labeling), reconstitute with 2.5 mL/vial (provides 50 units/mL). For I.M. administration, reconstitute with 1.25 mL/vial (provides 100 units/mL).

Storage/Stability Prior to reconstitution, store at 2°C to 8°C (36°F to 46°F); do not freeze. Following reconstitution, may store at 2°C to 8°C (36°F to 46°F) for up to 12 hours.

Mechanism of Action Antibodies obtained from pooled human plasma of individuals with high titers of varicella-zoster provide passive immunity.

Pharmacodynamics/Kinetics

Duration: ≥6 weeks

Metabolism: Metabolized in the reticuloendothelial system

Bioavailability: 100%

Half-life elimination: I.V.: 18-24 days; I.M.: 24-30 days

Time to peak, plasma: I.V.: <3 hours; I.M.: 2-7 days

Dosage

U.S. labeling: Postexposure prophylaxis: Children, Adolescents, and Adults: I.M.: Administer a single dose based on body weight. Dose may be repeated for high-risk patients with additional exposure >3 weeks after initial administration. The minimum dose is 62.5 int. units and the maximum dose is 625 int. units:

≤2 kg: 62.5 units

2.1-10 kg: 125 units

10.1-20 kg: 250 units

20.1-30 kg: 375 units

30.1-40 kg: 500 units

≥40.1 kg: 625 units

Note: Administration should begin as soon as possible and within 10 days after exposure (CDC, 2013).

Canadian labeling: Prevention or reduction of maternal infection: Adults: I.M., I.V.: 125 units/10 kg (minimum dose: 125 units; maximum dose: 625 units). Administer within 96 hours of exposure.

Administration

U.S. labeling: For I.M. administration. Administer into deltoid muscle or anterolateral aspect of upper thigh in ≥2 injections depending on patient size; avoid gluteal region. Do not use >3 mL per injection site.

Canadian labeling: For I.M. or I.V. administration. Bring to room temperature prior to use. Should be given as soon as possible following exposure; efficacy has not been established for use >96 hours following exposure. For I.M. injection, administer into deltoid muscle or anterolateral aspect of upper thigh; avoid gluteal region. For I.V. administration, inject over 3-5 minutes. Pre-existing I.V. lines should be flushed with normal saline prior to administration.

Monitoring Parameters Observe for adverse effects for 20 minutes following administration; baseline assessment of blood viscosity in patients at risk for hyperviscosity; signs and symptoms of varicella infection for 28 days after VZIG administration (CDC, 2013)

Test Interactions May cause false-positive test for immunity to VZV for 3 months following administration. May cause a false-positive Coomb's test.

Dosage Forms Excipient information presented when available (limited, particularly for generics); consult specific product labeling.

Solution Reconstituted, Injection [preservative free]:

VariZIG: 125 units (1 ea) [contains polysorbate 80]

◆ **Varicella-Zoster Virus (VZV) Vaccine (Varicella)** *see* Varicella Virus Vaccine *on page 2168*

◆ **Varilrix (Can)** *see* Varicella Virus Vaccine *on page 2168*

◆ **Varithena** *see* Polidocanol *on page 1666*

◆ **Varivax** *see* Varicella Virus Vaccine *on page 2168*

◆ **Varivax III (Can)** *see* Varicella Virus Vaccine *on page 2168*

◆ **VariZIG** *see* Varicella-Zoster Immune Globulin (Human) *on page 2171*

◆ **Vascepa** *see* Icosapent Ethyl *on page 1038*

◆ **Vascular Endothelial Growth Factor Trap** *see* Ziv-Aflibercept (Systemic) *on page 2233*

◆ **Vaseretic** *see* Enalapril and Hydrochlorothiazide *on page 704*

◆ **VasoClear [OTC]** *see* Naphazoline (Ophthalmic) *on page 1425*

◆ **VasoClear-A [OTC]** *see* Naphazoline (Ophthalmic) *on page 1425*

◆ **Vasocon® (Can)** *see* Naphazoline (Ophthalmic) *on page 1425*

◆ **Vasolex™** *see* Trypsin, Balsam Peru, and Castor Oil *on page 2133*

Vasopressin (vay soe PRES in)

Brand Names: U.S. Pitressin Synthetic

Brand Names: Canada Pressyn®; Pressyn® AR

Index Terms 8-Arginine Vasopressin; ADH; Antidiuretic Hormone; AVP

Pharmacologic Category Antidiuretic Hormone Analog; Hormone, Posterior Pituitary

Additional Appendix Information

Adult ACLS Algorithms *on page 2363*

Vasoactive Agents, Intravenous *on page 2315*

Use Treatment of central diabetes insipidus; differential diagnosis of diabetes insipidus

Unlabeled Use ACLS guidelines: Pulseless arrest (ventricular tachycardia [VT]/ventricular fibrillation [VF], asystole/pulseless electrical activity [PEA]); cardiac arrest secondary to anaphylaxis (unresponsive to epinephrine)

Adjunct in the treatment of GI hemorrhage and esophageal varices; adjunct in the treatment of vasodilatory shock (septic shock); donor management in brain-dead patients (hormone replacement therapy)

Pregnancy Risk Factor C

Pregnancy Considerations Animal reproduction studies have not been conducted. Vasopressin and desmopressin have been used safely during pregnancy based on case reports.

Breast-Feeding Considerations Based on case reports, vasopressin and desmopressin have been used safely during nursing.

Contraindications Hypersensitivity to vasopressin or any component of the formulation

Warnings/Precautions Use with caution in patients with seizure disorders, migraine, asthma, vascular disease, renal disease, cardiac disease; chronic nephritis with nitrogen retention, goiter with cardiac complications, or arteriosclerosis. I.V. administration (unlabeled route): Vesicant; ensure proper needle or catheter placement prior to and during infusion; extravasation may lead to severe vasoconstriction and localized tissue necrosis, gangrene of extremities, tongue, and ischemic colitis; avoid extravasation. May cause water intoxication; early signs include drowsiness, listlessness, and headache, these should be recognized to prevent coma and seizures. Elderly patients should be cautioned not to increase their fluid intake beyond that sufficient to satisfy their thirst in order to avoid water intoxication and hyponatremia; under experimental conditions, the elderly have shown to have a decreased responsiveness to vasopressin with respect to its effects on water homeostasis.

Adverse Reactions Frequency not defined.

Cardiovascular: Arrhythmia, asystole (>0.04 units/minute), blood pressure increased, cardiac output decreased (>0.04 units/minute), chest pain, MI, vasoconstriction (with higher doses), venous thrombosis

Central nervous system: Pounding in head, fever, vertigo

Dermatologic: Ischemic skin lesions, circumoral pallor, urticaria

Gastrointestinal: Abdominal cramps, flatulence, mesenteric ischemia, nausea, vomiting

Genitourinary: Uterine contraction

Neuromuscular & skeletal: Tremor

Respiratory: Bronchial constriction

Miscellaneous: Diaphoresis

Drug Interactions

Metabolism/Transport Effects None known.

Avoid Concomitant Use There are no known interactions where it is recommended to avoid concomitant use.

Increased Effect/Toxicity There are no known significant interactions involving an increase in effect.

Decreased Effect There are no known significant interactions involving a decrease in effect.

Ethanol/Nutrition/Herb Interactions Ethanol: Avoid ethanol (due to effects on ADH).

Storage/Stability Store injection at room temperature; do not freeze. Protect from heat. Use only clear solutions.

Mechanism of Action Increases cyclic adenosine monophosphate (cAMP) which increases water permeability at the renal tubule resulting in decreased urine volume and increased osmolality; causes peristalsis by directly stimulating the smooth muscle in the GI tract; direct vasoconstrictor without inotropic or chronotropic effects

Pharmacodynamics/Kinetics

Onset of action: Nasal: 1 hour

Duration: Nasal: 3-8 hours; I.M., SubQ: 2-8 hours

Metabolism: Nasal/Parenteral: Hepatic, renal

Half-life elimination: Nasal: 15 minutes; Parenteral: 10-20 minutes

Excretion: Nasal: Urine; SubQ: Urine (5% as unchanged drug) after 4 hours

Dosage

Central diabetes insipidus: **Note:** Dosage is highly variable; titrate based on serum and urine sodium and osmolality in addition to fluid balance and urine output. Use of vasopressin is impractical for chronic therapy.

I.M., SubQ:

Children: 2.5-10 units 2-4 times/day as needed

Adults: 5-10 units 2-4 times/day as needed

Continuous I.V. infusion (unlabeled route): **Note:** The optimum rate of infusion has not been well established; many protocols exist.

Children: Initial: 0.0005 units/kg/hour; increase dose by 0.0005 units/kg/hour increments every 5-10 minutes as needed to adequately reduce urine output (maximum dose: 0.01 unit/kg/hour) (Wise-Faberowski, 2004). **Note:** Although clinical trial titrated every 5-10 minutes, a reduced frequency of titration (eg, every 30 minutes) may be more appropriate given the half-life of vasopressin. To provide the infusion dose, the concentration used during the study was 20 units in 500 mL (0.04 units/mL) in D_5W.

Adults: Continuous infusion has not been formally evaluated in the post-neurosurgical adult. However, some convert I.M./SubQ requirement to an hourly continuous I.V. infusion rate.

Central diabetes insipidus, post-traumatic (unlabeled use): Adults: I.V.: Initial: 2.5 units/hour; titrate to adequately reduce urine output (Levitt, 1984)

Donor management in brain-dead patients (hormone replacement therapy) (unlabeled use): Adults: I.V.: Initial: 1 unit bolus followed by 0.5-4 units/hour (Rosendale, 2003; UNOS Critical Pathway, 2002)

GI/variceal hemorrhage (unlabeled use): Continuous I.V. infusion: Dilute in NS or D_5W to 0.1-1 unit/mL. **Note:** Other therapies may be preferred.

GI hemorrhage (unlabeled use): Children: Initial I.V. bolus: 0.3 unit/kg (maximum: 20 units) may be given. Continuous I.V. infusion: 0.001-0.01 units/kg/minute; titrate dose as needed; maximum: 0.01 unit/kg/minute; if bleeding controlled for 12-24 hours, then taper off over 24-36 hours

Variceal hemorrhage (unlabeled use) [AASLD guidelines, 2007]: Adults: Initial: 0.2-0.4 units/minute, may titrate dose as needed to a maximum dose of 0.8 units/minute; maximum duration: 24 hours at highest effective dose continuously (to reduce incidence of adverse effects). Patient should also receive I.V. nitroglycerin concurrently to prevent myocardial ischemic complications; monitor closely for signs/symptoms of ischemia (myocardial, peripheral, bowel)

Pulseless arrest (unlabeled use) [ACLS, 2010]: Adults: I.V., I.O.: 40 units; may give 1 dose to replace first or second dose of epinephrine. I.V./I.O. drug administration is preferred, but if no access, may give endotracheally. ACLS guidelines do not recommend a specific endotracheal dose; however, may be given endotracheally using the same I.V. dose (ACLS, 2010; Wenzel, 1997).

Vasodilatory shock/septic shock (unlabeled use): Adults: I.V.: 0.01-0.03 units/minute for the treatment of septic shock (Russell, 2008). **Note:** May be added to norepinephrine to raise MAP to target or to decrease norepinephrine dose (Dellinger, 2013). Doses >0.03 units/minute may have more cardiovascular side effects and should only be reserved for salvage therapy (ie, failure to achieve MAP goal with other vasopressors) (Dellinger, 2013). To prevent subsequent hypotension after withdrawal of vasopressors, vasopressin should be slowly tapered (eg, titrated down by 0.01 units/minute every 30 minutes) **after** the catecholamine(s) are discontinued until no longer required (Bauer, 2010).

Dosage adjustment in renal impairment: No dosage adjustment provided in manufacturer's labeling.

Dosage adjustment in hepatic impairment: No dosage adjustment provided in manufacturer's labeling.

Usual Infusion Concentrations: Adult I.V. infusion: 100 units in 500 mL (concentration: 0.2 unit/mL) **or** 100 units in 100 mL (concentration: 1 unit/mL) of D_5W or NS

Administration For I.M. or SubQ use (per manufacturer).

I.V. (unlabeled route): May administer as I.V. push over seconds (ACLS) or as a continuous I.V. infusion; when administered as a continuous I.V. infusion for vasodilatory shock, the use of a central venous catheter is recommended. Use extreme caution to avoid extravasation because of risk of necrosis and gangrene. In treatment of varices, infusions are often supplemented with nitroglycerin infusions to minimize cardiac effects.

Vesicant; ensure proper needle or catheter placement prior to and during infusion; avoid extravasation.

Extravasation management: If extravasation occurs, stop infusion immediately and disconnect (leave cannula/needle in place); gently aspirate extravasated solution (do **NOT** flush the line); remove needle/cannula; elevate extremity. Initiate phentolamine (or alternative antidote).

Phentolamine: Dilute 5-10 mg in 10-15 mL NS and administer into extravasation site as soon as possible after extravasation (Peberdy, 2010).

Alternatives to phentolamine (due to shortage):

Nitroglycerin topical 2% ointment (based on limited case reports in neonates/infants): Apply 4 mm/kg as a thin ribbon to the affected areas; may repeat after 8 hours if needed (Wong, 1992) **or** apply a 1-inch strip on the affected site (Denkler, 1989).

Terbutaline (based on limited case reports): Infiltrate extravasation area using a solution of terbutaline 1 mg diluted to 10 mL in NS (large extravasation site; administration volume varied from 3-10 mL) **or** 1 mg diluted in 1 mL NS (small/distal extravasation site; administration volume varied from 0.5-1 mL) (Stier, 1999).

Intranasal (topical administration on nasal mucosa; unlabeled route): Administer injectable vasopressin on cotton plugs, as nasal spray, or by dropper. Should not be inhaled.

Endotracheal (unlabeled route): If no I.V./I.O. access may give endotracheally. ACLS guidelines do not recommend a specific endotracheal dose; however, may be given endotracheally using the same I.V. dose (ACLS, 2010; Wenzel, 1997). Mix with 5-10 mL of water or normal saline, and administer down the endotracheal tube.

Monitoring Parameters Serum and urine sodium, urine specific gravity, urine and serum osmolality; urine output, fluid input and output, blood pressure, heart rate

Consult individual institutional policies and procedures.

Additional Information Vasopressin increases factor VIII levels and may be useful in hemophiliacs.

Dosage Forms Excipient information presented when available (limited, particularly for generics); consult specific product labeling.

Solution, Injection:

Pitressin Synthetic: 20 units/mL (1 mL) [contains chlorobutanol (chlorobutol)]

Generic: 20 units/mL (0.5 mL, 1 mL, 10 mL)

◆ Vasotec *see* Enalapril *on page 701*

◆ Vaxigrip (Can) *see* Influenza Virus Vaccine (Inactivated) *on page 1078*

◆ VCF Vaginal Contraceptive [OTC] *see* Nonoxynol 9 *on page 1471*

◆ Vectibix *see* Panitumumab *on page 1561*

◆ Vectical *see* Calcitriol *on page 314*

Vecuronium (vek ue ROE nee um)

Brand Names: Canada Norcuron®

Index Terms Norcuron; ORG NC 45

Pharmacologic Category Neuromuscular Blocker Agent, Nondepolarizing

Additional Appendix Information

Dosing Considerations for the Critically-Ill Patient With Morbid Obesity *on page 2379*

Use To facilitate endotracheal intubation and to relax skeletal muscles during surgery; to facilitate mechanical ventilation in ICU patients; does not relieve pain or produce sedation

Pregnancy Risk Factor C

Pregnancy Considerations There are no adequate and well-controlled studies in pregnant women. Use in cesarean section has been reported. Umbilical venous concentrations were 11% of maternal. Use only if the potential benefit justifies the potential risk to the fetus.

Breast-Feeding Considerations It is not known if vecuronium is excreted in breast milk. The manufacturer recommends that caution be exercised when administering vecuronium to nursing women.

Contraindications Hypersensitivity to vecuronium or any component of the formulation

Warnings/Precautions Ventilation must be supported during neuromuscular blockade. Vecuronium does not relieve pain or produce sedation; use should include appropriate anesthesia, pain control, and sedation. In patients requiring long-term administration, use of a peripheral nerve stimulator to monitor drug effects is strongly recommended. Additional doses of vecuronium or any other neuromuscular-blocking agent should be avoided unless nerve stimulation response suggests inadequate neuromuscular blockade. Certain clinical conditions may result in potentiation (dosage reduction may be necessary) or antagonism (dosage increase may be necessary) of neuromuscular blockade:

Antagonism: Alkalosis, hypercalcemia, demyelinating lesions, peripheral neuropathies, denervation, immobilization, infection, and muscle trauma

Potentiation: Electrolyte abnormalities, severe hyponatremia, severe hypocalcemia, severe hypokalemia, hypermagnesemia, cachexia, neuromuscular diseases, acidosis, Eaton-Lambert syndrome, and myasthenia gravis

Resistance may occur in burn patients (>30% of body) for period of 5-70 days postinjury. Hypothermia may prolong the duration of action. Use with caution in patients with hepatic impairment; clinical duration may be prolonged. Use with caution in patients who are anephric; clinical duration may be prolonged. Use with caution in patients who have underlying respiratory disease. Some patients may experience delayed recovery of neuromuscular function after administration (especially after prolonged use). Other factors associated with delayed recovery should be considered (eg, corticosteroid use, disease-related conditions). Cross-sensitivity with other neuromuscular-blocking agents may occur; use extreme caution in patients with previous anaphylactic reactions. Use caution in the elderly; dosage reduction may be considered. Children 1-10 years of age may require slightly higher initial doses and slightly more frequent supplementation. **[U.S. Boxed Warning]: Should be administered by adequately trained individuals familiar with its use.** Some dosage forms may contain benzyl alcohol which has been associated with "gasping syndrome" in neonates.

Adverse Reactions <1% (Limited to important or life-threatening): Acute quadriplegic myopathy syndrome (prolonged use), Bradycardia, circulatory collapse, edema, flushing; hypersensitivity reaction (hypotension, tachycardia, erythema, rash, urticaria); itching, myositis ossificans (prolonged use), rash

Drug Interactions

Metabolism/Transport Effects None known.

Avoid Concomitant Use

Avoid concomitant use of Vecuronium with any of the following: QuiNINE

Increased Effect/Toxicity

Vecuronium may increase the levels/effects of: Cardiac Glycosides; Corticosteroids (Systemic); OnabotulinumtoxinA; RimabotulinumtoxinB

The levels/effects of Vecuronium may be increased by: AbobotulinumtoxinA; Aminoglycosides; Calcium Channel Blockers; Capreomycin; Colistimethate; CycloSPORINE (Systemic); Dantrolene; Fosphenytoin-Phenytoin; Inhalational Anesthetics; Ketorolac (Nasal); Ketorolac (Systemic); Lincosamide Antibiotics; Lithium; Loop Diuretics; Magnesium Salts; Piperacillin; Polymyxin B; Procainamide; QuiNIDine; QuiNINE; Spironolactone; Tetracycline Derivatives; Vancomycin

Decreased Effect

The levels/effects of Vecuronium may be decreased by: Acetylcholinesterase Inhibitors; CarBAMazepine; Fosphenytoin-Phenytoin; Loop Diuretics

Preparation for Administration Reconstitute with compatible solution for injection to final concentration of 1 mg/mL. May further dilute reconstituted vial to 0.1-0.2 mg/mL in a compatible solution for I.V. infusion.

Storage/Stability Store intact vials of powder for injection at room temperature 20°C to 25°C (68°F to 77°F). Vials reconstituted with bacteriostatic water for injection (BWFI) may be stored for 5 days under refrigeration or at room temperature. Vials reconstituted with other compatible diluents (nonbacteriostatic) should be stored under refrigeration and used within 24 hours.

Mechanism of Action Blocks acetylcholine from binding to receptors on motor endplate inhibiting depolarization

Pharmacodynamics/Kinetics

Onset of action:

Good intubation conditions: Within 2.5-3 minutes

Maximum neuromuscular blockade: Within 3-5 minutes

Duration: Under balanced anesthesia (time to recovery to 25% of control): 25-40 minutes; recovery 95% complete ~45-65 minutes after injection of intubating dose

Distribution: V_d: 0.3-0.4 L/kg

Protein binding: 60% to 80%

Metabolism: Active metabolite: 3-desacetyl vecuronium (1/2 the activity of parent drug)

Half-life elimination: Healthy surgical patients and renal failure patients undergoing transplant surgery: 65-75 minutes; Late pregnancy: 35-40 minutes

Excretion: Primarily feces (40% to 75%); urine (30% as unchanged drug and metabolites)

Dosage Administer I.V.; dose to effect; doses will vary due to interpatient variability:

Children: ICU paralysis (eg, facilitate mechanical ventilation) in selected adequately sedated patients (unlabeled; Martin, 1999): Initial bolus dose: 0.1-0.15 mg/kg, then a continuous I.V. infusion of 1-2.5 **mcg**/kg/**minute** (0.06-0.15 **mg**/kg/**hour**); monitor depth of blockade using peripheral nerve stimulator every 2-3 hours initially until stable dose, then every 8-12 hours

Intermittent bolus dosing (Eldadah, 1989): 0.1 mg/kg every 1 hour as needed

Children ≥1 year and Adults: Surgical relaxation: **Note:** Children 1-10 years may require slightly higher initial doses and more frequent supplementation.

Tracheal intubation: I.V.: Initial: 0.08-0.1 mg/kg. **Note:** If intubation is performed using succinylcholine (not preferred agent in pediatric patients), the initial dose of vecuronium may be reduced to 0.04-0.06 mg/kg with inhalation anesthesia and 0.05-0.06 mg/kg with balanced anesthesia.

Obesity: For obese (≥130% of IBW) adult patients, may use ideal body weight (IBW) (Erstad, 2004; Schwartz, 1992; Weinstein, 1988); onset time may be slightly delayed using IBW.

Pretreatment/priming: Adults: 10% of intubating dose given 3-5 minutes before intubating dose

Maintenance for continued surgical relaxation (only after return of neuromuscular function): Intermittent dosing: 0.01-0.015 mg/kg **or** continuous infusion of 0.8-1.2 **mcg**/kg/**minute** (0.048-0.072 **mg**/kg/**hour**).

Note: Use lower end of the dosing range when anesthesia is maintained with an inhaled anesthetic agent, with the redosing interval guided by monitoring with a peripheral nerve stimulator.

Adults:

ICU paralysis (eg, facilitate mechanical ventilation) in selected adequately sedated patients (Darrah, 1989; Greenberg, 2013; Murray, 2002; Rudis, 1997): Initial bolus dose: 0.08-0.1 mg/kg, then a continuous I.V. infusion of 0.8-1.7 **mcg**/kg/**minute** (0.048-0.102 **mg**/kg/**hour**); monitor depth of blockade every 1-2 hours initially until stable dose, then every 8-12 hours. Usual maintenance infusion dose range: 0.8-1.2 **mcg**/kg/**minute** (0.048-0.072 **mg**/kg/**hour**).

Dosage adjustment (Rudis, 1996; Rudis, 1997): Adjust rate of administration in increments of 0.3 **mcg**/kg/**minute** (0.018 **mg**/kg/**hour**) or by 50% reductions of previous dose according to peripheral nerve stimulation response or desired clinical response. Discontinue infusion if neuromuscular function does not return.

Note: When possible, minimize depth and duration of paralysis. Stopping the infusion daily for some time until forced to restart based on patient condition is recommended to reduce post-paralytic complications (eg, acute quadriplegic myopathy syndrome [AQMS]) (Murray, 2002; Segredo, 1992).

Intermittent bolus dosing (Hunter, 1985): 0.1-0.2 mg/kg/dose; may be repeated when neuromuscular function returns

Control of refractory shivering in adequately sedated patients during therapeutic hypothermia after cardiac arrest (unlabeled use; Bernard, 2002; Nolan, 2003; Polderman, 2009): I.V.: 8-12 mg; redose as needed to control shivering. **Note:** Duration of action prolonged in hypothermic patients. May mask seizure activity.

Elderly: No specific guidelines available; refer to adult dosing. Dose selection should be cautious, at low end of dosage range, and titration should be slower to evaluate response.

Dosage adjustment in renal impairment: No dosage adjustment provided in manufacturer's labeling. However, patients with renal impairment do not experience clinically significant prolongation of neuromuscular blockade with vecuronium; however, in patients who are anephric, the clinical duration is prolonged.

Dosage adjustment in hepatic impairment: No dosage adjustment provided in manufacturer's labeling. However, dosage reduction may be necessary in patients with liver disease.

Usual Infusion Concentrations: Pediatric I.V. infusion: 0.1 mg/mL, 0.2 mg/mL, 1 mg/mL

Usual Infusion Concentrations: Adult I.V. infusion: 10 mg in 100 mL (concentration: 0.1 mg/mL), 20 mg in 100 mL (concentration: 0.2 mg/mL), **or** 50 mg in 50 mL (concentration: 1 mg/mL) of D_5W or NS

Administration Concentration of 1 mg/mL may be administered by rapid I.V. injection; may also be used for I.V. infusion in fluid-restricted patients.

Monitoring Parameters Blood pressure, heart rate; peripheral nerve stimulation (eg, train-of-four [TOF] count)

Additional Information Vecuronium is classified as an intermediate-duration neuromuscular-blocking agent. It produces minimal, if any, histamine release; does not relieve pain or produce sedation. It may produce cumulative effect on duration of blockade.

Dosage Forms Excipient information presented when available (limited, particularly for generics); consult specific product labeling.

Solution Reconstituted, Intravenous, as bromide:
Generic: 10 mg (1 ea); 20 mg (1 ea)

Solution Reconstituted, Intravenous, as bromide [preservative free]:
Generic: 10 mg (1 ea); 20 mg (1 ea)

◆ VEGF Trap *see* Aflibercept (Ophthalmic) *on page 56*

◆ VEGF Trap *see* Ziv-Aflibercept (Systemic) *on page 2233*

◆ VEGF Trap-Eye *see* Aflibercept (Ophthalmic) *on page 56*

◆ VEGF Trap R1R2 *see* Ziv-Aflibercept (Systemic) *on page 2233*

Velaglucerase Alfa (vel a GLOO ser ase AL fa)

Brand Names: U.S. Vpriv

Brand Names: Canada VPRIV

Index Terms Gene-Activated Human Acid-Beta-Glucosidase; GlcCerase

Pharmacologic Category Enzyme

Use Gaucher disease: For long-term enzyme replacement therapy for pediatric and adult patients with type 1 Gaucher disease.

Pregnancy Risk Factor B

Dosage Note: Pretreatment with antihistamines and/or corticosteroids can be considered for prevention of subsequent infusion reactions in patients with hypersensitivity reactions requiring symptomatic treatment; during clinical studies, patients were not routinely premedicated prior to infusion.

I.V.: Children ≥4 years, Adolescents, and Adults: Gaucher's disease (type 1): 60 units/kg every 2 weeks; adjust dose based upon disease activity (range: 15-60 units/kg evaluated in clinical trials)

Note: When switching from imiglucerase to velaglucerase alfa in stable patients, initiate treatment 2 weeks after the last imiglucerase dose and at the same dose.

Dosage adjustment in renal impairment: No dosage adjustment provided in manufacturer's labeling.

Dosage adjustment in hepatic impairment: No dosage adjustment provided in manufacturer's labeling.

Additional Information Complete prescribing information should be consulted for additional detail.

Dosage Forms Excipient information presented when available (limited, particularly for generics); consult specific product labeling.

Solution Reconstituted, Intravenous [preservative free]:
Vpriv: 400 units (1 ea)

◆ Velban *see* VinBLAStine *on page 2189*

◆ Velcade *see* Bortezomib *on page 270*

◆ Veletri *see* Epoprostenol *on page 727*

◆ Velivet *see* Ethinyl Estradiol and Desogestrel *on page 784*

◆ Veltin™ *see* Clindamycin and Tretinoin *on page 455*

Vemurafenib (vem ue RAF e nib)

Brand Names: U.S. Zelboraf

Brand Names: Canada Zelboraf

Index Terms BRAF(V600E) Kinase Inhibitor RO5185426; PLX4032; RG7204; RO5185426

Pharmacologic Category Antineoplastic Agent, BRAF Kinase Inhibitor

Use Melanoma:

U.S. labeling: Treatment of unresectable or metastatic melanoma in patients with a $BRAF^{V600E}$ mutation (as detected by an approved test); **Note:** Not recommended in patients with wild-type BRAF melanoma.

Canadian labeling: Treatment of unresectable or metastatic melanoma in patients with a $BRAF^{V600}$ mutation (as identified by a validated test)

Unlabeled Use Treatment of metastatic melanoma in patients with a $BRAF^{V600K}$ mutation

Pregnancy Risk Factor D

Pregnancy Considerations Adverse effects were not demonstrated in animal reproduction studies. Based on the mechanism of action, vemurafenib may cause fetal harm if administered during pregnancy or in patients who become pregnant during treatment. Women of childbearing potential and men of reproductive potential should use adequate contraception methods during and for at least 2 months after treatment (Canadian labeling recommends during and for at least 6 months after treatment).

Breast-Feeding Considerations It is not known if vemurafenib is excreted in breast milk. Due to the potential for serious adverse reactions in the nursing infant, the decision to discontinue vemurafenib or to discontinue breast-feeding during treatment should take into account the benefits of treatment to the mother.

Prescribing and Access Restrictions Available through specialty pharmacies. Further information may be obtained from the manufacturer, Genentech, at 1-888-249-4918, or at http://www.zelboraf.com.

Medication Guide Available Yes

Contraindications There are no contraindications listed within the manufacturer's labeling.

Canadian labeling: Hypersensitivity to vemurafenib or any component of the formulation.

Warnings/Precautions Hazardous agent - use appropriate precautions for handling and disposal (meets NIOSH, 2012 criteria). Only patients with a $BRAF^{V600}$ mutation-positive melanoma (including $BRAF^{V600E}$) will benefit from treatment; mutation must be detected and confirmed by an approved test prior to treatment. The cobas® 4800 BRAF V600 Mutation Test was used in clinical trials and is FDA-approved to detect $BRAF^{V600E}$ mutation.

Cutaneous squamous cell carcinomas (cuSCC), keratoacanthomas, and melanoma have been reported (at a higher rate in patients receiving vemurafenib compared to control). Cutaneous SCC generally occurs early in the treatment course (median onset: 7-8 weeks) and is managed with excision (while continuing vemurafenib treatment). Approximately one-third of patients experienced >1 cuSCC occurrence and the median time between occurrences was 6 weeks. Potential risk factors for cuSCC include age ≥65 years, history of skin cancer, or chronic sun exposure. Monitor for skin lesions (with dermatology evaluation) at baseline and every 2 months during treatment; consider continued monitoring for 6 months after treatment. Noncutaneous squamous cell carcinomas (SCC) of the head and neck have also been observed; monitor closely for signs/symptoms. Vemurafenib may promote malignancies correlated with RAS activation; monitor for signs/symptoms of other malignancies.

Dermatologic reactions have been observed, including case reports of Stevens-Johnson syndrome and toxic epidermal necrolysis; discontinue (permanently) for severe dermatologic toxicity. Photosensitivity ranging from mild to severe has been reported. Advise patients to avoid sun exposure and wear protective clothing and use effective UVA/UVB sunscreen and lip balm (SPF ≥30) when outdoors. Dosage modification are recommended for intolerable photosensitivity consisting of erythema ≥10% to 30% of body surface area. Uveitis cases have been reported;

monitor for signs and symptoms; may be managed with corticosteroid and mydriatic eye drops. Cases of blurred vision, iritis, photophobia, and a single case of retinal vein occlusion have been reported in clinical trials.

QT prolongation (dose-dependent) has been observed; may lead to increased risk for ventricular arrhythmia, including torsade de pointes. Monitor electrolytes (calcium, magnesium and potassium) at baseline and with dosage adjustments. Monitor ECG at baseline, 15 days after initiation, then monthly for 3 months, then every 3 months thereafter (more frequently if clinically appropriate); also monitor with dosage adjustments. Do not initiate treatment if baseline QT_c >500 msec. During treatment, if QT_c >500 msec, temporarily interrupt treatment; correct electrolytes and control other risk factors for QT prolongation. May reinitiate with a dose reduction once QT_c falls to <500 msec. Discontinue (permanently), if after correction of risk factors, both the QT_c continues to increase >500 msec and there is >60 msec change above baseline. Use is not recommended in patients with electrolyte abnormalities which are not correctable, long QT syndrome, or taking concomitant medication known to prolong the QT interval.

Increases in liver function tests have been reported. Monitor transaminases, alkaline phosphatase and bilirubin at baseline and monthly during therapy, or as clinically necessary. May require dosage reduction, therapy interruption, or discontinuation. Severe hypersensitivity (including anaphylaxis, rash [generalized], erythema, or hypotension), has been reported with use and following reinitiation of treatment. Discontinue (permanently) with severe hypersensitivity reaction. Elderly patients may be at increased risk for adverse effects; in clinical trials, there was an increased incidence of cuSCC and keratoacanthoma, atrial fibrillation, peripheral edema, and nausea/decreased appetite in patients ≥65 years of age. Potentially significant drug-drug interactions may exist, requiring dose or frequency adjustment, additional monitoring, and/or selection of alternative therapy.

Adverse Reactions

>10%:

Cardiovascular: Peripheral edema (17% to 23%)

Central nervous system: Fatigue (38% to 54%), headache (23% to 27%)

Dermatologic: Skin rash (37% to 52%; grade 3: 7% to 8%), skin photosensitivity (33% to 49%; grade 3: 3%), alopecia (36% to 45%), pruritus (23% to 30%), hyperkeratosis (24% to 28%; actinic: 8% to 17%; seborrheic: 10% to 14%; pilaris: ≤10%), maculopapular rash (9% to 21%), xeroderma (16% to 19%), sunburn (10% to 14%), erythema (8% to 14%), papular rash (5% to 13%)

Gastrointestinal: Nausea (35% to 37%; grade 3: 2%), diarrhea (28% to 29%; grade 3: <1%), vomiting (18% to 26%; grade 3: 1% to 2%), decreased appetite (18% to 21%), constipation (12% to 16%), dysgeusia (11% to 14%)

Hematologic & oncologic: Skin neoplasm (papilloma; 21% to 30%), squamous cell carcinoma of skin (24%; grade 3: 22% to 24%)

Hepatic: Increased gamma-glutamyl transferase (5% to 15%)

Neuromuscular & skeletal: Arthralgia (53% to 67%), myalgia (13% to 24%), limb pain (9% to 18%), back pain (8% to 11%), musculoskeletal pain (8% to 11%), weakness (2% to 11%)

Respiratory: Cough (8% to 12%)

Miscellaneous: Fever (17% to 19%)

≤10% and/or case reports:

Cardiovascular: Atrial fibrillation, hypotension, prolonged Q-T interval on ECG, retinal vein occlusion, vasculitis

Central nervous system: Cranial nerve palsy (facial), dizziness, peripheral neuropathy

Dermatologic: Erythema nodosum, folliculitis, palmar-plantar erythrodysesthesia, Stevens-Johnson syndrome, toxic epidermal necrolysis

Endocrine & metabolic: Weight loss

Hematologic & oncologic: Malignant melanoma (new primary), basal cell carcinoma, squamous cell carcinoma (oropharyngeal)

Hepatic: Increased serum alkaline phosphatase, increased serum ALT, increased serum AST, increased serum bilirubin

Hypersensitivity: Anaphylaxis, hypersensitivity

Neuromuscular & skeletal: Arthritis

Ophthalmic: Blurred vision, iritis, photophobia, uveitis

Renal: Increased serum creatinine

Drug Interactions

Metabolism/Transport Effects Substrate of BCRP, CYP3A4 (major), P-glycoprotein; **Note:** Assignment of Major/Minor substrate status based on clinically relevant drug interaction potential; **Inhibits** BCRP, CYP1A2 (moderate), CYP2D6 (weak), P-glycoprotein; **Induces** CYP3A4 (weak/moderate)

Avoid Concomitant Use

Avoid concomitant use of Vemurafenib with any of the following: Axitinib; Bosutinib; CYP3A4 Inducers (Strong); CYP3A4 Inhibitors (Strong); Fusidic Acid (Systemic); Highest Risk QTc-Prolonging Agents; Ivabradine; Mifepristone; Moderate Risk QTc-Prolonging Agents; Pirfenidone; Pomalidomide; Silodosin; Simeprevir; Topotecan; VinCRIStine (Liposomal)

Increased Effect/Toxicity

Vemurafenib may increase the levels/effects of: Afatinib; Agomelatine; ARIPiprazole; Bosutinib; Colchicine; CYP1A2 Substrates; Dabigatran Etexilate; Everolimus; Highest Risk QTc-Prolonging Agents; P-glycoprotein/ABCB1 Substrates; Pirfenidone; Pomalidomide; Porfimer; Prucalopride; Rivaroxaban; Silodosin; Topotecan; VinCRIStine (Liposomal); Vitamin K Antagonists

The levels/effects of Vemurafenib may be increased by: CYP3A4 Inhibitors (Moderate); CYP3A4 Inhibitors (Strong); Dasatinib; Fusidic Acid (Systemic); Ipilimumab; Ivabradine; Ivacaftor; Luliconazole; Mifepristone; Moderate Risk QTc-Prolonging Agents; P-glycoprotein/ABCB1 Inhibitors; QTc-Prolonging Agents (Indeterminate Risk and Risk Modifying); Simeprevir

Decreased Effect

Vemurafenib may decrease the levels/effects of: ARIPiprazole; Axitinib; Cardiac Glycosides; Ibrutinib; Saxagliptin; Simeprevir; Vitamin K Antagonists

The levels/effects of Vemurafenib may be decreased by: Bosentan; CYP3A4 Inducers (Strong); Dabrafenib; Deferasirox; Herbs (CYP3A4 Inducers); P-glycoprotein/ABCB1 Inducers; Tocilizumab

Storage/Stability Store at room temperature of 20°C to 25°C (68°F to 77°F); excursions permitted to 15°C and 30°C (59°F and 86°F). Store in the original container with the lid tightly closed.

Mechanism of Action BRAF kinase inhibitor (potent) which inhibits tumor growth in melanomas by inhibiting kinase activity of certain mutated forms of BRAF, including BRAF with V600E mutation, thereby blocking cellular proliferation in melanoma cells with the mutation. Does not have activity against cells with wild-type BRAF. $BRAF^{V600E}$ activating mutations are present in ~50% of melanomas; V600E mutation involves the substitution of glutamic acid for valine at amino acid 600. The cobas® 4800 BRAF V600 mutation test is approved to detect $BRAF^{V600E}$ mutation.

Pharmacodynamics/Kinetics

Distribution: V_d: ~106 L

Protein binding: >99%, to albumin and α_1-acid glycoprotein

Half-life, elimination: 57 hours (range: 30-120 hours)

Time to peak: ~3 hours

Excretion: Feces (~94%); urine (~1%)

Dosage

U.S. labeling: Melanoma, metastatic or unresectable (with $BRAF^{V600E}$ mutation): 960 mg twice daily; continue until disease progression or unacceptable toxicity.

Canadian labeling: Melanoma, metastatic or unresectable (with $BRAF^{V600}$ mutation): 960 mg twice daily; continue until disease progression or unacceptable toxicity.

Missed doses: A missed dose may be taken up to 4 hours prior to the next scheduled dose to maintain a twice daily schedule; both doses should not be taken at the same time.

Dosing adjustment for toxicity: Note: Do not dose reduce below 480 mg twice daily. NCI Common Terminology Criteria for Adverse Events (CTC-AE) version 4.0 used for adverse event grades.

Grade 1 or grade 2 (tolerable) toxicity: No dosage adjustment recommended.

Grade 2 (intolerable) or grade 3 toxicity:

First incident: Interrupt treatment until toxicity returns to grade 0 or 1, then resume at 720 mg twice daily.

Second incident: Interrupt treatment until toxicity returns to grade 0 or 1, then resume at 480 mg twice daily.

Third incident: Discontinue permanently

Grade 4 toxicity:

First incident: Interrupt treatment until toxicity returns to grade 0 or 1, then resume at 480 mg twice daily **or** discontinue permanently.

Second incident: Discontinue permanently.

Specific toxicities:

Severe hypersensitivity or severe dermatologic toxicity: Discontinue permanently.

QT_c interval changes:

QT_c >500 msec (grade ≥3): Temporarily withhold treatment, correct electrolytes and control risk factors for QT prolongation; may reinitiate with a dose reduction once QT_c <500 msec.

QT_c persistently >500 msec and >60 msec above baseline: Discontinue permanently.

QT_c interval changes: Canadian labeling:

QT_c >500 msec during treatment and <60 msec change from baseline:

First incident: Interrupt treatment until QT_c <500 msec, then resume at 720 mg twice daily or 480 mg twice daily if dose previously reduced.

Second incident: Interrupt treatment until QT_c <500 msec, then resume at 480 mg twice daily or discontinue permanently if dose previously reduced to 480 mg twice daily.

Third incident: Discontinue permanently.

QT_c >500 msec during treatment and >60 msec above baseline: Discontinue permanently.

Dosage adjustment in renal impairment:

Mild-to-moderate impairment (pre-existing): No dosage adjustment necessary.

Severe impairment (pre-existing): No dosage adjustment provided in manufacturer's labeling (data is insufficient to determine if dosage adjustment necessary); use with caution.

Dosage adjustment in hepatic impairment:

Mild-to-moderate impairment (pre-existing): No dosage adjustment necessary.

Severe impairment (pre-existing): No dosage adjustment provided in manufacturer's labeling (data is insufficient to determine if dosage adjustment necessary); use with caution.

Hepatotoxicity/lab abnormalities during treatment: Refer to dosage adjustment for toxicity and manage with dose reduction, treatment interruption, or discontinuation.

Dietary Considerations May be taken with or without food.

Administration Doses should be administered orally in the morning and evening, ~12 hours apart. Swallow whole with a glass of water; do not crush or chew. May be taken with or without a meal.

Hazardous agent; use appropriate precautions for handling and disposal (meets NIOSH, 2012 criteria).

Monitoring Parameters Liver transaminases, alkaline phosphatase and bilirubin at baseline and monthly during treatment (or as clinically appropriate). Electrolytes (calcium, magnesium and potassium) at baseline and after dosage modification. ECG at baseline, 15 days after initiation, then monthly for 3 months, then every 3 months thereafter (more frequently if clinically appropriate) and with dosage adjustments. Dermatology evaluation (for new skin lesions) at baseline and every 2 months during treatment; also consider continued monitoring for 6 months after completion of treatment. Signs/symptoms of hypersensitivity reactions, and uveitis, and malignancies.

Dosage Forms Excipient information presented when available (limited, particularly for generics); consult specific product labeling.

Tablet, Oral:

Zelboraf: 240 mg

Venlafaxine (ven la FAX een)

Brand Names: U.S. Effexor XR

Brand Names: Canada Apo-Venlafaxine XR; CO Venlafaxine XR; Dom-Venlafaxine XR; Effexor XR; GD-Venlafaxine XR; Mylan-Venlafaxine XR; PMS-Venlafaxine XR; Ran-Venlafaxine XR; Riva-Venlafaxine XR; Sandoz-Venlafaxine XR; Teva-Venlafaxine XR; Venlafaxine XR

Pharmacologic Category Antidepressant, Serotonin/Norepinephrine Reuptake Inhibitor

Additional Appendix Information

Antidepressant Agents *on page 2284*

Use Treatment of major depressive disorder, generalized anxiety disorder (GAD), social anxiety disorder (social phobia), panic disorder

Unlabeled Use Obsessive-compulsive disorder (OCD); hot flashes; neuropathic pain (including diabetic neuropathy); attention-deficit/hyperactivity disorder (ADHD); post-traumatic stress disorder (PTSD); migraine prophylaxis

Pregnancy Risk Factor C

Pregnancy Considerations Adverse events have been observed in some animal reproduction studies. Venlafaxine and its active metabolite ODV cross the human placenta. An increased risk of teratogenic effects following venlafaxine exposure during pregnancy has not been observed, based on available data. The risk of spontaneous abortion may be increased. Neonatal seizures and neonatal abstinence syndrome have been noted in case reports following maternal use of venlafaxine during pregnancy. Nonteratogenic effects in the newborn following SSRI/SNRI exposure late in the third trimester include respiratory distress, cyanosis, apnea, seizures, temperature instability, feeding difficulty, vomiting, hypoglycemia, hyper- or hypotonia, hyper-reflexia, jitteriness, irritability, constant crying, and tremor. Symptoms may be due to the toxicity of the SNRI or a discontinuation syndrome and may be consistent with serotonin syndrome associated with treatment. The long-term effects of *in utero* SNRI/SSRI exposure on infant development and behavior are not known.

Due to pregnancy-induced physiologic changes, some pharmacokinetic parameters of venlafaxine may be altered. Women should be monitored for decreased efficacy. The ACOG recommends that therapy with SSRIs or SNRIs during pregnancy be individualized; treatment of depression during pregnancy should incorporate the clinical expertise of the mental health clinician, obstetrician, primary healthcare provider, and pediatrician. According to the American Psychiatric Association (APA), the risks of medication treatment should be weighed against other treatment options and untreated depression. For women who discontinue antidepressant medications during pregnancy and who may be at high risk for postpartum depression, the medications can be restarted following delivery. Treatment algorithms have been developed by the ACOG and the APA for the management of depression in women prior to conception and during pregnancy.

Breast-Feeding Considerations Venlafaxine and ODV are found in breast milk and the serum of nursing infants. Adverse events have not been observed; however, it is recommended to monitor the infant for adverse events if the decision to breast-feed has been made. The long-term effects on neurobehavior have not been studied, thus one should prescribe venlafaxine to a mother who is breast-feeding only when the benefits outweigh the potential risks. The manufacturer does not recommend breast-feeding during therapy.

Medication Guide Available Yes

Contraindications Hypersensitivity to venlafaxine or any component of the formulation; use of MAO inhibitors intended to treat psychiatric disorders (concurrently or within 14 days of discontinuing the MAO inhibitor); initiation of MAO inhibitor intended to treat psychiatric disorders within 7 days of discontinuing venlafaxine; initiation of venlafaxine in a patient receiving linezolid or intravenous methylene blue

Warnings/Precautions [U.S. Boxed Warning]: Antidepressants increase the risk of suicidal thinking and behavior in children, adolescents, and young adults (18-24 years of age) with major depressive disorder (MDD) and other psychiatric disorders; consider risk prior to prescribing. Short-term studies did not show an increased risk in patients >24 years of age and showed a decreased risk in patients ≥65 years. Closely monitor for clinical worsening, suicidality, or unusual changes in behavior; the patient's family or caregiver should be instructed to closely observe the patient and communicate condition with healthcare provider. Reduced growth rate has been observed with venlafaxine therapy in children. A medication guide should be dispensed with each prescription. **Venlafaxine is not FDA approved for use in children.**

The possibility of a suicide attempt is inherent in major depression and may persist until remission occurs. Monitor for worsening of depression or suicidality, especially during initiation of therapy (generally first 1-2 months) or with dose increases or decreases. Use caution in high-risk patients. Worsening depression and severe abrupt suicidality that are not part of the presenting symptoms may require discontinuation or modification of drug therapy. The patient's family or caregiver should be alerted to monitor patients for the emergence of suicidality and associated behaviors (such as agitation, irritability, hostility, impulsivity, and hypomania) and call healthcare provider.

May worsen psychosis in some patients or precipitate a shift to mania or hypomania in patients with bipolar disorder. Patients presenting with depressive symptoms should be screened for bipolar disorder. Monotherapy in patients with bipolar disorder should be avoided. **Venlafaxine is not FDA approved for the treatment of bipolar depression.**

Potentially life-threatening serotonin syndrome (SS) has occurred with serotonergic agents (eg, SSRIs, SNRIs), particularly when used in combination with other serotonergic agents (eg, triptans, TCAs, fentanyl, lithium, tramadol, buspirone, St John's wort, tryptophan) or agents that impair metabolism of serotonin (eg, MAO inhibitors intended to treat psychiatric disorders, other MAO inhibitors [ie, linezolid and intravenous methylene blue]). Discontinue treatment (and any concomitant serotonergic agent) immediately if signs/symptoms arise.

May cause sustained increase in blood pressure or tachycardia; dose related and increases are generally modest (12-15 mm Hg diastolic). Control pre-existing hypertension prior to initiation of venlafaxine. Use caution in patients with recent history of MI, unstable heart disease, or hyperthyroidism; may cause increase in anxiety, nervousness, insomnia; may cause weight loss (use with caution in patients where weight loss is undesirable); may cause increases in serum cholesterol. Use caution with hepatic or renal impairment; dosage adjustments recommended. May cause hyponatremia/SIADH (elderly at increased risk); volume depletion (diuretics may increase risk).

Bleeding related to SSRI or SNRI use has been reported to range from relatively minor bruising and epistaxis to life-threatening hemorrhage. Interstitial lung disease and eosinophilic pneumonia have been rarely reported; may present as progressive dyspnea, cough, and/or chest pain. Prompt evaluation and possible discontinuation of therapy may be necessary. Venlafaxine may increase the risks associated with electroconvulsive therapy. Use cautiously in patients with a history of seizures. The risks of cognitive or motor impairment, as well as the potential for anticholinergic effects are very low. May cause or exacerbate sexual dysfunction. Bone fractures have been associated with antidepressant treatment. Consider the possibility of a fragility fracture if an antidepressant-treated patient presents with unexplained bone pain, point tenderness, swelling, or bruising (Rabenda, 2013; Rizzoli, 2012).

Use caution in elderly patients; may cause or exacerbate syndrome of inappropriate antidiuretic hormone secretion or hyponatremia; monitor sodium closely with initiation or dosage adjustments in older adults (Beers Criteria). Use caution in patients with increased intraocular pressure or at risk of acute narrow-angle glaucoma. Potentially significant drug-drug interactions may exist, requiring dose or frequency adjustment, additional monitoring, and/or selection of alternative therapy.

Abrupt discontinuation or interruption of antidepressant therapy has been associated with a discontinuation syndrome. Symptoms arising may vary with antidepressant however commonly include nausea, vomiting, diarrhea, headaches, lightheadedness, dizziness, diminished appetite, sweating, chills, tremors, paresthesias, fatigue, somnolence, and sleep disturbances (eg, vivid dreams, insomnia). Greater risks for developing a discontinuation syndrome have been associated with antidepressants with shorter half-lives, longer durations of treatment, and abrupt discontinuation. For antidepressants of short or intermediate half-lives, symptoms may emerge within 2-5 days after treatment discontinuation and last 7-14 days (APA, 2010; Fava, 2006; Haddad, 2001; Shelton, 2001; Warner, 2006).

Adverse Reactions Note: Actual frequency may be dependent upon formulation and/or indication

>10%:

Central nervous system: Headache (25% to 38%), somnolence (12% to 26%), dizziness (11% to 24%), insomnia (15% to 24%), nervousness (6% to 21%), anxiety (2% to 11%),

Gastrointestinal: Nausea (21% to 58%), xerostomia (12% to 22%), anorexia (8% to 17%), constipation (8% to 15%)

Genitourinary: Abnormal ejaculation/orgasm (2% to 19%)

Neuromuscular & skeletal: Weakness (8% to 19%)

Miscellaneous: Diaphoresis (7% to 19%)

1% to 10%:

Cardiovascular: Vasodilation (2% to 6%), hypertension (dose related; 3% in patients receiving <100 mg/day, up to 13% in patients receiving >300 mg/day), palpitation (3%), tachycardia (2%), chest pain (2%), orthostatic hypotension (1%), edema

Central nervous system: Yawning (3% to 8%), abnormal dreams (3% to 7%), chills (2% to 7%), agitation (2% to 5%), confusion (2%), abnormal thinking (2%), depersonalization (1%), depression (1% to 3%), fever, migraine, amnesia, hypoesthesia, vertigo

Dermatologic: Rash (3%), pruritus (1%), bruising

Endocrine & metabolic: Libido decreased (2% to 8%), hypercholesterolemia (5%), triglycerides increased

Gastrointestinal: Abdominal pain (8%), diarrhea (8%), vomiting (3% to 8%), dyspepsia (5% to 7%), weight loss (1% to 6%), flatulence (3% to 4%), taste perversion (2%), appetite increased, belching, weight gain

Genitourinary: Impotence (4% to 6%), urinary frequency (3%), urination impaired (2%), urinary retention (1%), metrorrhagia, prostatic disorder, vaginitis

Neuromuscular & skeletal: Tremor (1% to 10%), hypertonia (3%), paresthesia (2% to 3%), twitching (1% to 3%), arthralgia, neck pain, trismus

Ocular: Accommodation abnormal (6% to 9%), abnormal or blurred vision (4% to 6%), mydriasis (2%)

Otic: Tinnitus (2%)

Renal: Albuminuria

Respiratory: Pharyngitis (7%), sinusitis (2%), bronchitis, cough increased, dyspnea

Miscellaneous: Infection (6%), flu-like syndrome (2%), trauma (2%)

<1% (Limited to important or life-threatening): Agranulocytosis, anaphylaxis, anemia, aneurysm, angina pectoris, angioedema, anuria, aplastic anemia, appendicitis, arrhythmia (including atrial and ventricular tachycardia, fibrillation, and torsade de pointes), arteritis, asthma, ataxia, atelectasis, atrioventricular block, bacteremia, balance/coordination impaired, basophilia, bigeminy, biliary pain, bilirubinemia, bleeding time increased, bradycardia, bradykinesia, BUN increased, bundle branch block, carcinoma, cardiac arrest, cardiovascular disorder (mitral valve and circulatory disturbance), cataract, catatonia, cellulitis, cerebral ischemia, cholelithiasis, congestive heart failure, coronary artery disease, CPK increased, creatinine increased, crystalluria, cyanosis, deafness, DVT, dehydration, delusions, dementia, diabetes mellitus, dystonia, ECG abnormalities (including QT prolongation), embolus, eosinophilia, erythema multiforme, exfoliative dermatitis, extrapyramidal symptoms, extrasystoles, facial paralysis, fasciitis, fatty liver, gastrointestinal ulcer, glaucoma, glycosuria, granuloma, Guillain-Barré syndrome, hematemesis, hematoma, hemorrhage (eye, GI, mucocutaneous, rectal), hepatic necrosis, hepatic failure, hepatitis, homicidal ideation, hostility, hyperacusis, hypercalcinuria, hyperchlorhydria, hyper-/hypoglycemia, hyper-/hypokalemia, hyper-/hypophosphatemia, hyper-/hypothyroidism, hyperuricemia, hypocholesteremia, hyponatremia, hypoproteinemia, hypotension, interstitial lung disease (including eosinophilic pneumonia), intestinal obstruction, jaundice, kidney function abnormal, larynx edema, leukocytosis, leukoderma, leukopenia, liver enzymes increased, loss of consciousness, lymphadenopathy, lymphocytosis, maculopapular rash, menstrual abnormalities, MI, miliaria, moniliasis, multiple myeloma, myasthenia, myoclonus, myopathy, neck rigidity, neuroleptic malignant-like syndrome, neuropathy, neutropenia, osteoporosis, pancreatitis, pancytopenia, peripheral vascular disorder, pleurisy, pneumonia, pyelonephritis, pyuria, renal failure, rhabdomyolysis, rheumatoid arthritis, seizure, serotonin syndrome, SIADH, skin atrophy, Stevens-Johnson syndrome, suicidal ideation (reported at a frequency up to 2% in children/adolescents with major depressive disorder), suicide attempt, syncope, tendon rupture, thrombocythemia, thrombocytopenia, tongue edema, toxic epidermal necrolysis, withdrawal syndrome

Drug Interactions

Metabolism/Transport Effects Substrate of CYP2C19 (minor), CYP2C9 (minor), CYP2D6 (major), CYP3A4 (major); **Note:** Assignment of Major/Minor substrate status based on clinically relevant drug interaction potential; **Inhibits** CYP2B6 (weak), CYP2D6 (weak), CYP3A4 (weak)

Avoid Concomitant Use

Avoid concomitant use of Venlafaxine with any of the following: Conivaptan; Fusidic Acid (Systemic); Iobenguane I 123; Linezolid; MAO Inhibitors; Methylene Blue

Increased Effect/Toxicity

Venlafaxine may increase the levels/effects of: Agents with Antiplatelet Properties; Alpha-/Beta-Agonists; Anticoagulants; Antipsychotics; Aspirin; Collagenase (Systemic); Dabigatran Etexilate; Dofetilide; Highest Risk QTc-Prolonging Agents; Ibritumomab; Lomitapide; Methylene Blue; Moderate Risk QTc-Prolonging Agents; NSAID (Nonselective); Rivaroxaban; Salicylates; Serotonin Modulators; Thrombolytic Agents; Tositumomab and Iodine I 131 Tositumomab; TraZODone; Vitamin K Antagonists

The levels/effects of Venlafaxine may be increased by: Abiraterone Acetate; Alcohol (Ethyl); Antipsychotics; Conivaptan; CYP2D6 Inhibitors (Moderate); CYP2D6 Inhibitors (Strong); CYP3A4 Inhibitors (Moderate); CYP3A4 Inhibitors (Strong); Darunavir; Dasatinib; Fusidic Acid (Systemic); Glucosamine; Herbs (Anticoagulant/Antiplatelet Properties); Ibrutinib; Ivacaftor; Linezolid; Luliconazole; MAO Inhibitors; Metoclopramide; Mifepristone; Multivitamins/Fluoride (with ADE); Multivitamins/Minerals (with ADEK, Folate, Iron); Multivitamins/Minerals (with AE, No Iron); Nonsteroidal Anti-Inflammatory Agents; Omega-3 Fatty Acids; Pentosan Polysulfate Sodium; Pentoxifylline; Propafenone; Prostacyclin Analogues; Simeprevir; Tipranavir; Vitamin E; Voriconazole

Decreased Effect

Venlafaxine may decrease the levels/effects of: Alpha2-Agonists; Indinavir; Iobenguane I 123; Ioflupane I 123

The levels/effects of Venlafaxine may be decreased by: Bosentan; CYP3A4 Inducers (Strong); Dabrafenib; Deferasirox; Mitotane; Nonsteroidal Anti-Inflammatory Agents; Peginterferon Alfa-2b; Tocilizumab

Ethanol/Nutrition/Herb Interactions

Ethanol: May increase CNS depression; monitor for increased effects with coadministration. Caution patients about effects.

Herb/Nutraceutical: Avoid valerian, St John's wort, SAMe, kava kava, tryptophan (may increase risk of serotonin syndrome and/or excessive sedation).

Storage/Stability Store at controlled room temperature of 20°C to 25°C (68°F to 77°F).

Mechanism of Action Venlafaxine and its active metabolite, O-desmethylvenlafaxine (ODV), are potent inhibitors of neuronal serotonin and norepinephrine reuptake and weak inhibitors of dopamine reuptake. Venlafaxine and ODV have no significant activity for muscarinic cholinergic, H_1-histaminergic, or $alpha_2$-adrenergic receptors. Venlafaxine and ODV do not possess MAO-inhibitory activity.

Pharmacodynamics/Kinetics

Absorption: Oral: ≥92%; food has no significant effect on absorption or formation of active metabolite

Distribution: V_{dss}: Venlafaxine 7.5 ± 3.7 L/kg, ODV 5.7 ± 1.8 L/Kg

Protein binding: Venlafaxine 27% ± 2%, ODV 30% ± 12%

Metabolism: Hepatic via CYP2D6 to active metabolite, O-desmethylvenlafaxine (ODV); other metabolites include N-desmethylvenlafaxine and N,O-didesmethylvenlafaxine

Bioavailability: Oral: ~45%

Half-life elimination: Venlafaxine: 5 ± 2 hours; ODV: 11 ± 2 hours; prolonged with cirrhosis (venlafaxine: ~30%, ODV: ~60%), renal impairment (venlafaxine: ~50%, ODV: ~40%), and during dialysis (venlafaxine: ~180%, ODV: ~142%)

Time to peak:

Immediate release: Venlafaxine: 2 hours, ODV: 3 hours

Extended release: Venlafaxine: 5.5 hours, ODV: 9 hours

Excretion: Urine (~87%; 5% of total dose as unchanged drug; 29% of total dose as unconjugated ODV; 26% of total dose as conjugated ODV; 27% of total dose as minor inactive metabolites)

Dosage Oral:

Children and Adolescents:

Attention-deficit/hyperactivity disorder (unlabeled use; Olvera, 1996): Initial: 12.5 mg/day

Children <40 kg: Increase by 12.5 mg/week to maximum of 50 mg/day in 2 divided doses

Children ≥40 kg: Increase by 25 mg/week to maximum of 75 mg/day in 3 divided doses.

Mean dose: 60 mg or 1.4 mg/kg administered in 2-3 divided doses

Adults:

Depression:

Immediate-release tablets: Initial: 75 mg/day, administered in 2 or 3 divided doses; may increase in ≤75 mg/day increments at intervals of ≥4 days as tolerated (maximum daily dose: 225-375 mg)

Extended-release capsules or tablets: Initial: 37.5-75 mg once daily; in patients who are initiated at 37.5 mg once daily, may increase to 75 mg once daily after 4-7 days; dose may then be increased by ≤75 mg/day increments at intervals of ≥4 days as tolerated (maximum daily dose: 225 mg)

Generalized anxiety disorder: Extended-release capsules: Initial: 37.5-75 mg once daily; in patients who are initiated at 37.5 mg once daily, may increase to 75 mg once daily after 4-7 days; may then be increased by ≤75 mg/day increments at intervals of ≥4 days as tolerated (maximum daily dose: 225 mg)

Panic disorder: Extended-release capsules: Initial: 37.5 mg once daily for 1 week; may increase to 75 mg once daily after 7 days, may then be increased by ≤75 mg/day increments at intervals of ≥7 days (maximum daily dose: 225 mg).

Social anxiety disorder: Extended-release capsules or tablets: 75 mg once daily (maximum daily dose: 75 mg); no evidence that doses >75 mg/day offer any additional benefit

Obsessive-compulsive disorder (unlabeled use): Titrate to usual dosage range of 150-300 mg/day; however, doses up to 375 mg/day have been used; response may be seen in 4 weeks (Phelps, 2005)

Neuropathic pain (unlabeled use): Dosages evaluated varied considerably based on etiology of chronic pain, but efficacy has been shown for many conditions in the range of 75-225 mg/day; onset of relief may occur in 1-2 weeks, or take up to 6 weeks for full benefit (Grothe, 2004).

Diabetic neuropathy (unlabeled use): 75-225 mg/day (Bril, 2011)

Hot flashes (unlabeled use): Doses of 37.5-75 mg/day have demonstrated significant improvement of vasomotor symptoms after 4-8 weeks of treatment; in one study, doses >75 mg/day offered no additional benefit (Evans, 2005; Loprinzi, 2000); however, higher doses (225 mg/day) may be beneficial in patients with perimenopausal depression

Attention-deficit disorder (unlabeled use): Initial: Doses vary between 18.75 to 75 mg/day; may increase after 4 weeks to 150 mg/day; if tolerated, doses up to 225 mg/day have been used (Maidment, 2003)

Post-traumatic stress disorder (PTSD) (unlabeled use): Extended release formulation: 37.5-300 mg/day (Bandelow, 2008; Benedek, 2009)

Elderly: Refer to adult dosing. No specific recommendations for elderly, but may be best to start lower at 25-50 mg twice daily and increase as tolerated by 25 mg/dose. Extended-release formulation: 37.5 mg once daily, increase by 37.5 mg every 4-7 days as tolerated

Discontinuation of therapy: Upon discontinuation of antidepressant therapy, gradually taper the dose to minimize the incidence of withdrawal symptoms and allow for the detection of re-emerging symptoms. Evidence supporting ideal taper rates is limited. APA and NICE guidelines suggest tapering therapy over at least several weeks with consideration to the half-life of the antidepressant; antidepressants with a shorter half-life may need to be tapered more conservatively. In addition for long-term treated patients, WFSBP guidelines recommend tapering over 4-6 months. If intolerable withdrawal symptoms occur following a dose reduction, consider resuming the previously prescribed dose and/or decrease dose at a more gradual rate (APA, 2010; Bauer, 2002; Haddad, 2001; NCCMH, 2010; Schatzberg, 2006; Shelton, 2001; Warner, 2006).

MAO inhibitor recommendations:

Switching to or from an MAO inhibitor intended to treat psychiatric disorders:

Allow 14 days to elapse between discontinuing an MAO inhibitor intended to treat psychiatric disorders and initiation of venlafaxine.

Allow 7 days to elapse between discontinuing venlafaxine and initiation of an MAO inhibitor intended to treat psychiatric disorders.

Use with other MAO inhibitors (linezolid or I.V. methylene blue):

Do not initiate venlafaxine in patients receiving linezolid or I.V. methylene blue; consider other interventions for psychiatric condition.

If urgent treatment with linezolid or I.V. methylene blue is required in a patient already receiving venlafaxine and potential benefits outweigh potential risks, discontinue venlafaxine promptly and administer linezolid or I.V. methylene blue. Monitor for SS for 7 days or until 24 hours after the last dose of linezolid or I.V. methylene blue, whichever comes first. May resume venlafaxine 24 hours after the last dose of linezolid or I.V. methylene blue.

Dosing adjustment in renal impairment:

GFR: 10-70 mL/minute: Reduce total daily dose by 25% to 50%

Hemodialysis: Reduce total daily dose by 50%

Dosing adjustment in hepatic impairment: Mild-to-moderate hepatic impairment: Reduce total daily dose by 50%; further reductions may be necessary in some patients

Dietary Considerations Should be taken with food.

Administration Administer with food.

Extended-release formulations: Swallow capsule or tablet whole; do not crush or chew. Contents of capsule may be sprinkled on a spoonful of applesauce and swallowed immediately without chewing; followed with a glass of water to ensure complete swallowing of the pellets.

Monitoring Parameters Blood pressure should be regularly monitored, especially in patients with a high baseline blood pressure; may cause mean increase in heart rate of 4-9 beats/minute; cholesterol; mental status for depression, suicide ideation (especially at the beginning of therapy or when doses are increased or decreased), anxiety, social functioning, mania, panic attacks; signs/symptoms of serotonin syndrome; height and weight should be monitored in children

Test Interactions May interfere with urine detection of PCP and amphetamine (false-positives).

Dosage Forms Excipient information presented when available (limited, particularly for generics); consult specific product labeling.

Capsule Extended Release 24 Hour, Oral:
Effexor XR: 37.5 mg, 75 mg, 150 mg
Generic: 37.5 mg, 75 mg, 150 mg

Tablet, Oral:
Generic: 25 mg, 37.5 mg, 50 mg, 75 mg, 100 mg

Tablet Extended Release 24 Hour, Oral:
Generic: 37.5 mg, 75 mg, 150 mg, 225 mg

- Venlafaxine XR (Can) *see* Venlafaxine *on page 2178*
- Venofer *see* Iron Sucrose *on page 1121*
- Ventavis *see* Iloprost *on page 1047*
- Ventolin® (Can) *see* Albuterol *on page 61*
- Ventolin® Diskus (Can) *see* Albuterol *on page 61*
- Ventolin HFA *see* Albuterol *on page 61*
- Ventolin® HFA (Can) *see* Albuterol *on page 61*
- Ventolin® I.V. Infusion (Can) *see* Albuterol *on page 61*
- Ventolin® Nebules P.F. (Can) *see* Albuterol *on page 61*
- VePesid *see* Etoposide *on page 802*
- Vepesid™ (Can) *see* Etoposide *on page 802*
- Veramyst *see* Fluticasone (Nasal) *on page 896*

Verapamil (ver AP a mil)

Brand Names: U.S. Calan; Calan SR; Isoptin SR; Verelan; Verelan PM

Brand Names: Canada Apo-Verap®; Apo-Verap® SR; Covera-HS®; Covera®; Dom-Verapamil SR; Isoptin® SR; Mylan-Verapamil; Mylan-Verapamil SR; Novo-Veramil; Novo-Veramil SR; Nu-Verap; Nu-Verap SR; PHL-Verapamil SR; PMS-Verapamil SR; PRO-Verapamil SR; Riva-Verapamil SR; Verapamil Hydrochloride Injection, USP; Verapamil SR; Verelan®

Index Terms Iproveratril Hydrochloride; Verapamil Hydrochloride

Pharmacologic Category Antianginal Agent; Antiarrhythmic Agent, Class IV; Antihypertensive; Calcium Channel Blocker; Calcium Channel Blocker, Nondihydropyridine

Additional Appendix Information

Calcium Channel Blockers - Comparative Pharmacokinetics *on page 2296*

Dosing Considerations for the Critically-Ill Patient With Morbid Obesity *on page 2379*

Use

Oral: Treatment of hypertension; angina pectoris (vasospastic, chronic stable, unstable) (Calan®, Covera-HS®); supraventricular tachyarrhythmia (PSVT, atrial fibrillation/flutter [rate control])

I.V.: Supraventricular tachyarrhythmia (PSVT, atrial fibrillation/flutter [rate control])

Unlabeled Use Hypertrophic cardiomyopathy; bipolar disorder (manic manifestations)

Pregnancy Risk Factor C

Pregnancy Considerations Adverse events were observed in some animal reproduction studies in doses which also caused maternal toxicity. Verapamil crosses the placenta. Use during pregnancy may cause adverse fetal effects (bradycardia, heart block, hypotension) (Tan, 2001). Verapamil may be used to control atrial fibrillation in pregnant women (Fuster, 2006). Women with hypertrophic cardiomyopathy who are controlled with verapamil prior to pregnancy may continue therapy, but increased fetal monitoring is recommended (Gersh, 2011). Verapamil is not the preferred treatment for paroxysmal supraventricular tachycardia (PSVT) in pregnant women (Blomström-Lundqvist, 2003). Untreated chronic maternal hypertension is associated with adverse events in the fetus, infant, and mother. If treatment for hypertension during pregnancy is needed, other agents are preferred (ACOG, 2012; Chobanian, 2003).

Breast-Feeding Considerations Verapamil is excreted into breast milk; the estimated exposure to the nursing infant is <1% of the maternal dose. Breast-feeding is not recommended by some manufacturers. Breast-fed infants of mothers taking medications for hypertension should be monitored for adverse effects (Chobanian, 2003).

Contraindications Hypersensitivity to verapamil or any component of the formulation; severe left ventricular dysfunction; hypotension (systolic pressure <90 mm Hg) or cardiogenic shock; sick sinus syndrome (except in patients with a functioning artificial ventricular pacemaker); second- or third-degree AV block (except in patients with a functioning artificial ventricular pacemaker); atrial flutter or fibrillation and an accessory bypass tract (Wolff-Parkinson-White [WPW] syndrome, Lown-Ganong-Levine syndrome)

I.V.: Additional contraindications include concurrent use of I.V. beta-blocking agents; ventricular tachycardia

Warnings/Precautions Avoid use in heart failure; can exacerbate condition; use is contraindicated in severe left ventricular dysfunction. Symptomatic hypotension with or without syncope can rarely occur; blood pressure must be lowered at a rate appropriate for the patient's clinical condition. Rare increases in hepatic enzymes can be observed. Can cause first-degree AV block or sinus bradycardia; use is contraindicated in patients with sick sinus syndrome, second- or third-degree AV block (except in patients with a functioning artificial pacemaker), or an accessory bypass tract (eg, WPW syndrome). Other conduction abnormalities are rare. Considered contraindicated in patients with wide complex tachycardias unless known to be supraventricular in origin; severe hypotension likely to occur upon administration (ACLS, 2010). Use caution when using verapamil together with a beta-blocker. Administration of I.V. verapamil and an I.V. beta-blocker within a few hours of each other may result in asystole and should be avoided; simultaneous administration is contraindicated. Use with other agents known to reduce SA node function and/or AV nodal conduction (eg, digoxin) or reduce sympathetic outflow (eg, clonidine) may increase the risk of serious bradycardia. Verapamil significantly increases digoxin serum concentrations; adjust digoxin dose. Use with caution in patients with HCM with outflow tract obstruction (especially those with high gradients, advanced heart failure, or sinus bradycardia); may be used in patients who cannot tolerate beta-blockade. Verapamil should not be used in those with systemic hypotension or severe dyspnea at rest (Gersh, 2011; Nishimura, 2004).

Decreased neuromuscular transmission has been reported with verapamil; use with caution in patients with attenuated neuromuscular transmission (Duchenne's muscular dystrophy, myasthenia gravis); dosage reduction may be required. Use with caution in renal impairment; monitor hemodynamics and possibly ECG if severe impairment, particularly if concomitant hepatic impairment. Use with caution in patients with hepatic impairment; dosage reduction may be required; monitor hemodynamics and possibly ECG if severe impairment. May prolong recovery from nondepolarizing neuromuscular-blocking agents. Use Covera-HS® (extended-release delivery system) with caution in patients with severe GI narrowing. In patients with extremely short GI transit times (eg, <7 hours), dosage adjustment may be required; inadequate pharmacokinetic data. I.V. use for SVT for is not recommended in infants; use with caution in children as myocardial depression/hypotension may occur.

Adverse Reactions

>10%:

Central nervous system: Headache (1% to 12%)

Gastrointestinal: Gingival hyperplasia (≤19%), constipation (7% to 12%)

1% to 10%:

Cardiovascular: Peripheral edema (1% to 4%), hypotension (3%), CHF/pulmonary edema (2%), AV block (1% to 2%), bradycardia (HR <50 bpm: 1%), flushing (1%)

Central nervous system: Fatigue (2% to 5%), dizziness (1% to 5%), lethargy (3%), pain (2%), sleep disturbance (1%)

Dermatologic: Rash (1% to 2%)

Gastrointestinal: Dyspepsia (3%), nausea (1% to 3%), diarrhea (2%)

Hepatic: Liver enzymes increased (1%)

Neuromuscular & skeletal: Myalgia (1%), paresthesia (1%)

Respiratory: Dyspnea (1%)

Miscellaneous: Flu-like syndrome (4%)

Oral: ≤1%: Abdominal discomfort, alopecia, angina, arthralgia, atrioventricular dissociation, blurred vision, bruising, cerebrovascular accident, chest pain, claudication, confusion, diaphoresis, ECG abnormal, equilibrium disorders, erythema multiforme, exanthema, extrapyramidal symptoms, galactorrhea/hyperprolactinemia, gastrointestinal distress, gynecomastia, hyperkeratosis, impotence, insomnia, macules, MI, muscle cramps, palpitation, psychosis, purpura (vasculitis), shakiness, somnolence, spotty menstruation, Stevens-Johnson syndrome, syncope, tinnitus, urination increased, urticaria, weakness, xerostomia

I.V.: <1% (Limited to important or life-threatening): Bronchi/laryngeal spasm, depression, diaphoresis, itching, muscle fatigue, respiratory failure, rotary nystagmus, seizure, sleepiness, urticaria, vertigo

Postmarketing and/or case reports: Asystole, eosinophilia, EPS, exfoliative dermatitis, GI obstruction, hair color change, paralytic ileus, Parkinsonian syndrome, pulseless electrical activity, shock, ventricular fibrillation

Drug Interactions

Metabolism/Transport Effects Substrate of CYP1A2 (minor), CYP2B6 (minor), CYP2C9 (minor), CYP2E1 (minor), CYP3A4 (major), P-glycoprotein; **Note:** Assignment of Major/Minor substrate status based on clinically relevant drug interaction potential; **Inhibits** CYP1A2 (weak), CYP2C9 (weak), CYP2D6 (weak), CYP3A4 (moderate), P-glycoprotein

Avoid Concomitant Use

Avoid concomitant use of Verapamil with any of the following: Bosutinib; Conivaptan; Dantrolene; Disopyramide; Dofetilide; Fusidic Acid (Systemic); Ibrutinib; Ivabradine; Lomitapide; PAZOPanib; Pimozide; Pomalidomide; Simeprevir; Tolvaptan; Topotecan; Ulipristal; VinCRIStine (Liposomal)

Increased Effect/Toxicity

Verapamil may increase the levels/effects of: Afatinib; Alcohol (Ethyl); Aliskiren; Amifostine; Amiodarone; Antihypertensives; ARIPiprazole; AtorvaSTATin; Atosiban; Avanafil; Benzodiazepines (metabolized by oxidation); Beta-Blockers; Bosentan; Bosutinib; Budesonide (Systemic, Oral Inhalation); BusPIRone; Calcium Channel Blockers (Dihydropyridine); CarBAMazepine; Cardiac Glycosides; Colchicine; Corticosteroids (Systemic); CycloSPORINE (Systemic); CYP3A4 Substrates; Dabigatran Etexilate; Disopyramide; Dofetilide; Dronedarone; Eletriptan; Eplerenone; Everolimus; Fexofenadine; Fingolimod; Flecainide; Fosphenytoin; Halofantrine; Hypotensive Agents; Ibrutinib; Imatinib; Ivabradine; Ivacaftor; Lithium; Lomitapide; Lovastatin; Lurasidone; Magnesium Salts; Midodrine; Neuromuscular-Blocking Agents (Nondepolarizing); Nitroprusside; Obinutuzumab; OxyCODONE; PAZOPanib; P-glycoprotein/ABCB1 Substrates; Phenytoin; Pimecrolimus; Pimozide; Pomalidomide; Propafenone; Prucalopride; QuiNIDine; Ranolazine; Red Yeast Rice; RisperiDONE; RiTUXimab; Rivaroxaban; Salicylates; Salmeterol; Saxagliptin; Simeprevir; Simvastatin; Tacrolimus (Systemic); Tacrolimus (Topical); Tolvaptan; Topotecan; Ulipristal; Vilazodone; VinCRIStine (Liposomal); Zuclopenthixol

The levels/effects of Verapamil may be increased by: Alpha1-Blockers; Anilidopiperidine Opioids; Antifungal Agents (Azole Derivatives, Systemic); AtorvaSTATin; Brimonidine (Topical); Calcium Channel Blockers (Dihydropyridine); Cimetidine; CloNIDine; Conivaptan; CycloSPORINE (Systemic); CYP3A4 Inhibitors (Moderate); CYP3A4 Inhibitors (Strong); Dantrolene; Dasatinib; Diazoxide; Dronedarone; Fluconazole; Fusidic Acid (Systemic); Grapefruit Juice; Herbs (Hypotensive Properties); Ivabradine; Ivacaftor; Luliconazole; Macrolide Antibiotics; Magnesium Salts; MAO Inhibitors; Mifepristone; Pentoxifylline; P-glycoprotein/ABCB1 Inhibitors; Phosphodiesterase 5 Inhibitors; Prostacyclin Analogues; Protease Inhibitors; QuiNIDine; Regorafenib; Simeprevir; Telithromycin

Decreased Effect

Verapamil may decrease the levels/effects of: Clopidogrel; Ifosfamide

The levels/effects of Verapamil may be decreased by: Barbiturates; Bosentan; Calcium Salts; CarBAMazepine; CYP3A4 Inducers (Strong); Dabrafenib; Deferasirox; Herbs (CYP3A4 Inducers); Herbs (Hypertensive Properties); Methylphenidate; Mitotane; Nafcillin; P-glycoprotein/ABCB1 Inducers; Rifamycin Derivatives; Tocilizumab; Yohimbine

Ethanol/Nutrition/Herb Interactions

Ethanol: Verapamil may increase ethanol levels. Management: Avoid or limit ethanol.

Food: Grapefruit juice may increase the serum concentration of verapamil. Management: Avoid grapefruit juice or use with caution and monitor for effects. Calan® SR and Isoptin® SR products should be taken with food or milk; other formulations may be administered without regard to meals.

Herb/Nutraceutical: St John's wort may decrease levels of verapamil. Some herbal medications have hypertensive properties (eg, licorice); others may increase or decrease the antihypertensive effect of verapamil. Management: Avoid St John's wort, bayberry, blue cohosh, cayenne, ephedra, ginger, ginseng (American), kola, licorice, and yohimbe. Avoid black cohosh, California poppy, coleus, golden seal, hawthorn, mistletoe, periwinkle, quinine, and shepherd's purse.

Storage/Stability Store at controlled room temperature of 15°C to 30°C (59°F to 86°F). Protect from light.

Mechanism of Action Inhibits calcium ion from entering the "slow channels" or select voltage-sensitive areas of vascular smooth muscle and myocardium during depolarization; produces relaxation of coronary vascular smooth muscle and coronary vasodilation; increases myocardial oxygen delivery in patients with vasospastic angina; slows automaticity and conduction of AV node.

Pharmacodynamics/Kinetics

Onset of action: Peak effect: Oral: Immediate release: 1-2 hours; I.V.: 1-5 minutes

Duration: Oral: Immediate release tablets: 6-8 hours; I.V.: 10-20 minutes
Absorption: Well absorbed
Distribution: V_d: 3.89 L/kg (Storstein, 1984)
Protein binding: ~90%
Metabolism: Hepatic (extensive first-pass effect) via multiple CYP isoenzymes; primary metabolite is norverapamil (20% pharmacologic activity of verapamil)
Bioavailability: Oral: 20% to 35%
Half-life elimination: Infants: 4.4-6.9 hours; Adults: Single dose: 3-7 hours, Multiple doses: 4.5-12 hours; severe hepatic impairment: 14-16 hours
Time to peak, serum: Oral:
Immediate release: 1-2 hours
Extended release (Covera-HS®, Verelan PM®): ~11 hours, drug release delayed ~4-5 hours
Sustained release: 5.21 hours (Calan® SR, Isoptin® SR); 7-9 hours (Verelan®)
Excretion: Urine (70% as metabolites, 3% to 4% as unchanged drug); feces (16%)

Dosage

Children: **Note:** Verapamil is no longer included in the Pediatric Advanced Life Support (PALS) tachyarrhythmia algorithm.
Children: 1-15 years: SVT: I.V.: 0.1-0.3 mg/kg/dose over 2 minutes; maximum: 5 mg/dose, may repeat dose in 30 minutes if inadequate response; maximum for second dose: 10 mg

Adults:
SVT (ACLS, 2010): I.V.: 2.5-5 mg over 2 minutes; second dose of 5-10 mg (~0.15 mg/kg) may be given 15-30 minutes after the initial dose if patient tolerates, but does not respond to initial dose; maximum total dose: 20-30 mg
Angina: Oral: **Note:** When switching from immediate-release to extended/sustained release formulations, the total daily dose remains the same unless formulation strength does not allow for equal conversion.
Immediate release: Initial: 80-120 mg 3 times/day (elderly or small stature: 40 mg 3 times/day); Usual dose range (Gibbons, 2003): 80-160 mg 3 times/day
Extended release (Covera-HS®): Initial: 180 mg once daily at bedtime; if inadequate response, may increase dose at weekly intervals to 240 mg once daily, then 360 mg once daily, then 480 mg once daily; maximum dose: 480 mg/day
Chronic atrial fibrillation (rate-control), PSVT prophylaxis: Oral: Immediate release: 240-480 mg/day in 3-4 divided doses; Usual dose range (Fuster, 2006): 120-360 mg/day in divided doses
Hypertension: Oral: **Note:** When switching from immediate-release to extended/sustained release formulations, the total daily dose remains the same unless formulation strength does not allow for equal conversion.
Immediate release: 80 mg 3 times/day; usual dose range (JNC 7): 80-320 mg/day in 2 divided doses
Sustained release: Usual dose range (JNC 7): 120-480 mg/day in 1-2 divided doses; **Note:** There is no evidence of additional benefit with doses >360 mg/day.
Calan® SR, Isoptin® SR: Initial: 180 mg once daily in the morning (elderly or small stature: 120 mg/day); if inadequate response, may increase dose at weekly intervals to 240 mg once daily, then 180 mg twice daily (or 240 mg in the morning followed by 120 mg in the evening); maximum dose: 240 mg twice daily.
Verelan®: Initial: 180 mg once daily in the morning (elderly or small stature: 120 mg/day); if inadequate response, may increase dose at weekly intervals to 240 mg once daily, then 360 mg once daily, then 480 mg once daily; maximum dose: 480 mg/day
Extended release: Usual dose range (JNC 7): 120-360 mg once daily (once-daily dosing is recommended at bedtime)
Covera-HS®: Initial: 180 mg once daily at bedtime; if inadequate response, may increase dose at weekly intervals to 240 mg once daily, then 360 mg once daily, then 480 mg once daily; maximum dose: 480 mg/day
Verelan® PM: Initial: 200 mg once daily at bedtime (elderly or small stature: 100 mg/day); if inadequate response, may increase dose at weekly intervals to 300 mg once daily, then 400 mg once daily; maximum dose: 400 mg/day

Elderly: Hypertension: Oral: **Note:** When switching from immediate release to extended or sustained release formulations, the total daily dose remains the same unless formulation strength does not allow for equal conversion.
Manufacturer's recommendations:
Immediate release: Initial: 40 mg 3 times daily
Sustained release: Calan® SR, Isoptin® SR,Verelan®: Initial: 120 mg once daily in the morning
Extended release:
Covera-HS®: Initial: 180 mg once daily at bedtime
Verelan® PM: Initial: 100 mg once daily at bedtime
ACCF/AHA Expert Consensus recommendations: Consider lower initial doses and titrating to response (Aronow, 2011)

Dosing adjustment in renal impairment: Manufacturer recommends caution and additional ECG monitoring in patients with renal insufficiency. The manufacturer of Verelan PM® recommends an initial dose of 100 mg/day at bedtime. **Note:** A multiple dose study in adults suggests reduced renal clearance of verapamil and its metabolite (norverapamil) with advanced renal failure (Storstein, 1984). Additionally, several clinical papers report adverse effects of verapamil in patients with chronic renal failure receiving recommended doses of verapamil (Pritza, 1991; Váquez, 1996). In contrast, a number of single dose studies show no difference in verapamil (or norverapamil metabolite) disposition between chronic renal failure and control patients (Beyerlein, 1990; Hanyok, 1988; Mooy, 1985; Zachariah, 1991).
Dialysis: Not removed by hemodialysis (Mooy, 1985); supplemental dose is not necessary.

Dosing adjustment/comments in hepatic disease: In cirrhosis, reduce dose to 20% and 50% of normal for oral and intravenous administration, respectively, and monitor ECG (Somogyi, 1981). The manufacturer of Verelan PM® recommends an initial adult dose of 100 mg/day at bedtime. The manufacturers of Calan®, Calan® SR, Covera-HS®, Isoptin® SR, and Verelan® recommend giving 30% of the normal dose to patients with severe hepatic impairment.

Dietary Considerations Calan® SR and Isoptin® SR products may be taken with food or milk, other formulations may be administered without regard to meals; sprinkling contents of Verelan® or Verelan® PM capsule onto applesauce does not affect oral absorption.

Administration

Oral: Do not crush or chew sustained or extended release products.
Calan® SR, Isoptin® SR: Administer with food.
Verelan®, Verelan® PM: Capsules may be opened and the contents sprinkled on 1 tablespoonful of applesauce, then swallowed immediately without chewing. Do not subdivide contents of capsules.
I.V.: Rate of infusion: Over 2 minutes; over 3 minutes in older patients (ACLS, 2010)

Monitoring Parameters Monitor blood pressure and heart rate; periodic liver function tests; ECG, especially with renal and/or hepatic impairment

Consult individual institutional policies and procedures.

Test Interactions May interfere with urine detection of methadone (false-positive).

Dosage Forms Excipient information presented when available (limited, particularly for generics); consult specific product labeling. [DSC] = Discontinued product

Capsule Extended Release 24 Hour, Oral, as hydrochloride:
- Verelan: 120 mg [DSC]
- Verelan: 120 mg [contains fd&c red #40, methylparaben, propylparaben]
- Verelan: 180 mg [DSC]
- Verelan: 180 mg [contains fd&c red #40, methylparaben, propylparaben]
- Verelan: 240 mg [DSC]
- Verelan: 240 mg [contains brilliant blue fcf (fd&c blue #1), fd&c red #40, methylparaben, propylparaben]
- Verelan: 360 mg [DSC]
- Verelan: 360 mg [contains brilliant blue fcf (fd&c blue #1), fd&c red #40, methylparaben, propylparaben]
- Verelan PM: 100 mg [DSC]
- Verelan PM: 100 mg [contains brilliant blue fcf (fd&c blue #1), fd&c red #40]
- Verelan PM: 200 mg [DSC]
- Verelan PM: 200 mg [contains brilliant blue fcf (fd&c blue #1), fd&c red #40]
- Verelan PM: 300 mg [DSC]
- Verelan PM: 300 mg [contains brilliant blue fcf (fd&c blue #1), fd&c red #40]
- Generic: 100 mg, 120 mg, 180 mg, 200 mg, 240 mg, 300 mg, 360 mg

Solution, Intravenous, as hydrochloride:
- Generic: 2.5 mg/mL (2 mL, 4 mL)

Tablet, Oral, as hydrochloride:
- Calan: 80 mg, 120 mg [scored]
- Generic: 40 mg, 80 mg, 120 mg

Tablet Extended Release, Oral, as hydrochloride:
- Calan SR: 120 mg
- Calan SR: 180 mg [scored]
- Calan SR: 240 mg [scored; contains fd&c blue #2 aluminum lake, fd&c yellow #10 aluminum lake]
- Isoptin SR: 120 mg
- Isoptin SR: 180 mg [scored]
- Isoptin SR: 240 mg [scored; contains fd&c blue #2 aluminum lake, fd&c yellow #10 aluminum lake]
- Generic: 120 mg, 180 mg, 240 mg

Extemporaneous Preparations A 50 mg/mL oral suspension may be made with immediate release tablets and either a 1:1 mixture of Ora-Sweet® and Ora-Plus® or a 1:1 mixture of Ora-Sweet® SF and Ora-Plus® or cherry syrup. When using cherry syrup, dilute cherry syrup concentrate 1:4 with simple syrup, NF. Crush seventy-five verapamil hydrochloride 80 mg tablets in a mortar and reduce to a fine powder. Add small portions of chosen vehicle (40 mL total) and mix to a uniform paste; mix while adding the vehicle in incremental proportions to **almost** 120 mL; transfer to a calibrated bottle, rinse mortar with vehicle, and add quantity of vehicle sufficient to make 120 mL. Label "shake well", "refrigerate", and "protect from light". Stable for 60 days refrigerated (preferred) or at room temperature (Allen, 1996).

A 50 mg/mL oral suspension may be made with immediate release tablets, a 1:1 preparation of methylcellulose 1% and simple syrup, and purified water. Crush twenty 80 mg verapamil tablets in a mortar and reduce to a fine powder. Add 3 mL purified water USP and mix to a uniform paste; mix while adding the vehicle incremental proportions to **almost** 32 mL; transfer to a calibrated bottle, rinse mortar with vehicle, and add quantity of vehicle sufficient to make 32 mL. Label "shake well" and "refrigerate". Stable for 91 days refrigerated (preferred) or at room temperature (Nahata, 1997).

Allen LV Jr and Erickson MA 3rd, "Stability of Labetalol Hydrochloride, Metoprolol Tartrate, Verapamil Hydrochloride, and Spironolactone With Hydrochlorothiazide in Extemporaneously Compounded Oral Liquids," *Am J Health Syst Pharm*, 1996, 53(19):304-9.

Nahata MC, "Stability of Verapamil in an Extemporaneous Liquid Dosage Form," *J Appl Ther Res*, 1997,1(3):271-3.

◆ **Verapamil and Trandolapril** *see* Trandolapril and Verapamil *on page 2104*

◆ **Verapamil Hydrochloride** *see* Verapamil *on page 2182*

◆ **Verapamil Hydrochloride Injection, USP (Can)** *see* Verapamil *on page 2182*

◆ **Verapamil SR (Can)** *see* Verapamil *on page 2182*

◆ **Verdeso** *see* Desonide *on page 578*

◆ **Verdeso™ (Can)** *see* Desonide *on page 578*

◆ **Verelan** *see* Verapamil *on page 2182*

◆ **Verelan® (Can)** *see* Verapamil *on page 2182*

◆ **Verelan PM** *see* Verapamil *on page 2182*

◆ **Veripred 20** *see* PrednisoLONE (Systemic) *on page 1704*

◆ **Vermox** *see* Mebendazole *on page 1273*

◆ **Vermox® (Can)** *see* Mebendazole *on page 1273*

◆ **Versacloz** *see* CloZAPine *on page 477*

◆ **Versed** *see* Midazolam *on page 1359*

◆ **Versel® (Can)** *see* Selenium Sulfide *on page 1888*

◆ **Vertin-32 [OTC]** *see* Meclizine *on page 1277*

◆ **Verti-sulf** *see* Sulfur and Sulfacetamide *on page 1966*

◆ **Vesanoid** *see* Tretinoin (Systemic) *on page 2117*

◆ **Vesanoid® (Can)** *see* Tretinoin (Systemic) *on page 2117*

◆ **VESIcare** *see* Solifenacin *on page 1932*

◆ **Vestura™** *see* Ethinyl Estradiol and Drospirenone *on page 785*

◆ **Vexol** *see* Rimexolone *on page 1822*

◆ **Vexol® (Can)** *see* Rimexolone *on page 1822*

◆ **Vfend** *see* Voriconazole *on page 2203*

◆ **VFEND® (Can)** *see* Voriconazole *on page 2203*

◆ **Vfend IV** *see* Voriconazole *on page 2203*

◆ **Viagra** *see* Sildenafil *on page 1894*

◆ **Viagra® (Can)** *see* Sildenafil *on page 1894*

◆ **Vibativ** *see* Telavancin *on page 1999*

◆ **Vibramycin** *see* Doxycycline *on page 668*

◆ **Vibramycin® (Can)** *see* Doxycycline *on page 668*

◆ **Vibra-Tabs® (Can)** *see* Doxycycline *on page 668*

◆ **Vicks 44E [OTC]** *see* Guaifenesin and Dextromethorphan *on page 976*

◆ **Vicks DayQuil Mucus Control DM [OTC]** *see* Guaifenesin and Dextromethorphan *on page 976*

◆ **Vicks Nature Fusion Cough & Chest Congestion [OTC]** *see* Guaifenesin and Dextromethorphan *on page 976*

◆ **Vicks Pediatric Formula 44E [OTC]** *see* Guaifenesin and Dextromethorphan *on page 976*

◆ **Vicodin®** *see* Hydrocodone and Acetaminophen *on page 1006*

◆ **Vicodin ES®** *see* Hydrocodone and Acetaminophen *on page 1006*

◆ **Vicodin HP®** *see* Hydrocodone and Acetaminophen *on page 1006*

◆ **Vicoprofen** *see* Hydrocodone and Ibuprofen *on page 1008*

◆ **Victoza** *see* Liraglutide *on page 1223*
◆ **Victrelis** *see* Boceprevir *on page 267*
◆ **Victrelis® (Can)** *see* Boceprevir *on page 267*
◆ **Vidaza** *see* AzaCITIDine *on page 206*
◆ **Vidaza® (Can)** *see* AzaCITIDine *on page 206*
◆ **Videx** *see* Didanosine *on page 602*
◆ **Videx® (Can)** *see* Didanosine *on page 602*
◆ **Videx EC** *see* Didanosine *on page 602*
◆ **Videx® EC (Can)** *see* Didanosine *on page 602*

Vigabatrin (vye GA ba trin)

Brand Names: U.S. Sabril

Brand Names: Canada Sabril

Pharmacologic Category Anticonvulsant, Miscellaneous

Use

Infantile spasms: As monotherapy for pediatric patients 1 month to 2 years of age with infantile spasms for whom the potential benefits outweigh the potential risk of vision loss.

Refractory complex partial seizures: As adjunctive therapy for adults and pediatric patients 10 years and older with refractory complex partial seizures who have inadequately responded to several alternative treatments and for whom the potential benefits outweigh the risk of vision loss.

Canadian labeling: Additional uses (not in U.S. labeling): Active management of partial or secondary generalized seizures not controlled by usual treatments

Pregnancy Risk Factor C

Prescribing and Access Restrictions As a requirement of the REMS program, access to this medication is restricted. Vigabatrin is only available in the U.S. under a special restricted distribution program (SHARE). Under the SHARE program, only prescribers and pharmacies registered with the program are able to prescribe and distribute vigabatrin. Vigabatrin may only be dispensed to patients who are enrolled in and meet all conditions of SHARE. Contact the SHARE program at 1-888-45-SHARE.

Medication Guide Available Yes

Dosage

Infantile spasms: Oral: Infants and Children 1 month to 2 years: Initial dosing: 50 mg/kg/day divided twice daily; may titrate upwards by 25-50 mg/kg/day increments every 3 days to a maximum of 150 mg/kg/day divided twice daily

Note: To taper, decrease dose by 25-50 mg/kg/day increments every 3-4 days

Adjunctive treatment of seizures (Canadian labeling; not in U.S. labeling): Children: Oral: Initial: 40 mg/kg/day divided twice daily; maintenance dosages based on patient weight:

10-15 kg: 500-1000 mg daily divided twice daily
16-30 kg: 1000-1500 mg daily divided twice daily
31-50 kg: 1500-3000 mg daily divided twice daily
>50 kg: 2000-3000 mg daily divided twice daily

Refractory complex partial seizures: Oral:

Children and Adolescents 10 to <17 years and 25-60 kg: Initial: 250 mg twice daily; increase daily dose at weekly intervals based on response and tolerability. Recommended dose: 1000 mg twice daily

Note: To taper, decrease daily dose by one-third every week for 3 weeks.

Children ≥10 years and >60 kg, Adolescents ≥17 years, and Adults: Initial: 500 mg twice daily; increase daily dose by 500 mg increments at weekly intervals based on response and tolerability. Recommended dose: 1500 mg twice daily. (**Note:** Canadian labeling suggests that initial doses up to 2000 mg daily may be considered in patients with severe seizures.)

Note: To taper, decrease dose by 1000 mg daily on a weekly basis

Elderly: Initiate at low end of dosage range (refer to adult dosing); monitor closely for sedation and confusion

Dosage adjustment in renal impairment: Note: Renal function may be estimated using the Schwartz equation (children 10 to <12 years) and the Cockcroft-Gault formula (children ≥12 years, adolescents, and adults): Children ≥10 years, Adolescents, and Adults:

Cl_{cr} >50-80 mL/minute: Decrease dose by 25%
Cl_{cr} >30-50 mL/minute: Decrease dose by 50%
Cl_{cr} >10-30 mL/minute: Decrease dose by 75%

Dosage adjustment in hepatic impairment: No dosage adjustment provided in manufacturer's labeling; has not been studied. However, does not undergo appreciable hepatic metabolism.

Additional Information Complete prescribing information should be consulted for additional detail.

Dosage Forms Excipient information presented when available (limited, particularly for generics); consult specific product labeling.

Packet, Oral:
Sabril: 500 mg (50 ea)

Tablet, Oral:
Sabril: 500 mg [scored]

Dosage Forms: Canada Excipient information presented when available (limited, particularly for generics); consult specific product labeling.

Powder for suspension, oral [sachets]:
Sabril: 0.5 g

◆ **Vigamox** *see* Moxifloxacin (Ophthalmic) *on page 1406*
◆ **Vigamox® (Can)** *see* Moxifloxacin (Ophthalmic) *on page 1406*
◆ **VIGIV** *see* Vaccinia Immune Globulin (Intravenous) *on page 2143*
◆ **Viibryd** *see* Vilazodone *on page 2186*
◆ **Vilanterol and Fluticasone** *see* Fluticasone and Vilanterol *on page 899*
◆ **Vilanterol and Fluticasone Furoate** *see* Fluticasone and Vilanterol *on page 899*

Vilazodone (vil AZ oh done)

Brand Names: U.S. Viibryd

Index Terms EMD 68843; SB659746-A; Vilazodone Hydrochloride

Pharmacologic Category Antidepressant, Selective Serotonin Reuptake Inhibitor/5-HT_{1A} Receptor Partial Agonist

Additional Appendix Information

Antidepressant Agents *on page 2284*

Use Treatment of major depressive disorder

Pregnancy Risk Factor C

Pregnancy Considerations Adverse events have been observed in animal reproduction studies. An increased risk of teratogenic effects may be associated with maternal use of other SSRIs. However, available information is conflicting and information specific to the use of vilazodone has not been located. Nonteratogenic effects in the newborn following SSRI/SNRI exposure late in the third trimester include respiratory distress, cyanosis, apnea, seizures, temperature instability, feeding difficulty, vomiting, hypoglycemia, hypo- or hypertonia, hyper-reflexia, jitteriness, irritability, constant crying, and tremor. Symptoms may be due to the toxicity of the SSRIs/SNRIs or a discontinuation syndrome and may be consistent with serotonin syndrome associated with SSRI treatment. Persistent pulmonary hypertension of the newborn (PPHN) has also been reported with SSRI exposure. The long-term effects of *in* *utero* SSRI exposure on infant development and behavior are not known.

The ACOG recommends that therapy with SSRIs or SNRIs during pregnancy be individualized; treatment of depression during pregnancy should incorporate the clinical expertise of the mental health clinician, obstetrician, primary healthcare provider, and pediatrician. According to the American Psychiatric Association (APA), the risks of medication treatment should be weighed against other treatment options and untreated depression. For women who discontinue antidepressant medications during pregnancy and who may be at high risk for postpartum depression, the medications can be restarted following delivery. Treatment algorithms have been developed by the ACOG and the APA for the management of depression in women prior to conception and during pregnancy. Consideration should be given to using an agent with some safety information in pregnant women.

Breast-Feeding Considerations It is not known if vilazodone is excreted in breast milk. According to the manufacturer, the decision to continue or discontinue breast-feeding during therapy should take into account the risk of exposure to the infant and the benefits of treatment to the mother. Maternal use of an SSRI during pregnancy may cause delayed milk secretion. Long-term effects on development and behavior have not been studied.

Medication Guide Available Yes

Contraindications Use of MAO inhibitors intended to treat psychiatric disorders (concurrently or within 14 days of discontinuing either vilazodone or the MAO inhibitor); initiation of vilazodone in a patient receiving linezolid or intravenous methylene blue

Warnings/Precautions [U.S. Boxed Warning]: Antidepressants increase the risk of suicidal thinking and behavior in children, adolescents, and young adults (18-24 years of age) with major depressive disorder (MDD) and other psychiatric disorders; consider risk prior to prescribing. Short-term studies did not show an increased risk in patients >24 years of age and showed a decreased risk in patients ≥65 years. Closely monitor patients for clinical worsening, suicidality, or unusual changes in behavior, particularly during the initial 1-2 months of therapy or during periods of dosage adjustments (increases or decreases); the patient's family or caregiver should be instructed to closely observe the patient and communicate condition with healthcare provider. A medication guide concerning the use of antidepressants should be dispensed with each prescription. **Vilazodone is not FDA approved for use in children.**

The possibility of a suicide attempt is inherent in major depression and may persist until remission occurs. Use caution in high-risk patients. Worsening depression and severe abrupt suicidality that are not part of the presenting symptoms may require discontinuation or modification of drug therapy. The patient's family or caregiver should be alerted to monitor patients for the emergence of suicidality and associated behaviors (such as agitation, irritability, hostility, impulsivity, and hypomania) and call healthcare provider.

May worsen psychosis in some patients or precipitate a shift to mania or hypomania in patients with bipolar disorder. Patients presenting with depressive symptoms should be screened for bipolar disorder. Monotherapy in patients with bipolar disorder should be avoided. **Vilazodone is not FDA approved for the treatment of bipolar depression.**

Potentially life-threatening serotonin syndrome (SS) has occurred with serotonergic agents (eg, SSRIs, SNRIs), particularly when used in combination with other serotonergic agents (eg, triptans, TCAs, fentanyl, lithium, tramadol, buspirone, St John's wort, tryptophan) or agents that impair metabolism of serotonin (eg, MAO inhibitors intended to treat psychiatric disorders, other MAO inhibitors [ie, linezolid and intravenous methylene blue]). Discontinue treatment (and any concomitant serotonergic agent) immediately if signs/symptoms arise. May increase the risks associated with electroconvulsive therapy. Bone fractures have been associated with antidepressant treatment. Consider the possibility of a fragility fracture if an antidepressant-treated patient presents with unexplained bone pain, point tenderness, swelling, or bruising (Rabenda, 2013; Rizzoli, 2012). Has a low potential to impair cognitive or motor performance; caution operating hazardous machinery or driving. Potentially significant interactions may exist, requiring dose or frequency adjustment, additional monitoring, and/or selection of alternative therapy. Consult drug interactions database for more detailed information.

Use with caution in patients with hepatic impairment, seizure disorder (or with agents that lower the seizure threshold), or in elderly patients. May cause hyponatremia/SIADH (elderly at increased risk); volume depletion and diuretics may increase risk. May cause or exacerbate sexual dysfunction.

Abrupt discontinuation or interruption of antidepressant therapy has been associated with a discontinuation syndrome. Symptoms arising may vary with antidepressant however commonly include nausea, vomiting, diarrhea, headaches, light-headedness, dizziness, diminished appetite, sweating, chills, tremors, paresthesias, fatigue, somnolence, and sleep disturbances (eg, vivid dreams, insomnia). Greater risks for developing a discontinuation syndrome have been associated with antidepressants with shorter half-lives, longer durations of treatment, and abrupt discontinuation. For antidepressants of short or intermediate half-lives, symptoms may emerge within 2-5 days after treatment discontinuation and last 7-14 days (APA, 2010; Fava, 2006; Haddad, 2001; Shelton, 2001; Warner, 2006).

Adverse Reactions

>10%:

Gastrointestinal: Diarrhea (28%), nausea (23%)

1% to 10%:

Cardiovascular: Palpitation (2%)

Central nervous system: Dizziness (9%), insomnia (6%), dreams abnormal (4%), fatigue (4%), restlessness (3%), somnolence (3%), migraine (≥1%), sedation (≥1%)

Dermatologic: Hyperhidrosis (≥1%)

Endocrine & metabolic: Libido decreased (3% to 5%), orgasm abnormal (2% to 4%), sexual dysfunction (≤2%)

Gastrointestinal: Xerostomia (8%), vomiting (5%), dyspepsia (3%), flatulence (3%), gastroenteritis (3%), appetite increased (2%), appetite decreased (≥1%)

Genitourinary: Ejaculation delayed (2%), erectile dysfunction (2%)

Neuromuscular & skeletal: Arthralgia (3%), paresthesia (3%), jittery (2%), tremor (2%)

Ocular: Blurred vision (≥1%), dry eyes (≥1%)

Miscellaneous: Night sweats (≥1%)

<1% (Limited to important or life-threatening): Abnormal feeling, abnormal taste, cataracts, mania, panic attacks, pollakiuria, ventricular extrasystoles

Drug Interactions

Metabolism/Transport Effects Substrate of CYP2C19 (minor), CYP2D6 (minor), CYP3A4 (major); **Note:** Assignment of Major/Minor substrate status based on clinically relevant drug interaction potential; **Inhibits** CYP2C8 (weak), CYP2D6 (weak); **Induces** CYP2C19 (weak/moderate)

Avoid Concomitant Use

Avoid concomitant use of Vilazodone with any of the following: Dosulepin; Iobenguane I 123; Linezolid; MAO Inhibitors; Methylene Blue; Pimozide; Tryptophan

Increased Effect/Toxicity

Vilazodone may increase the levels/effects of: Agents with Antiplatelet Properties; Anticoagulants; Antidepressants (Serotonin Reuptake Inhibitor/Antagonist); Antipsychotics; Aspirin; Benzodiazepines (metabolized by oxidation); Beta-Blockers; BusPIRone; CarBAMazepine; CloZAPine; Collagenase (Systemic); Dabigatran Etexilate; Desmopressin; Dextromethorphan; Dosulepin; Galantamine; Hypoglycemic Agents; Ibritumomab; Methadone; Methylene Blue; Metoclopramide; Mexiletine; NSAID (COX-2 Inhibitor); NSAID (Nonselective); Pimozide; RisperiDONE; Rivaroxaban; Salicylates; Serotonin Modulators; Thiazide Diuretics; Thrombolytic Agents; Tositumomab and Iodine I 131 Tositumomab; TraMADol; Vitamin K Antagonists

The levels/effects of Vilazodone may be increased by: Alcohol (Ethyl); Analgesics (Opioid); Antipsychotics; BusPIRone; Cimetidine; CNS Depressants; Cobicistat; CYP3A4 Inhibitors (Moderate); CYP3A4 Inhibitors (Strong); Dasatinib; Glucosamine; Herbs (Anticoagulant/Antiplatelet Properties); Ibrutinib; Linezolid; Lithium; Macrolide Antibiotics; MAO Inhibitors; Metoclopramide; Metyrosine; Multivitamins/Fluoride (with ADE); Multivitamins/Minerals (with ADEK, Folate, Iron); Multivitamins/Minerals (with AE, No Iron); Omega-3 Fatty Acids; Pentosan Polysulfate Sodium; Pentoxifylline; Prostacyclin Analogues; Tipranavir; TraMADol; Tryptophan; Vitamin E

Decreased Effect

Vilazodone may decrease the levels/effects of: Iobenguane I 123; Ioflupane I 123; Thyroid Products

The levels/effects of Vilazodone may be decreased by: Bosentan; CarBAMazepine; CYP3A4 Inducers (Strong); Cyproheptadine; Dabrafenib; Deferasirox; Mitotane; NSAID (COX-2 Inhibitor); NSAID (Nonselective); Peginterferon Alfa-2b; Tocilizumab

Ethanol/Nutrition/Herb Interactions

Ethanol: Ethanol may increase CNS depression. Management: Avoid or limit use and monitor for increased effects.

Food: Management: Take with food.

Herb/Nutraceutical: Avoid valerian, St John's wort, tryptophan, SAMe, kava kava, gotu kola (may increase CNS depression and/or increase the risk of serotonin syndrome).

Storage/Stability Store at 25°C (77°F); excursions permitted to 15°C to 30°C (50°F to 86°F).

Mechanism of Action Vilazodone inhibits CNS neuron serotonin uptake; minimal or no effect on reuptake of norepinephrine or dopamine. It also binds selectively with high affinity to 5-HT_{1A} receptors and is a 5-HT_{1A} receptor partial agonist. 5-HT_{1A} receptor activity may be altered in depression and anxiety.

Pharmacodynamics/Kinetics

Protein binding: ~96% to 99%

Metabolism: Extensively hepatic, via CYP3A4 (major pathway) and 2C19 and 2D6 (minor pathways)

Bioavailability: 72% (with food); blood concentrations (AUC) may be decreased ~50% in the fasted state

Half-life elimination: Terminal: ~25 hours

Time to peak, serum: 4-5 hours

Excretion: Urine (1% as unchanged drug); feces (2% as unchanged drug)

Dosage Adults: Oral: Depression: Initial: 10 mg once daily for 7 days, then increase to 20 mg once daily for 7 days, then to recommended dose of 40 mg once daily

Discontinuation of therapy: Upon discontinuation of antidepressant therapy, gradually taper the dose to minimize the incidence of withdrawal symptoms and allow for the detection of re-emerging symptoms. Evidence supporting ideal taper rates is limited. APA and NICE guidelines suggest tapering therapy over at least several weeks with consideration to the half-life of the antidepressant; antidepressants with a shorter half-life may need to be tapered more conservatively. In addition for long-term treated patients, WFSBP guidelines recommend tapering over 4-6 months. If intolerable withdrawal symptoms occur following a dose reduction, consider resuming the previously prescribed dose and/or decrease dose at a more gradual rate (APA, 2010; Bauer, 2002; Haddad, 2001; NCCMH, 2010; Schatzberg, 2006; Shelton, 2001; Warner, 2006).

MAO inhibitor recommendations:

Switching to or from an MAO inhibitor intended to treat psychiatric disorders:

Allow 14 days to elapse between discontinuing an MAO inhibitor intended to treat psychiatric disorders and initiation of vilazodone.

Allow 14 days to elapse between discontinuing vilazodone and initiation of an MAO inhibitor intended to treat psychiatric disorders.

Use with other MAO inhibitors (linezolid or I.V. methylene blue):

Do not initiate vilazodone in patients receiving linezolid or I.V. methylene blue; consider other interventions for psychiatric condition.

If urgent treatment with linezolid or I.V. methylene blue is required in a patient already receiving vilazodone and potential benefits outweigh potential risks, discontinue vilazodone promptly and administer linezolid or I.V. methylene blue. Monitor for serotonin syndrome for 2 weeks or until 24 hours after the last dose of linezolid or I.V. methylene blue, whichever comes first. May resume vilazodone 24 hours after the last dose of linezolid or I.V. methylene blue.

Dosing adjustment for concomitant medications:

Strong CYP3A4 inhibitors: Reduce vilazodone dose to 20 mg once daily

Moderate CYP3A4 inhibitors (eg, erythromycin): Reduce vilazodone dose to 20 mg once daily in patients with intolerable side effects

Dosage adjustment in renal impairment: No dosage adjustment necessary.

Dosage adjustment in hepatic impairment:

Mild to moderate impairment (Child-Pugh class A or B): No dosage adjustment necessary

Severe impairment (Child-Pugh class C): No dosage adjustment provided in manufacturer's labeling (has not been studied).

Dietary Considerations Take with food.

Administration Administer with food.

Monitoring Parameters Monitor patient periodically for symptom resolution, mental status for depression, suicidal ideation (especially at the beginning of therapy or when doses are increased or decreased), anxiety, social functioning, mania, panic attacks, signs/symptoms of serotonin syndrome; akathisia

Dosage Forms Excipient information presented when available (limited, particularly for generics); consult specific product labeling.

Kit, Oral, as hydrochloride:

Viibryd: 10 & 20 & 40 MG [contains brilliant blue fcf (fd&c blue #1), fd&c red #40, fd&c yellow #6 (sunset yellow)]

Tablet, Oral, as hydrochloride:

Viibryd: 10 mg [contains fd&c red #40]

Viibryd: 20 mg [contains fd&c yellow #6 (sunset yellow)]

Viibryd: 40 mg [contains brilliant blue fcf (fd&c blue #1)]

◆ **Vilazodone Hydrochloride** *see* Vilazodone *on page 2186*

◆ **Vimpat** *see* Lacosamide *on page 1159*

◆ **Vimpat® (Can)** *see* Lacosamide *on page 1159*

VinBLAStine (vin BLAS teen)

Brand Names: Canada Vinblastine Sulphate Injection

Index Terms Velban; Vinblastine Sulfate; Vincaleukoblastine; VLB

Pharmacologic Category Antineoplastic Agent, Natural Source (Plant) Derivative; Antineoplastic Agent, Vinca Alkaloid

Use Treatment of Hodgkin's and non-Hodgkin's lymphoma; testicular cancer; breast cancer; mycosis fungoides; Kaposi's sarcoma; histiocytosis (Letterer-Siwe disease); choriocarcinoma

Unlabeled Use Treatment of bladder cancer, melanoma, nonsmall cell lung cancer (NSCLC), ovarian cancer, soft tissue sarcoma (desmoid tumors)

Pregnancy Risk Factor D

Pregnancy Considerations Animal studies have demonstrated resorption and teratogenic effects. There are no adequate and well-controlled studies in pregnant women. Women of childbearing potential should avoid becoming pregnant during vinblastine treatment. Aspermia has been reported in males who have received treatment with vinblastine.

Breast-Feeding Considerations Due to the potential for serious adverse reactions in the nursing infant, breast-feeding is not recommended.

Contraindications Significant granulocytopenia; presence of bacterial infection; I.T. administration is contraindicated (may result in death)

Warnings/Precautions Hazardous agent - use appropriate precautions for handling and disposal (NIOSH, 2012). **[U.S. Boxed Warning]: For I.V. use only. Intrathecal administration may result in death.** Must be dispensed in overwrap which bears the statement **"Do not remove covering until the moment of injection. Fatal if given intrathecally. For I.V. use only." [U.S. Boxed Warning]: Vinblastine is a vesicant; ensure proper needle or catheter placement prior to and during infusion. Avoid extravasation. Extravasation may cause significant irritation. Individuals administering should be experienced in vinblastine administration. If extravasation occurs, discontinue immediately and initiate appropriate extravasation management, including local injection of hyaluronidase and moderate heat application to the affected area. Use a separate vein to complete administration.** Leukopenia is common; granulocytopenia may be severe with higher doses. Leukopenia may be more pronounced in cachectic patients and patients with skin ulceration. Thrombocytopenia and anemia may occur rarely.

Use with caution in patients with hepatic impairment; toxicity may be increased; may require dosage modification. Neurotoxicity is rare at clinical doses; may occur with high doses (symptoms are similar to vincristine toxicity, including peripheral neuropathy, loss of deep tendon reflexes, headache, weakness, urinary retention, and GI symptoms). May rarely cause disabling neurotoxicity (usually reversible). Itraconazole may decrease the metabolism of vinblastine via CYP3A4 inhibition and may increase the effects of vinblastine via P-glycoprotein effects; severe myelosuppression and neurotoxicity may occur. Acute shortness of breath and severe bronchospasm have been reported, most often in association with concurrent administration of mitomycin; may occur within minutes to several hours following vinblastine administration or up to 14 days following mitomycin administration; use caution in patients with pre-existing pulmonary disease. Use with caution in patients with ischemic heart disease. **[U.S. Boxed Warning]: Should be administered under the supervision of an experienced cancer chemotherapy physician.** Some dosage forms may contain benzyl alcohol which has been associated with "gasping syndrome" in neonates.

Adverse Reactions Frequency not defined.

Common:

Cardiovascular: Hypertension
Central nervous system: Malaise
Dermatologic: Alopecia
Gastrointestinal: Constipation
Hematologic: Myelosuppression, leukopenia/granulocytopenia (nadir: 5-10 days; recovery: 7-14 days; dose-limiting toxicity)
Neuromuscular & skeletal: Bone pain, jaw pain, tumor pain

Less common:

Cardiovascular: Angina, cerebrovascular accident, coronary ischemia, ECG abnormalities, limb ischemia, MI, myocardial ischemia, Raynaud's phenomenon
Central nervous system: Depression, dizziness, headache, neurotoxicity (duration: >24 hours), seizure, vertigo
Dermatologic: Dermatitis, photosensitivity (rare), rash, skin blistering
Endocrine & metabolic: Aspermia, hyperuricemia, SIADH
Gastrointestinal: Abdominal pain, anorexia, diarrhea, gastrointestinal bleeding, hemorrhagic enterocolitis, ileus, metallic taste, nausea (mild), paralytic ileus, rectal bleeding, stomatitis, toxic megacolon, vomiting (mild)
Genitourinary: Urinary retention
Hematologic: Anemia, thrombocytopenia (recovery within a few days), thrombotic thrombocytopenic purpura
Local: Cellulitis (with extravasation), irritation, phlebitis (with extravasation), radiation recall
Neuromuscular & skeletal: Deep tendon reflex loss, myalgia, paresthesia, peripheral neuritis, weakness
Ocular: Nystagmus
Otic: Auditory damage, deafness, vestibular damage
Renal: Hemolytic uremic syndrome
Respiratory: Bronchospasm, dyspnea, pharyngitis

Drug Interactions

Metabolism/Transport Effects Substrate of CYP2D6 (minor), CYP3A4 (major), P-glycoprotein; **Note:** Assignment of Major/Minor substrate status based on clinically relevant drug interaction potential; **Inhibits** CYP2D6 (weak), CYP3A4 (weak); **Induces** P-glycoprotein

Avoid Concomitant Use

Avoid concomitant use of VinBLAStine with any of the following: BCG; CloZAPine; Conivaptan; Dabigatran Etexilate; Fusidic Acid (Systemic); Natalizumab; Pimecrolimus; Pimozide; Pomalidomide; Sofosbuvir; Tacrolimus (Topical); Tofacitinib; Vaccines (Live); VinCRIStine (Liposomal)

Increased Effect/Toxicity

VinBLAStine may increase the levels/effects of: ARIPiprazole; CloZAPine; Dofetilide; Leflunomide; Lomitapide; MitoMYcin (Systemic); Natalizumab; Pimozide; Tofacitinib; Tolterodine; Vaccines (Live)

The levels/effects of VinBLAStine may be increased by: Conivaptan; CYP3A4 Inhibitors (Moderate); CYP3A4 Inhibitors (Strong); Dasatinib; Denosumab; Fusidic Acid (Systemic); Itraconazole; Ivacaftor; Lopinavir; Luliconazole; Macrolide Antibiotics; MAO Inhibitors; Mifepristone; P-glycoprotein/ABCB1 Inhibitors; Pimecrolimus; Posaconazole; Ritonavir; Roflumilast; Simeprevir; Tacrolimus (Topical); Trastuzumab; Voriconazole

Decreased Effect

VinBLAStine may decrease the levels/effects of: Afatinib; BCG; Coccidioidin Skin Test; Dabigatran Etexilate; Linagliptin; P-glycoprotein/ABCB1 Substrates; Pomalidomide; Sipuleucel-T; Sofosbuvir; Vaccines (Inactivated); Vaccines (Live); VinCRIStine (Liposomal)

The levels/effects of VinBLAStine may be decreased by: Bosentan; CYP3A4 Inducers (Strong); Dabrafenib; Deferasirox; Echinacea; Herbs (CYP3A4 Inducers); Mitotane; Peginterferon Alfa-2b; P-glycoprotein/ABCB1 Inducers; Tocilizumab

Ethanol/Nutrition/Herb Interactions Herb/Nutraceutical: Avoid St John's wort (may decrease vinblastine levels). Avoid black cohosh, dong quai in estrogen-dependent tumors.

Preparation for Administration Hazardous agent; use appropriate precautions for handling and disposal (NIOSH, 2012). Reconstitute lyophilized powder to a concentration of 1 mg/mL with NS or bacteriostatic NS. For infusion, may dilute in 50 mL NS or D_5W; dilution in larger volumes (≥100 mL) of I.V. fluids is not recommended.

Storage/Stability Note: Must be dispensed in overwrap which bears the statement "Do not remove covering until the moment of injection. Fatal if given intrathecally. For I.V. use only." Syringes should be labeled: "Fatal if given intrathecally. For I.V. use only."

Store intact vials under refrigeration at 2°C to 8°C (36°F to 46°F). Protect from light. Solutions reconstituted in bacteriostatic NS are stable for 28 days under refrigeration.

Mechanism of Action Vinblastine binds to tubulin and inhibits microtubule formation, therefore, arresting the cell at metaphase by disrupting the formation of the mitotic spindle; it is specific for the M and S phases. Vinblastine may also interfere with nucleic acid and protein synthesis by blocking glutamic acid utilization.

Pharmacodynamics/Kinetics

Distribution: V_d: 27.3 L/kg; binds extensively to tissues; does not penetrate CNS or other fatty tissues; distributes to liver

Protein binding: 99%

Metabolism: Hepatic to active metabolite

Half-life elimination: Biphasic: Initial: 4 minutes; Terminal: 25 hours

Excretion: Feces (95%); urine (<1% as unchanged drug)

Dosage Details concerning dosing in combination regimens should also be consulted. **Note:** Frequency and duration of therapy may vary by indication, concomitant combination chemotherapy and hematologic response. **For I.V. use only.**

Children: I.V.:

Hodgkin's disease: Initial dose: 6 mg/m^2; do not administer more frequently than every 7 days

Letterer-Siwe disease: Initial dose: 6.5 mg/m^2; do not administer more frequently than every 7 days

Testicular cancer: Initial dose: 3 mg/m^2; do not administer more frequently than every 7 days

Adults: I.V.: Initial: 3.7 mg/m^2; adjust dose every 7 days (based on white blood cell response) up to 5.5 mg/m^2 (second dose); 7.4 mg/m^2 (third dose); 9.25 mg/m^2 (fourth dose); and 11.1 mg/m^2 (fifth dose); do not administer more frequently than every 7 days.

Usual range: 5.5-7.4 mg/m^2 every 7 days; Maximum dose: 18.5 mg/m^2; dosage adjustment goal is to reduce white blood cell count to ~3000/mm^3

Indication-specific dosing:

Hodgkin's disease: Usual dose: 6 mg/m^2 every 2 weeks (as part of a combination chemotherapy regimen) (Bartlett, 1995; Horning, 2002)

Testicular cancer: Usual dose: 0.11 mg/kg daily for 2 days every 3 weeks (as part of a combination chemotherapy regimen) (Loehrer, 1998) **or** 6 mg/m^2/day for 2 days every 3-4 weeks (as part of a combination chemotherapy regimen) (Clemm, 1986)

Bladder cancer (unlabeled use): Usual dose: 3 mg/m^2 every 7 days for 3 out of 4 weeks (as part of combination chemotherapy) (Sternberg, 2001) **or** 3 mg/m^2 days 2, 15, and 22 of a 28-day treatment cycle (as part of a combination chemotherapy regimen) (von der Maase, 2000)

Melanoma (unlabeled used): 2 mg/m^2 days 1-4 and 22-25 of a 6-week treatment cycle (as part of a combination chemotherapy regimen) (Eton, 2002)

Nonsmall cell lung cancer (unlabeled use): 4 mg/m^2 days 1, 8, 15, 22, and 29, then every 2 weeks (as part of combination chemotherapy) (Arriagada, 2004)

Ovarian cancer (unlabeled use): 0.11 mg/kg daily for 2 days every 3 weeks (as part of a combination chemotherapy regimen) (Loehrer, 1998)

Dosage adjustment in renal impairment: No dosage adjustment necessary.

Dosage adjustment in hepatic impairment:

The FDA-approved labeling recommends the following guidelines: Serum bilirubin >3 mg/dL: Administer 50% of dose

The following guidelines have been used by some clinicians:

Serum bilirubin >3.1 or transaminases >3 times ULN: Avoid use (Floyd, 2006) **or**

Serum bilirubin 1.5-3 mg/dL or AST 60-180 units: Administer 50% of dose

Serum bilirubin 3-5 mg/dL: Administer 25% of dose

Serum bilirubin >5 mg/dL or AST >180 units: Avoid use

Dosing in obesity: *ASCO Guidelines for appropriate chemotherapy dosing in obese adults with cancer:* Utilize patient's actual body weight (full weight) for calculation of body surface area- or weight-based dosing, particularly when the intent of therapy is curative; manage regimen-related toxicities in the same manner as for nonobese patients; if a dose reduction is utilized due to toxicity, consider resumption of full weight-based dosing with subsequent cycles, especially if cause of toxicity (eg, hepatic or renal impairment) is resolved (Griggs, 2012).

Administration For I.V. administration only. **Fatal if given intrathecally.** Administer usually as a slow (2-3 minutes) push, or a bolus (5-15 minutes) infusion; the manufacturer recommends an undiluted 1-minute infusion into a free flowing I.V. line to prevent venous irritation/extravasation. Prolonged administration times and/or increased administration volumes may increase the risk of vein irritation and extravasation.

Vesicant; ensure proper needle or catheter placement prior to and during infusion. Avoid extravasation.

Extravasation management: If extravasation occurs, stop infusion immediately and disconnect (leave cannula/needle in place); gently aspirate extravasated solution (do **NOT** flush the line); initiate hyaluronidase antidote; remove needle/cannula; apply dry warm compresses for 20 minutes 4 times a day for 1-2 days; elevate extremity (Perez Fidalgo, 2012). Remaining portion of the vinblastine dose should be infused through a separate vein.

Hyaluronidase: If needle/cannula still in place, administer 1-6 mL hyaluronidase (150 units/mL) into the existing I.V. line; the usual dose is 1 mL hyaluronidase for each 1 mL of extravasated drug (Perez Fidalgo, 2012; Schulmeister, 2011). If needle/cannula was removed, inject 1-6 mL (150 units/mL) subcutaneously in a clockwise manner using 1 mL for each 1 mL of drug extravasated (Schulmeister, 2011) **or** administer 1 mL (150 units/mL) as 5 separate 0.2 mL injections (using a 25-gauge needle) subcutaneously into the extravasation site (Polovich, 2009).

Hazardous agent; use appropriate precautions for handling and disposal (NIOSH, 2012).

Monitoring Parameters CBC with differential and platelet count, serum uric acid, hepatic function tests

Dosage Forms Excipient information presented when available (limited, particularly for generics); consult specific product labeling.

Solution, Intravenous, as sulfate:
Generic: 1 mg/mL (10 mL)

Solution Reconstituted, Intravenous, as sulfate:
Generic: 10 mg (1 ea)

- ◆ **Vinblastine Sulfate** *see* VinBLAStine *on page 2189*
- ◆ **Vinblastine Sulphate Injection (Can)** *see* VinBLAStine *on page 2189*
- ◆ **Vincaleukoblastine** *see* VinBLAStine *on page 2189*
- ◆ **Vincasar PFS** *see* VinCRIStine *on page 2191*

VinCRIStine (vin KRIS teen)

Brand Names: U.S. Vincasar PFS

Brand Names: Canada Vincristine Sulfate Injection; Vincristine Sulfate Injection USP

Index Terms Conventional Vincristine; Leurocristine Sulfate; Oncovin; Vincristine (Conventional); Vincristine Sulfate

Pharmacologic Category Antineoplastic Agent, Natural Source (Plant) Derivative; Antineoplastic Agent, Vinca Alkaloid

Additional Appendix Information

Beers Criteria – Potentially Inappropriate Medications for Geriatrics *on page 2368*

Use Treatment of acute lymphocytic leukemia (ALL), Hodgkin lymphoma, non-Hodgkin lymphomas, Wilms' tumor, neuroblastoma, rhabdomyosarcoma

Unlabeled Use Treatment of central nervous system tumors, chronic lymphocytic leukemia (CLL), Ewing's sarcoma, gestational trophoblastic tumors (high-risk), multiple myeloma, ovarian germ cell tumors, retinoblastoma, small cell lung cancer (SCLC); thymoma (advanced)

Pregnancy Risk Factor D

Pregnancy Considerations Animal reproduction studies have demonstrated teratogenicity and fetal loss. May cause fetal harm if administered during pregnancy. Women of childbearing potential should avoid becoming pregnant during treatment.

Breast-Feeding Considerations Due to the potential for serious adverse reactions in the nursing infant, the decision to discontinue vincristine or to discontinue breast-feeding should take into account the benefits of treatment to the mother.

Contraindications Patients with the demyelinating form of Charcot-Marie-Tooth syndrome

Warnings/Precautions Hazardous agent - use appropriate precautions for handling and disposal (NIOSH, 2012); avoid eye contamination.

[U.S. Boxed Warning]: For I.V. administration only; inadvertent intrathecal administration usually results in death. To prevent administration errors, the World Health Organization recommends dispensing vincristine diluted in a minibag (WHO, 2007), **if not dispensed in a minibag, affix an auxiliary label stating "For intravenous use only - fatal if given by other routes" and also place in an overwrap labeled "Do not remove covering until moment of injection."** Vincristine should **NOT** be prepared during the preparation of any intrathecal medications. After preparation, keep vincristine in a location **away** from the separate storage location recommended for intrathecal medications. Vincristine should **NOT** be delivered to the patient at the same time with any medications intended for central nervous system administration.

[U.S. Boxed Warning]: Vincristine is a vesicant; ensure proper needle or catheter placement prior to and during infusion. Avoid extravasation. Individuals administering should be experienced in vincristine administration. Extravasation may cause significant irritation. If extravasation occurs, discontinue immediately and initiate appropriate extravasation management, including local injection of hyaluronidase and moderate heat application to the affected area. Use a separate vein to complete administration.

Neurotoxicity, including alterations in mental status such as depression, confusion, or insomnia may occur; neurologic effects are dose-limiting (may require dosage reduction) and may be additive with those of other neurotoxic agents and spinal cord irradiation. Use with caution in patients with pre-existing neuromuscular disease and/or with concomitant neurotoxic agents. Constipation, paralytic ileus, intestinal necrosis and/or perforation may occur; constipation may present as upper colon impaction with an empty rectum (may require flat film of abdomen for diagnosis); generally responds to high enemas and laxatives. All patients should be on a prophylactic bowel management regimen.

Potentially significant drug-drug interactions may exist, requiring dose or frequency adjustment, additional monitoring, and/or selection of alternative therapy. Acute shortness of breath and severe bronchospasm have been reported with vinca alkaloids, usually when used in combination with mitomycin. Onset may be several minutes to hours after vincristine administration and up to 2 weeks after mitomycin. Progressive dyspnea may occur. Permanently discontinue vincristine if pulmonary dysfunction occurs.

Use with caution in patients with hepatic impairment; dosage modification required. May be associated with hepatic sinusoidal obstruction syndrome (SOS; formerly called veno-occlusive disease), increased risk in children <3 years of age; use with caution in hepatobiliary dysfunction. Monitor for signs or symptoms of hepatic SOS, including bilirubin >1.4 mg/dL, unexplained weight gain, ascites, hepatomegaly, or unexplained right upper quadrant pain (Arndt, 2004). Acute uric acid nephropathy has been reported with vincristine. Use with caution in the elderly; may cause or exacerbate syndrome of inappropriate antidiuretic hormone secretion or hyponatremia; monitor sodium closely with initiation or dosage adjustments in older adults (Beers Criteria).

Adverse Reactions Frequency not defined.

Cardiovascular: Edema, hyper-/hypotension, MI, myocardial ischemia

Central nervous system: Ataxia, coma, cranial nerve dysfunction (auditory damage, extraocular muscle impairment, laryngeal muscle impairment, paralysis, paresis, vestibular damage, vocal cord paralysis), dizziness, fever, headache, neurotoxicity (dose-related), neuropathic pain (common), seizure, vertigo

Dermatologic toxicity: Alopecia (common), rash

Endocrine & metabolic: Hyperuricemia, parotid pain, SIADH (rare)

Gastrointestinal: Abdominal cramps, abdominal pain, anorexia, constipation (common), diarrhea, intestinal necrosis, intestinal perforation, nausea, oral ulcers, paralytic ileus, vomiting, weight loss

Genitourinary: Bladder atony, dysuria, polyuria, urinary retention

Hematologic: Anemia (mild), leukopenia (mild), thrombocytopenia (mild), thrombotic thrombocytopenic purpura

Hepatic: Hepatic sinusoidal obstruction syndrome (SOS; veno-occlusive liver disease)

Local: Phlebitis, tissue irritation/necrosis (if infiltrated)

Neuromuscular & skeletal: Back pain, bone pain, deep tendon reflex loss, difficulty walking, foot drop, gait changes, jaw pain, limb pain, motor difficulties, muscle wasting, myalgia, paralysis, paresthesia, peripheral neuropathy (common), sensorimotor dysfunction, sensory loss

Ocular: Cortical blindness (transient), nystagmus, optic atrophy with blindness

Otic: Deafness

Renal: Acute uric acid nephropathy, hemolytic uremic syndrome

Respiratory: Bronchospasm, dyspnea, pharyngeal pain

Miscellaneous: Allergic reactions (rare), anaphylaxis (rare), hypersensitivity (rare)

Drug Interactions

Metabolism/Transport Effects Substrate of CYP3A4 (major), P-glycoprotein; **Note:** Assignment of Major/Minor substrate status based on clinically relevant drug interaction potential; **Inhibits** CYP3A4 (weak)

Avoid Concomitant Use

Avoid concomitant use of VinCRIStine with any of the following: BCG; Conivaptan; Fusidic Acid (Systemic); Natalizumab; Pimecrolimus; Pimozide; Tacrolimus (Topical); Tofacitinib; Vaccines (Live)

Increased Effect/Toxicity

VinCRIStine may increase the levels/effects of: ARIPiprazole; Dofetilide; Leflunomide; Lomitapide; MitoMYcin (Systemic); Natalizumab; Pimozide; Tofacitinib; Vaccines (Live); Vitamin K Antagonists

The levels/effects of VinCRIStine may be increased by: Conivaptan; CYP3A4 Inhibitors (Moderate); CYP3A4 Inhibitors (Strong); Dasatinib; Denosumab; Fusidic Acid (Systemic); Itraconazole; Ivacaftor; Lopinavir; Luliconazole; Macrolide Antibiotics; MAO Inhibitors; Mifepristone; NIFEdipine; P-glycoprotein/ABCB1 Inhibitors; Pimecrolimus; Posaconazole; Ritonavir; Roflumilast; Simeprevir; Tacrolimus (Topical); Teniposide; Trastuzumab; Voriconazole

Decreased Effect

VinCRIStine may decrease the levels/effects of: BCG; Cardiac Glycosides; Coccidioidin Skin Test; Fosphenytoin; Phenytoin; Sipuleucel-T; Vaccines (Inactivated); Vaccines (Live); Vitamin K Antagonists

The levels/effects of VinCRIStine may be decreased by: Bosentan; CYP3A4 Inducers (Strong); Dabrafenib; Deferasirox; Echinacea; Fosphenytoin; Herbs (CYP3A4 Inducers); Mitotane; P-glycoprotein/ABCB1 Inducers; Phenytoin; Tocilizumab

Ethanol/Nutrition/Herb Interactions Herb/Nutraceutical: St John's wort may decrease vincristine levels.

Preparation for Administration Hazardous agent; use appropriate precautions for handling and disposal (NIOSH, 2012).

Solutions for I.V. infusion may be mixed in NS or D_5W. **Note:** In order to prevent inadvertent intrathecal administration the World Health Organization (WHO) and the Institute for Safe Medical Practices (ISMP) recommend dispensing vincristine in a minibag (rather than a syringe). Vincristine should **NOT** be prepared during the preparation of any intrathecal medications. If dispensing vincristine in a syringe, affix an auxiliary label stating **"For intravenous use only - fatal if given by other routes"** to the syringe, and the syringe must also be packaged in the manufacturer-provided overwrap which bears the statement **"Do not remove covering until the moment of injection. For intravenous use only. Fatal if given intrathecally."**

Storage/Stability Store intact vials refrigerated at 2°C to 8°C (36°F to 46°F). Protect from light.

I.V. solution: Diluted in 25-50 mL NS or D_5W, stable for 7 days under refrigeration, or 2 days at room temperature. In ambulatory pumps, solution is stable for 7 days at room temperature. After preparation, keep vincristine in a location away from the separate storage location recommended for intrathecal medications.

Mechanism of Action Binds to tubulin and inhibits microtubule formation, therefore, arresting the cell at metaphase by disrupting the formation of the mitotic spindle; it is specific for the M and S phases. Vincristine may also interfere with nucleic acid and protein synthesis by blocking glutamic acid utilization.

Pharmacodynamics/Kinetics

Distribution: Rapidly removed from bloodstream and tightly bound to tissues; penetrates blood-brain barrier poorly

Metabolism: Extensively hepatic, via CYP3A4

Half-life elimination: Terminal: 85 hours (range: 19-155 hours)

Excretion: Feces (~80%); urine (10% to 20%; <1% as unchanged drug)

Dosage Note: Doses may be capped at a maximum of 2 mg/dose. Dosing and frequency may vary by protocol and/or treatment phase; refer to specific protocol.

Doses in the manufacturer's U.S. labeling: I.V.:

Children ≤10 kg: 0.05 mg/kg/dose once weekly

Children >10 kg: 1.5-2 mg/m²/dose; frequency may vary based on protocol

Adults: 1.4 mg/m²/dose; frequency may vary based on protocol

Additional dosing in combination therapy; indication-specific and/or unlabeled dosing: I.V.:

Children:

ALL: Induction phase: 1.5 mg/m²/dose days 0, 7, 14, and 21; Consolidation phase: 1.5 mg/m²/dose days 0, 28, and 56; Delayed intensification phase: 1.5 mg/m²/dose days 0, 7, and 14; Maintenance phase: 1.5 mg/m²/dose days 0, 28, and 56 (Bostrom, 2003) **or** Induction phase: 1.5 mg/m²/dose days 0, 7, 14, and 21; Consolidation phase: 1.5 mg/m²/dose days 0, 28, and 56; Interim maintenance phases: 1.5 mg/m²/dose days 0 and 28; Delayed intensification phase: 1.5 mg/m²/dose days 0, 7, and 14; Maintenance phase: 1.5 mg/m²/dose every 4 weeks (Avramis, 2002)

Burkitt lymphoma and B-cell ALL: 1.5 mg/m² (maximum dose: 2 mg) on days 4 and 11 of initial phase cycle (initial phase is in combination with cyclophosphamide, doxorubicin, and CNS prophylaxis; alternates with secondary phase) for a total of 4 cycles of each phase (Bowman, 1996) **or** 1.5 mg/m² (maximum dose: 2 mg) on day 1 of cycle AA (in combination with dexamethasone, ifosfamide, methotrexate, cytarabine, etoposide and CNS prophylaxis) and on day 1 of cycle BB (in combination with dexamethasone, cyclophosphamide, methotrexate, doxorubicin, and CNS prophylaxis) (Reiter, 1999)

Ewing's sarcoma (unlabeled use): 2 mg/m²/dose (maximum dose: 2 mg) on day 1 of a 21-day cycle, administer either every cycle or during odd-numbered cycles (Grier, 2003) **or** 0.67 mg/m²/day continuous infusion days 1, 2, and 3 (total 2 mg/m²/cycle; maximum dose/cycle: 2 mg) during cycles 1, 2, 3, and 6 (Kolb, 2003)

Hodgkin lymphoma: BEACOPP regimen: 2 mg/m²/dose (maximum dose: 2 mg) on day 7 of a 21-day treatment cycle (Kelly, 2002)

Neuroblastoma:

CE-CAdO regimen: 1.5 mg/m² (maximum dose: 2 mg) days 1 and 5 every 21 days for 2 cycles (Rubie, 1998) **or** 0.05 mg/kg days 1 and 5 for 2 cycles (Rubie, 2001)

CAV-P/VP regimen (unlabeled dosing): 0.033 mg/kg/day continuous infusion days 1, 2, and 3, then 1.5 mg/m² bolus day 9 of courses 1, 2, 4, and 6 (Kushner, 1994)

Retinoblastoma (unlabeled use):

Children: 0.05 mg/kg on day 1 every 21 days (in combination with carboplatin) for 8 cycles (Rodriguez-Galindo, 2003)

or

Children ≤36 months: 0.05 mg/kg on day 0 every 28 days (in combination with carboplatin and etoposide) for 6 cycles (Freidman, 2000)

or

Children >36 months: 1.5 mg/m^2 (maximum dose: 2 mg) on day 0 every 28 days (in combination with carboplatin and etoposide) for 6 cycles (Friedman, 2000)

Rhabdomyosarcoma:

VA regimen: 1.5 mg/m^2/dose (maximum dose: 2 mg) weeks 1-8, weeks 13-20, and weeks 25-32 (Crist, 2001)

VAC regimen: 1.5 mg/m^2/dose (maximum dose: 2 mg) weeks 0-12, week 16, weeks 20-25; Continuation therapy: Weeks 29-34, and weeks 38-43 (Crist, 2001)

Wilms' tumor:

Children <1 year: 0.75 mg/m^2/dose weekly for 10-11 weeks, then every 3 weeks for 15 additional weeks (total 25-26 weeks) (Pritchard, 1995)

Children ≥1 year: 1.5 mg/m^2/dose weekly for 10-11 weeks, then every 3 weeks for 15 additional weeks (total 25-26 weeks) (Pritchard, 1995)

or

Children ≤30 kg: 0.05 mg/kg/dose (maximum dose: 2 mg) weeks 1, 2, 4, 5, 6, 7, 8, 10, and 11, followed by 0.067 mg/kg/dose (maximum dose: 2 mg) weeks 12, 13, 18, and 24 (Green, 2007)

Children >30 kg: 1.5 mg/m^2/dose (maximum dose: 2 mg) weeks 1, 2, 4, 5, 6, 7, 8, 10, and 11, followed by 2 mg/m^2/dose (maximum dose: 2 mg) weeks 12, 13, 18, and 24 (Green, 2007)

Adults:

ALL:

Hyper-CVAD regimen: 2 mg/dose days 4 and 11 during odd-numbered cycles (cycles 1, 3, 5, 7) of an 8-cycle phase, followed by maintenance treatment (if needed) of 2 mg monthly for 2 years (Kantarjian, 2004)

Larson (CALBG 8811) regimen: Induction phase: 2 mg/dose days 1, 8, 15, and 22 (4-week treatment cycle); Early intensification phase: 2 mg/dose days 15, and 22 (4-week treatment cycle, repeat once); Late intensification phase: 2 mg/dose days 1, 8, 15 (8-week treatment cycle); Maintenance phase: 2 mg/dose day 1 every 4 weeks until 24 months from diagnosis (Larson, 1995)

Central nervous system tumors: PCV regimen: 1.4 mg/m^2/dose (maximum dose: 2 mg) on days 8 and 29 of a 6-week treatment cycle for a total of 6 cycles (van de Bent, 2006) **or** 1.4 mg/m^2/dose (no maximum dose) on days 8 and 29 of a 6-week treatment cycle for up to 4 cycles (Cairncross, 2006)

Hodgkin lymphoma:

BEACOPP regimen: 1.4 mg/m^2/dose (maximum dose: 2 mg) on day 8 of a 21-day treatment cycle (Diehl, 2003)

Stanford-V regimen: 1.4 mg/m^2/dose (maximum dose: 2 mg) in weeks 2, 4, 6, 8, 10, and 12 (Horning, 2000; Horning, 2002)

Non-Hodgkin lymphoma:

Burkitt lymphoma:

CODOX-M/IVAC: Cycles 1 and 3 (CODOX-M): 1.5 mg/m^2 (no maximum dose) days 1 and 8 of cycle 1 and days 1, 8, and 15 of cycle 3 (Magrath, 1996) **or** 1.5 mg/m^2 (maximum dose: 2 mg) days 1 and 8 of cycles 1 and 3 (Mead 2002; Mead 2008); CODOX-M is in combination with cyclophosphamide, doxorubicin, methotrexate, and CNS prophylaxis and alternates with IVAC (etoposide, ifosfamide, mesna, cytarabine, and CNS prophylaxis) for a total of 4 cycles

Hyper-CVAD: 2 mg (flat dose) days 4 and 11 of courses 1, 3, 5, and 7 (in combination with cyclophosphamide, doxorubicin, and dexamethasone) and alternates with even courses 2, 4, 6, and 8 (methotrexate and cytarabine) (Thomas, 2006)

Follicular lymphoma: CVP regimen: 1.4 mg/m^2/dose (maximum dose: 2 mg) on day 1 of a 21-day treatment cycle (in combination with cyclophosphamide and prednisone) for 8 cycles (Marcus, 2005)

Large B-cell lymphoma:

CHOP regimen: 1.4 mg/m^2/dose (maximum dose: 2 mg) on day 1 of a 21-day treatment cycle for 8 cycles (Coiffier, 2002)

EPOCH regimen: 0.4 mg/m^2/day continuous infusion for 4 days (over 96 hours) (total 1.6 mg/m^2/cycle; dose not usually capped) of a 21-day treatment cycle (Wilson, 2002)

Ewing's sarcoma (unlabeled use): VAC/IE regimen: VAC: 2 mg/m^2 (maximum dose: 2 mg) on day 1 of a 21-day treatment cycle (in combination with doxorubicin and cyclophosphamide), alternates with IE (ifosfamide and etoposide) for a total of 17 cycles (Grier, 2003)

Gestational trophoblastic tumors, high-risk (unlabeled use): EMA/CO regimen: 1 mg/m^2 on day 8 of 2-week treatment cycle (in combination with etoposide methotrexate, dactinomycin, and cyclophosphamide), continue for at least 2 treatment cycles after a normal hCG level (Escobar, 2003)

Multiple myeloma (unlabeled use):

DVD regimen: 1.4 mg/m^2/dose (maximum dose: 2 mg) on day 1 of a 28-day treatment cycle (Rifkin, 2006)

VAD regimen: 0.4 mg/day continuous infusion for 4 days (over 96 hours) (total 1.6 mg/cycle) of a 28-day treatment cycle (Rifkin, 2006)

Ovarian cancer (unlabeled use): VAC regimen: 1.5 mg/m^2/dose (maximum dose: 2 mg) weekly for 8-12 weeks (Slayton, 1985)

Small cell lung cancer (unlabeled use): CAV regimen: 1.4 mg/m^2/dose day 1 of a 21-day treatment cycle (Hong, 1989) **or** 2 mg/dose on day 1 of a 21-day treatment cycle (von Pawel, 1999)

Thymoma, advanced (unlabeled use): ADOC regimen: 0.6 mg/m^2 on day 3 every 3 weeks (in combination with cisplatin, doxorubicin, and cyclophosphamide) (Fornasiero, 1991)

Dosage adjustment in renal impairment: No dosage adjustment necessary (Kintzel, 1995).

Dosage adjustment in hepatic impairment:

The manufacturer's labeling recommends the following adjustment: Serum bilirubin >3 mg/dL: Administer 50% of normal dose.

The following adjustments have also been recommended:

Floyd, 2006: Serum bilirubin 1.5-3 mg/dL or transaminases 2-3 times ULN or alkaline phosphatase increased: Administer 50% of dose.

Superfin, 2007:

Serum bilirubin 1.5-3 mg/dL: Administer 50% of dose.

Serum bilirubin >3 mg/dL: Avoid use.

Dosing in obesity: *ASCO Guidelines for appropriate chemotherapy dosing in obese adults with cancer:* Adults: Dose should be capped at a maximum of 2 mg due to neurotoxicity concerns (Griggs, 2012).

Administration For I.V. administration only. FATAL IF GIVEN INTRATHECALLY.

Vincristine should **NOT** be delivered to the patient at the same time with any medications intended for central nervous system administration.

I.V.: Usually administered as short 5-10 minute infusion (preferred); may also be administered as a slow (1 minute) push or by a 24-hour continuous infusion (depending on the protocol).

Vesicant; ensure proper needle or catheter placement prior to and during infusion. Avoid extravasation.

Extravasation management: If extravasation occurs, stop infusion immediately and disconnect (leave cannula/needle in place); gently aspirate extravasated solution (do **NOT** flush the line); initiate hyaluronidase antidote; remove needle/cannula; apply dry warm compresses for 20 minutes 4 times a day for 1-2 days; elevate (Perez Fidalgo, 2012). Remaining portion of the vincristine dose should be infused through a separate vein.

Hyaluronidase: If needle/cannula still in place, administer 1-6 mL hyaluronidase (150 units/mL) into the existing I.V. line; the usual dose is 1 mL hyaluronidase for each 1 mL of extravasated drug (Perez Fidalgo, 2012; Schulmeister, 2011). If needle/cannula was removed, inject 1-6 mL (150 units/mL) subcutaneously in a clockwise manner using 1 mL for each 1 mL of drug extravasated (Schulmeister, 2011) **or** administer 1 mL (150 units/mL) as 5 separate 0.2 mL injections (using a 25-gauge needle) subcutaneously into the extravasation site (Polovich, 2009).

Hazardous agent; use appropriate precautions for handling and disposal (NIOSH, 2012).

Monitoring Parameters Serum electrolytes (sodium), hepatic function tests, CBC with differential, serum uric acid; monitor infusion site; neurologic examination, monitor for constipation/ileus and for signs/symptoms of peripheral neuropathy

Dosage Forms Excipient information presented when available (limited, particularly for generics); consult specific product labeling.

Solution, Intravenous, as sulfate:
Vincasar PFS: 1 mg/mL (1 mL, 2 mL)

Solution, Intravenous, as sulfate [preservative free]:
Generic: 1 mg/mL (1 mL, 2 mL)

VinCRIStine (Liposomal)

(vin KRIS teen lye po SO mal)

Brand Names: U.S. Marqibo

Index Terms Liposomal Vincristine; Liposome Vincristine; Vincristine Liposome; Vincristine Sulfate Liposome; VSLI

Pharmacologic Category Antineoplastic Agent, Natural Source (Plant) Derivative; Antineoplastic Agent, Vinca Alkaloid

Use Treatment of relapsed Philadelphia chromosome-negative (Ph-) acute lymphoblastic leukemia (ALL) in adult patients whose disease has progressed after two or more antileukemic therapies

Pregnancy Risk Factor D

Pregnancy Considerations Adverse events (fetal malformations, decreased fetal weight, and fetal loss) were observed in animal reproduction studies at doses less than the recommended human dose. Given the mechanism of action, adverse fetal events would be expected to occur with use in pregnant women. Women of childbearing potential should avoid becoming pregnant during therapy.

Breast-Feeding Considerations Due to the potential for adverse reactions in the nursing infant, the decision to discontinue breast-feeding or to discontinue liposomal vincristine should take into account the benefits of treatment to the mother.

Contraindications Hypersensitivity to vincristine, liposomal vincristine, or any component of the formulation; patients with Charcot-Marie-Tooth syndrome or other demyelinating conditions; administration via the intrathecal route

Warnings/Precautions Hazardous agent - use appropriate precautions for handling and disposal (NIOSH, 2012). **[U.S. Boxed Warning]: For I.V. administration only. Intrathecal administration is contraindicated; inadvertent intrathecal administration has resulted in death.** Liposomal vincristine should **NOT** be prepared during the preparation of any intrathecal medications. After preparation, keep liposomal vincristine in a location **away** from the separate storage location recommended for intrathecal medications. Liposomal vincristine should **NOT** be delivered to the patient at the same time with any medications intended for central nervous system administration.

[U.S. Boxed Warning]: Vincristine LIPOSOME and conventional vincristine are NOT interchangeable. Dosing differs between formulations; verify intended product and dose prior to preparation and administration to avoid overdoses. Avoid extravasation of liposomal vincristine (conventional vincristine is a vesicant). Only individuals experienced with vesicant administration should administer liposomal vincristine. Check for proper needle placement; if extravasation occurs, discontinue liposomal vincristine infusion immediately and institute appropriate extravasation management procedures.

Grade 3 and greater neutropenia, anemia, and thrombocytopenia were observed in clinical trials. Monitor blood counts closely and adjust dose or withhold therapy if necessary. Constipation, ileus, bowel obstruction, and colonic pseudo-obstruction have occurred with liposomal vincristine. Patients should be initiated on a prophylactic bowel regimen including a stool softener, dietary fiber, and hydration; laxative treatments may be considered. Severe fatigue was noted in clinical trials; treatment delay, dosage adjustment, or discontinuation may be necessary.

Neuropathies (sensory and motor) are common and cumulative. Neuropathy symptoms may include paresthesia, hyper-/hypoesthesia, hyporeflexia or areflexia, neuralgia, jaw pain, cranial neuropathy, ileus, arthralgia, myalgia, muscle spasm, and/or weakness. Evaluate neurologic status of patients closely prior to liposomal vincristine administration; neurologic toxicity risk is greater when given to patients with pre-existing neuromuscular conditions or when used concomitantly with other neurotoxic agents. Treatment delay, dosage adjustment, and/or discontinuation may be necessary. Tumor lysis syndrome may occur as a consequence of therapy; monitor closely for signs and symptoms and manage accordingly.

Hepatotoxicity (including fatal cases) and increased AST have been reported. Monitor hepatic function tests; reduce dose or interrupt therapy if necessary. Use caution in patients with hepatic impairment; liposomal vincristine has not been studied in patients with severe hepatic impairment. In a study in a limited number of melanoma patients with moderate (Child-Pugh class B) hepatic impairment secondary to liver metastases, C_{max} and AUC were comparable to those in patients with normal hepatic function; patients with hepatic impairment received a dose of 1 mg/m^2 every 2 weeks versus 2 mg/m^2 in subjects with normal hepatic function (Bedikian, 2011). Avoid concomitant therapy with strong CYP3A4 or P-glycoprotein (P-gp) inducers or inhibitors. Use with caution in the elderly patient population; conventional vincristine may cause or exacerbate hyponatremia or syndrome of inappropriate antidiuretic hormone secretion; monitor sodium closely with therapy initiation or dosage adjustments (Beers Criteria).

Adverse Reactions

>10%:

Central nervous system: Fever (43%), fatigue (41%), insomnia (32%)

Gastrointestinal: Constipation (57%), nausea (52%), diarrhea (37%), appetite decreased (33%)

Hematologic: Neutropenic fever (38%; grades 3/4: 31%), anemia (34%; grades 3/4: 17%), neutropenia (grades 3/4: 18%), thrombocytopenia (grades 3/4: 17%)
Hepatic: AST increased (grades 3/4: 6% to 11%)
Neuromuscular & skeletal: Peripheral neuropathy (39%; grades 3/4: 17%)

1% to 10%:

Cardiovascular: Cardiac arrest (grades 3/4: 6%), hypotension (grades 3/4: 6%)
Central nervous system: Pain (grades 3/4: 8%), mental status changes (grades 3/4: 4%)
Gastrointestinal: Abdominal pain (grades 3/4: 8%), ileus (grades 3/4: 6%)
Neuromuscular & skeletal: Weakness (grades 3/4: 5%), muscle weakness (grades 3/4: 1%)
Respiratory: Pneumonia (grades 3/4: 8%), respiratory distress (grades 3/4: 6%), respiratory failure (grades 3/4: 5%)
Miscellaneous: Septic shock (grades 3/4: 6%), staphylococcal bacteremia (grades 3/4: 6%)

Drug Interactions

Metabolism/Transport Effects Substrate of CYP3A4 (major), P-glycoprotein; **Note:** Assignment of Major/Minor substrate status based on clinically relevant drug interaction potential; **Inhibits** CYP3A4 (weak)

Avoid Concomitant Use

Avoid concomitant use of VinCRIStine (Liposomal) with any of the following: BCG; CloZAPine; CYP3A4 Inducers (Strong); CYP3A4 Inhibitors (Strong); Fusidic Acid (Systemic); Natalizumab; P-glycoprotein/ABCB1 Inducers; P-glycoprotein/ABCB1 Inhibitors; Pimecrolimus; Pimozide; St Johns Wort; Tacrolimus (Topical); Tofacitinib; Vaccines (Live)

Increased Effect/Toxicity

VinCRIStine (Liposomal) may increase the levels/effects of: ARIPiprazole; CloZAPine; Dofetilide; Leflunomide; Lomitapide; MitoMYcin (Systemic); Natalizumab; Pimozide; Tofacitinib; Vaccines (Live); Vitamin K Antagonists

The levels/effects of VinCRIStine (Liposomal) may be increased by: CYP3A4 Inhibitors (Moderate); CYP3A4 Inhibitors (Strong); Dasatinib; Denosumab; Fusidic Acid (Systemic); Ivacaftor; Luliconazole; Macrolide Antibiotics; MAO Inhibitors; Mifepristone; NIFEdipine; P-glycoprotein/ABCB1 Inhibitors; Pimecrolimus; Posaconazole; Roflumilast; Simeprevir; Tacrolimus (Topical); Teniposide; Trastuzumab; Voriconazole

Decreased Effect

VinCRIStine (Liposomal) may decrease the levels/effects of: BCG; Cardiac Glycosides; Coccidioidin Skin Test; Sipuleucel-T; Vaccines (Inactivated); Vaccines (Live); Vitamin K Antagonists

The levels/effects of VinCRIStine (Liposomal) may be decreased by: Bosentan; CYP3A4 Inducers (Strong); Dabrafenib; Deferasirox; Echinacea; P-glycoprotein/ABCB1 Inducers; St Johns Wort; Tocilizumab

Preparation for Administration Hazardous agent; use appropriate precautions for handling and disposal (NIOSH, 2012). Vincristine liposome preparation requires 60-90 minutes of dedicated time utilizing the manufacturer supplied kit. Do not reuse kit components with future doses.

1). Outside the sterile area, fill a water bath to a depth of at least 8 cm (3.2 inches); water should be heated to and maintained at **63°C to 67°C** (145.4°F to 152.6°F) for the entire procedure (use calibrated thermometer to monitor temperature). Maintain water depth of at least 8 cm (3.2 inches) throughout process. Water bath must remain outside the sterile area.

2). In a biological safety cabinet, vent the sodium phosphate vial with a sterile venting needle (with a 0.2 micron filter or other suitable venting device). Venting needle should always be kept above liquid level. Remove 1 mL of sphingomyelin/cholesterol liposome injection and inject into the sodium phosphate vial. Withdraw 5 mL of vincristine sulfate injection and inject into the sodium phosphate vial. Remove the venting needle and gently invert the sodium phosphate vial 5 times to mix (do **not** shake). Place flotation ring on the sodium phosphate vial.

3). Confirm the water bath is maintained between **63°C to 67°C** (145.4°F to 152.6°F). Outside the sterile area, place constituted sodium phosphate vial in the water bath for 10 minutes. Record constitution start and stop time, as well as starting and ending water temperature. After 10 minutes, remove the vial (with tongs), remove flotation ring, then dry the vial, affix vial overlabel, and gently invert 5 times to mix (do **not** shake). Allow the vial to equilibrate for at least 30 minutes at room temperature of 15°C to 30°C (59°F to 86°F), but for no longer than 12 hours. Once prepared, vincristine sulfate liposome concentration is 5 mg/31 mL (0.16 mg/mL).

4). Return vial to biologic safety cabinet. Calculate patient's vincristine liposome dose (based on actual BSA); remove corresponding volume from 100 mL NS or D_5W infusion bag. Inject vincristine liposome dose into the infusion bag (final volume of 100 mL). Do not use if a precipitate or other foreign matter is present in the vial or infusion bag. The amount contained in each vial may exceed the prescribed dose; use care with dosage and volume calculations. Discard unused portion of the vial. After preparation, keep liposomal vincristine in a location away from the separate storage location recommended for intrathecal medications.

Storage/Stability Store intact kit (containing vincristine vial, sphingomyelin/cholesterol liposome vial, and sodium phosphate vial) refrigerated at 2°C to 8°C (36°F to 46°F); do not freeze. Use appropriate precautions for handling and disposal. Once prepared, liposomal vincristine is stable for no more than 12 hours at room temperature. After preparation, keep liposomal vincristine in a location away from the separate storage location recommended for intrathecal medications.

Mechanism of Action Vincristine is a cell cycle specific agent which binds to tubulin, leading to microtubule depolymerization and cellular apoptosis. The liposomal formulation increases the half-life, allowing for enhanced cytotoxic activity in tumor cells.

Pharmacodynamics/Kinetics

Distribution: V_{dss}: 2.7 L (Bedikian, 2006)
Metabolism: Primarily hepatic
Half-life elimination: 45 hours (urinary half-life); dependent on rate of vincristine release from sphingosome (Bedikian, 2006)
Excretion: Feces (69%); urine (<8%)

Dosage Adults: **Note:** Vincristine liposomal and conventional vincristine are **NOT** interchangeable. Dosing differs between formulations; verify intended product and dose prior to preparation and administration. The liposomal vincristine dose is based on actual body surface area (BSA) and was not capped in studies (O'Brien, 2009; Rodriguez, 2009; Silverman, 2010).

Acute lymphoblastic leukemia (ALL; Philadelphia chromosome-negative), relapsed: I.V.: 2.25 mg/m^2 once every 7 days

Dosage adjustment for toxicity:

Fatigue, severe: Consider dose delay, reduction, or therapy discontinuation.
Hematologic toxicity: Grade 3 or 4 neutropenia, thrombocytopenia, or anemia: Consider dose reduction or modification.
Hepatic toxicity: Reduce dose or interrupt treatment.

Peripheral neuropathy:

Grade 3 or persistent grade 2 toxicity: Interrupt therapy until recovery to grade 1 or 2, then reduce dose to 2 mg/m^2. If grade 3 toxicity persists or if grade 4 toxicity occurs, discontinue liposomal vincristine.

Persistent grade 2 toxicity after first dose reduction to 2 mg/m^2: Interrupt therapy for up to 7 days until recovery to grade 1, then reduce dose to 1.825 mg/m^2. If neuropathy increases to grade 3 or 4, discontinue liposomal vincristine.

Persistent grade 2 toxicity after second dose reduction to 1.825 mg/m^2: Interrupt therapy for up to 7 days until recovery to grade 1, then reduce dose to 1.5 mg/m^2. If neuropathy increases to grade 3 or 4, discontinue liposomal vincristine.

Pre-existing neuropathy, severe: Assess treatment benefit versus risk.

Dosage adjustment in renal impairment: No dosage adjustment provided in manufacturer's labeling (has not been studied); however, liposomal vincristine is minimally excreted by the kidney and like the conventional formulation, likely does not require dosage adjustment in renal impairment.

Dosage adjustment in hepatic impairment:

Moderate impairment (Child-Pugh class B): In a study in a limited number of melanoma patients with moderate (Child-Pugh class B) hepatic impairment secondary to liver metastases, C_{max} and AUC were comparable to those in patients with normal hepatic function; patients with hepatic impairment received a dose of 1 mg/m^2 every 2 weeks versus 2 mg/m^2 in subjects with normal hepatic function (Bedikian, 2011).

Severe impairment (Child-Pugh class C): No dosage adjustment provided in manufacturer's labeling (has not been studied).

Hepatotoxicity during treatment: Reduce dose or interrupt treatment.

Dosing in obesity: *ASCO Guidelines for appropriate chemotherapy dosing in obese adults with cancer:* Utilize patient's actual body weight (full weight) for calculation of body surface area- or weight-based dosing, particularly when the intent of therapy is curative; manage regimen-related toxicities in the same manner as for nonobese patients; if a dose reduction is utilized due to toxicity, consider resumption of full weight-based dosing with subsequent cycles, especially if cause of toxicity (eg, hepatic or renal impairment) is resolved (Griggs, 2012).

Administration Conventional vincristine is a vesicant. Limited information is available regarding liposomal vincristine extravasation, but may cause inflammation if extravasated; avoid extravasation. **For I.V. administration only. FATAL IF GIVEN INTRATHECALLY.** Liposomal vincristine should **NOT** be delivered to the patient at the same time as any medications intended for central nervous system administration.

I.V.: Infuse over 1 hour. Do not administer I.V. push or bolus; do not use with in-line filters. Infusion must be completed within 12 hours of preparation.

Hazardous agent; use appropriate precautions for handling and disposal (NIOSH, 2012).

Monitoring Parameters CBC with differential and platelets; hepatic function; signs/symptoms of peripheral neuropathy or other neurologic toxicities; sodium (in elderly patients; conventional vincristine may cause or exacerbate hyponatremia or syndrome of inappropriate antidiuretic hormone secretion); signs/symptoms of tumor lysis syndrome; symptoms of constipation; monitor infusion site for extravasation

Additional Information The liposomal formulation of vincristine consists of vincristine encapsulated in sphingosomes, which are composed of sphingomyelin and cholesterol (Bedikian, 2006).

Dosage Forms Excipient information presented when available (limited, particularly for generics); consult specific product labeling.

Suspension, Intravenous, as sulfate:

Marqibo: 5 mg/31 mL (1 ea)

◆ **Vincristine (Conventional)** *see* VinCRIStine *on page 2191*

◆ **Vincristine Liposome** *see* VinCRIStine (Liposomal) *on page 2194*

◆ **Vincristine Sulfate** *see* VinCRIStine *on page 2191*

◆ **Vincristine Sulfate Injection (Can)** *see* VinCRIStine *on page 2191*

◆ **Vincristine Sulfate Injection USP (Can)** *see* VinCRIStine *on page 2191*

◆ **Vincristine Sulfate Liposome** *see* VinCRIStine (Liposomal) *on page 2194*

Vinorelbine (vi NOR el been)

Brand Names: U.S. Navelbine

Brand Names: Canada Navelbine®; Vinorelbine Injection, USP; Vinorelbine Tartrate for Injection

Index Terms Dihydroxydeoxynorvinkaleukoblastine; Vinorelbine Tartrate

Pharmacologic Category Antineoplastic Agent, Natural Source (Plant) Derivative; Antineoplastic Agent, Vinca Alkaloid

Use Treatment of nonsmall cell lung cancer (NSCLC)

Unlabeled Use Treatment of breast cancer (metastatic), cervical cancer (persistent or recurrent), Hodgkin lymphoma (relapsed or refractory), ovarian cancer (relapsed), malignant pleural mesothelioma, salivary gland cancer, small cell lung cancer, and soft tissue sarcoma (advanced)

Pregnancy Risk Factor D

Pregnancy Considerations Animal reproduction studies have demonstrated embryotoxicity, fetotoxicity, decreased fetal weight, and delayed ossification. May cause fetal harm if administered during pregnancy. Women of childbearing potential should avoid becoming pregnant during vinorelbine treatment.

Breast-Feeding Considerations It is not known if vinorelbine is excreted in breast milk. Due to the potential for serious adverse reactions in the nursing infant, breastfeeding should be discontinued during treatment.

Contraindications Pretreatment granulocyte counts <1000/mm^3

Warnings/Precautions Hazardous agent - use appropriate precautions for handling and disposal (NIOSH, 2012). **[U.S. Boxed Warning]: For I.V. use only; intrathecal administration of other vinca alkaloids has resulted in death. If dispensed in a syringe, should be labeled "for intravenous use only - fatal if given intrathecally". [U.S. Boxed Warning]: Vesicant; ensure proper needle or catheter placement prior to and during infusion. Avoid extravasation. Extravasation may cause local tissue necrosis and/or thrombophlebitis. [U.S. Boxed Warning]: Severe granulocytopenia may occur with treatment (may lead to infection); granulocyte counts should be ≥1000 cells/mm^3 prior to treatment initiation; dosage adjustment may be required based on blood counts (monitor blood counts prior to each dose).** Granulocytopenia is a dose-limiting toxicity; nadir is generally 7-10 days after administration and recovery occurs within the following 7-14 days. Monitor closely for infections and/or fever in patients with severe granulocytopenia. Use with extreme caution in patients with compromised marrow reserve due to prior chemotherapy or radiation therapy.

Fatal cases of interstitial pulmonary changes and ARDS have been reported (with single-agent therapy (mean onset of symptoms: 1 week); promptly evaluate changes in baseline pulmonary symptoms or any new onset pulmonary symptoms (eg, dyspnea, cough, hypoxia). Acute shortness of breath and severe bronchospasm have been reported with vinca alkaloids; usually associated with the concurrent administration of mitomycin.

Vinorelbine should **NOT** be prepared during the preparation of any intrathecal medications. After preparation, keep vinorelbine in a location **away** from the separate storage location recommended for intrathecal medications. Elimination is predominantly hepatic; while there is no evidence that toxicity is enhanced in patients with elevated transaminases, use with caution in patients with severe hepatic injury or impairment; dosage modification required for elevated total bilirubin. May cause new onset or worsening of pre-existing neuropathy; use with caution in patients with neuropathy; monitor for new or worsening sign/symptoms of neuropathy; dosage adjustment required. May cause severe constipation (grade 3-4), paralytic ileus, intestinal obstruction, necrosis, and/or perforation; some events were fatal. Potentially significant drug-drug interactions may exist, requiring dose or frequency adjustment, additional monitoring, and/or selection of alternative therapy. May have radiosensitizing effects with prior or concurrent radiation therapy; radiation recall reactions may occur in patients who have received prior radiation therapy. Avoid eye contamination (exposure may cause severe irritation). **[U.S. Boxed Warning]: Should be administered under the supervision of an experienced cancer chemotherapy physician.**

Adverse Reactions Note: Reported with single-agent therapy.

>10%:

Central nervous system: Fatigue (27%)

Dermatologic: Alopecia (12% to 30%)

Gastrointestinal: Nausea (31% to 44%; grade 3: 1% to 2%), constipation (35%; grade 3: 3%), vomiting (20% to 31%; grade 3: 1% to 2%), diarrhea (12% to 17%)

Hematologic: Leukopenia (83% to 92%; grade 4: 6% to 15%), granulocytopenia (90%; grade 4: 36%; nadir: 7-10 days; recovery 14-21 days), neutropenia (85%; grade 4: 28%), anemia (83%; grades 3/4: 9%)

Hepatic: AST increased (67%; grade 3: 5%; grade 4: 1%), total bilirubin increased (5% to 13%; grade 3: 4%; grade 4: 3%)

Local: Injection site reaction (22% to 28%; includes erythema, vein discoloration), injection site pain (16%)

Neuromuscular & skeletal: Weakness (36%), peripheral neuropathy (25%; grade 3: 1%; grade 4: <1%)

Renal: Creatinine increased (13%)

1% to 10%:

Cardiovascular: Chest pain (5%)

Dermatologic: Rash (<5%)

Gastrointestinal: Paralytic ileus (1%)

Hematologic: Neutropenic fever/sepsis (8%; grade 4: 4%), thrombocytopenia (3% to 5%; grades 3/4: 1%)

Local: Phlebitis (7% to 10%)

Neuromuscular & skeletal: Loss of deep tendon reflexes (<5%), myalgia (<5%), arthralgia (<5%), jaw pain (<5%)

Otic: Ototoxicity (≤1%)

Respiratory: Dyspnea (7%)

<1% (Limited to important or life-threatening): Abdominal pain, allergic reactions, anaphylaxis, angioedema, back pain, DVT, dysphagia, esophagitis, flushing, gait instability, headache, hemolytic uremic syndrome, hemorrhagic cystitis, hyper-/hypotension, hyponatremia, intestinal necrosis, intestinal obstruction, intestinal perforation, interstitial pulmonary changes, local rash, local urticaria, MI (rare), mucositis, muscle weakness, myocardial ischemia, pancreatitis, paralytic ileus, pneumonia, pruritus, pulmonary edema, pulmonary embolus, radiation recall (dermatitis, esophagitis), skin blistering, syndrome of inappropriate ADH secretion, tachycardia, thromboembolic events, thrombotic thrombocytopenic purpura, tumor pain, urticaria, vasodilation

Drug Interactions

Metabolism/Transport Effects Substrate of CYP2D6 (minor), CYP3A4 (major); **Note:** Assignment of Major/Minor substrate status based on clinically relevant drug interaction potential; **Inhibits** CYP2D6 (weak), CYP3A4 (weak)

Avoid Concomitant Use

Avoid concomitant use of Vinorelbine with any of the following: BCG; CloZAPine; Conivaptan; Fusidic Acid (Systemic); Natalizumab; Pimecrolimus; Pimozide; Tacrolimus (Topical); Tofacitinib; Vaccines (Live)

Increased Effect/Toxicity

Vinorelbine may increase the levels/effects of: ARIPiprazole; CloZAPine; Dofetilide; Leflunomide; Lomitapide; MitoMYcin (Systemic); Natalizumab; Pimozide; Tofacitinib; Vaccines (Live)

The levels/effects of Vinorelbine may be increased by: CISplatin; Conivaptan; CYP3A4 Inhibitors (Moderate); CYP3A4 Inhibitors (Strong); Dasatinib; Denosumab; Fusidic Acid (Systemic); Gefitinib; Itraconazole; Ivacaftor; Luliconazole; Macrolide Antibiotics; Mifepristone; PACLitaxel; PACLitaxel (Protein Bound); Pimecrolimus; Posaconazole; Roflumilast; Simeprevir; Tacrolimus (Topical); Trastuzumab; Voriconazole

Decreased Effect

Vinorelbine may decrease the levels/effects of: BCG; Coccidioidin Skin Test; Sipuleucel-T; Vaccines (Inactivated); Vaccines (Live)

The levels/effects of Vinorelbine may be decreased by: Bosentan; CYP3A4 Inducers (Strong); Dabrafenib; Deferasirox; Echinacea; Herbs (CYP3A4 Inducers); Mitotane; Peginterferon Alfa-2b; Tocilizumab

Ethanol/Nutrition/Herb Interactions Herb/Nutraceutical: Avoid St John's wort (may decrease vinorelbine levels).

Preparation for Administration Hazardous agent; use appropriate precautions for handling and disposal (NIOSH, 2012). Dilute in D_5W or NS to a final concentration of 1.5-3 mg/mL (for syringe) or D_5W, NS, $^1/_2$NS, $D_5{}^1/_2$NS, LR, or Ringer's to a final concentration of 0.5-2 mg/mL (for I.V. bag). Vinorelbine should **NOT** be prepared during the preparation of any intrathecal medications.

Storage/Stability Store intact vials refrigerated at 2°C to 8°C (36°F to 46°F); do not freeze. Protect from light. Intact vials are stable at room temperature of 25°C (77°F) for up to 72 hours. Solutions diluted for infusion in polypropylene syringes or polyvinyl chloride bags are stable for 24 hours at 5°C to 30°C (41°F to 86°F). After preparation, keep vinorelbine in a location **away** from the separate storage location recommended for intrathecal medications.

Mechanism of Action Semisynthetic vinca alkaloid which binds to tubulin and inhibits microtubule formation, therefore, arresting the cell at metaphase by disrupting the formation of the mitotic spindle; it is specific for the M and S phases. Vinorelbine may also interfere with nucleic acid and protein synthesis by blocking glutamic acid utilization.

Pharmacodynamics/Kinetics

Distribution: V_d: 25-40 L/kg; binds extensively to human platelets and lymphocytes (80% to 91%)

Protein binding: 80% to 91%

Metabolism: Extensively hepatic, via CYP3A4, to two metabolites, deacetylvinorelbine (active) and vinorelbine N-oxide

Half-life elimination: Triphasic: Terminal: 28-44 hours
Excretion: Feces (46%); urine (18%, 10% to 12% as unchanged drug)

Dosage Details concerning dosing in combination regimens should also be consulted. Adults: I.V.:

Nonsmall cell lung cancer (NSCLC):

Single-agent therapy: 30 mg/m^2 every 7 days until disease progression or unacceptable toxicity

Combination therapy: 25-30 mg/m^2 every 7 days (in combination with cisplatin)

Unlabeled dosing: 25 mg/m^2 days 1 and 8 every 21 days (in combination with cisplatin and cetuximab) for up to 6 cycles (Pirker, 2009) **or** 25-30 mg/m^2 days 1, 8, and 15 every 28 days (in combination with gemcitabine) for 6 cycles **or** until disease progression or unacceptable toxicity (Herbst, 2002; Greco, 2007)

Breast cancer, metastatic (unlabeled use): 25 mg/m^2 every 7 days (as a single agent) until disease progression or unacceptable toxicity (Zelek, 2001) **or** 25 mg/m^2 every 7 days (in combination with trastuzumab) until disease progression or unacceptable toxicity (Burstein, 2001) **or** 30 or 35 mg/m^2 days 1 and 8 every 21 days (in combination with trastuzumab) until disease progression or unacceptable toxicity (Andersson, 2011)

Cervical cancer (unlabeled use): 30 mg/m^2 days 1 and 8 of a of a 21-day treatment cycle (Muggia, 2004; Muggia, 2005)

Hodgkin lymphoma, relapsed or refractory (unlabeled use):

GVD regimen: 15 mg/m^2 (post-transplant patients) or 20 mg/m^2 (transplant-naïve patients) on days 1 and 8 of a 21-day cycle (in combination with gemcitabine and doxorubicin liposomal) for 2 to 6 cycles (Bartlett, 2007)

IGEV regimen: 20 mg/m^2 on day 1 of a 21-day cycle (in combination with ifosfamide, mesna, gemcitabine, and prednisolone) for 4 cycles (Santoro, 2007)

Malignant pleural mesothelioma (unlabeled use): 30 mg/m^2 (maximum dose: 60 mg) every 7 days per 6–week treatment cycle, continue until disease progression (Stebbing, 2009) **or** 30 mg/m^2 (maximum dose: 60 mg) every 7 days for 6 weeks, off 2 weeks, then repeat cycle (Muers, 2008)

Ovarian cancer, relapsed (unlabeled use): 25 mg/m^2 every 7 days (Bajetta, 1996) **or** 30 mg/m^2 days 1 and 8 of a 21-day treatment cycle (Rothenberg, 2004) until disease progression or unacceptable toxicity

Salivary gland cancer, recurrent (unlabeled use): 25 mg/m^2 on days 1 and 8 of a 21-day cycle (in combination with cisplatin) for up to 6 cycles (Airoldi, 2001) **or** 30 mg/m^2 every 7 days (monotherapy) for 9 weeks (Airoldi, 2001)

Small cell lung cancer, refractory (unlabeled use): 25 or 30 mg/m^2 every 7 days until disease progression or unacceptable toxicity (Furuse, 1996; Jessem, 1993)

Soft tissue sarcoma, advanced (unlabeled use): 25 mg/m^2 days 1 and 8 of a 21-day treatment cycle (in combination with gemcitabine) until disease progression or unacceptable toxicity (Dileo, 2007)

Dosage adjustment in hematological toxicity: Granulocyte counts should be ≥1000 cells/mm^3 prior to the administration of vinorelbine. Adjustments in the dosage of vinorelbine should be based on granulocyte counts obtained on the day of treatment as follows:

Granulocytes ≥1500 cells/mm^3 on day of treatment: Administer 100% of starting dose

Granulocytes 1000-1499 cells/mm^3 on day of treatment: Administer 50% of starting dose

Granulocytes <1000 cells/mm^3 on day of treatment: Do not administer. Repeat granulocyte count in one week; if 3 consecutive doses are held because granulocyte count is <1000 cells/mm^3, discontinue vinorelbine.

For patients who, during treatment, have experienced fever and/or sepsis while granulocytopenic or had 2 consecutive weekly doses held due to granulocytopenia, subsequent doses of vinorelbine should be:

75% of starting dose for granulocytes ≥1500 cells/mm^3

37.5% of starting dose for granulocytes 1000-1499 cells/mm^3

Dosage adjustment for neurotoxicity: Neurotoxicity ≥grade 2: Discontinue treatment

Dosage adjustment for other adverse events: Severe adverse events: Reduce dose or discontinue treatment

Dosage adjustment in renal impairment:

Renal insufficiency: No dosage adjustment necessary.

Hemodialysis: Initial: I.V.: Reduce dose to 20 mg/m^2/week; administer either after dialysis (on dialysis days) or on nondialysis days (Janus, 2010)

Dosing adjustment in hepatic impairment: Administer with caution in patients with hepatic insufficiency. In patients who develop hyperbilirubinemia during treatment with vinorelbine, the dose should be adjusted for total bilirubin as follows:

Serum bilirubin ≤2 mg/dL: Administer 100% of dose

Serum bilirubin 2.1-3 mg/dL: Administer 50% of dose (Ecklund, 2005; Floyd, 2006; Superfin, 2006)

Serum bilirubin >3 mg/dL: Administer 25% of dose (Ecklund, 2005; Floyd, 2006; Superfin, 2006)

Patients (breast cancer) with extensive liver metastases (>75% of liver volume): Administer 50% of dose (Ecklund, 2005; Superfin, 2006)

Dosing adjustment in patients with concurrent hematologic toxicity and hepatic impairment: Administer the lower of the doses determined from the adjustment recommendations.

Dosing in obesity: *ASCO Guidelines for appropriate chemotherapy dosing in obese adults with cancer:* Utilize patient's actual body weight (full weight) for calculation of body surface area- or weight-based dosing, particularly when the intent of therapy is curative; manage regimen-related toxicities in the same manner as for nonobese patients; if a dose reduction is utilized due to toxicity, consider resumption of full weight-based dosing with subsequent cycles, especially if cause of toxicity (eg, hepatic or renal impairment) is resolved (Griggs, 2012).

Administration For I.V. use only; FATAL IF GIVEN INTRATHECALLY. Administer as a direct intravenous push or rapid bolus, over 6-10 minutes (up to 30 minutes). Longer infusions may increase the risk of pain and phlebitis. Intravenous doses should be followed by at least 75-125 mL of saline or D_5W to reduce the incidence of phlebitis and inflammation.

Vesicant; ensure proper needle or catheter position prior to administration. Avoid extravasation.

Extravasation management: If extravasation occurs, stop infusion immediately and disconnect (leave cannula/needle in place); gently aspirate extravasated solution (do **NOT** flush the line); initiate hyaluronidase antidote; remove needle/cannula; apply dry warm compresses for 20 minutes 4 times a day for 1-2 days; elevate extremity (Perez Fidalgo, 2012). Remaining portion of the vinorelbine dose should be infused through a separate vein.

Hyaluronidase: If needle/cannula still in place, administer 1-6 mL hyaluronidase (150 units/mL) into the existing I.V. line; the usual dose is 1 mL hyaluronidase for each 1 mL of extravasated drug (Perez Fidalgo, 2012; Schulmeister, 2011). If needle/cannula was removed, inject 1-6 mL (150 units/mL) subcutaneously in a clockwise manner using 1mL for each 1 mL of drug extravasated (Schulmeister, 2011) **or** administer 1 mL (150 units/mL) as 5 separate 0.2 mL injections (using a 25-gauge needle) subcutaneously into the extravasation site (Polovich, 2009).

Hazardous agent; use appropriate precautions for handling and disposal (NIOSH, 2012).

Monitoring Parameters CBC with differential and platelet count (prior to each dose, and after treatment), hepatic function tests; monitor for new-onset pulmonary symptoms (or worsening from baseline); monitor for neuropathy (new or worsening symptoms; monitor infusion site; monitor for signs symptoms of constipation/ileus

Dosage Forms Excipient information presented when available (limited, particularly for generics); consult specific product labeling.

Solution, Intravenous:
Navelbine: 10 mg/mL (1 mL); 50 mg/5 mL (5 mL)
Generic: 10 mg/mL (1 mL); 50 mg/5 mL (5 mL)

Solution, Intravenous [preservative free]:
Generic: 10 mg/mL (1 mL); 50 mg/5 mL (5 mL)

◆ **Vinorelbine Injection, USP (Can)** *see* Vinorelbine *on page 2196*
◆ **Vinorelbine Tartrate** *see* Vinorelbine *on page 2196*
◆ **Vinorelbine Tartrate for Injection (Can)** *see* Vinorelbine *on page 2196*
◆ **Viokace** *see* Pancrelipase *on page 1558*
◆ **Viokase (Can)** *see* Pancrelipase *on page 1558*
◆ **Viorele** *see* Ethinyl Estradiol and Desogestrel *on page 784*
◆ **Viosterol** *see* Ergocalciferol *on page 733*
◆ **Viracept** *see* Nelfinavir *on page 1436*
◆ **Viramune** *see* Nevirapine *on page 1444*
◆ **Viramune® (Can)** *see* Nevirapine *on page 1444*
◆ **Viramune XR** *see* Nevirapine *on page 1444*
◆ **Viramune XR® (Can)** *see* Nevirapine *on page 1444*
◆ **Virazole** *see* Ribavirin *on page 1804*
◆ **Virdec [OTC]** *see* Chlorpheniramine and Phenylephrine *on page 412*
◆ **Virdec DM [OTC]** *see* Chlorpheniramine, Phenylephrine, and Dextromethorphan *on page 413*
◆ **Viread** *see* Tenofovir *on page 2012*
◆ **Viroptic** *see* Trifluridine *on page 2127*
◆ **Viroptic® (Can)** *see* Trifluridine *on page 2127*
◆ **Virtussin A/C** *see* Guaifenesin and Codeine *on page 976*
◆ **Virt-Vite Forte** *see* Folic Acid, Cyanocobalamin, and Pyridoxine *on page 908*
◆ **Viscoat®** *see* Sodium Chondroitin Sulfate and Sodium Hyaluronate *on page 1917*
◆ **Viscous Lidocaine** *see* Lidocaine (Topical) *on page 1212*
◆ **Visine-A [OTC]** *see* Naphazoline and Pheniramine *on page 1425*
◆ **Visine Advanced Allergy (Can)** *see* Naphazoline and Pheniramine *on page 1425*
◆ **Visken (Can)** *see* Pindolol *on page 1649*

Vismodegib (vis moe DEG ib)

Brand Names: U.S. Erivedge

Brand Names: Canada Erivedge

Index Terms GDC-0449; Hedgehog Antagonist GDC-0449

Pharmacologic Category Antineoplastic Agent, Hedgehog Pathway Inhibitor

Use Basal cell carcinoma: Treatment of metastatic basal cell carcinoma, or locally-advanced basal cell carcinoma that has recurred following surgery or in patients who are not candidates for surgery, and not candidates for radiation therapy

Pregnancy Risk Factor D

Pregnancy Considerations [U.S. Boxed Warning]: May result in severe birth defects or embryo-fetal death. Teratogenic effects (severe midline defects, missing digits, and other irreversible malformations), embryotoxic, and fetotoxic events were observed in animal reproduction studies when administered in doses less than the normal human dose. Based on its mechanism of action adverse effects on pregnancy would be expected. **[U.S. Boxed Warning]: Verify pregnancy status prior to initiating treatment and advise patients (female and male) of the risk of birth defects, the need for contraception and risk of exposure through semen.** In females of childbearing potential, obtain pregnancy test within 7 days prior to treatment initiation; after the negative pregnancy test, initiate highly effective contraception prior to the first vismodegib dose and continue during and for 7 months after treatment. During treatment (including treatment interruptions) and for 2 months after treatment, male patients should not donate sperm and should use condoms with spermicide (even after vasectomy) if their partner is of childbearing potential. Women exposed to vismodegib during pregnancy (directly or via seminal fluid) are encouraged to participate in the Erivedge Pregnancy Pharmacovigilance program by contacting the Genentech Adverse Event Line (1-888-835-2555). Pregnancies occurring during or within 7 months after treatment should be reported to the Genentech Adverse Event Line.

The Canadian labeling recommends that females of childbearing potential use 2 simultaneous forms of effective contraception beginning at least 4 weeks prior to treatment initiation, during treatment (including treatment interruptions), and for 24 months after discontinuation. Pregnancy testing should be performed within 7 days prior to treatment initiation, monthly during treatment (including treatment interruptions) and for 24 months after discontinuation. For females of child bearing potential, a new prescription is required each month to allow for monthly pregnancy testing. Any suspected exposure (directly or via seminal fluid) during pregnancy should be immediately reported to the Erivedge Pregnancy Prevention Program (EPPP) at 1-888-748-8926.

Breast-Feeding Considerations It is not known if vismodegib is excreted in human milk. Due to the potential for serious adverse reactions in the nursing infant or child, the decision to discontinue breast-feeding or to discontinue vismodegib should take into account the benefits of treatment to the mother. The Canadian labeling contraindicates use in women who are nursing and recommends that women abstain from nursing for 24 months after discontinuation of therapy.

Prescribing and Access Restrictions

U.S.: Available at specialty pharmacies through the Erivedge Access Solutions program. Further information may be obtained from the manufacturer, Genentech, at 1-888-249-4918, or at www.ErivedgeAccessSolutions.com

Canada: Available through a controlled distribution program called Erivedge Pregnancy Prevention Program (EPPP). Registration with the program is required for participating prescribers and pharmacies. Patients must also be registered with the program and meet all necessary requirements to receive vismodegib. Consult product monograph for detailed information regarding program requirements. Further information may also be obtained at 1-888-748-8926 or at www.erivedge.ca.

Medication Guide Available Yes

Contraindications

U.S. labeling: There are no contraindications listed within the manufacturer's labeling.

Canadian labeling: Hypersensitivity to vismodegib or any component of the formulation; pregnancy or females at risk of becoming pregnant; breast-feeding; male patients or female patients of childbearing potential who do not comply with the Erivedge Pregnancy Prevention Program; children and adolescents <18 years of age.

Warnings/Precautions Hazardous agent - use appropriate precautions for handling and disposal (meets NIOSH, 2012 criteria). **[U.S. Boxed Warnings]: May result in severe birth defects or embryo-fetal death. Teratogenic effects (severe midline defects, missing digits, and other irreversible malformations), embryotoxic, and fetotoxic events were observed in animal reproduction studies. Verify pregnancy status prior to initiating treatment and advise patients (female and male) of the risk of birth defects, the need for contraception and risk of exposure through semen.** Amenorrhea was observed in women of reproductive potential; it is unknown if this is reversible.

Cardiac events (eg, cardiac failure, atrial fibrillation, left ventricular dysfunction, restrictive cardiomyopathy, myocardial infarction) have been observed during treatment. All events ≥grade 3 occurred in patients with a history of significant cardiac disease. Cases of cutaneous squamous cell cancer (cuSCC) have been reported. Patients with advanced basal cell carcinoma are at risk for developing cuSCC; monitor during treatment. Vismodegib is associated with a moderate emetic potential; antiemetics may be needed to prevent nausea and vomiting. Diarrhea, constipation, abdominal pain, and decreased appetite may also occur.

Vismodegib metabolism is primarily hepatic; use with caution in patients with hepatic dysfunction. Elevated hepatic enzymes (mostly grades 1 and 2) have been observed with use; transient elevations ≥ grade 3 have been observed but did not require treatment interruption or discontinuation in most cases. Use with caution in patients with renal impairment (has not been studied). However, population pharmacokinetic analyses demonstrate that creatinine clearance (range: 30-80 mL/minute) does not have a clinically meaningful effect on systemic exposure; urinary excretion is <5%.

Advise patients not to donate blood or blood products during vismodegib treatment and for at least 7 months after the last vismodegib dose. The Canadian labeling recommends patients not donate blood or blood products during treatment (including treatment interruptions) and for 24 months after discontinuation.

Adverse Reactions

>10%:

Central nervous system: Fatigue (40%)

Dermatologic: Alopecia (64%)

Endocrine & metabolic: Amenorrhea (30%)

Gastrointestinal: Abnormal taste (55%), weight loss (45%), nausea (30%), diarrhea (29%), appetite decreased (25%), constipation (21%), vomiting (14%), loss of taste perception (11%)

Neuromuscular & skeletal: Muscle spasm (72%), arthralgia (16%)

1% to 10%:

Endocrine & metabolic: Hyponatremia (grade 3: 4%), hypokalemia (grade 3: 1%)

Renal: Azotemia (grade 3: 2%)

<1% (Limited to important or life-threatening): Abdominal pain, alkaline phosphatase increased, aspiration, atrial fibrillation, back pain, corneal abrasion, dehydration, dyspnea, hyperkalemia, hypocalcemia, keratitis, lymphopenia, pneumonia, urinary tract infection

Drug Interactions

Metabolism/Transport Effects Substrate of CYP2C9 (minor), CYP3A4 (minor), P-glycoprotein; **Note:** Assignment of Major/Minor substrate status based on clinically relevant drug interaction potential; **Inhibits** BCRP, CYP2C19 (weak), CYP2C8 (weak), CYP2C9 (weak)

Avoid Concomitant Use There are no known interactions where it is recommended to avoid concomitant use.

Increased Effect/Toxicity

The levels/effects of Vismodegib may be increased by: P-glycoprotein/ABCB1 Inhibitors

Decreased Effect

The levels/effects of Vismodegib may be decreased by: Antacids; H2-Antagonists; P-glycoprotein/ABCB1 Inducers; Proton Pump Inhibitors

Storage/Stability Store at 20°C to 25°C (68°F to 77°F); excursions permitted to 15°C to 30°C (59°F to 86°F).

Mechanism of Action Basal cell cancer is associated with mutations in Hedgehog pathway components. Hedgehog regulates cell growth and differentiation in embryogenesis; while generally not active in adult tissue, Hedgehog mutations associated with basal cell cancer can activate the pathway resulting in unrestricted proliferation of skin basal cells. Vismodegib is a selective Hedgehog pathway inhibitor which binds to and inhibits Smoothened homologue (SMO), the transmembrane protein involved in Hedgehog signal transduction.

Pharmacodynamics/Kinetics

Distribution: V_d: 16.4-26.6 L

Protein binding: >99%; primarily to serum albumin and $alpha_1$ acid glycoprotein (AAG)

Metabolism: Metabolized by oxidation, glucuronidation, and pyridine ring cleavage, although >98% of circulating components are as the parent drug

Bioavailability: ~32%

Half-life, elimination: Continuous daily dosing: ~4 days; Single dose: ~12 days

Time to peak: ~2.4 days (Graham, 2011)

Excretion: Feces (82%); urine (4%)

Dosage Basal cell cancer, metastatic or locally advanced: Adults: Oral: 150 mg once daily until disease progression or unacceptable toxicity. In clinical trials, treatment interruptions up to 4 weeks were allowed for toxicity recovery (Sekulik, 2012).

Missed doses: If a dose is missed, do not make up; resume dosing with the next scheduled dose.

Dosage adjustment in renal impairment: No dosage adjustment provided in manufacturer's labeling (has not been studied).

Dosage adjustment in hepatic impairment: No dosage adjustment provided in manufacturer's labeling (has not been studied).

Dietary Considerations May be taken without regard to food.

Administration Oral: May be taken with or without food. Swallow capsules whole; do not open or crush. Vismodegib is associated with a moderate emetic potential; antiemetics may be needed to prevent nausea and vomiting. Hazardous agent; use appropriate precautions for handling and disposal (meets NIOSH, 2012 criteria).

Monitoring Parameters Pregnancy test within 1 week prior to treatment initiation.

Canadian labeling: Pregnancy testing (minimum sensitivity of 25 mIU/mL) within 1 week prior to treatment initiation, monthly during treatment (including during treatment interruptions), and for 24 months after discontinuation; CBC with differential and comprehensive metabolic panel at baseline and every 4 weeks thereafter; skin examination routinely during therapy.

Additional Information In a study of vismodegib in patients with basal cell nevus syndrome (not an approved use), with discontinuation of vismodegib treatment, taste alteration and muscle cramps abated within 1 month, and scalp and body hair began to regrow within 3 months (Tang, 2012).

Dosage Forms Excipient information presented when available (limited, particularly for generics); consult specific product labeling.

Capsule, Oral:

Erivedge: 150 mg

- **Vistaril** *see* HydrOXYzine *on page 1025*
- **Vistide** *see* Cidofovir *on page 424*
- **Vistonuridine** *see* Uridine Triacetate *on page 2141*
- **VIT 45** *see* Ferric Carboxymaltose *on page 852*
- **Vita-C [OTC]** *see* Ascorbic Acid *on page 172*
- **Vitamin C** *see* Ascorbic Acid *on page 172*
- **Vitamin D_3 and Alendronate** *see* Alendronate and Cholecalciferol *on page 71*
- **Vitamin D and Calcium Carbonate** *see* Calcium and Vitamin D *on page 318*

Vitamin A (VYE ta min aye)

Brand Names: U.S. A+D Prevent [OTC]; A-25 [OTC]; AFirm 1X [OTC]; AFirm 2X [OTC]; AFirm 3X [OTC]; Aquasol A; Gordons-Vite A [OTC]; Vita-Ray [OTC]; Vitamin A Fish [OTC]

Index Terms Oleovitamin A

Pharmacologic Category Vitamin, Fat Soluble

Use Treatment and prevention of vitamin A deficiency; parenteral (I.M.) route is indicated when oral administration is not feasible or when absorption is insufficient (malabsorption syndrome); dietary supplement (OTC)

Unlabeled Use Treatment of xerophthalmia caused by vitamin A deficiency; supplement to prevent complications in children with measles in certain settings

Pregnancy Risk Factor X

Dosage

Oral:

Dietary Reference Intake for vitamin A (presented as retinol activity equivalent [RAE]) (IOM, 2000):

Adequate intake (AI):

1-6 months: 400 mcg/day (1330 units/day)

7-12 months: 500 mcg/day (1670 units/day)

Recommended dietary allowance (RDA):

1-3 years: 300 mcg/day (1000 units/day)

4-8 years: 400 mcg/day (1330 units/day)

9-13 years: 600 mcg/day (2000 units/day)

Males >13 years: 900 mcg/day (3000 units/day)

Females >13 years: 700 mcg/day (2330 units/day)

Pregnant females:

14-18 years: 750 mcg/day (2500 units/day)

≥19 years: 770 mcg/day (2560 units/day)

Lactating females:

14-18 years: 1200 mcg/day (4000 units/day)

≥19 years: 1300 mcg/day (4330 units/day)

Treatment of measles (unlabeled use) (WHO, 2004; WHO, 2010): **Note:** Repeat with single dose in 2-4 weeks if severe malnutrition exists or ophthalmic evidence of a vitamin deficiency is present:

Infants <6 months: 50,000 units once daily for 2 days

Infants 6-11 months: 100,000 units once daily for 2 days

Children >11 months to 5 years: 200,000 units once daily for 2 days

Treatment of xerophthalmia (unlabeled use):

Infants <6 months: 50,000 units once daily for 2 days; repeat with single dose after 2 weeks (WHO, 2010)

Infants 6-12 months: 100,000 units once daily for 2 days; repeat with single dose after 2 weeks (WHO, 2010)

Children >1 year and Adults (except females of reproductive age): 200,000 units once daily for 2 days; repeat with single dose after 2 weeks (WHO, 2008)

Females of reproductive age (WHO, 1997; WHO, 2008):

With night blindness or Bitot's spots (less severe xerophthalmia): 5000-10,000 units daily (maximum 10,000 units/day) or ≤25,000 units once weekly for ≥4 weeks

Severe xerophthalmia: Refer to adult dosing.

High-dose supplementation in patients at high risk for deficiency (unlabeled dose) (eg, persons living in developing areas of the world where deficiency is a public health problem, especially persons with severe infectious disease or malnutrition):

Infants <6 months: Not recommended (WHO, 2011a)

Infants 6-12 months: 100,000 units/dose; repeat every 4-6 months, but do not readminister within 30 days of previous dose (WHO, 1997; WHO, 2010)

Children >1 year: 200,000 units/dose; repeat every 4-6 months, but do not readminister within 30 days of previous dose (WHO, 1997; WHO, 2010)

Adults: 200,000 units/dose every 6 months (WHO, 2008)

Pregnant females: Maximum 10,000 units daily or 25,000 units once weekly. Administer for a minimum of 12 weeks during pregnancy or until delivery (WHO, 2008; WHO, 2011c)

Postpartum females: 200,000 units at delivery or within 8 weeks of delivery (WHO, 2008)

I.M.: **Deficiency (manufacturer recommendation): Note:** I.M. route is indicated when oral administration is not feasible or when absorption is insufficient (malabsorption syndrome):

Infants: 7500-15,000 units/day for 10 days

Children 1-8 years: 17,500-35,000 units/day for 10 days

Children >8 years and Adults: 100,000 units/day for 3 days, followed by 50,000 units/day for 2 weeks

Note: Follow-up therapy with an oral therapeutic multivitamin (containing additional vitamin A) is recommended: Oral:

Low Birth Weight Infants: Additional vitamin A is recommended; however, no dosage amount has been established.

Children ≤8 years: 5000-10,000 units/day for 2 months

Children >8 years and Adults: 10,000-20,000 units/day for 2 months

Additional Information Complete prescribing information should be consulted for additional detail.

Dosage Forms Excipient information presented when available (limited, particularly for generics); consult specific product labeling.

Capsule, Oral:

A-25: 25,000 units

Vitamin A Fish: 7500 units

Generic: 10,000 units

Capsule, Oral [preservative free]:

A-25: 25,000 units [dye free]

Generic: 8000 units

Cream, External:

AFirm 1X: 0.15% (30 g) [fragrance free; contains benzyl alcohol, cetyl alcohol, disodium edta, methylparaben, peg-10 soya sterol, trolamine (triethanolamine)]

AFirm 2X: 0.3% (30 g) [fragrance free; contains benzyl alcohol, cetyl alcohol, disodium edta, methylparaben, peg-10 soya sterol, trolamine (triethanolamine)]

AFirm 3X: 0.6% (30 g) [fragrance free; contains benzyl alcohol, cetyl alcohol, disodium edta, methylparaben, peg-10 soya sterol, trolamine (triethanolamine)]

Gordons-Vite A: 100,000 units/g (75 g, 120 g, 480 g, 2400 g)

Vita-Ray: 10-200000-3000 (15 g, 75 g)

Lotion, External:
Gordons-Vite A: 100,000 units (120 mL, 4000 mL)
Ointment, External:
A+D Prevent: (42.5 g, 113 g, 454 g)
Solution, Intramuscular:
Aquasol A: 50,000 units/mL (2 mL) [contains chlorobutanol (chlorobutol)]
Tablet, Oral:
Generic: 10,000 units, 15,000 units, 10000-1000 UNIT

◆ **Vitamin A Acid** *see* Tretinoin (Topical) *on page 2120*

Vitamin A and Vitamin D (Systemic)
(VYE ta min aye & VYE ta min dee)

Brand Names: U.S. A&D Jr. [OTC]; D-Natural-5 [OTC]
Index Terms Cod Liver Oil
Pharmacologic Category Vitamin, Fat Soluble
Use Dietary supplement
Dosage Oral: Adults: Dietary supplement: One tablet or capsule once daily.
Additional Information Complete prescribing information should be consulted for additional detail.
Dosage Forms Excipient information presented when available (limited, particularly for generics); consult specific product labeling.
Capsule, softgel, oral: Vitamin A 1250 units and vitamin D 130 units, Vitamin A 1250 units and vitamin D 135 units, Vitamin A 5,000 units and vitamin D 400 units, Vitamin A 10,000 units and vitamin D 400 units, Vitamin A 25,000 units and vitamin D 1000 units
A&D Jr.: Vitamin A 10,000 units and vitamin D 400 units [contains soybean oil]
D-Natural-5: Vitamin A 10,000 units and vitamin D 5000 units
Oil, oral: Vitamin A 5000 units and vitamin D 500 units per 5 mL (120 mL, 473 mL)
Tablet, oral: Vitamin A 10,000 units and vitamin D 400 units

Vitamin A and Vitamin D (Topical)
(VYE ta min aye & VYE ta min dee)

Brand Names: U.S. A+D® Original [OTC]; Baza® Clear [OTC]; Sween Cream® [OTC]
Index Terms Cod Liver Oil
Pharmacologic Category Topical Skin Product
Use Temporary relief of discomfort due to chapped skin or lips, cuts and scrapes, diaper rash, or minor burns
Dosage Topical: Children and Adults:
Diaper rash: Apply with each diaper change and any time prolonged exposure to wet diapers may occur (ie, at bedtime).
Skin protectant: Apply to affected areas as needed.
Additional Information Complete prescribing information should be consulted for additional detail.
Dosage Forms Excipient information presented when available (limited, particularly for generics); consult specific product labeling.
Cream, topical:
Sween Cream®: (57 g, 142 g)
Cream, topical [original formula]:
Sween Cream®: (2 g, 14 g, 85 g, 184 g, 339 g)
Ointment, topical: (5 g, 60 g, 120 g, 454 g)
A+D® Original: (42.5 g); (120 g); (454 g) [in lanolin-petrolatum base]
Baza® Clear: (50 g, 142 g, 227 g) [in petrolatum base]

◆ **Vitamin A Fish [OTC]** *see* Vitamin A *on page 2201*
◆ **Vitamin B_1** *see* Thiamine *on page 2045*
◆ **Vitamin B_2** *see* Riboflavin *on page 1809*
◆ **Vitamin B_3** *see* Niacin *on page 1447*
◆ **Vitamin B_3** *see* Niacinamide *on page 1450*
◆ **Vitamin B_6** *see* Pyridoxine *on page 1753*
◆ **Vitamin B_{12}** *see* Cyanocobalamin *on page 501*
◆ **Vitamin B_{12a}** *see* Hydroxocobalamin *on page 1017*
◆ **Vitamin D2** *see* Ergocalciferol *on page 733*

Vitamin E (VYE ta min ee)

Brand Names: U.S. Alph-E [OTC]; Alph-E-Mixed 1000 [OTC]; Alph-E-Mixed [OTC]; Aquasol E [OTC]; Aquavit-E [OTC]; Aqueous Vitamin E [OTC]; E-400 [OTC]; E-400-Clear [OTC]; E-400-Mixed [OTC]; E-Max-1000 [OTC]; E-Pherol [OTC]; Formula E 400 [OTC]; Gordons-Vite E [OTC]; Natural Vitamin E [OTC]; Nutr-E-Sol [OTC]; Vita-Plus E [OTC]; Vitamin E Beauty [OTC]; Vitec [OTC]; Xtra-Care [OTC]
Index Terms *d*-Alpha Tocopherol; *dl*-Alpha Tocopherol
Pharmacologic Category Vitamin, Fat Soluble
Use Dietary supplement
Dosage Vitamin E may be expressed as alpha-tocopherol equivalents (ATE), which refer to the biologically-active (R) stereoisomer content.
Oral:
Adequate intake (AI) (IOM, 2000): Infants (RDA not established):
1-6 months: 4 mg
7-12 months: 5 mg
Recommended daily allowance (RDA) (IOM, 2000):
Children:
1-3 years: 6 mg; upper limit of intake should not exceed 200 mg/day
4-8 years: 7 mg; upper limit of intake should not exceed 300 mg/day
9-13 years: 11 mg; upper limit of intake should not exceed 600 mg/day
14-18 years: 15 mg; upper limit of intake should not exceed 800 mg/day
Adults: 15 mg; upper limit of intake should not exceed 1000 mg/day
Pregnant female:
≤18 years: 15 mg; upper level of intake should not exceed 800 mg/day
19-50 years: 15 mg; upper level of intake should not exceed 1000 mg/day
Lactating female:
≤18 years: 19 mg; upper level of intake should not exceed 800 mg/day
19-50 years: 19 mg; upper level of intake should not exceed 1000 mg/day

Vitamin E deficiency:
Children (with malabsorption syndrome): 1 unit/kg/day of water miscible vitamin E (to raise plasma tocopherol concentrations to the normal range within 2 months and to maintain normal plasma concentrations)
Adults: 60-75 units/day
Cystic fibrosis supplementation (Borowitz 2002): Infants and Children:
1-12 months: 40-50 units/day
1-3 years: 80-150 units/day
4-8 years: 100-200 units/day
>8 years: 200-400 units/day

Topical: Adults: Apply a thin layer over affected area
Additional Information Complete prescribing information should be consulted for additional detail.
Dosage Forms Excipient information presented when available (limited, particularly for generics); consult specific product labeling.
Capsule, Oral:
Alph-E: 400 units
Alph-E-Mixed: 200 units
Alph-E-Mixed 1000: 1000 units

Alph-E-Mixed: 400 units [corn free, milk free, sugar free, wheat free, yeast free]
Formula E 400: 400 units
Vita-Plus E: 400 units
Generic: 100 units, 200 units, 400 units, 600 units, 1000 units

Capsule, Oral [preservative free]:
E-400: 400 units [corn free, gluten free, milk derivatives/products, no artificial color(s), no artificial flavor(s), sodium free, soy free, starch free, sugar free, yeast free]
E-400-Clear: 400 units [dye free]
E-400-Mixed: 400 units [dye free]
E-Max-1000: 1000 units [dye free]
Generic: 100 units, 400 units

Cream, External:
Gordons-Vite E: 1500 units/30 g (15 g, 75 g, 480 g, 2400 g)
Generic: 1000 units (112 g)

Liquid, External:
Generic: 920 units/mL (28.5 mL, 57 mL, 114 mL)

Liquid, Oral:
Nutr-E-Sol: 400 units/15 mL (473 mL) [color free, starch free, sugar free]

Lotion, External:
Vitec: (113 g)
Xtra-Care: (2 mL, 59 mL, 118 mL, 237 mL, 621 mL, 1000 mL, 3840 mL)

Oil, External:
Vitamin E Beauty: 24,000 units/52 mL (52 mL); 49,000 units/52 mL (52 mL)

Solution, Oral:
Aquasol E: 15 units/0.3 mL (12 mL, 30 mL) [contains polysorbate 80, propylene glycol, saccharin]
Aquavit-E: 15 units/0.3 mL (30 mL) [butterscotch flavor]
Aqueous Vitamin E: 15 units/0.3 mL (30 mL) [anise-butterscotch flavor]
Generic: 15 units/0.3 mL (12 mL)

Tablet, Oral:
E-Pherol: 400 units
Natural Vitamin E: 200 units, 400 units [animal products free, gelatin free, gluten free, kosher certified, lactose free, no artificial color(s), no artificial flavor(s), starch free, sugar free, yeast free]
Generic: 100 units, 200 units, 400 units

- **Vitamin E Beauty [OTC]** *see* Vitamin E *on page 2202*
- **Vitamin G** *see* Riboflavin *on page 1809*
- **Vitamin K** *see* Phytonadione *on page 1644*
- **Vitamin K_1** *see* Phytonadione *on page 1644*
- **Vita-Plus E [OTC]** *see* Vitamin E *on page 2202*
- **Vita-Ray [OTC]** *see* Vitamin A *on page 2201*
- **Vita-Respa®** *see* Folic Acid, Cyanocobalamin, and Pyridoxine *on page 908*
- **Vitec [OTC]** *see* Vitamin E *on page 2202*
- **Vituz** *see* Hydrocodone and Chlorpheniramine *on page 1007*
- **Vi Vaccine** *see* Typhoid Vaccine *on page 2135*
- **Vivactil** *see* Protriptyline *on page 1745*
- **Vivarin® [OTC]** *see* Caffeine *on page 309*
- **Vivelle-Dot** *see* Estradiol (Systemic) *on page 754*
- **Vivitrol** *see* Naltrexone *on page 1423*
- **Vivotif®** *see* Typhoid Vaccine *on page 2135*
- **VLB** *see* VinBLAStine *on page 2189*
- **VM-26** *see* Teniposide *on page 2012*
- **Volibris (Can)** *see* Ambrisentan *on page 94*
- **Voltaren** *see* Diclofenac (Systemic) *on page 597*
- **Voltaren Ophtha® (Can)** *see* Diclofenac (Ophthalmic) *on page 600*
- **Voltaren Rapide (Can)** *see* Diclofenac (Systemic) *on page 597*
- **Voltaren SR (Can)** *see* Diclofenac (Systemic) *on page 597*
- **Voltaren-XR** *see* Diclofenac (Systemic) *on page 597*
- **Volulyte (Can)** *see* Tetrastarch *on page 2036*
- **Voluven** *see* Tetrastarch *on page 2036*
- **von Willebrand Factor/Factor VIII Complex** *see* Antihemophilic Factor/von Willebrand Factor Complex (Human) *on page 146*
- **Voraxaze** *see* Glucarpidase *on page 961*

Voriconazole (vor i KOE na zole)

Brand Names: U.S. Vfend; Vfend IV

Brand Names: Canada VFEND®

Index Terms UK109496

Pharmacologic Category Antifungal Agent, Oral; Antifungal Agent, Parenteral

Additional Appendix Information
Antifungal Agents *on page 2286*

Use Treatment of invasive aspergillosis; treatment of esophageal candidiasis; treatment of candidemia (in non-neutropenic patients); treatment of disseminated *Candida* infections of the skin and viscera; treatment of serious fungal infections caused by *Scedosporium apiospermum* and *Fusarium* spp (including *Fusarium solani*) in patients intolerant of, or refractory to, other therapy

Unlabeled Use Fungal infection prophylaxis in intermediate or high risk neutropenic cancer patients with myelodysplastic syndrome (MDS) or acute myelogenous leukemia (AML), neutropenic allogeneic hematopoietic stem cell recipients, and patients with significant graft-versus-host disease; empiric antifungal therapy (second-line) for persistent neutropenic fever; empiric treatment of fungal meningitis or osteoarticular infections

Pregnancy Risk Factor D

Pregnancy Considerations Voriconazole can cause fetal harm when administered to a pregnant woman. Voriconazole was teratogenic and embryotoxic in animal studies, and lowered plasma estradiol in animal models. Women of childbearing potential should use effective contraception during treatment. Should be used in pregnant woman only if benefit to mother justifies potential risk to the fetus.

Breast-Feeding Considerations Excretion in breast milk has not been investigated; avoid breast-feeding until additional data are available.

Contraindications Hypersensitivity to voriconazole or any component of the formulation (cross-reaction with other azole antifungal agents may occur but has not been established, use caution); coadministration of CYP3A4 substrates which may lead to QT_c prolongation (cisapride, pimozide, or quinidine); coadministration with barbiturates (long acting), carbamazepine, efavirenz (with standard [eg, not adjusted] voriconazole and efavirenz doses), ergot derivatives, rifampin, rifabutin, ritonavir (≥800 mg/day), sirolimus, St John's wort

Warnings/Precautions Visual changes, including blurred vision, changes in visual acuity, color perception, and photophobia, are commonly associated with treatment; postmarketing cases of optic neuritis and papilledema (lasting >1 month) have also been reported. Patients should be warned to avoid tasks which depend on vision, including operating machinery or driving. Changes are reversible on discontinuation following brief exposure/treatment regimens (≤28 days).

Serious hepatic reactions (including hepatitis, cholestasis, and fulminant hepatic failure) have occurred during treatment, primarily in patients with serious concomitant medical conditions. However, hepatotoxicity has occurred in patients with no identifiable risk factors. Use caution in patients with pre-existing hepatic impairment (dose adjustment or discontinuation may be required).

Voriconazole tablets contain lactose; avoid administration in hereditary galactose intolerance, Lapp lactase deficiency, or glucose-galactose malabsorption. Suspension contains sucrose; use caution with fructose intolerance, sucrase-isomaltase deficiency, or glucose-galactose malabsorption. Avoid/limit use of intravenous formulation in patients with renal impairment; intravenous formulation contains excipient cyclodextrin (sulfobutyl ether beta-cyclodextrin), which may accumulate in renal insufficiency. Acute renal failure has been observed in severely ill patients; use with caution in patients receiving concomitant nephrotoxic medications. Anaphylactoid-type infusion-related reactions may occur with intravenous dosing. Consider discontinuation of infusion if reaction is severe.

Use caution in patients taking strong cytochrome P450 inducers, CYP2C9 inhibitors, and major 3A4 substrates (see Drug Interactions); consider alternative agents that avoid or lessen the potential for CYP-mediated interactions. QT interval prolongation has been associated with voriconazole use; rare cases of arrhythmia (including torsade de pointes), cardiac arrest, and sudden death have been reported, usually in seriously ill patients with comorbidities and/or risk factors (eg, prior cardiotoxic chemotherapy, cardiomyopathy, electrolyte imbalance, or concomitant QT_c-prolonging drugs). Use with caution in these patient populations; correct electrolyte abnormalities (eg, hypokalemia, hypomagnesemia, hypocalcemia) prior to initiating therapy. Do not infuse concomitantly with blood products or short-term concentrated electrolyte solutions, even if the two infusions are running in separate intravenous lines (or cannulas).

Rare cases of malignancy (melanoma, squamous cell carcinoma) have been reported in patients (mostly immunocompromised) with prior onset of severe photosensitivity reactions and exposure to long-term voriconazole therapy. Other serious exfoliative cutaneous reactions, including Stevens-Johnson syndrome, have also been reported. Patient should avoid strong, direct exposure to sunlight; may cause photosensitivity, especially with long-term use. Discontinue use in patients who develop an exfoliative cutaneous reaction or a skin lesion consistent with squamous cell carcinoma or melanoma. Periodic total body skin examinations should be performed, particularly with prolonged use.

Monitor pancreatic function in patients (children and adults) at risk for acute pancreatitis (eg, recent chemotherapy or hematopoietic stem cell transplantation); there have been postmarketing reports of pancreatitis in children.

Adverse Reactions

>10%:

- Central nervous system: Hallucination (2% to 12%; auditory and/or visual and likely serum concentration-dependent)
- Ophthalmic: Visual disturbance (19%)
- Renal: Increased serum creatinine (1% to 21%)

2% to 10%:

- Cardiovascular: Tachycardia (≤2%)
- Central nervous system: Chills (≤4%), headache (≤3%)
- Dermatologic: Skin rash (≤7%)
- Endocrine & metabolic: Hypokalemia (≤2%)
- Gastrointestinal: Nausea (1% to 5%), vomiting (1% to 4%)
- Hepatic: Increased serum alkaline phosphatase (4% to 5%), increased serum AST (2% to 4%), increased serum ALT (2% to 3%), cholestatic jaundice (1% to 2%)
- Ophthalmic: Photophobia (2%)
- Miscellaneous: Fever (≤6%)

<2%, postmarketing, and/or case reports (limited to important or life-threatening): Acute renal failure, adrenocortical insufficiency, agranulocytosis, alopecia, anaphylactoid reaction, anemia (aplastic, hemolytic, macrocytic, megaloblastic, or microcytic), angioedema, anorexia, anuria, arthritis, ascites, ataxia, atrial arrhythmia, atrial fibrillation, atrioventricular block, bacterial infection, bigeminy, blighted ovum, bone marrow depression, bradycardia, brain disease, bundle branch block, cardiac arrest, cardiac failure, cardiomegaly, cardiomyopathy, cellulitis, cerebral edema, cerebral hemorrhage, cerebral ischemia, cerebrovascular accident, chest pain, cholecystitis, cholelithiasis, cholestasis, chromatopsia, color blindness, coma, confusion, convulsions, corneal opacity, cyanosis, deafness, deep vein thrombophlebitis, deep vein thrombosis, delirium, dementia, dental fluorosis, depersonalization, depression, diabetes insipidus, diarrhea, discoid lupus erythematosus, disseminated intravascular coagulation, drowsiness, duodenal ulcer (active), duodenitis, dyspnea, eczema, edema, encephalitis, endocarditis, eosinophilia, erythema multiforme, esophageal ulcer, exfoliative dermatitis, extrapyramidal reaction, extrasystoles, fixed drug eruption, fungal infection, gastric ulcer, gastrointestinal hemorrhage, glucose tolerance decreased, graft versus host disease, Guillain-Barre syndrome, hematemesis, hemorrhagic cystitis, hepatic coma, hepatic failure, hepatitis, hepatomegaly, herpes simplex infection, hydronephrosis, hyperbilirubinemia, hypercholesterolemia, hyper-/hypocalcemia, hyper-/hypoglycemia, hyper-/hypomagnesemia, hyper-/hyponatremia, hyper-/hypotension, hyper-/hypothyroidism, hyperkalemia, hypersensitivity reaction, hyperuricemia, hypophosphatemia, hypoxia, impotence, increased blood urea nitrogen, increased gamma-glutamyl transferase, increased lactate dehydrogenase, increased susceptibility to infection, intestinal perforation, intracranial hypertension, jaundice, leukopenia, lymphadenopathy, lymphangitis, maculopapular rash, malignant melanoma, melanosis, multi-organ failure, myasthenia, myocardial infarction, myopathy, nephritis, nephrosis, neuropathy, nocturnal amblyopia, nodal arrhythmia, nodule, nystagmus, oculogyric crisis, optic atrophy, optic neuritis, orthostatic hypotension, osteomalacia, osteonecrosis, osteoporosis, otitis externa, palpitations, pancreatitis, pancytopenia, papilledema, paresthesia, perforated duodenal ulcer, periosteal disease, peripheral edema, peritonitis, petechia, pleural effusion, pneumonia, prolonged bleeding time, prolonged QT interval on ECG, pruritus, pseudomembranous colitis, pseudoporphyria, psoriasis, psychosis, pulmonary edema, pulmonary embolism, purpura, rectal hemorrhage, renal insufficiency, renal tubular necrosis, respiratory distress syndrome, respiratory tract infection, retinal hemorrhage, retinitis, seizure, sepsis, skin discoloration, skin photosensitivity, splenomegaly, squamous cell carcinoma, Stevens-Johnson syndrome, subconjunctival hemorrhage, substernal pain, suicidal ideation, supraventricular extrasystole, supraventricular tachycardia, syncope, thrombocytopenia, thrombophlebitis, thrombotic thrombocytopenic purpura, tongue edema, tonic-clonic seizures, torsades de pointes, toxic epidermal necrolysis, uremia, urinary incontinence, urinary retention, urinary tract infection, urticaria, uterine hemorrhage, uveitis, vaginal hemorrhage, vasodilation, ventricular arrhythmia, ventricular fibrillation, ventricular tachycardia, visual field defect

Drug Interactions

Metabolism/Transport Effects Substrate of CYP2C19 (major), CYP2C9 (major), CYP3A4 (minor); **Note:** Assignment of Major/Minor substrate status based on clinically relevant drug interaction potential; **Inhibits** CYP2C19 (moderate), CYP2C9 (moderate), CYP3A4 (strong)

Avoid Concomitant Use

Avoid concomitant use of Voriconazole with any of the following: Ado-Trastuzumab Emtansine; Alfuzosin; Apixaban; Astemizole; Atazanavir; Avanafil; Axitinib; Barbiturates; Bosutinib; Cabozantinib; CarBAMazepine; Cisapride; Conivaptan; Crizotinib; Darunavir; Dihydroergotamine; Dofetilide; Dronedarone; Eletriptan; Eplerenone; Ergoloid Mesylates; Ergonovine; Ergotamine; Everolimus; Fluconazole; Halofantrine; Highest Risk QTc-Prolonging Agents; Ibrutinib; Imatinib; Ivabradine; Lapatinib; Lomitapide; Lopinavir; Lovastatin; Lurasidone; Macitentan; Methylergonovine; Mifepristone; Nilotinib; Nisoldipine; Pimozide; Pomalidomide; QuiNIDine; Ranolazine; Red Yeast Rice; Regorafenib; Rifamycin Derivatives; Ritonavir; Rivaroxaban; Salmeterol; Silodosin; Simeprevir; Simvastatin; Sirolimus; St Johns Wort; Tamsulosin; Terfenadine; Ticagrelor; Tolvaptan; Toremifene; Ulipristal; Vemurafenib; VinCRIStine (Liposomal)

Increased Effect/Toxicity

Voriconazole may increase the levels/effects of: Ado-Trastuzumab Emtansine; Alfentanil; Alfuzosin; Almotriptan; Alosetron; Antineoplastic Agents (Vinca Alkaloids); Apixaban; ARIPiprazole; Astemizole; AtorvaSTATin; Avanafil; Axitinib; Bedaquiline; Benzodiazepines (metabolized by oxidation); Boceprevir; Bortezomib; Bosentan; Bosutinib; Brentuximab Vedotin; Brinzolamide; Budesonide (Nasal); Budesonide (Systemic, Oral Inhalation); BusPIRone; Busulfan; Cabozantinib; Calcium Channel Blockers; Carvedilol; Cilostazol; Cisapride; Cobicistat; Colchicine; Conivaptan; Contraceptives (Estrogens); Contraceptives (Progestins); Corticosteroids (Orally Inhaled); Corticosteroids (Systemic); Crizotinib; CycloSPORINE (Systemic); CYP2C19 Substrates; CYP2C9 Substrates; CYP3A4 Substrates; Diclofenac (Systemic); Diclofenac (Topical); Dienogest; Dihydroergotamine; DOCEtaxel; Dofetilide; Dronedarone; Dutasteride; Eletriptan; Elvitegravir; Enzalutamide; Eplerenone; Ergoloid Mesylates; Ergonovine; Ergotamine; Etravirine; Everolimus; FentaNYL; Fesoterodine; Fluticasone (Nasal); Fluticasone (Oral Inhalation); Fosamprenavir; Fosphenytoin; GuanFACINE; Halofantrine; Highest Risk QTc-Prolonging Agents; Ibrutinib; Ibuprofen; Iloperidone; Imatinib; Irinotecan; Ivabradine; Ivacaftor; Ixabepilone; Lacosamide; Lapatinib; Levomilnacipran; Lomitapide; Losartan; Lovastatin; Lumefantrine; Lurasidone; Macitentan; Macrolide Antibiotics; Maraviroc; Meloxicam; Methadone; Methylergonovine; MethylPREDNISolone; Mifepristone; Moderate Risk QTc-Prolonging Agents; Nelfinavir; Nilotinib; Nisoldipine; Ospemifene; OxyCODONE; Paricalcitol; PAZOPanib; Phenytoin; Pimecrolimus; Pimozide; Pomalidomide; PONATinib; Propafenone; Proton Pump Inhibitors; QUEtiapine; QuiNIDine; Ranolazine; Red Yeast Rice; Regorafenib; Repaglinide; Reverse Transcriptase Inhibitors (Non-Nucleoside); Rifamycin Derivatives; Rilpivirine; Rivaroxaban; RomiDEPsin; Ruxolitinib; Salmeterol; Saxagliptin; Sildenafil; Silodosin; Simeprevir; Simvastatin; Sirolimus; Solifenacin; SORAfenib; Sulfonylureas; SUNItinib; Tacrolimus (Systemic); Tacrolimus (Topical); Tadalafil; Tamsulosin; Telaprevir; Terfenadine; Ticagrelor; Tofacitinib; Tolterodine; Tolvaptan; Toremifene; Ulipristal; Vardenafil; Vemurafenib; Venlafaxine; Vilazodone; VinCRIStine (Liposomal); Vitamin K Antagonists; Zolpidem; Zuclopenthixol

The levels/effects of Voriconazole may be increased by: Atazanavir; Boceprevir; Chloramphenicol; Cobicistat; Contraceptives (Estrogens); Contraceptives (Progestins); CYP2C19 Inhibitors (Moderate); CYP2C19 Inhibitors (Strong); CYP2C9 Inhibitors (Moderate); CYP2C9 Inhibitors (Strong); Etravirine; Fluconazole; Fosamprenavir; Ivabradine; Luliconazole; Macrolide Antibiotics; Mifepristone; Proton Pump Inhibitors; QTc-Prolonging Agents (Indeterminate Risk and Risk Modifying); Telaprevir

Decreased Effect

Voriconazole may decrease the levels/effects of: Amphotericin B; Atazanavir; Clopidogrel; Ifosfamide; Prasugrel; Saccharomyces boulardii; Ticagrelor

The levels/effects of Voriconazole may be decreased by: Atazanavir; Barbiturates; CarBAMazepine; CYP2C19 Inducers (Strong); CYP2C9 Inducers (Strong); Dabrafenib; Darunavir; Didanosine; Etravirine; Fosphenytoin; Lopinavir; Peginterferon Alfa-2b; Phenytoin; Reverse Transcriptase Inhibitors (Non-Nucleoside); Rifamycin Derivatives; Ritonavir; St Johns Wort; Sucralfate; Telaprevir

Ethanol/Nutrition/Herb Interactions

Food: Food may decrease voriconazole absorption. Management: Oral voriconazole should be taken 1 hour before or 1 hour after a meal. Maintain adequate hydration unless instructed to restrict fluid intake.

Herb/Nutraceutical: St John's wort may decrease voriconazole levels. Management: Concurrent use of St John's wort with voriconazole is contraindicated.

Preparation for Administration

Powder for injection: Reconstitute 200 mg vial with 19 mL of sterile water for injection (use of automated syringe is not recommended). Resultant solution (20 mL) has a concentration of 10 mg/mL. Prior to infusion, must dilute to 0.5-5 mg/mL with NS, LR, D_5WLR, $D_5W^{1/2}$NS, D_5W, D_5W with KCl 20 mEq, $^{1/2}$NS, or D_5WNS. Do not dilute with 4.2% sodium bicarbonate infusion.

Powder for oral suspension: Add 46 mL of water to the bottle to make 40 mg/mL suspension. Discard unused portion after 14 days.

Storage/Stability

Powder for injection: Store at 15°C to 30°C (59°F to 86°F). Reconstituted solutions are stable for up to 24 hours under refrigeration at 2°C to 8°C (36°F to 46°F).

Powder for oral suspension: Store at 2°C to 8°C (36°F to 46°F). Reconstituted oral suspension may be stored at 15°C to 30°C (59°F to 86°F).

Tablets: Store at 15°C to 30°C (59°F to 86°F).

Mechanism of Action Interferes with fungal cytochrome P450 activity (selectively inhibits 14-alpha-lanosterol demethylation), decreasing ergosterol synthesis (principal sterol in fungal cell membrane) and inhibiting fungal cell membrane formation.

Pharmacodynamics/Kinetics

Absorption: Well absorbed after oral administration; administration of crushed tablets is considered bioequivalent to whole tablets

Distribution: V_d: 4.6 L/kg

Protein binding: 58%

Metabolism: Hepatic, via CYP2C19 (major pathway) and CYP2C9 and CYP3A4 (less significant); saturable (may demonstrate nonlinearity)

Bioavailability: 96%

Half-life elimination: Variable, dose-dependent

Time to peak: Oral: 1-2 hours; 0.5 hours (crushed tablet)

Excretion: Urine (as inactive metabolites; <2% as unchanged drug)

Dosage

Usual dosage ranges:

Children <12 years: Dosage not established

Children ≥12 years and Adults:

Oral: 100-300 mg every 12 hours

I.V.: 6 mg/kg every 12 hours for 2 doses; followed by maintenance dose of 4 mg/kg every 12 hours

Indication-specific dosing:

Children >2 to <12 years:

Aspergillosis, invasive including disseminated and extrapulmonary infection in HIV-exposed/-positive patients: (unlabeled; CDC, 2009):

Oral: Loading dose: 8 mg/kg/dose (maximum: 400 mg/dose) every 12 hours for 2 doses on day 1, followed by maintenance dose of 7 mg/kg/dose (maximum: 200 mg/dose) every 12 hours for ≥12 weeks

I.V.: Loading dose: 6-8 mg/kg/dose (maximum: 400 mg/dose) every 12 hours for 2 doses on day 1, followed by maintenance dose of 7 mg/kg/dose (maximum: 200 mg/dose) every 12 hours for ≥12 weeks

Children ≥12 years and Adults:

Aspergillosis, invasive, including disseminated and extrapulmonary infection: Duration of therapy should be a minimum of 6-12 weeks or throughout period of immunosuppression (Walsh, 2008):

I.V.: Initial: Loading dose: 6 mg/kg every 12 hours for 2 doses; followed by maintenance dose of 4 mg/kg every 12 hours

Oral: Maintenance dose:

Manufacturer's recommendations:

Patients <40 kg: 100 mg every 12 hours; maximum: 300 mg/day

Patients ≥40 kg: 200 mg every 12 hours; maximum: 600 mg/day

IDSA recommendations (Walsh, 2008): May consider oral therapy in place of I.V. with dosing of 4 mg/kg (rounded up to convenient tablet dosage form) every 12 hours; however, I.V. administration is preferred in serious infections since comparative efficacy with the oral formulation has not been established.

Scedosporiosis, fusariosis:

I.V.: Initial: Loading dose: 6 mg/kg every 12 hours for 2 doses; followed by maintenance dose of 4 mg/kg every 12 hours

Oral: Maintenance dose:

Patients <40 kg: 100 mg every 12 hours; maximum: 300 mg/day

Patients ≥40 kg: 200 mg every 12 hours; maximum: 600 mg/day

Candidemia and other deep tissue *Candida* infections: Treatment should continue for a minimum of 14 days following resolution of symptoms or following last positive culture, whichever is longer.

I.V.: Initial: Loading dose 6 mg/kg every 12 hours for 2 doses; followed by maintenance dose of 3-4 mg/kg every 12 hours

Oral:

Manufacturer's recommendations: Maintenance dose:

Patients <40 kg: 100 mg every 12 hours; maximum: 300 mg/day

Patients ≥40 kg: 200 mg every 12 hours; maximum: 600 mg/day

IDSA recommendations (Pappas, 2009): Initial: Loading dose: 400 mg every 12 hours for 2 doses; followed by 200 mg every 12 hours

Endophthalmitis, fungal (unlabeled use; Pappas, 2009): I.V.: 6 mg/kg every 12 hours for 2 doses, then 3-4 mg/kg every 12 hours

Esophageal candidiasis: Oral: Treatment should continue for a minimum of 14 days, and for at least 7 days following resolution of symptoms:

Patients <40 kg: 100 mg every 12 hours; maximum: 300 mg/day

Patients ≥40 kg: 200 mg every 12 hours; maximum: 600 mg/day

Meningitis (secondary to contaminated [eg, *Exserohilum rostratum*] steroid products) (unlabeled use) (CDC [parameningeal], 2012; Kauffman, 2013): Note: Consult an infectious disease specialist and current CDC guidelines for specific treatment recommendations. Therapy duration is ≥3 months; trough serum concentrations must be maintained between 2-5 mcg/mL.

I.V.: 6 mg/kg every 12 hours. If patient does not improve or has severe disease, consider adding amphotericin B (liposomal)

Oral (only in mild disease in adherent patients whose trough concentrations/response to therapy can be closely monitored): 6 mg/kg every 12 hours (CDC [parameningeal], 2012)

Osteoarticular infection involving the spine, discitis, epidural abscess or vertebral osteomyelitis (secondary to contaminated [eg, *Exserohilum rostratum*] steroid products) (unlabeled use) (CDC [osteoarticular], 2012; Kauffmann, 2013): I.V.: 6 mg/kg every 12 hours for ≥3 months. **Note:** Consult an infectious disease specialist and current CDC guidelines for specific treatment recommendations. Trough serum concentrations must be maintained between 2-5 mcg/mL. If patient has severe disease, consider adding amphotericin B (liposomal). Patients may be switched to oral therapy if condition has improved or stabilized.

Osteoarticular infection not involving the spine (secondary to contaminated [eg, *Exserohilum rostratum*] steroid products) (unlabeled use) (CDC [osteoarticular], 2012; Kauffman, 2013): Note: Consult an infectious disease specialist and current CDC guidelines for specific treatment recommendations. Therapy duration is ≥3 months. Trough serum concentrations must be maintained between 2-5 mcg/mL.

I.V.: 6 mg/kg every 12 hours for 2 doses, then 4 mg/kg every 12 hours. If patient has severe disease, consider adding amphotericin B (liposomal)

Oral (only in mild disease in adherent patients whose trough concentrations/response to therapy can be closely monitored): 6 mg/kg every 12 hours for 2 doses, then 4 mg/kg every 12 hours

Dosage adjustment in patients unable to tolerate treatment:

I.V.: Dose may be reduced to 3-4 mg/kg every 12 hours, depending upon condition

Oral: Dose may be reduced in 50 mg decrements to a minimum dosage of 200 mg every 12 hours in patients weighing ≥40 kg (100 mg every 12 hours in patients <40 kg)

Dosage adjustment in patients receiving concomitant CYP450 enzyme inducers or substrates:

Efavirenz: Oral: Increase maintenance dose of voriconazole to 400 mg every 12 hours and reduce efavirenz dose to 300 mg once daily; upon discontinuation of voriconazole, return to the initial dose of efavirenz

Phenytoin:

I.V.: Increase voriconazole maintenance dosage to 5 mg/kg every 12 hours

Oral: Increase voriconazole dose to 400 mg every 12 hours in patients ≥40 kg (200 mg every 12 hours in patients <40 kg)

Dosage adjustment in renal impairment: In patients with Cl_{cr} <50 mL/minute, accumulation of the intravenous vehicle (cyclodextrin) occurs. After initial I.V. loading dose, oral voriconazole should be administered to these patients, unless an assessment of the benefit:risk to the patient justifies the use of I.V. voriconazole. Monitor serum creatinine and change to oral voriconazole therapy when possible.

Oral: Poorly dialyzed; no supplemental dose or dosage adjustment necessary, including patients on intermittent hemodialysis, peritoneal dialysis, or continuous renal replacement therapy (eg, CVVHD).

Note: I.V. dosing **NOT** recommended since cyclodextrin vehicle is cleared at half the rate of voriconazole and may accumulate.

Dosage adjustment in hepatic impairment:

Mild-to-moderate hepatic dysfunction (Child-Pugh class A or B): Following standard loading dose, reduce maintenance dosage by 50%

Severe hepatic impairment: Should only be used if benefit outweighs risk; monitor closely for toxicity

Dietary Considerations Oral: Should be taken 1 hour before or 1 hour after a meal. Voriconazole tablets contain lactose; avoid administration in hereditary galactose intolerance, Lapp lactase deficiency, or glucose-galactose malabsorption. Suspension contains sucrose; use caution with fructose intolerance, sucrose-isomaltase deficiency, or glucose-galactose malabsorption.

Administration

Oral: Administer 1 hour before or 1 hour after a meal.

I.V.: Infuse over 1-2 hours (rate not to exceed 3 mg/kg/hour). Do not infuse concomitantly into same line or cannula with other drug infusions, including TPN.

Monitoring Parameters Hepatic function at initiation and during course of treatment; renal function; serum electrolytes (particularly calcium, magnesium and potassium) prior to therapy initiation; visual function (visual acuity, visual field and color perception) if treatment course continues >28 days; in meningitis or osteoarticular infections trough serum concentrations must be maintained between 2-5 mcg/mL; monitor trough serum concentrations on day 5 of therapy and weekly thereafter for 4-6 weeks or when dosing adjustments are made; for other infections, may consider obtaining voriconazole trough level in patients failing therapy or exhibiting signs of toxicity; pancreatic function (in patients at risk for acute pancreatitis); total body skin examination yearly (more frequently if lesions noted)

Dosage Forms Excipient information presented when available (limited, particularly for generics); consult specific product labeling.

Solution Reconstituted, Intravenous:

Generic: 200 mg (1 ea)

Solution Reconstituted, Intravenous [preservative free]:

Vfend IV: 200 mg (1 ea) [latex free]

Vfend IV: 200 mg (1 ea)

Suspension Reconstituted, Oral:

Vfend: 40 mg/mL (75 mL) [contains sodium benzoate; orange flavor]

Generic: 40 mg/mL (75 mL)

Tablet, Oral:

Vfend: 50 mg, 200 mg

Generic: 50 mg, 200 mg

Vorinostat (vor IN oh stat)

Brand Names: U.S. Zolinza

Brand Names: Canada Zolinza®

Index Terms SAHA; Suberoylanilide Hydroxamic Acid

Pharmacologic Category Antineoplastic Agent, Histone Deacetylase Inhibitor

Use Cutaneous T-cell lymphoma: Treatment of cutaneous manifestations of cutaneous T-cell lymphoma (CTCL) with progressive, persistent, or recurrent disease on or following 2 systemic treatments

Pregnancy Risk Factor D

Pregnancy Considerations Adverse events were observed in animal reproduction studies. Based on the mechanism of action, may cause fetal harm if administered during pregnancy. Inform patient of potential hazard if used during pregnancy or if pregnancy occurs during treatment.

Breast-Feeding Considerations It is not known if vorinostat is excreted in breast milk. Due to the potential for serious adverse reactions in the nursing infant, the decision to discontinue vorinostat or to discontinue breast-feeding should take into account the benefits of treatment to the mother.

Contraindications There are no contraindications in the manufacturer's U.S. labeling.

Canadian labeling: Hypersensitivity to vorinostat or any component of the formulation; severe hepatic impairment (total bilirubin ≥3 times ULN)

Warnings/Precautions Hazardous agent - use appropriate precautions for handling and disposal (NIOSH, 2012). Pulmonary embolism and deep vein thrombosis (DVT) have been reported; monitor for signs/symptoms; use caution in patients with a history of thrombotic events. Dose-related thrombocytopenia and/or anemia may occur; may require dosage adjustments or discontinuation; monitor blood counts (every 2 weeks for 2 months, then monthly). Gastrointestinal bleeding due to severe thrombocytopenia has been reported in patients receiving vorinostat in combination with other histone deacetylase inhibitors (eg, valproic acid); monitor platelet counts more frequently in patients receiving concomitant histone deacetylase inhibitor therapy. QT_c prolongation has been observed; baseline and periodic ECGs were done in clinical trials (Duvic, 2007; Olsen, 2007). Correct electrolyte abnormalities prior to treatment and monitor and correct potassium, calcium, and magnesium levels during therapy. Use caution in patients with a history of QT_c prolongation or with medications known to prolong the QT interval. May cause hyperglycemia (may be severe); monitor serum glucose and use with caution in diabetics; may require diet and/or therapy modifications. Nausea, vomiting, and diarrhea may occur; antiemetics and antidiarrheals may be required; control pre-existing nausea and vomiting prior to treatment initiation; replace fluids and electrolytes to avoid dehydration. Adverse anastomotic healing events have occurred in patients recovering from bowel surgery; use with caution in the perioperative period in patients requiring bowel surgery. May cause dizziness or fatigue; caution patients about performing tasks which require mental alertness (eg, operating machinery or driving). Use with caution in patients with hepatic impairment; dose reductions are recommended (elimination is predominantly hepatic). The Canadian labeling does not recommend use in patients with moderate hepatic impairment (total bilirubin 1.5-3 times ULN) and contraindicates use in severe hepatic impairment (bilirubin ≥3 times ULN). Potentially significant drug-drug interactions may exist, requiring dose or frequency adjustment, additional monitoring, and/or selection of alternative therapy.

Adverse Reactions

>10%:

Cardiovascular: Peripheral edema (13%)

Central nervous system: Fatigue (52%), chills (16%), dizziness (15%), headache (12%), fever (11%)

Dermatologic: Alopecia (19%), pruritus (12%)

Endocrine & metabolic: Hyperglycemia (8% to 69%; grade 3: 5%), dehydration (1% to 16%)

Gastrointestinal: Diarrhea (52%), nausea (41%), taste alteration (28%), anorexia (24%), weight loss (21%), xerostomia (16%), constipation (15%), vomiting (15%), appetite decreased (14%)

Hematologic: Thrombocytopenia (26%; grades 3/4: 6%), anemia (14%; grades 3/4: 2%)

Neuromuscular & skeletal: Muscle spasm (20%)

Renal: Proteinuria (51%), creatinine increased (16% to 47%)

Respiratory: Cough (11%), upper respiratory infection (11%)

1% to 10%:

Cardiovascular: QT_c prolongation (3% to 4%)

Dermatologic: Squamous cell carcinoma (4%)

Respiratory: Pulmonary embolism (5%)

<1% (Limited to important or life-threatening): Abdominal pain, angioneurotic edema, blurred vision, chest pain, cholecystitis, deafness, diverticulitis, dysphagia, DVT, enterococcal infection, exfoliative dermatitis, gastrointestinal bleeding, gastrointestinal hemorrhage, Guillain-Barré syndrome, hemoptysis, hypertension, hypokalemia, hyponatremia, infection, lethargy, leukopenia, MI, neutropenia, pneumonia, renal failure, sepsis, spinal cord injury, streptococcal bacteremia, stroke (ischemic), syncope, T-cell lymphoma, tumor hemorrhage, ureteric obstruction, ureteropelvic junction obstruction, urinary retention, vasculitis, weakness

Drug Interactions

Metabolism/Transport Effects None known.

Avoid Concomitant Use

Avoid concomitant use of Vorinostat with any of the following: CloZAPine

Increased Effect/Toxicity

Vorinostat may increase the levels/effects of: CloZAPine; Highest Risk QTc-Prolonging Agents; Moderate Risk QTc-Prolonging Agents; Vitamin K Antagonists

The levels/effects of Vorinostat may be increased by: Mifepristone; Valproic Acid and Derivatives

Decreased Effect There are no known significant interactions involving a decrease in effect.

Storage/Stability Store at 20°C to 25°C (68°F to 77°F); excursions permitted to 15°C to 30°C (59°F to 86°F).

Mechanism of Action Inhibits histone deacetylase enzymes, HDAC1, HDAC2, HDAC3, and HDAC6, which catalyze acetyl group removal from protein lysine residues (including histones and transcription factors). Histone deacetylase inhibition results in accumulation of acetyl groups, which alters chromatin structure and transcription factor activation; cell growth is terminated and apoptosis occurs.

Pharmacodynamics/Kinetics

Protein binding: ~71%

Metabolism: Glucuronidated and hydrolyzed (followed by beta-oxidation) to inactive metabolites

Bioavailability: Fasting: ~43%

Half-life elimination: ~2 hours

Time to peak, plasma: With high-fat meal: ~4 hours (range: 2-10 hours)

Excretion: Urine: 52% (~52% as inactive metabolites; <1% as unchanged drug)

Dosage Cutaneous T-cell lymphoma (CTCL): Adults: Oral: 400 mg once daily until disease progression or unacceptable toxicity

Dosage adjustment for toxicity:

Intolerance: Reduce dose to 300 mg once daily; if needed, may further reduce to 300 mg daily for 5 consecutive days per week

In clinical trials, **dose reductions** were instituted for the following adverse events: Increased serum creatinine, decreased appetite, hypokalemia, leukopenia, nausea, neutropenia, thrombocytopenia, and vomiting. Vorinostat was **discontinued** for the following adverse events: Anemia, angioneurotic edema, weakness, chest pain, exfoliative dermatitis, DVT, ischemic stroke, lethargy, pulmonary embolism, and spinal cord injury.

Treatment was withheld in clinical trials for grade 4 anemia or thrombocytopenia or other grade 3 or 4 drug related toxicity, until resolved to ≤grade 1. Treatment was reinitiated with dose reduction (Olsen, 2007).

Dosage adjustment in renal impairment: No dosage adjustment provided in manufacturer's labeling (has not studied). However, based on the minimal renal elimination, adjustment not expected. Use with caution.

Dosage adjustment in hepatic impairment:

U.S. labeling: Initial:

Mild-to-moderate impairment (total bilirubin 1-3 times ULN **or** AST >ULN): 300 mg once daily

Severe impairment (total bilirubin >3 times ULN): No dosage adjustment provided in manufacturer's labeling. Doses of 100-200 mg once daily were studied in a limited number of patients with severe impairment (Ramalingam, 2010); according to the manufacturer the maximum dose used was 200 mg once daily.

Canadian labeling:

Moderate impairment (total bilirubin 1.5-3 times ULN): Use is not recommended

Severe impairment (total bilirubin ≥3 times ULN): Use is contraindicated

Dietary Considerations Take with food.

Administration Administer with food. Do not open, crush or chew capsules. Maintain adequate hydration (≥2 L/day fluids) during treatment.

Hazardous agent; use appropriate precautions for handling and disposal (NIOSH, 2012). Avoid direct skin or mucous membrane contact with crushed or broken capsules and/or capsule contents.

Monitoring Parameters CBC with differential and serum chemistries, including calcium, magnesium, potassium, glucose and creatinine (baseline, then every 2 weeks for 2 months, then monthly, or as clinically necessary), hepatic function, INR (if on concomitant warfarin therapy), fluid status, signs/symptoms of thromboembolism. Baseline and periodic ECGs were done in clinical trials.

Dosage Forms Excipient information presented when available (limited, particularly for generics); consult specific product labeling.

Capsule, Oral:

Zolinza: 100 mg

Extemporaneous Preparations Hazardous agent: Use appropriate precautions for handling and disposal.

Although not recommended by the manufacturer, a 50 mg/mL oral suspension may be prepared with capsules. Add 20 mL Ora-Plus® into a glass bottle (≥4 oz). Add the contents of twenty 100 mg capsules and shake thoroughly to disperse (may take up to 3 minutes). Add 20 mL Ora-Sweet® and shake to disperse. Label "shake well". Stable for 14 days at room temperature.

Fouladi M, Park JR, Stewart CF, et al, "Pediatric Phase I Trial and Pharmacokinetic Study of Vorinostat: A Children's Oncology Group Phase I Consortium Report," *J Clin Oncol*, 2010, 28(22):3623-9.

Vortioxetine (vor tye OX e teen)

Brand Names: U.S. Brintellix

Index Terms Lu AA21004; Vortioxetine Hydrobromide

Pharmacologic Category Antidepressant, Selective Serotonin Reuptake Inhibitor; Serotonin 5-HT_{1A} Receptor Agonist; Serotonin 5-HT_3 Receptor Antagonist

Additional Appendix Information

Antidepressant Agents *on page 2284*

Use Major depressive disorder: Treatment of major depressive disorder (MDD)

Pregnancy Risk Factor C

Pregnancy Considerations Adverse events were observed in animal reproduction studies. Nonteratogenic effects in the newborn following SSRI/SNRI exposure late in the third trimester include respiratory distress, cyanosis, apnea, seizures, temperature instability, feeding difficulty, vomiting, hypoglycemia, hypo- or hypertonia, hyperreflexia, jitteriness, irritability, constant crying, and tremor. Symptoms may be due to the toxicity of the SSRIs/SNRIs or a discontinuation syndrome and may be consistent with serotonin syndrome associated with SSRI treatment. Persistent pulmonary hypertension of the newborn (PPHN) has also been reported with SSRI exposure.

The ACOG recommends that therapy with SSRIs or SNRIs during pregnancy be individualized; treatment of depression during pregnancy should incorporate the clinical expertise of the mental health clinician, obstetrician, primary healthcare provider, and pediatrician (ACOG, 2008). According to the American Psychiatric Association (APA), the risks of medication treatment should be weighed against other treatment options and untreated depression. For women who discontinue antidepressant medications during pregnancy and who may be at high risk for postpartum depression, the medications can be restarted following delivery (APA, 2010). Treatment algorithms have been developed by the ACOG and the APA for the management of depression in women prior to conception and during pregnancy (Yonkers, 2009).

Breast-Feeding Considerations It is not known if vortioxetine is excreted into breast milk. Due to the potential for serious adverse reactions in the nursing infant, the manufacturer recommends a decision be made whether to discontinue nursing or to discontinue the drug, taking into account the importance of treatment to the mother.

Medication Guide Available Yes

Contraindications Hypersensitivity to vortioxetine or any component of the formulation; use of MAO inhibitors intended to treat psychiatric disorders (concurrently or within 21 days of discontinuing vortioxetine or within 14 days of discontinuing the MAO inhibitor); initiation of vortioxetine in a patient receiving linezolid or intravenous methylene blue

Warnings/Precautions [U.S. Boxed Warning]: Antidepressants increase the risk of suicidal thinking and behavior in children, adolescents, and young adults (18-24 years of age) with major depressive disorder (MDD) and other psychiatric disorders; consider risk prior to prescribing. Short-term studies did not show an increased risk in patients >24 years of age and showed a decreased risk in patients ≥65 years. Closely monitor patients for clinical worsening, suicidality, or unusual changes in behavior, particularly during the initial 1-2 months of therapy or during periods of dosage adjustments (increases or decreases); the patient's family or caregiver should be instructed to closely observe the patient and communicate condition with healthcare provider. A medication guide concerning the use of antidepressants should be dispensed with each prescription. **Vortioxetine is not approved for use in children.**

The possibility of a suicide attempt is inherent in major depression and may persist until remission occurs. Use caution in high-risk patients. Worsening depression and severe abrupt suicidality that are not part of the presenting symptoms may require discontinuation or modification of drug therapy. The patient's family or caregiver should be alerted to monitor patients for the emergence of suicidality and associated behaviors (such as agitation, irritability, hostility, aggressiveness, impulsivity, and hypomania) and call healthcare provider.

May worsen psychosis in some patients or precipitate a mixed/manic episode in patients at risk for bipolar disorder. Use with caution in patients with a family history of bipolar disorder, mania, or hypomania. Patients presenting with depressive symptoms should be screened for bipolar disorder. **Vortioxetine is not FDA approved for the treatment of bipolar depression.**

Potentially life-threatening serotonin syndrome (SS) has occurred with serotonergic antidepressants (eg, SSRIs, SNRIs), particularly when used in combination with other serotonergic agents (eg, triptans, TCAs, fentanyl, lithium, tramadol, buspirone, St John's wort, tryptophan) or agents that impair metabolism of serotonin (eg, MAO inhibitors intended to treat psychiatric disorders, other MAO inhibitors [ie, linezolid and intravenous methylene blue]). Discontinue treatment (and any concomitant serotonergic agent) immediately if signs/symptoms arise.

May impair platelet aggregation resulting in increased risk of bleeding events, particularly if used concomitantly with aspirin, NSAIDs, warfarin or other anticoagulants. Bleeding related to antidepressant use has been reported to range from relatively minor bruising and epistaxis to life-threatening hemorrhage. May cause hyponatremia/SIADH (elderly at increased risk); volume depletion (diuretics may increase risk) may occur. Use caution in elderly patients; may cause or exacerbate syndrome of inappropriate antidiuretic hormone secretion or hyponatremia; monitor sodium closely with initiation or dosage adjustments in older adults. May cause CNS depression, which may impair physical or mental abilities; patients must be cautioned about performing tasks that require mental alertness (eg, operating machinery or driving). Angioedema has been reported. Potentially significant drug-drug interactions may exist, requiring dose or frequency adjustment, additional monitoring, and/or selection of alternative therapy. Use is not recommended in severe hepatic impairment.

Abrupt discontinuation or interruption of antidepressant therapy has been associated with a discontinuation syndrome. Symptoms arising may vary with antidepressant however commonly include nausea, vomiting, diarrhea, headaches, lightheadedness, dizziness, diminished appetite, sweating, chills, tremors, paresthesias, fatigue, somnolence, and sleep disturbances (eg, vivid dreams, insomnia). Greater risks for developing a discontinuation syndrome have been associated with antidepressants with shorter half-lives, longer durations of treatment, and abrupt discontinuation. For antidepressants of short or intermediate half-lives, symptoms may emerge within 2-5 days after treatment discontinuation and last 7-14 days (APA, 2010; Fava, 2006; Haddad, 2001; Shelton, 2001; Warner, 2006).

Adverse Reactions

>10%:

Central nervous system: Female sexual disorder (self-reporting: 1% to 2%; Arizona Sexual Experience Scale: 22% to 34%), male sexual disorder (self-reporting: 3% to 5%; Arizona Sexual Experience Scale: 10% to 29%)

Gastrointestinal: Nausea (dose-related, females >males, tolerance develops: 21% to 32%)

1% to 10%:

Central nervous system: Dizziness (8% to 9%), abnormal dreams (2% to 3%)

Dermatologic: Pruritus (2% to 3%)

Gastrointestinal: Diarrhea (7% to 10%), xerostomia (7% to 8%), constipation (5% to 6%), vomiting (3% to 6%), flatulence (2% to 3%)

<1% (Limited to important or life-threatening): Hypomania, hyponatremia, mania, serotonin syndrome, withdrawal syndrome

Drug Interactions

Metabolism/Transport Effects Substrate of CYP2A6 (minor), CYP2B6 (minor), CYP2C19 (minor), CYP2C8 (minor), CYP2C9 (minor), CYP2D6 (major), CYP3A4 (major); **Note:** Assignment of Major/Minor substrate status based on clinically relevant drug interaction potential

Avoid Concomitant Use

Avoid concomitant use of Vortioxetine with any of the following: Dosulepin; Iobenguane I 123; Linezolid; MAO Inhibitors; Methylene Blue; Pimozide; Tryptophan

Increased Effect/Toxicity

Vortioxetine may increase the levels/effects of: Agents with Antiplatelet Properties; Anticoagulants; Antidepressants (Serotonin Reuptake Inhibitor/Antagonist); Antipsychotics; Aspirin; Benzodiazepines (metabolized by oxidation); Beta-Blockers; BusPIRone; CarBAMazepine; CloZAPine; Collagenase (Systemic); Dabigatran Etexilate; Desmopressin; Dextromethorphan; Dosulepin; Galantamine; Hypoglycemic Agents; Ibritumomab; Methadone; Methylene Blue; Metoclopramide;

Mexiletine; NSAID (COX-2 Inhibitor); NSAID (Nonselective); Pimozide; QuiNIDine; RisperiDONE; Rivaroxaban; Salicylates; Serotonin Modulators; Thiazide Diuretics; Thrombolytic Agents; Tositumomab and Iodine I 131 Tositumomab; TraMADol; Vitamin K Antagonists

The levels/effects of Vortioxetine may be increased by: Abiraterone Acetate; Alcohol (Ethyl); Analgesics (Opioid); Antipsychotics; BuPROPion; BusPIRone; Cimetidine; CNS Depressants; Cobicistat; CYP2D6 Inhibitors (Moderate); CYP2D6 Inhibitors (Strong); Darunavir; Dasatinib; Glucosamine; Herbs (Anticoagulant/Antiplatelet Properties); Ibrutinib; Linezolid; Lithium; Macrolide Antibiotics; MAO Inhibitors; Metoclopramide; Metyrosine; Multivitamins/Fluoride (with ADE); Multivitamins/Minerals (with ADEK, Folate, Iron); Multivitamins/Minerals (with AE, No Iron); Omega-3 Fatty Acids; Pentosan Polysulfate Sodium; Pentoxifylline; Prostacyclin Analogues; TraMADol; Tryptophan; Vitamin E

Decreased Effect

Vortioxetine may decrease the levels/effects of: Iobenguane I 123; Ioflupane I 123; Thyroid Products

The levels/effects of Vortioxetine may be decreased by: Bosentan; CarBAMazepine; CYP3A4 Inducers (Strong); Cyproheptadine; Dabrafenib; Deferasirox; NSAID (COX-2 Inhibitor); NSAID (Nonselective); Peginterferon Alfa-2b; Tocilizumab

Ethanol/Nutrition/Herb Interactions Herb/Nutraceutical: Some herbal medications may increase risk of serotonin syndrome and/or excessive sedation. Management: Avoid valerian, St John's wort, SAMe, kava kava, and tryptophan.

Storage/Stability Store at 25°C (77°F); excursions are permitted between 15°C and 30°C (59°F and 86°F).

Mechanism of Action Inhibits reuptake of serotonin (5-HT); also has agonist activity at the 5-HT_{1A} receptor and antagonist activity at the 5-HT_3 receptor.

Pharmacodynamics/Kinetics

Absorption: Not affected by food

Distribution: V_d: 2600 L

Protein binding: 98%

Metabolism: Hepatic primarily through oxidation via CYP450 isoenzymes, primarily CYP2D6, and subsequent gluconic acid conjugation

Bioavailability: 75%

Half-life elimination: ~66 hours

Time to peak: 7-11 hours

Excretion: Urine (59%); feces (26%)

Dosage

Major depressive disorder: Adult: Oral: Initial: 10 mg once daily; increase to 20 mg once daily as tolerated; consider 5 mg once daily for patients who do not tolerate higher doses. Maintenance: 5-20 mg once daily.

Dosage adjustment for CYP2D6 poor metabolizers: Maximum dose: 10 mg once daily.

Dosage adjustment for concomitant therapy with strong CYP2D6 inhibitors: Reduce total daily dose by one half. Increase dose to original level when the CYP2D6 inhibitor is discontinued.

Dosage adjustment for concomitant strong CYP inducers: Consider increasing the dose when a strong CYP inducer (eg, rifampin, carbamazepine, phenytoin) is coadministered for >14 days. Maximum dose should not exceed three times the original dose. Reduce the dose to the original level within 14 days of discontinuing the CYP inducer.

Discontinuation of therapy: Upon discontinuation of antidepressant therapy, gradually taper the dose to minimize the incidence of withdrawal symptoms and allow for the detection of re-emerging symptoms. Evidence supporting ideal taper rates is limited. APA and NICE guidelines suggest tapering therapy over at least several weeks with consideration to the half-life of the antidepressant; antidepressants with a shorter half-life may need to be tapered more conservatively. In addition for long-term treated patients, WFSBP guidelines recommend tapering over 4-6 months. If intolerable withdrawal symptoms occur following a dose reduction, consider resuming the previously prescribed dose and/or decrease dose at a more gradual rate (APA, 2010; Bauer, 2002; Haddad, 2001; NCCMH, 2010; Schatzberg, 2006; Shelton, 2001; Warner, 2006).

Vortioxetine doses of 15 mg once daily or more are recommended by the manufacturer to be decreased to 10 mg once daily for one week before full discontinuation to prevent withdrawal symptoms.

MAO inhibitor recommendations:

Switching to or from an MAO inhibitor intended to treat psychiatric disorders:

Allow 14 days to elapse between discontinuing an MAO inhibitor intended to treat psychiatric disorders and initiation of vortioxetine.

Allow 21 days to elapse between discontinuing vortioxetine and initiation of an MAO inhibitor intended to treat psychiatric disorders.

Use with other MAO inhibitors (linezolid or I.V. methylene blue):

Do not initiate vortioxetine in patients receiving linezolid or I.V. methylene blue; consider other interventions for psychiatric condition.

If urgent treatment with linezolid or I.V. methylene blue is required in a patient already receiving vortioxetine and potential benefits outweigh potential risks, discontinue vortioxetine promptly and administer linezolid or I.V. methylene blue. Monitor for serotonin syndrome for 21 days or until 24 hours after the last dose of linezolid or I.V. methylene blue, whichever comes first. May resume vortioxetine 24 hours after the last dose of linezolid or I.V. methylene blue.

Dosage adjustment in renal impairment: No dosage adjustment necessary.

Dosage adjustment in hepatic impairment:

Mild-to-moderate impairment: No dosage adjustment necessary.

Severe impairment: Use not recommended (has not been studied).

Administration Administer without regard to meals.

Monitoring Parameters Mental status for depression, suicidal ideation (especially at the beginning of therapy or when doses are increased or decreased), anxiety, social functioning, mania, panic attacks; akathisia; signs/symptoms of serotonin syndrome and/or hyponatremia; hepatic function (baseline).

Dosage Forms Excipient information presented when available (limited, particularly for generics); consult specific product labeling.

Tablet, Oral:

Brintellix: 5 mg, 10 mg, 20 mg

- **Vortioxetine Hydrobromide** *see* Vortioxetine *on page 2208*
- **VoSol® HC** *see* Acetic Acid, Propylene Glycol Diacetate, and Hydrocortisone *on page 35*
- **VoSpire ER** *see* Albuterol *on page 61*
- **Votrient** *see* PAZOPanib *on page 1581*
- **VP-16** *see* Etoposide *on page 802*
- **VP-16-213** *see* Etoposide *on page 802*
- **Vpriv** *see* Velaglucerase Alfa *on page 2176*
- **VPRIV (Can)** *see* Velaglucerase Alfa *on page 2176*
- **VRT111950** *see* Telaprevir *on page 1996*
- **VSLI** *see* VinCRIStine (Liposomal) *on page 2194*

◆ **Vumon** *see* Teniposide *on page 2012*
◆ **Vumon® (Can)** *see* Teniposide *on page 2012*
◆ **VWF/FVIII Concentrate** *see* Antihemophilic Factor/von Willebrand Factor Complex (Human) *on page 146*
◆ **VWF:RCo** *see* Antihemophilic Factor/von Willebrand Factor Complex (Human) *on page 146*
◆ **vWF:RCof** *see* Antihemophilic Factor/von Willebrand Factor Complex (Human) *on page 146*
◆ **VX-770** *see* Ivacaftor *on page 1136*
◆ **VX-950** *see* Telaprevir *on page 1996*
◆ **Vyloma™ (Can)** *see* Imiquimod *on page 1057*
◆ **Vytone** *see* Iodoquinol and Hydrocortisone *on page 1109*
◆ **Vytorin®** *see* Ezetimibe and Simvastatin *on page 818*
◆ **Vyvanse** *see* Lisdexamfetamine *on page 1225*
◆ **VZIG** *see* Varicella-Zoster Immune Globulin (Human) *on page 2171*
◆ **VZV Vaccine (Varicella)** *see* Varicella Virus Vaccine *on page 2168*
◆ **VZV Vaccine (Zoster)** *see* Zoster Vaccine *on page 2247*

Warfarin (WAR far in)

Brand Names: U.S. Coumadin; Jantoven

Brand Names: Canada Apo-Warfarin®; Coumadin®; Mylan-Warfarin; Novo-Warfarin; Taro-Warfarin

Index Terms Warfarin Sodium

Pharmacologic Category Vitamin K Antagonist

Additional Appendix Information

Oral Anticoagulant Comparison Chart *on page 2307*
Reversal of Oral Anticoagulants *on page 2308*
Treatment of Elevated INR Due to Warfarin *on page 2377*

Use Prophylaxis and treatment of thromboembolic disorders (eg, venous, pulmonary) and embolic complications arising from atrial fibrillation or cardiac valve replacement; adjunct to reduce risk of systemic embolism (eg, recurrent MI, stroke) after myocardial infarction

Unlabeled Use Prevention of recurrent transient ischemic attacks

Pregnancy Risk Factor D (women with mechanical heart valves)/X (other indications)

Pregnancy Considerations Warfarin crosses the placenta; concentrations in the fetal plasma are similar to maternal values. Teratogenic effects have been reported following first trimester exposure and may include coumarin embryopathy (nasal hypoplasia and/or stippled epiphyses; limb hypoplasia may also be present). Adverse CNS events to the fetus have also been observed following exposure during any trimester and may include CNS abnormalities (including ventral midline dysplasia, dorsal midline dysplasia). Spontaneous abortion, fetal hemorrhage, and fetal death may also occur. Use is contraindicated during pregnancy (or in women of reproductive potential) except in women with mechanical heart valves who are at high risk for thromboembolism; use is also contraindicated in women with threatened abortion, eclampsia, or preeclampsia. Frequent pregnancy tests are recommended for women who are planning to become pregnant and adjusted-dose heparin or low molecular weight heparin (LMWH) should be substituted as soon as pregnancy is confirmed or adjusted-dose heparin or LMWH should be used instead of warfarin prior to conception.

In pregnant women with high-risk mechanical heart valves, the benefits of warfarin therapy should be discussed with the risks of available treatments; when possible avoid warfarin use during the first trimester and close to delivery. Adjusted-dose LMWH or adjusted-dose heparin may be used throughout pregnancy or until week 13 of gestation when therapy can be changed to warfarin. LMWH or heparin should be resumed close to delivery. In women who are at a very high risk for thromboembolism (older generation prothesis in mitral position or history of thromboembolism), warfarin can be used throughout pregnancy and replaced with LMWH or heparin near term; the use of low-dose aspirin is also recommended. Women who require long-term anticoagulation with warfarin and who are considering pregnancy, LMWH substitution should be done prior to conception when possible. When choosing therapy, fetal outcomes (ie, pregnancy loss, malformations), maternal outcomes (ie, VTE, hemorrhage), burden of therapy, and maternal preference should be considered (Bates, 2012).

Breast-Feeding Considerations Breast-feeding women may be treated with warfarin. Based on available data, warfarin does not pass into breast milk. Women who are breast-feeding should be carefully monitored to avoid excessive anticoagulation. According to the American College of Chest Physicians (ACCP), warfarin may be used in lactating women who wish to breast-feed their infants (Bates, 2012). Monitor nursing infants for bruising or bleeding (per manufacturer).

Medication Guide Available Yes

Contraindications Hypersensitivity to warfarin or any component of the formulation; hemorrhagic tendencies (eg, patients bleeding from the GI, respiratory, or GU tract; cerebral aneurysm; cerebrovascular hemorrhage; dissecting aortic aneurysm; spinal puncture and other diagnostic or therapeutic procedures with potential for significant bleeding; history of bleeding diathesis); recent or potential surgery of the eye or CNS; major regional lumbar block anesthesia or traumatic surgery resulting in large, open surfaces; blood dyscrasias; severe uncontrolled or malignant hypertension; pericarditis or pericardial effusion; bacterial endocarditis; unsupervised patients with conditions associated with a high potential for noncompliance; eclampsia/pre-eclampsia, threatened abortion, pregnancy (except in women with mechanical heart valves at high risk for thromboembolism)

Warnings/Precautions Hazardous agent - use appropriate precautions for handling and disposal (EPA, P-listed [>0.3%]; U-listed [<0.3%]). Use care in the selection of patients appropriate for this treatment. Ensure patient cooperation especially from the alcoholic, illicit drug user, demented, or psychotic patient; ability to comply with routine laboratory monitoring is essential. Use with caution in trauma, acute infection, moderate-severe renal insufficiency, prolonged dietary insufficiencies, moderate-severe hypertension, polycythemia vera, vasculitis, open wound, active TB, any disruption in normal GI flora, history of PUD, anaphylactic disorders, indwelling catheters, severe diabetes, and menstruating and postpartum women. Use with caution in patients with thyroid disease; warfarin responsiveness may increase (Ageno, 2012). Use with caution in protein C deficiency. Use with caution in patients with heparin-induced thrombocytopenia and DVT. Warfarin monotherapy is contraindicated in the initial treatment of active HIT. Reduced liver function, regardless of etiology, may impair synthesis of coagulation factors leading to increased warfarin sensitivity.

[U.S. Boxed Warning]: May cause major or fatal bleeding. Risk factors for bleeding include high intensity anticoagulation (INR >4), age (>65 years), variable INRs, history of GI bleeding, hypertension, cerebrovascular disease, serious heart disease, anemia, malignancy, trauma, renal insufficiency, drug-drug interactions, long duration of therapy, or known genetic deficiency in CYP2C9 activity. Patient must be instructed to report bleeding, accidents, or falls. Unrecognized bleeding sites (eg, colon cancer) may be uncovered by anticoagulation. Patient must also report any new or discontinued medications, herbal or alternative products used, or significant changes in smoking or dietary habits. Necrosis or gangrene of the skin and other tissue can occur, usually in conjunction with protein C or S deficiency. Consider alternative therapies if anticoagulation is necessary. Warfarin therapy may release atheromatous plaque emboli; symptoms depend on site of embolization, most commonly kidneys, pancreas, liver, and spleen. In some cases may lead to necrosis or death. "Purple toes syndrome," due to cholesterol microembolization, may rarely occur. The elderly may be more sensitive to anticoagulant therapy.

Presence of the CYP2C9*2 or *3 allele and/or polymorphism of the vitamin K oxidoreductase (VKORC1) gene may increase the risk of bleeding. Lower doses may be required in these patients; genetic testing may help determine appropriate dosing.

When temporary interruption is necessary before surgery, discontinue for approximately 5 days before surgery; when there is adequate hemostasis, may reinstitute warfarin therapy ~12-24 hours after surgery (evening of or next morning). Decision to safely continue warfarin therapy through the procedure and whether or not bridging of anticoagulation is necessary is dependent upon risk of perioperative bleeding and risk of thromboembolism, respectively. If risk of thromboembolism is elevated, consider bridging warfarin therapy with an alternative anticoagulant (eg, unfractionated heparin, LMWH) (Guyatt, 2012).

Adverse Reactions Bleeding is the major adverse effect of warfarin. Hemorrhage may occur at virtually any site. Risk is dependent on multiple variables, including the intensity of anticoagulation and patient susceptibility.

Cardiovascular: Vasculitis

Central nervous system: Signs/symptoms of bleeding (eg, dizziness, fatigue, fever, headache, lethargy, malaise, pain)

Dermatologic: Alopecia, bullous eruptions, dermatitis, rash, pruritus, urticaria

Gastrointestinal: Abdominal pain, diarrhea, flatulence, gastrointestinal bleeding, nausea, taste disturbance, vomiting

Genitourinary: Hematuria

Hematologic: Anemia, retroperitoneal hematoma, unrecognized bleeding sites (eg, colon cancer) may be uncovered by anticoagulation

Hepatic: Hepatitis (including cholestatic hepatitis), transaminases increased

Neuromuscular & skeletal: Osteoporosis (potential association with long-term use), paralysis, paresthesia, weakness

Respiratory: Respiratory tract bleeding, tracheobronchial calcification

Miscellaneous: Anaphylactic reaction, hypersensitivity/allergic reactions, skin necrosis, gangrene, "purple toes" syndrome

Drug Interactions

Metabolism/Transport Effects Substrate of CYP1A2 (minor), CYP2C19 (minor), CYP2C9 (major), CYP3A4 (minor); **Note:** Assignment of Major/Minor substrate status based on clinically relevant drug interaction potential; **Inhibits** CYP2C19 (weak), CYP2C9 (weak)

Avoid Concomitant Use

Avoid concomitant use of Warfarin with any of the following: Apixaban; Dabigatran Etexilate; Enzalutamide; Rivaroxaban; Tamoxifen

Increased Effect/Toxicity

Warfarin may increase the levels/effects of: Anticoagulants; Collagenase (Systemic); Deferasirox; Ethotoin; Fosphenytoin; Phenytoin; Regorafenib; Rivaroxaban; Sulfonylureas

The levels/effects of Warfarin may be increased by: Acetaminophen; Agents with Antiplatelet Properties; Allopurinol; Amiodarone; Androgens; Antineoplastic Agents; Apixaban; Atazanavir; Bicalutamide; Boceprevir; Capecitabine; Cephalosporins; Chloral Hydrate; Chloramphenicol; Cimetidine; Clopidogrel; Cloxacillin; Cobicistat; Corticosteroids (Systemic); Cranberry; CYP2C9 Inhibitors (Moderate); CYP2C9 Inhibitors (Strong); Dabigatran Etexilate; Desvenlafaxine; Dexmethylphenidate; Disulfiram; Dronedarone; Efavirenz; Erythromycin (Ophthalmic); Esomeprazole; Ethacrynic Acid; Ethotoin; Etoposide; Exenatide; Fenofibrate and Derivatives; Fenugreek; Fibric Acid Derivatives; Fluconazole; Fluorouracil (Systemic); Fluorouracil (Topical); Fosamprenavir; Fosphenytoin; Fusidic Acid (Systemic); Gefitinib; Ginkgo Biloba; Glucagon; Green Tea; Herbs (Anticoagulant/Antiplatelet Properties); HMG-CoA Reductase Inhibitors; Ibrutinib; Ifosfamide; Imatinib; Itraconazole; Ivermectin (Systemic); Ketoconazole (Systemic); Lansoprazole; Leflunomide; Levomilnacipran; Lomitapide; Macrolide Antibiotics; Methylphenidate; MetroNIDAZOLE (Systemic); Miconazole (Oral); Miconazole (Topical); Mifepristone; Milnacipran; Mirtazapine; Multivitamins/Fluoride (with ADE); Multivitamins/Minerals (with ADEK, Folate, Iron); Multivitamins/Minerals (with AE, No Iron); Nelfinavir; Neomycin; NSAID (COX-2 Inhibitor); NSAID (Nonselective); Omega-3 Fatty Acids; Omeprazole; Orlistat; Penicillins; Pentosan Polysulfate Sodium; Pentoxifylline; Phenytoin; Posaconazole; Proguanil; Propafenone; Prostacyclin Analogues; QuiNIDine; QuiNINE; Quinolone Antibiotics; Ranitidine; RomiDEPsin; Salicylates; Saquinavir; Selective Serotonin Reuptake Inhibitors; Sitaxentan; SORAfenib; Sugammadex; Sulfinpyrazone [Off Market]; Sulfonamide Derivatives; Sulfonylureas; Tamoxifen; Tegafur; Telaprevir; Tetracycline Derivatives; Thrombolytic Agents; Thyroid Products; Tibolone; Tigecycline; Tipranavir; Tolterodine; Toremifene; Torsemide; TraMADol; Tricyclic Antidepressants; Venlafaxine; Vitamin E; Voriconazole; Vorinostat; Zafirlukast; Zileuton

Decreased Effect

The levels/effects of Warfarin may be decreased by: Adalimumab; Aminoglutethimide; Antineoplastic Agents; Antithyroid Agents; Aprepitant; AzaTHIOprine; Barbiturates; Bile Acid Sequestrants; Boceprevir; Bosentan; CarBAMazepine; Cloxacillin; Coenzyme Q-10; Contraceptives (Estrogens); Contraceptives (Progestins); CYP2C9 Inducers (Strong); Darunavir; Dicloxacillin; Efavirenz; Elvitegravir; Enzalutamide; Eslicarbazepine; Estrogen Derivatives; Floxacillin; Fosaprepitant; Ginseng (American); Glutethimide; Green Tea; Griseofulvin; Lopinavir; Mercaptopurine; Multivitamins/Minerals (with ADEK, Folate, Iron); Nafcillin; Nelfinavir; Peginterferon Alfa-2b; Phytonadione; Progestins; Rifamycin Derivatives; Ritonavir; St Johns Wort; Sucralfate; Telaprevir; Teriflunomide; TraZODone

Ethanol/Nutrition/Herb Interactions

Ethanol: Acute ethanol ingestion (binge drinking) decreases the metabolism of warfarin and increases PT/INR. Chronic daily ethanol use increases the metabolism of warfarin and decreases PT/INR. Management: Avoid ethanol.

Food: The anticoagulant effects of warfarin may be decreased if taken with foods rich in vitamin K. Vitamin E may increase warfarin effect. Cranberry juice may increase warfarin effect. Management: Maintain a consistent diet; consult prescriber before making changes in diet. Take warfarin at the same time each day.

Herb/Nutraceutical: Some herbal medications (eg, St John's wort) may decrease warfarin levels and effects; many others can add additional antiplatelet activity to warfarin therapy. Management: Avoid ginseng (American), coenzyme Q_{10}, and St John's wort. Avoid cranberry, fenugreek, ginkgo biloba, glucosamine, alfalfa, anise, bilberry, bladderwrack, bromelain, cat's claw, celery, chamomile, coleus, cordyceps, dong quai, evening primrose oil, fenugreek, feverfew, garlic, ginger, ginkgo biloba, ginseng (Panax), ginseng (Siberian), grapeseed, green tea, guggul, horse chestnut seed, horseradish, licorice, omega-3-acids, prickly ash, red clover, reishi, SAMe (s-adenosylmethionine), sweet clover, turmeric, and white willow.

Preparation for Administration Reconstitute with 2.7 mL of sterile water (yields 2 mg/mL solution).

Hazardous agent; use appropriate precautions for handling and disposal (EPA, P-listed [>0.3%]; U-listed [<0.3%]).

Storage/Stability

Injection: Prior to reconstitution, store at 15°C to 30°C (59°F to 86°F). Following reconstitution with 2.7 mL of sterile water (yields 2 mg/mL solution), stable for 4 hours at 15°C to 30°C (59°F to 86°F). Protect from light.

Tablet: Store at 15°C to 30°C (59°F to 86°F). Protect from light.

Mechanism of Action Hepatic synthesis of coagulation factors II, VII, IX, and X, as well as proteins C and S, requires the presence of vitamin K. These clotting factors are biologically activated by the addition of carboxyl groups to key glutamic acid residues within the proteins' structure. In the process, "active" vitamin K is oxidatively converted to an "inactive" form, which is then subsequently reactivated by vitamin K epoxide reductase complex 1 (VKORC1). Warfarin competitively inhibits the subunit 1 of the multi-unit VKOR complex, thus depleting functional vitamin K reserves and hence reduces synthesis of active clotting factors.

Pharmacodynamics/Kinetics

Onset of action: Anticoagulation: Oral: 24-72 hours

Peak effect: Full therapeutic effect: 5-7 days; INR may increase in 36-72 hours

Duration: 2-5 days

Absorption: Oral: Rapid, complete

Distribution: 0.14 L/kg

Protein binding: 99%

Metabolism: Hepatic, primarily via CYP2C9; minor pathways include CYP2C8, 2C18, 2C19, 1A2, and 3A4

Genomic variants: Approximately 37% reduced clearance of S-warfarin in patients heterozygous for 2C9 (*1/*2 or *1/*3), and ~70% reduced in patients homozygous for reduced function alleles (*2/*2, *2/*3, or *3/*3)

Half-life elimination: 20-60 hours; Mean: 40 hours; highly variable among individuals

Time to peak, plasma: Oral: ~4 hours

Excretion: Urine (92%, primarily as metabolites)

Dosage Note: Labeling identifies genetic factors which may increase patient sensitivity to warfarin. Specifically, genetic variations in the proteins CYP2C9 and VKORC1, responsible for warfarin's primary metabolism and pharmacodynamic activity, respectively, have been identified as predisposing factors associated with decreased dose requirement and increased bleeding risk. Genotyping tests are available, and may provide guidance on initiation of anticoagulant therapy. The American College of Chest Physicians recommends against the use of routine pharmacogenomic testing to guide dosing (Guyatt, 2012). For management of elevated INRs as a result of warfarin therapy, see Additional Information for guidance.

Oral:

Infants and Children (unlabeled use): Initial loading dose (if baseline INR is 1-1.3): 0.2 mg/kg (maximum: 10 mg/dose); adjust dose based on INR (reported ranges to maintain INR of 2-3: 0.09-0.33 mg/kg/day). Infants <12 months of age may require doses at or near the high end of this range; consistent anticoagulation may be difficult to maintain in children <5 years of age (Monagle, 2012).

Adults: Initial dosing must be individualized. Consider the patient (hepatic function, cardiac function, age, nutritional status, concurrent therapy, risk of bleeding) in addition to prior dose response (if available) and the clinical situation. Start 2-5 mg once daily for 2 days **or** for healthy individuals, 10 mg once daily for 2 days; lower doses (eg, 5 mg once daily) recommended for patients with confirmed HIT once platelet recovery has occurred (Guyatt, 2012). In patients with acute venous thromboembolism, initiation may begin on the first or second day of low molecular weight heparin or unfractionated heparin therapy (Guyatt, 2012). Adjust dose according to INR results; usual maintenance dose ranges from 2-10 mg daily (individual patients may require loading and maintenance doses outside these general guidelines).

Note: Lower starting doses may be required for patients with hepatic impairment, poor nutrition, CHF, elderly, high risk of bleeding, or patients who are debilitated, or those with reduced function genomic variants of the catabolic enzymes CYP2C9 (*2 or *3 alleles) or VKORC1 (-1639 polymorphism); see table. Higher initial doses may be reasonable in selected patients (ie, receiving enzyme-inducing agents and with low risk of bleeding).

Range[1] of Expected Therapeutic Maintenance Dose Based on CYP2C9[2] and VKORC1[3] Genotypes

VKORC1	CYP2C9					
	*1/*1	*1/*2	*1/*3	*2/*2	*2/*3	*3/*3
GG	5-7 mg	5-7 mg	3-4 mg	3-4 mg	3-4 mg	0.5-2 mg
AG	5-7 mg	3-4 mg	3-4 mg	3-4 mg	0.5-2 mg	0.5-2 mg
AA	3-4 mg	3-4 mg	0.5-2 mg	0.5-2 mg	0.5-2 mg	0.5-2 mg

Note: Must also take into account other patient related factors when determining initial dose (eg, age, body weight, concomitant medications, comorbidities). The American College of Chest Physicians recommends against the use of routine pharmacogenomic testing to guide dosing (Guyatt, 2012).

[1]Ranges derived from multiple published clinical studies.

[2]Patients with CYP2C9 *1/*3, *2/*2, *2/*3, and *3/*3 alleles may take up to 4 weeks to achieve maximum INR with a given dose regimen.

[3]VKORC1 -1639G>A (rs 9923231) variant is used in this table; other VKORC1 variants may also be important determinants of dose.

I.V.: Adults: 2-5 mg/day administered as a slow bolus injection

Dosage adjustment in renal disease: No dosage adjustment necessary. However, patients with renal failure have an increased risk of bleeding complications; monitor closely.

Dosae adjustment in hepatic disease: No dosage adjustment provided in manufacturer's labeling. However, the response to oral anticoagulants may be markedly enhanced in obstructive jaundice, hepatitis, and cirrhosis. INR should be closely monitored.

Dietary Considerations Foods high in vitamin K (eg, beef liver, pork liver, green tea, and leafy green vegetables) inhibit anticoagulant effect. Do not change dietary habits once stabilized on warfarin therapy. A balanced diet with a consistent intake of vitamin K is essential. Avoid large amounts of alfalfa, asparagus, broccoli, Brussels sprouts, cabbage, cauliflower, green teas, kale, lettuce, spinach, turnip greens, and watercress; decreased efficacy of warfarin. It is recommended that the diet contain a CONSISTENT vitamin K content of 70-140 mcg/day. Check with healthcare provider before changing diet.

Administration

Oral: Administer with or without food. Take at the same time each day.

I.V.: Administer as a slow bolus injection over 1-2 minutes; avoid all I.M. injections

Hazardous agent; use appropriate precautions for handling and disposal (EPA, P-listed [>0.3%]; U-listed [<0.3%]).

Monitoring Parameters Prothrombin time, hematocrit; INR (frequency varies depending on INR stability); may consider genotyping of CYP2C9 and VKORC1 prior to initiation of therapy, if available

Reference Range

INR = patient prothrombin time/mean normal prothrombin time

ISI = international sensitivity index

INR should be increased by 2-3.5 times depending upon indication. An INR >4 does not generally add additional therapeutic benefit and is associated with increased risk of bleeding. **Note:** To prevent gastrointestinal bleeding events in patients receiving the combination of warfarin, aspirin, and clopidogrel, an INR of 2-2.5 is recommended unless condition requires a higher INR target (eg, certain mechanical heart valves) (Bhatt, 2008).

Adult Target INR Ranges Based Upon Indication

Indication	Targeted INR	Targeted INR Range
Cardiac		
Anterior myocardial infarction with LV thrombus or high risk for LV thrombus (EF<40%, anteroapical wall motion abnormality)[1,2]	2.5	2-3
Atrial fibrillation (nonvalvular)[3] or atrial flutter	2.5	2-3
LV systolic dysfunction (without established CAD) with an LV thrombus (eg, Takotsubo cardiomyopathy)	2.5	2-3
Valvular		
Carbomedics or St. Jude Medical bileaflet or Medtronic Hall tilting disk mechanical aortic valve in normal sinus rhythm and normal LA size[4]	2.5	2-3
Bileaflet or tilting disk mechanical mitral valve[4]	3	2.5-3.5
Caged ball or caged disk mechanical valve[4]	3	2.5-3.5
Mechanical aortic valve[5]	2.5	2-3
Mechanical mitral valve **or** mechanical valves in both the aortic and mitral positions[5]	3	2.5-3.5
Bioprosthetic mitral valve[6]	2.5	2-3
Rheumatic mitral valve disease (particularly mitral stenosis) and normal sinus rhythm (LA diameter >5.5 cm), AF, previous systemic embolism, or LA thrombus	2.5	2-3
Thromboembolism Treatment		
Venous thromboembolism[7]	2.5	2-3
Thromboprophylaxis		
Idiopathic pulmonary artery hypertension (IPAH)[8]	2	1.5-2.5
Antiphospholipid syndrome (no other risk factors)	2.5	2-3
Antiphospholipid syndrome and recurrent thromboembolism	2.5	2-3
Total hip or knee replacement or hip fracture surgery[9]	2.5	2-3
Other Indications		
Ischemic stroke due to AF[10]	2.5	2-3
Cryptogenic stroke (recurrent) and either patent foramen ovale (PFO) or atrial septal aneurysm	2.5	2-3

(continued)

Note: Unless otherwise noted, all recommendations derived from "Antithrombotic Therapy and Prevention of Thrombosis, 9th ed: American College of Chest Physicians Evidence-Based Clinical Practice Guidelines."

[1]If coronary stent placed, triple therapy (warfarin, low-dose aspirin, and clopidogrel) is recommended for 1 month (bare-metal stent) or 3-6 months (drug-eluting stent) followed by discontinuation of warfarin and use of dual antiplatelet therapy (eg, aspirin and clopidogrel) for up to 12 months.

[2]If coronary stent **not** placed, maintain anticoagulation (in combination with low-dose aspirin) for 3 months followed by discontinuation of warfarin and use of dual antiplatelet therapy (eg, aspirin and clopidogrel) for up to 12 months.

[3]Recommended for those patients with nonvalvular AF who are at moderate-to-high risk of stroke (Goldstein, 2011).

[4]Recommendation from Stein, 2001.

[5]If at low risk of bleeding, combine with aspirin 81 mg/day.

[6]Maintain anticoagulation for 3 months after valve insertion then switch to aspirin 81 mg/day if no other indications for warfarin exist or clinically reassess need for warfarin in patients with prior history of systemic embolism.

[7]Treat for 3 months in patients with provoked VTE due to transient reversible risk factor. Treat for a minimum of 3 months in patients with unprovoked VTE and evaluate for extended anticoagulant therapy (ie, >3 months of therapy without a scheduled stop date). Other risk groups (eg, cancer) may require extended anticoagulant therapy.

[8]Recommendation from the ACCF/AHA 2009 Expert Consensus Document on Pulmonary Hypertension (McLaughlin, 2009)

[9]Continue for at least 10-14 days; up to 35 days after surgery is suggested.

[10]Instead of adjusted dose warfarin, the use of dabigatran has been suggested. In either case, oral anticoagulation should be initiated within 1-2 weeks after stroke onset or earlier in patients at low bleeding risk; bridging with aspirin may be required.

Warfarin levels are not used for monitoring degree of anticoagulation. They may be useful if a patient with unexplained coagulopathy is using the drug surreptitiously or if it is unclear whether clinical resistance is due to true drug resistance or lack of drug intake.

Normal prothrombin time (PT): 10.9-12.9 seconds. Healthy premature newborns have prolonged coagulation test screening results (eg, PT, aPTT, TT) which return to normal adult values at approximately 6 months of age. Healthy prematures, however, do not develop spontaneous hemorrhage or thrombotic complications because of a balance between procoagulants and inhibitors.

Additional Information

Pharmacogenomic Testing: The American College of Chest Physicians recommends against the use of routine pharmacogenomic testing to guide dosing (Guyatt, 2012). However, prospective genotyping is available, and may provide guidance on initiation of anticoagulant therapy. Commercial testing with PGxPredict™: WARFARIN is available from PGxHealth™ (Division of Clinical Data, Inc, New Haven, CT). The test genotypes patients for presence of the CYP2C9*2 or *3 alleles and the VKORC1 -1639G>A polymorphism. The results of the test allow patients to be phenotyped as extensive, intermediate, or poor metabolizers (CYP2C9) and as low, intermediate, or high warfarin sensitivity (VKORC1). Ordering information is available at 888-592-7327 or warfarininfo@pgxhealth.com.

Management of Elevated INR:

If INR above therapeutic range to <4.5 (no evidence of bleeding): Lower or hold next dose and monitor frequently; when INR approaches desired range, resume dosing with a lower dose (Patriquin, 2011).

If INR 4.5-10 (no evidence of bleeding): The 2012 ACCP guidelines recommend against routine vitamin K administration in this setting (Guyatt, 2012). Previously, the 2008 ACCP guidelines recommended if no risk factors for bleeding exist, to omit next 1 or 2 doses, monitor INR more frequently, and resume with an appropriately adjusted dose when INR in desired range; may consider administering vitamin K orally 1-2.5 mg if other risk factors for bleeding exist (Hirsh, 2008). Others have recommended consideration of vitamin K 1 mg orally or 0.5 mg I.V. (Patriquin, 2011).

If INR >10 (no evidence of bleeding): The 2012 ACCP guidelines recommend administration of oral vitamin K (dose not specified) in this setting (Guyatt, 2012). Previously, the 2008 ACCP guidelines recommended to hold warfarin, administer vitamin K orally 2.5-5 mg, expect INR to be reduced within 24-48 hours, monitor INR more frequently and give additional vitamin K at an appropriate dose if necessary; resume warfarin at an appropriately adjusted dose when INR is in desired range (Hirsh, 2008). Others have recommended consideration of vitamin K 2-2.5 mg orally or 0.5-1 mg I.V. (Patriquin, 2011).

If minor bleeding at any INR elevation: Hold warfarin, may administer vitamin K orally 2.5-5 mg, monitor INR more frequently, may repeat dose after 24 hours if INR correction incomplete; resume warfarin at an appropriately adjusted dose when INR is in desired range (Patriquin, 2011).

If major bleeding at any INR elevation: The 2012 ACCP guidelines recommend administration of four-factor prothrombin complex concentrate (PCC) and I.V. vitamin K 5-10 mg in this setting (Guyatt, 2012). Four-factor PCCs include Beriplex P/N, Cofact, Kcentra (available in U.S.), or Octaplex (available in Canada). Previously, the 2008 ACCP guidelines recommended to hold warfarin, administer vitamin K 10 mg by slow I.V. infusion and supplement with PCC depending on the urgency of the situation; I.V. vitamin K may be repeated every 12 hours (Hirsh, 2008).

Note: Use of high doses of vitamin K (eg, 10-15 mg) may cause warfarin resistance for ≥1 week. During this period of resistance, heparin or low-molecular-weight heparin (LMWH) may be given until INR responds.

Dosage Forms Excipient information presented when available (limited, particularly for generics); consult specific product labeling.

Solution Reconstituted, Intravenous, as sodium:
- Coumadin: 5 mg (1 ea)

Tablet, Oral, as sodium:
- Coumadin: 1 mg [scored]
- Coumadin: 2 mg [scored; contains fd&c blue #2 aluminum lake, fd&c red #40 aluminum lake]
- Coumadin: 2.5 mg [scored; contains fd&c blue #1 aluminum lake, fd&c yellow #10 aluminum lake]
- Coumadin: 3 mg [scored; contains fd&c blue #2 aluminum lake, fd&c red #40 aluminum lake, fd&c yellow #6 aluminum lake]
- Coumadin: 4 mg [scored; contains fd&c blue #1 aluminum lake]
- Coumadin: 5 mg [scored; contains fd&c yellow #6 aluminum lake]
- Coumadin: 6 mg [scored; contains fd&c blue #1 aluminum lake, fd&c yellow #6 aluminum lake]
- Coumadin: 7.5 mg [scored; contains fd&c yellow #10 aluminum lake, fd&c yellow #6 aluminum lake]
- Coumadin: 10 mg [scored; dye free]
- Jantoven: 1 mg [scored; contains fd&c red #40 aluminum lake]
- Jantoven: 2 mg [scored; contains fd&c blue #2 aluminum lake, fd&c red #40 aluminum lake]
- Jantoven: 2.5 mg [scored; contains fd&c blue #1 aluminum lake, fd&c yellow #10 aluminum lake]
- Jantoven: 3 mg [scored]
- Jantoven: 4 mg [scored; contains fd&c blue #1 aluminum lake]
- Jantoven: 5 mg [scored; contains fd&c yellow #6 aluminum lake]
- Jantoven: 6 mg [scored; contains fd&c blue #1 aluminum lake]
- Jantoven: 7.5 mg [scored; contains fd&c yellow #10 aluminum lake, fd&c yellow #6 aluminum lake]
- Jantoven: 10 mg [scored]
- Generic: 1 mg, 2 mg, 2.5 mg, 3 mg, 4 mg, 5 mg, 6 mg, 7.5 mg, 10 mg

- ◆ **Warfarin Sodium** *see* Warfarin *on page 2211*
- ◆ **4-Way Saline [OTC]** *see* Sodium Chloride *on page 1914*
- ◆ **Welchol** *see* Colesevelam *on page 487*
- ◆ **Wellbutrin** *see* BuPROPion *on page 296*
- ◆ **Wellbutrin XL** *see* BuPROPion *on page 296*
- ◆ **Wellbutrin SR** *see* BuPROPion *on page 296*
- ◆ **Wera** *see* Ethinyl Estradiol and Norethindrone *on page 793*
- ◆ **Westcort** *see* Hydrocortisone (Topical) *on page 1011*
- ◆ **Westcort® (Can)** *see* Hydrocortisone (Topical) *on page 1011*
- ◆ **Westhroid** *see* Thyroid, Desiccated *on page 2052*
- ◆ **Westhroid-P [DSC]** *see* Thyroid, Desiccated *on page 2052*

Wheat Dextrin (weet DEKS trin)

Brand Names: U.S. Benefiber Drink Mix [OTC]; Benefiber For Children [OTC]; Benefiber Plus Calcium [OTC]; Benefiber [OTC]

Index Terms Dextrin; Resistant Dextrin; Resistant Maltodextrin

Pharmacologic Category Fiber Supplement; Laxative, Bulk-Producing

Additional Appendix Information

Laxatives, Classification and Properties *on page 2304*

Use OTC labeling: Dietary fiber supplement

Unlabeled Use Treatment of constipation; aid to enhance LDL lowering to reduce the risk of coronary heart disease

Dosage Oral: General dosing guidelines; consult specific product labeling.

Adequate intake for total fiber: **Note:** The definition of "fiber" varies; however, the soluble fiber in wheat dextrin is only one type of fiber which makes up the daily recommended intake of total fiber.
- Children 1-3 years: 19 g/day
- Children 4-8 years: 25 g/day
- Children 9-13 years: Male: 31 g/day; Female: 26 g/day
- Children 14-18 years: Male: 38 g/day; Female: 26 g/day
- Adults 19-50 years: Male: 38 g/day; Female: 25 g/day
- Adults ≥51 years: Male: 30 g/day; Female: 21 g/day
- Pregnancy: 28 g/day
- Lactation: 29 g/day

Additional Information Complete prescribing information should be consulted for additional detail.

Dosage Forms Excipient information presented when available (limited, particularly for generics); consult specific product labeling.

Packet, Oral:
- Benefiber Drink Mix: (28 ea) [flavor free, gluten free, grit free, sugar free]
- Benefiber Drink Mix: (8 ea) [sugar free; contains aspartame; raspberry tea flavor]
- Benefiber Drink Mix: (8 ea, 24 ea) [sugar free; contains aspartame, fd&c red #40; cherry pomegranate flavor]
- Benefiber Drink Mix: (16 ea, 24 ea) [sugar free; contains aspartame, fd&c red #40; kiwi strawberry flavor]

Benefiber Drink Mix: (16 ea) [sugar free; contains aspartame, fd&c yellow #6 (sunset yellow), soybean oil, tartrazine (fd&c yellow #5); citrus punch flavor]

Powder, Oral:

Benefiber: (80 g, 155 g, 245 g, 350 g, 477 g, 730 g) [gluten free, grit free, sugar free]

Benefiber: (267 g, 529 g) [grit free, sugar free; contains aspartame, fd&c red #40, fd&c yellow #6 (sunset yellow), lactose; orange flavor]

Benefiber For Children: (155 g) [grit free, sugar free; unflavored flavor]

Benefiber Plus Calcium: (423.8 g) [gluten free, grit free, sugar free]

Benefiber Plus Calcium: (305 g) [gluten free, grit free, sugar free; contains aspartame, fd&c red #40, fd&c yellow #6 (sunset yellow); orange flavor]

Tablet, Oral:

Benefiber:

Tablet Chewable, Oral:

Benefiber: [scored; gluten free, sugar free; contains aspartame, fd&c blue #1 aluminum lake, fd&c red #40 aluminum lake, fd&c yellow #6 aluminum lake; assorted fruit flavor]

Benefiber: [scored; gluten free, sugar free; contains aspartame, fd&c yellow #6 aluminum lake; orange cream flavor]

Benefiber Plus Calcium: [scored; sugar free; contains aspartame, fd&c blue #1 aluminum lake, fd&c red #40 aluminum lake, soybeans (glycine max); wild berry flavor]

- **Wilate®** *see* Antihemophilic Factor/von Willebrand Factor Complex (Human) *on page* 146
- **Winpred™ (Can)** *see* PredniSONE *on page* 1707
- **WinRho SDF** *see* Rh_o(D) Immune Globulin *on page* 1801
- **WinRho® SDF (Can)** *see* Rh_o(D) Immune Globulin *on page* 1801
- **Woman's Laxative [OTC] (Can)** *see* Bisacodyl *on page* 259
- **Womens Laxative [OTC]** *see* Bisacodyl *on page* 259
- **Wound Wash Saline [OTC]** *see* Sodium Chloride *on page* 1914
- **WP Thyroid** *see* Thyroid, Desiccated *on page* 2052
- **WR-2721** *see* Amifostine *on page* 96
- **WR-139007** *see* Dacarbazine *on page* 530
- **WR-139013** *see* Chlorambucil *on page* 403
- **WR-139021** *see* Carmustine *on page* 352
- **Wycillin** *see* Penicillin G Procaine *on page* 1610
- **Wycillin® (Can)** *see* Penicillin G Procaine *on page* 1610
- **Wymzya Fe** *see* Ethinyl Estradiol and Norethindrone *on page* 793
- **Xalatan** *see* Latanoprost *on page* 1178
- **Xalatan® (Can)** *see* Latanoprost *on page* 1178
- **Xalkori** *see* Crizotinib *on page* 497
- **Xamiol® (Can)** *see* Calcipotriene and Betamethasone *on page* 312
- **Xanax** *see* ALPRAZolam *on page* 81
- **Xanax® (Can)** *see* ALPRAZolam *on page* 81
- **Xanax TS™ (Can)** *see* ALPRAZolam *on page* 81
- **Xanax XR** *see* ALPRAZolam *on page* 81
- **Xarelto** *see* Rivaroxaban *on page* 1838
- **Xarelto® (Can)** *see* Rivaroxaban *on page* 1838
- **Xatral (Can)** *see* Alfuzosin *on page* 73
- **Xeljanz** *see* Tofacitinib *on page* 2082
- **Xeloda** *see* Capecitabine *on page* 329
- **Xenaderm®** *see* Trypsin, Balsam Peru, and Castor Oil *on page* 2133
- **Xenazine** *see* Tetrabenazine *on page* 2033
- **Xenical** *see* Orlistat *on page* 1516
- **Xeomin** *see* IncobotulinumtoxinA *on page* 1064
- **Xeomin® (Can)** *see* IncobotulinumtoxinA *on page* 106
- **Xeomin Cosmetic™ (Can)** *see* IncobotulinumtoxinA *on page* 1064
- **Xgeva** *see* Denosumab *on page* 568
- **Xiaflex** *see* Collagenase (Systemic) *on page* 490
- **Xifaxan** *see* Rifaximin *on page* 1815
- **Xilep** *see* Rufinamide *on page* 1865
- **Ximino™** *see* Minocycline *on page* 1373
- **Xodol® 5/300** *see* Hydrocodone and Acetaminophen *on page* 1006
- **Xodol® 7.5/300** *see* Hydrocodone and Acetaminophen *on page* 1006
- **Xodol® 10/300** *see* Hydrocodone and Acetaminophen *on page* 1006
- **Xolair** *see* Omalizumab *on page* 1502
- **Xolair® (Can)** *see* Omalizumab *on page* 1502
- **Xolegel** *see* Ketoconazole (Topical) *on page* 1149
- **Xolegel® (Can)** *see* Ketoconazole (Topical) *on page* 1149
- **Xopenex** *see* Levalbuterol *on page* 1192
- **Xopenex® (Can)** *see* Levalbuterol *on page* 1192
- **Xopenex Concentrate** *see* Levalbuterol *on page* 1192
- **Xopenex HFA** *see* Levalbuterol *on page* 1192
- **XP13512** *see* Gabapentin Enacarbil *on page* 936
- **Xpect [OTC]** *see* GuaiFENesin *on page* 974
- **XRP6258** *see* Cabazitaxel *on page* 307
- **Xtandi** *see* Enzalutamide *on page* 713
- **Xtra-Care [OTC]** *see* Vitamin E *on page* 2202
- **X-Viate** *see* Urea *on page* 2140
- **Xylac (Can)** *see* Loxapine *on page* 1253
- **Xylocaine** *see* Lidocaine (Systemic) *on page* 1210
- **Xylocaine** *see* Lidocaine (Topical) *on page* 1212
- **Xylocaine® (Can)** *see* Lidocaine (Topical) *on page* 1212
- **Xylocaine (Cardiac)** *see* Lidocaine (Systemic) *on page* 1210
- **Xylocaine-MPF** *see* Lidocaine (Systemic) *on page* 1210
- **Xylocaine® MPF With Epinephrine** *see* Lidocaine and Epinephrine *on page* 1213
- **Xylocaine Viscous** *see* Lidocaine (Topical) *on page* 1212
- **Xylocaine® With Epinephrine** *see* Lidocaine and Epinephrine *on page* 1213
- **Xylocard® (Can)** *see* Lidocaine (Systemic) *on page* 1210
- **Xyntha** *see* Antihemophilic Factor (Recombinant) *on page* 144
- **Xyntha® (Can)** *see* Antihemophilic Factor (Recombinant) *on page* 144
- **Xyntha Solofuse** *see* Antihemophilic Factor (Recombinant) *on page* 144
- **Xyrem** *see* Sodium Oxybate *on page* 1922
- **Xyrem® (Can)** *see* Sodium Oxybate *on page* 1922
- **Xyzal** *see* Levocetirizine *on page* 1197
- **Yasmin®** *see* Ethinyl Estradiol and Drospirenone *on page* 785

◆ **Yaz®** *see* Ethinyl Estradiol and Drospirenone *on page 785*

◆ **Yaz Plus (Can)** *see* Ethinyl Estradiol, Drospirenone, and Levomefolate *on page 797*

Yellow Fever Vaccine (YEL oh FEE ver vak SEEN)

Brand Names: U.S. YF-VAX®

Brand Names: Canada YF-VAX®

Pharmacologic Category Vaccine, Live (Viral)

Additional Appendix Information

Immunization Administration Recommendations *on page 2334*

Immunization Recommendations *on page 2339*

Use Induction of active immunity against yellow fever virus, primarily among persons traveling or living in areas where yellow fever infection exists and laboratory workers who may be exposed to the virus; vaccination may also be required for some international travelers

The Advisory Committee on Immunization Practices (ACIP) (CDC, 2010) recommends vaccination for:

- Persons traveling to or living in areas at risk for yellow fever transmission
- Persons traveling to countries which require vaccination for international travel
- Laboratory personnel who may be exposed to the yellow fever virus or concentrated preparations of the vaccine

Although the vaccine is approved for use in children ≥9 months of age, the CDC recommends use in children as young as 6 months under unusual circumstances (eg, travel to an area where exposure is unavoidable). Children <6 months of age should **never** receive the vaccine.

Pregnancy Risk Factor C

Pregnancy Considerations Animal reproduction studies have not been conducted. Adverse events were not observed in the mother or fetus following vaccination during the third trimester of pregnancy in Nigerian women; however, maternal seroconversion was reduced. Inadvertent exposure early in the first trimester of pregnancy in Brazilian women did not show decreased maternal seroconversion; no major congenital abnormalities were noted. Cord blood from an infant whose mother was vaccinated during the first trimester tested positive for IgM antibodies; no adverse events were noted in the infant. Vaccine should be administered if travel to an endemic area is unavoidable and the infant should be monitored after birth. Tests to verify maternal immune response may be considered. If a pregnant woman is to be vaccinated only to satisfy an international requirement (as opposed to decreasing risk of infection), efforts should be made to obtain a waiver letter. Women should wait 4 weeks after receiving vaccine before conceiving (CDC, 2010).

Breast-Feeding Considerations Laboratory confirmed transmission of 17DD yellow fever vaccine virus via breast-feeding has been documented. Yellow fever vaccine was administered to a nursing mother 15 days postpartum. She was exclusively breast-feeding her newborn. Eight days after maternal vaccination, the infant developed a fever, was irritable, refused to nurse, then was hospitalized for seizures the next day. Yellow fever virus specific to the vaccine and IgM antibodies were detected in the newborn CSF. The child was discharged after 24 days in the hospital; growth and neurodevelopment were normal through 6 months of age. Breast-feeding is contraindicated by the manufacturer, particularly in infants <9 months of age. If travel to an endemic area cannot be avoided or postponed, women who are nursing should be vaccinated. Breast-feeding does not adversely affect immunization (CDC, 2010; WHO, 2013).

Contraindications Hypersensitivity to egg or chick embryo protein, or any component of the formulation; children <9 months of age (per manufacturer); children <6 months of age (CDC guidelines); acute or febrile disease; immunosuppressed patients (eg, HIV infection, leukemia, lymphoma, thymic disease, generalized malignancy, or immunosuppression due to drugs or radiation); breast-feeding women

Warnings/Precautions Vaccination may not result in effective immunity in all patients. Response depends upon multiple factors (eg, type of vaccine, age of patient) and may be improved by administering the vaccine at the recommended dose, route, and interval. Vaccines may not be effective if administered during periods of altered immune competence (CDC, 2011). Malnourished persons may have a decreased response to vaccination (CDC, 2010). Patients who are immunosuppressed have a theoretical risk of encephalitis with yellow fever vaccine administration; consider delaying travel or obtaining a waiver letter. Patients on low-dose or short-term corticosteroids are not considered immunosuppressed and may be offered the vaccine. If vaccination is only to satisfy an international requirement (as opposed to decreasing risk of infection), efforts should be made to obtain a waiver letter. Per the ACIP guidelines, use is contraindicated in patients with symptomatic HIV infection or patients with CD4+ counts <200/mm^3 (or <15% of total lymphocytes in children <6 years of age); use caution when administering the vaccine to patients with asymptomatic infection with CD4+ counts 200-499/mm^3 (or 15% to 24% of total lymphocytes in children <6 years of age) (CDC, 2010). In general, household and close contacts of persons with altered immunocompetence may receive all age appropriate vaccines (CDC, 2011).

Immediate treatment (including epinephrine 1:1000) for anaphylactoid and/or hypersensitivity reactions should be available during vaccine use. Use is contraindicated in patients with immediate-type hypersensitivity reactions to eggs. Less severe or localized manifestations of allergy are not contraindications; in general, persons who are able to eat eggs or egg products may receive the vaccine. A hypersensitivity screening test and desensitization procedure is available for persons with suspected or known severe egg sensitivity. Consult manufacturer's labeling for details. Syncope has been reported with use of injectable vaccines and may be accompanied by transient visual disturbances, weakness, or tonic-clonic movements. Procedures should be in place to avoid injuries from falling and to restore cerebral perfusion if syncope occurs.

The vial stopper contains latex; product may contain gelatin. Immunization should be delayed during the course of an acute or febrile illness. The presence of a low-grade fever is generally not a reason to postpone vaccination (CDC, 2011). Due to an increased incidence of serious adverse events observed in older adults compared to younger adults, use with caution in the elderly ≥65 years (per manufacturer) or ≥60 years (per ACIP guidelines), particularly in patients who have not previously received the vaccine. The risk for vaccine-associated neurologic disease (YEL-AND) and vaccine-associated viscerotropic disease (YEL-AVD) is also increased. The ACIP guidelines note that if travel is unavoidable, the decision to vaccinate travelers ≥60 years should be made after weighing the risks vs benefits (CDC, 2011). Avoid use in pregnant women unless travel to high-risk areas is unavoidable. The manufacturer contraindicates use in infants <9 months of age due to risk of encephalitis. The CDC allows for use in infants 6-8 months of age when possible exposure with the yellow fever virus is unavoidable and the risk of infection exists. Infants <6 months of age should never be vaccinated (CDC, 2010). Transfusion-related transmission of yellow fever vaccine virus has been reported; wait 2 weeks after immunization with yellow fever vaccine to donate blood (CDC, 2010). In order to maximize vaccination rates, the ACIP recommends simultaneous administration of all age-appropriate vaccines (live or inactivated) for which a person is eligible at a single clinic visit, unless contraindications exist (CDC, 2011).

Adverse Reactions All serious adverse reactions must be reported to the U.S. Department of Health and Human Services (DHHS) Vaccine Adverse Event Reporting System (VAERS) 1-800-822-7967 or online at https://vaers.hhs.gov/esub/index. In Canada, adverse reactions may be reported to local provincial/territorial health agencies or to the Vaccine Safety Section at Public Health Agency of Canada (1-866-844-0018).

Frequency not defined (adverse reactions may be increased in patients <9 months or ≥60 years of age)

Central nervous system: Chills, fever (incidence of these reactions have been reported to be as low as <5% and as high as 10% to 30% depending on the study), focal neurological defects, headache, malaise, seizure

Dermatologic: Rash, urticaria

Local: Injection site reactions (edema, erythema, hypersensitivity, mass, pain, pruritus, rash, warmth)

Neuromuscular & skeletal: Myalgia, weakness

Miscellaneous: Guillain-Barré syndrome (GBS), hypersensitivity (immediate), vaccine-associated neurotropic disease (rare), viscerotropic disease (rare; may be associated with multiorgan failure)

Vaccine-associated neurologic disease (YEL-AND) may manifest as meningoencephalitis (neurotropic disease), GBS, acute disseminated encephalomyelitis, and bulbar palsy. Vaccine-associated viscerotropic disease (YEL-AVD) mimics naturally-acquired yellow fever disease; risk may be increased in older patients and those with a history of thymus disease or thymectomy.

Drug Interactions

Metabolism/Transport Effects None known.

Avoid Concomitant Use

Avoid concomitant use of Yellow Fever Vaccine with any of the following: Belimumab; Fingolimod; Immunosuppressants

Increased Effect/Toxicity

The levels/effects of Yellow Fever Vaccine may be increased by: AzaTHIOprine; Belimumab; Corticosteroids (Systemic); Dimethyl Fumarate; Fingolimod; Hydroxychloroquine; Immunosuppressants; Leflunomide; Mercaptopurine; Methotrexate

Decreased Effect

Yellow Fever Vaccine may decrease the levels/effects of: Tuberculin Tests

The levels/effects of Yellow Fever Vaccine may be decreased by: Dimethyl Fumarate; Fingolimod; Immunosuppressants

Preparation for Administration Reconstitute only with diluent provided. Inject diluent slowly into vial and allow to stand for 1-2 minutes. Gently swirl until a uniform suspension forms; swirl well before withdrawing dose. Avoid vigorous shaking to prevent foaming of suspension. Vaccine must be used within 60 minutes of reconstitution. Keep suspension refrigerated until used.

Storage/Stability Store at 2°C to 8°C (35°F to 46°F); do not freeze.

Pharmacodynamics/Kinetics

Onset of action: Seroconversion: 10-14 days

Duration: ≥30 years

Dosage SubQ:

Children ≥6 months (unlabeled use): One dose (0.5 mL) ≥10 days before travel; Booster: Every 10 years for those at continued risk of exposure (CDC, 2010)

Children ≥9 months (per manufacturer), Adolescents, and Adults: One dose (0.5 mL) ≥10 days before travel; Booster: Every 10 years for those at continued risk of exposure

Note: Based on currently available data, the World Health Organization (WHO) has determined that vaccine failure is rare and booster doses are not needed. Future studies may determine if there are specific risk groups who could benefit from a booster dose (WHO, 2013).

Elderly: Monitor closely due to an increased incidence of serious adverse events in patients ≥60 years of age, particularly in patients receiving their first dose. The ACIP guidelines note that if travel is unavoidable, the decision to vaccinate travelers ≥60 years should be made after weighing the risks vs benefits (CDC, 2010).

Dosage adjustment in renal impairment: No dosage adjustment provided in manufacturer's labeling.

Dosage adjustment in hepatic impairment: No dosage adjustment provided in manufacturer's labeling.

Administration For SubQ injection only. Do not administer I.M. or I.V.; if inadvertently administered I.M., the dose does not need repeated. Use of expired vaccine is not considered a valid dose and should be repeated after 28 days. For booster doses, if the date of previous vaccination cannot be determined and the patient requires vaccination, the booster dose can be given (CDC, 2010).

Blood donation following vaccine administration: Transfusion-related transmission of yellow fever vaccine virus has been reported; wait 2 weeks after immunization with yellow fever vaccine to donate blood (CDC, 2010).

Simultaneous administration of vaccines helps ensure the patients will be fully vaccinated by the appropriate age. Simultaneous administration of vaccines is defined as administering >1 vaccine on the same day at different anatomic sites. Separate vaccines should not be combined in the same syringe unless indicated by product specific labeling. Separate needles and syringes should be used for each injection. The ACIP prefers each dose of a specific vaccine in a series come from the same manufacturer when possible. Adolescents and adults should be vaccinated while seated or lying down. In general, preterm infants should be vaccinated at the same chronological age as full-term infants (CDC, 2011).

Antipyretics have not been shown to prevent febrile seizures. Antipyretics may be used to treat fever or discomfort following vaccination (CDC, 2011). One study reported that routine prophylactic administration of acetaminophen to prevent fever prior to vaccination decreased the immune response of some vaccines; the clinical significance of this reduction in immune response has not been established (Prymula, 2009).

Monitoring Parameters Monitor for syncope for 15 minutes following administration. If seizure-like activity associated with syncope occurs, maintain patient in supine or Trendelenburg position to reestablish adequate cerebral perfusion. Monitor for adverse effects 10 days after vaccination (specifically in the elderly) (CDC, 2010; CDC, 2011).

Additional Information U.S. federal law requires that the name of medication, date of administration, the vaccine manufacturer, lot number of vaccine, and the administering person's name, title, and address be entered into the patient's permanent medical record. Some countries require a valid International Certification of Vaccination or Prophylaxis (ICVP) showing receipt of vaccine. Certificate is valid beginning 10 days after and for 10 years following vaccination (booster doses received within 10 years are valid from the date of vaccination). The WHO requires revaccination every 10 years to maintain traveler's vaccination certificate. All travelers to endemic areas should be advised of the risks of yellow fever disease and all available methods to prevent it. All travelers should take protective measures to avoid mosquito bites.

The following CDC agencies may be contacted if serologic testing is needed or for advice when administering yellow fever vaccine to pregnant women, children <9 months, or patients with altered immune status:

Division of Vector-Borne Infectious Diseases: 970-221-6400 (CDC, 2010)

Division of Global Migration and Quarantine: 404-498-1600

Dosage Forms Excipient information presented when available (limited, particularly for generics); consult specific product labeling.

Injection, powder for reconstitution [17D-204 strain]:

YF-VAX®: ≥4.74 Log_{10} plaque-forming units (PFU) per 0.5 mL dose [single-dose or 5-dose vial; produced in chicken embryos; contains gelatin; packaged with diluent; vial stopper contains latex]

- ◆ **Yervoy** *see* Ipilimumab *on page 1109*
- ◆ **Yervoy® (Can)** *see* Ipilimumab *on page 1109*
- ◆ **YF-VAX®** *see* Yellow Fever Vaccine *on page 2217*
- ◆ **YM087** *see* Conivaptan *on page 491*
- ◆ **YM-178** *see* Mirabegron *on page 1378*
- ◆ **YM905** *see* Solifenacin *on page 1932*
- ◆ **YM-08310** *see* Amifostine *on page 96*
- ◆ **Yodoxin** *see* Iodoquinol *on page 1109*
- ◆ **Z4942** *see* Ifosfamide *on page 1041*
- ◆ **Zactima** *see* Vandetanib *on page 2162*
- ◆ **Zaditor [OTC]** *see* Ketotifen (Ophthalmic) *on page 1156*
- ◆ **Zaditor® (Can)** *see* Ketotifen (Ophthalmic) *on page 1156*

Zafirlukast (za FIR loo kast)

Brand Names: U.S. Accolate

Brand Names: Canada Accolate®

Index Terms ICI-204,219

Pharmacologic Category Leukotriene-Receptor Antagonist

Use Prophylaxis and chronic treatment of asthma

Pregnancy Risk Factor B

Pregnancy Considerations Adverse events were not observed in animal reproduction studies except with doses that were also maternally toxic. Based on limited data, an increased risk of teratogenic effects has not been observed with zafirlukast use in pregnancy (Bakhireva, 2007). Uncontrolled asthma is associated with adverse events on pregnancy (increased risk of perinatal mortality, pre-eclampsia, preterm birth, low birth weight infants). Zafirlukast may be considered for use in women who had a favorable response prior to becoming pregnant; however, initiating a leukotriene receptor antagonist during pregnancy is an alternative (but not preferred) treatment option for mild persistent asthma (NAEPP, 2005).

Breast-Feeding Considerations Zafirlukast is excreted into breast milk. In women receiving zafirlukast 40 mg twice daily, maternal serum concentrations were 225 ng/mL and breast milk concentrations were 50 ng/mL. Due to the potential for adverse reactions in the nursing infant, breast-feeding is not recommended by the manufacturer.

Contraindications Hypersensitivity to zafirlukast or any component of the formulation; hepatic impairment (including hepatic cirrhosis)

Canadian labeling: Additional contraindications (not in U.S. labeling): Patients in whom zafirlukast was discontinued due to treatment related hepatotoxicity

Warnings/Precautions Zafirlukast is not approved for use in the reversal of bronchospasm in acute asthma attacks, including status asthmaticus. Therapy with zafirlukast can be continued during acute exacerbations of asthma.

Hepatic adverse events (including hepatitis, hyperbilirubinemia, and hepatic failure) have been reported; female patients may be at greater risk. Periodic testing of liver function may be considered (early detection coupled with therapy discontinuation is generally believed to improve the likelihood of recovery). Advise patients to be alert for and to immediately report symptoms (eg, anorexia, right upper quadrant abdominal pain, nausea). If hepatic dysfunction is suspected (due to clinical signs/symptoms), discontinue use immediately and measure liver function tests (particularly ALT); resolution observed in most but not all cases upon discontinuation of therapy. Do not resume or restart if hepatic function studies indicate dysfunction. Use in patients with hepatic impairment (including hepatic cirrhosis) is contraindicated. Postmarketing reports of behavioral changes (ie, depression, insomnia) have been noted. Instruct patients to report neuropsychiatric symptoms/events during therapy.

Monitor INR closely with concomitant warfarin use. Rare cases of eosinophilic vasculitis (Churg-Strauss) have been reported in patients receiving zafirlukast (usually, but not always, associated with reduction in concurrent steroid dosage). No causal relationship established. Monitor for eosinophilic vasculitis, rash, pulmonary symptoms, cardiac symptoms, or neuropathy.

Clearance is decreased in elderly patients; C_{max} and AUC are increased approximately two- to threefold in adults ≥65 years compared to younger adults; however, no dosage adjustments are recommended in this age group. An increased proportion of zafirlukast patients >55 years of age reported infections as compared to placebo-treated patients. These infections were mostly mild or moderate in intensity and predominantly affected the respiratory tract. Infections occurred equally in both sexes, were dose-proportional to total milligrams of zafirlukast exposure, and were associated with coadministration of inhaled corticosteroids.

Adverse Reactions Incidence reported in children ≥12 years and adults unless otherwise specified.

>10%: Central nervous system: Headache (13%; children 5-11 years: 5%)

1% to 10%:

Central nervous system: Dizziness (2%), pain (2%), fever (2%)

Gastrointestinal: Nausea (3%), diarrhea (3%), abdominal pain (2%; children 5-11 years: 3%), vomiting (2%), dyspepsia (1%)

Hepatic: ALT increased (2%)

Neuromuscular & skeletal: Back pain (2%), myalgia (2%), weakness (2%)

Miscellaneous: Infection (4%)

<1% (Limited to important or life-threatening): Agranulocytosis, angioedema, arthralgia, bleeding, bruising, depression, edema, eosinophilia (systemic), eosinophilic pneumonia, hepatic failure, hepatitis, hyperbilirubinemia, hypersensitivity reactions, insomnia, malaise, pruritus, rash, urticaria, vasculitis with clinical features of Churg-Strauss syndrome (rare)

Drug Interactions

Metabolism/Transport Effects Substrate of CYP2C9 (major); **Note:** Assignment of Major/Minor substrate status based on clinically relevant drug interaction potential; **Inhibits** CYP1A2 (weak), CYP2C19 (weak), CYP2C8 (weak), CYP2C9 (moderate), CYP2D6 (weak), CYP3A4 (weak)

Avoid Concomitant Use

Avoid concomitant use of Zafirlukast with any of the following: Pimozide

Increased Effect/Toxicity

Zafirlukast may increase the levels/effects of: ARIPiprazole; Bosentan; Carvedilol; CYP2C9 Substrates; Dofetilide; Lomitapide; Pimozide; Theophylline Derivatives; Vitamin K Antagonists

The levels/effects of Zafirlukast may be increased by: CYP2C9 Inhibitors (Moderate); CYP2C9 Inhibitors (Strong); Mifepristone

Decreased Effect

The levels/effects of Zafirlukast may be decreased by: CYP2C9 Inducers (Strong); Dabrafenib; Erythromycin (Systemic); Peginterferon Alfa-2b; Theophylline Derivatives

Ethanol/Nutrition/Herb Interactions Food: Food decreases bioavailability of zafirlukast by 40%. Management: Take on an empty stomach 1 hour before or 2 hours after meals.

Storage/Stability Store tablets at controlled room temperature of 20°C to 25°C (68°F to 77°F). Protect from light and moisture; dispense in original airtight container.

Mechanism of Action Zafirlukast is a selectively and competitive leukotriene-receptor antagonist (LTRA) of leukotriene D4 and E4 (LTD4 and LTE4), components of slow-reacting substance of anaphylaxis (SRSA). Cysteinyl leukotriene production and receptor occupation have been correlated with the pathophysiology of asthma, including airway edema, smooth muscle constriction, and altered cellular activity associated with the inflammatory process, which contribute to the signs and symptoms of asthma.

Pharmacodynamics/Kinetics

Distribution: V_{dss}: ~70 L

Protein binding: >99%, primarily to albumin

Metabolism: Extensively hepatic via CYP2C9

Bioavailability: Reduced 40% with food

Half-life elimination: ~10 hours

Time to peak, serum: 3 hours

Excretion: Feces (~90%); Urine (~10%)

Dosage Oral:

U.S. labeling:

Children 5-11 years: 10 mg twice daily

Children ≥12 years and Adults: 20 mg twice daily

Canadian labeling: Children ≥12 years and Adults: 20 mg twice daily

Elderly: Refer to adult dosing.

Dosage adjustment in renal impairment: No dosage adjustment necessary.

Dosage adjustment in hepatic impairment: Use is contraindicated.

Dietary Considerations Should be taken on an empty stomach (1 hour before or 2 hours after meals).

Administration Administer at least 1 hour before or 2 hours after a meal.

Monitoring Parameters Monitor for improvements in air flow; monitor closely for sign/symptoms of hepatic injury; periodic monitoring of LFTs may be considered (not proved to prevent serious injury, but early detection may enhance recovery)

Dosage Forms Excipient information presented when available (limited, particularly for generics); consult specific product labeling.

Tablet, Oral:

Accolate: 10 mg, 20 mg

Generic: 10 mg, 20 mg

Zaleplon (ZAL e plon)

Brand Names: U.S. Sonata

Pharmacologic Category Hypnotic, Miscellaneous

Additional Appendix Information

Beers Criteria – Potentially Inappropriate Medications for Geriatrics *on page 2368*

Use Short-term (7-10 days) treatment of insomnia (has been demonstrated to be effective for up to 5 weeks in controlled trial)

Pregnancy Risk Factor C

Pregnancy Considerations Teratogenic effects were not observed in animal reproduction studies. Adverse effects, including stillbirth, postnatal mortality, and decreased growth and physical development, were observed near the end of gestation. A small study of pregnant women did not show an increased risk of teratogenic effects when used early in pregnancy (Wiker, 2011). Use during pregnancy is not recommended by the manufacturer.

Breast-Feeding Considerations Zaleplon is excreted in human milk with the highest concentration ~1 hour after administration; therefore, the manufacturer does not recommended use while breast-feeding.

Medication Guide Available Yes

Contraindications Hypersensitivity to zaleplon or any component of the formulation

Warnings/Precautions Symptomatic treatment of insomnia should be initiated only after careful evaluation of potential causes of sleep disturbance. Failure of sleep disturbance to resolve after 7-10 days may indicate psychiatric and/or medical illness.

Use with caution in patients with depression, particularly if suicidal risk may be present. Use with caution in patients with a history of drug dependence. Abrupt discontinuance may lead to withdrawal symptoms. Hypnotics/sedatives have been associated with abnormal thinking and behavior changes including decreased inhibition, aggression, bizarre behavior, agitation, hallucinations, and depersonalization. These changes may occur unpredictably and may indicate previously unrecognized psychiatric disorders; evaluate appropriately. May impair physical and mental capabilities. Patients must be cautioned about performing tasks which require mental alertness (operating machinery or driving). Use with caution in patients receiving other CNS depressants or psychoactive medications. Effects with other sedative drugs or ethanol may be potentiated. Postmarketing studies have indicated that the use of hypnotic/sedative agents for sleep has been associated with hypersensitivity reactions including anaphylaxis as well as angioedema. An increased risk for hazardous sleep-related activities such as sleep-driving, cooking and eating food, and making phone calls while asleep have been noted; amnesia may also occur. Evaluation is recommended in patients who report any sleep-related episodes.

Avoid chronic use (>90 days) in older adults; adverse events, including delirium, falls, fractures, has been observed with nonbenzodiazepine hypnotic use in the elderly similar to events observed with benzodiazepines. Data suggests improvements in sleep duration and latency are minimal (Beers Criteria).

Use with caution in the elderly, those with compromised respiratory function, or hepatic impairment (dosage adjustment recommended in mild-to-moderate hepatic impairment; use is not recommended in patients with severe impairment). Because of the rapid onset of action, zaleplon should be administered immediately prior to bedtime or after the patient has gone to bed and is having difficulty falling asleep. Capsules contain tartrazine (FDC yellow #5); avoid in patients with sensitivity (caution in patients with asthma).

Adverse Reactions

>10%: Central nervous system: Headache (30% to 42%)

1% to 10%:

Cardiovascular: Chest pain (≥1%), peripheral edema (≤1%)

Central nervous system: Dizziness (7% to 9%), drowsiness (5% to 6%), amnesia (2% to 4%), paresthesia (3%), altered sense of smell (<1% to 2%), depersonalization (<1% to 2%), hyperacusis (1% to 2%), hypoesthesia (<1% to 2%), malaise (<1% to 2%), abnormality in thinking (≥1%), anxiety (≥1%), depression (≥1%), migraine (≥1%), nervousness (≥1%), hypertonia (1%), confusion (≤1%), hallucination (≤1%), vertigo (≤1%)

Dermatologic: Pruritus (≥1%), skin rash (≥1%), skin photosensitivity (≤1%)

Gastrointestinal: Nausea (6% to 8%), abdominal pain (6%), anorexia (<1% to 2%), constipation (≥1%), dysgeusia (≥1%), dyspepsia (≥1%), xerostomia (≥1%), colitis (≤1%)

Genitourinary: Dysmenorrhea (3% to 4%)

Neuromuscular & skeletal: Weakness (5% to 7%), tremor (2%), arthralgia (≥1%), arthritis (≥1%), back pain (≥1%), myalgia (≥1%)

Ophthalmic: Eye pain (3% to 4%), visual disturbance (<1% to 2%), conjunctivitis (≥1%)

Otic: Otalgia (≤1%)

Respiratory: Bronchitis (≥1%), epistaxis (≤1%)

Miscellaneous: Fever (≥1%)

<1% (Limited to important or life-threatening): Abnormal gait, abnormal hepatic function tests, accommodation disturbance, ageusia, agitation, alopecia, anaphylactoid purpura, anaphylaxis, anemia, angina pectoris, apathy, aphthous stomatitis, apnea, asthma, ataxia, bigeminy, biliary colic, blepharitis, blepharoptosis, bruxism, bundle branch block, bursitis, cataract, central nervous system stimulation, cerebral ischemia, cholelithiasis, conjunctival hyperemia (subconjunctival hemorrhage), contact dermatitis, corneal erosion, cyanosis, cystitis, deafness, decreased libido, delusions, diabetes mellitus, diaphoresis, diplopia, dry eye syndrome, duodenal ulcer, dysarthria, dysarthria, dysphagia, dyspnea, dystonia, dysuria, ecchymoses, eczema, edema, emotional lability, eosinophilia, eructation, esophageal achalasia, esophagitis, euphoria, facial paralysis, flatulence, gastritis, gastroenteritis, gingival hemorrhage, gingivitis, glaucoma, glossitis, goiter, gout, hangover effect, hematuria, hemorrhage, hyperbilirubinemia, hypercholesterolemia, hyperesthesia, hyperglycemia, hyperkinesia, hypermenorrhea, hyperreflexia, hypertension, hyperuricemia, hyperventilation, hypoglycemia, hypokinesia, hyporeflexia, hypotension, hypothyroidism, hypotonia, impotence, increased appetite, increased bronchial secretions, increased serum ALT, increased serum AST, increased thirst, insomnia, intestinal obstruction, irregular menses, ketosis, lactose intolerance, laryngitis, leukocytosis, leukorrhea, lymphadenopathy, lymphocytosis, maculopapular rash, mastalgia, melanosis, melena, menstrual disease, myasthenia, myoclonus, myositis, neck stiffness, nephrolithiasis, neuralgia, neuropathy, nightmares, nystagmus, orthostatic hypotension, osteoporosis, palpitations, paradoxical central nervous system stimulation, peptic ulcer, pericardial effusion, photophobia, pleural effusion, pneumonia, psoriasis, psychomotor retardation, pulmonary embolism, purpura, pustular rash, rectal hemorrhage, renal pain, retinal detachment, sialorrhea, sinus bradycardia, skin discoloration, skin hypertrophy, skin rash, sleep talking, slurred speech, snoring, somnambulism (complex sleep-related behavior [sleep-driving, sleep- cooking, sleep-eating, sleep-talking on the phone]), stupor, substernal pain, syncope, tenosynovitis, thrombophlebitis, tinnitus, tongue discoloration, tongue edema, transient perioral paresthesia, trismus, urethritis, urinary frequency, urinary incontinence, urinary retention, urinary urgency, urticaria, vaginal hemorrhage, vaginitis, vasodilatation, ventricular premature contractions, ventricular tachycardia, vesicobullous dermatitis, visual field defect, voice disorder, weight gain, weight loss, xeroderma

Drug Interactions

Metabolism/Transport Effects Substrate of CYP3A4 (minor); **Note:** Assignment of Major/Minor substrate status based on clinically relevant drug interaction potential

Avoid Concomitant Use

Avoid concomitant use of Zaleplon with any of the following: Azelastine (Nasal); Paraldehyde; Sodium Oxybate

Increased Effect/Toxicity

Zaleplon may increase the levels/effects of: Alcohol (Ethyl); Azelastine (Nasal); Buprenorphine; CNS Depressants; Hydrocodone; Methotrimeprazine; Metyrosine; Mirtazapine; Paraldehyde; Pramipexole; ROPINIRole; Rotigotine; Selective Serotonin Reuptake Inhibitors; Sodium Oxybate; Zolpidem

The levels/effects of Zaleplon may be increased by: Brimonidine (Topical); Cimetidine; Doxylamine; Droperidol; HydrOXYzine; Magnesium Sulfate; Methotrimeprazine; Perampanel; Tapentadol

Decreased Effect

The levels/effects of Zaleplon may be decreased by: Flumazenil; Rifamycin Derivatives

Ethanol/Nutrition/Herb Interactions

Ethanol: Ethanol may increase CNS depression. Management: Avoid or limit use of ethanol and monitor for increased effects.

Food: High-fat meals prolong absorption; delay T_{max} by 2 hours, and reduce C_{max} by 35%. Management: Avoid taking after a high-fat meal.

Herb/Nutraceutical: St John's wort may decrease zaleplon levels. Some herbal medications may increase CNS depression. Management: Avoid St John's wort, valerian, kava kava, and gotu kola.

Storage/Stability Store at controlled room temperature of 20°C to 25°C (68°F to 77°F). Protect from light.

Mechanism of Action Zaleplon is unrelated to benzodiazepines, barbiturates, or other hypnotics. However, it interacts with the benzodiazepine GABA receptor complex. Nonclinical studies have shown that it binds selectively to the brain omega-1 receptor situated on the alpha subunit of the GABA-A receptor complex.

Pharmacodynamics/Kinetics

Onset of action: Rapid

Absorption: Rapid and almost complete; high-fat meal delays absorption

Distribution: V_d: ~1.4 L/kg

Protein binding: ~45% to 75%

Metabolism: Extensive, primarily via aldehyde oxidase to form 5-oxo-zaleplon and, to a lesser extent, by CYP3A4 to desethylzaleplon; all metabolites are pharmacologically inactive

Bioavailability: ~30%

Half-life elimination: 1 hour

Time to peak, serum: 1 hour

Excretion: Urine (~70% primarily metabolites, <1% as unchanged drug); feces (~17%)

Clearance: Plasma: Oral: 3 L/hour/kg

Dosage Oral:

Adults: 10 mg at bedtime (range: 5-20 mg); has been used for up to 5 weeks of treatment in controlled trial setting

Elderly: 5 mg at bedtime; maximum: 10 mg/day

Dosage adjustment in renal impairment:

Mild to moderate impairment: No dosage adjustment necessary.

Severe impairment: No dosage adjustment provided in manufacturer's labeling (has not been studied).

Dosage adjustment in hepatic impairment:

Mild to moderate impairment: 5 mg

Severe impairment: Use is not recommended

Dietary Considerations Avoid taking with or after a heavy, high-fat meal; reduces absorption.

Administration Immediately before bedtime or when the patient is in bed and cannot fall asleep

Additional Information Prescription quantities should not exceed a 1-month supply.

Dosage Forms Excipient information presented when available (limited, particularly for generics); consult specific product labeling.

Capsule, Oral:

Sonata: 5 mg, 10 mg [contains tartrazine (fd&c yellow #5)]

Generic: 5 mg, 10 mg

Controlled Substance C-IV

◆ Zaltrap *see* Ziv-Aflibercept (Systemic) *on page 2233*

◆ Zamicet™ *see* Hydrocodone and Acetaminophen *on page 1006*

◆ Zanaflex *see* TiZANidine *on page 2074*

Zanamivir (za NA mi veer)

Brand Names: U.S. Relenza Diskhaler

Brand Names: Canada Relenza®

Pharmacologic Category Antiviral Agent; Neuraminidase Inhibitor

Use Treatment of uncomplicated acute illness due to influenza virus A and B in patients who have been symptomatic for no more than 2 days; prophylaxis against influenza virus A and B

The Advisory Committee on Immunization Practices (ACIP) recommends that **treatment** be considered for the following:

- Persons with severe, complicated or progressive illness
- Hospitalized persons
- Persons at higher risk for influenza complications:
  - Children <2 years of age (highest risk in children <6 months of age)
  - Adults ≥65 years of age
  - Persons with chronic disorders of the pulmonary (including asthma) or cardiovascular systems (except hypertension)
  - Persons with chronic metabolic diseases (including diabetes mellitus), hepatic disease, renal dysfunction, hematologic disorders (including sickle cell disease), or immunosuppression (including immunosuppression caused by medications or HIV)
  - Persons with neurologic/neuromuscular conditions (including conditions such as spinal cord injuries, seizure disorders, cerebral palsy, stroke, mental retardation, moderate to severe developmental delay, or muscular dystrophy) which may compromise respiratory function, the handling of respiratory secretions, or that can increase the risk of aspiration
  - Pregnant or postpartum women (≤2 weeks after delivery)
  - Persons <19 years of age on long-term aspirin therapy
  - American Indians and Alaskan Natives
  - Persons who are morbidly obese (BMI ≥40)
  - Residents of nursing homes or other chronic care facilities
- Use may also be considered for previously healthy, nonhigh-risk outpatients with confirmed or suspected influenza based on clinical judgment when treatment can be started within 48 hours of illness onset.

The ACIP recommends that **prophylaxis** be considered for the following:

- Postexposure prophylaxis may be considered for family or close contacts of suspected or confirmed cases, who are at higher risk of influenza complications, and who have not been vaccinated against the circulating strain at the time of the exposure.
- Postexposure prophylaxis may be considered for unvaccinated healthcare workers who had occupational exposure without protective equipment.
- Pre-exposure prophylaxis should only be used for persons at very high risk of influenza complications who cannot be otherwise protected at times of high risk for exposure.
- Prophylaxis should also be administered to all eligible residents of institutions that house patients at high risk when needed to control outbreaks.

Pregnancy Risk Factor C

Pregnancy Considerations Adverse events were not observed in animal reproduction studies. Influenza infection may be more severe in pregnant women. Untreated influenza infection is associated with an increased risk of adverse events to the fetus and an increased risk of complications or death to the mother. Oseltamivir and zanamivir are currently recommended for the treatment or prophylaxis of influenza in pregnant women and women up to 2 weeks postpartum. Oseltamivir and zanamivir are currently recommended as an adjunct to vaccination and should not be used as a substitute for vaccination in pregnant women (consult current CDC guidelines).

Breast-Feeding Considerations It is not known if zanamivir is found in human milk and the manufacturer recommends that caution be exercised when administering zanamivir to nursing women. According to the CDC, breast-feeding while taking zanamivir can be continued. The CDC recommends that women infected with the influenza virus follow general precautions (eg, frequent hand washing) to decrease viral transmission to the child. Mothers with influenza-like illnesses at delivery should consider avoiding close contact with the infant until they have received 48 hours of antiviral medication, fever has resolved, and cough and secretions can be controlled. These measures may help decrease (but not eliminate) the risk of transmitting influenza to the newborn. During this time, breast milk can be expressed and bottle-fed to the infant by another person who is well. Protective measures, such as wearing a face mask, changing into a clean gown or clothing, and strict hand hygiene should be continued by the mother for ≥7 days after the onset of symptoms or until symptom-free for 24 hours. Infant care should be performed by a noninfected person when possible (consult current CDC guidelines). Influenza may cause serious illness in postpartum women and prompt evaluation for febrile respiratory illnesses is recommended.

Prescribing and Access Restrictions Zanamivir *aqueous solution* intended for nebulization or intravenous (I.V.) administration is **not** currently approved for use. Data on safety and efficacy via these routes of administration are limited. However, limited supplies of zanamivir aqueous solution may be made available through the Zanamivir Compassionate Use Program for qualifying patients for the treatment of serious influenza illness. For information, contact the GlaxoSmithKline Clinical Support Help Desk at 1-866-341-9160 or gskclinicalsupportHD@gsk.com.

Contraindications Hypersensitivity to zanamivir or any component of the formulation (contains milk proteins)

Warnings/Precautions Allergic-like reactions, including anaphylaxis, oropharyngeal edema, and serious skin rashes have been reported. Rare occurrences of neuropsychiatric events (including confusion, delirium, hallucinations, and/or self-injury) have been reported from postmarketing surveillance; direct causation is difficult to establish (influenza infection may also be associated with behavioral and neurologic changes). Patients must be instructed in the use of the delivery system. Antiviral treatment should begin within 48 hours of symptom onset. However, the CDC recommends that treatment may still be beneficial and should be started in hospitalized patients with severe, complicated or progressive illness if >48 hours. Treatment should not be delayed while awaiting results of laboratory tests for influenza. Nonhospitalized persons who are not at high risk for developing severe or complicated illness and who have a mild disease are not likely to benefit if treatment is started >48 hours after symptom onset. Nonhospitalized persons who are already beginning to recover do not need treatment. Effectiveness has not been established in patients with significant underlying medical conditions or for prophylaxis of influenza in nursing home patients (per manufacturer). The CDC recommends zanamivir to be used to control institutional outbreaks of influenza when circulating strains are suspected of being resistant to oseltamivir (refer to current guidelines). Not recommended for use in patients with underlying respiratory disease, such as asthma or COPD, due to lack of efficacy and risk of serious adverse effects. Bronchospasm, decreased lung function, and other serious adverse reactions, including those with fatal outcomes, have been reported in patients with and without airway disease; discontinue with bronchospasm or signs of decreased lung function. For a patient with an underlying airway disease where a medical decision has been made to use zanamivir, a fast-acting bronchodilator should be made available, and used prior to each dose. Not a substitute for annual flu vaccination; has not been shown to reduce risk of transmission of influenza to others. Consider primary or concomitant bacterial infections. Powder for oral inhalation contains lactose; use contraindicated in patients allergic to milk proteins. The inhalation powder should only be administered via inhalation using the provided Diskhaler® delivery device. The commercially available formulation is **not** intended to be solubilized or administered via any nebulizer/mechanical ventilator; inappropriate administration has resulted in death. Safety and efficacy of repeated courses or use with hepatic impairment or severe renal impairment have not been established. Indicated for children ≥5 years of age (for influenza prophylaxis) and children ≥7 years of age (for influenza treatment); children ages 5-6 years may have inadequate inhalation (via Diskhaler®) for the treatment of influenza.

Adverse Reactions Most adverse reactions occurred at a frequency which was less than or equal to the control (lactose vehicle).

>10%:

Central nervous system: Headache (prophylaxis 13% to 24%; treatment 2%)

Gastrointestinal: Throat/tonsil discomfort/pain (prophylaxis 8% to 19%)

Respiratory: Nasal signs and symptoms (prophylaxis 12% to 20%; treatment 2%), cough (prophylaxis 7% to 17%; treatment ≤2%)

Miscellaneous: Viral infection (prophylaxis 3% to 13%)

1% to 10%:

Central nervous system: Fever/chills (prophylaxis 5% to 9%; treatment <1.5%), fatigue (prophylaxis 5% to 8%; treatment <1.5%), malaise (prophylaxis 5% to 8%; treatment <1.5%), dizziness (treatment 1% to 2%)

Dermatologic: Urticaria (treatment <1.5%)

Gastrointestinal: Anorexia/appetite decreased (prophylaxis 2% to 4%), appetite increased (prophylaxis 2% to 4%), nausea (prophylaxis 1% to 2%; treatment ≤3%), diarrhea (prophylaxis 2%; treatment 2% to 3%), vomiting (prophylaxis 1% to 2%; treatment 1% to 2%), abdominal pain (treatment <1.5%)

Neuromuscular & skeletal: Muscle pain (prophylaxis 3% to 8%), musculoskeletal pain (prophylaxis 6%), arthralgia/articular rheumatism (prophylaxis 2%), arthralgia (treatment <1.5%), myalgia (treatment <1.5%)

Respiratory: Infection (ear/nose/throat; prophylaxis 2%; treatment 1% to 5%), sinusitis (treatment 3%), bronchitis (treatment 2%), nasal inflammation (prophylaxis 1%)

<1% (Limited to important or life-threatening): Allergic or allergic-like reaction (including oropharyngeal edema), arrhythmia, bronchospasm, consciousness altered, delusions, dyspnea, hallucinations, neuropsychiatric events (self-injury, confusion, delirium), nightmares, rash (including serious cutaneous reactions [eg, erythema multiforme, Stevens-Johnson syndrome, toxic epidermal necrolysis]), seizure, syncope

Drug Interactions

Metabolism/Transport Effects None known.

Avoid Concomitant Use There are no known interactions where it is recommended to avoid concomitant use.

Increased Effect/Toxicity There are no known significant interactions involving an increase in effect.

Decreased Effect

Zanamivir may decrease the levels/effects of: Influenza Virus Vaccine (Live/Attenuated)

Storage/Stability Store at 25°C (77°F); excursions permitted to 15°C to 30°C (59°F to 86°F). Do not puncture blister until taking a dose using the Diskhaler®.

Mechanism of Action Zanamivir inhibits influenza virus neuraminidase enzymes, potentially altering virus particle aggregation and release.

Pharmacodynamics/Kinetics

Absorption: Inhalation: Systemic: ~4% to 17%

Protein binding, plasma: <10%

Metabolism: None

Half-life elimination, serum: 2.5-5.1 hours; Mild-to-moderate renal impairment: 4.7 hours; Severe renal impairment: 18.5 hours

Time to peak, plasma: 1-2 hours

Excretion: Urine (as unchanged drug); feces (unabsorbed drug)

Dosage Oral inhalation: Influenza virus A and B:

Manufacturer's recommendations:

Prophylaxis, household setting: Children ≥5 years and Adults: Two inhalations (10 mg) once daily for 10 days. Begin within 36 hours following onset of signs or symptoms of index case.

Prophylaxis, community outbreak: Adolescents and Adults: Two inhalations (10 mg) once daily for 28 days. Begin within 5 days of outbreak.

Treatment: Children ≥7 years and Adults: Two inhalations (10 mg total) twice daily for 5 days. Doses on first day should be separated by at least 2 hours; on subsequent days, doses should be spaced by ~12 hours. Begin within 2 days of signs or symptoms. Longer treatment may be considered for patients who remain severely ill after 5 days.

Alternate recommendations:

Prophylaxis (household exposure, CDC, 2012): Children ≥5 years and Adults: Two inhalations (10 mg) once daily for 7 days after last known exposure

Prophylaxis (institutional outbreak, CDC, 2012): Children ≥5 years and Adults: Two inhalations (10 mg) once daily; continue for ≥2 weeks and until ~7 days after identification of illness onset in the last patient. Zanamivir is to be used to control institutional outbreaks of influenza when circulating strains are suspected of being resistant to oseltamivir.

Prophylaxis (community outbreak, IDSA/PIDS, 2011): Children ≥5 years and Adults: Two inhalations (10 mg) once daily; continue until influenza activity in community subsides or immunity obtained from immunization; up to 28 days has been well tolerated (CDC, 2011)

Dosage adjustment for renal impairment: Adjustment not necessary following a 5-day course of treatment due to low systemic absorption; however the potential for drug accumulation should be considered.

Dosage adjustment in hepatic impairment: No dosage adjustment provided in manufacturer's labeling (has not been studied).

Administration Inhalation: Must be used with Diskhaler® delivery device. The foil blister disk containing zanamivir inhalation powder should not be manipulated, solubilized, or administered via a nebulizer. Patients who are scheduled to use an inhaled bronchodilator should use their bronchodilator prior to zanamivir. With the exception of the initial dose when used for treatment, administer at the same time each day.

Additional Information Majority of patients included in clinical trials were infected with influenza A, however, a number of patients with influenza B infections were also enrolled. Patients with lower temperature or less severe symptoms appeared to derive less benefit from therapy. No consistent treatment benefit was demonstrated in patients with chronic underlying medical conditions.

The absence of symptoms does not rule out viral influenza infection and clinical judgment should guide the decision for therapy. Treatment should not be delayed while waiting for the results of diagnostic tests. Treatment should be considered for high-risk patients with symptoms despite a negative rapid influenza test when the illness cannot be contributed to another cause. Use of zanamivir is not a substitute for vaccination (when available); susceptibility to influenza infection returns once therapy is discontinued.

Dosage Forms Excipient information presented when available (limited, particularly for generics); consult specific product labeling.

Aerosol Powder Breath Activated, Inhalation:
Relenza Diskhaler: 5 mg/blister (20 ea) [contains lactose]

- **Zantac** *see* Ranitidine *on page* 1782
- **Zantac® (Can)** *see* Ranitidine *on page* 1782
- **Zantac 75 [OTC]** *see* Ranitidine *on page* 1782
- **Zantac 75® (Can)** *see* Ranitidine *on page* 1782
- **Zantac 150 Maximum Strength [OTC]** *see* Ranitidine *on page* 1782
- **Zantac EFFERdose [DSC]** *see* Ranitidine *on page* 1782
- **Zantac in NaCl [DSC]** *see* Ranitidine *on page* 1782
- **Zantac Maximum Strength Non-Prescription (Can)** *see* Ranitidine *on page* 1782
- **Zarah®** *see* Ethinyl Estradiol and Drospirenone *on page* 785
- **Zarontin** *see* Ethosuximide *on page* 798
- **Zarontin® (Can)** *see* Ethosuximide *on page* 798
- **Zaroxolyn** *see* Metolazone *on page* 1347
- **Zaroxolyn® (Can)** *see* Metolazone *on page* 1347
- **Zavesca** *see* Miglustat *on page* 1369
- **Zavesca® (Can)** *see* Miglustat *on page* 1369
- **Zazole** *see* Terconazole *on page* 2021
- **ZD1033** *see* Anastrozole *on page* 137
- **ZD1839** *see* Gefitinib *on page* 941
- **ZD6474** *see* Vandetanib *on page* 2162
- **ZD9238** *see* Fulvestrant *on page* 930
- **ZDV** *see* Zidovudine *on page* 2226
- **ZDV, Abacavir, and Lamivudine** *see* Abacavir, Lamivudine, and Zidovudine *on page* 20
- **ZDX** *see* Goserelin *on page* 970
- **Zeasorb-AF [OTC]** *see* Miconazole (Topical) *on page* 1358
- **Zebeta** *see* Bisoprolol *on page* 261
- **Zebutal** *see* Butalbital, Acetaminophen, and Caffeine *on page* 305
- **Zegerid®** *see* Omeprazole and Sodium Bicarbonate *on page* 1508
- **Zegerid OTC™ [OTC]** *see* Omeprazole and Sodium Bicarbonate *on page* 1508
- **Zelapar** *see* Selegiline *on page* 1884
- **Zelboraf** *see* Vemurafenib *on page* 2176
- **Zeldox** *see* Ziprasidone *on page* 2230
- **Zemplar** *see* Paricalcitol *on page* 1572
- **Zemuron** *see* Rocuronium *on page* 1846
- **Zemuron® (Can)** *see* Rocuronium *on page* 1846
- **Zenatane** *see* ISOtretinoin *on page* 1129
- **Zenchent** *see* Ethinyl Estradiol and Norethindrone *on page* 793
- **Zenchent Fe** *see* Ethinyl Estradiol and Norethindrone *on page* 793
- **Zencia** *see* Sulfur and Sulfacetamide *on page* 1966
- **Zenhale™ (Can)** *see* Mometasone and Formoterol *on page* 1395
- **Zenpep** *see* Pancrelipase *on page* 1558
- **Zenzedi** *see* Dextroamphetamine *on page* 588
- **Zephrex-D [OTC]** *see* Pseudoephedrine *on page* 1746
- **Zerit** *see* Stavudine *on page* 1949
- **Zerit® (Can)** *see* Stavudine *on page* 1949
- **Zestoretic** *see* Lisinopril and Hydrochlorothiazide *on page* 1229
- **Zestril** *see* Lisinopril *on page* 1226
- **Zetia** *see* Ezetimibe *on page* 817
- **Zetonna** *see* Ciclesonide (Nasal) *on page* 423
- **Ziac®** *see* Bisoprolol and Hydrochlorothiazide *on page* 262
- **Ziagen** *see* Abacavir *on page* 18
- **Ziagen® (Can)** *see* Abacavir *on page* 18
- **Ziana®** *see* Clindamycin and Tretinoin *on page* 455

Ziconotide (zi KOE no tide)

Brand Names: U.S. Prialt

Pharmacologic Category Analgesic, Nonopioid; Calcium Channel Blocker, N-Type

Use Management of severe chronic pain in patients requiring intrathecal (I.T.) therapy and who are intolerant or refractory to other therapies

Pregnancy Risk Factor C

Pregnancy Considerations Adverse events and maternal toxicity were observed in animal reproduction studies.

Breast-Feeding Considerations It is not known if ziconotide is excreted into breast milk. Due to the potential for serious adverse reactions in the nursing infant, the manufacturer recommends a decision be made whether to discontinue nursing or to discontinue the drug, taking into account the importance of treatment to the mother.

Contraindications Hypersensitivity to ziconotide or any component of the formulation; history of psychosis; I.V. administration

I.T. administration is contraindicated in patients with infection at the injection site, uncontrolled bleeding, or spinal canal obstruction that impairs CSF circulation

Warnings/Precautions [U.S Boxed Warning]: Severe psychiatric symptoms and neurological impairment have been reported; interrupt or discontinue therapy if cognitive impairment, hallucinations, mood changes, or changes in consciousness occur. May cause or worsen depression and/or risk of suicide. Cognitive impairment may appear gradually during treatment and is generally reversible after discontinuation (may take up to 2 weeks for cognitive effects to reverse). Use caution in the elderly; may experience a higher incidence of confusion. Patients should be instructed to use caution in performing tasks which require alertness (eg, operating machinery or driving). May have additive effects with opioids or other CNS-depressant medications; may potentiate opioid-induced decreased GI motility; does not interact with opioid receptors or potentiate opioid-induced respiratory depression. Will not prevent or relieve symptoms associated with opioid withdrawal and opioids should not be abruptly discontinued. Unlike opioids, ziconotide therapy can be interrupted abruptly or discontinued without evidence of withdrawal.

Meningitis may occur with use of I.T. pumps; monitor for signs and symptoms of meningitis; treatment of meningitis may require removal of system and discontinuation of intrathecal therapy. Elevated serum creatine kinase can occur, particularly during the first 2 months of therapy; consider dose reduction or discontinuing if combined with new neuromuscular symptoms (myalgias, myasthenia, muscle cramps, weakness) or reduction in physical activity. Safety and efficacy have not been established with renal or hepatic dysfunction, or in pediatric patients. Should not be used in combination with intrathecal opioids.

Adverse Reactions

>10%:

Central nervous system: Dizziness (46%), confusion (15% to 33%), memory impairment (7% to 22%), somnolence (17%), ataxia (14%), speech disorder (14%), headache (13%), aphasia (12%), hallucination (12%; including auditory and visual)

Gastrointestinal: Nausea (40%), diarrhea (18%), vomiting (16%)

Neuromuscular & skeletal: Creatine kinase increased (40%; ≥3 times ULN: 11%), weakness (18%), gait disturbances (14%)

Ocular: Blurred vision (12%)

2% to 10%:

Cardiovascular: Hypotension, orthostatic hypotension, peripheral edema

Central nervous system: Abnormal thinking (8%), amnesia (8%), anxiety (8%), vertigo (7%), insomnia (6%), fever (5%), paranoid reaction (3%), delirium (2%), hostility (2%), stupor (2%), agitation, attention disturbance, balance impaired, burning sensation, coordination abnormal, depression, disorientation, fatigue, fever, hypoesthesia, irritability, lethargy, mental impairment, mood disorder, nervousness, pain, sedation

Dermatologic: Pruritus (7%)

Gastrointestinal: Anorexia (6%), taste perversion (5%), abdominal pain, appetite decreased, constipation, xerostomia

Genitourinary: Urinary retention (9%), dysuria, urinary hesitance

Neuromuscular & skeletal: Dysarthria (7%), paresthesia (7%), rigors (7%), tremor (7%), muscle spasm (6%), limb pain (5%), areflexia, muscle cramp, muscle weakness, myalgia

Ocular: Nystagmus (8%), diplopia, visual disturbance

Respiratory: Sinusitis (5%)

Miscellaneous: Diaphoresis (5%)

<2% (Limited to important or life-threatening): Acute renal failure, aspiration pneumonia (<1%), atrial fibrillation, cerebral vascular accident, ECG abnormalities, incoherence, loss of consciousness, mania, meningitis, myoclonus, psychosis (1%), psychotic disorder, respiratory distress, rhabdomyolysis, seizure (clonic and grand mal), sepsis, suicidal ideation, suicide attempt (<1%)

Drug Interactions

Metabolism/Transport Effects None known.

Avoid Concomitant Use

Avoid concomitant use of Ziconotide with any of the following: Azelastine (Nasal); Paraldehyde

Increased Effect/Toxicity

Ziconotide may increase the levels/effects of: Alcohol (Ethyl); Azelastine (Nasal); Buprenorphine; CNS Depressants; Hydrocodone; Methotrimeprazine; Metyrosine; Mirtazapine; Paraldehyde; Pramipexole; ROPINIRole; Rotigotine; Selective Serotonin Reuptake Inhibitors; Zolpidem

The levels/effects of Ziconotide may be increased by: Brimonidine (Topical); Doxylamine; Droperidol; HydrOXYzine; Magnesium Sulfate; Methotrimeprazine; Perampanel; Sodium Oxybate; Tapentadol

Decreased Effect There are no known significant interactions involving a decrease in effect.

Ethanol/Nutrition/Herb Interactions Ethanol: May increase CNS depression; monitor for increased effects with coadministration. Caution patients about effects.

Preparation for Administration Preservative free NS should be used when dilution is needed.

CADD-Micro® ambulatory infusion pump: Initial fill: Dilute to final concentration of 5 mcg/mL.

Medtronic SynchroMed® EL or SynchroMed® II infusion system: Prior to initial fill, rinse internal pump surfaces with 2 mL ziconotide (25 mcg/mL), repeat twice. Only the 25 mcg/mL concentration (undiluted) should be used for initial pump fill.

Storage/Stability Prior to use, store vials at 2°C to 8°C (36°F to 46°F). Once diluted, may be stored at 2°C to 8°C (36°F to 46°F) for 24 hours; refrigerate during transit. Do not freeze. Protect from light.

When using the Medtronic SynchroMed® EL or SynchroMed® II Infusion System, solutions expire as follows:

25 mcg/mL: Undiluted:

Initial fill: Use within 14 days.

Refill: Use within 84 days.

100 mcg/mL:

Undiluted: Refill: Use within 84 days.

Diluted: Refill: Use within 40 days.

Mechanism of Action Ziconotide selectively binds to N-type voltage-sensitive calcium channels located on the nociceptive afferent nerves of the dorsal horn in the spinal cord. This binding is thought to block N-type calcium channels, leading to a blockade of excitatory neurotransmitter release and reducing sensitivity to painful stimuli.

Pharmacodynamics/Kinetics

Distribution: I.T.: V_d: ~140 mL

Protein binding: ~50%

Metabolism: Metabolized via endopeptidases and exopeptidases present on multiple organs including kidney, liver, lung; degraded to peptide fragments and free amino acids

Half-life elimination: I.V.: 1-1.6 hours (plasma); I.T.: 2.9-6.5 hours (CSF)

Excretion: I.V.: Urine (<1%)

Dosage I.T.:

Adults: Chronic pain: Initial dose: ≤2.4 mcg/day (0.1 mcg/hour)

Dose may be titrated by ≤2.4 mcg/day (0.1 mcg/hour) at intervals ≤2-3 times/week to a maximum dose of 19.2 mcg/day (0.8 mcg/hour) by day 21; average dose at day 21: 6.9 mcg/day (0.29 mcg/hour). A faster titration should be used only if the urgent need for analgesia outweighs the possible risk to patient safety.

Dosage adjustment for toxicity:

Cognitive impairment: Reduce dose or discontinue. Effects are generally reversible within 3-15 days of discontinuation.

Reduced level of consciousness: Discontinue until event resolves.

CK elevation with neuromuscular symptoms: Consider dose reduction or discontinuation.

Elderly: Refer to adult dosing; use with caution.

Dosage adjustment in renal impairment: No dosage adjustment provided in manufacturer's labeling (has not been studied).

Dosage adjustment in hepatic impairment: No dosage adjustment provided in manufacturer's labeling (has not been studied).

Administration Not for I.V. administration. For I.T. administration only using Medtronic SynchroMed® EL, SynchroMed® II Infusion System, or CADD-Micro® ambulatory infusion pump.

Medtronic SynchroMed® EL or SynchroMed® II Infusion Systems:

Naive pump priming (first time use with ziconotide): Use 2 mL of undiluted ziconotide 25 mcg/mL solution to rinse the internal surfaces of the pump; repeat twice for a total of 3 rinses

Initial pump fill: Use only undiluted 25 mcg/mL solution and fill pump after priming. Following the initial fill only, adsorption on internal device surfaces will occur, requiring the use of the undiluted solution and refill within 14 days.

Pump refills: Contents should be emptied prior to refill. Subsequent pump refills should occur at least every 40 days if using diluted solution or at least every 84 days if using undiluted solution.

CADD-Micro® ambulatory infusion pump: Refer to manufacturer's manual for initial fill and refill instructions

Monitoring Parameters Monitor for psychiatric or neurological impairment; signs and symptoms of meningitis or other infection; serum CPK (every other week for first month then monthly); pain relief

Dosage Forms Excipient information presented when available (limited, particularly for generics); consult specific product labeling.

Solution, Intrathecal, as acetate [preservative free]:

Prialt: 500 mcg/20 mL (20 mL); 100 mcg/mL (1 mL); 500 mcg/5 mL (5 mL)

◆ **Zictifa** *see* Vandetanib *on page* 2162

Zidovudine (zye DOE vyoo deen)

Brand Names: U.S. Retrovir

Brand Names: Canada Apo-Zidovudine®; AZT™; Novo-AZT; Retrovir®; Retrovir® (AZT™)

Index Terms Azidothymidine; AZT (error-prone abbreviation); Compound S; ZDV

Pharmacologic Category Antiretroviral, Reverse Transcriptase Inhibitor, Nucleoside (Anti-HIV)

Use Treatment of HIV infection in combination with at least two other antiretroviral agents; prevention of maternal/fetal HIV transmission

Unlabeled Use Postexposure prophylaxis for HIV exposure as part of a multidrug regimen

Pregnancy Risk Factor C

Pregnancy Considerations Adverse events have been observed in some animal reproduction studies. Zidovudine crosses the placenta and the placenta also metabolizes zidovudine to the active metabolite. No increased risk of overall birth defects has been observed following first trimester exposure according to data collected by the antiretroviral pregnancy registry. The pharmacokinetics of zidovudine are not significantly altered in pregnancy and dosing adjustment is not needed. The DHHS Perinatal HIV Guidelines consider zidovudine the preferred NRTI for use in combination regimens during pregnancy. The use of zidovudine has been shown to reduce the maternal-fetal transmission of HIV by ~70%. Zidovudine should be administered I.V. near delivery regardless of antepartum regimen or mode of delivery in women with HIV RNA >400 copies/mL or unknown HIV RNA status. In HIV-infected mothers not previously on antiretroviral therapy, and who do not need therapy for their own health, treatment may be delayed until after the first trimester; however, earlier initiation of therapy may be more effective in reducing perinatal transmission.

Cases of lactic acidosis/hepatic steatosis syndrome related to mitochondrial toxicity have been reported in pregnant women with prolonged use of nucleoside analogues. It is not known if pregnancy itself potentiates this known side effect; however, women may be at increased risk of lactic acidosis and liver damage. In addition, these adverse events are similar to other rare but life-threatening syndromes which occur during pregnancy (eg, HELLP syndrome). Hepatic enzymes and electrolytes should be monitored in women receiving nucleoside analogues and clinicians should watch for early signs of the syndrome. In addition, mitochondrial dysfunction may develop in infants following *in utero* exposure.

Regardless of CD4 count or HIV RNA copy number, all HIV-infected pregnant women should receive a combination antepartum antiretroviral (ARV) drug regimen; this includes women who require therapy for their own health, as well as women who do not yet require therapy for their own health. ARV therapy should be started as soon as possible if required for the woman's health. health. Although earlier initiation may be more effective in reducing the perinatal transmission of HIV), also consider maternal conditions (eg, nausea and vomiting) and the potential risks of first trimester fetal exposure for specific agents. Plasma HIV RNA levels should be assessed at ~34-36 weeks gestation in order to help determine mode of delivery. If ARV therapy must be interrupted for <24 hours during the peripartum period, stop then restart all medications simultaneously in order to decrease the chance of developing resistance. Long-term follow-up is recommended for all infants exposed to ARV medications.

Healthcare providers are encouraged to enroll pregnant women exposed to antiretroviral medications in the Antiretroviral Pregnancy Registry (1-800-258-4263 or www.-APRegistry.com). Healthcare providers caring for HIV-infected women and their infants may contact the National Perinatal HIV Hotline (888-448-8765) for clinical consultation (DHHS [perinatal], 2012).

Breast-Feeding Considerations Concentrations of zidovudine in breast milk are similar to those in the maternal serum. Maternal or infant antiretroviral therapy does not completely eliminate the risk of postnatal HIV transmission. In addition, multiclass-resistant virus has been detected in breast-feeding infants despite maternal therapy. Therefore, in the United States, where formula is accessible, affordable, safe, and sustainable, and the risk of infant mortality due to diarrhea and respiratory infections is low, complete avoidance of breast-feeding by HIV-infected women is recommended to decrease potential transmission of HIV (DHHS [perinatal], 2012).

Contraindications Life-threatening hypersensitivity to zidovudine or any component of the formulation

Canadian labeling: Additional contraindications (not in U.S. labeling): Neutrophil count <750/mm^3 or hemoglobin <7.5 g/dL (4.65 mmol/L)

Warnings/Precautions Hazardous agent - use appropriate precautions for handling and disposal (NIOSH, 2012). **[U.S. Boxed Warning]: Hematologic toxicity, including neutropenia and severe anemia have been reported with use.** Toxicity may be related to duration of use and prior bone marrow reserve. Use with caution in patients with bone marrow compromise (granulocytes <1000 cells/mm^3 or hemoglobin <9.5 mg/dL); dose interruption may be required in patients who develop anemia or neutropenia. **[U.S. Boxed Warning]: Lactic acidosis and severe hepatomegaly with steatosis have been reported, including fatal cases.** Risks may be increased with liver disease, obesity, pregnancy, prolonged exposure, or in females. Suspend treatment with zidovudine in any patient who develops clinical or laboratory findings suggestive of lactic acidosis (transaminase elevation may/may not accompany hepatomegaly and steatosis). Use caution in combination with interferon alfa with or without ribavirin in HIV/HCV coinfected patients; monitor closely for hepatic decompensation, anemia, or neutropenia; dose reduction or discontinuation of interferon and/or ribavirin may be required if toxicity evident. **[U.S. Boxed Warning]: Prolonged use has been associated with symptomatic myopathy and myositis.** May cause redistribution of fat (eg, buffalo hump, peripheral wasting with increased abdominal girth, cushingoid appearance). Immune reconstitution syndrome may develop resulting in the occurrence of an inflammatory response to an indolent or residual opportunistic infection during initial HIV treatment or activation of autoimmune disorders (eg, Graves' disease, polymyositis, Guillain-Barré syndrome) later in therapy; further evaluation and treatment may be required. Hematologic toxicity may be increased due to increased serum concentrations in patients with severe hepatic impairment. Use with caution in patients with severe renal impairment; dosage adjustment recommended. Reduce dose in patients with severe renal impairment. Do not administer with combination products that contain zidovudine as one of their components (eg, COMBIVIR® [lamivudine and zidovudine] or TRIZIVIR® [abacavir sulfate, lamivudine, and zidovudine]).

Adverse Reactions Note: Percentages noted with adults unless otherwise stated.

>10%:

Central nervous system: Headache (63%), malaise (53%), fever (children 25%)

Dermatologic: Rash (children 12%)

Gastrointestinal: Nausea (adults 51%; children 8%), anorexia (20%), vomiting (adults 17%; children 8%)

Hematologic: Macrocytosis (children >50%), anemia (neonates 22%; children 4%; adults 1%; onset 2-4 weeks)

Hepatic: Hepatomegaly (children 11%)

Respiratory: Cough (children 15%)

1% to 10%:

Cardiovascular: ECG abnormality (children <6%), edema (children <6%), heart failure (children <6%), left ventricular dilation (children <6%)

Central nervous system: Irritability (children <6%), nervousness (children <6%), chills (≥5%), fatigue (≥5%), insomnia (≥5%)

Gastrointestinal: Diarrhea (children 8%), constipation (6%), weight loss (children <6%), abdominal cramps (≥5%), abdominal pain (≥5%), dyspepsia (≥5%)

Genitourinary: Hematuria (children <6%)

Hematologic: Neutropenia (children 8%), granulocytopenia (2%; onset 6-8 weeks), thrombocytopenia (children 1%)

Hepatic: Transaminases increased (1% to 3%)

Neuromuscular & skeletal: Weakness (9%), arthralgia (≥5%), musculoskeletal pain (≥5%), myalgia (≥5%), neuropathy (≥5%)

Otic: Discharge/erythema/pain/swelling (7%)

Postmarketing and/or case reports: Allergic reactions, amblyopia, anaphylaxis, angioedema, anxiety, aplastic anemia, back pain, body fat redistribution, cardiomyopathy, confusion, CPK increased, depression, diabetes, dizziness, dyslipidemias, dyspnea, gynecomastia, hearing loss, hemolytic anemia, hepatitis, hepatomegaly with steatosis, immune reconstitution syndrome, insulin resistance, jaundice, lactic acidosis, LDH increased, leukopenia, loss of mental acuity, lymphadenopathy, macular edema, mania, myopathy, myositis, oral mucosa pigmentation, pancreatitis, pancytopenia with marrow hypoplasia, paresthesia, photophobia, pruritus, pure red cell aplasia, rhabdomyolysis, seizure, skin/nail pigmentation changes (blue), Stevens-Johnson syndrome, syncope, taste perversion, toxic epidermal necrolysis, tremor, urticaria, vertigo

Drug Interactions

Metabolism/Transport Effects Substrate of CYP2A6 (minor), CYP2C19 (minor), CYP2C9 (minor), CYP3A4 (minor); **Note:** Assignment of Major/Minor substrate status based on clinically relevant drug interaction potential

Avoid Concomitant Use

Avoid concomitant use of Zidovudine with any of the following: CloZAPine; Stavudine

Increased Effect/Toxicity

Zidovudine may increase the levels/effects of: CloZAPine; Ribavirin

The levels/effects of Zidovudine may be increased by: Acyclovir-Valacyclovir; Clarithromycin; DOXOrubicin; DOXOrubicin (Liposomal); Fluconazole; Ganciclovir-Valganciclovir; Interferons; Methadone; Probenecid; Raltegravir; Valproic Acid and Derivatives

Decreased Effect

Zidovudine may decrease the levels/effects of: Stavudine

The levels/effects of Zidovudine may be decreased by: Clarithromycin; DOXOrubicin; DOXOrubicin (Liposomal); Protease Inhibitors; Rifamycin Derivatives

Preparation for Administration Hazardous agent; use appropriate precautions for handling and disposal (NIOSH, 2012). Solution for injection should be diluted with D_5W to a concentration ≤4 mg/mL. Attempt to administer diluted solution within 8 hours if stored at room temperature or 24 hours if refrigerated to minimize potential for microbial-contaminated solutions (vials are single-use and do not contain preservative).

Storage/Stability

I.V.: Store undiluted vials at 15°C to 25°C (59°F to 77°F). Protect from light. When diluted, solution is physically and chemically stable for 24 hours at room temperature and 48 hours if refrigerated.

Tablets, capsules, syrup: Store at 15°C to 25°C (59°F to 77°F). Protect capsules from moisture.

Mechanism of Action Zidovudine is a thymidine analog which interferes with the HIV viral RNA-dependent DNA polymerase resulting in inhibition of viral replication; nucleoside reverse transcriptase inhibitor

Pharmacodynamics/Kinetics

Distribution: Significant penetration into the CSF

V_d: 1-2.2 L/kg

Relative diffusion from blood into CSF: Adequate with or without inflammation (exceeds usual MICs)

CSF:blood level ratio: Normal meninges: ~60%

Protein binding: 25% to 38%

Metabolism: Hepatic via glucuronidation to inactive metabolites; extensive first-pass effect
Bioavailability: 54% to 74%
Half-life elimination: Terminal: 0.5-3 hours
Time to peak, serum: 30-90 minutes
Excretion:
Oral: Urine (72% to 74% as metabolites, 14% to 18% as unchanged drug)
I.V.: Urine (45% to 60% as metabolites, 18% to 29% as unchanged drug)

Dosage Note: Patients should receive I.V. therapy only until oral therapy can be administered.

Prevention of maternal-fetal HIV transmission: **Note:** Start as soon as possible after birth, preferably within 6-12 hours of delivery. Continue dose from birth through 6 weeks of age. Use zidovudine in combination with nevirapine in select situations (eg, infants born to mothers with only intrapartum therapy or no therapy) (DHHS [perinatal], 2012).

Oral:

Manufacturer's labeling: Full-term infants: 2 mg/kg every 6 hours

DHHS [perinatal], 2012:

Infants ≥35 weeks: 4 mg/kg/dose twice daily

Infants ≥30 weeks and <35 weeks gestation at birth: 2 mg/kg/dose every 12 hours; at 15 days of age, advance to 3 mg/kg/dose every 12 hours

Infants <30 weeks gestation at birth: 2 mg/kg/dose every 12 hours; at 4 weeks of age, advance to 3 mg/kg/dose every 12 hours

I.V.: Infants unable to receive oral dosing (start as soon as possible after birth, preferably within 6-12 hours of delivery; continue dose from birth through 6 weeks of age): DHHS [perinatal], 2012:

Infants ≥35 weeks: 3 mg/kg/dose every 12 hours

Infants ≥30 weeks and <35 weeks gestation at birth: 1.5 mg/kg/dose every 12 hours; at 15 days of age, advance to 2.3 mg/kg/dose every 12 hours

Infants <30 weeks gestation at birth: 1.5 mg/kg/dose every 12 hours; at 4 weeks of age, advance to 2.3 mg/kg/dose every 12 hours

Maternal: Oral: Dose adjustment not required in pregnant women. Begin oral therapy with usual recommended dose based on current treatment guidelines. Zidovudine should be administered by continuous I.V. infusion near delivery regardless of antepartum regimen or mode of delivery in women with HIV RNA >400 copies/mL or unknown HIV RNA status. If oral zidovudine was part of the antepartum regimen, discontinue during intrapartum I.V. infusion. Other antiretroviral agents should be continued orally. Zidovudine I.V. is not required in women receiving combination antiretroviral therapy who have HIV RNA <400 copies/mL near delivery (DHHS [perinatal], 2012).

During labor and delivery, administer zidovudine I.V. at 2 mg/kg as loading dose followed by a continuous I.V. infusion of 1 mg/kg/hour until delivery. For scheduled cesarean delivery, begin I.V. zidovudine 3 hours before surgery.

Treatment of HIV infection:

Children 4 weeks to <18 years (U.S. labeling) or 3 months to ≤12 years (Canadian labeling):

Oral: Dose should be calculated by body weight (in kg) or body surface area and should not exceed the recommended adult dose. **Note:** Doses calculated by body weight may not be the same as those calculated by body surface area.

Dosing based on body surface area: 240 mg/m^2 twice daily (maximum: 300 mg twice daily) **or** 160 mg/m^2/dose 3 times daily (maximum: 200 mg 3 times daily)

Dosing based on weight (**Note:** 3 times daily dose i approved but rarely used in clinical practice):

4 to <9 kg: 12 mg/kg/dose twice daily **or** 8 mg/k dose 3 times/day

≥9 to <30 kg: 9 mg/kg/dose twice daily **or** 6 mg/k dose 3 times/day

≥30 kg: 300 mg twice daily **or** 200 mg 3 times/day

Children 3 months to ≤12 years (Canadian labeling): I.V intermittent infusion: 120 mg/m^2/dose every 6 hou (maximum: 160 mg/dose)

Children ≥12 years: I.V. intermittent infusion: 1 mg/k dose every 4 hours around-the-clock (5-6 doses/day)

Adults:

Oral: 300 mg twice daily or 200 mg 3 times/day

I.V.:

U.S. labeling: 1 mg/kg/dose administered every hours around-the-clock (5-6 doses/day)

Canadian labeling: 1-2 mg/kg/dose administere every 4 hours around-the-clock (6 doses/day)

Postexposure prophylaxis (unlabeled use): Adults: Ora 300 mg twice daily or 200 mg 3 times daily in combina tion with lamivudine or emtricitabine. A third agent ma be added for high risk exposures. Therapy should b started within hours of exposure and continued for weeks (CDC, 2005).

Dosage adjustment for hematologic toxicity: Conside dose interruption for significant anemia (hemoglobi <7.5 g/dL or >25% reduction from baseline) and/or ne tropenia (granulocyte count <750 cells/mm^3 or >50 reduction from baseline) until evidence of recovery. Ane mia associated with chronic zidovudine may warra dose reduction.

Dosage adjustment in renal impairment: Cl_{cr} <15 ml minute including hemo-/peritoneal dialysis (administe dose after dialysis on dialysis days [DHHS [adult], 2012]

Oral: 100 mg every 6-8 hours (manufacturers labeling 100 mg 3 times daily or 300 mg once daily (DHH [adult], 2012)

I.V.: 1 mg/kg every 6-8 hours

Continuous renal replacement therapy (CRRT): No adjus ment needed (Aronoff, 2007)

Dosage adjustment in hepatic impairment: No specifi dosage adjustment provided in manufacturer's labelin (has not been studied). However, adjustment may b necessary due to extensive hepatic metabolism.

Dietary Considerations May be taken without regard t meals.

Administration

Oral: Administer around-the-clock to promote less variatio in peak and trough serum levels; may be administere without regard to meals

I.M.: Do not administer I.M.

I.V.: Avoid rapid infusion or bolus injection

Neonates: Infuse over 30 minutes

Adults: Infuse over 1 hour; in pregnant women, infus loading dose over 1 hour followed by continuou infusion

Hazardous agent; use appropriate precautions for han dling and disposal (NIOSH, 2012).

Monitoring Parameters Monitor CD4 count (every 3- months; every 6-12 months once clinically stable); vira load (2-8 weeks after initiation/modification of therapy, an then every 3-6 months); CBC with differential (every 3- months); liver function tests (every 6-12 months); lipids glucose (yearly if normal); observe for appearance o opportunistic infections [DHHS [adult], 2012])

Additional Information Potential compliance problems frequency of administration, and adverse effects should b discussed with patients before initiating therapy to hel prevent the emergence of resistance.

Dosage Forms Excipient information presented when available (limited, particularly for generics); consult specific product labeling.
Capsule, Oral:
Retrovir: 100 mg [contains soybean lecithin]
Generic: 100 mg
Solution, Intravenous [preservative free]:
Retrovir: 10 mg/mL (20 mL)
Syrup, Oral:
Retrovir: 50 mg/5 mL (240 mL) [contains sodium benzoate; strawberry flavor]
Generic: 50 mg/5 mL (240 mL)
Tablet, Oral:
Generic: 300 mg

◆ **Zidovudine, Abacavir, and Lamivudine** *see* Abacavir, Lamivudine, and Zidovudine *on page 20*
◆ **Zidovudine and Lamivudine** *see* Lamivudine and Zidovudine *on page 1164*
◆ **Zilactin [OTC]** *see* Benzyl Alcohol *on page 245*
◆ **Zilactin-B® (Can)** *see* Benzocaine *on page 240*
◆ **Zilactin Baby [OTC]** *see* Benzocaine *on page 240*
◆ **Zilactin Baby® (Can)** *see* Benzocaine *on page 240*

Zileuton (zye LOO ton)

Brand Names: U.S. Zyflo; Zyflo CR
Pharmacologic Category 5-Lipoxygenase Inhibitor
Use Prophylaxis and chronic treatment of asthma
Pregnancy Risk Factor C
Dosage Oral: Children ≥12 years and Adults:
Immediate release: 600 mg 4 times/day
Extended release: 1200 mg twice daily

Dosage adjustment in renal impairment: No dosage adjustment necessary.
Dosage adjustment in hepatic impairment: Contraindicated with hepatic impairment.
Additional Information Complete prescribing information should be consulted for additional detail.
Dosage Forms Excipient information presented when available (limited, particularly for generics); consult specific product labeling.
Tablet, Oral:
Zyflo: 600 mg [scored]
Tablet Extended Release 12 Hour, Oral:
Zyflo CR: 600 mg

◆ **Zinacef** *see* Cefuroxime *on page 386*
◆ **Zinacef in D_5W [DSC]** *see* Cefuroxime *on page 386*
◆ **Zinacef in Sterile Water** *see* Cefuroxime *on page 386*
◆ **Zinc 15 [OTC]** *see* Zinc Sulfate *on page 2230*
◆ **Zinc-220 [OTC]** *see* Zinc Sulfate *on page 2230*

Zinc Acetate (zink AS e tate)

Brand Names: U.S. Galzin
Pharmacologic Category Trace Element
Use Maintenance treatment of Wilson's disease following initial chelation therapy
Pregnancy Risk Factor A
Dosage Oral: Wilson's disease: **Note:** Dose expressed in mg elemental zinc:
Children ≥10 years: 75 mg/day in 3 divided doses; may increase to 150 mg/day in 3 divided doses if inadequate response to lower dose
American Association for the Study of Liver Diseases (AASLD) practice guideline recommendations (Roberts, 2008):
Children <50 kg and >5 years: 75 mg/day in 3 divided doses
Children >50 kg: 150 mg/day in 3 divided doses
Adults:
Males and nonpregnant females: 150 mg/day in 3 divided doses
Pregnant females: 75 mg/day in 3 divided doses; may increase to 150 mg/day in 3 divided doses if inadequate response to lower dose

Dosage adjustment in renal impairment: No dosage adjustment provided in manufacturer's labeling.
Dosage adjustment in hepatic impairment: No dosage adjustment provided in manufacturer's labeling.
Additional Information Complete prescribing information should be consulted for additional detail.
Dosage Forms Considerations
Strength of Galzin capsule is expressed as elemental zinc
Dosage Forms Excipient information presented when available (limited, particularly for generics); consult specific product labeling.
Capsule, Oral:
Galzin: 25 mg, 50 mg

Zinc Chloride (zink KLOR ide)

Pharmacologic Category Trace Element
Use Cofactor for replacement therapy to different enzymes; helps maintain normal growth rates, normal skin hydration, and senses of taste and smell
Pregnancy Risk Factor C
Dosage Clinical response may not occur for up to 6-8 weeks
Supplemental to I.V. solutions:
Premature Infants <1500 g, up to 3 kg: 300 mcg/kg/day
Infants (full term) and Children ≤5 years: 100 mcg/kg/day
Adults:
Stable with fluid loss from small bowel: 12.2 mg zinc/L TPN or 17.1 mg zinc/kg (added to 1000 mL I.V. fluids) of stool or ileostomy output
Metabolically stable: 2.5-4 mg/day; add 2 mg/day for acute catabolic states

Dosage adjustment in renal impairment: No dosage adjustment provided in manufacturer's labeling. However, dosage adjustment may be necessary in severe impairment since zinc is primarily renally excreted. Additionally, aluminum accumulation may occur in the setting of renal impairment.
Dosage adjustment in hepatic impairment: No dosage adjustment provided in manufacturer's labeling.
Additional Information Complete prescribing information should be consulted for additional detail.
Dosage Forms Considerations
Strength of zinc chloride injection is expressed as elemental zinc
Dosage Forms Excipient information presented when available (limited, particularly for generics); consult specific product labeling.
Solution, Intravenous:
Generic: 1 mg/mL (10 mL)

Zinc Gelatin (zink JEL ah tin)

Brand Names: U.S. Gelucast®
Index Terms Dome Paste Bandage; Unna's Boot; Unna's Paste; Zinc Gelatin Boot
Pharmacologic Category Topical Skin Product
Use As a protectant and to support varicosities and similar lesions of the lower limbs

Dosage Topical: Apply externally as an occlusive boot

Additional Information Complete prescribing information should be consulted for additional detail.

Dosage Forms Excipient information presented when available (limited, particularly for generics); consult specific product labeling.

Bandage: 3" x 10 yards; 4" x 10 yards

◆ Zinc Gelatin Boot *see* Zinc Gelatin *on page 2229*

◆ Zincofax® (Can) *see* Zinc Oxide *on page 2230*

Zinc Oxide (zink OKS ide)

Brand Names: U.S. Ammens® Original Medicated [OTC]; Ammens® Shower Fresh [OTC]; Balmex® [OTC]; Boudreaux's® Butt Paste [OTC]; Critic-Aid Skin Care® [OTC]; Desitin® Creamy [OTC]; Desitin® [OTC]

Brand Names: Canada Zincofax®

Index Terms Base Ointment; Lassar's Zinc Paste

Pharmacologic Category Topical Skin Product

Use Protective coating for mild skin irritations and abrasions; soothing and protective ointment to promote healing of chapped skin, diaper rash

Dosage Infants, Children, and Adults: Topical: Apply as required for affected areas several times daily

Additional Information Complete prescribing information should be consulted for additional detail.

Dosage Forms Excipient information presented when available (limited, particularly for generics); consult specific product labeling.

Cream, topical:
- Balmex®: 11.3% (60 g, 120 g, 480 g) [contains aloe, benzoic acid, soybean oil, and vitamin E]

Cream, topical [stick]:
- Balmex®: 11.3% (56 g) [contains aloe, benzoic acid, soybean oil, and vitamin E]

Ointment, topical: 20% (30 g, 60 g, 454 g); 40% (120 g)
- Desitin®: 40% (30 g, 60 g, 90 g, 120 g, 270 g, 480 g) [contains cod liver oil and lanolin]
- Desitin® Creamy: 10% (60 g, 120 g)

Paste, topical:
- Boudreaux's® Butt Paste: 16% (30 g, 60 g, 120 g, 480 g) [contains castor oil, boric acid, mineral oil, and Peruvian balsam]
- Critic-Aid Skin Care®: 20% (71 g, 170 g)

Powder, topical:
- Ammens® Original Medicated: 9.1% (312 g)
- Ammens® Shower Fresh: 9.1% (312 g)

Zinc Sulfate (zink SUL fate)

Brand Names: U.S. Eye-Sed [OTC]; Orazinc [OTC]; Zinc 15 [OTC]; Zinc-220 [OTC]

Brand Names: Canada Anuzinc; Rivasol

Index Terms $ZnSO_4$ (error-prone abbreviation)

Pharmacologic Category Trace Element

Use Zinc supplement (oral and parenteral); may improve wound healing in those who are deficient

Pregnancy Risk Factor C

Dosage

Oral (dose expressed as elemental zinc):
- **Adequate intake (AI):** 1-6 months: 2.0 mg/day
- **Recommended daily allowance (RDA):**
  - 7-12 months: 3 mg/day
  - 1-3 years: 3 mg/day
  - 4-8 years: 5 mg/day
  - 9-13 years: 8 mg/day
  - 14-18 years:
    - Males: 11 mg/day
    - Females: 9 mg/day
      - Pregnancy: 12 mg/day
      - Lactation: 13 mg/day
  - ≥19 years:
    - Males: 11 mg/day
    - Females: 8 mg/day
      - Pregnancy: 11 mg/day
      - Lactation: 12 mg/day

Parenteral TPN: I.V.:
- Infants (premature, birth weight <1500 g up to 3 kg): 300 mcg/kg/day
- Infants (full term) and Children ≤5 years: 100 mcg/kg/day
- Adults:
  - Acute metabolic states: 4.5-6 mg/day
  - Metabolically stable: 2.5-4 mg/day
  - Replacement for small bowel fluid loss (metabolically stable): An additional 12.2 mg zinc/L of fluid lost, or an additional 17.1 mg zinc per kg of stool or ileostomy output

Additional Information Complete prescribing information should be consulted for additional detail.

Dosage Forms Considerations

Strength of zinc sulfate injection is expressed as elemental zinc

Oral zinc sulfate is approximately 23% elemental zinc

Dosage Forms Excipient information presented when available (limited, particularly for generics); consult specific product labeling.

Capsule, Oral:
- Orazinc: 220 mg
- Zinc-220: 220 mg
- Generic: 220 mg

Solution, Intravenous:
- Generic: 1 mg/mL (10 mL); 5 mg/mL (5 mL)

Solution, Ophthalmic:
- Eye-Sed: 0.217% (15 mL) [contains benzalkonium chloride, boric acid]

Tablet, Oral:
- Orazinc: 110 mg
- Zinc 15: 66 mg
- Generic: 50 mg, 220 (50 Zn) MG

Tablet, Oral [preservative free]:
- Generic: 220 (50 Zn) MG

◆ Zinda-Anastrozole (Can) *see* Anastrozole *on page 137*

◆ Zinda-Letrozole (Can) *see* Letrozole *on page 1185*

◆ Zinecard *see* Dexrazoxane *on page 587*

Ziprasidone (zi PRAS i done)

Brand Names: U.S. Geodon

Brand Names: Canada Zeldox

Index Terms Zeldox; Ziprasidone Hydrochloride; Ziprasidone Mesylate

Pharmacologic Category Antipsychotic Agent, Atypical

Additional Appendix Information

Antipsychotic Agents *on page 2290*

Beers Criteria – Potentially Inappropriate Medications for Geriatrics *on page 2368*

Use Treatment of schizophrenia; treatment of acute manic or mixed episodes associated with bipolar disorder with or without psychosis; maintenance treatment of bipolar disorder as an adjunct to lithium or valproate; acute agitation in patients with schizophrenia

Unlabeled Use Psychosis/agitation related to Alzheimer's dementia

Pregnancy Risk Factor C

Pregnancy Considerations Adverse events were observed in animal reproduction studies. Antipsychotic use during the third trimester of pregnancy has a risk for abnormal muscle movements (extrapyramidal symptoms [EPS]) and/or withdrawal symptoms in newborns following delivery. Symptoms in the newborn may include agitation, feeding disorder, hypertonia, hypotonia, respiratory distress, somnolence, and tremor; these effects may be self-limiting or require hospitalization. Ziprasidone may cause hyperprolactinemia, which may decrease reproductive function in both males and females.

The ACOG recommends that therapy during pregnancy be individualized; treatment with psychiatric medications during pregnancy should incorporate the clinical expertise of the mental health clinician, obstetrician, primary healthcare provider, and pediatrician. Safety data related to atypical antipsychotics during pregnancy is limited and routine use is not recommended. However, if a woman is inadvertently exposed to an atypical antipsychotic while pregnant, continuing therapy may be preferable to switching to a typical antipsychotic that the fetus has not yet been exposed to; consider risk:benefit (ACOG, 2008).

Healthcare providers are encouraged to enroll women 18-45 years of age exposed to ziprasidone during pregnancy in the Atypical Antipsychotics Pregnancy Registry (1-866-961-2388 or http://www.womensmentalhealth.org/pregnancyregistry).

Breast-Feeding Considerations It is not known if ziprasidone is excreted into breast milk. Breast-feeding is not recommended by the manufacturer.

Contraindications Hypersensitivity to ziprasidone or any component of the formulation; history of (or current) prolonged QT; congenital long QT syndrome; recent myocardial infarction; uncompensated heart failure; concurrent use of other QT_c-prolonging agents including arsenic trioxide, chlorpromazine, class Ia antiarrhythmics (eg, disopyramide, quinidine, procainamide), class III antiarrhythmics (eg, amiodarone, dofetilide, ibutilide, sotalol), dolasetron, droperidol, gatifloxacin, halofantrine, levomethadyl, mefloquine, mesoridazine, moxifloxacin, pentamidine, pimozide, probucol, sparfloxacin, tacrolimus, and thioridazine

Warnings/Precautions Hazardous agent - use appropriate precautions for handling and disposal (NIOSH, 2012). **[U.S. Boxed Warning]: Elderly patients with dementia-related behavioral disorders treated with antipsychotics are at an increased risk of death compared to placebo.** Most deaths appeared to be either cardiovascular (eg, heart failure, sudden death) or infectious (eg, pneumonia) in nature. Ziprasidone is not approved for the treatment of dementia-related psychosis.

May result in QT_c prolongation (dose related), which has been associated with the development of malignant ventricular arrhythmias (torsade de pointes) and sudden death. Note contraindications related to this effect. Observed prolongation was greater than with other atypical antipsychotic agents (risperidone, olanzapine, quetiapine), but less than with thioridazine. Correct electrolyte disturbances, especially hypokalemia or hypomagnesemia, prior to use and throughout therapy. Use caution in patients with bradycardia. Discontinue in patients found to have persistent QT_c intervals >500 msec. Patients with symptoms of dizziness, palpitations, or syncope should receive further cardiac evaluation. May cause orthostatic hypotension. Use is contraindicated in patients with recent acute myocardial infarction (MI), QT prolongation, or uncompensated heart failure. Avoid use in patients with a history of cardiac arrhythmias; use with caution in patients with history of MI or unstable heart disease. Dyslipidemia has been reported with atypical antipsychotics; risk profile may differ between agents.

Leukopenia, neutropenia, and agranulocytosis (sometimes fatal) have been reported in clinical trials and postmarketing reports with antipsychotic use; presence of risk factors (eg, pre-existing low WBC or history of drug-induced leuko-/neutropenia) should prompt periodic blood count assessment. Discontinue therapy at first signs of blood dyscrasias or if absolute neutrophil count <1000/mm^3.

May cause extrapyramidal symptoms (EPS). Risk of dystonia (and probably other EPS) may be greater with increased doses, use of conventional antipsychotics, males, and younger patients. Impaired core body temperature regulation may occur; caution with strenuous exercise, heat exposure, dehydration, and concomitant medication possessing anticholinergic effects; not reported in premarketing trials of ziprasidone. Antipsychotic use may also be associated with neuroleptic malignant syndrome (NMS). Use with caution in patients at risk of seizures.

Atypical antipsychotics have been associated with development of hyperglycemia. There is limited documentation with ziprasidone and specific risk associated with this agent is not known. Use caution in patients with diabetes or other disorders of glucose regulation; monitor for worsening of glucose control. May increase prolactin levels; clinical significance of hyperprolactinemia in patients with breast cancer or other prolactin-dependent tumors is unknown.

Use in elderly patients with dementia is associated with an increased risk of mortality and cerebrovascular accidents; avoid antipsychotic use for behavioral problems associated with dementia unless alternative nonpharmacologic therapies have failed and patient may harm self or others. In addition, use may cause or exacerbate syndrome of inappropriate antidiuretic hormone secretion or hyponatremia; monitor sodium closely with initiation or dosage adjustments in older adults (Beers Criteria).

Cognitive and/or motor impairment (sedation) is common with ziprasidone. Use with caution in disorders where CNS depression is a feature. Use with caution in Parkinson's disease. Antipsychotic use has been associated with esophageal dysmotility and aspiration; use with caution in patients at risk of pneumonia (ie, Alzheimer's disease). Use caution in hepatic impairment. Ziprasidone has been associated with a fairly high incidence of rash (5%). Significant weight gain has been observed with antipsychotic therapy; incidence varies with product. Monitor waist circumference and BMI. Rare cases of priapism have been reported. Use the intramuscular formulation with caution in patients with renal impairment; formulation contains cyclodextrin, an excipient which may accumulate in renal insufficiency.

The possibility of a suicide attempt is inherent in psychotic illness or bipolar disorder; use caution in high-risk patients during initiation of therapy. Prescriptions should be written for the smallest quantity consistent with good patient care.

Adverse Reactions Note: Although minor QT_c prolongation (mean: 10 msec at 160 mg/day) may occur more frequently (incidence not specified), clinically-relevant prolongation (>500 msec) was rare (0.06%) and less than placebo (0.23%).

>10%:

Central nervous system: Extrapyramidal symptoms (2% to 31%), somnolence (8% to 31%), headache (3% to 18%), dizziness (3% to 16%)

Gastrointestinal: Nausea (4% to 12%)

1% to 10%:

Cardiovascular: Orthostatic hypotension (5%), chest pain (3%), hypertension (2% to 3%), tachycardia (2%), bradycardia (≤2%), facial edema (1%), vasodilation (≤1%)

Central nervous system: Akathisia (2% to 10%), anxiety (2% to 5%), insomnia (3%), agitation (2%), speech disorder (2%), personality disorder (2%), akinesia (≥1%), amnesia (≥1%), ataxia (≥1%), confusion (≥1%), coordination abnormal (≥1%), delirium (≥1%), dystonia (≥1%), hostility (≥1%), oculogyric crisis (≥1%), vertigo (≥1%), chills (1%), fever (1%), hypothermia (1%), psychosis (1%)

Dermatologic: Rash (4% to 5%), fungal dermatitis (2%), photosensitivity reaction (1%)

Endocrine & metabolic: Dysmenorrhea (2%)

Gastrointestinal: Weight gain (6% to 10%), constipation (2% to 9%), dyspepsia (1% to 8%), diarrhea (3% to 5%), vomiting (3% to 5%), xerostomia (1% to 5%), salivation increased (4%), tongue edema (≤3%), anorexia (2%), abdominal pain (≤2%), dysphagia (≤2%), rectal hemorrhage (≤2%), buccoglossal syndrome (≥1%)

Genitourinary: Priapism (1%)

Local: Injection site pain (7% to 9%)

Neuromuscular & skeletal: Weakness (2% to 6%), hypoesthesia (2%), myalgia (2%), paresthesia (2%), abnormal gait (≥1%), choreoathetosis (≥1%), dysarthria (≥1%), dyskinesia (≥1%), hyper-/hypokinesia (≥1%), hypotonia (≥1%), neuropathy (≥1%), tremor (≥1%), twitching (≥1%), back pain (1%), cogwheel rigidity (1%), hypertonia (1%)

Ocular: Vision abnormal (3% to 6%), diplopia (≥1%)

Respiratory: Infection (8%), rhinitis (1% to 4%), cough (3%), pharyngitis (3%), dyspnea (2%)

Miscellaneous: Diaphoresis (2%), furunculosis (2%), withdrawal syndrome (≥1%), flank pain (1%), flu-like syndrome (1%)

<1% (Limited to important or life-threatening): Abnormal ejaculation, albuminuria, alkaline phosphatase increased, allergic reaction, alopecia, amenorrhea, anemia, angioedema, angina, anorgasmia, atrial fibrillation, AV block (first degree), basophilia, blepharitis, bruising, BUN increased, bundle branch block, cardiomegaly, cataract, cerebral infarction, cerebrovascular accident, cholestatic jaundice, circumoral paresthesia, conjunctivitis, contact dermatitis, CPK increased, creatinine (serum) increased, dehydration, depression, dry eyes, eczema, enuresis, eosinophilia, epistaxis, exfoliative dermatitis, facial droop, fatty liver, fecal impaction, galactorrhea, GGT increased, gingival bleeding, glycosuria, gout, gynecomastia, hematemesis, hemoptysis, hematuria, hepatitis, hepatomegaly, hyper-/hypochloremia, hyper-/hypocholesterolemia, hyper-/hypoglycemia, hyper-/hypokalemia, hyper-/hypothyroidism, hyperlipemia, hyperreflexia, hyperuricemia, hypocalcemia, hypomagnesemia, hyponatremia, hypoproteinemia, impotence, jaundice, keratitis, keratoconjunctivitis, ketosis, lactation (female), laryngismus, LDH increased, leukocytosis, leukopenia, leukoplakia (mouth), lymphadenopathy, lymphedema, lymphocytosis, maculopapular rash, mania/hypomania, melena, menorrhagia, metrorrhagia, monocytosis, myocarditis, myoclonus, myopathy, neuroleptic malignant syndrome, nocturia, nystagmus, ocular hemorrhage, oliguria, opisthotonos, paralysis, peripheral edema, phlebitis, photophobia, pneumonia, polycythemia, polyuria, pulmonary embolism, QT_c prolongation >500 msec, respiratory alkalosis, seizure, serotonin syndrome, sexual dysfunction (male and female), syncope, tardive dyskinesia, tenosynovitis, thirst, thrombocytopenia, thrombocythemia, thrombophlebitis, thyroiditis, tinnitus, torsade de pointes, torticollis, transaminases increased, trismus, urinary incontinence, urinary retention, urticaria, uterine hemorrhage, vaginal hemorrhage, vesiculobullous rash, visual field defect

Drug Interactions

Metabolism/Transport Effects Substrate of CYP1A (minor), CYP3A4 (minor); **Note:** Assignment of Majo Minor substrate status based on clinically relevant dru interaction potential; **Inhibits** CYP2D6 (weak), CYP3A (weak)

Avoid Concomitant Use

Avoid concomitant use of Ziprasidone with any of the following: Amisulpride; Azelastine (Nasal); FLUoxetine; Highest Risk QTc-Prolonging Agents; Ivabradine; Metoclopramide; Mifepristone; Moderate Risk QTc-Prolonging Agents; Paraldehyde; Sulpiride

Increased Effect/Toxicity

Ziprasidone may increase the levels/effects of: Alcoh (Ethyl); Amisulpride; ARIPiprazole; Azelastine (Nasa Buprenorphine; CNS Depressants; FLUoxetine; Highe Risk QTc-Prolonging Agents; Hydrocodone; Lomitapid Methotrimeprazine; Methylphenidate; Paraldehyd Serotonin Modulators; Sulpiride; Zolpidem

The levels/effects of Ziprasidone may be increased b Acetylcholinesterase Inhibitors (Central); Brimonidir (Topical); Doxylamine; FLUoxetine; HydrOXYzine; Ival radine; Lithium formulations; Magnesium Sulfate; Meth trimeprazine; Methylphenidate; Metoclopramid Metyrosine; Mifepristone; Moderate Risk QTc-Prolongir Agents; Perampanel; QTc-Prolonging Agents (Indeterm nate Risk and Risk Modifying); Serotonin Modulator Sodium Oxybate; Tetrabenazine

Decreased Effect

Ziprasidone may decrease the levels/effects of: Amphe amines; Anti-Parkinson's Agents (Dopamine Agonist Quinagolide

The levels/effects of Ziprasidone may be decreased b CarBAMazepine; Lithium formulations

Ethanol/Nutrition/Herb Interactions

Ethanol: May increase CNS depression; monitor fo increased effects with coadministration. Caution patien about effects.

Food: Administration with food increases serum leve twofold. Grapefruit juice may increase serum concentra tion of ziprasidone.

Herb/Nutraceutical: St John's wort may decrease seru levels of ziprasidone, due to a potential effect o CYP3A4. This has not been specifically studied. Som herbal medications may increase CNS depression. Ma agement: Avoid kava kava, gotu kola, valerian, and S John's wort.

Preparation for Administration Hazardous agent; us appropriate precautions for handling and disposal (NIOSH 2012). Each vial should be reconstituted with 1.2 m SWFI. Shake vigorously; will form a pale, pink solutio containing 20 mg/mL ziprasidone.

Storage/Stability

Capsule: Store at 25°C (77°F); excursion permitted t 15°C to 30°C (59°F to 86°F).

Vials for injection: Store at 25°C (77°F); excursion permi ted to 15°C to 30°C (59°F to 86°F). Protect from ligh Following reconstitution, injection may be stored at roo temperature up to 24 hours or under refrigeration for up t 7 days. Protect from light.

Mechanism of Action Ziprasidone is a benzylisothiazo lylpiperazine antipsychotic. The exact mechanism of actio is unknown. However, *in vitro* radioligand studies show tha ziprasidone has high affinity for D_2, D_3, $5\text{-}HT_{2A}$, $5\text{-}HT_{1A}$, $5\text{-}HT_{2C}$, $5\text{-}HT_{1D}$, and $alpha_1$-adrenergic; moderate affini for histamine H_1 receptors; and no appreciable affinity fo $alpha_2$-adrenergic receptors, beta-adrenergic, 5-HT, $5\text{-}HT_4$, cholinergic, mu, sigma, or benzodiazepine recep tors. Ziprasidone functions as an antagonist at the D, $5\text{-}HT_{2A}$, and $5\text{-}HT_{1D}$ receptors and as an agonist at th $5\text{-}HT_{1A}$ receptor. Ziprasidone moderately inhibits the reup take of serotonin and norepinephrine.

Pharmacodynamics/Kinetics

Absorption: Well absorbed

Distribution: V_d: 1.5 L/kg

Protein binding: >99%, primarily to albumin and alpha$_1$-acid glycoprotein

Metabolism: Extensively hepatic, primarily chemical and enzymatic reductions via glutathione and aldehyde oxidase, respectively; less than 1/3 of total metabolism via CYP3A4 and CYP1A2 (minor)

Bioavailability: Oral (with food): 60% (up to twofold increase with food); I.M.: 100%

Half-life elimination: Oral: Mean terminal half-life: 7 hours; I.M.: Mean half-life: 2-5 hours

Time to peak: Oral: 6-8 hours; I.M.: ≤60 minutes

Excretion: Feces (~66%; <4% of total dose as unchanged drug); urine (~20%; <1% of total dose as unchanged drug)

Dosage

Bipolar mania (acute): Adults: Oral: Initial: 40 mg twice daily

Adjustment: May increase to 60 mg or 80 mg twice daily on second day of treatment; average dose 40-80 mg twice daily

Bipolar disorder (maintenance; as adjunct to lithium or valproate): Adults: Oral: Continue ziprasidone dose at which the patient was initially stabilized; usual dosage range: 40-80 mg twice daily

Schizophrenia: Adults: Oral: Initial: 20 mg twice daily (U.S. labeling) or 20-40 mg twice daily (Canadian labeling)

Adjustment: Increases (if indicated) should be made no more frequently than every 2 days; ordinarily patients should be observed for improvement over several weeks before adjusting the dose

Maintenance: Range: 20-100 mg twice daily; however, dosages >80 mg twice daily are generally not recommended

Acute agitation (schizophrenia): Adults: I.M.: 10 mg every 2 hours **or** 20 mg every 4 hours; maximum: 40 mg daily; oral therapy should replace I.M. administration as soon as possible

Elderly: No dosage adjustment is recommended; consider initiating at a low end of the dosage range, with slower titration

Dosage adjustment in renal impairment:

Oral: No dosage adjustment is recommended

I.M.: Cyclodextrin, an excipient in the I.M. formulation, is cleared by renal filtration; use with caution.

Ziprasidone is not removed by hemodialysis.

Dosage adjustment in hepatic impairment:

U.S. labeling: No dosage adjustment is recommended; however, drug undergoes extensive hepatic metabolism and systemic exposure may be increased. Use with caution.

Canadian labeling: Manufacturer labeling suggests that dose reductions should be considered but does not provide specific dosing recommendations.

Dietary Considerations Capsule: Take with food.

Administration

Oral: Administer with food.

Injection: For I.M. administration only.

Hazardous agent; use appropriate precautions for handling and disposal (NIOSH, 2012).

Monitoring Parameters Blood pressure, heart rate; temperature; serum potassium and magnesium; fasting lipid profile and fasting blood glucose/Hb A_{1c} (prior to treatment, at 3 months, then annually); BMI; waist circumference; mental status, abnormal involuntary movement scale (AIMS), extrapyramidal symptoms. Weight should be assessed prior to treatment, at 4 weeks, 8 weeks, 12 weeks, and then at quarterly intervals. Consider titrating to a different antipsychotic agent for a weight gain ≥5% of the initial weight. The value of routine ECG screening or monitoring has not been established.

Additional Information The increased potential to prolong QT_c, as compared to other available antipsychotic agents, should be considered in the evaluation of available alternatives.

Dosage Forms Excipient information presented when available (limited, particularly for generics); consult specific product labeling.

Capsule, Oral, as hydrochloride:

Geodon: 20 mg, 40 mg, 60 mg, 80 mg

Generic: 20 mg, 40 mg, 60 mg, 80 mg

Solution Reconstituted, Intramuscular, as mesylate [strength expressed as base]:

Geodon: 20 mg (1 ea)

Extemporaneous Preparations Hazardous agent: Use appropriate precautions for handling and disposal.

A 2.5 mg/mL oral solution may be made with the injection. Use 8 vials of the 20 mg injectable powder. Add 1.2 mL of distilled water to each vial to make a 20 mg/mL solution. Once dissolved, transfer 7.5 mL to a calibrated bottle and add quantity of vehicle (Ora-Sweet®) sufficient to make 60 mL. Label "shake well" and "refrigerate". Stable for 14 days at room temperature or 42 days refrigerated (preferred).

Green K and Parish RC, "Stability of Ziprasidone Mesylate in an Extemporaneously Compounded Oral Solution," *J Pediatr Pharmacol Ther*, 2010, 15:138-41.

- **Ziprasidone Hydrochloride** *see* Ziprasidone *on page 2230*
- **Ziprasidone Mesylate** *see* Ziprasidone *on page 2230*
- **Zipsor** *see* Diclofenac (Systemic) *on page 597*
- **Zithranol** *see* Anthralin *on page 140*
- **Zithranol-RR** *see* Anthralin *on page 140*
- **Zithromax** *see* Azithromycin (Systemic) *on page 214*
- **Zithromax® (Can)** *see* Azithromycin (Systemic) *on page 214*
- **Zithromax® For Intravenous Injection (Can)** *see* Azithromycin (Systemic) *on page 214*
- **Zithromax TRI-PAK™** *see* Azithromycin (Systemic) *on page 214*
- **Zithromax Tri-Pak** *see* Azithromycin (Systemic) *on page 214*
- **Zithromax Z-PAK®** *see* Azithromycin (Systemic) *on page 214*
- **Zithromax Z-Pak** *see* Azithromycin (Systemic) *on page 214*

Ziv-Aflibercept (Systemic) (ziv a FLIB er sept)

Brand Names: U.S. Zaltrap

Index Terms Aflibercept I.V.; Vascular Endothelial Growth Factor Trap; VEGF Trap; VEGF Trap R1R2

Pharmacologic Category Antineoplastic Agent; Vascular Endothelial Growth Factor (VEGF) Inhibitor

Use Colorectal cancer, metastatic: Treatment of metastatic colorectal cancer (in combination with fluorouracil, leucovorin, and irinotecan [FOLFIRI]) in patients who are resistant to or have progressed on an oxaliplatin-based regimen

Pregnancy Risk Factor C

Pregnancy Considerations Adverse events were observed in animal reproduction studies with doses providing systemic exposure equivalent to ~30% of a human dose. The incidence of fetal malformations increased with increasing doses. Patients (male and female) should use effective contraception during therapy and for at least 3 months following treatment.

Breast-Feeding Considerations It is not known if ziv-aflibercept is excreted into breast milk. Due to the potential for adverse events in a nursing infant, the decision to discontinue breast-feeding during therapy or to discontinue aflibercept should take into account the benefits of treatment to the mother.

Contraindications There are no contraindications listed in the manufacturer's labeling.

Warnings/Precautions The risk for hemorrhage is increased with ziv-aflibercept. **[U.S. Boxed Warning]: Severe and occasionally fatal hemorrhage, including gastrointestinal (GI) bleeding, has been reported with ziv-aflibercept/FOLFIRI. Monitor for signs and symptoms of GI and other severe bleeding events; do not administer to patients with severe hemorrhage;** discontinue if severe hemorrhage develops. Hemorrhagic events have also included hematuria, postprocedural hemorrhage, intracranial hemorrhage, and pulmonary hemorrhage/hemoptysis.

[U.S. Boxed Warning]: Severe or fatal GI perforation is a possibility; discontinue ziv-aflibercept if GI perforation occurs; monitor for signs/symptoms of GI perforation. The risk for GI and non-GI fistulas is increased with ziv-aflibercept; fistula sites have included anal, enterovesical, enterocutaneous, colovaginal and intestinal; discontinue in patients who develop fistula. Severe diarrhea and dehydration have been reported; the incidence of diarrhea is increased in patients ≥65 years of age; monitor elderly patients closely for diarrhea.

Proteinuria, nephrotic syndrome, and thrombotic microangiopathy (TMA) have been associated with ziv-aflibercept. Evaluate for proteinuria during treatment with urine dipstick and/or urinary protein creatinine ratio (UPCR); if dipstick ≥2+ for protein or UPCR >1, obtain 24-hour urine collection. Withhold ziv-aflibercept for proteinuria ≥2 g/day; for recurrent proteinuria, withhold treatment until <2 g/day and then resume with permanent dose reduction. Discontinue treatment for nephrotic syndrome or TMA.

The risk for grades 3/4 hypertension is increased; onset is generally within the first 2 treatment cycles. Monitor blood pressure every 2 weeks (more frequently if clinically indicated); treat with appropriate antihypertensive therapy (may require adjustment of existing antihypertensives); temporarily withhold treatment with uncontrolled hypertension; may reinitiate with permanent dose reduction when controlled. Discontinue for hypertensive crisis or encephalopathy. Patients with NYHA class III or IV heart failure were excluded from clinical trials.

[U.S. Boxed Warning]: Severely compromised wound healing may occur with ziv-aflibercept/FOLFIRI. Discontinue ziv-aflibercept with compromised wound healing. Withhold ziv-aflibercept at least 4 weeks prior to elective surgery. Do not resume treatment until at least 4 weeks after major surgery AND until the surgical wound is completely healed. For minor surgeries (eg, central venous access port placement, biopsy, or tooth extraction), ziv-aflibercept may be resumed or initiated as soon as the surgical wound is fully healed.

A higher incidence of neutropenia and complications due to neutropenia (neutropenic fever and infection) occurred in patients receiving ziv-aflibercept; leukopenia and thrombocytopenia were also observed in clinical trials; monitor blood counts (baseline and prior to each cycle); delay treatment until ANC is ≥1500/mm^3. Cases of reversible posterior leukoencephalopathy syndrome (RPLS) have been reported; confirm diagnosis with MRI; discontinue ziv-aflibercept if verified; symptoms generally resolve or improve within days, although persistent neurologic symptoms and death have been reported. Arterial thrombotic events (ATE), including transient ischemic attack, cerebrovascular accidents, and angina have occurred. Discontinue ziv-aflibercept in patients who experience ATEs. Certain adverse events, such as diarrhea and dehydration, occurred at a higher incidence in elderly compared to younger adults; monitor closely during treatment.

Adverse Reactions Note: Reactions reported in combination therapy with fluorouracil, leucovorin, and irinotecan (FOLFIRI).

>10%:

- Cardiovascular: Hypertension (41%; grades 3/4: 19%)
- Central nervous system: Fatigue (48%), dysphonia (25%), headache (22%)
- Dermatologic: Palmar-plantar erythrodysesthesia (11%)
- Gastrointestinal: Diarrhea (69%), stomatitis (50%), appetite decreased (32%), weight loss (32%), abdominal pain (27%), upper abdominal pain (11%)
- Hematologic: Leukopenia (78%; grades 3/4: 16%), neutropenia (67%; grades 3/4: 37%), thrombocytopenia (48%; grades 3/4: 3%), bleeding (38%; grades 3/4: 3%)
- Hepatic: AST increased (62%), ALT increased (50%)
- Neuromuscular & skeletal: Weakness (18%)
- Renal: Proteinuria (62%; grades 3/4: 8%), creatinine increased (23%)
- Respiratory: Epistaxis (28%), dyspnea (12%)
- Miscellaneous: Infection (46%)

1% to 10%:

- Cardiovascular: Venous thromboembolic events (9%), arterial thromboembolic events (3%; grades 3/4: 2%)
- Central nervous system: Reversible posterior encephalopathy syndrome (RPLS) (1%)
- Dermatologic: Hyperpigmentation (8%)
- Endocrine & metabolic: Dehydration (9%)
- Gastrointestinal: Hemorrhoids (6%), proctalgia (5%), rectal hemorrhage (5%), gastrointestinal perforation (1%)
- Genitourinary: Urinary tract infection (9%)
- Hematologic: Neutropenic fever (grades 3/4: 4%), neutropenic infection/sepsis (grades 3/4: 2%)
- Renal: Nephrotic syndrome (1%)
- Respiratory: Oropharyngeal pain (8%), rhinorrhea (6%), pulmonary embolism (5%)
- Miscellaneous: Antibody formation (3%), fistula formation (2%; grades 3/4: <1%)

<1% (Limited to important or life-threatening): Hypersensitivity reactions, thrombotic microangiopathy, wound healing impaired

Drug Interactions

Metabolism/Transport Effects None known.

Avoid Concomitant Use

Avoid concomitant use of Ziv-Aflibercept (Systemic) with any of the following: CloZAPine

Increased Effect/Toxicity

Ziv-Aflibercept (Systemic) may increase the levels/effects of: Bisphosphonate Derivatives; CloZAPine

Decreased Effect There are no known significant interactions involving a decrease in effect.

Preparation for Administration Prior to infusion, dilute in D_5W or NS to a final concentration of 0.6-8 mg/mL. Use polyvinyl chloride (PVC) bags containing DEHP or polyolefin bags. After initial vial puncture, do not re-enter; discard unused portion of the vial. Do not mix with other medications.

Storage/Stability Store intact vials refrigerated at 2°C to 8°C (36°F to 46°F). Protect from light (store in original outer carton). Stable for up to 4 hours refrigerated after diluted for infusion.

Mechanism of Action Also known as VEGF-trap, ziv-aflibercept is a recombinant fusion protein which is comprised of portions of binding domains for vascular endothelial growth factor (VEGF) receptors 1 and 2, attached to the Fc portion of human IgG1. Ziv-aflibercept acts as a decoy receptor for VEGF-A, VEGF-B, and placental growth factor (PlGF) which prevent VEGF receptor binding/activation to their receptors (an action critical to angiogenesis), thus leading to antiangiogenesis and tumor regression.

Pharmacodynamics/Kinetics Half-life elimination: ~6 days (range: 4-7 days)

Dosage Colorectal cancer, metastatic: Adults: I.V.: 4 mg/kg every 2 weeks (in combination with fluorouracil, leucovorin, and irinotecan [FOLFIRI]), continue until disease progression or unacceptable toxicity

Dosage adjustment for toxicity:

Arterial thrombotic events: Discontinue treatment.

Fistula formation: Discontinue treatment.

Gastrointestinal perforation: Discontinue treatment.

Hemorrhage, severe: Discontinue treatment.

Hypertension:

Recurrent or severe hypertension: Temporarily withhold treatment until controlled, and then resume with a permanent dose reduction to 2 mg/kg every 2 weeks.

Hypertensive crisis or hypertensive encephalopathy: Discontinue treatment.

Neutropenia: Temporarily withhold treatment until ANC is ≥1500/mm^3.

Renal effects:

Proteinuria (≥2 g/24 hours): Temporarily withhold treatment until proteinuria <2 g/24 hours and then resume at previous dose.

Recurrent proteinuria: Temporarily withhold treatment until proteinuria <2 g/24 hours, and then resume with a permanent dose reduction to 2 mg/kg every 2 weeks.

Nephrotic syndrome or thrombotic microangiopathy: Discontinue treatment.

Reversible posterior leukoencephalopathy syndrome (RPLS): Discontinue treatment.

Surgery/wound healing impairment:

Elective surgery: Temporarily withhold treatment for at least 4 weeks prior to elective surgery; do not resume until at least 4 weeks after major surgery AND until wound is fully healed; for minor surgery (eg, biopsy, central venous port placement, tooth extraction), may be resumed after wound is fully healed.

Wound healing impaired: Discontinue treatment.

Note: For toxicities related to FOLFIRI, refer to individual Fluorouracil (Systemic) or Irinotecan monographs.

Dosage adjustment in renal impairment: No dosage adjustment provided in manufacturer's labeling; however, need for adjustment is not likely because exposure in patients with mild, moderate, and severe impairment was similar to that of patients with normal renal function.

Dosage adjustment in hepatic impairment:

Mild (total bilirubin >1-1.5 times ULN) to moderate (total bilirubin >1.5-3 times ULN) impairment: No dosage adjustment provided in manufacturer's labeling; however, need for adjustment is not likely because exposure was similar to that of patients with normal hepatic function.

Severe impairment (total bilirubin >3 times ULN): No dosage adjustment provided in the manufacturer's labeling (no data available).

Administration I.V.: Infuse over 1 hour. Do not administer I.V. push or bolus. Administer prior to any FOLFIRI component. Do not administer other medications through the same intravenous line.

Infuse via a 0.2 micron polyethersulfone filter; do not use filters made of polyvinylidene fluoride (PVDF) or nylon. Administer with one of the following types of infusion sets: Polyvinyl chloride (PVC) containing DEHP, DEHP-free PVC containing trioctyl-trimellitate (TOTM), polypropylene, polyethylene lined PVC, or polyurethane.

Monitoring Parameters CBC with differential (baseline and prior to each cycle); urine protein (dipstick analysis and/or urinary protein creatinine ratio [UPCR], obtain 24-hour urine collection if dipstick ≥2+ for protein or UPCR >1); blood pressure (every 2 weeks; more frequently if clinically indicated); monitor for signs/symptoms of hemorrhage or GI perforation; monitor elderly patients closely for diarrhea and/or dehydration. Monitor wounds for healing impairment.

Dosage Forms Excipient information presented when available (limited, particularly for generics); consult specific product labeling.

Solution, Intravenous [preservative free]:

Zaltrap: 100 mg/4 mL (4 mL); 200 mg/8 mL (8 mL) [contains mouse protein (murine) (hamster)]

◆ **Zmax** *see* Azithromycin (Systemic) *on page* 214

◆ **Zmax SR™ (Can)** *see* Azithromycin (Systemic) *on page* 214

◆ **ZnSO$_4$ (error-prone abbreviation)** *see* Zinc Sulfate *on page* 2230

◆ **Zocor** *see* Simvastatin *on page* 1899

◆ **Zofran** *see* Ondansetron *on page* 1510

◆ **Zofran® (Can)** *see* Ondansetron *on page* 1510

◆ **Zofran ODT** *see* Ondansetron *on page* 1510

◆ **Zofran® ODT (Can)** *see* Ondansetron *on page* 1510

◆ **Zol 446** *see* Zoledronic Acid *on page* 2235

◆ **Zoladex** *see* Goserelin *on page* 970

◆ **Zoladex® (Can)** *see* Goserelin *on page* 970

◆ **Zoladex® LA (Can)** *see* Goserelin *on page* 970

◆ **Zoledronate** *see* Zoledronic Acid *on page* 2235

Zoledronic Acid (zoe le DRON ik AS id)

Brand Names: U.S. Reclast; Zometa

Brand Names: Canada Aclasta; Zometa

Index Terms CGP-42446; Zol 446; Zoledronate

Pharmacologic Category Bisphosphonate Derivative

Use

Glucocorticoid-induced osteoporosis (Reclast): Treatment and prevention of glucocorticoid-induced osteoporosis in men and women who are initiating or continuing systemic glucocorticoids in a daily dose equivalent to 7.5 mg or more of prednisone and who are expected to remain on glucocorticoids for at least 12 months.

Hypercalcemia of malignancy (Zometa): Treatment of hypercalcemia (albumin-corrected serum calcium ≥12 mg/dL) of malignancy.

Multiple myeloma and bone metastases from solid tumors (Zometa): Treatment of patients with multiple myeloma and patients with documented bone metastases from solid tumors, in conjunction with standard antineoplastic therapy.

Osteoporosis in men (Reclast): To increase bone mass in men with osteoporosis.

Paget disease of bone (Reclast): Treatment of Paget disease of bone in men and women.

Postmenopausal osteoporosis (Reclast): Treatment and prevention of osteoporosis in postmenopausal women.

Unlabeled Use Prevention of bone loss associated with aromatase inhibitor therapy in postmenopausal women with breast cancer; prevention of bone loss associated with androgen deprivation therapy in prostate cancer

Pregnancy Risk Factor D

Pregnancy Considerations Adverse events were observed in animal reproduction studies. It is not known if bisphosphonates cross the placenta, but fetal exposure is expected (Djokanovic, 2008; Stathopoulos, 2011). Bisphosphonates are incorporated into the bone matrix and gradually released over time. The amount available in the systemic circulation varies by dose and duration of therapy. Theoretically, there may be a risk of fetal harm when pregnancy follows the completion of therapy; however, available data have not shown that exposure to bisphosphonates during pregnancy significantly increases the risk of adverse fetal events (Djokanovic, 2008; Levy, 2009; Stathopoulos, 2011). Until additional data is available, most sources recommend discontinuing bisphosphonate therapy in women of reproductive potential as early as possible prior to a planned pregnancy; use in premenopausal women should be reserved for special circumstances when rapid bone loss is occurring (Bhalla, 2010; Pereira, 2012; Stathopoulos, 2011). Because hypocalcemia has been described following *in utero* bisphosphonate exposure, exposed infants should be monitored for hypocalcemia after birth (Djokanovic, 2008; Stathopoulos, 2011). Use in pregnant women is contraindicated per the Canadian labeling.

Breast-Feeding Considerations It is not known if zoledronic acid is excreted into breast milk. Due to the potential for serious adverse reactions in the nursing infant, the U.S. manufacturer recommends a decision be made whether to discontinue nursing or to discontinue the drug, taking into account the importance of treatment to the mother. Use in nursing women is contraindicated per the Canadian labeling.

Medication Guide Available Yes

Contraindications

U.S. labeling:

Hypersensitivity to zoledronic acid or any component of the product; hypocalcemia (Reclast only); Cl_{cr}<35 mL/minute and in those with evidence of acute renal impairment (Reclast only).

Documentation of allergenic cross-reactivity for bisphosphonates is limited. However, because of similarities in chemical structure and/or pharmacologic actions, the possibility of cross-sensitivity cannot be ruled out with certainty.

Canadian labeling:

All indications: Hypersensitivity to zoledronic acid or other bisphosphonates, or any component of the formulation; uncorrected hypocalcemia at the time of infusion; pregnancy, breast-feeding

Nononcology uses: Additional contraindications: Use in patients with Cl_{cr} <35 mL/minute and use in patients with evidence of acute renal impairment due to an increased risk of renal failure

Warnings/Precautions Hazardous agent - use appropriate precautions for handling and disposal (NIOSH, 2012). Osteonecrosis of the jaw (ONJ) has been reported in patients receiving bisphosphonates. Risk factors include invasive dental procedures (eg, tooth extraction, dental implants, boney surgery); a diagnosis of cancer, with concomitant chemotherapy, radiotherapy, or corticosteroids; poor oral hygiene, ill-fitting dentures; and comorbid disorders (anemia, coagulopathy, infection, pre-existing dental disease). Most reported cases occurred after I.V. bisphosphonate therapy; however, cases have been reported following oral therapy. A dental exam and preventative dentistry should be performed prior to placing patients with risk factors on chronic bisphosphonate therapy. The manufacturer's labeling states that there are no data to suggest whether discontinuing bisphosphonates in patients requiring invasive dental procedures reduces the risk of ONJ. However, other experts suggest that there is no evidence that discontinuing therapy reduces the risk of developing ONJ (Assael, 2009). The benefit/risk must b assessed by the treating physician and/or dentist/surge prior to any invasive dental procedure. Patients developi ONJ while on bisphosphonates should receive care by a oral surgeon.

Atypical, low-energy, or low-trauma femur fractures ha been reported in patients receiving bisphosphonates. T fractures include subtrochanteric femur (bone just bel the hip joint) and diaphyseal femur (long segment of t thigh bone). Some patients experience prodromal pa weeks or months before the fracture occurs. It is uncle if bisphosphonate therapy is the cause for these fracture atypical femur fractures have also been reported patients not taking bisphosphonates, and in patien receiving glucocorticoids. Patients receiving long-ter (>3-5 years) bisphosphonate therapy may be at a increased risk. Patients presenting with thigh or groin pa with a history of receiving bisphosphonates should b evaluated for femur fracture. Consider interrupti bisphosphonate therapy in patients who develop a femo shaft fracture; assess for fracture in the contralateral lim

Infrequently, severe (and occasionally debilitating) musc loskeletal (bone, joint, and/or muscle) pain have bee reported during bisphosphonate treatment. The onset pain ranged from a single day to several months. Consid discontinuing therapy in patients who experience seve symptoms; symptoms usually resolve upon discontinu tion. Some patients experienced recurrence when recha lenged with same drug or another bisphosphonate; avo use in patients with a history of these symptoms in ass ciation with bisphosphonate therapy.

May cause a significant risk of hypocalcemia in patien with Paget's disease, in whom the pretreatment rate bone turnover may be greatly elevated. Hypocalcemi including severe and life-threatening hypocalcemia, ha also been reported with oncology-related uses. Hypoca cemia must be corrected before initiation of therapy patients with Paget's disease, osteoporosis, or oncolo indications. Ensure adequate calcium and vitamin D intak during therapy. Use caution in patients with disturbances calcium and mineral metabolism (eg, hypoparathyroidis thyroid/parathyroid, surgery, malabsorption syndrome excision of small intestine).

Nononcology indications: Use is contraindicated patients with Cl_{cr} <35 mL/minute and in patients wi evidence of acute renal impairment due to an increase risk of renal failure. Obtain serum creatinine and calcula creatinine clearance (using actual body weight) with th Cockcroft-Gault formula prior to each administration. In th management of osteoporosis, re-evaluate the need f continued therapy periodically; the optimal duration treatment has not yet been determined. Consider disco tinuing after 3-5 years of use in patients at low risk f fracture; following discontinuation, re-evaluate fracture ris periodically.

Oncology indications: Use caution in mild-to-modera renal dysfunction; dosage adjustment required. In canc patients, renal toxicity has been reported with dose >4 mg or infusions administered over 15 minutes. Ri factors for renal deterioration include pre-existing ren insufficiency and repeated doses of zoledronic acid a other bisphosphonates. Dehydration and the use of oth nephrotoxic drugs which may contribute to renal deteri ration should be identified and managed. Use is n recommended in patients with severe renal impairme (serum creatinine >3 mg/dL or Cl_{cr} <30 mL/minute) a bone metastases (limited data); use in patients with hype calcemia of malignancy and severe renal impairme (serum creatinine >4.5 mg/dL for hypercalcemia of mali nancy) should only be done if the benefits outweigh th risks. Diuretics should not be used before correcting hypovolemia. Renal deterioration, resulting in renal failure and dialysis has occurred in patients treated with zoledronic acid after single and multiple infusions at recommended doses of 4 mg over 15 minutes. Assess renal function prior to treatment and withhold for renal deterioration [increase in serum creatinine of 0.5 mg/dL (if baseline level normal) or increase of 1 mg/dL (if baseline level abnormal)]; treatment should be withheld until renal function returns to within 10% of baseline.

According to the American Society of Clinical Oncology (ASCO) guidelines for bisphosphonates in multiple myeloma, treatment with zoledronic acid is not recommended for asymptomatic (smoldering) or indolent myeloma or with solitary plasmacytoma (Kyle, 2007). The National Comprehensive Cancer Network (NCCN) multiple myeloma guidelines (v.2.2013) recommend bisphosphonates for all patients receiving treatment for symptomatic disease; the use of bisphosphonates in stage 1 or smoldering disease may be considered, although preferably as part of a clinical trial.

Adequate hydration is required during treatment (urine output ~2 L/day); avoid overhydration, especially in patients with heart failure. Pre-existing renal compromise, severe dehydration, and concurrent use with diuretics or other nephrotoxic drugs may increase the risk for renal impairment. Single and multiple infusions in patients with both normal and impaired renal function have been associated with renal deterioration, resulting in renal failure and dialysis or death (rare). Patients with underlying moderate-to-severe renal impairment, increased age, concurrent use of nephrotoxic or diuretic medications, or severe dehydration prior to or after zoledronic acid administration may have an increased risk of acute renal impairment or renal failure. Others with increased risk include patients with renal impairment or dehydration secondary to fever, sepsis, gastrointestinal losses, or diuretic use. If history or physical exam suggests dehydration, treatment should not be given until the patient is normovolemic. Transient increases in serum creatinine may be more pronounced in patients with impaired renal function; consider monitoring creatinine clearance in at-risk patients taking other renally-eliminated drugs.

Conjunctivitis, uveitis, episcleritis, iritis, scleritis, and orbital inflammation have been reported (infrequently) with use; further ophthalmic evaluation (and possibly therapy discontinuation) may be necessary in patients with complicated infection. Use caution in patients with aspirin-sensitive asthma (may cause bronchoconstriction) and the elderly (because decreased renal function occurs more commonly in elderly patients). Rare cases of urticaria and angioedema and very rare cases of anaphylactic reactions/shock have been reported. Do not administer Zometa and Reclast (Aclasta [Canadian brand]) to the same patient for different indications.

Adverse Reactions Note: An acute reaction (eg, arthralgia, fever, flu-like symptoms, myalgia) may occur within the first 3 days following infusion in up to 44% of patients; usually resolves within 3-4 days of onset, although may take up to 14 days to resolve. The incidence may be decreased with acetaminophen (prior to infusion and for 72 hours postinfusion).

Oncology indications:

>10%:

Cardiovascular: Lower extremity edema (5% to 21%), hypotension (11%)

Central nervous system: Fatigue (39%), headache (5% to 19%), dizziness (18%), insomnia (15% to 16%), anxiety (11% to 14%), depression (14%), agitation (13%), confusion (7% to 13%), hypoesthesia (12%), rigors (11%)

Dermatologic: Alopecia (12%), dermatitis (11%)

Endocrine & metabolic: Dehydration (5% to 14%), hypophosphatemia (13%), hypokalemia (12%), hypomagnesemia (11%)

Gastrointestinal: Nausea (29% to 46%), vomiting (14% to 32%), constipation (27% to 31%), diarrhea (17% to 24%), anorexia (9% to 22%), abdominal pain (14% to 16%), weight loss (16%), decreased appetite (13%)

Genitourinary: Urinary tract infection (12% to 14%)

Hematologic & oncologic: Anemia (22% to 33%), progression of cancer (16% to 20%), neutropenia (12%)

Infection: Candidiasis (12%)

Neuromuscular & skeletal: Ostealgia (55%), weakness (5% to 24%), myalgia (23%), arthralgia (5% to 21%), back pain (15%), paresthesia (15%), limb pain (14%), skeletal pain (12%)

Renal: Renal insufficiency (8% to 17%; up to 40% in patients with abnormal baseline creatinine)

Respiratory: Dyspnea (22% to 27%), cough (12% to 22%)

Miscellaneous: Fever (32% to 44%)

1% to 10%:

Cardiovascular: Chest pain (5% to 10%)

Central nervous system: Somnolence (5% to 10%)

Endocrine & metabolic: Hypocalcemia (5% to 10%; grades 3/4: ≤1%), hypermagnesemia (grade 3: 2%)

Gastrointestinal: Dyspepsia (10%), dysphagia (5% to 10%), mucositis (5% to 10%), stomatitis (8%), sore throat (8%)

Hematologic & oncologic: Granulocytopenia (5% to 10%), pancytopenia (5% to 10%), thrombocytopenia (5% to 10%)

Infection: Infection (nonspecific; 5% to 10%)

Renal: Increased serum creatinine (grades 3/4: ≤2%)

Respiratory: Upper respiratory tract infection (10%)

Nononcology indications:

>10%:

Cardiovascular: Hypertension (5% to 13%)

Central nervous system: Pain (2% to 24%), fever (9% to 22%), headache (4% to 20%), chills (2% to 18%), fatigue (2% to 18%)

Endocrine & metabolic: Hypocalcemia (≤3%; Paget's disease 21%)

Gastrointestinal: Nausea (5% to 18%)

Immunologic: Infusion related reaction (4% to 25%)

Neuromuscular & skeletal: Arthralgia (9% to 27%), myalgia (5% to 23%), back pain (4% to 18%), limb pain (3% to 16%), musculoskeletal pain (≤12%)

Respiratory: Flu-like symptoms (1% to 11%)

1% to 10%:

Cardiovascular: Chest pain (1% to 8%), peripheral edema (3% to 6%), atrial fibrillation (1% to 3%), palpitations (≤3%)

Central nervous system: Dizziness (2% to 9%), rigors (8%), malaise (1% to 7%), hypoesthesia (≤6%), lethargy (3% to 5%), vertigo (1% to 4%), paresthesia (2%), hyperthermia (≤2%)

Dermatologic: Skin rash (2% to 3%), hyperhidrosis (≤3%)

Gastrointestinal: Abdominal pain (1% to 9%), diarrhea (5% to 8%), vomiting (2% to 8%), constipation (6% to 7%), dyspepsia (2% to 7%), abdominal discomfort (1% to 2%), anorexia (1% to 2%)

Hematologic & oncologic: Change in serum protein (C-reactive protein increased; ≤5%)

Neuromuscular & skeletal: Ostealgia (3% to 9%), arthritis (2% to 9%), shoulder pain (≤7%), neck pain (1% to 7%), weakness (2% to 6%), muscle spasm (2% to 6%), stiffness (1% to 5%), jaw pain (2% to 4%), joint swelling (≤3%)

Ophthalmic: Eye pain (≤2%)

Renal: Increased serum creatinine (2%)

Respiratory: Dyspnea (5% to 7%)

All indications: <1% (Limited to important or life-threatening): Acute renal failure (requiring hospitalization/dialysis), anaphylactic shock, anaphylaxis, angioedema, arthralgia (sometimes severe and/or incapacitating), bradycardia, conjunctivitis, dysgeusia, episcleritis, exacerbation of asthma, femur fracture (diaphyseal or subtrochanteric), hematuria, hyperesthesia, hyperkalemia, hypernatremia, hyperparathyroidism, hypersensitivity, hypertension, injection site reaction (eg, itching, pain, redness), interstitial lung disease, iridocyclitis, iritis, myalgia (sometimes severe and/or incapacitating), osteonecrosis (primarily of the jaws), periorbital swelling, scleritis, toxic acute renal tubular necrosis, uveitis, weight gain

Drug Interactions

Metabolism/Transport Effects None known.

Avoid Concomitant Use There are no known interactions where it is recommended to avoid concomitant use.

Increased Effect/Toxicity

Zoledronic Acid may increase the levels/effects of: Deferasirox; Phosphate Supplements

The levels/effects of Zoledronic Acid may be increased by: Aminoglycosides; Nonsteroidal Anti-Inflammatory Agents; Systemic Angiogenesis Inhibitors; Thalidomide

Decreased Effect

The levels/effects of Zoledronic Acid may be decreased by: Proton Pump Inhibitors

Preparation for Administration Hazardous agent; use appropriate precautions for handling and disposal (NIOSH, 2012).

Solution for injection:

Reclast, Aclasta (Canadian brand): No further preparation is necessary.

Zometa concentrate vials: Further dilute in 100 mL NS or D_5W prior to administration.

Zometa ready-to-use bottles: No further preparation is necessary. If reduced doses are required for patients with renal impairment, withdraw the appropriate volume of solution and replace with an equal amount of NS or D_5W.

Storage/Stability Solution for injection:

Aclasta (Canadian brand): Store at room temperature of 15°C to 30°C (59°F to 86°F). Keep sealed in original package until administration.

Reclast: Store at room temperature of 25°C (77°F); excursions permitted to 15°C to 30°C (59°F to 86°F). After opening, stable for 24 hours at 2°C to 8°C (36°F to 46°F). If refrigerated, allow the refrigerated solution to reach room temperature before administration.

Zometa: Store concentrate vials and ready-to-use bottles at 25°C (77°F); excursions permitted to 15°C to 30°C (59°F to 86°F). Diluted solutions for infusion which are not used immediately after preparation should be refrigerated at 2°C to 8°C (36°F to 46°F). Infusion of solution must be completed within 24 hours of preparation. The ready-to-use bottles are for single use only; if any preparation is necessary (preparing reduced dosage for patients with renal impairment), the prepared, diluted solution may be refrigerated at 2°C to 8°C (36°F to 46°F) if not used immediately. Infusion of solution must be completed within 24 hours of preparation. The previously withdrawn volume from the ready-to-use solution should be discarded; do not store or reuse.

Mechanism of Action A bisphosphonate which inhibits bone resorption via actions on osteoclasts or on osteoclast precursors; inhibits osteoclastic activity and skeletal calcium release induced by tumors. Decreases serum calcium and phosphorus, and increases their elimination. In osteoporosis, zoledronic acid inhibits osteoclast-mediated resorption, therefore reducing bone turnover.

Pharmacodynamics/Kinetics

Distribution: Binds to bone

Protein binding: 23% to 53%

Metabolism: Primarily eliminated intact via the kidney; metabolism not likely

Half-life elimination: Triphasic; Terminal: 146 hours

Excretion: Urine (39% ± 16% as unchanged drug) within 24 hours; feces (<3%)

Dosage Note: Acetaminophen administration after the infusion may reduce symptoms of acute-phase reactions. Patients treated for multiple myeloma and Paget's disease should receive a daily calcium and vitamin D supplement, and patients with osteoporosis should receive calcium and vitamin D supplementation if dietary intake is inadequate.

Hypercalcemia of malignancy (albumin-corrected serum calcium ≥12 mg/dL) (Zometa): Adults: I.V.: 4 mg (maximum) given as a single dose. Wait at least 7 days before considering retreatment.

Multiple myeloma or metastatic bone lesions from solid tumors (Zometa): Adults: I.V.: 4 mg once every 3-4 weeks

Osteoporosis, glucocorticoid-induced, treatment and prevention (Reclast, Aclasta [Canadian brand]): Adults: I.V.: 5 mg once a year

Osteoporosis, prevention: Adults: I.V.:

Reclast: 5 mg once every 2 years

Aclasta (Canadian brand): 5 mg as a single (one-time) dose

Osteoporosis, treatment (Reclast, Aclasta [Canadian brand]): Adults: I.V.: 5 mg once a year; consider discontinuing after 3-5 years of use in patients at low risk for fracture

Paget's disease: Adults: I.V.:

Reclast: 5 mg as a single dose. **Note:** Data concerning retreatment is not available; retreatment may be considered for relapse (increase in alkaline phosphatase) if appropriate, for inadequate response, or in patients who are symptomatic.

Aclasta (Canadian brand): 5 mg as a single dose. Data concerning retreatment is limited; retreatment with 5 mg (single dose) may be considered for relapse after an interval of at least 1 year from initial treatment.

Prevention of aromatase inhibitor-induced bone loss in breast cancer (unlabeled use): Adults: I.V.: 4 mg once every 6 months for 5 years (Brufsky, 2012)

Prevention of androgen deprivation-induced bone loss in nonmetastatic prostate cancer (unlabeled use): Adults: I.V.: 4 mg once every 3 months for 1 year (Smith, 2003) or 4 mg once every 12 months (Michaelson, 2007)

Dosage adjustment in renal impairment (at treatment initiation): Note: Prior to each dose, obtain serum creatinine and calculate the creatinine clearance using the Cockcroft-Gault formula.

Nononcology uses: **Note:** Use actual body weight in the Cockcroft-Gault formula when calculating clearance for nononcology uses.

Cl_{cr} ≥35 mL/minute: No dosage adjustment required.

Cl_{cr} <35 mL/minute: Use is contraindicated.

Oncology uses:

Multiple myeloma and bone metastases:

Cl_{cr} >60 mL/minute: 4 mg (no dosage adjustment necessary)

Cl_{cr} 50-60 mL/minute: Reduce dose to 3.5 mg

Cl_{cr} 40-49 mL/minute: Reduce dose to 3.3 mg

Cl_{cr} 30-39 mL/minute: Reduce dose to 3 mg

Cl_{cr} <30 mL/minute: Use is not recommended.

Hypercalcemia of malignancy:

Mild-to-moderate impairment: No dosage adjustment necessary.

Severe impairment (serum creatinine >4.5 mg/dL):

U.S. labeling: Evaluate risk versus benefit

Canadian labeling: Use is not recommended.

Dosage adjustment for renal toxicity (during treatment):

Hypercalcemia of malignancy: Evidence of renal deterioration: Evaluate risk versus benefit.

Multiple myeloma and bone metastases: Evidence of renal deterioration: Withhold dose until renal function returns to within 10% of baseline; renal deterioration defined as follows:

Normal baseline creatinine: Increase of 0.5 mg/dL

Abnormal baseline creatinine: Increase of 1 mg/dL

Reinitiate therapy at the same dose administered prior to treatment interruption.

Multiple myeloma: Albuminuria >500 mg/24 hours (unexplained): Withhold dose until return to baseline, then reevaluate every 3-4 weeks; consider reinitiating with a longer infusion time of at least 30 minutes (Kyle, 2007).

Dosage adjustment in hepatic impairment: No dosage adjustment provided in the manufacturer's labeling (has not been studied); however, zoledronic acid is not metabolized hepatically.

Dietary Considerations

Multiple myeloma or metastatic bone lesions from solid tumors: Take daily calcium supplement (500 mg) and daily multivitamin (with 400 units vitamin D).

Osteoporosis: Ensure adequate calcium and vitamin D intake; if dietary intake is inadequate, dietary supplementation is recommended. Women and men should consume:

Calcium: 1000 mg/day (men: 50-70 years) **or** 1200 mg/day (women ≥51 years and men ≥71 years) (IOM, 2011; NOF, 2013)

Vitamin D: 800-1000 IU/day (men and women ≥50 years) (NOF, 2013). Recommended Dietary Allowance (RDA): 600 IU/day (men and women ≤70 years) **or** 800 IU/day (men and women ≥71 years) (IOM, 2011).

Paget's disease: Take elemental calcium 1500 mg/day (750 mg twice daily or 500 mg 3 times/day) and vitamin D 800 units/day, particularly during the first 2 weeks after administration.

Administration If refrigerated, allow solution to reach room temperature before administration. Infuse over at least 15 minutes. Flush I.V. line with 10 mL NS flush following infusion. Infuse in a line separate from other medications. Patients must be appropriately hydrated prior to treatment. Acetaminophen after administration may reduce the incidence of acute reaction (eg, arthralgia, fever, flu-like symptoms, myalgia).

Hazardous agent; use appropriate precautions for handling and disposal (NIOSH, 2012).

Monitoring Parameters Prior to initiation of therapy, dental exam and preventative dentistry for patients at risk for osteonecrosis, including all cancer patients

Nononcology uses: Serum creatinine prior to each dose, especially in patients with risk factors, calculate creatinine clearance before each treatment (consider interim monitoring in patients at risk for acute renal failure), evaluate fluid status and adequately hydrate patients prior to and following administration.

Osteoporosis: Bone mineral density (BMD) should be reevaluated every 2 years (or more frequently) after initiating therapy (NOF, 2013); in patients with combined zoledronic acid and glucocorticoid treatment, BMD should be made at initiation of therapy and repeated after 6-12 months; serum calcium and 25(OH)D; annual measurements of height and weight, assessment of chronic back pain; serum calcium and 25(OH)D; phosphorus and magnesium; may consider monitoring biochemical markers of bone turnover

Paget's disease: Alkaline phosphatase; pain; serum calcium and 25(OH)D; phosphorus and magnesium; symptoms of hypocalcemia

Oncology uses: Serum creatinine prior to each dose; serum electrolytes, phosphate, magnesium, and hemoglobin/hematocrit should be evaluated regularly. Monitor serum calcium to assess response and avoid overtreatment. In patients with multiple myeloma, monitor urine every 3-6 months for albuminuria.

Reference Range

Calcium (total): Adults: 9.0-11.0 mg/dL (2.05-2.54 mmol/L), may slightly decrease with aging

Phosphorus: 2.5-4.5 mg/dL (0.81-1.45 mmol/L)

Vitamin D: There is no clear consensus on a reference range for total serum 25(OH)D concentrations or the validity of this level as it relates clinically to bone health. In addition, there is significant variability in the reporting of serum 25(OH)D levels as a result of different assay types in use; however, the following ranges have been suggested:

Adults (IOM, 2011): Sufficient levels in practically all persons: ≥20 ng/mL (50 nmol/L); concern for risk of toxicity: >50 ng/mL (125 nmol/L)

Osteoporosis patients (NOF, 2013): Recommended level to reach and maintain: ~30 ng/mL (75 nmol/L)

Test Interactions Bisphosphonates may interfere with diagnostic imaging agents such as technetium-99m-diphosphonate in bone scans.

Additional Information Oncology Comment:

Metastatic breast cancer: The American Society of Clinical Oncology (ASCO) guidelines on the role of bone-modifying agents (BMAs) in the prevention and treatment of skeletal-related events for metastatic breast cancer patients were updated (Van Poznak, 2011). The guidelines recommend initiating a BMA (denosumab, pamidronate, zoledronic acid) in patients with a diagnosis of metastatic breast cancer to the bone. There is currently no literature indicating the superiority of one particular BMA over another. The optimal duration has yet to be defined; however, the guidelines recommend continuing therapy until substantial decline in patient's performance status. In patients with normal creatinine clearance (>60 mL/minute), no dosage/interval/infusion rate changes for pamidronate or zoledronic acid are necessary. For patients with Cl_{cr} <30 mL/minute, pamidronate and zoledronic acid are not recommended. While no renal dose adjustments are recommended for denosumab, close monitoring is advised for risk of hypocalcemia in patients with Cl_{cr} <30 mL/minute or on dialysis. The ASCO guidelines are in alignment with package insert guidelines for dosing, renal dose adjustments, infusion times, prevention and management of osteonecrosis of the jaw, and monitoring of laboratory parameter recommendations. BMAs are not the first-line therapy for pain. BMAs are to be used as adjunctive therapy for cancer-related bone pain associated with bone metastasis, demonstrating a modest pain control benefit. BMAs should be used in conjunction with agents such as NSAIDS, opioid and nonopioid analgesics, corticosteroids, radiation/surgery, interventional procedures.

Multiple myeloma: The American Society of Clinical Oncology (ASCO) also has guidelines published on the use of bisphosphonates for prevention and treatment of bone disease in multiple myeloma (Kyle, 2007). Pamidronate or zoledronic acid use is recommended in multiple myeloma patients with lytic bone destruction or compression spine fracture from osteopenia. Clodronate (not available in the U.S.; available in Canada), administered orally or I.V., is an alternative treatment. The use of the bisphosphonates pamidronate and zoledronic acid may be considered in patients with pain secondary to osteolytic disease, adjunct therapy to stabilize fractures or impending fractures, and I.V. bisphosphonates for multiple myeloma patients with osteopenia but no radiographic evidence of lytic bone disease. Bisphosphonates are not recommended in patients with solitary plasmacytoma, smoldering (asymptomatic) or indolent myeloma, or monoclonal gammopathy of undetermined significance. The guidelines recommend monthly treatment for a period of 2 years. At that time, physicians need to consider discontinuing in responsive and stable patients, and reinitiate if new-onset skeletal-related event occurs. The ASCO guidelines are in alignment with package insert guidelines for dosing, renal dose adjustments, infusion times, prevention and management of osteonecrosis of the jaw, and monitoring of laboratory parameter recommendations. The guidelines also state in patients with a serum creatinine >3 mg/dL or Cl_{cr} <30 mL/minute or extensive bone disease, pamidronate at a dose of 90 mg over 4-6 hours is recommended (unless pre-existing renal disease at which a reduced dose should be considered). The ASCO committee also recommends monitoring for the presence of albuminuria every 3-6 months. In patients with albuminuria >500 mg/24 hours, withhold the dose until level returns to baseline, then recheck every 3-4 weeks. Pamidronate may be reinitiated at a dose not to exceed 90 mg every 4 weeks with a longer infusion time of at least 4 hours. The committee also recommends considering increasing the infusion time of zoledronic acid to at least 30 minutes. However, one study has demonstrated that extending the infusion to 30 minutes did not change the safety profile (Berenson, 2011).

Dosage Forms Excipient information presented when available (limited, particularly for generics); consult specific product labeling.

Concentrate, Intravenous:
- Zometa: 4 mg/5 mL (5 mL)
- Generic: 4 mg/5 mL (5 mL)

Concentrate, Intravenous [preservative free]:
- Generic: 4 mg/5 mL (5 mL)

Solution, Intravenous:
- Reclast: 5 mg/100 mL (100 mL)
- Zometa: 4 mg/100 mL (100 mL)
- Generic: 5 mg/100 mL (100 mL)

Solution, Intravenous [preservative free]:
- Generic: 4 mg/100 mL (100 mL); 5 mg/100 mL (100 mL)

Solution Reconstituted, Intravenous:
- Generic: 4 mg (1 ea)

Dosage Forms: Canada Excipient information presented when available (limited, particularly for generics); consult specific product labeling.

Concentrate, Intravenous:
- Zometa: 4 mg/5 mL (5 mL)

Infusion, Solution [premixed]:
- Aclasta: 5 mg/100 mL (100 mL)

◆ Zolinza *see* Vorinostat *on page 2207*

◆ Zolinza® (Can) *see* Vorinostat *on page 2207*

ZOLMitriptan (zohl mi TRIP tan)

Brand Names: U.S. Zomig; Zomig ZMT

Brand Names: Canada Dom-Zolmitriptan; Mylan-Zolmitriptan; Mylan-Zolmitriptan ODT; PMS-Zolmitriptan; PMS-Zolmitriptan ODT; Riva-Zolmitriptan; Sandoz-Zolmitriptan; Sandoz-Zolmitriptan ODT; Teva-Zolmitriptan; Teva-Zolmitriptan OD; Zolmitriptan ODT; Zomig; Zomig Nasal Spray; Zomig Rapimelt

Index Terms 311C90

Pharmacologic Category Antimigraine Agent; Serotonin 5-$HT_{1B, 1D}$ Receptor Agonist

Additional Appendix Information

Antimigraine Drugs: 5-HT_1 Receptor Agonists *on page 2288*

Use Migraines: Acute treatment of migraine with or without aura in adults

Unlabeled Use Short-term prevention of menstrual migraines

Pregnancy Risk Factor C

Pregnancy Considerations Adverse events were observed in animal reproduction studies. Information related to zolmitriptan use in pregnancy is limited (Källén, 2011; Nezvalová-Henriksen, 2010; Nezvalová-Henriksen, 2012). Until additional information is available, other agents are preferred for the initial treatment of migraine in pregnancy (Da Silva, 2012; MacGregor, 2012; Williams, 2012).

Breast-Feeding Considerations It is not known if zolmitriptan is excreted in breast milk. Due to the potential for serious adverse reactions in the nursing infant, the decision to continue or discontinue breast-feeding during therapy should take into account the risk of exposure to the infant and the benefits of treatment to the mother.

Contraindications

Ischemic coronary artery disease (angina pectoris, history of myocardial infarction [MI], or documented silent ischemia); coronary artery vasospasm, including Prinzmetal variant angina, or other significant underlying cardiovascular disease; Wolff-Parkinson-White syndrome or arrhythmias associated with other cardiac accessory conduction pathway disorders; peripheral vascular disease; ischemic bowel disease; uncontrolled hypertension; recent use (within 24 hours) of treatment with another 5-HT_1 agonist, or an ergotamine-containing or ergot-type medication like dihydroergotamine or methysergide; history of stroke, transient ischemic attack, or history of hemiplegic or basilar migraine; coadministration of monoamine oxidase A (MAO A) inhibitors or use of zolmitriptan within 2 weeks of discontinuation of MAO A inhibitor therapy; hypersensitivity to zolmitriptan or any component of the formulation.

Documentation of allergenic cross-reactivity for triptans is limited. However, because of similarities in chemical structure and/or pharmacologic actions, the possibility of cross-sensitivity cannot be ruled out with certainty.

Warnings/Precautions Zolmitriptan is indicated only in patient populations with a clear diagnosis of migraine. If a patient does not respond to the first dose, the diagnosis of migraine should be reconsidered; rule out underlying neurologic disease in patients with atypical headache and in patients with no prior history of migraine. Not indicated for migraine prophylaxis (may be used off-label for menstrual migraine prophylaxis) or for the treatment of cluster headache. Acute migraine agents (eg, triptans, opioids, ergotamine, or a combination of the agents) used for 10 or more days per month may lead to worsening of headaches (medication overuse headache); withdrawal treatment may be necessary in the setting of overuse. Not for prophylactic treatment of migraine headaches. Cardiac events (coronary artery vasospasm, transient ischemia, myocardial infarction, ventricular tachycardia/fibrillation, cardiac arrest, and death) have been reported within a few hours of 5-HT_1 agonist administration; use in contraindicated in patients with ischemic or vasospastic coronary artery disease. Patients who experience sensations of chest pain/pressure/tightness or symptoms suggestive of angina following dosing should be evaluated for coronary artery disease or Prinzmetal's angina before receiving additional doses; if dosing is resumed and similar symptoms recur, monitor with ECG. Patients with Prinzmetal's variant angina, Wolff-Parkinson-White Syndrome or arrhythmias associated with other cardiac accessory conduction pathway disorders should not receive zolmitriptan. Should not be given to patients who have risk factors for CAD (eg, hypertension, hypercholesterolemia, smoker, obesity, diabetes, strong family history of CAD, menopause, male >40 years of age) without adequate cardiac evaluation. Patients with suspected CAD should have cardiovascular evaluation to rule out CAD before considering zolmitriptan's use; if cardiovascular evaluation negative, first dose would be safest if given in the healthcare provider's office (consider

ECG monitoring). Periodic evaluation of those without cardiovascular disease, but with continued risk factors, should be done. Significant elevation in blood pressure, including hypertensive crisis, has been reported in patients with and without a history of hypertension. Use is contraindicated in patients with uncontrolled hypertension. Peripheral vascular ischemia, gastrointestinal vascular ischemia, and infarction (presenting with abdominal pain and bloody diarrhea, splenic infarction, and Raynaud's syndrome have been reported with 5-HT_1 agonists. In patients who experience signs or symptoms suggestive of a vasospastic reaction following use of a 5-HT_1 agonist, rule out a vasospastic reaction before receiving additional doses. Cerebral/subarachnoid hemorrhage and stroke have been reported with 5-HT_1 agonist administration and some have resulted in fatalities. Do not administer to patients with a history of stroke or TIA; discontinue use if a cerebrovascular event occurs. Rarely, partial vision loss and blindness (transient and permanent) have been reported with 5-HT_1 agonists. Use with caution in patients with hepatic impairment. Zomig-ZMT tablets contain phenylalanine. Symptoms of agitation, confusion, hallucinations, labile blood pressure, hyper-reflexia, incoordination, myoclonus, shivering, and tachycardia (serotonin syndrome) may occur with concomitant proserotonergic drugs (eg, SSRIs, SNRIs, TCAs, MAO inhibitors, or triptans) or agents which reduce zolmitriptan's metabolism. Elderly patients are more likely to have underlying cardiovascular disease and hepatic or renal impairment; use with caution. Cardiovascular evaluation is recommended for elderly patients with other cardiovascular risk factors prior to initiation of therapy. Zomig-ZMT tablets contain phenylalanine.

Adverse Reactions

>10%: Gastrointestinal: Unpleasant taste (17% to 21%)

1% to 10%:

Cardiovascular: Chest pain (1% to 4%), palpitations (≤2%), facial edema (1% to <2%)

Central nervous system: Dizziness (6% to 10%), paresthesia (5% to 10%), drowsiness (4% to 8%), local alterations in temperature sensations (5% to 7%), sensation of pressure (2% to 5%), hyperesthesia (1% to 5%), hypoesthesia (1% to 5%), flushing sensation (≤4%), pain (2% to 4%), myasthenia (≤2%), vertigo (≤2%), chills (1% to <2%), depersonalization (1% to <2%), headache (1% to <2%), insomnia (1% to <2%)

Dermatologic: Application site irritation (nasal spray 3%), diaphoresis (≤3%)

Gastrointestinal: Nausea (4% to 9%), xerostomia (2% to 5%), dyspepsia (2% to 3%), dysphagia (≤2%), abdominal pain (1% to <2%), vomiting (1% to <2%)

Hypersensitivity: Hypersensitivity reaction (≤1%)

Local: Local pain (neck/throat/jaw; 4% to 10%)

Neuromuscular & skeletal: Weakness (3% to 9%), myalgia (1% to 2%), arthralgia (1% to <2%)

Respiratory: Nasal discomfort (nasal spray 3%), constriction of the pharynx (1% to 2%), pressure on pharynx (1% to <2%)

<1% (Limited to important or life-threatening): Amblyopia, anaphylactoid reaction, anaphylaxis, angina pectoris, apnea, arthritis, ataxia, atrial fibrillation, bradycardia, breast carcinoma, breast neoplasm, cardiac arrhythmia, cerebral ischemia, confusion, coronary artery vasospasm, cyanosis, eosinophilia, erythema multiforme, esophagitis, fibrocystic breast disease, gastrointestinal carcinoma, gastrointestinal infarction, gastrointestinal necrosis, genitourinary neoplasm, hallucination, hematemesis, hepatic neoplasm, hypertension, hypertensive crisis, hyperthyroidism, infection, intestinal obstruction, ischemic colitis, ischemic heart disease, mania, melena, myocardial infarction, neoplasm, pancreatitis, pneumonia, prolonged Q-T interval on ECG, psychosis, pyelonephritis, seizure, serotonin syndrome, sialadenitis, skin neoplasm, skin photosensitivity, splenic infarction, syncope, tardive dyskinesia, tetany, thrombocytopenia, ulcer, urinary tract infection, uterine fibroid enlargement, vaginitis, vasodilatation, visual field defect

Drug Interactions

Metabolism/Transport Effects Substrate of CYP1A2 (minor); **Note:** Assignment of Major/Minor substrate status based on clinically relevant drug interaction potential

Avoid Concomitant Use

Avoid concomitant use of ZOLMitriptan with any of the following: Ergot Derivatives; MAO Inhibitors

Increased Effect/Toxicity

ZOLMitriptan may increase the levels/effects of: Antipsychotics; Ergot Derivatives; Metoclopramide; Serotonin Modulators

The levels/effects of ZOLMitriptan may be increased by: Antipsychotics; Cimetidine; Ergot Derivatives; MAO Inhibitors; Propranolol

Decreased Effect There are no known significant interactions involving a decrease in effect.

Storage/Stability Store at 20°C to 25°C (68°F to 77°F). Protect tablets from light and moisture.

Mechanism of Action Selective agonist for serotonin (5-HT_{1B} and 5-HT_{1D} receptors) in cranial arteries and sensory nerves of the trigeminal system; causes vasoconstriction and reduces inflammation associated with antidromic neuronal transmission correlating with relief of migraine

Pharmacodynamics/Kinetics

Absorption: Well absorbed

Distribution: V_d: Oral: 7 L/kg; Nasal spray: 8.4 L/kg

Protein binding: 25%

Metabolism: Converted to an active N-desmethyl metabolite (2-6 times more potent than zolmitriptan at 5-HT_{1B} and 5-HT_{1D} receptors)

Bioavailability: 40% (not impacted by food); mean bioavailability of nasal spray compared with oral tablet: 102%

Half-life elimination: 3 hours

Time to peak, serum: Tablet: 1.5 hours; Orally-disintegrating tablet and nasal spray: 3 hours

Excretion: Urine (~60% to 65% total dose; 8% of total dose as unchanged drug; 4% of total dose as N-desmethyl metabolite); feces (30%)

Dosage Adults:

Migraine:

Initial dose: **Note:** Administer at the onset of migraine headache.

Nasal inhalation: 2.5 mg (maximum 5 mg)

Oral:

Tablet: 1.25-2.5 mg (maximum: 5 mg)

Orally-disintegrating tablet: 2.5 mg (maximum: 5 mg)

Second dose (either nasal inhalation or oral): May repeat in 2 hours if the migraine headache has not resolved or returns after transient improvement (maximum daily dose: 10 mg)

Menstrual migraine, prophylaxis (unlabeled use): Oral: 2.5 mg 2-3 times daily starting 2 days prior to the expected onset of menses and continued through to 5 days after the onset of menses (7 days total) (Tuchman, 2008)

Elderly: Initiate therapy at the low end of the dosing range.

Dosage adjustment for concomitant therapy with cimetidine: Maximum single dose: 2.5 mg (maximum daily dose: 5 mg)

Dosage adjustment in renal impairment: No dosage adjustment provided in manufacturer's labeling; however, zolmitriptan clearance is reduced in patients with severe renal impairment (Cl_{cr} 5-25 mL/minute).

Dosage adjustment in hepatic impairment:

Tablet: Moderate to severe impairment: Initial: 1.25 mg (maximum daily dose: 5 mg)

Orally disintegrating tablet: Not recommended in patients with moderate or severe hepatic impairment; oral disintegrating tablets should not be broken in half.

Nasal inhalation: Not recommended in patients with moderate or severe hepatic impairment

Dietary Considerations Some products may contain phenylalanine.

Administration Administer as soon as migraine headache starts.

Tablet: May be broken in half to achieve a smaller initial dose.

Orally-disintegrating tablet: Must be taken whole; do not break, crush, or chew. Place on tongue and allow to dissolve. Administration with liquid is not required.

Nasal spray: Blow nose gently prior to use. After removing protective cap, instill device into nostril. Block opposite nostril; breathe in gently through nose while pressing plunger of spray device. Breathe gently through mouth for 5-10 seconds.

Monitoring Parameters Headache severity, signs/symptoms suggestive of angina; blood pressure; ECG with first dose in patients with likelihood of unrecognized coronary disease, such as patients with significant hypertension, hypercholesterolemia, obese patients, patients with diabetes, smokers with other risk factors or strong family history of coronary artery disease

Dosage Forms Excipient information presented when available (limited, particularly for generics); consult specific product labeling.

Solution, Nasal:

Zomig: 2.5 mg (6 ea); 5 mg (6 ea)

Tablet, Oral:

Zomig: 2.5 mg [scored]

Zomig: 5 mg

Generic: 2.5 mg, 5 mg

Tablet Dispersible, Oral:

Zomig ZMT: 2.5 mg, 5 mg [contains aspartame; orange flavor]

Generic: 2.5 mg, 5 mg

◆ **Zolmitriptan ODT (Can)** *see* ZOLMitriptan *on page 2240*

◆ **Zoloft** *see* Sertraline *on page 1889*

Zolpidem (zole PI dem)

Brand Names: U.S. Ambien; Ambien CR; Edluar; Intermezzo; Zolpimist

Brand Names: Canada Sublinox

Index Terms Zolpidem Tartrate

Pharmacologic Category Hypnotic, Miscellaneous

Additional Appendix Information

Beers Criteria – Potentially Inappropriate Medications for Geriatrics *on page 2368*

Use

Ambien, Edluar, Zolpimist: Short-term treatment of insomnia (with difficulty of sleep onset)

Ambien CR: Treatment of insomnia (with difficulty of sleep onset and/or sleep maintenance)

Intermezzo: "As needed" treatment of middle-of-the-night insomnia with ≥4 hours of sleep time remaining.

Sublinox (Canadian availability; not available in U.S.): Short-term treatment of insomnia (with difficulty of sleep onset, frequent awakenings, and/or early awakenings)

Pregnancy Risk Factor C

Pregnancy Considerations Adverse events were observed in some animal reproduction studies. Zolpidem crosses the placenta (Juric, 2009). Severe neonatal respiratory depression has been reported when zolpidem was used at the end of pregnancy, especially when used concurrently with other CNS depressants. Children born of mothers taking sedative/hypnotics may be at risk for withdrawal; neonatal flaccidity has been reported in infants following maternal use of sedative/hypnotics during pregnancy. Additional adverse effects to the fetus/newborn have been noted in some studies (Wang, 2010; Wikner, 2011).

Breast-Feeding Considerations Zolpidem is excreted in breast milk. The manufacturer recommends that caution be exercised when administering zolpidem to nursing women.

Medication Guide Available Yes

Contraindications Hypersensitivity to zolpidem or any component of the formulation

Canadian labeling: Additional contraindications (not in U.S. labeling): Significant obstructive sleep apnea syndrome and acute and/or severe impairment of respiratory function; myasthenia gravis; severe hepatic impairment; personal or family history of sleepwalking

Warnings/Precautions Should be used only after evaluation of potential causes of sleep disturbance. Failure of sleep disturbance to resolve after 7-10 days may indicate psychiatric or medical illness. Hypnotics/sedatives have been associated with abnormal thinking and behavior changes including decreased inhibition, aggression, bizarre behavior, agitation, hallucinations, and depersonalization. These changes may occur unpredictably and may indicate previously unrecognized psychiatric disorders; evaluate appropriately. Sedative/hypnotics may produce withdrawal symptoms following abrupt discontinuation. Use with caution in patients with depression; worsening of depression, including suicide or suicidal ideation has been reported with the use of hypnotics. Intentional overdose may be an issue in this population. The minimum dose that will effectively treat the individual patient should be used. Prescriptions should be written for the smallest quantity consistent with good patient care. Causes CNS depression, which may impair physical and mental capabilities. Zolpidem should only be administered when the patient is able to stay in bed a full night (7-8 hours) before being active again. Potentially significant drug-drug interactions may exist, requiring dose or frequency adjustment, additional monitoring, and/or selection of alternative therapy. Consult drug interactions database for more detailed information. Effects with other sedative drugs or ethanol may be potentiated. Canadian labeling does not recommend concomitant use with alcohol.

Use caution in patients with myasthenia gravis (contraindicated in the Canadian labeling). Avoid use in patients with sleep apnea or a history of sedative-hypnotic abuse. Postmarketing studies have indicated that the use of hypnotic/sedative agents (including zolpidem) for sleep has been associated with hypersensitivity reactions including anaphylaxis as well as angioedema. An increased risk for hazardous sleep-related activities such as sleep-driving; cooking and eating food, and making phone calls while asleep have also been noted; amnesia may also occur. Discontinue treatment in patients who report any sleep-related episodes. Canadian labeling recommends avoiding use in patients with disorders (eg, restless legs syndrome, periodic limb movement disorder, sleep apnea) that may disrupt sleep and cause frequent awakenings, potentially increasing the risk of complex sleep-related behaviors. Use with caution in patients with a history of drug dependence. Risk of abuse is increased in patients with a history or family history of alcohol or drug abuse or mental illness.

Use caution with respiratory disease (Canadian labeling contraindicates use with acute and/or severe impairment of respiratory function). Use caution with hepatic impairment (Canadian labeling contraindicates use in severe impairment); dose adjustment required. Because of the rapid onset of action, administer immediately prior to bedtime, after the patient has gone to bed and is having difficulty falling asleep, or during the middle of the night when at least 4 hours are left before waking (Intermezzo).

Use caution in the elderly; dose adjustment recommended. Closely monitor elderly or debilitated patients for impaired cognitive and/or motor performance, confusion, and potential for falling. Avoid chronic use (>90 days) in older adults; adverse events, including delirium, falls, fractures, have been observed with nonbenzodiazepine hypnotic use in the elderly similar to events observed with benzodiazepines. Data suggests improvements in sleep duration and latency are minimal (Beers Criteria).

Dosage adjustment is recommended for females; pharmacokinetic studies involving zolpidem showed a significant increase in maximum concentration and exposure in females compared to males at the same dose. When studied for the unapproved use of insomnia associated with ADHD in children, a higher incidence (~7%) of hallucinations was reported. In addition, sleep latency did not decrease compared to placebo. Zolpidem is **not** FDA- or Health Canada-approved for use in pediatric patients.

Adverse Reactions Actual frequency may be dosage form, dose, and/or age dependent

>10%: Central nervous system: Headache (7% to 19%), drowsiness (2% to 15%), dizziness (5% to 12%)

1% to 10%:

Cardiovascular: Chest discomfort, increased blood pressure, palpitations

Central nervous system: Abnormal dreams, amnesia, anxiety, apathy, ataxia, burning sensation, confusion, depersonalization, depression, disinhibition, disorientation, drugged feeling, eating disorder (binge eating), emotional lability, equilibrium disturbance, euphoria, fatigue, hallucination, hypoesthesia, increased body temperature, insomnia, lack of concentration, lethargy, memory impairment, paresthesia, psychomotor retardation, sleep disorder, stress, vertigo

Dermatologic: Skin rash, urticaria, wrinkling of skin

Endocrine & metabolic: Hypermenorrhea

Gastrointestinal: Abdominal distress, abdominal tenderness, change in appetite, constipation, diarrhea, dyspepsia, flatulence, frequent bowel movements, gastroenteritis, gastroesophageal reflux disease, hiccups, nausea, vomiting, xerostomia

Genitourinary: Dysuria, urinary tract infection, vaginal dryness

Hypersensitivity: Hypersensitivity reaction

Neuromuscular & skeletal: Arthralgia, back pain, muscle cramps, muscle spasm, myalgia, neck pain, tremor, weakness

Ophthalmic: Accommodation disturbance, asthenopia, blurred vision, diplopia, eye redness, visual disturbance (including altered depth perception)

Otic: Labyrinthitis, tinnitus

Respiratory: Dry throat, flu-like symptoms, lower respiratory tract infection, pharyngitis, sinusitis, throat irritation, upper respiratory tract infection

Miscellaneous: Fever

<1% (Limited to important or life-threatening): Abnormal hepatic function tests, acute renal failure, aggressive behavior, anaphylaxis, anemia, angina pectoris, angioedema, anorexia, arteritis, arthritis, breast fibroadenosis, breast neoplasm, bronchitis, cardiac arrhythmia, cerebrovascular disease, circulatory shock, cognitive dysfunction, corneal ulcer, delusions, dementia, dermatitis, drug tolerance, dysarthria, dysphagia, edema, extrasystoles, glaucoma, hepatic insufficiency, hyperbilirubinemia, hyperglycemia, hyperlipidemia, hypertension, hypotension, hysteria, illusion, impotence, leukopenia, lymphadenopathy, migraine, myocardial infarction, neuralgia, neuritis, neuropathy, orthostatic hypotension, panic disorder, personality disorder, psychoneurosis, pulmonary edema, pulmonary embolism, pyelonephritis, respiratory depression, restless leg syndrome, rhinitis, scleritis, somnambulism, syncope, tachycardia, tenesmus, tetany, thrombosis, urinary incontinence, vaginitis, ventricular tachycardia

Drug Interactions

Metabolism/Transport Effects Substrate of CYP1A2 (minor), CYP2C19 (minor), CYP2C9 (minor), CYP2D6 (minor), CYP3A4 (major); **Note:** Assignment of Major/Minor substrate status based on clinically relevant drug interaction potential

Avoid Concomitant Use

Avoid concomitant use of Zolpidem with any of the following: Azelastine (Nasal); Conivaptan; Fusidic Acid (Systemic); Paraldehyde; Sodium Oxybate

Increased Effect/Toxicity

Zolpidem may increase the levels/effects of: Alcohol (Ethyl); Azelastine (Nasal); Buprenorphine; CarBAMazepine; Hydrocodone; Methotrimeprazine; Metyrosine; Mirtazapine; Paraldehyde; Pramipexole; ROPINIRole; Rotigotine; Selective Serotonin Reuptake Inhibitors; Sodium Oxybate

The levels/effects of Zolpidem may be increased by: Antifungal Agents (Azole Derivatives, Systemic); Brimonidine (Topical); CNS Depressants; Conivaptan; CYP3A4 Inhibitors (Moderate); CYP3A4 Inhibitors (Strong); Dasatinib; Doxylamine; Droperidol; Fluconazole; FluvoxaMINE; Fusidic Acid (Systemic); HydrOXYzine; Ivacaftor; Luliconazole; Magnesium Sulfate; Methotrimeprazine; Mifepristone; Perampanel; Simeprevir; Tapentadol

Decreased Effect

The levels/effects of Zolpidem may be decreased by: Bosentan; CarBAMazepine; CYP3A4 Inducers (Strong); Dabrafenib; Deferasirox; Flumazenil; Herbs (CYP3A4 Inducers); Mitotane; Peginterferon Alfa-2b; Rifamycin Derivatives; Telaprevir; Tocilizumab

Ethanol/Nutrition/Herb Interactions

Ethanol: May enhance the adverse/toxic effects of zolpidem. Management: Avoid use of ethanol.

Food: Maximum plasma concentration and bioavailability are decreased with food; time to peak plasma concentration is increased; half-life remains unchanged. Grapefruit juice may decrease the metabolism of zolpidem. Management: Avoid grapefruit juice.

Herb/Nutraceutical: St John's wort may decrease the levels/effects of zolpidem. Some herbal medications should be avoided due to the risk of increased CNS depression. Management: Avoid concomitant use of St John's wort. Avoid valerian, kava kava, and gotu kola.

Storage/Stability

Ambien, Edluar, Intermezzo: Store at 20°C to 25°C (68°F to 77°F). Protect sublingual tablets from light and moisture.

Ambien CR: Store at 15°C to 25°C (59°F to 77°F); limited excursions permitted up to 30°C (86°F).

Zolpimist: Store at 25°C (77°F); do not freeze. Avoid prolonged exposure to temperatures >30°C (86°F).

Sublinox (Canadian availability; not available in U.S.): Store at 15°C to 30°C (59°F to 86°F); protect from light and moisture.

Mechanism of Action Zolpidem, an imidazopyridine hypnotic that is structurally dissimilar to benzodiazepines, enhances the activity of the inhibitory neurotransmitter, γ-aminobutyric acid (GABA), via selective agonism at the benzodiazepine-1 (BZ_1) receptor; the result is increased chloride conductance, neuronal hyperpolarization, inhibition of the action potential, and a decrease in neuronal excitability leading to sedative and hypnotic effects. Because of its selectivity for the BZ_1 receptor site over the BZ_2 receptor site, zolpidem exhibits minimal anxiolytic, myorelaxant, and anticonvulsant properties (effects largely attributed to agonism at the BZ_2 receptor site).

Pharmacodynamics/Kinetics

Onset of action: Immediate release: 30 minutes

Duration: Immediate release: 6-8 hours

Absorption: Rapid; C_{max} and AUC is increased by ~45% in females compared to male subjects

Distribution: V_d: 0.54 L/kg after an I.V. dose (Holm, 2000)

Protein binding: ~93%

Metabolism: Hepatic methylation and hydroxylation via CYP3A4 (~60%), CYP2C9 (~22%), CYP1A2 (~14%), CYP2D6 (~3%), and CYP2C19 (~3%) to 3 inactive metabolites (Holm, 2000)

Bioavailability: Immediate-release tablet: 70% (Holm, 2000)

Half-life elimination:

Immediate release, Extended release: ~2.5 hours (range: 1.4-4.5 hours); Cirrhosis: Up to 9.9 hours; Elderly: Prolonged up to 32%

Spray: ~3 hours (range: 1.7-8.4)

Sublingual tablet (Edluar, Intermezzo): ~3 hours (range: 1.4-6.7 hours)

Time to peak, plasma:

Immediate release: 1.6 hours; 2.2 hours with food

Extended release: 1.5 hours; 4 hours with food

Spray: ~0.9 hours

Sublingual tablet: Edluar: ~1.4 hours, ~1.8 hours with food; Intermezzo: 0.6-1.3 hours, ~3 hours with food

Excretion: Urine (48% to 67%, primarily as metabolites); feces (29% to 42%, primarily as metabolites)

Dosage Oral:

Adults: **Note:** The lowest effective dose should be used; higher doses may be more likely to impair next morning activities.

Immediate release tablet, spray: 5 mg (females) or 5-10 mg (males) immediately before bedtime; maximum dose: 10 mg daily

Extended release tablet: 6.25 mg (females) or 6.25-12.5 mg (males) immediately before bedtime; maximum dose: 12.5 mg

Sublingual tablet:

Edluar: 5 mg (females) or 5-10 mg (males) immediately before bedtime; maximum dose: 10 mg daily

Sublinox (Canadian availability; not available in U.S.): 10 mg immediately before bedtime; maximum dose: 10 mg daily

Intermezzo: **Note:** Take in bed only if ≥4 hours left before waking and there is difficulty in returning to sleep.

Females: 1.75 mg once per night as needed (maximum: 1.75 mg/night)

Males: 3.5 mg once per night as needed (maximum: 3.5 mg/night)

Dosage adjustment with concomitant CNS depressants: Females and males: 1.75 mg once per night as needed; dose adjustment of concomitant CNS depressant(s) may be necessary.

Elderly:

Immediate release tablet, spray: 5 mg immediately before bedtime

Sublingual tablet:

Edluar, Sublinox (Canadian availability; not available in U.S.): 5 mg immediately before bedtime

Intermezzo: Females and males: 1.75 mg once per night as needed (maximum: 1.75 mg/night). **Note:** Take only if ≥4 hours left before waking and there is difficulty in returning to sleep.

Extended release tablet: 6.25 mg immediately before bedtime

Dosage adjustment in renal impairment: No dosage adjustment necessary. Use with caution and monitor patients with renal impairment closely. Not dialyzable.

Hemodialysis: Not dialyzable

Dosage adjustment in hepatic impairment:

U.S. labeling:

Immediate release tablet, spray: 5 mg immediately before bedtime

Extended release tablet: 6.25 mg immediately before bedtime

Sublingual tablet:

Edluar: 5 mg immediately before bedtime

Intermezzo: Females and males: 1.75 mg once per night as needed. **Note:** Take only if ≥4 hours left before waking and there is difficulty in returning to sleep.

Canadian labeling: Sublingual tablet: Sublinox:

Mild-to-moderate impairment: 5 mg immediately before bedtime; if therapy is well tolerated but ineffective, may increase to 10 mg in patients <65 years

Severe impairment: Use is contraindicated.

Dietary Considerations For faster sleep onset, do not administer with (or immediately after) a meal.

Administration Ingest immediately before bedtime due to rapid onset of action. Regardless of dosage form, do not administer with or immediately after a meal. Intermezzo should be taken in bed if patient awakes in the middle of the night (ie, if ≥4 hours left before waking) and there is difficulty in returning to sleep.

Ambien CR tablets should be swallowed whole; do not divide, crush, or chew.

Edluar, Intermezzo, or Sublinox (Canadian availability; not available in U.S.) sublingual tablets should be placed under the tongue and allowed to disintegrate; do not swallow or administer with water.

Zolpimist oral spray should be sprayed directly into the mouth over the tongue. Prior to initial use, pump should be primed by spraying 5 times. If pump is not used for at least 14 days, reprime pump with 1 spray.

Monitoring Parameters Daytime alertness; respiratory rate; behavior profile

Test Interactions Increased aminotransferase [ALT/AST], bilirubin (S); decreased RAI uptake

Additional Information Causes fewer disturbances in sleep stages as compared to benzodiazepines. Time spent in sleep stages 3 and 4 are maintained; zolpidem decreases sleep latency; should not be prescribed in quantities exceeding a 1-month supply.

Dosage Forms Excipient information presented when available (limited, particularly for generics); consult specific product labeling.

Solution, Oral, as tartrate:

Zolpimist: 5 mg/actuation (7.7 mL) [contains benzoic acid, propylene glycol; cherry flavor]

Tablet, Oral, as tartrate:

Ambien: 5 mg [contains fd&c red #40, polysorbate 80]

Ambien: 10 mg

Generic: 5 mg, 10 mg

Tablet Extended Release, Oral, as tartrate:

Ambien CR: 6.25 mg

Ambien CR: 12.5 mg [contains fd&c blue #2 (indigotine)]

Generic: 6.25 mg, 12.5 mg

Tablet Sublingual, Sublingual, as tartrate:

Edluar: 5 mg, 10 mg [contains saccharin sodium]

Intermezzo: 1.75 mg, 3.5 mg

Dosage Forms: Canada Excipient information presented when available (limited, particularly for generics); consult specific product labeling.

Tablet, sublingual, as tartrate:

Sublinox: 5 mg, 10 mg

Controlled Substance C-IV

◆ **Zolpidem Tartrate** *see* Zolpidem *on page* 2242

◆ **Zolpimist** *see* Zolpidem *on page* 2242

◆ **Zolvit®** *see* Hydrocodone and Acetaminophen *on page* 1006

- ◆ **Zometa** *see* Zoledronic Acid *on page 2235*
- ◆ **Zomig** *see* ZOLMitriptan *on page 2240*
- ◆ **Zomig Nasal Spray (Can)** *see* ZOLMitriptan *on page 2240*
- ◆ **Zomig Rapimelt (Can)** *see* ZOLMitriptan *on page 2240*
- ◆ **Zomig ZMT** *see* ZOLMitriptan *on page 2240*
- ◆ **Zonalon** *see* Doxepin (Topical) *on page 660*
- ◆ **Zonalon (Can)** *see* Doxepin (Systemic) *on page 658*
- ◆ **Zonalon® (Can)** *see* Doxepin (Topical) *on page 660*
- ◆ **Zonatuss** *see* Benzonatate *on page 243*
- ◆ **Zonegran** *see* Zonisamide *on page 2245*

Zonisamide (zoe NIS a mide)

Brand Names: U.S. Zonegran

Pharmacologic Category Anticonvulsant, Miscellaneous

Use Adjunct treatment of partial seizures in children >16 years of age and adults with epilepsy

Unlabeled Use Bipolar disorder

Pregnancy Risk Factor C

Pregnancy Considerations Teratogenic effects were observed in animal reproduction studies; therefore, zonisamide is classified as pregnancy category C. Zonisamide crosses the placenta and can be detected in the newborn following delivery. Although adverse fetal events have been reported, the risk of teratogenic effects following maternal use of zonisamide in not clearly defined. Other agents may be preferred until additional data is available. Newborns should be monitored for transient metabolic acidosis after birth. Zonisamide clearance may increase in the second trimester of pregnancy, requiring dosage adjustment. Women of childbearing potential are advised to use effective contraception during therapy.

Patients exposed to zonisamide during pregnancy are encouraged to enroll themselves into the AED Pregnancy Registry by calling 1-888-233-2334. Additional information is available at http://www.aedpregnancyregistry.org.

Breast-Feeding Considerations Zonisamide is excreted into breast milk in concentrations similar to those in the maternal plasma and has been detected in the plasma of a nursing infant. According to the manufacturer, the decision to continue or discontinue breast-feeding during therapy should take into account the risk of exposure to the infant and the benefits of treatment to the mother.

Medication Guide Available Yes

Contraindications Hypersensitivity to zonisamide, sulfonamides, or any component of the formulation

Warnings/Precautions Hazardous agent - use appropriate precautions for handling and disposal (NIOSH, 2012). Rare, but potentially fatal sulfonamide reactions have occurred following the use of zonisamide. These reactions include Stevens-Johnson syndrome, fulminant hepatic necrosis, agranulocytosis, aplastic anemia, and toxic epidermal necrolysis, usually appearing within 2-16 weeks of drug initiation. Discontinue zonisamide if rash develops. Chemical similarities are present among sulfonamides, sulfonylureas, carbonic anhydrase inhibitors, thiazides, and loop diuretics (except ethacrynic acid). Use in patients with sulfonamide allergy is specifically contraindicated in product labeling, however, a risk of cross-reaction exists in patients with allergy to any of these compounds; avoid use when previous reaction has been severe. Use may be associated with the development of metabolic acidosis (generally dose-dependent) in certain patients; predisposing conditions/therapies include renal disease, severe respiratory disease, diarrhea, surgery, ketogenic diet, and other medications. Pediatric patients may also be at an increased risk for and may have more severe metabolic acidosis. Serum bicarbonate should be monitored in all patients prior to and during use; if metabolic acidosis occurs, consider decreasing the dose or tapering the dose to discontinue. If use continued despite acidosis, alkali treatment should be considered. Untreated metabolic acidosis may increase the risk of developing nephrolithiasis, nephrocalcinosis, osteomalacia (or rickets in children), or osteoporosis; pediatric patients may also have decreased growth rates.

Pooled analysis of trials involving various antiepileptics (regardless of indication) showed an increased risk of suicidal thoughts/behavior (incidence rate: 0.43% treated patients compared to 0.24% of patients receiving placebo); risk observed as early as 1 week after initiation and continued through duration of trials (most trials ≤24 weeks). Monitor all patients for notable changes in behavior that might indicate suicidal thoughts or depression; notify healthcare provider immediately if symptoms occur.

Discontinue zonisamide in patients who develop acute renal failure or a significant sustained increase in creatinine/BUN concentration. Kidney stones have been reported. Do not use in patients with renal impairment (GFR <50 mL/minute); use with caution in patients with hepatic impairment.

Significant CNS effects include psychiatric symptoms, psychomotor slowing, and fatigue or somnolence. Fatigue and somnolence occur within the first month of treatment, most commonly at doses of 300-500 mg/day. Effects with other sedative drugs or ethanol may be potentiated. May cause sedation, which may impair physical or mental abilities; patients must be cautioned about performing tasks which require mental alertness (eg, operating machinery or driving). Abrupt withdrawal may precipitate seizures; discontinue or reduce doses gradually.

Safety and efficacy in children <16 years of age has not been established. Decreased sweating (oligohydrosis) and hyperthermia requiring hospitalization have been reported in children. Pediatric patients may also be at an increased risk and may have more severe metabolic acidosis.

Adverse Reactions Frequencies noted in patients receiving other anticonvulsants:

>10%:

Central nervous system: Somnolence (17%), dizziness (13%)

Gastrointestinal: Anorexia (13%)

1% to 10%:

Central nervous system: Headache (10%), agitation/irritability (9%), fatigue (8%), tiredness (7%), ataxia (6%), confusion (6%), concentration decreased (6%), memory impairment (6%), depression (6%), insomnia (6%), speech disorders (5%), mental slowing (4%), anxiety (3%), nervousness (2%), schizophrenic/schizophreniform behavior (2%), difficulty in verbal expression (2%), status epilepticus (1%), seizure (1%), hyperesthesia (1%), incoordination (1%)

Dermatologic: Rash (3%), bruising (2%), pruritus (1%)

Gastrointestinal: Nausea (9%), abdominal pain (6%), diarrhea (5%), dyspepsia (3%), weight loss (3%), constipation (2%), taste perversion (2%), xerostomia (2%), vomiting (1%)

Neuromuscular & skeletal: Paresthesia (4%), abnormal gait (1%), tremor (1%), weakness (1%)

Ocular: Diplopia (6%), nystagmus (4%), amblyopia (1%)

Otic: Tinnitus (1%)

Renal: Kidney stones (4%, children 3% to 8%)

Respiratory: Rhinitis (2%), pharyngitis (1%), increased cough (1%)

Miscellaneous: Flu-like syndrome (4%) accidental injury (1%)

<1% (Limited to important or life threatening): Agranulocytosis, allergic reaction, alopecia, amenorrhea, aplastic anemia, apnea, arthritis, atrial fibrillation, bladder calculus, bradycardia, cerebrovascular accident, cholangitis, cholecystitis, cholestatic jaundice, colitis, deafness, duodenitis, encephalopathy, fecal incontinence, gingivitis, GI ulcer, glaucoma, heart failure, hematuria, hemoptysis, hirsutism, hyper-/hypotension, hyperthermia, hypoglycemia, hyponatremia, immunodeficiency, impotence, iritis, leukopenia, lupus erythematosus, lymphadenopathy, mastitis, menorrhagia, metabolic acidosis, neuropathy, oculogyric crisis, oligohidrosis (children), pancreatitis, photophobia, pulmonary embolus, rectal hemorrhage, Stevens-Johnson syndrome, stroke, suicidal behavior/ideation, syncope, thrombocytopenia, thrombophlebitis, toxic epidermal necrolysis, urinary incontinence, ventricular extrasystoles

Drug Interactions

Metabolism/Transport Effects Substrate of CYP2C19 (minor), CYP3A4 (major); **Note:** Assignment of Major/Minor substrate status based on clinically relevant drug interaction potential

Avoid Concomitant Use

Avoid concomitant use of Zonisamide with any of the following: Azelastine (Nasal); Carbonic Anhydrase Inhibitors; Conivaptan; Fusidic Acid (Systemic); Paraldehyde

Increased Effect/Toxicity

Zonisamide may increase the levels/effects of: Alcohol (Ethyl); Alpha-/Beta-Agonists; Amphetamines; Anticonvulsants (Barbiturate); Anticonvulsants (Hydantoin); Azelastine (Nasal); Buprenorphine; CarBAMazepine; Carbonic Anhydrase Inhibitors; CNS Depressants; Flecainide; Hydrocodone; Memantine; MetFORMIN; Methotrimeprazine; Metyrosine; Mirtazapine; Paraldehyde; Pramipexole; Primidone; QuiNIDine; ROPINIRole; Rotigotine; Selective Serotonin Reuptake Inhibitors; Zolpidem

The levels/effects of Zonisamide may be increased by: Brimonidine (Topical); Conivaptan; CYP3A4 Inhibitors (Moderate); CYP3A4 Inhibitors (Strong); Dasatinib; Doxylamine; Droperidol; Fusidic Acid (Systemic); HydrOXYzine; Ivacaftor; Luliconazole; Magnesium Sulfate; Methotrimeprazine; Mifepristone; Perampanel; Salicylates; Simeprevir; Sodium Oxybate; Tapentadol

Decreased Effect

Zonisamide may decrease the levels/effects of: Lithium; Methenamine; Primidone

The levels/effects of Zonisamide may be decreased by: Bosentan; CYP3A4 Inducers (Strong); Dabrafenib; Deferasirox; Fosphenytoin; Herbs (CYP3A4 Inducers); Ketorolac (Nasal); Ketorolac (Systemic); Mefloquine; Mitotane; Orlistat; PHENobarbital; Phenytoin; Tocilizumab

Ethanol/Nutrition/Herb Interactions

Ethanol: May increase CNS depression; monitor for increased effects with coadministration. Caution patients about effects.

Food: Food delays time to maximum concentration, but does not affect bioavailability.

Storage/Stability Store at controlled room temperature 25°C (77°F). Protect from moisture and light.

Mechanism of Action The exact mechanism of action is not known. May stabilize neuronal membranes and suppress neuronal hypersynchronization through action at sodium and calcium channels. Does not affect GABA activity.

Pharmacodynamics/Kinetics

Distribution: V_d: 1.45 L/kg

Protein binding: 40%

Metabolism: Hepatic via CYP3A4; forms N-acetyl zonisamide and 2-sulfamoylacetyl phenol (SMAP)

Half-life elimination: Plasma: ~63 hours

Time to peak: 2-6 hours

Excretion: Urine (62%, 35% as unchanged drug, 65% as metabolites); feces (3%)

Dosage Oral:

Children >16 years and Adults:

Adjunctive treatment of partial seizures: Initial: 100 mg/day; dose may be increased to 200 mg/day after 2 weeks. Further dosage increases to 300 mg/day and 400 mg/day can then be made with a minimum of 2 weeks between adjustments, in order to reach steady state at each dosage level. Doses of up to 600 mg/day have been studied, however, there is no evidence of increased response with doses above 400 mg/day.

Mania (unlabeled use): Initial: 100-200 mg/day; maximum: 600 mg/day (Kanba, 1994)

Elderly: Data from clinical trials is insufficient for patients >65 years; begin dosing at the low end of the dosing range.

Dosage adjustment in renal impairment:

GFR ≥50 mL/minute: No dosage adjustment provided in manufacturer's labeling. However, slower titration and frequent monitoring are indicated in patients with renal disease; use with caution.

GFR <50 mL/minute: Use is not recommended.. Marked renal impairment (Cl_{cr} <20 mL/minute) was associated with a 35% increase in AUC.

Dosage adjustment in hepatic impairment: No dosage adjustment provided in manufacturer's labeling (has not been studied). However, slower titration and frequent monitoring are indicated in patients with hepatic impairment; use with caution.

Dietary Considerations May be taken without regard to meals.

Administration Capsules should be swallowed whole. Dose may be administered once or twice daily. Doses of 300 mg/day and higher are associated with increased side effects. Steady-state levels are reached in 14 days.

Hazardous agent; use appropriate precautions for handling and disposal (NIOSH, 2012).

Monitoring Parameters Metabolic profile, specifically BUN, serum creatinine; serum bicarbonate (prior to initiation and periodically during therapy); suicidality (eg, suicidal thoughts, depression, behavioral changes)

Dosage Forms Excipient information presented when available (limited, particularly for generics); consult specific product labeling.

Capsule, Oral:

Zonegran: 25 mg, 100 mg

Generic: 25 mg, 50 mg, 100 mg

Extemporaneous Preparations Hazardous agent; use appropriate precautions during preparation and disposal.

A 10 mg/mL suspension may be made using capsules and either simple syrup or methylcellulose 0.5%. Empty contents of ten 100 mg capsules into glass mortar. Reduce to a fine powder and add a small amount of Simple Syrup, NF and mix to a uniform paste; mix while adding the chosen vehicle in incremental proportions to **almost** 100 mL; transfer to an amber calibrated plastic bottle, rinse mortar with vehicle, and add quantity of vehicle sufficient to make 100 mL. Label "shake well" and "refrigerate". When using simple syrup vehicle, stable 28 days at room temperature or refrigerated (preferred). When using methylcellulose vehicle, stable 7 days at room temperature or 28 days refrigerated. **Note:** Although no visual evidence of microbial growth was observed, storage under refrigeration would be recommended to minimize microbial contamination.

Abobo CV, Wei B, and Liang D, "Stability of Zonisamide in Extemporaneously Compounded Oral Suspensions," *Am J Health Syst Pharm*, 2009, 66(12):1105-9.

◆ **Zorbtive** *see* Somatropin *on page* 1934

◆ **Zortress** *see* Everolimus *on page 807*

◆ **Zorvolex** *see* Diclofenac (Systemic) *on page 597*

◆ **Zostavax** *see* Zoster Vaccine *on page 2247*

Zoster Vaccine (ZOS ter vak SEEN)

Brand Names: U.S. Zostavax

Brand Names: Canada Zostavax

Index Terms Herpes Zoster Vaccine; HZV; Shingles Vaccine; VZV Vaccine (Zoster)

Pharmacologic Category Vaccine, Live (Viral)

Additional Appendix Information

Immunization Administration Recommendations *on page 2334*

Immunization Recommendations *on page 2339*

Use

Herpes zoster prevention: Prevention of herpes zoster (shingles) in patients ≥50 years of age

The Advisory Committee on Immunization Practices (ACIP) recommends:

Routine vaccination of **all patients ≥60 years of age, including** patients who report a previous episode of zoster; patients with chronic medical conditions (eg, chronic renal failure, diabetes mellitus, rheumatoid arthritis, chronic pulmonary disease) unless those conditions are contraindications; and residents of nursing homes and other long-term care facilities ≥60 years of age without contraindications (CDC, 2008).

Although not specifically recommended for their profession, healthcare providers within the recommended age group should also receive the zoster vaccine (CDC, 2013)

Limitations of use: Not indicated for treatment of zoster or postherpetic neuralgia (PHN); not indicated for prophylaxis of primary varicella infection (chickenpox).

Pregnancy Considerations Use during pregnancy is contraindicated. Women should avoid becoming pregnant for 3 months after vaccination (4 weeks per CDC). Risk to the fetus following exposure to wild-type varicella zoster virus is small and risk following exposure from the attenuated vaccine is probably even less (CDC, 2008). Based on information collected from 1995-2013 using the manufacturer's pregnancy registry, of 820 women who received a varicella-containing vaccine, there were no infants born with abnormalities consistent with congenital varicella syndrome. Any exposures to the vaccine during pregnancy or within 3 months prior to pregnancy should be reported to the manufacturer (Merck & Co, 877-888-4231) or to VAERS (800-822-7967) as suspected adverse reactions.

Breast-Feeding Considerations It is not known if virus from this vaccine is excreted into breast milk. Most live vaccines are not secreted into breast milk (CDC, 2011). The manufacturer recommends that caution be used if administered to a nursing woman.

Contraindications History of anaphylactic/anaphylactoid reaction to gelatin, neomycin (excluding contact dermatitis to neomycin), or any other component of the vaccine; immunosuppression or immunodeficiency, including individuals with leukemia, lymphomas, or other malignant neoplasms affecting the bone marrow or lymphatic systems; primary and acquired immunodeficiency states; AIDS or clinical manifestations of HIV; those receiving immunosuppressive therapy (including high-dose corticosteroids); pregnancy

In addition, ACIP recommends that the following immunocompromised patients should not receive zoster vaccine (CDC, 2008):

Patients undergoing hematopoietic stem cell transplant (limited data; assess risk:benefit, if needed, administer ≥24 months after transplantation);

Patients receiving recombinant human immune modulators, particularly antitumor necrosis factor agents (eg, adalimumab, infliximab, etanercept). Safety and efficacy of concurrent administration is unknown and not recommended. Defer vaccination for ≥1 month after discontinuation.

Patients with unspecified cellular immunodeficiency (exception, patients with impaired humoral immunity may receive vaccine).

Warnings/Precautions Zoster vaccine is not a substitute for varicella vaccine and should not be used in children and adolescents. Not for use in the treatment of active zoster outbreak, the treatment of postherpetic neuropathy (PHN), or prevention of primary varicella infection (chickenpox). Vaccination may not result in effective immunity in all patients. Response depends upon multiple factors (eg, type of vaccine, age of patient) and may be improved by administering the vaccine at the recommended dose, route, and interval. Vaccines may not be effective if administered during periods of altered immune competence (CDC, 2011). Avoid administration in patients with moderate to severe acute febrile illness; consider deferral of vaccination; may administer to patients with mild acute illness (with or without fever) (CDC, 2011). Defer treatment in patients with active untreated tuberculosis. May be used in patients with a history of zoster infection unless other contraindications to the vaccine exist (CDC, 2008).

Medications active against the herpesvirus family (eg, acyclovir, famciclovir, valacyclovir) may interfere with the zoster vaccine (CDC, 2008). In patients where immunosuppressant therapy is anticipated, zoster vaccine should be given at least 14 days to 1 month prior to beginning therapy when possible (CDC, 2008). Use is contraindicated in severely immunocompromised patients (eg, patients receiving chemo-/radiation therapy or other immunosuppressive therapy [including high-dose corticosteroids]); may have a reduced response to vaccination. Persons with AIDS or manifestations of HIV with CD4+ T-lymphocyte counts ≤200 cells/microliter or CD4+ T-lymphocyte percentages ≤15% should not be vaccinated. Persons with AIDS or manifestations of HIV with CD4+ T-lymphocyte counts ≤200 cells/microliter or CD4+ T-lymphocyte percentages ≤15% should not be vaccinated. Patients receiving corticosteroids in low-to-moderate doses, topical (inhaled, nasal, skin), local injection (intra-articular, bursal, tendon) may receive vaccine (CDC, 2008; CDC, 2011). Although transmission of the vaccine virus may occur between vaccinees and susceptible contacts, vaccinated individuals do not need to take precautions against spreading varicella following vaccination; transmission of virus following vaccination is rare unless rash develops. In case of rash, standard contact precautions should be followed. Persons with rash should avoid contact with persons at high risk for severe varicella infection until lesions have crusted (CDC, 2008). In general, household and close contacts of persons with altered immunocompetence may receive all age-appropriate vaccines (CDC, 2011).

Immediate treatment for anaphylactoid reaction should be available during vaccine use. Syncope has been reported with use of injectable vaccines and may be accompanied by transient visual disturbances, weakness, or tonic-clonic movements. Procedures should be in place to avoid injuries from falling and to restore cerebral perfusion if syncope occurs (CDC, 2011). Contains gelatin and neomycin; do not use in patients with a history of anaphylactic/anaphylactoid reaction. Contact dermatitis to neomycin is not a contraindication to the vaccine. Not for use in patients <50 years of age. The ACIP does not recommend zoster vaccination in patients of any age who have received the varicella vaccine (CDC, 2008). Use of this vaccine for specific medical and/or other indications (eg, immunocompromising conditions, hepatic or kidney disease, diabetes) is also addressed in the ACIP Recommended Immunization Schedule (CDC, 2013).

Adverse Reactions All serious adverse reactions must be reported to the U.S. Department of Health and Human Services (DHHS) Vaccine Adverse Event Reporting System (VAERS) 1-800-822-7967 or online at https://vaers.hhs.gov/esub/index.

>10%: Local: Injection site reaction (48% to 64%; includes erythema, tenderness, pain, swelling, hematoma, pruritus, and/or warmth)

1% to 10% (**Note:** Rates similar to placebo):

Central nervous system: Fever (2%), headache (1% to 9%)

Dermatologic: Skin disorder (1%)

Gastrointestinal: Diarrhea (2%)

Neuromuscular & skeletal: Weakness (1%)

Respiratory: Respiratory tract infection (2%), rhinitis (1%)

Miscellaneous: Flu-like syndrome (2%)

<1%, postmarketing, and/or case reports (Limited to important or life-threatening): Anaphylaxis, arthralgia, hypersensitivity reactions, injection site reactions (lymphadenopathy [transient], rash, urticaria), myalgia, nausea, rash (noninjection site)

Drug Interactions

Metabolism/Transport Effects None known.

Avoid Concomitant Use

Avoid concomitant use of Zoster Vaccine with any of the following: Acyclovir-Valacyclovir; Belimumab; Famciclovir; Fingolimod; Immunosuppressants

Increased Effect/Toxicity

The levels/effects of Zoster Vaccine may be increased by: AzaTHIOprine; Belimumab; Corticosteroids (Systemic); Dimethyl Fumarate; Fingolimod; Hydroxychloroquine; Immunosuppressants; Leflunomide; Mercaptopurine; Methotrexate

Decreased Effect

Zoster Vaccine may decrease the levels/effects of: Tuberculin Tests

The levels/effects of Zoster Vaccine may be decreased by: Acyclovir-Valacyclovir; Dimethyl Fumarate; Famciclovir; Fingolimod; Immune Globulins; Immunosuppressants; Pneumococcal Polysaccharide Vaccine (Polyvalent)

Preparation for Administration Reconstitute with supplied diluent only, immediately upon removal from the freezer; use only sterile syringes free of preservatives, antiseptics, and detergents. Withdraw entire contents of the vial containing the provided diluent to reconstitute vaccine. Gently agitate to mix thoroughly. Withdraw entire contents of reconstituted vaccine vial for administration. Discard if reconstituted vaccine is not used within 30 minutes.

Storage/Stability To maintain potency, the lyophilized vaccine must be stored frozen between -50°C to -15°C (-58°F to 5°F). Temperatures below -50°C (-58°F) may occur if stored in dry ice. Protect from light. Store diluent separately at room temperature of 20°C to 25°C (68°F to 77°F) or in refrigerator at 2°C to 8°C (36°F to 46°F). The lyophilized vaccine may also be stored and/or transported under refrigeration at temperatures of 2°C to 8°C (36°F to 46°F) for 72 continuous hours prior to reconstitution; discard if not used within 72 hours.

Mechanism of Action A decline in VZV-specific immunity increases the risk of developing zoster infection. As a live, attenuated vaccine (Oka/Merck strain of varicella-zoster virus), zoster virus vaccine stimulates active immunity to disease caused by the varicella-zoster virus. Administration has been demonstrated to protect against the development of herpes zoster, with the highest efficacy in patients 60-69 years of age. It may also reduce the severity of complications, including postherpetic neuralgia, in patients who develop zoster following vaccination.

Zoster vaccine reduced the incidence of zoster by ~70% in those 50 to 59 years of age, 64% in those 60-69 years of age, 41% in those 70-79 years of age, and 18% in those 80 years and older. The overall efficacy for those 60 years and older was 51%. Additional benefit was afforded to vaccine recipients who developed zoster by reduction in the incidence of PHN: 5% for those 60-69 years of age, 55% for those 70-79 years of age, and 26% for those 80 years and older. Other prespecified zoster-related complications were reported less frequently in subjects who received zoster vaccine compared with subjects who received placebo.

Pharmacodynamics/Kinetics

Onset of action: Seroconversion: ~6 weeks (CDC, 2008)

Duration: Not established; protection has been demonstrated for at least 4 years

Dosage SubQ: Adults ≥50 years: 0.65 mL administered as a single dose; there are no data to support readministration of the vaccine (CDC, 2008)

Dosage adjustment in renal impairment: No dosage adjustment provided in manufacturer's labeling.

Dosage adjustment in hepatic impairment: No dosage adjustment provided in manufacturer's labeling.

Administration Inject SubQ into the deltoid region of the upper arm. Do not administer I.V. or I.M.; inject immediately after reconstitution. In persons anticipating immunosuppression, give at least 14 days to 1 month prior to starting immunosuppressant (CDC, 2008).

Administration with chronic use of acyclovir, famciclovir, or valacyclovir: Discontinue ≥24 hours before administration of zoster vaccine. Do not use for ≥14 days after vaccination (CDC, 2008).

Simultaneous administration of vaccines helps ensure the patients will be fully vaccinated by the appropriate age. Simultaneous administration of vaccines is defined as administering >1 vaccine on the same day at different anatomic sites. Separate vaccines should not be combined in the same syringe unless indicated by product specific labeling. Separate needles and syringes should be used for each injection. The ACIP prefers each dose of a specific vaccine in a series come from the same manufacturer when possible. Adults should be vaccinated while seated or lying down (CDC, 2011).

Antipyretics have not been shown to prevent febrile seizures. Antipyretics may be used to treat fever or discomfort following vaccination (CDC, 2011). One study reported that routine prophylactic administration of acetaminophen to prevent fever prior to vaccination decreased the immune response of some vaccines; the clinical significance of this reduction in immune response has not been established (Prymula, 2009).

Monitoring Parameters Fever, rash; monitor for syncope for 15 minutes following administration. If seizure-like activity associated with syncope occurs, maintain patient in supine or Trendelenburg position to reestablish adequate cerebral perfusion (CDC, 2011).

Additional Information U.S. federal law requires that the name of medication, date of administration, the vaccine manufacturer, lot number of vaccine, and the administering person's name, title, and address be entered into the patient's permanent medical record.

The varicella-zoster virus (VZV) is capable of causing two distinct manifestations of infection. Primary infection results in chickenpox (varicella). These infections tend to occur in young children or younger adults. Reactivation of latent infection (painful vesicular cutaneous eruption usually in a dermatomal pattern) occurs in older patients or in immunosuppressed populations. This is commonly referred to as shingles (herpes zoster). Although the vaccines are directed against the same causative organism, healthcare workers should be aware of differences in indications, dosing, populations, and composition of the vaccine (the minimum potency of the zoster vaccine is ≥14 times the Varivax vaccine). Neither vaccine is intended for administration during active outbreaks (CDC, 2008).

Dosage Forms Excipient information presented when available (limited, particularly for generics); consult specific product labeling.

Solution Reconstituted, Subcutaneous [preservative free]:
Zostavax: 19,400 units/0.65 mL (1 ea)

APPENDIX TABLE OF CONTENTS

ABBREVIATIONS, ACRONYMS, AND SYMBOLS

Abbreviations Which May Be Used in This Reference

Abbreviation	Meaning
½NS	0.45% sodium chloride
5-HT	5-hydroxytryptamine
AACT	American Academy of Clinical Toxicology
AAP	American Academy of Pediatrics
AAPC	antibiotic-associated pseudomembranous colitis
ABG	arterial blood gases
ABMT	autologous bone marrow transplant
ABW	adjusted body weight
ACC	American College of Cardiology
ACE	angiotensin-converting enzyme
ACLS	advanced cardiac life support
ACOG	American College of Obstetricians and Gynecologists
ACTH	adrenocorticotrophic hormone
ADH	antidiuretic hormone
ADHD	attention-deficit/hyperactivity disorder
ADI	adequate daily intake
ADLs	activities of daily living
AED	antiepileptic drug
AHA	American Heart Association
AHCPR	Agency for Health Care Policy and Research
AIDS	acquired immunodeficiency syndrome
AIMS	Abnormal Involuntary Movement Scale
ALL	acute lymphoblastic leukemia
ALS	amyotrophic lateral sclerosis
ALT	alanine aminotransferase (formerly called SGPT)
AMA	American Medical Association
AML	acute myeloblastic leukemia
ANA	antinuclear antibodies
ANC	absolute neutrophil count
ANLL	acute nonlymphoblastic leukemia
aPTT	activated partial thromboplastin time
ARB	angiotensin receptor blocker
ARDS	acute respiratory distress syndrome
ASA-PS	American Society of Anesthesiologists – Physical Status P1: Normal, healthy patient P2: Patient having mild systemic disease P3: Patient having severe systemic disease P4: Patient having severe systemic disease which is a constant threat to life P5: Moribund patient; not expected to survive without the procedure P6: Patient declared brain-dead; organs being removed for donor purposes
AST	aspartate aminotransferase (formerly called SGOT)
ATP	adenosine triphosphate
AUC	area under the curve (area under the serum concentration-time curve)
A-V	atrial-ventricular
BDI	Beck Depression Inventory
BEC	blood ethanol concentration
BLS	basic life support
BMI	body mass index
BMT	bone marrow transplant
BP	blood pressure
BPD	bronchopulmonary disease or dysplasia
BPH	benign prostatic hyperplasia
BPRS	Brief Psychiatric Rating Scale
BSA	body surface area
BUN	blood urea nitrogen

Abbreviations Which May Be Used in This Reference *(continued)*

Abbreviation	Meaning
CABG	coronary artery bypass graft
CAD	coronary artery disease
CADD	computer ambulatory drug delivery
cAMP	cyclic adenosine monophosphate
CAN	Canadian
CAPD	continuous ambulatory peritoneal dialysis
CAS	chemical abstract service
CBC	complete blood count
CBT	cognitive behavioral therapy
CDC	Centers for Disease Control and Prevention
CF	cystic fibrosis
CFC	chlorofluorocarbons
CGI	Clinical Global Impression
CHD	coronary heart disease
CHF	congestive heart failure; chronic heart failure
CI	cardiac index
CIE	chemotherapy-induced emesis
C-II	schedule two controlled substance
C-III	schedule three controlled substance
C-IV	schedule four controlled substance
C-V	schedule five controlled substance
CIV	continuous I.V. infusion
CLL	chronic lymphocytic leukemia
C_{max}	maximum plasma concentration
C_{min}	minimum plasma concentration
CML	chronic myelogenous leukemia
CMV	cytomegalovirus
CNS	central nervous system or coagulase negative staphylococcus
COLD	chronic obstructive lung disease
COPD	chronic obstructive pulmonary disease
COX	cyclooxygenase
CPK	creatine phosphokinase
CPR	cardiopulmonary resuscitation
Cr_{cl}	creatinine clearance
CRF	chronic renal failure
CRP	C-reactive protein
CRRT	continuous renal replacement therapy
CSF	cerebrospinal fluid
CSII	continuous subcutaneous insulin infusion
CT	computed tomography
CVA	cerebrovascular accident
CVP	central venous pressure
CVVH	continuous venovenous hemofiltration
CVVHD	continuous venovenous hemodialysis
CVVHDF	continuous venovenous hemodiafiltration
CYP	cytochrome
$D_5{}^1\!/_4NS$	dextrose 5% in sodium chloride 0.2%
$D_5{}^1\!/_2NS$	dextrose 5% in sodium chloride 0.45%
D_5LR	dextrose 5% in lactated Ringer's
D_5NS	dextrose 5% in sodium chloride 0.9%
D_5W	dextrose 5% in water
$D_{10}W$	dextrose 10% in water
DBP	diastolic blood pressure
DEHP	di(3-ethylhexyl)phthalate
DIC	disseminated intravascular coagulation
DL_{co}	pulmonary diffusion capacity for carbon monoxide
DM	diabetes mellitus

Abbreviations Which May Be Used in This Reference *(continued)*

Abbreviation	Meaning
DMARD	disease modifying antirheumatic drug
DNA	deoxyribonucleic acid
DSC	discontinued
DSM-IV	Diagnostic and Statistical Manual
DVT	deep vein thrombosis
EBV	Epstein-Barr virus
ECG	electrocardiogram
ECHO	echocardiogram
ECMO	extracorporeal membrane oxygenation
ECT	electroconvulsive therapy
ED	emergency department
EEG	electroencephalogram
EF	ejection fraction
EG	ethylene glycol
EGA	estimated gestational age
EIA	enzyme immunoassay
ELBW	extremely low birth weight
ELISA	enzyme-linked immunosorbent assay
EPS	extrapyramidal side effects
ESR	erythrocyte sedimentation rate
ESRD	end stage renal disease
E.T.	endotracheal
EtOH	alcohol
FDA	Food and Drug Administration (United States)
FEV_1	forced expiratory volume exhaled after 1 second
FSH	follicle-stimulating hormone
FTT	failure to thrive
FVC	forced vital capacity
G-6-PD	glucose-6-phosphate dehydrogenase
GA	gestational age
GABA	gamma-aminobutyric acid
GAD	generalized anxiety disorder
GE	gastroesophageal
GERD	gastroesophageal reflux disease
GFR	glomerular filtration rate
GGT	gamma-glutamyltransferase
GI	gastrointestinal
GU	genitourinary
GVHD	graft versus host disease
HAM-A	Hamilton Anxiety Scale
HAM-D	Hamilton Depression Scale
HARS	HIV-associated adipose redistribution syndrome
HCAHPS	Hospital Consumer Assessment of Healthcare Providers and Systems
Hct	hematocrit
HDL-C	high density lipoprotein cholesterol
HF	heart failure
HFA	hydrofluoroalkane
HFSA	Heart Failure Society of America
Hgb	hemoglobin
HIV	human immunodeficiency virus
HMG-CoA	3-hydroxy-3-methylglutaryl-coenzyme A
HOCM	hypertrophic obstructive cardiomyopathy
HPA	hypothalamic-pituitary-adrenal
HPLC	high performance liquid chromatography
HSV	herpes simplex virus
HTN	hypertension
HUS	hemolytic uremic syndrome

Abbreviations Which May Be Used in This Reference *(continued)*

Abbreviation	Meaning
IBD	inflammatory bowel disease
IBS	irritable bowel syndrome
IBW	ideal body weight
ICD	implantable cardioverter defibrillator
ICH	intracranial hemorrhage
ICP	intracranial pressure
IDDM	insulin-dependent diabetes mellitus
IDSA	Infectious Diseases Society of America
IgG	immune globulin G
IHSS	idiopathic hypertrophic subaortic stenosis
ILCOR	International Liaison Committee on Resuscitation
I.M.	intramuscular
INR	international normalized ration
Int. unit	international unit
I.O.	intraosseous
I & O	input and output
IOP	intraocular pressure
IQ	intelligence quotient
I.T.	intrathecal
ITP	idiopathic thrombocytopenic purpura
IUGR	intrauterine growth retardation
I.V.	intravenous
IVH	intraventricular hemorrhage
IVP	intravenous push
IVPB	intravenous piggyback
JIA	juvenile idiopathic arthritis
JNC	Joint National Committee
JRA	juvenile rheumatoid arthritis
kg	kilogram
KIU	kallikrein inhibitor unit
KOH	potassium hydroxide
LAMM	L-α-acetyl methadol
LDH	lactate dehydrogenase
LDL-C	low density lipoprotein cholesterol
LE	lupus erythematosus
LFT	liver function test
LGA	large for gestational age
LH	luteinizing hormone
LP	lumbar posture
LR	lactated Ringer's
LV	left ventricular
LVEF	left ventricular ejection fraction
LVH	left ventricular hypertrophy
MAC	*Mycobacterium avium* complex
MADRS	Montgomery Asbery Depression Rating Scale
MAO	monoamine oxidase
MAOIs	monamine oxidase inhibitors
MAP	mean arterial pressure
MDD	major depressive disorder
MDRD	modification of diet in renal disease
MDRSP	multidrug resistant *streptococcus pneumoniae*
MI	myocardial infarction
MMSE	mini mental status examination
MOPP	mustargen (mechlorethamine), Oncovin® (vincristine), procarbazine, and prednisone
M/P	milk to plasma ratio
MPS I	mucopolysaccharidosis I
MRHD	maximum recommended human dose

Abbreviations Which May Be Used in This Reference *(continued)*

Abbreviation	Meaning
MRI	magnetic resonance imaging
MRSA	methicillin-resistant *Staphylococcus aureus*
MUGA	multiple gated acquisition scan
NAEPP	National Asthma Education and Prevention Program
NAS	neonatal abstinence syndrome
NCI	National Cancer Institute
ND	nasoduodenal
NF	National Formulary
NFD	Nephrogenic fibrosing dermopathy
NG	nasogastric
NIDDM	noninsulin-dependent diabetes mellitus
NIH	National Institute of Health
NIOSH	National Institute for Occupational Safety and Health
NKA	no known allergies
NKDA	No known drug allergies
NMDA	n-methyl-d-aspartate
NMS	neuroleptic malignant syndrome
NNRTI	non-nucleoside reverse transcriptase inhibitor
NRTI	nucleoside reverse transcriptase inhibitor
NS	normal saline (0.9% sodium chloride)
NSAID	nonsteroidal anti-inflammatory drug
NSF	nephrogenic systemic fibrosis
NSTEMI	Non-ST-elevation myocardial infarction
NYHA	New York Heart Association
OA	osteoarthritis
OCD	obsessive-compulsive disorder
OHSS	ovarian hyperstimulation syndrome
O.R.	operating room
OTC	over-the-counter (nonprescription)
PABA	para-aminobenzoic acid
PACTG	Pediatric AIDS Clinical Trials Group
PALS	pediatric advanced life support
PAT	paroxysmal atrial tachycardia
PCA	patient-controlled analgesia
PCP	*Pneumocystis jiroveci* pneumonia (also called *Pneumocystis carinii* pneumonia)
PCWP	pulmonary capillary wedge pressure
PD	Parkinson's disease; peritoneal dialysis
PDA	patent ductus arteriosus
PDE-5	phosphodiesterase-5
PE	pulmonary embolism
PEG tube	percutaneous endoscopic gastrostomy tube
P-gp	P-glycoprotein
PHN	post-herpetic neuralgia
PICU	Pediatric Intensive Care Unit
PID	pelvic inflammatory disease
PIP	peak inspiratory pressure
PMA	postmenstrual age
PMDD	premenstrual dysphoric disorder
PNA	postnatal age
PONV	postoperative nausea and vomiting
PPHN	persistent pulmonary hypertension of the neonate
PPN	peripheral parenteral nutrition
PROM	premature rupture of membranes
PSVT	paroxysmal supraventricular tachycardia
PT	prothrombin time
PTH	parathyroid hormone
PTSD	post-traumatic stress disorder

Abbreviations Which May Be Used in This Reference *(continued)*

Abbreviation	Meaning
PTT	partial thromboplastin time
PUD	peptic ulcer disease
PVC	premature ventricular contraction
PVD	peripheral vascular disease
PVR	peripheral vascular resistance
QT_c	corrected QT interval
QT_cF	corrected QT interval by Fredricia's formula
RA	rheumatoid arthritis
RAP	right arterial pressure
RDA	recommended daily allowance
REM	rapid eye movement
REMS	risk evaluation and mitigation strategies
RIA	radioimmunoassay
RNA	ribonucleic acid
RPLS	reversible posterior leukoencephalopathy syndrome
RSV	respiratory syncytial virus
SA	sinoatrial
SAD	seasonal affective disorder
SAH	subarachnoid hemorrhage
SBE	subacute bacterial endocarditis
SBP	systolic blood pressure
S_{cr}	serum creatinine
SERM	selective estrogen receptor modulator
SGA	small for gestational age
SGOT	serum glutamic oxaloacetic aminotransferase
SGPT	serum glutamic pyruvate transaminase
SI	International System of Units or Systeme international d'Unites
SIADH	syndrome of inappropriate antidiuretic hormone secretion
SLE	systemic lupus erythematosus
SLEDD	sustained low-efficiency daily diafiltration
SNRI	serotonin norepinephrine reuptake inhibitor
SSKI	saturated solution of potassium iodide
SSRIs	selective serotonin reuptake inhibitors
STD	sexually transmitted disease
STEM I	ST-elevation myocardial infarction
SVR	systemic vascular resistance
SVT	supraventricular tachycardia
SWFI	sterile water for injection
SWI	sterile water for injection
$T_{1/2}$	half-life
T_3	triiodothyronine
T_4	thyroxine
TB	tuberculosis
TC	total cholesterol
TCA	tricyclic antidepressant
TD	tardive dyskinesia
TG	triglyceride
TIA	transient ischemic attack
TIBC	total iron binding capacity
TMA	thrombotic microangiopathy
T_{max}	time to maximum observed concentration, plasma
TNF	tumor necrosis factor
TPN	total parenteral nutrition
TSH	thyroid stimulating hormone
TT	thrombin time
TTP	thrombotic thrombocytopenic purpura
UA	urine analysis

Abbreviations Which May Be Used in This Reference *(continued)*

Abbreviation	Meaning
UC	ulcerative colitis
ULN	upper limits of normal
URI	upper respiratory infection
USAN	United States Adopted Names
USP	United States Pharmacopeia
UTI	urinary tract infection
UV	ultraviolet
V_d	volume of distribution
V_{dss}	volume of distribution at steady-state
VEGF	vascular endothelial growth factor
VF	ventricular fibrillation
VLBW	very low birth weight
VMA	vanillylmandelic acid
VT	ventricular tachycardia
VTE	venous thromboembolism
vWD	von Willebrand disease
VZV	varicella zoster virus
WHO	World Health Organization
w/v	weight for volume
w/w	weight for weight
YBOC	Yale Brown Obsessive-Compulsive Scale
YMRS	Young Mania Rating Scale

Common Weights, Measures, or Apothecary Abbreviations

Abbreviation	Meaning
<[1]	less than
>[1]	greater than
≤	less than or equal to
≥	greater than or equal to
ac	before meals or food
ad	to, up to
ad lib	at pleasure
AM	morning
AMA	against medical advice
amp	ampul
amt	amount
aq	water
aq. dest.	distilled water
ASAP	as soon as possible
a.u.[1]	each ear
bid	twice daily
bm	bowel movement
C	Celsius, centigrade
cal	calorie
cap	capsule
cc[1]	cubic centimeter
cm	centimeter
comp	compound
cont	continue
d	day
d/c[1]	discharge
dil	dilute
disp	dispense
div	divide
dtd	give of such a dose

Common Weights, Measures, or Apothecary Abbreviations *(continued)*

Abbreviation	Meaning
Dx	diagnosis
elix, el	elixir
emp	as directed
et	and
ex aq	in water
F	Fahrenheit
f, ft	make, let be made
g	gram
gr	grain
gtt	a drop
h	hour
hs[1]	at bedtime
kcal	kilocalorie
kg	kilogram
L	liter
liq	a liquor, solution
M	molar
mcg	microgram
m. dict	as directed
mEq	milliequivalent
mg	milligram
microL	microliter
min	minute
mL	milliliter
mm	millimeter
mM	millimole
mm Hg	millimeters of mercury
mo	month
mOsm	milliosmoles
ng	nanogram
nmol	nanomole
no.	number
noc	in the night
non rep	do not repeat, no refills
NPO	nothing by mouth
NV	nausea and vomiting
O, Oct	a pint
o.d.[1]	right eye
o.l.	left eye
o.s.[1]	left eye
o.u.[1]	each eye
pc, post cib	after meals
PM	afternoon or evening
P.O.	by mouth
P.R.	rectally
prn	as needed
pulv	a powder
q	every
qad	every other day
qd[1,2]	every day, daily
qh	every hour
qid	four times a day
qod[1,2]	every other day
qs	a sufficient quantity
qs ad	a sufficient quantity to make
Rx	take, a recipe
S.L.	sublingual

Common Weights, Measures, or Apothecary Abbreviations *(continued)*

Abbreviation	Meaning
stat	at once, immediately
SubQ	subcutaneous
supp	suppository
syr	syrup
tab	tablet
tal	such
tid	three times a day
tr, tinct	tincture
trit	triturate
tsp	teaspoon
u.d.	as directed
ung	ointment
v.o.	verbal order
w.a.	while awake
x3	3 times
x4	4 times
y	year

[1]ISMP error-prone abbreviation

[2]JCAHO Do Not Use list

Additional abbreviations used and defined within a specific monograph or text piece may only apply to that text.

REFERENCES

The Institute for Safe Medication Practices (ISMP) list of Error-Prone Abbreviations, Symbols, and Dose Designations. Available at http://www.ismp.org/Tools/errorproneabbreviations.pdf

The Joint Commission Official "Do Not Use" list. Available at http://www.jointcommission.org/facts_about_the_official_/

APACHE II SCORING SYSTEM

The APACHE II score is the sum of the total acute physiology score (APS), age points, and chronic health points. Determination of these scores/points are outlined in the following tables.

APACHE II Score	Points
APS points	
+ Age points	
+ Chronic health points	
Total APACHE II Score	

Glasgow Coma Scale

(circle appropriate response)

Eyes open	**Verbal – nonintubated**
4 - Spontaneously	5 - Oriented and controversed
3 - To verbal	4 - Disoriented and talks
2 - To painful stimuli	3 - Inappropriate words
1 - No response	2 - Incomprehensible sounds
	1 - No response
Motor response	
6 - To verbal command	**Verbal – intubated**
5 - Localizes to pain	5 - Seems able to talk
4 - Withdraws to pain	3 - Questionable ability to talk
3 - Abnormal flexion (decorticate)	1 - Generally unresponsive
2 - Abnormal extension (decerebrate)	
1 - No response	

Age Points

Assign points to age as follows:	Points
≤44	0
45-54	2
55-64	3
65-74	5
≥75	6

Chronic Health Points

Liver Cardiovascular Pulmonary Kidney Immune	If the patient has a history of severe organ system insufficiency or is immunocompromised assign points as follows: a. for nonoperative or emergency postoperative patients - 5 points or b. for elective postoperative patients - 2 points **DEFINITIONS** Organ insufficiency or immunocompromised state must have been evident prior to this hospital admission and conform to the following criteria. **Liver:** Biopsy proven cirrhosis and documented portal hypertension; episodes of past upper GI bleeding attributed to portal hypertension; or prior episodes of hepatic failure/encephalopathy/coma **Cardiovascular:** New York Heart Association Class IV **Respiratory:** Chronic restrictive, obstructive, or vascular disease resulting in severe exercise restriction, ie, unable to climb stairs or perform household duties; or documented chronic hypoxia, hypercapnia, secondary polycythemia, severe pulmonary hypertension (>40 mm Hg), or respirator dependency **Renal:** Receiving chronic dialysis **Immunocompromised:** The patient has received therapy that suppresses resistance to infection, eg, immunosuppression, chemotherapy, radiation, long term or recent high dose steroids, or has a disease that is sufficiently advanced to suppress resistance to infection, eg, leukemia, lymphoma, AIDS **Chronic Health Points =**

REFERENCE

Knaus WA, Draper EA, Wagner DP, et al. APACHE II: a severity of disease classification system. *Crit Care Med.* 1985;13(10):818-829.

Total Acute Physiology Score (APS) (Choose the worst value in the past 24 hours)

	Physiologic Variable	High Abnormal Range								Low Abnormal Range
		+4	+3	+2	+1	0	+1	+2	+3	+4
1	Temperature rectal (°C)[1]	≥41	39-40.9		38.5-38.9	36-38.4	34-35.9	32-33.9	30-31.9	≤29.9
2	Mean arterial pressure (mm Hg)	≥160	130-159	110-129		70-109		50-69		≤49
3	Heart rate (ventricular response)	≥180	140-179	110-139		70-109		55-69	40-54	≤39
4	Respiratory rate (nonventilated or ventilated)	≥50	35-49		25-34	12-24	10-11	6-9		≤5
5	Oxygenation: A-a gradient or PaO_2 (mm Hg) a) FiO_2 ≥0.5: record A-a gradient	≥500	350-499	200-349		<200				
	b) FiO_2 <0.5: record only PaO_2					PO_2 >70	PO_2 61-70		PO_2 55-60	PO_2 <55
6*	Arterial pH	≥7.7	7.6-7.69		7.5-7.59	7.33-7.49		7.25-7.32	7.15-7.24	<7.15
7	Serum sodium (mmol/L)	≥180	160-179	155-159	150-154	130-149		120-129	111-119	≤110
8	Serum potassium (mmol/L)	≥7	6-6.9		5.5-5.9	3.5-5.4	3-3.4	2.5-2.9		<2.5
9	Serum creatinine (mg/100 mL) double point score for acute renal failure	≥3.5	2-3.4	1.5-1.9		0.6-1.4		<0.6		
10	Hematocrit (%)	≥60		50-59.9	46-49.9	30-45.9		20-29.9		<20
11	White blood count (total/mm³) (in 1000s)	≥40		20-39.9	15-19.9	3-14.9		1-2.9		<1
12	Glasgow coma score (GCS): Score = 15 minus actual GCS [see Glasgow Coma Scale table]									
A	Total acute physiology score (APS): Sum of the 12 individual variable points									
*	Serum HCO_3 (venous-mmol/L) Not preferred, use if no ABGs	≥52	41-51.9		32-40.9	22-31.9		18-21.9	15-17.9	<15

[1]Temperature may also be obtained by the following methods: Swan-Ganz core, bladder, tympanic membrane

APOTHECARY/METRIC EQUIVALENTS

Apothecary-Metric Exact Equivalents

1 gram (g)	=	15.43 grains (gr)
1 milliliter (mL)	=	16.23 minims
1 minim	=	0.06 mL
1 gr	=	64.8 milligrams (mg)
1 fluid ounce (fl oz)	=	29.57 mL
1 pint (pt)	=	473.2 mL
1 ounce (oz)	=	28.35 g
1 pound (lb)	=	453.6 g
1 kilogram (kg)	=	2.2 lb
1 quart (qt)	=	946.4 mL

0.1 mg	=	1/600 gr
0.12 mg	=	1/500 gr
0.15 mg	=	1/400 gr
0.2 mg	=	1/300 gr
0.3 mg	=	1/200 gr
0.4 mg	=	1/150 gr
0.5 mg	=	1/120 gr
0.6 mg	=	1/100 gr
0.8 mg	=	1/80 gr
1 mg	=	1/65 gr

Apothecary-Metric Approximate Equivalents[1]

Liquids

1 teaspoonful	=	5 mL
1 tablespoonful	=	15 mL

Solids

1/4 grain	=	15 mg
1/2 grain	=	30 mg
1 grain	=	60 mg
1 1/2 grain	=	100 mg
5 grains	=	300 mg
10 grains	=	600 mg

[1]Use exact equivalents for compounding and calculations requiring a high degree of accuracy.

BODY SURFACE AREA OF CHILDREN AND ADULTS

Calculating Body Surface Area in Children

In a child of average size, find weight and corresponding surface area on the boxed scale to the left or use the nomogram to the right. Lay a straightedge on the correct height and weight points for the child, then read the intersecting point on the surface area scale. (**Note:** 2.2 lb = 1 kg)

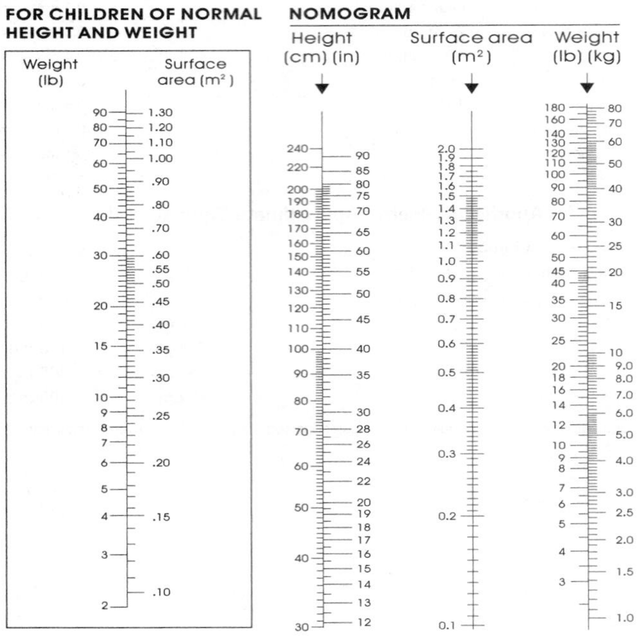

BODY SURFACE AREA FORMULA
(Adult and Pediatric)

$$\text{BSA (m}^2\text{)} = \sqrt{\frac{\text{ht (in)} \times \text{wt (lb)}}{3131}} \quad \text{or, in metric: BSA (m}^2\text{)} = \sqrt{\frac{\text{ht (cm)} \times \text{wt (kg)}}{3600}}$$

References

Lam TK and Leung DT, "More on Simplified Calculation of Body Surface Area," *N Engl J Med*, 1988, 318(17):1130 (letter).

Mosteller RD, "Simplified Calculation of Body Surface Area," *N Engl J Med*, 1987, 317(17):1098 (letter).

IDEAL BODY WEIGHT CALCULATION

Adults (18 years and older)

IBW (male) = 50 + (2.3 x height in inches over 5 feet)

IBW (female) = 45.5 + (2.3 x height in inches over 5 feet)

IBW is in kg.

Children

a. 1-18 years (Traub and Johnson, 1980)

$$IBW = \frac{(height^2 \times 1.65)}{1000}$$

IBW is in kg.

Height is in cm.

b. 5 feet and taller (Traub and Johnson, 1980)

IBW (male) = 39 + (2.27 x height in inches over 5 feet)

IBW (female) = 42.2 + (2.27 x height in inches over 5 feet)

IBW is in kg.

c. 1-17 years (Traub and Kichen, 1983)

$IBW = 2.396e^{0.01863\ (height)}$

IBW is in kg.

Height is in cm.

REFERENCES

Traub SL, Johnson CE. Comparison of methods of estimating creatinine clearance in children. *Am J Hosp Pharm.* 1980;37(2):195-201.

Traub SL, Kichen L. Estimating ideal body mass in children. *Am J Hosp Pharm.* 1983;40(1):107-110.

MILLIEQUIVALENT AND MILLIMOLE CALCULATIONS AND CONVERSIONS

DEFINITIONS AND CALCULATIONS

Definitions

mole	=	gram molecular weight of a substance (aka molar weight)
millimole (mM)	=	milligram molecular weight of a substance (a millimole is 1/1000 of a mole)
equivalent weight	=	gram weight of a substance which will combine with or replace 1 gram (1 mole) of hydrogen; an equivalent weight can be determined by dividing the molar weight of a substance by its ionic valence
milliequivalent (mEq)	=	milligram weight of a substance which will combine with or replace 1 milligram (1 millimole) of hydrogen (a milliequivalent is 1/1000 of an equivalent)

Calculations

$$\text{moles} = \frac{\text{weight of a substance (grams)}}{\text{molecular weight of that substance (grams)}}$$

$$\text{millimoles} = \frac{\text{weight of a substance (milligrams)}}{\text{molecular weight of that substance (milligrams)}}$$

$$\text{equivalents} = \text{moles x valence of ion}$$

$$\text{milliequivalents} = \text{millimoles x valence of ion}$$

$$\text{moles} = \frac{\text{equivalents}}{\text{valence of ion}}$$

$$\text{millimoles} = \frac{\text{milliequivalents}}{\text{valence of ion}}$$

$$\text{millimoles} = \text{moles x 1000}$$

$$\text{milliequivalents} = \text{equivalents x 1000}$$

Note: Use of equivalents and milliequivalents is valid only for those substances which have fixed ionic valences (eg, sodium, potassium, calcium, chlorine, magnesium, bromine, etc). For substances with variable ionic valences (eg, phosphorous), a reliable equivalent value cannot be determined. In these instances, one should calculate millimoles (which are fixed and reliable) rather than milliequivalents.

MILLIEQUIVALENT CONVERSIONS

To convert mg/100 mL to mEq/L the following formula may be used:

$$\frac{\text{(mg/100 mL) x 10 x valence}}{\text{atomic weight}} = \text{mEq/L}$$

To convert mEq/L to mg/100 mL the following formula may be used:

$$\frac{\text{(mEq/L) x atomic weight}}{\text{10 x valence}} = \text{mg/100 mL}$$

To convert mEq/L to volume of percent of a gas the following formula may be used:

$$\frac{\text{(mEq/L) x 22.4}}{10} = \text{volume percent}$$

Valences and Atomic Weights of Selected Ions

Substance	Electrolyte	Valence	Molecular Wt
Calcium	Ca^{++}	2	40
Chloride	Cl^{-}	1	35.5
Magnesium	Mg^{++}	2	24
Phosphate	HPO_4^{--} (80%)	1.8	96[1]
pH = 7.4	$H_2PO_4^{-}$ (20%)	1.8	96[1]
Potassium	K^{+}	1	39
Sodium	Na^{+}	1	23
Sulfate	SO_4^{--}	2	96[1]

[1]The molecular weight of phosphorus only is 31, and sulfur only is 32.

Approximate Milliequivalents — Weights of Selected Ions

Salt	mEq/g Salt	mg Salt/mEq
Calcium carbonate [$CaCO_3$]	20	50
Calcium chloride [$CaCl_2 \cdot 2H_2O$]	14	74
Calcium gluceptate [$Ca(C_7H_{13}O_8)_2$]	4	245
Calcium gluconate [$Ca(C_6H_{11}O_7)_2 \cdot H_2O$]	5	224
Calcium lactate [$Ca(C_3H_5O_3)_2 \cdot 5H_2O$]	7	154
Magnesium gluconate [$Mg(C_6H_{11}O_7)_2 \cdot H_2O$]	5	216
Magnesium oxide [MgO]	50	20
Magnesium sulfate [$MgSO_4$]	17	60
Magnesium sulfate [$MgSO_4 \cdot 7H_2O$]	8	123
Potassium acetate [$K(C_2H_3O_2)$]	10	98
Potassium chloride [KCl]	13	75
Potassium citrate [$K_3(C_6H_5O_7) \cdot H_2O$]	9	108
Potassium iodide [KI]	6	166
Sodium acetate [$Na(C_2H_3O_2)$]	12	82
Sodium acetate [$Na(C_2H_3O_2) \cdot 3H_2O$]	7	136
Sodium bicarbonate [$NaHCO_3$]	12	84
Sodium chloride [$NaCl$]	17	58
Sodium citrate [$Na_3(C_6H_5O_7) \cdot 2H_2O$]	10	98
Sodium iodine [NaI]	7	150
Sodium lactate [$Na(C_3H_5O_3)$]	9	112
Zinc sulfate [$ZnSO_4 \cdot 7H_2O$]	7	144

SELECTED CLINICAL EQUATIONS

CORRECTED SODIUM

Corrected Na^+ = measured Na^+ + [1.5 x (glucose – 150 divided by 100)]

Note: Do not correct for glucose <150.

WATER DEFICIT

Water deficit = 0.6 x body weight [1 – (140 divided by Na^+)]

Note: Body weight is estimated weight in kg when fully hydrated; **Na^+** is serum or plasma sodium. Use corrected Na^+ if necessary. Consult medical references for recommendations for replacement of deficit.

TOTAL SERUM CALCIUM CORRECTED FOR ALBUMIN LEVEL

[(Normal albumin – patient's albumin) x 0.8] + patient's measured total calcium

OSMOLALITY

Definition: The summed concentrations of all osmotically active solute particles.

Predicted serum osmolality =

$$\text{mOsm/L} = (2 \times \text{serum } Na^{++}) + \frac{\text{serum glucose}}{18} + \frac{\text{BUN}}{2.8}$$

The normal range of serum osmolality is 285-295 mOsm/L.

Calculated Osm

Note: Osm is a term used to reconcile osmolality and osmolarity

Osmol gap = measured Osm – calculated Osm

0 to +10: Normal
>10: Abnormal
<0: Probable lab or calculation error

Drugs Causing Osmolar Gap

(by freezing-point depression, gap is >10 mOsm)
Ethanol
Ethylene glycol
Glycerol
Iodine (questionable)
Isopropanol (acetone)
Mannitol
Methanol
Sorbitol

BICARBONATE DEFICIT

HCO_3^- deficit = (0.4 x wt in kg) x (HCO_3^- desired – HCO_3^- measured)

Note: In clinical practice, the calculated quantity may differ markedly from the actual amount of bicarbonate needed or that which may be safely administered.

ANION GAP

Definition: The difference in concentration between unmeasured cation and anion equivalents in serum.

Anion gap = $Na^+ - (Cl^- + HCO_3^-)$
(The normal anion gap is 10-14 mEq/L)

Differential Diagnosis of Increased Anion Gap Acidosis

Organic anions
- Lactate (sepsis, hypovolemia, seizures, large tumor burden)
- Pyruvate
- Uremia
- Ketoacidosis (β-hydroxybutyrate and acetoacetate)
- Amino acids and their metabolites
- Other organic acids

Inorganic anions
- Hyperphosphatemia
- Sulfates
- Nitrates

Differential Diagnosis of Decreased Anion Gap

Organic cations
- Hypergammaglobulinemia

Inorganic cations
- Hyperkalemia
- Hypercalcemia
- Hypermagnesemia

Medications and toxins
- Lithium

Hypoalbuminemia

RETICULOCYTE INDEX

(% retic divided by 2) x (patient's Hct divided by normal Hct) **or**
(% retic divided by 2) x (patient's Hgb divided by normal Hgb)

Normal index: 1.0
Good marrow response: 2.0-6.0

CORRECTED QT INTERVAL EQUATIONS

Bazett (B) Formula:

QT_cB: $QT_c = QT/(R - R\ interval^{0.5})$

or

QT_cB: QT_c = QT/Square root of (R - R interval)

Frederica (F) Formula:

QT_cF: $QT_c = QT/(R - R\ interval^{0.33})$

POUNDS/KILOGRAMS CONVERSION

1 pound = 0.45359 kilograms
1 kilogram = 2.2 pounds

lb	=	kg	lb	=	kg	lb	=	kg
1		0.45	70		31.75	140		63.50
5		2.27	75		34.02	145		65.77
10		4.54	80		36.29	150		68.04
15		6.80	85		38.56	155		70.31
20		9.07	90		40.82	160		72.58
25		11.34	95		43.09	165		74.84
30		13.61	100		45.36	170		77.11
35		15.88	105		47.63	175		79.38
40		18.14	110		49.90	180		81.65
45		20.41	115		52.16	185		83.92
50		22.68	120		54.43	190		86.18
55		24.95	125		56.70	195		88.45
60		27.22	130		58.91	200		90.72
65		29.48	135		61.24			

TEMPERATURE CONVERSION

Celsius to Fahrenheit = (°C x 9/5) + 32 = °F
Fahrenheit to Celsius = (°F - 32) x 5/9 = °C

°C	=	°F	°C	=	°F	°C	=	°F
100.0		212.0	39.0		102.2	36.8		98.2
50.0		122.0	38.8		101.8	36.6		97.9
41.0		105.8	38.6		101.5	36.4		97.5
40.8		105.4	38.4		101.1	36.2		97.2
40.6		105.1	38.2		100.8	36.0		96.8
40.4		104.7	38.0		100.4	35.8		96.4
40.2		104.4	37.8		100.1	35.6		96.1
40.0		104.0	37.6		99.7	35.4		95.7
39.8		103.6	37.4		99.3	35.2		95.4
39.6		103.3	37.2		99.0	35.0		95.0
39.4		102.9	37.0		98.6	0		32.0
39.2		102.6						

REFERENCE VALUES FOR ADULTS

CHEMISTRY

Test	Values	Remarks
Serum/Plasma		
Acetone	Negative	
Albumin	3.2-5 g/dL	
Alcohol, ethyl	Negative	
Aldolase	1.2-7.6 IU/L	
Ammonia	20-70 mcg/dL	Specimen to be placed on ice as soon as collected.
Amylase	30-110 units/L	
Bilirubin, direct	0-0.3 mg/dL	
Bilirubin, total	0.1-1.2 mg/dL	
Calcium	8.6-10.3 mg/dL	
Calcium, ionized	2.24-2.46 mEq/L	
Chloride	95-108 mEq/L	
Cholesterol, total	≤200 mg/dL	Fasted blood required – normal value affected by dietary habits. This reference range is for a general adult population.
HDL cholesterol	40-60 mg/dL	Fasted blood required – normal value affected by dietary habits.
LDL cholesterol	<160 mg/dL	If triglyceride is >400 mg/dL, LDL cannot be calculated accurately (Friedewald equation). Target LDL-C depends on patient's risk factors.
CO_2	23-30 mEq/L	
Creatine kinase (CK) isoenzymes		
CK-BB	0%	
CK-MB (cardiac)	0% to 3.9%	
CK-MM (muscle)	96% to 100%	
CK-MB levels must be both ≥4% and 10 IU/L to meet diagnostic criteria for CK-MB positive result consistent with myocardial injury.		
Creatine phosphokinase (CPK)	8-150 IU/L	
Creatinine	0.5-1.4 mg/dL	
Ferritin	13-300 ng/mL	
Folate	3.6-20 ng/dL	
GGT (gamma-glutamyltranspeptidase)		
male	11-63 IU/L	
female	8-35 IU/L	
GLDH	To be determined	
Glucose (preprandial)	<115 mg/dL	Goals different for diabetics.
Glucose, fasting	60-110 mg/dL	Goals different for diabetics.
Glucose, nonfasting (2-h postprandial)	<120 mg/dL	Goals different for diabetics.
Hemoglobin A_{1c}	<8	
Hemoglobin, plasma free	<2.5 mg/100 mL	
Hemoglobin, total glycosolated (Hb A_1)	4% to 8%	
Iron	65-150 mcg/dL	
Iron binding capacity, total (TIBC)	250-420 mcg/dL	
Lactic acid	0.7-2.1 mEq/L	Specimen to be kept on ice and sent to lab as soon as possible.
Lactate dehydrogenase (LDH)	56-194 IU/L	

CHEMISTRY *(continued)*

Test	Values	Remarks
Lactate dehydrogenase (LDH) isoenzymes		
LD_1	20% to 34%	
LD_2	29% to 41%	
LD_3	15% to 25%	
LD_4	1% to 12%	
LD_5	1% to 15%	
Flipped LD_1/LD_2 ratios (>1 may be consistent with myocardial injury) particularly when considered in combination with a recent CK-MB positive result.		
Lipase	23-208 units/L	
Magnesium	1.6-2.5 mg/dL	Increased by slight hemolysis.
Osmolality	289-308 mOsm/kg	
Phosphatase, alkaline		
adults 25-60 y	33-131 IU/L	
adults ≥61 y	51-153 IU/L	
infancy-adolescence	Values range up to 3-5 times higher than adults	
Phosphate, inorganic	2.8-4.2 mg/dL	
Potassium	3.5-5.2 mEq/L	Increased by slight hemolysis.
Prealbumin	>15 mg/dL	
Protein, total	6.5-7.9 g/dL	
AST	<35 IU/L (20-48)	
ALT (10-35)	<35 IU/L	
Sodium	134-149 mEq/L	
Thyroid stimulating hormone (TSH)		
adults ≤20 y	0.7-6.4 mIU/L	
21-54 y	0.4-4.2 mIU/L	
55-87 y	0.5-8.9 mIU/L	
Transferrin	>200 mg/dL	
Triglycerides	45-155 mg/dL	Fasted blood required.
Troponin I	<1.5 ng/mL	
Urea nitrogen (BUN)	7-20 mg/dL	
Uric acid		
male	2-8 mg/dL	
female	2-7.5 mg/dL	
Cerebrospinal Fluid		
Glucose	50-70 mg/dL	
Protein	15-45 mg/dL	CSF obtained by lumbar puncture.
Note: Bloody specimen gives erroneously high value due to contamination with blood proteins		
Urine (24-hour specimen is required for all these tests unless specified)		
Amylase	32-641 units/L	The value is in units/L and **not** calculated for total volume.
Amylase, fluid (random samples)		Interpretation of value left for physician, depends on the nature of fluid.
Calcium	Depends upon dietary intake	
Creatine		
male	150 mg/24 h	Higher value on children and during pregnancy.
female	250 mg/24 h	
Creatinine	1000-2000 mg/24 h	
Creatinine clearance (endogenous)		
male	85-125 mL/min	A blood sample must accompany urine specimen.
female	75-115 mL/min	

CHEMISTRY *(continued)*

Test	Values	Remarks
Glucose	1 g/24 h	
5-hydroxyindoleacetic acid	2-8 mg/24 h	
Iron	0.15 mg/24 h	Acid washed container required.
Magnesium	146-209 mg/24 h	
Osmolality	500-800 mOsm/kg	With normal fluid intake.
Oxalate	10-40 mg/24 h	
Phosphate	400-1300 mg/24 h	
Potassium	25-120 mEq/24 h	Varies with diet; the interpretation of urine electrolytes and osmolality should be left for the physician.
Sodium	40-220 mEq/24 h	
Porphobilinogen, qualitative	Negative	
Porphyrins, qualitative	Negative	
Proteins	0.05-0.1 g/24 h	
Salicylate	Negative	
Urea clearance	60-95 mL/min	A blood sample must accompany specimen.
Urea N	10-40 g/24 h	Dependent on protein intake.
Uric acid	250-750 mg/24 h	Dependent on diet and therapy.
Urobilinogen	0.5-3.5 mg/24 h	For qualitative determination on random urine, send sample to urinalysis section in Hematology Lab.
Xylose absorption test		
children	16% to 33% of ingested xylose	
Feces		
Fat, 3-day collection	<5 g/d	Value depends on fat intake of 100 g/d for 3 days preceding and during collection.
Gastric Acidity		
Acidity, total, 12 h	10-60 mEq/L	Titrated at pH 7.

Blood Gases

	Arterial	Capillary	Venous
pH	7.35-7.45	7.35-7.45	7.32-7.42
pCO_2 (mm Hg)	35-45	35-45	38-52
pO_2 (mm Hg)	70-100	60-80	24-48
HCO_3 (mEq/L)	19-25	19-25	19-25
TCO_2 (mEq/L)	19-29	19-29	23-33
O_2 saturation (%)	90-95	90-95	40-70
Base excess (mEq/L)	-5 to +5	-5 to +5	-5 to +5

HEMATOLOGY

Complete Blood Count

Age	Hgb (g/dL)	Hct (%)	RBC (mill/mm^3)	RDW
0-3 d	15.0-20.0	45-61	4.0-5.9	<18
1-2 wk	12.5-18.5	39-57	3.6-5.5	<17
1-6 mo	10.0-13.0	29-42	3.1-4.3	<16.5
7 mo to 2 y	10.5-13.0	33-38	3.7-4.9	<16
2-5 y	11.5-13.0	34-39	3.9-5.0	<15
5-8 y	11.5-14.5	35-42	4.0-4.9	<15
13-18 y	12.0-15.2	36-47	4.5-5.1	<14.5
Adult male	13.5-16.5	41-50	4.5-5.5	<14.5
Adult female	12.0-15.0	36-44	4.0-4.9	<14.5

Age	MCV (fL)	MCH (pg)	MCHC (%)	Plts (x 10^3/mm^3)
0-3 d	95-115	31-37	29-37	250-450
1-2 wk	86-110	28-36	28-38	250-450
1-6 mo	74-96	25-35	30-36	300-700
7 mo to 2 y	70-84	23-30	31-37	250-600
2-5 y	75-87	24-30	31-37	250-550
5-8 y	77-95	25-33	31-37	250-550
13-18 y	78-96	25-35	31-37	150-450
Adult male	80-100	26-34	31-37	150-450
Adult female	80-100	26-34	31-37	150-450

WBC and Differential

Age	WBC (x 10^3/mm^3)	Segs	Bands	Lymphs	Monos
0-3 d	9.0-35.0	32-62	<18	19-29	5-7
1-2 wk	5.0-20.0	14-34	<14	36-45	6-10
1-6 mo	6.0-17.5	13-33	<12	41-71	4-7
7 mo to 2 y	6.0-17.0	15-35	<11	45-76	3-6
2-5 y	5.5-15.5	23-45	<11	35-65	3-6
5-8 y	5.0-14.5	32-54	<11	28-48	3-6
13-18 y	4.5-13.0	34-64	<11	25-45	3-6
Adults	4.5-11.0	35-66	<11	24-44	3-6

Age	Eosinophils	Basophils	Atypical Lymphs	No. of NRBCs
0-3 d	0-2	0-1	0-8	0-2
1-2 wk	0-2	0-1	0-8	0
1-6 mo	0-3	0-1	0-8	0
7 mo to 2 y	0-3	0-1	0-8	0
2-5 y	0-3	0-1	0-8	0
5-8 y	0-3	0-1	0-8	0
13-18 y	0-3	0-1	0-8	0
Adults	0-3	0-1	0-8	0

Segs = segmented neutrophils.

Bands = band neutrophils.

Lymphs = lymphocytes.

Monos = monocytes.

Erythrocyte Sedimentation Rates and Reticulocyte Counts

Sedimentation rate, Westergren	Children	0-20 mm/h
	Adult male	0-15 mm/h
	Adult female	0-20 mm/h
Sedimentation rate, Wintrobe	Children	0-13 mm/h
	Adult male	0-10 mm/h
	Adult female	0-15 mm/h
Reticulocyte count	Newborns	2% to 6%
	1-6 mo	0% to 2.8%
	Adults	0.5% to 1.5%

ASSESSMENT OF LIVER FUNCTION

Child-Pugh Score

Component	Score Given for Observed Findings		
	1	2	3
Encephalopathy grade[1]	None	1-2	3-4
Ascites	None	Mild or controlled by diuretics	Moderate or refractory despite diuretics
Albumin (g/dL)	>3.5	2.8-3.5	<2.8
Total bilirubin (mg/dL)	<2 (<34 micromoles/L)	2-3 (34-50 micromoles/L)	>3 (>50 micromoles/L)
or			
Modified total bilirubin[2]	<4	4-7	>7
Prothrombin time (seconds prolonged)	<4	4-6	>6
or			
INR	<1.7	1.7-2.3	>2.3

[1]**Encephalopathy Grades**

Grade 0: Normal consciousness, personality, neurological examination, electroencephalogram
Grade 1: Restless, sleep disturbed, irritable/agitated, tremor, impaired handwriting, 5 cps waves
Grade 2: Lethargic, time-disoriented, inappropriate, asterixis, ataxia, slow triphasic waves
Grade 3: Somnolent, stuporous, place-disoriented, hyperactive reflexes, rigidity, slower waves
Grade 4: Unrousable coma, no personality/behavior, decerebrate, slow 2-3 cps delta activity

Alternative Encephalopathy Grades

Grade 1: Mild confusion, anxiety, restlessness, fine tremor, slowed coordination
Grade 2: Drowsiness, disorientation, asterixis
Grade 3: Somnolent but rousable, marked confusion, incomprehensible speech, incontinent, hyperventilation
Grade 4: Coma, decerebrate posturing, flaccidity

[2]Modified total bilirubin used to score patients who have Gilbert's syndrome or who are taking indinavir.

CHILD-PUGH CLASSIFICATION

Class A (mild hepatic impairment): Score 5-6
Class B (moderate hepatic impairment): Score 7-9
Class C (severe hepatic impairment): Score 10-15

REFERENCES

Centers for Disease Control and Prevention (CDC). Report of the NIH panel to define principles of therapy of HIV infection and guidelines for the use of antiretroviral agents in HIV-infected adults and adolescents. March 2004. Available at http://www.aidsinfo.nih.gov

U.S. Department of Health and Human Services Food and Drug Administration. Guidance for industry, pharmacokinetics in patients with impaired hepatic function: study design, data analysis, and impact on dosing and labeling. May 2003. Available at http://www.fda.gov/OHRMS/DOCKETS/98fr/99D-5047-GDL00002.pdf

RENAL FUNCTION ESTIMATION IN ADULT PATIENTS

Evaluation of a patient's renal function often includes the use of equations to estimate glomerular filtration rate (GFR) (eg, estimated GFR [eGFR] creatinine clearance [Cl_{Cr}]) using an endogenous filtration marker (eg, serum creatinine) and other patient variables. For example, the Cockcroft-Gault equation estimates renal function by calculating Cl_{Cr} and is typically used to steer medication dosing. Equations which calculate eGFR are primarily used to categorize chronic kidney disease (CKD) staging and monitor progression. The rate of creatinine clearance does not always accurately represent GFR; creatinine may be cleared by other renal mechanisms in addition to glomerular filtration and serum creatinine concentrations may be affected by nonrenal factors (eg, age, gender, race, body habitus, illness, diet). In addition, these equations were developed based on studies in limited populations and may either over- or underestimate the renal function of a specific patient.

Nevertheless, most clinicians estimate renal function using Cl_{Cr} as an indicator of actual renal function for the purpose of adjusting medication doses. For medications that require dose adjustment for renal impairment, utilization of eGFR (ie, Modification of Diet in Renal Disease [MDRD]) may overestimate renal function by up to 40% which may result in supra-therapeutic medication doses (Hermsen, 2009). These equations should only be used in the clinical context of patient-specific factors noted during the physical exam/work-up. The 2012 National Kidney Foundation (NKF)-Kidney Disease Improving Global Outcomes (KDIGO) CKD guidelines state that drug dosing should be based on an e-GFR which is **not** adjusted for body surface area (BSA) (ie, reported in units of mL/minute/1.73 m^2) since the effect of eGFR adjusted for BSA compared to eGFR without adjustments for BSA has not been extensively studied. **Decisions regarding drug therapy and doses must be based on clinical judgment.**

RENAL FUNCTION ESTIMATION EQUATIONS

Commonly used equations to estimate renal function utilizing the endogenous filtration marker serum creatinine include the Cockcroft-Gault, Jelliffe, four-variable Modification of Diet in Renal Disease (MDRD), six-variable MDRD (aka, MDRD extended), and Chronic Kidney Disease Epidemiology Collaboration (CKD-EPI). All of these equations, except for the CKD-EPI, were originally developed using a serum creatinine assay measured by the alkaline picrate-based (Jaffe) method. Many substances, including proteins, can interfere with the accuracy of this assay and overestimate serum creatinine concentration. The NKF and The National Kidney Disease Education Program (NDKEP) advocated for a universal creatinine assay, in order to ensure an accurate estimate of renal function in patients. As a result, a more specific enzymatic assay with an isotope dilution mass spectrometry (IDMS)-traceable international standard was developed. Compared to the older methods, IDMS-traceable assays may report lower serum creatinine values and may, therefore, overestimate renal function when used in the original equations not re-expressed for use with a standardized serum creatinine assay (eg, Cockcroft-Gault, Jelliffe, original MDRD). Updated four-variable MDRD and six-variable MDRD equations based on serum creatinine measured by the IDMS-traceable method has been proposed for adults (Levey, 2006); the Cockcroft-Gault and Jelliffe equations have not been re-expressed and may overestimate renal function when used with a serum creatinine measured by the IDMS-traceable method. However, at this point, all laboratories should be using creatinine methods calibrated to be IDMS traceable.

The CKD-EPI creatinine equation, published in 2009, uses the same four variables as the four-variable MDRD (serum creatinine, age, sex, and race), but allows for more precision when estimating higher GFR values (eg, eGFR >60 mL/minute/1.73 m^2) as compared to the MDRD equation. The NKDEP has not made a recommendation on the general implementation of the CKD-EPI equation but does suggest that laboratories which report numeric values for eGFR >60 mL/minute/1.73 m^2 should consider the use of CKD-EPI. The NKD-KDIGO 2012 CKD guidelines recommend that clinicians use a creatinine-derived equation for the evaluation and management of CKD and specifically recommend that clinical laboratories use the 2009 CKD-EPI equation when reporting eGFR in adults.

The following factors may contribute to an inaccurate estimation of renal function (Stevens, 2006):

- Increased creatinine generation (may underestimate renal function):
  - Black or African American patients
  - Muscular body habitus
  - Ingestion of cooked meats
- Decreased creatinine generation (may overestimate renal function):
  - Increased age
  - Female patients
  - Hispanic patients
  - Asian patients
  - Amputees
  - Malnutrition, inflammation, or deconditioning (eg, cancer, severe cardiovascular disease, hospitalized patients)
  - Neuromuscular disease
  - Vegetarian diet
- Rapidly changing serum creatinine (either up or down): In patients with rapidly rising serum creatinines (ie, increasing by >0.5-0.7 mg/dL/day), it is best to assume that the patient's renal function is severely impaired

Use extreme caution when estimating renal function in the following patient populations:

- Low body weight (actual body weight < ideal body weight)
- Liver transplant
- Elderly (>90 years of age)
- Dehydration
- Recent kidney transplantation (serum creatinine values may decrease rapidly and can lead to renal function underestimation; conversely, delayed graft function may be present)

Note: In most situations, the use of the patient's ideal body weight (IBW) is recommended for estimating renal function, except when the patient's actual body weight (ABW) is less than ideal. Use of actual body weight (ABW) in obese patients (and possibly patients with ascites) may significantly overestimate renal function. Some clinicians prefer to use an adjusted body weight in such cases [eg, IBW + 0.4 (ABW - IBW)]; the adjustment factor may vary based on practitioner and/or institutional preference.

IDMS-traceable methods

Method 1: MDRD equation[1]:

eGFR = 175 X $(\text{Creatinine})^{-1.154}$ X $(\text{Age})^{-0.203}$ X (Gender) X (Race)

where:

eGFR = estimated GFR; calculated in mL/minute/1.73 m^2
Creatinine is input in mg/dL
Age is input in years
Gender: Females: Gender = 0.742; Males: Gender = 1
Race: Black: Race = 1.212; White or other: Race = 1

Method 2: MDRD Extended equation:

eGFR = 161.5 X $(\text{Creatinine})^{-0.999}$ X $(\text{Age})^{-0.176}$ X $(\text{SUN})^{-0.170}$ X $(\text{Albumin})^{0.318}$ X (Gender) X (Race)

where:

eGFR = estimated GFR; calculated in mL/minute/1.73 m^2
Creatinine is input in mg/dL
Age is input in years
SUN = Serum Urea Nitrogen; input in mg/dL
Albumin = Serum Albumin; input in g/dL
Gender: Females: Gender = 0.762; Males: Gender = 1
Race: Black: Race = 1.18; White or other: Race = 1

Method 3: CKD-EPI equation[2]:

eGFR = 141 X $(\text{Creatinine/k})^{\text{Exp}}$ X $(0.993)^{\text{Age}}$ X (Gender) X (Race)

where:

eGFR = estimated GFR; calculated in mL/minute/1.73 m^2
(Creatinine/k):
Creatinine is input in mg/dL
k: Females: k = 0.7; Males: k = 0.9
Exp:
When (Creatinine/k) is ≤1: Females: Exp = -0.329; Males: Exp = -0.411
When (Creatinine/k) is >1: Exp = -1.209
Age is input in years
Gender: Females: Gender = 1.018; Males: Gender = 1
Race: Black: Race = 1.159; White or other: Race = 1

Alkaline picrate-based (Jaffe) methods

Note: These equations have not been updated for use with serum creatinine methods traceable to IDMS. Use with IDMS-traceable serum creatinine methods may overestimate renal function; use with caution.

Method 1: MDRD equation:

eGFR = 186 X $(\text{Creatinine})^{-1.154}$ X $(\text{Age})^{-0.203}$ X (Gender) X (Race)

where:

eGFR = estimated GFR; calculated in mL/minute/1.73 m^2
Creatinine is input in mg/dL
Age is input in years
Gender: Females: Gender = 0.742; Males: Gender = 1
Race: Black: Race = 1.212; White or other: Race = 1

Method 2: MDRD Extended equation:

$$eGFR = 170 \times (Creatinine)^{-0.999} \times (Age)^{-0.176} \times (SUN)^{-0.170} \times (Albumin)^{0.318} \times (Gender) \times (Race)$$

where:

eGFR = estimated GFR; calculated in mL/minute/1.73 m^2
Creatinine is input in mg/dL
Age is input in years
SUN = Serum Urea Nitrogen; input in mg/dL
Albumin = Serum Albumin; input in g/dL
Gender: Females: Gender = 0.762; Males: Gender = 1
Race: Black: Race = 1.18; White or other: Race = 1

Method 3: Cockroft-Gault equation[3]

Males: Cl_{Cr} = [(140 - Age) X Weight] / (72 X Creatinine)
Females: Cl_{Cr} = {[(140 - Age) X Weight] / (72 X Creatinine)} X 0.85
where:

Cl_{Cr} = creatinine clearance; calculated in mL/minute
Age is input in years
Weight is input in kg
Creatinine is input in mg/dL

Method 4: Jelliffe equation

Males: Cl_{Cr} = {98 - [0.8 X (Age - 20)]} / (Creatinine)
Females: Cl_{Cr} = Use above equation, then multiply result by 0.9
where:

Cl_{Cr} = creatinine clearance; calculated in mL/minute/1.73 m^2
Age is input in years
Creatinine is input in mg/dL

FOOTNOTES

[1]Preferred equation for CKD staging National Kidney Disease Education Program
[2]Recommended equation for the reporting of eGFR by the NKD-KDIGO guidelines
[3]Equation typically used for adjusting medication doses

REFERENCES

Cockcroft DW, Gault MH. Prediction of creatinine clearance from serum creatinine. *Nephron*. 1976;16(1):31-41.

Dowling TC, Matzke GR, Murphy JE, et al. Evaluation of renal drug dosing: prescribing information and clinical pharmacist approaches. *Pharmacotherapy*. 2010;30(8):776-786.

Hermsen ED, Maiefski M, Florescu MC, et al. Comparison of the modification of diet in renal disease and Cockcroft-Gault equations for dosing antimicrobials. *Pharmacotherapy*. 2009;29(6):649-655.

Jelliffe RW. Letter: creatinine clearance: bedside estimate. *Ann Intern Med*. 1973;79(4):604-605.

Kidney disease: improving global outcomes (KDIGO) CKD work group. KDIGO 2012 clinical practice guidelines for the evaluation and management of chronic kidney disease. *Kidney Inter*. 2013;3:1-150. http://www.kdigo.org/clinical_practice_guidelines/pdf/CKD/KDIGO_2012_CKD_GL.pdf

Levey AS, Bosch JP, Lewis JB, et al. A more accurate method to estimate glomerular filtration rate from serum creatinine: a new prediction equation. Modification of diet in renal disease study group. *Ann Intern Med*. 1999;16;130(6):461–470.

Levey AS, Coresh J, Greene T, et al. Using standardized serum creatinine values in the modification of diet in renal disease study equation for estimating glomerular filtration rate. *Ann Intern Med*. 2006;145(4):247-254.

Levey AS, Stevens LA, Schmid CH, et al. A new equation to estimate glomerular filtration rate. *Ann Intern Med*. 2009;150(9):604-612.

National Kidney Disease Education Program. GFR calculators. http://www.nkdep.nih.gov/professionals/gfr_calculators. Accessed April 24, 2013.

Stevens LA, Coresh J, Greene T, et al. Assessing kidney function – measured and estimated glomerular filtration rate. *N Engl J Med*. 2006;354 (23):2473-2483.

ANGIOTENSIN AGENTS

Comparison of Indications and Adult Dosages

Drug	Hypertension	HF	Renal Dysfunction	Dialyzable	Strengths (mg)
ACE Inhibitors					
Benazepril (Lotensin)	10-40 mg/day	Not FDA-approved	Cl_{cr} <30 mL/min: 5 mg/day initially Maximum: 40 mg/day	Yes	Tablets 5, 10, 20, 40
Captopril (Capoten)	25-100 mg/day bid-tid	6.25-100 mg tid Maximum: 450 mg/day	Cl_{cr} 10-50 mL/min: 75% of usual dose Cl_{cr} <10 mL/min: 50% of usual dose	Yes	Tablets 12.5, 25, 50, 100
Cilazapril (Inhibace) **Note:** Not available in U.S.	2.5-10 mg/day	0.5-2.5 mg/day	Cl_{cr} 10-40 mL/min: Initial: 0.5 mg/day (0.25-0.5 mg/day for HF) (maximum: 2.5 mg/day) Cl_{cr} <10 mL/minute: 0.25-0.5 mg once or twice weekly	Yes	Tablets 1, 2.5, 5
Enalapril (Vasotec)	2.5-40 mg/day qd-bid	2.5-20 mg bid Maximum: 20 mg bid	Cl_{cr} 30-80 mL/min: 5 mg/day initially Cl_{cr} <30 mL/min: 2.5 mg/day initially	Yes	Tablets 2.5, 5, 10, 20
Enalaprilat[1]	0.625 mg, 1.25 mg, 2.5 mg q6h Maximum: 5 mg q6h	Not FDA-approved	Cl_{cr} <30 mL/min: 0.625 mg q6h	Yes	1.25 mg/mL (1 mL, 2 mL vials)
Fosinopril (Monopril)	10-40 mg/day	10-40 mg/day	No dosage reduction necessary	Not well dialyzed	Tablets 10, 20, 40
Lisinopril (Prinivil, Zestril)	10-40 mg/day Maximum: 40 mg/day	5-40 mg/day	Cl_{cr} 10-30 mL/min: 5 mg/day initially Cl_{cr} <10 mL/min: 2.5 mg/day initially	Yes	Tablets 2.5, 5, 10, 20, 30, 40
Moexipril (Univasc)	7.5-30 mg/day qd-bid Maximum: 30 mg/day	LV dysfunction (post-MI): 7.5-30 mg/day	Cl_{cr} <40 mL/min: 3.75 mg/day initially Maximum: 15 mg/day	Unknown	Tablets 7.5, 15
Perindopril (Aceon)	4-8 mg/day	4-8 mg/day Maximum: 16 mg/day	Cl_{cr} 30-60 mL/min: 2 mg/day Cl_{cr} 15-29 mL/min: 2 mg qod Cl_{cr} <15 mL/min: 2 mg on dialysis days	Yes	Tablets 2, 4, 8
Quinapril (Accupril)	10-40 mg/day qd-bid	5-20 mg bid	Cl_{cr} 30-60 mL/min: 5 mg/day initially Cl_{cr} <10-30 mL/min: 2.5 mg/day initially	Not well dialyzed	Tablets 5, 10, 20, 40
Ramipril (Altace)	2.5-20 mg/day qd-bid	2.5-10 mg/day	Cl_{cr} <40 mL/min: 25% of normal dose	Unknown	Capsules 1.25, 2.5, 5, 10
Trandolapril (Mavik)	1-4 mg/day Maximum: 8 mg/day qd-bid	LV dysfunction (post-MI): 1-4 mg/day	Cl_{cr} <30 mL/min: 0.5 mg/day initially	No	Tablets 1, 2, 4

Comparison of Indications and Adult Dosages *continued*

Drug	Hypertension	HF	Renal Dysfunction	Dialyzable	Strengths (mg)
Angiotensin II Receptor Blockers					
Azilsartan (Edarbi)	40-80 mg/day	Not FDA-approved	No dosage adjustment necessary	Unknown	Tablets 40, 80
Candesartan (Atacand)	8-32 mg/day	Target: 32 mg once daily	No dosage adjustment necessary	No	Tablets 4, 8, 16, 32
Eprosartan (Teveten)	400-800 mg/day qd-bid	Not FDA-approved	No dosage adjustment necessary	Unknown	Tablets 400, 600
Irbesartan (Avapro)	150-300 mg/day	Not FDA-approved	No dosage reduction necessary	No	Tablets 75, 150, 300
Losartan (Cozaar)	25-100 mg qd or bid	Not FDA-approved	No dosage adjustment necessary	No	Tablets 25, 50, 100
Olmesartan (Benicar)	20-40 mg/day	Not FDA-approved	No dosage adjustment necessary	Unknown	Tablets 5, 20, 40
Telmisartan (Micardis)	20-80 mg/day	Not FDA-approved	No dosage reduction necessary	No	Tablets 20, 40, 80
Valsartan (Diovan)	80-320 mg/day	Target: 160 mg bid	Decrease dose only if Cl_{cr} <10 mL/minute	No	Tablets 40, 80, 160, 320
Renin Inhibitors					
Aliskiren (Tekturna)	150-300 mg once daily	Not FDA-approved	No dosage adjustment necessary in mild-to-moderate impairment; not adequately studied in severe impairment	Unknown	Tablets 150, 300

Dosage is based on 70 kg adult with normal hepatic and renal function.

[1]Enalaprilat is the only available ACE inhibitor in a parenteral formulation.

ACE Inhibitors: Comparative Pharmacokinetics

Drug	Prodrug	Absorption (%)	Serum $t_{1/2}$ (h) Normal Renal Function	Serum Protein Binding (%)	Elimination	Onset of BP Lowering Action (h)	Peak BP Lowering Effects (h)	Duration of BP Lowering Effects (h)
Benazepril	Yes	37		~97	Renal (32%), biliary (~12%)	1	2-4	24
Benazeprilat			10-11 (effective)	~95				
Captopril	No	60-75 (fasting)	1.9 (elimination)	25-30	Renal	0.25-0.5	1-1.5	~6
Enalapril	Yes	55-75	2	50-60	Renal (60% to 80%), fecal	1	4-6	12-24
Enalaprilat			11 (effective)			0.25	1-4	~6
Fosinopril		36			Renal (~50%), biliary (~50%)	1		24
Fosinoprilat			12 (effective)	>99				
Lisinopril	No	25	11-12	25	Renal	1	6	24
Moexipril	Yes		1	90	Fecal (53%), renal (8%)		1-2	>24
Moexiprilat			2-10	50				
Perindopril	Yes		1.5-3	60	Renal		3-7	
Perindoprilat			3-10 (effective)	10-20				
Quinapril	Yes	>60	0.8	97	Renal (~60%) as metabolite, fecal	1	2-4	24
Quinaprilat			3					
Ramipril	Yes	50-60	1-2	73	Renal (60%), fecal (40%)	1-2	3-6	24
Ramiprilat			13-17 (effective)	56				
Trandolapril	Yes		6	80	Renal (33%), fecal (66%)	1-2	6	≥24
Trandolaprilat			10	65-94				

Angiotensin II Receptor Blockers and Renin Inhibitors: Comparative Pharmacokinetics

Drug	Prodrug	Time to Peak	Bioavailability	Food "Area-Under-the-Curve"	Elimination Half-Life	Elimination Altered in Renal Dysfunction	Precautions in Severe Renal Dysfunction	Elimination Altered in Hepatic Dysfunction	Precautions in Hepatic Dysfunction	Protein Binding (%)
Angiotensin II Receptor Blockers										
Azilsartan (Edarbi)	Yes	1.5-3 h	60%	No effect	11 h	No	Yes	No	No	>99
Candesartan (Atacand)	Yes[1]	3-4 h	15%	No effect	9 h	Yes[2]	Yes	No	Yes	>99
Eprosartan (Teveten)	No	1-2 h	13%	No effect	5-9 h	No	Yes	No	Yes	98
Irbesartan (Avapro)	No	1.5-2 h	60% to 80%	No effect	11-15 h	No	Yes	No	No	90
Losartan (Cozaar)	Yes[3]	1 h/3-4 h[3]	33%	9% to 10%	1.5-2 h/6-9 h[3]	No	Yes	Yes	Yes	~99
Olmesartan (Benicar)	Yes	1-2 h	26%	No effect	13 h	Yes	Yes	Yes	No	99
Telmisartan (Micardis)	No	0.5-1 h	42% to 58%	9.6% to 20%	24 h	No	Yes	Yes	Yes	>99.5
Valsartan (Diovan)	No	2-4 h	25%	9% to 40%	6 h	No	Yes	Yes	Yes	95
Renin Inhibitors										
Aliskiren (Tekturna)	No	1-3 h	~3%	85% (high-fat meal)	16-32 h	Yes[4]	Yes	No	No	?

[1]Candesartan cilexetil: Active metabolite candesartan

[2]Dosage adjustments are not necessary.

[3]Losartan: Active metabolite E-3174

[4]No initial dosage adjustment in mild-to-moderate impairment

ANTIDEPRESSANT AGENTS

Comparison of Usual Adult Dosage, Mechanism of Action, and Adverse Effects

Drug	Initial Adult Dose	Usual Adult Dosage (mg/d)	Dosage Forms	Adverse Effects						Comments
				ACH	Drowsiness	Orthostatic Hypotension	Conduction Abnormalities	GI Distress	Weight Gain	
Tricyclic Antidepressants and Related Compounds[1]										
Amitriptyline	25-75 mg qhs	100-300	T	4+	4+	3+	3+	1+	4+	Also used in chronic pain, migraine, and as a hypnotic; contraindicated with cisapride
Amoxapine	50 mg bid	100-400	T	2+	2+	2+	2+	0	2+	May cause extrapyramidal symptom (EPS)
ClomiPRAMINE[2] (Anafranil)	25-75 mg qhs	100-250	C	4+	4+	2+	3+	1+	4+	Only approved for OCD
Desipramine (Norpramin)	25-75 mg qhs	100-300	T	1+	2+	2+	2+	0	1+	Blood levels useful for therapeutic monitoring
Doxepin	25-75 mg qhs	100-300	C, L	3+	4+	2+	2+	0	4+	
Imipramine (Tofranil, Tofranil-PM)	25-75 mg qhs	100-300	T, C	3+	3+	4+	3+	1+	4+	Blood levels useful for therapeutic monitoring
Maprotiline	25-75 mg qhs	100-225	T	2+	3+	2+	2+	0	2+	
Nortriptyline (Pamelor)	25-50 mg qhs	50-150	C, L	2+	2+	1+	2+	0	1+	Blood levels useful for therapeutic monitoring
Protriptyline (Vivactil)	15 mg qAM	15-60	T	2+	1+	2+	3+	1+	1+	
Trimipramine (Surmontil)	25-75 mg qhs	100-300	C	4+	4+	3+	3+	0	4+	
Selective Serotonin Reuptake Inhibitors[3]										
Citalopram (Celexa)	20 mg qAM	20-60	T, L	0	0	0	0	3+[4]	1+	
Escitalopram (Lexapro)	10 mg qAM	10-20	T, L	0	0	0	0	3+	1+	S-enantiomer of citalopram
FLUoxetine (PROzac, PROzac Weekly, Sarafem, Selfemra)	10-20 mg qAM	20-80	C, CDR, L, T	0	0	0	0	3+[4]	1+	CYP2B6 and 2D6 inhibitor
FluvoxaMINE[2] (Luvox CR)	50 mg qhs	100-300	T, CXR	0	0	0	0	3+[4]	1+	Contraindicated with pimozide, thioridazine, mesoridazine, CYP1A2, 2B6, 2C19, and 3A4 inhibitors
PARoxetine (Paxil, Paxil CR, Pexeva)	10-20 mg qAM	20-50	T, CXR, L	1+	1+	0	0	3+[4]	2+	CYP2B6 and 2D6 inhibitor
Sertraline (Zoloft)	25-50 mg qAM	50-200	T, L	0	0	0	0	3+[4]	1+	CYP2B6 and 2C19 inhibitor
Vilazodone (Viibryd)	10 mg qAM	10-40	T	0	0	0	0	3+	0	CYP2C8, 2C19, and 2D6 inhibitor; also is a 5-HT_{1A} partial agonist
Dopamine-Reuptake Blocking Compounds										
BuPROPion (Aplenzin, Buproban, Budeprion SR, Budeprion XL, Wellbutrin, Wellbutrin SR, Wellbutrin XL, Zyban)	100 mg bid-tid IR[5] 150 mg qAM-bid SR[6]	300-450	T, TSR, TXR	0	0	0	1+/0	1+	0	Contraindicated with seizures, bulimia, and anorexia; low incidence of sexual dysfunction IR: A 6-h interval between doses preferred SR: An 8-h interval between doses preferred XL: Administer once daily

Comparison of Usual Adult Dosage, Mechanism of Action, and Adverse Effects *continued*

Drug	Initial Adult Dose	Usual Adult Dosage (mg/d)	Dosage Forms	Adverse Effects						Comments
				ACH	Drowsiness	Orthostatic Hypotension	Conduction Abnormalities	GI Distress	Weight Gain	
Serotonin/Norepinephrine Reuptake Inhibitors[7]										
Desvenlafaxine (Pristiq)	50 mg/d	50-100	TXR	0	1+	1+	0	3+[4]	0	Active metabolite of venlafaxine
DULoxetine (Cymbalta)	40-60 mg/d	40-60	CDR	1+	1+	0	1+	3+	0	Also indicated for GAD, management of pain associated with diabetic neuropathy, and management of fibromyalgia
Levomilnacipran (Fetzima)	20 mg/d	20-120	CXR	1+	0	2+	1+	2+	0	1S,2R-enantiomer of milnacipram
Milnacipran[8] (Savella)	12.5 mg/d	100-200	T	2+	1+	0	1+	3+	0	Only indicated for fibromyalgia
Venlafaxine (Effexor, Effexor XR)	25 mg bid-tid IR 37.5 mg qd XR	75-375 IR 75-225 XR	T, TXR, CXR	1+	1+	0	1+	3+[4]	0	High-dose may be useful to treat refractory depression; frequency of hypertension increases with dosage >225 mg/d
5-HT_2 Receptor Antagonist Properties										
Nefazodone	100 mg bid	300-600	T	1+	1+	2+	1+	1+	0	Contraindicated with carbamazepine, pimozide, astemizole, cisapride, and terfenadine; caution with triazolam and alprazolam; low incidence of sexual dysfunction
TraZODone	50 mg tid	150-600	T	0	4+	3+	1+	1+	2+	
5-HT_3 Receptor Antagonist Properties										
Vortioxetine (Brintellix)	10 mg/d	5-20	T	0	0	0	0	3+	0	Also is a 5-HT_{1A} agonist; moderate incidence of sexual dysfunction
Noradrenergic Antagonist										
Mirtazapine (Remeron, Remeron SolTab)	15 mg qhs	15-45	T, TOD	1+	3+	1+	1+	0	3+	Dose >15 mg/d less sedating, low incidence of sexual dysfunction
Monoamine Oxidase Inhibitors										
Isocarboxazid (Marplan)	10 mg tid	10-30	T	2+	2+	2+	1+	1+	2+	Diet must be low in tyramine; contraindicated with sympathomimetics and other antidepressants
Phenelzine (Nardil)	15 mg tid	15-90	T	2+	2+	2+	0	1+	3+	
Tranylcypromine (Parnate)	10 mg bid	10-60	T	2+	1+	2+	1+	1+	2+	
Selegiline (EmSam)	6 mg/d	6-12	Trans-dermal	2+	1+	2+	0	1+	0	Low tyramine diet not required for 6 mg/d dosage

ACH = anticholinergic effects (dry mouth, blurred vision, urinary retention, constipation); 0 - 4+ = absent or rare - relatively common; T = tablet; TSR = tablet, sustained release; TXR = tablet, extended release; TOD = tablet, orally disintegrating; L = liquid; C = capsule; CDR = capsule, delayed release; CXR = capsule, extended release; IR = immediate release; SR = sustained release; XR = extended release

[1]**Important note:** A 1-week supply taken all at once in a patient receiving the maximum dose can be fatal.

[2]Not approved by FDA for depression; approved for OCD

[3]Flat dose response curve, headache, nausea, and sexual dysfunction are common side effects for SSRIs.

[4]Nausea is usually mild and transient.

[5]IR: 100 mg bid; may be increased to 100 mg tid no sooner than 3 days after beginning therapy

[6]SR: 150 mg qAM; may be increased to 150 mg bid as early as day 4 of dosing. To minimize seizure risk, do not exceed SR 200 mg/dose.

[7]Do not use with sibutramine; relatively safe in overdose

[8]Milnacipran is only approved for fibromyalgia.

ANTIFUNGAL AGENTS

Activities of Various Agents Against Specific Fungi

Organisms	Amphotericin B (Conventional)[1]	Caspofungin	Fluconazole	Flucytosine
Aspergillus spp	FA	FA	N	?
Blastomyces dermatitidis	FA	?	A	N
Candida albicans	FA	FA	FA	FA
Candida glabrata	A	A	?	A
Candida krusei	FA	A	?	A
Candida tropicalis	FA	A	?	A
Coccidioides immitis	FA	?	A	N
Cryptococcus spp	FA	N	FA	FA
Dermatophytes	A	?	A	?
Fusarium spp	A	N	N	N
Histoplasma capsulatum	FA	A?	A	N
Penicillium spp	A	?	?	A
Pseudoallescheria boydii	?	A	N	N
Sporothrix schenckii	A	?	?	?
Zygomycetes (Mucor, Rhizopus)	A	N	N	N

Organisms	Griseofulvin	Itraconazole	Ketoconazole	Micafungin
Aspergillus spp	N	FA	N	A
Blastomyces dermatitidis	N	FA	FA	?
Candida albicans	N	FA	FA	FA
Candida glabrata	N	?	?	FA
Candida krusei	N	A	?	A
Candida tropicalis	N	?	?	A
Coccidioides immitis	N	A	FA	?
Cryptococcus spp	N	A	A	N
Dermatophytes	FA	A	A	?
Fusarium spp	N	N	N	?
Histoplasma capsulatum	N	FA	FA	?
Penicillium spp	N	?	N	?
Pseudoallescheria boydii	N	N	N	?
Sporothrix schenckii	N	?	N	?
Zygomycetes (Mucor, Rhizopus)	N	N	N	N

Organisms	Miconazole	Nystatin	Terbinafine	Voriconazole
Aspergillus spp	N	A	N	FA
Blastomyces dermatitidis	N	A	N	A
Candida albicans	FA	FA	A	A
Candida glabrata	?	A	?	A
Candida krusei	?	A	?	A
Candida tropicalis	?	A	?	A
Coccidioides immitis	A	N	N	A
Cryptococcus spp	A	N	N	A
Dermatophytes	N	N	FA	?
Fusarium spp	N	N	N	FA
Histoplasma capsulatum	N	N	N	A
Penicillium spp	N	N	N	?
Pseudoallescheria boydii	N	N	N	FA
Sporothrix schenckii	?	N	N	?
Zygomycetes (Mucor, Rhizopus)	N	N	N	N?

Organisms	Anidulafungin	Posaconazole
Aspergillus spp	A	FA
Blastomyces dermatitidis	N	A
Candida albicans	FA	FA
Candida glabrata	FA	A
Candida krusei	A	A
Candida tropicalis	FA	A
Coccidioides immitis	?	A
Cryptococcus spp	N	A
Dermatophytes	N?	A
Fusarium spp	N	A
Histoplasma capsulatum	?	A
Penicillium spp	A	A
Pseudoallescheria boydii	?	A
Sporothrix schenckii	?	A
Zygomycetes (Mucor, Rhizopus)	N?	A

FA = FDA-approved indication, A = active, ? = unknown or questionable, N = not active

[1]Various lipid products have differing indications, but all have activity against the same organisms.

REFERENCES

Espinel-Ingroff A. Comparison of *in vitro* activities of the new triazole SCH56592 and the echinocandins MK-0991 (L-743,872) and LY303366 against opportunistic filamentous and dimorphic fungi and yeasts. *J Clin Microbiol.* 1998;36(10):2950-2956.

Sabatelli F, Patel R, Mann PA, et al. *in vitro* activities of posaconazole, fluconazole, itraconazole, voriconazole, and amphotericin B against a large collection of clinically important molds and yeasts. *Antimicrob Agents Chemother.* 2006;50(6):2009-2015.

Torres HA, Hachem RY, Chemaly RF, et al. Posaconazole: a broad-spectrum triazole antifungal. *Lancet Infect Dis.* 2005;5(12):775-785.

Vazquez JA. Anidulafungin: a new echinocandin with a novel profile. *Clin Ther.* 2005;27(6):657-673.

Zhanel GG, Karlowsky JA, Harding GA, et al. *in vitro* activity of a new semisynthetic echinocandin, LY-303366, against systemic isolates of *Candida* species, *Cryptococcus neoformans*, *Blastomyces dermatitidis*, and *Aspergillus* species. *Antimicrob Agents Chemother.* 1997;41(4):863-865.

ANTIMIGRAINE DRUGS: 5-HT_1 RECEPTOR AGONISTS

Pharmacokinetic Differences

Pharmacokinetic Parameter	Onset	Duration	Time to Peak Serum Concentration	Average Bioavailability (%)	Volume of Distribution (L)[1]	Half-life (h) Normal Renal Function	Fraction Excreted Unchanged in Urine (%)
Almotriptan (Axert) Tablet: 6.25 mg, 12.5 mg	<60 min	Short	1-3 h	70	180-200	3-4	40
Eletriptan (Relpax) Tablet: 20 mg, 40 mg	<2 h	Short	1.5-2 h	50	138	4, active metabolite ~13	–
Frovatriptan (Frova) Tablet: 2.5 mg	<2 h	Long	2-4 h	20-30	210-290	26	<10
Naratriptan (Amerge and generic) Tablet: 1 mg, 2.5 mg	1-2 h	Long	2-3 h	70	170	6	50
Rizatriptan (Maxalt and generic) Tablet: 5 mg, 10 mg	~30 min	Short	1-1.5 h	45	110-140	2-3	14
Rizatriptan (Maxalt-MLT and generic) Tablet, dispersible: 5 mg, 10 mg	~30 min	Short	0.7 h	45	110-140	2-3	14
SUMAtriptan (Alsuma, Imitrex, Sumavel, and generic) SubQ: 4 mg, 6 mg	10 min	Short	4-20 min	97	170	2-2.5	22
SUMAtriptan (Imitrex and generic) Tablet: 25 mg, 50 mg, 100 mg)	~30 min	Short	2-2.5 h	15	170	2-2.5[2]	3
SUMAtriptan (Imitrex and generic) Nasal: 5 mg, 20 mg	15-30 min	Short	1 h	17	170	2-2.5	3
SUMAtriptan (Zecuity) Transdermal: 6.5 mg over 4 h)	–	Short	1 h	–	168	3	11
ZOLMitriptan (Zomig and generic) Tablet: 2.5 mg, 5 mg	0.5-1 h	Short	1.5 h	40	490	3	8
ZOLMitriptan (Zomig ZMT and generic) Tablet, dispersible: 2.5 mg, 5 mg	0.5-1 h	Short	3 h	40	490	3	8
ZOLMitriptan (Zomig) Nasal: 2.5 mg, 5 mg	0.5-1 h	Short	3 h	100	588	3	8

[1]If reported as L/kg, used 70 kg to calculate

[2]With extended dosing, the half-life extends to 7 hours.

ANTIPARKINSONIAN AGENTS

Drugs Used for the Treatment of Parkinsonian Symptoms[1]

Drug	Mechanism	Initial Dose	Titration Schedule	Usual Daily Dosage	Recommended Dosing Schedule
Dopaminergic Agents					
Amantadine (Symmetrel)	NMDA receptor antagonist and inhibits neuronal reuptake of dopamine	100 mg every other day	100 mg/dose every week, up to 300 mg 3 times/day	100-200 mg	Twice daily
Apomorphine (Apokyn)	D_2 receptors (caudate-putamen)	1-2 mg	Complex; based on tolerance and response to test dose(s)	Variable; <20 mg	Individualized; 3-5 times/day prn
Bromocriptine (Parlodel)	Moderate affinity for D_2 and D_3 dopamine receptors	1.25 mg twice daily	2.5 mg/day every 2-4 wk	2.5-100 mg	3 times/day
Carbidopa/levodopa (Sinemet)	Converts to dopamine; binds to all CNS dopamine receptors	10-25/100 mg 2-4 times/day CR: 50/200 mg 2 times/day	0.5-1 tablet (10 or 25/100 mg) every 1-2 days	50/200 to 200/2000 mg (3-8 tablets)	3 times/day or twice daily (for controlled release)
Entacapone (Comtan)	COMT enzyme inhibitor	200 mg 3 times/day	Titrate down the doses of carbidopa/levodopa as required	600-1600 mg	3 times/day; up to 8 times/day
Levodopa/carbidopa/entacapone (Stalevo)	Converts to dopamine; binds to all CNS dopamine receptors; COMT enzyme inhibitor	1 tablet 3-4 times/day (to replace previous dosing with individual agents)	As tolerated based on response and presence of dyskinesias	3-8 tablets per day	3-4 times/day
Pramipexole (Mirapex)	High affinity for D_2 and D_3 dopamine receptors	0.125 mg 3 times/day	0.125 mg/dose every 5-7 days	1.5-4.5 mg	3 times/day
Rasagiline (Azilect)	Inhibits MAO-B	0.5-1 mg once daily	≤1 mg daily	0.5-1 mg	Once daily
Ropinirole (Requip)	High affinity for D_2 and D_3 dopamine receptors	0.25 mg 3 times/day	0.25 mg/dose weekly for 4 wk, then 1.5 mg/day every week up to 9 mg/day; 3 mg/day up to a max of 24 mg/day	0.75-24 mg	3 times/day
Rotigotine (Neupro)	D_3, D_2, D_1 dopamine receptor agonist	Early stage: 2 mg/24 hours transdermal patch once daily; Advanced stage: 4 mg/24 hours transdermal patch once daily	Increase by 2 mg/24 hours weekly; maximum: 6 mg/24 hours (early stage) or 8 mg/24 hours (advanced stage)	2 mg/24 hours, 4 mg/24 hours, or 6 mg/24 hours	Once daily patch
Selegiline (Eldepryl, Zelapar)	Inhibits MAO-B	Eldepryl: 5 mg twice daily Zelapar: 1.25 mg once daily	Titrate down the doses of carbidopa/levodopa as required	Eldepryl: 10 mg Zelapar: 1.25-2.5 mg	Eldepryl: Twice daily Zelapar: Once daily
Tolcapone (Tasmar)	COMT enzyme inhibitor	100 mg 3 times/day	Titrate down the doses of carbidopa/levodopa as required	300-600 mg	3 times/day
Anticholinergic Agents					
Benztropine (Cogentin)	Blocks cholinergic receptors, also has antihistamine effects	0.5-2 mg/day in 1-4 divided doses	0.5 mg/dose every 5-6 days	2-6 mg	1-2 times/day
Procyclidine (Kemadrin)	Blocks cholinergic receptors	2.5 mg 3 times/day	Gradually as tolerated	7.5-20 mg	3 times/day
Trihexyphenidyl (Artane)	Blocks cholinergic receptors; also some direct effects	1-2 mg/day	2 mg/d at intervals of 3-5 days	5-15 mg	3-4 times/day

[1]The medications listed in the table represent treatment options for both idiopathic Parkinson's disease, as well as Parkinsonian symptoms resulting from other drug therapy.

ANTIPSYCHOTIC AGENTS

Antipsychotic Agent	Dosage Forms	I.M./P.O. Potency	Equiv. Dosages (approx) (mg/d)	Usual Adult Daily Maintenance Dose (mg)	Sedation (Incidence)	Extrapyramidal Side Effects	Anticholinergic Side Effects	Orthostatic Hypotension	Comments
ARIPiprazole (Abilify)	Solution; tablet; tablet, orally disintegrating; injection		7.5	10-30	Low	Low	Very low	Very low	Low weight gain; activating
(Abilify Maintena)	Injection, long-acting			160-400**					
Asenapine (Saphris)	Tablet, sublingual			10-20	Moderate	Low	Very low	Low/moderate	Low weight gain; activating
ChlorproMAZINE	Injection; tablet	4:1	100	200-1000	High	Moderate	Moderate	Moderate/high	
CloZAPine (Clozaril, FazaClo, Versacloz)	Tablet; tablet, orally disintegrating		100	75-900	High	Very low	High	High	~1% incidence of agranulocytosis; weekly-biweekly CBC required; potential for weight gain, lipid abnormalities, and diabetes
FluPHENAZine	Solution, concentrate; injection; tablet	2:1	2	0.5-20	Low	High	Low	Low	
	Injection, long-acting			12.5-25*					
Haloperidol (Haldol)	Solution, concentrate; injection; tablet	2:1	2	0.5-20	Low	High	Low	Low	
(Haldol Decanoate)	Injection, long-acting			50-200*					
Iloperidone (Fanapt)	Tablet			12-24	Low	Low	Very low	Low/moderate	
Loxapine (Loxitane)	Capsule		10	25-250	Moderate	Moderate	Low	Low	
(Adasuve)	Inhaler			10					Potential for bronchospasm that can lead to respiratory distress; administer only in REMS-enrolled healthcare facility
Lurasidone (Latuda)	Tablet			20-160	Moderate	Low/moderate	Low	Low	Contraindicated with strong CYP3A4 inducers and inhibitors. Take with food.
OLANZapine (ZyPREXA)	Injection; tablet; tablet, orally disintegrating		5	5-20	Moderate/high	Low	Moderate	Moderate	Potential for weight gain, lipid abnormalities, diabetes
(ZyPREXA Relprew)	Injection, long-acting			210-405*					

continued

Antipsychotic Agent	Dosage Forms	I.M./P.O. Potency	Equiv. Dosages (approx) (mg/d)	Usual Adult Daily Maintenance Dose (mg)	Sedation (Incidence)	Extrapyramidal Side Effects	Anticholinergic Side Effects	Orthostatic Hypotension	Comments
Paliperidone (Invega)	Tablet, extended release			3-12	Low/moderate	Low	Very low	Moderate	Active metabolite of risperidone
(Invega Sustenna)	Injection, long-acting			39-234*					
Perphenazine	Tablet		10	16-64	Low	Moderate	Low	Low	
Pimozide (Orap)	Tablet		2	1-10	Moderate	High	Moderate	Low	Contraindicated with CYP3A inhibitors
QUEtiapine (SEROquel, SEROquel XR)	Tablet; tablet, extended release		75	50-800	Moderate/high	Very low	Moderate	Moderate	Moderate weight gain; potential for lipid abnormalities; diabetes
RisperiDONE (RisperDAL)	Solution; tablet; tablet, orally disintegrating		2	0.5-6	Low/moderate	Low	Very low	Moderate	Low to moderate weight gain; potential for diabetes
(RisperDAL Consta)	Injection, long-acting			25-50*					
Thioridazine	Tablet		100	200-800	High	Low	High	Moderate/high	May cause irreversible retinitis pigmentosa at doses >800 mg/d; prolongs QTc; use only in treatment of refractory illness
Thiothixene (Navane)	Capsule	4:1	4	15-30	Low	High	Low	Low/moderate	
Trifluoperazine	Tablet		5	2-40	Low	High	Low	Low	
Ziprasidone (Geodon)	Capsule; injection, powder	2:1	60	40-160	Low/moderate	Low	Very low	Low/moderate	Low weight gain; contraindicated with QTc-prolonging agents. Take with food.

*Administered every 2 or 4 weeks; consult drug monograph for specific dosage details

**Administered monthly; consult drug monograph for specific dosage details

Woods SW. Chlorpromazine equivalent doses for the newer atypical antipsychotics. *J Clin Psychiatry.* 2003;64(6):663-667.

BENZODIAZEPINE COMPARISON TABLE

Agent	FDA-Approved Indication	Dosage Forms	Relative Potency (mg)	Peak Blood Levels (oral) (h)	Protein Binding (%)	Volume of Distribution (L/kg)	Major Active Metabolite	Onset	Metabolism	Half-Life (parent) (h)	Half-Life[1] (metabolite) (h)	Elimination	Usual Initial Oral Dose	Adult Oral Dosage Range
Anxiolytic														
ALPRAZolam (Xanax XR; Xanax)	Anxiety, anxiety associated with depression, panic disorder treatment	Sol, tab	0.5	IR: 1-2 XR: 9	80	0.9-1.2	No	Intermediate	Hepatic via CYP3A4	12-15	—	Urine	0.25-0.5 tid	0.75-4 mg/d
ChlordiazePOXIDE (Librium)	Anxiety, EtOH withdrawal	Cap	10	2-4	90-98	0.3	Yes	Intermediate	Hepatic via CYP3A4	5-30	24-96	Urine	5-25 mg tid-qid	15-100 mg/d
Diazepam (Diastat, Valium)	Anxiety, EtOH withdrawal, adjunct to anesthesia (I.V.), anxiety/amnesiac during cardioversion (I.V.), anxiety/amnesia in endoscopic procedures, convulsions/status epilepticus (I.V.), adjunct in epilepsy (rectal gel), skeletal muscle spasms	Gel, inj, sol, tab	5	0.5-2	98	1.1	Yes	Rapid	Hepatic via 2C19 and 3A4	20-80	50-100	Urine	2-10 mg bid-qid	4-40 mg/d
LORazepam (Ativan)[2]	Anxiety, anxiety associated with depression, adjunct to anesthesia (I.V.), convulsions/status epilepticus (I.V.)	Inj, sol, tab	1	1-6	88-92	1.3	No	Intermediate	Hepatic	10-20	—	Urine and feces (minimal)	0.5-2 mg tid-qid	2-4 mg/d
Oxazepam (Serax)	Anxiety, anxiety associated with depression, EtOH withdrawal	Cap, tab	15-30	2-4	86-99	0.6-2	No	Slow	Hepatic via glucoronide conjugation	5-20	—	Urine as unchanged (50%) and glucoronide	10-30 mg tid-qid	30-120 mg/d
Sedative/Hypnotic														
Estazolam	Insomnia	Tab	0.3	2	93	—	No	Slow	Hepatic via CYP3A4	10-24	—	Urine	1 mg qhs	1-2 mg
Flurazepam (Dalmane)	Insomnia	Cap	5	0.5-2	97	—	Yes	Rapid	Hepatic via CYP3A4	Not significant	40-114	Urine	15 mg qhs	15-60 mg
Quazepam (Doral)	Insomnia	Tab	5	2	95	5	Yes	Intermediate	Hepatic via CYP3A4	25-41	28-114	Urine	15 mg qhs	7.5-15 mg
Temazepam (Restoril)	Insomnia	Cap	5	1.2-1.6	96	1.4	No	Slow	Hepatic via CYP2B6, 2C8/9, 2C19, 3A4	3.5-18.4	—	Urine as inactive metabolites	15-30 mg qhs	7.5-30 mg
Triazolam (Halcion)	Insomnia	Tab	0.1	1	89-94	0.8-1.3	No	Intermediate	Hepatic via CYP3A4	2.3	—	Urine as unchanged drug and metabolites	0.125-0.25 qhs	0.125-0.25 mg

continued

Agent	FDA-Approved Indication	Dosage Forms	Relative Potency (mg)	Peak Blood Levels (oral) (h)	Protein Binding (%)	Volume of Distribution (L/kg)	Major Active Metabolite	Onset	Metabolism	Half-Life (parent) (h)	Half-Life[1] (metabolite) (h)	Elimination	Usual Initial Oral Dose	Adult Oral Dosage Range
Miscellaneous														
Clobazam	Adjunct in Lennox-Gastaut syndrome	Tab	NA	0.5-4	80-90	—	Yes	NA	Hepatic via CYP3A4, 2C19, 2B6	36-42	71-82	Urine, primarily as metabolites	5 mg daily-bid	5-40 mg/d
ClonazePAM (Klonopin)	Adjunct in Lennox-Gastaut syndrome, akinetic seizures, myoclonic seizures, adjunct in absence seizures, panic disorder treatment	Tab	0.25-0.5	1-2	86	1.8-4	No	Intermediate	Hepatic via glucoronide and sulfate conjugation	18-50	—	Urine as glucoronide or sulfate conjugate	0.5 mg tid	1.5-20 mg/d
Clorazepate (Tranxene T-Tab)	Anxiety, EtOH withdrawal, adjunct in partial seizures	Cap, tab	7.5	1-2	80-95	—	Yes	Rapid	Decarboxylated in acidic stomach prior to absorption and hepatic via CYP3A4	Not significant	50-100	Urine	7.5-15 mg bid-qid	15-60 mg
Midazolam	Adjunct to anesthesia, anxiety/ amnesiac during cardioversion, anxiety/amnesia in endoscopic procedures	Inj	NA	0.4-0.7[3]	95	0.8-6.6	Yes	Rapid	Hepatic via CYP3A4	2-5 h	12 h	Urine	NA	NA

IR = immediate release, XR = extended release, NA = not available

Rapid = 15 minutes or less, intermediate = 15-30 minutes, slow = 30-60 minutes

[1]Significant metabolite

[2]Reliable bioavailability when given I.M.

[3]I.V. only

BETA-BLOCKERS

Agent	Adrenergic Receptor Blocking Activity	Intrinsic Sympathomimetic Activity (ISA)	Lipid Solubility	Protein Bound (%)	Half-Life (h)	Bioavailability (%)	Primary Site of Metabolism	Primary (Secondary) Route of Elimination	Indications	Usual Dosage
Acebutolol (Sectral)	$beta_1$	Yes	Low	15-25	3-4	40 7-fold[1]	Hepatic	Feces (renal)	Hypertension, arrhythmias	P.O.: 400-1200 mg/d
Atenolol (Tenormin)	$beta_1$	No	Low	<5-10	6-9	50-60 4-fold[1]	Hepatic (limited)	Feces (renal)	Hypertension, angina pectoris, acute MI	P.O.: 50-200 mg/d I.V.: Acute MI: 5 mg x 2 doses
Betaxolol (Kerlone)	$beta_1$	No	Low	50-55	14-22	84-94	Hepatic	Renal	Hypertension	P.O.: 5-20 mg/d
Bisoprolol (Zebeta)	$beta_1$	No	Low	26-33	9-12	80	Hepatic	Renal	Hypertension, heart failure	P.O.: HF: 2.5-10 mg/d HTN: 2.5-20 mg/d
Carvedilol (Coreg, Coreg CR)	$alpha_1$ $beta_1$ $beta_2$	No	ND	98	7-10	25-35	Hepatic	Feces	Hypertension, heart failure (mild to severe)	P.O.: 3.125-25 mg twice daily
Esmolol (Brevibloc)	$beta_1$	No	Low	55	0.15	NA 5-fold[1]	Red blood cell esterase	Renal	Supraventricular tachycardia, sinus tachycardia, atrial fibrillation/flutter, hypertension	I.V. infusion: 25-300 mcg/kg/min
Labetalol (Trandate)	$alpha_1$ $beta_1$ $beta_2$	No	Moderate	50	5.5-8	18-30 10-fold[1]	Hepatic	Renal	Hypertension	P.O.: 200-2400 mg/d I.V.: 20-80 mg at 10-min intervals up to a maximum of 300 mg **or** continuous infusion of 2-6 mg/min
Metoprolol (Lopressor, Toprol-XL)	$beta_1$	No	Moderate	10-12	3-7	50 7- to 10-fold[1] (Toprol XL: 77)	Hepatic	Renal	Hypertension, angina pectoris, acute MI, heart failure (mild to moderate; XL formulation only), atrial tachyarrhythmias (rate control)	P.O.: 100-450 mg/d HF: (Toprol-XL): 12.5-200 mg/d I.V.: Acute MI: 5 mg q2 min x 3 doses AF (rate control): 2.5-5 mg q2-5 min (max total dose: 15 mg over 0-15 min)
Nadolol (Corgard)	$beta_1$ $beta_2$	No	Low	25-30	20-24	30 5- to 8-fold[1]	None	Renal	Hypertension, angina pectoris	P.O.: 40-320 mg/d
Nebivolol (Bystolic)	$beta_1$	No	High	98	10-32	12-96	Hepatic	Renal (feces)	Hypertension	P.O.: 5-40 mg/d
Penbutolol (Levatol)	$beta_1$ $beta_2$	Yes	High	80-98	5	~100	Hepatic	Renal	Hypertension	P.O.: 20-80 mg/d
Pindolol	$beta_1$ $beta_2$	Yes	Moderate	57	3-4	90 2- to 2.5-fold[1]	Hepatic	Renal (feces)	Hypertension	P.O.: 20-60 mg/d
Propranolol (Inderal, various)	$beta_1$ $beta_2$	No	High	90	3-5	25 2- to 3-fold[1]	Hepatic	Renal	Hypertension, angina pectoris, arrhythmias, prophylaxis (post-MI)	P.O.: 40-480 mg/d I.V.: Tachyarrhythmias: 1-3 mg q2-5 min (max: 5 mg)

continued

Agent	Adrenergic Receptor Blocking Activity	Intrinsic Sympathomimetic Activity (ISA)	Lipid Solubility	Protein Bound (%)	Half-Life (h)	Bioavailability (%)	Primary Site of Metabolism	Primary (Secondary) Route of Elimination	Indications	Usual Dosage
Propranolol long-acting (Inderal-LA, InnoPran XL)	$beta_1$ $beta_2$	No	High	90	9-18	25 2- to 3-fold[1]	Hepatic	Renal	Hypertrophic cardiomyopathy with outflow tract obstruction, prophylaxis (post-MI)	P.O.: 180-240 mg/d
Sotalol (Betapace, Betapace AF, Sorine)	$beta_1$ $beta_2$	No	Low	0	12	90-100	None	Renal	Atrial and ventricular tachyarrhythmias	P.O.: 160-320 mg/d
Timolol (Blocadren)	$beta_1$ $beta_2$	No	Low to moderate	<10	4	75 7-fold[1]	Hepatic	Renal	Hypertension, prophylaxis (post-MI)	P.O.: 20-60 mg/d

Dosage is based on 70 kg adult with normal hepatic and renal function.

Note: All $beta_1$-selective agents will inhibit $beta_2$ receptors at higher doses.

[1]Interpatient variations in plasma levels

CALCIUM CHANNEL BLOCKERS – COMPARATIVE PHARMACOKINETICS

Agent	Bioavailability (%)	Protein Binding (%)	Onset of BP Effect (min)	Duration of BP Effect (h)	Half-Life (h)	Volume of Distribution	Route of Metabolism	Route of Excretion
Dihydropyridines								
AmLODIPine (Norvasc)	64-90	93-98	30-50	24	30-50	21 L/kg	Hepatic; inactive metabolites	Urine; 10% as parent
Clevidipine (Cleviprex)		>99.5	2-4	5-15 min	1-15 min	0.17 L/kg	Blood and extravascular tissue esterases	Urine (63% to 74%; as metabolites); feces (7% to 22%)
Felodipine (Plendil)	20	>99	2-5 h	24	11-16	10 L/kg	Hepatic; CYP3A4 substrate (major); inactive metabolites; extensive first pass	Urine (70%; as metabolites); feces 10%
Isradipine (DynaCirc)	15-24	95	2-3 h	>12	8	3 L/kg	Hepatic; CYP3A4 substrate (major); inactive metabolites; extensive first pass	Urine as metabolites
NiCARdipine (Cardene)	35	>95	30	≤8	2-4		Hepatic; CYP3A4 substrate (major); saturable first pass	Urine (60%; as metabolites); feces 35%
NIFEdipine (Procardia)	40-77	92-98	Within 20		2-5		Hepatic; CYP3A4 substrate (major); inactive metabolites	Urine as metabolites
NiMODipine (Nimotop)	13	>95	ND	4-6	1-2		Hepatic; CYP3A4 substrate (major); metabolites inactive or less active than parent; extensive first pass	Urine (50%; as metabolites); feces 32%
Nisoldipine (Sular)	5	>99	ND	6-12	7-12		Hepatic; CYP3A4 substrate (major); 1 active metabolite (10% of parent); extensive first pass	Urine as metabolites
Phenylalkylamines								
Verapamil (Calan, Verelan)	20-35	90	30	6-8	4.5-12		Hepatic; CYP3A4 substrate (major); 1 active metabolite (20% of parent); extensive first pass	Urine (70%; 3% to 4% as unchanged drug); feces 16%
Benzothiazepines								
Diltiazem (Cardizem)	~40	70-80	30-60	6-8	3-4.5	3-13 L/kg	Hepatic; CYP3A4 substrate (major); 1 major metabolite (20%-50% of parent); extensive first pass	Urine as metabolites

CORTICOSTEROIDS SYSTEMIC EQUIVALENCIES

Glucocorticoid	Approximate Equivalent Dose (mg)	Routes of Administration	Relative Anti-inflammatory Potency	Relative Mineralocorticoid Potency	Protein Binding (%)	Half-life Plasma (min)
Short-Acting						
Cortisone	25	P.O., I.M.	0.8	0.8	90	30
Hydrocortisone	20	I.M., I.V.	1	1	90	90
Intermediate-Acting						
MethylPREDNISolone[1]	4	P.O., I.M., I.V.	5	0	—	180
PrednisoLONE	5	P.O., I.M., I.V., intra-articular, intradermal, soft tissue injection	4	0.8	90-95	200
PredniSONE	5	P.O.	4	0.8	70	60
Triamcinolone[1]	4	I.M., intra-articular, intradermal, intrasynovial, soft tissue injection	5	0	—	300
Long-Acting						
Betamethasone	0.75	P.O., I.M., intra-articular, intradermal, intrasynovial, soft tissue injection	25	0	64	100-300
Dexamethasone	0.75	P.O., I.M., I.V., intra-articular, intradermal, soft tissue injection	25-30	0	—	100-300
Mineralocorticoids						
Fludrocortisone	—	P.O.	10	125	42	200

[1]May contain propylene glycol as an excipient in injectable forms

Asare K. Diagnosis and treatment of adrenal insufficiency in the critically ill patient. *Pharmacotherapy.* 2007;27(11):1512-1528.

INHALED CORTICOSTEROIDS

Estimated Comparative Daily Dosage

Children ≥12 Years of Age and Adults

Drug	Low Daily Dose	Medium Daily Dose	High Daily Dose
Beclomethasone HFA	80-240 mcg	>240-480 mcg	>480 mcg
Budesonide DPI	180-600 mcg	>600-1200 mcg	>1200 mcg
Flunisolide HFA	320 mcg	>320-640 mcg	>640 mcg
Fluticasone HFA	88-264 mcg	>264-440 mcg	>440 mcg
Fluticasone DPI	100-300 mcg	>300-500 mcg	>500 mcg
Mometasone DPI	200 mcg	400 mcg	>400 mcg

DPI = dry powder inhaler, HFA = hydrofluoroalkane

Children <12 Years of Age

Drug	Low Daily Dose	Medium Daily Dose	High Daily Dose
Beclomethasone HFA	0-4 years: NA 5-11 years: 80-160 mcg	0-4 years: NA 5-11 years: >160-320 mcg	0-4 years: NA 5-11 years: >320 mcg
Budesonide DPI	0-4 years: NA 5-11 years: 180-400 mcg	0-4 years: NA 5-11 years: >400-800 mcg	0-4 years: NA 5-11 years: >800 mcg
Budesonide nebulized	0-4 years: 0.25-0.5 mg 5-11 years: 0.5 mg	0-4 years: >0.5-1 mg 5-11 years: 1 mg	0-4 years: >1 mg 5-11 years: 2 mg
Flunisolide HFA	0-4 years: NA 5-11 years: 160 mcg	0-4 years: NA 5-11 years: 320 mcg	0-4 years: NA 5-11 years: ≥640 mcg
Fluticasone HFA	0-4 years: 176 mcg 5-11 years: 88-176 mcg	0-11 years: >176-352 mcg	0-11 years: >352 mcg
Fluticasone DPI	0-4 years: NA 5-11 years: 100-200 mcg	0-4 years: NA 5-11 years: >200-400 mcg	0-4 years: NA 5-11 years: >400 mcg
Mometasone	NA	NA	NA

DPI = dry powder inhaler, HFA = hydrofluoroalkane, NA = not approved for use in this age group or no data available

REFERENCE

Expert Panel Report 3. Guidelines for the diagnosis and management of asthma. *Clinical Practice Guidelines*, National Institutes of Health, National Heart, Lung, and Blood Institute, NIH Publication No. 08-4051. Available at http://www.nhlbi.nih.gov/guidelines/asthma/asthgdln.htm

TOPICAL CORTICOSTEROIDS

GUIDELINES FOR SELECTION AND USE OF TOPICAL CORTICOSTEROIDS

The quantity prescribed and the frequency of refills should be monitored to reduce the risk of adrenal suppression. In general, short courses of high-potency agents are preferable to prolonged use of low potency. After control is achieved, control should be maintained with a low potency preparation.

1. Low-to-medium potency agents are usually effective for treating thin, acute, inflammatory skin lesions; whereas, high or super-potent agents are often required for treating chronic, hyperkeratotic, or lichenified lesions.
2. Since the stratum corneum is thin on the face and intertriginous areas, low-potency agents are preferred but a higher potency agent may be used for 2 weeks.
3. Because the palms and soles have a thick stratum corneum, high or super-potent agents are frequently required.
4. Low potency agents are preferred for infants and the elderly. Infants have a high body surface area to weight ratio; elderly patients have thin, fragile skin.
5. The vehicle in which the topical corticosteroid is formulated influences the absorption and potency of the drug. Ointment bases are preferred for thick, lichenified lesions; they enhance penetration of the drug. Creams are preferred for acute and subacute dermatoses; they may be used on moist skin areas or intertriginous areas. Solutions, gels, and sprays are preferred for the scalp or for areas where a nonoil-based vehicle is needed.
6. In general, super-potent agents should not be used for longer than 2-3 weeks unless the lesion is limited to a small body area. Medium-to-high potency agents usually cause only rare adverse effects when treatment is limited to 3 months or less, and use on the face and intertriginous areas are avoided. If long-term treatment is needed, intermittent vs continued treatment is recommended.
7. Most preparations are applied once or twice daily. More frequent application may be necessary for the palms or soles because the preparation is easily removed by normal activity and penetration is poor due to a thick stratum corneum. Every-other-day or weekend-only application may be effective for treating some chronic conditions.

Relative Potency of Selected Topical Corticosteroids

Steroid		Dosage Form
	Very High Potency	
0.05%	Betamethasone dipropionate, augmented	Cream, gel, lotion, ointment
0.05%	Clobetasol propionate	Cream, foam, gel, lotion, ointment, shampoo, spray
0.05%	Diflorasone diacetate	Ointment
0.05%	Halobetasol propionate	Cream, ointment
	High Potency	
0.1%	Amcinonide	Cream, ointment, lotion
0.05%	Betamethasone dipropionate, augmented	Cream
0.05%	Betamethasone dipropionate	Cream, ointment
0.1%	Betamethasone valerate	Ointment
0.05%	Desoximetasone	Gel
0.25%	Desoximetasone	Cream, ointment
0.05%	Diflorasone diacetate	Cream, ointment
0.05%	Fluocinonide	Cream, ointment, gel
0.1%	Halcinonide	Cream, ointment
0.5%	Triamcinolone acetonide	Cream, spray
	Intermediate Potency	
0.05%	Betamethasone dipropionate	Lotion
0.1%	Betamethasone valerate	Cream
0.1%	Clocortolone pivalate	Cream
0.05%	Desoximetasone	Cream
0.025%	Fluocinolone acetonide	Cream, ointment
0.05%	Flurandrenolide	Cream, ointment, lotion, tape
0.005%	Fluticasone propionate	Ointment
0.05%	Fluticasone propionate	Cream, lotion
0.1%	Hydrocortisone butyrate[1]	Ointment, solution
0.2%	Hydrocortisone valerate[1]	Cream, ointment
0.1%	Mometasone furoate[1]	Cream, ointment, lotion
0.1%	Prednicarbate	Cream, ointment
0.025%	Triamcinolone acetonide	Cream, ointment, lotion
0.1%	Triamcinolone acetonide	Cream, ointment, lotion

Relative Potency of Selected Topical Corticosteroids *(continued)*

	Steroid	Dosage Form
	Low Potency	
0.05%	Alclometasone dipropionate[1]	Cream, ointment
0.05%	Desonide	Cream, ointment
0.01%	Fluocinolone acetonide	Cream, solution
0.5%	Hydrocortisone[1]	Cream, ointment, lotion
0.5%	Hydrocortisone acetate[1]	Cream, ointment
1%	Hydrocortisone acetate[1]	Cream, ointment
1%	Hydrocortisone[1]	Cream, ointment, lotion, solution
2.5%	Hydrocortisone[1]	Cream, ointment, lotion

[1]Not fluorinated

IMMUNE GLOBULIN PRODUCT COMPARISON

Brand Name	Concentration	pH	Initial Rate		Max Rate		IgA Content (mcg/mL)	Osmolarity/ Osmolality (mOsmol/kg)	Comments
			I.V.	SubQ[1]	I.V.[2]	SubQ[1]			
Bivigam	10%	4-4.6	0.3 mL/kg/h	–	3.6 mL/kg/h	–	≤200	Not available	Contains polysorbate 80
Carimune NF[3]	3%	6.4-6.8	1 mL/kg/h	–	6 mL/kg/h	–	Trace[4]	192-498[5]	Contains sucrose
	12%		0.24 mL/kg/h		1.5 mL/kg/h			768-1074[5]	
Flebogamma DIF	5%	5-6	0.6 mL/kg/h	–	6 mL/kg/h	–	<50	240-370	
	10%		0.6 mL/kg/h		4.8 mL/kg/h		<100		
GamaSTAN S/D	15% to 18%	6.4-7.2	–	–	–	–	Not available	Not available	For I.M. use
Gammagard S/D	5%	6.4-7.2	0.5 mL/kg/h	–	4 mL/kg/h	–	≤1[6]	636	Contains polysorbate 80
	10%		0.5 mL/kg/h		8 mL/kg/h		≤2[6]	1250	
Gammagard Liquid	10%	4.6-5.1	0.5 mL/kg/h	<40 kg: 15 mL/h/site with a maximum of 8 sites ≥40 kg: 20 mL/h/site with a maximum of 8 sites	5 mL/kg/h 5.4 mL/kg/h (MMN only)	<40 kg: 20 mL/h/site with a maximum of 8 sites; maximum **total** rate: 160 mL/h ≥40 kg: 30 mL/h/site with a maximum of 8 sites; maximum **total** rate: 240 mL/h	37	240-300	
Gammaked	10%	4-4.5	0.6 mL/kg/h 1.2 mL/kg/h (CIDP only)	20 mL/h/site with a maximum of 8 sites	4.8 mL/kg/h	Not determined	46	258	
Gammaplex	5%	4.8-5	0.6 mL/kg/h	–	4.8 mL/kg/h	–	<10	420-500	Contains polysorbate 80
Gamunex-C	10%	4-4.5	0.6 mL/kg/h 1.2 mL/kg/h (CIDP only)	20 mL/h/site with a maximum of 8 sites	4.8 mL/kg/h	Not determined	46	258	
Hizentra	20%	4.6-5.2	–	15 mL/h/site with a maximum of 4 sites	–	Up to 25 mL/h/site with a maximum of 4 sites; maximum **total** rate: 50 mL/h	≤50	380	Contains L-proline and polysorbate 80
Octagam	5%	5.1-6	0.6 mL/kg/h	–	4 mL/kg/h	–	≤200	310-380	Contains maltose
Privigen	10%	4.6-5	0.3 mL/kg/h	–	2.4 mL/kg/h (ITP) 4.8 mL/kg/h	–	≤25	240-440	Contains L-proline

CIDP = chronic inflammatory demyelinating polyneuropathy, ITP = immune (idiopathic) thrombocytopenic purpura, MMN = multifocal motor neuropathy

[1]Subcutaneous administration **only** for the treatment of primary humoral immunodeficiency (PI)

[2]Lower infusion rates should be used in patients at risk for renal dysfunction or thrombotic complications; see specific product information for details.

[3]Other concentrations may be prepared; see product information for additional details.

[4]Per product information; other sources list IgA content as 1000-2000 mcg/mL for 6% solution (Siegel J. Immune globulins: therapeutic, pharmaceutical, cost, and administration considerations. *Pharm Prac News*. 2013).

[5]Osmolarity depends on concentration and diluent used; see product information for details.

[6]Data presented is based on the maximum concentration that can be prepared. The 5% solution with IgA content <2.2 mcg/mL has been discontinued. The lower IgA product (ie, IgA <1 mcg/mL for the 5% prepared solution) is available by special request; contact manufacturer or see specific product information for details.

INJECTABLE AGENTS (NON-INSULIN) FOR TYPE 2 DIABETES

Generic Name (Brand Name)	Expected Decrease (%) in Hb A_{1c} With Monotherapy	Key Adverse Effects
Glucagon-Like Peptide 1 (GLP-1) Agonist		
Exenatide (Byetta)	0.5-1	Hypoglycemia, nausea, vomiting, pancreatitis, headache, jittery feeling
Liraglutide (Victoza)	1	**Thyroid C-cell Tumors [BOXED WARNING]**, nausea, vomiting, diarrhea, constipation, headache, pancreatitis
Amylin Agonists		
Pramlintide (Symlin)	0.4-0.6	**Coadministration with insulin may induce severe hypoglycemia [BOXED WARNING]**, nausea, vomiting, hypoglycemia, headache, anorexia

INSULIN PRODUCTS

Types of Insulin	Onset (h)	Peak Glycemic Effect (h)	Duration (h)
Rapid-Acting			
Insulin lispro (HumaLOG)	0.25-0.5	0.5-2.5	≤5
Insulin aspart (NovoLOG)	0.2-0.3	1-3	3-5
Insulin glulisine (Apidra)	0.2-0.5	1.6-2.8	3-4
Short-Acting			
Insulin regular (HumuLIN R, NovoLIN R)	0.5	2.5-5	4-12
Intermediate-Acting			
Insulin NPH (isophane suspension) (HumuLIN N, NovoLIN N)	1-2	4-12	14-24
Intermediate- to Long-Acting			
Insulin detemir (Levemir)	3-4	3-9	6-23 (duration is dose-dependent)
Long-Acting			
Insulin glargine (Lantus)	3-4	*	~11 to >24
Combinations			
Insulin aspart protamine suspension and insulin aspart (NovoLOG Mix 70/30)	0.17-0.33	1-4	18-24
Insulin lispro protamine and insulin lispro (HumaLOG Mix 75/25)	0.25-0.5	1-6.5	14-24
Insulin NPH suspension and insulin regular solution (NovoLIN 70/30)	0.5	2-12	18-24

*Insulin glargine has no pronounced peak.

LAXATIVES, CLASSIFICATION AND PROPERTIES

Laxative	Onset of Action	Site of Action	Mechanism of Action
Saline			
Magnesium citrate Magnesium hydroxide (Phillips' Milk of Magnesia)	30 min to 3 h	Small and large intestine	Attract/retain water in intestinal lumen increasing intraluminal pressure; cholecystokinin release
Sodium phosphates (Fleet Enema)	2-15 min	Colon	
Irritant/Stimulant			
Senna (Senokot)	6-10 h	Colon	Direct action on intestinal mucosa; stimulate myenteric plexus; alter water and electrolyte secretion
Bisacodyl (Dulcolax) tablets, suppositories	15 min to 1 h	Colon	
Castor oil	2-6 h	Small intestine	
Bulk-Producing			
Methylcellulose (Citrucel) Psyllium (Metamucil) Wheat dextrin (Benefiber)	12-24 h (up to 72 h) 24-48 h	Small and large intestine	Holds water in stool; mechanical distention
Lubricant			
Mineral oil	6-8 h	Colon	Lubricates intestine; retards colonic absorption of fecal water; softens stool
Surfactants/Stool Softener			
Docusate/senna (Peri-Colace)	8-12 h	Small and large intestine	Senna – mild irritant; docusate – stool softener
Docusate sodium (Colace) Docusate calcium (Surfak)	24-72 h	Small and large intestine	Detergent activity; facilitates admixture of fat and water to soften stool
Osmotic Laxatives			
Glycerin suppository	15-30 min	Colon	Local irritation; hyperosmotic action
Lactulose	24-48 h	Colon	Delivers osmotically active molecules to colon
Polyethylene glycol 3350 (GlycoLax, MiraLax)	48 h	Small and large intestine	Nonabsorbable solution which acts as an osmotic agent
Sodium sulfate, potassium sulfate, and magnesium sulfate (Suprep)	24 h	Small and large intestine	Hyperosmotic action
Sorbitol 70%	24-48 h	Colon	Delivers osmotically active molecules to colon
Combination Laxatives			
Sodium picosulfate, magnesium oxide, and citric acid (Prepopik)	3-6 h	Colon	Sodium picosulfate: Direct action on intestinal mucosa; stimulate myenteric plexus Magnesium oxide and citric acid: Combine to form magnesium citrate, which exhibits hyperosmotic action
Miscellaneous Laxatives			
Lubiprostone (Amitiza)	24-48 h	Apical membrane of the GI epithelium	Activates intestinal chloride channels increasing intestinal fluid

NITRATES

Nitrates[1]	Route/Dosage Form	Onset (min)	Duration
Nitroglycerin	I.V. (continuous)	1-2	Tolerance begins in 7-8 h
	Sublingual	1-3	≥25 min
	Translingual spray	2	≥25 min
	Oral, sustained release	40-60	4-8 h
	Topical ointment	20-60	Up to 7 h
	Transdermal	40-60	8-12 h
Isosorbide dinitrate	Sublingual	2-5	1-2 h
	Oral	~60	Up to 8 h
	Oral, sustained release	~60	Up to 8 h
Isosorbide mononitrate	Oral	~60	5-12 h
	Oral, extended release	30-60	12-24 h

[1]Hemodynamic and antianginal tolerance often develops within 24-48 hours of continuous nitrate administration; allow an adequate nitrate-free interval of 8-12 hours.

Adapted from Gibbons RJ, Abrams J, Chatterjee K, et al. ACC/AHA 2002 guideline update for the management of patients with chronic stable angina – summary article: a report of the American College of Cardiology/American Heart Association Task Force on Practice Guidelines (Committee on the Management of Patients With Chronic Stable Angina). *Circulation*. 2003;107(1):149-158.

OPIOID CONVERSION TABLE

This table serves as a general guide to opioid conversion. Utilization of a direct conversion without a detailed patients and medication assessment is not recommended and may result in over- or underdosing. Chronic administration may alter pharmacokinetics and change parenteral:oral ratio.

Opioid Analgesics – Initial Oral Dosing Commonly Used for Severe Pain

Drug	Equianalgesic Dose (mg)		Initial Oral Dose	
	Oral[1]	Parenteral[2]	Children[3] (mg/kg)	Adults (mg)
Buprenorphine	—	0.4	—	—
Butorphanol	—	2	—	—
FentaNYL	—	0.1	—	—
HYDROmorphone	7.5	1.5	0.06	4-8
Levorphanol	Acute: 4 Chronic: 1	Acute: 2 Chronic: 1	0.04	2-4
Meperidine[4]	300	75	Not recommended	
Methadone[5]	See Guidelines for Conversion to Oral Methadone in Adults	Variable	0.2	5-10
Morphine	30	10	0.3	15-30
Nalbuphine	—	10	—	—
OxyCODONE	20	—	0.2	10-20
Oxymorphone	10	1	—	5-10
Pentazocine	50	30	—	—

Guidelines for Conversion to Oral Methadone in Adults[5]

Oral Morphine Dose or Equivalent (mg/day)	Oral Morphine:Oral Methadone (Conversion Ratio)
<90	4:1
90-300	8:1
>300	12:1

[1]Elderly: Starting dose should be lower for this population group.

[2]Standard parenteral doses (I.M.) for acute pain in adults; can be used to convert doses for I.V. infusions and repeated small I.V. boluses. For single I.V. boluses, use half the I.M. dose.

[3]The pharmacokinetics of opioids in children and infants >6 months old are similar to adults, but infants <6 months old, especially premature or physically compromised ones, are at risk of apnea.

[4]Not recommended for routine use

[5]Conversion of higher doses may be guided by the following (consult a pain or palliative care specialist if unfamiliar with methadone prescribing): As the total daily chronic dose of morphine increases, the equianalgesic dose ratio (morphine:methadone) changes (American Pain Society, 2008). Total daily dose should be divided by 3; delivered every 8 hours. Methadone is significantly more potent with repetitive dosing (due to its active metabolite). Begin methadone at lower doses and gradually titrate. Applicability to pediatric patients is unknown.

REFERENCES

National Cancer Institute. Pain (PDQ). Last modified May 7, 2009. Available at http://www.cancer.gov/cancertopics/pdq/supportivecare/pain/HealthProfessional/page1

National Comprehensive Cancer Network (NCCN). Clinical practice guidelines in oncology: adult cancer pain. Version 1, 2009. Available at http://www.nccn.org/professionals/physician_gls/PDF/pain.pdf

Patanwala AE, Duby J, Waters D, et al. Opioid conversions in acute care. *Ann Pharmacother.* 2007;41(2):255-266.

Principles of Analgesic Use in the Treatment of Acute Pain and Cancer Pain. 6th ed. Glenview, IL: American Pain Society; 2008.

ORAL ANTICOAGULANT COMPARISON CHART

Medication	Mechanism of Action	Metabolism	Monitoring Parameters	Pharmacotherapy Pearls	Reversal Strategies[1]	Preoperative/Preprocedure Management (General Guide)
Warfarin	Inhibits formation of vitamin K-dependent clotting factors II, VII, IX, X, and proteins C and S	• CYP2C9 • CYP1A2 • CYP3A4 • CYP2C19	• PT/INR (individualized; depends on INR stability)	• CYP1A2, 3A4, 2C9, and 2C19 drug interactions and vitamin K-containing food interactions • Full therapeutic effect usually seen within 5-7 days • Half-life is ~40 hours	• Vitamin K (route and dose will depend on clinical situation and INR) • For major bleeding (at any INR): Consider PCC with vitamin K ± FFP	• Hold at least 5 days before surgery; depending on urgency of surgery/procedure, may administer low-dose I.V. or oral vitamin K • Minor dental and minor dermatological procedures or cataract surgery: Continue warfarin (with hemostatic agent [dental] or local hemostasis [dermatological]); may also discontinue use 2-3 days prior to dental procedures. Patients with prior stroke undergoing dental procedures should routinely continue warfarin.
Dabigatran (Pradaxa)	Directly inhibits thrombin	• Hepatic glucuronidation • P-gp substrate	• Routine lab monitoring not required; aPTT, ECT (if available), TT (most sensitive) may be used to detect presence of dabigatran • Renal function	• Compliance issues (BID dosing) • Specific conversions to/from warfarin, parenteral anticoagulants • Renal dosing adjustment required; per ACCP, contraindicated with Cl_{Cr} ≤30 mL/minute • Use with caution in patients ≥80 years of age • Dose reduction or avoidance required if used with dronedarone, ketoconazole, P-gp inhibitors • P-gp drug interactions • Half-life is 12-17 hours; considerably prolonged with severe renal impairment	• No specific antidote; for major bleeding, may consider activated PCC (ie, FEIBA NF), recombinant factor VIIa[2], or concentrates of factors II, IX, or X[3] • Use of a 4-factor PCC was shown **not** to be effective • Dabigatran is ~60% dialyzable • Activated charcoal may be used if ingestion occurred <2 hours prior to presentation	• Cl_{Cr} ≥50 mL/minute: Hold 1-2 days before surgery • Cl_{Cr} <50 mL/minute: Hold 3-5 days before surgery • May consider holding for >5 days in patients undergoing major surgery, spinal puncture, or insertion of a spinal or epidural catheter or port
Rivaroxaban (Xarelto)	Directly inhibits factor Xa	• CYP3A4 • CYP3A5 • CYP2J2 • P-gp substrate	• Routine lab monitoring not required; may use PT to detect presence of rivaroxaban • Renal and hepatic function	• Administer doses ≥15 mg/day with food • Dosing frequency depends on indication • Specific conversions to/from warfarin, parenteral anticoagulants • Renal dosing adjustment required • Avoid in moderate or severe hepatic impairment • CYP3A4 and P-gp drug interactions • Half-life is 5-9 hours; slightly prolonged with renal impairment	• No specific antidote; for major bleeding, may consider PCC, activated PCC (ie, FEIBA NF), or recombinant factor VIIa[3] • Rivaroxaban is **not** dialyzable	• Hold at least 24 hours before surgery; longer duration of treatment cessation may be necessary based on individual patient situation and physician clinical judgment
Apixaban (Eliquis)	Directly inhibits factor Xa	• CYP3A4 • P-gp substrate	• Routine lab monitoring not required; PT, INR, and aPTT may be used to detect presence of apixaban	• Compliance issues (BID dosing) • Specific conversions to/from warfarin, parenteral anticoagulants • Renal dosing adjustment required; the AHA/ASA recommends to avoid use with Cl_{Cr} <25 mL/minute • Not recommended in patients with severe liver impairment • CYP3A4 and P-gp drug interactions • Half-life is ~8-15 hours; slightly prolonged with renal impairment	• No specific antidote; for major bleeding, may consider PCC, activated PCC (ie, FEIBA NF), or recombinant factor VIIa • Apixaban is **not** dialyzable • Activated charcoal may be used if ingestion occurred within 2-6 hours of presentation	• Hold at least 24-48 hours, depending on risk or location of bleeding, before elective surgery or invasive procedures.

Abbreviations: ACCP = American College of Chest Physicians, AHA/ASA = American Heart Association/American Stroke Association, aPTT = activated partial thromboplastin time, BID = twice daily, ECT = ecarin clotting time, FFP = fresh frozen plasma, INR = international normalized ratio, PCC = prothrombin complex concentrate, P-gp = P-glycoprotein, PT = prothrombin time, TT = thrombin time

Note: Recommendations listed reflect only the U.S. labeling or U.S. clinical practice guidelines.

[1]Management of anticoagulant-associated bleeding requires careful consideration of the indication for anticoagulant therapy and bleeding extent (eg, epistaxis vs intracranial hemorrhage); minor bleeding may only require local hemostasis.

[2]The use of rFVIIa in healthy subjects treated with another direct thrombin inhibitor, melagatran (not FDA-approved), did not reverse the anticoagulant effects of melagatran.

[3]The evidence in support of these reversal strategies is limited; an exception to this may be the use of a 4-factor PCC for rivaroxaban reversal. The only available 4-factor PCC currently in the U.S. is Kcentra. Other 4-factor PCCs **not** available in the U.S. include Beriplex P/N, Cofact, and Octaplex. Bebulin VH and Profilnine SD **do not** contain adequate levels of factor VII and are considered 3-factor PCCs.

Armstrong MJ, Gronseth G, Anderson DC, et al. Summary of evidence-based guideline: periprocedural management of antithrombotic medications in patients with ischemic cerebrovascular disease: report of the Guideline Development Subcommittee of the American Academy of Neurology. *Neurology.* 2013;80(22):2065-2069.

Furie KL, Goldstein LB, Albers GW, et al. Oral antithrombotic agents for the prevention of stroke in nonvalvular atrial fibrillation: a science advisory for healthcare professionals from the American Heart Association/American Stroke Association. *Stroke.* 2012;43(12):3442-3453.

Guyatt GH, Akl EA, Crowther M, et al. Executive summary: antithrombotic therapy and prevention of thrombosis, 9th ed: American College of Chest Physicians evidence-based clinical practice guidelines. *Chest.* 2012;141(2 Suppl):7S-47S.

Kaatz S, Kouides PA, Garcia DA, et al. Guidance on the emergent reversal of oral thrombin and factor Xa inhibitors. *Am J Hematol.* 2012;87(Suppl 1):S141-S145.

Levi M, Eerenberg E, Kamphuisen PW. Bleeding risk and reversal strategies for old and new anticoagulants and antiplatelet agents. *J Thromb Haemost.* 2011;9(9):1705-1712.

Poulsen BK, Grove EL, Husted SE. New oral anticoagulants: a review of the literature with particular emphasis on patients with impaired renal function. *Drugs.* 2012;72(13):1739-1753.

Wolzt M, Levi M, Sarich TC, et al. Effect of recombinant factor VIIa on melagatran-induced inhibition of thrombin generation and platelet activation in healthy volunteers. *Thromb Haemost.* 2004;91(6):1090-1096.

REVERSAL OF ORAL ANTICOAGULANTS

Both oral and parenteral anticoagulants have established use in the prevention and treatment of a variety of thrombotic conditions (eg, acute coronary syndrome, venous thromboembolism, stroke). Although much has been done to prevent bleeding events associated with these agents, hemorrhagic events still continue to occur. Therefore, a thorough understanding of how best to reverse these agents when bleeding does occur is imperative. Information in this area is surfacing rapidly and recommendations may be changing. Refer to the most recent literature or guidelines for more detail and guidance. Reversal of parenteral anticoagulants, such as heparin and low molecular weight heparin (LMWH), and management of bleeding associated with these agents is established and beyond the focus of this piece.

For many years, vitamin K antagonists (eg, warfarin, acenocoumarol) were the only effective oral anticoagulants available. Recently, newer oral anticoagulants have been developed and are now marketed for prevention of stroke in patients with nonvalvular atrial fibrillation and prevention and treatment of venous thromboembolism. These include dabigatran, apixaban, and rivaroxaban. Dabigatran is an oral direct thrombin inhibitor. Apixaban and rivaroxaban are both oral factor Xa inhibitors.

VITAMIN K ANTAGONIST-INDUCED BLEEDING

Warfarin is the most common vitamin K antagonist (VKA) used in North America. The management of bleeding and reversal of other VKAs is the same. Therefore, the term VKA will be used here. VKAs interfere with the cyclic interconversion of vitamin K and vitamin K epoxide, ultimately resulting in lowered production of effective factors II, VII, IX, and X. VKAs also inhibit the production of proteins C, S, and Z which may result in procoagulation. The half-life of racemic warfarin ranges from 36-42 hours. Other VKAs, such as acenocoumarol, have significantly shorter half-lives. Warfarin, due to metabolism via the cytochrome P450 enzyme system (specifically CYP2C9, CYP3A4, CYP1A2, and CYP2C19), is subject to a number of drug-drug interactions which may occur by inhibiting these isoenzymes, leading to reduced metabolism and elevated warfarin concentrations. Intensity of anticoagulation with VKAs can predict the incidence of bleeding events. When the INR is greater than 5, the incidence of bleeding increases dramatically; patient factors also play a major role in risk of bleeding (eg, prior history of bleeding, advanced age, renal insufficiency) (Ageno, 2012).

Patients with elevated INR may not need reversal unless undergoing an invasive procedure. If the invasive procedure is elective, the procedure should be delayed until INR is acceptable for the procedure. In general, for patients with an INR of 6-10, up to ~2.5 days may elapse before the INR reduces to <4 (Patel, 2000). Some patients may require bridging with a parenteral anticoagulant during this time to prevent thrombosis.

Patients who are bleeding may require reversal with vitamin K (or phytonadione). Rapid reversal is necessary if the bleeding is life-threatening. In this case, the use of intravenous vitamin K and either fresh frozen plasma (FFP), prothrombin complex concentrates (PCC), or recombinant factor VIIa (rFVIIa) becomes imperative. Currently, the American College of Chest Physicians recommends an intravenous vitamin K dose of 5-10 mg administered slowly. Due to the occurrence of anaphylactoid reaction with rapid intravenous administration with vitamin K, intravenous vitamin K should always be diluted in a minimum of 50 mL of a compatible solution and infused over at least 20 minutes (Ageno, 2012). Reduction of INR with intravenous administration usually begins within 2 hours of administration. Subcutaneous administration of vitamin K is not recommended due to slower resolution of elevated INR.

The choice as to which coagulation factor (FFP, PCC, or rFVIIa) to use in addition to intravenous vitamin K for the patient who has life-threatening bleeding has not been established. Advantages and disadvantages exist with all the coagulation factors. Regardless of which one is chosen, the target INR for the patient with a life-threatening bleed is typically <1.5. FFP contains all of the factors inhibited by warfarin (factors II, VII, IX, and X) and would be an ideal agent to use for reversal. However, high volumes of FFP may be problematic in patients who are sensitive to rapid fluid shifts (eg, heart failure). FFP also has the disadvantages of possible allergic reaction, transfusion-related lung injury (TRALI), transmission of infection, and prolonged preparation time due to frozen storage. A new plasma substitute (OctaplaseLG) is now available. OctaplaseLG, labeled for the rapid reversal of VKA-induced anticoagulation, is solvent-detergent treated and has been shown to not cause TRALI and other side effects seen with FFP. PCCs, although more costly compared to FFP, are advantageous in that they have a lower infusion volume, lower transmission rate of infection, can be administered rapidly with rapid reversal of VKA-associated coagulopathy, do not require cross-matching, and are associated with less complications. Currently, the American College of Chest Physicians recommends the use of four-factor PCCs over FFP and rFVIIa. The only available four-factor PCC in the U.S. is Kcentra (known as Beriplex P/N outside the U.S.). Other four-factor PCCs not available in the U.S. include Cofact, Kanokad, and Octaplex. Bebulin VH and Profilnine SD do not contain adequate levels of factor VII and are considered three-factor PCCs (see table on next page).

Composition of Prothrombin Complex Concentrates

Prothrombin Complex Concentrate	Factor II	Factor VII	Factor IX	Factor X	Heparin	Human Antithrombin III	Protein C	Protein S	Protein Z
"Three-Factor (minimal factor VII component) PCCs"									
Bebulin VH	24-38 IU/mL	<5 IU/mL	24-38 IU/mL	24-38 IU/mL	<0.15 IU/IU FIX	–	–	–	–
Profilnine SD	NMT 150 units/ 100 FIX units	NMT 35 units/ 100 FIX units	100 units	NMT 100 units/ 100 FIX units	–	–	–	–	–
"Four-Factor PCCs"									
Cofact[a]	14-35 IU/mL	7-20 IU/mL	25 IU/mL	14-35 IU/mL	–	<0.6 IU/mL	11-39 IU/mL	1-8 IU/mL	–
Kanokad[a]	14-35 IU/mL	7-20 IU/mL	25 IU/mL	14-35 IU/mL	–	–	–	–	–
Kcentra (known as Beriplex P/N outside the U.S.)	19-40 IU/mL	10-25 IU/mL	20-31 IU/mL	25-51 IU/mL	0.4-2 IU/mL	0.2-1.5 IU/mL	21-41 IU/mL	12-34 IU/mL	–
Octaplex[a]	14-38 IU/mL	9-24 IU/mL	25 IU/mL	18-30 IU/mL	5-12.5 IU/mL	–	13-31 IU/mL	12-32 IU/mL	–
"Activated PCC"									
FEIBA NF	1.3 IU/IU[b]	0.9 IU/IU	1.4 IU/IU[b]	1.1 IU/IU[b]	–	–	1.1 IU/IU	–	–

FIX = Factor IX, NMT = not more than

[a]Not available in the U.S.

[b]Mainly nonactivated form

The use of rFVIIa gained some interest; however, it has not been shown to be superior to PCC or FFP and is the most expensive agent of the three. The combination of rFVIIa and three-factor PCC (along with intravenous vitamin K) has been used with some success (Sarode, 2012); however, the combination cannot be recommended at this time.

DABIGATRAN-INDUCED BLEEDING

Dabigatran is a new oral direct thrombin inhibitor with an elimination half-life of 12-17 hours. Dabigatran is 80% excreted in the urine as unchanged drug and therefore elimination half-life is prolonged in patients with renal impairment (up to 28 hours with severe impairment). Dabigatran is hepatically metabolized via glucuronidation to active acylglucuronide isomers. Although not a substrate for CYP450, dabigatran is a substrate of P-glycoprotein (gp). Therefore, P-gp inhibitors may increase dabigatran concentrations, resulting in a higher risk of bleeding events.

Similar to its parenteral counterparts (eg, argatroban), dabigatran does not have a specific reversal agent. Although the INR may be elevated with dabigatran use, vitamin K is not effective for dabigatran-induced bleeding. In addition, the aPTT rises as dabigatran concentrations increase; however, the use of protamine will not reverse these effects on the aPTT. Based on limited evidence for reversal strategies, several different recommendations have been put forth. Activated charcoal should be administered if oral intake was recent (ie, within a couple of hours of presentation). Hemodialysis, although this may be impractical, has been shown to remove 62% to 68% over 2-4 hours (Stangier, 2010). The use of a four-factor PCC (Cofact; not available in the U.S.) has been shown to be ineffective for dabigatran reversal (Eerenberg, 2011). In addition, other coagulation factors (eg, FFP, rFVIIa) have not adequately demonstrated benefit in humans and therefore cannot be formally recommended.

ORAL FACTOR XA INHIBITOR-INDUCED BLEEDING

Apixaban and rivaroxaban are oral factor Xa inhibitors. Apixaban has an elimination half-life of 8-15 hours and is metabolized to a minor degree via the cytochrome P450 system (specifically CYP2C19, CYP2C8, CYP2C9, and CYP3A4) and is a P-gp substrate. Apixaban is also partially excreted (~27%) as unchanged drug in the urine. Rivaroxaban has an elimination half-life of 5-9 hours and is excreted (~36%) as unchanged drug in the urine. Rivaroxaban is hepatically metabolized via CYP3A4/5 and CYP2J2 and is a substrate of P-gp as well.

The use of rFVIIa has been shown to decrease the bleeding time in animal models; however, it does not reverse the anticoagulant effect of rivaroxaban. The use of rFVIIa has not been formally evaluated in humans treated with rivaroxaban or apixaban. The use of a four-factor PCC (Cofact; not available in the U.S.) has been shown to reverse the anticoagulant effect of rivaroxaban in humans (Eerenberg, 2011). Therefore, because of the lack of data in humans, the use of PCC or rFVIIa cannot be formally recommended for rapid reversal in patients receiving apixaban or rivaroxaban.

CONCLUSION

The approach to the bleeding patient receiving oral anticoagulation is challenging. Unfortunately, data supporting specific reversal agents is lacking beyond the known antidotes used for specific therapies (eg, warfarin). Research in this area is expanding the knowledge; however, much research is still needed to further define specific approaches to patients receiving newer oral anticoagulants. Reversal agents for some of these new oral anticoagulants are being developed, such as the recombinant antidote PRT064445, and future oral anticoagulants will likely be released with a reversal agent (eg, betrixaban and its specific antidote PRT4445).

REFERENCES

Ageno W, Gallus AS, Wittkowsky A, et al. Oral anticoagulant therapy: antithrombotic therapy and prevention of thrombosis, 9th ed: American College of Chest Physicians evidence-based clinical practice guidelines. *Chest.* 2012;141(2 Suppl):e44S-e88S.

Bauer KA. Reversal of antithrombotic agents. *Am J Hematol.* 2012;87(Suppl 1):S119-S126.

Bechtel BF, Nunez TC, Lyon JA, et al. Treatments for reversing warfarin anticoagulation in patients with acute intracranial hemorrhage: a structured literature review. *Int J Emerg Med.* 2011;4(1):40.

Dager WE. Developing a management plan for oral anticoagulant reversal. *Am J Health Syst Pharm.* 2013;70(10 Suppl 1):S21-S31.

Dager WE, Gosselin RC, Kitchen S, et al. Dabigatran effects on the international normalized ratio, activated partial thromboplastin time, thrombin time, and fibrinogen: a multicenter, *in vitro* study. *Ann Pharmacother.* 2012;46(12):1627-1636.

Dumkow LE, Voss JR, Peters M, et al. Reversal of dabigatran-induced bleeding with a prothrombin complex concentrate and fresh frozen plasma. *Am J Health Syst Pharm.* 2012;69(19):1646-1650.

Eerenberg ES, Kamphuisen PW, Sijpkens MK, et al. Reversal of rivaroxaban and dabigatran by prothrombin complex concentrate: a randomized, placebo-controlled, crossover study in healthy subjects. *Circulation.* 2011;124(14):1573-1579.

Holbrook A, Schulman S, Witt DM, et al. Evidence-based management of anticoagulant therapy: antithrombotic therapy and prevention of thrombosis, 9th ed: American College of Chest Physicians evidence-based clinical practice guidelines. *Chest.* 2012;141(2 Suppl):e152S-e184S.

Kaatz S, Kouides PA, Garcia DA, et al. Guidance on the emergent reversal of oral thrombin and factor Xa inhibitors. *Am J Hematol.* 2012;87(Suppl 1): S141-S145.

Marlu R, Hodaj E, Paris A, et al. Effect of non-specific reversal agents on anticoagulant activity of dabigatran and rivaroxaban: a randomised crossover *ex vivo* study in healthy volunteers. *Thromb Haemost.* 2012;108(2):217-224.

Miesbach W, Seifried E. New direct oral anticoagulants – current therapeutic options and treatment recommendations for bleeding complications. *Thromb Haemost.* 2012;108(4):625-632.

Miyares MA, Davis K. Newer oral anticoagulants: a review of laboratory monitoring options and reversal agents in the hemorrhagic patient. *Am J Health Syst Pharm.* 2012;69(17):1473-1484.

Ortel TL. Perioperative management of patients on chronic antithrombotic therapy. *Hematology Am Soc Hematol Educ Program.* 2012;2012:529-535.

Patel RJ, Witt DM, Saseen JJ, et al. Randomized, placebo-controlled trial of oral phytonadione for excessive anticoagulation. *Pharmacotherapy.* 2000;20 (10):1159-1166.

Patriquin C, Crowther M. Treatment of warfarin-associated coagulopathy with vitamin K. *Expert Rev Hematol.* 2011;4(6):657-665.

Sarode R, Matevosyan K, Bhagat R, et al. Rapid warfarin reversal: a 3-factor prothrombin complex concentrate and recombinant factor VIIa cocktail for intracerebral hemorrhage. *J Neurosurg*. 2012;116(3):491-497.

Sarode R, Milling TJ Jr, Refaai MA, et al. Efficacy and safety of a four-factor prothrombin complex concentrate (4F-PCC) in patients on vitamin K antagonists presenting with major bleeding: a randomized, plasma-controlled, phase IIIb study. *Circulation*. 2013.

Siegal DM, Crowther MA. Acute management of bleeding in patients on novel oral anticoagulants. *Eur Heart J*. 2013;34(7):489-498b.

Stangier J, Rathgen K, Stähle H, et al. Influence of renal impairment on the pharmacokinetics and pharmacodynamics of oral dabigatran etexilate: an open-label, parallel-group, single-centre study. *Clin Pharmacokinet*. 2010;49(4):259-268.

van Ryn J, Stangier J, Haertter S, et al. Dabigatran etexilate – a novel, reversible, oral direct thrombin inhibitor: interpretation of coagulation assays and reversal of anticoagulant activity. *Thromb Haemost*. 2010;103(6):1116-1127.

Wanek MR, Horn ET, Elapavaluru S, et al. Safe use of hemodialysis for dabigatran removal before cardiac surgery. *Ann Pharmacother*. 2012;46(9):e21.

Weitz JI, Eikelboom JW, Samama MM, et al. New antithrombotic drugs: antithrombotic therapy and prevention of thrombosis, 9th ed: American College of Chest Physicians evidence-based clinical practice guidelines. *Chest*. 2012;141(2 Suppl):e120S-e151S.

ORAL ANTIDIABETIC AGENTS COMPARISON TABLE

Oral Antidiabetic Agents for Type 2 Diabetes

Generic Name (Brand Name)	Expected Decrease (%) in Hb A_{1c} With Monotherapy	Key Adverse Effects
Alpha-Glucosidase Inhibitors		
Acarbose (Precose)	0.5-0.8	GI distress, bloating, flatulence
Miglitol (Glyset)		
Antilipemic Agent (Adjunct Therapy)		
Colesevelam (WelChol)	0.5-1 (not for use as monotherapy)	Constipation, dyspepsia
Biguanide		
Metformin (Fortamet; Glucophage XR; Glucophage; Glumetza; Riomet)	1-2	**Lactic acidosis [BOXED WARNING]**, GI distress, weakness
Dipeptidyl Peptidase IV (DPP-IV) Inhibitors		
Linagliptin (Tradjenta)	0.4	Headache, nasopharyngitis, arthralgia, back pain
Saxagliptin (Onglyza)	0.4-0.5	Headache, UTI, sinusitis
Sitagliptin (Januvia)	0.5-0.8	Nasopharyngitis, GI distress, nausea, peripheral edema, hypoglycemia
Dopamine agonists		
Bromocriptine (Cycloset)	0.1	Nausea, dizziness, somnolence, postural hypotension, headache
Meglitinide Derivatives		
Nateglinide (Starlix)	0.5-1.5 (repaglinide may be more effective)	Upper respiratory infection, flu-like syndrome, headache, hypoglycemia
Repaglinide (Prandin)		
Sodium-Glucose Co-Transporter 2 (SGLT2) Inhibitors		
Canagliflozin (Invokana)	0.77-1.03	Genital mycotic infections, UTI, increased urination
Sulfonylurea, 1st Generation		
ChlorproPAMIDE (Diabinese)	1-2	Hypoglycemia, dizziness, headache, GI distress, SIADH
Tolazamide		
TOLBUTamide		
Sulfonylurea, 2nd Generation		
Glimepiride (Amaryl)	1-2	Hypoglycemia, dizziness, headache, GI distress, SIADH
GlipiZIDE (Glucotrol XL; Glucotrol)		
GlyBURIDE (DiaBeta; Glynase PresTab; Micronase)		
Thiazolidinediones		
Pioglitazone (Actos)	0.5-1.4	**May cause or exacerbate heart failure [BOXED WARNING]**, hepatic dysfunction, weight gain, edema, lipid changes
Rosiglitazone (Avandia)		

ORAL ANTIPLATELET COMPARISON CHART

Medication	Mechanism of Action	Reversible Platelet Inhibition	Prodrug	Metabolism	Pharmacotherapy Pearls	Reversal Strategies[1]	Preoperative/Preprocedure Management (General Guide)
Aspirin	Inhibits cyclooxygenase-1 and 2	No	No	• CYP2C9	• Chronic NSAID use can compromise antiplatelet effects • Monitor for GI ulceration	• No specific antidote • Consider platelet transfusion ± DDAVP • Normal platelet function returns within 7-10 days after discontinuation	• Hold 7-10 days before surgery • May be continued through surgery for CABG or noncardiac surgery in patients with moderate to high cardiac risk • Minor dental or dermatological procedures or cataract surgery: Continue through procedure. AAN recommends continuation when undergoing any dental procedure for patients taking aspirin for ischemic stroke prevention.
Cilostazol (Pletal)	Inhibits platelet phosphodiesterase III	Yes	No	• CYP3A4 • CYP2C19 • CYP1A2 • CYP2D6	• Administer before or 2 hours after meals • Contraindicated in patients with heart failure of any severity • CYP3A4 and 2C19 drug interactions	• No specific antidote • Normal platelet function returns within 4 days after discontinuation	• Hold 2-3 days before surgery
Clopidogrel (Plavix)	Inhibits $P2Y_{12}$ component of ADP receptors	No	Yes	• CYP2C19 • CYP3A4	• CYP2C19 inhibitors may reduce concentrations of active metabolite • CYP2C19 polymorphisms may affect clopidogrel efficacy	• No specific antidote • Consider platelet transfusion ± DDAVP • Normal platelet function returns within 7-10 days after discontinuation	• Hold 5-10 days before surgery[2]
Ticlopidine	Inhibits $P2Y_{12}$ component of ADP receptors	No	Yes	• CYP3A4	• Black Box warning on hematologic toxicities (aplastic anemia, TTP) • Frequent CBC monitoring required •BID dosing	• No specific antidote • Consider platelet transfusion ± DDAVP • Normal platelet function returns within 5-10 days after discontinuation	• Hold 10-14 days before surgery
Prasugrel (Effient)	Inhibits $P2Y_{12}$ component of ADP receptors	No	Yes	• CYP3A4 • CYP2B6	• Reduce maintenance dose to 5 mg in patients <60 kg • Contraindicated in patients with history of stroke, TIA • Not recommended in patients ≥75 years of age	• No specific antidote • Consider platelet transfusion ± DDAVP • Normal platelet function returns within 5-9 days after discontinuation	• Hold 5-7 days before surgery[2]
Ticagrelor (Brilinta)	Inhibits $P2Y_{12}$ component of ADP receptors	Yes	No	• CYP3A4 • CYP3A5	• Used in combination with aspirin; daily maintenance aspirin dose should not exceed 81 mg • CYP3A4 drug interactions • BID dosing • Monitor closely for dyspnea, bradyarrhythmia (including ventricular pauses)	• No specific antidote • Consider aminocaproic acid, tranexamic acid, recombinant factor VIIa • Normal platelet function returns within 3-5 days after discontinuation	• Hold at least 5 days before surgery[2]

[1]Management of antiplatelet-associated bleeding requires careful consideration of the indication for antiplatelet therapy and bleeding extent (eg, epistaxis vs intracranial hemorrhage); minor bleeding may only require local hemostasis.

[2]When urgent CABG is necessary, the ACCF/AHA CABG guidelines recommend discontinuation for at least 24 hours prior to surgery (Hillis, 2011).

Armstrong MJ, Gronseth G, Anderson DC, et al. Summary of evidence-based guideline: periprocedural management of antithrombotic medications in patients with ischemic cerebrovascular disease: report of the Guideline Development Subcommittee of the American Academy of Neurology. *Neurology.* 2013;80(22):2065-2069.

Hillis LD, Smith PK, Anderson JL, et al. 2011 ACCF/AHA guideline for coronary artery bypass graft surgery: executive summary: a report of the American College of Cardiology Foundation/American Heart Association task force on practice guidelines. *Circulation.* 2011;124(23):2610-2642.

Levi M, Eerenberg E, Kamphuisen PW. Bleeding risk and reversal strategies for old and new anticoagulants and antiplatelet agents. *J Thromb Haemost.* 2011;9(9):1705-1712.

Patrono C, Andreotti F, Arnesen H, et al. Antiplatelet agents for the treatment and prevention of atherothrombosis. *Eur Heart J.* 2011;32(23):2922-2932.

SELECTIVE SEROTONIN REUPTAKE INHIBITORS (SSRIS) PHARMACOKINETICS

SSRI	Half-Life (h)	Metabolite Half-Life	Peak Plasma Level (h)	% Protein Bound	Bioavailability (%)	Initial Dose
Citalopram (CeleXA)	35	S-desmethyl-citalopram: 59 hours	4	80	80	20 mg qAM
Escitalopram (Lexapro)	27-32	S-desmethyl-citalopram: 59 hours	5	56	80	10 mg qAM
FLUoxetine (PROzac, PROzac Weekly, Sarafem, Selfemra)	Initial: 24-72 Chronic: 96-144	Norfluoxetine: 4-16 days	6-8	95	72	10-20 mg qAM
FluvoxaMINE (Luvox CR)	16	N/A	3	80	53	50 mg qhs
PARoxetine (Paxil, Paxil CR, Pexeva)	21	N/A	5	95	>90	10-20 mg qAM
Sertraline (Zoloft)	26	N-desmethyl-sertraline: 62-104 hours	5-8	98	88	25-50 qAM

VASOACTIVE AGENTS, INTRAVENOUS

Drug	Dose	Hemodynamic Effects				
		HR	MAP	PAOP	CI	SVR
DOPamine	1-3 mcg/kg/min	↑	0	↓	0/↑	0/↓
	3-10 mcg/kg/min	↑	↑	0	↑	0
	>10-20 mcg/kg/min	↑↑	↑↑	0	↑	↑
EPINEPHrine	0.01-0.05 mcg/kg/min	↑	↑	0/↓	↑↑	0/↓
	>0.05 mcg/kg/min	↑↑	↑↑	↑	↑↑	↑↑
Norepinephrine	0.02-3 mcg/kg/min	0/↑	↑↑↑	↑↑	0/↓/↑	↑↑↑
Phenylephrine	0.5-9 mcg/kg/min	0/↓	↑	↑	0/↓/↑	↑↑↑
Vasopressin	0.04 units/min	0/↓	↑↑	↑	0/↓	↑↑
DOBUTamine	2-10 mcg/kg/min	0/↑	↑	↓	↑	0/↓
	>10-20 mcg/kg/min	↑↑	↓/↑	↓	↑↑	↓
Milrinone	0.375-0.75 mcg/kg/min	↑↑	0/↓/↑	↓	↑	↓↓
Nesiritide	2 mcg/kg bolus	0	↓	↓	0/↑	↓
	0.01-0.03 mcg/kg/min					
Nitroglycerin	0.1-2 mcg/kg/min	0/↑	0/↓	↓	0/↑	↓
Nitroprusside	0.25-10 mcg/kg/min	0/↑↑	0/↓↓	↓	↑/↑↑	↓/↓↓

HR = heart rate, MAP = mean arterial pressure, PAOP = pulmonary artery occlusion pressure, CI = cardiac index, SVR = systemic vascular resistance

↑ = increase, ↓ = decrease, 0 = no change

Drug	Dose	Receptor Activity						
		α_1	α_2	β_1	β_2	DA_1	V_1	V_2
DOBUTamine	2-10 mcg/kg/min	+	0	+++	++	0	0	0
	>10-20 mcg/kg/min	++	0	++++	+++	0	0	0
DOPamine	1-3 mcg/kg/min	0	0	+	0	++++	0	0
	3-10 mcg/kg/min	0/+	0	++++	++	++++	0	0
	>10-20 mcg/kg/min	+++	0	++++	+	0	0	0
EPINEPHrine	0.01-0.05 mcg/kg/min	++	++	++++	+++	0	0	0
	>0.05 mcg/kg/min	++++	++++	+++	+	0	0	0
Norepinephrine	0.02-3 mcg/kg/min	++++	++	++	0	0	0	0
Phenylephrine	0.5-9 mcg/kg/min	++++	+	0	0	0	0	0
Vasopressin	0.04 units/min	0	0	0	0	0	+++	+

Activity ranges from no activity (0) or maximal activity (++++)

DA = dopaminergic, V = vasopressin

REFERENCES

Biaggioni I, Robertson D. Adrenoceptor agonists & sympathomimetic drugs. *Basic and Clinical Pharmacology.* 11th ed. Katzung BG, Masters SB, Trevor AJ, eds. Stamford, CT: McGraw-Hill; 2009;127-148.

Hollenberg SM, Ahrens TS, Annane D, et al. Practice parameters for hemodynamic support of sepsis in adult patients: 2004 update. *Crit Care Med.* 2004;32(9):1928-1948.

Hollenberg SM. Vasopressor support in septic shock. *Chest.* 2007;132(5):1678-1687.

MacLaren R, Rudis MI, Dasta JF. Use of vasopressors and inotropes in the pharmacotherapy of shock. *Pharmacotherapy: A Pathophysiologic Approach.* 7th ed. Dipiro JT, Talbert RL, Yee GC, et al, eds. Stamford, CT: McGraw-Hill; 2008;417-439.

CYTOCHROME P450 ENZYMES: SUBSTRATES, INHIBITORS, AND INDUCERS

INTRODUCTION

Most drugs are eliminated from the body, at least in part, by being chemically altered to less lipid-soluble products (ie, metabolized), and thus are more likely to be excreted via the kidneys or the bile. Phase I metabolism includes drug hydrolysis, oxidation, and reduction, and results in drugs that are more polar in their chemical structure, while Phase II metabolism involves the attachment of an additional molecule onto the drug (or partially metabolized drug) in order to create an inactive and/or more water soluble compound. Phase II processes include (primarily) glucuronidation, sulfation, glutathione conjugation, acetylation, and methylation.

Virtually any of the Phase I and II enzymes can be inhibited by some xenobiotic or drug. Some of the Phase I and II enzymes can be induced. Inhibition of the activity of metabolic enzymes will result in increased concentrations of the substrate (drug), whereas induction of the activity of metabolic enzymes will result in decreased concentrations of the substrate. For example, the well-documented enzyme-inducing effects of phenobarbital may include a combination of Phase I and II enzymes. Phase II glucuronidation may be increased via induced UDP-glucuronosyltransferase (UGT) activity, whereas Phase I oxidation may be increased via induced cytochrome P450 (CYP) activity. However, for most drugs, the primary route of metabolism (and the primary focus of drug-drug interaction) is Phase I oxidation.

CYP enzymes may be responsible for the metabolism (at least partial metabolism) of approximately 75% of all drugs, with the CYP3A subfamily responsible for nearly half of this activity. Found throughout plant, animal, and bacterial species, CYP enzymes represent a superfamily of xenobiotic metabolizing proteins. There have been several hundred CYP enzymes identified in nature, each of which has been assigned to a family (1, 2, 3, etc), subfamily (A, B, C, etc), and given a specific enzyme number (1, 2, 3, etc) according to the similarity in amino acid sequence that it shares with other enzymes. Of these many enzymes, only a few are found in humans, and even fewer appear to be involved in the metabolism of xenobiotics (eg, drugs). The key human enzyme subfamilies include CYP1A, CYP2A, CYP2B, CYP2C, CYP2D, CYP2E, and CYP3A. However, the number of distinct isozymes (eg, CYP2C9) found to be functionally active in humans, as well as, the number of genetically variant forms of these isozymes (eg, CYP2C9*2) in individuals continues to expand.

CYP enzymes are found in the endoplasmic reticulum of cells in a variety of human tissues (eg, skin, kidneys, brain, lungs), but their predominant sites of concentration and activity are the liver and intestine. Though the abundance of CYP enzymes throughout the body is relatively equally distributed among the various subfamilies, the relative contribution to drug metabolism is (in decreasing order of magnitude) CYP3A4 (nearly 50%), CYP2D6 (nearly 25%), CYP2C8/9 (nearly 15%), then CYP1A2, CYP2C19, CYP2A6, and CYP2E1. Owing to their potential for numerous drug-drug interactions, those drugs that are identified in preclinical studies as substrates of CYP3A enzymes are often given a lower priority for continued research and development in favor of drugs that appear to be less affected by (or less likely to affect) this enzyme subfamily.

Each enzyme subfamily possesses unique selectivity toward potential substrates. For example, CYP1A2 preferentially binds medium-sized, planar, lipophilic molecules, while CYP2D6 preferentially binds molecules that possess a basic nitrogen atom. Some CYP subfamilies exhibit polymorphism (ie, genetic variation that results in a modified enzyme with small changes in amino acid sequences that may manifest differing catalytic properties). The best described polymorphisms involve CYP2C9, CYP2C19, and CYP2D6. Individuals possessing "wild type" genes exhibit normal functioning CYP capacity. Others, however, possess genetic variants that leave the person with a subnormal level of catalytic potential (so called "poor metabolizers"). Poor metabolizers would be more likely to experience toxicity from drugs metabolized by the affected enzymes (or less effects if the enzyme is responsible for converting a prodrug to it's active form as in the case of codeine). The percentage of people classified as poor metabolizers varies by enzyme and population group. As an example, approximately 7% of Caucasians and only about 1% of Asians appear to be CYP2D6 poor metabolizers.

CYP enzymes can be both inhibited and induced by other drugs, leading to increased or decreased serum concentrations (along with the associated effects), respectively. Induction occurs when a drug causes an increase in the amount of smooth endoplasmic reticulum, secondary to increasing the amount of the affected CYP enzymes in the tissues. This "revving up" of the CYP enzyme system may take several days to reach peak activity, and likewise, may take several days, even months, to return to normal following discontinuation of the inducing agent.

CYP inhibition occurs via several potential mechanisms. Most commonly, a CYP inhibitor competitively (and reversibly) binds to the active site on the enzyme, thus preventing the substrate from binding to the same site, and preventing the substrate from being metabolized. The affinity of an inhibitor for an enzyme may be expressed by an inhibition constant (Ki) or IC50 (defined as the concentration of the inhibitor required to cause 50% inhibition under a given set of conditions). In addition to reversible competition for an enzyme site, drugs may inhibit enzyme activity by binding to sites on the enzyme other than that to which the substrate would bind, and thereby cause a change in the functionality or physical structure of the enzyme. A drug may also bind to the enzyme in an irreversible (ie, "suicide") fashion. In such a case, it is not the concentration of drug at the enzyme site that is important (constantly binding and releasing), but the number of molecules available for binding (once bound, always bound).

Although an inhibitor or inducer may be known to affect a variety of CYP subfamilies, it may only inhibit one or two in a clinically important fashion. Likewise, although a substrate is known to be at least partially metabolized by a variety of CYP enzymes, only one or two enzymes may contribute significantly enough to its overall metabolism to warrant concern when used with potential inducers or inhibitors. Therefore, when attempting to predict the level of risk of using two drugs that may affect each other via altered CYP function, it is important to identify the relative effectiveness of the inhibiting/inducing drug on the CYP subfamilies that significantly contribute to the metabolism of the substrate. The contribution of a specific CYP pathway to substrate metabolism should be considered not only in light of other known CYP pathways, but also other nonoxidative pathways for substrate metabolism (eg, glucuronidation) and transporter proteins (eg, P-glycoprotein) that may affect the presentation of a substrate to a metabolic pathway.

HOW TO USE THIS TABLE

The following table provides a clinically relevant perspective on drugs that are affected by, or affect, cytochrome P450 (CYP) enzymes. Not all human, drug-metabolizing CYP enzymes are specifically (or separately) included in the table. Some enzymes have been excluded because they do not appear to significantly contribute to the metabolism of marketed drugs (eg, CYP2C18). In the case of CYP3A4, the industry routinely uses this single enzyme designation to represent all enzymes in the CYP3A subfamily. CYP3A7 is present in fetal livers. It is effectively absent from adult livers. CYP3A4 (adult) and CYP3A7 (fetal) appear to share similar properties in their respective hosts. The impact of CYP3A7 in fetal and neonatal drug interactions has not been investigated.

An enzyme that appears to play a clinically significant (major) role in a drug's metabolism is indicated by "S". A clinically significant designation is the result of a two-phase review. The first phase considered the contribution of each CYP enzyme to the overall metabolism of the drug. The enzyme pathway was considered potentially clinically relevant if it was responsible for at least 30% of the metabolism of the drug. If so, the drug was subjected to a second phase. The second phase considered the clinical relevance of a substrate's concentration being increased twofold, or decreased by one-half (such as might be observed if combined with an effective CYP inhibitor or inducer, respectively). If either of these changes was considered to present a clinically significant concern, the CYP pathway for the drug was designated "major." If neither change would appear to present a clinically significant concern, or if the CYP enzyme was responsible for a smaller portion of the overall metabolism (ie, <30%), then no association between the enzyme and the drug will appear in the table.

Enzymes that are strongly or moderately inhibited by a drug are indicated by "↓". Enzymes that are weakly inhibited are not identified in the table. The designations are the result of a review of published clinical reports, available Ki data, and assessments published by other experts in the field. As it pertains to Ki values set in a ratio with achievable serum drug concentrations ([I]) under normal dosing conditions, the following parameters were employed: [I]/Ki ≥1 = strong; [I]/Ki 0.1-1 = moderate; [I]/Ki <0.1 = weak.

Enzymes that appear to be effectively induced by a drug are indicated by "↑". This designation is the result of a review of published clinical reports and assessments published by experts in the field.

In general, clinically significant interactions are more likely to occur between substrates ("S") and either inhibitors or inducers of the same enzyme(s), which have been indicated by "↓" and "↑", respectively. However, these assessments possess a degree of subjectivity, at times based on limited indications regarding the significance of CYP effects of particular agents. An attempt has been made to balance a conservative, clinically-sensitive presentation of the data with a desire to avoid the numbing effect of a "beware of everything" approach. It is important to note that information related to CYP metabolism of drugs is expanding at a rapid pace, and thus, the contents of this table should only be considered to represent a "snapshot" of the information available at the time of publication.

SELECTED READINGS

Bjornsson TD, Callaghan JT, Einolf HJ, et al. The conduct of *in vitro* and *in vivo* drug-drug interaction studies: a PhRMA perspective. *J Clin Pharmacol.* 2003;43(5):443-469.

Drug-Drug Interactions. Rodrigues AD, ed. New York, NY: Marcel Dekker, Inc; 2002.

Metabolic Drug Interactions. Levy RH, Thummel KE, Trager WF, et al, eds. Philadelphia, PA: Lippincott Williams & Wilkins; 2000.

Michalets EL. Update: clinically significant cytochrome P-450 drug interactions. *Pharmacotherapy.* 1998;18(1):84-112.

Thummel KE, Wilkinson GR. *In vitro* and *in vivo* drug interactions involving human CYP3A. *Annu Rev Pharmacol Toxicol.* 1998;38:389-430.

Zhang Y, Benet LZ. The gut as a barrier to drug absorption: combined role of cytochrome P450 3A and P-Glycoprotein. *Clin Pharmacokinet.* 2001;40 (3):159-168.

SELECTED WEBSITES

http://www.imm.ki.se/CYPalleles

http://medicine.iupui.edu/flockhart

http://www.fda.gov/Drugs/DevelopmentApprovalProcess/DevelopmentResources/DrugInteractionsLabeling/ucm080499.htm

CYP: Substrates, Inhibitors, Inducers

S = substrate; ↓ = inhibitor; ↑ = inducer

Drug	1A2	2A6	2B6	2C8	2C9	2C19	2D6	2E1	3A4
Acenocoumarol	S				S				
Alfentanil									S
Alfuzosin									S
Alosetron	S								
ALPRAZolam									S
Ambrisentan						S			S
Aminophylline	S								
Amiodarone		↓		S	↓		↓		S, ↓
Amitriptyline							S		
AmLODIPine	↓								S
Amobarbital		↑							
Amoxapine							S		
Aprepitant									S, ↓
ARIPiprazole							S		S
Armodafinil						↓			S, ↑
Atazanavir									S, ↓
Atomoxetine							S		
Atorvastatin									S
Benzphetamine									S
Betaxolol	S						S		
Bisoprolol									S
Bortezomib						S, ↓			S
Bosentan					S, ↑				S, ↑
Bromazepam									S
Bromocriptine									S
Budesonide									S
Buprenorphine									S
BuPROPion			S						
BusPIRone									S
Busulfan									S
Caffeine	S								↓
Captopril							S		
CarBAMazepine	↑		↑	↑	↑	↑			S, ↑
Carisoprodol						S			
Carvedilol					S		S		
Celecoxib				↓	S				
ChlordiazePOXIDE									S
Chloroquine							S, ↓		S
Chlorpheniramine									S
ChlorproMAZINE							S, ↓		
Chlorzoxazone								S	
Ciclesonide									S
Cilostazol									S
Cimetidine	↓					↓	↓		↓
Cinacalcet							↓		
Ciprofloxacin	↓								
Cisapride									S
Citalopram						S			S

CYP: Substrates, Inhibitors, Inducers *(continued)*

Drug	1A2	2A6	2B6	2C8	2C9	2C19	2D6	2E1	3A4
Clarithromycin									S, ↓
Clobazam						S			S
ClomiPRAMINE	S					S	S, ↓		
ClonazePAM									S
Clorazepate									S
Clotrimazole									↓
CloZAPine	S						↓		
Cocaine							↓		S
Codeine[1]							S		
Colchicine									S
Conivaptan									S, ↓
Cyclobenzaprine	S								
Cyclophosphamide[2]			S						S
CycloSPORINE									S, ↓
Dacarbazine	S							S	
Dantrolene									S
Dapsone					S				S
Darifenacin							↓		S
Darunavir									S
Dasatinib									S
Delavirdine					↓	↓	↓		S, ↓
Desipramine		↓	↓				S, ↓		↓
Desogestrel						S			
Dexamethasone									S, ↑
Dexlansoprazole						S, ↓			S
Dexmedetomidine		S					↓		
Dextromethorphan							S		
Diazepam						S			S
Diclofenac	↓								
Dihydroergotamine									S
Diltiazem									S, ↓
DiphenhydrAMINE							↓		
Disopyramide									S
Disulfiram								↓	
DOCEtaxel									S
Doxepin							S		
DOXOrubicin			↓				S		S
Doxycycline									↓
DULoxetine	S						S, ↓		
Efavirenz[3]			S		↓	↓			S, ↓, ↑
Eletriptan									S
Enflurane								S	
Eplerenone									S
Ergoloid mesylates									S
Ergonovine									S
Ergotamine									S
Erlotinib									S
Erythromycin									S, ↓
Escitalopram						S			S
Esomeprazole						S, ↓			S
Estradiol	S								S
Estrogens, conjugated A/synthetic	S								S

CYP: Substrates, Inhibitors, Inducers *(continued)*

Drug	1A2	2A6	2B6	2C8	2C9	2C19	2D6	2E1	3A4
Estrogens, conjugated equine	S								S
Estrogens, esterified	S								S
Estropipate	S								S
Eszopiclone									S
Ethinyl estradiol									S
Ethosuximide									S
Etoposide									S
Exemestane									S
Felbamate									S
Felodipine				↓					S
FentaNYL									S
Flecainide							S		
Fluconazole					↓	↓			↓
Flunisolide									S
FLUoxetine	↓				S	↓	S, ↓		
FluPHENAZine							S		
Flurazepam									S
Flurbiprofen					↓				
Flutamide	S								S
Fluticasone									S
Fluvastatin					S, ↓				
FluvoxaMINE	S, ↓					↓	S		
Fosamprenavir (as amprenavir)									S, ↓
Fosaprepitant									S, ↓
Fosphenytoin (as phenytoin)			↑	↑	S, ↑	S, ↑			↑
Fospropofol	↓		S		S	↓			↓
Gefitinib									S
Gemfibrozil	↓			↓	↓	↓			
Glimepiride					S				
GlipiZIDE					S				
Guanabenz	S								
Haloperidol							S, ↓		S, ↓
Halothane								S	
Ibuprofen					↓				
Ifosfamide[4]		S				S			S
Imatinib							↓		S, ↓
Imipramine						S	S, ↓		
Indinavir									S, ↓
Indomethacin					↓				
Irbesartan				↓	↓				
Irinotecan			S						S
Isoflurane								S	
Isoniazid		↓				↓	↓	S, ↓	
Isosorbide dinitrate									S
Isosorbide mononitrate									S
Isradipine									S
Itraconazole									S, ↓
Ixabepilone									S
Ketamine			S		S				S
Ketoconazole	↓	↓			↓	↓	↓		S, ↓
Lansoprazole						S, ↓			S
Lapatinib									S

CYP: Substrates, Inhibitors, Inducers *(continued)*

Drug	1A2	2A6	2B6	2C8	2C9	2C19	2D6	2E1	3A4
Letrozole		↓							
Levonorgestrel									S
Lidocaine							S, ↓		S, ↓
Lomustine							S		
Lopinavir									S
Loratadine						↓			
Losartan				↓	S, ↓				S
Lovastatin									S
Maprotiline							S		
Maraviroc									S
MedroxyPROGESTERone									S
Mefenamic acid					↓				
Mefloquine									S
Mephobarbital						S			
Mestranol[5]					S				S
Methadone							↓		S
Methamphetamine							S		
Methoxsalen	↓	↓							
Methsuximide						S			
Methylergonovine									S
MethylPREDNISolone									S
Metoprolol							S		
MetroNIDAZOLE									↓
Mexiletine	S, ↓						S		
Miconazole	↓	↓			↓	↓	↓	↓	S, ↓
Midazolam									S
Mirtazapine	S						S		S
Moclobemide						S	S		
Modafinil						↓			S
Montelukast					S				S
Nafcillin									↑
Nateglinide					S				S
Nebivolol							S		
Nefazodone							S		S, ↓
Nelfinavir						S			S, ↓
Nevirapine			↑						S, ↑
NiCARdipine					↓	↓	↓		S, ↓
NIFEdipine	↓								S
Nilotinib									S
Nilutamide						S			
NiMODipine									S
Nisoldipine									S
Norethindrone									S
Norfloxacin	↓								↓
Norgestrel									S
Nortriptyline							S		
Ofloxacin	↓								
OLANZapine	S								
Omeprazole					↓	S, ↓			S
Ondansetron									S
OXcarbazepine									↑
PACLitaxel				S	S				S

CYP: Substrates, Inhibitors, Inducers *(continued)*

Drug	1A2	2A6	2B6	2C8	2C9	2C19	2D6	2E1	3A4
Pantoprazole						S, ↓			
Paricalcitol									S
PARoxetine			↓				S, ↓		
PAZOPanib									S
Pentamidine						S			
PENTobarbital		↑							↑
Perphenazine							S		
PHENobarbital	↑	↑	↑	↑	↑	S			↑
Phenytoin			↑	↑	S, ↑	S, ↑			↑
Pimozide	S								S
Pindolol							S		
Pioglitazone				S, ↓					
Piroxicam					↓				
Posaconazole									↓
Primaquine	↓								S
Primidone	↑		↑	↑	↑				↑
Procainamide							S		
Progesterone						S			S
Promethazine			S				S		
Propafenone							S		
Propofol	↓		S		S	↓			↓
Propranolol	S						S		
Protriptyline							S		
Pyrimethamine					↓				
Quazepam						S			S
QUEtiapine									S
QuiNIDine							↓		S, ↓
QuiNINE				↓	↓		↓		S
RABEprazole				↓		S, ↓			S
Ramelteon	S								
Ranolazine							↓		S
Rasagiline	S								
Repaglinide				S					S
Rifabutin									S, ↑
Rifampin	↑	↑	↑	↑	↑	↑			↑
Rifapentine				↑	↑				↑
Riluzole	S								
RisperiDONE							S		
Ritonavir				↓			S, ↓		S, ↓
ROPINIRole	S								
Ropivacaine	S								
Rosiglitazone				S, ↓					
Salmeterol									S
Saquinavir									S, ↓
Secobarbital		↑		↑	↑				
Selegiline			S						
Sertraline			↓			S, ↓	S, ↓		↓
Sevoflurane								S	
Sibutramine									S
Sildenafil									S
Simvastatin									S
Sirolimus									S

CYP: Substrates, Inhibitors, Inducers *(continued)*

Drug	1A2	2A6	2B6	2C8	2C9	2C19	2D6	2E1	3A4
Sitaxsentan					↓	↓			↓
Solifenacin									S
SORAfenib			↓	↓	↓				
Spiramycin									S
SUFentanil									S
SulfADIAZINE					S, ↓				
Sulfamethoxazole					S, ↓				
SUNItinib									S
Tacrine	S								
Tacrolimus									S
Tadalafil									S
Tamoxifen				↓	S		S		S
Tamsulosin							S		S
Telithromycin									S, ↓
Temsirolimus									S
Teniposide									S
Terbinafine							↓		
Tetracycline									S, ↓
Theophylline	S							S	S
Thiabendazole	↓								
Thioridazine							S, ↓		
Thiotepa			↓						
Thiothixene	S								
TiaGABine									S
Ticlopidine						↓	↓		S
Timolol							S		
Tinidazole									S
Tipranavir									S
TiZANidine	S								
TOLBUTamide					S, ↓				
Tolterodine							S		S
Toremifene									S
Torsemide					S				
TraMADol[1]							S		S
Tranylcypromine	↓	↓				↓	↓		
TraZODone									S
Tretinoin				S					
Triazolam									S
Trifluoperazine	S								
Trimethoprim				↓	S, ↓				S
Trimipramine						S	S		S
Vardenafil									S
Venlafaxine							S		S
Verapamil									S, ↓
VinBLAStine									S
VinCRIStine									S
Vinorelbine									S
Voriconazole					S	S			↓
Warfarin					S, ↓				

CYP: Substrates, Inhibitors, Inducers *(continued)*

Drug	1A2	2A6	2B6	2C8	2C9	2C19	2D6	2E1	3A4
Zafirlukast					S, ↓				
Zileuton	↓								
Zolpidem									S
Zonisamide									S
Zopiclone					S				S
Zuclopenthixol							S		

[1]This opioid analgesic is bioactivated *in vivo* via CYP2D6. Inhibiting this enzyme would decrease the effects of the analgesic. The active metabolite might also affect, or be affected by, CYP enzymes.

[2]Cyclophosphamide is bioactivated *in vivo* to acrolein via CYP2B6 and 3A4. Inhibiting these enzymes would decrease the effects of cyclophosphamide.

[3]Data have shown both induction (*in vivo*) and inhibition (*in vitro*) of CYP3A4.

[4]Ifosfamide is bioactivated *in vivo* to acrolein via CYP3A4. Inhibiting this enzyme would decrease the effects of ifosfamide.

[5]Mestranol is bioactivated *in vivo* to ethinyl estradiol via CYP2C8/9.

DESENSITIZATION PROTOCOLS

Desensitization should be performed under the supervision of a licensed healthcare professional. These protocols are potentially dangerous procedures and should be only performed in an area where immediate access to emergency drugs (eg, epinephrine) and equipment can be assured. Premedication with antihistamines or steroids is generally not recommended, as these drugs may mask early signs of reactivity that would otherwise result in a modification of the protocol (Cernadas, 2010). Prior to desensitization, medications such as beta-blockers should be discontinued unless required for certain indications. Desensitization is generally contraindicated in patients with severe idiosyncratic reactions, uncontrolled asthma, and prior anaphylaxis to the desensitizing agent. However, some clinicians may choose to perform desensitization in patients with a history of IgE-mediated reactions, including anaphylaxis. Under these circumstances, healthcare providers should proceed with caution.

During desensitization, breakthrough hypersensitivity reactions, such as pruritus, urticaria, rhinitis, or mild wheezing, may occur during the procedure. Breakthrough hypersensitivity reactions should be treated immediately and the desensitization protocol should be stopped. These reactions often are dose-dependent and can be managed with modifications to the protocol (Cernadas, 2010).

Note: Once desensitized, the patient's treatment with the desensitized agent must not lapse or the risk of an allergic reaction increases. If the patient requires treatment with the desensitized agent in the future and still remains skin test-positive, desensitization would be required again (Cunha, 2001).

The following desensitization protocols presented are examples of what has been reported/evaluated in literature. Only a summary of the protocol is presented; the complete reference should be reviewed prior to utilizing a desensitization protocol. The information provided in the tables below is often based on a single case report or a very limited number of patients. Both oral and parenteral medications have been used in desensitization protocols and both methods have been shown to be equally effective. Historically, oral dosage forms have been thought to be safer; however, parenteral dosage forms have been used when the oral route of administration is not feasible (Cernadas, 2010). These protocols are meant to be used as a guide with the knowledge that there are other methods of desensitization that may also be used successfully.

GENERAL INTRAVENOUS DESENSITIZATION PROTOCOL

For use with Ceftazidime, Ceftriaxone, Cefazolin, Imipenem, Nafcillin, Penicillin, Piperacillin/Tazobactam Sodium, and Vancomycin

Solution Preparation

Solution	Volume (mL)	Concentration (mg/mL)	Total Amount of Drug in Each Solution (mg)
1	250	0.040	10
2		0.40	100
3		3.969	992.13

Protocol for Administration

Step	Solution	Rate (mL/h)	Time (min)	Administered Dose (mg)	Cumulative Dose (mg)
1	1	2	15	0.02	0.02
2		5		0.05	0.07
3		10		0.1	0.17
4		20		0.2	0.37
5	2	5		0.5	0.87
6		10		1	1.87
7		20		2	3.87
8		40		4	7.87
9	3	10		9.9213	17.7913
10		20		19.8426	37.6339
11		40		39.6852	77.3191
12		75	186	922.6809	1000

Note: Total time = 351 minutes

Adapted from Castellas M. Rapid desensitization for hypersensitivity reactions to medications. *Immunol Allergy Clin N Am.* 2009;29:585-606.

PENICILLIN G

Parenteral Desensitization Protocol

Injection Number	Benzylpenicillin Concentration (units/mL)	Volume and Route (mL)[a]
1[b]	100	0.1 **I.D.**
2		0.2 SubQ
3		0.4 SubQ
4		0.8 SubQ
5[b]	1000	0.1 **I.D.**
6		0.3 SubQ
7		0.6 SubQ
8[b]	10,000	0.1 **I.D.**
9		0.2 SubQ
10		0.4 SubQ
11		0.8 SubQ
12[b]	100,000	0.1 **I.D.**
13		0.3 SubQ
14		0.6 SubQ
15[b]	1,000,000	0.1 **I.D.**
16		0.2 SubQ
17		0.2 SubQ
18		0.4 SubQ
19	Continuous SubQ infusion (1,000,000 units/h)	

I.D. = intradermal, SubQ = subcutaneous

[a]Administer progressive doses at intervals of not less than 20 minutes.

[b]Observe and record skin wheal and flare response to intradermal dose.

Adapted from Cunha BA. Antimicrobial selection in the penicillin-allergic. *Drugs Today.* 2001;37 (6):377-383.

Adapted from Castellas M. Rapid desensitization for hypersensitivity reactions to medications. *Immunol Allergy Clin N Am.* 2009;29:585-606.

PENICILLIN V

Oral Desensitization Protocol

Step[a]	Penicillin V Suspension (units/mL)	Amount[b] (mL)	Dose (units)	Cumulative Dosage (units)
1	1000	0.1	100	100
2		0.2	200	300
3		0.4	400	700
4		0.8	800	1500
5		1.6	1600	3100
6		3.2	3200	6300
7		6.4	6400	12,700
8	10,000	1.2	12,000	24,700
9		2.4	24,000	48,700
10		4.8	48,000	96,700
11	80,000	1	80,000	176,700
12		2	160,000	336,700
13		4	320,000	656,700
14		8	640,000	1,296,700
15	500,000	0.25	125,000	1,421,700
16		0.5	250,000	1,671,700
17		1	500,000	2,171,700
18		2.25	1,125,000	3,296,700

[a]Interval between steps = 15 minutes

[b]Amount of drug is diluted in ~30 mL of water and then given P.O.

Note: Observe patients for 30 minutes prior to parenteral administration of penicillin.

Adapted from Cunha BA. Antimicrobial selection in the penicillin-allergic. *Drugs Today.* 2001;37(6):377-383.

ALLOPURINOL

Oral Desensitization Protocol

Dosing Schedule	Oral Dose of Allopurinol
Days 1-3	50 mcg/day
Days 4-6	100 mcg/day
Days 7-9	200 mcg/day
Days 10-12	500 mcg/day
Days 13-15	1 mg/day
Days 16-18	5 mg/day
Days 19-21	10 mg/day
Days 22-24	25 mg/day
Days 25-27	50 mg/day
Day 28	100 mg/day

Note: For doses ≤1 mg, 1 mg/5 mL suspension was used; for doses 5-25 mg, 10 mg/5 mL suspension was used. For doses 50 mg and 100 mg, 1/2 tablet and 1 tablet of 100 mg allopurinol were used, respectively.

Note: High-risk patients should follow the modified desensitization protocol: Initial doses of 10 mcg and 25 mcg with dosage escalation every 5-10 days or longer

Adapted from Fam AG, Dunne SM, Iazzetta J, et al. Efficacy and safety of desensitization to allopurinol following cutaneous reactions. *Arthritis Rheum.* 2001;44(1):231-238.

AMPHOTERICIN B

Intravenous Desensitization Protocol

Step	Volume (mL)	Dose (mg)	Infusion time (min)
1	10	0.000001	10
2		0.00001	
3		0.0001	
4		0.001	
5		0.01	
6		1	30
7	250	30	240

Note: Mixtures were prepared in 5% dextrose. Patient was premedicated with methylprednisolone 60 mg I.V. and diphenhydramine 25 mg I.V.

Adapted from Kemp SF, Lockey RF. Amphotericin B: emergency challenge in a neutropenic, asthmatic patient with fungal sepsis. *J Allergy Clin Immunol.* 1995;96(3):425-427.

TRIMETHOPRIM-SULFAMETHOXAZOLE

Oral Desensitization Protocol

Dosing Level	Portion of Single-Strength TMP-SMZ (%)	Amount (Frequency) of Pediatric Suspension (mL)	Total TMP Dose (mg)	Total SMZ Dose (mg)
1	12.5	1.25 daily	10	50
2	25	1.25 bid	20	100
3	37.5	1.25 tid	30	150
4	50	2.5 bid	40	200
5	75	2.5 tid	60	300
6	100	1 single-strength tablet	80	400

Note: Each dosing level is a daily dose. For successful completion of the reintroduction phase, patients must have taken each dose level at least once. Patients were permitted to repeat dose levels once; dose levels were completed in increasing increments, and the level 6 dose was taken no later than day 13 of the reintroduction phase. Patients were permitted to withhold study drug for 2 days during the reintroduction phase (withholding study drug for >2 days during reintroduction resulted in permanent discontinuation). Patients were required to take an antihistamine during dose escalation.

Adapted from Leoung GS, Stanford JF, Giordano MF, et al. Trimethoprim-sulfamethoxazole (TMP-SMZ) dose escalation versus direct rechallenge for *Pneumocystis carinii* pneumonia, prophylaxis in human immunodeficiency virus-infected patients with previous adverse reaction to TMP-SMZ. *J Infect Dis.* 2001;184(8):992-997.

Alternate Oral Desensitization Protocol

Day	Morning Dose (g)	Evening Dose (g)
1	0.005	0.01
2	0.02	0.04
3	0.1	0.2
4	0.4	0.8
5	1	1

Note: A granular dosage form of trimethoprim-sulfamethoxazole was used in the protocol. A 0.005 g dose is equivalent to 0.4 mg of trimethoprim and 2 mg of sulfamethoxazole. On day 5, patients received a dose equivalent to one 80-400 mg trimethoprim-sulfamethoxazole tablet.

Adapted from Yoshizawa S, Yasuoka A, Kikuchi Y, et al. A 5-day course of oral desensitization to trimethoprim/sulfamethoxazole (T/S) in patients with human immunodeficiency virus type-1 infection who were previously intolerant to T/S. *Ann Allergy Asthma Imunol.* 2000;85:241-244.

VANCOMYCIN

Intravenous Desensitization Protocol

Infusion Number	Dilution	Vancomycin Dose (mg)	Concentration (mg/mL)
1	1:10,000	0.02	0.0002
2	1:1000	0.2	0.002
3	1:100	2	0.02
4	1:10	20	0.2
5	Standard	500	2

Adapted from Wazny LD, Daghigh B. Desensitization protocols for vancomycin hypersensitivity. *Ann Pharmacother.* 2001;35 (11):1458-1464.

Premedication: Generally not administered prior to desensitization protocols. However, the patients in this protocol were given diphenhydramine 50 mg I.V. and hydrocortisone 100 mg I.V. 15 minutes prior to initiation of protocol, then every 6 hours throughout protocol.

Infusion rate instructions:

Initiate infusion rate at 0.5 mL/minute (30 mL/hour) and increase by 0.5 mL/minute (30 mL/hour) as tolerated every 5 minutes to a maximum rate of 5 mL/minute (300 mL/hour). If pruritus, hypotension, rash, or difficulty breathing occurs, stop infusion and reinfuse the previously tolerated infusion at the highest tolerated rate. This step may be repeated up to three times for any given concentration.

Upon completion of infusion number 5, immediately administer the required dose of vancomycin in the usual dilution of NS or D_5W over 2 hours. Decrease rate if patient becomes symptomatic or, alternatively, increase rate if patient tolerates dose. Administer diphenhydramine 50 mg orally prior to each required dose of vancomycin.

CEFTRIAXONE

Intravenous Desensitization Protocol

Dose Number[a]	Concentration (mg/mL)	Flow Rate (mL/h)	Dose (mg)
1	0.01	6	0.015
2		12	0.03
3		24	0.06
4	0.1	5	0.125
5		10	0.25
6		20	0.5
7		40	1
8		80	2
9		160	4
10	10	3	7.5
11		6	15
12		12	30
13		25	62.5
14		50	125
15	100	10	250
16		20	500
17		40	1000

[a]Interval between doses = 15 minutes

Adapted from Solensky R. Drug desensitization. *Immunol Allergy Clin N Am.* 2004;24:425-443.

CIPROFLOXACIN

Intravenous Desensitization Protocol

Ciprofloxacin Concentration (mg/mL)	Volume Given (mL)	Dose (mg)	Cumulative Total Dose (mg)
0.1	0.1	0.01	0.01
	0.2	0.02	0.03
	0.4	0.04	0.07
	0.8	0.08	0.15
1	0.16	0.16	0.31
	0.32	0.32	0.63
	0.64	0.64	1.27
2	0.6	1.2	2.47
	1.2	2.4	4.87
	2.4	4.8	9.67
	5	10	19.67
	10	20	39.67
	20	40	79.67
	40	80	159.67
	120	240	399.67

Note: Patient was premedicated with diphenhydramine 50 mg I.V. and prednisone 10 mg I.V. 1 hour prior to desensitization. Doses were administered at 15-minute intervals. The total time for the desensitization procedure is 4 hours.

Note: Drug volumes <1 mL were mixed with normal saline solution to a final volume of 3 mL and then slowly infused; the other doses were administered over 10 minutes, except the last dose (240 mg in 120 mL), which was given with an infusion pump over 20 minutes.

Adapted from Gea-Banacloche JC, Metcalfe DD. Ciprofloxacin desensitization. *J Allergy Clin Immunol.* 1996;97:1426-1427.

IMIPENEM

Intravenous Desensitization Protocol

Time (min)	Concentration (mg/mL)	Fluid Infusion Rate (mL/min)
0	0.0001	1
30	0.0003	
60	0.001	
90	0.003	
120	0.01	
150	0.03	
180	0.1	
210	0.3	
240	0.7	1[a]

[a]Dosage reduction for renal dysfunction

Note: If rash or flushing occurs, return to previous step for 30 minutes and call physician.

Note: Total daily dosage of imipenem was 1008 mg (creatinine clearance 20-30 mL/min)

Adapted from Gorman SK, Zed PJ, Dhingra VK, et al. Rapid imipenem/cilastatin desensitization for multidrug-resistant acinetobacter pneumonia. *Ann Pharmacother.* 2003;37:513-516.

INSULIN

Parenteral Desensitization Protocol

Dosing Schedule	Time of Dose (min)	Dose (mL)	Dilution (units/mL)[a]	Units/Dose	Route of Administration
Day 1	0	0.1	0.001	1/10,000	Scratch
	15				I.D.
	20				SubQ
	45		0.01	1/1000	
	60		0.1	1/100	
	75		1	1/10	
	90		10	1	
	115 and q4h x 5				
Day 2	q4h	0.2		2	
Day 3	7 am and 4 pm			2 and 4	
Day 4			100	5 and 10	
Day 5				Individualize as needed	

[a]HumuLIN R insulin was used with diluent provided by manufacturer, Eli Lilly Co, with 1% human serum albumin incorporated into each diluent prepared.

Note: Patient was premedicated with antihistamines prior to initiation of desensitization protocol.

Adapted from Bodendofer TW, Brown ME, Frankel EH, et al. Desensitization with human (recombinant DNA) insulin. *Drug Intell Clin Pharm.* 1985;19:827-829.

NELFINAVIR

Oral Desensitization Protocol

Step	Time (min)	Nelfinavir Dose (mg)	
		q30min	Total
1	0	0.5	0.5
2	30	1	1.5
3	60	2	3.5
4	90	5	8.5
5	120	10	18.5
6	150	20	38.5
7	180	40	78.5
8	210	80	158.5
9	240	160	318.5
10	270	250	568.5
11	300	500	1068.5
12	330	750	1818.5

Note: Observe patient in ICU for 2 hours before discharge.

Note: One mg/mL and 10 mg/mL solutions were prepared to deliver the required dose.

Adapted from Abraham PE, Sorensen SJ, Baker WH, et al. Nelfinavir desensitization. *Ann Pharmacother.* 2001;35(5):553-556.

RIFAMPIN and ETHAMBUTOL

Oral Desensitization Protocol

Time from Start (h:min)	Rifampin (mg)	Ethambutol (mg)
0	0.1	0.1
00:45	0.5	0.5
01:30	1	1
02:15	2	2
03:00	4	4
03:45	8	8
04:30	16	16
05:15	32	32
06:00	50	50
06:45	100	100
07:30	150	200
11:00	300	400
Next day, starting at 6:30 am	300 mg twice daily	400 mg 3 times/day

Adapted from Matz J, Borish LC, Routes JM, et al. Oral desensitization to rifampin and ethambutol in mycobacterial disease. *Am J Respir Crit Care Med*. 1994;149:815-817.

RITUXIMAB

Intravenous Desensitization Protocol

Solution Preparation

Solution	Volume (mL)	Concentration (mg/mL)	Total Amount of Drug in Each Solution (mg)
1		0.034	8.51
2	250	0.34	85.1
3		3.377	844.303

Note: Total dose of rituximab used is 851 mg (less than prepared since solutions 1 and 2 are not completely infused)

Administration

Step	Solution	Rate (mL/h)	Time (min)	Volume Infused Per Step (mL)	Administered Dose (mg)	Cumulative Dose (mg)
1		2		0.5	0.017	0.017
2	1	5		1.25	0.0426	0.0596
3		10		2.5	0.0851	0.1447
4		20		5	0.1702	0.3149
5		5		1.25	0.4255	0.7404
6	2	10	15	2.5	0.851	1.5914
7		20		5	1.702	3.2934
8		40		10	3.404	6.6974
9		10		2.5	8.4443	15.1404
10	3	20		5	16.8861	32.0264
11		40		10	33.7721	65.7986
12		75	186	232.5	785.2014	851

Note: Total time = 351 minutes

Note: Patients developing reactions during the desensitization protocol developed them near step 12 and were treated with antihistamines. Additionally, antileukotriene therapy and prostaglandin blockade with aspirin may be beneficial in improving side effects.

Adapted from Castellas M. Rapid desensitization for hypersensitivity reactions to medications. *Immunol Allergy Clin N Am*. 2009;29:585-606.

CARBOPLATIN

Intravenous Desensitization Protocol

Solution Preparation

Solution	Volume (mL)	Concentration (mg/mL)	Total Dose in Each Solution (mg)
A	250	0.02	5
B		0.2	50
C		2	500

Note: Carboplatin was diluted in 250 mL of D_5W. The sum of doses in Solutions A through C is 555 mg; however, the total dose infused is 500 mg.

Administration

Step	Solution	Rate (mL/h)	Time (min)	Administered Dose (mg)	Cumulative Dose Infused (mg)
1	A	2	15	0.01	0.01
2		5		0.025	0.035
3		10		0.05	0.085
4		20		0.1	0.185
5	B	5		0.25	0.435
6		10		0.5	0.935
7		20		1	1.935
8		40		2	3.935
9	C	10		5	8.935
10		20		10	18.935
11		40		20	38.935
12		75	184.4	461.065	500

Note: Total time = ~6 hours

Adapted from Lee CW, Matulonis UA, Castells MC. Carboplatin hypersensitivity: a 6-H 12-step protocol effective in 35 desensitizations in patients with gynecological malignancies and mast cell/IgE-mediated reactions. *Gynecol Oncol*. 2004;95(2):370-376.

ASPIRIN

Oral Desensitization Protocol

Time (min)	Dose (mg)
0	0.1
20	0.3
40	1
60	3
80	10
100	30
120	40
140	81
160	162

Note: Aspirin was continued at 162 mg orally daily. Most patients were pretreated with an antihistamine (eg, diphenhydramine, hydroxyzine) prior to desensitization.

Adapted from Wong JT, Nagy CS, Krinzman SJ, et al. Rapid oral challenge-desensitization for patients with aspirin related urticaria-angioedema. *J Allergy Clin Immunol*. 2000;105(5):997-1001.

CLOPIDOGREL

Oral Desensitization Protocol

Dose Number[a]	Dose (mg)[b]	Day of Protocol
1	0.1	1
2	0.2	
3	0.5	
4	1	
5[c]	2	1 or 2
6	4	2
7	8	
8	16	
9	32	
10[d]	75	2 or 3

Note: Patients received clopidogrel as a 2-day protocol (doses 1-5 on day 1 and doses 6-10 on day 2) or a 3-day protocol (doses 1-4 on day 1, doses 5-9 on day 2, and dose 10 on day 3)

[a]Doses 1-9 were an oral clopidogrel 1 mg/mL solution; dose 10 was a clopidogrel tablet.

[b]Doses were given 1 hour apart.

[c]Dose 5 was given on day 1 in the 2-day protocol and on day 2 in the 3-day protocol.

[d]Dose 10 was given on day 2 in the 2-day protocol and on day 3 in the 3-day protocol.

Note: Patients were observed for 1 hour after the last dose of clopidogrel.

Adapted from Fajt M, Patrov A. Clopidogrel hypersensitivity: a novel muli-day outpatient oral desensitization regimen. *Ann Pharmacother.* 2010;44(1):11-18.

REFERENCES

Cernadas JR, Brockow K, Romano A, et al. General considerations on rapid desensitization for drug hypersensitivity – a consensus statement. *Allergy.* 2010;65(11):1357-1366.

Cunha BA. Antimicrobial selection in the penicillin-allergic patient. *Drugs Today (Barc).* 2001;37(6):377-383.

IMMUNIZATION ADMINISTRATION RECOMMENDATIONS

The following tables are taken from the General Recommendations on Immunization, 2011:

- Guidelines for Spacing of Live and Inactivated Antigens
- Guidelines for Administering Antibody-Containing Products and Vaccines
- Recommended Intervals Between Administration of Antibody-Containing Products and Measles- or Varicella-Containing Vaccine, by Product and Indication for Vaccination
- Vaccination of persons with Primary and Secondary Immunodeficiencies
- Needle length and Injection Site of I.M. injections

Guidelines for Spacing of Live and Inactivated Antigens

Antigen Combination	Recommended Minimum Interval Between Doses
Two or more inactivated[1]	May be administered simultaneously or at any interval between doses
Inactivated and live	May be administered simultaneously or at any interval between doses
Two or more live injectable[2]	28 days minimum interval, if not administered simultaneously

[1]Certain experts suggest a 28-day interval between tetanus toxoid, reduced diphtheria toxoid, and reduced acellular pertussis (Tdap) vaccine and tetravalent meningococcal conjugate vaccine if they are not administered simultaneously.

[2]Live oral vaccines (eg, Ty21a typhoid vaccine and rotavirus vaccine) may be administered simultaneously or at any interval before or after inactivated or live injectable vaccines.

Adapted from American Academy of Pediatrics. Pertussis. Pickering LK, Baker CJ, Kimberlin DW, et al, eds. *Red Book*: 2009 Report of the Committee on Infectious Diseases. 28th ed. Elk Grove Village, IL: American Academy of Pediatrics; 2009;22.

Guidelines for Administering Antibody-Containing Products[1] and Vaccines

Simultaneous Administration (during the same office visit)

Products Administered	Recommended Minimum Interval Between Doses
Antibody-containing products and inactivated antigen	Can be administered simultaneously at different anatomic sites or at any time interval between doses.
Antibody-containing products and live antigen	Should **not** be administered simultaneously.[2] If simultaneous administration of measles-containing vaccine or varicella vaccine is unavoidable, administer at different sites and revaccinate or test for seroconversion after the recommended interval.

Nonsimultaneous Administration

Products Administered: Administered first	Products Administered: Administered second	Recommended Minimum Interval Between Doses
Antibody-containing products	Inactivated antigen	No interval necessary
Inactivated antigen	Antibody-containing products	No interval necessary
Antibody-containing products	Live antigen	Dose-related[2,3]
Live antigen	Antibody-containing products	2 weeks[2]

[1]Blood products containing substantial amounts of immune globulin include intramuscular and intravenous immune globulin, specific hyperimmune globulin (eg, hepatitis B immune globulin, tetanus immune globulin, varicella zoster immune globulin, and rabies immune globulin), whole blood, packed red blood cells, plasma, and platelet products.

[2]Yellow fever vaccine, rotavirus vaccine, oral Ty21a typhoid vaccine, live-attenuated influenza vaccine, and zoster vaccine are exceptions to these recommendations. These live-attenuated vaccines can be administered at any time before, after, or simultaneously with an antibody-containing product.

[3]The duration of interference of antibody-containing products with the immune response to the measles component of measles-containing vaccine, and possibly varicella vaccine, is dose-related.

Recommended Intervals Between Administration of Antibody-Containing Products and Measles- or Varicella-Containing Vaccine, by Product and Indication for Vaccination

Product/Indication	Dose (mg IgG/kg) and Route[1]	Recommended Interval Before Measles- or Varicella-Containing Vaccine[2] Administration (mo)
Tetanus IG	I.M.: 250 units (10 mg IgG/kg)	3
Hepatitis A IG		
Contact prophylaxis	I.M.: 0.02 mL/kg (3.3 mg IgG/kg)	3
International travel	I.M.: 0.06 mL/kg (10 mg IgG/kg)	3
Hepatitis B IG	I.M.: 0.06 mL/kg (10 mg IgG/kg)	3
Rabies IG	I.M.: 20 int. units/kg (22 mg IgG/kg)	4
Varicella IG	I.M.: 125 units/10 kg (60-200 mg IgG/kg) (maximum: 625 units)	5
Measles prophylaxis IG		
Standard (ie, nonimmunocompromised) contact	I.M.: 0.25 mL/kg (40 mg IgG/kg)	5
Immunocompromised contact	I.M.: 0.50 mL/kg (80 mg IgG/kg)	6
Blood transfusion		
Red blood cells (RBCs), washed	I.V.: 10 mL/kg (negligible IgG/kg)	None
RBCs, adenine-saline added	I.V.: 10 mL/kg (10 mg IgG/kg)	3
Packed RBCs (hematocrit 65%)[3]	I.V.: 10 mL/kg (60 mg IgG/kg)	6
Whole blood cells (hematocrit 35% to 50%)[3]	I.V.: 10 mL/kg (80-100 mg IgG/kg)	6
Plasma/platelet products	I.V.: 10 mL/kg (160 mg IgG/kg)	7
Cytomegalovirus intravenous immune globulin (IGIV)	150 mg/kg maximum	6
IGIV		
Replacement therapy for immune deficiencies[4]	I.V.: 300-400 mg/kg[4]	8
Immune thrombocytopenic purpura treatment	I.V.: 400 mg/kg	8
Postexposure varicella prophylaxis[5]	I.V.: 400 mg/kg	8
Immune thrombocytopenic purpura treatment	I.V.: 1000 mg/kg	10
Kawasaki disease	I.V.: 2 g/kg	11
Monoclonal antibody to respiratory syncytial virus F protein (Synagis [Medimmune])[6]	I.M.: 15 mg/kg	None

HIV = human immunodeficiency virus, IG = immune globulin, IgG = immune globulin G, IGIV = intravenous immune globulin, mg IgG/kg = milligrams of immune globulin G per kilogram of body weight, I.M. = intramuscular, I.V. = intravenous, RBCs = red blood cells

[1]This table is not intended for determining the correct indications and dosages for using antibody-containing products. Unvaccinated persons might not be fully protected against measles during the entire recommended interval, and additional doses of IG or measles vaccine might be indicated after measles exposure. Concentrations of measles antibody in an IG preparation can vary by manufacturer's lot. Rates of antibody clearance after receipt of an IG preparation also might vary. Recommended intervals are extrapolated from an estimated half-life of 30 days for passively acquired antibody and an observed interference with the immune response to measles vaccine for 5 months after a dose of 80 mg IgG/kg.

[2]Does not include zoster vaccine. Zoster vaccine may be given with antibody-containing blood products.

[3]Assumes a serum IgG concentration of 16 mg/mL

[4]Measles and varicella vaccinations are recommended for children with asymptomatic or mildly symptomatic HIV infection but are contraindicated for persons with severe immunosuppression from HIV or any other immunosuppressive disorder.

[5]The investigational product VariZIG, similar to licensed varicella-zoster IG (VZIG), is a purified human IG preparation made from plasma containing high levels of anti-varicella antibodies (IgG). The interval between VariZIG and varicella vaccine (Var or MMRV) is 5 months.

[6]Contains antibody only to respiratory syncytial virus

Vaccination of Persons With Primary and Secondary Immunodeficiencies

Category	Specific Immunodeficiency	Contraindicated Vaccines[1]	Risk-Specific Recommended Vaccines[1]	Effectiveness and Comments
Primary				
B-lymphocyte (humoral)	Severe antibody deficiencies (eg, X-linked agammaglobulinemia and common variable immunodeficiency)	Oral poliovirus (OPV)[2] Smallpox Live-attenuated influenza vaccine (LAIV) BCG Ty21a (live oral typhoid) Yellow fever	Pneumococcal Consider measles and varicella vaccination	The effectiveness of any vaccine is uncertain if it depends only on the humoral response (eg, PPSV or MPSV4) IGIV interferes with the immune response to measles vaccine and possibly varicella vaccine
	Less severe antibody deficiencies (eg, selective IgA deficiency and IgG subclass deficiency)	OPV[2] BCG Yellow Fever Other live-vaccines appear to be safe	Pneumococcal	All vaccines likely effective; immune response may be attenuated
T-lymphocyte (cell-mediated and humoral)	Complete defects (eg, severe combined immunodeficiency [SCID] disease, complete DiGeorge syndrome)	All live vaccines[3,4,5]	Pneumococcal	Vaccines might be ineffective
	Partial defects (eg, most patients with DiGeorge syndrome, Wiskott-Aldrich syndrome, ataxia- telangiectasia)	All live vaccines[3,4,5]	Pneumococcal Meningococcal Hib (if not administered in infancy)	Effectiveness of any vaccine depends on degree of immune suppression
Complement	Persistent complement, properdin, or factor B deficiency	None	Pneumococcal Meningococcal	All routine vaccines likely effective
Phagocytic function	Chronic granulomatous disease, leukocyte adhesion defect, and myeloperoxidase deficiency	Live bacterial vaccines[3]	Pneumococcal[6]	All inactivated vaccines safe and likely effective; live viral vaccines likely safe and effective

Vaccination of Persons With Primary and Secondary Immunodeficiencies *continued*

Category	Specific Immunodeficiency	Contraindicated Vaccines[1]	Risk-Specific Recommended Vaccines[1]	Effectiveness and Comments
Secondary				
	HIV/AIDS	OPV[2] Smallpox BCG LAIV Withhold MMR and varicella in severely immunocompromised persons Yellow fever vaccine might have a contraindication or a precaution depending on clinical parameters of immune function[9]	Pneumococcal Consider Hib (if not administered in infancy) and meningococcal vaccination.	MMR, varicella, rotavirus, and all inactivated vaccines, including inactivated influenza, might be effective.[7]
	Malignant neoplasm, transplantation, immunosuppressive or radiation therapy	Live viral and bacterial, depending on immune status[3,4]	Pneumococcal	Effectiveness of any vaccine depends on degree of immune suppression
	Asplenia	None	Pneumococcal Meningococcal Hib (if not administered in infancy)	All routine vaccines likely effective
	Chronic renal disease	LAIV	Pneumococcal Hepatitis B[8]	All routine vaccines likely effective

AIDS = acquired immunodeficiency syndrome; BCG = bacille Calmette-Guerin; Hib = *Haemophilus influenzae* type b; HIV = human immunodeficiency virus; IG = immunoglobulin; IGIV = immune globulin intravenous; LAIV = live, attenuated influenza vaccine; MMR = measles, mumps, and rubella; MPSV4 = quadrivalent meningococcal polysaccharide vaccine; OPV = oral poliovirus vaccine (live); PPSV = pneumococcal polysaccharide vaccine; TIV = trivalent inactivated influenza vaccine

[1]Other vaccines that are universally or routinely recommended should be administered if not contraindicated.

[2]OPV is no longer available in the United States.

[3]Live bacterial vaccines: BCG and oral Ty21a *Salmonella typhi* vaccine

[4]Live viral vaccines: MMR, MMRV, OPV, LAIV, yellow fever, zoster, rotavirus, varicella, and vaccinia (smallpox). Smallpox vaccine is not recommended for children or the general public.

[5]Regarding T-lymphocyte immunodeficiency as a contraindication for rotavirus vaccine, data exist only for severe combined immunodeficiency.

[6]Pneumococcal vaccine is not indicated for children with chronic granulomatous disease beyond age-based universal recommendations for PCV. Children with chronic granulomatous disease are not at increased risk for pneumococcal disease.

[7]HIV-infected children should receive IG after exposure to measles and may receive varicella and measles vaccine if $CD4^+$ lymphocyte count is ≥15%.

[8]Indicated based on the risk from dialysis-based bloodborne transmission

[9]Symptomatic HIV infection or $CD4^+$ T-lymphocyte count of <200/mm^3 or <15% of total lymphocytes for children aged <6 years is a containdication to yellow fever vaccine administration. Asymptomatic HIV infection with $CD4^+$ T-lymphocyte count of 200-499/mm^3 for persons aged ≥6 years or 15% to 24% of total lymphocytes for children aged <6 years is a precaution for yellow fever vaccine administration. Details of yellow fever vaccine recommendations are available from the CDC. (CDC. Yellow fever vaccine: recommendations of the Advisory Committee on Immunization Practices [ACIP]. *MMWR Recomm Rep*. 2010;59[No. RR-7].)

Adapted from American Academy of Pediatrics. Passive immunization. Pickering LK, Baker CJ, Kimberline DW, et al, eds. *Red Book*: 2009 Report of the Committee on Infectious Diseases. 28th ed. Elk Grove Village, IL: American Academy of Pediatrics; 2009;74-75.

Needle Length and Injection Site of I.M. for Children Aged ≤18 years (by age) and Adults Aged ≥19 years (by sex and weight)

Age Group	Needle Length	Injection Site
Children (birth to 18 y)		
Neonates[1]	5/8" (16 mm)[2]	Anterolateral thigh
Infant 1-12 mo	1" (25 mm)	Anterolateral thigh
Toddler 1-2 y	1-1¼" (25-32 mm)	Anterolateral thigh[3]
	5/8[2]-1" (16-25 mm)	Deltoid muscle of the arm
Children 3-18 y	5/8[2]-1" (16-25 mm)	Deltoid muscle of the arm[3]
	1-1¼" (25-32 mm)	Anterolateral thigh
Adults ≥19 y		
Men and women <60 kg (130 lb)	1" (25 mm)[4]	Deltoid muscle of the arm
Men and women 60-70 kg (130-152 lb)	1" (25 mm)	
Men 70-118 kg (152-260 lb)	1-1½" (25-38 mm)	
Women 70-90 kg (152-200 lb)		
Men >118 kg (260 lb)	1½" (38 mm)	
Women >90 kg (200 lb)		

I.M. = intramuscular

[1]First 28 days of life

[2]If skin is stretched tightly and subcutaneous tissues are not bunched

[3]Preferred site

[4]Some experts recommend a 5/8" needle for men and women who weigh <60 kg.

Adapted from Poland GA, Borrud A, Jacobsen RM, et al. Determination of deltoid fat pad thickness: implications for needle length in adult immunization. *JAMA*. 1997;277:1709-1711.

RECOMMENDATIONS FOR TRAVELERS

The Centers for Disease Control and Prevention (CDC) also provides guidance to assist travelers and their healthcare providers in deciding the vaccines, medications, and other measures necessary to prevent illness and injury during international travel. Available at http://wwwnc.cdc.gov/travel

REFERENCE

Centers for Disease Control and Prevention (CDC). Recommendations of the Advisory Committee on Immunization Practices (ACIP): general recommendations on immunization. *MMWR Recomm Rep*. 2011;60(2):1-61.

IMMUNIZATION RECOMMENDATIONS

Recommended immunization schedule for persons aged 0 through 18 years —2013 (for those who fall behind or start late, see the catch-up schedule)

Vaccines	Birth	1 mo	2 mos	4 mos	6 mos	9 mos	12 mos	15 mos	18 mos	19-23 mos	2-3 yrs	**4-6 yrs**	7-10 yrs	**11-12 yrs**	13-15 yrs	16-18 yrs
Hepatitis B[1] (HepB)	←1st dose→	←2nd dose→					←3rd dose→									
Rotavirus[2] (RV) RV-1 (2-dose series); RV-5 (3-dose series)			←1st dose→	←2nd dose→	See footnote 2											
Diphtheria, tetanus, & acellular pertussis[3] (DTaP: <7 yrs)			←1st dose→	←2nd dose→	←3rd dose→			←4th dose→				←5th dose→				
Tetanus, diphtheria, & acellular pertussis[4] (Tdap: ≥7 yrs)														(Tdap)		
Haemophilus influenzae type b[5] (Hib)			←1st dose→	←2nd dose→	See footnote 5		←3rd or 4th dose→ see footnote 5									
Pneumococcal conjugate[6a,c] (PCV13)			←1st dose→	←2nd dose→	←3rd dose→		←4th dose→									
Pneumococcal polysaccharide[6b,c] (PPSV23)																
Inactivated poliovirus[7] (IPV) (<18years)			←1st dose→	←2nd dose→			←3rd dose→					←4th dose→				
Influenza[8] (IIV; LAIV) 2 doses for some : see footnote 8								Annual vaccination (IIV only)						Annual vaccination (IIV or LAIV)		
Measles, mumps, rubella[9] (MMR)							←1st dose→					←2nd dose→				
Varicella[10] (VAR)							←1st dose→					←2nd dose→				
Hepatitis A[11] (HepA)								←2 dose series see footnote 11→								
Human papillomavirus[12] (HPV2: females only; HPV4: males and females)														(3 dose series)		
Meningococcal[13] (Hib-MenCY ≥ 6 wks; MCV4-D≥9 mos; MCV4-CRM ≥ 2 yrs.)							see footnote 13							←1st dose→		booster

Range of recommended ages for all children	Range of recommended ages for catch-up immunization
Range of recommended ages for certain high-risk groups	Range of recommended ages during which catch-up is encouraged and for certain high-risk groups
Not routinely recommended	

This schedule includes recommendations in effect as of January 1, 2013. Any dose not administered at the recommended age should be administered at a subsequent visit, when indicated and feasible. The use of a combination vaccine generally is preferred over separate injections of its equivalent component vaccines. Vaccination providers should consult the relevant Advisory Committee on Immunization Practices (ACIP) statement for detailed recommendations, available at **http://www.cdc.gov/vaccines/pubs/acip-list.htm**. Clinically significant adverse events that follow vaccination should be reported to the Vaccine Adverse Event Reporting System (VAERS), available at http://vaers.hhs.gov/index or by telephone at **(800) 822-7967**. Suspected cases of vaccine-preventable diseases should be reported to the state or local health department. Additional information, including precautions and contraindications for vaccination, is available at http://www.cdc.gov/vaccines or by telephone at (800) 232-4636 [(800) CDC-INFO]. Also see the footnotes after the following "Catch-up Immunization Schedule" for more specific information about the vaccines.

Catch-up Immunization Schedule for Persons 4 Months to 18 Years of Age Who Start Late or Who Are >1 Month Behind – United States, 2013

This table provides catch-up schedules and minimum intervals between doses for children whose vaccinations have been delayed. A vaccine series does not need to be restarted, regardless of the time that has elapsed between doses. Use the section appropriate for the child's age. Always use this table in conjunction with the previous "Recommended immunization schedule for persons aged 0 through 18 years" and the footnotes that follow.

Vaccine	Minimum Age for Dose 1	Minimum Interval Between Doses			
		Dose 1 to Dose 2	Dose 2 to Dose 3	Dose 3 to Dose 4	Dose 4 to Dose 5
Catch-up Schedule for Persons 4 Months to 6 Years of Age					
Hepatitis B[1]	Birth	**4 weeks**	**8 weeks** and ≥16 weeks after first dose; minimum age for final dose is 24 weeks		
Rotavirus[2]	6 weeks	**4 weeks**	**4 weeks**[2]		
Diphtheria, tetanus, pertussis[3]	6 weeks	**4 weeks**	**4 weeks**	**6 months**	**6 months**[3]
Haemophilus influenzae type b[5]	6 weeks	**4 weeks** if first dose administered at <12 months of age **8 weeks** (as final dose) if first dose administered at 12-14 months of age **No further doses needed** if first dose administered at ≥15 months of age	**4 weeks**[5] if currently <12 months of age **8 weeks** (as final dose)[5] if currently ≥12 months of age and first dose administered at <12 months of age and second dose administered at <15 months of age **No further doses needed** if previous dose administered at ≥15 months of age	**8 weeks** (as final dose) This dose only necessary for children 12-59 months of age who received 3 doses before 12 months of age	
Pneumococcal[6]	6 weeks	**4 weeks** if first dose administered at <12 months of age **8 weeks** (as final dose for healthy children) if first dose administered at ≥12 months of age or currently 24-59 months of age **No further doses needed** for healthy children if first dose administered at ≥24 months of age	**4 weeks** if currently <12 months of age **8 weeks** (as final dose for healthy children) if currently ≥12 months of age **No further doses needed** for healthy children if previous dose administered at ≥24 months of age	**8 weeks** (as final dose) This dose only necessary for children 12-59 months of age who received 3 doses before 12 months of age or for children at high risk who received 3 doses at any age	
Inactivated poliovirus[7]	6 weeks	**4 weeks**	**4 weeks**	**6 months**[7] minimum 4 years of age for final dose	
Meningococcal[13]	6 weeks	**8 weeks**[13]	See footnote 13	See footnote 13	
Measles, mumps, rubella[9]	12 months	**4 weeks**			
Varicella[10]	12 months	**3 months**			
Hepatitits A[11]	12 months	**6 months**			
Catch-up Schedule for Persons 7-18 Years of Age					
Tetanus, diphtheria; tetanus, diphtheria, pertussis[4]	7 years[4]	**4 weeks**	**4 weeks** if first dose administered at <12 months of age **6 months** if first dose administered at ≥12 months of age	**6 months** if first dose administered at <12 months of age	
Human papillomavirus[12]	9 years	Routine dosing intervals are recommended[12]			
Hepatitis A[11]	12 months	**6 months**			
Hepatitis B[1]	Birth	**4 weeks**	**8 weeks** (and ≥16 weeks after first dose)		
Inactivated poliovirus[7]	6 weeks	**4 weeks**	**4 weeks**[7]	**6 months**[7]	
Meningococcal[13]	6 weeks	**8 weeks**[13]			
Measles, mumps, rubella[9]	12 months	**4 weeks**			
Varicella[10]	12 months	**3 months** if person is <13 years of age **4 weeks** if person is ≥13 years of age			

Footnotes to Recommended Immunization Schedule for Persons 0-18 Years of Age and the Catch-up Immunization Schedule

[1]**Hepatitis B vaccine (HepB)** *(Minimum age: Birth)*

Routine vaccination:

At birth:

- Administer monovalent HepB vaccine to all newborns before hospital discharge.
- For infants born to hepatitis B surface antigen (HB_sAg)-positive mothers, administer HepB vaccine and 0.5 mL of hepatitis B immune globulin (HBIG) within 12 hours of birth. These infants should be tested for HB_sAg and antibody to HB_sAg (anti-HBs) 1-2 months after completion of the HepB series at 9-18 months of age (preferably at the next well-child visit).
- If mother's HB_sAg status is unknown, within 12 hours of birth, administer HepB vaccine to all infants regardless of birth weight. For infants weighing <2000 grams, administer HBIG in addition to HepB within 12 hours of birth. Determine mother's HB_sAg status as soon as possible and, if she is HB_sAg-positive, also administer HBIG for infants weighing ≥2000 grams (no later than 1 week of age).

Doses following the birth dose:

- The second dose should be administered at 1 or 2 months of age. Monovalent HepB vaccine should be used for doses administered before 6 weeks of age.
- Infants who did not receive a birth dose should receive 3 doses of a HepB-containing vaccine on a schedule of 0, 1-2 months, and 6 months of age starting as soon as feasible. See **table below**.
- The minimum interval between dose 1 and 2 is 4 weeks, and between dose 2 and 3 is 8 weeks. The final (third or fourth) dose in the HepB vaccine series should be administered no earlier than 24 weeks of age and ≥16 weeks after the first dose.
- Administration of a total of 4 doses of HepB vaccine is recommended when a combination vaccine containing HepB is administered after the birth dose.

Catch-up vaccination:

- Unvaccinated persons should complete a 3-dose series.
- A 2-dose series (doses separated by at least 4 months) of adult formulation Recombivax HB is licensed for use in children 11-15 years of age.
- For other catch-up issues, see the previous "Catch-up Immunization Schedule".

[2]**Rotavirus vaccine (RV)** *(Minimum age: 6 weeks for both RV-1 [Rotarix] and RV-5 [RotaTeq])*

Routine vaccination:

- Administer a series of RV vaccine to all infants as follows:
  - If RV-1 is used, administer a 2-dose series at 2 and 4 months of age.
  - If RV-5 is used, administer a 3-dose series at ages 2, 4, and 6 months of age.
  - If any dose in series was RV-5 or vaccine product is unknown for any dose in the series, a total of 3 doses of RV vaccine should be administered.

Catch-up vaccination:

- The maximum age for the first dose in the series is 14 weeks, 6 days.
- Vaccination should not be initiated for infants ≥15 weeks, 0 days of age.
- The maximum age for the final dose in the series is 8 months, 0 days.
- If RV-1 (Rotarix) is administered for the first and second doses, a third dose is not indicated.
- For other catch-up issues, see the previous "Catch-up Immunization Schedule".

[3]**Diphtheria and tetanus toxoids and acellular pertussis vaccine (DTaP)** *(Minimum age: 6 weeks)*

Routine vaccination:

- Administer a 5-dose series of DTaP vaccine at 2, 4, 6, and 15-18 months of age, and at 4-6 years of age. The fourth dose may be administered as early as 12 months of age, provided at least 6 months have elapsed since the third dose.

Catch-up vaccination:

- The fifth (booster) dose of DTaP vaccine is not necessary if the fourth dose was administered at ≥4 years of age.
- For other catch-up issues, see the previous "Catch-up Immunization Schedule".

[4]**Tetanus and diphtheria toxoids and acellular pertussis (Tdap) vaccine**
(Minimum age: 10 years for Boostrix, 11 years for Adacel)

Routine vaccination:

- Administer 1 dose of Tdap vaccine to all adolescents 11-12 years of age.
- Tdap can be administered regardless of the interval since the last tetanus and diphtheria toxoid-containing vaccine.
- Administer 1 dose of Tdap vaccine to pregnant adolescents during each pregnancy (preferred during 27-36 weeks gestation) regardless of number of years from prior Td or Tdap vaccination.

Catch-up vaccination:

- Persons 7-10 years of age who are not fully immunized with the childhood DTaP vaccine series should receive Tdap vaccine as the first dose in the catch-up series; if additional doses are needed, use Td vaccine. For these children, an adolescent Tdap vaccine should not be given.
- Persons 11-18 years of age who have not received Tdap vaccine should receive a dose, followed by tetanus and diphtheria toxoids (Td) booster doses every 10 years thereafter.
- An inadvertent dose of DTaP vaccine administered to children 7-10 years of age can count as part of the catch-up series. This dose can count as the adolescent Tdap dose or the child can later receive a Tdap booster dose at 11-12 years of age.
- For other catch-up issues, see the previous "Catch-up Immunization Schedule".

[5]***Haemophilus influenzae* type b conjugate vaccine (Hib)** *(Minimum age: 6 weeks)*
Routine vaccination:

- Administer a Hib vaccine primary series and a booster dose to all infants. The primary series doses should be administered at 2, 4, and 6 months of age; however, if PRP-OMP (PedvaxHIB or Comvax) is administered at 2 and 4 months of age, a dose at 6 months of age is not indicated. One booster dose should be administered at 12-15 months of age.
- Hiberix (PRP-T) should only be used for the booster (final) dose in children 12 months to 4 years of age who have received at least 1 dose of Hib.

Catch-up vaccination:

- If dose 1 was administered at 12-14 months of age, administer booster (as final dose) at least 8 weeks after dose 1.
- If the first 2 doses were PRP-OMP (PedvaxHIB or Comvax) and were administered at ≤11 months of age, the third (and final) dose should be administered at 12-15 months of age and at least 8 weeks after the second dose.
- If the first dose was administered at 7-11 months of age, administer the second dose at least 4 weeks later and a final dose at 12-15 months of age, regardless of Hib vaccine (PRP-T or PRP-OMP) used for the first dose.
- For unvaccinated children ≥15 months of age, administer only 1 dose.
- For other catch-up issues, see the previous "Catch-up Immunization Schedule".

Vaccination of persons with high-risk conditions:

- Hib vaccine is not routinely recommended for patients >5 years of age. However, one dose of Hib vaccine should be administered to unvaccinated or partially vaccinated persons ≥5 years of age who have leukemia, malignant neoplasms, anatomic or functional asplenia (including sickle cell disease), human immunodeficiency virus (HIV) infection, or other immunocompromising conditions.

[6a]**Pneumococcal conjugate vaccine (PCV)** *(Minimum age: 6 weeks)*
Routine vaccination:

- Administer a series of PCV13 vaccine at 2, 4, and 6 months of age with a booster at 12-15 months of age.
- For children 14-59 months of age who have received an age-appropriate series of 7-valent PCV (PCV7), administer a single supplemental dose of 13-valent PCV (PCV13).

Catch-up vaccination:

- Administer 1 dose of PCV13 to all healthy children 24-59 months of age who are not completely vaccinated for their age.
- For other catch-up issues, see the previous "Catch-up Immunization Schedule".

Vaccination of persons with high-risk conditions:

- For children 24-71 months of age with certain underlying medical conditions (see footnote 6c), administer 1 dose of PCV13 if 3 doses of PCV were received previously, or administer 2 doses of PCV13 at least 8 weeks apart if fewer than 3 doses of PCV were received previously.
- A single dose of PCV13 may be administered to previously unvaccinated children 6-18 years of age who have anatomic or functional asplenia (including sickle cell disease), HIV infection or an immunocompromising condition, cochlear implant, or cerebrospinal fluid leak. See *MMWR*, 2010, 59(No. RR-11), available at http://www.cdc.gov/mmwr/pdf/rr/rr5911.pdf.
- Administer PPSV23 at least 8 weeks after the last dose of PCV to children ≥2 years of age with certain underlying medical conditions (see footnotes 6b and 6c).

[6b]**Pneumococcal polysaccharide vaccine (PPSV23)** *(Minimum age: 2 years)*
Vaccination of persons with high-risk conditions:

- Administer PPSV23 at least 8 weeks after the last dose of PCV to children ≥2 years of age with certain underlying medical conditions (see footnote 6c). A single revaccination with PPSV should be administered after 5 years to children with anatomic or functional asplenia (including sickle cell disease) or an immunocompromising condition.

[6c]Medical conditions for which PPSV23 is indicated in children ≥2 years of age and for which use of PCV13 is indicated in children 24-71 months of age

- Immunocompetent children with chronic heart disease (particularly cyanotic congenital heart disease and cardiac failure), chronic lung disease (including asthma if treated with high-dose oral corticosteroid therapy), diabetes mellitus, cerebrospinal fluid leaks, or cochlear implant.
- Children with anatomic or functional asplenia (including sickle cell disease and other hemoglobinopathies, congenital or acquired asplenia, or splenic dysfunction)
- Children with immunocompromising conditions: HIV infection; chronic renal failure and nephrotic syndrome; diseases associated with treatment with immunosuppressive drugs or radiation therapy, including malignant neoplasms, leukemias, lymphomas, and Hodgkin disease; solid organ transplantation; or congenital immunodeficiency

[7]Inactivated poliovirus vaccine (IPV) *(Minimum age: 6 weeks)*

Routine vaccination:

- Administer a series of IPV at 2, 4, and 6-18 months of age with a booster at 4-6 years of age. The final dose in the series should be administered on or after the fourth birthday and at least 6 months after the previous dose.

Catch-up vaccination:

- In the first 6 months of life, minimum age and minimum intervals are only recommended if the person is at risk for imminent exposure to circulating poliovirus (ie, travel to a polio-endemic region or during an outbreak).
- If ≥4 doses are administered before 4 years of age, an additional dose should be administered at 4-6 years of age.
- A fourth dose is not necessary if the third dose was administered at ≥4 years of age and at least 6 months after the previous dose.
- If both OPV and IPV were administered as part of a series, a total of 4 doses should be administered, regardless of the child's current age.
- IPV is not routinely recommended for U.S. residents ≥18 years of age.
- For other catch-up issues, see the previous "Catch-up Immunization Schedule".

[8]Influenza vaccines *(Minimum age: 6 months for inactivated influenza vaccine [IIV]; 2 years for live, attenuated influenza vaccine [LAIV])*

Routine vaccination:

- Administer influenza vaccine annually to all children beginning at 6 months of age. For most healthy, nonpregnant persons 2-49 years of age, either LAIV or IIV may be used. However, LAIV should **not** be administered to some persons, including 1) those with asthma, 2) children 2-4 years of age who had wheezing in the past 12 months, or 3) those who have any other underlying medical conditions that predispose them to influenza complications. For all other contraindications to use of LAIV, see *MMWR*, 2010, 59(No. RR-8), available at http://www.cdc.gov/mmwr/pdf/rr/rr5908.pdf.
- Administer 1 dose to persons ≥9 years of age.

For children 6 months to 8 years of age:

- For the 2012-13 season, administer 2 doses (separated by at least 4 weeks) to children who are receiving influenza vaccine for the first time. For additional guidance, follow dosing guidelines in the 2012 ACIP influenza vaccine recommendations. See *MMWR*, 2012, 61:613-8, available at http://www.cdc.gov/mmwr/pdf/wk/mm6132.pdf.
- For the 2013-14 season, follow dosing guidelines in the 2013 ACIP influenza vaccine recommendations.

[9]Measles, mumps, and rubella vaccine (MMR) *(Minimum age: 12 months for routine vaccination)*

Routine vaccination:

- Administer the first dose of MMR vaccine at 12-15 months of age and the second dose at 4-6 years of age. The second dose may be administered before 4 years of age, provided at least 4 weeks have elapsed since the first dose.
- Administer 1 dose of MMR vaccine to infants 6-11 months of age before departure from the United States for international travel. These children should be revaccinated with 2 doses of MMR vaccine, the first at 12-15 months of age (12 months if the child remains in an area where disease risk is high) and the second dose at least 4 weeks later.
- Administer 2 doses of MMR vaccine to children ≥12 months of age before departure from the United States for international travel. The first dose should be administered ≥12 months of age and the second dose at least 4 weeks later.

Catch-up vaccination:

- Ensure that all school-aged children and adolescents have had 2 doses of MMR vaccine; the minimum interval between the 2 doses is 4 weeks.
- For other catch-up issues, see the previous "Catch-up Immunization Schedule".

[10]Varicella vaccine (VAR) *(Minimum age: 12 months)*

Routine vaccination:

- Administer the first dose of VAR vaccine at 12-15 months of age and the second dose at 4-6 years of age. The second dose may be administered before 4 years of age, provided at least 3 months have elapsed since the first dose. If the second dose was administered at least 4 weeks after the first dose, it can be accepted as valid.

Catch-up vaccination:

- Ensure that all persons 7-18 years of age without evidence of immunity (see *MMWR*, 2007, 56[No. RR-4], available at http://www.cdc.gov/mmwr/pdf/rr/rr5604.pdf) have 2 doses of varicella vaccine. For children 7-12 years of age, the recommended minimum interval between doses is 3 months (if the second dose was administered at least 4 weeks after the first dose, it can be accepted as valid); for persons ≥13 years of age, the minimum interval between doses is 4 weeks.
- For other catch-up issues, see the previous "Catch-up Immunization Schedule".

[11]**Hepatitis A vaccine (HepA)** *(Minimum age: 12 months)*

Routine vaccination:

- Initiate the 2-dose HepA vaccine series for children 12-23 months of age; separate the 2 doses by 6-18 months.
- Children who have received 1 dose of HepA vaccine before 24 months of age should receive a second dose 6-18 months after the first dose.
- For any person ≥2 years of age who has not already received the HepA vaccine series, 2 doses of HepA vaccine separated by 6-18 months may be administered if immunity against hepatitis A virus infection is desired.

Catch-up vaccination:

- The minimum interval between the 2 doses is 6 months.
- For other catch-up issues, see the previous "Catch-up Immunization Schedule".

Special populations:

- Administer 2 doses of HepA vaccine at least 6 months apart to previously unvaccinated persons who live in areas where vaccination programs target older children or who are at increased risk for infection.

[12]**Human papillomavirus vaccines (HPV) (HPV4 [Gardasil] and HPV2 [Cervarix])** *(Minimum age: 9 years)*

Routine vaccination:

- Administer a 3-dose series of HPV vaccine on a schedule of 0, 1-2, and 6 months to all adolescents 11-12 years of age. Either HPV4 or HPV2 may be used for females and only HPV4 may be used for males.
- The vaccine series can be started beginning at 9 years of age.
- Administer the second dose 1-2 months after the **first** dose and administer the third dose 6 months after the **first** dose (at least 24 weeks after the first dose)

Catch-up vaccination:

- Administer the vaccine series to females (either HPV2 or HPV4) and males (HPV4) at 13-18 years of age if not previously vaccinated.
- Use recommended routine dosing intervals (see above) for vaccine series catch-up.
- For other catch-up issues, see the previous "Catch-up Immunization Schedule".

[13]**Meningococcal conjugate vaccines (MCV)** *(Minimum age: 6 weeks for Hib-MenCY, 9 months for Menactra [MCV4-D], 2 years for Menveo [MCV4-CRM])*

Routine vaccination:

- Administer MCV4 vaccine at 11-12 years of age with a booster dose at 16 years of age.
- Adolescents 11-18 years of age with human immunodeficiency virus (HIV) infection should receive a 2-dose primary series of MCV4 with at least 8 weeks between doses. See *MMWR*, 2011, 60:1018-9, available at http://www.cdc.gov/mmwr/pdf/wk/mm6030.pdf.
- For children 2 months to 10 years of age with high-risk conditions, see below.

Catch-up vaccination:

- Administer MCV4 vaccine at 13-18 years of age if not previously vaccinated.
- If the first dose is administered at 13-15 years of age, a booster dose should be administered at 16-18 years of age with a minimum interval of at least 8 weeks between doses.
- If the first dose is administered at ≥16 years of age, a booster dose is not needed.
- For other catch-up issues, see the previous "Catch-up Immunization Schedule".

Vaccination of persons with high-risk conditions:

- For children <19 months of age with anatomic or functional asplenia (including sickle cell disease), administer an infant series of Hib-MenCY at 2, 4, 6, and 12-15 months.
- For children 2-18 months of age with persistent complement component deficiency, administer either an infant series of Hib-MenCY at 2, 4, 6, and 12-15 months of age or a 2-dose primary series of MCV4-D starting at 9 months with at least 8 weeks between doses. For children 19-23 months of age with persistent complement component deficiency who have not received a complete series of Hib-MenCY or MCV4-D, administer 2 primary doses of MCV4-D at least 8 weeks apart.
- For children ≥24 months of age with persistent complement component deficiency or anatomic or functional asplenia (including sickle cell disease) who have not received a complete series of Hib-MenCY or MCV4-D, administer 2 primary doses of either MCV4-D or MCV4-CRM. If MCV4-D (Menactra) is administered to a child with asplenia (including sickle cell disease), do not administer MCV4-D until 2 years of age and at least 4 weeks after the completion of all PCV13 doses. See *MMWR*, 2011, 60:1391-2, available at http://www.cdc.gov/mmwr/pdf/wk/mm6040.pdf.

- For children ≥9 months of age who are residents of or travelers to countries in the African meningitis belt or to the Hajj, administer an age-appropriate formulation and series of MCV4 for protection against serogroups A and W-135. Prior receipt of Hib-MenCY is not sufficient for children traveling to the meningitis belt or the Hajj. See *MMWR*, 2011, 60:1391-2, available at http://www.cdc.gov/mmwr/pdf/wk/mm6040.pdf.
- For children who are present during outbreaks caused by a vaccine serogroup, administer or complete an age- and formulation-appropriate series of Hib-MenCY or MCV4.
- For booster doses among persons with high-risk conditions, refer to http://www.cdc.gov/vaccines/pubs/acip-list.-htm#mening.

This schedule is approved by the Advisory Committee on Immunization Practices (**http://www.cdc.gov/vaccines/acip/index.-html**), the American Academy of Pediatrics (**http://www.aap.org**), the American Academy of Family Physicians (**http://www.aafp.org**), and the American College of Obstetricians and Gynecologists (**http://www.acog.org**).

REFERENCE

Centers for Disease Control and Prevention (CDC). Advisory Committee on Immunization Practices (ACIP) recommended immunization schedules for persons aged 0 through 18 years and adults aged 19 years and older – United States, 2013. *MMWR Recomm Rep.* 2013;62(5). Available at http://www.cdc.gov/mmwr/pdf/wk/mm62e0128.pdf

Recommended adult immunization schedule, by vaccine and age group[1]

VACCINE ▼ AGE GROUP ▶	19-21 years	22-26 years	27-49 years	50-59 years	60-64 years	≥ 65 years
Influenza [2,*]	1 dose annually					
Tetanus, diphtheria, pertussis (Td/Tdap) [3,*]	Substitute 1-time dose of Tdap for Td booster; then boost with Td every 10 yrs					
Varicella [4,*]	2 doses					
Human papillomavirus (HPV) Female [5,*]	3 doses					
Human papillomavirus (HPV) Male [5,*]	3 doses					
Zoster [6]					1 dose	
Measles, mumps, rubella (MMR) [7,*]	1 or 2 doses					
Pneumococcal polysaccharide (PPSV23) [8,9]	1 or 2 doses					1 dose
Pneumococcal 13-valent conjugate (PCV13) [10]	1 dose					
Meningococcal [11,*]	1 or more doses					
Hepatitis A [12,*]	2 doses					
Hepatitis B [13,*]	3 doses					

*Covered by the Vaccine Injury Compensation Program

- For all persons in this category who meet the age requirements and who lack documentation of vaccination or have no evidence of previous infection; zoster vaccine recommended regardless of prior episode of zoster
- Recommended if some other risk factor is present (e.g., on the basis of medical, occupational, lifestyle, or other indication)
- No recommendation

Report all clinically significant postvaccination reactions to the Vaccine Adverse Event Reporting System (VAERS). Reporting forms and instructions on filing a VAERS report are available at www.vaers.hhs.gov or by telephone, 800-822-7967.
Information on how to file a Vaccine Injury Compensation Program claim is available at www.hrsa.gov/vaccinecompensation or by telephone, 800-338-2382. To file a claim for vaccine injury, contact the U.S. Court of Federal Claims, 717 Madison Place, N.W., Washington, D.C. 20005; telephone, 202-357-6400.
Additional information about the vaccines in this schedule, extent of available data, and contraindications for vaccination is also available at www.cdc.gov/vaccines or from the CDC-INFO Contact Center at 800-CDC-INFO (800-232-4636) in English and Spanish, 8:00 a.m. - 8:00 p.m. Eastern Time, Monday - Friday, excluding holidays.
Use of trade names and commercial sources is for identification only and does not imply endorsement by the U.S. Department of Health and Human Services.

The recommendations in this schedule were approved by the Centers for Disease Control and Prevention's (CDC) Advisory Committee on Immunization Practices (ACIP), the American Academy of Family Physicians (AAFP), the American College of Physicians (ACP), American College of Obstetricians and Gynecologists (ACOG) and American College of Nurse-Midwives (ACNM).

FIGURE 2. Recommended vaccinations indicated for adults based on medical and other indications[1]

VACCINE ▼ INDICATION ▶	Pregnancy	Immuno-compromising conditions (excluding human immunodeficiency virus [HIV])[4,6,7,10,15]	HIV infection CD4+ T lymphocyte count[4,6,7,10,14,15] < 200 cells/μL	HIV infection CD4+ T lymphocyte count ≥ 200 cells/μL	Men who have sex with men (MSM)	Heart disease, chronic lung disease, chronic alcoholism	Asplenia (including elective splenectomy and persistent complement component deficiencies)[10,14]	Chronic liver disease	Kidney failure, end-stage renal disease, receipt of hemodialysis	Diabetes	Healthcare personnel
Influenza [2,*]	1 dose IIV annually				1 dose IIV or LAIV annually	1 dose IIV annually					1 dose IIV or LAIV annually
Tetanus, diphtheria, pertussis (Td/Tdap) [3,*]	1 dose Tdap each pregnancy	Substitute 1-time dose of Tdap for Td booster; then boost with Td every 10 yrs									
Varicella [4,*]	Contraindicated			2 doses							
Human papillomavirus (HPV) Female [5,*]		3 doses through age 26 yrs				3 doses through age 26 yrs					
Human papillomavirus (HPV) Male [5,*]		3 doses through age 26 yrs				3 doses through age 21 yrs					
Zoster [6]	Contraindicated				1 dose						
Measles, mumps, rubella (MMR) [7,*]	Contraindicated			1 or 2 doses							
Pneumococcal polysaccharide (PPSV23) [8,9]	1 or 2 doses										
Pneumococcal 13-valent conjugate (PCV13) [10]		1 dose									
Meningococcal [11,*]	1 or more doses										
Hepatitis A [12,*]	2 doses										
Hepatitis B [13,*]	3 doses										

*Covered by the Vaccine Injury Compensation Program

- For all persons in this category who meet the age requirements and who lack documentation of vaccination or have no evidence of previous infection; zoster vaccine recommended regardless of prior episode of zoster
- Recommended if some other risk factor is present (e.g., on the basis of medical, occupational, lifestyle, or other indications)
- No recommendation

These schedules indicate the recommended age groups and medical indications for which administration of currently licensed vaccines is commonly indicated for adults ages 19 years and older, as of January 1, 2013. For all vaccines being recommended on the Adult Immunization Schedule: a vaccine series does not need to be restarted, regardless of the time that has elapsed between doses. Licensed combination vaccines may be used whenever any components of the combination are indicated and when the vaccine's other components are not contraindicated. For detailed recommendations on all vaccines, including those used primarily for travelers or that are issued during the year, consult the manufacturers' package inserts and the complete statements from the Advisory Committee on Immunization Practices (www.cdc.gov/vaccines/pubs/acip-list.htm). Use of trade names and commercial sources is for identification only and does not imply endorsement by the U.S. Department of Health and Human Services.

Footnotes to Recommended Adult Immunization Schedule

[1]Additional information

- Additional guidance for the use of the vaccines described in this supplement is available at http://www.cdc.gov/vaccines/pubs/acip-list.htm.
- Information on vaccination recommendations when vaccination status is unknown and other general immunization information can be found in the General Recommendations on Immunization at http://www.cdc.gov/mmwr/preview/mmwrhtml/rr6002a1.htm.
- Information on travel vaccine requirements and recommendations (eg, for hepatitis A and B, meningococcal, other vaccines) are available at http://wwwnc.cdc.gov/travel/page/vaccinations.htm.

[2]Influenza vaccine

- Annual vaccination against influenza is recommended for all persons ≥6 months of age.
- Persons ≥6 months of age, including pregnant women, can receive the inactivated influenza vaccine (IIV).
- Healthy, nonpregnant persons 2-49 years of age without high-risk medical conditions can receive either intranasally administered live, attenuated influenza vaccine (LAIV) (FluMist) or IIV. Healthcare personnel who care for severely immunocompromised persons (ie, those who require care in a protected environment) should receive IIV, rather than LAIV.
- The intramuscularly or intradermally administered IIV are options for adults 18-64 years of age.
- Adults ≥65 years of age can receive the standard-dose IIV or the high-dose IIV (Fluzone High-Dose).

[3]Tetanus, diphtheria, and acellular pertussis vaccine (Td/Tdap)

- Administer one dose of Tdap vaccine to pregnant women during each pregnancy (preferred during 27-36 weeks' gestation), regardless of number of years since prior Td or Tdap vaccination.
- Administer Tdap to all other adults who have not previously received Tdap or for whom vaccine status is unknown. Tdap can be administered regardless of interval since the most recent tetanus or diphtheria-toxoid-containing vaccine.
- Adults with an unknown or incomplete history of completing a 3-dose primary vaccination series with Td-containing vaccines should begin or complete a primary vaccination series, including a Tdap dose.
- For unvaccinated adults, administer the first 2 doses at least 4 weeks apart and the third dose 6-12 months after the second.
- For incompletely vaccinated adults (ie, <3 doses), administer remaining doses.
- Refer to the Advisory Committee on Immunization Practices (ACIP) statement for recommendations for administering Td/Tdap as prophylaxis in wound management (see footnote #1).

[4]Varicella vaccine

- All adults without evidence of immunity to varicella (as defined below) should receive 2 doses of single-antigen varicella vaccine or a second dose if they have received only 1 dose.
- Special consideration should be given to those who have close contact with persons at high risk for severe disease (eg, healthcare personnel and family contacts of persons with immunocompromising conditions) or those who are at high risk for exposure or transmission (eg, teachers; child care employees; residents and staff members of institutional settings, including correctional institutions; college students; military personnel; adolescents and adults living in households with children; nonpregnant women of childbearing age; international travelers).
- Pregnant women should be assessed for evidence of varicella immunity. Women who do not have evidence of immunity should receive the first dose of varicella vaccine upon completion or termination of pregnancy and before discharge from the healthcare facility. The second dose should be administered 4–8 weeks after the first dose.
- Evidence of immunity to varicella in adults includes any of the following:
  - Documentation of 2 doses of varicella vaccine ≥4 weeks apart
  - U.S.-born before 1980, except healthcare personnel and pregnant women
  - History of varicella based on diagnosis or verification of varicella disease by a healthcare provider
  - History of herpes zoster based on diagnosis or verification of herpes zoster disease by a healthcare provider, or
  - Laboratory evidence of immunity or laboratory confirmation of disease

[5]Human papillomavirus vaccine (HPV)

- Two vaccines are licensed for use in females, bivalent HPV vaccine (HPV2) and quadrivalent HPV vaccine (HPV4), and one HPV vaccine for use in males, HPV4.
- For females, either HPV4 or HPV2 is recommended in a 3-dose series for routine vaccination at 11 or 12 years of age, and for those 13-26 years of age, if not previously vaccinated.
- For males, HPV4 is recommended in a 3-dose series for routine vaccination at 11 or 12 years of age, and for those 13-21 years of age, if not previously vaccinated. Males 22-26 years of age may be vaccinated.
- HPV4 is recommended for men who have sex with men (MSM) through 26 years of age for those who did not get any of all doses when they were younger.

- Vaccination is recommended for immunocompromised persons (including those with HIV infection) through 26 years of age for those who did not get any or all doses when they were younger.
- A complete series for either HPV4 or HPV2 consists of 3 doses. The second dose should be administered 1–2 months after the first dose; the third dose should be administered 6 months after the first dose (≥24 weeks after the first dose).
- HPV vaccines are not recommended for use in pregnant women. However, pregnancy testing is not needed before vaccination. If a woman is found to be pregnant after initiating the vaccination series, no intervention is needed; the remainder of the 3-dose series should be delayed until completion of pregnancy.
- Although HPV vaccination is not specifically recommended for healthcare personnel (HCP) based on their occupation, HCP should receive the HPV vaccine as recommended (see above).

[6]Zoster vaccine

- A single dose of zoster vaccine is recommended for adults ≥60 years of age, regardless of whether they report a prior episode of herpes zoster. Although the vaccine is licensed by the Food and Drug Administration (FDA) for use among and can be administered to persons ≥50 years of age, ACIP recommendes that vaccination begin at 60 years of age.
- Persons ≥60 years of age with chronic medical conditions may be vaccinated, unless their condition constitutes a contraindication, such as pregnancy or severe immunodeficiency.
- Although zoster vaccination is not specifically recommended for healthcare personnel, they should receive the vaccine if they are in the recommended age group.

[7]Measles, mumps, rubella vaccine (MMR)

- Adults born before 1957 generally are considered immune to measles and mumps. All adults born in 1957 or later should have documentation of ≥1 dose of MMR vaccine, unless they have a medical contraindication to the vaccine or laboratory evidence of immunity to each of the three diseases. Documentation of provider-diagnosed disease is not considered acceptable evidence of immunity for measles, mumps, or rubella.
- **Measles component:**
  - A routine second dose of MMR vaccine, administered a minimum of 28 days after the first dose, is recommended for adults who:
    - Are students in postsecondary educational institutions
    - Work in a healthcare facility, or
    - Plan to travel internationally
  - Persons who received inactivated (killed) measles vaccine or measles vaccine of unknown type during 1963–1967 should be revaccinated with 2 doses of MMR vaccine.
- **Mumps component:**
  - A routine second dose of MMR vaccine, administered a minimum of 28 days after the first dose, is recommended for adults who:
    - Are students in postsecondary educational institutions
    - Work in a healthcare facility, or
    - Plan to travel internationally
  - Persons vaccinated before 1979 with either killed mumps vaccine or mumps vaccine of unknown type who are at high risk for mumps infection (eg, persons who are working in a healthcare facility) should be considered for revaccination with 2 doses of MMR vaccine.
- **Rubella component:** For women of childbearing age, regardless of birth year, rubella immunity should be determined. If there is no evidence of immunity, women who are not pregnant should be vaccinated. Pregnant women who do not have evidence of immunity should receive MMR vaccine upon completion or termination of pregnancy and before discharge from the healthcare facility.
- **Healthcare personnel born before 1957:** For unvaccinated healthcare personnel born before 1957 who lack laboratory evidence of measles, mumps, and/or rubella immunity or laboratory confirmation of disease, healthcare facilities should consider vaccinating personnel with 2 doses of MMR vaccine at the appropriate interval for measles and mumps or 1 dose of MMR vaccine for rubella.

[8]Pneumococcal polysaccharide vaccine (PPSV23)

- Vaccinate all persons with the following indications:
  - All adults ≥65 years of age
  - Adults <65 years of age with chronic lung disease (including chronic obstructive pulmonary disease, emphysema, and asthma), chronic cardiovascular diseases, diabetes mellitus, chronic renal failure, nephrotic syndrome, chronic liver disease (including cirrhosis), alcoholism, cochlear implants, cerebrospinal fluid leaks, immunocompromising conditions, and functional or anatomic asplenia (eg, sickle cell disease and other hemoglobinophathies, congenital or acquired asplenia, splenic dysfunction, or splenectomy [if elective splenectomy is planned, vaccinate ≥2 weeks before surgery])
  - Residents of nursing homes or long-term care facilities, and
  - Adults who smoke cigarettes

- Persons with immunocompromising conditions and other selected conditions are recommended to receive PCV13 and PPSV23 vaccines. See footnote #10 for information on timing of PCV13 and PPSV23 vaccinations.
- Persons with asymptomatic or symptomatic HIV infection should be vaccinated as soon as possible after their diagnosis.
- When cancer chemotherapy or other immunosuppressive therapy is being considered, the interval between vaccination and initiation of immunosuppresive therapy should be ≥2 weeks. Vaccination during chemotherapy or radiation therapy should be avoided.
- Routine use of PPSV23 is not recommended for American Indians/Alaska Natives or other persons <65 years of age, unless they have underlying medical conditions that are PPSV23 indications. However, public health authorities may consider recommending PPSV23 for American Indians/Alaska Natives who are living in areas where the risk for invasive pneumococcal disease is increased.
- When indicated, PPSV23 should be administered to patients who are uncertain of their vaccination status and there is no record of previous vaccination. When PCV13 is also indicated, a dose of PCV13 should be given first (see footnote #10).

[9]Revaccination with PPSV23

- One-time revaccination 5 years after the first dose is recommended for persons 19-64 years of age with chronic renal failure or nephrotic syndrome, those with functional or anatomic asplenia (eg, sickle cell disease, splenectomy), and those with immunocompromising conditions.
- Persons who received 1 or 2 doses of PPSV23 before 65 years of age for any indication should receive another dose of the vaccine at ≥65 years of age if at least 5 years have passed since their previous dose.
- No further doses are needed for persons vaccinated with PPSV23 at ≥65 years of age.

[10]Pneumococcal conjugate 13-valent vaccine (PCV13)

- Adults ≥19 years of age with immunocompromising conditions (including chronic renal failure and nephrotic syndrome), functional or anatomic asplenia, and CSF leaks or cochlear implants, as well as those who have not previously received PCF13 or PPSV23, should receive a single dose of PCV13, followed by a dose of PPSV23 at least 8 weeks later.
- Adults ≥19 years of age with the aforementioned conditions who have previously received ≥1 dose of PPSV23 should receive a dose of PCV13 ≥1 years after the last PPSV23 dose was received. For those who require additional doses of PPSV23, the first such dose should be given no sooner than 8 weeks after PCV13 and at least 5 years since the most recent dose of PPSV23.
- When indicated, PCV13 should be administered to patients who are uncertain of their vaccination status history and there is no record of previous vaccination.
- Although PCV13 is licensed by the Food and Drug Administration (FDA) for use among and can be administered to persons ≥50 years of age, ACIP recommends PCV13 for adults ≥19 years of age with the specific medical conditions noted above.

[11]Meningococcal vaccine

- Administer 2 doses of meningococcal conjugate vaccine quadrivalent (MCV4) ≥2 months apart to adults with functional asplenia or persistent complement component deficiencies.
- HIV-infected persons who are vaccinated should also receive 2 doses.
- Administer a single dose of meningococcal vaccine to microbiologists routinely exposed to isolates of *Neisseria meningitidis*, military recruits, and persons who travel to or live in countries in which meningococcal disease is hyperendemic or epidemic.
- First-year college students ≤21 years of age who are living in residence halls should be vaccinated if they have not received a dose on or after their 16th birthday.
- MCV4 is preferred for adults with any of the preceding indications who are ≤55 years of age; meningococcal polysaccharide vaccine (MPSV4) is preferred for adults ≥56 years of age.
- Revaccination with MCV4 every 5 years is recommended for adults previously vaccinated with MCV4 or MPSV4 who remain at increased risk for infection (eg, adults with anatomic or functional asplenia or persistent complement component deficiencies).

[12]Hepatitis A vaccine

- Vaccinate any person seeking protection from hepatitis A virus (HAV) infection and persons with any of the following indications:
  - Men who have sex with men and persons who use injection or noninjection illicit drugs
  - Persons working with HAV-infected primates or with HAV in a research laboratory setting
  - Persons with chronic liver disease and persons who receive clotting factor concentrates
  - Persons traveling to or working in countries that have high or intermediate endemicity of hepatitis A, and
  - Unvaccinated persons who anticipate close personal contatct (eg, household, regular babysitting) with an international adoptee during the first 60 days after arrival in the United States from a country with high or intermediate endemicity (see footnote #1 for more information on travel recommendations). The first dose of the 2-dose hepatitis A vaccine series should be administered as soon as adoption is planned, ideally ≥2 weeks before the arrival of the adoptee.

- Single-antigen vaccine formulations should be administered in a 2-dose schedule at either 0 and 6-12 months (Havrix) or 0 and 6-18 months (VAQTA). If the combined hepatitis A and hepatitis B vaccine (Twinrix) is used, administer 3 doses at 0, 1, and 6 months; alternatively, a 4-dose schedule may be used, administered on days 0, 7, and 21-30, followed by a booster dose at month 12.

[13]Hepatitis B vaccine

- Vaccinate persons with any of the following indications and any person seeking protection from hepatitis B virus (HBV) infection:
  - Sexually active persons who are not in a long-term, mutually monogamous relationship (eg, persons with more than one sex partner during the previous 6 months), persons seeking evaluation or treatment for a sexually transmitted disease (STD), current or recent injection-drug users, and men who have sex with men
  - Healthcare personnel and public-safety workers who are potentially exposed to blood or other infectious body fluids
  - Persons <60 years of age with diabetes as soon as feasible after diagnosis and persons with diabetes who are ≥60 years of age at the discretion of the treating clinician, based on increased need for assisted blood glucose monitoring in long-term care facilities; likelihood of acquiring hepatitis B infection, its complications, or chronic sequelae; and likelihood of immune response to vaccination
  - Persons with end-stage renal disease, including patients receiving hemodialysis; persons with HIV infection; and persons with chronic liver disease
  - Household contacts and sex partners of hepatitis B surface antigen-positive persons, clients and staff members of institutions for persons with developmental disabilities, and international travelers to countries with high or intermediate prevalence of chronic HBV infection, and
  - All adults in the following settings: STD treatment facilities, HIV testing and treatment facilities, facilities providing drug-abuse treatment and prevention services, healthcare settings targeting services to injection-drug users or men who have sex with men, correctional facilities, end-stage renal disease programs and facilities for chronic hemodialysis patients, and institutions and nonresidential daycare facilities for persons with developmental disabilities
- Administer missing doses to complete a 3-dose series of hepatitis B vaccine to those persons not vaccinated or not completely vaccinated. The second dose should be administered 1 month after the first dose; the third dose should be given ≥2 months after the second dose (and ≥4 months after the first dose). If the combined hepatitis A and hepatitis B vaccine (Twinrix) is used, give 3 doses at 0, 1, and 6 months; alternatively, a 4-dose Twinrix schedule, administered on days 0, 7, and 21-30, followed by a booster dose at month 12, may be used.
- Adult patients receiving hemodialysis or with other immunocompromising conditions should receive 1 dose of 40 μg/mL (Recombivax HB), administered on a 3-dose schedule, or 2 doses of 20 μg/mL (Engerix-B), administered simultaneously on a 4-dose schedule at 0, 1, 2, and 6 months.

[14]Selected conditions for which *Haemophilus influenzae* type b vaccine (Hib) may be used

- One dose of Hib vaccine should be considered for persons who have sickle cell disease, leukemia, or HIV infection, or who have anatomic or functional asplenia if they have not previously received Hib vaccine.

[15]Immunocompromising conditions

- Inactivated vaccines generally are acceptable (eg, pneumococcal, meningococcal, influenza [inactivated influenza vaccine]), and live vaccines generally are avoided in persons with immune deficiencies or immunocompromising conditions. Information on specific conditions is available at http://www.cdc.gov/vaccines/pubs/acip-list.htm.

REFERENCE

Centers for Disease Control and Prevention (CDC). Advisory Committee on Immunization Practices (ACIP) recommended immunization schedules for persons aged 0 through 18 years and adults aged 19 years and older – United States, 2013. *MMWR Recomm Rep.* 2013;62(5). Available at http://www.cdc.gov/mmwr/pdf/wk/mm62e0128.pdf

VACCINE INJURY TABLE

The Vaccine Injury Table makes it easier for some people to get compensation. The table lists and explains injuries/conditions that are presumed to be caused by vaccines. It also lists time periods in which the first symptom of these injuries/conditions must occur after receiving the vaccine. If the first symptom of these injuries/conditions occurs within the listed time period, it is presumed that the vaccine was the cause of the injury or condition, unless another cause is found. For example, if the patient received the tetanus vaccines and had a severe allergic reaction (anaphylaxis) within 4 hours after receiving the vaccine, then it is presumed that the tetanus vaccine caused the injury if no other cause is found.

If the injury/condition is not on the table or if the injury/condition did not occur within the time period on the table, it must be proven that the vaccine caused the injury/condition. Such proof must be based on medical records or opinion, which may include expert witness testimony.

Vaccine Injury Table[1]

Vaccine		Illness, Disability, Injury, or Condition Covered	Time Period for First Symptom or Manifestation of Onset or of Significant Aggravation After Vaccine Administration
Vaccines containing tetanus toxoid (eg, DTaP, DTP, DT, Td, TT)	A.	Anaphylaxis or anaphylactic shock	4 hours
	B.	Brachial neuritis	2-28 days
	C.	Any acute complication or sequela (including death) of above events	Not applicable
Vaccines containing whole cell pertussis bacteria, extracted or partial cell pertussis bacteria, or specific pertussis antigen(s) (eg, DTP, DTaP, P, DTP-Hib)	A.	Anaphylaxis or anaphylactic shock	4 hours
	B.	Encephalopathy (or encephalitis)	72 hours
	C.	Any acute complication or sequela (including death) of above events	Not applicable
Measles, mumps, and rubella vaccine or any of its components (eg, MMR, MR, M, R)	A.	Anaphylaxis or anaphylactic shock	4 hours
	B.	Encephalopathy (or encephalitis)	5-15 days
	C.	Any acute complication or sequela (including death) of above events	Not applicable
Vaccines containing rubella virus (eg, MMR, MR, R)	A.	Chronic arthritis	7-42 days
	B.	Any acute complication or sequela (including death) of above events	Not applicable
Vaccines containing measles virus (eg, MMR, MR, M)	A.	Thrombocytopenic purpura	7-30 days
	B.	Vaccine-strain measles viral infection in an immunodeficient recipient	6 months
	C.	Any acute complication or sequela (including death) of above events	Not applicable
Vaccines containing polio live virus (OPV)	A.	Paralytic polio	
		• In a nonimmunodeficient recipient	30 days
		• In an immunodeficient recipient	6 months
		• In a vaccine-associated community case	Not applicable
	B.	Vaccine-strain polio viral infection	
		• In a nonimmunodeficient recipient	30 days
		• In an immunodeficient recipient	6 months
		• In a vaccine-associated community case	Not applicable
	C.	Any acute complication or sequela (including death) of above events	Not applicable
Vaccines containing polio inactivated (eg, IPV)	A.	Anaphylaxis or anaphylactic shock	4 hours
	B.	Any acute complication or sequela (including death) of above events	Not applicable
Hepatitis B vaccines	A.	Anaphylaxis or anaphylactic shock	4 hours
	B.	Any acute complication or sequela (including death) of above events	Not applicable
Hemophilus influenzae type b polysaccharide conjugate vaccines	A.	No condition specified	Not applicable
Varicella vaccine	A.	No condition specified	Not applicable
Rotavirus vaccine	A.	No condition specified	Not applicable
Pneumococcal conjugate vaccines	A.	No condition specified	Not applicable

Vaccine Injury Table[1] *(continued)*

Vaccine		Illness, Disability, Injury, or Condition Covered	Time Period for First Symptom or Manifestation of Onset or of Significant Aggravation After Vaccine Administration
Hepatitis A vaccines	A.	No condition specified	Not applicable
Trivalent influenza vaccines	A.	No condition specified	Not applicable
Meningococcal vaccines	A.	No condition specified	Not applicable
Human papillomavirus (HPV) vaccines	A.	No condition specified	Not applicable
Any new vaccine recommended by the Centers for Disease Control and Prevention for routine administration to children, after publication by Secretary, HHS of a notice of coverage	A.	No condition specified	Not applicable

[1]Effective date: July 22, 2011; available at http://www.hrsa.gov/vaccinecompensation/vaccinetable.html

PREVENTION OF INFECTIVE ENDOCARDITIS

Recommendations by the American Heart Association

(*Circulation*. 2007;116(15):1736-1754.)

The recommendations were formulated by a writing group under the auspices of the American Heart Association (AHA), and included representation from the Infectious Diseases Society of America (IDSA), the American Academy of Pediatrics (AAP), and the American Dental Association (ADA). Additionally, input was received from both national and international experts on infective endocarditis (IE). These guidelines are based on expert interpretation and review of scientific literature from 1950 through 2006. The consensus statement was subsequently reviewed by outside experts not affiliated with the writing group and by the Science Advisory and Coordinating Committee of the American Heart Association. These guidelines are meant to aid practitioners but are not intended as the standard of care or as a substitute for clinical judgment.

In a major departure from the former recommendations, the current guidelines have been greatly simplified to place a much greater emphasis on a very limited number of underlying cardiac conditions (see Table 1). These specific conditions have been associated with the highest risk of adverse outcomes due to IE. Patients should receive IE prophylaxis only if they are undergoing certain invasive procedures (see Table 2) and have at least one of the underlying cardiovascular conditions specified below.

Common situations for which routine prophylaxis was previously, but no longer recommended, include mitral valve prolapse, general dental cleanings and local anesthetic administration (noninfected tissue), and bronchoscopy (see Table 2).

Table 1. Cardiac Conditions Associated With the Highest Risk of Adverse Outcome From Endocarditis

Prophylaxis With Dental Procedures Is Recommended
Previous infective endocarditis
Prosthetic cardiac valves
Congenital heart disease (CHD)
Unrepaired cyanotic CHD, including palliative shunts and conduits
Completely repaired congenital heart defect with prosthetic material or device, whether placed by surgery or by catheter intervention, during the first 6 months after the procedure[1]
Repaired CHD with residual defects at the site or adjacent to the site of a prosthetic patch or prosthetic device (which inhibit endothelialization)
Cardiac transplantation recipients who develop cardiac valvulopathy

[1]Prophylaxis is recommended because endothelialization of prosthetic material occurs within 6 months after the procedure.

Table 2. Guidance for Use of Prophylactic Antibiotic Therapy Based on Procedure or Condition[1]

Location of Procedure	Prophylaxis Recommended	Prophylaxis NOT Recommended
Dental	All invasive manipulations of the gingival or periapical region or perforation of oral mucosa (includes biopsies, suture removal, placement of orthodontic bands)	Anesthetic injections through noninfected tissue, radiographs, placement/adjustment/removal prosthodontics/orthodontic appliances or brackets, shedding of deciduous teeth, trauma-induced bleeding from lips, gums, or oral mucosa
Respiratory tract	Biopsy/incision of respiratory mucosa (eg, tonsillectomy/adenoidectomy); drainage of abscess or empyema[2]	Bronchoscopy (unless incision of mucosa required)
Gastrointestinal (GI) or genitourinary (GU) tract	Established GI/GU infection or prevention of infectious sequelae[3]; elective cystoscopy or other urinary tract procedure with established enterococci infection/ colonization[3,4]	Routine diagnostic procedures, including esophagogastroduodenoscopy or colonoscopy in the absence of active infection; vaginal delivery and hysterectomy
Skin, skin structure, or musculoskeletal	Any surgical procedure involving infected tissue	Procedures conducted in noninfected tissue; tattoos and ear/body piercing

[1]Patients should receive prophylactic antibiotic therapy if they meet the criteria for a specified procedure/condition in this table and they have a high-risk cardiovascular condition listed in the preceding text.

[2]If infection is known or suspected to be caused by *Staphylococcus aureus*, consider antistaphylococcal penicillin or cephalosporin, or vancomycin in beta-lactam-sensitive patients.

[3]Consider alternate agents with activity against enterococci (ampicillin, penicillin, piperacillin); vancomycin (for beta-lactam-sensitive patients)

[4]Eradication of enterococci from the urinary tract should be considered.

Table 3. Prophylactic Regimens for Dental Procedures

Situation	Agent	Regimen to Be Given 30-60 Minutes Before Procedure	
		Adults	Children[1]
Standard general prophylaxis	Amoxicillin	2000 mg P.O.	50 mg/kg P.O.
Unable to take oral medications	Ampicillin **or**	2000 mg I.M./I.V.	50 mg/kg I.M./I.V.
	CeFAZolin or cefTRIAXone	1000 mg I.M./I.V.	50 mg/kg I.M./I.V.
Allergic to penicillin	Clindamycin **or**	600 mg P.O.	20 mg/kg P.O.
	Cephalexin[2] or other dose-equivalent first/second generation cephalosporin[2] **or**	2000 mg P.O	50 mg/kg P.O.
	Azithromycin or clarithromycin	500 mg P.O.	15 mg/kg P.O.
Allergic to penicillin and unable to take oral medications	Clindamycin **or**	600 mg I.M./I.V.	20 mg/kg I.M./I.V.
	CeFAZolin[2] or cefTRIAXone[2]	1000 mg I.M./I.V.	50 mg/kg I.M./I.V.

[1]Total children's dose should not exceed adult dose.

[2]Cephalosporins should not be used in individuals with immediate-type hypersensitivity reaction (urticaria, angioedema, or anaphylaxis) to penicillins.

Gastrointestinal/Genitourinary/Respiratory Procedures and Surgery Involving Skin, Skin Structure, or Musculoskeletal Tissue

In general, antibiotic prophylaxis solely to prevent IE is **not** recommended in patients undergoing GI/GU procedures or surgery involving skin, skin structure, or musculoskeletal tissue, unless infection is present at the site where the procedure is to occur. For patients with conditions listed in Table 1 undergoing an invasive respiratory tract procedure to treat an established infection (eg, drainage of an abscess or empyema) and the infection is known or suspected to be caused by *Staphlococcus aureus* (*S. aureus*), an antistaphlococcal penicillin or cephalosporin is recommended. In those patients with infections of the GI or GU tract undergoing GI/GU procedures, it may be reasonable to administer an agent with activity against enterococci (eg, ampicillin, penicillin, piperacillin); amoxicillin or ampicillin is preferred. In patients with a condition listed in Table 1 undergoing surgery involving infected skin, skin structure, or musculoskeletal tissue, it is reasonable that the regimen contain an agent with activity against staphylococci and beta-hemolytic streptococci (eg, antistaphlococcal penicillin or cephalosporin). In any case, vancomycin (or clindamycin in the setting of infected skin, skin structure, or musculoskeletal tissue) may be administered to patients unable to tolerate a beta-lactam (eg, ampicillin). Vancomycin should be administered with any infection known or suspected to be caused by a methicillin-resistant *S. aureus*.

Table 4. Vancomycin Dosing

	Dosage for Adults	Dosage for Children
Vancomyin	1000 mg I.V. infused **slowly over 1 hour**; complete infusion within 30 minutes before procedure	20 mg/kg (maximum: 1000 mg) I.V. infused **slowly over 1 hour**; complete infusion within 30 minutes before procedure

If infection is caused by a known or suspected strain of resistant enterococcus, consult with an infectious diseases expert.

REFERENCE

Wilson W, Taubert KA, Gewitz M, et al. Prevention of infective endocarditis. Guidelines from the American Heart Association. A guideline from the American Heart Association Rheumatic Fever, Endocarditis, and Kawasaki Disease Committee, Council on Cardiovascular Disease in the Young, and the Council on Clinical Cardiology, Council on Cardiovascular Surgery and Anesthesia, and the Quality of Care and Outcomes Research Interdisciplinary Working Group. *Circulation*. 2007;116(15):1736-1754.

ANTIBIOTIC TREATMENT OF ADULTS WITH INFECTIVE ENDOCARDITIS

Table 1. Suggested Regimens for Therapy of Native Valve Endocarditis Due to Penicillin-Susceptible Viridans Streptococci and *Streptococcus bovis* (Minimum Inhibitory Concentration ≤0.12 mcg/mL)[1]

Antibiotic	Dosage and Route	Duration (wk)	Comments
Aqueous crystalline penicillin G sodium **or**	12-18 million units/24 h I.V. either continuously or in 4-6 equally divided doses	4	Preferred in most patients older than 65 y and in those with impairment of the 8th cranial nerve or renal function
CefTRIAXone sodium	2 g once daily I.V. or I.M.[2]	4	
Either penicillin or cefTRIAXone regimen above with gentamicin sulfate[3]	3 mg/kg/24 h I.M./I.V. as single daily dose	2	When using combination therapy, both β-lactam and aminoglycoside regimen duration is 2 weeks; 2-week regimen not intended if known cardiac or extracardiac abscess, Cl_{cr} <20 mL/min, 8th cranial nerve impairment or *Abiotrophia*, *Granulicatella*, or *Gemella* spp
Vancomycin hydrochloride[4]	30 mg/kg/24 h I.V. in 2 equally divided doses, not to exceed 2 g/24 h unless serum levels are monitored	4	Vancomycin therapy is recommended for patients allergic to β-lactams; peak serum concentrations of vancomycin should be obtained 1 h after completion of the infusion and should be in the range of 30-45 mcg/mL and trough of 10-15 mcg/mL for twice-daily dosing

[1]Dosages recommended are for patients with normal renal function. For nutritionally variant streptococci, see Table 3. I.V. indicates intravenous; I.M., intramuscular.

[2]Patients should be informed that I.M. injection of cefTRIAXone is painful.

[3]Dosing of gentamicin on a mg/kg basis will produce higher serum concentrations in obese patients than in lean patients. Therefore, in obese patients, dosing should be based on ideal body weight. (Ideal body weight for men is 50 kg + 2.3 kg per inch over 5 feet, and ideal body weight for women is 45.5 kg + 2.3 kg per inch over 5 feet.) Relative contraindications to the use of gentamicin are age >65 years, renal impairment, or impairment of the eighth nerve. Other potentially nephrotoxic agents (eg, nonsteroidal anti-inflammatory drugs) should be used cautiously in patients receiving gentamicin.

[4]Vancomycin dosage should be reduced in patients with impaired renal function. Vancomycin given on a mg/kg basis will produce higher serum concentrations in obese patients than in lean patients. Therefore, in obese patients, dosing should be based on ideal body weight. Each dose of vancomycin should be infused over at least 1 hour to reduce the risk of the histamine-release "red man" syndrome.

Table 2. Therapy for Native Valve Endocarditis Due to Strains of Viridans Streptococci and *Streptococcus bovis* Relatively Resistant to Penicillin G (Minimum Inhibitory Concentration >0.12 mcg/mL and ≤0.5 mcg/mL)[1]

Antibiotic	Dosage and Route	Duration (wk)	Comments
Aqueous crystalline penicillin G sodium	24 million units/24 h I.V. either continuously or in 4-6 equally divided doses	4	CeFAZolin or other first-generation cephalosporins may be substituted for penicillin in patients whose penicillin hypersensitivity is not of the immediate type.
With gentamicin sulfate[2]	3 mg/kg/24 h I.M./I.V. as single daily dose	2	
CefTRIAXone sodium	2 g once daily I.V. or I.M.[2]	4	
With gentamicin sulfate[2]	3 mg/kg/24 h I.M./I.V. as single daily dose	2	
Vancomycin hydrochloride[3]	30 mg/kg/24 h I.V. in 2 equally divided doses, not to exceed 2 g/24 h unless serum levels are monitored	4	Vancomycin therapy is recommended for patients allergic to β-lactams

[1]Dosages recommended are for patients with normal renal function. I.V. = intravenous, I.M. = intramuscular

[2]For specific dosing adjustment and issues concerning gentamicin (obese patients, relative contraindications), see Table 1 footnotes.

[3]For specific dosing adjustment and issues concerning vancomycin (obese patients, length of infusion), see Table 1 footnotes.

Table 3. Standard Therapy for Endocarditis Due to Enterococci[1]

Antibiotic	Dosage and Route	Duration (wk)	Comments
Aqueous crystalline penicillin G sodium	18-30 million units/24 h I.V. either continuously or in 6 equally divided doses	4-6	Native valve: 4-week therapy recommended for patients with symptoms ≤3 months in duration; 6-week therapy recommended for patients with symptoms >3 months in duration
With gentamicin sulfate[2]	1 mg/kg I.M. or I.V. every 8 h	4-6	
Ampicillin sodium	12 g/24 h I.V. in 6 equally divided doses	4-6	Prosthetic valve or other prosthetic material: 6-week minimum therapy recommended
With gentamicin sulfate[2]	1 mg/kg I.M. or I.V. every 8 hours	4-6	Target gentamicin peak concentration of 3-4 mcg/mL and trough of <1 mcg/mL
Vancomycin hydrochloride[2,3]	30 mg/kg/24 h I.V. in 2 equally divided doses, not to exceed 2 g/24 h unless serum levels are monitored	6	Vancomycin therapy is recommended for patients allergic to β-lactams; cephalosporins are not acceptable alternatives for patients allergic to penicillin
With gentamicin sulfate[2]	1 mg/kg I.M. or I.V. every 8 h	6	

[1]All enterococci causing endocarditis must be tested for antimicrobial susceptibility in order to select optimal therapy. This table is for endocarditis due to penicillin-, gentamicin-, and vancomycin-susceptible enterococci, viridans streptococci with a minimum inhibitory concentration of >0.5 mcg/mL, nutritionally variant viridans streptococci, or prosthetic valve endocarditis caused by viridans streptococci or *Streptococcus bovis*. If penicillin-resistant organisms, use vancomycin/gentamicin regimen above, or may use ampicillin/sulbactam (12 g/24 h in 4 divided doses) with gentamicin for 6 weeks. Antibiotic dosages are for patients with normal renal function. I.V. indicates intravenous; I.M., intramuscular.

[2]For specific dosing adjustment and issues concerning gentamicin (obese patients, relative contraindications), see Table 1 footnotes.

[3]For specific dosing adjustment and issues concerning vancomycin (obese patients, length of infusion), see Table 1 footnotes.

Table 4. Therapy for Native or Prosthetic Valve Endocarditis Due to Enterococci[1] Resistant to Vancomycin, Aminoglycosides, and Penicillin[2]

Antibiotic	Dosage and Route	Duration (wk)	Comments
E. faecium			
Linezolid	1200 mg/24 h P.O./I.V. in 2 divided doses	≥8	May cause severe, but reversible thrombocytopenia, particularly with extended therapy >2 weeks.
Quinupristin-dalfopristin	22.5 mg/kg/24 h I.V. in 3 divided doses	≥8	May cause severe myalgia; not effective against *E. faecalis*.
E. faecalis			
Imipenem/cilastatin	2 g/24 h I.V. in 4 divided doses	≥8	Limited patient experience with these regimens.
With ampicillin sodium	12 g/24 h in 6 divided doses	≥8	
or			
CefTRIAXone sodium	2 g/24 h I.V./I.M.[3] once daily	≥8	Limited patient experience with these regimens.
With ampicillin sodium	12 g/24 h in 6 divided doses	≥8	

[1]Endocarditis caused by the organisms should be treated in consultation with an infectious disease specialist; bacteriologic cure with antimicrobial therapy alone may be <50% and valve replacement may be required.

[2]Dosages recommended are for patients with normal renal function. I.V. = intravenous, I.M. = intramuscular

[3]Patients should be informed that I.M. injection of cefTRIAXone is painful.

Table 5. Therapy for Endocarditis Due to *Staphylococcus* in the Absence of Prosthetic Material[1]

Antibiotic	Dosage and Route	Duration	Comments
	Methicillin-Susceptible Staphylococci		
Regimens for non-β-lactam-allergic patients			
Nafcillin sodium or oxacillin sodium	12 g/24 h I.V. in 4-6 divided doses	6 wk	Uncomplicated right side endocarditis may be treated for 2 weeks.
With optional addition of gentamicin sulfate[2]	3 mg/kg/24 h I.M./I.V. in 2-3 divided doses	3-5 d	Benefit of additional aminoglycosides has not been established.
Regimens for β-lactam-allergic patients (nonanaphylactic)			
CeFAZolin (or other first-generation cephalosporins in equivalent dosages)	2 g I.V. every 8 h	6 wk	Cephalosporins should be avoided in patients with immediate-type hypersensitivity to penicillin; if penicillin-sensitive, vancomycin should be used.
With optional addition of gentamicin[2]	3 mg/kg/24 h I.M./I.V. in 2-3 divided doses	3-5 d	Benefit of additional aminoglycosides has not been established.
	Methicillin-Resistant Staphylococci		
Vancomycin hydrochloride[3]	30 mg/kg/24 h I.V. in 2 equally divided doses; not to exceed 2 g/24 h unless serum levels are monitored	4-6 wk	Vancomycin therapy is recommended for patients allergic to β-lactams; peak serum concentrations of vancomycin should be obtained 1 h after completion of the infusion and should be in the range of 30-45 mcg/mL and trough of 10-15 mcg/mL for twice-daily dosing.

[1]For treatment of endocarditis due to penicillin-susceptible staphylococci (minimum inhibitory concentration ≤0.1 mcg/mL and non-beta-lactamase producing), aqueous crystalline penicillin G sodium 24 million units/24 h can be used instead of nafcillin or oxacillin. Shorter antibiotic courses have been effective in some drug addicts with right-sided endocarditis due to *Staphylococcus aureus*. I.V. = intravenous, I.M. = intramuscular

[2]For specific dosing adjustment and issues concerning gentamicin (obese patients, relative contraindications), see Table 1 footnotes.

[3]For specific dosing adjustment and issues concerning vancomycin (obese patients, length of infusion), see Table 1 footnotes.

Table 6. Treatment of Staphylococcal Endocarditis in the Presence of a Prosthetic Valve or Other Prosthetic Material[1]

Antibiotic	Dosage and Route	Duration (wk)	Comments
	Methicillin-Susceptible Staphylococci		
Nafcillin sodium or oxacillin sodium[2]	12 g/24 h I.V. in 6 divided doses	≥6	First-generation cephalosporins or vancomycin should be used in patients allergic to β-lactam. Cephalosporins should be avoided in patients with immediate-type hypersensitivity to penicillin or with methicillin-resistant staphylococci.
With rifampin[3]	300 mg P.O./I.V. every 8 h	≥6	–
And with gentamicin sulfate[4,5]	3 mg/kg I.M./I.V. in 2-3 divided doses	2	Aminoglycoside should be administered in close proximity to vancomycin, nafcillin, or oxacillin.
	Methicillin-Resistant Staphylococci		
Vancomycin hydrochloride[6]	30 mg/kg/24 h I.V. in 2 equally divided doses, not to exceed 2 g/24 h unless serum levels are monitored	≥6	–
With rifampin[3]	300 mg P.O./I.V. every 8 h	≥6	Rifampin increases the amount of warfarin sodium required for antithrombotic therapy.
And with gentamicin sulfate[4,5]	3 mg/kg I.M./I.V. in 2-3 divided doses	2	Aminoglycoside should be administered in close proximity to vancomycin, nafcillin, or oxacillin.

[1]Dosages recommended are for patients with normal renal function. I.V. = intravenous, I.M. = intramuscular

[2]May use aqueous penicillin G 24 million units/24 h in 4-6 divided doses if strain is penicillin susceptible (MIC ≤0.1 mcg/mL and non-beta-lactamase producing).

[3]Rifampin plays a unique role in the eradication of staphylococcal infection involving prosthetic material; combination therapy is essential to prevent emergence of rifampin resistance.

[4]For a specific dosing adjustment and issues concerning gentamicin (obese patients, relative contraindications), see Table 1 footnotes.

[5]Use during initial 2 weeks.

[6]For specific dosing adjustment and issues concerning vancomycin (obese patients, relative contraindications), see Table 1 footnotes.

Table 7. Therapy for Native or Prosthetic Valve Endocarditis Due to HACEK Microorganisms (*Haemophilus parainfluenzae, Haemophilus aphrophilus, Actinobacillus actinomycetemcomitans, Cardiobacterium hominus, Eikenella corrodens,* and *Kingella kingae*)[1]

Antibiotic	Dosage and Route	Duration (wk)	Comments
CefTRIAXone sodium[2]	2 g once daily I.V. or I.M.[2]	4	Cefotaxime sodium or other third- or fourth-generation cephalosporins may be substituted.
Ampicillin/sulbactam[3]	12 g/24 h I.V. in 6 equally divided doses	4	
Ciprofloxacin	1000 mg/24 h orally or 800 mg/24 h I.V. in 2 divided doses	4	Use of fluoroquinolone recommended only if patient intolerant to ampicillin or cephalosporins; may substitute fluoroquinolone with equivalent coverage (eg, levofloxacin, moxifloxacin); if prosthetic material involved, treatment duration should be 6 weeks.

[1]Antibiotic dosages are for patients with normal renal function. I.V. = intravenous, I.M. = intramuscular

[2]Patients should be informed that I.M. injection of cefTRIAXone is painful.

[3]Ampicillin should not be used if laboratory tests show β-lactamase production.

REFERENCE

Baddour LM, Wilson WR, Bayer AS, et al. Infective endocarditis. Diagnosis, antimicrobial therapy, and management of complications. A statement for healthcare professionals from the Committee on Rheumatic Fever, Endocarditis, and Kawasaki Disease, Council on Cardiovascular Disease in the Young, and the Councils on Clinical Cardiology, Stroke, and Cardiovascular Surgery and Anesthesia, American Heart Association. *Circulation*. 2005;111(23):e394-e434.

PEDIATRIC ALS (PALS) ALGORITHMS

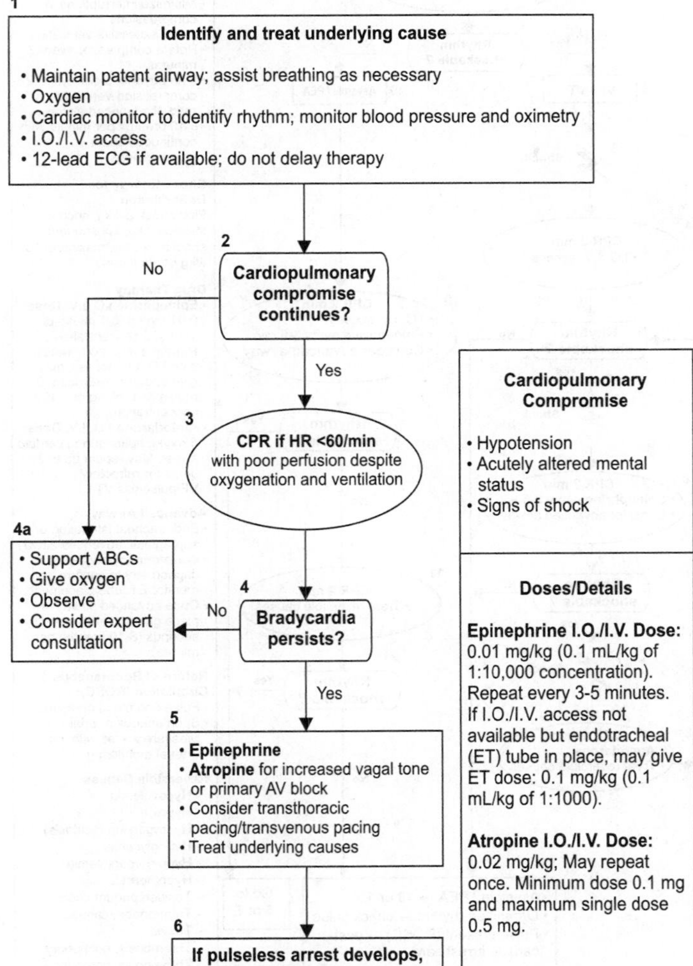

Pediatric Bradycardia
With a Pulse and Poor Perfusion
1
Identify and treat underlying cause
• Maintain patent airway; assist breathing as necessary
• Oxygen
• Cardiac monitor to identify rhythm; monitor blood pressure and oximetry
• I.O./I.V. access
• 12-lead ECG if available; do not delay therapy
2
Cardiopulmonary compromise continues?
No
Yes
3
CPR if HR <60/min with poor perfusion despite oxygenation and ventilation
4a
• Support ABCs
• Give oxygen
• Observe
• Consider expert consultation
4
Bradycardia persists?
No
Yes
5
• Epinephrine
• Atropine for increased vagal tone or primary AV block
• Consider transthoracic pacing/transvenous pacing
• Treat underlying causes
6
If pulseless arrest develops, go to Cardiac Arrest Algorithm
Cardiopulmonary Compromise
• Hypotension
• Acutely altered mental status
• Signs of shock
Doses/Details
Epinephrine I.O./I.V. Dose:
0.01 mg/kg (0.1 mL/kg of 1:10,000 concentration). Repeat every 3-5 minutes. If I.O./I.V. access not available but endotracheal (ET) tube in place, may give ET dose: 0.1 mg/kg (0.1 mL/kg of 1:1000).
Atropine I.O./I.V. Dose:
0.02 mg/kg; May repeat once. Minimum dose 0.1 mg and maximum single dose 0.5 mg.

Pediatric Cardiac Arrest

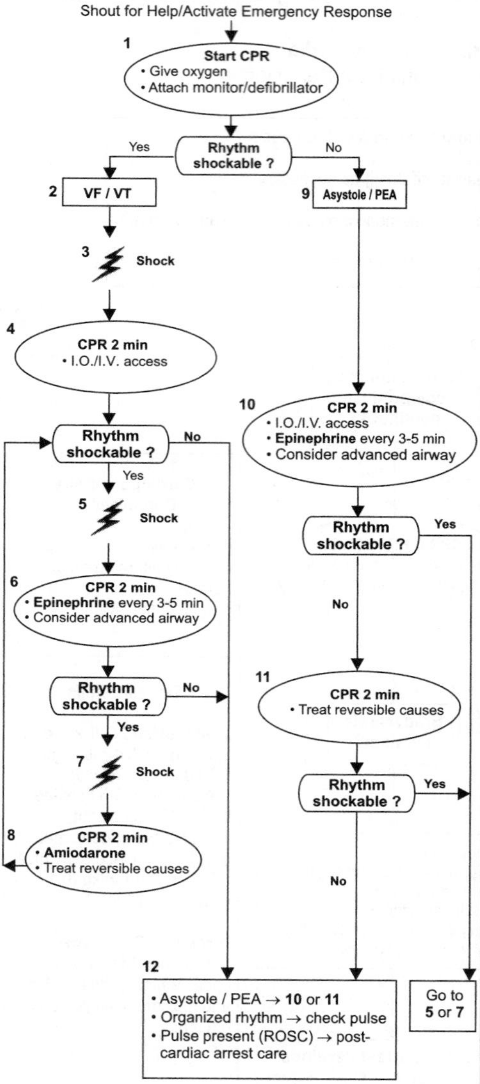

Shout for Help/Activate Emergency Response

1 **Start CPR**
- Give oxygen
- Attach monitor/defibrillator

Rhythm shockable ? — Yes → 2; No → 9

2 VF / VT

3 Shock

4 **CPR 2 min**
- I.O./I.V. access

Rhythm shockable ? — No → 12; Yes → 5

5 Shock

6 **CPR 2 min**
- **Epinephrine** every 3-5 min
- Consider advanced airway

Rhythm shockable ? — No → 12; Yes → 7

7 Shock

8 **CPR 2 min**
- **Amiodarone**
- Treat reversible causes

(→ back to Rhythm shockable ?)

9 Asystole / PEA

10 **CPR 2 min**
- I.O./I.V. access
- **Epinephrine** every 3-5 min
- Consider advanced airway

Rhythm shockable ? — Yes → Go to 5 or 7; No → 11

11 **CPR 2 min**
- Treat reversible causes

Rhythm shockable ? — Yes → Go to 5 or 7; No → 12

12
- Asystole / PEA → **10** or **11**
- Organized rhythm → check pulse
- Pulse present (ROSC) → post-cardiac arrest care

Go to **5** or **7**

Doses/Details

CPR Quality
- Push hard (≥1/3 of anterior-posterior diameter of chest) and fast (at least 100/min) and allow complete chest recoil
- Minimize interruptions in compressions
- Avoid excessive ventilation
- Rotate compressor every 2 minutes
- If no advanced airway, 15:2 compression-ventilation ratio. If advanced airway, 8-10 breaths per minute with continuous chest compressions

Shock Energy for Defibrillation
First shock 2 J/kg, second shock 4 J/kg, subsequent shocks ≥4 J/kg, maximum 10 J/kg or adult dose

Drug Therapy
- **Epinephrine I.O./I.V. Dose:** 0.01 mg/kg (0.1 mL/kg of 1:10,000 concentration). Repeat every 3-5 minutes. If no I.O./I.V. access, may give endotracheal dose: 0.1 mg/kg (0.1 mL/kg of 1:1000 concentration).
- **Amiodarone I.O./I.V. Dose:** 5 mg/kg bolus during cardiac arrest. May repeat up to 2 times for refractory VF/pulseless VT.

Advanced Airway
- Endotracheal intubation or supraglottic advanced airway
- Waveform capnography or capnometry to confirm and monitor ET tube placement
- Once advanced airway in place give 1 breath every 6-8 seconds (8-10 breaths per minute)

Return of Spontaneous Circulation (ROSC)
- Pulse and blood pressure
- Spontaneous arterial pressure waves with intra-arterial monitoring

Reversible Causes
- **H**ypovolemia
- **H**ypoxia
- **H**ydrogen ion (acidosis)
- **H**ypoglycemia
- **H**ypo-/hyperkalemia
- **H**ypothermia
- **T**ension pneumothorax
- **T**amponade, cardiac
- **T**oxins
- **T**hrombosis, pulmonary
- **T**hrombosis, coronary

Pediatric Tachycardia
With a Pulse and Poor Perfusion

1 Identify and Treat Underlying Cause
- Maintain patent airway; assist breathing as necessary
- Oxygen
- Cardiac monitor to identify rhythm; monitor blood pressure and oximetry
- I.O./I.V. access
- 12-lead ECG if available; do not delay therapy

2 Evaluate QRS duration

Narrow (≤0.09 sec) → 3; Wide (>0.09 sec) → 9

3 Evaluate rhythm with 12-lead ECG or monitor → 4 or 5

4 Probable Sinus Tachycardia
- Compatible history consistent with known cause
- P waves present/normal
- Variable R-R; constant PR
- Infants: Rate usually <220/min
- Children: Rate usually <180/min

5 Probable Supraventricular Tachycardia
- Compatible history (vague, nonspecific); history of abrupt rate changes
- P waves absent/abnormal
- HR not variable
- Infants: Rate usually ≥220/min
- Children: Rate usually ≥180/min

6 Search for and treat cause

7 Consider vagal maneuvers (no delays)

8
- If I.O./I.V. access present, give **adenosine**

OR

- If I.O./I.V. access not available or if adenosine ineffective, synchronized cardioversion

9 Possible ventricular tachycardia

10 Cardiopulmonary compromise?
- Hypotension
- Acutely altered mental status
- Signs of shock

Yes → 11; No → 12

11 Synchronized cardioversion

12 Consider adenosine if rhythm regular and QRS monomorphic

13 Expert consultation advised
- **Amiodarone**
- **Procainamide**

Doses/Details

Synchronized Cardioversion
Begin with 0.5-1 J/kg; if not effective, increase to 2 J/kg.
Sedate if needed, but do not delay cardioversion.

Adenosine I.O./I.V. Dose:
First dose: 0.1 mg/kg rapid bolus (maximum: 6 mg)
Second dose: 0.2 mg/kg rapid bolus (maximum second dose: 12 mg)

Amiodarone I.O./I.V. Dose:
5 mg/kg over 20-60 minutes

OR

Procainamide I.O./I.V. Dose:
15 mg/kg over 30-60 minutes

Do not routinely administer amiodarone and procainamide together.

MATERNAL CARDIAC ARREST

First Responder

- Activate maternal cardiac arrest team
- Document time of onset of maternal cardiac arrest
- Place the patient supine
- Start chest compressions as per BLS algorithm; place hands slightly higher on sternum than usual

Subsequent Responders

Maternal Interventions

Treat per BLS and ACLS Algorithms

- Do not delay defibrillation
- Give typical ACLS drugs and doses
- Ventilate with 100% oxygen
- Monitor waveform capnography and CPR quality
- Provide post-cardiac arrest care as appropriate

Maternal Modifications

- Start I.V. above the diaphragm
- Assess for hypovolemia and give fluid bolus when required
- Anticipate difficult airway; experienced provider preferred for advanced airway placement
- If patient receiving I.V./I.O. magnesium prearrest, stop magnesium and give I.V./I.O. calcium chloride 10 mL in 10% solution, or calcium gluconate 30 mL in 10% solution
- Continue all maternal resuscitative interventions (CPR, positioning, defribrillation, drugs, and fluids) during and after cesarean section

Obstetric Interventions for Patient With an Obviously Gravid Uterus*

- Perform manual left uterine displacement (LUD) - displace uterus to the patient's left to relieve aortocaval compression
- Remove both internal and external fetal monitors if present

Obstetric and neonatal teams should immediately prepare for possible emergency cesarean section

- If no ROSC by 4 minutes of resuscitative efforts, consider performing immediate emergency cesarean section
- Aim for delivery within 5 minutes of onset of resuscitative efforts

*An obviously gravid uterus is a uterus that is deemed clinically to be sufficiently large to cause aortocaval compression

Search for and Treat Possible Contributing Factors (BEAU-CHOPS)

Bleeding/DIC
Embolism: Coronary/pulmonary/amniotic fluid embolism
Anesthetic complications
Uterine atony
Cardiac disease (MI/ischemia/aortic dissection/cardiomyopathy)
Hypertension/pre-eclampsia/eclampsia
Other: Differential diagnosis of standard ACLS guidelines
Placenta abruptio/previa
Sepsis

ADULT ACLS ALGORITHMS

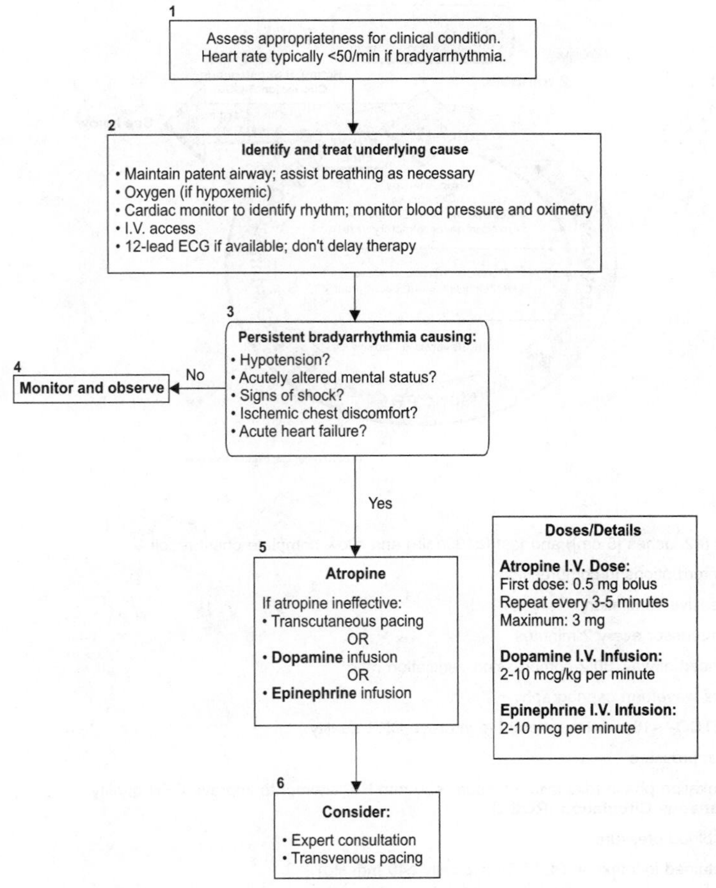

Adult Bradycardia
(With Pulse)
1
Assess appropriateness for clinical condition.
Heart rate typically <50/min if bradyarrhythmia.
2
Identify and treat underlying cause
• Maintain patent airway; assist breathing as necessary
• Oxygen (if hypoxemic)
• Cardiac monitor to identify rhythm; monitor blood pressure and oximetry
• I.V. access
• 12-lead ECG if available; don't delay therapy
3
Persistent bradyarrhythmia causing:
• Hypotension?
• Acutely altered mental status?
• Signs of shock?
• Ischemic chest discomfort?
• Acute heart failure?
No
4
Monitor and observe
Yes
5
Atropine
If atropine ineffective:
• Transcutaneous pacing
OR
• Dopamine infusion
OR
• Epinephrine infusion
Doses/Details
Atropine I.V. Dose:
First dose: 0.5 mg bolus
Repeat every 3-5 minutes
Maximum: 3 mg
Dopamine I.V. Infusion:
2-10 mcg/kg per minute
Epinephrine I.V. Infusion:
2-10 mcg per minute
6
Consider:
• Expert consultation
• Transvenous pacing

Adult Cardiac Arrest

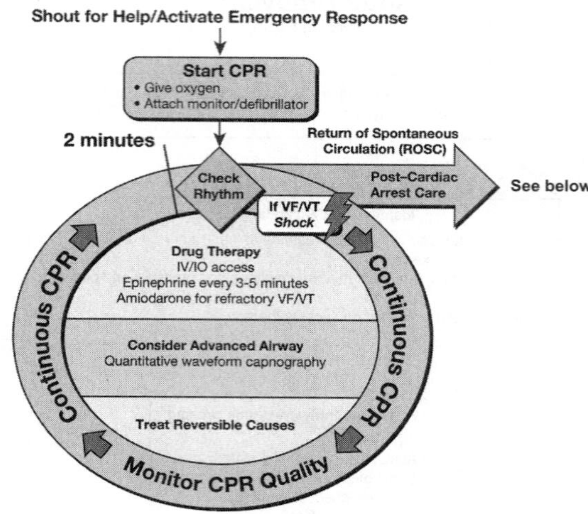

CPR Quality

- Push hard (≥2 inches [5 cm]) and fast (≥100/min) and allow complete chest recoil
- Minimize interruptions in compressions
- Avoid excessive ventilation
- Rotate compressor every 2 minutes
- If no advanced airway, 30:2 compression-ventilation ratio
- Quantitative waveform capnography
  - If $PETCO_2$ <10 mm Hg, attempt to improve CPR quality
- Intra-arterial pressure
  - If relaxation phase (diastolic) pressure <20 mm Hg, attempt to improve CPR quality

Return of Spontaneous Circulation (ROSC)

- Pulse and blood pressure
- Abrupt sustained increase in $PETCO_2$ (typically ≥40 mm Hg)
- Spontaneous arterial pressure waves with intra-arterial monitoring

Shock Energy

- **Biphasic:** Manufacturer recommendation (120-200 J); if unknown, use maximum available.

  Second and subsequent doses should be equivalent, and higher doses may be considered.
- **Monophasic:** 360 J

Drug Therapy

- Epinephrine I.V./I.O. Dose: 1 mg every 3-5 minutes
- Vasopressin I.V./I.O. Dose: 40 units can replace first or second dose of epinephrine
- Amiodarone I.V./I.O. Dose: First dose: 300 mg bolus; Second dose: 150 mg

Advanced Airway

- Supraglottic advanced airway or endotracheal intubation
- Waveform capnography to confirm and monitor ET tube placement
- 8-10 breaths per minute with continuous chest compressions

Reversible Causes

- **H**ypovolemia; **H**ypoxia; **H**ydrogen ion (acidosis); **H**ypo-/hyperkalemia; **H**ypothermia
- **T**ension pneumothorax; **T**amponade, cardiac; **T**oxins; **T**hrombosis, pulmonary; **T**hrombosis, coronary

Adult Tachycardia
(With Pulse)

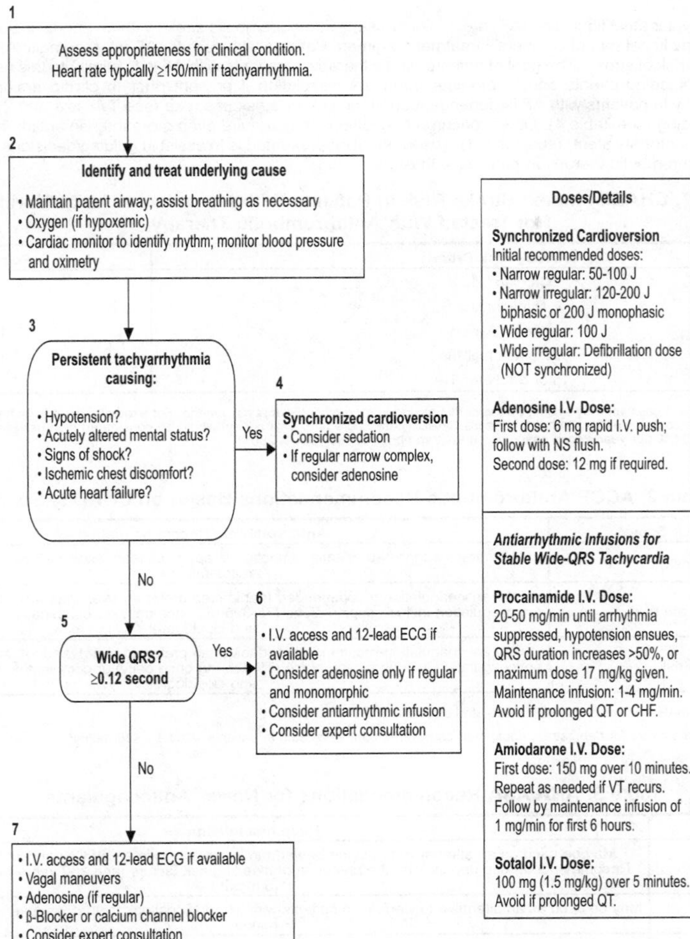
1
Assess appropriateness for clinical condition.
Heart rate typically ≥150/min if tachyarrhythmia.
2
Identify and treat underlying cause
• Maintain patent airway; assist breathing as necessary
• Oxygen (if hypoxemic)
• Cardiac monitor to identify rhythm; monitor blood pressure and oximetry
3
Persistent tachyarrhythmia causing:
• Hypotension?
• Acutely altered mental status?
• Signs of shock?
• Ischemic chest discomfort?
• Acute heart failure?
Yes
4
Synchronized cardioversion
• Consider sedation
• If regular narrow complex, consider adenosine
No
5
Wide QRS?
≥0.12 second
Yes
6
• I.V. access and 12-lead ECG if available
• Consider adenosine only if regular and monomorphic
• Consider antiarrhythmic infusion
• Consider expert consultation
No
7
• I.V. access and 12-lead ECG if available
• Vagal maneuvers
• Adenosine (if regular)
• ß-Blocker or calcium channel blocker
• Consider expert consultation
Doses/Details
Synchronized Cardioversion
Initial recommended doses:
• Narrow regular: 50-100 J
• Narrow irregular: 120-200 J biphasic or 200 J monophasic
• Wide regular: 100 J
• Wide irregular: Defibrillation dose (NOT synchronized)
Adenosine I.V. Dose:
First dose: 6 mg rapid I.V. push; follow with NS flush.
Second dose: 12 mg if required.
Antiarrhythmic Infusions for Stable Wide-QRS Tachycardia
Procainamide I.V. Dose:
20-50 mg/min until arrhythmia suppressed, hypotension ensues, QRS duration increases >50%, or maximum dose 17 mg/kg given.
Maintenance infusion: 1-4 mg/min.
Avoid if prolonged QT or CHF.
Amiodarone I.V. Dose:
First dose: 150 mg over 10 minutes.
Repeat as needed if VT recurs.
Follow by maintenance infusion of 1 mg/min for first 6 hours.
Sotalol I.V. Dose:
100 mg (1.5 mg/kg) over 5 minutes.
Avoid if prolonged QT.

ANTITHROMBOTIC THERAPY IN PATIENTS WITH ATRIAL FIBRILLATION

Patients with nonvalvular atrial fibrillation (AF) are at higher risk of thromboembolic stroke with an annual incidence of ~5% when antithrombotic therapy is not part of a patient's treatment regimen. Patients with valvular AF (ie, rheumatic AF, particularly mitral stenosis) are at high risk of stroke. The goal of antithrombotic therapy in patients with AF is to eliminate this risk of stroke without increasing serious bleeding events and to promote thrombus dissolution if present prior to cardioversion. The intensity of antithrombotic therapy in patients with AF is dependent upon the patient's risk of stroke (see Tables 1 and 2) balanced with the patient's risk of bleeding (see Table 4). Other concurrent conditions may require even more intense antithrombotic therapy (eg, placement of an intracoronary stent) (see Table 4). The information presented is to assist in guiding decisions regarding initiation and intensity of antithrombotic therapy in patients with AF.

Table 1. $CHADS_2$ Index: Stroke Risk in Patients With Nonvalvular Atrial Fibrillation Not Treated With Antithrombotic Therapy

$CHADS_2$ Risk Criteria	Point(s)
Cardiac failure	1
Hypertension	1
Age >75 years	1
Diabetes mellitus	1
Prior **S**troke or TIA	**2**

The $CHADS_2$ Risk Score is calculated by adding up the points assigned for each individual risk criteria. For example, if a patient has heart failure, is >75 years of age, and has diabetes mellitus, then the patient's $CHADS_2$ risk score is 3. This patient would be considered high-risk (see Table 2) with an adjusted stroke rate of 5.9% per year, which assumes no antithrombotic usage (Gage, 2001).

Table 2. ACCP Antithrombotic Recommendations Based on $CHADS_2$ Score

$CHADS_2$ Risk Score	Antithrombotic Recommendation
0 (low risk)	No therapy suggested; if antithrombotic therapy is chosen, aspirin 75-325 mg once daily is recommended
1 (intermediate risk)	Oral anticoagulation recommended (dabigatran preferred over warfarin); alternatives to oral anticoagulation include aspirin alone (75-325 mg once daily) or combination therapy with aspirin and clopidogrel
≥2 (high risk)	Oral anticoagulation recommended (dabigatran preferred over warfarin); alternatives to oral anticoagulation include aspirin alone (75-325 mg once daily) or combination therapy with aspirin and clopidogrel

$CHADS_2$ = Cardiac failure-Hypertension-Age-Diabetes-Stroke (doubled)

Note: No specific antidote exists for dabigatran; dabigatran considered contraindicated in patients with Cl_{Cr} <30 mL/min

Table 3. AHA/ASA Recommendations for Newer Anticoagulants

Drug	Recommendation
Apixaban	May be used as an alternative to aspirin or warfarin in patients with ≥1 additional risk factor for stroke. Recommended dose depends on the presence of bleeding risk factors (age ≥80 years, weight ≤60 kg, S_{Cr} ≥1.5 mg/dL)
Dabigatran	May be used as an alterntive to warfarin in patients with ≥1 additional risk factor for stroke whose Cl_{Cr} >30 mL/minute
Rivaroxaban	May be used as an alternative to warfarin in patients with moderate-to-high risk for stroke (prior history of TIA, stroke, or systemic embolism or ≥2 additional risk factors)

Table 4. Bleeding Risk Scores in Patients With Atrial Fibrillation

Bleeding Score	Low Risk	Moderate Risk	High Risk	Calculation
Outpatient Bleeding Risk Index (Beyth, 1998; Landefeld, 1989)	0	1-2	≥3	**1 point for each:** ≥65 years of age, GI bleed in past 2 weeks, previous stroke, comorbidities (recent MI, Hct <30%, DM, or S_{Cr} >1.5 mg/dL)
$HEMORR_2HAGES$ (Gage, 2006)	0-1	2-3	≥4	**1 point for each: H**epatic or renal disease, **E**thanol abuse, **M**alignancy, **O**lder age (>75 years), **R**educed platelet count or function, **H**ypertension (uncontrolled), **A**nemia, **G**enetic factors (CYP2C9 polymorphisms), **E**xcessive fall risk, **S**troke **2 points for:** Rebleeding risk (eg, prior bleed)
(Shireman, 2006)	≤1.07	>1.07 to <2.19	≥2.19	(0.49 x age >70) + (0.32 x female) + (0.58 x remote bleed) + (0.62 x recent bleed) + (0.71 x alcohol/drug abuse) + (0.27 x diabetes) + (0.86 x anemia) + (0.32 x antiplatelet drug use), **with 1 point for presence of each and 0 if absent**

Table 4. Bleeding Risk Scores in Patients With Atrial Fibrillation *(continued)*

Bleeding Score	Low Risk	Moderate Risk	High Risk	Calculation
HAS-BLED (Lip, 2011; Pisters, 2010)	0	1-2	≥3	**H**ypertension (ie, uncontrolled BP) **A**bnormal renal/liver function (1 point each) **S**troke **B**leeding history or predisposition **L**abile INR **E**lderly (eg, age >65 y) **D**rugs (eg, concomitant antiplatelet/NSAID) or alcohol (1 point each) **Maximum: 9 points**
ATRIA	0-3	4	5-10	**Anemia:** 3 points **Severe renal disease:** 3 points **Age ≥75 years:** 2 points **Any prior hemorrhage:** 1 point **Diagnosed hypertension:** 1 point

Note: These scores have not been extensively validated; ability to predict major bleeding events is modest. When patients have a $CHADS_2$ score of 0-1, patients who are at high risk of bleeding may be considered for no oral anticoagulation (You, 2012).

Table 5. Antithrombotic Recommendations for Patients With Atrial Fibrillation and Other Concurrent Conditions

Concurrent Condition	Antithrombotic Recommendation
Mitral stenosis	Adjusted dose warfarin therapy (target INR range: 2-3); alternatives include aspirin 75-325 mg once daily or combination therapy (preferred) with aspirin and clopidogrel
Stable coronary disease (no ACS within previous year)	Adjusted dose warfarin therapy (target INR range: 2-3) alone
ACS patients who do not undergo intracoronary stent placement	**$CHADS_2$ score 0:** 1st 12 months: Dual antiplatelet therapy (eg, aspirin and clopidogrel); after 1st 12 months, adjusted dose warfarin therapy (target INR range: 2-3) alone **$CHADS_2$ score ≥1:** Adjusted dose warfarin therapy (target INR range: 2-3) **plus** single antiplatelet therapy (eg, aspirin or clopidogrel); after 1st 12 months, adjusted dose warfarin therapy (target INR range: 2-3) alone
Placement of bare metal intracoronary stent	**$CHADS_2$ score ≥2:** During 1st month after placement: Triple therapy (eg, warfarin, aspirin, clopidogrel), followed by warfarin **plus** a single antiplatelet agent (eg, aspirin, clopidogrel); after 12 months of stent placement, adjusted dose warfarin (target INR range: 2-3)
Placement of drug eluting intracoronary stent	**$CHADS_2$ score ≥2:** During 1st 3-6 months after placement: Triple therapy (eg, warfarin, aspirin, clopidogrel), followed by warfarin **plus** a single antiplatelet agent (eg, aspirin, clopidogrel); after 12 months of stent placement, adjusted dose warfarin (target INR range: 2-3)
Placement of either bare metal or drug eluting intracoronary stent	**$CHADS_2$ score 0 or 1:** During 1st 12 months after placement: Dual antiplatelet therapy (eg, aspirin, clopidogrel), followed by adjusted dose warfarin

$CHADS_2$ = Cardiac failure-Hypertension-Age-Diabetes-Stroke (doubled)

Note: No specific antidote exists for dabigatran; dabigatran considered contraindicated in patients with Cl_{Cr} <30 mL/min

REFERENCES

Apostolakis S, Lane DA, Guo Y, et al. Performance of the HEMORR(2)HAGES, ATRIA, and HAS-BLED bleeding risk-prediction scores in patients with atrial fibrillation undergoing anticoagulation: the AMADEUS (Evaluating the Use of SR34006 Compared to Warfarin or Acenocoumarol in Patients With Atrial Fibrillation) study. *J Am Coll Cardiol*. 2012;60(9):861-867.

Beyth RJ, Quinn LM, Landefeld CS. Prospective evaluation of an index for predicting the risk of major bleeding in outpatients treated with warfarin. *Am J Med*. 1998;105(2):91-99.

Fang MC, Go AS, Chang Y, et al. A new risk scheme to predict warfarin-associated hemorrhage: the ATRIA (Anticoagulation and Risk Factors in Atrial Fibrillation) study. *J Am Coll Cardiol*. 2011;58(4):395-401.

Gage BF, Waterman AD, Shannon W, et al. Validation of clinical classification schemes for predicting stroke: results from the National Registry of Atrial Fibrillation. *JAMA*. 2001;285(22):2864-2870.

Gage BF, Yan Y, Milligan PE, et al. Clinical classification schemes for predicting hemorrhage: results from the National Registry of Atrial Fibrillation (NRAF). *Am Heart J*. 2006;151(3):713-719.

Guyatt GH, Akl EA, Crowther M, et al. Introduction to the ninth edition: antithrombotic therapy and prevention of thrombosis, 9th ed: American College of Chest Physicians evidence-based clinical practice guidelines. *Chest*. 2012;141(2 Suppl):48S-52S.

Landefeld CS, Goldman L. Major bleeding in outpatients treated with warfarin: incidence and prediction by factors known at the start of outpatient therapy. *Am J Med*. 1989;87(2):144-152.

Lip GY, Frison L, Halperin JL, et al. Comparative validation of a novel risk score for predicting bleeding risk in anticoagulated patients with atrial fibrillation: the HAS-BLED (Hypertension, Abnormal Renal/Liver Function, Stroke, Bleeding History or Predisposition, Labile INR, Elderly, Drugs/Alcohol Concomitantly) score. *J Am Coll Cardiol*. 2011;57(2):173-180.

Pisters R, Lane DA, Nieuwlaat R, et al. A novel user-friendly score (HAS-BLED) to assess 1-year risk of major bleeding in patients with atrial fibrillation: the Euro Heart Survey. *Chest*. 2010;138(5):1093-1100.

Shireman TI, Mahnken JD, Howard PA, et al. Development of a contemporary bleeding risk model for elderly warfarin recipients. *Chest*. 2006;130(5):1390-1396.

van Walraven C, Hart RG, Wells GA, et al. A clinical prediction rule to identify patients with atrial fibrillation and a low risk for stroke while taking aspirin. *Arch Intern Med*. 2003;163(8):936-943.

You JJ, Singer DE, Howard PA, et al. Antithrombotic therapy for atrial fibrillation: antithrombotic therapy and prevention of thrombosis, 9th ed: American College of Chest Physicians evidence-based clinical practice guidelines. *Chest*. 2012;141(2 Suppl):e531S-e575S.

BEERS CRITERIA – POTENTIALLY INAPPROPRIATE MEDICATIONS FOR GERIATRICS

Criteria for Medications That Should Be Avoided or Used With Caution in Older Adults: Independent of Diagnoses or Conditions

Applicable Medications	Summary of Prescribing Concerns	Recommendation	Quality of Evidence	Strength of Recommendation
$Alpha_1$-blockers: Doxazosin, prazosin, terazosin	High risk of orthostatic hypotension; alternative agents preferred due to a more favorable risk:benefit profile	Avoid use as an antihypertensive	Moderate	Strong
$Alpha_2$-agonists: CloNIDine, guanabenz, guanFACINE, methyldopa Central monoamine-depleting agent: Reserpine (>0.1 mg/day)	High risk of CNS adverse effects; may also cause orthostatic hypotension and bradycardia; not recommended for routine use as an antihypertensive	Avoid clonidine as a first-line antihypertensive. Avoid others as listed.	Low	Strong
Antiarrhythmic drugs (Class Ia, Ic, III): Amiodarone, dofetilide, dronedarone, flecainide, ibutilide, procainamide, propafenone, quinidine, sotalol	In older adults, data suggest rate control may provide more benefits than risks compared to rhythm control for most patients. Amiodarone is associated with numerous toxicities (eg, thyroid disease, QT prolongation, pulmonary disorders).	Avoid antiarrhythmic drugs as first-line treatment of atrial fibrillation	High	Strong
Antihistamines, first generation (alone or in combination products): Brompheniramine, carbinoxamine, chlorpheniramine, clemastine, cyproheptadine, dexchlorpheniramine, diphenhydrAMINE (oral), doxylamine, hydrOXYzine, promethazine, triprolidine	First generation antihistamines have potent anticholinergic properties; older adults are at increased risk for anticholinergic effects and toxicity. Diphenhydramine use may be appropriate in certain situations such as the acute treatment of severe allergic reactions.	Avoid	High (hydroxyzine, promethazine) Moderate (all others)	Strong
Antiparkinson agents: Benztropine (oral), trihexyphenidyl	Alternative, more-efficacious agents preferred for treatment of Parkinson's disease. Not recommended for prevention of extrapyramidal symptoms associated with antipsychotics.	Avoid	Moderate	Strong
Antipsychotics, first generation **and** second generation: ARIPiprazole, asenapine, chlorproMAZINE, cloZAPine, fluPHENAZine, haloperidol, iloperidone, loxapine, lurasidone, olanzapine, paliperidone, perphenazine, pimozide, QUEtiapine, risperiDONE, thioridazine, thiothixene, trifluoperazine, ziprasidone	Increased risk of stroke and mortality in patients with dementia. In addition, use may cause or exacerbate syndrome of inappropriate antidiuretic hormone secretion or hyponatremia; monitor sodium closely with initiation or dosage adjustments in older adults.	Avoid use for behavioral problems of dementia unless nonpharmacological options have failed and patient is threat to self or others; SIADH risk: Use with caution	Moderate	Strong
Antispasmodic drugs: Belladonna alkaloids, clidinium and chlordiazepoxide, dicyclomine, hyoscyamine, propantheline, scopolamine	Potent anticholinergic properties and uncertain efficacy	Avoid except in short-term palliative care to decrease oral secretions	Moderate	Strong
Barbiturates: Amobarbital, butabarbital, butalbital, mephobarbital, PENTobarbital, PHENobarbital, secobarbital	Risk of overdose with low dosages, tolerance to sleep effects, and increased risk of physical dependence	Avoid	High	Strong
Benzodiazepines, long-acting: Amitriptyline and chlordiazepoxide, chlorazepate, chlordiazePOXIDE, clidinium and chlordiazepoxide, clonazePAM, diazepam, flurazepam, quazepam	In older adults, benzodiazepines increase the risk of impaired cognition, delirium, falls, fractures, and motor vehicle accidents. Increased sensitivity to benzodiazepines in this age group and slower metabolism of long-acting agents.	Avoid benzodiazepines (any type) for treatment of insomnia, agitation, or delirium	High	Strong
Benzodiazepines, short-acting: ALPRAZolam, estazolam, LORazepam, oxazepam, temazepam, triazolam	In older adults, benzodiazepines increase the risk of impaired cognition, delirium, falls, fractures, and motor vehicle accidents. Increased sensitivity in this age group to benzodiazepines.	Avoid benzodiazepines (any type) for treatment of insomnia, agitation, or delirium	High	Strong

Criteria for Medications That Should Be Avoided or Used With Caution in Older Adults: Independent of Diagnoses or Conditions *continued*

Applicable Medications	Summary of Prescribing Concerns	Recommendation	Quality of Evidence	Strength of Recommendation
CarBAMazepine	Use may cause or exacerbate syndrome of inappropriate antidiuretic hormone secretion or hyponatremia; monitor sodium closely with initiation or dosage adjustments in older adults.	Use with caution	Moderate	Strong
CARBOplatin	Use may cause or exacerbate syndrome of inappropriate antidiuretic hormone secretion or hyponatremia; monitor sodium closely with initiation or dosage adjustments in older adults.	Use with caution	Moderate	Strong
Chloral hydrate	Potential risks exceed benefits; doses only 3 times the recommended dose are associated with overdosage potential; in addition, tolerance develops within 10 days of use.	Avoid	Low	Strong
ChlorproPAMIDE	Prolonged half-life in elderly patients which could cause prolonged hypoglycemia. Additionally, causes SIADH.	Avoid	High	Strong
CISplatin	Use may cause or exacerbate syndrome of inappropriate antidiuretic hormone secretion or hyponatremia; monitor sodium closely with initiation or dosage adjustments in older adults.	Use with caution	Moderate	Strong
Dabigatran	Greater risk of bleeding in older adults aged ≥75 years (exceeds warfarin bleeding risk); lack of safety and efficacy in patients with Cl_{cr} <30 mL/minute	Use with caution in adults aged ≥75 years of if Cl_{cr} <30mL/minute	Moderate	Weak
Desiccated thyroid	Concerns about cardiac effects; safer alternatives available	Avoid	Low	Strong
Digoxin >0.125 mg/day	Decreased renal clearance may lead to increased risk of toxic effects. Higher doses are associated with no additional benefit in heart failure patients, and may increase the risk of toxicity.	Avoid	Moderate	Strong
Dipyridamole, oral (short-acting)	May cause orthostatic hypotension; more-efficacious alternative agents available	Avoid	Moderate	Strong
Disopyramide	Potent negative inotrope and therefore may induce heart failure in elderly patients. It is also strongly anticholinergic. Other antiarrhythmic drugs should be used.	Avoid	Low	Strong
Dronedarone	In patient with permanent atrial fibrillation or heart failure, worse outcomes have been reported with use. In general, rate control is preferred over rhythm control for atrial fibrillation.	Avoid in patients with permanent atrial fibrillation or heart failure	Moderate	Strong
Ergot mesylates	Have not been shown to be effective	Avoid	High	Strong
Estrogens (with or without progestins)	Evidence of the carcinogenic (breast and endometrial cancer) potential of these agents and lack of cardioprotective effect in older women Evidence for vaginal estrogens for treatment of vaginal dryness to be safe and effective in women with breast cancer, particularly at estradiol doses <25 mcg twice weekly	Avoid oral and topical patch. Topical vaginal cream: Acceptable to use low-dose intravaginal estrogen for the management of dyspareunia, lower urinary tract infections, and other vaginal symptoms	High (oral and patch formulations) Moderate (topical formulations)	Strong (oral and patch formulations) Weak (topical formulations)
Glyburide	Increased risk of severe, prolonged hypoglycemia in older adults	Avoid	High	Strong

Criteria for Medications That Should Be Avoided or Used With Caution in Older Adults: Independent of Diagnoses or Conditions *continued*

Applicable Medications	Summary of Prescribing Concerns	Recommendation	Quality of Evidence	Strength of Recommendation
Indomethacin	Of all available NSAIDs, this drug produces the most adverse effects. Non-COX-selective oral NSAID use associated with an increased risk of GI bleeding and peptic ulcer disease in older adults in high-risk category (eg, >75 years or age or receiving concomitant oral/parenteral corticosteroids, anticoagulants, or antiplatelet agents). Proton pump inhibitors or misoprostol use reduces risk, but does not eliminate it. Longer duration of NSAID use correlates with a trend towards increasing incidence GI ulcers, bleeding, or perforation.	Avoid	Moderate	Strong
Insulin, sliding scale	Regardless of care setting, an increased risk of hypoglycemia without improvement in management of hyperglycemia	Avoid	Moderate	Strong
Isoxsuprine	Lack of efficacy	Avoid	High	Strong
Ketorolac (includes parenteral)	Associated with an increased risk of GI bleeding and peptic ulcer disease in older adults in high-risk category (eg, >75 years or age or receiving concomitant oral/parenteral corticosteroids, anticoagulants, or antiplatelet agents). Proton pump inhibitors or misoprostol use reduces risk, but does not eliminate it. Longer duration of NSAID use correlates with a trend towards increasing incidence GI ulcers, bleeding, or perforation.	Avoid	High	Strong
Megestrol	Increased risk of thrombotic events and possibly death; effect on weight is minimal	Avoid	Moderate	Strong
Meperidine	Not an effective oral analgesic in doses commonly used. Safer alternative agents preferred due to potential for neurotoxicity.	Avoid	High	Strong
Meprobamate	Highly sedating anxiolytic with a high rate of physical dependence	Avoid	Moderate	Strong
MethylTESTOSTERone	Potential for cardiac problems; contraindicated in men with prostate cancer	Avoid unless indicated for moderate-to-severe hypogonadism	Moderate	Weak
Metoclopramide	May cause extrapyramidal effects (including tardive dyskinesia), particularly in frail older adults	Avoid, unless for gastroparesis	Moderate	Strong
Mineral oil	Potential for aspiration and adverse effects; safer alternatives available	Avoid	Moderate	Strong
Mirtazapine	Use may cause or exacerbate syndrome of inappropriate antidiuretic hormone secretion or hyponatremia; monitor sodium closely with initiation or dosage adjustments in older adults.	Use with caution	Moderate	Strong
NIFEdipine, short-acting	Potential for hypotension; risk of precipitating myocardial ischemia	Avoid	High	Strong
Nitrofurantoin	Potential for pulmonary toxicity; safer alternatives available; renal impairment (Cl_{cr} <60 mL/minute) results in inadequate drug concentration in urine and lack of efficacy	Avoid for long-term suppression; avoid in patients with Cl_{cr} <60 mL/minute	Moderate	Strong
Nonbenzodiazepine hypnotics: Eszopiclone, zolpidem, zaleplon	Similar adverse events (eg, delirium, falls, fractures) in older adults to events seen with benzodiazepine use; minimal improvement seen with sleep latency and duration	Avoid chronic use (>90 days)	Moderate	Strong

Criteria for Medications That Should Be Avoided or Used With Caution in Older Adults: Independent of Diagnoses or Conditions *continued*

Applicable Medications	Summary of Prescribing Concerns	Recommendation	Quality of Evidence	Strength of Recommendation
Non-COX-selective NSAIDS (oral): Aspirin (>325 mg/day), diclofenac, diflunisal, etodolac, fenoprofen, ibuprofen, ketoprofen, meclofenamate, mefenamic acid, meloxicam, nabumetone, naproxen, oxaprozin, piroxicam, sulindac, tolmetin	Use associated with an increased risk of GI bleeding and peptic ulcer disease in older adults in high risk category (eg, >75 years or age or receiving concomitant oral/parenteral corticosteroids, anticoagulants, or antiplatelet agents). Proton pump inhibitors or misoprostol use reduce risk, but do not eliminate it. Longer duration of NSAID use correlates with a trend towards increasing incidence GI ulcers, bleeding, or perforation.	Avoid chronic use unless other alternatives are not effective and patient can take gastroprotective agent (proton pump inhibitor or misoprostol)	Moderate	Strong
Pentazocine	Opioid analgesic that causes more CNS adverse effects, including confusion and hallucinations, more commonly than other opioid drugs. Additionally, it is a mixed agonist and antagonist; safer alternative agents are available.	Avoid	Low	Strong
Prasugrel	Risk of bleeding is increased in older adults; risk may be offset by benefit in older adults at highest risk (eg, prior MI or diabetes)	Use with caution in adults aged ≥75 years	Moderate	Weak
Serotonin-norepinephrine reuptake inhibitors and selective serotonin reuptake inhibitors	Use may cause or exacerbate syndrome of inappropriate antidiuretic hormone secretion or hyponatremia; monitor sodium closely with initiation or dosage adjustments in older adults.	Use with caution	Moderate	Strong
Skeletal muscle relaxants: Carisoprodol, chlorzoxazone, cyclobenzaprine, metaxalone, methocarbamol, orphenadrine	Most muscle relaxants are poorly tolerated by elderly patients, since these cause anticholinergic adverse effects, sedation, and risk of fracture. Additionally, efficacy is questionable at dosages tolerated by elderly patients.	Avoid	Moderate	Strong
Somatropin (growth hormone)	Body composition effects are minimal and use associated with edema, arthralgia, carpal tunnel syndrome, gynecomastia, and impaired fasting glucose.	Avoid, except as hormone replacement after pituitary gland removal	High	Strong
Spironolactone (>25 mg/day)	Risk of hyperkalemia is increased for heart failure patients receiving >25 mg/day, particularly if taking concomitant medications such as NSAIDS, ACE inhibitors, angiotensin receptor blockers, or potassium supplements.	Avoid in patients with heart failure or with a Cl_{cr} <30 mL/minute	Moderate	Strong
Testosterone	Potential for cardiac problems; contraindicated in men with prostate cancer	Avoid unless indicated for moderate-to-severe hypogonadism	Moderate	Weak
Thioridazine	Potent anticholinergic properties; risk of QT-interval prolongation	Avoid	Moderate	Strong
Ticlopidine	Safer, more effective alternatives exist.	Avoid	Moderate	Strong
Tricyclic antidepressants	Use may cause or exacerbate syndrome of inappropriate antidiuretic hormone secretion or hyponatremia; monitor sodium closely with initiation or dosage adjustments in older adults.	Use with caution	High	Strong
Tricyclic antidepressants, tertiary (alone or in combination): Amitriptyline, amitriptyline and chlordiazepoxide, clomiPRAMINE, doxepin >6 mg/day, imipramine, perphenazine and amitriptyline, trimipramine	Potent anticholinergic properties, sedating, and potential for orthostatic hypotension; doxepin at doses ≤6 mg/day has safety profile comparable to placebo	Avoid	High	Strong
Trimethobenzamide	One of the least effective antiemetic drugs and may cause extrapyramidal adverse effects	Avoid	Moderate	Strong
VinCRIStine	Use may cause or exacerbate syndrome of inappropriate antidiuretic hormone secretion or hyponatremia; monitor sodium closely with initiation or dosage adjustments in older adults.	Use with caution	Moderate	Strong

Drugs with Potent Anticholinergic Properties

Class of Drug	Individual Agents
Antihistamines	Brompheniramine, carbinoxamine, chlorpheniramine, clemastine, cyproheptadine, dimenhydrinate, diphenhydrAMINE, hydrOXYzine, loratadine, meclizine
Antidepressants	Amitriptyline, amoxapine, clomiPRAMINE, desipramine, doxepin, imipramine, nortriptyline, PARoxetine, protriptyline, trimipramine
Antimuscarinics (urinary incontinence)	Darifenacin, fesoterodine, flavoxATE, oxybutynin, solifenacin, tolterodine, trospium
Antiparkinson agents	Benztropine, trihexyphenidyl
Antipsychotics	ChlorproMAZINE, cloZAPine, fluPHENAZine, loxapine, OLANZapine, perphenazine, pimozide, prochlorperazine, promethazine, thioridazine, thiothixene, trifluoperazine
Antispasmodics	Atropine products, belladonna alkaloids, dicyclomine, homatropine, hyoscyamine products, propantheline, scopolamine
Skeletal muscle relaxants	Carisoprodol, cyclobenzaprine, orphenadrine, tiZANidine

REFERENCE

American Geriatrics Society 2012 Beers Criteria Update Expert Panel. American Geriatrics Society updated beers criteria for potentially inappropriate medication use in older adults. *J Am Geriatr Soc*. 2012;60(4):616-631.

CONTRAST MEDIA REACTIONS, PREMEDICATION FOR PROPHYLAXIS

It is estimated that approximately 5% to 10% of patients will experience adverse reactions to the administration of contrast dye (less for nonionic contrast). In approximately 1000-2000 administrations, a life-threatening reaction will occur.

A variety of premedication regimens have been proposed, both for pretreatment of "at risk" patients who require contrast media and before the routine administration of the intravenous high-osmolality contrast media (HOCM). Such regimens have been shown in clinical trials to decrease the frequency of all forms of contrast medium reactions. Logistical and feasibility problems may preclude adequate premedication with this or any regimen for all patients. It is unclear at this time that steroid pretreatment prior to administration of ionic contrast media reduces the incidence of reactions to the same extent or less than that achieved with the use of nonionic contrast media alone. Information about the efficacy of nonionic contrast media combined with a premedication strategy, including steroids, is preliminary or not yet currently available. For high-risk patients (ie, previous contrast reactors), the combination of a pretreatment regimen with nonionic contrast media has empirical merit and may warrant consideration. Oral administration of steroids appears preferable to intravascular routes, and the drug may be prednisone or methylprednisolone. Supplemental administration of H_1 and H_2 antihistamine therapies, orally or intravenously, may reduce the frequency of urticaria, angioedema, and respiratory symptoms. Additionally, ephedrine administration has been suggested to decrease the frequency of contrast reactions, but caution is advised in patients with cardiac disease, hypertension, or hyperthyroidism. No premedication strategy should be a substitute for the ABC approach to preadministration preparedness listed above. Contrast reactions occur despite any and all premedication prophylaxis. The incidence can be decreased, however, in some categories of "at risk" patients receiving HOCM plus a medication regimen. For patients with previous contrast medium reactions, there is a slight chance that recurrence may be more severe or the same as the prior reaction; however, it is more likely that there will be no recurrence.

PREMEDICATION REGIMENS INCLUDE:

MethylPREDNISolone	32 mg orally 12 and 2 hours prior to the procedure
DiphenhydrAMINE	50 mg orally 1 hour prior to the procedure

OR

PredniSONE	50 mg orally 13, 7, and 1 hour before the procedure
DiphenhydrAMINE	50 mg orally 1 hour before the procedure

OR

PredniSONE	60 mg orally the night before and the morning of the procedure
DiphenhydrAMINE	50 mg orally 1 hour before the procedure

SUGGESTED REGIMEN FOR EMERGENT PROCEDURE (EG, PRIMARY PCI)

Hydrocortisone or MethylPREDNISolone or Dexamethasone	100 mg I.V. (hydrocortisone) **or** 80-125 mg I.V. (methylPREDNISolone) **or** 16 mg I.V. (dexamethasone) before the procedure
Cimetidine	300 mg I.V. before the procedure
DiphenhydrAMINE	25-50 mg I.V. or P.O. before the procedure

INDICATIONS FOR NONIONIC CONTRAST

- Previous reaction to contrast – premedicate. **Note:** For life-threatening reactions (throat swelling, laryngeal edema, etc), consider omitting the I.V. contrast
- Known allergy to iodine or shellfish
- Asthma, especially if on medication
- Myocardial instability or HF
- Risk for aspiration or severe nausea and vomiting
- Difficulty communicating or inability to give history
- Patients taking beta-blockers
- Small children at risk for electrolyte imbalance or extravasation
- Renal failure with diabetes, sickle cell disease, or myeloma
- At physician or patient request

CONTRAST-INDUCED NEPHROTOXICITY (CIN)

CIN is a common complication after exposure to I.V. radiocontrast agents. In the literature, CIN is defined as a rise in serum creatinine concentration of at least 0.5 mg/dL or an increase of 25% compared to baseline occurring after exposure to contrast medium. Most of the time, this increase in serum creatinine is transient; however, in some cases, the impairment may be permanent with some patients requiring dialysis. Many agents have been evaluated for prevention of this adverse event; however, only acetylcysteine, sodium bicarbonate, and sodium chloride have shown benefit. Of note, the Acetylcysteine for Contrast-induced Nephropathy Trial (ACT) demonstrated no benefit with acetylcysteine compared to placebo in patients undergoing coronary and vascular angiography. Use of acetylcysteine is no longer recommended in the prevention of CIN for patients undergoing percutaneous coronary intervention (PCI).

Risk Factors for CIN:

- Pre-existing renal impairment
- Diabetes nephropathy
- Age >70 years
- Hypovolemia
- Anemia
- Heart failure
- Hypotension
- Concomitant nephrotoxins (eg, aminoglycosides)
- Large contrast medium doses (eg, ≥140 mL)
- Type of contrast agent used (high-osmolality contrast media > low-osmolality contrast media)

STRATEGIES FOR THE PREVENTION OF CIN

General recommendations	1. Stratify all patients for risk of CIN prior to contrast exposure 2. Optimize volume status 3. Administer prehydration and prophylaxis using therapies with proven clinical benefit to all high-risk patients 4. Minimize contrast media volumes, especially in those with Cl_{Cr} <60 mL/minute; use of low- or iso-osmolality contrast agents has been suggested 5. Hold medications that adversely affect renal function before and after contrast exposure 6. Obtain follow-up serum creatinine between 24-72 hours after contrast exposure
Specific therapies:	
Acetylcysteine, P.O.[1]	600 mg orally twice daily on the day before and the day of the scan in addition to hydration with 0.45% saline intravenously
Sodium bicarbonate, I.V. (154 mEq/L)	3 mL/kg/hour for 1 hour prior to contrast injection, then 1 mL/kg/hour during contrast exposure and for 6 hours after procedure
Sodium chloride 0.9%, I.V.	1-1.5 mL/kg/hour for 3-12 hours prior to and for 6-24 hours after procedure

[1]The Acetylcysteine for Contrast-induced Nephropathy Trial (ACT) demonstrated no benefit in patients undergoing coronary and vascular angiography. Use is no longer recommended in the prevention of CIN for patients undergoing percutaneous coronary intervention (PCI).

REFERENCES

ACT Investigators. Acetylcysteine for prevention of renal outcomes in patients undergoing coronary and peripheral vascular angiography: main results from the randomized Acetylcysteine for Contrast-induced nephropathy Trial (ACT). *Circulation*. 2011;124(11):1250-1259.

American College of Radiology. Manual on contrast media, version 7.0. 2010. Available at http://gm.acr.org/SecondaryMainMenuCategories/quality_safety/contrast_manual.aspx

Klein LW, Sheldon MW, Brinker J, et al. The use of radiographic contrast media during PCI: a focused review: a position statement of the Society of Cardiovascular Angiography and Interventions. *Catheter Cardiovasc Interv*. 2009;74(5):728-746.

Levine GN, Bates ER, Blankenship JC, et al. 2011 ACCF/AHA/SCAI guideline for percutaneous coronary intervention: a report of the American College of Cardiology Foundation/American Heart Association Task Force on Practice Guidelines and the Society for Cardiovascular Angiography and Interventions. *J Am Coll Cardiol*. 2011;58(24):e44-e122.

Massicotte A. Contrast medium-induced nephropathy: strategies for prevention. *Pharmacotherapy*. 2008;28(9):1140-1150.

Merten GJ, Burgess WP, Gray LV, et al. Prevention of contrast-induced nephropathy with sodium bicarbonate: a randomized controlled trial. *JAMA*. 2004;291(19):2328-2334.

STATUS EPILEPTICUS

CONVULSIVE STATUS EPILEPTICUS

Treatment Guidelines

Convulsive status epilepticus is an emergency that is associated with high morbidity and mortality. Status epilepticus has been defined as a seizure that persists for a sufficient length of time or is repeated frequently enough that recovery between attacks does not occur (Meierkord, 2010). Seizures lasting >5 minutes are less likely to remit; therefore, if a seizure continues for >5 minutes, antiepileptic therapy is mandatory. The outcome largely depends on etiology, but prompt and appropriate pharmacological therapy can reduce morbidity and mortality. Etiology varies in children and adults and reflects the distribution of disease in these age groups. Immediate concerns include supporting respiration, maintaining blood pressure, gaining intravenous access, and identifying and treating the underlying cause. Initial therapeutic and diagnostic measures are conducted simultaneously. The goal of therapy is rapid termination of clinical and electrical seizure activity; the longer a seizure continues, the greater the likelihood of an adverse outcome. Several drug protocols now in use will terminate status epilepticus. Common to all patients is the need for a clear plan, prompt administration of appropriate drugs in adequate doses, and attention to the possibility of apnea, hypoventilation, or other metabolic abnormalities.

Management of Status Epilepticus

Time Since Seizure Onset	Drug Treatment		Evaluations/Actions
	Adults	Children	
Prolonged Seizure: Premonitory Stage (Out-of-Hospital)			
5 min	Diazepam 10 mg rectally; may repeat once if necessary	Diazepam 0.5 mg/kg rectally; may repeat once if necessary	• Airway/breathing • Monitor vital signs • Establish I.V. access • Blood glucose determination
If seizure continues ↓ **Early Status Epilepticus: First Stage (Out-of-Hospital or Inpatient)**[1]			
5-30 min	LORazepam 4 mg I.V. bolus (≤2 mg/min) **or** Diazepam 5-10 mg I.V. (≤5 mg/min; maximum dose: 30 mg) May repeat dose after 5-10 minutes	LORazepam 0.05-0.1 mg/kg I.V. (≤2 mg/min; maximum dose: 4 mg) **or** Diazepam 0.1-0.3 mg/kg I.V. (≤5 mg/min; maximum dose: 10 mg) May repeat dose after 5-10 minutes	• ABGs, oxygen/ventilation • CBC, electrolytes, renal/hepatic status • Cardiac monitoring, ECG • Neurologic assessment toxicology screen • Consider I.V. dextrose ± thiamine • AED concentrations
If seizure continues ↓ **Established Status Epilepticus: Second Stage**			
30-60 min	Fosphenytoin 15-20 mg PE/kg I.V. (maximum rate: 150 mg PE/min) **or** Phenytoin 15-20 mg/kg I.V. (maximum rate: 50 mg/min)	Fosphenytoin 15-20 mg PE/kg I.V. (maximum rate: 150 mg PE/min) **or** Phenytoin 20 mg/kg I.V. (maximum rate: 50 mg/min) **or** PHENobarbital 15-20 mg/kg I.V. (maximum rate: <100 mg/min[2])	• Intubation/mechanical ventilation • Cardiorespiratory function • Vasopressors if needed • Neurologic: CT, CSF, EEG • If no central venous access, fosphenytoin is preferred over phenytoin
If seizure continues ↓ **Refractory Status Epilepticus: Third Stage**			
>60 min	PHENobarbital 10-20 mg/kg I.V. (maximum rate: 100 mg/min[2]) **or** PENTobarbital 10-15 mg/kg I.V. over 1 hour[2], then initial infusion of 0.5-1 mg/kg/h (range: 0.5-10 mg/kg/h **or** Midazolam 0.2 mg/kg, followed by a continuous infusion of 0.05-0.6 mg/kg/h **or** Propofol[3] 1-2 mg/kg I.V. bolus (optional), then continuous infusion of 2-10 mg/kg/h **or** Valproic acid 15-45 mg/kg I.V. loading dose (maximum rate: 6 mg/kg/min) **or** LevETIRAcetam[4] 1-3 g I.V. over 15 min	PHENobarbital 15-20 mg/kg I.V. (maximum rate: <100 mg/min[2]) **or** PENTobarbital 5-15 mg/kg I.V. over 1 hour[2], then 0.5-5 mg/kg/h **or** Midazolam 0.15-0.5 mg/kg bolus (may repeat), then continuous infusion of 0.06-2 mg/kg/h	• ICU admission • Anesthesia monitoring/ hemodynamics • Therapeutic AED monitoring

AED = antiepileptic drug

[1]LORazepam is associated with a higher likelihood of seizure termination in the treatment of status epilepticus and, therefore, may be preferred (Alldredge, 2001).
[2]May induce hypotension; consider alternative agents in hemodynamically unstable patients. Monitor closely and reduce rate if hypotension develops. Fluids and/or vasopressors may be necessary to control significant hypotension.
[3]Doses >83 mcg/kg/minute (or >5 mg/kg/**hour**) may increase the risk of hypotension and propofol-related infusion syndrome (PRIS), especially if used for >48 hours; consider alternative therapies to avoid the risk of PRIS in longer-term propofol infusions.
[4]LevETIRAcetam 2500 mg has been safely administered over 5 minutes, as reported in one report (Uges, 2009). **Note:** Levetiracetam has not been well-studied in comparison to other agents routinely used in this setting.

REFERENCES

Abend NS, Dlugos DJ. Treatment of refractory status epilepticus: literature review and a proposed protocol. *Pediatr Neurol*. 2008;38(6):377-390.

Alldredge BK, Gelb AM, Isaacs SM, et al. A comparison of lorazepam, diazepam, and placebo for the treatment of out-of-hospital status epilepticus. *N Engl J Med*. 2001;345(9):631-637.

Claassen J, Hirsch LJ, Emerson RG, et al. Treatment of refractory status epilepticus with pentobarbital, propofol, or midazolam: a systematic review. *Epilepsia*. 2002;43(2):146-153.

Gaitanis JN, Drislane FW. Status epilepticus: a review of different syndromes, their current evaluation, and treatment. *Neurologist*. 2003;9(2):61-76.

Hanhan UA, Fiallos MR, Orlowski JP. Status epilepticus. *Pediatr Clin North Am*. 2001;48(3):683-694.

Hegenbarth MA. Preparing for pediatric emergencies: drugs to consider. *Pediatrics*. 2008;121(2):433-443.

Kälviäinen R, Eriksson K, Parviainen I. Refractory generalised convulsive status epilepticus: a guide to treatment. *CNS Drugs*. 2005;19(9):759-768.

Kälviäinen R. Status epilepticus treatment guidelines. *Epilepsia*. 2007;48(Suppl 8):99-102.

Limdi NA, Shimpi AV, Faught E, et al. Efficacy of rapid I.V. administration of valproic acid for status epilepticus. *Neurology*. 2005;64(2):353-355.

Lowenstein DH. Treatment options for status epilepticus. *Curr Opin Pharmacol*. 2005;5(3):334-339.

Meierkord H, Boon P, Engelsen B, et al. EFNS guideline on the management of status epilepticus. *Eur J Neurol*. 2010;17(3):348-355.

Misra UK, Kalita J, Patel R. Sodium valproate vs phenytoin in status epilepticus: a pilot study. *Neurology*. 2006;67(2):340-342.

Morrison G, Gibbons E, Whitehouse WP. High-dose midazolam therapy for refractory status epilepticus in children. *Intensive Care Med*. 2006;32(12):2070-2076.

Rivera R, Segnini M, Baltodano A, et al. Midazolam in the treatment of status epilepticus in children. *Crit Care Med*. 1993;21(7):991-994.

Rossetti AO, Reichhart MD, Schaller MD, et al. Propofol treatment of refractory status epilepticus: a study of 31 episodes. *Epilepsia*. 2004;45(7):757-763.

Sinha S, Naritoku DK. Intravenous valproate is well tolerated in unstable patients with status epilepticus. *Neurology*. 2000;55(5):722-724.

Uges JW, van Huizen MD, Engelsman J, et al. Safety and pharmacokinetics of intravenous levetiracetam infusion as add-on in status epilepticus. *Epilepsia*. 2009;50(3):415-421.

TREATMENT OF ELEVATED INR DUE TO WARFARIN

Management of Elevated INR in Patients Taking Warfarin

INR above therapeutic range to <4.5 No evidence of bleeding and rapid reversal unnecessary	**INR 4.5 to 10** No evidence of bleeding	**INR >10** No evidence of bleeding	**Minor bleeding at any INR elevation**	**Major bleeding at any INR elevation**
Lower or hold next dose and monitor frequently; when INR approaches desired range, resume dosing with a lower dose.	The 2012 ACCP guidelines recommend against routine vitamin K administration in this setting. Previously, the 2008 ACCP guidelines recommended if no risk factors for bleeding exist, to omit next 1 or 2 doses, monitor INR more frequently, and resume with an appropriately adjusted dose when INR in desired range; may consider administering vitamin K orally 1-2.5 mg if other risk factors for bleeding exist. Others have recommended consideration of vitamin K 1 mg orally or 0.5 mg I.V.	The 2012 ACCP guidelines recommend administration of oral vitamin K (dose not specified) in this setting. Previously, the 2008 ACCP guidelines recommended to hold warfarin, administer vitamin K orally 2.5-5 mg, expect INR to be reduced within 24-48 hours, monitor INR more frequently, and give additional vitamin K at an appropriate dose if necessary; resume warfarin at an appropriately adjusted dose when INR is in desired range. Others have recommended consideration of vitamin K 2-2.5 mg orally or 0.5-1 mg I.V.	Hold warfarin, may administer vitamin K orally 2.5-5 mg, monitor INR more frequently, may repeat dose after 24 hours if INR correction incomplete; resume warfarin at an appropriately adjusted dose when INR is in desired range.	The 2012 ACCP guidelines recommend administration of vitamin K 5-10 mg by slow I.V. infusion (may repeat in 12 hours if necessary) and four-factor prothrombin complex concentrate (PCC). The only available four-factor PCC in the U.S. is Kcentra. Other **four-factor** PCCs **not** available in the U.S. include Beriplex P/N, Cofact, and Octaplex. Bebulin VH and Profilnine SD **do not** contain adequate levels of factor VII and are considered **three-factor** PCCs.

INR = international normalized ratio

Note: Use of high doses of vitamin K (eg, 10-15 mg) may cause warfarin resistance for ≥1 week. During this period of resistance, heparin or low molecular weight heparin may be given until INR responds.

WARFARIN THERAPY

Patients should **not** receive loading doses of warfarin >10 mg as the steady-state INR is not achieved more quickly. In general, most patients should receive doses between 5-10 mg for the first 1-2 days with the addition of heparin or low molecular weight heparin when a more rapid anticoagulant effect is required. Initial warfarin doses of 5 mg usually results in an INR>2 in 4-5 days. Initial doses of 10 mg usually results in a therapeutic INR in 3-4 days; however, 10 mg doses may be associated with more excessive anticoagulation. Patients who are debilitated, malnourished, have heart failure, have had recent surgery, or are taking medications known to increase the effects of warfarin should begin treatment with a dose ≤5 mg. The intensity of anticoagulation therapy should be monitored closely until the patient has reached a stable PT/INR. Once the patient is stabilized on a fixed dose of warfarin, the PT/INR can be monitored on a monthly basis if the patient demonstrates a stable PT/INR on chronic therapy. If dosage adjustments are made, PT/INR should be evaluated in approximately 2 weeks.

Supratherapeutic INR values are managed based on the presence and severity of bleeding (see chart above). Determinants of bleeding due to warfarin therapy include intensity of treatment, patient characteristics, concomitant use of drugs that interfere with hemostasis, and the length therapy. The target INR should be established with consideration of these factors. Patients on warfarin should be warned to seek medical evaluation if they develop a very severe headache, abdominal pain, unusual bleeding, backache, or if they experience significant trauma, particularly head injuries. Please refer to the Warfarin monograph for complete drug information.

REFERENCES

Ansell J, Hirsh J, Hylek E, et al. Pharmacology and management of the vitamin K antagonists: American College of Chest Physicians evidence-based clinical practice guidelines (8th edition). *Chest.* 2008;133(6 Suppl):160S-198S.

Holbrook A, Schulman S, Witt DM, et al. Evidence-based management of anticoagulant therapy: antithrombotic therapy and prevention of thrombosis, 9th ed: American College of Chest Physicians evidence-based clinical practice guidelines. *Chest.* 2012;141(2 Suppl):e152-e184.

Patriquin C, Crowther M. Treatment of warfarin-associated coagulopathy with vitamin K. *Expert Rev Hematol.* 2011;4(6):657-665.

DOSING CONSIDERATIONS FOR THE CRITICALLY-ILL PATIENT WITH MORBID OBESITY

Most recent estimates from the World Health Organization (WHO) report that approximately 32% of the U.S. population is considered obese, defined as a body mass index (BMI) of ≥30 kg/m^2. Patients with morbid obesity (Obese class III), defined by the WHO as a BMI ≥40 kg/m^2, are challenging to care for especially when critically ill. Although obese class II (BMI 35 to <40 kg/m^2) are commonly encountered, patients with morbid obesity require dosage adjustment to achieve similar therapeutic results. Patients at the extremes of body weight are seldom included within clinical trials, forcing the clinician to use knowledge of pharmacokinetic principles (eg, volume of distribution) to properly dose the morbidly obese patient. Many drugs (eg, vasopressors, inotropes, neuromuscular blockers) used in the ICU are adjusted based on immediate measurable patient responses; however, many drugs (eg, antibiotics, LMWHs) do not have this advantage and inadequate dosing may lead to treatment failure. In the critical situation, the need to give the right dose to achieve an optimal clinical response is paramount.

Table 1. The International Classification of Adult Overweight and Obesity According to BMI

Classification	BMI (kg/m^2)
Normal range	18.5-24.99
Overweight	≥25
Pre-obese	25-29.99
Obese	≥30
Obese class I	30-34.99
Obese class II	35-39.99
Obese class III	≥40

BMI = Body mass index; defined as weight in kilograms divided by height in meters squared

IMPORTANT PHARMACOKINETIC CONSIDERATIONS

Several pharmacokinetic parameters are altered in the morbidly obese patient due to increases in cardiac output, blood volume, organ mass, lean body mass, and adipose tissue mass. Three pharmacokinetic parameters affected by obesity are distribution, metabolism, and excretion.

DISTRIBUTION

Distribution is altered due to a higher ratio of body fat to lean tissue and body water. This becomes important for drugs with lipophilic properties (eg, fentanyl, diazepam). Generally, as the octanol/water *log* partition coefficient (LPC) of the drug increases, distribution into adipose tissue increases. Exceptions to this include cyclosporine, digoxin, procainamide, and remifentanil. These agents may be highly lipophilic and have a high volume of distribution (V_d) but they are not significantly influenced by obesity. Therefore, it is not always possible to devise straightforward dosing schemes using volume of distribution alone. Clinical trials in obese and normal weight patients are necessary to determine whether or not the expected distribution for a particular drug actually occurs in the obese patient.

METABOLISM

Data on the relationship between obesity (especially morbid obesity) and alterations in drug metabolism/transport are inconclusive; however, evidence supports alterations in cytochrome P450 enzyme activity in the obese patient. CYP2E1 activity is increased and CYP3A4 and CYP1A activity may be decreased or unchanged. The effect of obesity on other CYP450 enzymes remains unclear. In general, increased glucuronidation and sulfation activity may occur with some drugs (eg, lorazepam) requiring more frequent administration of maintenance doses. Determinants of drug disposition may be altered in obesity, but the specific direction and magnitude of any such change is, at present, unclear. Increased monitoring seems prudent.

EXCRETION

Glomerular filtration rate (GFR) may be higher in patients who are obese compared to normal weight patients. It has been demonstrated that obese (BMI ≥30 kg/m^2) kidney donors have a significantly higher glomerular planar surface area compared to those kidneys of nonobese donors. Drugs dependant on GFR for excretion (eg, aminoglycosides) have been shown to have higher clearance rates in the obese patient. Therefore, maintenance dosing may be more frequent for agents which rely on glomerular filtration for excretion.

Although the Cockcroft-Gault formula used to estimate creatinine clearance (Cl_{Cr}) is the predominant equation used in clinical practice, choice of weight will often underestimate (eg, IBW) or overestimate (eg, TBW) Cl_{Cr}. The most precise formula estimation of Cl_{Cr} in the obese patient is the Salazar-Corcoran formula; however, this formula has not been validated in a large sample of obese subjects. The Modification of Diet in Renal Disease (MDRD) formula, although it does not incorporate weight, also has not been validated in a large sample of obese subjects. Of note, the result obtained with the MDRD equation may not correlate with Cl_{Cr} cutoffs for dosage adjustment for many drugs since evaluation of renal function for these agents used the

Cockcroft-Gault formula to develop dosing regimens in patients with renal impairment. Use of a timed 24-hour urine collection may be a more accurate method to determine Cl_{Cr}. Recently, the three equations used to determine glomerular filtration (GFR)/Cl_{Cr} were compared to results obtained using a timed 24-hour urine collection in morbidly obese patients. Use of the MDRD and IBW in the Cockcroft-Gault equation both underestimated Cl_{Cr}. The Salazar-Corcoran equation and the use of TBW or adjusted body weight (AdjBW) in the Cockcroft-Gault equation overestimated Cl_{Cr}. The authors concluded that the use of a lean body weight (LBW) estimate (see Table 2) based on TBW and BMI incorporated into the Cockcroft-Gault equation provides a relatively precise and accurate estimate of 24-hour measured Cl_{Cr} in morbidly obese patients.

DOSING MODIFICATIONS IN THE OBESE PATIENT

The importance of achieving similar concentrations in the critically ill obese patient as compared to the normal weight patient is imperative. However, dosing agents is not straightforward and requires pharmacokinetic evaluations in this patient population to define the optimal dose or dosing weight that should be used to determine an optimal dose for a particular agent. Many evaluations of this kind have been done but more clinical trials still need to be done. A summary of recommendations from various sources has been devised to assist the clinician in determining the most appropriate dosing weight or dosing strategy for this patient population (see Table 3). Equations for different body weight calculations are noted below.

Table 2. Body Weight Calculations

Ideal Body Weight (IBW)[1]	Male: 50 + (2.3 x height in inches over 5 feet) Female: 45.5 + (2.3 x height in inches over 5 feet)
Lean Body Weight (LBW)[1,2]	Male: (9270 x TBW)/(6680 + 216 x BMI) Female: (9270 x TBW)/(8780 + 244 x BMI)
Adjusted Body Weight (AdjBW) or Dosing Weight (DW)[1,3]	AdjBW or DW = IBW + 0.4 (TBW − IBW)

BMI = body mass index in kg/m^2, TBW = total body weight

[1]IBW, LBW, AdjBW, and DW are in kilograms

[2]Janmahasatian S, Duffull SB, Ash S, et al. Quantification of lean bodyweight. *Clin Pharmacokinet.* 2005;44(10):1051-1065.

[3]The difference between TBW and IBW is multiplied by a factor between 0.2-0.5. The factor most often used is 0.4; however, this may be modified for certain drugs (eg, ciprofloxacin).

Table 3. Selected Agents and Recommended Dosing Strategies in the Obese Patient

Drug	Recommendation for Dosing in Obese Patients	
	Loading Dose	Maintenance Dose[1]
Analgesics		
FentaNYL	Use TBW	Use: 0.8 x IBW; titrate to pain control
Morphine	Use IBW	Use IBW; titrate to pain control
Remifentanil	Use IBW	Use IBW; titrate to pain control
SUFentanil	Use TBW	Use: 0.8 x IBW; titrate to pain control
Antiarrhythmics		
Amiodarone	Use IBW or standard dose	IBW or standard dose
Lidocaine	Use TBW	IBW, standard infusion rate
Procainamide	Use IBW	Use IBW, standard infusion rate
Antibiotics		
Acyclovir	NA	IBW
Aminoglycosides[2]	Use IBW + 0.4 (TBW − IBW)	Use IBW + 0.4 (TBW − IBW)
CeFAZolin	Surgical prophylaxis: 2 g prior to induction	Not established
Ciprofloxacin	NA	Use IBW + 0.45 (TBW − IBW) or 800 mg q12h
DAPTOmycin	NA	Use TBW; concentrations expected to be higher; monitor closely for skeletal muscle toxicity
Fluconazole	NA	Prudent to use higher doses; none established[3]
Flucytosine	NA	Use IBW
Linezolid	NA	Use standard dosing
Meropenem	NA	Use standard dosing[4]
Quinupristin/ Dalfopristin	NA	Use TBW
Vancomycin	Use TBW	Use TBW; may require more frequent dosing

Table 3. Selected Agents and Recommended Dosing Strategies in the Obese Patient *(continued)*

Drug	Recommendation for Dosing in Obese Patients	
	Loading Dose	**Maintenance Dose[1]**
Anticoagulants		
Argatroban	NA	Use TBW (BMI <51 kg/m^2)
Enoxaparin (and other LMWHs)	Use TBW	Use TBW; monitor anti-Xa levels (if available) in patients >190 kg
Heparin	Not established	Not established; titrate to aPTT results
Antiepileptics		
Phenytoin	Use: DW = IBW + 1.33 x (TBW − IBW) or may give 14 mg/kg (IBW) + 19 mg/kg for weight in excess of IBW (maximum dose: 2 g)	Use IBW; monitor levels
Beta-Blockers		
Esmolol	Use IBW	Individualize
Labetalol	Use IBW or standard dose	Individualize
Metoprolol	Use IBW or standard dose	Individualize
Calcium Channel Blockers		
Diltiazem	Use TBW or standard dose	Individualize
Verapamil	Use TBW or standard dose	Individualize
Neuromuscular Blocking Agents[5]		
Atracurium	Use IBW	Use IBW
Rocuronium	Use IBW	Use IBW
Succinylcholine	Use TBW	NA
Vecuronium	Use IBW	Use IBW
Sedative/Hypnotic		
Etomidate	Use TBW	NA
Ketamine	Use IBW	Use IBW
Propofol	Use DW = IBW + 0.4 (TBW − IBW)	Use DW = IBW + 0.4 (TBW − IBW)
Thiopental	Use TBW	Use IBW
Other Agents		
Adenosine	Use IBW; standard dose	NA
Rasburicase	NA	Use IBW

BMI = body mass index, DW = dosing weight, IBW = ideal body weight, NA = not applicable, TBW = total body weight

[1]If therapeutic drug monitoring is available, it is recommended that this be done in all patients who are morbidly obese.

[2]Use once daily dosing regimens with caution in the morbidly obese patient as adequate studies have not been conducted in this patient population.

[3]It has been recommended that fluconazole be dosed using 6 mg/kg/day using TBW.

[4]May require higher doses for multidrug-resistant organisms

[5]Monitor clinical effects, peripheral nerve stimulation

REFERENCES

Arnold TM, Reuter JP, Delman BS, et al. Use of single-dose rasburicase in an obese female. *Ann Pharmacother.* 2004;38(9):1428-1431.

Bearden DT, Rodvold KA. Dosage adjustments for antibacterials in obese patients: applying clinical pharmacokinetics. *Clin Pharmacokinet.* 2000;38 (5):415-426.

Blouin RA, Bauer LA, Miller DD, et al. Vancomycin pharmacokinetics in normal and morbidly obese subjects. *Antimicrob Agents Chemother.* 1982;21 (4):575-580.

Blouin RA, Ensom MHH. Special pharmacokinetic considerations in the obese. *Applied Pharmacokinetics* & *Pharmacodynamics.* 4th ed. Burton ME, Shaw LE, Schentag JJ, et al, eds. Baltimore, MD: Lippincott Williams & Wilkins; 2006;231-241.

Brunette DD. Resuscitation of the morbidly obese patient. *Am J Emerg Med.* 2004;22(1):40-47.

Cheymol G. Effects of obesity on pharmacokinetics implications for drug therapy. *Clin Pharmacokinet.* 2000;39(3):215-231.

Demirovic JA, Pai AB, Pai MP. Estimation of creatinine clearance in morbidly obese patients. *Am J Health Syst Pharm.* 2009;66(7):642-648.

Dvorchik BH, Damphousse D. The pharmacokinetics of daptomycin in moderately obese, morbidly obese, and matched nonobese subjects. *J Clin Pharmacol.* 2005;45(1):48-56.

Erstad BL. Dosing of medications in morbidly obese patients in the intensive care unit setting. *Intensive Care Med.* 2004;30(1):18-32.

Galletti F, Fasano ML, Ferrara LA, et al. Obesity and beta-blockers: influence of body fat on their kinetics and cardiovascular effects. *J Clin Pharmacol.* 1989;29(3):212-216.

Hernandez JO, Norstrom J, Wysock G. Acyclovir-induced renal failure in an obese patient. *Am J Health Syst Pharm.* 2009;66(14):1288-1291.

Kotlyar M, Carson SW. Effects of obesity on the cytochrome P450 enzyme system. *Int J Clin Pharmacol Ther.* 1999;37(1):8-19.

Leykin Y, Pellis T, Lucca M, et al. The pharmacodynamic effects of rocuronium when dosed according to real body weight or ideal body weight in morbidly obese patients. *Anesth Analg.* 2004;99(4):1086-1089.

Meyhoff CS, Lund J, Jenstrup MT, et al. Should dosing of rocuronium in obese patients be based on ideal or corrected body weight? *Anesth Analg.* 2009;109(3):787-792.

Nutescu EA, Spinler SA, Wittkowsky A, et al. Low-molecular-weight heparins in renal impairment and obesity: available evidence and clinical practice recommendations across medical and surgical settings. *Ann Pharmacother.* 2009;43(6):1064-1083.

Pai MP, Bearden DT. Antimicrobial dosing considerations in obese adult patients. *Pharmacotherapy.* 2007;27(8):1081-1091.

Penzak SR, Gubbins PO, Rodvold KA, et al. Therapeutic drug monitoring of vancomycin in a morbidly obese patient. *Ther Drug Monit.* 1998;20(3):261-265.

Rea DJ, Heimbach JK, Grande JP, et al. Glomerular volume and renal histology in obese and nonobese living kidney donors. *Kidney Int.* 2006;70(9):1636-1641.

Rex JH, Bennett JE, Sugar AM, et al. A randomized trial comparing fluconazole with amphotericin B for the treatment of candidemia in patients without neutropenia. Candidemia Study Group and the National Institute. *N Engl J Med.* 1994;331(20):1325-1330.

Rice L, Hursting MJ, Baillie GM, et al. Argatroban anticoagulation in obese versus nonobese patients: implications for treating heparin-induced thrombocytopenia. *J Clin Pharmacol.* 2007;47(8):1028-1034.

Roberts JA, Lipman J. Pharmacokinetic issues for antibiotics in the critically ill patient. *Crit Care Med.* 2009;37(3):840-851.

Poirier P, Alpert MA, Fleisher LA, et al. Cardiovascular evaluation and management of severely obese patients undergoing surgery: a science advisory from the American Heart Association. *Circulation.* 2009;120(1):86-95.

Salazar DE, Corcoran GB. Predicting creatinine clearance and renal drug clearance in obese patients from estimated fat-free body mass. *Am J Med.* 1988;84(6):1053-1060.

Servin F, Farinotti R, Haberer JP, et al. Propofol infusion for maintenance of anesthesia in morbidly obese patients receiving nitrous oxide. A clinical and pharmacokinetic study. *Anesthesiology.* 1993;78(4):657-665.

Stein GE, Schooley SL, Peloquin CA, et al. Pharmacokinetics and pharmacodynamics of linezolid in obese patients with cellulitis. *Ann Pharmacother.* 2005;39(3):427-432.

Vance-Bryan K, Guay DR, Gilliland SS, et al. Effect of obesity on vancomycin pharmacokinetic parameters as determined by using a bayesian forecasting technique. *Antimicrob Agents Chemother.* 1993;37(3):436-440.

van Kralingen S, van de Garde EM, Knibbe CA, et al. Comparative evaluation of atracurium dosed on ideal body weight vs total body weight in morbidly obese patients. *Br J Clin Pharmacol.* 2011;71(1):34-40.

ORAL DOSAGES THAT SHOULD NOT BE CRUSHED

There are a variety of reasons for crushing tablets or capsule contents prior to administering to the patient. Patients may have nasogastric tubes which do not permit the administration of tablets or capsules, an oral solution for a particular medication may not be available from the manufacturer or readily prepared by pharmacy, patients may have difficulty swallowing capsules or tablets, or mixing of powdered medication with food or drink may make the drug more palatable.

Generally, medications which should not be crushed fall into one of the following categories:

- **Extended Release Products:** The formulation of some tablets is specialized as to allow the medication within it to be slowly released into the body. This may be accomplished by centering the drug within the core of the tablet, with a subsequent shedding of multiple layers around the core. Wax melts in the GI tract, releasing drug contained within the wax matrix (eg, OxyCONTIN). Capsules may contain beads which have multiple layers which are slowly dissolved with time.

  Common Abbreviations for Extended Release Products

CD	Controlled dose
CR	Controlled release
CRT	Controlled release tablet
LA	Long-acting
SR	Sustained release
TR	Timed release
TD	Time delay
SA	Sustained action
XL	Extended release
XR	Extended release

- **Medications Which Are Irritating to the Stomach:** Tablets which are irritating to the stomach may be enteric-coated which delays release of the drug until the time when it reaches the small intestine. Enteric-coated aspirin is an example of this.
- **Foul-Tasting Medication:** Some drugs are quite unpleasant to taste so the manufacturer coats the tablet in a sugar coating to increase its palatability. By crushing the tablet, this sugar coating is lost and the patient tastes the unpleasant tasting medication.
- **Sublingual Medication:** Medication intended for use under the tongue should not be crushed. While it appears to be obvious, it is not always easy to determine if a medication is to be used sublingually. Sublingual medications should indicate on the package that they are intended for sublingual use.
- **Effervescent Tablets:** These are tablets which, when dropped into a liquid, quickly dissolve to yield a solution. Many effervescent tablets, when crushed, lose their ability to quickly dissolve.
- **Potentially Hazardous Substances:** Certain drugs, including antineoplastic agents, hormonal agents, some antivirals, some bioengineered agents, and other miscellaneous drugs, are considered potentially hazardous when used in humans based on their characteristics. Examples of these characteristics include carcinogenicity, teratogenicity, reproductive toxicity, organ toxicity at low doses, genotoxicity, or new drugs with structural and toxicity profiles similar to existing hazardous drugs. Exposure to these substances can result in adverse effects and should be avoided. Crushing or breaking a tablet or opening a capsule of a potentially hazardous substance may increase the risk of exposure to the substance through skin contact, inhalation, or accidental ingestion. The extent of exposure, potency, and toxicity of the hazardous substance determines the health risk. Institutions have policies and procedures to follow when handling any potentially hazardous substance. **Note:** All potentially hazardous substances may not be represented in this table. Refer to institution-specific guidelines for precautions to observe when handling hazardous substances.

RECOMMENDATIONS

1. It is not advisable to crush certain medications.
2. Consult individual monographs prior to crushing capsule or tablet.
3. If crushing a tablet or capsule is contraindicated, consult with your pharmacist to determine whether an oral solution exists or can be compounded.

ORAL DOSAGES THAT SHOULD NOT BE CRUSHED

Drug Product	Dosage Form	Dosage Reasons/Comments
Accutane	Capsule	Mucous membrane irritant; teratogenic potential
Aciphex	Tablet	Slow release
Aciphex Sprinkle	Capsule	Slow release. Capsule may be opened and contents sprinkled on soft food (eg, applesauce, fruit- or vegetable-based baby food, yogurt) or emptied into a small amount of liquid (eg, infant formula, apple juice, pediatric electrolyte solution). Granules should not be chewed or crushed.
Actiq	Lozenge	Slow release. This lollipop delivery system requires the patient to dissolve it slowly.
Actoplus Met XR	Tablet	Slow release
Actonel	Tablet	Irritant. Chewed, crushed, or sucked tablets may cause oropharyngeal irritation.
Adalat CC	Tablet	Slow release
Adderall XR	Capsule	Slow release[1]
Adenovirus (Types 4, 7) Vaccine	Tablet	Teratogenic potential; enteric-coated; do not disrupt tablet to avoid releasing live adenovirus in upper respiratory tract
Advicor	Tablet	Slow release
Afeditab CR	Tablet	Slow release
Afinitor	Tablet	Mucous membrane irritant; teratogenic potential; hazardous substance[10]
Aggrenox	Capsule	Slow release. Capsule may be opened; contents include an aspirin tablet that may be chewed and dipyridamole pellets that may be sprinkled on applesauce.
Allegra-D	Tablet	Slow release
Alophen	Tablet	Enteric-coated
ALPRAZolam ER	Tablet	Slow release
Altoprev	Tablet	Slow release
Ambien CR	Tablet	Slow release
Amitiza	Capsule	Slow release
Amnesteem	Capsule	Mucous membrane irritant; teratogenic potential
Ampyra	Tablet	Slow release
Amrix	Capsule	Slow release
Aplenzin	Tablet	Slow release
Apriso	Capsule	Slow release[1]
Aptivus	Capsule	Taste. Oil emulsion within spheres
Aricept 23 mg	Tablet	Film-coated; chewing or crushing may increase rate of absorption
Arava	Tablet	Teratogenic potential; hazardous substance[10]
Arthrotec	Tablet	Enteric-coated
Asacol	Tablet	Slow release
Astagraf XL	Capsule	Slow release
Atelvia	Tablet	Slow release; tablet coating is an important part of the delayed release
Augmentin XR	Tablet	Slow release[2,8]
AVINza	Capsule	Slow release[1] (applesauce)
Avodart	Capsule	Capsule should not be handled by pregnant women due to teratogenic potential[9]; hazardous substance[10]
Azulfidine EN-tabs	Tablet	Enteric-coated
Bayer Aspirin EC	Caplet	Enteric-coated
Bayer Aspirin, Low Adult 81 mg	Tablet	Enteric-coated
Bayer Aspirin, Regular Strength 325 mg	Caplet	Enteric-coated
Biaxin XL	Tablet	Slow release
Biltricide	Tablet	Taste[8]
Bisac-Evac	Tablet	Enteric-coated[3]

(continued)

Drug Product	Dosage Form	Dosage Reasons/Comments
Bisacodyl	Tablet	Enteric-coated[3]
Boniva	Tablet	Irritant. Chewed, crushed, or sucked tablets may cause oropharyngeal irritation.
Bontril Slow-Release	Capsule	Slow release
Bosulif	Tablet	Hazardous substance[10]
Budeprion SR	Tablet	Slow release
Buproban	Tablet	Slow release
BuPROPion SR	Tablet	Slow release
Campral	Tablet	Enteric-coated; slow release
Calan SR	Tablet	Slow release[8]
Caprelsa	Tablet	Teratogenic potential; hazardous substance[10]
Carbatrol	Capsule	Slow release[1]
Cardene SR	Capsule	Slow release
Cardizem	Tablet	Not described as slow release but releases drug over 3 hours.
Cardizem CD	Capsule	Slow release
Cardizem LA	Tablet	Slow release
Cardura XL	Tablet	Slow release
Cartia XT	Capsule	Slow release
Casodex	Tablet	Teratogenic potential; hazardous substance[10]
CeeNU	Capsule	Teratogenic potential; hazardous substance[10]
Cefaclor extended release	Tablet	Slow release
Ceftin	Tablet	Taste[2]. Use suspension for children.
Cefuroxime	Tablet	Taste[2]. Use suspension for children.
CellCept	Capsule, tablet	Teratogenic potential; hazardous substance[10]
Charcoal Plus DS	Tablet	Enteric-coated
Chlor-Trimeton 12-Hour	Tablet	Slow release[2]
Claravis	Capsule	Mucous membrane irritant; teratogenic potential
Claritin-D 12-Hour	Tablet	Slow release
Claritin-D 24-Hour	Tablet	Slow release
Colace	Capsule	Taste[5]
Colestid	Tablet	Slow release
Cometriq	Capsule	Teratogenic potential; hazardous substance[10]
Commit	Lozenge	Integrity compromised by chewing or crushing
Concerta	Tablet	Slow release
ConZip	Capsule	Extended release; tablet disruption may cause overdose
Coreg CR	Capsule	Slow release[1]
Cotazym-S	Capsule	Enteric-coated[1]
Creon	Capsule	Slow release; enteric-coated contents
Crixivan	Capsule	Taste. Capsule may be opened and mixed with fruit puree (eg, banana).
Cymbalta	Capsule	Enteric-coated
Cytoxan	Tablet	Drug may be crushed, but manufacturer recommends using injection; hazardous substance[10]
Depakene	Capsule	Slow release; mucous membrane irritant[2]; hazardous substance[10]
Depakote	Tablet	Slow release; hazardous substance[10]
Depakote ER	Tablet	Slow release; hazardous substance[10]
Detrol LA	Capsule	Slow release
Dexedrine Spansule	Capsule	Slow release
Dexilant	Capsule	Slow release[1]
Diamox Sequels	Capsule	Slow release

ORAL DOSAGES THAT SHOULD NOT BE CRUSHED

(continued)

Drug Product	Dosage Form	Dosage Reasons/Comments
Dibenzyline	Capsule	Hazardous substance[10]
Diclegis	Tablet	Slow release; manufacturer recommendation
Dilacor XR	Capsule	Slow release
Dilatrate-SR	Capsule	Slow release
Dilt-CD	Capsule	Slow release
Dilt-XR	Capsule	Slow release
Diltia XT	Capsule	Slow release
Ditropan XL	Tablet	Slow release
Divalproex ER	Tablet	Slow release
Donnatal Extentab	Tablet	Slow release[2]
Doxidan	Tablet	Enteric-coated[3]
Drisdol	Capsule	Liquid filled[4]
Droxia	Capsule	May be opened; wear gloves to handle; hazardous substance[10]
Duavee	Tablet	Manufacturer recommendation
Dulcolax	Capsule	Liquid-filled
Dulcolax	Tablet	Enteric-coated[3]
EC-Naprosyn	Tablet	Enteric-coated
Ecotrin Adult Low Strength	Tablet	Enteric-coated
Ecotrin Maximum Strength	Tablet	Enteric-coated
Ecotrin Regular Strength	Tablet	Enteric-coated
E.E.S.	Tablet	Enteric-coated[2]
Effer-K	Tablet	Effervescent tablet[6]
Effexor XR	Capsule	Slow release
E-Mycin	Tablet	Enteric-coated
Enablex	Tablet	Slow release
Entocort EC	Capsule	Enteric-coated[1]
Equetro	Capsule	Slow release[1]
Ergomar	Tablet	Sublingual form[7]
Erivedge	Capsule	Teratogenic potential[10]
Ery-Tab	Tablet	Enteric-coated
Erythromycin Stearate	Tablet	Enteric-coated
Erythromycin Base	Tablet	Enteric-coated
Erythromycin Delayed-Release	Capsule	Enteric-coated pellets[1]
Etoposide	Capsule	Hazardous substance[10]
Evista	Tablet	Taste; teratogenic potential; hazardous substance[10]
Exalgo	Tablet	Slow release; breaking, chewing, crushing, or dissolving before ingestion increases the risk of overdose
Fareston	Tablet	Teratogenic potential; hazardous substance[10]
Feldene	Capsule	Mucous membrane irritant
Fentora	Tablet	Buccal tablet
Feosol	Tablet	Enteric-coated[2]
Fergon	Tablet	Enteric-coated
Ferro-Sequels	Tablet	Slow release
Flagyl ER	Tablet	Slow release
Flomax	Capsule	Slow release
Focalin XR	Capsule	Slow release[1]
Forfivo XL	Capsule	Slow release
Fosamax	Tablet	Mucous membrane irritant
Fosamax Plus D	Tablet	Mucous membrane irritant
Fulyzaq	Tablet	Slow release

(continued)

Drug Product	Dosage Form	Dosage Reasons/Comments
Gengraf	Capsule	Teratogenic potential; hazardous substance[10]
Geodon	Capsule	Hazardous substance[10]
Gleevec	Tablet	Taste[8]. May be dissolved in water or apple juice; hazardous substance[10]
GlipiZIDE ER	Tablet	Slow release
Glucophage XR	Tablet	Slow release
Glucotrol XL	Tablet	Slow release
Glumetza	Tablet	Slow release
Gralise	Tablet	Slow release
Guaifenex PSE	Tablet	Slow release[8]
Halfprin	Tablet	Enteric coated
Hexalen	Capsule	Teratogenic potential; hazardous substance[10]
Horizant	Tablet	Slow release
Hycamtin	Capsule	Teratogenic potential; hazardous substance[10]
Hydrea	Capsule	Can be opened and mixed with water; wear gloves to handle; hazardous substance[10]
Iclusig	Tablet	Teratogenic potential; hazardous substance[10]
Imbruvica	Capsule	Teratogenic potential; hazardous substance[10]
Imdur	Tablet	Slow release[8]
Inderal LA	Capsule	Slow release
Indocin SR	Capsule	Slow release[1,2]
Inlyta	Tablet	Teratogenic potential; hazardous substance[10]
InnoPran XL	Capsule	Slow release
Intelence	Tablet	Tablet should be swallowed whole and not crushed; tablet may be dispersed in water
Intuniv	Tablet	Slow release
Invega	Tablet	Slow release
Ionamin	Capsule	Slow release
Isoptin SR	Tablet	Slow release[8]
Isosorbide Dinitrate Sublingual	Tablet	Sublingual form[7]
Jalyn	Capsule	Capsule should not be handled by pregnant women due to teratogenic potential[9]; hazardous substance[10]
Janumet XR	Tablet	Slow release
Juxtapid	Capsule	Manufacturer recommendation
Kadian	Capsule	Slow release[1]. Do not give via NG tubes.
Kaletra	Tablet	Film coated
Kaon-Cl 10	Tablet	Slow release[2]
Kapidex	Capsule	Slow release[1]
Kapvay	Tablet	Slow release
K-Dur	Tablet	Slow release
Keppra	Tablet	Taste[2]
Keppra XR	Tablet	Slow release
Ketek	Tablet	Slow release
Klor-Con	Tablet	Slow release[2]
Klor-Con M	Tablet	Slow release[2]; some strengths are scored
K-Lyte/Cl	Tablet	Effervescent tablet[6]
Kombiglyze XR	Tablet	Slow release; tablet matrix may remain in stool
K-Tab	Tablet	Slow release[2]
LaMICtal XR	Tablet	Slow release
Lescol XL	Tablet	Slow release

(continued)

Drug Product	Dosage Form	Dosage Reasons/Comments
Letairis	Tablet	Film coated; hazardous substance[10]
Leukeran	Tablet	Teratogenic potential; hazardous substance[10]
Levbid	Tablet	Slow release[8]
Lialda	Tablet	Delayed release, enteric coated
Linzess	Capsule	Slow release
Lithobid	Tablet	Slow release
Lovaza	Capsule	Contents of capsule may erode walls of styrofoam or plastic materials
Luvox CR	Capsule	Slow release
Lysodren	Tablet	Hazardous substance[10]
Mag-Tab SR	Tablet	Slow release
Matulane	Capsule	Teratogenic potential; hazardous substance[10]
Maxifed-G	Tablet	Slow release
Maxiphen DM	Tablet	Slow release[8]
Mestinon Timespan	Tablet	Slow release[2]
Metadate CD	Capsule	Slow release[1]
Metadate ER	Tablet	Slow release
Metoprolol ER	Tablet	Slow release
MicroK Extencaps	Capsule	Slow release[1,2]
Minocin	Capsule	Slow release
Morphine sulfate extended-release	Tablet	Slow release
Motrin	Tablet	Taste[5]
Moxatag	Tablet	Slow release
MS Contin	Tablet	Slow release[2]
Mucinex	Tablet	Slow release
Mucinex DM	Tablet	Slow release[2]
Multaq	Tablet	Hazardous substance[10]
Myfortic	Tablet	Slow release; teratogenic potential; hazardous substance[10]
Myrbetriq	Tablet	Slow release
Naprelan	Tablet	Slow release
Neoral	Capsule	Teratogenic potential; hazardous substance[10]
NexIUM	Capsule	Slow release[1]
Niaspan	Tablet	Slow release
Nicotinic Acid	Capsule, Tablet	Slow release[8]
Nifediac CC	Tablet	Slow release
Nifedical XL	Tablet	Slow release
NIFEdipine ER	Tablet	Slow release
Nitrostat	Tablet	Sublingual route[7]
Norflex	Tablet	Slow release
Norpace CR	Capsule	Slow release
Norvir	Tablet	Crushing tablets has resulted in decreased bioavailability of drug[2]
Noxafil	Tablet	Slow release
Nucynta ER	Tablet	Slow release; tablet disruption may cause a potentially fatal overdose
Oleptro	Tablet	Slow release[8]
Onglyza	Tablet	Film coated
Opana ER	Tablet	Slow release; tablet disruption may cause a potentially fatal overdose
Opsumit	Tablet	Teratogenic potential; hazardous substance[10]

(continued)

Drug Product	Dosage Form	Dosage Reasons/Comments
Oracea	Capsule	Slow release
Oramorph SR	Tablet	Slow release[2]
Oravig	Tablet	Buccal tablet
Orphenadrine citrate ER	Tablet	Slow release
Oxtellar XR	Tablet	Slow release
OxyCONTIN	Tablet	Slow release; surrounded by wax matrix; tablet disruption may cause a potentially fatal overdose
Pancrease MT	Capsule	Enteric-coated[1]
Pancreaze	Capsule	Slow-release; enteric-coated contents
Pancrelipase	Capsule	Slow-release; enteric-coated contents
Paxil CR	Tablet	Slow release
Pentasa	Capsule	Slow release
Pertzye	Capsule	Slow-release; enteric-coated contents
Plendil	Tablet	Slow release
Pomalyst	Capsule	Teratogenic potential; hazardous substance[10]; healthcare workers should avoid contact with capsule contents/body fluids
Pradaxa	Capsule	Bioavailability increases by 75% when the pellets are taken without the capsule shell
Prevacid	Capsule	Slow release[1]
Prevacid	Suspension	Slow release. Contains enteric-coated granules. Not for use in NG tubes.
Prevacid SoluTab	Tablet	Orally disintegrating. Do not swallow; dissolve in water only and dispense via dosing syringe or NG tube.
PriLOSEC	Capsule	Slow release
PriLOSEC OTC	Tablet	Slow release
Pristiq	Tablet	Slow release
Procardia XL	Tablet	Slow release
Procysbi	Capsule	Slow release
Propecia	Tablet	Women who are, or may become, pregnant should not handle crushed or broken tablets due to teratogenic potential[9]; hazardous substance[10]
Proscar	Tablet	Women who are, or may become, pregnant should not handle crushed or broken tablets due to teratogenic potential[9]; hazardous substance[10]
Protonix	Tablet	Slow release
PROzac Weekly	Capsule	Enteric coated
Purinethol	Tablet	Teratogenic potential[9]; hazardous substance[10]
QuiNIDine ER	Tablet	Slow release[8]; enteric-coated
Ranexa	Tablet	Slow release
Rapamune	Tablet	Taste; hazardous substance[10]
Razadyne ER	Capsule	Slow release
Renagel	Tablet	Expands in liquid if broken/crushed.
Renvela	Tablet	Enteric-coated
Requip XL	Tablet	Slow release
Rescriptor	Tablet	If unable to swallow, may dissolve 100 mg tablets in water and drink; 200 mg tablets must be swallowed whole
Revlimid	Capsule	Teratogenic potential; hazardous substance[10]; healthcare workers should avoid contact with capsule contents/body fluids
RisperDAL M-Tab	Tablet	Orally disintegrating. Do not chew or break tablet; after dissolving under tongue, tablet may be swallowed
Ritalin LA	Capsule	Slow release[1]
Ritalin-SR	Tablet	Slow release
Rybix ODT	Tablet	Orally disintegrating. Do not chew, break, or split tablet; after dissolving on the tongue, may swallow.

(continued)

Drug Product	Dosage Form	Dosage Reasons/Comments
Rythmol SR	Capsule	Slow release
Ryzolt	Tablet	Slow release; tablet disruption may cause overdose
SandIMMUNE	Capsule	Teratogenic potential; hazardous substance[10]
Saphris	Tablet	Sublingual form[7]
Sensipar	Tablet	Tablets are not scored and cutting may cause inaccurate dosage
SEROquel XR	Tablet	Slow release
Sinemet CR	Tablet	Slow release
Slo-Niacin	Tablet	Slow release[8]
Slow-Mag	Tablet	Slow release
Solodyn	Tablet	Slow release
Somnote	Capsule	Liquid filled
Soriatane	Capsule	Teratogenic potential; hazardous substance[10]
Sotret	Capsule	Mucous membrane irritant; teratogenic potential
Sprycel	Tablet	Film coated. Active ingredients are surrounded by a wax matrix to prevent healthcare exposure. Women who are, or may become pregnant, should not handle crushed or broken tablets; teratogenic potential; hazardous substance[10]
Stavzor	Capsule	Slow release; hazardous substance[10]
Stivarga	Tablet	Manufacturer recommendation; teratogenic potential; hazardous substance[10]
Strattera	Capsule	Capsule contents can cause ocular irritation.
Sudafed 12-Hour	Capsule	Slow release[2]
Sudafed 24-Hour	Capsule	Slow release[2]
Sulfazine EC	Tablet	Delayed release, enteric coated
Sular	Tablet	Slow release
Sustiva	Tablet	Tablets should not be broken (capsules should be used if dosage adjustment needed)
Symax Duotab	Tablet	Slow release
Symax SR	Tablet	Slow release
Syprine	Capsule	Potential risk of contact dermatitis
Tabloid	Tablet	Teratogenic potential; hazardous substance[10]
Tafinlar	Capsule	Teratogenic potential; hazardous substance[10]
Tamoxifen	Tablet	Teratogenic potential; hazardous substance[10]
Targretin	Capsule	Teratogenic potential; hazardous substance[10]
Tasigna	Capsule	Hazardous substance[10]; altering capsule may lead to high blood levels, increasing the risk of toxicity
Taztia XT	Capsule	Slow release[1]
Tecfidera	Capsule	Manufacturer recommendation; delayed release; irritant
TEGretol-XR	Tablet	Slow release
Temodar	Capsule	Teratogenic potential; hazardous substance[10]. **Note:** If capsules are accidentally opened or damaged, rigorous precautions should be taken to avoid inhalation or contact of contents with the skin or mucous membranes.
Tessalon	Capsule	Swallow whole; pharmacologic action may cause choking if chewed or opened and swallowed.
Tetracycline	Capsule	Hazardous substance[10]
Thalomid	Capsule	Teratogenic potential; hazardous substance[10]
Theo-24	Tablet	Slow release[2]
Tiazac	Capsule	Slow release[1]
Topamax	Capsule	Taste[1]
Topamax	Tablet	Taste
Toprol XL	Tablet	Slow release[8]

(continued)

Drug Product	Dosage Form	Dosage Reasons/Comments
Toviaz	Tablet	Slow release
Tracleer	Tablet	Teratogenic potential; hazardous substance[9,10]
TRENtal	Tablet	Slow release
Treximet	Tablet	Unique formulation enhances rapid drug absorption
TriLipix	Capsule	Slow release
Trokendi XR	Capsule	Slow release
Tylenol Arthritis Pain	Caplet	Slow release
Tylenol 8 Hour	Caplet	Slow release
Uceris	Tablet	Slow release
Ultram ER	Tablet	Slow release. Tablet disruption my cause a potentially fatal overdose.
Ultresa	Capsule	Slow release; enteric-coated contents
Ultrase	Capsule	Enteric-coated[1]
Ultrase MT	Capsule	Enteric-coated[1]
Uniphyl	Tablet	Slow release
Urocit-K	Tablet	Wax-coated
Uroxatral	Tablet	Slow release
Valcyte	Tablet	Irritant potential; teratogenic potential; hazardous substance[10]
Vascepa	Capsule	Manufacturer recommendation
Verapamil SR	Tablet	Slow release[8]
Verelan	Capsule	Slow release[1]
Verelan PM	Capsule	Slow release[1]
Vesanoid	Capsule	Teratogenic potential; hazardous substance[10]
VESIcare	Tablet	Enteric-coated
Videx EC	Capsule	Slow release
Vimovo	Tablet	Slow release
Viokace	Tablet	Mucous membrane irritant
Viramune XR	Tablet	Slow release[2]
Voltaren-XR	Tablet	Slow release
VoSpire ER	Tablet	Slow release
Votrient	Tablet	Crushing significantly increases AUC and T_{max}; hazardous substance[10]
Wellbutrin SR	Tablet	Slow release
Wellbutrin XL	Tablet	Slow release
Xalkori	Capsule	Teratogenic potential; hazardous substance[10]
Xanax XR	Tablet	Slow release
Xeloda	Tablet	Teratogenic potential; hazardous substance[10].
Xtandi	Capsule	Teratogenic potential; hazardous substance[10]
Zegerid OTC	Capsule	Slow release
Zelboraf	Tablet	Teratogenic potential; hazardous substance[10]
Zenpep	Capsule	Slow release; enteric-coated contents
Zolinza	Capsule	Irritant; avoid contact with skin or mucous membranes; use gloves to handle; teratogenic potential; hazardous substance[10]
Zomig-ZMT	Tablet	Sublingual form[7]
Zortress	Tablet	Mucous membrane irritant; teratogenic potential; hazardous substance[10]
Zyban	Tablet	Slow release

ORAL DOSAGES THAT SHOULD NOT BE CRUSHED

(continued)

Drug Product	Dosage Form	Dosage Reasons/Comments
Zyflo CR	Tablet	Slow release
ZyrTEC-D Allergy & Congestion	Tablet	Slow release
Zytiga	Tablet	Teratogenic potential; hazardous substance[10]

[1]Capsule may be opened and the contents taken without crushing or chewing; soft food, such as applesauce or pudding, may facilitate administration; contents may generally be administered via nasogastric tube using an appropriate fluid, provided entire contents are washed down the tube.

[2]Liquid dosage forms of the product are available; however, dose, frequency of administration, and manufacturers may differ from that of the solid dosage form.

[3]Antacids and/or milk may prematurely dissolve the coating of the tablet.

[4]Capsule may be opened and the liquid contents removed for administration.

[5]The taste of this product in a liquid form would likely be unacceptable to the patient; administration via nasogastric tube should be acceptable.

[6]Effervescent tablets must be dissolved in the amount of diluent recommended by the manufacturer.

[7]Tablets are made to disintegrate under (or on) the tongue.

[8]Tablet is scored and may be broken in half without affecting release characteristics.

[9]Prescribing information recommends that women who are, or may become, pregnant should not handle medication, especially if crushed or broken; avoid direct contact.

[10]Potentially hazardous or hazardous substance; refer to institution-specific guidelines for precautions to observe when handling this substance.

REFERENCES

Mitchell JF. Oral dosage forms that should not be crushed. Available at http://www.ismp.org/tools/DoNotCrush.pdf. Accessed November 11, 2011.

National Institute for Occupational Safety and Health (NIOSH). NIOSH list of antineoplastic and other hazardous drugs in healthcare settings 2012. Available at http://www.cdc.gov/niosh/docs/2012-150/pdfs/2012-150.pdf. Accessed July 11, 2012.

PATIENT INFORMATION FOR DISPOSAL OF UNUSED MEDICATIONS

Federal guidelines and the Food and Drug Administration (FDA) recommend that disposal of most unused medications should NOT be accomplished by flushing them down the toilet or drain unless specifically stated in the drug label prescribing information. (See "Disposal of Unused Medications Not Specified to be Flushed" below.)

However, certain drugs can potentially harm an individual for whom it is not intended, even in a single dose, depending on the size of the individual and strength of the medication. Accidental (or intentional) ingestion of one of these drugs by an unintended individual (eg, child or pet) can cause hypotension, somnolence, respiratory depression, or other severe adverse events that could lead to coma or death. For this reason, certain unused medications **should** be disposed of by flushing them down a toilet or sink.

Disposal by flushing of these medications is not believed to pose a risk to human health or the environment. Trace amounts of medicine in the water system have been noted, mainly from the body's normal elimination through urine or feces, but there has been no evidence of these small amounts being harmful. Disposal by flushing of these select, few medications contributes a small fraction to the amount of medicine in the water system. The FDA believes that the benefit of avoiding a potentially life-threatening overdose by accidental ingestion outweighs the potential risk to the environment by flushing these medications.

Medications Recommended for Disposal by Flushing

Medication	Active Ingredient
Actiq, oral transmucosal lozenge	FentaNYL citrate
AVINza, capsule (extended release)	Morphine sulfate
Daytrana, transdermal patch	Methylphenidate
Demerol, tablet[1]	Meperidine hydrochloride
Demerol, oral solution[1]	Meperidine hydrochloride
Diastat/Diastat AcuDial, rectal gel	Diazepam
Dilaudid, tablet[1]	HYDROmorphone hydrochloride
Dilaudid, oral liquid[1]	HYDROmorphone hydrochloride
Dolophine, tablet (as hydrochloride)[1]	Methadone hydrochloride
Duragesic, patch (extended release)[1]	FentaNYL
Embeda, capsule (extended release)	Morphine sulfate and naltrexone hydrochloride
Fentora, tablet (buccal)	FentaNYL citrate
Kadian, capsule (extended release)	Morphine sulfate
Methadone hydrochloride (oral solution)[1]	Methadone hydrochloride
Methadose, tablet[1]	Methadone hydrochloride
Morphine sulfate, tablet (immediate release)[1]	Morphine sulfate
Morphine sulfate, oral solution[1]	Morphine sulfate
MS Contin, tablet (extended release)[1]	Morphine sulfate
Onsolis, soluble film (buccal)	FentaNYL citrate
Opana, tablet (immediate release)	Oxymorphone hydrochloride
Opana ER, tablet (extended release)	Oxymorphone hydrochloride
Oramorph SR, tablet (sustained release)	Morphine sulfate
OxyCONTIN, tablet (extended release)[1]	OxyCODONE hydrochloride
Percocet, tablet[1]	Oxycodone hydrochloride and acetaminophen
Percodan, tablet[1]	Oxycodone hydrochloride and aspirin
Xyrem, oral solution	Sodium oxybate

[1]Medications available in generic formulations

DISPOSAL OF UNUSED MEDICATIONS NOT SPECIFIED TO BE FLUSHED

The majority of medications should be disposed of without flushing them down a toilet or drain. These medications should be removed from the original container, mixed with an unappealing substance (eg, coffee grounds, cat litter), sealed in a plastic bag or other closable container, and disposed of in the household trash.

Another option for disposal of unused medications is through drug take-back programs. For information on availability of drug take-back programs in your area, contact city or county trash and recycling service.

For more information on unused medication disposal, see specific drug product labeling information or call the FDA at (888) INFO-FDA (1-888-463-6332).

REFERENCE

U.S. Food and Drug Administration (FDA). Disposal by flushing of certain unused medicines: what you should know. Available at: http://www.fda.gov/Drugs/ResourcesForYou/Consumers/BuyingUsingMedicineSafely/EnsuringSafeUseofMedicine/SafeDisposalofMedicines/ucm186187.htm Accessed October 20, 2009.

TYRAMINE CONTENT OF FOODS

Food[1]	Allowed	Minimize Intake	Not Allowed
Beverages	Decaffeinated beverages (eg, coffee, tea, soda); milk, soy milk, chocolate beverage	Caffeine-containing drinks, clear spirits, wine, bottled/canned beers	**Tap** beer
Breads/cereals	All except those containing cheese	None	Cheese bread and crackers
Dairy products	Cottage cheese, farmers or pot cheese, cream cheese, ricotta cheese, all milk, eggs, ice cream, pudding, yogurt, sour cream, processed cheese, mozzarella	None	All other cheeses (**aged** cheese, Camembert, cheddar, Gouda, gruyere, parmesan, provolone, romano, Roquefort, stilton)
Meat, fish, and poultry	All fresh packaged or processed (eg, hot dogs, bologna), or frozen	Pepperoni	**Aged** chicken and beef liver, dried and pickled fish, shrimp paste, summer or dry sausage, dried meats (eg, salami, cacciatore), meat extracts, liverwurst
Starches — potatoes/rice	All	None	Soybean (including paste), tofu
Vegetables	All fresh, frozen, canned, or dried vegetable juices except those not allowed	Chili peppers, Chinese pea pods	Sauerkraut, broad or fava bean pods (not beans)
Fruit	Fresh, frozen, or canned fruits and fruit juices	Avocado, figs	Banana peel, avocado (over-ripened)
Soups	All soups not listed to limit or avoid	None	Soups which contain **aged** cheese, **tap** beer, any made with flavor cubes or meat extract, miso soup, broad or fava bean pods (not beans)
Fats	All except fermented	None	None
Sweets	Sugar, hard candy, honey, molasses, syrups, chocolate candy	None	None
Desserts	Cakes, cookies, gelatin, pastries, sherbets, sorbets, chocolate desserts	None	None
Miscellaneous	Salt, nuts, spices, herbs, flavorings, Worcestershire sauce, Brewer's or Baker's yeast, monosodium glutamate, vitamins with Brewer's yeast	Peanuts	Soy sauce, all aged and fermented products, marmite and other concentrated yeast extracts

[1]Freshness is of primary importance. Food that is spoiled or improperly stored should be avoided.

REFERENCES

Shulman KI, Walker SE. A reevaluation of dietary restrictions for irreversible monoamine oxidase inhibitors. *Psychiatr Ann*. 2001;31(6):378-384.

Shulman KI, Walker SE. Refining the MAOI diet: tyramine content of pizza and soy products. *J Clin Psychiatry*. 1999;60(3):191-193.

Walker SE, Shulman KI, Tailor SAN, et al. Tyramine content of previously restricted foods in monoamine oxidase inhibitor diets. *J Clin Psychopharmacol*. 1996;16(5):383-388.

VITAMIN K CONTENT IN SELECTED FOODS

The following list describes the relative amounts of vitamin K in foods generally considered high in vitamin K. This is a partial listing of foods with estimated portions. For more complete information, refer to the USDA National Nutrient Database for Standard Reference, Release 25, at https://www.ars.usda.gov/SP2UserFiles/Place/12354500/Data/SR25/nutrlist/sr25a430.pdf

Foods	Portion Size	Vitamin K Content (mcg)
Asparagus	1 cup	144
Asparagus	4 spears	30-48
Beet greens	1 cup	697
Broccoli	1 cup	90-220
Brussels sprouts	1 cup	219-300
Cabbage	1 cup	27-163
Collards	1 cup	773-1059
Cucumber	1 large	49
Dandelion greens	1 cup	579
Endive	1 cup	116
Kale	1 cup	1062-1147
Lettuce	1 head	130-167
Mustard greens	1 cup	830
Noodles	1 cup	162
Oil, canola	1 Tbsp	10
Oil, olive, salad, or cooking	1 Tbsp	8
Okra	1 cup	64-88
Onions	1 cup	207
Parsley	10 sprigs	164
Peas	1 cup	10-63
Spinach	1 cup	145-1027
Turnip greens	1 cup	529-851

PHARMACOLOGIC CATEGORY INDEX

NOTES

NOTES

NOTES

NOTES

Other Solutions Offered by Lexicomp

Anesthesiology & Critical Care Drug Handbook

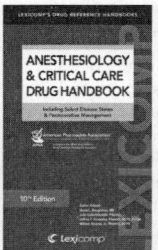

Designed for anesthesiologists, critical care practitioners, and all healthcare professionals involved in the treatment of surgical or ICU patients.

Includes: extensive drug information to ensure appropriate clinical management of patients; intensivist and anesthesiologist perspective; over 2000 medications most commonly used in the preoperative and critical care setting; Special Topics/Issues addressing frequently encountered patient conditions.

Drug Information Handbook with International Trade Names Index

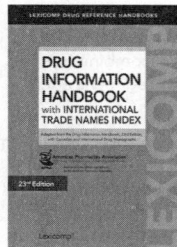

The *Drug Information Handbook with International Trade Names Index* includes the content of our *Drug Information Handbook*, plus international drug monographs for use worldwide! This easy-to-use reference is complied especially for the pharmacist, physician, or other healthcare professional seeking quick access to comprehensive drug information.

Drug Information Handbook for Advanced Practice Nursing

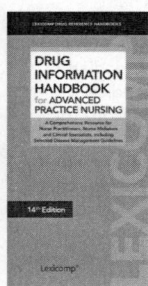

Designed to assist the advanced practice nurse with prescribing, monitoring and educating patients.

Includes: over 4800 generic and brand names cross-referenced by page number; generic drug names and cross-references highlighted in RED; labeled and investigational indications; adult, geriatric, and pediatric dosing; and up to 75 fields of information per monograph, including Patient Education and Physical Assessment.

Drug Information Handbook for Nursing

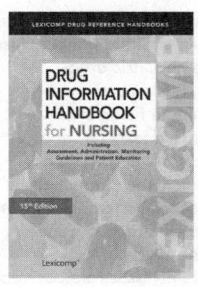

Designed for registered professional nurses and upper-division nursing students requiring dosing, administration, monitoring and patient education information.

Includes: Over 4800 generic and brand name drugs, cross-referenced by page number; drug names and specific nursing fields highlighted in RED for easy reference, Nursing Actions field includes Physical Assessment and Patient Education guidelines.

To order, call Customer Service at 1-866-397-3433 or visit www.lexi.com.
Outside of the U.S., call +1-330-650-6506 or visit www.lexi.com.

Other Solutions Offered by Lexicomp

Drug Information Handbook for Oncology

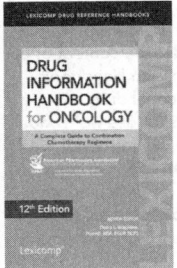

Designed for oncology professionals requiring information on combination chemotherapy regimens and dosing protocols.

Includes: monographs containing warnings, adverse reaction profiles, drug interactions, dosing for specific indications, vesicant, emetic potential, combination regimens, and more; where applicable, a special Combination Chemotherapy field links to specific oncology monographs; Special Topics such as Cancer Treatment Related Complications, Bone Marrow Transplantation, and Drug Development.

Geriatric Dosage Handbook

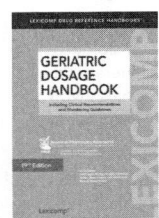

Designed for healthcare professionals managing geriatric patients.

Includes: a wide range of adult and geriatric dosing; special geriatric considerations; up to 44 key fields of information in each monograph, including Medication Safety Issues; extensive information on drug interactions, as well as dosing for patients with renal/hepatic impairment.

Pediatric Dosage Handbook

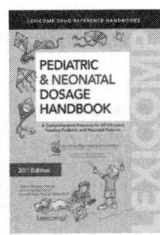

This book is designed for healthcare professionals requiring quick access to extensive pediatric drug information. Each monograph contains multiple fields of content, including usual dosage by age group, indication, and route of administration. Drug interactions, adverse reactions, extemporaneous preparations, pharmacodynamics/pharmacokinetics data, and medication safety issues are covered.

Pediatric Dosage Handbook with International Trade Names Index

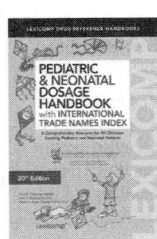

The *Pediatric Dosage Handbook with International Trade Names Index* is the trusted pediatric drug resource of medical professionals worldwide. The international edition contains all the content of the Lexicomp *Pediatric Dosage Handbook,* plus an International Trade Names Index including trade names from over 100 countries.

To order, call Customer Service at 1-866-397-3433 or visit www.lexi.com.
Outside of the U.S., call +1-330-650-6506 or visit www.lexi.com.

Other Solutions Offered by Lexicomp

Lexicomp® Mobile Apps

Apps for smartphones and tablets

At Lexicomp, we take pride in creating quality drug information for use at the point of care. Our content is not subject to third-party recommendations, but based on the contributions of our respected authors and editors, internal clinical team and thousands of professionals within the healthcare industry who continually review and validate our data.

With Lexicomp Mobile Apps, you can be confident you are accessing the most timely drug information available for mobile devices. All updates are included with your annual subscription.

Lexicomp Mobile Apps databases include:

- Lexi-Drugs®
- Pediatric & Neonatal Lexi-Drugs™
- Lexi-Drugs® para Pediatría (Spanish Version)
- Lexi-Interact™
- Lexi-Natural Products™
- Lexi-Tox™
- Household Products
- Lexi-Infectious Diseases™
- Lexi-Lab & Diagnostic Procedures™
- Nursing Lexi-Drugs™
- Dental Lexi-Drugs™
- Oral Soft Tissue Diseases
- Lexi-Pharmacogenomics™
- Lexi-Patient Education™
- Lexi-Drug ID™
- Lexi-CALC™
- Lexi-I.V. Compatibility™*
- Lexi-Companion Guides™
- Drug Allergy & Idiosyncratic Reactions
- Lexi-Pregnancy & Lactation™
- The 5-Minute Clinical Consult
- The 5-Minute Pediatric Consult
- AHFS DI® Essentials™
- Stedman's Medical Dictionary for the Health Professions and Nursing
- Stedman's Medical Abbreviations

* I.V. compatibility information © copyright King Guide Publications, Inc.

Visit www.lexi.com for more information and device compatibility!

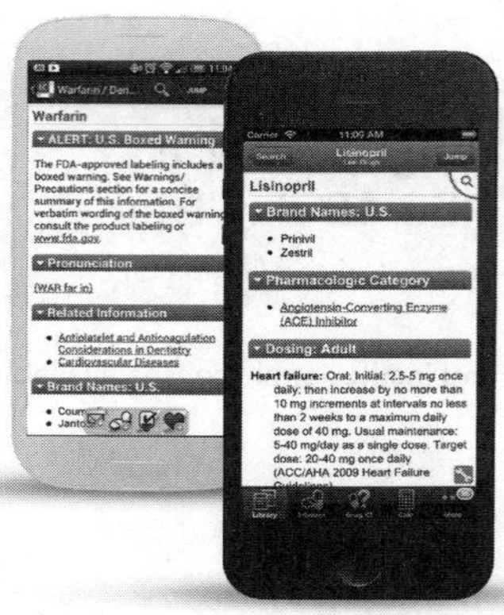

To order, call Customer Service at 1-866-397-3433 or visit www.lexi.com.
Outside of the U.S., call +1-330-650-6506 or visit www.lexi.com.